D1587540

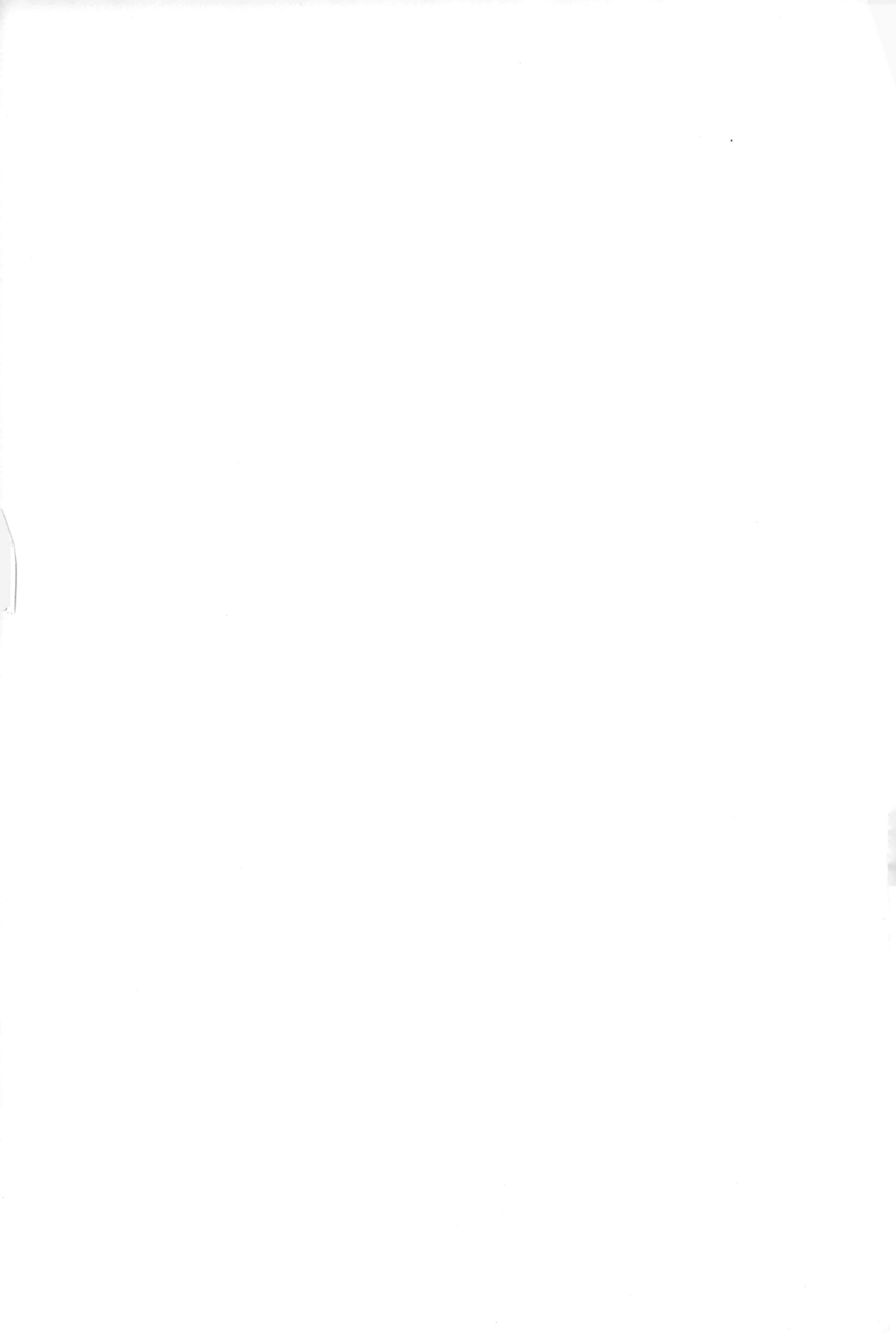

ABPI COMPENDIUM OF DATA SHEETS

AND

SUMMARIES OF PRODUCT CHARACTERISTICS

1999–2000

With The Code of Practice for the Pharmaceutical Industry

Datapharm Publications Limited
12 Whitehall, London SW1A 2DY

Responsibility for Data Sheets and Summaries of Product Characteristics

The data sheets and summaries of product characteristics in this Compendium are prepared independently by each participating company and each proof is checked and the text confirmed as correct by the participant concerned. Neither Datapharm Publications Limited nor The Association of the British Pharmaceutical Industry (ABPI) gives any guarantee whatsoever as to the accuracy of the information contained in the data sheets or summaries of product characteristics and accepts no liability whatsoever in respect of any loss, damage or expense arising from any such information or for any error or omission in the data sheets or summaries of product characteristics and in particular (but without prejudice to the generality of the foregoing) shall not be liable for any consequential damages or expenses or any loss of profit or any liability to third parties incurred by anyone relying on the information contained in the data sheets and summaries of product characteristics appearing in this Compendium.

Published by Datapharm Publications Limited

ISBN 0 907102 18 2
ISSN 1364–5005

Typeset, printed and bound in Great Britain
by William Clowes Limited, Beccles and London

THE COMPENDIUM

This is the third edition of the Compendium in which summaries of product characteristics (SPCs) appear. New requirements came into effect in 1995 replacing data sheets with SPCs for new products and those products coming up for licence renewal. There will be a period of about five years during which data sheets will coexist with SPCs and this edition of the Compendium reflects that fact.

Both data sheets and SPCs are prepared by the individual companies concerned and, in consequence, vary somewhat in style, but all follow either the requirements laid down by 'The Medicines (Data Sheet) Regulations 1972' (for data sheets) or the European Commission's Committee for Proprietary Medicinal Products (CPMP) Note for Guidance (for SPCs).

Participation in the Compendium is open to all companies supplying medicinal products intended for use under medical supervision.

Data sheets and SPCs are intended for members of the medical and pharmaceutical professions and are written with them in mind. Any member of the public who reads them should bear in mind the need to take professional advice before making any decision affecting his or her own medication based upon their contents.

DATE OF PREPARATION

The data sheets included in this Compendium were finalised during the fourth quarter of 1998 and the Compendium itself was published in April 1999. Summaries of product characteristics have individual dates of approval/revision.

REVISED DATA SHEETS/SPCs

Individual participating companies may issue loose leaf data sheets/summaries of product characteristics (SPCs) which supersede those included in this Compendium.

It is advisable to retain any such revised data sheets/SPCs which are received and to indicate that fact on the corresponding data sheets or SPCs in the Compendium.

LEGAL CATEGORY

The following abbreviations are used under the heading 'Legal category' in data sheets and summaries of product characteristics in the Compendium.

- GSL A preparation which is included in the General Sale List.
- P A pharmacy sale medicine which can be sold only from a retail pharmacy.
- POM A prescription only medicine.
- CD A preparation controlled by the Misuse of Drugs Act 1971 and Regulations. The CD is followed by (Sch 1), (Sch 2), (Sch 3), (Sch 4) or (Sch 5) depending on the schedule to the Misuse of Drugs Regulations 1985, as amended, in which the preparation is included.

Doctors are reminded that certain of the particulars must be in their own handwriting on prescriptions for preparations coming within Schedule 2 and Schedule 3 (except phenobarbitone) to the Misuse of Drugs Regulations 1985, as amended.

SYMBOLS AND ABBREVIATIONS

An asterisk (*) by the name of a product indicates that the name is a trade mark. The company symbols which appear in certain participants' sections are also trade marks.

An inverted triangle (▼) by the name of a product indicates that that product is newly introduced and there are special requirements as to the reporting of adverse reactions (see page iv).

OP in the 'Package quantities' section of a data sheet indicates that the pack is an 'original pack'.

FURTHER INFORMATION

The regulations which relate to data sheets restrict the scope of the material which may be given under the heading 'Further information' and require insertion of the word 'Nil' in any data sheet where there is no entry under that heading. Companies are, of course, none the less always willing to provide additional information on their products upon request.

Enquiries should be directed to the companies concerned. Addresses and telephone numbers are provided in the Directory of Participants in the coloured section at the end of the Compendium.

The reporting of adverse reactions

Any drug may produce unwanted or unexpected adverse reactions. Detection and recording of these is of vital importance. Doctors and hospital pharmacists† are urged to help by reporting adverse reactions to:

Medicines Control Agency
CSM Freepost
London SW8 5BR
(0800 731 6789)

Suspected adverse reactions to *any* therapeutic agent should be reported, including drugs (those taken for *self-medication* as well as those *prescribed*), blood products, vaccines, X-ray contract media, dental or surgical materials, intra-uterine devices, and herbal products.

† A demonstration scheme will also allow community pharmacists within the CSM's Monitoring Centres in Cardiff, Birmingham, Liverpool and Newcastle to report suspected reactions. All pharmacists must discuss the particular case with the patient's doctor before sending a yellow card report. Whilst it is not recommended for a report to be made against the advice of the patient's doctor, the pharmacist may wish to exercise professional judgement in sending such a report.

Newer drugs marked ▼

Doctors and hospital pharmacists are asked to report *all* suspected reactions (i.e. any adverse or any unexpected event, however minor, which could conceivably be attributed to the drug). Reports should be made despite uncertainty about a causal relationship, irrespective of whether the reaction is well recognised, and even if other drugs have been given concurrently.

Established drugs

Doctors and hospital pharmacists are asked to report *all* serious suspected reactions including those that are fatal, life-threatening, disabling, incapacitating, or which result in or prolong hospitalisation; they should be reported even if the effect is well recognised.

Examples include anaphylaxis, blood disorders, endocrine disturbances, effects on fertility, haemorrhage from any site, renal impairment, jaundice, ophthalmic disorders, severe CNS effects, severe skin reactions, reactions in pregnant women, and any drug interactions. Reports of serious adverse reactions are required to enable risk/benefit ratios to be compared with other drugs of a similar class. For established drugs doctors are asked not to report well known, relatively minor side-effects, such as dry mouth with tricyclic antidepressants, constipation with opioids, or nausea with digoxin.

Special problems

(i) Delayed drug effects Doctors are reminded that some reactions (e.g., the development of cancers, chloroquine retinopathy and retroperitoneal fibrosis) may become manifest months or years after drug exposure. Please report any suspicion of such an association.

(ii) Drugs in the elderly Doctors are asked to be particularly alert to the possibility of adverse reactions when drugs are given to the elderly.

(iii) Congenital abnormalities When an infant is born with a congenital abnormality or there is a malformed aborted fetus, doctors are asked to consider the possibility that this might be an adverse reaction to a drug and to report all drugs (including self-medication) take[n] by the mother during pregnancy.

Yellow Cards

Prepaid Yellow Cards for reporting are available from the above address and forms for doctors are also included at the back of the Compendium.

A 24-hour Freefone service is available to all parts of the United Kingdom. For advice and information on adverse reactions contact the National Yellow Card Information Service at the Medicines Control Agency on 0800 7316789. Outside office hours a telephone-answering machine will take messages.

The following regional centres also collect data:

CSM Mersey
Freepost
Liverpool L3 3AB
(0151 794 8113)

CMS Wales
Freepost
Cardiff CF4 1ZZ
(01222 744181
Direct Line)

CSM Northern
Freepost
Newcastle upon Tyne
NE1 1BR
(0191-232 1525
Direct Line)

CSM West Midlands
Freepost
Birmingham
B18 7BR

The above statement and the symbols marking certain products have been included in the Compendium at the request of the Medicines Control Agency.

The individual companies concerned would find it helpful to be informed by practitioners of any adverse reactions to their products which are reported.

Contents

Abbott Laboratories Limited
Queenborough
Kent ME11 5EL

☎ 01628 773355 📠 01628 644185

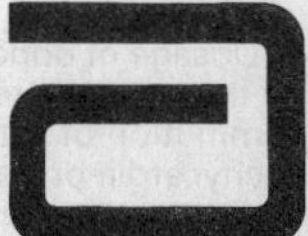

CALCIJEX*

Presentation Calcijex (calcitriol injection) is a sterile, isotonic, clear, aqueous solution for intravenous injection. It is available in 1 ml ampoules each containing calcitriol (1 microgram/ml or 2 micrograms/ml).

Uses Calcijex is indicated in the management of hypocalcaemia in patients undergoing dialysis for chronic renal failure. It has been shown to significantly reduce elevated parathyroid hormone (PTH) levels. Reduction of PTH has been shown to result in an improvement in renal osteodystrophy.

Actions: Calcitriol is the active form of vitamin D_3 (cholecalciferol). It is produced in the kidney from the vitamin D metabolite 25-hydroxyvitamin D_3 (calcifediol). A vitamin D-resistant state may exist in uremic patients because of the failure of the kidney to adequately produce the active compound, calcitriol.

The known sites of action of calcitriol are intestine, bone, kidney and parathyroid gland. Calcitriol is the most active known form of vitamin D_3 in stimulating intestinal calcium absorption. In bone, calcitriol, in conjunction with parathyroid hormone, stimulates resorption of calcium; and in the kidney, calcitriol increases the tubular reabsorption of calcium. *In-vitro* and *in-vivo* studies have shown that calcitriol directly suppresses secretion and synthesis of PTH by the parathyroids.

Calcitriol when administered by bolus injection is rapidly available in the blood stream. Vitamin D metabolites are known to be transported in blood, bound to specific plasma proteins. The pharmacological activity of an administered dose of calcitriol lasts approximately 3 to 5 days.

Dosage and administration The optimal dose of Calcijex must be carefully determined for each patient.

The recommended initial dose of Calcijex is 0.50 µg (approximately 0.01 µg/kg) administered three times weekly, approximately every other day. If a satisfactory response in the biochemical parameters and clinical manifestations of the disease state is not observed, the dose may be increased by 0.25 to 0.50 µg increments at two to four week intervals. During this titration period, serum calcium and phosphate levels should be obtained at least twice weekly, and if hypercalcaemia is noted, the drug should be immediately discontinued until normocalcaemia ensues. Most patients undergoing haemodialysis respond to doses of between 0.5 and 3.0 µg three times weekly.

Parenteral drug products such as Calcijex should be inspected visually for particulate matter prior to administration. Although calcitriol itself is a colourless, crystalline compound, the sodium ascorbate added as an antioxidant in Calcijex is white or very faintly yellow, and can turn yellow as it combines with oxygen.

Calcijex should be drawn up into a plastic 1 ml tuberculin syringe and administered as a bolus dose intravenously at the end of dialysis. It may be administered through the catheter at the end of haemodialysis.

The effectiveness of Calcijex therapy is predicted on the assumption that each patient is receiving an adequate and appropriate daily intake of calcium. To ensure that each patient receives an adequate daily intake of calcium, the physician should either prescribe a calcium supplement, or instruct the patient in proper dietary measures. Patients should be informed of the symptoms of hypercalcaemia (see *Side-effects*).

Use in children: Safety and efficacy of Calcijex in children have not been established.

Use in pregnancy and lactation: There are no adequate and well-controlled studies in pregnant women. Calcijex should be used during pregnancy only if the potential benefit justifies the potential risk to the foetus.

It is not known whether this drug is excreted in human milk. Because of the potential for serious adverse reaction in nursing infants due to calcitriol, breast feeding cannot be recommended.

Contra-indications, warnings, etc

Contra-indications: Calcijex should not be given to patients with hypercalcaemia or evidence of vitamin D toxicity.

Calcijex injection should not be given to patients with previous hypersensitivity to calcitriol or any of its excipients.

Warnings: Since calcitriol is the most potent metabolite of vitamin D available, vitamin D and its derivatives should be withheld during treatment.

In patients undergoing dialysis who have high serum phosphate levels, appropriate serum phosphate binders should be used. Overdosage of any form of vitamin D is dangerous (see also *Overdosage*). Progressive hypercalcaemia due to overdosage of vitamin D and its metabolites may be so severe as to require emergency attention. Chronic hypercalcaemia can lead to generalised vascular calcification, nephrocalcinosis and other soft-tissue calcification. The serum calcium times phosphate (Ca×P) product should not be allowed to exceed 70. Radiographic evaluation of suspect anatomical regions may be useful in the early detection of this condition.

Precautions: Excessive dosage of Calcijex induces hypercalcaemia, and in some instances hypercalciuria. Therefore, serum calcium and phosphate should be determined at least twice weekly early in treatment during dosage adjustment. Should hypercalcaemia develop, the drug should be discontinued immediately.

Renal transplantation: The rate of bone loss can be excessive and may exceed 5% per year in the immediate post-transplant period. Recommendations for treating post-transplant bone loss with calcitriol have not been established.

Interactions:

Magnesium-containing antacids: Magnesium-containing antacids and Calcijex should not be used concomitantly, because such use may lead to the development of hypermagnesaemia.

Cardiac glycosides: Calcijex should be given cautiously to patients on cardiac glycosides, because hypercalcaemia in such patients may precipitate cardiac arrhythmias.

Barbiturates and anticonvulsants: Higher doses of Calcijex may be required for patients taking barbiturates or anticonvulsants as these may reduce its effects.

Corticosteroids: The effects of Calcijex may be counteracted by corticosteroids.

Side-effects: Adverse effects of Calcijex are, in general, similar to those encountered with excessive vitamin D intake. The early symptoms of vitamin D intoxication associated with hypercalcaemia include weakness, headache, somnolence, nausea, vomiting, dry mouth, constipation, muscle pain, bone pain and metallic taste. Late signs include polyuria, polydipsia, anorexia, weight loss, nocturia, conjunctivitis (calcific), pancreatitis, photophobia, rhinorrhea, pruritus, hyperthermia, decreased libido, elevated BUN, albuminuria, hypercholesterolaemia, elevated SGOT and SGPT, ectopic calcification, hypertension, cardiac arrhythmias and, rarely, overt psychosis.

Rare cases of hypersensitivity reactions have been reported including anaphylaxis and localised redness at the injection site.

Overdosage: Administration of Calcijex to patients in excess of their requirements can cause hypercalcaemia, hypercalciuria and hyperphosphataemia. High intake of calcium and phosphate concomitant with Calcijex may lead to similar abnormalities.

General treatment of hypercalcaemia (greater than 1 mg/dl above the upper limit of normal range) consists of immediate discontinuation of Calcijex therapy, institution of a low calcium diet and withdrawal of calcium supplements. Serum calcium levels should be determined daily until normocalcaemia (8.5 to 10.5 mg/dl) ensues. Hypercalcaemia usually resolves in two to seven days. When serum calcium levels have returned to within normal limits, Calcijex therapy may be reinstituted at a dose 0.5 µg less than prior therapy. Serum calcium levels should be obtained at least twice weekly after all dosage changes.

Persistent or markedly elevated serum calcium levels may be corrected by dialysis against a calcium-free dialysate.

The treatment of acute accidental overdosage of Calcijex should consist of general supportive measures. Serial serum electrolyte determinations (especially calcium), rate of urinary calcium excretion and assessment of electrocardiographic abnormalities due to hypercalcaemia should be obtained. Such monitoring is critical in patients receiving digitalis. Discontinuation of supplemental calcium and initiation of low calcium diet are also indicated in accidental overdosage. Due to the pharmacological action of calcitriol lasting only 3–5 days, further measures are probably unnecessary. However, should persistent and markedly elevated serum calcium levels occur, there are a variety of therapeutic alternatives which may be considered, depending on the patient's underlying condition. These include the use of drugs such as biphosphonates, mithramycin, calcitonin, gallium nitrate and corticosteroids as well as measures to induce an appropriate forced diuresis. The use of peritoneal dialysis and haemodialysis against a calcium-free dialysate has also been reported.

Pharmaceutical precautions Calcitriol is known to be adsorbed onto PVC containers and tubing. It should therefore not be infused with the dialysate during CAPD as the dose could be significantly reduced due to drug adsorption to the PVC bag and tubing. See *Dosage and Administration* for recommended dosage method.

Store at room temperature and protect from light.

Discard any unused solution immediately after use.

Legal category POM.

Package quantities Calcijex is supplied in 1 ml amber glass ampoules containing calcitriol (1 microgram/ml or 2 micrograms/ml).

Further information Nil.

Product licence numbers

1 microgram ampoule 0037/0245
2 microgram ampoule 0037/0246.

DOPAMINE HYDROCHLORIDE 400 mg in 5% DEXTROSE INJECTION DOPAMINE HYDROCHLORIDE 800 mg in 5% DEXTROSE INJECTION

Qualitative and quantitative composition Each 250 ml of the injection contains either 400 mg or 800 mg of Dopamine Hydrochloride USP, sodium metabisulphite, dextrose anhydrous or hydrous, water for injections and hydrochloric acid or sodium hydroxide.

Pharmaceutical form A clear, sterile solution for intravenous infusion.

Clinical particulars

Therapeutic indications: Dopamine administered intravenously is a positive myocardial inotropic agent, which also may increase mesenteric and renal blood flow plus urinary output.

Dopamine hydrochloride in 5% Dextrose is indicated for the correction of haemodynamic imbalances present in shock due to myocardial infarction, trauma, endotoxic septicaemia, open heart surgery, renal failure and chronic cardiac decompensation as in refractory congestive failure.

Posology and method of administration:

Adults: Where appropriate, restoration of the circulatory volume should be instituted or completed with a suitable plasma expander or whole blood, prior to administration of dopamine hydrochloride.

Begin infusion of dopamine hydrochloride solution at doses of 2.5 micrograms/kg/min in patients who are likely to respond to modest increments of heart force and renal perfusion.

In more seriously ill patients, begin infusion of dopamine hydrochloride at doses of 5 micrograms/kg/min and increase gradually using 5 to 10 micrograms/kg/min increments up to a rate of 20 to 50 micrograms/kg/min as needed. If doses in excess of 50 micrograms/kg/min are required, it is advisable to check urine output frequently. Should urinary flow begin to decrease in the absence of hypotension, reduction of dopamine dosage should be considered. It has been found that more than 50% of patients have been satisfactorily maintained on doses less than 20 micrograms/kg/min.

As with all potent intravenously administered drugs, care should be taken to control the rate of infusion so as to avoid inadvertent administration of a bolus drug.

In patients who do not respond to these doses with adequate arterial pressures or urine flow, additional increments of dopamine may be given in an effort to produce an appropriate arterial pressure and central perfusion.

Dosage of dopamine should be adjusted according to the patient's response, with particular attention to diminution of established urine flow rate, increasing tachycardia or development of new dysrhythmias as indications for decreasing or temporarily suspending the dosage.

Children: Safety and effectiveness in children have not been established.

Contra-indications: Use in patients with phaeochromocytoma.

Dextrose solution without electrolytes should not administered simultaneously with blood through the same infusion set because of the possibility that pseudo-agglutination of the red blood cells may occur.

Dopamine should not be administered in the presence of uncorrected tachyarrhythmias or ventricular fibrillation.

Special warnings and special precautions for use: Hypovolemia should be corrected where necessary prior to treatment with dopamine.

Avoid bolus administration of the drug.

Excess administration of potassium-free solutions may result in significant hypokalaemia.

The intravenous administration of these solutions can cause a fluid and/or solute overload resulting in dilution of serum electrolyte concentrations, overhydration, congested states or pulmonary oedema.

Hypoxia, hypercapnia and acidosis may reduce the effectiveness and/or increase the incidence of adverse effects of dopamine and must be identified and corrected prior to, or concurrently with, administration of dopamine.

If a tachyarrhythmia or an increased number of ectopic beats are observed, the dose of dopamine should be reduced if possible.

If a disproportionate rise in diastolic pressure (i.e. a marked decrease in pulse pressure) is observed, the infusion rate should be decreased and the patient observed carefully for further evidence of predominant vasoconstriction activity, unless such an effect is desired.

At lower infusion rates, if hypotension occurs, the infusion rate should be rapidly increased until adequate blood pressure is obtained. If hypotension persists, dopamine hydrochloride should be discontinued and alternative therapies should be instituted.

Patients with a history of peripheral vascular disease should be closely monitored for any changes in colour or temperature of the skin of the extremities. If a change of skin colour or temperature occurs, and is thought to be the result of compromised circulation to the extremities, the benefits of continued dopamine infusion should be weighed against the risk of possible necrosis. These changes may be reversed by decreasing the rate or discontinuing the infusion.

Dopamine hydrochloride in 5% Dextrose injection should be infused into a large vein whenever possible to prevent the possibility of infiltration of perivascular tissue adjacent to the infusion site. Extravasation may cause necrosis and sloughing of the surrounding tissue. Ischaemia can be reversed by infiltration of the affected area with 10–15 ml of saline containing 5 to 10 mg phentolamine mesylate. A syringe with a fine hypodermic needle should be used to liberally infiltrate the ischaemic area as soon as extravasation is noted.

Dopamine hydrochloride in 5% Dextrose contains sodium metabisulphite which may cause allergic type reactions, including anaphylactic symptoms and life threatening or less severe asthmatic episodes in certain susceptible people.

Dextrose solutions should be used with caution in patients with known subclinical or overt diabetes mellitus.

When discontinuing the infusion, it may be necessary to gradually decrease the dose of dopamine hydrochloride while expanding blood volume, if appropriate, with intravenous fluids, since sudden cessation may result in marked hypotension.

Interaction with other medicaments and other forms of interaction: Patients who have been treated with monoamine oxidase (MAO) inhibitors prior to administration of dopamine should receive a substantially reduced dosage of the latter. The starting dose in such patients should be reduced to at least one tenth of the usual dose.

Dopamine should be used with extreme caution in patients inhaling cyclopropane or halogenated hydrocarbon anaesthetics.

Concurrent administration of dopamine and diuretics may produce an additive or potentiating effect on urine flow.

Pregnancy and lactation: Animal studies have shown no evidence of teratogenic effects with dopamine. The drug may be used in pregnant women when, in the judgement of the physician, the expected benefits outweigh the potential risk to the foetus.

Effects on ability to drive and use machines: None.

Undesirable effects: The most frequently reported adverse reactions to dopamine have been ectopic beats, tachycardia, nausea, vomiting, anginal pain, palpitations, dyspnoea, headache, hypotension and vasoconstriction.

Very rarely reported reactions include aberrant conduction, bradycardia, piloerection, widened QRS complex, azotaemia and elevated blood pressure.

Overdosage: Accidental overdosage as evidenced by excessive blood pressure elevation can be controlled by dose reduction or discontinuing the administration for a short period until the patient's condition stabilises.

If these measures fail, an infusion of phentolamine mesylate should be considered.

Pharmacological properties
Pharmacodynamic properties: Dopamine is a sympathomimetic agent with both direct and indirect effects. It dilates renal and mesenteric blood vessels and increases urine output. Dopamine also stimulates beta adrenergic receptors in the myocardium.

Pharmacokinetic properties: Dopamine is metabolised in the liver, kidney and plasma by MAO and catechol-O-methyl transferase to inactive compounds; homovanillic acid (HVA) and 3,4-dihydroxyphenyl-acetic acid. About 25% of the dose is taken up into specialised neurosecretory vesicles where it is hydroxylated to form noradrenaline.

It has been reported that about 80% of the drug is excreted within 24 hours, primarily as HVA. A very small portion is excreted unchanged.

Preclinical safety data: There are no pre-clinical data of relevance to the prescriber which are additional to that already included in other sections of the SPC.

Pharmaceutical particulars
List of excipients: Dextrose; sodium metabisulphite; hydrochloric acid, and/or sodium hydroxide; water for injections.

Incompatibilties: Do not add sodium bicarbonate or other alkaline substances, since dopamine is inactivated in alkaline solution.

Shelf life: 2 years.

Special precautions for storage: Store away from heat and protect from freezing.

Nature and contents of container: A flexible, copolyester 250 ml blow moulded container or 150 ml fabricated container, within an aluminium foil overwrap.

Instructions for use/handling: Use only if solution is clear and container is intact. For single use only. Discard unused portion.

Other drugs should not be added to this solution.

Marketing authorisation numbers
Dopamine 400 mg 0037/0146
Dopamine 800 mg 0037/0147

Date of approval/revision of SPC September 1997.

Legal category POM.

ENFLURANE

Presentation Enflurane is an inhalation anaesthetic with a pleasant ethereal odour. No additives or stabilisers are present.

Uses Enflurane may be used for induction and maintenance of general anaesthesia. Adequate data are not available yet to establish its full place in obstetric anaesthesia other than in caesarean section. High concentrations of enflurane may produce marked uterine relaxation.

Enflurane may be used for outpatient and dental anaesthesia in view of the rapidity of action and recovery, with stability of the cardiovascular system. Enflurane can be used in children.

Actions: Induction and recovery are rapid. It does not stimulate excessive salivation, tracheobronchial secretions or cause bronchial constriction. Pharyngeal and laryngeal reflexes are diminished quickly. The level of anaesthesia changes rapidly with enflurane. Tachypnoea does not usually occur. Spontaneous respiration becomes depressed as the depth of anaesthesia increases.

Enflurane provokes a 'sigh' response reminiscent of that seen with diethyl ether.

During induction there is a decrease in blood pressure followed by a return to near normal levels, which may or may not be associated with surgical stimulation.

Blood pressure tends to fall in direct relation to the depth of anaesthesia but cardiac rate and rhythm remain stable. Enflurane appears to 'sensitise' the myocardium to adrenaline in man to a lesser extent than halothane. Available data indicate that subcutaneous injections of adrenaline may be safely administered to humans in concentrations of 1:100,000 or less at a dose of 10 ml in any given 10 minute period and not more than 30 ml/hour. All the usual precautions in the use of vasoconstrictor substances must be observed.

Good muscular relaxation is obtained with enflurane, but should greater relaxation be necessary minimal doses of an intravenous muscle relaxant may be used with measures to ensure adequate ventilation.

All commonly used intravenous muscle relaxants are compatible with enflurane.

Note: Enflurane potentiates the effect of the non-depolarising muscle relaxants which should therefore be used in reduced dosage. Neostigmine does not reverse the direct effect of enflurane.

Enflurane produces little post-operative analgesia.

Metabolism of enflurane in the human body proceeds at a low rate; inorganic fluoride is formed but serum levels in healthy individuals have not been shown to rise to significant levels.

Dosage and administration Vaporisers calibrated specifically for enflurane should be used so that the concentration being delivered is known.

The inspired concentration required to achieve clinical anaesthesia depends upon the age of the patient and to a minimal extent on body temperature. The MAC value is higher in children and decreases with advancing age, falling from an average in oxygen of 2.4% in the newborn and 2.5% at puberty, to 1.9% in young adults, and 1.7% at middle age. As with other agents, lesser concentrations of enflurane are normally required to maintain surgical anaesthesia in elderly patients. MAC values increase with increasing body temperature.

Premedication: Drugs used for premedication should be selected for each individual patient. The use of anticholinergic drugs is a matter of choice.

Induction: To avoid excitement a short-acting barbiturate or other intravenous induction agent should be administered, followed by inhalation of the enflurane mixture. Enflurane and oxygen alone or oxygen-nitrous oxide mixtures may be used.

It is recommended that enflurane induction be initiated at a concentration of 0.4% and gradually increased by 0.5% increments after every few breaths until surgical anaesthesia is achieved.

The maximum inspired concentration during induction should be no more than 4.5%. High inspired concentrations should be lowered as rapidly as possible to maintenance levels to prevent overdosage, and the blood pressure carefully observed.

Maintenance: In conjunction with nitrous oxide, surgical levels of anaesthesia may be maintained with a 0.5%–3% concentration of enflurane. A 3% concentration should not be exceeded for maintenance during spontaneous respiration. With controlled respiration techniques, during prolonged operations, single or supplementary doses of muscle relaxants may be used if required, bearing in mind the possibility of some slight potentiation. Ventilation to maintain the carbon dioxide tension in arterial blood in the the 4.7–6.0 kPa (35–45 mmHg) range is preferred to hyper- or hypoventilation, in order to minimise the possibility of CNS excitation.

Blood pressure levels during maintenance depend on enflurane concentration in the absence of other complicating factors. Excessive decreases (unless related to hypovolaemia) may be due to depth of anaesthesia and in such instances should be corrected by reducing the inspired enflurane concentration.

Elderly: As with other agents, lesser concentrations of enflurane are normally required to maintain surgical anaesthesia in elderly patients.

Contra-indications, warnings, etc
Contra-indications: Known sensitivity to enflurane and in patients with known or suspected genetic susceptability to malignant hyperthermia.

Precautions: Enflurane should be used with caution in patients who, by virtue of medical or drug history, may be considered more susceptible to cerebral stimulation produced by this drug. Increasing depth of anaesthesia with enflurane may produce changes in the electroencephalogram characterised by high voltage, fast frequency waves progressing through spike-dome complexes alternating with periods of electrical silence to frank seizure activity patterns. The latter may or may not be associated with motor movement. Motor activity, when encountered, generally consists of twitching or 'jerks' of various muscle groups; it is self-limiting and can be terminated by lowering the anaesthetic concentration. This electroencephalographic pattern associated with deep anaesthesia may be exacerbated by hyperventilation producing low arterial carbon dioxide tension. The pattern serves as a warning that depth of anaesthesia is excessive. Cerebral blood flow and metabolism studies in normal volunteers during seizure patterns show no evidence of cerebral hypoxia, and recovery appears to be uncomplicated.

In susceptible individuals, enflurane anaesthesia may trigger a skeletal muscle hypermetabolic state and the clinical syndrome known as malignant hyperthermia. The syndrome includes non-specific features such as muscle rigidity, tachycardia, tachypnoea, cyanosis, arrhythmias and unstable blood pressure.

Treatment includes discontinuing enflurane anaesthesia, administration of dantrolene sodium and supportive therapy. Renal failure may appear later and urine flow should be sustained if possible.

Since levels of anaesthesia may be altered easily and rapidly, only vaporisers which deliver a predictable output with reasonable accuracy should be used. Hypotension and respiratory exchange can serve as a guide to anaesthetic depth. With deep levels of anaesthesia, more marked hypotension and respiratory depression are encountered.

The action of non-depolarising relaxants is augmented by enflurane, so less than the usual amounts of those drugs should be used.

Overdosage or unduly rapid absorption of adrenaline administered topically or by subcutaneous or submucosal injection during enflurane anaesthesia may give rise to cardiac arrhythmias (see 'Actions' section). Care must be taken to avoid intravenous injection.

Bromsulphthalein (BSP) retention is mildly raised post-operatively in some cases. There is some elevation of blood glucose and white blood cell count intra-operatively.

Enflurane has been reported to interact with dry carbon dioxide absorbents to form carbon monoxide. In order to minimise the risk of formation of carbon monoxide in rebreathing circuits and the possibility of elevated carboxyhaemoglobin levels, carbon dioxide absorbents should not be allowed to dry out.

Use in pregnancy: Reproduction studies have been performed in rats and rabbits. Following single and multiple maternal administrations, no evidence of teratogenicity due to enflurane was found in the developing foetuses in these species. The relevance of these studies to the human is not known. Since there is no adequate experience in pregnant women who have received the drug, safety in pregnancy has not been established.

It is not known whether enflurane is excreted in breast milk and caution should therefore be exercised when enflurane is administered to a nursing mother.

Adverse reactions:

1. Motor activity exemplified by movement of various muscle groups and seizures may be encountered with deep levels of enflurane anaesthesia, particularly with hyperventilation.

2. Hypotension, respiratory depression and arrhythmias have been reported.

3. Elevation of the white blood cell count has been observed. It has not been determined whether this is related to enflurane or to surgical stress.

4. A mild increase in serum glucose concentration has been observed in some normal and diabetic patients, as with other anaesthetic agents. There seems to be no contra-indication to the use of the agent in these patients for whom rapid recovery is advantageous.

5. Hepatic enzyme changes occur less frequently and to a lesser degree after multiple enflurane anaesthetics when compared with multiple exposures to halothane. While jaundice and significant hepatic enzyme increases occasionally occur after halothane anaesthesia, this is extremely rare after the administration of enflurane in the absence of complicating factors such as blood transfusion or concomitant administration of hepatotoxic drugs.

6. Increased serum inorganic fluoride levels have been found during and immediately after enflurane anaesthesia due to biodegradation of the agent. These levels normally remain well below the postulated threshold for nephrotoxicity and, after reaching a peak within eight hours of the end of the anaesthetic, rapidly return to preoperative values.

Although there is no evidence that enflurane anaesthesia adversely affects the normal or diseased kidney it may be prudent to avoid its use in cases of chronic renal failure.

Side-effects: Nausea, vomiting, hiccups or shivering may occur occasionally.

Pharmaceutical precautions Store away from heat. Keep well closed.

Legal category P.

Package quantities Enflurane is supplied in bottles of 250 ml.

Further information Nil.

Product licence number 0037/0053.

ERYTHROCIN* 250
ERYTHROCIN* 500

Qualitative and quantitative composition
Erythrocin 250 contains Erythromycin as erythromycin stearate 250 mg/tablet.

Erythrocin 500 contains Erythromycin as erythromycin stearate 500 mg/tablet.

Pharmaceutical form Film coated tablet.

Clinical particulars
Therapeutic indications: For the prophylaxis and treatment of infections caused by erythromycin-sensitive organisms.

Erythromycin is highly effective in the treatment of a great variety of clinical infections such as:

1. Upper Respiratory Tract infections: tonsillitis, peritonsillar abscess, pharyngitis, laryngitis, sinusitis, secondary infections in influenza and common colds.
2. Lower Respiratory Tract infections: tracheitis, acute and chronic bronchitis, pneumonia (lobar pneumonia, bronchopneumonia, primary atypical pneumonia), bronchiectasis, Legionnaire's disease.
3. Ear infection: otitis media and otitis externa, mastoiditis.
4. Oral infections: gingivitis, Vincent's angina.
5. Eye infections: blepharitis.
6. Skin and soft tissue infections: boils and carbuncles, paronychia, abscesses, pustular acne, impetigo, cellulitis, erysipelas.
7. Gastrointestinal infections: cholecystitis, staphylococcal enterocolitis.
8. Prophylaxis: pre- and post-operative trauma, burns, rheumatic fever, bacterial endocarditis in patients allergic to penicillin with congenital heart disease, or rheumatic or other acquired valvular heart disease when undergoing dental procedures or surgical procedures of the upper respiratory tract.
9. Other infections: osteomyelitis, urethritis, gonorrhoea, syphilis, lymphogranuloma venereum, diphtheria, prostatitis, scarlet fever.

Posology and method of administration:
Adults and children over 8 years: 1–2 g/day in divided doses. For severe infections up to 4 g/day in divided doses.

Elderly: No special dosage recommendations.

Children under 8 years: Erythroped suspension is recommended.

Contra-indications: Known hypersensitivity to erythromycin. Erythromycin is contra-indicated in patients taking astemizole, terfenadine, cisapride or pimozide.

Erythromycin is contra-indicated with ergotamine and dihydroergotamine.

Special warnings and special precautions for use: Erythromycin is excreted principally by the liver, so caution should be exercised in administering the antibiotic to patients with impaired hepatic function or concomitantly receiving potentially hepatotoxic agents. Hepatic dysfunction including increased liver enzymes and/or cholestatic hepatitis, with or without jaundice, has been infrequently reported with erythromycin.

There have been reports suggesting erythromycin does not reach the foetus in adequate concentrations to prevent congenital syphilis. Infants born to women treated during pregnancy with oral erythromycin for early syphilis should be treated with an appropriate penicillin regimen.

There have been reports that erythromycin may aggravate the weakness of patients with myasthenia gravis.

Erythromycin interferes with the fluorometric determination of urinary catecholamines.

As with other broad spectrum antibiotics, pseudomembranous colitis has been reported rarely with erythromycin.

Rhabdomyolysis with or without renal impairment has been reported in seriously ill patients receiving erythromycin concomitantly with lovastatin.

Interaction with other medicaments and other forms of interaction: Concomitant use of erythromycin with terfenadine or astemizole is likely to result in an enhanced risk of cardiotoxicity with these drugs. The concomitant use of erythromycin with either astemizole or terfenadine is therefore contra-indicated.

The metabolism of terfenadine and astemizole is significantly altered when either are taken concomitantly with erythromycin. Rare cases of serious cardiovascular events have been observed, including torsades de pointes, other ventricular arrhythmias and cardiac arrest. Death has been reported with the terfenadine/erythromycin combination.

Elevated cisapride levels have been reported in patients receiving erythromycin and cisapride concomitantly. This may result in QT prolongation and cardiac arrhythmias including ventricular tachycardia, ventricular fibrillation and torsades de pointes. Similar effects have been observed with concomitant administration of pimozide and clarithromycin, another macrolide antibiotic.

Concurrent use of erythromycin and ergotamine or dihydroergotamine has been associated in some patients with acute ergot toxicity characterised by the rapid development of severe peripheral vasospasm and dysaesthesia.

Increases in serum concentrations of the following drugs metabolised by the cytochrome P450 system may occur when administered concurrently with erythromycin: alfentanil, astemizole, bromocriptine, carbamazepine, cyclosporin, digoxin, dihydroergotamine, disopyramide, ergotamine, hexobarbitone, midazolam, phenytoin, quinidine, tacrolimus, terfenadine, theophylline, triazolam, valproate, and warfarin. Appropriate monitoring should be undertaken and dosage should be adjusted as necessary.

Erythromycin has been reported to decrease the clearance of zopiclone and thus may increase the pharmacodynamic effects of this drug.

When oral erythromycin is given concurrently with theophylline, there is also a significant decrease in erythromycin serum concentrations. The decrease could result in subtherapeutic concentrations of erythromycin.

Pregnancy and lactation: There is no evidence of hazard from erythromycin in human pregnancy. It has been in widespread use for a number of years without apparent ill consequence. Animal studies have shown no hazard.

Erythromycin has been reported to cross the placental barrier in humans, but foetal plasma levels are generally low.

Erythromycin is excreted in breast milk, therefore, caution should be exercised when erythromycin is administered to a nursing mother.

Effects on ability to drive and to use machines: None reported.

Undesirable effects: Occasional side effects such as nausea, abdominal discomfort, vomiting and diarrhoea may be experienced. Reversible hearing loss associated with doses of erythromycin usually greater than 4 g per day has been reported. Allergic reactions are rare and mild, although anaphylaxis has occurred. Skin reactions ranging from mild eruptions to erythema multiforme, Stevens-Johnson syndrome and toxic epidermal necrolysis have rarely been reported. There are no reports implicating erythromycin products with abnormal tooth development, and only rare reports of damage to the blood, kidneys or central nervous system.

Cardiac arrhythmias have been very rarely reported in patients receiving erythromycin therapy. There have been isolated reports of chest pain, dizziness and palpitations, however, a cause and effect relationship has not been established.

Symptoms of hepatitis, hepatic dysfunction and/or abnormal liver function test results may occur.

Overdosage:
Symptoms: hearing loss, severe nausea, vomiting and diarrhoea.

Treatment: gastric lavage, general supportive measures.

Pharmacological properties
Pharmacodynamic properties: Erythromycin exerts its antimicrobial action by binding to the 50S ribosomal sub-unit of susceptible microorganisms and suppresses protein synthesis. Erythromycin is usually active against most strains of the following organisms both *in vitro* and in clinical infections:

Gram positive bacteria – *Listeria monocytogenes, Corynebacterium diphtheriae* (as an adjunct to antitoxin), Staphylococci spp, Streptococci spp (including Enterococci).

Gram negative bacteria – *Haemophilus influenzae, Neisseria meningitidis, Neisseria gonorrhoeae, Legionella pneumophila, Moraxella (Branhamella) catarrhalis, Bordetella pertussis,* Campylobacter spp.

Mycoplasma – *Mycoplasma pneumoniae, Ureaplasma urealyticum.*

Other organisms – *Treponema pallidum,* Chlamydia spp, Clostridia spp, L-forms, the agents causing trachoma and lymphogranuloma venereum.

Note: The majority of strains of Haemophilus influenzae are susceptible to the concentrations reached after ordinary doses.

Pharmacokinetic particulars: None stated.

Preclinical safety data: There are no pre-clinical data of relevance to the prescriber which are additional to that already included in other sections of the SPC.

Pharmaceutical particulars
List of excipients: Povidone, maize starch, magnesium hydroxide, polacrilin potassium, polyethylene glycol 8000, polyethylene glycol 400, hydroxypropyl methyl cellulose, sorbic acid.

Incompatibilities: None stated.

Shelf life: 60 months.

Special precautions for storage: None stated.

Nature and contents of container: Erythrocin 250: High density polyethylene bottle with urea cap with 100 tablets, securitainer or snap-secure container with 50, 100 or 1000 tablets. Blister packs containing 28 tablets: PVC, heat sealed with 20 micron hard tamper aluminium foil.

Erythrocin 500: High density polyethylene bottle with urea cap with 100 tablets, securitainer or snap-secure container with 50, 100 or 1000 tablets. Blister packs containing 10, 14, 15, 28 or 56 tablets: PVC, heat sealed with 20 micron hard tamper aluminium foil.

Instructions for use/handling: Not applicable.

Marketing authorisation numbers

Erythrocin 250	PL 0037/5079R
Erythrocin 500	PL 0037/5044R

Date of first authorisation/renewal of authorisation 16/06/97

Date of (partial) revision of text August 1997

Legal category POM

ERYTHROMID*

Presentation Erythromid is an white to off-white, enteric-coated, film-coated tablet containing 250 mg of Erythromycin BP. They are Erythromycin Tablets BP.

Uses For the prophylaxis and treatment of infections caused by erythromycin-sensitive organisms. Erythromycin is highly effective in the treatment of a great variety of clinical infections such as:

1. Upper Respiratory Tract infections: tonsillitis, peritonsillar abscess, pharyngitis, laryngitis, sinusitis, secondary infections in influenza and common colds.
2. Lower Respiratory Tract infections: tracheitis, acute and chronic bronchitis, pneumonia (lobar pneumonia, bronchopneumonia, primary atypical pneumonia), bronchiectasis, Legionnaire's disease.
3. Ear infection: otisis media and otitis externa, mastoiditis.
4. Oral infections: gingivitis, Vincent's angina.
5. Eye infections: blepharitis.
6. Skin and soft tissue infections: boils and carbuncles, paronychia, abscesses, pustular acne, impetigo, cellulitis, erysipelas.
7. Gastrointestinal infections: cholecystitis, staphylococcal enterocolitis.
8. Prophylaxis: pre- and post-operative trauma, burns, rheumatic fever.
9. Other infections: osteomyelitis, urethritis, gonorrhoea, syphilis, lymphogranuloma venereum, diphtheria, prostatitis, scarlet fever.

Note: Erythromycin has also proved to be of value in endocarditis and septicaemia, but in these conditions initial administration of erythromycin lactobionate by the intravenous route is advisable.

Pharmacological properties: Erythromycin exerts its antimicrobial action by binding to the 50S ribosomal sub-unit of susceptible microorganisms and suppresses protein synthesis. Erythromycin is usually active against most strains of the following organisms both *in vitro* and in clinical infections:

Gram positive bacteria – *Listeria monocytogenes, Corynebacterium diphtheriae* (as an adjunct to antitoxin), Staphylococci spp, Streptococci spp (including Enterococci).

Gram negative bacteria – *Haemophilus influenzae, Neisseria meningitidis, Neisseria gonorrhoeae, Legionella pneumophila, Moraxella (Branhamella) catarrhalis, Bordetella pertussis,* Campylobacter spp.

Mycoplasma – *Mycoplasma pneumoniae, Ureaplasma urealyticum.*

Other organisms – *Treponema pallidum,* Chlamydia spp, Clostridia spp, L-forms, the agents causing trachoma and lymphogranuloma venereum.

Note: The majority of strains of *Haemophilus influenzae* are susceptible to the concentrations reached after ordinary doses.

Pharmacokinetic particulars:

Absorption and Fate: Erythromycin is adversely affected by gastric acid. For this reason erythromycin tablets are enteric coated.

It is absorbed from the small intestine. It is widely distributed throughout body tissues. Little metabolism occurs and only about 5% is eliminated in the urine. It is excreted principally by the liver.

Dosage and administration

Adults and children over 8 years: For mild to moderate infections 1–2 g daily in divided doses. For severe infections this may be increased to 4 g daily in divided doses. Tablets should be taken before or with meals.

Elderly: No special dosage recommendations.

Children under 8 years: Erythroped suspension is recommended.

Period of dosing with regard to indication: Duration of dosing should be related to the severity and site of infection, but generally lies within the range of 5–14 days. However, the duration may need to be longer in certain cases, e.g. NGU and syphilis 10–21 days or longer, chlamydial inclusion conjunctivitis up to 21 days, acne may require prolonged treatment. Prophylaxis prior to dental or surgical procedures should begin 1½ to 2 hours before the procedure and continued every 6 hours for 8 doses.

Contra-indications, warnings, etc

Contra-indications: Known hypersensitivity to erythromycin. Erythromycin is contra-indicated in patients taking astemizole or terfenadine, cisapride or pimozide. Erythromycin is contra-indicated with ergotamine and dihydroergotamine.

Precautions: Erythromycin is excreted principally by the liver, so caution should be exercised in administering the antibiotic to patients with impaired hepatic function or concomitantly receiving potentially hepatotoxic agents. Hepatic dysfunction including increased liver enzymes and/or cholestatic hepatitis, with or without jaundice, has been infrequently reported with erythromycin.

There have been reports suggesting erythromycin does not reach the foetus in adequate concentrations to prevent congenital syphilis. Infants born to women treated during pregnancy with oral erythromycin for early syphilis should be treated with an appropriate penicillin regimen.

There have been reports that erythromycin may aggravate the weakness of patients with myasthenia gravis.

Erythromycin interferes with the fluorometric determination or urinary catecholamines.

As with other broad spectrum antibiotics, pseudomembraneous colitis has been reported rarely with erythromycin.

Rhabdomyolysis with or without renal impairment has been reported in seriously ill patients receiving erythromycin concomitantly with lovastatin.

Interactions: Concomitant use of erythromycin with terfenadine or astemizole is likely to result in an enhanced risk of cardiotoxicity with these drugs. The concomitant use of erythromycin with either astemizole or terfenadine is therefore contra-indicated.

The metabolism of terfenadine and astemizole is significantly altered when either are taken concomitantly with erythromycin. Rare cases of serious cardiovascular events have been observed, including Torsades de pointes, other ventricular arrhythmias and cardiac arrest. Death has been reported with the terfenadine/erythromycin combination. Elevated cisapride levels have been reported in patients receiving erythromycin and cisapride concomitantly. This may result in QT prolongation and cardiac arrhythmias including ventricular tachycardia, ventricular fibrillation and Torsades de pointes. Similar effects have been observed with concomitant administration of pimozide and clarithromycin, another macrolide antibiotic.

Concurrent use of erythromycin and ergotamine or dihydroergotamine has been associated in some patients with acute ergot toxicity characterised by the rapid development of severe peripheral vasospasm and dysethesia.

Increases in serum concentrations of the following drugs metabolised by the cytochrome P450 system may occur when administered concurrently with erythromycin: alfentanil, astemizole, bromocriptine, carbamazepine, cyclosporin, digoxin, dihydroergotamine, disopyramide, ergotamine, hexobarbitone, midazolam, phenytoin, quinidine, tacrolimus, terfenadine, theophylline, triazolam, valproate, and warfarin. Appropriate monitoring should be undertaken and dosage should be adjusted as necessary.

Erythromycin has been reported to decrease the clearance of zopiclone and thus may increase the pharmacodynamic effects of this drug.

When oral erythromycin is given concurrently with theophylline, there is also a significant decrease in erythromycin serum concentrations. The decrease could result in subtherapeutic concentrations of erythromycin.

Use in pregnancy and nursing mothers: There is no evidence of hazard from erythromycin in human pregnancy. It has been in wide use for many years without apparent ill consequence. Animal studies have shown no hazard.

Erythromycin has been reported to cross the placental barrier in humans, but foetal plasma levels are generally low.

Erythromycin is excreted in breast milk, therefore, caution should be exercised when erythromycin is administered to a nursing mother.

Side-effects: Occasional side-effects such as nausea, abdominal discomfort, vomiting and diarrhoea may be experienced. Reversible hearing loss associated with doses of erythromycin usually greater than 4 g per day has been reported. Allergic reactions are rare and mild, although anaphylaxis has occurred. Skin reactions ranging from mild eruptions to erythema multiforme, Stevens-Johnson syndrome and toxic epidermal neurolysis have rarely been reported. There are no reports implicating erythromycin products with abnormal tooth development and only rare reports of damage to the blood, kidneys, liver or central nervous system.

Cardiac arrhythmias have been very rarely reported in patients receiving erythromycin therapy. There have been isolated reports of chest pain, dizziness and palpitations; however, a cause and effect relationship has not been established.

Symptoms of hepatitis, hepatic dysfunction and/or abnormal liver function test results may occur.

Overdosage: Symptoms: Hearing loss, severe nausea, vomiting and diarrhoea. Treatment: Gastric lavage, general supportive measures.

Pharmaceutical precautions Keep bottle tightly closed. Protect from light. Store below 25°C.

Legal category POM.

Package quantities Erythromid: Containers of 100, 500 and 1000 tablets.

Further information No metabolisable carbohydrate is present.

Product licence number

Erythromid 0037/5019R.

ERYTHROMYCIN LACTOBIONATE I.V.

Presentation A sterile, white, lyophilised presentation of 1.0 g of erythromycin as erythromycin lactobionate in a vial.

When reconstituted with 20 ml Water for Injections BP provides 22 ml of solution. Deliberate overage ensures that each 20 ml of this solution contains 1.0 g of erythromycin as erythromycin lactobionate.

The solution must be further diluted prior to intravenous administration (see dosage and administration).

Erythromycin Lactobionate is not suitable for intramuscular use. It is intended for intravenous use.

Uses

Clinical indications: Erythromycin lactobionate is indicated in severe and immunocompromised cases of infections caused by sensitive organisms where high blood levels are required at the earliest opportunity or when the oral route is compromised.

1. Upper Respiratory Tract infections: tonsillitis, peritonsillar abscess, pharyngitis, laryngitis, sinusitis, secondary infections in influenza and common colds.
2. Lower Respiratory Tract infections: tracheitis, acute and chronic bronchitis, pneumonia (lobar pneumonia, bronchopneumonia, primary atypical pneumonia), bronchiectasis, Legionnaire's disease.
3. Ear infection: otitis media and otitis externa, mastoiditis.
4. Oral infections: gingivitis, Vincent's angina.
5. Eye infections: blepharitis.
6. Skin and soft tissue infections: boils and carbuncles, paronychia, abscesses, pustular acne, impetigo, cellulitis, erysipelas.
7. Gastrointestinal infections: cholecystitis, staphylococcal enterocolitis.
8. Prophylaxis: peri-operative secondary infection prophylaxis, severe trauma and burns secondary infection prophylaxis, endocarditis prophylaxis (dental procedures).
9. Septicaemia.
10. Endocarditis.
11. Other infections: osteomyelitis, urethritis, gonorrhoea, syphilis, lymphogranuloma venereum, diphtheria, prostatitis, scarlet fever.

Pharmacodynamic properties: Erythromycin exerts its antimicrobial action by binding to the 50S ribosomal sub-unit of susceptible microorganisms and suppresses protein synthesis. Erythromycin is usually active against most strains of the following organisms both *in vitro* and in clinical infections:

Gram positive bacteria – *Listeria monocytogenes, Corynebacterium diphtheriae* (as an adjunct to antitoxin), Staphylococci spp, Streptococci spp (including Enterococci).

Gram negative bacteria – *Haemophilus influenzae, Neisseria meningitidis, Neisseria gonorrhoea, Legionella pneumophila, Moraxella (Branhamella) catarrhalis, Bordetella pertussis,* Campylobacter spp.

Mycoplasma – *Mycoplasma pneumoniae, Ureaplasma urealyticum.*

Other organisms – *Treponema pallidum,* Chlamydia spp, Clostridia spp, L-forms, the agents causing trachoma and lymphogranuloma venereum.

Note: The majority of strains of *Haemophilus influenzae* are susceptible to the concentrations reached after ordinary doses.

Pharmacokinetic particulars: Following intravenous infusion, erythromycin is widely distributed throughout body tissues, including lung tissues.

Dosage and administration

Recommended dosage

Adults, children and neonates: Severe and immunocompromised infections, 50 mg/kg/day, preferably by continuous infusion (equivalent to 4 g per day for adults).

Mild to moderate infections (oral route compromised) 25 mg/kg/day.

Elderly: No special dosage recommendations.

Recommended administration: Continuous intravenous infusion with an erythromycin concentration of 1 mg/ml (0.1% solution) is recommended.

If required, solution strengths up to 5 mg/ml (0.5% solution) may be used, but should not be exceeded. Higher concentrations may result in pain along the vein.

Bolus injection is not recommended.

However, if it is decided to administer the daily dose as 4 doses once every 6 hours, then the erythromycin concentration should not exceed 5 mg/ml and the time of each infusion should be between 20 and 60 minutes.

Intravenous therapy should be replaced by oral administration at the appropriate time.

Preparation of solution for intravenous administration

Step 1: Inject 20 ml of Water for Injections BP into the vial and shake to dissolve contents. Do not use saline or other diluents. This will give 22 ml of solution.

20 ml of this solution will contain 1.0 g erythromycin (50 mg erythromycin/ml).

Use within 24 hours of preparation. Keep in a refrigerator between 2°C and 8°C.

This solution must be further diluted before administration, see Step 2.

Step 2: Solutions for administration are prepared with Sodium Chloride Intravenous Infusion BP 0.9% w/v (see also below).

Dose required	*Volume from Step 1*	*Volume of sterile 0.9% saline*	*Total volume*	*Erythromycin concentration*
1.0 g	20 ml	1000 ml	1020 ml	1.0 mg/ml
500 mg	10 ml	500 ml	510 ml	
1.0 g	20 ml	500 ml	520 ml	1.9 mg/ml
500 mg	10 ml	250 ml	260 ml	
1.0 g	20 ml	200 ml	220 ml	4.6 mg/ml
500 mg	10 ml	100 ml	110 ml	

If, for clinical reasons, 0.9% saline is not suitable, then neutralised Glucose Intravenous Infusion BP 5% w/v may be used. Neutralised glucose solution is prepared by the addition of 5 ml of sterile 8.4% w/v sodium bicarbonate solution to each litre of Glucose Intravenous Injection BP 5% w/v.

It is necessary to buffer the glucose solution in this way because the stability of Erythromycin Lactobionate is adversely affected below pH 5.5.

To ensure potency, all solutions for administration should be used within 8 hours of preparation.

Contra-indications, warnings, etc

Contra-indications: Known hypersensitivity to erythromycin. Erythromycin is contra-indicated in patients taking astemizole, terfenadine, cisapride or pimozide. Erythromycin is contra-indicated with ergotamine and dihydroergotamine.

Precautions: Extravasation should be avoided. The injection should be slow to avoid pain along the vein.

Erythromycin is excreted principally by the liver, so caution should be exercised in administering the antibiotic to patients with impaired hepatic function or concomitantly receiving potentially hepatotoxic agents. Hepatic dysfunction including increased liver enzymes and/or cholestatic hepatitis, with or without jaundice, has been infrequently reported with erythromycin.

There have been reports suggesting erythromycin does not reach the foetus in adequate concentrations to prevent congenital syphilis. Infants born to women treated during pregnancy with oral erythromycin for early syphilis should be treated with an appropriate penicillin regimen.

There have been reports that erythromycin may aggravate the weakness of patients with myasthenia gravis.

Erythromycin interferes with the fluorometric determination or urinary catecholamines.

As with other broad spectrum antibiotics, pseudomembraneous colitis has been reported rarely with erythromycin.

Rhabdomyolysis with or without renal impairment has been reported in seriously ill patients receiving erythromycin concomitantly with lovastatin.

Prolonged QTc interval and ventricular arrhythmias have rarely been reported in patients receiving erythromycin IV.

Interactions: Concomitant use of erythromycin with terfenadine or astemizole is likely to result in an enhanced risk of cardiotoxicity with these drugs. The concomitant use of erythromycin with either astemizole or terfenadine is therefore contra-indicated.

The metabolism of terfenadine and astemizole is significantly altered when either are taken concomitantly with erythromycin. Rare cases of serious cardiovascular events have been observed, including torsades de pointes, other ventricular arrhythmias and cardiac arrest. Death has been reported with the terfenadine/erythromycin combination.

Elevated cisapride levels have been reported in patients receiving erythromycin and cisapride concomitantly. This may result in QT prolongation and cardiac arrhythmias including ventricular trachycardia, ventricular fibrillation and Torsades de pointes. Similar effects have been observed with concomitant administration of pimozide and clarithromycin, another macrolide antibiotic.

Concurrent use of erythromycin and ergotamine or dihydroergotamine has been associated in some patients with acute ergot toxicity characterised by the rapid development of severe peripheral vasospasm and dysethesia.

Increases in serum concentrations of the following drugs metabolised by the cytochrome P450 system may occur when administered concurrently with erythromycin: alfentanil, astemizole, bromocriptine, carbamazepine, cyclosporin, digoxin, dihydroergotamine, disopyramide, ergotamine, hexobarbitone, midazolam, phenytoin, quinidine, tacrolimus, terfenadine, theophylline, triazolam, valproate, and warfarin. Appropriate monitoring should be undertaken and dosage should be adjusted as necessary.

Erythromycin has been reported to decrease the clearance of zopiclone and thus may increase the pharmacodynamic effects of this drug.

When oral erythromycin is given concurrently with theophylline, there is also a significant decrease in erythromycin serum concentrations. The decrease could result in subtherapeutic concentrations of erythromycin.

Use in pregnancy and nursing mothers: There is no evidence of hazard from erythromycin in human pregnancy. It has been in wide use for many years without apparent ill consequence. Animal studies have shown no hazard.

Erythromycin has been reported to cross the placental barrier in humans, but foetal plasma levels are generally low.

Erythromycin is excreted in breast milk, therefore, caution should be exercised when erythromycin is administered to a nursing mother.

Side-effects: Occasional venous irritation has been encountered, but if the infusion is given slowly, in dilute solution, as recommended above, pain and vessel trauma are minimised.

Occasional side-effects such as nausea, abdominal discomfort, vomiting and diarrhoea may be experienced. Reversible hearing loss associated with doses of erythromycin usually greater than 4 g per day has been reported. Allergic reactions are rare and mild, although anaphylaxis has occurred extremely rarely. Skin reactions ranging from mild eruptions to erythema multiforme, Stevens-Johnson syndrome and toxic epidermal neurolysis have rarely been reported. There are no reports implicating erythromycin products with abnormal tooth development and only rare reports of damage to the blood, kidneys, liver or central nervous system.

Cardiac arrhythmias have been very rarely reported in patients receiving erythromycin therapy. There have been isolated reports of chest pain, dizziness and palpitations; however, a cause and effect relationship has not been established.

Symptoms of hepatitis, hepatic dysfunction and/or abnormal liver function test results may occur.

Overdosage: Symptoms: Hearing loss, severe nausea, vomiting and diarrhoea.

Treatment: General supportive measures.

Pharmaceutical precautions The powder is stable at room temperature.

Legal category POM.

Package quantities 1 g vials of Erythromycin Lactobionate.

Further information Contains no sodium. Compatibility with other IV additives has not been established.

Product licence number 0037/0092.

ERYTHROPED* A

Qualitative and quantitative composition Erythromycin as Erythromycin Ethylsuccinate PhEur 500 mg/tablet.

Pharmaceutical form Tablets.

Clinical particulars

Therapeutic indications: For the prophylaxis and treatment of infections caused by erythromycin-sensitive organisms.

Erythromycin is highly effective in the treatment of a great variety of clinical infections such as:

1. Upper Respiratory Tract infections: tonsillitis, peritonsillar abscess, pharyngitis, laryngitis, sinusitis, secondary infections in influenza and common colds
2. Lower Respiratory Tract infections: tracheitis, acute and chronic bronchitis, pneumonia (lobar pneumonia, bronchopneumonia, primary atypical pneumonia), bronchiectasis, Legionnaire's disease
3. Ear infection: otitis media and otitis externa, mastoiditis
4. Oral infections: gingivitis, Vincent's angina
5. Eye infections: blepharitis
6. Skin and soft tissue infections: boils and carbuncles, paronychia, abscesses, pustular acne, impetigo, cellulitis, erysipelas
7. Gastrointestinal infections: cholecystitis, staphylococcal enterocolitis
8. Prophylaxis: pre- and post- operative trauma, burns, rheumatic fever
9. Other infections: osteomyelitis, urethritis, gonorrhoea, syphilis, lymphogranuloma venereum, diphtheria, prostatitis, scarlet fever.

Posology and method of administration: For oral administration.

Adults and children over 8 years: For mild to moderate infections 2 g daily in divided doses. Up to 4 g daily in severe infections.

Elderly: No special dosage recommendations.

Children: Age 2–8: For mild to moderate infections 1 g daily in divided doses.

Infants and babies up to 2 years: For mild to moderate infections 500 mg daily in divided doses.

For severe infections doses may be doubled.

Note: For younger children, infants and babies, Erythroped, erythromycin ethylsuccinate suspensions, are normally recommended.

Contra-indications: Known hypersensitivity to erythromycin. Erythromycin is contraindicated in patients taking astemizole, terfenadine, cisapride or pimozide.

Erythromycin is contraindicated with ergotamine and dihydroergotamine.

Special warnings and special precautions for use: Erythromycin is excreted principally by the liver, so caution should be exercised in administering the antibiotic to patients with impaired hepatic function or concomitantly receiving potentially hepatotoxic agents. Hepatic dysfunction including increased liver enzymes and/or cholestatic hepatitis, with or without jaundice, has been infrequently reported with erythromycin.

There have been reports suggesting erythromycin does not reach the foetus in adequate concentrations to prevent congenital syphilis. Infants born to women treated during pregnancy with oral erythromycin for early syphilis should be treated with an appropriate penicillin regimen.

There have been reports that erythromycin may aggravate the weakness of patients with myasthenia gravis.

Erythromycin interferes with the fluorometric determination of urinary catecholamines.

As with other broad spectrum antibiotics, pseudomembranous colitis has been reported rarely with erythromycin.

Rhabdomyolysis with or without renal impairment has been reported in seriously ill patients receiving erythromycin concomitantly with lovastatin.

Interaction with other medicaments and other forms of interaction: Concomitant use of erythromycin with terfenadine or astemizole is likely to result in an enhanced risk of cardiotoxicity with these drugs. The concomitant use of erythromycin with either astemizole or terfenadine is therefore contraindicated.

The metabolism of terfenadine and astemizole is significantly altered when either are taken concomitantly with erythromycin. Rare cases of serious cardiovascular events have been observed, including Torsades de pointes, other ventricular arrhythmias and cardiac arrest. Death has been reported with the terfenadine / erythromycin combination.

Elevated cisapride levels have been reported in patients receiving erythromycin and cisapride concomitantly. This may result in QT prolongation and cardiac arrhythmias including ventricular tachycardia, ventricular fibrillation and Torsades de pointes. Similar effects have been observed with concomitant administration of pimozide and clarithromycin, another macrolide antibiotic.

Concurrent use of erythromycin and ergotamine or dihydroergotamine has been associated in some patients with acute ergot toxicity characterised by the rapid development of severe peripheral vasospasm and dysaesthesia.

Increases in serum concentrations of the following drugs metabolised by the cytochrome P450 system may occur when administered concurrently with erythromycin: alfentanil, astemizole, bromocriptine, carbamazepine, cyclosporin, digoxin, dihydroergotamine, disopyramide, ergotamine, hexobarbitone, midazolam, phenytoin, quinidine, tacrolimus, terfenadine, theophylline, triazolam, valproate, and warfarin. Appropriate monitoring should be undertaken and dosage should be adjusted as necessary.

Erythromycin has been reported to decrease the clearance of zopiclone and thus may increase the pharmacodynamic effects of this drug.

When oral erythromycin is given concurrently with theophylline, there is also a significant decrease in erythromycin serum concentrations. The decrease could result in subtherapeutic concentrations of erythromycin.

Pregnancy and lactation: There is no evidence of hazard from erythromycin in human pregnancy. It has been in widespread use for a number of years without apparent ill consequence. Animal studies have shown no hazard.

Erythromycin has been reported to cross the placental barrier in humans, but foetal plasma levels are generally low.

Erythromycin is excreted in breast milk, therefore, caution should be exercised when erythromycin is administered to a nursing mother.

Effects on ability to drive and use machines: None stated.

Undesirable effects: Occasional side effects such as nausea, abdominal discomfort, vomiting and diarrhoea may be experienced. Reversible hearing loss associated with doses of erythromycin usually greater than 4 g per day has been reported. Allergic reactions are rare and mild, although anaphylaxis has occurred. Skin reactions ranging from mild eruptions to erythema multiforme, Stevens-Johnson syndrome and toxic epidermal necrolysis have rarely been reported. There are no reports implicating erythromycin products with abnormal tooth development, and only rare reports of damage to the blood, kidneys or central nervous system.

Cardiac arrhythmias have been very rarely reported in patients receiving erythromycin therapy. There have been isolated reports of chest pain, dizziness and palpitations, however, a cause and effect relationship has not been established.

Symptoms of hepatitis, hepatic dysfunction and/or abnormal liver function test results may occur.

Overdose: Symptoms: hearing loss, severe nausea, vomiting and diarrhoea.

Treatment: gastric lavage, general supportive measures.

Pharmacological properties

Pharmacodynamic Properties: Erythromycin exerts its antimicrobial action by binding to the 50S ribosomal sub-unit of susceptible microorganisms and suppresses protein synthesis. Erythromycin is usually active against most strains of the following organisms both *in vitro* and in clinical infections:

Gram positive bacteria – *Listeria monocytogenes, Corynebacterium diphtheriae* (as an adjunct to antitoxin), Staphylococci spp, Streptococci spp (including Enterococci).

Gram negative bacteria – *Haemophilus influenzae, Neisseria meningitidis, Neisseria gonorrhoeae, Legionella pneumophila, Moraxella (Branhamella) catarrhalis, Bordetella pertussis,* Campylobacter spp.

Mycoplasma – *Mycoplasma pneumoniae, Ureaplasma urealyticum.*

Other organisms – Treponema pallidum, Clostridia spp, Chlamydia spp, L-forms, the agents causing trachoma and lymphogranuloma venereum.

Note: The majority of strains of *Haemophilus influenzae* are susceptible to the concentrations reached after ordinary doses.

Pharmacokinetic properties: Peak blood levels normally occur within 1 hour of dosing of erythromycin ethylsuccinate granules. The elimination half life is approximately 2 hours. Doses may be administered 2, 3 or 4 times a day.

Erythromycin ethylsuccinate is less susceptible than erythromycin to the adverse effect of gastric acid. It is absorbed from the small intestine. It is widely distributed throughout body tissues. Little metabolism occurs and only about 5% is excreted in the urine. It is excreted principally by the liver.

Preclinical safety data: There are no pre-clinical data of relevance to the prescriber which are additional to that already included in other sections of the SPC.

Pharmaceutical particulars

List of excipients: Calcium hydrogen phosphate, sodium starch glycollate, starch maize, povidone, magnesium stearate, hydroxypropyl methylcellulose, polyethylene glycol, titanium dioxide, quinoline yellow (E104), sorbic acid.

Incompatibilities: None stated.

Shelf life: 24 months.

Special precautions for storage: None.

Nature and contents of container: Polypropylene bottles of 50, 100 or 500 tablets.

Blister: PVC/aluminium of 4 or 28 tablets.

Instructions for use/handling: Not applicable.

Marketing authorisation number PL 0037/0137

Date of first authorisation/renewal of authorisation 19/05/95

Date of (partial) revision of the text July 1998

ERYTHROPED* PI SF
ERYTHROPED* SF
ERYTHROPED* FORTE SF

Qualitative and quantitative composition

Erythroped PI SF contains 125 mg erythromycin as erythromycin ethylsuccinate per 5 ml.

Erythroped SF contains 250 mg erythromycin as erythromycin ethylsuccinate per 5 ml.

Erythroped Forte SF contains 500 mg erythromycin as erythromycin ethylsuccinate per 5 ml.

Pharmaceutical form Granules for reconstitution.

Clinical particulars

Therapeutic indications: For the prophylaxis and treatment of infections caused by erythromycin-sensitive organisms.

Erythromycin is highly effective in the treatment of a great variety of clinical infections such as:

1. Upper Respiratory Tract infections: tonsillitis, peritonsillar abscess, pharyngitis, laryngitis, sinusitis, secondary infections in influenza and common colds.
2. Lower Respiratory Tract infections: tracheitis, acute and chronic bronchitis, pneumonia (lobar pneumonia, bronchopneumonia, primary atypical pneumonia), bronchiectasis, Legionnaire's disease.
3. Ear infection: otitis media and otitis externa, mastoiditis.
4. Oral infections: gingivitis, Vincent's angina.
5. Eye infections: blepharitis.
6. Skin and soft tissue infections: boils and carbuncles, paronychia, abscesses, pustular acne, impetigo, cellulitis, erysipelas.
7. Gastrointestinal infections: cholecystitis, staphylococcal enterocolitis.
8. Prophylaxis: pre- and post-operative trauma, burns, rheumatic fever.
9. Other infections: osteomyelitis, urethritis, gonorrhoea, syphilis, lymphogranuloma venereum, diphtheria, prostatitis, scarlet fever.

Note: Erythromycin has also proved to be of value in endocarditis and septicaemia, but in these conditions initial administration of erythromycin lactobionate by the intravenous route is advisable.

Posology and method of administration:

Adults and children over 8 years: 2 g/day in divided doses. For severe infections up to 4 g/day in divided doses.

Children 2–8 years: 30 mg/kg/day in divided doses. For severe infections up to 50 mg/kg/day in divided doses.

Normal dose: 250 mg four times a day or 500 mg twice daily.

Children up to 2 years: 30 mg/kg/day in divided doses. For severe infections up to 50 mg/kg/day in divided doses.

Normal dose: 125 mg four times a day or 250 mg twice daily.

Presentations are available for adults and children over 8 years, children aged 2–8 years, and for children under 2 years.

Contra-indications: Known hypersensitivity to erythromycin. Erythromycin is contra-indicated in patients taking astemizole, terfenadine, cisapride or pimozide.

Erythromycin is contra-indicated with ergotamine and dihydroergotamine.

Special warnings and special precautions for use: Erythromycin is excreted principally by the liver, so caution should be exercised in administering the antibiotic to patients with impaired hepatic function or concomitantly receiving potentially hepatotoxic agents. Hepatic dysfunction including increased liver enzymes and/or cholestatic hepatitis, with or without jaundice, has been infrequently reported with erythromycin.

There have been reports suggesting erythromycin does not reach the foetus in adequate concentrations to prevent congenital syphilis. Infants born to women treated during pregnancy with oral erythromycin for early syphilis should be treated with an appropriate penicillin regimen.

There have been reports that erythromycin may aggravate the weakness of patients with myasthenia gravis.

Erythromycin interferes with the fluorometric determination of urinary catecholamines.

As with other broad spectrum antibiotics, pseudomembranous colitis has been reported rarely with erythromycin.

Rhabdomyolysis with or without renal impairment has been reported in seriously ill patients receiving erythromycin concomitantly with lovastatin.

Interaction with other medicaments and other forms of interaction: Concomitant use of erythromycin with terfenadine or astemizole is likely to result in an enhanced risk of cardiotoxicity with these drugs. The concomitant use of erythromycin with either astemizole or terfenadine is therefore contra-indicated.

The metabolism of terfenadine and astemizole is significantly altered when either are taken concomitantly with erythromycin. Rare cases of serious cardiovascular events have been observed, including torsades de pointes, other ventricular arrhythmias and cardiac arrest. Death has been reported with the terfenadine/erythromycin combination.

Elevated cisapride levels have been reported in patients receiving erythromycin and cisapride concomitantly. This may result in QT prolongation and cardiac arrhythmias including ventricular trachycardia, ventricular fibrillation and torsades de pointes. Similar effects have been observed with concomitant administration of pimozide and clarithromycin, another macrolide antibiotic.

Concurrent use of erythromycin and ergotamine or dihydroergotamine has been associated in some patients with acute ergot toxicity characterised by the rapid development of severe peripheral vasospasm and dysaesthesia.

Increases in serum concentrations of the following drugs metabolised by the cytochrome P450 system may occur when administered concurrently with erythromycin: alfentanil, astemizole, bromocriptine, carbamazepine, cyclosporin, digoxin, dihydroergotamine, disopyramide, ergotamine, hexobarbitone, midazolam, phenytoin, quinidine, tacrolimus, terfenadine, theophylline, triazolam, valproate, and warfarin. Appropriate monitoring should be undertaken and dosage should be adjusted as necessary.

Erythromycin has been reported to decrease the clearance of zopiclone and thus may increase the pharmacodynamic effects of this drug.

When oral erythromycin is given concurrently with theophylline, there is also a significant decrease in erythromycin serum concentrations. The decrease could result in subtherapeutic concentrations of erythromycin.

Pregnancy and lactation: There is no evidence of hazard from erythromycin in human pregnancy. It has been in widespread use for a number of years without apparent ill consequence. Animal studies have shown no hazard.

Erythromycin has been reported to cross the placental barrier in humans, but foetal plasma levels are generally low.

Erythromycin is excreted in breast milk, therefore, caution should be exercised when erythromycin is administered to a nursing mother.

Effects on ability to drive and to use machines: None reported.

Undesirable effects: Occasional side effects such as nausea, abdominal discomfort, vomiting and diarrhoea may be experienced. Reversible hearing loss associated with doses of erythromycin usually greater than 4 g per day has been reported. Allergic reactions are rare and mild, although anaphylaxis has occurred. Skin reactions ranging from mild eruptions to erythema multiforme, Stevens-Johnson syndrome and toxic epidermal necrolysis have rarely been reported. There are no reports implicating erythromycin products with abnormal tooth development, and only rare reports of damage to the blood, kidneys or central nervous system.

Cardiac arrhythmias have been very rarely reported in patients receiving erythromycin therapy. There have been isolated reports of chest pain, dizziness and palpitations, however, a cause and effect relationship has not been established.

Symptoms of hepatitis, hepatic dysfunction and/or abnormal liver function test results may occur.

Overdosage:

Symptoms: hearing loss, severe nausea, vomiting and diarrhoea.

Treatment: gastric lavage, general supportive measures.

Pharmacological properties

Pharmacodynamic properties: Erythromycin exerts its antimicrobial action by binding to the 50S ribosomal sub-unit of susceptible microorganisms and suppresses protein synthesis. Erythromycin is usually active against most strains of the following organisms both *in vitro* and in clinical infections:

Gram positive bacteria – *Listeria monocytogenes, Corynebacterium diphtheriae* (as an adjunct to antitoxin), Staphylococci spp, Streptococci spp (including Enterococci).

Gram negative bacteria – *Haemophilus influenzae, Neisseria meningitidis, Neisseria gonorrhoea, Legionella pneumophila, Moraxella (Branhamella) catarrhalis, Bordetella pertussis,* Campylobacter spp.

Mycoplasma – *Mycoplasma pneumoniae, Ureaplasma urealyticum.*

Other organisms – Treponema pallidum, Chlamydia spp, Clostridia spp, L-forms, the agents causing trachoma and lymphogranuloma venereum.

Note: The majority of strains of *Haemophilus influenzae* are susceptible to the concentrations reached after ordinary doses.

Pharmacokinetic particulars: Peak blood levels normally occur within 1 hour of dosing of erythromycin ethylsuccinate granules. The elimination half life is approximately 2 hours. Doses may be administered 2, 3 or 4 times a day.

Erythromycin ethylsuccinate is less susceptible than erythromycin to the adverse effect of gastric acid. It is absorbed from the small intestine. It is widely distributed throughout body tissues. Little metabolism occurs and only about 5% is excreted in the urine. It is excreted principally by the liver.

Preclinical safety data: There are no pre-clinical data of relevance to the prescriber which are additional to that already included in other sections of the SPC.

Pharmaceutical particulars

List of excipients: Sorbitol, xanthan gum, sodium citrate, surfactant poloxamer 188, acesulfame (K), sodium saccharin, purified water, sodium methylhydroxybenzoate, sodium propylhydroxybenzoate, colloidal silicon dioxide, imitation banana flavour entrapped No. 2, entrapped artificial cream.

Incompatibilities: None stated.

Shelf life:

Erythroped PI SF, Erythroped SF and Erythroped Forte SF. Bottles – 24 months. Once reconstituted the suspensions should be used within 7 days.

Erythroped PI SF and Erythroped SF. Sachets – 24 months.

Special precautions for storage: None.

Nature and contents of container: Erythroped PI SF, Erythroped SF and Erythroped Forte SF. High density polyethylene bottles, 100 ml or 140 ml, with polypropylene cap which may be a child resistant cap.

Erythroped PI SF and Erythroped SF. Sachet: 44 GSM paper/12 GSM LDPE/9 μm Al foil/34 GSM LDPE.

Instructions for use/handling: Not applicable.

Marketing authorisation numbers

Erythroped PI SF	PL 0037/0223
Erythroped SF	PL 0037/0224
Erythroped Forte SF	PL 0037/0225

Date of first authorisation/renewal of authorisation 25/03/97

Date of (partial) revision of text July 1997

Legal category POM

FERROGRAD*

Presentation Each red Filmtab* (film-coated tablet Abbott) contains Dried Ferrous Sulphate BP 325 mg (equivalent to 105 mg elemental iron) in a controlled release form (Gradumet*).

Uses For the prevention and treatment of iron-deficiency anaemia.

The Gradumet device allows controlled release of ferrous sulphate over a number of hours and reduces gastro-intestinal intolerance. The device consists of an inert plastic matrix, honeycombed by thousands of narrow passages which contain ferrous sulphate together with a water soluble channelling agent. As the tablet passes down the gastro-intestinal tract the iron is leached out. The spent matrix is finally excreted in the stools.

Dosage and administration

Recommended adult oral dosage: One tablet a day before food. Patients should be advised to swallow tablets whole. As gastro intestinal intolerance is not a problem with Ferrograd, it should be given on an empty stomach when iron is most effectively absorbed.

Children: Not recommended for children under 12 years of age.

Elderly: The controlled release tablet and its inert plastic matrix may cause a safety hazard in some elderly or other patients suffering from delayed intestinal transit.

Contra-indications, warnings, etc

Contra-indications: Intestinal diverticula or any intestinal obstruction.

Iron preparations are contra-indicated in patients with haemochromatosis and haemosiderosis.

Iron is contra-indicated in patients receiving repeated blood transfusions.

Oral iron preparations are contra-indicated when used concomitantly with parenteral iron therapy.

Precautions: Ferrograd tablets should be kept out of children's reach.

Acute iron poisoning occurs rarely in adults, however it could happen if childen swallow this medication.

The controlled release tablet and its inert plastic matrix may cause a safety hazard in some elderly or other patients suffering from delayed intestinal transit.

Iron preparations colour the faeces black, which may interfere with tests used for detection of occult blood in the stools. The guaiac test occasionally yields false positive tests for blood.

Interaction with other medicaments and other forms of interaction: Iron interacts with tetracyclines, magnesium trisilicate, trientine and zinc salts and absorption of all these agents may be impaired.

Iron inhibits the absorption of tetracyclines from the gastrointestinal tract and tetracycline inhibits the absorption of iron. If both drugs must be given, tetracycline should be administered three hours after or two hours before oral iron supplements.

Concurrent administration of oral iron preparations with antacids, calcium supplements, (calcium carbonate or phosphate), tea, coffee, eggs, food or medications containing bicarbonates, carbonate, oxalates or phosphates, milk or milk products, wholegrain breads and cereals and dietary fibre, may decrease iron absorption. Therefore, oral iron preparations should not be taken within one hour before or two hours after ingestion of such items.

Concurrent administration of oral iron preparations may interfere with the oral absorption of some quinolone anti-infective agents (e.g. ciprofloxacin, norfloxacin, ofloxacin), resulting in decreased serum and urine concentrations of the quinolones. Therefore, oral iron preparations should not be ingested with or within two hours of a dose of an oral quinolone.

Iron can decrease gastrointestinal absorption of penicillamines. Therefore, administration should be at least two hours apart if both drugs must be co-administered.

Chloramphenicol may delay response to iron therapy.

Pregnancy and lactation: Ferrograd tablets are not appropriate for use during pregnancy since they do not contain folic acid.

Side-effects: Side-effects reported are similar to those associated with conventional oral iron preparations, ie. nausea, vomiting, abdominal pain or discomfort, blackening of stools, diarrhoea and/or constipation, but the incidence of side-effects is less owing to the controlled release of nature of the formulation.

Isolated cases of allergic reaction have been reported ranging from rash to anaphylaxis.

Overdosage: Symptoms: Initial symptoms of iron overdosage include nausea, vomiting, diarrhoea, abdominal pain, haematemesis, rectal bleeding, lethargy and circulatory collapse. Hyperglycaemia and metabolic acidosis may also occur. The controlled release characteristic may delay excessive absorption of iron, and thus allow more time for counter measures to be implemented. However, initial symptoms of overdosage may be absent due to the controlled release formulation. Therefore, if overdosage is suspected, treatment should be implemented immediately. In severe cases, after a latent phase, relapse may occur after 24–48 hours, manifested by hypotension, coma and hepatocellular necrosis and renal failure.

Treatment: The following steps are recommended to minimise or prevent further absorption of the medication:

Children

1. Administer an emetic such as syrup of ipecacuanha.

2. Emesis should be followed by gastric lavage with desferrioxamine solution (2 g/l). This should then be followed by the instillation of desferrioxamine 5 g in 50–100 ml water, to be retained in the stomach. Inducing diarrhoea in children may be dangerous and should not be undertaken in young children. Keep the patient under constant surveillance to detect possible aspiration of vomitus – maintain suction apparatus and standby emergency oxygen in case of need.

3. Unleached tablets are radio-opaque. Therefore, an abdominal x-ray should be taken to determine the number of tablets retained in the stomach following emesis and gastric lavage.

4. Severe poisoning: in the presence of shock and/or coma with high serum iron levels (serum iron >90 μmol/l) immediate supportive measures plus i.v infusion of desferrioxamine should be instituted. Desferrioxamine 15 mg/kg body weight should be administered every hour by slow i.v infusion to a maximum 80 mg/kg/24 hours. Warning: hypotension may occur if the infusion rate is too rapid.

5. Less severe poisoning: i.m desferrioxamine 1 g 4–6 hourly is recommended.

6. Serum iron levels should be monitored throughout.

Adults

1. Administer an emetic.

2. Gastric lavage may be necessary to remove drug already released into the stomach. This should be undertaken using desferrioxamine solution (2 g/l). Desferrioxamine 5 g in 50–100 ml water should be introduced into the stomach following gastric emptying. Keep the patient under constant surveillance to detect possible aspiration of vomitus; maintain suction apparatus and standby emergency oxygen in case of need.

3. Unleached tablets are radio-opaque. Therefore, an abdominal x-ray of the patient should be taken to determine the number of tablets retained in the stomach following emesis and gastric lavage. The risk/benefit ratio of x-raying pregnant women must be carefully weighed but should be avoided if possible.

4. A drink of mannitol or sorbitol should be given to induce small bowel emptying.

5. Severe poisoning: in the presence of shock and/or coma with high serum iron levels (>142 μmol/l) immediate supportive measures plus i.v infusion of desferrioxamine should be instituted. The recommended dose of desferrioxamine is 5 mg/kg/h by slow i.v infusion up to a maximum of 80 mg/kg/24 hours. Warning: hypotension may occur if the infusion rate is too rapid.

6. Less severe poisoning: i.m desferrioxamine 50 mg/kg up to a maximum dose of 4 g should be given.

7. Serum iron levels should be monitored throughout.

Pharmaceutical precautions Store in a cool dry place.

Legal category P.

Package quantities Ferrograd is supplied in 5 carton packs, each containing 30 (3×10) tablets (OP).

Further information Ferrograd Folic tablets are available for the prevention and treatment of anaemia in pregnancy and for the prophylaxis of megaloblastic anaemia of pregnancy.

Product licence number 0037/5000R.

FERROGRAD* FOLIC

Presentation A two-layered (red and yellow), round, bi-convex Filmtab* (film-coated tablet Abbott). Each tablet contains Dried Ferrous Sulphate BP 325 mg (equivalent to 105 mg elemental iron) in a controlled release form (red half – Gradumet*) and 350 micrograms Folic Acid BP (yellow half).

Uses Ferrograd Folic is indicated:

1. For the prevention and treatment of iron-deficiency anaemia of pregnancy.

2. For the prophylaxis of megaloblastic anaemia of pregnancy.

Folic acid requirements in pregnancy can be met with supplements of between 300 and 400 micrograms daily. Without such supplements folate deficiency may develop leading to megaloblastic anaemia with attendant obstetric risks. Doses over 400 micrograms may mask undiagnosed primary B_{12} deficiency. In the extremely unlikely event of this condition occurring in a pregnant woman, the safe prophylactic dose is considered to be 350 micrograms.

The Gradumet device allows controlled release of ferrous sulphate over a number of hours, and reduces gastro-intestinal intolerance. The device consists of an inert plastic matrix, honeycombed by thousands of narrow passages which contain the ferrous sulphate together with water-soluble channelling agent. As the tablet passes down the gastro-intestinal tract the iron is leached out. The spent matrix is finally excreted in the stools.

Dosage and administration

Recommended adult oral dosage: One tablet daily before food throughout pregnancy and during the first month of the puerperium. Patients should be advised to swallow tablets whole.

Children: Not recommended for children under 12 years of age.

Elderly: The controlled release tablet and its inert plastic matrix may cause a safety hazard in some elderly or other patients suffering from delayed intestinal transit.

Contra-indications, warnings, etc

Contra-indications: Megaloblastic anaemia due to primary vitamin B_{12} deficiency.

Ferrograd Folic is contra-indicated in patients with pernicious anaemia.

Intestinal diverticula or any intestinal obstruction.

Iron preparations are contra-indicated in patients with haemochromatosis and haemosiderosis.

Iron is contra-indicated in patients receiving repeated blood transfusions.

Oral iron preparations are contra-indicated when used concomitantly with parenteral iron therapy.

Ferrograd Folic is contra-indicated in the rare instance of hypersensitivity to folic acid.

Precautions: Ferrograd Folic tablets should be kept out of children's reach. The controlled release tablet and its inert plastic matrix may cause a safety hazard in some elderly or other patients suffering from delayed intestinal transit.

Acute iron poisoning occurs rarely in adults, however it could happen if childen swallow this medication.

Pernicious anaemia is rare in women of childbearing age and less likely in pregnancy as Vitamin B_{12} deficiency reduces fertility. However, folic acid, at the recommended dosage may obscure the neurological manifestations of pernicious anaemia.

Iron preparations colour the faeces black, which may interfere with tests used for detection of occult blood in the stools. The guaiac test occasionally yields false positive tests for blood.

Interaction with other medicaments and other forms of interaction: Iron interacts with tetracyclines, magnesium trisilicate, trientine and zinc salts and absorption of all these agents may be impaired.

Concurrent administration of oral iron preparations with antacids, calcium supplements, (calcium carbonate or phosphate), tea, coffee, eggs, food or medications containing bicarbonates, carbonate, oxalates or phosphates, milk or milk products, wholegrain breads and cereals and dietary fibre, may decrease iron absorption. Therefore, oral iron preparations should not be taken within one hour before or two hours after ingestion of such items.

Iron inhibits the absorption of tetracyclines from the gastrointestinal tract and tetracycline inhibits the absorption of iron. If both drugs must be given, tetracycline should be administered three hours after or two hours before oral iron supplements.

Iron can decrease gastrointestinal absorption of penicillamines. Therefore, administration should be at least two hours apart if both drugs must be co-administered.

Chloramphenicol may delay response to iron therapy.

Concomitant administration of oral iron preparations may interfere with the oral absorption of some quinolone anti-infective agents (e.g. ciprofloxacin, norfloxacin, ofloxacin), resulting in decreased serum and urine concentrations of the quinolones. Therefore, oral iron preparations should not be ingested concomitantly with or within two hours of a dose of an oral quinolone.

Pregnancy and lactation: Ferrograd Folic is indicated for the prevention and treatment of iron deficiency anaemia of pregnancy and for prophylaxis of megaloblastic anaemia of pregnancy.

Folic acid is excreted in breast milk.

Side-effects: Side-effects reported are similar to those associated with conventional oral iron preparations, ie. nausea, vomiting, abdominal pain or discomfort, blackening of stools, diarrhoea and/or constipation, but the incidence of side-effects is less owing to the controlled release nature of the formulation.

Isolated cases of allergic reaction have been reported ranging from rash to anaphylaxis.

Allergic sensitisation has been reported following both oral and parenteral administration of folic acid.

Overdosage: Symptoms: initial symptoms of iron overdosage include nausea, vomiting, diarrhoea, abdominal pain, haematemesis, rectal bleeding, lethargy and circulatory collapse. Hyperglycaemia and metabolic acidosis may also occur. The controlled release characteristic may delay excessive absorption of iron, and thus allow more time for counter measures to be implemented. However, initial symptoms of overdosage may be absent due to the controlled release formulation. Therefore, if overdosage is suspected, treatment should be implemented immediately. In severe cases, after a latent phase, relapse may occur after 24–48 hours, manifested by hypotension, coma and hepatocellular necrosis and renal failure.

Treatment: The following steps are recommended to minimise or prevent further absorption of the medication:

Children

1. Administer an emetic such as syrup of ipecacuanta.
2. Emesis should be followed by gastric lavage with desferrioxamine solution (2 g/l). This should then be followed by the instillation of desferrioxamine 5 g in 50–100 ml water, to be retained in the stomach. Inducing diarrhoea in children may be dangerous and should not be undertaken in young children. Keep the patient under constant surveillance to detect possible aspiration of vomitus – maintain suction apparatus and standby emergency oxygen in case of need.
3. Unleached tablets are radio-opaque. Therefore, an abdominal x-ray should be taken to determine the number of tablets retained in the stomach following emesis and gastric lavage.
4. Severe poisoning: in the presence of shock and/or coma with high serum iron levels (serum iron >90 μmol/l) immediate supportive measures plus i.v infusion of desferrioxamine should be instituted. Desferrioxamine 15 mg/kg body weight should be administered every hour by slow i.v infusion to a maximum 80 mg/kg/24 hours. Warning: hypotension may occur if the infusion rate is too rapid.
5. Less severe poisoning: i.m desferrioxamine 1 g 4–6 hourly is recommended.
6. Serum iron levels should be monitored throughout.

Adults

1. Administer an emetic.
2. Gastric lavage may be necessary to remove drug already released into the stomach. This should be undertaken using desferrioxamine solution (2 g/l). Desferrioxamine 5 g in 50–100 ml water should be introduced into the stomach following gastric emptying. Keep the patients under constant surveillance to detect possible aspiration of vomitus; maintain suction apparatus and standby emergency oxygen in case of need.
3. Unleached tablets are radio-opaque. Therefore, an abdominal x-ray of the patient should be taken to determine the number of tablets retained in the stomach following emesis and gastric lavage. The risk/benefit ratio of x-raying pregnant women must be carefully weighed but should be avoided if possible.
4. A drink of mannitol or sorbitol should be given to induce small bowel emptying.
5. Severe poisoning: in the presence of shock and/or coma with high serum iron levels (>142 μmol/l) immediate supportive measures plus i.v infusion of desferrioxamine should be instituted. The recommended dose of desferrioxamine is 5 mg/kg/h by slow i.v infusion up to a maximum of 80 mg/kg/24 hours. Warning: hypotension may occur if the infusion rate is too rapid.
6. Less severe poisoning: i.m desferrioxamine 50 mg/kg up to a maximum dose of 4 g should be given.
7. Serum iron levels should be monitored throughout.

Pharmaceutical precautions Store in a cool dry place.

Legal category P.

Package quantities Ferrograd Folic is supplied in 5 carton packs, each containing 30 (3×10) tablets (OP).

Further information Nil.

Product licence number 0037/5002R.

HYTRIN* TABLETS

Qualitative and quantitative composition Terazosin as monohydrochloride dihydrate 1 mg, 2 mg, 5 mg or 10 mg per tablet.

Pharmaceutical form Round, flat bevelled tablets embossed with [logo] logo and triangular facets on one face and plain on the other. Hytrin tablets are coloured as follows: 1 mg (white); 2 mg (yellow); 5 mg (tan); 10 mg (blue).

Clinical particulars

Therapeutic indications: Orally administered Hytrin is indicated in the treatment of mild to moderate hypertension. It may be used in combination with thiazide diuretics and/or other antihypertensive drugs or as sole therapy where other agents are inappropriate or ineffective. The hypotensive effect is most pronounced on the diastolic pressure. Although the exact mechanism of the hypotensive action of terazosin is not established, the relaxation of peripheral blood vessels appears to be produced mainly by competitive antagonism of post-synaptic $alpha_1$-adrenoceptors. Hytrin usually produces an initial gradual decrease in blood pressure followed by a sustained antihypertensive action.

Posology and method of administration:

Adults:

Initial dose – 1 mg before bedtime is the starting dose for all patients and should not be exceeded. Compliance with this initial dosage recommendation should be strictly observed to minimise potential for acute first-dose hypotensive episodes.

Subsequent doses – The single daily dosage may be increased by approximately doubling the dosage at weekly intervals to achieve the desired blood pressure response.

The usual maintenance dose is 2 mg to 10 mg once daily. Doses over 20 mg rarely improve efficacy and doses over 40 mg have not been studied.

Use with thiazide diuretics and other antihypertensive agents: When adding a thiazide diuretic or another antihypertensive agent to a patient's regimen the dose of Hytrin should be reduced and retitration carried out if necessary. Caution should be observed when Hytrin is administered with thiazides or other antihypertensive agents as hypotension may develop.

Use in renal insufficiency: Pharmacokinetic studies indicate that patients with impaired renal function need no alteration in recommended dosage.

Use in children: Safety and efficacy in children has not been established.

Use in the elderly: Pharmacokinetic studies in the elderly indicate that no alteration in dosage recommendation is required.

Contra-indications: Known sensitivity to alpha-adrenoceptor antagonists.

Special warnings and special precautions for use: As with other alpha adrenoceptor antagonists, terazosin is not recommended in patients with a history of micturition syncope.

In clinical trials, the incidence of postural hypotension was greater in BPH patients than those with hypertension. In these cases, the incidence of postural hypotension events was greater in patients aged 65 years and over (5.6%) than those aged less than 65 years (2.6%).

If administration is discontinued for more than several days, therapy should be re-instituted using the initial dosing regimen.

Interaction with other medicaments and other forms of interaction: In patients receiving terazosin plus ACE inhibitors or diuretics the proportion reporting dizziness or related side effects was greater than in the total population of terazosin treated patients from clinical trials.

Caution should be observed when terazosin is administered with other antihypertensive agents, to avoid the possibility of significant hypotension. When adding terazosin to a diuretic or other antihypertensive agent, dosage reduction and retitration may be necessary.

Terazosin has been given without interaction with analgesics/anti-inflammatories, cardiac glycosides, hypoglycemics, antiarrhythmics, anxiolytics/sedatives, antibacterials, hormone/steroids and drugs used for gout.

Pregnancy and lactation: Although no teratogenic effects were seen in animal testing, the safety of Hytrin use during pregnancy or during lactation has not yet been established. Hytrin should not be used therefore in pregnancy unless the potential benefit outweighs the risk.

Effects on ability to drive and use machines: Dizziness, light-headedness or drowsiness may occur with the initial dose or in association with missed doses and subsequent reinitiation of Hytrin therapy. Patients should be cautioned about these possible adverse effects and the circumstances in which they may occur and advised to avoid driving or hazardous tasks for approximately 12 hours after initial dose or when the dose is increased.

Undesirable effects: Hytrin in common with other alpha-adrenoceptor antagonists may cause syncope. Syncopal episodes have occurred within 30 or 90 minutes of the initial dose of the drug. Syncope has occasionally occurred in association with rapid dosage increases or the introduction of another antihypertensive agent.

In clinical trials in hypertension, the incidence of syncopal episodes was approximately one per cent. In most cases this was believed to be due to an excessive postural hypotensive effect although occasionally the syncopal episode has been preceded by a bout of tachycardia with heart rates of 120 to 160 beats per minute.

If syncope occurs the patient should be placed in a recumbent position and supportive treatment applied as necessary.

Dizziness, light-headedness or fainting may occur when standing up quickly from a lying or sitting position. Patients should be advised of this possibility and instructed to lie down if these symptoms appear and then sit for a few minutes before standing up to prevent their recurrence.

These adverse effects are self limiting and in most cases do not recur after the initial period of therapy or during subsequent re-titration.

Adverse events reported with terazosin: The most common events were asthenia, palpitations, nausea, peripheral oedema, dizziness, somnolence, nasal congestion/rhinitis and blurred vision/amblyopia.

In addition, the following have been reported: back pain; headache; tachycardia; postural hypotension; syncope; oedema; weight gain; pain in extremities; decreased libido; depression; nervousness; paraesthesia; vertigo; dyspnoea; sinusitis and impotence.

Additional adverse reactions reported in clinical trials or reported during marketing experience but not clearly associated with the use of terazosin include the following: chest pain; facial oedema; fever; abdominal pain; neck pain; shoulder pain; vasodilatation; arrhythmia; constipation; diarrhoea; dry mouth; dyspepsia; flatulence; vomiting; gout; arthralgia; arthritis; joint disorders; myalgia; anxiety; insomnia; bronchitis; epistaxis; flu symptoms; pharyngitis; rhinitis; cold symptoms; pruritis; rash; increased cough; sweating; abnormal vision; conjunctivitis; tinnitus; urinary frequency; urinary tract infection and urinary incontinence primarily reported in post-menopausal women.

At least two cases of anaphylactoid reactions have been reported with the administration of terazosin.

Post marketing experience: Thrombocytopenia and priapism have been reported. Atrial fibrillation has been reported: however, a cause and effect relationship has not been established.

Laboratory tests: Small but statistically significant decreases in haemotocrit, haemoglobin, white blood cells, total protein and albumin were observed in controlled clinical trials. These laboratory findings suggest the possibility of haemodilution. Treatment with terazosin for up to 24 months had no significant effect on prostate specific antigen (PSA) levels.

Overdosage: Should administration of Hytrin lead to acute hypotension, cardiovascular support is of first importance. Restoration of blood pressure and normalisation of heart rate may be accomplished by keeping the patient in a supine position. If this measure is inadequate, shock should first be treated with volume expanders and if necessary, vasopressors could then be used. Renal function should be monitored and general supportive measures applied as required. Dialysis may not be of benefit since laboratory data indicate that terazosin is highly protein bound.

Pharmacological properties

Pharmacodynamics: Although the exact mechanism of the hypotensive action is not established, the relaxation of peripheral blood vessels appears to be produced mainly by competitive antagonism of post-synaptic alpha-adrenoceptors. Hytrin usually produces an initial gradual decrease in blood pressure followed by a sustained antihypertensive action.

Clinical experience indicates that a 2–5% decrease in total cholesterol plasma concentration and a 3–7% decrease in the combined LDL_c+VLDL_c fraction plasma concentration from pretreatment values are associated with the administration of therapeutic doses of terazosin.

In clinical trials, plasma concentrates of total cholesterol and combined low density and very low density lipoproteins were found to be slightly reduced following Hytrin administration. Additionally, the increase in total cholesterol seen with other hypertensive agents did not occur when these were used in combination with Hytrin.

Pharmacokinetics: The plasma concentration of the parent drug is a maximum about 1 hour post administration and declines with a half-life of approximately 12 hours. Food has little or no effect on bioavailability. Approximately 40% of the administered dose is eliminated in the urine and 60% in the faeces. The drug is highly bound to plasma proteins.

Preclinical safety data: Carcinogenicity: Hytrin has been shown to produce tumours in male rats when administered at a high dose over a long period of time. No such occurrences were seen in female rats or in a similar study in mice. The relevance of these findings with respect to the clinical use of the drug in man is unknown.

Pharmaceutical particulars

List of excipients: Lactose, maize starch, purified talc, magnesium stearate and purified water; quinoline yellow (E104) 2 mg tablet only; iron oxide burnt sienna (E172) 5 mg tablet only; FD&C No 2 blue (E132) 10 mg tablet only.

Incompatibilities: None known.

Shelf life: 36 months.

Special precautions for storage: None.

Nature and contents of container: Tablets in a blister original pack. Blisters are packaged in a carton with a pack insert. Starter pack: 7×1 mg+21×2 mg tablets. Maintenance packs: 28×2 mg; 28×5 mg; 28×10 mg.

Instructions for use/handling: Not applicable.

Marketing authorisation numbers

1 mg	0037/0159
2 mg	0037/0160
5 mg	0037/0161
10 mg	0037/0162

Date of approval/revision of SPC May 1997.

Legal category POM.

HYTRIN* BPH 1 mg TABLETS
HYTRIN* BPH 2 mg TABLETS
HYTRIN* BPH 5 mg TABLETS
HYTRIN* BPH 10 mg TABLETS

Qualitative and quantitative composition

Tablet	*Active*	*mg/Tablet*
Hytrin BPH 1 mg	Terazosin as monohydrochloride dihydrate	1.0
Hytrin BPH 2 mg	Terazosin as monohydrochloride dihydrate	2.0
Hytrin BPH 5 mg	Terazosin as monohydrochloride dihydrate	5.0
Hytrin BPH 10 mg	Terazosin as monohydrochloride dihydrate	10.0

Pharmaceutical form Tablet.

Clinical particulars

Therapeutic indications: Orally administered Hytrin BPH is indicated as a therapy for the symptomatic treatment of urinary obstruction caused by benign prostatic hyperplasia (BPH). Terazosin is a selective post synaptic alpha-1-adrenoreceptor antagonist. Antagonism of alpha-1-receptors on prostatic and urethral smooth muscle has been shown to improve urinary tract flow and relieve the urinary obstruction caused by BPH.

Posology and method of administration:

Adults only: The dose of terazosin should be adjusted according to the patient's response. The following is a guide to administration:

Initial dose: 1 mg before bedtime is the starting dose for all patients and should not be exceeded. Strict compliance with this recommendation should be observed to minimise acute first-dose hypotensive episodes.

Subsequent dose: The dose may be increased by approximately doubling at weekly or bi-weekly intervals to achieve the desired reduction in symptoms. The maintenance dose is usually 5 to 10 mg once daily. Improvements in symptoms have been detected as early as two weeks after starting treatment with terazosin.

At present there are insufficient data to suggest additional symptomatic relief with doses above 10 mg once daily.

Treatment should be initiated using the Hytrin BPH Starter Pack and response to treatment reviewed at four weeks. Transient side effects may occur at each titration step. If any side effects persist, consideration should be given to reducing the dose.

Use in renal insufficiency: Pharmacokinetic studies indicate that patients with impaired renal function need no alteration in the recommended dosages.

Use in children: Use in children for BPH is not applicable.

Use in the elderly: Pharmacokinetic studies in the elderly indicate that no alteration in dosage recommendation is required.

Postural hypotension: Postural hypotension has been reported to occur in patients receiving terazosin for the symptomatic treatment of urinary obstruction caused by BPH. In these cases, the incidence of postural hypotensive events was greater in patients aged 65 years and over (5.6%) than those aged less than 65 years (2.6%).

Contra-indications: Terazosin is contra-indicated in patients known to be hypersensitive to alpha-adrenoreceptor antagonists.

Special warnings and precautions for use: As with other alpha adrenoreceptor antagonists, terazosin is not recommended in patients with a history of micturition syncope.

In clinical trials, the incidence of postural hypotension was greater in patients who received terazosin for BPH than in patients who received terazosin for hypertension. In this indication the incidence of postural hypotensive events was greater in patients aged 65 years and over (5.6%) than those aged less than 65 years (2.6%).

If administration is discontinued for more than several days, therapy should be re-instituted using the initial dosing regimen.

Interaction with other medicaments and other forms of interaction: In patients receiving terazosin for BPH, plus ACE inhibitors or diuretics, the proportion reporting dizziness or related side effects was greater than in the total population of terazosin treated patients from clinical trials.

Caution should be observed when terazosin is administered with other antihypertensive agents, to avoid the possibility of significant hypotension. When adding terazosin to a diuretic or other antihypertensive agent, dosage reduction and retitration may be necessary.

Terazosin has been given without interaction with analgesics/anti-inflammatories, cardiac glycosides, hypoglycaemics, antiarrhythmics, anxiolytics/sedatives, antibacterials, hormones/steroids and drugs used for gout.

Pregnancy and lactation: Although no teratogenic effects were seen in animal testing, the safety during pregnancy and lactation has not yet been established. Hytrin should not be used therefore in pregnancy unless the potential benefit outweighs the risk.

Effects on ability to drive and use machines: Dizziness, light-headedness or drowsiness may occur with the initial dose or in association with missed doses and subsequent reinitiation of Hytrin therapy. Patients should be cautioned about these possible adverse events and the circumstances in which they may occur and advised to avoid driving or hazardous tasks for approximately the first 12 hours after the initial dose or when the dose is increased.

Undesirable effects: Hytrin, in common with other alpha-adrenoreceptor antagonists, may cause syncope. Syncopal episodes have occurred within 30 to 90 minutes of the initial dose of the drug. Syncope has occasionally occurred in association with rapid dosage increases or the introduction of another antihypertensive agent.

In clinical studies in hypertension, the incidence of syncopal episodes was approximately one percent. In most cases, this was believed to be due to an excessive postural hypotensive effect although occasionally the syncopal episode has been preceded by a bout of tachycardia with heart rates of 120 to 160 beats per minute.

If syncope occurs the patient should be placed in a recumbent position and given supportive treatment as necessary.

Dizziness, light-headedness or fainting may occur when standing up quickly from a lying or sitting position. Patients should be advised of this possibility and instructed to lie down if these symptoms appear and then sit for a few minutes before standing to prevent re-occurrence.

These adverse effects are self limiting and, in most cases, do not recur after the initial period of therapy or during subsequent titration.

Adverse events reported with terazosin: The most common events were asthenia, palpitations, nausea, peripheral oedema, dizziness, somnolence, nasal congestion/rhinitis and blurred vision/amblyopia.

In addition, the following have been reported: back pain; headache; tachycardia; postural hypotension; syncope; oedema; weight gain; pain in extremities; decreased libido; depression; nervousness; paraesthesia; vertigo; dyspnoea; sinusitis and impotence.

Additional adverse reactions reported in clinical trials or reported during marketing experience but not clearly associated with the use of terazosin include the following: chest pain; facial oedema; fever; abdominal pain; neck pain; shoulder pain; vasodilation; arrhythmia; constipation; diarrhoea; dry mouth; dyspepsia; flatulence; vomiting; gout; arthralgia; arthritis; joint disorders; myalgia; anxiety; insomnia; bronchitis; epistaxis; flu symptoms; pharyngitis; rhinitis; cold symptoms; pruritus; rash; increased cough; sweating; abnormal vision; conjunctivitis; tinnitus; urinary frequency; urinary tract infection and urinary incontinence primarily reported in post-menopausal women.

At least two cases of severe anaphylactoid reactions have been reported with the administration of terazosin.

Post marketing experience: Thrombocytopenia and priapism have been reported. Atrial fibrillation has been reported: however, a cause and effect relationship has not been established.

Laboratory tests: Small but statistically significant decreases in haematocrit, haemoglobin, white blood cells, total protein and albumin were observed in controlled clinical trials. These laboratory findings suggest the possibility of haemodilution. Treatment with terazosin for up to 24 months had no significant effect on prostate specific antigen (PSA) levels.

Overdose: Should administration of terazosin lead to acute hypotension, cardiovascular support is of first importance. Restoration of blood pressure and normalisation of heart rate may be accomplished by keeping the patient in a supine position. If this measure is inadequate, shock should first be treated with volume expanders and, if necessary, vasopressors could then be used. Renal function should be monitored and general supportive measures applied as required. Dialysis may not be of benefit since laboratory data indicate that terazosin is highly protein bound.

Pharmacological properties

Pharmacodynamic properties: Studies suggest that alpha-1-adrenoreceptor antagonism is useful in improving the urodynamics in patients with chronic bladder obstruction such as in benign prostatic hyperplasia (BPH).

The symptoms of BPH are caused mainly by the presence of an enlarged prostate and by the increased smooth muscle tone of the bladder outlet and prostate, which is regulated by alpha-1-adrenergic receptors.

In *in-vitro* experiments, terazosin has been shown to antagonise phenylephrine-induced contractions of human prostatic tissue. In clinical trials terazosin has been shown to improve the urodynamics and symptomatology in patients with BPH.

Pharmacokinetic properties: The plasma concentration of the parent drug is a maximum 1 hour post administration and declines with a half-life of approximately 12 hours. Food has little or no effect on bioavailability. Approximately 40% of the administered dose is eliminated in the urine and 60% in the faeces. The drug is highly bound to plasma proteins.

Preclinical safety data: Carcinogenicity: terazosin has been shown to produce benign adrenal medullary tumours in male rats when administered in very high doses over a long period of time. No such findings were seen in female rats or in a similar study in mice. The relevance of these findings with respect to the clinical use of the drug in man is unknown.

Pharmaceutical particulars

List of excipients: Lactose, maize starch, purified talc, magnesium stearate and purified water.

In addition: Hytrin BPH 2 mg tablets contains dye yellow (quinoline yellow, E104); Hytrin BPH 5 mg tablets contain dye (iron oxide burnt sienna, E172); Hytrin BPH 10 mg tablets contain dye blue (FD&C No. 2 lake).

Incompatibilities: None known.

Shelf life: 36 months.

Special precautions for storage: None.

Nature and contents of container: Tablets in a blister pack. The 1 mg tablets are only available as part of a starter pack. The starter pack consists of 7×1 mg, 14×2 mg and 7×5 mg tablets. The 2 mg and 5 mg tablets are available as part of a starter pack and are also supplied in packs of 28 tablets. The 10 mg tablets are supplied in packs of 28 tablets. The blisters, of PVC/PVdC, are heat sealed with 20 micron hard tempered aluminium foil and packaged in a carton with a pack insert.

Instruction for use/handling: Not applicable.

Marketing authorisation numbers

Hytrin BPH 1 mg Tablets PL 0037/0234
Hytrin BPH 2 mg Tablets PL 0037/0235
Hytrin BPH 5 mg Tablets PL 0037/0236
Hytrin BPH 10 mg Tablets PL 0037/0237

Date of first authorisation/renewal of authorisation 20/05/93, 20/05/98

Date of (partial) revision of text February 1998

Legal category POM

ISOFLURANE

Presentation Isoflurane is an inhalation anaesthetic with a mildly pungent ethereal odour. No additive or stabiliser is present.

Uses Inhalation anaesthesia.

Actions: Induction and particularly recovery are rapid. Although slight pungency may limit the rate of induction, excessive salivation and tracheobronchial secretions are not stimulated. Pharyngeal and laryngeal reflexes are diminished quickly. Levels of anaesthesia change rapidly with Isoflurane. Heart rhythm remains stable. Spontaneous respiration becomes depressed as depth of anaesthesia increases and should be closely monitored.

During induction there is a decrease in blood pressure which returns towards normal with surgical stimulation.

Blood pressure tends to fall during maintenance in direct relation to depth of anaesthesia, due to peripheral vasodilation, but cardiac rhythm remains stable. With controlled respiration and normal $PaCO_2$, cardiac output tends to be maintained despite increasing depth of anaesthesia, primarily through a rise in heart rate. With spontaneous respiration, the resulting hypercapnia may increase heart rate and cardiac output above awake levels.

Cerebral blood flow remains unchanged during light Isoflurane anaesthesia but tends to rise at deeper levels. Increases in cerebrospinal fluid pressure may be prevented or reversed by hyperventilating the patient before or during anaesthesia.

Electroencephalographic changes and convulsions are extremely rare with Isoflurane.

Isoflurane appears to sensitise the myocardium to adrenaline to an even lesser extent than enflurane. Limited data suggest that subcutaneous infiltration of up to 50 ml of 1:200,000 solution adrenaline does not induce ventricular arrhythmias in patients anaesthetised with Isoflurane.

Muscular relaxation may be adequate for some intra-abdominal operations at normal levels of anaesthesia, but should greater relaxation be required small doses of intravenous muscle relaxants may be used. All commonly used muscle relaxants are markedly potentiated by Isoflurane, the effect being most profound with non-depolarising agents. Neostigmine reverses the effects of non-depolarising muscle relaxants but has no effect on the relaxant properties of Isoflurane itself. All commonly used muscle relaxants are compatible with Isoflurane.

Isoflurane may be used for the induction and maintenance of general anaesthesia. Adequate data are not available to establish its place in pregnancy or obstetrics anaesthesia other than for caesarian section.

Relatively little metabolism of Isoflurane occurs in the human body. In the post-operative period only 0.17% of the isoflurane taken up can be recovered as urinary metabolites. Peak serum inorganic fluoride values usually average less than 5 micromol/litre and occur about four hours after anaesthesia, returning to normal levels within 24 hours. No signs of renal injury have been reported after Isoflurane administration.

Dosage and administration Vaporisers specially calibrated for Isoflurane should be used so that the concentration of anaesthetic delivered can be accurately controlled.

MAC values for Isoflurane vary with age. The table below indicates average MAC values for different age groups:

Age	*Average MAC value in oxygen*
0–1 month	1.6%
1–6 months	1.87%
6–12 months	1.8%
1–5 years	1.6%
mid-twenties	1.28%
mid-forties	1.15%
mid-sixties	1.05%

Premedication: Drugs used for premedication should be selected for the individual patient, bearing in mind the respiratory depressant effect of Isoflurane. The use of anticholinergic drugs is a matter of choice but may be advisable for inhalation induction in paediatrics.

Induction: A short-acting barbiturate or other intravenous induction agent is usually administered followed by inhalation of the Isoflurane mixture. Alternatively, Isoflurane with oxygen or with an oxygen/nitrous oxide mixture may be used.

It is recommended that induction with Isoflurane be initiated at a concentration of 0.5%. Concentrations of 1.5 to 3.0% usually produce surgical anaesthesia in 7 to 10 minutes.

Maintenance: Surgical levels of anaesthesia may be maintained with 1.0–2.5% Isoflurane in oxygen/nitrous oxide mixtures. An additional 0.5–1.0% Isoflurane may be required when given with oxygen alone.

For caesarian section, 0.5–0.75% Isoflurane in a mixture of oxygen/nitrous oxide is suitable to maintain anaesthesia for this procedure.

Arterial pressure levels during maintenance tend to be inversely related to alveolar Isoflurane concentrations in the absence of other complicating factors. Excessive falls in blood pressure may be due to depth of anaesthesia and, in these circumstances, should be corrected by reducing the inspired Isoflurane concentration.

Elderly: As with other agents, lesser concentrations of Isoflurane are normally required to maintain surgical anaesthesia in elderly patients. See above for MAC values related to age.

Contra-indications, warnings, etc

Contra-indications: Known sensitivity to Isoflurane, or history of malignant hyperpyrexia following its administration should be considered contra-indications.

Precautions: Since levels of anaesthesia may be altered quickly and easily with Isoflurane, only vaporisers which deliver a predictable output with reasonable accuracy, or techniques during which inspired or expired concentrations can be monitored, should be used. The degree of hypotension and respiratory depression may provide some indication of anaesthetic depth.

Clinical data demonstrate that Isoflurane may produce hepatic injury in very rare instances.

As with other halogenated agents, Isoflurane must be used with caution in patients with increased intracranial pressure. In such cases hyperventilation may be necessary.

The action of non-depolarising relaxants is markedly potentiated with Isoflurane.

Isoflurane has been reported to interact with dry carbon dioxide absorbents to form carbon monoxide. In order to minimise the risk of formation of carbon monoxide in rebreathing circuits and the possibility of elevated carboxyhaemoglobin levels, carbon dioxide absorbents should not be allowed to dry out.

Use in pregnancy: Reproduction studies have been carried out on animals after repeated exposure to anaesthetic concentrations of Isoflurane. Studies with the rat demonstrated no effect on fertility, pregnancy or delivery or on the viability of the offspring. No evidence of teratogenicity was revealed. Comparable experiments in rabbits produced similar negative results. The relevance of these studies to the human is not known. As there is insufficient experience in the use of Isoflurane in pregnant women, safety in human pregnancy has not been established. Blood losses comparable with those found following anaesthesia with other inhalation agents have been observed with Isoflurane in patients undergoing induced abortion. Adequate data have not been developed to establish the safety of Isoflurane in obstetric anaesthesia, other than for caesarian section.

Side effects:

1. Arrhythmias have been occasionally reported.
2. Elevation of the white blood cell count has been observed, even in the absence of surgical stress.
3. Minimally raised levels of serum inorganic fluoride occur during and after Isoflurane anaesthesia, due to biodegradation of the agent. It is unlikely that the low levels of serum inorganic fluoride observed (mean 4.4 micromol/l in one study) could cause renal toxicity, as these are well below the proposed threshold levels for kidney toxicity.
4. Undesirable effects during recovery (shivering, nausea and vomiting) are minor in nature and comparable in incidence with those found with other anaesthetics.

Overdosage: As with other halogenated anaesthetics, hypotension and respiratory depression have been observed. Close monitoring of blood pressure and respiration is recommended. Supportive measures may be necessary to correct hypotension and respiratory depression resulting from excessively deep levels of anaesthesia.

Pharmaceutical precautions Store below 25°C. Keep container well closed.

Legal category P.

Package quantities Isoflurane is supplied in bottles of 250 ml.

Further information Nil.

Product licence number 0037/0115.

KLARICID*

Qualitative and quantitative composition Clarithromycin 250 mg per tablet.

Pharmaceutical form A yellow, ovaloid film-coated tablet containing 250 mg of clarithromycin.

Clinical particulars

Therapeutic indications: Klaricid is indicated in the treatment of infections caused by susceptible organisms. Indications include:

Lower respiratory tract infections for example, acute and chronic bronchitis, and pneumonia.

Upper respiratory tract infections for example, sinusitis and pharyngitis.

Klaricid is appropriate for initial therapy in community acquired respiratory infections and has been shown to be active *in vitro* against common and atypical respiratory pathogens as listed in the microbiology section.

Klaricid is also indicated in skin and soft tissue infections of mild to moderate severity.

Klaricid in the presence of acid suppression effected by omeprazole or lansoprazole is also indicated for the eradication of *H pylori* in patients with duodenal ulcers. See *Dosage and administration* section.

Klaricid is usually active against the following organisms *in vitro:*

Gram-positive bacteria: Staphylococcus aureus (methicillin susceptible); *Streptococcus pyogenes* (Group A beta-haemolytic streptococci); alpha-haemolytic streptococci (viridans group); *Streptococcus (Diplococcus) pneumoniae; Streptococcus agalactiae; Listeria monocytogenes.*

Gram-negative bacteria: Haemophilus influenzae, Haemophilus parainfluenzae, Moraxella (Branhamella) catarrhalis, Neisseria gonorrhoeae; Legionella pneumophila, Bordetella pertussis, Helicobacter pylori; Campylobacter jejuni.

Mycoplasma: Mycoplasma pneumoniae; Ureaplasma urealyticum.

Other organisms: Chlamydia trachomatis; Mycobacterium avium; Mycobacterium leprae.

Anaerobes: Macrolide-susceptible *Bacteroides fragilis; Clostridium perfringens; Peptococcus* species;

Peptostreptococcus species; *Propionibacterium acnes*.

Clarithromycin also has bactericidal activity against several bacterial strains. These organisms include *Haemophilus influenzae, Streptococcus pneumoniae, Streptococcus pyogenes, Streptococcus agalactiae, Moraxella (Branhamella) catarrhalis, Neisseria gonorrhoeae, H. pylori* and *Campylobacter* spp.

The activity of clarithromycin against *H pylori* is greater at neutral pH than at acid pH.

Posology and method of administration
Patients with respiratory tract/skin and soft tissue infections:
Adults: The usual dose is 250 mg twice daily for 7 days although this may be increased to 500 mg twice daily for up to 14 days in severe infections.

Children older than 12 years: As for adults.
Children younger than 12 years: Use Klaricid Paediatric Suspension.

Eradication of H pylori in patients with duodenal ulcers (Adults):

Triple therapy (7–14 days): Klaricid 500 mg twice daily and lansoprazole 30 mg twice daily should be given with amoxycillin 1000 mg twice daily for 7–14 days.

Triple therapy (7 days): Klaricid (500 mg) twice daily and omeprazole 40 mg daily should be given with amoxycillin 1000 mg twice daily for 7 days.

Triple therapy (10 days): Klaricid (500 mg) twice daily should be given with amoxycillin 1000 mg twice daily and omeprazole 20 mg daily for 10 days.

Dual therapy (14 days): The usual dose of Klaricid is 500 mg three times daily for 14 days. Klaricid should be administered with oral omeprazole 40 mg once daily. The pivotal study was conducted with omeprazole 40 mg once daily for 28 days. Supportive studies have been conducted with omeprazole 40 mg once daily for 14 days.

For further information on the dosage for omeprazole see the Astra data sheet.

Elderly: As for adults.

Renal impairment: Dosage adjustments are not usually required except in patients with severe renal impairment (creatinine clearance <30 ml/min). If adjustment is necessary, the total daily dosage should be reduced by half, e.g. 250 mg once daily or 250 mg twice daily in more severe infections.

Klaricid may be given without regard to meals as food does not affect the extent of bioavailability.

Contra-indications: Clarithromycin is contra-indicated in patients with known hypersensitivity to macrolide antibiotic drugs.

Clarithromycin and ergot derivates should not be co-administered.

Concomitant administration of clarithromycin and any of the following drugs is contra-indicated: cisapride, pimozide and terfenadine. Elevated cisapride, pimozide and terfenadine levels have been reported in patients receiving either of these drugs and clarithromycin concomitantly. This may result in QT prolongation and cardiac arrhythmias including ventricular tachycardia, ventricular fibrillation and Torsade de Pointes. Similar effects have been observed with concomitant administration of astemizole and other macrolides.

Special warnings and special precautions for use: Clarithromycin is principally excreted by the liver and kidney. Caution should be exercised in administering this antibiotic to patients with impaired hepatic or renal function.

Prolonged or repeated use of clarithromycin may result in an overgrowth of non-susceptible bacteria or fungi. If super-infection occurs, clarithromycin should be discontinued and appropriate therapy instituted.

H pylori organisms may develop resistance to clarithromycin in a small number of patients.

Interaction with other medicaments and other forms of interaction: Clarithromycin has been shown not to interact with oral contraceptives.

As with other macrolide antibiotics the use of clarithromycin in patients concurrently taking drugs metabolised by the cytochrome p450 system (e.g. warfarin, ergot alkaloids, triazolam, midazolam, disopyramide, lovastatin, rifabutin, phenytoin and cyclosporin) may be associated with elevations in serum levels of these other drugs. Rhabdomyolysis, coincident with the co-administration of clarithromycin and HMG-CoA reductase inhibitors, such as lovastatin and simvastatin has been reported.

The administration of clarithromycin to patients who are receiving theophylline has been associated with an increase in serum theophylline levels and potential theophylline toxicity.

The use of clarithromycin in patients receiving warfarin may result in potentiation of the effects of warfarin. Prothrombin time should be frequently monitored in these patients. The effects of digoxin may be potentiated with concomitant administration of Klaricid. Monitoring of serum digoxin levels should be considered.

Clarithromycin may potentiate the effects of carbamazepine due to a reduction in the rate of excretion.

Simultaneous oral administratioin of clarithromycin tablets and zidovudine to HIV infected adult patients may result in decreased steady-state zidovudine levels. This can be largely avoided by staggering the doses of Klaricid and zidovudine by 1 to 2 hours. No such reaction has been reported in children.

Ritonavir increases the area under the curve (AUC), C_{max} and C_{min} of clarithromycin when administered concurrently. Because of the large therapeutic window for clarithromycin, no dosage reduction should be necessary in patients with normal renal function. However, for patients with renal impairment, the following dosage adjustments should be considered: For patients with CL_{CR} 30 to 60 ml/min the dose of clarithromycin should be reduced by 50%. For patients with CL_{CR} <30 ml/min the dose of clarithromycin should be decreased by 75%. Doses of clarithromycin greater than 1 g/day should not be coadministered with ritonavir.

Although the plasma concentrations of clarithromycin and omeprazole may be increased when they are administered concurrently, no adjustment to the dosage is necessary. At the dosages recommended, there is no clinically significant interaction between clarithromycin and lansoprazole. Increased plasma concentrations of clarithromycin may also occur when it is co-administered with Maalox or ranitidine. No adjustment to the dosage is necessary.

Pregnancy and lactation: The safety of clarithromycin during pregnancy and breast feeding of infants has not been established. Klaricid should thus not be used during pregnancy or lactation unless the benefit is considered to outweigh the risk. Some animal studies have suggested an embryotoxic effect, but only at dose levels which are clearly toxic to mothers. Clarithromycin has been found in milk of lactating animals and in human breast milk.

Effects on ability to drive and use machines: None known.

Undesirable effects: Clarithromycin is generally well tolerated. Side effects include nausea, dyspepsia, diarrhoea, vomiting and abdominal pain. Stomatitis, glossitis, oral monilia and tongue discolouration have been reported. Other side-effects include headache, arthralgia, myalgia and allergic reactions ranging from urticaria, mild skin eruptions and angioedema to anaphylaxis and rarely Stevens-Johnson syndrome.

Reports of alteration of the sense of smell, usually in conjunction with taste perversion have also been received. There have been reports of tooth discolouration in patients treated with clarithromycin. Tooth discolouration is usually reversible with professional dental cleaning.

There have been reports of transient central nervous system side-effects including dizziness, vertigo, anxiety, insomnia, bad dreams, tinnitus, confusion, disorientation, hallucinations, psychosis and depersonalisation. There have been reports of hearing loss with clarithromycin which is usually reversible upon withdrawal of therapy. Pseudomembranous colitis has been reported rarely with clarithromycin, and may range in severity from mild to life threatening. There have been rare reports of hypoglycaemia, some of which have occurred in patients on concomitant oral hypoglycaemic agents or insulin. Isolated cases of thrombocytopenia have been reported.

As with other macrolides, hepatic dysfunction (which is usually reversible) including altered liver function tests, hepatitis and cholestasis with or without jaundice, has been reported. Dysfunction may be severe and very rarely fatal hepatic failure has been reported.

Cases of increased serum creatinine, interstitial nephritis and renal failure have been reported rarely.

As with other macrolides, QT prolongation, ventricular tachycardia and torsade de pointes have been rarely reported with clarithromycin.

Overdosage: Reports indicate that the ingestion of large amounts of clarithromycin can be expected to produce gastro-intestinal symptoms. One patient who had a history of bipolar disorder ingested 8 g of clarithromycin and showed altered mental status, paranoid behaviour, hypokalemia and hypoxemia. Allergic reactions accompanying overdosage should be treated by gastric lavage and supportive measures. As with other macrolides, clarithromycin serum levels are not expected to be appreciably affected by haemodialysis or peritoneal dialysis.

Pharmacological properties
Pharmacodynamic properties: Clarithromycin is a semi-synthetic derivative of erythromycin A. It exerts its antibacterial action by binding to the 50s ribosomal sub-unit of susceptible bacteria and suppresses protein synthesis. It is highly potent against a wide variety of aerobic and anaerobic gram-positive and gram-negative organisms. The minimum inhibitory concentrations (MICs) of clarithromycin are generally two-fold lower than the MICs of erythromycin.

The 14-hydroxy metabolite of clarithromycin also has antimicrobial activity. The MICs of this metabolite are equal or two-fold higher than the MICs of the parent compound, except for *H influenzae* where the 14-hydroxy metabolite is two-fold more active than the parent compound.

Klaricid is usually active against the following organisms *in vitro*:

Gram-positive bacteria: Staphylococcus aureus (methicillin susceptible); *Streptococcus pyogenes* (Group A beta-hemolytic streptococci); alpha-hemolytic streptoccci (viridans group); *Streptococcus (Diplococcus) pneumoniae; Streptococcus agalactiae; Listeria monocytogenes.*

Gram-negative bacteria: Haemophilus influenzae; Haemophilus parainfluenzae; Moraxella (Branhamella) catarrhalis; Neisseria gonorrhoeae; Legionella pneumophila; Bordetella pertussis; Helicobacter pylori; Campylobacter jejuni.

Mycoplasma: Mycoplasma pneumoniae; Ureaplasma urealyticum.

Other organisms: Chlamydia trachomatis; Mycobacterium avium; Mycobacterium leprae.

Anaerobes: Macrolide-susceptible *Bacteroides fragilis; Clostridium perfringens; Peptococcus* species; *Peptostreptococcus* species; *Propionibacterium acnes*.

Clarithromycin has bactericidal activity against several bacterial strains. The organisms include *Haemophilus influenzae, Streptococcus pneumoniae, Streptococcus pyogenes, Streptococcus agalactiae, Moraxella (Branhamella) catarrhalis, Neisseria gonorrhoeae* and *Helicobacter pylori* and *Campylobacter* spp.

Pharmacokinetics: Helicobacter pylori (H pylori) is associated with acid peptic disease including duodenal ulcer and gastric ulcer in which about 95% and 80% of patients respectively are infected with the agent. *H pylori* is also implicated as a major contribution factor in the development of gastritis and ulcer recurrence in such patients. Recent evidence further suggests a causative link between *H pylori* and gastric carcinoma.

Clarithromycin has been used in small numbers of patients in other treatment regimens. Possible kinetic interactions have not been fully investigated. These regimens include: clarithromycin plus tinidazole and omeprazole; clarithromycin plus tetracycline, bismuth subsalicylate and ranitidine; clarithromycin plus ranitidine alone.

Clinical studies using various different *H pylori* eradication regimens (including clarithromycin plus omeprazole) have shown that eradication of *H pylori* prevents ulcer recurrence.

Clarithromycin is rapidly and well absorbed from the gastro-intestinal tract after oral administration of Klaricid tablets. The microbiologically active metabolite 14-hydroxyclarithromycin is formed by first pass metabolism. Klaricid may be given without regard to meals as food does not affect the extent of bioavailability of Klaricid tablets. Food does slightly delay the onset of absorption of clarithromycin and formation of the 14-hydroxymetabolite. The pharmacokinetics of clarithromycin are non linear; however, steady-state is attained within 2 days of dosing. At 250 mg b.i.d. 15–20% of unchanged drug is excreted in the urine. With 500 mg b.i.d. daily dosing urinary excretion is greater (approximately 36%). The 14-hydroxy-clarithromycin is the major urinary metabolite and accounts for 10–15% of the dose. Most of the remainder of the dose is eliminated in the faeces, primarily via the bile. 5–10% of the parent drug is recovered from the faeces.

When clarithromycin 500 mg is given three times daily, the clarithromycin plasma concentrations are increased with respect to the 500 mg twice daily dosage.

Klaricid provides tissue concentrations that are several times higher than the circulating drug levels. Increased levels have been found in both tonsillar and lung tissue. Clarithromycin is 80% bound to plasma proteins at therapeutic levels.

Klaricid also penetrates the gastric mucus. Levels of clarithromycin in gastric mucus and gastric tissue are higher when clarithromycin is co-administered with omeprazole than when clarithromycin is administered alone.

Preclinical safety data: In acute mouse and rat studies, the median lethal dose was greater than the highest feasible dose for administration (5 g/kg).

In repeated dose studies, toxicity was related to dose, duration of treatment and species. Dogs were more sensitive than primates or rats. The major clinical signs at toxic doses included emesis, weakness, reduced food consumption and weight gain, salivation, dehydration and hyperactivity. In all species the liver was the primary target organ at toxic doses. Hepatotoxicity was detectable by early elevations of liver function tests. Discontinuation of the drug generally resulted in a return to or toward normal results. Other tissues less commonly affected included the stomach, thymus and other lymphoid tissues and the kidneys. At near therapeutic doses, conjunctival injection and lacrimation occurred only in dogs. At a massive dose of 400 mg/kg/day, some dogs and monkeys developed corneal opacities and/or oedema.

Fertility and reproduction studies in rats have shown no adverse effects. Teratogenicity studies in rats (Wistar (p.o.) and Sprague-Dawley (p.o. and i.v.)), New Zealand White rabbits and cynomolgous monkeys failed to demonstrate any teratogenicity from clarithromycin. However, a further similar study in Sprague-Dawley rats indicated a low (6%) incidence of cardiovascular abnormalities which appeared to be due to spontaneous expression of genetic changes. Two mouse studies revealed a variable incidence (3–30%) of cleft palate and embryonic loss was seen in monkeys but only at dose levels which were clearly toxic to the mothers.

Pharmaceutical particulars

List of excipients: Croscarmellose sodium, starch pregelatinised, cellulose microcrystalline, silica gel, povidone, stearic acid, magnesium stearate, talc, hypromellose, hydroxypropylcellulose, propylene glycol, sorbitan monooleate, titanium dioxide, sorbic acid, vanillin, quinoline yellow E104.

Incompatibilities: None known.

Shelf life: The recommended shelf life is 24 months.

Special precautions for storage: Protect from light. Store in a dry place.

Nature and contents of container: 2/14/56 tablets in a blister original pack. The blisters are packaged in a carton with a pack insert.

Instructions for use/handling: Not applicable.

Marketing authorisation number 0037/0211.

Date of approval/revision of SPC September 1998.

Legal category POM.

KLARICID* 500

Qualitative and quantitative composition Clarithromycin 500 mg/tablet.

Pharmaceutical form A yellow, ovaloid film-coated tablet containing 500 mg of clarithromycin.

Clinical particulars

Therauputic indications: Klaricid is indicated for treatment of infections caused by susceptible organisms. Indications include:

Lower respiratory tract infections for example, acute and chronic bronchitis, and pneumonia.

Upper respiratory tract infections for example, sinusitis and pharyngitis.

Klaricid is appropriate for initial therapy in community acquired respiratory infections and has been shown to be active *in vitro* against common and atypical respiratory pathogens as listed in the microbiology section.

Klaricid is also indicated in skin and soft tissue infections of mild to moderate severity.

Klaricid in the presence of acid suppression effected by omeprazole or lansoprazole is also indicated for the eradication of *H pylori* in patients with duodenal ulcers. See *Posology and method of administration* section.

Klaricid is usually active against the following organisms *in vitro*:

Gram-positive bacteria: *Staphylococcus aureus* (methicillin susceptible); *Streptococcus pyogenes* (Group A beta-hemolytic streptococci) alpha-hemolytic streptococci (viridans group); *Streptococcus* (*Diplococcus*) *pneumoniae*; *Streptococcus agalactiae, Listeria monocytogenes.*

Gram-negative bacteria: *Haemophilus influenzae, Haemophilus parainfluenzae, Moraxella (Branhamella) catarrhalis, Neisseria gonorrhoeae; Legionella pneumophila, Bordetella pertussis, Helicobacter pylori; Campylobacter jejuni.*

Mycoplasma: *Mycoplasma pneumoniae; Ureaplasma urealyticum.*

Other organisms: *Chlamydia trachomatis; Mycobacterium avium; Mycobacterium leprae; Mycobacterum Kansasaii; Mycobacterium chelonae; Mycobacterium fortuitum; Mycobacterium intracellulare.*

Anaerobes: Macrolide-susceptible *Bacteroides fragilis; Clostridium perfringens; Peptococcus* species; *Peptostreptococcus* species; *Propionibacterium acnes.*

Clarithromycin has bactericidal activity against several bacterial strains. The organisms include *Haemophilus influenzae, Streptococcus pneumoniae, Streptococcus pyogenes, Streptococcus agalactiae, Moraxella (Branhamella) catarrhalis, Neisseria gonorrhoeae, H. pylori* and *Campylobacter* spp.

The activity of clarithromycin against *H. pylori* is greater at neutral pH than at acid pH.

Posology and method of administration

Patients with respiratory tract/skin and soft tissue infections

Adults: The usual dose is 250 mg twice daily for 7 days although this may be increased to 500 mg twice daily for up to 14 days in severe infections.

Children older than 12 years: As for adults.

Children younger than 12 years: Use Klaricid Paediatric Suspension.

Eradication of H pylori in patients with duodenal ulcers (Adults):

Triple therapy (7–14 days): Klaricid 500 mg twice daily and lansoprazole 30 mg twice daily should be given with amoxycillin 1000 mg twice daily for 7–14 days.

Triple therapy (7 days): Klaricid (500 mg) twice daily and omeprazole 40 mg daily should be given with amoxycillin 1000 mg twice daily for 7 days.

Triple therapy (10 days): Klaricid (500 mg) twice daily should be given with amoxycillin 1000 mg twice daily and omeprazole 20 mg daily for 10 days.

Dual therapy (14 days): The usual dose of Klaricid is 500 mg three times daily for 14 days. Klaricid should be administered with oral omeprazole 40 mg once daily. The pivotal study was conducted with omeprazole 40 mg once daily for 28 days. Supportive studies have been conducted with omeprazole 40 mg once daily for 14 days.

For further information on the dosage for omeprazole see the Astra data sheet.

Elderly: As for adults.

Renal impairment: Dosage adjustments are not usually required except in patients with severe renal impairment (creatinine clearance <30 ml/min). If adjustment is necessary, the total daily dosage should be reduced by half, e.g. 250 mg once daily or 250 mg twice daily in more severe infections.

Klaricid may be given without regard to meals as food does not affect the extent of bioavailability.

Contra-indications: Clarithromycin is contra-indicated in patients with known hypersensitivity to macrolide antibiotic drugs.

Clarithromycin and ergot derivatives should not be co-administered.

Concomitant administration of clarithromycin and any of the following drugs is contra-indicated: cisapride, pimozide and terfenadine. Elevated cisapride, pimozide and terfenadine levels have been reported in patients receiving either of these drugs and clarithromycin concomitantly. This may result in QT prolongation and cardiac arrhythmias including ventricular tachycardia, ventricular fibrillation and Torsade de Pointes. Similar effects have been observed with concomitant administration of astemizole and other macrolides.

Special warnings and special precautions for use: Clarithromycin is principally excreted by the liver and kidney. Caution should be exercised in administering this antibiotic to patients with impaired hepatic or renal function.

Prolonged or repeated use of clarithromycin may result in an overgrowth of non-susceptible bacteria or fungi. If super-infection occurs, clarithromycin should be discontinued and appropriate therapy instituted.

H pylori organisms may develop resistance to clarithromycin in a small number of patients.

Interaction with other medicaments and other forms of interaction: Clarithromycin has been shown not to interact with oral contraceptives.

As with other macrolide antibiotics the use of clarithromycin in patients concurrently taking drugs metabolised by the cytochrome p450 system (e.g. warfarin, ergot alkaloids, triazolam, midazolam, disopyramide, lovastatin, rifabutin, phenytoin and cyclosporin) may be associated with elevations in serum levels of these other drugs. Rhabdomyolysis, coincident with the co-administration of clarithromycin, and HMG-CoA reductase inhibitors, such as lovastatin and simvastatin has been reported.

The administration of clarithromycin to patients who are receiving theophylline has been associated with an increase in serum theophylline levels and potential theophylline toxicity.

The use of clarithromycin in patients receiving warfarin may result in potentiation of the effects of warfarin. Prothrombin time should be frequently monitored in these patients. The effects of digoxin may be potentiated with concomitant administration of Klaricid. Monitoring of serum digoxin levels should be considered.

Clarithromycin may potentiate the effects of carbamazepine due to a reduction in the rate of excretion.

Simultaneous oral administration of clarithromycin tablets and zidovudine to HIV infected adult patients may result in decreased steady-state zidovudine levels. This can be largely avoided by staggering the doses of Klaricid and zidovudine by 1–2 hours. No such reaction has been reported in children.

Ritonavir increases the area under the curve (AUC), C_{max} and C_{min} of clarithromycin when administered concurrently. Because of the large therapeutic window for clarithromycin, no dosage reduction should be necessary in patients with normal renal function. However, for patients with renal impairment, the following dosage adjustments should be considered: For patients with CL_{CR} 30 to 60 ml/min the dose of clarithromycin should be reduced by 50%. For patients with CL_{CR} <30 ml/min the dose of clarithromycin should be decreased by 75%. Doses of clarithromycin greater than 1 g/day should not be coadministered with ritonavir.

Although the plasma concentrations of clarithromycin and omeprazole may be increased when they are administered concurrently, no adjustment to the dosage is necessary. At the dosages recommended, there is no clinically significant interaction between clarithromycin and lansoprazole. Increased plasma concentrations of clarithromycin may also occur when it is co-administered with Maalox or ranitidine. No adjustment to the dosage is necessary.

Pregnancy and lactation: The safety of clarithromycin during pregnancy and breast feeding of infants has not been established. Klaricid should thus not be used during pregnancy or lactation unless the benefit is considered to outweigh the risk. Some animal studies have suggested an embryotoxic effect, but only at dose levels which are clearly toxic to mothers. Clarithromycin has been found in the milk of lactating animals and in human breast milk.

Effects on ability to drive and use machines: None known.

Undesirable effects: Clarithromycin is generally well tolerated. Side effects include nausea, dyspepsia, diarrhoea, vomiting and abdominal pain. Stomatitis, glossitis, oral monilia and tongue discolouration have been reported. Other side-effects include headache, arthralgia, myalgia and allergic reactions ranging from urticaria and mild skin eruptions and angioedema to anaphylaxis and rarely Stevens-Johnson syndrome. Reports of alteration of the sense of smell, usually in conjunction with taste perversion have also been received. There have been reports of tooth discolouration in patients treated with clarithromycin. Tooth discolouration is usually reversible with professional dental cleaning. There have been reports of transient central nervous system side-effects including dizziness, vertigo, anxiety, insomnia, bad dreams, tinnitus, confusion, disorientation, hallucinations, psychosis and depersonalisation. There have been reports of hearing loss with clarithromycin which is usually reversible on withdrawal of therapy. Pseudomembranous colitis has been reported rarely with clarithromycin, and may range in severity from mild to life threatening. There have been rare reports of hypoglycaemia, some of which have occurred in patients on concomitant oral hypoglycaemic agents or insulin. Isolated cases of thrombocytopenia have been reported. As with other macrolides, hepatic dysfunction (which is usually reversible) including altered liver function tests, hepatitis and cholestasis with or without jaundice, has been reported. Dysfunction may be severe and very rarely fatal hepatic failure has been reported. Cases of increased serum creatinine, interstitial nephritis and renal failure have been reported rarely. As with other macrolides, QT prolongation, ventricular tachycardia and Torsade de Pointes have been rarely reported with clarithromycin.

Overdosage: Reports indicate that the ingestion of large amounts of clarithromycin can be expected to produce gastro-intestinal symptoms. One patient who had a history of bipolar disorder ingested 8 grams of clarithromycin and showed altered mental status, paranoid behaviour, hypokalemia and hypoxemia. Allergic reactions accompanying overdosage should be treated by gastric lavage and supportive measures. As with other macrolides, clarithromycin serum levels are not expected to be appreciably affected by haemodialysis or peritoneal dialysis.

Pharmacological properties

Pharmacodynamic properties: Clarithromycin is a semi-synthetic derivative of erythromycin A. It exerts its antibacterial action by binding to the 50s ribosomal sub-unit of susceptible bacteria and suppresses protein synthesis. It is highly potent against a wide variety of aerobic and anaerobic gram-positive and gram-negative organisms. The minimum inhibitory concentrations (MICs) of clarithromycin are generally two-fold lower than the MICs of erythromycin.

The 14-hydroxy metabolite of clarithromycin also has antimicrobial activity. The MICs of the metabolite are equal or two-fold higher than the MICs of the parent compound, except for H influenzae where the 14-hydroxy metabolite is two-fold more active than the parent compound.

Klaricid is usually active against the following organisms in vitro:

Gram-positive bacteria: *Staphylococcus aureus*

(methicillin susceptible); *Streptococcus pyogenes* (Group A beta-hemolytic streptococci) alpha-hemolytic streptococci (viridans group); *Streptococcus (Diplococcus) pneumoniae; Streptococcus agalactiae, Listeria monocytogenes.*

Gram-negative bacteria: *Haemophilus influenzae, Haemophilus parainfluenzae, Moraxella (Branhamella) catarrhalis, Neisseria gonorrhoeae; Legionella pneumophila, Bordetella pertussis, Helicobacter pylori; Campylobacter jejuni.*

Mycoplasma: *Mycoplasma pneumoniae; Ureaplasma urealyticum.*

Other organisms: *Chlamydia trachomatis; Mycobacterium avium; Mycobacterium leprae; Mycobacterium Kansasaii; Mycobacterium chelonae; Mycobacterium fortuitum; Mycobacterium intracellulare.*

Anaerobes: Macrolide-susceptible *Bacteroides fragilis; Clostridium perfringens; Peptococcus* species; *Peptostreptococcus* species; *Propionibacterium acnes.*

Clarithromycin has bactericidal activity against several bacterial strains. The organisms include *Haemophilus influenzae, Streptococcus pneumoniae, Streptococcus pyogenes, Streptococcus agalactiae, Moraxella (Branhamella) catarrhalis, Neisseria gonorrhoeae, Helicobacter pylori* and *Campylobacter* spp.

Pharmacokinetics: H. pylori is associated with acid peptic disease including duodenal ulcer and gastric ulcer in which about 95% and 80% of patients respectively are infected with the agent. *H. pylori* is also implicated as a major contribution factor in the development of gastritis and ulcer recurrence in such patients.

Clarithromycin has been used in small numbers of patients in other treatment regimens. Possible kinetic interactions have not been fully investigated. These regimens include: clarithromycin plus tinidazole and omeprazole; clarithromycin plus tetracycline; bismuth subsalicylate and ranitidine; clarithromycin plus ranitidine alone.

Clinical studies using various different *H. pylori* eradication regimens have shown that eradication of *H. pylori* prevents ulcer recurrence.

Clarithromycin is rapidly and well absorbed from the gastro-intestinal tract after oral administration of Klaricid tablets. The microbiologically active metabolite 14-hydroxyclarithromycin is formed by first pass metabolism. Klaricid may be given without regard to meals as food does not affect the extent of bioavailability of Klaricid tablets. Food does slightly delay the onset of absorption of clarithromycin and formation of the 14-hydroxymetabolite. The pharmacokinetics of clarithromycin are non linear; however, steady-state is attained within 2 days of dosing. At 250 mg b.i.d. 15–20% of unchanged drug is excreted in the urine. With 500 mg b.i.d. daily dosing urinary excretion is greater (approximately 36%). The 14-hydroxy-clarithromycin is the major urinary metabolite and accounts for 10–15% of the dose. Most of the remainder of the dose is eliminated in the faeces, primarily via the bile. 5–10% of the parent drug is recovered from the faeces.

When clarithromycin 500 mg is given three times daily, the clarithromycin plasma concentrations are increased with respect to the 500 mg twice daily dosage.

Klaricid provides tissue concentrations that are several times higher than the circulating drug levels. Increased levels have been found in both tonsillar and lung tissue. Clarithromycin is 80% bound to plasma proteins at therapeutic levels.

Klaricid also penetrates the gastric mucus. Levels of clarithromycin in gastric mucus and gastric tissue are higher when clarithromycin is co-administered with omeprazole than when clarithromycin is administered alone.

Preclinical safety data: In acute mouse and rat studies, the median lethal dose was greater than the highest feasible dose for administration (5 g/kg).

In repeated dose studies, toxicity was related to dose, duration of treatment and species. Dogs were more sensitive than primates or rats. The major clinical signs at toxic doses included emesis, weakness, reduced food consumption and weight gain, salivation, dehydration and hyperactivity. In all species the liver was the primary target organ at toxic doses. Hepatotoxicity was detectable by early elevations of liver function tests. Discontinuation of the drug generally resulted in a return to or toward normal results. Other tissues less commonly affected included the stomach, thymus and other lymphoid tissues and the kidneys. At near therapeutic doses, conjunctival injection and lacrimation occurred only in dogs. At a massive dose of 400 mg/kg/day, some dogs and monkeys developed corneal opacities and/or oedema.

Fertility and reproduction studies in rats have shown no adverse effects. Teratogenicity studies in rats (Wistar (p.o.) and Sprague-Dawley (p.o. and i.v.)), New Zealand White rabbits and cynomolgous monkeys failed to demonstrate any teratogenicity from clarithromycin. However, a further similar study in Sprague-Dawley rats indicated a low (6%) incidence of cardiovascular abnormalities which appeared to be due to spontaneous expression of genetic changes. Two mouse studies revealed a variable incidence (3–30%) of cleft palate and embryonic loss was seen in monkeys but only at dose levels which were clearly toxic to the mothers.

Pharmaceutical particulars

List of excipients: Croscarmellose sodium, cellulose microcrystalline, silicon dioxide, povidone, stearic acid, magnesium stearate, talc, hypromellose, hydroxypropylcellulose, propylene glycol, sorbitan monooleate, titanium dioxide, sorbic acid, vanillin, quinoline yellow E104.

Incompatibilities: None known.

Shelf life: 36 months.

Special precautions for storage: Store in a dry place, protected from light.

Nature and contents of container: Tablets in a blister original pack. Pack sizes are 14, 20, 28, 42, 84, 168 tablets. The blisters are packaged in a carton with a patient leaflet.

Tablets in HDPE bottle with a patient leaflet. Pack sizes are 100, 250, 500, 1000 tablets.

Instructions for use/handling: Not applicable.

Marketing authorisation number 0037/0254.

Date of approval/revision of SPC September 1998.

Legal category POM.

KLARICID* IV

Presentation A sterile, white to off white lyophilised powder containing 500 mg clarithromycin per vial and lactobionic acid as a solubilising agent.

When reconstituted with 10 ml Sterilised Water for Injections, each ml of the resulting solution contains 50 mg clarithromycin. This solution must be further diluted prior to intravenous administration (see dosage and administration).

Uses Klaricid IV is indicated whenever parenteral therapy is required for treatment of infections caused by susceptible organisms in the following conditions: Lower respiratory tract infections for example, acute and chronic bronchitis, and pneumonia; upper respiratory tract infections for example, sinusitis and pharyngitis; skin and soft tissue infections.

Microbiology: Clarithromycin is a semi-synthetic derivative of erythromycin A. It exerts its anti-bacterial action by binding to the 50s ribosomal sub-unit of susceptible bacteria and suppresses protein synthesis. It is highly potent against a wide variety of aerobic and anaerobic gram-positive and gram-negative organisms. The minimum inhibitory concentrations (MICs) of clarithromycin are generally two-fold lower than the MICs of erythromycin. The 14-hydroxy metabolite of clarithromycin also has anti-microbial activity. The MICs of this metabolite are equal or two-fold higher than the MICs of the parent compound, except for *H. influenzae* where the 14-hydroxy metabolite is two-fold lower than the parent compound.

Klaricid is usually active against the following organisms *in vitro*: Gram-positive bacteria: Staphylococcus aureus (methicillin susceptible); *Streptococcus pyogenes* (Group A beta-haemolytic streptococci); alpha-haemolytic streptococci (viridans group); *Streptococcus (Diplococcus) pneumoniae: Streptococcus agalactiae; Listeria monocytogenes.*

Gram-negative bacteria: *Haemophilus influenzae, Haemophilus parainfluenzae, Moraxella (Branhamella) catarrhalis, Neisseria gonorrhoeae; Legionella pneumophila, Bordetella pertussis, Helicobacter pylori; Campylobacter jejuni.*

Mycoplasma: Mycoplasma pneumoniae; Ureaplasma urealyticum.

Other Organisms: *Chlamydia trachomatis; Mycobacterium avium; Mycobacterium leprae.*

Anaerobes: Macrolide-susceptible *Bacteroides fragilis; Clostridium perfringens; Peptococcus* species; *Peptostreptococcus* species; *Propionibacterium acnes.*

Clarithromycin has bactericidal activity against several bacterial strains. These organisms include *H. influenzae, Streptococcus pneumoniae, Streptococcus pyogenes, Streptococcus agalactiae, Moraxella (Branhamella) catarrhalis, Neisseria gonorrhoeae* and *Campylobacter* spp.

The activity of clarithromycin against *Helicobacter pylori* is greater at neutral pH than at acid pH.

Dosage and administration

Recommended dosage: Intravenous therapy may be given for 2 to 5 days and should be changed to oral clarithromycin therapy when appropriate.

Adults: The recommended dosage of Klaricid IV is 1.0 gram daily, divided into two 500 mg doses, appropriately diluted as described below.

Children: At present, there are insufficient data to recommend a dosage regimen for routine use in children.

Elderly: As for adults.

Renal impairment: In patients with renal impairment who have creatinine clearance less than 30 ml/min, the dosage of clarithromycin should be reduced to one half of the normal recommended dose.

Recommended administration: Klaricid IV should be administered into one of the larger proximal veins as an IV infusion over 60 minutes, using a solution concentration of about 2 mg/ml. Clarithromycin should not be given as a bolus or an intramuscular injection.

Preparation of the solution for intravenous administration

Step 1: Inject 10 ml Sterilised Water for Injections into the vial and shake to dissolve the contents. Do not use diluents containing preservatives or inorganic salts. Each ml of reconstituted solution contains 50 mg clarithromycin. Use within 24 hours. Can be stored from 5°C up to room temperature (25°C).

Step 2: Add the reconstituted product (500 mg in 10 ml Water for Injections) to 250 ml of one of the following diluents before administration: 5% dextrose in Lactated Ringer's solution, 5% dextrose, Lactated Ringer's, 5% dextrose in 0.3% sodium chloride, Normosol-M in 5% dextrose, Normosol-R in 5% dextrose, 5% dextrose in 0.45% sodium chloride, or 0.9% sodium chloride.

The final diluted product (concentration about 2 mg/ml) should be used within 6 hours if stored at room temperature (25°C), or within 24 hours if stored at 5°C.

Compatibility with other IV additives has not been established.

Contra-indications, warnings, etc

Contra-indications: Klaricid IV is contra-indicated in patients with known hypersensitivity to macrolide antibiotic drugs.

Klaricid and ergot derivatives should not be co-administered.

Concomitant administration of clarithromycin and any of the following drugs is contra-indicated: cisapride, pimozide and terfenadine. Elevated cisapride, pimozide and terfenadine levels have been reported in patients receiving either of these drugs and clarithromycin concomitantly. This may result in QT prolongation and cardiac arrhythmias including ventricular fibrillation and Torsade de Pointes. Similar effects have been observed with concomitant administration of astemizole and other macrolides.

Precautions: Clarithromycin is principally excreted by the liver and kidney. Caution should be exercised in administering this antibiotic to patients with impaired hepatic and renal function.

Prolonged or repeated use of clarithromycin may result in an overgrowth of non-susceptible bacteria or fungi. If super-infection occurs, clarithromycin should be discontinued and appropriate therapy instituted.

Interactions: Clarithromycin has been shown not to interact with oral contraceptives.

As with other macrolide antibiotics, the use of clarithromycin in patients concurrently taking drugs metabolised by the cytochrome p450 system (e.g. warfarin, ergot alkaloids, triazolam, midazolam, disopyramide, lovastatin, rifabutin, phenytoin and cyclosporin) may be associated with elevations in serum levels of these other drugs. Rhabdomyolysis, co-incident with the co-administration of clarithromycin, and HMG-CoA reductase inhibitors, such as lovastatin and simvastatin has been reported.

The administration of Klaricid to patients who are receiving theophylline has been associated with an increase of serum theophylline levels and potential theophylline toxicity.

The use of Klaricid in patients receiving warfarin may result in a potentiation of the effects of warfarin. Prothrombin time should be frequently monitored in these patients. The effects of digoxin may be potentiated with concomitant administration of Klaricid. Monitoring of serum digoxin levels should be considered.

Klaricid may potentiate the effects of carbamazepine due to a reduction in the rate of excretion.

Simultaneous oral administration of clarithromycin tablets and zidovudine to HIV-infected adult patients may result in decreased steady-state zidovudine concentrations. Since this interaction in adults is thought to be due to interference of clarithromycin with simultaneously administered oral zidovudine, this interaction should not be a problem when clarithromycin is administered intravenously.

With oral clarithromycin, the interaction can be largely avoided by staggering doses; see SPC for Klaricid tablets for further information.

No similar reaction has been reported in children.

Ritonavir increases the area under the curve (AUC), C_{max} and C_{min} of clarithromycin when administered concurrently. Because of the large therapeutic window for clarithromycin, no dosage reduction should be necessary in patients with normal renal function. However, for patients with renal impairment, the following dosage adjustments should be considered: For patients with CL_{CR} 30 to 60 ml/min the dose of clarithromycin should be decreased by 50%. For patients with CL_{CR} <30 ml/min the dose of clarithromycin should be decreased by 75%. Doses of clarithromycin greater than 1 g/day should not be coadministered with ritonavir.

Other undesirable effects: The most frequently reported infusion-related adverse events in clinical studies were injection-site inflammation, tenderness, phlebitis and pain. The most common non-infusion-related adverse event reported was taste perversion.

During clinical studies with *oral* Klaricid, the drug was generally well tolerated. Side-effects included nausea, vomiting, diarrhoea, dyspepsia and abdominal pain. Stomatitis, glossitis and oral monilia have been reported. Other side-effects include headache, tooth and tongue discolouration, arthralgia, myalgia and allergic reactions ranging from urticaria and mild skin eruptions and angioedema to anaphylaxis and rarely, Stevens-Johnson syndrome. Reports of alteration of the sense of smell, usually in conjunction with taste perversion has also been received. There have been transient reports of increased central nervous system side-effects including dizziness, vertigo, anxiety, insomnia, bad dreams, tinnitus, confusion, disorientation, hallucinations, psychosis and depersonalisation. There have been reports of hearing loss with clarithromycin which is usually reversible upon withdrawal of therapy.

Pseudomembranous colitis has been reported rarely with clarithromycin and may range in severity from mild to life threatening.

There have been reports of hypoglycaemia, some of which have occurred in pateints on concomitant oral hypoglycaemic agents or insulin. Isolated cases of thrombocytopenia have been reported.

As with other macrolides, hepatic dysfunction (which is usually reversible) including altered liver function tests, hepatitis and cholestasis with or without jaundice, has been reported. Dysfunction may be severe and very rarely fatal hepatic failure has been reported.

Cases of increased serum creatinine, interstitial nephritis and renal failure have been reported rarely.

As with other macrolides, QT prolongation, ventricular tachycardia and Torsade de Pointes have been rarely reported with clarithromycin.

Use in pregnancy and lactating women: The safety of clarithromycin during pregnancy and breast feeding of infants has not been established. Some animal studies have suggested an embryotoxic effect but only at dose levels which are clearly toxic to mothers. Therefore, if a patient of post-pubertal age becomes pregnant, clarithromycin should not be used during pregnancy or lactation unless the benefit is considered to outweigh the risk. Clarithromycin has been found in the milk of lactating animals and in human breast milk.

Overdosage: There is no experience of overdosage after I.V. administration of clarithromycin. However, reports indicate that the ingestion of large amounts of clarithromycin orally can be expected to produce gastro-intestinal symptoms. Allergic reactions accompanying overdosage should be treated by gastric lavage and supportive measures.

As with other macrolides, clarithromycin serum levels are not expected to be appreciably affected by haemodialysis or peritoneal dialysis.

One patient who had a history of bipolar disorder ingested 8 grams of clarithromycin and showed altered mental status, paranoid behaviour, hypokalaemia and hypoxaemia.

Pharmaceutical precautions Store at up to 30°C and protect from light.

Legal category POM.

Package quantities Packs of 1.

Further information Nil.

Product licence number 0037/0251.

KLARICID* PAEDIATRIC SUSPENSION

Qualitative and quantitative composition Clarithromycin 125 mg/5 ml.

Pharmaceutical form White to off-white granules for reconstitution.

Clinical particulars

Therapeutic indications: Klaricid Paediatric Suspension is indicated for the treatment of infections caused by susceptible organisms. Indications include: Lower respiratory tract infections; upper respiratory tract infections; skin and skin structure infections; acute otitis media.

Klaricid Paediatric Suspension is usually active against the following organisms *in vitro*:

Gram-positive bacteria: *Staphylococcus aureus* (methicillin susceptible); *Streptococcus pyogenes* (Group A beta-haemolytic streptococci); alpha-haemolytic streptococci (viridans group); *Streptococcus (Diplococcus) pneumoniae; Streptococcus agalactiae; Listeria monocytogenes.*

Gram-negative bacteria: *Haemophilus influenzae, Haemophilus parainfluenzae, Moraxella (Branhamella) catarrhalis, Neisseria gonorrhoeae; Legionella pneumophila, Bordetella pertussis, Helicobacter pylori; Campylobacter jejuni.*

Mycoplasma: *Mycoplasma pneumoniae; Ureaplasma urealyticum.*

Other organisms: Chlamydia trachomatis; Mycobacterium avium; Mycobacterium leprae; Chlamydia pneumoniae.

Anaerobes: Macrolide-susceptible *Bacteroides fragilis; Clostridium perfringens; Peptococcus* species; *Peptostreptococcus* species; *Propionibacterium acnes.*

Klaricid Paediatric Suspension has bactericidal activity against several bacterial strains. These organisms include *H. influenzae, Streptococcus pneumoniae, Streptococcus pyogenes, Streptococcus agalactiae, Moraxella (Branhamella) catarrhalis, Neisseria gonorrhoeae, Helicobacter pylori* and *Campylobacter* species.

The activity of clarithromycin against *H. pylori* is greater at neutral pH than at acid pH.

Posology and method of administration: Recommended doses and dosage schedules: The usual duration of treatment is for 5 to 10 days depending on the pathogen involved and the severity of the condition. The recommended daily dosage of Klaricid Paediatric Suspension in children is given in the following table and is based on a 7.5 mg/kg b.i.d. regime. Doses up to 500 mg b.i.d. have been used in the treatment of severe infection.

Klaricid Paediatric Suspension dosage in children

Dosage based on body weight (kg)			
Weight (kg)*	*Approx. age (yrs)*	*Dosage (ml) bid*	*Dosage per 5 ml teaspoonful twice daily*
8–11	1–2	2.5	½
12–19	3–6	5	1
20–29	7–9	7.5	1½
30–40	10–12	10	2

* Children <8 kg should be dosed on a per kg basis (approx. 7.5 mg/kg bid)

Preparation for use:

140 ml bottle: 74 ml of water should be added to the granules in the bottle and shaken to yield 140 ml of reconstituted suspension. The concentration of clarithromycin in the reconstituted suspension is 125 mg per 5 ml.

100 ml bottle: 53 ml of water should be added to the granules in the bottle and shaken to yield 100 ml of reconstituted suspension. The concentration of clarithromycin in the reconstituted suspension is 125 mg per 5 ml.

70 ml bottle: 37 ml of water should be added to the granules in the bottle and shaken to yield 70 ml of reconstituted suspension. The concentration of clarithromycin in the reconstituted suspension is 125 mg per 5 ml.

50 ml bottle: 27 ml of water should be added to the granules in the bottle and shaken to yield 50 ml of reconstituted suspension. The concentration of clarithromycin in the reconstituted suspension is 125 mg per 5 ml.

Sachet: After cutting along the dotted line, empty contents of sachet into a glass, half fill the sachet with cold water. Add to glass and stir thoroughly before taking.

Contra-indications: Klaricid Paediatric Suspension is contra-indicated in patients with known hypersensitivity to macrolide antibiotic drugs and other ingredients.

Klaricid Paediatric Suspension and ergot derivatives should not be co-administered.

Concomitant administration of clarithromycin and any of the following drugs is contra-indicated: cisapride, pimozide and terfenadine. Elevated cisapride, pimozide and terfenadine levels have been reported in patients receiving either of these drugs and clarithromycin concomitantly. This may result in QT prolongation and cardiac arrhythmias including ventricular tachycardia, ventricular fibrillation and Torsade de Pointes. Similar effects have been observed with concomitant administration of astemizole and other macrolides.

Special warnings and special precautions for use: Clarithromycin is principally excreted by the liver and kidneys. This antibiotic should not be administered to paediatric patients with hepatic or renal failure.

Prolonged or repeated use of clarithromycin may result in an overgrowth of non-susceptible bacteria or fungi. If super-infection occurs, clarithromycin should be discontinued and appropriate therapy instituted.

Interaction with other medicaments and other forms of interaction As with other macrolide antibiotics, the use of clarithromycin in patients concurrently taking drugs metabolized by the cytochrome P450 system (e.g. warfarin, ergot alkaloids, triazolam, midazolam, disopyramide, lovastatin, rifabutin, phenytoin and cyclosporin) may be associated with elevations in serum levels of these other drugs. Rhabdomyolysis, co-incident with the co-administration of clarithromycin, and HMG-CoA reductase inhibitors, such as lovastatin and simvastatin has been reported.

The administration of clarithromycin to patients who are receiving theophylline has been associated with an increase of serum theophylline levels and potential theophylline toxicity.

The use of Klaricid Paediatric Suspension in patients receiving digoxin, warfarin and carbamazepine may result in potentiation of their effects due to a reduction in the rate of excretion. Prothrombin time should be frequently monitored in patients receiving warfarin. Monitoring of serum digoxin levels should be considered.

Ritonavir increases the AUC (area under the curve), of clarithromycin when administered concurrently. Because of the large therapeutic window for clarithromycin, no dosage reduction should be necessary in patients with normal renal function. However, for patients with renal impairment, the following dosage adjustments should be considered: For patients with CL_{CR} 30 to 60 ml/min the dose of clarithromycin should be reduced by 50%. For patients with CL_{CR} <30 ml/min the dose of clarithromycin should be decreased by 75%. Doses of clarithromycin greater than 1 g/day should not be coadministered with ritonavir.

Simultaneous oral administration of clarithromycin tablets and zidovudine to HIV-infected adult patients may result in decreased steady-state zidovudine levels. To date, this interaction does not appear to occur in paediatric HIV-infected patients taking Klaricid Paediatric Suspension with zidovudine or dideoxyinosine.

Pregnancy and lactation: The safety of clarithromycin during pregnancy and breast feeding of infants has not been established. Some animal studies have suggested an embryotoxic effect, but only at dose levels which are clearly toxic to mothers. Therefore, if a patient of post-pubertal age becomes pregnant, clarithromycin should not be used during pregnancy or lactation unless the benefit outweighs the risk. Clarithromycin has been found in the milk of lactating animals and in human breast milk.

Effects on ability to drive and use machines: None known.

Undesirable effects: Clarithromycin is generally well tolerated. Side-effects reported include nausea, dyspepsia, diarrhoea, vomiting and abdominal pain. Stomatitis, glossitis, oral monilia and tongue discolouration have been reported. Other side-effects include headache, arthralgia, myalgia and allergic reactions ranging from urticaria, mild skin eruptions and angioedema to anaphylaxis and rarely, Stevens-Johnson syndrome. Reports of alteration of the sense of smell, usually in conjunction with taste perversion have also been received. There have been reports of tooth discolouration in patients treated with clarithromycin. Tooth discolouration is usually reversible with professional dental cleaning. There have been reports of transient central nervous system side-effects including dizziness, vertigo, anxiety, insomnia, bad dreams, tinnitus, confusion, disorientation, hallucinations, psychosis and depersonalisation. There have been reports of hearing loss with clarithromycin which is usually reversible upon withdrawal of therapy. Pseudomembranous colitis has been reported rarely with clarithromycin and may range in severity from mild to life threatening. There have been rare reports of hypoglycaemia, some of which have occurred in patients on concomitant oral hypoglycaemic agents or insulin. As with other macrolides, hepatic dysfunction (which is usually reversible) including altered liver function tests, hepatitis and cholestasis with or without jaundice has been reported. Dysfunction may be severe, and very rarely, fatal hepatic failure has been reported.

Cases of increased serum creatinine, interstitial nephritis and renal failure have been reported rarely.

As with other macrolides, QT prolongation, ventricular tachycardia and torsade de pointes have been rarely reported with clarithromycin.

Overdosage: Reports indicate that the ingestion of large amounts of clarithromycin can be expected to produce gastro-intestinal symptoms. Allergic reactions accompanying overdosage should be treated by gastric lavage and supportive measures. One patient who had a history of bipolar disorder ingested 8 grams of clarithromycin and showed altered mental status, paranoid behaviour, hypokalaemia and hypoxemia.

Pharmacological properties

Microbiology: Clarithromycin is a semi-synthetic derivative of erythromycin A. It exerts its anti-bacterial action by binding to the 50s ribosomal sub-unit of susceptible bacteria and suppresses protein synthesis. Clarithromycin demonstrates excellent *in-vitro* activity against standard strains of clinical isolates. It is highly potent against a wide variety of aerobic and anaerobic gram-positive and gram-negative organisms. The minimum inhibitory concentrations (MICs) of clarithromycin are generally two-fold lower than the MICs of erythromycin.

The 14-(R)-hydroxy metabolite of clarithromycin formed in man by first pass metabolism also has antimicrobial activity. The MICs of this metabolite are equal or two-fold higher than the MICs of the parent compound, except for *H. influenzae* where the 14-hydroxy metabolite is two-fold more active than the parent compound. Clarithromycin is also bactericidal against several bacterial strains.

Clarithromycin is usually active against the following organisms *in vitro*: Gram-positive bacteria: *Staphylococcus aureus* (methicillin susceptible); *Streptococcus pyogenes* (Group A beta-haemolytic streptococci); alpha-haemolytic streptococci (viridans group); *Streptococcus (Diplococcus) pneumoniae; Streptococcus agalactiae; Listeria monocytogenes.*

Gram-negative bacteria: *Haemophilus influenzae, Haemophilus parainfluenzae, Moraxella (Branhamella) catarrhalis, Neisseria gonorrhoeae; Legionella pneumophila, Bordetella pertussis, Helicobacter pylori; Campylobacter jejuni.*

Mycoplasma: *Mycoplasma pneumoniae; Ureaplasma urealyticum.*

Other organisms: *Chlamydia trachomatis; Mycobacterium avium; Mycobacterium leprae; Chlamydia pneumoniae.*

Anaerobes: Macrolide-susceptible *Bacteroides fragilis; Clostridium perfringens; Peptococcus* species; *Peptostreptococcus* species; *Propionibacterium acnes.*

Clarithromycin also has bactericidal activity against several bacterial strains. These organisms include *H. influenzae, Streptococcus pneumoniae, Streptococcus pyogenes, Streptococcus agalactiae, Moraxella (Branhamella) catarrhalis, Neisseria gonorrhoeae, Helicobacter pylori* and *Campylobacter* species.

Pharmacokinetics: Clarithromycin is rapidly and well absorbed from the gastro-intestinal tract after oral administration. The microbiologically active 14(R)-hydroxyclarithromycin is formed by first pass metabolism. Clarithromycin, may be given without regard to meals as food does not affect the extent of bioavailability. Food does slightly delay the onset of absorption of clarithromycin and formation of the 14-hydroxy metabolite. Although the pharmacokinetics of clarithromycin are non linear, steady state is attained within 2 days of dosing. 14-Hydroxyclarithromycin is the major urinary metabolite and accounts for 10–15% of the dose. Most of the remainder of the dose is eliminated in the faeces, primarily via the bile. 5–10% of the parent drug is recovered from the faeces.

Clarithromycin provides tissue concentrations that are several times higher than circulating drug level. Increased levels of clarithromycin have been found in both tonsillar and lung tissue. Clarithromycin penetrates into the middle ear fluid at concentrations greater than in the serum. Clarithromycin is 80% bound to plasma proteins at therapeutic levels.

Klaricid Paediatric Suspension does not contain tartrazine or other azo dyes, lactose or gluten.

Preclinical safety data: The acute oral LD_{50} values for a clarithromycin suspension administered to 3-day old mice were 1290 mg/kg for males and 1230 mg/kg for females. The LD_{50} values in 3-day old rats were 1330 mg/kg for males and 1270 mg/kg for females. For comparison, the LD_{50} of orally-administered clarithromycin is about 2700 mg/kg for adult mice and about 3000 mg/kg for adult rats. These results are consistent with other antibiotics of the penicillin group, cephalosporin group and macrolide group in that the LD_{50} is generally lower in juvenile animals than in adults.

In both mice and rats, body weight was reduced or its increase suppressed and suckling behaviour and spontaneous movements were depressed for the first few days following drug administration. Necropsy of animals that died disclosed dark-reddish lungs in mice and about 25% of the rats; rats treated with 2197 mg/kg or more of a clarithromycin suspension were also noted to have a reddish-black substance in the intestines, probably because of bleeding. Deaths of these animals were considered due to debilitation resulting from depressed suckling behaviour or bleeding from the intestines.

Pre-weaning rats (5 days old) were administered a clarithromycin suspension formulation for two weeks at doses of 0, 15, 55 and 200 mg/kg/day. Animals from the 200 mg/kg/day group had decreased body-weight gains, decreased mean haemoglobin and haematocrit values, and increased mean relative kidney weights compared to animals from the control group. Treatment-related minimal to mild multifocal vacuolar degeneration of the intrahepatic bile duct epithelium and an increased incidence of nephritic lesions were also observed in animals from this treatment group. The 'no-toxic effect' dosage for this study was 55 mg/kg/day.

An oral toxicity study was conducted in which immature rats were administered a clarithromycin suspension (granules for suspension) for 6 weeks at daily dosages of 0, 15, 50 and 150 mg base/kg/day. No deaths occurred and the only clinical sign observed was excessive salivation for some of the animals at the highest dosage from 1 to 2 hours after administration during the last 3 weeks of treatment. Rats from the 150 mg/kg dose group had lower mean body weights during the first three weeks, and were observed to have decreased mean serum albumin values and increased mean relative liver weight compared to the controls. No treatment-related gross or microscopic histopathological changes were found. A dosage of 150 mg/kg/day produced slight toxicity in the treated rats and the 'no effect dosage' was considered to be 50 mg/kg/day.

Juvenile beagle dogs, 3 weeks of age, were treated orally daily for four weeks with 0, 30, 100, or 300 mg/kg of clarithromycin, followed by a 4-week recovery period. No deaths occurred and no change in the general condition of the animals were observed. Necropsy revealed no abnormalities. Upon histological examination, fatty deposition of centrilobular hepatocytes and cell infiltration of portal areas were observed by light microscopy and an increase in hepatocellular fat droplets was noted by electron microscopy in the 300 mg/kg dose group. The toxic dose in juvenile beagle dogs was considered to be greater than 300 mg/kg and the 'no effect dose' 100 mg/kg.

Fertility, reproduction and teratogenicity: Fertility and reproduction studies have shown daily dosages of 150–160 mg/kg/day to male and female rats caused no adverse effects on the oestrus cycle, fertility, parturition and number and viability of offspring. Two teratogenicity studies in both Wistar (p.o.) and Sprague-Dawley (p.o. and i.v.) rats, one study in New Zealand white rabbits and one study in cynomolgus monkeys failed to demonstrate any teratogenicity from clarithromycin.

Pharmaceutical particulars

List of excipients: Carbopol 974P, povidone K90, water purified, hydroxypropylmethylcellulose phthalate (HP-55), castor oil, acetone, ethanol, silicon dioxide, sucrose, xanthan gum, flavour – fruit punch, potassium sorbate, citric acid, titanium dioxide and maltodextrin.

Incompatibilities: None known.

Shelf life: bottles: The recommended shelf life is 24 months stored at room temperature at 15–30°C. Once reconstituted, Klaricid Paediatric Suspension should be used within 14 days.

Sachets: The recommended shelf life is 18 months stored at room temperature (15° to 30°C).

Special precautions for storage: None stated.

Nature and contents of container: Granules for reconstitution in a HDPE bottle. Pack sizes of 50, 70, 100 and 140 ml.

Granules for reconstitution in paper/LDPE/Al foil/LDPE sachet. Packs of 2 sachets.

Instructions for use/handling: Not applicable.

Marketing authorisation number 0037/0264.

Date of approval/revision of SPC September 1998.

Legal category POM.

KLARICID* XL

Qualitative and quantitative composition Clarithromycin 500 mg per tablet.

Pharmaceutical form A yellow, ovaloid tablet containing 500 mg of clarithromycin in a modified-release preparation.

Clinical particulars

Therapeutic indications: Klaricid XL is indicated for treatment of infections caused by susceptible organisms. Indications include:

Lower respiratory tract infections for example, acute and chronic bronchitis, and pneumonia.

Upper respiratory tract infections for example, sinusitis and pharyngitis.

Klaricid XL is also indicated in skin and soft tissue infections of mild to moderate severity, for example folliculitis, cellulitis and erysipelas.

Posology and method of administration:

Adults: The usual recommended dosage of Klaricid XL in adults is one 500 mg modified-release tablet daily to be taken with food. In more severe infections, the dosage can be increased to two 500 mg modified-release tablets daily. The usual duration of treatment is 7 to 14 days.

Children older than 12 years: As for adults.

Children younger than 12 years: Use Klaricid Paediatric Suspension.

Klaricid XL should not be used in patients with renal impairment (creatinine clearance less than 30 ml/min). Klaricid immediate release tablets may be used in this patient population (see *Contra-indications*).

Contra-indications: Clarithromycin is contra-indicated in patients with known hypersensitivity to macrolide antibiotic drugs.

Clarithromycin and ergot derivates should not be co-administered.

As the dose cannot be reduced from 500 mg daily, Klaricid XL is contra-indicated in patients with creatinine clearance less than 30 ml/min.

Concomitant administration of clarithromycin and any of the following drugs is contra-indicated: cisapride, pimozide and terfenadine. Elevated cisapride, pimozide and terfenadine levels have been reported in patients receiving either of these drugs and clarithromycin concomitantly. This may result in QT prolongation and cardiac arrhythmias including ventricular tachycardia, ventricular fibrillation and torsade de pointes. Similar effects have been observed with concomitant administration of astemizole and other macrolides.

Special warnings and special precautions for use: Clarithromycin is principally excreted by the liver and kidney. Caution should be exercised in administering this antibiotic to patients with impaired hepatic or renal function.

Prolonged or repeated use of clarithromycin may result in an overgrowth of non-susceptible bacteria or fungi. If super-infection occurs, clarithromycin should be discontinued and appropriate therapy instituted.

Interaction with other medicaments and other forms of interaction: Clarithromycin has been shown not to interact with oral contraceptives.

As with other macrolide antibiotics the use of clarithromycin in patients concurrently taking drugs metabolised by the cytochrome P450 system (e.g. warfarin, ergot alkaloids, triazolam, midazolam, disopyramide, rifabutin, lovastatin, phenytoin and cyclosporin) may be associated with elevations in serum levels of these other drugs. Rhabdomyolysis, coincident with the co-administration of clarithromycin, and HMG-CoA reductase inhibitors, such as lovastatin and simvastatin has been reported.

The administration of clarithromycin to patients who are receiving theophylline has been associated with an increase in serum theophylline levels and potential theophylline toxicity.

The use of clarithromycin in patients receiving warfarin may result in potentiation of the effects of warfarin. Prothrombin time should be frequently monitored in these patients.

The effects of digoxin may be potentiated with concomitant administration of clarithromycin. Monitoring of serum digoxin levels should be considered.

Clarithromycin may potentiate the effects of carbamazepine due to a reduction in the rate of excretion.

Interaction studies have not been conducted with Klaricid XL and zidovudine. If concomitant administration of clarithromycin and zidovudine is required, then an immediate release formulation of clarithromycin should be used.

Ritonavir increases the area under the curve (AUC), C_{max} and C_{min} of clarithromycin when administered concurrently. Because of the large therapeutic window for clarithromycin, no dosage reduction should be necessary in patients with normal renal function. However, for patients with renal impairment an immediate release form of clarithromycin should be used. Doses of clarithromycin greater than 1 g/day should not be coadministered with ritonavir.

Pregnancy and lactation: The safety of clarithromycin during pregnancy and breast feeding of infants has not been established. Clarithromycin should thus not be used during pregnancy or lactation unless the benefit is considered to outweigh the risk. Some animal studies have suggested an embryotoxic effect, but only at dose levels which are clearly toxic to mothers. Clarithromycin has been found in milk of lactating animals and in human breast milk.

Effects on ability to drive and use machines: The medicine is unlikely to produce an effect.

Undesirable effects: Clarithromycin is generally well tolerated. Side effects reported include nausea, dyspepsia, diarrhoea, vomiting and abdominal pain. Stomatitis, glossitis, oral monilia and tongue discolouration have been reported. Other side-effects include headache, arthralgia, myalgia and allergic reactions ranging from urticaria, mild skin eruptions and angioedema to anaphylaxis and rarely Stevens-Johnson syndrome. Reports of alteration of the sense of smell, usually in conjunction with taste perversion have also been received. There have been reports of tooth discolouration in patients treated with clarithromycin. Tooth discolouration is usually reversible with professional dental cleaning. There have been reports of transient central nervous system side-effects including dizziness, vertigo, anxiety, insomnia, bad dreams, tinnitus, confusion, disorientation, hallucinations, psychosis and depersonalisation. There have been reports of hearing loss with clarithromycin which is usually reversible on withdrawal of therapy. Pseudomembranous colitis has been reported rarely with clarithromycin, and may range in severity from mild to life threatening. There have been rare reports of hypoglycaemia, some of which have occurred in patients on concomitant oral hypoglycaemic agents or insulin. Isolated cases of thrombocytopenia have been reported.

As with other macrolides, hepatic dysfunction (which is usually reversible) including altered liver function tests, hepatitis and cholestasis with or without jaundice, has been reported. Dysfunction may be severe and very rarely fatal hepatic failure has been reported. Cases of increased serum creatinine, interstitial nephritis and renal failure have been reported rarely. As with other macrolides, QT prolongation, ventricular tachycardia and Torsade de Pointes have been rarely reported with clarithromycin.

Overdosage: Reports indicate that the ingestion of large amounts of clarithromycin can be expected to produce gastro-intestinal symptoms. One patient who had a history of bipolar disorder ingested 8 g of clarithromycin and showed altered mental status, paranoid behaviour, hypokalaemia and hypoxaemia. Allergic reactions accompanying overdosage should be treated by gastric lavage and supportive measures. As with other macrolides, clarithromycin serum levels are not expected to be appreciably affected by haemodialysis or peritoneal dialysis.

Pharmaceutical properties

Microbiology: Clarithromycin is a semi-synthetic derivative of erythromycin A. It exerts its antibacterial action by binding to the 50s ribosomal sub-unit of susceptible bacteria and suppresses protein synthesis. It is highly potent against a wide variety of aerobic and anaerobic gram-positive and gram-negative organisms. The minimum inhibitory concentrations (MICs) of clarithromycin are generally two-fold lower than the MICs of erythromycin.

The 14-hydroxy metabolite of clarithromycin also has antimicrobial activity. The MICs of this metabolite are equal or two-fold higher than the MICs of the parent compound, except for *H influenzae* where the 14-hydroxy metabolite is two-fold more active than the parent compound.

Clarithromycin is usually active against the following organisms *in vitro*:

Gram-positive bacteria: Staphylococcus aureus (methicillin susceptible); *Streptococcus pyogenes* (Group A beta-hemolytic streptococci); alpha-hemolytic streptococci (viridans group); *Streptococcus (Diplococcus) pneumoniae; Streptococcus agalactiae; Listeria monocytogenes.*

Gram-negative bacteria: Haemophilus influenza; Haemophilus parainfluenza; Moraxella (Branhamella) catarrhalis; Neisseria gonorrhoeae; Legionella pneumophila; Bordetella pertussis; Campylobacter jejuni.

Mycoplasma: Mycoplasma pneumoniae; Ureaplasma urealyticum.

Other organisms: Chlamydia trachomatis; Mycobacterium avium; Mycobacterium leprae; Mycobacterium kansasaii; Mycobacterium chelonae; Mycobacterium fortuitum; Mycobacterium intracellularis; Chlamydia pneumoniae.

Anaerobes: Clostridium perfringens; Peptococcus species; *Peptostreptococcus* species; *Propionibacterium* acnes.

Clarithromycin has bactericidal activity against several bacterial strains. The organisms include *Haemophilus influenzae, Streptococcus pneumoniae, Streptococcus pyogenes, Streptococcus agalactiae, Moraxella (Branhamella) catarrhalis, Neisseria gonorrhoeae* and *Campylobacter* spp.

Pharmacokinetics: The kinetics of orally administered modified-release clarithromycin have been studied in adult humans and compared with clarithromycin 250 mg and 500 mg immediate release tablets. The extent of absorption was found to be equivalent when equal total daily doses were administered. The absolute bioavailability is approximately 50%. Little or no unpredicted accumulation was found and the metabolic disposition did not change in any species following multiple dosing. Based upon the finding of equivalent absorption the following *in vitro* and *in vivo* data are applicable to the modified-release formulation.

In vitro: Results of *in vitro* studies showed that the protein binding of clarithromycin in human plasma averaged about 70% at concentrations of 0.45–4.5 mcg/ml. A decrease in binding to 41% at 45.0 mcg/ml suggested that the binding sites might become saturated, but this only occurred at concentrations far in excess of therapeutic drug levels.

In vivo: Clarithromycin levels in all tissues, except the central nervous system, were several times higher than the circulating drug levels. The highest concentrations were found in the liver and lung tissue, where the tissue to plasma ratios reached 10 to 20.

The pharmacokinetic behaviour of clarithromycin is non-linear. In fed patients given 500 mg clarithromycin modified-release daily, the peak steady state plasma concentration of clarithromycin and 14 hydroxy clarithromycin were 1.3 and 0.48 mcg/ml, respectively. When the dosage was increased to 1000 mg daily, these steady-state values were 2.4 mcg/ml and 0.67 mcg/ml respectively. Elimination half-lives of the parent drug and metabolite were approximately 5.3 and 7.7 hours respectively. The apparent half-lives of both clarithromycin and its hydroxylated metabolite tended to be longer at higher doses.

Urinary excretion accounted for approximately 40% of the clarithromycin dose. Faecal elimination accounts for approximately 30%.

Preclinical safety data: In repeated dose studies, clarithromycin toxicity was related to dose and duration of treatment. The primary target organ was the liver in all species, with hepatic lesions seen after 14 days in dogs and monkeys. Systemic exposure levels associated with this toxicity are not known but toxic mg/kg doses were higher than the dose recommended for patient treatment.

No evidence of mutagenic potential of clarithromycin was seen during a range of *in vitro* and *in vivo* tests.

Fertility and reproduction studies in rats have shown no adverse effects. Teratogenicity studies in rats (Wistar (p.o.) and Sprague-Dawley (p.o. and i.v.)), New Zealand White rabbits and cynomolgous monkeys failed to demonstrate any teratogenicity from clarithromycin. However, a further similar study in Sprague-Dawley rats indicated a low (6%) incidence of cardiovascular abnormalities which appeared to be due to spontaneous expression of genetic changes. Two mouse studies revealed a variable incidence (3–30%) of cleft palate and in monkeys embryonic loss was seen but only at dose levels which were clearly toxic to the mothers.

No other toxicological findings considered to be of relevance to the dose level recommended for patient treatment have been reported.

Pharmaceutical particulars

List of excipients: Citric acid anhydrous, sodium alginate, sodium calcium alginate, lactose, povidone K30, talc, stearic acid, magnesium stearate, methyl hydroxypropylcellulose 6 cps, polyethylene glycol 400, polyethylene glycol 800, titanium dioxide (E171), sorbic acid, quinoline yellow (dye) aluminium lake (E104).

Incompatibilities: None known.

Shelf life: The shelf life is 18 months when stored in HDPE or glass bottles and in PVC/PVdC blisters.

Special precautions for storage: Store between 15°C and 30°C. Protect from light.

Nature and contents of container: 1, 4, 5, 6, 7 or 14 tablets in a blister original pack or in bottles. The blisters, of PVC/PVdC, are heat sealed with 20 micron hard tempered aluminium foil and packaged in a cardboard carton with a pack insert. The bottles, of HDPE or glass, are packaged in a cardboard carton with a pack insert.

Instructions for use/handling: Not applicable.

Marketing authorisation number 0037/0275.

Date of approval/revision of SPC September 1998.

Legal category POM.

NORVIR* ▼

Qualitative and quantitative composition Norvir oral solution contains 80 mg of ritonavir per ml.

Pharmaceutical form Oral solution.

Clinical particulars

Therapeutic indications: Norvir is indicated in combination with antiretroviral nucleoside analogue(s) for the treatment of HIV-1 infected adult patients with advanced or progressive immunodeficiency.

Clinical endpoint data are only available in patients with advanced HIV-disease. In patients with less advanced HIV-disease only data based on biological markers such as viral load and CD4 cell count are yet available. In these patients studies on the effect of ritonavir on clinical endpoints are ongoing.

See *Pharmacodynamic properties* for the results of the important studies.

Posology and method of administration: Norvir solution is administered orally and should preferably be ingested with food. The recommended dosage of Norvir solution is 600 mg (7.5 ml) twice daily by mouth.

The bitter taste of Norvir solution may be lessened if mixed with chocolate milk.

Paediatric use: The safety and efficacy of ritonavir in children below the age of 12 have not been established.

Renal and hepatic impairment: Currently, there are no data specific to these patient populations and therefore specific dosage recommendations cannot be made. Ritonavir is principally metabolised and eliminated by the liver. Norvir should not be given to patients with severe hepatic insufficiency (see *Contra-indications*). Because ritonavir is highly protein bound it is unlikely that it will be significantly removed by haemodialysis or peritoneal dialysis.

Contra-indications: Patients with known hypersensitivity to ritonavir or any of its excipients. Patients with severe hepatic insufficiency.

In vitro and *in vivo* studies have demonstrated that ritonavir is a potent inhibitor of CYP3A- and CYP2D6-mediated biotransformations. Based primarily on literature review, ritonavir is expected to produce large increases in the plasma concentrations of the following drugs: amiodarone, astemizole, bepridil, bupropion, cisapride, clozapine, dihydroergotamine, encainide, ergotamine, flecainide, meperidine, pimozide, piroxicam, propafenone, propoxyphene, quinidine, and terfenadine. These agents have recognized risks of arrhythmias, hematologic abnormalities, seizures, or other potentially serious adverse effects. Additionally, severe ergotism, characterised by peripheral vasospasm and ischaemia of the extremities, has been associated with co-administration of ritonavir and ergotamine or dihydroergotamine. These drugs should not be co-administered with ritonavir. Ritonavir in addition is likely to produce large increases in these highly metabolized sedatives and hypnotics: clorazepate, diazepam, estazolam, flurazepam, midazolam, triazolam and zolpidem. Due to the potential for extreme sedation and respiratory depression from these agents, they should not be co-administered with ritonavir.

Concomitant use of ritonavir and rifabutin is contra-indicated because of clinical consequences such as uveitis resulting from a multifold increase of rifabutin serum concentrations.

Special warnings and special precautions for use: There are no data on the pharmacokinetics and safety of ritonavir in patients with significant hepatic or renal dysfunction. Ritonavir is principally metabolized and eliminated by the liver. Therefore, caution should be exercised when administering this drug to patients with impaired hepatic function (see *Contra-indications*).

The safety and efficacy of ritonavir in children below the age of 12 have not been established. Therefore, ritonavir should be used in children below the age of 12 only when the potential benefits clearly outweigh the potential risks.

Human pharmacokinetic data for combination of Norvir with antiretroviral drugs other than zidovudine and didanosine (ddI) are not yet available. Although the clinical use of combinations with zalcitabine (ddC) and stavudine (d4T) in a relatively limited number of patients did not seem to be associated with unfavorable effects, the use of combinations of Norvir with other nucleoside analogues should be guided by cautious therapeutic and safety monitoring.

Extra monitoring is recommended when diarrhoea occurs. The relatively high frequency of diarrhoea during treatment with ritonavir may compromise the absorption and efficacy (due to decreased compliance) of ritonavir or other concurrent medications. Serious persistent vomiting and/or diarrhoea associated with ritonavir use might also compromise renal function. It is advisable to monitor renal function in patients with renal function impairment.

A pharmacokinetic study demonstrated that ritonavir extensively inhibits the metabolism of saquinavir resulting in greatly increased saquinavir plasma concentrations (see *Interactions*). Doses greater than 400 mg bid of either drug were associated with an increased incidence of adverse events.

Norvir oral solution contains 43% ethanol, therefore concomitant administration of Norvir with disulfiram or drugs with disulfiram-like reactions (e.g. metronidazole) should be avoided.

There have been reports of increased bleeding, including spontaneous skin haematomas and haemarthroses, in haemophiliac patients type A and B treated with protease inhibitors. In some patients additional factor VIII was given. In more than a half of the reported cases, treatment with protease inhibitors was continued or reintroduced if treatment had been discontinued. A causal relationship has been evoked, although the mechanism of action has not been elucidated. Haemophiliac patients should therefore be made aware of the possibility of increased bleeding.

There may be an increased risk for transaminase elevations in patients with underlying hepatitis B or C, therefore, caution should be exercised when administering ritonavir alone or in combination with other antiretrovirals to patients with pre-existing liver disease, liver enzyme abnormalities, or hepatitis.

New onset diabetes mellitus, hyperglycaemia or exacerbation of existing diabetes mellitus has been reported in patients receiving protease inhibitors. In some of these the hyperglycaemia was severe and in some cases also associated with ketoacidosis. Many patients had confounding medical conditions, some of which required therapy with agents that have been associated with the development of diabetes mellitus of hyperglycaemia.

Interaction with other medicaments and other forms of interaction: Refer also to *Contra-indications.*

Ritonavir has a high affinity for several cytochrome P450 (CYP) isoforms with the following ranked order: CYP3A > CYP2D6 > CYP2C9. In addition to the drugs listed in the *Contra-indications* section, the following drugs or drug classes are known or suspected to be metabolized by these same cytochrome P450 isozymes: immunosuppressants (e.g. cyclosporine, tacrolimus), macrolide antibiotics (e.g. erythromycin), various steroids (e.g. dexamethasone, prednisolone), other HIV-protease inhibitors, nonsedating antihistamines (e.g. loratidine), calcium channel antagonists, several tricyclic antidepressants (e.g. desipramine, imipramine, amitriptyline, nortriptyline), other antidepressants (e.g., fluoxetine, paroxetine, sertraline), neuroleptics (e.g. haloperidol, risperidone, thioridazine), antifungals (e.g. ketoconazole, itraconazole), morphinomimetics (e.g. methadone, fentanyl), carbamazepine, warfarin, tolbutamide. Due to the potential for significant elevation of serum levels of these drugs they should not be used concomitantly with ritonavir without a careful assessment of the potential risks and benefits. Careful monitoring of therapeutic and adverse effects is recommended when these drugs are concomitantly administered with ritonavir.

There are no pharmacokinetic data available on the concomitant use of morphine with ritonavir. On the basis of the metabolism of morphine (glucoronidation) lower levels of morphine may be expected.

Norvir increases the AUCs (area under the curve) of the following drugs when administered concomitantly:

Clarithromycin: because of the large therapeutic window for clarithromycin, no dosage reduction should be necessary in patients with normal renal function. For patients with renal impairment the following dosage adjustment should be considered: for creatinine clearance (CL_{CR}) of 30 to 60 ml/min. the clarithromycin dose should be reduced by 50%, for CL_{CR} < 30 ml/min. the clarithromycin dose should be reduced by 75%. Doses of clarithromycin > 1 g/day should not be coadministered with Norvir.

Desipramine: dosage reduction of desipramine should be considered in patients taking the combination.

Rifabutin and its active metabolite 25-O-desacetyl rifabutin: concomitant use with ritonavir has resulted in a multifold increase in the AUC of rifabutin and its active metabolite 25-O-desacetyl rifabutin with clinical consequences. Therefore, the concomitant use of ritonavir and rifabutin is contraindicated. (see Section 4.3 Contra-indications).

Saquinavir: data from pharmacokinetic studies in patients indicate that co-administration of ritonavir 400 mg twice daily produce multifold increases in saquinavir steady state blood levels (AUC; 17 fold: C_{max}, 14 fold increase). Doses greater than 400 mg bid of either drug were associated with an increased incidence of adverse events.

Norvir decreases the AUCs of the following drugs when administered concomitantly:

Zidovudine (AZT) and ddI: zidovudine and ddI have little if any effect on ritonavir pharmacokinetics. Ritonavir decreased the mean zidovudine AUC by approx. 25% in a study which has not been of sufficient duration to reach steady state for ritonavir. Ritonavir resulted in a reduction of the mean ddI AUC by 13% when given 2.5 hours apart from ritonavir. Dose alteration of AZT or ddI during concomitant Norvir therapy should usually not be necessary. However, dosing of ritonavir and ddI should be separated by 2.5 hours to avoid formulation incompatibilities. Human pharmacokinetic data for combination with antiretroviral drugs other than zidovudine and ddI are not yet available (see also *Special warnings and special precautions for use*).

Ethinyl estradiol: because concomitant administration of ritonavir with a fixed combination oral contraceptive resulted in a reduction of the ethinyl estradiol mean AUC by 41%, increased doses of oral contraceptives containing ethinyl estradiol, or alternate methods of contraception should be considered.

Theophylline: an increased dosage of theophylline may be required, as concomitant use with ritonavir caused an approx. 45 % decrease in the AUC of theophylline.

Fixed combination of sulfamethoxazole/trimethoprim: the concomitant administration of Norvir and sulfamethoxazole/trimethoprim resulted in a 20 % reduction of the sulfamethoxazole AUC and a 20% increase of the trimethoprim AUC. Dose alteration of sulfamethoxazole/trimethoprim during concomitant Norvir therapy should not be necessary.

Because ritonavir is highly protein bound, the possibility of increased therapeutic and toxic effects due to protein binding displacement of concomitant medications should be considered.

Cardiac and neurologic events have been reported when ritonavir has been co-administered with disopyramide, mexiletine, nefazadone, or fluoxetine. The possibility of drug interaction cannot be excluded.

Use during pregnancy and lactation: No treatment-related malformations were observed with ritonavir in either rats or rabbits. Developmental toxicity observed in rats (embryolethality, decreased foetal body weight and ossification delays and visceral changes, including delayed testicular descent) occurred mainly at a maternally toxic dosage. Developmental toxicity in rabbits (embryolethality, decreased litter size and decreased foetal weights) occurred at a maternally toxic dosage. There are no studies in pregnant women. This drug should be used during pregnancy only if the potential benefits clearly outweigh the potential risks.

It is not known whether this drug is excreted in human milk. Milk excretion has not been measured in the animal studies, however a study in rats showed some effects on offspring development during lactation which are compatible with excretion of ritonavir in milk in that species. HIV-infected women should not breast feed their infants under any circumstances to avoid transmission of HIV.

Effects on ability to drive and use machines: Norvir has not specifically been tested for its possible effects on the ability to drive a car or operate machines. As somnolence and dizziness are known undesirable effects, this should be taken into account when driving or using machinery.

Norvir oral solution contains 43% alcohol.

Undesirable effects: In clinical studies (Phase II/III), the following adverse events with possible, probable or unknown relationship to ritonavir have been reported in ≥2% of 1033 patients:

Gastrointestinal: Nausea (47.5%), diarrhea (44.9%), vomiting (23.6%), abdominal pain (11.6%), taste perversion (11.4%); frequently dyspepsia, anorexia, local throat irritation; occasionally flatulence, dry mouth, eructation, mouth ulcer.

Nervous system: circumoral paresthesia (26.6%), peripheral paresthesia (15.4%); frequently dizziness, paresthesia, hyperesthesia, somnolence; occasionally insomnia, anxiety.

Skin: Frequently rash; occasionally pruritus, sweating.

Respiratory system: occasionally pharyngitis, cough increased.

Cardiovascular: Frequently vasodilation.

Others: Asthenia (22.3%), headache (15.5%); occasionally fever, pain, hyperlipemia, myalgia, weight loss, decrease of free and total thyroxine (T_4) values.

Nausea, diarrhoea, vomiting, asthenia, taste perversion, circumoral and peripheral paresthesia, and vasodilatation have been observed most frequently and are felt to be clearly related to ritonavir.

Allergic reactions including urticaria, mild skin eruptions, bronchospasm, and angioedema have been reported. Rare cases of anaphylaxis have been reported

There have been spontaneous reports of seizure. Hyperglycemia has been reported in individuals with and without a known history of diabetes. Cause and effect relationship has not been established.

Dehydration usually associated with gastrointestinal symptoms, and sometimes resulting in hypotension, syncope, or renal insufficiency has been reported. Syncope, orthostatic hypotension and renal insufficiency have also been reported without known dehydration.

Hepatic transaminase elevations exceeding five times the upper limit of normal, clinical hepatitis, and jaundice have occurred in patients receiving ritonavir alone or in combination with other antiretrovirals.

Clinical chemistry: High gamma-glutamyl transpeptidase (GGT) (12%); frequently high creatine phosphokinase (CPK), high triglycerides, high alanine transaminase (SGPT); occasionally high aspartate transaminase (SGOT), high amylase, high uric acid, low potassium, high glucose, low total calcium, high magnesium, high total bilirubin, high alkaline phosphatase.

Hypertriglyceridemia, hypercholesterolemia and hyperuricemia were clearly related to ritonavir therapy.

Hematology: Low white blood cell (WBC) (16%); occasionally low hemoglobin, low neutrophils, high eosinophils, high WBC, high neutrophils, high prothrombin time.

Overdose: Human experience of acute overdose with ritonavir is limited. One patient in clinical trials took ritonavir 1500 mg/day for two days and reported paresthesia which resolved after the dose was decreased. A case of renal failure with eosinophilia has been reported.

The signs of toxicity observed in animals (mice and rats) included decreased activity, ataxia, dyspnea and tremors.

There is no specific antidote for overdose with ritonavir. Treatment of overdose with ritonavir should consist of general supportive measures including monitoring of vital signs and observation of the clinical status of the patient. Due to the solubility characteristics and possibility of transintestinal elimination, it is proposed that management of overdose could entail gastric lavage and administration of activated charcoal. Since ritonavir is extensively metabolized by the liver and is highly protein bound, dialysis is unlikely to be beneficial in significant removal of the drug.

Pharmacological properties

Pharmacodynamic properties: Pharmaco-therapeutic group: antiviral for systemic use. ATC code: JO5A EO3.

Ritonavir is an orally active peptidomimetic inhibitor of the HIV-1 and HIV-2 aspartyl proteases. Inhibition of HIV protease renders the enzyme incapable of processing the *gag-pol* polyprotein precursor which leads to the production of HIV particles with immature morphology that are unable to initiate new rounds of infection. Ritonavir has selective affinity for the HIV protease and has little inhibitory activity against human aspartyl proteases.

In vitro data indicates that ritonavir is active against all strains of HIV tested in a variety of transformed and primary human cell lines. The concentration of drug that inhibits 50% and 90% of viral replication *in vitro* is approximately 0.02 μM and 0.11μM, respectively. Similar potencies were found with both AZT-sensitive and AZT-resistant strains of HIV. Studies which measured direct cell toxicity of ritonavir on several cell lines showed no direct toxicity at concentrations up to 25 μM, with a resulting *in vitro* therapeutic index of at least 1000.

Resistance: Ritonavir-resistant isolates of HIV-1 have been selected *in vitro*. The resistant isolates showed reduced susceptibility to ritonavir and genotypic analysis showed that the resistance was attributable primarily to specific amino acid substitutions in the HIV-1 protease at codons 82 and 84.

Susceptibility of clinical isolates to ritonavir was monitored in controlled clinical trials. Some patients receiving ritonavir monotherapy developed HIV strains with decreased susceptibility to drug. Serial genotypic and phenotypic analysis indicated that susceptibility to ritonavir declined in an ordered and stepwise fashion. Initial mutations occurred at position 82 from wildtype valine to usually alanine or phenylalanine (V82A/F). Viral strains isolated *in vivo* without a change at codon 82 did not have decreased susceptibility to ritonavir.

Cross-resistance to other antiretrovirals: Serial HIV isolates obtained from six patients during ritonavir therapy showed a decrease in ritonavir susceptibility *in vitro* but did not demonstrate a concordant decrease in susceptibility to saquinavir in vitro when compared to matched baseline isolates. However, isolates from two of these patients demonstrated decrease susceptibility to indinavir *in vitro* (8-fold). Cross-resistance between ritonavir and reverse transcriptase inhibitors is unlikely because of the different enzyme targets involved. One ZDV-resistant HIV isolate tested *in vitro* retained full susceptibility to ritonavir.

Clinical pharmacodynamic data: The effects of ritonavir (alone or combined with other antiretroviral agents) on biological markers of disease activity such as CD4 cell count and viral RNA were evaluated in several studies involving HIV-1 infected patients. The following studies are the most important.

A controlled study with ritonavir as add-on therapy in HIV-1 infected patients extensively pre-treated with nucleoside analogues and baseline CD4 cell counts ≤100 cells/μl showed a reduction in mortality and AIDS defining events. The mean average change from baseline over 16 weeks for HIV RNA levels was -0.79 $\log_{10}$ (maximum mean decrease: 1.29 $\log_{10}$) in the ritonavir group vs -0.01 $\log_{10}$ in the control group. The most frequently used nucleosides in this study were zidovudine, stavudine, didanosine and zalcitabine.

In a study recruiting less advanced HIV-1 infected patients (CD4 200-500 cells/μl) without previous antiretroviral therapy, ritonavir in combination with zidovudine or alone reduced viral load in plasma and increased CD4 count. The effects of ritonavir monotherapy seemed unexpectedly to be at least as large as the combination therapy, a finding which has not been explained adequately. The mean average change from baseline over 48 weeks for HIV RNA levels was -0.88 $\log_{10}$ in the ritonavir group vs -0.66 $\log_{10}$ in the ritonavir+zidovudine group vs -0.42 $\log_{10}$ in the zidovudine group. The continuation of ritonavir therapy should be evaluated by viral load because of the possibility of emergence of resistance as described under *Therapeutic indications.*

In an open label trial in 32 antiretroviral naive HIV-1 infected patients the combination of ritonavir with zidovudine and zalcitabine decreased the viral load (mean decrease at week 20 of -1.76 $\log_{10}$).

Studies investigating optimal combinations and the long term efficacy and safety of ritonavir are ongoing.

Pharmacokinetic properties: There is no parenteral formulation of ritonavir, therefore the extent of absorption and absolute bioavailability have not been determined. The pharmacokinetics of ritonavir during multiple dose regimens were studied in non-fasting HIV positive adult volunteers. Upon multiple dosing, ritonavir accumulation is slightly less than predicted from a single dose due to a time and dose-related increase in apparent clearance (Cl/F). Trough concentrations of ritonavir were observed to decrease over time, possibly due to enzyme induction, but appeared to stabilize by the end of 2 weeks. At steady state with a 600 mg bid dose, maximal concentration (Cmax) and trough concentration (Ctrough) values of 11.2 ± 3.6 and 3.7 ± 2.6 µg/ml (mean ± SD) were observed, respectively. The half life (t1/2) of ritonavir was approximately 3 to 5 hours. The steady-state apparent clearance in patients treated with 600 mg bid has averaged 8.8 + 3.2 L/h. Renal clearance averaged less than 0.1 L/h and was relatively constant throughout the dosage range. The time to maximum concentration (Tmax) remained constant at approximately 4 hours with increasing dose.

The pharmacokinetics of ritonavir are dose-dependent: more than proportional increases in the AUC and C_{max} were reported with increasing dose. Ingestion with food results in higher ritonavir exposure than ingestion in the fasted state.

No clinically significant differences in AUC or C_{max} were noted between males and females. Ritonavir pharmacokinetic parameters were not statistically significantly associated with body weight or lean body mass.

The apparent volume of distribution (V_B/F) of ritonavir is approximately 20-40 L after a single 600 mg dose. The protein binding of ritonavir in human plasma was noted to be approximately 98-99%. Ritonavir binds to both human alpha 1-acid glycoprotein (AAG) and human serum albumin (HSA) with comparable affinities. Plasma protein binding is constant over the concentration range of 0.1-100 mg/ml.

Tissue distribution studies with ^{14}C-labeled ritonavir in rats showed the liver, adrenals, pancreas, kidneys and thyroid to have the highest concentrations of drug. Tissue to plasma ratios of approximately 1 measured in rat lymph nodes suggests that ritonavir distributes into lymphatic tissues. Ritonavir penetrates minimally into the brain.

Ritonavir was noted to be extensively metabolized by the hepatic cytochrome P450 system, primarily isozyme CYP3A4 and to a lesser extent CYP2D6. Animal studies as well as *in vitro* experiments with human hepatic microsomes indicated that ritonavir primarily underwent oxidative metabolism. Four ritonavir metabolites have been identified in man. The isopropylthiazole oxidation metabolite (M-2) is the major metabolite and has antiviral activity similar to that of parent drug. However, the AUC of the M-2 metabolite was approximately 3% of the AUC of parent drug.

Human studies with radiolabeled ritonavir demonstrated that the elimination of ritonavir was primarily via the hepatobiliary system; approximately 86% of radiolabel was recovered from stool, part of which is expected to be unabsorbed ritonavir. In these studies renal elimination was not found to be a major route of elimination of ritonavir. This was consistent with the observations in animal studies.

Preclinical safety data: Repeated dose toxicity studies in animals identified major target organs as the liver, retina, thyroid gland and kidney. Hepatic changes involved hepatocellular, biliary and phagocytic elements and were accompanied by increases in hepatic enzymes. Hyperplasia of the retinal pigment epithelium (RPE) and retinal degeneration have been seen in all of the rodent studies conducted with ritonavir, but have not been seen in dogs. Ultrastructural evidence suggests that these retinal changes may be secondary to phospholipidosis. However, clinical trials revealed no evidence of drug-induced ocular changes in humans. All thyroid changes were reversible upon discontinuation of drug. Clinical investigation in humans has revealed no clinically significant alteration in thyroid function tests. Renal changes including tubular degeneration, chronic inflammation and proteinurea were noted in rats and are felt to be attributable to species-specific spontaneous disease. Furthermore, no clinically significant renal abnormalities were noted in clinical trials.

Long-term carcinogenicity studies of ritonavir in animal systems have not been completed. However, ritonavir was not found to be mutagenic or clastogenic in a battery of *in vitro* and *in vivo* assays including the Ames bacterial reverse mutation assay using *S. typhimurium* and *E. coli*, the mouse lymphoma assay, the mouse micronucleus test and chromosomal aberration assays in human lymphocytes.

Pharmaceutical particulars

List of excipients: Norvir oral solution contains: ethanol, purified water, polyoxyl 35 castor oil, propylene glycol, anhydrous citric acid, saccharin sodium, peppermint oil, creamy caramel flavour, and dye E110.

Incompatibilities: Norvir oral solution should not be diluted with water.

Shelf life: 6 months.

Special precautions for storage: Norvir oral solution should be stored at room temperature between 20°-25°C and should be used within 30 days of dispensing. Norvir oral solution should not be refrigerated and should be shaken well before each use. If, after shaking, particles or precipitate can be seen in the solution, the patient should take the next dose and see their doctor about a fresh supply.

Avoid exposure to excessive heat.

Nature and contents of container: Norvir oral solution is supplied in amber coloured multiple-dose polyethylene terephthalate (PET) bottles in a 90 ml size. Each commercial pack contains 5 bottles of 90 ml (450 ml). A dosage cup containing graduations at 3.75 ml (300 mg dose), 5 ml (400 mg dose), 6.25 ml (500 mg dose) and 7.5 ml (600 mg dose) is provided.

Instructions for use/handling: The dosage cup should be cleaned immediately with hot water and dish soap after use. When cleaned immediately, drug residue is removed. The device must be dry prior to use

Marketing authorisation number EU/1/96/016/001

Date of approval/revision of SPC July 1998

Legal category POM

SELSUN* SUSPENSION

Presentation Selsun suspension is presented as a viscous yellow suspension of Selenium Sulphide BP 2.5%.

Uses

Indications: For the treatment of simple dandruff and seborrhoeic dermatitis of the scalp.

Main pharmacological action: Selenium sulphide appears to have a cytostatic effect on cells of the epidermis and follicular epithelium, thus reducing corneocyte production. Selsun acts as an antiseborrhoeic agent which effectively controls itching and scaling dandruff. It has activity against certain dermatophytes including *Pityrosporum orbiculare* the organism causing pityriasis versicolor (tinea versicolor).

Dosage and administration

Adults and the elderly: A liberal application should be made twice a week for the first two weeks and then once a week for the next two weeks to control condition. After this initial course of treatment Selsun should not be used more often than necessary.

Children aged 5–14 years: Treatment as for adults.

Children under 5 years: Not recommended.

Contra-indications, warnings, etc

Contra-indications: Hypersensitivity to any of the ingredients. Do not allow contact with broken or inflamed skin.

Precautions: Gold, silver and other metallic jewellery should be removed prior to use, since discolouration may be caused.

Selsun should be very thoroughly rinsed from the hair before dyeing, tinting or waving the hair. It should not be applied for a period of two days before or after any of these procedures. Contact with eyes should be avoided.

Use in pregnancy: It is not known whether Selsun can cause foetal harm when applied to the body surfaces of a pregnant woman or can affect reproductive capacity. Its effect on the milk of a lactating woman is unknown. As with all medications, avoid during the first 3 months of pregnancy.

Side-effects: Application to skin or scalp may produce irritation or sensitisation, and an increase in the amount of normal hair loss. Discolouration of the hair may occur; this can be avoided or minimised by thorough washing of the hair after treatment.

As with other shampoos, oiliness or dryness of hair and scalp may occur.

Overdosage

Topical application: None known.

Ingestion: Symptoms: Nausea and vomiting. Treatment: Vomiting should be provoked or gastric lavage undertaken. General supportive measures are required. A purgative may be administered to hasten elimination.

Pharmaceutical precautions Do not store above 25°C.

Legal category P.

Package quantities Selsun suspension is available in bottles of 50, 100 and 150 ml.

Further information Nil.

Product licence number 0037/5010R.

SEVOFLURANE ▼

Qualitative and quantitative composition The finished product comprises only the active ingredient sevoflurane.

Pharmaceutical form Sevoflurane is a nonflammable volatile liquid. Sevoflurane is administered via inhalation of the vaporised liquid.

Clinical particulars

Therapeutic indications: Sevoflurane is indicated for induction and maintenance of general anaesthesia in adult and paediatric patients for inpatient and outpatient surgery.

Posology and method of administration: Sevoflurane should be delivered via a vaporiser specifically calibrated for use with sevoflurane so that the concentration delivered can be accurately controlled. MAC (minimum alveolar concentration) values for sevoflurane decrease with age and with the addition of nitrous oxide. The table below indicates average MAC values for different age groups:

Effect of age on MAC of sevoflurane

Age of patient (years)	*Sevoflurane in oxygen*	*Sevoflurane in 65% N_2O/ 35%O_2 **
<3	3.3–2.6%	2.0%
3–<5	2.5%	Not available
5–12	2.4%	Not available
25	2.5%	1.4%
35	2.2%	1.2%
40	2.05%	1.1%
50	1.8%	0.98%
60	1.6%	0.87%
80	1.4%	0.70%

* In paediatric patients 60%N_2O/40%O_2 was used.

Induction: Dosage should be individualised and titrated to the desired effect according to the patient's age and clinical status. A short acting barbiturate or other intravenous induction agent may be administered followed by inhalation of sevoflurane. Induction with sevoflurane may be achieved in oxygen or in combination with oxygen-nitrous oxide mixtures. In adults inspired concentrations of up to 5% sevoflurane usually produce surgical anaesthesia in less than 2 minutes. In children, inspired concentrations of up to 7% sevoflurane usually produce surgical anaesthesia in less than 2 minutes. Alternatively, for induction of anaesthesia in unpremedicated patients, inspired concentrations of up to 8% sevoflurane may be used.

Maintenance: Surgical levels of anaesthesia may be sustained with concentrations of 0.5–3% sevoflurane with or without the concomitant use of nitrous oxide.

Elderly: As with other inhalation agents, lesser concentrations of sevoflurane are normally required to maintain surgical anaesthesia.

Emergence: Emergence times are generally short following sevoflurane anaesthesia. Therefore, patients may require early post operative pain relief.

Contra-indications: Sevoflurane should not be used in patients with known sensitivity to sevoflurane. Sevoflurane is also contraindicated in patients with known or suspected genetic susceptibility to malignant hyperthermia.

Special warnings and special precautions for use: Sevoflurane should be administered only by persons trained in the administration of general anaesthesia. Facilities for maintenance of a patent airway, artificial ventilation, oxygen enrichment and circulatory resuscitation must be immediately available. Sevoflurane should be delivered via a vaporiser specifically calibrated for use with sevoflurane so that the concentration delivered can be accurately controlled. Hypotension and respiratory depression increase as anaesthesia is deepened.

During the maintenance of anaesthesia, increasing the concentration of sevoflurane produces dose-dependent decreases in blood pressure. Excessive decrease in blood pressure may be related to depth of anaesthesia and in such instances may be corrected by decreasing the inspired concentration of sevoflurane. The recovery from general anaesthesia should be assessed carefully before patients are discharged from the recovery room.

Malignant hyperthermia: In susceptible individuals, potent inhalation anaesthetic agents may trigger a skeletal muscle hypermetabolic state leading to high oxygen demand and the clinical syndrome known as malignant hyperthermia. Treatment includes discontinuation of triggering agents (e.g. sevoflurane), administration of intravenous dantrolene sodium, and application of supportive therapy. Renal failure may appear later, and urine flow should be monitored and sustained if possible.

Because of the small number of patients with renal insufficiency (baseline serum creatinine greater than 133 mcmol/l) studied, the safety of Sevoflurane administration in this group has not been fully established. Therefore, Sevoflurane should be used with caution in patients with renal insufficiency.

Sevoflurane produces low levels of Compound A (pentafluoroisopropenyl fluoromethyl ether (PIFE)) and trace amounts of Compound B (pentafluoromethoxy isopropyl fluoromethyl ether (PMFE)), when in direct contact with CO_2 absorbents. Levels of Compound A increase with: increase in canister temperature; increase in anaesthetic concentration; decrease in gas flow rate and increase more with the use of Baralyme rather than soda lime (see also '*Pharmaceutical particulars*').

In some studies in rats, nephrotoxicity was seen in animals exposed to levels of Compound A in excess of those usually seen in routine clinical practice. The mechanism of this renal toxicity in rats is unknown and its relevance to man has not been established (see '*Preclinical safety data*' for further details).

Experience with repeat exposure to sevoflurane is very limited. However, there were no obvious differences in adverse events between first and subsequent exposures.

Interactions with other medicaments and other forms of interaction: The action of non-depolarising muscle relaxants is markedly potentiated with sevoflurane, therefore, when administered with sevoflurane, dosage adjustments of these agents should be made.

Sevoflurane is similar to isoflurane in the sensitisation of the myocardium to the arrhythmogenic effect of exogenously administered adrenaline.

MAC values for sevoflurane decrease with the addition of nitrous oxide as indicated in the table on 'Effect of age on MAC of sevoflurane' (see '*Posology and method of administration*').

As with other agents, lesser concentrations of sevoflurane may be required following use of an intravenous anaesthetic e.g. propofol.

The metabolism of sevoflurane may be increased by known inducers of CYP2E1 (e.g. isoniazid and alcohol) but it is not inducible by barbiturates.

Pregnancy and lactation: With the exception of one study in Caesarean Section, there are no other studies in pregnant women, including in labour and delivery. Experience in Caesarean Section is limited to one trial in a small number of patients.

Reproduction studies have been performed in rats and rabbits at doses up to 1 MAC. No effects on male and female reproductive capabilities were observed. Reduced foetal body weights concomitant with increased skeletal variations were noted in rats only at maternally toxic concentrations. No adverse foetal effects were observed in rabbits. Sevoflurane was not teratogenic.

Therefore, sevoflurane should be used during pregnancy only if clearly needed.

It is not known whether sevoflurane is excreted in human milk therefore caution should be exercised when sevoflurane is administered to a nursing woman.

Effects on ability to drive and use machines: As with other agents, patients should be advised that performance of activities requiring mental alertness, such as operating hazardous machinery, may be impaired for some time after general anaesthesia.

Patients should not be allowed to drive for a suitable period after sevoflurane anaesthesia.

Undesirable effects: As with all potent inhaled anaesthetics, sevoflurane may cause dose-dependent cardio-respiratory depression. Most adverse events are mild to moderate in severity and are transient. Nausea and vomiting are commonly observed in the post-operative period, at a similar incidence to those found with other inhalation anaesthetics. These effects are common sequelae of surgery and general anaesthesia which may be due to the inhalational anaesthetic, other agents administered intra-operatively or post-operatively and to the patient's response to the surgical procedure.

Adverse event data are derived from controlled clinical trials conducted in the United States and Europe in over 3,200 patients. The type, severity and frequency of adverse events in sevoflurane patients were comparable to adverse events in patients treated with other inhalational anaesthetics.

The most frequent adverse events associated with sevoflurane overall were nausea (24%) and vomiting (17%). Agitation occurred frequently in children (23%). Other frequent adverse events (≥10%) associated with sevoflurane administration overall were: increased cough and hypotension.

In addition to nausea and vomiting, other frequent adverse events (≥10%) by age listings were: in adults, hypotension; in elderly, hypotension and bradycardia; in children, agitation and increased cough.

Less frequent adverse events (1–<10% overall) associated with sevoflurane administration were: agitation, somnolence, chills, bradycardia, dizziness, increased salivation, respiratory disorder, hypertension, tachycardia, laryngismus, fever, headache, hypothermia, increased SGOT.

Occasional (<1% overall) adverse events occurring during clinical trials included: arrhythmias, increased LDH, increased SGPT, hypoxia, apnoea, leukocytosis, ventricular extrasystoles, supra-ventricular extrasystoles, asthma, confusion, increased creatinine, urinary retention, glycosuria, atrial fibrillation, complete AV block, bigeminy, leucopenia.

Malignant hyperthermia and acute kidney failure have been reported very rarely.

Rare reports of post-operative hepatitis exist, but with an uncertain relationship to Sevoflurane.

As with other anaesthetic agents, cases of twitching and jerking movements with spontaneous resolution have been reported in children receiving Sevoflurane for induction of anaesthesia with an uncertain relationship to Sevoflurane.

Laboratory findings: Transient elevations in glucose and white blood cell count may occur as with use of other anaesthetic agents.

Occasional cases of transient changes in hepatic function tests were reported with sevoflurane.

Overdose: In the event of overdosage, the following action should be taken. Stop drug administration, establish a clear airway and initiate assisted or controlled ventilation with pure oxygen and maintain adequate cardiovascular function.

Pharmacological properties

Pharmacodynamic properties: Changes in the clinical effects of sevoflurane rapidly follow changes in the inspired concentration.

Cardiovascular effects: As with all other inhalation agents sevoflurane depresses cardiovascular function in a dose related fashion. In one volunteer study, increases in sevoflurane concentration resulted in decrease in mean arterial pressure, but there was no change in heart rate. Sevoflurane did not alter plasma noradrenaline concentrations in this study.

Nervous system effects: No evidence of seizure was observed during the clinical development programme.

In patients with normal intracranial pressure (ICP), sevoflurane had minimal effect on ICP and preserved CO_2 responsiveness. The safety of sevoflurane has not been investigated in patients with a raised ICP. In patients at risk for elevations of ICP, sevoflurane should be administered cautiously in conjunction with ICP-reducing manoeuvres such as hyperventilation.

Pharmacokinetic properties: The low solubility of sevoflurane in blood should result in alveolar concentrations which rapidly increase upon induction and rapidly decrease upon cessation of the inhaled agent.

In humans, <5% of the absorbed sevoflurane is metabolised. The rapid and extensive pulmonary elimination of sevoflurane minimises the amount of anaesthetic available for metabolism. Sevoflurane is defluorinated via cytochrome P450 (CYP)2E1 resulting in the production of hexafluoroisopropanol (HFIP) with release of inorganic fluoride and carbon dioxide (or a one carbon fragment). HFIP is then rapidly conjugated with glucuronic acid and excreted in the urine.

The metabolism of sevoflurane may be increased by known inducers of CYP2E1 (e.g. isoniazid and alcohol), but it is not inducible by barbiturates.

Transient increases in serum inorganic fluoride levels may occur during and after sevoflurane anaesthesia. Generally, concentrations of inorganic fluoride peak within 2 hours of the end of sevoflurane anaesthesia and return within 48 hours to pre-operative levels.

Preclinical safety data: Animal studies have shown that hepatic and renal circulation are well maintained with sevoflurane.

Sevoflurane decreases the cerebral metabolic rate for oxygen ($CMRO_2$) in a fashion analogous to that seen with isoflurane. An approximately 50% reduction of $CMRO_2$ is observed at concentrations approaching 2.0 MAC. Animal studies have demonstrated that sevoflurane does not have a significant effect on cerebral blood flow.

In animals, sevoflurane significantly suppresses electroencephalographic (EEG) activity comparable to equipotent doses of isoflurane. There is no evidence that sevoflurane is associated with epileptiform activity during normocapnia or hypocapnia. In contrast to enflurane, attempts to elicit seizure-like EEG activity during hypopcapnia with rhythmic auditory stimuli have been negative.

Compound A was minimally nephrotoxic at concentrations of 50–114 ppm for 3 hours in a range of studies in rats. The toxicity was characterised by sporadic single cell necrosis of the proximal tubule cells. The mechanism of the renal toxicity in rats is unknown and its relevance to man has not been established. Comparable human threholds for Compound A-related nephrotoxicty would be predicted to be 150–200 ppm. The concentrations of Compound A found in routine clinical practice are on average 19 ppm in adults (maximum 32 ppm) with use of soda lime as the CO_2 absorbent.

Pharmaceutical particulars

List of excipients: None.

Incompatibilities: Sevoflurane is chemically stable. No discernible degradation occurs in the presence of strong acids or heat. The only known degradation reaction in the clinical setting is through direct contact with CO_2 absorbents (soda lime and Baralyme) producing low levels of Compound A (pentafluoroisopropenyl fluoromethyl ether (PIFE)), and trace amounts of Compound B (pentafluoromethoxy isopropyl fluoromethyl ether (PMFE)).

The interaction with CO_2 absorbents is not unique to sevoflurane. The production of degradants in the anaesthesia circuit results from the extraction of the acidic proton in the presence of a strong base (KOH and/or NaOH) forming an alkene (Compound A) from sevoflurane, similar to formation of 2-bromo-2-chloro-1, 1-difluoro ethylene (BCDFE) from halothane. No dose adjustment or change in clinical practice is necessary when rebreathing circuits are used.

Higher levels of Compound A are obtained when using Baralyme rather than soda lime.

Shelf life: The recommended shelf life is 24 months.

Special precautions for storage: None.

Nature and contents of container: 100 ml and 250 ml amber glass bottles.

Instructions for use/handling: Sevoflurane should be administered via a vaporiser calibrated specifically for sevoflurane using a key filler system designed for sevoflurane specific vaporisers or other appropriate sevoflurane specific vaporiser filling systems.

Some halogenated anaesthetics have been reported to interact with dry carbon dioxide absorbent to form carbon monoxide. To date there is no evidence that this can occur with sevoflurane. However, in order to minimise the risk of formation of carbon monoxide in re-breathing circuits and the possibility of elevated carboxyhaemoglobin levels, carbon dioxide absorbents should not be allowed to dry out.

Marketing authorisation number 0037/0258.

Date of approval/revision of SPC August 1997.

Legal category POM.

SURVANTA*

Qualitative and quantitative composition Each ml contains Beractant equivalent to:

Phospholipids	25 mg/ml
(including disaturated phosphatidylcholines 11.0–15.5 mg/ml)	
Triglycerides	0.5–1.75 mg/ml
Free Fatty Acids	1.4–3.5 mg/ml
Protein	0.1–1.0 mg/ml

Pharmaceutical form Sterile suspension for intratrachael administration.

Clinical particulars

Therapeutic indications: Survanta is indicated for treatment of Respiratory Distress Syndrome (RDS) (hyaline membrane disease) in new born premature infants with a birth weight of 700 g or greater and who are intubated and are receiving mechanical ventilation.

Posology and method of administration:

Dosage in infants: 100 mg phosholipid/kg birth weight in a volume not exceeding 4 ml/kg.

Treatment of RDS should be administered early in the course of RDS, i.e. preferably less than 8 hours of age. Depending on clinical course, this dose may be repeated within 48 hours at intervals of at least six hours for up to 4 doses.

Method of Administration Survanta should be administered by intratracheal administration (i.e. drug should be conducted into the lungs via an endotracheal tube) using a 5 Fr catheter. The tip of the catheter should lie at the end of the endotracheal tube. Infants should not be intubated solely for the administration of Survanta.

Survanta should be warmed to room temperature before administration (see *Precautions*).

Before administering Survanta to infants on mechanical ventilation, set the respiratory frequency at 60/minute–with inspiration time 0.5s and F_iO_2 at 1.0. Inspiratory pressure needs no change at this point.

To ensure distribution of Survanta throughout the lungs, each dose is divided into fractional doses. Each dose can be administered as either two half-doses or four quarter-doses. Each fractional dose is administered with the infant in different positions as given below. Between each position the infant should be ventilated for 30 seconds.

For four quarter-doses, the recommended positions are:

Right Lateral Position with the head lowered (i.e. head and body slanting down at an angle of approximately 15°).

Left Lateral Position with the head lowered (i.e. head and body slanting down at an angle of approximately 15°).

Right Lateral Position with head elevated (i.e. head and body slanting up at an angle of approximately 15°).

Left Lateral Position with head elevated (i.e. head and body slanting up at an angle of approximately 15°).

For administration of each quarter dose, the ventilator is disconnected, the catheter inserted, the dose administered then the ventilator reconnected. Between each quarter dose the infant is ventilated for 30 seconds.

For two half-doses, the recommended positions are:

With infant supine, the head and body turned approximately 45° to the right.

With infant supine, the head and body turned approximately 45° to the left.

When two half-doses of Survanta are being administered there are 2 alternative methods of administration:

Installation with disconnection from the ventilator

Each half dose is administered by disconnecting the endotracheal tube from the ventilator, inserting the catheter and administering the half dose. Between the half doses, the ventilator is reconnected for 30 seconds.

Alternatively, instillation without disconnection from the ventilator (through a suction port connector).

The first half dose is administered by inserting the catheter through a suction port connector without disconnection from the ventilator. There should be at least 30 seconds between the half doses during which time the catheter is retracted from the endotracheal tube but not removed from the connector. The catheter is then reinserted into the endotracheal tube and the second half dose administered. The catheter is then withdrawn completely.

Dosage in adults: Not applicable.

Dosage in elderly: Not applicable.

Contra-indications: No specific contraindications for Survanta have been defined by the clinical studies.

Special warnings and precautions for use: Survanta should only be administered with adequate facilities for ventilation and monitoring of babies with RDS.

Marked improvements in oxygenation may occur within minutes of the administration of Survanta. Therefore, frequent and careful monitoring of systemic oxygenation is essential to avoid hyperoxia. Following Survanta administration, monitoring of the arterial blood gases, the fraction of inspired oxygen and ventilatory change is required to ensure appropriate adjustments.

During the dosing procedure, transient episodes of bradycardia and/or oxygen desaturation have been reported. If these occur, dosing should be stopped and appropriate measures to alleviate the condition should be initiated. After stabilisation, the dosing procedure should be resumed.

Survanta is stored refrigerated (2–8°C). Before administration, Survanta should be warmed by standing at room temperature for 20 minutes or warmed in the hand for 8 minutes. ARTIFICIAL WARMING METHODS SHOULD NOT BE USED. Discard each vial if not used within 8 hours of rewarming to room temperature. Vials should not be returned to the refrigerator once warmed.

Each vial of Survanta is for single use only. Used vials with residual drug should be discarded.

Survanta should be inspected visually for discolouration prior to administration. The colour of Survanta is off-white to light brown. Some settling may occur during storage. If this occurs, gently invert the vial several times (DO NOT SHAKE) to redisperse.

Interactions with other medicaments and other forms of Interaction: None known to date.

Pregnancy and lactation: Not applicable.

Effects on ability to drive and use machines: Not applicable.

Undesirable effects: Intracranial haemorrhage has been observed in patients who received either Survanta or placebo. The incidence of intracranial haemorrhage in all patients is similar to that reported in the literature in this patient population. Pulmonary haemorrhage has also been reported. No other serious adverse reactions have been reported. No antibody production to Survanta proteins has been observed.

Overdose: If an excessively large dose of Survanta is given, observe the infant for signs of acute airway obstruction. Treatment should be symptomatic and supportive. Rales and moist breath sounds can transiently occur after Survanta is given, and do not indicate overdosage. Endotracheal suction or other remedial action is not required unless clear-cut signs of airway obstruction are present.

Pharmacological properties

Pharmacodynamic properties: The mode of action of Survanta is biophysical rather than biochemical, i.e. it reduces surface tension and concomitantly increases lung compliance.

Intratracheally administered Survanta distributes rapidly to the alveolar surfaces and stabilises the alveoli against collapse during respiration thereby increasing alveolar ventilation.

In clinical studies of premature infants with Respiratory Distress Syndrome (RDS), a significant improvement in oxygenation was demonstrated after treatment with a single dose of Survanta.

These infants showed a decreased need for supplemental oxygen and an increase in the arterial/alveolar oxygen ratio (a/ApO_2). Significantly decreased need for respiratory support, as indicated by a lower mean airway pressure, was also observed. In most cases these effects were maintained for at least 72 hours after the administration of the single dose of Survanta.

Pharmacokinetic properties: In preclinical studies using radiolabelled phosphatidylcholine, the clearance rate of Survanta in the lung of three day old rabbits has been shown to be similar to that of natural calf and sheep surfactants (approximately 13% within 24 hours). In addition some re-uptake and secretion of Survanta was shown, implying its entry into a metabolically active surfactant pool.

Since an exogenous preparation of Survanta is delivered directly to the lung, classical clinical pharmocokinetic parameters (blood levels, plasma half-life etc.) have not been studied.

Preclinical safety data: There are no pre-clinical data of relevance to the prescriber which are additional to that already included in other sections of the SPC.

Pharmaceutical particulars

List of excipients: Sodium chloride and water for injection.

Incompatibilities: None experienced to date, as product administration is unique.

Shelf life: 18 months.

Special precautions for storage: Store under refrigerated conditions (2-8°C) protected from light.

Nature and contents of container: 21 ml glass bottle with a 20 mm rubber stopper and a 20 mm aluminium seal finish containing 8 ml of product.

Pack sizes: 1, 3 and 10

Instructions for use/handling: Do not freeze. Any inadvertently frozen product should be discarded.

Marketing Authorisation Number 0037/0218

Date of First Authorisation/Renewal of Authorisation 3rd February 1993/13th October 1998

Date of (Partial) Revision Of The Text October 1997

**Trade Mark*

Akita Pharmaceuticals Limited
33 Moyle House
Churchill Gardens
Westminster
London SW1V 3BE
☎ 0870 6071260 🗋 0870 6071261

SECTRAL*

Qualitative and quantitative composition Sectral Capsules 100 mg contains Acebutolol hydrochloride 111.0 mg (equivalent to 100 mg of base). Sectral Capsules 200 mg contains Acebutolol hydrochloride 222.0 mg (equivalent to 200 mg of base). Sectral Tablets 400 mg contains Acebutolol hydrochloride 443.4 mg (equivalent to 400 mg of base).

Pharmaceutical form

Sectral 100 capsules are hard gelatin capsules, the bodies being opaque yellowish-buff and the caps opaque white in colour. Length approximately 17 mm, diameter of body appoximately 6 mm. Both body and cap are printed in black 'Sectral 100'. The capsules contain a white or almost white powder. *Sectral 200 capsules* are hard gelatin capsules, the bodies being opaque yellowish-buff and the caps opaque pink in colour. Length approximately 17 mm, diameter of body approximately 6 mm. Both body and cap are printed in black 'Sectral 200'. The capsules contain a white or almost white power. *Sectral 400 tablets* are white to off-white, circular, biconvex, film-coated tablets with bevel edges, one face impressed 'Sectral 400'. Plain reverse.

Clinical particulars

Therapeutic indications: Sectral is indicated for the management of all grades of hypertension, angina pectoris and the control of tachyarrhythmias.

Posology and method of administration:

Hypertension: Initial dosage of 400 mg orally once daily at breakfast or 200 mg orally twice daily. If response is not adequate within two weeks, dosage may be increased up to 400 mg orally twice daily; if the hypertension is still not adequately controlled consideration should be given to adding a second antihypertensive agent such as the calcium antagonist nifedipine or small doses of a thiazide diuretic.

Angina pectoris: Initial dosage of 400 mg orally once daily at breakfast or 200 mg twice daily. In severe forms up to 300 mg three times daily may be required. Up to 1200 mg daily has been used.

Cardiac arrhythmias: Maximal anti-arrhythmic effect may not be achieved until up to 3 hours after oral administration.

The daily dose requirement for long term anti-arrhythmic activity should lie between 400 and 1200 mg daily. The dose can be gauged by response. Since the presence of more consistent beta-blockade may be necessary for the control of arrhythmias, better control may be achieved by divided doses rather than single daily doses.

Elderly: There are no specific dosage recommendations for the elderly with normal glomerular filtration rate. Dose reduction is necessary if moderate to severe renal impairment is present.

Children: Paediatric dose has not been established.

Contra-indications: Cardiogenic shock is an absolute contra-indication and caution is required in patients with blood pressures of the order of 100/60 mmHg or below. Sectral is also contra-indicated in patients with atrioventricular block, hypersensitivity to acebutolol or beta blockers, marked bradycardia and uncontrolled heart failure. Although cardio-selective beta blockers may have less effect on lung function than non-selective beta blockers as with all beta blockers these should be avoided in patients with obstructive airways disease unless there are compelling clinical reasons for their use.

Special warnings and special precautions for use: Renal impairment is not a contra-indication to the use of Sectral which has both renal and non-renal excretory pathways. Some caution should be exercised when administering high doses to patients with severe renal failure as cumulation could possibly occur in these circumstances. The dosage frequency should not exceed once daily in patients with renal impairment. As a guide, the dosage should be reduced by 50% when glomerular filtration rates are between 25–50 ml/min and by 75% when they are below 25 ml/min. Drug-induced bronchospasm is usually at least partially reversible by the use of a suitable agonist. Withdrawal of treatment by beta blockers should be achieved by gradual dosage reduction. Beta blockers may mask signs of thyrotoxicosis and hypoglycaemia. *Caution should be exercised if using in patients with a history of wheezing or asthma.*

Interaction with other medicaments and other forms of interaction: Sectral should not be used with Verapamil or within several days of Verapamil therapy (and vice versa).

Although nifedipine has been successfully combined with beta blockers, the risk of hypotension is increased. There is also a risk of cardiac failure in patients with a latent or an uncontrolled cardiac insufficiency. Blood pressure should be closely monitored in cases of coadministration with dihydropyridine derivatives especially when initiating therapy.

Diltiazem should be used with caution in combination with beta blockers.

In patients with labile and insulin-dependent diabetes, the dosage of the hypoglycaemic agent may need to be reduced. However beta blockers have also been known to blunt the effect of glibenclamide. Cross reactions due to displacement of other drugs from plasma protein binding sites are unlikely due to the low degree of plasma protein binding exhibited by acebutolol and diacetolol. If a beta-adrenoceptor antagonist is used concurrently with clonidine the latter should not be withdrawn until several days after the former is discontinued. Acebutolol is a cardioselective beta blocker and it may antagonise the effect of sympathomimetic and xanthine bronchodilators but to a lesser extent than non-cardio selective beta blockers. Concurrent use of digoxin and beta blockers may occasionally induce serious bradycardia. The antihypertensive effects of beta blockers may be attenuated by non-steroidal anti-inflammatory agents. There is a theoretical risk that concurrent administration of monoamine oxidase inhibitors and high doses of beta blockers, even if they are cardio-selective can produce hypertension. Sectral therapy should be brought to the attention of the anaesthetist prior to general anaesthesia. If treatment is continued, special care should be taken when using anaesthetic agents such as ether, cyclopropane and trichlorethylene.

Pregnancy and lactation:

Pregnancy: Sectral should not be administered to female patients during the first trimester of pregnancy unless the physician considers it essential. Beta blockers administered in late pregnancy may give rise to bradycardia and hypoglycaemia of the foetus/neonate. Animal studies have shown no teratogenic hazard.

Lactation: Acebutolol and its active metabolite are excreted in breast milk and the half life of acebutolol in the neonate is double that in adults. The risks of hypoglycaemia and bradycardia occurring in the nursing infant have not been evaluated. Therefore, breast-feeding is not recommended during treatment.

Effects on ability to drive and use machines: None stated.

Undesirable effects: Sectral possesses antihypertensive effects but these are unlikely to be noted in normotensive subjects. Those common to beta-blockade: bradycardia, gastrointestinal effects, cold extremities, dizziness, headaches, shortness of breath, nightmares, loss of libido and lethargy have been met with infrequency. The low lipid solubility and lack of cumulation in CNS tissues of acebutolol and its active metabolite reduce the likelihood of sleep disturbances, depression or other central effects and such occurrences are rare. There have been reports of skin rashes and/or dry eyes associated with the use of beta-adrenoceptor blocking drugs. The reported incidence is small and in most cases the symptoms have cleared when treatment was withdrawn. Discontinuation of the drug should be considered if any such reaction is not otherwise explicable. Cessation of therapy with a beta blocker should be gradual. Although some patients have developed anti-nuclear factor titres, the incidence of associated clinical symptoms is rare and when present, these clear promptly on discontinuation of treatment. Bronchospasm has occurred rarely during treatment with acebutolol.

Overdose: In the rare event of excessive bradycardia or hypotension, 1 mg atropine sulphate administered intravenously should be given without delay. If this is insufficient it should be followed by a slow intravenous injection of isoprenaline (5 mcg per minute) with constant monitoring until a response occurs. In severe cases of self-poisoning with circulatory collapse unresponsive to atropine and catecholamines the intravenous injection of glucagon 10–20 mg may produce a dramatic improvement. Cardiac pacing may be employed if bradycardia becomes severe.

Judicious use of vasopressors, diazepam, phenytoin, lidocaine, digoxin and bronchodilators should be considered depending on the presentation of the patient. Acebutolol can be removed from blood by haemodialysis. Other symptoms and signs of overdosage include cardiogenic shock, AV block, conduction defects, pulmonary oedema, depressed level of consciousness, bronchospasm, hypoglycaemia and rarely hyperkalaemia.

Pharmacological properties

Pharmacodynamic properties: Mode of action: Sectral is a beta adrenoceptor antagonist which is cardioselective, i.e. acts preferentially on beta-1 adrenergic receptors in the heart. Its principal effects are to reduce heart rate especially on exercise and to lower blood pressure in hypertentive subjects. Sectral and its equally active metabolite, diacetolol have anti-arrhythmic activity, the combined plasma half-life of the active drug and metabolite being 7–10 hours. Both have partial agonist activity (PAA) also known as intrinsic sympathomimetic activity (ISA). This property ensures that some degree of stimulation of beta receptors is maintained. Under conditions of rest, this tends to balance the negative chronotropic and negative inotropic effects. Sectral blocks the effects of excessive catecholamine stimulation resulting from stress.

Pharmacokinetic properties: After oral administration, acebutolol is rapidly and almost completely absorbed. Absorption appears to be unaffected by the presence of food in the gut. There is rapid formation of a major equiactive metabolite, diacetolol, which possesses a similar pharmacological profile to acebutolol. Peak plasma concentrations of active material (i.e. acebutolol plus diacetolol) are achieved within 2–4 hours and the terminal plasma elimination half-life is around 8–10 hours. Because of biliary excretion and direct transfer across the gut wall from the systemic circulation to the gut lumen, more than 50% of an oral dose of Sectral is recovered in the faeces with acebutolol and diacetolol in equal proportions; the rest of the dose is recovered in the urine, mainly as diacetolol. Both acebutolol and diacetolol are hydrophilic and exhibit poor penetration of the CNS.

Pharmaceutical particulars

List of excipients: Sectral 100 and 200 capsules contain Starch potato, Aerosil (Silicon dioxide (E551)), Magnesium stearate (E572). Opadry OY-L-28900 containing Titanium dioxide (E171) PhEur, Lactose PhEur, HPMC 2910 15cP, and Polyethylene glycol 4000NF. The Capsule shell contains Yellow Iron Oxide (E172), Titanium dioxide (E171), Gelatin, Black ink (Opacode S-24-8109). Sectral 200 also contains red iron oxide (E172).

The tablets contain lactose BP, Starch maize BP, French chalk powdered (E553b), aerosil (silicon dioxide E551), Povidone K30 BP, Magnesium stearate (E572) BP, Opadry OY-L-28900 (contains titanium dioxide (E171) PhEur, Lactose PhEur, HPMC 2190 15cP (E464), Polyethylene glycol 4000 NF).

Incompatibilities: Not applicable.

Shelf life: The shelf life of Sectral capsules is 60 months.

The shelf life of Sectral tablets is 36 months.

Special precautions for storage: Capsules only: Store in a dry place below 25°C. Protect from light.

Nature and contents of container:

Sectral capsules 100 mg aluminium foil/UPVC blister strip packs of 84 capsules.

Sectral capsules 200 mg aluminium foil/UPVC blister strip packs of 56 capsules.

Sectral tablets 400 mg aluminium foil/UPVC blister strip packs of 28 tablets.

Instructions for use/handling: None.

Marketing authorisation numbers
Sectral capsules 100 mg PL 16951/0002
Sectral capsules 200 mg PL 16951/0003
Sectral tablets 400 mg PL 16951/0004

Date of approval/revision of SPC July 1998

Legal category POM

SECADREX*

Qualitative and quantitative composition Each tablet contains the equivalent of 200 mg acebutolol (in the form of the hydrochloride) and 12.5 mg hydrochlorothiazide. The tablets also contain lactose.

Pharmaceutical form Secadrex tablets are white, round, slightly biconvex, and film-coated, imprinted 'SECADREX' on one face.

Clinical particulars

Therapeutic indications: Secadrex tablets are indicated for the control of mild and moderate hypertension.

Posology and method of administration: One tablet once daily, usually in the morning. If response is inadequate, dosage may be increased to two tablets daily. Secadrex is not intended for use in children.

Contra-indications: Cardiogenic shock is an absolute contra-indication to beta-blockade and caution is required in patients with blood pressures of the order of 100/60 mmHg or below. Heart block: Administration of any beta-adrenoceptor blocking agent is considered inadvisable (except perhaps in first degree block).

Severe kidney and liver failure. Hypersensitivity to hydrocholorthiazide.

Secadrex tablets should not be used with verapamil or within several days of verapamil therapy (and vice versa). Insulin-dependent diabetes. Use in non-insulin dependent diabetics may be inadvisable since thiazide diuretics may cause further impairment of glucose tolerance. Gout or hyperuricaemia.

Reversible obstructive airways disease. Although cardio-selective beta blockers may have less effect on lung function than non-selective beta blockers as with all beta blockers these should be avoided in patients with reversible obstructive airways disease unless there are compelling clinical reasons for their use.

Special warnings and special precautions for use: Caution should be exercised: If Secadrex tablets are administered in the presence of bradycardia (depending on the circumstances). If Secadrex tablets are to be prescribed with a catecholamine-depleting drug, such as reserpine. In the presence of signs of heart failure, since acebutolol has a slight but acceptable cardiodepressant action. In anaesthesia, some anaesthetists prefer to discontinue therapy 48 hours before anaesthesia, others do not consider this essential. Withdrawal should be made gradually. Thiazides may increase responsiveness to tubocurarine. If Secadrex and clonidine are given concurrently, clonidine should not be discontinued until several days after withdrawal of the beta blocker. *If used in patients with a history of asthma and wheezing.* All patients receiving hydrochlorothiazide therapy (as in Secadrex tablets) should be monitored periodically for clinical signs of fluid or electrolyte imbalance, hypokalaemia, hyponatraemia and hypochloraemic alkalosis. Hypokalaemia can sensitise or exaggerate the response of the heart to the toxic effects of digitalis (e.g. increased venticular irritability). With the low dose of hydrochlorothiazide present in Secadrex tablets, the possibility of significant imbalance becomes less likely.

Interaction with other medicaments and other forms of interaction: Tricyclic antidepressants and MAO inhibitors should not be used with Secadrex tablets. Lithium should generally not be given to patients receiving diuretics since the risk of lithium toxicity is very high in such patients.

Pregnancy and lactation: Secadrex should not be administered to female patients during the first trimester of pregnancy unless the physician considers it essential. Animal studies with acebutolol have shown no teratogenic hazard. Thiazides are not generally recommended in the treatment of pregnancy hypertension; it may be preferable to use monotherapy with Sectral or another suitable antihypertensive drug in pregnant patients.

Effects on ability to drive and use machines: Secadrex has no effect on patients' ability to drive and operate machines.

Undesirable effects: No serious side effects have been reported with Secadrex treatment. The most common i.e. those related to beta-blockade – hypotension, bradycardia, gastrointestinal effects and depression – have been met with infrequently, and usually do not require interruption or withdrawal of therapy.

There have been reports of skin rashes and/or dry eyes associated with the use of beta-adrenoceptor antagonists. The reported incidence is small and in most cases the symptoms have cleared when treatment was withdrawn. Discontinuation of the drug should be considered if any such reaction is not explicable. Cessation of treatment with a beta blocker should be gradual. Bronchospasm has occurred rarely with usage of acebutolol.

Skin rashes and photosensitivity due to hydrochlorothiazide have been reported as have blood dyscrasias including thrombocytopenia, but these are rare.

Overdose: In the rare event of excessive bradycardia or hypotension, 1 mg atropine sulphate administered intravenously should be given without delay. If this proves insufficient, it should be followed by a slow intravenous injection of isoprenaline (5 mcg per minute) with constant monitoring until a response occurs. In cases of severe poisoning with beta-adrenoceptor antagonists an injection of 10 mg glucagon intravenously has produced rapid improvement. If bradycardia becomes severe, electrical pacing may be necessary.

Pharmacological properties

Pharmacodynamic properties: Acebutolol is a cardioselective beta-adrenoceptor antagonist. Hydrochlorothiazide is a thiazide diuretic/antihypertensive agent.

Pharmacokinetic properties: Acebutolol reaches a peak plasma level 2 to 4 hours after dosing, for hydrochlorothiazide the average time to peak plasma levels is about two hours after dosing.

Pharmaceutical particulars

List of excipients: Lactose, Starch maize, Povidone K30, Magnesium stearate.

Incompatibilities: Not applicable.

Shelf life: 36 months.

Special precautions for storage: Store in a dry place below 25°C.

Nature and contents of container: Secadrex is packed in blister strips of 28 tablets.

Instructions for use/handling: Secadrex should always be kept out of the reach of children.

Marketing authorisation number PL 16951/0001

Date of approval/revision of SPC July 1998

Legal category POM

**Trade Mark*

Alcon Laboratories (U.K.) Limited

Pentagon Park
Boundary Way
Hemel Hempstead
Hertfordshire, HP2 7UD

☎ 01442 (Int +44 1442) 341234   🗋 01442 (Int +44 1442) 341200

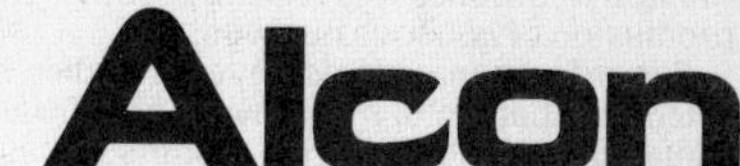

ALOMIDE* OPHTHALMIC SOLUTION

Qualitative and quantitative composition Lodoxamide trometamol 0.178% HSE (equivalent to 0.1% w/v lodoxamide).

Pharmaceutical form Eye drops.

Clinical particulars

Therapeutic indications: Alomide Ophthalmic Solution is indicated in the treatment of non-infectious allergic conjunctivitis (vernal conjunctivitis, giant papillary conjunctivitis, and allergic-atopic conjunctivitis). The etiologic factors are unknown, but common airborne allergens and contact lenses have been implicated. Lodoxamide trometamol may be effective against other ocular diseases where type I immediate hypersensitivity (or mast cells) play a major role in the inflammatory process.

Posology and method of administration:

Adults and children: One or two drops in each eye four times a day at regular intervals. Patients should be advised that the effect of Alomide therapy is dependent upon its administration at regular intervals, as directed. Improvements in signs and symptoms in response to Alomide therapy (decreased discomfort, itching, foreign body sensation, photophobia, acute ocular pain, tearing, discharge, erythema/swelling, conjunctival redness, limbal reaction, epithelial disease, ptosis) are usually evident within a few days, but longer treatment for up to four weeks is sometimes required. Once symptomatic improvement has been established, therapy should be continued for as long as needed to sustain improvement. Patients should also be advised that instillation of eye drops in allergic conjunctivitis may cause discomfort initially and that this will decline with improvement of the disease (see *Undesirable effects*).

Children less than 4 years: The safety and effectiveness of Alomide in children below the age of four years have not been established.

Elderly: There are no special precautions to be followed in prescribing Alomide for the elderly.

If required, corticosteroids may be used concomitantly with Alomide.

Contra-indications: Alomide is contra-indicated in those persons who have a known hypersensitivity to lodoxamide or any component of the medicament.

Special warnings and precautions for use: Alomide is not for injection. The recommended frequency of administration should not be exceeded. As with all preparations containing benzalkonium chloride, users of soft (hydrophilic) contact lenses should refrain from wearing lenses while under treatment with Alomide. Lenses may be worn within a few hours of discontinuation of treatment.

Interaction with other medicaments and other forms of interaction: None known.

Pregnancy and lactation: Reproduction studies with lodoxamide trometamol administered orally to rats and rabbits in doses of 100 mg/kg/day (more than 5000 times the proposed human dose) produced no evidence of developmental toxicity. However, there are no adequate and well-controlled studies in pregnant women. Since animal reproduction studies are not always predictive of human response, Alomide should be used during pregnancy only if clearly needed.

It is not known whether lodoxamide is secreted in human milk. Because many drugs are excreted in human milk, caution should be exercised when Alomide is administered to nursing mothers.

Effect on ability to drive and use machines: Alomide is unlikely to affect a patient's ability to drive or to use machinery.

Undesirable effects: During clinical studies of Alomide, the most frequently reported ocular adverse experiences were transient burning, stinging or discomfort upon instillation, which occurred in 13% of patients. Other ocular events occurring in 1 to 5% of the patients included ocular pruritus, blurred vision, lid margin crusting, dry eye, tearing and hyperaemia. Events that occurred in less than 1% of the patients included foreign body sensation, ocular pain, discharge, ocular edema, ocular fatigue, ocular warming sensation, lid edema, chemosis, anterior chamber cells, epitheliopathy, keratopathy/keratitis, blepharitis, sticky sensation, corneal erosion, dim vision, corneal abrasion and allergy. Non-ocular events are rare and reported at incidences below 1%; these included warm sensation, headache, nausea, stomach discomfort, dizziness, somnolence, dry nose, sneezing and rash.

Overdose: In the event of a topical overdose, flush from the eye with running water. Accidental overdose of an oral preparation of 120 to 180 mg of lodoxamide resulted in temporary sensation of warmth, profuse sweating, diarrhoea, light-headedness and a feeling of stomach distension; no permanent adverse effects were observed. Consideration may be given by the physician to emesis in the event of accidental ingestion.

Pharmacological properties

Pharmacodynamic properties: Lodoxamide, a mast cell stabiliser inhibits the *in vivo* Type I immediate hypersensitivity reaction in animals and man.

In vitro studies have demonstrated the ability of lodoxamide to stabilise mast cells and prevent the antigen specific induced release of histamine. In addition, lodoxamide prevents the release of other mast cell inflammatory mediators (i.e. SRS-A, slow reacting substances of anaphylaxis also known as the peptido-leukotrienes). Lodoxamide inhibits histamine release *in vitro* by preventing the movement of calcium into the mast cell after stimulation.

Pharmacokinetic properties: The oral bioavailability of ^{14}C-lodoxamide in man is 71%, approximately 87% of the absorbed drug undergoes biotransformation. The metabolic transformation of lodoxamide results from stepwise hydrolysis of the oxylamide groups to form the monoxamate and the diamine. The diamine undergoes further hydroxylation followed by conjugation to either the O-glucuronide or O-sulphate. The O-glucuronide and O-sulphate metabolites account for 79% of the biotransformed lodoxamide, with the monoxamate and diamine accounting for 5% and 3% of the excreted metabolites. Only 2.7% of the absorbed dose is recovered as unchanged drug in the urine.

Preclinical safety data: There are no preclinical data of relevance to the prescriber which were additional to that already included in other sections of the SPC.

Pharmaceutical particulars

List of excipients: Benzalkonium chloride, mannitol, methylhydroxypropylcellulose PhEur, sodium citrate, citric acid, disodium edetate, tyloxapol sodium hydroxide and/or hydrochloric acid (to adjust pH), purified water.

Incompatibilities: None known.

Shelf life: 24 months. The contents and bottle should be discarded one month after opening the container for the first time.

Special precautions for storage: Store upright below 25°C.

Nature and contents of container: Alomide is supplied in 5 ml, 10 ml and 15 ml natural, low-density polyethylene bottles with natural, low density polyethylene dispensing plugs and tamper evident polypropylene screw caps. Only 5 ml and 10 ml are currently marketed.

Instructions for use/handling: The dispensing tip should not be touched with the fingers or by the conjunctiva when drops are instilled. The container should be kept tightly closed.

Marketing authorisation number 0649/0117.

Date of approval/revision of SPC 25 March 1997.

Legal category POM.

BETOPTIC*

Qualitative and quantitative composition Betaxolol hydrochloride USP 0.56% w/v.

Pharmaceutical form Sterile ophthalmic solution.

Clinical particulars

Therapeutic indications: Betoptic is indicated for the reduction of elevated intraocular pressure in patients with ocular hypertension and chronic open angle glaucoma.

Posology and method of administration:

Adults (including the elderly): The usual dose is one drop to be instilled into the affected eye(s) twice daily.

Children: Betoptic is not recommended for use in children.

Contra-indications: Betoptic is contra-indicated in patients with sinus bradycardia greater than a first degree block, cardiogenic shock or a history of overt cardiac failure and in patients with hypersensitivity to any component.

Special warnings and special precautions for use: Patients who are receiving a beta-adrenergic blocking agent orally and Betoptic should be observed for potential additive effect either on intraocular pressure or the known systemic effects of beta-blockade.

While Betoptic has demonstrated a low potential for systemic effects, it should be used with caution in patients with diabetes (especially labile diabetes) or in patients suspected of developing thyrotoxicosis.

Consideration should be given to the gradual withdrawal of beta-adrenergic blocking agents prior to general anaesthesia because of the reduced ability of the heart to respond to beta-adrenergically mediated sympathetic reflex stimuli.

Betoptic, a cardioselective beta-blocker, has produced only minimal effects in patients with reversible airway obstruction, however, caution should be exercised in the treatment of patients with a history of obstructive pulmonary disease.

In patients with angle-closure glaucoma, the immediate treatment objective is to re-open the angle by constriction of the pupil with a miotic agent, betaxolol has no effect on the pupil; therefore, Betoptic should be used with a miotic to reduce elevated intraocular pressure in angle-closure glaucoma.

This product contains benzalkonium chloride and is not recommended for use when soft contact lenses are being worn.

Interaction with other medicaments and other forms of interaction: Although Betoptic used alone has little or no effect on pupil size, mydriasis resulting from concomitant therapy with Betoptic and adrenaline has been reported occasionally.

Close observation of the patient is recommended when a beta blocker is administered to patients receiving catecholamine-depleting drugs such as reserpine, because of possible additive effects and the production of hypotension and/or bradycardia. Caution should be exercised in patients using concomitant adrenergic psychotropic drugs.

Pregnancy and lactation: Although animal studies have not demonstrated any specific hazard there are no adequate and well-controlled studies in pregnant women. Because animal studies are not always predictive of human response this drug should be used during pregnancy only if clearly indicated.

It is not known whether Betoptic is excreted in human milk, caution should therefore be exercised when Betoptic is administered to nursing mothers.

Effects on ability to drive and use machines: No effects on ability to drive and use machines have been reported.

Undesirable effects: Although Betopic is generally well tolerated, discomfort of short duration may be experienced by some patients upon instillation and occasional tearing has been reported. Rare instances of decreased corneal sensitivity, erythema, itching, corneal punctate staining, keratitis, anisocoria and photophobia have been reported.

Systemic reactions following topical administration of Betoptic (e.g. insomnia and depressive neurosis) have only rarely been reported.

Overdosage: A topical overdose of Betoptic may be flushed from the eye(s) with warm tap water.

Pharmacological properties
Pharmacodynamic properties: Betaxolol is a cardioselective Beta$_1$ receptor blocker which, when applied topically to the eye, lowers intraocular pressure. It is thought to produce this effect by reducing the rate of production of aqueous humour.

Clinical pharmacology: Several studies have indicated that betaxolol may have a beneficial effect on visual function for up to 48 months in patients with chronic open-angle glaucoma and up to 60 months in patients with ocular hypertension. Moreover there is evidence that betaxolol maintains or increases ocular blood flow/perfusion.

Pharmacokinetic properties: Betaxolol is highly lipophylic which results in good permeation of the cornea, allowing high intraocular levels of the drug. Betaxolol is characterised by its good oral absorption, low first pass loss and a relatively long half-life of approx 16–22 hours. The elimination of Betaxolol is primarily by the renal rather than faecal route. The major metabolic pathways yield two carboxylic acid forms plus unchanged betaxolol in the urine (approx. 16% of the administered dose).

Preclinical safety data: There are no preclinical data of relevance to the prescriber which are additional to that already in other sections of the SPC.

Pharmaceutical particulars
List of excipients: Disodium edetate, sodium chloride, benzalkonium chloride, sodium hydroxide, hydrochloric acid, purified water.

Incompatibilities: None known.

Shelf life: Unopened 36 months, after opening 28 days.

Special precautions for storage: Store below 25°C.

Nature and contents of container: 5 ml and 10 ml LDPE bottles (10 ml present in 15 ml container) with LDPE plug and white polystyrene or polypropylene cap.

Instructions for use/handling: Do not touch the top of the bottle to any surface as this may contaminate the contents.

Marketing authorisation number 0649/0097.

Date of approval/revision of SPC 13 August 1997.

Legal category POM.

BETOPTIC SUSPENSION*

Qualitative and quantitative composition BETOPTIC SUSPENSION contains, per mL, betaxolol hydrochloride PhEur 2.8 mg (equivalent to 2.5 mg betaxolol base).

Pharmaceutical form BETOPTIC SUSPENSION is a sterile, multidose, preserved suspension for topical ocular administration.

Clinical particulars
Therapeutic indication: BETOPTIC SUSPENSION lowers the intraocular pressure and is indicated in patients with chronic open-angle glaucoma and ocular hypertension.

Posology and method administration:
Adults (including Elderly): The recommended dose is one drop in the affected eye(s) twice daily. In some patients, the intraocular pressure lowering responses to BETOPTIC SUSPENSION may require a few weeks to stabilise. As with any new medication, careful monitoring of patients is advised.

If the intraocular pressure of the patient is not adequately controlled on this regimen, concomitant therapy with pilocarpine and other miotics and/or adrenaline (epinephrine) and/or carbonic anhydrase inhibitors can be instituted.

Children: Safety and effectiveness in children have not been established.

The volume of each drop dispensed is 24 μl.

Contra-indications: Hypersensitivity to any component of this medication. BETOPTIC SUSPENSION is contraindicated in patients with sinus bradycardia, second or third degree heart block,cardiogenic shock, or a history of overt cardiac failure.

Special warnings and special precautions for use: Ophthalmic betaxolol has been shown to have a minor effect on heart rate and blood pressure in clinical studies. Caution should be used in treating patients with a history of cardiac failure or heart block. Treatment with BETOPTIC SUSPENSION should be discontinued at the first signs of cardiac failure.

Diabetes Mellitus: Beta-adrenergic blocking agents should be administered with caution in patients subject to spontaneous hypoglycemia or to diabetic patients (especially those with labile diabetes) who are receiving insulin or oral hypoglycemic agents. Beta-adrenergic receptor blocking agents may mask the signs and symptoms of acute hypoglycemia.

Thyrotoxicosis: Beta-adrenergic blocking agents may mask certain clinical signs (e.g., tachycardia) of hyperthyroidism. Patients suspected of developing thyrotoxicosis should be managed carefully to avoid abrupt withdrawal of beta-adrenergic blocking agents, which might precipitate a thyroid storm.

Major Surgery: Consideration should be given to the gradual withdrawal of beta-adrenergic blocking agents prior to general anesthesia because of the reduced ability of the heart to respond to beta-adrenergically mediated sympathetic reflex stimuli.

Respiratory: Although cardioselective beta-blockers have less effect on lung function than non-selective beta-blockers, caution should be exercised in the treatment of glaucoma patients with obstructive airway disease. There have been reports of asthmatic attacks and respiratory distress during Betoptic treatment in such patients. In individual cases, the risk to benefit ratio for each patient should be considered. An increase in airway resistance can be relieved by inhaled beta$_2$-mimetics.

In controlled clinical studies, ophthalmic betaxolol has shown little effect on respiratory and cardiovascular function.

Ocular: In patients with angle-closure glaucoma, the immediate treatment objective is to reopen the angle by constriction of the pupil with a miotic agent. Betaxolol has little or no effect on the pupil. When BETOPTIC SUSPENSION is used to reduce elevated intraocular pressure in angle-closure glaucoma, it should be used with a miotic and not alone.

There have been reports of dry eyes associated with the topical ocular use of beta-blocking agents. Caution should be exercised in the use of beta-blocking agents in patients with Sicca Syndrome or similar tear film abnormalities.

Contact lens wearers must remove their lenses prior to instillation of BETOPTIC SUSPENSION and wait for 15 minutes after dosing before reinserting the contact lenses.

Interactions: Patients who are receiving a beta-adrenergic blocking agent orally and BETOPTIC SUSPENSION should be observed for potential additive effect either on the intraocular pressure or on the known systemic effects of beta blockade.

Close observation of the patient is recommended when a beta-blocker is administered to patients receiving catecholamine-depleting drugs such as reserpine, because of possible additive effects and the production of hypotension and/or bradycardia.

Betaxolol is an adrenergic blocking agent; therefore, caution should be exercised in patients using concomitant adrenergic psychotropic drugs.

Use during pregnancy and lactation: Reproduction studies have been conducted with orally administered betaxolol HCl in rats and rabbits. There was evidence of drug related postimplantation loss in rabbits and rats at dose levels above 12 mg/kg and 128 mg/kg (1500 and 16,000 times the maximum recommended human ocular dose), respectively. Betaxolol HCl was not shown to be teratogenic, however, and there were no other adverse effects on reproduction at subtoxic dose levels. However, there are no adequate and well controlled studies in pregnant women. BETOPTIC SUSPENSION should be used during pregnancy only if the potential benefit justifies the potential risk to the foetus.

It is not known whether betaxolol HCl is excreted in human milk. Caution should be exercised when BETOPTIC SUSPENSION is administered to nursing women.

Effects on ability to drive and use machines: The ability to drive and use machines is unlikely to be affected, other than any problems associated with transient blurred vision following the use of BETOPTIC SUSPENSION.

Undesirable Effects: Topically applied beta-adrenergic blocking agents may be absorbed systemically. Adverse reactions found with systemic administration of beta$_1$-adrenergic blocking agents may occur with topical administration (see Special Warnings).

Ocular: Transient ocular discomfort, such as ocular stinging and burning, blurred vision, corneal disease, such as corneal punctate staining, superficial punctate keratitis, foreign body sensation, photophobia, tearing, itching, erythema, may occur occasionally.

Systemic: Systemic reactions following topical administration of betaxolol have been rarely reported. These include: bradycardia, dyspnea, asthma, insomnia, headaches, depression, alopecia.

Overdosage: No information is available on overdosage of humans after ocular application. The oral LD_{50} of the drug ranged from 350–920 mg/kg in mice and 860–1050 mg/kg in rats. The symptoms which might be expected with an overdose of systemically administered beta$_1$-adrenergic receptor blocking agent are hypotension, bradycardia and acute cardiac failure.

No information is available on overdosage after ocular administration. A topical overdose of BETOPTIC SUSPENSION may be flushed from the eye(s) with warm tap water.

Pharmacological properties
Pharmacodynamic properties: Betaxolol, a cardioselective (beta$_1$-adrenergic) receptor blocking agent, does not have significant membrane-stabilising (local anaesthetic) activity and is devoid of intrinsic sympathomimetic action. Orally administered beta-adrenergic blocking agents may reduce cardiac output in healthy subjects and patients with heart disease. In patients with severe impairment of myocardial function, beta-adrenergic receptor antagonists may inhibit the sympathetic stimulatory effect necessary to maintain adequate cardiac function.

Betaxolol has no significant effect on pulmonary function as measured by FEV_1, Forced Vital Capacity (FVC), FEV_1/FVC and no evidence of cardiovascular beta-adrenergic-blockade during exercise was observed.

When instilled in the eye, betaxolol has the action of reducing elevated as well as normal intraocular pressure (IOP), whether or not accompanied by glaucoma. It is thought to produce this effect by reducing the rate of production of aqueous humour as demonstrated by tonography and aqueous fluorophotometry. BETOPTIC SUSPENSION provides IOP lowering activity equivalent to that demonstrated by BETOPTIC Ophthalmic Solution 0.5%. Ophthalmic betaxolol has little or no effect on the constriction of the pupil and little effect on respiratory and cardiovascular function.

Several studies have indicated that Betaxolol may have a beneficial effect on visual function for up to 48 months in patients with chronic open angle glaucoma and up to 60 months in patients with ocular hypertension. Moreover there is evidence that betaxolol maintains or increases ocular blood flow/perfusion.

Pharmacokinetic properties: Betaxolol is highly lipophilic which results in good permeation of the cornea, allowing high intraocular levels of the drug. Betaxolol is characterised by its good oral absorption, low first pass loss and a relatively long half-life of approximately 16–22 hours. The elimination of betaxolol is primarily by the renal rather than faecal route. The major metabolic pathways yield two carboxylic acid forms plus unchanged betaxolol in the urine (approximately 16% of the administered dose).

The onset of action of betaxolol can generally be noted within 30 minutes and the maximal effect can usually be detected 2 hours after topical administration. A single dose provides a 12-hour reduction in intraocular pressure.

The polar nature of betaxolol can produce apparent ocular discomfort. In this formulation, betaxolol molecules are ionically bound to the amberlite resin. Upon instillation the betaxolol molecules are displaced by ions in the tear film. This displacement process occurs over several minutes and enhances the ocular comfort observed for Betoptic Suspension.

Pre-clinical Safety Data: There are no pre-clinical data of relevance to the prescriber which are additional to that already included in other sections of the SPC.

Pharmaceutical particulars
List of excipients: Benzalkonium Chloride; Poly (styrene divinylbenzene) sulphonic acid; Carbomer; Boric Acid; Mannitol; Disodium Edetate; N-Lauroylsarcosine; Hydrochloric acid and/or Sodium Hydroxide; Purified Water.

Incompatibilities: Not Applicable.

Shelf life: 24 months.

Special precautions for storage: There are no special storage requirements for Betoptic Suspension.

Nature and contents of container: BETOPTIC SUSPENSION is packaged as a 5 mL label fill in a 5 mL natural low density polyethylene (LDPE), DROP-TAINER* with a LDPE dispensing plug and a 15 mm white polypropylene closure. The DROP-TAINER* utilises a tamper evident closure with a break away ring.

Instructions for use/handling: Shake before each use. Discard product 1 month after first opening.

Marketing authorisation number PL 0649/0145

Date of approval/revision of SPC 22 August 1997/ 16 April 1998

Legal category POM

BSS* STERILE IRRIGATING SOLUTION

Description BSS Sterile Irrigating Solution is a sterile balanced salt solution, each mL containing Sodium Chloride 0.64%, Potassium Chloride 0.075%, Calcium Chloride Dihydrate 0.048%, Magnesium Chloride Hexahydrate 0.03%, Sodium Acetate Trihydrate 0.39%, Sodium Citrate Dihydrate 0.17%, Sodium Hydroxide and/or Hydrochloric Acid (to adjust pH), and Water for Injection.

Clinical applications BSS Sterile Irrigating solution is an isotonic solution for use in irrigating tissues of the eyes.

Indications and usage: For use as an extraocular and intraocular irrigating solution.

Warnings:

- NOT FOR INJECTION OF INTRAVENOUS INFUSION.
- DO NOT USE ADDITIVES WITH THIS PRODUCT; TISSUE DAMAGE COULD RESULT.
- Do not use unless product is clear, seal is intact, vacuum is present and container is undamaged.
- Do not use if product is discoloured or contains a precipitate.
- SINGLE patient use only. The contents of this bottle or bag should not be used in more than one patient.
- This solution contains no preservative, unused contents should be discarded.

Precautions: Open under aseptic conditions only. Studies suggest that intraocular irrigating solutions which are iso-osmotic with normal aqueous fluids should be used with caution in diabetic patients undergoing vitrectomy since intraoperative lens changes have been observed.

There have been reports of corneal clouding or oedema following ocular sugery in which BSS Sterile Irrigating Solution was used as an irrigating solution.

Adverse reactions: Irrigation or any trauma to the corneal endothelium may result in corneal swelling or bullous keratopathy.

Postoperative inflammatory reactions as well as incidents or corneal oedema and corneal decompensation have been reported.

Dosage and administration: This irrigating solution should be used according to standard format for each surgical procedure.

15 ml Steri-Unit Drop-Tainer dispensers: If the blister or paper backing is damaged or broken, sterility of the enclosed bottle cannot be assured.

Open under aseptic conditions only.

The adaptor plug is designed to accept an ophthalmic irrigating needle. Intra-ocular tissue may be irrigated by attaching the needle to the Steri-Unit Drop-Tainer Bottle as follows:

1. Aseptically remove the Drop-Tainer by peeling off the paper backing.
2. Snap on surgical irrigator needle. Push well to ensure it is firmly in place.
3. Test patency of the assembly.

Squeeze out several drops before inserting into the anterior chamber. The needle should be removed from the chamber prior to releasing pressure to prevent suction.

250 ml and 500 ml glass bottles and 250 ml and 500 ml Viaflex containers:

Bottles: Use an administration set with an air inlet in the plastic spike since the bottle does not contain a separate airway tube. Follow directions of the particular administration set to be used. Pull the tab to remove the outer aluminium ring and dust cover. Insert the spike aseptically into the bottle through the target area of the rubber stopper. Allow the fluid to flow and remove air from the tubing before irrigation begins.

Viaflex container:

1. Tear overwrap down side at slit and remove solution container.
2. Suspend container from eyelet support.
3. Remove plastic protector from outlet port at bottom of container. Attach administration set.
4. Attach administration set. Follow directions of the particular administration set to be used.
5. Allow the fluid to flow and remove air from the tubing before irrigation begins.

How supplied: 15 ml Steri-Unit Drop-Tainer dispensers, 250 and 500 ml glass infusion bottles and 500 ml Viaflex Containers (polyvinyl chloride).

All sterilised by steam.

Storage: Store at 8–27°C.
CE 0123

BSS PLUS*

Presentation STERILE INTRAOCULAR IRRIGATING SOLUTION

(Balanced Salt Solution Enriched with Bicarbonate, Dextrose and Glutathione)

Description BSS PLUS is a sterile intraocular irrigating solution for use during all intraocular surgical procedures, even those requiring a relatively long intraocular perfusion time (e.g., pars plana vitrectomy, phacoemulsification, extracapsular cataract extraction/lens aspiration, anterior segment reconstruction, etc.). The solution does not contain a preservative and should be prepared just prior to use in surgery.

Part I: Part I is a sterile 480 ml solution in a 500 ml single-dose bottle to which the Part II concentrate is added.

Each ml of Part I contains: Sodium Chloride 7.44 mg, Potassium Chloride 0.395 mg, Dibasic Sodium Phosphate 0.433 mg, Sodium Bicarbonate 2.19 mg, Hydrochloric Acid and/or Sodium Hydroxide (to adjust pH), in Water for Injection.

Part II: Part II is a sterile concentrate in a (20 ml) single-dose vial for addition to Part I.

Each ml of Part II contains: Calcium Chloride Dihydrate 3.85 mg, Magnesium Chloride Hexahydrate 5 mg, Dextrose 23 mg, Glutathione Disulfide (Oxidized Glutathione) 4.6 mg, in Water for Injection.

After addition of BSS PLUS Part II to the Part I bottle, each ml of the reconstituted product contains: Sodium Chloride 7.14 mg, Potassium Chloride 0.38 mg, Calcium Chloride Dihydrate 0.154 mg, Magnesium Chloride Hexahydrate 0.2 mg, Dibasic Sodium Phosphate 0.42 mg, Sodium Bicarbonate 2.1 mg, Dextrose 0.92 mg, Glutathione Disulfide (Oxidized Glutathione) 0.184 mg, Hydrochloric Acid and/or Sodium Hydroxide (to adjust pH), in water for injection. The reconstituted product has a pH of approximately 7.4. Osmolality is approximately 305 mOsm.

Clinical applications None of the components of BSS PLUS are foreign to the eye, and BSS PLUS has no pharmacological action. Human perfused cornea studies have shown BSS PLUS to be an effective irrigation solution for providing corneal detumescence and maintaining corneal endothelial integrity during intraocular perfusion. An *in vivo* study in rabbits has shown that BSS PLUS is more suitable than normal saline or Balanced Salt Solution for intravitreal irrigation because BSS PLUS contains the appropriate bicarbonate, pH, and ionic composition necessary for the maintenance of normal retinal electrical activity. Human *in vivo studies* have demonstrated BSS PLUS to be safe and effective when used during surgical procedures such as pars plana vitrectomy, phacoemulsification, cataract extraction/lens aspiration, and anterior segment reconstruction.

Indications and usage: BSS PLUS is indicated for use as an intraocular irrigating solution during intraocular surgical procedures involving perfusion of the eye.

Contra-indications: There are no specific contraindications to the use of BSS PLUS. However, contraindications for the surgical procedure during which BSS PLUS is to be used should be strictly adhered to.

Warnings: For IRRIGATION during ophthalmic surgery only. Not for injection or intravenous infusion. Do not use unless product is clear, seal is intact, vacuum is present and container is undamaged. Do not use if product is discolored or contains a precipitate.

Precautions: DO NOT USE BSS PLUS UNTIL PART I IS FULLY RECONSTITUTED WITH PART II. Discard unused contents. BSS PLUS does not contain a preservative. Therefore, do not use this container for more than one patient. Do not use additives other than BSS PLUS Concentrate Part II with this product. Tissue damage could result if other drugs are added to product. DISCARD ANY UNUSED PORTION SIX HOURS AFTER PREPARATION. Studies suggest that intraocular irrigating solutions which are iso-osmotic with normal aqueous fluids should be used with caution in diabetic patients undergoing vitrectomy since intraoperative lens changes have been observed.

There have been reports of corneal clouding or edema following ocular surgery in which BSS PLUS was used as an irrigating solution. As in all surgical procedures appropriate measures should be taken to minimize trauma to the cornea and other ocular tissues.

Preparation: Reconstitute BSS PLUS Sterile Intraocular Irrigating Solution just prior to use in surgery. Follow the same strict aseptic procedures in the reconstitution of BSS PLUS as is used for intravenous additives. Pull the tab to remove the outer aluminium ring and dust cover from the BSS PLUS Part I (480 ml) bottle. Remove the blue flip-off seal from the BSS PLUS Part II (20 ml) vial, respectively. Clean and disinfect the rubber stoppers on both containers by using sterile alcohol wipes. Transfer the contents of the Part II vial to the Part I bottle using a BSS PLUS Vacuum Transfer Device (provided). Gently agitate the contents to mix the solution. Place a sterile cap on the bottle. Remove the tear-off portion of the label. Record the time and date of reconstitution and the patient's name on the bottle label.

Adverse reactions: Postoperative inflammatory reactions as well as incidents of corneal edema and corneal decompensation have been reported. Their relationship to the use of BSS PLUS has not been established.

Overdosage: The solution has no pharmacological action and thus no potential for overdosage. However, as with any intraocular surgical procedure, the duration of intraocular manipulation should be kept to a minimum.

Dosage and administration: The solution should be used according to the technique standardly employed by the operating surgeon. Use an administration set with an air inlet in the plastic spike since the bottle does not contain a separate airway tube. Follow the directions for the particular administration set to be used. Insert the spike aseptically into the bottle through the target area of the rubber stopper. Allow the fluid to flow to remove air from the tubing before intraocular irrigation begins. If a second bottle is necessary to complete the surgical procedure ensure that the vacuum is vented from the second bottle BEFORE attachment to the administration set.

How supplied: BSS PLUS is supplied in two packages for reconstitution prior to use:
a 500 ml bottle containing 480 ml, (Part I) sterilized by steam and 20 ml vial (PartII) sterilized by filtration.

See the *Precautions* and *Preparation* section for information concerning reconstitution of the solution.

Storage: Store Part I and Part II at 8° -27°C. Discard prepared solution after six hours.
CE 0123

CILOXAN*

Presentation A sterile ophthalmic solution containing 0.35% w/v ciprofloxacin hydrochloride (equivalent to 0.3% w/v ciprofloxacin base) and preserved with benzalkonium chloride 0.006% w/v.

Uses Ciloxan is indicated for the treatment of corneal ulcers and superficial infections of the eye and adnexa caused by susceptible strains of bacteria.

Dosage and administration

Adults:

Superficial ocular infection: The usual dose is one or two drops in the affected eye(s) four times a day. In severe infections, the dosage for the first two days may be one or two drops every two hours during waking hours.

Corneal ulcers: Ciloxan must be administered in the following intervals, even during night time: On the first day, instill 2 drops into the affected eye every 15 minutes for the first six hours and then 2 drops into the affected eye every 30 minutes for the remainder of the day. On the second day, instill 2 drops in the affected eye hourly.

On the third through the fourteenth day, place two drops in the affected eye every 4 hours. If the patient needs to be treated longer than 14 days, the dosing regimen is at the discretion of the attending physician.

For either indication a maximum duration of therapy of 21 days is recommended.

Children: The safety and efficacy of Ciloxan in children under the age of 1 year has not been established.

Elderly: There are no special prescribing instructions for the elderly.

Contra-indications, warnings, etc

Contra-indications: Hypersensitivity to any component of this medication. The use of Ciloxan is also contra-indicated in patients with hypersensitivity to other quinolones.

Precautions: As with other antibacterial preparations, prolonged use of ciprofloxacin may result in overgrowth of nonsusceptible organisms, including fungi. If superinfection occurs, appropriate therapy should be initiated. Whenever clinical judgement dictates, the patient should be examined with the aid of magnification, such as slit lamp biomicroscopy and, where appropriate, fluorescein staining.

Ciprofloxacin should be discontinued at the first appearance of a skin rash or any other sign of hypersensitivity reaction.

Serious and occasionally fatal hypersensitivity (anaphylactic) reactions, some following the first dose, have been reported in patients receiving systemic quinolone therapy. Some reactions were accompanied by cardiovascular collapse, loss of consciousness, tingling, pharyngeal or facial edema, dyspnea, urticaria, and itching. Only a few patients had a history of hypersensitivity reactions. Serious anaphylactic reactions require immediate emergency treatment with epinephrine and other resuscitation measures, including oxygen, intravenous fluids, intravenous antihistamines, corticosteroids, pressor amines and airway management, as clinically indicated.

During therapy, soft contact lenses should not be worn.

Use in pregnancy: As there are no controlled studies in pregnancy women Ciloxan should be used during pregnancy only if the potential benefit justifies the potential risk to the foetus.

Use by nursing mothers: Orally administered ciprofloxacin is excreted in the human milk. Excretion of ciprofloxacin into human milk following topical ophthalmic administration has not been investigated. Therefore caution should be exercised when Ciloxan is administered to nursing mothers.

Adverse reactions: Local burning and ocular discomfort may occur as well as itching, foreign body sensation, lid margin crusting, crystals/scales, conjunctival hyperemia and bad taste following installation. Additionally, corneal staining, keratopathy/keratitis, allergic reactions, lid edema, tearing, photophobia, corneal infiltrates, nausea and decreased vision have been reported. Hypersensitivity reactions cannot be excluded.

In patients with corneal ulcer and frequent administration of the drug white precipitates have been observed which resolved after continuous application of the Ciloxan. The precipitate does not preclude the continued use of Ciloxan nor does it adversely affect the clinical course of the ulcer or the visual outcome. The onset of the precipitate was within 24 hours to 7 days after starting therapy. Resolution of the precipitate varied from immediately to 13 days after therapy commencing.

Drug interactions: Specific drug interaction studies have not been conducted with ophthalmic ciprofloxacin. However, the systemic administration of some quinolones has been shown to elevate plasma concentrations of theophylline, to interfere with the metabolism of caffeine, and to enhance the effect of the oral anticoagulant, warfarin, and its derivatives. Transient elevations in serum creatinine has been reported in patients receiving cyclosporin concomitantly with systemic ciprofloxacin.

Treatment of overdosage: A topical overdose of Ciloxan may be flushed from the eyes with warm tap water.

Pharmaceutical precautions Incompatible with alkaline solutions. Keep the container tightly closed. Store at room temperature (below 25°C). Discard contents one month after opening.

Legal category POM.

Package quantities 5 ml containers.

Further information Ciprofloxacin has cidal and inhibitory activities against bacteria which result from an interference with DNA gyrase, an enzyme needed by the bacterium for the synthesis of DNA. Thus, vital information from the bacterial chromosomes cannot be transcribed, which causes a break-down of bacterial metabolism.

Ciprofloxacin has a very high *in vitro* activity against almost all Gram negative microorganisms including *Pseudomonas aeruginosa*. It is also effective against Gram positive bacteria, such as staphylococci and streptococci. Anaerobes are in general less susceptible.

Resistance development against ciprofloxacin occurs infrequently. A plasmid mediated bacterial resistance does not appear to occur with the fluoroquinolone class of antibiotics.

The arthropathogenic potential of some quinolones in immature animals after oral administration is recognised. Topical ocular administration of ciprofloxacin to immature animals did not cause any arthopathy and there is no evidence that the ophthalmic dosage form has any effect on the weight bearing points.

Product licence number 0649/0125.

ILUBE* EYE DROPS

Qualitative and quantitative composition Acetylcysteine BP 5% w/v.

Pharmaceutical form Sterile Ophthalmic Solution.

Clinical particulars
Therapeutic indications: Ilube Eye Drops are artificial tears with mucolytic and lubricant properties, indicated for the relief of dry eye syndromes associated with deficient tear secretion, impaired or abnormal mucus production.

Posology and method of administration: Ilube Eye Drops are administered by topical instillation into the conjunctival sac. The usual dose is 1 or 2 drops instilled into the affected eye three or four times daily.

Contra-indications: Known hypersensitivity to any component.

Special warnings and precautions for use: Ilube Eye Drops contain benzalkonium chloride as preservative and, therefore, should not be used to treat patients who wear soft contact lenses. Discontinue use if discomfort, increased reddening or irritation occurs and persists.

Interactions with other medicaments and other forms of interaction: None known.

Pregnancy and lactation: Not applicable.

Effects on ability to drive and use machinery: None known.

Undesirable effects: None known.

Overdose: None known.

Pharmacological properties
Pharmacodynamic properties: Acetylcysteine, a derivative of the naturally occurring amino acid L-cysteine, is neither an enzyme nor a detergent. Acetylcysteine has been shown to dramatically reduce the viscosity and tenacity of sputum. The liquefying action is due to the presence of a free sulphydryl group which opens up disulphide bonds present in mucus. This pharmacological action of acetylcysteine is of benefit to patients suffering from ocular mucus abnormality.

Acetylcysteine has marked mucolytic properties which reduce the viscosity and tenacity of mucus in the eyes. This combined with the emollient properties of hypromellose, ensures lubrication and soothing relief for dry eye syndrome.

Pharmacokinetic properties: No specific work has been carried out on the pharmacokinetic properties of acetylcysteine when used as a topical preparation for the eye. Acetylcysteine has marked mucolytic properties which reduce the viscosity and tenacity of mucus in the eye. This, combined with the emollient properties of hypromellose, ensures lubrication and soothing relief for dry eye syndromes.

Preclinical safety data: There are no preclinical data of relevance to the prescriber which are additional to that already included in other sections of the SPC.

Pharmaceutical particulars
List of excipients: Inactive excipients: Disodium edetate PhEur, hydroxypropylmethylcellulose USP, benzalkonium chloride BP, sodium hydroxide BP, purified water PhEur.

Incompatibilities: None known.

Shelf life: 24 months (unopened), 1 month (after first opening).

Special precautions for storage: Store below 25°C. Protect from light. Discard 28 days after first opening the pack.

Nature and contents of container: 15 ml or 10 ml amber type 1 glass bottle with polypropylene screw cap lined with a rubber wad. The bottle and cap are closed with a tamper evident shrink-sleeve (alternatively tamper evidency is provided by the presence of a sticker covering the opening edge of the outer carton). The dropper assembly comprises a rubber teat, a plastic cap and a polycarbonate pipette.

Instructions for use/handling: Do not touch dropper to any surface as this may contaminate the contents. Keep tightly closed after first opening.

Marketing authorisation number PL 00649/0144

Date of approval/revision of SPC 18 June 1997

Legal category POM.

IOPIDINE 0.5% OPHTHALMIC SOLUTION*

Qualitative and quantitative composition Iopidine 0.5% Ophthalmic Solution contains apraclonidine hydrochloride 0.5% (as base) and benzalkonium chloride 0.01% as preservative, sodium acetate (trihydrate) 0.07%, sodium chloride 0.757%, hydrochloric acid/sodium hydroxide q.s. to pH 5.3 and purified water to 100%.

Pharmaceutical form Iopidine 0.5% Ophthalmic Solution is a sterile, buffered isotonic ophthalmic solution.

Clinical particulars
Therapeutic indications: Iopidine 0.5% Ophthalmic Solution is indicated for short-term adjunctive therapy of chronic glaucoma in patients on maximally tolerated medical therapy who require additional IOP reduction to delay laser treatment or glaucoma surgery.

The IOP lowering efficacy of Iopidine 0.5% Ophthalmic Solution diminishes over time in most patients. Although some patients have received successful treatment with Iopidine 0.5% Ophthalmic Solution for longer periods, the benefit for most patients is less than one month.

The addition of Iopidine 0.5% Ophthalmic Solution to patients already using two aqueous suppressing drugs (i.e. beta-blockers plus carbonic anhydrase inhibitor) as part of their maximally tolerated medical therapy may not provide additional benefit. This is because Iopidine 0.5% Ophthalmic Solution is an aqueous suppressing drug and the addition of a third aqueous suppressant may not significantly reduce IOP.

Posology and method of administration: One drop of Iopidine 0.5% Ophthalmic Solution should be instilled into the affected eye(s) three times per day (t.i.d.). Since Iopidine 0.5% Ophthalmic Solution will be used with other ocular glaucoma therapies, an approximate five minute interval between instillation of each medication should be observed to prevent washout of the previous dose. The maximum recommended duration of therapy is one month due to loss of effect over time. However, some patients may benefit from treatment with Iopidine 0.5% Ophthalmic Solution for longer periods.

Clinical studies to establish safety and efficacy in children have not been conducted and, therefore, Iopidine 0.5% Ophthalmic Solution is not recommended for use in children.

There are no special precautions for administration to the elderly.

Contra-indications: Iopidine 0.5% Ophthalmic Solution is contra-indicated in patients with a history of severe or unstable and uncontrolled cardiovascular disease.

Iopidine 0.5% Ophthalmic Solution is contra-indicated in patients with hypersensitivity to any component of the formulation or to systemic clonidine and in patients receiving monoamine oxidase inhibitors, systemic sympathomimetics or tricyclic antidepressants.

Iopidine 0.5% Ophthalmic Solution is preserved with benzalkonium chloride and should not be used whilst the patient is wearing soft contact lenses.

Special warnings and special precautions for use
Warnings: For topical ophthalmic use only. Not for injection or oral ingestion. While the topical administration of Iopidine 0.5% Ophthalmic Solution had minimal effect on heart rate or blood pressure in clinical studies evaluating glaucoma patients including those with cardiovascular disease, the possibility of a vasovagal attack should be considered and caution should be exercised in patients with a history of such episodes. Iopidine 0.5% Ophthalmic Solution should be used with caution in patients with a history of angina, severe coronary insufficiency, recent myocardial infarction, overt cardiac failure, cerebrovascular disease, chronic renal failure, Raynaud's disease or thromboangiitis obliterans. Caution in and monitoring of depressed patients are advised since apraclonidine has been rarely associated with depression.

In end-stage glaucoma, if reduction in vision occurs immediately following Iopidine 0.5% Ophthalmic Solution therapy, treatment should be suspended.

Precautions: As with all glaucoma patients on maximally tolerated medical therapy, those who are treated with Iopidine 0.5% Ophthalmic Solution to delay surgery should have frequent follow-up examinations and treatment should be discontinued if the intraocular pressure rises significantly. The loss of effect which occurs over time in most patients appears to be an individual occurrence with a variable time of onset and should be closely monitored. Furthermore, these patients should have their visual fields evaluated periodically.

No data are available on the topical use of apraclonidine in patients with renal or hepatic failure. Systemic absorption of apraclonidine following topical administration is low, resulting in plasma levels less than 1.0 ng/ml. Nonetheless, since the structurally related compound clonidine is partly metabolized in the liver and undergoes a significant increase in half-life in patients with severe renal impairment, close monitoring of patients with impaired renal or hepatic function is advised. Close monitoring of cardiovascular parameters in patients with impaired liver function is also advised as the systemic dosage form of clonidine is partly metabolised in the liver.

Use of Iopidine 0.5% Ophthalmic Solution can result in an ocular intolerance reaction characterised wholly or in part by the symptoms of ocular hyperaemia, pruritis, discomfort, tearing, foreign body sensation, and oedema of the lids and conjunctiva. If such ocular symptoms occur, Iopidine 0.5% Ophthalmic Solution therapy should be discontinued. Also, preclinical data suggest that there may be patients who develop a contact sensitisation response with repeated use of the drug. Ocular intolerance responses are more common in patients treated for more than one month.

Discontinuation of therapy in the event of rising intraocular pressure should coincide with the initiation of alternative therapy, or pressure-relieving surgery. Since apraclonidine is a potent depressor of intraocular pressure, patients who develop an exaggerated reduction in intraocular pressure should be closely monitored.

Interaction with other medicaments and other forms of interaction: No drug interactions were reported in those patients who were receiving concomitant medication for glaucoma or for other ocular disorders or for any systemic disease present during clinical studies.

Although no specific drug interactions with topical glaucoma drugs or systemic medicaments were identified in clinical studies of Iopidine 0.5% Ophthalmic Solution, the possibility of an additive or potentiating effect with CNS depressants (alcohol, barbiturates, opiates, sedatives, anaethetics) should be considered. Iopidine 0.5% Ophthalmic Solution has been used as additive therapy with topical epinephrine and dipivefrin without evidence of adverse interaction. However, there is a theoretical possibility that use of Iopidine 0.5% Ophthalmic Solution in conjunction with topical sympathomimetics may give rise to a systemic pressor response and blood pressure should be checked initially in patients receiving these drug combinations.

The possibility exists for an additive or potentiating effect with CNS depressants; tricyclic antidepressants have been reported to blunt the hypotensive effect of systemic clonidine. It is not known whether or not the concurrent use of these agents with Iopidine 0.5% Ophthalmic Solution can lead to a reduction in IOP lowering effect. No data on the level of circulating catecholamines after apraclonidine withdrawal are available. Caution, however, is advised in patients taking tricyclic antidepressants which can affect the metabolism and uptake of circulating amines.

An additive hypotensive effect has been reported with the combination of systemic clonidine and neuroleptic therapy. Systemic clonidine may inhibit the production of catecholamine in response to insulin-induced hypoglycaemia and mask the signs and symptoms of hypoglycaemia.

Since apraclonidine may reduce pulse and blood pressure, caution in using drugs such as beta-blockers (ophthalmic and systemic), antihypertensives, and cardiac glycosides is advised. Patients using cardiovascular drugs concurrently with Iopidine 0.5% Ophthalmic Solution should have pulse and blood pressure frequently monitored. Caution should be exercised with simultaneous use of clonidine and other similar pharmacologic agents.

Pregnancy and lactation: There are no studies of Iopidine 0.5% Ophthalmic Solution in pregnant women. Iopidine 0.5% Ophthalmic Solution should be used during pregnancy only if the potential benefit to the mother justifies the potential risk to the fetus.

Animal studies have been conducted which have demonstrated an absence of teratogenic effects in rats and rabbits. Slight fetal toxicity has been observed when pregnant animals were dosed systemically with apraclonidine over the entire period of organogenesis at exposure levels (mg/kg/d) of 60 times the recommended dosage regimen for Iopidine 0.5% Ophthalmic Solution. It is not known if topically applied apraclonidine is excreted in human milk. Since many drugs are excreted in human milk, caution should be exercised when Iopidine 0.5% Ophthalmic Solution is administered to nursing women.

Effects on ability to drive and use machines: since clonidine-like drugs may cause drowsiness, patients so affected are advised not drive or operate machinery.

Undesirable effects: Use of Iopidine 0.5% Ophthalmic Solution can lead to an ocular intolerance reaction characterised wholly or in part by the symptoms of hyperaemia, pruritus, discomfort, tearing, foreign body sensation, and oedema of the lids and conjunctiva. The pattern of the reactions was thought to be allergy-like. The mean onset of these reactions was 44 days (range 1–127 days). If such ocular intolerance symptoms occur, Iopidine 0.5% Ophthalmic Solution should be discontinued.

In clinical studies, the overall discontinuation rate related to Iopidine 0.5% Ophthalmic Solution was 15%. The most commonly reported events leading to discontinuation included (in decreasing order of frequency) hyperaemia, pruritus, tearing, discomfort, lid oedema, dry mouth, and foreign body sensation.

The following adverse reactions (incidences) were reported in clinical studies of Iopidine 0.5% Ophthalmic Solution as being possibly, probably, or definitely related to therapy:

Ocular: Hyperaemia (13%), pruritus (10%), discomfort (6%), tearing (4%). The following adverse reactions were reported in less than 3% of the patients: lid oedema, blurred vision, foreign body sensation, dry eye, conjunctivitis, discharge, blanching. The following adverse reactions were reported in less than 1% of patients: lid margin crusting, conjunctival follicles, conjunctival oedema, oedema, abnormal vision, pain, lid disorder, keratitis, blepharitis, photophobia, corneal staining, lid erythema, blepharoconjunctivitis, irritation, corneal erosion, corneal infiltrate, keratopathy, lid scales, lid retraction.

Nonocular: Body as a whole: The following adverse reactions were reported in less than 3% of the patients: headache, asthenia. The following adverse reactions (incidences) were reported in less than 1% of the patients: chest pain, abnormal coordination, malaise, facial oedema.

Cardiovasular: The following adverse reactions were reported in less than 1% of the patients: peripheral oedema, arrhythmia. Although there were no reports of bradycardia related to Iopidine 0.5% Ophthalmic Solution from clinical studies, the possibility of its occurrence based on apraclonidine's alpha-2-adrenergic agonist effect should be considered.

Central nervous system: The following adverse reactions were reported in less than 1% of the patients: somnolence, dizziness, nervousness, depression, insomnia, paraesthesia.

Digestive system: Dry mouth (10%). The following adverse reactions were reported in less than 1% of the patients: constipation, nausea.

Musculoskeletal: Myalgia (0.2%).

Respiratory system: Dry nose (2%). The following adverse reactions were reported in less than 1% of the patients: rhinitis, dyspnea, pharyngitis, asthma.

Skin: The following adverse reactions were reported in less than 1% of the patients: contact dermatitis, dermatitis.

Special senses: Taste perversion (3%), parosmia (0.2%).

Overdose: Iopidine 0.5% Ophthalmic Solution may be flushed from the eyes with water. While no instances of human ingestion of Iopidine 0.5% Ophthalmic Solution are known, overdose with the oral form of clonidine has been reported to cause hypotension, transient hypertension, asthenia, vomiting, irritability, diminished or absent reflexes, lethargy, somnolence, sedation or coma, pallor, hypothermia, bradycardia, conduction defects, arrhythmias, dryness of the mouth, miosis, apnoea, respiratory depression, hypoventilation, and seizure. Treatment of a oral overdose includes supportive and symptomatic therapy; a patent airway should be maintained. Haemodialysis is of limited value, since a maximum of 5% of circulating drug is removed.

Pharmacological properties

Pharmacodynamic properties: Apraclonidine is a relatively selective alpha-2-adrenergic agonist which does not possess significant membrane stabilising (local anaesthetic) activity. When instilled into the eye, apraclonidine has the action of reducing intraocular pressure. Ophthalmic apraclonidine has minimal effect on cardiovascular parameters. Aqueous fluorophotometry studies in man suggest that the mechanism of the ocular hypotensive action of apraclonidine is related to a reduction in aqueous formation. The onset of action of apraclonidine can usually be noted within one hour and the maximum intraocular pressure reduction usually occurs three to five hours after application of a single dose.

Pharmacokinetic properties: Following topical ocular administration to New Zealand White rabbits, apraclonidine reached peak concentrations after two hours in the aqueous humour, iris, ciliary body and lens. The cornea exhibited the greatest concentration and peaked at the earliest time point (20 minutes). The tissue distribution of apraclonidine from highest to lowest concentration in microgram equivalents per gram of tissue was cornea, iris-ciliary body, aqueous humour, lens and vitreous humour. The elimination half-life of apraclonidine from the aqueous humour was determined to be approximately two hours.

Plasma concentration of apraclonidine following three times daily, bilateral, topical ocular dosing of Iopidine 0.5% Ophthalmic Solution to normal human volunteers was less than 1.0 ng/ml. A steady state level was attained after five days of dosing. The half-life of the drug was calculated to be eight hours.

Preclinical safety data: Administration of apraclonidine intravenously and via the topical ocular route to both cats and monkeys resulted in a reduced anterior segment blood flow, whereas flow to the posterior segment, i.e. retina, choroid or optic nerve head, was not affected. Chronic treatment of primates with apraclonidine hydrochloride 1.5% ocularly three times a day for one year did not result in morphologic effects which would be indicative of vasoconstriction of the anterior or posterior segments of the eye. Although ocular blood flow studies have not been conducted in humans, the animal studies provide a basis for the safe use of this drug in the treatment of chronic glaucoma.

Acute toxicity: Acute toxicity was evaluated intravenously and orally in rats and mice and orally in primates. The approximate oral LD_{50} ranged from 5.04 mg/kg (mice) to 63.9 mg/kg (rats); no lethalities were observed in primates at 55 mg/kg. In rodents toxic signs included lethargy, hypothermia, corneal cloudiness, and haemorrhagic areas as well as distension of the gastrointestinal tract. Pronounced inhibition of gastrointestinal motility is considered the cause of mortality in mice. The reduced intestinal motility was observed in mice after intravenous administration of 0.1 mg/kg. Lethargy and disturbed defecation were found in monkeys after oral administration of 55 mg/kg. The normal human dose from ophthalmic use is 0.03 mg/kg/d in divided doses.

Subchronic and chronic toxicity: Rabbits tolerated apraclonidine hydrochloride solutions of 0.5%, 1% or 1.5% (2 drops t.i.d.), over a period of one month without signs of systemic toxicity. Conjunctival irritation and minimal corneal cloudiness (at 1.5%) were sporadic observations.

Rats and mice received daily oral doses of up to 1.2 mg/kg and 2 mg/kg, respectively, over a period of 13 weeks. Mortalities occurred in rats at 1.2 mg/kg/d and in mice at 1.6 mg/kg/d. Pharmacotoxic reactions included disturbed defecation and distended abdomen plus corneal cloudiness in female mice of the high-dose group. Rats in the high-dose group that died before the end of the study showed toxic effects on the immune system, but these effects were not seen in animals which survived to the end of the study. No drug-related toxic or ophthalmic findings were observed when monkeys received apraclonidine hydrochloride solutions of 0.5%, 1% and 1.5% by topical ocular administration t.i.d. for one year. Mild hepatocyte vacuolisation was observed in the group receiving the 1.5% solution.

Local tolerance: The topical ocular administration of apraclonidine hydrochloride solutions of 0.5%, 1% and 1.5% (2 drops instilled at 30 min intervals into one eye for 6 h) led to dose-dependent conjunctival and corneal irritation in the rabbit.

Assessment of the sensitisation potential in the guinea pig proved apraclonidine hydrochloride to be moderately sensitising.

Mutagenic and tumorigenic potential: Mutagenicity testing of apraclonidine hydrochloride using different standard systems all produced negative results.

Two-year long-term studies evaluating the carcinogenic potential in rats (at doses of 0.1, 0.3 and 1.0 mg/kg/d) and mice (at doses of 0.1, 0.3 and 0.6 mg/kg/d) revealed no signs of a tumorigenic potential of apraclonidine hydrochloride. After 18 months of oral treatment both species (rats from 0.3 mg/kg/d and mice from 0.6 mg/kg/d) showed an increased incidence of ocular changes (mineralisation and vascularisation of the cornea, and keratitis). In addition, renal changes (mineralisation) were found in rats from 0.3 mg/kg/d onward.

Reproduction toxicity: Studies performed in rats and rabbits did not suggest any teratogenic action. Slight fetal toxicity was observed in pregnant animals which during the whole period of morphogenesis were systemically exposed to 60 times the apraclonidine hydrochloride dosage proposed for treatment with Iopidine 0.5% Ophthalmic Solution.

Pharmaceutical particulars

List of excipients: Inactive excipients in Iopidine 0.5% Ophthalmic Solution are sodium acetate (trihydrate), 0.07% sodium chloride 0.757%, hydrochloric acid and/or sodium hydroxide q.s. to pH 5.3 and purified water to 100%. The solution is preserved with benzalkonium chloride 0.01%.

Incompatibilities: None known.

Shelf life: Twenty four months (unopened), one month (after bottle is opened).

Special precautions for storage: Store at room temperature (15–25°C). Protect from light.

Nature and contents of container: Iopidine 0.5% Ophthalmic Solution will be packaged as 5 ml in a 5 ml, and 10 ml in a 10 ml, white LDPE Drop-Tainer* with a natural LDPE dispensing plug and white polypropylene closure.

Instructions for use/handling: Do not touch dropper tip to any surface as this may contaminate the contents. If the drop of medication is not retained in the eye upon dosing for any reason, instil another drop.

Marketing authorisation number 0649/0132.

Date of approval/revision of SPC 29 December 1994.

Legal category POM.

IOPIDINE* 1.0% OPHTHALMIC SOLUTION

Qualitative and quantitative composition Iopidine 1.0% Ophthalmic Solution contains apraclonidine hydrochloride 1.15% w/v HSE (equivalent to apraclonidine 1% w/v).

Pharmaceutical form Eye drops.

Clincal particulars

Therapeutic indications: Iopidine 1.0% Ophthalmic Solution is indicated to control or prevent postsurgical elevations in intraocular pressure that occur in patients after anterior segment laser surgery. (Clinical trials have been conducted in trabeculoplasty, iridotomy and capsulotomy).

Posology and method of administration:

Adults: One drop of Iopidine 1.0% Ophthalmic Solution should be instilled into the eye scheduled for operation one hour before initiating anterior segment laser surgery. A second drop should be instilled to the same eye immediately upon completion of the laser surgical procedure.

Children: Safety and effectiveness of Iopidine in children have not been established and therefore Iopidine 1.0% Ophthalmic Solution is not recommended for use in children.

Elderly: There are no special precautions for administration to the elderly.

Contra-indications: Iopidine 1.0% Ophthalmic Solution is contraindicated in patients with a history of severe or unstable and uncontrolled cardiovascular disease.

Iopidine 1.0% Ophthalmic Solution is contraindicated for children, for patients receiving monoamine oxidase inhibitor therapy, systemic sympathomimetic agents, tricyclic antidepressants, and for patients with hypersensitivity to any component of the preparation or to clonidine.

Special warnings and special precautions for use: *Warnings:* For topical ophthalmic use only. Not for injection or oral ingestion. While the topical administration of two drops of Iopidine 1.0% Ophthalmic Solution had minimal effect on heart rate or blood pressure in clinical studies evaluating patients undergoing anterior segment laser surgery, including those with cardiovascular disease, the possibility of a vasovagal attack should be considered and caution should be exercised in patients with a history of such episodes. Iopidine 1.0% Ophthalmic Solution should be used with caution in patients with a history of angina, severe coronary insufficiency, recent myocardial infarction, chronic renal failure, overt cardiac failure, cerebrovascular disease, Raynaud's disease or thromboangiitis obliterans. Caution in and monitoring of depressed patients are advised since apraclonidine has been rarely associated with depression.

Precautions: No data are available on the topical use of apraclonidine in patients with renal or hepatic failure. Systemic absorption of apraclonidine following topical administration is low, resulting in plasma levels less than 1.0 ng/ml. Nonetheless, since the structurally related compound clonidine is partly metabolised in the liver and undergoes a significant increased in half-life in patients with severe renal impairment, close monitoring of patients with impaired renal or hepatic function is advised. Close monitoring of cardiovascular parameters in patients with impaired liver function is also advised as the systemic dosage form of clonidine is partly metabolised in the liver.

Since apraclonidine is a potent depressor of intraocular pressure, patients who develop an exaggerated reduction in intraocular pressure should be closely monitored.

Interactions with other medicaments and other forms of interactions: No drug interactions were reported in those patients who were receiving concomitant medication for glaucoma or for other ocular disorders or for any systemic disease present during clinical studies.

Although no specific drug interactions with topical glaucoma drugs or systemic medicaments were identified in clinical studies of Iopidine 1.0% Ophthalmic Solution, the possibility of an additive or potentiating effect with CNS depressants (alcohol, barbiturates, opiates, sedatives, anaesthetics) should be considered. There is a theoretical possibility that use of Iopidine 1.0% Ophthalmic Solution in conjunction with topical sympathomimetics may give rise to a systemic pressor response and blood pressure should be checked initially in patients receiving these drug combinations.

The possibility exists for an additive or potentiating effect with CNS depressants; tricyclic antidepressants have been reported to blunt the hypotensive effect of systemic clonidine. It is not known whether or not the concurrent use of these agents with Iopidine 1.0% Ophthalmic Solution can lead to a reduction in IOP lowering effect. No data on the level of circulating catecholamines after apraclonidine withdrawal are available. Caution, however, is advised in patients taking tricyclic antidepressants which can affect the metabolism and uptake of circulating amines.

An additive hypotensive effect has been reported with the combination of systemic clonidine and neuroleptic therapy. Systemic clonidine may inhibit the production of catecholamine in response to insulin-induced hypoglycaemia and mask the signs and symptoms of hypoglycaemia.

Since apraclonidine may reduce pulse and blood pressure, caution in using drugs such as beta-blockers (ophthalmic and systemic), antihypertensives, and cardiac glycosides is advised. Patients using cardiovascular drugs concurrently with Iopidine 1.0% Ophthalmic Solution should have pulse and blood pressure frequently monitored. Caution should be exercised with simultaneous use of clonidine and other similar pharmacologic agents.

Pregnancy and lactation: There are no well controlled studies of Iopidine 1.0% Ophthalmic Solution in pregnant women. Iopidine 1.0% Ophthalmic Solution should be used in pregnancy only if the potential benefit to the mother justifies the potential risk to the foetus.

Animal studies have been conducted which have demonstrated an absence of teratogenic effects in rats and rabbits. Embryotoxicity has been observed when pregnant rabbits were dosed orally with doses of apraclonidine (doses >1.25 mg/kg/day) that were maternally toxic, and administered over the entire period of organogenesis at exposure levels >100 times the recommended daily dosage regimen for Iopidine 1.0% Ophthalmic Solution based on a 50 kg person. It is not known if topically applied apraclonidine is excreted in human milk. Because many drugs are excreted in human milk, caution should be exercised when Iopidine 1.0% Ophthalmic Solution is administered to nursing women.

Effects on ability to drive and use machines: Clonidine-like drugs may cause drowsiness; patients if so affected should not drive or operate machinery.

Undesirable effects: The following adverse reactions (incidences) were reported in clinical studies in Iopidine 1.0% Ophthalmic Solution in laser surgery as being possible, probably, or definitely related to therapy:

Ocular: Ocular hyperaemia (1.3%). The following adverse reactions were reported in less than 1% of the patients: upper lid elevation, ocular inflammation, conjunctival bleeding, mydriasis.

Nonocular: The following adverse reactions were reported in less than 1% of the patients: irregular heart rate, nasal decongestion. The following adverse events were observed in investigational studies dosing Iopidine 1.0% Ophthalmic Solution once or twice daily for up to 28 days in nonlaser studies:

Ocular: Conjunctival blanching, upper lid elevation, mydriasis, burning, discomfort, foreign body sensation, dryness, itching, hypotony, blurred or dimmed vision, allergic response, conjunctival microhaemorrhage.

Gastrointestinal: Abdominal pain, diarrhoea, stomach discomfort, emesis.

Cardiovascular: Bradycardia, vasovagal attacks, palpitations, orthostatic episode.

Central nervous system: Insomnia, dream disturbances, irritability, decreased libido.

Other: Taste abnormalities, dry mouth, nasal burning or dryness, headache, heat cold sensation, chest heaviness or burning, clammy or sweaty palms, body heat sensation, shortness of breath, increased pharyngeal secretion, extremity pain or numbness, fatigue, paresthesia, pruritus not associated with rash.

Overdose: In the case of accidental overdose, Iopidine 1% can be removed by rinsing the eye with water. While no instances of accidental or intentional ingestion of ophthalmic apraclonidine are known, overdose with the oral form of clonidine has been reported to cause hypotension, transient hypertension, asthenia, vomiting, irritability, diminished or absent reflexes, lethargy, somnolence, sedation or coma, pallor, hypothermia, bradycardia, conduction defects, arrhythmias, dryness of the mouth, miosis, apnea, respiratory depression, hypoventilation, and seizure. Treatment of an oral overdose includes supportive and symptomatic therapy, a patent airway should be maintained. Haemodialysis is of limited value since a maximum of 5% of circulating drug is removed.

Pharmacological properties

Pharmacodynamic properties: Apraclonidine is a relatively selective alpha-2-adrenergic agonist which does not possess significant membrane stabilising (local anaesthetic) activity. When instilled into the eye, apraclonidine has the action of reducing intraocular pressure. Ophthalmic apraclonidine has minimal effect on cardiovascular parameters. Aqueous fluorophotometry studies in man suggest that the mechanism of the ocular hypotensive action of apraclonidine is related to reduction in aqueous formation. The onset of action of Iopidine 1.0% Ophthalmic Solution can usually be noted within one hour and the maximum intraocular pressure reduction usually occurs three to five hours after application of a single dose.

Pharmacokinetic properties: Following topical ocular administration to New Zealand albino rabbits, apraclonidine reached peak concentrations after two hours in the aqueous humor, iris, ciliary body and lens. The cornea exhibited the greatest concentration and peaked at the earliest time point (20 minutes). The tissue distribution of apraclonidine from highest to lowest concentration in microgram equivalents per gram of tissue was cornea, iris-ciliary body, aqueous humour, lens and vitreous humour. The elimination half-life of apraclonidine from the aqueous humour was determined to be approximately two hours.

Plasma concentration of apraclonidine following three times daily, bilateral, topical ocular dosing of 0.5% apraclonidine ophthalmic solution to normal human volunteers was less than 1.0 ng/ml. A steady state level was attained after five days of dosing. The systemic elimination half-life of apraclonidine was approximately 8 hours.

Preclinical safety data: Administration of apraclonidine intravenously and via the topical ocular route to both cats and monkeys resulted in a reduced anterior segment blood flow whereas flow to the posterior segment (i.e. retina, choroid or optic nerve head) was not affected. Chronic treatment of primates with apraclonidine hydrochloride 1.5% ocularly three times a day for one year did not result in morphological effects.

Acute toxicity: Acute toxicity was evaluated intravenously and orally in rats and mice and orally in primates. The approximate oral LD_{50} ranged from 5.04 mg/kg (mice) to 63.9 mg/kg (rats); no lethalities were observed in primates at 55 mg/kg. In rodents toxic signs included lethargy, hypothermia, corneal cloudiness, and haemorrhagic areas as well as distension of the gastrointestinal tract. Pronounced inhibition of gastrointestinal motility is considered the cause of mortality in mice. The reduced intestinal motility was observed in mice after intravenous administration of 0.1 mg/kg. Lethargy and disturbed defecation were found in monkeys after oral administration of 55 mg/kg. The normal human dose from ophthalmic use is approximately 0.01 mg/kg/d.

Subchronic and chronic toxicity: Rabbits tolerated apraclonidine hydrochloride solutions of 0.5%, 1% or 1.5% (2 drops t.i.d.) over a period of one month without signs of systemic toxicity. Minimal corneal cloudiness was observed sporadically in some eyes receiving the 1.5% apraclonidine hydrochloride solution.

Rats and mice received daily oral doses of up to 1.2 mg/kg and 2 mg/kg, respectively, over a period of 13 weeks. Mortalities occurred in rats at 1.2 mg/kg/d and in mice at 1.6 mg/kg/d. Pharmacotoxic reactions included disturbed defecation and distended abdomen plus corneal cloudiness predominantly in female mice of the high-dose group. Rats in the high-dose group that died before the end of the study showed lymphocytic effects in the spleen and thymus, but these effects were not seen in animals which survived to the end of the study. No drug-related toxic or ophthalmic findings were observed when monkeys received apraclonidine hydrochloride solutions of 0.5%, 1% and 1.5% by topical ocular administration t.i.d. for one year.

Local tolerance: The topical ocular administration of apraclonidine hydrochloride solutions of 0.5%, 1% and 1.5% (2 drops instilled at 30 min intervals into one eye for 6 h) led to dose-dependent conjunctival and corneal irritation in the rabbit.

Assessment of the sensitisation potential in the guinea pig proved apraclonidine hydrochloride to be moderately sensitising.

Mutagenic and tumorigenic potential: Mutagenicity testing of apraclonidine hydrochloride using different standard systems all produced negative results.

Two-year long-term studies evaluating the carcinogenic potential in rats (at doses of 0.1, 0.3 and 1.0 mg/kg/d) and mice (at doses of 0.1, 0.3 and 0.6 mg/kg/d) revealed no signs of a carcinogenic potential of apraclonidine hydrochloride. Both species showed an increased incidence of ocular changes (mineralisation and neo-vascularisation of the cornea, and keratitis), which are considered related to the pharmacological effect of the drug in reducing the tear film. In addition, renal changes (mineralisation) were found in rats from 0.3 mg/kg/d onward.

Reproduction toxicity: Studies performed in rats and rabbits did not suggest any teratogenic effects of apraclonidine. Embryotoxicity has been observed when pregnant rabbits were dosed orally with doses of apraclonidine (doses >1.25 mg/kg/day) that were maternally toxic, and administered over the entire period of organogenesis at exposure levels >100 times the recommended daily dosage regimen for Iopidine 1.0% Ophthalmic Solution based on a 50 kg person.

Pharmaceutical particulars

List of excipients: Inactive excipients in Iopidine 1.0% Ophthalmic Solution are Sodium acetate (trihydrate), sodium chloride, hydrochloric acid and/or sodium hydroxide (to adjust pH), purified water.

Incompatibilities: None known.

Shelf life: 24 months.

Special precautions for storage: Store below 25°C. Protect from light.

Nature and contents of container: Two sealed LDPE form/fill/seal single-dose containers each containing 0.25 ml and wrapped in a foil pouch. Preservative free.

Instructions for use/handling: If the drop of medication is not retained in the eye upon dosing for any reason, instil another drop. Discard any unused contents immediately after use.

Marketing authorisation number 0649/0120.

Date of approval/revision of SPC 19 September 1996.

Legal category POM.

ISOPTO* ALKALINE

Qualitative and quantitative composition Hydroxypropylmethyl Cellulose PhEur 1.0% w/v.

Pharmaceutical form Sterile eye drops for topical ocular administration.

Clinical particulars
Therapeutic indications: Used topically to provide tear-like lubrication for the symptomatic relief of dry eyes and eye irritation associated with deficient tear production. (Usually in cases of rheumatoid arthritis, keratoconjunctivitis sicca and xerophthalmia.) Also used as an ocular lubricant for artificial eyes.

Posology and method of administration:
Adults, children and the elderly: The dose depends on the need for lubrication. Usually one to two drops to each eye three times daily, or as prescribed.

Contra-indications: Hypersensitivity to any component of the product. This product contains benzalkonium chloride and should not be used when soft contact lenses are worn.

Special warnings and special precautions for use: If irritation persists or worsens, or headache, eye pain, vision changes or continued redness occur, discontinue use and consult a physician. To preserve sterility do not allow the dropper to touch the eye or any other surface.

Interaction with other medicaments and other forms of interaction: None known.

Pregnancy and lactation: There is insufficient evidence as to safety in pregnancy and this product should, therefore, only be used in pregnancy if it is considered essential by the physician.

Effects on ability to drive and use machines: May cause transient blurring of vision on instillation. Do not drive or operate hazardous machinery unless vision is clear.

Undesirable effects: May cause transient mild stinging or temporarily blurred vision.

Overdose: Not applicable.

Pharmacological properties
Pharmacodynamic properties: Hydroxylpropylmethylcellulose is an inert substance. It has no pharmacological activity.

Pharmacokinetic properties: Hydroxylpropylmethylcellulose is an inert substance. It has no pharmacological activity and, hence, the pharmacokinetic properties have not been studied.

Preclinical safety data: There are no preclinical data of relevance to the prescriber which are additional to that already included in other sections of the SPC.

Pharmaceutical particulars
List of excipients: Sodium citrate dihydrate PhEur, sodium phosphate dried USP, sodium biphosphate USP, sodium chloride PhEur, benzalkonium chloride PhEur, purified water PhEur.

Incompatabilities: None known.

Shelf life: 36 months (unopened), 1 month (after first opening).

Special precautions for storage: Store at a temperature not exceeding 25°C. Do not refrigerate. Keep container tightly closed. Discard 1 month after opening.

Nature and contents of container: Drop-Tainer – Natural Low Density Polyethylene Bottle and Plug. Polystyrene or Polypropylene cap.

Instructions for use/handling: Do not touch dropper tip to any surface as this may contaminate the contents. If the drop of medication is not retained in the eye upon dosing for any reason, instill another drop.

Marketing authorisation number 0649/5900R.

Date of approval/revision of SPC 29 July 1996.

Legal category POM.

ISOPTO* ATROPINE

Qualitative and quantitative composition Atropine Sulphate PhEur 1.0% w/v.

Pharmaceutical form Sterile ophthalmic solution for topical ocular administration.

Clinical particulars
Therapeutic indications: Atropine is a powerful and long-acting anti-cholinergic agent used for producing cycloplegia and mydriasis. It is indicated for: Cycloplegic refraction, particularly in the determination of refraction in children below the age of six and in children with convergent strabismus.

In the treatment of iritis and uveitis to immobilise the ciliary muscle and iris and to prevent or breakdown adhesions.

Posology and method of administration:
Adults and the Elderly: For refraction, instil one drop into each eye twice daily for one or two days before examination. For uveitis, instil one or two drops into the eye(s) four times daily, or as required.

Atropine should be used with particular caution in the elderly who are prone to systemic adverse effects and to the precipitation and exacerbation of glaucoma.

Children: For refraction, instil one drop twice daily for one to three days before examination and one hour before examination.

Usage in children: Do not use during the first three months of life due to possible association with the development of amblyopia. Safety and efficacy for use in children has not been established therefore use with extreme caution.

Contra-indications: Glaucoma or a tendency towards glaucoma (e.g. narrow anterior chamber angle). Hypersensitivity to any component. This product contains benzalkonium chloride and should not be used when soft contact lenses are worn.

Special warnings and special precautions for use: To reduce systemic absorption the lacrimal sac should be compressed at the medial canthus by digital pressure for at least one minute after instillation of the drops.

Extreme caution is advised for use in childen and individuals susceptible to belladonna alkaloids because of the increased risk of systemic toxicity. Parents should be warned of the oral toxicity of this preparation for children and advised to wash their hands after use.

Interaction with other medicaments and other forms of interaction: The effects of anti-muscarinic agents may be enhanced by the concomitant administration of other drugs with anti-muscarinic properties such as amantadine, some anti-histamines, butyrophenones, phenothiazines and tricyclic anti-depressants.

Pregnancy and lactation: There is insufficient evidence as to drug safety in pregnancy and lactation, this product should not be used during pregnancy unless it is considered essential by a physician.

Effects on ability to drive and use machines: May cause blurred vision and sensitivity to light. Patients should be warned not to drive or engage in other hazardous activities unless vision is clear. Complete recovery from the effects of Atropine eye drops may take up to seven days.

Undesirable effects: Local: Increased intraocular pressure, transient stinging, and sensitivity to light secondary to pupillary dilation. Prolonged administration may lead to local irritation, hyperaemia, oedema and conjunctivitis.

Systemic: Systemic anti-cholinergic toxicity is manifested by dryness in the mouth, flushing, dryness of the skin, bradycardia followed by tachycardia with palpitations and arrhythmias, urinary urgency, difficulty and retention, reduction in the tone and motility of the gastrointestinal tract leading to constipation.

Vomiting, giddiness and staggering may occur, a rash may be present in children and abdominal distension in infants.

Toxic doses cause rapid respiration, hyperpyrexia and CNS stimulation or depression marked by restlessness, confusion, hallucinations and occasionally convulsions. In severe toxicity coma may lead to circulatory and respiratory failure and death.

Overdose: Systemic toxicity may occur following topical use, particularly in children. It is manifested by flushing and dryness of the skin (a rash may be present in children), blurred vision, a rapid and irregular pulse, fever, abdominal distention in infants, convulsions and hallucinations and the loss of neuromuscular co-ordination.

Treatment is supportive (there is no evidence that physostigmine is superior to supportive management). In infants and small children the body surface must be kept moist. If accidentally ingested, induce emesis or perform gastric lavage.

Pharmacological properties
Pharmacodynamic properties: Atropine blocks the response of the sphincter muscle to the iris and the accommodative muscle of the ciliary body to cholinergic stimulation producing pupillary dilatation – mydriasis and paralysis of accommodation – cycloplegia.

The ocular effects of topically applied atropine are prolonged accommodation and pupillary reflexes may not fully recover for 7–12 days.

Pharmacokinetic properties: Atropine is readily absorbed transconjunctivally and is distributed throughout the body. It is mainly metabolised in the liver and some is excreted. Unchanged in the urine.

Preclinical safety data: No specific preclinical studies have been conducted with Isopto Atropine. The reported, oral LD_{50} in mice is 75 mg/kg and in rats is 500 mg/kg.

Pharmaceutical particulars
List of excipients: Boric acid, benzalkonium chloride, hydroxypropyl methyl cellulose, sodium hydroxide and/or hydrochloric (to adjust pH), purified water.

Incompatibilities: None known.

Shelf life: 36 months (unopened), 1 month (after first opening).

Special precautions for storage: Store at a temperature not exceeding 25°C away from direct sunlight. Do not refrigerate. Keep container tightly closed. Discard 1 month after opening.

Nature and contents of container: Drop-Tainer – natural low density polyethylene bottle and plug. Polystyrene or polypropylene cap.

Instructions for use/handling: Do not touch dropper tip to any surface as this may contaminate the contents. If the drop of medication is not retained in the eye upon dosing for any reason, instill another drop.

Marketing authorisation number 0649/5901R.

Date of approval/revision of SPC 23 July 1996.

Legal category POM.

ISOPTO* CARBACHOL

Qualitative and quantitative composition Carbachol USP 3.0% w/v.

Pharmaceutical form Sterile eye drop for topical administration to humans.

Clinical particulars
Therapeutic indications: A directly acting miotic used for the treatment of glaucoma. May be used topically to control intraocular pressure in patients who become refractory to pilocarpine alone and in patients who are unable to tolerate pilocarpine.

Posology and method of administration
Adults and the elderly: One or two drops up to four times daily. The frequency of instillation is determined by the severity of the glaucoma and the response to treatment.

Children: Not recommended for use in chidlren. The safety and efficacy of use in children has not been established.

Contra-indications: Conditions where pupillary constriction is undesirable, e.g. acute iritis, anterior uveitis and some forms of secondary glaucoma. Hypersensitivity to any component of the preparation. This product contains benzalkonium chloride and should not be used when soft contact lenses are worn.

Special warnings and special precautions for use: Although systemic reactions rarely occur in the treatment of chronic simple glaucoma with the usual doses used, in the treatment of acute closed-angle glaucoma the possibility of systemic reactions must be considered because of the higher doses given. Caution is particularly advised with patients with acute heart failure, bronchial asthma, peptic ulceration, hypertension or hypotension, urinary tract obstruction, gastro-intestinal spasm, recent myocardial infarct and Parkinson's disease.

Carbachol penetrates the intact cornea poorly. To reduce the risk of systemic toxicity, use carbachol with caution in the presence of a corneal abrasion or damage to the epithelial barrier of the conjunctiva or cornea caused by topical anaesthesia or tonometry.

Retinal detachments have been caused in susceptible individuals and those with pre-existing retinal disease, therefore, fundus examination is advised in all patients prior to the initiation of therapy.

Interaction with other medicaments and other forms of interaction: None known.

Pregnancy and lactation: Safety for use in pregnancy and lactation has not been established, therefore, use only when clearly indicated.

Effects on ability to drive and use machines: Causes difficulty with dark adaptation, therefore, caution is necessary with night driving and when hazardous tasks are undertaken in poor illumination. May cause accommodation spasm. Patients should be advised not to drive or use machinery.

Undesirable effects
Local: Burning, itching, smarting, blurring, ciliary spasm, conjunctival vascular congestion, induced myopia, sensitisation of the lids and conjunctiva, reduced visual acuity in poor illumination, lens changes with chronic use, increased pupillary block, retinal detachments and vitreous haemorrhages.

Systemic: Systemic reactions following ocular use are rare but they may include hypotension, bradycardia, bronchial spasm, pulmonary oedema, salivation, sweating, nausea, vomiting, diarrhoea and lacrimation, cardiac arrhythmia, gastro-intestinal cramping, asthma, frequent urgency to urinate.

CNS: Browache and headache (especially in younger patients who have recently started therapy).

Overdose: If accidentally ingested induce emesis or perform gastric lavage. Observe for signs of toxicity (salivation, lacrimation, sweating, nausea, vomiting and diarrhoea). If these occur, therapy with anti-cholinergic agents, such as atropine, may be necessary.

Pharmacological properties
Pharmacodynamic properties: Carbachol is the car-

bamyl ester of choline, it is a parasympathomimetic agent and its pharmacological properties are similar to those of acetylcholine. Carbachol is totally resistant to hydrolysis by acetylcholinesterase or non-specific cholinesterase. Carbachol has, therefore, a two-phase physiological action, direct and indirect which is advantageous in the treatment of glaucoma. In the eye, topical administration of carbachol produces miosis and accommodative spasm, more intense and of longer duration than that produced by pilocarpine.

Pharmacokinetic properties: Carbachol is not lipid soluble at any pH and thus penentration of the intact corneal epithelium is poor. Hydroxypropylmethylcellulose is present in Isopto Carbachol to reduce the surface tension of the formulation and to aid penetration of carbachol across the cornea. Studies with Isopto Carbachol formulated in a hydroxypropylmethylcellulose vehicle have provided evidence of intraocular penetration as demonstrated by miotic activity in animal studies.

Preclinical safety data: There are no preclinical safety data of relevance to the prescriber which are not already covered by the clinical section of the SPC.

Pharmaceutical particulars
List of excipients: Benzalkonium Chloride 0.005% w/v; boric acid; sodium borate; sodium chloride; HPMC 2910; sodium hydroxide; hydrochloric acid; purified water.

Incompatibilities: None known.

Shelf life: 48 months unopened 28 days after opening.

Special precautions for storage: Store at 8–25°C away from direct sunlight.
Keep the container tightly closed.
Discard 1 month after opening.

Nature and contents of container: Drop-Tainer – Natural low density polyethylene bottle and plug. Polystyrene or polypropylene cap.

Instructions for use/handling: Do not touch dropper tip to any surface as this may contaminate the contents.

If the drop of medication is not retained in the eye upon dosing for any reason then instil another drop.

Marketing authorisation number 0649/5902R.

Date of approval/revision of SPC 30 January 1997.

Legal category POM.

ISOPTO* FRIN 0.12%

Presentation Isopto Frin is a clear, colourless sterile solution, containing Phenylephrine Hydrochloride BP 0.12% and Hydroxypropylmethylcellulose (Hypromellose) USP 0.5%, and preserved with Benzethonium Chloride USP 0.01%.

Uses For the temporary relief of redness of the eye due to minor eye irritations.

Dosage and administration One or two drops instilled topically into the eye up to four times a day. Isopto Frin is suitable for use by both adults and children.

Contra-indications, warnings, etc
Contra-indications: Not to be used by contact lens wearers except under medical supervision.

Interactions: Phenylephrine may interfere with the actions of antihypertensive agents while monoamine oxidase inhibitors and tricyclic antidepressants can exacerbate the systemic effects of phenylephrine.

Effects on ability to drive and to use machines: As with other eyedrops blurring of vision may occur immediately after instillation. Patients should be advised not to drive until any effects on vision have cleared.

Warnings and precautions: Patients being treated for high blood pressure or depression should consult their doctor before using these drops. If eye pain, changes in vision, continued redness of the eye are experienced or if the condition worsens or persists for more than 24 hours, patients should consult their doctor. Isopto Frin should not be used in patients with any eye disease or who have had eye surgery except under the advice and supervision of a doctor. Continued use of this product may increase redness of the eye. Care should be exercised in its use in small children, pressure should be put on the inner canthus of the eye for a few minutes after instillation to decrease systemic absorption through the conjunctiva. Use with caution on an inflamed eye, as hyperaemia greatly increases the rate of systemic absorption through the conjunctiva. Slight dilation of the pupil may occur in some patients. For this reason it should be used with care where narrow angle glaucoma may be present since its use may precipitate angle closure or in those with a shallow anterior chamber.

Pregnancy Warning: This product should only be used during pregnancy if considered essential by the physician.

Treatment of overdose: An overdose from a 0.12% solution of phenylephrine hydrochloride is extremely unlikely. Symptoms would however be those of acute hypertension. In such an event a quick acting adrenergic blocking agent such as 5 to 10 mg phentolamine mesylate, followed by a β-blocking agent such as 2.5 to 5 mg propranolol should be given.

Pharmaceutical precautions Isopto Frin eye drops should be stored in a cool place away from direct sunlight. Keep the container tightly closed. Contents should be discarded one month after opening. If the solution changes colour or becomes cloudy, do not use.

Legal category P.

Package quantities 10 ml containers.

Further information Isopto Frin eye drops are contained in an unbreakable semi-rigid plastic dropper bottle with screw-on cap.

Product licence number 0649/5911.

ISOPTO* PLAIN

Qualitative and quantitative composition Hydroxypropylmethyl Cellulose Ph.Eur. 0.5% w/v

Pharmaceutical form Sterile eye drops for topical ocular administration.

Clinical particulars
Therapeutic indications: Used topically to provide tear-like lubrication for the symptomatic relief of dry eyes and eye irritation associated with deficient tear production. (Usually in cases of rheumatoid arthritis, keratoconjunctivitis sicca and xerophthalmia.

Also used as an ocular lubricant for artificial eyes.

Posology and method of administration
Adults, children and the elderly: The dose depends on the need for lubrication. Usually one to two drops to each eye three times daily or as prescribed.

Contra-indications: Hypersensitivity to any component of the product. The product contains benzalkonium chloride and should not be used when soft contact lenses are worn.

Special warnings and special precautions for use: If irritation persists or worsens, or headache, eye pain, vision changes or continued redness occur, discontinue use and consult a physician.

To preserve sterility do not allow the dropper to touch the eye or any other surface.

Interaction with other medicaments and other forms of interaction: None known

Pregnancy and lactation: There is insufficient evidence as to safety in pregnancy and this product should, therefore, only be used in pregnancy if it is considered essential by the physician.

Effects on ability to drive and use machines: May cause transient blurring of vision on instillation. Do not drive or operate hazardous machinery unless vision is clear.

Undesirable effects: May cause transient mild stinging or temporarily blurred vision.

Overdose: Not applicable

Pharmacological properties
Pharmacodynamic properties: Hydroxypropylmethylcellulose is an inert substance. It has no pharmacological activity.

Pharmacokinetic properties: Hydroxypropylmethylcellulose is an inert substance. It has no pharmacological activity and, hence, the pharmacokinetic properties have not been studied.

Preclinical safety data: Hydroxypropylmethylcellulose is an inert substance and is not expected to be absorbed systemically. Hence, although no systemic toxicity studies have been conducted it is not expected to demonstrate any systemic toxicity or to have any effect on reproductive processes.

Similarly no specific local ocular toxicity or irritation studies have been conducted, however, no adverse effects are anticipated. Indeed, hydroxypropylmethylcellulose ophthalmic solution is used as a control in some ophthalmic drug studies because of the acknowledged low level of toxicity.

Pharmaceutical particulars
List of excipients: Sodium citrate dihydrate Ph.Eur., Sodium phosphate dried USP, Sodium biphosphate USP, Sodium chloride Ph.Eur., Benzalkonium chloride Ph.Eur, Purified water Ph.Eur.

Incompatibilities: None known

Shelf life: 36 months (unopened), 1 month (after first opening).

Special precautions for storage: Store at a temperature not exceeding 25°C. Do not refrigerate. Keep container tightly closed. Discard 1 month after opening.

Nature and contents of container: Drop-Tainer–Natural Low Density Polyethylene Bottle and Plug. Polystyrene or Polypropylene cap.

Instructions for use/handling: Do not touch dropper tip to any surface as this may contaminate the contents. If the drop of medication is not retained in the eye upon dosing for any reason, instill another drop.

Marketing authorisation number PL 0649/5920R

Date of approval/revision of SPC 21st May 1996

Legal category P

LUBRI-TEARS*

Presentation Pale yellow, sterile ophthalmic ointment containing active ingredients: Wool Fat PhEur 10% w/w, White Soft Paraffin BP 60% w/w, Liquid Paraffin PhEur 30% w/w. No preservatives are included in the formulation.

Uses As adjunctive therapy to lubricate and protect the eye in conditions such as exposure keratitis, decreased corneal sensitivity, recurrent corneal erosions, keratitis sicca, ophthalmic surgery and non-ophthalmic surgery.

Dosage and administration Pull down the lower eye lid and place a small quantity in the conjunctival sac. Use as required. There is no variation of dosage for age.

Contra-indications, warnings, etc
Contra-indications: Hypersensitivity to the active ingredients.

Precautions and warnings: Application of the ointment may cause blurring of vision. Patients should be advised not to drive or operate machinery if affected.

Use in pregnancy and lactation: Suitable for use in pregnancy and lactation.

Pharmaceutical precautions Store below 30°C. To avoid contamination during use, do not allow the tube tip to touch any surface. Close the tube after each application.

Legal category P.

Package quantities Ophthalmic ointment tubes of 5 g.

Further information Nil.

Product licence number 0649/0143.

MAXIDEX*

Qualitative and quantitative composition Dexamethasone Ph.Eur. 0.1% w/v

Pharmaceutical form Eye drops, suspension.

Clinical particulars
Therapeutic indications: Indicated for treatment of steroid responsive inflammatory conditions of the conjunctiva, cornea and anterior segment of the eye such as: anterior uveitis, iritis, cyclitis, allergic and vernal conjunctivitis, herpes zoster keratitis, superficial punctate keratitis and non-specific superficial keratitis.

Also indicated for the treatment of corneal injury from chemical, radiation or thermal burns or following penetration by foreign bodies. Indicated for post-operative use to reduce inflammatory reactions and suppress graft reaction.

Posology and method of administration: The frequency of instillation of drops and the duration of treatment will vary depending upon the severity of the underlying condition and the response to treatment.

Severe inflammations require one to two drops instilled into the eye every thirty to sixty minutes until a satisfactory response occurs.

Subconjunctival or systemic steroid therapy should be considered if there is no response. When a favourable response has been observed reduce the dosage towards one drop every four hours.

Contra-indications: Herpes simplex and other viral diseases of the cornea and conjunctiva, fungal disease, ocular tuberculosis, untreated purulent infections and hypersensitivity to any component of the preparation. Patients with soft contact lenses should not use this preparation.

Special warnings and special precautions for use: Topical corticosteroids should never be given for an undiagnosed red eye as inappropriate use is potentially blinding.
Because of the risk of 'steroid glaucoma' and cataract formation the intraocular pressure and the lens must be checked frequently during use of this preparation.

To avoid the risk of enhancement of herpetic corneal disease, frequent slit-lamp examination is essential.

Topical steroids may mask or enhance the activity of acute purulent eye infections. In such cases antibiotic therapy is mandatory.

Persistent corneal ulceration following long-term topical steroid use may be due to fungal invasion.

Topical corticosteroids are not effective in mustard gas keratitis or Sjogren's keratoconjunctivitis.

Interaction with other medicaments and other forms of interaction: None relevant to topical use.

Pregnancy and lactation: There is inadequate evidence of safety in human pregnancy. Topical administration of corticosteroids to pregnant animals can cause abnormalities of foetal development including cleft palate and intra-uterine growth retardation. There may therefore be a very small risk of such effects in the human pregnancy.

Effects on ability to drive and use machines: May cause transient stinging on instillation or sensitivity to bright light. Warn patients not to drive or use hazardous machinery if vision is not clear.

Undesirable effects: Topical steroid use may result in increased intraocular pressure leading to optic nerve damage, reduced visual acuity and visual field defects.

Intensive or prolonged use of topical corticosteroids may lead to the formation of posterior subcapsular cataracts. In those diseases causing thinning of the cornea or sclera, perforation of the globe may occur. Viral and fungal infections may be exacerbated by steroids. Transient stinging or burning may occur on instillation of the drops. Systemic side effects may occur with extensive use.

Overdose: Long-term intensive topical use may lead to systemic effects. Oral ingestion of the contents of the bottle (up to 10 mls) is unlikely to lead to any serious adverse effects.

Pharmacological properties

Pharmacodynamic properties: Dexamethasone has been demonstrated by animal and human studies based on oral application to possess approximately six to seven times the potency of prednisolone and at least 30 times the potency of cortisone. The potency of the compound is accomplished by the addition of a methyl radical and a fluorine atom to the prednisolone radical.

Pharmacokinetic properties: Dexamethasone is absorbed rapidly after oral administration with a half-life of about 190 minutes. Sufficient absorption may occur after topical application to the skin and eye to produce systemic effects. In plasma dexamethasone protein binding is less than for most other corticosteroids. Corticosteroids diffuse into tissue fluids and cerebrospinal fluid but transplacental diffusion in significant amounts has not been demonstrated. Corticosteroids are metabilised in the liver the kidney and excrete in the urine. Metabolism is similar to other corticosteroids. Intraocular penetration occurs in significant amounts and contributes to the effectiveness of dexamethasone in anterior segment inflammatory disease.

Preclinical safety data: There are no preclinical data of relevance to the presciber which are additional to that already included in other sections of the SPC.

Pharmaceutical particulars

List of excipients: Sodium phosphate USP, Polysorbate 80 Ph.Eur., Disodium edetate Ph.Eur., Sodium chloride Ph.Eur., Benzalkonium chloride Ph.Eur., Hydroxy propyl methyl cellulose Ph. Eur., Citric acid Ph.Eur., Purified water Ph.Eur.

Incompatibilities: None known

Shelf life: 36 months (unopened), 1 month (after first opening)

Special precautions for storage: Store at a temperature not exceeding 25°C away from direct sunlight. Do not refrigerate. Keep container tightly closed. Discard 1 month after opening.

Nature and contents of container: Drop-Tainer–5 ml and 10 ml Natural Low Density Polyethylene Bottles and Plugs. Polystyrene or Polypropylene cap.

Instructions for use/handling: Do not touch dropper tip to any surface as this may contaminate the contents.

If the drop of medication is not retained in the eye upon dosing for any reason then instill another drop.

Marketing authorisation number PL 0649/5914R

Date of approval/revision of SPC 16th October 1997/ 6th January 1998

Legal category POM

MAXITROL* EYE DROPS

Qualitative and quantitative composition Dexamethasone PhEur 0.1% w/v, *Polymyxin B Sulphate PhEur 6000.0 U, *Neomycin Sulphate (as base) 3500.0 U.

*The quantity of ingredient is expressed per ml of product.

Pharmaceutical form White sterile suspension for topical ocular administration.

Clinical particulars

Therapeutic indications: Maxitrol Eye Drops is indicated for the short-term treatment of steroid responsive conditions of the eye when prophylactic antibiotic treatment is also required, after excluding the presence of fungal and viral disease.

Posology and method of administration

Children and adults (including the elderly): Apply one or two drops to each affected eye up to six times daily or, more frequently if required. (Severe infections may require one or two drops every 15–20 minutes initially, reducing the frequency of instillation gradually as the infection is controlled.)

Contra-indications: Hypersensitivity to neomycin or to any component of the preparation. (Cross-sensitivity with other aminoglycoside antibiotics may occur.) Herpes simplex and other viral diseases of the cornea and conjunctiva, fungal disease, ocular tuberculosis, untreated purulent infections. This product contains benzalkonium chloride and should not be used when soft contact lenses are worn.

Special warning and special precautions for use: In severe infections topical use should be supplemented with appropriate systemic treatment.

Prolonged use should be avoided as it may lead to skin sensitisation and the emergence of resistant organisms.

Neomycin may cause irreversible partial or total deafness when given systemically or when applied topically to open wounds or damaged skin. This effect is dose-related and is enhanced by renal or hepatic impairment. Although this effect has not been reported following topical ocular use the possibility should be considered when high dose topical treatment is given to small children or infants. Topical corticosteroids should never be given for an undiagnosed red eye as inappropriate use is potentially blinding.

Because of the risk of 'steroid glaucoma' and cataract formation the intraocular pressure and the lens must be checked frequently during use of this preparation.

To avoid the risk of enhancement of herpetic corneal disease, frequent slip lamp examination is essential.

Topical steroids may mask or enhance the activity of acute purulent eye infections. In such cases antibiotic therapy is mandatory. Persistent corneal ulceration following long-term topical steroid use may be due to fungal invasion.

Topical corticosteroids are not effective in mustard gas keratitis or Sjorgren's keratoconjunctivitis.

Interaction with other medicaments and other forms of interaction: None relevant to topical use.

Pregnancy and lactation: Safety for use in pregnancy and lactation has not been established. Topical administration of corticosteroids to pregnant animals can cause abnormalities of foetal development including cleft palate and intra-uterine growth with retardation. There may therefore be a very small risk of such effects in human pregnancy. Use only when it is considered essential by the physician.

Effects on ability to drive and use machines: May cause transient blurring of vision on instillation. Warn patients not to drive or operate hazardous machinery unless vision is clear.

Undesirable effects: Hypersensitivity reactions, usually of the delayed type, occur frequently with local treatment with neomycin. Irritation, burning, stinging, itching and dermatitis may occur. Topical steroid use may result in increased intraocular pressure leading to optic nerve disease, reduced visual acuity and visual field defects. Intensive or prolonged use of topical corticosteroids may lead to formation of posterior subcapsular cataracts. In those diseases causing thinning of the cornea or sclera, perforation of the globe may occur. Viral and fungal infections may be exacerbated by steroids. Systemic side effects may occur with extensive use.

Overdose: Long-term intensive topical use may lead to systemic effects. Oral ingestion of the contents of one bottle (up to 10 ml) is unlikely to lead to any serious adverse effects.

Pharmacological properties

Pharmacodynamic properties: Maxitrol contains dexamethasone, neomycin sulphate and polymyxin B sulphate as active constituents.

Dexamethasone is a synthetic glucocorticoid with a potent anti-inflammatory activity. The relative anti-inflammatory potency of dexamethasone is 25 times that of cortisone, but its effects on sodium and water retention, potassium loss and abnormal sugar metabolism are minimal.

Neomycin is a broad spectrum antibiotic, highly sensitive gram negative organisms include: *E. coli, Enterobactor aerogenes, K. pneumoniae,* Pasteurella, *Pr. vulgaris,* Salmonella, Shigella, *Haemophilus influenzae, Neisseria meningitidis, Vibrio cholerae,* and *Bordetella pertussis.*

Gram positive microorganisms that are inhibited include: *Bacillus anthracis, Corynebacterium diptheriae, Staph. aureus, Strep. facecalis, Listeria monocytogenes* and *M. tuberculosis. Borrelia* and *Leptospira interrogans (icterohaemorrhagiae)* are also suppressed. Strains of *Pseudomonas aeruginosa* are resitant to neomycin.

Polymyxin B sulphate is active only against gram negative bacteria and is particularly active against *Pseudomonas aeruginosa.* Other sensitive organisms are: Enterobacter, *Escherichia coli,* Klebsiella, Salmonella, Pasteurella, Bordetella and Shigella. However, protens and most strains of Neisseria, Providentia and Serratia are resistant to Polymyxin B. Most sensitive organisms are inhibited by 0.1 to 0.2 units/ml.

Pharmacokinetic properties: Dexamethasone, like other corticosteroids, is absorbed rapidly after oral administration and has a biological half-life of about 190 minutes. Sufficient absorption may occur after topical application to the skin and eye to produce systemic effects. Intraocular penetration of dexamethasone occurs in significant amounts and contributes to the effectiveness of dexamethasone in anterior segment inflammatory disease.

Polymyxin B sulphate is not absorbed from the gastrointestinal tract or through intact skin, although the intact corneal epithelium prevents penetration into the corneal stroma, therapeutic concentrations do enter the stroma after epithelial damage. Good stromal penetration occurs after epithelial abrasion following topical instillation, subconjunctival injection, or corneal bath. No significant polymyxin B penetration into the vitrous is demonstrable after parenteral or local administration of the drug.

Neomycin is poorly absorbed from the gastrointestinal tract and after topical administration insufficient is absorbed to produce systemic effects. Absorption has been reported to occur from wounds and inflamed skin. After absorption neomycin is rapidly excreted by the kidneys in active form.

Preclinical safety data: There are no preclinical data of relevance to the prescriber which are additional to that already included in other sections of the SPC.

Pharmaceutical particulars

List of excipients: Sodium chloride, polysorbate 20, benzalkonium chloride, hydroxypropyl methylcellulose, hydrochloric acid/sodium hydroxide, purified water.

Incompatibilities: None known.

Shelf life: Unopened 24 months, after opening 28 days.

Special precautions for storage: Store at 8–25°C away from direct sunlight. Keep the container tightly closed.

Nature and contents of container: 5 ml and 10 ml Drop-Tainers, natural LDPE bottle and plug with a polystyrene or polypropylene cap.

Instructions for use/handling: Do not touch the tip of the bottle to any surface as this contaminate the contents.

Marketing authorisation number 0649/5915R.

Date of approval/revision of SPC 24 January 1996.

Legal category POM.

MAXITROL* OINTMENT

Qualitative and quantitative composition Dexamethasone PhEur 0.1% w/w; *Polymyxin B Sulphate PhEur 6000.0 U; *Neomycin Sulphate (as base) 3500.0 U.

*The quantity of ingredient is expressed per gram of product.

Pharmaceutical form White to very pale yellow greasy homogeneous ointment for topical administration.

Clinical particulars

Therapeutic indications: Maxitrol Ointment is indicated for the short-term treatment of steroid responsive conditions of the eye when prophylactic antibiotic treatment is also required, after excluding the presence of fungal and viral disease.

Posology and method of administration

Children and adults (including the elderly): Apply a small amount into the conjunctival sac(s) up to three or four times daily or, may be used adjunctively with drops at bedtime.

Contra-indications: Hypersensitivity to neomycin or to any component of the preparation. (Cross-sensitivity with other aminoglycoside antibiotics may occur.)

Herpes simplex and other viral diseases of the cornea and conjunctiva, fungal disease, ocular tuberculosis, untreated purulent infections.

Special warnings and special precautions for use: In severe infections topical use should be supplemented with appropriate systemic treatment.

Prolonged use should be avoided as it may lead to skin sensitisation and the emergence of resistant organisms.

Neomycin may cause irreversible partial or total deafness when given systemically or when applied topically to open wounds or damaged skin. This effect is dose-related and is enhanced by renal or hepatic impairment. Although this effect has not been reported following topical ocular use the possibility should be considered when high dose topical treatment is given to small children or infants.

Topical corticosteroids should never be given for an undiagnosed red eye as inappropriate use is potentially blinding.

Because of the risk of 'steroid glaucoma' and cataract formation the intraocular pressure and the lens must be checked frequently during use of this preparation.

To avoid the risk of enhancement of herpetic corneal disease, frequent slip lamp examination is essential.

Topical steroids may mask or enhance the activity of acute purulent eye infections. In such cases antibiotic therapy is mandatory. Persistent corneal ulceration following long-term topical steroid use may be due to fungal invasion.

Topical corticosteroids are not effective in mustard gas keratitis or Sjorgren's keratoconjunctivitis.

Interaction with other medicaments and other forms of interaction: None relevant to topical use.

Pregnancy and lactation: Safety for use in pregnancy and lactation has not been established. Topical administration of corticosteroids to pregnant animals can cause abnormalities of foetal development including cleft palate and intra-uterine growth with retardation. There may therefore be a very small risk of such effects in human pregnancy. Use only when it is considered essential by the physician.

Effects on ability to drive and use machines: May cause transient blurring of vision on instillation. Warn patients not to drive or operate hazardous machinery unless vision is clear.

Undesirable effects: Hypersensitivity reactions, usually of the delayed type, occur frequently with local treatment with neomycin. Irritation, burning, stinging, itching and dermatitis may occur. Topical steroid use may result in increased intraocular pressure leading to optic nerve disease, reduced visual acuity and visual field defects. Intensive or prolonged use of topical corticosteroids may lead to formation of posterior subcapsular cataracts. In those diseases causing thinning of the cornea or sclera, perforation of the globe may occur. Viral and fungal infections may be exacerbated by steroids. Systemic side effects may occur with extensive use.

Overdose: Long-term intensive topical use may lead to systemic effects. Oral ingestion of the contents of one tube is unlikely to lead to any serious adverse effects.

Pharmacological properties

Pharmacodynamic properties: Maxitrol contains dexamethasone, neomycin sulphate and polymyxin B sulphate as active constituents.

Dexamethasone is a synthetic glucocorticoid with a potent anti-inflammatory activity. The relative anti-inflammatory potency of dexamethasone is 25 times that of cortisone, but its effects on sodium and water retention, potassium loss and abnormal sugar metabolism are minimal.

Neomycin is a broad spectrum antibiotic, highly sensitive gram negative organisms include: *E. coli, Enterobacter aerogenes, K. pneumoniae,* Pasteurella, *Pr. vulgaris,* Salmonella, Shigella, *Haemophilus influenzae, Neisseria meningitidis, Vibrio cholerae,* and *Bordetella pertussis.*

Gram positive microorganisms that are inhibited include: *Bacillus anthracis, Corynebacterium diptheriae, Staph. aureus, Strep. facecalis, Listeria monocytogenes* and *M. tuberculosis. Borrelia* and *Leptospira interrogans (icterohaemorrhagiae)* are also suppressed. Strains of *Pseudomonas aeruginosa* are resitant to neomycin.

Polymyxin B sulphate is active only against gram negative bacteria and is particularly active against *Pseudomonas aeruginosa.* Other sensitive organisms are: *Enterobacter, Escherichia coli,* Klebsiella, Salmonella, Pasteurella, Bordetella and Shigella. However, proteus and most strains of Neisseria, Providentia and Serratia are resistant to Polymyxin B. Most sensitive organisms are inhibited by 0.1 to 0.2 units/ml.

Pharmacokinetic properties: Dexamethasone, like other corticosteroids, is absorbed rapidly after oral administration and has a biological half-life of about 190 minutes. Sufficient absorption may occur after topical application to the skin and eye to produce systemic effects. Intraocular penetration of dexamethasone occurs in significant amounts and contributes to the effectiveness of dexamethasone in anterior segment inflammatory disease.

Polymyxin B sulphate is not absorbed from the gastrointestinal tract or through intact skin, although the intact corneal epithelium prevents penetration into the corneal stroma, therapeutic concentrations do enter the stroma after epitherlial damage. Good stromal penetration occurs after epithelial abrasion following topical instillation, subconjunctival injection, or corneal bath. No significant polymyxin B penetration into the vitreous is demonstrable after parenteral or local administration of the drug.

Neomycin is poorly absorbed from the gastrointestinal tract and after topical administration insufficient is absorbed to produce systemic effects. Absorption has been reported to occur from wounds and inflamed skin. After absorption neomycin is rapidly excreted by the kidneys in active form.

Preclinical safety data: There are no preclinical data of relevance to the prescriber which are additional to that already included in other sections of the SPC.

Pharmaceutical particulars

List of excipients: Methylparaben, propylparaben, liquid lanolin (Lantrol), petrolatum (Penndrake No. 4).

Incompatibilities: None known.

Shelf life: Unopened 30 months, after opening 28 days.

Special precautions for storage: Store at 8–25°C away from direct sunlight. Keep the container tightly closed.

Nature and contents of container: 3.5 g metal tube with nozzle and screw cap.

Instructions for use/handling: Do not touch the top of the tube to any surface as this may contaminate the contents.

Marketing authorisation number 0649/5916R.

Date of approval/revision of SPC 18 January 1996.

Legal category POM.

MYDRIACYL* 0.5% and 1.0%

Qualitative and quantitative composition Tropicamide BP 0.5% w/v and 1.0% w/v.

Pharmaceutical form Sterile eye drops for topical ocular administration.

Clincal particulars

Therapeutic indications: Tropicamide is a short acting anticholinergic agent used as a mydriatic and cycloplegic. It is indicated for topical use for: Diagnostic purposes for fundoscopy and cycloplegic refraction. Use in pre- and post-operative states where a short acting mydriatic is required.

Posology and method of administration:

Adults, elderly and children: Fundoscopy: One or two drops of 0.5% solution instilled into the eyes 15 to 20 minutes prior to examination.

Cycloplegic refraction: One or two drops of 1% solution repeated after 5 minutes. If the patient is not seen within 20 to 30 minutes an additional drop may be instilled to prolong the effect.

Use in children: Tropicamide has been reported to be inadequate for cycloplegia in children. A more powerful cycloplegic agent, such as atropine, may be required.

Contra-indications: Glaucoma or a tendency towards glaucoma (e.g. Narrow anterior chamber angle). Hypersensitivity to any component. This preparation contains benzalkonium chloride and should not be used where soft contact lenses are worn.

Special warnings and special precautions for use: Because of the risk of precipitating angle-closure glaucoma in the elderly and others prone to raised intraocular pressure, an estimate of the depth of the angle of the anterior chamber should be made before use.

Extreme caution is advised for use in children and individuals susceptible to belladonna alkaloids because of the increased risk of systemic toxicity. Parents should be warned of the oral toxicity of this preparation for children and advised to wash their hands after use.

Use with caution in an inflamed eye as the hyperaemia greatly increases the rate of systemic absorption through the conjunctiva.

To reduce systemic absorption the lacrimal sac should be compressed at the medial canthus by digital pressure for at least one minute after instillation of the drops.

Interaction with other medicaments and other forms of interaction: The effect of anti-muscarinic agents may be enhanced by the concomitant administration of other drugs with anti-muscarinic properties such as amantadine, some anti-histamines, butyrophenones, phenothiazines and tricyclic anti-depressants.

Pregnancy and lactation: There is insufficient evidence as to drug safety in pregnancy and lactation. This product should be used during pregnancy only when it is considered essential by a physician.

Effects on ability to drive and use machines: May cause blurred vision and sensitivity to light. Patients should be warned not to drive or engage in other hazardous activities unless vision is clear. Complete recovery from the effects of tropicamide eyedrops may take up to six hours.

Undesirable effects: Local: Increased intraocular pressure, transient stinging and sensitivity to light secondary to pupillary dilation. Prolonged administration may lead to local irritation, hyperaemia, oedema and conjunctivitis.

Systemic: Systemic anti-cholinergic toxicity is manifested by dryness of the mouth, flushing, dryness of the skin, bradycardia followed by tachycardia with palpitations and arrhythmias, urinary urgency, difficulty and retention, reduction in the tone and motility of the gastrointestinal tract leading to constipation.

Vomiting, giddiness and staggering may occur, a rash may be present in children and abdominal distention in infants.

Psychotic reactions, behavioural disturbances and cardio-respiratory collapse may occur in children.

Overdose: Systemic toxicity may occur following topical use, particularly in children, it is manifested by flushing and dryness of the skin (a rash may be present in children), blurred vision, a rapid and irregular pulse, fever, abdominal distention in infants, convulsions and hallucinations and the loss of neuromuscular co-ordination.

Treatment is supportive (there is no evidence that physostigmine is superior to supportive management). In infants and small children the body surface must be kept moist. If accidentally ingested, induce emesis or perform gastric lavage.

Pharmacological properties

Pharmacodynamic properties: Tropicamide is an anticholinergic which blocks the responses of the sphincter muscle of the iris and the ciliary muscle to cholinergic stimulation thus dilating the pupil (mydriasis). At higher concentrations (1%), tropicamide also paralyses accommodation. This preparation acts rapidly and has a relatively short duration of action.

Pharmacokinetic properties: Tropicamide administered topically to the human eye does not bind to tissues as firmly as does atropine. The wash out time for half recovery of carbachol responsiveness was shown to be less than 15 minutes for non-pigmented iris and 30 minutes for pigmented iris.

Preclinical safety data: There are no preclinical data of relevance to the prescriber which are additional to that already included in other sections of the SPC.

Pharmaceutical particulars

List of excipients: Benzalkonium chloride, disodium edetate, sodium chloride, sodium hydroxide and/or hydrochloric acid (to adjust pH), purified water.

Incompatibilities: None known.

Shelf life: 36 months (unopened). 1 month (after first opening).

Special precautions for storage: Store at a temperature not exceeding 25°C away from direct sunlight. Do not refrigerate. Keep container tightly closed. Discard contents one month after opening.

Nature and contents of container: Pack size – 5 ml. Drop-Tainer – Natural Low Density Polyethylene Bottle and Plug. Polystyrene or Polypropylene cap.

Instructions for use/handling: Do not touch dropper tip to any surface as this may contaminate the contents.

Marketing authorisation numbers

0.5% 0649/5917R
1.0% 0649/5918R

Date of approval/revision of SPC 6 February 1997.

Legal category POM.

PILOGEL*

Qualitative and quantitative composition Pilogel contains active ingredient Pilocarpine Hydrochloride PhEur 40 mg, 4.0% w/w and Benzalkonium Chloride PhEur 0.008% w/w as preservative, Carbomer 940 3.5% w/w, Edetate Disodium PhEur 0.01% w/w, Sodium Hydroxide PhEur and/or Hydrochloric acid PhEur q.s. to pH 4.7–5.1, Purified Water PhEur to 100%.

Pharmaceutical form Sterile ophthalmic gel.

Clinical particulars

Therapeutic indications: Pilogel is indicated for the control of intraocular pressure in patients with ocular hypertension and chronic open-angle glaucoma. It may be used in combination with other miotics, beta-blockers, carbonic anhydrase inhibitors, sympathomimetics or hyperosmotic agents.

Posology and method of administration

Adults: Apply a 1.0–1.5 cm (½ inch) ribbon of gel under the lower eyelid of the eye(s) to be treated once a day at bedtime. After the gel has been instilled, close the eye, hold the lid shut and move the eye in several different directions.

Elderly: There are no special dosage modifications required for the elderly.

Children: Pilogel is not recommended for use in children.

Contra-indications: Miotics are contra-indicated where constriction of the pupil is undesirable such as in acute iritis, in those persons showing hypersensitivity to any of the components and in pupillary block glaucoma.

Special warnings and special precautions for use: For topical use only. This product contains benzalkonium chloride and is not recommended for use when soft contact lenses are worn. As with all miotics rare cases of retinal detachment have been reported when used in certain susceptible individuals and those with pre-existing retinal disease, therefore, fundus examination is advised in all patients prior to the initiation of therapy. The miosis usually causes difficulty in dark adaptation. Patients should be advised to exercise caution in night driving and other hazardous occupations in poor illumination.

Interaction with other medicaments and other forms of interactions: Although clinically not proven, the miotic effects of pilocarpine may be antagonised by long term topical or systemic corticosteroid therapy, systemic anticholinergics, antihistamines, pethidine, sympathomimetics, or tricyclic antidepressants. Concomitant administration of two different miotic drugs is not recommended because of potential interdrug antagonism, and potential development of unresponsiveness to both drugs.

Pregnancy and lactation: There is insufficient evidence as to the drug safety in human pregnancy. This product should, therefore, only be used during pregnancy if considered essential by the physician.

Effects on ability to drive and use machines: Pilogel causes miosis which usually results in difficulty in dark adaptation. Patients should be advised to exercise caution in night driving and other hazardous occupations in poor illumination.

Undesirable effects: The following adverse reactions associated with pilocarpine therapy have been reported:

Local: Burning, itching, smarting, blurring, ciliary spasm, conjunctival vascular congestion, induced myopia, sensitisation of the lids and conjunctiva, reduced visual acuity in poor illumination, lens changes with chronic use, increased pupillary block, retinal detachments and vitreous haemorrhages. Ocular reactions usually occur during initiation of therapy and often will not persist with continued therapy.

CNS: Browache and headache, especially in younger patients who have recently started therapy.

Systemic: Systemic reactions following ocular use are rare but they may include hypotension, bradycardia, bronchial spasm, pulmonary oedema, salivation, sweating, nausea, vomiting, diarrhoea and lacrimation.

Overdose: Systemic reactions following topical administration are extremely rare. If accidentally ingested, induce emesis or perform gastric lavage. Observe for signs of toxicity (salivation, lacrimation, sweating, nausea, vomiting and diarrhoea). If these occur, therapy with anti-cholinergic agents, such as atropine, may be necessary.

Pharmacological properties Pilocarpine is a direct acting cholinergic parasympathomimetic agent. It acts through a direct stimulation of muscarinic receptors in the iris sphincter pupillae muscle and the ciliary muscle both of which receive parasympathetic innervation. Contraction of the sphincter pupillae muscle causes miosis (constriction of the pupil) whilst contraction of the ciliary muscle increases tension on the scleral spur, opening trabecular meshwork spaces to facilitate outflow of aqueous humor and thus lower intraocular pressure. Pilocarpine has been used as an ophthalmic medication for many years and the toxicity profile of pilocarpine has been well docmented. All the excipients used in Pilogel have been widely used in pharmaceutical preparations. In addition acute, sub-acute and chronic ocular toxicity studies have demonstrated that Pilogel has a low potential for ocular irritation and toxicity.

Pharmaceutical particulars

List of excipients: Benzalkonium chloride, Carbomer 940, edetate disodium, sodium hydroxide and/or hydrochloric acid, purified water.

Incompatibilities: None known.

Shelf life: 24 months.

Special precaution for storage: Store at a temperature not exceeding 25°C. Do not freeze. Avoid excessive heat. Discard product 28 days after opening. Keep out of the reach of children.

Nature and contents of container: Polyfoil laminate collapsible tube with an HDPE closure and dispensing tip containing 5 g.

Instructions for use/handling: Instructions for patients are as follows:

1. Wash your hands before using pilogel.
2. Sit down in front of a mirror so that you can see what you are doing.
3. Remove the cap from the tube.
4. Make sure the tube tip does not touch anything as this may contaminate the contents.
5. Hold the tube upside down in one hand between your fingers.
6. Using the forefinger of your other hand, gently pull down the lower eyelid of the affected eye.
7. Place the tube tip close to, but not touching, your eye and gently squeeze the tube with your fingers so that a 1 to 1.5 cm (½ inch) strip is applied into the gap between the eye and the lower lid.
8. Now release the lower eyelid, close your eye and hold the eyelids shut while moving your eye around in several different directions.
9. Repeat steps 5 to 8 above, for the other eye, if necessary.
10. Replace and tightly close the cap on the tube.

Marketing authorisation number 0649/0115.

Date of approval/revision of SPC 31 July 1997.

Legal category POM.

PROVISC

Description Provisc Viscoelastic Material is a sterile, non-pyrogenic, high molecular weight, non-inflammatory highly purified fraction of sodium hyaluronate, dissolved in physiological sodium chloride phosphate buffer. Each ml of Provisc contains 10.0 mg sodium hyaluronate; 0.56 mg dibasic sodium phosphate, anhydrous; 0.04 mg monobasic sodium phosphate, monohydrate; 8.4 mg sodium chloride; hydrochloric acid and/or sodium hydroxide to adjust pH; and water for injection.

Characteristics: Sodium hyaluronate is a high molecular weight polysaccharide, composed of sodium glycuronate and N-acetyl-glucosamine which forms a repeating disaccharide unit by linking alternately beta 1-3 and beta 1-4 glycosidic bonds. The 1 % viscous and transparent material, Provisc, is a specific fraction of sodium hyaluronate, developed as an aid in ophthalmic surgery. It acts as a space occupying fluid that replaces the body's natural fluids.

Indications: Provisc is indicated for use as an ophthalmic surgical aid in the anterior segment during cataract extraction and intraocular lens (IOL) implantation.

Ophthalmic viscoelastic materials serve to maintain a deep anterior chamber during anterior segment surgery allowing reduced trauma to the corneal endothelium and surrounding ocular tissues. They help to push back the vitreous face and prevent formation of a flat chamber during the surgical procedure.

Contra-indications: At present there are no known contraindications to the use of Provisc when used as recommended; care should be used in patients with hypersensitivity to any components in this material (see *Precautions*).

Precautions:

(a) Precautions normally associated with anterior segment surgical procedures should be observed.
(b) Postoperative increases in intraocular pressure have been reported with sodium hyaluronate products, The IOP should be carefully monitored and appropriate therapy instituted if significant increases occur.
(c) It is recommended that Provisc be removed by irrigation and/or aspiration at the close of surgery. Do not overfill the anterior chamber.
(d) Provisc is obtained from microbial fermentation by a proprietary purification process. Although precautions have been taken to make this device protein-free and it has been tested in animals for allergenic response, this device, used in susceptible persons, may produce allergenic responses.
(e) In addition to the above, the following precautions should be observed:
 –Use only the cannula provided with the syringe.
 –Do not reuse the cannula provided.
 –Use only if material is clear.
 –Avoid trapping air bubble.

Adverse reactions:

(a) Provisc is tolerated after injection into human eyes during ophthalmic surgical procedures. As with most viscoelastic ophthalmic materials, a transient rise in intraocular pressure has been reported in some cases.
(b) Postoperative inflammatory reactions such as hypopyon and iritis have been reported with the use of ophthalmic viscoelastic materials, as well as incidents of corneal edema and cornea decompensation. Their relationship to the use of sodium hyaluronate (Provisc Viscoelastic Material) has not been established.

Applications:

Cataract **Surgery–IOL** Implantation

The cannula provided is used to slowly and carefully inject an amount of Provisc into the anterior chamber. The injection may be performed before or after removal of the crystalline lens. Provisc also possesses physicochemical properties that make it well suited for tissue manipulation, such as expansion of the capsular bag and facilitation of intraocular lens implantation following cataract extraction. Provisc facilitates viscoelastic removal at the conclusion of surgery.

Provisc may also be used to coat surgical instruments and the intraocular lens prior to implantation. Additional Provisc can be injected during surgery to replace any Provisc viscoelastic material lost during surgical manipulation (see *Precautions)*.

How supplied:

Provisc Viscoelastic Material is a sterile, non-pyrogenic viscoelastic material (sodium hyaluronate, 10 mg/ml, dissolved in physiological sodium chloride phosphate buffer) supplied in disposable glass syringes delivering 0.55 ml or 0.85 ml.

Each ml of Provisc contains 10.0 mg sodium hyaluronate; 0.56 mg dibasic sodium phosphate, anhydrous; 0.04 mg monobasic sodium phosphate, monohydrate; 8.4 mg sodium chloride; hydrochloric acid and/or sodium hydroxide to adjust pH and QS water for injection. Provisc syringes are aseptically packaged in blister packs also containing a 27-gauge, blunt tip cannula and terminally sterilized.

Refrigerated Provisc should be allowed to attain room temperature prior to use (approximately 20-40 minutes depending on quantity).

- Store in a refrigerator between 2° and 8° C.
- Protect from freezing.
- Protect from light.

Caution:

Do not use this product after the expiry date which is provided on the syringe label, backing label and outer carton.

CE 0123

TEARS Naturale*

Presentation Tears Naturale is a clear, colourless sterile solution, presented in a 15 ml Drop-Tainer Dispenser, and contains the Duasorb water soluble polymeric system Dextran 70 0.1% and Hydroxypropyl Methylcellulose (Hypromellose) USP 0.3%, and preserved with Benzalkonium Chloride PhEur 0.01% and Disodium Edetate PhEur 0.05%.

Uses A soothing solution for use as an artificial tear and lubricant in the relief of dry eye syndromes associated with deficient tear secretion or deficient mucous.

Dosage and administration Instill 1 or 2 drops into the eye(s), as frequently as to relieve eye irritation symptoms.

Contra-indications, warnings, etc

Contra-indications: This product contains benzalkonium chloride, and should not be used when soft contact lenses are being worn.

Precautions: If irritation persists, discontinue use.

Pharmaceutical precautions To avoid contaminating the solution, do not let the dropper tip touch any surface. Store at a temperature not exceeding 25°C. Do not refrigerate. Keep the container tightly closed. Discard the contents 1 month after opening.

Legal category P.

Package quantities 15 ml.

Further information Tears Naturale eye-drops are contained in an unbreakable semi-rigid plastic dropper bottle with a screw-on cap.

Product licence number 0649/0031.

VISCOAT*

Ophthalmic viscosurgical device *Description:* Viscoat ophthalmic viscosurgical device is a sterile, non-pyrogenic, viscoelastic solution of highly purified, non-inflammatory medium molecular weight sodium chondroitin sulphate and sodium hyaluronate.

Each 1 ml of Viscoat ophthalmic viscosurgical device contains not more than 40 mg sodium chondroitin sulphate, 30 mg sodium hyaluronate, 0.45 mg monobasic sodium phosphate, monohydrate, 2.00 mg dibasic sodium phosphate, anhydrous, 4.3 mg sodium chloride with water for injection.

Sodium chondroitin sulphate and sodium hyaluronate are quite similar in regard to chemical and physical composition, as each occurs as a large, unbranched chain structure of medium to high molecular weight.

The sodium chondroitin sulphate used in the preparation of the Viscoat ophthalmic viscosurgical device has a mean molecular weight of approximately 22,500 daltons, while the sodium hyaluronate exhibits a molecular weight of over 500,000 daltons.

The sugar moieties of these two compounds occur as repeating disaccharide subunits consisting of glucuronic acid in b1→3 linkage with N-acetylgalactosamine for sodium chondroitin sulphate and N-acetyl-glucosamine for sodium hyaluronate. The subunits are then combined by b1→4 linkage of the amino sugar residue to the glucuronic residue of the next subunit to form large polymers. The two compounds differ in that sodium chondroitin sulphate possesses a sulphate group and a double, rather than a single, negative charge (as in the case of sodium hyaluronate) per repeating disaccharide subunit.

Sodium chondroitin sulphate and sodium hyaluronate are biological polymers found in the extracellular matrix of animals and humans. The cornea is the ocular tissue having the greatest concentration of sodium chondroitin sulphate, while the vitreous and aqueous humor contain the greatest concentration of sodium hyaluronate.

Viscoat is a specific formulation of sodium chondroitin sulphate-sodium hyaluronate that has been developed for use as an aid in ophthalmic surgery.

Viscoat is completely transparent and exhibits excellent flow properties.

Indications: Viscoat is indicated for use as a surgical aid in anterior segment procedures including cataract extraction and intraocular lens implantation. Viscoat maintains a deep chamber during anterior segment surgeries, enhances visualization during the surgical procedure, and protects the corneal endothelium and other ocular tissues. The viscoelasticity of the solution maintains the normal position of the vitreous face and prevents formation of a flat chamber during surgery.

Contra-indications: At the present time, there are no known contraindications to the use of Viscoat when used as recommended.

Warnings: Failure to follow all of the assembly instructions in 'Directions for Use' or use of an alternate cannula may result in cannula detachment and the possibility of serious injury.

Precautions: Precautions are limited to those normally associated with the surgical procedure being performed. Although sodium hyaluronate and sodium chondroitin sulphate are highly purified biological polymers, the physician should be aware of the potential allergic risks inherent in the use of any biological material.

In addition to the above, the following cautions should be observed:

- Do not reuse cannulas.
- Use only if material is clear.
- Avoid trapping air bubbles within Viscoat before injection.

Adverse reactions Viscoat has been extremely well tolerated in human and animal studies. A transient rise in intraocular pressure may be expected due to the presence of sodium hyaluronate, which has been shown to effect such a rise if left in the eye.

Clinical applications For cataract surgery and intraocular lens implantation, Viscoat should be carefully injected using standard aseptic techniques (and using only the 27-gauge cannula provided with the syringe) into the anterior chamber prior to capsulotomy. Viscoat may be injected into the chamber prior to or following removal of the crystalline lens. Instillation of Viscoat prior to lens removal will provide additional protection to the corneal endothelium. Instillation of the solution at this point is significant, in that a coating of Viscoat may protect the corneal endothelium from possible damage arising from surgical instrumentation during cataract extraction surgery. Viscoat may also be used to coat an intraocular lens as well as the tips of surgical instruments prior to implantation. Additional Viscoat may be injected during anterior segment surgery to fully maintain the chamber or replace any volume lost during the surgical procedure. At the end of the surgical procedure, it is recommended that Viscoat be removed from the eye as completely as practical by thoroughly irrigating and aspirating with a balanced salt solution.

How supplied: VISCOAT is a non-pyrogenic, single-use ophthalmic viscosurgical device sterilized by filtration supplied in a disposable syringe delivering 0.5 ml or 0.75 ml. A sterile 27-gauge, disposable, bent, blunt-tip cannula and cannula locking ring are provided separately. The cannula sheath should be used to firmly attach the cannula to the syringe, followed by attachment of the cannula locking ring.

Store in a refrigerator between 2°and 8°C.
Protect from freezing and light.
Store upright.
CE 0123

**Trade Mark*

Allen & Hanburys
Stockley Park West,
Uxbridge, Middlesex UB11 1BT

☎ 0181 990 9000 📠 0181 990 4321

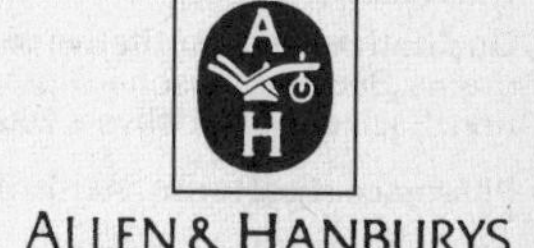

ALLEN & HANBURYS

BECLOFORTE* DISKHALER*

Qualitative and quantitative composition Double-foil disks comprising eight regularly spaced blisters each delivering a mixture of 400 micrograms beclomethasone dipropionate (as the monohydrate) and lactose, used in a Diskhaler device.

Pharmaceutical form Inhalation powder.

Clinical particulars

Therapeutic indications: Beclomethasone dipropionate given by inhalation offers preventative treatment for asthma. It provides effective anti-inflammatory action in the lungs with a lower incidence and severity of adverse effects than those observed when corticosteroids are administered systemically.

Becloforte Diskhaler is indicated in the prophylactic management of severe asthma in adults.

Severe asthma: Patients with severe chronic asthma and those who are dependent on systemic corticosteroids for adequate control of symptoms. Many patients who are dependent on systemic corticosteroids for adequate control of symptoms may be able to reduce significantly, or eliminate, their requirement for oral corticosteroids when they are transferred to high dose inhaled beclomethasone dipropionate.

Becloforte Diskhaler is particularly useful in patients who have difficulty with co-ordinating the effective use of metered-dose inhalers.

Posology and method of administration Beclomethasone Diskhaler is for oral inhalation use only. Patients should be given a starting dose of inhaled beclomethasone dipropionate appropriate to the severity of their disease. The dose may then be adjusted until control is achieved and should be titrated to the lowest dose at which effective control of asthma is maintained.

Adults (including the elderly): 400 micrograms twice daily which may be increased to 800 micrograms twice daily.

For optimum results Becloforte Diskhaler should be used regularly, even when patients are asymptomatic.

Children: Not recommended.

Contra-indications: Hypersensitivity to any of the components.

Special care is necessary in patients with active or quiescent pulmonary tuberculosis.

Special warnings and precautions for use: Becloforte Diskhaler is not designed to relieve acute asthma symptoms for which an inhaled short-acting bronchodilator is required. Patients should be advised to have such relief medication available.

Severe asthma requires regular medical assessment, including lung-function testing, as patients are at risk of severe attacks and even death. Patients must be instructed to seek medical attention if short-acting relief bronchodilator treatment becomes less effective, or more inhalations than usual are required, as this may indicate deterioration of asthma control. In this situation, patients should be assessed and the need for increased anti-inflammatory therapy (e.g. higher doses of inhaled corticosteroid or a course of oral corticosteroid) considered.

Severe exacerbations of asthma must be treated in the normal way, e.g. by increasing the dose of inhaled beclomethasone dipropionate and, if necessary, by giving a systemic steroid, and/or an antibiotic if there is an infection, and by use of β-agonist therapy.

Treatment with **Becloforte Diskhaler** should not be stopped abruptly.

Systemic effects of inhaled corticosteroids may occur, particularly at high doses prescribed for prolonged periods. These effects are much less likely to occur than with oral corticosteroids. Possible systemic effects include adrenal suppression, growth retardation in children and adolescents, decrease in bone mineral density, cataract and glaucoma. It is important therefore that the dose of inhaled corticosteroid is titrated to the lowest dose at which effective control of asthma is maintained.

It is recommended that the height of children receiving prolonged treatment with inhaled corticosteroids is regularly monitored. If growth is slowed, therapy should be reviewed with the aim of reducing the dose of inhaled corticosteroid, if possible, to the lowest dose at which effective control of asthma is maintained. In addition, consideration should be given to referring the patient to a paediatric respiratory specialist.

Prolonged treatment with high doses of inhaled corticosteroids, particularly higher than recommended doses, may result in clinically significant adrenal suppression. Additional systemic corticosteroid cover should be considered during periods of stress or elective surgery.

The transfer to Becloforte Diskhaler of patients who have been treated with systemic steroids for long periods of time, or at a high dose, needs special care, since recovery from any adrenocortical suppression sustained may take a considerable time. Approximately one week after initiating treatment with Becloforte Diskhaler reduction of the dose of systemic steroid can be commenced. The size of the reduction should correspond to the maintenance dose of systemic steroid. Reductions in dose of not more than 1 mg are suitable for patients receiving maintenance doses of 10 mg daily or less of prednisolone or its equivalent. Larger reductions in dose may be appropriate for higher maintenance doses. The reductions in dose should be introduced at not less than weekly intervals. Adrenocortical function should be monitored regularly as the dose of systemic steroid is gradually reduced.

Some patients feel unwell in a non-specific way during the withdrawal phase despite maintenance or even improvement of the respiratory function. They should be encouraged to persevere with inhaled beclomethasone dipropionate and to continue withdrawal of systemic steroid, unless there are objective signs of adrenal insufficiency.

Patients weaned off oral steroids whose adrenocortical function is impaired should carry a steroid warning card indicating that they may need supplementary systemic steroid during periods of stress, e.g. worsening asthma attacks, chest infections, major intercurrent illness, surgery, trauma, etc.

Replacement of systemic steroid treatment with inhaled therapy sometimes unmasks allergies such as allergic rhinitis or eczema previously controlled by the systemic drug. These allergies should be symptomatically treated with antihistamine and/or topical preparations, including topical steroids.

As with all inhaled corticosteroids, special care is necessary in patients with active or quiescent pulmonary tuberculosis.

Interaction with other medicaments and other forms of interaction
None reported.

Pregnancy and lactation
There is inadequate evidence of safety in human pregnancy. Administration of corticosteroids to pregnant animals can cause abnormalities of fetal development including cleft palate and intra-uterine growth retardation. There may therefore be a very small risk of such effects in the human fetus. It should be noted, however, that the fetal changes in animals occur after relatively high systemic exposure. Becloforte Diskhaler delivers the drug directly to the lungs by the inhaled route and so avoids the high level of exposure that occurs when corticosteroids are given by systemic routes.

The use of beclomethasone dipropionate in pregnancy requires that the possible benefits of the drug be weighed against the possible hazards.

No specific studies examining the transference of beclomethasone dipropionate into the milk of lactating animals have been performed. It is reasonable to assume that beclomethasone dipropionate is secreted in milk, but at the dosages used for direct inhalation there is low potential for significant levels in breast milk.

The use of beclomethasone dipropionate in mothers breast feeding their babies requires that the therapeutic benefits of the drug be weighed against the potential hazards to the mother and baby.

Effect on ability to drive and use machines: None reported.

Undesirable effects: Systemic effects of inhaled corticosteroids may occur, particularly at high doses prescribed for prolonged periods. These may include adrenal suppression, growth retardation in children and adolescents, decrease in bone mineral density, cataract and glaucoma.

As with other inhalation therapy, paradoxical bronchospasm may occur with an immediate increase in wheezing after dosing. This responds to a fast-acting inhaled bronchodilator. The preparation should be discontinued immediately, the patient assessed, and if necessary alternative therapy instituted.

Hypersensitivity reactions including rashes, urticaria, pruritus and erythema, and oedema of the eyes, face, lips and throat, have been reported.

Candidiasis of the mouth and throat (thrush) occurs in some patients, the incidence increasing with doses greater than 400 micrograms beclomethasone dipropionate per day. Patients with high blood levels of *Candida precipitins*, indicating a previous infection, are most likely to develop this complication. Patients may find it helpful to rinse their mouth thoroughly with water after using Becloforte Diskhaler. Symptomatic candidiasis can be treated with topical antifungal therapy whilst still continuing with the treatment.

In some patients inhaled beclomethasone dipropionate may cause hoarseness or throat irritation. It may be helpful to rinse out the mouth with water immediately after inhalation.

Overdose

Acute: Inhalation of the drug in doses in excess of those recommended may lead to temporary suppression of adrenal function. This does not require emergency action.

In these patients treatment should be continued at a dose sufficient to control asthma; adrenal function recovers in a few days and can be verified by measuring plasma cortisol.

Chronic: Use of inhaled beclomethasone dipropionate in daily doses in excess of 1,500 micrograms over prolonged periods may lead to adrenal suppression. Monitoring of adrenal reserve may be indicated. Treatment should be continued at a dose sufficient to control asthma.

Pharmacological properties

Pharmacodynamic properties: Beclomethasone dipropionate given by inhalation has a potent glucocorticoid anti-inflammatory action within the lungs.

Pharmacokinetic properties: Beclomethasone dipropionate is rapidly metabolised in the lung to beclomethasone 17-monopropionate and more slowly to free beclomethasone. Irrespective of route of administration the principal route of excretion is faeces. Less than 10% of the drug and its metabolites is excreted in the urine. In humans, 12% to 15% of an orally administered dose of Beclomethasone Dipropionate was excreted in the urine as both conjugated and free metabolites of the drug.

Preclinical safety data: There are no pre-clinical data of relevance to the prescriber which are additional to that already included in other sections of the SPC.

Pharmaceutical particulars

List of excipients: Lactose BP.

Incompatibilities: None reported.

Shelf life: 36 months when stored below 30°C.

Special precautions for storage: Store below 30°C.

A disk may be kept in the Diskhaler device but the blisters must only be pierced immediately prior to use.

Nature and contents of container: A circular double-foil disk with 8 blisters containing the powder mix of beclomethasone dipropionate and lactose. The foil disk is inserted into the Diskhaler device.

Becloforte Diskhaler is supplied as a carton containing 14 disks with a Diskhaler or Refill pack of 14 disks alone.

Instructions for use/handling: The powdered medicine is inhaled through the mouth into the lungs. The Diskhaler device is loaded with a disk which contains the medicine in individual blisters which are opened as the device is manipulated.

For detailed instructions for use refer to the Patient Information Leaflet in every pack.

Marketing authorisation number PL 10949/0066.

Date of approval/revision of SPC August 1998

Legal status POM.

BECLOFORTE* EASI-BREATHE* INHALER

Qualitative and quantitative composition 250 micrograms Beclomethasone Dipropionate BP per actuation. Each canister delivers 200 actuations.

Pharmaceutical form Aerosol.

Clinical particulars
Therapeutic indications: Beclomethasone dipropionate given by inhalation offers preventative treatment for asthma. It provides effective anti-inflammatory action in the lungs without the problems of systemic corticosteroid treatment.

Becloforte Easi-Breathe Inhaler is indicated in the prophylactic management of severe asthma in adults.

Severe asthma: Patients with severe chronic asthma and those who are dependent on systemic corticosteroids for adequate control of symptoms. Many patients who are dependent on systemic corticosteroids for adequate control of symptoms may be able to reduce significantly, or eliminate, their requirement for oral corticosteroids when they are transferred to high dose inhaled beclomethasone dipropionate.

Posology and method of administration: Becloforte Easi-Breathe Inhaler is for oral inhalation use only. The inhaler can be used alone or in combination with the Optimiser* spacer device.

Patients should be given a starting dose of inhaled beclomethasone dipropionate appropriate to the severity of their disease. Those demonstrating a need for high dose inhaled steroid therapy should start on 1,000 micrograms daily. The dose may then be adjusted until control is achieved, or reduced to the minimum effective dose according to individual response.

Adults (including the elderly): 1,000 micrograms daily which may be increased to 2,000 micrograms daily. This may then be reduced when the patient's asthma has stabilised. The total daily dose may be administered as two, three, or four divided doses.

Becloforte Easi-Breathe Inhaler is not recommended for children.

Contra-indications: Hypersensitivity to any of the components.

Special care is necessary in patients with active or quiescent pulmonary tuberculosis.

Special warnings and special precautions for use: Patients should be instructed in the proper use of the inhaler, and their technique checked, to ensure that the drug reaches the target areas within the lungs. They should also be made aware that Becloforte Easi-Breathe Inhaler has to be used regularly, every day, even when they are asymptomatic, for optimum benefit.

Becloforte Easi-Breathe Inhaler is not designed to relieve acute asthma symptoms for which an inhaled short-acting bronchodilator is required. Patients should be advised to have such relief medication available.

Severe asthma requires regular medical assessment, including lung-function testing, as patients are at risk of severe attacks and even death. Patients must be instructed to seek medical attention if short-acting relief bronchodilator treatment becomes less effective, or more inhalations than usual are required as this may indicate deterioration of asthma control. In this situation, patients should be assessed and the need for increased anti-inflammatory therapy (e.g. higher doses of inhaled corticosteroid or a course of oral corticosteroid) considered.

Severe exacerbations of asthma must be treated in the normal way, e.g. by increasing the dose of inhaled beclomethasone dipropionate and, if necessary, by giving a systemic steroid, and/or an antibiotic if there is an infection, and by use of β-agonist therapy.

Treatment with Becloforte Easi-Breathe Inhaler should not be stopped abruptly.

Significant adrenal suppression rarely occurs before doses of 1,500 micrograms per day of inhaled beclomethasone dipropionate are exceeded. Reduction of plasma cortisol levels has been reported in some patients taking 2,000 micrograms per day. In such patients, the risks of developing adrenal suppression should be balanced against the therapeutic advantages, and precautions taken to provide systemic steroid cover in situations of prolonged stress. Prolonged suppression of the hypothalamic-pituitary-adrenal (HPA) axis may eventually lead to systemic effects, including growth retardation in children and adolescents.

The transfer to Becloforte Easi-Breathe Inhaler of patients who have been treated with systemic steroids for long periods of time, or at a high dose, needs special care, since recovery from any adrenocortical suppression sustained may take a considerable time. Approximately one week after initiating treatment with Becloforte Easi-Breathe Inhaler, reduction of the dose of systemic steroid can be commenced.

The size of the reduction should correspond to the maintenance dose of systemic steroid. Reductions in dose of not more than 1 mg are suitable for patients receiving maintenance doses of 10 mg daily or less of prednisolone or its equivalent. Larger reductions in dose may be appropriate for higher maintenance doses. The reductions in dose should be introduced at not less than weekly intervals. Adrenocortical function should be monitored regularly as the dose of systemic steroid is gradually reduced.

Some patients feel unwell in a non-specific way during the withdrawal phase despite maintenance or even improvement of the respiratory function. They should be encouraged to persevere with inhaled beclomethasone dipropionate and to continue withdrawal of systemic steroid, unless there are objective signs of adrenal insufficiency.

Patients weaned off oral steroids whose adrenocortical function is impaired should carry a steroid warning card indicating that they may need supplementary systemic steroid during periods of stress, e.g. worsening asthma attacks, chest infections, major intercurrent illness, surgery, trauma, etc.

Replacement of systemic steroid treatment with inhaled therapy sometimes unmasks allergies such as allergic rhinitis or eczema previously controlled by the systemic drug. These allergies should be symptomatically treated with antihistamine and/or topical preparations, including topical steroids.

As with all inhaled corticosteroids, special care is necessary in patients with active or quiescent pulmonary tuberculosis.

Interaction with other medicaments and other forms of interaction: None reported.

Pregnancy and lactation: There is inadequate evidence of safety in human pregnancy. Administration of corticosteroids to pregnant animals can cause abnormalities of fetal development including cleft palate and intra-uterine growth retardation. There may therefore be a very small risk of such effects in the human fetus. It should be noted, however, that the fetal changes in animals occur after relatively high systemic exposure. Becloforte Easi-Breathe Inhaler delivers the drug directly to the lungs by the inhaled route and so avoids the high level of exposure that occurs when corticosteroids are given by systemic routes.

The use of beclomethasone dipropionate in pregnancy requires that the possible benefits of the drug be weighed against the possible hazards.

No specific studies examining the transference of beclomethasone dipropionate into the milk of lactating animals have been performed. It is reasonable to assume that beclomethasone dipropionate is secreted in milk, but at the dosages used for direct inhalation there is low potential for significant levels in breast milk.

The use of beclomethasone dipropionate in mothers breast feeding their babies requires that the therapeutic benefits of the drug be weighed against the potential hazards to the mother and baby.

Effects on the ability to drive and use machines: None reported.

Undesirable effects: As with other inhalation therapy, paradoxical bronchospasm may occur with an immediate increase in wheezing after dosing. This should be treated immediately with a fast-acting inhaled bronchodilator. The Becloforte Easi-Breathe Inhaler should be discontinued immediately, the patient assessed and, if necessary, alternative therapy instituted.

Hypersensitivity reactions including rashes, urticaria, pruritus and erythema, and oedema of the eyes, face, lips and throat, have been reported.

Candidiasis of the mouth and throat (thrush) occurs in some patients, the incidence increasing with doses greater than 400 micrograms beclomethasone dipropionate per day. Patients with high blood levels of *Candida precipitins*, indicating a previous infection, are most likely to develop this complication. Patients may find it helpful to rinse their mouth thoroughly with water after using the inhaler. The Optimiser spacer can be used to reduce oropharyngeal deposition. Symptomatic candidiasis can be treated with topical anti-fungal therapy whilst still continuing with Becloforte Easi-Breathe Inhaler.

In some patients inhaled beclomethasone dipropionate may cause hoarseness or throat irritation. It may be helpful to rinse the mouth out with water immediately after inhalation. Alternatively, the Optimiser spacer can be used to reduce oropharyngeal deposition.

Overdose:
Acute: Inhalation of the drug in doses in excess of those recommended may lead to temporary suppression of adrenal function. This does not require emergency action. In these patients treatment should be continued at a dose sufficient to control asthma; adrenal function recovers in a few days and can be verified by measuring plasma cortisol.

Chronic: Use of inhaled beclomethasone dipropionate in daily doses in excess of 1,500 micrograms over prolonged periods may lead to some degree of adrenal suppression. Monitoring of adrenal reserve may be indicated. Treatment should be continued at a dose sufficient to control asthma.

Pharmacological properties
Pharmacodynamic properties: Beclomethasone dipropionate given by inhalation has a potent glucocorticoid anti-inflammatory action within the lungs.

Pharmacokinetic properties: Beclomethasone 17,21-dipropionate (BDP) administered intravenously is cleared rapidly with a half-life of approximately 30 minutes. Beclomethasone 17-monopropionate (BMP) appears rapidly in the plasma after intravenous administration of BDP and is itself cleared with a half-life again of about 30 minutes. BDP is bound to plasma proteins to the extent of 87%. Up to 14% of an intravenous dose of BDP is excreted in the urine in 96 hours, mainly as polar metabolites, a proportion of which are conjugated. Up to 64% of the dose is excreted in faeces in this time, again primarily as free and conjugated metabolites.

After inhalation about 25% of the dose reaches the lungs and is available for absorption from this site. The remainder is deposited on the delivery device or in the oropharynx. That portion deposited in the mouth or upper airways will ultimately be swallowed.

There is rapid metabolic inactivation of most of the swallowed portion of BDP during its first passage through the liver. An oral dose (4 mg) of tritium-labelled BDP was absorbed slowly with peak levels of radioactivity equivalent to 20 ng drug/ml plasma being reached 5 hours after dosing. Excretion was mainly in the faeces (35–76% of the dose in 96 hours) and primarily as polar metabolites although the presence of BDP and BMP in faeces suggested incomplete absorption of the dose. Up to 14% of the dose was excreted as polar metabolites in urine.

The lung tissue rapidly hydrolyses BDP to BMP which in turn is hydrolysed more slowly to beclomethasone. The liver also metabolises BDP and BMP and further converts it to polar metabolites.

Preclinical safety data: BDP has low acute oral, subcutaneous and intraperitoneal toxicity in mice and rats, and repeat dose toxicity studies showed findings characteristic of glucocorticoids, with no evidence of irritancy to the respiratory tract. The main findings, at above therapeutic doses, were depression of corticosterone levels in rats and cortisol levels in dogs. BDP is non-genotoxic, and demonstrated no oncogenic potential following combined inhalation/oral administration to rats. Susceptibility of fetuses to cleft palate, noted in the mouse organogenesis study, is considered to have no relevance for therapeutic use.

Pharmaceutical particulars
List of excipients: Oleic acid, dichlorodifluoromethane, trichlorofluoromethane.

Incompatibilities: None reported.

Shelf life: Two years when stored below 30°C.

Special precautions for storage: Store below 30°C.

As with most inhaled medicines in aerosol canisters, the therapeutic effect may decrease when the canister is cold.

Protect from frost and direct sunlight.

The canister should not be broken, punctured or burnt, even when apparently empty.

Nature and contents of container: An inhaler comprising an aluminium can fitted with a breath-operated, metering valve, actuator and dust cap. Each canister contains 200 metered actuations of 250 micrograms beclomethasone dipropionate.

Instructions for use/handling: The aerosol spray is inhaled through the mouth into the lungs. After shaking the inhaler, open the cap and place the mouthpiece in the mouth with the lips closed around it. Suck in slowly through the mouthpiece, this releases a spray. The inhaler can be used with the Optimiser spacer device.

For detailed instructions for use refer to the patient information leaflet in every pack.

Marketing authorisation number 10949/0270.

Date of approval/revision of SPC December 1996.

Legal category POM.

BECLOFORTE INTEGRA

Qualitative and quantitative composition Beclomethasone Dipropionate 250 micrograms per puff.

Pharmaceutical form Metered Dose Aerosol.

Clinical particulars
Therapeutic indications: Beclomethasone Dipropionate provides effective anti-inflammatory action in the lungs, with a lower incidence and severity of adverse effects than those observed when corticosteroids are

administered systemically. It also offers preventative treatment of asthma.

Adults: Becloforte Integra is indicated in the prophylactic management of severe asthma.

Patients with severe chronic asthma and those who are dependent on systemic corticosteroids for adequate control of symptoms. On transfer to high dose inhaled beclomethasone dipropionate, many patients who are dependent on systemic corticosteroids for adequate control of symptoms may be able to reduce significantly or eliminate their requirement for oral corticosteroids.

Posology and method of administration: Patients should be given a starting dose of inhaled beclomethasone dipropionate which is appropriate for the severity of their disease. The dose may then be adjusted until control is achieved and should be titrated to the lowest dose at which effective control of asthma is maintained.

Patients demonstrating a need for high dose inhaled steroid therapy should start on 1000 micrograms daily.

Adults: Two inhalations (500 micrograms) twice daily, or one inhalation (250 micrograms) four times daily is the recommended maintenance dosage. If necessary, dosage may be increased to two inhalations (500 micrograms) three or four times daily, according to response.

Children: Becloforte Integra is not indicated for use in children.

There is no need to adjust the dose in elderly patients or in those with hepatic or renal impairment.

Route of administration: Becloforte Integra is for inhalation use only.

Some patients find difficulty in co-ordinating the firing of an inhaler with inspiration and therefore fail to maximise the potential benefit offered by treatment. Becloforte Integra may be used in patients who find it difficult to synchronise aerosol actuation with inspiration of breath. Patients should inhale straight away after discharging the dose into the spacer device.

Contra-indications: Becloforte Integra is contra-indicated in patients with a history of hypersensitivity to any of its components. Special care is necessary in patients with active or quiescent pulmonary tuberculosis.

Special warnings and precautions for use: Patients should be instructed in the proper use of the inhaler to ensure that the drug reaches the target areas within the lungs. They should also be made aware that Becloforte has to be used regularly, every day, for optimum benefits.

Patients should be made aware of the prophylactic nature of therapy with Becloforte and that they should use it regularly even when they are asymptomatic.

Becloforte Integra is not designed to relieve acute asthmatic symptoms for which an inhaled short-acting bronchodilator is required. Patients should be advised to have such rescue medication available.

Severe asthma requires regular medical assessment including lung function testing as patients are at risk of severe attacks and even death.

Increasing use of bronchodilators, in particular short-acting inhaled β_2 agonists to relieve symptoms indicates deterioration of asthma control. If patients find that short acting relief bronchodilator treatment becomes less effective or they need more inhalations than usual, medical attention must be sought. In this situation, patients should be reassessed and consideration given to the need for increased anti-inflammatory therapy (e.g. higher doses of inhaled corticosteroids or a course of oral corticosteroids). Severe exacerbations of asthma must be treated in the normal way.

Systemic effects of inhaled corticosteroids may occur, particularly at high doses prescribed for prolonged periods. These effects are much less likely to occur than with oral corticosteroids. Possible systemic effects include adrenal suppression, growth retardation in children and adolescents, decrease in bone mineral density, cataract and glaucoma. It is important therefore that the dose of inhaled corticosteroid is titrated to the lowest dose at which effective control of asthma is maintained.

It is recommended that the height of children receiving prolonged treatment with inhaled corticosteroids is regularly monitored. If growth is slowed, therapy should be reviewed with the aim of reducing the dose of inhaled corticosteroid, if possible, to the lowest dose at which effective control of asthma is maintained. In addition, consideration should be given to referring the patient to a paediatric respiratory specialist.

Prolonged treatment with high doses of inhaled corticosteroids, particularly higher than recommended doses, may result in clinically significant adrenal suppression. Additional systemic corticosteroid cover should be considered during periods of stress or elective surgery.

Lack of response or severe exacerbations of asthma should be treated by increasing the dose of inhaled beclomethasone dipropionate and if necessary, by giving a systemic steroid and/or an antibiotic if there is an infection and with beta-agonist therapy.

For the transfer of patients being treated with oral corticosteroids:

The transfer of oral steroid-dependent patients to inhaled beclomethasone dipropionate and their subsequent management needs special care as recovery from impaired adrenocortical function, caused by prolonged systemic steroid therapy, may take a considerable time.

Patients who have been treated with systemic steroids for long periods of time or at a high dose, may have adrenocortical suppression. With these patients, adrenocortical function should be monitored regularly and their dose of systemic steroid reduced cautiously.

After approximately a week, gradual withdrawal of the systemic steroid is commenced. Decrements in dosages should be appropriate to the level of maintenance systemic steroid and introduced at not less than weekly intervals. For maintenance doses of prednisolone (or equivalent) of 10 mg daily or less, the decrements in dose should not be greater than 1 mg per day, at not less than weekly intervals. For maintenance doses of prednisolone in excess of 10 mg daily, it may be appropriate to employ cautiously, larger decrements in dose at weekly intervals.

Some patients feel unwell in a non-specific way during the withdrawal phase despite maintenance or even improvement of the respiratory function. They should be encouraged to persevere with inhaled beclomethasone dipropionate and to continue withdrawal of systemic steroid, unless there are objective signs of adrenal insufficiency.

Patients weaned off oral steroids whose adrenocortical function is impaired should carry a steroid warning card indicating that they may need supplementary systemic steroid during periods of stress, i.e. worsening asthma attacks, chest infections, major intercurrent illness, surgery, trauma, etc.

Replacement of systemic steroid treatment with inhaled therapy sometimes unmasks allergies such as allergic rhinitis or eczema previously controlled by the systemic drug. These allergies should be symptomatically treated with antihistamine and/or topical preparations, including topical steroids.

Treatment with Becloforte Integra should not be stopped abruptly.

As with all inhaled corticosteroids, special care is necessary in patients with active or quiescent pulmonary tuberculosis.

Interaction with other medicaments and other forms of interaction: None known.

Pregnancy and lactation: There is inadequate evidence of safety in human pregnancy. Administration of corticosteroids to pregnant animals can cause abnormalities of foetal development including cleft palate and intra-uterine growth retardation. There may therefore be a very small risk of such effects in the human foetus. It should be noted, however, that the foetal changes in animals occur after relatively high systemic exposure. Because beclomethasone dipropionate is delivered directly to the lungs by the inhaled route, it avoids the high level of exposure that occurs when corticosteroids are given by systemic routes.

The use of beclomethasone dipropionate in pregnancy requires that the possible benefits of the drug be weighed against the possible hazards. It should be noted that the drug has been in widespread use for many years without apparent ill consequence.

No specific studies examining the transference of beclomethasone dipropionate into the milk of lactating animals have been performed. It is reasonable to assume that beclomethasone dipropionate is secreted in milk but at the dosages used for direct inhalation, there is low potential for significant levels in breast milk. The use of beclomethasone dipropionate in mothers breast feeding their babies, requires that the therapeutic benefits of the drug be weighed against the potential hazards to the mother and baby.

Effect on ability to drive and use machines: None known.

Undesirable effects: Systemic effects of inhaled corticosteroids may occur, particularly at high doses prescribed for prolonged periods. These may include adrenal suppression, growth retardation in children and adolescents, decrease in bone mineral density, cataract and glaucoma.

Candidiasis of the mouth and throat (thrush) occurs in some patients, the incidence of which is increased with doses greater than 400 micrograms beclomethasone dipropionate per day. Patients with high blood levels of *Candida precipitins*, indicating a previous infection, are most likely to develop this complication. Patients may find it helpful to rinse their mouth thoroughly with water after using the inhaler. Symptomatic candidiasis can be treated with topical antifungal therapy whilst still continuing with the Becloforte Integra.

In some patients, inhaled beclomethasone dipropionate may cause hoarseness or throat irritation. It may be helpful to rinse the mouth out with water after inhalation.

As with other inhalation therapy, paradoxical bronchospasm may occur with an immediate increase in wheezing after dosing. This responds to a fast-acting inhaled bronchodilator. Becloforte Integra should be discontinued immediately, the patient assessed and if necessary, alternative therapy (e.g. Becloforte Diskhaler) instituted.

Hypersensitivity reactions including rashes, urticaria, pruritus and erythema and oedema of the eyes, face, lips and throat, have been reported.

Overdose

Acute: Inhalation of the drug in doses in excess of those recommended may lead to temporary suppression of adrenal function. This does not necessitate emergency action being taken. In these patients, treatment with beclomethasone dipropionate by inhalation should be continued at a dose sufficient to control asthma; adrenal function recovers in a few days and can be verified by measuring plasma cortisol.

Chronic: Use of inhaled beclomethasone dipropionate in daily doses in excess of 1500 micrograms over prolonged periods may lead to adrenal suppression. Monitoring of adrenal reserve may be indicated. Treatment with inhaled beclomethasone dipropionate should be continued at a dose sufficient to control asthma.

Pharmacological properties

Pharmacodynamic properties: Beclomethasone dipropionate given by inhalation has a potent glucocorticoid anti-inflammatory action within the lungs.

Pharmacokinetic properties: Beclomethasone 17,21-dipropionate (BDP) administered intravenously is cleared rapidly with a half-life of approximately 30 minutes. Beclomethasone 17-monopropionate (BMP) appears rapidly in the plasma after intravenous BDP and is itself cleared with a half-life again of about 30 minutes. BDP is bound to plasma proteins to the extent of 87%. Up to 14% of an intravenous dose of BDP is excreted in the urine in 96 hours, mainly as polar metabolites, a proportion of which are conjugated. Up to 64% of the dose is excreted in faeces in this time, again primarily as free and conjugated metabolites.

After an inhaled dose, the majority of the dose will be deposited in the oropharynx or on the delivery device, with only a fraction reaching the lungs and available for absorption from this site. That portion deposited in the mouth or upper airways will ultimately be swallowed.

There is rapid metabolic inactivation of the majority of the swallowed portion of BDP during its first passage through the liver. An oral dose (4 mg) of tritium labelled BDP was absorbed slowly with peak levels of radioactivity equivalent to 20 ng drug/ml plasma being reached 5 hours after dosing. Excretion was mainly in the faeces (35–76% of the dose in 96 hours) and primarily as polar metabolites although the presence of BDP and BMP in faeces suggested incomplete absorption of the dose. Up to 14% of the dose was excreted as polar metabolites in urine.

The lung tissue rapidly hydrolyses BDP to BMP which in turn is hydrolysed more slowly to beclomethasone. The liver also metabolises BDP and BMP and further converts it to polar metabolites.

Preclinical safety data: There are no pre-clinical data of relevance to the prescriber which are additional to that already included in other sections of the SmPC.

Pharmaceutical particulars

List of excipients:

Oleic acid	HSE
Trichlorofluoromethane	BP
Dichlorodifluoromethane	BP

Incompatibilities: None known.

Shelf life: 36 months.

Special precautions for storage: Becloforte Integra (80 actuations) should be stored at temperatures below 25°C (2–25°C). Becloforte Integra (200 actuations) should be stored at temperatures below 30°C (2–30°C). Direct sunlight and heat should be avoided. The canister should not be punctured, broken or burnt even when apparently empty.

Nature and contents of container: Combination pack of an aluminium aerosol can with valve (200 actuations) and integral actuator with the compatible spacer device. Refill pack containing aluminium aerosol can with valve (200 actuations) and integral actuator.

Instructions for use/handling: Detailed instructions for use/handling can be found on the Patient Information Leaflet.

Marketing authorisation number PL 10949/0041.

Date of approval/revision of SPC July 1998.

Legal classification POM.

BECLOFORTE* INHALER

Qualitative and quantitative composition 250 micrograms Beclomethasone Dipropionate BP per actuation. Each canister delivers 200 actuations.

Pharmaceutical form Aerosol.

Clinical particulars

Therapeutic indications: Beclomethasone dipropionate given by inhalation offers preventative treatment for asthma. It provides effective anti-inflammatory action in the lungs with a lower incidence and severity of adverse effects than those observed when corticosteroids are administered systemically.

Becloforte Inhaler is indicated in the prophylactic management of severe asthma in adults.

Severe asthma: Patients with severe chronic asthma and those who are dependent on systemic corticosteroids for adequate control of symptoms. Many patients who are dependent on systemic corticosteroids for adequate control of symptoms may be able to reduce significantly, or eliminate, their requirement for oral corticosteroids when they are transferred to high dose inhaled beclomethasone dipropionate.

Posology and method of administration: Becloforte Inhaler is for oral inhalation use only.

Some patients find difficulty in co-ordinating the firing of an inhaler with inspiration and therefore fail to maximise the potential benefit offered by treatment. Becloforte Inhaler may be used with a Volumatic* spacer device in patients who find it difficult to synchronise aerosol actuation with inspiration.

Patients should be given a starting dose of inhaled beclomethasone dipropionate appropriate to the severity of their disease. Those demonstrating a need for high dose inhaled steroid therapy should start on 1,000 micrograms daily. The dose may then be adjusted until control is achieved and should be titrated to the lowest dose at which effective control of asthma is maintained.

Adults (including the elderly): 1,000 micrograms daily which may be increased to 2,000 micrograms daily. This may then be reduced when the patient's asthma has stabilised. The total daily dose may be administered as two, three, or four divided doses.

For optimum results Becloforte Inhaler should be used regularly, even when patients are asymptomatic.

Children: Not recommended.

Contra-indications: Hypersensitivity to any of the components.

Special care is necessary in patients with active or quiescent pulmonary tuberculosis.

Special warnings and precautions for use: Patients' inhaler technique should be checked to make sure that aerosol actuation is synchronised with inspiration of breath for optimum delivery of drug to the lungs.

Patients should be made aware of the prophylactic nature of therapy with Becloforte and that, for optimum benefits, they should use it regularly, every day, even when they are asymptomatic.

Becloforte Inhaler is not designed to relieve acute asthmatic symptoms for which an inhaled short-acting bronchodilator is required. Patients should be advised to have such rescue medication available.

Severe asthma requires regular medical assessment, including lung function testing, as patients are at risk of severe attacks and even death.

Increasing use of bronchodilators, in particular short-acting inhaled Beta$_2$ agonists to relieve symptoms indicates deterioration of asthma control. If patients find that short acting relief bronchodilator treatment becomes less effective or they need more inhalations than usual, medical attention must be sought. In this situation patients should be reassessed and consideration given to the need for increased anti-inflammatory therapy (e.g. higher doses of inhaled corticosteroids or a course of oral corticosteroids). Severe exacerbations of asthma must be treated in the normal way.

Systemic effects of inhaled corticosteroids may occur, particularly at high doses prescribed for prolonged periods. These effects are much less likely to occur than with oral corticosteroids. Possible systemic effects include adrenal suppression, growth retardation in children and adolescents, decrease in bone mineral density, cataract and glaucoma. It is important therefore that the dose of inhaled corticosteroid is titrated to the lowest dose at which effective control of asthma is maintained.

It is recommended that the height of children receiving prolonged treatment with inhaled corticosteroids is regularly monitored. If growth is slowed, therapy should be reviewed with the aim of reducing the dose of inhaled corticosteroid, if possible, to the lowest dose at which effective control of asthma is maintained. In addition, consideration should be given to referring the patient to a paediatric respiratory specialist.

Prolonged treatment with high doses of inhaled corticosteroids, particularly higher than recommended doses, may result in clinically significant adrenal suppression. Additional systemic corticosteroid cover should be considered during periods of stress or elective surgery.

Lack of response of severe exacerbations of asthma should be treated by increasing the dose of inhaled beclomethasone dipropionate and, if necessary, by giving a systemic steroid and/or an antibiotic if there is an infection, and with Beta-agonist therapy.

For the transfer of patients being treated with oral corticosteroids: The transfer of oral steroid-dependent patients to inhaled beclomethasone dipropionate and their subsequent management needs special care as recovery from impaired adrenocortical function caused by prolonged systemic steroid therapy, may take a considerable time.

Patients who have been treated with systemic steroids for long periods of time or at a high dose may have adrenocortical suppression. With these patients adrenocortical function should be monitored regularly and their dose of systemic steroid reduced cautiously.

After approximately a week, gradual withdrawal of the systemic steroid is commenced. Decrements in dosages should be appropriate to the level of maintenance systemic steroid, and introduced at not less than weekly intervals. For maintenance doses of prednisolone (or equivalent) of 10 mg daily or less, the decrements in dose should not be greater than 1 mg per day, at not less than weekly intervals. For maintenance doses of prednisolone in excess of 10 mg daily, it may be appropriate to employ cautiously, larger decrements in dose at weekly intervals.

Some patients feel unwell in a non-specific way during the withdrawal phase despite maintenance or even improvement of the respiratory function. They should be encouraged to persevere with inhaled beclomethasone dipropionate and to continue withdrawal of systemic steroid, unless there are objective signs of adrenal insufficiency.

Patients weaned off oral steroids whose adrenocortical function is impaired should carry a steroid warning card indicating that they may need supplementary systemic steroid during periods of stress e.g. worsening asthma attacks, chest infections, major intercurrent illness, surgery, trauma etc.

Replacement of systemic steroid treatment with inhaled therapy sometimes unmasks allergies such as allergic rhinitis or eczema previously controlled by the systemic drug. These allergies should be treated with antihistamine and/or topical preparations, including topical steroids.

Treatment with Becloforte Inhaler should not be stopped abruptly.

As with all inhaled corticosteroids, special care is necessary in patients with active quiescent pulmonary tuberculosis.

Interaction with other medicaments and other forms of interaction: None reported.

Pregnancy and lactation: There is inadequate evidence of safety in human pregnancy. Administration of corticosteroids to pregnant animals can cause abnormalities of fetal development including cleft palate and intra-uterine growth retardation. There may therefore be a very small risk of such effects in the human fetus. It should be noted, however, that the fetal changes in animals occur after relatively high systemic exposure. Becloforte Inhaler delivers the drug directly to the lungs by the inhaled route and so avoids the high level of exposure that occurs when corticosteroids are given by systemic routes.

The use of beclomethasone dipropionate in pregnancy requires that the possible benefits of the drug be weighed against the possible hazards.

No specific studies examining the transference of beclomethasone dipropionate into the milk of lactating animals have been performed. It is reasonable to assume that beclomethasone dipropionate is secreted in milk, but at the dosages used for direct inhalation there is low potential for significant levels in breast milk.

The use of beclomethasone dipropionate in mothers breast feeding their babies requires that the therapeutic benefits of the drug be weighed against the potential hazards to the mother and baby.

Effect on the ability to drive and use machines: None reported.

Undesirable effects: Systemic effects of inhaled corticosteroids may occur, particularly at high doses prescribed for prolonged periods. These may include adrenal suppression, growth retardation in children and adolescents, decrease in bone mineral density, cataract and glaucoma.

As with other inhalation therapy, paradoxical bronchospasm may occur with an immediate increase in wheezing after dosing. This responds to a fast-acting inhaled bronchodilator. The preparation should be discontinued immediately, the patient assessed, and if necessary alternative therapy instituted.

Hypersensitivity reactions including rashes, urticaria, pruritus and erythema, and oedema of the eyes, face, lips and throat, have been reported.

Candidiasis of the mouth and throat (thrush) occurs in some patients, the incidence increasing with doses greater than 400 micrograms beclomethasone dipropionate per day. Patients with high blood levels of *Candida precipitins*, indicating a previous infection, are most likely to develop this complication. Patients may find it helpful to rinse their mouth thoroughly with water after using Becloforte Inhaler. Symptomatic candidiasis can be treated with topical antifungal therapy whilst still continuing with the treatment.

In some patients inhaled beclomethasone dipropionate may cause hoarseness or throat irritation. It may be helpful to rinse out the mouth with water immediately after inhalation. The use of the Volumatic spacer device may also be considered.

Overdose:

Acute: Inhalation of the drug in doses in excess of those recommended may lead to temporary suppression of adrenal function. This does not require emergency action.

In these patients treatment should be continued at a dose sufficient to control asthma; adrenal function recovers in a few days and can be verified by measuring plasma cortisol.

Chronic: Use of inhaled beclomethasone dipropionate in daily doses in excess of 1,500 micrograms over prolonged periods may lead to adrenal suppression. Monitoring of adrenal reserve may be indicated. Treatment should be continued at a dose sufficient to control asthma.

Pharmacological properties

Pharmacodynamic properties: Beclomethasone dipropionate given by inhalation has a potent glucocorticoid anti-inflammatory action within the lungs.

Pharmacokinetic properties: Beclomethasone 17,21-dipropionate (BDP) administered intravenously is cleared rapidly with a half-life of approximately 30 minutes. Beclomethasone 17-monopropionate (BMP) appears rapidly in the plasma after intravenous administration of BDP and is itself cleared with a half-life again of about 30 minutes. BDP is bound to plasma proteins to the extent of 87%. Up to 14% of an intravenous dose of BDP is excreted in the urine in 96 hours, mainly as polar metabolites, a proportion of which are conjugated. Up to 64% of the dose is excreted in faeces in this time, again primarily as free and conjugated metabolites.

After an inhaled dose, the majority of the dose will be deposited in the oropharynx or on the delivery device, with only a fraction reaching the lungs and available for absorption from this site. That portion deposited in the mouth or upper airways will ultimately be swallowed.

There is rapid metabolic inactivation of most of the swallowed portion of BDP during its first passage through the liver. An oral dose (4 mg) of tritium-labelled BDP was absorbed slowly with peak levels of radioactivity equivalent to 20 ng drug/ml plasma being reached 5 hours after dosing. Excretion was mainly in the faeces (35–76% of the dose in 96 hours) and primarily as polar metabolites although the presence of BDP and BMP in faeces suggested incomplete absorption of the dose. Up to 14% of the dose was excreted as polar metabolites in urine.

The lung tissue rapidly hydrolyses BDP to BMP which in turn is hydrolysed more slowly to beclomethasone. The liver also metabolises BDP to BMP and further converts it to polar metabolites.

Preclinical safety data: There are no pre-clinical data of relevance to the prescriber which are additional to that already included in other sections of the SPC.

Pharmaceutical particulars

List of excipients:
Oleic Acid.
Dichlorodifluoromethane.
Trichlorofluoromethane.

Incompatibilities: None reported.

Shelf life: 3 years when stored below 30°C. 3 years when stored below 25°C (80 actuations only).

Special precautions for storage: Store below 30°C.

Store below 25°C (80 actuations only).

As with most inhaled medicines in aerosol canisters, the therapeutic effect may decrease when the canister is cold.

Protect from frost and direct sunlight.

The canister should not be broken, punctured or burnt, even when apparently empty.

Nature and contents of container: An inhaler comprising an aluminium can sealed with a metering valve, with an actuator and dust cap. Each canister provides 200 metered actuations of 250 micrograms beclomethasone dipropionate.

Instructions for use/handling: The aerosol spray is inhaled through the mouth into the lungs. After shaking the inhaler, the mouthpiece is placed in the mouth and the lips closed around it. The actuator is depressed to release a spray, which must coincide with inspiration of breath.

For detailed instructions for use refer to the Patient Information Leaflet in every pack.

Marketing authorisation number PL 10949/0065.

Date of approval/revision of SPC August 1998.

Legal status POM.

BECODISKS*

Presentation: The active ingredient is presented in a disk comprising eight regularly spaced double-foil blisters each containing either 100 micrograms or 200 micrograms of Beclomethasone Dipropionate BP, or 400 micrograms of beclomethasone dipropionate as the monohydrate, and larger particle lactose. Each dosage strength is identified in the centre of the disk as 'Becodisk 100 mcg', or 'Becodisk 200 mcg', or 'Becodisk 400 mcg' respectively.

Becodisks are intended only for use in a specific drug delivery device known as the Diskhaler*. The contents of each blister are deposited in the Diskhaler device when pierced with an integral needle. The contents are then available to the patient to inhale by breath operation which allows the drug to be fully available even at low inspiratory flow rates.

Becodisks therefore provide reliable drug delivery for many patients.

Uses Beclomethasone dipropionate provides effective anti-inflammatory action in the lungs, with a lower incidence and severity of adverse effects than those observed when corticosteroids are administered systemically. It also offers preventative treatment of asthma.

Becodisks are particularly useful in patients who have difficulty with co-ordinating the effective use of metered-dose inhalers.

Therapeutic indications: Becodisks are indicated for a wide range of patients with asthma.

Adults: Prophylactic management in:

mild asthma: Patients requiring symptomatic bronchodilator asthma medication on a regular basis.

moderate asthma: Patients with unstable or worsening asthma despite prophylactic therapy or bronchodilator alone.

severe asthma: Patients with severe chronic asthma and those who are dependent on systemic corticosteroids for adequate control of symptoms. On transfer to high dose inhaled beclomethasone dipropionate, many patients who are dependent on systemic corticosteroids for adequate control of symptoms may be able to reduce significantly, or eliminate, their requirement for oral corticosteroids.

Children: Any child who requires prophylactic asthma medication.

Dosage and administration Becodisks are for inhalation use only, using a Becotide* Diskhaler. Patients should be made aware of the prophylactic nature of therapy with inhaled beclomethasone dipropionate and that it should be taken regularly every day even when they are asymptomatic. Patients should be given a starting dose of inhaled beclomethasone dipropionate which is appropriate to the severity of their disease. The dose may then be adjusted until control is achieved and should be titrated to the lowest dose at which effective control of asthma is maintained.

Adults: 400 micrograms twice daily is the usual starting dose. One 400 micrograms blister or two 200 micrograms blisters twice daily is the usual maintenance dose. Alternatively, 200 micrograms may be administered three or four times daily.

Children: 100 micrograms two, three or four times a day according to the response. Alternatively the usual starting dose of 200 micrograms twice daily may be administered.

There is no need to adjust the dose in elderly patients or in those with hepatic or renal impairment.

Contra-indications, warnings, etc

Contra-indications: Becodisks are contra-indicated in patients with a history of hypersensitivity to any of the components. Special care is necessary in patients with active or quiescent pulmonary tuberculosis.

Precautions: Patients should be instructed in the proper use of the Diskhaler to ensure that the drug reaches the target areas within the lungs. They should also be made aware that Becodisks have to be used regularly, every day, for optimum benefit. Patients should be made aware of the prophylactic nature of therapy with Becodisks and that they should be used regularly, even when they are asymptomatic.

Becodisks are not designed to relieve acute asthmatic symptoms for which an inhaled short-acting bronchodilator is required. Patients should be advised to have such rescue medication available.

Severe asthma requires regular medical assessment, including lung-function testing, as patients are at risk of severe attacks and even death.

Increasing use of bronchodilators, in particular short-acting inhaled β_2-agonists, to relieve symptoms indicates deterioration of asthma control. If patients find that short-acting relief bronchodilator treatment becomes less effective, or they need more inhalations than usual, medical attention must be sought. In this situation patients should be reassessed and consideration given to the need for increased anti-inflammatory therapy (e.g. higher doses of inhaled corticosteroids or a course of oral corticosteroids). Severe exacerbations of asthma must be treated in the normal way.

Systemic effects of inhaled corticosteroids may occur, particularly at high doses prescribed for prolonged periods. These effects are much less likely to occur than with oral corticosteroids. Possible systemic effects include adrenal suppression, growth retardation in children and adolescents, decrease in bone mineral density, cataract and glaucoma. It is important therefore that the dose of inhaled corticosteroid is titrated to the lowest dose at which effective control of asthma is maintained.

It is recommended that the height of children receiving prolonged treatment with inhaled corticosteroids is regularly monitored. If growth is slowed, therapy should be reviewed with the aim of reducing the dose of inhaled corticosteroid, if possible, to the lowest dose at which effective control of asthma is maintained. In addition, consideration should be given to referring the patient to a paediatric respiratory specialist.

Prolonged treatment with high doses of inhaled corticosteroids, particularly higher than the recommended doses, may result in clinically significant adrenal suppression. Additional systemic corticosteroid cover should be considered during periods of stress or elective surgery.

Lack of response or severe exacerbations of asthma should be treated by increasing the dose of inhaled beclomethasone dipropionate and, if necessary, by giving a systemic steroid and/or antibiotic if there is an infection, and by use of β-agonist therapy.

For the transfer of patients being treated with oral corticosteroids: The transfer of oral steroid-dependent patients to Becodisks, and their subsequent management, needs special care as recovery from impaired adrenocortical function, caused by prolonged systemic steroid therapy, may take a considerable time.

Patients who have been treated with systemic steroids for long periods of time or at a high dose may have adrenocortical suppression. With these patients adrenocortical function should be monitored regularly and their dose of systemic steroid reduced cautiously.

After approximately a week, gradual withdrawal of the systemic steroid is commenced. Decrements in dosages should be appropriate to the level of maintenance systemic steroid, and introduced at not less than weekly intervals. For maintenance doses of prednisolone (or equivalent) of 10 mg daily or less, the decrements in dose should be not greater than 1 mg per day, at not less than weekly intervals. For maintenance doses of prednisolone in excess of 10 mg daily, it may be appropriate to employ cautiously, larger decrements in dose at weekly intervals.

Some patients feel unwell in a non-specific way during the withdrawal phase despite maintenance or even improvement of the respiratory function. They should be encouraged to persevere with the Diskhaler and withdrawal of systemic steroid continued, unless there are objective signs of adrenal insufficiency.

Patients weaned off oral steroids whose adrenocortical function is impaired should carry a steroid warning card indicating that they may need supplementary systemic steroid during periods of stress, e.g. worsening asthma attacks, chest infections, major intercurrent illness, surgery, trauma, etc.

Replacement of systemic steroid treatment with inhaled therapy sometimes unmasks allergies such as allergic rhinitis or eczema previously controlled by the systemic drug. These allergies should be symptomatically treated with antihistamine and/or topical preparations, including topical steroids.

Treatment with Becodisks should not be stopped abruptly.

As with all inhaled corticosteroids, special care is necessary in patients with active or quiescent pulmonary tuberculosis.

Pregnancy: There is inadequate evidence of safety in human pregnancy. Administration of corticosteroids to pregnant animals can cause abnormalities of fetal development including cleft palate and intra-uterine growth retardation. There may therefore be a very small risk of such effects in the human fetus. It should be noted, however, that the fetal changes in animals occur after relatively high systemic exposure. Because beclomethasone dipropionate is delivered directly to the lungs by the inhaled route it avoids the high level of exposure that occurs when corticosteroids are given by systemic routes.

The use of beclomethasone dipropionate in pregnancy requires that the possible benefits of the drug be weighed against the possible hazards. It should be noted that the drug has been in widespread use for many years without apparent ill consequence.

Lactation: No specific studies examining the transference of beclomethasone dipropionate into the milk of lactating animals have been performed. It is reasonable to assume that beclomethasone dipropionate is secreted in milk, but at the dosages used for direct inhalation there is low potential for significant levels in breast milk.

The use of beclomethasone dipropionate in mothers breast feeding their babies requires that the therapeutic benefits of the drug be weighed against the potential hazards to the mother and baby.

Side-effects: Systemic effects of inhaled corticosteroids may occur, particularly at high doses prescribed for prolonged periods. These may include adrenal suppression, growth retardation in children and adolescents, decrease in bone mineral density, cataract and glaucoma.

Candidiasis of the mouth and throat (thrush) occurs in some patients, the incidence increasing with doses greater than 400 micrograms beclomethasone dipropionate per day. Patients with high blood levels of *Candida precipitins*, indicating a previous infection, are more likely to develop this complication. Some patients may find it helpful to rinse their mouth thoroughly with water after using Becodisks. Symptomatic candidiasis can be treated with topical antifungal therapy whilst still continuing with the treatment.

In some patients inhaled beclomethasone dipropionate may cause hoarseness or throat irritation. It may be helpful to rinse the mouth out with water immediately after inhalation.

As with other inhalation therapy, paradoxical bronchospasm may occur with an immediate increase in wheezing after dosing. This responds to a fast-acting inhaled bronchodilator. The preparation should be discontinued immediately, the patient assessed, and if necessary alternative therapy instituted.

Hypersensitivity reactions including rashes, urticaria, pruritus and erythema, and oedema of the eyes, face, lips and throat, have been reported.

Overdosage: Acute. Inhalation of the drug in doses in excess of those recommended may lead to temporary suppression of adrenal function. This does not necessitate emergency action being taken. In these patients treatment with beclomethasone dipropionate by inhalation should be continued at a dose sufficient to control asthma; adrenal function recovers in a few days and can be verified by measuring plasma cortisol.

Chronic. Use of inhaled beclomethasone dipropionate in daily doses in excess of 1,500 micrograms over prolonged periods may lead to adrenal suppression. Monitoring of adrenal reserve may be indicated. Treatment with inhaled beclomethasone dipropionate should be continued at a dose sufficient to control asthma.

Pharmaceutical precautions Whilst the disks provide a good protection to the blister contents from the effects of the atmosphere they should not be exposed to extremes of temperature and should be stored below 30°C. A disk may be kept in the Diskhaler at all times but a blister should only be pierced immediately prior to use. Failure to observe this instruction may affect the operation of the Diskhaler.

Legal category POM.

Package quantities Becodisks 100 micrograms and 200 micrograms are supplied in cartons of 14, together with a Diskhaler device. Becodisks 400 micrograms are supplied in cartons of 7 with a Diskhaler device.

Further information Nil.

Product licence numbers

Becodisks 100 micrograms 10949/0055
Becodisks 200 micrograms 10949/0056
Becodisks 400 micrograms 10949/0057

BECONASE* AQUEOUS NASAL SPRAY

Qualitative and quantitative composition Beclomethasone Dipropionate 50 mcg (as monohydrate, micronised).

Pharmaceutical form Aqueous suspension for intranasal inhalation via metered dose atomising pump.

Clinical particulars

Therapeutic indications: Beconase Aqueous Nasal Spray is indicated for the prophylaxis and treatment of perennial and seasonal allergic rhinitis including hayfever, and vasomotor rhinitis. Beclomethasone dipropionate has a potent, anti-inflammatory effect within the respiratory tract, with a lower incidence and severity of adverse events than those observed when corticosteroids are administered systemically.

Posology and method of administration: Beconase Aqueous Nasal Spray is for administration by the intranasal route only.

Adults and children over six years of age: The recommended dosage is two sprays into each nostril twice daily (400 micrograms/day). Once control has been established it may be possible to maintain control with fewer sprays. A dosage regimen of one spray into each nostril morning and evening has been shown to be efficacious in some patients. However, should symptoms recur, patients should revert to the recommended dosage of two sprays into each nostril morning and evening. The minimum dose should be used at which effective control of symptoms is maintained. Total daily administration should not normally exceed eight sprays.

For full therapeutic benefit regular usage is essential. The co-operation of the patient should be sought to comply with the regular dosage schedule and it should be explained that maximum relief may not be obtained within the first few applications.

For children under six years old, there are insufficient clinical data to recommend use.

Contra-indications: Beconase Aqueous Nasal Spray is contra-indicated in patients with a history of hypersensitivity to any of its components.

Special warnings and precautions for use: Systemic effects of nasal corticosteroids may occur, particularly at high doses prescribed for prolonged periods. Growth retardation has been reported in children receiving nasal corticosteroids at licensed doses.

It is recommended that the height of children receiving prolonged treatment with nasal corticosteroids is regularly monitored. If growth is slowed, therapy should be reviewed with the aim of reducing the dose of nasal corticosteroid, if possible to the lowest dose at which effective control of symptoms is maintained. In addition, consideration should be given to referring the patient to a paediatric specialist.

Treatment with higher than recommended doses may result in clinically significant adrenal suppression. If there is evidence for higher than recommended doses being used then additional systemic corticosteroid cover should be considered during periods of stress or elective surgery.

Care must be taken while transferring patients from systemic steroid treatment to Beconase Aqueous Nasal Spray if there is any reason to suppose that their adrenal function is impaired.

Infections of the nasal passages and paranasal sinuses should be appropriately treated but do not constitute a specific contra-indication to treatment with Beconase Aqueous Nasal Spray.

Although Beconase Aqueous Nasal Spray will control seasonal allergic rhinitis in most cases, an abnormally heavy challenge of summer allergens may in certain instances necessitate appropriate additional therapy particularly to control eye symptoms.

Interaction with other medicaments and other forms of interaction: Not applicable.

Pregnancy and lactation: There is inadequate evidence of safety in human pregnancy. Administration of corticosteroids to pregnant animals can cause abnormalities of foetal development including cleft palate and intra-uterine growth retardation. There may therefore be a very small risk of such effects in the human foetus. It should be noted, however, that the foetal changes in animals occur after relatively high systemic exposure. Beconase Aqueous Nasal Spray delivers beclomethasone dipropionate directly to the nasal mucosa and so minimises systemic exposure.

The use of beclomethasone dipropionate should be avoided during pregnancy unless thought essential by the doctor.

No specific studies examining the transference of beclomethasone dipropionate into the milk of lactating animals have been performed. It is reasonable to assume that beclomethasone dipropionate is secreted in milk, but at the dosages used for direct intranasal administration there is low potential for significant levels in breast milk. The use of beclomethasone dipropionate in mothers breast feeding their babies requires that the therapeutic benefits of the drug be weighed against the potential hazards to the mother and baby.

Effect on ability to drive and use machines: Not applicable.

Undesirable effects: Systemic effects of nasal corticosteroids may occur particularly when presented at high doses for prolonged periods.

Rare cases of nasal septal perforation have been reported following the use of intranasal corticosteroids.

As with other nasal sprays, dryness and irritation of the nose and throat, unpleasant taste and smell and epistaxis have been reported rarely.

Rare cases of raised intraocular pressure or glaucoma in association with intranasal formulations of beclomethasone have been reported.

Hypersensitivity reactions including rashes, urticaria, pruritus and erythema, and oedema of the eyes, face, lips and throat, have been reported.

Overdose: The only harmful effect that follows inhalation of large amounts of the drug over a short time period is suppression of Hypothalamic-Pituitary-Adrenal (HPA) function. No special emergency action need be taken. Treatment with Beconase Aqueous Nasal Spray should be continued at the recommended dose. HPA function recovers in a day or two.

Pharmacological properties

Pharmacodynamic properties: Beclomethasone dipropionate BP given by inhalation has a potent glucocorticoid anti-inflammatory action within the lungs with a lower incidence and severity of adverse effects than those when corticosteroids are administered systemically.

Extensive studies have been performed in animals on the pharmacology of beclomethasone dipropionate.

Pharmacokinetic properties: Inhaled beclomethasone dipropionate BP has been shown to have a satisfactory pharmacokinetic profile through many years of successful clinical experience.

Irrespective of the route of administration less than 10% of the drug and its metabolites are excreted in the urine. The principal route of excretion is in the faeces, following biliary conjugation.

In humans, 12% to 15% of an orally administered dose of beclomethasone dipropionate was excreted in the urine as both the conjugated and free metabolites of the drug.

Preclinical safety data: No clinically relevant findings were observed in preclinical studies.

Pharmaceutical particulars

List of excipients: Avicel RC 591 (Microcrystalline Cellulose And Carboxymethylcellulose Sodium) US NF, Anhydrous Dextrose BP, Benzalkonium Chloride BP, Phenylethyl Alcohol USP, Polysorbate 80 BP, Purified Water BP.

Incompatibilities: Not applicable.

Shelf life: 24 months below 30°C.

Special precautions for storage: Beconase Aqueous Nasal Spray should be protected from light and stored below 30°C. Do not refrigerate.

Nature and contents of container: A 25 ml amber neutral glass bottle fitted with a metering atomising pump. Pack size: 200 Metered Spray.

Instructions for use/handling: Refer to Patient Information Leaflet.

Marketing authorisation number PL 10949/0104.

Date of approval/revision of SPC September 1998.

BECOTIDE* 50 EASI-BREATHE* INHALER
BECOTIDE* 100 EASI-BREATHE* INHALER

Qualitative and quantitative composition 50 or 100 micrograms Beclomethasone Dipropionate BP per actuation. Each canister delivers 200 actuations.

Pharmaceutical form Aerosol.

Clinical particulars

Therapeutic indications: Beclomethasone dipropionate given by inhalation offers preventative treatment for asthma. It provides effective anti-inflammatory action in the lungs without the problems of systemic corticosteroid treatment.

Becotide Easi-Breathe Inhalers are indicated in the prophylactic management of mild, moderate, or severe asthma in adults or children.

Mild asthma: Patients requiring symptomatic bronchodilator asthma medication on a regular basis.

Moderate asthma: Patients with unstable or worsening asthma despite prophylactic therapy or bronchodilator alone.

Severe asthma: Patients with severe chronic asthma and those who are dependent on systemic corticosteroids for adequate control of symptoms. Many patients who are dependent on systemic corticosteroids for adequate control of symptoms may be able to reduce significantly, or eliminate, their requirement for oral corticosteroids when they are transferred to high dose inhaled beclomethasone dipropionate.

Posology and method of administration: Becotide Easi-Breathe Inhalers are for oral inhalation use only. The inhalers can be used alone or in combination with the Optimiser* spacer device.

Patients should be given a starting dose of inhaled beclomethasone dipropionate appropriate to the severity of their disease. The dose may than be adjusted until control is achieved, or reduced to the minimum effective dose according to individual response.

Adults (including the elderly): The usual starting dose is 200 micrograms twice a day. In more severe cases the starting dose may need to increase to 600 to 800 micrograms per day which may then be reduced when the patient's asthma has stabilised. The total daily dose may be administered as two, three, or four divided doses.

Children: The usual starting dose is 100 micrograms twice a day. This may be increased to 400 micrograms per day according to the response, administered as two, three, or four divided doses.

Contra-indications: Hypersensitivity to any of the components.

Special care is necessary in patients with active or quiescent pulmonary tuberculosis.

Special warnings and special precautions for use: Patients should be instructed in the proper use of the inhaler, and their technique checked, to ensure that the drug reaches the target areas within the lungs. They should also be made aware that Becotide Easi-Breathe Inhaler has to be used regularly, every day, even when they are asymptomatic, for optimum benefit.

Becotide Easi-Breathe Inhaler is not designed to relieve acute asthma symptoms for which an inhaled short-acting bronchodilator is required. Patients should be advised to have such relief medication available.

Severe asthma requires regular medical assessment, including lung-function testing, as patients are at risk of severe attacks and even death. Patients must be instructed to seek medical attention if short-acting relief bronchodilator treatment becomes less effective, or more inhalations than usual are required as this may indicate deterioration of asthma control. In this situation, patients should be assessed and the need for increased anti-inflammatory therapy (e.g. higher doses of inhaled corticosteroid or a course of oral corticosteroid) considered.

Severe exacerbations of asthma must be treated in the normal way, e.g. by increasing the dose of inhaled beclomethasone dipropionate and, if necessary by giving a systemic steroid, and/or an antibiotic if there is an infection, and by use of β-agonist therapy.

Treatment with Becotide Easi-Breathe Inhaler should not be stopped abruptly.

Significant adrenal suppression rarely occurs before doses of 1,500 micrograms per day of inhaled beclomethasone dipropionate are exceeded. Reduction of plasma cortisol levels has been reported in some patients taking 2,000 micrograms per day. In such patients, the risks of developing adrenal suppression should be balanced against the therapeutic advantages, and precautions taken to provide systemic steroid cover in situations of prolonged stress. Prolonged suppression of the hypothalamic-pituitary-adrenal (HPA) axis may eventually lead to systemic effects, including growth retardation in children and adolescents.

The transfer to Becotide Easi-Breathe Inhaler of patients who have been treated with systemic steroids for long periods of time, or at a high dose, needs special care, since recovery from any adrenocortical suppression sustained may take a considerable time. Approximately one week after initiating treatment with Becotide Easi-Breathe Inhaler, reduction of the dose of systemic steroid can be commenced. The size of the reduction should correspond to the maintenance dose of systemic steroid. Reductions in dose of not more than 1 mg are suitable for patients receiving maintenance doses of 10 mg daily or less of prednisolone or its equivalent. Larger reductions in dose may be appropriate for higher maintenance doses. The reductions in dose should be introduced at not less than weekly intervals. Adrenocortical function should be monitored regularly as the dose of systemic steroid is gradually reduced.

Some patients feel unwell in a non-specific way during the withdrawal phase despite maintenance or even improvement of the respiratory function. They should be encouraged to persevere with inhaled beclomethasone dipropionate and to continue withdrawal of systemic steroid, unless there are objective signs of adrenal insufficiency.

Patients weaned off oral steroids whose adrenocortical function is impaired should carry a steroid warning card indicating that they may need supplementary systemic steroid during periods of stress, e.g. worsening asthma attacks, chest infections, major intercurrent illness, surgery, trauma, etc.

Replacement of systemic steroid treatment with inhaled therapy sometimes unmasks allergies such as allergic rhinitis or eczema previously controlled by the systemic drug. These allergies should be symptomatically treated with antihistamine and/or topical preparations, including topical steroids.

As with all inhaled corticosteroids, special care is necessary in patients with active or quiescent pulmonary tuberculosis.

Interaction with other medicaments and other forms of interaction: None reported.

Pregnancy and lactation: There is inadequate evidence of safety in human pregnancy. Administration of corticosteroids to pregnant animals can cause abnormalities of fetal development including cleft palate and intra-uterine growth retardation. There may therefore be a very small risk of such effects in the human fetus. It should be noted, however, that the fetal changes in animals occur after relatively high systemic exposure. Becotide Easi-Breathe Inhaler delivers the drug directly to the lungs by the inhaled route and so avoids the high level of exposure that occurs when corticosteroids are given by systemic routes.

The use of beclomethasone dipropionate in pregnancy requires that the possible benefits of the drug be weighed against the possible hazards.

No specific studies examining the transference of beclomethasone dipropionate into the milk of lactating animals have been performed. It is reasonable to assume that beclomethasone dipropionate is secreted in milk, but at the dosages used for direct inhalation there is low potential for significant levels in breast milk.

The use of beclomethasone dipropionate in mothers breast feeding their babies requires that the therapeutic benefits of the drug be weighed against the potential hazards to the mother and baby.

Effects on the ability to drive and use machines: None reported.

Undesirable effects: As with other inhalation therapy, paradoxical bronchospasm may occur with an immediate increase in wheezing after dosing. This should be treated immediately with a fast-acting inhaled bronchodilator. The Becotide Easi-Breathe Inhaler should be discontinued immediately, the patient assessed and, if necessary, alternative therapy instituted.

Hypersensitivity reactions including rashes, urticaria, pruritus and erythema, and oedema of the eyes, face, lips and throat, have been reported.

Candidiasis of the mouth and throat (thrush) occurs in some patients, the incidence increasing with doses greater than 400 micrograms beclomethasone dipropionate per day. Patients with high blood levels of *Candida precipitins*, indicating a previous infection, are most likely to develop this complication. Patients may find it helpful to rinse their mouth thoroughly with water after using the inhaler. The Optimiser spacer can be used to reduce oropharyngeal deposition. Symptomatic candidiasis can be treated with topical anti-fungal therapy whilst still continuing with Becotide Easi-Breathe Inhaler.

In some patients inhaled beclomethasone dipropionate may cause hoarseness or throat irritation. It may be helpful to rinse the mouth out with water immediately after inhalation. Alternatively, the Optimiser spacer can be used to reduce oropharyngeal deposition.

Overdose:

Acute: Inhalation of the drug in doses in excess of those recommended may lead to temporary suppression of adrenal function. This does not require emergency action. In these patients treatment should be continued at a dose sufficient to control asthma; adrenal function recovers in a few days and can be verified by measuring plasma cortisol.

Chronic: Use of inhaled beclomethasone dipropionate in daily doses in excess of 1,500 micrograms over prolonged periods may lead to some degree of adrenal suppression. Monitoring of adrenal reserve may be indicated. Treatment should be continued at a dose sufficient to control asthma.

Pharmacological properties
Pharmacodynamic properties: Beclomethasone dipropionate given by inhalation has a potent glucocorticoid anti-inflammatory action within the lungs.

Pharmacokinetic properties: Beclomethasone 17,21-dipropionate (BDP) administered intravenously is cleared rapidly with a half-life of approximately 30 minutes. Beclomethasone 17-monopropionate (BMP) appears rapidly in the plasma after intravenous administration of BDP and is itself cleared with a half-life again of about 30 minutes. BDP is bound to plasma proteins to the extent of 87%. Up to 14% of an intravenous dose of BDP is excreted in the urine in 96 hours, mainly as polar metabolites, a proportion of which are conjugated. Up to 64% of the dose is excreted in faeces in this time, again primarily as free and conjugated metabolites.

After inhalation about 25% of the dose reaches the lungs and is available for absorption from this site. The remainder is deposited on the delivery device or in the oropharynx. That portion deposited in the mouth or upper airways will ultimately be swallowed.

There is rapid metabolic inactivation of most of the swallowed portion of BDP during its first passage through the liver. An oral dose (4 mg) of tritium-labelled BDP was absorbed slowly with peak levels of radioactivity equivalent to 20 ng drug/ml plasma being reached 5 hours after dosing. Excretion was mainly in the faeces (35–76% of the dose in 96 hours) and primarily as polar metabolites although the presence of BDP and BMP in faeces suggested incomplete absorption of the dose. Up to 14% of the dose was excreted as polar metabolites in urine.

The lung tissue rapidly hydrolyses BDP to BMP which in turn is hydrolysed more slowly to beclomethasone. The liver also metabolises BDP to BMP and further converts it to polar metabolites.

Preclinical safety data: BDP has low acute oral, subcutaneous and intraperitoneal toxicity in mice and rats, and repeat dose toxicity studies showed findings characteristic of glucocorticoids, with no evidence of irritancy to the respiratory tract. The main findings, at above therapeutic doses, were depression of corticosterone levels in rats and cortisol levels in dogs. BDP is non-genotoxic, and demonstrated no oncogenic potential following combined inhalation/oral administration to rats. Susceptibility of fetuses to cleft palate, noted in the mouse organogenesis study, is considered to have no relevance for therapeutic use.

Pharmaceutical particulars
List of excipients: Oleic acid, dichlorodifluoromethane, trichlorofluoromethane.

Incompatibilities: None reported.

Shelf life: Two years when stored below 30°C.

Special precautions for storage: Store below 30°C.

As with most inhaled medicines in aerosol canisters, the therapeutic effect may decrease when the canister is cold.

Protect from frost and direct sunlight.

The canister should not be broken, punctured or burnt, even when apparently empty.

Nature and contents of container: An inhaler comprising an aluminium can fitted with a breath-operated metering valve, actuator and dust cap. Each canister contains 200 metered actuations of 50 or 100 micrograms beclomethasone dipropionate.

Instructions for use/handling: The aerosol spray is inhaled through the mouth into the lungs. After shaking the inhaler, open the cap and place the mouthpiece in the mouth with the lips closed around it. Suck in slowly through the mouthpiece, this releases a spray.

The inhaler can be used with the Optimiser spacer device.

For detailed instructions for use refer to the patient information leaflet in every pack.

Marketing authorisation numbers
Becotide 50 Easi-Breathe Inhaler 10949/00268
Becotide 100 Easi-Breathe Inhaler 10949/00269

Date of approval/revision of SPC December 1996.

Legal category POM.

BECOTIDE* INHALERS

Presentation Becotide 50 Inhaler is a metered-dose aerosol which delivers 50 micrograms Beclomethasone Dipropionate BP per actuation into the mouthpiece of a specially designed actuator.

Becotide 100 Inhaler is a metered-dose aerosol which delivers 100 micrograms Beclomethasone Dipropionate BP per actuation into the mouthpiece of a specially designed actuator.

Becotide 200 Inhaler is a metered-dose aerosol which delivers 200 micrograms Beclomethasone Dipropionate BP per actuation into the mouthpiece of a specially designed actuator.

Other ingredients: Oleic acid, dichlorodifluoromethane and trichlorofluoromethane.

Uses Beclomethasone dipropionate given by inhalation offers preventative treatment for asthma. It provides effective anti-inflammatory action in the lungs with a lower incidence and severity of adverse effects than those observed when corticosteroids are administered systemically.

Becotide Inhaler is indicated for a wide range of patients with asthma.

Therapeutic indications:
Adults: Prophylactic management in:

mild asthma: Patients requiring intermittent symptomatic bronchodilator asthma medication on a regular basis.

moderate asthma: Patients with unstable or worsening asthma despite prophylactic therapy or bronchodilator alone.

severe asthma: Patients with severe chronic asthma and those who are dependent on systemic corticosteroids for adequate control of symptoms. On transfer to high dose inhaled beclomethasone dipropionate, many patients who are dependent on systemic corticosteroids for adequate control of symptoms may be able to reduce significantly, or eliminate, their requirement for oral corticosteroids.

Children: Any child who requires prophylactic asthma medication.

Dosage and administration Becotide Inhalers are for inhalation use only. A Volumatic* spacer device may be used in patients who find it difficult to synchronise aerosol actuation with inspiration of breath.

Patients should be given a starting dose of inhaled beclomethasone dipropionate which is appropriate for the severity of their disease. The dose may then be adjusted until control is achieved and should be titrated to the lowest dose at which effective control of asthma is maintained.

Adults: The usual starting dose is 200 micrograms twice a day. In more severe cases dosage may be started at, or increased to, 600 to 800 micrograms per day, and subsequently reduced when the patient's asthma has stabilised. The total daily dose may be administered as two, three or four divided doses.

Children: 50 to 100 micrograms, two, three or four times daily, according to the response. Alternatively, 100 micrograms or 200 micrograms twice daily may be administered. The usual starting dose is 100 micrograms twice a day.

The Babyhaler* spacer device may be used with Becotide 50 Inhaler to facilitate administration to children under 5 years of age.

Becotide 200 Inhaler is not suitable for children.

There is no need to adjust the dose in elderly patients or in those with hepatic or renal impairment.

If patients find that short-acting relief bronchodilator treatment becomes less effective or they need more inhalations than usual, medical attention must be sought.

Contra-indications, warnings, etc
Contra-indications: Becotide Inhaler is contra-indicated in patients with a history of hypersensitivity to any of its components.

Special care is necessary in patients with active or quiescent pulmonary tuberculosis.

Precautions: Patients should be instructed in the proper use of the inhaler to ensure that the drug reaches the target areas within the lungs. They should also be made aware that Becotide Inhaler has to be used regularly, every day, for optimum benefit. Patients should be made aware of the prophylactic nature of therapy with Becotide Inhaler and that it should be taken regularly, even when they are asymptomatic.

Becotide Inhaler is not designed to relieve acute asthma symptoms for which an inhaled short-acting bronchodilator is required. Patients should be advised to have such relief medication available.

Severe asthma requires regular medical assessment, including lung-function testing, as patients are at risk of severe attacks and even death. Increasing use of bronchodilators, in particular short-acting inhaled β_2-agonists, to relieve symptoms indicates deterioration of asthma control. If patients find that short-acting relief bronchodilator treatment becomes less effective, or they need more inhalations than usual, medical attention must be sought. In this situation patients should be reassessed and consideration given to the need for increased anti-inflammatory therapy (e.g. higher doses of inhaled corticosteroids or a course of oral corticosteroids). Severe exacerbations of asthma must be treated in the normal way.

Systemic effects of inhaled corticosteroids may occur, particularly at high doses prescribed for prolonged periods. These effects are much less likely to occur than with oral corticosteroids. Possible systemic effects include adrenal suppression, growth retardation in children and adolescents, decrease in bone mineral density, cataract and glaucoma. It is important therefore that the dose of inhaled corticosteroid is titrated to the lowest dose at which effective control of asthma is maintained.

It is recommended that the height of children receiving prolonged treatment with inhaled corticosteroids is regularly monitored. If growth is slowed, therapy should be reviewed with the aim of reducing the dose of inhaled corticosteroid, if possible, to the lowest dose at which effective control of asthma is maintained. In addition, consideration should be given to referring the patient to a paediatric respiratory specialist.

Prolonged treatment with high doses of inhaled corticosteroids, particularly higher than the recommended doses, may result in clinically significant adrenal suppression. Additional systemic corticosteroid cover should be considered during periods of stress or elective surgery.

Lack of response or severe exacerbations of asthma

should be treated by increasing the dose of inhaled beclomethasone dipropionate and, if necessary, by giving a systemic steroid and/or an antibiotic if there is an infection, and by use of β-agonist therapy.

For the transfer of patients being treated with oral corticosteroids: The transfer of oral steroid-dependent patients to inhaled beclomethasone dipropionate, and their subsequent management, needs special care as recovery from impaired adrenocortical function, caused by prolonged systemic steroid therapy, may take a considerable time.

Patients who have been treated with systemic steroids for long periods of time, or at a high dose, may have adrenocortical suppression. With these patients adrenocortical function should be monitored regularly and their dose of systemic steroid reduced cautiously.

After approximately a week, gradual withdrawal of the systemic steroid is commenced. Reductions in dosage should be appropriate to the level of maintenance systemic steroid, and introduced at not less than weekly intervals. For maintenance doses of prednisolone, or its equivalent, of 10 mg daily or less, the reductions in dose should be not greater than 1 mg per day, at not less than weekly intervals. For maintenance doses of prednisolone in excess of 10 mg daily, it may be appropriate to employ cautiously larger reductions in dose at weekly intervals.

Some patients feel unwell in a non-specific way during the withdrawal phase despite maintenance or even improvement of the respiratory function. They should be encouraged to persevere with inhaled beclomethasone dipropionate and to continue withdrawal of systemic steroid, unless there are objective signs of adrenal insufficiency.

Patients weaned off oral steroids whose adrenocortical function is impaired should carry a steroid warning card indicating that they may need supplementary systemic steroid during periods of stress, e.g. worsening asthma attacks, chest infections, major intercurrent illness, surgery, trauma, etc.

Replacement of systemic steroid treatment with inhaled therapy sometimes unmasks allergies such as allergic rhinitis or eczema previously controlled by the systemic drug. These allergies should be symptomatically treated with antihistamine and/or topical preparations, including topical steroids.

Treatment with Becotide Inhaler should not be stopped abruptly.

As with all inhaled corticosteroids, special care is necessary in patients with active or quiescent pulmonary tuberculosis.

Pregnancy: There is inadequate evidence of safety in human pregnancy. Administration of corticosteroids to pregnant animals can cause abnormalities of fetal development including cleft palate and intra-uterine growth retardation. There may therefore be a very small risk of such effects in the human fetus. It should be noted, however, that the fetal changes in animals occur after relatively high systemic exposure. Beclomethasone dipropionate is delivered directly to the lungs by the inhaled route and so avoids the high level of exposure that occurs when corticosteroids are given by systemic routes.

The use of beclomethasone dipropionate in pregnancy requires that the possible benefits of the drug be weighed against the possible hazards. It should be noted that the drug has been in widespread use for many years without apparent ill consequence.

Lactation: No specific studies examining the transference of beclomethasone dipropionate into the milk of lactating animals have been performed. It is reasonable to assume that beclomethasone dipropionate is secreted in milk, but at the dosages used for direct inhalation there is low potential for significant levels in breast milk.

The use of beclomethasone dipropionate in mothers breast feeding their babies requires that the therapeutic benefits of the drug be weighed against the potential hazards to the mother and baby.

Side-effects: Systemic effects of inhaled corticosteroids may occur, particularly at high doses prescribed for prolonged periods. These may include adrenal suppression, growth retardation in children and adolescents, decrease in bone mineral density, cataract and glaucoma.

Candidiasis of the mouth and throat (thrush) occurs in some patients, the incidence increases with doses greater than 400 micrograms beclomethasone dipropionate per day. Patients with high blood levels of *Candida precipitins,* indicating a previous infection, are most likely to develop this complication. Patients may find it helpful to rinse their mouth thoroughly with water after using the inhaler. Symptomatic candidiasis can be treated with topical anti-fungal therapy whilst still continuing with Becotide Inhaler.

In some patients inhaled beclomethasone dipropionate may cause hoarseness or throat irritation. It may be helpful to rinse the mouth out with water immediately after inhalation. The use of the Volumatic spacer device may be considered.

As with other inhalation therapy, paradoxical bronchospasm may occur with an immediate increase in wheezing after dosing. This responds to a fast-acting inhaled bronchodilator. The preparation should be discontinued immediately, the patient assessed and, if necessary, alternative therapy (e.g. Becodisks*) instituted.

Hypersensitivity reactions including rashes, urticaria, pruritus and erythema, and oedema of the eyes, face, lips and throat, have been reported.

Overdosage: Acute. Inhalation of the drug in doses in excess of those recommended may lead to temporary suppression of adrenal function. This does not necessitate emergency action being taken. In these patients treatment with beclomethasone dipropionate by inhalation should be continued at a dose sufficient to control asthma; adrenal function recovers in a few days and can be verified by measuring plasma cortisol.

Chronic. Use of inhaled beclomethasone dipropionate in daily doses in excess of 1,500 micrograms over prolonged periods may lead to adrenal suppression. Monitoring of adrenal reserve may be indicated. Treatment with inhaled beclomethasone dipropionate should be continued at a dose sufficient to control asthma.

Pharmaceutical precautions Becotide Inhaler should be stored at a temperature below 30°C.

As with most inhaled medications in aerosol canisters, the therapeutic effect of this medication may decrease when the canister is cold.

Protect from frost and direct sunlight.

The canister should not be punctured, broken or burnt even if it is apparently empty.

Legal category POM.

Package quantities Becotide 50 Inhaler, Becotide 100 Inhaler and Becotide 200 Inhaler provide 200 metered actuations.

Further information Nil.

Product licence numbers
Becotide 50 Inhaler 10949/0058
Becotide 100 Inhaler 10949/0059
Becotide 200 Inhaler 10949/0060

BECOTIDE* ROTACAPS*

Presentation Becotide Rotacaps capsules, an alternative inhalation form of beclomethasone dipropionate to Becotide Inhaler, are especially valuable for treating patients who are unable to use pressurised inhalers effectively, or who might use them incorrectly.

Becotide Rotacaps contain a mixture of microfine beclomethasone dipropionate and large particle lactose in coloured, hard gelatin capsules. Each Rotacaps capsule contains 100 micrograms (buff/colourless), 200 micrograms (brown/colourless) or 400 micrograms (dark brown/colourless) beclomethasone dipropionate, and is marked Becotide 100, Becotide 200 or Becotide 400, respectively.

The contents of the Rotacaps capsule are inhaled using a specially developed device called a Rotahaler* inhaler which separates the capsule into halves that rotate and release the drug when the patient inhales. This breath actuation is very sensitive and so the drug is fully available even at the lowest inspiratory flow rates. The Rotahaler device is therefore a reliable drug delivery system for many patients.

Uses Beclomethasone dipropionate provides effective anti-inflammatory action in the lungs, with a lower incidence and severity of adverse effects than those observed when corticosteroids are administered systemically. It also offers preventative treatment of asthma. Becotide Rotacaps are indicated for a wide range of patients with asthma.

Therapeutic indications:
Adults: Prophylactic management in:

mild asthma: Patients requiring symptomatic bronchodilator asthma medication on a regular basis.

moderate asthma: Patients with unstable or worsening asthma despite prophylactic therapy or bronchodilator alone.

severe asthma: Patients with severe chronic asthma and those who are dependent on systemic corticosteroids for adequate control of symptoms. On transfer to high dose inhaled beclomethasone dipropionate, many patients who are dependent on systemic corticosteroids for adequate control of symptoms may be able to reduce significantly, or eliminate, their requirement for oral corticosteroids.

Children: Any child who requires prophylactic asthma medication.

Dosage and administration Patients should be made aware of the prophylactic nature of therapy with inhaled beclomethasone dipropionate and that it should be taken regularly every day even when they are asymptomatic.

Becotide Rotacaps are for inhalation use only, using a Becotide Rotahaler. For optimum results Becotide Rotacaps should be used regularly. Patients should be given a starting dose of inhaled beclomethasone dipropionate which is appropriate for the severity of their disease. The dose may then be adjusted until control is achieved and should be titrated to the lowest dose at which effective control of asthma is maintained.

Adults: 400 micrograms twice daily is the usual starting dose. One 400 micrograms Rotacaps capsule or two 200 micrograms Rotacaps capsules twice a day is the usual maintenance dose. Alternatively, one 200 micrograms Rotacaps capsule may be given three or four times daily.

Children: One 100 micrograms Rotacaps capsule two, three or four times a day, according to the response. Alternatively, the usual starting dose of 200 micrograms twice daily may be administered.

There is no need to adjust the dose in elderly patients or in those with hepatic or renal impairment.

Contra-indications, warnings, etc
Contra-indications: Becotide Rotacaps are contra-indicated in patients with a history of hypersensitivity to any of the components. Special care is necessary in patients with active or quiescent pulmonary tuberculosis.

Precautions: Patients should be instructed in the proper use of the Rotahaler to ensure that the drug reaches the target areas within the lungs. They should also be made aware that Becotide Rotacaps have to be used regularly, every day, for optimum benefit. They should be made aware of the prophylactic nature of therapy with inhaled beclomethasone dipropionate and that it should be taken regularly, even when they are asymptomatic.

Becotide Rotacaps are not designed to relieve acute asthmatic symptoms for which an inhaled short-acting bronchodilator is required. Patients should be advised to have such rescue medication available.

Severe asthma requires regular medical assessment, including lung-function testing, as patients are at risk of severe attacks and even death.

Increasing use of bronchodilators, in particular short-acting inhaled β_2-agonists, to relieve symptoms indicates deterioration of asthma control. If patients find that short-acting relief bronchodilator treatment becomes less effective, or they need more inhalations than usual, medical attention must be sought. In this situation patients should be reassessed and consideration given to the need for increased anti-inflammatory therapy (e.g. higher doses of inhaled corticosteroids or a course of oral corticosteroids). Severe exacerbations of asthma must be treated in the normal way.

Systemic effects of inhaled corticosteroids may occur, particularly at high doses prescribed for prolonged periods. These effects are much less likely to occur than with oral corticosteroids. Possible systemic effects include adrenal suppression, growth retardation in children and adolescents, decrease in bone mineral density, cataract and glaucoma. It is important therefore that the dose of inhaled corticosteroid is titrated to the lowest dose at which effective control of asthma is maintained.

It is recommended that the height of children receiving prolonged treatment with inhaled corticosteroids is regularly monitored. If growth is slowed, therapy should be reviewed with the aim of reducing the dose of inhaled corticosteroid, if possible, to the lowest dose at which effective control of asthma is maintained. In addition, consideration should be given to referring the patient to a paediatric respiratory specialist.

Prolonged treatment with high doses of inhaled corticosteroids, particularly higher than the recommended doses, may result in clinically significant adrenal suppression. Additional systemic corticosteroid cover should be considered during periods of stress or elective surgery.

Lack of response or severe exacerbations of asthma should be treated by increasing the dose of inhaled beclomethasone dipropionate and, if necessary, by giving a systemic steroid and/or antibiotic if there is an infection, and by use of β-agonist therapy.

For the transfer of patients being treated with oral corticosteroids: The transfer of oral steroid-dependent patients to Becotide Rotacaps, and their subsequent management, needs special care as recovery from impaired adrenocortical function, caused by prolonged systemic steroid therapy, may take a considerable time.

Patients who have been treated with systemic steroids for long periods of time, or at a high dose, may have adrenocortical suppression. With these patients adrenocortical function should be monitored regularly and their dose of systemic steroid reduced cautiously.

After approximately a week, gradual withdrawal of the systemic steroid is commenced. Decrements in dosage should be appropriate to the level of maintenance systemic steroid, and introduced at not less than weekly intervals. For maintenance doses of prednisolone, or its equivalent, of 10 mg daily or less, the decrements in dose should not be greater than 1 mg per day, at not less than weekly intervals. For maintenance doses of prednisolone in excess of 10 mg daily, it may be appropriate to employ cautiously larger decrements in dose at weekly intervals.

Some patients feel unwell in a non-specific way during the withdrawal phase despite maintenance or even improvement of the respiratory function. They should be encouraged to persevere with the Rotahaler and withdrawal of systemic steroid continued, unless there are objective signs of adrenal insufficiency.

Patients weaned off oral steroids whose adrenocortical function is impaired should carry a steroid warning card indicating that they may need supplementary systemic steroid during periods of stress, e.g. worsening asthma attacks, chest infections, major intercurrent illness, surgery, trauma, etc.

Replacement of systemic steroid treatment with inhaled therapy sometimes unmasks allergies such as allergic rhinitis or eczema previously controlled by the systemic drug. These allergies should be symptomatically treated with antihistamine and/or topical preparations, including topical steroids.

Treatment with Becotide Rotacaps should not be stopped abruptly.

As with all inhaled corticosteroids, special care is necessary in patients with active or quiescent pulmonary tuberculosis.

Pregnancy: There is inadequate evidence of safety in human pregnancy. Administration of corticosteroids to pregnant animals can cause abnormalities of fetal development including cleft palate and intra-uterine growth retardation. There may therefore be a very small risk of such effects in the human fetus. It should be noted, however, that the fetal changes in animals occur after relatively high systemic exposure. Because beclomethasone dipropionate is delivered directly to the lungs by the inhaled route it avoids the high level of exposure that occurs when corticosteroids are given by systemic routes.

The use of beclomethasone dipropionate in pregnancy requires that the possible benefits of the drug be weighed against the possible hazards. It should be noted that the drug has been in widespread use for many years without apparent ill consequence.

Lactation: No specific studies examining the transference of beclomethasone dipropionate into the milk of lactating animals have been performed. It is reasonable to assume that beclomethasone dipropionate is secreted in milk, but at the dosages used for direct inhalation there is low potential for significant levels in breast milk.

The use of beclomethasone dipropionate in mothers breast feeding their babies requires that the therapeutic benefits of the drug be weighed against the potential hazards to the mother and baby.

Side-effects: Systemic effects of inhaled corticosteroids may occur, particularly at high doses prescribed for prolonged periods. These may include adrenal suppression, growth retardation in children and adolescents, decrease in bone mineral density, cataract and glaucoma.

Candidiasis of the mouth and throat (thrush) occurs in some patients, the incidence increases with doses greater than 400 micrograms beclomethasone dipropionate per day. Patients with high blood levels of *Candida precipitins,* indicating a previous infection, are more likely to develop this complication. Some patients may find it helpful to rinse their mouth thoroughly with water after using the Rotahaler. Symptomatic candidiasis can be treated with topical anti-fungal therapy whilst still continuing with the treatment.

In some patients inhaled beclomethasone dipropionate may cause hoarseness or throat irritation. It may be helpful to rinse the mouth out with water immediately after inhalation.

As with other inhalation therapy, paradoxical bronchospasm may occur with an immediate increase in wheezing after dosing. This responds to a fast-acting inhaled bronchodilator. The preparation should be discontinued immediately, the patient assessed and, if necessary, alternative therapy instituted.

Hypersensitivity reactions including rashes, urticaria, pruritus and erythema, and oedema of the eyes, face, lips and throat, have been reported.

Overdosage: Acute. Inhalation of the drug in doses in excess of those recommended may lead to temporary suppression of adrenal function. This does not necessitate emergency action being taken. In these patients treatment with beclomethasone dipropionate by inhalation should be continued at a dose sufficient to control asthma; adrenal function recovers in a few days and can be verified by measuring plasma cortisol.

Chronic. Use of inhaled beclomethasone dipropionate in daily doses in excess of 1,500 micrograms over prolonged periods may lead to adrenal suppression. Monitoring of adrenal reserve may be indicated. Treatment with inhaled beclomethasone dipropionate should be continued at a dose sufficient to control asthma.

Pharmaceutical precautions To keep the Rotacaps capsules in good condition it is important that they are stored in a dry place below 30°C where they will not be exposed to extremes of temperature. A convenient supply may be carried in the special container for the Rotahaler device. The Rotacaps capsules should be inserted into the Rotahaler immediately prior to use to avoid softening. Failure to observe this instruction may affect the delivery of the drug. The Rotacaps must only be used in the Rotahaler.

Legal category POM.

Package quantities Becotide Rotacaps 100 micrograms, 200 micrograms and 400 micrograms are supplied in packs of 112.

Further information Nil.

Product licence numbers
Becotide Rotacaps 100 micrograms 10949/0061
Becotide Rotacaps 200 micrograms 10949/0062
Becotide Rotacaps 400 micrograms 10949/0063

FLIXONASE* AQUEOUS NASAL SPRAY

Presentation Flixonase Aqueous Nasal Spray is an aqueous suspension of microfine fluticasone propionate (0.05% w/w) for topical administration to the nasal mucosa by means of a metering, atomising spray pump. Each 100 mg of spray delivered by the nasal adaptor contains 50 micrograms of fluticasone propionate.

Other ingredients: Microcrystalline cellulose, sodium carboxymethylcellulose, dextrose, polysorbate 80, purified water, benzalkonium chloride and phenylethylalcohol.

Uses Flixonase Aqueous Nasal Spray is indicated for the prophylaxis and treatment of seasonal allergic rhinitis including hayfever, and perennial rhinitis. Fluticasone propionate has potent anti-inflammatory activity but when used topically on the nasal mucosa has no detectable systemic activity.

Dosage and administration Flixonase Aqueous Nasal Spray is for administration by the intranasal route only.

Adults and children over 12 years of age: For the prophylaxis and treatment of seasonal allergic rhinitis and perennial rhinitis: two sprays into each nostril once a day, preferably in the morning. In some cases two sprays into each nostril twice daily may be required. The maximum daily dose should not exceed four sprays into each nostril.

Elderly: The normal adult dosage is applicable.

Children under 12 years of age: For the prophylaxis and treatment of seasonal allergic rhinitis and perennial rhinitis in children aged 4 to 11 years a dose of one spray into each nostril once daily is recommended. In some cases one spray into each nostril twice daily may be required. The maximum daily dose should not exceed two sprays into each nostril.

For full therapeutic benefit regular usage is essential. The absence of an immediate effect should be explained to the patient as maximum relief may not be obtained until after 3 to 4 days of treatment.

Contra-indications, warnings, etc
Contra-indications: Flixonase Aqueous Nasal Spray is contra-indicated in patients with hypersensitivity to any of its ingredients.

Precautions: Infections of the nasal airways should be appropriately treated but do not constitute a specific contra-indication to treatment with Flixonase Aqueous Nasal Spray.

The full benefit of Flixonase Aqueous Nasal Spray may not be achieved until treatment has been administered for several days.

Care must be taken while transferring patients from systemic steroid treatment to Flixonase Aqueous Nasal Spray if there is any reason to suppose that their adrenal function is impaired.

Although Flixonase Aqueous Nasal Spray will control seasonal allergic rhinitis in most cases, an abnormally heavy challenge of summer allergens may in certain instances necessitate appropriate additional therapy, particularly to control eye symptoms.

Pregnancy: There is inadequate evidence of safety in human pregnancy. Administration of corticosteroids to pregnant animals can cause abnormalities of fetal development, including cleft palate and intra-uterine growth retardation. There may therefore be a very small risk of such effects in the human fetus. It should be noted, however, that the fetal changes in animals occur after relatively high systemic exposure; direct intranasal application ensures minimal systemic exposure.

As with other drugs the use of Flixonase Aqueous Nasal Spray during human pregnancy requires that the possible benefits of the drug be weighed against the possible hazards.

Lactation: The secretion of fluticasone propionate in human breast milk has not been investigated. Subcutaneous administration of fluticasone propionate to lactating laboratory rats produced measurable plasma levels and evidence of fluticasone propionate in the milk. However, following intranasal administration to primates, no drug was detected in the plasma, and it is therefore unlikely that the drug would be detectable in milk. When fluticasone propionate is used in breast feeding mothers the therapeutic benefits must be weighed against the potential hazards to mother and baby.

Side-effects: Extremely rare cases of nasal septal perforation have been reported following the use of intranasal corticosteroids, usually in patients who have had previous nasal surgery.

As with other nasal sprays, dryness and irritation of the nose and throat, unpleasant taste and smell and epistaxis have been reported.

Hypersensitivity reactions including skin rash and oedema of the face or tongue have been reported.

There have also been rare reports of anaphylaxis/anaphylactoid reactions and bronchospasm.

Overdosage: There are no data available on the effects of acute or chronic overdosage with Flixonase Aqueous Nasal Spray. Intranasal administration of 2 mg fluticasone propionate twice daily for seven days to healthy human volunteers had no effect on hypothalamic-pituitary-adrenal (HPA) axis function. Inhalation or oral administration of high doses of corticosteroids over a long period may lead to suppression of HPA function.

Pharmaceutical precautions Shake gently before use. Flixonase Aqueous Nasal Spray should be stored below 30°C.

Legal category POM.

Package quantities Flixonase Aqueous Nasal Spray is supplied in an amber glass bottle fitted with a metering, atomising pump, nasal adaptor and a dust cover. Each bottle provides approximately 120 metered sprays, when used as recommended.

Further information Nil.

Product licence number 10949/0036

FLIXOTIDE* ACCUHALER*

Qualitative and quantitative composition Flixotide Accuhaler is a moulded plastic device containing a foil strip with 60 regularly placed blisters each containing a mixture of microfine fluticasone propionate (50 micrograms, 100 micrograms, 250 micrograms or 500 micrograms) and larger particle size lactose.

Pharmaceutical form Multi-dose dry powder inhalation device.

Clinical particulars
Therapeutic indications: Fluticasone propionate given by inhalation offers preventative treatment for asthma. At recommended doses it has a potent glucocorticoid anti-inflammatory action within the lungs, with a lower incidence and severity of adverse effects than those observed when corticosteroids are administered systemically. In the majority of patients it has no effect on adrenal function or reserve at recommended doses.
Adults: Prophylactic management in:

Mild asthma: Patients requiring intermittent symptomatic bronchodilator asthma medication on a regular daily basis.

Moderate asthma: Patients with unstable or worsening asthma despite prophylactic therapy or bronchodilator alone.

Severe asthma: Patients with severe chronic asthma and those who are dependent on systemic corticosteroids for adequate control of symptoms. On introduction of inhaled fluticasone propionate many of these patients may be able to reduce significantly, or to eliminate, their requirement for oral corticosteroids.

Children: Any child who requires prophylactic medication, including patients not controlled on currently available prophylactic medication.

Posology and method of administration: Flixotide Accuhaler is for oral inhalation use only. Flixotide Accuhaler is suitable for many patients, including those who cannot use a metered-dose inhaler successfully.

Patients should be made aware of the prophylactic nature of therapy with Flixotide Accuhaler and that it should be taken regularly even when they are asymptomatic. The onset of therapeutic effect is within 4 to 7 days.

Adults and children over 16 years: 100 to 1,000 micrograms twice daily.

Patients should be given a starting dose appropriate to the severity of their disease. Equivalent disease control is usually obtained at half the daily dose of other currently available inhaled steroids.

Typical starting doses are:

Mild asthma: 100 to 250 micrograms twice daily.

Moderate asthma: 250 to 500 micrograms twice daily.

Severe asthma: 500 to 1,000 micrograms twice daily.

The dose should be titrated to the lowest dose at which effective control of asthma is maintained.

Children aged 4 years and over: 50 to 100 micrograms twice daily.

The starting dose should be appropriate to the severity of the disease. The dose should be titrated to the lowest dose at which effective control of asthma is maintained.

Flixotide Accuhaler 250 micrograms and Flixotide Accuhaler 500 micrograms are not suitable for use in children.

Special patient groups: There is no need to adjust the dose in elderly patients or in those with hepatic or renal impairment.

Contra-indications: Hypersensitivity to any ingredient of the preparation.

Special warnings and special precautions for use:

Flixotide Accuhaler is not designed to relieve acute symptoms for which an inhaled short acting bronchodilator is required. Patients should be advised to have such rescue medication available.

Severe asthma requires regular medical assessment, including lung-function testing, as patients are at risk of severe attacks and even death. Increasing use of short-acting inhaled β_2-agonists to relieve symptoms indicates deterioration of asthma control. If patients find that short-acting relief bronchodilator treatment becomes less effective, or they need more inhalations than usual, medical attention must be sought. In this situation patients should be reassessed and consideration given to the need for increased anti-inflammatory therapy (e.g. higher doses of inhaled corticosteroids or a course of oral corticosteroids). Severe exacerbations of asthma must be treated in the normal way.

Systemic effects of inhaled corticosteroids may occur, particularly at high doses prescribed for prolonged periods. These effects are much less likely to occur than with oral corticosteroids. Possible systemic effects include adrenal suppression, growth retardation in children and adolescents, decrease in bone mineral density, cataract and glaucoma. It is important therefore that the dose of inhaled corticosteroid is titrated to the lowest dose at which effective control of asthma is maintained.

It is recommended that the height of children receiving prolonged treatment with inhaled corticosteroids is regularly monitored. If growth is slowed, therapy should be reviewed with the aim of reducing the dose of inhaled corticosteroid, if possible, to the lowest dose at which effective control of asthma is maintained. In addition, consideration should be given to referring the patient to a paediatric respiratory specialist.

Prolonged treatment with high doses of inhaled corticosteroids, particularly higher than recommended doses, may result in clinically significant adrenal suppression. Additional systemic corticosteroid cover should be considered during periods of stress or elective surgery.

The benefits of inhaled fluticasone propionate should minimise the need for oral steroids. However, patients transferred from oral steroids, remain at risk of impaired adrenal reserve for a considerable time after transferring to inhaled fluticasone propionate. The possibility of adverse effects may persist for some time. These patients may require specialised advice to determine the extent of adrenal impairment before elective procedures. The possibility of residual impaired adrenal response should always be considered in emergency (medical or surgical) and elective situations likely to produce stress, and appropriate corticosteroid treatment considered.

Lack of response or severe exacerbations of asthma should be treated by increasing the dose of inhaled fluticasone propionate and, if necessary, by giving a systemic steroid and/or an antibiotic if there is an infection.

Replacement of systemic steroid treatment with inhaled therapy sometimes unmasks allergies such as allergic rhinitis or eczema previously controlled by the systemic drug. These allergies should be symptomatically treated with antihistamine and/or topical preparations, including topical steroids.

As with all inhaled corticosteroids, special care is necessary in patients with active or quiescent pulmonary tuberculosis.

Treatment with Flixotide Accuhaler should not be stopped abruptly.

For the transfer of patients being treated with oral corticosteroids: The transfer of oral steroid-dependent patients to Flixotide Accuhaler and their subsequent management needs special care as recovery from impaired adrenocortical function, caused by prolonged systemic steroid therapy, may take a considerable time.

Patients who have been treated with systemic steroids for long periods of time or at a high dose may have adrenocortical suppression. With these patients adrenocortical function should be monitored regularly and their dose of systemic steroid reduced cautiously.

After approximately a week, gradual withdrawal of the systemic steroid is commenced. Decrements in dosages should be appropriate to the level of maintenance systemic steroid, and introduced at not less than weekly intervals. For maintenance doses of prednisolone (or equivalent) of 10 mg daily or less, the decrements in dose should not be greater than 1 mg per day, at not less than weekly intervals. For maintenance doses of prednisolone in excess of 10 mg daily, it may be appropriate to employ cautiously, larger decrements in dose at weekly intervals.

Some patients feel unwell in a non-specific way during the withdrawal phase despite maintenance or even improvement of the respiratory function. They should be encouraged to persevere with inhaled fluticasone propionate and to continue withdrawal of systemic steroid, unless there are objective signs of adrenal insufficiency.

Patients weaned off oral steroids whose adrenocortical function is still impaired should carry a steroid warning card indicating that they need supplementary systemic steroid during periods of stress, e.g. worsening asthma attacks, chest infections, major intercurrent illness, surgery, trauma, etc.

Interaction with other medicaments and other forms of interaction: No specific drug interaction studies have been performed. However, because of the very low plasma drug concentrations achieved after inhaled dosing, there are unlikely to be any implications for displacement drug interactions.

There were no reports of suspected drug interactions in the clinical programme.

Pregnancy and lactation: There is inadequate evidence of safety of fluticasone propionate in human pregnancy. Administration of corticosteroids to pregnant animals can cause abnormalities of fetal development, including cleft palate and intra-uterine growth retardation. There may therefore be a very small risk of such effects in the human fetus. It should be noted, however, that the fetal changes in animals occur after relatively high systemic exposure. Because Flixotide Accuhaler delivers fluticasone propionate directly to the lungs by the inhaled route it avoids the high level of exposure that occurs when corticosteroids are given by systemic routes. Administration of fluticasone propionate during pregnancy should only be considered if the expected benefit to the mother is greater than any possible risk to the fetus.

The secretion of fluticasone propionate in human breast milk has not been investigated. Subcutaneous administration of fluticasone propionate to lactating laboratory rats produced measurable plasma levels and evidence of fluticasone propionate in the milk. However, plasma levels in humans after inhalation at recommended doses are likely to be low.

When fluticasone propionate is used in breast feeding mothers the therapeutic benefits must be weighed against the potential hazards to mother and baby.

Effects on ability to drive and use machines: Fluticasone propionate is unlikely to produce an effect.

Undesirable effects: As with other inhalation therapy, paradoxical bronchospasm may occur with an immediate increase in wheezing after dosing. This should be treated immediately with a fast-acting, inhaled bronchodilator. Flixotide Accuhaler should be discontinued immediately, the patient assessed and, if necessary, alternative therapy instituted.

Candidiasis of the mouth and throat (thrush) occurs in some patients. Such patients may find it helpful to rinse out their mouth with water after inhalation. Symptomatic candidiasis can be treated with topical anti-fungal therapy whilst still continuing with Flixotide Accuhaler.

In some patients inhaled fluticasone propionate may cause hoarseness. It may be helpful to rinse out the mouth with water immediately after inhalation.

Systemic effects of inhaled corticosteroids may occur, particularly at high doses prescribed for prolonged periods. These may include adrenal suppression, growth retardation in children and adolescents, decrease in bone mineral density, cataract and glaucoma.

There have been rare reports of peripheral oedema and cutaneous hypersensitivity reactions such as skin rash.

There have been very rare reports of dyspepsia and arthralgia although a causal link with fluticasone propionate has not been established.

Overdose:

Acute: Inhalation of the drug in doses in excess of those recommended may lead to temporary suppression of adrenal function. This does not necessitate emergency action being taken. In these patients treatment with fluticasone propionate by inhalation should be continued at a dose sufficient to control asthma; adrenal function recovers in a few days and can be verified by measuring plasma cortisol.

Chronic: Use of inhaled fluticasone propionate in daily doses in excess of 2 milligrams over prolonged periods may lead to adrenal suppression. Monitoring of adrenal reserve may be indicated. Treatment with inhaled fluticasone propionate should be continued at a dose sufficient to control asthma.

Pharmacological properties

Pharmacodynamic properties: Fluticasone propionate given by inhalation at recommended doses has a potent glucocorticoid anti-inflammatory action within the lungs, resulting in reduced symptoms and exacerbations of asthma, with a lower incidence and severity of adverse effects than those observed when corticosteroids are administered systemically.

Pharmacokinetic properties: Systemic absolute bioavailability of fluticasone propionate is estimated at 12–26% of an inhaled dose, dependent on presentation. Systemic absorption occurs mainly through the lungs and is initially rapid then prolonged. The remainder of the dose may be swallowed.

Absolute oral bioavailability is negligible (<1%) due to a combination of incomplete absorption from the GI tract and extensive first-pass metabolism.

87–100% of an oral dose is excreted in the faeces, up to 75% as parent compound. There is also a non-active major metabolite.

After an intravenous dose, fluticasone propionate is extensively distributed in the body. The very high clearance rate indicates extensive hepatic clearance.

Preclinical safety data: Toxicology has shown only those class effects typical of potent corticosteroids, and these only at doses greatly in excess of that proposed for therapeutic use. No novel effects were identified in repeat dose toxicity tests, reproductive studies or teratology studies. Fluticasone propionate is devoid of mutagenic activity *in vitro* and *in vivo* and showed no tumorigenic potential in rodents. It is both non-irritant and non-sensitising in animal models.

Pharmaceutical particulars

List of excipients: Lactose.

Incompatibilities: None reported.

Shelf life: 18 months when stored below 30°C.

Special precautions for storage: Store below 30°C (86°F). Store in a dry place.

Nature and contents of container: The powder mix of fluticasone propionate and lactose is filled into a blister strip consisting of a formed base foil with a peelable foil laminate lid. The foil strip is contained within the Accuhaler device.

Instructions for use/handling: The powdered medicine is inhaled through the mouth into the lungs.

The Accuhaler device contains the medicine in individual blisters which are opened as the device is manipulated.

For detailed instructions for use refer to the Patient Information Leaflet in every pack.

Marketing authorisation numbers

Flixotide Accuhaler 50 micrograms 10949/0226
Flixotide Accuhaler 100 micrograms 10949/0227
Flixotide Accuhaler 250 micrograms 10949/0228
Flixotide Accuhaler 500 micrograms 10949/0229

Date of approval/ revision of SPC July 1998.

Legal category POM.

FLIXOTIDE* DISKHALER*

Presentation The active ingredient is presented in a disk comprising four regularly spaced double-foil blisters each delivering a mixture of fluticasone propionate and lactose. Flixotide Diskhaler is available in four strengths containing 50 micrograms, 100 micrograms, 250 micrograms or 500 micrograms fluticasone propionate per blister.

Uses Fluticasone propionate given by inhalation offers preventative treatment for asthma. At recommended doses it has a potent glucocorticoid anti-inflammatory action within the lungs, with a lower incidence and severity of adverse effects than those observed when corticosteroids are administered systemically.

Therapeutic indications:

Adults: Prophylactic management in:

mild asthma: Patients requiring intermittent symptomatic bronchodilator asthma medication on a regular daily basis.

moderate asthma: Patients with unstable or worsening asthma despite prophylactic therapy or bronchodilator alone.

severe asthma: Patients with severe chronic asthma and those who are dependent on systemic corticosteroids for adequate control of symptoms. On introduction of inhaled fluticasone propionate many of these patients may be able to reduce significantly, or to eliminate, their requirement for oral corticosteroids.

Children: Any child who requires prophylactic medication, including patients not controlled on currently available prophylactic medication.

Dosage and administration Flixotide Diskhaler is for oral inhalation use only. Flixotide Diskhaler is suitable for many patients, including those who cannot use a metered-dose inhaler successfully.

Patients should be made aware of the prophylactic nature of therapy with Flixotide Diskhaler and that it should be taken regularly even when they are asymptomatic. The onset of therapeutic effect is within 4 to 7 days.

Adults and children over 16 years: 100 to 1,000 micrograms twice daily.

Patients should be given a starting dose appropriate to the severity of their disease.

Equivalent disease control is usually obtained at half the daily dose of other currently available inhaled steroids.

Typical starting doses are:

mild asthma: 100 to 250 micrograms twice daily,

moderate asthma: 250 to 500 micrograms twice daily,

severe asthma: 500 to 1,000 micrograms twice daily.

The dose should be titrated to the lowest dose at which effective control of asthma is maintained.

Children aged 4 and over: 50 to 100 micrograms twice daily.

The starting dose should be appropriate to the severity of the disease. The dose should be titrated to the lowest dose at which effective control of asthma is maintained.

Flixotide Diskhaler 250 micrograms and Flixotide Diskhaler 500 micrograms are not suitable for use in children.

Special patient groups: There is no need to adjust the dose in elderly patients or in those with hepatic or renal impairment.

Contra-indications, warnings, etc

Contra-indications: Flixotide Diskhaler is contra-indicated in patients with a history of hypersensitivity to any of its components.

Precautions: Flixotide Diskhaler is not designed to relieve acute symptoms, for which an inhaled short-acting bronchodilator is required. Patients should be advised to have such rescue medication available.

Severe asthma requires regular medical assessment, including lung-function testing, as patients are at risk of severe attacks and even death. Increasing use of short-acting inhaled β_2-agonists to relieve symptoms indicates deterioration of asthma control. If patients find that short-acting relief bronchodilator treatment becomes less effective, or they need more inhalations than usual, medical attention must be sought. In this situation patients should be reassessed and consideration given to the need for increased anti-inflammatory therapy (e.g. higher doses of inhaled corticosteroids or a course of oral corticosteroids). Severe exacerbations of asthma must be treated in the normal way.

Systemic effects of inhaled corticosteroids may occur, particularly at high doses prescribed for prolonged periods. These effects are much less likely to occur than with oral corticosteroids. Possible systemic effects include adrenal suppression, growth retardation in children and adolescents, decrease in bone mineral density, cataract and glaucoma. It is important therefore that the dose of inhaled corticosteroid is titrated to the lowest dose at which effective control of asthma is maintained.

It is recommended that the height of children receiving prolonged treatment with inhaled corticosteroids is regularly monitored. If growth is slowed, therapy should be reviewed with the aim of reducing the dose of inhaled corticosteroid, if possible, to the lowest dose at which effective control of asthma is maintained. In addition, consideration should be given to referring the patient to a paediatric respiratory specialist.

Prolonged treatment with high doses of inhaled corticosteroids, particularly higher than the recommended doses, may result in clinically significant adrenal suppression. Additional systemic corticosteroid cover should be considered during periods of stress or elective surgery.

The benefits of inhaled fluticasone propionate should minimise the need for oral steroids. However patients transferred from oral steroids, remain at risk of impaired adrenal reserve for a considerable time after transferring to inhaled fluticasone propionate. The possibility of adverse effects may persist for some time.

These patients may require specialised advice to determine the extent of adrenal impairment before elective procedures. The possibiity of residual impaired adrenal response should always be considered in emergency (medical or surgical) and elective situations likely to produce stress, and appropriate corticosteroid treatment considered.

Lack of response or severe exacerbations of asthma should be treated by increasing the dose of inhaled fluticasone propionate and, if necessary, by giving a systemic steroid and/or an antibiotic if there is an infection.

For the transfer of patients being treated with oral corticosteroids: The transfer of oral steroid-dependent patients to Flixotide Diskhaler, and their subsequent management, needs special care as recovery from impaired adrenocortical function, caused by prolonged systemic steroid therapy, may take a considerable time.

Patients who have been treated with systemic steroids for long periods of time, or at a high dose, may have adrenocortical suppression. With these patients, adrenocortical function should be monitored regularly and their dose of systemic steroid reduced cautiously.

After approximately a week, gradual withdrawal of the systemic steroid is started by reducing the daily dose by 1 mg prednisolone, or its equivalent, at not less than weekly intervals. For maintenance doses of prednisolone in excess of 10 mg daily, it may be appropriate to cautiously use larger reductions in dose at weekly intervals.

Some patients feel unwell in a non-specific way during the withdrawal phase despite maintenance or even improvement of respiratory function. They should be encouraged to persevere with Flixotide Diskhaler and to continue withdrawal of systemic steroid, unless there are objective signs of adrenal insufficiency.

Patients transferred from oral steroids whose adrenocortical function is still impaired should carry a steroid warning card indicating that they need supplementary systemic steroid during periods of stress, e.g. worsening asthma attacks, chest infections, major intercurrent illness, surgery, trauma, etc.

Replacement of systemic steroid treatment with inhaled therapy sometimes unmasks allergies such as allergic rhinitis or eczema previously controlled by the systemic drug. These allergies should be symptomatically treated with antihistamine and/or topical preparations, including topical steroids.

Treatment with Flixotide Diskhaler should not be stopped abruptly.

Special care is necessary in patients with active or quiescent pulmonary tuberculosis.

Pregnancy and lactation: There is inadequate evidence of safety of fluticasone propionate in human pregnancy. Administration of corticosteroids to pregnant animals can cause abnormalities of fetal development, including cleft palate and intra-uterine growth retardation. There may therefore be a very small risk of such effects in the human fetus. It should be noted, however, that the fetal changes in animals occur after relatively high systemic exposure. Because fluticasone propionate is delivered directly to the lungs by the inhaled route it avoids the high level of exposure that occurs when corticosteroids are given by systemic routes. Administration of fluticasone propionate during pregnancy should only be considered if the expected benefit to the mother is greater than any possible risk to the fetus. The secretion of fluticasone propionate in human breast milk has not been investigated.

Subcutaneous administration of fluticasone propionate to lactating laboratory rats produced measurable plasma levels and evidence of fluticasone propionate in the milk. However plasma levels in humans after inhalation at recommended doses are likely to be low. When fluticasone propionate is used in breast feeding mothers the therapeutic benefits must be weighed against the potential hazards to mother and baby.

Side-effects: As with other inhalation therapy, paradoxical bronchospasm may occur with an immediate increase in wheezing after dosing. This should be treated immediately with a fast-acting inhaled bronchodilator. Flixotide Diskhaler should be discontinued immediately, the patient assessed and, if necessary, alternative therapy instituted.

Candidiasis of the mouth and throat (thrush) occurs in some patients. Such patients may find it helpful to rinse out their mouth with water after using the Inhaler. Symptomatic candidiasis can be treated with topical anti-fungal therapy whilst still continuing with inhaled fluticasone propionate.

In some patients inhaled fluticasone propionate may cause hoarseness. It may be helpful to rinse out the mouth with water immediately after inhalation.

Systemic effects of inhaled corticosteroids may occur, particularly at high doses prescribed for prolonged periods. These may include adrenal suppression, growth retardation in children and adolescents, decrease in bone mineral density, cataract and glaucoma.

There have been rare reports of peripheral oedema and cutaneous hypersensitivity reactions such as skin rash.

There have been very rare reports of dyspepsia and arthralgia although a causal link with fluticasone propionate has not been established.

Overdosage: Acute. Inhalation of the drug in doses in excess of those recommended may lead to temporary suppression of adrenal function. This does not necessitate emergency action being taken. In these patients treatment with fluticasone propionate by inhalation should be continued at a reduced dose to control asthma; adrenal function recovers in a few days and can be verified by measuring plasma cortisol.

Chronic. Use of inhaled fluticasone propionate in daily doses in excess of 2 mg over prolonged periods may lead to adrenal suppression. Monitoring of adrenal reserve may be indicated. Treatment with Flixotide Diskhaler should be continued at a dose sufficient to control asthma.

Pharmaceutical precautions Whilst the disks provide good protection to the blister contents from the effect of the atmosphere, they should not be exposed to extremes of temperature and should be stored below 30°C.

Disks may be kept in the Diskhaler at all times but a blister should only be pierced immediately prior to use. Failure to observe this instruction will affect operation of the Diskhaler.

Legal category POM.

Package quantities Flixotide Diskhaler is supplied in cartons containing 14 disks (14 x 4 blisters), together with a Diskhaler inhaler.

Further information Nil.

Product licence numbers
Flixotide Diskhaler 50 micrograms 10949/0005
Flixotide Diskhaler 100 micrograms 10949/0006
Flixotide Diskhaler 250 micrograms 10949/0007
Flixotide Diskhaler 500 micrograms 10949/0008

FLIXOTIDE* INHALER

Presentation Flixotide Inhaler is a pressurised metered-dose inhaler available in four strengths delivering 25 micrograms, 50 micrograms, 125 micrograms or 250 micrograms fluticasone propionate per actuation.

Other ingredients: trichlorofluoromethane, dichlorodifluoromethane and lecithin.

Uses Fluticasone propionate given by inhalation offers preventative treatment for asthma. At recommended doses it has a potent glucocorticoid anti-inflammatory action within the lungs, with a lower incidence and severity of adverse effects than those observed when corticosteroids are administered systemically.

Therapeutic indications:

Adults: Prophylactic management in:

mild asthma: Patients requiring intermittent symptomatic bronchodilator asthma medication on a regular daily basis.

moderate asthma: Patients with unstable or worsening asthma despite prophylactic therapy or bronchodilator alone.

severe asthma: Patients with severe chronic asthma and those who are dependent on systemic corticosteroids for adequate control of symptoms. On introduction of inhaled fluticasone propionate many of these patients may be able to reduce significantly or to eliminate their requirement for oral corticosteroids.

Children: Any child who requires prophylactic medication, including patients not controlled on currently available prophylactic medication.

Dosage and administration Flixotide Inhaler is for oral inhalation use only. A Volumatic* spacer device may be used in patients who find it difficult to synchronise aerosol actuation with inspiration of breath.

Patients should be made aware of the prophylactic nature of therapy with Flixotide Inhaler and that it should be taken regularly even when they are asymptomatic. The onset of therapeutic effect is within 4 to 7 days.

Adults and children over 16 years: 100 to 1,000 micrograms twice daily, usually as two inhalations twice daily.

Patients should be given a starting dose appropriate to the severity of their disease.

Equivalent disease control is usually obtained at half the daily dose of other currently available inhaled steroids.

Typical starting doses are:

mild asthma: 100 to 250 micrograms twice daily,

moderate asthma: 250 to 500 micrograms twice daily,

severe asthma: 500 to 1,000 micrograms twice daily.

The dose should be titrated to the lowest dose at which effective control of asthma is maintained.

Children aged 4 and over: 50 to 100 micrograms twice daily.

The starting dose should be appropriate to the severity of the disease. The dose should be titrated to the lowest dose at which effective control of asthma is maintained.

Flixotide Inhaler 125 micrograms and Flixotide Inhaler 250 micrograms are not suitable for use in children.

Special patient groups: There is no need to adjust the dose in elderly patients or those with hepatic or renal impairment.

Contra-indications, warnings, etc

Contra-indications: Flixotide Inhaler is contra-indicated in patients with a history of hypersensitivity to any of its components.

Precautions: Patients' inhaler technique should be checked regularly to make sure that inhaler actuation is synchronised with inspiration to ensure optimum delivery of the drug to the lungs.

Flixotide Inhaler is not designed to relieve acute symptoms, for which an inhaled short-acting bronchodilator is required. Patients should be advised to have such rescue medication available.

Severe asthma requires regular medical assessment, including lung-function testing, as patients are at risk of severe attacks and even death. Increasing use of short-acting inhaled β_2-agonists to relieve symptoms indicates deterioration of asthma control. If patients find that short-acting relief bronchodilator treatment becomes less effective, or they need more inhalations than usual, medical attention must be sought. In this situation patients should be reassessed and consideration given to the need for increased anti-inflammatory therapy (e.g. higher doses of inhaled corticosteroids or a course of oral corticosteroids). Severe exacerbations of asthma must be treated in the normal way.

Systemic effects of inhaled corticosteroids may occur, particularly at high doses prescribed for prolonged periods. These effects are much less likely to occur than with oral corticosteroids. Possible systemic effects include adrenal suppression, growth retardation in children and adolescents, decrease in bone mineral density, cataract and glaucoma. It is important therefore that the dose of inhaled corticosteroid is titrated to the lowest dose at which effective control of asthma is maintained.

It is recommended that the height of children receiving prolonged treatment with inhaled corticosteroids is regularly monitored. If growth is slowed, therapy should be reviewed with the aim of reducing the dose of inhaled corticosteroid, if possible, to the lowest dose at which effective control of asthma is maintained. In addition, consideration should be given to referring the patient to a paediatric respiratory specialist.

Prolonged treatment with high doses of inhaled corticosteroids, particularly higher than the recommended doses, may result in clinically significant adrenal suppression. Additional systemic corticosteroid cover should be considered during periods of stress or elective surgery.

The benefits of inhaled fluticasone propionate should minimise the need for oral steroids. However, patients transferred from oral steroids, remain at risk of impaired adrenal reserve for a considerable time after transferring to inhaled fluticasone propionate. The possibility of adverse effects may persist for some time.

These patients may require specialised advice to determine the extent of adrenal impairment before elective procedures. The possibility of residual impaired adrenal response should always be considered in emergency (medical or surgical) and elective situations likely to produce stress, and appropriate corticosteroid treatment considered.

Lack of response or severe exacerbations of asthma should be treated by increasing the dose of inhaled fluticasone propionate and, if necessary, by giving a systemic steroid and/or an antibiotic if there is an infection.

For the transfer of patients being treated with oral corticosteroids: The transfer of oral steroid-dependent patients to Flixotide Inhaler, and their subsequent management, needs special care as recovery from impaired adrenocortical function, caused by prolonged systemic steroid therapy, may take a considerable time.

Patients who have been treated with systemic steroids for long periods of time, or at a high dose, may have adrenocortical suppression. With these patients adrenocortical function should be monitored regularly and their dose of systemic steroid reduced cautiously.

After approximately a week, gradual withdrawal of the systemic steroid is started by reducing the daily dose by 1 mg prednisolone, or its equivalent. For maintenance doses of prednisolone in excess of 10 mg daily, it may be appropriate to cautiously use larger reductions in dose at weekly intervals.

Some patients feel unwell in a non-specific way during the withdrawal phase despite maintenance or even improvement of respiratory function. They should be encouraged to persevere with Flixotide Inhaler and to continue withdrawal of systemic steroid, unless there are objective signs of adrenal insufficiency.

Patients transferred from oral steroids whose adrenocortical function is still impaired should carry a steroid warning card indicating that they need supplementary systemic steroid during periods of stress, e.g. worsening asthma attacks, chest infections, major intercurrent illness, surgery, trauma, etc.

Replacement of systemic steroid treatment with inhaled therapy sometimes unmasks allergies such as allergic rhinitis or eczema previously controlled by the systemic drug. These allergies should be symptomatically treated with antihistamine and/or topical preparations, including topical steroids.

Treatment with Flixotide Inhaler should not be stopped abruptly.

Special care is necessary in patients with active or quiescent pulmonary tuberculosis.

Pregnancy and lactation: There is inadequate evidence of safety of fluticasone propionate in human pregnancy. Administration of corticosteroids to pregnant animals can cause abnormalities of fetal development, including cleft palate and intra-uterine growth retardation. There may therefore be a very small risk of such effects in the human fetus. It should be noted, however, that the fetal changes in animals occur after relatively high systemic exposure. Because fluticasone propionate is delivered directly to the lungs by the inhaled route it avoids the high level of exposure that occurs when corticosteroids are given by systemic routes. Administration of fluticasone propionate during pregnancy should only be considered if the expected benefit to the mother is greater than any possible risk to the fetus.

The secretion of fluticasone propionate in human breast milk has not been investigated. Subcutaneous administration of fluticasone propionate to lactating laboratory rats produced measurable plasma levels and evidence of fluticasone propionate in the milk. However plasma levels in humans after inhalation at recommended doses are likely to be low. When fluticasone propionate is used in breast feeding mothers the therapeutic benefits must be weighed against the potential hazards to mother and baby.

Side-effects: As with other inhalation therapy, paradoxical bronchospasm may occur with an immediate increase in wheezing after dosing. This should be treated immediately with a fast-acting inhaled bronchodilator. Flixotide Inhaler should be discontinued immediately, the patient assessed and, if necessary, alternative therapy instituted.

Candidiasis of the mouth and throat (thrush) occurs in some patients. Such patients may find it helpful to rinse out their mouth with water after using the Inhaler. Symptomatic candidiasis can be treated with topical anti-fungal therapy whilst still continuing with inhaled fluticasone propionate.

In some patients inhaled fluticasone propionate may cause hoarseness. It may be helpful to rinse out the mouth with water immediately after inhalation.

Systemic effects of inhaled corticosteroids may occur, particularly at high doses prescribed for prolonged periods. These may include adrenal suppression, growth retardation in children and adolescents, decrease in bone mineral density, cataract and glaucoma.

There have been rare reports of peripheral oedema and cutaneous hypersensitivity reactions such as skin rash.

There have been very rare reports of dyspepsia and arthralgia although a causal link with fluticasone propionate has not been established.

Overdosage: Acute. Inhalation of the drug in doses in excess of those recommended may lead to temporary suppression of adrenal function. This does not necessitate emergency action being taken. In these patients treatment with fluticasone propionate by inhalation should be continued at a reduced dose to control asthma; adrenal function recovers in a few days and can be verified by measuring plasma cortisol.

Chronic. Use of inhaled fluticasone propionate in daily doses in excess of 2 mg over prolonged periods may lead to adrenal suppression. Monitoring of adrenal reserve may be indicated. Treatment with Flixotide Inhaler should be continued at a dose sufficient to control asthma.

Pharmaceutical precautions Flixotide Inhaler should be stored between 2°C and 30°C.

As with most inhaled medications in pressurised canisters, the therapeutic effect of this medication may decrease when the canister is cold.

Protect from frost and direct sunlight.

The canister should not be punctured, broken or burnt even when apparently empty.

Legal category POM.

Package quantities Flixotide Inhaler is a pressurised metered-dose inhaler with a specially designed actuator. Each canister provides 120 inhalations.

Further information Nil.

Product licence numbers

Flixotide Inhaler 25 micrograms 10949/0001

Flixotide Inhaler 50 micrograms 10949/0002

Flixotide Inhaler 125 micrograms 10949/0003

Flixotide Inhaler 250 micrograms 10949/0004

FLIXOTIDE* NEBULES* 0.5 mg/2 ml ▼
FLIXOTIDE* NEBULES* 2 mg/2 ml ▼

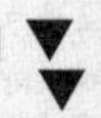

Qualitative and quantitative composition Plastic ampoules containing 2 ml of a buffered, isotonic saline suspension containing either 0.5 mg or 2 mg fluticasone propionate.

Pharmaceutical form Inhalation suspension for nebulisation.

Clincal particulars

Therapeutic indications: In adults and adolescents over 16 years Flixotide Nebules can be used:

For prophylactic management of severe chronic asthma in patients requiring high dose inhaled or oral corticosteroid therapy. On introduction of inhaled fluticasone propionate many patients currently treated with oral corticosteroids may be able to reduce significantly, or eliminate, their oral dose.

Flixotide Nebules are not licensed for use in children under 16 years and therefore should not be used in this patient population. Current clinical data do not allow appropriate dosage recommendations to be made in this patient population.

Fluticasone propionate given by inhalation has a potent glucocorticoid anti-inflammatory action within the lungs. It reduces symptoms and exacerbations of asthma in patients previously treated with bronchodilators alone or with other prophylactic therapy. Relatively brief symptomatic episodes can generally be relieved by the use of fast-acting bronchodilators, but longer-lasting exacerbations require, in addition, the use of corticosteroid therapy as soon as possible to control the inflammation.

Posology and method of administration:

Adults and adolescents over 16 years: 500–2,000 micrograms twice daily. Patients should receive a dose appropriate to the severity of their disease. The dose should be titrated to the lowest dose at which effective control of asthma is maintained.

Children 16 years and under: Flixotide Nebules are not licensed for use in children under 16 years and therefore should not be used in this patient population. Current clinical data do not allow appropriate dosage recommendations to be made in this patient population.

Special patient groups: There is no need to adjust the dose in elderly patients or those with hepatic or renal impairment.

Flixotide Nebules are for inhalation use only. They should be administered as an aerosol produced by a jet nebuliser, as directed by a physician. As drug delivery from nebulisers is variable, the manufacturer's instructions for using the nebuliser must be followed.

Use of Flixotide Nebules with ultrasonic nebulisers is not generally recommended.

Flixotide Nebules should not be injected or administered orally.

Patients should be made aware of the prophylactic nature of therapy with inhaled fluticasone propionate and that it should be taken regularly.

It is advisable to administer Flixotide Nebules via a mouthpiece to avoid the possibility of atrophic changes to facial skin which may occur with prolonged use with a face-mask. When a face-mask is used, the exposed skin should be protected using a barrier cream, or the face should be thoroughly washed after treatment.

Contra-indications: Hypersensitivity to any ingredient of the preparation.

Special warnings and precautions for use: Flixotide Nebules are not designed to relieve acute symptoms for which an inhaled short-acting bronchodilator is required. Patients should be advised to have such rescue medication available. Flixotide Nebules are intended for regular daily prophylactic treatment.

Flixotide Nebules are not a substitute for injectable or oral corticosteroids in an emergency.

Severe asthma requires regular medical assessment, including lung function testing, as patients are at risk of severe attacks and even death. Increasing use of short-acting inhaled β_2-agonists to relieve symptoms indicates deterioration of asthma control. If patients find that short-acting relief bronchodilator treatment becomes less effective, or they need more inhalations than usual, medical attention must be sought. In this situation patients should be reassessed and consideration given to the need for increased anti-inflammatory therapy (e.g. higher doses of inhaled corticosteroids or a course of oral corticosteroids). Severe exacerbations of asthma must be treated in the normal way.

Systemic effects of inhaled corticosteroids may occur, particularly at high doses prescribed for prolonged periods. These effects are much less likely to occur than with oral steroids. Possible systemic effects include adrenal suppression, growth retardation in children and adolescents, decrease in bone mineral density, cataract and glaucoma. It is important therefore that the dose of inhaled corticosteroid is titrated to the lowest dose at which effective control of asthma is maintained.

It is recommended that the height of children receiving prolonged treatment with inhaled corticosteroids is regularly monitored. If growth is slowed, therapy should be reviewed with the aim of reducing the dose of inhaled corticosteroid, if possible to the lowest dose at which effective control of asthma is maintained. In addition, consideration should be given to referring the patient to a paediatric respiratory specialist.

Prolonged treatment with high doses of inhaled corticosteroids, particularly higher than recommended doses, may result in clinically significant adrenal suppression. Additional systemic corticosteroid cover should be considered during periods of stress or elective surgery.

The benefits of inhaled fluticasone propionate should minimise the need for oral steroids. However, patients transferred from oral steroids, remain at risk of impaired adrenal reserve for a considerable time after transferring to inhaled fluticasone propionate. The possibility of adverse effects may persist for some time. These patients may require specialised advice to determine the extent of adrenal impairment before elective procedures. The possibility of residual impaired adrenal response should always be considered in emergency (medical or surgical) and elective situations likely to produce stress, and appropriate corticosteroid treatment considered.

Patients should receive a dose appropriate to the severity of their disease; the dose should be titrated to the lowest dose at which effective control of asthma is maintained. If control cannot be maintained, the use of a systemic steroid and/or an antibiotic may be necessary.

Replacement of systemic steroid treatment with inhaled therapy sometimes unmasks allergies such as allergic rhinitis or eczema previously controlled by the systemic drug. These allergies should be symptomatically treated with antihistamine and/or topical preparations, including topical steroids.

As with all inhaled corticosteroids, special care is necessary in patients with active or quiescent pulmonary tuberculosis.

Treatment with Flixotide Nebules should not be stopped abruptly.

For the transfer of patients being treated with oral corticosteroids: The transfer of oral steroid-dependent patients to Flixotide Nebules and their subsequent management needs special care as recovery from impaired adrenocortical function, caused by prolonged systemic steroid therapy, may take a considerable time.

Patients who have been treated with systemic steroids for long periods of time or at a high dose, may have adrenocortical suppression. With these patients adrenocortical function should be monitored regularly and their dose of systemic steroid reduced cautiously.

After approximately a week, gradual withdrawal of the systemic steroid is commenced. Dosage reductions should be appropriate to the level of maintenance systemic steroid, and introduced at not less than weekly intervals. In general, for maintenance doses of prednisolone (or equivalent) of 10 mg daily or less, the dosage reductions should not be greater than 1 mg per day, at not less than weekly intervals. For maintenance doses of prednisolone in excess of 10 mg daily, it may be appropriate to employ cautiously, larger reductions in dose at weekly intervals.

Some patients feel unwell in a non-specific way during the withdrawal phase despite maintenance or even improvement of the respiratory function. They should be encouraged to persevere with inhaled fluticasone propionate and to continue withdrawal of systemic steroid, unless there are objective signs of adrenal insufficiency.

Patients weaned off oral steroids whose adrenocortical function is still impaired should carry a steroid warning card indicating that they need supplementary systemic steroid during periods of stress, e.g. worsening asthma attacks, chest infections, major intercurrent illness, surgery, trauma, etc.

Interaction with other medicaments and other forms of interaction: There are unlikely to be any implications for displacement drug interactions because of the very low plasma drug concentrations achieved after inhaled dosing.

There were no reports of suspected drug interactions in the clinical programme.

Pregnancy and lactation: There is inadequate evidence of safety of fluticasone propionate in human pregnancy. Administration of corticosteroids to pregnant animals can cause abnormalities of fetal development, including cleft palate and intra-uterine growth retardation. There may therefore be a very small risk of such effects in the human fetus. It should be noted, however, that the fetal changes in animals occur after relatively high systemic exposure. Because Flixotide Nebules deliver fluticasone propionate directly to the lungs by the inhaled route the high level of exposure that occurs when corticosteroids are given by systemic routes is avoided. Administration of fluticasone propionate during pregnancy should only be considered if the expected benefit to the mother is greater than any possible risk to the fetus.

The secretion of fluticasone propionate in human breast milk has not been investigated. Subcutaneous administration of fluticasone propionate to lactating laboratory rats produced measurable plasma levels and evidence of fluticasone propionate in the milk. However, plasma levels in humans after inhalation at recommended doses are likely to be low. When fluticasone propionate is used in breast-feeding mothers the therapeutic benefits must be weighed against the potential hazards to mother and baby.

Effects on ability to drive and operate machinery: Fluticasone propionate is unlikely to produce an effect.

Undesirable effects: As with other inhalation therapy, paradoxical bronchospasm may occur with an immediate increase in wheezing after dosing. This should be treated immediately with a fast-acting inhaled bronchodilator. Flixotide Nebules should be discontinued immediately, the patient assessed, and if necessary, alternative therapy instituted.

Candidiasis of the mouth and throat (thrush) occurs in some patients. Such patients may find it helpful to rinse out their mouth with water after using the nebuliser. Symptomatic candidiasis can be treated with topical anti-fungal therapy whilst still continuing to use Flixotide Nebules.

In some patients inhaled fluticasone propionate may cause hoarseness. It may be helpful to rinse out the mouth with water immediately after inhalation.

Systemic effects of inhaled corticosteroids may occur particularly at high doses prescribed for prolonged periods. These may include adrenal suppression, growth retardation in children and adolescents, decrease in bone mineral density, cataract and glaucoma.

There have been rare reports of peripheral oedema and cutaneous hypersensitivity reactions such as skin rash.

There have been very rare reports of dyspepsia and arthralgia although a causal link with fluticasone propionate has not been established.

Overdose:

Acute: Inhalation of the drug in doses in excess of those recommended may lead to temporary suppression of adrenal function. This does not necessitate emergency action being taken. In these patients treatment with fluticasone propionate by inhalation should be continued at a dose sufficient to control asthma; adrenal function recovers in a few days and can be verified by measuring plasma cortisol.

Chronic: Use of inhaled fluticasone propionate in daily doses in excess of those recommended over prolonged periods may lead to adrenal suppression. Monitoring of adrenal reserve may be indicated. Treatment with inhaled fluticasone propionate should be continued at a dose sufficient to control asthma.

Pharmacological properties

Pharmacodynamic properties: Fluticasone propionate given by inhalation at recommended doses has a potent glucocorticoid anti-inflammatory action within the lungs, which results in reduced symptoms and exacerbations of asthma.

Pharmacokinetic properties: Following inhaled dosing, systemic availability of the nebulised fluticasone propionate in healthy volunteers is estimated at 8% as compared with up to 26% received from the metered dose inhaler presentation. Systemic absorption occurs mainly through the lungs and is initially rapid then prolonged. The remainder of the dose may be swallowed. Absolute oral bioavailability is negligible (<1%) due to a combination of incomplete absorption from the GI tract and extensive first-pass metabolism.

87–100% of an oral dose is excreted in the faeces, up to 75% as parent compound. There is also a non-active major metabolite.

After an intravenous dose, fluticasone propionate is extensively distributed in the body. The very high clearance rate indicates extensive hepatic clearance.

Preclinical safety data: Toxicology has shown only those class effects typical of potent corticosteroids, and these only at doses greatly in excess of that proposed for therapeutic use. No novel effects were identified in repeat dose toxicity tests, reproductive studies or teratology studies. Fluticasone propionate is devoid of mutagenic activity *in vitro* and *in vivo* and showed no tumorigenic potential in rodents. It is both non-irritant and non-sensitising in animal models.

Pharmaceutical particulars

List of excipients:
Polysorbate 20 PhEur.
Sorbitan monolaurate PhEur.
Monosodium phosphate dihydrate PhEur.
Dibasic sodium phosphate anhydrous USP.
Sodium Chloride PhEur.
Water for Injection PhEur.

Incompatibilities: None reported.

Shelf life: 24 months unopened.

Special precautions for storage: Flixotide Nebules should be stored below 30°C, protected from light and freezing. Store upright. The blister pack should be opened immediately before use. Opened Nebules should be refrigerated and used within 12 hours of opening.

Nature and contents of container: 2.5 ml low density polyethylene ampoules wrapped in a double foil blister, in boxes of 10.

The foil blister pack consists of a base and lidding foil. The base foil of the blister consists of aluminium (60 microns) coated on the outside with polyamide and on the inside with polyvinylchloride. The lidding consists of paper bonded to polyethyleneterephthalate bonded to aluminium (20 microns), with a coating of vinyl/acrylate lacquer on the inner surface.

Instructions for use/handling: It is important to ensure that the contents of the Nebule are well mixed before use. While holding the Nebule horizontally by the labelled tab, 'flick' the other end a few times and shake. Repeat this process several times until the entire contents of the Nebule are completely mixed. To open the Nebule, twist off the tab.

Dilution: Flixotide Nebules may be diluted with Sodium Chloride Injection BP if required, to aid administration of small volumes or if a prolonged delivery time is desirable. Any unused suspension remaining in the nebuliser should be discarded.

For detailed instructions please refer to the Patient Information Leaflet in every pack.

The nebuliser must be used according to the manufacturer's instructions. It is advisable to administer Flixotide Nebules via a mouthpiece (see *Posology and method of administration*). As many nebulisers operate on a continuous flow basis, it is likely that some nebulised drug will be released into the local environment. Flixotide Nebules should therefore be administered in a well-ventilated room, particularly in hospitals where several patients may be using nebulisers at the same time.

Marketing authorisation numbers
Flixotide Nebules 0.5 mg/2 ml 10949/0297.
Flixotide Nebules 2 mg/2 ml 10949/0298.

Date of approval/revision of SPC November 1998.

Legal category POM.

RESPONTIN* NEBULES*

Qualitative and quantitative composition 1 ml or 2 ml plastic ampoules containing 0.25 mg/ml of Ipratropium Bromide PhEur.

Pharmaceutical form Oral inhalation solution via a nebuliser.

Clinical particulars

Therapeutic indications: Respontin Nebules are indicated for the treatment of reversible airways obstruction.

Posology and method of administration: The recommended dose is:

Adults: 0.4 to 2 ml solution (100–500 micrograms) up to four times daily.

Children (3 to 14 years): 0.4 to 2 ml solution (100–500 micrograms) up to three times daily.

The volume of ipratropium bromide solution may need to be diluted in order to obtain a final volume suitable for the particular nebuliser used. If dilution is necessary use only sterile sodium chloride 0.9% solution.

There is no specific information on the use of the isotonic nebuliser solution in the elderly. Clinical trials with the previously available hypotonic formulation included patients over 65 years and no adverse reactions specific to this age group were reported.

Contra-indications: Known hypersensitivity to any components of the formulation or to atropine.

Special warnings and precautions for use: Use of the nebuliser solution should be subject to close medical supervision during initial dosing. There have been rare reports of paradoxical bronchospasm associated with the administration of ipratropium bromide nebuliser solution. The patient should be advised to seek medical advice should a reduced response become apparent.

Patients must be instructed in the correct administration of Respontin Nebules and warned not to allow the solution or mist to enter the eyes. Acute angle-closure glaucoma has been reported rarely when ipratropium bromide has been used in conjunction with nebulised β_2-agonist bronchodilators. Protection of the eyes appears to prevent any increase in intraocular pressure and patients who may be susceptible to glaucoma should be warned specifically of the need for ocular protection. Inhaled doses of ipratropium bromide up to 1 mg have not been associated with elevation of intra-ocular pressure.

Use anticholinergic agents with caution in patients with prostatic hypertrophy.

Interaction with other medicaments and other forms of interaction: There is evidence that the concurrent administration of ipratropium bromide and sympathomimetic drugs produces a greater relief of bronchospasm than either drug given alone. Ipratropium bromide has been shown to produce effective bronchodilatation in patients receiving β-adrenergic blocking agents.

Pregnancy and lactation: Ipratropium bromide has been in general use for several years and there is no definite evidence of ill-consequence during pregnancy. Animal studies have shown no hazard. Nevertheless, medicines should not be used in pregnancy, especially during the first trimester, unless the expected benefit is thought to outweigh any possible risk to the fetus.

Effect on ability to drive and use machines: None stated.

Undesirable effects: Anticholinergic side-effects are unlikely at therapeutic doses, but some patients may experience a dry mouth. Urinary retention and constipation have only rarely been reported with ipratropium bromide. There is no evidence that in the therapeutic dose range, ipratropium bromide has any adverse effect on bronchial secretion.

Overdose: Inhaled doses of 5 mg produce an increase in heart rate and palpitation but single doses at 2 mg have been given to adults and 1 mg to children without causing side-effects. Single doses of ipratropium bromide 30 mg by mouth cause anticholinergic side-effects but these are not severe and do not require specific reversal.

Pharmacological properties

Pharmacodynamic properties: Ipratropium bromide is an anticholinergic bronchodilator which affects airways function primarily through its neural effects on the parasympathetic nervous system. Ipratropium bromide blocks the acetylcholine receptors on smooth muscle in the lung. Stimulation of these receptors normally produces contraction and depending on the degree of activation, bronchoconstriction. Thus ipratropium bromide will cause bronchodilatation.

Pharmacokinetic properties: Ipratropium bromide is a quaternary ammonium compound which is poorly absorbed from the gastro-intestinal tract, and is slow to cross mucous membranes and the blood/brain barrier. Following inhalation, uptake into the plasma is minimal, a peak blood concentration is obtained $1\frac{1}{2}$ to 3 hours after inhalation. Excretion is chiefly via the kidneys.

Preclinical safety data: There are no pre-clinical data of relevance to the prescriber which are additional to that already included in other sections of the SmPC.

Pharmaceutical particulars

List of excipients:

Sodium Chloride PhEur, Diluted Phosphoric Acid PhEur, Purified Water PhEur.

Incompatibilities: None stated.

Shelf life: 24 months.

Special precautions for storage: Store below 25°C. Protect from light.

This product contains no preservative. A new Nebule should be used for each dose. A Nebule should be opened immediately before administration and any remaining solution should be discarded. Any unused Nebules should be discarded four weeks after opening the foil pack.

Nature and contents of container: 1 or 2 ml low density polyethylene ampoules in boxes of 20 in strips of 5.

Instructions for use/handling: The nebulised solution may be inhaled through a face mask, T-piece or via an endotracheal tube. Intermittent positive pressure ventilation (IPPV) may be used but is rarely necessary. When there is a risk of anoxia through hypoventilation, oxygen should be added to the inspired air.

As many nebulisers operate on a continuous flow basis, it is likely that some nebulised drug will be released into the local environment. Ipratropium bromide should therefore be administered in a well-ventilated room, particularly in hospitals where several patients may be using nebulisers at the same time. Do not allow the solution or mist to enter the eyes.

Marketing authorisation number PL 10949/0275.

Date of approval/revision of SPC April 1998.

Legal category POM.

SEREVENT* ACCUHALER*

Qualitative and quantitative composition Serevent Accuhaler is a moulded plastic device containing a foil strip with 60 regularly spaced blisters each containing 50 micrograms of salmeterol (as xinafoate) and lactose.

Pharmaceutical form Inhalation powder.

Clinical particulars

Therapeutic indications: Salmeterol is a selective β_2-agonist providing long-acting (usually 12 hours) bronchodilatation with a relatively slow onset (within 10–20 minutes) in reversible airways obstruction.

Serevent Accuhaler can be used to treat reversible airways obstruction in patients requiring long-term regular bronchodilator therapy, including those with asthma and with chronic obstructive pulmonary disease (COPD).

It is particularly useful in the treatment of nocturnal asthma and in the prevention of exercise-induced symptoms.

Serevent Accuhaler should not be used to treat acute asthma symptoms (see *Special warnings*).

Patients with asthma should normally also be receiving regular and adequate doses of inhaled anti-inflammatory agents (e.g. corticosteroids, and/or in children, sodium cromoglycate), or oral corticosteroids. Serevent Accuhaler is not a replacement for these treatments which should be continued at the same dose, and not stopped or reduced, when treatment with Serevent Accuhaler is initiated.

Posology and method of administration: Serevent Accuhaler is for inhalation use only.

Serevent Accuhaler should be used regularly. The full benefits of treatment will be apparent after several doses of the drug.

In reversible airways obstruction such as asthma

Adults (including the elderly): One inhalation (50 micrograms) twice daily, increasing to two inhalations (2 × 50 micrograms) twice daily if required.

Children 4 years and over: One inhalation (50 micrograms) twice daily.

The dosage or frequency of administration should only be increased on medical advice.

There are insufficient clinical data to recommend the use of Serevent Accuhaler in children under the age of four.

In chronic obstructive pulmonary disease

Adults (including the elderly): One inhalation (50 micrograms) twice daily.

Children: Not appropriate.

Special patient groups: There is no need to adjust the dose in patients with impaired renal function.

Contra-indications: Hypersensitivity to any ingredient of the preparation.

Special warnings and special precautions for use: Serevent Accuhaler should not be initiated in patients with significantly worsening or acutely deteriorating asthma.

Sudden and progressive deterioration in asthma control is potentially life-threatening and consideration should be given to starting or increasing corticosteroid therapy. Under these circumstances, daily peak flow monitoring may be advisable.

Serevent Accuhaler is not a replacement for inhaled or oral corticosteroids or sodium cromoglycate (see *Therapeutic indications*). Patients with asthma must be warned not to stop steroid therapy (and for children, sodium cromoglycate therapy), and not to reduce it without medical advice, even if they feel better on Serevent Accuhaler.

With its relatively slow onset of action Serevent Accuhaler should not be used to relieve acute asthma symptoms, for which an inhaled short-acting bronchodilator is required. Patients should be advised to have such rescue medication available.

Bronchodilators should not be the only or the main treatment in patients with severe or unstable asthma. Severe asthma requires regular medical assessment, including lung-function testing, as patients are at risk of severe attacks and even death. Physicians should consider using the maximum recommended dose of inhaled corticosteroid and/or oral corticosteroid therapy in these patients.

Increasing use of bronchodilators, in particular short-acting inhaled β_2-agonists to relieve symptoms, indicates deterioration of asthma control. The patient should be instructed to seek medical advice if short-acting relief bronchodilator treatment becomes less effective, or more inhalations than usual are required. In this situation the patient should be assessed and consideration given to the need for increased anti-inflammatory therapy (e.g. higher doses of inhaled corticosteroid or a course of oral corticosteroid). Severe exacerbations of asthma must be treated in the normal way.

Salmeterol should be administered with caution in patients with thyrotoxicosis.

Potentially serious hypokalaemia may result from β_2-agonist therapy. Particular caution is advised in acute severe asthma as this effect may be potentiated by hypoxia and by concomitant treatment with xanthine derivatives, steroids and diuretics. Serum potassium levels should be monitored in such situations.

Interaction with other medicaments and other forms of interaction: Both non-selective and selective β-blockers should be avoided in patients with reversible obstructive airways disease, unless there are compelling reasons for their use.

Pregnancy and lactation: In animal studies, some effects on the fetus, typical for a β_2-agonist, occurred at exposure levels substantially higher than those that occur with therapeutic use. Extensive experience with other β_2-agonists has provided no evidence that such effects are relevant for women receiving clinical doses. As yet, experience of the use of salmeterol during pregnancy is limited. As with any medicine, use during pregnancy should be considered only if the expected benefit to the mother is greater than any possible risk to the fetus.

Plasma levels of salmeterol after inhaled therapeutic doses are negligible, and therefore levels in milk should be correspondingly low. Nevertheless, as there is limited experience of the use of salmeterol in nursing mothers, its use in such circumstances should only be considered if the expected benefit to the mother is greater than any possible risk to the infant.

Studies in lactating animals support the view that salmeterol is likely to be secreted in only very small amounts into breast milk.

Effects on ability to drive and use machines: None reported.

Undesirable effects: As with other inhalation therapy, paradoxical bronchospasm may occur with an immediate increase in wheezing and drop in peak expiratory flow rate (PEFR) after dosing. This responds to a fast-acting inhaled bronchodilator. Serevent Accuhaler should be discontinued immediately, the patient assessed, and if necessary an alternative presentation or therapy should be instituted.

The pharmacological side effects of β_2-agonist treatment, such as tremor, subjective palpitations and headache, have been reported, but tend to be transient and to reduce with regular therapy. Tachycardia may occur in some patients. In common with other β_2 agonists, cardiac arrhythmias (including atrial fibrillation, supraventricular tachycardia and extrasystoles) have been reported in association with the use of salmeterol, usually in susceptible patients.

Potentially serious hypokalaemia may result from β_2-agonist therapy.

There have been reports of the following: hypersensitivity reactions such as rash and oedema including angioedema; muscle cramps; non-specific chest pain; local irritation; arthralgia.

Overdose: The symptoms and signs of salmeterol overdosage are tremor, headache and tachycardia. The preferred antidote for overdosage with Serevent Accuhaler is a cardioselective β-blocking agent. Cardioselective β-blocking drugs should be used with caution in patients with a history of bronchospasm.

Pharmacological properties

Pharmacodynamic properties: Salmeterol is a selective long-acting (usually 12 hours) β_2-adrenoceptor agonist with a long side-chain which binds to the exo-site of the receptor. These pharmacological properties of salmeterol offer more effective protection against histamine-induced bronchoconstriction and produce a longer duration of bronchodilatation, lasting for at least 12 hours, than recommended doses of conventional short-acting β_2-agonists. *In vitro* tests have shown that salmeterol is a potent and long-lasting inhibitor of the release from the human lung of mast cell mediators, such as histamine, leukotrienes and prostaglandin D_2. In man, salmeterol inhibits the early and late phase response to inhaled allergen; the latter persisting for over 30 hours after a single dose when the bronchodilator effect is no longer evident. Single dosing with salmeterol attenuates bronchial hyper-responsiveness. These properties indicate that salmeterol has additional non-bronchodilator activity, but the full clinical significance is not yet clear. The mechanism is different from the anti-inflammatory effect of corticosteroids, which should not be stopped or reduced when Serevent Accuhaler is prescribed.

Salmeterol has been studied in the treatment of conditions associated with COPD, and has been shown to improve symptoms and pulmonary function, and quality of life. Salmeterol acts as a β_2-agonist on the reversible component of the disease. *In vitro* salmeterol has also been shown to increase cilial beat frequency of human bronchial epithelial cells, and also reduce a ciliotoxic effect of *Pseudomonas* toxin on the bronchial epithelium of patients with cystic fibrosis.

Pharmacokinetic properties: Salmeterol acts locally in the lung, therefore plasma levels are not predictive of therapeutic effects. In addition there are only limited data available on the pharmacokinetics of salmeterol because of the technical difficulty of assaying the drug in plasma because of the very low plasma concentrations at therapeutic doses (approximately 200 pg/ml or less) achieved after inhaled dosing. After regular dosing with salmeterol xinafoate, xinafoic acid can be detected in the systemic circulation, reaching steady state concentrations of approximately 100 ng/ml. These concentrations are up to 1000-fold lower than steady state levels observed in toxicity studies. These concentrations in long term regular dosing (more than 12 months) in patients with airways obstruction, have been shown to produce no ill effects.

Preclinical safety data: In reproduction studies in animals, some effects on the fetus, typical of a β_2-agonist, have been observed at very high doses.

Salmeterol xinafoate produced no genetic toxicity in a range of studies using either prokaryotic or eukaryotic cell systems *in vitro* or *in vivo* in the rat.

Long term studies with salmeterol xinafoate, induced class-related benign tumours of smooth muscle in the mesovarium of rats and the uterus of mice. The scientific literature and our own pharmacological studies provide good evidence that these effects are species-specific and have no relevance for clinical use.

Pharmaceutical particulars

List of excipients: Lactose.

Incompatibilities: None reported.

Shelf life: 24 months when stored below 30°C for moderate climates.

18 months when stored below 30°C for tropical climates.

Special precautions for storage: Store below 30°C in a dry place.

Nature and contents of container: The powder mix of salmeterol xinafoate and lactose is filled into a blister strip consisting of a formed base foil with a peelable foil laminate lid. The foil strip is contained within the Accuhaler device.

Instructions for use/handling: The powdered medicine is inhaled through the mouth into the lungs.

The Accuhaler device contains the medicine in individual blisters which are opened as the device is manipulated.

For detailed instructions for use refer to the Patient Information Leaflet in every pack.

Marketing authorisation number 10949/0214

Date of approval/revision of SPC June 1998.

Legal category POM.

SEREVENT* DISKHALER*

Qualitative and quantitative composition Disks comprising four regularly spaced double-foil blisters each delivering a mixture of 50 micrograms salmeterol (as xinafoate) and lactose used in a Diskhaler device.

Pharmaceutical form Inhalation powder.

Clinical particulars

Therapeutic indications: Salmeterol is a selective β_2-agonist providing long-acting (usually 12 hours) bronchodilatation with a relatively slow onset (within 10–20 minutes) in reversible airways obstruction.

Serevent Diskhaler can be used to treat reversible airways obstruction in patients requiring long-term regular bronchodilator therapy, including those with asthma and with chronic obstructive pulmonary disease (COPD).

It is particularly useful in the treatment of nocturnal asthma and in the prevention of exercise-induced symptoms.

Serevent Diskhaler should not be used to treat acute asthma symptoms (see *Special warnings*).

Patients with asthma should normally also be receiving regular and adequate doses of inhaled anti-inflammatory agents (e.g. corticosteroids, and/or in children, sodium cromoglycate), or oral corticosteroids. Serevent Diskhaler is not a replacement for these treatments which should be continued at the same dose, and not stopped or reduced, when treatment with Serevent Diskhaler is initiated.

Posology and method of administration: Serevent Diskhaler is for inhalation use only.

Serevent Diskhaler should be used regularly. The full benefits of treatment will be apparent after several doses of the drug.

In reversible airways obstruction such as asthma:

Adults (including the elderly): One blister (50 micrograms) twice daily, increasing to two blisters (2 × 50 micrograms) twice daily if required.

Children 4 years and over: One blister (50 micrograms) twice daily.

The dosage or frequency of administration should only be increased on medical advice.

There are insufficient clinical data to recommend the use of Serevent Diskhaler in children under the age of four.

In chronic obstructive pulmonary disease:

Adults (including the elderly): One blister (50 micrograms) twice daily.

Children: Not appropriate.

Special patient groups: There is no need to adjust the dose in patients with impaired renal function.

Contra-indications: Hypersensitivity to any ingredient of the preparation.

Special warnings and special precautions for use: Serevent Diskhaler should not be initiated in patients with significantly worsening or acutely deteriorating asthma.

Sudden and progressive deterioration in asthma control is potentially life-threatening and consideration should be given to starting or increasing corticosteroid therapy. Under these circumstances, regular peak flow monitoring may be advisable.

Serevent Diskhaler is not a replacement for inhaled or oral corticosteroids or sodium cromoglycate (see *Therapeutic indications*). Patients with asthma must be warned not to stop steroid therapy (and for children, sodium cromoglycate therapy), and not to reduce it without medical advice, even if they feel better on Serevent Diskhaler.

With its relatively slow onset of action Serevent Diskhaler should not be used to relieve acute asthma symptoms, for which an inhaled short-acting bronchodilator is required. Patients should be advised to have such rescue medication available.

Bronchodilators should not be the only or the main treatment in patients with severe or unstable asthma. Severe asthma requires regular medical assessment, including lung-function testing, as patients are at risk of severe attacks and even death. Physicians should consider using the maximum recommended dose of inhaled corticosteroid and/or oral corticosteroid therapy in these patients.

Increasing use of bronchodilators, in particular short-acting inhaled β_2-agonists to relieve symptoms, indicates deterioration of asthma control. The patient should be instructed to seek medical advice if short-acting relief bronchodilator treatment becomes less effective, or more inhalations than usual are required. In this situation the patient should be assessed and consideration given to the need for increased anti-inflammatory therapy (e.g. higher doses of inhaled corticosteroid or a course of oral corticosteroid). Severe exacerbations of asthma must be treated in the normal way.

Salmeterol should be administered with caution in patients with thyrotoxicosis.

Potentially serious hypokalaemia may result from β_2-agonist therapy. Particular caution is advised in acute severe asthma as this effect may be potentiated by hypoxia and by concomitant treatment with xanthine derivatives, steroids and diuretics. Serum potassium levels should be monitored in such situations.

Interaction with other medicaments and other forms of interaction: Both non-selective and selective β-blockers should be avoided in patients with reversible obstructive airways disease, unless there are compelling reasons for their use.

Pregnancy and lactation: In animal studies, some effects on the fetus, typical for a β_2-agonist occurred at exposure levels substantially higher than those that occur with therapeutic use. Extensive experience with other β_2-agonists has provided no evidence that such effects are relevant for women receiving clinical doses. As yet, experience of the use of salmeterol during pregnancy is limited. As with any medicine, use during pregnancy should be considered only if the expected benefit to the mother is greater than any possible risk to the fetus.

Plasma levels of salmeterol after inhaled therapeutic doses are negligible, and therefore levels in milk should be correspondingly low. Nevertheless, as there is limited experience of the use of salmeterol in nursing mothers, its use in such circumstances should only be considered if the expected benefit to the mother is greater than any possible risk to the infant.

Studies in lactating animals support the view that salmeterol is likely to be secreted in only very small amounts into breast milk.

Effects on the ability to drive and use machines: None reported.

Undesirable effects: As with other inhalation therapy, paradoxical bronchospasm may occur with an immediate increase in wheezing and drop in peak expiratory flow rate (PEFR) after dosing. This responds to a fast-acting inhaled bronchodilator. Serevent Diskhaler should be discontinued immediately, the patient assessed, and if necessary an alternative presentation or therapy should be instituted.

The pharmacological side-effects of β_2-agonist treatment, such as tremor, subjective palpitations and headache, have been reported, but tend to be transient and to reduce with regular therapy. Tachycardia may occur in some patients. In common with other β_2 agonists, cardiac arrhythmias (including atrial fibrillation, supraventricular tachycardia and extrasystoles) have been reported in association with the use of salmeterol, usually in susceptible patients.

Potentially serious hypokalaemia may result from β_2-agonist therapy.

There have been reports of the following: hypersensitivity reactions such as rash and oedema including angioedema; muscle cramps; non-specific chest pain; local irritation; arthralgia.

Overdose: The symptoms and signs of salmeterol overdosage are tremor, headache and tachycardia. The preferred antidote for overdosage with Serevent Diskhaler is a cardioselective β-blocking agent. Cardioselective β-blocking drugs should be used with caution in patients with a history of bronchospasm.

Pharmacological properties

Pharmacodynamic properties: Salmeterol is a selective long-acting (usually 12 hours) β_2-adrenoceptor agonist with a long side-chain which binds to the exo-site of the receptor. These pharmacological properties of salmeterol offer more effective protection against histamine-induced bronchoconstriction and produce a longer duration of bronchodilatation, lasting for at least 12 hours, than recommended doses of conventional short-acting β_2-agonists. *In vitro* tests have shown that salmeterol is a potent and long-lasting inhibitor of the release from the human lung of mast cell mediators, such as histamine, leukotrienes and prostaglandin D_2. In man, salmeterol inhibits the early and late phase response to inhaled allergen; the latter persisting for over 30 hours after a single dose when the bronchodilator effect is no longer evident. Single dosing with salmeterol attenuates bronchial hyper-responsiveness. These properties indicate that salmeterol has additional non-bronchodilator activity, but the full clinical significance is not yet clear. The mechanism is different from the anti-inflammatory effect of corticosteroids, which should not be stopped or reduced when Serevent Diskhaler is prescribed.

Salmeterol has been studied in the treatment of conditions associated with COPD, and has been shown to improve symptoms and pulmonary function, and quality of life. Salmeterol acts as a β_2-agonist on the reversible component of the disease. *In vitro* salmeterol has also been shown to increase cilial beat frequency of human bronchial epithelial cells, and also reduce a ciliotoxic effect of *Pseudomonas* toxin on the bronchial epithelium of patients with cystic fibrosis.

Pharmacokinetic properties: Salmeterol acts locally in the lung, therefore plasma levels are not predictive of therapeutic effect. In addition there are only limited data available on the pharmacokinetics of salmeterol because of the technical difficulty of assaying the drug in plasma because of the very low plasma concentrations (approximately 200 pg/ml or less) achieved after inhaled dosing. After regular dosing with salmeterol xinafoate, xinafoic acid can be detected in the systemic circulation, reaching steady state concentrations of approximately 100 ng/ml. These concentrations are up to 1000-fold lower than steady state levels observed in toxicity studies. These concentrations in long term regular dosing (more than 12 months) in patients with airways obstruction, have been shown to produce no ill effects.

Preclinical safety data: In reproduction studies in animals, some effects on the fetus, typical of a β_2-agonist, have been observed at very high doses.

Salmeterol xinafoate produced no genetic toxicity in a range of studies using either prokaryotic or eukaryotic cell systems *in vitro* or *in vivo* in the rat.

Long-term studies with salmeterol xinafoate, induced class-related benign tumours of smooth muscle in the mesovarium of rats and the uterus of mice. The scientific literature and our own pharmacological studies provide good evidence that these effects are species-specific and have no relevance for clinical use.

Pharmaceutical particulars
List of excipients: Lactose.

Incompatibilities: None reported.

Shelf life: 2 years when stored below 25°C.

Special precautions for storage: Store below 25°C.
A disk may be kept in the Diskhaler device but the blisters must only be pierced immediately prior to use.

Nature and contents of container: A circular double-foil disk with four blisters containing the powder mix of salmeterol (as xinafoate) and lactose. The foil disk is inserted into the Diskhaler device.
The following packs are available: 14 disks alone or with a Diskhaler.

Instructions for use/handling: The powdered medicine is inhaled through the mouth into the lungs. The Diskhaler device is loaded with a disk which contains the medicine in individual blisters which are opened as the device is manipulated.
For detailed instructions for use refer to the Patient Information Leaflet in every pack.

Marketing authorisation number 10949/0069

Date of approval/revision of SPC June 1998.

Legal category POM.

SEREVENT* INHALER

Qualitative and quantitative composition Each metered dose actuation delivers 25 micrograms salmeterol (as xinafoate). Each canister delivers 60/120 actuations.

Pharmaceutical form Pressurised metered-dose aerosol.

Clinical particulars
Therapeutic indications: Salmeterol is a selective β_2-agonist providing long-acting (usually 12 hours) bronchodilatation with a relatively slow onset (within 10–20 minutes) in reversible airways obstruction.
Serevent Inhaler can be used to treat reversible airways obstruction in patients requiring long-term regular bronchodilator therapy, including those with asthma and with chronic obstructive pulmonary disease (COPD).
It is particularly useful in the treatment of nocturnal asthma and in the prevention of exercise-induced symptoms.
Serevent Inhaler should not be used to treat acute asthma symptoms (see *Special warnings*).
Patients with asthma should normally also be receiving regular and adequate doses of inhaled anti-inflammatory agents (e.g. corticosteroids, and/or in children, sodium cromoglycate), or oral corticosteroids. Serevent Inhaler is not a replacement for these treatments which should be continued at the same dose, and not stopped or reduced, when treatment with Serevent Inhaler is initiated.

Posology and method of administration: Serevent Inhaler is for inhalation use only. A Volumatic* spacer device may be used in patients who find it difficult to synchronise aerosol actuation with inspiration of breath.
Serevent Inhaler should be used regularly. The full benefits of treatment will be apparent after several doses of the drug.

In reversible airways obstruction such as asthma:
Adults (including the elderly): Two inhalations (2 × 25 micrograms) twice daily, increasing to four inhalations (4 × 25 micrograms) twice daily if required.
Children aged 4 years and over: Two inhalations (2 × 25 micrograms) twice daily.
The dosage or frequency of administration should only be increased on medical advice.
There are insufficient clinical data to recommend the use of Serevent Inhaler in children under the age of four.

In chronic obstructive pulmonary disease:
Adults (including the elderly): Two inhalations (2 × 25 micrograms) twice daily.
Children: Not appropriate.

Special patient groups: There is no need to adjust the dose in patients with impaired renal function.

Contra-indications: Hypersensitivity to any ingredient of the preparation.

Special warnings and special precautions for use: Serevent Inhaler should not be initiated in patients with significantly worsening or acutely deteriorating asthma.
Sudden and progressive deterioration in asthma control is potentially life-threatening and consideration should be given to starting or increasing corticosteroid therapy. Under these circumstances, regular peak flow monitoring may be advisable.
Serevent Inhaler is not a replacement for inhaled or oral corticosteroids or sodium cromoglycate (see *Therapeutic indications*). Patients with asthma must be warned not to stop steroid therapy (and for children, sodium cromoglycate therapy), and not to reduce it without medical advice, even if they feel better on Serevent Inhaler.
With its relatively slow onset of action Serevent Inhaler should not be used to relieve acute asthma symptoms, for which an inhaled short-acting bronchodilator is required. Patients should be advised to have such rescue medication available.
Bronchodilators should not be the only or the main treatment in patients with severe or unstable asthma. Severe asthma requires regular medical assessment, including lung-function testing, as patients are at risk of severe attacks and even death. Physicians should consider using the maximum recommended dose of inhaled corticosteroid and/or oral corticosteroid therapy in these patients.
Increasing use of bronchodilators, in particular short-acting inhaled β_2-agonists to relieve symptoms, indicates deterioration of asthma control. The patient should be instructed to seek medical advice if short-acting relief bronchodilator treatment becomes less effective, or more inhalations than usual are required. In this situation the patient should be assessed and consideration given to the need for increased anti-inflammatory therapy (e.g. higher doses of inhaled corticosteroid or a course of oral corticosteroid). Severe exacerbations of asthma must be treated in the normal way.
Salmeterol should be administered with caution in patients with thyrotoxicosis.
Potentially serious hypokalaemia may result from β_2-agonist therapy. Particular caution is advised in acute severe asthma as this effect may be potentiated by hypoxia and by concomitant treatment with xanthine derivatives, steroids and diuretics. Serum potassium levels should be monitored in such situations.

Interaction with other medicaments and other forms of interaction: Both non-selective and selective β-blockers should be avoided in patients with reversible obstructive airways disease, unless there are compelling reasons for their use.

Pregnancy and lactation: In animal studies, some effects on the fetus, typical for a β_2-agonist, occurred at exposure levels substantially higher than those that occur with therapeutic use. Extensive experience with other β_2-agonists has provided no evidence that such effects are relevant for women receiving clinical doses. As yet, experience of the use of salmeterol during pregnancy is limited. As with any medicine, use during pregnancy should be considered only if the expected benefit to the mother is greater than any possible risk to the fetus.
Plasma levels of salmeterol after inhaled therapeutic doses are negligible, and therefore levels in milk should be correspondingly low. Nevertheless, as there is limited experience of the use of salmeterol in nursing mothers, its use in such circumstances should only be considered if the expected benefit to the mother is greater than any possible risk to the infant.
Studies in lactating animals support the view that salmeterol is likely to be secreted in only very small amounts into breast milk.

Effects on the ability to drive and use machines: None reported.

Undesirable effects: As with other inhalation therapy, paradoxical bronchospasm may occur with an immediate increase in wheezing and drop in peak expiratory flow rate (PEFR) after dosing. This responds to a fast-acting inhaled bronchodilator, Serevent Inhaler should be discontinued immediately, the patient assessed, and if necessary an alternative presentation (e.g. Serevent Diskhaler*) or therapy should be instituted.
In a study involving 11,000 patients a very low percentage (1.1%) of patients experienced a drop of 20% or more in PEFR whilst taking Serevent Inhaler. This occurred most frequently in patients over 60 and those with a poor baseline peak flow. This drop in PEFR occurred in a similar percentage in a control group of patients taking placebo.
The pharmacological side-effects of β_2-agonist treatment, such as tremor, subjective palpitations and headache, have been reported, but tend to be transient and to reduce with regular therapy. Tachycardia may occur in some patients. In common with other β_2 agonists, cardiac arrhythmias (including atrial fibrillation, supraventricular tachycardia and extrasystoles) have been reported in association with the use of salmeterol, usually in susceptible patients.
Potentially serious hypokalaemia may result from β_2-agonist therapy.
There have been reports of the following: hypersensitivity reactions such as rash and oedema including angioedema; muscle cramps; non-specific chest pain; local irritation; arthralgia.

Overdose: The symptoms and signs of salmeterol overdosage are tremor, headache and tachycardia. The preferred antidote for overdosage with Serevent Inhaler is a cardioselective β-blocking agent. Cardioselective β-blocking drugs should be used with caution in patients with a history of bronchospasm.

Pharmacological properties
Pharmacodynamic properties: Salmeterol is a selective long-acting (usually 12 hours) β_2-adrenoceptor agonist with a long side-chain which binds to the exo-side of the receptor. These pharmacological properties of salmeterol offer more effective protection against histamine-induced bronchoconstriction and produce a longer duration of bronchodilatation, lasting for at least 12 hours, than recommended doses of conventional short-acting β_2-agonists. *In vitro* tests have shown that salmeterol is a potent and long-lasting inhibitor of the release from the human lung of mast cell mediators, such as histamine, leukotrienes and prostaglandin D_2. In man, salmeterol inhibits the early and late phase response to inhaled allergen; the latter persisting for over 30 hours after a single dose when the bronchodilator effect is no longer evident. Single dosing with salmeterol attenuates bronchial hyper-responsiveness. These properties indicate that salmeterol has additional non-bronchodilator activity, but the full clinical significance is not yet clear. The mechanism is different from the anti-inflammatory effect of corticosteroids, which should not be stopped or reduced when Serevent Inhaler is prescribed.
Salmeterol has been studied in the treatment of conditions associated with COPD, and has been shown to improve symptoms and pulmonary function, and quality of life. Salmeterol acts as a β_2-agonist on the reversible component of the disease. *In vitro* salmeterol has also been shown to increase cilial beat frequency of human bronchial epithelial cells, and also reduce a ciliotoxic effect of *Pseudomonas* toxin on the bronchial epithelium of patients with cystic fibrosis.

Pharmacokinetic properties: Salmeterol acts locally in the lung, therefore plasma levels are not predictive of therapeutic effect. In addition there are only limited data available on the pharmacokinetics of salmeterol because of the technical difficulty of assaying the drug in plasma because of the very low plasma concentrations (approximately 200 pg/ml or less) achieved after inhaled dosing. After regular dosing with salmeterol xinafoate, xinafoic acid can be detected in the systemic circulation, reaching steady state concentrations of approximately 100 ng/ml. These concentrations are up to 1000-fold lower than steady state levels observed in toxicity studies. These concentrations in long term regular dosing (more than 12 months) in patients with airways obstruction, have been shown to produce no ill effects.

Preclinical safety data: In reproduction studies in animals, some effects on the fetus, typical of a β_2-agonist, have been observed at very high doses.
Salmeterol xinafoate produced no genetic toxicity in a range of studies using either prokaryotic or eukaryotic cell systems *in vitro* or *in vivo* in the rat.
Long-term studies with salmeterol xinafoate, induced class-related benign tumours of smooth muscle in the mesovarium of rats and the uterus of mice. The scientific literature and our own pharmacological studies provide good evidence that these effects are species-specific and have no relevance for clinical use.

Pharmaceutical particulars
List of excipients: Lecithin, dichlorodifluoromethane, trichlorofluoromethane.

Incompatibilities: None reported.

Shelf life: 2 years when stored below 30°C.

Special precautions for storage: Salmeterol Inhaler should be stored below 30°C.
Protect from frost and direct sunlight.
As with most inhaled medications in aerosol canisters, the therapeutic effect of this medication may decrease when the canister is cold.
The canister should not be broken, punctured or burnt, even when apparently empty.

Nature and contents of container: An inhaler comprising an aluminium alloy can fitted with a metering valve, actuator and dust cap. Each canister contains 120 metered actuations of 25 micrograms salmeterol (as xinafoate).

Instructions for use/handling: The aerosol spray is inhaled through the mouth into the lungs. After shaking the inhaler, the mouthpiece is placed in the mouth and the lips closed around it. The actuator is depressed to release a spray, which must coincide with inspiration of breath.
For detailed instructions for use refer to the Patient Information Leaflet in every pack.

Marketing authorisation number 10949/0068

Date of approval/revision of SPC June 1998.

Legal category POM.

VENTIDE* INHALER

Presentation Ventide Inhaler is a pressurised metered-dose inhaler which delivers 100 micrograms Salbutamol BP and 50 micrograms Beclomethasone Dipropionate BP per actuation.

Other ingredients: Oleic acid, dichlorodifluoromethane, trichlorofluoromethane.

Uses Salbutamol is a selective β_2-agonist providing short-acting (4-6 hour) bronchodilatation with a fast onset (within 5 minutes) in reversible airways obstruction.

Beclomethasone dipropionate given by inhalation offers effective anti-inflammatory action in the lungs with a lower incidence and severity of adverse effects than those observed when corticosteroids are administered systemically.

Ventide Inhaler is suitable for those patients who require regular doses of both drugs for treatment of reversible airways obstruction.

Ventide Inhaler is not intended for use as a first-line treatment but after the need for inhaled corticosteroid therapy has been established.

Dosage and administration Ventide Inhaler is for inhalation use only. A Volumatic* spacer device may be used in patients who find it difficult to synchronise aerosol actuation with inspiration of breath.

The dose should be titrated to the lowest dose at which effective control of asthma is maintained.

Adults (including the elderly): Two inhalations (200 micrograms salbutamol and 100 micrograms beclomethasone dipropionate) three or four times a day.

Children: One or two inhalations (100 or 200 micrograms salbutamol and 50 or 100 micrograms beclomethasone dipropionate) two, three or four times a day.

Contra-indications, warnings, etc

Contra-indications: Although intravenous salbutamol, and occasionally salbutamol tablets, are used in the management of premature labour uncomplicated by conditions such as placenta praevia, ante-partum haemorrhage or toxaemia of pregnancy, inhaled salbutamol preparations are not appropriate for managing premature labour. Salbutamol preparations should not be used for threatened abortion.

Ventide Inhaler is contra-indicated in patients with a history of hypersensitivity to any of the components.

Precautions: Patients should be instructed in the proper use of the inhaler to ensure that the drug reaches the target area within the lungs. They should also be made aware that Ventide Inhaler must be used regularly, every day, for optimum benefit. Patients should be regularly reassessed so that their continuing need for corticosteroid therapy can also be reviewed.

Ventide Inhaler is not for use in acute attacks but for routine long-term management, so patients will require a fast- and short-acting inhaled bronchodilator to relieve acute symptoms. However, should the effect of the additional inhaled bronchodilator or the relief provided by the Ventide Inhaler last for less than three hours, patients should be advised that this may indicate that their condition is worsening and to seek medical advice, in case treatment with inhaled corticosteroid needs to be increased, or treatment with systemic corticosteroid needs to be started or increased. As there may be adverse effects associated with excessive dosing, the dosage or frequency of administration should only be increased on medical advice.

Severe asthma requires regular medical assessment, including lung-function testing, as patients are at risk of severe attacks and even death. Increasing use of short-acting inhaled β_2-agonists to relieve symptoms, indicates deterioration of asthma control. If patients find that short-acting relief bronchodilator treatment becomes less effective, or they need more inhalations than usual, medical attention must be sought.

For those patients who are steroid-dependent it is advisable to commence therapy with beclomethasone dipropionate alone.

Patients who have been weaned in the previous few months from long-term systemic corticosteroids need special consideration until the hypothalamic-pituitary-adrenal (HPA) system has recovered sufficiently to enable the patient to cope with emergencies such as trauma, surgery or infections. Such patients should carry a steroid warning card indicating that they may need supplementary systemic steroid during periods of stress, until their adrenocortical function has become normal. These patients should also be given a supply of oral steroid to use in emergency when their airways obstruction worsens.

Systemic effects of inhaled corticosteroids may occur, particularly at high doses prescribed for prolonged periods. These effects are much less likely to occur than with oral corticosteroids. Possible systemic effects include adrenal suppression, growth retardation in children and adolescents, decrease in bone mineral density, cataract and glaucoma. It is important therefore that the dose of inhaled corticosteroid is titrated to the lowest dose at which effective control of asthma is maintained.

It is recommended that the height of children receiving prolonged treatment with inhaled corticosteroids is regularly monitored. If growth is slowed, therapy should be reviewed with the aim of reducing the dose of inhaled corticosteroid, if possible, to the lowest dose at which effective control of asthma is maintained. In addition, consideration should be given to referring the patient to a paediatric respiratory specialist.

Prolonged treatment with high doses of inhaled corticosteroids, particularly higher than the recommended doses, may result in clinically significant adrenal suppression. Additional systemic corticosteroid cover should be considered during periods of stress or elective surgery.

As with all inhaled corticosteroids, special care is necessary in patients with active or quiescent pulmonary tuberculosis.

Salbutamol should be administered cautiously to patients suffering from thyrotoxicosis.

Salbutamol and non-selective β-blocking drugs, such as propranolol, should not normally be prescribed together.

Potentially serious hypokalaemia may result from β_2-agonist therapy, mainly from parenteral and nebulised administration. Particular caution is advised in acute severe asthma, as this effect may be potentiated by hypoxia and by concomitant treatment with xanthine derivatives, steroids and diuretics. Serum potassium levels should be monitored in such situations.

Treatment should not be stopped abruptly.

Pregnancy: Administration of drugs during pregnancy should only be considered if the expected benefit to the mother is greater than any possible risk to the fetus. As with the majority of drugs, there is little published evidence of the safety of salbutamol in the early stages of human pregnancy, but in animal studies there was evidence of some harmful effects on the fetus at very high dose levels.

There is inadequate evidence of safety of beclomethasone dipropionate in human pregnancy. Administration of corticosteroids to pregnant animals can cause abnormalities of fetal development including cleft palate and intra-uterine growth retardation. There may therefore be a very small risk of such effects on the human fetus. It should be noted however, that the fetal changes in animals occur after relatively high systemic exposure. Because beclomethasone dipropionate is delivered directly to the lungs by the inhaled route it avoids the high level of exposure that occurs when corticosteroids are given by systemic routes.

The use of Ventide Inhaler in pregnancy requires that the possible benefit of the drugs be weighed against the possible hazards.

Lactation: No specific studies examining the transference of beclomethasone dipropionate into the milk of lactating animals have been performed. It is reasonable to assume that beclomethasone dipropionate is secreted in milk, but at the dosages used for direct inhalation there is low potential for significant levels in breast milk. As salbutamol is probably also secreted in breast milk the use of Ventide Inhaler in nursing mothers should be restricted to situations where it is felt that the expected benefit to the mother is likely to outweigh any potential risk to the neonate.

Side-effects: Systemic effects of inhaled corticosteroids may occur, particularly at high doses prescribed for prolonged periods. These may include adrenal suppression, growth retardation in children and adolescents, decrease in bone mineral density, cataract and glaucoma.

As with other inhalation therapy, paradoxical bronchospasm may occur with an immediate increase in wheezing after dosing. This should be treated immediately with a fast-acting inhaled bronchodilator. Ventide Inhaler should be discontinued immediately, the patient assessed and, if necessary, alternative therapy instituted.

Hoarseness, mouth and throat irritation may occur. It may be helpful to rinse the mouth with water immediately after inhalation.

Hypersensitivity reactions, including angioedema, bronchospasm, hypotension and collapse have been reported very rarely. Rashes, urticaria, pruritus and erythema and oedema of the eyes, face, lips and throat, have also been reported.

Salbutamol: Salbutamol may cause a fine tremor of skeletal muscle, usually the hands are most obviously affected. This effect is dose related and is common to all β-adrenergic stimulants. Headaches have occasionally been reported. Tachycardia, with or without peripheral vasodilatation, may rarely occur.

In common with other β_2 agonists, cardiac arrhythmias (including atrial fibrillation, supraventricular tachycardia and extrasystoles) have been reported in association with the use of salbutamol, usually in susceptible patients.

There have been very rare reports of muscle cramps. Potentially serious hypokalaemia may result from β_2-agonist therapy.

As with other β_2-agonists, hyperactivity in children has been reported rarely.

Beclomethasone dipropionate: Candidiasis of the mouth and throat (thrush) occurs in some patients inhaling beclomethasone dipropionate, the incidence increases with doses greater than 400 micrograms beclomethasone dipropionate per day. Patients with high blood levels of *Candida precipitins,* indicating a previous infection, are most likely to develop this complication. Such patients may find it helpful to rinse their mouth with water after using the inhaler. The condition usually responds to topical anti-fungal therapy without discontinuing treatment with Ventide Inhaler.

Overdosage:

Salbutamol: The preferred antidote for overdosage with salbutamol is a cardioselective, β-blocking agent, but β-blocking drugs should be used with caution in patients with a history of bronchospasm. Hypokalaemia may occur following overdose with salbutamol. Serum potassium levels should be monitored.

Beclomethasone dipropionate: Acute. Inhalation of the drug in doses in excess of those recommended may lead to temporary suppression of adrenal function. This does not require emergency action. In these patients treatment should be continued at a dose sufficient to control asthma; adrenal function recovers in a few days and can be verified by measuring plasma cortisol.

Chronic. Use of inhaled beclomethasone dipropionate in daily doses in excess of 1,500 micrograms over prolonged periods may lead to adrenal suppression. Monitoring of adrenal reserve may be indicated. Treatment should be continued at a dose sufficient to control asthma.

Pharmaceutical precautions Ventide Inhaler should be stored below 30°C, protected from direct sunlight, heat and frost. The canister should not be punctured, broken or burnt even if it is apparently empty.

As with most inhaled medications in aerosol canisters, the therapeutic effect of this medication may decrease when the canister is cold.

Legal category POM.

Package quantities Ventide Inhaler is a metered-dose aerosol with a specially designed actuator. Each canister provides 200 inhalations.

Further information Products containing salbutamol do not cause difficulty in micturition because, unlike sympathomimetic drugs such as ephedrine, salbutamol does not stimulate alpha-adrenoceptors.

Salbutamol products are not contra-indicated in patients under treatment with monoamine oxidase inhibitors (MAOIs).

Product licence number 10949/0076

VENTIDE* ROTACAPS*
VENTIDE* PAEDIATRIC ROTACAPS*

Presentation Ventide Rotacaps capsules contain a mixture of microfine salbutamol sulphate, microfine beclomethasone dipropionate and larger particle lactose in grey/colourless hard gelatin capsules. Each light grey Rotacaps capsule contains 200 micrograms salbutamol (as sulphate) plus 100 micrograms beclomethasone dipropionate. Each dark grey Rotacaps capsule contains 400 micrograms salbutamol (as sulphate) plus 200 micrograms beclomethasone dipropionate. The capsules are marked 'Ventide Paed' or 'Ventide' respectively. The contents of a capsule are inhaled using a specific drug delivery device called a Ventide Rotahaler*.

Uses Salbutamol is a selective β_2-agonist providing short-acting (4-6 hour) bronchodilatation with a fast onset (within 5 minutes) in reversible airways obstruction. Beclomethasone dipropionate given by inhalation offers effective anti-inflammatory action in the lungs with a lower incidence and severity of adverse effects than those observed when corticosteroids are administered systemically.

Ventide Rotacaps and Ventide Paediatric Rotacaps are suitable for those patients who require regular doses of both drugs for treatment of reversible airways obstruction.

Ventide Rotacaps and Ventide Paediatric Rotacaps are not intended for use as a first-line treatment but after the need for inhaled corticosteroid therapy has been established.

Dosage and administration Ventide Rotacaps and Ventide Paediatric Rotacaps are for inhalation use only, using a Ventide Rotahaler. They are suitable for many patients including those who cannot use a metered-dose inhaler successfully.

The dose should be titrated to the lowest dose at which effective control of asthma is maintained.

Adults (including the elderly): One Ventide Rotacaps capsule (400 micrograms salbutamol and 200 micrograms beclomethasone dipropionate) three or four times a day.

Children: One Ventide Paediatric Rotacaps capsule (200 micrograms salbutamol and 100 micrograms beclomethasone dipropionate) two, three or four times a day.

Contra-indications, warnings, etc

Contra-indications: Although intravenous salbutamol, and occasionally salbutamol tablets, are used in the management of premature labour uncomplicated by conditions such as placenta praevia, ante-partum haemorrhage or toxaemia of pregnancy, inhaled salbutamol preparations are not appropriate for managing premature labour. Salbutamol preparations should not be used for threatened abortion.

Ventide Rotacaps and Ventide Paediatric Rotacaps are contra-indicated in patients with a history of hypersensitivity to any of the components.

Precautions: Patients should be instructed in the proper use of the Rotahaler device to ensure that the drug reaches the target area within the lungs. They should also be made aware that Ventide Rotacaps or Ventide Paediatric Rotacaps must be used regularly, every day, for optimum benefit. Patients should be regularly reassessed so that their continuing need for corticosteroid therapy can also be reviewed.

Ventide Rotacaps or Ventide Paediatric Rotacaps are not for use in acute attacks but for routine long-term management, so patients will require a fast- and short-acting inhaled bronchodilator to relieve acute symptoms. However, should the effect of the additional inhaled bronchodilator, or the relief provided by Ventide Rotacaps or Ventide Paediatric Rotacaps, last for less than three hours, patients should be advised that this may indicate that their condition is worsening and to seek medical advice, in case treatment with inhaled corticosteroid needs to be increased, or treatment with systemic corticosteroid needs to be started or increased. As there may be adverse effects associated with excessive dosing, the dosage or frequency of administration should only be increased on medical advice.

Severe asthma requires regular medical assessment, including lung-function testing, as patients are at risk of severe attacks and even death. Increasing use of bronchodilators, in particular short-acting inhaled β_2-agonists to relieve symptoms, indicates deterioration of asthma control. If patients find that short-acting relief bronchodilator treatment becomes less effective, or they need more inhalations than usual, medical attention must be sought.

For those patients who are steroid-dependent it is advisable to commence therapy with beclomethasone dipropionate alone.

Patients who have been weaned in the previous few months from long-term systemic corticosteroid need special consideration until the hypothalamic-pituitary-adrenal (HPA) system has recovered sufficiently to enable the patient to cope with emergencies such as trauma, surgery or infections. Such patients should carry a steroid warning card indicating that they may need supplementary systemic steroid during periods of stress, until their adrenocortical function has become normal. These patients should also be given a supply of oral steroid to use in emergency when their airways obstruction worsens.

Systemic effects of inhaled corticosteroids may occur, particularly at high doses prescribed for prolonged periods. These effects are much less likely to occur than with oral corticosteroids. Possible systemic effects include adrenal suppression, growth retardation in children and adolescents, decrease in bone mineral density, cataract and glaucoma. It is important therefore that the dose of inhaled corticosteroid is titrated to the lowest dose at which effective control of asthma is maintained.

It is recommended that the height of children receiving prolonged treatment with inhaled corticosteroids is regularly monitored. If growth is slowed, therapy should be reviewed with the aim of reducing the dose of inhaled corticosteroid, if possible, to the lowest dose at which effective control of asthma is maintained. In addition, consideration should be given to referring the patient to a paediatric respiratory specialist.

Prolonged treatment with high doses of inhaled corticosteroids, particularly higher than the recommended doses, may result in clinically significant adrenal suppression. Additional systemic corticosteroid cover should be considered during periods of stress or elective surgery.

As with all inhaled corticosteroids special care is necessary in patients with active or quiescent pulmonary tuberculosis.

Salbutamol should be administered cautiously to patients suffering from thyrotoxicosis.

Salbutamol and non-selective β-blocking drugs, such as propranolol, should not normally be prescribed together.

Potentially serious hypokalaemia may result from β_2-agonist therapy, mainly from parenteral and nebulised administration. Particular caution is advised in acute severe asthma, as this effect may be potentiated by hypoxia and by concomitant treatment with xanthine derivatives, steroids and diuretics. Serum potassium levels should be monitored in such situations.

Treatment should not be stopped abruptly.

Pregnancy: Administration of drugs during pregnancy should only be considered if the expected benefit to the mother is greater than any possible risk to the fetus. As with the majority of drugs, there is little published evidence of the safety of salbutamol in the early stages of human pregnancy, but in animal studies there was evidence of some harmful effects on the fetus at very high dose levels.

There is inadequate evidence of safety of beclomethasone dipropionate in human pregnancy. Administration of corticosteroids to pregnant animals can cause abnormalities of fetal development including cleft palate and intra-uterine growth retardation. There may therefore, be a very small risk of such effects on the human fetus. It should be noted however, that the fetal changes in animals occur after relatively high systemic exposure. Because beclomethasone dipropionate is delivered directly to the lungs by the inhaled route it avoids the high level of exposure that occurs when corticosteroids are given by systemic routes.

The use of Ventide Rotacaps in pregnancy requires that the possible benefit of the drugs be weighed against the possible hazards.

Lactation: No specific studies examining the transference of beclomethasone dipropionate into the milk of lactating animals have been performed. It is reasonable to assume that beclomethasone dipropionate is secreted in milk, but at the dosages used for direct inhalation there is low potential for significant levels in breast milk. As salbutamol is probably also secreted in breast milk the use of Ventide Rotacaps in nursing mothers should be restricted to situations where it is felt that the expected benefit to the mother is likely to outweigh any potential risk to the neonate.

Side-effects: Systemic effects of inhaled corticosteroids may occur, particularly at high doses prescribed for prolonged periods. These may include adrenal suppression, growth retardation in children and adolescents, decrease in bone mineral density, cataract and glaucoma.

As with other inhalation therapy, paradoxical bronchospasm may occur with an immediate increase in wheezing after dosing. This should be treated immediately with a fast-acting inhaled bronchodilator. The preparation should be discontinued immediately, the patient assessed and, if necessary, alternative therapy instituted.

Hoarseness, mouth and throat irritation may occur. It may be helpful to rinse the mouth with water immediately after inhalation.

Hypersensitivity reactions, including angioedema, bronchospasm, hypotension and collapse have been reported very rarely. Rashes, urticaria, pruritus and erythema and oedema of the eyes, face, lips and throat, have also been reported.

Salbutamol: Salbutamol may cause a fine tremor of skeletal muscle, usually the hands are most obviously affected. This effect is dose related and common to all β-adrenergic stimulants. Headaches have occasionally been reported. Tachycardia, with or without peripheral vasodilatation, may rarely occur.

In common with other β_2 agonists, cardiac arrhythmias (including atrial fibrillation, supraventricular tachycardia and extrasystoles) have been reported in association with the use of salbutamol, usually in susceptible patients.

There have been very rare reports of muscle cramps. Potentially serious hypokalaemia may result from β_2-agonist therapy.

As with other β_2-agonists, hyperactivity in children has been reported rarely.

Beclomethasone dipropionate: Candidiasis of the mouth and throat (thrush) occurs in some patients; the incidence increases with doses greater than 400 micrograms beclomethasone dipropionate per day. Patients with high blood levels of *Candida precipitins*, indicating a previous infection, are more likely to develop this complication. Such patients may find it helpful to rinse their mouth with water after using the Rotahaler device. The condition usually responds to topical anti-fungal therapy without discontinuing treatment with Ventide Rotacaps or Ventide Paediatric Rotacaps.

Overdosage:

Salbutamol: The preferred antidote for overdosage with salbutamol is a cardioselective, β-blocking agent, but β-blocking drugs should be used with caution in patients with a history of bronchospasm. Hypokalaemia may occur following overdose with salbutamol. Serum potassium levels should be monitored.

Beclomethasone dipropionate: Acute. Inhalation of the drug in doses in excess of those recommended may lead to temporary suppression of adrenal function. This does not require emergency action. In these patients treatment should be continued at a dose sufficient to control asthma; adrenal function recovers in a few days and can be verified by measuring plasma cortisol.

Chronic. Use of inhaled beclomethasone dipropionate in daily doses in excess of 1,500 micrograms over prolonged periods may lead to adrenal suppression. Monitoring of adrenal reserve may be indicated. Treatment should be continued at a dose sufficient to control asthma.

Pharmaceutical precautions To keep the Rotacaps capsules in good condition it is important that they are stored in a dry place, below 30°C, where they will not be exposed to extremes of temperature. A convenient supply may be carried in the special container for the Rotahaler. A capsule should only be inserted into the Rotahaler immediately prior to use. Failure to observe this instruction may affect the operation of the Rotahaler.

Legal category POM.

Package quantities Ventide Rotacaps and Ventide Paediatric Rotacaps are supplied in containers of 112.

Further information Products containing salbutamol do not cause difficulty in micturition because, unlike sympathomimetic drugs such as ephedrine, salbutamol does not stimulate alpha-adrenoceptors.

Salbutamol products are not contra-indicated in patients under treatment with monoamine oxidase inhibitors (MAOIs).

Product licence numbers
Ventide Rotacaps 10949/0077
Ventide Paediatric Rotacaps 10949/0078

VENTODISKS*

Presentation Ventodisks is a dry powder inhalation device available in two strengths providing 200 micrograms or 400 micrograms salbutamol per blister. The active ingredient is presented in a disk comprising eight regularly spaced double-foil blisters each containing a mixture of microfine salbutamol (as sulphate) and larger particle lactose.

The disks are intended only for use in a specific drug delivery device known as the Ventolin* Diskhaler*.

Uses Salbutamol is a selective β_2-agonist providing short-acting (4-6 hour) bronchodilatation with a fast onset (within 5 minutes) in reversible airways obstruction.

Ventodisks can be used in the management of asthma, bronchospasm and/or reversible airways obstruction.

Ventodisks is particularly suitable for the relief of asthma symptoms. It should be used to relieve symptoms when they occur, and to prevent them in those circumstances recognised by the patient to precipitate an asthma attack (e.g. before exercise or unavoidable allergen exposure).

Ventodisks is particularly valuable as relief medication in mild, moderate or severe asthma, provided that reliance on it does not delay the introduction and use of regular inhaled corticosteroid therapy.

Dosage and administration Ventodisks is for inhalation use only, using a Ventolin Diskhaler. Ventodisks is suitable for many patients including those who cannot use a metered-dose inhaler successfully.

Adults (including the elderly): For the relief of acute bronchospasm 200 micrograms or 400 micrograms should be taken as a single dose. The maximum daily dose is 400 micrograms four times a day.

To prevent allergen- or exercise-induced symptoms, 400 micrograms should be taken 10-15 minutes before challenge.

Children: The recommended dose for relief of acute bronchospasm or before allergen exposure or exercise is 200 micrograms. The maximum daily dose is 200 micrograms four times a day.

On-demand use of Ventodisks should not exceed four times daily. Reliance on such frequent supplementary use, or a sudden increase in dose, indicates poorly controlled or deteriorating asthma (see *Precautions*).

Contra-indications, warnings, etc

Contra-indications: Although intravenous salbutamol, and occasionally salbutamol tablets, are used in the management of premature labour uncomplicated by conditions such as placenta praevia, ante-partum haemorrhage, or toxaemia of pregnancy, inhaled salbutamol preparations are not appropriate for managing premature labour. Salbutamol preparations should not be used for threatened abortion.

Ventodisks is contra-indicated in patients with a history of hypersensitivity to any of the components.

Precautions: Bronchodilators should not be the only or main treatment in patients with severe or unstable asthma. Severe asthma requires regular medical assessment, including lung-function testing, as patients are at risk of severe attacks and even death. Physicians should consider using the maximum recommended dose of inhaled corticosteroid and/or oral corticosteroid therapy in these patients.

The dosage or frequency of administration should only be increased on medical advice.

Increasing use of bronchodilators, in particular short-acting inhaled β_2-agonists to relieve symptoms, indicates deterioration of asthma control. The patient should be instructed to seek medical advice if short-acting relief bronchodilator treatment becomes less effective, or more inhalations than usual are required. In this situation the patient should be assessed and consideration given to the need for increased anti-inflammatory therapy (e.g. higher doses of inhaled corticosteroid or a course of oral corticosteroid).

Severe exacerbations of asthma must be treated in the normal way.

Salbutamol should be administered cautiously to patients suffering from thyrotoxicosis.

Salbutamol and non-selective β-blocking drugs such as propranolol, should not usually be prescribed together.

Potentially serious hypokalaemia may result from β_2-agonist therapy, mainly from parenteral and nebulised administration. Particular caution is advised in acute severe asthma as this effect may be potentiated by hypoxia and by concomitant treatment with xanthine derivatives, steroids and diuretics. Serum potassium levels should be monitored in such situations.

Pregnancy: Administration of drugs during pregnancy should only be considered if the expected benefit to the mother is greater than any possible risk to the fetus. As with the majority of drugs, there is little published evidence of the safety of salbutamol in the early stages of human pregnancy, but in animal studies there was evidence of some harmful effects on the fetus at very high dose levels.

Lactation: As salbutamol is probably secreted in breast milk, its use in nursing mothers requires careful consideration. It is not known whether salbutamol has a harmful effect on the neonate, and so its use should be restricted to situations where it is felt that the expected benefit to the mother is likely to outweigh any potential risk to the neonate.

Side-effects: As with other inhalation therapy, paradoxical bronchospasm may occur with an immediate increase in wheezing after dosing. This should be treated immediately with an alternative presentation or a different fast-acting inhaled bronchodilator. The preparation should be discontinued immediately, the patient assessed and, if necessary, alternative therapy instituted.

Hypersensitivity reactions including angioedema, urticaria, bronchospasm, hypotension and collapse have been reported very rarely.

Potentially serious hypokalaemia may result from β_2-agonist therapy.

Ventodisks may cause a fine tremor of skeletal muscle, usually the hands are most obviously affected. This effect is dose-related and is common to all β-adrenergic stimulants.

Tachycardia, with or without peripheral vasodilatation, may rarely occur.

In common with other β_2 agonists, cardiac arrhythmias (including atrial fibrillation, supraventricular tachycardia and extrasystoles) have been reported in association with the use of salbutamol, usually in susceptible patients.

Headaches have occasionally been reported.

Mouth and throat irritation may occur with inhaled salbutamol.

As with other β_2-agonists hyperactivity in children has been reported rarely.

There have been very rare reports of muscle cramps.

Overdosage: The preferred antidote for overdosage with salbutamol is a cardioselective β-blocking agent, but β-blocking drugs should be used with caution in patients with a history of bronchospasm.

Hypokalaemia may occur following overdose with salbutamol. Serum potassium levels should be monitored.

Pharmaceutical precautions Whilst the disks provide a good protection to the blister contents from the effects of the atmosphere, they should not be exposed to extremes of temperature and should be stored below 30°C. A disk may be kept in the Diskhaler at all times but a blister should only be pierced immediately prior to use. Failure to observe this instruction may affect the operation of the Diskhaler.

Legal category POM.

Package quantities Ventodisks 200 micrograms and 400 micrograms are supplied in cartons containing 14 disks (14 x 8 blisters), together with a Diskhaler device.

Further information Ventodisks does not cause difficulty in micturition because unlike sympathomimetic drugs such as ephedrine, salbutamol does not stimulate alpha-adrenoceptors. Ventodisks is not contra-indicated in patients under treatment with monoamine oxidase inhibitors (MAOIs).

Product licence numbers
Ventodisks 200 micrograms 10949/0079
Ventodisks 400 micrograms 10949/0080

VENTOLIN* ACCUHALER*

Qualitative and quantitative composition Ventolin Accuhaler is a plastic inhaler device containing a foil strip with 60 regularly spaced blisters each containing a mixture of 200 micrograms of microfine salbutamol (as sulphate) and larger particle lactose.

Pharmaceutical form Multi-dose dry powder inhalation device.

Clinical particulars

Therapeutic indications: Ventolin Accuhaler can be used in the management of asthma, bronchospasm and/or reversible airways obstruction.

Ventolin Accuhaler is particularly suitable for the relief of asthma symptoms. It should be used to relieve symptoms when they occur, and to prevent them in those circumstances recognised by the patient to precipitate an asthma attack (e.g. before exercise or unavoidable allergen exposure).

Ventolin Accuhaler is particularly valuable as relief medication in mild, moderate or severe asthma, provided that reliance on it does not delay the introduction and use of regular inhaled corticosteroid therapy.

Posology and method of administration: Ventolin Accuhaler is for inhalation use only. Ventolin Accuhaler is suitable for many patients including those who cannot use a metered-dose inhaler successfully.

Adults (including the elderly): For the relief of acute bronchospasm, 200 micrograms as a single dose. The maximum daily dose is 200 micrograms four times a day.

To prevent allergen- or exercise-induced symptoms, 200 micrograms should be taken 10-15 minutes before challenge.

Children: The recommended dose for relief of acute bronchospasm or before allergen exposure or exercise is 200 micrograms. The maximum daily dose is 200 micrograms four times a day.

On-demand use of Ventolin Accuhaler should not exceed four times daily. Reliance on such frequent supplementary use, or a sudden increase in dose, indicates poorly controlled or deteriorating asthma (see *Precautions*).

Contra-indications: Although intravenous salbutamol, and occasionally salbutamol tablets, are used in the management of premature labour uncomplicated by conditions such as placenta praevia, ante-partum haemorrhage, or toxaemia of pregnancy, inhaled salbutamol preparations are not appropriate for managing premature labour. Salbutamol preparations should not be used for threatened abortion.

Ventolin Accuhaler is contra-indicated in patients with a history of hypersensitivity to any of the components.

Special warnings and precautions for use: Bronchodilators should not be the only or main treatment in patients with severe or unstable asthma. Severe asthma requires regular medical assessment, including lung-function testing, as patients are at risk of severe attacks and even death. Physicians should consider using the maximum recommended dose of inhaled corticosteroid and/or oral corticosteroid therapy in these patients.

The dosage or frequency of administration should only be increased on medical advice.

Increasing use of bronchodilators, in particular short-acting inhaled β_2-agonists to relieve symptoms, indicates deterioration of asthma control. The patient should be instructed to seek medical advice if short-acting relief bronchodilator treatment becomes less effective, or more inhalations than usual are required. In this situation the patient should be assessed and consideration given to the need for increased anti-inflammatory therapy (e.g. higher doses of inhaled corticosteroid or a course of oral corticosteroid).

Severe exacerbations of asthma must be treated in the normal way.

Salbutamol should be administered cautiously to patients suffering from thyrotoxicosis.

Potentially serious hypokalaemia may result from β_2-agonist therapy, mainly from parenteral and nebulised administration. Particular caution is advised in acute severe asthma as this effect may be potentiated by hypoxia and by concomitant treatment with xanthine derivatives, steroids and diuretics. Serum potassium levels should be monitored in such situations.

Interaction with other medicaments and other forms of interaction: Salbutamol and non-selective β-blocking drugs such as propranolol, should not usually be prescribed together.

Pregnancy and lactation:

Pregnancy: Administration of drugs during pregnancy should only be considered if the expected benefit to the mother is greater than any possible risk to the fetus. As with the majority of drugs, there is little published evidence of the safety of salbutamol in the early stages of human pregnancy, but in animal studies there was evidence of some harmful effects on the fetus at very high dose levels.

Lactation: As salbutamol is probably secreted in breast milk, its use in nursing mothers requires careful consideration. It is not known whether salbutamol has a harmful effect on the neonate, and so its use should be restricted to situations where it is felt that the expected benefit to the mother is likely to outweigh any potential risk to the neonate.

Effects on ability to drive and use machines: None reported.

Undesirable effects: As with other inhalation therapy, paradoxical bronchospasm may occur with an immediate increase in wheezing after dosing. This should be treated immediately with an alternative presentation or a different fast-acting inhaled bronchodilator. The preparation should be discontinued immediately, the patient assessed and, if necessary, alternative therapy instituted.

Hypersensitivity reactions including angioedema, urticaria, bronchospasm, hypotension and collapse have been reported very rarely.

Potentially serious hypokalaemia may result from β_2-agonist therapy.

Ventolin Accuhaler may cause a fine tremor of skeletal muscle, usually the hands are most obviously affected. This effect is dose-related and is common to all β-adrenergic stimulants.

Tachycardia, with or without peripheral vasodilatation, may rarely occur.

In common with other β_2 agonists, cardiac arrhythmias (including atrial fibrillation, supraventricular tachycardia and extrasystoles) have been reported in association with the use of salbutamol, usually in susceptible patients.

Headaches have occasionally been reported.

Mouth and throat irritation may occur with inhaled salbutamol.

As with other β_2-agonists hyperactivity in children has been reported rarely.

There have been very rare reports of muscle cramps.

Overdose: The preferred antidote for overdosage with salbutamol is a cardioselective β-blocking agent, but β-blocking drugs should be used with caution in patients with a history of bronchospasm.

Hypokalaemia may occur following overdose with salbutamol. Serum potassium levels should be monitored.

Pharmacological properties

Pharmacodynamic properties: Salbutamol is a selective β_2-adrenoceptor agonist. At therapeutic doses it acts on the β_2-adrenoceptors of bronchial muscle, with little or no action on the β_1-adrenoceptors of cardiac muscle.

Salbutamol provides short-acting (4-6 hour) bronchodilatation with a fast onset (within 5 minutes) in reversible airways obstruction.

Pharmacokinetic properties: Salbutamol administered intravenously has a half-life of 4 to 6 hours and is cleared partly renally, and partly by metabolism to the inactive 4'-O-sulphate (phenolic sulphate) which is also excreted primarily in the urine. The faeces are a minor route of excretion. After administration by the inhaled route between 10 and 20% of the dose reaches the lower airways. The remainder is retained in the delivery system or is deposited in the oropharynx from where it is swallowed. The fraction deposited in the airways is absorbed into the pulmonary tissues and circulation, but is not metabolised by the lung. On reaching the systemic circulation it becomes accessible to hepatic metabolism and is excreted, primarily in the urine, as unchanged drug and as the phenolic sulphate. The swallowed portion of an inhaled dose is absorbed from the gastrointestinal tract and undergoes considerable first-pass metabolism to the phenolic sulphate. Both unchanged drug and conjugate are excreted primarily in the urine. Almost all of a dose of salbutamol given intravenously, orally or by inhalation is excreted within 72 hours. Salbutamol is bound to plasma proteins to the extent of 10%.

Preclinical safety data: In common with other potent selective β_2-receptor agonists, salbutamol has been shown to be teratogenic in mice when given subcutaneously. In a reproductive study, 9.3% of fetuses were found to have cleft palate at 2.5 mg/kg, 4 times the maximum human oral dose. In rats, treatment at the levels of 0.5, 2.32, 10.75 and 50 mg/kg/day orally throughout pregnancy resulted in no significant fetal abnormalities. The only toxic effect was an increase in neonatal mortality at the highest dose level as the result of lack of maternal care. A reproductive study in rabbits revealed cranial malformations in 37% of fetuses at 50 mg/kg/day, 78 times the maximum human oral dose.

Pharmaceutical particulars
List of excipients: Lactose.

Incompatibilities: None reported.

Shelf life: 24 months.

Special precautions for storage: Store below 30°C (86°F). Store in a dry place.

Nature and contents of container: The powder mix of salbutamol (as sulphate) and lactose is filled into a blister strip consisting of a formed base foil with a peelable foil laminate lid. The foil strip is contained within the Accuhaler device.

Instructions for use/handling: The powdered medicine is inhaled through the mouth into the lungs.

The Accuhaler device contains the medicine in individual blisters which are opened as the device is manipulated.

For detailed instructions for use refer to the Patient Information Leaflet in every pack.

Marketing authorisation number 10949/0252

Date of approval/revision of SPC June 1998

Legal category POM.

VENTOLIN* EASI-BREATHE* INHALER

Qualitative and quantitative composition 100 micrograms Salbutamol BP per actuation. Each canister delivers 200 actuations.

Pharmaceutical form Aerosol.

Clinical particulars
Therapeutic indications: Ventolin Easi-Breathe Inhaler provides short-acting (4 to 6 hour) bronchodilatation with fast onset (within 5 minutes) in reversible airways obstruction.

It is particularly suitable for the relief and prevention of asthma symptoms. It should be used to relieve symptoms when they occur, and to prevent them in those circumstances recognised by the patient to precipitate an asthma attack (e.g. before exercise or unavoidable allergen exposure).

Ventolin Easi-Breathe Inhaler is particularly valuable as relief medication in mild, moderate or severe asthma, provided that reliance on it does not delay the introduction and use of regular inhaled corticosteroid therapy.

Posology and method of administration: Ventolin Easi-Breathe Inhaler is for oral inhalation use only.

Adults (including the elderly): For the relief of acute asthma symptoms including bronchospasm, one inhalation (100 micrograms) may be administered as a single minimum starting dose. This may be increased to two inhalations if necessary. To prevent allergen- or exercise-induced symptoms, two inhalations should be taken 10–15 minutes before challenge.

For chronic therapy, two inhalations up to four times a day.

Children: For the relief of acute asthma symptoms including bronchospasm, or before allergen exposure or exercise, one inhalation, or two if necessary.

For chronic therapy, two inhalations up to four times a day.

On-demand use of Ventolin Easi-Breathe Inhaler should not exceed 8 inhalations in any 24 hours. Reliance on such frequent supplementary use, or a sudden increase in dose, indicates poorly controlled or deteriorating asthma (see *Special warnings and precautions for use*).

Contra-indications: Although intravenous salbutamol, and occasionally salbutamol tablets, are used in the management of premature labour uncomplicated by conditions such as placenta praevia, ante-partum haemorrhage or toxaemia of pregnancy, inhaled salbutamol preparations are not appropriate for managing premature labour. Salbutamol preparations should not be used for threatened abortion.

Ventolin Easi-Breathe Inhaler is contra-indicated in patients with a history of hypersensitivity to any of the components.

Special warnings and special precautions for use: Patients should be instructed in the proper use of the inhaler, and their technique checked, to ensure that the drug reaches the target areas within the lungs. Bronchodilators should not be the only or main treatment in patients with severe or unstable asthma. Severe asthma requires regular medical assessment, including lung-function testing, as patients are at risk of severe attacks and even death. Physicians should consider using the maximum recommended dose of inhaled corticosteroid and/or oral corticosteroid therapy in these patients.

The dosage or frequency of administration should only be increased on medical advice. If a previously effective dose of inhaled salbutamol fails to give relief lasting at least three hours, the patient should be advised to seek medical advice.

Increasing use of bronchodilators, in particular short-acting inhaled β_2-agonists, to relieve symptoms, indicates deterioration of asthma control. The patient should be instructed to seek medical advice if short-acting relief bronchodilator treatment becomes less effective, or more inhalations than usual are required. In this situation the patient should be assessed and consideration given to the need for increased anti-inflammatory therapy (e.g. higher doses of inhaled corticosteroid or a course of oral corticosteroid).

Severe exacerbations of asthma must be treated in the normal way.

Salbutamol should be administered cautiously to patients with thyrotoxicosis. Potentially serious hypokalaemia may result from β_2-agonist therapy, mainly from parenteral and nebulised administration. Particular caution is advised in acute severe asthma as this effect may be potentiated by hypoxia and by concomitant treatment with xanthine derivatives, steroids and diuretics. Serum potassium levels should be monitored in such situations.

Interaction with other medicaments and other forms of interaction: Salbutamol and non-selective β-blocking drugs such as propranolol, should not usually be prescribed together.

Pregnancy and lactation: Administration of drugs during pregnancy should only be considered if the expected benefit to the mother is greater than any possible risk to the fetus. As with the majority of drugs, there is little published evidence of the safety of salbutamol in the early stages of human pregnancy, but in animal studies there was evidence of some harmful effects on the fetus at very high dose levels.

As salbutamol is probably secreted in breast milk, its use in nursing mothers requires careful consideration. It is not known whether salbutamol has a harmful effect on the neonate, and so its use should be restricted to situations where it is felt that the expected benefit to the mother is likely to outweigh any potential risk to the neonate.

Effects on the ability to drive and use machines: None reported.

Undesirable effects: As with other inhalation therapy, paradoxical bronchospasm may occur with an immediate increase in wheezing after dosing. This should be treated immediately with an alternative presentation or a different fast-acting inhaled bronchodilator. Ventolin Easi-Breathe Inhaler should be discontinued immediately, the patient assessed and, if necessary, alternative therapy instituted.

Hypersensitivity reactions including angioedema, urticaria, bronchospasm, hypotension and collapse have been reported very rarely.

Potentially serious hypokalaemia may result from β_2-agonist therapy.

Ventolin Easi-Breathe Inhaler may cause a fine tremor of skeletal muscle, usually the hands are most obviously affected. This effect is dose-related and is common to all β-adrenergic stimulants.

Tachycardia, with or without peripheral vasodilatation, may rarely occur.

Headaches have occasionally been reported.

Mouth and throat irritation may occur with inhaled salbutamol.

As with other β_2-agonists hyperactivity in children has been reported rarely.

There have been very rare reports of muscle cramps.

Overdose: The preferred antidote for overdosage with salbutamol is a cardioselective β-blocking agent, but β-blocking drugs should be used with caution in patients with a history of bronchospasm.

Hypokalaemia may occur following overdose with salbutamol. Serum potassium levels should be monitored.

Pharmacological properties
Pharmacodynamic properties: Salbutamol is a selective β_2-adrenoceptor agonist. At therapeutic doses it acts on the β_2-adrenoceptors of bronchial muscle providing short-acting (4–6 hour) bronchodilatation with a fast onset (within 5 minutes) in reversible airways obstruction.

Pharmacokinetic properties: Salbutamol administered intravenously has a half-life of 4 to 6 hours and is cleared, partly renally and partly by metabolism, to the inactive 4′-O-sulphate (phenolic sulphate) which is also excreted primarily in the urine. The faeces are a minor route of excretion.

After administration by the inhaled route between 10 and 20% of the dose reaches the lower airways. The remainder is retained in the delivery system or is deposited in the oropharynx from where it is swallowed. The fraction deposited in the airways is absorbed into the pulmonary tissues and circulation, but is not metabolised by the lung. On reaching the systemic circulation it becomes accessible to hepatic metabolism and is excreted, primarily in the urine, as unchanged drug and as the phenolic sulphate.

The swallowed portion of an inhaled dose is absorbed from the gastrointestinal tract and undergoes considerable first-pass metabolism to the phenolic sulphate. Both unchanged drug and conjugate are excreted primarily in the urine. Most of a dose of salbutamol given intravenously, orally or by inhalation is excreted within 72 hours. Salbutamol is bound to plasma proteins to the extent of 10%.

Preclinical safety data: In common with other potent selective β_2-agonists, salbutamol has been shown to be teratogenic in mice when given subcutaneously. In a reproductive study, 9.3% of fetuses were found to have cleft palate at 2.5 mg/kg dose. In rats, treatment at the levels of 0.5, 2.32, 10.75 and 50 mg/kg/day orally throughout pregnancy resulted in no significant fetal abnormalities. The only toxic effect was an increase in neonatal mortality at the highest dose level as the result of lack of maternal care. Reproductive studies in the rabbit at doses of 50 mg/kg/day (i.e. much higher than the normal human dose) have shown fetuses with treatment related changes; these included open eyelids (ablepharia), secondary palate clefts (palatoschisis), changes in ossification of the frontal bones of the cranium (cranioschisis) and limb flexure.

Pharmaceutical particulars
List of excipients: Oleic acid, dichlorodifluoromethane, trichlorofluoromethane.

Incompatibilities: None reported.

Shelf life: Three years when stored below 30°C.

Special precautions for storage: Store below 30°C.

Protect from frost and direct sunlight.

As with most inhaled medications in aerosol canisters, the therapeutic effect of this medication may decrease when the canister is cold.

The canister should not be broken, punctured or burnt, even when apparently empty.

Nature and contents of container: An inhaler comprising an aluminium can fitted with a breath-operated metering valve, actuator and dust cap. Each canister contains 200 metered actuations providing 100 micrograms Salbutamol BP.

Instructions for use/handling: The aerosol spray is inhaled through the mouth into the lungs. After shaking the inhaler, open the cap and place the mouthpiece in the mouth with the lips closed around it. Suck in slowly through the mouthpiece, this releases a spray.

For detailed instructions for use refer to the Patient Information Leaflet in every pack.

Marketing authorisation number 10949/0267.

Date of approval/revision of SPC December 1996.

Legal category POM.

VENTOLIN* EVOHALER* 

Qualitative and quantitative composition Ventolin Evohaler is a pressurised metered-dose inhaler delivering 100 micrograms of salbutamol (as Salbutamol Sulphate BP) per actuation. Ventolin Evohaler contains a new propellant (HFA 134a) and does not contain any chlorofluorocarbons.

Pharmaceutical form Aerosol.

Clinical particulars
Therapeutic indications: Ventolin Evohaler provides short-acting (4 to 6 hour) bronchodilatation with fast onset (within 5 minutes) in reversible airways obstruction.

It is particularly suitable for the relief and prevention of asthma symptoms. It should be used to relieve symptoms when they occur, and to prevent them in those circumstances recognised by the patient to precipitate an asthma attack (e.g. before exercise or unavoidable allergen exposure).

Ventolin Evohaler is particularly valuable as relief medication in mild, moderate or severe asthma, provided that reliance on it does not delay the introduction and use of regular inhaled corticosteroid therapy.

Posology and method of administration: Ventolin Evohaler is for oral inhalation use only. A Volumatic* spacer device may be used in patients who find it difficult to synchronise aerosol actuation with inspiration of breath.

Adults (including the elderly): For the relief of acute asthma symptoms including bronchospasm, one inhalation (100 micrograms) may be administered as a single minimum starting dose. This may be increased to two inhalations if necessary. To prevent allergen- or exercise-induced symptoms, two inhalations should be taken 10–15 minutes before challenge.

For chronic therapy, two inhalations up to four times a day.

Children: For the relief of acute asthma symptoms including bronchospasm, or before allergen exposure or exercise, one inhalation, or two if necessary.

For chronic therapy, two inhalations up to four times a day.

The Babyhaler* spacer device may be used to facilitate administration to children under 5 years of age.

On-demand use of Ventolin Evohaler should not exceed 8 inhalations in any 24 hours. Reliance on such frequent supplementary use, or a sudden increase in dose, indicates poorly controlled or deteriorating asthma (see *Special warnings and precautions for use*).

Contra-indications: Although intravenous salbutamol, and occasionally salbutamol tablets, are used in the management of premature labour uncomplicated by conditions such as placenta praevia, ante-partum haemorrhage or toxaemia of pregnancy, inhaled salbutamol preparations are not appropriate for managing premature labour. Salbutamol preparations should not be used for threatened abortion.

Ventolin Evohaler is contra-indicated in patients with a history of hypersensitivity to any of the components.

Special warnings and special precautions for use: Patients inhaler technique should be checked to make sure that aerosol actuation is synchronised with inspiration of breath for optimum delivery of drug to the lungs. Patients should be warned that they may experience a different taste upon inhalation compared to their previous inhaler.

Bronchodilators should not be the only or main treatment in patients with severe or unstable asthma. Severe asthma requires regular medical assessment, including lung-function testing, as patients are at risk of severe attacks and even death. Physicians should consider using the maximum recommended dose of inhaled corticosteroid and/or oral corticosteroid therapy in these patients.

The dosage or frequency of administration should only be increased on medical advice. If a previously effective dose of inhaled salbutamol fails to give relief lasting at least three hours, the patient should be advised to seek medical advice.

Increasing use of bronchodilators, in particular short-acting inhaled β_2-agonists, to relieve symptoms, indicates deterioration of asthma control. The patient should be instructed to seek medical advice if short-acting relief bronchodilator treatment becomes less effective, or more inhalations than usual are required. In this situation the patient should be assessed and consideration given to the need for increased anti-inflammatory therapy (e.g. higher doses of inhaled corticosteroid or a course of oral corticosteroid).

Severe exacerbations of asthma must be treated in the normal way.

Salbutamol should be administered cautiously to patients with thyrotoxicosis. Potentially serious hypokalaemia may result from β_2-agonist therapy, mainly from parenteral and nebulised administration. Particular caution is advised in acute severe asthma as this effect may be potentiated by hypoxia and by concomitant treatment with xanthine derivatives, steroids and diuretics. Serum potassium levels should be monitored in such situations.

Interaction with other medicaments and other forms of interaction: Salbutamol and non-selective β-blocking drugs such as propranolol, should not usually be prescribed together.

Pregnancy and lactation: Administration of drugs during pregnancy should only be considered if the expected benefit to the mother is greater than any possible risk to the fetus. As with the majority of drugs, there is little published evidence of the safety of salbutamol in the early stages of human pregnancy, but in animal studies there was evidence of some harmful effects on the fetus at very high dose levels. A full range of reproductive studies with the non-chlorofluorocarbon propellant HFA 134a, have shown no effect on fetal development in animals.

Specific teratology studies with Ventolin Evohaler have shown no effects over and above those consistent with the known effects of high doses of beta-agonists. However, there is no experience on use in pregnancy and lactation in humans.

As salbutamol is probably secreted in breast milk, its use in nursing mothers requires careful consideration. It is not known whether salbutamol has a harmful effect on the neonate, and so its use should be restricted to situations where it is felt that the expected benefit to the mother is likely to outweigh any potential risk to the neonate.

Effects on the ability to drive and use machines: None reported.

Undesirable effects: As with other inhalation therapy, paradoxical bronchospasm may occur with an immediate increase in wheezing after dosing. This should be treated immediately with an alternative presentation or a different fast-acting inhaled bronchodilator. Ventolin Evohaler should be discontinued immediately, the patient assessed, and, if necessary, alternative therapy instituted.

Hypersensitivity reactions including angioedema, urticaria, bronchospasm, hypotension and collapse have been reported very rarely.

Potentially serious hypokalaemia may result from β_2-agonist therapy.

Ventolin Evohaler may cause a fine tremor of skeletal muscle, usually the hands are most obviously affected. This effect is dose-related and is common to all β-adrenergic stimulants.

Tachycardia, with or without peripheral vasodilatation, may rarely occur. In common with other B_2-agonists, cardiac arrhythmias (including atrial fibrillation, supraventricular tachycardia and extrasystoles) have been reported in association with the use of salbutamol, usually in susceptible patients.

Headaches have occasionally been reported.

Mouth and throat irritation may occur with inhaled salbutamol.

As with other β_2-agonists hyperactivity in children has been reported rarely.

There have been very rare reports of muscle cramps.

Overdose: The preferred antidote for overdosage with salbutamol is a cardioselective β-blocking agent, but β-blocking drugs should be used with caution in patients with a history of bronchospasm.

Hypokalaemia may occur following overdose with salbutamol. Serum potassium levels should be monitored.

Pharmacological properties

Pharmacodynamic properties: Salbutamol is a selective β_2-adrenoceptor agonist. At therapeutic doses it acts on the β_2-adrenoceptors of bronchial muscle providing short-acting (4–6 hour) bronchodilatation with a fast onset (within 5 minutes) in reversible airways obstruction.

Pharmacokinetic properties: Salbutamol administered intravenously has a half-life of 4 to 6 hours and is cleared partly renally and partly by metabolism to the inactive 4'-O-sulphate (phenolic sulphate) which is also excreted primarily in the urine. The faeces are a minor route of excretion.

After administration by the inhaled route between 10 and 20% of the dose reaches the lower airways. The remainder is retained in the delivery system or is deposited in the oropharynx from where it is swallowed. The fraction deposited in the airways is absorbed into the pulmonary tissues and circulation, but is not metabolised by the lung. On reaching the systemic circulation it becomes accessible to hepatic metabolism and is excreted, primarily in the urine, as unchanged drug and as the phenolic sulphate.

The swallowed portion of an inhaled dose is absorbed from the gastrointestinal tract and undergoes considerable first-pass metabolism to the phenolic sulphate. Both unchanged drug and conjugate are excreted primarily in the urine. Most of a dose of salbutamol given intravenously, orally or by inhalation is excreted within 72 hours. Salbutamol is bound to plasma proteins to the extent of 10%.

Preclinical safety data: In common with other potent selective β_2-agonists, salbutamol has been shown to be teratogenic in mice when given subcutaneously. In a reproductive study, 9.3% of fetuses were found to have cleft palate at 2.5 mg/kg dose. In rats, treatment at the levels of 0.5, 2.32, 10.75 and 50 mg/kg/day orally throughout pregnancy resulted in no significant fetal abnormalities. The only toxic effect was an increase in neonatal mortality at the highest dose level as the result of lack of maternal care. Reproductive studies in the rabbit at doses of 50 mg/kg/day orally (i.e. much higher than the normal human dose) have shown fetuses with treatment related changes; these included open eyelids (ablepharia), secondary palate clefts (palatoschisis), changes in ossification of the frontal bones of the cranium (cranioschisis) and limb flexure. Reformulation of the Ventolin Evohaler has not altered the known toxicological profile of salbutamol. The non-CFC propellant, HFA 134a, has been shown to have no toxic effect at very high vapour concentrations, far in excess of those likely to be experienced by patients, in a wide range of animal species exposed daily for periods of two years.

Pharmaceutical particulars

List of excipients: HFA 134a.

Incompatibilities: None reported.

Shelf life: 24 months when stored below 30°C.

Special precautions for storage: Store below 30°C (86°F).

Protect from frost and direct sunlight.

As with most inhaled medications in aerosol canisters, the therapeutic effect of this medication may decrease when the canister is cold.

The canister should not be broken, punctured or burnt, even when apparently empty.

Nature and contents of container: An inhaler comprising an aluminium alloy can internally coated with fluoropolymer, and sealed with a metering valve, actuator and dust cap. Each canister contains 200 metered actuations providing 100 micrograms of salbutamol (as Salbutamol Sulphate BP).

Instructions for use/handling: The aerosol spray is inhaled through the mouth into the lungs. After shaking the inhaler, the mouthpiece is placed in the mouth and the lips closed around it. The actuator is depressed to release a spray, which must coincide with inspiration of breath.

For detailed instructions for use refer to the Patient Information Leaflet in every pack.

Marketing authorisation number PL 10949/0274.

Date of approval/revision of SPC August 1998.

Legal category POM.

VENTOLIN* INHALER

Presentation Ventolin Inhaler is a pressurised metered-dose inhaler delivering 100 micrograms Salbutamol BP per actuation.

Other ingredients: Oleic acid, dichlorodifluoromethane, trichlorofluoromethane.

Uses Salbutamol is a selective β_2-agonist providing short-acting (4-6 hour) bronchodilatation with a fast onset (within 5 minutes) in reversible airways obstruction.

Ventolin Inhaler can be used in the management of asthma, bronchospasm and/or reversible airways obstruction.

Ventolin Inhaler is particularly suitable for the relief of asthma symptoms. It should be used to relieve symptoms when they occur, and to prevent them in those circumstances recognised by the patient to precipitate an asthma attack (e.g. before exercise or unavoidable allergen exposure).

Ventolin Inhaler is particularly valuable as relief medication in mild, moderate or severe asthma, provided that reliance on it does not delay the introduction and use of regular inhaled corticosteroid therapy.

Dosage and administration Ventolin Inhaler is for inhalation use only. A Volumatic* spacer device may be used in patients who find it difficult to synchronise aerosol actuation with inspiration of breath.

Adults (including the elderly): For the relief of acute bronchospasm, one or two inhalations (100 or 200 micrograms) as necessary. To prevent allergen- or exercise-induced symptoms, two inhalations should be taken 10-15 minutes before challenge.

Children: One or two inhalations for the relief of acute bronchospasm, or before allergen exposure or exercise.

The Babyhaler* spacer device may be used to facilitate administration to children under 5 years of age.

On-demand use of Ventolin Inhaler should not exceed 8 inhalations in any 24 hours. Reliance on such frequent supplementary use, or a sudden increase in dose, indicates poorly controlled or deteriorating asthma (see *Precautions*).

Contra-indications, warnings, etc

Contra-indications: Although intravenous salbutamol, and occasionally salbutamol tablets, are used in the management of premature labour uncomplicated by conditions such as placenta praevia, ante-partum haemorrhage or toxaemia of pregnancy, inhaled salbutamol preparations are not appropriate for managing premature labour. Salbutamol preparations should not be used for threatened abortion.

Ventolin Inhaler is contra-indicated in patients with a history of hypersensitivity to any of the components.

Precautions: Patients' inhaler technique should be checked to make sure that aerosol actuation is synchronised with inspiration of breath for optimum delivery of drug to the lungs.

Bronchodilators should not be the only or main treatment in patients with severe or unstable asthma. Severe asthma requires regular medical assessment, including lung-function testing, as patients are at risk of severe attacks and even death. Physicians should consider using the maximum recommended dose of inhaled corticosteroid and/or oral corticosteroid therapy in these patients.

The dosage or frequency of administration should only be increased on medical advice.

Increasing use of bronchodilators, in particular short-acting inhaled β_2-agonists, to relieve symptoms, indicates deterioration of asthma control. The patient should be instructed to seek medical advice if short-acting relief bronchodilator treatment becomes less effective, or more inhalations than usual are required. In this situation the patient should be assessed and consideration given to the need for increased anti-inflammatory therapy (e.g. higher doses of inhaled corticosteroid or a course of oral corticosteroid).

Severe exacerbations of asthma must be treated in the normal way.

Salbutamol should be administered cautiously to patients suffering from thyrotoxicosis.

Salbutamol and non-selective β-blocking drugs such as propranolol, should not usually be prescribed together.

Potentially serious hypokalaemia may result from β_2-agonist therapy, mainly from parenteral and nebulised administration. Particular caution is advised in acute severe asthma as this effect may be potentiated by hypoxia and by concomitant treatment with xanthine derivatives, steroids and diuretics. Serum potassium levels should be monitored in such situations.

Pregnancy: Administration of drugs during pregnancy should only be considered if the expected benefit to the mother is greater than any possible risk to the fetus. As with the majority of drugs, there is little published evidence of the safety of salbutamol in the early stages of human pregnancy, but in animal studies there was evidence of some harmful effects on the fetus at very high dose levels.

Lactation: As salbutamol is probably secreted in breast milk, its use in nursing mothers requires careful consideration. It is not known whether salbutamol has a harmful effect on the neonate, and so its use should be restricted to situations where it is felt that the expected benefit to the mother is likely to outweigh any potential risk to the neonate.

Side-effects: As with other inhalation therapy, paradoxical bronchospasm may occur with an immediate increase in wheezing after dosing. This should be treated immediately with an alternative presentation or a different fast-acting inhaled bronchodilator. Ventolin Inhaler should be discontinued immediately, the patient assessed and, if necessary, alternative therapy instituted.

Hypersensitivity reactions including angioedema, urticaria, bronchospasm, hypotension and collapse have been reported very rarely.

Potentially serious hypokalaemia may result from β_2-agonist therapy.

Ventolin Inhaler may cause a fine tremor of skeletal muscle, usually the hands are most obviously affected. This effect is dose-related and is common to all β-adrenergic stimulants.

Tachycardia, with or without peripheral vasodilatation, may rarely occur.

In common with other β_2 agonists, cardiac arrhythmias (including atrial fibrillation, supraventricular tachycardia and extrasystoles) have been reported in association with the use of salbutamol, usually in susceptible patients.

Headaches have occasionally been reported.

Mouth and throat irritation may occur with inhaled salbutamol.

As with other β_2-agonists hyperactivity in children has been reported rarely.

There have been very rare reports of muscle cramps.

Overdosage: The preferred antidote for overdosage with salbutamol is a cardioselective β-blocking agent, but β-blocking drugs should be used with caution in patients with a history of bronchospasm.

Hypokalaemia may occur following overdose with salbutamol. Serum potassium levels should be monitored.

Pharmaceutical precautions Ventolin Inhaler should be stored below 30°C protected from direct sunlight, heat and frost. The canister should not be broken, punctured or burnt, even when apparently empty.

As with most inhaled medications in aerosol canisters, the therapeutic effect of this medication may decrease when the canister is cold.

Legal category POM.

Package quantities Ventolin Inhaler is a metered-dose aerosol with a specially designed actuator. Each canister provides 200 inhalations.

Further information Ventolin Inhaler does not cause difficulty in micturition because, unlike sympathomimetic drugs such as ephedrine, salbutamol does not stimulate alpha-adrenoceptors. Ventolin Inhaler is not contra-indicated in patients under treatment with monoamine oxidase inhibitors (MAOIs).

Product licence number 0045/5022R

Product licence holder: Allen & Hanburys Ltd, Greenford, Middlesex UB6 0HB.

VENTOLIN* INJECTION 250 micrograms (0.25 mg) in 5 ml VENTOLIN* INJECTION 500 micrograms (0.5 mg) in 1 ml

Qualitative and quantitative composition Ventolin Injection 250 micrograms (0.25 mg) in 5 ml (50 micrograms/ml) is presented as ampoules of 5 ml, each containing 250 micrograms salbutamol as Salbutamol Sulphate BP in a sterile isotonic solution.

Ventolin Injection 500 micrograms (0.5 mg) in 1 ml (500 micrograms/ml) is presented as ampoules of 1 ml, each containing 500 micrograms salbutamol as Salbutamol Sulphate BP in a sterile isotonic solution.

Pharmaceutical form Clear, colourless or pale straw-coloured solution for injection.

Clinical particulars

Therapeutic indications: Ventolin Injection is indicated for the relief of severe bronchospasm.

Posology and method of administration: Ventolin Injection may be administered by the subcutaneous, intramuscular or intravenous route, under the direction of a physician.

Adults: Subcutaneous route: 500 micrograms (8 micrograms/kg body weight) and repeated every four hours as required.

Intramuscular route: 500 micrograms (8 micrograms/kg body weight) and repeated every four hours as required.

Intravenous route: 250 micrograms (4 micrograms/kg body weight) injected slowly. If necessary the dose may be repeated.

Ventolin Injection 250 micrograms in 5 ml (50 micrograms/ml) is a suitably dilute preparation for slow intravenous injection, but if Ventolin Injection 500 micrograms in 1 ml (500 micrograms/ml) is used, the injection may be facilitated by dilution with Water for Injections BP.

Children: There are insufficient data to recommend a dosage regime for routine use.

Contra-indications: Although intravenous salbutamol, and occasionally salbutamol tablets, are used in the management of premature labour uncomplicated by conditions such as placenta praevia, ante-partum haemorrhage or toxaemia of pregnancy, salbutamol preparations should not be used for threatened abortion.

Ventolin Injection is contra-indicated in patients with a history of hypersensitivity to any of the components.

Special warnings and precautions for use: Bronchodilators should not be the only or main treatment in patients with severe or unstable asthma. Severe asthma requires regular medical assessment, including lung-function testing, as patients are at risk of severe attacks and even death. Physicians should consider using the maximum recommended dose of inhaled corticosteroid and/or oral corticosteroid therapy in these patients.

The dosage or frequency of administration should only be increased on medical advice.

Patients being treated with Ventolin Injection may also be receiving short-acting inhaled bronchodilators to relieve symptoms. Increasing use of bronchodilators, in particular short-acting inhaled β_2-agonists to relieve symptoms, indicates deterioration of asthma control. The patient should be instructed to seek medical advice if short-acting relief bronchodilator treatment becomes less effective, or more inhalations than usual are required. In this situation the patient should be assessed and consideration given to the need for increased anti-inflammatory therapy (e.g. higher doses of inhaled corticosteroid or a course of oral corticosteroid).

Severe exacerbations of asthma must be treated in the normal way.

The use of Ventolin Injection in the treatment of severe bronchospasm does not obviate the requirement for corticosteroid therapy as appropriate. When practicable, administration of oxygen concurrently with Ventolin Injection is recommended. In common with other β-adrenoceptor agonists, salbutamol can induce reversible metabolic changes such as hypokalaemia and increased blood glucose levels. Diabetic patients may be unable to compensate for the increase in blood glucose and the development of ketoacidosis has been reported. Concurrent administration of corticosteroids can exaggerate this effect.

Salbutamol should be administered cautiously to patients suffering from thyrotoxicosis.

Potentially serious hypokalaemia may result from β_2-agonist therapy, mainly from parenteral and nebulised administration. Particular caution is advised in acute severe asthma as this effect may be potentiated by hypoxia and by concomitant treatment with xanthine derivatives, steroids and diuretics. Serum potassium levels should be monitored in such situations.

Interaction with other medicaments and other forms of interaction: Ventolin Injection should not be administered in the same syringe as any other medication.

Salbutamol and non-selective β-blocking drugs such as propranolol, should not usually be prescribed together.

Pregnancy and lactation: Administration of drugs during pregnancy should only be considered if the expected benefit to the mother is greater than any possible risk to the fetus. As with the majority of drugs, there is little published evidence of the safety of salbutamol in the early stages of human pregnancy, but in animal studies there was evidence of some harmful effects on the fetus at very high dose levels.

As salbutamol is probably secreted in breast milk, its use in nursing mothers requires careful consideration. It is not known whether salbutamol has a harmful effect on the neonate, and so its use should be restricted to situations where it is felt that the expected benefit to the mother is likely to outweigh any potential risk to the neonate.

Effect on ability to drive and use machines: None reported.

Undesirable effects: Hypersensitivity reactions including angioedema, urticaria, bronchospasm, hypotension and collapse have been reported very rarely.

Enhancement of physiological tremor may occur with Ventolin Injection. This effect is caused by a direct action on skeletal muscle and is common to all β-adrenergic stimulants.

Tachycardia, with or without dilatation of peripheral arterioles leading to a small reduction in arterial pressure, may occur. Increases in heart rate are more likely to occur in patients with normal heart rates and these increases are dose-dependent. In patients with pre-existing sinus tachycardia, especially those in status asthmaticus, the heart rate tends to fall as the condition of the patient improves.

In common with other β_2 agonists, cardiac arrhythmias (including atrial fibrillation, supraventricular tachycardia and extrasystoles) have been reported in association with the use of salbutamol, usually in susceptible patients.

Headaches have occasionally been reported.

There have been very rare reports of muscle cramps.

Potentially serious hypokalaemia may result from β_2-agonist therapy.

Intramuscular use of the undiluted injection may produce slight pain or stinging.

Overdose: The preferred antidote for overdosage with salbutamol is a cardioselective β-blocking agent, but β-blocking drugs should be used with caution in patients with a history of bronchospasm.

Hypokalaemia may occur following overdose with salbutamol. Serum potassium levels should be monitored.

Pharmacological properties

Pharmacodynamic properties: Salbutamol is a selective β_2-agonist providing short-acting (4-6 hour) bronchodilatation with a fast onset (within 5 minutes) in reversible airways obstruction.

Pharmacokinetic properties: Salbutamol administered intravenously has a half-life of 4 to 6 hours and is cleared partly renally and partly by metabolism to the inactive 4'-0-sulphate (phenolic sulphate) which is also excreted primarily in the urine. The faeces are a minor route of excretion. Most of a dose of salbutamol given intravenously, orally or by inhalation is excreted within 72 hours. Salbutamol is bound to plasma proteins to the extent of 10%.

Preclinical safety data: No additional preclinical safety data are included here.

Pharmaceutical particulars

List of excipients: Sodium chloride, sodium hydroxide, sulphuric acid and Water for Injections.

Incompatibilities: None stated.

Shelf life: 36 months.

Special precautions for storage: Store below 30°C and protect from light.

Nature and contents of container: Clear, neutral glass ampoules.

Ventolin Injection 250 micrograms in 5 ml is available in packs of 10.

Ventolin Injection 500 micrograms in 1 ml is available in packs of 5.

Instructions for use/handling: The only recommended diluents for Ventolin Injection are Water for Injections

BP, Sodium Chloride Injection BP, Sodium Chloride and Dextrose Injection BP or Dextrose Injection BP.

All unused admixtures of Ventolin Injection should be discarded twenty-four hours after preparation.

Marketing authorisation numbers
Ventolin Injection 250 micrograms in 5 ml 10949/0083
Ventolin Injection 500 micrograms in 1 ml 10949/0084

Date of approval/revision of SPC June 1998.

Legal category POM.

VENTOLIN* NEBULES* 2.5 mg
VENTOLIN* NEBULES* 5 mg

Qualitative and quantitative composition Plastic ampoule containing 2.5 ml of either a sterile 0.1% or 0.2% w/v solution of salbutamol (as Salbutamol Sulphate BP) in normal saline.

Pharmaceutical form Solution for inhalation via a nebuliser.

Clinical particulars
Therapeutic indications: Salbutamol is a selective β_2-agonist providing short-acting (4–6 hour) bronchodilatation with a fast onset (within 5 minutes) in reversible airways obstruction.

Ventolin Nebules are indicated for use in the routine management of chronic bronchospasm unresponsive to conventional therapy, and in the treatment of acute severe asthma.

Posology and method of administration: Ventolin Nebules are for inhalation use only under the direction of a physician, using a suitable nebuliser.

The solution should not be injected or administered orally.

Adults (including the elderly): 2.5 mg to 5 mg salbutamol up to four times a day. Up to 40 mg per day can be given under strict medical supervision in hospital.

Children: 2.5 mg to 5 mg up to four times a day.

In infants under 18 months old the clinical efficacy of nebulised salbutamol is uncertain. As transient hypoxia may occur supplemental oxygen therapy should be considered.

Ventolin Nebules are intended to be used undiluted. However, if prolonged delivery time (more than 10 minutes) is required, the solution may be diluted with sterile normal saline.

Contra-indications: Although intravenous salbutamol, and occasionally salbutamol tablets, are used in the management of premature labour uncomplicated by conditions such as placenta praevia, ante-partum haemorrhage or toxaemia of pregnancy, inhaled salbutamol preparations are not appropriate for managing premature labour. Salbutamol preparations should not be used for threatened abortion.

Ventolin Nebules are contra-indicated in patients with a history of hypersensitivity to any of the components.

Special warnings and precautions for use: Bronchodilators should not be the only or main treatment in patients with severe or unstable asthma. Severe asthma requires regular medical assessment, including lung-function testing, as patients are at risk of severe attacks and even death. Physicians should consider using the maximum recommended dose of inhaled corticosteroid and/or oral corticosteroid therapy in these patients.

Patients receiving treatment at home should seek medical advice if treatment with Ventolin Nebules becomes less effective. The dosage or frequency of administration should only be increased on medical advice.

Patients being treated with Ventolin Nebules may also be receiving other dosage forms of short-acting inhaled bronchodilators to relieve symptoms. Increasing use of bronchodilators, in particular short-acting inhaled β_2-agonists to relieve symptoms, indicates deterioration of asthma control. The patient should be instructed to seek medical advice if short-acting relief bronchodilator treatment becomes less effective or more inhalations than usual are required. In this situation patients should be assessed and consideration given to the need for increased anti-inflammatory therapy (e.g. higher doses of inhaled corticosteroid or a course of oral corticosteroid).

Severe exacerbations of asthma must be treated in the normal way.

Salbutamol should be administered cautiously to patients suffering from thyrotoxicosis.

Ventolin Nebules should be used with care in patients known to have received large doses of other sympathomimetic drugs.

Potentially serious hypokalaemia may result from β_2-agonist therapy, mainly from parenteral and nebulised administration. Particular caution is advised in acute severe asthma as this effect may be potentiated by hypoxia and by concomitant treatment with xanthine derivatives, steroids and diuretics. Serum potassium levels should be monitored in such situations.

In common with other β-adrenoceptor agonists, salbutamol can induce reversible metabolic changes such as increased blood glucose levels. Diabetic patients may be unable to compensate for the increase in blood glucose and the development of ketoacidosis has been reported. Concurrent administration of corticosteroids can exaggerate this effect.

A small number of cases of acute angle-closure glaucoma have been reported in patients treated with a combination of nebulised salbutamol and ipratropium bromide. A combination of nebulised salbutamol with nebulised anticholinergics should therefore be used cautiously. Patients should receive adequate instruction in correct administration and be warned not to let the solution or mist enter the eye.

Interaction with other medicaments and other forms of interaction: Salbutamol and non-selective β-blocking drugs such as propranolol, should not usually be prescribed together.

Pregnancy and lactation: Administration of drugs during pregnancy should only be considered if the expected benefit to the mother is greater than any possible risk to the fetus. As with the majority of drugs, there is little published evidence of the safety of salbutamol in the early stages of human pregnancy, but in animal studies there was evidence of some harmful effects on the fetus at very high dose levels.

As salbutamol is probably secreted in breast milk, its use in nursing mothers requires careful consideration. It is not known whether salbutamol has a harmful effect on the neonate, and so its use should be restricted to situations where it is felt that the expected benefit to the mother is likely to outweigh any potential risk to the neonate.

Effect on ability to drive and use machines: None reported.

Undesirable effects: As with other inhalation therapy, paradoxical bronchospasm may occur with an immediate increase in wheezing after dosing. This should be treated immediately with an alternative presentation or a different fast-acting inhaled bronchodilator. The preparation should be discontinued immediately, the patient assessed, and, if necessary, alternative therapy instituted.

Solutions which are not of neutral pH may rarely cause bronchospasm.

Hypersensitivity reactions including angioedema, urticaria, bronchospasm, hypotension and collapse have been reported very rarely.

Potentially serious hypokalaemia may result from β_2-agonist therapy.

Ventolin Nebules may cause a fine tremor of skeletal muscle, usually the hands are most obviously affected. This effect is dose-related and is common to all β-adrenergic stimulants.

Tachycardia, with or without peripheral vasodilatation, may rarely occur.

In common with other β_2 agonists, cardiac arrhythmias (including atrial fibrillation, supraventricular tachycardia and extrasystoles) have been reported in association with the use of salbutamol, usually in susceptible patients.

Headaches have occasionally been reported.

Mouth and throat irritation may occur with inhaled salbutamol.

As with other β_2-agonists hyperactivity in children has been reported rarely.

There have been very rare reports of muscle cramps.

Overdose: The preferred antidote to overdosage with salbutamol is a cardioselective β-blocking agent, but β-blocking drugs should be used with caution in patients with a history of bronchospasm.

Hypokalaemia may occur following overdose with salbutamol. Serum potassium levels should be monitored.

Pharmacological properties
Pharmacodynamic properties: Salbutamol is a selective β_2-agonist providing short-acting (4–6 hour) bronchodilatation with a fast onset (within 5 minutes) in reversible airways obstruction. At therapeutic doses it acts on the β_2-adrenoceptors of bronchial muscle. With its fast onset of action, it is particularly suitable for the management and prevention of attack in asthma.

Pharmacokinetic properties: Salbutamol administered intravenously has a half-life of 4 to 6 hours and is cleared partly renally, and partly by metabolism to the inactive 4'-O-sulphate (phenolic sulphate) which is also excreted primarily in the urine. The faeces are a minor route of excretion. Most of a dose of salbutamol given intravenously, orally or by inhalation is excreted within 72 hours. Salbutamol is bound to plasma proteins to the extent of 10%.

After administration by the inhaled route between 10 and 20% of the dose reaches the lower airways. The remainder is retained in the delivery system or is deposited in the oropharynx from where it is swallowed. The fraction deposited in the airways is absorbed into the pulmonary tissues and circulation, but is not metabolised by the lung. On reaching the systemic circulation it becomes accessible to hepatic metabolism and is excreted, primarily in the urine, as unchanged drug and as the phenolic sulphate.

The swallowed portion of an inhaled dose is absorbed from the gastrointestinal tract and undergoes considerable first-pass metabolism to the phenolic sulphate. Both unchanged drug and conjugate are excreted primarily in the urine.

Preclinical safety data: No additional preclinical safety data are included here.

Pharmaceutical particulars
List of excipients: Sodium chloride. Sulphuric acid if required to adjust pH. Purified water.

Incompatibilities: None known.

Shelf life: 3 years if unopened. 3 months after removal from the foil overwrap (see below).

Special precautions for storage: Ventolin Nebules should be stored below 30°C. The Nebules should be protected from light after removal from the foil tray.

Nature and contents of container: Low density polyethylene ampoules available in boxes of 20 in strips of 5.

Instructions for use/handling: The nebulised solution may be inhaled through a face mask, T-piece or via an endotracheal tube. Intermittent positive pressure ventilation (IPPV) may be used but is rarely necessary. When there is a risk of anoxia through hypoventilation, oxygen should be added to the inspired air.

As many nebulisers operate on a continuous flow basis, it is likely that some nebulised drug will be released into the local environment. Ventolin Nebules should therefore be administered in a well-ventilated room, particularly in hospitals when several patients may be using nebulisers at the same time.

Dilution: Ventolin Nebules may be diluted with Sodium Chloride Injection BP (normal saline). Solutions in nebulisers should be replaced daily.

Marketing authorisation numbers
Ventolin Nebules 2.5 mg 10949/0085
Ventolin Nebules 5.0 mg 10949/0086

Date of approval/revision of SPC June 1998.

Legal classification POM.

VENTOLIN* RESPIRATOR SOLUTION

Qualitative and quantitative composition Aqueous, colourless to light yellow solution, pH 3.5, providing 5 mg/ml of salbutamol (as Salbutamol Sulphate BP).

Pharmaceutical form Solution for nebulisation.

Clinical particulars
Therapeutic indications: Ventolin Respirator Solution is indicated for use in the routine management of chronic bronchospasm unresponsive to conventional therapy, and in the treatment of acute severe asthma.

Posology and method of administration: Ventolin Respirator Solution is for inhalation use only under the direction of a physician, using a suitable nebuliser.

The solution should not be injected or administered orally.

Ventolin Respirator Solution may be administered intermittently or continuously.

Salbutamol has a duration of action of 4 to 6 hours in most patients.

1. Intermittent administration
Adults: Ventolin Respirator Solution 0.5 ml (2.5 mg of salbutamol) should be diluted to a final volume of 2 ml with normal saline for injection. This may be increased to 1 ml (5 mg of salbutamol) diluted to a final volume of 2.5 ml. The resulting solution is inhaled from a suitably driven nebuliser until aerosol generation ceases. Using a correctly matched nebuliser and driving source this should take about ten minutes.

Ventolin Respirator Solution may be used undiluted for intermittent administration. For this, 2 ml of Ventolin Respirator Solution (10 mg of salbutamol) is placed in the nebuliser and the patient allowed to inhale the nebulised solution until bronchodilatation is achieved. This usually takes 3–5 minutes.

Some adult patients may require higher doses of salbutamol up to 10 mg, in which case nebulisation of the undiluted solution may continue until aerosol generation ceases.

Children: The same mode of administration for intermittent administration is also applicable to children. The minimum starting dosage for children under the age of twelve years is 0.5 ml (2.5 mg of salbutamol) diluted to 2 to 2.5 ml with normal saline for injection. Some children may, however, require higher doses of salbutamol up to 5 mg.

Intermittent treatment may be repeated up to four times daily.

2. Continuous administration

Ventolin Respirator Solution is diluted with normal saline for injection to contain 50–100 micrograms of salbutamol per ml, (1–2 ml solution made up to 100 ml with diluent). The diluted solution is administered as an aerosol by a suitably driven nebuliser. The usual rate of administration is 1–2 mg per hour.

Delivery of the aerosol may be by face mask, T-piece or via an endotracheal tube. Intermittent positive pressure ventilation (IPPV) may be used, but is rarely necessary. When there is a risk of anoxia through hypoventilation, oxygen should be added to the inspired air. In infants under 18 months the clinical efficacy of nebulised salbutamol is uncertain. As transient hypoxaemia may occur supplemental oxygen therapy should be considered.

Contra-indications: Hypersensitivity. Threatened abortion.

Special warnings and precautions for use: Bronchodilators should not be the only or main treatment in patients with severe or unstable asthma. Severe asthma requires regular medical assessment, including lung-function testing, as patients are at risk of severe attacks and even death. Physicians should consider using the maximum recommended dose of inhaled corticosteroid and/or oral corticosteroid therapy in these patients.

Patients receiving treatment at home should be warned to seek medical advice if treatment with Ventolin Respirator Solution becomes less effective. As there may be adverse effects associated with excessive dosing the dosage or frequency of administration should only be increased on medical advice.

Patients being treated with Ventolin Respirator Solution may also be receiving other dosage forms of short-acting inhaled bronchodilators to relieve symptoms.

Increasing use of bronchodilators, in particular short-acting inhaled β_2-agonists, to relieve symptoms, indicates deterioration of asthma control. The patient should be instructed to seek medical advice if short-acting relief bronchodilator treatment becomes less effective, or more inhalations than usual are required. In this situation the patient should be assessed and consideration given to the need for increased anti-inflammatory therapy (e.g. higher doses of inhaled corticosteroid or a course of oral corticosteroid).

Severe exacerbations of asthma must be treated in the normal way.

Salbutamol should be administered cautiously to patients suffering from thyrotoxicosis.

Ventolin Respirator Solution should be used with care in patients known to have received large doses of other sympathomimetic drugs.

Potentially serious hypokalaemia may result from β_2-agonist therapy, mainly from parenteral and nebulised administration. Particular caution is advised in acute severe asthma as this effect may be potentiated by hypoxia and by concomitant treatment with xanthine derivatives, steroids and diuretics. Serum potassium levels should be monitored in such situations.

In common with other β-adrenoceptor agonists, salbutamol can induce reversible metabolic changes such as increased blood glucose levels. Diabetic patients may be unable to compensate for the increase in blood glucose and the development of ketoacidosis has been reported. Concurrent administration of corticosteroids can exaggerate this effect.

A small number of cases of acute angle-closure glaucoma have been reported in patients treated with a combination of nebulised salbutamol and ipratropium bromide. A combination of nebulised salbutamol with nebulised anticholinergics should therefore be used cautiously. Patients should receive adequate instruction in correct administration and be warned not to let the solution or mist enter the eye.

Interaction with other medicaments and other forms of interaction: Should not normally be prescribed with non-selective β-blocking drugs such as propranolol.

Use during pregnancy and lactation: Administration of drugs during pregnancy should only be considered if the expected benefit to the mother is greater than any possible risk to the fetus. As with the majority of drugs, there is little published evidence of the safety of salbutamol in the early stages of human pregnancy, but in animal studies there was evidence of some harmful effects on the fetus at very high dose levels.

As salbutamol is probably secreted in breast milk, its use in nursing mothers requires careful consideration. It is not known whether salbutamol has a harmful effect on the neonate, and so its use should be restricted to situations where it is felt that the expected benefit to the mother is likely to outweigh any potential risk to the neonate.

Effect on the ability to drive and use machines: None reported.

Undesirable effects: As with other inhalation therapy, paradoxical bronchospasm may occur with an immediate increase in wheezing after dosing. This should be treated immediately with an alternative presentation or a different fast-acting inhaled bronchodilator. The preparation should be discontinued immediately, the patient assessed and, if necessary, alternative therapy instituted.

Non-isotonic solutions, or solutions which are not of neutral pH, or which contain benzalkonium chloride, may rarely cause paradoxical bronchospasm.

Hypersensitivity reactions including angioedema, urticaria, bronchospasm, hypotension and collapse have been reported very rarely.

Potentially serious hypokalaemia may result from β_2-agonist therapy.

Ventolin Respirator Solution may cause a fine tremor of skeletal muscle, usually the hands are most obviously affected. This effect is dose-related and is common to all β-adrenergic stimulants.

Tachycardia, with or without peripheral vasodilatation, may rarely occur.

In common with other β_2 agonists, cardiac arrhythmias (including atrial fibrillation, supraventricular tachycardia and extrasystoles) have been reported in association with the use of salbutamol, usually in susceptible patients.

Headaches have occasionally been reported.

Mouth and throat irritation may occur with inhaled salbutamol.

As with other β_2-agonists hyperactivity in children has been reported rarely.

There have been very rare reports of muscle cramps.

Overdose: Discontinue administration of Ventolin Respirator Solution if there are any signs of overdosage.

The preferred antidote for overdosage with salbutamol is a cardioselective β-blocking agent, but β-blocking drugs should be used with caution in patients with a history of bronchospasm.

Hypokalaemia may occur following overdose with salbutamol. Serum potassium levels should be monitored.

Pharmacological properties

Pharmacodynamic properties: Salbutamol is a selective β_2-agonist providing short-acting (4–6 hours) bronchodilatation with a fast onset (within 5 minutes) in reversible airways obstruction. At therapeutic doses it acts on the β_2-adrenoceptors of bronchial muscle. With its fast onset of action, it is particularly suitable for the management and prevention of attack in asthma.

Pharmacokinetic properties: Salbutamol administered intravenously has a half-life of 4 to 6 hours and is cleared partly renally and partly by metabolism to the inactive 4'-0-sulphate (phenolic sulphate) which is also excreted primarily in the urine. The faeces are a minor route of excretion. Most of a dose of salbutamol given intravenously, orally or by inhalation is excreted within 72 hours. Salbutamol is bound to plasma proteins to the extent of 10%.

After administration by the inhaled route between 10 and 20% of the dose reaches the lower airways. The remainder is retained in the delivery system or is deposited in the oropharynx from where it is swallowed. The fraction deposited in the airways is absorbed into the pulmonary tissues and circulation, but is not metabolised by the lung. On reaching the systemic circulation it becomes accessible to hepatic metabolism and is excreted, primarily in the urine, as unchanged drug and as the phenolic sulphate.

The swallowed portion of an inhaled dose is absorbed from the gastrointestinal tract and undergoes considerable first-pass metabolism to the phenolic sulphate. Both unchanged drug and conjugate are excreted primarily in the urine.

Preclinical safety data: No additional preclinical safety data are included here.

Pharmaceutical particulars

List of excipients: Preservative: Benzalkonium chloride. Sulphuric acid if required to adjust to pH 3.5. Purified water.

Incompatibilities: None known.

Shelf life: Unopened: 3 years. Following opening for the first time: 28 days.

Special precautions for storage: Store below 25°C. Protect from light. Discard any contents remaining one month after opening the bottle.

Nature and contents of container: Screw-capped 20 ml amber glass bottle.

Instructions for use/handling: Inhalation use only, using a suitable nebuliser.

As many nebulisers operate on a continuous flow basis, it is likely that nebulised drug will be released into the local environment. Ventolin Respirator Solution should therefore be administered in a well ventilated room, particularly in hospitals when several patients may be using nebulisers at the same time.

Marketing authorisation number 10949/0244

Date of approval/revision of SPC June 1998.

Legal category POM.

VENTOLIN* ROTACAPS* 200 mcg
VENTOLIN* ROTACAPS* 400 mcg

Qualitative and quantitative composition

Ventolin Rotacaps 200 mcg: 200 mcg microfine salbutamol (as sulphate) in each light blue capsule, marked Ventolin 200.

Ventolin Rotacaps 400 mcg: 400 mcg microfine salbutamol (as sulphate) in each dark blue capsule, marked Ventolin 400.

Pharmaceutical form Hard gelatin capsule containing powder for inhalation.

Clinical particulars

Therapeutic indications: Salbutamol is a selective β_2-agonist providing short-acting (4–6 hour) bronchodilatation with a fast onset (within 5 minutes) in reversible airways obstruction.

Ventolin Rotacaps can be used in the management of asthma, bronchospasm and/or reversible airways obstruction.

Ventolin Rotacaps are particularly suitable for the relief of asthma symptoms. They should be used to relieve symptoms when they occur, and to prevent them in those circumstances recognised by the patient to precipitate an asthma attack (e.g. before exercise or unavoidable allergen exposure).

Ventolin Rotacaps are particularly valuable as relief medication in mild, moderate or severe asthma, provided that reliance on them does not delay the introduction and use of regular inhaled corticosteroid therapy.

Posology and method of administration: Ventolin Rotacaps are for oral inhalation use only, using a Ventolin Rotahaler*. Ventolin Rotacaps are suitable for many patients including those who cannot use a metered-dose inhaler successfully.

Adults (including the elderly): For the relief of acute bronchospasm: 200 micrograms or 400 micrograms as a single dose. The maximum daily dose is 400 micrograms four times a day.

To prevent allergen- or exercise-induced symptoms: 400 micrograms 10–15 minutes before challenge.

Children: The recommended dose for the relief of acute bronchospasm or before allergen exposure or exercise is 200 micrograms. The maximum daily dose is 200 micrograms four times a day.

On-demand use of Ventolin Rotacaps should not exceed four times daily. Reliance on such frequent supplementary use, or a sudden increase in dose, indicates poorly controlled or deteriorating asthma (see *Special warnings and precautions for use*).

Contra-indications: Although intravenous salbutamol, and occasionally salbutamol tablets, are used in the management of premature labour uncomplicated by conditions such as placenta praevia, ante-partum haemorrhage or toxaemia of pregnancy, inhaled salbutamol preparations are not appropriate for managing premature labour. Salbutamol preparations should not be used for threatened abortion.

Ventolin Rotacaps are contra-indicated in patients with a history of hypersensitivity to any of the components.

Special warnings and precautions for use: Patients should be instructed in the proper use of the Rotahaler device to ensure that the drug reaches the target area within the lungs.

Bronchodilators should not be the only or main treatment in patients with severe or unstable asthma. Severe asthma requires regular medical assessment, including lung-function testing, as patients are at risk of severe attacks and even death. Physicians should consider using the maximum recommended dose of inhaled corticosteroid and/or oral corticosteroid therapy in these patients.

The dosage or frequency of administration should only be increased on medical advice.

Increasing use of bronchodilators, in particular short-acting inhaled β_2-agonists to relieve symptoms, indicates deterioration of asthma control. The patient should be instructed to seek medical advice if short-acting relief bronchodilator treatment becomes less effective, or more inhalations than usual are required. In this situation the patient should be assessed, and consideration given to the need for increased anti-inflammatory therapy (e.g. higher doses of inhaled corticosteroid or a course of oral corticosteroid).

Severe exacerbations of asthma must be treated in the normal way.

Salbutamol should be administered cautiously to patients suffering from thyrotoxicosis.

Potentially serious hypokalaemia may result from β_2-agonist therapy, mainly from parenteral and nebulised administration. Particular caution is advised in acute severe asthma as this effect may be potentiated by hypoxia and by concomitant treatment with xanthine derivatives, steroids and diuretics. Serum potassium levels should be monitored in such situations.

Interaction with other medicaments and other forms of interaction: Salbutamol and non-selective β-blocking drugs such as propranolol, should not usually be prescribed together.

Pregnancy and lactation: Administration of drugs during pregnancy should only be considered if the expected benefit to the mother is greater than any possible risk to the fetus. As with the majority of drugs, there is little published evidence of the safety of salbutamol in the early stages of human pregnancy, but in animal studies there was evidence of some harmful effects on the fetus at very high dose levels.

As salbutamol is probably secreted in breast milk, its use in nursing mothers requires careful consideration. It is not known whether salbutamol has a harmful effect on the neonate, and so its use should be restricted to situations where it is felt that the expected benefit to the mother is likely to outweigh any potential risk to the neonate.

Effect on ability to drive and operate machinery: None reported.

Undesirable effects: As with other inhalation therapy, paradoxical bronchospasm may occur with an immediate increase in wheezing after dosing. This should be treated immediately with an alternative presentation or a different fast-acting inhaled bronchodilator. The preparation should be discontinued immediately, the patient assessed and, if necessary, alternative therapy instituted.

Hypersensitivity reactions including angioedema, urticaria, bronchospasm, hypotension and collapse have been reported very rarely.

Potentially serious hypokalaemia may result from β_2-agonist therapy.

Ventolin Rotacaps may cause a fine tremor of skeletal muscle, usually the hands are most obviously affected. This effect is dose-related and is common to all β-adrenergic stimulants.

Tachycardia, with or without peripheral vasodilatation, may rarely occur.

In common with other β_2 agonists, cardiac arrhythmias (including atrial fibrillation, supraventricular tachycardia and extrasystoles) have been reported in association with the use of salbutamol, usually in susceptible patients.

Headaches have occasionally been reported.

Mouth and throat irritation may occur with inhaled salbutamol.

As with other β_2-agonists hyperactivity in children has been reported rarely.

There have been very rare reports of muscle cramps.

Overdose: The preferred antidote for overdosage with salbutamol is a cardioselective β-blocking agent, but β-blocking drugs should be used with caution in patients with a history of bronchospasm.

Hypokalaemia may occur following overdose with salbutamol. Serum potassium levels should be monitored.

Pharmacological properties
Pharmacodynamic properties: Salbutamol is a selective β_2-adrenoceptor agonist. At therapeutic doses it acts on the β_2-adrenoceptors of bronchial muscle providing short acting (4–6 hours) bronchodilatation with a fast onset (within 5 minutes) in reversible airways obstruction.

Pharmacokinetic properties: Salbutamol administered intravenously has a half-life of 4 to 6 hours and is cleared partly renally and partly by metabolism to the inactive 4′-O-sulphate (phenolic sulphate) which is also excreted primarily in the urine. The faeces are a minor route of excretion.

After administration by the inhaled route between 10 and 20% of the dose reaches the lower airways. The remainder is retained in the delivery system or is deposited in the oropharynx from where it is swallowed. The fraction deposited in the airways is absorbed into the pulmonary tissues and circulation, but is not metabolised by the lung. On reaching the systemic circulation it becomes accessible to hepatic metabolism and is excreted, primarily in the urine, as unchanged drug and as the phenolic sulphate.

The swallowed portion of an inhaled dose is absorbed from the gastrointestinal tract and undergoes considerable first-pass metabolism to the phenolic sulphate. Both unchanged drug and conjugate are excreted primarily in the urine. Most of a dose of salbutamol given intravenously, orally or by inhalation is excreted within 72 hours. Salbutamol is bound to plasma proteins to the extent of 10%.

Preclinical safety data: There are no pre-clinical data of relevance to the prescriber which are additional to that already included in other sections of the SPC.

Pharmaceutical particulars
List of excipients: Lactose.

Incompatibilities: None reported.

Shelf life: 3 years.

Special precautions for storage: Store in a dry place below 30°C.

Nature and contents of container: Ventolin Rotacaps 200 mcg and 400 mcg are supplied in polypropylene containers with snap-on tamper-evident polyethylene caps containing 112 capsules.

Instructions for use/handling: The contents of the Rotacaps capsule are inhaled through the mouth into the lungs. The capsule is inserted into a Rotahaler device which separates the two halves. The drug is released as the patient inhales through the mouth.

A capsule should only be inserted into the Rotahaler device when required for use.

For detailed instructions for use refer to the Patient Information Leaflet in every pack.

Marketing authorisation numbers
Ventolin Rotacaps 200 mcg 10949/0072
Ventolin Rotacaps 400 mcg 10949/0073

Date of approval/revision of SPC June 1998.

Legal category POM.

VENTOLIN* SOLUTION FOR INTRAVENOUS INFUSION 5 mg in 5 ml (1 mg/ml)

Qualitative and quantitative composition Ventolin Solution for Intravenous Infusion 5 mg in 5 ml (1 mg/ml) is presented as ampoules of 5 ml, each containing 5 mg salbutamol as Salbutamol Sulphate BP in a sterile isotonic solution.

Pharmaceutical form Clear, colourless or pale straw-coloured solution for intravenous infusion.

Clinical particulars

Therapeutic indications: Ventolin Solution for Intravenous Infusion should be administered under the direction of a physician. It is indicated for two distinct clinical situations:

(1) For the relief of severe bronchospasm.

(2) In the management of premature labour; to arrest uncomplicated labour between 24 and 33 weeks of gestation in patients with no medical or obstetric contra-indication to tocolytic therapy. Data suggest that the main effect of tocolytic therapy is a delay in delivery of up to 48 hours. This delay may be used to administer glucocorticoids or to implement other measures known to improve perinatal health.

Posology and method of administration: Ventolin Solution for Intravenous Infusion is used to prepare an infusion solution. It should not be injected undiluted. Ventolin Solution for Intravenous Infusion should not be administered in the same syringe or infusion as any other medication.

1. *In severe bronchospasm.*
Adults: A suitable solution for infusion providing 10 micrograms salbutamol/ml is prepared by diluting 5 ml Ventolin Solution for Intravenous Infusion to 500 ml with an infusion solution such as Sodium Chloride and Dextrose Injection BP. Other suitable diluents are Water for Injections BP, Sodium Chloride Injection BP or Dextrose Injection BP.

Infusion rates providing 3 to 20 micrograms salbutamol/minute (0.3 to 2 ml/minute of the above infusion solution) are usually adequate. Higher doses have been used with success in patients with respiratory failure.

Children: There are insufficient data to recommend a dosage regime for routine use.

2. *In the management of premature labour.*
The infusion, prepared as described below, should be administered as early as possible after the diagnosis of premature labour, and after evaluation of the patient to eliminate any contra-indications to the use of salbutamol (see *Contra-indications*).

During infusion the maternal pulse rate should be monitored and the infusion rate adjusted to avoid excessive maternal heart rate (above 140 beats/minute).

It is essential that the volume of infusion fluid is kept to a minimum to control the level of hydration and so avoid the risk of maternal pulmonary oedema (see *Undesirable effects*). A controlled infusion device, preferably a syringe pump, should be used.

Infusion rates providing 10 to 45 micrograms salbutamol/minute are generally adequate to control uterine contractions. A starting rate of 10 micrograms/minute is recommended, increasing the rate at 10-minute intervals until there is evidence of patient response shown by diminution in strength, frequency or duration of contractions. Thereafter the infusion rate may be increased slowly until contractions cease.

Once uterine contractions have ceased the infusion rate should be maintained at the same level for one hour and then reduced by 50% decrements at six-hourly intervals. If labour progresses despite treatment the infusion should be stopped. If contractions have been successfully inhibited by the infusion, treatment may be continued orally with Ventolin Tablets 4 mg given three or four times daily.

Dilution: The recommended diluent is 5% Dextrose (see precautions for use in diabetic patients).

For use in a syringe pump: Prepare a solution providing 200 micrograms salbutamol/ml by diluting 10 ml Ventolin Solution for Intravenous Infusion with 40 ml diluent. An infusion rate of 10 to 45 micrograms/minute is equivalent to 0.05 to 0.225 ml/minute of this solution.

Other infusion methods: Prepare a solution providing 20 micrograms salbutamol/ml by diluting 10 ml Ventolin Solution for Intravenous Infusion with 490 ml diluent. An infusion rate of 10 to 45 micrograms/minute is equivalent to 0.5 to 2.25 ml/minute of this solution.

Contra-indications: Although Ventolin Solution for Intravenous Infusion and occasionally salbutamol tablets, are used in the management of premature labour uncomplicated by conditions such as placenta praevia, ante-partum haemorrhage or toxaemia of pregnancy, salbutamol preparations should not be used for threatened abortion.

Ventolin Solution for Intravenous Infusion is contra-indicated in patients with a history of hypersensitivity to any of the components.

Special warnings and precautions for use: Bronchodilators should not be the only or main treatment in patients with severe or unstable asthma. Severe asthma requires regular medical assessment, including lung-function testing, as patients are at risk of severe attacks and even death. Physicians should consider using the maximum recommended dose of inhaled corticosteroid and/or oral corticosteroid therapy in these patients.

The dosage or frequency of administration should only be increased on medical advice.

Patients being treated with Ventolin Solution for Intravenous Infusion may also be receiving short-acting inhaled bronchodilators to relieve symptoms. Increasing use of bronchodilators, in particular short-acting inhaled β_2-agonists to relieve symptoms, indicates deterioration of asthma control. The patient should be instructed to seek medical advice if short-acting relief bronchodilator treatment becomes less effective, or more inhalations than usual are required. In this situation the patient should be assessed and consideration given to the need for increased anti-inflammatory therapy (e.g. higher doses of inhaled corticosteroid or a course of oral corticosteroid).

Severe exacerbations of asthma must be treated in the normal way.

The use of Ventolin Solution for Intravenous Infusion in the treatment of severe bronchospasm does not obviate the requirement for corticosteroid therapy as appropriate. When practicable, administration of oxygen concurrently with parenteral Ventolin is recommended, particularly when it is given by intravenous infusion to hypoxic patients. In common with other β-adrenoceptor agonists, salbutamol can induce reversible metabolic changes such as hypokalaemia and increased blood glucose levels. Diabetic patients may be unable to compensate for the increase in blood glucose and the development of ketoacidosis has been reported. Concurrent administration of corticosteroids can exaggerate this effect.

Therefore, diabetic patients and those concurrently receiving corticosteroids should be monitored frequently during intravenous infusion of Ventolin so that remedial steps (e.g. an increase in insulin dosage) can be taken to counter any metabolic change occurring. For these patients it may be preferable to dilute Ventolin Solution for Intravenous Infusion in Sodium Chloride Injection BP rather than in diluents containing dextrose.

Salbutamol should be administered cautiously to patients suffering from thyrotoxicosis.

Potentially serious hypokalaemia may result from β_2-agonist therapy, mainly from parenteral and nebulised administration. Particular caution is advised in acute severe asthma as this effect may be potentiated by hypoxia and by concomitant treatment with xanthine derivatives, steroids and diuretics. Serum potassium levels should be monitored in such situations.

As maternal pulmonary oedema has been reported during or following treatment of premature labour with β_2-agonists, careful attention should be given to fluid balance and cardio-respiratory function monitored. In patients being treated for premature labour by intravenous infusion of salbutamol, increases in maternal heart rate of the order of 20 to 50 beats per minute usually accompany the infusion. The maternal pulse rate should be monitored and not normally allowed to exceed a steady rate of 140 beats per minute. Maternal blood pressure may fall slightly during the infusion; the effect being greater on diastolic than on systolic pressure. Falls in diastolic pressure are usually within the range of 10 to 20 mmHg. The effect of infusion on fetal heart rate is less marked, but increases of up to 20 beats per minute may occur. In the treatment of premature labour, before Ventolin Solution for Intravenous Infusion is given to any patient with known heart disease, an adequate assessment of the patient's cardiovascular status should be made by a physician experienced in cardiology. In order to minimise the risk of hypotension associated with tocolytic therapy, special care should be taken to avoid caval compression by keeping the patient in the left or right lateral positions throughout the infusion.

Interaction with other medicaments and other forms of interaction: Ventolin Solution for Intravenous Infusion should not be administered in the same syringe or infusion as any other medication.

Salbutamol and non-selective β-blocking drugs such as propranolol, should not usually be prescribed together.

Pregnancy and lactation: Administration of drugs during pregnancy should only be considered if the expected benefit to the mother is greater than any possible risk to the fetus. As with the majority of drugs, there is little published evidence of the safety of salbutamol in the early stages of human pregnancy, but in animal studies there was evidence of some harmful effects on the fetus at very high dose levels.

As salbutamol is probably secreted in breast milk, its use in nursing mothers requires careful consideration. It is not known whether salbutamol has a harmful effect on the neonate, and so its use should be restricted to situations where it is felt that the expected benefit to the mother is likely to outweigh any potential risk to the neonate.

Effect on ability to drive and use machines: None reported.

Undesirable effects: Hypersensitivity reactions including angioedema, urticaria, bronchospasm, hypotension and collapse have been reported very rarely.

Enhancement of physiological tremor may occur with Ventolin Solution for Intravenous Infusion. This effect is caused by a direct action on skeletal muscle and is common to all β-adrenergic stimulants.

Tachycardia, with or without dilatation of peripheral arterioles leading to a small reduction in arterial pressure, may occur. Increases in heart rate are more likely to occur in patients with normal heart rates and these increases are dose-dependent. In patients with pre-existing sinus tachycardia, especially those in status asthmaticus, the heart rate tends to fall as the condition of the patient improves.

In common with other β_2 agonists, cardiac arrhythmias (including atrial fibrillation, supraventricular tachycardia and extrasystoles) have been reported in association with the use of salbutamol, usually in susceptible patients.

Maternal pulmonary oedema has been reported in association with use of β-agonists, including salbutamol, for the management of premature labour; in some cases this has proved fatal. Predisposing factors include fluid overload, multiple pregnancy, pre-existing cardiac disease and maternal infection. Close monitoring of the patient's state of hydration is essential. If signs of pulmonary oedema develop (e.g. cough, shortness of breath), treatment should be discontinued immediately and diuretic therapy instituted.

Headaches have occasionally been reported.

There have been very rare reports of muscle cramps.

Potentially serious hypokalaemia may result from β_2-agonist therapy.

In the management of premature labour, intravenous infusion of Ventolin has occasionally been associated with nausea, vomiting and headaches.

Overdose: The preferred antidote for overdosage with salbutamol is a cardioselective β-blocking agent, but β-blocking drugs should be used with caution in patients with a history of bronchospasm.

Hypokalaemia may occur following overdose with salbutamol. Serum potassium levels should be monitored.

Pharmacological properties
Pharmacodynamic properties: Salbutamol is a selective β_2-agonist which acts on the β_2-adrenoceptors of the bronchi and uterus.

Pharmacokinetic properties: Salbutamol administered intravenously has a half-life of 4 to 6 hours and is cleared partly renally and partly by metabolism to the inactive 4'-0-sulphate (phenolic sulphate) which is also excreted primarily in the urine. The faeces are a minor route of excretion. Most of a dose of salbutamol given intravenously, orally or by inhalation is excreted within 72 hours. Salbutamol is bound to plasma proteins to the extent of 10%.

Preclinical safety data: No additional preclinical safety data are included here.

Pharmaceutical particulars
List of excipients: Sodium chloride, sodium hydroxide, sulphuric acid and Water for Injections.

Incompatibilities: None stated.

Shelf life: 36 months.

Special precautions for storage: Store below 30°C and protect from light.

Nature and contents of container: Clear, neutral glass ampoules, available in boxes of 10.

Instructions for use/handling: Ventolin Solution for Intravenous Infusion must be diluted before use. The recommended diluents are Water for Injections BP, Sodium Chloride Injection BP, Sodium Chloride and Dextrose Injection BP and Dextrose Injection BP. (See *Posology and method of administration.*)

All unused admixtures of Ventolin Solution for Intravenous Infusion with infusion fluids should be discarded twenty-four hours after preparation.

Marketing authorisation number 10949/0087

Date of approval/revision of SPC June 1998.

Legal category POM.

VENTOLIN* SYRUP

Presentation Salbutamol 2 mg as Salbutamol Sulphate BP in each 5 ml of a fruit-flavoured, sugar-free syrup.

Other ingredients: Water, Sodium citrate, citric acid, hydroxypropylmethylcellulose, saccharin sodium, sodium chloride, sodium benzoate and orange flavour.

Uses Salbutamol is a selective β_2-agonist providing short-acting (4-6 hour) bronchodilatation in reversible airways obstruction.

Ventolin Syrup can be used in the management of asthma, bronchospasm and/or reversible airways obstruction.

Ventolin Syrup is suitable for children and adults who are unable to use an inhaler device.

Dosage and administration
Adults: The minimum starting dose is 2 mg (5 ml syrup) three times a day. The usual effective dose is 4 mg (10 ml syrup) three or four times a day, which may be increased to a maximum of 8 mg (20 ml syrup) three or four times a day if adequate bronchodilatation is not obtained.

In elderly patients, or in those known to be unusually sensitive to β-adrenergic stimulant drugs, it is advisable to initiate treatment with the minimum starting dose.

Children 2–6 years: The minimum starting dose is 1 mg (2.5 ml syrup) three times daily. This may be increased to 2 mg (5 ml syrup) three or four times daily.

6–12 years: The minimum starting dose is 2 mg (5 ml syrup) three times daily. This may be increased to four times daily.

Over 12 years: The minimum starting dose is 2 mg (5 ml syrup) three times daily. This may be increased to 4 mg (10 ml syrup) three or four times daily.

Contra-indications, warnings, etc
Contra-indications: Although intravenous salbutamol, and occasionally salbutamol tablets, are used in the management of premature labour uncomplicated by conditions such as placenta praevia, ante-partum haemorrhage or toxaemia of pregnancy, salbutamol preparations should not be used for threatened abortion.

Ventolin Syrup is contra-indicated in patients with a history of hypersensitivity to any of the components.

Precautions: Bronchodilators should not be the only or main treatment in patients with severe or unstable asthma. Severe asthma requires regular medical assessment, including lung-function testing, as patients are at risk of severe attacks and even death. Physicians should consider using the maximum recommended dose of inhaled corticosteroid and/or oral corticosteroid therapy in these patients.

Patients should seek medical advice if treatment with Ventolin Syrup becomes less effective.

The dosage or frequency of administration should only be increased on medical advice.

Patients taking Ventolin Syrup may also be receiving short-acting inhaled bronchodilators to relieve symptoms. Increasing use of bronchodilators, in particular short-acting inhaled β_2-agonists to relieve symptoms, indicates deterioration of asthma control. The patient should be instructed to seek medical advice if short-acting relief bronchodilator treatment becomes less effective, or more inhalations than usual are required. In this situation the patient should be assessed and consideration given to the need for increased anti-inflammatory therapy (e.g. higher doses of inhaled corticosteroid or a course of oral corticosteroid).

Severe exacerbations of asthma must be treated in the normal way.

Salbutamol should be administered cautiously to patients suffering from thyrotoxicosis.

Salbutamol and non-selective β-blocking drugs such as propranolol, should not usually be prescribed together.

Potentially serious hypokalaemia may result from β_2-agonist therapy, mainly from parenteral and nebulised administration. Particular caution is advised in acute severe asthma as this effect may be potentiated by hypoxia and by concomitant treatment with xanthine derivatives, steroids and diuretics. Serum potassium levels should be monitored in such situations.

In common with other β-adrenoceptor agonists, salbutamol can induce reversible metabolic changes such as increased blood glucose levels. Diabetic patients may be unable to compensate for the increase in blood glucose and the development of ketoacidosis has been reported. Concurrent administration of corticosteroids can exaggerate this effect.

Pregnancy: Administration of drugs during pregnancy should only be considered if the expected benefit to the mother is greater than any possible risk to the fetus. However, as with the majority of drugs, there is little published evidence of the safety of salbutamol in the early stages of human pregnancy, but in animal studies there was evidence of some harmful effects on the fetus at very high dose levels.

Lactation: As salbutamol is probably secreted in breast milk, its use in nursing mothers requires careful consideration. It is not known whether salbutamol has a harmful effect on the neonate and so its use should be restricted to situations where it is felt that the expected benefit to the mother is likely to outweigh any potential risk to the neonate.

Side-effects: Hypersensitivity reactions including angioedema, urticaria, bronchospasm, hypotension and collapse have been reported very rarely.

Potentially serious hypokalaemia may result from β_2-agonist therapy.

Ventolin Syrup may cause a fine tremor of skeletal muscle, usually the hands are most obviously affected. This effect is dose-related and is common to all β-adrenergic stimulants. A few patients feel tense. This is also due to the effects on skeletal muscle and not to direct CNS stimulation.

Tachycardia, with or without peripheral vasodilatation, may rarely occur.

In common with other β_2 agonists, cardiac arrhythmias (including atrial fibrillation, supraventricular tachycardia and extrasystoles) have been reported in association with the use of salbutamol, usually in susceptible patients.

Headaches have occasionally been reported.

As with other β_2-agonists hyperactivity in children has been reported rarely.

There have been very rare reports of muscle cramps.

Overdosage: The preferred antidote for overdosage with salbutamol is a cardioselective β-blocking agent, but β-blocking drugs should be used with caution in patients with a history of bronchospasm.

Hypokalaemia may occur following overdose with salbutamol. Serum potassium levels should be monitored.

Pharmaceutical precautions Ventolin Syrup should be stored at a temperature not exceeding 30°C. Ventolin Syrup should be protected from light.

Dilution: Ventolin Syrup does not contain sugars. It may be diluted with Purified Water BP. The resulting mixture should be protected from light and used within 28 days. A 50% v/v dilution of Ventolin Syrup has been shown to be adequately preserved against microbial contamination. However, to avoid the possibility of introducing excessive microbial contamination, the Purified Water used for dilution should be recently prepared or alternatively it should be boiled and cooled immediately before use. Dilution of Ventolin Syrup with Syrup BP or Sorbitol solutions is not recommended as this may result in precipitation of the cellulose thickening agent. Admixture of Ventolin Syrup with other liquid preparations is not recommended.

Legal category POM.

Package quantities Ventolin Syrup is supplied in bottles of 150 ml.

Further information Ventolin Syrup preparation does not contain sugars, so it is unlikely to predispose to dental caries with long-term use. It does not contain any artificial colouring agent.

Ventolin Syrup does not cause difficulty in micturition because, unlike sympathomimetic drugs such as ephedrine, salbutamol does not stimulate alpha-adrenoceptors.

Ventolin Syrup is not contra-indicated in patients under treatment with monoamine oxidase inhibitors (MAOIs).

Product licence number 10949/0088

VOLMAX* TABLETS

Presentation *Volmax Tablets 4 mg*: White hexagonal controlled-release tablets each containing 4 mg salbutamol as Salbutamol Sulphate BP. Printed 4 on one side.

Volmax Tablets 8 mg: White hexagonal controlled-release tablets each containing 8 mg salbutamol as Salbutamol Sulphate BP. Printed 8 on one side.

Other ingredients: The tablet core contains sodium chloride, silica gel, povidone, croscarmellose sodium and magnesium stearate. The outer coats contain cellulose acetate, hydroxypropylmethylcellulose and E171 (titanium dioxide). The numbers '4' or '8' are printed with E132 (indigo carmine).

The tablets consist of an outer semi-permeable membrane and an inner core containing salbutamol sulphate. There is a hole in the outer coat which allows a gradual osmotically controlled release of the drug.

Uses Salbutamol is a selective β_2-adrenoceptor agonist.

Volmax Tablets are indicated for the treatment of asthma, bronchospasm and/or reversible airways obstruction.

Volmax Tablets are suitable oral therapy for children and adults who are unable to use an inhaler device. In these patients the controlled-release formulation makes Volmax Tablets helpful in the management of nocturnal asthma.

Dosage and administration Volmax Tablets must be swallowed whole with a glass of water and not chewed or crushed.

Volmax Tablets sustain bronchodilatation over a period of 12 hours.

Adults (including the elderly): One 8 mg tablet twice daily.

Children aged 3-12 years: One 4 mg tablet twice daily.

Contra-indications, warnings, etc

Contra-indications: Although intravenous salbutamol, and occasionally salbutamol tablets, are used in the management of premature labour uncomplicated by conditions such as placenta praevia, ante-partum haemorrhage or toxaemia of pregnancy, salbutamol preparations should not be used for threatened abortion.

Volmax Tablets are contra-indicated in patients with a history of hypersensitivity to any of the components.

Precautions: Bronchodilators should not be the only or main treatment in patients with severe or unstable asthma. Severe asthma requires regular medical assessment, including lung-function testing, as patients are at risk of severe attacks and even death. Physicians should consider using the maximum recommended dose of inhaled corticosteroid and/or oral corticosteroid therapy in these patients.

Patients should seek medical advice if treatment with Volmax Tablets becomes less effective.

The dosage or frequency of administration should only be increased on medical advice.

Patients taking Volmax Tablets may also be receiving short-acting inhaled bronchodilators to relieve symptoms. Increasing use of bronchodilators, in particular short-acting inhaled β_2-agonists to relieve symptoms, indicates deterioration of asthma control. The patient should be instructed to seek medical advice if short-acting relief bronchodilator treatment becomes less effective, or more inhalations than usual are required. In this situation the patient should be assessed and consideration given to the need for increased anti-inflammatory therapy (e.g. higher doses of inhaled corticosteroid or a course of oral corticosteroid).

Severe exacerbations of asthma must be treated in the normal way.

Salbutamol should be administered cautiously to patients suffering from thyrotoxicosis.

Salbutamol and non-selective β-blocking drugs such as propranolol, should not usually be prescribed together.

Potentially serious hypokalaemia may result from β_2-agonist therapy, mainly from parenteral and nebulised administration. Particular caution is advised in acute severe asthma as this effect may be potentiated by hypoxia and by concomitant treatment with xanthine derivatives, steroids and diuretics. Serum potassium levels should be monitored in such situations.

In common with other β-adrenoceptor agonists, salbutamol can induce reversible metabolic changes such as increased blood glucose levels. Diabetic patients may be unable to compensate for the increase in blood glucose and the development of ketoacidosis has been reported. Concurrent administration of corticosteroids can exaggerate this effect.

Pregnancy: Administration of drugs during pregnancy should only be considered if the expected benefit to the mother is greater than any possible risk to the fetus. As with the majority of drugs, there is little published evidence of the safety of salbutamol in the early stages of human pregnancy, but in animal studies there was evidence of some harmful effects on the fetus at very high dose levels.

Lactation: As salbutamol is probably secreted in breast milk, its use in nursing mothers requires careful consideration. It is not known whether salbutamol has a harmful effect on the neonate and so its use should be restricted to situations where it is felt that the expected benefit to the mother is likely to outweigh any potential risk to the neonate.

Side-effects: Hypersensitivity reactions including angioedema, urticaria, bronchospasm, hypotension and collapse have been reported very rarely.

Potentially serious hypokalaemia may result from β_2-agonist therapy.

Volmax Tablets may cause a fine tremor of skeletal muscle, usually the hands are most obviously affected. This effect is common to all β-adrenergic stimulants. A few patients feel tense. This is also due to the effects on skeletal muscle and not to direct CNS stimulation.

Tachycardia, with or without peripheral vasodilatation, may rarely occur.

In common with other β_2 agonists, cardiac arrhythmias (including atrial fibrillation, supraventricular tachycardia and extrasystoles) have been reported in association with the use of salbutamol, usually in susceptible patients.

Headaches have occasionally been reported.

As with other β_2-agonists hyperactivity in children has been reported rarely.

There have been very rare reports of muscle cramps.

Overdosage: The preferred antidote for overdosage with salbutamol is a cardioselective beta-blocking agent, but β-blocking drugs should be used with caution in patients with a history of bronchospasm.

Hypokalaemia may occur following overdose with salbutamol. Serum potassium levels should be monitored.

Pharmaceutical precautions Volmax Tablets should be stored at a temperature not exceeding 30°C. Volmax Tablets should not be removed from their foil pack until required.

Legal category POM.

Package quantities Volmax Tablets are supplied in double-foil blisters of 14 in cartons of 56.

Further information Volmax Tablets do not cause difficulty in micturition because, unlike sympathomimetic drugs such as ephedrine, salbutamol does not stimulate alpha-adrenoceptors.

Volmax Tablets are not contra-indicated in patients under treatment with monoamine oxidase inhibitors (MAOIs).

Product licence numbers
Volmax Tablets 4 mg 10949/0089
Volmax Tablets 8 mg 10949/0090

**Trade Mark*

Allergan Ltd
Coronation Road
High Wycombe
Bucks HP12 3SH

☎ 01494 444722 🗋 01494 473593, 01494 436871

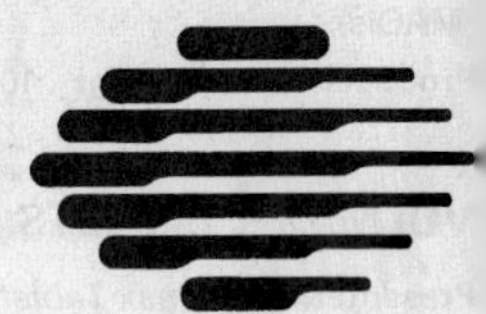

ACULAR* ▼

Qualitative and quantitative composition Ketorolac trometamol 0.5% w/v.

Pharmaceutical form Eye drops.

Clinical particulars

Therapeutic indications: Acular is indicated for the prophylaxis and reduction of inflammation and associated symptoms following ocular surgery.

Posology and method of administration

Route of administration: Ocular.

One drop instilled into the eye three times daily starting 24 hours pre-operatively and continuing for up to three weeks post-operatively.

No special dosage for the elderly.

Contra-indications: Acular is contra-indicated in individuals hypersensitive to any component of the medication.

The potential exists for cross-sensitivity to acetylsalicylic acid and other non-steroidal anti-inflammatory drugs. Acular is contra-indicated in individuals who have previously exhibited sensitivities to these drugs.

Acular is contra-indicated in children and during pregnancy or lactation.

Special warnings and special precautions for use: It is recommended that Acular be used with caution in patients with known bleeding tendencies or who are receiving other medications which may prolong bleeding time, or patients with a known history of peptic ulceration.

In common with other anti-inflammatory drugs, Acular may mask signs of infection.

Acular contains benzalkonium chloride as a preservative and should not be used in patients continuing to wear soft (hydrophilic) contact lenses.

Interactions with other medicaments and other forms of interaction: Acular has been safely administered with systemic and ophthalmic medications such as antibiotics, sedatives, beta blockers, carbonic anhydrase inhibitors, miotics, mydriatics, cycloplegics and corticosteroids.

Pregnancy and lactation: There was no evidence of teratogenicity in rats or rabbits studied at maternally-toxic doses of ketorolac. Prolongation of the gestation period and/or delayed parturition were seen in the rat. Ketorolac and its metabolites have been shown to pass into the foetus and milk of animals. Ketorolac has been detected in human milk at low levels. Safety in human pregnancy has not been established. Ketorolac is therefore contra-indicated during pregnancy, labour or delivery, or in mothers who are breast feeding.

Effects on ability to drive and use machines: Transient blurring of vision may occur on installation of eye drops. Do not drive or use hazardous machinery unless vision is clear.

Undesirable effects: The most frequent adverse events reported with the use of Acular are transient stinging and burning on instillation and other minor symptoms of ocular irritation.

Blurring and/or diminished vision have been reported with the use of Acular and other non-steroidal anti-inflammatory drugs.

None of the typical adverse reactions reported with the systemic non-steroidal anti-inflammatory agents (including ketorolac trometamol) have been observed at the doses used in topical ophthalmic therapy.

Overdose: There is no experience of overdose by the ophthalmic route. Overdose is unlikely to occur via the recommended method of administration.

Pharmacological properties

Pharmacodynamic properties: Pharmacotherapeutic classification (ATC): SO1B C.

Acular (ketorolac trometamol) is a non-steroidal anti-inflammatory agent demonstrating analgesic and anti-inflammatory activity. Ketorolac trometamol inhibits the cyclo-oxygenase enzyme essential for biosynthesis of prostaglandins. Acular has been shown to reduce prostaglandin levels in the aqueous humour after topical ophthalmic administration.

Ketorolac trometamol given systemically does not cause pupil constriction. Results from clinical studies indicate that Acular has no significant effect on intraocular pressure.

Pharmacokinetic properties

(a) *General characteristics*

Absorption

Rabbit aqueous humour bioavailability:

Mean concentration of total radioactivity	
	0.856 g-equiv./ml @ 0.5 hr
	1.607 g-equiv./ml @ 2 hr
T_{max}	3.38 hr
C_{max}	1.905 g-equiv./ml
AUC (0–8 hr)	9.39 g-equiv. hr/ml
Total AUC	13.53 g-equiv. hr/ml
Half-life	3.77 hr
Absolute ocular bioavailability	3.7%

After topical ocular doses in the rabbit the half life of total radioactivity in aqueous humour was longer than after intracameral injection. This suggests that topical dosing may lead to a 'reservoir' effect in the corneal epithelium and continued flux of drug from the reservoir into the aqueous humour.

Distribution: After ophthalmic doses were administered to rabbits, peak concentrations of radioactivity were achieved within 1 hour in the ocular tissues and were highest in the cornea (6.06 mcg-eq./ml). At 1 hour, the majority of the radioactivity (0.9% of administered dose) was recovered from the sclera (0.58%) and cornea (0.24%), and smaller amounts were recovered from the aqueous humour (0.026%), vitreous humour (0.023%), retina-choroid (0.018%), irisciliary body (0.007%) and lens (0.002%).

Relative to plasma AUC values, the AUC's in rabbits were higher for cornea (104 fold), sclera (27 fold), irisciliary body (5.8 fold), retin-choroid (5.6 fold) aqueous humour (3.3 fold) and approximately one-half in the vitreous humour and lens. After ophthalmic administration, concentrations of drug-related radioactivity were higher in the ocular tissues and lower in plasma compared with those after IV dosing.

Systemic absorption: After ophthalmic doses in the rabbit, ketorolac was absorbed rapidly into the systemic circulation (T_{max}, 15 min). Plasma half-lives after ophthalmic doses (6.6–6.9 hr) were longer than those after IV administration (1.1 hr), suggesting that removal of drug from eye into the venous circulation may be rate-limiting. By comparison of drug levels in aqueous humour after intracameral injection vs. plasma levels after IV administration, ketorolac was shown to clear more rapidly from plasma (6 ml/min) than from the anterior chamber (11 mcl/min).

In the cynomolgus monkey, peak plasma levels of ketorolac occurred at 1.1 hr after the ophthalmic dose. The plasma half-life of ketorolac was similar after ophthalmic (1.8 hr) and IV doses (1.6 hr).

The majority of the ophthalmic dose was excreted in urine (66% in rabbit and 75% in monkey) and a small amount in faeces (11% in rabbit and 2% in monkey). The extent of systemic absorption after ophthalmic dosing averaged 73% in the rabbit and 76% in the cynomolgus monkey.

Metabolism: After ophthalmic administration in rabbits, ketorolac represented the major component (more than 90%) of radioactivity in aqueous humour and plasma and the p-hydroxy metabolite accounted for 5% of radioactivity in plasma. Ketorolac was also the major component (96%) of plasma radioactivity after ophthalmic dosing in monkeys.

After ophthalmic dosing in the rabbit, 72%, 17% and 6% of the total radioactivity in urine was comprised of intact ketorolac, p-hydroxy ketorolac and other polar metabolites, respectively. After IV dosing, the relative proportions of total radioactivity in urine averaged 6% as intact ketorolac, 68% as p-hydroxy ketorolac and 22% as polar metabolites.

In the monkey, intact ketorolac and its polar metabolite accounted for 32% and 65% of the total radioactivity in urine, respectively, after ophthalmic dosing, and 50% and 49% of the radioactivity in urine, respectively, after IV dosing. Thus, the metabolism of ketorolac was qualitatively similar after ophthalmic and IV administration in the monkey and rabbit.

(b) *Characteristics in patients:* Ketorolac tromethamine solutions (0.1% or 0.5%) or vehicle were instilled into the eyes of patients approximately 12 hours and 1 hour prior to surgery. Concentrations of ketorolac in aqueous humor sampled at the time of surgery were at the lower limit of detection (40 ng/ml) in 1 patient and below the quantitation limit in 7 patients dosed with 0.1% ketorolac tromethamine. The average aqueous humor level of ketorolac in patients treated with 0.5% ketorolac tromethamine was 95/ng/ml. Concentrations of PGE_2 in aqueous humor were 80 pg/ml, 40 pg/ml and 28 pg/ml in patients treated with vehicle, 0.1% ketorolac tromethamine and 0.5% ketorolac tromethamine, respectively.

In the 21-day multiple dose (TID) tolerance study in healthy subjects, only 1 of 13 subjects had a detectable plasma level pre-dose (0.21 μg/ml). In another group of 13 subjects, only 4 subjects showed very low plasma levels of ketorolac (0.011 to 0.023 μg/ml) 15 minutes after the ocular dose.

Thus, higher levels of ketorolac in the aqueous humor and very low or no detectable plasma levels after ophthalmic doses, suggest that the use of ketorolac tromethamine by the ophthalmic route in treatment of ocular disorders results in quite low systemic absorption in patients.

Preclinical safety data: Acute, sub-acute and chronic studies of Acular in experimental animals have established the safety of the drug. In addition, octoxynol 40 was separately evaluated for its ocular safety. Acular was found to be non-irritating, it did not demonstrate a local anaesthetic effect, it did not influence the healing of experimental corneal wounds in rabbits, it did not enhance the spread of experimental ocular infections of *Candida albicans, Herpes simplex* virus type one, or *Pseudomonas aeruginosa* in rabbits, and it did not increase the ocular pressure of normal rabbit eyes.

Pharmaceutical particulars

List of excipients: Sodium chloride PhEur, Benzalkonium chloride PhEur, Edetate disodium PhEur, Octoxynol 40, 1 N sodium hydroxide PhEur or 1 N hydrochloric acid PhEur, to adjust pH, Purified water PhEur.

Incompatibilities: None known.

Shelf life: 24 months, unopened. Discard any unused contents 28 days after opening the bottle.

Special precautions for storage: None.

Nature and contents of container: Bottle with dropper applicator, containing clear, colourless to slightly yellow, sterile ophthalmic solution. Pack size: 5 ml.

Instruction for use/handling: None.

Marketing authorisation number PL 0426/0082

Date of approval/revision of SPC March 1996

ALPHAGAN* 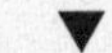

Qualitative and quantitative composition Brimonidine tartrate 0.2% (2.0 mg/ml) (equivalent to brimonidine base 0.13%, 1.3 mg/ml); 1 drop of Alphagan*=approximately 35 μl=70 μg brimonidine tartrate.

Pharmaceutical form Eye drops, solution.

Clinical particulars

Therapeutic indications: Alphagan may be used as monotherapy for the lowering of intraocular pressure (IOP) in patients with open angle glaucoma or ocular hypertension, who are known, or thought likely to be intolerant of topical betablocker therapy and/or in whom topical betablocker therapy is contra-indicated. Alphagan may be used as adjunctive therapy when IOP is not adequately controlled by a topical betablocking agent.

Posology and method of administration: The recommended dose is one drop of Alphagan in the affected eye(s) twice daily, approximately 12 hours apart. No dosage adjustment is required for use in elderly patients.

As with any eye drops, to reduce possible systemic absorption, it is recommended that the lachrymal sac be compressed at the medial canthus (punctal occlusion) for one minute. This should be performed immediately following the instillation of each drop.

If more than one topical ophthalmic drug is to be used, the different drugs should be instilled 5–15 minutes apart.

Alphagan has not been studied in patients with hepatic or renal impairment – see *Special warnings and special precautions for use.*

The safety and effectiveness of Alphagan in children has not been established (see *Special warnings and special precautions for use*).

Contra-indications: Alphagan is contra-indicated in patients with hypersensitivity to brimonidine tartrate or any component of this medication. Alphagan is also contra-indicated in patients receiving monoamine oxidase (MAO) inhibitor therapy and patients on antidepressants which affect noradrenergic transmission (e.g. tricyclic antidepressants and mianserin).

Special warnings and special precautions for use: Symptoms of brimonidine overdose have been reported in a few neonates receiving Alphagan as part of medical treatment of congenital glaucoma.

Caution should be exercised in treating patients with severe or unstable and uncontrolled cardiovascular disease.

Some (12.7%) patients in clinical trials experienced an ocular allergic type reaction with Alphagan (see *Undesirable effects*). If allergic reactions are observed, treatment with Alphagan should be discontinued.

Alphagan should be used with caution in patients with depression, cerebral or coronary insufficiency, Raynaud's phenomenon, orthostatic hypotension or thromboangiitis obliterans.

Alphagan has not been studied in patients with hepatic or renal impairment; caution should be used in treating such patients.

The preservative in Alphagan, benzalkonium chloride, may be absorbed by soft contact lenses. Patients wearing soft (hydrophilic) contact lenses should be instructed to wait at least 15 minutes before inserting soft contact lenses after instilling Alphagan.

Interaction with other medicaments and other forms of interaction: Although specific drug interaction studies have not been conducted with Alphagan, the possibility of an additive or potentiating effect with CNS depressants (alcohol, barbiturates, opiates, sedatives, or anaesthetics) should be considered.

No data on the level of circulating catecholamines after Alphagan administration are available. Caution, however, is advised in patients taking medications which can affect the metabolism and uptake of circulating amines e.g. chlorpromazine, methylphenidate, reserpine.

After the application of Alphagan, clinically insignificant decreases in blood pressure were noted in some patients. Caution is advised when using drugs such as antihypertensives and/or cardiac glycosides concomitantly with Alphagan.

Caution is advised when initiating (or changing the dose of) a concomitant systemic agent (irrespective of the pharmaceutical form) which may interact with alpha-adrenergic agonists or interfere with their activity i.e. agonists or antagonists of the adrenergic receptor e.g. (isoprenaline, prazosin).

Pregnancy and lactation: The safety of use during human pregnancy has not been established. In animal studies, brimonidine tartrate did not cause any teratogenic effects. In rabbits, brimonidine tartrate, at plasma levels higher than are achieved during therapy in humans, has been shown to cause increased preimplantation loss and postnatal growth reduction. Alphagan should be used during pregnancy only if the potential benefit to the mother justifies the potential risk to the foetus.

Use during lactation: It is not known brimonidine is excreted in human milk. The compound is excreted in the milk of the lactating rat. Alphagan should not be used by women nursing infants.

Effects on ability to drive and use machines: Alphagan may cause fatigue and/or drowsiness, which may impair the ability to drive or operate machinery.

Undesirable effects:

Ocular effects: The most frequently reported ocular adverse events (in descending order of incidence) were ocular hyperaemia, ocular burning/stinging, blurring, foreign body sensation, conjunctival follicles, ocular allergic reactions and ocular pruritus. Some patients experienced several of these symptoms and/or signs which collectively were considered to be an ocular allergic reaction. This occurred in 12.7% of subjects (causing withdrawal in 11.5% of subjects) in clinical trials and the onset was between 3 and 9 months in the majority of patients. Where data are available in subjects who withdrew from the studies due to ocular allergic reactions, all the symptoms resolved without long term sequelae upon discontinuation of therapy.

Ocular events occurring occasionally included: corneal erosion/staining, photophobia, eyelid hyperaemia, ocular ache/pain, ocular dryness, tearing, eyelid oedema, conjunctival oedema, blepharitis, conjunctival blanching, ocular irritation, abnormal vision, conjunctival discharge and conjunctivitis.

Systemic effects: The most frequently reported systemic effects were oral dryness, headache and fatigue/drowsiness.

Occasional reports included upper respiratory symptoms, dizziness, gastrointestinal symptoms, asthenia and abnormal taste.

Rarely reported systemic events included depression, systemic allergic reaction, nasal dryness and palpitations. However, symptoms of brimonidine overdose such as hypotension, bradycardia, hypothermia and apnea have been reported in a few neonates receiving Alphagan as part of medical treatment of congenital glaucoma.

Overdose: Ophthalmic overdose: There is no experience with the unlikely case of an overdosage via the ophthalmic route.

Systemic overdose resulting from accidental ingestion: No incidences of human adult ingestion of Alphagan are known. Oral overdoses of other alpha-2-agonists have been reported to cause symptoms such as hypotension, asthenia, vomiting, lethargy, sedation, bradycardia, arrhythmias, miosis, apnae, hypotonia, hypothermia, respiratory depression and seizure.

Pharmacological properties

Pharmacodynamic properties: Brimonidine is an alpha-2 adrenergic receptor agonist that is 1000-fold more selective for the alpha-2 adrenoreceptor than the alpha-1 adrenoreceptor.

This selectivity results in no mydriasis and the absence of vasoconstriction in microvessels associated with human retinal xenografts.

Topical administration of brimonidine decreases intraocular pressure (IOP) in humans with minimal effect on cardiovascular or pulmonary parameters. Limited data are available for patients with bronchial asthma showing no adverse effects.

Alphagan has a rapid onset of action, with peak ocular hypotensive effect seen at two hours post-dosing. In two 1 year studies, Alphagan lowered IOP by mean values of approximately 4–6 mmHg.

Fluorophotometric studies in animals and humans suggest that brimonidine tartrate has a dual mechanism of action. It is thought that Alphagan may lower IOP by reducing aqueous humour formation and enhancing uveoscleral outflow.

Pharmacokinetic properties:

a) General characteristics: After ocular administration of a 0.2% solution twice daily for 10 days, plasma concentrations were low (mean Cmax was 0.06 ng/ml). There was a slight accumulation in the blood after multiple (2 times daily for 10 days) instillations. The area under the plasma concentration-time curve over 12 hours at steady state (AUC_{0-12h}) was 0.31 ng·hr/ml, as compared to 0.23 ng·hr/ml after the first dose. The mean apparent half-life in the systemic circulation was approximately 3 hours in humans after topical dosing.

The plasma protein binding of brimonidine after topical dosing in humans is approximately 29%.

Brimonidine binds reversibly to melanin in ocular tissues, in vitro and in vivo. Following 2 weeks of ocular instillation, the concentrations of brimonidine in iris, ciliary body and choroid-retina were 3- to 17-fold higher than those after a single dose. Accumulation does not occur in the absence of melanin.

The significance of melanin binding in humans is unclear. However, no significant ocular adverse reaction was found during biomicroscopic examination of eyes in patients treated with Alphagan for up to one year, nor was significant ocular toxicity found during a one year ocular safety study in monkeys given approximately four times the recommended dose of brimonidine tartrate.

Following oral administration to man, brimonidine is well absorbed and rapidly eliminated. The major part of the dose (around 75% of the dose) was excreted as metabolites in urine within five days; no unchanged drug was detected in urine. In vitro studies, using animal and human liver, indicate that the metabolism is mediated largely by aldehyde oxidase and cytochrome P450. Hence, the systemic elimination seems to be primarily hepatic metabolism.

Kinetics profile: No great deviation from dose proportionality for plasma C_{max} and AUC was observed following a single topical dose of 0.08%, 0.2% and 0.5%.

b) Characteristics in elderly patients: The C_{max}, AUC, and apparent half-life of brimonidine are similar in the elderly (subjects 65 years or older) after a single dose compared with young adults, indicating that its systemic absorption and elimination are not affected by age.

Based on data from a 3 month clinical study, which included elderly patients, system exposure to brimonidine was very low.

Preclinical safety data: The available mutagenicity and carcinogenicity data indicate that Alphagan will not exert neither mutagenic nor carcinogenic activities under the conditions of clinical use.

Pharmaceutical particulars

List of excipients: Benzalkonium Chloride (Preservative) 0.005% (0.05 mg/ml); Polyvinyl alcohol 1.4% (14 mg/ml); Sodium chloride; Sodium citrate, dihydrate; Citric acid, monohydrate; Purified water; Hydrochloric acid/or Sodium hydroxide to adjust pH.

Incompatibilities: Physical and chemical incompatibilities have not been observed.

Shelf life: Alphagan has a shelf life of 36 months in the unopened 5.0 container. Use within 28 days after first opening.

Special precautions for storage: Alphagan should be stored at or below 25°C (77°F).

Nature and contents of container: White low density polyethylene dropper bottles with a 35 microlitre tip. The cap is either a conventional screw cap or a Compliance Cap (C-Cap). Alphagan is available as 5 ml pack.

Instructions for use/handling: None.

Marketing authorisation number PL 00426/0088

Date of approval/revision of SPC September 1998

Legal category POM

BETAGAN*

Presentation Betagan is a clear, colourless to light yellow, sterile ophthalmic solution containing levobunolol hydrochloride 0.5% (w/v). Also contains Liquifilm* (polyvinyl alcohol USP) 1.4% (w/v), benzalkonium chloride PhEur 0.004% (w/v), disodium edetate PhEur 0.0127% (w/v), with sodium metabisulphite BP, sodium phosphate dibasic USP, potassium phosphate monobasic USP, sodium chloride PhEur and purified water PhEur.

Uses Betagan is indicated for the reduction of intraocular pressure in chronic open-angle glaucoma and ocular hypertension.

Dosage and administration The recommended adult dose is one drop of Betagan in the affected eye(s) once or twice daily.

In common with other topical ophthalmic beta-adrenergic blocking agents, full clinical response may take several weeks to occur. Intraocular pressure should, therefore, be measured approximately four weeks after starting treatment. Because of diurnal variations in intraocular pressure satisfactory response is best determined by measuring the intraocular pressure at different times during the day.

Use in the elderly: The recommended dosage is suitable for use in the elderly.

Use in children: Betagan is not currently recommended for use in children.

Concomitant administration: If the patient's intraocular pressure is not satisfactory on this regimen, concomitant therapy with dipivefrin or adrenaline, and/or pilocarpine and other miotics, and/or systemically administered carbonic anhydrase inhibitors can be instituted.

Contra-indications, warnings, etc

Contra-indications: Bronchial asthma; history of bronchial asthma; chronic obstructive pulmonary disease; sinus bradycardia; second and third degree atrioventricular block; cardiac failure; cardiogenic shock; hypersensitivity to any component.

Warnings: As with other topically applied ophthalmic drugs, Betagan may be absorbed systemically and adverse reactions typical of oral beta-adrenoceptor blocking agents may occur.

Respiratory and cardiac reactions have been reported including, rarely, death due to bronchospasm or associated with cardiac failure.

Congestive heart failure should be adequately controlled before commencing therapy with Betagan. In patients with a history of cardiac disease pulse rates should be monitored.

Diabetic control should be monitored during Betagan therapy in patients with labile diabetes.

Betagan contains benzalkonium chloride and should not be used in patients continuing to wear hydrophilic (soft) contact lenses.

Betagan has little or no effect on pupil size and if administered in angle-closure glaucoma, for reduction of intraocular pressure, must only be given in combination with a miotic.

Use in pregnancy: Betagan has not been studied in human pregnancy. It is recommended that Betagan be avoided in pregnancy.

Use during lactation: If treatment with Betagan during lactation is considered necessarily for the benefit of the mother, consideration should be given to the cessation of breast feeding.

Interactions: Use with caution in patients receiving oral beta-adrenergic blocking agents, because of the potential for additive effects on systemic blockade.

Side effects:

Ocular: Transient burning and stinging on instillation; blepharoconjunctivitis and iridocyclitis have been reported occasionally. The pharmacological and physical properties of levobunolol indicate a potential for post-instillation reduction in corneal sensitivity: this potential has not been confirmed in clinical studies with Betagan.

Cardiovascular: Bradycardia and hypotension have been reported occasionally.

Respiratory: There have been reports of dyspnoea and asthma.

CNS: Headache, transient ataxia and dizziness, and lethargy have been reported occasionally.

Dermatological: Urticaria and pruritis have been rarely reported.

Overdosage: There are no data available on human overdosage with Betagan, which is unlikely to occur via the ocular route. Should accidental ocular overdosage occur, flush the eye(s) with water or normal saline. If accidentally ingested, systemic symptoms may result.

The symptoms associated with systemic overdosage are most likely to be bradycardia, hypotension, bronchospasm and cardiac failure. Therapy for overdosage of a beta-adrenergic blocking agent should be instituted, such as intravenous administration of atropine sulphate 0.25 to 2 mg to induce vagal blockade. Conventional therapy for hypotension, bronchospasm, heart block and cardiac failure may be necessary.

Pharmaceutical precautions Betagan should be stored at or below 25°C and protected from light. Discard any unused contents 28 days after opening the bottle. Keep out of the reach of children.

Legal category POM.

Package quantities Betagan is supplied in plastic dropper bottles containing 5 ml of 0.5% w/v solution or in a triple pack (3×5 ml bottles).

Further information In controlled clinical studies of approximately two years duration, intraocular pressure was well controlled in approximately 80% of subjects treated with Betagan 0.5% b.i.d. No significant effect on pupil size, tear production or corneal sensitivity was observed.

In a 3 month study, one drop once-a-day of Betagan 0.5% controlled intraocular pressure in 72% of subjects.

The onset of action is detected within one hour of instillation, with maximum effect seen between 2 and 6 hours.

A significant decrease in intraocular pressure can be maintained for up to 24 hours following a single dose.

Diminished response after prolonged therapy has been reported in some patients.

Product licence number PL 0426/0060

Legal category POM

BETAGAN* UNIT DOSE

Qualitative and quantitative composition Levobunolol hydrochloride 0.5% USP.

Pharmaceutical form Sterile aqueous ophthalmic solution.

Clinical particulars

Therapeutic indications: Reduction of intraocular pressure in chronic open-angle glaucoma and ocular hypertension

Posology and method of administration

Adults including the elderly: The recommended adult dose is one drop of Betagan Unit Dose once or twice daily in the affected eye(s). Discard product after use.

Children: Use in children is not currently recommended.

Contra-indications: Bronchial asthma; history of bronchial asthma; chronic obstructive pulmonary disease; sinus bradycardia; second and third degree atrioventricular block; cardiac failure; cardiogenic shock; hypersensitivity to any component.

Special warnings and special precautions for use: As with other topically applied ophthalmic drugs, Betagan may be absorbed systemically.

Interactions: Betagan may have additive effects in patients taking systemic antihypertensive drugs. These possible effects may include hypotension, including orthostatic hypotension, bradycardia, dizziness and/or syncope. Conversely, systemic beta-adrenoceptor blocking agents may potentiate the ocular hypotensive effect of Betagan.

Betagan may potentially add to the effects of oral calcium antagonists, rauwolfia alkaloids or beta blockers to induce hypotension and/or marked bradycardia.

Pregnancy and Lactation: There are no adequate and well-controlled studies in pregnant women. Levobunolol should be used during pregnancy only if the potential benefit justifies the potential risk to the foetus.

It is not known whether this drug is excreted in human milk. Systemic beta-blockers and topical Timolol maleate are known to be excreted in human milk. Because similar drugs are excreted in human milk, caution should be exercised when Betagan is administered to a nursing woman.

Effects on ability to drive and use machines: None known.

Undesirable effects: Blepharoconjunctivitis, transient ocular burning, stinging, and decreases in heart rate and blood pressure have been reported occasionally with the use of Betagan. Urticaria has been reported rarely with the use of Betagan.

The following adverse effects have been reported rarely and a definite relationship with the use of Betagan has not been established: change in heart rhythm, iridocyclitis, browache, headache, transient ataxia, lethargy, urticaria, elevated liver enzymes, eructation, dizziness and itching.

The following additional adverse reactions have been reported with opthalmic use of $beta_1$ and $beta_2$ non selective blocking agents:

Special senses: conjunctivitis, blepharitis, keratitis and decreased corneal sensitivity, visual disturbances, including refractory changes, diplopia and ptosis.

Cardiovascular: bradycardia, hypotension, sycope, heartblock, cerebrovascular accident, cerebral ischaemia, congestive heart failure, palpitation and cardiac arrest.

Respiratory: bronchospasm, respiratory failure and dyspnea.

Body as a whole: asthenia, nausea and depression.

Overdosage: There are no data available on human overdosage with Betagan which is unlikely to occur via the ocular route. Should accidental ocular overdosage occur, flush the eye(s) with water or normal saline. If accidentally ingested, efforts to decrease further absorption may be appropriate.

Pharmacological properties

Pharmacodynamic properties: Levobunolol is a non-cardioselective beta-adrenoceptor blocking agent, equipotent at both $beta_1$ and $beta_2$ receptors. Levobunolol is greater than 60 times more potent than its dextro isomer in its beta-blocking activity. In order to obtain the highest degree of beta-blocking potential without increasing the potential for direct myocardial depression, the levo isomer, levobunolol, is used. Levobunolol does not have significant local anaesthetic (membrane-stabilising) or intrinsic sympathomimetic activity. Betagan has shown to be as effective as Timolol in lowering intraocular pressure.

Betagan when instilled in the eye will lower elevated intraocular pressure as well as normal intraocular pressure, whether or not accompanied by glaucoma. Elevate intraocular pressure presents a major risk factor in the pathogenesis of glaucomatous field loss. The higher the level of intraocular pressure, the likelihood of optic nerve damage and visual field loss.

The primary mechanism of action of levobunolol in reducing intraocular pressure is most likely a decrease in aqueous humor production. Betagan reduces intraocular pressure with little or no effect on pupil size in contrast to the miosis which cholinergic agents are known to produce.

The blurred vision and night blindness are often associated with miotics would not be expected with the use of Betagan. Patients with cateracts avoid the inability to see around lenticular opacities caused by pupil constriction.

Pharmacokinetic properties: The onset of action with one drop of Betagan can be detected within one hour of treatment, with maximum effect seen between two and six hours. A significant decrease can be maintained for up to 24 hours following a single dose.

Preclinical safety data: Not applicable.

Pharmaceutical particulars

List of excipients: Polyvinyl alcohol USP; Sodium chloride EP; Disodium edetate EP; Sodium phosphate dibasic, heptahydrate USP; Potassium phosphate monobasic NF; Sodium hydroxide or hydrochloride acid (to adjust pH) EP; Purified water EP.

Incompatibilities: No major incompatibilities have been reported from topical use of levobunolol.

Shelf life: 24 months.

Special precautions for storage: Store at or below 25°C. Protect from light. Discard after use.

Nature and content of containers: Low density polyethylene (LDPE) blow-fill-seal unit dose container (0.9 ml volume) filled with 0.4 ml solution. Unit dose containers are packaged into a foil covered pouch (5 containers per pouch). Pouches are packaged into carton such that each carton contains 30 or 60 unit dose containers.

Instructions for use/handling: None.

Marketing authorisation number PL 00426/0072.

Date of first authorisation 20 April 1993.

Date of approval/revision of SPC 16 April 1998.

Legal category POM

BOTOX* ▼

Qualitative and quantitative composition *Clostridium botulinum* type A neurotoxin complex, 100 units.

Pharmaceutical form Powder for solution for injection.

Clinical particulars

Therapeutic indications: Botox* is indicated for the symptomatic relief of blepharospasm, hemifacial spasm and idiopathic cervical dystonia (spasmodic torticollis). Botox is also indicated for the treatment, in hospital specialist centres with appropriately trained personnel, of dynamic equinus foot deformity due to spasticity in ambulant paediatric cerebral palsy patients, two years of age or older. The safety and effectiveness of Botox in the treatment of blepharospasm, hemifacial spasm, or idiopathic cervical dystonia in children have not been demonstrated.

Posology and method of administration: **Doses recommended for Botox are not interchangeable with other preparations of botulinum toxin.**

There is no difference in dose between adults and the elderly.

Blepharospasm: After reconstitution, Botox is injected using a sterile, 27–30 gauge needle. Electromyographic guidance is not necessary. The initial recommended dose is 1.25–2.5 U (0.05–0.1 ml volume at each site) injected into the medial and lateral orbicularis oculi of the upper lid and the lateral orbicularis oculi of the lower lid. Additional sites in the brow area, the lateral orbicularis and in the upper facial area may also be injected if spasms here interfere with vision. In general, the initial effect of the injections is seen within three days and reaches a peak at one to two weeks post-treatment. Each treatment lasts approximately three months, following which the procedure can be repeated indefinitely. At repeat treatment sessions, the dose may be increased up to two-fold if the response from the initial treatment is considered insufficient – usually defined as an effect that does not last longer than two months. However, there appears to be little benefit obtainable from injecting more than 5.0 U per site. The intial dose should not exceed 25 U per eye. Normally no additional benefit is conferred by treating more frequently than every three months. It is rare for the effect to be permanent.

In the management of blepharospasm total dosing should not exceed 100 U every 12 weeks.

Hemifacial spasm: Patients with hemifacial spasm or VIIth nerve disorders should be treated as for unilateral blepharospasm, with other affected facial muscles being injected as needed. Electromyographic control may be necessary to identify affected small circumoral muscles.

Cervical dystonia: Several dosing regimens have been used in clinical trials for treatment of cervical dystonia with Botox. Dosing must be tailored to the individual patient based on the patient's head and neck position, location of pain, muscle hypertrophy, patient's body weight, and patient response.

In practice, the maximum total dose is not usually more than 200 U. No more than 50 U should be given at any one injection site. The dilutions suggested are indicated in the following table:

Dilution table

Diluent added	*Resulting dose in units per 0.1 ml*
0.5 ml	20.0 U
1.0 ml	10.0 U
2.0 ml	5.0 U
4.0 ml	2.5 U
8.0 ml	1.25 U

The treatment of cervical dystonia typically may include injection of Botox into the sternocleidomastoid, levator scapulae, scalene, splenius capitis, and/or the trapezius muscle(s). The muscle mass and the degree of hypertrophy are factors to be taken into consideration when selecting the appropriate dose.

The sternocleidomastoid muscle should not be injected bilaterally as there is an increased risk of adverse effects (in particular dysphagia) when bilateral injections or doses in excess of 100 U are administered to this muscle.

A 25, 27 or 30 gauge needle may be used for superficial muscles, and a 22 gauge needle may be used for deeper musculature. For cervical dystonia, localisation of the involved muscles with electromyographic guidance may be useful.

Multiple injection sites allow Botox to have more uniform contact with the innervation areas of the dystonic muscle and are especially useful in larger muscles. The optimal number of injection sites is

The following doses are recommended:

Cervical dystonia classification	*Muscle groupings*	*Total dosage (No. of Units)*	*No. of sites*
Type I Head *rotated* toward side of shoulder elevation	Sternomastoid	50–100	At least 2 sites
	Levator scapulae	50	1–2 sites
	Scalene	25–50	1–2 sites
	Splenius capitis	25–75	1–3 sites
	Trapezius	25–100	1–8 sites
Type II Head rotation only	Sternomastoid	25–100	At least 2 sites if >25 U given
Type III Head *tilted* toward side of shoulder elevation	Sternomastoid	25–100 at posterior border	At least 2 sites if >25 U given
	Levator scapulae	25–100	at least 2 sites
	Scalene	25–75	at least 2 sites
	Trapezius	25–100	1–8 sites
Type IV Bilateral posterior cervical muscle spasm with elevation of the face	Splenius capitis and cervicis	50–200	2–8 sites, treat bilaterally (This is the total dose and not the dose for each side of the neck)

dependent upon the size of the muscle to be chemically denervated.

Paediatric cerebral palsy: Diluted Botox is injected using a sterile 23–26 gauge needle. It is administered into each of two sites in the medial and lateral heads of the affected gastrocnemius muscle. The recommended total dose is 4 units/kg body weight. When both lower limbs are to be injected on the same occasion this dose should be divided between the two limbs.

Clinical improvement generally occurs within the first two weeks after injection. Repeat doses should be administered when the clinical effect of a previous injection diminishes but not more frequently than every two months.

Contra-indications: Botox is contra-indicated (a) in individuals with a known hypersensitivity to any component of the formulation; (b) when there are generalised disorders of muscle activity (e.g. myasthenia gravis); (c) when aminoglycoside antibiotics or spectinomycin are already being used or are likely to be used; (d) when there are bleeding disorders of any type, in case of anticoagulant therapy and whenever there is any reason to avoid intramuscular injections, and (e) during pregnancy or lactation.

Special warnings and special precautions for use: The relevant anatomy, and any alterations to the anatomy due to prior surgical procedures, must be understood prior to administering Botox. Extra caution should be paid in the case of injection sites close to structures such as the carotid artery and pleural apices.

The recommended dosages and frequency of administration of Botox should not be exceeded.

Adrenaline and other treatments for anaphylaxis should be available.

Reconstituted Botox is for intramuscular injection ONLY.

Blepharospasm: Reduced blinking following Botox injection of the orbicularis muscle can lead to corneal exposure, persistent epithelial defect and corneal ulceration, especially in patietns with VIIth nerve disorders. Careful testing of corneal sensation in eyes previously operated upon, avoidance of injection into the lower lid area to avoid ectropion, and vigorous treatment of any epithelial defect should be employed. This may require protective drops, ointment, bandage soft contact lenses, or closure of the eye by patching or other means.

Cervical dystonia: Limiting the dose injected into the sternocleidomastoid muscle to less than 100 U may decrease the occurrence of dysphagia. Patients with smaller neck muscle mass, or patients who require bilateral injections into the sternocleidomastoid muscle, have been reported to be at greater risk of dysphagia. Dysphagia is attributable to the spread of the toxin to the oesophageal musculature.

Interactions with other medicaments and other forms of interaction: The effect of botulinum toxin may be potentiated by aminoglycoside antibiotics or other drugs that interfere with neuromuscular transmission e.g. tubocurarine-type muscle relaxants. Concomitant use of Botox with aminoglycosides or spectinomycin is contra-indicated. Polymyxins, tetracyclines and lincomycin should be used with caution in the Botox-treated patient. Muscle relaxants should also be used with caution, perhaps reducing the starting dose of relaxant, or using an intermediate-action drug, such as vecuronium or atracurium, rather than those with longer lasting effects.

Pregnancy and lactation: Botox has been shown to produce abortions and effects at daily doses of 0.125 U/kg/day and at 2 U/kg and higher in rabbits, the most sensitive species; whereas in rats and mice, no abortions or effects were observed when up to 4 U/kg of Botox were injected. Doses of 8 and 16 U/kg in rats and mice have been shown to be associated with reduced foetal body weight and/or delayed ossification of the hyoid bone, which may be reversible.

Botox is contra-indicated in pregnancy and lactation.

Effects on the ability to drive and use machines: Due to the nature of the disease being treated, the effects of Botox on the ability to drive or to operate machines cannot be predicted. Some of the post-therapy and/or unwanted effects may temporarily impair the ability to drive or operate machinery and consequently an affected person should avoid these tasks until faculties are fully recovered.

Undesirable effects: Side-effects may occur from misplaced injections of Botox temporarily paralysing nearby muscle groups. Execessive doses may cause paralysis in muscles distant to the injection site.

Blepharospasm: The most commonly-reported side-effects are ptosis, lacrimation, irritation (including dry eye and photophobia) and lagophthalmos. Ectropion. keratitis, diplopia and entropion have been reported rarely. Ecchymosis occurs easily in the soft eyelid tissues. This can be minimised by applying gentle pressure at the injection site immediately after the injection.

One case of angle-closure glaucoma following treatment with botulinum toxin has been reported.

Cervical dystonia: In an evaluation of 710 patients, dysphagia was observed in 15.8% of the patients. Other frequently reported adverse reactions were pain and soreness at the injection site (16.3%), and local weakness (12.8%). Less frequent adverse reactions (1–5%) included bruising at the injection site, general weakness, malaise and nausea.

Rare adverse events observed during clinical trials in <1% of patients with Botox injection include drowsiness, numbness, stiffness, diplopia, ptosis, headache, dyspnea, fever, and flu syndrome.

Further possible adverse events which may be associated with treatment for cervical dystonia are neck weakness and instability, head tremor, dysphonia and interference with local autonomic system functions (e.g. dry mouth) and allergic reactions such as mild fever and/or the development of a local or more generalised maculo-papular rash.

Dysphagia ranges in severity from very mild to severe, with potential for aspiration, and in rare instances may require medical intervention. It may persist for two or three weeks after injection, but has been reported in one case to last five months post-injection. Dysphagia appears to be dose-related and has been reported in clinical trials to occur less frequently with total doses below 200 U in one treatment session.

Paediatric cerebral palsy: The safety of Botox used for the treatment of dynamic equinus foot deformity due to spasticity in paediatric cerebral palsy patients was evaluated. As is expected for any intramuscular injection procedure, localised pain was associated with the injection in these patients. All treatment-related adverse events were mild-to-moderate in severity.

The adverse reactions most frequently reported as related to treatment include falling, leg pain, leg (local) weakness, and general weakness. The percentage of patients who experienced these events at least once during the study are summarised below:

	Botox, n=215
Falling	9.3%
Leg pain	2.3%
Weakness, local	2.3%
Weakness, general	2.3%

Falling may be attributable to a change in ankle position and gait pattern and/or local weakness. Local weakness represents the expected pharmacological action of botulinum toxin.

Other treatment-related adverse reactions reported in 1% of patients were: leg cramps, fever, knee pain, ankle pain, pain at the injection site post-treatment, and lethargy.

General: Following injection of Botox some distant muscles can show increased electrophysiologic jitter which is not associated with clinical weakness or other types of electrophysiologic abnormalities.

This product contains a small amount of human albumin.

The viral safety of the human albumin used as excipient in Botox is documented through the several steps of its preparation. Particular care is given to the controls of the donors, to the manufacturing process and to the virus removal/inactivation process. Concerning this last point, a high margin of safety from the risk of viral transmission is achieved by using a combination of removal by the Cohn ethanol fractionation process and inactivation by pasteurisation (10 hours at 60°C).

Botox has not been known to transmit hepatitis or human immunodeficiency virus.

Overdosage: Based on reports on individual human cases of intoxication, the lethal dose for humans is estimated to be 3,000 to 30,000 U or higher after oral administration.

A case of peripheral neuropathy has been reported in a large adult male who received 1800 U of Botox intramuscularly (for neck and back spasm, and severe pain) in an 11 week period. There have not been any reported instances of systemic toxicity resulting from accidental injection or oral ingestion of Botox. Should overdosage occur, the patient should be medically supervised for several days for signs or symptoms of systemic weakness or muscle paralysis. The entire content of one vial is below the estimated dose for systemic toxicity in humans weighing 6 kg or greater.

Pharmacological properties

Pharmacodynamic properties: ATC class MO3A X01.

The active constituent in Botox is a protein complex derived from *Clostridium botulinum*. The protein consists of type A neurotoxin and several other proteins. Under physiological conditions it is presumed that the complex dissociates and releases the pure neurotoxin.

Clostridium botulinum toxin type A blocks cholinergic transport at the neuromuscular junction by preventing the release of acetylcholine. The nerve endings of the neuromuscular junction no longer respond to nerve impulses and secretion of the chemotransmitter is prevented (chemical denervation). Re-establishment of impulse transmission is by newly formed nerve endings and motor end plates.

Pharmacokinetic properties:

(a) General characteristics of the active substance: Classical absorption, distribution, biotransformation and elimination studies on the active substance have not been performed due to the extreme toxicity of botulinum toxin type A.

(b) Characteristics in patients: Human ADME studies have not been performed due to the nature of the product. It is believed that little systemic distribution of therapeutic doses of Botox occurs. Botox is probably metabolised by proteases and the molecular components recycled through normal metabolic pathways.

Preclinical safety data:

Acute toxicity: In monkeys receiving a single intramuscular (i.m.) injection of Botox, the No Observed Effect Level (NOEL) ranged from 4 to 24 U/kg. The i.m. LD_{50} was reported to be 39 U/kg.

Toxicity on repeated injection: In three different studies (six months in rats; 20 weeks in juvenile monkeys; 1 year in monkeys) where the animals received i.m. injections, the NOEL was at the following respective Botox dosage levels: <4 U/kg, 8 U/kg and 4 U/kg. The main systemic effect was a transient decrease in body weight gain.

There was no indication of a cumulative effect in the animal studies when Botox was given at dosage intervals of 1 month or greater.

Local toxicity: Botox was shown not to cause ocular or dermal irritation, or give rise to toxicity when injected into the vitreous body in rabbits.

Allergic or inflammatory reactions in the area of the injection sites are rarely observed after Botox administration. However, formation of haematoma may occur.

Reproduction toxicology:
Teratogenic effects: When pregnant mice and rats were injected intramuscularly during the period of organogenesis, the developmental NOEL of Botox was at 4 U/kg. Reductions in ossification were observed at 8 and 16 U/kg (mice) and reduced ossification of the hyoid bone at 16 U/kg (rats). Reduced foetal body weights were observed at 8 and 16 U/kg (rats).

In a range finding study in rabbits, daily injections at dosages of 0.5 U/kg/day (days 6 to 18 of gestation), and 4 and 6 U/kg (administered on days 6 and 13 of gestation), caused death and abortions among surviving dams. External malformations were observed in one foetus each in the 0.125 U/kg/day and the 2 U/kg dosage groups. The rabbit appears to be a very sensitive species to Botox treatment.

Impairment of fertility and reproduction: The reproductive NOEL following i.m. injection of Botox was 4 U/kg in male rats and 8 U/kg in female rats. Higher dosages were associated with dose-dependent reductions in fertility. Provided impregnation occurred, there were no adverse effects on the numbers or viability of the embryos sired or conceived by treated male or female rats.

Pre- and post-natal developmental effects: In female rats, the reproductive NOEL was 16 U/kg. The developmental NOEL was 4 U/kg.

Mutagenicity: Botox has been evaluated and shown to be non-mutagenic in a number of *in vitro* and *in vivo* systems including the Ames test, the AS52/XPRT Mammalian Cell Forward Gene Mutation assay and the CHO test, and non-clastogenic in the mouse PCE test.

Carcinogenicity: No animal studies have been conducted.

Antigenicity: Botox showed antigenicity in mice only in the presence of adjuvant. Botox was found to be slightly antigenic in the guinea pig.

Blood compatibility: No haemolysis was detected up to 100 U/ml of Botox in normal human blood.

Pharmaceutical particulars
List of excipients: Human serum albumin; sodium chloride.

Incompatibilities: None known, other than described under *Interactions with other medicaments and other forms of interaction*, above.

Shelf life: Unopened vial – 24 months. Reconstituted vial – 4 hours.

Special precautions for storage: Unopened vials should be stored in a freezer at or below –5°C. After reconstitution Botox may be stored in a refrigerator (2–8°C) for up to 4 hours prior to use.

Nature and contents of containers: Clear glass vial, with rubber stopper and tamper-proof aluminium seal, containing white powder for solution for injection.

Instructions for use/handling: Botox is reconstituted prior to use with sterile unpreserved normal saline (0.9% sodium chloride for injection). It is good practice to perform vial reconstitution and syringe preparation over plastic-lined paper towels to catch any spillage. An appropriate amount of diluent (see dilution table below) is drawn up into a syringe. The exposed portion of the rubber septum of the vial is cleaned with alcohol (70%) prior to insertion of the needle. Since Botox is denatured by bubbling or similar violent agitation, the diluent should be injected gently into the vial. Discard the vial if a vacuum does not pull the diluent into the vial. Reconstituted Botox is a clear colourless to slightly yellow solution free of particulate matter. When reconstituted, Botox may be stored in a refrigerator (2–8°C) for up to 4 hours prior to use. After this period used or unused vials should be discarded.

Dilution table

Diluent added	*Resulting dose in units per 0.1 ml*
0.5 ml	20.0 U
1.0 ml	10.0 U
2.0 ml	5.0 U
4.0 ml	2.5 U
8.0 ml	1.25 U

The 'unit' by which the potency of preparations of Botox is measured should be used to calculate dosages of Botox only and is not transferable to other preparations of botulinum toxin.

An injection volume of approximately 0.1 ml is recommended. A decrease or increase in the Botox dose is possible by administering a smaller or larger injection volume. The smaller the injection volume the less discomfort and less spread of toxin in the injected muscle occurs. This is of benefit in reducing effects on nearby muscles when small muscle groups are being injected.

For safe disposal, unused vials should be reconstituted with a small amount of water then autoclaved. Any used vials, syringes, and spillages etc. should be autoclaved, or the residual Botox inactivated using dilute hypochlorite solution (0.5%).

Marketing authorisation number PL 0426/0074.

Date of approval/revision of SPC October 1998

Legal category POM

LACRI-LUBE*

Presentation Off-white, smooth, preservative-free sterile ophthalmic ointment containing White Soft Paraffin BP 57.3% (w/w), Mineral Oil USP 42.5% (w/w) and Lanolin Alcohols NF 0.2% (w/w).

Uses Useful as adjunctive therapy to lubricate and protect the eye in conditions such as exposure keratitis, decreased corneal sensitivity, recurrent corneal erosions, keratitis sicca, and also in ophthalmic and non-ophthalmic surgery.

Dosage and administration For topical administration. Pull lower lid down to form a pocket and apply a small amount as required. There is no variation of dose for age.

Contra-indications, warnings, etc Do not use in patients hypersensitive to lanolin alcohols.

Pharmaceutical precautions Store away from heat. To avoid contamination during use, do not touch tube tip to any surface.

Legal category P.

Package quantities Lacri-Lube is available in 3.5 g and 5 g ophthalmic ointment tubes.

Further information Dry eye symptoms commonly persist at night – Lacri-Lube has been specifically formulated to lubricate and protect the dry eye during sleep.

Lacri-Lube can provide prophylactic ocular care during general surgical procedures as an adjunct to taping of the eyelids.

Product licence number PL 0426/0041

Legal category P

LIQUIFILM* TEARS

Qualitative and quantitative composition Polyvinyl alcohol 1.4% w/v USP

Pharmaceutical form Eye drops.

Clinical particulars
Therapeutic indications: As an ocular lubricant for the relief of dry eye and dry eye symptoms.

Posology and method of administration: For all ages. One or two drops administered topically to the affected eye(s) as required.

Contra-indications: Sensitivity to any of the ingredients. Not for use with soft contact lenses.

Special warnings and precautions for use: None.

Interactions with other medicaments and other forms of interaction: None known.

Pregnancy and lactation: No untoward effect is anticipated (product contains no pharmacologically active ingredient).

Effects on ability to drive and use machines: None.

Undesirable effects: None.

Overdose: None.

Pharmocological properties
Pharmacodynamic properties: Not applicable. Liquifilm Tears contains no pharmacologically active ingredient.

Pharmocokinetic properties: Not applicable. Liquifilm Tears contains no pharmacologically active ingredient.

Preclinical safety data: The constituents of Liquifilm Tears have been used safely in pharmaceutical products for many years. Topical administration in animal studies showed no untoward effects.

Pharmaceutical particulars
List of excipients: Sodium chloride EP; Sodium phosphate dibasic USP; Sodium phosphate monobasic USP; Benzalkonium chloride EP; Edetate disodium EP; Hydrochloride acid or sodium hydroxide (to adjust pH) EP; Purified water EP

Incompatibilities: None known.

Shelf life: 24 months unopened. Discard 28 days after opening.

Special precautions for storage: None.

Nature and contents of container: Low density polyethylene (LDPE) bottle and tip and medium impact polystrene (MIPS) screw cap. Safety seal to ensure integrity of the container.

Liquifilm Tears is available in 15 ml bottles.

Instructions for use/handling: Not applicable.

Marketing authorisation number PL 00426/0009R

Date of approval/revision of SPC September 1998.

Legal category P

LIQUIFILM* TEARS PRESERVATIVE FREE

Qualitative and quantitative composition Polyvinyl alcohol 1.4% w/v.

Pharmaceutical form Sterile ophthalmic solution.

Clinical particulars
Therapeutic indications: Symptomatic relief of dry eye and symptomatic relief of eye irritation associated with deficient tear production.

Posology and method of administration:
Dosage schedule: Apply one or two drops in each eye as needed, or as directed. No special dosage for the elderly or for children.

Route of administration: Ocular installation.

Contra-indications: Hypersensitivity to any component of the formulation.

Special warnings and precautions for use: If symptoms worsen or persist or other adverse effects occur, discontinue use and consult a doctor.

In order to avoid contamination, dropper should not be allowed to touch the eye or any other surface.

Use immediately after opening.

Do not store opened container.

Interaction with other medications and other forms of interaction: None known.

Pregnancy and lactation: The constituents of Liquifilm Tears Preservative Free have been used as pharmaceutical agents for many years with no untoward effects. No special precautions are necessary for the use of Liquifilm Tears Preservative Free in pregnancy and lactation.

Effects on ability to drive and use machines: May cause transient blurring. Do not drive or use hazardous machinery unless vision is clear.

Undesirable effects: May cause transient stinging or irritation on installation.

Overdose: Accidental overdose will not present any hazard.

Pharacological properties
Pharmacodynamic properties: Liquifilm Tears Preservative Free exerts a mechanical, not a pharmacological action. The viscosity enhancing agent is polyvinyl alcohol and the lubricating-enhancing agent is povidone.

Pharmacokinetic properties: Not applicable.

Preclinical safety data: The constituents of Liquifilm Tears Preservative Free have been used safely in pharmaceutical products for many years. Topical administration in animal studies showed untoward effects.

Pharmaceutical particulars
List of excipients: Povidone; Sodium chloride; Sodium hydroxide or hydrochloric acid (to adjust pH); Purified water.

Incompatibilities: None known.

Shelf life: 24 months (unopened).

Do not store opened container.

Special precautions for storage: Store below 25°C.

Nature and contents of container: Low density polyethylene unit dose vials containing 0.4 ml of Liquifilm Tears Preservative Free.

Cartons contain 30 units per pack.

Instructions for use/handling: Ensure container is intact. Twist off tab and apply eyedrops.

Marketing authorisation number PL 00426/0063.

Date of approval/revision of SPC November 1997.

Legal category P

ZORAC* ▼

Qualitative and quantitative composition 1 g gel contains: Zorac 0.05% (tazarotene 0.5 mg) or Zorac 0.1% (tazarotene 1.0 mg).

Pharmaceutical form Aqueous gel.

Clinical particulars
Therapeutic indications: For the topical treatment of mild to moderate plaque psoriasis involving up to 10% body surface area.

Posology and method of administration: Zorac gel is available in two concentrations. Treatment with the higher concentration gel gives a faster and numerically higher response rate. Treatment with the lower concentration gel is associated with a somewhat lower incidence of local adverse events (see *Undesirable effects* and *Pharmacological properties*). The physician should choose the concentration to be used based on clinical circumstances and the principle of using the least concentration of drug to achieve the desired effect.

Individual variations with respect to efficacy and tolerability are possible. It is thus advisable for patients to consult their physician on a weekly basis when initiating therapy.

A thin film of the gel should be applied once daily in the evening; care should be taken to apply it only to areas of affected skin, avoiding application to healthy skin or in skin folds. Treatment is limited to 10% body surface area (approximately equivalent to the total skin area of one arm).

If the patient experiences more drying or irritation, an effective greasy emollient (without pharmaceutically active ingredients) can be applied to the areas of the skin to be treated to improve tolerability. Healthy skin around the psoriatic plaques can be covered by using zinc paste, for example, to prevent irritation.

Usually, the treatment period is up to 12 weeks. Clinical experience, particularly on tolerability, is available on periods of use of up to 12 months.

Contra-indications: Hypersensitivity to any ingredient of the medication.

Pregnancy or in women planning a pregnancy.

Breast-feeding mothers

Since there is, as yet, no clinical experience, Zorac should not be used in the treatment of psoriasis pustulosa and psoriasis exfoliativa, and the gel should not be applied to intertriginous areas, to the face, or to hair-covered scalp.

Special warnings and special precautions for use: Care should be taken to ensure that Zorac is applied only to psoriatic lesions, as application to normal, eczematous or inflamed skin or skin affected by other pathologies may cause irritation. Patients should be advised to wash their hands after application of the gel to avoid accidental transfer to the eyes.

If psoriatic areas on the skin of the hands are being treated, particular care should be taken to ensure that no gel is transferred to facial skin or the eyes.

If skin irritation develops, treatment with Zorac should be interrupted.

The safety of use on more than 10% of the body surface areas has not been established. There is limited experience of application to up to 20% of the body surface area.

Patients should be advised to avoid excessive exposure to UV light (including sunlight, use of a solarium, PUVA or UVB therapy) during treatment with Zorac (see *Preclinical safety data*).

No therapeutic studies using Zorac under occlusion or concomitantly with other antipsoriatic agents (including tar shampoos) have been carried out. To minimise interference with absorption and to avoid unnecessary spreading of the medication, topical application of emollients and cosmetics should not be applied within 1 hour of applying Zorac.

The safety and efficacy of Zorac have not been established in patients under the age of 18 years.

Interactions with other medicaments and other forms of interaction: Concomitant use of pharmaceutical and cosmetic preparations which cause irritation or have a strong drying effect should be avoided.

Pregnancy and lactation

Pregnancy: Although in animals no malformations were observed after dermal application, skeletal alterations were seen in the foetuses, which may be attributable to systemic retinoid effects. Teratogenic effects were observed after oral administration.

In view of these findings Zorac gel must not be used by pregnant women or women planning a pregnancy.

Women of childbearing potential should be informed of the potential risk and adopt adequate birth control measures when Zorac is used.

Lactation: Although no data are available on the excretion of tazarotene in human milk, animal data indicate that excretion into milk is possible. For that reason Zorac gel should not be used during breast feeding.

Effects on ability to drive and use machines: None known.

Undesirable effects: The most frequently reported adverse reactions in controlled clinical trials of Zorac in the treatment of psoriasis were pruritus (incidence 20–25%), burning, erythema, and irritation (10–20%), desquamation, non-specific rash, irritant contact dermatitis, skin pain, and a worsening of psoriasis (5–10%). More rarely observed were stinging and inflamed and dry skin (1–3%). The incidence of adverse reactions appears to be concentration-related and dependent on duration of use. The higher concentration gel (0.1%) may cause up to 5% more cases of severe skin irritation than the lower concentration gel (0.05%), especially during the first 4 weeks of use.

Overdosage: Excessive dermal use of Zorac may result in marked redness, peeling or local discomfort.

Inadvertent ingestion of Zorac is a theoretical possibility. In such a case, the signs and symptoms associated with hypervitaminosis A (severe headache, nausea, vomiting, drowsiness, irritability and pruritus) may occur. However, it is likely that these symptoms would prove to be reversible.

Pharmacological properties Both gels have demonstrated therapeutic effects as early as 1 week after commencement of a course of treatment. A good clinical response was seen in up to 65% of the patients after 12 weeks of treatment. The therapeutic effect of the higher concentration gel is more rapidly apparent and the efficacy more marked. In various studies in which patients were also evaluated for 12 weeks following cessation of therapy, it was found that patients continued to show a certain clinical benefit, however, no difference between the higher and lower concentrations with regard to this effect was observed.

Pharmacodynamic properties: Topical antipsoriatic agent (D05A).

Tazarotene, a member of the acetylenic class of retinoids, is a prodrug which is converted to its active free form, tazarotenic acid, by de-esterification in the skin area. Tazarotenic acid is the only known metabolite of tazarotene to have retinoid activity.

The active metabolite specifically regulates gene expression, thus modulating cell proliferation, hyperplasia, and differentiation in a wide range of tissues, as has been demonstrated in *in vitro* and *in vivo* trials.

The exact mechanism of action of tazarotene in psoriasis is, as yet, unknown. Improvement in psoriatic patients occurs in association with restoration of normal cutaneous morphology, and reduction of the inflammatory markers ICAM-1 and HLA-DR, and of markers of epidermal hyperplasia and abnormal differentiation, such as elevated keratinocyte transglutaminase, involucrin, and keratin 16.

Pharmacokinetic properties:

(a) General characteristics

Absorption: Systemic absorption is limited. Results of a pharmacokinetic study of single topical application of 0.1% ^{14}C-tazarotene gel show that approximately 5% is absorbed when applied to normal skin under occlusion.

After a single topical application of tazarotene gel to 20% body surface area for 10 hours in healthy volunteers, tazarotene was not detectable in the plasma. Maximum plasma levels for the active metabolite tazarotenic acid of 0.3±0.2 ng/ml (for the 0.05% strength) and 0.5±0.3 ng/ml (0.1% gel) were measured after approximately 15 hours. The AUC was 40% higher for the 0.1% gel compared with the 0.05% gel. Thus, the two strengths of the gel are not strictly dose proportional with respect to systemic absorption. Repeated topical application of the 0.1% gel over 7 days led to maximum plasma levels for tazarotenic acid of 0.7±0.6 ng/ml after 9 hours.

Biotransformation: After dermal application, tazarotene undergoes esterase hydrolysis to form its free acid, tazarotenic acid, and oxidative metabolism to form inactive sulphoxide and sulphone derivatives.

Elimination: Secondary metabolites of tazarotenic acid (the sulphoxide, the sulphone and an oxygenated derivative of tazarotenic acid) have been detected in human urine and faeces. The elimination half-life of tazarotenic acid after dermal application of tazarotene is approximately 18 hours in normal and psoriatic subjects.

After intravenous administration, the half-life of tazarotene was approximately 6 hours and that of tazarotenic acid 14 hours.

(b) Characteristics after use in patients: After single topical application of 0.1% ^{14}C-tazarotene gel for 10 hours to psoriatic lesions (without occlusion), 4.5% of the dose was recovered in the stratum corneum and 2.4% in the epidermal/dermal layers. Less than 1% of the dose was absorbed systemically. More than 75% of drug elimination was completed within 72 hours.

In a small five patient study, repeated topical application of tazarotene 0.1% gel over 13 days resulted in a mean peak plasma level of tazarotenic acid of 12±8 ng/ml. these patients had psoriatic lesions on 8–18% of body surface area. In a larger 24 psoriatic patient study, tazarotene 0.05% and 0.1% gels were applied for 3 months and yielded a Cmax of 0.45±0.78 ng/ml and 0.83±1.22 ng/ml, respectively.

In a 1 year clinical study with 0.05% and 0.1% tazarotene gel, tazarotene was detected in 3 out of 112 patients at plasma concentrations below 1 ng/ml, while its active metabolite tazarotenic acid was found in 31 patients. Only four patients had plasma concentrations of tazarotenic acid greater than or equal to 1 ng/ml (maximum 2.8 ng/ml).

Preclinical safety data:

Subacute/chronic toxicity: The safety of daily dermal application of tazarotene gel was tested in mouse, rat and mini-pig over periods of up to one year. The main observation was reversible skin irritation. In the case of the mini-pig, an incomplete healing of the dermal irritation was observed after an 8 week recovery period. The rat appears to be the most sensitive species to tazarotene, as is the case with other retinoids. Here, dermal application induced severe skin reactions and clinically significant retinoid-like systemic effects. No adverse systemic effects were observed in the other species.

After oral administration of 0.025 mg/kg/day for 1 year in the cynomolgus monkey, no toxic effects were observed. At higher doses, typical symptoms of retinoid toxicity were seen.

Reproductive toxicity: Safety of use during pregnancy has not been established. Teratogenic and embryotoxic effects were observed after oral administration in the rat and rabbit. In dermal application studies during foetal development, skeletal alterations and decreased pup weight at birth and at the end of the lactation period were observed.

Animal tests suggest that tazarotene or its active metabolite is excreted in breast milk and passes the placenta barrier.

No effects on fertility are reported after topical application in the male and female rat.

Mutagenicity/Carcinogenicity: No evidence of a mutagenic potential of tazarotene has been reported in *in vitro* and *in vivo* trials.

In long term investigations of the effects of dermal and oral administration in animals, no carcinogenic effects were observed.

There was an increased incidence of photocarcinogenic effects in the hairless mouse when exposed to UV light after topical application of tazarotene.

Local tolerability: Tazarotene gel has a considerable irritative potential on skin in all animal species investigated.

Instillation of tazarotene gel in the eye of the rabbit resulted in irritation with marked hyperaemia of the conjunctiva, but there was no corneal damage.

Pharmaceutical particulars

List of excipients: Benzyl alcohol, macrogol 400, hexylene glycol (2-methylpentane-2,4-diol), carbomer, trometamol, poloxamer 407, polysorbate 40, ascorbic acid, butyl hydroxyanisole, butyl hydroxytoluene, disodium edetate dihydrate, purified water.

Incompatibilities: Tazarotene is susceptible to oxidising agents and may undergo ester hydrolysis when in contact with bases.

Shelf life: Finished product in the unopened container: 36 months. Finished product after first opening of the container: 180 days.

Special precautions for storage: Zorac gel should not be stored at temperatures over 30°C.

Nature and contents of container: Aluminium tube, internally lacquered, with seal and polypropylene screw cap containing a colourless to light yellow, translucent to cloudy, homogeneous gel.

Pack sizes: 30 g and 60 g.

Instructions for use/handling: To break the seal, use the top of the cap. Keep tube tightly closed when not in use.

Marketing authorisation numbers

Zorac 0.05% PL 00426/0096
Zorac 0.1% PL 00426/0097

Date of approval/revision of SPC September 1998.

Legal category POM.

**Trade Mark*

Alliance Pharmaceuticals UK Ltd

Avonbridge House
2 Bath Road
Chippenham
Wiltshire SN15 2BB

☎ +44 01249 466966 ☐ +44 01249 466977

ALLIANCE

APRESOLINE* AMPOULES 20 mg

Qualitative and quantitative composition Hydralazine hydrochloride PhEur 20mg per 2ml ampoule.

Pharmaceutical form Powder for injection contained in a 2ml glass ampoule.

Clinical particulars

Therapeutic indications:

1. Hypertensive emergencies, particularly those associated with pre-eclampsia and toxaemia of pregnancy.
2. Hypertension with renal complications.

Posology and method of administration: The contents of the vial should be reconstituted by dissolving in 1ml of Water for Injection PhEur. This should then be further diluted with 10 ml of Sodium Chloride Injection BP 0.9% and be administered by slow intravenous injection. The injection must be given immediately and any remainder discarded.

Adults: Initially 5 to 10 mg by slow intravenous injection, to avoid precipitous decreases in arterial pressure with a critical reduction in cerebral or utero-placental perfusion. If necessary a repeat injection can be given after an interval of 20 to 30 minutes, throughout which blood pressures and heart rate should be monitored. A satisfactory response can be defined as a decrease in diastolic blood pressure to 90/100 mmHg.

Apresoline may also be given by continuous iv infusion, beginning with a flow rate of 200 to 300 µg/min. Maintenance flow rates must be determined individually and are usually within the range 50 to 150 µg/min.

The product reconstituted as for direct iv injection may be added via the infusion container to 500 ml of Sodium Chloride Injection BP 0.9% and given by continuous infusion. The addition should be made immediately before administration and the mixture should not be stored. Apresoline for infusion can also be used with 5% sorbitol solution or isotonic inorganic infusion solutions such as Ringer's solution.

Children: Not recommended.

Elderly: Clinical evidence would indicate that no special dosage regime is necessary. Advancing age does not affect either blood concentration or systemic clearance. Renal elimination may however be affected as kidney function diminishes with age.

Contra-indications: Known hypersensitivity to hydralazine or dihydralazine.

Idiopathic systemic lupus erythematosus (SLE) and related diseases.

Severe tachycardia and heart failure with a high cardiac output (e.g., in thyrotoxicosis).

Myocardial insufficiency due to mechanical obstruction (e.g., in the presence of aortic or mitral stenosis or constrictive pericarditis).

Isolated right ventricular failure due to pulmonary hypertension (cor pulmonale).

Dissecting aortic aneurysm.

Special warnings and special precautions for use:

Warnings: The overall 'hyperdynamic' state of the circulation induced by hydralazine may accentuate certain clinical conditions. Myocardial stimulation may provoke or aggravate angina pectoris. Patients with suspected or confirmed coronary artery disease should therefore be given Apresoline only under cover of a beta-blocker or in combination with other suitable sympatholytic agents. It is important that the beta-blocker medication should be commenced a few days before the start of treatment with Apresoline.

Patients who have survived a myocardial infarction should not receive Apresoline until a post-infarction stabilisation phase has been achieved.

Prolonged treatment with hydralazine (i.e., usually for more than 6 months) may provoke a lupus erythematosus (LE) like syndrome, especially where doses exceed 100 mg daily. First symptoms are likely to be arthralgia, sometimes associated with fever and rash, and are reversible after withdrawal of the drug. In its more severe form it resembles acute SLE, and in rare cases renal and ocular involvement have been reported. Long term treatment with corticosteroids may be required to reverse these changes. Since such reactions tend to occur more frequently the higher the dose and the longer its duration, and since they are also more common in slow acetylators, it is recommended that for maintenance therapy the lowest effective dose should be used. If 100 mg daily fails to elicit an adequate clinical effect, the patient's acetylator status should be evaluated. Slow acetylators and women run a greater risk of developing the LE-like syndrome and every effort should therefore be made to keep the dosage below 100 mg daily and a careful watch kept for signs and symptoms suggestive of this syndrome. If such symptoms do develop the drug should be gradually withdrawn. Rapid acetylators often respond inadequately even to doses of 100 mg daily and therefore the dose can be raised with only a slightly increased risk of an LE-like syndrome.

During long-term treatment with Apresoline it is advisable to determine the antinuclear factors and conduct urine analysis at intervals of approximately 6 months. Microhaematuria and/or proteinuria, in particular together with positive titres of ANF, may be initial signs of immuno-complex glomerulonephritis associated with the SLE-like syndrome. If overt clinical signs or symptoms develop, the drug should be withdrawn immediately.

Skin rash, febrile reactions and changes in blood count occur rarely and the drug should be withdrawn. Peripheral neuritis in the form of paraesthesia has been reported, and may respond to pyridoxine administration or drug withdrawal.

Precautions: In patients with renal impairment (creatinine clearance <30 ml/min or serum creatinine concentrations >2.5 mg/100 ml or 221 µmol/l) and in patients with hepatic dysfunction, the dose or interval between doses should be adjusted according to clinical response, in order to avoid accumulation of the 'apparent' active substance.

Apresoline should be used with caution in patients with coronary artery disease (since it may increase angina) or cerebrovascular disease.

When undergoing surgery, patients treated with Apresoline may show a fall in blood pressure. Adrenaline should not be used to correct the hypotension, since it enhances the cardiac-accelerating effects of hydralazine.

Interaction with other medicaments and other forms of interaction: Potentiation of effects: Concurrent therapy with other antihypertensives (vasodilators, calcium antagonists, ACE inhibitors, diuretics), anaesthetics, tricyclic antidepressants, major tranquillisers or drugs exerting central depressant actions (including alcohol).

Administration of Apresoline shortly before or after diazoxide may give rise to marked hypotension.

MAO inhibitors should be used with caution in patients receiving Apresoline.

Concurrent administration of Apresoline with beta-blockers subject to a strong first-pass effect (e.g., propranolol) may increase their bioavailability. Downward adjustment of these drugs may be required when they are given concomitantly with Apresoline.

Pregnancy and lactation: Use of Apresoline in pregnancy before the third trimester should be avoided, but the drug may be employed in later pregnancy if there is no safer alternative or when the disease itself carries serious risks for the mother or child e.g., pre-eclampsia and/or eclampsia.

No serious adverse effects in human pregnancy have been reported to date with Apresoline, although experience in the third trimester is extensive.

Hydralazine passes into breast milk but reports available so far have not shown adverse effects on the infant. Where use of Apresoline proves unavoidable, mothers may breast feed their infant, provided that the infant is observed for possible adverse effects.

Effects on ability to drive and use machines: Patients should be warned of the potential hazards when driving or operating machinery if they suffer from side effects such as dizziness or blurred vision.

Undesirable effects: Some of the adverse effects listed below e.g., tachycardia, palpitation, anginal symptoms, flushing, headache, dizziness, nasal congestion and gastro-intestinal disturbances are commonly seen at the start of the treatment, especially if the dose is raised quickly. However such effects generally subside in the further course of treatment.

(The following frequency estimates are used: frequent >10%, occasional 1-10%, rare 0.001-1%, isolated cases <0.001%).

Cardiovascular system: Frequent: tachycardia, palpitation. Occasional: Flushing, hypotension, anginal symptoms. Rare: oedema, heart failure. Isolated cases: paradoxical pressor responses.

Central and peripheral nervous system: Frequent: headache. Rare: dizziness. Isolated cases: peripheral neuritis, polyneuritis, paraesthesiae (these unwanted effects may be reversed by administering pyridoxine).

Musculo-skeletal system: Occasional: arthralgia, joint swelling, myalgia.

Skin and appendages: Rare: rash.

Urogenital system: Rare: proteinuria, increased plasma creatinine, haematuria sometimes in association with glomerulonephritis. Isolated cases: acute renal failure, urinary retention.

Gastro-intestinal: Occasional: gastro-intestinal disturbance, diarrhoea, nausea, vomiting. Rare: jaundice, liver enlargement, abnormal liver function sometimes in association with hepatitis. Isolated cases: paralytic ileus.

Blood: Rare: anaemia, leucopenia, neutropenia, thrombocytopenia with or without purpura. Isolated cases: haemolytic anaemia, leucocytosis, lymphadenopathy, pancytopenia, splenomegaly, agranulocytosis.

Psyche: Rare: agitation, anorexia, anxiety. Isolated cases: depression, hallucinations.

Sense organs: Rare: increased lacrimation, conjunctivitis, nasal congestion.

Hypersensitivity reactions: Occasional: SLE-like syndrome (see *Special warnings and special precautions for use*). Rare: hypersensitivity reactions such as pruritus, urticaria, vasculitis, eosinophilia, hepatitis.

Respiratory tract: Rare: dyspnoea, pleural pain.

Miscellaneous: Rare: fever, weight decrease, malaise. Isolated cases: exophthalmos.

Overdose

Signs and symptoms: Hypotension, tachycardia, myocardial ischaemia, dysrrhythmias and coma.

Treatment: Supportive measures including intravenous fluids are indicated. If hypotension is present, an attempt should be made to raise the blood pressure without increasing the tachycardia. Adrenaline should be avoided.

Pharmacological properties

Pharmacodynamic properties: Hydralazine is a direct acting peripheral vasodilator, which exerts its effects principally on the arterioles. Its precise mode of action is not known. Administration of hydralazine produces a fall in peripheral resistance and a decrease in arterial blood pressure, effects which induce reflex sympathetic cardiovascular responses. The concomitant use of a beta-blocker will reduce these reflex effects and enhance the anti-hypertensive effect. The use of hydralazine can result in sodium and fluid retention, producing oedema and reduced urinary volume. These effects can be prevented by concomitant administration of a diuretic.

Pharmacokinetic properties: Apresoline is rapidly distributed in the body and displays a particular affinity for the blood-vessel walls. Plasma protein binding is of the order of 90%.

Plasma half-life averages 2 to 3 hours but is prolonged up to 16 hours in severe renal failure (creatinine clearance less than 20 ml/min) and shortened to approximately 45 minutes in rapid acetylators.

Preclinical safety data: Hydralazine has been found to be teratogenic in mice, producing a small incidence of cleft palate and certain other bony malformations, in oral doses ranging from 20 to 120 mg/kg i.e., 20 to 30 times the maximum human daily dose. It was not teratogenic in rats or rabbits.

In high (cyto-) toxic concentrations, hydralazine induces gene mutations in single cell organisms and in mammalian cells *in vitro*. No unequivocally mutagenic effects have been detected *in vivo* in a great number of test systems.

Hydralazine, in lifetime carcinogenicity studies, caused, towards the end of the experiments, small but statistically significant increases in lung tumours in mice and in hepatic and testicular tumours in rats. These tumours also occur spontaneously with fairly high frequency in aged rodents.

With due consideration of these animal and *in vitro* toxicological findings, hydralazine in therapeutic doses does not appear to bear a risk that would necessitate a limitation of its administration. Many years of clinical experience have not suggested that human cancer is associated with hydralazine use.

Pharmaceutical particulars
List of excipients: Hydrochloric acid.

Incompatibilities: Dextrose infusion solutions are not compatible as contact between hydralazine and glucose causes hydralazine to be rapidly broken down.

Shelf life: Five years for the unopened container.

Special precautions for storage: The ampoules should be protected from light and stored below 30°C. The reconstituted solution should be stored below 25°C and used within 24 hours.

Nature and contents of container: Colourless type I glass 2ml ampoule. Five ampoules are packed in a cardboard printed carton.

Instructions for use/handling: See *Posology and method of administration*.

Marketing authorisation number PL 16853/0001

Date of first authorisation 25 June 1998

Date of (partial) revision of the text June 1998

Legal status POM

APRESOLINE* TABLETS 25 mg

Qualitative and quantitative composition Hydralazine hydrochloride Ph.Eur. 25 mg.

Pharmaceutical form Round, biconvex, pale yellow sugar-coated tablet marked 'CG' on one side and 'GF' on the other.

Clinical particulars
Therapeutic indications: Moderate to severe hypertension as an adjunct to other anti-hypertensive agents.

In combination with long acting nitrates in moderate to severe chronic congestive cardiac failure, in patients in whom optimal doses of diuretics and cardiac glycosides have proved insufficient.

Posology and method of administration: See *Precautions* before use.

Adults:
Hypertension: The dose should be adjusted to the individual requirements of the patient. Treatment should begin with low doses of Apresoline which, depending on the patient's response, should be increased stepwise to achieve optimal therapeutic effect whilst keep unwanted effects to a minimum.

Initially 25 mg bid. This can be increased gradually to a dose not exceeding 200 mg daily. The dose should not be increased beyond 100 mg daily without first checking the patient's acetylator status.

Chronic congestive heart failure: Treatment with Apresoline should always be initiated in hospital, where the patient's individual haemodynamic values can be reliably determined with the help of invasive monitoring. It should then be continued in hospital until the patient has become stabilised on the requisite maintenance dose. Doses vary greatly between individual patients and are generally higher than those used for treating hypertension. After progressive titration (initially 25 mg tid or qid, increasing every second day) the maintenance dosage averages 50-75 mg qid.

Children: Not recommended.

Elderly: Clinical evidence would indicate that no special dosage regime is necessary. Advancing age does not affect either blood concentration or systemic clearance. Renal elimination may however be affected insofar as kidney function diminishes with age.

Contra-indications: Known hypersensitivity to hydralazine or dihydralazine.

Idiopathic systemic lupus erythematosus (SLE) and related diseases.

Severe tachycardia and heart failure with a high cardiac output (e.g. in thyrotoxicosis).

Myocardial insufficiency due to mechanical obstruction (e.g. in the presence of aortic or mitral stenosis or constrictive pericarditis).

Isolated right ventricular failure due to pulmonary hypertension (cor pulmonale).

Special warnings and special precautions for use: The overall 'hyperdynamic' state of the circulation induced by hydralazine may accentuate certain clinical conditions. Myocardial stimulation may provoke or aggravate angina pectoris. Patients with suspected or confirmed coronary artery disease should therefore be given Apresoline only under cover of beta-blockers or in combination with other suitable sympatholytic agents. It is important that the beta-blocker medication should be commenced a few days before the start of treatment with Apresoline.

Patients who have survived a myocardial infarction should not receive Apresoline until a post-infarction stabilisation phase has been achieved.

Prolonged treatment with hydralazine (i.e. usually for more than 6 months) may provoke a lupus erythematosus (LE) like syndrome, especially where doses exceed 100 mg daily. First symptoms are likely to be arthralgia, sometimes associated with fever and rash, and are reversible after withdrawal of the drug. In its more severe form it resembles acute SLE, and in rare cases renal and ocular involvement have been reported. Long term treatment with corticosteroids may be required to reverse these changes. Since such reactions tend to occur more frequently the higher the dose and the longer its duration, and since they are also more common in slow acetylators, it is recommended that for maintenance therapy the lowest effective dose should be used. If 100 mg daily fails to elicit an adequate clinical effect, the patient's acetylator status should be evaluated. Slow acetylators and women run a greater risk of developing the LE-like syndrome and every effort should therefore be made to keep the dosage below 100 mg daily and a careful watch kept for signs and symptoms suggestive of this syndrome. If such symptoms do develop the drug should be gradually withdrawn. Rapid acetylators often respond inadequately even to doses of 100mg daily and therefore the dose can be raised with only a slightly increased risk of an LE-like syndrome.

During long-term treatment with Apresoline it is advisable to determine the antinuclear factors and conduct urine analysis at intervals of approximately 6 months. Microhaematuria and/or proteinuria, in particular together with positive titres of ANF, may be initial signs of immune-complex glomerulonephritis associated with the SLE-like syndrome. If overt clinical signs or symptoms develop, the drug should be withdrawn immediately.

Skin rash, febrile reactions and changes in blood count occur rarely; the drug should be withdrawn in these cases. Peripheral neuritis in the form of paraesthesia has been reported, and may respond to pyridoxine administration or drug withdrawal.

In patients with renal impairment (creatinine clearance <30 ml/min or serum creatinine concentrations >2.5 mg/100 ml or 221 μmol/l) and in patients with hepatic dysfunction the dose or interval between doses should be adjusted according to clinical response, in order to avoid accumulation of the 'apparent' active substance.

Apresoline should be used with caution in patients with coronary artery disease (since it may increase angina) or cerebrovascular disease.

When undergoing surgery, patients treated with Apresoline may show a fall in blood pressure, in which case adrenaline should not be used to correct the hypotension, since it enhances the cardiac-accelerating effects of hydralazine.

When initiating therapy in heart failure, particular caution should be exercised and the patient kept under surveillance and/or haemodynamic monitoring for early detection of postural hypotension or tachycardia. Where discontinuation of therapy in heart failure is indicated, Apresoline should be withdrawn gradually (except in serious situations, such as SLE-like syndrome or blood dyscrasias) in order to avoid precipitation and/or exacerbation of heart failure.

Interaction with other medicaments and other forms of interaction: Potentiation of effects: Concurrent therapy with other antihypertensives (vasodilators, calcium antagonists, ACE inhibitors, diuretics), anaesthetics, tricyclic antidepressants, major tranquillisers or drugs exerting central depressant actions (including alcohol).

Administration of Apresoline shortly before or after diazoxide may give rise to marked hypotension.

MAO inhibitors should be used with caution in patients receiving Apresoline.

Concurrent administration of Apresoline with beta-blockers subject to a strong first-pass effect (e.g. propranolol) may increase their bioavailability. Downward adjustment of these drugs may be required when they are given concomitantly with Apresoline.

Pregnancy and lactation: Use of Apresoline in pregnancy before the third trimester should be avoided, but the drug may be used in later pregnancy if there is no safer alternative or when the disease itself carries serious risks for the mother or child e.g. pre-eclampsia and/or eclampsia.

No serious adverse effects in human pregnancy have been reported to date with Apresoline, although experience in the third trimester is extensive.

Hydralazine passes into breast milk but reports available so far have not shown adverse effects on the infant. Where use of Apresoline proves unavoidable, mothers may breast feed their infant, provided that the infant is observed for possible adverse effects.

Effects on ability to drive and use machines: Patients should be warned of the potential hazards when driving or operating machinery if they suffer from side effects such as dizziness.

Undesirable effects: Some of the adverse effects listed below e.g. tachycardia, palpitation, anginal symptoms, flushing, headache, dizziness, nasal congestion and gastro-intestinal disturbances are commonly seen at the start of treatment, especially if the dose is raised quickly. However such effects generally subside in the further course of treatment. (The following frequency estimates are used: frequent > 10%, occasional 1-10%, rare 0.001-1%, isolated cases < 0.001%)

Cardiovascular system: Frequent: tachycardia, palpitation. Occasional: flushing, hypotension, anginal symptoms. Rare: oedema, heart failure. Isolated cases: paradoxical pressor responses.

Central and peripheral nervous system: Frequent: headache. Rare: dizziness. Isolated cases: peripheral neuritis, polyneuritis, paraesthesiae (these unwanted effects may be reversed by administering pyridoxine).

Musculo-skeletal system: Occasional: arthralgia, joint swelling, myalgia.

Skin and appendages: Rare: rash.

Urogenital system: Rare: proteinuria, increased plasma creatinine, haematuria sometimes in association with glomerulonephritis. Isolated cases: acute renal failure, urinary retention.

Gastro-intestinal tract: Occasional: gastro-intestinal disturbances, diarrhoea, nausea, vomiting. Rare: jaundice, liver enlargement, abnormal liver function sometimes in association with hepatitis. Isolated cases: paralytic ileus.

Blood: Rare: anaemia, leucopenia, neutropenia, thrombocytopenia with or without purpura. Isolated cases: haemolytic anaemia, leucocytosis, lymphadenopathy, pancytopenia, splenomegaly, agranulocytosis.

Psyche: Rare: agitation, anorexia, anxiety. Isolated cases: depression, hallucinations.

Sense organs: Rare: increased lacrimation, conjunctivitis, nasal congestion.

Hypersensitivity reactions: Occasional: SLE-like syndrome (see *Special warnings and special precautions for use*). Rare: hypersensitivity reactions such as pruritus, urticaria, vasculitis, eosinophilia, hepatitis.

Respiratory tract: Rare: dyspnoea, pleural pain.

Miscellaneous: Rare: fever, weight decrease, malaise. Isolated cases: exophthalmos.

Overdose:
Signs and symptoms: Symptoms include hypotension, tachycardia, myocardial ischaemia, dysrrhythmias and coma.

Treatment: Gastric lavage should be instituted as soon as possible. Supportive measures including intravenous fluids are also indicated. If hypotension is present, an attempt should be made to raise the blood pressure without increasing the tachycardia. Adrenaline should be avoided.

Pharmacological particulars
Pharmacodynamic properties: Hydralazine is a direct acting peripheral vasodilator that exerts its effects principally on the arterioles. Its precise mode of action is not known. Administration of hydralazine produces a fall in peripheral resistance and a decrease in arterial blood pressure, effects which induce reflex sympathetic cardiovascular responses. The concomitant use of a beta-blocker will reduce these reflex effects and enhance the anti-hypertensive effect. The use of hydralazine can result in sodium and fluid retention, producing oedema and reduced urinary volume. These effects can be prevented by concomitant administration of a diuretic.

Pharmacokinetic properties: Orally administered Apresoline is rapidly and completely absorbed but is subject to a dose-dependent first pass effect (systemic bioavailability: 26-55%) which is dependent upon the individual's acetylator status. Peak plasma concentrations are attained after 0.5 to 1.5 hours. Apresoline is rapidly distributed in the body and displays a particular affinity for the blood-vessel walls. Plasma protein binding is of the order of 90%. Within 24 hours after an oral dose, the quantity recovered in the urine averages 80% of the dose. Apresoline appears in the plasma chiefly in the form of a readily hydrolysable conjugate with pyruvic acid. Plasma half-life averages 2-3 hours but is prolonged up to 16 hours in severe renal failure (creatinine clearance less than 20 ml/min) and shortened to approximately 45 minutes in rapid acetylators. The bulk of the dose is excreted as acetylated and hydroxylated metabolites, some of which are conjugated with glucuronic acid.

Preclinical safety data: Hydralazine has been found to be teratogenic in mice, producing a small incidence of cleft palate and certain other bony malformations, in oral doses ranging from 20-120 mg/kg i.e. 20-30 times the maximum human daily dose. It was not teratogenic in rats or rabbits.

In high (cyto-) toxic concentrations, hydralazine induces gene mutations in single cell organisms and in mammalian cells *in-vitro*. No unequivocally mutagenic effects have been detected *in-vivo* in a great number of test systems.

Hydralazine, in lifetime carcinogenicity studies, caused, towards the end of the experiments, small but statistically significant increases in lung tumours in mice and in hepatic and testicular tumours in rats. These tumours also occur spontaneously with fairly high frequency in aged rodents.

With due consideration of these animal and *in-vitro* toxicological findings, hydralazine in therapeutic doses does not appear to bear a risk that would necessitate a limitation of its administration. Many years of clinical experience have not suggested that human cancer is associated with hydralazine use.

Pharmaceutical particulars
List of excipients: Silicon dioxide, microcrystalline cellulose, magnesium stearate, polyvinylpyrrolidone, wheat starch, hydroxypropylmethylcellulose, povidone, talc, titanium dioxide (E171), polyethylene glycol, sucrose and yellow iron oxide (E172).

Incompatibilities: None.

Shelf life: Four years.

Special precautions for storage: Protect from moisture and heat (store below 30°C).

Nature and contents of container: Securitainers of 84 tablets.

Instructions for use/handling: None.

Marketing authorisation number PL 16853/0002

Date of first authorisation 26 June 1998.

Date of (partial) revision of the text June 1998.

Legal status POM.

CAFERGOT* SUPPOSITORIES 2mg

Qualitative and quantitative composition
Ergotamine tartrate PhEur 2 mg and caffeine PhEur 100 mg.

Pharmaceutical form
Off-white suppositories, 3 cm in length, 1 cm in diameter.

Clinical particulars
Therapeutic indications: Acute attacks of migraine and migraine variants unresponsive to simple analgesics.

Posology and method of administration
Adults: There is considerable inter-individual variation in the sensitivity of patients to ergotamine. Care should therefore be exercised in selecting the optimum therapeutic dose for an individual patient which will not give rise to unwanted effects, either acutely or chronically. The maximum recommended dosages should not be exceeded and ergotamine treatment should not be administered at intervals of less than 4 days.

For maximum efficacy, the optimal dose (in the preferred presentation) should be administered immediately prodromal symptoms are experienced.

One suppository should be administered at the first warning of an attack. This dose is normally sufficient, although some individuals may require higher dosages which should never exceed 2 suppositories (4 mg ergotamine) in 24 hours. It is essential to use the minimum effective dose.

The maximum recommended weekly dosage of 4 suppositories (8 mg ergotamine) should never be exceeded.

Children under 12 years: Not recommended.

Elderly: Whilst there is no evidence to suggest that the elderly require different dosages of Cafergot, the contra-indications of this drug are common in the elderly, e.g. coronary heart disease, renal impairment, hepatic impairment and severe hypertension. Caution should therefore be exercised when prescribing for this age group.

Contra-indications: Patients with peripheral vascular disease, coronary heart disease, obliterative vascular disease and Raynaud's Syndrome, in view of the increased risk of peripheral vasospasm secondary to ergotamine. Impaired hepatic or renal function, sepsis and severe hypertension, pregnancy or nursing mothers.

Cafergot should not be used for migraine prophylaxis nor should the recommended dosage be exceeded. Frequent attacks of migraine may be an indication for the use of a suitable prophylactic agent.

Special warnings and precautions for use: If symptoms such as tingling in the fingers or toes occur, the drug should be discontinued at once and the physician consulted.

Interactions with other medicaments and other forms of interaction: Concomitant use of erythromycin and ergotamine should be avoided, as this can result in an elevated concentration of ergotamine in the plasma.

As vasospastic reactions have been reported with beta-blockers alone and in a few patients treated concomitantly with ergotamine and propranolol, caution is advised in the concomitant use of these agents with Cafergot.

Pregnancy and lactation: Ergotamine-containing products are contra-indicated in pregnancy due to oxytocic effects on the pregnant uterus, and in breast feeding mothers due to the risk of the infant developing ergotism. Repeated doses of ergotamine may inhibit lactation.

Effects on ability to drive and use machinery: None known.

Undesirable effects: The caffeine component of Cafergot may give rise to unwanted stimulant effects.

Side-effects of Cafergot are related in the main to the ergotamine component. Acutely, these may include nausea, vomiting and abdominal pain. Paraesthesia and peripheral vasoconstriction or pain and weakness in the extremities may develop after both acute and chronic dosing. Numbness and tingling of the extremities can be indicative of peripheral vasospasm and treatment must be stopped immediately if signs of circulatory impairment appear. Failure to observe this precaution can lead to the development of ergotism. Due to its vasoconstrictor properties ergotamine may cause precordial pain, myocardial ischaemia, or, in rare cases, infarction, even in patients with no known history of coronary heart disease.

Excessive use of ergotamine-containing products for prolonged periods may result in fibrotic changes, in particular of the pleura and retroperitoneum.

Overdosage
Symptoms: Nausea, vomiting, drowsiness, confusion, tachycardia, dizziness, tingling and numbness in the extremities due to ischaemia, respiratory depression, coma.

Treatment: Should be directed to the elimination of ingested material by aspiration and gastric lavage.

Rarely, headache may be provoked either by chronic overdosage or by rapid withdrawal of the product. Caffeine is a weak stimulant and excessive use of Cafergot may lead to a state of arousal and anxiety.

If severe arteriospasms occur, vasodilators such as nitroprusside sodium should be administered. General supportive measures should be applied with particular reference to the respiratory and cardiovascular systems.

Pharmacological properties
Pharmacodynamic properties: Ergotamine is a highly vasoactive ergot alkaloid having characteristically complex pharmacological actions. It is a partial tryptaminic agonist in certain blood vessels and both a partial agonist and antagonist of α-adrenergic receptors of blood vessels.

Although its exact mode of action in migraine is not known, its therapeutic effects have been attributed to its ability to cause vasoconstriction, thereby eliminating the painful dilation/pulsation of branches of the external carotid artery.

Pharmacokinetic properties: There is great interindividual variation in the absorption of ergotamine in patients and volunteers. Bioavailability is of the order of 5% or less by oral or rectal administration. After im or iv administration, plasma concentrations decay in a bi-exponential fashion. The elimination half life is 2 to 2.5 hours and clearance is about 0.68L/h/kg. Metabolism occurs in the liver and the primary route of excretion is biliary.

Preclinical safety data: There are no pre-clinical data of relevance to the prescriber which are additional to those already included in other sections of the Summary of Product Characteristics.

Pharmaceutical particulars
List of excipients: Tartaric acid, lactose, Suppocire AM.

Incompatibilities: None.

Shelf life: 3 years.

Special precautions for storage: Store below 25°C.

Nature and contents of container: Carton of 30 suppositories in an aluminium blister pack.

Instructions for use/handling: None.

Administrative data
Marketing authorisation holder Alliance Pharmaceuticals Ltd, Avonbridge House, Bath Road, Chippenham, Wiltshire, SN15 2BB.

Marketing authorisation number PL16853/0003.

Date of first authorisation 25 June 1998.

Date of (partial) revision of the text June 1998.

Legal status POM.

CAFERGOT* TABLETS

Qualitative and quantitative composition
Ergotamine tartrate PhEur 1 mg and caffeine PhEur 100 mg.

Pharmaceutical form
White, round, sugar coated tablets.

Clinical particulars
Therapeutic indications: Acute attacks of migraine and migraine variants unresponsive to simple analgesics.

Posology and method of administration
Adults: There is considerable inter-individual variation in the sensitivity of patients to ergotamine. Care should therefore be exercised in selecting the optimum therapeutic dose for an individual patient which will not give rise to unwanted effects, either acutely or chronically. The maximum recommended dosages should not be exceeded and ergotamine treatment should not be administered at intervals of less than 4 days.

For maximum efficacy, the optimal dose (in the preferred presentation) should be administered immediately prodromal symptoms are experienced.

One or two tablets taken at the first warning of an attack are normally sufficient to obtain migraine relief. Some individuals may require higher dosages which should never exceed 4 tablets (4 mg ergotamine) in 24 hours. It is essential to use the minimum effective dose.

The maximum recommended weekly dosage of 8 tablets (8 mg ergotamine) should not be exceeded.

Children under 12 years: Not recommended.

Elderly: Whilst there is no evidence to suggest that the elderly require different dosages of Cafergot, the contra-indications of this drug are common in the elderly, e.g. coronary heart disease, renal impairment, hepatic impairment and severe hypertension. Caution should therefore be exercised when prescribing for this age group.

Contra-indications: Patients with peripheral vascular disease, coronary heart disease, obliterative vascular disease and Raynaud's Syndrome, in view of the increased risk of peripheral vasospasm secondary to ergotamine. Impaired hepatic or renal function, sepsis and severe hypertension. Pregnancy or nursing mothers.

Cafergot should not be used for migraine prophylaxis nor should the recommended dosage be exceeded. Frequent attacks of migraine may be an indication for the use of a suitable prophylactic agent.

Special warnings and precautions for use: If symptoms such as tingling in the fingers or toes occur, the drug should be discontinued at once and the physician consulted.

Interactions with other medicaments and other forms of interaction: Concomitant use of erythromycin and ergotamine should be avoided, as this can result in an elevated concentration of ergotamine in the plasma.

As vasospastic reactions have been reported with beta-blockers alone and in a few patients treated concomitantly with ergotamine and propranolol, caution is advised in the concomitant use of these agents with Cafergot.

Pregnancy and lactation: Ergotamine-containing products are contra-indicated in pregnancy due to oxytocic effects on the pregnant uterus, and in breast feeding mothers due to the risk of the infant developing ergotism. Repeated doses of ergotamine may inhibit lactation.

Effects on ability to drive and use machinery: None known.

Undesirable effects: The caffeine component of Cafergot may give rise to unwanted stimulant effects.

Side-effects of Cafergot are related in the main to the ergotamine component. Acutely, these may include nausea, vomiting and abdominal pain. Paraesthesia and peripheral vasoconstriction or pain and weakness in the extremities may develop after both acute and chronic dosing. Numbness and tingling of the extremities can be indicative of peripheral vasospasm and treatment must be stopped immediately if signs of circulatory impairment appear. Failure to observe this precaution can lead to the development of ergotism. Due to its vasoconstrictor properties, ergotamine may cause precordial pain, myocardial ischaemia, or, in rare cases, infarction, even in patients with no known history of coronary heart disease.

Excessive use of ergotamine-containing products for prolonged periods may result in fibrotic changes, in particular of the pleura and retroperitoneum.

Overdosage
Symptoms: Nausea, vomiting, drowsiness, confusion, tachycardia, dizziness, tingling and numbness in the

extremities due to ischaemia, respiratory depression, coma.

Treatment: Should be directed to the elimination of ingested material by aspiration and gastric lavage.

Rarely, headache may be provoked either by chronic overdosage or by rapid withdrawal of the product. Caffeine is a weak stimulant and excessive use of Cafergot may lead to a state of arousal and anxiety.

If severe arteriospasms occur, vasodilators such as nitroprusside sodium should be administered. General supportive measures should be applied with particular reference to the respiratory and cardiovascular systems.

Pharmacological properties

Pharmacodynamic properties: Ergotamine is a highly vasoactive ergot alkaloid having characteristically complex pharmacological actions. It is a partial tryptaminic agonist in certain blood vessels and both a partial agonist and antagonist of α-adrenergic receptors of blood vessels.

Although its exact mode of action in migraine is not known, its therapeutic effects have been attributed to its ability to cause vasoconstriction, thereby eliminating the painful dilation/pulsation of branches of the external carotid artery.

Pharmacokinetic properties: There is great interindividual variation in the absorption of ergotamine in patients and volunteers. Bioavailability is of the order of 5% or less by oral or rectal administration. After im or iv administration, plasma concentrations decay in a bi-exponential fashion. The elimination half life is 2 to 2.5 hours and clearance is about 0.68L/h/kg. Metabolism occurs in the liver and the primary route of excretion is biliary.

Preclinical safety data: There are no pre-clinical data of relevance to the prescriber which are additional to those already included in other sections of the Summary of Product Characteristics.

Pharmaceutical particulars

List of excipients: Tartaric acid, gelatin, stearic acid, lactose, starch, talc, gum acacia, sugar and carnauba wax.

Incompatibilities: None.

Shelf life: 2 years.

Special precautions for storage: None.

Nature and contents of container: Cartons of 30 tablets in opaque aluminium/PVDC blister packs.

Instructions for use/handling: None.

Marketing authorisation number PL 16853/0004.

Date of first authorisation 25 June 1998.

Date of (partial) revision of the text June 1998.

Legal status POM.

CALCIUM-SANDOZ* SYRUP

Presentation

Calcium-Sandoz Syrup: Colourless to pale straw coloured, fruit flavoured syrup. Each 15 ml contains 3.27 g calcium glubionate and 2.18 g calcium lactobionate. Three 5 ml spoonfuls provide 325 mg calcium (8.1 mmol: 16.2 mEq Ca^{++}).

Uses

Principal action: Calcium is an essential body electrolyte. It is involved in the maintenance of normal muscle and nerve function, is essential for normal cardiac function and is essential to blood coagulation. There is a dynamic equilibrium between the calcium in blood and that in the skeleton. Homeostasis is mainly regulated by parathyroid hormone, by calcitonin and by vitamin D.

Indications

1. As an adjunct to conventional therapy in the arrest or slowing down of bone demineralisation in osteoporosis.

2. In the arrest or slowing down of bone demineralisation in osteoporosis where other effective treatment is contra-indicated.

3. As a supplemental source of calcium in the correction of dietary deficiencies or when normal requirements are high.

4. Treatment of neonatal hypocalcaemia.

Signs of hypocalcaemia may occur when the serum calcium concentration falls below 2.25 mmol per litre (or 4.5 mEq per litre). Symptoms may include paraesthesia, laryngospasm, muscle cramps, increased muscle excitability leading to tetany, prolongation of the Q-T interval on the ECG, convulsions and mental changes (e.g. anxiety, depression, delusions). Also ectodermal changes including loss of hair, grooved and brittle fingernails, defects of dental enamel and fungal infections, typically generalised candidiasis.

Dosage and administration In health the concentration of calcium in serum is maintained close to 2.5 mmol per litre (normal range 2.25–2.75 mmol or 4.5–5.5 mEq per litre). Treatment or therapeutic supplementation should aim to restore or maintain this level.

Indication	*Daily Dose 5 ml spoonfuls syrup*
Adults	
Osteoporosis	11–15
Therapeutic supplement (dose dependent upon severity)	3–15
Children	
Calcium deficiency	6–9
Dietary supplementation	2–6

Neonatal hypocalcaemia: Calcium-Sandoz syrup may be given at a dose of 1 mmol calcium/kg/24 hours in divided doses. Serum calcium levels should be monitored and the dosage adjusted if necessary. Doses may be mixed with the first (small) part of milk feeds. Note: 1 mmol of calcium is equivalent to 1.85 ml Calcium-Sandoz syrup.

Use in the elderly: No evidence exists that tolerance is directly affected by advanced age; however, elderly patients should be supervised as factors sometimes associated with ageing, such as poor diet or impaired renal function, may indirectly affect tolerance and may require dosage reduction.

Contra-indications, warnings, etc

Contra-indications: Hypercalcaemia (e.g. in hyperparathyroidism, vitamin D overdosage, decalcifying tumours such as plasmocytoma, severe renal failure, bone metastases), severe hypercalciuria, and renal calculi.

Due to its galactose component Calcium-Sandoz syrup should not be given to patients with galactosaemia.

Precautions: In mild hypercalciuria (exceeding 300 mg (7.5 mmol)/24 hours) or renal failure, or where there is evidence of stone formation in the urinary tract, adequate checks must be kept on urinary calcium excretion; if necessary the dosage should be reduced or calcium therapy discontinued. High vitamin D intake should be avoided during calcium therapy, unless especially indicated.

Thiazide diuretics reduce urinary calcium excretion so the risk of hypercalcaemia should be considered.

Oral calcium supplementation is aimed at restoring normal serum calcium levels. Although it is extremely unlikely that high enough levels will be achieved to adversely affect digitalised patients, this theoretical possibility should be considered.

The sugar content of Calcium-Sandoz syrup should be taken into account in diabetic patients.

Oral calcium administration may reduce the absorption of oral tetracycline or fluoride preparations. An interval of 3 hours should be observed if the two are to be given.

Use in pregnancy and lactation: The likelihood of hypercalcaemia is increased in pregnant women in whom calcium and vitamin D are co-administered. Epidemiological studies with calcium have shown no increase in the teratogenic hazard to the foetus if used in the doses recommended. Although supplemental calcium may be excreted in breast milk, the concentration is unlikely to be sufficient to produce any adverse effect on the neonate.

Side-effects: Mild gastrointestinal disturbances have occurred rarely (e.g. constipation, diarrhoea). Although hypercalcaemia would not be expected in patients unless their renal function were impaired, the following symptoms could indicate the possibility of hypercalcaemia: nausea, vomiting, anorexia, constipation, abdominal pain, bone pain, thirst, polyuria, muscle weakness, drowsiness or confusion.

Overdosage: The amount of calcium absorbed following overdosage will depend on the individual's calcium status. It might cause gastrointestinal disturbances but would not be expected to cause hypercalcaemia except in patients treated with excessive doses of vitamin D. Treatment should be aimed at lowering serum calcium levels, e.g. administration of oral phosphates.

Pharmaceutical precautions Calcium-Sandoz Syrup may be diluted with Syrup BP; the diluted syrup should be used within 14 days.

Legal category P.

Package quantities Bottles of 300 ml.

Further information Calcium-Sandoz Syrup contains 1.512 g sucrose per 5 ml (4.536 g sucrose per 15 ml dose). Approximate calorific value of 13 kcals per 5 ml (39 kcals per 15 ml dose).

Product licence number 16853/0005

DESERIL* TABLETS 1 mg

Qualitative and quantitative composition

Methysergide maleate BP 1.33 mg.

Pharmaceutical form

White, biconvex, sugar-coated tablet, branded DSL on one side.

Clinical particulars

Therapeutic indications: Prophylactic treatment of migraine, cluster headache and other vascular headaches in patients who, despite attempts at control, experience headaches of such severity or regularity that social or economic life is seriously disrupted. (Note: Deseril is not recommended for treatment of the acute attack.)

Control of profuse diarrhoea associated with carcinoid disease.

Posology and method of administration

Prophylactic treatment of headache: 1 or 2 tablets three times a day with meals. Treatment should start with one tablet at bedtime and dosage should then be increased gradually over about two weeks until effective levels are reached. The minimum effective dose should be used, often that which will prevent 75% of attacks rather than all headaches.

From the outset, patients should understand that regular clinical supervision and periodic withdrawal of treatment are essential so that adverse effects can be recognised and minimised.

Carcinoid syndrome: High doses are usually necessary. In most reported cases, dosage ranged between 12 and 20 tablets daily.

Children: Not recommended.

Elderly: No evidence exists that elderly patients require different dosages from younger patients.

Contra-indications: Hypersensitivity to the drug, pregnancy, lactation, peripheral vascular disorders, progressive arteriosclerosis, severe hypertension, coronary heart disease, valvular heart disease, phlebitis or cellulitis of the lower extremities, pulmonary disease, collagen disease, impaired kidney or liver function, disease of the urinary tract, cachectic or septic conditions.

Special warnings and precautions for use: Continuous Deseril administration should not exceed six months without a drug-free interval of at least one month for re-assessment; dosage should be reduced gradually over two to three weeks to avoid rebound headaches. In patients undergoing treatment with Deseril the dose of ergotamine required to control acute attacks may have to be reduced.

Regular clinical supervision of patients treated with Deseril is essential. Particular attention should be paid to complaints of urinary dysfunction, pain in the loin, flank or chest, and pain, coldness or numbness in the limbs. Patients should be regularly examined for the presence of cardiac murmurs, vascular bruits, pleural or pericardial friction rubs and abdominal or flank masses or tenderness. Treatment with Deseril should be stopped should any of these symptoms or signs occur. Caution is also advised during drug administration to patients with a past history of peptic ulceration.

In carcinoid syndrome the risk of adverse reactions due to the higher dosage must be weighed against the therapeutic benefit.

Interactions with other medicaments and other forms of interaction: Concomitant use of Deseril and vasoconstrictors or vasopressors may result in enhanced vasoconstriction.

Pregnancy and lactation: Deseril is contra-indicated during pregnancy or lactation.

Effects on ability to drive and use machines: Patients should be warned of the potential hazards of driving or operating machinery if they experience side-effects such as dizziness or drowsiness.

Undesirable effects

General: The most commonly reported side-effects are nausea, heartburn, abdominal discomfort, vomiting, dizziness, lassitude and drowsiness. These side-effects can often be minimised by taking Deseril with food. Tissue oedema, insomnia, leg cramps and weight gain have occurred, and skin eruptions or loss of scalp hair have occasionally been reported. Mental and behavioural disturbances have occurred in isolated instances.

Inflammatory fibrosis: Retroperitoneal fibrosis: Continuous long-term Deseril administration has been associated with the development of retroperitoneal fibrosis. This is very rare when continuous treatment has not exceeded 6 months. Retroperitoneal fibrosis usually presents with symptoms of urinary tract obstruction such as persistent loin or flank pain, oliguria, dysuria, increased blood nitrogen and vascular insufficiency of the lower limbs. Deseril must be withdrawn if retroperitoneal fibrosis develops; drug withdrawal is often associated with clinical improvement over a few days to several weeks.

Fibrosis in other areas: Fibrotic processes involving lungs, pleura, heart valves and major vessels have been reported in a small number of patients. Presenting symptoms include chest pain, dyspnoea or pleural friction rub and pleural effusion. Cardiac murmurs or vascular bruits have also been reported. Appearance of these symptoms demands immediate withdrawal of Deseril. These fibrotic manifestations are often reversible although less readily so than retroperitoneal fibrosis.

Vascular: Vascular reactions, including arterial spasm, have been seen in some patients. The following have all been described: arterial spasm in a limb causing coldness, numbness, pain or intermittent claudication; renal artery spasm giving rise to transitory hypertension; mesenteric artery spasm causing abdominal pain; retinal artery spasm causing reversible loss of vision; coronary artery spasm causing angina and questionably resulting in myocardial infarction. Arterial spasm is rapidly reversible following drug withdrawal.

Overdose: Treatment should be directed to elimination of the ingested material by aspiration and gastric lavage. General supportive measures should be applied. The patient should be carefully observed for peripheral vasospasm which may be treated by warmth, care being taken to protect ischaemic limbs. If there is evidence of impending tissue damage vasodilators may be used.

Pharmacological properties

Pharmacodynamic properties: Deseril is effective in the prevention of migraine chiefly on account of two properties: Its marked serotonin antagonism (inhibition of pain-facilitation and permeability-increasing actions of serotonin), and its potentiating effect on vasoconstrictor stimuli.

Pharmacokinetic properties: Methysergide is rapidly and well absorbed. The parent drug is metabolised in the liver mainly to methylergometrine. Unchanged parent drug and metabolites are excreted predominantly via the kidney; the elimination is biphasic, with a half-life of 2.7 hours for the α-phase and 10 hours for the β-phase. Protein binding is moderate (66%).

Preclinical safety data: None stated.

Pharmaceutical particulars

List of excipients: Maleic acid, gelatin, stearic acid, talc, starch, lactose. The coating constituents are gum acacia, sugar, talc, titanium dioxide, colloidal anhydrous silica, carnauba wax and printing ink.

Incompatibilities: None.

Shelf life: 5 years.

Special precautions for storage: None.

Nature and contents of container: Aluminium/PVDC blister strips of 60 tablets.

Instruction for use/handling: None.

Marketing authorisation number PL16853/0006.

Date of first authorisation 25 June 1998.

Date of (partial) revision of the text June 1998.

Legal status POM.

HYGROTON* TABLETS 50 mg

Qualitative and quantitative composition

Chlorthalidone PhEur 50 mg.

Pharmaceutical form

Pale yellow, round, flat tablets with bevelled edges, impressed Geigy on one side with a breakline, and the letters Z/A on the other side.

Clinical particulars

Therapeutic indications: Treatment of arterial hypertension, essential or nephrogenic or isolated systolic. Treatment of stable, chronic heart failure of mild to moderate degree (New York Heart Association, NYHA: functional class II or III).

Oedema of specific origin

- Ascites due to cirrhosis of the liver in stable patients under close control.
- Oedema due to nephrotic syndrome.

Diabetes insipidus.

Posology and method of administration

The dosage of Hygroton should be individually titrated to give the lowest effective dose; this is particularly important in the elderly. Hygroton should be taken orally, preferably as a single daily dose at breakfast time.

Adults

Hypertension: The recommended starting dose is 25 mg/day. This is sufficient to produce the maximum hypotensive effect in most patients. If the decrease in blood pressure proves inadequate with 25 mg/day, then the dose can be increased to 50 mg/day. If a further reduction in blood pressure is required, additional hypertensive therapy may be added to the dosage regime.

Stable, chronic heart failure (NYHA: functional class II/III): The recommended starting dose is 25 to 50 mg/day, in severe cases it may be increased up to 100 to 200 mg/day. The usual maintenance dose is the lowest effective dose, e.g. 25 to 50 mg/day either daily or every other day. If the response proves inadequate, digitalis or an ACE inhibitor, or both, may be added (see *Special warnings and precautions for use*).

Oedema of specific origin (see Therapeutic indications): The lowest effective dose is to be identified by titration and administered over limited periods only. It is recommended that doses should not exceed 50 mg/day.

Diabetes insipidus: Initially 100 mg twice daily but reducing where possible to a daily maintenance dose of 50 mg.

Children: The lowest effective dose should also be used in children. For example, an initial dose of 0.5 to 1 mg/kg/48 hours and a maximum dose of 1.7 mg/kg/48 hours have been used.

Elderly patients and patients with renal impairment: The lowest effective dose of Hygroton is also recommended for patients with mild renal insufficiency and for elderly patients (see *Pharmacokinetic properties*).

In elderly patients, the elimination of chlorthalidone is slower than in healthy young adults, although absorption is the same. Therefore, a reduction in the recommended adult dosage may be needed. Close medical observation is indicated when treating patients of advanced age with chlorthalidone.

Hygroton and the thiazide diuretics lose their diuretic effect when the creatinine clearance is <30 ml/min.

Contra-indications: Anuria, severe hepatic or renal failure (creatinine clearance <30 ml/min), hypersensitivity to chlorthalidone and other sulphonamide derivatives, refractory hypokalaemia, hyponatraemia and hypercalcaemia, symptomatic hyperuricaemia (history of gout or uric acid calculi), hypertension during pregnancy, untreated Addison's disease and concomitant lithium therapy.

Special warnings and precautions for use

Warnings: Hygroton should be used with caution in patients with impaired hepatic function or progressive liver disease since minor changes in the fluid and electrolyte balance due to thiazide diuretics may precipitate hepatic coma, especially in patients with liver cirrhosis (see *Contra-indications*).

Hygroton should also be used with caution in patients with severe renal disease. Thiazides may precipitate azotaemia in such patients, and the effects of repeated administration may be cumulative.

Precautions

Electrolytes: Treatment with thiazide diuretics has been associated with electrolyte disturbances such as hypokalaemia, hypomagnesaemia, hyperglycaemia and hyponatraemia. Since the excretion of electrolytes is increased, a very strict low-salt diet should be avoided.

Hypokalaemia can sensitise the heart or exaggerate its response to the toxic effects of digitalis.

Like all thiazide diuretics, kaluresis induced by Hygroton is dose dependent and varies in extent from one subject to another. With 25 to 50 mg/day, the decrease in serum potassium concentrations averages 0.5 mmol/l. Periodic serum electrolyte determinations should be carried out, particularly in digitalised patients.

If necessary, Hygroton may be combined with oral potassium supplements or a potassium-sparing diuretic (e.g. triamterene).

If hypokalaemia is accompanied by clinical signs (e.g. muscular weakness, paresis and ECG alteration), Hygroton should be discontinued.

Combined treatment consisting of Hygroton and a potassium salt or a potassium-sparing diuretic should be avoided in patients also receiving ACE inhibitors.

Monitoring of serum electrolytes is particularly indicated in the elderly, in patients with ascites due to liver cirrhosis, and in patients with oedema due to nephrotic syndrome. There have been isolated reports of hyponatraemia with neurological symptoms (e.g. nausea, debility, progressive disorientation and apathy) following thiazide treatment.

For nephrotic syndrome, Hygroton should be used only under close control in normokalaemic patients with no signs of volume depletion.

Metabolic effects: Hygroton may raise the serum uric acid level, but attacks of gout are uncommon during chronic treatment.

As with the use of other thiazide diuretics, glucose intolerance may occur; this is manifest as hyperglycaemia and glycosuria. Hygroton may very seldom aggravate or precipitate diabetes mellitus; this is usually reversible on stopping therapy.

Small and partly reversible increases in plasma concentrations of total cholesterol, triglycerides, or low-density lipoprotein cholesterol were reported in patients during long-term treatment with thiazides and thiazide-like diuretics. The clinical relevance of these findings is a matter for debate.

Hygroton should not be used as a first-line drug for long-term treatment in patients with overt diabetes mellitus or in subjects receiving therapy for hypercholesterolaemia (diet or combined).

As with all antihypertensive agents, a cautious dosage schedule is indicated in patients with severe coronary or cerebral anteriosclerosis.

Other effects: The antihypertensive effect of ACE inhibitors is potentiated by agents that increase plasma renin activity (diuretics). It is recommended that the diuretic be reduced in dosage or withdrawn for 2 to 3 days and/or that the ACE inhibitor therapy be started with a low initial dose of the ACE inhibitor. Patients should be monitored for several hours after the first dose.

Interactions with other medicaments and other forms of interaction: Diuretics potentiate the action of curare derivatives and antihypertensive drugs (e.g. guanethidine, methyldopa, β-blockers, vasodilators, calcium antagonists and ACE inhibitors).

The hypokalaemic effect of diuretics may be potentiated by corticosteroids, ACTH, β_2-agonists, amphotericin and carbenoxolone.

It may prove necessary to adjust the dosage of insulin and oral anti-diabetic agents.

Thiazide-induced hypokalaemia or hypomagnesaemia may favour the occurrence of digitalis-induced cardiac arrhythmias (see *Special warnings and precautions for use*).

Concomitant administration of certain non-steroidal anti-inflammatory drugs (e.g. indomethacin) may reduce the diuretic and antihypertensive activity of Hygroton; there have been isolated reports of a deterioration in renal function in predisposed patients.

The bioavailability of thiazide-type diuretics may be increased by anticholinergic agents (e.g. atropine, biperiden), apparently due to a decrease in gastrointestinal motility and stomach-emptying rate.

Absorption of thiazide diuretics is impaired in the presence of anionic exchange resins such as cholestyramine. A decrease in the pharmacological effect may be expected.

Concurrent administration of thiazide diuretics may increase the incidence of hypersensitivity reactions to allopurinol, increase the risk of adverse effects caused by amantadine, enhance the hyperglycaemic effect of diazoxide, and reduce renal excretion of cytotoxic agents (e.g. cyclophosphamide, methotrexate) and potentiate their myelosuppressive effects.

The pharmacological effects of both calcium salts and vitamin D may be increased to clinically significant levels if given with thiazide diuretics. The resultant hypercalcaemia is usually transient but may be persistent and symptomatic (weakness, fatigue, anorexia) in patients with hyperparathyroidism.

Concomitant treatment with cyclosporin may increase the risk of hyperuricaemia and gout-type complications.

Pregnancy and lactation: Diuretics are best avoided for the management of oedema or hypertension in pregnancy as their use may be associated with hypovolaemia, increased blood viscosity and reduced placental perfusion. There have been reports of foetal bone marrow depression, thrombocytopenia, and foetal and neonatal jaundice associated with the use of thiazide diuretics.

Chlorthalidone passes into the breast milk; mothers taking Hygroton should refrain from breast-feeding their infants.

Effects on ability to drive and use machines: Patients should be warned of the potential hazards of driving or operating machinery if they experience side-effects such as dizziness.

Undesirable effects: Frequency estimate: very rare <0.01%, rare ≥0.01% to ≤0.1%; uncommon ≥0.1% to <1%; common ≥1% to <10%; very common ≥10%.

Electrolytes and metabolic disorders: Very common: mainly at higher doses, hypokalaemia, hyperuricaemia, and rise in blood lipids.

Common: hyponatraemia, hypomagnesaemia and hyperglycaemia.

Uncommon: gout.

Rare: hypercalcaemia, glycosuria, worsening of diabetic metabolic state.

Very rare: hypochloraemic alkalosis.

Skin: Common: urticaria and other forms of skin rash.

Rare: photosensitisation.

Liver: Rare: intrahepatic cholestasis or jaundice.

Cardiovascular system: Common: postural hypotension.

Rare: cardiac arrhythmias.

Central nervous system: Common: dizziness.

Rare: paraesthesia, headache.

Gastro-intestinal tract: Common: loss of appetite and minor gastrointestinal distress.

Rare: mild nausea and vomiting, gastric pain, constipation and diarrhoea.

Very rare: pancreatitis.

Blood: Rare: thrombocytopenia, leucopenia, agranulocytosis and eosinophilia.

Other effects: Common: impotence.

Rare: Idiosyncratic pulmonary oedema (respiratory disorders), allergic interstitial nephritis.

Overdose

Signs and symptoms: In poisoning due to an overdosage the following signs and symptoms may occur: dizziness, nausea, somnolence, hypovolaemia, hypotension and electrolyte disturbances associated with cardiac arrhythmias and muscle spasms.

Treatment: There is no specific antidote to Hygroton. Gastric lavage, emesis or activated charcoal should be employed to reduce absorption. Blood pressure and fluid and electrolyte balance should be monitored and appropriate corrective measures taken. Intravenous fluid and electrolyte replacement may be indicated.

Pharmacological properties

Pharmacodynamic properties: Chlorthalidone is a benzothiadiazine (thiazide)-related diuretic with a long duration of action.

Thiazide and thiazide-like diuretics act primarily on the distal renal tubule (early convoluted part), inhibiting NaCl⁻ reabsorption (by antagonising the Na^+Cl^- cotransporter) and promoting Ca^{++} reabsorption (by an unknown mechanism). The enhanced delivery of Na^+ and water to the cortical collection tubule and/or the increased flow rate leads to increased secretion and excretion of K^+ and H^+.

In persons with normal renal function, diuresis is induced after the administration of 12.5 mg Hygroton. The resulting increase in urinary excretion of sodium and chloride and the less prominent increase in urinary potassium are dose dependent and occur both in normal and in oedematous patients. The diuretic effect sets in after 2 to 3 hours, reaches its maximum after 4 to 24 hours, and may persist for 2 to 3 days.

Thiazide-induced diuresis initially leads to decreases in plasma volume, cardiac output and systemic blood pressure. The renin-angiotensin-aldosterone system may possibly become activated.

In hypertensive individuals, chlorthalidone gently reduces blood pressure. On continued administration, the hypotensive effect is maintained, probably due to the fall in peripheral resistance; cardiac output returns to pretreatment values, plasma volume remains somewhat reduced and plasma renin activity may be elevated.

On chronic administration, the antihypertensive effect of Hygroton is dose dependent between 12.5 and 50 mg/day. Raising the dose above 50 mg increases metabolic complications and is rarely of therapeutic benefit.

As with other diuretics, when Hygroton is given as monotherapy, blood pressure control is achieved in about half of patients with mild to moderate hypertension. In general, elderly and black patients are found to respond well to diuretics given as primary therapy. Randomised clinical trials in the elderly have shown that treatment of hypertension or predominant systolic hypertension in older persons with low-dose thiazide diuretics, including chlorthalidone, reduces cerebrovascular (stroke), coronary heart and total cardiovascular morbidity and mortality.

Combined treatment with other antihypertensives potentiates the blood-pressure lowering effects. In the large proportion of patients failing to respond adequately to monotherapy, a further decrease in blood pressure can thus be achieved.

In renal diabetes insipidus, Hygroton paradoxically reduces polyuria. The mechanism of action has not been elucidated.

Pharmacokinetic properties

Absorption and plasma concentration: The bioavailability of an oral dose of 50 mg Hygroton is approximately 64%, peak blood concentrations being attained after 8 to 12 hours. For doses of 25 and 50 mg, C_{max} values average 1.5µg/ml (4.4µmol/L) and 3.2µg/ml (9.4µmol/L) respectively. For doses up to 100 mg there is a proportional increase in AUC. On repeated daily doses of 50 mg, mean steady-state blood concentrations of 7.2µg/ml (21.2µmol/L), measured at the end of the 24 hour dosage interval, are reached after 1 to 2 weeks.

Distribution: In blood, only a small fraction of chlorthalidone is free, due to extensive accumulation in erythrocytes and binding to plasma proteins. Owing to the large degree of high affinity binding to the carbonic anhydrase of erythrocytes, only some 1.4% of the total amount of chlorthalidone in whole blood was found in plasma at steady state during treatment with 50 mg doses. *In vitro*, plasma protein binding of chlorthalidone is about 76% and the major binding protein is albumin.

Chlorthalidone crosses the placental barrier and passes into the breast milk. In mothers treated with 50 mg chlorthalidone daily before and after delivery, chlorthalidone levels in fetal whole blood are about 15% of those found in maternal blood. Chlorthalidone concentrations in amniotic fluid and in the maternal milk are approximately 4% of the corresponding maternal blood level.

Metabolism: Metabolism and hepatic excretion into bile constitute a minor pathway of elimination. Within 120 hours, about 70% of the dose is excreted in the urine and the faeces, mainly in unchanged form.

Elimination: Chlorthalidone is eliminated from whole blood and plasma with an elimination half-life averaging 50 hours. The elimination half-life is unaltered after chronic administration. The major part of an absorbed dose of chlorthalidone is excreted by the kidneys, with a mean renal clearance of 60 ml/min.

Special patient groups: Renal dysfunction does not alter the pharmacokinetics of chlorthalidone, the rate-limiting factor in the elimination of the drug from blood or plasma being most probably the affinity of the drug to the carbonic anhydrase of erythrocytes.

No dosage adjustment is needed in patients with impaired renal function.

In elderly patients, the elimination of chlorthalidone is slower than in healthy young adults, although absorption is the same. Therefore, close medical observation is indicated when treating patients of advanced age with chlorthalidone.

Preclinical safety data: There are no pre-clinical data of relevance to the prescriber which are additional to those already included in other sections of the Summary of Product Characteristics.

Pharmaceutical particulars

List of excipients: Microcrystalline cellulose, silicon dioxide, maize starch, magnesium stearate, sodium carboxymethyl cellulose, yellow iron oxide (E172).

Incompatibilities: None known.

Shelf life: Five years.

Special precautions for storage: None.

Nature and contents of container: Aluminium/PVC blister packs of 28 tablets.

Instructions for use/handling: None.

Marketing authorisation number PL16853/0007.

Date of first authorisation 25 June 1998.

Date of (partial) revision of the text June 1998.

Legal status POM.

ISMELIN* AMPOULES 10 mg/ml

Qualitative and quantitative composition Guanethidine monosulphate Ph.Eur. 10mg/ml

Pharmaceutical form A colourless solution in a clear glass 1ml ampoule, for intramuscular administration.

Clinical particulars

Therapeutic indications: Control of hypertensive crises, and to obtain more rapid blood pressure control.

Posology and method of administration:

Adults: Ismelin should be given by intramuscular injection. One injection of 10 to 20mg will generally cause a fall in blood pressure within 30 minutes which reaches a maximum in one to two hours and is maintained for four to six hours. If a further dose of 10 to 20mg is deemed necessary, then three hours should be allowed to elapse between doses.

In hypertensive patients with moderate renal insufficiency, the intervals between dosing should be extended or the dosage reduced to avoid accumulation as the drug is renally excreted. (For patients with renal failure, see *Contra-indications*).

Children: Not recommended.

Elderly: Clinical evidence would indicate that no special dosage regime is necessary, but concurrent coronary or cerebral insufficiency should be taken into account.

Contra-indications: Cases of phaeochromocytoma and patients previously treated with monoamine oxidase inhibitors (see *Interactions with other medicaments and other forms of interaction*); in such cases, Ismelin may lead to the release of large quantities of catecholamines, which may cause a hypertensive crisis.

Patients with known hypersensitivity to guanethidine and related derivatives. Heart failure due to causes other than hypertension. Renal failure (creatinine clearance 10 to 40 ml/min).

Special warnings and special precautions for use: Heat and physical exertion may increase the anti-hypertensive effect of Ismelin.

Ismelin should be used with caution in patients with moderate renal insufficiency (creatinine clearance 41 to 65 ml/min), or with coronary and/or cerebral arteriosclerosis; abrupt lowering of blood pressure should be avoided. Caution should be exercised in asthmatic patients or in patients with a history of gastro-intestinal ulceration.

The concurrent administration of guanethidine and β-blockers may provoke severe bradycardia.

When patients have to undergo surgery, it is recommended that treatment with Ismelin be withdrawn a few days before the operation. To avoid excessive bradycardia during anaesthesia, it is advisable to premedicate with larger than usual doses of atropine.

After prolonged treatment with Ismelin, latent heart failure may develop. This is due to salt and water retention, and mild negative inotropic and chronotropic effects. Concomitant administration of diuretics can readily correct this condition.

If patients develop fever, the dose of Ismelin should be lowered.

Interaction with other medicaments and other forms of interaction: Monoamine oxidase inhibitors should be withdrawn at least fourteen days before starting treatment with Ismelin (See *Contra-indications*).

Concurrent administration of Ismelin with anti-arrhythmic agents and digitalis may lead to sinus bradycardia.

The anti-hypertensive action of Ismelin may be enhanced by other anti-hypertensive agents such as reserpine, methyldopa, vasodilators (especially minoxidil), calcium antagonists, β-blockers, ACE inhibitors and alcohol.

The anti-hypertensive action of Ismelin may be reduced by chlorpromazine, phenothiazine derivatives, tricyclic antidepressants and related anti-psychotic drugs, and oral contraceptives. Consequently if larger doses of Ismelin are prescribed, care must be taken upon the withdrawal of any of the drugs listed, as severe hypotension may ensue if the dose of Ismelin is not adjusted in advance.

After prolonged treatment with Ismelin, it may be necessary to adjust the dosage of insulin or oral anti-diabetic drugs.

Patients on Ismelin may become hypersensitive to adrenaline, amphetamines or other sympathomimetic agents. Therefore caution should be exercised when taking or using preparations containing these drugs.

Pregnancy and lactation: No foetal toxicity or fertility studies have been carried out in animals. Therefore the drug should only be used if there is no safer alternative. However, in particular, it should not be used during the first trimester of pregnancy nor within at least two weeks prior to the birth or during labour since it may induce paralytic ileus in the newborn infant.

In mothers receiving Ismelin in therapeutic doses, the active substance passes into the breast milk, but in quantities so small that no undesirable effects on the infant are to be expected.

Effects on ability to drive and use machines: Patients should be warned of the potential hazards of driving or operating machinery if they experience side effects such as dizziness, blurred vision or drowsiness.

Undesirable effects: Side effects are often an indication of excessive dosage. The following effects may occur:

Central nervous system: Particularly at the start of treatment: dizziness, tiredness, lethargy, paraesthesia and headache. Occasional: blurred vision and depression. Rare: myalgia and muscular tremor.

Cardiovascular system: Postural hypotension (which may be associated with cerebral or myocardial ischaemia in severe cases) especially when getting up in the morning or after physical exertion, sick-sinus syndrome, oedema, exacerbation of intermittent claudication and bradycardia. Occasional: heart failure. Rare: angina pectoris.

Gastro-intestinal tract: Diarrhoea and gaseous distension. Occasional: vomiting, nausea and dry mouth. Rare: swelling of parotid glands.

Respiratory tract: Nasal congestion. Rare: asthma.

Urogenital system: Raised BUN levels or uraemia in patients with latent or manifest renal failure, and ejaculation disturbances.

Skin and hair: Occasional: dermatitis. Rare: hair loss.

Blood: Isolated reports of anaemia, leucopenia, and/or thrombocytopenia.

Overdose: Symptoms: May include postural hypotension which may cause syncope, sinus bradycardia (although tachycardia has been observed), tiredness, dizziness, blurring of vision, muscular weakness, nausea, vomiting, severe diarrhoea and oliguria.

Treatment: Postural hypotension may be overcome by keeping the patient recumbent, or by instituting fluid and electrolyte replacement, and if necessary, by cautious administration of pressor agents (see *Interactions with other medicaments and other forms of interaction*). Sinus bradycardia can be treated with atropine, and diarrhoea with an anticholinergic agent.

Pharmacological properties

Pharmacodynamic properties: Ismelin is a peripheral sympathetic blocking drug which lowers blood pressure by depleting and inhibiting reformation of noradrenaline in postganglionic nerve endings. Guanethidine, being highly polar, does not cross the blood-brain barrier and is unlikely therefore to exert any effect on the central nervous system. In addition, guanethidine has no effect on the parasympathetic nervous system.

Pharmacokinetic properties: Guanethidine may be excreted more slowly in those patients with moderate to severely compromised renal function, therefore the potential for accumulation of the drug will be higher.

Preclinical safety data: There are no pre-clinical data of relevance to the prescriber which are additional to those already included in other sections of the Summary of Product Characteristics.

Pharmaceutical particulars
List of excipients: Sodium chloride, sulphuric acid and water for injections.

Incompatibilities: None known.

Shelf life: 5 years.

Special precautions for storage: Protect from light.

Nature and contents of container: Clear glass type I, 1ml ampoules containing 10 mg/ml: Boxes of 5.

Instructions for use/handling: None.

Marketing authorisation number PL 16853/0008

Date of first authorisation 25 June 1998.

Date of (partial) revision of the text July 1998.

Legal status POM.

LAMPRENE* CAPSULES 100 mg

Qualitative and quantitative composition Clofazimine BP 100mg.

Pharmaceutical form Brown, opaque, oblong soft gelatin capsules containing a brown viscous mass with a vanilla odour. One side has the imprint 'GEIGY' and the other 'GM' in white.

Clinical particulars
Therapeutic indications: Lamprene, given in combination with dapsone and rifampicin, can be used to treat the multibacillary forms of leprosy. These include lepromatous, borderline lepromatous and mid-borderline leprosy. In addition, this combination of drugs may be used to treat the lepra reaction, erythema nodosum leprosum. Combined chemotherapy should be employed to prevent the emergence of resistant strains of M. leprae.

Posology and method of administration: Lamprene should be taken at meal-times or together with milk.

Lamprene should be used in combination with rifampicin and dapsone. The following dosage regimen is recommended by the World Health Organisation:

Adults: The dosage of Lamprene should be adjusted according to body weight, but for adults weighing approximately 60 kg, the following doses are recommended:

For the treatment of multibacillary forms of leprosy:

Lamprene:	300 mg once a month under surveillance and 100 mg once every 2 days.
Rifampicin:	600 mg once a month under surveillance.
	Dapsone: 100 mg once a day.

This combined therapy should be given for at least 2 years, and whenever possible, until such time as the skin smears become negative.

For the treatment of erythema nodosum leprosum:

Lamprene:	a maximum of 300 mg once a day for not longer than 3 months.
Rifampicin:	600 mg once a month under surveillance.
Dapsone:	100 mg once a day.

Children: Children should receive lower doses, according to their body weight.

Elderly: Clinical evidence would indicate that no special dosage regime is necessary, but concurrent renal or hepatic insufficiency should be taken into account.

Contra-indications: Hypersensitivity to clofazimine or the excipients of Lamprene.

Special warnings and special precautions for use: After prolonged administration in high doses, clofazimine may accumulate in tissue, e.g. the wall of the small bowel, and precipitate. Enteropathy may develop if crystals are deposited in the lamina propria of the jejunal mucosa and the mesenteric lymph nodes, sometimes leading to intestinal obstruction. If gastrointestinal symptoms develop during treatment, the dosage should be reduced or the interval between doses prolonged. Symptoms may slowly regress on withdrawal of the drug.

In the event of persistent diarrhoea or vomiting, the patient should be confined to hospital.

Lamprene should not be used to treat leprosy patients suffering from repeated attacks of abdominal pain and diarrhoea, or in patients with renal or hepatic damage, unless absolutely necessary.

Patients should be kept under medical supervision when treated with daily doses of Lamprene exceeding 100mg; this dosage should not be continued for longer than 3 months.

Physicians should be aware that skin discolouration due to Lamprene may result in depression (two cases of depression with suicide have been reported in patients being treated for leprosy with Lamprene). Patients should be warned that Lamprene may cause discolouration of the conjunctiva, lacrimal fluid, sweat, sputum, urine, faeces, nasal secretions, semen, breast milk and reddish to brownish-black discolouration of the skin. Patients should be told that discolouration of the skin, although reversible, may take several months or years to disappear after the end of therapy with Lamprene.

Interaction with other medicaments and other forms of interaction: Lamprene seems to have no important effects on the pharmacokinetics of dapsone, although a transient increase in the urinary excretion of dapsone occurred in a few patients. Preliminary data suggesting that dapsone inhibits the anti-inflammatory activity of Lamprene have not been confirmed. If leprosy-associated inflammatory reactions develop in patients being treated with dapsone and Lamprene, it is still advisable to continue treatment with both drugs.

Clofazimine reduces rifampicin absorption in leprosy patients, increasing the time it takes for peak serum concentration to be reached and prolonging the half-life. Bioavailability was not affected, so this interaction is unlikely to be clinically significant.

In patients receiving high doses of clofazimine (300 mg daily) and isoniazid (300 mg daily), elevated concentrations of clofazimine were detected in plasma and urine, although skin concentrations were found to be lower.

Pregnancy and lactation: Experience with Lamprene in pregnancy is limited. Clofazimine crosses the placenta, and skin discolouration in neonates has been observed. Lamprene should be used during pregnancy only if the potential benefit justifies the risk to the fetus. Since leprosy is exacerbated during pregnancy, the WHO recommends that treatment with Lamprene should be continued during pregnancy.

Clofazimine passes into the breast milk, and skin discolouration may occur in the infant. Lamprene should be administered to a breast-feeding woman only if clearly indicated.

Effects on ability to drive and use machines: Patients should be warned of the potential hazards of driving or operating machinery if they experience side effects such as dimness of vision, tiredness or headache.

Undesirable effects: Frequency estimates: frequent >10%, occasional 1–10%, rare 0.001%–1%, isolated cases <0.001%.

Skin and appendages: Frequent: reddish to brownish-black discolouration of the skin and leprous lesions, particularly in fair-skinned patients at sites exposed to light, and discolouration of the hair (in 75–100% of patients). This discolouration is reversible, although in the case of the skin it may take several months to disappear after the end of treatment. Ichthyosis and dry skin. Occasional: rash, pruritus. Rare: photosensitivity, acneiform eruptions.

Gastrointestinal tract: Frequent: nausea, vomiting, abdominal pain, diarrhoea (in 40–50% of patients). Rare: anorexia, eosinophilic enteropathy. Isolated cases: bowel obstruction.

Eyes: Frequent to occasional: discolouration of the conjunctiva, cornea and lacrimal fluid. Occasional: dry, irritated eyes. Dimness of vision. Rare: pigmentation of the macula. Subepithelial corneal brownish pigmented lines due to crystal deposits, reversible on discontinuation of Lamprene.

Central nervous system: Rare: headache, tiredness. Isolated cases: depression due to skin discolouration.

Laboratory values: Rare: elevated levels of blood sugar.

Others: Frequent: discolouration of body fluids and secretions e.g. sweat, sputum, urine, faeces. Occasional: weight loss. Isolated cases: splenic infarction, lymphadenopathy.

Overdose: No specific data are available on the treatment of overdosage with Lamprene. In cases of acute overdose the stomach should be emptied by inducing vomiting or performing gastric lavage, and symptomatic treatment should be given as required.

Pharmacological properties
Pharmacodynamic properties: Clofazimine exerts a bacteriostatic and weakly bactericidal effect in man on *Mycobacterium leprae* (M. leprae, Hansen's bacillus). Its precise mechanism of action against mycobacteria remains to be elucidated. Clofazimine appears to bind preferentially to mycobacterial DNA and inhibit mycobacterial replication and growth.

No cross-resistance occurs with dapsone and rifampicin, probably because clofazimine has a different mode of action. *M. leprae* resistant to clofazimine have been reported only in isolated cases.

The minimum inhibitory concentration of clofazimine for *M. leprae* in mouse tissue has been estimated at between 0.1 and 1 μg/g; uneven tissue distribution precludes a more accurate estimate. In patients with lepromatous leprosy, the overall antibacterial effect of Lamprene is comparable to that of dapsone. However, the onset of antimicrobial activity of Lamprene is slow and can only be demonstrated after about 50 days of therapy.

Clofazimine also displays an anti-inflammatory effect, which may contribute to the efficacy of Lamprene in controlling ENL reactions.

Pharmacokinetic properties: Clofazimine is absorbed relatively slowly. Bioavailability of the micronised suspension in an oil-wax base is up to 70% after a dose of 100 mg, and decreases with higher doses. Peak plasma concentrations of the unchanged active substance are reached 8–12 hours after a single oral dose. Administering the drug with food increases bioavailability in terms of AUC (area under the concentration-time curve) by about 60% and tends to accelerate the absorption rate. After administration of a single oral dose of 200 mg clofazimine at breakfast, mean peak plasma concentrations of 861 (±289) pmol/g were measured in healthy volunteers. When clofazimine is taken on an empty stomach, the peak plasma concentration is approximately 20% lower.

After repeated administration of clofazimine to leprosy patients in daily doses of 50 mg and 100 mg, mean morning trough concentrations of 580 pmol/g and 910 pmol/g, respectively, were measured after 42 consecutive days. Steady-state concentrations were not reached within this time period.

Clofazimine is strongly lipophilic and accumulates mainly in fatty tissue and in macrophages of the reticuloendothelial system. After long-term treatment, clofazimine has been detected in the following organs and tissues and body fluids: subcutaneous fat, mesenteric lymph nodes, bile and gall bladder, adrenals, spleen, small intestine, liver, muscle tissue, bones, and skin, but never in the brain. Clofazimine does not appear to cross the intact blood-brain barrier.

Clofazimine crosses the placenta and passes into the breast milk in sufficient quantities to colour the milk.

Clofazimine is eliminated slowly from the plasma. The mean elimination half-life of the unchanged substance following a single dose of 200mg in healthy volunteers is 10.6 (±4.0) days. After repeated administration of 50 mg and 100 mg daily to leprosy patients, the elimination half-life as estimated from the concentration/time curve was about 25 days.

Unchanged clofazimine is excreted via the bile mainly in the faeces. Within 3 days on average 35% of the dose is recovered. Information on the metabolism of clofazimine is limited. Three metabolites, two glucuronides, have been identified in urine. No more than 0.4% of the dose is found in the urine as unchanged clofazimine after 24 hours. The urinary metabolites account for about 0.6% of the daily dose.

Preclinical safety data: No mutagenic activity was detected in the Ames test and in cytogenic tests in patients treated with Lamprene. No teratogenic effect was observed in rabbits or rats given clofazimine doses 8 and 25 times the usual human dose, respectively. However, with doses 12 to 25 times those given to humans, retardation of fetal skull ossification and fetotoxicity were observed in mice.

Pharmaceutical particulars
List of excipients: Butylated hydroxytoluene, citric acid, propylene glycol, rapeseed oil, soybean lecithin, wax blend (beeswax, hydrogenated soybean oil and other partially hydrogenated plant oils), sodium ethyl paraben, ethyl vanillin, gelatin, glycerin, black iron oxide, red iron oxide, p-methoxy acetophenone and sodium propylparaben.

Incompatibilities: None known.

Shelf life: 5 years

Special precautions for storage: Protect from moisture. Store below 25°C.

Nature and contents of container: White plastic containers with white plastic tops and yellow tamper evident seals, containing 100 capsules.

Instructions for use/handling: None.

Marketing authorisation number PL 16853/0009

Date of first authorisation 25 June 1998

Date of (partial) revision of the text June 1998

Legal status POM

METOPIRONE* CAPSULES 250 mg

Qualitative and quantitative composition Metyrapone BP 250 mg.

Pharmaceutical form Yellowish-white, oblong, opaque, soft gelatin capsules printed 'CIBA' on one side and 'LN' on the other in brown ink.

Clinical particulars
Therapeutic indications: A diagnostic aid in the differential diagnosis of ACTH-dependent Cushing's syndrome. The management of patients with Cushing's syndrome. In conjunction with glucocorticosteroids in the treatment of resistant oedema due to increased aldosterone secretion in patients suffering from cirrhosis, nephrosis and congestive heart failure.

Posology and method of administration: Adults: The capsules should be taken with milk or after a meal, to minimise nausea and vomiting, which can lead to impaired absorption.

For use as a diagnostic aid: The patient must be hospitalised. Urinary 17-oxygenic steroid excretion is measured over 24 hours on each of 4 consecutive days. The first 2 days serve as a control period. On the third day, 750 mg Metopirone (3 capsules) must be given at four-hourly intervals to give a total of 6 doses (i.e. 4.5 g). Maximum urine steroid excretion may occur on the fourth day. If urinary steroid excretion increases in response to Metopirone, this suggests the high levels of circulatory cortisol are due to adrenocortical hyperplasia following excessive ACTH production rather than a cortisol-producing adrenal tumour.

For therapeutic use: For the management of Cushing's syndrome, the dosage must be adjusted to meet the patient's requirements; a daily dosage from 250 mg to 6 g may be required to restore normal cortisol levels.

For the treatment of resistant oedema: The usual daily dose of 3 g (12 capsules) should be given in divided doses in conjunction with a glucocorticoid.

Children: Children should be given a smaller amount based upon 6 four-hourly doses of 15 mg/kg, with a minimum dose of 250 mg every four hours.

Elderly: Clinical evidence would indicate that no special dosage regimen is necessary.

Contra-indications: Primary adrenocorticol insufficiency. Hypersensitivity to Metopirone or to any of the excipients. Pregnancy.

Special warnings and special precautions for use:
In relation to use as a diagnostic aid: Anticonvulsants (eg phenytoin, barbiturates), anti-depressants and neuroleptics (e.g. amitriptyline, chlorpromazine), hormones that affect the hypothalamo-pituitary axis and anti-thyroid agents may influence the results of the Metopirone test. If these drugs cannot be withdrawn, the necessity of carrying out the Metopirone test should be reviewed.

If adrenocortical or anterior pituitary function is more severely compromised than indicated by the results of the test, Metopirone may trigger transient adrenocortical insufficiency. This can be rapidly corrected by giving appropriate doses of corticosteroids.

Long-term treatment with Metopirone can cause hypertension as the result of excessive secretion of desoxycorticosterone.

The ability of the adrenal cortex to respond to exogenous ACTH should be demonstrated before Metopirone is employed as a test, as Metopirone may induce acute adrenal insufficiency in patients with reduced adrenal secretory capacity, as well as in patients with gross hypopituitarism.

Patients with liver cirrhosis often show a delayed response to Metopirone, due to liver damage delaying the metabolism of cortisol.

In cases of thyroid hypofunction, urinary steroid levels may rise very slowly, or not at all, in response to Metopirone.

Interaction with other medicaments and other forms of interaction: In some cases concomitant medication may affect the results of the Metopirone test (see *Special warnings and special precautions for use*).

Pregnancy and lactation: No data are available from animal reproduction studies. Metopirone should not be administered during pregnancy since the drug can impair the biosynthesis of foetal-placental steroids. It is not known whether metyrapone passes into the breast milk, therefore nursing mothers should refrain from breast-feeding their infants during treatment with Metopirone.

Effects on ability to drive and use machines: Patients should be warned of the potential hazards of driving or operating machinery. If they experience side effects such as dizziness and sedation.

Undesirable effects:
Gastrointestinal tract: Occasional: nausea, vomiting. Rare: abdominal pain.

Central nervous system: Occasional: dizziness, sedation, headache.

Cardiovascular system: Occasional: hypotension.

Skin: Rare: allergic skin reactions.

Endocrine system: Rare: hypoadrenalism, hirsutism.

Overdose:
Signs and symptoms: The clinical picture of acute Metopirone poisoning is characterised by gastrointestinal symptoms and acute adrenocortical insufficiency. Laboratory findings: hyponatraemia, hypochloraemia, hyperkalaemia. In patients under treatment with insulin or oral antidiabetics, the signs and symptoms of acute poisoning with Metopirone may be aggravated or modified.

Treatment: There is no specific antidote. Gastric lavage and forced emesis should be employed to reduce the absorption of the drug. In addition to general measures, a large dose of hydrocortisone should be administered at once, together with iv saline and glucose. This should be repeated as necessary in accordance with the patient's clinical condition. For a few days, blood pressure and fluid and electrolyte balance should be monitored.

Pharmacological particulars
Pharmacodynamic properties: Metopirone inhibits the enzyme responsible for the 11β-hydroxylation stage in the biosynthesis of cortisol and to a lesser extent, aldosterone. The fall in plasma concentration of circulating glucocorticoids stimulates ACTH secretion, via the feedback mechanism which accelerates steroid biosynthesis. As a result, 11-desoxycortisol, the precursor of cortisol, is released into the circulation, metabolised by the liver and excreted in the urine. Unlike cortisol, 11-desoxycortisol does not suppress ACTH secretion and its urinary metabolites may be measured.

These metabolites can easily be determined by measuring urinary 17-hydroxycorticosteroids (17-OHCS) or 17-ketogenic steroids (17-KGS). Metopirone is used as a diagnostic test on the basis of these properties, with plasma 11-desoxycortisol and urinary 17-OHCS measured as an index of pituitary ACTH responsiveness. Metopirone may also suppress biosynthesis of aldosterone, resulting in mild natriuresis.

Pharmacokinetic properties: Metyrapone is rapidly absorbed and eliminated from the plasma. Peak plasma levels usually occur one hour after ingestion of Metopirone; after a dose of 750 mg Metopirone, plasma drug levels average 3.7 μg/ml. Plasma drug levels decrease to a mean value of 0.5 μg/ml 4 hours after dosing. The half-life of elimination of Metopirone from the plasma is 20 to 26 minutes.

Metyrapol, the reduced form of metyrapone, is the main active metabolite. Eight hours after a single oral dose, the ratio of metyrapone to metyrapol in the plasma is 1:1.5. Metyrapol takes about twice as long as metyrapone to be eliminated in the plasma.

Seventy-two hours after a first daily dose of 4.5 g Metopirone (750 mg every 4 hours), 5.3% of the total dose was excreted in the urine as metyrapone (9.2% in free form and 90.8% conjugated with glucuronic acid), and 38.5% in the form of metyrapol (8.1% in free form and 91.9% conjugated with glucuronic acid).

Preclinical safety data: There are no pre-clinical data of relevance to the prescriber which are additional to those already included in other sections of the Summary of Product Characteristics.

Pharmaceutical particulars
List of excipients:
Capsule contents: Glycerin, polyethylene glycol 400, polyethylene glycol 4000 and water.

Capsule shell: Sodium ethylparaben, ethyl vanillin, gelatin, glycerin 85%, p-methoxy acetophenone, sodium propylparaben and titanium oxide (E171).

Incompatibilities: None stated.

Shelf life: 5 years

Special precautions for storage: Protect from moisture and heat. Store below 30°C.

Nature and contents of container: Polypropylene tubs of 100 capsules.

Instructions for use/handling: None stated.

Marketing authorisation number PL 16853/0010

Date of first authorisation 25 June 1998

Date of (partial) revision of the text June 98

Legal status POM

NAVIDREX* TABLETS 0.5 mg

Qualitative and quantitative composition Cyclopenthiazide BP 0.5 mg.

Pharmaceutical form White, flat, round tablets with bevelled edges, pressed 'CIBA' on one side, and the letters AO on each side of a breakline on the other.

Clinical particulars
Therapeutic indications: Treatment of mild to moderate hypertension; in more severe hypertension Navidrex may be used in conjunction with other antihypertensive agents.

Stable, chronic heart failure of mild to moderate degree (functional class II, III), as long as creatinine clearance is >30 ml/min.

Oedema of specific origin:

- fluid retention in pre-menstrual syndrome only as short-term therapy and only if the gain in weight is the main symptom and is well documented,
- ascites due to cirrhosis of the liver in stable patients under close control.
- oedema associated with renal disease.

Posology and method of administration: The dosage of Navidrex should be individually titrated to give the lowest effective dose; this is particularly important in the elderly. Navidrex should be taken orally: a single dose of up to 1 mg given in the morning is recommended.

Adults: Hypertension: Initially 0.25 mg daily; if necessary the dosage may be raised to 0.5 mg daily. For a given dose, the full effect is reached after 4 to 6 weeks. If the decrease in blood pressure proves inadequate with 0.5 mg/day, combined treatment with other antihypertensive drugs such as a β-blocker (if necessary, a β-blocker and vasodilator), or an ACE inhibitor is recommended. It is recommended that diuretics (Navidrex) should be withdrawn for several days before starting the ACE inhibitor.

Stable, chronic heart failure (NYHA class II, III): Initially 0.25 to 0.5 mg daily. If necessary the dose may be titrated up to 1 mg/day; higher doses rarely achieve any further benefit. The lowest effective dose should be used for maintenance therapy. If the response proves inadequate, a positive inotropic drug (e.g. digitalis), possibly combined with an ACE inhibitor may be added. In the latter case a reduction in the dose of Navidrex may be necessary.

Oedema: The lowest effective dose should be determined by titration and administered over limited periods only. Doses should not exceed 0.5 mg/day.

Children: Adequate experience regarding the dosage in children is lacking.

Elderly: Particular caution should be exercised since the elderly are more susceptible to electrolyte imbalances (see *Special warnings and special precautions for use*).

Patients with renal impairment: There is no evidence on the effect of renal impairment on the excretion of cyclopenthiazide, but experience with other thiazide diuretics indicates that a 50% reduction of the normal adult dose may be appropriate.

Contra-indications: Anuria, severe renal and hepatic failure. Hypersensitivity to cyclopenthiazide and other sulphonamide derivatives. Refractory hypokalaemia, hyponatraemia and hypercalcaemia. Symptomatic hyperuricaemia (history of gout or uric acid calculi). Hypertension during pregnancy. Creatinine clearance lower than 30 ml/min. Conditions involving enhanced potassium loss, e.g. salt-losing nephropathies and prerenal (cardiogenic) impairment of kidney function. Untreated Addison's disease. Concomitant lithium therapy.

Special warnings and special precautions for use: Navidrex should be used with caution in patients with renal disease or with impaired hepatic function (see *Contra-indications* and below under *other precautions*).

Electrolytes: As with all thiazide diuretics, potassium loss induced by Navidrex is dose dependent. With daily doses of 125 and 500 μg given for 8 weeks, the decreases in serum potassium concentrations averaged 0.2 and 0.6 mmol/l, respectively. For chronic treatment, serum potassium concentrations should be checked initially and then after 3 to 4 weeks. Thereafter (if the potassium balance is not disturbed by additional factors, e.g. vomiting, diarrhoea, change in renal function etc.) checks should be carried out every 4 to 6 months.

Titrated co-administration of an oral potassium salt (e.g. KCl) may be considered in patients receiving digitalis, glucocorticoids or ACTH; in patients exhibiting signs of coronary heart disease, unless they are also receiving an ACE inhibitor; in patients on high doses of a β-adrenergic agonist; and in all cases where plasma concentrations are <3.0 nmol/l. If oral potassium preparations are not tolerated, Navidrex may be combined with a potassium-sparing diuretic (e.g. amiloride). Combined treatment consisting of Navidrex and a potassium salt or a potassium-sparing diuretic must be avoided in patients also receiving ACE inhibitors.

In all cases of combined treatment, maintenance or normalisation of the potassium balance should be checked closely. If hypokalaemia is accompanied by clinical signs (e.g. muscular weakness, paresis and ECG alteration), Navidrex should be discontinued.

There have been isolated reports of hyponatraemia with neurological symptoms (e.g. nausea, debility, progressive disorientation and apathy).

Serum electrolyte levels should be monitored particularly in the elderly, and in patients with ascites due to liver cirrhosis and in patients with oedema due to nephrotic syndrome. For the latter condition, Navidrex should be used only under close control in normokalaemic patients with no signs of volume depletion or severe hypoalbuminaemia.

As with other diuretics, Navidrex may cause disturbances in the electrolyte balance during prolonged treatment. Since the excretion of electrolytes is increased, a very strict low salt diet should be avoided.

Metabolic effects: Navidrex may raise the serum uric acid level and provoke attacks of gout in predisposed patients. Glucose intolerance may occur (this may manifest as hypoglycaemia and glycosuria) but diabetes mellitus very seldom occurs under treatment.

In patients with hyperlipidaemia, serum lipids should be monitored regularly. Small and partly reversible increases in plasma concentrations of total cholesterol, triglycerides or low density lipoprotein cholesterol have been reported in patients during long term treatments with thiazides and thiazide-like diuretics. The clinical relevance of these findings is not clear. Withdrawal of Navidrex should be considered if serum lipids rise further.

Navidrex should not be used as first line therapy for long-term treatment in patients with overt diabetes mellitus or in subjects receiving therapy for hypercholesterolaemia (diet or combined).

Other precautions: Navidrex may accumulate in patients with impaired renal function. At creatinine clearance levels of <30 ml/min (or at serum creatinine levels of >2.5 mg/100 ml), cyclopenthiazide will not exert a diuretic effect. In such cases, loop diuretics are indicated.

The antihypertensive effect of ACE inhibitors is potentiated by diuretics that increase plasma renin activity. A cautious dosage schedule should therefore be adopted when an ACE inhibitor is added to a diuretic agent.

As with all antihypertensive agents, a cautious dosage schedule is indicated in patients with severe coronary or cerebral arteriosclerosis.

Lupus erythematosus may possibly become activated under treatment with thiazides.

Interactions with other medicaments and other forms of interaction
Curare derivatives and antihypertensive drugs: Diuretics potentiate the action of these drugs (e.g. guanethidine, methyldopa, β-blockers, vasodilators, calcium antagonists and ACE inhibitors).

Lithium: Diuretics raise the blood level of lithium. Where lithium has produced polyuria, diuretics may exert a paradoxical antidiuretic effect. (see *Contra-indications*).

Corticosteroids, ACTH, amphotericin and carbenoxolone: These may increase the hypokalaemic effect of diuretics.

Anti-diabetic agents: It may prove necessary to adjust the dosage of insulin and oral anti-diabetic agents.

Digitalis: Hypokalaemia or hypomagnesaemia possibly occurring as unwanted effects may cause onset of digitalis-induced cardiac arrhythmias.

Non-steroidal anti-inflammatory agents: Concomitant administration of certain NSAIDs (e.g. indomethacin) may reduce the diuretic and antihypertensive activity of Navidrex; there have been isolated reports of a deterioration in renal function in predisposed patients.

Allopurinol: Co-administration of thiazide diuretics may increase the incidence of hypersensitivity reactions to allopurinol. (see *Contra-indications*).

Amantadine: Co-administration of thiazide diuretics may increase the risk of adverse effects from amantadine.

Antineoplastic agents (e.g. cyclophosphamide, methotrexate): Concomitant use of thiazide diuretics may reduce renal excretion of cytotoxic agents and enhance the myelosuppresive effects.

Anticholinergic agents (e.g. atropine, biperiden): The bioavailability of thiazide type diuretics may be increased by anticholinergic agents, apparently due to a decrease in gastro-intestinal motility and stomach emptying rate.

Cholestyramine: Absorption of thiazide diuretics is decreased by cholestyramine. A decrease of the pharmacological effect may be expected.

Vitamin D: Concomitant use of thiazide diuretics may decrease urinary excretion of calcium, and coadministration of Vitamin D may potentiate the increase in serum calcium.

Cyclosporin: Concomitant treatment with diuretics may increase the risk of hyperuricaemia and gout type complications.

Calcium salts: Concomitant use of thiazide type diuretics may cause hypercalcaemia by increasing tubular calcium resorption.

Diazoxide: Thiazide diuretics may enhance the hyperglycaemic effect of diazoxide.

Methyldopa: There have been reports in the literature of haemolytic anaemia occurring with concomitant use of a thiazide diuretic and methyldopa.

Pregnancy and lactation: Diuretics are best avoided for the management of oedema or hypertension in pregnancy as their use may be associated with hypovolaemia, increased blood viscosity and reduced placental perfusion.

Diuretics do not prevent or alter the course of oedema, proteinuria or hypertension during pregnancy (pre-eclampsia). Cyclopenthiazide must not be used to treat hypertension during pregnancy (see *Contra-indications*), and the use of Navidrex for other indications (e.g. heart disease) during pregnancy should be avoided unless there are no safer alternatives. There have been reports of foetal bone marrow depression, thrombocytopenia, and foetal and neonatal jaundice associated with the use of thiazide diuretics.

Cyclopenthiazide may be excreted into the breast milk and thus mothers taking Navidrex should refrain from breast-feeding their infants.

Effects on ability to drive and use machines: Patients should be warned of the potential hazards of driving or operating machinery if they experience side effects such as dizziness, sleep disturbances or visual disturbances.

Undesirable effects
Electrolytes and metabolic disorders: Frequent: mainly at higher doses, hypokalaemia, and rise in blood lipids (see *Special warnings and special precautions for use*). Occasional: hyponatraemia, hypomagnesaemia and hyperuricaemia. Rare: hypercalcaemia, hyperglycaemia, glycosuria, worsening of diabetic metabolic state. Isolated cases: hypochloraemic alkalosis.

Skin: Occasional: urticaria and other forms of skin rash. Rare: photosensitisation. Isolated cases: necrotising vasculitis and toxic epidermal necrolysis, cutaneous lupus erythematosus-like reactions, reactivation of cutaneous lupus erythematosus.

Gastro-intestinal tract: Occasional: loss of appetite, mild nausea and vomiting. Rare: abdominal distress, constipation, diarrhoea and gastro-intestinal discomfort. Isolated cases: pancreatitis.

Liver: Rare: intrahepatic cholestasis.

Cardiovascular system: Occasional: postural hypotension, which may be aggravated by alcohol, anaesthetics or sedatives. Rare: cardiac arrhythmias.

Central nervous system: Rare: headache, dizziness or muzziness, sleep disturbance, depression and paraesthesia.

Special senses: Visual disturbances, particularly in the first few weeks of treatment.

Blood: Rare: thrombocytopenia, sometimes with purpura. Isolated cases: leucopenia, agranulocytosis, bone marrow depression and haemolytic anaemia.

Other effects: Occasional: impotence. Isolated cases: hypersensitivity reactions - respiratory distress including pneumonitis and pulmonary oedema. Gout may be precipitated or aggravated in susceptible patients or those with a history of the illness, but there have been only isolated reports of attacks occurring during chronic therapy.

Overdose:
Symptoms: Dizziness, nausea, somnolence, hypovolaemia, hypotension and electrolyte disturbances associated with cardiac arrhythmias and muscle spasms.

Treatment: There is no specific antidote to Navidrex. Gastric lavage, emesis or activated charcoal should be employed to reduce absorption. Blood pressure and fluid and electrolyte balance should be monitored and appropriate corrective measures taken. Intravenous fluid and electrolyte replacement may be indicated.

Pharmacological properties
Pharmacodynamic properties: Cyclopenthiazide is a benzothiadiazine (thiazide) diuretic.

Thiazide diuretics act primarily on the distal renal tubule (early convoluted part), inhibiting NaCl reabsorption (by antagonising the Na^{+} Cl^{-} cotransporter), promoting Ca^{++} reabsorption (by an unknown mechanism). The enhanced delivery of Na^{+} and water to the cortical collecting tubule and/or the increased flow rate leads to increased secretion and excretion of K^{+} and H^{+}.

In healthy volunteers or in patients with oedema, cyclopenthiazide administration results in a dose dependent increase in urinary excretion of sodium and chloride and a less prominent dose dependent increase in potassium excretion. The diuretic and natriuretic effect appears within 1 to 3 hours and subsides within 24 hours.

Thiazide-induced diuresis initially leads to a decrease in plasma volume, cardiac output and systemic blood pressure. The renin-angiotensin-aldosterone system may possibly become activated. On continued administration the hypotensive effect is maintained, probably due to the fall in peripheral resistance; cardiac output returns to pretreatment values, plasma volume remains somewhat reduced and plasma renin activity may be elevated.

During repeated administration of Navidrex the antihypertensive effect is dose dependent from 125 to 500 µg/day. The maximum hypotensive effect is reached with 500 µg in most patients. In chronic heart failure, daily doses of 1mg may enhance the therapeutic benefit but at higher doses the expected benefit must be balanced by the increased risk of side-effects.

As with other diuretics, when Navidrex is given as monotherapy, blood pressure control is achieved in about half of patients with mild to moderate hypertension. In general the elderly and black patients are found to respond well to diuretics as primary therapy.

Combined treatment with other antihypertensives has an additive effect and in a large proportion of patients failing to respond to monotherapy, a further decrease in blood pressure can thus be achieved.

Pharmacokinetic properties: Based on limited pharmacokinetic data, the variability of the amount of cyclopenthiazide absorbed appears to be low. After oral administration of single doses of 0.5 or 1.0 mg cyclopenthiazide, peak plasma levels of about 3 and 7 ng/ml respectively were reached after an average of 3 to 4 hours. Twelve hours after the administration of 1mg cyclopenthiazide, the plasma concentration decreases to about 25% of the peak concentration.

In rats, cyclopenthiazide is excreted mainly by tubular secretion. In humans receiving cyclopenthiazide the drug can be detected in the urine. At 24 hours after the administration of a 0.5mg dose, for instance, the concentration in the urine is about 400 ng/ml.

Preclinical safety data: There are no pre-clinical data of relevance to the prescriber which are additional to those already included in other sections of the Summary of Product Characteristics.

Pharmaceutical particulars
List of excipients: Lactose, wheat starch, gelatin, stearic acid and talc.

Incompatibilities: None known

Shelf life: 3 Years.

Special precautions for storage: Protect from heat and moisture. Store below 25°C.

Nature and contents of container: PVC/PVdC/Aluminium blister packs of 28 tablets.

Instructions for use/handling: None.

Marketing authorisation number PL 16853/0011

Date of first authorisation 25 June 1998

Date of (partial) revision of the text June 1998

Legal status POM

ROGITINE* AMPOULES 10mg

Qualitative and quantitative composition Phentolamine mesylate PhEur 10 mg.

Pharmaceutical form Colourless to pale yellow solution in 1 ml Water for Injections PhEur.

Clinical particulars
Therapeutic indications: Management of hypertensive episodes that may occur in patients with phaeochromocytoma, for example during pre-operative preparation and surgical manipulation.

Diagnosis of phaeochromocytoma by Rogitine blocking test if other more specific tests are not available.

Posology and method of administration
Adults: Management of hypertensive episodes in patients with phaeochromocytoma

For the management of hypertensive crises that arise during the pre-operative phase or during induction of anaesthesia, intubation, or surgical removal of the tumour, 2 to 5 mg of Rogitine is injected intravenously and repeated if necessary. The blood pressure response should be monitored.

Diagnosis of phaeochromocytoma–Rogitine blocking test: The test is most reliable in detecting phaeochromocytoma in patients with sustained hypertension and least reliable in those with paroxysmal hypertension. False-positive tests may occur in patients with hypertension without phaeochromocytoma.

Preparation for the test: Sedatives, analgesics and all other medications except those that might be deemed essential (such as digitalis and insulin) are withheld for at least 24 hours, and preferably 48 to 72 hours, prior to the test. Antihypertensive drugs are withheld until blood pressure returns to the untreated, hypertensive level. This test is not performed on a patient who is normotensive.

Procedure: (intravenous) The patient is kept at rest in the supine position throughout the test, preferably in a quiet, darkened room. Injection of Rogitine is delayed until blood pressure is stabilised, as evidenced by blood pressure readings taken every 10 minutes for at least 30 minutes.

The dose for adults is 5 mg. The syringe needle is inserted into the vein and injection delayed until the pressor response to venepuncture has subsided.

Rogitine is injected rapidly. Blood pressure is recorded immediately after injection, at 30-second intervals for the first 3 minutes, and at 60-second intervals for the next 7 minutes.

Interpretation: A positive response, suggestive of phaeochromocytoma, is indicated when the blood pressure is reduced by more than 35 mmHg systolic and by 25 mmHg diastolic. A typical positive response is a reduction in pressure of 60 mmHg systolic and 25 mmHg diastolic. Usually, the maximal effect is evident within 2 minutes after injection. A return to preinjection pressure commonly occurs within 15 to 20 minutes but may occur more rapidly.

If blood pressure decreases to a dangerous level, the patient should be treated as outlined under *Overdose*.

A negative response is indicated when the blood pressure is elevated, unchanged, or reduced by less than 35 mmHg systolic and 25 mmHg diastolic after injection of Rogitine. A negative response to this test does not exclude the diagnosis of phaeochromocytoma, especially in patients with paroxysmal hypertension, in whom the incidence of false-negative responses is high.

Procedure: (intramuscular) A dose of 5 mg is administered intramuscularly.

Interpretation: Blood pressure is recorded every 5 minutes for 30 to 45 minutes following injection. A positive response is indicated when the blood pressure is reduced by 35 mmHg systolic and by 25 mmHg diastolic, or more, within 20 minutes following injection.

Children: Management of hypertensive episodes in patients with phaeochromocytoma: The dosage is 1mg given intravenously.

Diagnosis of phaeochromocytoma - Rogitine blocking test: The dosage is 1 mg given intravenously or 3 mg given intramuscularly.

Elderly: In elderly patients, it is advisable to use the lowest dose or a low infusion rate in case of undiagnosed coronary insufficiency, (see *Contra-indications*).

Patients with renal impairment: Since no pharmacokinetic studies with Rogitine have been performed in patients with renal impairment, use caution in administering Rogitine to these patients.

Contra-indications: Known hypersensitivity to phentolamine and related compounds. Known hypersensitivity to sulphites. Hypotension. Myocardial infarction, history of myocardial infarction, coronary insufficiency, angina, or other evidence of coronary artery disease.

Special warnings and special precautions for use: Monitoring of the blood pressure is necessary for appropriate selection of patient, dosage, and duration of therapy. Myocardial infarction, cerebrovascular spasm, and cerebrovascular occlusion have been reported following the administration of Rogitine, usually in association with marked hypotensive episodes.

The presence of sulphites in Rogitine ampoules can lead to isolated hypersensitivity reactions especially in patients with bronchial asthma, which may become manifest as an acute asthma attack, shock, or clouding of consciousness.

For screening tests in patients with hypotension, the generally available urinary assay of catecholamines or other biochemical assays have largely replaced the Rogitine blocking test and other pharmacological tests for reasons of accuracy and safety. Therefore the Rogitine blocking test is not the procedure of choice and should be used only when these other specific tests are not available.

Tachycardia and cardiac arrhythmias may occur with the use of Rogitine.

Due to its stimulatory effect on the gastro-intestinal tract, including gastric secretion, Rogitine should be used with caution in patients with gastritis and peptic ulcer. Excessive cardiac stimulation and hypertensive crisis may occur during surgical removal of a tumour due to manipulation of the phaeochromocytoma, despite the fact that phentolamine had been given as pre-medication to prevent such an occurrence. In the event of this complication, use a β_1-selective, β-adrenergic blocking agent in slow i.v. injection.

Interactions with other medicaments and other forms of interaction: Rogitine may augment the hypotensive effect of other antihypertensive agents. Antipsychotics may enhance the hypotensive effect of α-adrenergic blocking agents.

Pregnancy and lactation: Experience with Rogitine in pregnant women is not available. Do not use in pregnancy unless treatment is considered essential. No information is available as to whether phentolamine passes into breast milk. For safety reasons, it is not recommended to use Rogitine during lactation.

Effects on ability to drive and use machines: Patients should be warned of the potential hazards of driving or operating machinery if they experience side effects such as dizziness and sedation.

Undesirable effects

Cardiovascular system: Frequent: Orthostatic hypotension and tachycardia. Occasional: Acute or prolonged hypotensive episodes (flushing, sweating and feelings of apprehension). Myocardial infarction, cerebrospasm, and cerebrovascular occlusion may occur under these circumstances. Rare: Anginal pain and cardiac arrhythmias.

Central nervous system: Occasional: Dizziness and weakness.

Gastro-intestinal tract: Occasional: Nausea, vomiting and diarrhoea.

Other organ systems: Occasional: Nasal stuffiness and flushing. Rare: Chest pain.

Overdose

Symptoms: Arterial hypotension, reflex tachycardia, cardiac stimulation, arrhythmia, increase of systemic venous capacity, and possibly shock. These effects may be accompanied by headache, hyperexcitability and disturbances of vision, sweating, increased gastric motility, vomiting and diarrhoea, hypoglycaemia.

Treatment: Hypotension, excessive peripheral vasodilation: noradrenaline, in cautiously titrated continuous i.v. infusion, can be considered the physiological antagonist; the effect of Rogitine may wear off in a short time, and administration of noradrenaline may have to be adjusted accordingly. When a pressor agent is used, ECG should be monitored, as major arrhythmias may occur. Alternative measures such as keeping the patient's legs raised and administering a plasma expander should be implemented concomitantly. Do not use adrenaline since this may cause a further fall of blood pressure under the given conditions.

Disturbances of cardiac rhythm: adjust treatment to the nature of the arrhythmia.

Hypoglycaemia: Provide glucose iv until reaction is compensated.

Pharmacological properties

Pharmacodynamic properties: Phentolamine is a competitive non-selective α_1 and α_2-adrenergic receptor blocker of relatively short duration. It causes vasodilation and a fall in blood pressure which is based upon the blockade of both postjunctional vascular α_1 and α_2-adrenoceptors. It also antagonises the vasoconstrictor response to noradrenaline and adrenaline infusions. Enhanced neural release of noradrenaline due to presynaptic α_2-blockade may contribute to the positive inotropic and chronotropic effects of Rogitine on cardiac muscle.

The administration of Rogitine intravenously to man produces transient declines in mean systemic vascular resistance and mean systemic arterial pressure as a result of dilatation in the arterial as well as in the venous vascular bed. These effects of Rogitine are accompanied by tachycardia, triggered by the baroreceptor reflex system and the autonomic nervous system.

Pharmacokinetic properties: The elimination of phentolamine from blood is rapid and does not follow first order kinetics. After two to four hours the concentration has fallen to about 15% of the peak value. At concentrations of 0.02 to 109 μg/ml, 54% of phentolamine is bound to human serum proteins. Phentolamine is extensively metabolised, on average about 13% of a dose given by intravenous infusion is excreted unchanged in the urine. Phentolamine metabolism is more pronounced following oral administration than after intravenous administration.

Preclinical safety data: According to the experimental data available, phentolamine did not reveal either a mutagenic or a teratogenic potential. Long-term carcinogenicity studies have not been conducted with phentolamine.

Pharmaceutical particulars

List of excipients: Water, sodium metabisulphite and glucose.

Incompatibilities: Rogitine should not be mixed with alkaline solutions.

Shelf life: 5 Years

Special precautions for storage: Protect from light and heat. Store below 25°C.

Nature and contents of container: Glass ampoules in boxes of 5.

Instructions for use/handling: None

Marketing authorisation number PL 16853/0012

Date of first authorisation 25 June 1998

Date of (partial) revision of the text June 1998

Legal status POM

SINTHROME*

Qualitative and quantitative composition Each tablet contains 1 mg of nicoumalone BP.

Pharmaceutical form White, round, flat tablets, with slightly bevelled edges, one side bearing the imprint 'CG', the other the imprint 'AA'.

Clinical particulars

Therapeutic indications: Sinthrome is an oral anticoagulant for the treatment and prevention of thromboembolic diseases.

Posology and method of administration

Oral route of administration: Sensitivity to anticoagulants varies from patient to patient and may also fluctuate during the course of treatment. Therefore it is essential to perform regular coagulation tests and to adjust the patient's dosage accordingly. If this is not possible, Sinthrome should not be used.

Sinthrome should be given in a single dose at the same time every day.

Adults: Initial dosage: If the thromboplastin time before starting treatment is within the normal range, the following dosage schedule is recommended:

First day: 8 to 12 mg

Second day: 4 to 8 mg

If the initial thromboplastin time is abnormal, treatment should be instituted with caution.

Maintenance therapy: The maintenance dose of Sinthrome varies from patient to patient and must be determined on the basis of regular laboratory estimations of the patient's blood coagulation time.

Adjustment of the maintenance dose can only be made by monitoring the Quick value or International Normalised Ratio (INR) at regular intervals so that dosage remains within the therapeutic range. Depending on the individual, the maintenance dose generally lies between 1 to 8 mg daily.

Before the start of treatment, up to the time when the coagulation valency is stabilised within the optimum range, routine measurement of the thromboplastin time should be carried out daily in hospital. Blood samples for laboratory tests should always be taken at the same time of day.

The INR is the ratio of the patient's plasma thromboplastin time and the normal thromboplastin time raised to a power determined for a reference thromboplastin. As the Quick value decreases, the patient's thromboplastin time increases and the INR is greater. The therapeutic range generally lies between INR values of 2 to 4.5.

Generally after withdrawal of Sinthrome, there is usually no danger of reactive hypercoagulability and therefore it is not necessary to give gradually diminishing doses. However, in extremely rare cases in some high risk patients (e.g. after myocardial infarction) withdrawal should be gradual.

Use in children: Not recommended.

Use in the elderly: A dose lower than the recommended adult dose may be sufficient in elderly patients. (See *Precautions*).

Contra-indications: Sinthrome is contra-indicated in patients with a known hypersensitivity to nicoumalone and related coumarin derivatives, and in patients unable to co-operate (e.g. unsupervised and senile patients, alcoholics and patients with psychiatric disorders).

Sinthrome is also contra-indicated in all conditions where the risk of haemorrhage exceeds possible clinical benefit e.g. haemorrhagic diathesis and/or blood dyscrasia, immediately prior to, or after surgery on the central nervous system or eyes and traumatising surgery involving extensive exposure of the tissues, peptic ulceration or haemorrhage in the gastro-intestinal tract, urogenital tract or respiratory system, cerebrovascular haemorrhages, pericarditis, pericardial effusion, subacute bacterial endocarditis, severe hypertension (due to occult risks), severe hepatic or renal disease, and in cases of increased fibrinolytic activity following operations on the lung, prostate and uterus.

Special warnings and special precautions for use: Strict medical supervision should be given in cases where the disease or condition may reduce the protein binding of Sinthrome (e.g. thyrotoxicosis, tumours, renal disease, infections and inflammation).

Particular care should be taken in patients with hepatic dysfunction since the synthesis of blood coagulation factors may be impaired. Disorders affecting gastro-intestinal absorption may alter the anticoagulant activity of Sinthrome. In severe heart failure, a very cautious dosage schedule must be adopted, since hepatic congestion may reduce the activation of γ-carboxylation of coagulation factors.

However with reversal of the hepatic congestion, it may be necessary to raise the dosage.

In elderly patients, anticoagulant medication should be monitored with special care (see 'Pharmacokinetics' and 'Dosage' recommendations).

Since nicoumalone is extensively metabolised by the liver, impaired renal function will not greatly affect the elimination of the drug although care should be taken due to the possibility of underlying platelet dysfunction.

During treatment with anticoagulants, intramuscular injections may cause haematomas and should be avoided. Subcutaneous and intravenous injections may be given without such complications.

Meticulous care should be taken where it is necessary to shorten the thromboplastin time for diagnostic or therapeutic procedures (e.g. angiography, lumbar puncture, minor surgery, tooth extractions, etc.).

Interaction with other medicaments and other forms of interaction: There are many possible interactions between coumarins and other drugs; the interactions of clinical relevance are given below. The mechanisms of these interactions include disturbances of absorption, inhibition or induction of liver microsomal enzyme systems and reduced availability of vitamin K necessary for γ-carboxylation of coagulation factors. Every form of therapy may involve the risk of an interaction although not all will be significant. Thus careful surveillance is important and frequent coagulation tests (e.g. twice weekly) should be carried out when initially prescribing any drug in combination with Sinthrome or withdrawing a concomitantly administered drug.

The anticoagulant effect may be potentiated by concomitant administration of the following drugs:

Allopurinol, anabolic steroids, androgens, anti-arrhythmic agents (e.g. amiodarone, quinidine), antibiotics (e.g. erythromycin, tetracyclines, neomycin, chloramphenicol), clofibric acid, its derivatives and structural analogues, disulfiram, ethacrynic acid, glucagon, histamine H_2-receptor antagonists, imidazole derivatives (e.g. metronidazole and, even when administered locally, miconazole), long-acting sulphonamides (including co-trimoxazoles), oral antidiabetics, thyroid hormones (incl. dextrothyroxine), sulphinpyrazone.

Drugs altering haemostasis may potentiate the anticoagulant activity of Sinthrome and thereby increase the risk of gastro-intestinal haemorrhage. Consequently, Sinthrome should not be prescribed with such drugs, which include heparin, salicylic acid and its derivatives.

When Sinthrome is prescribed in combination with NSAIDs, coagulation tests should be performed more frequently.

The anticoagulant effect may be diminished by concomitant administration of the following drugs:

Aminoglutethimide, barbiturates, carbamazepine, cholestyramine (see below), griseofulvin, oral contraceptives, rifampicin, and thiazide diuretics.

During concomitant treatment with hydantoin derivatives, the serum hydantoin concentration may rise.

Sinthrome may potentiate the hypoglycaemic effect of sulphonylurea derivatives.

Patients being treated with Sinthrome (especially those suffering from hepatic dysfunction), should limit their alcohol intake since it is not possible to predict the severity of any drug interactions nor identify any early signs of such interactions.

Pregnancy and lactation: Sinthrome, like other coumarin derivatives may be associated with congenital malformations of the embryo. Therefore Sinthrome is contra-indicated for use in pregnancy. Women of child-bearing potential should take contraceptive measures during treatment with Sinthrome.

Sinthrome active substance passes into the breast milk of lactating mothers, but in quantities so small that no undesirable effects on the infant are to be expected. However, as a precaution, the infant should be given 1 mg vitamin K_1 per week as a prophylactic measure.

Effects on ability to drive and use machines: None known.

Undesirable effects: Haemorrhage, in various organs, is the most common side-effect associated with Sinthrome; its occurrence is related to the dosage of the drug, the patient's age and the nature of the underlying disease (but not the duration of treatment).

Possible sites of haemorrhage include the gastro-intestinal tract, brain, urogenital tract, uterus, liver, gall bladder and the eye.

If haemorrhage occurs in a patient with a thromboplastin time within the therapeutic range, diagnosis of their condition must be clarified.

Rare effects noted with similar coumarin derivatives include gastro-intestinal disorders (loss of appetite, nausea, vomiting), allergic reactions (urticaria, dermatitis and fever) and reversible alopecia.

Isolated cases of haemorrhagic skin necrosis (usually associated with congenital protein C deficiency) and liver damage have also been reported.

Overdose: Clinical manifestations of overdosage are unlikely with large single doses but more likely following prolonged use of daily doses exceeding those required therapeutically.

Symptoms: The onset and severity of the symptoms are dependent on the individual's sensitivity to oral anticoagulants, the size of the overdose and the duration of treatment.

Haemorrhage is the prominent feature of an overdose and may occur within 1 to 5 days after ingestion. Nose-bleeds, haematemesis, haemoptysis, gastro-intestinal haemorrhage, vaginal bleeding, haematuria (with renal colic), cutaneous haemorrhages, bleeding into the joints or menorrhagia may be experienced.

Further symptoms include tachycardia, hypotension, peripheral circulatory disorders due to loss of blood, nausea, vomiting, diarrhoea, and abdominal pains.

Laboratory tests will show an extremely low Quick value (or high INR value) pronounced prolongation of the recalcification time or thromboplastin time and disturbed γ-carboxylation of factors II, VII, IX and X.

Treatment: If, at the time of overdosage, the patient's thromboplastin time was normal, drug absorption may be reduced by emesis or gastric lavage in combination with giving activated charcoal or a fast-acting laxative. Cholestyramine may markedly enhance the drug's elimination by inhibiting the enterohepatic circulation.

A temporary reduction of the dose of Sinthrome is often sufficient to control slight bleeding.

Vitamin K_1 may antagonise the effect of Sinthrome within 3 to 5 hours. In cases of moderate haemorrhage, 2 to 5 mg vitamin K_1 should be given orally; in severe haemorrhage, 1 to 10 mg vitamin K_1 should be injected very slowly (at a rate less than 1 mg/min) intravenously. Additional doses (up to a maximum dose of 40 mg daily) should be given at 4-hour intervals. Vitamin K_1 should not be given by intramuscular injection.

Doses of vitamin K_1 in excess of 5 mg can cause resistance to further anticoagulant therapy for several days. If an anticoagulant is required, heparin may be used temporarily, although oral anticoagulant therapy should be resumed at the same time and heparin withdrawn once the therapeutic range has been reached.

In the case of life-threatening haemorrhage, intravenous transfusions of fresh frozen plasma or whole blood can abolish the effects of Sinthrome.

Pharmacological properties

Pharmacodynamic properties: To initiate blood clotting, vitamin K causes γ-carboxylation of certain glutamic acid molecules on the coagulation factors II, VII, IX and X. Coumarin derivatives such as Sinthrome prevent γ-carboxylation of these proteins by vitamin K although the precise nature of this antagonism has yet to be established.

Depending on the initial dosage, Sinthrome prolongs the thromboplastin time within approximately 36 to 72 hours. Following withdrawal of Sinthrome, the thromboplastin time usually reverts to normal after a few days.

Pharmacokinetic properties: Following oral administration, Sinthrome is rapidly absorbed; at least 60% of the administered dose is systemically available. Peak plasma concentrations are achieved within 1 to 3 hours after a single dose of 10 mg and AUC values are proportional to the size of the dose over a dosage range of 8 to 16 mg.

No correlation between plasma concentrations of Sinthrome active substance (nicoumalone) and the apparent prothrombin levels can be established due to the variation of plasma drug concentrations between patients.

Plasma drug concentrations are generally higher in patients of 70 years or over when compared with younger patients, after the same dose.

Over 98% of nicoumalone is protein-bound, mainly to albumin. The calculated apparent volume of distribution is 0.16 to 0.18 l/kg for the R(+) enantiomer and 0.22 to 0.34 l/kg for the S(-) enantiomer.

Nicoumalone is extensively metabolised although the metabolites appear to be pharmacologically inactive in man.

The elimination half-life of nicoumalone from the plasma is 8 to 11 hours. Less than 0.2% of the dose is renally excreted unchanged with 60% being excreted in the urine and 29% in the faeces.

Preclinical safety data: None stated.

Pharmaceutical particulars

List of excipients: Aerosil 200 (silica aerogel), cellulose HP-M603 (hydroxypropylmethylcellulose), Lactose ground, magnesium stearate, maize starch, talc pH, de-ionised water.

Incompatibilities: None stated.

Shelf life: 36 months.

Special precautions for storage: None stated.

Nature and contents of container: Blister packs of 100 tablets.

Instructions for use/handling: None stated.

Marketing authorisation number PL 16853/0013

Date of first authorisation 25 June 1998

Date of (partial) revision of the text June 1998

Legal status POM

SLOW-K* TABLETS 600 mg

Qualitative and quantitative composition Potassium chloride 600 mg Ph.Eur.

Pharmaceutical form Pale orange, round, biconvex, polished, sugar-coated modified release tablets. Printed Slow-K in black on one side.

Clinical particulars

Therapeutic indications: The correction and/or prevention of hypokalaemia in those patients who cannot tolerate and/or refuse to take liquid or effervescent potassium chloride, or when there is a problem of compliance with these preparations.

Posology and method of administration: Slow-K is taken orally. It is important that the tablets should be swallowed whole, with fluid, during meals, whilst the patient is sitting upright.

Adults: The dosage of Slow-K should be adapted to the cause, degree and duration of potassium depletion. 2 to 3 tablets daily are usually an adequate supplement. In states of severe potassium deficiency, a higher dose of 9 to 12 tablets daily may be needed.

If the dosage exceeds 16mmol K^+ (2 tablets) it should be taken in divided doses. Where intermittent diuretic therapy is being used, it is advisable to give Slow-K on intervening days between administration of the diuretic. The response to treatment should preferably be monitored by repeat determination of plasma potassium and Slow-K continued until the hypokalaemia has been corrected.

Children: Not recommended.

Elderly: No special dosage regime is usually necessary, but concurrent renal insufficiency should be taken into account (See *Special warnings and special precautions for use*).

Contra-indications: Hypersensitivity to potassium administration, eg hyperkalaemic periodic paralysis, congenital paramyotonia. Marked renal failure (even when not yet associated with manifest hyperkalaemia), untreated Addison's Disease, hyporeninaemic hypoaldosteronism, acute dehydration, hyperkalaemia and conditions involving extensive cell destruction (e.g. severe burns).

All solid forms of potassium medication are contra-indicated in the presence of obstructions in the digestive tract (eg resulting from compression of the oesophagus due to dilation of the left atrium or from stenosis of the gut).

In cases of metabolic acidosis, the hypokalaemia should be treated not with potassium chloride but with an alkaline potassium salt (e.g. potassium bicarbonate).

Concomitant treatment with potassium sparing diuretics (eg spironolactone, triamterene, amiloride).

Special warnings and special precautions for use: If a patient under treatment with Slow-K develops severe vomiting, severe abdominal pains or flatulence, or gastro-intestinal haemorrhage, the preparation should be withdrawn at once, because in the presence of an obstruction it could conceivably give rise to ulceration or perforation.

Oral potassium preparations should be prescribed with particular caution in patients with a history of peptic ulcer.

Caution should be exercised when prescribing solid oral potassium preparations, particularly in high dosage, in patients concurrently receiving anticholinergics, because of their potential to slow gastro-intestinal motility.

Patients with ostomies may have altered intestinal transit times and are better treated with other forms of potassium salts.

In patients suffering from impaired renal function, special care should be exercised when prescribing potassium salts owing to the risk of their producing hyperkalaemia. Monitoring of the serum electrolytes is particularly necessary in patients with diseases of the heart or kidneys.

In some patients, diuretic-induced magnesium deficiency will prevent restoration of intracellular deficits of potassium, so that hypomagnesaemia should be corrected at the same time as hypokalaemia.

Interaction with other medicaments and other forms of interaction: Combined treatment with the following increase the risk of hyperkalaemia: ACE inhibitors, cyclosporin, NSAIDs, β-blockers, heparin, digoxin, potassium sparing diuretics (see *Contra-indications*).

Pregnancy and lactation: Because of gastro-intestinal hypomotility associated with pregnancy, solid forms of oral potassium preparations should be given to pregnant women only if clearly needed.

The normal K^+ content of human milk is about 13 mmol/litre. Since oral potassium becomes part of the body's potassium pool, provided this is not excessive, Slow-K can be expected to have little or no effect on the potassium level in human milk.

Effects on ability to drive and use machines: None known.

Undesirable effects: Side effects are rare with Slow-K, as any excess potassium is rapidly excreted in the urine.

Gastrointestinal tract: Rare: oral potassium preparations may provoke gastro-intestinal disturbances (nausea, vomiting, abdominal pains, diarrhoea) necessitating either a reduction in dosage or withdrawal of medication (see *Special warnings and special precautions for use*). Isolated cases: obstruction, bleeding and ulceration, with or without perforation of the upper or lower GIT, have been reported, usually associated with other factors known to predispose a patient to these effects (e.g. delayed GIT transit time, obstruction of GIT).

Skin: Rare: Pruritus and/or skin rash, urticaria.

Electrolytes: Hyperkalaemia may develop in patients having difficulty with either renal potassium excretion or potassium metabolism.

Overdose

Signs and symptoms: Mainly cardiovascular (hypotension, shock, ventricular arrhythmias, bundle-branch block, ventricular fibrillation leading possibly to cardiac arrest) and neuromuscular (paraesthesiae, convulsions, areflexia, flaccid paralysis of striated muscle leading possibly to respiratory paralysis). Beside elevation of serum potassium concentration, typical ECG changes are also encountered (increasing amplitude and peaking of T waves, disappearance of P wave, widening of QRS complex and S-T segment depression).

Treatment: Gastric lavage, administration of cation exchange agents, infusion of glucose and insulin, forced diuresis and possibly peritoneal dialysis or haemodialysis.

Pharmacological particulars

Pharmacodynamic properties: The potassium chloride in Slow-K is finely distributed in a neutral wax base, from which it is gradually released over a period of 3 to 6 hours during its passage through the digestive tract. This special form of potassium substitution therapy is designed to avoid high localised concentrations of potassium chloride which might irritate or damage the mucosa. The potassium chloride in Slow-K is completely absorbed in the intestinal tract.

Pharmacokinetic properties: The potassium chloride in Slow-K has been shown to be completely absorbed; occasionally patients may notice "ghost" tablet cores in the faeces, these do not contain any potassium.

Following a single dose of Slow-K, potassium chloride is released over a period of approximately 4 hours. Renal excretion of potassium chloride following ingestion of Slow-K occurs 30 to 60 minutes later than when the same dose is given in the form of a solution. In the presence of a normal potassium balance, 90% of the potassium supplied by Slow-K is excreted renally within 8 hours, and more than 98% by 24 hours.

Preclinical safety data: There are no pre-clinical data of relevance to the prescriber which are additional to those already included in other sections of the Summary of Product Characteristics.

Pharmaceutical particulars

List of excipients: Cetostearyl alcohol, gelatin, magnesium stearate, acacia, titanium dioxide (E171), talc, sucrose, polyethylene glycol 6000, red iron oxide (E172), yellow iron oxide (E172) and printing ink (Opacode black S-1-27708 or Opacode black S-1-8015 consisting of methylated spirit, shellac, propylene glycol, vegetable carbon E153, water and dimethylpolysiloxane).

Incompatibilities: None known.

Shelf life: 5 years.

Special precautions for storage: Protect from heat and moisture.

Nature and contents of container: Polypropylene Securitainer with polyethylene cap containing 100 tablets.

Instructions for use/handling: None.

Marketing authorisation number PL 16853/0014

Date of first authorisation 25 June 1998

Date of (partial) revision of the text November 1998

Legal status Pharmacy

SYMMETREL*

Qualitative and quantitative composition The active ingredient is 1-Adamantanamine hydrochloride (=amantadine hydrochloride).

The capsules contain 100 mg Amantadine Hydrochloride PhEur.

The syrup contains 50 mg/5 ml Amantadine Hydrochloride PhEur.

Pharmaceutical form Capsules and syrup.

Clinical particulars

Therapeutic indications: Parkinson's disease.

Herpes zoster.

Note: Herpes zoster: It is recommended that the drug be given to elderly or debilitated patients in whom the physician suspects that a severe and painful rash could occur. Symmetrel can significantly reduce the proportion of patients experiencing pain of long duration.

Prophylaxis and treatment of signs and symptoms of infection caused by influenza A virus.

Influenza A: It is suggested that Symmetrel be given to patients suffering from clinical influenza in whom complications might be expected to occur. In addition, Symmetrel is recommended prophylactically in cases particularly at risk, for example those with chronic respiratory disease or debilitating conditions, the elderly, those living in crowded conditions and for individuals in families where influenza has already been diagnosed, control of institutional outbreaks or those in essential services who are unvaccinated or when vaccination is unavailable or contra-indicated.

Symmetrel does not completely prevent the host immune response to influenza A infection so individuals who take this drug still develop immune responses to the natural disease or vaccination and may be protected when later exposed to antigenically related viruses. Symmetrel may also be used in post-exposure prophylaxis in conjunction with inactivated vaccine during an outbreak until protective antibodies develop or in patients who are not expected to have a substantial antibody response (immunosuppression).

Posology and method of administration:

Parkinson's disease: Initially 100 mg daily for the first week, increasing to 100 mg twice daily.

The dose can be titrated against signs and symptoms. In some cases amounts exceeding 200 mg daily may provide some additional relief but may also be associated with increasing toxicity. A dose of 400 mg/day should not be exceeded. The dose should be increased gradually, at intervals of not less than 1 week. Since patients over 65 years of age tend to show lower renal clearance and consequently higher plasma concentrations, the recommended dose for elderly patients with parkinsonism is 100 mg daily.

Amantadine acts within a few days but sometimes appears to lose some of its efficacy within a few months of continuous treatment.

The effectiveness of amantadine may be prolonged by a temporary withdrawal of three to four weeks, which seems to restore activity. During this time existing concomitant antiparkinsonian therapy should be continued or low dose L-dopa treatment initiated if clinically necessary.

Treatment with Symmetrel must be reduced gradually, e.g. at a rate of half the dose at weekly intervals because abrupt discontinuation may exacerbate Parkinson's syndrome, regardless of the patient's response to therapy (see *Special warnings and precautions for use*).

Combined treatment: any antiparkinson drug with which the patient is already being treated should be continued during the first stage of treatment with Symmetrel. In many cases it is then possible gradually to reduce the dosage of the other drug without prejudicing the treatment response. If increased side effects occur, however, its dosage should be reduced more quickly. In patients already receiving large doses of anticholinergic agents or L-dopa the initial low-dosage phase of treatment with Symmetrel should be extended to 15 days.

Herpes zoster: Treatment should be started as soon as possible after the diagnosis has been made. The dosage is 100 mg twice daily for 14 days. If post-herpetic pain persists after this period it is recommended that treatment be continued for a further 14 days.

Treatment of influenza A: It is advisable to start treating influenza as early as possible and to continue for 4 to 5 days. When amantadine is started within 48 hours of symptoms appearing the duration of fever and other effects is reduced by one or two days and the inflammatory reaction of the bronchial tree that usually accompanies influenza resolves more quickly.

Prophylaxis of influenza A: Treatment daily for as long as protection from influenza infection is required. In most instances this is expected to be for 6 weeks but when used with inactivated influenza A vaccine amantadine is continued for 2 to 3 weeks following inoculation.

Adults: 100 mg daily for the recommended period.

Use in children aged 10–15 years: 100 mg daily for the recommended period.

Use in children under 10 years of age: Dosage not established.

Adults over 65 years of age: Plasma amantadine concentrations are influenced by renal function. In elderly patients, the elimination half-life is longer and renal clearance of the compound is diminished in comparison to young people. Therefore a daily dose of less than 100 mg or 100 mg given at intervals of greater than one day may be appropriate.

Use in patients with renal impairment: in patients with compromised renal function, the dose of amantadine should be reduced accordingly. This can be achieved by reducing the daily dose or prolonging the dosage interval in accordance with the creatinine clearance. For example:

Creatinine clearance [ml/(min. 1.73 m²)]	*Dose*
<15	Symmetrel contra-indicated
15–35	100 mg/2–3 days
>35	100 mg/day

The above recommendations are for guidance only and physicians should continue to monitor their patients for signs of unwanted effects.

Contra-indications: It is not recommended that Symmetrel be used to treat individuals who are subject to convulsions, or who have a history of gastric ulceration.

Symmetrel should not be used in patients with severe renal disease. Pregnancy.

Known hypersensitivity to amantadine, or any of the excipients of the capsules and syrup.

Special warnings and precautions for use: Symmetrel should be used with caution in patients with confusional or hallucinatory states or underlying psychiatric disorders.

Particular care is called for in patients suffering from, or who have a history of, cardiovascular disorders.

Symmetrel should be used cautiously in patients with liver or kidney disorders.

Discontinuation of treatment. Abrupt discontinuation of amantadine may result in worsening of symptoms.

There have been isolated reports of a possible association with the occurrence or aggravation of neuroleptic malignant syndrome or neuroleptic-induced catatonia in patients treated concurrently with neuroleptics and amantadine, following abrupt cessation of the latter. Treatment should not be stopped abruptly in such patients.

Because of the possibility of serious adverse effects, caution should be observed when prescribing Symmetrel to patients being treated with drugs having CNS effects, or for whom the potential risks outweigh the benefit of treatment. Because some patients have attempted suicide on amantadine, prescriptions should be written for the smallest quantity consistent with good patient management.

Peripheral oedema thought to be due to an alteration in the responsiveness of peripheral vessels may occur in some patients during treatment with Symmetrel. This should be considered when the drug is prescribed for those with congestive heart failure.

Resistance to amantadine occurs during serial passage of influenza virus strains *in vitro* or *in vivo* in the presence of the drug. Apparent transmission of drug-resistant viruses may have been the cause of failure of prophylaxis and treatment in household contacts and in nursing-home patients. However, there is no evidence to date that the resistant virus produces a disease that is in any way different from that produced by sensitive viruses.

Interaction with other medicaments and other forms of interaction: Concurrent administration of amantadine and anticholinergic agents or L-dopa may increase confusion, hallucinations, nightmares, gastro-intestinal disturbances, or other atropine-like side effects (see also *Overdose*).

In isolated cases psychotic decompensation has been reported in patients receiving amantadine and concomitant neuroleptic medication.

Psychotic reactions have been observed in patients receiving amantadine and L-dopa.

Concurrent administration of amantadine and drugs or substances (e.g. alcohol) acting on the central nervous system may result in additive CNS toxicity. Close observation is recommended (see also *Overdose*).

There have been isolated reports of a suspected interaction between amantadine and combination diuretics (hydrochlorothiazide+potassium sparing diuretics). One or both of the components apparently reduce the clearance of amantadine, leading to higher plasma concentrations and toxic effects (confusion, hallucinations, ataxia, myoclonus).

Pregnancy and lactation: Reproductive toxicity studies were performed in rats and rabbits. In rat oral doses of 50 and 100 mg/kg proved to be teratogenic.

Amantadine-related complications during pregnancy have been reported. Symmetrel is contra-indicated during pregnancy and in women wishing to become pregnant.

Amantadine passes into breast milk. Undesirable effects have been reported in breast-fed infants. Nursing mothers should not take Symmetrel.

Effects on ability to drive or use machines: Patients who note CNS effects or blurring of vision should be advised to avoid situations where alertness is essential.

Undesirable effects: Amantadine's undesirable effects are often of mild and transient nature. They usually appear within the first 2 to 4 days of treatment and promptly disappear in 24 to 48 hours after discontinuation of amantadine.

A direct relationship between dose and incidence of side effects has not been demonstrated; however, there seems to be a tendency towards more frequent undesirable effects (particularly affecting the CNS) with increasing doses.

Frequency estimates: frequent>10%, occasional 1%–10%, rare 0.001%–1%, isolated cases<0.001%.

Central nervous system: Occasional: depression, anxiety, elevation of mood, agitation, nervousness, difficulty in concentrating, dizziness, lightheadedness, headache, insomnia, lethargy, hallucinations, nightmares, ataxia, slurred speech, blurred vision. Hallucinations, confusion, and nightmares are more common when amantadine is administered concurrently with anticholinergic agents or when the patient has an underlying psychiatric disorder. Rare: confusion, disorientation, psychosis, tremor, dyskinesia, convulsions. Delirium, hypomanic state, and mania have been reported but their incidence cannot be readily deduced from the literature.

Cardiovascular system: Frequent: oedema of ankles, livedo reticularis. Occasional: palpitations, orthostatic hypotension. Isolated cases: heart insufficiency/failure.

Blood: Isolated cases: leucopenia, reversible elevation of liver enzymes.

Gastrointestinal tract: Occasional: dry mouth, anorexia, nausea, vomiting, constipation. Rare: diarrhoea.

Skin and appendages: Occasional: diaphoresis. Rare: exanthema. Isolated cases: photosensitisation.

Sense organs: Rare: corneal lesions, e.g. punctate subepithelial opacities which might be associated with superficial punctate keratitis, corneal epithelial oedema, and markedly reduced visual acuity.

Urogenital tract: Rare: urinary retention, urinary incontinence.

Overdose: Signs and symptoms: neuromuscular disturbances and symptoms of acute psychosis are prominent features of acute poisoning with amantadine.

Central nervous system: Hyperreflexia, motor restlessness; convulsions; extrapyramidal signs: torsion spasms, dystonic posturing: dilated pupils. Confusion, disorientation, delirium, visual hallucinations.

Respiratory system: hyperventilation, pulmonary oedema, respiratory distress, including adult respiratory distress syndrome.

Cardiovascular system: sinus tachycardia, arrhythmia.

Gastrointestinal system: nausea, vomiting, dry mouth.

Renal function: urine retention, renal dysfunction, including increases in BUN and decreased creatinine clearance.

Overdose from combined drug treatment: the peripheral and central adverse effects of anticholinergic drugs are increased by the concomitant use of amantadine, and acute psychotic reactions, which may be identical to those caused by atropine poisoning, may occur when large doses of anticholinergic agents are used. Where alcohol or central nervous stimulants have been taken at the same time, the signs and symptoms of acute poisoning with amantadine may be aggravated and/or modified.

Management: There is no specific antidote. Removal and/or activation of poisoning agent(s): induction of vomiting and/or gastric aspiration and lavage if patient is conscious, activated charcoal, saline cathartic, if judged appropriate. Since amantadine is excreted for a large part unchanged in the urine, maintenance of renal excretory function, copious diuresis, and forced diuresis if necessary, are effective ways to remove it from the blood stream. Acidification of the urine favours the excretion of amantadine in the urine. Haemodialysis does not remove significant amounts of amantadine.

Monitoring of blood pressure, heart rate, ECG, respiration, body temperature and treatment for possible hypotension and cardiac arryhthmias, as necessary.

Convulsions and excessive motor restlessness: administer anticonvulsants such as diazepam i.v., paraldehyde i.m. or per rectum, or phenobarbital i.m.

Acute psychotic symptoms, delirium, dystonic posturing, myoclonic manifestations: physostigmine by slow intravenous infusion (1 mg doses in adults, 0.5 mg in children) repeated administration according to the initial response and the subsequent need, has been reported.

Retention of urine: bladder should be catheterised; an indwelling catheter can be left in place for the time required.

Pharmacological properties Pharmacotherapeutic group: Antiparkinson agent and anti-influenza virostatic.

Pharmacodynamic properties;

Parkinson's disease: Symmetrel probably acts by enhancing the release of dopamine and delaying the reuptake into synaptic vesicles. It may also exert some anticholinergic activity. When administered either alone or in combination with other drugs, amantadine produces an improvement in the cardinal signs and symptoms of parkinsonism and improves functional capacity in about 60% of patients.

The effect generally sets in two to five days after the start of treatment. It exerts a positive effect particularly on akinesia, rigidity and tremor.

Herpes zoster: The mechanism of action of Symmetrel in herpes zoster has not been fully characterised.

Influenza: Amantadine specifically inhibits the replication of influenza A viruses at low concentrations. Using a sensitive plaque-reduction assay human influenza viruses including H_1N_1, H_2N_2, H_3N_2 subtypes, are inhibited by 0.4 mcg/ml of amantadine or less. The exact mechanism of action of amantadine is unclear but it appears to inhibit an early stage in viral replication. Effects on late replicative steps have been found for representative avian influenza viruses.

Data from tests with representative strains of influenza A virus indicate that Symmetrel is likely to be active against previously unknown strains and could be used in the early stages of an epidemic before a vaccine against the causative strain is generally available.

Pharmacokinetic properties:

Absorption: Amantadine is absorbed slowly but almost completely. Peak plasma concentrations of approximately 250 ng/ml and 500 ng/ml are attained within 3 to 4 hours after single oral administration of 100 mg and 200 mg amantadine, respectively.

Following repeated administration of 200 mg daily the steady-state plasma concentration settles at 300 ng/ml within 3 days.

Distribution: In vitro, 67% of amantadine is bound to plasma proteins. A substantial amount of amantadine is bound to red blood cells. The concentration of amantadine in erythrocytes in normal healthy volunteers is 2.66 times the plasma concentration.

The apparent volume of distribution of the drug is 5 to 10 litres/kg, suggesting extensive tissue binding. It declines with increasing doses. The concentration of amantadine in the lung, heart, kidney, liver and spleen is higher than in the blood.

The drug accumulates after several hours in nasal secretions.

Amantadine passes the blood-brain barrier; it is, however, not possible to quantify this event.

Biotransformation: Amantadine is metabolised to a minor extent, principally by N-acetylation.

Elimination: The drug is eliminated in healthy young adults with a mean plasma elimination half-life of 15 hours (10 to 31 hours).

The total plasma clearance is about the same as renal clearance (250 ml/min). The renal amantadine clearance is much higher than the creatinine clearance, suggesting renal tubular secretion.

A single dose of amantadine is excreted over 72 hours as follows: 65 to 85% unchanged, 5 to 15% as acetyl metabolite in urine, and 1% in stools. After 4 to 5 days 90% of the dose appears unchanged in urine. The rate is considerably influenced by urinary pH. A rise in pH brings about a fall in excretion.

Characteristics in special patient populations: Elderly patients: compared with healthy young adults, the half-life may be doubled and renal clearance diminished. Tubular secretion diminishes more than glomerular filtration in the elderly. In elderly patients repeated administration of 100 mg daily may raise the plasma concentration into the toxic range.

Renal impairment: accumulation of amantadine may occur in renal failure causing severe adverse drug reactions. The rate of elimination of amantadine from plasma is correlated to creatinine clearance values divided by body surface area (1.73 m²) but total renal elimination exceeds this value, possibly due to tubular secretion. The effects of reduced kidney function on elimination are dramatic (a reduction in creatinine clearance to 40 ml/min/1.73 m² may result in a five-fold increase in elimination half-life). The urine remains the almost exclusive route of excretion even in cases of renal failure, where amantadine may persist in the plasma for several days.

Haemodialysis: little amantadine is removed by haemodialysis; this inefficiency may be related to extensive tissue binding. Less than 5% of a dose is eliminated in 4 hours and the mean dialysis time taken to remove half of the dose is 24 hours.

Preclinical safety data: There are no pre-clinical data of relevance to the prescriber which are additional to that already included in other sections of the SPC.

Pharmaceutical particulars

List of excipients: The capsules also contain lactose, polyvinylpyrrolidone, magnesium stearate, red iron oxide, titanium dioxide, gelatin and white printer's ink.

The syrup also contains methyl hydroxybenzoate, propyl hydroxybenzoate, sorbitol, disodium hydrogen citrate, lemon flavouring, strawberry flavouring and water.

Incompatibilities: None known.

Shelf life: Five years.

Special precautions for storage: Capsules: Protect from moisture. Syrup: Protect from heat and light. Keep container closed.

Nature and contents of container: The capsules of 100 mg (brownish-red, hard gelatin capsules, imprinted GEIGY in white on both cap and body) are packed in PVC/PVdC blister packs of 56 capsules.

The clear, citrus flavoured syrup is contained in 150 ml amber glass bottles with child proof closures.

Instruction for use/handling: There is no specific instruction for use/handling.

Marketing authorisation numbers

Capsules PL 16853/0015
Syrup PL 16853/0016

Date of first authorisation 25 June 1998.

Date of approval/revision of SPC June 1998.

Legal status POM.

SYNACTHEN* AMPOULES 250 mcg

Qualitative and quantitative composition Tetracosactrin acetate PhEur. 250 micrograms per ampoule.

Pharmaceutical form A clear colourless sterile solution in a clear glass ampoule.

Clinical particulars

Therapeutic indications: Diagnostic test for the investigation of adrenocortical insufficiency.

Posology and method of administration

Adults: This preparation of Synacthen is intended for administration for diagnostic purposes only as a single intramuscular or intravenous dose; it is not to be used for repeated therapeutic administration.

The 30-minute Synacthen diagnostic test: This test is based on measurement of the plasma cortisol concentration immediately before and exactly 30 minutes after an intramuscular or intravenous injection of 250 micrograms (1 ml) Synacthen. Adrenocortical function can be regarded as normal if the post-injection rise in plasma cortisol concentration amounts to at least 200 nmol/litre (70 micrograms/litre).

Where the 30-minute test has yielded inconclusive results, or where it is desired to determine the functional reserve of the adrenal cortex, a 5-hour test can be performed with Synacthen Depot (see separate Summary of Product Characteristics). Furthermore, a 3-day test with Synacthen Depot may be used to differentiate between primary and secondary adrenocortical insufficiency.

Children: An intravenous dose of 250 micrograms/1.73m² body surface area has been suggested. Thus for children aged 5 to 7 years, approximately half the adult dose will be adequate. For more accurate dosing of other ages, standard body surface area tables should be consulted.

Elderly: There is no evidence to suggest that dosage should be different in the elderly.

Contra-indications: History of hypersensitivity to ACTH, Synacthen or Synacthen Depot. Synacthen is contra-indicated in patients with allergic disorders (e.g. asthma).

Special warnings and special precautions for use: Before using Synacthen, the doctor should make every effort to find out whether the patient is suffering from, or has a history of, allergic disorders (see *Contra-indications*). In particular, he should enquire whether the patient has previously experienced adverse reactions to ACTH, Synacthen or other drugs.

Synacthen should only be administered under the

supervision of appropriate senior hospital medical staff (e.g. consultants).

If local or systemic hypersensitivity reactions occur after the injection (for example, marked redness and pain at the injection site, urticaria, pruritus, flushing, faintness or dyspnoea), Synacthen or other ACTH preparations should be avoided in the future. Hypersensitivity reactions tend to occur within 30 minutes of an injection. The patient should therefore be kept under observation during this time.

Preparation should be made in advance to combat any anaphylactic reaction that may occur after an injection of Synacthen. In the event of a serious anaphylactic reaction occurring, the following measures must be taken immediately: administer adrenaline (0.4 to 1ml of a 0.1% solution intramuscularly or 0.1 to 0.2 ml of a 0.1% solution in 10 ml physiological saline slowly intravenously) as well as a large intravenous dose of a corticosteroid (for example 100mg to 500 mg hydrocortisone, three or four times in 24 hours), repeating the dose if necessary.

The hydrocortisone product information prepared by the manufacturer should also be consulted.

Interaction with other medicaments and other forms of interaction: None known.

Pregnancy and lactation: The Synacthen test should not be utilised during pregnancy and lactation unless there are compelling reasons for doing so.

Effects on ability to drive and use machines: Patients should be warned of the potential hazards of driving or operating machinery if they experience side effects such as dizziness.

Undesirable effects

Hypersensitivity reactions: Synacthen may provoke hypersensitivity reactions. In patients suffering from, or susceptible to, allergic disorders (especially asthma) this may take the form of anaphylactic shock (see *Contra-indications*).

Hypersensitivity may be manifested as skin reactions at the injection site, dizziness, nausea, vomiting, urticaria, pruritus, flushing, malaise, dyspnoea, angioneurotic oedema and Quinke's oedema.

Other side effects are unlikely to be observed with short-term use of Synacthen as a diagnostic tool. For an extended list of side effects reported with long-term use of tetracosactrin acetate, see Synacthen Depot Summary of Product Characteristics.

Overdose: Overdosage is unlikely to be a problem when the product is used as a single dose for diagnostic purposes.

Pharmacodynamic properties: Tetracosactrin acetate consists of the first 24 amino acids occurring in the natural corticotrophic hormone (ACTH) sequence and displays the same physiological properties as ACTH. In the adrenal cortex, it stimulates the biosynthesis of glucocorticoids, mineralocorticoids, and, to a lesser extent androgens.

The site of action of ACTH is the plasma membrane of the adrenocortical cells, where it binds to a specific receptor. The hormone-receptor complex activates adenylate cyclase, stimulating the production of cyclic AMP (adenosine monophosphate) and so promoting the synthesis of pregnenolone from cholesterol. From pregnenolone the various corticosteroids are produced via different enzymatic pathways.

Pharmacokinetic properties: Following an intravenous injection, elimination of tetracosactrin acetate from the plasma consists of 3 phases. The half-lives of these phases are approximately 7 minutes (0 to 1 hour), 37 minutes (1 to 2 hours) and 3 hours thereafter.

Tetracosactrin acetate has an apparent volume of distribution of approximately 0.4 L/kg.

In the serum, tetracosactrin acetate is broken down by serum endopeptidases into inactive oligopeptides and then by aminopeptidases into free amino acids. The rapid elimination from plasma is probably not attributable to this relatively slow cleavage process, but rather to the rapid concentration of the active substance in the adrenal glands and kidneys.

Following an iv dose of ^{131}I-labelled tetracosactrin acetate, 95 to 100% of the radioactivity is excreted in the urine within 24 hours.

Preclinical safety data: There are no pre-clinical data of relevance to the prescriber, which are additional to those already included in other sections of the Summary of Product Characteristics.

Pharmaceutical particulars

List of excipients: Acetic acid, sodium acetate, sodium chloride and water.

Incompatibilities: None known.

Shelf life: 5 years.

Special precautions for storage: Synacthen should be protected from light and stored in a refrigerator (2 - 8°C).

Nature and contents of container: The ampoules are colourless glass PhEur type I. Five ampoules are packed in a cardboard box.

Instructions for use/handling: Shake well before use.

Marketing authorisation number PL 16853/0017

Date of first authorisation 25 June 1998

Date of (partial) revision of the text June 1998

Legal status POM

SYNACTHEN* DEPOT

Presentation Tetracosactrin Acetate BP is absorbed on to zinc phosphate. A sterile, white suspension, which settles on standing, containing 1 mg of Synacthen per ml and 10 mg benzyl alcohol per ml. This preparation is available in 1 ml ampoules.

The ampoules contain zinc, sodium phosphate, benzyl alcohol, sodium chloride, sodium hydroxide and water.

Uses

Indications:

Therapeutic use: Synacthen Depot should normally only be used for short-term therapy in conditions for which glucocorticoids are indicated in principle, for example, in ulcerative colitis and Crohn's disease, juvenile rheumatoid arthritis, or as adjunct therapy in patients with rheumatoid arthritis and osteoarthrosis. Synacthen Depot may be particularly useful in patients unable to tolerate oral glucocorticoid therapy or in patients where normal therapeutic doses of glucocorticoids have been ineffective.

Diagnostic use: As a diagnostic aid for the investigation of adrenocortical insufficiency.

Mode of action: Tetracosactrin, the active substance of Synacthen, consists of the first 24 amino acids occurring in the natural corticotrophic hormone (ACTH) sequence and displays the same physiological properties as ACTH. Like ACTH, it stimulates adrenocortical production of glucocorticoids and mineralocorticoids, and to a lesser extent androgens, which explains its therapeutic effect in conditions responsive to glucocorticoid treatment.

However, its pharmacological activity is not comparable to that of corticosteroids, because under ACTH treatment (in contrast to treatment with a single glucocorticoid) the tissues are exposed to a physiological spectrum of corticosteroids.

The site of action of ACTH is the plasma membrane of the adrenocortical cells, where it binds to a specific receptor. The hormone-receptor complex activates adenylate cyclase, stimulating the production of cyclic AMP (adenosine monophosphate) and so promoting the synthesis of pregnenolone from cholesterol. From pregnenolone the various corticosteroids are produced via different enzymatic pathways.

Pharmacokinetics: Tetracosactrin is absorbed on to a zinc phosphate complex which ensures the sustained release of the active substance from the intramuscular injection site. After an intramuscular injection of 1 mg Synacthen Depot, the radioimmunologically determined plasma concentrations of tetracosactrin range between 200-300 pg/ml and are maintained for 12 hours.

Tetracosactrin has an apparent volume of distribution of approximately 0.4 litres/kg.

In the serum, tetracosactrin is broken down by serum endopeptidases into inactive oligopeptides and then by aminopeptidases into free amino acids.

Following an intravenous dose of ^{131}I-labelled tetracosactrin, 95 to 100% of the radioactivity is excreted in the urine within 24 hours.

Dosage and administration Synacthen Depot is intended for intramuscular injection. The ampoule should be shaken before use.

Therapeutic use: Initially, daily doses of Synacthen Depot should be given but after approximately 3 days, intermittent doses may be given.

Adults: Initially 1 mg intramuscularly daily or 1 mg every 12 hours in acute cases. After the acute symptoms of the disease have disappeared, treatment may be continued at a dose of 1 mg every 2 to 3 days; in patients who respond well, the dosage may be reduced to 0.5 mg every 2 to 3 days or 1 mg per week.

Infants aged 1 month to 2 years: Initially 0.25 mg intramuscularly daily; the maintenance dose is 0.25 mg every 2 to 8 days.

Children aged 2 to 5 years: Initially 0.25 to 0.5 mg intramuscularly daily; the maintenance dose is 0.25 to 0.5 mg every 2 to 8 days.

Children aged 5 to 12 years: Initially 0.25 to 1 mg intramuscularly daily; the maintenance dose is 0.25 to 1 mg every 2 to 8 days.

Elderly: There is no evidence to suggest that dosage should be different in the elderly.

Diagnostic use: In cases of suspected adrenocortical insufficiency, where the 30-minute diagnostic test with Synacthen ampoules (see Synacthen SmPC) has yielded inconclusive results or where it is desired to determine the functional reserve of the adrenal cortex, a 5-hour test with Synacthen Depot may be performed.

Adults: This test is based on measurement of the plasma cortisol concentration before and exactly 30 minutes, 1, 2, 3, 4 and 5 hours after an intramuscular injection of 1 mg Synacthen Depot. Adrenocortical function can be regarded as normal if the post-injection rise in plasma cortisol concentration increases 2-fold in the first hour, and continues to rise steadily. The values expected would be 600 to 1,250 nmol/l in the first hour increasing slowly up to 1,000 to 1,800 nmol/l by the fifth hour. Lower concentrations of plasma cortisol may be attributable to Addison's disease, secondary adrenocortical insufficiency due to a disorder of hypothalamo-pituitary function or overdosage of corticosteroids.

A 3-day test with Synacthen Depot may be used to differentiate between primary and secondary adrenocortical insufficiency.

Children: No paediatric dosage has been established.

Elderly: There is no evidence to suggest that dosage should be different in the elderly.

Contra-indications, warnings, etc

Contra-indications: History of hypersensitivity to ACTH, Synacthen or Synacthen Depot. Synacthen Depot therapy is also contra-indicated in acute psychoses, in infectious diseases, in Cushing's syndrome, in patients with peptic ulcer, refractory heart failure, adrenogenital syndrome, pregnancy and lactation and for therapeutic use in adrenocortical insufficiency.

In view of the increased risk of anaphylactic reactions, Synacthen Depot should not be used in patients known to have asthma and/or other forms of allergy.

Synacthen Depot is contra-indicated for use in neonates (especially premature infants) since it contains benzyl alcohol which can cause severe poisoning.

Synacthen Depot must not be administered intravenously.

Warnings: Patients should be made aware that very occasionally they may suffer from side effects which could interfere with their ability to drive a car or operate machinery.

Precautions: Before using Synacthen Depot, the doctor should make every effort to find out whether the patient is suffering from, or has a history of allergic disorders. In particular, he should enquire whether the patient has previously experienced adverse reactions to ACTH, Synacthen Depot or other drugs.

Synacthen Depot should only be administered under medical supervision.

If local or systemic hypersensitivity reactions occur during or after an injection (for example, marked redness and pain at the injection site, urticaria, pruritus, flushing, faintness or dyspnoea), Synacthen Depot or other ACTH preparations should be avoided in the future. Hypersensitivity reactions tend to occur within 30 minutes of the injection. The patient should therefore be kept under observation during this time.

In the event of a serious anaphylactic reaction occurring, despite these precautions, the following measures must be taken immediately: administer adrenaline (0.4 to 1 ml of a 0.1% solution intramuscularly or 0.1 to 0.2 ml of a 0.1% solution in 10 ml physiological saline *slowly* intravenously) as well as a large intravenous dose of a corticosteroid (for example 100 to 500 mg hydrocortisone, three or four times in 24 hours) repeating the dose if necessary.

The hydrocortisone product information prepared by the manufacturer should also be consulted.

Synacthen Depot should not be used in the presence of active infectious or systemic diseases, when the use of live vaccine is contemplated or in the presence of a reduced immune response, unless adequate disease specific therapy is being given.

Use with care in patients with non-specific ulcerative colitis, diverticulitis, recent intestinal anastomosis, renal insufficiency, hypertension, thromboembolic tendencies, osteoporosis and myasthenia gravis.

The increased production of adrenal steroids may result in corticosteroid type effects:

- Salt and water retention can occur and may respond to a low salt diet. Potassium supplementation may be necessary during long term treatment
- Psychological disturbances may be triggered or aggravated
- Latent infections (e.g. amoebiasis, tuberculosis) may become activated
- Ocular effects may be produced (e.g. glaucoma, cataracts)
- Provided the dose is chosen to meet the individual's needs, Synacthen Depot is unlikely to inhibit growth in children. Nevertheless, growth should be monitored in children undergoing long-term treatment. In infants and children aged up to 5 years, reversible myocardial hypertrophy may occur in rare

cases following long-term treatment with high doses. Therefore echocardiographic recordings should be made regularly.
- Dosage adjustments may be necessary in patients being treated for diabetes or hypertension
An enhanced effect of tetracosactrin therapy may occur in patients with hypothyroidism and in those with cirrhosis of the liver.

Use in pregnancy: Synacthen Depot is contra-indicated for therapeutic use during pregnancy and lactation and should not be used as a diagnostic tool unless there are compelling reasons for doing so.

Drug interactions: Interactions are likely with drugs whose actions are affected by adrenal steroids (See Precautions).

Side-effects: Since Synacthen Depot stimulates the adrenal cortex to increase the output of glucocorticoids and mineralocorticoids, side-effects associated with excessive adrenocorticotrophic activity may be encountered.
Hypersensitivity reactions: Synacthen Depot may provoke hypersensitivity reactions, which in patients suffering from, or susceptible to allergic disorders (especially asthma) may take the form of anaphylactic shock. (See Precautions). Hypersensitivity may be manifested as a skin reaction at the injection site, dizziness, nausea, vomiting, urticaria, pruritus, flushing, malaise, dyspnoea, angioneurotic oedema and Quincke's oedema. In rare cases, the benzyl alcohol in Synacthen Depot may provoke hypersensitivity reactions.
The following side-effects have also been reported during corticotrophin/corticosteroid therapy, although not necessarily observed during tetracosactrin therapy:
Musculoskeletal system: Osteoporosis, muscle weakness, steroid myopathy, loss of muscle mass, vertebral compression fractures, aseptic necrosis of femoral and humeral heads, pathologic fracture of long bones and tendon rupture.
Gastro-intestinal tract: Peptic ulceration with possible perforation and haemorrhage, pancreatitis, abdominal distension and ulcerative oesophagitis.
Skin and appendages: Impaired wound healing, thin fragile skin, petechia and ecchymosis, facial erythema, increased sweating, suppression of skin test reactions, acne and skin pigmentation.
Central and peripheral nervous system: Convulsions, increased intracranial pressure with papilloedema (pseudotumour cerebri) usually after treatment, vertigo, headache and psychic changes.
Endocrine system: Sodium retention, fluid retention, potassium loss, hypokalaemic alkalosis and calcium loss. Menstrual irregularities, Cushing's syndrome, suppression of growth in children, secondary adrenocortical and pituitary unresponsiveness, particularly in times of stress, as in trauma, surgery or illness; decreased carbohydrate tolerance, hyperglycaemia, manifestations of latent diabetes mellitus, hirsutism.
Ophthalmic: Posterior subcapsular cataracts, increased intraocular pressure, glaucoma and exophthalmos.
Metabolism: Negative nitrogen balance due to protein catabolism.
Cardiovascular system: A rise in blood pressure, necrotising angiitis and congestive heart failure. In infants and small children treated over a prolonged period with high doses, reversible myocardial hypertrophy may occur in isolated cases.
Miscellaneous: Increased susceptibility to infection, abscess, thromboembolism, weight gain, increased appetite, leucocytosis.

Overdosage:
Relating to therapeutic usage of Synacthen Depot: Overdosage may lead to fluid retention and signs of excessive adrenocorticotrophic activity (Cushing's Syndrome). In such cases, Synacthen Depot should either be withdrawn temporarily, given in lower doses or the interval between injections should be prolonged (e.g. 5 to 7 days).
Treatment: There is no known antidote. Treatment should be symptomatic.

Pharmaceutical precautions Synacthen Depot should be protected from light and stored in a refrigerator (2 to 8°C).

Legal category POM.

Package quantities Boxes of 10.

Further information Nil.

Product licence number 16853/0018

SYNTOCINON* AMPOULES 5 IU/ml
SYNTOCINON* AMPOULES 10 IU/ml

Qualitative and quantitative composition Oxytocin PhEur 5 or 10 units in 1 ml.

Pharmaceutical form A clear, colourless, sterile solution in 1ml clear glass ampoules.

Clinical particulars
Therapeutic indications: Induction of labour for medical reasons; stimulation of labour in hypotonic uterine inertia; during caesarean section, following delivery of the child; prevention and treatment of postpartum uterine atony and haemorrhage.
Early stages of pregnancy as a adjunctive therapy for the management of incomplete, inevitable, or missed abortion.

Posology and method of administration
Induction or enhancement of labour: Syntocinon should be administered as an iv drip infusion or, preferably, by means of a variable-speed infusion pump. For drip infusion it is recommended that 5 IU of Syntocinon be added to 500 ml of a physiological electrolyte solution. For patients in whom infusion of sodium chloride must be avoided, 5% dextrose solution may be used as the diluent (see *Special warnings and special precautions for use*). To ensure even mixing, the bottle or bag must be turned upside down several times before use.
The initial infusion rate should be set at 1 to 4 mU/min (2 to 8 drops/min). It may be gradually increased at intervals not shorter than 20 min, until a contraction pattern similar to that of normal labour is established. In pregnancy near term this can often be achieved with an infusion of less than 10 mU/min (20 drops/min), and the recommended maximum rate is 20 mU/min (40 drops/min). In the unusual event that higher rates are required, as may occur in the management of foetal death *in utero* or for induction of labour at an earlier stage of pregnancy, when the uterus is less sensitive to oxytocin, it is advisable to use a more concentrated Syntocinon solution, e.g., 10 IU in 500 ml.
When using a motor-driven infusion pump which delivers smaller volumes than those given by drip infusion, the concentration suitable for infusion within the recommended dosage range must be calculated according to the specifications of the pump.
The frequency, strength, and duration of contractions as well as the foetal heart rate must be carefully monitored throughout the infusion. Once an adequate level of uterine activity is attained, the infusion rate can often be reduced. In the event of uterine hyperactivity and/or foetal distress, the infusion must be discontinued immediately.
If, in women who are at term or near term, regular contractions are not established after the infusion of a total amount of 5 IU, it is recommended that the attempt to induce labour be ceased; it may be repeated on the following day, starting again from a rate of 1 to 4 mU/min.
Caesarean section: 5 IU by slow iv injection immediately after delivery.
Prevention of postpartum uterine haemorrhage: The usual dose is 5 IU slowly iv after delivery of the placenta. In women given Syntocinon for induction or enhancement of labour, the infusion should be continued at an increased rate during the third stage of labour and for the next few hours thereafter.
Treatment of postpartum uterine haemorrhage: 5 IU slowly iv, followed in severe cases by iv infusion of a solution containing 5 to 20 IU of oxytocin in 500 ml of a non-hydrating diluent, run at the rate necessary to control uterine atony.
Incomplete, inevitable, or missed abortion: 5 IU slowly iv, if necessary followed by iv infusion at a rate of 20 to 40 mU/min or higher.

Children: Not applicable.

Elderly: Not applicable.
Route of administration: Intravenous infusion or intravenous injection.

Contra-indications: Hypersensitivity to the drug. Hypertonic uterine contractions, mechanical obstruction to delivery, foetal distress. Any condition in which, for foetal or maternal reasons, spontaneous labour is inadvisable and/or vaginal delivery is contra-indicated: e.g., significant cephalopelvic disproportion; foetal malpresentation; placenta praevia and vasa praevia; placental abruption; cord presentation or prolapse; overdistension or impaired resistance of the uterus to rupture as in multiple pregnancy; polyhydramnios; grand multiparity and in the presence of a uterine scar resulting from major surgery including classical caesarean section.
Syntocinon should not be used for prolonged periods in patients with oxytocin-resistant uterine inertia, severe pre-eclamptic toxaemia or severe cardiovascular disorders.

Special warnings and special precautions for use: The induction of labour by means of oxytocin should be attempted only when strictly indicated for medical reasons. Administration should only be under hospital conditions and qualified medical supervision. When given for induction and enhancement of labour, Syntocinon must only be administered as an iv infusion and never by iv bolus injection. Careful monitoring of foetal heart rate and uterine motility (frequency, strength, and duration of contractions) is essential, so that the dosage may be adjusted to individual response.
When Syntocinon is given for induction or enhancement of labour, particular caution is required in the presence of borderline cephalopelvic disproportion, secondary uterine inertia, mild or moderate degrees of pregnancy-induced hypertension or cardiac disease, and in patients above 35 years of age or with a history of lower-uterine-segment caesarean section.
In the case of foetal death *in utero*, and/or in the presence of meconium-stained amniotic fluid, tumultous labour must be avoided, as it may cause amniotic fluid embolism.
Because oxytocin possesses slight antidiuretic activity, its prolonged iv administration at high doses in conjunction with large volumes of fluid, as may be the case in the treatment of inevitable or missed abortion or in the management of postpartum haemorrhage, may cause water intoxication associated with hyponatraemia. To avoid this rare complication, the following precautions must be observed whenever high doses of oxytocin are administered over a long time: an electrolyte-containing diluent must be used (not dextrose); the volume of infused fluid should be kept low (by infusing oxytocin at a higher concentration than recommended for the induction or enhancement of labour at term); fluid intake by mouth must be restricted; a fluid balance chart should be kept, and serum electrolytes should be measured when electrolyte imbalance is suspected.
When Syntocinon is used for prevention or treatment of uterine haemorrhage, rapid iv injection should be avoided, as it may cause an acute short-lasting drop in blood pressure.

Interaction with other medicaments and other forms of interaction: Prostaglandins may potentiate the uterotonic effect of oxytocin and vice versa; therefore, concomitant administration requires very careful monitoring.
Some inhalation anaesthetics, e.g., cyclopropane or halothane, may enhance the hypotensive effect of oxytocin and reduce its oxytocic action. Their concurrent use with oxytocin has also been reported to cause cardiac rhythm disturbances.
When given during or after caudal block anaesthesia, oxytocin may potentiate the pressor effect of sympathomimetic vasoconstrictor agents.

Pregnancy and lactation: See *Therapeutic indications.*

Effects on ability to drive and use machines: None known.

Undesirable effects: As there is a wide variation in uterine sensitivity, uterine spasm may be caused in some instances by what are normally considered to be low doses. When oxytocin is used by iv infusion for the induction or enhancement of labour, administration at too high doses results in uterine overstimulation which may cause foetal distress, asphyxia, and death, or may lead to hypertonicity, tetanic contractions, soft tissue damage or rupture of the uterus.
Water intoxication associated with maternal and neonatal hyponatraemia has been reported in cases where high doses of oxytocin together with large amounts of electrolyte-free fluid have been administered over a prolonged period of time (see *Special warnings and special precautions for use*). Symptoms of water intoxication include:

1. Headache, anorexia, nausea, vomiting and abdominal pain.
2. Lethargy, drowsiness, unconsciousness and grand-mal type seizures.
3. Low blood electrolyte concentration.

Rapid iv bolus injection of oxytocin at doses amounting to several IU may result in acute short-lasting hypotension accompanied with flushing and reflex tachycardia.
Oxytocin may occasionally cause nausea, vomiting, or cardiac arrhythmias. In a few cases, skin rashes and anaphylactoid reactions associated with dyspnoea, hypotension, or shock have been reported.

Overdose: The fatal dose of Syntocinon has not been established. Syntocinon is subject to inactivation by proteolytic enzymes of the alimentary tract. Hence it is not absorbed from the intestine and is not likely to have toxic effects when ingested.
The symptoms and consequences of overdosage are those mentioned under *Undesirable effects.* In addition, as a result of uterine overstimulation, placental abruption and/or amniotic fluid embolism have been reported.
Treatment: When signs or symptoms of overdosage occur during continuous iv administration of Syntocinon, the infusion must be discontinued at once and oxygen should be given to the mother. In cases of water intoxication it is essential to restrict fluid intake, promote diuresis, correct electrolyte imbalance, and control convulsions that may eventually occur, by

judicious use of diazepam. In the case of coma, a free airway should be maintained with routine measures normally employed in the nursing of the unconscious patient.

Pharmacological properties
Pharmacodynamic properties: The active principle of Syntocinon is a synthetic nonapeptide identical with oxytocin, a hormone released by the posterior lobe of the pituitary. It exerts a stimulatory effect on the smooth musculature of the uterus, particularly towards the end of pregnancy, during labour, after delivery, and in the puerperium, i.e., at times when the number of specific oxytocin receptors in the myometrium is increased.

When given by low-dose iv infusion, Syntocinon elicits rhythmic uterine contractions that are indistinguishable in frequency, force, and duration from those observed during spontaneous labour. At higher infusion dosages, or when given by single injection, the drug is capable of causing sustained uterine contractions.

Being synthetic, Syntocinon does not contain vasopressin, but even in its pure form oxytocin possess some weak intrinsic vasopressin-like antidiuretic activity.

Another pharmacological effect observed with high doses of oxytocin, particularly when administered by rapid iv bolus injection, consists of a transient direct relaxing effect on vascular smooth muscle, resulting in brief hypotension, flushing and reflex tachycardia.

Pharmacokinetic properties: The plasma half-life of oxytocin is of the order of five minutes, hence the need for continuous iv infusion. Elimination is via the liver, kidney, functional mammary gland and oxytocinase.

Preclinical safety data: There are no pre-clinical data of relevance to the prescriber which are additional to those already included in other sections of the Summary of Product Characteristics.

Pharmaceutical particulars
List of excipients: Sodium acetate tri-hydrate, acetic acid, chlorbutanol, ethanol and water for injections.

Incompatibilities: Syntocinon should not be infused via the same apparatus as blood or plasma, because the peptide linkages are rapidly inactivated by oxytocin-inactivating enzymes. Syntocinon is incompatible with solutions containing sodium metabisulphite as a stabiliser.

Shelf life: Five years

Special precautions for storage: Store betwen 2° and 8°C. Syntocinon may be stored for up to 3 months up to 30°C but must then be discarded..

Nature and contents of container: Clear glass 1ml ampoules. Boxes of 5 ampoules.

Instructions for use/handling: Snap ampoules: no file required.

Syntocinon is compatible with the following infusion fluids, but due attention should be paid to the advisability of using electrolyte fluids in individual patients: sodium/potassium chloride (103mmol Na^+ and 51mmol K^+), sodium bicarbonate 1.39%, sodium chloride 0.9%, sodium lactate 1.72%, dextrose 5%, laevulose 20%, macrodex 6%, rheomacrodex 10%, ringer's solution.

Marketing authorisation numbers

Syntocinon 5 IU/ml	PL 16853/0019
Syntocinon 10 IU/ml	PL 16853/0020

Date of first authorisation 25 June 1998

Date of (partial) revision of the text November 1998

Legal status POM

SYNTOMETRINE* AMPOULES

Qualitative and quantitative composition Each 1 ml ampoule contains 5.0 IU Oxytocin PhEur and 0.5 mg of Ergometrine Maleate PhEur.

Pharmaceutical form Injection.

Clinical particulars
Therapeutic indications: Syntometrine is indicated in the active management of the third stage of labour, or routinely, following the birth of the placenta, to prevent or treat postpartum haemorrhage.

Posology and method of administration
Adults:
Active management of third stage of labour: Intramuscular injection of 1 ml after delivery of the anterior shoulder, or at the latest, immediately after delivery of the child. Expulsion of the placenta, which is normally separated by the first strong uterine contraction, should be assisted by gentle suprapubic pressure and controlled cord traction.

Prevention and treatment of postpartum haemorrhage: Intramuscular injection of 1 ml following expulsion of the placenta, or when bleeding occurs.

Third stage of labour and postpartum haemorrhage: Syntometrine may also be administered by a slow intravenous injection in a dose of 0.5 to 1 ml. This route of administration is not generally recommended.

Children: Not applicable.

Use in the elderly: Not applicable.

Method of administration: Intramuscular, intravenous.

Contra-indications: Hypersensitivity to any of the components.

Pregnancy, first stage of labour, primary or secondary uterine inertia.

Second stage of labour before crowning of the head.

Severe disorders of cardiac, liver or kidney functions; occlusive vascular disease, sepsis, severe hypertension, pre-eclampsia, eclampsia.

Special warnings and precautions for use: When the intravenous route is employed, care should be exercised in patients of doubtful cardiac status.

In breech presentations and other abnormal presentations, Syntometrine should not be given until after delivery of the child, and in multiple births not until the last child has been delivered. In postpartum haemorrhage, if bleeding is not arrested by the injection of Syntometrine, the possibility of retained placental fragments, of soft tissue injury (cervical or vaginal laceration), or of a clotting defect, should be excluded before a further injection is given. Caution should be exercised in the presence of mild or moderate hypertension, or with mild or moderate degrees of cardiac, liver or kidney disease.

Interaction with other medicaments and other forms of interaction: Halothane anesthesia may diminish the uterotonic effect of Syntometrine. Syntometrine may enhance the effects of vasoconstrictors and of prostaglandins.

Pregnancy and lactation: See indications.

Effects on ability to drive and to use machines: Not applicable.

Undesirable effects: Nausea, vomiting, abdominal pain, headache, dizziness and skin rashes. On rare occasions hypertension, bradycardia, cardiac arrhythmias, chest pain or anaphylactoid reactions associated with dyspnoea, hypotension, collapse or shock.

Overdose: No case of maternal intoxication with Syntometrine has been reported to the company. If such a case were to occur the most likely symptoms would be those of ergometrine intoxication: nausea, vomiting, hypertension or hypotension, vasospastic reactions, respiratory depression, convulsions, coma. Treatment would have to be symptomatic.

Accidental administration to the newborn infant has been reported and has proved fatal. In these accidental neonatal overdosage cases, symptoms such as respiratory depression, convulsions, hypertonia, heart arrhythmia have been reported. Treatment has been symptomatic in most cases, respiratory and cardiovascular support have been required.

Pharmacological properties
Pharmacodynamic properties: Syntometrine combines the known sustained oxytocic action of ergometrine with the more rapid action of oxytocin on the uterus.

Pharmacokinetic properties: Ergometrine is reported to be rapidly and completely absorbed after an intramuscular injection. Uterine stimulation occurs within 7 minutes of i.m. injection and immediately after intravenous injection. Oxytocin is also rapidly absorbed and is rapidly metabolised by the liver and the kidneys.

Preclinical safety data: There are no pre-clinical data of relevance to the prescriber which are additional to that already included in other sections of the SPC.

Pharmaceutical particulars
List of excipients: Sodium chloride, maleic acid and water for injections.

Incompatibilities: None.

Shelf life: 36 months.

Special precautions for storage: For prolonged periods store between 2° and 8°C. Protect from light. Syntometrine may be stored at temperatures up to 25°C for 2 months when protected from light.

Nature and contents of container: Uncoloured borosilicate glass Type I snap ampoule. Pack of 5 ampoules.

Instructions for use/handling: None.

Marketing authorisation number 16853/0021.

Date of first authorisation 25 June 1998.

Date of revision of text June 1998.

Legal category POM.

**Trade Mark*

AMGEN Ltd

240 Cambridge Science Park
Milton Road
Cambridge CB4 0WD

☎ +44 01223 420305 🗋 +44 01223 423049 420319

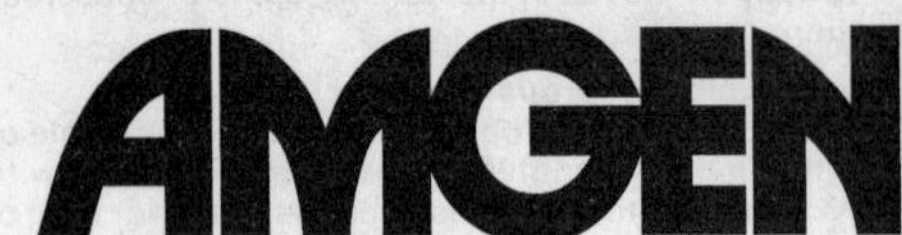

NEUPOGEN ▼
Filgrastim

Qualitative and quantitative composition Neupogen is a sterile, clear, colourless liquid. Each single use vial and each single use pre-filled syringe of Neupogen contains 30 million units/ml (300 μg/ml) of filgrastim formulated in an aqueous sodium acetate buffer at pH 4.0. The quantitative composition (per ml) of Neupogen is:

Filgrastim (pINN)	30 million units (MU)
Acetate	0.59 mg
Sorbitol	50.0 mg
Polysorbate 80	0.04 mg
Sodium	0.035 mg
Water for injections (qs ad)	to 1.0 ml

Filgrastim is produced in a laboratory strain of *Escherichia coli* bacteria which has been genetically altered by the addition of a gene for the granulocyte-colony stimulating factor.

Pharmaceutical form Neupogen is a sterile, clear, colourless liquid for subcutaneous or intravenous injection presented in vials and pre-filled syringes.

Neupogen 30 contains 30 million units (300 μg) of active substance in 1.0 ml.

Neupogen 48 contains 48 million units (480 μg) of active substance in 1.6 ml.

Clinical particulars

Therapeutic indications: Neupogen is indicated for the reduction in the duration of neutropenia and the incidence of febrile neutropenia in patients treated with established cytotoxic chemotherapy for malignancy (with the exception of chronic myeloid leukaemia and myelodysplastic syndromes) and for the reduction in the duration of neutropenia in patients undergoing myeloablative therapy followed by bone marrow transplantation considered to be at increased risk of prolonged severe neutropenia.

Neupogen is indicated for the mobilisation of autologous peripheral blood progenitor cells alone, or following myelosuppressive chemotherapy in order to accelerate haematopoietic recovery by infusion of such cells, after myelosuppressive or myeloablative therapy.

The safety and efficacy of Neupogen are similar in adults and children receiving cytotoxic chemotherapy.

In patients, children or adults, with severe congenital, cyclic, or idiopathic neutropenia with an ANC of $\leq 0.5 \times 10^9$/L, and a history of severe or recurrent infections, long term administration of Neupogen is indicated to increase neutrophil counts and to reduce the incidence and duration of infection-related events.

Posology and method of administration of Neupogen: Established cytotoxic chemotherapy: The recommended dose of Neupogen is 0.5 MU (5 μg)/kg/day. The first dose of Neupogen should not be administered less than 24 hours following cytotoxic chemotherapy. Neupogen may be given as a daily subcutaneous injection or as a daily intravenous infusion diluted in 5% glucose solution given over 30 minutes (see *Instructions for use/handling*). The subcutaneous route is preferred in most cases. There is some evidence from a study of single dose administration that intravenous dosing may shorten the duration of effect. The clinical relevance of this finding to multiple dose administration is not clear. The choice of route should depend on the individual clinical circumstance. In randomised clinical trials, a subcutaneous dose of 230 μg/m²/day (4.0 to 8.4 μg/kg/day) was used.

Daily dosing with Neupogen should continue until the expected neutrophil nadir is passed and the neutrophil count has recovered to the normal range. Following established chemotherapy for solid tumours it is expected that the duration of treatment required to fulfill these criteria will be up to 14 days. Following induction and consolidation treatment for acute myeloid leukaemia the duration of treatment may be substantially longer (up to 38 days) depending on the type, dose and schedule of cytotoxic chemotherapy used.

In patients receiving cytotoxic chemotherapy, a transient increase in neutrophil counts is typically seen 1 to 2 days after initiation of Neupogen therapy. However, for a sustained therapeutic response, Neupogen therapy should not be discontinued before the expected nadir has passed and the neutrophil count has recovered to the normal range. Premature discontinuation of Neupogen therapy, prior to the time of the expected neutrophil nadir, is not recommended.

In patients treated with myeloablative therapy followed by bone marrow transplantation: The recommended starting dose of Neupogen is 1.0 MU (10 μg)/kg/day given as a 30 minute or 24 hour intravenous infusion or 1.0 MU (10 μg)/kg/day given by continuous 24 hour subcutaneous infusion. Neupogen should be diluted in 20 mL of 5% glucose solution (see *Instructions for use/handling*).

The first dose of Neupogen should not be administered less than 24 hours following cytotoxic chemotherapy and within 24 hours of bone marrow infusion.

Once the neutrophil nadir has been passed, the daily dose of Neupogen should be titrated against the neutrophil response as follows:

Neutrophil count	*Neupogen dose adjustment*
$>1.0 \times 10^9$/L for 3 consecutive days	Reduce to 0.5 MU/kg/day
Then, if ANC remains $>1.0 \times 10^9$/L for 3 more consecutive days	Discontinue Neupogen
If the ANC decreases to $<1.0 \times 10^9$/L during the treatment period the dose of Neupogen should be re-escalated according to the above steps	

ANC = absolute neutrophil count

For the mobilisation of PBPCs in patients undergoing myelosuppressive or myeloablative therapy followed by autologous PBPC transplantation with or without bone marrow transplantation: The recommended dose of Neupogen for PBPC mobilisation when used alone is 1.0 MU (10 μg)/kg/day as a 24 hour subcutaneous continuous infusion or a single daily subcutaneous injection for 6 consecutive days. For infusions Neupogen should be diluted in 20 ml of 5% glucose solution (see *Instructions for use/handling*). Timing of leukapheresis: a total of three consecutive collections is recommended, on days 5, 6 and 7.

The recommended dose of Neupogen for PBPC mobilisation after myelosuppressive chemotherapy is 0.5 MU (5 μg)/kg/day given daily by subcutaneous injection from the first day after completion of chemotherapy until the expected neutrophil nadir is passed and the neutrophil count has recovered to the normal range. Leukapheresis should be performed during the period when the ANC rises from $<0.5 \times 10^9$/L to $>5.0 \times 10^9$/L. For patients who have not had extensive chemotherapy, one leukapheresis is often sufficient. In other circumstances, additional leukaphereses are recommended.

In patients with severe chronic neutropenia: Congenital neutropenia: the recommended starting dose is 1.2 MU (12 μg)/kg/day) subcutaneously as a single dose or in divided doses.

Idiopathic or cyclic neutropenia: The recommended starting dose is 0.5 MU (5 μg)/kg/day subcutaneously as a single dose or in divided doses.

Dose adjustment: Neupogen should be administered daily by subcutaneous injection until the neutrophil count has reached and can be maintained at more than 1.5×10^9/L. When the response has been obtained the minimal effective dose to maintain this level should be established. Long term daily administration is required to maintain an adequate neutrophil count. After one to two weeks of therapy, the initial dose may be doubled or halved depending upon the patient's response. Subsequently the dose may be individually adjusted every 1 to 2 weeks to maintain the average neutrophil count between 1.5×10^9/L and 10×10^9/L. A faster schedule of dose escalation may be considered in patients presenting with severe infections. In clinical trials, 97% of patients who responded had a complete response at doses ≤24 μg/kg/day. The long-term safety of Neupogen administration above 24 μg/kg/day in patients with severe chronic neutropenia has not been established.

Other particulars: Neupogen therapy should only be given in collaboration with an oncology centre which has experience in G-CSF treatment and haematology and has the necessary diagnostic facilities. The mobilisation and apheresis procedures should be performed in collaboration with an oncology-haematology centre with acceptable experience in this field and where the monitoring of haematopoietic progenitor cells can be correctly performed.

Clinical trials with Neupogen have included a small number of elderly patients but special studies have not been performed in this group and therefore specific dosage recommendations cannot be made.

Paediatric use in the severe chronic neutropenia (SCN) and cancer settings: Sixty-five percent of the patients studied in the SCN trial program were under 18 years of age. The efficacy of treatment was clear for this age group, which included most patients with congenital neutropenia. There were no differences in the safety profiles for paediatric patients treated for severe chronic neutropenia.

Data from clinical studies in paediatric patients indicate that the safety and efficacy of Neupogen are similar in both adults and children receiving cytotoxic chemotherapy.

The dosage recommendations in paediatric patients are the same as those in adults receiving myelosuppressive cytotoxic chemotherapy.

Contra-indications: Neupogen should not be administered to patients with known hypersensitivity to the product or its constituents. Neupogen should not be used to increase the dose of cytotoxic chemotherapy beyond established dosage regimens.

Neupogen should not be administered to patients with severe congenital neutropenia (Kostman's syndrome) with abnormal cytogenetics (see also *Special precautions in SCN patients*).

Special warnings and special precautions for use: Malignant cell growth: Granulocyte-colony stimulating factor can promote growth of myeloid cells in vitro and similar effects may be seen on some non-myeloid cells in vitro.

The safety and efficacy of Neupogen administration in patients with myelodysplastic syndrome, or chronic myelogenous leukaemia have not been established. Neupogen is not indicated for use in these conditions. Particular care should be taken to distinguish the diagnosis of blast transformation of chronic myeloid leukaemia from acute myeloid leukaemia.

Other special precautions: Monitoring of bone density may be indicated in patients with underlying osteoporotic bone diseases who undergo continuous therapy with Neupogen for more than 6 months.

Studies of Neupogen in patients with severe impairment of renal or hepatic function demonstrate that it exhibits a similar pharmacokinetic and pharmacodynamic profile to that seen in normal individuals. Dose adjustment is not required in these circumstances.

Special precautions in cancer patients:

Leucocytosis: White blood cell counts of 100×10^9/L or greater have been observed in less than 5% of patients receiving Neupogen at doses above 0.3 MU/kg/day (3 μg/kg/day). No adverse events directly attributable to this degree of leucocytosis have been reported. However, in view of the potential risks associated with severe leucocytosis, a white blood cell count should be performed at regular intervals during Neupogen therapy. If leucocyte counts exceed 50×10^9/L after the expected nadir, Neupogen should be discontinued immediately. However, during the period of administration of Neupogen for PBPC mobilisation, discontinuation of Neupogen is appropriate if the leukocyte counts rise to $>100 \times 10^9$/L.

Risks associated with increased doses of chemotherapy: Special caution should be used when treating patients with high dose chemotherapy, because improved tumour outcome has not been demonstrated and intensified doses of chemotherapeutic agents may lead to increased toxicities including cardiac, pulmonary, neurologic, and dermatologic effects (please refer to the prescribing information of the specific chemotherapy agents used).

Treatment with Neupogen alone does not preclude thrombocytopenia and anaemia due to myelosuppressive chemotherapy. Because of the potential of receiving higher doses of chemotherapy (e.g., full doses on the prescribed schedule) the patient may be at greater risk of thrombocytopenia and anaemia. Regular monitoring of platelet count and haematocrit is recommended. Special care should be taken when administering single or combination chemotherapeutic agents which are known to cause severe thrombocytopenia.

The use of Neupogen-mobilised PBPCs has been shown to reduce the depth and duration of thrombocytopenia following myelosuppressive or myeloablative chemotherapy.

Other special precautions: The effects of Neupogen in patients with substantially reduced myeloid progenitors have not been studied. Neupogen acts primarily on neutrophil precursors to exert it's effect in elevating neutrophil counts. Therefore in patients with reduced precursors neutrophil response may be diminished (such as those treated with extensive radiotherapy or chemotherapy, or those with bone marrow infiltration by tumour).

The effect of Neupogen on graft versus host disease has not been defined.

Known cases of Hereditary Fructose Intolerance. Neupogen contains sorbitol as an excipient at a concentration of 50 mg/ml. It is unlikely that as a consequence of treatment with Neupogen alone that sufficient sorbitol will be infused to result in clinically relevant toxicity in affected individuals. However, in cases of HFI caution is advised.

Special precautions in patients undergoing peripheral blood progenitor cell mobilisation:
Mobilisation: There are no prospectively randomised comparisons of the two recommended mobilisation methods (filgrastim alone, or in combination with myelosuppressive chemotherapy) within the same patient population. The degree of variation between individual patients and between laboratory assays of CD34+ cells mean that direct comparison between different studies is difficult. It is therefore difficult to recommend an optimum method. The choice of mobilisation method should be considered in relation to the overall objectives of treatment for an individual patient.

Prior exposure to cytotoxic agents: Patients who have undergone very extensive prior myelosuppressive therapy may not show sufficient mobilisation of PBPC to achieve the recommended minimum yield ($\geq 2.0 \times 10^6$ CD34+ cells/kg) or acceleration of platelet recovery, to the same degree.

Some cytotoxic agents exhibit particular toxicities to the haematopoietic progenitor pool, and may adversely affect progenitor mobilisation. Agents such as melphalan, carmustine (BCNU), and carboplatin, when administered over prolonged periods prior to attempts at progenitor mobilisation may reduce progenitor yield. However, the administration of melphalan, carboplatin or BCNU together with Neupogen, has been shown to be effective for progenitor mobilisation. When a peripheral blood progenitor cell transplantation is envisaged it is advisable to plan the stem cell mobilisation procedure early in the treatment course of the patient. Particular attention should be paid to the number of progenitors mobilised in such patients before the administration of high-dose chemotherapy. If yields are inadequate, as measured by the criteria above, alternative forms of treatment, not requiring progenitor support should be considered.

Assessment of progenitor cell yields: In assessing the number of progenitor cells harvested in patients treated with Neupogen, particular attention should be paid to the method of quantitation. The results of flow cytometric analysis of CD34+ cell numbers vary depending on the precise methodology used and recommendations of numbers based on studies in other laboratories need to be interpreted with caution.

Statistical analysis of the relationship between the number of CD34+ cells re-infused and the rate of platelet recovery after high-dose chemotherapy indicates a complex but continuous relationship.

Currently the minimum yield of CD34+ cells is not well defined. The recommendation of a minimum yield of $\geq 2.0 \times 10^6$ CD34+ cells/kg is based on published experience resulting in adequate haematologic reconstitution. Yields in excess of this appear to correlate with more rapid recovery, those below with slower recovery.

Special precautions in severe chronic neutropenia (SCN) patients:
Blood cell counts: Platelet counts should be monitored closely, especially during the first few weeks of Neupogen therapy. Consideration should be given to intermittent cessation or decreasing the dose of Neupogen in patients who develop thrombocytopenia, i.e. platelets consistently < 100,000/mm³.

Other blood cell changes occur, including anaemia and transient increases in myeloid progenitors, which require close monitoring of cell counts.

Transformation to leukaemia or myelodysplastic syndrome: Special care should be taken in the diagnosis of severe chronic neutropenias to distinguish them from other haematopoietic disorders such as aplastic anaemia, myelodysplasia, and myeloid leukaemia. Complete blood cell counts with differential and platelet counts, and an evaluation of bone marrow morphology and karyotype should be performed prior to treatment.

There was a low frequency (approximately 3%) of myelodysplastic syndromes (MDS) or leukaemia in clinical trial patients with severe chronic neutropenia treated with Neupogen. This observation has only been made in patients with congenital neutropenia. MDS and leukaemias are natural complications of the disease and are of uncertain relation to Neupogen therapy. A subset of approximately 12% of patients who had normal cytogenetic evaluations at baseline were subsequently found to have abnormalities, including monosomy 7, on routine repeat evaluation. If patients with severe chronic neutropenia develop abnormal cytogenetics, the risks and benefits of continuing Neupogen should be carefully weighed; Neupogen should be discontinued if MDS or leukaemia occur. It is currently unclear whether long-term treatment of patients with severe chronic neutropenia will predispose patients to cytogenetic abnormalities, MDS or leukaemic transformation. It is recommended to perform morphologic and cytogenetic bone marrow examinations in patients at regular intervals (approximately every 12 months).

Other special precautions: Causes of transient neutropenia, such as viral infections should be excluded.

Splenic enlargement is a direct effect of treatment with Neupogen. Thirty-one percent (31%) of patients in studies were documented as having palpable splenomegaly. Increases in volume, measured radiographically, occurred early during Neupogen therapy and tended to plateau. Dose reductions were noted to slow or stop the progression of splenic enlargement, and in 3% of patients a splenectomy was required. Spleen size should be evaluated regularly. Abdominal palpation should be sufficient to detect abnormal increases in splenic volume.

Haematuria/proteinuria occurred in a small number of patients. Regular urinanalysis should be performed to monitor this event.

The safety and efficacy in neonates and patients with autoimmune neutropenia have not been established.

Interaction with other medicaments and other forms of interaction: The safety and efficacy of Neupogen given on the same day as myelosuppressive cytotoxic chemotherapy have not been definitively established. In view of the sensitivity of rapidly dividing myeloid cells to myelosuppressive cytotoxic chemotherapy, the use of Neupogen is not recommended in the period from 24 hours before to 24 hours after chemotherapy. Preliminary evidence from a small number of patients treated concomitantly with Neupogen and 5-Fluorouracil indicate that the severity of neutropenia may be exacerbated.

Possible interactions with other haematopoietic growth factors and cytokines have not yet been investigated in clinical trials.

Since lithium promotes the release of neutrophils, lithium is likely to potentiate the effect of Neupogen. Although this interaction has not been formally investigated, there is no evidence that such an interaction is harmful.

Use during pregnancy and lactation: The safety of Neupogen has not been established in pregnant women. There is no evidence from studies in rats and rabbits that Neupogen is teratogenic. An increased incidence of embryo-loss has been observed in rabbits, but no malformation has been seen. In pregnancy, the possible risk of Neupogen use to the foetus must be weighed against the expected therapeutic benefit.

It is not known whether Neupogen is excreted in human milk. Neupogen is not recommended for use in nursing women.

Effects on ability to drive and use machines: No effects have been reported.

Undesirable effects:
In cancer patients: In clinical trials the most frequent clinical adverse events attributable to Neupogen at the recommended dose were mild or moderate musculoskeletal pain, occurring in 10%, and severe musculoskeletal pain in 3% of patients. Musculoskeletal pain is usually controlled with standard analgesics. Less frequent adverse events include urinary abnormalities predominantly mild or moderate dysuria.

In randomised, placebo-controlled clinical trials, Neupogen did not increase the incidence of clinical adverse events associated with cytotoxic chemotherapy. Adverse events reported with equal frequency in patients treated with Neupogen/chemotherapy and placebo/chemotherapy included nausea and vomiting, alopecia, diarrhoea, fatigue, anorexia, mucositis, headache, cough, skin rash, chest pain, generalised weakness, sore throat, constipation and unspecified pain.

Reversible, dose-dependent and usually mild or moderate elevations of lactate dehydrogenase, alkaline phosphatase, serum uric acid, and gamma-glutamyl transpeptidase occurred with Neupogen in approximately 50%, 35%, 25%, and 10% of patients, respectively at recommended doses.

Transient decreases in blood pressure, not requiring clinical treatment, have been reported occasionally.

Vascular disorders, including veno-occlusive disease and fluid volume disturbances, have been reported occasionally in patients undergoing high dose chemotherapy followed by autologous bone marrow transplantation. The causal association with Neupogen has not been established.

Very rare events of cutaneous vasculitis have been reported in patients treated with Neupogen. The mechanism of vasculitis in patients receiving Neupogen is unknown.

The occurrence of Sweet's syndrome (acute febrile dermatosis) has been reported occasionally. However, since a significant percentage of these patients were suffering from leukaemia, a condition known to be associated with Sweet's syndrome, a causal relationship with Neupogen has not been established.

Exacerbation of rheumatoid arthritis has been observed in individual cases.

There are occasional reports of the occurrence of adult respiratory distress syndrome (ARDS) in patients receiving Neupogen. In view of the presence of multiple risk factors in these patients a causal relationship with Neupogen use is unclear.

Symptoms suggestive of allergic-type reactions have been reported in rare cases, approximately half of these were associated with the initial dose. Overall, reports were more common after IV administration. In some cases, rechallenge resulted in a recurrence of symptoms.

In severe chronic neutropenia (SCN) patients: Adverse reactions related to Neupogen therapy in SCN patients have been reported and for some their frequency tend to decrease with time.

The most frequent clinical adverse events attributable to Neupogen were bone pain, and general musculoskeletal pain.

Other events seen include splenic enlargement, which may be progressive in a minority of cases, and thrombocytopenia. Headache, and diarrhoea have been reported shortly after starting Neupogen therapy, typically in less than 10% of patients. Anaemia and epistaxis have also been reported with a similar incidence but only following sustained administration.

Transient increases with no clinical symptoms were observed in serum uric acid, lactic dehydrogenase, and alkaline phosphatase. Transient, moderate decreases in non-fasting blood glucose have also been seen.

Adverse events possibly related to Neupogen therapy and typically occurring in < 2% of SCN patients were injection site reaction, headache, hepatomegaly, arthralgia, alopecia, osteoporosis, and rash.

During long term use cutaneous vasculitis has been reported in 2% of SCN patients. There have been very few instances of proteinuria/haematuria.

Overdosage: The effects of Neupogen overdosage have not been established. Discontinuation of Neupogen therapy usually results in a 50% decrease in circulating neutrophils within 1 to 2 days, with a return to normal levels in 1 to 7 days.

Pharmacological properties
Pharmacodynamic properties: Human G-CSF is a glycoprotein which regulates the production and release of functional neutrophils from the bone marrow. Neupogen containing r-metHuG-CSF causes marked increases in peripheral blood neutrophil counts within twenty-four hours, with minor increases in monocytes. In some severe chronic neutropenia patients Neupogen can also induce a minor increase in the number of circulating eosinophils and basophils relative to baseline; some of these patients may present with eosinophilia or basophilia already prior to treatment. Elevations of neutrophil counts are dose-dependent at recommended doses. Neutrophils produced in response to Neupogen show normal or enhanced function as demonstrated by tests of chemotactic and phagocytic function. Following termination of Neupogen therapy, circulating neutrophil counts decrease by 50% within 1 to 2 days, and to normal levels within 1 to 7 days.

Use of Neupogen in patients undergoing cytotoxic chemotherapy leads to significant reductions in the incidence, severity and duration of neutropenia and febrile neutropenia. Treatment with Neupogen significantly reduces the durations of febrile neutropenia, antibiotic use and hospitalisation after induction chemotherapy for acute myelogenous leukaemia or myeloablative therapy followed by bone marrow transplantation. The incidence of fever and documented infections were not reduced in either setting. The duration of fever was not reduced in patients undergoing myeloablative therapy followed by bone marrow transplantation.

Use of Neupogen, either alone, or after chemotherapy, mobilises haematopoietic progenitor cells into the peripheral blood. These autologous peripheral blood progenitor cells (PBPCs) may be harvested and infused after high-dose cytotoxic therapy, either in place of, or in addition to bone marrow transplantation. Infusion of PBPCs accelerates haematopoietic recovery reducing the duration of risk for haemorrhagic complications and the need for platelet transfusions.

Use of Neupogen in patients, children or adults, with severe chronic neutropenia (severe congenital, cyclic, and idiopathic neutropenia) induces a sustained increase in absolute neutrophil counts in peripheral blood and a reduction of infection and related events.

Pharmacokinetic properties: Clearance of r-metHuG-CSF has been shown to follow first-order pharmacokinetics after both subcutaneous and intravenous administration. The serum elimination half-life of r-metHuG-CSF is approximately 3.5 hours, with a clearance rate of approximately 0.6 mL/min/kg. Continuous infusion with Neupogen over a period of up to 28 days, in patients recovering from autologous bone-marrow transplantation, resulted in no evidence of drug accumulation and comparable elimination half-lives. There is a positive linear correlation between the dose and the serum concentration of r-metHuG-CSF, whether administered intravenously or subcutaneously. Following subcutaneous administration of recommended doses, serum concentrations were maintained above 10 ng/mL for 8 to 16 hours. The volume of distribution in blood is approximately 150 ml/kg.

Preclinical safety data: There are no preclinical data of relevance to the prescriber which are additional to that already included in other sections of the SmPC.

Pharmaceutical particulars

List of excipients: Neupogen is a sterile, clear, colourless liquid. Each single use vial and each single use pre-filled syringe of Neupogen contains 30 million units/ml (300 µg/ml) of filgrastim formulated in a sterile preservative free solution containing acetate (0.59 mg/ml), sorbitol (50 mg/ml), polysorbate 80 (0.04 mg/ml), and sodium (0.035 mg/ml) in Water for Injection.

Incompatibilities: Neupogen should not be diluted with saline solutions.

Shelf life: Under recommended storage conditions, Neupogen is stable for up to 24 months.

Special precautions for storage: Neupogen 30 and Neupogen 48 should be stored in a refrigerator at 2 to 8°C. Accidental exposure to freezing temperatures does not adversely affect the stability of Neupogen.

Neupogen should not be used after the given expiry date.

Diluted Neupogen solutions should not be prepared more than 24 hours before administration and should be stored refrigerated at 2 to 8°C.

Neupogen contains no preservative. In view of the possible risk of microbial contamination, Neupogen vials and syringes are for single use only. Remaining solution should be discarded after dose withdrawal.

Nature and contents of container: Neupogen 30 is supplied in colourless glass vials with rubber stoppers or pre-filled syringes containing 30 million units, equivalent to 300 µg of filgrastim.

Neupogen 48 is supplied in colourless glass vials with rubber stoppers or pre-filled syringes containing 48 million units, equivalent to 480 µg of filgrastim.

Instructions for use/handling: If required, Neupogen may be diluted in 5% glucose.

Dilute Neupogen may be adsorbed to glass and plastic materials. Dilution to a final concentration less than 0.2. MU (2 µg) per ml is not recommended at any time.

For patients treated with Neupogen diluted to concentrations below 1.5 MU (15 µg) per ml, human serum albumin (HSA) should be added to a final concentration of 2 mg/ml.

Example: In a final injection volume of 20 ml, total doses of Neupogen less than 30 MU (300 µg) should be given with 0.2 ml of 20% human albumin solution PhEur added.

When diluted in 5% glucose solution, Neupogen is compatible with glass and a variety of plastics including PVC, polyolefin (a co-polymer of polypropylene and polyethylene) and polypropylene.

Marketing authorisation holder: Roche Products Limited, PO Box 8, Welwyn Garden City, Hertfordshire AL7 3AY.

Marketing authorisation numbers

Vials	0031/0268
Syringes 30 MU	0031/0450
Syringes 48 MU	0031/0451

Date of first authorisation/renewal of authorisation First authorised in UK and Ireland in 1991.

Date of approval/revision of SPC March 1998

Legal category POM

***Trade Mark*

Approved Prescription Services Ltd

Brampton Road
Hampden Park
Eastbourne
East Sussex
BN22 9AG

☎ 01323 501111

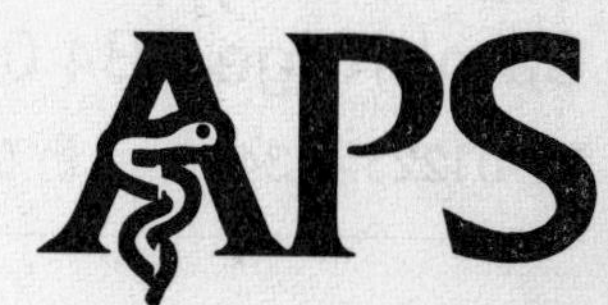

APSTIL

Stilboestrol Tablets BP

Qualitative and quantitative composition Each tablet contains either 1 mg or 5 mg of Stilboestrol BP.

Pharmaceutical form Tablets.

Clinical particulars

Therapeutic indications: Stilboestrol tablets are indicated for the treatment of carcinoma of the prostate and metastatic post-menopausal carcinoma of the breast.

Stilboestrol is a synthetic non-steroidal oestrogen hormone. It has been in use for many years. However, due to its carcinogenic potential, the use of stilboestrol is now only justified in the management of malignant disease.

It may be used to suppress androgenic hormonal activity in the management of androgen-dependent carcinomas such as carcinoma of the prostate in males and some post-menopausal carcinomas such as breast cancer in females.

Posology and method of administration: For oral administration.

Adults: Management of prostatic carcinoma: 1–3 mg daily.

Management of post-menopausal breast carcinoma: 10–20 mg daily.

Children: Stilboestrol should not be used in children.

Elderly: The recommended adult dose is appropriate.

Contra-indications: Stilboestrol is contra-indicated in those who are pregnant (it is not suitable for pre-menopausal women); and children. It is also contra-indicated in the following conditions; oestrogen-dependent neoplasms especially of the genital tract; pre-menopausal carcinoma of the breast; endometrial hyperplasia or uterine fibromyomata (fibroids). Stilboestrol should not be given where there is undiagnosed vaginal bleeding; a history of herpes gestationis; porphyria; moderate to severe hypertension; severe or active liver disease; hyperlipoproteinaemia; any cardiovascular or cerebrovascular disorder or a history of thrombo-embolism or conditions predisposing to it such as sickle cell anaemia, untreated polycythaemia and pulmonary hypertension.

Special warnings and special precautions for use: Stilboestrol should not be used in children or young adults because it has carcinogenic potential.

Care should be taken when administering stilboestrol preparations to patients with cardiac failure; hypertension; diabetes; epilepsy; migraine; depression; contact lenses; cholelithiasis; any evidence of renal dysfunction; a history of, or with cholestatic jaundice from any cause e.g. jaundice of pregnancy or following the use of oral contraceptives.

During treatment with stilboestrol blood pressure should be monitored at regular intervals and if hypertension develops treatment should be stopped. In addition, if surgery is contemplated or signs or symptoms of thrombosis develop treatment should be discontinued. This is because of the significant increase in risk of deep vein thrombosis in the presence of high oestrogen activity.

In patients who suffer from diabetes, glucose tolerance may be lowered, and the need for insulin or other anti-diabetic drugs may be increased.

In thyroid disease or investigations of thyroid function, thyroid hormone binding globulin may be increased leading to increased circulating total thyroid hormone, which may lead to difficulty in interpreting thyroid function tests.

Interaction with other medicaments and other forms of interaction: Oestrogens may antagonise diuretics and reduce the effect of anti-hypertensives.

Pregnancy and lactation: Stilboestrol is contra-indicated in pre-menopausal women.

Effects on ability to drive and use machines: None known.

Undesirable effects: As high doses of stilboestrol in early pregnancy have caused vaginal carcinoma in female offspring 16-20 years later, it should not be used in pre-menopausal women.

As with other oestrogens the following hormonal disturbances may occur, fluid retention, headache, nausea and vomiting, weight gain, hypertension, breast discomfort, chloasma, skin rashes, erythema nodosum, cholelithiasis and cholestatic jaundice. Venous thrombosis, thromboembolism and possibly cerebral and coronary thrombosis are also risks.

In women, stilboestrol may cause an increase in the size of uterine fibromyomata, endometrial proliferation and/or an aggravation or recurrence of endometriosis and an excessive production of cervical mucous. The risk of endometrial neoplasia is increased significantly.

In both sexes the use of stilboestrol may cause tenderness, pain, enlargement and secretion of milk like fluid from the breast. It also may aggravate corneal discomfort in patients with contact lenses and be associated with fluctuating moods (both elation and depression) and headaches including an increase in incidence of migraine.

The general metabolic effects of stilboestrol include sodium and water retention, reduced glucose tolerance and changes in body weight (usually increases).

In men there will be some feminization, e.g. gynaecomastia and testicular atrophy, and impotence.

Other effects may be withdrawal bleeding in women and an increased incidence of cholelithiasis. In the event of prolonged usage there is an increased risk of endometrial carcinoma.

Overdose: There is no specific antidote to stilboestrol. The commonest symptoms of overdosage are nausea and vomiting. Management may include gastric lavage associated with special care of plasma electrolytes and any other appropriate symptomatic relief. Should the overdose (abuse) be in female children, an oestrogen-withdrawal bleed may be induced.

Pharmacological properties

Pharmacodynamic properties: Like other oestrogens action of stilboestrol is intracellular. It is bound to a receptor protein in the cytoplasm and translocated to the nucleus where binding to chromatin occurs. Specific mRNA and specific proteins are then synthesised.

The pharmacological action of oestrogens is complex and not fully understood, but is believed that oestrogen receptors contained in tumour cells account for the palliative action of stilboestrol.

Pharmacokinetic properties: Following oral administration, stilboestrol is readily absorbed through the gastro intestinal tract. It is metabolised slowly in the liver and enterohepatic recycling has been reported.

Preclinical safety data: Not applicable.

Pharmaceutical particulars

List of excipients: Magnesium Stearate PhEur, Maize Starch PhEur, Methylhydroxypropylcellulose PhEur, Talc PhEur, Anhydrous Lactose USP and colouring agents E110, E127, E132 and E171.

Incompatibilities: None known.

Shelf life: 48 months.

Special precautions for storage: Store in a dry place below 25°C, protect from light.

Nature and contents of container: Stilboestrol Tablets BP 1 mg–blister strips in packs of 28 and 56 tablets.

Stilboestrol Tablets BP 5 mg–blister strips in packs of 28 tablets.

Instructions for use/handling: Not applicable.

Marketing authorisation holder: Approved Prescription Services Limited, Eastbourne BN22 9AG England.

Marketing authorisation numbers
Stilboestrol Tablets BP 1 mg–PL 0289/5188R
Stilboestrol Tablets BP 5 mg–PL 0289/5189R

Date of first authorisation/renewal of authorisation
Stilboestrol Tablets BP 1 mg
Date MA granted : 25.07.90
Last renewal date : 13.12.95
Stilboestrol Tablets BP 5 mg
Date MA granted : 23.07.90
Last renewal date : 13.12.95

Date of (partial) revision of the text November 1996.

Legal category POM.

**Trade Mark*

ASTA Medica Limited
168 Cowley Road
Cambridge CB4 0DL

☎ 01223 423434 🗋 01223 420943

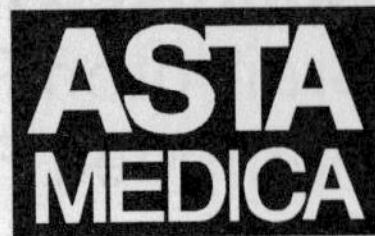

CYCLO-PROGYNOVA* 1 mg
CYCLO-PROGYNOVA* 2 mg

Qualitative and quantitative composition
Cyclo-Progynova 1 mg

Beige tablets	1 mg oestradiol valerate
Pale brown tablets	250 micrograms levonorgestrel 1 mg oestradiol valerate

Cyclo-Progynova 2 mg

White Tablets	2 mg oestradiol valerate
Pale Brown Tablets	500 micrograms norgestrel 2 mg oestradiol valerate

Pharmaceutical form Sugar-coated tablets.

Clinical particulars
Therapeutic indications:
Cyclo-Progynova 1 mg and 2 mg: Hormone replacement therapy for the treatment of the climacteric syndrome.

Cyclo-Progynova 1 mg and 2 mg: Prevention of postmenopausal osteoporosis in women considered at risk of developing fractures. Epidemiological studies suggest a number of risk factors may contribute to postmenopausal osteoporosis including:

- early menopause (either natural or surgically induced)
- family history of osteoporosis
- recent corticosteroid therapy
- thin
- a small frame
- cigarette consumption

For maximum prophylactic benefit treatment should commence as soon as possible after the menopause.

Bone mineral density measurements may help to confirm the presence of low bone mass.

Posology and method of administration: For all indications, Cyclo-Progynova 1 mg or 2 mg is to be taken orally at the following doses:

Adult Women: one tablet per day for 21 days with a 7-day tablet-free interval between courses

Contraindications:
- pregnancy
- severe disturbances of liver function
- previous or existing liver tumours
- jaundice or general pruritus during a previous pregnancy
- Dubin-Johnson Syndrome
- Rotor syndrome
- Active deep venous thrombosis, thromboembolic disorders, or a history of confirmed venous thromboembolism
- sickle-cell anaemia
- suspected or existing hormone-dependent disorders or tumours of the uterus and breast
- undiagnosed irregular vaginal bleeding
- congenital disturbances of lipid metabolism
- a history of herpes gestationis
- otosclerosis with deterioration in previous pregnancies
- endometriosis
- severe diabetes with vascular changes
- mastopathy

Special warnings and special precautions for use: Before starting treatment, pregnancy must be excluded. If withdrawal bleeding fails to occur at about 28-day intervals, treatment should be stopped until pregnancy has been ruled out.

Before starting Cyclo-Progynova, patients should have a thorough general medical and gynaecological examination with special emphasis on the body-weight, blood pressure, heart, breasts, pelvic organs with an endometrial assessment if indicated, the legs and skin.

Follow up examinations are recommended at least six-monthly during treatment.

Treatment should be stopped at once if migrainous or frequent and unusually severe headaches occur for the first time, or if there are other symptoms that are possible prodromata of vascular occlusion.

Treatment should also be stopped if trauma, illness or impending surgery is considered to entail a risk of thrombosis.

Treatment should be stopped at once if jaundice or pregnancy occurs, or if there is a significant rise in blood-pressure, the occurrence of thromboembolic disease or if there are exacerbations of epileptic seizures.

Pre-existing fibroids may increase in size under the influence of oestrogens. If this is observed, treatment should be discontinued.

In patients with mild chronic liver disease, liver function should be checked every 8-12 weeks.

Persistent breakthrough bleeding during treatment is an indication for endometrial assessment which may include biopsy.

Prolonged exposure to unopposed oestrogens may increase the risk of development of endometrial carcinoma. The general consensus of opinion is that the addition of 10 days progestogen towards the end of the cycle, as in Cyclo-Progynova, diminishes the possibility of such a risk, and some investigators consider that it might be protective. At the present time there is some evidence which suggests a slight increase in the relative risk of breast cancer in postmenopausal women receiving long-term hormone replacement therapy. A careful appraisal of the risk/benefit ratio should be undertaken before treating for longer than 5 to 10 years.

Some women are predisposed to cholestasis during steroid therapy. Diseases that are known to be subject to deterioration during pregnancy (e.g. multiple sclerosis, epilepsy, diabetes, benign breast disease, hypertension, cardiac or renal dysfunction, asthma, porphyria, tetany and otosclerosis) and women with a strong family history of breast cancer should be carefully observed during treatment.

In rare cases benign, and in even rarer cases, malignant liver tumours leading in isolated cases to life-threatening intra-abdominal haemorrhage have been observed after the use of hormonal substances such as those contained in Cyclo-Progynova. If severe upper abdominal complaints, liver enlargement or signs of intra-abdominal haemorrhage occur, a liver tumour should be included in the differential diagnostic considerations.

Epidemiological studies have suggested that hormone replacement therapy (HRT) is associated with an increased relative risk of developing venous thromboembolism (VTE) ie deep vein thrombosis or pulmonary embolism. The studies find a 2-3 fold increase for users compared with non-users which for healthy women amounts to a low risk of one extra case of VTE each year for every 5000 patients taking HRT.

Generally recognised risk factors for VTE include a personal or family history and severe obesity (Body Mass Index >30 kg/m²). In women with these factors the benefits of treatment with HRT need to be carefully weighed against risks.

The risk of VTE may be temporarily increased with prolonged immobilisation, major trauma or major surgery. In women on HRT scrupulous attention should be given to prophylactic measures to prevent VTE following surgery. Where prolonged immobilisation is liable to follow elective surgery, particularly abdominal or orthopaedic surgery to the lower limbs, consideration should be given to temporarily stopping HRT 4 weeks earlier, if this is possible.

If venous thromboembolism develops after initiating therapy the drug should be discontinued.

Interaction with other medicaments and other forms of interaction: Hormonal contraception should be stopped when treatment with Cyclo-Progynova is started and the patient should be advised to take non-hormonal contraceptive precautions.

Drugs which induce hepatic microsomal enzyme systems e.g. barbiturates, phenytoin, rifampicin accelerate the metabolism of oestrogen/progestogen combinations such as Cyclo-Progynova and may reduce their efficacy.

The requirement for oral antidiabetics or insulin can change.

Use in pregnancy and lactation: Contra-indicated.

Effects on ability to drive and to use machinery: None known.

Undesirable effects: During the first few months treatment, breakthrough bleeding, spotting and breast tenderness or enlargement can occur. These are usually temporary and normally disappear after continued treatment. Other symptoms known to occur are: anxiety, increased appetite, bloating, palpitations, depressive symptoms, dizziness, dyspepsia, leg pains and oedema, altered libido, headache, nausea, rashes, vomiting and altered weight.

Overdose: There have been no reports of ill-effects from overdosage which it is, therefore, generally unnecessary to treat. There are no specific antidotes, and treatment should be symptomatic.

Pharmacological properties
Pharmacodynamic properties: Cyclo-Progynova contains oestradiol valerate, (the valeric-acid ester of the endogenous female oestrogen, oestradiol) and the synthetic progestogen, (levo)norgestrel.

Oestradiol valerate provides hormone replacement during and after the climacteric. The addition of (levo)norgestrel in the second half of each course of tablets helps to provide good cycle control and opposes the development of endometrial hyperplasia.

Pharmacokinetic properties: Following oral administration to man, oestradiol valerate is split into the biologically-active oestradiol and the valerate which is rapidly degraded. Oestradiol is metabolised in the liver with the formation of sulphuric acid and glucuronic acid esters (conjugated oestrogens) which are excreted in the urine.

(Levo)norgestrel is similarly absorbed from the gastrointestinal tract, metabolised by the liver and excreted in the urine and faeces as glucuronide and sulphate conjugates.

Preclinical safety data: There are no preclinical safety data which could be of relevance to the prescriber and which is not already included in other relevant sections of the SPC.

Pharmaceutical particulars
List of excipients: Lactose, maize starch, povidone, talc, magnesium stearate [E572], sucrose, calcium carbonate [E170], polyethylene glycol 6000, montan glycol wax, titanium dioxide [E171], yellow ferric oxide [E172], red brown ferric oxide [E172], glycerin.

Incompatibilities: None stated.

Shelf Life: 5 years.

Special Precautions for Storage: Not applicable.

Nature and Contents of container: Cardboard outer containing either: one circular blister pack or three circular blister packs. Each pack consists of aluminium foil and PVC and contains 21 tablets.

Instructions for use/handling: None stated.

Marketing authorisation numbers

Cyclo-Progynova 1 mg	PL 08336/0087
Cyclo-Progynova 2 mg	PL 08336/0088

Date of (partial) revision of the text April 1998

ENDOXANA* INJECTION
ENDOXANA* TABLETS

Presentation
Tablets: White, sugar-coated tablets containing Cyclophosphamide Monohydrate BP 53.5 mg (equivalent to 50 mg anhydrous cyclophosphamide).

Injection: White powder for injection in vials containing Cyclophosphamide Monohydrate BP 213.8 mg, 534.5 mg or 1,069 mg (equivalent to 200 mg, 500 mg or 1,000 mg anhydrous cyclophosphamide respectively) and sodium chloride sufficient to render isotonic when diluted with water for injections using the volume recommended for each strength.

Uses
Action: Cyclophosphamide is inert until activated by microsomal enzymes. This occurs mainly in the liver, producing potent alkylating cytotoxic metabolites.

Indications: Endoxana is a cytotoxic drug for the treatment of malignant disease. As a single agent it has successfully produced an objective remission in a wide range of malignant conditions. Endoxana is also frequently used in combination with other cytotoxic drugs, radiotherapy or surgery.

Dosage and administration Endoxana should only be used by clinicians experienced in the use of cancer chemotherapy.

Dosage: The dose, route of administration and frequency of administration should be determined by the tumour type, tumour stage, the general condition of the patient, previous cytotoxic chemotherapy and whether other chemotherapy or radiotherapy is to be administered concurrently. A guide to dosage regimens used for most indications is given below:

a. 100-300 mg daily as an oral dose. This dose may be divided.

or

b. 80-300 mg/m² as single iv dose daily.

or

c. 300-600 mg/m² as a single iv dose weekly.

or

d. 600-1500 mg/m² as a single iv dose, or short infusion at 10–20 day intervals.

With single doses of cyclophosphamide over 10 mg/kg, mesna should be given concurrently, in addition to a good fluid intake, to avoid urothelial toxicity.

Endoxana tablets should be swallowed with sufficient fluid without chewing.

Elderly: No specific information on the use of this product in the elderly is available. Clinical trials have included patients over 65 years and no adverse reactions specific to this age group have been reported.

Children: No specific information. Children have received Endoxana, no adverse reactions specific to this group have been reported.

Administration: Endoxana is inert until activated by enzymes in the liver. However, safe handling is required and advice is included under 'Pharmaceutical precautions'. The dry contents of a vial should be dissolved in water for injections (5 ml per 100 mg Endoxana) and used within eight hours. The pH of an aqueous solution is between 4.0 and 6.0.

Endoxana is usually given directly into the tubing of a fast running iv infusion with the patient supine. Care should be taken that extravasation does not take place, however, should it occur, no specific measures need be taken.

Endoxana injection may also be given intraperitoneally or intrapleurally, but these routes offer no therapeutic advantages over the iv route. Endoxana has been given intra-arterially and by local perfusion. These routes should be used only by clinicians experienced in these procedures.

A minimum urine output of 100 ml/hr should be maintained during therapy with conventional doses to avoid cystitis. If the larger doses are used, an output of at least this level should be maintained for 24 hours following administration, if necessary by forced diuresis. Alkalinisation of the urine is not recommended. Endoxana should be given early in the day and the bladder voided frequently. The patient should be well hydrated and maintained in fluid balance.

Mesna (Uromitexan) can be used concurrently with Endoxana to reduce urotoxic effects (for dosage see Uromitexan data sheet). If mesna (Uromitexan) is used to reduce urothelial toxicity, frequent emptying of the bladder should be avoided.

Endoxana should be avoided in patients with cystitis from any cause until it has been treated.

Anti-emetics given before and during therapy may reduce nausea and vomiting.

If the leucocyte count is below 4,000/mm³ or the platelet count is below 100,000/mm³, treatment with Endoxana should be temporarily withheld until the blood count returns to normal levels.

For oral administration an elixir may be prepared by dissolving the contents of the dry powder vials in Aromatic Elixir USP shortly before oral administration.

Contra-indications, warnings, etc

Contra-indications: Endoxana should only be administered where there are facilities for regular monitoring of clinical, biochemical and haematological parameters before, during and after administration and under the direction of a specialist oncology service.

Endoxana is contra-indicated in patients with known hypersensitivity to cyclophosphamide, with acute infections, with bone marrow aplasia, or with acute urothelial toxicity from cytotoxic chemotherapy or radiation therapy.

Endoxana should not be used in the management of non-malignant disease, except for immunosuppression in life-threatening situations.

Use in pregnancy and lactation: Endoxana should not be used in pregnancy, especially the first trimester, unless the expected benefit is thought to outweigh the substantial risk to the foetus. Mothers should not breast-feed while being treated with Endoxana or for 36 hours after stopping treatment.

Precautions: Care should be exercised in patients who are elderly, debilitated, have diabetes mellitus or evidence of myelosuppression or who have recently received or are receiving concurrent treatment with radiotherapy or cytotoxic agents.

Endoxana is not recommended in patients with a plasma creatinine greater than 120μ mol/l (1.5 mg/100 ml) bilirubin greater than 17μ mol/l (1 mg/100 ml); or serum transaminases or alkaline phosphatase more than 2-3 times the upper limit of normal.

Cardiotoxicity may be induced in patients who have had or are receiving mediastinal irradiation, doxorubicin or high doses of cyclophosphamide. In such instances cyclophosphamide therapy should be stopped and appropriate treatment instituted.

Contraception in both sexes is advised during and for at least 3 months after Endoxana therapy. Patients should receive counselling with respect of subsequent pregnancies.

Endoxana may have an adverse effect on prepubertal gonads and amenorrhoea and azoospermia often occur. Appropriate counselling should be given.

Interactions: The following clinically significant interactions of cyclophosphamide with other drugs have been reported: allopurinol (increased incidence of bone marrow depression), sulfonylureas (enhanced hypoglycaemic effect) and suxamethonium (prolonged apnoea).

Increased myelosuppression may be seen following concurrent administration of other bone marrow depressant drugs.

Side-effects: During Endoxana therapy, the reticulo-endothelial system is depressed, granulopoiesis and lymphopoiesis being more affected than thrombopoiesis and erythropoiesis, but this depression is reversible. When a single dose is given, the fall in the peripheral white cell count reaches its nadir within 5 to 10 days. Recovery is seen at 10-14 days following administration, with full recovery in most cases by 21-28 days. The fall in the peripheral count and the time taken to recover may increase with increasing doses of Endoxana.

Haematuria may occur during or after therapy with Endoxana. Acute sterile haemorrhagic cystitis may occur in up to 10% of patients not given mesna (Uromitexan) in conjunction with Endoxana. Late sequelae of this cystitis are bladder contracture and fibrosis.

An alteration in carbohydrate metabolism may been seen in patients on Endoxana; hyperglycaemia has been reported.

Azoospermia often occurs in men and is dose dependent. Spontaneous recovery of fertility may occur, and is also dependent on dose. Menstruation in women commonly ceases during therapy, and may be permanent, particularly in older women. Endoxana may have an adverse effect on prepubertal gonads.

Cardiotoxicity may be induced in patients who have had or are receiving mediastinal irradiation or doxorubicin. It has also been reported with high doses of cyclophosphamide. This mainly occurs as a tachyarrhythmia and may progress in severe cases to intractable heart failure. Following large doses, ECG changes and elevation of LDH, SGOT and CPK have been reported in some patients.

There is evidence that, like other alkylating agents, cyclophosphamide is a human carcinogen. In certain laboratory tests, it has been shown to be mutagenic, teratogenic and carcinogenic and as with other cytotoxic drugs there have been reports of possible drug-induced neoplasia. There is an excess risk of acute leukaemia and bladder cancer following cyclophosphamide therapy.

Anorexia, nausea, vomiting and mucosal ulceration can occur. Nausea and vomiting may be reduced by administration of an anti-emetic agent, before, during and after therapy.

Alopecia occurs to some degree in about 20% of patients receiving over 100 mg daily and is inevitable following high doses. Epilation usually commences after the first three weeks of treatment but regrowth is evident after three months in most patients even though they remain on treatment.

Cyclophosphamide therapy may lead to inappropriate secretion of anti-diuretic hormone, fluid retention and hyponatraemia, with subsequent water intoxication. Should this occur, diuretic therapy should be instigated.

Other side-effects include: Pigmentation of the fingernails and the skin (mainly the palms of the hands and the soles of the feet), macrocytosis, and induction of hyperglycaemia or hypoglycaemia. Pneumonitis and interstitial pulmonary fibrosis may also occur.

Side-effects have occasionally occurred after cessation of treatment.

Overdosage: The most serious consequences of overdosage are profound myelosuppression, haemorrhagic cystitis, and cardiotoxicity in the form of arrhythmias and severe heart failure. Myelosuppression usually recovers spontaneously. Myelosuppression may be alleviated by transfusion of red cells, platelets or white cells. Broad spectrum antibiotic cover may be necessary.

If the overdose is recognised within the first 24 hours and possibly up to 48 hours, iv mesna may be beneficial in ameliorating damage to the urinary system. Normal supportive measures such as analgesics and maintenance of fluid balance should be instituted. If, despite these measures the cystitis does not resolve, more intensive treatment may be necessary and a urological opinion should be sought. No further courses should be given until the patient has fully recovered.

Endoxana is dialysable.

Pharmaceutical precautions: The following protective recommendations are advised during handling due to the toxic nature of the substance.

Reconstitution and administration must be undertaken only by trained personnel. Pregnant staff and breast feeding mothers should be excluded.

Protective clothing, goggles, masks and disposable PVC or Latex gloves should be worn.

A designated area should be defined for reconstitution (preferably under a laminar-airflow system). The work surface should be protected by a disposable, plastic-backed, absorbent paper. Accidental contact with the skin or eyes should be treated immediately by copious lavage with water. Soap and water should then be used on non-mucous membranes. Spillages should be removed with dry or moist disposable towels.

Care must be taken in the disposal of all waste materials (syringes, needles and disposable towels etc). Used items should be placed in appropriate secure containers, in readiness for destruction in a chemical incinerator equipped with an after-burner.

Store below 25°C. Vials should on no account be stored above the recommended temperature as this can cause degradation of the active ingredient, identifiable by a yellow melted appearance to the vial contents. Vials containing melted material should not be used.

Endoxana injection is compatible with dextrose and saline infusion solutions. Endoxana injection is chemically stable for 6 days at room temperature in saline and 48 hours at room temperature in dextrose. As Endoxana does not contain a preservative, the above solutions should be used within eight hours unless prepared under strict aseptic technique.

Legal category POM.

Package quantities Cartons containing 10 blister packs, each of 10 x 50 mg tablets.
200 mg dry vials in packs of 10
500 mg dry vials, singles
1 g, dry vials, singles

Further information The dosage regimen for mesna (Uromitexan) varies according to the dose of Endoxana administered. In general, i.v. Uromitexan is given as 60% w/w of the dose of i.v. Endoxana in three equal doses of 20% at 0, 4 and 8 hours. With the higher doses of Endoxana, the dose and frequency of administration may need to be increased. Uromitexan Tablets are also available; full prescribing information for both presentations is available on the appropriate data sheet.

Product licence numbers

50 mg Tablets	8336/0016
200 mg Vials	8336/0012
500 mg Vials	8336/0013
1,000 mg Vials	8336/0014

HONVAN* INJECTION
HONVAN* TABLETS

Qualitative and quantitative composition

Honvan Injection–300 mg fosfestrol tetrasodium BP in 5 ml solution.

Honvan Tablets–120 mg fosfestrol tetrasodium BP

Pharmaceutical form Sterile aqueous solution for injection. Film-coated tablets for oral use.

Clinical particulars

Therapeutic indications: Honvan is a synthetic oestrogen used for the treatment of prostatic carcinoma. Honvan may be used as an adjuvant to surgery, in inoperable cases and for the reduction of pain due to metastases. Patients who are resistant to conventional hormone therapy have responded to Honvan. Where acute retention has occurred the use of Honvan may reduce the need for transurethral resection.

Posology and method of administration

Route of administration: Intravenous injection.

The patient should preferably by lying down and the injection given slowly into the vein. Slow infusions are not recommended as high local cytotoxic levels may not be achieved.

Dosage: The dosage should be according to clinical and biochemical findings. Response to treatment with Honvan may be objectively assessed by the reduction of plasma acid phosphatase concentrations and the degree of reduction in size of the primary prostatic tumour, cutaneous, subcutaneous or lymph node metastases, bone lesions or visceral metastases. Subjective improvement may be made by the reduction of pain, improvement in urinary function and improvement in patient well-being.

Adults: Initial therapy: acute retention of urine and relapse: 2-4 ampoules Honvan intravenous as a single injection daily for at least five days or until a response has been obtained (seven to ten days). Maintenance: 1 ampoule intravenously one to four times weekly.

Route of administration: Oral.

Dosage: The dosage should be according to clinical and biochemical findings. Response to treatment with Honvan may be objectively assessed by the reduction of plasma acid phosphatase concentrations and the degree of reduction in size of the primary prostatic tumour, cutaneous, subcutaneous or lymph node metastases, bone lesions or visceral metastases. Subjective improvement may be made by the reduction of pain, improvement in urinary function and improvement in patient well being.

Oral maintenance therapy is usually 1-6 tablets daily in divided doses. The initial dose should be up to 2 tablets three times daily for the first week, reducing over the next two weeks to the lowest dose that will control the disease which is usually 1-3 tablets daily in divided doses.

Oral and intravenous

Children: Not recommended.

Elderly: No specific information on the use of this product in the elderly is available. Clinical trials have included patients over 65 and no adverse reactions specific to this group have been included.

Contra-indications: History of hypersensitivity to Honvan or other synthetic oestrogens.

Special warnings and special precautions for use: Honvan should only be administered under the direction of a specialist oncology service having facilities for the regular monitoring of clinical biochemical and haematological effects during and after administration.

Caution is advised when using Honvan in patients with poor cardiac reserve or fluid retention and in those cases concomitant diuretic therapy may be indicated. Caution is also advised for patients with active thrombophlebitis or thromboembolic disorders, cardiac failure, hypertension or cerebrovascular disease.

Particular care should be taken in patients over 70 years of age, those on long-term Honvan therapy and those having had recent surgery. Caution is also advised in patients with a history of liver disease and diabetic patients. Glucose tolerance may be impaired in the latter and their urine should be carefully monitored.

In rare cases hypersensitivity to Honvan has been noted. Honvan Injection is non-irritant to the veins and should an injection accidentally enter the paravenous tissue no specific action is necessary.

Interaction with other medicaments and other forms of interaction: Honvan is not known to interact with any other drugs, food or alcohol.

Pregnancy and lactation: Honvan should not be administered to pregnant women as oestrogens have been shown to be teratogenic to the foetus.

Effects on ability to drive and use machines: None known.

Undesirable effects: Pain in bony metastases may occur during or immediately after administration of Honvan. A burning in the perineum may occur during or immediately after i.v. injection. Perineal discomfort may be reduced by prior administration of a sedative.

Anorexia, nausea, vomiting, dizziness, fever, rigor, abdominal cramps and abdominal bloating may occur. Skin rash and disturbances of vision have been reported.

Transient rises in transferase and aspartate levels have been reported. A moderate hypophosphataemia may occur and there may be a transient rise in alkaline phosphatase. Fluid retention and hypernatraemia have been reported, fluid retention may lead to congestive cardiac failure. There is an increased risk of pulmonary embolism, deep vein thrombosis and cerebrovascular accidents reported with oestrogens.

Androgen reduction may lead to impotence, mental disturbance and mood changes, gynaecomastia and testicular atrophy.

Overdose: In the event of overdosage, monitoring for fluid retention should be undertaken and in patients with cardiac disease, the administration of diuretics and digitalis should be considered.

Pharmacological properties

Pharmacodynamic properties: Fosfestrol Tetrasodium is a water soluble synthetic oestrogen which is inert. The active principle is diethylstilboestrol which becomes liberated through enzymatic cleavage as soon as it enters the body.

Diethylstilboestrol has three principal effects in man:

(i) oestrogen-like effects in hormone sensitive tissues

(ii) oestrogen-like negative feedback on the endocrine system, thereby reducing the production of male sexual hormones

(iii) at high doses indirect interference with cellular reproductive functions, i.e. some cytotoxic activity.

Pharmacokinetic properties: Following i.v. infusion, plasma levels of Fosfestrol Tetrasodium and DES (DES = Diethylstilboestrol) monophosphate rise steeply for 1.5 hours, thereafter more slowly. Both these compounds have short half lives, 5 minutes and 30 minutes respectively. DES appears gradually during the infusion as does DES monoglucuronide; the latter reaches greater concentration than the DES.

The main metabolites of Fosfestrol Tetrasodium are conjugates: DES monoglucuronide, DES monosulphate, DES glucuronide sulphate. Oxidative metabolism also takes place but does not play a major role.

Tetrasodium Fosfestrol→DES monophosphate→DES→conjugates and other metabolites.

These DES conjugates may also behave as prodrugs.

The metabolism of Tetrasodium Fosfestrol after oral administration follows the same time course for DES. After oral administration, unchanged fosfestrol could not be detected. This is due to extensive first pass metabolism by phosphatase enzymes in the gut wall.

Plasma protein binding has been shown to be concentration dependent. DES is 95% protein bound.

Elimination studies show that only DES glucuronide and DES glucuronide-sulphate can be found in urine following either i.v. or oral administration. The other conjugates as well as free DES appear in the faeces.

90-95% of the dose given is trapped in the enterohepatic cycle from where it escapes over a period of 24 hours.

Preclinical safety data: Not relevant.

Pharmaceutical particulars

List of excipients:

Honvan Injection: Water for injections; sodium hydroxide, Nitrogen.

Honvan Tablets:

Lactose	42.74–31.86 mg
Maize starch	11.20 mg
Talc	4.0 mg
Magnesium stearate	2.7 mg
Aerosil 200v	2.0 mg
Gelatine	1.0 mg
Lactose monohydrate	0.98 mg
Eudragit NE30D	0.23 mg
Polyethylene glycol 6000	0.23 mg
Carboxymethylcellulose sodium	0.06 mg
Purified water	-

Incompatibilities: Honvan Injection is incompatible with aqueous solutions of pH less than 7 and solutions containing calcium or magnesium ions.

Shelf life: 3 years.

Special precautions for storage: Store at up to 25°C

Nature and contents of container:

Injection: Clear glass ampoules in a folded cardboard box.

Tablets: PVC/PVDC–aluminium blister pack, in a folded cardboard box.

Instructions for use and handling: These medicines should not be handled by pregnant women.

Marketing authorisation numbers

Honvan Injection 8336/0048
Honvan Tablets 8336/0047

Date of approval/revision of SPC March 1996.

Legal category POM.

MITOXANA* INJECTION

Qualitative and quantitative composition

1 vial of 1 g Mitoxana Injection contains 1 g of ifosfamide.

1 vial of 2 g Mitoxana Injection contains 2 g of ifosfamide.

Pharmaceutical form Dry powder for injection after reconstitution.

Clinical particulars

Therapeutic indications: Mitoxana is a cytotoxic drug for the treatment of malignant disease. As a single agent is has successfully produced an objective remission in a wide range of malignant conditions. Mitoxana is also frequently used in combination with other cytotoxic drugs, radiotherapy and surgery.

Posology and method of administration: For intravenous use as a diluted solution only–by infusion, or if solution is less than 4% by direct injection. Mitoxana should only be used by clinicians experienced in the use of cancer chemotherapy.

Dosage: Mitoxana should not be used without the concurrent administration of Uromitexan (mesna) to protect against urothelial toxicity that can occur with the oxazaphosphorine alkylating agents. The dose and frequency of administration should be determined by the tumour type, tumour stage, the general condition of the patient, any previous cytotoxic therapy, and whether other chemotherapy or radiotherapy is to be administered concurrently.

A guide to the dosage regimens used for most indications is given below:

(a) 8–12 g/m² equally fractionated as single daily doses over 3–5 days every 2–4 weeks.

(b) 5–6 g/m² (maximum 10 g) given as a 24 hour infusion every 3–4 weeks.

The frequency of dosage is determined by the degree of myelosuppression and the time taken to recover adequate bone marrow function. The usual number of courses given is 4, but up to 7 (6 by 24 hour infusion) courses have been given. Re-treatment has been given following relapse.

Children: In children, the dosage and administration should be determined by the tumour type, tumour stage, the general condition of the patient, any previous cytotoxic therapy, and whether chemotherapy or radiotherapy is to be administered concurrently. Clinical trials have involved doses of:

(a) 5 g/m² over 24 hours

(b) 9 g/m² equally fractionated as single daily doses over 5 days

(c) 9 g/m² as a continuous infusion over 72 hours repeated at three weekly intervals.

Elderly: No specific information on the use of this product in the elderly is available. Clinical trials have included patients over 65 years and no adverse reactions specific to this age group have been reported.

Administration: Mitoxana is inert until activated by enzymes in the liver. However, safe handling is required and advice is included under Pharmaceutical Precautions. The dry contents of a vial should be dissolved in Water for Injections as follows:
1 g vial: add 12.5 ml of Water for Injections
2 g vial: add 25 ml of Water for Injections

The resultant solution of 8% of ifosfamide should not be injected directly into the vein. The solution may be:

1. diluted to less than a 4% solution and injected directly into the vein, with the patient supine.
2. infused in 5% dextrose-saline or normal saline over 30-120 mins.
3. injected directly into a fast-running infusion.
4. made up in 3 litres of dextrose-saline or normal saline and infused over 24 hours. Each litre should be given over eight hours, and should be freshly made up immediately before infusion.

Care should be taken that extravasation does not take place, however should it occur, local tissue damage is unlikely and no specific measures need be taken. Repeated intravenous injections of large doses of Mitoxana have resulted in local irritation.

Mesna (Uromitexan) should be used to prevent urothelial toxicity.

Where Mitoxana is used as an i.v. bolus, increased dosages of mesna are recommended in children, patients whose urothelium may be damaged from previous therapies and those who are not adequately protected by the standard dose of mesna.

The patient should be well hydrated and maintained in fluid balance, replacement fluids being given as necessary to achieve this. The fluid intake of patients on the intermittent regimen should be at least 2 litres in 24 hours. As Mitoxana may exert an antidiuretic effect, a diuretic may be necessary to ensure an adequate urinary output.

Urine should be sent for laboratory analysis before, and at the end of, each course of treatment, and the patient should be monitored for output and evidence of proteinuria and haematuria at regular intervals (4-hourly if possible) throughout the treatment period. The patient should be instructed to report any signs or symptoms of cystitis. Mitoxana should be avoided in patients with cystitis from any cause until it has been treated.

Antiemetics given before, during and after therapy may reduce nausea and vomiting. Oral hygiene is important.

If leucocyte count is below 4,000/mm³ or the platelet count is below 100,000/mm³, treatment with Mitoxana should be withheld until the blood count returns to normal.

There should be no signs or symptoms of urothelial toxicity or renal or hepatic impairment prior to the start of each course of Mitoxana.

Contra-indications: Mitoxana should only be administered when there are facilities for regular monitoring of clinical, biochemical and haematological parameters before, during and after administration and under the direction of a specialist oncology service.

Mitoxana is contra-indicated in patients with known hypersensitivity to ifosfamide, bone marrow aplasia, myelosuppression, urinary tract obstruction, acute infections including urinary tract infection, or with acute urothelial toxicity from cytotoxic chemotherapy or radiation therapy.

Mitoxana is contra-indicated in patients with renal impairment (serum creatinine greater than 120μ mol/l or 1.5 mg/100 ml) or hepatic impairment (bilirubin greater than 17μ mol/l or 1 mg/100 ml), or serum transaminases or alkaline phosphatase more than 2.5 times the upper limit of normal.

Contraception in both sexes is advised during and for at least 6 months after Mitoxana therapy. Patients should receive counselling with respect to subsequent pregnancies.

Special warnings and special precautions for use: Care should be exercised in patients who are elderly, debilitated, have diabetes mellitus or evidence of myelosuppression or who have recently received or are receiving concurrent treatment with radiotherapy or cytotoxic agents. Any electrolyte imbalances should be corrected before treatment is started.

Caution is necessary in patients who have previously received platinum compounds or undergone a nephrectomy.

In children, high cumulative doses of ifosfamide and continued treatment in the presence of renal tubular dysfunction may be associated with increased frequency or severity of renal damage.

Mitoxana is a potent immunuosuppressive drug and the increased risk to the patient should be borne in mind.

Amenorrhoea and azoospermia can occur. Patients should be warned of a potential risk to future progeny.

Mitoxana has been shown to be mutagenic, teratogenic and carcinogenic in laboratory tests and there is a risk of drug-induced neoplasia following long-term treatment.

Interaction with other medicaments and other forms of interaction: Concurrent administration of anticoagulants, especially Warfarin, can result in disturbance of anticoagulant control and an increased risk of bleeding. Concurrent administration of antidiabetic agents, sulfonylureas for instance and ifosfamide may enhance the hypoglycaemic effects of the former drugs. Theoretical interactions of ifosfamide and allopurinol resulting in an increased severity of bone marrow depression may occur. Prior treatment with enzyme inducing drugs may result in a faster metabolism of ifosfamide.

Pregnancy and lactation: Contraception is advised in both sexes during Mitoxana therapy and for at least six months following treatment. Patients should receive counselling with respect to subsequent pregnancies. Mothers should not breast-feed while being treated with Mitoxana as ifosfamide has been shown to be teratogenic in animals and is excreted in breast milk.

Mitoxana should not be used in pregnancy especially the first trimester, unless the expected benefit is thought to outweigh the substantial risk to the foetus.

Effects on ability to drive and use machines: Potential side-effects on the central nervous system may transiently impair the ability to operate machinery and motor vehicles.

Undesirable effects: Treatment with ifosfamide may be associated with the following dose-related, generally reversible side-effects.

Urogenital tract–Urothelial toxicity is the usual dose-limiting factor. This can be largely prevented by the concurrent administration of mesna. Urotoxicity involving the efferent urinary tract as well as the bladder can lead to haemorrhagic cystitis and dysuria.

Nephrotoxicity may occur with oliguria, raised uric acid, increased blood urea and serum creatinine and decreased creatinine clearance. Glycosuria, proteinuria, aminoaciduria and hyperphosphaturia which may lead to renal rickets have been reported with changes in serum proteins and electrolytes. Nephrotoxicity is usually reversible, especially in the early stages but severe cases are recorded. Delay in the diagnosis and treatment of renal toxicity may, especially in children, lead to a full picture of Fanconi's Syndrome or diabetes insipidus. Patients with pre-existing renal dysfunction and/or prior treatment with nephrotoxic drugs such as cisplatin may be predisposed to nephrotoxicity.

Haematological reactions–large doses of ifosfamide give rise to a predictable bone marrow toxicity and consequent immunosuppression. The white cell count reaches its nadir 5-10 days after commencing treatment, recovery commencing after 10-14 days and usually returning to normal within 2-3 weeks. About 30% of patients would be expected to have a fall in haemoglobin of greater than 2 g/100 ml and a white cell count less than 2000/mm³, but only 5% would be expected to have a platelet count less than 100,000/mm³. There have been only occasional reports of coagulation disorders.

Central nervous system side-effects may occur. These may present as drowsiness, confusion, disorientation, restlessness, depressive psychoses and/or hallucinations, rarely convulsions. These will rarely persist beyond 2 days, and will usually resolve spontaneously after cessation of treatment. Occasionally tonic-clonic spasms, motor unrest and emotional lability have been noted.

A severe encephalopathy occurs less frequently. The symptoms may be preceded by EEG abnormalities. Clumsiness, confusion, disorientation, logorrhoea, echolalia, perseveration, aggression and depression of conscious level have been reported. Fever and tachycardia may be present. Occasionally recovery has been incomplete with persistent psychological disturbances, coma and death.

If central nervous system toxicity is suspected, ifosfamide should be stopped and supportive therapy given. There are indications of a higher incidence of CNS effects in elderly patients and those with cerebral metastases. Special care should be taken in giving Mitoxana to patients with reduced plasma albumin levels and/or impaired kidney function.

Gastrointestinal reactions–frequently nausea and vomiting, very occasionally anorexia, diarrhoea or constipation. Nausea and vomiting may be reduced by the prior administration of an anti-emetic.

Other side-effects include: frequent but reversible alopecia, stomatitis, dermatitis, impairment of gonadal function and hypersensitivity reactions. More rarely hepatic dysfunction (including jaundice and increased liver enzyme and/or bilirubin levels), thrombophlebitis at site of injection or syndrome of inappropriate antidiuretic hormone secretion may occur.

There have been isolated reports of cardiac arrhythmia or heart failure after very high doses of ifosfamide and/or prior or concurrent treatment with anthracyclines. As is the case with cytotoxic therapy in general, treatment with ifosfamide involves the risk of secondary tumours as late sequelae.

Overdose: The most serious consequences of overdosage are haemorrhagic cystitis and myelosuppression. The latter usually recovers spontaneously, but until it does, administration of a broad spectrum antibiotic may be advisable. Transfusion of whole blood should be given as necessary. If the overdosage is recognised within the first 24 hours, i.v. mesna may be beneficial in ameliorating damage to the urinary system.

Normal supportive measures such as analgesics and maintenance of fluid balance should be instituted. If despite these measures the cystitis does not resolve, more intensive treatment may be necessary and a urological opinion should be sought. No further courses should be given until the patient has fully recovered.

Pharmacological properties

Pharmacodynamic properties: Mitoxana is an antineoplastic, a cytotoxic alkylating agent. It is a prodrug and shows no in vitro cytotoxic activity until activated by microsomal enzymes. The cytotoxic activity of Mitoxana (alkylation of the nucleophilic centres in the cells) is associated with the activated oxazaphosphorine ring hydroxylated at the C4 atom which interacts with DNA-DNA cross linking. This activity manifests itself by blocking the late S and early G2 phases of the cell cycle.

Pharmacokinetic properties: Mitoxana is rapidly absorbed from the site of administration, activation of Mitoxana is primarily in the liver by microsomal mixed function oxidases. Elimination of metabolised Mitoxana is primarily via the kidneys. The serum half-life ranges between 4–8 hours depending on the dose and dosage regimen. Over 80% of a single dose of ifosfamide was excreted in the urine within 24 hours. Approximately 80% of the dose was excreted as parent compound. Significant quantities of unchanged ifosfamide were found in the cerebrospinal fluid consistent with the high lipid solubility of the drug.

Preclinical safety data: Not relevant.

Pharmaceutical particulars

List of excipients: None.

Incompatibilities: None known.

Shelf life: Five years.

The reconstituted solution should be used immediately. The product does not contain a preservative, therefore microbial stability cannot be guaranteed. When prepared under strict aseptic conditions, ifosfamide is, as a 4% solution, however, chemically stable for 7 days at room temperature with Water for Injections, 0.9% saline, dextrose/saline and dextrose solutions. Ifosfamide and mesna when prepared under strict aseptic conditions at the recommended dilutions are chemically stable with:

(i) 0.9% saline and dextrose/saline solution for one week at room temperature.

(ii) Water for Injection for one week under refrigeration.

(iii) 5% dextrose solution for 24 hours at room temperature.

(iv) 0.9% saline solution for 28 days at room temperature.

Special precautions for storage: The vials should be stored below 25°C, protected from light.

Nature and contents of container: Glass injection vial with rubber closure and beading cap. Packed in a cardboard box.

Instructions for use and handling: The following protective recommendations are advised during handling due to the toxic nature of the substance:

Reconstitution and administration must be undertaken only by trained personnel. Pregnant staff and breastfeeding mothers should be excluded.

Protective clothing, goggles, masks and disposable PVC or latex gloves should be worn.

A designated area should be defined for reconstitution (preferably under a laminar-airflow system). The work surface should be protected by a disposable, plastic backed absorbent paper. Accidental contact with the skin or eyes should be treated immediately by copious lavage with water. Soap and water should then be used on non-mucous membranes. Spillage should be removed by dry or moist disposable towels.

Care must be taken in the disposal of all waste material (syringes, needles and disposable towels etc.) Used items should be placed in appropriate secure containers in readiness for destruction in a chemical incinerator equipped with an after-burner.

Marketing authorisation numbers

1 g Mitoxana Injection	8336/0031
2 g Mitoxana Injection	8336/0032

Date of approval/revision of SPC December 1994.

Legal category POM.

OPTILAST* ▼

Qualitative and quantitative composition

Sterile, clear, colourless, aqueous solution containing azelastine hydrochloride 0.05%. Each drop contains 0.015 mg azelastine hydrochloride.

Pharmaceutical form Eye drops.

Clinical particulars

Therapeutic Indications: Symptomatic treatment and prevention of seasonal allergic conjunctivitis.

Posology and method of administration: The usual dosage for adults and children over 12 years is one drop in each eye twice daily.

During periods of severe allergen challenge, the dosage can be increased to one drop in each eye four times daily.

Treatment should be continued as long as required for relief of symptoms.

Contra-indications: Proven allergy to any of the components of Optilast.

Special warnings and precautions for use: As with other ophthalmic solutions, Optilast is not recommended for use whilst wearing contact lenses.

Optilast is not intended for treatment of eye infections. Further warnings see *Pregnancy and Lactation* sections.

Interactions with other medicaments and other forms of interaction: No specific interaction studies with Optilast have been performed.

Interaction studies at high *oral* doses have been performed however they bear no relevance to Optilast, as systemic levels, after administration of the eye drops, are in the picogram range.

Pregnancy and lactation: Due to the low locally administered dose, minimal systemic exposure to azelastine can be expected.

There is insufficient information available about the use of azelastine in human pregnancy and lactation, therefore as with all medicines caution should be exercised when using Optilast during pregnancy and lactation.

Effects on ability to drive and use machines: None.

Undesirable effects: Occasionally, a mild, transient irritation in the eye after application of Optilast is experienced. Less frequently reported is a bitter taste.

Overdose: No specific reactions after ocular overdosage are known, and with the ocular route of administration, overdosage reactions are not anticipated.

Pharmacological properties

Pharmacodynamic properties: Azelastine, a phthalazinone derivative of novel structure is classified as a potent long-acting anti-allergic compound with particularly strong, selective H_1 antagonist properties. An additional anti-inflammatory effect could be detected after topical ocular administration (higher local concentrations).

Data from in vivo (pre-clinical) and in vitro studies show that azelastine inhibits the synthesis or release of the chemical mediators known to be involved in early and late stage allergic reactions e.g. leukotriene, histamine, PAF inhibitors and serotonin.

To date, long term therapy ECG evaluations of

patients treated with high oral doses of azelastine, have shown that in multiple dose studies, there is no clinically significant effect of azelastine on the corrected QT (QTc) interval.

No association of azelastine with ventricular arrhythmia or torsade de pointes was observed in over 3700 patients treated with oral azelastine.

Pharmacokinetic properties

General characteristics (systemic pharmacokinetics): Following oral administration azelastine is rapidly absorbed showing an absolute bioavailability of 81%. Food has no influence on absorption. The volume of distribution is high indicating distribution predominantly into the periphery. The level of protein binding is relatively low (80–90%, a level too low to give concern over drug displacement reactions).

Plasma elimination half-lives after a single dose of azelastine are approximately 20 hours for azelastine and about 45 hours for the therapeutically active metabolite N-Desmethyl azelastine. Excretion occurs mainly via the faeces. The sustained excretion of small amounts of the dose in the faeces suggests that some entero-hepatic circulation may take place.

Characteristics in patients (ocular pharmacokinetics): After repeated ocular application of Optilast (up to one drop in each eye, four times daily), C_{max} steady state plasma levels of azelastine hydrochloride were very low and were detected at or below the limit of quantification.

Preclinical safety data: Azelastine hydrochloride displayed no sensitising potential in the guinea pig. Azelastine demonstrated no genotoxic potential in a battery of in vitro and in vivo tests, nor any carcinogenic potential in rats or mice.

In male and female rats, azelastine at oral doses greater than 3.0 mg/kg/day caused a dose-related decrease in the fertility index; no substance-related alterations were found in the reproductive organs of males or females during chronic toxicity studies, however. Embryotoxic and teratogenic effects in rats, mice and rabbits occurred only at maternal toxic doses (for example, skeletal malformations were observed in rats and rabbits at doses of 50 mg/kg/day).

Pharmaceutical particulars

List of excipients: Benzalkonium chloride (preservative), disodium edetate, hypromellose, sorbitol, sodium hydroxide and water for injections.

Incompatibilities: None known.

Shelf life: 30 months. Do not use for longer than 4 weeks after first opening.

Special precautions for storage: None.

Nature and contents of container: White 10 ml HDPE bottle with LDPE dropper and HDPE screw cap. Volume of Optilast 6 ml and 10 ml.

Instruction for use/handling: Not relevant.

Marketing authorisation number
PL 8336/0075

Date of (partial) revision of the text
November 1997

RHINOLAST* NASAL SPRAY

Qualitative and quantitative composition Azelastine hydrochloride 0.1% w/v.

Pharmaceutical form Nasal spray.

Clinical particulars

Therapeutic Indications: For the treatment of both seasonal allergic rhinitis (e.g. Hay fever) and perennial allergic rhinitis.

Posology and method of administration: Route of application is topical–nasal mucosa.

Adults: One application (0.14 ml) in each nostril twice daily (0.56 mg of azelastine hydrochloride).

Elderly: There have been no specific studies in the elderly.

Children: For children aged 5 years and older, one application (0.14 ml) in each nostril twice daily (0.56 mg of azelastine hydrochloride).

Contra-indications: Proven allergy against azelastine hydrochloride or benzalkonium chloride.

Special warnings and precautions for use: None.

Interactions with other medicaments and other forms of interaction: No specific interactions have been studied.

Pregnancy and lactation: At high oral doses in animals, 500 times the proposed oral human daily dose, foetal death, growth retardation and an increased incidence of skeletal abnormalities occurred during reproduction toxicity testing. Due to the nasal route of administration and the low dose administered, minimal systemic exposure can be expected. However as with all medicines caution should be exercised with use during pregnancy and lactation.

Effects on ability to drive and use machines: None.

Undesirable effects: Occasionally the nasal mucosa may become irritated (level of incidence 5%). A bitter taste can occur after administration (level of incidence 3%) due to incorrect method of application i.e. head tilting too far backwards.

Overdose: The results of animal studies show that toxic doses can product CNS symptoms, e.g. excitation, tremor, convulsions. Should these occur in humans symptomatic and supportive treatment should be instigated as there is no specific antidote. Gastric lavage is recommended if the overdose is recent.

With the nasal route of administration overdosage reactions are not anticipated.

Pharmacological properties

Pharmacodynamic properties: Azelastine, a phthalazinone derivative of novel structure, is classified as a potent long acting anti-allergic compound with particularly strong H1 antagonist properties.

Data from animal studies show that where high levels of azelastine are achieved both inhibition and release of chemical mediators (e.g. leukotriene, histamine, serotonin) involved in allergic reaction occurs.

Pharmacokinetic properties: After repeated nasal application (0.14 mg) into each nostril twice daily, the plasma levels of azelastine were about 0.26ng/ml. The levels of the active metabolite desmethylazelastine were detected at or below the lower limit of quantification (0.12ng/ml).

After repeated oral administration, the mean C_{max} steady state plasma levels were determined giving 3.9 ng/ml for azelastine and 1.86 ng/ml for desmethylazelastine after 2.2 mg b.i.d. azelastine which represents the therapeutic oral dose for the treatment of allergic rhinitis.

Following oral administration azelastine is rapidly absorbed showing an absolute bioavailability of 81%. Food has no influence on absorption. The volume of distribution is high indicating distribution predominantly to the peripheral tissues. The level of protein binding is low, (80-95% a level too low to give concern over drug displacement reactions).

Plasma elimination half lives after a single dose of azelastine are approximately 20 hours for azelastine and about 45 hours for N desmethylazelastine (a therapeutically active metabolite). Excretion occurs mainly via the faeces. The sustained excretion of small amounts of the dose in the faeces suggest that some enterohepatic circulation may take place.

Preclinical safety data: Not relevant.

Pharmaceutical particulars

List of excipients: Methylhydroxypropyl cellulose, sodium edetate, benzalkonium chloride, citric acid, sodium phosphate, sodium chloride, purified water.

Incompatibilities: None.

Shelf life: Three years unopened.

Special precautions for storage: Do not store below 8°C. Do not refrigerate.

Nature and contents of container:

10 ml or 20 ml polyethylene bottle with polypropylene cap and polyethylene seal.

10 ml or 20 ml glass bottle with screw closure and polypropylene seal.

10 ml or 20 ml glass bottle with pump attached.

10 ml glass bottle with pump attached, containing 5 ml aqueous solution.

10 ml polyethylene bottle with polypropylene cap and polyethylene seal, containing 5 ml aqueous solution.

Instruction for use/handling:

For separate bottle and pump: Open the bottle by unscrewing the cap. Place the spray pump nozzle in the bottle and screw the pump onto the bottle. Remove the protective cap. Before first using, squeeze down the collar several times until an even spray emerges. The Rhinolast spray is now ready to use.

For attached pump and bottle: Remove the protective cap. Before first using, squeeze down the collar several times until an even spray emerges. The Rhinolast spray is now ready to use.

Marketing authorisation number 8336/0039

Date of approval/revision of SPC July 1996.

Legal category POM.

UROMITEXAN* INJECTION

Presentation Clear, glass ampoules containing a clear, colourless, aqueous solution of mesna (sodium 2-mercapto-ethanesulphonate) 400 mg in 4 ml and 1000 mg in 10 ml.

Uses

Action: Mesna is a sulphydryl-containing compound which is excreted in the urine. Co-administration with oxazaphosphorine alkylating agents such as ifosfamide (Mitoxana) and cyclophosphamide (Endoxana) significantly reduces their urotoxic effects by reacting with the causal metabolites, including acrolein, in the urinary system. No reduction in the antitumour activity of these oxazaphosphorine compounds has been detected.

Indications: For the prophylaxis of urothelial toxicity including haemorrhagic cystitis, microhaematuria and macrohaematuria in patients treated with ifosfamide or cyclophosphamide, in doses considered to be urotoxic.

Dosage and administration

Dosage: Sufficient mesna must be given to protect the patient adequately from the urotoxic effects of the oxazaphosphorine. The duration of mesna treatment should equal that of the oxazaphosphorine treatment plus the time taken for the urinary concentration of metabolites to fall to non-toxic levels. This usually occurs within 8-12 hours after the end of oxazaphosphorine treatment but may vary depending on the scheduling of the oxazaphosphorine. Urinary output should be maintained at 100 ml/hr (as required for oxazaphosphorine treatment) and the urine monitored for haematuria and proteinuria throughout the treatment period.

Intravenous usage of mesna

Where ifosfamide or cyclophosphamide is used as an iv bolus: Mesna is given by intravenous injection over 15-30 minutes at 20% of the simultaneously administered oxazaphosphorine on a weight for weight basis (w/w). The same dose of mesna is repeated after 4 and 8 hours. The total dose of mesna is 60% (w/w) of the oxazaphosphorine dose. This is repeated on each occasion that the cytotoxic agents are used.

e.g.

	0 hrs	*4 hrs*	*8 hrs*
Mitoxana/Endoxana	2 g	-	-
Uromitexan	400 mg	400 mg	400 mg

If necessary the dose of mesna can be increased to 40% of the oxazaphosphorine dose given four times at three hourly intervals (0, 3, 6 and 9 hours). (Total dose = 160% (w/w) of the oxazaphosphorine dose). This larger dose is recommended in children, or in patients whose urothelium may be damaged from previous treatment with oxazaphosphorine or pelvic irradiation, or in patients who are not adequately protected by the standard dose of mesna.

e.g.

	0 hrs	*3 hrs*	*6 hrs*	*9 hrs*
Mitoxana/Endoxana	2 g	-	-	-
Uromitexan	800 mg	800 mg	800 mg	800 mg

Where cyclophosphamide is used orally: The same dose regimen of mesna applies as though cyclophosphamide were used as an iv bolus.

Where ifosfamide is used as a 24-hour infusion: Mesna can be used as a concurrent infusion. An initial 20% (w/w) of the total ifosfamide dose is given as an i.v. bolus, then an infusion of 100% (w/w) of the ifosfamide over 24 hours, followed by a further 12-hour infusion of 60% (w/w) of the ifosfamide dose. (Total mesna dose = 180% of the ifosfamide dose) (see Table 1).

The final 12-hour infusion of mesna after 24 hour infusion of ifosfamide and mesna, can be replaced by boluses at 28, 32 and 36 hours, each of 20% (w/w) of the 24 hour ifosfamide dose, or by oral mesna.

Where ifosfamide is used as a long-term infusion: Mesna is given initially as an i.v. bolus of 20% (w/w) of the first 24-hour ifosfamide infusion dose as the infusion starts, then as concurrent infusions of 100% (w/w) of the daily ifosfamide dose. This is followed by a further 12-hour infusion of 60% (w/w) of the *final 24 hour* dose (see Table 2).

As above, the final 12-hour infusion of mesna, after long-term infusion of ifosfamide and mesna, can be replaced by boluses each of 20% (w/w) of the 24 hour ifosfamide dose, or by oral mesna.

Mesna can be mixed in the same infusion bag as the ifosfamide.

Oral use of mesna ampoules: Mesna has been shown to be effective when taken orally. Compared with intravenous administration, overall availability of mesna in urine after oral administration is approximately 50%; the onset of urinary excretion is delayed by up to 2 hours and is more prolonged than following intravenous dosing.

For intermittent oxazaphosphorine therapy, oral mesna 40% (w/w) of the oxazaphosphorine dose should be given 2 hours prior to the oxazaphosphorine

Table 1: Where ifosfamide is used as a 24-hour infusion

	0 hrs	0-24 hrs	24 hrs	28 hrs	32 hrs	36 hrs
Mitoxana	-	5 g/m² infusion	-	-	-	-
Uromitexan	1 g/m² iv	5 g/m² infusion	← 3 g/m² infusion →			
				1 g/m² iv	1 g/m² iv	1 g/m² iv

Table 2: Where ifosfamide is used as a long-term infusion

	Day 1		Day 2	Day 3		Day 4		
	0 hrs	0-24 hrs	0-24 hrs	0-24 hrs	24 hrs	4 hrs	8 hrs	12 hrs
Mitoxana	-	2 g/m² infusion	2 g/m² infusion	2 g/m² infusion	-	-	-	-
Uromitexan	0.4 g/m² iv	2 g/m² infusion	2 g/m² infusion	2 g/m² infusion	← 1.2 g/m² → infusion			
						0.4 g/m² iv	0.4 g/m² iv	0.4 g/m² iv

dose, and repeated at 2 and 6 hours. Alternatively, an initial intravenous dose of mesna 20% (w/w) of the oxazaphosphorine dose could be given with the cytotoxic dose. Additional oral mesna 40% (w/w) of the oxazaphosphorine dose can then be given at 2 and 6 hours.

e.g.

	-2 hrs	0 hrs	2 hrs	6 hrs
Mitoxana/Endoxana	-	1 g iv	-	-
Uromitexan	400 mg po	-	400 mg po	400 mg po
		200 mg iv	400 mg po	400 mg po

Oral mesna may also be used following a 24-hour infusion of ifosfamide and mesna. The first dose of 40% (w/w) of the ifosfamide is given as the infusion is stopped, and repeated after 2 and 6 hours.

e.g.

	0 hrs	0-24 hrs	24 hrs	26 hrs	30 hrs
Mitoxana	-	5 g/m² infusion	-	-	-
Uromitexan	1 g/m² iv	5 g/m² infusion	2 g/m² po	2 g/m² po	2 g/m² po

If mesna is to be taken orally, it should be added to a flavoured drink such as orange juice or cola. This may be stored in the refrigerator for up to 24 hours in a sealed container.

Mesna tablets are also available for oral administration. The dose of mesna tablets is the same as for oral use of mesna injection outlined above. Further information on the use of mesna tablets can be found on a separate datasheet or from ASTA Medica Ltd.

Elderly: No specific information on the use of this product in the elderly is available. Clinical trials have included patients over 65 years and no adverse reactions specific to this age group have been reported.

Children: Because of greater frequency of micturition, children may require shorter intervals between doses. (e.g. 3 hourly, see above, under *Dosage*)

Contra-indications, warnings, etc

Contra-indications: Known hypersensitivity to mesna or any thiol containing compounds.

Use in pregnancy and lactation: Pregnancy and lactation are contraindications for cytostatic treatment and consequently Uromitexan is not likely to be used under these circumstances.

Should an individual patient be undergoing oxazaphosphorine therapy during pregnancy then Uromitexan should be administered to this patient.

Animal studies have shown no evidence of embryotoxic or teratogenic effects of Uromitexan.

Precautions: As mesna counteracts only the urotoxic side-effects of oxazaphosphorines, other side-effects of cytotoxic therapy e.g. myelosuppression, nausea, vomiting, alopecia, may still be expected. No other interaction between mesna and these alkylating agents has been demonstrated.

The prevention of urotoxicity with Uromitexan should only be undertaken after medical guidance and careful consideration of the risks and benefits.

Interactions: There are no known in vivo interactions of mesna with other agents.

Side-effects: Because patients receive potent cytotoxic agents concurrently, the side-effect profile of mesna is difficult to define. However, in healthy volunteers the following side-effects occurred at single doses of 60-70 mg/kg per day: nausea, vomiting, colic, diarrhoea, headache, fatigue, limb and joint pains, depression, irritability, lack of energy, rash, hypotension and tachycardia.

In rare cases, pseudoallergic reactions (rash, pruritus, blistering of skin and mucous membranes, fever, urticarial oedema, sudden hypotension and tachycardia and a transient rise of liver transaminases) have been reported. These pseudoallergic reactions appear to be more common in patients with autoimmune disorders.

Overdosage: Healthy volunteers given single bolus doses of 70 mg/kg mesna showed no evidence of major toxic side-effects. A specific antidote to mesna is not known.

Pharmaceutical precautions Protect from light, store below 30°C.

Mesna is chemically compatible with 0.9% saline for 24 hours. Mesna and ifosfamide are chemically compatible with 0.9% saline for 24 hours

Mesna is incompatible with platinum derivatives and nitrogen mustard and must not be mixed in the same infusion solution.

Legal category POM.

Package quantities
4 ml ampoules in boxes of 15.
10 ml ampoules in boxes of 15.

Further information There is evidence that the long-term urothelial toxicity of the oxazaphosphorines can be almost totally prevented by the concurrent administration of mesna in the appropriate dosage. Mesna only exerts this protective effect on the urinary tract and other precautionary measures recommended for the use of oxazaphosphorines are not affected and should continue to be used. A false positive test of urinary ketones (e.g. Rothera's test, N-Multistix reagent strip) may arise in patients treated with mesna. The colour is red-violet rather than violet and it will fade immediately on the addition of glacial acetic acid. A false negative or false positive reaction in the dipstick tests for erythrocytes in the urine of patients treated with mesna may occur, therefore use of urinary microscopy is recommended.

Product licence numbers
4 ml ampoules Uromitexan
Injection 400 mg 8336/0033
10 ml ampoules Uromitexan
Injection 1 g 8336/0033

UROMITEXAN TABLETS*

Presentation White, oblong biconvex film-coated tablets containing 400 mg and 600 mg of mesna (sodium 2-mercaptoethanesulphonate).

Uses

Action: Mesna is a sulphydryl-containing compound which is excreted in the urine. Co-administration with oxazaphosphorine alkylating agents such as ifosfamide (Mitoxana) and cyclophosphamide (Endoxana) significantly reduces their urotoxic effects by reacting with the causal metabolites, including acrolein, in the urinary system. No reduction in the antitumour activity of these oxazaphosphorine compounds has been detected.

Indications: For the prophylaxis of urothelial toxicity including haemorrhagic cystitis, microhaematuria and macrohaematuria in patients treated with ifosfamide and cyclophosphamide, in doses considered to be urotoxic.

Dosage and administration

Dosage: Sufficient Uromitexan must be given to protect the patient adequately from the urotoxic effects of the oxazaphosphorine. The duration of Uromitexan treatment should equal that of the oxazaphosphorine treatment plus the time taken for the urinary concentration of oxazaphosphorine metabolites to fall to non-toxic levels. This usually occurs within 8-12 hours after the end of oxazaphosphorine treatment but may vary depending on the scheduling of oxazaphosphorine. When calculating the dose of Uromitexan the quantity should be rounded down to the nearest whole tablet. Urinary output should be maintained at 100 ml/hr (as required for oxazaphosphorine treatment) and the urine monitored for haematuria and proteinuria throughout the treatment period.

Compared with intravenous administration, overall availability of mesna in urine after oral administration is approximately 50%; and the onset of urinary excretion is delayed by up to 2 hours and is more prolonged than following intravenous dosing.

For intermittent oxazaphosphorine therapy: oral mesna 40% (w/w) of the oxazaphosphorine dose should be given 2 hours prior to, and repeated 2 hours and 6 hours after the oxazaphosphorine dose. Alternatively, an initial intravenous dose of mesna (20% (w/w) of the oxazaphosphorine dose) can be given with the cytotoxic dose, additional oral mesna 40% (w/w) of the oxazaphosphorine dose should then be given at 2 and 6 hours.

e.g.

	-2 hrs	0 hrs	2 hrs	6 hrs
Cyclophosphamide/ Ifosfamide	-	1 g iv	-	-
Uromitexan	400 mg po	-	400 mg po	400 mg po
		200 mg iv	400 mg po	400 mg po

Following 24-hour infusion of ifosfamide and Uromitexan: the first oral Uromitexan dose of 40% (w/w) of the ifosfamide dose is given as the infusion is stopped, and the same dose is repeated at 2 and 6 hours.

e.g.

	0 hrs	0-24 hrs	24 hrs	26 hrs	30 hrs
Ifosfamide	-	5 g/m² infusion	-	-	-
Uromitexan	1 g/m² iv	5 g/m² infusion	2 g/m² po	2 g/m² po	2 g/m²

Following long-term infusion: the first oral Uromitexan dose should be 40% (w/w) of the ifosfamide dose taken in the FINAL 24 HOURS, and is given as the infusion is stopped and the same dose repeated at 2 and 6 hours (see Table 1).

Higher doses of Uromitexan can be given if urothelial toxicity occurs.

Elderly: No specific information on the use of this product in the elderly is available. Clinical trials have included patients over 65 years and no adverse reactions specific to this age group have been reported.

Children: Due to increased micturition, children may require shorter intervals between doses and/or an increased number of individual doses.

High risk patients: Those who have had previous irradiation of the small pelvis, occurrence of cystitis during previous cyclophosphamide, ifosfamide or trofosfamide therapy, history of urinary tract lesions, may also require shorter intervals between doses and/ or an increased number of doses.

Contra-indications, warnings, etc

Contra-indications: Known hypersensitivity to mesna or any thiol containing compounds.

Use in pregnancy and lactation: Cytostatic treatment is contra-indicated during pregnancy and lactation, and consequently Uromitexan is not likely to be used under these circumstances.

Should an individual patient be undergoing oxazaphosphorine therapy during pregnancy then Uromitexan should be administered to this patient.

Animal studies have shown no evidence of embryotoxic or teratogenic effects of Uromitexan.

Precautions: As Uromitexan counteracts only the urotoxic side-effects of oxazaphosphorines, other side-effects of cytotoxic therapy eg myelosuppression, nausea, vomiting, alopecia, may still be expected. No other interaction between Uromitexan and these alkylating agents has been demonstrated.

Oral Uromitexan should be replaced by i.v. Uromitexan in patients experiencing vomiting.

The prevention of urotoxicity with Uromitexan tablets should only be undertaken after medical guidance and careful consideration of the risks and benefits.

Interactions: There are no known in-vivo interactions of Uromitexan with other agents. There is no interaction with food.

Table 1: Following long-term infusion

	Day 1		Day 2	Day 3		Day 4	
	0 hrs	0-24 hrs	0-24 hrs	0-24 hrs	24 hrs	26 hrs	30 hrs
Ifosfamide	-	2 g/m² infusion	2 g/m² infusion	2 g/m² infusion	-	-	-
Uromitexan	0.4 g/m² iv	2 g/m² infusion	2 g/m² infusion	2 g/m² infusion	0.8 g/m² po	0.8 g/m² po	0.8 g/m² po

Side effects: Because patients receive potent cytotoxic agents concurrently, the side-effect profile of Uromitexan is difficult to define. However, in healthy volunteers the following side effects occurred at single doses of 60-70 mg/kg per day: nausea, vomiting, colic, diarrhoea, headache, fatigue, limb and joint pains, depression, irritability, lack of energy, rash, hypotension and tachycardia.

In rare cases, pseudoallergic reactions (rash, pruritus, blistering of skin and mucous membranes, urticarial oedema, sudden hypotension, tachycardia and a transient rise of liver transaminases) have been reported. These pseudoallergic reactions appear to be more common in patients with autoimmune disorders.

Overdosage: Healthy volunteers given single bolus doses of 70 mg/kg Uromitexan showed no evidence of major toxic side-effects.

A specific antidote to Uromitexan is not known.

Pharmaceutical precautions None necessary.

Legal category POM.

Package quantities Ten tablets in a blister strip. Pack size–10 tablets.

Further information There is evidence that the long term urothelial toxicity of the oxazaphosphorines can be almost totally prevented by the concurrent administration of Uromitexan in the appropriate dosage. Uromitexan only exerts this protective effect on the urinary tract and other precautionary measures recommended for the use of oxazaphosphorine are not affected and should continue to be used.

A false positive test for urinary ketones (eg Rothera's test, N-Multistix reagent strip) may arise in patients treated with Uromitexan. The colour is red-violet rather than violet and it will fade immediately on the addition of glacial acetic acid.

A false positive or false negative reaction in the dipstick test for erythrocytes in the urine of patients treated with Uromitexan may occur, therefore use of urinary microscopy is recommended.

Product licence numbers
400 mg film coated tablets 8336/0049
600 mg film coated tablets 8336/0050

ZAMADOL* CAPSULES 50 mg ▼

Qualitative and quantitative composition
Tramadol hydrochloride 50 mg

Pharmaceutical form Hard gelatin capsules.

Clinical particulars
Therapeutic indications: For the treatment and prevention of moderate to severe pain.

Posology and method of administration: The capsules are for oral administration. As with all analgesic drugs the dosing of Zamadol Capsules 50 mg should be adjusted depending on the severity of the pain and the individual clinical response of the patient.
Adults: For acute pain–an initial dose of 100 mg is usually necessary. This can be followed by doses of 50 mg or 100 mg not more frequently than 4 hourly, and duration of therapy should be matched to clinical need.

For pain associated with chronic conditions–use in an initial dose of 50 mg and then titrate dose according to pain severity. The need for continued treatment should be assessed at regular intervals as withdrawal symptoms and dependence have been reported, although rarely (See *Special Warnings and Precautions for Use* section).

A total oral daily dose of over 400 mg should not be exceeded except in special clinical circumstances.
Elderly patients: Dosing as for adults but it should be noted that in a study in elderly volunteers (aged over 75 years) the elimination half-life for orally administered tramadol was increased by 17%.
Patients with renal insufficiency: The usual initial adult doses should be employed, but the elimination of tramadol may be prolonged in patients with renal impairment and therefore the dosage interval should be adjusted.

For creatinine clearance <30 ml/min the dosing should be increased to 12 hourly intervals.

For creatinine clearance <10 ml/min (severe renal impairment) tramadol is not recommended.

Tramadol is removed very slowly by haemodialysis or haemofiltration and therefore post-dialysis dosing to maintain analgesia is usually unnecessary.

Patients with hepatic insufficiency: The usual adult doses should be used, but it should be noted that elimination of tramadol may be prolonged in severe hepatic impairment and dosing should be at 12 hourly intervals.

Children: Over 12 years: Dosage as for adults. Under 12 years : Not recommended for children under 12 years

Contra-indications: Zamadol Capsules 50 mg should not be given to patients who have previously shown hypersensitivity to the product.

The product should not be administered to patients suffering from acute intoxication with hypnotics, centrally acting analgesics, opioids, psychotropic drugs or alcohol.

In common with other opioid analgesics, tramadol should not be administered to patients who are receiving monoamine oxidase inhibitors or within 2 weeks of their withdrawal.

Special warnings and precautions for use
Warnings: At therapeutic doses, tramadol has the potential to cause withdrawal symptoms. Rarely cases of dependence and abuse have been reported.

At therapeutic doses withdrawal symptoms have been reported at a reporting frequency of 1 in 8,000. Reports of dependence and abuse have been less frequent. Because of this potential the clinical need for continued analgesic treatment should be reviewed regularly.

In patients with a tendency to drug abuse or dependence, treatment should be for short periods and under strict medical supervision.

Zamadol Capsules 50 mg are not a suitable substitute in opioid dependent patients. The product does not suppress morphine withdrawal symptoms although it is an opioid agonist.

Convulsions have been reported at therapeutic doses and the risk may be increased at doses exceeding the usual upper daily dose limit. Patients with a history of epilepsy or those susceptible to seizures should only be treated with tramadol if there are compelling reasons. The risk of convulsions may increase in patients taking tramadol and concomitant medication that can lower the seizure threshold (see *Interactions* section).

Precautions: In patients with severe renal or hepatic impairment, head injury, increased intracranial pressure, or patients in shock or at risk of convulsions, Zamadol Capsules 50 mg should be used with caution.

At present Zamadol Capsules 50 mg should not be used during light planes of anaesthesia as enhanced intra-operative recall was reported in a study of the use of tramadol during anaesthesia with enflurane and nitrous oxide.

At therapeutic doses of tramadol respiratory depression has been reported infrequently. Therefore care should be taken when administering Zamadol Capsules 50 mg to patients with existing respiratory depression or to patients taking concomitant CNS depressant drugs.

Interaction with other medicaments and other forms of interaction: Zamadol Capsules 50 mg may potentiate the CNS depressant effects of other centrally acting drugs (including alcohol) when administered concomitantly with such drugs.

Tramadol may increase the potential for both selective serotonin re-uptake inhibitors (SSRIs) and tricyclic antidepressants (TCAs) to cause convulsions (See *Special Warnings and Precautions* and *Pharmacokinetic Properties* sections).

Administration of Zamadol Capsules 50 mg together with carbamazepine results in markedly decreased serum concentrations of tramadol which may reduce analgesic effectiveness and shorten the duration of action.

Changes in serum concentrations of tramadol have been associated with the simultaneous dosing of cimetidine. However, such changes are clinically insignificant and therefore no dosage adjustment for Zamadol Capsules 50 mg is recommended in patients receiving chronic cimetidine therapy.

Theoretically, tramadol could interact with noradrenaline, 5-HT or lithium, due to their mechanisms of action, and thus potentiate their anti-depressant effect. However there have been no reports of such interactions.

Pregnancy and lactation
Pregnancy: Zamadol Capsules 50 mg should not be used in pregnancy as there is inadequate evidence available to assess the safety of tramadol in pregnant women.

Studies of tramadol in rats and rabbits have revealed no teratogenic effects. However, embryotoxicity was shown in the form of delayed ossification. Fertility, reproductive performance and development of offspring were unaffected.

Lactation: Zamadol Capsules 50 mg should not be administered during breast feeding as tramadol and its metabolites have been detected in breast milk. An infant could ingest 0.1% of the dose administered to the mother.

Effects on ability to drive and use machines: Zamadol Capsules 50 mg may cause drowsiness and this effect may be potentiated by alcohol and other CNS depressants. Patients should be warned not to drive or operate machinery if affected.

Undesirable effects: Somnolence, fatigue, dizziness, headache, confusion, constipation, pruritis, urticaria, skin rashes, hallucinations, dysphoria and infrequently respiratory depression have been reported.

Dependence, abuse and withdrawal reactions have been reported. Typical opiate withdrawal reactions include agitation, anxiety, nervousness, insomnia, hyperkinesia, tremor and gastro-intestinal symptoms (see *Posology and Method of Administration* and *Special Warnings and Precautions* sections).

Convulsions have been reported rarely (see *Interactions* section).

Tachycardia, bradycardia, increase in blood pressure, orthostatic hypotension, syncope, anaphylaxis, flushing and diaphoresis have rarely been reported. There have been rare cases of blood dyscrasias observed with tramadol treatment but direct causality has not been confirmed.

Nausea, vomiting and occasionally dry mouth have been reported. Allergy to tramadol is characterised by dyspnoea, wheezing, bronchospasm and a worsening of existing asthma.

Overdose: Symptoms of tramadol overdose include vomiting, miosis, sedation, coma, seizures, cardiovascular collapse and respiratory depression. Such symptoms are typical of opioid analgesics.

Treatment of overdose requires the maintenance of the airway and cardiovascular functions. Respiratory depression may be reversed using naloxone and fits controlled with diazepam.

The treatment of acute overdose of tramadol using haemodialysis or haemofiltration alone is not sufficient or suitable due to the slow elimination of tramadol from the serum by these routes.

Pharmacological properties
Pharmacodynamic properties: Tramadol, a cyclohexanol derivative, is a centrally acting analgesic which possesses opioid agonist properties. Tramadol appears to modify the transmission of pain impulses by inhibition of monoamine reuptake. The duration of analgesia with orally administered tramadol has been shown to be 3-6 hours with maximum pain relief at 1-4 hours post-dosing. Tramadol also has an antitussive action but has no effect on gastrointestinal motility. At the recommended dosages, the effects of tramadol given orally on the respiratory and cardiovascular systems appear to be clinically insignificant.

Pharmacokinetic properties
General: Following oral dosing, tramadol is rapidly and almost completely absorbed. After oral administration as capsules or tablets, tramadol appears in the plasma within 15-45 minutes, reaching peak plasma concentrations at a mean of 2 hours. The mean oral bioavailability of tramadol is approximately 68% after single doses and increases to 90 to 100% on multiple administration.

The half-life of absorption for oral tramadol (solid dose formulation) is 0.38 ± 0.18 hours with a peak plasma concentration of 280 ± 49 ng/ml 2 hours after oral dosing with 100 mg tramadol (solid dose formulation). Tramadol has a high tissue affinity with an apparent volume of distribution of 306 litres after oral dosing in healthy volunteers.

Tramadol undergoes hepatic metabolism with approximately 85% of an oral dose being metabolised in young healthy volunteers. Tramadol is biotransformed primarily by N- and O-demethylation and by glucuronidation of the O-demethylation products. Eleven metabolites have so far been identified in man.

Only one metabolite, O-demethyl tramadol (M1), is pharmacologically active showing analgesic activity.

The mean elimination half-life of tramadol following oral administration is 5-6 hours. Approximately 90% of an oral dose is excreted by the kidneys.

Characteristics in patients: Effect of age: Tramadol

pharmacokinetics show little age-dependence in volunteers up to the age of 75 years. In volunteers aged over 75 years, the terminal elimination half-life was 7.0 ± 1.6 h compared to 6.0 ± 1.5 h in young volunteers after oral administration.

Effect of hepatic or renal impairment: As both tramadol and its pharmacologically active metabolite, O-demethyl tramadol, are eliminated both metabolically and renally, the terminal half-life of elimination ($t_{\frac{1}{2}}$) may be prolonged in patients with hepatic or renal dysfunction. However, the increase in $t_{\frac{1}{2}}$ is relatively small if either excretory organ is functioning normally. In liver cirrhosis patients, the mean $t_{\frac{1}{2}}$ of tramadol was 13.3 ± 4.9 hours. In patients with renal failure (creatinine clearance < 5 mL/min) the $t_{\frac{1}{2}}$ of tramadol was 11.0 ± 3.2 hours and that of M1 was 16.9 ± 3.0 hours. Extreme values observed to date are 22.3 hours (tramadol) and 36.0 hours (M1) in liver cirrhosis patients and 19.5 hours (tramadol) and 43.2 hours (M1) in renal failure patients.

Preclinical Safety Data: The standard range of pharmacodynamic, pharmacokinetic and toxicological tests have been carried out for Tramadol and the effects observed from these investigations that are relevant to the prescriber are mentioned in other sections.

Pharmaceutical particulars

List of excipients: Capsule Contents: Dibasic calcium phosphate anhydrous, magnesium stearate, colloidal anhydrous silica.

Capsule Shell: Gelatin, titanium dioxide (E171)

Incompatibilities: No pharmaceutical incompatibilities reported.

Shelf-life: Two years, as packaged for sale.

Special precautions for storage: No special requirements.

Nature and contents of container: White opaque PVC/PVDC and aluminium foil blister strips. Each strip contains 10 capsules. The blister strips are packed in cartons containing 100 capsules.

Instructions for use/handling: None.

Marketing authorisation number PL 8336/0061

Date of (partial) revision of the text 19 March 1997

ZAMADOL* INJECTION ▼

Qualitative and quantitative composition Tramadol hydrochloride 50 mg/ml of injection solution (100 mg per ampoule)

Pharmaceutical form Clear, colourless sterile solution for injection. Zamadol Injection has an osmolarity of 320-380 mOsmol, whereas normal serum is 285-290 mOsmol. Zamadol Injection therefore is slightly hypertonic.

Clinical particulars

Therapeutic Indications: For the treatment and prevention of moderate to severe pain.

Posology and method of administration: The injection is for parenteral administration either intramuscularly, by slow intravenous injection or, when diluted in solution, by infusion or patient controlled analgesia. As with all analgesic drugs the dosing of Zamadol Injection should be adjusted depending on the severity of the pain and the individual clinical response of the patient.

Adults: A dose of 50 or 100 mg 4-6 hourly is usually required. Intravenous injections must be given slowly over 2-3 minutes.

In post-operative pain, an initial bolus of 100 mg is administered. For the 60 minutes following this initial bolus, 50 mg doses may be given every 10-20 minutes up to a total dose of 250 mg including the initial bolus.

Subsequent doses should be 50 or 100 mg 4-6 hourly up to a total daily dose of 600 mg.

A total parenteral daily dose of over 600 mg should not be exceeded except in special circumstances.

Elderly patients: Dosing as for adults but it should be noted that in a study in elderly volunteers (aged over 75 years) the elimination half-life for orally administered tramadol was increased by 17%.

Patients with renal insufficiency/renal dialysis: As the elimination of tramadol may be prolonged in patients with renal impairment, the usual initial adult doses should be employed, but the dosage interval should be adjusted.

For creatinine clearance <30 ml/min the dosing should be increased to 12 hourly intervals.

For creatinine clearance <10 ml/min (severe renal impairment) tramadol is not recommended.

Tramadol is removed very slowly by haemodialysis or haemofiltration and therefore post dialysis dosing to maintain analgesia is usually unnecessary.

Patients with hepatic insufficiency: It should be noted that as the elimination of tramadol may be prolonged in severe hepatic impairment, although the usual initial adult doses should be used, dosing should be at 12 hourly intervals.

Children: Over 12 years: Dosage as for adults. Under 12 years : Not recommended for children under 12 years

Contra-indications: Zamadol Injection should not be given to patients who have previously shown hypersensitivity to the product.

The product should not be administered to patients suffering from acute intoxication with hypnotics, centrally acting analgesics, opioids, psychotropic drugs or alcohol.

In common with other opioid analgesics, tramadol should not be administered to patients who are receiving monoamine oxidase inhibitors or within 2 weeks of their withdrawal.

Special warnings and precautions for use:
Warnings: At therapeutic doses, tramadol has the potential to cause withdrawal symptoms.

Rarely cases of dependence and abuse have been reported.

At therapeutic doses withdrawal symptoms have been reported at a reporting frequency of 1 in 8,000. Reports of dependence and abuse have been less frequent. Because of this potential the clinical need for continued analgesic treatment should be reviewed regularly.

In patients with a tendency to drug abuse or dependence, treatment should be for short periods and under strict medical supervision.

Zamadol Injection is not a suitable substitute in opioid dependent patients. The product does not suppress morphine withdrawal symptoms although it is an opioid agonist.

Convulsions have been reported at therapeutic doses and the risk may be increased at doses exceeding the usual upper daily dose limit. Patients with a history of epilepsy or those susceptible to seizures should only be treated with tramadol if there are compelling reasons. The risk of convulsions may increase in patients taking tramadol and concomitant medication that can lower the seizure threshold (see *Interactions* section).

Precautions: In patients with severe renal or hepatic impairment, head injury, increased intracranial pressure, or patients in shock or at risk of convulsions, Zamadol Injection should be used with caution.

At present Zamadol Injection should not be used during light planes of anaesthesia as enhanced intra-operative recall was reported in a study of the use of tramadol during anaesthesia with enflurane and nitrous oxide.

At therapeutic doses of tramadol respiratory depression has been reported infrequently. Therefore care should be taken when administering Zamadol Injection to patients with existing respiratory depression or to patients taking concomitant CNS depressant drugs.

Interaction with other medicaments and other forms of interaction: Zamadol Injection may potentiate the CNS depressant effects of other centrally acting drugs (including alcohol) when administered concomitantly with such drugs.

Tramadol may increase the potential for both selective serotonin re-uptake inhibitors (SSRIs) and tricyclic antidepressants (TCAs) to cause convulsions (See *Special Warnings and Precautions for Use* and *Pharmacokinetic Properties* sections).

Administration of Zamadol Injection together with carbamazepine results in markedly decreased serum concentrations of tramadol which may reduce analgesic effectiveness and shorten the duration of action.

Changes in serum concentrations of tramadol have been associated with simultaneous dosing of cimetidine. However, such changes are clinically insignificant and therefore no dosage adjustment for Zamadol Injection is recommended in patients receiving chronic cimetidine therapy.

Theoretically, tramadol could interact with noradrenaline, 5-HT or lithium due to their respective mechanisms of action, and thus potentiate the antidepressant effect of lithium. However there have been no reports of such interactions.

Pregnancy and lactation
Pregnancy: Zamadol Injection should not be used throughout pregnancy as there is inadequate evidence available to assess the safety of tramadol in pregnant women. Studies of tramadol in rats and rabbits have revealed no teratogenic effects. However, embryo toxicity was shown in the form of delayed ossification. Fertility, reproductive performance and development of offspring were unaffected.

Lactation: Zamadol Injection should not be administered during breast feeding as tramadol and its metabolites have been detected in breast milk. An infant could ingest 0.1% of the dose administered to the mother.

Effects on ability to drive and use machines: Zamadol Injection may cause drowsiness and this effect may be potentiated by alcohol and other CNS depressants. Patients
should be warned not to drive or operate machinery if affected.

Undesirable effects: Somnolence, fatigue, dizziness, headache, confusion, constipation, pruritis, urticaria, skin rashes, hallucinations, dysphoria and infrequently respiratory depression have been reported.

Dependence, abuse and withdrawal reactions have been reported. Typical opiate withdrawal reactions include agitation, anxiety, nervousness, insomnia, hyperkinesia, tremor and gastro-intestinal symptoms (see *Posology and Method of Administration* and *Special Warnings and Precautions for Use* sections).

Convulsions have been reported rarely (see *Interactions* section). Tachycardia, bradycardia, increase in blood pressure, orthostatic hypotension, syncope, anaphylaxis, flushing and diaphoresis have rarely been reported. There have been rare cases of blood dyscrasias observed with tramadol treatment but direct causality has not been confirmed. Nausea, vomiting and occasionally dry mouth have been reported. Allergy to tramadol is characterised by dyspnoea, wheezing, bronchospasm and a worsening of existing asthma.

Overdose: Symptoms of tramadol overdose include vomiting, miosis, sedation, coma, seizures, cardiovascular collapse and respiratory depression. Such symptoms are typical of Opioid analgesics.

Treatment of overdose requires the maintenance of the airway and cardiovascular functions. Respiratory depression may be reversed using naloxone and fits controlled with diazepam.

The treatment of acute overdose of tramadol using haemodialysis or haemofiltration alone is not sufficient or suitable due to the slow elimination of tramadol from the serum by these routes.

Pharmacological properties

Pharmacodynamic properties: Tramadol, a cyclohexanol derivative, is a centrally acting analgesic which possesses Opioid agonist properties. Tramadol appears to modify the transmission of pain impulses by inhibition of monoamine reuptake. The analgesic activity of tramadol has been demonstrated in both animal models and human subjects.

Tramadol also has an antitussive action but has no effect on gastrointestinal motility. At the recommended dosages, the effects of tramadol given parenterally on the respiratory and cardiovascular systems appear to be clinically insignificant.

Pharmacokinetic properties
General: The mean absolute bioavailability after intramuscular administration was found to be 100%.

The distribution of tramadol following intravenous administration is rapid and in two phases with different half-lives of 0.31 ± 0.17 hours (initial rapid phase) and 1.7 ± 0.4 hours (slower phase) respectively.

After intravenous administration of 100 mg tramadol, the serum concentration was 613 ± 221 ng/ml at 15 minutes post dosing and 409 ± 79 ng/ml at 2 hours post dosing. Tramadol has a high tissue affinity with an apparent volume of distribution of 203 L after intravenous dosing in healthy volunteers.

Tramadol undergoes hepatic metabolism with approximately 85% of an intravenous dose being metabolised in young healthy volunteers. Tramadol is biotransformed primarily by N- and O-demethylation and by glucuronidation of the O-demethylation products. Eleven metabolites have so far been identified in man.

Only one metabolite, O-demethyl tramadol (M1), is pharmacologically active showing analgesic activity.

Tramadol is essentially excreted via the kidneys. The mean elimination half-life of tramadol following intravenous administration is 5-6 hours. Total clearance of tramadol was 28.0 L/h following intravenous administration.

Characteristics in patients: Effect of age: Tramadol pharmacokinetics show little age-dependence in volunteers up to the age of 75 years. In volunteers aged over 75 years, the terminal elimination half-life was 7.0 ± 1.6 h compared to 6.0 ± 1.5 h in young volunteers after oral administration.

Effect of hepatic or renal impairment: As both tramadol and its pharmacologically active metabolite, O-demethyl tramadol, are eliminated both metabolically and renally, the terminal half-life of elimination ($t_{\frac{1}{2}}$) may be prolonged in patients with hepatic or renal dysfunction. However, the increase in $t_{\frac{1}{2}}$ is relatively small if either excretory organ is functioning normally. In liver cirrhosis patients, the mean $t_{\frac{1}{2}}$ of tramadol was 13.3 ± 4.9 hours. In patients with renal failure (creatinine clearance < 5 mL/min) the $t_{\frac{1}{2}}$ of tramadol was 11.0 ± 3.2 hours and that of M1 was 16.9 ± 3.0 hours. Extreme values observed to date are 22.3 hours (tramadol) and 36.0 hours (M1) in liver cirrhosis patients and 19.5 hours (tramadol) and 43.2 hours (M1) in renal failure patients.

Preclinical safety data: The standard range of pharmacodynamic, pharmacological and toxicological tests have been carried out for tramadol and the effects observed from these investigations that are relevant to the prescriber are mentioned in other sections.

Pharmaceutical particulars

List of excipients: Sodium acetate, Water for injection, Nitrogen (insert head space gas)

Incompatibilities: Precipitation will occur if Zamadol Injection is mixed in the same syringe with injections of diazepam, diclofenac sodium, indomethacin, midazolam and piroxicam.

Shelf-life: Thirty six months, as packaged for sale.

Special precautions for storage: No special requirements.

Nature and contents of container: A colourless glass ampoule containing 2 ml of injection solution. Ampoules are contained in a pre-fabricated blister strip, (5 ampoules per strip) which is enclosed in a cardboard outer carton. Cartons contain either 5 or 10 ampoules.

Instructions for use/handling: Zamadol Injection is physically and chemically compatible for up to 24 hours with the following infusion solutions: Ringer-Lactate solution, 5% Glucose.

The prepared infusion solution should be made immediately before use.

Marketing authorisation number PL 8336/0066

Date of (partial) revision of the text August 1997

ZAMADOL* SR CAPSULES 50 mg ▼
ZAMADOL* SR CAPSULES 100 mg ▼
ZAMADOL* SR CAPSULES 150 mg ▼
ZAMADOL* SR CAPSULES 200 mg ▼

Qualitative and quantitative composition

Zamadol SR Capsule 50 mg contains 50 mg tramadol hydrochloride; Zamadol SR Capsule 100 mg contains 100 mg tramadol hydrochloride; Zamadol SR Capsule 150 mg contains 150 mg tramadol hydrochloride; Zamadol SR Capsule 200 mg contains 200 mg tramadol hydrochloride

Pharmaceutical form

Prolonged release capsule, hard. 50 mg capsules are dark green, 100 mg capsules are white, 150 mg capsules are dark green and 200 mg capsules are yellow. The capsules are marked T50SR, T100SR, T150SR and T200SR.

Clinical particulars

Therapeutic indications: Treatment of moderate to severe pain.

Posology and method of administration: The capsules are intended for twice daily oral administration and can be taken independently of meal times, swallowed whole with water.

As with all analgesic drugs the dosing of Zamadol SR Capsules should be adjusted depending on the severity of the pain and the individual clinical response of the patient. The dose used should be the lowest dose that provides pain relief.

Adults: The usual initial dose is 50-100 mg twice daily, morning and evening. This dose may be titrated up to 150-200 mg twice daily according to pain severity.

If long-term pain treatment with tramadol is necessary in view of the nature and severity of the illness, then careful and regular monitoring should be carried out (if necessary with breaks in treatment) to establish whether and to what extent further treatment is necessary.

A total oral daily dose of over 400 mg should not be exceeded except in special clinical circumstances.

Elderly patients: Dosing as for adults, however it should be noted that in patients over 75 years there tends to be an increase in absolute bioavailability of 17% and a prolongation of the terminal half-life of tramadol. An adjustment of the dosage or the dose interval may be required.

Patients with renal or hepatic insufficiency: As the elimination of tramadol may be prolonged in patients with severe renal and/or hepatic impairment, the use of Zamadol SR is not recommended. In moderate cases an adjustment of the dosage interval may be required.

Patients who have difficulty in swallowing: Zamadol SR Capsules can be opened, carefully, so that the pellets are deposited on a spoon. The spoon and pellets should be taken into the mouth, followed by a drink of water to rinse the mouth of *all* pellets. The pellets must not be chewed or crushed.

Children: Over 12 years: Dosage as for adults. Under 12 years : Zamadol SR has not been studied in children. Therefore, safety and efficacy have not been established and the product should not be used in children.

Contra-indications: Zamadol SR Capsules should not be given to patients who have previously shown hypersensitivity to tramadol.

The product should not be administered to patients suffering from acute intoxication with hypnotics, centrally acting analgesics, opioids, psychotropic drugs or alcohol.

Tramadol should not be administered to patients who are receiving monoamine oxidase inhibitors or within 2 weeks of their withdrawal.

Tramadol must not be used for narcotic withdrawal treatment.

Special warnings and precautions for use

Warnings: Tramadol has a low dependence potential. On long-term use tolerance, psychic and physical dependence may develop. In patients with a tendency to drug abuse or dependence, treatment should be for short periods under strict medical supervision. In rare cases at therapeutic doses, tramadol has the potential to cause withdrawal symptoms.

Zamadol SR Capsules are not a suitable substitute in opioid dependent patients. The product does not suppress morphine withdrawal symptoms although it is an opioid agonist. Convulsions have been reported at therapeutic doses and the risk may be increased at doses exceeding the usual upper daily dose limit. Patients with a history of epilepsy or those susceptible to seizures should only be treated with tramadol if there are compelling reasons. The risk of convulsions may increase in patients taking tramadol and concomitant medication that can lower the seizure threshold (see section 4.5).

Precautions: Zamadol SR Capsules should be used with prudence in patients who have shown previous hypersensitivity to opiates, and in patients with severe renal or hepatic impairment, head injury, decreased level of consciousness, increased intracranial pressure, or patients in shock or at risk of convulsions.

At recommended therapeutic doses Zamadol SR Capsules are unlikely to produce clinically relevant respiratory depression. Care should however be taken when administering Zamadol SR Capsules to patients with existing respiratory depression or excessive bronchial secretion and in those patients taking concomitant CNS depressant drugs.

Interaction with other medicaments and other forms of interaction: Tramadol should not be administered to patients who are receiving monoamine oxidase inhibitors or within 2 weeks of their withdrawal.

Tramadol may potentiate the CNS depressant effects of other centrally acting drugs (including alcohol) when administered concomitantly with such drugs.

Co-administered Ritonavir may increase serum concentration of tramadol resulting in tramadol toxicity.

Digoxin toxicity has occurred rarely during co-administration of digoxin and tramadol.

Tramadol may increase the potential for selective serotonin re-uptake inhibitors (SSRIs), tricyclic anti-depressants (TCAs), anti-psychotics and other seizure threshold lowering drugs to cause convulsions (See sections 4.4 and 5.2).

Administration of Zamadol SR Capsules together with carbamazepine results in markedly decreased serum concentrations of tramadol which may reduce analgesic effectiveness and shorten the duration of action.

Although changes in serum concentrations of tramadol have been associated with simultaneous dosing of cimetidine, such changes are clinically insignificant and a dose adjustment for Zamadol SR Capsules is not recommended.

Drugs such as ketoconazole and erythromycin which are known to inhibit CYP3A4, may inhibit the metabolism of tramadol (N-demethylation) and the metabolism of the active O-demethylated metabolite. No studies have been performed on the clinical significance of such an interaction.

There is no interaction with food.

Pregnancy and lactation

Pregnancy: Zamadol SR Capsules should not be used during pregnancy as there is inadequate evidence available to assess the safety of tramadol in pregnant women. Tramadol–administered before or during birth–does not affect uterine contractility. In neonates it may induce changes in the respiratory rate which are usually not clinically relevant.

Lactation: Zamadol SR Capsules should not be administered during breast feeding as tramadol and its metabolites have been detected in breast milk. 0.1% of the dose administered to the mother may be excreted in milk.

Effects on ability to drive and use machines: Zamadol SR Capsules may cause drowsiness and this effect may be potentiated by alcohol, anti-histamines and other CNS depressants. If patients are affected they should be warned not to drive or operate machinery.

Undesirable effects: Frequently (more than 10%) nausea and dizziness have been reported.

Occasionally (1-10%) headache, constipation, vomiting, sweating, dry mouth and muzziness may occur.

In rare cases (< 1%) there may be effects on cardiovascular regulation (palpitation, tachycardia, postural hypotension or cardiovascular collapse). These adverse effects may occur especially on intravenous administration and in patients who are physically stressed. Retching, gastrointestinal irritation (a feeling of pressure in the stomach, bloating) and dermal reactions (e.g. pruritus, rash, urticaria) may occur.

In very rare cases (< 0.1%) motorial weakness, changes in appetite and micturition disorders have been observed. In very rare cases various psychic side-effects may occur following administration of Zamadol SR which vary individually in intensity and nature (depending on personality and duration of medication). These include changes in mood (usually elation, occasionally dysphoria), changes in activity (usually suppression, occasionally increase) and changes in cognitive and sensorial capacity (e.g. decision behaviour, perception disorders).

Allergic reactions (e.g. dyspnoea, bronchospasm, wheezing, angioneurotic oedema) and anaphylaxis have also been reported in very rare cases.

Very rarely epileptiform convulsions have been reported. They occurred mainly after administration of high doses of tramadol or after concomitant treatment with drugs which can lower the seizure threshold or themselves induce cerebral convulsions (e.g. anti-depressants or anti-psychotics).

Increase in blood pressure and bradycardia have been reported in very rare cases.

Worsening of asthma has also been reported, though a causal relationship has not been established.

Respiratory depression has been reported. If the recommended doses are considerably exceeded and other centrally depressant substances are administered concomitantly, respiratory depression may occur.

Dependence may occur. Symptoms of withdrawal reactions, similar to those occurring during opiate withdrawal, may occur as follows: agitation, anxiety, nervousness, insomnia, hyperkinesia, tremor and gastrointestinal symptoms.

Overdose: Symptoms of tramadol overdose include vomiting, miosis, sedation, seizures, respiratory depression and hypotension, with circulatory failure and coma. Respiratory failure may also occur. Such symptoms are typical of opioid analgesics.

Treatment of overdose requires the maintenance of the airway and cardiovascular functions. Respiratory depression may be reversed using naloxone and fits controlled with diazepam. Naloxone administration may increase the risk of seizures.

The treatment of acute overdose of tramadol using haemodialysis or haemofiltration alone is not suffi cient or suitable due to the slow elimination o tramadol from the serum by these routes.

Pharmacological properties

Pharmacodynamic properties: Tramadol is a centrall acting analgesic which possesses opioid agonis properties. Tramadol consists of two enantiomers the (+)-isomer is predominantly active as an opiate with preferential activity for the μ-receptor. The (-) isomer potentiates the analgesic effect of the (+) isomer and is active as an inhibitor of noradrenalin and serotonin uptake thereby modifying the transmis sion of pain impulses. The duration of analgesia wit orally administered normal release tramadol has bee shown to be 3-6 hours with maximum pain relief at 1 4 hours post-dosing.

Tramadol also has an antitussive action. At th recommended dosages, the effects of tramadol give orally on the respiratory and cardiovascular system appear to be clinically insignificant. The potency c tramadol is reported to be 1/10 to 1/6 of morphine.

Pharmacokinetic properties: About 90% of Tramadc released from Zamadol SR Capsules is absorbed afte oral administration. The mean absolute bioavailabilit is approximately 70%, irrespective of concomitar intake of food.

The difference between absorbed and non-meta bolised available Tramadol is probably due to lov first-pass effect. The first pass-effect after oral admir istration is a maximum of 30%.

Tramadol has a high tissue affinity with an apparer volume of distribution of 203 ± 40 litres after or dosing in healthy volunteers. Protein binding is limite to 20%.

After single dose administration of Zamadol S Capsules 50 mg the peak plasma concentration C_{m} 70 ± 16 ng/ml is reached after 5.3 h. After administra tion of Zamadol SR Capsules 100 mg C_{max} 137 ±27 n ml is reached after 5.9 h. Following administration Zamadol SR Capsules 200 mg C_{max} 294 ± 82 ng/ml reached after 6.5 h. The reference product (Tramad Immediate Release Capsules, given as a total dose

200 mg Tramadol hydrochloride) reached a peak concentration of C_{max} 640 ± 143 ng/ml after 2.0 hours.

The relative bioavailability for the slow release formulation after single dose administration is 89% and increases to 100% after multiple dose administration in comparison to the reference product.

Tramadol passes the blood-brain and placenta barriers. Very small amounts of the substance and its O-demethyl derivative are found in the breast-milk (0.1% and 0.02% respectively of the applied dose.)

Elimination of half-life $t_{\frac{1}{2}}\beta$ is approximately 6 h, irrespective of the mode of administration. In patients above 75 years of age it may be prolonged by a factor of 1.4.

In humans tramadol is mainly metabolised by means of N- and O-demethylation and conjugation of the O-demethylation products with glucuronic acid. Only O-desmethyl-tramadol is pharmacologically active. There are considerable interindividual quantitative differences between the other metabolites. So far, eleven metabolites have been found in the urine. Animal experiments have shown that O-desmethyltramadol is more potent than the parent substance by the factor 2-4. Its half life $t_{\frac{1}{2}}\beta$ (6 healthy volunteers) is 7.9 h (range 5.4-9.6 h) and is approximately that of tramadol.

Tramadol and its metabolites are almost completely excreted via the kidneys. cumulative urinary excretion is 90% of the total radioactivity of the administered dose. In cases of impaired hepatic and renal function the half-life may be slightly prolonged. In patients with cirrhosis of the liver, elimination half-lives of 13.3 ± 4.9 h (tramadol) and 18.5 ± 9.4 h (O-desmethyltramadol), in an extreme case 22.3 h and 36 h respectively have been determined. In patients with renal insufficiency (creatinine clearance < 5 ml/min) the values were 11 ± 3.2 h and 16.9 ± 3 h, in an extreme case 19.5 h and 43.2 h, respectively.

Tramadol has a linear pharmacokinetic profile within the therapeutic dosage range.

The relationship between serum concentrations and the analgesic effect is dose-dependent, but varies considerably in isolated cases. A serum concentration of 100–300 ng/ml is usually effective.

Preclinical safety data: Pre-clinical data reveal no special hazard for humans based on conventional studies of safety pharmacology, repeated dose toxicity, genotoxicity or carcinogenic potential. Studies of tramadol in rats and rabbits have revealed no teratogenic effects. However, embryo toxicity was shown in the form of delayed ossification. Fertility, reproductive performance and development of offspring were unaffected.

Pharmaceutical particulars

List of excipients: Capsule Contents: Sugar spheres (sucrose and maize starch), colloidal anhydrous silica, ethylcellulose, shellac, talc.

Capsule Shell: Gelatin and titanium dioxide (E171). 50 mg, 150 mg and 200 mg capsules contain Iron Oxide Yellow (E172), 50 mg and 150 mg capsules contain Indigotin (E132). Printing ink contains shellac, iron oxide black (E172), soya lecithin and antifoam DC 1510.

Incompatibilities: No pharmaceutical incompatibilities reported.

Shelf-life: Two years.

Special precautions for storage: Store in a dry place at room temperature (below 25°C).

Nature and contents of container: White opaque PVC/PVDC and aluminium foil blister strips. Each strip contains 10 capsules. The blister strips are packed in cartons containing 30 or 60 capsules. 50 mg capsules are dark green, 100 mg capsules are white, 150 mg capsules are dark green and 200 mg capsules are yellow.

Instructions for use/handling: None.

Marketing authorisation numbers

Zamadol™SR Capsules 50 mg	PL 8336/0079
Zamadol™ SR Capsules 100 mg	PL 8336/0080
Zamadol™ SR Capsules 150 mg	PL 8336/0081
Zamadol™ SR Capsules 200 mg	PL 8336/0082

Date of (partial) revision of the text

January 1998.

**Trade Mark*

Astra Pharmaceuticals Limited
Home Park
Kings Langley
Herts WD4 8DH

☎ 01923 266191 🗋 01923 260431

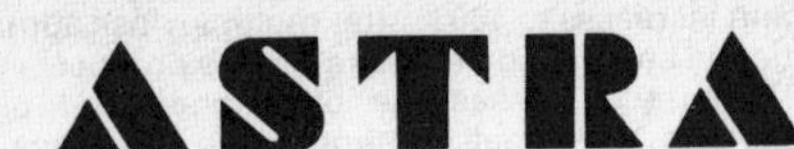

AMIAS* TABLETS ▼

Qualitative and quantitative composition Each tablet contains 2 mg, 4 mg, 8 mg or 16 mg candesartan cilexetil.

Pharmaceutical form Tablets.

Clinical particulars
Therapeutic indications: Essential hypertension.

Posology and method of administration
Dosage: A suggested starting dose of Amias is 4 mg once daily. The usual maintenance dose is 8 mg once daily. The maximum dose is 16 mg once daily.

Therapy should be adjusted according to blood pressure response. Most of the antihypertensive effect is attained within 4 weeks of initiation of treatment.

Administration: Amias should be taken once daily with or without food.

Use in the elderly: The starting dose is 4 mg in elderly patients with normal renal and hepatic function. In the presence of renal or hepatic impairment an initial dose of 2 mg is recommended. The dose may be adjusted according to response.

Use in impaired renal function: No dosage adjustment is necessary in patients with mild renal impairment. In patients with moderate to severe renal impairment, an initial dose of 2 mg once daily is recommended. The dose may be adjusted according to response. Due to limited experience, Amias is not recommended in patients with very severe or end-stage renal impairment ($Cl_{creatinine}$<15 ml/min).

Use in impaired hepatic function: An initial dose of 2 mg once daily is recommended in patients with mild to moderate hepatic impairment. The dose may be adjusted according to response. There is no experience in patients with severe hepatic impairment.

Concomitant therapy: Addition of a thiazide-type diuretic such as hydrochlorothiazide has been shown to have an additive antihypertensive effect with Amias.

Use in children: The safety and efficacy of Amias have not been established in children.

Contra-indications: Hypersensitivity to any component of Amias.

Pregnancy and lactation (see section *Pregnancy and lactation*).

Severe hepatic impairment and/or cholestasis.

Special warnings and special precautions for use
Renal artery stenosis: Other drugs that affect the renin-angiotensin-aldosterone system, i.e. angiotensin converting enzyme (ACE) inhibitors, may increase blood urea and serum creatinine in patients with bilateral renal artery stenosis or stenosis of the artery to a solitary kidney. While this is not reported with Amias, a similar effect may be anticipated with angiotensin II receptor antagonists.

Intravascular volume depletion: In patients with intravascular volume depletion (such as those receiving high dose diuretics) symptomatic hypotension may occur, as described for other agents acting on the renin-angiotensin-aldosterone system. Therefore, these conditions should be corrected prior to administration of Amias.

Renal impairment: When Amias is used in patients with severe renal impairment, periodic monitoring of serum potassium and creatinine levels should be considered. There is limited experience in patients with very severe or end-stage renal impairment ($Cl_{creatinine}$<15 ml/min).

Kidney transplantation: There is no experience regarding the administration of Amias in patients with a recent kidney transplantation.

Aortic and mitral valve stenosis (obstructive hypertrophic cardiomyopathy): As with other vasodilators, special caution is indicated in patients suffering from haemodynamically relevant aortic or mitral valve stenosis, or obstructive hypertrophic cardiomyopathy.

Primary hyperaldosteronism: Patients with primary hyperaldosteronism will not generally respond to antihypertensive drugs acting through inhibition of the renin-angiotensin-aldosterone system. Therefore, the use of Amias is not recommended.

Hyperkalaemia: Based on experience with the use of other drugs that affect the renin-angiotensin-aldosterone system, concomitant use of potassium-sparing diuretics, potassium supplements, salt substitutes containing potassium, or other drugs that may increase potassium levels (e.g. heparin) may lead to increases in serum potassium.

General: In patients whose vascular tone and renal function depend predominantly on the activity of the renin-angiotensin-aldosterone system (e.g. patients with severe congestive heart failure or underlying renal disease, including renal artery stenosis), treatment with other drugs that affect this system has been associated with acute hypotension, azotaemia, oliguria or, rarely, acute renal failure. Although the possibility of similar effects cannot be excluded with angiotensin II receptor antagonists, these effects are not reported with Amias. As with any antihypertensive agent, excessive blood pressure decrease in patients with ischaemic cardiopathy or ischaemic cerebrovascular disease could result in a myocardial infarction or stroke.

Interaction with other medicaments and other forms of interaction: No drug interactions of clinical significance have been identified.

Compounds which have been investigated in clinical pharmacokinetic studies include hydrochlorothiazide, warfarin, digoxin, oral contraceptives (i.e. ethinylestradiol/ levonorgestrel), glibenclamide and nifedipine.

Candesartan is eliminated only to a minor extent by hepatic metabolism (CYP2C9). Available interaction studies indicate no effect on CYP2C9 and CYP3A4 but the effect on other cytochrome P450 isoenzymes is presently unknown.

The antihypertensive effect of Amias may be enhanced by other antihypertensives.

Based on experience with the use of other drugs that affect the renin-angiotensin-aldosterone system, concomitant use of potassium-sparing diuretics, potassium supplements, salt substitutes containing potassium, or other drugs that may increase potassium levels (e.g. heparin) may lead to increases in serum potassium.

Reversible increases in serum lithium concentrations and toxicity have been reported during concomitant administration of lithium with ACE inhibitors. While not reported with Amias the possibility of a similar effect cannot be excluded and careful monitoring of serum lithium levels is recommended during concomitant use.

The bioavailability of candesartan is not affected by food.

Pregnancy and lactation
Pregnancy: There is no experience with the use of Amias in pregnant women, but animal studies with candesartan cilexetil have demonstrated late foetal and neonatal injury in the kidney. The mechanism is believed to be pharmacologically mediated through effects on the renin-angiotensin-aldosterone system.

In humans, foetal renal perfusion, which is dependent upon the development of the renin-angiotensin-aldosterone system, begins in the second trimester. Thus risk to the foetus increases if Amias is administered during the second or third trimesters of pregnancy.

Based on the above information, Amias should not be used in pregnancy. If pregnancy is detected during treatment, Amias should be discontinued (see section *Contra-indications*).

Lactation: It is not known whether candesartan is excreted in human milk. However, candesartan is excreted in the milk of lactating rats. Because of the potential for adverse effects on the nursing infant, breast feeding should be discontinued if the use of Amias is considered essential (see section *Contra-indications*).

Effects on ability to drive and use machines: The effect of Amias on the ability to drive and use machines has not been studied, but based on its pharmacodynamic properties Amias is unlikely to affect this ability. When driving vehicles or operating machines, it should be taken into account that occasionally dizziness or weariness may occur during treatment of hypertension.

Undesirable effects: In controlled clinical studies adverse events were mild and transient and comparable to placebo. The overall incidence of adverse events showed no association with dose or age. Withdrawals from treatment due to adverse events were similar with candesartan cilexetil (2.4%) and placebo (2.6%).

Clinical adverse events regardless of causal relationship occurring with an incidence of ≥1% on Amias in double-blind placebo controlled studies are presented in the following table:

	Placebo (n=573) %	*Cand. cil. (n=1388) %*
Headache	10.3	10.4
URTI*	3.8	5.1
Back pain	0.9	3.2
Dizziness	2.3	2.5
Nausea	1.3	1.9
Coughing	1.1	1.6
Influenza-like symptoms	0.8	1.5
Fatigue	1.6	1.5
Abdominal pain	1.3	1.5
Diarrhoea	1.9	1.5
Pharyngitis	0.4	1.1
Peripheral oedema	0.7	1.0
Vomiting	1.2	1.0
Bronchitis	2.2	1.0
Rhinitis	0.4	1.0

* Upper respiratory tract infection

Laboratory findings: In general, there were no clinically important influences of Amias on routine laboratory variables. Increases in S-ALAT (S-GPT) were reported as adverse events slightly more often with Amias than with placebo (1.3% vs 0.5%). No routine monitoring of laboratory variables is usually necessary for patients receiving Amias. However, in patients with severe renal impairment, periodic monitoring of serum potassium and creatinine levels should be considered.

Overdose: Symptoms: Based on pharmacological considerations, the main manifestation of an overdose is likely to be symptomatic hypotension and dizziness. In a case report of an overdose of 160 mg candesartan cilexetil, the patient's recovery was uneventful.

Management: If symptomatic hypotension should occur, symptomatic treatment should be instituted and vital signs monitored. The patient should be placed supine with the legs elevated. If this is not sufficient, plasma volume should be increased by infusion of, for example, isotonic saline solution. Sympathomimetic drugs may be administered if the above-mentioned measures are not sufficient.

Candesartan is unlikely to be removed by haemodialysis.

Pharmacological properties
Pharmacodynamic properties: Pharmaco-therapeutic group: Angiotensin II antagonists, ATC code C09C A.

Angiotensin II is the primary vasoactive hormone of the renin-angiotensin-aldosterone system and plays a significant role in the pathophysiology of hypertension and other cardiovascular disorders. It also has an important role in the pathogenesis of end organ hypertrophy and damage. The major physiological effects of angiotensin II, such as vasoconstriction, aldosterone stimulation, regulation of salt and water homeostasis and stimulation of cell growth, are mediated via the type 1 (AT_1) receptor.

Amias is a prodrug suitable for oral use. It is rapidly converted to the active drug, candesartan, by ester hydrolysis during absorption from the gastrointestinal tract. Candesartan is an angiotensin II receptor antagonist, selective for AT_1 receptors, with tight binding to and slow dissociation from the receptor. It has no agonist activity.

Candesartan does not inhibit ACE, which converts angiotensin I to angiotensin II and degrades bradykinin. There is no effect on, ACE and no potentiation of bradykinin or substance P. In controlled clinical trials comparing Amias with ACE inhibitors, the incidence of cough was lower in patients receiving Amias. Candesartan does not bind to or block other hormone receptors or ion channels known to be important in cardiovascular regulation. The antagonism of the angiotensin II (AT_1) receptors results in dose related increases in plasma renin levels, angiotensin I and angiotensin II levels, and a decrease in plasma aldosterone concentration.

In hypertension, Amias causes a dose-dependent, long-lasting reduction in arterial blood pressure. The antihypertensive action is due to decreased systemic peripheral resistance, without reflex increase in heart rate. There is no indication of serious or exaggerated first dose hypotension or rebound effect after cessation of treatment.

After administration of a single dose of Amias, onset of antihypertensive effect generally occurs within 2 hours. With continuous treatment, most of the reduction in blood pressure with any dose is generally attained within four weeks and is sustained during long-term treatment. Amias once daily provides effective and smooth blood pressure reduction over 24 hours, with little difference between maximum and trough effects during the dosing interval. When Amias is used together with hydrochlorothiazide, the reduction in blood pressure is additive. Concomitant administration of Amias with hydrochlorothiazide or amlodipine is well tolerated.

Amias is similarly effective in patients irrespective of age and gender.

Amias increases renal blood flow and either has no effect on, or increases glomerular filtration rate while renal vascular resistance and filtration fraction are reduced. In hypertensive patients with type II diabetes mellitus, 12 weeks treatment with candesartan cilexetil 8 mg to 16 mg had no adverse effects on blood glucose or lipid profile.

Currently there are no data regarding the effects of candesartan cilexetil on morbidity and mortality in hypertensive patients.

Pharmacokinetic properties

Absorption and distribution: Following oral administration, candesartan cilexetil is converted to the active drug candesartan. The absolute bioavailability of candesartan is approximately 40% after an oral solution of candesartan cilexetil. The relative bioavailability of the tablet formulation compared with the same oral solution is approximately 34% with very little variability. The estimated absolute bioavailability of the tablet is therefore 14%. The mean peak serum concentration (C_{max}) is reached 3-4 hours following tablet intake. The candesartan serum concentrations increase linearly with increasing doses in the therapeutic dose range. No gender related differences in the pharmacokinetics of candesartan have been observed. The area under the serum concentration *versus* time curve (AUC) of candesartan is not significantly affected by food.

Candesartan is highly bound to plasma protein (more than 99%). The apparent volume of distribution of candesartan is 0.1 l/kg.

Metabolism and elimination: Candesartan is mainly eliminated unchanged via urine and bile and only to a minor extent eliminated by hepatic metabolism. The terminal half-life of candesartan is approximately 9 hours. There is no accumulation following multiple doses.

Total plasma clearance of candesartan is about 0.37 ml/min/kg, with a renal clearance of about 0.19 ml/min/kg. The renal elimination of candesartan is both by glomerular filtration and active tubular secretion. Following an oral dose of ^{14}C-labelled candesartan cilexetil, approximately 26% of the dose is excreted in the urine as candesartan and 7% as an inactive metabolite while approximately 56% of the dose is recovered in the faeces as candesartan and 10% as the inactive metabolite.

Pharmacokinetics in special populations: In the elderly (over 65 years) C_{max} and AUC of candesartan are increased by approximately 50% and 80%, respectively in comparison to young subjects. However, the blood pressure response and the incidence of adverse events are similar after a given dose of Amias in young and elderly patients (see section *Posology and method of administration*).

In patients with mild to moderate renal impairment C_{max} and AUC of candesartan increased during repeated dosing by approximately 50% and 70%, respectively, but $t_{1/2}$ was not altered, compared to patients with normal renal function. The corresponding changes in patients with severe renal impairment were approximately 50% and 110%, respectively. The terminal $t_{1/2}$ of candesartan was approximately doubled in patients with severe renal impairment. The pharmacokinetics in patients undergoing haemodialysis were similar to those in patients with severe renal impairment.

In patients with mild to moderate hepatic impairment, there was a 23% increase in the AUC of candesartan (see section 4.2 Posology and method of administration).

Preclinical safety data: There was no evidence of abnormal systemic or target organ toxicity at clinically relevant doses. In preclinical safety studies candesartan had effects on the kidneys and on red cell parameters at high doses in mice, rats, dogs and monkeys. Candesartan caused a reduction of red blood cell parameters (erythrocytes, haemoglobin, haematocrit). Effects on the kidneys (such as interstitial nephritis, tubular distension, basophilic tubules; increased plasma concentrations of urea and creatinine) were induced by candesartan which could be secondary to the hypotensive effect leading to alterations of renal perfusion. Furthermore, candesartan induced hyperplasia/hypertrophy of the juxtaglomerular cells. These changes were considered to be caused by the pharmacological action of candesartan. For therapeutic doses of candesartan in humans, the hyperplasia/hypertrophy of the renal juxtaglomerular cells does not seem to have any relevance.

Foetotoxicity has been observed in late pregnancy (see section *Pregnancy and lactation*).

Data from *in vitro* and *in vivo* mutagenicity testing indicates that candesartan will not exert mutagenic or clastogenic activities under conditions of clinical use. There was no evidence of carcinogenicity.

Pharmaceutical particulars

List of excipients: Carmellose calcium, hydroxypropyl cellulose, lactose monohydrate, magnesium stearate, maize starch, polyethylene glycol and iron oxide red E172 (8 mg only).

Incompatibilities: None stated.

Shelf life: Three years.

Special precautions for storage: Store below 30°C.

Nature and contents of container: Amias Tablets 2 mg are round white tablets. Amias Tablets 4 mg are round white tablets with a single score line on both sides.
Amias Tablets 8 mg are round pale pink tablets with a single score line on both sides.
Amias Tablets 16 mg are round white tablets with a single score line on both sides.
2 mg tablet: Polypropylene blister packs of 7 tablets.
4 mg tablet: Polypropylene blister packs of 7 and 28 tablets.
8 mg tablet: Polypropylene blister packs of 28 tablets.
16 mg tablet: Polypropylene blister packs of 28 tablets.

Instructions for use/handling: Not applicable.

Marketing authorisation holder: Takeda UK Limited, 3, The Courtyard, Meadowbank, Furlong Road, Bourne End, Buckinghamshire SL8 5AJ, United Kingdom

Marketing authorization numbers
Amias Tablets 2 mg PL 16189/0001
Amias Tablets 4 mg PL 16189/0002
Amias Tablets 8 mg PL 16189/0003
Amias Tablets 16 mg PL 16189/0004

Date of approval/revision of SPC 26 March 1998

Legal category POM.

*Registered trademark owned by Takeda Chemical Industries Ltd.

BAMBEC* TABLETS

Qualitative and quantitative composition Bambuterol hydrochloride INN 10 mg; bambuterol hydrochloride INN 20 mg.

Pharmaceutical form Tablet

Clinical particulars

Therapeutic indications: Management of asthma, bronchospasm and/or reversible airways obstruction.

Posology and method of administration: Bambec is formulated as a tablet and should be taken orally. Bambec Tablets 20 mg are effective once daily.

Adults: The recommended starting doses are 10 mg-20 mg. The 10 mg dose may be increased to 20 mg if necessary after 1-2 weeks, depending on the clinical effect.

In patients who have previously tolerated β_2-agonists well, the recommended starting as well as maintenance, dose is 20 mg.

Children: Until the clinical documentation has been completed, Bambec should not be used in children.

Elderly: Dose adjustment is not required in the elderly.

Significant hepatic dysfunction: Not recommended because of unpredictable conversion to terbutaline.

Moderate to severely impaired renal function (GFR <50 ml/min): It is recommended that the starting dose of Bambec should be halved in these patients.

Contra-indications: Bambec tablets are contra-indicated in patients with a history of hypersensitivity to any of their ingredients. Bambec is presently not recommended for children due to limited clinical data in this age group.

Special warnings and special precautions for use: Care should be taken with patients suffering from myocardial insufficiency or thyrotoxicosis. Due to the hyperglycaemic effects of β_2-stimulants additional blood glucose measurements are recommended initially when Bambec therapy is commenced in diabetic patients. If diabetic treatment becomes less effective or shorter acting the patient's general condition should be reviewed.

Due to the positive inotropic effects of β_2-agonists these drugs should not be used in patients with hypertrophic cardiomyopathy.

β-agonists may be arrhythmogenic and this must be considered in the treatment of the individual patient. Unpredictable interindividual variation in the metabolism of bambuterol to terbutaline has been shown in subjects with liver cirrhosis. The use of another β-agonist is recommended in patients with cirrhosis and other forms of severely impaired liver function.

Potentially serious hypokalaemia may result from β_2-agonist therapy. Particular caution is advised in severe asthma as this effect may be potentiated by concomitant treatment with xanthine derivatives, steroids, diuretics and by hypoxia. It is recommended that serum potassium levels are monitored in such situations.

Interaction with other medicaments and other forms of interaction: Bambuterol may interact with suxamethonium (succinyl choline). A prolongation of the muscle-relaxing effect of suxamethonium of up to 2-fold has been observed in some patients after taking Bambec 20 mg on the evening prior to surgery. The interaction is dose dependent. It is due to the fact that plasma cholinesterase, which inactivates suxamethonium, is partly, but fully reversibly, inhibited by bambuterol. In extreme situations, the interaction may result in a prolonged apnoea time which may be of clinical importance.

Bambuterol may also interact with other muscle relaxants metabolised by plasma cholinesterases.

Beta-receptor blocking agents, especially non-selective ones, may partly or totally inhibit the effect of beta-stimulants.

Pregnancy and lactation: Unless there are compelling reasons, avoid in pregnancy, lactation and women of child-bearing potential who are not taking adequate contraceptive precautions. Although no teratogenic effects have been observed in animals after administration of bambuterol there is no experience of use in human pregnancy. Terbutaline, the active metabolite of bambuterol has been in widespread clinical use for many years and may be considered in such patients. Terbutaline should be used with caution in the first trimester of pregnancy. Maternal β_2-agonist treatment may result in transient hypoglycaemia in pre-term new-born infants.

It is not known whether bambuterol or intermediary products pass into breast milk. Terbutaline does pass into breast milk, but an effect on the infant is unlikely at therapeutic doses.

Effects on ability to drive and use machines: No effects are known.

Undesirable effects: Side effects which have been reported e.g. tremor, headache, cramps and palpitations are all characteristic of sympathomimetic amines. The intensity of the side effects is dose dependent and the majority of these effects have reversed spontaneously within the first 1-2 weeks of treatment.

Potentially serious hypokalaemia may result from β_2-agonist therapy.

Urticaria and exanthema may occur.

Overdosage: No cases of overdosage with Bambec have yet been reported.

Pharmacological properties

Pharmacodynamic properties: Bambuterol is an active precursor of the selective β_2-adrenergic agonist terbutaline. Bambuterol is the bis-dimethylcarbamate of terbutaline, and is present in the formulation as a 1:1 racemate.

Pharmacodynamic studies have shown that after oral administration of bambuterol to guinea pigs, a sustained protective effect was achieved against histamine induced bronchoconstriction. At equipotent doses, the duration of the relaxing activity was more prolonged than after plain terbutaline. Bambuterol, or the monocarbamate ester, did not exert any smooth muscle relaxing properties. The bronchoprotective effects seen after oral administration of bambuterol are related to the generation of terbutaline, as were the secondary effects (effects on other organs).

Pharmacodynamic studies have been conducted in asthmatics and healthy volunteers. The effects observed were bronchodilation, tremor and increases in heart rate. The metabolic effects included a small increase in blood glucose, while the effect on serum potassium was negligible. In short-term studies on lipoprotein metabolism, an increase in HDL cholesterol, has been observed. In conclusion, all pharmacodynamic effects observed can be ascribed to the active metabolite terbutaline.

Pharmacokinetic properties: On average, 17.5% of an oral dose is absorbed. Approximately 70-90% of the absorption occurs in the first 24 hours.

Bambuterol is metabolised in the liver and terbutaline is formed by both hydrolysis and oxidation. After absorption from the gut, about 2/3 of terbutaline is first-pass metabolised, bambuterol escapes this first-pass metabolism. Of the absorbed amount, about 65% reaches the circulation. Bambuterol therefore has a bioavailability of about 10%.

Protein binding of bambuterol is low, 40-50% at therapeutic concentrations.

The terminal half-life of bambuterol after an oral dose is 9-17 hours.

Studies on the effects on plasma cholinesterase showed that bambuterol inhibited activity, but that this was reversible.

All categories of subjects studied were able to form terbutaline in a predictive way except for liver cirrhotics.

Preclinical safety data: Bambuterol has not revealed any adverse effects which pose a risk to man at therapeutic dosages in the toxicity studies.

Bambuterol is given as a racemate: (-)-bambuterol is responsible for the pharmacodynamic effects via generation of (-)-terbutaline. (+)-bambuterol generates the pharmacodynamic inactive (+)-terbutaline. Both (+) and (-)-bambuterol are equally active as plasma cholinesterase inhibitors. This inhibition is reversible.

The toxicity studies showed that bambuterol has β_2-stimulatory effects, expressed as cardiotoxicity in dogs, and at high doses, observed in the acute toxicity studies, cholinergic effects.

There is no evidence from the preclinical safety data to indicate that bambuterol cannot be used in man for the intended indications with sufficient safety.

Pharmaceutical particulars

List of excipients: lactose; maize starch; povidone; microcrystalline cellulose; magnesium stearate; water, purified.

Incompatibilities: Not applicable.

Shelf-life: 3 years.

Special precautions for storage: Store below 30°C.

Nature and contents of container: PVC blisters: 7 or 28 tablets.

Instructions for use/handling: Bambec should be taken once daily, shortly before bedtime.

Marketing authorisation numbers

Bambec 10 mg	PL 0017/0313
Bambec 20 mg	PL 0017/0314

Date of approval/revision of SPC March 1995

Legal category POM.

BETALOC* TABLETS 50 mg and 100 mg

Presentation White tablets containing either 50 mg (coded A/BB) or 100 mg (coded A/ME) metoprolol tartrate PhEur.

Inactive ingredients: Microcrystalline cellulose, lactose, sodium starch glycolate, colloidal silica, polyvidone, magnesium stearate.

Uses In the management of hypertension and angina pectoris. Cardiac arrhythmias, especially supraventricular tachyarrhythmias.

Adjunct to the treatment of hyperthyroidism.

Early intervention with Betaloc in acute myocardial infarction reduces infarct size and the incidence of ventricular fibrillation. Pain relief may also decrease the need for opiate analgesics.

Betaloc has been shown to reduce mortality when administered to patients with acute myocardial infarction.

Prophylaxis of migraine.

Dosage and administration The dose must always be adjusted to the individual requirements of the patient. The following are guidelines:

Hypertension: Total daily dosage Betaloc 100–400 mg to be given as a single or twice daily dose. The starting dose is 100 mg per day. This may be increased by 100 mg per day at weekly intervals. If full control is not achieved using a single daily dose, a b.d. regimen should be initiated. Combination therapy with a diuretic or other anti-hypertensive agent may also be considered.

Angina: Usually Betaloc 50–100 mg twice or three times daily.

Cardiac arrhythmias: Betaloc 50 mg b.i.d. or t.i.d. should usually control the condition. If necessary the dose can be increased up to 300 mg per day in divided doses.

Following the treatment of an acute arrhythmia with Betaloc injection, continuation therapy with Betaloc tablets should be initiated 4–6 hours later. The initial oral dose should not exceed 50 mg t.i.d.

Hyperthyroidism: Betaloc 50 mg four times a day. The dose should be reduced as the euthyroid state is achieved.

Myocardial infarction: Early intervention – to achieve optimal benefits from intravenous Betaloc, suitable patients should present within 12 hours of the onset of chest pain. Therapy should commence with 5 mg i.v. every 2 minutes to a maximum of 15 mg total as determined by blood pressure and heart rate. The second or third dose should not be given if the systolic blood pressure is <90 mmHg, the heart rate is <40 beats/min and the P-Q time is >0.26 seconds, or if there is any aggravation of dyspnoea or cold sweating. Orally, therapy should commence 15 minutes after the last injection with 50 mg every 6 hours for 48 hours. Patients who fail to tolerate the full intravenous dose should be given half the suggested oral dose.

Maintenance – The usual maintenance dose is 200 mg daily, given in divided doses.

Migraine prophylaxis: Betaloc 100–200 mg daily, given in divided doses.

Elderly: There are no special dosage requirements in otherwise healthy elderly patients.

Significant hepatic dysfunction: A reduction in dosage may be necessary.

Contra-indications, warnings, etc

Contra-indications: AV block. Uncontrolled heart failure. Severe bradycardia. Sick-sinus syndrome. Cardiogenic shock. Severe peripheral arterial disease. Known hypersensitivity to Betaloc or other β-blockers.

Betaloc is also contra-indicated when myocardial infarction is complicated by significant bradycardia, first degree heart block, systolic hypotension (<100 mmHg) and/or severe heart failure.

Warnings: Betaloc may aggravate bradycardia, symptoms of peripheral arterial circulatory disorders and anaphylactic shock.

Abrupt interruption of β-blockers is to be avoided. When possible, Betaloc should be withdrawn gradually over a period of 10 days, in diminishing doses to 25 mg daily for the last 6 days. During its withdrawal patients should be kept under close surveillance, especially those with known ischaemic heart disease.

Betaloc may be administered when heart failure has been controlled. Digitalisation and/or diuretic therapy should also be considered for patients with a history of heart failure, or patients known to have a poor cardiac reserve.

Although cardioselective β-blockers may have less effect on lung function than non-selective β-blockers, as with all β-blockers these should be avoided in patients with reversible obstructive airways disease unless there are compelling clinical reasons for their use. When administration is necessary, use of a β_2-bronchodilator (e.g. terbutaline) may be advisable in some patients.

The label shall state – 'If you have a history of wheezing, asthma or any other breathing difficulties, you must tell your doctor before you take this medicine'.

In labile and insulin-dependent diabetes it may be necessary to adjust the hypoglycaemic therapy.

In patients with a phaeochromocytoma, an α-blocker should be given concomitantly.

In the presence of liver cirrhosis the bioavailability of Betaloc may be increased.

The administration of adrenaline to patients undergoing β-blockade can result in an increase in blood pressure and bradycardia, although this is less likely to occur with β_1-selective drugs.

Betaloc therapy must be reported to the anaesthetist prior to general anaesthesia. If withdrawal of Betaloc is considered desirable, this should if possible be completed at least 48 hours before general anaesthesia. However, in some patients it may be desirable to employ a β-blocker as premedication. By shielding the heart against the effects of stress the β-blocker may prevent excessive sympathetic stimulation provoking cardiac arrhythmias or acute coronary insufficiency. If a β-blocker is given for this purpose, an anaesthetic with little negative inotropic activity should be selected to minimise the risk of myocardial depression.

Pregnancy: Betaloc should not be used in pregnancy or nursing mothers unless the physician considers that the benefit outweighs the possible hazard to the foetus/infant. As with all β-blockers Betaloc may cause side-effects e.g. bradycardia, hypoglycaemia in the foetus, and in the newborn and breast-fed infant. Betaloc has, however, been used in pregnancy associated hypertension under close supervision, after 20 weeks gestation. Although Betaloc crosses the placental barrier and is present in cord blood, no evidence of foetal abnormalities has been reported.

Lactation: The amount of Betaloc ingested via breast milk should not produce significant β-blocking effects in the neonate if the mother is treated with normal therapeutic doses.

Interactions: The effects of Betaloc and other anti-hypertensive drugs on blood pressure are usually additive, and care should be taken to avoid hypotension. However, combinations of antihypertensive drugs may often be used with benefit to improve control of hypertension.

Betaloc can reduce myocardial contractility and impair intracardiac conduction. Care should be exercised when drugs with similar activity, e.g. antiarrhythmic agents, general anaesthetics, are given concurrently. Like all other β-blockers, Betaloc should not be given in combination with verapamil since this may cause bradycardia, hypotension and asystole. Care should also be exercised when β-blockers are given in combination with sympathetic ganglion blocking agents, other β-blockers (i.e. eye drops) or MAO inhibitors. If combination treatment with clonidine is to be discontinued, Betaloc should be withdrawn several days before clonidine.

As β-blockers may affect the peripheral circulation, care should be exercised when drugs with similar activity e.g. ergotamine are given concurrently.

Betaloc will antagonise the β_1-effects of sympathomimetic agents but should have little influence on the bronchodilator effects of β_2-agonists at normal therapeutic doses. Enzyme inducing agents (e.g. rifampicin) may reduce plasma concentrations of Betaloc, whereas enzyme inhibitors (e.g. cimetidine) may increase plasma concentrations. Betaloc may impair the elimination of lignocaine.

Indomethacin may reduce the antihypertensive effect of β-blockers.

Side-effects: These are usually mild and infrequent. The most common appear to be lassitude, GI disturbances (nausea, vomiting or abdominal pain) and disturbances of sleep pattern. In many cases these effects have been transient or have disappeared after a reduction in dosage.

Effects related to the CNS which have been reported occasionally are dizziness and headache and rarely paraesthesia, muscle cramps, depression and decreased mental alertness. There have also been isolated reports of personality disorders like amnesia, memory impairment, confusion, hallucination, nervousness and anxiety.

Cardiovascular effects which have been reported occasionally are bradycardia, postural hypotension and rarely, heart failure, palpitations, cardiac arrhythmias, Raynaud's phenomenon, peripheral oedema and precordial pain. There have also been isolated reports of cardiac conduction abnormalities, and gangrene in patients with pre-existing severe peripheral circulatory disorders.

Common gastro-intestinal disturbances have been described above but rarely diarrhoea or constipation also occur and there have been isolated cases of dry mouth and abnormal liver function.

Skin rashes (urticaria, psoriasiform, dystrophic skin lesions) and positive anti-nuclear antibodies (not associated with SLE) occur rarely. Isolated cases of photosensitivity, psoriasis exacerbation, increased sweating and alopecia have been reported. Respiratory effects include occasional reports of dyspnoea on exertion and rare reports of bronchospasm and isolated cases of rhinitis.

Rarely impotence/sexual dysfunction. Isolated cases of weight gain, thrombocytopenia, disturbances of vision, conjunctivitis, tinnitus, dry or irritated eyes, taste disturbance and arthralgia have also been reported.

The reported incidence of skin rashes and/or dry eyes is small and in most cases the symptoms have cleared when treatment was withdrawn. Discontinuation of the drug should be considered if any such reaction is not otherwise explicable.

Overdosage: Poisoning due to an overdose of Betaloc may lead to severe hypotension, sinus bradycardia, atrioventricular block, heart failure, cardiogenic shock, cardiac arrest, bronchospasm, impairment of consciousness, coma, nausea, vomiting, cyanosis, hypoglycaemia and, occasionally, hyperkalaemia. The first manifestations usually appear 20 minutes to 2 hours after drug ingestion.

Treatment should include close monitoring of cardiovascular, respiratory and renal function, and blood glucose and electrolytes. Further absorption may be prevented by induction of vomiting, gastric lavage or administration of activated-charcoal if ingestion is recent. Cardiovascular complications should be treated symptomatically, which may require the use of sympathomimetic agents (e.g. noradrenaline, metaraminol), atropine or inotropic agents (e.g. dopamine, dobutamine). Temporary pacing may be required for AV block. Glucagon can reverse the effects of excessive β-blockade, given in a dose of 1–10 mg intravenously. Intravenous β_2-stimulants e.g. terbutaline may be required to relieve bronchospasm.

Betaloc cannot be effectively removed by haemodialysis.

Pharmaceutical precautions Store below 25°C.

Legal category POM.

Package quantities PVC/Aluminium blister strips (10 tablets per strip) in a cardboard outer, pack size 100.

Further information Betaloc is well absorbed after oral administration, peak plasma concentrations occurring 1.5–2 hours after dosing. The bioavailability of a single dose is approximately 50%, increasing to approximately 70% during repeated administration. The bioavailability also increases if metoprolol is given with food.

Elimination is mainly by hepatic metabolism and the average elimination half-life is 3.5 hours (range 1 to 9 hours). Rates of metabolism vary between individuals, with poor metabolisers (approximately 10%) showing higher plasma concentrations and slower elimination than extensive metabolisers. Within individuals, however, plasma concentrations are stable and reproducible.

Because of variation in rates of metabolism, the dose of Betaloc should always be adjusted to the individual requirements of the patient. As the therapeutic response, adverse effects and relative cardioselectivity are related to plasma concentration, poor metabolisers may require lower than normal doses. Dosage adjustment is not routinely required in the elderly or in patients with renal failure, but dosage may need to be reduced in patients with significant hepatic dysfunction when Betaloc elimination may be impaired.

Product licence numbers
Betaloc Tablets 50 mg 0017/0073R
Betaloc Tablets 100 mg 0017/0074R

BETALOC* I.V. INJECTION

Presentation
Ampoules: Each ampoule of 5 ml contains 5 mg metoprolol tartrate Ph Eur and sodium chloride.

Inactive ingredients: Sodium chloride, water for injection.

Uses Control of tachyarrhythmias, especially supraventricular tachyarrhythmias.

Early intervention with Betaloc in acute myocardial infarction reduces infarct size and the incidence of ventricular fibrillation. Pain relief may also decrease the need for opiate analgesics.

Betaloc has been shown to reduce mortality when administered to patients with acute myocardial infarction.

Dosage and administration
Control of tachyarrhythmias: Initially up to 5 mg injected i.v. at a rate of 1–2 mg per minute. The injection can be repeated at 5 minute intervals until a satisfactory response has been obtained. A total dose of 10–15 mg generally proves sufficient.

Because of the risk of a pronounced drop of blood pressure, the i.v. administration of Betaloc to patients with a systolic blood pressure below 100 mmHg should only be given with special care.

During anaesthesia: 2–4 mg injected slowly i.v. at induction is usually sufficient to prevent the development of arrhythmias during anaesthesia. The same dosage can also be used to control arrhythmias developing during anaesthesia. Further injections of 2 mg may be given as required to a maximum overall dose of 10 mg.

Myocardial infarction: Early intervention. To achieve optimal benefits from intravenous Betaloc, suitable patients should present within 12 hours of the onset of chest pain. Therapy should commence with 5 mg i.v. every 2 minutes to a maximum of 15 mg total as determined by blood pressure and heart rate. The second or third dose should not be given if the systolic blood pressure is <90 mmHg, the heart rate is <40 beats/min and the P-Q time is >0.26 seconds, or if there is any aggravation of dyspnoea or cold sweating. Orally, therapy should commence 15 minutes after the injection with 50 mg every 6 hours for 48 hours. Patients who fail to tolerate the full intravenous dose should be given half the suggested oral dose.

Elderly: There are no special dosage requirements in otherwise healthy elderly patients.

Significant hepatic dysfunction: A reduction in dosage may be necessary.

Contra-indications, warnings, etc
Contra-indications: AV Block. Uncontrolled heart failure. Severe bradycardia. Sick sinus syndrome. Cardiogenic shock. Severe peripheral arterial disease. Known hypersensitivity to Betaloc or other β-blockers.

Betaloc i.v. is also contra-indicated when myocardial infarction is complicated by significant bradycardia, first degree heart block, systolic hypotension (<100 mmHg) and/or severe heart failure.

Warnings: Betaloc i.v. may aggravate bradycardia, symptoms of peripheral arterial circulatory disorders and anaphylactic shock.

Betaloc i.v. may be administered when heart failure has been controlled. Digitalisation and/or diuretic therapy should also be considered for patients with a history of heart failure, or patients known to have a poor cardiac reserve.

Although cardioselective β-blockers may have less effect on lung function than non-selective β-blockers, as with all β-blockers these should be avoided in patients with reversible obstructive airways disease unless there are compelling clinical reasons for their use. When administration is necessary, use of a β_2-bronchodilator (e.g. terbutaline) may be advisable in some patients.

The label shall state – 'Use with caution in patients with a history of wheezing, asthma or any other breathing difficulties, see enclosed user leaflet'.

In labile and insulin-dependent diabetes it may be necessary to adjust the hypoglycaemic therapy.

In patients with a phaeochromocytoma, an α-blocker should be given concomitantly.

The administration of adrenaline to patients undergoing β-blockade can result in an increase in blood pressure and bradycardia although this is less likely to occur with β_1-selective drugs.

Betaloc i.v. therapy must be reported to the anaesthetist prior to general anaesthesia. However, in some patients it may be desirable to employ a β-blocker as premedication. By shielding the heart against the effects of stress the β-blocker may prevent excessive sympathetic stimulation provoking cardiac arrhythmias or acute coronary insufficiency. If a β-blocker is given for this purpose, an anaesthetic with little negative inotropic activity should be selected to minimise the risk of myocardial depression.

Pregnancy: Betaloc i.v. should not be used in pregnancy or nursing mothers unless the physician considers that the benefit outweighs the possible hazard to the foetus/infant. As with all β-blockers metoprolol may cause side-effects e.g. bradycardia, hypoglycaemia in the foetus, and in the newborn and breast-fed infant. Metoprolol has, however, been used in pregnancy associated hypertension under close supervision, after 20 weeks gestation. Although Betaloc i.v. crosses the placental barrier and is present in cord blood, no evidence of foetal abnormalities has been reported.

Lactation: The amount of Betaloc i.v. ingested via breast milk should not produce significant β-blocking effects in the neonate if the mother is treated with normal therapeutic doses.

Interactions: The effects of Betaloc i.v. and other antihypertensive drugs on blood pressure are usually additive, and care should be taken to avoid hypotension.

Betaloc i.v. can reduce myocardial contractility and impair intracardiac conduction. Care should be exercised when drugs with similar activity, e.g. antiarrhythmic agents, general anaesthetics, are given concurrently. Like all other β-blockers, Betaloc i.v. should not be given in combination with verapamil since this may cause bradycardia, hypotension and asystole. Care should also be exercised when β-blockers are given in combination with sympathetic ganglion blocking agents, other β-blockers (i.e. eye drops) or MAO inhibitors.

As β-blockers may affect the peripheral circulation, care should be exercised when drugs with similar activity e.g. ergotamine are given concurrently.

Betaloc i.v. will antagonise the β_1-effects of sympathomimetic agents but should have little influence on the bronchodilator effects of β_2-agonists at normal therapeutic doses. Enzyme inducing agents (e.g. rifampicin) may reduce plasma concentrations of Betaloc, whereas enzyme inhibitors (e.g. cimetidine) may increase plasma concentrations. Betaloc i.v. may impair the elimination of lignocaine.

Side-effects: As in the case of other β-blockers, a marked fall in blood pressure may sometimes occur following intravenous injection of Betaloc. Other side-effects are usually mild and infrequent. The most common appear to be lassitude, GI disturbances (nausea, vomiting or abdominal pain) and disturbances of sleep pattern. In many cases these effects have been transient or have disappeared after a reduction in dosage.

Effects related to the CNS which have been reported occasionally are dizziness and headache and rarely paraesthesia, muscle cramps, depression and decreased mental alertness. There have also been isolated reports of personality disorders, like amnesia, memory impairment, confusion, hallucination, nervousness and anxiety.

The label shall state – 'If you have a history of wheezing, asthma or any other breathing difficulties, you must tell your doctor before you take this medicine'.

Cardiovascular effects which have been reported occasionally are bradycardia, postural hypotension and rarely, heart failure, palpitations, cardiac arrhythmias, Raynaud's phenomenon, peripheral oedema and precordial pain. There have also been isolated reports of cardiac conduction abnormalities, and gangrene in patients with pre-existing severe peripheral circulatory disorders.

Common gastro-intestinal disturbances have been described above but rarely diarrhoea or constipation also occur and there have been isolated cases of dry mouth and abnormal liver function.

Skin rashes (urticaria, psoriasiform, dystrophic skin lesions) and positive anti-nuclear antibodies (not associated with SLE) occur rarely. Isolated cases of photosensitivity, psoriasis exacerbation, increased sweating and alopecia have been reported. Respiratory effects include occasional reports of dyspnoea on exertion and rare reports of bronchospasm and isolated cases of rhinitis.

Rarely impotence/sexual dysfunction. Isolated cases of weight gain, thrombocytopenia, disturbances of vision, conjunctivitis, tinnitus, dry or irritated eyes, taste disturbance and arthralgia have also been reported.

The reported incidence of skin rashes and/or dry eyes is small and in most cases the symptoms have cleared when treatment was withdrawn. Discontinuation of the drug should be considered if any such reaction is not otherwise explicable.

Overdosage: Poisoning due to an overdose of Betaloc i.v. may lead to severe hypotension, sinus bradycardia, atrioventricular block, heart failure, cardiogenic shock, cardiac arrest, bronchospasm, impairment of consciousness, coma, nausea, vomiting, cyanosis, hypoglycaemia and, occasionally, hyperkalaemia.

Treatment should include close monitoring of cardiovascular, respiratory and renal function, and blood glucose and electrolytes. Cardiovascular complications should be treated symptomatically, which may require the use of sympathomimetic agents (e.g. noradrenaline, metaraminol), atropine or inotropic agents (e.g. dopamine, dobutamine). Temporary pacing may be required for AV block. Glucagon can reverse the effects of excessive β-blockade, given in a dose of 1–10 mg intravenously. Intravenous β_2-stimulants e.g. terbutaline may be required to relieve bronchospasm.

Betaloc i.v. cannot be effectively removed by haemodialysis.

Pharmaceutical precautions Protect from light. Store below 25°C.

Legal category POM.

Package quantities 5×5 ml ampoules.

Further information Betaloc is a cardioselective β_1-receptor blocker exhibiting no intrinsic sympathomimetic activity. Elimination is mainly by hepatic metabolism and the average elimination half-life is 3.5 hours (range 1 to 9 hours). Rates of metabolism vary between individuals, with poor metabolisers (approximately 10%) showing higher plasma concentrations and slower elimination than extensive metabolisers. Within individuals, however, plasma concentrations are stable and reproducible.

Product licence number 0017/0072

BETALOC* SA

Presentation White tablets (coded A/MD) containing 200 mg metoprolol tartrate PhEur, extended release formulation (Durules*).

Inactive ingredients: Sodium aluminium silicate, paraffin, magnesium stearate, ethylcellulose, hydroxypropyl methylcellulose, polyethylene glycol, titanium dioxide.

Uses In the management of angina pectoris and hypertension.

Prophylaxis of migraine.

Dosage and administration
Angina pectoris and hypertension: One tablet daily, in the morning. In rare cases two tablets may be indicated.

Migraine Prophylaxis: One tablet daily, in the morning.

Betaloc SA tablets must not be chewed or crushed. They should be swallowed whole with half a glass of water.

Elderly: There are no special dosage requirements in otherwise healthy elderly patients.

Significant hepatic dysfunction: A reduction in dosage may be necessary.

Contra-indications, warnings, etc
Contra-indications: AV block. Uncontrolled heart failure. Severe bradycardia. Sick-sinus syndrome. Cardiogenic shock. Severe peripheral arterial disease. Known hypersensitivity to Betaloc SA or other β-blockers.

Warnings: Betaloc SA may aggravate bradycardia, symptoms of peripheral arterial circulatory disorders and anaphylactic shock.

Abrupt interruption of β-blockers is to be avoided.

When possible, Betaloc SA should be withdrawn gradually over a period of 10 days. During its withdrawal patients should be kept under close surveillance, especially those with known ischaemic heart disease.

Betaloc SA may be administered when heart failure has been controlled. Digitalisation and/or diuretic therapy should also be considered for patients with a history of heart failure, or patients known to have a poor cardiac reserve.

Although cardioselective β-blockers may have less effect on lung function than non-selective β-blockers, as with all β-blockers these should be avoided in patients with reversible obstructive airways disease unless there are compelling clinical reasons for their use. When administration is necessary, use of a β_2-bronchodilator (e.g. terbutaline) may be advisable in some patients.

In labile and insulin-dependent diabetes it may be necessary to adjust the hypoglycaemic therapy.

In patients with phaeochromocytoma, an α-blocker should be given concomitantly.

In the presence of liver cirrhosis the bioavailability of Betaloc SA may be increased.

The administration of adrenaline to patients undergoing β-blockade can result in an increase in blood pressure and bradycardia although this is less likely to occur with β_1-selective drugs.

Betaloc SA therapy must be reported to the anaesthetist prior to general anaesthesia. If withdrawal of metoprolol is considered desirable, this should if possible be completed at least 48 hours before general anaesthesia. However, in some patients it may be desirable to employ a β-blocker as premedication. By shielding the heart against the effects of stress the β-blocker may prevent excessive sympathetic stimulation provoking cardiac arrhythmias or acute coronary insufficiency. If a β-blocker is given for this purpose, an anaesthetic with little negative inotropic activity should be selected to minimise the risk of myocardial depression.

Pregnancy: Betaloc SA should not be used in pregnancy or nursing mothers unless the physician considers that the benefit outweighs the possible hazard to the foetus/infant. As with all β-blockers metoprolol may cause side-effects e.g. bradycardia, hypoglycaemia in the foetus, and in the newborn and breast-fed infant. Metoprolol has, however, been used in pregnancy associated hypertension under close supervision, after 20 weeks gestation. Although Betaloc SA crosses the placental barrier and is present in cord blood, no evidence of foetal abnormalities has been reported.

Lactation: The amount of metoprolol ingested via breast milk should not produce significant β-blocking effects in the neonate if the mother is treated with normal therapeutic doses.

Interactions: The effects of Betaloc SA and other antihypertensive drugs on blood pressure are usually additive, and care should be taken to avoid hypotension. However, combinations of antihypertensive drugs may often be used with benefit to improve control of hypertension.

Betaloc SA can reduce myocardial contractility and impair intracardiac conduction. Care should be exercised when drugs with similar activity, e.g. antiarrhythmic agents, general anaesthetics, are given concurrently. Like all other β-blockers, Betaloc SA should not be given in combination with verapamil since this may cause bradycardia, hypotension and asystole. Care should also be exercised when β-blockers are given in combination with sympathetic ganglion blocking agents, other β-blockers (i.e. eye drops) or MAO inhibitors. If combination treatment with clonidine is to be discontinued, Betaloc SA should be withdrawn several days before clonidine.

As β-blockers may affect the peripheral circulation, care should be exercised when drugs with similar activity e.g. ergotamine are given concurrently.

Betaloc SA will antagonise the β_1-effects of sympathomimetic agents but should have little influence on the bronchodilator effects of β_2-agonists at normal therapeutic doses. Enzyme inducing agents (e.g. rifampicin) may reduce plasma concentrations of Betaloc SA, whereas enzyme inhibitors (e.g. cimetidine) may increase plasma concentrations. Betaloc SA may impair the elimination of lignocaine.

Indomethacin may reduce the antihypertensive effect of β-blockers.

Side-effects: These are usually mild and infrequent. The most common appear to be lassitude, GI disturbances (nausea, vomiting or abdominal pain) and disturbances of sleep pattern. In many cases these effects have been transient or have disappeared after a reduction in dosage.

Effects related to the CNS which have been reported occasionally are dizziness and headache and rarely paraesthesia, muscle cramps, depression and decreased mental alertness. There have also been isolated reports of personality disorders like amnesia, memory impairment, confusion, hallucination, nervousness and anxiety.

Cardiovascular effects which have been reported occasionally are bradycardia, postural hypotension and rarely, heart failure, palpitations, cardiac arrhythmias, Raynaud's phenomenon, peripheral oedema and precordial pain. There have also been isolated reports of cardiac conduction abnormalities, and gangrene in patients with pre-existing severe peripheral circulatory disorders.

Common gastro-intestinal disturbances have been described above but rarely diarrhoea or constipation also occur and there have been isolated cases of dry mouth and abnormal liver function.

Skin rashes (urticaria, psoriasiform, dystrophic skin lesions) and positive anti-nuclear antibodies (not associated with SLE) occur rarely. Isolated cases of photosensitivity, psoriasis exacerbation, increased sweating and alopecia have been reported. Respiratory effects include occasional reports of dyspnoea on exertion and rare reports of bronchospasm and isolated cases of rhinitis.

Rarely impotence/sexual dysfunction. Isolated cases of weight gain, thrombocytopenia, disturbances of vision, conjunctivitis, tinnitus, dry or irritated eyes, taste disturbance and arthralgia have also been reported.

The reported incidence of skin rashes and/or dry eyes is small and in most cases the symptoms have cleared when treatment was withdrawn. Discontinuation of the drug should be considered if any such reaction is not otherwise explicable.

Overdosage: Poisoning due to an overdose of Betaloc SA may lead to severe hypotension, sinus bradycardia, atrioventricular block, heart failure, cardiogenic shock, cardiac arrest, bronchospasm, impairment of consciousness, coma, nausea, vomiting, cyanosis, hypoglycaemia and, occasionally, hyperkalaemia. The first manifestations usually appear 20 minutes to 2 hours after drug ingestion.

Treatment should include close monitoring of cardiovascular, respiratory and renal function, and blood glucose and electrolytes. Further absorption may be prevented by induction of vomiting, gastric lavage or administration of activated-charcoal if ingestion is recent. Cardiovascular complications should be treated symptomatically, which may require the use of sympathomimetic agents (e.g. noradrenaline, metaraminol), atropine or inotropic agents (e.g. dopamine, dobutamine). Temporary pacing may be required for AV block. Glucagon can reverse the effects of excessive β-blockade, given in a dose of 1–10 mg intravenously. Intravenous β_2-stimulants e.g. terbutaline may be required to relieve bronchospasm.

Metoprolol cannot be effectively removed by haemodialysis.

Pharmaceutical precautions Store below 25°C.

Legal category POM.

Package quantities Blister strips (press through packs of thermoformed PVC) 7 tablets per strip – pack size 28.

Further information Administration of Betaloc SA results in a controlled release of active substance which means that the peak plasma levels are reduced. Compared to Betaloc tablets the absorption phase is prolonged and the duration of effect is extended. The substance is completely absorbed and the maximal β-blocking effect is reached after about four hours.

These factors may lead to a more convenient dosage and an improved degree of β_1-selectivity.

The effect on the pulse and blood pressure remain pronounced 24 hours after administration.

Elimination is mainly by hepatic metabolism and the average elimination half-life is 3.5 hours (range 1 to 9 hours). Rates of metabolism vary between individuals, with poor metabolisers (approximately 10%) showing higher plasma concentrations and slower elimination than extensive metabolisers. Within individuals, however, plasma concentrations are stable and reproducible.

Product licence number 0017/0093

BRICANYL* INHALER
BRICANYL* SPACER INHALER

Presentation
Bricanyl Inhaler: Metered dose aerosol delivering 0.25 mg terbutaline sulphate per actuation.

Bricanyl spacer inhaler: Metered dose aerosol with extended mouthpiece delivering 0.25 mg terbutaline sulphate per actuation.
Inactive Ingredients: Sorbitan trioleate and chlorofluorocarbons 11, 12 and 114.

Nebuhaler: 750 ml plastic cone with a one-way valve. For use in conjunction with Bricanyl aerosol.

Both the Bricanyl Spacer Inhaler and the Nebuhaler are recommended to enable patients with difficulty co-ordinating conventional aerosols to derive greater therapeutic benefit. A package insert is provided giving simple operating instructions.

Uses Terbutaline is a selective β_2-adrenergic agonist recommended for the relief and prevention of bronchospasm in bronchial asthma and in chronic bronchitis, emphysema and other bronchopulmonary disorders in which bronchospasm is a complicating factor.

Dosage and administration
Bricanyl Inhaler: Adults and children: Prophylaxis and relief of acute attacks: One or two inhalations as required, with a short interval between each inhalation at 6 hourly intervals. Not more than 8 inhalations should be necessary in any 24 hours, but medical advice should be sought and treatment reviewed if condition fails to improve.

Bricanyl Spacer Inhaler: Adults and children: Prophylaxis and relief of acute attacks: One or two inhalations as required, with a short interval between each inhalation at 6 hourly intervals. Not more than 8 inhalations should be necessary in any 24 hours, but medical advice should be sought and treatment reviewed if condition fails to improve.

Nebuhaler: Adults and children: The dose must always be adjusted to patient response and severity of the bronchospasm. Patients must be instructed to actuate the aerosol and breathe in slowly and deeply through the mouthpiece. Ideally two inspirations per actuation are required to empty the Nebuhaler.

Prophylaxis and relief of acute attacks: One or two inhalations as required, with a short interval between each inhalation at 6 hourly intervals. Not more than 8 inhalations should be necessary in any 24 hours, but medical advice should be sought and treatment reviewed if condition fails to improve.

Bricanyl via the Nebuhaler may also be used in conditions such as severe bronchospasm and severe acute asthma which are normally managed by administration of nebulised bronchodilators.

For hospital use in acute asthma: Adults: The initial dose should be 2 mg (8 actuations); this may be repeated up to a total dose of 8 mg in one hour. Thereafter a dose of up to 4 mg may be given four times daily.

A similar dose range may be used for domiciliary use, but patients should be warned that if either the usual relief or duration of action is diminished, they should seek medical advice immediately.

Children over 5 years: Dosage must be individualised but clinical studies have shown that when used for the management of acute asthma in children, the following dosages given over a 15 minute period have been as effective as equal doses administered by nebuliser.

Children under 25 kg	1.25–2.5 mg (5–10 puffs)
Children over 25 kg	2.5–5.0 mg (10–20 puffs)

Elderly: Dosage as for adults. Because of the difficulty experienced by many elderly patients in co-ordinating inhalation with actuation, Bricanyl Spacer Inhaler or use via the Nebuhaler will provide a more certain delivery of drug.

Contra-indications, warnings, etc
Contra-indications: Bricanyl preparations are contra-indicated in patients with a history of hypersensitivity to any of their constituents.

Precautions: Care should be taken with patients suffering from myocardial insufficiency or thyrotoxicosis. Due to the hyperglycaemic effects of β_2-stimulants, additional blood glucose measurements are initially recommended when Bricanyl therapy is commenced in diabetic patients. If treatment becomes less effective or shorter acting the patients general condition should be reviewed.

Due to the positive inotropic effect of β_2-agonists, these drugs should not be used in patients with hypertrophic cardiomyopathy.

Potentially serious hypokalaemia may result from β_2-agonist therapy. Particular caution is advised in severe asthma as this effect may be potentiated by concomitant treatment with xanthine derivatives, steroids, diuretics and by hypoxia. It is recommended that serum potassium levels are monitored in such situations.

Interactions: Beta-blocking agents, especially the non-selective ones such as propranolol, may partially or totally inhibit the effect of β-stimulants. Therefore Bricanyl and non-selective β-blockers should not normally be administered concurrently. Bricanyl should be used with caution in patients receiving other sympathomimetics.

Pregnancy and lactation: Although no teratogenic effects have been observed in animals or in patients, Bricanyl should only be administered with caution during the Ist trimester of pregnancy.

Terbutaline is secreted via breast milk, but effect on the infant is unlikely at therapeutic doses.

Side-effects: The frequency of side-effects is low at the recommended doses. Side-effects which have been recorded such as tremor, tonic cramp and palpitations are all characteristic of sympathomimetic amines. A few patients feel tense; this is also due to the effects on skeletal muscle and not to direct CNS stimulation. Whenever these side-effects have occurred the majority have usually been spontaneously reversible within the first week of treatment. Rare cases of bronchospasm have occurred. The chlorofluorocarbons used as propellants may in some asthmatics cause a fall in FEV_1 immediately after exposure.

Potentially serious hypokalaemia may result from β_2-agonist therapy.

Overdose

(i) *Possible symptoms and signs:* Headache, anxiety, tremor, tonic cramp, palpitations, arrhythmia. A fall in blood pressure sometimes occurs. Laboratory findings: hypokalaemia, hyperglycaemia and lactic acidosis sometimes occur.

(ii) *Treatment: Mild and moderate cases:* Reduce the dose.

Severe cases: Determination of acid-base balance, blood sugar and electrolytes. Monitoring of heart rate and rhythm and blood pressure. Metabolic changes should be corrected. A cardioselective β-blocker (e.g. metoprolol) is recommended for the treatment of arrhythmias causing haemodynamic deterioration. The β-blocker should be used with care because of the possibility of inducing bronchoconstriction. If the β_2-mediated reduction in peripheral vascular resistance significantly contributes to the fall in blood pressure, a volume expander should be given.

Pharmaceutical precautions Store at temperatures not exceeding 25°C.

Legal category POM.

Package quantities Bricanyl Inhaler: Aerosol containing 400 metered doses.

Bricanyl Spacer Inhaler: Aerosol containing 400 metered doses complete with extended mouthpiece.

Nebuhaler: 750 ml plastic cone with a one-way valve.

Further information Bricanyl is also available as Respirator Solution, Tablets, Syrup and Injection.

Product licence number 0017/0061R

BRICANYL* INJECTION

Presentation Clear aqueous solution for injection containing 0.5 mg terbutaline sulphate per ml, sodium chloride and water for injection.

Bricanyl Injection is available in 1 ml and 5 ml ampoules. Bricanyl Injection in 1 ml ampoules is intended for subcutaneous, intramuscular or intravenous injection. Bricanyl Injection in 5 ml ampoules is intended for infusion after dilution with infusion solutions.

Uses

1. *For bronchodilation:* Terbutaline is a selective β_2-adrenergic agonist recommended for the relief of bronchospasm in bronchial asthma and other bronchopulmonary disorders in which bronchospasm is a complicating factor.

2. *For the management of uncomplicated premature labour:* To arrest labour between 24 and 33 weeks of gestation in patients with no medical or obstetric contra-indication to tocolytic therapy. The main effect of tocolytic therapy is a delay in delivery of up to 48 hours; no statistically significant effect on perinatal mortality or morbidity has as yet been observed in randomised-controlled trials. The greatest benefit from tocolytic therapy is gained by using the delay in delivery to administer glucocorticoids or to implement other measures known to improve perinatal health.

Dosage and administration The dosage should be individual.

1. *For bronchodilation:* When a rapid therapeutic response is required, Bricanyl can be administered by any of the three standard parenteral routes: subcutaneous, intramuscular, or i.v. bolus. The preferred routes will usually be subcutaneous or intramuscular. When given as an i.v. bolus the injection must be made slowly noting patient response.

Adults: 0.5 ml–1 ml (0.25–0.50 mg) up to four times a day.

Children: 2–15 years. 0.01 mg/kg body weight to a maximum of 0.3 mg total.

Age	*Average weight* kg	*(lb)*	*mg terbutaline*	*ml volume*
<3	10	(22)	0.1	0.2
3	15	(33)	0.15	0.3
6	20	(44)	0.2	0.4
8	25	(55)	0.25	0.5
10+	30+	(66+)	0.3	0.6

By infusion: 3–5 ml (1.5–2.5 mg) in 500 ml dextrose, saline or dextrose/saline given by continuous intravenous infusion at a rate of 10–20 drops (0.5–1 ml) per minute for 8 to 10 hours. A corresponding reduction in dosage should be made for children.

Elderly: Dosages as for adults.

2. *For the management of premature labour. Procedure:* To be administered as early as possible after the diagnosis of premature labour, and after evaluation of the patient to rule out contra-indications to the use of terbutaline (see Contra-indications).

Initially 5 microgram/min should be infused during the first 20 minutes increasing by 2.5 micrograms/min at 20 minute intervals until contractions stop. More than 10 micrograms/min should seldom be given, 20 micrograms/min should not be exceeded.

The infusion should be stopped if labour progresses despite treatment at the maximum dose. **If successful**, the infusion should continue for 1 hour at the chosen rate and then be decreased by 2.5 micrograms/min every 20 minutes to the lowest dose that produces suppression of contractions. Keep the infusion at this rate for 12 hours and then continue with oral maintenance therapy.

As an alternative, subcutaneous injections (0.25 mg) should be given four times a day for a few days before oral treatment is commenced.

Oral treatment may be continued for as long as the physician considers it desirable to prolong pregnancy.

Special cautions for infusion: The dose must be individually titrated with reference to suppression of contractions, increase in pulse rate and changes in blood pressure, which are limiting factors. These parameters should be carefully monitored during treatment. A maternal heart rate of more than 135 beats/min should be avoided.

Careful control of the level of hydration is essential to avoid the risk of maternal pulmonary oedema (see *Side-effects*). The volume of fluid in which the drug is administered should thus be kept to a minimum. A controlled infusion device should be used preferably a syringe pump.

Dilution: The recommended infusion fluid is 5% dextrose.

If a syringe pump is available, the concentration of the drug infused should be 0.1 mg/ml (10 ml Bricanyl Injection should be added to 40 ml of 5% dextrose). At this dilution, 5 micrograms/min equates with 0.05 ml/min, and 10 micrograms/min equates with 0.1 ml/min. If no syringe pump is available, the concentration of the drug should be 0.01 mg/ml (10 ml Bricanyl Injection should be added to 490 ml of 5% dextrose). At this dilution, 5 micrograms/min equates with 0.5 ml/min and 10 micrograms/min equates with 1 ml/min.

Contra-indications, warnings, etc

Contra-indications: Bricanyl preparations are contra-indicated in patients with a history of hypersensitivity to any of their constituents.

Although Bricanyl Injection and Tablets are used in the management of uncomplicated premature labour, their use in the following conditions is contra-indicated: Any condition of the mother or foetus in which prolongation of the pregnancy is hazardous e.g. severe toxaemia, ante-partum haemorrhage, intrauterine infection, abruptio placentae, threatened abortion during the first and second trimesters or cord compression.

Precautions: Care should be taken with patients suffering from myocardial insufficiency or thyrotoxicosis. Due to the hyperglycaemic effects of β_2-stimulants, additional blood glucose measurements are initially recommended when Bricanyl therapy is commenced in diabetic patients. If treatment becomes less effective or shorter-acting, the patients' general condition should be reviewed.

Due to the positive inotropic effect of β_2-agonists these drugs should not be used in patients with hypertrophic cardiomyopathy.

Potentially serious hypokalaemia may result from β_2-agonist therapy. Particular caution is advised in severe asthma as this effect may be potentiated by concomitant treatment with xanthine derivatives, steroids, diuretics and by hypoxia. It is recommended that serum potassium levels are monitored in such situations.

In premature labour in a patient with known or suspected cardiac disease a physician experienced in cardiology should assess the suitability of treatment before i.v. infusion with Bricanyl.

In order to minimise the risk of hypotension associated with tocolytic therapy, special care should be taken to avoid caval compression by keeping the patient in the left or right lateral positions throughout the infusion.

Warnings: In treatment of premature labour, hyperglycaemia and ketoacidosis have been found in pregnant women with diabetes after treatment with β_2-stimulants. It may therefore be necessary to adjust the insulin dose when β_2-stimulants are used in the treatment.

Increased tendency to uterine bleeding has been reported in connection with Caesarean section. However, this can be effectively stopped by propranolol 1–2 mg injected intravenously.

Interactions: β-blocking agents especially the non-selective ones such as propranolol may partially or totally inhibit the effect of β-stimulants. Therefore Bricanyl and non-selective β-blockers should not normally be administered concurrently. Bricanyl should be used with caution in patients receiving other sympathomimetics.

Pregnancy and lactation: Although no teratogenic effects have been observed in animals or in patients, Bricanyl should only be administered with caution during the first trimester of pregnancy.

Terbutaline is secreted into breast milk, but effects on the infant are unlikely at therapeutic doses.

Side-effects: When used as a bronchodilator the frequency of side-effects is low. Side-effects which have been recorded such as tremor, tonic cramp and palpitations are all characteristics of sympathomimetic amines. A few patients feel tense; this is also due to the effects on skeletal muscle and not to direct CNS stimulation. Whenever these side-effects have occurred the majority have usually been spontaneously reversible within the first week of treatment. Urticaria and exanthema may occur.

Potentially serious hypokalaemia may result from β_2-agonist therapy.

In common with other β_2-agonists maternal pulmonary oedema has been reported in association with the use of terbutaline for the management of premature labour; in some cases this has proved fatal. Predisposing factors include fluid overload, multiple pregnancy, pre-existing cardiac disease and maternal infection. Close monitoring of the patient's state of hydration is essential. If signs of pulmonary oedema develop (e.g. cough, shortness of breath), treatment should be discontinued immediately and diuretic therapy instituted.

Overdosage: Possible symptoms and signs: Headache, anxiety, tremor, tonic cramp, palpitations, arrhythmia. A fall in blood pressure sometimes occurs. Laboratory findings: hypokalaemia, hyperglycaemia and lactic acidosis sometimes occur.

Treatment:

(a) Mild and moderate cases: Reduce the dose.

(b) Severe cases: Determination of acid-base balance, blood sugar and electrolytes. Monitoring of heart rate and rhythm and blood pressure. Metabolic changes should be corrected. A cardioselective β-blocker (e.g. metoprolol) is recommended for the treatment of arrhythmias causing haemodynamic deterioration. The β-blocker should be used with care because of the possibility of inducing bronchoconstriction. If the β_2-mediated reduction in peripheral vascular resistance significantly contributes to the fall in blood pressure, a volume expander should be given.

(c) In preterm labour: Pulmonary oedema: discontinue administration of Bricanyl. A normal dose of loop diuretic (e.g. frusemide) should be given intravenously.

Increased bleeding in connection with Caesarian section: Propranolol, 1–2 mg intravenously.

Pharmaceutical precautions Store below 25°C. Protect from light.

Bronchodilation: The recommended diluent is water for injection, or dextrose. Saline should be avoided due to the risk of pulmonary oedema. If saline is used the patient should be carefully monitored.

In the management of premature labour the recommended infusion fluid is 5% dextrose.

Legal category POM.

Package quantities Packs of 5×1 ml ampoules and 10×5 ml ampoules.

Further information Nil

Product licence number 0017/0048R

BRICANYL* RESPULES*

Presentation A clear aqueous isotonic solution for nebulisation. Single dose plastic units (Respules) containing 5 mg terbutaline sulphate in 2 ml.

Inactive ingredients: Sodium chloride, sodium edetate.

Uses Terbutaline is a selective β_2-adrenergic agonist recommended for the relief of severe bronchospasm in bronchial asthma and in chronic bronchitis, emphysema and other bronchopulmonary disorders in which bronchospasm is a complicating factor.

Dosage and administration In most patients the use of terbutaline sulphate, based on the doses below, given 2–4 times daily will be sufficient to relieve bronchospasm. In acute severe asthma additional doses may be necessary.

Bricanyl Respules:
Adults: 1 or 2 Respules (5 or 10 mg)
Children: (>25 kg) 1 Respule (5 mg)
Children: (<25 kg) use multidose bottles.

Multidose bottles:
Adults: 0.5 to 1 ml (5 to 10 mg) diluted to required nebuliser volume with sterile physiological saline.

Children: 0.2 to 0.5 ml (2 to 5 mg), see table, diluted to required nebuliser volume with sterile physiological saline.

Table illustrating ml undiluted solution from multidose bottle required for administration to children

Age	Average weight kg	lb	mg terbutaline	ml undiluted solution
<3	10	22	2.0	0.2
3	15	33	3.0	0.3
6	20	44	4.0	0.4
8+	25+	55+	5.0	0.5

Elderly: Dosage as for adults.

Contra-indications, warnings, etc
Contra-indications: Bricanyl preparations are contra-indicated in patients with a history of hypersensitivity to any of their constituents.

Precautions: Care should be taken with patients suffering from myocardial insufficiency or thyrotoxicosis. Due to the hyperglycaemic effects of β_2-stimulants, additional blood glucose measurements are initially recommended when Bricanyl therapy is commenced in diabetic patients. If treatment becomes less effective or shorter acting, the patients general condition should be reviewed.

Due to the positive inotropic effect of the β_2-agonists, these drugs should not be used in patients with hypertrophic cardiomyopathy.

Potentially serious hypokalaemia may result from β_2-agonist therapy. Particular caution is advised in severe asthma as this effect may be potentiated by concomitant treatment with xanthine derivatives, steroids, diuretics and by hypoxia. It is recommended that serum potassium levels are monitored in such situations.

Interactions: β-blocking agents especially the non-selective ones such as propranolol may partially or totally inhibit the effect of β-stimulants. Therefore Bricanyl and non-selective β-blockers should not normally be administered concurrently. Bricanyl should be used with caution in patients receiving other sympathomimetics.

Pregnancy and lactation: Although no teratogenic effects have been observed in animals or in patients, Bricanyl should only be administered with caution during the first trimester of pregnancy.

Terbutaline is excreted in breast milk, but effect on the infant is unlikely at therapeutic doses.

Side-effects: The frequency of side-effects is low. Side-effects which have been recorded, such as tremor, tonic cramps and palpitations, are all characteristic of sympathomimetic amines. A few patients feel tense; this is also due to effects on skeletal muscle and not to direct CNS stimulation. Whenever these side-effects have occurred, the majority have been spontaneously reversible within the first week of treatment. Rare cases of bronchospasm have occurred

Potentially serious hypokalaemia may result from β_2-agonist therapy.

Overdosage:
(i) Possible symptoms and signs: Headache, anxiety, tremor, tonic cramp, palpitations and arrhythmia. A fall in blood pressure sometimes occurs.

Laboratory findings: Hypokalaemia, hyperglycaemia and metabolic acidosis sometimes occur.

(ii) Treatment: Mild and moderate cases: Reduce the dose.

Severe cases: Determination of acid-base balance, blood sugar and electrolytes. Monitoring of heart rate and rhythm and blood pressure. Metabolic changes should be corrected. A cardioselective β-blocker (e.g. metoprolol) is recommended for the treatment of arrhythmias causing haemodynamic deterioration. The β-blocker should be used with care because of the possibility of inducing bronchoconstriction. If the β_2-mediated reduction in peripheral vascular resistance significantly contributes to the fall in blood pressure, a volume expander should be given.

Pharmaceutical precautions Store below 30°C. Away from light.

Single dose plastic units (Respules) in an opened foil envelope must be used within 3 months. Bricanyl Respules will not normally require dilution at recommended doses. The pH of Bricanyl Respules is 3–4.5.

Legal category POM.

Package quantities Single dose units (Respules): Packs of 20×2 ml. (Strips of 5 units wrapped in a foil envelope).

Further information Bricanyl Respules Solution contains 0.1 mg/ml sodium edetate, which has been shown to cause bronchoconstriction at levels above 1.2 mg/ml.

Product licence numbers 0017/0228

BRICANYL* RESPIRATOR SOLUTION

Qualitative and quantitative composition Terbutaline sulphate PhEur 10 mg/ml

Pharmaceutical form Solution for nebulisation

Clinical particulars
Therapeutic indications: Terbutaline is a selective β_2-adrenergic agonist recommended for the relief of severe bronchospasm in bronchial asthma and in chronic bronchitis, emphysema and other bronchopulmonary disorders in which bronchospasm is a complicating factor.

Posology and method of administration: In most patients the use of terbutaline sulphate, based on the doses below, given 2–4 times daily will be sufficient to relieve bronchospasm. In acute severe asthma additional doses may be necessary.
Adults: 0.5 to 1 ml (5 to 10 mg) diluted to required nebuliser volume with sterile physiological saline.

Elderly: Dosage as for adults.

Children: 0.2 to 0.5 ml (2 to 5 mg), see table, diluted to required nebuliser volume with sterile physiological saline.

Table illustrating ml undiluted solution required for administration to children

Age	Average weight kg	lb	mg terbutaline	ml undiluted solution	drops undiluted solution
<3	10	22	2.0	0.2	6
3	15	33	3.0	0.3	8
6	20	44	4.0	0.4	11
8+	25 +	55+	5.0	0.5	use mark on the dropper

Chronic usage: If Bricanyl Respirator Solution is to be used in a continuous ventilation system, a suitable dosage is 1–2 mg/hour at a dilution of 100 microgram/ml (1:100 dilution) for adults, with a pro rata reduction in dosage for children.

Contra-indications: Bricanyl preparations are contra-indicated in patients with a history of hypersensitivity to any of their constituents.

Interactions with other medicaments: Non–selective β-blocking agents such as propranolol may partially or totally inhibit the effect of β-stimulants. Therefore Bricanyl preparations and non-selective β-blockers should not normally be administered concurrently. Bricanyl should be used with caution in patients receiving other sympathomimetics.

Precautions: Care should be taken with patients suffering form myocardial insufficiency or thyrotoxicosis. Due to the hyperglycaemic effects of β_2–stimulants, additional blood glucose measurements are initially recommended when Bricanyl therapy is commenced in diabetic patients. If treatment becomes less effective or shorter acting, the patients general condition should be reviewed.

Due to the positive inotropic effect of the β_2–agonists, these drugs should not be used in patients with hypertrophic cardiomyopathy.

Potentially serious hypokalaemia may result from β_2-agonist therapy. Particular caution is advised in severe asthma as this effect may be potentiated by concomitant treatment with xanthine derivatives, steroids, diuretics and by hypoxia. It is recommended that serum potassium levels are monitored in such situations.

Pregnancy and lactation: Although no teratogenic effects have been observed in animals or in patients, Bricanyl should only be administered with caution during the first trimester of pregnancy.

Terbutaline is secreted via breast milk but effect on the infant is unlikely at therapeutic doses.

Effect on ability to drive and use machines: Bricanyl does not affect the ability to drive or use machines.

Undesirable effects: The frequency of side-effects is low. Side effects which have been recorded, such as tremor, tonic cramp and palpitations, are all characteristics of sympathomimetic amines. A few patients feel tense; this is also due to effects on skeletal muscle and not to direct CNS stimulation.

Whenever these side-effects have occurred, the majority have been spontaneously reversible within the first week of treatment. Rare cases of bronchospasm have occurred.

Potentially serious hypokalaemia may result from β_2–agonist therapy.

Overdosage: i) *Possible symptoms and signs:* Headache, anxiety, tremor, tonic cramp, palpitations and arrhythmia. A fall in blood pressure sometimes occurs. Laboratory findings: Hypokalaemia, hyperglycaemia and metabolic acidosis sometimes occur.

ii)Treatment: Mild and moderate cases: Reduce the dose.

Severe cases: Determination of acid-base balance, blood sugar and electrolytes. Monitoring of heart rate and rhythm and blood pressure. Metabolic changes should be corrected. A cardioselective β–blocker (e.g. metoprolol) is recommended for the treatment of arrhythmias causing haemodynamic deterioration. The β–blocker should be used with care because of the possibility of inducing bronchoconstriction. If the β–mediated reduction in peripheral vascular resistance significantly contributes to the fall in blood pressure, a volume expander should be given.

Pharmacological properties
Pharmacodynamic properties: Terbutaline is a selective β_2–adrenergic stimulant having the following pharmacological effects:

i) In the lung: bronchodilation, increase in mucociliary clearance, suppression of oedema and anti-allergic effects.

ii) In skeletal muscle: stimulates Na^+/K^+ transport and also causes depression of subtetanic contractions in slow-contracting muscle.

iii) In uterine muscle: inhibition of uterine contractions.

iv) In the C.N.S: low penetration into the blood-brain barrier at therapeutic doses, due to the highly hydrophilic nature if the molecule.

v) In the C.V.S: administration of terbutaline results in cardiovascular effects mediated through β_2–receptors in the peripheral arteries and in the heart e.g. in healthy subjects, 0.25-0.5 mg injected s.c., is associated with an increase in cardiac output (up to 85% over controls) due to an increase in heart rate and a larger stroke volume. The increase in heart rate is probably due to a combination of a reflex tachycardia via a fall in peripheral resistance and a direct positive chronotropic effect of the drug.

Pharmacokinetic properties: Basic parameters have been evaluated in man after i.v. and oral administration of therapeutic doses, e.g.
I.V. single dose:
Volume distribution (VSS) – 114 L.
Total body clearance (CL)– 213 ml/min.
Mean residence time (MRT) – 9.0 h.
Renal clearance (CLR) – 149 ml/min (males)
Oral dose:
Renal clearance (CLR) – 1.925 ml/min (males)
Renal clearance (CLR) – 2.32 ml/min (females)

The plasma concentration/time curve after i.v. administration is characterised by a fast distribution phase, an intermediate elimination phase and a late elimination phase.

Terminal half-life $t_{1/2}$ has been determined after single and multiple dosing (mean values varied between 16–20 h).

Bioavailability: Food reduces bioavailability following oral dose (10% on average) fasting values of 14–15% have been obtained.

Metabolism: The main metabolite after oral dosing is the sulphate conjugate and also some glucoronide conjugate can be found in the urine.

Pre-clinical safety data: —

Pharmaceutical particulars
List of excipients: Sodium chloride, chlorobutanol, disodium edetate, hydrochloric acid and purified water.

Incompatibilities: (major) – Not known.

Shelf-life: The contents of the bottle should be used within 3 months of opening.

Special precautions for storage: Store below 25°C.

Nature and content of container: 20 ml amber, Type II (PhEur) glass bottles with a polypropylene screw cap.

Instructions for use and handling: Bricanyl Respirator Solution must be used with a nebuliser. The mist produced is then inhaled through the mouthpiece of the mask.

To take your medicine, follow these steps:

1. Remove the screw cap from the Bricanyl Respirator Solution bottle and replace it with the graduated dropper, which is included in the pack.
2. Empty the prescibed volume of Bricanyl Respirator Solution into the nebuliser cup.
3. Next, dilute your Bricanyl Respirator Solution to the required nebuliser volume using sterile physiological saline. Your doctor may prescribe another drug to be used for the dilution instead of the sterile physiological saline, if so follow your doctor's instructions. Replace the nebuliser top on the nebuliser cup.

4. Connect one end of the cup to the mask or mouthpiece and the other ent to the air pump, which should be connected to the compressor unit.
5. Start to nebulise. During nebulising, breathe in the mist of nebulised medicine calmly and deeply.
6. The length of nebulisation time will vary with the type of medicine or nebuliser you use, but, when no mist comes out of the mouthpiece or nebuliser, your treatment is completed.
7. You must wash the nebuliser cup and mouthpiece (or face mask) in warm soapy water and rinse well after each use. Then dry these parts by connecting up to the air outlet or compressor and blow air through them.

Additional information: Bricanyl Respirator Solution in multidose bottles contains preservative and may be diluted before use with sterile physiological saline. Solution in nebulisers should be replaced daily. The pH of Bricanyl Respirator Solution is 2.5–3.5.

Marketing authorisation number PL0017/0078R

Date of approval/revision of SPC January 1998

Legal category POM.

BRICANYL* SA

Presentation White tablet with engraving $\frac{A}{BD}$ containing 7.5 mg Terbutaline Sulphate PhEur in a sustained-release formulation.

Inactive ingredients: Polyvinyl chloride, colloidal silicon dioxide, tartaric acid, ethyl cellulose, stearyl alcohol.

Uses Terbutaline is a selective β_2-adrenergic agonist recommended for relief and prevention of bronchospasm in bronchial asthma and in chronic bronchitis, emphysema and other bronchopulmonary disorders in which bronchospasm is a complicating factor.

Dosage and administration
Adults: 1 tablet morning and evening. The tablet may not be divided or chewed, but must be swallowed whole together with liquid.

Elderly: Dosage as for adults.

Contra-indications, warnings, etc
Contra-indications: Bricanyl oral preparations are contra-indicated in patients with a history of hypersensitivity to any of their constituents.

Precautions: Care should be taken with patients suffering from myocardial insufficiency or thyrotoxicosis. Due to the hyperglycaemic effects of β_2-stimulants, additional blood glucose measurements are initially recommended when Bricanyl therapy is commenced in diabetic patients. If treatment becomes less effective or shorter acting the patient's general condition should be reviewed.

Potentially serious hypokalaemia may result from β_2-agonist therapy. Particular caution is advised in severe asthma as this effect may be potentiated by concomitant treatment with xanthine derivatives, steroids, diuretics and by hypoxia. It is recommended that serum potassium levels are monitored in such situations.

Due to the positive inotropic effect of β_2-agonists, these drugs should not be used in patients with hypertrophic cardiomyopathy.

Interactions: β-blocking agents especially the non-selective ones such as propranolol may partially or totally inhibit the effect of β-stimulants. Therefore, Bricanyl oral preparations and non-selective β-blockers should not normally be administered concurrently. Bricanyl should be used with caution in patients receiving other sympathomimetics.

Use in pregnancy and lactation: Although no teratogenic effects have been observed in animals or in patients, terbutaline should only be administered with caution during the first trimester of pregnancy.

Terbutaline is secreted via breast milk, but effect on the infant is unlikely at therapeutic doses.

Side-effects: The frequency of side-effects is low at the recommended doses. Side-effects which have been recorded such as tremor, headache, tonic cramp and palpitations are all characteristic of sympathomimetic amines. A few patients feel tense; this is also due to the effects on skeletal muscle and not to direct CNS stimulation. Whenever these side-effects have occurred the majority have usually been spontaneously reversible within the first week of treatment. Urticaria and exanthema may occur. In children, sleep disturbances and disturbances of behavioural effects have been observed.

Potentially serious hypokalaemia may result from β_2-agonist therapy.

Overdosage: Possible symptoms and signs: Headache, anxiety, tremor, tonic cramp, palpitations, arrhythmia. A fall in blood pressure sometimes occurs. Laboratory findings: hypokalaemia, hyperglycaemia and lactic acidosis sometimes occur.

Treatment: (a) *Mild and moderate cases:* Reduce the dose.

(b) *Severe cases:* Gastric lavage, activated charcoal. Determination of acid-base balance, blood sugar and electrolytes. Monitoring of heart rate and rhythm and blood pressure. Metabolic changes should be corrected. A cardioselective β-blocker (e.g. metoprolol) is recommended for the treatment of arrhythmias causing haemodynamic deterioration. The β-blocker should be used with care because of the possibility of inducing bronchoconstriction. If the β_2-mediated reduction in peripheral vascular resistance significantly contributes to the fall in blood pressure, a volume expander should be given.

Pharmaceutical precautions No special storage conditions are necessary.

Legal category POM.

Package quantities Glass bottles containing 60 tablets.

Further information The inactive components in Bricanyl SA form a matrix which is insoluble in the digestive juices. The empty matrix may sometimes pass through the digestive system unchanged and be excreted.

Product licence number 0017/0110

BRICANYL* TABLETS
BRICANYL* SYRUP

Presentation
Bricanyl Tablets 5 mg: Off white tablet, engraved with A/BT and scored on one side, symbol '5' on the reverse containing Terbutaline Sulphate PhEur 5 mg.

Inactive ingredients: Lactose, maize starch, povidone, microcrystalline cellulose, magnesium stearate.

Bricanyl Syrup: A clear, colourless raspberry-flavoured aqueous syrup containing 0.30 mg Terbutaline Sulphate PhEur per ml.

Inactive ingredients: Citric acid, disodium edetate, ethanol, glycerol, sodium hydroxide, sorbitol, sodium benzoate, flavour raspberry, flavour lemon limette, water.

Uses *1. For bronchodilation:* Terbutaline is a selective β_2-adrenergic agonist recommended for the relief and prevention of bronchospasm in bronchial asthma and other bronchopulmonary disorders in which bronchospasm is a complicating factor.

2. For the management of uncomplicated premature labour.

Dosage and administration
(1) *Use in bronchospasm*
Bricanyl Tablets and Syrup have a duration of action of 7 to 8 hours. The minimum recommended dosage interval is therefore 7 hours.

Adults:
Tablets: During the first 1–2 weeks 2.5 mg (half a tablet) 3 times in a 24 hour period is recommended. The dose may then be increased to 5 mg (1 tablet) 3 times in 24 hours to achieve adequate bronchodilation.

Syrup: The starting dose should be 2×5 ml spoonfuls 3 times in 24 hours. The dose may then be increased to 3×5 ml spoonfuls 3 times in 24 hours if necessary.

Elderly: Dosage as for adults.

Children: Tablets: 7–15 years, the starting dose should normally be 2.5 mg (half a tablet) 2 times in 24 hours. However, in some patients, the dose may need to be increased to 2.5 mg 3 times in 24 hours.
Syrup: The following dosage is recommended – 0.075 mg (0.25 ml)/kg body weight 3 times in a 24 hour period e.g.

Body weight (kg)	*Dosage*
14	3.5 ml×3
16	4 ml×3
18	4.5 ml×3
20	5 ml×3
24	6 ml×3
28	7 ml×3
32	8 ml×3
36	9 ml×3
40	10 ml×3

(2) *Use in the management of premature labour:* Oral treatment should not be used initially in an attempt to arrest premature labour. After uterine contractions have been controlled by intravenous infusion of Bricanyl Injection, (see Bricanyl Injection data sheet) or subcutaneous injections (0.25 mg, 4 times in a 24 hour period for a few days) maintenance therapy can be continued with oral treatment (5 mg, 3 times in a 24 hour period). Oral treatment may be continued for as long as the physician considers it desirable to prolong pregnancy.

Contra-indications, warnings, etc
Contra-indications: Bricanyl oral preparations are contra-indicated in patients with a history of hypersensitivity to any of their constituents.

Although Bricanyl Injection and Tablets are used in the management of uncomplicated premature labour, their use in the following conditions is contra-indicated:

Any condition of the mother or foetus in which prolongation of the pregnancy is hazardous, e.g. severe toxaemia, ante-partum haemorrhage, intra-uterine infection, abruptio placentae, threatened abortion during the first and second trimesters, or cord compression.

Precautions: Care should be taken with patients suffering from myocardial insufficiency or thyrotoxicosis. Due to the hyperglycaemic effects of β_2-stimulants, additional blood glucose measurements are initially recommended when Bricanyl therapy is commenced in diabetic patients. If a previously effective dosage regimen no longer gives the same symptomatic relief the patient should seek further medical advice, for reassessment of asthma therapy, as soon as possible.

Potentially serious hypokalaemia may result from β_2-agonist therapy. Particular caution is advised in severe asthma as this effect may be potentiated by concomitant treatment with xanthine derivatives, steroids, diuretics and by hypoxia. It is recommended that serum potassium levels are monitored in such situations.

Due to the positive inotropic effect of β_2-agonists, these drugs should not be used in patients with hypertrophic cardiomyopathy.

Warnings: During infusion treatment in pregnant women with β_2-stimulants in combination with corticosteroids a rare complication with a pathological picture resembling pulmonary oedema, has been reported.

Increased tendency to uterine bleeding has been reported in connection with Caesarian section. However, this can be effectively stopped by propranolol 1–2 mg injected intravenously.

Interactions: β-blocking agents, especially the non-selective ones such as propranolol, may partially or totally inhibit the effect of β-stimulants. Therefore Bricanyl preparations and non-selective β-blockers should not normally be administered concurrently. Bricanyl should be used with caution in patients receiving other sympathomimetics.

Use in pregnancy and lactation: Although no teratogenic effects have been observed in animals or in patients, Bricanyl should only be administered with caution during the first trimester of pregnancy.

Terbutaline is secreted via breast milk, but effect on the infant is unlikely at therapeutic doses.

Side-effects: The frequency of side-effects is low at the recommended doses. Side-effects which have been recorded such as tremor, headache, tonic cramp and palpitations are all characteristic of sympathomimetic amines. A few patients feel tense; this is also due to the effects on skeletal muscle and not to direct CNS stimulation. Whenever these side-effects have occurred the majority have usually been spontaneously reversible within the first week of treatment. Urticaria and exanthema may occur.

In children sleep disturbances and disturbances of behavioural effects have been observed.

Potentially serious hypokalaemia may result from β_2-agonist therapy.

Overdosage:
Possible symptoms and signs: Headache, anxiety, tremor, tonic cramp, palpitations, arrhythmia. A fall in blood pressure sometimes occurs. Laboratory findings: hypokalaemia, hyperglycaemia and lactic acidosis sometimes occur.

Treatment: (a) Mild and moderate cases: Reduce the dose.

(b) *Severe cases:* Gastric lavage, administration of activated charcoal. Determination of acid-base balance, blood sugar and electrolytes. Monitoring of heart rate and rhythm and blood pressure. Metabolic changes should be corrected. A cardioselective β-blocker (e.g. metoprolol) is recommended for the treatment of arrhythmias causing haemodynamic deterioration. The β_2-blocker should be used with care because of the possibility of inducing bronchoconstriction. If the β_2-mediated reduction in peripheral vascular resistance significantly contributes to the fall in blood pressure, a volume expander should be given.

(c) *In preterm labour:* Pulmonary oedema: discontinue administration of Bricanyl. A normal dose of loop diuretic (e.g. frusemide) should be given intravenously.

Increased bleeding in connection with Caesarian section: Propranolol, 1–2 mg intravenously.

Pharmaceutical precautions
Bricanyl Tablets: Store below 25°C.
Bricanyl Syrup: Store below 25°C.

Legal category POM.

Package quantities
Bricanyl Tablets: Securitainers of 100.
Bricanyl Syrup: Bottles of 300 ml.

Further information Bricanyl Tablets and Syrup exert a prolonged bronchodilation, in clinical trials demonstrated for up to 8 hours. Maximum plasma concentration is reached 1–4 hours after dosing.

Bricanyl oral preparations contain no colouring agents and are sugar-free.

A suitable regimen for providing eight-hourly oral administration is: on rising, in the mid-afternoon, on retiring.

Product licence numbers
Bricanyl Tablets 0017/0047R
Bricanyl Syrup 0017/0058R

BRICANYL* TURBOHALER*

Presentation Breath-actuated metered dose powder inhaler delivering 0.5 mg terbutaline sulphate per actuation. Each inhaler contains 100 doses. Bricanyl Turbohaler is free from propellants, lubricants, preservatives, carrier substances or other additives.

Uses Terbutaline is a selective β_2-adrenergic agonist recommended for the relief and prevention of bronchospasm in bronchial asthma and other bronchopulmonary disorders in which bronchospasm or reversible airways obstruction is a complicating factor.

Dosage and administration
Adults and children: One inhalation (0.5 mg) as required. Not more than 4 inhalations should be necessary in any 24 hour period.

The duration of action of a single dose is up to 6 hours.

Elderly: Dosage as for adults.

Contra-indications, warnings, etc
Contra-indications: Bricanyl preparations are contra-indicated in patients with a history of sensitivity to terbutaline sulphate.

Precautions: Care should be used in patients suffering from myocardial insufficiency or thyrotoxicosis. Due to the hyperglycaemic effects of β_2-stimulants, additional blood glucose measurements are initially recommended when Bricanyl therapy is commenced in diabetic patients. If a previously effective dosage regimen no longer gives the same symptomatic relief the patient should seek further medical advice, for reassessment of asthma therapy, as soon as possible.

Due to the positive inotropic effect of β_2-agonists, these drugs should not be used in patients with hypertrophic cardiomyopathy.

Potentially serious hypokalaemia may result from β_2-agonist therapy. Particular caution is advised in severe asthma as this effect may be potentiated by concomitant treatment with xanthine derivatives, steroids, diuretics and by hypoxia. It is recommended that serum potassium levels are monitored in such situations.

Use in pregnancy and lactation: Although no teratogenic effects have been observed in animals or in patients Bricanyl should only be administered with caution during the first trimester of pregnancy.

Terbutaline is secreted via breast milk, but effect on the infant is unlikely at therapeutic doses.

Interactions: β-blocking agents especially the non-selective ones such as propranolol may partially or totally inhibit the effect of β-stimulants. Therefore Bricanyl preparations and non-selective β-blockers should not normally be administered concurrently. Bricanyl should be used with caution in patients receiving other sympathomimetics.

Side-effects: The frequency of side-effects is low. Side-effects which have been recorded such as tremor, tonic cramp and palpitations are all characteristic of sympathomimetic amines. A few patients feel tense; this is also due to the effects on skeletal muscle and not to direct CNS stimulation. Whenever these have occurred, the majority have usually been spontaneously reversible within the first week of treatment.

Potentially serious hypokalaemia may result from β_2-agonist therapy.

Overdosage: (i) *Possible symptoms and signs:* Headache, anxiety, tremor, tonic cramp, palpitations and arrhythmia. A fall in blood pressure sometimes occurs.
Laboratory findings: Hypokalaemia, hyperglycaemia and metabolic acidosis sometimes occur.

(ii) Treatment: Mild and moderate cases: Reduce the dose.

Severe cases: Determination of acid-base balance, blood sugar and electrolytes. Monitoring of heart rate and rhythm and blood pressure. Metabolic changes should be corrected. A cardioselective β-blocker (e.g. metoprolol) is recommended for the treatment of arrhythmias causing haemodynamic deterioration. The β-blocker should be used with care because of the possibility of inducing bronchoconstriction. If the β_2-mediated reduction in peripheral vascular resistance significantly contributes to the fall in blood pressure, a volume expander should be given.

Pharmaceutical precautions Store below 30°C.

Legal category POM.

Package quantities Powder inhaler containing 100 doses.

Further information Bricanyl Turbohaler is breath-actuated and therefore there is no need to co-ordinate the release of the dose and the inhalation. Treatment with Bricanyl Turbohaler is effective even at low inspiratory flow rates, such as those present during an acute asthmatic attack.

Product licence number 0017/0241

CITANEST* 0.5% SINGLE DOSE VIALS

Presentation Glass vials containing a sterile, clear, aqueous solution of prilocaine hydrochloride 5 mg/ml.

Inactive ingredients: Sodium chloride, sodium hydroxide and water for injections. No preservative is added.

Uses Citanest 0.5% is a local anaesthetic solution for use in infiltration anaesthesia, intravenous regional anaesthesia and nerve blocks.

Dosage and administration The dose is adjusted according to the response of the patient and the site of administration. The lowest concentration and smallest dose to produce the required effect should be given.

In children over 6 months of age the dosage can be calculated on a weight basis, up to 5 mg/kg.

The maximum dose for healthy adults should not exceed 400 mg.

Elderly or debilitated patients require smaller doses, commensurate with age and physical status.

Citanest 0.5% is a single dose vial for use on one patient during one treatment only. The remaining contents should be discarded.

Contra-indications, warnings, etc
Contra-indications: Known hypersensitivity to anaesthetics of the amide type or to any other component of the solution.

Citanest should be avoided in patients with anaemia or congenital or acquired methaemoglobinaemia.

Precautions and warnings: Great caution should be exercised to avoid accidental intravascular injection of this compound since it may give rise to the rapid onset of toxicity, with marked restlessness, twitching or convulsions, followed by coma with apnoea and cardiovascular collapse.

Use cautiously in the elderly, patients in poor health, in patients with epilepsy, severe or untreated hypertension, impaired cardiac conduction, severe heart disease, impaired respiratory function and in patients with liver or kidney damage, if the dose or site of administration is likely to result in high blood levels.

Facilities for resuscitation should be available when local anaesthetics are administered.

Local anaesthetics should be avoided when there is inflammation in the region of the proposed injection.

Adverse reactions: In common with other local anaesthetics, adverse reactions to Citanest are rare and are usually the result of excessively high blood concentrations, due to inadvertent intravascular injection, excessive dosage, rapid absorption or occasionally to hypersensitivity, idiosyncrasy or diminished tolerance on the part of the patient. In such circumstances systemic effects occur involving the central nervous system and/or the cardiovascular system.

CNS reactions are excitatory and/or depressant, and may be characterised by nervousness, dizziness, blurred vision and tremors, followed by drowsiness, convulsions, unconsciousness and possibly respiratory arrest. The excitatory reactions may be very brief or may not occur at all, in which case the first manifestations of toxicity may be drowsiness, merging into unconsciousness and respiratory arrest.

Cardiovascular reactions are depressant, and may be characterised by hypotension, myocardial depression, bradycardia and possibly cardiac arrest.

Allergic reactions are extremely rare. They may be characterised by cutaneous lesions, urticaria, oedema or anaphylactoid reactions. Detection of sensitivity by skin testing is of doubtful value.

Hypotension may occur as a physiological response to central nerve blocks.

This product gives rise to methaemoglobinaemia in a dose related fashion.

Clinically significant levels of methaemoglobin may occur with cyanosis when doses of prilocaine exceed 600 mg.

Methaemoglobinaemia may occur at lower doses of prilocaine in patients suffering from anaemia, from congenital or acquired haemoglobinopathy (including methaemoglobinaemia), or in patients receiving concomitant therapy e.g. sulphonamides, known to cause such conditions. Infants are particularly susceptible, due to a lower activity of the enzyme which reduces methaemoglobin to haemoglobin.

Methaemoglobinaemia may be treated by the intravenous administration of a 1% solution of methylene blue in a dose of 1 mg/kg, over a 5 minute period.

Use in pregnancy and lactation: Although there is no evidence from animal studies of harm to the foetus, as with all drugs, Citanest should not be given during early pregnancy unless the benefits are considered to outweigh the risks. Prilocaine enters mothers milk but there is generally no risk of effects on the infant at recommended doses.

Interactions: Patients receiving concomitant sulphonamide therapy with prilocaine e.g. cotrimoxazole are at increased risk of developing methaemoglobinaemia. Prilocaine should be used with caution in patients receiving other local anaesthetics or agents structurally related to amide-type anaesthetics, since the toxic effects are additive.

Overdosage: Treatment of a patient with systemic toxicity consists of arresting convulsions and ensuring adequate ventilation with oxygen, if necessary by assisted or controlled ventilation (respiration). If convulsions occur they must be treated promptly by intravenous injection of thiopentone 100 to 200 mg or diazepam 5 to 10 mg. Alternatively succinylcholine 50 to 100 mg i.v. may be used providing the clinician is capable of performing endotracheal intubation and managing a fully paralysed patient. If cardiac arrest occurs effective cardiopulmonary resuscitation must be instituted. This should include external cardiac compression, artificial ventilation with oxygen, adrenaline and sodium bicarbonate.

Pharmaceutical precautions Store below 25°C.

Legal category POM.

Package quantities Single dose vial: 0.5%: 50 ml.

Further information Citanest 0.5% SDV (single dose vial) is preservative free and should therefore be used on one occasion only.

Product licence numbers PL 0017/0208

CITANEST* 0.5% MULTI DOSE VIALS

Qualitative and quantitative composition Each ml of sterile, clear, aqueous solution contains prilocaine hydrochloride 5 mg.

Pharmaceutical form Aqueous solution for injection.

Clinical particulars
Therapeutic indications: Citanest is a local anaesthetic for use in infiltration anaesthesia, intravenous regional anaesthesia and nerve blocks.

Posology and method of administration: The dose is adjusted according to the response of the patient and the site of administration.

The lowest concentration and smallest dose producing the required effect should be given.

The maximum dose of Citanest for healthy adults should not exceed 400 mg.

Elderly or debilitated patients require smaller doses, commensurate with age and physical status.

In children over 6 months of age the dosage can be calculated on a weight basis up to 5 mg/kg.

Contra-indications: Known hypersensitivity to anaesthetics of the amide type or to any component of the solution.

Citanest should be avoided in patients with anaemia or congenital or acquired methaemoglobinaemia.

Special warnings and special precautions for use: Great caution must be exercised to avoid accidental intravascular injection of this compound, since it may give rise to the rapid onset of toxicity, with marked restlessness, twitching, or convulsions, followed by coma with apnoea and cardiovascular collapse.

In common with other local anaesthetics, Citanest should be used cautiously in the elderly, patients in poor health, patients with epilepsy, severe or untreated hypertension, impaired cardiac conduction, severe heart disease, impaired respiratory function, and in patients with liver or kidney damage, if the dose or site of administration is likely to result in high blood levels.

Facilities for resuscitation should be available when

local anaesthetics are administered. Local anaesthetics should be avoided when there is inflammation at the site of the proposed injection.

Interaction with other medicaments and other forms of interaction: Patients receiving concomitant sulphonamide therapy with prilocaine e.g. cotrimoxazole are at increased risk of developing methaemoglobinaemia.

Prilocaine should be used with caution in patients receiving other local anaesthetics or agents structurally related to amide-type anaesthetics, since the toxic effects are additive.

Use during pregnancy and lactation: Although there is no evidence from animal studies of harm to the foetus, as with all drugs Citanest should not be given in early pregnancy unless the benefits are considered to outweigh the risks.

Prilocaine enters the mothers milk but there is generally no risk of effects on the infant at recommended doses.

Effects on ability to drive and use machines: No effects are foreseen.

Undesirable effects: In common with other local anaesthetics, adverse reactions to Citanest are extremely rare and are usually the result of excessively high blood concentrations due to inadvertent intravascular injection, excessive dosage, rapid absorption or occasionally to hypersensitivity, idiosyncrasy or diminished tolerance on the part of the patient. In such circumstances systemic effects occur involving the central nervous system and/or the cardiovascular system.

CNS reactions are excitatory and/or depressant and may be characterised by nervousness, dizziness, blurred vision and tremors, followed by drowsiness, convulsions , unconsciousness and possibly respiratory arrest. The excitatory reactions may be very brief or may not occur at all, in which case the first manifestations of toxicity may be drowsiness, merging into unconsciousness and respiratory arrest. Cardiovascular reactions are depressant and may be characterised by hypotension, myocardial depression, bradycardia and possibly cardiac arrest. Allergic reactions are extremely rare. They may be characterised by cutaneous lesions, urticaria, oedema or anaphylactoid reactions. Detection of sensitivity by skin testing is of doubtful value.

Hypotension may occur as a physiological response to central nerve blocks.

This product gives rise to methaemoglobinaemia in a dose related fashion.

Clinically significant levels occur with cyanosis when doses of prilocaine exceed 600 mg.

Methaemoglobinaemia may occur at lower doses of prilocaine in patients suffering from anaemia, from congenital or acquired haemoglobinopathy (including methaemoglobinaemia), or in patients receiving concomitant therapy e.g. sulphonamides, known to cause such conditions. Infants are particularly susceptible, due to a lower activity of the enzyme which reduces methaemoglobin to haemoglobin.

Methaemoglobinaemia may be treated by the intravenous administration of a 1% solution of methylene blue in a dose of 1 mg/kg, over a 5 minute period.

Overdosage: Treatment of a patient with systemic toxicity consists of arresting convulsions and ensuring adequate ventilation with oxygen, if necessary by assisted or controlled ventilation (respiration). If convulsions occur they must be treated promptly by intravenous injection of thiopentone 100 to 200 mg or diazepam 5 to 10 mg. Alternatively succinylcholine 50 to 100 mg i.v. may be used providing the clinician is capable of performing endotracheal intubation and managing a fully paralysed patient. If cardiac arrest occurs effective cardiopulmonary resuscitation must be instituted. This should include external cardiac compression, artificial ventilation with oxygen, adrenaline and sodium bicarbonate.

Pharmacological properties

Pharmacodynamic properties: Prilocaine is a local anaesthetic of the amide type. Local anaesthetics act by preventing transmission of impulses along nerve fibres and at nerve endings; depolarisation and ion-exchange are inhibited. The effects are reversible.

Pharmacokinetic properties: Prilocaine hydrochloride is absorbed more slowly than lignocaine (lidocaine) because of its slight vasoconstrictor action but its half life in blood is less than that of lidocaine (lidocaine half life approximately 10 minutes, elimination half life approximately 2 hours).

Amidases in the liver and kidney metabolise prilocaine directly.

Preclinical safety data: Prilocaine hydrochloride is a well established active ingredient.

Pharmaceutical particulars

List of excipients: Sodium chloride, sodium hydroxide, methyl parahydroxybenzoate and water for injections.

Incompatibilities: None known.

Shelf-life: The shelf-life is 36 months.

Special precautions for storage: Store below 25°C.

Nature and contents of container: Multi–dose glass vials of 20 ml and 50 ml.

Instructions for use/handling: Not applicable.

Marketing authorisation number PL 0017/5047R

Date of approval/revision of SPC October 1997.

Legal category POM.

CITANEST* 1% MULTI DOSE VIALS

Qualitative and quantitative composition Each ml of sterile, clear, aqueous solution contains prilocaine hydrochloride 10 mg.

Pharmaceutical form Aqueous solution for injection.

Clinical particulars

Therapeutic indications: Citanest is a local anaesthetic for use in infiltration anaesthesia, intravenous regional anaesthesia and nerve blocks.

Posology and method of administration: The dose is adjusted according to the response of the patient and the site of administration.

The lowest concentration and smallest dose producing the required effect should be given.

The maximum dose of Citanest for healthy adults should not exceed 400 mg.

Elderly or debilitated patients require smaller doses, commensurate with age and physical status.

In children over 6 months of age the dosage can be calculated on a weight basis up to 5 mg/kg.

Contra-indications: Known hypersensitivity to anaesthetics of the amide type or to any component of the solution.

Citanest should be avoided in patients with anaemia or congenital or acquired methaemoglobinaemia.

Special warnings and special precautions for use: Great caution must be exercised to avoid accidental intravascular injection of this compound, since it may give rise to the rapid onset of toxicity, with marked restlessness, twitching, or convulsions, followed by coma with apnoea and cardiovascular collapse.

In common with other local anaesthetics, Citanest should be used cautiously in the elderly, patients in poor health, patients with epilepsy, severe or untreated hypertension, impaired cardiac conduction, severe heart disease, impaired respiratory function, and in patients with liver or kidney damage, if the dose or site of administration is likely to result in high blood levels.

Facilities for resuscitation should be available when local anaesthetics are administered. Local anaesthetics should be avoided when there is inflammation at the site of the proposed injection.

Interaction with other medicaments and other forms of interaction: Patients receiving concomitant sulphonamide therapy with prilocaine e.g. cotrimoxazole are at increased risk of developing methaemoglobinaemia.

Prilocaine should be used with caution in patients receiving other local anaesthetics or agents structurally related to amide-type anaesthetics, since the toxic effects are additive.

Use during pregnancy and lactation: Although there is no evidence from animal studies of harm to the foetus, as with all drugs Citanest should not be given in early pregnancy unless the benefits are considered to outweigh the risks.

Prilocaine enters the mothers milk but there is generally no risk of effects on the infant at recommended doses.

Effects on ability to drive and use machines: No effects are foreseen.

Undesirable effects: In common with other local anaesthetics, adverse reactions to Citanest are extremely rare and are usually the result of excessively high blood concentrations due to inadvertent intravascular injection, excessive dosage, rapid absorption or occasionally to hypersensitivity, idiosyncrasy or diminished tolerance on the part of the patient. In such circumstances systemic effects occur involving the central nervous system and/or the cardiovascular system.

CNS reactions are excitatory and/or depressant and may be characterised by nervousness, dizziness, blurred vision and tremors, followed by drowsiness, convulsions, unconsciousness and possibly respiratory arrest. The excitatory reactions may be very brief or may not occur at all, in which case the first manifestations of toxicity may be drowsiness, merging into unconsciousness and respiratory arrest. Cardiovascular reactions are depressant and may be characterised by hypotension, myocardial depression, bradycardia and possibly cardiac arrest. Allergic reactions are extremely rare. They may be characterised by cutaneous lesions, urticaria, oedema or anaphylactoid reactions. Detection of sensitivity by skin testing is of doubtful value.

Hypotension may occur as a physiological response to central nerve blocks.

This product gives rise to methaemoglobinaemia in a dose related fashion.

Clinically significant levels occur with cyanosis when doses of prilocaine exceed 600 mg.

Methaemoglobinaemia may occur at lower doses of prilocaine in patients suffering from anaemia, from congenital or acquired haemoglobinopathy (including methaemoglobinaemia), or in patients receiving concomitant therapy e.g. sulphonamides, known to cause such conditions. Infants are particularly susceptible, due to a lower activity of the enzyme which reduces methaemoglobin to haemoglobin.

Methaemoglobinaemia may be treated by the intravenous administration of a 1% solution of methylene blue in a dose of 1 mg/kg, over a 5 minute period.

Overdosage: Treatment of a patient with systemic toxicity consists of arresting convulsions and ensuring adequate ventilation with oxygen, if necessary by assisted or controlled ventilation (respiration). If convulsions occur they must be treated promptly by intravenous injection of thiopentone 100 to 200 mg or diazepam 5 to 10 mg. Alternatively succinylcholine 50 to 100 mg i.v. may be used providing the clinician is capable of performing endotracheal intubation and managing a fully paralysed patient. If cardiac arrest occurs effective cardiopulmonary resuscitation must be instituted. This should include external cardiac compression, artificial ventilation with oxygen, adrenaline and sodium bicarbonate.

Pharmacological properties

Pharmacodynamic properties: Prilocaine is a local anaesthetic of the amide type. Local anaesthetics act by preventing transmission of impulses along nerve fibres and at nerve endings; depolarisation and ion-exchange are inhibited. The effects are reversible.

Pharmacokinetic properties: Prilocaine hydrochloride is absorbed more slowly than lidocaine (lignocaine) because of its slight vasoconstrictor action but its half life in blood is less than that of lidocaine (lidocaine half life approximately 10 minutes, elimination half life approximately 2 hours).

Amidases in the liver and kidney metabolise prilocaine directly.

Preclinical safety data: Prilocaine hydrochloride is a well established active ingredient.

Pharmaceutical particulars

List of excipients: Sodium chloride, sodium hydroxide, methyl parahydroxybenzoate and water for injections.

Incompatibilities: None known.

Shelf-life: The shelf-life is 36 months.

Special precautions for storage: Store below 25°C.

Nature and contents of container: Multi-dose glass vials of 20 ml and 50 ml.

Instructions for use/handling: Not applicable.

Marketing authorisation number PL 0017/5048R

Date of approval/revision of SPC October 1997.

Legal category POM.

CITANEST* 2% SOLUTION

Qualitative and quantitative composition Each ml of sterile, clear, aqueous solution contains prilocaine hydrochloride 20 mg.

Pharmaceutical form Aqueous solution for injection.

Clinical particulars

Therapeutic indications: Citanest 2% is a local anaesthetic for use in infiltration anaesthesia, epidurals, nerve blocks and analgesia.

Posology and method of administration: The dose is adjusted according to the response of the patient and the site of administration.

The smallest dose to produce the required effect should be given.

In children over 6 months of age the dosage can be calculated on a weight basis of up to 5 mg/kg.

Elderly or debilitated patients require smaller doses, commensurate with age and physical status.

The maximum dose of Citanest for healthy adults should not exceed 400 mg.

Citanest 2% is a single dose vial for use on one patient during one treatment only. The remaining contents should be discarded.

Contra-indications: Known hypersensitivity to anaesthetics of the amide type or to any other component of the solution.

Citanest should be avoided in patients with anaemia or congenital or acquired methaemoglobinaemia.

Special warnings and special precautions for use: Great caution must be exercised to avoid accidental intravascular injection of this compound, since it may give rise to the rapid onset of toxicity, with marked restlessness, twitching, or convulsions, followed by coma with apnoea and cardiovascular collapse.

In common with other local anaesthetics, Citanest should be used cautiously in the elderly, patients in poor health, patients with epilepsy, severe or untreated hypertension, impaired cardiac conduction, severe heart disease, impaired respiratory function, and in patients with liver or kidney damage, if the dose or site of administration is likely to result in high blood levels.

In epidural anaesthesia, careful monitoring of the foetal heart rate is necessary and caution should be taken in patients with impaired cardiovascular function.

Facilities for resuscitation should be available when local anaesthetics are administered.

Local anaesthetics should be avoided when there is inflammation at the site of the proposed injection.

Interaction with other medicaments and other forms of interaction: Patients receiving concomitant sulphonamide therapy with prilocaine e.g. cotrimoxazole are at increased risk of developing methaemoglobinaemia.

Prilocaine should be used with caution in patients receiving other local anaesthetics or agents structurally related to amide-type anaesthetics since the toxic effects are additive.

Use during pregnancy and lactation: Although there is no evidence from animal studies of harm to the foetus, as with all drugs Citanest should not be given in early pregnancy unless the benefits are considered to outweigh the risks. Prilocaine enters the mother's milk but there is generally no risk of effects on the infant at recommended doses.

Effects on ability to drive and use machines: No effects are foreseen.

Undesirable effects: In common with other local anaesthetics, adverse reactions to Citanest are extremely rare and are usually the result of excessively high blood concentrations due to inadvertent intravascular injection, excessive dosage, rapid absorption or occasionally to hypersensitivity, idiosyncrasy or diminished tolerance on the part of the patient. In such circumstances systemic effects occur involving the central nervous system and/or the cardiovascular system.

CNS reactions are excitatory and/or depressant and may be characterised by nervousness, dizziness, blurred vision and tremors, followed by drowsiness, convulsions, unconsciousness and possibly respiratory arrest. The excitatory reactions may be very brief or may not occur at all, in which case the first manifestations of toxicity may be drowsiness, merging into unconsciousness and respiratory arrest. Cardiovascular reactions are depressant and may be characterised by hypotension, myocardial depression, bradycardia and possibly cardiac arrest.

Allergic reactions are extremely rare. They may be characterised by cutaneous lesions, urticaria, oedema or anaphylactoid reactions. Detection of sensitivity by skin testing is of doubtful value.

Hypotension may occur as a physiological response to central nerve blocks.

This product gives rise to methaemoglobinaemia in a dose related fashion.

Clinically significant levels occur with cyanosis when doses of prilocaine exceed 600 mg.

Methaemoglobinaemia may occur at lower doses of prilocaine in patients suffering from anaemia, from congenital or acquired haemoglobinopathy (including methaemoglobinaemia), or in patients receiving concomitant therapy e.g. sulphonamides, known to cause such conditions. Infants are particularly susceptible, due to a lower activity of the enzyme which reduces methaemoglobin to haemoglobin.

Methaemoglobinaemia may be treated by the intravenous administration of a 1% solution of methylene blue in a dose of 1 mg/kg, over a 5 minute period.

Overdosage: Treatment of a patient with systemic toxicity consists of arresting convulsions and ensuring adequate ventilation with oxygen, if necessary by assisted or controlled ventilation (respiration). If convulsions occur they must be treated promptly by intravenous injection of thiopentone 100 to 200 mg or diazepam 5 to 10 mg. Alternatively succinylcholine 50 to 100 mg i.v. may be used providing the clinician is capable of performing endotracheal intubation and managing a fully paralysed patient. If cardiac arrest occurs effective cardiopulmonary resuscitation must be instituted. This should include external cardiac compression, artificial ventilation with oxygen, adrenaline and sodium bicarbonate.

Pharmacological properties

Pharmacodynamic properties: Prilocaine is a local anaesthetic of the amide type. Local anaesthetics act by preventing transmission of impulses along nerve fibres and at nerve endings; depolarisation and ion-exchange are inhibited. The effects are reversible.

Pharmacokinetic properties: Prilocaine hydrochloride is absorbed more slowly than lignocaine (lidocaine) because of its slight vasoconstrictor action but its half life in blood is less than that of lignocaine (lignocaine half-life approximately 10 minutes, elimination half-life approximately 2 hours).

Amidases in the liver and kidney metabolise prilocaine directly.

Preclinical safety data: Prilocaine hydrochloride is a well established active ingredient.

Pharmaceutical particulars

List of excipients: Sodium chloride, sodium hydroxide and water for injections.

Incompatibilities: None known.

Shelf-life: 3 years.

Special precautions for storage: Store below 25°C.

Nature and contents of container: Single dose, glass vials; 10 ml and 20 ml.

Instructions for use/handling: Use on one patient during one treatment only.

Marketing authorisation number PL 0017/0090

Date of approval/revision of SPC 8th September 1997.

Legal category POM.

CITANEST* 3% WITH OCTAPRESSIN

Qualitative and quantitative composition A sterile aqueous solution containing prilocaine hydrochloride 30 mg per ml and octapressin corresponding to felypressin 0.03IU per ml.

Pharmaceutical form Sterile solution for injection.

Clinical particulars

Therapeutic indications: Citanest with Octapressin is a local anaesthetic solution for use in dental infiltration and all dental nerve block techniques.

Posology and method of administration: In normal healthy adults the usual dose is 1-5 ml. Children under 10 years of age require approximately 1-2 ml. A dose of 10 ml (5 cartridges) of Citanest with Octapressin should not be exceeded.

Elderly or debilitated patients require smaller doses.

Contra-indications: Known hypersensitivity to anaesthetics of the amide type or to any other component of the solution.

Citanest should be avoided in patients with anaemia or congenital or acquired methaemoglobinaemia.

Special warnings and special precautions for use: Great caution must be exercised to avoid accidental intravascular injection of this compound, since it may give rise to the rapid onset of toxicity, with marked restlessness, twitching, or convulsions, followed by coma with apnoea and cardiovascular collapse.

In common with other local anaesthetics, Citanest should be used cautiously in the elderly, patients in poor health, in patients with epilepsy, severe or untreated hypertension, impaired cardiac conduction, severe heart disease, impaired respiratory function and in patients with liver or kidney damage, if the dose or site of administration is likely to result in high blood levels.

Facilities for resuscitation should be available when local anaesthetics are administered.

Local anaesthetics should be avoided when there is inflammation in the region of the proposed injection.

Interaction with other medicaments and other forms of interaction: Patients receiving concomitant therapy with sulphonamides e.g. cotrimoxazole are at increased risk of developing methaemoglobinaemia.

The vasopressor properties of octapressin should be borne in mind.

Prilocaine should be used with caution in patients receiving other local anaesthetics or agents structurally related to amide-type anaesthetics, since the toxic effects are additive.

Pregnancy and lactation: Although there is no evidence of harm to the foetus, as with all drugs Citanest with Octapressin should not be given in early pregnancy unless the benefits are considered to outweigh the risks. Prilocaine enters the mothers milk, but there is generally no risk of effects on the infant at recommended doses.

Effects on ability to drive and use machines: No effects are foreseen.

Undesirable effects: In common with other local anaesthetics, adverse reactions to Citanest are extremely rare in dental practice and are usually the result of excessively high blood concentrations due to inadvertent intravascular injection, excessive dosage, rapid absorption or occasionally to hypersensitivity, idiosyncrasy or diminished tolerance on the part of the patient.

In such circumstances systemic effects occur involving the central nervous system and/or the cardiovascular system.

CNS reactions are excitatory and/or depressant, and may be characterised by nervousness, dizziness, blurred vision and tremors, followed by drowsiness, convulsions, unconsciousness and possibly respiratory arrest. The excitatory reactions may be brief or may not occur at all, in which case the first manifestations of toxicity may be drowsiness, merging into unconsciousness and respiratory arrest. Cardiovascular reactions are depressant, and may be characterised by hypotension, myocardial depression, bradycardia and possibly cardiac arrest.

Allergic reactions are extremely rare. They may be characterised by cutaneous lesions, urticaria, oedema or anaphylactoid reactions. Detection of sensitivity by skin testing is of doubtful value.

This product gives rise to methaemoglobinaemia in a dose related fashion. Clinically significant levels of methaemoglobin may occur with cyanosis when doses of prilocaine exceed 600 mg.

Methaemoglobinaemia may occur at lower doses of prilocaine in patients suffering from anaemia, from congenital or acquired haemoglobinopathy (including methaemoglobinaemia), or in patients receiving concomitant therapy e.g. sulphonamides, known to cause such conditions. Infants are particularly susceptible, due to a lower activity of the enzyme which reduces methaemoglobin to haemoglobin.

Methaemoglobinaemia may be treated by the intravenous administration of a 1% solution of methylene blue at a dose of 1 mg/kg, over a 5 minute period.

Overdosage: Treatment of a patient with systemic toxicity consists of arresting convulsions and ensuring adequate ventilation with oxygen, if necessary by assisted or controlled ventilation (respiration). If convulsions occur they must be treated promptly by intravenous injection of thiopentone 100 to 200 mg or diazepam 5 to 10 mg. If cardiac arrest occurs effective cardiopulmonary resuscitation must be instituted. This should include external cardiac compression, artificial ventilation with oxygen, adrenaline and sodium bicarbonate.

Pharmacological properties

Pharmacodynamic properties: Prilocaine is a local anaesthetic of the amide type. Local anaesthetics act by preventing transmission of impulses along nerve fibres and at nerve endings; depolarisation and ion-exchange are inhibited. The effects are reversible.

Pharmacokinetic properties: Prilocaine hydrochloride is absorbed more slowly than lignocaine (lidocaine) because of its slight vasoconstrictor action but its half life in blood is less than that of lignocaine (lignocaine half life approximately 10 minutes, elimination half life approximately 2 hours).

Amidases in the liver and kidney metabolise prilocaine directly.

Preclinical safety data: Prilocaine hydrochloride is a well established active ingredient.

Pharmaceutical particulars

List of excipients: Sodium chloride, hydrochloric acid and water for injections.

Incompatibilities: None known.

Shelf life: Plastic cartridges: 2 years. Glass cartridges: 3 years.

Special precautions for storage: Store below 25°C.

Nature and contents of container: Polypropylene (2.2 ml) or glass (1.8 ml and 2.2 ml) standard or self-aspirating cartridges in boxes of 100.

Instructions for use/handling: Use on one patient during one treatment only. Discard unused contents.

Marketing authorisation number PL 0017/5003R

Date of approval/revision of SPC 19th August 1997.

Legal category POM.

CITANEST* 4% SOLUTION FOR INJECTION

Presentation 2.2 ml glass or polypropylene cartridge containing a colourless, sterile, clear, aqueous solution. Each millilitre contains prilocaine hydrochloride 40 mg.

Inactive ingredients: Sodium chloride, sodium hydroxide.

Uses Citanest 4% is a local anaesthetic solution for use in dental infiltration anaesthesia and all dental nerve block techniques.

Dosage and administration In normal healthy adults the usual dose is 1 ml to 2 ml. Children under 10 years of age require approximately 1 ml.

The maximum dose of Citanest should not exceed 400 mg (5 cartridges, 10 ml) for healthy adults.

Citanest 4% is a single dose cartridge for use on one patient during one treatment only. The remaining contents should be discarded.

Elderly or debilitated patients require smaller doses.

Contra-indications, warnings, etc
Contra-indications: Known hypersensitivity to anaesthetics of the amide type or to any other component of the solution.

Citanest should be avoided in patients with anaemia or congenital or acquired methaemoglobinaemia.

Precautions and warnings: Great caution must be exercised to avoid accidental intravascular injection of this compound, since it may give rise to the rapid onset of toxicity, with marked restlessness, twitching, or convulsions, followed by coma with apnoea and cardiovascular collapse.

In common with other local anaesthetics, Citanest should be used cautiously in the elderly, patients in poor health, in patients with epilepsy, severe or untreated hypertension, impaired cardiac conduction, severe heart disease, impaired respiratory function and in patients with liver or kidney damage, if the dose or site of administration is likely to result in high blood levels.

Facilities for resuscitation should be available when local anaesthetics are administered.

Local anaesthetics should be avoided when there is inflammation in the region of the proposed injection.

Adverse Reactions: In common with other local anaesthetics, adverse reactions to Citanest are extremely rare in dental practice and are usually the result of excessively high blood concentrations due to inadvertent intravascular injection, excessive dosage, rapid absorption or occasionally to hypersensitivity, idiosyncrasy or diminished tolerance on the part of the patient.

In such circumstances systemic effects occur involving the central nervous system and/or the cardiovascular system.

CNS reactions are excitatory and/or depressant, and may be characterised by nervousness, dizziness, blurred vision and tremors, followed by drowsiness, convulsions, unconsciousness and possibly respiratory arrest. The excitatory reactions may be brief or may not occur at all, in which case the first manifestations of toxicity may be drowsiness, merging into unconsciousness and respiratory arrest. Cardiovascular reactions are depressant, and may be characterised by hypotension, myocardial depression, bradycardia and possibly cardiac arrest.

Allergic reactions are extremely rare. They may be characterised by cutaneous lesions, urticaria, oedema or anaphylactoid reactions. Detection of sensitivity by skin testing is of doubtful value.

This product gives rise to methaemoglobinaemia in a dose related fashion.

Clinically significant levels of methaemoglobin may occur with cyanosis when doses of prilocaine exceed 600 mg.

Methaemoglobinaemia may occur at lower doses of prilocaine in patients suffering from anaemia, from congenital or acquired haemoglobinopathy (including methaemoglobinaemia), or in patients receiving concomitant therapy e.g. sulphonamides, known to cause such conditions. Infants are particularly susceptible, due to a lower activity of the enzyme which reduces methaemoglobin to haemoglobin.

Methaemoglobinaemia may be treated by the intravenous administration of a 1% solution of methylene blue in a dose of 1 mg/kg, over a period of 5 minutes.

Use in Pregnancy and Lactation: Although there is no evidence of harm to the foetus, as with all drugs Citanest should not be given in early pregnancy unless the benefits are considered to outweigh the risks.

Prilocaine enters the mothers milk but there is generally no risk of effects on the infant at recommended doses.

Interactions: Patients receiving concomitant sulphonamide therapy with prilocaine e.g. cotrimoxazole are at increased risk of developing methaemoglobinaemia. Prilocaine should be used with caution in patients receiving other local anaesthetics or agents structurally related to amide-type local anaesthetics since the toxic effects are additive.

Overdosage: Treatment of a patient with systemic toxicity consists of arresting convulsions and ensuring adequate ventilation with oxygen, if necessary by assisted or controlled ventilation (respiration). If convulsions occur they must be treated promptly by intravenous injection of thiopentone 100 to 200 mg or diazepam 5 to 10 mg. If cardiac arrest occurs effective cardiopulmonary resuscitation must be instituted. This should include external cardiac compression, artificial ventilation with oxygen, adrenaline and sodium bicarbonate.

Pharmaceutical precautions Store below 25°C.

Legal category POM.

Package quantities Glass or polypropylene cartridges of 2.2 ml in boxes of 100.

Further information Nil

Product licence number 0017/5050R

CO-BETALOC*

Presentation White scored tablets (coded A/MH) containing 100 mg metoprolol tartrate PhEur and 12.5 mg hydrochlorothiazide PhEur.

Inactive ingredients: Lactose, microcrystalline cellulose, sodium starch glycolate, polyvinylpyrrolidone, colloidal silicon dioxide, magnesium stearate.

Uses In the management of mild or moderate hypertension. Co-Betaloc may be suitable for use when satisfactory control of arterial blood pressure cannot be obtained with either a diuretic or a β-adrenoreceptor blocking drug used alone.

Dosage and administration The dose will depend on patient response. Usually 1–3 tablets per day as a single or divided dose.

Elderly: There are no special dosage requirements in otherwise healthy elderly patients.

Significant hepatic dysfunction: A reduction in dosage may be necessary.

Contra-indications, warnings, etc
Contra-indications: AV block. Uncontrolled heart failure. Severe bradycardia. Sick sinus syndrome. Cardiogenic shock. Severe peripheral arterial disease. Known hypersensitivity to Betaloc or other β-blockers.

Severe kidney and liver failure. Therapy resistant hypokalaemia and hyponatraemia. Hypercalcaemia, symptomatic hyperuricaemia. Anuria. Known hypersensitivity to hydrochlorothiazide or other sulphonamide derivatives.

An anti-diuretic effect has been reported following concomitant treatment with diuretics and lithium. As with all products which contain diuretics, Co-Betaloc is contra-indicated during lithium therapy.

Warnings: Metoprolol may aggravate bradycardia, symptoms of peripheral arterial circulatory disorders and anaphylactic shock.

Abrupt interruption of β-blockers is to be avoided. When possible, Co-Betaloc should be withdrawn gradually over a period of 10 days. During its withdrawal patients should be kept under close surveillance, especially those with known ischaemic heart disease.

Co-Betaloc may be administered when heart failure has been controlled. Digitalisation and/or additional diuretic therapy should also be considered for patients with a history of heart failure, or patients known to have a poor cardiac reserve.

Although cardioselective β-blockers may have less effect on lung function than non-selective β-blockers, as with all β-blockers these should be avoided in patients with reversible obstructive airways disease unless there are compelling clinical reasons for their use. When administration is necessary, use of a β_2-bronchodilator (e.g. terbutaline) may be advisable in some patients.

The label shall state – 'If you have a history of wheezing, asthma or any other breathing difficulties, you must tell your doctor before you take this medicine'.

In labile and insulin-dependent diabetes it may be necessary to adjust the hypoglycaemic therapy.

In patients with a phaeochromocytoma, an α-blocker should be given concomitantly.

In the presence of liver cirrhosis the bioavailability of metoprolol may be increased.

The administration of adrenaline to patients undergoing β-blockade can result in an increase in blood pressure and bradycardia although this is less likely to occur with β_1-selective drugs.

Co-Betaloc therapy must be reported to the anaesthetist prior to general anaesthesia. If withdrawal of metoprolol is considered desirable, this should if possible be completed at least 48 hours before general anaesthesia.

Co-Betaloc does not interfere with potassium balance. However, at higher doses of hydrochlorothiazide disturbances in the electrolyte and water balance may be experienced. Hyperuricaemia may occur or frank gout may be precipitated in certain patients receiving higher doses of thiazide therapy. Latent diabetes may become manifest during thiazide therapy.

Diuretics in higher doses may precipitate azotemia in patients with renal disease. Cumulative effects of hydrochlorothiazide may develop in patients with impaired renal function. If renal impairment becomes evident metoprolol/hydrochlorothiazide therapy should be discontinued.

Pregnancy: Co-Betaloc should not be used in pregnancy or nursing mothers unless the physician considers that the benefit outweighs the possible hazard to the foetus/infant. As with all β-blockers metoprolol may cause side-effects e.g. bradycardia, hypoglycaemia in the foetus, and in the newborn and breast-fed infant. Metoprolol has, however, been used in pregnancy associated hypertension under close supervision, after 20 weeks gestation. Although Betaloc crosses the placental barrier and is present in cord blood, no evidence of foetal abnormalities has been reported.

Hydrochlorothiazide can reduce the plasma volume as well as the uteroplacental blood circulation.

Lactation: The amount of metoprolol ingested via breast milk should not produce significant β-blocking effects in the neonate if the mother is treated with normal therapeutic doses.

As hydrochlorothiazide passes into breast milk, consideration should be given to withdrawal of Co-Betaloc, replacement by metoprolol in monotherapy or breast-feeding stopped.

Interactions: The effects of Co-Betaloc and other antihypertensive drugs on blood pressure are usually additive, and care should be taken to avoid hypotension. However, combinations of antihypertensive drugs may often be used with benefit to improve control of hypertension.

Metoprolol can reduce myocardial contractility and impair intracardiac conduction. Care should be exercised when drugs with similar activity, e.g. antiarrhythmic agents, general anaesthetics, are given concurrently. Like all other β-blockers, metoprolol should not be given in combination with verapamil since this may cause bradycardia, hypotension and asystole. Care should also be exercised when β-blockers are given in combination with sympathetic ganglion blocking agents, other β-blockers (i.e. eye drops) or MAO inhibitors. If combination treatment with clonidine is to be discontinued, metoprolol should be withdrawn several days before clonidine.

As β-blockers may affect the peripheral circulation, care should be exercised when drugs with similar activity e.g. ergotamine are given concurrently.

Metoprolol will antagonise the β_1-effects of sympathomimetic agents but should have little influence on the bronchodilator effects of β_2-agonists at normal therapeutic doses. Enzyme inducing agents (e.g. rifampicin) may reduce plasma concentrations of metoprolol, whereas enzyme inhibitors (e.g. cimetidine) may increase plasma concentrations. Metoprolol may impair the elimination of lignocaine.

Indomethacin may reduce the antihypertensive effect of β-blockers.

In general reported interactions have occurred with doses of hydrochlorothiazide higher than those used in this combination. Insulin requirements in diabetic patients may be altered and lithium renal clearance is reduced, increasing the risk of lithium toxicity. Responsiveness to tubocurarine may be increased and arterial responsiveness to noradrenaline may be decreased, but not enough to preclude effectiveness of the pressor agent for therapeutic use. Hypokalaemia may develop during concomitant use of steroids or ACTH, and may sensitise or exaggerate the response of the heart to toxic effects of digitalis.

Side-effects: Side-effects to metoprolol are usually mild and infrequent. The most common appear to be lassitude, GI disturbances (nausea, vomiting or abdominal pain) and disturbances of sleep pattern. In many cases these effects have been transient or have disappeared after a reduction in dosage.

Effects related to the CNS which have been reported occasionally are dizziness and headache and rarely paraesthesia, muscle cramps, depression and decreased mental alertness. There have also been isolated reports of personality disorders like amnesia, memory impairment, confusion, hallucination, nervousness and anxiety.

Cardiovascular effects which have been reported occasionally are bradycardia, postural hypotension and rarely, heart failure, palpitations, cardiac arrhythmias, Raynaud's phenomenon, peripheral oedema and precordial pain. There have also been isolated reports of cardiac conduction abnormalities, and gangrene in patients with pre-existing severe peripheral circulatory disorders.

Common gastro-intestinal disturbances have been described above but rarely diarrhoea or constipation also occur and there have been isolated cases of dry mouth and abnormal liver function.

Skin rashes (urticaria, psoriasiform, dystrophic skin lesions) and positive anti-nuclear antibodies (not associated with SLE) occur rarely. Isolated cases of photosensitivity, psoriasis exacerbation, increased sweating and alopecia have been reported. Respiratory effects include occasional reports of dyspnoea on exertion and rare reports of bronchospasm and isolated cases of rhinitis.

Rarely impotence/sexual dysfunction. Isolated cases of weight gain, thrombocytopenia, disturbances of vision, conjunctivitis, tinnitus, dry or irritated eyes, taste disturbance and arthralgia have also been reported.

The reported incidence of skin rashes and/or dry eyes is small and in most cases the symptoms have cleared when treatment was withdrawn. Discontinuation of the drug should be considered if any such reaction is not otherwise explicable.

Hydrochlorothiazide is generally well tolerated at the dose used (12.5 mg) in the combination. However the familiar side-effects of thiazide diuretics may be expected e.g. gastro-intestinal disturbances, metabolic and electrolyte changes, disturbances in sleep pattern, skin rashes and effects relating to the CNS.

Overdosage: Poisoning due to an overdose of Co-Betaloc may lead to severe hypotension, sinus bradycardia, atrioventricular block, heart failure, cardiogenic shock, cardiac arrest, bronchospasm, impairment of consciousness, coma, nausea, vomiting, cyanosis, hypoglycaemia and, occasionally, hyperkalaemia. The first manifestations usually appear 20 minutes to 2 hours after drug ingestion.

The most prominent feature of poisoning due to hydrochlorothiazide is acute loss of fluid and electrolytes. The following symptoms may also be observed: dizziness, sedation/impairment of consciousness, hypotension and muscle cramps.

Treatment should include close monitoring of cardiovascular, respiratory and renal function, and blood glucose and electrolytes. Further absorption may be prevented by induction of vomiting, gastric lavage or administration of activated-charcoal if ingestion is recent. Cardiovascular complications should be treated symptomatically, which may require the use of sympathomimetic agents (e.g. noradrenaline, metaraminol), atropine or inotropic agents (e.g. dopamine, dobutamine). Temporary pacing may be required for AV block. Glucagon can reverse the effects of excessive β-blockade, given in a dose of 1–10 mg intravenously. Intravenous β_2-stimulants e.g. terbutaline may be required to relieve bronchospasm.

Intravenous volume and electrolyte-replacement may be necessary.

Metoprolol cannot be effectively removed by haemodialysis.

Pharmaceutical precautions Store below 25°C in a dry place.

Legal category POM.

Package quantities PVC blister strips in an outer carton (7 tablets per strip). Pack size 28.

Further information Metoprolol is well absorbed after oral administration, peak plasma concentrations occurring 1.5–2 hours after dosing. The bioavailability of a single dose is approximately 50%, increasing to approximately 70% during repeated administration. The bioavailability also increases if metoprolol is given with food.

Elimination is mainly by hepatic metabolism and the average elimination half-life is 3.5 hours (range 1 to 9 hours). Rates of metabolism vary between individuals, with poor metabolisers (approximately 10%) showing higher plasma concentrations and slower elimination than extensive metabolisers. Within individuals, however, plasma concentrations are stable and reproducible.

Because of variation in rates of metabolism, the dose of metoprolol should always be adjusted to the individual requirements of the patient. As the therapeutic response, adverse effects and relative cardioselectivity are related to plasma concentration, poor metabolisers may require lower than normal doses. Dosage adjustment is not routinely required in the elderly or in patients with renal failure, but dosage may need to be reduced in patients with significant hepatic dysfunction when metoprolol elimination may be impaired.

Product licence number 0017/0092

CO-BETALOC* SA

Presentation Yellow, biconvex, film coated tablets engraved A/MC.

Each tablet contains metoprolol tartrate 200 mg embedded in a white tablet layer, from which release takes place slowly, and hydrochlorothiazide 25 mg, in a yellow layer, which is rapidly released.

Inactive ingredients: Sodium aluminium silicate, paraffin, ethyl cellulose, magnesium stearate, lactose, microcrystalline cellulose, maize starch, polyvinylpyrrolidone, riboflavin, sodium stearyl fumarate, hydroxypropyl methylcellulose, polyethylene glycol, iron oxide yellow, titanium dioxide.

Uses In the management of mild or moderate hypertension. Co-Betaloc SA may be suitable for use when satisfactory control of arterial blood pressure cannot be obtained with either a diuretic or a β-adrenoreceptor blocking drug used alone.

Dosage and administration The dose will depend on patient response. Usually one tablet daily, taken whole and swallowed with water.

Elderly: There are no special dosage requirements in otherwise healthy elderly patients.

Significant hepatic dysfunction: A reduction in dosage may be necessary.

Contra-indications, warnings, etc
Contra-indications: AV block. Uncontrolled heart failure. Severe bradycardia. Sick sinus syndrome. Cardiogenic shock. Severe peripheral arterial disease. Known hypersensitivity to metoprolol or other β-blockers.

Severe kidney and liver failure. Therapy resistant hypokalaemia and hyponatraemia. Hypercalcaemia, symptomatic hyperuricaemia. Anuria. Known hypersensitivity to hydrochlorothiazide or other sulphonamide derivatives.

An anti-diuretic effect has been reported following concomitant treatment with diuretics and lithium. As with all products which contain diuretics, Co-Betaloc SA is contra-indicated during lithium therapy.

Warnings: Metoprolol may aggravate bradycardia, symptoms of peripheral arterial circulatory disorders and anaphylactic shock.

Abrupt interruption of Co-Betaloc SA is to be avoided. When possible, the drug should be withdrawn gradually over a period of 10 days using Co-Betaloc to help reduce the dose. During withdrawal from treatment patients should be kept under close surveillance, especially those with known ischaemic heart disease.

Co-Betaloc SA may be administered when heart failure has been controlled. Digitalisation and/or diuretic therapy should also be considered for patients with a history of heart failure, or patients known to have a poor cardiac reserve.

Although cardioselective β-blockers may have less effect on lung function than non-selective β-blockers, as with all β-blockers these should be avoided in patients with reversible obstructive airways disease unless there are compelling clinical reasons for their use. When administration is necessary, use of a β_2-bronchodilator (e.g. terbutaline) may be advisable in some patients.

The label shall state – 'If you have a history of wheezing, asthma or any other breathing difficulties, you must tell your doctor before you take this medicine'.

In labile and insulin dependent diabetes, it may be necessary to adjust the hypoglycaemic therapy.

In patients with phaeochromocytoma, an α-blocker should be given concomitantly.

The bioavailability of metoprolol may be increased in the presence of liver cirrhosis.

The administration of adrenaline to patients undergoing β-blockade can result in an increase in blood pressure and bradycardia although this is less likely to occur with β_1-selective drugs.

Metoprolol therapy must be reported to the anaesthetist prior to general anaesthetic. If it is desirable to withdraw metoprolol in patients who are to undergo anaesthesia the withdrawal should if possible be completed at least 48 hours before the anaesthesia.

Co-Betaloc SA does not interfere with potassium balance. However, at higher doses of hydrochlorothiazide disturbances in the electrolyte and water balance may be experienced. Hyperuricaemia may occur or frank gout may be precipitated in certain patients receiving higher doses of thiazide therapy. Latent diabetes may manifest itself during thiazide therapy.

Diuretics in higher doses may precipitate azotemia in patients with renal disease. Cumulative effects of hydrochlorothiazide may develop in patients with impaired renal function. If renal impairment becomes evident metoprolol/hydrochlorothiazide therapy should be discontinued.

Pregnancy: Co-Betaloc SA should not be used in pregnancy or nursing mothers unless the physician considers that the benefit outweighs the possible hazard to the foetus/infant. As with all β-blockers metoprolol may cause side-effects e.g. bradycardia, hypoglycaemia in the foetus, and in the newborn and breast-fed infant. Metoprolol has, however, been used in pregnancy associated hypertension under close supervision, after 20 weeks gestation. Although metoprolol crosses the placental barrier and is present in cord blood, no evidence of foetal abnormalities has been reported.

Hydrochlorothiazide can reduce the plasma volume as well as the uteroplacental blood circulation.

Lactation: The amount of metoprolol ingested via breast milk should not produce significant β-blocking effects in the neonate if the mother is treated with normal therapeutic doses.

As hydrochlorothiazide passes into breast milk, consideration should be given to either the withdrawal of Co-Betaloc SA, replacement with metoprolol monotherapy or instructing the patient to stop breast-feeding.

Interactions: The effects of metoprolol and other antihypertensive drugs on blood pressure are usually additive, and care should be taken to avoid hypotension. However, combinations of antihypertensive drugs may often be used with benefit to improve control of hypertension.

Metoprolol can reduce myocardial contractility and impair intracardiac conduction. Care should be exercised when drugs with similar activity, e.g. antiarrhythmic agents, general anaesthetics, are given concurrently. Like all other β-blockers, metoprolol should not be given in combination with verapamil since this may cause bradycardia, hypotension and asystole. Care should also be exercised when β-blockers are given in combination with sympathetic ganglion blocking agents, other β-blockers (i.e. eye drops) or MAO inhibitors. If combination treatment with clonidine is to be discontinued, metoprolol should be withdrawn several days before clonidine.

As β-blockers may affect the peripheral circulation, care should be exercised when drugs with similar activity e.g. ergotamine are given concurrently.

Metoprolol will antagonise the β_1-effects of sympathomimetic agents but should have little influence on the bronchodilator effects of β_2-agonists at normal therapeutic doses. Enzyme inducing agents (e.g. rifampicin) may reduce plasma concentrations of metoprolol, whereas enzyme inhibitors (e.g. cimetidine) may increase plasma concentrations. Metoprolol may impair the elimination of lignocaine.

Indomethacin may reduce the antihypertensive effect of β-blockers.

In general reported interactions have occurred with doses of hydrochlorothiazide higher than those used in this combination. Insulin requirements in diabetic patients may be altered and lithium renal clearance is reduced, increasing the risk of lithium toxicity. Responsiveness to tubocurarine may be increased and arterial responsiveness to noradrenaline may be decreased, but not enough to preclude effectiveness of the pressor agent for therapeutic use. Hypokalaemia may develop during concomitant use of steroids or ACTH, and may sensitise or exaggerate the response of the heart to toxic effects of digitalis.

Side-effects: Side-effects to metoprolol are usually mild and infrequent. The most common appear to be lassitude, GI disturbances (nausea, vomiting or abdominal pain) and disturbances of sleep pattern. In many cases these effects have been transient or have disappeared after a reduction in dosage.

Effects related to the CNS which have been reported occasionally are dizziness and headache and rarely paraesthesia, muscle cramps, depression and decreased mental alertness. There have also been isolated reports of personality disorders like amnesia, memory impairment, confusion, hallucination, nervousness and anxiety.

Cardiovascular effects which have been reported occasionally are bradycardia, postural hypotension and rarely, heart failure, palpitations, cardiac arrhythmias, Raynaud's phenomenon, peripheral oedema and precordial pain. There have also been isolated reports of cardiac conduction abnormalities, and gangrene in patients with pre-existing severe peripheral circulatory disorders.

Common gastro-intestinal disturbances have been described above but rarely diarrhoea or constipation also occur and there have been isolated cases of dry mouth and abnormal liver function.

Skin rashes (urticaria, psoriasiform, dystrophic skin lesions) and positive anti-nuclear antibodies (not associated with SLE) occur rarely. Isolated cases of photosensitivity, psoriasis exacerbation, increased sweating and alopecia have been reported. Respiratory effects include occasional reports of bronchospasm and isolated cases of rhinitis.

Rarely impotence/sexual dysfunction. Isolated cases of weight gain, thrombocytopenia, disturbances of vision, conjunctivitis, tinnitus, dry or irritated eyes, taste disturbance and arthralgia have also been reported.

The reported incidence of skin rashes and/or dry eyes is small and in most cases the symptoms have cleared when treatment was withdrawn. Discontinuation of the drug should be considered if any such reaction is not otherwise explicable.

Hydrochlorothiazide is generally well tolerated at the dose used (25 mg) in the combination. However the familiar side-effects of thiazide diuretics may be expected e.g. gastro-intestinal disturbances, metabolic and electrolyte changes, disturbances in sleep pattern, skin rashes and effects relating to the CNS.

Overdosage: Poisoning due to an overdose of metoprolol may lead to severe hypotension, sinus bradycardia, atrioventricular block, heart failure, cardiogenic shock, cardiac arrest, bronchospasm, impairment of consciousness, coma, nausea, vomiting, cyanosis, hypoglycaemia and, occasionally, hyperkalaemia. The first manifestations usually appear 20 minutes to 2 hours after drug ingestion.

The most prominent feature of poisoning due to

hydrochlorothiazide is acute loss of fluid and electrolytes. The following symptoms may also be observed: dizziness, sedation/impairment of consciousness, hypotension and muscle cramps.

Treatment should include close monitoring of cardiovascular, respiratory and renal function, and blood glucose and electrolytes. Further absorption may be prevented by induction of vomiting, gastric lavage or administration of activated-charcoal if ingestion is recent. Cardiovascular complications should be treated symptomatically, which may require the use of sympathomimetic agents (e.g. noradrenaline, metaraminol), atropine or inotropic agents (e.g. dopamine, dobutamine). Temporary pacing may be required for AV block. Glucagon can reverse the effects of excessive β-blockade, given in a dose of 1–10 mg intravenously. Intravenous β_2-stimulants e.g. terbutaline may be required to relieve bronchospasm.

Intravenous volume and electrolyte-replacement may be necessary.

Metoprolol cannot be effectively removed by haemodialysis.

Pharmaceutical precautions Store below 25°C in a dry place.

Legal category POM.

Package quantities Packs of 28 tablets.

Further information
Metoprolol Tartrate: Metoprolol is well absorbed after oral administration, peak plasma concentrations occurring 1.5–2 hours after dosing. The bioavailability of a single dose is approximately 50%, increasing to approximately 70% during repeated administration. The bioavailability also increases if metoprolol is given with food.

Elimination is mainly by hepatic metabolism and the average elimination half-life is 3.5 hours (range 1 to 9 hours). Rates of metabolism vary between individuals, with poor metabolisers (approximately 10%) showing higher plasma concentrations and slower elimination than extensive metabolisers. Within individuals, however, plasma concentrations are stable and reproducible.

Because of variation in rates of metabolism, the dose of metoprolol should always be adjusted to the individual requirements of the patient. As the therapeutic response, adverse effects and relative cardioselectivity are related to plasma concentrations, poor metabolisers may require lower than normal doses. Dosage adjustment is not routinely required in the elderly or in patients with renal failure, but dosage may need to be reduced in patients with significant hepatic dysfunction when metoprolol elimination may be impaired.

Hydrochlorothiazide: Hydrochlorothiazide is incompletely but rapidly absorbed from the gastrointestinal tract. It is estimated to have a plasma half-life of 3-4 hours with a biological half-life up to 12 hours. It is excreted unchanged in the urine. It crosses the placental barrier and is excreted in breast milk.

Product licence number 0017/0202

COLAZIDE* ▼

Qualitative and quantitative composition Balsalazide disodium 750 mg. INN: balsalazide. Each capsule contains balsalazide disodium 750 mg corresponding to balsalazide 612.8 mg and to mesalazine 262.5 mg.

Pharmaceutical form Capsule, hard. Size 00 beige gelatin capsules.

Clinical particulars
Therapeutic indications: Colazide is indicated for:

Treatment of mild–to–moderate active ulcerative colitis.

Posology and method of administration: To be swallowed whole after food.

Adults: 2.25 g Balsalazide disodium (3 capsules) three times daily (6.75 g daily) until remission or for 12 weeks maximum. Rectal or oral steroids can be given concomitantly if necessary.

Elderly: No dose adjustment is anticipated.

Children: Colazide is not recommended in children.

Contra-indications: Hypersensitivity to any component of the product or its metabolites, including mesalazine. History of hypersensitivity to salicylates.

Severe hepatic impairment, moderate-severe renal impairment.

Pregnant and breast feeding women.

Special warnings and special precautions for use: Colazide should be used with caution in patients with asthma, bleeding disorders, active ulcer disease, mild renal impairment or those with established hepatic disease.

During treatment with Colazide blood counts, BUN/creatinine and urine analysis should be performed. Patients receiving balsalazide should be advised to report any unexplained bleeding, bruising, purpura, sore throat, fever or malaise that occurs during treatment. A blood count should be performed and the drug stopped immediately if there is suspicion of a blood dyscrasia.

Interaction with other medicaments and other forms of interaction: Formal interaction studies have not been performed with Colazide. Available data suggest that the systemically available amounts of balsalazide and its metabolites may be increased if Colazide is administered in the fasting as compared with the fed state. Therefore, Colazide should preferably be administered with food.

The acetylated metabolites of balsalazide are actively secreted in the renal tubule to a high degree. Therefore, plasma levels of co–prescribed drugs also eliminated by this route may be raised and this should be noted in the case of those with a narrow therapeutic range, such as methotrexate.

Pharmacodynamic interactions have not been studied. However, while balsalazide, mesalazine, and N–acetylmesalazine are salicylates chemically, their properties and kinetics make classical salicylate interactions such as those found with acetylsalicylic acid very unlikely.

The uptake of digoxin has been impaired in some individuals by concomitant treatment with sulphasalazine. Even if it is not known whether this would occur also during treatment with balsalazide, it is recommended that plasma levels of digoxin should be monitored in digitalised patients starting Colazide.

Pregnancy and lactation: Animal studies on fertility and reproductive function did not reveal adverse effects of balsalazide. Human experience with balsalazide is limited, therefore Colazide should not be given to pregnant women. Colazide should not be given to breast feeding women as the active metabolite mesalazine has produced adverse effects in nursing infants.

Effects on ability to drive and use machines: No evidence of any relevant effect. Presumed to be safe.

Undesirable effects: The adverse effects are expected to be those of mesalazine. In clinical trials of active ulcerative colitis, headache (8.6%), gastrointestinal symptoms such as abdominal pain (7.4%), diarrhoea (5.1%), nausea (4.0%) and vomiting (3.4%) have been reported as adverse events. Four per cent (4%) of patients were withdrawn, usually early in treatment.

With oral mesalazine, rare reports of exacerbation of colitis, interstitial nephritis, acute pancreatitis, hepatitis, blood dyscrasias and allergic reactions, bronchospasm, allergic alveolitis, lupus erythematodes-like syndrome, arthralgia, myalgia, neuropathia, alopecia, myo- and pericarditis have been recorded.

Serious blood dyscrasias (which include aplastic anaemia, leucopenia, neutropenia, agranulocytosis and thrombocytopenia) have been reported very rarely with mesalazine–see *Special warnings and precautions for use.*

Overdose: To date, there are no reports of overdosage with mesalazine-releasing products. Overdose with large amounts of balsalazide may result in symptoms resembling mild salicylate intoxication. Treatment should be symptomatic.

Pharmacological properties
Pharmacodynamic properties: ATC-code: A07 EC. Balsalazide consists of mesalazine linked to a carrier molecule (4-aminobenzoyl-β-alanine) via an azo bond.

Bacterial azo-reduction releases mesalazine as an active metabolite in the colon. Mesalazine is an intestinal anti-inflammatory agent acting locally on the colonic mucosa. Its precise mechanism of action is unknown. Balsalazide and the carrier do not contribute to the pharmacodynamic action.

Pharmacokinetic properties: The pharmacokinetics of balsalazide and its metabolites have been studied in healthy subjects and patients in remission. The systemic uptake of balsalazide itself is low (<1%) and the major part of the dose is split in the colon by bacterial azoreductase. This cleavage results in the primary metabolites 5-aminosalicylic acid (5-ASA), responsible for the anti-inflammatory action, and 4-aminobenzoyl-beta-alanine (4-ABA), considered to be an inert carrier.

Most of the dose is eliminated via the faeces but about 25% of the released 5-ASA appears systemically predominantly as the N–acetylated metabolite (NASA) after inactivation in the colonic mucosa and liver. The systemic uptake of 4-ABA is only 10-15% of that of 5-ASA and also this metabolite is grossly N–acetylated (to NABA) in the first pass.

In urine, virtually only NASA and NABA are recovered and their renal clearances are high: 0.2-0.3 litre/min and 0.4-0.5 litre/min, respectively. The half–life of NASA is in the order of 6-9 hours. The half-life of 5-ASA itself is very short: about 1 hour.

Because of the great importance of renal clearance for the elimination, Colazide should be used with caution in renal impairment. No studies have been performed in patients with hepatic disease.

Protein binding of 5-ASA is about 40% and that of NASA about 80%. Available data suggest that the pharmacokinetics of balsalazide is not affected by genetic polymorphism, nor does age seem to be an important factor. Fasting slightly increases the systemic uptake of balsalazide and its metabolites.

Preclinical safety data: Preclinical data reveal no special hazard for humans based on conventional studies of genotoxicity, carcinogenic potential, toxicity to reproduction, safety pharmacology and validating kinetics and metabolism. In repeated dose toxicity studies, nephrotoxicity, an effect known to occur following mesalazine, was observed particularly in rats.

Pharmaceutical particulars
List of excipients: Magnesium stearate, colloidal anhydrous silica, gelatin, shellac, titanium dioxide (E171), yellow, red and black iron oxide (E172).

Incompatibilities: Not relevant.

Shelf life: 3 years.

Special precautions for storage: None.

Nature and contents of container: High density polyethylene container fitted with tamper-evident, child-resistant, high density polyethylene screw caps.

Pack sizes are 50, 56, 100, 112, **130**, 224 (2 x 112), 260 (2 x 130), 300 (3 x 100), 500 (10 x 50), 672 (6 x 112) & 780 (6 x 130) capsules.

Instructions for use/handling: None.

Marketing authorisation number PL 0017/0394

Date of approval/revision of the SPC June 1998

Legal category POM.

DIRYTHMIN* SA

Presentation White, film-coated extended release formulation (Durules*), engraved A/DR on one side containing 150 mg disopyramide base as the phosphate.

Inactive ingredients: Paraffin, polyvinyl acetate, carboxypolymethylene, magnesium stearate, ethanol 95%, hydroxypropyl methylcellulose, polyethylene glycol 6000, titanium dioxide.

Uses Dirythmin SA is a Class IA antiarrhythmic drug, indicated for treatment of a wide range of supraventricular and ventricular arrhythmias including:
Atrial or ventricular ectopic beats.
Paroxysmal atrial or ventricular tachycardia.
Arrhythmias associated with myocardial infarction.
Wolff-Parkinson-White syndrome.
Maintenance of sinus rhythm following electroconversion.

Dirythmin SA can be used in both digitalised and non-digitalised patients.

Dosage and administration Initiation of treatment, as with other antiarrhythmic agents used to treat life-threatening ventricular arrhythmias, should be carried out in hospital.

The dosage should be adjusted dependant on the patient response and tolerance. The normal adult dosage is 2 tablets 12 hourly (600 mg daily). Dosage should not normally exceed 750 mg daily.

Patients should be digitalised prior to Dirythmin SA administration for the treatment of atrial flutter/fibrillation or blocked supraventricular tachycardia.

In patients with moderate renal insufficiency (creatinine clearance >40 ml/min) or hepatic insufficiency, dosage should be limited to 1 Dirythmin SA tablet b.d. In patients with creatinine clearance <40 ml/min Dirythmin SA tablets are not advised.

For patients with cardiomyopathy or compensated cardiac failure, the initial dosage should be limited to 1 tablet b.d. (300 mg daily). Subsequent dosage adjustment should be made with caution.

Patients treated with conventional disopyramide capsules q.i.d. can be transferred to the equivalent dosage of Dirythmin SA e.g. 150 mg disopyramide q.i.d. is equivalent to 2×150 mg Dirythmin SA tablets b.d.

Transferring to disopyramide from quinidine sulphate or procainamide therapy: Disopyramide may be started 6–12 hours after the last dose of quinidine sulphate or 3–6 hours after the last dose of procainamide.

Elderly: The renal function of the patient must be considered in relation to the dose as above.

Children: The safety and efficacy of Dirythmin SA in children has not been established.

Patients with renal or hepatic impairment: Hepatic impairment causes an increase in the plasma half-life of Dirythmin SA. Dosage should be reduced for such patients. If treatment is warranted, patients should be closely monitored.

Disopyramide is eliminated predominantly by glomerular filtration. The dose administered to patients with significant renal impairment may consequently require adjustment.

Dirythmin SA tablets must not be chewed or crushed. They should be swallowed whole with half a glass of water.

Contra-indications, warnings, etc
Contra-indications: Dirythmin SA is contra-indicated in patients with second or third degree AV block if no pacemaker is present, cardiomyopathy, cardiogenic shock and hypersensitivity to disopyramide phosphate.

Patients with heart failure or who are susceptible to heart failure should be fully digitalised before Dirythmin SA therapy in order to ensure its mild negative inotropic effect does not contribute to any cardiac insufficiency.

Dirythmin SA should not be administered to patients with hypotension.

Warnings and precautions: Disopyramide should not be administered to patients with hypotension, cardiomyopathy or congestive cardiac failure unless cardiac failure is adequately treated.

Severe hypotension has been observed following disopyramide administration primarily in patients with primary cardiomyopathy or inadequately controlled congestive cardiac failure. If hypotension develops, disopyramide should be discontinued. Treatment may later be restarted at a lower dosage and the patient should be closely monitored. In patients with bifascicular bundle branch block, intravenous administration of disopyramide has been reported to induce AV-block in some patients.

If first-degree heart block develops in a patient receiving disopyramide, dosage should be reduced. If the block persists despite reduction of dosage, continuation of the drug must depend upon assessment of benefit vs risk. Development of second or third degree AV-block or significant intraventricular conduction abnormality requires discontinuation of therapy, unless the ventricular rate is adequately controlled by a temporary or permanent ventricular pacemaker.

Like other antiarrhythmic drugs disopyramide may worsen arrhythmias. Disopyramide should be discontinued in the presence of significant (greater than 25%) QRS-widening. QT-prolongation and worsening of the arrhythmia may occur, particularly at high doses. If QT-prolongation of more than 25% appears or the ectopy persists, the patient should be carefully monitored and disopyramide discontinued if necessary.

Disopyramide should not be given simultaneously with other Class I antiarrhythmic agents and/or β-blockers unless life-threatening arrhythmias demonstrably unresponsive to single drug therapy are present. Patients receiving more than one antiarrhythmic agent must be carefully monitored. Caution should be observed during concomitant treatment with other drugs with a negative inotropic action.

There have been reports of hypoglycaemia in association with disopyramide administration, usually in patients with impaired liver function of other conditions predisposing to disturbance of glucoregulatory mechanisms.

Disopyramide may be given to patients with glaucoma if it appears that the overall potential benefits of therapy outweigh the risk of treatment with regard to the glaucoma. Careful monitoring and aggressive therapy of the glaucoma should then be undertaken.

Administration of disopyramide to patients who have or develop urinary retention is possible, but appropriate corrective measures e.g. catheterisation may be necessary. The potential life-saving effects of disopyramide should be weighed against the disadvantages of treatment in such patients.

Disopyramide should be used with caution in patients with benign prostatic hypertrophy, because its anticholinergic action may precipitate urinary retention.

Disopyramide should be used with extreme caution in the presence of digitalis intoxication. AV-conduction should be monitored carefully in such circumstances.

Antiarrhythmic drugs may be ineffective in patients with hypokalaemia. Significant potassium deficit should be corrected prior to initiating disopyramide therapy.

Disopyramide should be used with caution in patients with myasthenia gravis.

Administration to children cannot be recommended owing to the lack of clinical studies verifying safety and effect.

Pregnancy and lactation: The safety of Dirythmin SA in pregnancy has not been established. Animal teratology and reproduction studies have demonstrated no adverse effects. The benefits of Dirythmin SA therapy must be weighed against the possible hazards to the mother and foetus. Dirythmin SA has been reported to stimulate contractions of the pregnant uterus. However, it is not known whether the use of Dirythmin SA during labour has any effect on either the foetus or the course of labour and delivery.

Disopyramide phosphate is excreted in breast milk, and at the therapeutic doses used, effects on the child are likely.

Side-effects: The adverse reactions are mostly dose-related and attributed to the anticholinergic effect or the effect on the cardiovascular system.

Anticholinergic: Occur in about 30% of patients, mainly in the form of dry mouth, urinary retention, constipation and blurred vision.

Cardiovascular: Arrhythmias. In isolated cases hypotension and heart failure.

Gastrointestinal: Nausea, vomiting and diarrhoea.

Metabolic: In isolated cases hypoglycaemia and hypokalaemia.

Miscellaneous: Rarely fatigue, myalgia, muscular weakness and dizziness. In isolated cases acute psychosis and cholestatic jaundice.

Interactions: Rifampicin and phenytoin induce the metabolism of disopyramide, leading to reduced plasma concentrations of disopyramide and increased concentrations of the dealkylated metabolite. Atenolol reduces the clearance of disopyramide.

Overdosage: Poisoning due to an overdose of Dirythmin SA may lead to widening of the QRS complex and prolongation of the QT interval, atrioventricular block, sinoatrial block or arrest, asystole, paroxysmal ventricular tachycardia, flutter or fibrillation, myocardial depression, severe hypotension and cardiac arrest. Cinchonism, nausea, vomiting, drowsiness and sometimes convulsions also occur. Metabolic acidosis and hypokalaemia may complicate severe poisoning.

Treatment should include close monitoring of cardiovascular, respiratory and renal function, electrolytes and continuous ECG monitoring. Further absorption may be prevented by induction of vomiting or gastric lavage, or administration of activated charcoal if ingestion is recent. Cardiovascular complications should be treated symptomatically, which may require the use of sympathomimetic agents (e.g. noradrenaline, metaraminol), or inotropic agents (e.g. dopamine, dobutamine). Temporary pacing may be required for AV block. Glucagon may be used to treat hypotension, and intravenous sodium bicarbonate to correct acidosis and intravenous diazepam for convulsions.

Disopyramide and its metabolites cannot be removed effectively by peritoneal or haemodialysis, or charcoal column haemoperfusion but repeated oral administration of activated charcoal may enhance elimination. Forced acid diuresis is not recommended.

As Dirythmin SA is an extended release formulation, treatment of overdosage may be required for a longer period.

In case of any impaired renal function, measures to increase the glomerular filtration rate may reduce the toxicity (disopyramide is excreted primarily by the kidney). Altering the urinary pH in humans does not affect the plasma half-life or the amount of disopyramide excreted in the urine.

Pharmaceutical precautions Store below 30°C.

Legal category POM.

Package quantities Press-through packages of thermoformed PVC (10 tablets per press-through strip). Pack size 100.

Further information Nil.

Product licence number 0017/0100

EMLA* CREAM 5%

Presentation White cream. Each gramme contains lidocaine base 25 mg and prilocaine base 25 mg in a eutectic mixture as an oil water emulsion also containing arlatone, carboxypolymethylene, sodium hydroxide and purified water.

Uses Local anaesthetic for topical use to produce surface anaesthesia of the skin.

For topical use on the genital mucosa to facilitate the removal of warts in adults.

Dosage and administration
Adults (including elderly) and children > 1 year:

Surface	*Procedure*	*Application*
Skin (apply a thick layer of cream under an occlusive dressing)	Minor dermatological procedures e.g. needle insertion and surgical treatment of localised lesions	Approximately 2 g EMLA applied for a minimum of 60 minutes, maximum 5 hours
	Dermal procedures on larger areas e.g. split skin grafting	Approximately 1.5-3 g/10cm² EMLA applied for a minimum of 2 hours, maximum 5 hours

Surface	*Procedure*	*Application*
Genital mucosa (Adults) (No occlusive dressing required)	Surgical treatment of localised lesions	Apply up to 10 g EMLA for 5-10 minutes. Commence procedure immediately thereafter

Analgesic efficacy may decline if the skin application time is more than 5 hours. Procedures on intact skin should begin soon after the occlusive dressing is removed.

On the genital mucosa analgesic efficacy declines after 10–15 minutes and therefore the procedure should be commenced immediately.

Not recommended in infants under one year of age.

Contra-indications, warnings, etc
Contra-indications: Known hypersensitivity to anaesthetics of the amide type.

Precautions: Until further clinical experience is available, EMLA Cream should not be applied to wounds, mucous membranes or in areas of atopic dermatitis.

EMLA Cream should not be applied to genital mucosa in children.

EMLA causes corneal irritation and should not be applied to or near the eyes. EMLA, like other local anaesthetics may be ototoxic and should not be instilled in the middle ear nor should it be used for procedures which might allow penetration into the middle ear.

Although the systemic availability of prilocaine by percutaneous absorption of EMLA is low, caution should be exercised in patients with anaemia, congenital or acquired methaemoglobinaemia or patients on concomitant therapy known to produce such conditions.

Pregnancy and lactation: Lidocaine and prilocaine cross the placental barrier. However, both drugs have been in widespread clinical use for many years and a large number of women of childbearing age have been exposed to them. No specific effects on the reproductive process have been reported.

Lidocaine and prilocaine are excreted in breast milk in small amounts.

Adverse events: Transient paleness, redness and oedema have been reported.

Prilocaine has been known to cause methaemoglobinaemia when given parenterally.

In rare cases local anaesthetics have been associated with allergic reactions including anaphylactic shock.

Interactions: Methaemoglobinaemia may be accentuated in patients already taking drugs known to induce the condition, e.g. sulphonamides.

The risk of additional systemic toxicity should be considered when large doses of EMLA are applied to patients already using other local anaesthetics or structurally related drugs e.g. tocainide.

Overdosage: Overdosage with EMLA is unlikely but signs of systemic toxicity will be similar in nature to those observed after administration of other local anaesthetics.

Pharmaceutical precautions Store below 30°C.

Legal category POM.

Package quantities 'Pre-medication pack' containing 10×5 g tubes EMLA and 25 occlusive dressings. 30 g tube EMLA. 1×5 g tube EMLA without dressing.

Further information Nil.

Product licence number 0017/0213

ENTOCORT* CR 3 mg CAPSULES

Qualitative and quantitative composition Each capsule contains budesonide 3 mg.

Pharmaceutical form Entocort CR 3 mg Capsules: Hard gelatin capsules for oral administration with an opaque, light grey body and opaque, pink cap marked $\frac{\text{CIR}}{\text{3 mg}}$ in black radial print. Each capsule contains budesonide 3 mg as gastro-resistant, prolonged release granules.

Clinical particulars
Therapeutic Indications: Entocort CR Capsules are indicated for the induction of remission in patients with mild to moderate Crohn's disease affecting the ileum and/or the ascending colon.

Posology and method of administration:
Adults: Active Crohn's disease: The recommended daily dose for induction of remission is 9 mg once daily in the morning, taken before breakfast, for up to eight weeks.

When treatment is to be discontinued, the dose

should normally be reduced for the last 2 to 4 weeks of therapy.

Children: There is presently no experience with Entocort CR Capsules in children. Entocort is not recommended for use in children.

Elderly: No special dose adjustment is recommended. However, experience with Entocort CR Capsules in the elderly is limited.

Contra-indications: Bacterial, fungal or viral infections. Known hypersensitivity to any of the ingredients.

Special warnings and special precautions for use: Treatment with Entocort CR Capsules results in lower systemic steroid levels than conventional oral steroid therapy. Transfer from other steroid therapy may result in symptoms related to the change in systemic steroid levels. The following warnings apply, in common with other oral steroids.

Use with caution in patients with tuberculosis, hypertension, diabetes mellitus, osteoporosis, peptic ulcer, glaucoma or cataracts or with a family history of diabetes or glaucoma or with any other condition where the use of glucocorticosteroids may have unwanted effects.

Chicken pox and measles may follow a more serious course in patients on oral glucocorticosteroids. Particular care should be taken to avoid exposure in patients who have not previously had these diseases.

Corticosteroids may cause suppression of the HPA axis and reduce the stress response. Where patients are subject to surgery or other stresses, supplementary systemic glucocorticoid treatment is recommended.

In patients with compromised liver function, blood levels of glucocorticosteroid may increase, as with other drugs which are metabolised via the liver.

When treatment is to be discontinued, the dose should normally be reduced for the last 2 to 4 weeks of therapy.

Interactions with other medicaments and other forms of interaction: Although not studied, concomitant administration of cholestyramine may reduce Entocort uptake, in common with other drugs.

Pregnancy and lactation:
Pregnancy: "The ability of corticosteroids to cross the placenta varies between individual drugs, however, in mice, budesonide and/or its metabolites have been shown to cross the placenta."

Administration of corticosteroids to pregnant animals can cause abnormalities of foetal development including cleft palate, intra-uterine growth retardation and affects on brain growth and development. There is no evidence that corticosteroids result in an increased incidence of congenital abnormalities, such as cleft palate/lip in man. However, when administered for prolonged periods or repeatedly during pregnancy, corticosteroids may increase the risk of intra-uterine growth retardation. Hypoadrenalism may, in theory, occur in the neonate following prenatal exposure to corticosteroids but usually resolves spontaneously following birth and is rarely clinically important. As with all drugs, corticosteroids should only be prescribed when the benefits to the mother and child outweigh the risks. When corticosteroids are essential however, patients with normal pregnancies may be treated as though they were in the non-gravid state.

Lactation: Corticosteroids are secreted in small amounts in breast milk, however, budesonide given at the clinically recommended dose is unlikely to cause systematic effects in the infant. Infants of mothers taking higher than recommended doses of budesonide may have a degree of adrenal suppression but the benefits of breast feeding are likely to outweigh any theoretical risk."

Effects on ability to drive and use machines: No effects are known.

Undesirable Effects: Undesirable effects characteristic of systemic corticosteroid therapy, such as Cushingoid features, may occur.

In clinical trials other adverse events: dyspepsia, muscle cramps, tremor, palpitations, nervousness, blurred vision, skin reactions (rash, pruritus) and menstrual disorders have been reported. Most of these adverse events were classed as mild to moderate and were not considered serious. In clinical studies, at recommended doses, the incidence of adverse events was comparable to placebo.

Clinical studies showed the frequency of steroid associated side-effects for Entocort CR Capsules to be approximately half that of conventional prednisolone treatment, at equipotent doses. In studies of patients with active disease, receiving Entocort 9 mg daily, the incidence of adverse events was comparable to placebo.

Overdose: Acute overdosage with Entocort CR Capsules even at very high doses, is not expected to lead to an acute clinical crisis. Use supportive therapy as required.

Chronic overdosage may lead to systemic corticosteroid effects, such as Cushingoid features. If such changes occur, the dose of Entocort CR Capsules should be gradually reduced until treatment is discontinued, in accordance with normal procedures for the discontinuation of prolonged oral steroid therapy.

Pharmacological properties
Pharmacodynamic properties: The exact mechanism of budesonide in the treatment of Crohn's disease is not fully understood. Data from clinical pharmacology studies and controlled clinical trials strongly indicate that the mode of action of Entocort CR Capsules is based, at least partly, on a local action in the gut. Budesonide is a glucocorticosteroid with a high local anti-inflammatory effect. At doses clinically equivalent to prednisolone, budesonide gives significantly less HPA axis suppression and has a lower impact on inflammatory markers.

At recommended doses, Entocort CR Capsules caused significantly less effect than prednisolone 20-40 mg daily on: morning plasma cortisols; 24 hour plasma cortisol (AUC 0-24h) and 24 hour urine cortisol levels.

ACTH tests have shown Entocort CR Capsules to have significantly less effect than prednisolone on adrenal functions.

Pharmacokinetic properties: Budesonide has a high volume of distribution (about 3 litre/kg) and a high systemic clearance (about 1.2 litre/min). Plasma protein binding averages 85-90%. After oral dosing of plain micronized compound, absorption is rapid and seems to be complete. Budesonide then undergoes extensive biotransformation in the liver (approximately 90%) to metabolites of low glucocorticosteroid activity. The glucocorticosteroid activity of the major metabolites, 6β-hydroxybudesonide and 16α-hydroxyprednisolone, is less than 1% of that of budesonide.

In healthy volunteers mean maximal plasma concentrations of 5-10 nmol/litre were seen at 3-5 hours following a single oral dose of Entocort CR Capsules 9 mg, taken before breakfast.

Systemic availability in healthy subjects is approximately 10% for Entocort CR Capsules similar to the systemic availability of plain micronised budesonide, indicating complete absorption.

In patients with active Crohn's disease systemic availability is approximately 20% at the start of treatment, and reduces to around 15% after 8 weeks treatment.

A large proportion of the drug is absorbed from the ileum and ascending colon. Elimination is rate limited by absorption. The average terminal half-life is 4 hours.

Preclinical safety data: Results from acute, subacute and chronic toxicity studies show that the systemic effects of budesonide are less severe or similar to those observed after administration of other glucocorticosteroids, e.g. decreased body-weight gain and atrophy of lymphoid tissues and adrenal cortex.

Budesonide, evaluated in six different test systems, did not show any mutagenic or clastogenic effects.

An increased incidence of brain gliomas in male rats in a carcinogenicity study could not be verified in a repeat study, in which the incidence of gliomas did not differ between any of the groups on active treatment (budesonide, prednisolone, triamcinolone acetonide) and the control groups.

Liver changes (primary hepatocellular neoplasms) found in male rats in the original carcinogenicity study were noted again in the repeat study with budesonide as well as the reference glucocorticosteroids. These effects are most probably related to a receptor effect and thus represent a class effect.

Available clinical experience shows that there are no indications that budesonide or other glucocorticosteroids induce brain gliomas or primary hepatocellular neoplasms in man.

The toxicity of Entocort CR Capsules, with focus on the gastrointestinal tract, has been studied in cynomolgus monkeys in doses up to 5 mg/kg after repeated oral administration for up to 6 months. No effects were observed in the gastrointestinal tract, neither at gross pathology nor in the histopathological examination.

Pharmaceutical particulars
List of excipients: Ethylcellulose, Acetyltributyl citrate, Methacrylic acid copolymer, Triethylcitrate, Antifoam M, Polysorbate 80, Talc, Sucrose, Maize starch, Gelatine, Titanium dioxide (E171), Iron-oxide (E172).

Incompatibilities: No known incompatibilities.

Shelf life: Entocort CR Capsules have a shelf-life of 2 years when stored below 30°C in the original container.

Special precautions for storage: Store in the original container. Replace cap firmly after use. Store out of reach of children.

Nature and contents of container: White polyethylene bottles of 100 capsules, having either a tamper evident or child resistant polypropylene screw cap, with an integral desiccant.

Instructions for use/handling: The capsules should be swallowed whole with water. The capsules must not be chewed.

Marketing authorisation number PL 0017/0359

Date of approval/revision of SPC June 1998

Legal category POM.

ENTOCORT* ENEMA

Qualitative and quantitative composition 0.02 mg/ml budesonide INN (2 mg budesonide INN/100 ml).

Pharmaceutical form Enema.

Clinical particulars
Therapeutic indications: Ulcerative colitis involving rectal and recto-sigmoid disease.

Posology and method of administration: Adults: One Entocort Enema nightly for 4 weeks.

Children: Not recommended.

Elderly: Dosage as for adults.

No dosage reduction is necessary in patients with reduced liver function.

Contra-indications: Local bacterial and viral infection. Hypersensitivity to any of the ingredients.

Special warnings and special precautions for use: Special care is needed in treatment of patients transferred from systemic steroids to Entocort Enema, as disturbances in the hypothalamic-pituitary-adrenal axis could be expected in these patients.

Interaction with other medicaments and other forms of interaction: Information on possible interactions with rectal administration of budesonide is not available presently.

Pregnancy and lactation:
Pregnancy: "The ability of corticosteroids to cross the placenta varies between individual drugs, however, in mice, budesonide and/or its metabolites have been shown to cross the placenta."

Administration of corticosteroids to pregnant animals can cause abnormalities of foetal development including cleft palate, intra-uterine growth retardation and affects on brain growth and development. There is no evidence that corticosteroids result in an increased incidence of congenital abnormalities, such as cleft palate/lip in man. However, when administered for prolonged periods or repeatedly during pregnancy, corticosteroids may increase the risk of intra-uterine growth retardation. Hypoadrenalism may, in theory, occur in the neonate following prenatal exposure to corticosteroids but usually resolves spontaneously following birth and is rarely clinically important. As with all drugs, corticosteroids should only be prescribed when the benefits to the mother and child outweigh the risks. When corticosteroids are essential however, patients with normal pregnancies may be treated as though they were in the non-gravid state.

Lactation: Corticosteroids are secreted in small amounts in breast milk, however, budesonide given at the clinically recommended dose is unlikely to cause systematic effects in the infant. Infants of mothers taking higher than recommended doses of budesonide may have a degree of adrenal suppression but the benefits of breast feeding are likely to outweigh any theoretical risk."

Effects on ability to drive and use machines: Entocort Enema does not affect the ability to drive and operate machinery.

Undesirable effects: The most common adverse reactions are gastrointestinal disturbances e.g. flatulence, nausea, diarrhoea. Skin reactions (e.g. rash, pruritus) may occur. Less common adverse reactions include agitation and insomnia.

Overdose: Acute overdosage with Entocort Enema, even in excessive doses, is not expected to be a clinical problem. The dosage form and route of administration make any prolonged overdosage unlikely.

Pharmacological properties
Pharmacodynamic properties: Budesonide is a glucocorticosteroid with a high local anti-inflammatory effect. Budesonide undergoes an extensive degree (~90%) of biotransformation in the liver to metabolites of low glucocorticosteroid activity. The glucocorticosteroid activity of the major metabolites, 6β-hydroxybudesonide and 16α-hydroxyprednisolone, is less than 1% of that of budesonide.

Pharmacokinetic properties: At recommended doses, budesonide causes no or small suppression of plasma cortisol.

The mean maximal plasma concentration after

rectal administration of 2 mg budesonide is 3 nmol/litre (range 1–9 nmol/litre), reached within 1.5 hours.

Preclinical safety data: Budesonide is a well established active ingredient.

Pharmaceutical particulars
List of excipients:
Tablet: Lactose anhydrous, riboflavin sodium phosphate, lactose, crosslinked polyvidone, colloidal anhydrous silica and magnesium stearate.
Vehicle: Sodium chloride, methyl parahydroxybenzoate, propyl parahydroxybenzoate, and water, purified.

Incompatibilities: None stated.

Shelf-life: 24 months.

Special precautions for storage: Store below 30°C.

Nature and contents of container: Entocort Enema 0.02 mg/ml consists of 2 components: A dispersible tablet and a vehicle.

The primary package for the tablets is an aluminium blister package consisting of polyamide 25 micrometre/Al 43 micrometre / polyvinylchloride 60 micrometre / Al 20 micrometre.

The primary package for the vehicle is a polyethylene bottle equipped with a combined seal gasket and non-return valve, a rectal nozzle and a protective cap for the nozzle.

The bottle, the nozzle and the protective cap are made of LD-polyethylene. The combined seal gasket and non-return valve is made of thermoplastic rubber.

Instructions for use/handling: None stated.

Marketing authorisation number PL 0017/0332

Date of approval/revision of SPC June 1998

Legal category POM.

FOSCAVIR*

Presentation Solution for intravenous infusion containing foscarnet 24 mg/ml.

1 ml contains 24 mg (80 micromol) foscarnet trisodium hexahydrate for injection, hydrochloric acid for pH adjustment and water for injection. The solution is sterile, clear and isotonic with a pH of 7.4.

Uses Therapeutic conditions: Foscavir is indicated for the treatment of cytomegalovirus (CMV) retinitis in patients with AIDS. Induction therapy of mucocutaneous Herpes Simplex Virus (HSV) infections unresponsive to acyclovir in immunocompromised patients.

Following induction therapy over 2–3 weeks Foscavir produced stabilisation of retinal lesions in approximately 80% of cases treated. However, since CMV causes latent infections and since Foscavir exerts a virustatic activity, relapses are likely in the majority of patients with persistent immunodeficiency once treatment is discontinued. Following completion of induction therapy, maintenance therapy should be instituted with a once daily regimen at an initial dose of 60 mg/kg increasing to 90-120 mg/kg if tolerated. A number of patients have received 90 mg/kg over a two hour period as a maintenance therapy starting dose. Maintenance therapy has produced a delay in time to retinitis progression. In patients experiencing progression of retinitis while receiving maintenance therapy or off therapy, reinstitution of induction therapy has shown efficacy equivalent to that of the initial course.

Foscavir is also indicated for the treatment of mucocutaneous HSV infections, clinically unresponsive to acyclovir in immunocompromised patients. The safety and efficacy of Foscavir for the treatment of other HSV infections (e.g. retinitis, encephalitis); congenital or neonatal disease; or HSV in immunocompetent individuals has not been established.

The diagnosis of acyclovir unresponsiveness can be made either clinically by treatment with intravenous acyclovir (5-10 mg/kg t.i.d) for 10 days without response or by *in vitro* testing.

For treatment of acyclovir unresponsive mucocutaneous infections Foscavir was administered at 40 mg/kg every 8 hours over 2–3 weeks or until healing. In a prospective randomised study in patients with AIDS, Foscavir treated patients healed within 11–25 days, had a complete relief of pain within 9 days and stopped shedding HSV virus within 7 days.

Foscavir is not recommended for treatment of CMV infections other than retinitis or HSV or for use in non-AIDS or non-immunocompromised patients.

Dosage and administration
Method of administration: Foscavir should be administered by the intravenous route only, either by a central venous line or in a peripheral vein.

When peripheral veins are used, the solution of foscarnet 24 mg/ml must be diluted. Individually dispensed doses of foscarnet should be aseptically transferred and diluted with equal parts of 0.9% sodium chloride (9 mg/ml) or 5% dextrose (50 mg/ml) by the hospital pharmacy. The diluted solutions should be used as soon as possible after preparation but can be stored for up to 24 hours if kept refrigerated.

The solution of foscarnet 24 mg/ml may be given without dilution via a central vein.

Adults: Induction therapy for CMV retinitis: Foscavir is administered over 2-3 weeks depending on the clinical response, as intermittent infusions every 8 hours at a dose of 60 mg/kg in patients with normal renal function.

Dosage must be individualised for patients' renal function (see dosing chart below). The infusion time should not be shorter than 1 hour.

Maintenance therapy: For maintenance therapy, following induction therapy of CMV retinitis, Foscavir is administered seven days a week as long as therapy is considered appropriate. In patients with normal renal function it is a recommended to initiate therapy at 60 mg/kg. Increase to a dose range of 90-120 mg/kg may then be considered in patients tolerating the initial dose level and/or those with progressive retinitis. A number of patients have received 90 mg/kg over a 2 hour period as a starting dose for maintenance therapy. Dosage must be reduced in patients with renal insufficiency (see dosing chart at the end of the dosage section).

Patients who experience progression of retinitis while receiving maintenance therapy may be retreated with the induction regimen.

Induction therapy of mucocutaneous HSV infections unresponsive to acyclovir: Foscavir is administered for 2–3 weeks or until healing of lesions, as intermittent infusions at a dose of 40 mg/kg over one hour every 8 hours in patients with normal renal function. Dosage must be individualised for patient's renal function (see dosing chart below). The infusion time should not be shorter than 1 hour.

Efficacy of Foscavir maintenance therapy following induction therapy of acyclovir unresponsive HSV infections has not been established.

Caution – do not administer Foscavir by rapid intravenous injection.

Foscavir Dosing Chart
Induction Therapy

Creatinine clearance (ml/kg/min)	*CMV every 8 hrs (mg/kg)*	*HSV every 8 hrs (mg/kg)*
>1.6	60	40
1.6-1.4	55	37
1.4-1.2	49	33
1.2-1.0	42	28
1.0-0.8	35	24
0.8-0.6	28	19
0.6-0.4	21	14
<0.4	Treatment not recommended	

CMV Maintenance Therapy

Creatinine clearance (ml/kg/min)	*One infusion dose: mg/kg/day in not less than one hour*
>1.6	60*
1.6-1.4	55
1.4-1.2	49
1.2-1.0	42
1.0-0.8	35
0.8-0.6	28
0.6-0.4	21
<0.4	Treatment not recommended

* A number of patients have received 90 mg/kg as a starting dose for maintenance therapy

Foscavir is not recommended in patients undergoing haemodialysis since dosage guidelines have not been established.

Hydration: Renal toxicity of Foscavir can be reduced by adequate hydration of the patient. It is recommended to establish diuresis by hydration with 0.5-1.0 litre of normal saline at each infusion.

Elderly: As for adults.

Children: There is very limited experience in treating children.

Renal or hepatic insufficiency: The dose must be reduced in patients with renal insufficiency, according to the creatinine clearance level as described in the table above. Dose adjustment is not required in patients with hepatic insufficiency.

Instructions for use/handling: Foscarnet contains no preservatives and once the sterility seal of a bottle has been broken the solution should be used within 24 hours.

Individually dispensed doses of foscarnet can be aseptically transferred to plastic infusion bags by the hospital pharmacy. The physico-chemical stability of foscarnet and dilutions thereof in equal parts with 0.9% sodium chloride (9 mg/ml) or 5% dextrose (50 mg/ml) in PVC bags is 7 days. However, diluted solutions should be refrigerated and storage restricted to 24 hours.

Accidental skin and eye contact with the foscarnet sodium solution may cause local irritation and burning sensation. If accidental contact occurs the exposed area should be rinsed with water.

Each bottle of Foscavir should only be used to treat one patient with a single infusion. Unused solution should be discarded.

Contra-indications, warnings, etc
Contra-indications: Hypersensitivity to Foscavir, pregnancy and lactation.

Precautions and Warnings: Foscavir should be used with caution in patients with reduced renal function. Since renal functional impairment may occur at any time during foscarnet administration, serum creatinine should be monitored every second day during induction therapy and once weekly during maintenance therapy and appropriate dose adjustments should be performed according to renal function. Adequate hydration should be maintained in all patients. (See Dosage and Administration).

Due to Foscavir's propensity to chelate bivalent metal ions, such as calcium, Foscavir administration may be associated with an acute decrease of ionised serum calcium, which may not be reflected in total serum calcium levels. The electrolytes, especially calcium and magnesium, should be assessed prior to and during Foscavir therapy and deficiencies corrected.

Foscavir has local irritating properties and when excreted in high concentrations in the urine it may induce genital irritation or even ulcerations. Close attention to personal hygiene is recommended after micturition to lessen the potential of local irritation.

When diuretics are indicated, thiazides are recommended.

Following treatment with foscarnet, clinical unresponsiveness can appear which may be due to appearance of virus strains with decreased sensitivity towards foscarnet. Termination of treatment with foscarnet should then be considered.

Mutagenicity studies showed that foscarnet has a genotoxic potential. The possible explanation for the observed effect in the mutagenicity studies is an inhibition of the DNA polymerase in the cell line used. Foscarnet therapeutically acts by inhibition of the herpes virus specific DNA polymerase. The human cellular polymerase α is about 100 times less sensitive to foscarnet. The carcinogenicity studies performed did not disclose any oncogenic potential.

Side-effects: In different patient populations Foscavir has been administered to more than 11,500 patients, the majority severely immunocompromised and suffering from serious viral infections.

The patient's physical status, the severity of the underlying disease, other infections and concurrent therapy also contribute to the observed adverse event profile of Foscavir.

Consistent findings associated with Foscavir administration are renal function impairment, impact on serum electrolytes and haemoglobin concentration, convulsions and local genital irritation/ulceration.

The adverse events discussed and tabulated below refer to results for 188 AIDS patients studied in prospective clinical trials and include those events related, unrelated and of unknown relationship to Foscavir. The adverse event profile from marketed use is similar to that reported in clinical studies.

Renal function impairment: Twenty-seven percent of the above 188 study patients experienced renal functional impairment recorded as a rise in serum creatinine (19%), decreases in creatinine clearance (6%), abnormal renal function (9%), acute renal failure (2%), uraemia (1%) and polyuria in 2%. Metabolic acidosis was seen in 1%. The overall pattern of these symptoms is consistent with previous experiences although the incidence may vary. Most patients with increased serum creatinine have shown normalisation or a return to pre-treatment levels within 1-10 weeks of treatment discontinuation.

Electrolytes: Among the above 188 patients, hypocalcaemia was recorded in 14%. Also, hypomagnesaemia was recorded in 15%. Frequently recorded were also hypokalaemia in 16% and hypophosphataemia and hyperphosphataemia in 8 and 6% respectively. Foscarnet chelates with metal ions (Ca^{2+}, Mg^{2+}, Fe^{2+}, Zn^{2+}) and acute hypocalcaemia, sometimes symptomatic, has been a common observation in some 30% of AIDS patients receiving foscarnet. Experimental and clinical data have shown that foscarnet acutely decreases ionised calcium in a dose-related manner. The drop in serum calcium is reversible. It is reasonable to assume that the infusion rate significantly affects the decrease rate of ionised calcium.

Convulsions: Among the AIDS patients referred to above, convulsions including grand mal were recorded in 10%. Based on the occurrence of convulsions among immunocompromised patients receiving foscarnet, an association between foscarnet induced hypocalcaemia or a direct action of foscarnet per se and convulsions has been discussed. Although many of the patients experiencing convulsions had pre-existing CNS abnormalities such as cryptococcal meningitis, space occupying lesions or other CNS tumours, an association with foscarnet can not be excluded.

Haemoglobin concentration: Decreases of the haemoglobin concentration have been observed in 25-33% of patients. Generally, there has been no consistent pattern of simultaneous decreases in white blood cell and platelet counts. Some 30% of the above study patients were also on concurrent AZT treatment. Many AIDS patients were anaemic already before foscarnet administration.

Local irritation in terms of thrombophlebitis in peripheral veins following infusion of undiluted foscarnet solution and genital irritation/ulcerations have been observed. Since foscarnet is excreted in high concentrations in the urine local irritation/ulceration may ensue especially during induction therapy when high doses of foscarnet are being administered.

Other adverse events: Other adverse events that were recorded in the 188 study patients include a variety of symptoms varying in frequency from 1% to approximately 60%, the latter being the incidence for fever. Subgrouped by body system the following adverse events, related, unrelated or of unknown relationship to foscarnet therapy were recorded.

Body as a whole: Asthenia, fatigue, malaise and chills were observed in 12, 20, 7 and 13% respectively and sepsis in 7%.

Gastro-intestinal system disorders: Nausea and vomiting were observed in 45 and 25% respectively and diarrhoea in 32%. Abdominal pain and occasionally dyspepsia and constipation were observed in 10, 3, and 6% respectively. Isolated cases of pancreatitis have been reported from marketed use.

Metabolic and nutritional disorders: Hyponatraemia and oedema in legs were seen in 4 and 1% respectively and increase in LDH and alkaline phosphatases in 2 and 3% respectively. Increased levels of amylase have been reported from marketed use.

Central/peripheral nervous system disorders: Paraesthesia was observed in 18%, headache in 25% and dizziness in 12%. Involuntary muscle contractions and tremor were seen in 9 and 5% respectively. Hypoaesthesia, ataxia and neuropathy were observed in 7, 4 and 6% respectively.

Psychiatric disorders: Anorexia, anxiety and nervousness were observed in 15 and 5% respectively and depression in 10%, confusion in 7%, psychosis in 1%, agitation in 3% and aggressive reaction in 2%.

White blood cells: Adverse events related to white blood cells included leukopenia 9%, granulocytopenia 17%. In these patients over 90% had some degree of leukopenia already before foscarnet administration, in 8% severe or even life-threatening. Moreover in some patients, it is noteworthy that mean WBC counts increased during treatment with foscarnet. Although a few patients worsened in this respect, there is no clear evidence to indicate that foscarnet is myelosuppressive.

Platelet, bleeding, clotting disorders: Thrombocytopenia was observed in 4%.

Skin and appendages: Rash was observed in 16%.

Liver and biliary system disorders: Abnormal liver function was observed in 4% and increase in serum ALAT and ASAT in 3 and 2% respectively and gamma GT in 2%.

Cardiovascular disorders: Abnormal ECG, hypertension, and hypotension were observed in 1, 4 and 2% respectively.

Heart rate and rhythm disorders: Ventricular arrhythmia has been reported in 2 patients from marketed use.

Urinary system disorders: A few cases of diabetes insipidus, usually of the nephrogenic type, have been reported from marketed use.

Musculo-skeletal disorders: Muscle weakness has been reported from marketed use.

Use during pregnancy and lactation: Foscavir is contra-indicated in pregnancy. Breast feeding should be discontinued before starting Foscavir treatment.

Interactions: Since Foscavir can impair renal function, additive toxicity may occur when used in combination with other nephrotoxic drugs such as aminoglycosides and amphotericin B. Moreover, since Foscavir can reduce serum levels of ionised calcium, extreme caution is advised when used concurrently with other drugs known to influence serum calcium levels, like intravenous pentamidine. Renal impairment and symptomatic hypocalcaemia (Trousseau's and Chvostek's signs) have been observed during concurrent treatment with Foscavir and intravenous pentamidine.

The elimination of Foscavir may be impaired by drugs which inhibit renal tubular secretion.

There is no evidence of an increased myelotoxicity when foscarnet is used in combination with zidovudine (AZT). Neither is there any pharmacokinetic interaction between the two drugs.

Overdose: Overdose has been reported in 33 patients, the highest dose being about 10 times the prescribed dose. Twenty-eight of the patients experienced adverse events and five patients suffered no ill effects in connection with foscarnet overdosing. Four patients died, one from respiratory/cardiac arrest 3 days after stopping foscarnet, one from progressive AIDS and renal failure approximately 2 months after the last foscarnet dose, one from end stage AIDS and bacteraemia 2 weeks after overdosing and one from multi-organ failure 11 days after stopping foscarnet. The pattern of adverse events reported in connection with overdose was in correspondence with the symptoms previously observed during foscarnet therapy.

Haemodialysis increases foscarnet elimination and may be of benefit in severe overdosage.

Effects on ability to drive and use machines: Adverse effects such as dizziness and convulsions may occur during Foscavir therapy. The physician is advised to discuss this issue with the patient, and based upon the condition of the disease and the tolerance of medication, give his recommendation in the individual case.

Pharmaceutical Particulars

Foscavir is not compatible with dextrose 30% solution, amphotericin B, acyclovir sodium, ganciclovir, pentamidine isethionate, trimethoprimsulfamtoxazole and vancomycin hydrochloride. Neither is foscarnet compatible with solutions containing calcium. It is recommended that other drugs should not be infused concomitantly in the same line until further experience is gained.

Special precautions for storage: Store below 30°C. Do not refrigerate. If refrigerated or exposed to temperatures below freezing point precipitation may occur. By keeping the bottle at room temperature with repeated shaking the precipitate can be brought into solution again.

Legal category POM.

Package quantities 250 ml or 500 ml glass bottles.

Further information Nil.

Product licence number 0017/0248

HEMINEVRIN* CAPSULES

Qualitative and quantitative composition 192 mg Chlormethiazole(base)/per capsule.

Pharmaceutical form Capsules.

Clinical particulars

Therapeutic indications: Heminevrin is a short acting hypnotic and sedative with anticonvulsant effect. It is used for the: management of restlessness and agitation in the elderly, short term treatment of severe insomnia in the elderly and treatment of alcohol withdrawal symptoms where close hospital supervision is also provided.

Posology and method of administration: Management of restlessness and agitation in the elderly: one capsule three times daily.

Severe insomnia in the elderly: 1-2 capsules before going to bed. The lower dose should be tried first. As with all psychotropic drugs, treatment should be kept to a minimum, reviewed regularly and discontinued as soon as possible.

Alcohol withdrawal states: Heminevrin is not a specific 'cure' for alcoholism. Alcohol withdrawal should be treated in hospital or, in exceptional circumstances, on an outpatient basis by specialist units when the daily dosage of Heminevrin must be monitored closely by community health staff. The dosage should be adjusted to patient response. The patient should be sedated but rousable. A suggested regimen is:

Initial dose: 2 to 4 capsules, if necessary repeated after some hours.

Day 1, first 24 hours: 9 to 12 capsules, divided into 3 or 4 doses.

Day 2: 6 to 8 capsules, divided into 3 or 4 doses.

Day 3: 4 to 6 capsules, divided into 3 or 4 doses.

Days 4 to 6: A gradual reduction in dosage until the final dose.

Administration for more than nine (9) days is not recommended.

Contra-indications: Known sensitivity to chlormethiazole. Acute pulmonary insufficiency.

Special warnings and special precautions for use: Heminevrin should be used cautiously in patients with chronic pulmonary insufficiency. Heminevrin may potentiate or be potentiated by centrally acting depressant drugs including alcohol and benzodiazepines. Fatal cardiorespiratory collapse has been reported when chlormethiazole was combined with other CNS depressant drugs. When used concomitantly dosage should be appropriately reduced.

Hypoxia, resulting from, for example, cardiac and/or respiratory insufficiency, can manifest itself as an acute confusional state. Recognition and specific treatment of the cause is essential in such patients and in such cases sedatives/hypnotics should be avoided.

Moderate liver disorders associated with alcoholism do not preclude the use of chlormethiazole, though an associated increase in systemic availability of oral doses and delayed elimination of the drug may require reduced dosage. Great caution should be observed in patients with gross liver damage and decreased liver function, particularly as sedation can mask the onset of liver coma.

Caution should be observed in patients with chronic renal disease.

Caution must be exercised in prescribing for individuals known to be addiction prone or for those whose histories suggest they may increase the dose on their own initiative since chlormethiazole is not free from the risk of producing psychological and/or physical dependence. After prolonged administration of high doses, physical dependence has been reported with withdrawal symptoms such as convulsions, tremors, and organic psychosis. These reports have mainly been associated with indiscriminate prescribing to outpatient alcoholics and Heminevrin should not be prescribed to patients who continue to abuse alcohol.

Alcoholism: Alcohol combined with chlormethiazole particularly in alcoholics with cirrhosis can lead to fatal respiratory depression even with short term use. It should not therefore be prescribed for alcoholics who continue to drink alcoholic beverages.

Elderly: Caution is advised as there may be increased bioavailability and delayed elimination of chlormethiazole.

Children: Oral Heminevrin is not recommended for use in children.

Interactions with other medications and other forms of interaction: A combination of chlormethiazole and diazoxide should be avoided as an adverse neonatal reaction suspected to be due to the maternal administration of this combination has been reported.

The combination of propranolol and chlormethiazole has produced profound bradycardia in one patient possibly due to increased bioavailability of propranolol.

There is evidence to indicate that the metabolism of chlormethiazole is inhibited by cimetidine, thus the co-administration of these drugs may lead to increased blood/plasma levels of chlormethiazole.

Pregnancy and lactation: Do not use in pregnancy especially during the first and last trimesters, unless there are compelling reasons. There is no evidence of safety in human pregnancy, nor is there evidence from animal studies that it is entirely free from hazard.

Chlormethiazole is excreted into the breast milk. The effect of even small quantities of sedative/hypnotic and anticonvulsant drugs on the infant brain is not established.

Chlormethiazole should only be used in nursing mothers where the physician considers that the benefit outweighs the possible hazard to the infant.

Effect on ability to drive and use machines: As with all centrally acting depressant drugs, the driving of vehicles and the operating of machinery are to be avoided when under treatment.

Undesirable effects: The most common side-effect is nasal congestion and irritation, which may occur 15 to 20 minutes after drug ingestion. Conjunctival irritation has also been noted in some cases. Occasionally, these symptoms may be severe and may be associated with severe headache. This is commonest with the initial dose following which it decreases in severity with subsequent doses. Increased nasopharyngeal/bronchial secretions can occur.

Rash and urticaria have been reported. In rare cases, bullous skin eruptions have been reported.

Gastrointestinal disturbances have been reported.

Reversible increases of transaminases or bilirubin have been reported.

In rare cases anaphylactic reactions have occurred.

When Heminevrin has been given at higher than recommended doses for other than recommended indications over prolonged periods of time, physical dependence, tolerance and withdrawal reactions have been reported.

Great caution is required in prescribing Heminevrin for patients with a history of chronic alcoholism, drug abuse or marked personality disorder.

When used as a night-time hypnotic, hangover effects in the elderly may occur but are uncommon due to the short half-life.

Excessive sedation may occur, especially with higher doses or when given to the elderly for daytime sedation. Paradoxical excitement or confusion may occur rarely.

Overdosage: The main effects to be expected with overdose of Heminevrin are: coma, respiratory depression, hypotension and hypothermia.

Hypothermia is thought to be due to a direct central effect as well as a result of lying unconscious for several hours. In addition, patients have increased secretion in the upper airways, which in one series was associated with a high incidence of pneumonia. The effects of overdosage are not usually severe in patients with no evidence of alcoholic liver disease, but they may be exacerbated when chlormethiazole is taken in combination with alcohol and/or CNS depressant drugs, particularly those that are metabolised by the liver. There is no specific antidote to chlormethiazole. Treatment of overdosage should therefore be carried out on a symptomatic basis, applying similar principles to those used in the treatment of barbiturate overdosage.

Charcoal column haemoperfusion is not and cannot be expected to be effective in treating chlormethiazole poisoning.

Pharmacological properties

Pharmacodynamic properties: Chlormethiazole is pharmacologically distinct from both the benzodiazepines and the barbiturates.

Chlormethiazole has sedative, muscle relaxant and anticonvulsant properties. It is used for hypnosis in elderly and institutionalised patients, for preanaesthetic sedation and especially in the management of withdrawal from ethanol. Given alone its effects on respiration are slight and the therapeutic index high.

Pharmacokinetic properties: Chlormethiazole has a short half-life, low oral bioavailability, high plasma clearance and shows no evidence of accumulation or altered pharmacokinetics after repeated dosage. It is excreted in urine after extensive metabolism in the liver. The rate of elimination is decreased by about 30% in liver cirrhosis.

Pre-clinical safety data: Extensive clinical use and experience with chlormethiazole has provided a well established safety profile for this drug.

Pharmaceutical particulars

List of excipients: Coconut oil fractionated, Gelatin, Glycerin, Sorbitol, Mannitol, Non hydrogenated Starch hydrolysate, Titanium Dioxide, Brown Iron Oxide Paste (E172).

Incompatibilities: Not applicable.

Shelf-life: Amber glass bottles: 36 months. Aluminium foil blister packs: 24 months.

Special precautions for storage: Store below 25°C.

Nature and content of container: **Amber glass bottle with** either a screw cap or **clic-loc cap containing 60** or 100 **capsules**. Transparent plastic bag in a cardboard outer for bulk packaging of 20,000 capsules. Aluminium foil blister packs each containing 10 capsules.

Instructions for use and handling: The capsules should remain in the container in which they are supplied. The capsules should be swallowed whole.

Legal category POM.

Marketing authorisation number PL0017/5009R

Date of approval / revision of SPC Revised February 1997.

HEMINEVRIN* SYRUP

Qualitative and quantitative composition 50 mg/ml Chlormethiazole edisylate.

Pharmaceutical form Syrup.

Clinical particulars

Therapeutic indications: Heminevrin is a short acting hypnotic and sedative with anticonvulsant effect. It is used for the: management of restlessness and agitation in the elderly, short term treatment of severe insomnia in the elderly and treatment of alcohol withdrawal symptoms where close hospital supervision is also provided.

Posology and method of administration: Management of restlessness and agitation in the elderly: 5 ml of syrup three times daily.

Severe insomnia in the elderly: 5-10 ml of the syrup before going to bed. The lower dose should be tried first. As with all psychotropic drugs, treatment should be kept to a minimum, reviewed regularly and discontinued as soon as possible.

Alcohol withdrawal states: Heminevrin is not a specific 'cure' for alcoholism. Alcohol withdrawal should be treated in hospital or, in exceptional circumstances, on an outpatient basis by specialist units when the daily dosage of Heminevrin must be monitored closely by community health staff. The dosage should be adjusted to patient response. The patient should be sedated but rousable. A suggested regimen is:

Initial dose: 10 to 20 ml, if necessary repeated after some hours.

Day 1, first 24 hours: 45 to 60 ml, divided into 3 or 4 doses.

Day 2: 30 to 40 ml, divided into 3 or 4 doses.

Day 3: 20 to 30 ml, divided into 3 or 4 doses.

Days 4 to 6: A gradual reduction in dosage until the final dose.

Administration for more than nine (9) days is not recommended.

Contra-indications: Known sensitivity to chlormethiazole. Acute pulmonary insufficiency.

Special warnings and special precautions for use: Heminevrin should be used cautiously in patients with chronic pulmonary insufficiency. Heminevrin may potentiate or be potentiated by centrally acting depressant drugs including alcohol and benzodiazepines. Fatal cardiorespiratory collapse has been reported when chlormethiazole was combined with other CNS depressant drugs. When used concomitantly dosage should be appropriately reduced.

Hypoxia, resulting from, for example, cardiac and/or respiratory insufficiency, can manifest itself as an acute confusional state. Recognition and specific treatment of the cause is essential in such patients and in such cases sedatives/hypnotics should be avoided.

Moderate liver disorders associated with alcoholism do not preclude the use of chlormethiazole, though an associated increase in systemic availability of oral doses and delayed elimination of the drug may require reduced dosage. Great caution should be observed in patients with gross liver damage and decreased liver function, particularly as sedation can mask the onset of liver coma.

Caution should be observed in patients with chronic renal disease.

Caution must be exercised in prescribing for individuals known to be addiction prone or for those whose histories suggest they may increase the dose on their own initiative since chlormethiazole is not free from the risk of producing psychological and/or physical dependence. After prolonged administration of high doses, physical dependence has been reported with withdrawal symptoms such as convulsions, tremors, and organic psychosis. These reports have mainly been associated with indiscriminate prescribing to outpatient alcoholics and Heminevrin should not be prescribed to patients who continue to abuse alcohol.

Alcoholism: Alcohol combined with chlormethiazole particularly in alcoholics with cirrhosis can lead to fatal respiratory depression even with short term use. It should not therefore be prescribed for alcoholics who continue to drink alcoholic beverages.

Elderly: Caution is advised as there may be increased bioavailability and delayed elimination of chlormethiazole.

Children: Oral Heminevrin is not recommended for use in children.

Interactions with other medications and other forms of interaction: A combination of chlormethiazole and diazoxide should be avoided as an adverse neonatal reaction suspected to be due to the maternal administration of this combination has been reported.

The combination of propranolol and chlormethiazole has produced profound bradycardia in one patient possibly due to increased bioavailability of propranolol.

There is evidence to indicate that the metabolism of chlormethiazole is inhibited by cimetidine, thus the co-administration of these drugs may lead to increased blood/plasma levels of chlormethiazole.

Pregnancy and lactation: Do not use in pregnancy especially during the first and last trimesters, unless there are compelling reasons. There is no evidence of safety in human pregnancy, nor is there evidence from animal studies that it is entirely free from hazard.

Chlormethiazole is excreted into the breast milk. The effect of even small quantities of sedative/hypnotic and anticonvulsant drugs on the infant brain is not established.

Chlormethiazole should only be used in nursing mothers where the physician considers that the benefit outweighs the possible hazard to the infant.

Effect on ability to drive and use machines: As with all centrally acting depressant drugs, the driving of vehicles and the operating of machinery are to be avoided when under treatment.

Undesirable effects: The most common side-effect is nasal congestion and irritation, which may occur 15 to 20 minutes after drug ingestion. Conjunctival irritation has also been noted in some cases. Occasionally, these symptoms may be severe and may be associated with severe headache. This is commonest with the initial dose following which it decreases in severity with subsequent doses. Increased nasopharyngeal/bronchial secretions can occur.

Rash and urticaria have been reported. In rare cases, bullous skin eruptions have been reported.

Gastrointestinal disturbances have been reported.

Reversible increases of transaminases or bilirubin have been reported.

In rare cases anaphylactic reactions have occurred.

When Heminevrin has been given at higher than recommended doses for other than recommended indications over prolonged periods of time, physical dependence, tolerance and withdrawal reactions have been reported.

Great caution is required in prescribing Heminevrin for patients with a history of chronic alcoholism, drug abuse or marked personality disorder.

When used as a night-time hypnotic, hangover effects in the elderly may occur but are uncommon due to the short half-life.

Excessive sedation may occur, especially with higher doses or when given to the elderly for daytime sedation. Paradoxical excitement or confusion may occur rarely.

Overdosage: The main effects to be expected with overdose of Heminevrin are: coma, respiratory depression, hypotension and hypothermia.

Hypothermia is thought to be due to a direct central effect as well as a result of lying unconscious for several hours. In addition, patients have increased secretion in the upper airways, which in one series was associated with a high incidence of pneumonia. The effects of overdosage are not usually severe in patients with no evidence of alcoholic liver disease, but they may be exacerbated when chlormethiazole is taken in combination with alcohol and/or CNS depressant drugs, particularly those that are metabolised by the liver. There is no specific antidote to chlormethiazole. Treatment of overdosage should therefore be carried out on a symptomatic basis, applying similar principles to those used in the treatment of barbiturate overdosage.

Charcoal column haemoperfusion is not and cannot be expected to be effective in treating chlormethiazole poisoning.

Pharmacological properties

Pharmacodynamic properties: Chlormethiazole is pharmacologically distinct from both the benzodiazepines and the barbiturates.

Chlormethiazole has sedative, muscle relaxant and anticonvulsant properties. It is used for hypnosis in elderly and institutionalised patients, for preanaesthetic sedation and especially in the management of withdrawal from ethanol. Given alone its effects on respiration are slight and the therapeutic index high.

Pharmacokinetic properties: Chlormethiazole has a short half-life, low oral bioavailability, high plasma clearance and shows no evidence of accumulation or altered pharmacokinetics after repeated dosage. It is excreted in urine after extensive metabolism in the liver. The rate of elimination is decreased by about 30% in liver cirrhosis.

Pre-clinical safety data: Extensive clinical use and experience with chlormethiazole has provided a well established safety profile for this drug.

Pharmaceutical particulars

List of excipients: Sorbitol 70%, Cineole, Menthol, Ethanol 99.5% vol, Sodium hydroxide, Purified water.

Incompatibilities: Not applicable.

Shelf-life: 36 months.

Special precautions for storage: Store at 2-8°C (refrigerate). Do not freeze.

Nature and content of container: 300 ml soda-glass bottle with a white polypropylene cap.

Instructions for use and handling: Not Applicable.

Legal category POM.

Marketing authorisation number PL0017/0063R

Date of approval/revision SPC February 1997.

HEMINEVRIN* 0.8% INFUSION

Presentation Colourless aqueous solution containing Chlormethiazole Edisylate BP 8 mg/ml.

Inactive ingredients: Dextrose anhydrous, sodium hydroxide.

Uses Heminevrin is a short acting hypnotic and sedative with anticonvulsant effects used for the treatment of: Pre-eclamptic toxaemia, eclampsia, status epilepticus, acute alcohol withdrawal symptoms where oral administration is not practicable; as a sedative during regional anaesthesia.

Dosage and administration When Heminevrin is given by i.v. infusion, the dosage should always be controlled by the desired effect and the patient's response. Exact recommendations on dosage cannot be given because of individual patient variation and the presence or absence of other CNS depressant drugs such as diazepam, paraldehyde or alcohol. The doses given below therefore are guides only and due account must be taken of the patient's age (i.e. children and the very elderly), the general condition and any previous medication.

In general, the infusion should be given as a loading dose to produce the required effect, followed by a maintenance dose. As is the case with intravenous anaesthetics, Heminevrin's brief action is due to redistribution of the drug and not to rapid elimination. Thus stopping the drug, will allow rapid reversal of its sedative effect initially, but after large and prolonged dosage, recovery may be considerably delayed. The patient should be closely and constantly observed.

Pre-eclamptic toxaemia: Heminevrin is used to sedate the patient and raise the threshold for eclamptic convulsions.

It is indicated in moderate or severe pre-eclamptic toxaemia under the following circumstances: rapid progression of the disease, symptoms and signs associated with impending eclampsia, when labour is to be induced, during labour and post-partum (a) for up to 12 hours in patients with adequate urine output or (b) until recovery of diuresis in patients with poor urinary output.

During labour most patients will require an average of 0.5 to 0.75 ml/min of Heminevrin 0.8%. As the majority of patients are delivered within 24 hours, prolonged infusion is not necessary. Heminevrin has no analgesic properties and pain relief must be given as necessary. After delivery the intravenous infusion is maintained at 0.5 ml/min for 12 hours. Thereafter oral therapy is continued.

Eclampsia: Heminevrin is used to control eclamptic fits or to prevent their recurrence. It is used in conjunction with antihypertensive drugs. If seizures are occurring, Heminevrin 0.8% should be started at an infusion rate of 5–10 ml/min until the fits stop. Once this is achieved the infusion rate is decreased to 0.5–1 ml/min, though this may be varied to suit the individual patient, who should be well sedated but communicative.

If the patient is not having a fit at the start of treatment then Heminevrin is given at 3–5 ml/min until deep sedation occurs. Once the desired level of sedation is achieved this is maintained with an infusion rate of 0.5 to 1 ml/min, though this may be varied to suit the individual patient.

The patient should be lying on one side and adequate oxygenation assured. Loss of the airway, pulmonary aspiration of gastric contents, ventilatory failure and circulatory collapse may occur unless the patient is constantly monitored by experienced staff with oxygen and resuscitation equipment available.

Status epilepticus: Adults: 5–15 ml/min should be infused intravenously up to a total of 40–100 ml of Heminevrin 0.8%. This will usually stop convulsions. Thereafter the infusion rate will depend on the patient's response but in most cases 0.5–1 ml/min will be required. The patient should be nursed in the lateral position, to avoid airway obstruction, and turned every 2 hours. The sedation must be maintained until the epileptic convulsions do not recur if the infusion is slowed or stopped. If a prolonged infusion is necessary, fluid and electrolyte balance must be checked.

Children: An initial infusion rate of 0.01 ml/kg/min (0.08 mg/kg/min). If seizures continue, the dose is increased every 2 to 4 hours until seizures are abolished or drowsiness occurs. When seizures have ceased for 2 days the rate of infusion may be gradually reduced every 4 to 6 hours. If seizures recur the dose should be increased to the previous level at which they were controlled.

Acute alcohol withdrawal symptoms; including delirium tremens: Most patients can be treated with oral Heminevrin but in severe cases an i.v. infusion will give rapid control. The dosing principles mentioned previously, that is, a loading dose for a short period of time followed by maintenance infusion should be used. The initial drip rate should be set in the range of 3 to 7.5 ml/min until shallow sleep is induced from which the patient can easily be awakened. Thereafter, the drip rate should be reduced to a maintenance level, usually 0.5 to 1.0 ml/min, to achieve the lowest possible rate to maintain shallow sleep and adequate spontaneous breathing.

The patients should be nursed on their side to prevent airway obstruction and turned every 2 hours.

For those patients who urgently require deep sedation, an alternative is to give intravenously 40–100 ml of the 0.8% solution over a period of 3–5 minutes. Such treatment should only be given under direct medical supervision. Thereafter maintenance therapy can be established as indicated above.

Because there is a risk of producing unconsciousness with too high a rate of infusion, special attention should be paid to 'Precautions' regarding intravenous administration.

Intravenous administration is usually carried out over a period of 6 to 12 hours during which time usually 500 to 1000 ml of the 0.8% infusion is given. The level of consciousness and the effect of therapy on symptoms should be checked by interrupting the drip flow at intervals. The level of consciousness should lighten rapidly on stopping the drip flow but the longer the administration lasts, the longer the recovery will take. It is desirable to limit the period of intravenous use and to transfer the patient to oral therapy as soon as possible. During prolonged intravenous administration careful attention should be paid to fluid balance and nutrition.

Sedative during regional anaesthesia: Pre-medication with atropine or similar antisialogogues will help to prevent nasal congestion and upper airway mucus secretion that otherwise may occur with chlormethiazole. As judged by unresponsiveness to sound and loss of eyelash reflex, unconsciousness should be induced by a fast running intravenous infusion (approx. 25 ml/min) for 1–2 minutes. Thereafter, maintenance must be judged on the patient's reaction but the dose required is of the order of 1–4 ml/min.

If being used as an intravenous sedative in association with regional block anaesthesia e.g. spinal or epidural, the block must be fully effective before surgery begins. Chlormethiazole has no analgesic properties and the patient will respond to painful stimuli by moving.

If the regional block does not fully relieve the pain of operation it is better to give an i.v. opioid analgesic or convert to a volatile inhalation anaesthetic rather than try to increase the dosage of chlormethiazole.

At the end of an operation, stopping the chlormethiazole allows the patient to awaken usually in 1–5 minutes.

Elderly: Caution is advised as there may be delayed elimination of chlormethiazole.

Contra-indications, warnings, etc

Contra-indications: Known sensitivity to chlormethiazole. Acute pulmonary insufficiency.

Precautions and warnings: Heminevrin should be used cautiously in patients with chronic pulmonary insufficiency because there is a risk of respiratory depression.

Heminevrin may potentiate or be potentiated by centrally acting depressant drugs, including alcohol and benzodiazepines. Fatal cardiorespiratory collapse has been reported when chlormethiazole was combined with other CNS depressant drugs. When used concomitantly, dosage should be appropriately reduced.

The patient should be kept under close and constant observation by a nurse during the period of continuous infusion. With too high a rate of infusion the sleep induced with Heminevrin can pass unnoticed into deep unconsciousness with the consequent risk of mechanical airway obstruction. With overdosage there is always the possibility of causing centrally induced respiratory depression and circulatory collapse.

Because of the possible danger of mechanical airway obstruction occurring in deep sedation during Heminevrin therapy, the patient's airway may be maintained where necessary by the use of an oral airway tube. In addition, facilities for intubation and resuscitation equipment should always be close at hand.

Hypoxia resulting from, for example, respiratory insufficiency, can manifest itself as an acute confusional state. Recognition and specific treatment of the cause is essential in such patients and other sedative/hypnotics should be avoided.

Moderate liver disorders associated with alcoholism do not preclude the use of chlormethiazole, but delayed elimination of the drug may require reduced dosage. Great caution should be observed in patients with gross liver damage and decreased liver function, particularly as sedation can mask the onset of liver coma.

Caution should be observed in patients with chronic renal disease.

Paradoxical worsening may occur in the Lennox Gastaut syndrome.

Nasopharyngeal/bronchial secretions may be increased at a time when the heavily sedated patient may be unable to cough or maintain the airway.

There has been a report of thrombophlebitis, fever and headache in young children during prolonged Heminevrin infusion. This may have been due to interaction with plastic i.v. infusion sets and silastic i.v. cannulae. For administration in small children a motor driven glass syringe should be used in preference to a drip set. A teflon intravenous cannula should be used which can be connected to the syringe by a polythene extension tube. If an infusion set is used it should be changed at least every 24 hours.

As Heminevrin is sorbed by PVC giving sets, there may be some loss in concentration before the drug reaches the patient. Dosage must therefore be adjusted to the patient's response and not given on a fixed milligram basis.

When i.v. Heminevrin is given for longer than 24 hours, there is a possibility of electrolyte imbalance due to the water load involved with the glucose vehicle. Electrolytes such as Na^+, K^+, $Ca2^+$ and Cl^- can be added to the infusion bottle to produce physiological concentrations. They will not affect the stability of chlormethiazole over a 24 hour period. Other drugs however, must not be added.

Interactions: A combination of chlormethiazole and diazoxide should be avoided as an adverse neonatal reaction suspected to be due to the maternal administration of this combination has been reported.

There is evidence to indicate that the metabolism of chlormethiazole is inhibited by cimetidine, thus the co-administration of these drugs may lead to increased blood/plasma levels of chlormethiazole.

Pregnancy and lactation: Do not use in pregnancy, especially during the first trimester, unless there are compelling reasons. There is no evidence of safety in human pregnancy nor is there evidence from animal studies that it is entirely free from hazard.

Chlormethiazole is excreted into breast milk. The effects of even small quantities of sedative/hypnotic and anticonvulsant drugs on the infant brain is not established.

Adverse effects: The most common side-effect appears to be a tingling sensation in the nose and sneezing occurring immediately after the start of the intravenous infusion. Conjunctival irritation has also been noted in some cases. Occasionally these symptoms may be severe and may be associated with severe headache. Increased nasopharyngeal/bronchial secretions can occur. Rash and urticaria have also been reported. In rare cases anaphylactic reactions have occurred.

Intravenous administration of Heminevrin solution may be followed by moderate tachycardia and a slight but temporary decrease in blood pressure, which is less pronounced the slower the infusion is given. Rapid infusion may cause transient apnoea and hypotension. Care is needed in patients in whom these events may cause cerebral or cardiac complications e.g. elderly. Thrombophlebitis may occur at the site of injection with intravenous infusion. Neither heparin nor cortisone has been shown to be helpful in preventing such reactions.

Overdosage: Overdosage can produce unconsciousness with deep coma accompanied by respiratory and cardiovascular depression similar to that seen with barbiturate overdosage. Treatment consists of securing the airway, giving oxygen (with assisted or controlled ventilation if necessary) and supporting the circulation.

Legal category POM.

Pharmaceutical Precautions Store between 5°C–8°C.

Package quantities Bottles of 500 ml.

Further information Nil.

Product licence number 0017/5007R

IMDUR*

Presentation Yellow oval biconvex film coated tablet, scored both sides and coded A/ID. Each tablet contains 60 mg isosorbide mononitrate in an extended release formulation based on Durules*.

Uses Prophylactic treatment of angina pectoris.

Dosage and administration

Adults: Imdur 60 mg (one tablet) once daily to be taken in the morning. The dose may be increased to 120 mg (two tablets) daily, both to be taken once daily in the morning. The dose can be titrated to minimise the possibility of headache by initiating treatment with 30 mg (half a tablet) for the first 2–4 days.

Imdur tablets must not be chewed or crushed. They should be swallowed whole with half a glass of water.

Children: The safety and efficacy of Imdur in children has not been established.

Elderly: No evidence of a need for routine dosage adjustment in the elderly has been found, but special care may be needed in those with increased susceptibility to hypotension or marked hepatic or renal insufficiency.

The core of the tablet is insoluble in the digestive juices but disintegrates into small particles when all active substance has been released. Very occasionally the matrix may pass through the gastrointestinal tract without disintegrating and be found visible in the stool, but all active substance has been released.

Contra-indications, warnings, etc

Contra-indications: Severe cerebrovascular insufficiency or hypotension are relative contra-indications to the use of Imdur.

Precautions: Imdur is not indicated for relief of acute angina attacks; in the event of an acute attack, sublingual or buccal glyceryl trinitrate tablets should be used.

Pregnancy and lactation: The safety and efficacy of Imdur during pregnancy or lactation has not been established.

Side-effects: Most of the adverse reactions are pharmacodynamic mediated and dose dependent. Headache may occur when treatment is initiated but usually disappears after continued treatment. Hypotension with symptoms such as dizziness and nausea has occasionally been reported. These symptoms generally disappear during long-term treatment.

Overdosage:
Symptoms: Pulsing headache. More serious symptoms are excitation, flushing, cold perspiration, nausea, vomiting, vertigo, syncope, tachycardia and a fall in blood pressure.

Treatment: Induction of emesis, activated charcoal. In case of pronounced hypotension the patient should first be placed in the supine position with legs raised. If necessary intravenous administration of fluid.

Pharmaceutical precautions Store below 30°C.

Legal category POM.

Package quantities PVC blister strips (7 tablets per strip) 28, 98.

Further information Isosorbide mononitrate is an active metabolite of isosorbide dinitrate and exerts qualitatively similar effects. Isosorbide mononitrate is completely absorbed and not metabolised during the first passage through the liver. This reduces the fluctuations in plasma levels and leads to predictable and reliable clinical effects.

Administration of Imdur results in a controlled release of active substance leading to reduced peak plasma levels. Compared to ordinary tablets the absorption phase is prolonged and the duration of effect is extended.

With Imdur 60 mg or 120 mg once daily no development of tolerance with respect to antianginal effects has been detected. The phenomenon of rebound angina between doses as described with intermittent nitrate therapy has not been seen with Imdur.

Product licence number 0017/0226

JECTOFER*

Presentation Dark brown liquid for intramuscular injection; Iron Sorbitol Injection BP (contains 50 mg elemental iron per ml).

Uses For the treatment of iron-deficiency anaemia and the rapid replenishment of iron stores.

Dosage and administration The recommended single dose of Jectofer is 1.5 mg per kg body weight by intramuscular injection to a maximum of 100 mg per injection. A series of daily injections of this single dose should be given to restore haemoglobin levels to normal and replenish iron stores based on the following table.

Hb gm/100 ml	5.0	6.0	7.0	8.0	9.0	10.0	11.0
Hb%	33	40	46	53	60	66	73
No. of injections	24	22	20	17	14	12	10

In elderly or debilitated patients or patients who have a low tolerance threshold to intramuscular iron the injections should be given on alternate days. Not recommended in children under 3 kg (7 lb) body weight.

Contra-indications, warnings, etc
Contra-indications: Severe liver damage, acute kidney infection, untreated urinary tract infection. Early pregnancy. Intravenous use. Known hypersensitivity to iron or Jectofer.

Precautions: Jectofer should not be used to treat anaemias other than iron deficiency anaemia.

Care should be taken when treating patients with iron-storage diseases or haemoglobinopathies.

The importance of using the correct recommended dose in relation to body weight is emphasised, especially in patients who are already markedly underweight.

Warnings: Oral iron should be discontinued 24 hours before Jectofer is administered.

Jectofer should not be given intravenously.

Use in pregnancy and lactation: Administration is contra-indicated in early pregnancy.

Side-effects: Initial local discomfort or temporary discolouration may occur at the site of injection. A transient metallic taste or loss of taste may occur. Nausea, sometimes vomiting, dizziness and flushing may also occur. Occasionally palpitations and pressure sensations in the chest have been reported.

A few cases have been reported of serious reactions of a cardiovascular type with cardiac arrhythmia.

Interactions: The concomitant administration of chloramphenicol may delay the response to iron therapy in patients with iron deficiency anaemia.

Overdosage: Systemic reactions have been observed when doses higher than recommended are given, especially to patients who are significantly underweight. Similar reactions may rarely occur in debilitated or sensitive patients given recommended doses. See *Side-effects* above.

Pharmaceutical precautions Store at 25°C, do not refrigerate.

Legal category POM.

Package quantities 10×2 ml ampoules for intramuscular use.

Further information Nil.

Product licence number 0017/5011R

KINIDIN* DURULES*

Qualitative and quantitative composition Each tablet contains 250 mg quinidine bisulphate (hydrate) equivalent to quinidine sulphate BP 200 mg.

Pharmaceutical form Film coated white to off-white oval tablet in an extended–release formulation (Durules).

Clinical particulars
Therapeutic indications: Maintenance of sinus rhythm following cardioversion of atrial fibrillation. Suppression of supraventricular and ventricular tachyarrhythmias.

Posology and method of administration: Initiation of treatment, as with other antiarrhythmic agents used to treat life-threatening ventricular arrhythmias, should be carried out in hospital.

An initial test dose of one tablet should be given to detect hypersensitivity.

Dosage is adjusted according to individual patient requirements. The quinidine dose should preferably be established by determination of the serum concentration after about one week of treatment. The therapeutic plasma concentration range is 1–6 mg/L (3–18 μmol/L). The QT-time should be checked before and during treatment. The normal dose is 2–5 tablets (0.4–1.0 g) morning and evening. The normal dose for maintenance treatment after conversion of atrial fibrillation is 3 tablets (0.6 g) morning and evening.

Concomitant food intake may increase the tolerability.

Kinidin Durules must not be chewed or crushed. They should be swallowed whole with half a glass of water.

Contra-indications: Kinidin Durules are contra-indicated in patients with known hypersensitivity to quinidine, a history of quinidine induced thrombocytopenia or complete heart block.

Quinidine should be used with extreme caution in patients with incomplete atrio-ventricular block, uncompensated cardiac failure, digitalis toxicity, myocarditis, severe myocardial damage or myasthenia gravis.

The use of Kinidin Durules is contra-indicated in pregnancy.

Special warnings and special precautions for use: The patient should be observed after the first dose with special attention to hypersensitivity reactions. Quinidine should be administered with caution to patients with prolonged AV-conduction, sustained cardiac decompensation, cardiogenic shock, hypotension, bradycardia or disturbed potassium balance.

Caution is indicated in combined therapy with other class I antiarrhythmic drugs, β-blockers and digitalis glycosides (see further interaction with digoxin and digitoxin). Myocarditis or severe myocardial damage also requires caution.

Heart failure and hypokalaemia should be corrected before quinidine treatment is started. In patients treated with digoxin, the digoxin dosage should be halved if quinidine is given in addition.

Like other antiarrhythmic drugs quinidine may worsen arrhythmias.

At toxic quinidine concentrations, and in some patients even at therapeutic levels, the QT-interval may be considerably prolonged, which increases the risk of ventricular tachycardia, often of the torsades de pointes type and in some cases also ventricular fibrillation.

Kinidin Durules should be used with caution in the presence of obstructive changes in the digestive tract, oesophagus, when there is a potential risk of oesophageal complications.

Interaction with other medicaments and other forms of interaction:
Digoxin: The plasma concentration of digoxin increases (may be doubled) when quinidine is given in addition. This is due to reduced renal clearance and a reduced distribution volume of digoxin. When quinidine is administered, the dose of digoxin should be halved and the plasma concentration of digoxin checked.

This recommendation is based on the assumption that the digoxin concentration is within the therapeutic range when quinidine treatment is started.

Digitoxin: The interaction between digitoxin and quinidine is a controversial issue. Several studies indicate, however, that quinidine increases the plasma concentration of digitoxin.

Cimetidine: Cimetidine decreases the clearance of quinidine, thereby increasing the plasma level.

Coumarin derivatives: Quinidine may enhance the anticoagulant effect of coumarin derivatives.

Rifampicin, barbituric acid derivatives and phenytoin: These drugs increase the metabolism of quinidine, thereby reducing the plasma concentration to sub-therapeutic levels if the normal dosage is maintained.

Verapamil, amiodarone and nifedipine: Concomitant administration of verapamil or amiodarone can produce clinically important increases in serum quinidine concentrations. Conversely, simultaneous administration of nifedipine has been reported to significantly reduce plasma quinidine levels.

Appropriate quinidine dose changes and ECG monitoring should be carried out when these drugs are added or discontinued. During quinidine therapy 30–50% change in quinidine dosage may be required in order to avoid systemic toxicity or lack of efficacy.

Desipramine and imipramine: Quinidine inhibits the metabolism of desipramine and imipramine in rapid hydroxylators resulting in increased plasma concentrations. In addition they have additive antiarrhythmic properties. The combination should be avoided.

Procainamide: One case-report indicates that the plasma concentration of procainamide and its main metabolite N-acetyl-procainamide may increase significantly if quinidine is given simultaneously.

Metoprolol: In rapid hydroxylators quinidine may inhibit the metabolism of metoprolol resulting in increased plasma concentrations of metoprolol.

Pregnancy and lactation: The use of Kinidin Durules is contra-indicated in pregnancy.

Quinidine is excreted in breast milk but is unlikely to cause effects at therapeutic doses.

Effects on ability to drive and use machines: None known.

Undesirable effects: Gastrointestinal adverse reactions are frequent and occur in approximately 30% of the patients.

Gastrointestinal: Diarrhoea, nausea and vomiting.

Central and peripheral nervous system: Rarely signs of cinchonism e.g. tinnitus, blurred vision, headache and dizziness.

Cardiovascular: Arrhythmias such as ventricular tachycardia, mostly of the torsades de pointes type or ventricular fibrillation. Rarely hypotension and bradycardia, which may lead to cardiac arrest.

Hypersensitivity reactions: Rarely urticaria, skin rash and fever. In isolated cases hepatitis, thrombocytopenia, pancytopenia, agranulocytosis, photosensitisation, lupus erythematosus-like syndrome, myalgia and arthralgia.

Overdose: Poisoning due to an overdose of Kinidin Durules may lead to widening of the QRS complex and prolongation of the QT interval, atrioventricular block, sinoatrial block or arrest, asystole, paroxysmal ventricular tachycardia, flutter or fibrillation, myocardial depression, severe hypotension and cardiac arrest. Cinchonism, nausea, vomiting, drowsiness and sometimes convulsions also occur. Metabolic acidosis and hypokalaemia may complicate severe poisoning.

Treatment should include close monitoring of cardiovascular, respiratory and renal function, electrolytes and continuous ECG monitoring. Further absorption may be prevented by induction of vomiting or gastric lavage, or administration of activated charcoal if ingestion is recent. Cardiovascular complications should be treated symptomatically, which may require the use of sympathomimetic agents (e.g. noradrenaline, metaraminol), or inotropic agents (e.g. dopamine, dobutamine). Temporary pacing may be required for AV block. Glucagon may be used to treat hypotension, and intravenous sodium bicarbonate to correct acidosis and intravenous diazepam for convulsions.

Quinidine and its metabolites cannot be removed effectively by peritoneal or haemodialysis, or charcoal column haemoperfusion but repeated oral administration of activated charcoal may enhance elimination. Forced acid diuresis is not recommended.

As Kinidin Durules is an extended release formulation, treatment of overdosage may be required for a longer period.

Pharmacological properties
Pharmacodynamic properties: Quinidine reduces the excitability, automaticity and conduction velocity in the atrium, AV node and ventricle and increases the duration of the action potential and the effective refractory period. These effects are closely related to the blockade of the 'fast sodium channels' in the cell membranes, resulting in a reduced rate of the rise of action potential and thus a slower conduction and reduced automaticity in the purkinje fibres. The effect is considerably diminished when the extracellular potassium concentration is reduced and enhanced when it is increased.

The direct electrophysiological effects are modified by a relatively pronounced anticholinergic effect dominating particularly at lower plasma concentrations.

Pharmacokinetic properties: Oral bioavailability of quinidine is 70%–80%, the absorption is not influenced by concomitant intake of food. Plasma protein binding is 70%–95%. Half-life in the elimination phase is approximately 6 hours and the dose is almost entirely excreted in the urine, 10%–20% as unchanged drug. Alkaline urine prolongs the elimination time.

The Durules formulation provides gradual release of active substance, thereby reducing the plasma concentration peaks. The absorption phase is prolonged compared to ordinary tablets and a more constant and prolonged effect is achieved, reducing the number of doses needed per day. The peak serum concentration is reached 4 hours after intake of Kinidin Durules.

Preclinical safety data: Quinidine bisulphate is an established active ingredient.

Pharmaceutical particulars
List of excipients: Hydoxypropyl methylcellulose, Polyethylene glycol, Paraffin, Polyvinyl chloride, Polyvinyl acetate, Magnesium stearate and Colour (E171).

Incompatibilities: None Known.

Shelf-life: Glass bottle–Press-through packages–60 months.

Special precautions for storage: PVC press-through packs–store below 25°C.

Nature and contents of container: Press-through packages of thermoformed PVC (10 tablets per strip) 100 tablets.

Instructions for use/handling: None.

Marketing authorisation number PL 0017/5015R

Date of approval/revision of SPC 20th August 1997

LIGNOSTAB* A

Presentation Local anaesthetic injection of lidocaine (lignocaine) 2% with adrenaline 1:80,000. A clear sterile aqueous solution for injection supplied in polypropylene cartridges for use with dental type syringes. Each cartridge contains 2.2 ml of solution.

Each ml of solution contains lidocaine hydrochloride BP 21.3 mg equivalent to lidocaine hydrochloride anhydrous 20.0 mg and Adrenaline BP 12.5 micrograms.

Inactive ingredients: Sodium chloride, disodium edetate, sodium metabisulphite, Water for Injections.

Lidocaine is synonymous with lignocaine.

Uses Local anaesthetic solution for use mainly in dental procedures.

Lignostab-A contains adrenaline. The effect of vasoconstrictors is to prolong the local anaesthesia by delaying the diffusion of the anaesthetic in the surrounding tissues. If lidocaine without adrenaline is required, Xylocaine 2% Plain should be used.

Dosage and administration The dosage is adjusted according to the response of the patient and the site of administration. The lowest concentration and smallest dose producing the required effect should be given. The maximum single dose of lidocaine hydrochloride is 500 mg or 25 ml when given with a vasoconstrictor. This is equivalent to 11.3 cartridges containing 2.2 ml.

Children and elderly or debilitated patients require smaller doses, commensurate with age and physical status.

Contra-indications, warnings, etc
Contra-indications: Known hypersensitivity to anaesthetics of the amide type or the other constituents.

The use of a vasoconstrictor is contra-indicated for anaesthesia of fingers, toes, tip of nose, ears and penis.

Intravenous use.

Precautions: As for other local anaesthetics, use cautiously in patients with epilepsy, impaired cardiac conduction, impaired respiratory function, and in patients with impaired hepatic function, if the dose or site of administration is likely to result in high blood levels.

Facilities for resuscitation should be available when local anaesthetics are administered.

The effect of local anaesthetics may be reduced if an injection is made into an inflamed or infected area.

Solutions containing a vasoconstrictor should be used with caution in patients with hypertension, cardiac disease, cerebrovascular insufficiency, thyrotoxicosis, in patients taking tricyclic antidepressants, monoamine oxidase inhibitors, or receiving potent general anaesthetic agents.

Solutions containing adrenaline should be used where possible so as to prolong anaesthesia and reduce systemic absorption. This is particularly important in highly vascular areas.

Use on one patient during one treatment only. Discard unused contents.

Use in pregnancy: Although this product crosses the placenta, the low doses used in dental anaesthesia would not be expected to give rise to signs of toxicity in the foetus.

Side-effects: In common with other local anaesthetics, adverse reactions are rare and are usually the result of excessively high blood concentrations due to inadvertent intravascular injection, excessive dosage, rapid absorption or diminished tolerance on the part of the patient. In such circumstances systemic effects occur involving the central nervous system and/or the cardiovascular system.

CNS reactions are excitatory and/or depressant, and may be characterised by nervousness, dizziness, blurred vision and tremors, followed by drowsiness, convulsions, unconsciousness and possibly respiratory arrest. The excitatory reactions may be very brief or may not occur at all, in which case the first manifestations of toxicity may be drowsiness, merging into unconsciousness and respiratory arrest.

Cardiovascular reactions are depressant, and may be characterised by hypotension, myocardial depression, bradycardia and possibly cardiac arrest.

Allergic reactions are extremely rare. They may be characterised by cutaneous lesions, urticaria, oedema or anaphylactoid reactions. Detection of sensitivity by skin testing is of doubtful value.

Hypotension may occur as a physiological response to central nerve blocks.

Symptoms and treatment of overdosage: The injection of excessive amounts of Lignostab-A may, due to the vasoconstrictor, cause ischaemia. This can be followed by a reactive hyperaemia resulting in post extraction bleeding. Respiratory failure may need assisted ventilation. The circulation can be maintained with electrolyte or plasma infusions. Should convulsions develop these can be controlled with diazepam or a short acting barbiturate.

In cases of overdosage with adrenaline containing solutions, intravenous phentolamine and a β-blocker may be required to control blood pressure.

Pharmaceutical precautions Store below 25°C.

Legal category: POM.

Package quantities: Boxes of 500 cartridges (polypropylene).

Further information Nil.

Product licence numbers PL 0017/0257

LOSEC* CAPSULES 10 mg 20 mg and 40 mg

Presentation Losec Capsules 10 mg: hard gelatin capsules with an opaque pink body, marked 10 and an opaque pink cap marked A/OS in black ink. Each capsule contains omeprazole 10 mg as enteric-coated granules, with an aqueous based coating.

Losec Capsules 20 mg: hard gelatin capsules with an opaque pink body, marked 20 and an opaque reddish-brown cap marked A/OM in black ink. Each capsule contains omeprazole 20 mg as enteric-coated granules, with an aqueous based coating.

Losec Capsules 40 mg: hard gelatin capsules with an opaque reddish-brown body, marked 40 and an opaque reddish-brown cap marked A/OL in black ink. Each capsule contains omeprazole 40 mg as enteric-coated granules, with an aqueous based coating.

Uses Treatment of oesophageal reflux disease. In reflux oesophagitis the majority of patients are healed after 4 weeks. Symptom relief is rapid.

Treatment of duodenal and benign gastric ulcers including those complicating NSAID therapy.

Relief of reflux-like symptoms (e.g. heartburn) and/or ulcer-like symptoms (e.g. epigastric pain) associated with acid-related dyspepsia.

Treatment and prophylaxis of NSAID-associated benign gastric ulcers, duodenal ulcers, and gastroduodenal erosions in patients with a previous history of gastroduodenal lesions who require continued NSAID treatment.

Relief of associated dyspeptic symptoms.

Helicobacter pylori eradication: Omeprazole should be used in combination with antibiotics for eradication of *Helicobacter pylori (Hp)* in peptic ulcer disease.

Relief of associated dyspeptic symptoms.

Prophylaxis of acid aspiration.

Zollinger-Ellison syndrome.

Dosage and administration *Oesophageal reflux disease including reflux oesophagitis:* The usual dosage is 20 mg Losec once daily. The majority of patients are healed after 4 weeks. For those patients not fully healed after the initial course, healing usually occurs during a further 4–8 weeks treatment. Losec has also been used in a dose of 40 mg once daily in patients with reflux oesophagitis refractory to other therapy. Healing usually occurred within 8 weeks. Patients can be continued at a dosage of 20 mg once daily.

Acid reflux disease: For long-term management Losec 10 mg once daily is recommended, increasing to 20 mg if symptoms return.

Duodenal and benign gastric ulcers: The usual dose is 20 mg Losec once daily. The majority of patients with duodenal ulcer are healed after 4 weeks. The majority of patients with benign gastric ulcer are healed after 8 weeks. In severe or recurrent cases the dose may be increased to 40 mg Losec daily. Long-term therapy for patients with a history of recurrent duodenal ulcer is recommended at a dosage of 20 mg Losec once daily.

For prevention of relapse in patients with duodenal ulcer the recommended dose is Losec 10 mg, once daily, increasing to 20 mg, once daily if symptoms return.

The following groups are at risk from recurrent ulcer relapse; those with *Helicobacter pylori* infection, younger patients (<60 years), those whose symptoms persist for more than one year and smokers. These patients will require initial long-term therapy with Losec 20 mg once daily, reducing to 10 mg once daily, if necessary.

Acid-related dyspepsia: The usual dosage is Losec 10 mg or 20 mg once daily for 2–4 weeks depending on the severity and persistence of symptoms. Patients who do not respond after 4 weeks or who relapse shortly afterwards, should be investigated.

For the treatment of NSAID-associated gastric ulcers, duodenal ulcers or gastroduodenal erosions: The recommended dosage of Losec is 20 mg once daily. Symptom resolution is rapid and in most patients healing occurs within 4 weeks. For those patients who may not be fully healed after the initial course, healing usually occurs during a further 4 weeks treatment.

For the prophylaxis of NSAID-associated gastric ulcers, duodenal ulcers, gastroduodenal erosions and dyspeptic symptoms in patients with a previous history of gastroduodenal lesions who require continued NSAID treatment: The only recommended dosage of Losec is 20 mg once daily.

Helicobacter pylori (Hp) eradication regimens in peptic ulcer disease: Losec is recommended at a dose of 40 mg once daily or 20 mg twice daily in association with antimicrobial agents as detailed below:

Triple therapy regimens in duodenal ulcer disease: Losec and the following antimicrobial combinations:

Amoxycillin 500 mg and metronidazole 400 mg both three times a day for one week, **or** Clarithromycin 250 mg and metronidazole 400 mg (or tinidazole 500 mg) both twice a day for one week, **or** Amoxycillin 1 g and clarithromycin 500 mg both twice a day for one week.

Dual therapy regimens in duodenal ulcer disease: Losec and amoxycillin 750 mg to 1 g twice daily for two weeks. Alternatively Losec and clarithromycin 500 mg three times a day for two weeks.

Dual therapy regimens in gastric ulcer disease: Losec and amoxycillin 750 mg to 1 g twice daily for two weeks.

In each regimen if symptoms return and the patient is *Hp* positive therapy may be repeated or one of the alternative regimens can be used: if the patient is *Hp* negative then see dosage instructions for acid reflux disease.

To ensure healing in patients with active peptic ulcer disease, see further dosage recommendations for duodenal and benign gastric ulcer.

Prophylaxis of acid aspiration: For patients considered to be at risk of aspiration of the gastric contents during general anaesthesia, the recommended dosage is Losec 40 mg on the evening before surgery followed by Losec 40 mg 2–6 hours prior to surgery.

Zollinger-Ellison syndrome: The recommended initial dosage is 60 mg Losec once daily. The dosage should be adjusted individually and treatment continued as long as clinically indicated. More than 90% of patients with severe disease and inadequate response to other therapies have been effectively controlled on doses of 20–120 mg daily. With doses above 80 mg daily, the dose should be divided and given twice daily.

Elderly: Dose adjustment is not required in the elderly.

Children: Experience of the use of Losec in children is limited. In children over 2 years with severe ulcerating reflux oesophagitis, Losec is recommended for healing and symptom relief within the dose range of 0.7-1.4 mg/kg daily, to a maximum of 40 mg/day, for 4-12 weeks. Data suggest that approximately 65% of children will experience pain relief with this dose regimen. Treatment should be initiated by a hospital-based paediatrician.

For children aged 2–6 years, the capsule may be opened, see section: "Patients with Swallowing Difficulties."

Impaired renal function: Dose adjustment is not required in patients with impaired renal function.

Impaired hepatic function: As bioavailability and half-life can increase in patients with impaired hepatic function, the dose requires adjustment with a maximum daily dose of 20 mg.

Patients with swallowing difficulties: The capsules may be opened and the contents swallowed alone or suspended in a small amount of fruit juice or yoghurt after gentle mixing. Actual capsules may be sucked and then swallowed. It is important that the contents of the capsules should not be crushed or chewed.

Contra-indications, warnings, etc.
Contra-indications: Known hypersensitivity to omeprazole. When gastric ulcer is suspected, the possibility of malignancy should be excluded before treatment with Losec is instituted, as treatment may alleviate symptoms and delay diagnosis.

Warnings: Decreased gastric acidity, due to any means – including proton-pump inhibitors, increases gastric counts of bacteria normally present in the gastrointestinal tract. Treatment with acid-reducing drugs may lead to slightly increased risk of gastrointestinal infections such as Salmonella and Campylobacter.

Use in pregnancy and lactation: There is no evidence on the safety of Losec in human pregnancy. Animal studies have revealed no teratogenic effect, but reproduction studies have revealed reduced litter weights. Avoid in pregnancy unless there is no safer alternative.

There is no information available on the passage of Losec into breast milk or its effects on the neonate. Breast feeding should therefore be discontinued if the use of Losec is considered essential.

Adverse reactions: Losec is well tolerated and adverse reactions have generally been mild and reversible. The following have been reported as adverse events in clinical trials or reported from routine use but in many cases a relationship to treatment with omeprazole has not been established.

Skin rash, urticaria and pruritus have been reported, usually resolving after discontinuation of treatment. In addition photosensitivity, bullous eruption, erythema multiforme, angioedema and alopecia have been reported in isolated cases.

Diarrhoea and headache have been reported and may be severe enough to require discontinuation of therapy in a small number of patients. In the majority of cases the symptoms resolved after discontinuation of therapy.

Other gastrointestinal reactions have included constipation, nausea/vomiting, flatulence and abdominal pain. Dry mouth, stomatitis and candidiasis have been reported as isolated cases.

Paraesthesia has been reported. Dizziness, light-headedness and feeling faint have been associated with treatment, but all usually resolve on cessation of therapy. Also reported are somnolence, insomnia and vertigo. Reversible mental confusion, agitation, depression and hallucinations have occurred predominantly in severely ill patients.

Arthritic and myalgic symptoms have been reported and have usually resolved when therapy is stopped.

In isolated cases, the following have been reported: blurred vision, taste disturbance, aggression, peripheral oedema, hyponatraemia, increased sweating, gynaecomastia, impotence, leucopenia, thrombocytopenia, agranulocytosis, pancytopenia, anaphylactic shock, malaise, fever, bronchospasm, encephalopathy in patients with pre-existing severe liver disease, hepatitis with or without jaundice, rarely hepatic failure and interstitial nephritis which has resulted in acute renal failure.

Increases in liver enzymes have been observed.

Interactions: Due to the decreased intragastric acidity the absorption of ketoconazole may be reduced during omeprazole treatment as it is during treatment with other acid secretion inhibitors. As Losec is metabolised in the liver through cytochrome P450 it can delay the elimination of diazepam, phenytoin and warfarin. Monitoring of patients receiving warfarin or phenytoin is recommended and a reduction of warfarin or phenytoin dose may be necessary. However concomitant treatment with Losec 20 mg daily did not change the blood concentration of phenytoin in patients on continuous treatment with phenytoin. Similarly concomitant treatment with Losec 20 mg daily did not change coagulation time in patients on continuous treatment with warfarin. Plasma concentrations of omeprazole and clarithromycin are increased during concomitant administration. This is considered to be a useful interaction during *H. pylori* eradication. There is no evidence of an interaction with phenacetin, theophylline, caffeine, propranolol, metoprolol, cyclosporin, lidocaine, quinidine, estradiol, amoxycillin or antacids. The absorption of Losec is not affected by alcohol or food.

There is no evidence of an interaction with piroxicam, diclofenac or naproxen. This is considered useful when patients are required to continue these treatments.

Simultaneous treatment with omeprazole and digoxin in healthy subjects lead to a 10% increase in the bioavailability of digoxin as a consequence of the increased intragastric pH.

Animal toxicology: Gastric ECL-cell hyperplasia and carcinoids have been observed in life-long studies in rats treated with omeprazole or subjected to partial fundectomy. These changes are the result of sustained hypergastrinaemia secondary to acid inhibition, and not from a direct effect of any individual drug.

Overdosage: There is no information available on the effects of overdosage in man and specific recommendations for treatment cannot be given. Single oral doses of up to 400 mg have not resulted in any severe symptoms; elimination remained first order and no specific treatment was needed.

Pharmaceutical precautions Store below 30°C.

Legal category POM.

Package quantities
Blisters of 7, 14 or 28 capsules.

Further information Losec is a specific inhibitor of the gastric proton pump (H^+,K^+ ATPase) in the parietal cell. There it produces dose-dependent inhibition of acid secretion by binding to the enzyme, and effectively reduces gastric acid secretion. Oral dosing with 20 mg Losec once daily produces inhibition of gastric acid secretion within 1–2 hours of the first dose. The maximum effect is achieved within 4 days of starting treatment after which the degree of acid inhibition remains constant. The mean decrease in pentagastrin-stimulated peak acid output twenty-four hours after dosing with Losec is about 70%. The inhibition of acid secretion is directly related to the area under the plasma concentration-time curve (AUC) but not to the plasma concentration at any given time. Available data from children (1 year and older) suggest that the pharmacokinetics within the recommended doses are similar to those reported in adults. At steady state, lower plasma levels of omeprazole were seen in some children.

Clinical data for omeprazole in the prophylaxis of NSAID induced gastroduodenal lesions are derived from studies of up to 6 months duration.

Helicobacter pylori (*Hp*) is associated with acid peptic disease including duodenal ulcer (DU) and gastric ulcer (GU) in which about 95% and 80% of patients respectively are infected with this bacterium. *Hp* is implicated as a major contributing factor in the development of gastritis and ulcers in such patients. Recent evidence also suggests a causative link between *Hp* and gastric carcinoma.

Omeprazole has been shown to have a bactericidal effect on *Hp* in vitro.

Eradication of *Hp* with omeprazole and antimicrobials is associated with rapid symptom relief, high rates of healing of any mucosal lesions, and long-term remission of peptic ulcer disease, thus reducing complications such as gastrointestinal bleeding as well as the need for prolonged anti-secretory treatment.

In recent clinical data in patients with acute peptic ulcer omeprazole *Hp* eradication therapy improved patients' quality of life.

During long-term treatment an increased frequency of gastric glandular cysts have been reported. These changes are a physiological consequence of pronounced inhibition of acid secretion. The cysts are benign and appear to be reversible. No other treatment related mucosal changes have been observed in patients treated continuously with omeprazole for periods up to 5 years.

Product licence number
PL 0017/0337 Losec Capsules 10 mg
PL 0017/0238 Losec Capsules 20 mg
PL 0017/0320 Losec Capsules 40 mg

MARCAIN* WITH ADRENALINE 0.25%

Qualitative and quantitative composition Bupivacaine hydrochloride 2.5 mg/ml, adrenaline tartrate 10.0 microgram/ml.

Pharmaceutical form Solution for injection.

Clinical particulars
Therapeutic indications: Marcain 0.25% and 0.5% solutions are used for the production of local anaesthesia by percutaneous infiltration, peripheral nerve block(s) and central neural block (caudal or epidural), that is, for specialist use in situations where prolonged anaesthesia is required. Because sensory nerve block is more marked than motor block, Marcain is especially useful in the relief of pain, e.g. during labour.

Posology and method of administration: The utmost care should be taken to prevent an accidental intravascular injection, always including careful aspiration. For epidural anaesthesia, a test dose of 3-5 ml of bupivacaine containing adrenaline should be administered, since an intravascular injection of adrenaline will be quickly recognised by an increase in heart rate. Verbal contact and repeated measurement of heart rate should be maintained throughout a period of 5 minutes following the test dose. Aspiration should be repeated prior to administration of the total dose. The main dose should be injected slowly, 25-50 mg/min, in incremental doses under constant contact with the patient. If mild toxic symptoms occur, the injection should be stopped immediately.

The dosage varies and depends upon the area to be anaesthetised, the vascularity of the tissues, the number of neuronal segments to be blocked, individual tolerance and the technique of anaesthesia used. The lowest dosage needed to provide effective anaesthesia should be administered. For most indications, the duration of anaesthesia with Marcain solutions is such that a single dose is sufficient.

The maximum dosage must be determined by evaluating the size and physical status of the patient and considering the usual rate of systemic absorption from a particular injection site. Experience to date indicates a single dose of up to 150 mg bupivacaine hydrochloride. Doses of up to 50 mg 2-hourly may subsequently be used. The dosages in the table overleaf are recommended as a guide for use in the average adult. For young, elderly or debilitated patients, these doses should be reduced.

Contra-indications: Bupivacaine hydrochloride solutions are contra-indicated in patients with a known hypersensitivity to local anaesthetic agents of the amide type or to other components of the injectable formulation.

Solutions of bupivacaine hydrochloride are contra-indicated for intravenous regional anaesthesia (Bier's-block).

Solutions containing adrenaline are contra-indicated in patients with thyrotoxicosis or severe heart disease, particularly when tachycardia is present.

Solutions of bupivacaine hydrochloride with adrenaline should not be used in connection with anaesthesia in areas of the body supplied by end arteries or otherwise having a compromised blood supply such as digits, nose, external ear, penis, etc.

0.75% solution is contra-indicated for epidural use in obstetrics.

Epidural anaesthesia, regardless of the local anaesthetic used, has its own contra-indications which include:

Active disease of the central nervous system such as meningitis, poliomyelitis, intracranial haemorrhage, sub-acute combined degeneration of the cord due to pernicious anaemia and cerebral and spinal tumours. Tuberculosis of the spine. Pyogenic infection of the skin at or adjacent to the site of lumbar puncture. Cardiogenic or hypovolaemic shock. Coagulation disorders or ongoing anticoagulation treatment.

Special warnings and special precautions for use: There have been reports of cardiac arrest with difficult resuscitation or death during use of bupivacaine for epidural anaesthesia in obstetric patients. In most cases, this has followed use of the 0.75% concentration. Resuscitation has been difficult or impossible despite apparently adequate preparation and appropriate management. Cardiac arrest has occurred after convulsions resulting from systemic toxicity, presumably following unintentional intravascular injection. The 0.75% concentration should be reserved for surgical procedures where a high degree of muscle relaxation and prolonged effect are necessary.

Epidural blockade and large nerve plexus blocks should only be employed by those with the necessary training and experience.

Adequate resuscitation equipment should be available whenever local or general anaesthesia is administered. Overdosage or accidental intravenous injection may give rise to toxic reactions.

Injection of repeated doses of bupivacaine hydrochloride may cause significant increases in blood levels with each repeated dose due to slow accumulation of the drug. Tolerance varies with the status of the patient. Debilitated, elderly or acutely ill patients should be given reduced doses commensurate with their physical status.

Only in rare cases have amide local anaesthetics been associated with allergic reactions (in most severe instances anaphylactic shock).

Patients allergic to ester-type local anaesthetic drugs (procaine, tetracaine, benzocaine, etc.) have not shown cross-sensitivity to agents of the amide type such as bupivacaine.

Local anaesthetics should be used with caution for epidural anaesthesia in patients with impaired cardiovascular function since they may be less able to compensate for functional changes associated with the prolongation of A-V conduction produced by these drugs.

Since bupivacaine is metabolised in the liver, it should be used cautiously in patients with liver disease or with reduced liver blood flow.

Epidural anaesthesia with any local anaesthetic can cause hypotension and bradycardia which should be

Type of block	% Conc	Each dose ml	mg	Motor block†
Local infiltration	0.25	up to 60	up to 150	–
Lumbar epidural				
Surgical operations	0.50	10 to 20	50 to 100	Moderate to complete
	0.75	10 to 20	75 to 150	Complete
Analgesia in labour	0.50	6 to 12	30 to 60	Moderate to complete
	0.25	6 to 12	15 to 30	Minimal
Caudal epidural				
Surgical operations	0.50	15 to 30	75 to 150	Moderate to complete
Children (aged up to 10yrs):				
Up to lower thoracic (T10)	0.25	0.3–0.4 ml/kg	0.75–1.0 mg/kg	
Up to mid-thoracic (T6)	0.25	0.4–0.6 ml/kg	1.0–1.5 mg/kg	
If total amount greater than 20 ml reduce concentration to 0.2%.				
Analgesia in labour	0.50	10 to 20	50 to 100	Moderate to complete
	0.25	10 to 20	25 to 50	Moderate
Peripheral Nerves	0.50	up to 30	up to 150	Moderate to complete
	0.25	up to 60	up to 150	Slight to moderate
Sympathetic blocks	0.25	20 to 50	50 to 125	–

†With continuous (intermittent) techniques, repeat doses increase the degree of motor block. The first repeat dose of 0.5% may produce complete motor block for intra-abdominal surgery.

anticipated and appropriate precautions taken. These may include pre-loading the circulation with crystalloid or colloid solution. If hypotension develops it should be treated with a vasopressor such as ephedrine 10-15 mg intravenously. Severe hypotension may result from hypovolaemia due to haemorrhage or dehydration, or aorto-caval occlusion in patients with massive ascites, large abdominal tumours or late pregnancy. Marked hypotension should be avoided in patients with cardiac decompensation.

Patients with hypovolaemia due to any cause can develop sudden and severe hypotension during epidural anaesthesia.

Epidural anaesthesia can cause intercostal paralysis and patients with pleural effusions may suffer respiratory embarrassment. Septicaemia can increase the risk of intraspinal abscess formation in the postoperative period.

Paracervical block may have a greater adverse effect on the foetus than other nerve blocks used in obstetrics. Due to the systemic toxicity of bupivacaine special care should be taken when using bupivacaine for paracervical block.

Small doses of local anaesthetics injected into the head and neck, including retrobulbar, dental and stellate ganglion blocks, may produce systemic toxicity due to inadvertent intra-arterial injection.

Clinicians who perform retrobulbar blocks should be aware that there have been reports of respiratory arrest following local anaesthetic injection. Prior to retrobulbar block, necessary equipment, drugs and personnel should be immediately available as with all other regional procedures.

Solutions containing adrenaline should be used with caution in patients with hypertension, arteriosclerotic heart disease, cerebrovascular insufficiency or diabetes.

Interaction with other medicaments and other forms of interaction: Bupivacaine should be used with care in patients receiving anti-arrhythmic drugs with local anaesthetic activity, e.g. lidocaine since their toxic effects may be additive.

Solutions containing adrenaline should be used with caution in those patients receiving drugs known to produce blood pressure alterations, i.e. MAO inhibitors, tricyclic antidepressants, phenothiazines, etc., as severe and sustained hypotension or hypertension may occur.

Pregnancy and Lactation: Bupivacaine enters the mother's milk, but in such small quantities that there is no risk of affecting the child at therapeutic dose levels.

There is no evidence of untoward effects in human pregnancy. In large doses there is evidence of decreased pup survival in rats and an embryological effect in rabbits if Marcain is administered in pregnancy. Marcain should not therefore be given in early pregnancy unless the benefits are considered to outweigh the risks.

Effects on ability to drive and use machines: None stated.

Undesirable effects: Serious systemic adverse reactions are rare, but may occur in connection with overdosage or unintentional intravascular injection.

Bupivacaine causes systemic toxicity similar to that observed with other local anaesthetic agents. It is caused by high plasma concentrations as a result of excessive dosage, rapid absorption or, most commonly, inadvertent intravascular injection. Pronounced acidosis or hypoxia may increase the risk and severity of toxic reactions. Such reactions involve the central nervous system and the cardiovascular system. CNS reactions are characterised by numbness of the tongue, lightheadedness, dizziness, blurred vision and muscle twitch, followed by drowsiness, convulsions, unconsciousness and possibly respiratory arrest.

Cardiovascular reactions are related to depression of the conduction system of the heart and myocardium leading to decreased cardiac output, heart block, hypotension, bradycardia and sometimes ventricular arrhythmias, including ventricular tachycardia, ventricular fibrillation and cardiac arrest. Usually these will be preceded or accompanied by major CNS toxicity, i.e. convulsions, but in rare cases cardiac arrest has occurred without prodromal CNS effects.

Epidural anaesthesia itself can cause adverse reactions regardless of the local anaesthetic agent used. These include hypotension and bradycardia due to sympathetic blockade and/or vasovagal fainting.

In severe cases cardiac arrest may occur.

Accidental sub-arachnoid injection can lead to very high spinal anaesthesia possibly with apnoea and severe hypotension.

Neurological damage is a rare but well recognised consequence of regional and particularly epidural and spinal anaesthesia. It may be due to several causes, e.g. direct injury to the spinal cord or spinal nerves, anterior spinal artery syndrome, injection of an irritant substance, or an injection of a non-sterile solution.

These may result in localised areas of paraesthesia or anaesthesia, motor weakness, loss of sphincter control and paraplegia. Occasionally these are permanent.

Overdose:

Treatment of side effects: Treatment of a patient with systemic toxicity consists of arresting convulsions and ensuring adequate ventilation with oxygen, if necessary by assisted or controlled ventilation (respiration). If convulsions occur they must be treated promptly by intravenous injection of thiopentone 100 to 200 mg or diazepam 5 to 10 mg. Alternatively succinylcholine 50 mg-100 mg i.v. may be used providing the clinician is capable of performing endotracheal intubation and managing a fully paralysed patient.

Once convulsions have been controlled and adequate ventilation of the lungs ensured, no other treatment is generally required. If hypotension is present, however, a vasopressor, preferably one with inotropic activity, e.g. ephedrine 15 to 30 mg, should be given intravenously.

Cardiac arrest due to bupivacaine can be resistant to electrical defibrillation and resuscitation must be continued energetically for a prolonged period.

High or total spinal blockade causing respiratory paralysis and hypotension during epidural anaesthesia should be treated by ensuring and maintaining a patent airway and giving oxygen by assisted or controlled ventilation.

Hypotension should be treated by the use of vasopressors, e.g. ephedrine 10-15 mg intravenously and repeated until the desired level of arterial pressure is reached. Intravenous fluids, both electrolytes and colloids, given rapidly can also reverse hypotension.

Pharmacological properties

Pharmacodynamic properties: Bupivacaine is a potent amide local anaesthetic with a prolonged duration of action. It affects sensory nerves more than motor nerves and is ideal for producing analgesia without motor blockade.

Pharmacokinetic properties: In adults, the terminal half-life of bupivacaine is 3.5 hours. The maximum blood concentration varies with the site of injection and is highest after intercostal nerve blockade.

Total dose, rather than concentration, is an important determinant of peak blood levels.

Bupivacaine is biodegraded in the liver and only 6% is excreted unchanged in the urine.

Preclinical safety data: Bupivacaine hydrochloride and adrenaline tartrate are well established active ingredients.

Pharmaceutical particulars

List of excipients: Sodium metabisulphite, sodium chloride, hydrochloric acid and water for injection.

Incompatibilities: None known.

Shelf-life: 10 ml ampoules – 18 months, 20 ml vials – 30 months.

Special precautions for storage: 10 ml ampoules–store below 25°C. 20 ml vials–store below 15°C.

Nature and contents of container: **10 ml glass ampoules–blister packed.** 20 ml single dose glass vials.

Instructions for use/handling: None.

Marketing authorisation number PL 0017/0118

Date of approval/revision of SPC 23rd July 1997

Legal category POM.

MARCAIN* WITH ADRENALINE 0.5%

Qualitative and quantitative composition Bupivacaine hydrochloride 5.0 mg/ml, adrenaline tartrate 10.0 microgram/ml.

Pharmaceutical form Solution for injection.

Clinical particulars

Therapeutic indications: Marcain 0.25% and 0.5% solutions are used for the production of local anaesthesia by percutaneous infiltration, peripheral nerve block(s) and central neural block (caudal or epidural), that is, for specialist use in situations where prolonged anaesthesia is required. Because sensory nerve block is more marked than motor block, Marcain is especially useful in the relief of pain, e.g. during labour.

Posology and method of administration: The utmost care should be taken to prevent an accidental intravascular injection, always including careful aspiration. For epidural anaesthesia, a test dose of 3-5 ml of bupivacaine containing adrenaline should be administered, since an intravascular injection of adrenaline will be quickly recognised by an increase in heart rate. Verbal contact and repeated measurement of heart rate should be maintained throughout a period of 5 minutes following the test dose. Aspiration should be repeated prior to administration of the total dose. The main dose should be injected slowly, 25-50 mg/min, in incremental doses under constant contact with the patient. If mild toxic symptoms occur, the injection should be stopped immediately.

The dosage varies and depends upon the area to be anaesthetised, the vascularity of the tissues, the number of neuronal segments to be blocked, individual tolerance and the technique of anaesthesia used. The lowest dosage needed to provide effective anaesthesia should be administered. For most indications, the duration of anaesthesia with Marcain solutions is such that a single dose is sufficient.

The maximum dosage must be determined by evaluating the size and physical status of the patient and considering the usual rate of systemic absorption from a particular injection site. Experience to date indicates a single dose of up to 150 mg bupivacaine hydrochloride. Doses of up to 50 mg 2-hourly may subsequently be used. The dosages in the table overleaf are recommended as a guide for use in the average adult. For young, elderly or debilitated patients, these doses should be reduced.

Contra-indications: Bupivacaine hydrochloride solutions are contra-indicated in patients with a known hypersensitivity to local anaesthetic agents of the amide type or to other components of the injectable formulation.

Solutions of bupivacaine hydrochloride are contra-indicated for intravenous regional anaesthesia (Bier's-block).

Solutions containing adrenaline are contra-indicated in patients with thyrotoxicosis or severe heart disease, particularly when tachycardia is present.

Solutions of bupivacaine hydrochloride with adrenaline should not be used in connection with anaesthesia in areas of the body supplied by end arteries or otherwise having a compromised blood supply such as digits, nose, external ear, penis, etc.

0.75% solution is contra-indicated for epidural use in obstetrics.

Epidural anaesthesia, regardless of the local anaesthetic used, has its own contra-indications which include:

Active disease of the central nervous system such

Type of block	% Conc	Each dose ml	mg	Motor block†
Local infiltration	0.25	up to 60	up to 150	–
Lumbar epidural				
Surgical operations	0.50	10 to 20	50 to 100	Moderate to complete
	0.75	10 to 20	75 to 150	Complete
Analgesia in labour	0.50	6 to 12	30 to 60	Moderate to complete
	0.25	6 to 12	15 to 30	Minimal
Caudal epidural				
Surgical operations	0.50	15 to 30	75 to 150	Moderate to complete
Children (aged up to 10yrs):				
Up to lower thoracic (T10)	0.25	0.3–0.4 ml/kg	0.75–1.0 mg/kg	
Up to mid-thoracic (T6)	0.25	0.4–0.6 ml/kg	1.0–1.5 mg/kg	
If total amount greater than 20 ml reduce concentration to 0.2%				
Analgesia in labour	0.50	10 to 20	50 to 100	Moderate to complete
	0.25	10 to 20	25 to 50	Moderate
Peripheral Nerves	0.50	up to 30	up to 150	Moderate to complete
	0.25	up to 60	up to 150	Slight to moderate
Sympathetic blocks	0.25	20 to 50	50 to 125	–

† With continuous (intermittent) techniques, repeat doses increase the degree of motor block. The first repeat dose of 0.5% may produce complete motor block for intra-abdominal surgery.

as meningitis, poliomyelitis, intracranial haemorrhage, sub-acute combined degeneration of the cord due to pernicious anaemia and cerebral and spinal tumours. Tuberculosis of the spine. Pyogenic infection of the skin at or adjacent to the site of lumbar puncture. Cardiogenic or hypovolaemic shock. Coagulation disorders or ongoing anticoagulation treatment.

Special warnings and special precautions for use: There have been reports of cardiac arrest with difficult resuscitation or death during use of bupivacaine for epidural anaesthesia in obstetric patients. In most cases, this has followed use of the 0.75% concentration. Resuscitation has been difficult or impossible despite apparently adequate preparation and appropriate management. Cardiac arrest has occurred after convulsions resulting from systemic toxicity, presumably following unintentional intravascular injection. The 0.75% concentration should be reserved for surgical procedures where a high degree of muscle relaxation and prolonged effect are necessary.

Epidural blockade and large nerve plexus blocks should only be employed by those with the necessary training and experience.

Adequate resuscitation equipment should be available whenever local or general anaesthesia is administered. Overdosage or accidental intravenous injection may give rise to toxic reactions.

Injection of repeated doses of bupivacaine hydrochloride may cause significant increases in blood levels with each repeated dose due to slow accumulation of the drug. Tolerance varies with the status of the patient. Debilitated, elderly or acutely ill patients should be given reduced doses commensurate with their physical status.

Only in rare cases have amide local anaesthetics been associated with allergic reactions (in most severe instances anaphylactic shock).

Patients allergic to ester-type local anaesthetic drugs (procaine, tetracaine, benzocaine, etc.) have not shown cross-sensitivity to agents of the amide type such as bupivacaine.

Local anaesthetics should be used with caution for epidural anaesthesia in patients with impaired cardiovascular function since they may be less able to compensate for functional changes associated with the prolongation of A-V conduction produced by these drugs.

Since bupivacaine is metabolised in the liver, it should be used cautiously in patients with liver disease or with reduced liver blood flow.

Epidural anaesthesia with any local anaesthetic can cause hypotension and bradycardia which should be anticipated and appropriate precautions taken. These may include pre-loading the circulation with crystalloid or colloid solution. If hypotension develops it should be treated with a vasopressor such as ephedrine 10-15 mg intravenously. Severe hypotension may result from hypovolaemia due to haemorrhage or dehydration, or aorto-caval occlusion in patients with massive ascites, large abdominal tumours or late pregnancy. Marked hypotension should be avoided in patients with cardiac decompensation.

Patients with hypovolaemia due to any cause can develop sudden and severe hypotension during epidural anaesthesia.

Epidural anaesthesia can cause intercostal paralysis and patients with pleural effusions may suffer respiratory embarrassment. Septicaemia can increase the risk of intraspinal abscess formation in the postoperative period.

Paracervical block may have a greater adverse effect on the foetus than other nerve blocks used in obstetrics. Due to the systemic toxicity of bupivacaine special care should be taken when using bupivacaine for paracervical block.

Small doses of local anaesthetics injected into the head and neck, including retrobulbar, dental and stellate ganglion blocks, may produce systemic toxicity due to inadvertent intra-arterial injection.

Clinicians who perform retrobulbar blocks should be aware that there have been reports of respiratory arrest following local anaesthetic injection. Prior to retrobulbar block, necessary equipment, drugs and personnel should be immediately available as with all other regional procedures.

Solutions containing adrenaline should be used with caution in patients with hypertension, arteriosclerotic heart disease, cerebrovascular insufficiency or diabetes.

Interaction with other medicaments and other forms of interaction: Bupivacaine should be used with care in patients receiving anti-arrhythmic drugs with local anaesthetic activity, e.g. lidocaine since their toxic effects may be additive.

Solutions containing adrenaline should be used with caution in those patients receiving drugs known to produce blood pressure alterations, i.e. MAO inhibitors, tricyclic antidepressants, phenothiazines, etc., as severe and sustained hypotension or hypertension may occur.

Pregnancy and Lactation: Bupivacaine enters the mother's milk, but in such small quantities that there is no risk of affecting the child at therapeutic dose levels.

There is no evidence of untoward effects in human pregnancy. In large doses there is evidence of decreased pup survival in rats and an embryological effect in rabbits if Marcain is administered in pregnancy. Marcain should not therefore be given in early pregnancy unless the benefits are considered to outweigh the risks.

Effects on ability to drive and use machines: None stated.

Undesirable effects: Serious systemic adverse reactions are rare, but may occur in connection with overdosage or unintentional intravascular injection.

Bupivacaine causes systemic toxicity similar to that observed with other local anaesthetic agents. It is caused by high plasma concentrations as a result of excessive dosage, rapid absorption or, most commonly, inadvertent intravascular injection. Pronounced acidosis or hypoxia may increase the risk and severity of toxic reactions. Such reactions involve the central nervous system and the cardiovascular system. CNS reactions are characterised by numbness of the tongue, lightheadedness, dizziness, blurred vision and muscle twitch, followed by drowsiness, convulsions, unconsciousness and possibly respiratory arrest.

Cardiovascular reactions are related to depression of the conduction system of the heart and myocardium leading to decreased cardiac output, heart block, hypotension, bradycardia and sometimes ventricular arrhythmias, including ventricular tachycardia, ventricular fibrillation and cardiac arrest. Usually these will be preceded or accompanied by major CNS toxicity, i.e. convulsions, but in rare cases cardiac arrest has occurred without prodromal CNS effects.

Epidural anaesthesia itself can cause adverse reactions regardless of the local anaesthetic agent used. These include hypotension and bradycardia due to sympathetic blockade and/or vasovagal fainting.

In severe cases cardiac arrest may occur.

Accidental sub-arachnoid injection can lead to very high spinal anaesthesia possibly with apnoea and severe hypotension.

Neurological damage is a rare but well recognised consequence of regional and particularly epidural and spinal anaesthesia. It may be due to several causes, e.g. direct injury to the spinal cord or spinal nerves, anterior spinal artery syndrome, injection of an irritant substance, or an injection of a non-sterile solution.

These may result in localised areas of paraesthesia or anaesthesia, motor weakness, loss of sphincter control and paraplegia. Occasionally these are permanent.

Overdose:
Treatment of side effects: Treatment of a patient with systemic toxicity consists of arresting convulsions and ensuring adequate ventilation with oxygen, if necessary by assisted or controlled ventilation (respiration). If convulsions occur they must be treated promptly by intravenous injection of thiopentone 100 to 200 mg or diazepam 5 to 10 mg. Alternatively succinylcholine 50 mg-100 mg i.v. may be used providing the clinician is capable of performing endotracheal intubation and managing a fully paralysed patient.

Once convulsions have been controlled and adequate ventilation of the lungs ensured, no other treatment is generally required. If hypotension is present, however, a vasopressor, preferably one with inotropic activity, e.g. ephedrine 15 to 30 mg, should be given intravenously.

Cardiac arrest due to bupivacaine can be resistant to electrical defibrillation and resuscitation must be continued energetically for a prolonged period.

High or total spinal blockade causing respiratory paralysis and hypotension during epidural anaesthesia should be treated by ensuring and maintaining a patent airway and giving oxygen by assisted or controlled ventilation.

Hypotension should be treated by the use of vasopressors, e.g. ephedrine 10-15 mg intravenously and repeated until the desired level of arterial pressure is reached. Intravenous fluids, both electrolytes and colloids, given rapidly can also reverse hypotension.

Pharmacological properties
Pharmacodynamic properties: Bupivacaine is a potent amide local anaesthetic with a prolonged duration of action. It affects sensory nerves more than motor nerves and is ideal for producing analgesia without motor blockade.

Pharmacokinetic properties: In adults, the terminal half-life of bupivacaine is 3.5 hours. The maximum blood concentration varies with the site of injection and is highest after intercostal nerve blockade.

Total dose, rather than concentration, is an important determinant of peak blood levels.

Bupivacaine is biodegraded in the liver and only 6% is excreted unchanged in the urine.

Preclinical safety data: Bupivacaine hydrochloride and adrenaline tartrate are well established active ingredients.

Pharmaceutical particulars
List of excipients: Sodium metabisulphite, sodium chloride, hydrochloric acid and water for injection.

Incompatibilities: None known.

Shelf-life: 10 ml ampoules–18 months, 20 ml vials–30 months.

Special precautions for storage: 10 ml ampoules–store below 25°C. 20 ml vials–store below 15°C.

Nature and contents of container: **10 ml glass ampoules–blister packed.** 20 ml single dose glass vials.

Instructions for use/handling: None.

Marketing authorisation number PL 0017/0119

Date of approval/revision of SPC 23rd July 1997.

Legal category POM.

MARCAIN* HEAVY

Presentation Clear, colourless solution containing Bupivacaine Hydrochloride BP 5.28 mg/ml equivalent to bupivacaine hydrochloride anhydrous 5 mg per ml, Dextrose Anhydrous PhEur 72.7 mg/ml equivalent to dextrose monohydrate 80 mg/ml. The specific gravity of the solution is 1.026 at 20°C.

Inactive ingredients: Sodium hydroxide and water.

Uses Spinal anaesthesia for surgery (urological and lower limb surgery lasting 2–3 hours, abdominal surgery lasting 45–60 minutes). Bupivacaine is a long acting local anaesthetic agent of the amide type. Marcain Heavy has rapid onset of action and long duration. The duration of analgesia in the T10–T12 segments is 2–3 hours.

Marcain Heavy produces a moderate muscular relaxation of the lower extremities lasting 2–2.5 hours. The motor blockade of the abdominal muscles makes the solution suitable for performance of abdominal surgery lasting 45–60 minutes. The duration of motor blockade does not exceed the duration of analgesia. The cardiovascular effects of Marcain Heavy are similar or less than those seen with other spinal agents. Bupivacaine 5 mg/ml with glucose 80 mg/ml is exceptionally well tolerated by all tissues with which it comes in contact.

Dosage and administration The doses recommended below should be regarded as a guide for use in the average adult.

Spinal anaesthesia for surgery: 2–4 ml (10–20 mg bupivacaine hydrochloride).

The spread of anaesthesia obtained with Marcain Heavy, depends on several factors, including the volume of solution and the position of the patient during and following the injection. When injected at the L3-L4 intervertebral space with the patient in the sitting position, 3 ml of Marcain Heavy spreads to the T7-T10 spinal segments. With the patient receiving the injection in the horizontal position and then turned supine, the blockade spreads to T4-T7 spinal segments. It should be understood that the level of spinal anaesthesia achieved with any local anaesthetic can be unpredictable in a given patient.

The effects of injections of Marcain Heavy exceeding 4 ml have not yet been studied and such volumes can therefore not be recommended.

Contra-indications, warnings, etc

Contra-indications: Known hypersensitivity to local anaesthetics of the amide type.

Spinal anaesthesia, regardless of the local anaesthetic used, has its own contra-indications which include: Active disease of the central nervous system such as meningitis, poliomyelitis, intracranial haemorrhage, sub-acute combined degeneration of the cord due to pernicious anaemia and cerebral and spinal tumours. Tuberculosis of the spine. Pyogenic infection of the skin at or adjacent to the site of lumbar puncture. Cardiogenic or hypovolaemic shock. Coagulation disorders or ongoing anticoagulation treatment.

Precautions: Spinal anaesthesia should only be undertaken by clinicians with the necessary knowledge and experience. Resuscitative equipment and drugs should be immediately available and the anaesthetist should remain in constant attendance. Spinal anaesthesia with any local anaesthetic can cause hypotension and bradycardia which should be anticipated and appropriate precautions taken. These may include pre-loading the circulation with crystalloid or colloid solution. If hypotension develops it should be treated with a vasopressor such as ephedrine 10–15 mg intravenously. Severe hypotension may result from hypovolaemia due to haemorrhage or dehydration, or aorto-caval occlusion in patients with massive ascites, large abdominal tumours or late pregnancy. Marked hypotension should be avoided in patients with cardiac decompensation.

Patients with hypovolaemia due to any cause can develop sudden and severe hypotension during spinal anaesthesia.

Spinal anaesthesia can cause intercostal paralysis and patients with pleural effusions may suffer respiratory embarrassment. Septicaemia can increase the risk of intraspinal abscess formation in the postoperative period.

Pregnancy and lactation: Bupivacaine enters the mother's milk but in such small quantities that there is generally no risk of affecting the child at therapeutic dose levels.

There is no evidence of untoward effects in human pregnancy. In large doses there is evidence of decreased pup survival in rats and an embryological effect in rabbits if Marcain is administered in pregnancy. Marcain should not therefore be given in early pregnancy unless the benefits are considered to outweigh the risks.

Drug interactions: Bupivacaine should be used with care in patients receiving antiarrhythmic drugs with local anaesthetic activity, as their toxic effects may be additive.

Side-effects: The safety of Marcain Heavy is comparable to that of other local anaesthetics used for spinal anaesthesia.

In rare cases bupivacaine has been associated with allergic reactions and anaphylactic shock.

Spinal anaesthesia itself can cause adverse reactions regardless of the local anaesthetic agent used. These include hypotension and bradycardia due to sympathetic blockade and/or vasovagal fainting.

In severe cases cardiac arrest can occur.

High spinal anaesthesia may result in paralysis of all respiratory muscles.

Postoperatively a post lumbar puncture headache can occur.

Neurological damage is a rare but well recognised consequence of regional and particularly spinal anaesthesia. It may be due to several causes, e.g. direct injury to the spinal cord or spinal nerves, anterior spinal artery syndrome, injection of an irritant substance, or an injection of a non-sterile solution. These may result in localised areas of paraesthesia or anaesthesia, motor weakness, loss of sphincter control and paraplegia. Occasionally these are permanent. Neurological complications of this type have been reported after the use of all local anaesthetics used for spinal anaesthesia.

Systemic toxicity: is rarely associated with spinal anaesthesia but might occur after accidental intravascular injection. Systemic adverse reactions are characterised by numbness of the tongue, lightheadedness, dizziness and tremors, followed by convulsions and cardiovascular disorders.

Treatment of side-effects: High or total spinal blockade causing respiratory paralysis should be treated by ensuring and maintaining a patent airway and giving oxygen by assisted or controlled ventilation.

Hypotension should be treated by the use of vasopressors, e.g. ephedrine 10–15 mg intravenously and repeated until the desired level of arterial pressure is reached. Intravenous fluids, both electrolytes and colloids, given rapidly can also reverse hypotension.

Treatment of systemic toxicity: No treatment is required for milder symptoms of systemic toxicity but if convulsions occur then it is important to ensure adequate oxygenation and to arrest the convulsions if they last more than 15–30 seconds. Oxygen should be given by face mask and the respiration assisted or controlled if necessary. Convulsions can be arrested by injection of thiopentone 100–150 mg intravenously or with diazepam 5–10 mg intravenously. Alternatively, succinylcholine 50–100 mg intravenously may be given but only if the clinician has the ability to perform endotracheal intubation and to manage a totally paralysed patient.

Pharmaceutical precautions The solution must not be stored in contact with metals, e.g. needles or metal parts of syringes, as dissolved metal ions may cause swelling at the site of the injection.

The solution should be used immediately after opening of the ampoule. Any remaining solution should be discarded.

Store below 25°C.

Legal category POM.

Package quantities **Sterile wrapped ampoules 5×4 ml.** Sterile wrapped ampoules 4×4 ml.

Further information Nil.

Product licence number PL 0017/0139.

MARCAIN* POLYAMP* STERIPACK 0.25%
MARCAIN* POLYAMP* STERIPACK 0.375%
MARCAIN* POLYAMP* STERIPACK 0.5%
MARCAIN* POLYAMP* STERIPACK 0.75%

Qualitative and quantitative composition Marcain Polyamp Steripack 0.25% contains Bupivacaine Hydrochloride BP 2.64 mg/ml equivalent to bupivacaine hydrochloride anhydrous 2.5 mg/ml.

Marcain Polyamp Steripack 0.375% contains Bupivacaine Hydrochloride BP 3.96 mg/ml equivalent to bupivacaine hydrochloride anhydrous 3.75 mg/ml.

Marcain Polyamp Steripack 0.5% contains Bupivacaine Hydrochloride BP 5.28 mg/ml equivalent to bupivacaine hydrochloride anhydrous 5.0 mg/ml.

Marcain Polyamp Steripack 0.75% contains Bupivacaine Hydrochloride BP 7.92 mg/ml equivalent to bupivacaine hydrochloride anhydrous 7.5 mg/ml.

Pharmaceutical form Injection.

Clinical particulars

Therapeutic indications: Marcain 0.25%, 0.375% and 0.5% solutions are used for the production of local anaesthesia by percutaneous infiltration, peripheral nerve block(s) and central neural block (caudal or epidural), that is, for specialist use in situations where prolonged anaesthesia is required. Because sensory nerve block is more marked than motor block, Marcain is especially useful in the relief of pain, e.g. during labour.

A list of indications and the suggested dose and strength of solution appropriate for each are shown in the table overleaf.

Marcain 0.75% solution produces a more prolonged motor block than 0.25%, 0.375% or 0.5% solutions and is, therefore, recommended for epidural anaesthesia for surgical purposes. Epidural anaesthesia is usually maintained for 3 to 4 hours.

Posology and method of administration: The utmost care should be taken to prevent an accidental intravascular injection, always including careful aspiration. For epidural anaesthesia, a test dose of 3–5 ml of bupivacaine containing adrenaline should be administered, since an intravascular injection of adrenaline will be quickly recognised by an increase in heart rate. Verbal contact and repeated measurement of heart rate should be maintained throughout a period of 5 minutes following the test dose. Aspiration should be repeated prior to administration of the total dose. The main dose should be injected slowly, **25–50 mg/min**, in incremental doses under constant contact with the patient. If mild toxic symptoms occur, the injection should be stopped immediately.

The dosage varies and depends upon the area to be anaesthetised, the vascularity of the tissues, the number of neuronal segments to be blocked, individual tolerance and the technique of anaesthesia used. The lowest dosage needed to provide effective anaesthesia should be administered. For most indications, the duration of anaesthesia with Marcain solutions is such that a single dose is sufficient.

The maximum dosage must be determined by evaluating the size and physical status of the patient and considering the usual rate of systemic absorption from a particular injection site. Experience to date indicates a single dose of up to 150 mg bupivacaine hydrochloride. Doses of up to 50 mg 2-hourly may subsequently be used. The dosages in the following table are recommended as a guide for use in the average adult. For young, elderly or debilitated patients, these doses should be reduced.

Contra-indications: Bupivacaine hydrochloride solutions are contra-indicated in patients with a known hypersensitivity to local anaesthetic agents of the amide type or to other components of the injectable formulation.

Solutions of bupivacaine hydrochloride are contra-indicated for intravenous regional anaesthesia (Bier's-block).

0.75% solution is contra-indicated for epidural use in obstetrics.

Epidural anaesthesia, regardless of the local anaesthetic used, has its own contra-indications which include:

Active disease of the central nervous system such as meningitis, poliomyelitis, intracranial haemorrhage, sub-acute combined degeneration of the cord due to pernicious anaemia and cerebral and spinal tumours. Tuberculosis of the spine. Pyogenic infection of the skin at or adjacent to the site of lumbar puncture. Cardiogenic or hypovolaemic shock. Coagulation disorders or ongoing anticoagulation treatment.

Special warnings and special precautions for use: There have been reports of cardiac arrest with difficult resuscitation or death during use of bupivacaine for epidural anaesthesia in obstetrical patients. In most cases, this has followed use of the 0.75% concentration. Resuscitation has been difficult or impossible despite apparently adequate preparation and appropriate management. Cardiac arrest has occurred after convulsions resulting from systemic toxicity, presumably following unintentional intravascular injection. The 0.75% concentration should be reserved for surgical procedures where a high degree of muscle relaxation and prolonged effect are necessary.

Epidural blockade and large nerve plexus blocks should only be employed by those with the necessary training and experience.

Adequate resuscitation equipment should be available whenever local or general anaesthesia is administered. Overdosage or accidental intravenous injection may give rise to toxic reactions.

Injection of repeated doses of bupivacaine hydrochloride may cause significant increases in blood levels with each repeated dose due to slow accumulation of the drug. Tolerance varies with the status of the patient. Debilitated, elderly or acutely ill patients should be given reduced doses commensurate with their physical status.

Only in rare cases have amide local anaesthetics been associated with allergic reactions (in most severe instances anaphylactic shock).

Patients allergic to ester-type local anaesthetic drugs (procaine, tetracaine, benzocaine, etc.) have not shown cross-sensitivity to agents of the amide type such as bupivacaine.

Local anaesthetics should be used with caution for epidural anaesthesia in patients with impaired cardiovascular function since they may be less able to compensate for functional changes associated with the prolongation of A-V conduction produced by these drugs.

Since bupivacaine is metabolised in the liver, it should be used cautiously in patients with liver disease or with reduced liver blood flow.

Epidural anaesthesia with any local anaesthetic can cause hypotension and bradycardia which should be anticipated and appropriate precautions taken. These may include pre-loading the circulation with crystalloid or colloid solution. If hypotension develops it should be treated with a vasopressor such as ephe-

Type of block	*% Conc*	*Each dose ml*	*mg*	*Motor block†*
Local infiltration	0.25	up to 60	up to 150	–
Lumbar epidural				
Surgical operations	0.50	10 to 20	50 to 100	Moderate to complete
	0.75	10 to 20	75 to 150	Complete
Analgesia in labour	0.50	6 to 12	30 to 60	Moderate to complete
	0.375	6 to 12	22.5 to 45	Moderate to minimal
	0.25	6 to 12	15 to 30	Minimal
Caudal epidural				
Surgical operations	0.50	15 to 30	75 to 150	Moderate to complete
Children (aged up to 10yrs):				
Up to lower thoracic (T10)	0.25	0.3–0.4 ml/kg	0.75–1.0 mg/kg	
Up to mid-thoracic (T6)	0.25	0.4–0.6 ml/kg	1.0–1.5 mg/kg	
If total amount greater than 20 ml reduce concentration to 0.2%				
Analgesia in labour	0.50	10 to 20	50 to 100	Moderate to complete
	0.375	10 to 20	37.5 to 75	Moderate
	0.25	10 to 20	25 to 50	Moderate
Peripheral Nerves	0.50	up to 30	up to 150	Moderate to complete
	0.375	up to 40	up to 150	Moderate
	0.25	up to 60	up to 150	Slight to moderate
Sympathetic blocks	0.25	20 to 50	50 to 125	–

† With continuous (intermittent) techniques, repeat doses increase the degree of motor block. The first repeat dose of 0.5% may produce complete motor block for intra-abdominal surgery.

drine 10–15 mg intravenously. Severe hypotension may result from hypovolaemia due to haemorrhage or dehydration, or aorto-caval occlusion in patients with massive ascites, large abdominal tumours or late pregnancy. Marked hypotension should be avoided in patients with cardiac decompensation.

Patients with hypovolaemia due to any cause can develop sudden and severe hypotension during epidural anaesthesia.

Epidural anaesthesia can cause intercostal paralysis and patients with pleural effusions may suffer respiratory embarrassment. Septicaemia can increase the risk of intraspinal abscess formation in the postoperative period.

Paracervical block may have a greater adverse effect on the foetus than other nerve blocks used in obstetrics. Due to the systemic toxicity of bupivacaine special care should be taken when using bupivacaine for paracervical block.

Small doses of local anaesthetics injected into the head and neck, including retrobulbar, dental and stellate ganglion blocks, may produce systemic toxicity due to inadvertent intra-arterial injection.

Clinicians who perform retrobulbar blocks should be aware that there have been reports of respiratory arrest following local anaesthetic injection. Prior to retrobulbar block, necessary equipment, drugs and personnel should be immediately available as with all other regional procedures.

Interaction with other medicaments and other forms of interaction: Bupivacaine should be used with care in patients receiving anti-arrhythmic drugs with local anaesthetic activity, e.g. lidocaine, since their toxic effects may be additive.

Serious cardiac arrhythmias may occur if preparations containing a vasoconstrictor drug are employed in patients during or following the administration of chloroform, halothane, cyclopropane, trichlorethylene or other related agents.

Pregnancy and lactation: There is no evidence of untoward effects in human pregnancy. In large doses there is evidence of decreased pup survival in rats and an embryological effect in rabbits if Marcain is administered in pregnancy. Marcain should not therefore be given in early pregnancy unless the benefits are considered to outweigh the risks.

Bupivacaine enters the mother's milk, but in such small quantities that there is no risk of affecting the child at therapeutic dose levels.

Effects on ability to drive and use machines: None stated.

Undesirable effects: Serious systemic adverse reactions are rare, but may occur in connection with overdosage or unintentional intravascular injection.

Bupivacaine causes systemic toxicity similar to that observed with other local anaesthetic agents. It is caused by high plasma concentrations as a result of excessive dosage, rapid absorption or, most commonly, inadvertent intravascular injection. Pronounced acidosis or hypoxia may increase the risk and severity of toxic reactions. Such reactions involve the central nervous system and the cardiovascular system. CNS reactions are characterised by numbness of the tongue, light-headedness, dizziness, blurred vision and muscle twitch, followed by drowsiness, convulsions, unconsciousness and possibly respiratory arrest.

Cardiovascular reactions are related to depression of the conduction system of the heart and myocardium leading to decreased cardiac output, heart block, hypotension, bradycardia and sometimes ventricular arrhythmias, including ventricular tachycardia, ventricular fibrillation and cardiac arrest. Usually these will be preceded or accompanied by major CNS toxicity, i.e. convulsions, but in rare cases cardiac arrest has occurred without prodromal CNS effects.

Epidural anaesthesia itself can cause adverse reactions regardless of the local anaesthetic agent used. These include hypotension and bradycardia due to sympathetic blockade and/or vasovagal fainting.

In severe cases cardiac arrest may occur.

Accidental sub-arachnoid injection can lead to very high spinal anaesthesia possibly with apnoea and severe hypotension.

Neurological damage is a rare but well recognised consequence of regional and particularly epidural and spinal anaesthesia. It may be due to several causes, e.g. direct injury to the spinal cord or spinal nerves, anterior spinal artery syndrome, injection of an irritant substance, or an injection of a non-sterile solution. These may result in localised areas of paraesthesia or anaesthesia, motor weakness, loss of sphincter control and paraplegia. Occasionally these are permanent.

Overdose: Treatment of a patient with systemic toxicity consists of arresting convulsions and ensuring adequate ventilation with oxygen, if necessary by assisted or controlled ventilation (respiration). If convulsions occur they must be treated promptly by intravenous injection of thiopentone 100 to 200 mg or diazepam 5 to 10 mg. Alternatively succinylcholine 50 mg–100 mg i.v. may be used providing the clinician is capable of performing endotracheal intubation and managing a fully paralysed patient.

Once convulsions have been controlled and adequate ventilation of the lungs ensured, no other treatment is generally required. If hypotension is present, however, a vasopressor, preferably one with inotropic activity, e.g. ephedrine 15 to 30 mg, should be given intravenously.

Cardiac arrest due to bupivacaine can be resistant to electrical defibrillation and resuscitation must be continued energetically for a prolonged period.

High or total spinal blockade causing respiratory paralysis and hypotension during epidural anaesthesia should be treated by ensuring and maintaining a patent airway and giving oxygen by assisted or controlled ventilation.

Hypotension should be treated by the use of vasopressors, e.g. ephedrine 10–15 mg intravenously and repeated until the desired level of arterial pressure is reached. Intravenous fluids, both electrolytes and colloids, given rapidly can also reverse hypotension.

Pharmacological properties

Pharmacodynamic properties: Bupivacaine is a potent amide local anaesthetic with a prolonged duration of action. It affects sensory nerves more than motor nerves and is ideal for producing analgesia without motor blockade.

Pharmacokinetic properties: In adults, the terminal half-life of bupivacaine is 3.5 hours. The maximum blood concentration varies with the site of injection and is highest after intercostal nerve blockade.

Total dose, rather than concentration, is an important determinant of peak blood levels.

Bupivacaine is biodegraded in the liver and only 6% is excreted unchanged in the urine.

Preclinical safety data: Bupivacaine hydrochloride is a well established active ingredient.

Pharmaceutical precautions

List of excipients: Sodium chloride, sodium hydroxide and water for injections.

Incompatibilities: None stated.

Shelf-life: 24 months.

Special precautions for storage: Store below 30°C.

Nature and contents of container: 10 ml polypropylene ampoules (Steripack).

Instructions for use/handling: For single use only. Discard any unused solution.

Marketing authorisation numbers

Marcain Polyamp Steripack 0.25%	**PL 0017/0305**
Marcain Polyamp Steripack 0.375%	**PL 0017/0306**
Marcain Polyamp Steripack 0.5%	**PL 0017/0307**
Marcain Polyamp Steripack 0.75%	**PL 0017/0308.**

Date of approval/revision of SPC September 1998.

MUSE* ▼

Qualitative and quantitative composition *Active ingredient:* Alprostadil USP: 125 micrograms, 250 micrograms, 500 micrograms or 1000 micrograms.

Pharmaceutical form Urethral stick.

MUSE is a sterile, single-use transurethral system for the delivery of alprostadil to the male urethra. Alprostadil is suspended in macrogol and is formed into a urethral stick (1.4 mm in diameter by 3 mm or 6 mm in length) which is contained in the tip of the polypropylene applicator.

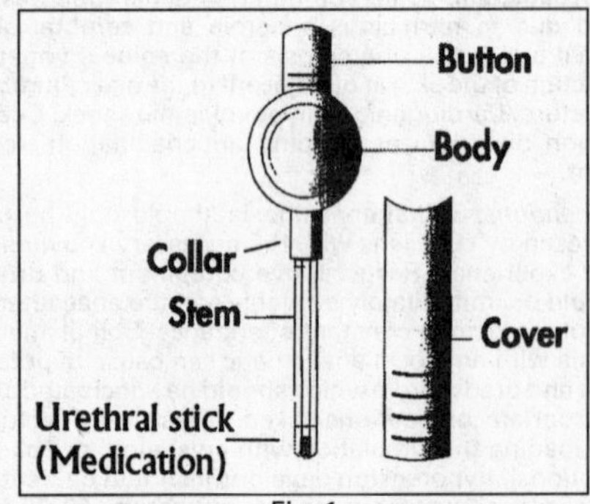

Fig. 1

Clinical particulars

Therapeutic indications: 1. Treatment of erectile dysfunction of primarily organic etiology.

2. Adjunct to other tests in the diagnosis and management of erectile dysfunction.

Posology and method of administration: 1. Treatment of erectile dysfunction.

It is important for the patient to urinate before administration since a moist urethra makes administration of MUSE easier and is essential to dissolve the drug. To administer MUSE, remove the protective cover from the MUSE applicator, stretch the penis upward to its full length, and insert the applicator stem into the urethra. Depress the applicator button to release the medication from the applicator and remove the applicator from the urethra, (rocking the applicator gently prior to removal will ensure that the medication is separated from the applicator stem). Roll the penis between the hands for at least 10 seconds to ensure that the medication is adequately distributed along the wall of the urethra. If the patient feels a burning sensation it may help to roll the penis for an additional 30 to 60 seconds or until the burning subsides. The erection will develop within 5–10 minutes after administration and lasts approximately 30–60 minutes. After administration of the MUSE, it is important to sit, or preferably, stand or walk for about 10 minutes while the erection is developing. More detailed information is given under "*Instructions for use/handling*" and in the Patient Information Leaflet.

Not more than 2 doses are recommended to be used in any 24-hour period.

Initiation of therapy: A medical professional should instruct each patient on the correct use of MUSE. The recommended starting dose is 250 micrograms. Dosage may be increased in a stepwise manner (from 500 to 1000 micrograms), or decreased (to 125 micrograms) under medical supervision until the patient achieves a satisfactory response. After an assessment of the patient's skill and competence with the procedure, the chosen dose may then be prescribed for home use.

2. Adjunct to other tests in the diagnosis and management of erectile dysfunction.

MUSE can be used as an adjunct in evaluating penile vascular function using Doppler duplex ultrasonography. It has been shown that a 500 microgram dose of MUSE has a comparable effect on penile arterial dilatation and peak systolic velocity flow to 10 microgram of alprostadil given by intracavernosal injection. At the time of discharge from the clinic, the erection should have subsided.

Elderly: No adjustment for age is required

Children: Not recommended.

Contra-indications: MUSE is contra-indicated in men with any of the following conditions:

Known hypersensitivity to alprostadil.

Abnormal penile anatomy (urethral stricture, severe hypospadia or severe curvature), balanitis, acute or chronic urethritis.

Conditions with an increased risk of priapism (sickle cell anaemia or trait, thrombocythaemia, polycythaemia, multiple myeloma, predisposition to venous thrombosis).

MUSE should not be used in men for whom sexual activity is inadvisable.

Special warnings and special precautions for use: Underlying treatable medical causes of erectile dysfunction should be diagnosed and treated prior to initiation of treatment with MUSE.

Incorrect insertion of MUSE may cause urethral abrasion and minor urethral bleeding. Patients on anticoagulants or with bleeding disorders may have an increased risk of urethral bleeding.

Patients should be asked to report to a physician any erections lasting 4 hours or more. In clinical trials of MUSE, priapism (rigid erections lasting $\geq$ 6 hours) and prolonged erection (rigid erection lasting 4 hours and < 6 hours) were reported infrequently (<0.1% and 0.3% of patients, respectively). Nevertheless, these events are a potential risk of pharmacologic therapy. It may be necessary to reduce the dose or discontinue treatment in any patient who develops priapism.

Patients and their partners should be advised that MUSE offers no protection from transmission of sexually transmitted diseases. They should be counselled about the protective measures that are necessary to guard against the spread of sexually transmitted agents, including the human immunodeficiency virus (HIV). The use of MUSE will not affect the integrity of condoms. Since MUSE may add small amounts of alprostadil to the naturally occurring PGE_1 already present in the semen, it is recommended that adequate contraception is used if the woman is of child-bearing potential. MUSE should not be used if the female partner is pregnant unless the couple uses a condom barrier.

Interaction with other medicaments and other forms of interaction: Systemic interactions are unlikely because of the low levels of alprostadil in the peripheral venous circulation, however, the presence of medication affecting erectile function may influence the response to MUSE. Decongestants and appetite suppressants may diminish the effect of MUSE. Patients on anticoagulants or with bleeding disorders may have an increased risk of urethral bleeding.

The use of MUSE in patients with penile implants has not been studied.

Pregnancy and lactation: MUSE may add small amounts of alprostadil to the naturally occurring PGE_1 already present in the semen. A condom barrier should therefore be used during sexual intercourse if the female partner is pregnant to avoid irritation of the vagina and guard against any risk to the foetus.

Effects on ability to drive and use machines: Patients should be cautioned to avoid activities, such as driving or hazardous tasks, where injury could result if hypotension or syncope were to occur after MUSE administration. In patients experiencing hypotension and/or syncope, these events have usually occurred during initial titration and within one hour of drug administration.

Undesirable effects: The most frequently reported local adverse events in clinical trials of home treatment with MUSE are (% of patients):

Penile pain (32%), urethral burning (12%), minor urethral bleeding (5%), testicular pain (5%). Swelling of the leg veins, leg and perineal pain have been observed.

During a supervised initiation of treatment, symptomatic hypotension occurred in 3% of patients. Dizziness was reported in 4% of patients. Syncope was reported by 0.4% of patients. Patients should be advised about the symptoms of hypotension. Rapid pulse has also been reported. These same effects have been reported, although less frequently, during home treatment.

Vaginal burning/itching was reported by approximately 6% of partners of patients on active treatment. This may be a result of resuming sexual intercourse.

Overdosage: Symptoms: Overdosage has not been reported with MUSE.

Symptomatic hypotension, persistent penile pain and in rare instances, priapism may occur with alprostadil overdosage. Patients should be kept under medical supervision until systemic or local symptoms have resolved.

Treatment: Should a prolonged erection lasting 4 or more hours occur, the patient should be advised to seek medical help. The following actions can be taken:

1. The patient should be supine or lying on his side. Apply an ice pack alternately for two minutes to each upper inner thigh (this may cause a reflex opening of venous valves). If there is no response after 10 minutes, discontinue treatment.

2. If this treatment is ineffective and a rigid erection has lasted for more than 6 hours, penile aspiration should be performed. Using aseptic technique, insert a 19–21 gauge butterfly needle into the corpus cavernosum and aspirate 20–50 ml of blood. This may detumesce the penis. If necessary, the procedure may be repeated on the opposite side of the penis.

3. If still unsuccessful, intracavernous injection of α-adrenergic medication is recommended. Although the usual contra-indication to intrapenile administration of a vasoconstrictor does not apply in the treatment of priapism, caution is advised when this option is exercised. Blood pressure and pulse should be continuously monitored during the procedure. Extreme caution is required in patients with coronary heart disease, uncontrolled hypertension, cerebral ischaemia, and in subjects taking monoamine oxidase inhibitors. In the latter case, facilities should be available to manage a hypertensive crisis. A 200 microgram/ml solution of phenylephrine should be prepared, and 0.5 to 1.0 ml of the solution injected every 5–10 minutes. Alternatively, a 20 microgram/ml solution of adrenaline should be used. If necessary, this may be followed by further aspiration of blood through the same butterfly needle. The maximum dose of phenylephrine should be 1 mg, or adrenaline 100 micrograms (5 ml of the solution).

4. As an alternative, metaraminol may be used but it should be noted that fatal hypertensive crises have been reported. If this still fails to resolve the priapism, the patient should immediately be referred for surgical management.

Pharmacological properties

Pharmacodynamic properties: Alprostadil is chemically identical to prostaglandin E_1, the actions of which include vasodilatation of blood vessels in the erectile tissues of the corpora cavernosa and increase in cavernosal artery blood flow, causing penile rigidity.

Pharmacokinetic properties: Approximately 80% of the alprostadil delivered by MUSE is absorbed through the urethral mucosa within 10 minutes. The half-life is less than 10 minutes and peripheral venous plasma concentrations are low or undetectable. Alprostadil is rapidly metabolised, both locally and in the pulmonary capillary bed; metabolites are excreted in the urine (90% within 24 hours) and the faeces. There is no evidence of tissue retention of alprostadil or its metabolites.

Pre-clinical safety data: In rats, high doses of prostaglandin E_1 increased foetal resorption, presumably due to maternal stress. High concentrations of alprostadil (400 microgram/ml) had no effect on human sperm motility or viability *in vitro*. In rabbits, there was no foetal damage or effect on reproductive function at the maximum tested intravaginal dose of 4 mg.

In the majority of *in vitro* and *in vivo* genotoxicity test systems in which alprostadil has been evaluated it produced negative results. These tests include the bacterial reversion test using *Salmonella typhimurium*, unscheduled DNA synthesis in rat primary hepatocytes, forward mutation assay at the hprt locus in cultured ovary cells from Chinese hamsters, alkaline elution test, sister chromatid exchange assay (all *in vitro* tests) and the micronucleus test in both mice and rats (*in vivo* tests). In two other *in vitro* tests, the mouse lymphoma forward mutation assay and the Chinese hamster ovary chromosomal aberration assay, alprostadil produced borderline positive and positive evidence, respectively, for chromosomal damage. In view of the number of negative *in vitro* results and the lack of evidence for genotoxicity in two *in vivo* tests, it is considered that the positive results obtained in these two *in vitro* tests are of doubtful biological significance. Overall, the presently available evidence suggests that alprostadil is unlikely to exert any significant genotoxic activity in humans at the dosage levels used in the present product.

Pharmaceutical particulars

List of excipients: Macrogol.

Incompatibilities (major): Not known.

Shelf-life: 2 years.

Special precautions for storage: Store unopened foil pouches in a refrigerator at 2°–8°C. Do not expose to temperatures above 30°C. MUSE may be kept by the patient at room temperature (below 30°C) for up to 14 days prior to use.

Nature and contents of container: MUSE is supplied as cartons of 6 individual foil pouches, with each pouch containing one delivery system. Packs containing 1 delivery system will also be available.

The pouches are composed of foil/laminate. The applicators are made from radiation-resistant medical-grade polypropylene.

Instructions for use/handling: Immediately prior to administration, the patient should urinate, and gently shake the penis to remove excess urine. A moist urethra makes administration of MUSE easier and is essential to dissolve the medication.

Open the foil pouch and allow MUSE to slide out of the pouch. Save the pouch for discarding the MUSE applicator. Remove the protective cover from the applicator stem by holding the body of the applicator, twisting and pulling it from the cover. Be careful not to push in or pull out the applicator button, and avoid touching the applicator stem and tip. Examine the MUSE and observe the medication at the end of the stem. Save the cover for discarding the MUSE applicator later. With the patient sitting, or standing, pull the penis upright and stretch to its full length (this is necessary to straighten the urethra). Slowly insert the stem into the urethra up to the collar. If there is any discomfort or a pulling sensation, withdraw the applicator slightly and then gently re-insert. Once inserted, gently and completely push down the button at the top of the applicator until it is fully depressed. It is important to do this to ensure that the medication is completely released. Hold the applicator in this position for 5 seconds. Gently rock the applicator from side to side, then remove the applicator whilst keeping the penis upright. If too much pressure is applied, the lining of the urethra may be scratched causing it to bleed. After removal of the applicator, observe the tip of the stem to ensure that the medication has been delivered. If there is some residual medication in the end of the applicator, gently re-insert into the urethra and repeat the procedure. Holding the penis upright and stretched to its full length, roll the penis firmly between the hands for at least 10 seconds. If the patient feels a burning sensation it may help to continue rolling the penis for an additional 30–60 seconds or until the burning subsides. After administration of the MUSE, it is important to sit, or preferably, stand or walk for about 10 minutes while the erection is developing. Replace the cover on the empty MUSE applicator, place in the opened foil pouch, fold and discard as normal household waste.

Marketing authorisation holder VIVUS UK, Providence House, River Street, Windsor, Berkshire SL4 1QT. Distributed and marketed in the UK by Astra Pharmaceuticals Ltd.

Marketing authorisation numbers

125 micrograms	PL 15504/0001
250 micrograms	PL 15504/0002
500 micrograms	PL 15504/0003
1000 micrograms	PL 15504/0004

Date of approval/revision of SPC November 1997

Legal category POM.

NAROPIN* POLYAMP*2 mg/ml, 7.5 mg/ml and 10 mg/ml ▼ NAROPIN* INFUSION 2 mg/ml ▼

Qualitative and quantitative composition Ropivacaine hydrochloride monohydrate

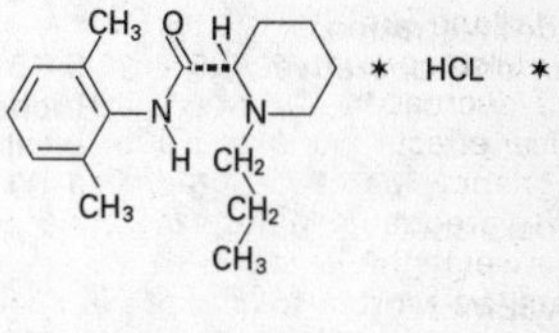

* HCL * H_2O

Molecular formula $C_{17}H_{26}N_2O{*}HCl{*}H_2O$
m.w.:328.9

Naropin 2 mg/ml: 2 mg/ml ropivacaine hydrochloride
Naropin 7.5 mg/ml: 7.5 mg/ml ropivacaine hydrochloride
Naropin 10 mg/ml: 10 mg/ml ropivacaine hydrochloride

Pharmaceutical form Solution for injection for perineural and epidural administration (10–20 ml).

Solution for epidural infusion (100 and 200 ml).

Clinical particulars

Therapeutic indications: Naropin is indicated for:

1. Surgical anaesthesia:

Epidural blocks for surgery, including Caesarean section.

Field blocks.

2. Acute pain management:

Continuous epidural infusion or intermittent bolus administration during postoperative or labour pain.

Field blocks.

Posology and method of administration: Naropin should only be used by, or under the supervision of, clinicians experienced in regional anaesthesia.

Posology: The table below is a guide to dosage for the more commonly used blocks. The smallest dose required to produce an effective block should be used. The clinician's experience and knowledge of the patient's physical status are of importance when deciding the dose.

In general, surgical anaesthesia (e.g. epidural administration) requires the use of the higher concentrations and doses. Naropin 10 mg/ml is recommended for epidural anaesthesia in which a profound motor block is essential for surgery. For analgesia (e.g. epidural administration for acute pain management) the lower concentrations and doses are recommended.

Method of administration: Careful aspiration before and during injection is recommended to prevent intravascular injection. When a large dose is to be injected, e.g. in epidural block, a test dose of 3-5 ml lidocaine (lignocaine) with adrenaline (Xylocaine* 2% with Adrenaline 1:200,000) is recommended. An inadvertent intravascular injection may be recognised by a temporary increase in heart rate and an accidental intrathecal injection by signs of a spinal block.

Aspiration should be repeated prior to and during administration of the main dose, which should be injected slowly or in incremental doses, at a rate of 25-50 mg/min, while closely observing the patient's vital functions and maintaining verbal contact. If toxic symptoms occur, the injection should be stopped immediately.

In epidural block for surgery, single doses of up to 250 mg ropivacaine have been used and well tolerated.

When prolonged blocks are used, either through continuous epidural infusion or through repeated bolus administration, the risks of reaching a toxic plasma concentration or inducing local neural injury must be considered. Experience to date indicates that a cumulative dose of up to 675 mg ropivacaine administered over 24 hours is well tolerated in adults. In a limited number of patients higher doses of up to 800 mg/day have been administered with relatively few adverse reactions. However higher doses may be associated with an increased risk of adverse reactions.

For treatment of postoperative pain, the following technique can be recommended: Unless preoperatively instituted, an epidural block with Naropin 7.5 mg/ml is induced via an epidural catheter. Analgesia is maintained with Naropin 2 mg/ml infusion. Infusion rates of 6-10 ml (12-20 mg) per hour provide adequate analgesia with only slight and non-progressive motor block in most cases of moderate to severe postoperative pain. If some patients do not react adequately, higher doses with an infusion rate of up to 12-14 ml (24-28 mg ropivacaine) per hour may be used.

With this technique a significant reduction in the need for opioids has been observed. Clinical experience supports the use of Naropin epidural infusions for up to 24 hours.

Concentrations above 7.5 mg/ml Naropin have not been documented for Caesarean section.

Contra-indications: Naropin solutions are contra-indicated in patients with known hypersensitivity to anaesthetics of the amide type.

General contra-indications related to epidural anaesthesia, regardless of the local anaesthetic used, should be taken into account.

Intravenous regional anaesthesia.

Obstetric paracervical anaesthesia.

Hypovolaemia.

Special warnings and special precautions for use: Regional anaesthetic procedures should always be performed in a properly equipped and staffed area. Equipment and drugs necessary for monitoring and emergency resuscitation should be immediately available. For emergency medication, patients receiving major blocks should have an intravenous line inserted before the blocking procedure. The clinician responsible should be appropriately trained and familiar with diagnosis and treatment of side-effects, systemic toxicity and other complications (see *"Overdosage"*).

Certain local anaesthetic procedures, such as injections in the head and neck regions, may be associated with a higher frequency of serious adverse reactions, regardless of the local anaesthetic used. Care should be taken to avoid injections in infected areas.

Naropin cannot be recommended for use in children below the age of 12 years as there is no data with regard to efficacy and safety in this group of patients.

Patients in poor general condition due to ageing or other compromising factors such as partial or complete heart conduction block, advanced liver disease or severe renal dysfunction require special attention, although regional anaesthesia is frequently indicated in these patients.

Patients with hypovolaemia due to any cause can develop sudden and severe hypotension during epidural anaesthesia, regardless of the local anaesthetic used.

Ropivacaine is metabolised in the liver and should therefore be used with caution in patients with severe liver disease. Repeated doses may need to be reduced due to delayed elimination. Normally there is no need to modify the dose in patients with impaired renal function when used for single dose or short term treatment. Acidosis and reduced plasma protein concentration, frequently seen in patients with chronic renal failure, may increase the risk of systemic toxicity.

A possible cross-hypersensitivity with other amide-type local anaesthetics should be taken into account.

Interaction with other medicaments and other forms of interaction: Naropin should be used with caution in patients receiving other local anaesthetics or agents structurally related to amide-type local anaesthetics, e.g. certain antiarrhythmics, since the toxic effects are additive. Simultaneous use of Naropin with general anaesthetics or opioids may potentiate each others (adverse) effects.

There is a potential risk for metabolic interaction when Naropin is used in combination with CYP1A-inhibitors, e.g. fluvoxamine and verapamil, which may result in increased plasma levels of Naropin.

	Conc. mg/ml	*Volume ml*	*Dose mg*	*Onset minutes*	*Duration hours*
SURGICAL ANAESTHESIA					
Lumbar Epidural Administration					
Surgery	7.5	15–25	113–188	10–20	3–5
	10	15–20	150–200	10–20	4–6
Caesarean Section	7.5	15–20	113–150(1)	10–20	3–5
Thoracic Epidural Administration					
To establish block for post-operative pain relief	7.5	5–15 (depending on the level of injection)	38–113	10–20	n/a(2)
Field Block (e.g. minor nerve blocks and infiltration)	7.5	1–30	7.5–225	1–15	2–6
ACUTE PAIN MANAGEMENT					
Lumbar Epidural Administration					
Bolus	2	10–20	20–40	10–15	0.5–1.5
Intermittent injections (top up) (e.g. labour pain management)	2	10–15 (minimum interval 30 mins)	20–30		
Continuous infusion (labour pain and postoperative pain management)	2	6–10 ml/h	12–20 mg/h	n/a(2)	n/a(2)
Thoracic Epidural Administration					
Continuous infusion (postoperative pain management)	2	4–8 ml/h	8–16 mg/h	n/a(2)	n/a(2)
Field Block (e.g. minor nerve blocks and infiltration)	2	1–100	2–200	1–5	2–6

The doses in the table are those considered to be necessary to produce a successful block and should be regarded as guidelines for use in adults. Individual variations in onset and duration occur. The figures in the column 'Dose' reflect the expected average dose range needed. For other local anaesthetic techniques standard textbooks should be consulted.

(1) Incremental dosing should be applied, the starting dose of about 100 mg (97.5 mg = 13 ml; 105 mg = 14 ml) to be given over 3–5 minutes. Two additional doses, each of 25 mg, may be administered as needed. The total administered dose should not exceed 150 mg.

(2) n/a = not applicable

Pregnancy and lactation:

Pregnancy: The safety of ropivacaine for use in human pregnancy has not been established. Evaluation of experimental animal studies does not indicate direct or indirect harmful effects. The use of ropivacaine at recommended doses during child birth has not shown any harmful effects.

Lactation: There is no data available concerning the excretion of ropivacaine into human milk.

Effects on ability to drive and use machines: No data is available. Depending on the dose, local anaesthetics may have a very mild effect on mental function and co-ordination even in the absence of overt CNS toxicity and may temporarily impair locomotion and alertness.

Undesirable effects:

General: The adverse reaction profile for Naropin is similar to those for other long acting local anaesthetics of the amide type.

Adverse reactions to local anaesthetics are very rare in the absence of overdose or inadvertent intravascular injection. They should be distinguished from the physiological effects of the nerve block itself e.g. a decrease in blood pressure and bradycardia during epidural anaesthesia. The effects of systemic overdose and unintentional intravascular injections can be serious (see *"Overdosage"*).

Allergic reactions: Allergic reactions (in the most severe instances anaphylactic shock) to local anaesthetics of the amide type are rare.

Neurological complications: Neuropathy and spinal cord dysfunction (e.g. anterior spinal artery syndrome, arachnoiditis, cauda equina syndrome) have been associated with regional anaesthesia, regardless of the local anaesthetic drug used.

Acute systemic toxicity: Naropin may cause acute toxic effects following high doses or if very rapidly rising blood levels occur due to accidental intravascular injection or overdose. (See *"Overdosage"* and *"Pharmacodynamic properties"*).

One case of convulsions has been observed after an unintended intravascular injection during an attempted brachial plexus block with 200 mg.

Most common adverse reactions: A large number of adverse reactions have been reported during the clinical development, the great majority of which are related to the expected effects of the block and to the clinical situation rather than reactions to the drug. Thus hypotension and nausea have been reported as the most frequent adverse reactions.

The following other reported adverse reactions are considered to be of clinical importance regardless of causal relationship: Bradycardia, vomiting, paraesthesia, temperature elevation, headache, urinary retention, dizziness, hypertension, rigors (chills), tachycardia, anxiety, hypoesthesia.

Overdosage:

Symptoms: Acute systemic toxicity: Accidental intravascular injections of local anaesthetics may cause immediate toxic effects. In the event of overdose, peak plasma concentrations may not be reached for one to two hours, depending on the site of the injection, and signs of toxicity may thus be delayed. Systemic toxic reactions may involve the central nervous system and the cardiovascular system. Such complications can also occur with accidental sub-arachnoid injection.

Central nervous system: Central nervous system toxicity is a graded response with symptoms and signs of escalating severity. Initially symptoms such as visual or hearing disturbances, perioral numbness, dizziness, light-headedness, tingling and paraesthesia are seen. Dysarthria, muscular rigidity and muscular twitching are more serious and may precede the onset of generalised convulsions. These signs must not be mistaken for neurotic behaviour. Unconsciousness and grand mal convulsions may follow, which may last from a few seconds to several minutes. Hypoxia and hypercarbia occur rapidly during convulsions due to the increased muscular activity, together with the interference with respiration. In severe cases even apnoea may occur. The respiratory and metabolic acidosis increases and extends the toxic effects of local anaesthetics.

Recovery follows the redistribution of the local anaesthetic drug from the central nervous system and subsequent metabolism and excretion. Recovery may be rapid unless large amounts of the drug have been injected. However, permanent neurological damage after accidental sub-arachnoid injection can occur.

Cardiovascular toxicity: Cardiovascular toxicity indicates a more severe situation. Hypotension, bradycardia, arrhythmia and even cardiac arrest may occur as a result of high systemic concentrations of local anaesthetics. In volunteers the intravenous infusion of ropivacaine resulted in signs of depression of conductivity and contractility.

Cardiovascular toxicity effects are generally preceded by signs of toxicity in the central nervous system, unless the patient is receiving a general anaesthetic or is heavily sedated with drugs such as benzodiazepines or barbiturates.

Treatment of acute toxicity: Equipment and drugs necessary for monitoring and emergency resuscitation should be immediately available. If signs of acute systemic toxicity appear, injection of the local anaesthetic should be stopped immediately.

In the event of convulsions, treatment will be required. The objectives of treatment are to maintain oxygenation, stop the convulsions and support the circulation. Oxygen must be given and ventilation assisted, when necessary (mask and bag). An anticonvulsant should be given intravenously if the convulsions do not stop spontaneously in 15–20 seconds. Thiopentone 100–150 mg intravenously will abort the convulsions rapidly. Alternatively diazepam 5–10 mg intravenously may be used, although its action is slower. Suxamethonium will stop the muscle convulsions rapidly, but the patient will require controlled ventilation and tracheal intubation.

If cardiovascular depression is evident (hypotension, bradycardia), ephedrine 5–10 mg intravenously should be given and repeated, if necessary, after 2–3 minutes.

Should circulatory arrest occur, immediate cardiopulmonary resuscitation should be instituted. Optimal oxygenation and ventilation and circulatory support as well as treatment of acidosis are of vital importance.

Pharmacological properties

Pharmacodynamic properties: Ropivacaine is a long-acting amide-type local anaesthetic developed as a pure enantiomer. It has both anaesthetic and analgesic effects. At high doses it produces surgical anaesthesia, while at lower doses it produces sensory block with limited and non-progressive motor block.

The mechanism is a reversible reduction of the membrane permeability of the nerve fibre to sodium ions. Consequently the depolarisation velocity is decreased and the excitable threshold increased, resulting in a local blockade of nerve impulses.

The most characteristic property of ropivacaine is the long duration of action. Onset and duration of the local anaesthetic efficacy are dependant upon the administration site, but are not influenced by the presence of a vasoconstrictor (e.g. adrenaline). For details concerning the onset and duration of action, see table under *"Posology and method of administration"*.

Healthy volunteers exposed to intravenous infusions tolerated ropivacaine well. The clinical experience with this drug indicates a good margin of safety.

Pharmacokinetic properties: The plasma concentration of ropivacaine depends upon the dose, the route of administration and the vascularity of the injection site. Ropivacaine follows linear pharmacokinetics and the C_{max} is proportional to the dose.

Ropivacaine shows complete and biphasic absorption from the epidural space with half-lives of the two phases of the order of 14 min and 4 h. The slow absorption is the rate-limiting factor in the elimination of ropivacaine, which explains why the apparent elimination half-life is longer after epidural than after intravenous administration.

Ropivacaine has a total plasma clearance in the order of 440 ml/min, a renal clearance of 1 ml/min, a volume of distribution at steady state of 47 litres and a terminal half-life of 1.8 h. Ropivacaine has an intermediate hepatic extraction ratio of about 0.4. It is mainly bound to α_1-acid glycoprotein in plasma with an unbound fraction of about 6%.

An increase in total plasma concentrations during continuous epidural infusion has been observed, related to a postoperative increase of α_1-acid glycoprotein.

Variations in unbound, i.e. pharmacologically active, concentration have been much less than in total plasma concentration.

Ropivacaine readily crosses the placenta and equilibrium in regard to unbound concentration will be rapidly reached. The degree of plasma protein binding in the foetus is less than in the mother, which results in lower total plasma concentrations in the foetus than in the mother.

Ropivacaine is extensively metabolised, predominantly by aromatic hydroxylation. In total, 86% of the dose is excreted in the urine after intravenous administration, of which only about 1% relates to unchanged drug. The major metabolite is 3-hydroxy-ropivacaine, about 37% of which is excreted in the urine, mainly conjugated. Urinary excretion of 4-hydroxy-ropivacaine, the N-dealkylated metabolite and the 4-hydroxy-dealkylated accounts for 1-3%. Conjugated+unconjugated 3-hydroxy-ropivacaine shows only detectable concentrations in plasma. 3-hydroxy and 4-hydroxy-ropivacaine have a local anaesthetic activity although less than that of ropivacaine.

There is no evidence of *in vivo* racemisation of ropivacaine.

Preclinical safety data: Results from mutagenicity studies do not give indications of a relevant mutagenicity potential of ropivacaine.

Pharmaceutical particulars

List of excipients: All forms: Sodium chloride, hydrochloric acid, sodium hydroxide, water for injections.

Incompatibilities: Naropin should not be diluted or mixed with other solutions. In alkaline solutions precipitation may occur as ropivacaine shows poor solubility at pH > 6.0.

Shelf life: Ampoule (Polyamp):*

Naropin Polyamp	2 mg/ml	3 years
Naropin Polyamp	7.5 mg/ml	3 years
Naropin Polyamp	10 mg/ml	3 years

The expiry date is shown on the package.

Infusion bag (Polybag):*

Naropin Infusion 2 mg/ml: 2 years. The expiry date is shown on the package.

Special precautions for storage: Store between 15–30°C. Avoid freezing. Store out of reach of children.

Nature and contents of containers:

Naropin Polyamp 2 mg/ml:

10 ml polypropylene ampoules (Polyamp) in packs of 5 and 10

10 ml polypropylene ampoules (Polyamp) in sterile blister packs of 5 and **10†**

20 ml polypropylene ampoules (Polyamp) in packs of 5 and 10

20 ml polypropylene ampoules (Polyamp) in sterile blister packs of 5 and *10*

Naropin Polyamp 7.5 mg/ml:

10 ml polypropylene ampoules (Polyamp) in packs of 5 and 10

10 ml polypropylene ampoules (Polyamp) in sterile blister packs of 5 and **10†**

20 ml polypropylene ampoules (Polyamp) in packs of 5 and 10

20 ml polypropylene ampoules (Polyamp) in sterile blister packs of 5 and 10

Naropin Polyamp 10 mg/ml:

10 ml polypropylene ampoules (Polyamp) in packs of 5 and 10

10 ml polypropylene ampoules (Polyamp) in sterile blister packs of 5 and **10†**

20 ml polypropylene ampoules (Polyamp) in packs of 5 and 10

20 ml polypropylene ampoules (Polyamp) in sterile blister packs of 5 and 10

Naropin Infusion 2 mg/ml:

100 ml polypropylene bags (Polybag) in sterile blister packs of 5†

200 ml polypropylene bags (Polybag) in sterile blister packs of 5†

The polypropylene ampoules (Polyamp) are specially designed to fit Luer lock and Luer fit syringes.

† Only those pack sizes highlighted in bold are available in the UK.

Instructions for use/handling: Naropin products are preservative free and are intended for single use only. Discard any unused solution.

The intact container must not be re-autoclaved. A blistered container should be chosen when a sterile outside is required.

Marketing authorisation number(s)

Naropin Polyamp 2 mg/ml	PL 0017/0375
Naropin Polyamp 7.5 mg/ml	PL 0017/0377
Naropin Polyamp 10 mg/ml	PL 0017/0378
Naropin Infusion 2 mg/ml	PL 0017/0376

Date of approval/revision of SPC 17 May 1996

Legal category POM.

OXIS* TURBOHALER* 6 ▼

Qualitative and quantitative composition Each delivered dose (i.e. the dose leaving the mouthpiece) from Oxis Turbohaler 6 contains 4.5 micrograms formoterol fumarate dihydrate which is derived from a metered dose of 6 micrograms.

Formoterol INN is also known as eformoterol BAN.

Pharmaceutical form Inhalation powder.

Clinical particulars

Therapeutic indications: Oxis Turbohaler is indicated for the relief of broncho-obstructive symptoms in asthmatics when adequate treatment with corticosteroids is not sufficient.

Posology and method of administration:

Adults: Normal dosage: 1 or 2 actuations once or twice daily. The dose can be administered in the morning and/or at night. Some patients may need 4 actuations once or twice daily. The maximum daily dose is 8 actuations. In the case of nocturnal asthma symptoms the dosage may be given as a single administration at night. The duration of action has in clinical studies been shown to last for about 12 hours. The treatment should always aim for the lowest effective dose. **NB** A higher strength is available as an alternative for patients requiring 2 or more actuations.

Children: The use of Oxis Turbohaler in children has not been documented.

Special patient groups: No adjustment of dose should be required in the elderly, or in patients with renal or hepatic impairment at the recommended normal doses. (See Special warnings and special precautions for use.)

Contra-indications: Hypersensitivity to formoterol or to inhaled lactose.

Special warnings and special precautions for use: Asthmatic patients who require therapy with β_2-agonists, should also receive optimal anti-inflammatory therapy with corticosteroids. Oxis Turbohaler should only be used in patients requiring long-term regular bronchodilator therapy and not as an alternative to short-acting β-agonists used "on demand" or in the event of an acute attack. Patients must be advised to continue taking their anti-inflammatory therapy after the introduction of Oxis Turbohaler even when symptoms decrease. Should symptoms persist, or treatment with β_2-agonists need to be increased, this indicates a worsening of the underlying condition and warrants a reassessment of the asthma therapy. Therapy should not be initiated or the dose increased during an exacerbation. In the event of an acute attack, a β-agonist with a short duration of action should be used.

Caution should be observed when treating patients with thyrotoxicosis phaeochromocytoma, hypertrophic obstructive cardiomyopathy, idiopathic subvalvular aortic stenosis, severe hypertension, aneurysm or other severe cardiovascular disorders, such as ischaemic heart disease, tachyarrhythmias or severe heart failure.

Caution should be observed when treating patients with prolongation of the QTc-interval. Formoterol itself may induce prolongation of the QTc-interval.

Due to the hyperglycaemic effects of β_2-agonists, additional blood glucose monitoring is recommended initially in diabetic patients.

Potentially serious hypokalaemia may result from β_2-agonist therapy. Particular caution is recommended in acute severe asthma as the associated risk may be augmented by hypoxia. The hypokalaemic effect may be potentiated by concomitant treatment with xanthine-derivatives, steroids and diuretics. The serum potassium levels should therefore be monitored.

As with other inhalation therapy, the potential for paradoxical bronchospasm should be considered.

Oxis Turbohaler contains lactose 450 micrograms per delivered dose (corresponding to 600 micrograms per metered dose). This amount does not normally cause problems in lactose intolerant people.

Children up to the age of 12 years should not be treated with Oxis Turbohaler, as insufficient experience is available for this group.

The effect of decreased liver or kidney function on the pharmacokinetics of formoterol and the pharmacokinetics in the elderly is not known. As formoterol is primarily eliminated via metabolism an increased exposure can be expected in patients with severe liver cirrhosis.

Interaction with other medicaments and other forms of interaction: No specific interaction studies have been carried out with Oxis Turbohaler.

Concomitant treatment with other sympathomimetic substances may potentiate the undesirable effects of Oxis Turbohaler.

Concomitant treatment with xanthine derivatives, steroids or diuretics may potentiate a possible hypokalaemic effect of β_2-agonists. Hypokalaemia may increase the disposition towards arrhythmias in patients who are treated with digitalis glycosides.

Concomitant treatment with quinidine, disopyramide, procainamide, phenothiazines, antihistamines (terfenadine), monoamine oxidase inhibitors and tricyclic antidepressants can prolong the QTc-interval and increase the risk of ventricular arrhythmias.

In addition L-Dopa, L-thyroxine, oxytocin and alcohol can impair cardiac tolerance towards β_2-sympathomimetics.

Concomitant treatment with monoamine oxidase inhibitors including agents with similar properties such as furazolidone and procarbazine may precipitate hypertensive reactions.

There is an elevated risk of arrhythmias in patients receiving concomitant anaesthesia with halogenated hydrocarbons.

β-adrenergic blockers can weaken or inhibit the effect of Oxis Turbohaler. Oxis Turbohaler should therefore not be given together with β-adrenergic blockers (including eye drops) unless there are compelling reasons.

Pregnancy and lactation: Clinical experience in pregnant women is limited. In animal studies formoterol has caused implantation losses as well as decreased early postnatal survival and birth weight. The effects appeared at considerably higher systemic exposures than those reached during clinical use of Oxis Turbohaler. During pregnancy, Oxis Turbohaler should, until further experience is available, only be used after special consideration, especially during the first three months and shortly before delivery.

It is not known whether formoterol passes into human breast milk. Oxis Turbohaler should therefore not be given to mothers who are breast feeding their infants. In rats, small amounts of formoterol have been detected in maternal milk.

Effects on the ability to drive and use machines: Oxis Turbohaler does not affect the ability to drive or use machines.

Undesirable effects:

Common (>1/100)	*Central nervous system:*	Headache
	Cardiovascular system:	Palpitations
	Musculoskeletal system:	Tremor
Uncommon	*Central nervous system:*	Agitation, restlessness, sleep disturbances
	Musculoskeletal system:	Muscle cramps
	Cardiovascular system:	Tachycardia
Very rare (<1/1000)	*Skin:*	Exanthema, urticaria, pruritus
	Respiratory tract:	Bronchospasm
	Metabolic:	Hypokalaemia/ hyperkalaemia

Tremor and palpitations may occur, but tend to be transient and reduce with regular therapy. As with all inhalation therapy, paradoxical bronchospasm may occur in very rare cases.

In isolated cases the following undesirable effects have been reported: Nausea, taste disturbances, dizziness, angina pectoris, variations in the blood pressure, and hyperglycaemia.

Treatment with β_2-sympathomimetics may result in an increase in blood levels of insulin, free fatty acids, glycerol and ketone bodies.

Overdose: There is no clinical experience on the management of overdose. An overdose would likely lead to effects that are typical of β_2-agonists: tremor, headache, palpitations, and tachycardia. Hypotension, metabolic acidosis, hypokalaemia and hyperglycaemia may also occur. Supportive and symptomatic treatment is indicated.

Use of cardioselective β-blockers may be considered, but only subject to extreme caution since the use of β-adrenergic blocker medication may provoke bronchospasm. Serum potassium should be monitored.

Pharmacological properties

Pharmacodynamic properties: Formoterol is a selective β_2-adrenoceptor agonist that produces relaxation of bronchial smooth muscle. Formoterol thus has a bronchodilating effect in patients with reversible airways obstruction. The bronchodilating effect sets in rapidly, within 1–3 minutes after inhalation and has a mean duration of 12 hours after a single dose.

Pharmacokinetic properties: Absorption: Inhaled formoterol is rapidly absorbed. Peak plasma concentration is reached about 15 minutes after inhalation.

In studies the mean lung deposition of formoterol after inhalation via Turbohaler ranged from 28–49% of the delivered dose (corresponding to 21–37% of the metered dose). The total systemic availability for the higher lung deposition was around 61% of the delivered dose (corresponding to 46% of the metered dose).

Distribution and metabolism: Plasma protein binding is approximately 50%.

Formoterol is metabolised via direct glucuronidation and O-demethylation. The enzyme responsible for O-demethylation has not been identified. Total plasma clearance and volume of distribution has not been determined.

Elimination: The major part of the dose of formoterol is eliminated via metabolism. After inhalation 8–13% of the delivered dose (corresponding to 6–10% of the metered dose) of formoterol is excreted unmetabolised in the urine. About 20% of an intravenous dose is excreted unchanged in the urine. The terminal half-life after inhalation is estimated to be 8 hours.

Preclinical safety data: The effects of formoterol seen in toxicity studies in rats and dogs were mainly on the cardiovascular system and consisted of hyperaemia, tachycardia, arrhythmias and myocardial lesions. These effects are known pharmacological manifestations seen after the administration of high doses of β_2-agonists.

A somewhat reduced fertility in male rats was observed at high systemic exposure to formoterol.

No genotoxic effects of formoterol have been observed in *in-vitro* or *in-vivo* tests. In rats and mice a slight increase in the incidence of benign uterine leiomyomas has been observed. This effect is looked upon as a class-effect observed in rodents after long exposure to high doses of β_2-agonists.

Pharmaceutical particulars

List of excipients: Lactose monohydrate.

Incompatibilities: None stated.

Shelf life: 2 years.

Special precautions for storage: Should be stored with cover tightened.

Nature and contents of container: Oxis Turbohaler is a multidose, inspiratory flow driven, dry powder inhaler. The inhaler is made of plastic parts.

Each inhaler contains 60 doses.

Instructions for use/handling: Oxis Turbohaler is inspiratory flow driven which means that, when the patient inhales through the mouthpiece, the substance will follow the inspired air into the airways.

NOTE. It is important to instruct the patient to breathe in forcefully and deeply through the mouthpiece to ensure that an optimal dose is obtained.

The patient may not taste or feel any medication when using Oxis Turbohaler due to the small amount of drug dispensed.

Detailed instructions for use are packed together with each inhaler.

Marketing authorisation number PL 00017/0386

Date of approval/revision of SPC March 1997

Legal Category POM.

OXIS* TURBOHALER* 12 ▼

Qualitative and quantitative composition Each delivered dose (i.e. the dose leaving the mouthpiece) from Oxis Turbohaler 12 contains 9 micrograms formoterol fumarate dihydrate which is derived from a metered dose of 12 micrograms.

Formoterol INN is also known as eformoterol BAN.

Pharmaceutical form Inhalation powder.

Clinical particulars

Therapeutic indications: Oxis Turbohaler is indicated for the relief of broncho-obstructive symptoms in asthmatics when adequate treatment with corticosteroids is not sufficient.

Posology and method of administration:

Adults: Normal dosage: 1 actuation once or twice daily. The dose can be administered in the morning and/or at night. Some patients may need 2 actuations once or twice daily. The maximum daily dose is 4 actuations. In the case of nocturnal asthma symptoms the dosage may be given as a single administration at night. The duration of action has in clinical studies been shown to last for about 12 hours. The treatment should always aim for the lowest effective dose. **NB** A lower strength is also available.

Children: The use of Oxis Turbohaler in children has not been documented.

Special patient groups: No adjustment of dose should be required in the elderly, or in patients with renal or hepatic impairment at the recommended normal doses. (See Special warnings and special precautions for use.)

Contra-indications: Hypersensitivity to formoterol or to inhaled lactose.

Special warnings and special precautions for use: Asthmatic patients who require therapy with β_2-agonists, should also receive optimal anti-inflammatory therapy with corticosteroids. Oxis Turbohaler should only be used in patients requiring long-term regular bronchodilator therapy and not as an alternative to short-acting β-agonists used "on demand" or in the event of an acute attack. Patients must be advised to continue taking their anti-inflammatory therapy after the introduction of Oxis Turbohaler even when symptoms decrease. Should symptoms persist, or treatment with β_2-agonists need to be increased, this indicates a worsening of the underlying condition and warrants a reassessment of the asthma therapy. Therapy should not be initiated or the dose increased during an exacerbation. In the event of an acute attack, a β-agonist with a short duration of action should be used.

Caution should be observed when treating patients with thyrotoxicosis phaeochromocytoma, hypertrophic obstructive cardiomyopathy, idiopathic subvalvular aortic stenosis, severe hypertension, aneurysm or other severe cardiovascular disorders, such as ischaemic heart disease, tachyarrhythmias or severe heart failure.

Caution should be observed when treating patients with prolongation of the QTc-interval. Formoterol itself may induce prolongation of the QTc-interval.

Due to the hyperglycaemic effects of β_2-agonists, additional blood glucose monitoring is recommended initially in diabetic patients.

Potentially serious hypokalaemia may result from β_2-agonist therapy. Particular caution is recommended in acute severe asthma as the associated risk may be augmented by hypoxia. The hypokalaemic effect may be potentiated by concomitant treatment with xanthine-derivatives, steroids and diuretics. The serum potassium levels should therefore be monitored.

As with other inhalation therapy, the potential for paradoxical bronchospasm should be considered.

Oxis Turbohaler contains lactose 450 micrograms per delivered dose (corresponding to 600 micrograms per metered dose). This amount does not normally cause problems in lactose intolerant people.

Children up to the age of 12 years should not be treated with Oxis Turbohaler, as insufficient experience is available for this group.

The effect of decreased liver or kidney function on the pharmacokinetics of formoterol and the pharmacokinetics in the elderly is not known. As formoterol is primarily eliminated via metabolism an increased exposure can be expected in patients with severe liver cirrhosis.

Interaction with other medicaments and other forms of interaction: No specific interaction studies have been carried out with Oxis Turbohaler.

Concomitant treatment with other sympathomimetic substances may potentiate the undesirable effects of Oxis Turbohaler.

Concomitant treatment with xanthine derivatives, steroids or diuretics may potentiate a possible hypokalaemic effect of β_2-agonists. Hypokalaemia may increase the disposition towards arrhythmias in patients who are treated with digitalis glycosides.

Concomitant treatment with quinidine, disopyramide, procainamide, phenothiazines, antihistamines (terfenadine), monoamine oxidase inhibitors and tricyclic antidepressants can prolong the QTc-interval and increase the risk of ventricular arrhythmias.

In addition L-Dopa, L-thyroxine, oxytocin and alcohol can impair cardiac tolerance towards β_2-sympathomimetics.

Concomitant treatment with monoamine oxidase inhibitors including agents with similar properties such as furazolidone and procarbazine may precipitate hypertensive reactions.

There is an elevated risk of arrhythmias in patients receiving concomitant anaesthesia with halogenated hydrocarbons.

β-adrenergic blockers can weaken or inhibit the effect of Oxis Turbohaler. Oxis Turbohaler should therefore not be given together with β-adrenergic blockers (including eye drops) unless there are compelling reasons.

Pregnancy and lactation: Clinical experience in pregnant women is limited. In animal studies formoterol has caused implantation losses as well as decreased early postnatal survival and birth weight. The effects appeared at considerably higher systemic exposures than those reached during clinical use of Oxis Turbohaler. During pregnancy Oxis Turbohaler should, until further experience is available, only be used after special consideration, especially during the first three months and shortly before delivery.

It is not known whether formoterol passes into human breast milk. Oxis Turbohaler should therefore not be given to mothers who are breast feeding their infants. In rats, small amounts of formoterol have been detected in maternal milk.

Effects on the ability to drive and use machines: Oxis Turbohaler does not affect the ability to drive or use machines.

Undesirable effects:

Common (>1/100)	*Central nervous system:*	Headache
	Cardiovascular system:	Palpitations
	Musculoskeletal system:	Tremor
Uncommon	*Central nervous system:*	Agitation, restlessness, sleep disturbances
	Musculoskeletal system:	Muscle cramps
	Cardiovascular system:	Tachycardia
Very rare (<1/1000)	*Skin:*	Exanthema, urticaria, pruritus
	Respiratory tract:	Bronchospasm
	Metabolic:	Hypokalaemia/ hyperkalaemia

Tremor and palpitations may occur, but tend to be transient and reduce with regular therapy. As with all inhalation therapy, paradoxical bronchospasm may occur in very rare cases.

In isolated cases the following undesirable effects have been reported: Nausea, taste disturbances, dizziness, angina pectoris, variations in the blood pressure, and hyperglycaemia.

Treatment with β_2-sympathomimetics may result in an increase in blood levels of insulin, free fatty acids, glycerol and ketone bodies.

Overdose: There is no clinical experience on the management of overdose. An overdose would likely lead to effects that are typical of β_2-agonists: tremor, headache, palpitations, and tachycardia. Hypotension, metabolic acidosis, hypokalaemia and hyperglycaemia may also occur. Supportive and symptomatic treatment is indicated.

Use of cardioselective β-blockers may be considered, but only subject to extreme caution since the use of β-adrenergic blocker medication may provoke bronchospasm. Serum potassium should be monitored.

Pharmacological properties

Pharmacodynamic properties: Formoterol is a selective β_2-adrenoceptor agonist that produces relaxation of bronchial smooth muscle. Formoterol thus has a bronchodilating effect in patients with reversible airways obstruction. The bronchodilating effect sets in rapidly, within 1–3 minutes after inhalation and has a mean duration of 12 hours after a single dose.

Pharmacokinetic properties: Absorption: Inhaled formoterol is rapidly absorbed. Peak plasma concentration is reached about 15 minutes after inhalation.

In studies the mean lung deposition of formoterol after inhalation via Turbohaler ranged from 28–49% of the delivered dose (corresponding to 21–37% of the metered dose). The total systemic availability for the higher lung deposition was around 61% of the delivered dose (corresponding to 46% of the metered dose).

Distribution and metabolism: Plasma protein binding is approximately 50%.

Formoterol is metabolised via direct glucuronidation and O-demethylation. The enzyme responsible for O-demethylation has not been identified. Total plasma clearance and volume of distribution has not been determined.

Elimination: The major part of the dose of formoterol is eliminated via metabolism. After inhalation 8–13% of the delivered dose (corresponding to 6–10% of the metered dose) of formoterol is excreted unmetabolised in the urine. About 20% of an intravenous dose is excreted unchanged in the urine. The terminal half-life after inhalation is estimated to be 8 hours.

Preclinical safety data: The effects of formoterol seen in toxicity studies in rats and dogs were mainly on the cardiovascular system and consisted of hyperaemia, tachycardia, arrhythmias and myocardial lesions. These effects are known pharmacological manifestations seen after the administration of high doses of β_2-agonists.

A somewhat reduced fertility in male rats was observed at high systemic exposure to formoterol.

No genotoxic effects of formoterol have been observed in *in-vitro* or *in-vivo* tests. In rats and mice a slight increase in the incidence of benign uterine leiomyomas has been observed. This effect is looked upon as a class-effect observed in rodents after long exposure to high doses of β_2-agonists.

Pharmaceutical particulars

List of excipients: Lactose monohydrate.

Incompatibilities: None stated.

Shelf life: 2 years.

Special precautions for storage: Should be stored with cover tightened.

Nature and contents of container: Oxis Turbohaler is a multidose, inspiratory flow driven, dry powder inhaler. The inhaler is made of plastic parts.

Each inhaler contains 60 doses.

Instructions for use/handling: Oxis Turbohaler is inspiratory flow driven which means that, when the patient inhales through the mouthpiece, the substance will follow the inspired air into the airways.

NOTE. It is important to instruct the patient to breathe in forcefully and deeply through the mouthpiece to ensure that an optimal dose is obtained.

The patient may not taste or feel any medication when using Oxis Turbohaler due to the small amount of drug dispensed.

Detailed instructions for use are packed together with each inhaler.

Marketing authorisation number PL00017/0387

Date of approval/revision of SPC March 1997

Legal Category POM.

PLENDIL* 2.5 mg, 5 mg and 10 mg

Qualitative and quantitative composition

Plendil 2.5 mg contains Felodipine PhEur 2.5 mg.
Plendil 5 mg contains Felodipine PhEur 5 mg.
Plendil 10 mg contains Felodipine PhEur 10 mg.

Pharmaceutical form Circular bi-convex film coated extended-release tablets.

Plendil 2.5 mg - yellow tablets coded A/FL and 2.5 on the reverse.

Plendil 5 mg - pink tablets coded A/FM and 5 on the reverse.

Plendil 10 mg - red-brown tablets coded A/FE and 10 on the reverse.

Clinical particulars

Therapeutic indications: In the management of hypertension and prophylaxis of chronic stable angina pectoris.

Posology and method of administration: For oral administration

Hypertension:

Adults (including elderly): The dose should be adjusted to the individual requirements of the patient. The recommended starting dose is 5 mg once daily. If necessary the dose may be further increased or another antihypertensive agent added. The usual maintenance dose is 5–10 mg once daily. Doses higher than 20 mg daily are not usually needed. For dose titration purposes a 2.5 mg tablet is available. In elderly patients an initial treatment with 2.5 mg daily should be considered.

Angina pectoris:

Adults: The dose should be adjusted individually. Treatment should be started with 5 mg once daily and if needed be increased to 10 mg once daily.

Administration: The tablets should be taken in the morning irrespective of food intake. Plendil tablets must not be chewed or crushed. They should be swallowed whole with half a glass of water.

Children: The safety and efficacy of Plendil in children has not been established.

Plendil can be used in combination with β-blockers, ACE inhibitors or diuretics. The effects on blood pressure are likely to be additive and combination therapy will usually enhance the antihypertensive effect. Care should be taken to avoid hypotension. In patients with severely impaired liver function the dose of felodipine should be low. The pharmacokinetics are not significantly affected in patients with impaired renal function.

Contra-indications:

Unstable angina pectoris.

Pregnancy.

Patient with a previous allergic reaction to Plendil or other dihydropyridines because of the theoretical risk of cross-reactivity.

Plendil should not be used in patients with clinically significant aortic stenosis, and during or within one month of a myocardial infarction.

As with other calcium channel blockers, Plendil should be discontinued in patients who develop cardiogenic shock.

Special warnings and special precautions for use: As with other vasodilators, Plendil may, in rare cases, precipitate significant hypotension with tachycardia which in susceptible individuals may result in myocardial ischaemia.

There is no evidence that Plendil is useful for secondary prevention of myocardial infarction.

The efficacy and safety of Plendil in the treatment of malignant hypertension has not been studied.

Plendil should be used with caution in patients with severe left ventricular dysfunction.

Interaction with other medicaments and other forms of interaction: Concomitant administration of substances which interfere with the cytochrome P450 system may affect plasma concentrations of felodipine. Enzyme inhibitors such as cimetidine, erythromycin and itraconazole impair the elimination of felodipine, and Plendil dosage may need to be reduced when drugs are given concomitantly. Conversely, powerful enzyme inducing agents such as some anticonvulsants (phenytoin, carbamazepine, phenobarbitone) can increase felodipine elimination and higher than normal Plendil doses may be required in patients taking the drugs.

No dosage adjustment is required when Plendil is given concomitantly with digoxin.

Felodipine does not appear to affect the unbound fraction of other extensively plasma protein bound drugs such as warfarin.

Grapefruit juice results in increased peak plasma levels and bioavailability possibly due to an interaction with flavonoids in the fruit juice. This interaction has been seen with other dihydropyridine calcium antagonists and represents a class effect. Therefore grapefruit juice should not be taken together with Plendil tablets.

Pregnancy and lactation: Felodipine should not be given during pregnancy.

In a study on fertility and general reproductive performance in rats, a prolongation of parturition resulting in difficult labour, increased foetal deaths and early postnatal deaths were observed in the medium- and high-dose groups. Reproductive studies in rabbits have shown a dose-related reversible enlargement of the mammary glands of the parent animals and dose-related digital abnormalities in the foetuses when felodipine was administered during stages of early foetal development.

Felodipine has been detected in breast milk, but it is unknown whether it has harmful effects on the newborn.

Effects on ability to drive and use machines: None.

Undesirable effects: As with other calcium antagonists, flushing, headache, palpitations, dizziness and fatigue may occur. These reactions are usually transient and are most likely to occur at the start of treatment or after an increase in dosage.

As with other calcium antagonists ankle swelling, resulting from precapillary vasodilation, may occur. The degree of ankle swelling is dose related.

In patients with gingivitis/periodontitis, mild gingival enlargement has been reported with Plendil, as with other calcium antagonists. The enlargement can be avoided or reversed by careful dental hygiene.

As with other dihydropyridines, aggravation of angina has been reported in a small number of individuals especially after starting treatment. This is more likely to happen in patients with symptomatic ischaemic heart disease.

The following adverse events have been reported from clinical trials and from Post Marketing Surveillance. In the great majority of cases a causal relationship between these events and treatment with felodipine has not been established.

Skin: rarely – rash and/or pruritus, and isolated cases of photosensitivity.

Musculoskeletal: in isolated cases arthralgia and myalgia.

Central and peripheral nervous system: headache, dizziness. In isolated cases paraesthesia.

Gastrointestinal: in isolated cases nausea, gum hyperplasia.

Hepatic: in isolated cases increased liver enzymes.

Cardiovascular: rarely – tachycardia, palpitations and syncope.

Vascular (extracardiac): peripheral oedema, flush.

Other: rarely – fatigue, in isolated cases hypersensitivity reactions e.g. urticaria, angiooedema.

Overdose: Symptoms: Overdosage may cause excessive peripheral vasodilatation with marked hypotension which may sometimes be accompanied by bradycardia.

Management: Severe hypotension should be treated symptomatically, with the patient placed supine and the legs elevated. Bradycardia, if present, should be treated with atropine 0.5–1 mg i.v. If this is not sufficient, plasma volume should be increased by infusion of e.g. glucose, saline or dextran. Sympathomimetic drugs with predominant effect on the α_1-adrenoceptor may be given e.g. metaraminol or phenylephrine.

Pharmacological properties

Pharmacodynamic properties: Felodipine is a vascular selective calcium antagonist, which lowers arterial blood pressure by decreasing peripheral vascular resistance. Due to the high degree of selectivity for smooth muscle in the arterioles, felodipine in therapeutic doses has no direct effect on cardiac contractility or conduction.

It can be used as monotherapy or in combination with other antihypertensive drugs, e.g. β-receptor blockers, diuretics or ACE-inhibitors, in order to achieve an increased antihypertensive effect. Felodipine reduces both systolic and diastolic blood pressure and can be used in isolated systolic hypertension. In a study of 12 patients, felodipine maintained its antihypertensive effect during concomitant therapy with indomethacin.

Because there is no effect on venous smooth muscle or adrenergic vasomotor control, felodipine is not associated with orthostatic hypotension.

Felodipine has anti-anginal and anti-ischaemic effects due to improved myocardial oxygen supply/demand balance. Coronary vascular resistance is decreased and coronary blood flow as well as myocardial oxygen supply are increased by felodipine due to dilation of both epicardial arteries and arterioles. Felodipine effectively counteracts coronary vasospasm. The reduction in systemic blood pressure caused by felodipine leads to decreased left ventricular afterload.

Felodipine improves exercise tolerance and reduces anginal attacks in patients with stable effort induced angina pectoris. Both symptomatic and silent myocardial ischaemia are reduced by felodipine in patients with vasospastic angina. Felodipine can be used as monotherapy or in combination with β-receptor blockers in patients with stable angina pectoris.

Felodipine possesses a mild natriuretic/diuretic effect and generalised fluid retention does not occur.

Felodipine is well tolerated in patients with concomitant disease such as congestive heart failure well-controlled on appropriate therapy, asthma and other obstructive pulmonary diseases, diabetes, gout, hyperlipideamia, impaired renal function, renal transplant recipients and Raynaud's disease. Felodipine has no significant effect on blood glucose levels or lipid profiles.

Haemodynamic effects: The primary haemodynamic effect of felodipine is a reduction of total peripheral vascular resistance which leads to a decrease in blood pressure. These effects are dose-dependent. In patients with mild to moderate essential hypertension, a reduction in blood pressure usually occurs 2 hours after the first oral dose and lasts for at least 24 hours with a trough/peak ratio usually above 50%.

Plasma concentration of felodipine and decrease in total peripheral resistance and blood pressure are positively correlated.

Electrophysiological and other cardiac effects: Felodipine in therapeutic doses has no effect on cardiac contractility or atrioventricular conduction or refractoriness.

Renal effects: Felodipine has a natriuretic and diuretic effect. Studies have shown that the tubular reabsorption of filtered sodium is reduced. This counteracts the salt and water retention observed for other vasodilators. Felodipine does not affect the daily potassium excretion. The renal vascular resistance is decreased by felodipine. Normal glomerular filtration rate is unchanged. In patients with impaired renal function glomerular filtration rate may increase.

Felodipine is well tolerated in renal transplant recipients.

Site and mechanism of action: The predominant pharmacodynamic feature of felodipine is its pronounced vascular versus myocardial selectivity. Myogenically active smooth muscles in arterial resistance vessels are particularly sensitive to felodipine.

Felodipine inhibits electrical and contractile activity of vascular smooth muscle cells via an effect on the calcium channels in the cell membrane.

Pharmacokinetic properties: Absorption and distribution: Felodipine is completely absorbed from the gastrointestinal tract after administration of felodipine extended release tablets.

The systemic availability of felodipine is approximately 15% in man and is independent of dose in the therapeutic dose range.

With the extended-release tablets the absorption phase is prolonged. This results in even felodipine plasma concentrations within the therapeutic range for 24 hours.

The plasma protein binding of felodipine is approximately 99%. It is bound predominantly to the albumin fraction.

Elimination and metabolism: The average half-life of felodipine in the terminal phase is 25 hours. There is no significant accumulation during long-term treatment. Felodipine is extensively metabolised by the liver and all identified metabolites are inactive. Elderly patients and patients with reduced liver function have an average higher plasma concentration of felodipine than younger patients.

About 70% of a given dose is excreted as metabolites in the urine; the remaining fraction is excreted in the faeces. Less than 0.5% of a dose is recovered unchanged in the urine.

The kinetics of felodipine are not changed in patients with renal impairment.

Preclinical safety data: Felodipine is a calcium antagonist and lowers arterial blood pressure by decreasing vascular resistance. In general a reduction in blood pressure is evident 2 hours after the first oral dose and at steady state lasts for at least 24 hours after dose.

Felodipine exhibits a high degree of selectivity for smooth muscles in the arterioles and in therapeutic doses has no direct effect on cardiac contractility. Felodipine does not affect venous smooth muscle and adrenergic vasomotor control.

Electrophysiological studies have shown that felodipine has no direct effect on conduction in the specialised conducting system of the heart and no effect on the AV nodal refractories.

Plendil possesses a mild natriuretic/diuretic effect and does not produce general fluid retention, nor affect daily potassium excretion. Plendil is well tolerated in patients with congestive heart failure.

Pharmaceutical particulars

List of Excipients: Polyoxyl 40 hydrogenated castor oil, Hydroxypropyl cellulose, Propyl gallate, Hydroxypropyl methylcellulose, Sodium aluminium silicate, Microcrystalline cellulose, Lactose anhydrous, Sodium stearyl fumarate, Polyethylene glycol, Colour Titanium dioxide (E171), Colour Iron oxide yellow (E172) and Carnauba wax.

Incompatibilities: None stated.

Shelf-life: 3 years.

Special precautions for storage: Store below 30°C.

Nature and contents of container: PVC/PVDC Blisters: Press through blister package of PVC/PVDC form foil with an aluminium foil as enclosure web. Each blister strip contains 7 tablets. A single pack contains 28 tablets as multiples of blisters of 7.

Marketing authorisation number

Plendil 2.5 mg	PL 0017/0349
Plendil 5 mg	PL 0017/0301
Plendil 10 mg	PL 0017/0302

Date of approval/revision of SPC Plendil 2.5 mg, 5 mg and 10 mg February 1997

PULMICORT*

Presentation Pulmicort Inhaler is a metered dose aerosol delivering 200 micrograms budesonide per actuation via a standard or Spacer adapter. Pulmicort L.S. Inhaler is a metered dose aerosol delivering 50 micrograms budesonide per actuation via a standard or L.S. Spacer adapter.

Inactive ingredients: Sorbitan trioleate and chlorofluorocarbons 11, 12 and 114.

Uses Pulmicort Inhaler and Pulmicort LS Inhaler contain the potent, non-halogenated corticosteroid budesonide. Inhaled budesonide possesses a local anti-inflammatory action in the lungs with a lower incidence and severity of adverse effects than those seen with oral corticosteroids.

Pulmicort is recommended in patients with bronchial asthma.

The specially designed Spacer adapter permits the aerosol propellants to evaporate and the particle velocity to decrease, resulting in reduced drug deposition in the oral cavity. In addition the Spacer adapter diminishes the need for co-ordination between aerosol actuation and inhalation, making this inhaler suitable for patients who have difficulty using conventional inhalers.

Dosage and administration *Adults:* 200 micrograms twice daily, in the morning and in the evening. During periods of severe asthma the daily dosage can be increased to up to 1600 micrograms.

In patients well controlled the daily dose may be reduced below 400 micrograms, but should not go below 200 micrograms.

The dose should be reduced to the minimum needed to maintain good asthma control.

Children: 50 to 400 micrograms to be given twice daily. During periods of severe asthma the daily dose can be increased up to 800 micrograms.

The dose should be reduced to the minimum needed to maintain good asthma control.

Elderly: Dosage as for adults.

Contra-indications, warnings, etc

Contra-indications: Hypersensitivity to any of the constituents. No other specific contra-indications are known, but special care is needed in patients with lung tuberculosis, fungal and viral infections in the airways.

Special warnings and precautions:

Pregnancy and breast feeding: In pregnant animals, administration of budesonide causes abnormalities of foetal development. The relevance of this finding to man has not been established. Administration during pregnancy should be avoided unless there are compelling reasons. As yet there is no information regarding the passage of budesonide into breast milk.

Patients not dependent on steroids: Treatment with the recommended doses of Pulmicort usually gives a therapeutic benefit within 7 days. However, certain patients may have an excessive collection of mucous secretion in the bronchi, which reduces penetration of the active substance into the airways. In these cases a short course of oral corticosteroids (usually 1 to 2 weeks) should be given in addition to the aerosol. After the course of the oral drug the inhaler alone should be sufficient therapy. Exacerbations of asthma caused by bacterial infections are usually controlled by appropriate antibiotic treatment and possibly increasing the Pulmicort dosage or if necessary, by giving systemic steroids.

Steroid dependent patients: Transfer of patients dependent upon oral steroids to treatment with Pulmicort demands special care mainly due to the slow restitution of the disturbed hypothalamic-pituitary function caused by extended treatment with oral corticosteroids. When the Pulmicort treatment is initiated the patient should be in a relatively stable phase. Pulmicort is then given in combination with the previously used oral steroid dose for about 10 days.

After this period of time the reduction of the oral corticoid dose can be started with a dose reduction corresponding to about 1 mg prednisolone per day every week. The oral dose is thus reduced to the lowest level which in combination with Pulmicort gives a stable respiratory capacity.

In many cases it may eventually be possible to withdraw completely the oral steroid with Pulmicort treatment, but other cases may have to be maintained on a low oral steroid dosage.

Some patients may experience uneasiness during the withdrawal period due to a decreased steroid effect. The physician may have to explain the reason for the Pulmicort treatment in order to encourage the patient to continue. The length of time needed for the body to regain its natural production of corticosteroid in sufficient amounts is often extensive. Prolonged treatment with high doses of inhaled corticosteroids, particularly higher than the recommended doses, may result in clinically significant adrenal suppression. Additional systemic corticosteroid cover should be considered during periods of stress or elective surgery.

Acute exacerbations, accompanied by increased mucous viscosity and mucous plugging, require complementary treatment with a short course of oral corticosteroids.

During transfer from oral therapy to Pulmicort a generally lower systemic steroid action will be experienced which may result in the appearance of allergic or arthritic symptoms such as rhinitis, eczema and muscle and joint pain. Specific treatment should be initiated for these conditions.

Systemic effects of inhaled corticosteroids may occur, particularly at high doses prescribed for prolonged periods. These effects are much less likely to occur than with oral corticosteroids. Possible systemic effects include adrenal suppression, growth retardation in children and adolescents, decrease in bone mineral density, cataract and glaucoma.

It is important therefore that the dose of inhaled corticosteroid is titrated to the lowest dose at which effective control of asthma is maintained.

It is recommended that the height of children receiving prolonged treatment with inhaled corticosteroids is regularly monitored. If growth is slowed, therapy should be reviewed with the aim of reducing the dose of inhaled corticosteroid, if possible, to the lowest dose at which effective control of asthma is maintained. In addition, consideration should be given to referring the patient to a paediatric respiratory specialist.

Side-effects: Occasional cases of mild irritation in the throat and hoarseness have been reported. Due to drug deposition in the oral cavity candidiasis of the mouth and throat occurs in some patients. However, the incidence should be less with the Spacer adapter or Nebuhaler as these reduce oral deposition. Advising the patient to rinse the mouth with water after each dosing occasion is also recommended. In most cases this condition responds to topical anti-fungal therapy without discontinuing treatment with Pulmicort.

Systemic effects of inhaled corticosteroids may occur, particularly at high doses prescribed for prolonged periods. These may include adrenal suppression, growth retardation in children and adolescents, decrease in bone mineral density, cataract and glaucoma.

Overdosage: The only harmful effect that follows inhalation of large amounts of the drug over a short period is suppression of hypothalamic–pituitary–adrenal (HPA) function. No special emergency action needs to be taken. Treatment with Pulmicort inhaler should be continued at the recommended dose to control the asthma.

Pharmaceutical precautions Store below 30°C.

Legal category POM.

Package quantities Pulmicort Inhaler (200 micrograms/actuation). Aerosol canister containing 200 metered doses complete with standard and Spacer delivery systems.

Pulmicort L.S. Inhaler (50 micrograms/puff). Aerosol canister containing 200 metered doses complete with standard and Spacer delivery systems.

Pulmicort (200 dose, 200 micrograms/puff) and Pulmicort L.S. (200 dose, 50 micrograms/puff).

Further information Pulmicort and Pulmicort L.S. may also be administered via the Nebuhaler.

Product licence numbers

(200 micrograms/puff)	0017/0128
(50 micrograms/puff)	0017/0113

PULMICORT* RESPULES* 0.5 mg

Qualitative and quantitative composition Budesonide, 0.25 mg/ml

Pharmaceutical form A white to off-white suspension for nebulisation. Each 2 ml single dose unit contains 0.5 mg of budesonide

Clinical particulars

Therapeutic indications: Pulmicort Respules contain the potent non-halogenated corticosteroid, budesonide for use in bronchial asthma in patients where use of a pressurised inhaler or dry powder formulation is unsatisfactory or inappropriate.

Pulmicort Respules are also recommended for use in infants and children with acute larygnotracheobronchitis–croup.

Posology and method of administration:

Dosage schedules: Pulmicort Respules should be administered from suitable nebulisers. The dose delivered to the patient varies depending on the nebulising equipment used. The nebulisation time and the dose delivered is dependent on flow rate, volume of nebuliser chamber and volume fill. An airflow rate of 6- 8 litres per minute through the device should be employed. A suitable volume fill for most nebulisers is 2-4 ml. The dosage of Pulmicort Respules should be adjusted to the need of the individual.

The dose should be reduced to the minimum needed to maintain good asthma control.

Bronchial Asthma: Initiation of therapy:

When treatment is started, during periods of severe asthma and while reducing or discontinuing oral glucocorticosteroids the recommended dose of Pulmicort Respules is:

Adults (including elderly): Usually 1-2 mg twice daily. In very severe cases the dosage may be further increased.

Children 12 years and older: Dosage as for adults.

Children 3 months to 12 years: 0.5-1 mg twice daily.

Maintenance: The maintenance dose should be individualised and be the lowest dose which keeps the patient symptom-free.

Adults (including elderly and children 12 years and older): 0.5-1 mg twice daily.

Children (3 months–12 years): 0.25- 0.5 mg twice daily.

Recommended dosage table:

	Pulmicort Respule Presentation
Dose (mg)	0.5 mg Volume (ml)
0.25	1
0.5	2
0.75	3
1.0	4
1.5	6
2.0	8

Where an increased therapeutic effect is desired, especially in those patients without major mucus secretion in the airways, an increased dose of Pulmicort is recommended rather than combined treatment with oral corticosteroids because of the lower risk of systemic effects.

Acute laryngotracheobronchitis–croup:

In infants and children with croup the usual dose is 2 mg of nebulised budesonide. This dose is given as a single administration or as two 1 mg doses separated by 30 minutes.

Contra-indications: Hypersensitivity to any of the constituents.

Special warnings and special precautions for use: Special care is needed in patients with pulmonary tuberculosis and viral infections of the airways.

Non-steroid dependent patients: A therapeutic effect is usually reached within 10 days. In patients with excessive mucus secretion in the bronchi a short (about 2 weeks) additional oral corticosteroid regimen can be given initially. After the course of the oral drug Pulmicort Respules alone should be sufficient therapy.

Steroid dependent patients: When transfer from oral corticosteroid to treatment with Pulmicort is initiated the patient should be in a relatively stable phase. Pulmicort is then given in combination with the previously used oral steroid dose for about 10 days.

After that the oral dose should be gradually reduced (by for example 2.5 mg prednisolone or the equivalent each month) to the lowest possible level. In many cases, it is possible to completely substitute Pulmicort for the oral corticosteroid.

During transfer from oral therapy to Pulmicort a generally lower systemic corticosteroid action will be experienced which may result in the appearance of allergic or arthritic symptoms such as rhinitis, eczema and muscle and joint pain. Specific treatment should be initiated for these conditions.

Prolonged treatment with high doses of inhaled corticosteroids, particularly higher than the recommended doses, may result in clinically significant adrenal suppression. Additional systemic corticosteroid cover should be considered during periods of stress or elective surgery.

Acute exacerbations of asthma may need additional treatment with a short course of oral corticosteroid.

The nebuliser chamber should be cleaned after every administration. Wash the nebuliser chamber and mouthpiece or face-mask in hot water using a mild detergent. Rinse well and dry by connecting the nebuliser chamber to the compressor or air inlet.

Acute exacerbations of asthma may need additional treatment with a short course of oral corticosteroid.

The nebuliser chamber should be cleaned after every administration. Wash the nebuliser chamber and mouthpiece or face-mask in hot water using a mild detergent. Rinse well and dry by connecting the nebuliser chamber to the compressor or air inlet.

Systemic effects of inhaled corticosteroids may occur, particularly at high doses prescribed for prolonged periods. These effects are much less likely to occur than with oral corticosteroids. Possible systemic effects include adrenal suppression, growth retardation in children and adolescents, decrease in bone mineral density, cataract and glaucoma.

It is important therefore that the dose of inhaled corticosteroid is titrated to the lowest dose at which effective control of asthma is maintained.

It is recommended that the height of children receiving prolonged treatment with inhaled corticosteroids is regularly monitored. If growth is slowed, therapy should be reviewed with the aim of reducing the dose of inhaled corticosteroid, if possible, to the lowest dose at which effective control of asthma is maintained. In addition, consideration should be given to referring the patient to a paediatric respiratory specialist.

Interaction with other medicaments and other forms of interaction: None Known

Pregnancy and Lactation: In pregnant animals administration of budesonide causes abnormalities of foetal development. The relevance of this finding to man has not been established. Administration during pregnancy should be avoided unless there are compelling reasons. As yet there is no information regarding the passage of budesonide into breast milk.

Effects on ability to drive and use machines: Pulmicort does not affect the ability to drive or use machinery.

Undesirable effects: Mild irritation in the throat, coughing and hoarseness. Candida infection in the oropharynx has been reported. To minimise oropharyngeal thrush the mouth should be rinsed with water after administration. In rare cases inhaled drugs may provoke bronchoconstriction in hyperreactive patients. Facial skin irritation has occurred in a few cases when a nebuliser with a face mask has been used. To prevent irritation facial skin should be washed after use of the face mask. Coughing can usually be prevented by inhaling a β_2-agonist (e.g. terbutaline) 5-10 minutes before inhalation of Pulmicort Respules.

Systemic effects of inhaled corticosteroids may occur, particularly at high doses prescribed for prolonged periods. These may include adrenal suppression, growth retardation in children and adolescents, decrease in bone mineral density, cataract and glaucoma.

Overdosage: Pulmicort Respules contains 0.1 mg/ml disodium edetate which has been shown to cause bronchoconstriction at levels above 1.2 mg/ml. Acute overdosage with Pulmicort should not present a clinical problem.

Pharmacological properties

Pharmacodynamic properties: Budesonide is a glucocorticosteroid which possesses a high local anti-inflammatory action with a lower incidence and severity of adverse effects than those seen with oral corticosteroids.

Budesonide has shown anti-anaphylactic and anti-inflammatory effects in provocation studies in animals and patients, manifested as decreased bronchial obstruction in the immediate as well as the late allergic reaction.

Budesonide has also been shown to decrease airway reactivity to histamine and methacholine in hyperreactive patients. Therapy with inhaled budesonide has effectively been used for prevention of exercise induced asthma.

After a single dose of orally inhaled budesonide, delivered via dry powder inhaler, improvement of the lung function is achieved within a few hours. However, after therapeutic use of orally inhaled budesonide, several weeks may pass before full effect is obtained.

Pharmacokinetic properties: Budesonide undergoes an extensive biotransformation in the liver to metabolites of low glucocorticosteroid activity. The glucocorticosteroid activity of the major metabolites, 6β-hydroxybudesonide and 16α-hydroxyprednisolone, is less than 1% of that of budesonide.

Of the fraction of budesonide which is swallowed, approximately 90% is inactivated at first passage through the liver. The maximal plasma concentration after inhalation of 1 mg budesonide, delivered with dry powder inhaler, is about 3.5nmol/L and is reached after about 20 minutes.

Preclinical safety data: The acute toxicity of budesonide is low and of the same order of magnitude and type as that of the reference glucocorticosteroids studied (beclomethasone dipropionate, fluocinolone acetonide).

Results from subacute and chronic toxicity studies show that the systemic effects of budesonide are less severe or similar to those observed after administration of other glucocorticosteroids, e.g. decreased body-weight gain and atrophy of lymphoid tissues and adrenal cortex.

An increased incidence of brain gliomas in male rats in a carcinogenicity study could not be verified in a repeat study, in which the incidence of gliomas did not differ between any of the groups with active treatment (budesonide, prednisolone, triamcinolone acetonide) and the control groups.

Liver changes (primary hepatocellular neoplasms) found in male rats in the original carcinogenicity study were noted again in the repeat study with budesonide as well as with the reference glucocorticosteroids. These effects are most probably related to a receptor effect and thus represent a class-effect.

Available clinical experience shows that there are no indications that budesonide or other glucocorticosteroids induce brain gliomas or primary hepatocellular neoplasms in man.

Pharmaceutical particulars

List of excipients: Other constituents: Disodium edetate, Sodium chloride, Polysorbate 80, Citric acid anhydrous, Sodium citrate, Water purified.

Incompatibilities: None known.

Shelf-life: 24 months

Special precautions for storage: Store below 30°C. Use within 3 months of opening the foil envelope. Protect opened ampoule from light. Use within 12 hours of opening.

Nature and contents of container: Single dose unit made of LD-polyethylene and each single dose unit contains 2 ml of suspension. Sheets of 5 units are packed in a heat sealed envelope of foil laminate. 4 heat sealed envelopes are packed into a carton.

Instructions for use/handling: Pulmicort Respules can be mixed with 0.9% saline and with solutions of terbutaline, salbutamol, sodium cromoglycate or ipratropium bromide.

Marketing authorisation number PL 0017/0309

Date of approval / revision of SPC September 1998

Legal category POM.

PULMICORT* RESPULES* 1 mg

Qualitative and quantitative composition Budesonide, 0.5 mg/ml

Pharmaceutical form A white to off-white suspension for nebulisation. Each 2 ml single dose unit contains 1 mg of budesonide

Clinical particulars

Therapeutic indications: Pulmicort Respules contain the potent non-halogenated corticosteroid, budesonide for use in bronchial asthma in patients where use of a pressurised inhaler or dry powder formulation is unsatisfactory or inappropriate.

Pulmicort Respules are also recommended for use in infants and children with acute larygnotracheobronchitis–croup.

Posology and method of administration:

Dosage schedules: Pulmicort Respules should be administered from suitable nebulisers. The dose delivered to the patient varies depending on the nebulising equipment used. The nebulisation time and the dose delivered is dependent on flow rate, volume of nebuliser chamber and volume fill. An airflow rate of 6- 8 litres per minute through the device should be employed. A suitable volume fill for most nebulisers is 2-4 ml. The dosage of Pulmicort Respules should be adjusted to the need of the individual.

The dose should be reduced to the minimum needed to maintain good asthma control.

Bronchial Asthma: Initiation of therapy:

When treatment is started, during periods of severe asthma and while reducing or discontinuing oral glucocorticosteroids the recommended dose of Pulmicort Respules is:

Adults (including elderly): Usually 1-2 mg twice daily. In very severe cases the dosage may be further increased.

Children 12 years and older: Dosage as for adults.

Children 3 months to 12 years: 0.5-1 mg twice daily.

Maintenance: The maintenance dose should be individualised and be the lowest dose which keeps the patient symptom-free.

Adults (including elderly and children 12 years and older): 0.5-1 mg twice daily.

Children (3 months–12 years): 0.25- 0.5 mg twice daily.

Recommended dosage table:

Pulmicort Respule Presentation	
Dose (mg)	1 mg Volume (ml)
0.25	-
0.5	1
0.75	-
1.0	2
1.5	3
2.0	4

Where an increased therapeutic effect is desired, especially in those patients without major mucus secretion in the airways, an increased dose of Pulmicort is recommended rather than combined treatment with oral corticosteroids because of the lower risk of systemic effects.

Acute laryngotracheobronchitis–croup:

In infants and children with croup the usual dose is 2 mg of nebulised budesonide. This dose is given as a single administration or as two 1 mg doses separated by 30 minutes.

Contra-indications: Hypersensitivity to any of the constituents.

Special warnings and special precautions for use: Special care is needed in patients with pulmonary tuberculosis and viral infections of the airways.

Non-steroid dependent patients: A therapeutic effect is usually reached within 10 days. In patients with excessive mucus secretion in the bronchi a short (about 2 weeks) additional oral corticosteroid regimen can be given initially. After the course of the oral drug Pulmicort Respules alone should be sufficient therapy.

Steroid dependent patients: When transfer from oral corticosteroid to treatment with Pulmicort is initiated the patient should be in a relatively stable phase. Pulmicort is then given in combination with the previously used oral steroid dose for about 10 days.

After that the oral dose should be gradually reduced (by for example 2.5 mg prednisolone or the equivalent each month) to the lowest possible level. In many cases, it is possible to completely substitute Pulmicort for the oral corticosteroid.

During transfer from oral therapy to Pulmicort a generally lower systemic corticosteroid action will be experienced which may result in the appearance of allergic or arthritic symptoms such as rhinitis, eczema and muscle and joint pain. Specific treatment should be initiated for these conditions.

Prolonged treatment with high doses of inhaled corticosteroids, particularly higher than the recommended doses, may result in clinically significant adrenal suppression. Additional systemic corticosteroid cover should be considered during periods of stress or elective surgery.

Acute exacerbations of asthma may need additional treatment with a short course of oral corticosteroid.

The nebuliser chamber should be cleaned after every administration. Wash the nebuliser chamber and mouthpiece or face-mask in hot water using a mild detergent. Rinse well and dry by connecting the nebuliser chamber to the compressor or air inlet.

Acute exacerbations of asthma may need additional treatment with a short course of oral corticosteroid.

The nebuliser chamber should be cleaned after every administration. Wash the nebuliser chamber and mouthpiece or face-mask in hot water using a mild detergent. Rinse well and dry by connecting the nebuliser chamber to the compressor or air inlet.

Systemic effects of inhaled corticosteroids may occur, particularly at high doses prescribed for prolonged periods. These effects are much less likely to occur than with oral corticosteroids. Possible systemic effects include adrenal suppression, growth retardation in children and adolescents, decrease in bone mineral density, cataract and glaucoma.

It is important therefore that the dose of inhaled corticosteroid is titrated to the lowest dose at which effective control of asthma is maintained.

It is recommended that the height of children receiving prolonged treatment with inhaled corticosteroids is regularly monitored. If growth is slowed, therapy should be reviewed with the aim of reducing the dose of inhaled corticosteroid, if possible, to the lowest dose at which effective control of asthma is maintained. In addition, consideration should be given to referring the patient to a paediatric respiratory specialist.

Interaction with other medicaments and other forms of interaction: None Known

Pregnancy and Lactation: In pregnant animals administration of budesonide causes abnormalities of foetal development. The relevance of this finding to man has not been established. Administration during pregnancy should be avoided unless there are compelling reasons. As yet there is no information regarding the passage of budesonide into breast milk.

Effects on ability to drive and use machines: Pulmicort does not affect the ability to drive or use machinery.

Undesirable effects: Mild irritation in the throat, coughing and hoarseness. Candida infection in the oropharynx has been reported. To minimise oropharyngeal thrush the mouth should be rinsed with water after administration. In rare cases inhaled drugs may provoke bronchoconstriction in hyperreactive patients. Facial skin irritation has occurred in a few cases when a nebuliser with a face mask has been used. To prevent irritation facial skin should be washed after use of the face mask. Coughing can usually be prevented by inhaling a β2-agonist (e.g. terbutaline) 5-10 minutes before inhalation of Pulmicort Respules.

Systemic effects of inhaled corticosteroids may occur, particularly at high doses prescribed for prolonged periods. These may include adrenal suppression, growth retardation in children and adolescents, decrease in bone mineral density, cataract and glaucoma.

Overdosage: Pulmicort Respules contains 0.1 mg/ml disodium edetate which has been shown to cause bronchoconstriction at levels above 1.2 mg/ml. Acute overdosage with Pulmicort should not present a clinical problem.

Pharmacological properties

Pharmacodynamic properties: Budesonide is a glucocorticosteroid which possesses a high local anti-inflammatory action with a lower incidence and severity of adverse effects than those seen with oral corticosteroids.

Budesonide has shown anti-anaphylactic and anti-inflammatory effects in provocation studies in animals and patients, manifested as decreased bronchial obstruction in the immediate as well as the late allergic reaction.

Budesonide has also been shown to decrease airway reactivity to histamine and methacholine in hyperreactive patients. Therapy with inhaled budesonide has effectively been used for prevention of exercise induced asthma.

After a single dose of orally inhaled budesonide, delivered via dry powder inhaler, improvement of the lung function is achieved within a few hours. However, after therapeutic use of orally inhaled budesonide, several weeks may pass before full effect is obtained.

Pharmacokinetic properties: Budesonide undergoes an extensive biotransformation in the liver to metabolites of low glucocorticosteroid activity. The glucocorticosteroid activity of the major metabolites, 6β-hydroxybudesonide and 16α-hydroxyprednisolone, is less than 1% of that of budesonide.

Of the fraction of budesonide which is swallowed, approximately 90% is inactivated at first passage through the liver. The maximal plasma concentration after inhalation of 1 mg budesonide, delivered with dry powder inhaler, is about 3.5nmol/L and is reached after about 20 minutes.

Preclinical safety data: The acute toxicity of budesonide is low and of the same order of magnitude and type as that of the reference glucocorticosteroids studied (beclomethasone dipropionate, fluocinolone acetonide).

Results from subacute and chronic toxicity studies show that the systemic effects of budesonide are less severe or similar to those observed after administration of other glucocorticosteroids, e.g. decreased body-weight gain and atrophy of lymphoid tissues and adrenal cortex.

An increased incidence of brain gliomas in male rats in a carcinogenicity study could not be verified in a repeat study, in which the incidence of gliomas did not differ between any of the groups with active treatment (budesonide, prednisolone, triamcinolone acetonide) and the control groups.

Liver changes (primary hepatocellular neoplasms) found in male rats in the original carcinogenicity study were noted again in the repeat study with budesonide as well as with the reference glucocorticosteroids. These effects are most probably related to a receptor effect and thus represent a class-effect.

Available clinical experience shows that there are no indications that budesonide or other glucocorticosteroids induce brain gliomas or primary hepatocellular neoplasms in man.

Pharmaceutical particulars

List of excipients: Other constituents: Disodium edetate, Sodium chloride, Polysorbate 80, Citric acid anhydrous, Sodium citrate, Water purified.

Incompatibilities: None known.

Shelf-life: 24 months

Special precautions for storage: Store below 30°C. Use within 3 months of opening the foil envelope. Protect opened ampoule from light. Use within 12 hours of opening.

Nature and contents of container: Single dose unit made of LD-polyethylene and each single dose unit contains 2 ml of suspension. Sheets of 5 units are packed in a heat sealed envelope of foil laminate. 4 heat sealed envelopes are packed into a carton.

Instructions for use/handling: Pulmicort Respules can be mixed with 0.9% saline and with solutions of terbutaline, salbutamol, sodium cromoglycate or ipratropium bromide.

Marketing authorisation number PL 0017/0310

Date of approval/revision of SPC September 1998

Legal category POM.

PULMICORT* TURBOHALER*

Presentation Pulmicort Turbohaler 100 is a breath-actuated metered dose powder inhaler delivering 100 micrograms budesonide per actuation.

Pulmicort Turbohaler 200 is a breath-actuated metered dose powder inhaler delivering 200 micrograms budesonide per actuation.

Pulmicort Turbohaler 400 is a breath-actuated metered dose powder inhaler delivering 400 micrograms budesonide per actuation.

Pulmicort Turbohaler 100, Pulmicort Turbohaler 200 and Pulmicort Turbohaler 400 are free from propellants, lubricants, preservatives, carrier substances or other additives.

Uses Pulmicort Turbohaler 100, Pulmicort Turbohaler 200 and Pulmicort Turbohaler 400 contain the potent, non-halogenated corticosteroid budesonide. Clinical studies have shown inhaled budesonide to possess a local anti-inflammatory action in the lungs with a lower incidence and severity of adverse effects than those seen with oral corticosteroids. Investigations with Pulmicort have documented good therapeutic results in bronchial asthma, whilst being well tolerated during prolonged treatment.

Pulmicort is, therefore, recommended in patients with bronchial asthma.

Dosage and administration

Adults: The dosage of Pulmicort Turbohaler 100, Pulmicort Turbohaler 200 and Pulmicort Turbohaler 400 should be individualised. When starting treatment, during periods of severe asthma and while reducing or discontinuing oral glucocorticosteroids the dosage in adults should be 200–1600 micrograms daily in divided doses. In less severe cases 200–800 micrograms daily in divided doses may be used; during periods of severe asthma the daily dosage can be increased to up to 1600 micrograms in divided doses.

Mild to moderate stable asthmatics: Adults (including elderly and children over 12 years): A once daily regimen of up to 800 micrograms may be used by patients already controlled on inhaled steroids (e.g. budesonide or beclomethasone dipropionate) administered twice daily. The patient should be transferred to once daily dosing at the same equivalent total daily dose. The dose should subsequently be reduced to the minimum needed to maintain good asthma control.

Patients should be instructed to take the once daily dose in the evening. It is important the dose is taken consistently and at a similar time each evening.

There are insufficient data to make recommendations for the transfer of patients from newer inhaled steroids to once daily Pulmicort Turbohaler.

In keeping with accepted medical practice, when transferring patients to Turbohaler from other devices treatment should be individualised and consideration given to the drug and the method of delivery.

Children: 200–800 micrograms daily in divided doses. During periods of severe asthma the daily dose can be increased up to 800 micrograms.

A once daily regimen is not recommended for children under 12 years.

Elderly: Dosage as for adults.

The maintenance dose should be individualised and should be the lowest possible, whether once or twice daily dosing is being used.

Patients, in particular those receiving once daily treatment should be advised that if their asthma deteriorates (e.g. increased frequency of bronchodilator use or persistent respiratory symptoms) to double their steroid dose, by administering twice daily and advised to contact their doctor as soon as possible.

In patients where an increased therapeutic effect is desired, an increased dose of Pulmicort is recommended because of the lower risk of systemic effects as compared with a combined treatment with oral glucocorticosteroids.

In order to reduce the risk of oral candidiasis and hoarseness, patients should brush their teeth and rinse their mouths out with water after each administration.

When transferring patients to Turbohaler from other devices, treatment should be individualised. The drug and method of delivery should be considered.

Patients should be reminded of the importance of taking prophylactic therapy regularly even when they are asymptomatic.

Contra-indications, warnings, etc
Contra-indications: Active pulmonary tuberculosis. Hypersensitivity to budesonide.

Special warnings and precautions: Special care is needed in patients with quiescent lung tuberculosis, fungal and viral infections in the airways.

Precautions:
Non-steroid dependent patients: A therapeutic effect is usually reached within 10 days. In patients with excessive mucus secretion in the bronchi a short (about 2 weeks) additional oral corticosteroid regimen can be given initially.

Steroid dependent patients: When transfer from oral steroids to Pulmicort Turbohaler is started, the patient should be in a relatively stable phase. A high dose of Pulmicort Turbohaler is given in combination with the previously used oral steroid for about 10 days. After that the oral dose should be gradually reduced (by for example 2.5 mg prednisolone or the equivalent each month) to the lowest possible level. In many cases, it is possible to completely substitute Pulmicort for the oral steroid.

Note: During transfer from oral therapy to Pulmicort a generally lower systemic steroid action will be experienced which may result in the appearance of allergic or arthritic symptoms such as rhinitis, eczema and muscle and joint pain. Specific treatment should be initiated for these conditions.

Acute exacerbations of asthma may need an increase in the dose of Pulmicort or additional treatment with a short course of oral corticosteroids and/or an antibiotic if there is an infection.

Patients, who have previously been dependant on oral steroids may, as a result of prolonged systemic steroid therapy experience the effects of impaired adrenal function. Recovery may take a considerable amount of time after cessation of oral steroid therapy hence oral steroid dependant patients transferred to budesonide may remain at risk from impaired adrenal function for some considerable time. In such circumstances HPA axis functions should be monitored regularly.

Prolonged treatment with high doses of inhaled corticosteroids, particularly higher than the recommended doses, may result in clinically significant adrenal suppression. Additional systemic corticosteroid cover should be considered during periods of stress or elective surgery. These patients should be instructed to carry a steroid warning card indicating their needs. Treatment with supplementary systemic steroids or Pulmicort should not be stopped abruptly.

Systemic effects of inhaled steroids may occur, particularly at high doses prescribed for prolonged periods. These effects are much less likely to occur than with oral corticosteroids. Possible systemic effects include adrenal suppression, growth retardation in children and adolescents, decrease in bone mineral density, cataract and glaucoma.

It is important therefore that the dose of inhaled steroid is titrated to the lowest dose at which effective control of asthma is maintained.

It is recommended that the height of children receiving prolonged treatment with inhaled corticosteroids is regularly monitored. If growth is slowed, therapy should be reviewed with the aim of reducing the dose of inhaled corticosteroid, if possible, to the lowest dose at which effective control of asthma is maintained. In addition, consideration should be given to referring the patient to a paediatric respiratory specialist.

Pregnancy and breast feeding: In pregnant animals, administration of budesonide causes abnormalities of foetal development. The relevance of this finding to man has not been established. Administration during pregnancy should be avoided unless there are compelling reasons. If treatment with glucocorticosteroids during pregnancy is unavoidable, inhaled glucocorticosteroids should be preferred because of their lower systemic effect compared with equipotent anti-asthmatic doses of oral glucocorticosteroids. There is no information regarding the passage of budesonide into breast milk.

Side-effects: Mild irritation in the throat and hoarseness. Candida infection in the oropharynx has been reported. Advising the patient to rinse the mouth with water after each administration is recommended. In most cases this condition responds to topical antifungal therapy without discontinuing treatment with Pulmicort.

Skin reactions such as a rash may occur in rare cases.

As with other inhalation therapy, the potential for paradoxical bronchospasm should be kept in mind. If it occurs treatment should be discontinued immediately and if necessary, alternative treatment initiated. Paradoxical bronchospasm responds to a fast acting inhaled bronchodilator.

Systemic effects of inhaled corticosteroids may occur, particularly at high doses prescribed for prolonged periods. These may include adrenal suppression, growth retardation in children and adolescents, decrease in bone mineral density, cataract and glaucoma.

Overdosage: The only harmful effect that follows inhalation of large amounts of the drug over a short period is suppression of hypothalamic-pituitary-adrenal (HPA) function. No special emergency action needs to be taken. Treatment with Pulmicort Turbohaler should be continued at the recommended dose to control the asthma.

Pharmaceutical precautions Store below 30°C.

Legal category POM.

Package quantities
Pulmicort Turbohaler 100: containing 200 actuations.
Pulmicort Turbohaler 200: containing 100 actuations.
Pulmicort Turbohaler 400: containing 50 actuations.

Further information Pulmicort Turbohaler is breath-actuated and therefore there is no need to co-ordinate the release of the dose and the inhalation.

Treatment with Pulmicort Turbohaler is effective even at low inspiratory flow rates.

Product licence numbers
Pulmicort Turbohaler 100 0017/0319
Pulmicort Turbohaler 200 0017/0272
Pulmicort Turbohaler 400 0017/0271

RHINOCORT* AQUA

Presentation Rhinocort Aqua is a metered pump spray for nasal application delivering 100 micrograms budesonide per actuation. Also contains disodium edetate, potassium sorbate, glucose, microcrystalline cellulose carboxymethyl cellulose sodium, polysorbate 80, hydrochloric acid and water.

Uses Seasonal and perennial allergic rhinitis and vasomotor rhinitis. Treatment of nasal polyps.

Dosage and administration
Adults: Rhinitis: The recommended daily dose is 400 mcg. Rhinocort Aqua may be given once daily for nasal inhalation (two applications into each nostril in the morning). When good effect has been achieved the dosage may be reduced to one application into each nostril. Rhinocort Aqua may also be given twice daily (one application into each nostril morning and evening).

Nasal polyps: The recommended dose is 200 mcg twice daily (one application into each nostril morning and evening). This is the maximum recommended total daily dose. Treatment can be continued for up to 3 months.

Children: There are insufficient data to recommend the use of Rhinocort Aqua in children. However, it is unlikely that the risk/benefit ratio in children is different from that in adults.

Patients should be reminded of the importance of taking this medicine regularly.

The minimum dose should be used at which effective control of symptoms is maintained.

Contra-indications, warnings, etc
Contra-indications: Hypersensitivity to any of the ingredients.

Precautions and warnings: Special care is demanded in treatment of patients transferred from oral steroids to Rhinocort where disturbance in the hypothalamic-pituitary-adrenal (HPA) axis could be expected.

Special care is needed in patients with fungal and viral infections in the airways, and in patients with lung tuberculosis.

Systemic effects of nasal corticosteroids may occur, particularly at high doses prescribed for prolonged periods. Growth retardation has been reported in children receiving nasal corticosteroids at licensed doses.

It is recommended that the height of children receiving prolonged treatment with nasal corticosteroids is regularly monitored. If growth is slowed, therapy should be reviewed with the aim of reducing the dose of nasal corticosteroid, if possible, to the lowest dose at which effective control of symptoms is maintained. In addition, consideration should also be given to referring the patient to a paediatric specialist.

Treatment with higher than recommended doses may result in clinically significant adrenal suppression. If there is evidence for higher than recommended doses being used then additional systemic corticosteroid cover should be considered during periods of stress or elective surgery.

The patient should be informed that full effect of Rhinocort is not achieved until after a few days treatment. Treatment of seasonal rhinitis should, if possible, start before exposure to the allergens.

Concomitant treatment may sometimes be necessary to counteract eye symptoms caused by the allergy. In continuous long-term treatment, the nasal mucosa should be inspected regularly e.g. every 6 months.

Rhinocort Aqua does not affect the ability to drive and operate machinery.

Pregnancy and lactation: Administration during pregnancy should be avoided unless there are compelling reasons. In pregnant animals administration of budesonide causes abnormalities of foetal development. The relevance of this to man has not been established. There is no information available regarding the passage of budesonide into breast milk. Use in lactation requires that the therapeutic benefit to the mother be weighed against any potential risk to the neonate.

Side effects: Occasionally sneezing, nasal stinging and dryness may follow immediately after the use of the spray. Slight haemorrhagic secretion/epistaxis may occur.

Contact allergy (rash, urticaria, dermatitis) involving the skin of the face may also occur, but is rare.

Ulceration of mucous membrane and nasal septal perforation have been reported following the use of intranasal aerosol corticosteroids, but these are extremely rare.

Note: This statement was omitted in error from the Data Sheet submitted to the MCA.

Rare cases of raised intraocular pressure or glaucoma have been reported following the use of intranasal steroid formulations.

Systemic effects of nasal corticosteroids may occur, particularly when prescribed at high doses for prolonged periods.

Overdosage: Acute overdose with Rhinocort should not present clinical problems.

Inhalation of high doses of corticosteroids may lead to suppression of the hypothalamic–pituitary–adrenal (HPA) axis function.

Pharmaceutical precautions Store below 30°C. Use within 2 months of starting treatment.

Legal status POM.

Package quantities Rhinocort Aqua is a nasal spray containing 100 × 100 microgram actuations budesonide.

Further information In pharmacological investigations and investigations in human beings budesonide (a non-halogenated corticosteroid) has shown a favourable relationship between anti-inflammatory effects and systemic effects due to the fact that budesonide is inactivated very rapidly in the liver after systemic absorption.

With the recommended dosage of Rhinocort Aqua an effective corticosteroid treatment of the nasal mucous membrane is attained with very little risk of systemic side effects.

Product licence number 0017/0304

THEO-DUR*

Presentation An extended release formulation (Durules) containing Theophylline Anhydrous PhEur, designed to give therapeutic blood levels over 8–12 hours.

200 mg tablet: A white, mottled, biconvex, elliptical tablet with the engraving Theo-Dur/200 on one side and a score in the transverse direction on the opposite side.

300 mg tablet: A white, mottled, biconvex, elliptical tablet with the engraving Theo-Dur/300 on one side and a score in the transverse direction on the opposite side.

Uses As a bronchodilator in the symptomatic or prophylactic treatment of bronchospasm associated with chronic obstructive airways disease including asthma and chronic bronchitis.

Dosage and administration
Standard dosing: Adults: the usual maintenance dose is one 300 mg tablet 12 hourly.

Children: <35 kg body weight: 100 mg (half a 200 mg tablet) 12 hourly. >35 kg body weight: 200 mg 12 hourly.

Elderly and patients with liver disease: Plasma half-life of theophylline may be prolonged and individual dosing should be adopted (see below).

Theophylline clearance is increased in cigarette

smokers and such patients may require increased doses of Theo-Dur to achieve a therapeutic effect.

Individual dosing: If sufficient therapeutic effect is not achieved or if side-effects occur, the dose of Theo-Dur may be increased or decreased by 100 mg (half a 200 mg tablet) or 150 mg (half a 300 mg tablet) stages. If doses higher than the usual maintenance doses are to be given, it is recommended that the patient's serum theophylline level is determined and the dose adjusted to maintain this level between 10-20 micrograms/ml (55–110 micromols/litre). The following procedure is recommended.

Adults: 150 mg (half a 300 mg tablet) 12 hourly for 4–7 days then 300 mg 12 hourly for 7–10 days.

Children: <35 kg body weight: 100 mg (half a 200 mg tablet) 12 hourly for 7–14 days. >35 kg body weight: 100 mg (half a 200 mg tablet) 12 hourly for 4–7 days then 200 mg 12 hourly for 7–10 days.

Blood for theophylline assay should be taken 3–8 hours after a dose when there has been no dosage adjustment for at least 4 days and no doses have been missed for 48 hours. The dose of Theo-Dur may be adjusted as follows:

Peak serum theophylline level	*Dosage adjustment*
<7.9 micrograms/ml	Increase dose by 50%.*
8–9.9 micrograms/ml	Increase dose by 20%* to the nearest 50 mg.
10–13.9 micrograms/ml	If the patient's symptoms persist, increase the dose by 10% to the nearest 50 mg.
14–19.9 micrograms/ml	Do not adjust the dose unless side-effects occur in which case a 10% decrease, to the nearest 50 mg may be necessary.
20–24.9 micrograms/ml	Decrease dose by 10% to the nearest 50 mg.
25–29.9 micrograms/ml	Miss next dose and decrease maintenance dose by 25%.*
>30 micrograms/ml	Miss next two doses and decrease maintenance dose by 50%*.

* With patients falling into these categories it is advisable to re-check the serum theophylline concentration 3–5 days after dosage adjustment.

Nocturnal asthma: For the control of symptoms of nocturnal asthma the appropriately individualised dosage of Theo-Dur should be administered once daily at approximately 8 p.m.

Note:

1. The tablet must not be crushed or chewed but swallowed whole or as a half.
2. Any previous therapy with theophylline, aminophylline or other theophylline salts should be discontinued.
3. If a patient has not previously been treated with theophylline or aminophylline or other theophylline salts, it is advisable to give half the maintenance dose of Theo-Dur (100 mg or 150 mg) for the first 4–7 days of treatment. This procedure should reduce the incidence of side-effects.

It is not possible to ensure bioequivalence between different extended release theophylline products. It should therefore be emphasised that patients once titrated to an effective dose should not be changed from Theo-Dur tablets to other extended release preparations or vice versa without retitration and clinical assessment.

After an effective therapeutic regime is attained it is important that practitioners, pharmacists and patients are aware of the possible dangers of inefficacy or toxicity if an alternative extended release theophylline preparation is substituted. This may be a particular hazard because the products are available without prescription. Likewise there may be a hazard if the doctor prescribes "generically" or if the preparation used in hospital is unknown by the general practitioner.

Contra-indications, warnings, etc
Contra-indications: None known.

Precautions: Theophylline should be given with caution to patients with congestive heart failure, liver disease or viral infections, and in the elderly. Plasma half-life of theophylline is prolonged in most of these patients, and the drug may accumulate to toxic concentrations.

Consideration should be given to advising alternative treatment in patients with a history of seizures.

Use in pregnancy and lactation: Caution is recommended during pregnancy and lactation. When theophylline is prescribed to pregnant and nursing women, the risk-benefit of the treatment must be taken into account.

Theophylline crosses the placenta, but no influence on foetal development or reproductive capacity has been established. Theophylline should not be used routinely in nursing women even though only very small amounts of theophylline are excreted into breast milk.

Premature children with low birthweight have an extremely prolonged theophylline half-life, which may lead to high theophylline plasma levels causing insomnia, agitation and/or anxiety. Full capacity to eliminate theophylline is not reached until the age of 6–12 months. Caution should be used when theophylline is given to infants who cannot complain of minor adverse reactions.

Side-effects: Side-effects of theophylline depend to a great extent on serum concentration and are frequent only at theophylline concentration exceeding 20 micrograms/ml. The Theo-Dur extended release formulation reduces fluctuation in serum levels of theophylline, thereby reducing the incidence of side-effects.

The most common side-effects are gastro-intestinal disturbances (nausea, vomiting and anorexia) which, in most cases, disappear on reducing the dose. Monitoring of the serum concentration of theophylline is recommended.

The CNS stimulating effect of theophylline can cause restlessness, irritability, anxiety and insomnia in some patients. Cardiovascular effects such as palpitations and tachycardia may appear.

Severe side-effects (cramps, convulsions and cardiac arrythmias) may appear at very high serum concentration, in which case the medication should be discontinued.

Drug interactions: The serum theophylline concentration may increase in patients receiving cimetidine, quinolone derivatives such as ciprofloxacin or macrolide antibiotics such as erythromycin and troleandomycin, concurrently with theophylline preparations. Increase in the theophylline serum concentration is also seen with oestrogen, allopurinol and propranolol. The serum theophylline concentration may be reduced during concurrent therapy with phenobarbitone, phenytoin and rifampicin as these drugs increase theophylline clearance. Theophylline has been shown to decrease the serum concentration of lithium.

Concurrent administration of ketamine with theophylline may reduce the threshold value for inducing convulsions.

Xanthines may potentiate hypokalaemia resulting from β_2-agonist therapy, steroids, diuretics and hypoxia. Particular caution is advised in severe asthma. It is recommended that serum potassium levels are monitored in such situations.

The concomitant use of theophylline and fluvoxamine should usually be avoided. Where this is not possible, patients should have their theophylline dose halved and plasma theophylline should be monitored closely.

Changes in serum theophylline concentration have been reported in patients concurrently taking the calcium channel antagonists diltiazem or verapamil.

Occasionally, the serum theophylline concentration may rise in patients who receive concomitant vaccination against influenza.

Treatment of overdosage: Gastric lavage and symptomatic treatment to maintain fluid and electrolyte balance and correct hypokalaemia. Give oxygen as necessary. Monitor serum theophylline levels. Oral activated charcoal may reduce serum theophylline concentration. In severe cases charcoal haemoperfusion may be required. Tablets in the intestine may continue to release theophylline for several hours.

Possible signs and symptoms of overdosage are insomnia, anorexia, agitation, anxiety, nausea, vomiting, convulsions, hypotension, palpitations, tachycardia and cardiac arrhythmias. Serious toxicity is not always preceded by less severe adverse effects.

Pharmaceutical precautions Store below 30°C.

Legal category P.

Package quantities 100 tablets.

Further information Nil.

Product licence numbers
0017/0098 200 mg
0017/0099 300 mg

XYLOCAINE* VIALS 0.5%, 1% and 2%

Presentation A sterile clear aqueous solution of Lidocaine Hydrochloride BP. Each ml contains:

0.5% solution:	Lidocaine Hydrochloride PhEur 5.35 mg equivalent to lidocaine hydrochloride anhydrous 5 mg.
1.0% solution:	Lidocaine Hydrochloride PhEur 10.7 mg equivalent to lidocaine hydrochloride anhydrous 10 mg.
2.0% solution:	Lidocaine Hydrochloride PhEur 21.4 mg equivalent to lidocaine hydrochloride anhydrous 20 mg.

All the above contain sodium chloride to produce isotonic solutions.

Uses Xylocaine is a local anaesthetic solution for use in infiltration anaesthesia, intravenous regional anaesthesia and nerve blocks.

Dosage and administration The dosage is adjusted according to the response of the patient and site of administration. The lowest concentration and smallest dose producing the required effect should be given. The maximum dose for healthy adults should not exceed 200 mg.

Children and elderly or debilitated patients require smaller doses, commensurate with age and physical status.

Contra-indications, warnings, etc
Contra-indications: Known hypersensitivity to anaesthetics of the amide type.

Precautions: In common with other local anaesthetics, Xylocaine should be used cautiously in patients with epilepsy, impaired cardiac conduction, bradycardia, impaired respiratory function, and in patients with impaired hepatic function, if the dose or site of administration is likely to result in high blood levels.

Facilities for resuscitation should be available when local anaesthetics are administered.

The effect of local anaesthetics may be reduced if an injection is made into an inflamed or infected area.

Pregnancy and lactation: Although there is no evidence from animal studies of harm to the foetus, as with all drugs, Xylocaine should not be given during early pregnancy unless the benefits are considered to outweigh the risks.

Side-effects: In common with other local anaesthetics, adverse reactions to Xylocaine are rare and are usually the result of excessively high blood concentrations due to inadvertent intravascular injection, excessive dosage, rapid absorption or occasionally to hypersensitivity, idiosyncrasy or diminished tolerance on the part of the patient. In such circumstances systemic effects occur involving the central nervous system and/or the cardiovascular system.

CNS reactions are excitatory and/or depressant, and may be characterised by nervousness, dizziness, blurred vision and tremors, followed by drowsiness, convulsions, unconsciousness and possibly respiratory arrest. The excitatory reactions may be very brief or may not occur at all, in which case the first manifestations of toxicity may be drowsiness, merging into unconsciousness and respiratory arrest. Cardiovascular reactions are depressant, and may be characterised by hypotension, myocardial depression, bradycardia and possibly cardiac arrest.

Allergic reactions are extremely rare. They may be characterised by cutaneous lesions, urticaria, oedema or anaphylactoid reactions. Detection of sensitivity by skin testing is of doubtful value.

Hypotension may occur as a physiological response to central nerve blocks.

Interactions: Cimetidine can impair the metabolism of lidocaine absorbed into the circulation. Elimination will be delayed and the risk of adverse reactions increased.

Overdosage: Treatment of a patient with systemic toxicity consists of arresting convulsions and ensuring adequate ventilation with oxygen, if necessary by assisted or controlled ventilation (respiration). If convulsions occur they must be treated promptly by intravenous injection of thiopentone 100 to 200 mg or diazepam 5 to 10 mg. Alternatively succinylcholine 50 mg–100 mg i.v. may be used providing the clinician is capable of performing endotracheal intubation and managing a fully paralysed patient,

Once convulsions have been controlled and adequate ventilation of the lungs ensured, no other treatment is generally required. If hypotension is present, however, a vasopressor, preferably one with inotropic activity, e.g. ephedrine 15 to 30 mg, should be given intravenously.

Pharmaceutical precautions Store below 25°C.

Legal category POM.

Package quantities
0.5% solution – 20 ml. Pack of 5 vials.
1.0% solution – 20 ml. Pack of 5 vials.
2.0% solution – 20 ml. Pack of 5 vials.

Further information Multidose vial preparations of Xylocaine contain Methyl Parahydroxybenzoate PhEur 1 mg/ml.

Product licence numbers
0.5% 0017/5031R
1.0% 0017/5032R
2.0% 0017/5034R

XYLOCAINE* 2% WITH ADRENALINE 1:80,000

Presentation Sterile, clear aqueous solution. Each ml contains Lidocaine Hydrochloride 21.4 mg equivalent to lidocaine hydrochloride anhydrous 20.0 mg and Adrenaline Tartrate PhEur 22.7 micrograms equivalent to adrenaline 12.5 micrograms.

Inactive ingredients: sodium chloride to produce an isotonic solution, sodium metabisulphite, hydrochloric acid and water for injections.

Uses Xylocaine 2% with Adrenaline is a local anaesthetic solution for use in dental infiltration anaesthesia and all dental nerve block techniques.

Dosage and administration Infiltration – usual dose is 1 ml. Nerve block – usual dose is 1.5 to 2 ml.

The recommended maximum dose for Xylocaine when given with adrenaline is 500 mg.

Children and elderly or debilitated patients require smaller doses.

Contra-indications, warnings, etc
Contra-indications: Known hypersensitivity to anaesthetics of the amide type.

The use of a vasoconstrictor is contra-indicated for anaesthesia of fingers, toes, tip of nose, ears and penis.

Xylocaine with Adrenaline should not be given intravenously.

Precautions: In common with other local anaesthetics, Xylocaine with Adrenaline should be used cautiously in patients with epilepsy, impaired cardiac conduction, impaired respiratory function, and in patients with impaired hepatic function if the dose or site of administration is likely to result in high blood levels.

Facilities for resuscitation should be available when local anaesthetics are administered.

The effect of local anaesthetics may be reduced if an injection is made into an inflamed or infected area. Solutions containing adrenaline should be used with caution in patients with hypertension, cardiac disease, cerebrovascular insufficiency or thyrotoxicosis.

Solutions containing adrenaline should be used where possible so as to prolong anaesthesia and reduce systemic absorption. This is particularly important in highly vascular areas.

Use on one patient during one treatment only.

Use in pregnancy and lactation: Although there is no evidence from animal studies of harm to the foetus, as with all drugs lidocaine should not be given in early pregnancy unless the benefits are considered to outweigh the risks.

Interactions: Use with caution in patients taking tricyclic antidepressants, MAOI's or receiving potent general anaesthetic agents.

Adverse reactions: In common with other local anaesthetics, adverse reactions to Xylocaine with Adrenaline are extremely rare in dental practice and are usually the result of excessively high blood concentrations due to inadvertent intravascular injection, excessive dosage, rapid absorption or occasionally to hypersensitivity, idiosyncrasy or diminished tolerance on the part of the patient. In such circumstances systemic effects occur involving the central nervous system and/or the cardiovascular system.

CNS reactions are excitatory and/or depressant, and may be characterised by nervousness, dizziness, blurred vision and tremors, followed by drowsiness, convulsions, unconsciousness and possibly respiratory arrest. The excitatory reactions may be very brief or may not occur at all, in which case the first manifestations of toxicity may be drowsiness, merging into unconsciousness and respiratory arrest.

Cardiovascular reactions are depressant, and may be characterised by hypotension, myocardial depression, bradycardia and possibly cardiac arrest.

Allergic reactions are extremely rare. They may be characterised by cutaneous lesions, urticaria, oedema or anaphylactoid reactions. Detection of sensitivity by skin testing is of doubtful value.

Pharmaceutical precautions Store below 25°C.

Legal category POM.

Package quantities Glass cartridges of 2 ml standard and 2 ml self-aspirating, in boxes of 100.

Further information Dental cartridges of Xylocaine 2% with Adrenaline 1:80,000 do not contain an antimicrobial agent.

Product licence number 0017/5027R

XYLOCAINE* 0.5% WITH ADRENALINE 1:200,000
XYLOCAINE* 1% WITH ADRENALINE 1:200,000
XYLOCAINE* 2% WITH ADRENALINE 1:200,000

Qualitative and quantitative composition *Xylocaine 0.5% with Adrenaline 1:200,000*

Each ml of solution contains Lidocaine Hydrochloride Monohydrate PhEur equivalent to 5 mg of lidocaine hydrochloride, Adrenaline Tartrate PhEur equivalent to 5 microgram of adrenaline.

Xylocaine 1% with Adrenaline 1:200,000

Each ml of solution contains Lidocaine Hydrochloride Monohydrate PhEur equivalent to 10 mg of lidocaine hydrochloride, Adrenaline Tartrate PhEur equivalent to 5 microgram of adrenaline.

Xylocaine 2% with Adrenaline 1:200,000

Each ml of solution contains Lidocaine Hydrochloride Monohydrate PhEur equivalent to 20 mg of lidocaine hydrochloride, Adrenaline Tartrate PhEur equivalent to 5 microgram of adrenaline.

Pharmaceutical form Injection

Clinical particulars
Therapeutic indications: Xylocaine with Adrenaline is a local anaesthetic solution for use in infiltration anaesthesia and nerve blocks.

Posology and method of administration: The dosage is adjusted according to the response of the patient and the site of administration. The lowest concentration and smallest dose producing the required effect should be given. The maximum single dose of Xylocaine when given with adrenaline is 500 mg.

Children and elderly or debilitated patients require smaller doses, commensurate with age and physical status.

Contra-indications: Known hypersensitivity to anaesthetics of the amide type.

The use of a vasoconstrictor is contra-indicated for anaesthesia of fingers, toes, tip of nose, ears and penis.

Special warnings and special precautions for use: In common with other local anaesthetics, Xylocaine with Adrenaline should be used cautiously in patients with epilepsy, impaired cardiac conduction, impaired respiratory function and in patients with impaired hepatic function, if the dose or site of administration is likely to result in high blood levels.

Xylocaine with Adrenaline should not be given intravenously.

Facilities for resuscitation should be available when local anaesthetics are administered.

The effect of local anaesthetics may be reduced if an injection is made into an inflamed or infected area.

Solutions containing adrenaline should be used with caution in patients with hypertension, cardiac disease, cerebrovascular insufficiency or thyrotoxicosis.

Interaction with other medicaments and other forms of interaction: Solutions containing adrenaline should be used cautiously in patients taking tricyclic antidepressants, monoamine oxidase inhibitors or receiving potent general anaesthetic agents.

Pregnancy and lactation: Although there is no evidence from animal studies of harm to the foetus, as with all drugs, Xylocaine should not be given during early pregnancy unless the benefits are considered to outweigh the risks.

Effects on ability to drive and use machines: None known.

Undesirable effects: In common with other local anaesthetics, adverse reactions to Xylocaine with Adrenaline are rare and are usually the result of excessively high blood concentrations due to inadvertent intravascular injection, excessive dosage, rapid absorption or occasionally to hypersensitivity, idiosyncrasy or diminished tolerance on the part of the patient. In such circumstances systemic effects occur involving the central nervous system and/or the cardiovascular system.

CNS reactions are excitatory and/or depressant, and may be characterised by nervousness, dizziness, blurred vision and tremors, followed by drowsiness, convulsions, unconsciousness and possibly respiratory arrest. The excitatory reactions may be very brief or may not occur at all, in which case the first manifestations of toxicity may be drowsiness, merging into unconsciousness and respiratory arrest.

Cardiovascular reactions are depressant, and may be characterised by hypotension, myocardial depression, bradycardia and possibly cardiac arrest.

Allergic reactions are extremely rare. They may be characterised by cutaneous lesions, urticaria, oedema or anaphylactoid reactions. Detection of sensitivity by skin testing is of doubtful value.

Hypotension may occur as a physiological response to central nerve blocks.

Overdose: None stated.

Pharmacological properties
Pharmacodynamic properties: Lidocaine is a local anaesthetic of the amide type. At high doses lidocaine has a quinidine like action on the myocardium i.e. cardiac depressant. All local anaesthetics stimulate the CNS and may produce anxiety, restlessness and tremors.

Pharmacokinetic properties: Lidocaine is readily absorbed from the gastrointestinal tract, from mucous membranes and through damaged skin. It is rapidly absorbed from injection sites including muscle.

Elimination half-life is 2 hours.

Lidocaine undergoes first pass metabolism in the liver.

Less than 10% of a dose is excreted unchanged via the kidneys.

The speed of onset and duration of action of lidocaine are increased by the addition of a vasoconstrictor and absorption into the site of injection is reduced.

Preclinical safety data: Lidocaine and adrenaline are well established active ingredients.

Pharmaceutical particulars
List of excipients: Sodium chloride, sodium metabisulphite, methyl parahydroxybenzoate and water for injections.

Incompatibilities: None.

Shelf-life: Two years.

Special precautions for storage: Store between 2°C and 8°C.

Nature and contents of container: Multiple dose vials–20 ml and 50 ml.

Instructions for use/handling: None.

Marketing authorisation numbers

Xylocaine 0.5% with Adrenaline 1:200,000	PL 0017/5028R
Xylocaine 1% with Adrenaline 1:200,000	PL 0017/5029R
Xylocaine 2% with Adrenaline 1:200,000	PL 0017/5030R

Dates of approval/revision of SPC February 1998

Legal category POM.

XYLOCAINE* 2% PLAIN

Presentation A clear sterile aqueous solution for injection supplied in polypropylene cartridges for use with dental type syringes. Each cartridge contains 2.2 ml of solution.

Each ml of solution contains Lidocaine Hydrochloride BP 21.3 mg equivalent to lidocaine hydrochloride anhydrous 20.0 mg.

Inactive ingredients: sodium chloride and water for injections.

Lidocaine is synonymous with lignocaine.

Uses Local anaesthetic solution for use mainly in dental procedures.

NOTE: If a vasoconstrictor is needed to prolong the local anaesthesia by delaying the diffusion of the anaesthetic in the surrounding tissues a product containing lidocaine and adrenaline such as Lignostab-A should be used.

Dosage and administration The dosage is adjusted according to the response of the patient and the site of administration. The lowest concentration and smallest dose producing the required effect should be given. The maximum single dose of lidocaine hydrochloride is 200 mg when given alone. This is equivalent to 4 cartridges containing 2.2 ml.

Children and elderly or debilitated patients require smaller doses, commensurate with age and physical status.

Contra-indications, warnings, etc
Contra-indications: Known hypersensitivity to anaesthetics of the amide type or the other constituents.

Intravenous use.

Precautions: As for other local anaesthetics, use cautiously in patients with epilepsy, impaired cardiac conduction, impaired respiratory function, and in patients with impaired hepatic function, if the dose or site of administration is likely to result in high blood levels.

Facilities for resuscitation should be available when local anaesthetics are administered.

The effect of local anaesthetics may be reduced if an injection is made into an inflamed or infected area.

Use on one patient during one treatment only. Discard unused contents.

Use in Pregnancy: Although this product crosses the placenta, the low doses used in dental anaesthesia would not be expected to give rise to signs of toxicity in the foetus.

Side-effects: In common with other local anaesthetics, adverse reactions are rare and are usually the result of excessively high blood concentrations due to inadvertent intravascular injection, excessive dosage, rapid absorption or diminished tolerance on the part of the patient. In such circumstances systemic effects occur involving the central nervous system and/or the cardiovascular system.

CNS reactions are excitatory and/or depressant, and

may be characterised by nervousness, dizziness, blurred vision and tremors, followed by drowsiness, convulsions, unconsciousness and possibly respiratory arrest. The excitatory reactions may be very brief or may not occur at all, in which case the first manifestations of toxicity may be drowsiness, merging into unconsciousness and respiratory arrest.

Cardiovascular reactions are depressant, and may be characterised by hypotension, myocardial depression, bradycardia and possibly cardiac arrest.

Allergic reactions are extremely rare. They may be characterised by cutaneous lesions, urticaria, oedema or anaphylactoid reactions. Detection of sensitivity by skin testing is of doubtful value. Hypotension may occur as a physiological response to central nerve blocks.

Pharmaceutical precautions Store below 25°C.

Legal category POM.

Package quantities Boxes of 100 (polypropylene) cartridges.

Further information Nil.

Product licence no PL 0017/0256

XYLOCAINE* ANTISEPTIC GEL 2% XYLOCAINE* ACCORDION ANTISEPTIC GEL 2%

Presentation A topical anaesthetic/antiseptic gel.

1 g Xylocaine Antiseptic Gel 2% contains:
Active constituents: Lidocaine Hydrochloride BP 21.6 mg (equivalent to 20 mg lidocaine hydrochloride anhydrous), Chlorhexidine Gluconate Solution BP 2.7 mg.
Inactive ingredients: Hydroxypropyl methylcellulose, sodium hydroxide and water, purified.

1 g Xylocaine Accordion Antiseptic Gel 2% contains:
Active constituents: Lidocaine Hydrochloride PhEur 21.6 mg (equivalent to lidocaine hydrochloride anhydrous 20 mg), Chlorhexidine Digluconate BP 2.7 mg.
Inactive constituents: Hydroxypropyl methylcellulose, sodium hydroxide q.s., water purified q.s. Lidocaine is synonymous with lignocaine.

Both Xylocaine Antiseptic Gel 2% and Xylocaine Accordion Antiseptic Gel 2% provide prompt and profound anaesthesia of mucous membranes and lubrication which reduces friction. The water miscible base, characterised by high viscosity and low surface tension, brings the anaesthetic into intimate and prolonged contact with the tissue for effective anaesthesia of long duration (approx. 20–30 mins.). Anaesthesia usually occurs rapidly (within 5 minutes depending upon area of application).

The anaesthetic ingredient of both Xylocaine Antiseptic Gel 2% and Xylocaine Accordion Antiseptic Gel 2% is lidocaine, which stabilises the neuronal membrane and prevents the initiation and conduction of nerve impulses, thereby affecting local anaesthetic action. Lidocaine is absorbed following application to mucous membranes. The absorption occurs most rapidly after intratracheal administration. Blood concentrations of lidocaine after instillation in urethra of doses up to 800 mg are of low range and below toxic levels. The metabolism of lidocaine takes place in the liver and metabolites and unchanged drug are excreted by the kidney.

Uses For anaesthesia of the urethra and topical application on mucous membranes wherever an anaesthetic/antiseptic effect is required.

Dosage and administration As with any local anaesthetic, reactions and complications are best averted by employing the minimal effective dosage. Debilitated, elderly patients and children should be given doses commensurate with their age and physical condition.

Urethral anaesthesia:
Surface anaesthesia of the male adult urethra: 10 ml injected initially followed by 3–5 ml.

Surface anaesthesia of the female adult urethra: Instil 5–10 ml in small portions to fill the whole urethra.

In order to obtain adequate anaesthesia, several minutes should be allowed prior to performing urological procedures.

Contra-indications, warnings, etc
Contra-indications: Known history of hypersensitivity to local anaesthetics of the amide type or other components of the gel.

Precautions and warnings: Absorption from wound surfaces and mucous membranes is relatively high, especially in the bronchial tree. Xylocaine Antiseptic Gel 2% and Xylocaine Accordion Antiseptic Gel 2% should be used with caution in patients with traumatised mucosa and/or sepsis in the region of the proposed application.

If the dose or site of administration is likely to result in high blood levels, lidocaine, in common with other local anaesthetics, should be used cautiously in patients with epilepsy, impaired cardiac conduction, bradycardia, impaired hepatic function and in severe shock.

The oropharyngeal use of topical anaesthetic agents may interfere with swallowing and thus enhance the danger of aspiration. This is particularly important in children because of their frequency of eating. Numbness of the tongue or buccal mucosa may increase the danger of biting trauma.

Care should be taken to avoid instillation of excessive amounts of Xylocaine Antiseptic Gel 2% or Xylocaine Accordion Antiseptic Gel 2% into the rectum. This is of particular importance in infants and children. Systemic absorption of lidocaine may occur from the rectum, and large doses may result in CNS side-effects. On rare occasions convulsions have occurred in children.

Use in Pregnancy and Lactation: Although there is no evidence from animal studies of harm to the foetus, as with all drugs, Xylocaine should not be given during early pregnancy unless the benefits are considered to outweigh the risks. Lidocaine enters the mother's milk, but in such small quantities that there is generally no risk of the child being affected at therapeutic dose levels.

Side-effects: In extremely rare cases local anaesthetic preparations have been associated with allergic reactions (in the most severe instances anaphylactic shock).

Systemic adverse reactions are extremely rare and may result from high plasma levels due to excessive dosage or rapid absorption or from hypersensitivity, idiosyncrasy or reduced tolerance on the part of the patient. Such reactions are systemic in nature and involve the central nervous system and/or the cardiovascular system.

CNS reactions are excitatory and/or depressant and may be characterised by nervousness, dizziness, convulsions, unconsciousness and, possibly, respiratory arrest. The excitatory reactions may be very brief or may not occur at all, in which case the first manifestations of toxicity may be drowsiness, merging into unconsciousness and respiratory arrest.

Cardiovascular reactions are depressant and may be characterised by hypotension, myocardial depression, bradycardia and possibly cardiac arrest.

Interactions: Lidocaine should be used with caution in patients receiving antiarrhythmic drugs, such as tocainide, since the toxic effects are additive.

Overdosage: Treatment of a patient with systemic toxicity consists of arresting convulsions and ensuring adequate ventilation with oxygen, if necessary by assisted or controlled ventilation (respiration). If convulsions occur they must be treated promptly by intravenous injection of thiopentone 100 to 200 mg or diazepam 5 to 10 mg. Alternatively succinylcholine 50 to 100 mg i.v. may be used providing the clinician is capable of performing endotracheal intubation and managing a fully paralysed patient. If ventricular fibrillation or cardiac arrest occurs, effective cardiovascular resuscitation must be instituted. Adrenaline in repeated doses and sodium bicarbonate should be given as rapidly as possible.

Pharmaceutical precautions Store below 25°C. Xylocaine Accordion Antiseptic Gel 2% is sterile and is meant for single use only.

Legal category P.

Package quantities Xylocaine Antiseptic Gel 2%: 20 g tubes.

Xylocaine Accordion Antiseptic Gel 2%: blister packs containing 10 syringes. Each syringe contains 20 g of gel.

Further information Nil.

Product licence numbers

Xylocaine Antiseptic Gel 2%	0017/0244R
Xylocaine Accordion Antiseptic Gel 2%	0017/5035R

XYLOCAINE* GEL 2% XYLOCAINE* ACCORDION GEL 2%

Presentation A topical anaesthetic for urological procedures and lubrication of endotracheal tubes.

1 g Xylocaine Gel 2% contains:
Active constituent: Lidocaine Hydrochloride PhEur 21.6 mg (equivalent to 20 mg lidocaine hydrochloride anhydrous).
Inactive constituents: Hydroxypropyl methylcellulose PhEur, Methyl parahydroxybenzoate PhEur, Propyl parahydroxybenzoate PhEur, sodium hydroxide, hydrochloric acid and Water, purified PhEur.

1 g Xylocaine Accordion Gel 2% contains:
Active constituent: Lidocaine Hydrochloride PhEur corresponding to lidocaine hydrochloride 20 mg.
Inactive constituents: Hydroxypropyl methylcellulose PhEur, sodium hydroxide q.s., hydrochloric acid q.s., Water, purified PhEur q.s.

Both Xylocaine Gel 2% and Xylocaine Accordion Gel 2% provide prompt and profound anaesthesia of mucous membranes and lubrication which reduces friction. The water miscible base, characterised by high viscosity and low surface tension, brings the anaesthetic into intimate and prolonged contact with the tissue for effective anaesthesia of long duration (approx. 20–30 min).

Anaesthesia usually occurs rapidly (within 5 minutes depending upon area of application).

The active ingredient of both Xylocaine Gel 2% and Xylocaine Accordion Gel 2% is lidocaine, which stabilises the neuronal membrane and prevents the initiation and conduction of nerve impulses, thereby affecting local anaesthetic action. Lidocaine is absorbed following application to mucous membranes. The absorption occurs most rapidly after intratracheal administration. Blood concentrations of lidocaine after instillation in urethra of doses up to 800 mg are of low range and below toxic levels. The metabolism of lidocaine takes place in the liver and metabolites and unchanged drug are excreted by the kidneys.

Uses Surface anaesthesia and lubrication:
- the male and female urethra during cystoscopy, catheterisation, exploration by sound and other endourethral operations.
- nasal and pharyngeal cavities in endoscopic procedures such as gastroscopy and bronchoscopy.
- during proctoscopy and rectoscopy.
- intubation.

Symptomatic treatment of pain in connection with cystitis and urethritis.

Dosage and administration As with any local anaesthetic, reactions and complications are best averted by employing the minimal effective dosage. Debilitated, elderly patients and children should be given doses commensurate with their age and physical condition.

Urethral anaesthesia: Surface anaesthesia of the male adult urethra: For adequate analgesia in males 20 ml (=400 mg lidocaine hydrochloride) jelly is required. The jelly is instilled slowly until the patient has a feeling of tension or until almost half the syringe tube (10 ml=200 mg lidocaine hydrochloride) is emptied. A penile clamp is then applied for several minutes at the corona; then the rest of the jelly is instilled.

When anaesthesia is especially important, e.g. during sounding or cystoscopy, a larger quantity of jelly, for example 30–40 ml , may be instilled in 3–4 portions and allowed to work for 10–12 minutes before insertion of the instrument.

Surface anaesthesia of the female adult urethra: Instil 5–10 ml in small portions to fill the whole urethra. In order to obtain adequate anaesthesia, several minutes should be allowed prior to performing urological procedures.

Endoscopy: Instillation of 10–20 ml is recommended for adequate analgesia and a small amount should be applied on the instrument for lubrication.

Lubrication for endotracheal intubation: About 5 ml applied on the surface of the tube just prior to insertion. Care should be taken to avoid introducing the product into the lumen of the tube.

Contra-indications, warnings, etc
Contra-indications: Known history of hypersensitivity to local anaesthetics of the amide type or other components of the gel.

Precautions: Absorption from wound surfaces and mucous membranes is relatively high, especially in the bronchial tree. Xylocaine Gel 2%/Accordion Gel 2% should be used with caution in patients with traumatised mucosa and/or sepsis in the region of the proposed application.

If the dose or site of administration is likely to result in high blood levels, lidocaine, in common with other local anaesthetics, should be used cautiously in patients with epilepsy, impaired cardiac conduction, bradycardia, impaired hepatic function and in severe shock.

The oropharyngeal use of topical anaesthetic agents may interfere with swallowing and thus enhance the danger of aspiration. This is particularly important in children because of their frequency of eating. Numbness of the tongue or buccal mucosa may increase the danger of biting trauma.

When used for endotracheal tube lubrication care should be taken to avoid introduction of the jelly into the lumen of the tube. The jelly may dry on the inner surface leaving residue which tend to clump with flexion, narrowing the lumen. There have been rare reports in which this residue has caused the lumen to occlude.

Care should be taken to avoid instillation of excessive amounts of Xylocaine Gel 2%/Accordion Gel 2% into the rectum. This is of particular importance in infants and children. Systemic absorption of lidocaine may occur from the rectum, and large doses may result in CNS side-effects. On rare occasions convulsions have occurred in children.

Pregnancy: Although there is no evidence from animal studies of harm to the foetus, as with all drugs, Xylocaine should not be given during early pregnancy unless the benefits outweigh the risks.

Lactation: Lidocaine enters the mother's milk, but in such small quantities that there is generally no risk of affecting the child at therapeutic dose levels.

Side-effects: In extremely rare cases local anaesthetic preparations have been associated with allergic reactions (in the most severe instances anaphylactic shock).

Systemic adverse reactions are rare and may result from high plasma levels due to excessive dosage, rapid absorption or may result from hypersensitivity, idiosyncrasy or diminished tolerance on the part of the patient. Such reactions involve the central nervous system and/or the cardiovascular system.

CNS reactions are excitatory and/or depressant and may be characterised by nervousness, dizziness, convulsions, unconsciousness and, possibly, respiratory arrest. The excitatory reactions may be very brief or may not occur at all, in which case the first manifestations of toxicity may be drowsiness, merging into unconsciousness and respiratory arrest.

Cardiovascular reactions are depressant and may be characterised by hypotension, myocardial depression, bradycardia and possibly cardiac arrest.

Interactions: Lidocaine should be used with caution in patients receiving antiarrhythmic drugs, such as tocainide, since the toxic effects are additive.

Overdosage: Treatment of a patient with systemic toxicity consists of arresting convulsions and ensuring adequate ventilation with oxygen, if necessary by assisted or controlled ventilation (respiration). If convulsions occur, they should be treated rapidly by intravenous injection of thiopentone 100 to 200 mg or diazepam 5 to 10 mg. Alternatively succinylcholine 50 to 100 mg i.v. may be used providing the clinician is capable of performing endotracheal intubation and managing a fully paralysed patient. If ventricular fibrillation or cardiac arrest occurs effective cardiovascular resuscitation must be instituted. Adrenaline in repeated doses and sodium bicarbonate should be given as rapidly as possible.

Pharmaceutical precautions Xylocaine Gel 2% contains preservatives (see **Presentation**). Store below 25°C.

Xylocaine Accordion Gel 2% is sterile and is meant for single use only. Store below 25°C.

Legal category P.

Package quantities Xylocaine Gel 2%: Packs of 10 x 20 g tubes.

Xylocaine Accordion Gel 2%: Packs of 10 × 20 g Accordion syringes.

Further information Nil

Product licence numbers

Xylocaine Gel 2%	0017/0242R
Xylocaine Accordion Gel 2%	0017/5037R

XYLOCAINE* OINTMENT 5%

Presentation A water-soluble topical anaesthetic ointment.

1 g Xylocaine ointment contains: lignocaine 50 mg, propylene glycol, polyethylene glycols, water purified.

Xylocaine ointment contains lignocaine which is dissolved in a vehicle consisting of carbowaxes and propylene glycol. Lignocaine penetrates the tissues and exerts a topical anaesthetic effect. The onset of action is 3–5 minutes on mucous membrane. It is ineffective when applied to intact skin. Propylene glycol in the ointment base has an antibacterial effect against many pathogenic micro-organisms. The carbowax base melts readily at body temperature and spreads evenly. The ointment is easily removed with water.

Lignocaine stabilises the neuronal membrane and prevents the initiation and conduction of nerve impulses effecting local anaesthetic action. Lignocaine is absorbed following the application to mucous membranes. The absorption occurs most rapidly after intratracheal administration. The metabolism of lignocaine takes place in the liver and metabolites and unchanged drug are excreted by the kidney.

Uses Temporary relief of pain associated with minor burns and abrasions of the skin, e.g. sunburn, herpes zoster and labialis, pruritus, sore nipples, insect bites.

Anaesthesia of mucous membranes, e.g. various anal conditions such as haemorrhoids and fissures.

For the alleviation of pain during examination and instrumentation, e.g. proctoscopy, sigmoidoscopy, cystocopy, endotracheal intubation.

Dentistry: Surface anaesthesia of the gums prior to injection, before deep scaling and in conjunction with the fitting of new dentures.

Dosage and administration As with any local anaesthetic, reactions and complications are best averted by employing the minimal effective dosage. Debilitated, elderly patients and children should be given dosage commensurate with their age and physical condition.

The ointment should be applied in a thin layer for adequate control of symptoms. A sterile gauze pad is suggested for application to broken and burned tissue.

Apply to tube prior to endotracheal intubation.

In dentistry, apply to previously dried oral mucosa, allow at least 3-5 minutes for anaesthesia to become effective. When inserting new dentures, apply to all denture surfaces contacting mucosa.

For tender nipples, apply on a small piece of gauze; the ointment must be washed away before next feeding.

Not more than 35 g of the ointment should be administered in any 24 hour period.

Contra-indications, warnings, etc

Contra-indications: Known history of hypersensitivity to local anaesthetics of the amide type or to other components of the ointment.

Precautions: Absorption from wound surfaces and mucous membranes is relatively high, especially in the bronchial tree. This should be taken into special consideration when the ointment is used in children for treatment of large areas.

Xylocaine ointment should be used with caution in patients with traumatised mucosa and/or sepsis in the region of the proposed application.

If the dose or site of administration is likely to result in high blood levels, lignocaine, in common with other local anaesthetics should be used cautiously in patients with epilepsy, impaired cardiac conduction, bradycardia, impaired hepatic function and in severe shock.

The use of oral topical anaesthetic agents may interfere with swallowing and thus enhance the danger of aspiration. This is particularly important in children because of their frequency of eating. Numbness of the tongue or buccal mucosa may increase the danger of biting trauma.

When used for endotracheal tube lubrication care should be taken to avoid introduction of the ointment into the lumen of the tube. The ointment may dry on the inner surface leaving residue which tend to clump with flexion, narrowing the lumen. There have been rare reports in which this residue has caused the lumen to occlude.

Pregnancy: There is no or inadequate evidence of safety of the drug in human pregnancy but it has been in wide use for many years without apparent ill consequence, animal studies have shown no hazard. If drug therapy is needed in pregnancy, this drug can be used if there is no safer alternative.

Lactation: Lignocaine enters the mother's milk, but in such small quantities that there is generally no risk of affecting the child at therapeutic dose levels.

Side-effects: In extremely rare cases local anaesthetic preparations have been associated with allergic reactions (in the most severe instances anaphylactic shock).

Systemic adverse reactions are rare and may result from high plasma levels due to excessive dosage, rapid absorption or may result from hypersensitivity, idiosyncrasy or diminished tolerance on the part of the patient. Such reactions involve the central nervous system and/or the cardiovascular system.

CNS reactions are excitatory and/or depressant, and may be characterised by nervousness, dizziness, convulsions, unconsciousness and possible respiratory arrest. The excitatory reactions may be very brief or may not occur at all, in which case the first manifestations of toxicity may be drowsiness, merging into unconsciousness and respiratory arrest.

Cardiovascular reactions are depressant, and may be characterised by hypotension, myocardial depression, bradycardia and possibly cardiac arrest.

Interactions: Lignocaine should be used with caution in patients receiving antiarrhythmic drugs, such as tocainide, since the toxic effects are additive.

Overdosage: Treatment of a patient with toxic manifestations consists of ensuring adequate ventilation and arresting convulsions. Ventilation should be maintained with oxygen by assisted or controlled respiration as required. If convulsions occur, they should be treated rapidly by intravenous administration of succinylcholine 50–100 mg and/or 5–15 mg diazepam. As succinylcholine will arrest respiration it should only be used if the clinician has the ability to perform endotracheal intubation and to manage a totally paralysed patient. Thiopentone may also be used to abort convulsions in dosage 100–200 mg. If ventricular fibrillation or cardiac arrest occurs, effective cardiovascular resuscitation must be instituted. Adrenaline in repeated doses and sodium bicarbonate should be given as rapidly as possible.

Pharmaceutical precautions Store at room temperature.

Legal category P.

Package quantities 15 g tubes.

Further information Nil.

Product licence number 0017/5038R

XYLOCAINE* SPRAY

Presentation Topical anaesthetic pump spray containing lidocaine 10 mg/dose.

Inactive ingredients: Ethanol, polyethylene glycol 400, essence of banana, menthol natural, saccharin and purified water.

Uses For the prevention of pain associated with the following procedures:

Otorhinolaryngology: Puncture of the maxillary sinus and minor surgical procedures in the nasal cavity, pharynx and epipharynx.

Paracentesis.

Obstetrics: During the final stages of delivery and before episiotomy and perineal suturing as supplementary pain control.

Introduction of instruments and catheters into the respiratory and digestive tract: Provides surface anaesthesia for the oropharyngeal and tracheal areas to reduce reflex activity, attenuate haemodynamic response and to facilitate insertion of the tube or the passage of instruments during endotracheal intubation, laryngoscopy, bronchoscopy and oesophagoscopy.

Dental practice: Before injections, dental impressions, X-ray photography, removal of calculus.

Dosage and administration As with any local anaesthetic, reactions and complications are best averted by employing the minimal effective dosage. Debilitated or elderly patients and children should be given doses commensurate with their age and physical condition.

Each activation of the metered dose valve delivers 10 mg lidocaine base. It is unnecessary to dry the site prior to application. No more than 20 spray applications should be used in any adult to produce the desired anaesthetic effect.

The number of sprays depend on the extent of the area to be anaesthetised.

Dental practice: 1–5 applications to the mucous membranes.

Otorhinolaryngology: 3 applications for puncture of the maxillary sinus.

During delivery: Up to 20 applications (200 mg lidocaine base).

Introduction of instruments and catheters into the respiratory and digestive tract: Up to 20 applications (200 mg lidocaine base) for procedures in pharynx, larynx, and trachea.

Contra-indications, warnings, etc

Contra-indications: Known history of hypersensitivity to local anaesthetics of the amide type or to other components of the spray solution.

Precautions: Absorption from wound surfaces and mucous membranes is relatively high, especially in the bronchial tree. Xylocaine Spray should be used with caution in patients with traumatised mucosa and/or sepsis in the region of the proposed application.

If the dose or site of administration is likely to result in high blood levels, lidocaine, in common with other local anaesthetics, should be used with caution in patients with epilepsy, impaired cardiac conduction, bradycardia, impaired hepatic function and in severe shock.

The oropharyngeal use of topical anaesthetic agents may interfere with swallowing and thus enhance the danger of aspiration. This is particularly important in children because of their frequency of eating. Numbness of the tongue or buccal mucosa may increase the danger of biting trauma.

Avoid contact with the eyes.

Effect on ability to drive and use machines: Depending on the dose, local anaesthetics may have a very mild effect on mental function and may temporarily impair locomotion and co-ordination.

Use in pregnancy and lactation: There is no or inadequate evidence of safety of the drug in human pregnancy but it has been in wide use for many years without apparent ill consequence, animal studies having shown no hazard. If drug therapy is needed in pregnancy, this drug can be used if there is no safer alternative.

Lidocaine enters the mother's milk, but in such

small quantities that there is generally no risk of the child being affected at therapeutic dose levels.

Side-effects: In extremely rare cases local anaesthetic preparations have been associated with allergic reactions (in the most severe instances anaphylactic shock).

Systemic adverse reactions are rare and may result from high plasma levels due to excessive dosage or rapid absorption or from hypersensitivity, idiosyncrasy or reduced tolerance on the part of the patient. Such reactions involve the central nervous system and/or the cardiovascular system.

CNS reactions are excitatory and/or depressant and may be characterised by nervousness, dizziness, convulsions, unconsciousness and possibly respiratory arrest. The excitatory reactions may be very brief or may not occur at all, in which case the first manifestations of toxicity may be drowsiness, merging into unconsciousness and respiratory arrest.

Cardiovascular reactions are depressant and may be characterised by hypotension, myocardial depression, bradycardia and possibly cardiac arrest.

Interactions: Lidocaine should be used with caution in patients receiving antiarrhythmic drugs, such as tocainide, since the toxic effects are additive.

Overdosage: The treatment of a patient with toxic manifestations consists of ensuring adequate ventilation and arresting convulsions. Ventilation should be maintained with oxygen by assisted or controlled respiration as required. If convulsions occur, they should be treated rapidly by the intravenous administration of succinylcholine 50–100 mg and/or 5–15 mg diazepam. As succinylcholine will arrest respiration, it should only be used if the clinician has the ability to perform endotracheal intubation and to manage a totally paralysed patient. Thiopentone may also be used to abort convulsions in the dosage 100–200 mg. If ventricular fibrillation or cardiac arrest occurs, effective cardiopulmonary resuscitation must be instituted. Adrenaline in repeated doses and sodium bicarbonate should be given as rapidly as possible.

Pharmaceutical precautions Each depression of the metered valve delivers 10 mg lidocaine base. The contents of the spray bottle are sufficient to provide approximately 500 sprays.

Store below 25°C. During storage at temperatures below +8°C precipitation may occur. The precipitate dissolves on warming up to room temperature.

Legal category P.

Package quantities 50 ml spray bottles (approx. 500 spray doses) with a metering valve with applicator.

Further information The nozzle must not be shortened, as it will affect spray function. To clean the nozzle submerge in boiling water for 5 minutes. The nozzle may also be autoclaved.

Product licence number 0017/5039R

XYLOCAINE* 4% TOPICAL

Qualitative and quantitative composition Lidocaine Hydrochloride PhEur 42.8 mg/ml, corresponding to anhydrous lidocaine hydrochloride 40 mg/ml.

Pharmaceutical form Solution for topical anaesthesia.

Clinical particulars
Therapeutic indications: Anaesthesia of mucous membranes of the oropharyngeal, tracheal and bronchial areas e.g. in bronchography, bronchoscopy, laryngoscopy, oesophagoscopy and endotracheal intubation.

Biopsy in the mouth and throat: puncture of the maxillary sinus or polypectomy.

Tonsillectomy: resection of nasal turbinates.

In dentistry.

Surface anaesthesia may be achieved by instillation into a cavity or by spraying, e.g. using an atomiser or nebulizer. Xylocaine 4% Topical may also be applied from a swab.

Posology and method of administration: As with any local anaesthetic, reactions and complications are best averted by employing the minimal effective dosage. Debilitated or elderly patients and children should be given doses commensurate with their age and physical condition.

The recommended dosage for adults is 1-7.5 ml Xylocaine 4% Topical (= 40-300 mg lidocaine HCl). Doses exceeding 7.5 ml (= 300 mg lidocaine) may result in plasma levels associated with toxic manifestations.

In children, smaller amounts should be administered depending on their age and weight.

Biopsy: 3-4 ml may be sprayed on the area or the solution may be applied for a few minutes with a swab. Adrenaline may be added to this solution in order to produce vasoconstriction (add 1-2 drops, 0.05 ml, 1:1,000 solution to 5 ml Xylocaine 4% Topical).

Puncture of maxillary sinus or polypectomy: A swab soaked in the solution may be applied for two to three minutes. The addition of adrenaline is advised in these procedures, made up as indicated under 'Biopsy' above.

Xylocaine 4% Topical may be applied from a swab, which should be discarded after use. Surface anaesthesia may also be achieved by instillation into a cavity or on to a surface. When spraying, the solution should be transferred from the original container to an atomiser.

Contra-indications: Known history of hypersensitivity to local anaesthetics of the amide type or other components of the solution.

Special warnings and special precautions for use: Absorption from wound surfaces and mucous membranes is relatively high, especially in the bronchial tree. Xylocaine 4% Topical should be used with caution in patients with traumatised mucosa and/or sepsis in the region of the proposed application.

If the dose or site of administration is likely to result in high blood levels, lidocaine, in common with other local anaesthetics, should be used with caution in patients with epilepsy, impaired cardiac conduction, bradycardia, impaired hepatic function and in severe shock.

The oropharyngeal use of topical anaesthetic agents may interfere with swallowing and thus enhance the danger of aspiration. This is particularly important in children because of their frequency of eating. Numbness of the tongue or buccal mucosa may increase the danger of biting trauma.

Interaction with other medicaments and other forms of interaction: Lidocaine should be used with caution in patients receiving antiarrhythmic drugs, such as tocainide, since the toxic effects are additive.

Pregnancy and lactation: There is no or inadequate evidence of safety of the drug in human pregnancy but it has been in wide use for many years without apparent ill consequence, animal studies have shown no hazard. If drug therapy is needed in pregnancy, this drug can be used if there is no safer alternative.

Lidocaine enters the mother's milk, but in such small quantities that there is generally no risk of affecting the child at therapeutic dose levels.

Effects on ability to drive and use machines: Depending on the dose, local anaesthetics may have a very mild effect on mental function and may temporarily impair locomotion and co-ordination.

Undesirable effects: In extremely rare cases, local anaesthetic preparations have been associated with allergic reactions (in the most severe instances anaphylactic shock).

Systemic adverse reactions are rare and may result from high plasma levels due to excessive dosage or rapid absorption or from hypersensitivity, idiosyncrasy or reduced tolerance on the part of the patient. Such reactions involve the central nervous system and/or the cardiovascular system.

CNS reactions are excitatory and/or depressant and may be characterised by nervousness, dizziness, convulsions, unconsciousness and possibly respiratory arrest. The excitatory reactions may be very brief or may not occur at all, in which case the first manifestations of toxicity may be drowsiness, merging into unconsciousness and respiratory arrest.

Cardiovascular reactions are depressant and may be characterised by hypotension, myocardial depression, bradycardia and possibly cardiac arrest.

Overdose: The treatment of a patient with toxic manifestations consists of ensuring adequate ventilation and arresting convulsions. Ventilation should be maintained with oxygen by assisted or controlled respiration as required. If convulsions occur, they should be treated rapidly by the intravenous administration of succinylcholine 50-100 mg and/or 5-15 mg diazepam. As succinylcholine will arrest respiration, it should only be used if the clinician has the ability to perform endotracheal intubation and to manage a totally paralysed patient. Thiopentone may also be used to abort convulsions in the dosage 100-200 mg. If ventricular fibrillation or cardiac arrest occurs, effective cardiovascular resuscitation must be instituted. Adrenaline in repeated doses and sodium bicarbonate should be given as rapidly as possible.

Pharmacological properties
Pharmacodynamic properties: Lidocaine stabilises the neuronal membrane and prevents the initiation of nerve impulses, thereby affecting local anaesthetic action.

When applied topically to accessible mucous membranes anaesthesia occurs within 1-5 minutes and persists for 15-30 minutes.

Pharmacokinetic properties: Lidocaine is absorbed systemically when applied to mucous membranes; absorption occurs most rapidly after intratacteal administration.

The drug is extensively metabolised in the liver, and metabolites and a small amount of unchanged drug are excreted by the kidneys.

Preclinical safety data: Lidocaine hydrochloride is a well established active ingredient.

Pharmaceutical particulars
List of excipients: methyl parahydroxybenzoate, sodium hydroxide, water for injections.

Incompatibilities: None stated.

Shelf-life: 36 months.

Special precautions for storage: Store below 25°C. Avoid freezing.

Nature and contents of container: 30 ml brown soda glass bottles with pilfer-proof caps.

Instructions for use/handling: None stated.

Marketing authorisation number PL 0017/5040R

Date of approval/revision of SPC 21-11-97

Legal category P.

XYLOCARD*

Presentation *Xylocard 100 mg intravenous bolus injection:* Clear aqueous sterile solution in pre-loaded 5 ml syringe: lidocaine hydrochloride anhydrous 20 mg/ml, equivalent to 21.2 mg Lidocaine Hydrochloride Monohydrate for Injection PhEur.

Uses Prevention of ventricular tachyarrhythmias in patients with suspected or proven acute myocardial infarction. Treatment of ventricular tachyarrhythmias associated with acute myocardial infarction. Ventricular extrasystoles and ventricular tachycardia. As anti-arrhythmic cover in cases of ventricular fibrillation being DC converted.

Dosage and administration
Adults: Xylocard 100 mg i.v. bolus injection 1 mg/kg body weight. Normal dose 50–100 mg (2.5–5 ml) as initial treatment to be injected slowly over a period of two minutes. When necessary injection can be repeated once or twice at 5–10 minute intervals. Effect can be observed within two minutes and usually persists for 15–20 minutes. Not more than 200–300 mg should be administered during one hour.

Children: The safety and efficacy of lidocaine in children has not been established.

Elderly: In patients with cardiac failure, total plasma clearance will be reduced and lower dosages may be required.

Contra-indications, warnings, etc
Contra-indications: Known hypersensitivity to lidocaine (extremely rare). Known hypersensitivity to the local anaesthetics of the amide type, such as prilocaine, mepivacaine or bupivacaine.

Atrioventricular block is an absolute or relative contra-indication, according to severity and in the absence of pacemaker. Second or third degree AV-block. Other serious conduction disturbances, and cardiac decompensation not dependent on treatable tachyarrhythmias, are also contra-indicated.

Precautions: ECG-monitoring should be instituted when lidocaine is administered as an intravenous infusion.

Caution should be observed in patients with cardiac decompensation and hypotension or posterior diaphragmal infarction with a tendency towards heart block.

Lidocaine should be administered with caution to patients with bradycardia, untreated first-degree AV-block with bifascicular block or hypokalaemia.

Severely impaired liver or kidney function may mean a risk of accumulation and toxic reactions as lidocaine is mainly metabolised in the liver and the metabolites are excreted by the kidneys. Caution should be observed during repeated treatment with lidocaine in patients with these functional disorders.

When high doses are used and the patients myocardial function is impaired, combination with other drugs which reduce the excitability of cardiac muscle requires caution. Lidocaine treatment may aggravate arrhythmias.

The potassium concentration should be normalised before lidocaine treatment is started.

In patients with bradycardia complicated by ventricular tachyarrhythmia, lidocaine may have to be combined with atropine or atropine-like drugs or pacemaker treatment.

Pregnancy and lactation: Lidocaine has been used by a large number of pregnant women and women of child-bearing age. No specific disturbances to the reproductive process have so far been reported, e.g. an increased incidence of malformations or direct or indirect harmful effects on the foetus.

It is not known whether lidocaine is excreted in breast milk.

Side-effects: Most frequent are adverse reactions from the central and peripheral nervous system. They occur in 5–10% of the patients and are mostly dose-related.
Central and peripheral nervous system: Dizziness, paraesthesia and drowsiness. Rarely persistent dizziness, tinnitus, confusion, blurred vision, tremor, convulsions, loss of consciousness and respiratory depression.

Cardiovascular: Rarely hypotension and bradycardia, which may lead to cardiac arrest.

Interactions: Propranolol and cimetidine can impair the metabolism of lidocaine. Elimination will be delayed, the duration of action prolonged and the risk of adverse reactions increased.

Overdosage: Poisoning due to an overdose of lidocaine may lead to CNS excitation with paraesthesia, muscle twitching and convulsions, atrioventricular block, sinoatrial block or arrest, asystole, myocardial depression, severe hypotension and cardiac arrest.

Treatment should include close monitoring of cardiovascular and respiratory function and electrolytes. If convulsions occur, maintenance of a patent airway is mandatory and assisted or controlled ventilation with oxygen may be required. Convulsions may be controlled with intravenous diazepam or a short-acting barbiturate.

Cardiovascular complications should be treated symptomatically, which may require the use of sympathomimetic agents (e.g. noradrenaline, metaraminol), or inotropic agents (e.g. dopamine, dobutamine). Temporary pacing may be required for AV block.

Lidocaine is usually eliminated rapidly from the body, but elimination may be delayed in severe hypotension, cardiac failure or cardiogenic shock.

Pharmaceutical precautions Store below 25°C.

Legal category POM.

Further information All Xylocard syringes are free of bacteriostat and preservatives.

Product licence number 0017/5018R

XYLOPROCT* OINTMENT

Qualitative and quantitative composition Composition for 100 g: Lidocaine 5 g, Hydrocortisone acetate micro PhEur 0.275 g.

Pharmaceutical form Ointment.

Clinical particulars
Therapeutic indications: For the relief of symptoms such as anal and peri-anal pruritus, pain and inflammation associated with haemorrhoids, anal fissure, fistulas and proctitis. Pruritus vulva.

Posology and method of administration: To be applied several times daily according to the severity of the condition.

Contra-indications: Known hypersensitivity to local anaesthetics of the amide type or any of the other ingredients. Use on atrophic skin.

Special warnings and special precautions for use: Xyloproct is intended for use for limited periods.

Appropriate antibacterial, antiviral or antifungal therapy should be given with Xyloproct if infection is present at the site of application.

The possibility of malignancy should be excluded before use.

If irritation or rectal bleeding develops treatment should be discontinued.

When using the special applicator, care should be taken to avoid instillation of excessive amounts of Xyloproct Ointment into the rectum. This is of particular importance in infants and children.

Systemic absorption of lidocaine may occur from the rectum, and large doses may result in CNS side-effects. On rare occasions convulsions have occurred in children. Xyloproct Suppositories should be used in preference to ointment for treatment of proctitis or internal haemorrhoids.

Interaction with other medicaments and other forms of interaction: Lidocaine should be used with caution in patients receiving antiarrhythmic drugs, such as tocainide, since the toxic effects are additive.

Pregnancy and lactation: Do not use in pregnancy unless considered essential by the physician.

Lidocaine and hydrocortisone acetate are excreted into breast milk but in such small quantities that adverse effects on the child are unlikely at therapeutic doses.

Effects on ability to drive and use machines: None known.

Undesirable effects: Local reactions such as dermatitis have been reported with the use of Xyloproct ointment.

Overdosage: When using the special applicator care should be taken to avoid instillation of excessive amounts of Xyloproct Ointment into the rectum. This is of particular importance in infants and children.

Systemic absorption of lidocaine may occur from the rectum, and large doses may result in CNS side effects. On rare occasions convulsions have occurred in children. Xyloproct Suppositories should be used in preference to ointment for treatment of proctitis or internal haemorrhoids.

Pharmacological properties
Pharmacodynamic properties: Lidocaine exerts a local anaesthetic effect by stabilising the neural membrane and preventing the initiation and conduction of nerve impulses.

Hydrocortisone acetate belongs to the mild group of corticosteroids and is effective because of its anti-inflammatory and anti-pruritic action.

Pharmacokinetic properties: The onset of action of lidocaine is 3–5 minutes on mucous membranes. Lidocaine can be absorbed following application to mucous membranes with metabolism taking place in the liver. Metabolites and unchanged drug are excreted by the kidney.

Absorption of hydrocortisone may occur from normal intact skin and mucous membranes. Locally applied hydrocortisone acetate is mainly transformed in dermis or epidermis to inactive metabolites.

Preclinical safety data: Lidocaine hydrochloride and hydrocortisone acetate are well established active ingredients.

Pharmaceutical particulars
List of excipients: Zinc oxide, Aluminium acetate, Stearyl alcohol, cetyl alcohol, water purified, polyethylene glycol 3350, polyethylene glycol 400.

Incompatibilities: None known.

Shelf-life: The shelf-life of this product is 2 years when stored below 5°C and 2 months when stored at 25°C.

Special precautions for storage: Store in a refrigerator. The patient may store the ointment at 25°C for 2 months. The product should be discarded 2 months after opening.

Nature and contents of container: Aluminium tube 30 g.

Instructions for use/handling: None.

Marketing authorisation number PL 0017/5023R

Date of approval/revision of SPC 25-04-97.

Product licence number 0017/5023R

XYLOPROCT* SUPPOSITORIES

Qualitative and quantitative composition Lidocaine 60 mg, Hydrocortisone acetate PhEur 5 mg.

Pharmaceutical form Suppositories.

Clinical particulars
Therapeutic indications: For the treatment of symptoms associated with haemorrhoids and other disorders of the anal canal such as proctitis, anal fissure and anal fistula.

Posology and method of administration: Remove protective foil, use one suppository at night before retiring and repeat the treatment after each bowel action.

Contra-indications: Known hypersensitivity to local anaesthetics of the amide type or any of the other ingredients. Use on atrophic skin.

Special warnings and special precautions for use: Xyloproct is intended for use for limited periods.

Appropriate antibacterial, antiviral or antifugal therapy should be given with Xyloproct if infection is present at the site of application.

The possibility of malignancy should be excluded before use.

If irritation or rectal bleeding develops, treatment should be discontinued.

Xyloproct suppositories should be used in preference to ointment for the treatment of proctitis or internal haemorrhoids.

Interaction with other medicaments and other forms of interaction: Lidocaine should be used with caution in patients receiving antiarrhythmic drugs, such as tocainide, since the toxic effects are additive.

Pregnancy and Lactation: Do not use in pregnancy unless considered essential by the physician.

Lidocaine and hydrocortisone acetate are excreted into breast milk but in such small quantities that adverse effects on the child are unlikely at therapeutic doses.

Effects on ability to drive and use machines: None known.

Undesirable effects: Local reactions such as dermatitis have been reported with the use of Xyloproct ointment.

Overdose: Care should be taken to avoid application of excessive quantities of Xyloproct suppositories into the rectum. This is of particular importance in infants and children. Systemic absorption of lidocaine may occur from the rectum and large doses may result in CNS side effects. On rare occasions convulsions have occurred in children.

Pharmacological properties
Pharmacodynamic properties: Lidocaine exerts a local anaesthetic effect by stabilising the neural membrane and preventing the initiation and conduction of nerve impulses.

Hydrocortisone acetate belongs to the mild group of corticosteroids and is effective because of its anti-inflammatory and anti-pruritic action.

Pharmacokinetic properties: The onset of action of lidocaine is 3-5 minutes on mucous membranes. Lidocaine can be absorbed following application to mucous membranes with metabolism taking place in the liver. Metabolites and unchanged drug are excreted by the kidney.

Absorption of hydrocortisone may occur from normal intact skin and mucous membranes. Locally applied hydrocortisone acetate is mainly transformed in dermis or epidermis to inactive metabolites.

Preclinical safety data: Lidocaine and hydrocortisone acetate are well established active ingredients.

Pharmaceutical particulars
List of excipients: Zinc oxide powder 40 PhEur, Aluminium acetate basic powder, Hard fat (Witepsol W25) PhEur.

Incompatibilities: None known.

Shelf-life: The shelf-life of this product is 2.5 years.

Special precautions for storage: Store in a fridge (below 5°C). The patient may store the product at room temperature (25°C) for 2 months. The remaining suppositories should then be discarded. Avoid freezing.

Nature and contents of container: Polypropylene coated aluminium foil packs of 10 suppositories.

Instructions for use/handling: None.

Marketing authorisation number PL 0017/5024R

Date of approval/revision of SPC 08-09-97

Legal category POM.

XYLOTOX* 2% E80

Presentation Xylotox 2% E80 is a sterile clear aqueous solution of lidocaine hydrochloride monohydrate 24.65 mg equivalent to lidocaine base 20 mg and adrenaline tartrate 25.0 micrograms corresponding to adrenaline 12.5 micrograms.

Xylotox 2% E80 is supplied in polypropylene cartridges for use in dental type syringes.

Inactive ingredients: Sodium chloride, calcium chloride, potassium chloride and sodium metabisulphite.

Uses Local anaesthetic solution with vasoconstrictor for dental infiltration anaesthesia where a vasoconstrictor is indicated.

Dosage and administration Infiltration – 0.5 to 2 ml. Nerve block – 1.5 to 2 ml. Extensive surgery – 3 to 10 ml. Adult maximum dose 500 mg.

In children the maximum dose is considerably less and should be calculated in relation to the body weight.

Contra-indications, warnings, etc
Contra-indications: Known hypersensitivity to anaesthetics of the amide type.

Xylotox 2% E80 should not be given intravenously.

The use of a vasoconstrictor is contra-indicated for anaesthesia of the fingers, toes, tip of nose and penis.

Precautions: In common with other local anaesthetics, Xylotox 2% E80 should be used cautiously in patients with epilepsy, cardiac disease particularly with arrhythmia or hypertension, impaired respiratory function, thyrotoxicosis, hypovolaemia, acute porphyria and impaired hepatic function.

Adequate resuscitation equipment must be available whenever local or general anaesthesia is administered. Though clinical tolerance is remarkably good, overdosage or accidental intravenous injection may give rise to toxic reactions.

These are best avoided by aspiration before making an injection in order to avoid accidental intravascular injection.

Use in pregnancy and lactation: There is no or inadequate evidence of safety of the drug in human pregnancy but it has been in wide use for many years without apparent ill consequence, animal studies have shown no hazard. If drug therapy is needed in pregnancy this drug can be used if there is no safer alternative.

Lidocaine enters the mother's milk but in such small quantities that there is generally no risk of affecting the child at therapeutic dose levels.

Side-effects: The type of toxic reaction is unpredictable and depends on dosage, route of administration and state of patient, the reactions are primarily of two types, typified by stimulation and depression of the cerebral cortex and medulla respectively. Slow onset – stimulation leading to nervousness, dizziness, blurred vision, nausea, tremor, convulsions and respiratory arrest. Rapid onset – depression leading primarily to respiratory arrest, cardiovascular collapse and cardiac arrest. Symptoms occur rapidly and with little warning.

Interactions: Care should be observed in patients taking tricyclic anti-depressants.

Overdose: Toxicity is initially manifested as CNS excitation and may be characterised by nervousness, dizziness, blurred vision and tremors followed by drowsiness, convulsions, unconsciousness and possible respiratory arrest. Toxic cardiovascular reactions to local anaesthetics are usually depressant in nature and are characterised by peripheral vasodilation, hypotension, myocardial depression, bradycardia and possibly cardiac arrest.

Treatment of a patient with toxic symptoms consists of assuring a patent airway and supporting ventilation with oxygen and assisted or controlled respiration as required. This usually will be sufficient in the management of most reactions.

Should a convulsion persist despite ventilation therapy, small increments of a benzodiazepine (e.g. diazepam) or an ultra-short acting barbiturate (e.g. thiopentone) may be given intravenously.

Cardiovascular depression may require circulatory assistance in the form of intravenous fluids and/or vasopressor agents as dictated by the clinical situation.

Pharmaceutical precautions Store below 25°C (polypropylene).

Legal category POM.

Package quantities Polypropylene cartridges of 2.2 ml in boxes of 100.

Further information Nil.

Product licence number PL 0017/0141

**Trade Mark*

Athena Neurosciences
1 Meadway Court
Rutherford Close
Stevenage
Herts SG1 2EF

☎ 01438 730200   🗋 01438 741452

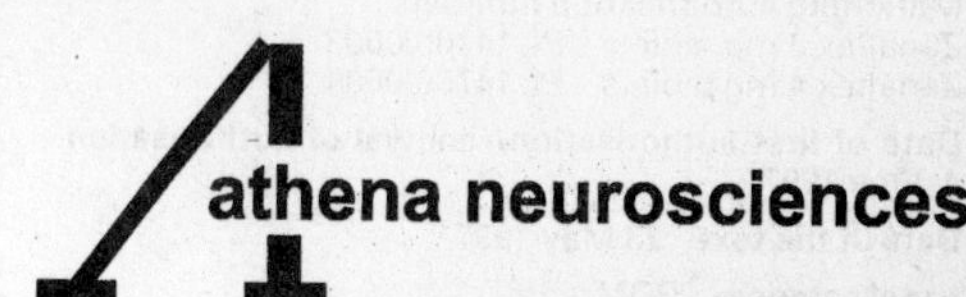

ZANAFLEX* ▼

Qualitative and quantitative composition Zanaflex tablets containing 2 mg or 4 mg of tizanidine as the hydrochloride.

Pharmaceutical form Tablets for oral administration.

Clinical particulars

Therapeutic indications: Treatment of spasticity associated with multiple sclerosis or with spinal cord injury or disease.

Posology and method of administration: For oral administration

The effect of Zanaflex on spasticity is maximal within 2-3 hours of dosing and it has a relatively short duration of action. The timing and frequency of dosing should therefore be tailored to the individual, and Zanaflex should be given in divided doses, up to 3-4 times daily, depending on the patient's needs. There is considerable variation in response between patients so careful titration is necessary. Care should be taken not to exceed the dose producing the desired therapeutic effect. It is usual to start with a single dose of 2 mg increasing by 2 mg increments at no less than half-weekly intervals.

The total daily dose should not exceed 36 mg, although it is usually not necessary to exceed 24 mg daily. Secondary pharmacological effects (see section 4.8 Undesirable Effects) may occur at therapeutic doses but these can be minimised by slow titration so that in the large majority of patients they are not a limiting factor.

Elderly: Experience in the elderly is limited and use of Zanaflex is not recommended unless the benefit of treatment clearly outweighs the risk. Pharmacokinetic data suggest that renal clearance in the elderly may be decreased by up to three fold.

Children: Experience with Zanaflex in patients under the age of 18 years is limited. Zanaflex is not recommended for use in children.

Patients with renal impairment: In patients with renal insufficiency (creatinine clearance < 25 mL/min) treatment should be started with 2 mg once daily with slow titration to achieve the effective dose. Dosage increases should be in increments of no more than 2 mg according to tolerability and effectiveness. It is advisable to slowly increase the once-daily dose before increasing the frequency of administration. Renal function should be monitored as appropriate in these patients.

Patients with hepatic impairment: Zanaflex is contraindicated in patients with significantly impaired hepatic function.

Contra-indications: Hypersensitivity to tizanidine or any other component of the product.

The use of Zanaflex in patients with significantly impaired hepatic function is contraindicated, because tizanidine is extensively metabolised by the liver.

Special warnings and special precautions for use:
Use in renal impairment: Patients with renal impairment may require lower doses and therefore caution should be exercised when using Zanaflex in these patients (see section 4.2 Posology and Method of Administration).

Liver function: Hepatic dysfunction has been reported in association with Zanaflex. It is recommended that liver function tests should be monitored monthly for the first four months in all patients and in those who develop symptoms suggestive of liver dysfunction such as unexplained nausea, anorexia or tiredness. Treatment with Zanaflex should be discontinued if serum levels of SGPT and/or SGOT are persistently above three times the upper limit of normal range.

Zanaflex should be kept out of the reach of children.

Interaction with other medicaments and other forms of interaction: As Zanaflex may induce hypotension it may potentiate the effect of antihypertensive drugs, including diuretics, and caution should therefore be exercised in patients receiving blood pressure lowering drugs. Caution should also be exercised when Zanaflex is used concurrently with β-adrenoceptor blocking drugs or digoxin as the combination may potentiate hypotension or bradycardia.

Pharmacokinetic data following single and multiple doses of Zanaflex suggested that clearance of Zanaflex was reduced by approximately 50% in women who were concurrently taking oral contraceptives. Although no specific pharmacokinetic study has been conducted to investigate a potential interaction between oral contraceptives and Zanaflex, the possibility of a clinical response and/or adverse effects occurring at lower doses of Zanaflex should be borne in mind when prescribing Zanaflex to a patient taking the contraceptive pill. Clinically significant drug-drug interactions have not been reported in clinical trials.

Alcohol or sedatives may enhance the sedative action of Zanaflex.

Pregnancy and lactation: Reproductive studies in rats and rabbits indicate that Zanaflex does not have embryotoxic or teratogenic potential but at maternally toxic doses of 10-100 mg/kg per day Zanaflex can retard foetal development due to its pharmacodynamic effects. Zanaflex and/or its metabolites have been found in the milk of rodents (see section 5.3 preclinical safety data). The safety of Zanaflex in pregnancy has not been established and its safety in breast-fed infants of mothers receiving Zanaflex is not known. Therefore Zanaflex should not be used in pregnant or nursing mothers unless the likely benefit clearly outweighs the risk.

Effects on ability to drive and use machines: Patients experiencing drowsiness should be advised against activities requiring a high degree of alertness, eg. driving a vehicle or operating machinery.

Undesirable effects: The most frequently reported adverse events occurring in association with Zanaflex include drowsiness, fatigue, dizziness, dry mouth, nausea, gastrointestinal disturbances, and a reduction in blood pressure. With slow upward titration of the dose of Zanaflex these effects are usually not severe enough to require discontinuation of treatment. Insomnia, bradycardia and hallucinations have also been reported. The hallucinations are self-limiting, without evidence of psychosis, and have invariably occurred in patients concurrently taking potentially hallucinogenic drugs, eg. anti-depressants. Increases in hepatic serum transaminases, which are reversible on stopping treatment, have occurred. Infrequent cases of acute hepatitis have been reported. Muscle weakness has been reported infrequently, although in controlled clinical trials it was clearly demonstrated that Zanaflex does not adversely affect muscle strength.

Overdose: Clinical experience is limited. In one adult case, who ingested 400 mg Zanaflex, recovery was uneventful. This patient received mannitol and frusemide.

Symptoms: nausea, vomiting, hypotension, dizziness, miosis, respiratory distress, coma, restlessness, somnolence.

Treatment: General supportive measures are indicated and an attempt should be made to remove uningested drug from the gastro-intestinal tract using gastric lavage or activated charcoal. The patient should be well hydrated.

Pharmacological properties

Pharmacodynamic properties: Tizanidine is an α_2-adrenergic receptor agonist within the central nervous system at supra-spinal and spinal levels. This effect results in inhibition of spinal polysynaptic reflex activity. Tizanidine has no direct effect on skeletal muscle, the neuromuscular junction or on monosynaptic spinal reflexes.

In humans, tizanidine reduces pathologically increased muscle tone, including resistance to passive movements and alleviates painful spasms and clonus.

Pharmacokinetic properties: Tizanidine is rapidly absorbed, reaching peak plasma concentration in approximately 1 hour. Tizanidine is only about 30% bound to plasma proteins and, in animal studies, was found to readily cross the blood-brain barrier. Although tizanidine is well absorbed, first pass metabolism limits plasma availability to 34% of that of an intravenous dose. Tizanidine undergoes rapid and extensive metabolism in the liver and the pattern of biotransformation in animals and humans is qualitatively similar. The metabolites are primarily excreted via the renal route (approximately 70% of the administered dose) and appear to be inactive. Renal excretion of the parent compound is approximately 53% after a single 5 mg dose and 66% after dosing with 4 mg three times daily. The elimination half-life of tizanidine from plasma is 2-4 hours in patients.

Concomitant food intake has no influence on the pharmacokinetic profile of tizanidine tablets.

Preclinical safety data:
Acute toxicity: Tizanidine possesses a low order of acute toxicity. Signs of overdosage were seen after single doses >40 mg/kg in animals and are related to the pharmacological action of the drug.

Repeat dose toxicity: The toxic effects of tizanidine are mainly related to its pharmacological action. At doses of 24 and 40 mg/kg per day in subchronic and chronic rodent studies, the α_2-agonist effects resulted in CNS stimulation, eg. motor excitation, aggressiveness, tremor and convulsions.

Signs related to centrally mediated muscle relaxation, eg. sedation and ataxia, were frequently observed at lower dose levels in subchronic and chronic oral studies with dogs. Such signs, related to the myotonolytic activity of the drug, were noted at 1 to 4 mg/kg per day in a 13 week dog study, and at 1.5 mg/kg per day in a 52- week dog study.

Prolongation of the QT interval and bradycardia were noted in chronic toxicity studies in dogs at doses of 1.0 mg/kg per day and above.

Slight increases in hepatic serum transaminases were observed in a number of toxicity studies at higher dose levels. They were not consistently associated with histopathological changes in the liver.

Mutagenicity: Various in vitro assays as well as in vivo assays produced no evidence of mutagenic potential of tizanidine.

Carcinogenicity: No evidence for carcinogenicity was demonstrated in two long-term dietary studies in mice (78 weeks) and rats (104 weeks), at dose levels up to 9 mg/kg per day in rats and up to 16 mg/kg per day in mice. At these dose levels, corresponding to the maximum tolerated dose, based on reductions in growth rate, no neoplastic or pre-neoplastic pathology, attributable to treatment, was observed.

Reproductive toxicity: No embryotoxicity or teratogenicity occurred in pregnant rats and rabbits at dose levels up to 30 mg/kg per day of tizanidine. However, doses of 10-100 mg/kg per day in rats were maternally toxic and resulted in developmental retardation of foetuses as seen by lower foetal body weights and retarded skeletal ossification.

In female rats, treated prior to mating through lactation or during late pregnancy until weaning of the young, a dose-dependent (10 and 30 mg/kg per day) prolongation of gestation time and dystocia occurred, resulting in an increased foetal mortality and delayed development. These effects were attributed to the pharmacological effect of tizanidine. No developmental effects occurred at 3 mg/kg per day although sedation was induced in the treated dams. Passage of tizanidine and/or its metabolites into milk of rodents is known to occur.

Pharmaceutical particulars

List of excipients
Zanaflex tablets: silica, colloidal anhydrous; stearic acid; cellulose, microcrystalline; lactose, anhydrous.

Incompatibilities: None known

Shelf life: Zanaflex tablets: 5 years in both temperate and hot climates, and 5 years in tropical climate.

Special precautions for storage: None

Nature and contents of container:
2 mg tablets: Carton of 120, in blister strips (PVC/PVDC Alfoil) of 30.
4 mg tablets: Carton of 120, in blister strips (PVC/PVDC Alfoil) of 30.

Instructions for use/handling: Not applicable

Marketing authorisation holder Athena Neurosciences (Europe) Ltd, Stevenage.

Marketing authorisation numbers
Zanaflex 2 mg tablets PL 14700/0003
Zanaflex 4 mg tablets PL 14700/0001

Date of first authorisation/renewal of authorisation
4 June 1997

Date of the text 23 May 1997

Legal category POM

ZELAPAR*

Qualitative and quantitative composition Each Zelapar tablet contains 1.25 mg of selegiline hydrochloride, equivalent to 1.05 mg selegiline free base.

Pharmaceutical form Oral lyophilisate (freeze dried tablet).

Clinical particulars
Therapeutic indications: Adjunctive therapy in combination with levodopa (with or without a peripheral decarboxylase inhibitor or other treatment of Parkinson's disease) in the treatment of Parkinson's disease and symptomatic parkinsonism. Zelapar in combination with maximal levodopa therapy is indicated particularly in patients who experience fluctuations in their condition such as 'end-dose' type fluctuations, 'on-off' symptoms or other dyskinesias.

Zelapar may be used alone in early Parkinson's disease for symptomatic relief and/or to delay the need for levodopa.

Zelapar is particularly indicated in those patients with Parkinson's disease who experience difficulties in swallowing.

Posology and method of administration: When prescribed as monotherapy for the first time in the early stage of Parkinson's disease or as an adjuvant to levodopa, the initial dose of Zelapar is one 1.25mg unit placed on the tongue in the morning before breakfast and allowed to dissolve. The unit will dissolve rapidly (in less than 10 seconds) in the mouth. The patient should not drink, rinse or wash-out out their mouth for five minutes after taking their medicine to enable selegiline to be absorbed pre-gastrically.

When Zelapar adjunctive therapy is prescribed a reduction (10 to 30%) in the dose of levodopa is usually required. Reduction of the levodopa dose should be gradual in steps of 10% every 3 to 4 days.

Patients already receiving 10mg conventional selegiline tablets can be switched to Zelapar 1.25mg.

No dosage adjustment is required for patients with renal or hepatic impairment.

Contra-indications: Zelapar is contra-indicated in patients with known hypersensitivity (including severe dizziness or hypotension) to conventional selegiline tablets or liquid.
Selegiline is also contra-indicated for concomitant use with pethidine, other opioids and fluoxetine (and, as a precaution, other selective serotonin reuptake inhibitors).

Selegiline should not be used in patients with other extrapyramidal disorders not related to dopamine deficiency.

Selegiline should not be used in patients with active duodenal or gastric ulcer.

Selegiline should not be used in patients who are being treated with antidepressant drugs or other monoamine oxidase inhibitors.

Selegiline in combination with levodopa is contra-indicated in severe cardiovascular disease, arterial hypertension, hyperthyroidism, phaeochromocytoma, narrow-angle glaucoma, prostatic adenoma with appearance of residual urine, tachycardia, arrhythmias, severe angina pectoris, psychoses, advanced dementia and thyrotoxicosis.

Special warnings and precautions for use: Special care should be taken when administering selegiline to patients who have labile hypertension, cardiac arrhythmias, severe angina pectoris, psychosis or a history of peptic ulceration.

Although serious hepatic toxicity has not been observed, caution is recommended in patients with a history of hepatic dysfunction. Transient or continuing abnormalities with a tendency for elevated plasma concentrations of liver enzymes have been described during long-term therapy with conventional tablets of selegiline.

The selectivity for MAO-B following administration of conventional selegiline tablets may be diminished with doses above 10mg/day. A non-selective dose of Zelapar above 10mg/day has not been determined. The precise dose at which selegiline becomes a non-selective inhibitor of all MAO has not been determined, but with doses higher than 10mg/day there is a theoretical risk of hypertension after ingestion of tyramine-rich food.

Concomitant treatment with medicines which inhibit MAO-A, (or non-selective MAO inhibitors) can cause hypotensive reactions. Hypotension, sometimes sudden in onset, has been reported with conventional selegiline.

Since selegiline potentiates the effects of levodopa, the adverse effects of levodopa may be increased. When selegiline is added to the maximum tolerated dose of levodopa, involuntary movements and agitation may occur. Levodopa should be reduced by about 10 to 30% when selegiline is added to the treatment (see section 4.2 Posology and Method of Administration). When an optimum dose of levodopa is reached, adverse effects from the combination are less than those observed with levodopa on its own.

Although conventional tablets of selegiline, at doses of 5 to 10mg/day, have been in widespread use for many years, the full spectrum of possible responses to Zelapar may not have been observed to date. Therefore patients should be observed closely for atypical responses.

Interaction with other medicaments and other forms of interaction: Serious reactions with signs and symptoms that may include diaphoresis, flushing, ataxia, tremor, hyperthermia, hyper/hypotension, seizures, palpitation, dizziness and mental changes that include agitation, confusion and hallucinations progressing to delirium and coma have been reported in some patients receiving a combination of selegiline and fluoxetine.

Similar experience has been reported in patients receiving selegiline and two other serotonin reuptake inhibitors, sertraline and paroxetine. Since the mechanisms of these reactions are not fully understood, it is recommended to avoid the combination of selegiline and fluoxetine, sertraline or paroxetine.

Death has been reported to occur following the initiation of therapy with non-selective MAO inhibitors shortly after discontinuation of fluoxetine. Because of the long half-lives of fluoxetine and its active metabolite, at least 5 weeks (approximately 5 half-lives) should elapse between discontinuation of fluoxetine and initiation of MAO inhibitor therapy. Based on experience with the combined use of MAO inhibitors and tricyclic antidepressants, at least 14 days should elapse between discontinuation of an MAO inhibitor and initiation of treatment with fluoxetine. Accordingly, selegiline should not be given in conjunction with non-specific MAO inhibitors.

Selegiline should not be administered with any type of antidepressants.

Severe CNS toxicity has been reported in patients with the combination of tricyclic antidepressants and selegiline. In one patient receiving amitriptyline and selegiline this included hyperpyrexia and death, and another patient receiving protriptyline and selegiline experienced tremor, agitation, and restlessness followed by unresponsiveness and death two weeks after selegiline was added.

Other adverse reactions occasionally reported in patients receiving a combination of selegiline with various tricyclic antidepressants include hyper/hypotension, dizziness, diaphoresis, tremor, seizures and changes in behavioural and mental status.

Concomitant use of sympathomimetics, nasal decongestants, hypertensive agents, antihypertensives, psychostimulants, central suppressant drugs (sedatives, hypnotics) and alcohol should be avoided.

Foodstuffs containing tyramine have not been found to cause hypertensive reactions during therapy with conventional selegiline tablets at dosages recommended for the treatment of Parkinson's disease. As the selectivity of action of Zelapar for MAO-B is identical to that of conventional tablets of selegiline given in the same dosage (10mg), no adverse interactions with foodstuffs containing tyramine are anticipated with Zelapar.

Concomitant administration of amantadine and anticholinergic drugs can lead to an increased occurrence of side-effects.

In view of the high degree of binding to plasma proteins by selegiline particular attention must be given to patients who are being treated with medicines with a narrow therapeutic margin such as digitalis and/or anticoagulants.

Interactions between non-selective MAO-inhibitors and pethidine as well as selegiline and pethidine have been described. The mechanism of this interaction is not fully understood and therefore, use of pethidine concomitantly with selegiline should be avoided (see contra-indications).

Pregnancy and lactation: Selegiline is indicated for the treatment of Parkinson's disease and symptomatic parkinsonism, which, in most cases, is a disease occurring after childbearing age. As no work has been done to assess the effects of selegiline on pregnancy and lactation, it should not be used in such cases.

Information is lacking concerning whether selegiline passes into breast milk.

Effects on ability to drive and use machines: Even when used correctly, this medicine can affect reaction capacity to the extent that driving or operating machinery is affected and therefore patients should avoid these activities. This effect is potentiated further by alcohol.

Undesirable effects: In clinical trials, Zelapar was associated with the following adverse events in 5% or more of patients: back pain, dizziness, tremor, sore throat. Adverse events occurring with Zelapar at a frequency of less than 5% include stomatitis, mouth ulceration, impaired balance, muscle cramps, joint pain, falling, insomnia, abnormal dreams, hallucinations, nasal congestion, constipation, diarrhoea and pharyngitis.

Serious adverse reactions with selegiline in monotherapy have been reported as follows: depression, chest pain, myopathy, hypotension and diarrhoea. Other reported adverse reactions included dry mouth, insomnia, tiredness, headache, nausea, dizziness and vertigo. Transient increases in liver enzyme values have also been observed.

As selegiline potentiates the effect of levodopa, the side-effects of levodopa may be emphasised unless the dosage of levodopa is reduced. When selegiline is added to the maximal levodopa therapy tolerated by the patient, the patient may experience, for example, involuntary movements, agitation, insomnia and confusion. The most common undesirable effect reported for conventional tablets is hyperkinesia (10 to 15% of patients). Commonly reported undesirable effects for selegiline (>1%): dizziness, hypotension, problems in sleeping, dry mouth, nausea, transient transaminase increase (ALAT), confusion, hallucinations and psychoses. Other side-effects reported for selegiline include loss of appetite and other gastrointestinal disorders, headache, agitation, anxiety, irritability, micturition disorders, dyspnoea, palpitations, arrhythmias, angina pectoris, tiredness, depression, loss of balance, hypertension, syncope, excessive perspiration, ankle oedema, hair loss and blurred vision. The dosage of levodopa may be reduced by about 10 to 30% when selegiline is added to the therapy. Once the optimum levodopa dose level has been established, the side-effects produced by this combination will usually be less than those caused by the levodopa therapy on its own.

Overdose: Zelapar is rapidly metabolised and the metabolites rapidly excreted. In cases of suspected overdosage the patient should be kept under observation for 24 to 48 hours.

No specific information is available about clinically significant overdoses with Zelapar. However, experience gained in use of conventional tablets of selegiline reveals that some individuals exposed to doses of 60mg/day suffered severe hypotension and psychomotor agitation.

Since the selective inhibition of MAO-B by selegiline hydrochloride is achieved only at doses in the range recommended for the treatment of Parkinson's disease, overdoses are likely to cause significant inhibition of both MAO-A and MAO-B. Consequently, the signs and symptoms of overdose may resemble those observed with non-selective MAOIs (e.g. tranylcypromine, isocarboxazide and phenelzine) and are dizziness, ataxia, irritability, pyrexia, tremor, convulsions, hypomania, psychosis, convulsions, euphoria, respiratory depression, hypotension, hypertension (sometimes with sub-arachnoid haemorrhage), coma and extra-pyramidal symptoms.

Pharmacological properties
Pharmacodynamic properties: Zelapar selectively inhibits MAO-B. It prevents dopamine and β-phenylethylamine breakdown in the brain. Selegiline can be used as monotherapy and permits the initiation of treatment with levodopa to be significantly postponed. It potentiates and prolongs the effect of concomitantly administered levodopa. Since it does not interfere with the breakdown of 5-hydroxytryptamine (serotonin) or noradrenaline, it does not cause any hypertensive crises or changes in the plasma or urinary metabolites of these monoamines. Although dietary restrictions are not necessary during Zelapar treatment, the inhibition of MAO-B in blood platelets can lead to a slight potentiation of the circulatory effects of any tyramine not broken down by gastrointestinal MAO-A during absorption. This effect is no greater with Zelapar than with conventional selegiline in equal doses.

The magnitude of increase in the urinary excretion of β-phenylethylamine over 24 hours is simply related to the area under the selegiline plasma concentration-time curve after any selegiline product. Urinary β-phenylethylamine increase reflects the degree of inhibition of MAO-B. Zelapar gives rise to a similar increase in β-phenylethylamine as 10mg conventional selegiline tablets.

Combined with levodopa therapy selegiline reduces, in particular, fluctuation in the condition of patients who suffer from parkinsonism, e.g. on-off symptoms or end-of-dose akinesia.

Pharmacokinetic properties: Zelapar dissolves completely within 10 seconds of placing on the tongue and, in contrast to conventional tablets, selegiline is absorbed primarily pregastrically.

The plasma concentrations of selegiline following single doses of Zelapar 1.25mg are similar to those obtained with conventional 10mg tablets of selegiline, but are much less variable. The range of AUCs for plasma selegiline is 0.22 to 2.82 ng.h/ml for Zelapar 1.25mg and 0.05 to 23.64 ng.h/ml for conventional 10mg tablets. The Cmax ranges are 0.32 to 4.58 ng/ml and 0.07 to 16.0 ng/ml respectively.

After Zelapar 1.25mg, plasma concentrations of selegiline metabolites, *N*-desmethylselegiline, *l*-metamphetamine and *l*-amphetamine, were reduced by between 88% and 92% in comparison with the concentrations reached after conventional selegiline tablets 10mg.

Ninety-four per cent of plasma selegiline is reversibly bound to protein. Selegiline is excreted mainly in the urine as metabolites (mainly *l*-metamphetamine) and the remainder in the faeces.

Pre-clinical safety data: The acute toxic range for rats, mice and dogs is approximately 800-3000 times that of the recommended therapeutic dose of conventional tablets of selegiline (5-10mg/day). The corresponding therapeutic margin from subchronic and chronic toxicity studies is 20-40 times, with only the reactions being attributable to the pharmacological effect, i.e. no organ-toxic effects being detected. There is also no evidence of mutagenic or teratogenic effects or changes influencing fertility or reproduction with non-toxic doses. After long-term administration, no accumulation reactions and no morphological signs of progressive organ alterations were observed.

Studies have not been performed to date to evaluate the carcinogenic potential of selegiline, but chronic human use of conventional selegiline appears to have given no cause for concern in this respect.

Pharmaceutical particulars

List of excipients: Gelatin, Mannitol, Glycine, Aspartame, Citric Acid, Grapefruit flavour, Yellow colouring (E172)

Incompatibilities: None.

Shelf life: Sealed sachets - 24 months

Opened sachets - 3 months.

Special precautions for storage: Store below 25°C.

Nature and contents of container: PVC (200µm)/PE(30µm)/PVdC(90gsm) blister packs sealed with aluminium foil (20µm) enclosed in a paper(44gsm)/PE(10gsm)/foil (8µm)/PE (25gsm) sachet.

Each pack contains 30 tablets.

Instructions for use/handling: Do not push the Zelapar tablet through the foil blister. Peel back the foil and carefully remove the unit.

Marketing authorisation holder: Elan Pharma International Limited, W.I.L. House, Shannon Business Park, Shannon, County Clare, Ireland

Product licence number PL 16804/0001

Date of first authorisation 18 September 1998

Date of (partial) revision of the text September 1998

Legal category POM

**Trade Mark*

Baker Norton (Division of Norton Healthcare Ltd)

Albert Basin
Royal Docks
London
E16 2QJ

☎ 0990 020304 📠 08705 323334

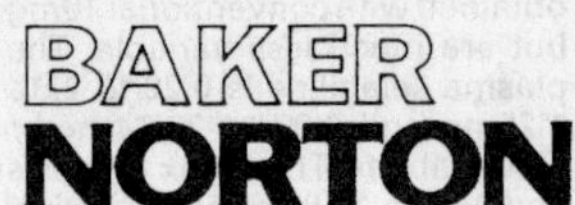

AMIL-CO*

Presentation Flat, pale peach, bisected tablets with bevelled edges, 8.5 mm diameter, coded 'AMILCO' around the circumference on one side and bearing a twin triangle logo on the reverse, and containing Amiloride Hydrochloride BP equivalent to 5 mg anhydrous amiloride hydrochloride and 50 mg Hydrochlorothiazide BP.

Uses Antihypertensive and diuretic with potassium conserving properties. Indicated in the care of patients with hypertension, congestive heart failure, or hepatic cirrhosis with ascites, or where potassium depletion may occur. The amiloride hydrochloride in Amil-Co reduces the possibility of excessive potassium loss during prolonged and vigorous diuresis. Amil-Co is recommended in those conditions where potassium balance is particularly important, for example in patients with congestive heart failure receiving digitalis.

In hepatic cirrhosis with ascites, Amil-Co is likely to provide satisfactory diuresis with diminished potassium loss, thus lessening the risk of metabolic alkalosis.

Dosage and administration The rate of weight loss and the level of serum electrolytes should determine the dosage. The ideal target for weight loss after initiation of diuresis being in the range of 0.5–1.0 kg per day in adults. Amil-Co is not recommended for children.

Hypertension: Usually 1 or 2 tablets once a day or in divided doses, which may be increased up to a maximum of 4 tablets per day.

Amil-Co may be used alone or in conjunction with other antihypertensive drugs. Since Amil-Co enhances the actions of such agents, the antihypertensive dosage regimen may have to be altered to obviate any hypotensive reaction.

Hepatic cirrhosis with ascites: Starting with 1 tablet per day, dosage may be increased if required until there is effective diuresis provided the dose does not exceed 4 tablets per day. Ideally, a gradual weight loss is preferred in cirrhotic patients to minimise the occurrence of untoward reactions associated with diuretic therapy (your attention is drawn to the precautions section). Maintenance doses are sometimes less than the dosage necessary to initiate diuresis; consequently, attempts should be made to reduce the dosage when the patient's weight is stable.

Congestive heart failure: The starting dose is 1 or 2 tablets per day, which may be altered if necessary to a maximum of 4 tablets per day. Serum potassium levels and diuretic response will establish the optimal dosage. On the establishment of initial diuresis, maintenance therapy is possible with a dosage reduction, or by the use of intermittent therapy.

The preparation should be used with care in elderly patients. Dosage should be monitored.

Contra-indications, warnings, etc

Contra-indications: Hyperkalaemia (serum potassium over 5.5 mmol/litre); other potassium-conserving diuretics e.g. spironolactone or triamterene, and potassium supplements; acute renal failure, severe progressive renal disease, severe hepatic failure, diabetic nephropathy; precoma associated with hepatic cirrhosis, hypercalcaemia or Addison's disease; anuria; patients with blood urea over 60 mg per 100 ml or serum creatinine over 1.5 mg per 100 ml, in whom serum electrolyte and blood urea levels cannot be monitored with satisfaction and frequency; a known sensitivity to amiloride hydrochloride or hydrochlorothiazide and related sulphonamides. In renal impairment, use of potassium-conserving agents may result in rapid development of hyperkalaemia.

The safety of amiloride hydrochloride for use in children has not been established; Amil-Co is therefore not recommended in children. For use in pregnancy and the nursing mother see 'Precautions'.

Precautions: Patients who are being treated with this preparation require regular supervision with monitoring of fluid and electrolyte state to avoid inadequate potassium supplementation or excessive loss of fluid.

The preparation should be used with care in elderly patients, or those with potential obstructions of the urinary tract.

Diabetes mellitus: Hyperkalaemia has been widely reported in diabetic patients on amiloride; mainly associated with chronic renal disease or pre-renal azotaemia. Renal function status should be established before prescribing Amil-Co to known or suspected diabetics. The taking of Amil-Co should be stopped prior to giving a glucose-tolerance test. Restabilising the insulin requirements of diabetic patients may be necessary. Latent diabetes mellitus may become manifest during thiazide therapy.

Metabolic or respiratory acidosis: Severely ill patients likely to experience respiratory or metabolic acidosis on introduction of potassium-conserving therapy, should be treated with caution. Categories such as decompensated diabetics or cardiopulmonary cases should be assessed for shifts in acid-base balance which may alter the balance of extracellular-intracellular potassium; the development of acidosis may be associated with a market rise in serum potassium.

Blood urea increases and electrolyte imbalance: Very infrequently, amiloride and hydrochlorothiazide, as combined in Amil-Co, fail to overcome the advent of hypokalaemia. In this instance, the use of potassium supplements should be carefully monitored.

Hyponatraemia and hypochloraemia are possible although the likelihood of hypochloraemic alkalosis is reduced with Amil-Co. Ammonium chloride (except in patients with hepatic complications) may be used to overcome any chloride deficit. Normal salt intake will, in the main, prevent any problem in this area.

Hyperkalaemia (serum potassium level over 5.5 mmol/litre): It has been noted that hyperkalaemia may be present in patients receiving amiloride either alone or in combination with other diuretics, especially in such categories as diabetics; the aged; congestive heart failure cases with known renal involvement; patients suffering from hepatic cirrhosis, or those subjected to vigorous diuretic therapy or the seriously ill. Careful observation of such categories of patients for manifestation of hyperkalaemia, using clinical, laboratory and ECG evidence should be undertaken as hyperkalaemia is not always accompanied by an abnormal ECG. In any development of hyperkalaemia, Amil-Co therapy should be stopped forthwith and, should it be desirable, reduction of serum potassium levels to normal values should be actively instituted.

Reversible increases in blood urea have been reported in association with vigorous diuresis, notably in cases of hepatic cirrhosis with ascites and metabolic alkalosis or resistant oedema. In these cases, serum electrolyte and blood urea levels should be carefully monitored. Caution is advised with the use of Amil-Co in patients suffering renal impairment (see 'Contra-indications'). Care should be taken to avoid cumulative or toxic effects due to a reduced excretion of its components. Azotaemia may be precipitated or increased by hydrochlorothiazide. Amil-Co should be discontinued if increased azotaemia and oliguria occur during treatment.

Effects in cirrhotic patients: Patients with hepatic cirrhosis and ascites are more likely to experience adverse reactions during oral diuretic therapy owing to the fact that these patients are intolerant of acute shifts in electrolyte balance and because they may be subject to pre-existing hypokalaemia due to associated aldosteronism. Hepatic encephalopathy as characterised by coma, confusion and tremors has been reported with patients receiving amiloride and subjects with liver disease on Amil-Co should be observed for this complication. A tenuous relationship between amiloride and a deepening of jaundice in cirrhotic patients has been postulated.

Hepatic disease: Thiazide should be used with caution in patients with impaired hepatic function or progressive liver disease.

Additional precautions: Thiazides may produce sensitivity reactions in patients with or without a record of allergy or bronchial asthma. The action of other antihypertensive agents is potentiated by hydrochlorothiazide and a reduced dosage may be necessary at the introduction of Amil-Co. The risk of lithium toxicity with patients combined on lithium and diuretics is very high and lithium should not be administered concurrently with Amil-Co. Reports indicate that there exists a possibility that thiazides may activate or exacerbate systemic lupus erythematosus.

Magnesium excretion is increased and calcium excretion is decreased by hydrochlorothiazide.

Hydrochlorothiazide may reduce arterial responsiveness to noradrenaline, but not to such a degree as to prevent the effectiveness of noradrenaline in therapeutic usage. Thiazides may enhance the responsiveness of tubocurarine. In post-sympathectomy patients, the antihypertensive action of thiazides may be enhanced. Should orthostatic hypotension occur, it may be potentiated by narcotics, barbiturates and alcohol.

Concomitant administration of potassium-sparing agents such as amiloride with ACE inhibitors may increase serum potassium levels and is not recommended. However, if the concomitant use of these agents is deemed appropriate, they should be used with caution and with frequent monitoring of plasma potassium. Non-steroidal anti-inflammatory drugs may attenuate the antihypertensive effect of thiazide diuretics.

Indomethacin (and possibly other NSAIDs), potassium supplements and trilostane may cause hyperkalaemia.

In some patients receiving thiazides, gout may be precipitated or hyperuricaemia may occur.

The concomitant administration of this preparation with cardiac glycosides or hypotensive agents may necessitate adjustment of the dosage of those drugs.

There is an increased risk of hypokalaemia when corticosteroids are given with loop diuretics and thiazides and an increased risk of hyponatraemia when chlorpropamide is given with Amil-Co.

There have been isolated reports of pathological changes in parathyroid glands accompanied by hypophosphataemia and hypercalcaemia following prolonged thiazide therapy. Serum concentrations of plasma bound iodine may increase without signs of thyroid disturbance during thiazide therapy. To establish parathyroid function, first discontinue Amil-Co.

As with any recently introduced preparation, patients should be monitored for possible signs of blood dyscrasias, liver dysfunction and idiosyncratic reactions.

Administration during pregnancy and for the nursing mother: The use of Amil-Co is not recommended during pregnancy since the use of diuretics may be associated with hypovolaemia, increased blood viscosity and decreased placental perfusion.

Diuretics do not prevent toxaemia of pregnancy and there is no conclusive evidence that they are useful for its treatment. Hazards to the foetus may include foetal or neonatal jaundice, thrombocytopenia, bone marrow depression and possibly other side-effects known to occur in adults. There is no indication for the use of diuretics on a routine basis in the healthy pregnant woman whether or not mild oedema is present.

Thiazides are excreted in breast milk. If continuation of Amil-Co is thought to be essential then the patient should be instructed to stop breast feeding.

Side-effects:

Related to diuresis: Orthostatic hypotension, muscle cramps, susceptibility to fatigue, weakness, dizziness, vertigo, salivary gland inflammation, transient blurred vision, paraesthesiae, thirst, dry mouth, minor psychiatric changes, e.g. confusion, depression, insomnia.

Gastro-intestinal: Constipation and diarrhoea, pain, cramps, gastric irritation, abdominal fullness, vomiting, nausea, anorexia.

Additional side-effects: Side-effects associated with thiazide therapy are hyperuricaemia, glycosuria, hyperglycaemia, yellow vision, pancreatitis, renal dysfunction and interstitial nephritis, jaundice (intrahepatic cholestatic jaundice), restlessness, headache. Fever, necrotising angitiis (vasculitis, cutaneous vasculitis), photosensitivity, urticaria, rash, purpura, haemolytic anaemia, aplastic anaemia, agranulocytosis, leucopenia, thrombocytopenia, respiratory distress including pneumonitis and anaphylactic reactions have also been reported.

Impotence has been reported in patients taking hydrochlorothiazide.

There have been a few reports of gastro-intestinal bleeding in subjects with a background of gastro-intestinal disease receiving amiloride hydrochloride alone; a casual relationship to amiloride, however, has not been established. Rare reversible abnormalities, possibly relating to amiloride hydrochloride, have been noted in liver function tests.

In the case of moderate or severe side-effects, the dosage of Amil-Co should be reduced or withdrawn altogether.

Treatment of overdosage: There is no specific antidote. Dehydration, electrolyte imbalance and hepatic coma are treated by the established procedures. Symptoms of fluid or electrolyte imbalance include dry mouth, weakness, lethargy, drowsiness, restlessness, muscle pain or cramps, hypotension, gastro-intestinal disturbances, low urine output. If ingestion is recent, gastric lavage should be performed or emesis induced. Treatment is symptomatic and supportive. Blood pressure, fluid and electrolyte balance should be monitored. If hyperkalaemia occurs, prompt measures should be taken to lower the serum potassium levels. For respiratory impairment, oxygen or artificial respiration should be administered.

Pharmaceutical precautions Keep container tightly closed; store in a cool, dry place below 25°C and protect from light.

Legal category POM.

Package quantities Containers and blister packs of 7, 14, 21, 28, 30, 50, 56, 60, 84, 90, 100, 112, 120, 250, 500 and 5000 tablets.

Further information Oral potassium supplements and potassium conserving diuretics must not be given with Amil-Co.

Onset of diuretic action begins within two to four hours after administration of Amil-Co, and reaches a peak at about the fourth hour; there is detectable activity for about 24 hours.

Product licence number 0530/0070

Product licence holder: Norton Healthcare Limited, Albert Basin, Royal Docks, London E16 2QJ.

BECLAZONE* 50 INHALER
BECLAZONE* 100 INHALER
BECLAZONE* 200 INHALER
BECLAZONE* 250 INHALER

Qualitative and quantitative composition
Beclazone 50 Inhaler: 50 µg Beclomethasone Dipropionate per dose.
Beclazone 100 Inhaler: 100 µg Beclomethasone Dipropionate per dose.
Beclazone 200 Inhaler: 200 µg Beclomethasone Dipropionate per dose.
Beclazone 250 Inhaler: 250 µg Beclomethasone Dipropionate per dose.

Pharmaceutical form Metered-dose aerosol inhaler.

Clinical particulars
Therapeutic indications:
BECLAZONE 50, 100 AND 200 INHALERS:

(i) For the prophylactic treatment of patients with worsening asthma and where there is no satisfactory control of symptoms with bronchodilators.

(ii) For patients inadequately controlled with sodium cromoglycate in addition to bronchodilators.

(iii) For patients with severe chronic asthma and those who are dependant on systemic corticosteroids.

BECLAZONE 250 INHALER:

(i) Beclazone 250 Inhaler is indicated for those asthmatic patients who have been shown to require high doses (greater than 800–1000 micrograms daily) of beclomethasone dipropionate BP to control their symptoms.

(ii) It may also be indicated for those patients whose asthma is no longer controlled by maximum maintenance doses of bronchodilators and low doses of beclomethasone dipropionate BP (less than 800 micrograms daily). Some patients with severe asthma require oral corticosteroid therapy in addition to low doses of beclomethasone dipropionate BP (less than 800 micrograms daily) for the adequate control of their symptoms. Many of these patients may, on transfer to Beclazone 250 Inhaler, be able to reduce significantly or eliminate their requirement for additional oral corticosteroids.

Posology and method of administration:
BECLAZONE 50, 100 AND 200 INHALERS:

(i) Adults: The usual starting dose is 200 micrograms twice a day. In more severe cases dosage may be started at, or increased to, 600 to 800 micrograms per day, and subsequently reduced when the patient's asthma has stabilised. The total daily dose may be administered as two, three or four divided doses.

(ii) Elderly: There is no need to adjust the dose in elderly patients.

(iii) Children: 50–100 micrograms should be given two, three or four times daily according to response. Alternatively, 100 or 200 micrograms twice daily may be administered. The usual starting dose is 100 micrograms twice a day.

Beclazone 200 inhaler is not indicated for use in children.

(iv) Patients with hepatic or renal impairment: There is no need to adjust the dose.

BECLAZONE 250 INHALER:

(i) Adults: Patients should be given a starting dose of inhaled beclomethasone dipropionate which is appropriate for the severity of their disease. The dose may then be adjusted until control is achieved, or reduced to the minimum effective dose according to individual response.

Patients demonstrating a need for high dose inhaled steroid therapy should start on 1,000 micrograms daily.

The usual maintenance dose is two inhalations (500 micrograms) twice daily, or one inhalation (250 micrograms) four times daily. If necessary, dosage may be increased to two inhalations (500 micrograms) three or four times daily according to response.

(ii) Elderly: There is no need to adjust the dose in elderly patients.

(iii) Children: Beclazone 250 Inhaler is not indicated for use in children.

(iv) Patients with hepatic or renal impairment: There is no need to adjust the dose.

Method of administration: Oral inhalation.

Contra-indications: Beclazone Inhaler is contra-indicated in patients with a history of hypersensitivity to any of its components. Furthermore, it is contra-indicated in patients with pulmonary tuberculosis (active or quiescent).

Beclazone Inhaler is not indicated in the treatment of acute asthmatic attacks.

Special warnings and special precautions for use: Patients should be instructed on the proper use of the inhaler to ensure that the drug reaches the target areas within the lungs. They should also be made aware that Beclazone Inhaler has to be used regularly for optimum benefit. Patients should be made aware of the prophylactic nature of therapy with Beclazone Inhaler and that it should be taken regularly, even when they are asymptomatic.

BECLAZONE 50, 100 AND 200 INHALERS: The maximum daily intake of Beclazone 50, 100 or 200 Inhaler in adults should not exceed 1 mg. Significant reduction of plasma cortisol levels has been reported in patients who received twice this amount.

The maximum daily intake of Beclazone 50 or 100 Inhalers in children should not exceed 500 micrograms.

Systemic effects of inhaled corticosteroids may occur, particularly at high doses prescribed for long periods. These effects are much less likely to occur than with oral corticosteroids. Possible systemic effects include adrenal suppression, growth retardation in children and adolescents, decrease in bone mineral density, cataract and glaucoma. It is important therefore that the dose of inhaled corticosteroid cover should be considered during periods of stress or elective surgery.

In the majority of patients, no significant adrenal suppression occurs until doses of 1,500 micrograms per day are exceeded. Some patients receiving 2,000 micrograms of beclomethasone dipropionate per day may show a degree of adrenocortical suppression although short term adrenal reserve remains intact. In such patients the risks of developing adrenal suppression should be balanced against the therapeutic advantages and precautions should be taken to provide systemic steroid cover in situations of prolonged stress.

Patients inadequately controlled by brochodilator therapy: The use of Beclazone 50, 100 or 200 Inhaler in patients who have never taken steroids, or taken only occasional courses of steroids is straightforward. An improvement in respiratory function is normally obvious within a week. The few patients who do not respond during this period usually have excessive mucus in their bronchi so that the drug is unable to penetrate to its site of action. In such cases, a short course of systemic steroid in relatively high dosage should be given to control secretion of mucus and other inflammatory changes in the lungs. Continuation of treatment with Beclazone 50 Inhaler usually maintains the improvement achieved, the oral steroid being gradually withdrawn. Exacerbations of asthma caused by infections is usually controlled by appropriate antibiotic treatment, by increasing the dose of inhaled beclomethasone dipropionate and, if necessary, by giving a systemic steroid. Use of a β_2-agonist may also be required.

Oral steroid-dependent patients: The transfer of oral steroid-dependent patients to Beclazone 50, 100 or 200 Inhaler and their subsequent management needs special care mainly because recovery from impaired adrenocortical function caused by prolonged systemic steroid therapy is slow. The patient should be in a reasonably stable state before being given Beclazone 50, 100 or 200 Inhaler in addition to his usual maintenance dose of systemic steroid. After about a week, gradual withdrawal of the systemic steroid is started by reducing the daily dose by 1 mg prednisolone, or its equivalent of other corticosteroids, at not less than weekly intervals. Patients treated with systemic steroids for long periods of time, or who have received high doses may have adrenocortical suppression. With these patients adrenocortical function should be monitored regularly and their dose of systemic steroid reduced cautiously. Some patients feel unwell during the withdrawal phase despite maintenance or even improvement of respiratory function. They should be encouraged to persevere with the inhaler and withdrawal of systemic steroid continued unless there are objective signs of adrenal insufficiency. Most patients can be successfully transferred to Beclazone 50 or 100 Inhaler with maintenance of good respiratory function, but special care is necessary for the first months after the transfer until the pituitary-adrenal system has sufficiently recovered to enable the patient to cope with emergencies such as trauma, surgery or infections.

Transferred patients whose adrenocortical function is impaired should carry a warning card indicating that they need supplementary systemic steroids during periods of stress, e.g. surgery, chest infection or worsening asthma attacks, but that this can be reduced again after the stress has been resolved. They should also be given a supply of oral steroid to use in emergency, for example when the asthma worsens as a result of a chest infection. The dose of beclomethasone should be increased at this time and then reduced to the maintenance level after the systemic steroid has been discontinued.

Replacement of systemic steroid treatment with Beclazone 50 Inhaler sometimes unmasks allergies such as allergic rhinitis or eczema previously controlled by the systemic drug. These allergies should be symptomatically treated with antihistamine and/or topical preparations.

BECLAZONE 250 INHALER: Patients should be instructed on the proper use of the inhaler to ensure that the drug reaches the target areas within the lungs. They should also be made aware that Beclazone 250 Inhaler has to be used regularly for optimum benefit. Patients should be made aware of the prophylactic nature of therapy with Beclazone 250 Inhaler and that it should be taken regularly, even when they are asymptomatic.

Patients being treated with the low doses of beclomethasone dipropionate BP (less than 800 micrograms daily) may be transferred directly to treatment with Beclazone 250 Inhaler.

Increasing use of bronchodilators, in particular short-acting inhaled β_2-agonists, to relieve symptoms indicates deterioration of asthma control. If patients find that short-acting relief bronchodilator treatment becomes less effective, or they need more inhalations than usual, medical attention must be sought. In this situation patients should be reassessed and consideration given to the need for increased anti-inflammatory therapy (e.g. higher doses of inhaled corticosteroids or a course of oral corticosteroids). Severe exacerbations of asthma must be treated in the normal way. Exacerbations of asthma caused by infections are usually controlled by appropriate antibiotic treatment, by increasing the dose of inhaled beclomethasone dipropionate and, if necessary, by giving a systemic steroid. Use of a β_2-agonist may also be required.

In the majority of patients, no significant adrenal suppression occurs until doses of 1,500 micrograms per day are exceeded. Some patients receiving 2,000 micrograms of beclomethasone dipropionate per day may show a degree of adrenocortical suppression although short term adrenal reserve remains intact. In such patients the risks of developing adrenal suppression should be balanced against the therapeutic advantages and precautions should be taken to provide systemic steroid cover in situations of prolonged stress.

Patients being treated with oral corticosteroids should be in a stable state before having Beclazone 250 Inhaler added to their current therapy. After about a week, gradual withdrawal of the systemic steroid is started by reducing the daily dose by 1 mg prednisolone, or its equivalent of other corticosteroids, at not less than weekly intervals. Patients who have been treated with systemic steroids for long periods of time or at a high dose may have adrenocortical suppression. With these patients adrenocortical function should be monitored regularly and their dose of systemic steroid reduced cautiously. Some patients feel unwell during the withdrawal phase despite maintenance or even improvement of respiratory function. They should be encouraged to persevere with the inhaler and withdrawal of systemic steroid continued unless there are objective signs of adrenal insufficiency. Most patients can be successfully transferred to Beclazone 250 Inhaler with maintenance of good respiratory function, but special care is necessary for the first months after the transfer until the pituitary-adrenal system has sufficiently recovered to enable the patient to cope with emergencies such as trauma, surgery or infections. Patients recently transferred from oral steroids to Beclazone 250 Inhaler together with those still receiving oral steroids should carry a warning card indicating that they may need to start or increase the dosage of oral steroids during periods of stress, e.g. surgery, chest infection or worsening asthmatic attacks, but that this can be reduced again after the stress has been resolved. A small supply of oral steroids can be given to them for emergency use.

Treatment with Beclazone 250 Inhaler should not be stopped abruptly.

Replacement of systemic steroid treatment with Beclazone 250 Inhaler sometimes unmasks allergies such as allergic rhinitis or eczema previously controlled by the systemic drugs. These allergies should be symptomatically treated with antihistamine and/or topical preparations.

Interaction with other medicaments and other forms of interaction: None reported for inhaled beclomethasone dipropionate.

Pregnancy and lactation: Beclazone Inhaler should only be used in pregnancy or lactation if the potential benefit outweighs the risk. There is insufficient data regarding safety in human pregnancy. High doses of systemic corticosteroids in pregnant animals can cause abnormalities in foetal development, including cleft palate and intra-uterine growth retardation.

No data regarding excretion of beclomethasone dipropionate in human breast milk is available.

Effects on ability to drive and use machines: On the basis of the pharmacodynamic profile, reported adverse drug reactions (ADR) and/or impairment of performance related to driving, Beclazone Inhaler is presumed to be safe or unlikely to produce an effect.

Undesirable effects: Systemic effects of inhaled corticosteroids may occur, particularly at high doses prescribed for long periods. These may include adrenal suppression, growth retardation in children and adolescents, decrease in bone mineral density, cataract and glaucoma.

In some patients hoarseness or throat irritation may occur. Rinsing the mouth and throat with water after each dose to remove residual medication may be helpful.

Paradoxical bronchospasm may occur, in which case use of the inhaler should cease immediately and medical advice should be sought. Alternative therapy should be introduced.

Hypersensitivity reactions including rashes, urticaria, pruritus and erythema, and oedema of the eyes, face, lips and throat, have been reported.

Candidiasis of the mouth and throat (thrush) occurs in some patients; the incidence of which is increased with doses greater than 400 micrograms beclomethasone dipropionate per day. Patients with high blood levels of *Candida precipitins*, indicating a previous infection, are more likely to develop this complication. Such patients may find it helpful to rinse their mouth with water after using the inhaler. Symptomatic candidiasis can be treated with topical anti-fungal therapy whilst still continuing with Beclazone Inhaler.

Overdose: The acute toxicity of beclomethasone dipropionate is low. The only harmful effect that follows inhalation of large amounts of the drug over a short period is suppression of hypothalamic-pituitary-adrenal (HPA) function. No special emergency action need be taken. Treatment with Beclazone Inhaler should be continued at the recommended dose to control asthma; HPA function recovers in a day or two.

Reduction of plasma cortisol levels has been reported in patients who received twice the daily recommended maximum dose of beclomethasone dipropionate. In the unlikely event of excessive intake of beclomethasone dipropionate for weeks or months on end, a degree of adrenocortical atrophy could occur in addition to suppression of HPA function. The patient should be treated as steroid-dependent and transferred to a suitable maintenance dose of a systemic steroid such as prednisolone. Once the patient's condition has stabilised he should be transferred to Beclazone Inhaler by the method described in *Special warnings and precautions for use* above.

To guard against the unexpected event of adrenal suppression, regular tests of adrenal function are advised.

Pharmacological properties

Pharmacodynamic properties: Beclomethasone dipropionate by inhalation has a potent glucocorticoid anti-inflammatory action within the lungs, but at recommended dosage, is without significant systemic activity.

Beclomethasone dipropionate also has vasoconstrictor effects and it inhibits the late responses to antigen challenge.

Pharmacokinetic properties: The pharmacokinetics of beclomethasone dipropionate have not been extensively studied. The current available methods are not of sufficient sensitivity to measure the therapeutically relevant plasma concentrations, particularly those occurring following inhalation.

Beclomethasone dipropionate is readily absorbed after oral administration.

About 25% of an inhaled dose reaches the lungs.

The drug and its metabolites are excreted chiefly in the faeces via biliary elimination and to a lesser extent in the urine.

Preclinical safety data: Preclinical data were confined to those associated with over-stimulation of the recognised pharmacological action of corticosteroids, which is the only safety concern for human use derived from animal studies. However, information concerning genotoxicity is lacking. See above for further guidance.

Pharmaceutical particulars

List of excipients: Oleic Acid BP; Trichlorofluoromethane BP 1988; Dichlorodifluoromethane BP 1988.

Incompatibilities: None known.

Shelf life: 24 months in the container packaged for sale.

Special precautions for storage: Store below 30°C. Protect from frost and direct sunlight. The canister is pressurised, it must not be burnt, punctured or broken even when apparently empty. The therapeutic effect of the medication may decrease when the canister is cold.

Nature and contents of container: A pressurised aluminium container with a metered dispensing valve.

Instructions for use/handling: The instructions for use/handling that appear in the patient information leaflet are as follows:

1. Remove the cap from the inhaler. Make sure the mouthpiece is clean and clear of fluff and dirt.
2. Hold the inhaler upright, with your thumb on the base and your first finger on the top of the can.
   Now shake the inhaler vigorously up and down.
3. Breathe out fully to empty the lungs, then place the mouthpiece firmly between the lips.
4. Now breathe in slowly and deeply. At the same time, press the aerosol can with your first finger to fire the aerosol and release Beclomethasone Dipropionate.
5. Remove the inhaler from your mouth and hold your breath for 10 seconds, or as long as possible. Breathe out slowly.
6. If more than one puff is required, wait at least one minute and repeat the procedure from step 2. Replace the cap.

Important: Do not rush steps 3 and 4. It is important that you start to breathe in as slowly as possible just before operating your inhaler. Practice in the mirror for the first few times. If you see 'mist' coming from the top of the inhaler or the sides of your mouth you should start again from step 2.

Cleaning the inhaler: Your inhaler should be cleaned reguarly, usually at least once a week. To clean, remove the metal canister from the plastic body and rinse the plastic body and the mouthpiece cover in warm water. Dry thoroughly, then replace the canister and mouthpiece cover. Avoid excessive heat. Do not put the metal canister into water.

Marketing authorisation holder: Norton (Waterford) Limited, IDA Estate, Waterford, Eire.

Marketing authorisation numbers

Beclazone 50 Inhaler	8142/0003
Beclazone 100 Inhaler	8142/0004
Beclazone 200 Inhaler	0530/0535
Beclazone 250 Inhaler	8142/0005

Date of approval/revision of SPC June 1998

Legal category POM

CARDILATE MR* 20 mg TABLETS

Qualitative and quantitative composition Active ingredient: Nifedipine (INN) PhEur 20 mg.

Pharmaceutical form Modified release tablet for oral administration.

Clinical particulars

Therapeutic indications: Cardilate MR 20 mg is indicated for the treatment of hypertension and for prophylaxis of chronic stable angina pectoris.

Posology and method of administration: Cardilate MR 20 mg tablets should be taken with a little water.

Tablets must be swallowed whole and not broken or chewed.

The recommended starting dose of nifedipine is 10 mg every 12 hours swallowed with water, with subsequent titration of dosage according to response. The dose may be adjusted to 40 mg every 12 hours.

The pharmacokinetics of nifedipine are altered in the elderly so that lower maintenance doses of nifedipine may be required compared to younger patients.

Cardilate MR 20 mg (Nifedipine) is not recommended for treatment of children.

Nifedipine is metabolised primarily by the liver and therefore patients with liver dysfunction should be carefully monitored. Patients with renal impairment should not require adjustment of dosage.

Route of administration: Oral.

Contra-indications: Cardilate MR 20 mg should not be given to patients with known hypersensitivity to nifedipine, other tablet constituents, or other dihydropyridines, because of the theoretical risk of cross reactivity.

It is contra-indicated in women of child-bearing potential and those breast-feeding their babies.

Cardilate MR 20 mg is contra-indicated in patients with clinically significant aortic stenosis, unstable angina, porphyria, or those in cardiogenic shock. It should not be used during or within one month of a myocardial infarction.

Cardilate MR 20 mg tablets should not be used for the treatment of acute attacks of angina.

The safety of nifedipine in malignant hypertension has not been established.

Cardilate MR 20 mg tablets should not be used for secondary prevention of myocardial infarction.

Cardilate MR 20 mg tablets should not be administered concomitantly with rifampicin since effective plasma levels of nifedipine may not be achieved owing to enzyme induction.

Special warnings and special precautions for use: Cardilate MR 20 mg should be administered to patients with low cardiac reserve or with severe hypotension with caution. Patients at risk of hypotensive crisis should begin any therapy under close medical supervision.

Interaction with other medicaments and other forms of interaction: As with other dihydropyridines, nifedipine should not be taken with grapefruit juice, because bioavailability is increased.

Cardilate MR 20 mg can be administered concomitantly with other antihypertensives including beta-receptor blockers. These may have additive antihypertensive effects and postural hypotension may therefore occur. Cardilate MR 20 mg will not prevent the possibility that there might be a rebound effect when other antihypertensive treatment is stopped. Concomitant therapy with cimetidine may potentiate the antihypertensive action of nifedipine. Nifedipine adminstration may suppress serum levels of quinidine.

The simultaneous administration of nifedipine and digoxin may lead to reduced digoxin clearance, and hence an increase in the plasma digoxin. Digoxin levels should be monitored and if necessary, the digoxin dose reduced.

Cardilate MR 20 mg may modify insulin and glucose responses, requiring adjustment in therapy of treated diabetics.

Cardilate MR 20 mg tablets should not be administered concomitantly with rifampicin since effective plasma levels of nifedipine may not be achieved owing to enzyme induction (see *Contra-indications*).

Pregnancy and lactation: Cardilate MR 20 mg is contra-indicated in pregnant women and women of child-bearing potential because fetal risks, observed in animal experiments and during human use, far outweigh the potential benefits.

Nifedipine is secreted into breast milk, so Cardilate MR 20 mg should not be administered during lactation.

Effects on ability to drive and use machines: Infrequently, Cardilate MR 20 mg may cause headaches, dizziness, nausea and tiredness to such a degree that reaction time is affected. These effects can be aggravated by concurrent alcohol. If this occurs, the patient should not be allowed to drive or operate machines.

Undesirable effects: Cardilate MR 20 mg may cause headaches, facial reddening and dizziness and leg oedema. These effects are secondary to vasodilation. Less common side-effects include rash, nausea, lethargy and urinary frequency. Rarely, gingival hyperplasia may occur; this may resolve when treatment is discontinued. Chest pain due to myocardial ischaemia may occur 1–4 hours after ingestion of Cardilate MR

20 mg. A 'steal' effect has not been observed up to now with Cardilate MR 20 mg, but treatment should be discontinued in patients in which this does occur. Cases of hypersensitivity to nifedipine resulting in jaundice have been reported.

Exacerbation of angina pectoris may occur rarely at the start of treatment with sustained release formulations of nifedipine. The occurrence of myocardial infarction has been described, although it is not possible to distinguish such an event from the natural course of ischaemic heart disease.

Overdose: Toxic affects arise from the three main actions of nifedipine in overdose: dilatation of vascular smooth muscles (predominant effect); decreased myocardial contractility; and depression of AV nodal conduction. Hypotension and tachycardia or bradycardia are the most likely manifestations of overdose. Other toxic effects include nausea, vomiting, drowsiness, dizziness, confusion, lethargy, flushing, coma and convulsions. Cardiac effects may include heart block, AV dissociation and asystole; metabolic disturbances include hyperglycaemia, acidosis, hypo- or hyperkalaemia and hypocalcaemia; pulmonary oedema has been reported.

Primary treatment involves removal of nifedipine by gastric lavage or ipecac and administration of activated charcoal (50 g adults; 10–15 g children). Cardilate MR 20 mg is a modified release product, therefore activated charcoal should be repeated at 4-hourly intervals (25 g adults; 10 g children). The patient should be closely monitored and treated according to predominating signs:

- for hypotension: the feet should be raised and plasma expanders given. If this is not effective, 10% calcium gluconate or chloride can be given intravenously (calcium chloride should not be given to acidotic patients). If this fails, dopamine may be tried (large doses may be needed). Glucagon may also be of value.
- for bradycardia: treatment with atropine, isoprenaline and cardiac pacing should be given as required.

The value of extracorporeal methods of removal of nifedipine have not been established.

Pharmacological properties

Pharmacodynamic properties: Nifedipine inhibits the influx of calcium into myocardial cells, the smooth muscle cells of the coronary arteries and the peripheral capillaries. Nifedipine brings about a substantial improvement in the oxygen supply to the myocardium while reducing oxygen demand. It has been shown to exhibit anti-anginal properties. High blood pressure is normalised due to a reduction in the peripheral resistance (vasodilation).

Pharmacokinetic properties

Absorption: Nifedipine is absorbed rapidly and almost completely following oral administration. Nifedipine can be detected in plasma 30–60 minutes after administration of Cardilate MR 20 mg and reaches maximal concentration between 0.75 and 5 hours.

Distribution: Nifedipine is more than 90% serum protein bound. Animal studies with labelled nifedipine have shown that distribution of the fraction not protein bound is throughout all organs and tissues, with higher concentrations in myocardium than in skeletal muscle. Neither nifedipine nor its metabolites are stored selectively in any tissue.

Metabolism: Nifedipine is converted almost compeltely to inactive metabolites.

Elimination: 70 to 80% of administered nifedipine is excreted as metabolites by the kidneys with an elimination half-life of approximately 10 hours.

Elimination may be retarded by renal failure or insufficiency.

Preclinical safety data: None stated.

Pharmaceutical particulars

List of excipients: Microcrystalline cellulose; carboxymethyl sodium starch; mannitol; colloidal anhydrous silica; polyvidone; magnesium stearate; sodium lauryl sulphate; methylhydroxypropyl cellulose; polyoxyethelene glycol 6000; polyoxyethylene glycol 400; red ferric oxide (E172); titanium dioxide (E171); talc. Purified water; alcohol (industrial) – not detected in finished product.

Incompatibilities: None known.

Shelf life: Three years.

Special precautions for storage: Cardilate MR 20 mg should be stored in the original pack below 25°C, in a dry place and protected from light.

Nifedipine is highly sensitive to light and is therefore protected both by materials in the tablet and in the packaging. Nonetheless tablets should not be exposed to direct sunlight and should only be removed from the blister pack when about to be taken.

Nature and contents of container: Thermoformed blister packs of PVC/red transparent PVdC/aluminium in boxes of 7, 14, 20, 21, 28, 30, 56, 60, 84, 90, 100, 112 and 120 tablets.

Instructions for use/handling: None.

Marketing authorisation holder: Norton Healthcare Ltd, Albert Basin, Royal Docks, London E16 2QJ.

Marketing authorisation number 0530/0488.

Date of approval/revision of SPC 17 January 1997.

Legal category POM.

CORDILOX* IV

Presentation Colourless glass 2 ml ampoules with breakline containing 5 mg Verapamil Hydrochloride BP per ampoule.

Uses The treatment of supraventricular arrhythmias.

Mode of action: Cordilox is a calcium channel blocker which inhibits the inward movement of calcium in smooth muscle cells of the systemic and coronary arteries and in the cells of cardiac muscle and the intracardiac conduction system.

Because of its effect on the movement of calcium in the intracardiac conduction system, it reduces automaticity, decreases conduction velocity and increases the refractory period.

Dosage and administration

Acute (IV injection)

Adults: For the treatment of tachyarrhythmias, 5–10 mg (1–2 ampoules) should be injected intravenously over a period of 30 seconds with continuous observation of the patient and, preferably, with simultaneous ECG monitoring.

In cases of paroxysmal tachyarrhythmias a further 5 mg may, if necessary, be injected 5–10 minutes after the first injection with the same precautions being observed. Higher doses are not usually necessary.

Children:

Newborn: 0.75–1 mg (0.3–0.4 ml)
Infants: 0.75–2 mg (0.3–0.8 ml)
1–5 years: 2–3 mg (0.8–1.2 ml)
6–15 years: 2.5–5 mg (1.0–2.0 ml)

In many cases smaller doses than those mentioned above are sufficient. The injection should be stopped at the onset of the desired effect.

For concomitant administration with beta-blockers see 'Precautions'.

Elderly: No special dosage recommendations except:

(a) In those patients with impaired liver function, particular attention should be paid to dosage because of reduced drug metabolism.

(b) In cardiac conduction disturbances, the effects of Cordilox and beta-blockers or other cardio-depressive drugs may be additive.

(see 'Precautions')

Contra-indications, warnings, etc

Contra-indications: Hypotension, marked bradycardia (less than 50 beats/minute), second and third degree atrioventricular block, sick sinus syndrome, uncompensated heart failure. Combination with beta-blockers is contra-indicated in patients with poor ventricular function.

Precautions: Cordilox may affect impulse conduction and should be used with caution in patients with first degree atrioventricular block. The effects of Cordilox and beta blockers or other drugs with a cardio-depressive action may be additive both with respect to conduction and contraction, therefore care must be exercised when these are administered concurrently or closely together. This is especially true when either drug is administered intravenously.

Patients with atrial fibrillation/flutter and an accessory pathway (eg W-P-W syndrome) may rarely develop increased conduction across the anomalous pathway and ventricular tachycardia may be precipitated.

If there are signs of tachycardia-induced heart failure (energetic exhaustion of the myocardium) digitalisation is necessary before intravenous administration of Cordilox.

Drug interactions: Cordilox may have an additive effect with other antihypertensive drugs. Thus, in many cases, with Cordilox, a reduction in the dose of the other antihypertensive drug may be possible.

There is a possibility of an interaction between verapamil and quinidine, causing hypotension, when Cordilox is administered by the intravenous route.

Verapamil hydrochloride has been shown to increase the serum concentration of digoxin and caution should be exercised with regard to digitalis toxicity. The effects of beta-blockers, anti-arrhythmics and general anaesthetics with verapamil may be additive both with respect to conduction and contraction of cardiac muscle.

There is a risk of nephrotoxicity if lithium is given at the same time as Cordilox due to increased lithium levels. Cordilox has also been reported to decrease lithium serum levels.

An increase in serum verapamil levels is possible if cimetidine is given concurrently. The effect of Cordilox may be reduced if given to patients already taking phenytoin, phenobarbitone or rifampicin, due to an increase in its metabolism. Plasma concentrations of carbamazepine, theophylline and cyclosporin may be increased when these drugs are given concurrently with Cordilox.

Cordilox may affect left ventricular contractility as a result of its mode of action. This effect is small and normally not important but cardiac failure may be precipitated or aggravated if it exists. In cases of poor ventricular function therefore, Cordilox should only be given after appropriate therapy for cardiac failure such as digitalis, etc.

Caution should be observed in the acute phase of myocardial infarction.

In patients with impaired liver function, particular attention should be paid to the dosage because of reduced drug metabolism.

Long term verapamil therapy may give rise to potentiation of neuromuscular blocking agents during anaesthesia.

Use in pregnancy and lactation: Verapamil is excreted into the breast milk in small amounts and is unlikely to be harmful. However, hypersensitivity reactions have been reported rarely with verapamil and therefore it should only be used during lactation if in the clinician's judgement it is essential to the welfare of the patient.

Animal studies have not shown any teratogenic effect. Cordilox should not be given during the first trimester of pregnancy unless, in the clinician's judgement, it is essential for the welfare of the patient. The possibility that Cordilox can cause relaxation of the uterine muscle should be considered at term.

Side-effects: Cordilox is well tolerated and does not exert a bronchoconstrictor effect.

Due to its mode of action, undesired effects on atrioventricular conduction and blood pressure are possible. This applies particularly to patients with atrioventricular block and/or considerably impaired myocardial function. On rare occasions the intravenous administration of Cordilox may lead to an undesired blocking of conduction and, in extreme cases, to asystole. The asystole is usually of short duration and normally sinus rhythm returns spontaneously after a few seconds. However, if on rare occasions asystole persists, treatment should be carried out as described below.

Intravenous administration of Cordilox may lead to a slight transient fall in blood pressure due to a reduction in peripheral resistance. Rarely this may result in severe hypotension.

Treatment of acute cardiovascular side-effects: If acute complications occur after intravenous injection of Cordilox (asystole, atrioventricular block or ventricular fibrillation) the usual emergency measures should be applied, e.g. cardiac massage, mechanical ventilation, the intravenous injection of adrenaline, and the intravenous injection of 10–20 ml of calcium gluconate 10% solution. Hypotension following intravenous injection of Cordilox may, if necessary, be controlled without difficulty by the use of vasoconstrictor substances.

Overdosage: Symptoms include hypotension, shock, first and second degree AV block, total AV block, asystole, sinus bradycardia and sinus arrest. Bradycardia may be treated with atropine, isoprenaline or cardiac pacing.

Pharmaceutical precautions Cordilox IV is incompatible with alkaline solutions (eg Sodium Bicarbonate Intravenous Infusion BP) as this may lead to a precipitation of the verapamil base.

Legal category POM.

Package quantities Containers of 5×2 ml ampoules.

Further information Metabolisable carbohydrate: Nil.

Sodium content: 0.30 mmol/ampoule (0.15 mmol/ml).

Product licence number 0530/0387

Product licence holder: Norton Healthcare Limited, Albert Basin, Royal Docks, London E16 2QJ.

CORDILOX TABLETS 40 mg, 80 mg and 120 mg

Qualitative and quantitative composition

Cordilox Tablets: Verapamil Hydrochloride BP 40 mg.
Cordilox Tablets: Verapamil Hydrochloride BP 80 mg.
Cordilox Tablets: Verapamil Hydrochloride BP 120 mg.

Pharmaceutical form Tablets.

Clinical particulars

Therapeutic indications:

1. The treatment of prophylaxis of paroxysmal supraventricular tachycardia and of atrial flutter/fibrillation. Verapamil should not be used when atrial flutter/fibrillation complicates Wolff-Parkinson-White syndrome.
2. The treatment of prophylaxis of angina pectoris.

3. The treatment of mild to moderate hypertension and renal hypertension.

Posology and method of administration:
(Note: n40 mg, 80 mg, 120 mg, 160 mg and 240 mg presentations of Cordilox are available.)

1. Supraventricular tachycardia:
Adults: 40 to 120 mg t.d.s. according to the severity of the condition.
Children: Up to 2 years: half of a 40 mg tablet 2 to 3 times a day.
2 years and above: 40 to 120 mg 2 to 3 times a day according to age and effectiveness.

2. Angina pectoris:
Adults: 120 mg t.d.s. In some patients with angina of effort 80 mg t.d.s. can be completely satisfactory. Less than 120 mg t.d.s. is not likely to be effective in angina at rest and variant angina.
Children: No data available.

3. Hypertension:
Adults: The usual dosage is 160 mg twice a day. However, a minority of patients may be successfully controlled on 120 mg twice a day while others may require up to 480 mg daily given in divided doses.
Children: Up to 10 mg/kg/day in divided doses, according to severity of disease.

Elderly dosages: No special recommendations except:
(a) In those patients with impaired liver function, particular attention should be paid to dosage because of reduced drug metabolism.
(b) In cardiac conduction disturbances, the effects of Cordilox and beta-blockers or other cardio-depressive drugs may be additive.

Route of administration: Oral.

Contra-indications: Hypotension associated with cardiogenic shock.
Marked bradycardia (less than 50 beats/minute).
Second or third degree atrioventricular block.
Sick sinus syndrome.
Uncompensated heart failure.
Sino-atrial block.
Concomitant ingestion of grapefruit juice.

Special warnings and precautions for use: Cordilox may affect impulse conduction and should be used with caution in patients with first degree atrioventricular block. The effects of Cordilox and beta blockers or other drugs with a cardio-depressive action may be additive both with respect to conduction and contraction, therefore care must be exercised when these are administered concurrently or closely together. This is especially true when either drug is administered intravenously.

Patients with atrial flutter/fibrillation in association with an accessory pathway (e.g. W-P-W syndrome), may rarely develop increased conduction across the anomalous pathway and ventricular tachycardia may be precipitated.

If there are signs of tachycardia-induced heart failure (energetic exhaustion of the myocardium) digitalisation is necessary before intravenous administration of Cordilox.

Cordilox may affect left ventricular contractility as a result of its mode of action. This effect is small and normally not important but cardiac failure may be precipitated or aggravated if it exists. In case of poor ventricular function therefore, Cordilox should only be given after appropriate therapy for cardiac failure such as digitalis, etc.

Caution should be observed in the acute phase of myocardial infarction.

In patients with impaired liver function, particular attention should be paid to the dosage because of reduced drug metabolism. The disposition of verapamil in patients with renal impairment has not been fully established and careful patient monitoring is recommended. Verapamil is not removed during dialysis.

Interactions with other medicaments and other forms of interaction: The effects of Cordilox and beta-blockers, anti-arrhythmics, general anaesthetics or other drugs with a cardio-depressive action may be additive with respect to conduction and contraction. Cordilox may have an additive effect with other antihypertensive drugs. Thus, in many cases with Cordilox, a reduction in the dose of other antihypertensive drugs may be possible.

The effect of Cordilox may be reduced when combined with phenytoin, phenobarbitone or rifampicin due to an increase in its metabolism.

There is a possibility of an interaction between verapamil and quinidine, causing hypotension when Cordilox is administered by the intravenous route.

Plasma concentrations of carbamazepine, theophylline and cyclosporin may be increased when these drugs are given concurrently with Cordilox.

Verapamil hydrochloride has been shown to increase the serum concentration of digoxin and caution should be exercised with regard to digitalis toxicity.

There is a risk of neurotoxicity when lithium is given at the same time as Cordilox. Cordilox has also been reported to decrease lithium serum levels.

Long term verapamil therapy may give rise to potentiation of neuromuscular blocking agents during anaesthesia.

An increase in serum Verapamil levels is possible when Cimetidine is given concurrently. Grapefruit juice – an increase in verapamil serum levels has been reported.

Pregnancy and lactation: Pregnancy: Although animal studies have not shown any teratogenic effects, Cordilox should not be given during the first trimester of pregnancy unless, in the clinician's judgement, it is essential for the welfare of the patients. The possibility that Cordilox can cause relaxation of the uterine muscle should be considered at term.

Lactation: Verapamil is excreted into the breast milk in small amounts and is unlikely to be harmful. However, hypersensivity reactions have been reported rarely with verapamil and therefore it should only be used during lactation if in the clinician's judgement it is essential to the welfare of the patient.

Effects on ability to drive and use machines: None stated.

Undesirable effects: Constipation (mild) – not common.
Flushing (mild) – occasional.
Headache (mild), dizziness, fatigue and ankle oedema – rare.
Nausea and vomiting (mild) – seldom.
Allergic reaction (mild) – very rare.
Impairment of liver function (reversible).
Characterised increase in transaminase and/or alkaline phosphatase – very rare.
Rash and pruritus, alopecia and urticaria – a possible side effect.
Rarely, reversible gynaecomastia and gingival hyperplasia.

Overdose: Symptoms include hypotension, shock, first and second degree AV block, total AV block, asystole, sinus bradycardia and sinus arrest.

For acute cardio-vascular side-effects, gastric lavage, taking the usual precautionary measures, may be appropriate. The usual emergency measure should be followed, e.g. cardiac massage, mechanical ventilation, the intravenous injection of adrenaline, the intravenous injection of 10–20 ml of calcium gluconate 10% solution.

In the case of second or third degree AV block, atropine, isoprenaline or a temporary pacemaker may be necessary. If myocardial insufficiency occurs, dopamine, dobutamine, cardiac glycosides or calcium gluconate (10–20 ml of a 10% solution) may be required. Appropriate positioning of the patient and vasoconstrictor drugs may be indicated in the case of hypotension.

Bradycardia may be treated with atropine, isoprenaline or cardiac pacing.

Pharmacological properties

Pharmacodynamic properties: Cordilox is a calcium channel blocker which inhibits the inward movement of calcium in cardiac muscle cells of the systemic and coronary arteries and in the cells of cardiac muscle and the intracardiac conduction system.

Cordilox lowers peripheral vascular resistance with little or no reflex tachycardia. Its efficacy in reducing both raised systolic and diastolic blood pressure is thought to be primarily due to this mode of action.

The decrease in systemic and coronary vascular resistance and the sparing effect on intracellular oxygen consumption appear to explain the anti-anginal properties of the product.

Because of its effect on the movement of calcium in the intracardiac conduction system, it reduces automaticity, decreases conduction velocity and increases the refractory period.

Pharmacokinetic properties: More than 90% of the orally administered dose of Cordilox is absorbed. Because of rapid biotransformation of verapamil during its first pass through the portal circulation, absolute bioavailability ranges from 20% to 35%. Peak plasma concentrations are reached between 1 and 2 hours after oral administration.

A close relationship exists between verapamil plasma concentration and prolongation of the PR interval. The mean elimination half-life in single dose studies ranged from 2.8 to 7.4 hours. In these same studies, after repetitive dosing, the half-life increased to a range from 4.5 to 12 hours (after less then 10 consecutive doses given 6 hours apart). Half-life may increase during titration due to saturation of hepatic enzyme systems as plasma verapamil levels rise.

Most of the drug in healthy subjects is eliminated in the urine (about 70% of dose in 5 days) and only about 15% in faeces. 12 different metabolites have been identified. Norverapamil is the major metabolite (25% of recovered products) and is the only metabolite with pharmacological activity (dogs). Approximately 90% is bound to plasma proteins.

Preclinical safety data: Not applicable.

Pharmaceutical particulars

List of excipients: Calcium Phosphate Dibasic Dihydrate USP; Sodium Starch Glycollate BP; Maize Starch BP; Magnesium Stearate PhEur; Water Purified PhEur.
Coating: Hydroxypropylmethylcellulose 2910 15CPS USP; Titanium Dioxide (E171) BP; Polyethylene Glycol 8000 NF; Polyethylene Glycol 400; Dye, Yellow D&C No. 110 A1 Lake (E104); Dye, Yellow FD&C No. 6 A1 Lake (E110); Acid Sorbic BP; Alcohol 3A; Water Purified PhEur.

Incompatibilities: None stated.

Shelf life: 5 years for Securitainer, 'Snap-Secure' Container, Tampertainer or Duma Container.
2 years for PVdC coated PVC/Aluminium blisters.

Special precautions for use: None stated.

Nature and contents of container: Securitainer, 'Snap-Secure' Container, Tampertainer, Duma Container or PVdC coated PVC/Aluminium blister packs (60 mg/m² PVdC on 250 μ PVC/20 μ A1) in pack sizes of 7, 14, 21, 28, 30, 50, 56, 60, 84, 90, 100, 112, 120 tablets.

Instructions for use/handling: None.

Marketing authorisation holder: Norton Healthcare Limited, Albert Basin, Royal Docks, London E16 2QJ.

Marketing authorisation numbers

Cordilox Tablets 40 mg	0503/0382
Cordilox Tablets 80 mg	0503/0383
Cordilox Tablets 120 mg	0503/0384

Date of approval/revision of SPC 24 April 1997

Legal category POM

CORDILOX TABLETS 160 mg

Qualitative and quantitative composition Verapamil Hydrochloride BP 160 mg.

Pharmaceutical form Tablets.

Clinical particulars

Therapeutic indications: The treatment of mild to moderate hypertension and renal hypertension, used alone or in conjunction with other antihypertensive therapy.

Posology and method of administration:
Hypertension:
Adults: The usual dosage is 160 mg twice a day. However, a minority of patients may be successfully controlled on 120 mg twice a day while others may require up to 480 mg daily given in divided doses.

Children: Up to 10 mg/kg/day in divided doses, according to severity of disease.

Elderly dosages: No special recommendations except:
- in those patients with impaired liver function, particular attention should be paid to dosage because of reduced drug metabolism.
- in cardiac conduction disturbances, the effects of Cordilox and beta-blockers or other cardio-depressive drugs may be additive.

Route of administration: Oral.

Contra-indications: Hypotension associated with cardiogenic shock.
Marked bradycardia (less than 50 beats/minute).
Second or third degree atrioventricular block.
Sick sinus syndrome.
Uncompensated heart failure.
Sino-atrial block.
Concomitant ingestion of grapefruit juice.

Special warnings and precautions for use: Cordilox may affect impulse conduction and should be used with caution in patients with first degree atrioventricular block. The effects of Cordilox and beta blockers or other drugs with a cardio-depressive action may be additive both with respect to conduction and contraction, therefore care must be exercised when these are administered concurrently or closely together. This is especially true when either drug is administered intravenously.

Patients with atrial flutter/fibrillation in association with an accessory pathway (e.g. W-P-W syndrome), may rarely develop increased conduction across the anomalous pathway and ventricular tachycardia may be precipitated.

If there are signs of tachycardia-induced heart failure (energetic exhaustion of the myocardium) digitalisation is necessary before intravenous administration of Cordilox.

Cordilox may affect left ventricular contractility as a result of its mode of action. This effect is small and normally not important but cardiac failure may be precipitated or aggravated if it exists. In case of poor ventricular function therefore, Cordilox should only be given after appropriate therapy for cardiac failure such as digitalis, etc.

Caution should be observed in the acute phase of myocardial infarction.

In patients with impaired liver function, particular attention should be paid to the dosage because of reduced drug metabolism. The disposition of verapamil in patients with renal impairment has not been fully established and careful patient monitoring is recommended. Verapamil is not removed during dialysis.

Interactions with other medicaments and other forms of interaction: The effects of Cordilox and beta-blockers, anti-arrhythmics, general anaesthetics or other drugs with a cardio-depressive action may be additive with respect to conduction and contraction. Cordilox may have an additive effect with other antihypertensive drugs. Thus, in many cases with Cordilox, a reduction in the dose of other antihypertensive drugs may be possible. The effect of Cordilox may be reduced when combined with phenytoin, phenobarbitone or rifampicin due to an increase in its metabolism.

There is a possibility of an interaction between verapamil and quinidine, causing hypotension when Cordilox is administered by the intravenous route.

Plasma concentrations of carbamazepine, theophylline and cyclosporin may be increased when these drugs are given concurrently with Cordilox.

Verapamil hydrochloride has been shown to increase the serum concentration of digoxin and caution should be exercised with regard to digitalis toxicity.

There is a risk of neurotoxicity when lithium is given at the same time as Cordilox. Cordilox has also been reported to decrease lithium serum levels.

Long term verapamil therapy may give rise to potentiation of neuromuscular blocking agents during anaesthesia.

An increase in serum Verapamil levels is possible when Cimetidine is given concurrently.

Grapefruit juice – an increase in verapamil serum levels has been reported.

Pregnancy and lactation:

Pregnancy: Although animal studies have not shown any teratogenic effects, Cordilox should not be given during the first trimester of pregnancy unless, in the clinician's judgement, it is essential for the welfare of the patients. The possibility that Cordilox can cause relaxation of the uterine muscle should be considered at term.

Lactation: Verapamil is excreted into the breast milk in small amounts and is unlikely to be harmful. However, hypersensivity reactions have been reported rarely with verapamil and therefore it should only be used during lactation if in the clinician's judgement it is essential to the welfare of the patient.

Effects on ability to drive and use machines: None stated.

Undesirable effects: Constipation (mild) – not common.

Flushing (mild) – occasional.

Headache (mild), dizziness, fatigue and ankle oedema – rare.

Nausea and vomiting (mild) – seldom.

Allergic reaction (mild) – very rare.

Impairment of liver function (reversible).

Characterised increase in transminase and/or alkaline phosphatase – very rare.

Rash and pruritus, alopecia and urticaria – a possible side effect.

Rarely, reversible gynaecomastia and gingival hyperplasia.

Overdose: Symptoms include hypotension, shock, first and second degree AV block, total AV block, asystole, sinus brachycardia and sinus arrest.

For acute cardio-vascular side-effects, gastric lavage, taking the usual precautionary measures, may be appropriate. The usual emergency measure should be followed, e.g. cardiac massage, mechanical ventilation, the intravenous injection of adrenaline, the intravenous injection of 10–20 ml of calcium gluconate 10% solution.

In the case of second or third degree AV block, atropine, isoprenaline or a temporary pacemaker may be necessary. If myocardial insufficiency occurs, dopamine, dobutamine, cardiac glycosides or calcium gluconate (10–20 ml of a 10% solution) may be required. Appropriate positioning of the patient and vasoconstrictor drugs may be indicated in the case of hypotension.

Bradycardia may be treated with atropine, isoprenaline or cardiac pacing.

Pharmacological properties

Pharmacodynamic properties: Cordilox is a calcium channel blocker which inhibits the inward movement of calcium in cardiac muscle cells of the systemic and coronary arteries and in the cells of cardiac muscle and the intracardiac conduction system.

Cordilox lowers peripheral vascular resistance with little or no reflex tachycardia. Its efficacy in reducing both raised systolic and diastolic blood pressure is thought to be primarily due to this mode of action.

The decrease in systemic and coronary vascular resistance and the sparing effect on intracellular oxygen consumption appear to explain the anti-anginal properties of the product.

Because of its effect on the movement of calcium in the intracardiac conduction system, it reduces automaticity, decreases conduction velocity and increases the refractory period.

Pharmacokinetic properties: More than 90% of the orally administered dose of Cordilox is absorbed. Because of rapid biotransformation of verapamil during its first pass through the portal circulation, absolute bioavailability ranges from 20% to 35%. Peak plasma concentrations are reached between 1 and 2 hours after oral administration.

A close relationship exists between verapamil plasma concentration and prolongation of the PR interval. The mean elimination half-life in single dose studies ranged from 2.8 to 7.4 hours. In these same studies, after repetitive dosing, the half-life increased to a range from 4.5 to 12 hours (after less then 10 consecutive doses given 6 hours apart). Half-life may increase during titration due to saturation of hepatic enzyme systems as plasma verapamil levels rise.

Most of the drug in healthy subjects is eliminated in the urine (about 70% of dose in 5 days) and only about 15% in faeces. 12 different metabolites have been identified. Norverapamil is the major metabolite (25% of recovered products) and is the only metabolite with pharmacological activity (dogs). Approximately 90% is bound to plasma proteins.

Preclinical safety data: Not applicable.

Pharmaceutical particulars

List of excipients: Maize Starch BP; Calcium Hydrogen Phosphage BP; Sodium Starch Glycollate BP; Magnesium Stearate BP.

Coating: Hydroxypropylmethylcellulose USP; Polyethylene Glycol 8000 NF; Polyethylene Glycol 400; Titanium Dioxide (E171) BP; Dye, Yellow Lake (E104); Dye, Yellow Lake (E110); Sorbic Acid BP.

Incompatibilities: None stated.

Shelf life: 5 years.

Special precautions for use: None stated.

Nature and contents of container: Blister Pack, Securitainer, 'Snap-Secure' Container, Tampertainer, Duma Container containing 7, 14, 21, 28, 30, 50, 56, 60, 84, 90, 100, 112 and 120 tablets.

Instruction for use/handling: None.

Marketing authorisation holder: Norton Healthcare Limited, Albert Basin, Royal Docks, London E16 2QJ.

Marketing authorisation number 0503/0385

Date of approval/revision of SPC 7 March 1997

Legal category POM

CROMOGEN* 5 mg INHALER

Qualitative and quantitative composition Sodium cromoglycate 5 mg (INN sodium cromoglycate).

Pharmaceutical form Metered-dose aerosol inhaler.

Clinical particulars

Therapeutic indications: Cromogen 5 mg Inhaler is indicated for the preventative treatment of mild to moderate bronchial asthma, including the prevention of exercise-induced asthma.

Posology and method of administration:

Adults and children: Initial dose is two inhalations of the aerosol four times daily. Once adequate control of symptoms has been achieved it may be possible to reduce to a maintenance dose of one inhalation four times daily. However, the dose may be increased to two inhalations six or eight times daily in more severe cases or during periods of severe antigen challenge. Additional doses before exercise may also be taken.

Elderly patients: No current evidence for alteration of the recommended adult dose.

Contra-indications: Cromogen 5 mg Inhaler is contra-indicated in patients with known sensitivity to any of its ingredients.

Special warnings and special precautions for use:

Concomitant bronchodilator therapy: Where a concomitant aerosol bronchodilator is prescribed, it is recommended that this be administered prior to the Cromogen 5 mg Inhaler.

Concomitant steroid therapy: In patients currently treated with steroids the addition of Cromogen 5 mg Inhaler to the regimen may make it possible to reduce the maintenance dose or discontinue steroids completely. The patient must be carefully supervised while the steroid dose is reduced, a rate of reduction of 10% weekly is suggested. If reduction of steroid dosage has been possible Cromogen 5 mg Inhaler should not be withdrawn until cover has been re-instituted.

Since the therapy is prophylactic it is important to continue therapy in those patients who benefit. If it is necessary to withdraw this treatment, it should be done progressively over a period of one week. Symptoms of asthma may recur.

Cromogen 5 mg Inhaler is not indicated for the treatment of acute asthma attack.

Interaction with other medicaments and other forms of interaction: No major interactions are anticipated with the proposed usage of the product. See *Special warnings and special precautions for use.*

Pregnancy and lactation: As with all medication caution should be exercised especially during the first trimester of pregnancy. Cumulative experience with sodium cromoglycate suggest that it has no adverse effects on foetal development. It should only be used in pregnancy where there is a clear need.

It is not known whether sodium cromoglycate is excreted in breast milk but on the basis of its physico-chemical properties this is considered unlikely. There is no evidence to suggest that the use of sodium cromoglycate has any undesirable effects on the baby.

Effects on ability to drive and use machines: No known effects.

Undesirable effects: Sodium cromoglycate is well-tolerated, mild throat irritation, coughing and transient bronchospasm may occur. Very rarely severe bronchospasm associated with a marked fall in pulmonary function has been reported. In such cases treatment should be stopped and should not be re-introduced. Reactions sometimes occurring after several months treatment include aggravation of existing asthma, gastroestinal symptoms (nausea, vomiting), myositis, dizziness, urticaria, rashes and pulmonary infiltration with eosinophilia.

Overdose: No action other than medical observation should be necessary.

Pharmacological properties

Pharmacodynamic properties: Sodium cromoglycate has no intrinsic bronchodilator, anti-histaminic or anti-inflammatory activity.

In vitro and *in vivo* studies have consistently suggested that sodium cromoglycate inhibits the release of inflammatory mediators from sensitised mast cells. It appears to inhibit reactions caused by both antigenic and non-antigenic stimuli and prevents both the immediate and late asthmatic responses. Most evidence suggests that the effects of sodium cromoglycate are due to a stabilisation of mast cell membranes, although the precise mechanism of action remains unknown.

Pharmacokinetic properties: Sodium cromoglycate is poorly absorbed from the gastrointestinal tract. Following inhalation as a fine powder from sodium cromoglycate capsules, about 8% of the total dose administered is deposited in the lungs from where it is rapidly and completely absorbed and excreted unchanged in the urine and bile. The elimination half-life is 1.5–2 hours and the protein binding is 65%. The majority of an inhaled dose is swallowed and excreted unchanged in the faeces.

Preclinical safety data: No relevant information.

Pharmacological particulars

List of excipients: Sorbitan trioleate, trichlorofluoromethane, dichlorodifluoromethane.

Incompatibilities: No incompatibilities are anticipated with the proposed usage of the product.

Shelf life: Shelf life of the product as packaged for sale is 24 months.

Special precautions for storage: Store below 30°C. The canister is pressurised and should be protected from direct sunlight and frost. It must not be punctured or burnt, even when empty.

Nature and contents of container: The container consists of an aluminium can with a metered dispensing valve crimped to it. The can is inserted into a plastic oral inhalation applicator with a dust cap.

Each metered-dose aerosol inhaler contains at least 112 actuations.

Instructions for use/handling:

1. Remove the cap from the inhaler. Make sure the mouthpiece is clean and clear of fluff or dirt.
2. Hold the inhaler upright, with your thumb on the base and your first finger on the top of the can. Now shake vigorously, up and down.
3. Breathe out fully to empty the lungs, then place the mouthpiece firmly between the lips.
4. Now breathe in slowly and deeply. At the same time, press the aerosol can with your first finger to fire the aerosol and release sodium cromoglycate.
5. Remove the inhaler from your mouth and hold your breath for 10 seconds, or as long as possible. Breathe out slowly.
6. If more than one puff is required, wait at least one minute and repeat the procedure from step 2. Replace the cap.

Cleaning your inhaler: Your inhaler should be cleaned regularly, usually at least once a week. To clean, remove the metal canister from the plastic body and rinse the plastic body and mouthpiece cover in warm water. Dry thoroughly, then replace the canister and mouthpiece cover. Avoid excessive heat. Do not put the metal canister into water.

Important: Do not rush steps 3 and 4. It is important that you start to breathe in as slowly as possible just before operating your inhaler. Practice in front of the mirror for the first few times. If you see 'mist' coming from the top of the inhaler or the sides of your mouth you should start again from step 2.

Marketing authorisation holder: Norton Healthcare Limited, Albert Basin, Royal Docks, London E16 2QJ.

Marketing authorisation number 0530/0319

Date of approval/revision of SPC March 1997

Legal category POM.

CROMOGEN* 5 mg EASI-BREATHE INHALER

Qualitative and quantitative composition Sodium cromoglycate 5 mg (INN cromoglicate acid).

Pharmaceutical form Breath-operated metered dose aerosol inhaler.

Clinical particulars

Therapeutic indications: Cromogen 5 mg Easi-Breathe Inhaler is indicated for the treatment of bronchial asthma, including the prevention of exercise-induced asthma.

Posology and method of administration:

Adults and children: Initial dose is two inhalations of the aerosol four times daily. Once adequate control of symptoms has been achieved it may be possible to reduce to a maintenance dose of one inhalation four times daily. However, the dose may be increased to two inhalations six or eight times daily in more severe cases or during periods of severe antigen challenge. Additional doses before exercise may also be taken.

Elderly patients: No current evidence for alteration of the recommended adult dose.

Contra-indications: Cromogen 5 mg Easi-Breathe Inhaler is contra-indicated in patients with known sensitivity to any of its ingredients.

Special warnings and special precautions for use:

Concomitant bronchodilator therapy: Where a concomitant aerosol bronchodilator is prescribed, it is recommended that this be administered prior to the Cromogen 5 mg Easi-Breathe Inhaler.

Concomitant steroid therapy: In patients currently treated with steroids the addition of Cromogen 5 mg Easi-Breathe Inhaler to the regimen may make it possible to reduce the maintenance dose or to discontinue steroids completely. The patient must be carefully supervised while the steroid dose is reduced, a rate of reduction of 10% weekly is suggested. If reduction of steroid dosage has been possible Cromogen 5 mg Easi-Breathe Inhaler should not be withdrawn until steroid cover has been re-instituted.

Since the therapy is prophylactic it is important to continue therapy in those patients who benefit. If it is necessary to withdraw this treatment, it should be done progressively over a period of one week. Symptoms of asthma may recur.

Interaction with other medicaments and other forms of interaction: No major interactions are anticipated with the proposed usage of the product. See *Special warnings and special precautions for use.*

Pregnancy and lactation: As with all medication, caution should be exercised especially during the first trimester of pregnancy. Cumulative experience with sodium cromoglycate suggests that it has no adverse effects on foetal development. It should only be used in pregnancy where there is a clear need.

It is not known whether sodium cromoglycate is excreted in the breast milk but on the basis of its physico-chemical properties this is considered unlikely. There is no evidence to suggest that the use of sodium cromoglycate has any undesirable effects on the baby.

Effects on ability to drive and use machines: No known effects.

Undesirable effects: Sodium cromoglycate is well-tolerated, mild throat irritation, coughing and transient bronchospasm may occur. Very rarely severe bronchospasm associated with a marked fall in pulmonary function has been reported. In such cases treatment should be stopped and should not be re-introduced. Reactions sometimes occurring after several months treatment include aggravation of existing asthma, urticaria, rashes and pulmonary infiltration with eosinophilia.

Overdose: No action other than medical observation should be necessary.

Pharmacological properties

Pharmacodynamic properties: Sodium Cromoglycate has no intrinsic bronchodilator, anti-histaminic or anti-inflammatory activity.

In vitro and *in vivo* studies have consistently suggested that sodium cromoglycate inhibits the release of inflammatory mediators from sensitised mast cells. It appears to inhibit reactions caused by both antigenic and non-antigenic stimuli and prevents both the immediate (Type I) and late (Type II) asthmatic responses. Most evidence suggests that the effects of sodium cromoglycate are due to a stabilisation of mast cell membranes, although the precise mechanism of action remains unknown.

Pharmacokinetic properties: Sodium cromoglycate is poorly absorbed from the gastrointestinal tract. Following inhalation as a fine powder from sodium cromoglycate capsules, about 8% of the total dose administered is deposited in the lungs from where it is rapidly absorbed and excreted unchanged in the urine and bile. The majority of an inhaled dose is swallowed and excreted unchanged in the faeces.

Preclinical safety data: See *Posology, Contra-indications, Special warnings, Interactions, Pregnancy and lactation, Undesirable effects* and *Overdose* sections above.

Pharmaceutical particulars

List of excipients: Sorbitan trioleate, trichlorofluoromethane, dichlorodifluoromethane.

Incompatibilities: No incompatibilities are anticipated with the proposed usage of the product.

Shelf life: Shelf life of the product as packaged for sale is 24 months.

Special precautions for storage: Store below 30°C. The canister is pressurised and should be protected from direct sunlight and frost. It must not be punctured or burnt, even when empty.

Nature and contents of container: Breath operated metered dose aerosol inhaler containing at least 112 actuations.

Instructions for use/handling:

1. Before use shake the inhaler vigorously.
2. Then, holding the inhaler upright, open the cap.
3. Breathe out normally. Place the mouthpiece firmly between your lips. Make sure that your hand is not blocking the airholes and that you are still holding the inhaler upright.
4. Breathe in slowly through the mouthpiece. Don't stop breathing when the inhaler puffs the dose into your mouth. Carry on until you have taken a deep breath.
5. Hold your breath for 10 seconds or as long as is comfortable, then breathe out slowly.
6. After use, hold the inhaler upright and immediately close the cap.
7. If you need to take more than one puff, wait at least one minute between doses and repeat from Step 1.
8. It is very important to keep the inhaler clean, especially in the mouthpiece area, to prevent build-up of deposits from the aerosol. Washing once a week is recommended.

How to clean your inhaler

A. Unscrew the top of the inhaler. Keep this top dry at all times.
B. Remove metal canister.
C. Rinse inhaler body in warm water and dry. Replace canister.
D. Close cap and screw top of inhaler back onto body. Do not wash the top part of the inhaler.

Marketing authorisation holder: Norton Healthcare Limited, Albert Basin, Royal Docks, London E16 2QJ.

Marketing authorisation number 0530/0404

Date of approval/revision of SPC February 1997.

Legal category POM.

CROMOGEN* STERI-NEB*

Presentation Cromogen Steri-Neb is a sterile sodium cromoglycate solution for inhalation via a power operated nebuliser. Each polyethylene ampoule contains 20 mg of sodium cromoglycate in 2 ml of water.

Uses Cromogen Steri-Neb is indicated for the preventive treatment of bronchial asthma which may be due to allergy, exercise, cold air or chemical and occupational irritants. Sodium cromoglycate has no intrinsic bronchodilator, anti-histaminic or anti-inflammatory activity. Most evidence suggests that the effects of sodium cromoglycate are due to a stabilisation of mast cell membranes, although the precise mechanism of action remains unknown.

Dosage and administration Cromogen Steri-Neb must only be administered by a power operated nebuliser, via a face mask or a mouthpiece.

Dosage: Since Cromogen Steri-Neb therapy is essentially preventive, it is important to continue therapy in those patients who benefit.

Adults, children and the elderly: The normal dose is the contents of 1 ampoule (20 mg), four times a day at intervals of 3–6 hours. In severe cases this may be increased to 5 or 6 times daily but with at least a 3 hour interval between administration of each ampoule.

Contra-indications, warnings, etc

Contra-indications: Cromogen Steri-Neb should not be administered by injection or administered to those patients with a known hypersensitivity to sodium cromoglycate.

Concomitant steroid therapy: In patients currently treated with steroids, the addition of Cromogen Steri-Neb to the regime may make it possible to reduce the maintenance dose or to discontinue steroids completely. The patient must be carefully supervised while the steroid dose is reduced; a rate of reduction of 10% weekly is suggested. An increase in steroid dosage may be necessary if symptoms increase and at times of infection, severe antigen challenge or stress. If reduction in steroid dosage has been possible Cromogen Steri-Neb should not be withdrawn until steroid cover has been reinstituted.

Concomitant bronchodilator therapy: If bronchodilators are used concomitantly patients may find that the frequency of bronchodilator usage can be reduced as their asthma is stabilised with Cromogen Steri-Neb.

Side effects: Sodium cromoglycate is well tolerated, mild throat irritation, coughing and transient bronchospasm may occur. Very rarely, severe bronchospasm associated with a marked fall in pulmonary function has been reported. In such cases treatment should be stopped and should not be re-introduced. Reactions sometimes occurring after several months treatment include aggravation of existing asthma, urticaria, rashes and pulmonary infiltration with eosinophilia.

Overdosage: No action other than medical observation should be necessary.

Pharmacological properties

Pharmacodynamic properties: Sodium cromoglycate has no intrinsic bronchodilator, anti-histaminic or anti-inflammatory activity.

In vitro and *in vivo* studies have consistently suggested that sodium cromoglycate inhibits the release of inflammatory mediators from sensitised most cells. It appears to inhibit reactions caused by both antigenic and non-antigenic stimuli and prevents both the immediate (Type I) and late (Type II) asthmatic responses. Most evidence suggests that the effects of sodium cromoglycate are due to stabilisation of most cell membranes although the precise mechanism of action remains unknown.

Pharmacokinetic properties: Sodium cromoglycate is poorly absorbed from the gastro-intestinal tract. Following inhalation as a fine powder from sodium cromoglycate capsules, about 8% of the total dose administered is deposited in the lungs from where it is rapidly absorbed and excreted unchanged in the urine and bile. The majority of an inhaled dose is swallowed and excreted unchanged in the faeces.

Withdrawal of therapy: Since Cromogen Steri-Neb acts prophylactically, it is important to continue treatment in those patients who benefit. The withdrawal of Cromogen Steri-Neb should be done progressively over a period of one week. Symptoms of asthma may recur.

Use in pregnancy and lactation: As with all medication, particular caution must be exercised during the first trimester of pregnancy. Cumulative experience with sodium cromoglycate suggest that it has no adverse effects on foetal development. It should only be used in pregnancy where there is a clear need.

It is not known whether sodium cromoglycate is excreted in the breast-milk but on the basis of its physico-chemical properties this is considered unlikely. There is no evidence to suggest that the use of sodium cromoglycate has any undersirable effects on the baby.

Pharmaceutical precautions Store in the box below 25°C protected from light. Cromogen Steri-Neb should not be diluted or mixed with other preparations due to possible incompatibility problems.

Legal category POM.

Package quantities Packs containing 60 Cromogen Steri-Neb ampoules in strips of 5.

Further information Nil.

Product licence number 0530/0349.

Product licence holder: Norton Healthcare Limited, Albert Basin, Royal Docks, London E16 2QJ.

FRU-CO*

Qualitative and quantitative composition Frusemide BP 40 mg and Amiloride Hydrochloride (anhydrous) BP 5 mg.

Pharmaceutical form Tablets for oral administration.

Clinical particulars
Therapeutic indications: Co-amilofruse is indicated where a prompt diuresis is required. It is of particular value in conditions where potassium conservation is important: congestive cardiac failure, nephrosis, corticosteroid therapy, oestrogen therapy, ascites associated with cirrhosis.

Posology and method of administration:
Adults: One to two tablets taken in the morning.

Elderly: The dosage should be adjusted according to diuretic response: serum electrolytes and urea should be carefully monitored.

Children: Not recommended.

Route of administration: Oral.

Contra-indications: Hyperkalaemia (serum potassium >5.3 mmol/litre), Addison's disease, acute renal failure, anuria, severe progressive renal disease, electrolyte imbalance, precomatose states associated with cirrhosis, concomitant potassium supplements, known sensitivity to frusemide or amiloride.

Special warnings and precautions for use: Patients who are being treated with this preparation require regular supervision, with monitoring of fluid and electrolyte states to avoid excessive loss of fluid.

Co-amilofruse should be used with particular caution in elderly patients or those with potential obstruction of the urinary tract or disorders rendering electrolyte balance precarious.

Hyponatraemia, hypochloraemia and raised blood urea nitrogen may occur during vigorous diuresis, especially in seriously ill patients. Careful monitoring of serum electrolytes and urea should therefore be undertaken in these patients.

The dosage of concurrently administered cardiac glycosides or antihypertensive agents may require adjustment.

Co-amilofruse should be discontinued before a glucose tolerance test.

Interaction with other medicaments and other forms of interaction: ACE inhibitors should be avoided in patients receiving co-amilofruse as serum potassium levels may be increased. If concomitant use of ACE inhibitors is considered essential, serum electrolytes and clinical condition must be monitored carefully. Concomitant administration of potassium supplements may cause severe hyperkalaemia and is contraindicated.

Nephrotoxicity caused by cephalosporins may be increased by concomitant administration of co-amilofruse.

In common with other diuretics, serum lithium levels may be increased when lithium is given concomitantly with frusemide, necessitating adjustment of the lithium dosage.

Certain non-steroidal anti-inflammatory agents (e.g. indomethacin) may attenuate the action of frusemide and may cause renal failure in cases of pre-existing hypovolaemia.

The effects of curariform muscle relaxants may be enhanced by frusemide, whilst the effects of antidiabetics may be reduced.

The diuretic effects of frusemide may be reduced by concurrent administraiton of phenytoin.

Interactions have also been reported with ototoxic antibiotics. In cases of concomitant glucocorticoid therapy or abuse of laxatives, the risk of an increased potassium loss should be borne in mind.

Pregnancy and lactation: The safety of co-amilofruse has not been established during pregnancy and lactation.

Effects on ability to drive and use machines: Reduced mental alertness may impair ability to drive or operate dangerous machinery.

Undesirable effects: As with other diuretics, electrolytes and water balance may be disturbed as a result of diuresis after prolonged therapy. This may cause symptoms such as headache, hypotension and muscle cramps.

Hyperkalaemia has been observed in patients receiving amiloride hydrochloride.

Frusemide may cause latent diabetes to become manifest. It may be necessary to increase the dose of hypoglycaemic agents in diabetic patients.

Patients with prostatic hypertrophy or inmpairment of micturition have an increased risk of developing acute urinary retention during diuretic therapy.

Serum uric acid levels may rise during treatment with co-amilofruse and acute attacks of gout may be precipitated.

Malaise, gastric upset, nausea, vomiting, diarrhoea, and constipation may occur.

If skin rashes or pruritus occur, treatment should be withdrawn.

Rare complications may include minor psychiatric disturbances, disturbances in liver function tests and ototoxicity.

Bone marrow depression occasionally complicates treatment, necessitating withdrawal of the product.

The haematopoietic state should be regularly monitored during treatment.

Serum calcium level may be reduced; in very rare cases tetany has been observed.

Serum cholesterol and triglyceride levels may rise during frusemide treatment but usually return to normal within six months during long term therapy.

Overdose: Treatment of overdosage should be aimed at reversing dehydration and correcting electrolyte imbalance, particularly hyperkalaemia. Emesis should be induced or gastric lavage performed. Treatment is symptomatic and supportive. If hyperkalaemia is seen, appropriate measures to reduce serum potassium must be instituted.

Pharmacological properties:
Pharmacodynamic properties:
Amiloride: Amiloride is a mild diuretic which appears to act mainly on the distal renal tubules. It is described as potassium-sparing since, like spironolactone, it increases the excretion of sodium and chloride and reduces the excretion of potassium. Unlike spironolactone, however, it does not act by inhibiting aldosterone. Amiloride does not inhibit carbonic anhydrase. It takes effect about 2 hours after administration by mouth and its diuretic action has been reported to persist for about 24 hours. The full effect may be delayed until several days of treatment.

Frusemide: Frusemide is a potent diuretic with a rapid action. Its effects are evident within 30 minutes to 1 hour after a dose by mouth and lasts for about 4 to 6 hours. After intravenous injection its effects are evident in about 5 minutes and last for about 2 hours. Frusemide inhibits the reabsorption of electrolytes in the ascending limb of the loop of Henle and also in the distal renal tubules. It may also have a direct effect in the proximal tubules. Excretion of sodium, potassium, and chloride ions is increased and water excretion enhanced. It has no clinically significant effect on carbonic anhydrase.

Pharmacokinetic properties:
Amiloride: Amiloride is incompletely absorbed from the gastro-intestinal tract; bioavailability of about 50% is reported and is reduced by food. It is not bound to plasma proteins and has a half-life of 6 to 9 hours. It is excreted unchanged by the kidneys.

Frusemide: Frusemide is incompletely but fairly rapidly absorbed from the gastro-intestinal tract; bioavailability has been reported to be about 60 to 70% but is reduced in renal failure. It has a biphasic half-life in the plasma with a terminal elimination phase that has been estimated to range up to about 1½ hours although it is prolonged in renal and hepatic insufficiency. It is up to 99% bound to plasma proteins, and is mainly excreted in the bile, non-renal elimination being considerably increased in renal failure. Frusemide crosses the placental barrier and is excreted in milk.

Preclinical safety data: Not applicable.

Pharmaceutical particulars
List of excipients: Lactose BP, Starch BP, Anstead dispersed orange 11348 (E110), Starch (pre-gelatinised) BP, Croscarmellose sodium USP, Magnesium sterate BP, Talc BP.

Incompatibilities: None known.

Shelf life: 36 months.

Special precautions for storage: Store in a dry place below 25°C and protect from light.

Nature and contents of container: Polypropylene tubular container with an open end equipped to accept a polyethylene closure with a tamper-evident tear strip, tampertainers or duma containers. Pack sizes 7, 14, 21, 28, 30, 50, 56, 60, 84, 90, 100, 112, 120, 500 and 1000 tablets, or

250 μm opaque UPVC/20 μm hard temper aluminium foil strip packs or PVdC coated PVC/Aluminium blisters (60 g/m² PVdC on 250 μm PVC/20 μm Al) containing 7, 14, 21, 28, 30, 50, 56, 60, 84, 90, 100, 112 and 120 tablets.

Instructions for use/handling: No special instructions.

Marketing authorisation holder: Norton Healthcare Ltd, Albert Basin, Royal Docks, London E16 2QJ.

Marketing authorisation number 0530/0348

Date of approval/revision of SPC June 1997

Legal category POM

HAY-CROM AQUEOUS* EYE DROPS

Presentation A clear pale straw coloured solution of Sodium Cromoglycate PhEur 2.0% w/v, with benzalkonium chloride 0.01% w/v. Other constituents: Disodium Edetate BP, Purified Water BP.

Uses Hay-Crom Aqueous Eye Drops are indicated for the prophylaxis and treatment of acute and chronic allergic conjunctivitis, including hay fever and seasonal kerato conjunctivitis. Most evidence suggests that the effects of sodium cromoglycate are due to stabilisation of sensitised mast cells, although the precise mechanism of action remains unknown.

Dosage and administration
Adults, children and the elderly: One or two drops into each affected eye up to four times daily.

Contra-indications, warnings, etc
Contra-indications: Hypersensitivity to sodium cromoglycate, benzalkonium chloride or disodium edetate.

Precautions: Since sodium cromoglycate is essentially prophylactic, patients should be advised not to discontinue using the medication unless advised to do so.

Side-effects: Following instillation of the drops, transient blurring of vision, burning, stinging or other transient symptoms may occur. Patients should be advised not to drive or operate machinery until clarity of vision is restored.

Overdosage or ingestion: Sodium cromoglycate is poorly absorbed through the gastro-intestinal tract. In case of overdosage, no action other than medical observation should be necessary.

Use in pregnancy and lactation: Caution should be exercised with respect to administration during pregnancy, especially during the first trimester. No adverse effects on foetal development have been reported with sodium cromoglycate. Hay-Crom Aqueous Eye Drops should be used in pregnancy only where there is a clear need. No data are available on the excretion of sodium cromoglycate in breast milk, but on the basis of its physico-chemical properties it is considered unlikely.

Pharmaceutical precautions Store below 30°C protected from light. Dispose of any unused solution 28 days after opening the pack. The product contains benzalkonium chloride as preservative. The eye drops should not be used whilst wearing soft contact lenses. Not for injection. Do not use if the pack is open when supplied or if any cloudiness is evident.

Pharmacological properties
Pharmacodynamic properties: Both *in-vitro* and *in-vivo* studies have consistently suggested that sodium cromoglycate prevents the release of granules that produce the allergen-mediated inflammatory reaction in the eye. Sodium cromoglycate appears to inhibit reactions caused by both antigenic and non antigenic stimuli. Sodium cromoglycate has no intrinsic antihistaminic or anti-inflammatory activity. Most evidence suggests that the effects of sodium cromoglycate are due to a stabilisation of mast cell membranes, although the precise mechanism remains unknown.

Pharmacokinetic properties: Due to lipid insolubility, sodium cromoglycate is effective only by topical application and only very small amounts are systemically absorbed in man. Any systemically absorbed drug is excreted unchanged in the bile and urine.

Preclinical safety data: None available.

List of excipients:
Benzalkonium Chloride 50% Solution 1980* BP
Benzalkonium Chloride* BP
Disodium Edetate BP
Purified water BP.

* equivalent to 0.01% w/v Benzalkonium Chloride in final product.

Incompatibilities: None known.

Shelf life: 3 years. 28 days after opening the bottle.

Nature and contents of container: Sterile, blow filled seal polyethylene eye dropper bottle with a two piece dropper assembly consisting of a white or translucent main body and white nozzle together with a blue nozzle cap. The eye dropper assembly is composed of a styrene acrylonitrile co-polymer. The pack size for the POM product is 13.5 ml and 10.0 ml for the P product.

Legal category POM.

Package quantities 13.5 ml.

Further information Full instructions for use by patients are provided with each pack. As with other ophthalmic preparations, discard any solution remaining 28 days after opening.

Since the product contains benzalkonium chloride as preservative, the eye drops should not be used whilst wearing soft contact lenses.

Product licence number 0530/0356

Product licence holder: Norton Healthcare Ltd, Albert Basin, Royal Docks, London E16 2QJ.

Date of approval/revision of SPC January 1998.

IPRATROPIUM STERI-NEB*

Presentation Sterile, unit dose, low density polyethylene vial containing a clear, colourless isotonic solution of ipratropium bromide 0.025% w/v (250 micrograms/ml) for administration by inhalation. Two vial sizes are available:

(i) a Steri-Neb vial containing 250 micrograms ipratropium bromide in 1 ml solution;

(ii) a Steri-Neb vial containing 500 micrograms ipratropium bromide in 2 ml solution.

Uses
Ipratropium bromide is an anticholinergic bronchodilator. It is indicated for the treatment of reversible airways obstruction.

Dosage and administration
The solution may be administered from an intermittent positive pressure ventilator or from suitable nebulisers using the following recommended doses:

Adult (including the elderly): 0.4–2.0 ml solution (100–500 micrograms) up to four times daily.

Children (3–14 years): 0.4–2.0 ml solution (100–500 micrograms) up to three times daily.

The dose of nebuliser solution may need to be diluted in order to obtain a final volume suitable for the particular nebuliser being used. If dilution is necessary only sterile Sodium Chloride 0.9% PhEur, such as Saline Steri-Neb (Sodium Chloride 0.9% PhEur) should be used.

Use in the elderly: No special precautions are required.

Contra-indications, warnings, etc
Contra-indications: Known hypersensitivity to atropine. Hypersensitivity to any of the components of Ipratropium Steri-Neb.

Warnings and precautions: Occasional reports of paradoxical bronchospasm following administration of nebulised solutions of ipratropium bromide have occurred during early treatment. Therefore, use of Ipratropium Steri-Neb should always be initiated in hospital and be subject to close medical supervision during the first week of treatment. The patient should be advised to seek medical advice should a reduced response to treament become apparent.

Patients must be instructed in the correct administration of the nebuliser solution and be warned not to allow the solution or mist to enter the eyes. Caution is advised in the use of anticholinergic agents in patients with glaucoma.

Anticholinergic agents can precipitate acute urinary retention in patients with prostatic hypertrophy should sufficient plasma concentrations be achieved. However, urinary retention has rarely been reported. Nevertheless, caution is advised in patients with prostatic hypertrophy.

Use in pregnancy: Animal teratology and reproduction studies have demonstrated no adverse effects. The safety of ipratropium bromide in human pregnancy has not been established.

As with all medicines, Ipratropium Steri-Neb should not be used in pregnancy, especially during the first trimester, unless the expected benefit is thought to outweigh any possible risk to the foetus.

Use in breast-feeding. It is not known to what extent ipratropium bromide passes into breast milk. The product should not be administered to nursing mothers unless considered essential by the physician.

Side-effects: Anticholinergic side-effects are unlikely at therapeutic doses, but some patients may complain of a dry mouth. Urinary retention and constipation have rarely been reported.

No adverse effect on bronchial secretion has been shown within the therapeutic dose range.

Overdosage: Inhaled doses of 5 mg produced an increase in heart rate with palpitations but single inhaled doses of 2 mg in adults and 1 mg in children did not cause side-effects. Single oral doses of ipratropium bromide 30 mg caused anticholinergic side-effects but these were not severe and did not require treatment.

Pharmacological properties
Pharmacodynamic properties: Ipratropium Bromide is a competitive muscarinic acetyl choline receptor antagonist selective for bronchial receptors.

Pharmacokinetic properties: The plasma half-life following iv administration is 3.6 hours. After iv dosing approximately 70% is excreted in the urine.

Ipratropium has a wide therapeutic range and only a small amount of drug is absorbed following inhalation of high therapeutic doses (0.5 mg). Hence the altered pharmacokinetics which may be present in patients with renal or hepatic impairment, or in elderly patients, is not likely to be clinically significant. Therefore, no special dosage recommendations are required in these populations.

Pharmaceutical precautions The vials should be stored at a temperature not exceeding 25°C. Protect from light. The vial should be opened immediately before use and any solution remaining after use should be discarded.

Legal category POM

Package quantities Packs containing 20 Steri-Nebs in strips of 5.

Further information Ipratropium Steri-Neb is an isotonic, sterile, preservative free solution for single use administration.

Product licence number 4544/0018

Product licence holder: Steripak Limited, Goddard Road, Runcorn, Cheshire WA7 1QE.

NASOBEC* AQUEOUS

Qualitative and quantitative composition Each 100 milligram spray contains 50 micrograms Beclomethasone Dipropionate BP.

Pharmaceutical form Nasal spray.

Clinical particulars
Therapeutic indications: Beclomethasone Dipropionate Aqueous Nasal Spray is indicated for the prophylaxis and treatment of seasonal and perennial allergic rhinitis and vasomotor rhinitis. Beclomethasone Diproprionate BP has anti-inflammatory glucocorticoid properties without significant systemic activity at recommended doses.

Posology and method of administration:
Adults and children over six years old: Two sprays twice daily into each nostril (400 micrograms beclomethasone dipropionate per day) is the recommended dosage. It may be preferable for some patients to administer a single spray into each nostril three to four times daily.

It should be made clear to patients that full therapeutic benefit will only be achieved after a few days treatment.

Elderly: Dosage as for adults.

Children less than twelve years old: Beclomethasone Dipropionate Aqueous Nasal Spray is not indicated for children under twelve years old, due to insufficient clinical data.

The total dosage for any 24 hour period should not normally exceed eight sprays, i.e. 400 micrograms of beclomethasone dipropionate.

Contra-indications: Patients with a history of hypersensitivity to any of its ingredients.

Special warnings and precautions for use: Systemic effects rarely occur. These include hypothalamic-pituitary-adrenal (HPA) suppression and growth retardation in children.

Care must be taken while transferring patients from systemic steroid treatment to Beclomethasone Dipropionate Aqueous Nasal Spray where disturbances in the hypothalamic-pituitary-adrenal (HPA) axis could be expected.

Beclomethasone Dipropionate Aqueous Nasal will control seasonal allergic rhinitis in the majority of cases, concomitant therapy to control eye symptoms may be necessary during a heavy challenge to allergens.

Interactions with other medicaments and other forms of interaction: None known.

Pregnancy and lactation: There is inadequate evidence of safety in human pregnancy. Early studies in animals have demonstrated an increase in foetal cleft palate and growth retardation following maternal ingestion of high corticosteroid doses. However, direct intranasal application at the recommended doses ensures minimal systemic exposure.

Use during lactation: It is probable that beclomethasone dipropionate is excreted in milk. However, given the relatively low dose used by the nasal route, the levels are likely to be low. In mothers breast feeding their baby the therapeutic benefits of the drug should be weighed against the potential hazards to mother and baby.

Effects on ability to drive and use machines: Beclomethasone Dipropionate Aqueous Nasal Spray does not affect the ability to operate and drive machines.

Undesirable effects: In very rare cases septal perforation can develop during therapy.

Dryness and irritation of the nose and throat as well as blood stained crusts in the nose can occur when taking nasal sprays but these conditions are not progressive and are seldom troublesome. An unpleasant smell and taste are rarely reported.

Rare cases of intraocular pressure or glaucoma in association with intranasal formulations of the beclomethasone dipropionate have been reported.

Widespread use of beclomethasone dipropionate for a decade has shown no serious local damage to mucous membranes.

Overdose: Suppression of the HPA function is the only harmful effect that would arise from taking large amounts of beclomethasone dipropionate over a short period of time. No emergency procedure need be undertaken and treatment with Beclomethasone Dipropionate Aqueous Nasal Spray should continue at the recommended dose. The HPA function reverts back to normal within a day or two.

Pharmacological properties
Pharmacodynamic properties: Beclomethasone dipropionate is the diester of beclomethasone, a synthetic glucocorticoid which demonstrates anti-inflammatory and immunosuppressant properties. This drug is stated to exert a topical effect on the lungs without significant systemic activity at recommended doses, although the mechanisms of action are as yet unknown.

Pharmacokinetic properties: The pharmacokinetics of beclomethasone dipropionate have not been extensively studied. The currently available chemical methods are not of sufficient sensitivity to measure therapeutically relevant plasma concentrations, particularly those occurring following inhalation.

(a) General characteristics of the active substance
Absorption: Beclomethasone dipropionate is readily absorbed from the gastro-intestinal tract. It is also well absorbed from sites of local application. When administered by topical application, as in the case of Beclomethasone Dipropionate Aqueous Nasal Spray, sufficient beclomethasone dipropionate may be absorbed to give systemic effects.

Distribution: The drug is rapidly distributed to all body tissues. It crosses the placenta and may be excreted in small amounts in breast milk.

Elimination: After metabolism in the liver and kidney, the drug is excreted in the urine.

(b) Characteristics in patients: As above.

Preclinical safety data: See *Contra-indications, Special warnings, Interactions, Pregnancy and lactation, Undesirable effects* and *Overdose* sections above.

Pharmaceutical particulars
List of excipients: Benzalkonium Chloride Solution BP, Phenylethylalcohol USP, Polysorbate 80 BP, Dextrose Anhydrous BP, Dispersible Cellulose BP, Hydrochloric Acid BP (if necessary – to adjust pH), Purified Water BP.

Incompatibilities: None known.

Shelf life: 24 months, unopened, for all three pack sizes.

Special precautions for storage: Protect from light. Do not refrigerate. Store below 30°C. Discard three months after first using the spray.

Nature and contents of container: Beclomethasone Dipropionate Aqueous Nasal Spray is supplied in polyethylene bottles of 30 ml capacity containing a nominal 200 doses. Each bottle is fitted with a metering pump designed to deliver a nominal 100 milligrams of suspension per spray.

Instructions for use/handling: No special instructions.

Marketing authorisation holder: Norton Healthcare Limited, Albert Basin, Royal Docks, London E16 2QJ.

Marketing authorisation number 00530/0492

Date of approval/revision of SPC August 1996.

Legal category POM.

PEPTAC* LIQUID

Presentation Peptac Liquid is a pink suspension with a flavour of aniseed. Each 5 ml contains Sodium Alginate BP 250 mg, Sodium Bicarbonate BP 133.5 mg, Calcium Carbonate BP 80 mg in a base containing Carbopol 974P, Sodium Hydroxide BP, Saccharin Sodium BP, Ethyl Hydroxy Benzoate BP, Propyl Hydroxy Benzoate BP, Butyl Hydroxy Benzoate BP, Isopropyl Alcohol BP, Erythrosine Colour (E127), Aniseed Oil BP, Purified Water BP.

Uses Peptac alleviates the painful conditions resulting from the reflux of gastric acid and bile into the oesophagus by suppressing the reflux itself. It is indicated in heartburn, including heartburn of pregnancy, dyspepsia associated with gastric reflux, hiatus hernia, reflux oesophagitis, regurgitation and all cases of epigastric and retrosternal distress where the underlying cause is gastric reflux.

Dosage and administration For oral use.

Adults and children over 12 years: Two to four 5 ml spoonfuls.

Children 6–12 years: One to two 5 ml spoonfuls.

Not recommended in children under six years of age.

Doses should be taken after meals and at bedtime.

Contra-indications, warnings, etc There are no specific contra-indications.

Each 10 ml dose of Peptac Liquid contains 141 mg (6.2 mEq) of sodium and therefore care should be exercised in patients on a sodium restricted diet.

Peptac Liquid should not be taken within 1–2 hours of taking other medicines by mouth, or for more than 2 weeks if symptoms persist.

Peptac Liquid should not be used by patients allergic to any of it's constiuents.

Drug interactions: Antacids may interact with other drugs as they alter the gastric pH which may affect dissolution, solubility or ionisation of the other drug. Antacids reduce the absorption of certain drugs from the following groups: ACE Inhibitors, Analgesics, Antibacterials, Antiepileptics, Antifungals, Antimalarials, Antipsychotics, Biphosphonates, Penicillamine.

Antacids may increase the pH of the urine and affect the rate of drug elimination. Excretion of basic drugs is decreased whereas acidic drugs are eliminated more rapidly.

Due to effects at the renal level sodium bicarbonate may reduce plasma lithium levels and increase plasma quinidine levels.

Use in pregnancy: Peptac Liquid is indicated for heartburn of pregnancy and may be used during lactation.

Undesirable effects: Constipation, flatulence, stomach cramps or belching may occasionally occur.

Treatment of overdosage: As Peptac Liquid's mode of action is physical, overdosage in terms of the alginate content is virtually no hazard. The only consequence is abdominal distension which is best treated conservatively. The relatively low concentrations of sodium and calcium carbonate in Peptac Liquid would also make serious consequences from overdosage very unlikely.

Pharmacological properties
Pharmacodynamic properties: When taken after a meal Sodium Alginate forms a rigid raft of alginic acid in the stomach reducing gastric reflux. This raft formed is maintained in the stomach for two hours. Sodium bicarbonate reacts with gastric acid to produce carbon dioxide which is retained in the gel and allows the raft to rise to the surface of the gastric contents. Calcium ions from calcium carbonate link the alginic acid molecules and strengthen the raft.

Pharmacokinetic properties: Alginic acid is not absorbed into the systemic circulation.

Preclinical safety data: There is no preclinical safety data.

Pharmaceutical particulars
Special precautions for storage: Store below 25°C. Do no refrigerate.

Shelf life:
2 years – amber glass bottles.
18 months – HDPE bottles.

Nature and contents of container: Pharmaceutical Grade III amber glass bottles with pilfer proof caps and virgin/white high density polyethylene bottles with tamper evident screw caps.

Pack sizes: 100, 150, 200, 250, 300 and 500 ml.

Instructions for use/handling: Not applicable.

Marketing authorisation holder: Pinewood Laboratories Limited, Ballymacarbry, Clonmel, Co. Tipperary.

Marketing authorisation number PL 4917/0021

Date of first authorisation/renewal of authorisation 25/03/1998

Date of (partial) revision of text September 1998

SALAMOL* STERI-NEB* 2.5 mg and 5 mg

Presentation Salamol Steri-Nebs 2.5 mg are unit dose polyethylene ampoules containing a sterile, clear, colourless to light yellow aqueous solution of Salbutamol Sulphate BP. Each Steri-Neb contains 2.5 ml of solution equivalent to 2.5 mg salbutamol, i.e. a concentration of 0.1%. The solution is adjusted to a pH of 4.

Salamol Steri-Nebs 5 mg are unit dose polyethylene ampoules containing a sterile, clear, colourless to light yellow aqueous solution of Salbutamol Sulphate BP. Each Steri-Neb contains 2.5 ml of solution equivalent to 5 mg salbutamol, i.e. a concentration of 0.2%. The solution is adjusted to a pH of 4.

Uses For use in the routine management of chronic bronchospasm unresponsive to conventional therapy and the treatment of acute severe asthma.

Dosage and administration
Adults: The usual dose is 2.5 mg given up to three to four times a day by a nebuliser. This may be increased to 5 mg up to three to four times a day if necessary.

In domiciliary practice, however, the benefits of increasing the dose of nebulised salbutamol sulphate should be weighed against the risk that a deterioration in the patient's underlying condition may be masked. In such circumstances a medical assessment should be considered, since alternative therapy may be indicated.

Children: The same dosage as for adults.

Infants: The clinical efficacy of nebulised salbutamol sulphate in infants under 18 months is uncertain. As transient hypoxaemia may occur, supplemental oxygen therapy should be considered.

Elderly: The same dosage as for other adults.

Delivery of the aerosol may be by face mask or 'T' piece.

Salamol Steri-Nebs should be used undiluted. However, if a delivery time in excess of 10 minutes is required, they should be diluted with Sodium Chloride Injection BP or Saline Steri-Neb.

Contra-indications, warnings, etc
Contra-indications: Hypersensitivity to any of the components of Salamol Steri-Nebs.

Although some forms of salbutamol sulphate have been used for the management of premature labour, Salamol Steri-Nebs should not be used for this purpose.

Salamol Steri-Nebs should not be used in threatened abortion.

Warnings: The use of nebulised anti-cholinergic agents and nebulised salbutamol sulphate in combination has been reported to precipitate acute angle closure glaucoma. This combination should be used with caution when giving nebuliser therapy to patients with actual or potential glaucoma.

The patient should be warned not to allow the solution or mist to enter the eyes.

Precautions: Salamol Steri-Nebs should be used with caution in patients with thyrotoxicosis or in patients known to have received large doses of other sympathomimetic drugs.

Salamol Steri-Nebs are for use with a nebuliser under the direction of a physician. The solution should not be injected or administered orally. Patients who use Salamol Steri-Nebs at home should be warned that if their usual dose is less effective or its duration of action reduced, they should not increase either the dose or frequency of treatment, but should consult their doctor.

As with other inhalation therapy, the potential for paradoxical bronchospasm should be considered. If it occurs the preparation should be discontinued immediately and alternative therapy given. Solutions which are not of neutral pH may rarely cause paradoxical bronchospasm in some patients.

Salbutamol and non-selective beta blocking drugs such as propranolol should not usually be prescribed together.

Potentially serious hypokalaemia may result from $beta_2$ agonist therapy. Particular caution is advised in acute severe asthma as this effect may be potentiated by concomitant treatment with xanthine derivatives, steroids, diuretics and by hypoxia. It is recommended that serum potassium levels are monitored in such situations.

Pregnancy: Administration of the drug during pregnancy should only be considered if the expected benefit to the mother is greater than any possible risk to the foetus. Salbutamol has been in widespread use for many years in human beings without apparent ill consequence; this includes its well established use in the management of premature labour. However, as with the majority of drugs, there is little published evidence of its safety in the early stages of human pregnancy, but in animal studies there was evidence of some harmful effects on the foetus at very high dose levels.

Lactation: As salbutamol is probably secreted in breast milk, its use in nursing mothers requires careful consideration. It is not known whether salbutamol has a harmful effect on the neonate and so its use should be restricted to situations where it is felt that the expected benefit to the mother is likely to outweigh any potential risk to the neonate.

Side-effects: A small increase in heart rate may occur in patients who inhale large doses of salbutamol sulphate. This is not usually accompanied by any other changes in the electrocardiogram.

Solutions which are not of neutral pH may rarely cause paradoxical bronchospasm in some patients. As with other inhalation therapy, the potential for paradoxical bronchospasm should be considered. If it occurs, the preparation should be discontinued immediately and alternative therapy given.

Other side-effects which occur with very high doses of salbutamol sulphate by inhalation are peripheral vasodilation and fine tremor of skeletal muscle.

Headaches have been rarely reported. They usually disappear with continued treatment.

There have been rare reports of transient muscle cramps.

Hypersensitivity reactions including angioedema and urticaria, bronchospasm, hypotension and collapse have been reported very rarely. Potentially serious hypokalaemia may result from $beta_2$ agonist therapy.

As with other $beta_2$ agonists, hyperactivity in children has been reported rarely.

Overdosage: The most significant symptom of a large overdosage would be a reflex tachycardia. The recommended antidote to overdosage with salbutamol sulphate is a cardioselective beta blocking agent. However, all beta blocking agents should be used with caution in patients with a history of bronchospasm.

Pharmacological properties
Pharmacodynamic properties: Salbutamol is a direct acting sympathomimetic agent with predominately beta adrenergic activity and a selective action on $beta_2$ receptors, it is used as a bronchodilator in the treatment of asthma.

Pharmacokinetic properties: Salbutamol does not appear to be metabolised in the lung therefore its ultimate metabolism and excretion following inhalation depends upon delivery method used, which is determined by the proportion of drug inhaled relative to the proportion inadvertently swallowed.

Pharmaceutical precautions
Storage: Salamol Steri-Nebs should be stored at a temperature not exceeding 25°C and protected from light.

Dilution: Salamol Steri-Nebs may be diluted if required with Sodium Chloride Injection BP or Saline Steri-Neb. Nebuliser solutions should be replaced daily.

Legal category POM.

Package quantities Salamol Steri-Nebs 2.5 mg and 5 mg are available in boxes containing 20 Steri-Nebs in 4 strips of 5.

Further information Nil.

Product licence numbers
Salamol Steri-Neb 2.5 mg: 4544/0013
Salamol Steri-Neb 5.0 mg: 4544/0017

Product licence holder: Steripak Limited, Goddard Road, Astmoor, Runcorn, Cheshire WA7 1QE.

SALINE STERI-NEB*

Presentation Saline Steri-Nebs are unit dose polyethylene ampoules containing a clear, colourless solution of Sodium Chloride PhEur. Each Steri-Neb contains 2.5 ml of a 0.9% w/v solution of sodium chloride.

Uses For the dilution of solutions for nebulisation.

Dosage and administration
Adults, children and the elderly: As directed by the physician.

Contra-indications, warnings, etc
Contra-indications: Not for injection.

Side-effects: Substantial oral ingestion may require the use of a diuretic to remove excess sodium.

Precautions: Do not use unless the product is clear and the pack intact. Discard any surplus after use.

Use in pregnancy: As with all medication, particular caution must be exercised during the first trimester of pregnancy.

Pharmaceutical precautions
Storage: Saline Steri-Nebs should be stored between 5°C and 25°C and protected from light. When diluting nebuliser solutions, make up freshly according to the manufacturer's instructions.

Legal category POM.

Package quantities Saline Steri-Nebs are available in boxes containing 20 Steri-Nebs in 4 strips of 5.

Further information Nil.

Product licence number 4544/0015

Product licence holder: Steripak Limited, Goddard Road, Astmoor, Runcorn, Cheshire, WA7 1QE.

SERENACE* AMPOULES

Qualitative and quantitative composition
Serenace 5 mg Ampoules: Haloperidol BP 5 mg.
Serenace 20 mg Ampoules: Haloperidol BP 20 mg.

Pharmaceutical form Solution for intramuscular or intravenous injection.

Clinical particulars
Therapeutic indications: Psychotic disorders – schizophrenia, mania and hypomania, especially paranoid psychoses.

Mental or behavioural problems such as aggression, hyperactivity and self-mutilation in the mentally retarded.

Moderate to severe psychomotor agitation, excitement, violent or dangerously impulsive behaviour.

Gilles de la Tourette syndrome and severe tics.

Restlessness and agitation in the elderly.

Serenace 5 mg Ampoules: Nausea and vomiting. Intractable hiccup.

Posology and method of administration: There is

considerable variation from patient to patient in the response to treatment and the dosage required. As with all antipsychotics, dosage should be individualised according to the needs and response of each patient.

To determine the initial dosage, consideration should be given to the patient's age, severity of symptoms and previous response to other antipsychotic therapy. Oral dosage may be given in single or divided doses. Administration twice daily is sufficient in most cases.

Adults: Psychotic behaviour; Mental or behavioural problems; Moderate to severe psychomotor agitation or impulsive behaviour.

Initial treatment: For rapid emergency treatment 5 or 10 mg, or infrequently up to 30 mg by intramuscular injection may be required. Depending on the response of the patient, subsequent doses may be given as frequently as every 30 to 60 minutes although 6–12 hourly intervals may be satisfactory. There is a wide variation among individual patients so that cumulative dosage is not predictable in advance. Some patients may have an optimal early response after as little as 10 mg, whereas others may require up to 40 or 50 mg. Higher doses are not usually necessary. Serenace injection may also be administered intravenously.

Maintenance treatment: Once a satisfactory therapeutic response has been achieved, dosage should be reduced gradually to the lowest effective maintenance level which is often as low as 3 to 10 mg daily dependent on the characteristics and response of each individual patient. If possible, maintenance treatment should be oral.

Gilles de la Tourette syndrome: Initial dosage is usually 2 mg daily. During the acute phase of treatment, dosage can be increased gradually to obtain maximum control of symptoms and may range between 6 and 50 mg or, exceptionally up to 180 mg daily.

Once a satisfactory therapeutic response has been achieved, dosage should be reduced gradually to the lowest effective maintenance level which for most patients is 4 mg daily.

Serenace 5 mg Ampoules:

Nausea and vomiting: 0.5 to 1 mg I.M. daily.

Intractable hiccup: 3 to 15 mg daily in divided doses parenterally has proved useful.

Elderly: Half the recommended adult starting dose may be sufficient for therapeutic response in the elderly. The maximum and maintenance dose will generally be lower for debilitated or geriatric patients who may be more sensitive to serenace.

Children: Parenteral administration is not recommended for children.

Route of administration: By intramuscular or intravenous injection.

Contra-indications: Comatose states, patients with Parkinson's disease or a sensitivity to haloperidol and use during lactation.

Special warnings and precautions for use: Liver disease, renal failure, phaeochromocytoma, conditions predisposing to epilepsy (e.g. alcohol withdrawal or brain damage). May be given to epileptics, but usual anticonvulsant therapy could be continued.

Use cautiously in thyrotoxic patients and those with arteriosclerosis who may have occult or manifest lesions of the basal ganglia. Such patients may be more prone to develop extrapyramidal symptoms.

Administer with care to patients with severe cardiovascular disorders, because of the possibility of transient hypotension. Should hypotension occur and a vasopressor be required, adrenaline should not be used since haloperidol may block its vasopressor activity and paradoxical further lowering of the blood pressure may occur.

Interactions with other medicaments and other forms of interaction: Serenace may potentiate the central nervous system depression produced by other CNS-depressant drugs including alcohol, hypnotics, sedatives or strong analgesics. Enhanced CNS effects (sedation, mental disturbances) have been reported with the combined use of methyldopa and haloperidol. Severe neuromuscular symptoms with impairment of consciousness and fever have been reported with combined use of lithium and haloperidol. A causal relationship has not been established. However, patients receiving such combined therapy should be carefully observed for early evidence of neurological toxicity and treatment should be discontinued if such signs appear.

Serenace may antagonise the action of adrenaline and other sympathomimetic agents.

Possible interactions have been reported between haloperidol and carbamazepine. Haloperidol levels have been shown to be reduced by approximately 50% when carbamazepine is administered concurrently. The psychotic symptoms in some patients have been exacerbated in association with these lowered haloperidol levels but in some instances increased efficacy was seen, possibly as a result of the central action of carbamazepine itself. The mechanism for this interaction is thought to be enzyme induction and increased hepatic metabolism of haloperidol.

Pregnancy and lactation: Pregnancy: The safety of serenace in pregnancy has not been established. Reproduction studies in rodents have shown an increased incidence of resorption, reduced fertility and pup mortality. No specific teratogenic effect has been reported in rats, rabbit or dogs, but cleft palate and open eye syndrome have been observed in mice.

No well-controlled studies of haloperidol use in pregnant women have been conducted. Two cases of foetal limb malformation have been reported following maternal use of haloperidol, combined with other drugs during the first trimester. No causal relationship has been established. Use of haloperidol during pregnancy requires that the anticipated benefit be weighed against the possible hazards to mother and foetus.

Lactation: Haloperidol has been detected in breast milk. If use of haloperidol is considered essential, breast feeding should be discontinued.

Effects on ability to drive and use machines: Haloperidol may impair alertness, especially at the start of treatment. These effects may be potentiated by alcohol. Patients should be warned of the risks of sedation and advised not to drive or operate machinery during treatment, until their susceptibility is known.

Undesirable effects: Extrapyramidal symptoms such as Parkinson-like symptoms, akinesia, akathisia, dyskinesia, dystonia may develop during haloperidol treatment, very rarely dystonia has been reported to produce laryngeal/pharyngeal spasm associated with gagging, respiratory distress and asphyxia.

In common with other antipsychotics haloperidol has been associated with persistent dyskinesia. Tardive dyskinesia may develop in some patients on long term therapy, possibly in relation to total cumulative dose, or may develop after drug therapy has been discontinued. The risk is reported to be greater in elderly patients on high dose therapy. Characteristic symptoms are rhythmical involuntary movements of the tongue, face, mouth or jaw sometimes accompanied by involuntary movements of the extremities. They may persist for many months or even years and, while they gradually disappear in some patients, they appear to be permanent in others.

At the first signs of tardive dyskinesia which may be orofacial dyskinesia the benefit of continued treatment should be carefully assessed against the risk of the development of persistent dyskinesia. Withdrawal of treatment with careful observation of the dyskinesia and psychotic condition has been suggested in order to assess the need for continued neuroleptic therapy and to reveal persisting dyskinesia. Should it be necessary to reinstate treatment, the antipsychotic agent may mask the syndrome. Anti-Parkinsonian agents have proved of little value in this syndrome. In schizophrenia, the response to antipsychotic drug treatment may be delayed. If drugs are withdrawn, recurrence of symptoms may not become apparent for several weeks or months.

Some degree of sedation may occur, particularly with higher doses and at the start of treatment. The elderly appear more susceptible. At low doses in susceptible (especially non-psychotic) individuals, haloperidol may cause unpleasant subjective feelings of being mentally dulled or slowed down, dizziness, headaches or paradoxical effects of excitement, agitation or insomnia.

Other adverse effects reported include gastrointestinal symptoms, nausea, loss of appetite, dyspepsia, autonomic effects such as blurring of vision and, infrequently, tachycardia. Dose-related hypotension is uncommon, but can occur, particularly in the elderly or after parenteral administration. Impairment of sexual function, including erection and ejaculation, oedema; blood dyscrasias, including agranulocytosis and transient leucopenia; skin reactions including exfoliative dermatitis, erythema multiforme and photosensitisation and jaundice, are rarely reported. Transient abnormalities of liver function tests may occur in the absence of jaundice.

Impairment of body temperature could occur at high doses. In common with other antipsychotics, hormonal effects include hyperprolactinaemia which could cause galactorrhoea, gynaecomastia and oligo- or amenorrhoea. Abrupt discontinuation of high doses of antipsychotics has very rarely resulted in acute withdrawal symptoms, including nausea, vomiting and insomnia. Gradual withdrawal is advisable.

Rare cases of sudden and unexplained death have been reported in psychiatric patients receiving treatment with antipsychotics including haloperidol. The nature of the evidence makes it impossible to determine the contributory role, if any, of the drug.

In common with other antipsychotics haloperidol has been associated with rare cases of neuroleptic malignant syndrome, an idiosyncratic response characterised by hyperthermia, muscle rigidity, autonomic instability, altered consciousness and coma. Signs of autonomic dysfunction such as tachycardia, labile arterial pressure and sweating may precede the onset of hyperthermia, acting as early warning signs. Recovery usually occurs within five to seven days of antipsychotic withdrawal. Affected patients should be carefully monitored.

Overdose: Intensification of the known pharmacological and adverse effects may occur. The most prominent would be severe extrapyramidal symptoms, hypotension or sedation. The patient may appear comatose with respiratory depression and hypotension which could be severe enough to produce a shock-like state.

Extrapyramidal reactions may include muscular weakness or rigidity and a generalised or localised tremor. With accidental overdosage hypothermia, bradycardia, sinus arrhythmia and hypertension have been reported in young children. No specific antidote has been identified.

In the event of overdosage the stomach should be emptied by aspiration and lavage. Emetics should not be used. Establishment of patent airway and artificial ventilation may be needed. Hypotension may be counteracted by placing the patient in the head-down position and by the use of a plasma expander and careful use of a vasopressor agent such as noradrenaline. Adrenaline should not be used. Severe extrapyramidal reactions should be treated with parenteral antihistamines or antiparkinsonian drugs. The relatively long plasma elimination half-life of haloperidol should be considered.

Pharmacological properties

Pharmacodynamic properties: Haloperodol is a butyrophenone. Its pharmacological profile of activity includes a pronounced capacity to induce extrapyramidal reactions and a low incidence of autonomic side-effects, such as hypotension.

Pharmacokinetic properties: The pharmacokinetics of haloperidol have been studied in healthy volunteers and patients. In volunteers, following a single intravenous or oral dose, serum elimination half-life ranged from 10–19 hours and 12–38 hours respectively. Similar elimination half-lives were observed in patients after administration of a single oral or intramuscular dose of the drug or after withdrawal of the drug from patients who were in a steady state. Steady state serum levels were usually achieved within 6 days on a fixed oral dosage.

Preclinical safety data: Not applicable.

Pharmaceuticl particulars

List of excipients: Lactic Acid BP; Sodium Hydroxide BP; Water for Injections PhEur.

Incompatibilities: None.

Shelf life: 3 years.

Special precautions for storage: Store in a dry place below 30°C. Protect from light.

Nature and contents of container:

Serenace 5 mg Ampoules: 1 ml printed clear, neutral glass ampoules with a yellow band around the neck constriction, 6 or 10 packed into cardboard cartons.

Serenace 20 mg Ampoules: 2 ml printed, clear, neutral glass ampoules with a yellow band around the neck constriction; 10 packed in cardboard cartons.

Instructions for use/handling: No special instructions.

Marketing authorisation holder: Norton Healthcare Limited, Albert Basin, Royal Docks, London E16 2QJ.

Marketing authorisation numbers

Serenace 5 mg Ampoules 0530/0368
Serenace 20 mg Ampoules 0530/0369

Date of approval/revision of SPC 30 September 1996

Legal category POM

SERENACE* TABLETS
SERENACE* LIQUID
SERENACE* CAPSULUES

Qualitative and quantitative composition

Serenace 1.5 mg Tablets: Haloperidol BP 1.5 mg.
Serenace 5 mkg Tablets: Haloperidol BP 5 mg.
Serenace 10 mg Tablets: Haloperidol BP 10 mg.
Serenace 20 mg Tablets: Haloperidol BP 20 mg.
Serenace Liquid: Haloperidol BP 10 mg/5 ml.
Serenace Capsules: Haloperidol BP 0.5 mg.

Pharmaceutical form Tablets, hard gelatin capsules or liquid.

Clinical particulars

Therapeutic indications: Psychotic disorders – schizophrenia, mania and hypomania, especially paranoid psychoses.

Mental or behavioural problems such as aggression, hyperactivity and self-mutilation in the mentally retarded.

Moderate to severe psychomotor agitation, excitement, violent or dangerously impulsive behaviour.

Gilles de la Tourette syndrome and severe tics.

Childhood behaviour disorders, especially when associated with hyperactivity and aggression.

Restlessness and agitation in the elderly.

Serenace 1.5 mg, 5 mg, and 10 mg Tablets and Serenace Liquid 2 mg/ml: Intractable hiccup.

Serenace Liquid 2 mg/ml and Serenace 500 mg Capsules: Nausea and vomiting.

Serenace 500 mg Capsules: Adjunct to short-term management of anxiety.

Posology and method of administration: There is considerable variation from patient to patient in the response to treatment and the dosage required. As with all antipsychotics, dosage should be individualised according to the needs and response of each patient.

To determine the initial dosage, consideration should be given to the patient's age, severity of symptoms and previous response to other antipsychotic therapy. Oral dosage may be given in single or divided doses. Administration twice daily is sufficient in most cases.

Adults: Psychotic behaviour; Mental or behavioural problems; Moderate to severe psychomotor agitation or impulsive behaviour.

Initial treatment: Initial dosage may range from as little as 1.5 mg daily to 20 mg daily, dependent on the characteristics, severity of symptoms and response of each individual patient. It may be necessary to increase the dosage gradually to obtain maximum control of symptoms. In severely disturbed or resistant patients, the maximum daily dose is 30 mg.

Maintenance treatment: Once a satisfactory therapeutic response has been achieved, dosage should be reduced gradually to the lowest effective maintenance level which is often as low as 3 to 10 mg daily dependent on the characteristics and response of each individual patient.

Gilles de la Tourette syndrome: Initial dosage is usually 2 mg daily. During the acute phase of treatment, dosage can be increased gradually to obtain maximum control of symptoms and may range between 6 and 30 mg daily.

Once a satisfactory therapeutic response has been achieved, dosage should be reduced gradually to the lowest effective maintenance level which for most patients is 4 mg daily.

Serenace 1.5 mg, 5 mg, and 10 mg Tablets and Serenace Liquid 2 mg/ml
Intractable hiccup: 3 to 15 mg daily in divided doses, orally has proven useful.

Serenace Liquid 2 mg/ml and Serenace 500 mg Capsules
Nausea and vomiting: 1 mg daily orally has proved useful.

Serenace 500 microgram Capsules
Anxiety: 500 micrograms twice daily.

Elderly: Half the recommended adult starting dose may be sufficient for therapeutic response in the elderly. The maximum and maintenance dose will generally be lower for debilitated or geriatric patients who may be more sensitive to serenace.

Children: (Oral administration): 25 to 50 micrograms per kg body weight per day to a maximum of 10 mg, although, exceptionally, adolescents may require up to 30 mg daily.

Route of administration: Oral.

Contra-indications: Comatose states, patients with Parkinson's disease or a sensitivity to haloperidol and use during lactation.

Special warnings and special precautions for use: Liver disease, renal failure, phaeochromocytoma, conditions predisposing to epilepsy (e.g. alcohol withdrawal or brain damage). May be given to epileptics, but usual anticonvulsant therapy should be continued.

Use cautiously in thyrotoxic patients and those with arteriosclerosis who may have occult or manifest lesions of the basal ganglia. Such patients may be more prone to develop extrapyramidal symptoms.

Administer with care to patients with severe cardiovascular disorders, because of the possibility of transient hypotension. Should hypotension occur and a vasopressor be required, adrenaline should not be used since haloperidol may block its vasopressor activity and further lowering of the blood pressure may occur.

Interactions with other medicaments and other forms of interaction: Serenace may potentiate the central nervous system depression produced by other CNS-depressant drugs including alcohol, hypnotics, sedatives or strong analgesics. Enhanced CNS effects (sedation, mental disturbances) have been reported with the combined use of methyldopa and haloperidol. Severe neuromuscular symptoms with impairment of consciousness and fever have been reported with combined use of lithium and haloperidol. A causal relationship has not been established. However, patients receiving such combined therapy should be carefully observed for early evidence of neurological toxicity and treatment should be discontinued if such signs appear.

Serenace may antagonise the action of adrenaline and other sympathomimetic agents.

Possible interactions have been reported between haloperidol and carbamazepine. Haloperidol levels have been shown to be reduced by approximately 50% when carbamazepine is administered concurrently. The psychotic symptoms in some patients have been exacerbated in association with these lowered haloperidol levels but in some instances increased efficacy was seen, possibly as a result of the central action of carbamazepine itself. The mechanism for this interaction is thought to be enzyme induction and increased hepatic metabolism of haloperidol.

Pregnancy and lactation: Pregnancy: The safety of Serenace in pregnancy has not been established. Reproduction studies in rodents have shown an increased incidence of resorption, reduced fertility and pup mortality. No specific teratogenic effect has been reported in rats, rabbit or dogs, but cleft palate and open eye syndrome have been observed in mice.

No well-controlled studies of haloperidol use in pregnant women have been conducted. Two cases of foetal limb malformation have been reported following maternal use of haloperidol, combined with other drugs during the first trimester. No causal relationship has been established. Use of haloperidol during pregnancy requires that the anticipated benefit be weighed against the possible hazards to mother and foetus.

Lactation: Haloperidol has been detected in breast milk. If use of haloperidol is considered essential, breast feeding should be discontinued.

Effects on ability to drive and use machines: Haloperidol may impair alertness, especially at the start of treatment. These effects may be potentiated by alcohol. Patients should be warned of the risks of sedation and advised not to drive or operate machinery during treatment, until their susceptibility is known.

Undesirable effects: Extrapyramidal symptoms such as Parkinson-like symptoms, akinesia, akathisia, dyskinesia, dystonia may develop during haloperidol treatment, very rarely dystonia has been reported to produce laryngeal/pharyngeal spasm associated with gagging, respiratory distress and asphyxia.

In common with other antipsychotics haloperidol has been associated with persistent dyskinesia. Tardive dyskinesia may develop in some patients on long term therapy, possibly in relation to total cumulative dose, or may develop after drug therapy has been discontinued. The risk is reported to be greater in elderly patients on high dose therapy. Characteristic symptoms are rhythmical involuntary movements of the tongue, face, mouth or jaw sometimes accompanied by involuntary movements of the extremities. They may persist for many months or even years and, while they gradually disappear in some patients, they appear to be permanent in others.

At the first signs of tardive dyskinesia which may be orofacial dyskinesia the benefit of continued treatment should be carefully assessed against the risk of the development of persistent dyskinesia. Withdrawal of treatment with careful observation of the dyskinesia and psychotic condition has been suggested in order to assess the need for continued neuroleptic therapy and to reveal persisting dyskinesia. Should it be necessary to reinstate treatment, the antipsychotic agent may mask the syndrome. Anti-Parkinsonian agents have proved of little value in this syndrome. In schizophrenia, the response to antipsychotic drug treatment may be delayed. If drugs are withdrawn, recurrence of symptoms may not become apparent for several weeks or months.

Some degree of sedation may occur, particularly with higher doses and at the start of treatment. The elderly appear more susceptible. At low doses in susceptible (especially non-psychotic) individuals, haloperidol may cause unpleasant subjective feelings of being mentally dulled or slowed down, dizziness, headaches or paradoxical effects of excitement, agitation or insomnia.

Other adverse effects reported include gastrointestinal symptoms, nausea, loss of appetite, dyspepsia, autonomic effects such as blurring of vision and, infrequently, tachycardia. Dose-related hypotension is uncommon, but can occur, particularly in the elderly or after parenteral administration. Impairment of sexual function, including erection and ejaculation, oedema; blood dyscrasias, including agranulocytosis and transient leucopenia; skin reactions including exfoliative dermatitis, erythema multiforme and photosensitisation and jaundice, are rarely reported. Transient abnormalities of liver function tests may occur in the absence of jaundice.

Impairment of body temperature could occur at high doses. In common with other antipsychotics, hormonal effects include hyperprolactinaemia which could cause galactorrhoea, gynaecomastia and oligo- or amenorrhoea. Abrupt discontinuation of high doses of antipsychotics has very rarely resulted in acute withdrawal symptoms, including nausea, vomiting and insomnia. Gradual withdrawal is advisable.

Rare cases of sudden and unexplained death have been reported in psychiatric patients receiving treatment with antipsychotics including haloperidol. The nature of the evidence makes it impossible to determine the contributory role, if any, of the drug.

In common with other antipsychotics haloperidol has been associated with rare cases of neuroleptic malignant syndrome, an idiosyncratic response characterised by hyperthermia, muscle rigidity, autonomic instability, altered consciousness and coma. Signs of autonomic dysfunction such as tachycardia, labile arterial pressure and sweating may precede the onset of hyperthermia, acting as early warning signs. Recovery usually occurs within five to seven days of antipsychotic withdrawal. Affected patients should be carefully monitored.

Overdose: Intensification of the known pharmacological and adverse effects may occur. The most prominent would be severe extrapyramidal symptoms, hypotension or sedation. The patient may appear comatosed with respiratory depression and hypotension which could be severe enough to produce a shock-like state.

Extrapyramidal reactions may include muscular weakness or rigidity and a generalised or localised tremor. With accidental overdosage hypothermia, bradycardia, sinus arrhythmia and hypertension have been reported in young children. No specific antidote has been identified.

In the event of overdosage the stomach should be emptied by aspiration and lavage. Emetics should not be used. Establishment of patent airway and artificial ventilation may be needed. Hypotension may be counteracted by placing the patient in the head-down position and by the use of a plasma expander and careful use of a vasopressor agent such as noradrenaline. Adrenaline should not be used. Severe extrapyramidal reactions should be treated with parenteral antihistamines or antiparkinsonian drugs. The relatively long plasma elimination half-life of haloperidol should be considered.

Pharmacological properties
Pharmacodynamic properties: Haloperodol is a butyrophenone. Its pharmacological profile of activity includes a pronounced capacity to induce extrapyramidal reactions and a low incidence of autonomic side-effects, such as hypotension.

Pharmacokinetic properties: The pharmacokinetics of haloperidol have been studied in healthy volunteers and patients. In volunteers, following a single intravenous or oral dose, serum elimination half-life ranged from 10–19 hours and 12–38 hours respectively. Similar elimination half-lives were observed in patients after administration of a single oral or intramuscular dose of the drug or after withdrawal of the drug from patients who were in a steady state. Steady state serum levels were usually achieved within 6 days on a fixed oral dosage.

Preclinical safety data: Not applicable.

Pharmaceutical particulars
List of excipients: Serenace Tablets: Lactose PhEur; Corn Starch PhEur; Pregelatinised Maize Starch BP; Magnesium Stearate PhEur.

Serenace 5 mg and 10 mg Tablets Additional Excipient: FD&C Red No. 3 Lake (E127).

Serenace 20 mg Tablet Additional Excipient: Anstead Dispersed Red 11652 (E124).

Serenace Liquid: Polypropylene Glycol BP; Methyl Hydroxybenzoate BP; Propyl Hydroxybenzoate BP; Lactic Acid BP; Purified Water BP.

Serenace Capsule: Lactose PhEur; Corn Starch PhEur. *Hard Gelatin Shell:* Tartrazine (E102); Patent Blue V (E131); Titanium Dioxide (E171).

Incompatibilities: None.

Shelf life:
Serenace 1.5 mg and 5 mg Tablets: 5 years.

Serenace 10 mg and 20 mg Tablets: 5 years. 3 years in blister packs.

Serenace Liquid: 3 years.

Serenace Capsules: 5 years.

Special precautions for storage:
Serenace Tablets and Capsules: Store in a dry place below 30°C.

Serenace Liquid: Store between 15 and 25°C. Protect from light.

Nature and contents of container:
Serenace Tablets: Ward pack sizes of 50.

High density polyethylene bottles with tamper-evident snap closure, or amber glass bottles with metal screw cap in pack sizes of 7, 14, 21, 28, 30, 50, 56, 60, 84, 90, 100, 112, 120, 250, 1000 and 5000 tablets. PVC/Aluminium blisters, or PVdC coated PVC/Aluminium blisters in pack sizes of 7, 14, 21, 28, 30, 50, 56, 60, 84, 90, 100, 112 and 120 tablets.

Serenace Liquid: Amber glass bottles with ROPP closures containing 100 ml or 500 ml.

Serenace Capsules: Ward pack sizes of 50.

High density polyethylene bottles with tamper-evident snap closure, or amber glass bottles with metal screw cap in pack sizes of 7, 14, 21, 28, 30, 50, 56, 60, 84, 90, 100, 112, 120, 250, 1000 and 5000.

PVC/Aluminium blisters, or PVdC coated PVC/Aluminium blisters in pack sizes of 7, 14, 21, 28, 30, 50, 56, 60, 84, 90, 100, 112 and 120.

Instructions for use/handling: No special instructions.

Marketing authorisation holder: Norton Healthcare Limited, Albert Basin, Royal Docks, London E16 2QJ.

Marketing authorisation numbers

Serenace 1.5 mg Tablet	0530/0370
Serenace 5 mg Tablet	0530/0371
Serenace 10 mg Tablet	0530/0372
Serenace 20 mg Tablet	0530/0373
Serenace Liquid 2 mg/ml	0530/0374
Serenace 500 micrograms Capsules	0530/0375

Date of approval/revision of SPC February 1997

Legal category POM

TEMAZEPAM 10 mg TABLETS
TEMAZEPAM 20 mg TABLETS

Presentation Temazepam 10 mg and 20 mg tablets are white, flat bevel-edged tablets containing 10 mg and 20 mg temazepam. The 10 mg tablets are embossed 'TMZ 10' with a breakline on one side and a twin triangle logo on the reverse. The 20 mg tablets are embossed 'TMZ 20' with a breakline on one side and a twin triangle logo on the reverse.

Uses Temazepam is a benzodiazepine; it has anxiolytic, sedative and hypnotic characteristics as well as possible muscle relaxant and anticonvulsant characteristics.

1. As an hypnotic for the short-term management of insomnia only when it is severe, disabling or subjecting the individual to extreme distress.
2. For pre-medication prior to minor surgery or other related procedures.

Dosage and administration Treatment should be as short as possible. Generally the duration of treatment varies from a few days to two weeks with a maximum (including tapering off) of four weeks. The tapering off process should be tailored to the individual. In certain cases, extension beyond the maximum treatment period may be necessary; if so, it should not take place without re-evaluation of the patient's status. The product should be taken on retiring or up to 30 minutes before going to bed.

Insomnia: Adults: 10–20 mg. In exceptional circumstances, the dose may be increased to 30–40 mg.

Elderly: 10 mg. In exceptional circumstances, the dose may be increased to 20 mg.

Premedication: The usual dose is 20–40 mg 30–60 minutes before the procedure.

Children: Not recommended for use in children.

Treatment should be started with the lowest recommended dose. The maximum dose should not be exceeded. Patients with impaired liver or kidney function should have a reduced dose.

A lower dose is also recommended for patients with chronic respiratory insufficiency due to the risk of respiratory depression.

Contra-indications, warnings, etc

Contra-indications: Myasthenia gravis; hypersensitivity to benzodiazepines; severe respiratory insufficiency; sleep apnoea syndrome; children; severe hepatic insufficiency.

Precautions and warnings: An underlying cause for insomnia should be sought before deciding on the use of benzodiazepines for symptomatic relief.

Some loss of efficacy to the hypnotic effects of short-acting benzodiazepines may develop after repeated use for a few weeks.

The duration of treatment should be as short as possible. Treatment should not exceed 4 weeks, including the tapering off process. Extension beyond this period should not take place without re-evaluation of the situation. It may be useful to inform the patient when treatment is started that it will be of limited duration and to explain precisely how the dosage will be progressively decreased. Moreover, it is important that the patient should be aware of the possibility of rebound phenomena, thereby minimising anxiety over such symptoms should they occur while the medicinal product is being discontinued. There are indications that, in the case of benzodiazepines with a short duration of action, withdrawal phenomena can become manifest within the dosage interval, especially when the dosage is high.

Benzodiazepines may induce anterograde amnesia. The condition occurs most often several hours after ingesting the product, and therefore to reduce the risk, patients should ensure that they will be able to have an uninterrupted sleep of 7–8 hours.

Benzodiazepines are not indicated to treat patients with severe hepatic insufficiency as it may precipitate encephalopathy. Benzodiazepines are not recommended for the primary treatment of psychotic illness.

Benzodiazepines should not be used alone to treat depression or anxiety associated with depression (suicide may be precipitated in such patients).

Benzodiazepines should also be used with extreme caution in patients with a history of alcohol or drug abuse.

Sedation, amnesia, impaired concentration and impaired muscular function may adversely affect the ability to drive or to use machines. If insufficient sleep duration occurs, the likelihood of impaired alertness may be increased.

After medication with temazepam for surgical or other procedures, patients should be accompanied home afterwards.

Special precautions: Use of benzodiazepines may lead to the development of physical and psychic dependence upon these products. The risk of dependence increases with dose and duration of treatment; it is also greater in patients with a history of alcohol or drug abuse or marked personality disorders.

Once physical dependence has developed, abrupt termination of treatment will be accompanied by withdrawal symptoms. These may consist of headaches, muscle pain, extreme anxiety, tension, restlessness, confusion and irritability. In severe cases the following symptoms may occur: derealisation; depersonalisation; hyperacusis; numbness and tingling of the extremities; hypersensitivity to light, noise and physical contact; hallucinations or epileptic seizures.

'Rebound insomnia' a transient syndrome whereby the symptoms that led to treatment with a benzodiazepine recur in an enhanced form, may occur on withdrawal of hypnotic treatment. It may be accompanied by other reactions, including mood changes, anxiety and restlessness.

Since the risk of withdrawal phenomena/rebound phenomena is greater after abrupt discontinuation of treatment, it is recommended that the dosage is decreased gradually.

Use in pregnancy and lactation: Insufficient data are available on temazepam to assess its safety during pregnancy and lactation. Therefore temazepam is not recommended for administration during pregnancy and lactation. If the product is prescribed to a woman of childbearing potential, she should be warned to contact her physician regarding stopping the product if she intends to become or suspects that she is pregnant.

If, for compelling medical reasons, temazepam is administered during the late phase of pregnancy, or during labour, effects on the neonate, such as hypothermia, hypotonia and moderate respiratory depression, can be expected due to the pharmacological action of the product.

Moreover, infants born to mothers who took benzodiazepines chronically during the latter stages of pregnancy may have developed physical dependence and may be at some risk of developing withdrawal symptoms in the postnatal period.

Since benzodiazepines are found in the breast milk, temazepam should not be administered to breast-feeding mothers.

Effects on ability to drive and use machines: Sedation, amnesia and impaired muscular function may adversely affect the ability to drive or operate machinery.

Side-effects: Side-effects include the following: Drowsiness during the day, numbed emotions, reduced alertness, confusion, fatigue, headache, dizziness, muscle weakness, ataxia, or double vision. These phenomena occur predominantly at the start of the therapy and usually disappear with repeated administration. However, sedation, amnesia and impaired muscular function may adversely affect the ability to drive or use machines. Other side effects like gastrointestinal disturbances, changes in libido, skin reactions, vivid dreams/nightmares, dry mouth, restless sleep and palpitations have been reported occasionally.

Anterograde amnesia may occur using therapeutic dosages, the risk increasing at higher dosages. Amnesia may be associated with inappropriate behaviour.

Pre-existing depression may be unmasked during benzodiazepine use.

Reactions like restlessness, agitation, irritability, aggressiveness, delusion, rages, nightmares, hallucinations, psychoses, inappropriate behaviour and other adverse behavioural effects are known to occur with use of benzodiazepines. These reactions are more likely to occur in the elderly. Should this occur, use of the product should be discontinued.

On rare occasions, visual disturbances, urinary retention, blood dyscrasias, increased liver enzymes and jaundice have been reported with some benzodiazepines. If any of these occur, use of the product should be discontinued.

Interactions: Not recommended: Concomitant intake with alcohol. The sedative effect may be enhanced when the product is used in combination with alcohol. This affects the ability to drive or use machines.

Take into account: Combination with CNS depressants. Enhancement of the central depressive effect may occur in cases in concomitant use with antipsychotics (neuroleptics), hypnotics, anxiolytics/sedatives, antidepressant agents, narcotic analgesics, antiepileptic drugs, anaesthetics and sedative antihistamines. In the case of narcotic analgesics, enhancement of euphoria may also occur leading to an increase in dependence.

Overdosage: As with other benzodiazepines, overdose should not present a threat to life unless combined with other CNS depressants (including alcohol). In the management of overdose with any medicinal product, it should be borne in mind that multiple agents may have been taken. Following overdose with oral benzodiazepines, vomiting should be induced (within one hour) if the patient is conscious or gastric lavage undertaken with the airway protected if the patient is unconscious. If there is no advantage in emptying the stomach, activated charcoal should be given to reduce absorption. The value of dialysis has not been determined for temazepam.

3-hydroxy benzodiazepines are, as a rule, not dialysable and their metabolites (glucuronides) only dialysable with difficulty. Special attention should be paid to respiratory and cardiovascular functions in intensive care. Overdose of benzodiazepines is usually manifested by degrees of central nervous system depression ranging from drowsiness to coma. In mild cases, symptoms include drowsiness, mental confusion and lethargy. In more serious cases symptoms may include ataxia, hypotonia, hypotension, respiratory depression, rarely coma and very rarely death. Flumazenil may be useful as an antidote.

Pharmacological properties

Pharmacodynamic properties: Temazepam is a 1,4 benzodiazepine. Benzodiazepines have anxiolytic, hypnotic, sedative, anticonvulsant and muscle relaxing properties.

Temazepam hastens the onset of sleep, increases the duration of sleep, improves its quality and decreases awakenings.

Pharmacokinetic properties: Pharmacokinetic studies have shown that temazepam is well-absorbed (90–100% and the first pass effect is slight (about 5%)). The time to reach peak plasma levels is usually about 50 minutes when given orally. Maximum plasma levels observed after doses of 20 mg are 660–1100 ng/ml. With multiple dosing steady state is obtained by the third day and there is little or no accumulation of parent drug or metabolites.

Volume of distribution. The volume of distribution volume is 1.3 to 1.5 L/kg bodyweight; for the unbound fraction, 43–68 L/kg. Approximately 96% of unchanged drug is bound to plasma proteins.

Temazepam is metabolised principally in the liver where most of the unchanged drug is directly conjugated to the glucuronide and excreted in the urine. Less than 5% of drug is demethylated to oxazepam and eliminated as the glucuronide. The glucuronide of temazepam have no demonstrable CNS activity.

Temazepam is rapidly eliminated, most studies showing an elimination half life in the range of 7–11 hrs. (Mean 8 hrs). Following a single dose, 80% of the dose appears in the urine, mostly as the conjugates and 12% of the dose appears in the faeces. Less than 2% of the dose is excreted unchanged in the urine.

In established renal insufficiency the metabolic clearance of temazepam as well as the plasma level of the non-protein bound temazepam remain within the normal range. The elimination half-life for temazepam glucuronide is however increased by which this inactive metabolite accumulates. As stated under 'Overdose' it is unlikely that temazepam may be significantly removed by dialysis.

List of excipients: Mannitol BP, Lactose (spray dried) BP, Polyethylene Glycol 1540 BP, Crospovidone USP, Magnesium Stearate BP.

Incompatibilities: None known.

Shelf life: 3 years.

Nature and contents of container: Polypropylene tubular container with an open end equipped to accept a polyethylene closure with a tamper-evident tear strip or tampertainers or amber glass bottles with metal or plastic screw-caps with liners. The pack sizes are 30, 50, 100, 250, 500, 1000 or 5000 tablets.

Pharmaceutical precautions: Store in a cool dry place.

Legal category POM

Package quantities 10 mg: Containers of 30, 100, 250, 500 and 1000 tablets and 5000 tablets.
20 mg: Containers of 30, 100, 250, 500 and 1000 tablets and 5000 tablets.

Further information The risk of benzodiazepine related dependence may be minimised by adopting the following guidelines for treatment:

(1) Select patients carefully taking into account the precautions and warnings stated in this data sheet.
(2) Adopt short-term or intermittent therapy.
(3) Use lowest dose possible to achieve effective treatment.
(4) Review treatment regularly; and especially before repeating prescriptions.
(5) Discontinue treatment gradually taking into account patient reaction at each stage, i.e. 'titrate downwards'.

Product licence numbers
10 mg: 0530/0255
20 mg: 0530/0256

Product licence holder: Norton Healthcare Limited, Albert Basin, Royal Docks, London E16 2QJ.

TRIAM-CO* TABLETS

Qualitative and quantitative composition Each tablet contains Triamterene BP 50 mg and Hydrochlorothiazide BP 25 mg.

Pharmaceutical form Peach-yellow FBE tablets.

Clinical particulars

Therapeutic indications: Anti-hypertensive and diuretic with potassium conserving properties indicated in patients for the control of oedema in cardiac failure, cirrhosis of the liver or the nephrotic syndrome and in drug-induced and premenstrual oedema. Triam-co may be used in the treatment of mild to moderate hypertension, alone or in combination with other anti-hypertensive drugs.

Posology and method of administration:

Adults and elderly: Triam-co should be administered to adults only. However in the case of elderly patients the normally occurring reduction in glomerular filtration with age should be considered when prescribing Triam-co.

Hypertension: Starting with 1 tablet a day following the morning meal and thereafter adjusting to the patient's needs but not exceeding 4 tablets. When Triam-co is used in addition to another anti-hypertensive drug the dosage of the latter should be reduced and adjusted if necessary. However, the addition of another anti-hypertensive drug to Triam-co therapy will not normally require reduction of the Triam-co dosage.

Oedema: Starting dose: 1 tablet twice a day after meals. The maximum dosage may be 3 tablets a day, 2 after breakfast and 1 after lunch. Adverse reactions have been reported on a dosage of 4 tablets daily therefore this dosage level should not be exceeded.

Maintenance dose: Dosage should be reduced to one tablet daily or 2 tablets on alternate days as soon as diuresis has been established.

Children: Not recommended.

Route of administration: Oral.

Contra-indications: Triam-co should not be given to patients with hyperkalaemia. Progressive renal or hepatic dysfunction, hypercalcaemia, Addison's disease, diabetic ketoacidosis, or known hypersensitivity to the product's constituents. The use of potassium supplements or other potassium-conserving drugs with Triam-co is not recommended.

Special warnings and special precautions for use: Triam-co should be used with caution in patients with hepatic or renal insufficiency. As both triamterene and hydrochlorothiazide can elevate uric acid levels Triam-co should be used with caution in patients who may suffer from gout.

Thiazides may provoke hyperglycaemia and glycosuria and should be prescribed with caution in diabetic patients. Patients with diabetic nephropathy should be treated with care due to possible hyperkalaemia; concomitant sulphonylurea dosage may need increasing. Pancreatitis may be aggravated by Triam-co.

Serum potassium levels, blood urea and electrolytes should be monitored periodically. This is important in the elderly, or renally impaired patients and those receiving concomitant treatment with NSAIDs.

Triam-co may interfere with laboratory tests for thyroid and parathyroid function, and folic acid biossay.

Interaction with other medicaments and other forms of interaction: Care should be taken in patients being treated with lithium as reduction in lithium excretion can occur with resultant toxicity. There have been occasional reports of decreased renal function when triamterene has been administered with indomethacin. Triam-co may reduce arterial responsiveness to noradrenaline and may enhance the responsiveness to tubocurarine.

The action of other anti-hypertensive agents is potentiated and a reduced dosage may be necessary at the introduction of Triam-co. The concurrent use of potassium supplements or potassium conserving drugs may cause hyperkalaemia.

Due to the risk of excess potassium loss, care should be taken when Triam-co is taken in conjunction with corticosteroids; also with cardiac glycosides and antiarrhythmic drugs whose toxicity may be enhanced by hypokalaemia.

Carbenoxolone may antagonise the diuretic action of Triam-co and cholestyramine may delay or reduce its absorption.

Concomitant folate antagonists are inadvisable in pregnant women or patients with hepatic cirrhosis because of the risk of folate deficiency.

Pregnancy and lactation: Animal studies have indicated that triamterene crosses the placental barrier and is excreted in breast milk.

In humans, hydrochlorothiazide crosses the placental barrier, and appears in milk.

There are no signficiant reports citing foetal abnormalities when using the combination of triamterene and hydrochlorothiazide; however in isolated instances new-born infants of mothers treated with thiazides have been found to be suffering from thrombocytopenia, pancreatitis or hypoglycaemia. The use of Triam-co in pregnant women or nursing mothers should therefore be avoided unless considered essential.

Effects on ability to drive and use machines: Patients should be warned that dizziness may occur and therefore should take care when driving or operating machines.

Undesirable effects: Nausea, vomiting, diarrhoea, muscle cramps, weakness, headache, dry mouth, undesirable decreases in blood pressure and rash have been reported. Photosensitivity is rare. Renal failure, reversed on stopping treatment, has been reported very rarely. Anaphylaxis is a possibility.

Consideration should be given to the possibility of minor serum electrolyte changes, metabolic acidosis and fluctuation in serum potassium levels. Large doses may induce electrolyte imbalance although this imbalance could be secondary to the condition being treated. Hyperglycaemia, hyperlipidaemia, raised uric acid levels and hypercalcaemia have been reported. Reduction of glomerular filtration rate causing a temporary increase in blood urea and creatinine levels may occur with Triam-co.

Reports of rare cases of thrombocytopenic purpura and megaloblastic anaemia when using triamterene have appeared in the literature as have reports of thiazides causing jaundice, acute pancreatitis and blood dyscrasias including agranulocytosis, thrombocytopenia and leucopenia. Systemic lupus erythematosus has been very rarely reported with this diuretic combination. Triamterene, under certain light conditions, has been known to cause a blue fluorescence in the urine.

Overdose: Symptoms of electrolyte imbalance, especially hyperkalaemia, are likely. These include gastro-intestinal disturbance, weakness, lassitude, hypotension and cardiac arrhythmias. Treatment consists of gastric lavage with correction of electrolyte imbalance and fluid depletion. Cardiac monitoring is advised as are appropriate measures to correct hyperkalaemia as necessary. There is no specific antidote; however, if hypotension persists after adequate fluid replacement dopamine may be used. In cases of severe overdosage renal dialysis may be of some benefit.

Pharmaceutical properties

Pharmacodynamic properties: Triam-co is a combination of a thiazide diuretic, hydrochlorothiazide, and a potassium sparing diuretic, triamterene.

Hydrochlorothiazide acts on the distal convulted tubule of the kidney and diuresis is initiated in about two hours and lasts up to twelve hours.

Triamterene causes potassium retention and is used in this particular combination as an alteranative to giving potassium supplements.

Pharmacokinetic properties: Hydrochlorothiazide is incompletely but fairly rapidly absorbed from the gastro-intestinal tract. It has been estimated to have a half-life of about 3 to 4 hours with a subsequent longer terminal phase; its biological half-life is up to about 12 hours. It appears to be preferentially bound to red blood cells. It is excreted unchanged in the urine. Hydrochlorothiazide crosses the placental barrier and is excreted in breast milk.

Triamterene is incompletely but fairly rapidly absorbed from the gastro-intestinal tract. It has been estimated to have half-life of about 2 hours. It is extensively metabolised and is mainly excreted in the urine in the form of metabolites with some unchanged triamterene; variable amounts are also excreted in the bile. Animal studies have indicated that triamterene crosses the placental barrier and is excreted in breast milk.

Preclinical safety data: Not applicable.

Pharmaceutical particulars

List of excipients: Avicel PH 101 (E460) NF, Explotab NF, Sodium Lauryl Sulphate NF, Cab-O-Sil NF, Magnesium Stearate NF, F.D. & C. Yellow No. 6 (E110).

Incompatibilities: None known.

Shelf life: 5 years.

Special precautions for storage: Store in a cool dry place.

Nature and contents of container: Polypropylene tubular container with an open end equipped to accept a polyethylene closure, with tamper-evident tear strip.

Tampertainers – 250 m opaque UPVC/20 μ, hard temper aluminium foil.

Duma Container – PVdC coated PVC/Aluminium blisters (60 g/m² PVdC on 250 mm PVC/20 mm A1).

Of the appropriate size to accommodate 7, 14, 21, 28, 30, 50, 56, 60, 84, 90, 100, 112, 120, 250, 500 or 1000 tablets.

Instructions for use/handling: No special instructions.

Marketing authorisation holder: Norton Healthcare Ltd, Albert Basin, Royal Docks, London E16 2QJ.

Marketing authorisation number 0530/0177

Date of approval/revision of SPC 2 December 1996

**Trade Mark*

Bayer plc
Pharmaceutical Division
Bayer House
Strawberry Hill
Newbury, Berkshire, RG14 1JA

☎ 01635 563000 🗋 01635 563393

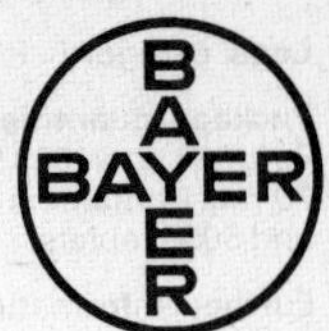

ADALAT*
ADALAT* 5

Presentation *Adalat capsules:* Orange, soft gelatin ovoid capsules containing a yellow viscous fluid. Each capsule is overprinted with 'ADALAT' and the Bayer cross and contains 10 mg nifedipine.

Adalat 5 capsules: Orange, soft gelatin ovoid capsules containing a yellow viscous fluid. Each capsule is overprinted with 'ADALAT 5' and the Bayer cross and contains 5 mg nifedipine.

Uses
Mode of action: As a specific and potent calcium antagonist, the main action of Adalat is to relax arterial smooth muscle both in the coronary and peripheral circulation.

In angina pectoris, Adalat capsules relax peripheral arteries so reducing the load on the left ventricle. Additionally, Adalat dilates submaximally both clear and pre-stenotic, stenotic and post-stenotic coronary arteries, thus protecting the heart against coronary artery spasm and improving perfusion to the ischaemic myocardium.

Adalat capsules reduce the frequency of painful attacks and ischaemic ECG changes, irrespective of the relative contribution from coronary artery spasm or atherosclerosis.

Adalat causes a reduction in blood pressure such that the percentage lowering is directly related to its initial level. In normotensive individuals, Adalat has little or no effect on blood pressure.

Indications: For the prophylaxis of chronic stable angina pectoris, the treatment of Raynaud's phenomenon and hypertension.

Dosage and administration The capsules should be taken orally with a little water. The recommended starting dose is 5 mg every eight hours with subsequent titration of dose according to response. The dose can be increased to 20 mg every eight hours.

The pharmacokinetics of nifedipine are altered in the elderly so that lower maintenance doses of nifedipine may be required compared to younger patients.

Nifedipine is metabolised primarily by the liver and therefore patients with liver dysfunction should be carefully monitored.

Patients with renal impairment should not require adjustment of dosage.

Treatment may be continued indefinitely.

Nifedipine is not recommended for use in children.

Contra-indications, warnings, etc
Contra-indications: Adalat should not be administered to patients with known hypersensitivity to nifedipine or other dihydropyridines because of the theoretical risk of cross-reactivity.

Adalat should not be administered to women capable of child-bearing or to nursing mothers.

Adalat should not be used in cardiogenic shock, clinically significant aortic stenosis, unstable angina, or during or within one month of a myocardial infarction.

Adalat should not be used for the treatment of acute attacks of angina.

The safety of Adalat in malignant hypertension has not been established.

Adalat should not be used for secondary prevention of myocardial infarction.

Adalat should not be administered concomitantly with rifampicin since effective plasma levels of nifedipine may not be achieved owing to enzyme induction.

Warnings and precautions: Adalat may be used in combination with beta-blocking drugs and other antihypertensive agents but the possibility of an additive effect resulting in postural hypotension should be borne in mind. Adalat will not prevent possible rebound effects after cessation of other antihypertensive therapy.

Adalat should be used with caution in patients whose cardiac reserve is poor. Deterioration of heart failure has occasionally been observed with nifedipine.

At doses higher than those recommended, there is some concern about increased mortality and morbidity in the treatment of ischaemic heart disease, in particular after myocardial infarction.

Treatment with short-acting nifedipine may induce an exaggerated fall in blood pressure and reflex tachycardia which can cause cardiovascular complications such as myocardial and cerebrovascular ischaemia.

Caution should be exercised in patients with severe hypotension.

Ischaemic pain has been reported in a small proportion of patients within 30 to 60 minutes of the introduction of Adalat therapy. Although a 'steal' effect has not been demonstrated, patients experiencing this effect should discontinue Adalat.

Diabetic patients taking Adalat may require adjustment of their control.

In dialysis patients with malignant hypertension and hypovolaemia, a marked decrease in blood pressure can occur.

Interactions: The antihypertensive effect of Adalat may be potentiated by simultaneous administration of cimetidine.

When used in combination with nifedipine, serum quinidine levels have been shown to be suppressed regardless of dosage of quinidine.

The simultaneous administration of nifedipine and digoxin may lead to reduced digoxin clearance and hence an increase in the plasma digoxin level. Plasma digoxin levels should be monitored and, if necessary, the digoxin dose reduced.

Diltiazem decreases the clearance of nifedipine and hence increases plasma nifedipine levels. Therefore, caution should be taken when both drugs are used in combination and a reduction of the nifedipine dose may be necessary.

Nifedipine may increase the spectrophotometric values of urinary vanillylmandelic acid falsely. However, HPLC measurements are unaffected.

Adalat should not be administered concomitantly with rifampicin since effective plasma levels of nifedipine may not be achieved owing to enzyme induction.

As with other dihydropyridines, nifedipine should not be taken with grapefruit juice because bioavailability is increased.

Side-effects: Most side-effects are consequences of the vasodilatory effects of nifedipine. Headache, flushing, tachycardia and palpitations may occur, most commonly in the early stages of treatment with nifedipine. Gravitational oedema, not associated with heart failure or weight gain, may also occur.

Paraesthesia, dizziness, lethargy and gastro-intestinal symptoms such as nausea and altered bowel habit may occur occasionally.

There are reports of skin reactions such as rash, pruritus and urticaria.

Other less frequently reported side-effects include myalgia, tremor and visual disturbances. Impotence may occur rarely.

Increased frequency of micturition may occur.

As with the use of other short-acting dihydropyridines in patients with ischaemic heart disease, exacerbation of angina pectoris may occur frequently at the start of treatment with nifedipine capsules. The occurrence of myocardial infarction has been described although it is not possible to distinguish such an event from the natural course of ischaemic heart disease.

There are reports of gingival hyperplasia and, in older men on long-term therapy, gynaecomastia, which usually regress upon withdrawal of therapy.

Mood changes may occur rarely.

Side-effects which may occur in isolated cases are photosensitivity, exfoliative dermatitis, systemic allergic reactions and purpura. Usually, these regress after discontinuation of the drug.

Rare cases of hypersensitivity-type jaundice have been reported. In addition, disturbances of liver function such as intra-hepatic cholestasis may occur. These regress after discontinuation of therapy.

Overdosage: Clinical effects: Reports of nifedipine overdosage are limited and symptoms are not necessarily dose-related. Severe hypotension due to vasodilatation, and tachycardia or bradycardia are the most likely manifestations of overdose.

Metabolic disturbances include hyperglycaemia, metabolic acidosis and hypo- or hyperkalaemia.

Cardiac effects may include heart block, AV dissociation and asystole, and cardiogenic shock with pulmonary oedema.

Other toxic effects include nausea, vomiting, drowsiness, dizziness, confusion, lethargy, flushing, hypoxia and unconsciousness to the point of coma.

Treatment: As far as treatment is concerned, elimination of nifedipine and the restoration of stable cardiovascular conditions have priority.

After oral ingestion, gastric lavage is indicated, if necessary in combination with irrigation of the small intestine. Ipecacuanha should be given to children.

Activated charcoal should be given, 50 g for adults, 10–15 g for children.

Blood pressure, ECG, central arterial pressure, pulmonary wedge pressure, urea and electrolytes should be monitored.

Hypotension as a result of cardiogenic shock and arterial vasodilatation should be treated with elevation of the feet and plasma expanders. If these measures are ineffective, hypotension may be treated with 10% calcium gluconate 10–20 ml intravenously over 5–10 minutes. If the effects are inadequate, the treatment can be continued, with ECG monitoring. In addition, beta-sympathomimetics may be given, e.g. isoprenaline 0.2 mg slowly i.v. or as a continuous infusion of 5 µg/min. If an insufficient increase in blood pressure is achieved with calcium and isoprenaline, vasoconstricting sympathomimetics such as dopamine or noradrenaline should be administered. The dosage of these drugs should be determined by the patient's response.

Bradycardia may be treated with atropine, beta-sympathomimetics or a temporary cardiac pacemaker, as required.

Additional fluids should be administered with caution to avoid cardiac overload.

Pharmaceutical precautions The capsules should be protected from strong light and stored in the manufacturer's original container at temperatures below 25°C.

Legal category POM.

Package quantities Adalat and Adalat 5 capsules are available in foil strips of 10 in packs of 90. Hospital packs containing 500 Adalat 10 mg capsules are also available.

Further information Adalat has no therapeutic antiarrhythmic effect. Since Adalat does not cause a rise in intraocular pressure, it can be used in patients with glaucoma. Adalat can be used in patients with obstructive airways disease with coexisting hypertension or angina pectoris. Long-term metabolic disturbances have not been observed.

Product licence numbers

Adalat	0010/0021
Adalat 5	0010/0079

ADALAT* LA 30
ADALAT* LA 60

Presentation Pink lacquered tablets each containing 30 mg or 60 mg nifedipine in a modified (extended) release formulation, one side marked Adalat 30 or Adalat 60.

Uses
Mode of action: As a specific and potent calcium antagonist, the main action of nifedipine is to relax arterial smooth muscle both in the coronary and peripheral circulation. The Adalat LA tablet is formulated to achieve controlled delivery of nifedipine in a release profile sufficient to enable once-daily administration to be effective in clinical use.

In hypertension, the main action of nifedipine is to cause peripheral vasodilatation and thus reduce peripheral resistance. Nifedipine administered once-daily provides 24-hour control of raised blood pressure. Nifedipine causes reduction in blood pressure such that the percentage lowering is proportional to its initial level. In normotensive individuals, nifedipine has little or no effect on blood pressure.

In angina, nifedipine reduces peripheral and coronary vascular resistance, leading to an increase in coronary blood flow, cardiac output and stroke volume, whilst decreasing after-load. Additionally, nifedipine dilates submaximally both clear and atherosclerotic coronary arteries, thus protecting the heart against coronary artery spasm and improving perfusion to the ischaemic myocardium. Nifedipine reduces the frequency of painful attacks and the ischaemic ECG changes irrespective of the relative contribution from coronary artery spasm or atherosclerosis.

Indications: For the treatment of mild to moderate hypertension.

For the prophylaxis of chronic stable angina pectoris either as monotherapy or in combination with a beta-blocker.

Dosage and administration For oral administration, the tablets should be swallowed whole with a glass of water. The tablets should be taken at approximately 24-hour intervals, i.e. at the same time each day, preferably during the morning. Adalat LA tablets must be swallowed whole; under no circumstances should they be bitten, chewed or broken up.

In hypertension and angina pectoris, the recommended initial dose is one 30 mg tablet once-daily. If necessary, the dosage can be increased according to individual requirements up to a maximum of 90 mg once-daily.

Patients in whom hypertension or anginal symptoms are controlled on Adalat capsules or Adalat retard may be switched safely to Adalat LA. Prophylactic anti-anginal efficacy is maintained when patients are switched from other calcium antagonists such as diltiazem or verapamil to Adalat LA. Patients switched from other calcium antagonists should initiate therapy at the recommended initial dose of 30 mg Adalat LA once-daily. Subsequent titration to a higher dose may be initiated as warranted clinically.

The pharmacokinetics of nifedipine are altered in the elderly so that lower maintenance doses of nifedipine may be required compared to younger patients.

Patients with renal impairment should not require adjustment of dosage.

Treatment may be continued indefinitely.

Nifedipine is not recommended for use in children.

Contra-indications, warnings, etc

Contra-indications: Adalat LA should not be administered to patients with known hypersensitivity to nifedipine or other dihydropyridines because of the theoretical risk of cross-reactivity.

Adalat LA should not be administered to women capable of child-bearing or to nursing mothers.

Adalat LA should not be used in cardiogenic shock, clinically significant aortic stenosis, unstable angina, or during or within one month of a myocardial infarction.

Adalat LA should not be used for the treatment of acute attacks of angina.

The safety of Adalat LA in malignant hypertension has not been established.

Adalat LA should not be used for secondary prevention of myocardial infarction.

Owing to the duration of action of the formulation, Adalat LA should not be administered to patients with hepatic impairment.

Adalat LA should not be administered to patients with a history of gastro-intestinal obstruction, oesophageal obstruction, or any degree of decreased lumen diameter of the gastro-intestinal tract.

Adalat LA is contra-indicated in patients with inflammatory bowel disease or Crohn's disease.

Adalat LA should not be administered concomitantly with rifampicin since effective plasma levels of nifedipine may not be achieved owing to enzyme induction.

Warnings and precautions: Adalat LA tablets must be swallowed whole; under no circumstances should they be bitten, chewed or broken up.

The outer membrane of the Adalat LA tablet is not digested and, therefore, what appears to be the complete tablet may be seen in the toilet or associated with the patient's stools.

Caution should be exercised in patients with hypotension as there is a risk of further reduction in blood pressure.

Adalat LA may be used in combination with beta-blocking drugs and other antihypertensive agents but the possibility of an additive effect resulting in postural hypotension should be borne in mind. Adalat LA will not prevent possible rebound effects after cessation of other antihypertensive therapy.

Adalat LA should be used with caution in patients whose cardiac reserve is poor. Deterioration of heart failure has occasionally been observed with nifedipine.

Ischaemic pain has been reported in a small proportion of patients following the introduction of nifedipine therapy. Although a 'steal' effect has not been demonstrated, patients experiencing this effect should discontinue nifedipine therapy.

Diabetic patients taking Adalat LA may require adjustment of their control.

In dialysis patients with malignant hypertension and hypovolaemia, a marked decrease in blood pressure can occur.

Interactions: The antihypertensive effect of Adalat LA may be potentiated by simultaneous administration of cimetidine.

When used in combination with nifedipine, serum quinidine levels have been shown to be suppressed regardless of dosage of quinidine.

The simultaneous administration of nifedipine and digoxin may lead to reduced digoxin clearance and hence an increase in the plasma digoxin level. Plasma digoxin levels should be monitored and, if necessary, the digoxin dose reduced.

Diltiazem decreases the clearance of nifedipine and, hence, increases plasma nifedipine levels. Therefore, caution should be taken when both drugs are used in combination and a reduction of the nifedipine dose may be necessary.

Nifedipine may increase the spectrophotometric values of urinary vanillylmandelic acid falsely. However, HPLC measurements are unaffected.

Adalat LA should not be administered concomitantly with rifampicin since effective plasma levels of nifedipine may not be achieved owing to enzyme induction.

As with other dihydropyridines, nifedipine should not be taken with grapefruit juice because bioavailability is increased.

Side-effects: Most side-effects are consequences of the vasodilatory effects of nifedipine. Headache, flushing, tachycardia and palpitations may occur, most commonly in the early stages of treatment with nifedipine. Gravitational oedema, not associated with heart failure or weight gain, may also occur.

Paraesthesia, dizziness, lethargy and gastro-intestinal symptoms such as nausea and altered bowel habit may occur occasionally.

There are reports of skin reactions such as rash, pruritus and urticaria.

Other less frequently reported side-effects include myalgia, tremor and visual disturbances. Impotence may occur rarely.

Increased frequency of micturition may occur.

As with other sustained release dihydropyridines, exacerbation of angina pectoris may occur rarely at the start of treatment with sustained release formulations of nifedipine. The occurrence of myocardial infarction has been described although it is not possible to distinguish such an event from the natural course of ischaemic heart disease.

There are reports of gingival hyperplasia and, in older men on long-term therapy, gynaecomastia, which usually regress upon withdrawal of therapy.

Mood changes may occur rarely.

Side-effects which have been observed in isolated cases are photosensitivity, exfoliative dermatitis, systemic allergic reactions and purpura. Usually, these regress after discontinuation of the drug.

Rare cases of hypersensitivity-type jaundice have been reported. In addition, disturbances of liver function such as intra-hepatic cholestasis may occur. These regress after discontinuation of therapy.

Overdosage: There are no reports of overdosage with Adalat LA.

Clinical effects: Reports of nifedipine overdosage are limited and symptoms are not necessarily dose-related. Severe hypotension due to vasodilatation, and tachycardia or bradycardia are the most likely manifestations of overdose.

Metabolic disturbances include hyperglycaemia, metabolic acidosis and hypo- or hyperkalaemia.

Cardiac effects may include heart block, AV dissociation and asystole, and cardiogenic shock with pulmonary oedema.

Other toxic effects include nausea, vomiting, drowsiness, dizziness, confusion, lethargy, flushing, hypoxia and unconsciousness to the point of coma.

Treatment: As far as treatment is concerned, elimination of nifedipine and the restoration of stable cardiovascular conditions have priority.

After oral ingestion, gastric lavage is indicated, if necessary in combination with irrigation of the small intestine. Ipecacuanha should be given to children.

Elimination must be as complete as possible, including the small intestine, to prevent the otherwise inevitable subsequent absorption of the active substance.

Activated charcoal should be given in 4-hourly doses of 25 g for adults, 10 g for children.

Blood pressure, ECG, central arterial pressure, pulmonary wedge pressure, urea and electrolytes should be monitored.

Hypotension as a result of cardiogenic shock and arterial vasodilatation should be treated with elevation of the feet and plasma expanders. If these measures are ineffective, hypotension may be treated with 10% calcium gluconate 10–20 ml intravenously over 5–10 minutes. If the effects are inadequate, the treatment can be continued, with ECG monitoring. In addition, beta-sympathomimetics may be given, e.g. isoprenaline 0.2 mg slowly i.v. or as a continuous infusion of 5 μg/min. If an insufficient increase in blood pressure is achieved with calcium and isoprenaline, vasoconstricting sympathomimetics such as dopamine or noradrenaline should be administered. The dosage of these drugs should be determined by the patient's response.

Bradycardia may be treated with atropine, beta-sympathomimetics or a temporary cardiac pacemaker, as required.

Additional fluids should be administered with caution to avoid cardiac overload.

Pharmaceutical precautions The tablets should be protected from strong light and stored in the manufacturer's original container.

Legal category POM.

Package quantities Adalat LA 30 and Adalat LA 60: calendar packs containing 28 tablets.

Further information Adalat LA has no therapeutic antiarrhythmic effect. Since Adalat LA does not cause a rise in intraocular pressure, it can be used in patients with glaucoma. Adalat LA can be used in patients with obstructive airways disease with coexisting hypertension or angina. Long-term metabolic disturbances have not been observed.

Product licence numbers
Adalat LA 30 0010/0174
Adalat LA 60 0010/0175

ADALAT* RETARD
ADALAT* RETARD 10

Presentation *Adalat retard:* Pink-grey lacquered tablets each containing 20 mg nifedipine, one side marked 1U and the reverse side with the Bayer cross. *Adalat retard 10:* Pink-grey lacquered tablets each containing 10 mg nifedipine, one side marked A10 and the reverse side with the Bayer cross.

Uses

Mode of action: Nifedipine is a specific and potent calcium antagonist. In hypertension, the main action of Adalat retard is to cause peripheral vasodilatation and thus reduce peripheral resistance.

In angina, Adalat retard reduces peripheral and coronary vascular resistance, leading to an increase in coronary blood flow, cardiac output and stroke volume, whilst decreasing after-load.

Adalat retard administered twice-daily provides 24-hour control of raised blood pressure. Adalat retard causes reduction in blood pressure such that the percentage lowering is directly related to its initial level. In normotensive individuals, Adalat retard has little or no effect on blood pressure.

Indications: For the prophylaxis of chronic stable angina pectoris and the treatment of hypertension.

Dosage and administration The recommended starting dose of Adalat retard is 10 mg every 12 hours swallowed with water with subsequent titration of dosage according to response. The dose may be adjusted to 40 mg every 12 hours.

Adalat retard 10 permits titration of initial dosage. The recommended dose is one Adalat retard 10 tablet (10 mg) every 12 hours.

The pharmacokinetics of nifedipine are altered in the elderly so that lower maintenance doses of nifedipine may be required compared to younger patients.

Nifedipine is metabolised primarily by the liver and therefore patients with liver dysfunction should be carefully monitored.

Patients with renal impairment should not require adjustment of dosage.

Treatment may be continued indefinitely.

Nifedipine is not recommended for use in children.

Contra-indications, warnings, etc

Contra-indications: Adalat retard should not be administered to patients with known hypersensitivity to nifedipine or other dihydropyridines because of the theoretical risk of cross-reactivity.

Adalat retard should not be administered to women capable of child-bearing or to nursing mothers.

Adalat retard should not be used in cardiogenic shock, clinically significant aortic stenosis, unstable angina, or during or within one month of a myocardial infarction.

Adalat retard should not be used for the treatment of acute attacks of angina.

The safety of Adalat retard in malignant hypertension has not been established.

Adalat retard should not be used for secondary prevention of myocardial infarction.

Adalat retard should not be administered concomitantly with rifampicin since effective plasma levels of nifedipine may not be achieved owing to enzyme induction.

Warnings and precautions: Adalat retard may be used in combination with beta-blocking drugs and other antihypertensive agents but the possibility of an additive effect resulting in postural hypotension should be borne in mind. Adalat retard will not prevent possible rebound effects after cessation of other antihypertensive therapy.

Adalat retard should be used with caution in patients whose cardiac reserve is poor. Deterioration of heart failure has occasionally been observed with nifedipine.

Caution should be exercised in patients with severe hypotension.

Ischaemic pain has been reported in a small proportion of patients within one to four hours of the introduction of Adalat retard therapy. Although a 'steal' effect has not been demonstrated, patients experiencing this effect should discontinue Adalat retard.

Diabetic patients taking Adalat retard may require adjustment of their control.

In dialysis patients with malignant hypertension and hypovolaemia, a marked decrease in blood pressure can occur.

Interactions: The antihypertensive effect of Adalat retard may be potentiated by simultaneous administration of cimetidine.

When used in combination with nifedipine, serum quinidine levels have been shown to be suppressed regardless of dosage of quinidine.

The simultaneous administration of nifedipine and digoxin may lead to reduced digoxin clearance and hence an increase in the plasma digoxin level. Plasma digoxin levels should be monitored and, if necessary, the digoxin dose reduced.

Diltiazem decreases the clearance of nifedipine and hence increases plasma nifedipine levels. Therefore, caution should be taken when both drugs are used in combination and a reduction of the nifedipine dose may be necessary.

Nifedipine may increase the spectrophotometric values of urinary vanillylmandelic acid falsely. However, HPLC measurements are unaffected.

Adalat retard should not be administered concomitantly with rifampicin since effective plasma levels of nifedipine may not be achieved owing to enzyme induction.

As with other dihydropyridines, nifedipine should not be taken with grapefruit juice because bioavailability is increased.

Side-effects: Most side-effects are consequences of the vasodilatory effects of nifedipine. Headache, flushing, tachycardia and palpitations may occur, most commonly in the early stages of treatment with nifedipine. Gravitational oedema, not associated with heart failure or weight gain, may also occur.

Paraesthesia, dizziness, lethargy and gastro-intestinal symptoms such as nausea and altered bowel habit may occur occasionally.

There are reports of skin reactions such as rash, pruritus and urticaria.

Other less frequently reported side-effects include myalgia, tremor and visual disturbances. Impotence may occur rarely.

Increased frequency of micturition may occur.

As with other sustained release dihydropyridines, exacerbation of angina pectoris may occur rarely at the start of treatment with sustained release formulations of nifedipine. The occurrence of myocardial infarction has been described although it is not possible to distinguish such an event from the natural course of ischaemic heart disease.

There are reports of gingival hyperplasia and, in older men on long-term therapy, gynaecomastia, which usually regress upon withdrawal of therapy.

Mood changes may occur rarely.

Side-effects which may occur in isolated cases are photosensitivity, exfoliative dermatitis, systemic allergic reactions and purpura. Usually, these regress after discontinuation of the drug.

Rare cases of hypersensitivity-type jaundice have been reported. In addition, disturbances of liver function such as intra-hepatic cholestasis may occur. These regress after discontinuation of therapy.

Overdosage: Clinical effects: Reports of nifedipine overdosage are limited and symptoms are not necessarily dose-related. Severe hypotension due to vasodilatation, and tachycardia or bradycardia are the most likely manifestations of overdose.

Metabolic disturbances include hyperglycaemia, metabolic acidosis and hypo- or hyperkalaemia.

Cardiac effects may include heart block, AV dissociation and asystole, and cardiogenic shock with pulmonary oedema.

Other toxic effects include nausea, vomiting, drowsiness, dizziness, confusion, lethargy, flushing, hypoxia and unconsciousness to the point of coma.

Treatment: As far as treatment is concerned, elimination of nifedipine and the restoration of stable cardiovascular conditions have priority.

After oral ingestion, gastric lavage is indicated, if necessary in combination with irrigation of the small intestine. Ipecacuanha should be given to children.

Elimination must be as complete as possible, including the small intestine, to prevent the otherwise inevitable subsequent absorption of the active substance.

Activated charcoal should be given in 4-hourly doses of 25 g for adults, 10 g for children.

Blood pressure, ECG, central arterial pressure, pulmonary wedge pressure, urea and electrolytes should be monitored.

Hypotension as a result of cardiogenic shock and arterial vasodilatation should be treated with elevation of the feet and plasma expanders. If these measures are ineffective, hypotension may be treated with 10% calcium gluconate 10–20 ml intravenously over 5–10 minutes. If the effects are inadequate, the treatment can be continued, with ECG monitoring. In addition, beta-sympathomimetics may be given, e.g. isoprenaline 0.2 mg slowly i.v. or as a continuous infusion of 5 μg/min. If an insufficient increase in blood pressure is achieved with calcium and isoprenaline, vasoconstricting sympathomimetics such as dopamine or noradrenaline should be administered. The dosage of these drugs should be determined by the patient's response.

Bradycardia may be treated with atropine, beta-sympathomimetics or a temporary cardiac pacemaker, as required.

Additional fluids should be administered with caution to avoid cardiac overload.

Pharmaceutical precautions The tablets should be protected from strong light and stored in the manufacturer's original container.

Legal category POM.

Package quantities Adalat retard tablets: strips of 14 in packs of 56.

Adalat retard 10 tablets: strips of 14 in packs of 56.

Further information Adalat retard has no therapeutic antiarrhythmic effect. Since Adalat retard does not cause a rise in intraocular pressure, it can be used in patients with glaucoma. Adalat retard can be used in patients with obstructive airways disease with coexisting hypertension or angina pectoris. Long-term metabolic disturbances have not been observed.

Product licence numbers
Adalat retard 0010/0078
Adalat retard 10 0010/0151

BAYCARON*

Presentation A white scored tablet 7 mm × 2 mm, one side scored L/1 and the reverse side with the Bayer cross, containing 25 mg mefruside.

Uses Baycaron is a diuretic agent and is intended for the treatment of hypertension and oedema.

Dosage and administration Baycaron is best taken with a little fluid after meals.

Hypertension: 25 mg to 50 mg initially for 10 to 14 days, then maintenance dose of 25 mg each morning. Alternate day dosage may also be used.

Oedema: 25 mg to 50 mg every morning increasing if necessary to 75 mg to 100 mg to obtain the desired response. For long-term therapy intermittent dosage is preferable, e.g. 25 mg to 50 mg every second or third day.

Daily doses in excess of 100 mg do not usually increase diuresis further.

Paediatric dosage has not been established.

Contra-indications, warnings, etc
Contra-indications: Severe renal failure, hepatic coma, Addisons disease, severe hypercalcaemia.

Warnings and precautions: It is often necessary to give extra potassium during treatment with diuretics and potassium supplements may be necessary during long-term treatment with Baycaron, especially in patients with impaired liver function or in those also receiving digoxin and other cardiac glycosides.

Particular care is necessary in the elderly because of their susceptibility to electrolyte imbalance.

Although there is no short-term alteration of carbohydrate metabolism in normal subjects on a 50 mg daily dose, the glucose tolerance curve may be prolonged in some diabetics. After Baycaron administration serum uric acid may be raised and therefore it should be used with caution in potential cases of gout.

Baycaron is not suitable for the treatment of acute conditions of fluid excess such as pulmonary and cerebral oedema and glaucoma.

Baycaron should not be administered concurrently with lithium carbonate. Patients with known sulphonamide sensitivity may show allergic reactions to Baycaron. Care should be exercised when prescribed with non-steroidal anti-inflammatory drugs. It is always advisable to monitor renal function. Thiazide and thiazide-like diuretics have been implicated in blood dyscrasias and pancreatitis.

Pregnancy warning: Baycaron has not been shown to produce teratogenic effects, either after administration to animals, or when used to treat toxaemia of pregnancy. However, the benefits should be carefully weighed against possible risks in the first trimester of pregnancy.

Diuretics are best avoided for the management of oedema of pregnancy or hypertension in pregnancy as their use may be associated with hypovolaemia, increased blood viscosity and reduced placental perfusion.

There is inadequate evidence of safety in human pregnancy and some workers have described foetal bone marrow depression and thrombocytopenia. Foetal and neonatal jaundice have also been described.

Lactation warning: As diuretics pass into breast milk they should be avoided in mothers who wish to breast feed.

Side-effects: Baycaron is very well tolerated. Occasionally, with daily doses of up to 100 mg, dyspepsia and nausea are encountered initially, but usually subside on continued treatment. There are no reports of postural hypotension nor of any impairment of micturition or bowel habit. Due to its profile of diuretic action, Baycaron does not precipitate acute retention of urine in, for example, cases of prostatic hypertrophy. Impotence is rarely associated with mefruside.

Overdosage: There is no special antidote and general supportive measures should be offered together with monitoring of blood pressure, fluid and electrolyte balance, correcting when necessary.

Pharmaceutical precautions There are no special precautions or requirements regarding the storage of Baycaron.

Legal category POM.

Package quantities Bottles of 150 tablets.

Further information
Hypertension: Baycaron, with its powerful natriuretic effect is particularly suited to the treatment of hypertension, especially in the long term. Baycaron may be administered alone or in combination with other antihypertensive agents.

Oedema: By virtue of its prolonged and smooth natriuretic action, Baycaron is suitable for the long-term treatment of oedematous conditions, for example: oedema of cardiac, hepatic, or renal origin, and premenstrual tension. Its profile of action leads to minimum patient inconvenience. Diuresis begins two to four hours following oral administration and is maximal between six and twelve hours after administration.

Product licence number 0010/5903R

BETA-ADALAT*

Presentation Beta-Adalat is presented as reddish brown capsules bearing the name Beta-Adalat with the Bayer cross. Each capsule contains nifedipine retard 20 mg and atenolol 50 mg.

Uses
Mode of action: Atenolol effects a marked negative inotropic and chronotropic effect thereby reducing cardiac output, myocardial oxygen demand and blood pressure, particularly during exercise. Nifedipine is a powerful coronary and peripheral vasodilator which increases myocardial oxygen supply and reduces blood pressure (afterload) and peripheral resistance. Concomitant use of beta$_1$-blockade, therefore, ameliorates the reflex sympathetic response to nifedipine monotherapy by blocking the rise in heart rate, while atenolol's tendency to increase peripheral resistance is balanced by the vasodilation and increased sympathetic tone induced by the calcium antagonist. Consequently, greater antihypertensive or antianginal efficacy is achieved by the concomitant use of nifedipine and atenolol than either drug alone.

Indications: Management of hypertension and of chronic stable angina pectoris where therapy with either a calcium channel blocker or a beta-blocker proves inadequate.

Dosage and administration

Adults: Hypertension: One capsule daily swallowed with water. If necessary, the dosage may be increased to one capsule dosed every 12 hours. Patients can be transferred to the combination from other antihypertensive treatments with the exception of clonidine (see *Precautions* below).

Angina: One capsule every 12 hours swallowed with water. Where additional efficacy is necessary, prophylactic nitrate therapy or additional nifedipine may be of benefit.

Children: There is no paediatric experience with Beta-Adalat and, therefore, this preparation should not be used in children.

Elderly: Dosage should not exceed one capsule daily in hypertension or one capsule twice daily in angina.

The pharmacokinetics of nifedipine are altered in the elderly so that lower maintenance doses of nifedipine may be required compared to younger patients.

Contra-indications, warnings, etc

Contra-indications: Beta-Adalat should not be administered to patients with known hypersensitivity to nifedipine or other dihydropyridines because of the theoretical risk of cross-reactivity.

Beta-Adalat should not be administered to patients with a history of wheezing or asthma.

Beta-Adalat must not be administered to women capable of child-bearing or to nursing mothers.

Beta-Adalat must not be used in the presence of second or third degree heart block, or in patients with evidence of overt heart failure.

Beta-Adalat should not be used in cardiogenic shock, clinically significant aortic stenosis, unstable angina, or during or within one month of a myocardial infarction.

Beta-Adalat should not be used for the treatment of acute attacks of angina.

The safety of Beta-Adalat in malignant hypertension has not been established.

Beta-Adalat should not be used for secondary prevention of myocardial infarction.

Beta-Adalat must not be used in conjunction with other drugs with a cardio-depressant action, e.g. verapamil, as conduction disturbances may ensue.

Beta-Adalat should not be administered concomitantly with rifampicin since effective plasma levels of nifedipine may not be achieved owing to enzyme induction.

Precautions

Cardiac: Particular care should be taken with patients with conduction defects or whose cardiac reserve is poor. However, in patients already treated with a beta-adrenoceptor antagonist, and/or where signs of cardiac failure have been controlled, Beta-Adalat may be substituted with care if necessary.

Care should be taken in prescribing a beta-adrenoceptor blocking drug with Class 1 antidysrhythmic agents such as disopyramide.

One of the pharmacological actions of beta-adrenoceptor blocking drugs is to reduce heart rate. In the rare instances where symptoms may be attributable to the slow heart rate at a dose of one capsule daily, the drug should be discontinued.

Cessation of therapy with a beta-adrenoceptor blocking drug in patients with ischaemic heart disease should be gradual.

Caution should be exercised when transferring patients from clonidine to beta-adrenoceptor blocking drugs. If beta-adrenoceptor blocking drugs are given concurrently, clonidine should not be discontinued until several days after withdrawal of the beta-adrenoceptor blocking drug.

Obstructive airways disease: Although cardioselective ($beta_1$) beta-blockers may have less effect on lung function than non-selective beta-blockers, as with all beta-blockers these should not be administered to patients with reversible obstructive airways disease.

Renal impairment: In patients with marked renal impairment (i.e. creatinine clearance below 15 ml/min/1.73 m^2, serum creatinine greater than 600 micromol/litre), the use of the combination is considered inappropriate.

Hepatic impairment: Care should be taken in patients with marked hepatic impairment. Although no dosage adjustment is suggested from the systemic availability of the monocomponents in patients with cirrhosis, hypertensive patients with clinically significant liver disease have not been studied. Nifedipine is metabolised primarily by the liver and therefore patients with liver dysfunction should be carefully monitored.

Anaesthesia: It is not advisable to withdraw beta-adrenoceptor blocking drugs prior to surgery in the majority of patients. However, care should be taken when using anaesthetic agents such as ether, cyclopropane and trichloroethylene. Vagal dominance, if it occurs, may be corrected with atropine (1–2 mg i.v.).

Diabetes: The use of nifedipine in diabetic patients may require adjustment of their control.

Beta-Adalat modifies the tachycardia of hypoglycaemia.

Interactions: The antihypertensive effect of nifedipine can be potentiated by simultaneous administration of cimetidine.

When used in combination with nifedipine, serum quinidine levels may be suppressed regardless of dosage of quinidine.

The simultaneous administration of nifedipine and digoxin may lead to reduced digoxin clearance and hence an increase in the plasma digoxin level. Plasma digoxin levels should be monitored and, if necessary, the digoxin dose reduced.

Beta-Adalat should not be administered concomitantly with rifampicin since effective plasma levels of nifedipine may not be achieved owing to enzyme induction.

As with other dihydropyridines, nifedipine should not be taken with grapefruit juice because bioavailability is increased.

Side-effects: Side-effects which have been reported during treatment with the combination include headache, flushing, fatigue, dizziness and oedema. Side-effects of nifedipine such as flushing and headache may occur at the beginning of the treatment. They are, however, mostly slight and diminish with continuous use.

Impotence may occur rarely as a side-effect of nifedipine.

Rare cases of hypersensitivity-type jaundice have been reported with nifedipine.

There are reports of gingival hyperplasia with nifedipine which may regress on withdrawal of therapy.

There have been reports of skin rashes and/or dry eyes associated with the use of beta-adrenoceptor blocking drugs. The reported incidence is small. Discontinuance of the drug should be considered if any such reaction is not otherwise explicable.

As with other sustained release dihydropyridines, exacerbation of angina pectoris may occur rarely at the start of treatment with sustained release formulations of nifedipine. The occurrence of myocardial infarction has been described although it is not possible to distinguish such an event from the natural course of ischaemic heart disease.

Overdosage: Excessive bradycardia can be countered with atropine 1–2 mg intravenously. If necessary, this may be followed by a bolus dose of glucagon 10 mg intravenously. If required, this may be repeated or followed by an intravenous infusion of glucagon 1–10 mg/hour depending on response. If no response to glucagon occurs or if glucagon is unavailable, a beta-adrenoceptor stimulant such as prenalterol 5 mg intravenously, followed if necessary by an intravenous infusion of 5 mg/hour or dobutamine 2.5 to 10 microgram/kg/minute by intravenous infusion may be given.

There is a possibility of hypotension occurring following the use of beta-adrenoceptor agonists but this will be reduced by the more selective agents, prenalterol and dobutamine. In severe cases, cardiac pacing with appropriate cardiorespiratory support may be necessary.

Intravenous calcium gluconate combined with metaraminol may be beneficial for hypotension induced by nifedipine.

Pharmaceutical precautions Beta-Adalat should be stored at room temperature, protected from light and moisture.

Legal category POM.

Package quantities Packs of 28 capsules.

Further information When the combined antihypertensive effect or anti-anginal effect of a beta-adrenoceptor antagonist and calcium antagonist is required, Beta-Adalat is a convenient and acceptable therapy. The combination of atenolol and nifedipine retard, given once daily, provides control of raised blood pressure over a 24 hour period and may be expected to improve patient compliance. Given twice daily, the combination provides control of angina.

Product licence number 0010/0155

CANESTEN* GYNAECOLOGICAL PRODUCTS

Presentation

Pessaries: White convex pessaries measuring 25 mm×6.5 mm×10 mm containing Clotrimazole BP.

Canesten 100 mg Pessary is marked 'Bayer' on one side and 'AD' on the other.

Canesten 200 mg Pessary is marked 'Bayer' on one side and 'F9' on the other.

Canesten Pessary (500 mg) is marked 'Bayer' on one side and 'MU' on the other.

10% VC (Canesten Once): A white cream containing 10.0% Clotrimazole BP.

Combi: A combination pack comprising one Canesten Pessary (500 mg) plus a 20 g tube of Canesten 1% cream (containing 1.0% Clotrimazole BP).

Uses

Pessaries: The pessaries are indicated for the treatment of candidal vaginitis.

10% VC: As for pessaries.

Combi: Pessary for candidal vaginitis; cream for associated vulvitis and to treat the sexual partner to prevent re-infection.

Dosage and administration

Adults

100 mg Pessaries: Two pessaries should be inserted daily, preferably at night, for three consecutive days. Alternatively, one pessary daily for six days may be inserted, preferably at night.

200 mg Pessaries: One pessary should be inserted daily, preferably at night, for three consecutive days.

500 mg Pessary: The single pessary should be inserted, preferably at night.

10% VC: Insert the contents of the filled applicator (5 g) intravaginally, preferably at night. A second treatment may be carried out if necessary.

Combi: The single pessary should be inserted, preferably at night.

The cream should be applied night and morning to the vulva and surrounding area and/or to the partner's penis to prevent re-infection.

Using the applicator provided, each pessary or dose of vaginal cream should be inserted as deeply as is comfortable into the vagina. This is best achieved when lying back with the legs bent up.

Children: As the above products are used with an applicator, paediatric usage is not recommended.

Contra-indications, warnings, etc

Contra-indications: Hypersensitivity to clotrimazole.

Warnings and precautions: Medical advice should be sought if this is the first time the patient has experienced symptoms of candidal vaginitis. Before using the pessaries or cream, medical advice must be sought if any of the following are applicable:

- More than two infections of candidal vaginitis in the last six months.
- Previous history of a sexually transmitted disease or exposure to partner with sexually transmitted disease.
- Pregnancy or suspected pregnancy.
- Aged under 16 or over 60 years.
- Known hypersensitivity to imidazoles or other vaginal anti-fungal products.

Canesten pessaries and cream should not be used if the patient has any of the following symptoms, whereupon medical advice should be sought:

- Irregular vaginal bleeding.
- Abnormal vaginal bleeding or a blood-stained discharge.
- Vulval or vaginal ulcers, blisters or sores.
- Lower abdominal pain or dysuria.
- Any adverse events such as redness, irritation or swelling associated with the treatment.
- Fever or chills.
- Nausea or vomiting.
- Diarrhoea.
- Foul smelling vaginal discharge.

If no improvement in symptoms is seen after seven days, the patient should consult their doctor.

Side-effects: Rarely patients may experience local mild burning or irritation immediately after applying the cream or inserting the pessaries. Very rarely, the patient may find this irritation intolerable and stop treatment. Hypersensitivity reactions may occur.

Use in pregnancy: In animal studies, clotrimazole has not been associated with teratogenic effects but following oral administration of high doses to rats there was evidence of foetotoxicity. The relevance of this effect to topical application in humans is not known. However, clotrimazole has been used in pregnant patients for over a decade without attributable adverse effects. It is therefore recommended that clotrimazole should be used in pregnancy only when considered necessary by the clinician. If used during pregnancy, extra care should be taken when using the applicator to prevent the possibility of mechanical trauma.

Accidental oral ingestion: In the event, routine measures such as gastric lavage should be performed as soon as possible after ingestion.

Pharmaceutical precautions No special storage precautions are necessary for the pessaries. Canesten 10% VC (Canesten Once) and Combi should be stored below 25°C.

Legal category P.

Package quantities

Pessaries: 6×100 mg pessaries packed in a blister strip.

3×200 mg pessaries packed in a blister strip.
1×500 mg pessary packed in foil.
An applicator and a patient information leaflet are included.

Canesten 10% VC (Canesten Once): A prefilled applicator containing 5 g cream. A patient information leaflet is included.

Combi: 1×500 mg pessary packed in foil, plus a 20 g tube of Canesten 1% cream. An applicator for the pessary and a patient information leaflet are included.

Further information Nil.

Product licence numbers

100 mg Pessaries	0010/0015R
200 mg Pessaries	0010/0072
500 mg Pessary	0010/0083
10% VC (Canesten Once)	0010/0136
Combi: Cream 1%	0010/0016R
500 mg Pessary	0010/0083

CANESTEN* TOPICAL PRODUCTS

Presentation
Cream: A white cream containing 1.0% Clotrimazole BP.

Atomiser spray: A clear spray containing 1.0% Clotrimazole BP in 30% isopropanol. The spray is produced by an atomiser and contains no propellant.

Solution: A clear solution containing 1.0% Clotrimazole BP in polyethylene glycol 400.

Powder: A white powder containing 1.0% Clotrimazole BP.

Uses Clotrimazole is a broad spectrum antifungal. It also exhibits activity against *Trichomonas*, staphylococci, streptococci and *Bacteroides*.

Clotrimazole is recommended for the treatment of skin infections due to dermatophytes (e.g. *Trichophyton* species), yeasts (e.g. *Candida* species), moulds and other fungi. These include ringworm (tinea) infections, athlete's foot, paronychia, pityriasis versicolor, erythrasma and intertrigo.

Cream: The cream may also be used for the treatment of fungal nappy rash, candidal vulvitis and candidal balanitis.

Atomiser Spray: The spray is recommended in particular for infections covering large and/or hairy areas.

Solution: The solution is particularly suitable for use on hairy skin and in fungal infections of the outer and middle ear (otitis externa and otomycoses).

Powder: The powder is to be used as an adjunct to treatment with cream or atomiser spray and as a prophylactic against re-infection, particularly in infections such as athlete's foot. The powder should be applied to the lesions simultaneously and dusted inside articles of clothing in contact with infected areas.

Dosage and administration
Cream: Canesten cream should be thinly and evenly applied to the affected area two to three times daily and rubbed in gently.

Treatment should be continued for at least one month for dermatophyte infections, or for at least two weeks for candidal infections.

If the feet are infected, they should be thoroughly washed and dried, especially between the toes, before applying the cream.

Atomiser Spray: Canesten atomiser spray should be applied to the affected area two to three times daily. Treatment should be continued for at least one month for dermatophyte infections, or for at least two weeks for candidal infections and pityriasis versicolor infections.

Solution: Canesten solution should be thinly and evenly applied to the affected area two to three times daily. To prevent relapse treatment should be continued for at least two weeks after the disappearance of all signs of infection.

Powder: Sprinkle onto the affected areas two to three times daily after using the cream or atomiser spray. The powder may also be dusted inside articles of clothing and footwear which are in contact with the infected area.

Contra-indications, warnings, etc
Contra-indications: Hypersensitivity to clotrimazole or, (in the case of the atomiser spray), propylene glycol.

Warnings and precautions: Canesten atomiser spray should not be used near a naked flame, should not be allowed to come into contact with the eyes, ears or mucous membranes and should not be inhaled.

Side-effects: Rarely patients may experience local mild burning or irritation immediately after applying the cream, solution, atomiser spray or powder. Very rarely, the patient may find this irritation intolerable and stop treatment. Hypersensitivity reactions may occur.

Use in pregnancy: In animal studies clotrimazole has not been associated with teratogenic effects but following oral administration of high doses to rats there was evidence of foetotoxicity. The relevance of this effect to topical application in humans is not known. However, clotrimazole has been used in pregnant patients for over a decade without attributable adverse effects. It is therefore recommended that clotrimazole should be used in pregnancy only when considered necessary by the clinician.

Accidental oral ingestion: In the event, routine measures such as gastric lavage should be performed as soon as possible after ingestion.

Pharmaceutical precautions Cream: Store below 25°C. Atomiser spray, Solution, Powder: No special storage precautions are necessary.

Legal category P.

Package quantities
Cream: Tubes containing 20 g or 50 g.
Atomiser Spray: Bottles containing 40 ml.
Solution: Dropper bottles containing 20 ml.
Powder: Packs containing 30 g.

Further information Nil.

Product licence numbers

Cream	0010/0016R
Atomiser Spray	0010/0060R
Solution	0010/0082
Powder	0010/0067

CANESTEN*HC

Presentation A white cream containing 1.0% Clotrimazole BP and 1.0% Hydrocortisone PhEur.

Uses Clotrimazole is a broad spectrum antifungal agent. It also exhibits activity against *Trichomonas*, staphylococci, streptococci and *Bacteroides*. It has no effect on lactobacilli.

Hydrocortisone has a vasoconstrictive effect, thus reducing inflammation and oedema and also has an antipruritic effect.

Canesten HC is indicated for the treatment of the following skin infections where co-existing symptoms of inflammation, e.g. itching, require rapid relief:

1. All dermatomycoses due to dermatophytes, (e.g. Trichophyton species), moulds and other fungi.
2. All dermatomycoses due to yeasts (Candida species).
3. Skin diseases showing secondary infection with these fungi.
4. The treatment of nappy rash where infection due to *Candida albicans* is present. Candidal vulvitis, candidal balanitis and candidal intertrigo.

Dosage and administration Canesten HC should be thinly and evenly applied to the affected area twice daily and rubbed in gently.

Contra-indications, warnings, etc
Contra-indications: Hypersensitivity to any of the ingredients.

Warnings and precautions: As with all corticosteroids, long term continuous therapy to extensive areas of skin should be avoided, particularly in infants and children. In infants the napkin may act as an occlusive dressing and increase absorption.

Treatment should be for a maximum period of seven days.

Side-effects: Rarely patients may experience local mild burning or irritation immediately after applying the cream. Very rarely, the patient may find this irritation intolerable and stop treatment. Hypersensitivity reactions may occur.

Use in pregnancy: Topical administration of corticosteroids to pregnant animals can cause abnormalities of foetal development. The relevance of this to humans has not been established.

In animal studies clotrimazole has not been associated with teratogenic effects but following oral administration of high doses to rats there was evidence of foetotoxicity. The relevance of this effect to topical application in humans is not known. However, clotrimazole has been used in pregnant patients for over a decade without attributable adverse effects.

It is therefore recommended that Canesten HC should be used in pregnancy only when considered necessary by the clinician.

Accidental oral ingestion: In the event, routine measures such as gastric lavage should be performed as soon as possible after ingestion.

Pharmaceutical precautions Store in a cool place.

Legal category POM.

Package quantities Tubes containing 30 g.

Further information Nil.

Product licence number 0010/0120

CANESTEN* HYDROCORTISONE

Qualitative and quantitative composition 15 g of cream contains Clotrimazole BP 150 mg (1%) and Hydrocortisone PhEur 150 mg (1%).

Pharmaceutical form Cream.

Clinical particulars
Therapeutic Indications: Canesten Hydrocortisone is indicated for the treatment of the following skin infections where co-existing symptoms of inflammation, e.g. itching, require rapid relief:
(i) Athlete's foot.
(ii) Candidal intertrigo.

Posology and method of administration: Canesten Hydrocortisone should be thinly and evenly applied to the affected area twice daily and rubbed in gently. The maximum period of treatment is seven days.

Contra-indications: Canesten Hydrocortisone is contra-indicated in the following cases:

- Use on broken skin.
- Use on large areas of skin.
- Use for periods of longer than seven days.
- Hypersensitivity to any of the ingredients.
- To treat cold sores or acne.
- Use on the face, eyes, mouth or mucous membranes.
- Children under 10 years of age, unless prescribed by a doctor.
- Pregnancy and lactation, unless prescribed by a doctor.
- Use on the ano-genital area, unless prescribed by a doctor.
- To treat ringworm, unless prescribed by a doctor.
- To treat secondarily infected skin conditions, unless prescribed by a doctor.

Special warnings and special precautions for use: As with all corticosteroids, long-term continuous therapy to extensive areas of skin should be avoided. Therefore, treatment should be for a maximum period of seven days.

Care should be taken not to cover the treated area with a tight bandage or dressing as this may increase absorption of hydrocortisone.

Interaction with other medicaments and other forms of interaction: None.

Pregnancy and lactation: Topical administration of corticosteroids to pregnant animals can cause abnormalities of foetal development. The relevance of this to humans has not been established. In animal studies, clotrimazole has not been associated with teratogenic effects but following oral administration of high doses to rats, there was evidence of foetotoxicity. The relevance of this effect to topical application in humans is not known. However, clotrimazole has been used in pregnant patients for over a decade without attributable adverse effects. It is therefore recommended that Canesten Hydrocortisone should be used in pregnancy and lactation only when considered necessary by the clinician.

Effects on ability to drive and use machines: None applicable.

Undesirable effects: Rarely patients may experience local, mild burning or irritation immediately after applying the cream. Very rarely, patients may find this irritation intolerable and stop treatment. Hypersensitivity reactions may occur.

Overdose: In the event of accidental oral ingestion, routine measures such as gastric lavage should be performed as soon as possible after ingestion.

Pharmacological properties
Pharmacodynamic properties: Clotrimazole has a broad spectrum of activity (yeast, dermatophytes, moulds and a number of other fungi). It also exhibits activity against *Trichomonas vaginalis*, staphylococci, streptococci and *Bacteroides*.

Hydrocortisone has a vasoconstrictive effect thus reducing inflammation and oedema. It also has an antipruritic effect.

Pharmacokinetic properties: Following application of 1% ^{14}C-clotrimazole cream (8 mg clotrimazole–200cm^2 with occlusive dressing for six hours) to five healthy volunteers, urinary excretion within six days amounted to a maximum of 0.2% of the activity applied. Maximum equivalent concentrations of clotrimazole in the serum remained below 0.0001μg/ml.

A study in 16 healthy volunteers following topical application of 1.5–2.5 g Canesten Hydrocortisone cream (doses of 15–25 mg hydrocortisone) resulted in no measurably effective levels of hydrocortisone in the blood or urine (analytical method used was Amerlex Cortisol ^{125}I RIA).

Preclinical safety data: The maximum oral dose of Canesten Hydrocortisone that could be administered to mice was not lethal.

Topical administration of the cream to rabbits produced dermatitis. However, the cream is well tolerated in man and the skin irritation seen in rabbits does not apply to human use.

Pharmaceutical particulars
List of excipients: Canesten Hydrocortisone contains the following excipients: Hostaphosphate KW solid; Cetylstearyl alcohol DAB; Myritol 318 DAB; Benzyl alcohol PhEur; Purified water PhEur.

Incompatibilities: None stated.

Shelf life: 30 months.

Special precautions for storage: The cream should be stored in a cool place.

Nature and contents of container: Aluminium tube with internal lacquer coating and HDPE screw-on cap containing 15 g of cream.

Instructions for use/handling: Not applicable.

Marketing authorisation number 0010/0216

Date of approval/revision of SPC January 1997.

Legal category P

CIPROXIN*

Presentation
Infusion: Clear, almost colourless to pale yellow solution containing 254.4 mg ciprofloxacin lactate (equivalent to 200 mg ciprofloxacin) per 100 ml solution.

Tablets: White, round, film-coated tablets marked on one side with the Bayer cross and "CIP 100" on the reverse side. Each tablet contains 116.4 mg ciprofloxacin hydrochloride monohydrate (equivalent to 100 mg ciprofloxacin).

White, scored, round, film-coated tablets, marked on one side with the Bayer cross, and with "CIP 250" on the reverse side. Each tablet contains 291 mg ciprofloxacin hydrochloride monohydrate (equivalent to 250 mg ciprofloxacin).

White, scored, oblong, film-coated tablets marked "BAYER" on one side and "CIP 500" on the reverse side. Each tablet contains 582 mg ciprofloxacin hydrochloride monohydrate (equivalent to 500 mg ciprofloxacin).

White, oblong, film-coated tablets marked "BAYER" on one side and "CIP 750" on the reverse side. Each tablet contains 873 mg ciprofloxacin hydrochloride monohydrate (equivalent to 750 mg ciprofloxacin).

Uses Ciprofloxacin is a synthetic, 4-quinolone derivative with bactericidal activity against a wide range of Gram-negative and Gram-positive organisms.

Ciprofloxacin is indicated for the treatment of single infections or mixed infections caused by two or more susceptible organisms. It may be used for infections caused by organisms resistant to other antibiotics, including aminoglycosides, penicillins and cephalosporins.

The extensive tissue penetration of ciprofloxacin combined with its enhanced antibacterial activity (including anti-pseudomonal activity), enables ciprofloxacin to be used alone (pending sensitivity results) or in combination with an aminoglycoside or with beta-lactam antibiotics, for instance when severe neutropenia is present, or with an antibiotic active against anaerobes where the presence of these organisms is suspected.

Microbiology: In-vitro studies have shown that the antibacterial action of ciprofloxacin results from the inhibition of bacterial DNA gyrase.

This mode of action differs from that of penicillins, cephalosporins, aminoglycosides and tetracyclines and, therefore, organisms resistant to these antibiotics are generally sensitive to ciprofloxacin.

Ciprofloxacin is active *in-vitro* against the following Gram-negative and Gram-positive organisms: *Citrobacter* spp., *Edwardsiella tarda, Enterobacter* spp., *Escherichia coli, Hafnia alvei, Klebsiella* spp., *Morganella morganii, Proteus* spp. (indole positive and indole negative), *Providencia* spp., *Salmonella* spp., *Serratia* spp., *Shigella* spp., *Yersinia* spp., *Aeromonas* spp., *Campylobacter coli, Campylobacter jejuni, Plesiomonas shigelloides, Pseudomonas aeruginosa, Vibrio* spp., *Haemophilus* spp., *Branhamella catarrhalis, Pasteurella multocida, Moraxella* spp., *Neisseria* spp., *Legionella* spp., *Brucella melitensis, Staphylococcus* spp., *Listeria monocytogenes, Corynebacterium* spp.

Ciprofloxacin is less active against the following organisms. Sensitivity testing should be performed before treatment is commenced: *Acinetobacter* spp., *Alcaligenes* spp., *Flavobacterium* spp., non-*aeruginosa Pseudomonas* spp., *Gardnerella vaginalis, Chlamydia* spp., *Mycoplasma* spp., *Mycobacterium tuberculosis, Mycobacterium fortuitum, Enterococcus faecalis, Streptococcus agalactiae, Streptococcus pneumoniae, Streptococcus pyogenes,* viridans group streptococci.

Anaerobes vary in their susceptibility from being moderately sensitive to resistant. In particular, the *Bacteroides fragilis* group and *Clostridium difficile* are resistant.

In addition, the following organisms are resistant to ciprofloxacin: *Ureaplasma urealyticum, Nocardia asteroides, Enterococcus faecium.*

Ciprofloxacin is not active against *Treponema pallidum.*

In-vitro studies have shown that additive activity often results when ciprofloxacin is used concomitantly with other antibacterial agents.

Indications: Ciprofloxacin is indicated for the treatment of the following infections caused by sensitive bacteria:

Adults: Severe systemic infection: e.g. septicaemia, bacteraemia, peritonitis, infections in immunosuppressed patients with haematological or solid tumours and in patients in intensive care units with specific problems such as infected burns.

Respiratory tract infections: e.g. lobar and bronchopneumonia, acute and chronic bronchitis, acute exacerbation of cystic fibrosis, bronchiectasis, empyema. Ciprofloxacin is not recommended as first-line therapy for the treatment of pneumococcal pneumonia. Ciprofloxacin may be used for treating Gram-negative pneumonia.

Ear, nose and throat infections: e.g. otitis media, sinusitis and mastoiditis, especially if due to Gram-negative bacteria (including *Pseudomonas* spp.). Ciprofloxacin is not recommended for the treatment of acute tonsillitis.

Urinary tract infections: e.g. uncomplicated and complicated urethritis, cystitis, pyelonephritis, prostatitis, epididymitis.

Skin and soft tissue infections: e.g. infected ulcers, wound infections, abscesses, cellulitis, otitis externa, erysipelas, infected burns.

Gastro-intestinal infections: e.g. enteric fever, infective diarrhoea.

Eye infections: e.g. bacterial conjunctivitis.

Infections of the biliary tract: e.g. cholangitis, cholecystitis, empyema of the gall bladder.

Intra-abdominal infections: e.g. peritonitis, intra-abdominal abscesses.

Bone and joint infections: e.g. osteomyelitis, septic arthritis.

Pelvic infections: e.g. salpingitis, endometritis, pelvic inflammatory disease.

Gonorrhoea: including urethral, rectal and pharyngeal gonorrhoea caused by beta-lactamase-producing organisms or organisms moderately sensitive to penicillin.

Ciprofloxacin is also indicated for prophylaxis against infection in elective upper gastro-intestinal surgery and endoscopic procedures where there is an increased risk of infection.

Children: For the treatment of acute pulmonary exacerbation of cystic fibrosis associated with *P. aeruginosa* infection in paediatric patients aged 5–17 years.

Dosage and administration General dosage recommendations: the dosage of ciprofloxacin is determined by the severity and type of infection, the sensitivity of the causative organism(s) and the age, weight and renal function of the patient.

Adults
Ciproxin Infusion: Ciproxin Infusion in 50 ml (100 mg) infusion bottles may be infused directly and should be administered by short-term infusion over periods of 30–60 minutes. The dosage range for adults is 100–400 mg twice daily. The 400 mg dose should be administered over a period of 60 minutes.

In gonorrhoea, a single dose of 100 mg.

Infections of the lower and upper urinary tract, 100 mg twice daily.

For both upper and lower respiratory tract infections, 200–400 mg twice daily depending on the severity of the infection and the sensitivity of the causative organism (see Indications).

Although ciprofloxacin is not recommended as first-line treatment for pneumococcal pneumonia, where it is considered to be appropriate, oral ciprofloxacin may be used (see below).

Cystic fibrosis: In adults with pseudomonal infections of the lower respiratory tract, the dose should be 400 mg twice daily, although, as the pharmacokinetics of ciprofloxacin remain unchanged in patients with cystic fibrosis, the low body weight of these patients should be taken into consideration when determining dosage.

In the majority of other infections, 200–400 mg twice daily depending on the severity of the infection.

Initial intravenous administration may be followed by oral treatment.

Ciproxin Tablets: Ciproxin Tablets should be swallowed whole with an adequate amount of liquid. The dosage range for adults is 100–750 mg twice daily.

In gonorrhoea, a single dose of 250 mg.

In acute, uncomplicated cystitis in women, 100 mg twice daily. In other infections of the lower and upper urinary tract (depending on severity), 250–500 mg twice daily.

In respiratory tract infections, 250–750 mg twice daily for both upper and lower respiratory tract infections, depending on severity. Although ciprofloxacin is not recommended as first-line treatment for pneumococcal pneumonia, where it is considered to be appropriate, a dosage of 750 mg twice daily should be used.

Cystic fibrosis: In adults with pseudomonal infections of the lower respiratory tract, the normal dose is 750 mg twice daily. As the pharmacokinetics of ciprofloxacin remain unchanged in patients with cystic fibrosis, the low body weight of these patients should be taken into consideration when determining dosage.

In the majority of other infections, 500–750 mg twice daily should be administered. In severe infections, particularly due to *Pseudomonas*, staphylococci and streptococci, the higher dosage of 750 mg twice daily should be used.

For surgical prophylaxis, a single 750 mg dose given 60–90 minutes before the procedure. The tablet may be given with an oral premedicant (but see interactions). In cases of suspected gastro-oesophageal obstructive lesions, ciprofloxacin should be administered in combination with an appropriate antibiotic effective against anaerobes.

Impaired renal function: Dosage adjustments are not usually required, except in patients with severe renal impairment (serum creatinine >265 micromole/l or creatinine clearance <20 ml/minute). If adjustment is necessary, this may be achieved by reducing the total daily dose by half, although monitoring of drug serum levels provides the most reliable basis for dose adjustment.

Impaired hepatic function: No adjustment of dosage is necessary.

Elderly: Although higher ciprofloxacin serum levels are found in the elderly, no adjustment of dosage is necessary.

Adolescents and children: As with other drugs in its class, ciprofloxacin has been shown to cause arthropathy in weight-bearing joints of immature animals. Although analysis of available safety data from ciprofloxacin use in patients less than 18 years of age, the majority of whom had cystic fibrosis, did not disclose any evidence of drug-related cartilage or articular damage, its use in the paediatric patient population is generally not recommended.

Clinical and pharmacokinetic data support the use of ciprofloxacin in paediatric cystic fibrosis patients (aged 5–17 years) with acute pulmonary exacerbation associated with *P. aeruginosa* infection, at a dose of 20 mg/kg orally twice daily (maximum daily dose 1500 mg) or 10 mg/kg iv three times daily (maximum daily dose 1200 mg). The infusion should be administered over 60 minutes.

Sequential therapy can also be used. Dosage as follows: 10 mg/kg iv three times daily (maximum daily dose 1200 mg) followed by 20 mg/kg orally twice daily (maximum daily dose 1500 mg).

For indications other than treatment of pulmonary exacerbation in cystic fibrosis, ciprofloxacin may be used in children and adolescents where the benefit is considered to outweigh the potential risks. In these cases a dosage of 4–8 mg/kg iv twice daily or 5–15 mg/kg orally twice daily should be administered depending upon the severity of the infection.

Dosing in children with impaired renal and/or hepatic function has not been studied.

Duration of treatment: The duration of treatment depends upon the severity of infection, clinical response and bacteriological findings.

In acute, uncomplicated cystitis, the treatment period is 3 days.

In other acute infections the usual treatment period is 5 to 7 days with Ciproxin Infusion or 5 to 10 days with Ciproxin Tablets.

Generally, acute and chronic infections (e.g. osteomyelitis and prostatitis, etc), where the causative organism is known to be sensitive to ciprofloxacin, should be treated for at least 3 days after the signs and symptoms of the infection have disappeared.

For acute pulmonary exacerbation of cystic fibrosis associated with *P. aeruginosa* infection in paediatric patients (aged 5–17 years), the duration of treatment is 10–14 days.

Contra-indications, warnings, etc
Contra-indications: Ciprofloxacin is contra-indicated in patients who have shown hypersensitivity to ciprofloxacin or other quinolones.

Except in cases of exacerbation of CF associated with *P. aeruginosa* (in patients aged 5–17 years), ciprofloxacin is contra-indicated in children and growing adolescents unless the benefits of treatment are considered to outweigh the risks.

Warnings and precautions: Ciprofloxacin should be used with caution in epileptics and patients with a history of CNS disorders and only if the benefits of treatment are considered to outweigh the risk of possible CNS side-effects.

Ciprofloxacin could result in an impairment of the patient's ability to drive or operate machinery, particularly in conjunction with alcohol.

Crystalluria related to the use of ciprofloxacin has been reported. Patients receiving ciprofloxacin should be well hydrated and excessive alkalinity of the urine should be avoided.

Patients with a family history of or actual defects in glucose-6-phosphate dehydrogenase activity are prone to haemolytic reactions with quinolones, and so ciprofloxacin should be used with caution in these patients.

Tendon inflammation and rupture may occur with quinolone antibiotics. Such reactions have been observed particularly in older patients and in those treated concurrently with corticosteroids. At the first sign of pain or inflammation, patients should discontinue Ciproxin and rest the affected limbs.

Drug interactions: Ciproxin Tablets should not be administered within 4 hours of medications containing magnesium, aluminium, calcium or iron salts as interference with absorption may occur. When appropriate, patients should be advised not to self-medicate with preparations containing these compounds during therapy with Ciproxin.

Phenytoin levels may be altered when Ciproxin is used concomitantly.

Increased plasma levels of theophylline have been observed following concurrent administration with ciprofloxacin. It is recommended that the dose of theophylline should be reduced and plasma levels of theophylline monitored. Where monitoring of plasma levels is not possible, the use of ciprofloxacin should be avoided in patients receiving theophylline. Particular caution is advised in those patients with convulsive disorders.

Prolongation of bleeding time has been reported during concomitant administration of ciprofloxacin and oral anticoagulants.

Animal data have shown that high doses of quinolones in combination with some non-steroidal anti-inflammatory drugs (e.g. fenbufen, but not acetylsalicylic acid) can lead to convulsions.

Transient increases in serum creatinine have been seen following concomitant administration of ciprofloxacin and cyclosporin. Therefore, monitoring of serum creatinine levels is advisable.

The simultaneous administration of quinolones and glibenclamide can on occasion potentiate the effect of glibenclamide, resulting in hypoglycaemia.

Concomitant use with probenecid reduces the renal clearance of ciprofloxacin, resulting in increased quinolone plasma levels.

The use of metoclopramide with ciprofloxacin may accelerate the absorption of ciprofloxacin.

When ciprofloxacin is used for surgical prophylaxis, it is recommended that opiate premedicants (e.g. papaveretum) or opiate premedicants used with anticholinergic premedicants (e.g. atropine or hyoscine) are not used, as the serum levels of ciprofloxacin are reduced and adequate cover may not be obtained during surgery. Co-administration of ciprofloxacin and benzodiazepine premedicants has been shown not to affect ciprofloxacin plasma levels.

Use in pregnancy and lactation: Reproduction studies performed in mice, rats and rabbits using parenteral and oral administration did not reveal any evidence of teratogenicity, impairment of fertility or impairment of peri-/post-natal development. However, as with other quinolones, ciprofloxacin has been shown to cause arthropathy in immature animals, and therefore its use during pregnancy is not recommended. Studies have indicated that ciprofloxacin is secreted in breast milk. Administration to nursing mothers is thus not recommended.

Side-effects: Ciprofloxacin is generally well tolerated. The most frequently reported adverse reactions are: nausea, diarrhoea, vomiting, dyspepsia, abdominal pain, headache, restlessness, rash, dizziness and pruritus.

The following adverse reactions have been observed:

Gastro-intestinal disturbances, e.g. nausea, diarrhoea, vomiting, dyspepsia, abdominal pain, anorexia, flatulence, dysphagia. Rarely, pseudomembranous colitis.

CNS disturbances, e.g. headache, restlessness, depression, dizziness, tremor, convulsions, confusion, hallucinations, somnolence. Very rarely, sleep disorders and anxiety states. Isolated cases of ciprofloxacin-induced psychoses have been reported. There are isolated reports of intracranial hypertension associated with quinolone therapy. Paraesthesia has been reported.

Hypersensitivity/skin, e.g. rash, pruritus, urticaria, photosensitivity, drug-induced fever, anaphylactic/anaphylactoid reactions including angioedema and dyspnoea. Rarely, erythema nodosum and erythema multiforme. Very rarely, petechiae, haemorrhagic bullae, vasculitis, Stevens-Johnson Syndrome and Lyells Syndrome. Treatment with ciprofloxacin should be discontinued if any of the above occur upon first administration.

Hepatic disturbances, e.g. transient increases in liver enzymes or serum bilirubin (particularly in patients with previous liver damage), hepatitis, jaundice and major liver disorders including hepatic necrosis, which may rarely progress to hepatic failure.

Renal disturbances, e.g. transient increases in blood urea or serum creatinine, renal failure, crystalluria and nephritis.

Musculoskeletal disturbances, e.g. reversible arthralgia, joint swelling and myalgia. Rarely, tenosynovitis. Isolated cases of tendon inflammation have been reported, which may lead to tendon rupture. Treatment should be discontinued immediately if these symptoms occur.

Effects on haematological parameters, e.g. eosinophilia, leucopenia, granulocytopenia, thrombocytopenia, thrombocytosis, altered prothrombin levels and very rarely, haemolytic anaemia or agranulocytosis.

Special sense disturbances, e.g. very rarely, visual disturbances, impaired taste and smell, tinnitus and transient impairment of hearing, particularly at high frequencies.

Tachycardia has been reported.

In addition with Ciproxin Infusion, local irritation including pain at the site of injection has been reported, accompanied in a small number of patients by phlebitis or thrombophlebitis.

Overdosage: Based on the limited information available, in two cases of ingestion of over 18 g of ciprofloxacin, reversible renal toxicity has occurred. Therefore, apart from routine emergency measures, it is recommended to monitor renal function, including urinary pH and acidify, if required, to prevent crystalluria. Patients must be kept well hydrated and in the case of renal damage resulting in prolonged oliguria, dialysis should be initiated.

Calcium or magnesium antacids may be administered as soon as possible after ingestion of Ciproxin Tablets in order to reduce the absorption of ciprofloxacin.

Serum levels of ciprofloxacin are reduced by dialysis.

Pharmaceutical precautions Ciproxin Infusion is compatible with sodium chloride 0.9% solution, Ringer's Solution, glucose 5% and 10% solutions, glucose/saline and fructose 10% solution.

Ciproxin Infusion is incompatible with injection solutions (e.g. penicillins, heparin solutions) which are chemically or physically unstable at its pH of 3.9–4.5.

Unless compatibility is proven, the infusion should always be administered separately.

Since Ciproxin Infusion is light-sensitive, the bottles should always be stored in the cardboard outer container. No special precautions are required during the normal 30–60 minute infusion period.

Do not refrigerate Ciproxin Infusion. If the product is inadvertently refrigerated, crystals may form. Do not use if crystals are present. These crystals will, however, redissolve at room temperature and do not adversely affect the quality of the product.

No special storage precautions are necessary for Ciproxin Tablets.

Legal category POM.

Package quantities Ciproxin Infusion, bottle of 50 ml.

Ciproxin Tablets 250 mg, 500 mg and 750 mg, blister strips of 10 in packs of 10, 20 and 100 tablets. Ciproxin Tablets 100 mg are available in blister packs of six.

Further information Ciproxin Infusion contains 0.01% w/v lactic acid plus 0.9% w/v sodium chloride, equivalent to approximately 154 mmol sodium per litre.

Product licence numbers

Ciproxin Infusion	0010/0150
Ciproxin Tablets 100 mg	0010/0145
Ciproxin Tablets 250 mg	0010/0146
Ciproxin Tablets 500 mg	0010/0147
Ciproxin Tablets 750 mg	0010/0148

CIPROXIN* I.V. FLEXIBAG

Qualitative and quantitative composition Ciprofloxacin (INN).

Quantitative composition per presentation:

(i) 100 ml: One flexible container with 100 ml infusion solution contains Ciprofloxacin USP 200 mg in the form of ciprofloxacin lactate 254.4 mg, and 5% w/v dextrose.

(ii) 200 ml: One flexible container with 200 ml infusion solution contains Ciprofloxacin USP 400 mg in the form of ciprofloxacin lactate 508.8 mg, and 5% w/v dextrose.

Pharmaceutical form Solution for intravenous infusion.

Clinical particulars

Therapeutic indications: Ciprofloxacin is indicated for the treatment of the following infections caused by sensitive bacteria:

Adults: Severe systemic infections: e.g. septicaemia, bacteraemia, peritonitis, infections in immunosuppressed patients with haematological or solid tumours and in patients in intensive care units with specific problems such as infected burns.

Respiratory tract infections: e.g. lobar and bronchopneumonia, acute and chronic bronchitis, acute exacerbation of cystic fibrosis, bronchiectasis, empyema. Ciprofloxacin is not recommended as first-line therapy for the treatment of pneumococcal pneumonia. Ciprofloxacin may be used for treating Gram-negative pneumonia.

Ear, nose and throat infections: e.g. mastoiditis, otitis media and sinusitis, especially if due to Gram-negative bacteria (including *Pseudomonas* spp.). Ciprofloxacin is not recommended for the treatment of acute tonsillitis.

Eye infections: e.g. bacterial conjunctivitis.

Urinary tract infections: e.g. uncomplicated and complicated urethritis, cystitis, pyelonephritis, prostatitis, epididymitis.

Skin and soft tissue infections: e.g. infected ulcers, wound infections, abscesses, cellulitis, otitis externa, erysipelas, infected burns.

Bone and joint infections: e.g. osteomyelitis, septic arthritis.

Intra-abdominal infections: e.g. peritonitis, intra-abdominal abscesses.

Infections of the biliary tract: e.g. cholangitis, cholecystitis, empyema of the gall bladder.

Gastro-intestinal infections: e.g. enteric fever, infective diarrhoea.

Pelvic infections: e.g. salpingitis, endometritis, pelvic inflammatory disease.

Gonorrhoea: including urethral, rectal and pharyngeal gonorrhoea caused by β-lactamase producing organisms or organisms moderately sensitive to penicillin.

Children: For the treatment of acute pulmonary exacerbation of cystic fibrosis associated with *P. aeruginosa* infection in paediatric patients aged 5–17 years.

In-vitro investigations have indicated that ciprofloxacin is active against the following Gram-negative and Gram-positive organisms: *Citrobacter* spp., *Edwardsiella tarda*, *Enterobacter* spp., *Escherichia coli*, *Hafnia alvei*, *Klebsiella* spp., *Morganella morganii*, *Proteus* spp. (indole positive and indole negative), *Providencia* spp., *Salmonella* spp., *Serratia* spp., *Shigella* spp., *Yersinia* spp., *Aeromonas* spp., *Campylobacter coli*, *Campylobacter jejuni*, *Plesiomonas shigelloides*, *Pseudomonas aeruginosa*, *Vibrio* spp., *Haemophilus* spp., *Branhamella catarrhalis*, *Pasteurella multocida*, *Moraxella* spp., *Neisseria* spp., *Legionella* spp., *Brucella melitensis*, *Staphylococcus* spp., *Listeria monocytogenes*, *Corynebacterium* spp.

Ciprofloxacin is less active against the following organisms. Sensitivity testing should be performed before treatment is commenced: *Acinetobacter* spp., *Alcaligenes* spp., *Flavobacterium* spp., non-aeruginosa *Pseudomonas* spp., *Gardnerella vaginalis*, *Chlamydia* spp., *Mycoplasma* spp., *Mycobacterium tuberculosis*, *Mycobacterium fortuitum*, *Enterococcus faecalis*, *Streptococcus agalactiae*, *Streptococcus pneumoniae*, *Streptococcus pyogenes*, *viridans* group streptococci.

Anaerobes vary in their susceptibility from being moderately sensitive to resistant. In particular, the *Bacteroides fragilis* group and *Clostridium difficile* are resistant.

In addition, the following organisms are resistant to ciprofloxacin: *Ureaplasma urealyticum*, *Nocardia asteroides*, *Enterococcus faecium*.

Ciprofloxacin is not active against *Treponema pallidum*.

In-vitro studies have shown that additive activity often results when ciprofloxacin is used concomitantly with other antibacterial agents.

Posology and method of administration: The dosage of intravenous ciprofloxacin is determined by the severity and type of infection, the sensitivity of the causative organism(s) and the age, weight and renal function of the patient.

The dosage range for adults is 100–400 mg twice daily. The product should be infused directly and administered by short-term infusion over periods of 30–60 minutes. The 400 mg dose should be administered over a period of 60 minutes. Initial intravenous administration may be followed by oral treatment.

Adults: The following dosages for specific types of infection are recommended:

Table 1: Recommended adult dosage

Indication	*Dosage i.v. (mg ciprofloxacin)*
Treatment	
Gonorrhoea	100 mg single dose
Upper and lower urinary tract infections	100 mg b.d.
Upper and lower respiratory tract infections (depending on severity and sensitivity of causative organism)	200–400 mg b.d.
Pneumococcal pneumonia (second-line PL 0010/0148)	No recommended i.v. dosage, 750 mg p.o. b.d.
Cystic fibrosis patients with pseudomonal lower RTI†	400 mg b.d.
Other infections as detailed under *Therapeutic indications*	200–400 mg b.d.

† Although the pharmacokinetics of ciprofloxacin remains unchanged in patients with cystic fibrosis, the low bodyweight of these patients should be taken into consideration when determining dosage.

Impaired renal function: Dosage adjustments are not usually required, except in patients with severe renal impairment (serum creatinine >265 micromole/l or creatinine clearance <20 ml/minute). If adjustment is necessary, this may be achieved by reducing the total daily dose by half, although monitoring of drug serum levels provides the most reliable basis for dose adjustment.

Impaired hepatic function: No adjustment of dosage is necessary.

Elderly: Although higher ciprofloxacin serum levels are found in the elderly, no adjustment of dosage is necessary.

Adolescents and children: As with other drugs in its class, ciprofloxacin has been shown to cause arthropathy in weight-bearing joints of immature animals. Although analysis of available safety data from ciprofloxacin use in patients less than 18 years of age, the majority of whom had cystic fibrosis, did not disclose any evidence of drug-related cartilage or articular damage, its use in the paediatric patient population is generally not recommended.

Clinical and pharmacokinetic data support the use of ciprofloxacin in paediatric cystic fibrosis patients (aged 5–17 years) with acute pulmonary exacerbation associated with *P. aeruginosa* infection, at a dose of 10 mg/kg iv three times daily (maximum daily dose 1200 mg). The infusion should be administered over 60 minutes.

Sequential therapy can also be used. Dosage as follows: 10 mg/kg iv three times daily (maximum daily dose 1200 mg) followed by 20 mg/kg orally twice daily (maximum daily dose 1500 mg).

For indications other than treatment of pulmonary exacerbation in cystic fibrosis, ciprofloxacin may be used in children and adolescents where the benefit is considered to outweigh the potential risks. In these cases a dosage of 4–8 mg/kg iv twice daily or 5–15 mg/kg orally twice daily should be administered depending upon the severity of the infection.

Dosing in children with impaired renal and/or hepatic function has not been studied.

Duration of treatment: The duration of treatment depends upon the severity of infection, clinical response and bacteriological findings. The usual treatment period for acute infections is 5–7 days.

Generally, acute and chronic infections (e.g. osteomyelitis and prostatitis, etc), where the causative organism is known to be sensitive to ciprofloxacin, should be treated for at least three days after the signs and symptoms of the infection have disappeared.

For acute pulmonary exacerbation of cystic fibrosis associated with *P. aeruginosa* infection in paediatric patients (aged 5–17 years), the duration of treatment is 10–14 days.

Contra-indications: Ciprofloxacin is contra-indicated in patients who have shown hypersensitivity to ciprofloxacin or other quinolone anti-infectives.

Except in cases of exacerbation of CF associated with *P. aeruginosa* (in patients aged 5–17 years), ciprofloxacin is contra-indicated in children and growing adolescents unless the benefits of treatment are considered to outweigh the risks.

Special warnings and precautions for use: Ciprofloxacin should be used with caution in epileptics and patients with a history of CNS disorders and only if the benefits of treatment are considered to outweigh the risk of possible CNS side-effects.

Crystalluria related to the use of ciprofloxacin has been reported. Patients receiving ciprofloxacin should be well hydrated and excessive alkalinity of the urine should be avoided.

Patients with a family history of or actual defects in glucose-6-phosphate dehydrogenase activity are prone to haemolytic reactions with quinolones, and so ciprofloxacin should be used with caution in these patients.

Tendon inflammation and rupture may occur with quinolone antibiotics. Such reactions have been observed particularly in older patients and in those treated concurrently with corticosteroids. At the first sign of pain or inflammation, patients should discontinue ciprofloxacin and rest the affected limbs.

Interactions with other medicaments and other forms of interaction: Increased plasma levels of theophylline have been observed following concurrent administration with ciprofloxacin. It is recommended that the dose of theophylline should be reduced and plasma levels of theophylline monitored. Where monitoring of plasma levels is not possible, the use of ciprofloxacin should be avoided in patients receiving theophylline. Particular caution is advised in those patients with convulsive disorders.

Phenytion levels may be altered when Ciproxin is used concomitantly.

Prolongation of bleeding time has been reported during concomitant administration of ciprofloxacin and oral anti-coagulants.

Animal data have shown that high doses of quinolones in combination with some non-steroidal anti-inflammatory drugs (e.g. fenbufen, but not acetylsalicylic acid) can lead to convulsions.

Transient increases in serum creatinine have been seen following concomitant administration of ciprofloxacin and cyclosporin. Therefore, monitoring of serum creatinine levels is advisable.

The simultaneous administration of quinolones and glibenclamide can on occasion potentiate the effect of glibenclamide resulting in hypoglycaemia.

Concomitant use with probenecid reduces the renal clearance of ciprofloxacin, resulting in increased quinolone plasma levels.

Pregnancy and lactation: Reproduction studies performed in mice, rats and rabbits using parenteral and oral administration did not reveal any evidence of teratogenicity, impairment of fertility or impairment of peri-/post-natal development. However, as with other quinolones, ciprofloxacin has been shown to cause arthropathy in immature animals, and therefore its use during pregnancy is not recommended. Studies have indicated that ciprofloxacin is secreted in breast milk. Administration to nursing mothers is thus not recommended.

Effects on ability to drive and use machines: Ciprofloxacin could result in impairment of the patient's ability to drive or operate machinery, particularly in conjunction with alcohol.

Undesirable effects: Ciprofloxacin is generally well tolerated. The most frequently reported adverse reactions are: nausea, diarrhoea, vomiting, dyspepsia, abdominal pain, headache, restlessness, rash, dizziness and pruritus.

The following adverse reactions have been observed:

Local irritation including pain at the site of injection accompanied in a small number of patients by phlebitis or thrombophlebitis.

Gastro-intestinal disturbances, e.g. nausea, diarrhoea, vomiting, dyspepsia, abdominal pain, anorexia, flatulence, dysphagia. Rarely, pseudomembranous colitis.

CNS disturbances, e.g. headache, restlessness, depression, dizziness, tremor, convulsions, confusion, hallucinations, somnolence. Very rarely, sleep disorders and anxiety states. Isolated cases of ciprofloxacin-induced psychoses have been reported. There are isolated reports of intracranial hypertension associated with quinolone therapy. Paraesthesia has been reported.

Hypersensitivity/skin, e.g. rash, pruritus, urticaria, photosensitivity, drug-induced fever, anaphylactic/anaphylactoid reactions including angioedema and dyspnoea. Rarely, erythema nodosum and erythema multiforme. Very rarely, petechiae, haemorrhagic bullae, vasculitis, Stevens-Johnson Syndrome and Lyells Syndrome. Treatment with ciprofloxacin should be discontinued if any of the above occur upon first administration.

Hepatic disturbances, e.g. transient increases in liver enzymes or serum bilirubin (particularly in patients with previous liver damage), hepatitis, jaundice and major liver disorders including hepatic necrosis, which may rarely progress to hepatic failure.

Renal disturbances, e.g. transient increases in blood urea or serum creatinine, renal failure, crystalluria, nephritis.

Musculoskeletal disturbances, e.g. reversible arthralgia, joint swelling and myalgia. Rarely, tenosynovitis. Isolated cases of tendon inflammation have been reported which may lead to tendon rupture. Treatment should be discontinued immediately if these symptoms occur.

Effects on haematological parameters, e.g. eosinophilia, leucopenia, granulocytopenia, thrombocytopenia, thrombocytosis, altered prothrombin levels, and, very rarely, haemolytic anaemia or agranulocytosis.

Special sense disturbances, e.g. very rarely, visual disturbances, impaired taste and smell, tinnitus, transient impairment of hearing particularly at high frequencies.

Tachycardia has been reported.

Overdose: Based on the limited information available in two cases of ingestion of over 18 g of ciprofloxacin, reversible renal toxicity has occurred. Therefore, apart from routine emergency measures, it is recommended to monitor renal function, including urinary pH and acidify, if required, to prevent crystalluria. Patients must be kept well hydrated, and in the case of renal damage resulting in prolonged oliguria, dialysis should be initiated.

Serum levels of ciprofloxacin are reduced by dialysis.

Pharmacological properties

Pharmacodynamic properties: Ciprofloxacin is a synthetic 4-quinolone derivative, with bactericidal activity. It acts via inhibition of bacterial DNA gyrase, ultimately resulting in interference with DNA function. Ciprofloxacin is highly active against a wide range of Gram-positive and Gram-negative organisms and has shown activity against some anaerobes, *Chlamydia* spp. and *Mycoplasma* spp. Killing curves demonstrate the rapid bactericidal effect against sensitive organisms and it is often found that minimum bactericidal concentrations are in the range of minimum inhibitory concentrations. Ciprofloxacin has been shown to have no activity against *Treponema pallidum*, and *Ureaplasma urealyticum*, *Nocardia asteroides* and *Enterococcus faecium* are resistant.

Plasmid-related transfer of resistance has not been observed with ciprofloxacin and the overall frequency of development of resistance is low (10^{-9}–10^{-7}). Cross-resistance to penicillins, cephalosporins, aminoglycosides and tetracyclines has not been observed and organisms resistant to these antibiotics are generally sensitive to ciprofloxacin.

Ciprofloxacin is also suitable for use in combination with these antibiotics, and additive behaviour is usually observed.

Pharmacokinetic properties: Absorption of oral doses of ciprofloxacin 250 mg, 500 mg and 750 mg tablet formulation occurs rapidly, mainly from the small intestine, the half-life of absorption being 2–15 minutes. Plasma levels are dose-related and peak 0.5–1.5 hours after dosing. The AUC also increases dose proportionately after administration of both single and repeated oral (tablet) and intravenous doses. The pharmacokinetic profile of intravenous ciprofloxacin was shown to be linear over the dose range (100 mg–400 mg). Following intravenous administration of ciprofloxacin, the mean maximum plasma concentrations were achieved at the end of the infusion period. That is, for a 100 mg or 200 mg dose, 30 minutes, and for a 400 mg dose, 60 minutes. Reported plasma levels at this time point were 1.8 mg/l, 3.4 mg/l and 3.9 mg/l, respectively. The absolute bioavailability is reported to be 52–83% and ciprofloxacin is subject to only slight first-pass metabolism.

Distribution of ciprofloxacin within tissues is wide and the volume of distribution high, though slightly lower in the elderly. Protein binding is low (between 19–40%). Ciprofloxacin is present in plasma largely in a non-ionised form.

Only 10–20% of a single oral or intravenous dose is eliminated as metabolites (which exhibit lower activity than the parent drug). Four different antimicrobially active metabolites have been reported, desethyleneciprofloxacin (M1), sulphociprofloxacin (M2), oxaciprofloxacin (M3) and formylciprofloxacin (M4). M2 and M3 account for one third each of metabolised substance and M1 is found in small amounts (1.3–2.6% of the dose). M4 has been found in very small quantities (<0.1% of the dose). M1–M3 have antimicrobial activity comparable to nalidixic acid and M4 found in the smallest quantity has antimicrobial activity similar to that of norfloxacin.

Elimination of ciprofloxacin and its metabolites occurs rapidly, primarily by the kidney. After single oral and intravenous doses of ciprofloxacin, 55% and 75% respectively are eliminated by the kidney and 39% and 14% in the faeces within 5 days. Renal elimination takes place mainly during the first 12 hours after dosing and renal clearance levels suggest that active secretion by the renal tubules occurs in addition to normal glomerular filtration. Renal clearance is between 0.18–0.3 l/h.kg and total body clearance between 0.48–0.60 l/h.kg. Approximately 1% of a ciprofloxacin dose is excreted via the biliary route. The elimination kinetics are linear and after repeated dosing at 12 hourly intervals, no further accumulation is detected after the distribution equilibrium is attained (at 4–5 half-lives). The elimination half-life of unchanged ciprofloxacin over a period of 24–48 hours post-dose is 3.1–5.1 hours. A total body clearance of approximately 35 l/h was observed after intravenous administration.

Some studies carried out with ciprofloxacin in severely renally impaired patients (serum creatinine >265 micromole/l or creatinine clearance <20 ml/minute) demonstrated either a doubling of the elimination half-life, or fluctuations in half-life in comparison with healthy volunteers, whereas other studies showed no significant correlation between elimination half-life and creatinine clearance. However, it is recommended that in severely renally impaired patients, the total daily dose should be reduced by half, although monitoring of drug serum levels provides the most reliable basis for dose adjustment as necessary.

Results of pharmacokinetic studies in paediatric cystic fibrosis patients have shown dosages of 20 mg/kg orally twice daily or 10 mg/kg iv three times daily are recommended to achieve plasma concentration/time profiles comparable to those achieved in the adult population at the currently recommended dosage regimen.

Preclinical safety data: Following extensive oral and intravenous toxicology testing with ciprofloxacin, only two findings which may be considered relevant to the use of ciprofloxacin in man were observed. Crystalluria was noted in those species of animals which had a normally alkaline urine. Kidney damage without the presence of crystalluria was not observed. This effect is considered a secondary inflammatory foreign-body reaction, due to the precipitation of a crystalline complex of ciprofloxacin, magnesium and protein in the distal tubule system of the kidneys. This is considered not to be a problem in man, because the urine is normally acidic. However, to avoid the occurrence of crystalluria, patients should be well hydrated and excessive alkalinity of the urine avoided.

As with other quinolones, damage to the weight-bearing joints of only juvenile rats and dogs treated with ciprofloxacin was noted in repeat dose toxicity testing. This was more noticeable in the dog. Although analysis of available safety data from ciprofloxacin use in paediatric patients did not disclose any evidence of drug related cartilage or articular damage, the use of ciprofloxacin in children and growing adolescents is generally not recommended (with the exception of treatment of cystic fibrosis), unless the benefits are considered to outweigh the potential risks. Additionally, because of the potential of arthropathy, the use of ciprofloxacin during pregnancy and lactation is not recommended.

Pharmaceutical particulars

List of excipients: Lactic Acid 20%, prepared from Lactic Acid PhEur and Water for Injections PhEur, Dextrose (hydrous) PhEur, Hydrochloric Acid PhEur and Water for Injections PhEur.

Incompatibilities: The Ciproxin I.V. Flexibag should not be mixed with any other drug product or the co-infusion solution 10% Laevulose (D-fructose) since compatibility has not been established with these products. For compatible co-infusion solutions see *Instructions for use/handling.*

Shelf-life: For both the 100 ml and 200 ml presentations, the shelf-life is two years.

Special precautions for storage: Store between 5–25°C, protected from light; avoid excessive heat and protect from freezing.

Nature and contents of container: Clear PVC flexible container, with PVC administration port closure with a butadienestyrene copolymer cap, containing 100 ml or 200 ml of Ciproxin I.V. Flexibag solution, with an aluminium foil overwrap.

Instructions for use/handling: The Ciproxin I.V. Flexibag should be infused directly and be administered by short-term intravenous infusion over a period of 30–60 minutes. The 400 mg/200 ml dose should be administered over 60 minutes. The product should not be mixed with other drug products or the co-infusion solution 10% Laevulose (D-fructose). However, Ciproxin I.V. Flexibag has been shown to be compatible with Ringer's solution, 5% fructose solution, isotonic sodium chloride solution and 10% glucose solution. Unless compatibility is proven, the infusion solution should always be administered separately. In addition, discard any unused portion of product immediately after use.

Marketing authorisation number 0010/0220.

Date of approval/revision of SPC August 1998.

Legal category POM.

CIPROXIN* SUSPENSION

Qualitative and quantitative composition
Qualitative composition: Ciprofloxacin (INN)
Quantitative composition:

(i) **Per presentation**
5 g/100 ml (5% w/v)
1 bottle containing 7.95 g of film-coated granules containing 5.0 g ciprofloxacin (base form).
1 bottle containing 99.20 g of a non-aqueous diluent to prepare 100 ml of ready-to-use suspension.

(ii) **Per standard 5 ml dosage**
Each nominal 5 ml graduated measuring spoon (supplied with the product) contains 250 mg of ciprofloxacin.

Pharmaceutical form Gastro-resistant granules and non-aqueous diluent for reconstitution as a ready-to-use suspension for oral administration.

Clinical particulars
Therapeutic indications: Ciprofloxacin is indicated for the treatment of the following infections caused by sensitive bacteria:

Adults: Respiratory tract infections: e.g. lobar and bronchopneumonia, acute and chronic bronchitis, acute exacerbation of cystic fibrosis, bronchiectasis, empyema. Ciprofloxacin is not recommended as first-line therapy for the treatment of pneumococcal pneumonia. Ciprofloxacin may be used for treating Gram-negative pneumonia.

Ear, nose and throat infections: e.g. mastoiditis, otitis media and sinusitis, especially if due to Gram-negative bacteria (including *Pseudomonas* spp.). Ciprofloxacin is not recommended for the treatment of acute tonsillitis.

Eye infections: e.g. bacterial conjunctivitis.

Urinary tract infections: e.g. uncomplicated and complicated urethritis, cystitis, pyelonephritis, prostatitis, epididymitis.

Skin and soft tissue infections: e.g. infected ulcers, wound infections, abscesses, cellulitis, otitis externa, erysipelas, infected burns.

Bone and joint infections: e.g. osteomyelitis, septic arthritis.

Intra-abdominal infections: e.g. peritonitis, intra-abdominal abscesses.

Infections of the biliary tract: e.g. cholangitis, cholecystitis, empyema of the gall bladder.

Gastro-intestinal infections: e.g. enteric fever, infective diarrhoea.

Pelvic infections: e.g. salpingitis, endometritis, pelvic inflammatory disease.

Severe systemic infections: e.g. septicaemia, bacteraemia, peritonitis, infections in immuno-suppressed patients.

Gonorrhoea: including urethral, rectal and pharyngeal gonorrhoea caused by β-lactamase producing organisms or organisms moderately sensitive to penicillin.

Ciprofloxacin is also indicated for prophylaxis against infection in elective upper gastro-intestinal tract surgery and endoscopic procedures, where there is an increased risk of infection.

Children: For the treatment of acute pulmonary exacerbation of cystic fibrosis associated with *P. aeruginosa* infection in paediatric patients aged 5–17 years.

In-vitro investigations have indicated that ciprofloxacin is active against the following Gram-negative and Gram-positive organisms: *Citrobacter* spp., *Edwardsiella tarda, Enterobacter* spp., *Escherichia coli, Hafnia alvei, Klebsiella* spp., *Morganella morganii, Proteus* spp. (indole positive and indole negative), *Providencia* spp., *Salmonella* spp., *Serratia* spp., *Shigella* spp., *Yersinia* spp., *Aeromonas* spp., *Campylobacter coli, Campylobacter jejuni, Plesiomonas shigelloides, Pseudomonas aeruginosa, Vibrio* spp., *Haemophilus* spp., *Branhamella catarrhalis, Pasteurella multocida, Moraxella* spp., *Neisseria* spp., *Legionella* spp., *Brucella melitensis, Staphylococcus* spp., *Listeria monocytogenes, Corynebacterium* spp.

Ciprofloxacin is less active against the following organisms. Sensitivity testing should be performed before treatment is commenced: *Acinetobacter* spp., *Alcaligenes* spp., *Flavobacterium* spp., non-aeruginosa *Pseudomonas* spp., *Gardnerella vaginalis, Chlamydia* spp., *Mycoplasma* spp., *Mycobacterium tuberculosis, Mycobacterium fortuitum, Enterococcus faecalis, Streptococcus agalactiae, Streptococcus pneumoniae, Streptococcus pyogenes, viridans* streptococci.

Anaerobes vary in their susceptibility from being moderately sensitive to resistant. In particular, the *Bacteroides fragilis* group and *Clostridium difficile* are resistant.

In addition, the following organisms are resistant to ciprofloxacin: *Ureaplasma urealyticum, Nocardia asteroides, Enterococcus faecium.*

Ciprofloxacin is not active against *Treponema pallidum.*

In-vitro studies have shown that additive activity often results when ciprofloxacin is used concomitantly with other antibacterial agents.

Posology and method of administration: The dosage of Ciproxin Suspension is determined by the severity and type of infection, the sensitivity of the causative organism(s) and the age, weight and renal function of the patient.

The reconstituted suspension should be swallowed whole and the granules should not be chewed. A glass of water may be taken after dosing.

The dosage range for adults is 250–750 mg twice daily. The reconstituted suspension should always be dosed with the graduated measuring spoon provided. Each nominal 5.0 ml spoonful will deliver 250 mg ciprofloxacin. The ½ marking on the spoon will dose a nominal 2.5 ml of product. The 1/1 marking on the spoon will dose a nominal 5.0 ml of product.

Impaired renal function: Dosage adjustments are not usually required, except in patients with severe renal impairment (serum creatinine >265 micromole/l or creatinine clearance <20 ml/minute). If adjustment is necessary, this may be achieved by reducing the total daily dose by half, although monitoring of drug serum levels provides the most reliable basis for dose adjustment.

Impaired hepatic function: No adjustment of dosage is necessary.

Elderly: Although higher ciprofloxacin serum levels are found in the elderly, no adjustment of dosage is necessary.

Adolescents and children: As with other drugs in its class, ciprofloxacin has been shown to cause arthropathy in weight-bearing joints of immature animals.

Adults: The following dosages for specific types of infection are recommended.

Table 1: Recommended adult dosage

Indication	*Dosage (mg ciprofloxacin)*	*No. of spoonfuls (5 ml) of reconstituted Ciproxin Suspension**
Treatment		
Gonorrhoea	250 mg single dose	1 s.d.
Acute, uncomplicated cystitis	250 mg b.d.	1 b.d.
Upper and lower urinary tract infections (depending on severity)	250–500 mg b.d.	1 or 2 b.d.
Upper and lower respiratory tract infections (depending on severity)	250–750 mg b.d.	1, 2 or 3 b.d.
Pneumococcal pneumonia (second-line)	750 mg b.d.	3 b.d.
Cystic fibrosis patients with pseudomonal lower RTI**	750 mg b.d.	3 b.d.
Other infections as detailed under *Therapeutic indications*	500–750 mg b.d.	2 or 3 b.d.
Severe infections, particularly due to Pseudomonas, staphylococci and streptococci	750 mg b.d.	3 b.d.
Prophylaxis		
Elective upper gastro-intestinal surgical and endoscopic procedures	750 mg single dose 60–90 minutes prior to the procedure. If gastro-oesophageal obstructive lesions are suspected use with an anti-infective effective against anaerobes	3 s.d.

* For correct dosing always use the graduated measuring spoon supplied with the product.
** Although the pharmacokinetics of ciprofloxacin remains unchanged in patients with cystic fibrosis, the low bodyweight of these patients should be taken into consideration when determining dosage.

Although analysis of available safety data from ciprofloxacin use in patients less than 18 years of age, the majority of whom had cystic fibrosis, did not disclose any evidence of drug-related cartilage or articular damage, its use in the paediatric patient population is generally not recommended.

Clinical and pharmacokinetic data support the use of ciprofloxacin in paediatric cystic fibrosis patients (aged 5–17 years) with acute pulmonary exacerbation associated with *P. aeruginosa* infection, at a dose of 20 mg/kg orally twice daily (maximum daily dose 1500 mg).

For indications other than treatment of pulmonary exacerbation in cystic fibrosis, ciprofloxacin may be used in children and adolescents where the benefit is considered to outweigh the potential risks. In these cases a dosage of 4–8 mg/kg iv twice daily or 5–15 mg/kg orally twice daily should be administered depending upon the severity of infection. N.B. Ciproxin Suspension should not be used in children of less than two years of age (see *Special warnings and precautions for use*).

Dosing in children with impaired renal and/or hepatic function has not been studied.

Duration of treatment: The duration of treatment depends upon the severity of infection, clinical response and bacteriological findings.

In acute, uncomplicated cystitis the treatment period is three days.

In other acute infections the usual treatment period is 5–10 days. Generally, acute and chronic infections (e.g. osteomyelitis and prostatitis, etc), where the causative organism is known to be sensitive to ciprofloxacin, should be treated for at least three days after the signs and symptoms of the infection have disappeared.

For acute pulmonary exacerbation of cystic fibrosis associated with *P. aeruginosa* infection in paediatric patients (aged 5–17 years), the duration of treatment is 10–14 days.

Contra-indications: Ciprofloxacin is contra-indicated in patients who have shown hypersensitivity to ciprofloxacin or other quinolone anti-infectives.

Except in cases of exacerbation of CF associated with *P. aeruginosa* (in patients aged 5–17 years), ciprofloxacin is contra-indicated in children and growing adolescents unless the benefits of treatment are considered to outweigh the risks.

Ciproxin Suspension should not be used in children of less than two years of age (see *Special warnings and precautions for use*).

Special warnings and precautions for use: Ciprofloxacin should be used with caution in epileptics and patients with a history of CNS disorders and only if the benefits of treatment are considered to outweigh the risk of possible CNS side-effects.

Crystalluria related to the use of ciprofloxacin has been reported. Patients receiving ciprofloxacin should be well hydrated and excessive alkalinity of the urine should be avoided.

Patients with a family history of or actual defects in glucose-6-phosphate dehydrogenase activity are prone to haemolytic reactions with quinolones, and so ciprofloxacin should be used with caution in these patients.

Tendon inflammation and rupture may occur with quinolone antibiotics. Such reactions have been observed particularly in older patients and in those treated concurrently with corticosteroids. At the first sign of pain or inflammation, patients should discontinue ciprofloxacin and rest the affected limbs.

The tolerability of Ciproxin Suspension has not been investigated in children or adolescents. In addition, owing to the presence of lecithin in the suspension formulation, there is a theoretical possibility of increased gastro-intestinal side-effects in children of less than two years of age. Therefore, the product is not recommended for use in this patient group.

Interactions with other medicaments and other forms of interaction: Increased plasma levels of theophylline have been observed following concurrent administration with ciprofloxacin. It is recommended that the dose of theophylline should be reduced and plasma levels of theophylline monitored. Where monitoring of plasma levels is not possible, the use of ciprofloxacin should be avoided in patients receiving theophylline. Particular caution is advised in those patients with convulsive disorders.

Phenytion levels may be altered when Ciproxin is used concomitantly.

Ciproxin Suspension should not be administered within 4 hours of medications containing magnesium, aluminium, calcium or iron salts as interference with absorption may occur. When appropriate, patients should be advised not to self-medicate with preparations containing these compounds during therapy with ciprofloxacin.

Prolongation of bleeding time has been reported during concomitant administration of ciprofloxacin and oral anti-coagulants.

Animal data have shown that high doses of quinolones in combination with some non-steroidal anti-inflammatory drugs (e.g. fenbufen, but not acetysalicylic acid), can lead to convulsions.

Transient increases in serum creatinine have been seen following concomitant administration of ciprofloxacin and cyclosporin. Therefore, monitoring of serum creatinine levels is advisable.

The simultaneous administration of quinolones and glibenclamide can on occasion potentiate the effect of glibenclamide resulting in hypoglycaemia.

Concomitant use with probenecid reduces the renal clearance of ciprofloxacin, resulting in increased quinolone plasma levels.

The use of metoclopramide with ciprofloxacin may accelerate the absorption of ciprofloxacin.

When Ciproxin Suspension is used for surgical prophylaxis, it is recommended that opiate premedicants (e.g. papaveretum), or opiate premedicants used with anticholinergic pre-medicants (e.g. atropine, or hyoscine), are not used, as the serum levels of ciprofloxacin are reduced and adequate cover may not be obtained during surgery. Co-administration of ciprofloxacin and benzodiazepine premedicants has been shown not to affect ciprofloxacin plasma levels.

Pregnancy and lactation: Reproduction studies performed in mice, rats and rabbits using parenteral and oral administration did not reveal any evidence of teratogenicity, impairment of fertility or impairment of peri-/post-natal development. However, as with other quinolones, ciprofloxacin has been shown to cause arthropathy in immature animals, and therefore its use during pregnancy is not recommended. Studies have indicated that ciprofloxacin is secreted in breast milk. Administration to nursing mothers is thus not recommended.

Effects on ability to drive and use machines: Ciprofloxacin could result in impairment of the patient's ability to drive or operate machinery, particularly in conjunction with alcohol.

Undesirable effects: Ciprofloxacin is generally well tolerated. The most frequently reported adverse reactions are: nausea, diarrhoea, vomiting, dyspepsia, abdominal pain, headache, restlessness, rash, dizziness and pruritus.

The following adverse reactions have been observed:

Gastro-intestinal disturbances, e.g. nausea, diarrhoea, vomiting, dyspepsia, abdominal pain, anorexia, flatulence, dysphagia. Rarely, pseudomembranous colitis.

CNS disturbances, e.g. headache, restlessness, depression, dizziness, tremor, convulsions, confusion, hallucinations, somnolence. Very rarely, sleep disorders and anxiety states. Isolated cases of ciprofloxacin-induced psychoses have been reported. There are isolated reports of intracranial hypertension associated with quinolone therapy. Paraesthesia has been reported.

Hypersensitivity/skin, e.g. rash, pruritus, urticaria, photosensitivity, drug-induced fever, anaphylactic/anaphylactoid reactions including angioedema or dyspnoea. Rarely, erythema nodosum and erythema multiforme. Very rarely, petechiae, haemorrhagic bullae, vasculitis, Stevens-Johnson Syndrome and Lyells Syndrome. Treatment with ciprofloxacin should be discontinued if any of the above occur upon first administration.

Hepatic disturbances, e.g. transient increases in liver enzymes or serum bilirubin (particularly in patients with previous liver damage), hepatitis, jaundice and major liver disorders including hepatic necrosis, which may rarely progress to hepatic failure.

Renal disturbances, e.g. transient increases in blood urea or serum creatinine, renal failure, crystalluria, nephritis.

Musculoskeletal disturbances, e.g. reversible arthralgia, joint swelling and myalgia. Rarely, tenosynovitis. Isolated cases of tendon inflammation have been reported which may lead to tendon rupture. Treatment should be discontinued immediately if these symptoms occur.

Effects on haematological parameters, e.g. eosinophilia, leucopenia, granulocytopenia, thrombocytopenia, thrombocytosis, altered prothrombin levels, and, very rarely, haemolytic anaemia or agranulocytosis.

Special sense disturbances, e.g. very rarely, visual disturbances, impaired taste and smell, tinnitus, transient impairment of hearing particularly at high frequencies.

Tachycardia has been reported.

Overdose: Based on the limited information available in two cases of ingestion of over 18 g of ciprofloxacin, reversible renal toxicity has occurred. Therefore, apart from routine emergency measures, it is recommended to monitor renal function, including urinary pH and acidify, if required, to prevent crystalluria. Patients must be kept well hydrated, and in the case of renal damage resulting in prolonged oliguria, dialysis should be initiated.

Calcium or magnesium antacids may be administered as soon as possible after ingestion of Ciproxin Suspension in order to reduce the absorption of ciprofloxacin.

Serum levels of ciprofloxacin are reduced by dialysis.

Pharmacological properties

Pharmacodynamic properties: Ciprofloxacin is a synthetic 4-quinolone derivative, with bactericidal activity. It acts via inhibition of bacterial DNA gyrase, ultimately resulting in interference with DNA function. Ciprofloxacin is highly active against a wide range of Gram-positive and Gram-negative organisms and has shown activity against some anaerobes, *Chlamydia* spp. and *Mycoplasma* spp. Killing curves demonstrate the rapid bactericidal effect against sensitive organisms and it is often found that minimum bactericidal concentrations are in the range of minimum inhibitory concentrations. Ciprofloxacin has been shown to have no activity against *Treponema pallidum*, and *Ureaplasma urealyticum, Nocardia asteroides* and *Enterococcus faecium* are resistant.

Plasmid-related transfer of resistance has not been observed with ciprofloxacin and the overall frequency of development of resistance is low (10^{-9}–10^{-7}). Cross-resistance to penicillins, cephalosporins, aminoglycosides and tetracyclines has not been observed and organisms resistant to these antibiotics are generally sensitive to ciprofloxacin. Ciprofloxacin is also suitable for use in combination with these antibiotics, and additive behaviour is usually observed.

Pharmacokinetic properties: Absorption of oral doses of ciprofloxacin 250 mg, 500 mg and 750 mg tablet formulation occurs rapidly, mainly from the small intestine, the half-life of absorption being 2–15 minutes. Plasma levels are dose-related and peak 0.5–2.0 hours after dosing. The AUC also increases dose proportionately after administration of both single and repeated oral (tablet) and intravenous doses. Bioequivalence of the same dose of the tablet formulation with that of the suspension formulation has been demonstrated. Plasma levels peak approximately 1.5–2.5 hours after dosing and the $AUC_{0-\infty}$ is in the range of 5–12 mg.h/l. The absolute bioavailability is reported to be 52–83% and ciprofloxacin is subject to only slight first pass metabolism. The oral bioavailability is approximately 70–80%.

The intake of food at the same time as administration of oral ciprofloxacin (tablet of suspension) has a marginal but clinically not relevant effect on the pharmacokinetic parameters C_{max} and AUC. In a food effect study with the suspension formulation, C_{max} was decreased by 11% and the AUC increased by 13% after administration of the suspension with food. However, there was no significant decrease in the rate and extent of absorption compared with administration of the suspension without food. Therefore, no specific recommendations are necessary with regard to time of administration of the suspension relative to food intake.

Distribution of ciprofloxacin within tissues is wide and the volume of distribution high, though slightly lower in the elderly. Protein binding is low (between 19–40%).

Only 10–20% of a single oral or intravenous dose is eliminated as metabolites (which exhibit lower activity than the parent drug). Four different antimicrobially active metabolites have been reported, desethyleneciprofloxacin (M1), sulphociprofloxacin (M2), oxaciprofloxacin (M3) and formylciprofloxacin (M4). M2 and M3 account for one third each of metabolised substance and M1 is found in small amounts (1.3–2.6% of the dose). M4 has been found in very small quantities (<0.1% of the dose). M1–M3 have antimicrobial activity comparable to nalidixic acid and M4 found in the smallest quantity has antimicrobial activity similar to that of norfloxacin.

Elimination of ciprofloxacin and its metabolites occurs rapidly, primarily by the kidney. After single oral and intravenous doses of ciprofloxacin, 55% and 75% respectively are eliminated by the kidney and 39% and 14% in the faeces within 5 days. Renal elimination takes place mainly during the first 12 hours after dosing and renal clearance levels suggest that active secretion by the renal tubules occurs in addition to normal glomerular filtration. Renal clearance is between 0.18–0.3 l/h.kg and total body clearance between 0.48–0.60 l/h.kg. Approximately 1% of a ciprofloxacin dose is excreted via the biliary route. The elimination kinetics are linear and after repeated dosing at 12 hourly intervals, no further accumulation is detected after the distribution equilibrium is attained (at 4–5 half-lives). The elimination half-life of unchanged ciprofloxacin over a period of 24–48 hours post-dose is 3.1–5.1 hours.

Some studies carried out with ciprofloxacin in severely renally impaired patients (serum creatinine >265 micromole/l or creatinine clearance <20 ml/

minute) demonstrated either a doubling of the elimination half-life, or fluctuations in half-life in comparison with healthy volunteers, whereas other studies showed no significant correlation between elimination half-life and creatinine clearance. However, it is recommended that in severely renally impaired patients, the total daily dose should be reduced by half, although monitoring of drug serum levels provides the most reliable basis for dose adjustment as necessary.

Results of pharmacokinetic studies in paediatric cystic fibrosis patients have shown dosages of 20 mg/kg orally twice daily or 10 mg/kg iv three times daily are recommended to achieve plasma concentration/time profiles comparable to those achieved in the adult population at the currently recommended dosage regimen.

Preclinical safety data: Following extensive oral and intravenous toxicology testing with ciprofloxacin, only two findings which may be considered relevant to the use of ciprofloxacin in man were observed. Crystalluria was noted in those species of animals which had a normally alkaline urine. Kidney damage without the presence of crystalluria was not observed. This effect is considered a secondary inflammatory foreign-body reaction, due to the precipitation of a crystalline complex of ciprofloxacin, magnesium and protein in the distal tubule system of the kidneys. This is considered not to be a problem in man, because the urine is normally acidic. However, to avoid the occurrence of crystalluria, patients should be well hydrated and excessive alkalinity of the urine avoided.

As with other quinolones, damage to the weight-bearing joints of only juvenile rats and dogs treated with ciprofloxacin was noted in repeat dose toxicity testing. This was more noticeable in the dog. Although analysis of available safety data from ciprofloxacin used in paediatric patients did not disclose any evidence of drug related cartilage or articular damage, the use of ciprofloxacin in children and growing adolescents is generally not recommended, unless the benefits are considered to outweigh the potential risks (with the exception of treatment of cystic fibrosis). Additionally, because of the potential of arthropathy, the use of ciprofloxacin during pregnancy and lactation is not recommended.

Pharmaceutical particulars

List of excipients:

(i) *Film-coated granules*
Copolymer of ethyl acrylate and methyl methacrylate, magnesium stearate, methylhydroxypropylcellulose, polysorbate 20, polyvidone 25.

(ii) *Diluent*
Lecithin, medium chain triglycerides, sucrose, purified water, strawberry flavours.

Incompatibilities: No other products should be added to the re-constituted suspension.

Shelf-life:

(i) *Shelf-life of packaged product*
Film-coated granules: 2 years
Diluent: 2 years

(ii) *Shelf-life of re-constituted suspension*
In a refrigerator (2–8°C), 14 days
At room temperature (up to 30°C), 14 days.

Special precautions for storage

(i) *Packaged product*
Film-coated granules: Do not store above 25°C.
Diluent: Protect from freezing. Do not store above 25°C. Avoid inverted storage. Occasionally a slight yellow layer is observed on the surface of the sucrose in the diluent prior to resuspending. However, upon shaking, this layer is dispersed and has been shown to have no influence on the quality of the product.

(ii) *Re-constituted suspension*
Avoid inverted storage.

Nature and contents of container

(i) *Film-coated granules:* Brown glass Type III narrow-necked bottle with a PP/PE child resistant closure.

(ii) *Diluent:* Plastic PE white transparent bottle with sealing insert and white opaque PP child resistant screw cap.

(iii) *Re-constituted suspension:* This is the same container as is used for the diluent prior to reconstitution.

(iv) *Measuring spoon:* Blue opaque PE with graduation marks.

The above (iii) contains a nominal 100 ml of re-constituted ready-to-use suspension. For quantities of (i) and (ii) see *Qualitative and quantitative composition.*

Instructions for use/handling

(i) *Preparation of the re-constituted suspension*

The re-constituted suspension is prepared for use as follows:

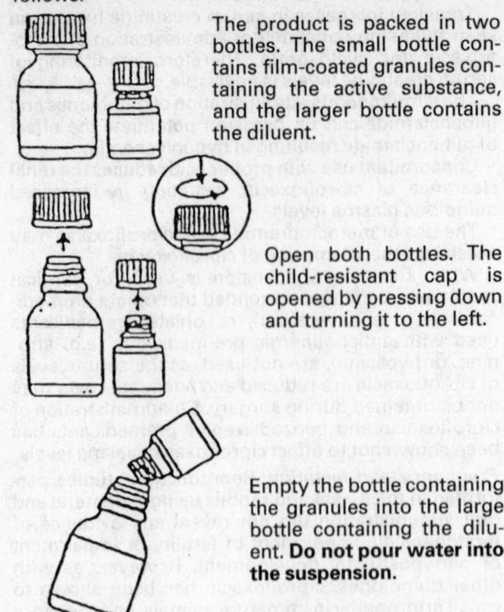

The product is packed in two bottles. The small bottle contains film-coated granules containing the active substance, and the larger bottle contains the diluent.

Open both bottles. The child-resistant cap is opened by pressing down and turning it to the left.

Empty the bottle containing the granules into the large bottle containing the diluent. **Do not pour water into the suspension.**

Re-close the large bottle and shake it vigorously **horizontally** for approx. 15 seconds. The suspension is now ready for use.

(ii) *Dosing the re-constituted suspension*

The re-constituted suspension should be shaken vigorously for approx. 15 seconds prior to each dosage. In order to ensure correct dosing, each dose should be measured into the graduated measuring spoon provided with the product. The ½ marking will dose a nominal 2.5 ml of product, the $\frac{1}{1}$ marking will dose a nominal 5.0 ml of product. The re-constituted suspension should be swallowed whole and the granules should **not** be chewed. A glass of water may be taken after dosing of the suspension. Reclose the bottle properly after use according to the instructions on the cap.

After the treatment period, the re-constituted suspension should not be stored and re-used. It should be disposed of.

Marketing authorisation holder

Bayer plc, Bayer House, Strawberry Hill, Newbury, Berkshire RG14 1JA

Trading as: Bayer plc, Pharmaceutical Division, Bayer House, Strawberry Hill, Newbury, Berkshire RG14 1JA, or Baypharm.

Marketing authorisation number PL 0010/0211

Date of first authorisation/renewal of authorisation
19 April 1996.

Date of revision of the text August 1998.

Legal category POM.

DTIC-DOME 200 mg

Qualitative and quantitative composition Each vial contains 200 mg dacarbazine citrate equivalent to 200 mg of dacarbazine USP.

Pharmaceutical form DTIC-DOME is a sterile, colourless to ivory-coloured solid to be reconstituted with Water for Injections BP for intravenous administration.

Clinical particulars

Therapeutic indications: The treatment of metastatic malignant melanoma, sarcoma and Hodgkin's disease. In addition, dacarbazine has been shown, when used in combination with other cytotoxic agents, to be of value in treatment of other malignant diseases, including: carcinoma of the colon, ovary, breast, lung, testicular teratoma, and solid tumours in children.

Posology and method of administration

Dosage:

Adults: The following standard dosage schedules are recommended:

1. 2.0 to 4.5 mg/kg/day for 10 days, which may be repeated at four week intervals.
2. 250 mg/m²/day for five days, which may be repeated at three week intervals.
3. A further alternative is to administer the total schedule on the first day.

Other schedules may be used at the discretion of the physician.

Children: The dosage for children is calculated on a mg/kg or mg/m² basis as per the standard adult dose.

Administration: DTIC/DOME 200 mg vials are reconstituted with 19.7 ml of Water for Injections BP. The resulting solution contains dacarbazine 10 mg/ml, citric acid and mannitol, at pH 3.0 to 4.0. After the solution has been prepared, the calculated dose is drawn into a syringe and injected intravenously. Injection may be completed in approximately one minute.

If desired, the reconstituted solution may be diluted further with 125 to 250 ml of Dextrose Injection BP 5% or Sodium Chloride Injection BP 0.9% and administered by intravenous infusion over a period of 15 to 30 minutes.

Contra-indications: Patients who are hypersensitive to dacarbazine.

Special warnings and precautions for use: DTIC-DOME should be administered preferably to patients who are hospitalised and who can be observed carefully and frequently during and after therapy, with particular reference to the haemopoeitic system.

Care must be taken to avoid extravasation of the drug subcutaneously during intravenous administration as this may result in tissue damage and severe pain.

It is recommended that DTIC-DOME be administered under the supervision of a physician experienced in the use of cancer chemotherapeutic agents. Since facilities for necessary laboratory studies must be available, hospitalisation is recommended.

Interactions with other medicaments and other forms of interaction: None known.

Pregnancy and lactation: DTIC-DOME is teratogenic. DTIC-DOME should not normally be administered to patients who are pregnant or to mothers who are breast feeding.

Effects on ability to drive and use machines: None known.

Undesirable effects: Haemopoietic depression is the most common toxic side-effect of dacarbazine and involves primarily the leucocytes and platelets, although mild anaemia may sometimes occur. Leucopenia and thrombocytopenia may be severe enough to cause death. The possible bone marrow depression requires careful monitoring of white blood cell, red blood cell and platelet levels. Haemopoietic toxicity may warrant temporary suspension or cessation of dacarbazine therapy.

Symptoms of anorexia, nausea and vomiting are the most frequently noticed side-effects. Over 90% of patients are affected with the first few doses. The vomiting lasts for 1–12 hours and may be completely but unpredictably palliated by prochlorperazine. Rarely, dacarbazine causes diarrhoea in which case restricting the patient's oral intake of fluids and food four to six hours prior to treatment may be helpful. The rapid toleration of these symptoms suggests a central nervous system mechanism, and usually these symptoms subside after the first one or two days.

Infrequently, some patients have experienced an influenza-like syndrome of fever to 39°C, myalgias and malaise. This syndrome occurs usually after large single doses and approximately seven days after treatment with dacarbazine and lasts 7–21 days, and may recur with successive treatments.

Alopecia has been noted, as has facial flushing and facial paraesthesia.

Hepatic toxicity, accompanied by hepatic vein thrombosis and hepatocellular necrosis resulting in death, has been reported. The incidence of such reactions has been low; approximately 0.01% of patients treated. This toxicity has been observed mostly when dacarbazine has been administered concomitantly with other anti-neoplastic drugs; however, it has also been reported in some patients treated with dacarbazine alone.

Anaphylaxis can occur very rarely following administration of dacarbazine.

Erythematous and urticarial rashes have been observed infrequently after administration of dacarbazine.

Rarely, photosensitivity reactions may occur.

Overdose: No information available.

Pharmacological properties

Pharmacodynamic properties: Dacarbazine is a cell cycle non-specific antineoplastic agent.

Although the exact mechanism of action of dacarbazine is unknown, three hypotheses have been proposed:

1. Inhibition of DNA synthesis by acting as a purine analogue.
2. Action as an alkylating agent.
3. Interaction with sulphydryl groups.

Pharmacokinetic properties: A pharmacokinetic study in 6 patients at a dose range of 4.8–9 mg/kg body weight (single intravenous injection) showed an average plasma half-life of 38 minutes. A further study in 6 patients at a dose of 4.5 mg/kg body weight by single intravenous administration resulted in a mean plasma half-life of 75 minutes, and after an oral dose of 4.5 mg/kg body weight to four patients the plasma half-life was 66 minutes. Dacarbazine is not significantly protein bound (approximately 5%).

Preclinical safety data: The drug has been shown to be teratogenic and carcinogenic in animals.

Pharmaceutical particulars
List of excipients: Citric acid, Mannitol.

Incompatibilities: None known.

Shelf-life: DTIC-DOME can be stored for up to 48 months under refrigeration (2°C to 8°C) and protected from light.

After reconstitution with Water for Injections BP, the solution may be stored, suitably protected from light, at 4°C to 72 hours or at normal room temperature (20°C) for up to 8 hours.

Following reconstitution, if the solution is diluted further in Dextrose Injection BP 5% or Sodium Chloride Injection BP 0.9%, the resulting solution may be stored at 4°C for up to 24 hours.

Special precautions for storage: The product should be protected from light and stored in the manufacturer's original container in a refrigerator between 2°C and 8°C.

The reconstituted solution should be protected from light.

Nature and contents of container: 20 ml amber glass vial with butyl rubber stopper and aluminium seal containing 200 mg DTIC-DOME as sterile dacarbazine.

Instructions for use/handling: Users should avoid contact of DTIC-DOME with the skin and eyes when reconstituting or administering.

Marketing authorisation holder
Bayer plc, Bayer House, Strawberry Hill, Newbury, Berkshire RG14 1JA.

Trading as: Phamaceutical Division, Baypharm or Baymet.

Marketing authorisation number PL 0010/0128

Date of first authorisation/renewal of authorisation
Date of first authorisation: 12 March 1984
Date of last renewal: 30 October 1992

Date of (partial) revision of the text January 1998

Legal category POM.

GLUCOBAY* 50
GLUCOBAY* 100

Presentation *Glucobay 50:* Off-white round tablets of diameter 7 mm, each containing 50 mg acarbose. One side marked G50 and the reverse side marked with the Bayer cross.

Glucobay 100: Off-white round tablets of diameter 9 mm, each containing 100 mg acarbose. One side marked G100 with a scoreline and the reverse side marked with the Bayer cross.

Uses
Mode of action: Glucobay is a competitive inhibitor of intestinal alpha-glucosidases with maximum specific inhibitory activity against sucrase. Under the influence of Glucobay, the digestion of starch and sucrose into absorbable monosaccharides in the small intestine is dose-dependently delayed. In diabetic subjects, this results in a lowering of postprandial hyperglycaemia and a smoothing effect on fluctuations in the daily blood glucose profile.

In contrast to sulphonylureas Glucobay has no stimulatory action on the pancreas.

Treatment with Glucobay also results in a reduction of fasting blood glucose and to modest changes in levels of glycated haemoglobin (HbA_1, HbA_{1c}). The changes may be a reduction or reduced deterioration in HbA_1 or HbA_{1c} levels, depending upon the patient's clinical status and disease progression. These parameters are affected in a dose-dependent manner by Glucobay.

Following oral administration, only 1–2% of the active inhibitor is absorbed.

Indications: Glucobay is recommended for the treatment of non-insulin dependent (NIDDM) diabetes mellitus in patients inadequately controlled on diet alone, or on diet and oral hypoglycaemic agents.

Dosage and administration Glucobay tablets are taken orally and should be chewed with the first mouthful of food, or swallowed whole with a little liquid directly before the meal. Owing to the great individual variation of glucosidase activity in the intestinal mucosa, there is no fixed dosage regimen, and patients should be treated according to clinical response and tolerance of intestinal side-effects.

Adults: The recommended initial dose is 50 mg three times a day. However, some patients may benefit from more gradual initial dose titration to minimise gastro-intestinal side-effects. This may be achieved by initiating treatment at 50 mg once or twice a day with subsequent titration to a three times a day regimen.

If after six to eight weeks' treatment patients show an inadequate clinical response, the dosage may be increased to 100 mg three times a day. A further increase in dosage to a maximum of 200 mg three times a day may occasionally be necessary. Patients receiving the maximum dose require careful monitoring (see Warnings and Precautions).

Glucobay is intended for continuous long-term treatment.

Elderly patients: No modification of the normal adult dosage regimen is necessary.

Contra-indications, warnings, etc
Contra-indications: Hypersensitivity to acarbose or any of the excipients, use in children aged less than 12 years, pregnancy and in nursing mothers. Glucobay is also contra-indicated in patients with inflammatory bowel disease, colonic ulceration, partial intestinal obstruction or in patients predisposed to intestinal obstruction. In addition, Glucobay should not be used in patients who have chronic intestinal diseases associated with marked disorders of digestion or absorption and in patients who suffer from states which may deteriorate as a result of increased gas formation in the intestine, e.g. larger hernias.

Glucobay is contra-indicated in patients with hepatic impairment.

As Glucobay has not been studied in patients with severe renal impairment, it should not be used in patients with a creatinine clearance of <25 ml/min/1.73 m².

Warnings and precautions
Hypoglycaemia: When administered alone, Glucobay does not cause hypoglycaemia. It may, however, act to potentiate the hypoglycaemic effects of insulin and sulphonylurea drugs, and the dosages of these agents may need to be modified accordingly. Episodes of hypoglycaemia occurring during therapy must, where appropriate, be treated by the administration of glucose, not sucrose. This is because acarbose will delay the digestion and absorption of disaccharides, but not monosaccharides.

Transaminases: Patients treated with acarbose may, on rare occasions, experience an idiosyncratic response with either symptomatic or asymptomatic hepatic dysfunction. In the majority of cases this dysfunction is reversible on discontinuation of acarbose therapy. It is recommended that liver enzyme monitoring is considered during the first six to twelve months of treatment. If elevated transaminases are observed, withdrawal of therapy may be warranted, particularly if the elevations persist. In such circumstances, patients should be monitored at weekly intervals until normal values are established.

Intestinal adsorbents (e.g. charcoal) and digestive enzyme preparations containing carbohydrate splitting enzymes (e.g. amylase, pancreatin) may reduce the effect of Glucobay and should not therefore be taken concomitantly.

The concomitant administration of neomycin may lead to enhanced reductions of postprandial blood glucose and to an increase in the frequency and severity of gastro-intestinal side-effects. If the symptoms are severe, a temporary dose reduction of Glucobay may be warranted.

The concomitant administration of cholestyramine may enhance the effects of Glucobay, particularly with respect to reducing postprandial insulin levels. In the rare circumstance that both acarbose and cholestyramine therapy are withdrawn simultaneously, care is needed as a rebound phenomenon has been observed with respect to insulin levels in non-diabetic subjects.

In a pilot study to investigate a possible interaction between Glucobay and nifedipine, no significant or reproducible changes were observed in the plasma nifedipine profiles.

Side-effects: Owing to its mode of action, Glucobay results in a greater proportion of dietary carbohydrate being digested in the large bowel. This carbohydrate may also be utilised by the intestinal flora, resulting in the increased formation of intestinal gas. The majority of patients are therefore likely to experience one or more symptoms related to this, particularly flatulence, borborygmi and a feeling of fullness. Abdominal distension, abdominal pain, softer stools and diarrhoea may occur, particularly after sugar or sucrose-containing foods have been ingested. Rarely, these gastrointestinal reactions may be severe and might be confused with paralytic ileus.

The symptoms are both dose and dietary substrate related, and may subside with continued treatment. Symptoms can be reduced by adherence to the prescribed diabetic diet and the avoidance of sucrose or foodstuffs containing sugar. If symptoms are poorly tolerated, a reduction in dosage is recommended.

Should diarrhoea persist, patients should be closely monitored and the dosage reduced, or therapy withdrawn, if necessary.

The administration of antacid preparations containing magnesium and aluminium salts, e.g. hydrotalcite, has been shown not to ameliorate the acute gastrointestinal symptoms of Glucobay and should therefore not be recommended to patients for this purpose.

Rarely, a transient elevation of serum hepatic transaminases may be observed. Very rarely, jaundice and hepatitis have been reported. Skin reactions may occur rarely.

Overdosage: No information on overdosage is available. No specific antidotes to Glucobay are known.

Intake of carbohydrate-containing meals or beverages should be avoided for 4–6 hours.

Diarrhoea should be treated by standard conservative measures.

Pharmaceutical precautions The tablets should be stored in the manufacturer's original container in a dry place at temperatures below 25°C.

Legal category POM.

Package quantities Blister packs in a cardboard outer containing:
Glucobay 50: 90 tablets
Glucobay 100: 90 tablets.

Product licence numbers
Glucobay 50 0010/0171
Glucobay 100 0010/0172

KOGENATE* 250
KOGENATE* 500
KOGENATE* 1000

Presentation Kogenate is a sterile, lyophilised recombinant human Factor VIII preparation for reconstitution with Water for Injections. Kogenate is available as single-dose vials containing 250, 500 or 1000 I.U. octocog alfa (Factor VIII (rDNA) (bhk)). Glycine, sodium chloride, calcium chloride and human albumin are present as excipients.

A vial containing a suitable volume of Water for Injections for reconstitution, a sterile administration set and two alcohol swabs are also provided.

Uses Kogenate is indicated in congenital Factor VIII deficiency (haemophilia A) for the treatment and prophylaxis of bleeding in both untreated and previously treated patients without inhibitors. Treatment can be continued in patients who develop Factor VIII inhibitors (neutralising antibodies, less than 10 Bethesda Units (B.U.)) who continue to respond to Kogenate.

Kogenate does not contain von Willebrand Factor and hence is not indicated in von Willebrand's disease.

Dosage and administration
Dosage: Clinical studies have demonstrated a mean rise of about 2% in Factor VIII activity for each unit of Kogenate administered per kg body weight. The following formulae may be used to estimate (I) the appropriate dose required for a given response, or (II) the response to be expected from a given dose:

I. Required I.U. = body weight (kg) × desired Factor VIII rise (% of normal) × 0.5

II. Expected Factor VIII rise (% of normal) = $\dfrac{2 \times \text{administered I.U.}}{\text{body weight (kg)}}$

The dosage and duration of the substitution therapy should be based upon the patient's body weight, the degree of Factor VIII deficiency, the site and extent of the bleeding, the titre of inhibitors, the Factor VIII level desired and the clinical course. The following provides a guide for Factor VIII minimum blood levels.

Treatment of haemorrhage: The required Factor VIII minimum activity (in % of normal) is set out below. These minimal values should be maintained for the specified duration:

Minor haemorrhage (haemorrhage into joints): The therapeutically required plasma level of Factor VIII activity is 30% of normal, maintained for at least one day, and is dependent on the severity of haemorrhage.

Moderate to major haemorrhage (e.g. haemorrhage into muscles or into the oral cavity), surgery (e.g. tooth extraction, operations of medium duration) and mild cranial trauma: The therapeutically required plasma level of Factor VIII activity is 40–50% of normal maintained for three to four days or until adequate wound healing.

Major to life-threatening haemorrhage (e.g. intracranial, intra-abdominal or intrathoracic haemorrhages, gastro-intestinal bleeding), major operations (e.g. cardiovascular, orthopaedic surgery) and fractures: The therapeutically required plasma level of Factor VIII activity is 60–100% of normal, maintained for seven days, then therapy for another seven days to maintain the Factor VIII level at 30–50% of normal.

Note: The dose and the frequency of administration should be adapted according to the clinical effectiveness in each individual case. Larger amounts than those calculated may be required, especially at the beginning of treatment.

Prophylaxis of haemophilia A: In short or long-term prophylaxis of haemophilia A, doses of 10 to 50 I.U. Kogenate per kg body weight administered at intervals of two to three days have been successful in limiting the number of recurrent bleeding episodes. In some cases, especially in younger patients, shorter dosage intervals or higher doses may be necessary.

Patients with Factor VIII inhibitors: Kogenate remains efficacious in patients who have developed Factor VIII inhibitors (neutralising antibodies, less than 10 Bethesda Units (B.U.)), during treatment with Kogenate.

Factor VIII levels and inhibitor titres must be assessed to ensure adequate replacement therapy. The control of bleeding in patients with a high titre of inhibitors (typically above 10 Bethesda Units) may require extensive Factor VIII concentrate infusion therapy but might be impractical because of the very large dose needed to maintain adequate Factor VIII levels. If haemostasis cannot be achieved with Factor VIII concentrate in the presence of high-titre inhibitors, the use of (activated) prothrombin complex concentrate (PCC) should be considered. Such therapy should be undertaken by physicians experienced in the care of patients with haemophilia A.

Reconstitution and administration: Sterile conditions are required. Kogenate is intended for intravenous administration only and must be administered within four hours of reconstitution. Do not refrigerate after reconstitution.

Prior to use, clean the rubber stoppers of each vial with the alcohol swabs provided. Ensure that the solvent and the concentrate are warmed to room temperature first (maximum 37°C). To reconstitute the lyophilised powder, add the Water for Injections to the vial containing the lyophilised powder, using the transfer device provided. Use only the solvent provided. Ensure that all the solvent is drawn into the other vial. Remove the solvent vial and transfer device. Swirl continuously until the powder is completely dissolved. **Ensure** that Kogenate is completely dissolved before administration, i.e. a clear liquid is obtained.

Attach the filter needle to the syringe, insert into the rubber stopper of the vial containing the diluted Kogenate after swabbing the stopper, and fill the syringe as required. Remove the filled syringe from the filter needle (which should remain attached to the vial). Attach the venepuncture set to the syringe. Once ready to infuse, transfer Kogenate solution into the venepuncture set by depressing the syringe plunger until the tube is two-thirds full. Puncture vein and secure venepuncture set. Ensure no blood enters the syringe. The reconstituted Kogenate solution should be administered slowly, at not more than 1–2 ml per minute. Discard any unused solution.

If a further dose is required, leave the syringe connected to the venepuncture set until administration of the further dose. Fill a new syringe with reconstituted Kogenate and administer (as above). Remove venepuncture set once all doses have been given, apply pressure to injection site (for approximately two minutes) and apply a small pressure dressing.

Contra-indications, warnings, etc

Contra-indications: Known hypersensitivity to mouse or hamster protein (see Warnings).

Caution is advised in patients with known allergic reactions to the constituents of Kogenate.

Warnings: Kogenate should only be administered intravenously.

Patients should be made aware that the appearance of chest tightness, dizziness, mild hypotension and nausea can constitute an early warning for hypersensitivity and anaphylactic reactions. Symptomatic treatment and therapy for hypersensitivity reactions should be instituted as appropriate.

If allergic or anaphylactic reactions occur, administration of Kogenate should be stopped immediately and the patient treated for shock.

The required dose can only be calculated approximately. The plasma level of Factor VIII activity should be monitored therefore by appropriate clotting tests. A continuous monitoring of the plasma Factor VIII activity is recommended strongly especially in the case of major surgery or other operations. If bleeding cannot be controlled or the plasma Factor VIII level does not reach calculated values, the presence of Factor VIII inhibitors should be suspected and verified by appropriate tests.

The formation of neutralising antibodies, inhibitors, to Factor VIII is a known complication in the management of haemophilia A (see Side-effects). Patients should be carefully monitored for the development of inhibitory antibodies by appropriate tests.

Animal reproduction studies have not been conducted with Kogenate. Based on the very rare occurrence of haemophilia A in women, experience regarding the use of Kogenate during pregnancy and lactation is not available. Kogenate should only be used during pregnancy and the breast feeding period if clearly necessary.

Precautions: No interaction of Factor VIII with other drugs is known.

There are no indications that Factor VIII may impair the ability to drive or to use machines.

Kogenate should not be mixed with other medicinal products or infusion solutions, as this could change its blood clotting activity.

Kogenate should be used promptly and always within four hours of reconstitution. Reconstituted Kogenate should not be refrigerated. Any unused solution must be discarded.

Side-effects: Following administration of Kogenate, mild to moderate adverse events have been observed rarely. These include burning, transient erythema and rash at the injection site, hypersensitivity reactions, chest tightness, dizziness, mild hypotension and nausea. In addition, the possibility of anaphylactic shock cannot be completely excluded.

Development of Factor VIII inhibitors has been observed, predominantly in previously untreated haemophiliacs receiving Kogenate. Patients should be carefully monitored for the development of inhibitors by appropriate clinical observations and laboratory tests.

No patient in clinical studies with Kogenate developed clinically relevant antibody titres against the trace amounts of mouse and hamster protein present in Kogenate. Caution is advised in patients with known allergic reactions to the constituents of Kogenate.

Overdosage: No information on symptoms of overdosage is available.

Pharmaceutical precautions For both Kogenate and the solvent Water for Injections, store at +2°C to +8°C.

Do not freeze, since the solvent vial may break.

Do not use after the expiry date.

Do not refrigerate after reconstitution and use within four hours.

In exceptional cases, Kogenate and the solvent Water for Injections may be kept at room temperature (up to 25°C) for a limited period of up to three months. In this case, the expiry date **must** be observed and the date of the end of the three-month period must be noted on the vial and/or the outer packaging.

Legal category POM.

Package quantities Kogenate 250, Kogenate 500 and Kogenate 1000 are supplied as single dose vials containing 250, 500 or 1000 I.U. octocog alfa (Factor VIII (rDNA) (bhk)) together with one vial of Water for Injections for parenteral use containing 2.5, 5.0 or 10.0 ml of solvent, respectively, and two sterile alcohol swabs. A sterile administration set is also provided for single use comprising one transfer device, one filter needle, one venepuncture set and one plastic syringe 5 ml (Kogenate 250 and 500) or 10 ml (Kogenate 1000).

Further information Kogenate is a recombinant human antihaemophilic Factor VIII preparation produced from genetically engineered baby hamster kidney cells containing a cloned Human Factor VIII gene. The INN for the active ingredient Factor VIII (rDNA) (bhk) is octocog alfa.

Product licence numbers

Kogenate 250, 500, 1000	0010/0194–0196
Water for Injections	0010/0095

Date of preparation October 1997.

LIPOBAY* 100 MICROGRAM TABLETS ▼
LIPOBAY* 200 MICROGRAM TABLETS ▼
LIPOBAY* 300 MICROGRAM TABLETS ▼

Qualitative and quantitative composition

Lipobay 100 Microgram Tablets: Each tablet contains 95.4 micrograms cerivastatin in the form of 100 micrograms cerivastatin sodium.

Lipobay 200 Microgram Tablets: Each tablet contains 190.8 micrograms cerivastatin in the form of 200 micrograms cerivastatin sodium.

Lipobay 300 Microgram Tablets: Each tablet contains 286.2 micrograms cerivastatin in the form of 300 micrograms cerivastatin sodium.

Pharmaceutical form Film-coated tablet for oral administration.

Clinical particulars

Therapeutic indications: Primary hypercholesterolaemia (Types IIA + IIB): The treatment of hypercholesterolaemia in patients who have not responded adequately to an appropriate diet.

Posology and method of administration: Prior to initiating Lipobay, secondary causes of hypercholesterolaemia should be excluded. Patients should continue on their standard cholesterol-lowering diet during treatment.

Adults: Lipobay should be taken once a day in the evening (at dinner or bed time).

The initial dose is 100 mcg once daily. At intervals of at least 4 weeks, the dosage may be increased by increments of 100 mcg depending on the response. The maximum recommended dose is 300 mcg once daily.

Administration with food does not influence the effect of cerivastatin.

A response to Lipobay is seen within two weeks and the maximum therapeutic response occurs within four weeks. The response is maintained during continuation of therapy.

Elderly patients: There is no clinical evidence to suggest the dosage needs to be different in these patients. In common with other agents, treatment should be initiated at the lower end of the dosage range.

Renal impairment: Patients with moderate to severe renal disease should initiate treatment at a once daily dose of 100 mcg. Subsequent titration, up to a maximum dose of 200 mcg once daily should be performed with caution.

Children: Owing to an absence of clinical experience, use in children is not recommended.

Concomitant administration: Whilst Lipobay is effective in lowering total and LDL cholesterol as monotherapy, efficacy may be enhanced when combined with a bile-acid sequestrant (e.g. cholestyramine, see *Interaction with other medicaments and other forms of interaction*).

Contra-indications: Known hypersensitivity to any component of Lipobay.

Myopathy, hepatic impairment or unexplained, persistent elevations in serum transaminases.

Pregnancy, lactation or women of childbearing potential unless adequately protected by non-hormonal contraceptive methods.

Special warnings and precautions for use:

Liver function: As with other statins, increases in liver enzymes have occurred during therapy with Lipobay. In the majority of cases these elevations were minor and asymptomatic. As with other lipid lowering agents, it is recommended that liver function tests be performed before treatment begins and periodically thereafter. Attention should be paid to patients who develop increased transaminase levels and therapy should be discontinued if increases in ALT and AST exceed three times the upper limit of normal (ULN).

Caution should be exercised when Lipobay is administered to patients with a history of heavy alcohol ingestion or a past history of liver disease (active liver disease or unexplained transaminase elevations are contra-indications to the use of Lipobay).

Muscle: As with other statins, sporadic elevations of creatine phosphokinase (CPK) have been observed in patients receiving Lipobay. These have usually been of no clinical significance. Rarely, myopathy, associated with marked elevations of CPK (≥ 10 times the ULN) and/or with diffuse myalgias, muscle tenderness or weakness, has been reported with HMG-CoA reductase inhibitors. Patients should be asked to report promptly muscle pain, tenderness or weakness especially if accompanied by malaise or fever. Lipobay should be discontinued if markedly elevated CPK levels occur, or if myopathy is diagnosed or suspected. The risk of myopathy is known to increase in those patients receiving HMG-CoA reductase inhibitors who are concomitantly treated with cyclosporin, fibric acid derivatives, erythromycin, itraconazole and nicotinic acid.

There have been rare cases of renal dysfunction secondary to rhabdomyolysis with drugs of this class. Hence therapy with Lipobay should be temporarily withheld in any patient experiencing a condition predisposing to the development of renal failure secondary to rhabdomyolysis.

Ophthalmological: New subcapsular and nuclear opacities have been reported although, as with some other statins, a causal relationship with Lipobay has not been established.

Interaction with other medicaments and other forms of interaction: The involvement of cytochrome P450 isozyme CYP 3A4, besides others, in the metabolism of cerivastatin could be demonstrated by *in-vitro* experiments.

The co-administration of the non-specific cytochrome P450 inhibitor cimetidine did not lead to any significant changes in cerivastatin pharmacokinetics. Interaction studies with cytochrome P450 3A4 inhibitors (i.e. erythromycin, itraconazole, cyclosporin) have not been performed and therefore caution should be exercised when these products are co-prescribed. The effect of cytochrome P450 3A4 inducers (e.g. rifampicin or phenytoin) on cerivastatin pharmacokinetics is unknown.

The possible interaction with other substrates of this isozyme is unknown but should be considered for other drugs with a narrow therapeutic index (e.g. antiarrythmic agents class III including amiodarone).

No clinically significant effects were seen in a range of other interaction studies with drugs commonly prescribed in hypercholesterolaemic patients (e.g. warfarin, digoxin, antacids, cimetidine).

Bile acid sequestering agents: Lipobay should be administered at least four hours after the resin (e.g. cholestyramine) to avoid an interaction due to drug binding to the resin.

Pregnancy and lactation: There have been no teratogenic effects observed in animal studies. There are no data available on the use of Lipobay in pregnant women. Both cholesterol and other products of cholesterol biosynthesis are essential components of foetal development. Therefore HMG-CoA reductase inhibitors are contra-indicated during pregnancy and in women of child-bearing potential not taking adequate non-hormonal contraceptive precautions.

Lipobay should not be prescribed to nursing mothers.

Effects on ability to drive and use machines: None known.

Undesirable effects: In placebo controlled clinical studies of cerivastatin 100 mcg to 300 mcg the following events showed an increase over placebo – sinusitis (placebo subtracted incidence 3.8%), headache (2.2%), rhinitis (1.8%), increased cough (1.8%), insomnia (1.6%), flu syndrome (1.4%), myalgia (1.2%), abdominal pain (0.8%), arthralgia (0.7%), back pain (0.5%).

As with other statins, an increase of serum transaminases was observed in patients treated with Lipobay. The majority of the transaminase elevations seen in all treatment groups were mild (less than twice the upper limit of normal). In patients treated with cerivastatin 100 – 300 mcg, 0.46% developed clinically significant elevations of greater than three times the upper limit of normal for aspartate transaminase, and 0.44% similar elevations of alanine transaminase.

Elevated levels of creatine phosphokinase (CPK) greater than three times the upper limit of normal were seen in 1.7% of patients under treatment with cerivastatin for one year, and 2.1% for two years. In patients treated with cerivastatin doses 100–300 mcg, 0.18% of patients with normal CPK levels at baseline showed CPK elevations more than ten times the upper limit of normal.

Overdose: There is no experience with cerivastatin overdose. No specific antidotes to cerivastatin are known. Should overdose occur, treat symptomatically and institute appropriate supportive measures as required.

Pharmacological properties

Pharmacodynamic properties: Cerivastatin is a synthetic, pure enantiomeric competitive cholesterol synthesis inhibitor which specifically inhibits the enzyme HMG-CoA reductase (hydroxy-methyl-glutaryl coenzyme A). This enzyme catalyses the rate-determining step in the synthesis of cholesterol, the conversion of HMG-CoA to mevalonic acid.

The primary site of action of cerivastatin is the liver.

By reducing intracellular cholesterol content, HMG-CoA reductase inhibitors cause secondary up-regulation of hepatic LDL receptors with increased LDL cholesterol clearance and reduction of both total, and LDL cholesterol in the serum.

Pharmacokinetic properties:

Absorption and bioavailability: cerivastatin is readily and almost completely absorbed from the gastrointestinal tract reaching maximum plasma concentrations (C_{max}) 2 – 3 h after oral administration. Maximum concentration and area under the concentration/time curve (AUC) increase dose-proportionally over the dosing range of 50 to 400 mcg.

The absolute bioavailability of cerivastatin is about 60%. Lipobay tablets show the same bioavailability as a solution (i.e. relative bioavailability is equal to 100%) with similar results for C_{max} and t_{max} The pharmacokinetics of cerivastatin are not influenced by concomitant administration of food.

Distribution: cerivastatin is highly bound to plasma proteins (99.1 – 99.5%). The volume of distribution at steady-state of about 0.3 l/kg body weight indicates that the drug penetrates only moderately into tissues. No accumulation is observed on repeated administration.

Metabolism: Two metabolic pathways are equally important in humans: demethylation of the benzylic methyl ether moiety and hydroxylation at one methyl group of the 6-isopropyl substituent. The product from the combined biotransformation reactions is observed as a minor metabolite. All three metabolites are active inhibitors of HMG-CoA reductase at a similar ED_{50} value as the parent drug, contributing to the overall activity of the drug. The involvement of cytochrome P450 isozyme CYP 3A4, besides others, could be demonstrated by *in-vitro* experiments.

Elimination: Cerivastatin is exclusively cleared via cytochrome P450 mediated biotransformation (CYP 3A4 and others) with a plasma elimination half-life of approximately 2 – 3 h. Thirty percent of the dose is excreted as metabolites in urine, and 70% via the faeces. With a clearance of about 13 l/h cerivastatin can be regarded as a low clearance drug.

Cerivastatin intersubject variability for AUC and C_{max} is described by coefficients of variation of approximately 30 to 40 %.

Age and gender have no clinically significant effects on the pharmacokinetics of cerivastatin. Comparable pharmacokinetic data have been found for different ethnic groups investigated.

A single 300 mcg oral dose of cerivastatin was administered to 18 patients with varying degrees of renal impairment (as determined by creatinine clearance ranging from 9 to 84 ml/min) and to 6 healthy young males. For cerivastatin, mean AUC, C_{max}, $t_{1/2}$, and unbound plasma fraction values tended to be higher in the renally impaired patients. The AUC and $t_{1/2}$ of the main active metabolite also tended to be higher in the renally impaired patients, although C_{max} was lower in those severely impaired.

As cerivastatin is contra-indicated in patients with active liver disease, no pharmacokinetic investigations have been performed in this patient group.

Preclinical safety data: Increase in stillbirths and delays in bone development were found in the foetuses of rats treated with an oral dose of 0.3 mg/kg.

In a battery of *in vivo* and *in vitro* tests for the detection of point mutations, chromosomal aberrations and DNA-damage, cerivastatin has not been associated with mutagenic properties.

Liver tumours, known to occur in rodents with other statins, have been observed with cerivastatin in mice at oral doses of 6.75 mg/kg/day (males) and 11.5 mg/kg/day (females). These doses well exceed the therapeutic dose in man. Due to an almost completely different metabolism of cerivastatin in mice, these findings are not considered to be of relevance for man. No tumours have been found in rats.

Pharmaceutical particulars

List of excipients: Lipobay tablets contain the following excipients: Mannitol PhEur, Crospovidone PhEur, Povidone 25 PhEur, Magnesium Stearate PhEur, and Sodium Hydroxide PhEur.

The tablets are film-coated with a mixture comprising Hypromellose PhEur, Macrogol 4000 PhEur, titanium dioxide (E171) and yellow ferric oxide (E172).

Incompatibilities: Not applicable.

Shelf life: The shelf life of Lipobay is 24 months.

Special precautions for storage: The tablets should be stored in the manufacturer's original container, in a dry place at temperatures up to 25°C.

Nature and contents of container: Blister strips in hard outers comprising: 300 μm polypropylene foil sealed with a 20 μm aluminium backing foil. Pack sizes: 14, 20, 28, 30, 50, 98, 100 and 160 (10 by 16).

Instructions for use/handling: None stated.

Marketing authorisation numbers

Lipobay 100 Microgram Tablets	0010/0226
Lipobay 200 Microgram Tablets	0010/0227
Lipobay 300 Microgram Tablets	0010/0228

Date of approval/revision of SPC July 1997

Legal category POM

NIMOTOP*

Presentation

Nimotop tablets: Yellow film-coated tablets marked with the Bayer cross on one side and with the letters SK on the reverse. Each tablet contains 30 mg nimodipine.

Nimotop solution: Vials for intravenous infusion, each containing 10 mg nimodipine in 50 ml (0.02%) of sterile aqueous alcoholic solvent.

Uses

Mode of action: Nimodipine is a calcium channel blocker of the dihydropyridine group with preferential activity on cerebral vessels. Nimodipine increases cerebral perfusion, particularly in poorly perfused areas, by arterial dilatation, an effect which is proportionately greater in smaller than in larger vessels.

Indications: Nimotop tablets are recommended for the prevention of ischaemic neurological deficits following aneurysmal or traumatic subarachnoid haemorrhage.

Nimotop solution is recommended for the treatment of ischaemic neurological deficits following aneurysmal or traumatic subarachnoid haemorrhage.

Dosage and administration

Aneurysmal subarachnoid haemorrhage

Prophylactic administration: The recommended dose is two tablets at 4-hourly intervals (total daily dose 360 mg), to be taken with water. Prophylactic administration should commence within four days of onset of subarachnoid haemorrhage and should be continued for 21 days.

In the event of surgical intervention, administration of Nimotop tablets should be continued (dose as above) to complete the 21 days treatment period.

Therapeutic administration: For the first two hours of treatment 1 mg of nimodipine, i.e. 5 ml Nimotop solution (about 15 μg/kg bw/h), should be infused each hour via a central catheter.

The dose should be increased after two hours to 2 mg nimodipine, i.e. 10 ml Nimotop solution per hour (about 30 μg/kg bw/h), providing no severe decrease in blood pressure is observed.

Patients of body-weight less than 70 kg or with unstable blood pressure should be started on a dose of 0.5 mg nimodipine per hour (2.5 ml of Nimotop solution), or less if necessary.

Therapeutic administration should commence as soon as cerebral ischaemia occurs, and should continue for at least five days up to a maximum of 14 days.

In the event of surgical intervention during treatment, administration of Nimotop solution should be continued (dose as above) for at least five days.

If cerebral ischaemia occurs during prophylactic administration, tablet treatment may be continued to complete the 21-day treatment period or substituted by Nimotop solution (dosage as above). Nimotop solution may be used with or without pre-treatment with Nimotop tablets. In the event of Nimotop tablets and Nimotop solution being administered sequentially the total duration of treatment should not exceed 21 days. Nimotop solution should not be administered for longer than 14 days. Nimotop solution and tablets should not be used concomitantly.

For administration, Nimotop solution must be drawn up into a 50 ml syringe and connected to a three-way stopcock using the infusion line provided. (The stopcock must allow for concomitant flow of the Nimotop solution and a co-infusion solution.) Nimotop solution must be administered with a co-infusion running at a rate of 40 ml/hr of either sodium chloride 0.9%, glucose 5%, Ringer's lactate solution, dextran 40, human albumin 5% or mannitol 10% which is connected to the second port of the three-way stopcock prior to its connection with the central line catheter.

Nimotop solution must not be added to an infusion bag or bottle and must not be mixed with other drugs.

Nimotop solution may be used during anaesthesia or surgical procedures.

Traumatic subarachnoid haemorrhage: Intravenous therapy should be started no later than 12 hours after trauma, as soon as possible after the presence of subarachnoid blood has been diagnosed. Administration of Nimotop solution should be continued for seven to ten days (dosage as for aneurysmal subarachnoid haemorrhage).

On completion of the intravenous therapy, it is recommended that oral administration of Nimotop tablets be continued for eleven to fourteen days, i.e. to complete the 21 day period (dosage as for aneurysmal subarachnoid haemorrhage).

The total duration of treatment with Nimotop should not exceed 21 days.

Special precautions: Nimotop solution reacts with polyvinylchloride (PVC). Polyethylene or polypropylene are the recommended plastic materials to be used during nimodipine infusion (see also 'Pharmaceutical precautions').

Polyethylene tubes are supplied with Nimotop solution 50 ml vials.

Contra-indications, warnings, etc

Contra-indications: Nimodipine should not be administered to patients during or within one month of a myocardial infarction or an episode of unstable angina.

Warnings: Nimotop tablets and solution should be used with care when cerebral oedema or severely raised intracranial pressure are present.

Nimotop tablets should not be administered concomitantly with Nimotop solution.

Nimodipine may potentiate the hypotensive effect of anti-hypertensives. Where concomitant administration of other calcium channel blockers (e.g. nifedipine, diltiazem, verapamil), α-methyldopa or beta-blockers is necessary, blood pressure must be monitored, and careful dose titration of nimodipine should be undertaken with possible reduction or discontinuation of the anti-hypertensive agent.

Nimotop solution must be used with caution in hypotensive patients.

Patients with known renal disease and/or receiving nephrotoxic drugs, should have renal function monitored closely during intravenous treatment with Nimotop solution.

Decreased drug clearance may occur in cirrhotic patients receiving Nimotop and therefore close monitoring of blood pressure is recommended in these patients.

Drug interactions: Concomitant administration of anti-epileptic drugs (phenobarbitone, phenytoin or carbamazepine) markedly reduces the bioavailability of orally administered nimodipine.

The simultaneous administration of cimetidine or sodium valproate may lead to an increase in the plasma nimodipine concentration.

Nimotop tablets should not be administered concomitantly with rifampicin since the efficacy of nimodipine could be reduced owing to enzyme induction.

The intake of grapefruit juice is not recommended in combination with nimodipine as it can result in increased plasma nimodipine concentrations due to the inhibition of the oxidative metabolism of dihydropyridines.

Use in pregnancy: No reproductive toxicology studies following parenteral administration are available. Reproductive toxicology studies in animals after oral administration showed no teratogenic effect. Nimotop tablets and solution should be used with caution in pregnant women, and only when the benefit of treatment is considered to outweigh the risk.

Side-effects

Nimotop solution and tablets: The following have been reported: decrease in blood pressure, slight increase or decrease in heart rate, flushing, headache, dizziness, gastro-intestinal disorders, nausea, sweating and feeling of warmth. Very rarely thrombocytopenia and ileus have been reported.

Nimotop solution: A transient rise in liver enzymes may occur during intravenous administration; this usually reverts to normal on completion of treatment. The infusion contains 20% ethanol and 17% polyethylene glycol-400; this should be taken into account during treatment.

Overdosage

Nimotop Tablets: If overdosage occurs, gastric lavage should be carried out and activated charcoal administered. If blood pressure is low, a vasopressor should be administered.

Nimotop Solution: If overdosage occurs, treatment should be discontinued immediately. If there is a large drop in blood pressure an intravenous injection of dopamine or noradrenaline may be indicated.

Pharmaceutical precautions *Nimotop tablets* should be stored in the manufacturer's original container in a dry place at a temperature not exceeding 25°C.

Nimotop solution is light sensitive and therefore should be stored only in the manufacturer's light-protective container within the cardboard carton at a temperature not exceeding 25°C. The solution when in the syringe must be protected from direct sunlight during administration, but it is stable in diffuse daylight and artificial light for up to 10 hours.

The solution should not be allowed to come into contact with PVC. The only plastic materials suitable for use are polyethylene or polypropylene. Nimotop solution is compatible with glass infusion bottles and infusion packs made of polyethylene (e.g. Polyfusor, Boots).

Nimotop solution 50 ml vials should be infused using a glass or rigid plastic (polyethylene or polypropylene) syringe and giving set (Gillette Sabre syringe; BD plastipak syringe; Monoject disposable syringe, Sherwood Medical Ltd; Combidyn tubes, Braun; Nitrocassette giving set, Imed Ltd.). Nimotop solution is incompatible with infusion bags and any giving sets made of PVC (e.g. Viaflex, Travenol; Steriflex, Boots).

Legal category POM.

Package quantities *Nimotop tablets:* Each pack contains 100×30 mg tablets in foil strips of 10.

Nimotop solution: Each pack contains 5×50 ml (0.02% solution) vials and 5 polyethylene infusion lines.

Further information Pharmacokinetic studies have shown the area under the curve to be similar following oral or intravenous administration of Nimotop at the recommended doses.

Product licence numbers
Nimotop tablets 0010/0137
Nimotop solution 0010/0138

NYSTAFORM*-HC OINTMENT NYSTAFORM*-HC CREAM

Presentation *Nystaform-HC ointment:* Yellow ointment containing Nystatin BP 100,000 Units/g, Chlorhexidine acetate BP 1.0% w/w and Hydrocortisone Ph Eur 1.0% w/w in a water-repellent base.

Nystaform-HC cream: Light yellow cream containing Nystatin BP 100,000 Units/g, Chlorhexidine hydrochloride BP 1.0% w/w and Hydrocortisone Ph Eur 0.5% w/w in a water-miscible base.

Uses Nystatin is a fungistatic and fungicidal antibiotic primarily effective against *Candida albicans*. Chlorhexidine has activity against a wide range of bacteria. Hydrocortisone exercises a vasoconstrictive effect, thus reducing inflammation and oedema. Hydrocortisone also has an antipruritic effect.

Nystaform-HC preparations are indicated for the treatment of infected dermatoses where fungal (particularly monilial) and/or bacterial infections are present. The choice of cream or ointment depends upon the severity, physical characteristics and site of the condition, and upon the physician's preference.

Dosage and administration
Adults and children: For topical application only. Apply to the infected areas 2–3 times daily. Treatment should be for a maximum period of 7 days.

Contra-indications, warnings, etc
Contra-indications: Tuberculous lesions of the skin. Known sensitivity to any of the ingredients.

Warnings and precautions: For external use only. Avoid contact with eyes. If sensitivity occurs, or if new infection appears, discontinue use and institute alternative therapy.

In infants, long-term continuous topical steroid therapy should be avoided. Adrenal suppression can occur even without occlusion. As with other topical corticosteroids, systemic absorption may occur when extensive areas are treated, particularly under occlusion.

Use in pregnancy: Topical administration of corticosteroids to pregnant animals can cause abnormalities of foetal development including cleft palate and intra-uterine growth retardation. The relevance of this finding to humans has not been established. However, topical steroids should not be used extensively in the first trimester of pregnancy and nystatin only with caution. The use of Nystaform-HC products requires that the anticipated benefits outweigh the possible risks.

Side-effects: Side-effects are uncommon. Hypersensitivity type reactions including application site reaction and allergic reactions are rarely reported.

Accidental oral ingestion: Nystatin is poorly absorbed from the gastro-intestinal tract. In the event, routine measures such as gastric lavage should be performed as soon as possible after ingestion.

Pharmaceutical precautions *Storage:* Store in a cool place.

Legal category POM.

Package quantities Nystaform-HC cream 15 g and 30 g tubes. Nystaform-HC ointment 30 g tubes.

Further information The water-miscible base of Nystaform-HC cream is particularly easy to apply to inflamed and tender skin. It is pleasant to use and does not leave the skin feeling greasy. The water-repellent base of Nystaform-HC ointment spreads easily and helps to protect against urine when used in the nappy rash area.

Product licence numbers
Nystaform-HC ointment 0010/0124
Nystaform-HC cream 0010/0123

NYSTAFORM* CREAM

Presentation Light yellow cream containing Nystatin BP 100,000 Units/g and Chlorhexidine hydrochloride BP 1.0% w/w in a water-miscible base.

Uses Nystatin is a fungistatic and fungicidal antibiotic primarily effective against *Candida albicans*. Chlorhexidine has activity against a wide range of bacteria.

Nystaform preparations are indicated for the treatment of infected skin conditions where fungal (particularly monilial) and/or bacterial infections are present.

Dosage and administration
Adults and children: For topical application only. Apply to the infected areas 2–3 times daily. Continue application for one week after lesions have healed.

The patient should be advised that if the condition has not improved within seven days, to return to the surgery for further consultation. If the condition does not improve within 14 days of starting treatment, then an alternative treatment should be substituted.

Contra-indications, warnings, etc
Contra-indications: Known sensitivity to any of the ingredients.

Warnings and precautions: For external use only. Avoid contact with eyes. If sensitivity occurs, or if new infection appears, discontinue use and institute alternative therapy.

Use in pregnancy: As with all drugs nystatin should be administered with caution during the early months of pregnancy and its use requires that the anticipated benefits outweigh the possible risks.

Side-effects: Side-effects are uncommon. Hypersensitivity-type reactions including application site reaction and allergic reactions are rarely reported.

Accidental oral ingestion: Nystatin is poorly absorbed from the gastro-intestinal tract. In the event, routine measures such as gastric lavage should be performed as soon as possible after ingestion.

Pharmaceutical precautions *Storage:* Store in a cool place.

Legal category POM.

Package quantities 30 g tubes.

Further information The water-miscible base of Nystaform cream is particularly easy to apply to inflamed and tender skin. It is pleasant to use and does not leave the skin feeling greasy.

Product licence number 0010/0121

SECUROPEN*

Presentation Vials containing 1.0 g, 2.0 g azlocillin as azlocillin sodium. Infusion vials containing 5.0 g azlocillin as azlocillin sodium. Securopen infusion sets containing 3×5.0 g azlocillin, 3×50 ml Water for Injections, 3 transfer needles and 3 hanging bags.

Uses Azlocillin is a broad spectrum antibiotic with especially significant anti-pseudomonal activity. In addition to *Pseudomonas* strains the spectrum of activity of azlocillin includes the following Gram-negative and Gram-positive pathogens: *Escherichia coli, Klebsiella/Enterobacter/Serratia* group, *Proteus* (indole-positive and indole-negative), *Providencia, Citrobacter, Salmonella* and *Shigella*, enterococci, staphylococci (penicillin sensitive), *Haemophilus influenzae*, gonococci, meningococci, pneumococci, streptococci and *Corynebacterium*. The spectrum also includes the anaerobic organisms *Clostridia* and *Bacteroides* species, including *Bacteroides fragilis*.

Azlocillin is indicated for the treatment of systemic and/or local infections due to sensitive organisms, especially infections of the respiratory and urinary tracts, and for septicaemia.

Azlocillin may be administered concomitantly with an aminoglycoside or with beta-lactamase stable isoxazolyl-penicillin, since there is evidence of synergy with these compounds.

Dosage and administration
Adult Dosage:
Patients with normal renal function: Life-threatening infections 5.0 g every 8 hours. In non-life-threatening and urinary tract infections 2.0 g every 8 hours.

Children's Dosage:

Age	*Bodyweight (kg)*	*Daily dose (mg/kg bodyweight)*	*(g)*
6–14 years	20–40	3×75	3×1.5–3.0
2–6 years	13–20	3×75	3×1.0–1.5
1–2 years	10–13	3×75	3×0.75–1.0
Infants			
7 days–1 year	3–10	3×100	3×0.3–1.0
Neonates			
up to 7 days	3	2×100	2×0.3
Premature	2.5	2×50	2×0.125
babies	2.0	2×50	2×0.100
	1.5	2×50	2×0.075

Patients with impaired renal function: i.e. with serum creatinine above 177 micromol/l (2 mg/dl) or with creatinine clearance less than 30 ml/minute, the unit dose should be as above but at 12-hourly intervals.

In patients presenting with severe impairment of both renal and hepatic functions, a further reduction of the dose may be necessary.

Patients on haemodialysis: Azlocillin is dialysable. On non-dialysing days, patients should receive the recommended unit dose of azlocillin twice daily. Before each dialysis an additional unit dose may be given to compensate for the amount of azlocillin removed by dialysis.

Duration of treatment: The duration of treatment depends upon the severity of the infection and also the clinical and bacteriological course of the disease.

In principle, treatment should be maintained for at least 3 days after fever or clinical symptoms have disappeared. This, on average, requires 7–10 days therapy.

Administration: Azlocillin is administered intravenously as a 10% solution in Water for Injections. For doses of 2.0 g or less it is administered as a bolus injection and for higher doses it should be infused over 20–30 minutes.

Supplementary drugs should be injected through the drip tubing and not introduced into the bag or bottle containing azlocillin. In patients already receiving intravenous infusion therapy with other drugs, azlocillin should be infused during the intervening periods or as a parallel infusion. In order to achieve higher initial concentrations in the serum and tissues, up to half of the appropriate dose of azlocillin may be injected slowly through the tubing of the existing infusion.

Combination therapy: aminoglycosides, injectable tetracycline derivatives, ciprofloxacin, and metronidazole have proved to be incompatible with azlocillin and must therefore be administered separately. Before administering rarely used solutions or drugs, the compatibility of the individual components must be ascertained; precipitation, cloudiness or discolouration indicate possible incompatibility.

Contra-indications, warnings, etc
Contra-indications: A history of allergy to other penicillins and cephalosporins. Azlocillin is inactivated by beta-lactamases (penicillinases).

Use in pregnancy: Animal studies have shown no evidence of teratogenic or embryotoxic effects of azlocillin. However, as with all drugs, it should be administered with caution during the early months of pregnancy and its use requires that the anticipated benefits outweigh the possible risks.

Side-effects: Side-effects are uncommon and typical of other injectable penicillins. These may include: local irritation including pain at the site of injection; gastro-intestinal disturbances e.g. nausea, diarrhoea, vomiting, and occasionally pseudomembranous colitis; hypersensitivity reactions e.g. skin rashes, pruritus. Anaphylactic reactions may also occur.

Since very high serum levels of penicillins may induce seizures, dose adjustment is necessary in patients with severely impaired renal function.

Abnormal clinico-chemical and blood values, may be seen during therapy.

During treatment with high doses of azlocillin a prolongation of bleeding time may occur as a result of a dose-dependent disturbance of thrombocyte function.

Interactions: The duration of neuromuscular blockade due to vecuronium may be prolonged if azlocillin is administered at the end of the operation.

Patients being treated with azlocillin and concomitant heparin or other anticoagulants need more frequent control of coagulation parameters.

Overdosage: Overdosage should be treated by standard monitoring and supportive measures. Serum levels of azlocillin may be reduced by dialysis.

Pharmaceutical precautions *Storage:* Azlocillin should not be stored in temperatures exceeding 25°C. The expiry date is printed on the packaging.

Dilution and compatibility: Azlocillin should be freshly prepared immediately before administration by shaking the powder with a suitable volume of Water for Injections until completely dissolved to make a 10% solution – that is, 1.0 g in 10 ml, 2.0 g in 20 ml and 5.0 g in 50 ml. If azlocillin has to be prepared in advance of administration, it may be kept as the 10% solution at room temperature for 6 hours without loss of efficacy. Any unused solution should be discarded.

Azlocillin is compatible and stable in the common infusion fluids provided that the solutions are freshly prepared as above. These include 5% and 10% glucose solutions, fructose 5%, Ringer's solution and sodium chloride 0.9%. Compatibility with rarely used solutions must be ascertained prior to administration; possible incompatibility is indicated by precipitation, cloudiness or discolouration.

Legal category POM.

Package quantities 1.0 g, 2.0 g vials packed in boxes of 5.
5.0 g vial packed singly.
Infusion pack of 3 × 5.0 g with diluent, transfer needles and hanging bags.

Further information
Sodium content:
Each 5.0 g vial contains 10.84 mEq sodium (249.1 mg)
Each 2.0 g vial contains 4.33 mEq sodium (99.6 mg)
Each 1.0 g vial contains 2.17 mEq sodium (49.8 mg)
Displacement value 0.74 ml/g

Product licence numbers
Securopen 0010/0075
Water for Injections BP 0010/0095

TRASYLOL*

Presentation Colourless glass vials containing a solution of aprotinin for injection, each 50 ml vial containing 70 mg aprotinin (=500,000 Kallikrein Inactivator Units, KIU, =277.8 European Pharmacopoeia Units, PhEur units) in 0.9% sodium chloride solution.

Uses Trasylol is an inhibitor of proteolytic enzymes including human trypsin, plasmin, and both plasma and tissue kallikrein.

Trasylol is indicated for the treatment of patients at high risk of major blood loss during and following open heart surgery with extracorporeal circulation. These include:

Patients requiring re-operation through a previous median sternotomy.

Patients with septic endocarditis.

Patients with known blood dyscrasias and coagulopathy, e.g. haemophiliacs, patients with von Willebrand's disease, patients receiving treatment with aspirin.

Trasylol is also indicated for the treatment of patients in whom optimal blood conservation during open heart surgery is an absolute priority. These include:

Jehovah's Witnesses who are to undergo open heart surgery with extracorporeal circulation.

Patients who require open heart surgery and are known carriers of a highly infectious virus, e.g. Hepatitis B, HIV.

Patients with rare blood groups who require open heart surgery.

Since Trasylol can contribute to the re-establishment of haemostasis by inactivating free plasmin, it is indicated for the treatment of life-threatening haemorrhage due to hyperplasminaemia. Such haemorrhage has occasionally been observed during the mobilisation and dissection of malignant tumours, in acute promyelocytic leukaemia, and following thrombolytic therapy. Trasylol also inhibits the fibrinolytic activity of the plasmin-streptokinase complex formed following thrombolytic therapy with streptokinase.

Dosage and administration
Open heart surgery
Adults: The recommended regimen involves a loading dose, maintenance dose, and a pump prime dose, administered as follows:

(i) Loading dose: The loading dose of 200 ml (2 million KIU) should be administered intravenously after induction of anaesthesia and prior to sternotomy. The initial 5 ml (50,000 KIU) should be administered slowly, over several minutes, due to the small risk of allergic or pseudo-allergic reactions. The remainder of the loading dose should then be given as a slow intravenous infusion or injection over a period of 20 minutes.

(ii) Maintenance dose: The loading dose should be followed by the administration of a continuous infusion of 50 ml (500,000 KIU) per hour until the end of the operation except in patients with septic endocarditis where it may be continued into the early postoperative period.

(iii) Pump prime dose: An additional 200 ml (2 million KIU) should be added to the priming volume of the extracorporeal circuit. In patients with septic endocarditis 300 ml (3 million KIU) should be added to the pump prime.

Elderly: No dosage adjustment in the elderly is necessary.

Children: The dosage has not been established.

Hyperplasminaemia
Adults: Initially 50 ml (500,000 KIU) to 100 ml (1 million KIU) should be given by slow intravenous injection or infusion (maximum rate 10 ml/min). If necessary, this should be followed by 20 ml (200,000 KIU) hourly until bleeding stops.

Children: The dose should be calculated in proportion to the adult dose on the basis of body weight.

Contra-indications, warnings, etc
Contra-indications: Known hypersensitivity to aprotinin.

Side-effects: Trasylol is generally well tolerated but when given through a peripheral line may occasionally cause local thrombophlebitis.

Hypersensitivity or pseudo-allergic reactions can occur, not only after repeated courses of treatment but also with first administration. These include skin eruptions, tachycardia, pallor or cyanosis, dyspnoea, nausea and anaphylactic shock.

Trasylol should be administered slowly (maximum 10 ml/min) intravenously to the supine patient. If a hypersensitivity reaction occurs during the injection, administration should be stopped immediately and the appropriate therapeutic measures instituted, e.g. adrenaline, antihistamines and intravenous corticosteroids. Intravenous fluids, bronchodilators, and respiratory support may also be needed.

Warnings: The addition of Trasylol to heparinised blood will prolong the activated clotting time (ACT). Thus, the ACT should not be taken as a reliable indicator of the need to administer additional heparin during a prolonged period of cardiopulmonary bypass. Furthermore, a prolonged ACT in the presence of Trasylol does not necessarily signify excess heparin requiring additional protamine. It is therefore not necessary to adjust the usual heparin/protamine regimen during treatment with Trasylol.

Use in pregnancy and lactation: No evidence of teratogenic or embryotoxic effects has been seen in animals. Experience in human pregnancy and lactation is limited and inadequate to assess safety. As hyperplasminaemia is a life-threatening condition, Trasylol may be used during pregnancy and lactation when the benefit of treatment is considered to outweigh the risk.

Overdosage: There is no special antidote or other action to be taken.

Pharmaceutical precautions Any unused solution should be discarded immediately. Trasylol vials are stable at room temperature. However, if the contents are cloudy, the product must not be used. Do not use the contents of the vials after the expiry date shown on the label.

Trasylol has been shown to be incompatible with corticosteroids, heparin, nutrient solutions containing amino acids or fat emulsions, and tetracyclines. Administration of Trasylol in mixed infusions (particularly with beta-lactam antibiotics) should be avoided. Trasylol is compatible with electrolyte and sugar solutions.

Legal category POM.

Package quantities Trasylol is supplied as 50 ml vials each containing aprotinin 500,000 KIU (277.8 PhEur units).

Further information Nil.

Product licence number 0010/5900R

YOMESAN*

Presentation Yellowish tablets measuring 13 mm × 4 mm, each tablet containing 500 mg Niclosamide BP. One side marked FE, the reverse side with the Bayer cross. The tablets are flavoured with vanilla.

Uses An anthelmintic for treatment of tapeworm infections:

Taenia saginata	(beef tapeworm)
Taenia solium	(pork tapeworm)
Diphyllobothrium latum	(fish tapeworm)
Hymenolepis nana	(dwarf tapeworm)

It has no effect in cysticercosis and echinococcosis due to cestode larvae (cysticerci) lodging in extra intestinal tissues.

Dosage and administration *Taenia saginata, Taenia solium, Diphyllobothrium latum.*

Adults and children over 6 years:	4 tablets
Children 2 to 6 years:	2 tablets
Children under 2 years:	1 tablet

In *Taenia solium* the tablets should be taken as a single dose after a light breakfast but in the case of *Taenia saginata* and *Diphyllobothrium latum* the dose may be divided, half being taken after breakfast and the remainder one hour later.

An aperient should be administered two hours later and in the case of *Taenia solium* a drastic purge should be given.

Infection due to *Hymenolepsis nana* should be treated for 7 days:

First day:

Adults and children over 6 years:	4 tablets
Children from 2 to 6 years:	2 tablets
Children under 2 years:	1 tablet

The subsequent 6 days:

Adults and children over 6 years:	2 tablets
Children from 2 to 6 years:	1 tablet
Children under 2 years:	½ tablet

It is important that the tablets are chewed thoroughly before washing down with water. In the case of small children the tablets should be ground up before administration.

Contra-indications, warnings, etc
Contra-indications: Hypersensitivity to niclosamide.

Side-effects: Very rarely the drug may cause mild transient GI disturbances (such as nausea, retching and abdominal pain), light headedness and pruritus.

Overdosage: Yomesan is not absorbed and no cases of overdosage have occurred. In the event of overdose a fast acting laxative and enema may be given. Vomiting should not be induced.

Use in Pregnancy: In common with most drugs it is wise to avoid treatment in the first trimester of pregnancy. Healthy children have been born to women treated with Yomesan in the first trimester of pregnancy.

Experimental studies in rats showed no embryotoxic or teratogenic effects.

Warning: In infections with *Taenia solium* there is always a danger of cysticercosis. A drastic purge is therefore recommended after treatment to eject the lower segment of the tapeworm containing mature eggs.

The hands should be thoroughly scrubbed after defaecation not only on the treatment day but for several days afterwards to avoid reinfection.

The consumption of alcohol during treatment must be avoided.

In the event of constipation it is imperative to restore regular bowel movements before Yomesan treatment.

Pharmaceutical precautions The tablets are light sensitive and should only be stored in the original foil.

Legal category P.

Package quantities Packs of 4 tablets of 0.5 g.

Further information Unless the tapeworm is expelled by a drastic purgative, residual parts of it may be eliminated with the stools during the next two or three days. Thereafter, neither tapeworm segments nor ova should be present in the stools. In re-infection with *Taenia saginata* and *Taenia solium* new tapeworm segments or ova should only appear after three months.

In infections with *Hymenolepis nana* the follow-up period is only 14 days as surviving scolices regenerate very rapidly to sexually mature tapeworms and accordingly, after approx. 10 days, ova are eliminated with the stools.

Product licence number 0010/5910R

**Trade Mark*

Beecham Research
Welwyn Garden City
Hertfordshire AL7 1EY

☎ 01707 325111 🗋 01707 325600

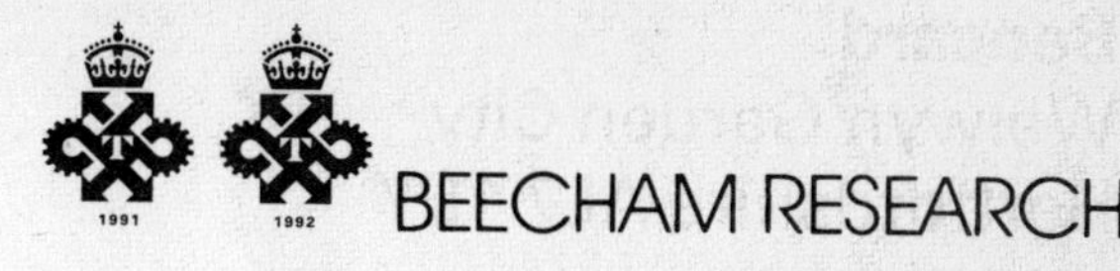

Please refer to SmithKline Beecham Pharmaceuticals.

Bencard
Welwyn Garden City
Hertfordshire AL7 1EY

☎ 01707 325111 🗋 0181 913 4560

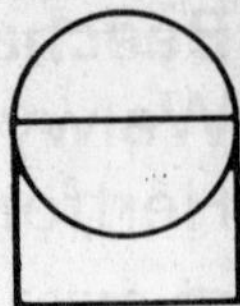

AMOXIL* CAPSULES 250 mg and 500 mg
AMOXIL* DISPERSIBLE TABLETS
AMOXIL* SYRUPS SUCROSE-FREE 125 and 250 mg/5 ml
AMOXIL* SACHETS 750 mg and 3 g SUCROSE-FREE
AMOXIL* PAEDIATRIC SUSPENSION
AMOXIL* VIALS FOR INJECTION 250 mg, 500 mg and 1 g

Qualitative and quantitative composition
Amoxil Capsules 250 mg contain 250 mg amoxycillin per capsule
Amoxil Capsules 500 mg contain 500 mg amoxycillin per capsule
Amoxil Dispersible Tablets contain 500 mg amoxycillin per tablet
Amoxil Syrup Sucrose-Free 125 mg/5 ml contains 125 mg amoxycillin per 5 ml dose
Amoxil Syrup Sucrose-Free 250 mg/5 ml contains 250 mg amoxycillin per 5 ml dose
Amoxil Sachets 750 mg Sucrose-Free contain 750 mg amoxycillin per sachet
Amoxil Sachets 3 g Sucrose-Free contain 3 g amoxycillin per sachet
Amoxil Paediatric Suspension contains 125 mg amoxycillin per 1.25 ml dose
Amoxil Vials For Injection 250 mg contain 250 mg amoxycillin
Amoxil Vials For Injection 500 mg contain 500 mg amoxycillin
Amoxil Vials For Injection 1 g contain 1 g amoxycillin

The amoxycillin is present as the trihydrate in Amoxil oral preparations and as the sodium salt in Amoxil injections (each 1 g vial contains approximately 3.3 mmol of sodium).

Pharmaceutical form Amoxil Capsules: maroon and gold capsules overprinted 'Amoxil 250' or 'Amoxil 500'.

Amoxil Dispersible Tablets: flat white circular tablets engraved 'Amoxil 500'.

Amoxil Syrups Sucrose-Free: citrus-flavoured sucrose-free suspensions in a sorbitol base. Presented as powder in bottles for preparing 100 ml.

Amoxil Sachets Sucrose-Free: sucrose-free sachets in a sorbitol base, for reconstitution in water. Each sachet carries instructions for preparation.

Amoxil Paediatric Suspension: citrus flavoured suspension. Presented as powder in bottles for preparing 20 ml.

Amoxil Vials: vials containing sterile powder for reconstitution.

Clinical particulars
Therapeutic indications:
Treatment of infection: Amoxil is a broad spectrum antibiotic indicated for the treatment of commonly occurring bacterial infections such as:
Upper respiratory tract infections
Otitis media
Acute and chronic bronchitis
Chronic bronchial sepsis
Lobar and bronchopneumonia
Cystitis, urethritis, pyelonephritis
Bacteriuria in pregnancy
Gynaecological infections including puerperal sepsis and septic abortion
Gonorrhoea
Peritonitis
Intra-abdominal sepsis
Septicaemia
Bacterial endocarditis
Typhoid and paratyphoid fever
Skin and soft tissue infections
Osteomyelitis
Dental abscess (as an adjunct to surgical management)
Helicobacter pylori eradication in peptic (duodenal and gastric) ulcer disease.

In children with urinary tract infection the need for investigation should be considered.

Prophylaxis of endocarditis: Amoxil may be used for the prevention of bacteraemia, associated with procedures such as dental extraction, in patients at risk of developing bacterial endocarditis.

The wide range of organisms sensitive to the bactericidal action of Amoxil include:

Gram-positive	Gram-negative
Streptococcus faecalis	*Haemophilus influenzae*
Streptococcus pneumoniae	*Escherichia coli*
Streptococcus pyogenes	*Proteus mirabilis*
Streptococcus viridans	*Salmonella* species
Staphylococcus aureus (penicillin-sensitive)	*Shigella* species
	Bordetella pertussis
Clostridium species	*Brucella* species
Corynebacterium species	*Neisseria gonorrhoeae*
Bacillus anthracis	*Neisseria meningitidis*
Listeria monocytogenes	*Vibrio cholerae*
	Pasteurella septica
	Helicobacter pylori

Posology and method of administration:
Treatment of infection:
Adult dosage (including elderly patients): Oral:
Standard adult dosage: 250 mg three times daily, increasing to 500 mg three times daily for more severe infections.

High-dosage therapy (maximum recommended oral dosage 6 g daily in divided doses): A dosage of 3 g twice daily is recommended in appropriate cases for the treatment of severe or recurrent purulent infection of the respiratory tract.

Short-course therapy: Simple acute urinary tract infection: two 3 g doses with 10-12 hours between the doses. Dental abscess: two 3 g doses with 8 hours between the doses. Gonorrhoea: single 3 g dose.

Helicobacter eradication in peptic (duodenal and gastric) ulcer disease: Amoxil is recommended at a dose of twice daily in association with a proton pump inhibitor and antimicrobial agents as detailed below:

Omeprazole 40 mg daily, Amoxycillin 1G BID, Clarithromycin 500 mg BID x 7 days
or
Omeprazole 40 mg daily, Amoxycillin 750 mg-1G BID, Metronidazole 400 mg TID x 7 days

Injectable: 500 mg IM eight hourly (or more frequently if necessary) in moderate infections. (This dose may be given by slow IV injection if more convenient.)

1 g IV six hourly in severe infections.

Children's dosage (up to 10 years of age): Oral:
Standard children's dosage: 125 mg three times daily, increasing to 250 mg three times daily for more severe infections.

Amoxil Paediatric Suspension is recommended for children under six months of age.

In severe or recurrent acute otitis media, especially where compliance may be a problem, 750 mg twice a day for two days may be used as an alternative course of treatment in children aged 3 to 10 years. The use of Amoxil 750 mg Sachets Sucrose-Free is recommended.

Injectable: 50–100 mg/kg body weight a day, in divided doses.

Parenteral therapy is indicated if the oral route is considered impracticable or unsuitable, and particularly for the urgent treatment of severe infection.

In renal impairment the excretion of the antibiotic will be delayed and, depending on the degree of impairment, it may be necessary to reduce the total daily dosage.

Prophylaxis of endocarditis: see table.

Administration: Oral: Using capsules, dispersible tablets, syrups, sachets or paediatric suspension.

Intravenous injection, intravenous infusion, intramuscular: Using vials for injection (see *Instructions for use/handling*).

Contra-indications: Amoxil is a penicillin and should not be given to penicillin-hypersensitive patients. Attention should be paid to possible cross-sensitivity with other beta-lactam antibiotics eg. cephalosporins.

Special warnings and special precautions for use: Serious and occasionally fatal hypersensitivity (anaphylactoid) reactions have been reported in patients on penicillin therapy. These reactions are more likely to occur in individuals with a history of hypersensitivity to beta-lactam antibiotics (see *Contra-indications*).

Erythematous (morbilliform) rashes have been associated with glandular fever in patients receiving amoxycillin.

Prolonged use may also occasionally result in overgrowth of non-susceptible organisms.

At high doses relative to urinary output, adequate fluid intake and urinary output must be maintained to minimise the possibility of amoxycillin crystalluria.

Dosage should be adjusted in patients with renal impairment (see *Posology and method of administration*).

When prepared for intramuscular or direct intravenous injection, Amoxil should be administered immediately after reconstitution. The stability of Amoxil in various infusion fluids is given in the Package Enclosure Leaflet.

Interaction with other medicaments and other forms of interaction: In common with other broad spectrum antibiotics, amoxycillin may reduce the efficacy of oral contraceptives and patients should be warned accordingly.

Concurrent administration of allopurinol during treatment with amoxycillin can increase the likelihood of allergic skin reactions.
Prolongation of prothrombin time has been reported rarely in patients receiving amoxycillin. Appropriate monitoring should be undertaken when anticoagulants are prescribed concurrently.

It is recommended that when testing for the presence of glucose in urine during amoxycillin treatment, enzymatic glucose oxidase methods should be used. Due to the high urinary concentrations of amoxycillin, false positive readings are common with chemical methods.

Pregnancy and lactation:
Use in pregnancy: Animal studies with Amoxil have shown no teratogenic effects. The product has been in extensive clinical use since 1972 and its suitability in human pregnancy has been well documented in clinical studies. When antibiotic therapy is required during pregnancy, Amoxil may be considered appropriate when the potential benefits outweigh the potential risks associated with treatment.

Use in lactation: Amoxycillin may be given during lactation. With the exception of the risk of sensitisation associated with the excretion of trace quantities of amoxycillin in breast milk, there are no known detrimental effects for the breast-fed infant.

Effects on ability to drive and use machines: Adverse effects on the ability to drive or operate machinery have not been observed.

Undesirable effects: Side-effects, as with other penicillins, are uncommon and mainly of a mild and transitory nature.

Hypersensitivity reactions: If any hypersensitivity reaction occurs, the treatment should be discontinued.

Skin rash, pruritis and urticaria have been reported occasionally. Rarely, skin reactions such as erythema multiforme and Stevens-Johnson syndrome, toxic epidermal necrolysis and bullous and exfoliative dermatitis have been reported.

As with other antibiotics, severe allergic reactions including angioneurotic oedema, anaphylaxis (see *Special warnings and special precautions for use*), serum sickness and hypersensitivity vasculitis have been reported rarely.

Interstitial nephritis can occur rarely.

Gastrointestinal reactions: Minor gastrointestinal upsets (e.g. nausea, vomiting and diarrhoea) may occur during treatment. Mucocutaneous candidiasis and antibiotic associated colitis including pseudomembranous colitis and haemorrhagic colitis have been reported rarely.

Superficial tooth discolouration has been reported rarely and mostly with the suspension and chewable tablets. It can usually be removed by brushing.

Hepatic effects: A moderate rise in AST and/or ALT has been occasionally noted but the significance of this is unclear. As with other beta-lactam antibiotics, hepatitis and cholestatic jaundice have been reported rarely.

Haematological effects: As with other beta-lactams, reversible leucopenia (including severe neutropenia or agranulocytosis), reversible thrombocytopenia and haemolytic anaemia have been reported rarely. Prolongation of bleeding time and prothrombin time have also been reported rarely (see *Interaction with other medicaments and other forms of interaction*).

CNS effects: CNS effects have been seen rarely. They include hyperkinesia, dizziness and convulsions. Convulsions may occur in patients with impaired renal function or in those receiving high doses.

Overdose: Problems of overdosage with amoxycillin

Prophylaxis of Endocarditis:

Condition		*Adults' Dosage (including elderly)*	*Children's Dosage*	*Notes*
Dental Procedures: Prophylaxis for patients undergoing extraction, scaling or surgery involving gingival tissues, and who have not received a penicillin in the previous month. (N.B. Patients with prosthetic heart valves should be referred to hospital – see below.)	Patient not having general anaesthetic.	3 g Amoxil orally, 1 hour before procedure. A second dose may be given 6 hours later, if considered necessary.	Under 10: Half adult dose. Under 5: Quarter adult dose The use of Amoxil 500 mg Dispersible Tablets or 750 mg Sachets SF is recommended.	*Note 1.* If prophylaxis with Amoxil is given twice within one month, emergence of resistant streptococci is unlikely to be a problem. Alternative antibiotics are recommended if more frequent prophylaxis is required, or if the patient has received a course of treatment with a penicillin during the previous month. *Note 2.* To minimise pain on injection, Amoxil may be given as two injections of 500 mg dissolved in sterile 1% lignocaine solution (see 'Administration').
	Patient having general anaesthetic: if oral antibiotics considered to be appropriate.	Initially 3 g Amoxil orally 4 hours prior to anaesthesia, followed by 3 g orally (or 1 g IV or IM if oral dose not tolerated) as soon as possible after the operation.		
	Patient having general anaesthetic: if oral antibiotics not appropriate.	1 g Amoxil IV or IM immediately before induction; with 500 mg orally, 6 hours later.		
Dental Procedures: Patients for whom referral to hospital is recommended: (a) patients to be given a general anaesthetic who have been given a penicillin in the previous month. (b) patients to be given a general anaesthetic who have a prosthetic heart valve. (c) patients who have had one or more attacks of endocarditis.		Initially: 1 g Amoxil IV or IM with 120 mg gentamicin IV or IM, immediately prior to anaesthesia (if given) or 15 minutes prior to dental procedure. Followed by (6 hours later): 500 mg Amoxil orally.	Under 10: The doses of Amoxil should be half the adult dose; the dose of gentamicin should be 2 mg/kg. Under 5: The doses of Amoxil should be quarter the adult dose: the dose of gentamicin should be 2 mg/kg.	See Note 2. *Note 3.* Amoxil and gentamicin should not be mixed in the same syringe. *Note 4.* Please consult the appropriate data sheet for full prescribing information on gentamicin.
Genito-urinary Surgery or Instrumentation: Prophylaxis for patients who have no urinary tract infection and who are to have genito-urinary surgery or instrumentation under general anaesthesia. *Obstetric and Gynaecological Procedures* } Routine prophylaxis is recommended only for patients with prosthetic heart valves. *Gastro-intestinal Procedures*		Initially: 1 g Amoxil IV or IM with 120 mg gentamicin IV or IM, immediately before induction. Followed by (6 hours later): 500 mg Amoxil orally or IV or IM according to clinical condition.		See Notes 2, 3 and 4 above.
Surgery or Instrumentation of the Upper Respiratory Tract	Patients other than those with prosthetic heart valves.	1 g Amoxil IV or IM immediately before induction; 500 mg Amoxil IV or IM 6 hours later.	Under 10: Half adult dose. Under 5: Quarter adult dose.	See Note 2 above. *Note 5.* The second dose of Amoxil may be administered orally as Amoxil Syrup SF.
	Patients with prosthetic heart valves.	Initially: 1 g Amoxil IV or IM with 120 mg gentamicin IV or IM, immediately before induction; followed by (6 hours later) 500 mg Amoxil IV or IM.	Under 10: The dose of Amoxil should be half the adult dose; the gentamicin dose should be 2 mg/kg. Under 5: The dose of Amoxil should be quarter the adult dose; the dose of gentamicin should be 2 mg/kg.	See Notes 2, 3, 4 and 5 above.

are unlikely to occur. If encountered, gastrointestinal effects such as nausea, vomiting and diarrhoea may be evident and should be treated symptomatically with attention to the water/electrolyte balance. Crystalluria may also occur.

Amoxycillin may be removed from the circulation by haemodialysis.

Pharmacological properties

Pharmacodynamic properties: Amoxil is a broad spectrum antibiotic.

It is rapidly bactericidal and possesses the safety profile of a penicillin.

Pharmacokinetic properties Amoxil is well absorbed by the oral and parenteral routes. Oral administration, usually at convenient t.d.s. dosage, produces high serum levels independent of the time at which food is taken. Amoxil gives good penetration into bronchial secretions and high urinary concentrations of unchanged antibiotic.

Preclinical safety data: There are no preclinical data of relevance to the prescriber which are additional to those already stated in other sections of the SPC.

Pharmaceutical particulars

List of excipients:

AMOXIL CAPSULES 250 AND 500 MG

Each capsule contains magnesium stearate (E572) and erythrosine (E127), indigo carmine (E132), titanium dioxide (E171), yellow iron oxide (E172) and gelatin.

AMOXIL DISPERSIBLE TABLETS 500 MG

Each tablet contains magnesium stearate (E572), polyvinylpyrrolidone cross-linked, monoammonium glycyrrhizinate, saccharin sodium, colloidal silica (E551), lemon, honey and menthol dry flavours and microcrystalline cellulose (E460).

AMOXIL SYRUPS SUCROSE-FREE

The syrups contain quinoline yellow (E104), disodium edetate, sodium benzoate (E211), saccharin sodium, silica (E551), xanthan gum (E415), peach, strawberry and lemon dry flavours and sorbitol (E420).

AMOXIL SACHETS SUCROSE-FREE

Each sachet contains quinoline yellow (E104), saccharin sodium, xanthan gum (E415), peach, strawberry and lemon dry flavours and sorbitol (E420).

AMOXIL PAEDIATRIC SUSPENSION

The powder contains sodium benzoate (E211), sodium carboxymethyllcellulose (E466), quinoline yellow (E104), peach, strawberry and lemon dry flavours and sucrose (0.6 g per 1.25 ml dose).

AMOXIL VIALS FOR INJECTION

None

Incompatibilities: Amoxil should not be mixed with blood products, other proteinaceous fluids such as protein hydrolysates, or with intravenous lipid emulsions.

If Amoxil is prescribed concurrently with an aminoglycoside, the antibiotics should not be mixed in the syringe, intravenous fluid container or giving set because loss of activity of the aminoglycoside can occur under these conditions.

Shelf-life

Capsules	60M
Dispersible Tablets	36M
Syrups Sucrose-Free	60M (once reconstituted: 14 days)
Sachets Sucrose-Free	36M
Paediatric Suspension	36M (once reconstituted: 14 days)
Injection Vials	18M

Special precautions for storage: Amoxil Sachets Sucrose-Free should be stored in a dry place below 25°C. Prior to use, other oral presentations of Amoxil should be stored in a dry place. Amoxil Vials for Injection should be stored in a cool, dry place.

Once dispensed, Amoxil Syrups Sucrose-Free and Amoxil Paediatric Suspension should be stored at 25°C or below and used within 14 days. If dilution of the reconstituted Sucrose-Free product is required, water should be used. Amoxil Paediatric Suspension may be diluted with water or Syrup BP.

When prepared for intramuscular or direct intravenous injection, Amoxil should be administered immediately after reconstitution. The stability of Amoxil in various infusion fluids is dependent upon the concentration and temperature: stability times are given in the Package Enclosure Leaflet.

Nature and contents of container:

Amoxil Capsules: 250 mg Original Pack of 21 with Patient Information Leaflet; also container of 500. 500 mg Original Pack of 21 with Patient Information Leaflet; also container of 100.

Amoxil Dispersible Tablets: 500 mg: Original Pack of 21 with Patient Information Leaflet.

Amoxil Syrups Sucrose-Free: 125 mg/5 ml and 250 mg/5 ml: Original Pack of 100 ml with Patient Information Leaflet.

Amoxil 750 mg Sachet Sucrose-Free: Original Pack of 4. Each sachet carries instructions for preparation and each pack contains a Patient Information Leaflet.

Amoxil 3 g Sachet Sucrose-Free: Original Packs of 2 and 14. Each sachet carries instructions for preparation and each pack contains a Patient Information Leaflet.

Amoxil Paediatric Suspension: 125 mg per 1.25 ml: Original Pack of 20 ml with pipette and Patient Information Leaflet.

Amoxil Vials for Injection: Clear glass vials fitted with a butyl rubber closure and an aluminium seal. 250 mg, 500 mg and 1 g: packs of 10, 10 and 5 respectively. Each pack carries instructions for use.

Instructions for use/handling:

Sachets: To be taken immediately following reconstitution.

Intravenous injection: Dissolve 250 mg in 5.0 ml Water for Injections BP (Final volume=5.2 ml).

Dissolve 500 mg in 10 ml Water for Injections BP (Final volume=10.4 ml).

Dissolve 1 g in 20 ml Water for Injections BP (Final volume=20.8 ml).

Amoxil injection, suitably diluted, may be injected directly into a vein or the infusion line over a period of 3–4 minutes.

Intravenous infusion: Solutions may be prepared as described for intravenous injections and then added to an intravenous solution in a minibag or in-line burette and administered over a period of half to one hour. Alternatively, using a suitable reconstitution device, the appropriate volume of intravenous fluid may be transferred from the infusion bag into the vial and then drawn back into the bag after dissolution.

Intramuscular:

250 mg: Add 1.5 ml Water for Injections BP † and shake vigorously (Final volume=1.7 ml).

500 mg: Add 2.5 ml Water for Injections BP † and shake vigorously (Final volume=2.9 ml).

1 g: Add 2.5 ml Water for Injections BP ‡ and shake vigorously (Final volume=3.3 ml).

† If pain is experienced on intramuscular injection, a sterile 1% solution of lignocaine hydrochloride or 0.5% solution of procaine hydrochloride may be used in place of Water for Injections.

‡ The 1 g vial will not dissolve in sterile 1% solution

of lignocaine hydrochloride at the required concentration. To minimise pain on injection, 1 g of Amoxil may be given as two separate injections of 500 mg dissolved in a sterile solution of 1% lignocaine hydrochloride (see above).

A transient pink colouration or slight opalescence may appear during reconstitution. Reconstituted solutions are normally a pale straw colour.

Marketing authorisation holder Beecham Group plc, SB House, Brentford, Middlesex TW8 1BD.
Trading as Bencard, Mundells Welwyn Garden City, Hertfordshire, AL7 1EY.

Marketing authorisation numbers

Amoxil Capsules 250 mg	0038/0103
Amoxil Capsules 500 mg	0038/0105
Amoxil Dispersible Tablets 500 mg	0038/0277
Amoxil Syrup Sucrose-Free 125 mg/5 ml	0038/0326
Amoxil Syrup Sucrose-Free 250 mg/5 ml	0038/0327
Amoxil 750 mg Sachet Sucrose-Free	0038/0332
Amoxil 3 g Sachet Sucrose-Free	0038/0334
Amoxil Paediatric Suspension	0038/0107
Amoxil Vials for Injection 250 mg	0038/0221
Amoxil Vials for Injection 500 mg	0038/0222
Amoxil Vials for Injection 1 g	0038/0225

Date of renewal of authorisation

Amoxil Capsules 250 mg	13.01.98
Amoxil Capsules 500 mg	13.01.98
Amoxil Dispersible Tablets 500 mg	12.12.96
Amoxil Syrup Sucrose-Free 125 mg/5 ml	16.01.98
Amoxil Syrup Sucrose-Free 250 mg/5 ml	16.01.98
Amoxil 750 mg Sachet Sucrose-Free	17.03.97
Amoxil 3 g Sachet Sucrose-Free	17.03.97
Amoxil Paediatric Suspension	13.01.98
Amoxil Vials for Injection 250 mg	13.10.98
Amoxil Vials for Injection 500 mg	13.10.98
Amoxil Vials for Injection 1 g	13.10.98

Date of (partial) revision of the text October 1998

Legal category POM.

**Trade Mark*

Berk Pharmaceuticals Limited
Brampton Road
Hampden Park
Eastbourne
East Sussex
BN22 9AG

☎ 01323 501111 🗋 01323 520306

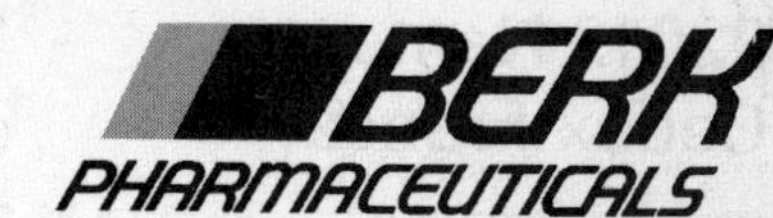

AlfaD*

Presentation AlfaD 0.25 mcg are pink soft gelatin capsules printed '0.25' containing alfacalcidol (1-α hydroxyvitamin D_3) 0.25 micrograms.

AlfaD 1 mcg are orange soft gelatin capsules printed '1.0' containing alfacalcidol (1-α hydroxyvitamin D_3) 1 microgram.

The capsules also contain arachnis (peanut) oil, sodium ethyl hydroxybenzoate (E215) and sodium propyl hydroxybenzoate (E217). The 0.25 mcg capsules contain the colours erythrosine (E127) and black iron oxide (E172). The 1 mcg capsules contain the colours sunset yellow (E110) and black iron oxide (E172).

Uses
Action: Alfacalcidol undergoes rapid hepatic conversion to 1,25-dihydroxyvitamin D_3, the Vitamin D_3 metabolite which acts as a regulator of calcium and phosphate metabolism.

When 1-α hydroxylation by the kidneys is impaired, endogenous 1,25-dihydroxyvitamin D_3 production is reduced. Disorders in which this can occur include renal bone disease, hypoparathyroidism and Vitamin D-dependent rickets. Such conditions require high doses of Vitamin D for their correction but will respond to small doses of AlfaD, which does not depend on the renal 1-α hydroxylation process.

When using parent Vitamin D, the high dose and variable response time can lead to unpredictable hypercalcaemia which may take many weeks, sometimes months, to reverse. With AlfaD, the more rapid onset of response allows better titration of dose and, if hypercalcaemia does occur, it can be reversed within days of stopping treatment.

AlfaD is used for treating conditions in which calcium metabolism is disturbed due to impaired 1-α hydroxylation and other disorders associated with Vitamin D resistance.

The main indications are: Renal osteodystrophy; hypoparathyroidism; hyperparathyroidism (with bone disease); nutritional and malabsorptive rickets and osteomalacia; hypophosphataemic vitamin-D resistant rickets and osteomalacia; pseudo-deficiency (D-dependent Type I) rickets and osteomalacia.

Dosage and administration
All indications: Starting dose:
Children 20 kg and over: 1 microgram/day
Adults: 1 microgram/day
Elderly patients: 0.5 microgram/day.

The dose should subsequently be adjusted according to the biochemical response. Plasma calcium levels (preferably corrected for protein binding) should initially be measured weekly. The dose of AlfaD can be increased by increments of 0.25 to 0.5 micrograms/day. Most adults respond to doses of 1 to 3 micrograms/day. Once the dose is stabilised, calcium levels may be measured every 2-4 weeks.

Indices of response, in addition to plasma calcium, may include alkaline phosphatase, parathyroid hormone levels, bone radiography and histological investigations. When there is biochemcial or radiographic evidence of bone healing (or in hypoparathyroidism when calcium levels have normalised) the dose required for maintenance generally decreases to around 0.25 to 1 microgram/day. Should hypercalcaemia occur, AlfaD should be stopped until plasma calcium returns to normal (usually about a week) then restarted at one half of the previous dose.

Renal osteodystrophy: Patients with already high plasma calcium levels may have autonomous hyperparathyroidism. In this situation they may not respond to alfacalcidol and other therapeutic measures may be indicated.

In patients with chronic renal disease it is particularly important to check the plasma calcium frequently because prolonged hypercalcaemia may further impair renal function.

Before and during AlfaD treatment, the use of phosphate binding agents to prevent hyperphosphataemia may also be considered.

Hypoparathyroidism: Low plasma calcium levels can be dangerous and may be restored to normal more quickly with AlfaD than with parent Vitamin D. Severe hypocalcaemia is corrected more rapidly with higher doses of AlfaD (e.g. 3-5 micrograms) together with calcium supplements.

Hyperparathyroidism: In patients needing surgery for primary or tertiary hyperparathyroidism, pre-operative treatment with AlfaD for 2-3 weeks can reduce bone pain and myopathy without aggravating hypercalcaemia. To decrease the risk of post-operative hypocalcaemia, AlfaD should be continued until the plasma alkaline phophatase falls to normal or hypercalcaemia occurs.

Nutritional and malabsorptive rickets and osteomalacia: Malabsorptive osteomalacia, which responds to large doses of IM or IV parent Vitamin D, will respond to small oral doses of AlfaD. Nutritional rickets and osteomalacia can also be rapidly cured with AlfaD.

Hypophosphataemic vitamin D-resistant rickets and osteomalacia: Normal doses of AlfaD rapidly relieve myopathy, when present, and increase calcium and phosphate retention. Phosphate supplements may also be required in some patients. Neither large doses of parent Vitamin D nor phosphate supplements are entirely satisfactory in these conditions.

Pseudo-deficiency (D-dependent Type I) rickets and osteomalacia: As with the nutritional conditions, similar oral doses of AlfaD are effective in circumstances which would require high doses of parent Vitamin D.

Contra-indications, warnings, etc
Contra-indications: Alfacalcidol should not be used in patients with evidence of Vitamin D toxicity or known hypersensitivity to the effects of Vitamin D or any of its analogues.

Precautions: Alfacalcidol increases the intestinal absorption of calcium and phosphate, serum levels of which should be monitored, particularly in patients with renal failure.

If hypercalcaemia or hypercalciuria occur this can be corrected rapidly by stopping treatment with AlfaD and any calcium supplements until plasma calcium levels return to normal, usually in about a week. AlfaD may then be restarted at half the last dose used.

Response to alfacalcidol may be impaired if the diet is markedly deficient in calcium.

Healing of bone lesions often indicates a decreased requirement for AlfaD in which case appropriate dose adjustments should be made (see Dosage and administration section).

Use in pregnancy and lactation: There is insufficient evidence on which to assess the safety of alfacalciol use during pregnancy, although it has been widely used for many years without apparent adverse effects. Animal studies have not revealed any hazard but as with all drugs, AlfaD should only be used during pregnancy if treatment is essential and no better alternative is available.

Although not definitely established, it is likely that increased levels of 1,25-dihydroxyvitamin D_3 will be found in the breast milk of mothers treated with alfacalcidol. This might have an influence on calcium metabolism in a breast-fed infant.

Use in children: AlfaD capsules are not indicated in children under 20 kg as the dosage cannot be titrated adequately.

Use in the elderly: Initiation of therapy requires a lower dose in elderly patients. The clinical manifestations of hypo- or hypercalcaemia should be considered especially in elderly patients with pre-existing renal or heart conditions.

Drug interactions: Hypercalcaemia in patients taking digitalis preparations may precipitate cardiac arrhythmias. Patients taking digitalis concurrently with alfacalcidol must therefore be closely monitored.

Patients on barbiturates or other anticonvulsants may require an increased dose of AlfaD to produce the desired effect.

Absorption of alfacalcidol may be impaired by concurrent use of mineral oil (prolonged use), cholestyramine, colestipol, sucralfate or large amounts of aluminium-based antacids.

Caution should be exercised in the use of magnesium based antacids or laxatives for patients taking alfacalcidol who are on chronic renal dialysis. Hypermagnesaemia may occur.

The risk of hypercalcaemia is increased in patients taking calcium-containing preparations or thiazide diuretics concurrently with alfacalcidol.

Alfacalcidol is a potent derivative of Vitamin D. Pharmacological doses of Vitamin D or its analogues should not be given during alfacalcidol treatment because of the possibility of additive effects and an increased risk of hypercalcaemia.

Adverse effects: Adverse effects generally relate to abnormally elevated serum calcium levels and, in the case of renal impairment, elevated serum phosphate levels which may be induced by AlfaD therapy. The dosage should be adjusted to the patient's requirements.

Overdosage: Administration of AlfaD should be stopped if hypercalcaemia occurs. Severe hypercalcaemia may require treatment with general supporting measures, with intravenous fluids, with a loop diuretic or with corticosteroids.

In acute overdosage, early treatment with gastric lavage and/or the administration of mineral oil may reduce absorption and promote faecal elimination.

Pharmaceutical precautions Store below 25°C.

Legal category POM.

Package quantities

AlfaD 0.25 mcg:	Containers of 100 capsules
AlfaD 1 mcg:	Containers of 30 or 100 capsules

Further information Nil

Product licence numbers

AlfaD 0.25 mcg	6468/0001
AlfaD 1 mcg	6468/0002

Product licence holder: TEVA Pharmaceutical Industries Limited, PO Box 3190, Petah Tikva, Israel.

*Trade Mark

Biogen Europe
55 Avenue des Champs Pierreux
92012 Nanterre
Cedex-France

☎ 33 141 379595 📠 33 141 372400

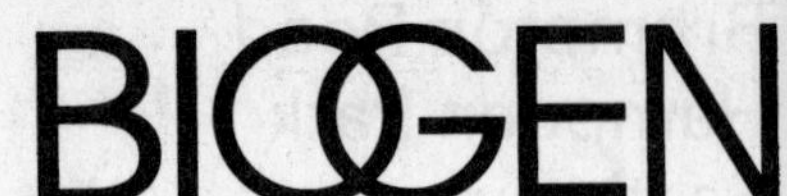

AVONEX*

Qualitative and quantitative composition Avonex (Interferon beta-1a) contains a 30 µg (6 million IU) dose of Interferon beta-1a per vial.

Using the World Health Organisation (WHO) natural interferon beta standard, Second International Standard for Interferon, Human Fibroblast (Gb-23-902-531), 30 µg of Avonex contains 6 million IU of antiviral activity. The activity against other standards is not known.

Pharmaceutical form Avonex (Interferon beta-1a) is a powder and solvent for solution for injection.

Clinical particulars

Therapeutic indications: Avonex (Interferon beta-1a) is indicated for the treatment of ambulatory patients with relapsing multiple sclerosis (MS) characterised by at least 2 recurrent attacks of neurologic dysfunction (relapses) over the preceding 3-year period without evidence of continuous progression between relapses. Avonex slows the progression of disability and decreases the frequency of relapses over a 2-year period.

Avonex has not yet been investigated in patients with progressive multiple sclerosis, and should be discontinued in patients who develop progressive multiple sclerosis.

Not all patients respond to treatment with Avonex. No clinical criteria that would predict the response to treatment have been identified.

Posology and method of administration: The recommended dosage of Avonex (Interferon beta-1a) for the treatment of relapsing MS is 30 µg injected (1 ml solution) IM once a week (see *Instructions for use and handling, and disposal (if appropriate)*). Treatment should be initiated under supervision of a physician experienced in the treatment of the disease.

The safety and efficacy of doses other than 30 µg given IM once weekly in patients with MS have not been evaluated. Therefore, the optimal dose of Interferon beta-1a in MS may not have been established.

The IM injection site should be varied each week (see *Preclinical safety data*).

Prior to injection and for an additional 24 hours after each injection, an antipyretic analgesic is advised to decrease flu-like symptoms associated with Avonex administration. These symptoms are usually present during the first few months of treatment.

There is no experience with Avonex in patients aged 16 years or less. Therefore, Avonex should not be used in children.

At the present time, it is not known for how long patients should be treated. There is currently no clinical experience with Avonex beyond 2 years of treatment. Patients should be clinically evaluated after 2 years of treatment and longer-term treatment should be decided on an individual basis by the treating physician. Treatment should be discontinued if the patient develops chronic progressive multiple sclerosis.

Contra-indications: Avonex (Interferon beta-1a) is contra-indicated in patients with a history of hypersensitivity to natural or recombinant interferon beta, human serum albumin, or any other component of the formulation.

Avonex is contra-indicated in pregnant patients (also see *Use during pregnancy and lactation*), patients with severe depressive disorders and/or suicidal ideation, and in epileptic patients with a history of seizures not adequately controlled by treatment.

Special warnings and special precautions for use: There is limited long-term safety experience with Avonex (Interferon beta-1a). To date, a limited number of patients have been followed for up to 2 years.

Patients should be informed of the most common adverse events associated with interferon beta administration, including symptoms of the flu-like syndrome (see *Undesirable effects*). These symptoms tend to be most prominent at the initiation of therapy and decrease in frequency and severity with continued treatment.

Avonex should be used with caution in patients with depression. Depression and suicidal ideation are known to occur in association with interferon use and to occur at an increased frequency in the MS population. Patients treated with Avonex should be advised to immediately report any symptom of depression and/or suicidal ideation to their prescribing physician. Patients exhibiting depression should be monitored closely during therapy with Avonex and treated appropriately. Cessation of therapy with Avonex should be considered.

Caution should be exercised when administering Avonex to patients with pre-existing seizure disorder. For patients without a pre-existing seizure disorder who develop seizures during therapy with Avonex, an aetiologic basis should be established and appropriate anti-convulsant therapy instituted prior to resuming Avonex treatment.

Caution should be used and close monitoring considered when administering Avonex to patients with severe renal and hepatic failure and to patients with severe myelosuppression.

Patients with cardiac disease, such as angina, congestive heart failure or arrhythmia, should be closely monitored for worsening of their clinical condition during initiation of therapy with Avonex. Symptoms of the flu-like syndrome associated with Avonex therapy may prove stressful to patients with cardiac conditions.

Patients should be advised about the abortifacient potential of interferon beta (see *Use during pregnancy and lactation* and *Preclinical safety data*).

Laboratory abnormalities are associated with the use of interferons. Therefore, in addition to those laboratory tests normally required for monitoring patients with multiple sclerosis, complete and differential white blood cell counts, platelet counts, and blood chemistries, including liver function tests, are recommended during Avonex therapy. Patients with myelosuppression may require more intensive monitoring of complete blood cell counts, with differential and platelet counts.

Patients may develop antibodies to Avonex. The antibodies of some of those patients reduce the activity of interferon beta-1a *in vitro* (neutralising antibodies). Neutralising antibodies are associated with a reduction in the *in vivo* biological effects of Avonex and may potentially be associated with a reduction of clinical efficacy. It is estimated that the plateau for the incidence of neutralising antibody formation is reached after 12 months of treatment. Data from patients treated up to two years with Avonex suggests that approximately 8% develop neutralising antibodies.

The use of various assays to detect serum antibodies to interferons limits the ability to compare antigenicity among different products.

Interactions with other medicinal products and other forms of interaction: No formal drug interaction studies have been conducted with Avonex (Interferon beta-1a) in humans.

The interaction of Avonex with corticosteroids or ACTH has not been studied systematically. The clinical studies indicate that multiple sclerosis patients can receive Avonex and corticosteroids or ACTH during relapses.

Interferons have been reported to reduce the activity of hepatic cytochrome P450-dependent enzymes in humans and animals. The effect of high-dose Avonex administration on P450-dependent metabolism in monkeys was evaluated and no changes in liver metabolising capabilities were observed. Caution should be exercised when Avonex is administered in combination with medicinal products that have a narrow therapeutic index and are largely dependent on the hepatic cytochrome P450 system for clearance, e.g. antiepileptics and some classes of antidepressants.

Use during pregnancy and lactation: Because of the potential hazards to the foetus, Avonex (Interferon beta-1a) is contra-indicated in pregnancy. There are no studies of Interferon beta-1a in pregnant women. At high doses, in rhesus monkeys, abortifacient effects were observed. It cannot be excluded that such effects will be observed in humans.

Fertile women receiving Avonex should take appropriate contraceptive measures. Patients planning for pregnancy and those becoming pregnant should be informed of the potential hazards and Avonex should be discontinued.

Nursing mothers: It is not known whether Avonex is excreted in human milk. Because of the potential for serious advserse reactions in nursing infants, a decision should be made either to discontinue nursing or to discontinue Avonex therapy.

Effects on the ability to drive and use machines: Certain less commonly reported undesirable effects on the central nervous system (see *Undesirable effects*) may influence the ability to drive and operate a machine in susceptible patients.

Undesirable effects: The highest incidence of adverse events associated with the interferon therapy are related to flu syndrome. The most commonly reported symptoms of the flu syndrome are muscle ache, fever, chills, asthenia, headache, and nausea. Symptoms of the flu syndrome tend to be most prominent at the initiation of therapy and decrease in frequency with continued treatment.

Other less common adverse events include: diarrhoea, anorexia, vomiting, arthralgia, insomnia, dizziness, anxiety, rash, injection site reaction, vasodilation, palpitations, alopecia, metrorrhagia and/or menorrhagia. A syncope episode may occur after Avonex injection; it is normally a single episode that usually appears at the beginning of the treatment and does not recur with subsequent injections.

Hypersensitivity reactions may occur and appropriate treatment should be initiated.

Seizures and arrhythmia can rarely occur during treatment with Avonex (Interferon beta-1a, see *Special warnings and special precautions for use*).

Depression and suicide have been reported, therefore Avonex should be used with caution in patient with depression (see *Special warnings and special precautions for use*).

Transient episodes of hypertonia and/or severe muscle weakness that prevent voluntary movements may occur early in the course of therapy. These episodes are of limited duration, temporally related to the injections and may recur after subsequent injections. In some cases these symptoms are associated with flu-like symptoms.

Although not usually requiring treatment, certain laboratory abnormalities may occur during treatment with Avonex. Decreases in circulating lymphocytes, white blood cell count, platelet count, neutrophils and hematocrit may occur. With interferons in general, transient increases in creatinine, potassium, urea nitrogen, alanine transaminase and aspartate transaminase may occur. Transient moderate increases in urinary calcium may also occur.

Overdose: There are no reports of overdosage. However, in case of overdosage, patients should be hospitalised for observation and appropriate supportive treatment given.

Pharmacological properties

Pharmacodynamic properties: Pharmacotherapeutic Group: Cytokines, ATC code L03 AA.

Interferons are a family of naturally occurring proteins that are produced by eukaryotic cells in response to viral infection and other biological inducers. Interferons are cytokines that mediate antiviral, antiproliferative, and immunomodulatory activities. Three major forms of interferons have been distinguished: alpha, beta, and gamma. Interferons alpha and beta are classified as Type I interferons, and interferon gamma is a Type II interferon. These interferons have overlapping but clearly distinguishable biological activities. They can also differ with respect to their cellular sites of synthesis.

Interferon beta is produced by various cell types including fibroblasts and macrophages. Natural interferon beta and Avonex (Interferon beta-1a) are glycosylated and have a single N-linked complex carbohydrate moiety. Glycosylation of other proteins is known to affect their stability, activity, biodistribution, and half-life in blood. However, the effects of interferon beta that are dependent on glycosylation are not fully defined.

Avonex exerts its biological effects by binding to specific receptors on the surface of human cells. This binding initiates a complex cascade of intracellular events that leads to the expression of numerous interferon-induced gene products and markers. These include MHC Class I, Mx protein, 2′/5′-oligoadenylate synthetase, β_2-microglobulin, and neopterin. Some of these products have been measured in the serum and cellular fractions of blood collected from patients treated with Avonex. After a single IM dose of Avonex, serum levels of these products remain elevated for at least 4 days and up to 1 week.

Whether the mechanism of action of Avonex in multiple sclerosis is mediated by the same pathway as the biological effects described above is not known because the pathophysiology of multiple sclerosis is not well established.

The effects of Avonex in the treatment of multiple sclerosis were demonstrated in a single placebo-controlled study of 301 patients (Avonex, n=158; placebo, n=143) with relapsing MS. Due to the design of the study, patients were followed for variable lengths of time. One hundred and fifty Avonex-treated patients completed 1 year on study and 85 completed 2 years on study. In the study, the cumulative percentage of patients who developed disability progression (by Kaplan-Meier life table analysis) by the end of 2 years was 35% for placebo-treated patients and 22% for Avonex-treated patients. Disability progression was measured as an increase in the Expanded Disability Status Scale (EDSS) of 1.0 point, sustained for at least 6 months. It was also shown that there was a one-third reduction in annual relapse rate. This latter clinical effect was observed after more than one year of treatment.

Pharmacokinetic properties: The pharmacokinetic profile of Avonex (Interferon beta-1a) has been investigated indirectly with an assay that measures interferon antiviral activity. This assay is limited in that it is sensitive for interferon but lacks specificity for interferon beta. Alternative assay techniques are not sufficiently sensitive.

Following IM administration of Avonex, serum antiviral activity levels peak between 5 and 15 hours post-dose and decline with a half-life of approximately 10 hours. With appropriate adjustment for the rate of absorption from the injection site, the calculated bioavailability is approximately 40%. The calculated bioavailability is greater without such adjustments. Intramuscular bioavailability is three-fold higher than subcutaneous bioavailability. Subcutaneous administration cannot be substituted for IM administration.

Preclinical safety data: Carcinogenesis: No carcinogenicity data for Interferon beta-1a are available in animals or humans.

Chronic toxicity: No chronic toxicity data for Interferon beta-1a is available in animals.

Local tolerance: IM irritation has not been evaluated in animals following repeated administration to the same injection site.

Mutagenesis: Limited but relevant mutagenesis tests have been carried out. The results have been negative.

Impairment of fertility: Fertility and developmental studies in rhesus monkeys have been carried out with a related form of interferon beta-1a. At very high doses, anovulatory and abortifacient effects in test animals were observed. Similar reproductive dose-related effects have also been observed with other forms of alpha and beta interferons.

No teratogenic effects or effects on foetal development have been observed, but the available information on the effects of interferon beta-1a in the peri- and postnatal periods is limited.

No information is available on the effects of the interferon beta-1a on male fertility.

Pharmaceutical particulars

List of excipients: Human serum albumin, di- and monobasic sodium phosphate, sodium chloride.

Incompatibilities: None known.

Shelf life: Two years.

Special precautions for storage: Avonex (Interferon beta-1a) can be stored at temperatures up to 25°C. DO NOT FREEZE lyophilised or reconstituted product.

Nature and contents of container: Avonex (Interferon beta-1a) is available as a package of four individual doses of: Avonex in a 3 ml clear glass vial with a 13 mm bromobutyl rubber stopper and aluminium seal. It is provided with a 1 ml pre-filled glass syringe of solvent for reconstitution and 2 needles.

Instructions for use and handling, and disposal (if appropriate): Avonex should be administered after reconstitution. However, the reconstituted solution can be stored at 2–8°C for up to 6 hours, prior to injection.

To reconstitute Avonex for injection, the supplied pre-filled syringe of solvent is used. No other solvent should be used. The content of the syringe is injected into the vial of Avonex using the green reconstitution needle. The contents in the vial are gently swirled until all materials are dissolved. DO NOT SHAKE. The reconstituted product is inspected and if it contains particulate matter or is other than colourless to slightly yellow in colour, the vial should be discarded. After reconstitution, 1 ml is drawn from the vial (guidance mark on the pre-filled syringe) for the administration of 30 µg Avonex. The needle for IM injection (blue) is provided. The formulation does not contain a preservative. Each vial of Avonex contains a single dose only. The unused portion of any vial should be discarded.

Marketing authorisation holder: Biogen France SA, 55, avenue des Champs Pierreux, 92012 Nanterre, France.

Number in the community register of medicinal products EU/1/97/033/001

Date of first authorisation/renewal of the authorisation 13 March 1997.

Date of revision of the text 23 October 1998

Legal category POM.

**Trade Mark*

Bioglan Laboratories Limited
5 Hunting Gate
Hitchin
Herts SG4 0TJ

☎ 01462 438444 🗋 01462 421242

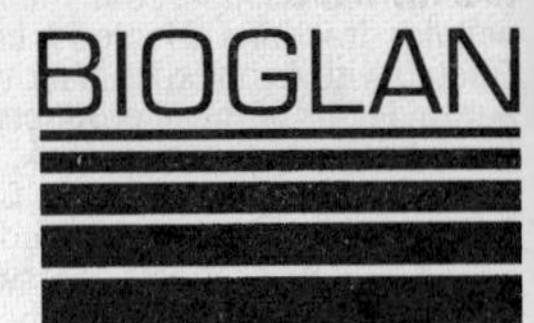

AXSAIN ▼

Qualitative and quantitative composition Capsaicin 0.075% w/w HSE

Pharmaceutical Form Cream for topical application.

Clinical Particulars
Therapeutic indications:

1. For the symptomatic relief of neuralgia associated with the following Herpes Zoster infections (post-herpetic neuralgia) after open skin lesions have healed.
2. For the symptomatic management of painful diabetic peripheral polyneuropathy.

Posology and method of administration
Adults and the elderly: For topical administration to unbroken skin. Apply to the affected area 3 or 4 times daily. Axsain may cause transient burning on application. The burning is observed more frequently when application schedules of less than 3 or 4 times daily are used. Hands should be washed immediately after application of Axsain with the fingers. Do not apply near the eyes.

Patients using Axsain for the treatment of painful diabetic peripheral polyneuropathy should only do so under the direct supervision of a hospital consultant who has access to specialist resources. The recommended duration of use in the first instance is 8 weeks, since there is no clinical trial evidence of efficacy for treatment of more than 8 weeks duration. After this time, it is recommended that the patient's condition should be fully clinically assessed prior to continuation of treatment, and regularly re-evaluated thereafter, by the supervising consultant.

Not suitable for children.

Contra-indications: Axsain cream is contra-indicated for use on broken or irritated skin.

Special warnings and special precautions for use: Keep away from the eyes.

After applying Axsain cream with the fingers, hands should be washed immediately. If the condition worsens, seek medical advice.

Interactions with other medicaments and other forms of interaction: Not applicable

Pregnancy and lactation: The safety of Axsain during pregnancy or lactation has not been established in either humans or animals. However, in the small amounts absorbed transdermally from Axsain Cream, it is considered unlikely that capsaicin will cause any adverse effects in humans.

Effects on ability to drive and use machines: Not applicable

Undesirable effects: Axsain may cause transient burning on application. This burning is observed more frequently when application schedules of less than 3-4 times daily are utilised.

Overdose: Not applicable

Pharmacological properties
Pharmacodynamic properties: Although the precise mechanism of action of capsaicin is not fully understood, current evidence suggests that capsaicin renders skin insensitive to pain by depleting and preventing reaccumulation of substance P in peripheral sensory neurons. Substance P is thought to be the principal chemomediator of pain impulses from the periphery to the Central Nervous System.

Pharmacokinetic properties: Absorption after topical application is unknown. Average consumption of dietary spice from capsicum fruit has been estimated as 2.5 g/person/day in India and 5.0 g/person/day in Thailand. Capsaicin content in capsicum fruit is approximately 1% therefore daily dietary intake of capsaicin may range from 0.5–1 mg/kg/day for a 50 kg person. Application of two tubes of Axsain Cream 0.075% (90 g) each week results in a 9.6 mg/day topical exposure. Assuming 100% absorption in a 50 kg person, daily exposure would be 0.192 mg/kg which is approximately one third to one quarter of the above mentioned dietary intake.

Preclinical safety data: The available animal toxicity data relating to capsicum, capsicum extracts and capsaicin do not suggest that, in usual doses, they pose any significant toxicity hazard to man. Thus, in both single and repeat dosing studies which have been reported, capsicum extracts and capsicum are generally well tolerated at many times even the highest estimated human intakes. The safety of Axsain for use in human pregnancy has not been established since no formal reproduction studies have been performed on either animals or man. However, there is no reason to suspect from human or animal studies currently available that any adverse effects in humans are likely.

Studies reported in the published literature, which relate to potential genotoxic and carcinogenic action of capsaicin have produced inconclusive and conflicting data. However, it is unlikely that capsaicin, in the quantities absorbed transdermally from Axsain Cream, will pose any significant hazard to humans.

Pharmaceutical particulars
List of excipients: Purified water USP, Sorbitol solution USP, Isopropyl myristate NF, Cetyl alcohol NF, Petrolatum (white) USP, Glyceryl stearate and PEG-100 stearate (Arlacel 165) HSE, Benzyl alcohol NF.

Incompatibilities: Not applicable

Shelf Life: 3 years

Special precautions for storage: Store below 25°C

Nature and contents of container: Aluminium tubes with S-22 epoxyphenolic lining and high density polyethylene spiked cap containing 45 g Axsain Cream or 7.5 g for use as professional sample.

Instruction for use/handling: Not applicable

Marketing authorisation number
PL 0041/0067

Date of first authorisation/renewal of authorisation
18 December 1997

Date of (partial) revision of the text 2 December 1997

Legal Category POM

BARITOP* 100

Qualitative and quantitative composition Barium Sulphate PhEur 100% w/v.

Pharmaceutical form Barium Sulphate Suspension.

Clinical particulars
Therapeutic indications: Baritop 100 is an x-ray contrast medium for use in the radiological examination of the gastrointestinal tract.

Posology and method of administration: Oral or by enema in accordance with the parts to be examined and examination methods

Adults and the elderly:

Part of GI Tract	*Method*	*Volume (ml)*	*Concentration (% w/v)*
Oesophagus	Oral	10-150	50-100
Stomach and duodenum	Oral, double contrast, distension filling and relief	10-300	30-100
Small intestine	Oral	100-300	30-100
Colon	Enema	200-2000	20-100

Children: As for adults but in proportion to body weight.

Infants: As for adults but in proportion to body weight.

Contra-indications:

Oral use:	Suspected perforation of intestinal organs: Haemorrhage in digestive organs
Enema use:	Suspected perforation of intestinal organs: Haemorrhage in digestive organs: Extreme exhaustion

Special warnings and precautions for use: Baritop 100 should be used with great caution in:

Oral use:	Suspected or known fistula in digestive organs: stricture or signs suggesting obstruction. Suffering from extreme exhaustion.
Enema use:	Suspected or known fistula in digestive organs: stricture or signs suggesting obstruction: diseases of internal organs that could lead to perforation (e.g. appendicitis, diverticulitis, ulcerative colitis, invagination tumour, parasitic disease etc).

Interaction with other medicaments and other forms of interaction: None stated.

Pregnancy and lactation: At the discretion of the physician.

Effects on ability to drive and use machines: None stated.

Undesirable effects: May cause constipation, transient diarrhoea, abdominal pain, anal pain and bleeding.

Overdose: Treat symptomatically.

Pharmacological properties
Pharmacodynamic properties: Not applicable.

Pharmacokinetic properties: Not applicable.

Preclinical safety data: No formal preclinical studies have been undertaken. Barium sulphate is a well established pharmaceutical substance that has been available for many years. It is also the subject of a recognised Pharmacopoeial Monograph.

Pharmaceutical particulars
List of excipients: In addition to the active ingredient, Baritop 100 contains: Sodium Carboxymethylcellulose BP, Tragacanth HSE, Sodium Saccharin HSE, Glycine BP, Sodium Ascorbate HSE, Silicon Resin Emulsion HSE, Sodium Benzoate BPC, Sodium Dehydroacetate USNF, Cream Soda Essence Flavour HSE, Purified Water BP.

Incompatabilities: None known.

Shelf life: 24 months.

Special precautions for storage: None stated.

Nature and contents of container: 300 ml sealed can. Tin free steel coated internally with vinyl resin on epoxy resin.

Instructions for use/handling: None stated.

Marketing authorisation number: 0041/0024

Date of approval/revision of SPC January 1996.

Legal category P

BARITOP* PLUS

Qualitative and quantitative composition Barium sulphate JP 94.6% w/w

Pharmaceutical form Granules to prepare an aqueous suspension for oral or rectal use as a radiopaque.

Clinical particulars
Therapeutic indications: Baritop Plus is an x-ray contrast medium for use in the radiological examination of the gastrointestinal tract.

Posology and method of administration: After reconstitution with water to make a suspension, Baritop Plus is either taken orally as a barium meal or given rectally as an enema.

Adult:

Part of GI Tract	*Method*	*Volume (ml)*	*Concentration (% w/v)*
Oesophagus	Oral	10-150	50-200
Stomach and duodenum	Oral, double contrast, distension filling and relief	10-300	30-200
Small intestine	Oral	100-300	30-150
Colon	Enema	200-2000	20-130

Children and infants: As for adults but in proportion to body weight.

Contra-indications:

Oral use:	Suspected perforation of intestinal organs: Haemorrhage in digestive organs
Enema use:	Suspected perforation of intestinal organs: Haemorrhage in digestive organs: Extreme exhaustion

Special warnings and precautions for use: Baritop Plus should be used with great caution in:

Oral use:	Suspected or known fistula in digestive organs: stricture or signs suggesting obstruction.
Enema use:	Suspected or known fistula in digestive organs: stricture or signs suggesting obstruction: diseases of internal organs that could lead to perforation (e.g. appendicitis, diverticulitis, ulcerative colitis, invagination tumour, parasitic disease etc).

Interaction with other medicaments and other forms of interaction: None stated.

Pregnancy and lactation: At the discretion of the physician.

Effects on ability to drive and use machines: None stated.

Undesirable effects: May cause constipation.

Overdose: Treat symptomatically.

Pharmacological properties

Pharmacodynamic properties: Not applicable – barium sulphate is not absorbed from the gastrointestinal tract.

Pharmacokinetic properties: Not applicable – barium sulphate is not absorbed from the gastro-intestinal tract.

Preclinical safety data: No formal preclinical studies have been undertaken. Barium sulphate is a well established pharmaceutical substance that has been available for many years. It is also the subject of a recognised pharmacopoeial monograph.

Pharmaceutical particulars

List of excipients: In addition to the active ingredient, Baritop Plus contains: Potato Starch (soluble) HSE, Powdered Acacia JP, Silicon Resin Emulsion HSE, Sodium Benzoate JP, Strawberry Oil HSE, Sodium Carboxymethyl Cellulose JSFA, Hydrogenated Maltose Starch Syrup HSE, Purified Water BP.

Incompatabilities: None known.

Shelf life: 24 months.

Special precautions for storage: None stated.

Nature and contents of container: Polyethylene – cellulose bags 200 gm pack. Polyethylene – Nylon bags 1000 gm pack.

Instructions for use/handling: None stated.

Marketing authorization number: 0041/0025

Date of approval/revision of SPC January 1996.

Legal category P

BENZAMYCIN* GEL

Presentation Benzamycin Gel is presented in a plastic jar containing 20 or 40 g of gel and a separate plastic vial containing (Erythro-pak) containing 0.8 or 1.6 g of erythromycin, which is dissolved in IMS 96 and added to the gel at the time of dispensing by the pharmacist.

When dispensed Benzamycin Gel is a white gel containing benzoyl peroxide 5% w/w and Erythromycin BP 3% w/w.

Uses For the topical treatment of acne vulgaris.

Pharmacology: Benzamycin provides an antimicrobial agent with mild keratolytic properties and antibiotic effects. Erythromycin inhibits lipase production whilst benzoyl peroxide reduces the comedone count and has antibacterial action.

Dosage and administration Benzamycin should be applied twice daily, morning and evening, to areas usually affected by acne or as directed by the physician. These areas should first be gently washed, rinsed with lukewarm water, and patted dry. Benzamycin should be applied with the fingertips and the hands washed after application.

Contra-indications, warnings, etc

Contra-indications: Benzamycin is contra-indicated in persons who have shown hypersensitivity to benzoyl peroxide or erythromycin.

Warnings: For external use only. Keep away from the eyes, nose, mouth and other mucous membranes. Very fair individuals should begin with a single application at bedtime allowing overnight medication. May bleach hair or dyed fabrics.

Interactions: Concomitant topical acne therapy should be used with caution to avoid a possible cumulative irritancy effect. Antagonism has been demonstrated between clindamycin and erythromycin.

Use in pregnancy and lactation: The safe use of Benzamycin during pregnancy and lactation has not been established.

Side effects: Reported adverse rections have been dryness of the skin and uriticaria.

Overdose: Due to the topical administration of this product, overdose is unlikely to occur.

Pharmaceutical precautions Prior to reconstitution store at or below 25°C. After reconstitution, store between 2° and 8°C in the refrigerator. Do not freeze.

Legal category POM

Package quantities 23.3 g and 46.6 g as dispensed.

Further information Nil.

Product licence number 0041/0077

BIORPHEN*

Qualitative and quantitative composition Orphenadrine Hydrochloride BP 25 mg/5 ml.

Pharmaceutical form Aqueous liquid.

Therapeutic indications: Parkinsonism, particularly with apathy and depression, and drug induced extrapyramidal syndrome.

Posology and method of administration: Oral dose.
Adults and elderly: 150 mg daily in divided doses. Maximum dose 400 mg daily. Optimal dose range 150–300 mg and this is usually achieved by raising the dose by 50 mg every two to three days.
Children: Not recommended.

Contra-indications: Glaucoma, prostatic hypertrophy, urinary retention.

Special warnings and precautions for use: Caution in renal and hepatic disease.

Interaction with other medicaments and other forms of interaction: Amantidine, antidepressants, antihistamines, disopyramide, phenothiazines, terodiline. May additionally increase anticholinergic activity.

Pregnancy and lactation: Caution must be observed.

Effects on ability to drive and use machines: None known.

Undesirable effects: Dry mouth, blurred vision.

Overdose: Gastric lavage, emetic and high enema is recommended. Cholinergics may be useful.

Pharmacological properties

Pharmacodynamic properties: Orphenadrine is an antimuscarinic agent.

Pharmacokinetic properties: No formal pharmacokinetic studies have been performed. The product is an oral solution and the active material is therefore immediately available for absorption.

Preclinical safety data: No formal preclinical studies have been undertaken. Orphenadrine hydrochloride is a well-established pharmaceutical substance that has been available for many years. It is also the subject of a recognised pharmacopoeial monograph.

Pharmaceutical particulars

List of excipients: In addition to the active ingredients Biorphen contains: Sorbitol PhEur, Glycerol PhEur, Anise Water Concentrated BP, Saccharin Sodium BP, Tween 20 PhEur, Benzoic Acid Solution BP, Water Purified PhEur.

Incompatibilities: None known.

Shelf life: 24 months.

Special precautions for storage: None stated.

Marketing authorization number 0041/0028

Date of approval/revision of SPC January 1996.

Legal category POM.

BROFLEX*

Qualitative and quantitive composition Benzhexol Hydrochloride BP 5 mg/5 ml.

Pharmaceutical form Syrup.

Clinical particulars

Therapeutic indications: Parkinsonism and drug induced extrapyramidal syndrome.

Posology and method of administration: Oral administration.

Adults and elderly: Initial dose 2 mg subsequent doses up to 20 mg as recommended by a physician.
Children: Not recommended.

Contra-indications: Incipient glaucoma may be precipitated. The following are not absolute contra-indications, nevertheless caution must be observed in patients with: hypertension, cardiac, liver or kidney dysfunction, glaucoma, obstructive diseases of the gastro-intestinal or genito-urinary tracts and in males with prostatic hypertrophy.

Special warnings and special precautions for use: None stated.

Interaction with other medicaments and other forms of interaction: Monoamine oxidase inhibitors (MAOIs), antihistamines, disopyramide, phenothiazines, tricyclic antidepressants increase the side-effects of blurred vision and dry mouth, constipation, urinary retention, MAOIs and amantadine and some tricyclic antidepressants may also cause excitation, confusion and hallucination.

Pregnancy and lactation: At the discretion of the physician.

Effects on the ability to drive and use machines: None known.

Undesirable effects: Dry mouth, constipation and blurred vision occur and this is more frequent in the elderly but reduces with tolerance.

Overdose: There is no specific antidote. Gastric lavage, emetics and high enemas are recommended. Forced fluid intake and general supportive measures are necessary. Atropine antagonists may be helpful.

Pharmacological properties

Pharmacodynamic properties: None stated.

Pharmacokinetic properties: None stated.

Preclinical safety data: No formal preclinical studies have been undertaken. Benzhexol Hcl is a well-established pharmaceutical substance that has been available for many years. It is also the subject of a recognised pharmacopoeial monograph.

Pharmaceutical particulars

List of excipients: In addition to the active ingredients Broflex contains: Anhydrous Citric Acid PhEur, Benzoic Acid PhEur, Propylene Glycol PhEur, Amaranth E123 HSE, Glycerol PhEur, Chloroform Spirit BP, Blackcurrant Flavour A402 HSE, Syrup BP, Purified Water PhEur.

Incompatibilities: None known.

Shelf life: 24 months.

Special precautions for storage: None.

Nature and contents of container: 200 ml and 1000 ml pack size in amber glass bottle with polycone lined closure.

Instructions for use/handling: None stated.

Marketing authorization number 0041/0029

Date of approval/revision of SPC December 1996.

Legal category POM.

CITRAMAG*

Presentation A sachet containing a white, effervescent powder which produces 17.7 g magnesium citrate in aqueous solution, equivalent in alkalinity to 5 g magnesium oxide.

Uses For preparation of the patient for all radiological examinations requiring a completely evacuated bowel. May also be used for colorectal surgery.

Dosage and administration

Dosage:
Adults: The contents of one sachet are to be used as required before the radiological examinations or colorectal surgery. The dose may be reduced for very ill, very thin or elderly patients who may tolerate vigorous purgation poorly.
Children (over 10 years): Reduce the dose to half the adult dose. (5-9 years): Reduce the dose to one third of adult dose

Administration: A low residue or a fluid only diet, according to the instructions of the prescribing clinician, is begun thirty six hours before the examination. At 7.30 a.m. on the day before the examination, the aqueous solution is prepared and allowed to dissolve and cool. It is taken orally at 8.00am. Plenty of clear fluids should be drunk between taking Citramag and the examination.

Contra-indications, warnings etc. There are no contra-indications. For some patients, particularly those in renal failure, it may be necessary to modify the routine instructions supplied with Citramag.

When any doubts exist about the suitability of the routine instructions, the advice of the treating physician should be obtained. It should be noted that fruit juice, which has a high content of potassium, should be avoided in conditions in which hyperkalaemia can occur, such as Addison's disease, selective hypoaldosteronism, and treatment with spironolactones, triamterene or amiloride.

Similarly, the risk of toxic hypermagnesaemia indicates the need for caution in the administration of magnesium citrate to patients in renal failure.

Use in pregnancy and lactation: Use at the discretion of the physician.

Pharmaceutical precautions Store in a cool, dry place– below 25C

Legal category P

Package quantities Sachets containing 29.5 g

Further information Nil

Product licence number 0041/0030.

ISOTRATE* 20

Presentation Isotrate 20 tablets are white, round biconvex uncoated tablets engraved 'B20 ISMN' on one side and plain on the reverse. Each tablet contains isosorbide mononitrate 20 mg.

Uses Isotrate is indicated for the prophylaxis of angina pectoris.

Isotrate is not indicated in the management of acute attacks of angina pectoris.

Mode of action: Isosorbide-5-mononitrate is an active metabolite of isosorbide dinitrate and from an oral dose exerts qualitatively similar effects. However, unlike the dinitrate which is subject to extensive 'first pass' hepatic metabolism, it has virtually complete systemic availability from an oral dose. Isosorbide mononitrate thus achieves predictable and sustained blood levels. Onset of pharmacological effects occur within 20 minutes of an oral dose and are maintained for more than 8 hours. Isosorbide-5-mononitrate is mainly eliminated via metabolism in the liver. The inactive metabolites are mainly excreted via the kidneys.

Dosage and administration

Adults: Usually one tablet twice or three times daily. Patients already accustomed to prophylactic nitrate therapy (for example with isosorbide dinitrate) may normally be transferred directly to a therapeutic dose of Isotrate. For patients not receiving prophylactic nitrate therapy, it is recommended that the initial dose should be one Isotrate tablet daily. Maintenance dose in individual patients will be between 20 mg and 120 mg daily.

Elderly patients: As for adults, but particular care is required because of susceptibility to hypotension.

The tablets should be swallowed whole with a little fluid.

Children: Safety and efficacy in children has not been established.

Contra-indications, warnings, etc A known sensitivity to the drug or to isosorbide dinitrate, acute myocardial infarction with low filling pressures, acute circulatory failure (shock), severe hypotension or cerebral trauma, marked anaemia or hypovolaemia.

Precautions and warnings: Side-effects include hypotension, headache, dizziness and nausea. Usually, these respond to temporary reduction in dose on continued therapy.

Nitrates may give rise to symptoms of collapse after the first dose in patients with labile circulation. These symptoms can largely be avoided if the treatment is started with a low dose.

Isosorbide mononitrate should be used with caution in patients who are predisposed to closed angle glaucoma.

Headache may occur at the onset of treatment but will usually subside after a few days; if the headache persists dosage should be temporarily decreased.

Isosorbide mononitrate should be used with caution in patients suffering from hypothyroidism, hypothermia, malnutrition, severe liver or renal disease.

Pregnancy and lactation: As with other drugs, nitrates should not be administered to pregnant women and nursing mothers unless essential.

Overdosage: Overdosage should be treated symptomatically. The main symptom is likely to be hypotension and this may be treated by elevation of the legs to promote venous return.

Pharmaceutical precautions Store at room temperature. Protect from moisture.

Legal category P

Package quantities Isotrate is blister packed in cartons of 60 sachets.

Further information Isosorbide mononitrate is the British Approved Name for Isosorbide-5-mononitrate.

Product licence number 0041/0006.

METAZEM*

Qualitative and quantitative composition Diltiazem hydrochloride HSE 60 mg per tablet

Pharmaceutical form Tablets intended for internal use.

Clinical particulars

Therapeutic indications: Prophylaxis and treatment of angina pectoris.

Posology and method of administration: Adults: 60 mg three times daily. As patient response may vary, the dose can be increased to a maximum of 360 mg daily in divided doses. Higher doses up to 480 mg/day have been used with benefit in some patients especially in unstable angina.

Elderly patients with impaired hepatic or renal function: Initially 60 mg twice daily. Monitoring of the heart rate should be carried out. The dose should not be increased if the rate falls below 50 beats per minute.

Children: Not recommended.

Contra-indications: Bradycardia, second or third degree heart block, uncontrolled left ventricular failure, sick sinus syndrome. Also contraindicated in pregnancy and in women of childbearing potential.

Special warnings and precautions for use: The product should be used with caution in patients with reduced ventricular function. Patients with mild bradycardia, first degree AV block or prolonged PR interval should be observed closely.

Interaction with other medicaments and other forms of interaction: The doses of both Metazem and beta-blockers should be reduced when both drugs are used concurrently. Metazem may increase the levels of beta-blockers which have a low bioavailability. Metazem may cause small increases in the plasma levels of digitalis. The blood levels of carbamazipine, cyclosporin and theophylline may be increased when given concurrently with diltiazem hydrochloride. Concurrent administration of H_2 antagonists may increase the blood level of Metazem. Concurrent use of Metazem with alpha blockers such as prazosin should be strictly monitored because of the possible synergistic hypotensive effect of this combination.

Metazem treatment has been continued with problem during anaesthesia, but the anaesthetist should be informed that the patient is receiving a calcium antagonist. Metazem, like any calcium antagonist, should not be administered concurrently with dantrolene infusion because of the risk of ventricular fibrillation.

Pregnancy and lactation: Metazem is teratogenic in some animal species and therefore should not be used in pregnancy or in women of childbearing potential.

Metazem is excreted in breast milk and therefore should not be used in nursing mothers until an alternative method of infant feeding has been instituted.

Effects on ability to drive and use machines: None known.

Undesirable effects: Metazem is generally well tolerated. Occasional undesirable effects are nausea, headache, skin rashes, oedema of the legs, flushing, hypotension and fatigue which disappear on cessation of treatment. Metazem may cause depression of atrioventricular nodal conduction and bradycardia. Changes in liver function tests and renal function have been reported in a few cases.

Overdose: The clinical syndromes of acute intoxication may include pronounced hypotension or even collapse, and sinus bradycardia with or without atrioventricular conduction defects.

The patient should be closely monitored in hospital to exclude arrhythmias or atrioventricular conduction defects. Gastric lavage and osmotic diuresis should be undertaken when considered appropriate. Symptomatic bradycardia and high grade atrioventricular block may respond to atropine, isoprenaline or occasionally temporary cardiac pacing. Hypotension may require correction with plasma volume expanders, intravenous calcium gluconate and positive inotropic agents.

Pharmacological properties

Pharmacodynamic properties: Metazem is a calcium antagonist. It restricts the slow channel entry of calcium ions into the cell and so reduces the liberation of calcium from stores in the sarcoplasmic reticulum. This results in a reduction in the amount of available intracellular calcium and consequently a (1) reduction of myocardial oxygen consumption (2) dilation of small and large coronary arteries (3) mild peripheral vasodilation (4) negative dromotropic effects (5) reflex positive chronotrophic and inotropic effects due to reflex sympathetic activity are partially inhibited and result in a slight reduction or no change in heart rate.

The antianginal effect is due to reduction in cardiac oxygen demand with maintenance of coronary blood flow. Cardiac contractility and ventricular ejection fraction are unchanged. Metazem increases exercise capacity and improves indices of myocardial ischaemia in the angina patient. Metazem relieves the spasm of vasospastic (Prinzmetal's) angina.

Pharmacokinetic properties: Metazem is rapidly and almost completely absorbed from gastrointestinal tract following oral administration, but undergoes extensive first-pass hepatic metabolism. The bioavailability has been reported to be about 40%, although there is considerable inter-individual variation in plasma concentration. Metazem is about 80% bound to plasma proteins. It is extensively metabolised in the liver; one of the metabolites, desacetyldiltiazem has been reported to have 25 to 50% of the activity of the parent compound. The half-life is reported to be about 3 to 5 hours. Approximately 2 to 4% of a dose is excreted in urine as unchanged diltiazem with the remainder excreted as metabolites in bile and urine.

Preclinical safety data: There are no pre-clinical data of relevance to the prescriber which are additional to that already included in other sections of the SPC.

Pharmaceutical particulars

List of excipients: In addition to the active ingredient, Metazem contains: Lactose Monohydrate PhEur, Hydrogenated Castor Oil USNF, Polyethylene Glycol 6000 USNF, Magnesium Stearate PhEur.

Incompatibilities: None known.

Shelf life: 3 years.

Special precautions for storage: Store below 25°C in a dry place. Keep out of the reach of children.

Nature and contents of container: The product is blister packed (10s) in 250μ PVC film faced with 48 g PVDC and sealed with hard tempered aluminium lidding foil. The blister strips are subsequently packed in printed boxboard cartons, in pack sizes of 60, 100 and 500 tablets.

Instructions for use/handling: No special precautions.

Marketing authorization number 0041/0011

Date of approval/revision of SPC October 1995.

Legal category POM

PRAGMATAR* CREAM

Presentation Pragmatar Cream is a pale, buff-coloured, oil-in-water cream containing 4% w/w cetyl alcohol-coal tar distillate, 3% w/w precipitated sulphur and 3% w/w salicylic acid.

Uses Pragmatar has mild antipruritic, antiseptic and keratolytic properties. It is indicated in the treatment of dandruff, other seborrhoeic conditions, and common scaly skin disorders.

Dosage and administration

Adults and children: For mild dandruff, apply the cream once a week when the hair is washed. For more severe cases, treat the entire scalp daily at bedtime, applying lightly but thoroughly with the fingertips. The cream can be washed out the next morning or when convenient. For other indicated subacute or chronic skin disorders, apply daily in small quantities to affected areas only.

For use in infants, the cream may be diluted by mixing with a few drops of water in the palm of the hand.

Contra-indications, warnings, etc Do not use in patients who are sensitive to sulphur, or in the presence of acute local infection.

Warnings (caution): Use with care near the eyes, mucous membranes, or on acutely inflamed areas. If any cream should accidentally enter the eye, flush with normal saline solution.

Adverse reactions: No side effects are to be expected if the cream is used accordingly to directions. Excessive use, however, may cause erythema and irritation.

Overdosage: If ingestion occurs, gastro-intestinal disturbances may follow. Treatment consists of rinsing out the mouth together with symptomatic measures if necessary. Even with massive ingestion, salicylate poisoning seems unlikely.

Pharmaceutical precautions Store in a cool place.

Legal category P

Package quantities Tubes containing 25 g and 100 g with applicator.

Ingredients: Cetyl alcohol-coal tar distillate, Precipitated Sulphur BP, Salicylic Acid BP, Sodium Carboxymethyl cellulose 7MF, Glycerol PhEur, Sodium Lauryl

Sulphate BP, Cetyl Alcohol, light Liquid Paraffin BP, Perfume Bouquet 3522, Purified Water PhEur.

Product licence number 0041/0066.

XEPIN*

Qualitative and quantitative composition Doxepin hydrochloride 5% w/w

Pharmaceutical form Cream for topical application to the skin.

Clinical particulars

Therapeutic indications: For the relief of pruritus associated with eczema.

Posology and method of administration:

Adults and children over 12 years: A thin film of Xepin should be applied three to four times daily, to the affected area only. Clinical experience has shown that drowsiness is significantly more common in patients applying cream to more than 10% of the body surface area, therefore, the maximum coverage should be less than 10% of body surface area. For an average sized patient, this would equate to 3 g of Xepin per application and not more than 12 g of Xepin per day. If excessive drowsiness does occur, it may be necessary to reduce the number of applications, the amount of cream applied and/or the percentage of body surface area treated.

Occlusive dressings or clothing may increase the absorption of any topically applied drug, including Xepin; therefore, caution must be exercised when utilising occlusive dressings.

Children under 12 years: There are insufficient data to enable dosage recommendations to be made for children.

Elderly: There are no specific dosage recommendations for elderly patients.

Contra-indications: Xepin is contra-indicated in individuals who have shown previous hypersensitivity to any of its components.

Special warnings and precautions for use: Drowsiness may occur with the use of Xepin. Clinical trial data demonstrate that drowsiness is observed principally in patients receiving treatment to greater than 10% of body surface area and that drowsiness is transient, usually remitting after the first few days of treatment. Patients should, therefore be warned of this possibility and cautioned against driving or operating machinery if they become drowsy while being treated with Xepin. Patients should also be warned that the effects of alcohol could be potentiated.

Xepin should be used with caution in patients with glaucoma, a tendency to urinary retention, severe liver disease or mania, in view of the known adverse effects of orally administered doxepin hydrochloride.

Interactions with other medicaments and other forms of interaction: Alcohol ingestion may exacerbate the potential sedative effects of Xepin particularly in those individuals who use alcohol excessively.

MAO inhibitors should be discontinued at least two weeks prior to the initiation of treatment with Xepin since serious interactions have been reported between orally administered doxepin hydrochloride and MAO inhibitors. As doxepin is metabolised via hepatic microsomal enzymes, care should be taken when co-prescribing any other medicines which are also metabolised by this route.

Caution should also be exercised in patients being treated with cimetidine since it has been found to affect serum concentrations of orally administered tricyclic antidepressants, such as doxepin hydrochloride.

Pregnancy and lactation: There is inadequate evidence of safety in human pregnancy and lactation. Reproductive studies performed in rats, rabbits, monkeys and dogs with oral doxepin showed no evidence of harm to the animal foetus.

As with all drugs, Xepin should only be used in pregnancy and lactation if, in the clinician's judgement, the benefits outweigh the risks.

Effects on ability to drive and use machines: Patients should be advised not to drive a motor vehicle or operate machinery whilst using Xepin. Particular caution should be exercised during the first few days of treatment.

Undesirable effects: Drowsiness has been reported in clinical trials, with an incidence of 12–19%. However, it is generally of mild to moderate severity and of short duration. Limiting the body surface treated to less than 10% is important in minimising the risk of drowsiness.

Local adverse reactions have been reported with the use of Xepin and may occur more frequently with the use of occlusive dressings. Local reactions, in decreasing order of frequency, include burning, stinging, irritation, and tingling and local rash. Dry mouth has been reported in some patients, but other systemic effects which have been observed with orally administered doxepin such as anticholinergic effects, central nervous effects (other than drowsiness) and gastrointestinal effects are less frequently observed with topical Xepin.

Overdose:

Symptoms: Symptoms of overdosage of orally administered doxepin hydrochloride include an increase of any of the reported reactions, primarily excessive sedation and anticholinergic effects such as blurred vision and dry mouth. Other effects may be pronounced tachycardia, hypotension and extrapyramidal symptoms, but these are unlikely to be seen following topical use.

Treatment: Excess cream should be washed off immediately. Treatment of overdosage is essentially symptomatic. Supportive therapy may be necessary if hypotension and/or excessive sedation occur.

Pharmacological properties

Pharmacodynamic properties: Doxepin hydrochloride is a dibenzoxepin tricyclic compound structurally related to tricyclic antidepressant drugs such as amitriptyline. Doxepin hydrochloride has potent H_1 and H_2 receptor blocking actions. Histamine is considered to be an important chemical mediator in the pathogenesis of pruritus. Histamine blocking drugs appear to compete at histamine receptor sites and inhibit the biological activation of histamine receptors.

Pharmacokinetic properties: There is a small but noteworthy amount of systemic absorption following topical administration, with wide inter-individual variations in plasma levels and in the handling of doxepin. Orally administered doxepin undergoes extensive first-pass metabolism but topical administration avoids this initial clearance. Plasma doxepin levels following topical administration are generally low, although in a few subjects they may approach the lower limit of the therapeutic range (for depression) of orally administered doxepin.

Preclinical safety data: Doxepin, which is given orally as a tricyclic antidepressant, has been shown to have potent antihistamine activity in animal models. Acute and chronic toxicity of doxepin has been fully evaluated following oral administration to rats and dogs, and these studies revealed the expected effects for this class of drug.

The local toxicity of Xepin has been studied in healthy volunteers. It has been shown to be neither irritant nor allergenic, although it caused local irritation in a small number of cases.

Pharmaceutical particulars

List of excipients: Inactive ingredients in the cream are; sorbitol, cetyl alcohol, isopropyl myristate, glyceryl stearate, PEG 100 stearate, petrolatum, benzyl alcohol, titanium dioxide and purified water.

Incompatibilities: None known

Shelf life: 3 years

Special precautions for storage: Store below 25°C

Nature and contents of container: Aluminium tubes with S-22 epoxyphenolic lining and a high density polyethylene spiked screw cap containing 30 g, 60 g or 120 g Xepin. A 6.0 g pack is available as a professional sample.

Instruction for use/handling: Not applicable.

Marketing authorisation number PL 00041/0075

Date of first authorisation/renewal of authorisation 27 April 1998

Date of (partial) revision of the text February 1998

Legal Category POM

ZACIN CREAM 0.025%

Qualitative and quantitative composition Capsaicin 0.025% w/w HSE

Pharmaceutical form Cream for topical application.

Clinical particulars

Therapeutic indications: For the symptomatic relief of pain associated with osteoarthritis

Posology and method of administration

Adults and the elderly: For topical administration to unbroken skin. Apply to affected area 4 times daily. Hands should be washed immediately after application of Zacin unless hands and fingers are being treated. Zacin should not be applied near the eyes. Pain relief usually begins within the first week of treatment and increases with continuing regular application for the next two to eight weeks.

Not suitable for use in children.

Contra-indications: Zacin Cream is contra-indicated on broken or irritated skin.

Special warnings and precautions for use: Keep Zacin away from the eyes. Medical advice should be sought if the condition worsens, or clears up then recurs.

Tight bandages should not be applied on top of Zacin Cream.

Interactions with other medicaments and other forms of interaction: Not applicable.

Pregnancy and lactation: The safety of Zacin during pregnancy and lactation has not been established, in either humans or animals. However, in the small amounts absorbed transdermally from Zacin Cream, it is considered unlikely that capsaicin will cause any adverse effects in humans.

Effects on ability to drive and use machines: Not applicable.

Undesirable effects: Zacin may cause transient burning following application. This burning sensation generally disappears after several days of treatment, but may persist particularly when application schedules of less than four times daily are used.

Overdose: Not applicable.

Pharmacological properties

Pharmacodynamic properties: Although the precise mechanism of action of capsaicin is not fully understood, current evidence suggests that capsaicin exerts an analgesic effect by depleting and preventing reaccumulation of Substance P in peripheral sensory neurons. Substance P is thought to be the principal chemomediator of pain impulses from the periphery to the central nervous system.

Pharmacokinetic properties: Absorption after topical application is unknown. Average consumption of dietary spice from capsicum fruit has been estimated at 2.5 g/person/day in India and 5.0 g/person/day in Thailand. Capsaicin content in capsicum fruit is approximately 1% therefore dietary intake of capsaicin may range from 0.5–1 mg/kg/day for a 50 kg person. Application of two tubes of Zacin Cream 0.025% (90 g) each week results in 3.21 mg/day topical exposure. Assuming 100% absorption in a 50 kg person, daily exposure would be 0.064 mg/kg which is approximately one seventh to one eighth of the above mentioned dietary intake.

Preclinical safety data: The available animal toxicity relating to capsicum, capsicum extracts and capsaicin do not suggest that, in usual doses, they pose any significant toxicity hazard to man. Thus, in both single and repeat dosing studies which have been reported, capsicum extracts and capsicum are generally well-tolerated at many times even the highest estimated human intakes. The safety of Zacin for use in human pregnancy has not been established since no formal reproduction studies have been performed in either animals or man. However, there is no reason to suspect from human or animal studies currently available that any adverse effects in humans are likely.

Studies reported in the published literature which relate to potential genotoxic and carcinogenic action of capsaicin have produced inconclusive and conflicting data. However, it is unlikely that capsaicin, in the quantities absorbed transdermally from Zacin Cream, will pose any significant hazard to humans.

Pharmaceutical particulars

List of excipients: Purified water PhEur, Sorbitol solution PhEur, Isopropyl myristate PhEur, Cetyl alcohol PhEur, Petrolatum (white) BP, Glyceryl stearate and Peg-100 stearate (arlacel 165) HSE, Benzyl alcohol PhEur.

Incompatibilities: Not applicable.

Shelf life: 3 years.

Special precautions for storage: Store below 25°C.

Return any unused cream to your doctor or pharmacist.

Nature and contents of container: Aluminium tubes with S-22 epoxyphenolic lining and high density polyethylene spiked cap containing 45 g of Zacin Cream 0.025%.

Instruction for use/handling: Not applicable.

Marketing authorisation number PL 00041/0076

Date of first authorisation/renewal of authorisation 16 January 1998

Date of (partial) revision of the text December 1996

Legal category POM

**Trade Mark*

Boehringer Ingelheim Limited
Ellesfield Avenue
Bracknell
Berkshire RG12 8YS

☎ +44 01344 424600 📠 +44 01344 741444

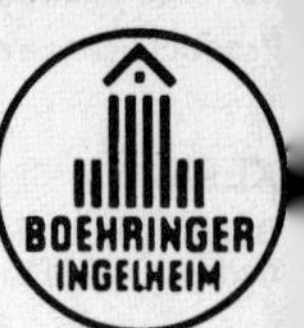

ALUPENT* METERED AEROSOL

Qualitative and quantitative composition Each metered dose contains 750 micrograms of orciprenaline sulphate.

Pharmaceutical form Metered Aerosol for oral inhalation.

Clinical particulars
Therapeutic indications: Alupent is indicated for the relief of reversible airways obstruction.

Posology and method of administration
Adults: The usual starting dose is 1 puff. This may be increased to 2 puffs as necessary. The maximum daily dose should not exceed 12 puffs in 24 hours. Doses should not be repeated within 30 minutes.

Children 6–12 years: As for adults. The maximum daily dose should, however, not exceed 8 puffs in 24 hours. Doses should not be repeated within 30 minutes.

Children under 6 years: The usual dose is 1 puff. The maximum daily dose should not exceed 4 puffs in 24 hours. Doses should not be repeated within 30 minutes.

Elderly: No specific information on the use of this product in the elderly is available. Clinical trials have included patients over 65 years and no adverse reactions specific to this age group have been reported.

Contra-indications: Hypersensitivity to orciprenaline sulphate or the inactive ingredients of the metered aerosol.

Special warnings and special precautions for use: In patients suffering from bronchial asthma, on demand or symptom-oriented treatment may be preferable to regular use. A chronic requirement for treatment would suggest the need for clinical review of the management of the patient's asthma. The use of inhaled corticosteroids as anti-inflammatory treatment should be considered.

Patients must be instructed in the correct use of a metered aerosol and warned not to exceed the prescribed dose. In the case of acute rapidly worsening dyspnoea a doctor should be consulted immediately. In the event of a previously effective dose of inhaled Alupent failing to give relief lasting at least three hours, the patient should be advised to seek medical advice in order that any necessary additional steps may be taken.

Sympathomimetic agents can cause unwanted effects. The concomitant use of other sympathomimetic drugs should be avoided or only used under strict medical supervision. Alupent and anticholinergic bronchodilators have been administered concurrently in reversible airways obstruction. In some situations, co-administered sympathomimetic agents and anticholinergics have been shown to produce greater bronchodilatation than the use of either agent alone (but see *Interactions*).

In the following conditions Alupent should only be used after careful risk/benefit assessment, especially when doses higher than those recommended are used:

Insufficiently controlled diabetes mellitus, recent myocardial infarction, severe organic heart or vascular disorders, such as hypertrophic obstructive cardiomyopathy and tachyarrhythmia; hyperthyroidism.

Potentially serious hypokalaemia may result from excessive beta-agonist therapy. This effect may be potentiated by concomitant treatment with xanthine derivatives, glucocorticosteroids and diuretics. Additionally, hypoxia may aggravate the effects of hypokalaemia on cardiac rhythm. It is recommended that serum potassium levels are monitored in such situations.

Interaction with other medicaments and other forms of interaction: In view of the possible interaction between beta-adrenergics and monoamine oxidase inhibitors or tricyclic anti-depressants, care should be exercised if it is proposed to administer these compounds concurrently with Alupent.

Beta-adrenergics, anticholinergics and xanthine derivatives may enhance the bronchodilator effect of orciprenaline.

The concurrent administration of the other beta-adrenergics, systemically absorbed anticholinergics and xanthine derivatives may increase the frequency and severity of unwanted effects.

$Beta_2$-receptor blockers counteract the action of Alupent.

Potentially serious bronchospasm may occur during concurrent administration of beta-blockers to patients with reversible airways obstruction.

Pregnancy and lactation: Although orciprenaline sulphate has been in general use for several years, there is no definite evidence of ill-consequence following administration of the drug during human pregnancy. Only in doses far in excess of the equivalent maximum human dose were effects on foetal development seen in animals.

Alupent should only be used during pregnancy, especially the first trimester, if the potential benefit outweighs the potential risk to the foetus.

The inhibitory effect of orciprenaline sulphate on uterine contraction should be taken into account.

Safety in breast-fed infants has not been established.

Effect on ability to drive and use machines: None stated.

Undesirable effects: The most frequently reported undesirable effects observed with Alupent are tremor and nervousness, headache, dizziness, tachycardia, palpitations, gastro-intestinal discomfort, nausea and vomiting. Some patients have experienced a feeling of tightness of chest.

In rare cases, local irritation or allergic reactions have been reported.

As with other inhaled bronchodilators, paradoxical broncho-constriction has been reported.

Overdose
Symptoms: The expected symptoms of overdosage with Alupent are those of excessive beta-stimulation such as flushing, tremor, nausea, restlessness, tachycardia, palpitation, dizziness, headache, hypotension, hypertension, a feeling of pressure in the chest, excitation, angina, increased pulse pressure and arrhythmia. Hypokalaemia may occur following overdose with orciprenaline. Serum potassium levels should be monitored.

Therapy: Treatment of overdosage should primarily be supportive and symptom-oriented.

If specific therapy is considered necessary, cardioselective beta-blockers are to be preferred. These should be administered with extreme caution to patients with asthma because of the risk of precipitating severe bronchospasm.

Pharmacological properties
Pharmacodynamic properties: Alupent is a sympathomimetic amine with bronchodilator properties. The duration of action of a single dose is 3–6 hours.

Pharmacokinetic properties: Alupent contains orciprenaline sulphate. Following oral administration orciprenaline is absorbed from the GI tract and undergoes extensive first-pass metabolism; about 40% of an oral dose is reported to reach the circulation unchanged. It is excreted in the urine primarily as glucuronide conjugates.

Pharmaceutical particulars
List of excipients:
Soya Lecithin
Monofluorotrichloromethane
Difluorodichloromethane
Tetrafluorodichloroethane

Incompatibilities: None stated.

Shelf life: The shelf life expiry date for this product is 5 years from the date of its manufacture.

Special precautions for storage: Protect from heat, including direct sunlight. Protect from frost.

The vials should not be opened, punctured or incinerated even when apparently empty.

Nature and contents of container: Alupent Metered Aerosol contains 15 ml homogeneous cream coloured suspension contained in a one-piece aluminium vial with a 50 µl metering valve. Each vial contains approximately 300 doses. A plastic mouthpiece is provided. A 15 ml refill pack is also available.

Instructions for use/handling: The correct administration of the metered aerosol is essential for successful therapy.

To make sure that your inhaler is working, test fire it twice into the air before using it for the first time and whenever your inhaler has not been used for a week or more.

1. Remove the dustcap from the mouthpiece and **shake the inhaler vigorously.**
2. Holding the inhaler as shown, breathe out gently and then immediately . . .
3. . . . place the mouthpiece in the mouth and close your lips around it. After starting to breathe in slowly and deeply, through your mouth, press the inhaler firmly as shown to release the Alupent. *Continue to breathe in as deeply as you can.*
4. Hold your breath for 10 seconds, or as long as is comfortable, before breathing out slowly.
5. If you are to take more than one puff you should wait at least one minute before shaking the inhaler again and repeating steps 2, 3 and 4.
6. After use, replace the dustcap on the mouthpiece.

Marketing authorisation number PL 0015/5002R

Date of renewal of authorisation 16/09/97

Date of revision of the text 8 October 1996

Legal category POM.

ALUPENT* SYRUP

Qualitative and quantitative composition Clear, colourless syrup with a vanilla-like flavour. Each 5 ml contains orciprenaline sulphate 10 mg.

Pharmaceutical form Syrup for oral administration.

Clinical particulars
Therapeutic indications: Alupent is indicated for the relief of reversible airways obstruction.

Alupent Syrup is suggested for maintenance therapy.

Posology and method of administration:
Adults: The usual dose is 2 x 5 ml four times daily. The maximum recommended daily dosage is 8 x 5 ml spoonfuls.

Children 3-12 years: The usual starting dose is 1 x 5 ml four times daily. This may be increased to 2 x 5 ml three times daily as necessary. The maximum recommended daily dosage is 6 x 5 ml spoonfuls.

Children 1-3 years: The usual starting dose is ½ x 5 ml four times daily. This may be increased to 1 x 5 ml four times daily as necessary. The maximum recommended daily dosage is 4 x 5 ml spoonfuls.

Children 0-1 year: The usual starting dose is ½ x 5 ml three times daily. This may be increased to 1 x 5 ml three times daily as necessary. The maximum recommended daily dosage is 3 x 5 ml spoonfuls.

Diluents: Alupent Syrup may be diluted with either Syrup BP or Sorbitol Solution BP

No specific information on the use of this product in the elderly is available. Clinical trials have included patients over 65 years and no adverse reactions specific to this age group have been reported.

Contra-indications: Hypersensitivity to any of the ingredients in Alupent Syrup.

Special warnings and special precautions for use: A chronic requirement for treatment would suggest the need for clinical review of the management of the patient's asthma. The patient's need for anti-inflammatory therapy (e.g. corticosteroids), or the adequacy of such therapy in patients already receiving it should be assessed.

Patients must be warned not to exceed the prescribed dose. In the case of acute rapidly worsening dyspnoea a doctor should be consulted immediately.

Sympathomimetic agents can cause unwanted effects. The concomitant use of other sympathomimetic drugs should be avoided or only used under strict medical supervision. Alupent and anticholinergic bronchodilators have been administered concurrently in reversible airways obstruction. In some situations, co-administered sympathomimetic agents and anticholinergics have been shown to produce greater bronchodilatation than the use of either agent alone (but see Interactions).

In the following conditions Alupent should only be used after careful risk/benefit assessment, especially when doses higher than those recommended are used: Insufficiently controlled diabetes mellitus, recent myocardial infarction, severe organic heart or vascular disorders, such as hypertrophic obstructive cardiomyopathy and tachyarrhythmia; hyperthyroidism.

Potentially serious hypokalaemia may result from excessive beta-agonist therapy. This effect may be potentiated by concomitant treatment with xanthine derivatives, glucocorticosteroids and diuretics.

Additionally, hypoxia may aggravate the effects of hypokalaemia on cardiac rhythm. It is recommended that serum potassium levels are monitored in such situations.

Interaction with other medicaments and other forms of interaction: In view of the possible interaction between beta-adrenergics and monoamine oxidase inhibitors or tricyclic anti-depressants, care should be exercised if it is proposed to administer these compounds concurrently with Alupent.

Beta-adrenergics, anticholinergics and xanthine derivatives may enhance the bronchodilator effect of orciprenaline.

The concurrent administration of the other beta-adrenergics, systemically absorbed anticholinergics and xanthine derivatives may increase the frequency and severity of unwanted effects.

$Beta_2$-receptor blockers counteract the action of Alupent.

Potentially serious bronchospasm may occur during concurrent administration of beta-blockers to patients with reversible airways obstruction.

Pregnancy and lactation: Although orciprenaline sulphate has been in general use for several years, there is no definite evidence of ill-consequence following administration of the drug during human pregnancy. Only in doses far in excess of the equivalent maximum human dose were effects on foetal development seen in animals.

Alupent should only be used during pregnancy, especially the first trimester, if the potential benefit outweighs the potential risk to the foetus.

The inhibitory effect of orciprenaline sulphate on uterine contraction should be taken into account.

Safety in breast-fed infants has not been established.

Effects on ability to drive and use machines: None stated.

Undesirable effects: The most frequently reported undesirable effects observed with Alupent are tremor and nervousness, headache, dizziness, tachycardia, palpitations, gastro-intestinal discomfort, nausea and vomiting. Some patients have experienced a feeling of tightness of chest.

In rare cases, local irritation or allergic reactions have been reported.

Overdose: Symptoms: The expected symptoms of overdosage with Alupent are those of excessive beta-stimulation such as flushing, tremor, nausea, restlessness, tachycardia, palpitation, dizziness, headache, hypotension, hypertension, a feeling of pressure in the chest, excitation, angina, increased pulse pressure and arrhythmia. Hypokalaemia may occur following overdose with orciprenaline. Serum potassium levels should be monitored.

Therapy: Treatment of overdosage should primarily be supportive and symptom-oriented.

If specific therapy is considered necessary, cardioselective beta-blockers are to be preferred. These should be administered with extreme caution to patients with asthma because of the risk of precipitating severe bronchospasm.

Pharmacological properties

Pharmacodynamic properties: Alupent is a sympathomimetic amine with bronchodilator properties. The duration of action of a single dose is 3-6 hours.

Pharmacokinetic properties: Following oral administration orciprenaline is absorbed from the GI tract and undergoes extensive first-pass metabolism; about 40% of an oral dose is reported to reach the circulation unchanged. It is excreted in the urine primarily as glucuronide conjugates.

Pharmaceutical particulars

List of excipients: Sodium metabisulphite; disodium edetate dihydrate; methyl parahydroxybenzoate; propyl parahydroxybenzoate; hydroxyethylcellulose; saccharin; sorbitol solution ; woodruff aroma ; sodium hydroxide; purified water.

Incompatibilities: None stated.

Shelf life: 5 years.

Special precautions for storage: Store below 25°C. Protect from light.

Nature and contents of container: 300 ml amber glass bottle (type III glass) with an aluminium roll-on pilfer proof cap.

Instructions for use/handling: None stated

Marketing authorisation number 0015/0001R

Date of approval/revision of SPC October 1996

Legal category POM

ALUPENT* TABLETS

Qualitative and quantitative composition Round, white/off-white compressed tablets scored and impressed with $\frac{20A}{20A}$ on one side and the Boehringer Ingelheim Company logo on the reverse.

Each tablet contains 20 mg of orciprenaline sulphate.

Pharmaceutical form Tablets for oral administration.

Clinical particulars

Therapeutic indications: Alupent is indicated for the relief of reversible airways obstruction. Alupent Tablets are suggested for maintenance therapy.

Posology and method of administration:

Adults: The usual dose is 1 tablet four times daily. The maximum recommended daily dosage is 4 tablets.

Children 3–12 years: The usual starting dose is ½ tablet four times daily. This may be increased to 1 tablet three times daily as necessary. The maximum recommended daily dosage is 3 tablets.

Children under 3 years: The syrup is recommended.

Elderly: No specific information on the use of this product in the elderly is available. Clinical trials have included patients over 65 years and no adverse reactions specific to this age group have been reported.

Contra-indications: Hypersensitivity to any of the ingredients in Alupent Tablets.

Special warnings and special precautions for use: A chronic requirement for treatment would suggest the need for clinical review of the management of the patient's asthma. The patient's need for anti-inflammatory therapy (e.g. corticosteroids), or the adequacy of such therapy in patients already receiving it should be assessed.

Patients must be warned not to exceed the prescribed dose. In the case of acute rapidly worsening dyspnoea a doctor should be consulted immediately.

Sympathomimetic agents can cause unwanted effects. The concomitant use of other sympathomimetic drugs should be avoided or only used under strict medical supervision. Alupent and anticholinergic bronchodilators have been administered concurrently in reversible airways obstruction. In some situations, co-administered sympathomimetic agents and anticholinergics have been shown to produce greater bronchodilatation than the use of either agent alone (but see *Interactions*).

In the following conditions Alupent should only be used after careful risk/benefit assessment, especially when doses higher than those recommended are used:

Insufficiently controlled diabetes mellitus, recent myocardial infarction, severe organic heart or vascular disorders, such as hypertrophic obstructive cardiomyopathy and tachyarrhythmia; hyperthyroidism.

Potentially serious hypokalaemia may result from excessive beta-agonist therapy. This effect may be potentiated by concomitant treatment with xanthine derivatives, glucocorticosteroids and diuretics.

Additionally, hypoxia may aggravate the effects of hypokalaemia on cardiac rhythm. It is recommended that serum potassium levels are monitored in such situations.

Interaction with other medicaments and other forms of interaction: In view of the possible interaction between beta-adrenergics and monoamine oxidase inhibitors or tricyclic anti-depressants, care should be exercised if it is proposed to administer these compounds concurrently with Alupent.

Beta-adrenergics, anticholinergics and xanthine derivatives may enhance the bronchodilator effect of orciprenaline.

The concurrent administration of the other beta-adrenergics, systemically absorbed anticholinergics and xanthine derivatives may increase the frequency and severity of unwanted effects.

$Beta_2$-receptor blockers counteract the action of Alupent.

Potentially serious bronchospasm may occur during concurrent administration of beta-blockers to patients with reversible airways obstruction.

Pregnancy and lactation: Although orciprenaline sulphate has been in general use for several years, there is no definite evidence of ill-consequence following administration of the drug during human pregnancy. Only in doses far in excess of the equivalent maximum human dose were effects on foetal development seen in animals.

Alupent should only be used during pregnancy, especially the first trimester, if the potential benefit outweighs the potential risk to the foetus.

The inhibitory effect of orciprenaline sulphate on uterine contraction should be taken into account.

Safety in breast-fed infants has not been established.

Effect on ability to drive and use machines: None stated.

Undesirable effects: The most frequently reported undesirable effects observed with Alupent are tremor and nervousness, headache, dizziness, tachycardia, palpitations, gastro-intestinal discomfort, nausea and vomiting. Some patients have experienced a feeling of tightness of chest.

In rare cases, local irritation or allergic reactions have been reported.

Overdose: Symptoms: The expected symptoms of overdosage with Alupent are those of excessive beta-stimulation such as flushing, tremor, nausea, restlessness, tachycardia, palpitation, dizziness, headache, hypotension, hypertension, a feeling of pressure in the chest, excitation, angina, increased pulse pressure and arrhythmia. Hypokalaemia may occur following overdose with orciprenaline. Serum potassium levels should be monitored.

Therapy: Treatment of overdosage should primarily be supportive and symptom-oriented. If specific therapy is considered necessary, cardioselective beta-blockers are to be preferred. These should be administered with extreme caution to patients with asthma because of the risk of precipitating severe bronchospasm.

Pharmacological properties

Pharmacodynamic properties: Orciprenaline sulphate is a $beta_2$-adrenergic agonist bronchodilator which decreases reversible bronchospasm. Following oral administration, the effect is usually noted within 30 minutes. The peak effect of bronchodilator activity following orciprenaline sulphate generally occurs within 60–90 minutes, and lasts for 1 to 5 hours.

It is postulated that $beta_2$-adrenergic agonists produce many of their pharmacological effects by activation of adenylcyclase, the enzyme that catalyses the conversion of adenosine triphosphate to adenosine monophosphate.

Orciprenaline sulphate has been shown to inhibit antigen-induced histamine release both *in vitro* in human lung tissue and in isolated mast cells.

Furthermore, an increase in the rate of bronchial ciliary movement has been demonstrated with adrenergic agonists. This enhances mucociliary clearance, a phenomenon that has also been described for orciprenaline sulphate.

Pharmacokinetic properties: Oral administration of Alupent Tablets is followed by a rapid absorption with a plasma level maximum between 0.75–3 hours and a half-life of 2.1 hours.

After intravenous administration (1 mg/40 min), the plasma level can be described by a mammalian compartment model; the distribution volume in the steady state is about 60 litres and the total clearance 500 ml. The half-life of the terminal elimination is about 2.7 hours.

The p.o./i.v. quotient of the renally excreted radioactivity of tritium-labelled orciprenaline sulphate is 0.6; from this one can infer an absorption of about 60% of the orally administered dose. The renal excretion of radioactivity after oral administration of tritium-labelled orciprenaline sulphate is 45%.

The active substance is not metabolised by the catechol-0-methyl transferase or monoamine oxidase; it is excreted mainly as the sulphuric acid conjugate.

Pharmaceutical particulars

List of excipients: Calcium hydrogen phosphate; phosphoric acid 85%; lactose, fine; maize starch, dried; colloidal silica; soluble maize starch; magnesium stearate.

Incompatibilities: None stated.

Shelf life: The shelf life expiry date for this product is 5 years from the date of its manufacture, when packed in polypropylene securitainers with polythene lids.

The shelf life expiry date for this product is 3 years from the date of its manufacture, when packed in PVC/PVDC blister packs.

Special precautions for storage: Store below 25°C. Protect from light. Tablets packed in blister packs should also be stored in a dry place.

Nature and contents of container: Polypropylene securitainers with polythene lids containing 28, 50, 112, 250 and 1000 tablets. PVC/PVDC blister packs of 100 tablets.

Instructions for use/handling: None stated.

Marketing authorisation number 0015/0046R

Date of approval/revision of SPC October 1996

Legal category POM

ASASANTIN* RETARD ▼

Qualitative and quantitative composition Each capsule contains dipyridamole 200 mg and aspirin 25 mg.

Pharmaceutical form Capsule containing aspirin in standard release form and dipyridamole in modified release form.

Clinical particulars

Therapeutic indications: Secondary prevention of ischaemic stroke and transient ischaemic attacks.

Posology and method of administration: For oral administration.

Adults, including the elderly: The recommended dose is one capsule twice daily, usually one in the morning and one in the evening preferably with meals.

The capsules should be swallowed whole without chewing.

Children: Asasantin Retard is not recommended for children.

Contra-indications: Hypersensitivity to any component of the product or salicylates.

Patients with active gastric or duodenal ulcers or with bleeding disorders.

Patients in the last trimester of pregnancy.

Special warnings and special precautions for use: Among other properties dipyridamole acts as a vasodilator. It should be used with caution in patients with severe coronary artery disease (e.g. unstable angina or recently sustained myocardial infarction), subvalvular aortic stenosis, or haemodynamic instability (e.g. decompensated heart failure).

Asasantin Retard should be used in caution in patients with coagulation disorders.

In patients with myasthenia gravis readjustment of therapy may be necessary after changes in dipyridamole dosage. (See *Interactions*.)

Due to the aspirin component, Asasantin Retard should be used in caution in patients with asthma, allergic rhinitis, nasal polyps, chronic or recurring gastric or duodenal complaints, impaired renal (avoid if severe) or hepatic function or glucose-6-phosphate dehydrogenase deficiency.

In addition, caution is advised in patients hypersensitive to other non-steroidal anti-inflammatory drugs.

Interaction with other medicaments and other forms of interaction: Dipyridamole increases the plasma levels and cardiovascular effects of adenosine. Adjustment of adenosine dosage should therefore be considered if use with dipyridamole is unavoidable.

Dipyridamole may increase the hypotensive effect of blood pressure lowering drugs and may counteract the anticholinesterase effect of cholinesterase inhibitors thereby potentially aggravating myasthenia gravis.

Aspirin may enhance the effect of anticoagulants (e.g. coumarin derivatives and heparin) and increase the risk of gastrointestinal side effects when administered simultaneously with NSAIDs or corticosteroids. Addition of dipyridamole to aspirin does not increase the incidence of bleeding events. When dipyridamole was administered concomitantly with warfarin, bleeding was no greater in frequency or severity than that observed when warfarin was administered alone.

The effect of hypoglycaemic agents and the toxicity of methotrexate may be increased by the concomitant administration of aspirin.

Aspirin may decrease the natriuretic effect of spironolactone and inhibit the effect of uricosuric agents (e.g. probenecid, sulphinpyrazone).

Pregnancy and lactation: There is inadequate evidence of safety of Asasantin Retard in human pregnancy.

Animal studies performed with the drug combination revealed no increased teratogenic risk over the individual components alone. Fertility studies and studies covering the peri-postnatal period have not been performed with the combination.

Asasantin Retard should be used with caution in the first and second trimester, and, since aspirin is associated with delayed and prolonged labour and an increased risk of bleeding, its use is contraindicated in the third trimester.

Dipyridamole and salicylates are excreted in breast milk. Therefore Asasantin Retard should only be administered to nursing mothers if clearly needed.

Effects on ability to drive and use machines: None stated.

Undesirable effects: Adverse reactions at therapeutic doses are usually mild. Vomiting, diarrhoea and symptoms such as dizziness, nausea, dyspepsia, headache and myalgia have been observed following treatment with dipyridamole. These tend to occur early after initiating treatment and may disappear with continued treatment.

As a result of its vasodilating properties, dipyridamole may cause hypotension, hot flushes and tachycardia. In rare cases, worsening of the symptoms of coronary heart disease has been observed.

Hypersensitivity reactions like rash and urticaria have been reported for dipyridamole.

Aspirin produces a prolongation of the bleeding time and in very rare cases increased bleeding during or after surgery has been observed following administration of dipyridamole.

Aspirin may produce epigastric distress, nausea and vomiting, gastro or duodenal ulcers and erosive gastritis which may lead to serious gastrointestinal bleeding. These side effects are more likely to occur when higher doses are administered although they may also occur when low doses are used.

Iron deficiency anaemia may develop as a result of occult gastrointestinal bleeding when aspirin is used for long periods of time.

Hypersensitivity reactions such as rhinitis, angioedema, severe cutaneous skin eruptions, pre-orbital oedema and bronchoconstriction have been reported for aspirin. Very rarely a reduction in platelet count (thrombocytopenia) may occur. Dizziness and tinnitus can, particularly in elderly patients, be symptoms of aspirin overdosage.

Overdose: Due to the low number of observations, experience with dipyridamole overdose is limited.

Symptoms such as a warm feeling, flushes, sweating, accelerated pulse, restlessness, feeling of weakness, dizziness, drop in blood pressure and anginal complaints can be expected.

The signs and symptoms of mild acute aspirin overdose are hyperventilation, tinnitus, nausea, vomiting, impairment of vision and hearing, dizziness and confusional states. In severe poisoning, delirium, tremor, dyspnoea, sweating, bleedings, dehydration, disturbances of the acid base balance and electrolyte composition of the plasma, hypothermia and coma may be seen.

Administration of xanthine derivatives (e.g. aminophylline) may reverse the haemodynamic effects of dipyridamole overdose. Due to its wide distribution to tissues and its predominantly hepatic elimination, dipyridamole is not likely to be accessible to enhanced removal procedures.

Apart from general measures (e.g. gastric lavage), treatment of aspirin overdosage consists chiefly of measures to accelerate the excretion of aspirin (forced alkaline diuresis) and to restore the acid-base and electrolyte balance. Infusions of sodium bicarbonate and potassium chloride solutions may be given. In severe cases haemodialysis may be necessary.

Pharmacological properties

Pharmacodynamic properties: The antithrombotic action of dipyridamole is based on its ability to modify various aspects of platelet function such as inhibition of platelet adhesion and aggregation, which have been shown to be factors associated with the initiation of thrombus formation, as well as lengthening shortened platlet survival time.

Aspirin inhibits platelet aggregation by its inhibitory effect on cyclo-oxygenase in thrombocytes. Dipyridamole does not affect cyclo-oxygenase activity in human platelets and when given simultaneously with aspirin, does not reduce the inhibitory effect on cyclo-oxygenase activity which is obtained with aspirin alone.

The anti-thrombotic effects of dipyridamole and aspirin are additive.

Pharmacokinetic properties: Peak plasma concentrations of dipyridamole are reached 2–3 hours after administration. Steady state conditions are reached within 3 days.

Metabolism of dipyridamole occurs in the liver predominantly by conjugation with glucuronic acid to form a monoglucuronide. In plasma about 70–80% of the total amount is present as parent compound and 20–30% as the monoglucuronide.

Renal excretion is very low (1–5%).

Aspirin is well absorbed from the upper gastrointestinal tract after oral administration and is rapidly distributed throughout the whole body.

Salicylates are mainly eliminated by hepatic metabolism although unchanged salicylate is also excreted in the urine.

In Asasantin Retard the pharmacokinetics of the individual components remain unchanged.

Preclinical safety data: Dipyridamole and aspirin separately have been extensively investigated in animal models and no clinically significant findings have been observed at doses equivalent to therapeutic doses in humans. Toxicokinetic evaluations were not included in these studies.

Studies with the drug combination dipyridamole/aspirin in a ratio of 1:4 revealed additive, but no potentiating toxic effects. A single dose study in rats using dipyridamole/aspirin in a ratio of 1:0.125 gave comparable results to studies with the 1:4 combination.

Pharmaceutical particulars

List of excipients:
Tartaric acid
Povidone
Eudragit S 100
Talc
Acacia
Methylhydroxypropylcellulose phthalate
Methylhydroxypropylcellulose
Triacetin
Dimethicone 300
Stearic acid
Lactose
Aluminium stearate
Colloidal silica
Maize starch
Microcrystalline cellulose
Sucrose
Titanium dioxide; E171
and in the capsule shells:
Gelatin
Erythrosine; E127
Titanium dioxide; E171
Red and yellow iron oxides; E172

Incompatibilities: None stated.

Shelf life: 30 months.

Special precautions for storage: Store below 25°C. Discard any capsules remaining 6 weeks after first opening.

Nature and contents of container: White polypropylene tubes with low-density polyethylene Air-sec stoppers filled with desiccating agent (90% white silicon gel/10% molecular sieves). Packs contain 60 capsules.

Instructions for use/handling: None stated.

Marketing authorisation number PL 0015/0224

Date of first authorisation 12 May 1998

Date of (partial) revision of the text April 1998

Legal category POM.

ATROVENT* AEROCAPS*

Qualitative and quantitative composition Dark olive/light olive opaque size 3 hard gelatin capsules containing 40 micrograms of ipratropium bromide powder.

Pharmaceutical form Capsules containing powder for inhalation.

Clinical particulars

Therapeutic indications: Atrovent Aerocaps are indicated in the treatment of chronic reversible airways obstruction, particularly in asthma and chronic bronchitis.

Posology and method of administration: For inhalation use only. The specially developed Aerohaler* device pierces the capsules making the contents available for inhalation.

Adults: 1 capsule three or four times daily. This dose may be doubled safely in patients who are less responsive.

Children under 12 years: There is limited experience of the use of Atrovent Aerocaps in children, therefore the product is not recommended for use in children.

Elderly: There are no special dosage recommendations in the elderly. Clinical trials have included patients over 65 years and no adverse reactions specific to this age group have been reported.

One Atrovent Aerocap is equivalent to two puffs of Atrovent Inhaler or one puff of Atrovent Forte.

Contra-indications: Known hypersensitivity to atropine.

Special warnings and special precautions for use: As with other agents, powder-induced bronchoconstriction has been reported occasionally and may occur as wheeze or cough.

The patient should be warned to seek medical advice should a reduced response become apparent.

Patients must be instructed in the correct administration of Atrovent Aerocaps. Generally caution is advocated in the use of anticholinergic agents in patients with glaucoma or prostatic hypertrophy. However, specific studies with Atrovent in patients with glaucoma showed that inhaling cumulative doses of 160 micrograms had no effect on the eye.

Interaction with other medicaments and other forms of interaction: There is evidence that the concurrent administration of Atrovent and sympathomimetic drugs produces a greater relief of bronchospasm than either drug given alone.

Atrovent has been shown to produce effective bronchodilation in patients receiving beta-adrenergic blocking agents.

Pregnancy and lactation: Atrovent has been in wide general use for many years without apparent ill-consequence during pregnancy: Animal studies have shown no hazard. Nevertheless, medicines should not be used in pregnancy, especially the first trimester, unless the expected benefit is thought to outweigh any possible risk to the foetus.

Effects on ability to drive and use machines: None stated.

Undesirable effects: Anticholinergic side-effects are unlikely at therapeutic doses, but some patients may complain of a dry mouth. Urinary retention and constipation have only rarely been reported with Atrovent. There is no evidence that in the therapeutic dose range Atrovent has any adverse effect on bronchial secretion.

Overdose: Inhaled doses of 5 mg ipratropium bromide have produced an increase in heart rate and palpitation. Single doses of ipratropium bromide 30 mg by mouth caused anticholinergic side effects but these were not severe and did not require specific reversal.

Pharmacological properties
Pharmacodynamic properties: Ipratropium bromide affects airway function primarily through its neural effect on the para-sympathetic nervous system. Ipratropium bromide blocks the acetylcholine receptors on smooth muscle in the lung. Stimulation of these receptors normally produces contraction and, depending on the degree of activation, bronchoconstriction. Thus, even in normal subjects, ipratropium bromide will cause bronchodilation.

Pharmacokinetic properties: Ipratropium bromide is a quaternary ammonium compound which is poorly absorbed from the gastro-intestinal tract and is slow to cross mucous membranes and the blood brain barrier. Following inhalation, uptake into the plasma is minimal; a peak blood concentration is attained 1½ to 3 hours after inhalation (and similarly for oral administration). Excretion is chiefly via the kidneys.

Preclinical safety data: There are no pre-clinical data of relevance to the prescriber which are additional to that already included in other sections of the SPC.

Pharmaceutical particulars
List of excipients: Glucose (ground anhydrous). *Capsule shell:* Titanium dioxide (E171), indigo carmine (E132), iron oxide yellow (E172), iron oxide black (E172), gelatin.

Incompatibilities: None stated.

Shelf life: 24 months.

Special precautions for storage: Store below 25°C. Keep away from heat, including the sun.

Nature and contents of container: PVC/Aluminium blister packs containing 30, 50, 60, 90, 100, 120, 180, 240, 300 or 360 Aerocaps (currently only the 100 pack size is marketed: Pack containing 100 Aerocaps and 1 Aerohaler device and refill pack containing 100 Aerocaps).

Instructions for use/handling: Full instructions for use are given in the Patient Information Leaflet enclosed in the pack.

Marketing authorisation number 0015/0156

Date of approval/revision of SPC April 1997

Legal category POM

ATROVENT* METERED DOSE INHALER

Qualitative and quantitative composition Atrovent Metered Dose Aerosol is a 10 ml homogeneous cream coloured suspension contained in a 17 ml one-piece aluminium container with a 50 mcl metering valve. Each metered dose delivers 20 micrograms of ipratropium bromide.

Pharmaceutical form Metered dose aerosol.

Clinical particulars
Therapeutic indications: Atrovent Metered Dose Inhaler is indicated in the treatment of chronic reversible airways obstruction, particularly in chronic bronchitis.

Posology and method of administration:
Adults: Usually 1 or 2 puffs three or four times daily, although some patients may need up to 4 puffs at a time to obtain maximum benefit during early treatment.

Children:
6–12 years: Usually 1 or 2 puffs three times daily.
Under 6 years: Usually 1 puff three times daily.
In order to ensure that the inhaler is used correctly, administration should be supervised by an adult.
Some patients may find it beneficial to use the metered dose inhaler with an extension tube.

Elderly: No specific information on the use of this product in the elderly is available. Clinical trials have included patients over 65 years and no adverse reactions specific to this age group have been reported.

Contra-indications: Known hypersensitivity to atropine.

Special warnings and special precautions for use: The patient should be warned to seek medical advice should a reduced response become apparent.

Patients must be instructed in the correct use of a metered dose inhaler and warned against the accidental release of the contents into the eye. Generally, caution is advocated in the use of anticholinergic agents in patients with glaucoma or prostatic hypertrophy. However, specific studies with Atrovent in patients with glaucoma showed that inhaling cumulative doses of 0.16 mg had no effect on the eye. Patients should be informed when starting treatment that onset of action of Atrovent is slower than that of inhaled sympathomimetic bronchodilators.

Interaction with other medicaments and other forms of interaction: There is evidence that the concurrent administration of Atrovent and sympathomimetic drugs produces a greater relief of bronchospasm than either drug given alone.

Atrovent has been shown to produce effective bronchodilatation in patients receiving beta adrenergic blocking agents.

There are no serious drug interactions known.

Pregnancy and lactation: Atrovent has been in general use for several years and there is no definite evidence of ill-consequence during pregnancy; animal studies have shown no hazard. Nevertheless, medicines should not be used in pregnancy, especially during the first trimester, unless the expected benefit is thought to outweigh any possible risk to the foetus.

Effect on ability to drive and use machines: None known.

Undesirable effects: Anticholinergic side-effects are unlikely to occur at therapeutic doses although dry mouth has occasionally been reported. Urinary retention and constipation have only rarely been reported with Atrovent.

There is no evidence that in the therapeutic dose range Atrovent has any adverse effect on bronchial secretion.

Overdose: Inhaled doses of 5 mg produce an increase in heart rate and palpitation. Single doses of ipratropium bromide 30 mg by mouth caused anticholinergic side-effects but these were not severe and did not require specific reversal.

Pharmacological properties
Pharmacodynamic properties: Ipratropium bromide affects airway function primarily through its neural effects on the parasympathetic nervous system. Ipratropium bromide blocks the acetylcholine receptors on smooth muscle in the lung. Stimulation of these receptors normally produces contraction and, depending on the degree of activation, bronchoconstriction. Thus, even in normal subjects ipratropium bromide will cause bronchodilatation.

Pharmacokinetic properties: Ipratropium bromide is a quaternary ammonium compound which is poorly absorbed from the gastro-intestinal tract, and is slow to cross mucous membranes and the blood-brain barrier. Following inhalation, uptake into the plasma is minimal; a peak blood concentration is attained 1½ to 3 hours after inhalation (and similarly for oral administration). Excretion is chiefly via the kidneys.

Pharmaceutical particulars
List of excipients: Soya lecithin; monofluorotrichloromethane; difluorotrichloromethane; tetrafluorodichloroethane.

Incompatibilities: None known.

Shelf life: The shelf life expiry date for this product is 5 years from the date of its manufacture.

Special precautions for storage: Protect from heat, including the sun. Protect from frost. The vials should not be opened, punctured or incinerated even when apparently empty.

Nature and contents of container: 10 ml of a homogeneous cream coloured suspension in a 17 ml one-piece aluminium container with a 50 mcl metering valve.

Instructions for use/handling: To make sure that your inhaler is working, test fire it into the air before using it for the first time and whenever your inhaler has not been used for a week or more.

1. Remove the dustcap from the mouthpiece and **shake the inhaler vigorously.**
2. Holding the inhaler as shown, breathe out gently and then immediately . . .
3. . . . place the mouthpiece in the mouth and close your lips around it. After starting to breathe in slowly and deeply, through your mouth, press the inhaler firmly as shown to release the Atrovent. *Continue to breathe in as deeply as you can.*
4. Hold your breath for 10 seconds, or as long as is comfortable, before breathing out slowly.
5. If you are to take more than one puff you should wait at least one minute before shaking the inhaler again and repeating steps 2, 3 and 4.
6. After use, replace the dustcap on the mouthpiece.

Marketing authorisation number 00015/0043R

Date of approval/revision of SPC May 1996

Legal category POM

ATROVENT* AUTOHALER*

Qualitative and quantitative composition Each metered dose contains ipratropium bromide 20 micrograms.

Pharmaceutical form A breath-actuated pressurised aerosol for inhalation therapy.

Clinical particulars
Therapeutic indications: Atrovent Autohaler is indicated in the treatment of chronic reversible airways obstruction, particularly in chronic bronchitis.

Posology and method of administration: By inhalation.

Adults: Usually 1 or 2 puffs three or four times daily, although some patients may need up to 4 puffs at a time to obtain maximum benefit during early treatment.

Children: 6–12 years: Usually 1 or 2 puffs three times daily.
Under 6 years: Usually 1 puff three times daily.
In order to ensure that the Autohaler is used correctly, administration should be supervised by an adult.

Elderly: No specific information on the use of this product in the elderly is available. Clinical trials have included patients over 65 years and no adverse reactions specific to this age group have been reported.

Contra-indications: Known hypersensitivity to atropine.

Special warnings and special precautions for use:
Precautions: The patient should be warned to seek medical advice should a reduced response become apparent.

Patients must be instructed in the correct use of the Autohaler device. Generally, caution is advocated in the use of anticholinergic agents in patients with glaucoma or prostatic hypertrophy. However, specific studies with Atrovent in patients with glaucoma showed that inhaling cumulative doses of 0.16 mg had no effect on the eye.

Patients should be informed when starting treatment that onset of action of Atrovent is slower than that of inhaled sympathomimetic bronchodilators.

Interaction with other medicaments and other forms of interaction: There is evidence that the concurrent administration of Atrovent and sympathomimetic drugs produces a greater relief of bronchospasm than either drug given alone.

Atrovent has been shown to produce effective bronchodilatation in patients receiving beta adrenergic blocking agents. There are no serious drug interactions known.

Pregnancy and lactation: Atrovent has been in general use for several years, there is no definite evidence of ill-consequence during pregnancy; animal studies have shown no hazard. Nevertheless, medicines should not be used in pregnancy, especially during the first trimester, unless the expected benefit is thought to outweigh any possible risk to the foetus.

Effect on ability to drive and use machines: None known.

Undesirable effects: Anticholinergic side-effects are unlikely to occur at therapeutic doses, although dry mouth has occasionally been reported. Urinary retention and constipation have only rarely been reported with Atrovent. There is no evidence that in the therapeutic dose range Atrovent has any adverse effect on bronchial secretion.

Overdose: Inhaled doses of 5 mg produce an increase in heart rate and palpitation. Single doses of ipratropium bromide 30 mg by mouth caused anticholinergic side-effects but these were not severe and did not require specific reversal.

Pharmacological properties
Pharmacodynamic properties: Ipratropium bromide affects airway function primarily through its neural effects on the parasympathetic nervous system. Ipratropium bromide blocks the acetylcholine receptors on smooth muscle in the lung. Stimulation of these receptors normally produces contraction and, depending on the degree of activation, bronchoconstriction. Thus, even in normal subjects ipratropium bromide will cause bronchodilatation.

Pharmacokinetic properties: Ipratropium bromide is a quaternary ammonium compound which is poorly absorbed from the gastro-intestinal tract, and is slow to cross mucous membranes and the blood-brain barrier. Following inhalation, uptake into the plasma is minimal; a peak blood concentration is attained 1.5

to 3 hours after inhalation (and similarly for oral administration). Excretion is chiefly via the kidneys.

Preclinical safety data: There are no pre-clinical data of relevance to the prescriber which are additional to that already included in other sections of the SPC.

Pharmaceutical particulars
List of excipients: Soya lecithin, monofluorotrichloromethane, difluorotrichloromethane, tetrafluorodichloroethane.

Incompatibilities: None stated.

Shelf life: 5 years.

Special precautions for storage: Store below 25°C. Protect from direct sunlight. Protect from frost. The vials should not be opened, punctured or incinerated even when apparently empty.

Nature and contents of container: 17 ml aluminium aerosol can with metering valve (200 metered doses). Pack size: 10 ml.

Instructions for use/handling:
1. To remove the mouthpiece cover, pull down on the lip at the back.
2. Hold the Autohaler upright as shown. Push the lever up so that it stays up.
3. With the lever still up, shake the Autohaler.
4. Continue to hold the Autohaler device upright, making sure that your hand is not blocking the air vents at the bottom. Breathe out normally and close your lips firmly around the mouthpiece.
5. Breathe in through the mouthpiece. When you hear the slight click, continue to breathe in. This click lets you know you have received your puff of medication. Hold your breath for 10 seconds, or as long as is comfortable, and then breathe out normally.
6. The lever must be lowered after each puff. If your doctor has prescribed more than one puff, wait one minute before repeating steps 2–6. Replace the mouthpiece cover after use.

Marketing authorisation number 0015/0160

Date of approval/revision of SPC May 1997

Legal category POM

ATROVENT* 250 UDVs*, 1 ml
ATROVENT* UDVs*, 2 ml

Qualitative and quantitative composition Each single dose unit contains 0.025% w/v ipratropium bromide i.e. 250 micrograms in 1 ml and 500 micrograms in 2 ml.

Pharmaceutical form Inhalation solution presented in single dose units of 1 ml and 2 ml.

Clinical particulars
Therapeutic indications: Atrovent 250 UDVs, 1 ml and Atrovent UDVs, 2 ml, are indicated in the treatment of reversible airways obstruction.

Posology and method of administration: By inhalation from an intermittent positive pressure ventilator or from suitable nebulisers.

Adults: 0.4–2.0 ml solution (100–500 micrograms) up to 4 times daily.

Children (3–14 years): 0.4–2.0 ml solution (100–500 micrograms) up to 3 times daily.

There is no specific information on the use of the isotonic nebuliser solution in the elderly. Clinical trials with the previously available hypotonic formulation included patients over 65 years and no adverse reactions specific to this age group were reported.

The dose of nebuliser solution may need to be diluted in order to obtain a final volume suitable for the particular nebuliser being used; if dilution is necessary use only sterile sodium chloride 0.9% solution.

Contra-indications: Known hypersensitivity to atropine.

Special warnings and precautions for use: Use of the nebuliser solution should be subject to close medical supervision during initial dosing. There have been rare reports of paradoxical bronchospasm associated with the administration of Atrovent nebuliser solution. The patient should be advised to seek mecical advice should a reduced response become apparent.

Patients must be instructed in the correct administration of Atrovent UDVs and warned not to allow the solution or mist to enter the eyes. Acute angle-closure glaucoma has been reported rarely when Atrovent UDVs have been used in conjunction with nebulised β_2-agonist bronchodilators. Protection of the eyes appears to prevent any increase in intra-ocular pressure and patients who may be susceptible to glaucoma should be warned specifically on the need for ocular protection. Inhaled doses of Atrovent UDVs up to 1 mg have not been associated with elevation of intra-ocular pressure.

Caution is advocated in the use of anticholinergic agents in patients with prostatic hypertrophy.

Interaction with other medicaments and other forms of interaction: There is evidence to suggest that the concurrent administration of Atrovent and sympathomimetic drugs produces a greater relief of bronchospasm than either drug given alone.

Atrovent has been shown to produce effective bronchodilatation in patients receiving beta-blocking agents.

Pregnancy and lactation: Atrovent has been in general use for several years and there is no definite evidence of ill-consequence during pregnancy; animal studies have shown no hazard. Nevertheless, medicines should not be used in pregnancy, especially during the first trimester, unless the expected benefit is thought to outweigh any possible risk to the foetus.

Effect on ability to drive and use machines: None stated.

Undesirable effects: Anticholinergic side-effects are unlikely at therapeutic doses, but some patients may complain of a dry mouth. Urinary retention and constipation have only rarely been reported with Atrovent.

There is no evidence that in the therapeutic dose range Atrovent has any adverse effect on bronchial secretion.

Overdose: Inhaled doses of 5 mg produce an increase in heart rate and palpitation but single doses of 2 mg have been given to adults and 1 mg to children without causing side-effects. Single doses of ipratropium bromide 30 mg by mouth cause anticholinergic side-effects but these are not severe and do not require reversal.

Pharmacological properties
Pharmacodynamic properties: Ipratropium bromide is an anticholinergic bronchodilator.

Pharmacokinetic properties: Ipratropium bromide is poorly absorbed from the gastro-intestinal tract. It has been reported to be partly metabolised following oral administration and to be excreted in the urine and faeces as unchanged drug and metabolites. Little or none is absorbed from the lungs following inhalation.

Pharmaceutical particulars
List of excipients: Sodium chloride, 1N Hydrochloric acid, Purified water.

Incompatibilities: None stated.

Shelf life: 3 years.

As the product contains no preservative, a fresh vial should be used for each dose and the vial should be opened immediately before administration. Any solution left in the vial should be discarded.

Special precautions for storage: Store below 25°C. Protect from direct light.

Nature and contents of container: Polyethylene single dose units packed in cartons. Each single dose unit contains either 1 ml or 2 ml of solution in pack sizes of 10, 20, 30, 50, 60, 80, 100, 120, 150, 200, 300, 500 and 1000.

Pack sizes of 20 and 60 are currently marketed.

Instructions for use/handling: Atrovent 250 UDVs, 1 ml and Atrovent UDVs, 2 ml, should only be used in a nebuliser approved by your doctor.

1. Get your nebuliser ready by following the manufacturer's instructions and the advice of your doctor.
2. Carefully separate a new dose unit from the strip. NEVER use one which has been opened already.
3. Open by simply twisting off the top, always taking care to hold it in an upright position.
4. Unless otherwise instructed by your doctor, squeeze all the contents into the nebuliser chamber. If dilution is necessary this should be carried out using ONLY sterile sodium chloride 0.9% solution and as instructed by your doctor.
5. Use your nebuliser as directed by your doctor.
6. After you have finished, throw away any leftover solution.

Follow the manufacturer's instructions for cleaning your nebuliser. It is important that your nebuliser is kept clean.

Marketing authorisation number PL 0015/0108

Date of first authorisation/renewal of authorisation 27 August 1986/17 January 1997

Date of revision of the text July 1998

Legal category POM.

ATROVENT* FORTE

Qualitative and quantitative composition Each metered dose contains ipratropium bromide 40 micrograms.

Pharmaceutical form A metered dose inhaler for inhalation therapy.

Clinical particulars
Therapeutic indications: Atrovent Forte is indicated for the treatment of chronic reversible airways obstruction, particularly in chronic bronchitis.

Posology and method of administration: For administration by inhalation only.

Adults: Usually 1 puff three or four times daily, although some patients may need 2 puffs at a time to obtain maximum benefit during early treatment.

Children 6–12 years: Usually 1 puff three times daily. In order to ensure that the inhaler is used correctly, administration should be supervised by an adult.

No specific information on the use of this product in the elderly is available. Clinical trials have included patients over 65 years and no adverse reactions specific to this age group have been reported.

Contra-indications: Known hypersensitivity to any components of the formulation or atropine. Since the formulation contains soya lecithin, patients who are hypersensitive to related food products such as soya bean or peanuts are also contra-indicated.

Special warnings and special precautions for use: The patient should be warned to seek medical advice should a reduced response become apparent.

Patients must be instructed in the correct use of a metered dose inhaler and warned against accidental release of the contents into the eye.

Generally, caution is advocated in the use of anticholinergic agents in patients with glaucoma or prostatic hypertrophy. However, specific studies with Atrovent in patients with glaucoma showed that inhaling cumulative doses of 160 micrograms had no effect on the eye.

Interaction with other medicaments and other forms of interaction: There is evidence that the concurrent administration of Atrovent and sympathomimetic drugs produce a greater relief of bronchospasm than either drug given alone. Atrovent has been shown to produce effective bronchodilatation in patients receiving beta-adrenergic blocking agents.

Pregnancy and lactation: Atrovent has been in general use for several years, there is no definite evidence of ill-consequence during pregnancy; animal studies have shown no hazard. Nevertheless, medicines should not be used in pregnancy, especially during the first trimester, unless the expected benefit is thought to outweigh any possible risk to the foetus.

Effects on ability to drive and use machines: None stated.

Undesirable effects: Anticholinergic side-effects are unlikely to occur at therapeutic doses, although dry mouth has occasionally been reported. Urinary retention and constipation have only rarely been reported with Atrovent. There is no evidence that in the therapeutic dose range Atrovent has any adverse effect on bronchial secretion.

Overdose: Inhaled doses of 5 mg produce an increase in heart rate and palpitation. Single doses of ipratropium bromide 30 mg by mouth caused anticholinergic side-effects but these were not severe and did not require specific reversal.

Pharmacological properties
Pharmacodynamic properties: Ipratropium bromide is an anticholinergic bronchodilator which affects airway function primarily through its neural effects on the parasympathetic nervous system. Ipratropium bromide blocks the acetylcholine receptors on smooth muscle in the lung. Stimulation of these receptors normally produces contraction and depending on the degree of activation, bronchoconstriction. Thus ipratropium bromide will cause bronchodilatation.

Pharmacokinetic properties: Ipratropium bromide is a quaternary ammonium compound which is poorly absorbed from the gastro-intestinal tract, and is slow to cross mucous membranes and the blood brain barrier. Following inhalation, uptake into the plasma is minimal, a peak blood concentration is attained 1½ to 3 hours after inhalation (and similarly for oral administration). Excretion is chiefly via the kidneys.

Pharmaceutical particulars
List of excipients:
Soya lecithin
Monofluorotrichloromethane
Difluorodichloromethane
Tetrafluorodichloroethane

Incompatibilities: None stated.

Shelf life: 5 years.

Special precautions for storage: Store below 25°C. Protect from heat, including the sun. Protect from frost. The vials should not be opened, punctured or incinerated even when apparently empty.

Nature and contents of container: A 17 ml one piece aluminium vial (fill volume 10 ml) with a 50 µl metering valve containing 200 metered doses.

Instructions for use/handling
Correct use of the inhaler:
1. Remove the dustcap from the mouthpiece and **shake the inhaler vigorously**.
2. Holding the inhaler as shown, breathe out gently and then immediately . . .
3. . . . place the mouthpiece in the mouth and close your lips around it. After starting to breathe in slowly and deeply, through your mouth, press the inhaler firmly as shown to release the Atrovent Forte. *Continue to breathe in as deeply as you can.*
4. Hold your breath for 10 seconds, or as long as is comfortable, before breathing out slowly.
5. If you are to take more than one puff you should wait at least one minute before shaking the inhaler again and repeating steps 2, 3 and 4.
6. After use, replace the dustcap on the mouthpiece.

How to clean and care for the inhaler: Remove the canister and dustcap. Wash and clean the grey mouthpiece in warm soapy water, rinse in warm water, dry.

Marketing authorisation number PL 0015/0107

Date of renewal of authorisation 06/07/95

Date of revision of the text May 1996

Legal category POM.

BEROTEC* 100 METERED DOSE INHALER

Qualitative and quantitative composition Each actuation delivers 100 micrograms of fenoterol hydrobromide.

Pharmaceutical form Pressurised metered aerosol.

Clinical particulars
Therapeutic indications: For the treatment of reversible airways obstruction in bronchial asthma and chronic obstructive pulmonary disease.

Posology and method of administration: By inhalation.

Adults: The recommended dose of Berotec 100 is one to two puffs given as a single dose. This may be given 1–3 times daily. Dosing should not exceed two puffs every six hours (i.e. the maximum dose is 800 micrograms daily). Patients with persistent bronchospasm and those who require higher doses may be prescribed Berotec 200.

Children: Children aged 6–12 years will normally require one puff. This may be given 1–3 times daily. Dosing should not exceed two puffs every six hours (i.e. the maximum dose is 800 micrograms daily). It is recommended that administration of Berotec 100 to children should be supervised by a responsible adult.

Elderly: No specific information on the use of this product in the elderly is available. Clinical trials have included patients over 65 years and no adverse reactions specific to this age group have been reported.

Contra-indications: Hypersensitivity to fenoterol hydrobromide or inactive ingredients of the metered aerosol.

Special warnings and special precautions for use: In patients suffering from bronchial asthma, on demand or symptom-oriented treatment may be preferable to regular use. A chronic requirement for treatment would suggest the need for clinical review of the management of the patient's asthma. The use of inhaled corticosteroids as anti-inflammatory treatment should be considered.

Patients must be instructed in the correct use of a metered aerosol and warned not to exceed the prescribed dose. In the case of acute rapidly worsening dyspnoea (difficulty in breathing) a doctor should be consulted immediately.

Excessive use of sympathomimetic agents can cause unwanted effects. The concomitant use of other sympathomimetic drugs should be avoided or only used under strict medical supervision. Concurrent administration of Berotec with anticholinergic bronchodilators in reversible airways obstruction has been shown to produce greater bronchodilatation than the use of either agent alone (but see Interactions).

In the following conditions Berotec 100 should only be used after careful risk/benefit assessment, especially when doses higher than those recommended are used:

Insufficiently controlled diabetes mellitus, recent myocardial infarction, severe organic heart or vascular disorders, such as hypertrophic obstructive cardiomyopathy and tachyarrhythmia; hyperthyroidism.

Potentially serious hypokalaemia may result from excessive beta$_2$-agonist therapy. This effect may be potentiated by concomitant treatment with xanthine derivatives, glucocorticosteroids and diuretics. Additionally, hypoxia may aggravate the effects of hypokalaemia on cardiac rhythm. It is recommended that serum potassium levels are monitored in such situations.

Interaction with other medicaments and other forms of interaction: In view of the possible interaction between sympathomimetic amines and monoamine oxidase inhibitors or tricyclic anti-depressants, care should be exercised if it is proposed to administer these compounds concurrently with Berotec.

Beta-adrenergics, anticholinergics, xanthine derivatives and corticosteroids may enhance the bronchodilator effect of fenoterol. The concurrent administration of the other beta-mimetics, systemically absorbed anticholinergics and xanthine derivatives may increase the frequency and severity of unwanted effects.

Potentially serious bronchospasm may occur during concurrent administration of beta-blockers to patients with reversible airways obstruction.

Pregnancy and lactation: Although fenoterol hydrobromide has been in general use for several years, there is no definite evidence of ill-consequence following administration of the drug during human pregnancy; animal studies have shown no hazard.

Nonetheless, the usual precautions regarding the use of drug during pregnancy, especially during the first trimester, should be exercised.

The inhibitory effect of fenoterol on uterine contraction should be taken into account.

Preclinical studies have shown that fenoterol is secreted in breast milk.

Safety in breast-fed infants has not been established.

Effect on ability to drive and use machines: None stated.

Undesirable effects: Frequent undesirable effects observed with Berotec 100 are tremor, nervousness, headache, dizziness, tachycardia, palpitations and oropharyngeal irritation. Allergic reactions have also been reported.

As with other inhaled bronchodilators, cough and paradoxical bronchospasm have been reported.

Overdose: Symptoms: Flushing, tremor, nausea, restlessness, tachycardia, palpitation, dizziness, headache, increase in systolic blood pressure, fall in diastolic blood pressure, a feeling of pressure in the chest, excitation and extra systoles may occur following overdose. Hypokalaemia may occur following overdose with fenoterol. Serum potassium levels should be monitored.

Therapy: Treatment of overdosage should primarily be supportive and symptom oriented.

If specific therapy is considered necessary, cardioselective beta-blockers are to be preferred. These should be administered with extreme caution to patients with asthma because of the risk of precipitating severe bronchospasm.

Pharmacological properties
Pharmacodynamic properties: Berotec is highly effective adrenergic exerting a selective effect on the beta$_2$-receptors of the bronchial tree. The active ingredient, fenoterol hydrobromide, is a sympathomimetic amine where the catechol nucleus of isoprenaline has been replaced by a resorcinol nucleus, and the substituent moiety on the amino group is larger. This substitution has the effect of depressing the affinity of the molecule towards beta$_1$ (cardiac and lipolytic) adrenergic receptors and enhancing the affinity towards the beta$_2$ (bronchial vascular and intestinal) adrenergic receptors.

Pharmacokinetic properties: Fenoterol hydrobromide is readily absorbed orally in the dog (90%) and maximum blood levels achieved in 30 minutes to one hour. About 78% is excreted in the urine of the dog, with the remainder eliminated by the bile duct or directly through the gastrointestinal tract. No significant enterohepatic circulation was detected in the dog.

The absorbed compound is very rapidly taken up by the tissues and detoxified via the formation of acid conjugates. Excretion of the conjugates is also very rapid. Excretion of the drug by the kidneys is essentially complete after 12 hours.

Renal excretion accounts for 1% after oral administration to rats with 79% in the faeces.

In man fenoterol is very rapidly distributed through the tissues following intravenous administration. The kidneys excrete up to 65% mainly in the form of acidic conjugates. Following oral administration, the plasma levels reach their maximum 2 hours after ingestion and then drop exponentially. The renal excretion is 39% following peroral administration and over 98% of the renal excretory products consist of acidic conjugates. The half life for total excretion is 7.2 hours and absorption was calculated to be 60%.

The duration of action following the use of a metered aerosol is considerably larger and can be explained by the dose independent absorption in the upper bronchial tree. The concentration-independent absorption at this site, from the depot produced by the metered aerosol is maintained for several hours.

Pharmaceutical particulars
List of excipients: Sorbitan trioleate; monofluorotrichloromethane; difluorodichloromethane; tetrafluorodichloroethane.

Incompatibilities: None stated.

Shelf life: 5 years.

Special precautions for storage: Protect from heat, including the sun. Protect from frost.

The vials should not be opened, punctured or incinerated even when apparently empty.

Nature and contents of container: A one piece aluminium vial fitted with a 50 mcl metering valve and containing 10 ml (100 doses) of a white homogeneous suspension, complete with mouthpiece.

Instructions for use/handling: The correct administration of the metered aerosol is essential for successful therapy.

To make sure that your inhaler is working, test fire it twice into the air before using it for the first time and whenever your inhaler has not been used for a week or more.

1. Remove the dustcap from the mouthpiece and shake the inhaler vigorously.
2. Holding the inhaler as shown, breathe out gently and then immediately . . .
3. . . . place the mouthpiece in the mouth and close your lips around it. After starting to breathe in slowly and deeply, through your mouth, press the inhaler firmly as shown to release the Berotec. *Continue to breathe in as deeply as you can.*
4. Hold your breath for 10 seconds, or as long as is comfortable, before breathing out slowly.
5. If you are to take more than one puff you should wait at least one minute before shaking the inhaler again and repeating steps 2, 3 and 4.
6. After use, replace the dustcap on the mouthpiece.

Marketing authorisation number 0015/0150

Date of approval/revision of SPC August 1996

Legal category POM

BEROTEC* 200 METERED DOSE INHALER

Qualitative and quantitative composition Each actuation delivers 200 micrograms of fenoterol hydrobromide.

Pharmaceutical form Pressurised metered aerosol.

Clinical particulars
Therapeutic indications: For the treatment of reversible airways obstruction in bronchial asthma and chronic obstructive pulmonary disease.

Posology and method of administration:
By inhalation:
Adults: The recommended dose of Berotec 200 is two puffs given as a single dose. This may be given 1–3 times daily. Patients who can be controlled with lower doses should be prescribed Berotec 100. Dosing must not exceed two puffs every six hours (i.e. the maximum daily dose is 1600 micrograms).

Children: Berotec 200 is not recommended for children under 16 years of age.

Elderly: No specific information on the use of this product in the elderly is available. Clinical trials have included patients over 65 years and no adverse reactions specific to this age group have been reported.

Contra-indications: Hypersensitivity to fenoterol hydrobromide or inactive ingredients of the metered aerosol.

Special warnings and special precautions for use: In patients suffering from bronchial asthma, on demand or symptom-oriented treatment may be preferable to regular use. A chronic requirement for treatment would suggest the need for clinical review of the management of the patient's asthma. The use of inhaled corticosteroids as anti-inflammatory treatment should be considered.

Patients must be instructed in the correct use of a metered aerosol and warned not to exceed the prescribed dose. In the case of acute rapidly worsening dyspnoea (difficulty in breathing) a doctor should be consulted immediately.

Excessive use of sympathomimetic agents can cause unwanted effects. The concomitant use of other sympathomimetic drugs should be avoided or only used under strict medical supervision. Concurrent administration of Berotec with anticholinergic bronchodilators in reversible airways obstruction has been shown to produce greater bronchodilatation than the use of either agent alone (but see *Interactions*).

In the following conditions Berotec 200 should only be used after careful risk/benefit assessment, especially when doses higher than those recommended are used: Insufficiently controlled diabetes mellitus, recent myocardial infarction, severe organic heart or vascular disorders, such as hypertrophic obstructive cardiomyopathy and tachyarrhythmia; hyperthyroidism.

Potentially serious hypokalaemia may result from excessive $beta_2$-agonist therapy. This effect may be potentiated by concomitant treatment with xanthine derivatives, glucocorticosteroids and diuretics. Additionally, hypoxia may aggravate the effects of hypokalaemia on cardiac rhythm. It is recommended that serum potassium levels are monitored in such situations.

Interaction with other medicaments and other forms of interaction: In view of the possible interaction between sympathomimetic amines and monoamine oxidase inhibitors or tricyclic anti-depressants, care should be exercised if it is proposed to administer these compounds concurrently with Berotec.

Beta-adrenergics, anticholinergics, xanthine derivatives and corticosteroids may enhance the bronchodilator effect of fenoterol. The concurrent administration of the other beta-mimetics, systemically absorbed anticholinergics and xanthine derivatives may increase the frequency and severity of unwanted effects.

Potentially serious bronchospasm may occur during concurrent administration of beta-blockers to patients with reversible airways obstruction.

Pregnancy and lactation: Although fenoterol hydrobromide has been in general use for several years, there is no definite evidence of ill-consequence following administration of the drug during human pregnancy; animal studies have shown no hazard.

Nonetheless, the usual precautions regarding the use of drugs during pregnancy, especially during the first trimester, should be exercised.

The inhibitory effect of fenoterol on uterine contraction should be taken into account.

Preclinical studies have shown that fenoterol is secreted in breast milk.

Safety in breast-fed infants has not been established.

Effect on ability to drive and use machines: None stated.

Undesirable effects: Frequent undesirable effects observed with Berotec 200 are tremor, nervousness, headache, dizziness, tachycardia, palpitations and oropharyngeal irritation. Allergic reactions have also been reported. As with other inhaled bronchodilators, cough and paradoxical bronchospasm have been reported.

Overdose

Symptoms: Flushing, tremor, nausea, restlessness, tachycardia, palpitation, dizziness, headache, increase in systolic blood pressure, fall in diastolic blood pressure, a feeling of pressure in the chest, excitation and extra systoles may occur following overdose. Hypokalaemia may occur following overdose with fenoterol. Serum potassium levels should be monitored.

Therapy: Treatment of overdosage should primarily be supportive and symptom oriented.

If specific therapy is considered necessary, cardioselective beta-blockers are to be preferred. These should be administered with extreme caution to patients with asthma because of the risk of precipitating severe bronchospasm.

Pharmacological properties

Pharmacodynamic properties: Fenoterol hydrobromide is a sympathetic amine, having high affinity for $beta_2$ (bronchial/vascular/intestinal) receptors. Fenoterol acts as a bronchodilator, increasing the rate of ciliary activity and speed of mucus transport, while having no effect on the heart and peripheral circulation. Animal studies have shown that this selective effect is further improved by inhalation of the drug. Lung function studies in man have shown fenoterol to be efficacious in the reduction of airways resistance and in protection against induced bronchospasm.

Pharmacokinetic properties: Pharmacokinetic studies show that the effect of the inhalation is due to the local effect in the bronchial muscle and does not correlate with plasma levels. Compared with equivalent oral doses, the plasma levels after inhalation are lower by a factor of 500–1000 and show a delayed course similar to that after oral administration. In contrast, the onset of the effect after inhalation is much more rapid.

Pharmaceutical particulars

List of excipients:

Sorbitan Trioleate
Monofluorotrichloromethane
Difluorodichloromethane
Tetrafluorodichloroethane

Incompatibilities: None known.

Shelf life: 5 years.

Special precautions for storage: Protect from heat, including the sun. Protect from frost.

The vials should not be opened, punctured or incinerated even when apparently empty.

Nature and contents of container: A one-piece aluminium vial fitted with a 50 µl metering valve and containing 10 ml (200 doses) of a white homogeneous suspension, complete with mouthpiece.

Instructions for use/handling: The correct administration of the metered aerosol is essential for successful therapy.

To make sure that your inhaler is working, test fire it twice into the air before using it for the first time and whenever your inhaler has not been used for a week or more.

1. Remove the dustcap from the mouthpiece and **shake the inhaler vigorously.**
2. Holding the inhaler as shown, breathe out gently and then immediately . . .
3. . . . place the mouthpiece in the mouth and close your lips around it. After starting to breathe in slowly and deeply, through your mouth, press the inhaler firmly as shown to release the Berotec. *Continue to breathe in as deeply as you can.*
4. Hold your breath for 10 seconds, or as long as is comfortable, before breathing out slowly.
5. If you are to take more than one puff you should wait at least one minute before shaking the inhaler again and repeating steps 2, 3 and 4.
6. After use, replace the dustcap on the mouthpiece.

Marketing authorisation numbers

UK:	PL 0015/0034
Ireland:	PA 7/33/1

Date of first authorisation

UK Product Licence	08.03.77
Irish Product Authorisation	28.01.82

Date of revision of the text December 1996.

Legal category POM.

BUSCOPAN* AMPOULES

Qualitative and quantitative composition Each 1 ml ampoule contains hyoscine-N-butylbromide 20 mg.

Pharmaceutical form Ampoules for intramuscular or intravenous injection.

Clinical particulars

Therapeutic indications: Buscopan Ampoules are indicated in acute spasm, as in renal or biliary colic, in radiology for differential diagnosis of obstruction and to reduce spasm and pain in pyelography, and in other diagnostic procedures where spasm may be a problem, e.g. gastro-duodenal endoscopy.

Posology and method of administration:

Not recommended for children.

Adults: One ampoule (20 mg) intramuscularly or intravenously, repeated after half an hour if necessary. When used in endoscopy this dose may need to be repeated more frequently.

Diluent: Buscopan injection solution may be diluted with dextrose or with sodium chloride 0.9% injection solutions. It is also miscible and compatible with most of the commonly used aqueous radiological contrast media such as sodium diatrizoate.

No specific information on the use of this product in the elderly is available. Clinical trials have included patients over 65 years and no adverse reactions specific to this age group have been reported.

Contra-indications: Buscopan Ampoules should not be administered to patients with myasthenia gravis, megacolon, glaucoma, tachycardia, benign prostatic hypertrophy with urinary retention and mechanical stenoses in the region of the gastrointestinal tract.

In addition, Buscopan should not be used in patients with a known sensitivity to hyoscine-N-butylbromide.

Special warnings and special precautions for use: Buscopan Ampoules should be used with caution in conditions characterised by tachycardia such as thyrotoxicosis, cardiac insufficiency or failure and in cardiac surgery where it may further accelerate the heart rate.

Because of the possibility that anticholinergics may reduce sweating, Buscopan should be administered with caution to patients with pyrexia and in situations where the ambient temperature is high.

Interaction with other medicaments and other forms of interaction: The anticholinergic effect of tricyclic antidepressants, antihistamines, quinidine, amantadine, phenothiazines, butyrophenones and disopyramide may be intensified by Buscopan.

The tachycardic effects of beta-adrenergic agents may be enhanced by Buscopan.

Pregnancy and lactation: Although Buscopan has been in wide general use for many years, there is no definitive evidence of ill-consequence during human pregnancy; animal studies have shown no hazard. Nevertheless, medicines should not be used in pregnancy, especially the first trimester, unless the expected benefit is thought to outweigh any possible risk to the foetus.

Safety during lactation has not yet been established.

Effect on ability to drive and use machines: Because of visual accommodation disturbances patients should not drive or operate machinery after parenteral administration of Buscopan until vision has normalised.

Undesirable effects: Anticholinergic side-effects including dry mouth, visual accommodation disturbances, tachycardia, dizziness, constipation and potentially urinary retention may occur but are generally mild and self-limiting.

Allergic reactions including skin reactions, anaphylactoid reactions and anaphylactic shock have been reported very rarely.

There have been extremely rare reports of dyspnoea in patients with a history of bronchial asthma or allergy.

Injection site pain, particularly after intramuscular use, occurs infrequently.

Overdose

Symptoms: Serious signs of poisoning following acute overdosage have not been observed in man. In the case of overdosage, anticholinergic symptoms such as urinary retention, dry mouth, tachycardia, drowsiness, orthostatic hypotension and transient visual disturbances may occur, and Cheynes-Stokes respiration has been reported.

Therapy: Symptoms of Buscopan overdosage respond to parasympathomimetics. For patients with glaucoma, pilocarpine should be given locally. Circulation can be supported with sympathomimetics. In the case of orthostatic fall in blood pressure, it is sufficient for the patient to lie flat. Catheterisation may be required for urinary retention.

In addition, appropriate supportive measures should be used as required.

Pharmacological properties

Pharmacodynamic properties: Buscopan is an antispasmodic agent, which relaxes smooth muscle of the organs of the abdominal and pelvic cavities. It is believed to act predominantly on the intramural parasympathetic ganglia of these organs.

Pharmacokinetic properties: i.v. administration of tritiated hyoscine butylbromide (HBB) resulted in very rapid disappearance of radioactivity from plasma.

Following i.v. administration of 8 mg tritiated HBB it was found that 42% of the activity was eliminated via the urine and 37% via the faeces. Other studies using 20 mg i.v. has shown that 54% and 52.5%, were excreted in the urine and 35–55% and 10% were excreted in the faeces.

The renal excretion of i.v. HBB was found to be rapid.

Pharmaceutical particulars

List of excipients: Sodium chloride, Distilled water.

Incompatibilities: None stated.

Shelf life: 5 years.

Special precautions for storage: Store below 30°C. Protect from light.

Nature and contents of container: 1 ml clear glass ampoules containing a clear colourless sterile solution for parenteral administration to human beings, packed in cartons containing 10 ampoules.

Instructions for use/handling: None stated.

Marketing authorisation number PL 0015/5005R

Date of first authorisation/renewal of authorisation 19 July 1985/11 December 1997

Date of (partial) revision of the text December 1997

Legal category POM.

BUSCOPAN* TABLETS

Qualitative and quantitative composition Each tablet contains hyoscine-N-butylbromide 10 mg.

Pharmaceutical form Tablet for oral administration.

Clinical particulars

Therapeutic indications: Buscopan Tablets are indicated for the relief of spasm of the genito-urinary tract or gastrointestinal tract, for the symptomatic relief of Irritable Bowel Syndrome, and in the prevention and treatment of spasmodic dysmenorrhoea.

Posology and method of administration: Buscopan Tablets should be swallowed whole with adequate water.

Adults: 2 tablets four times daily.

For the symptomatic relief of Irritable Bowel Syndrome, the recommended starting dose is 1 tablet three times daily; this can be increased up to 2 tablets four times daily if necessary. In spasmodic dysmenorrhoea, treatment should commence two days before the expected onset of the period and continue for three days after menstruation has begun.

Children 6–12 years: 1 tablet three times daily.

No specific information on the use of this product in the elderly is available. Clinical trials have included patients over 65 years and no adverse reactions specific to this age group have been reported.

Contra-indications: Buscopan Tablets should not be administered to patients with myasthenia gravis, megacolon and glaucoma. In addition, they should not be given to patients with a known sensitivity to hyoscine-N-butylbromide.

Special warnings and special precautions for use: Due to the risk of anticholinergic complications, caution should be used in patients susceptible to intestinal or urinary outlet obstructions and in those inclined to tachycardia.

Because of the possibility that anticholinergics may reduce sweating, Buscopan should be administered with caution to patients with pyrexia and in situations where the ambient temperature is high.

Additional warnings for the patient information leaflet for the pharmacy only pack size (in relation to the Irritable Bowel Syndrome Indication).

Special warnings if you are taking Buscopan Tablets for Irritable Bowel Syndrome.

If this is the first time you have had symptoms of Irritable Bowel Syndrome, consult your doctor before using any treatment.

If any of the following apply to you do not take Buscopan Tablets. It may not be the right treatment for you. See your doctor as soon as possible.

- you are aged over 40 years or over
- you have passed blood from the bowel
- you are feeling sick or vomiting
- you have lost your appetite or lost weight
- you are looking pale and feeling tired
- you are suffering from severe constipation
- you have a fever
- you have recently travelled abroad
- you have abnormal vaginal bleeding or discharge
- you have difficulty or pain passing urine

Consult your doctor if you have developed new symptoms, or if your symptoms worsen, or if they do not improve after 2 weeks of treatment.

Interaction with other medicaments or other forms of interaction: The anticholinergic effect of other drugs, for example tricyclic antidepressants, antihistamines, quinidine, amantadine, butyrophenones, phenothiazines and disopyramide may be intensified by Buscopan.

Concomitant treatment with dopamine antagonists such as metoclopramide may result in diminution of the effects of both drugs on the gastrointestinal tract.

The tachycardic effects of beta-adrenergic agents may be enhanced by Buscopan.

Pregnancy and lactation: Although Buscopan has been in wide general use for many years, there is no definitive evidence of ill-consequence during human pregnancy; animal studies have shown no hazard. Medicines should not be used in pregnancy, especially during the first trimester, unless the expected benefit is thought to outweigh any possible risk to the foetus.

Safety during lactation has not yet been established.

Effects on ability to drive and use machines: Because of possible visual accommodation disturbances patients should not drive or operate machinery if affected.

Undesirable effects: Anticholinergic side-effects including dry mouth, visual accommodation disturbances, tachycardia, constipation and potentially urinary retention, may occur but are generally mild and self-limiting.

Allergic reactions, particularly skin reactions, have been reported very rarely.

There have been extremely rare reports of dyspnoea in patients with a history of bronchial asthma or allergy.

Overdose

Symptoms: Serious signs of poisoning following acute overdosage have not been observed in man. In the case of overdosage, anticholinergic effects such as urinary retention, dry mouth, tachycardia, drowsiness, orthostatic hypotension and transient visual disturbances, may occur, and Cheynes-Stokes respiration has been reported.

Therapy: In the case of oral poisoning, gastric lavage with medicinal charcoal should be followed by magnesium sulphate (15%). Symptoms of Buscopan overdosage respond to parasympathomimetics. For patients with glaucoma, pilocarpine should be given locally. Circulation can be supported with sympathomimetics. In the case of orthostatic fall in blood pressure, it is sufficient for the patient to lie flat. Catheterisation may be required for urinary retention.

In addition, appropriate supportive measures should be administered as required.

Pharmacological properties

Pharmacodynamic properties: Buscopan exerts a spasmolytic action on the smooth muscle of the gastrointestinal, biliary and genito-urinary tracts. Peripheral anticholinergic action results from a ganglion-blocking action within the visceral wall as well as from anti-muscarinic activity.

Pharmacokinetic properties: Following oral and intravenous administration, hyoscine-N-butylbromide concentrates in the tissue of the gastrointestinal tract, liver and kidneys. As a quaternary ammonium derivative, hyoscine-N-butylbromide does not pass the blood-brain barrier or enter the central nervous system.

Following oral administration, hyoscine-N-butylbromide is only partially absorbed. Nevertheless, despite the briefly measurable low blood levels, hyoscine-N-butylbromide remains available at the site of action because of its high tissue affinity.

Preclinical safety data: There are no pre-clinical data of relevance to the prescriber which are additional to that already included in other sections of the SPC.

Pharmaceutical particulars

List of excipients:

Calcium hydrogen phosphate	Sucrose
	Talc
Maize starch, dried	Gum arabic
Starch, soluble	Titanium dioxide
Colloidal silica	Polyethylene glycol 6000
Tartaric acid	Carnauba wax
Stearic/Palmitic acid	White beeswax
Ethanol	Povidone
Water, purified	

Incompatibilities: None stated.

Shelf life: Five years.

Special precautions for storage: Store in a dry place below 25°C. Protect from light.

Nature and contents of container: Buscopan Tablets are registered in blister packs of 56, 100, 500 and 560 with a Prescription Only status and blister packs of 20 and 24 with a Pharmacy Only status. However, currently the marketed packs in the UK are blister packs of 56 (POM) and 20 (P) tablets.

Instructions for use/handling: None stated.

Marketing authorisation number PL 0015/0047R

Date of first authorisation/renewal of authorisation 31 May 1990

Date of revision of the text September 1996

Legal category
56 pack: POM
20 pack: P

CATAPRES* AMPOULES

Qualitative and quantitative composition 1 ml colourless glass ampoules containing 0.150 mg clonidine hydrochloride in each 1 ml of solution.

Pharmaceutical form Ampoules for injection.

Clinical particulars

Therapeutic indications: Catapres is indicated for the treatment of hypertensive crises.

Posology and method of administration: In hypertensive crises 1 or 2 Catapres Ampoules should be given by slow intravenous injection.

An effect is usually seen within 10 minutes and reaches a maximum about 30 minutes to 1 hour after administration. The duration of effect depends upon the severity of the condition and is commonly of the order of 3-7 hours. Up to 5 ampoules may be given in 24 hours to achieve and maintain the required blood pressure.

Patients undergoing anaesthesia should continue their Catapres treatment before, during and after anaesthesia using oral or intravenous administration according to individual circumstances.

Intravenous injection of Catapres should be given slowly over 10-15 minutes to avoid a possible transient pressor effect.

Catapres injection solution is compatible with 0.9% sodium chloride solution and with 5% Dextrose solution.

No specific information on the use of this product in the elderly is available. Clinical trials have included patients over 65 years and no adverse reactions specific to this age group have been reported.

Contra-indications: There are no absolute contra-indications to the use of Catapres.

Special warnings and special precautions for use: Sudden withdrawal of Catapres, particularly in those patients receiving high doses may result in rebound hypertension. Termination of long-term therapy with Catapres for any reason should therefore be performed gradually. With Catapres PL this may be achieved by increasing progressively the interval between doses. If a hypertensive episode should nevertheless occur conventional oral or intravenous Catapres should reverse any such effect.

Patients known with a history of depression should be carefully supervised while under long-term treatment with Catapres as there have been occasional reports of further depressive episodes during oral treatment in such patients.

Cautions should be exercised in patients with Raynaud's disease or other peripheral vascular occlusive disease. As with all drugs used in hypertension, Catapres should be used with caution in patients with cerebrovascular, coronary or renal insufficiency.

Interaction with other medicaments and other forms of interaction: Concomitant use of diuretics or other antihypertensive agents will usually result in an increased hypotensive effect.

Concomitant administration of tricyclic antidepressants may reduce the hypotensive effect of Catapres.

Alpha-adrenergic blocking drugs antagonise the acute effects of Catapres.

Pregnancy and lactation: This product should only be used in pregnancy or lactating women if considered essential by the physician.

Effects on ability to drive and use machines: This product may cause drowsiness. Patients who are affected should not drive or operate machinery. Sedation due to the drug may be increased by the concomitant use of other central nervous depressants.

Undesirable effects: There are occasional reports of fluid retention during initial stages of oral treatment with clonidine hydrochloride. This is usually transitory and can be corrected by the addition of a diuretic.

A single case of toxic hepatitis has been reported, but the authors commented that the role of clonidine in hepatotoxicity in this patient remains questionable.

Acute administration of clonidine hydrochloride in animals or in man has occasionally induced a transient elevation of blood sugar. This is believed to be due to the initial pharmacological effect of alpha-adrenergic stimulation. Investigators agree that this has no clinical significance. The inclusion of diabetic patients in many clonidine hydrochloride investigations has confirmed its suitability as an antihypertensive agent for such patients.

Overdose: Accidental overdosage may cause hypotension, bradycardia, sedation and coma. Transient hypertension may be seen if the total dose is over 10 mg.

Gastric lavage should be performed. In most cases all that is required are general supportive measures. Forced diuresis has been employed. Where bradycardia is severe atropine will increase the heart rate. If hypotension is giving rise to concern the administration of an alpha-adrenergic blocking drug such as phentolamine may help.

Pharmacological properties

Pharmacodynamic properties: Catapres has been shown to have both central and peripheral sites of action. With long-term treatment Catapres reduces the responsiveness of peripheral vessels to vasoconstrictor and vasodilator substances and to synthetic nerve stimulation. Early in treatment, however, blood pressure reduction is associated with a central reduction of sympathetic outflow and increased vagal tone.

Clinically, there may be reduced venous return and slight bradycardia resulting in reduced cardiac output. Although initially peripheral resistance may be unchanged, it tends to be reduced as treatment continues. There is no interference with myocardial contractility. Studies have shown that cardiovascular reflexes, as shown by the lack of postural hypotension and exercise hypotension, are preserved.

Pharmacokinetic properties: Peak plasma concentrations are observed 3-5 hours after administration, declining with a half-life up to about 23 hours. Clonidine is metabolised in the liver. About 65% is excreted in the urine, partly as unchanged clonidine and about 20% is excreted in the faeces.

Pharmaceutical particulars

List of excipients: Sodium chloride; water for injections.

Incompatibilities: None stated.

Shelf life: 5 years

Special precautions for storage: Store below 30°C. Protect from light.

Nature and contents of container: 1 ml colourless glass (PhEur Type I) ampoules, marketed in packs of 5.

Instructions for use/handling: None stated.

Marketing authorisation number 0015/5008

Date of first authorisation/renewal of authorisation 23.08.95

Date of approval/revision of SPC August 1995.

Legal category POM

CATAPRES* TABLETS

Qualitative and quantitative composition

Catapres Tablets 100 micrograms: White compressed tablets impressed with the motif $\frac{01C}{01C}$ on one side and with the Company symbol on the reverse.

Each tablet contains 100 micrograms of clonidine hydrochloride.

Catapres Tablets 300 micrograms: White compressed tablets impressed with the motif $\frac{03C}{03C}$ on one side and with the Company symbol on the reverse.

Each tablet contains 300 micrograms of clonidine hydrochloride.

Pharmaceutical form Tablets for oral administration.

Clinical particulars

Therapeutic indications: Catapres is indicated for the treatment of all grades of essential and secondary hypertension.

Posology and method of administration: Oral treatment should commence with 0.05-0.10 mg three times daily. This dose should be increased gradually every second or third day until control is achieved. Most patients will be controlled on divided daily doses of 0.30-1.2 mg. However, some patients may require higher doses, e.g. 1.8 mg or more.

Catapres may be added to an existing antihypertensive regimen where blood pressure control has not been satisfactorily achieved. If side-effects with existing therapy are troublesome the concomitant use of Catapres may allow a lower dose of the established regimen to be employed. Patients changing treatment should have their existing therapy reduced gradually whilst Catapres is added to their regimen.

Patients undergoing anaesthesia should continue their Catapres treatment before, during and after anaesthesia using oral or i.v. administration according to individual circumstances.

No specific information on the use of this product in the elderly is available. Clinical trials have included patients over 65 years and no adverse reactions specific to this age group have been reported.

Contra-indications: There are no absolute contra-indications to the use of Catapres.

Special warnings and special precautions for use: Initially, sedation or dry mouth are encountered in a few patients. These effects usually subside as treatment continues. Other drug related side-effects which have been mentioned in the literature include dizziness, headache, nocturnal unrest, nausea, euphoria, rash, constipation, impotence (rarely) and agitation on withdrawal of long-term therapy.

There are occasional reports of fluid retention during initial stages of oral treatment. This is usually transitory and can be corrected by the addition of a diuretic.

A single case of toxic hepatitis has been reported, but the authors commented that the role of Catapres in hepatotoxicity in this patient remains questionable.

Acute administration in animals or in man has occasionally induced a transient elevation of blood sugar. This is believed to be due to the initial pharmacological effect of alpha-adrenergic stimulation. Investigators agree that this has no clinical significance. The inclusion of diabetic patients in many Catapres investigations has confirmed its suitability as an antihypertensive agent for such patients.

Interaction with other medicaments and other forms of interaction: Concomitant use of diuretics or other antihypertensive agents will usually result in an increased hypotensive effect.

Concomitant administration of tricyclic antidepressants may reduce the hypotensive effect of Catapres.

Alpha-adrenergic blocking drugs antagonise acute effects of Catapres.

Pregnancy and lactation: Although clonidine has been in wide general use for many years, there is no definite evidence of hazard during human pregnancy. In animal studies involving doses higher than the equivalent maximum therapeutic dose in man, effects on foetal development were only seen in one species. Foetal malformations did not occur. Medicines should not be used in pregnancy, especially the first trimester, unless the expected benefit is thought to outweigh any possible risk to the foetus.

Catapres should only be given to breast feeding women if considered essential by the physician. There is as yet insufficient experience to enable Catapres to be recommended for children.

Effects on ability to drive and use machines: This product may cause drowsiness. Patients who are affected should not drive or operate machinery. Sedation due to the drug may be increased by the concomitant use of other central nervous depressants.

Undesirable effects: Sudden withdrawal of Catapres, particularly in those patients receiving high doses, may result in rebound hypertension. As with other antihypertensives, doctors should warn their patients not to stop medication themselves. Termination of long-term therapy with Catapres for any reason should therefore be performed gradually. If a hypertensive episode should nevertheless occur, reintroduction of oral or intravenous Catapres should reverse any such effect. If the use of Catapres is not practical then an alpha-adrenergic blocking drug, such as phentolamine, should be used.

If Catapres is being given concurrently with a beta-blocker, Catapres should not be discontinued until several days after the withdrawal of the beta-blocker.

Patients known with a history of depression should be carefully supervised while under long-term treatment with Catapres as there have been occasional reports of further depressive episodes during oral treatment in such patients.

Caution should be exercised in patients with Raynaud's disease or other peripheral vascular occlusive disease. As with all drugs used in hypertension, Catapres should be used with caution in patients with cerebrovascular, coronary or renal insufficiency.

Overdose: Accidental overdosage may cause hypotension, bradycardia, sedation and coma. Transient hypertension may be seen if the total dose is over 10 mg. Gastric lavage should be performed where appropriate. In most cases all that is required are general supportive measures. Forced diuresis has been employed. Where bradycardia is severe atropine will increase the heart rate.

Pharmacological properties

Pharmacodynamic properties: Catapres has been shown to have both central and peripheral sites of action. With long-term treatment Catapres reduces the responsiveness of peripheral vessels to vasoconstrictor and vasodilator substances and to synthetic nerve stimulation. Early in treatment, however, blood pressure reduction is associated with a central reduction of sympathetic outflow and increased vagal tone.

Clinically, there may be reduced venous return and slight bradycardia resulting in reduced cardiac output. Although initially peripheral resistance may be unchanged, it tends to be reduced as treatment continues. There is no interference with myocardial contractility. Studies have shown that cardiovascular reflexes, as shown by the lack of postural hypotension and exercise hypotension, are preserved.

Pharmacokinetic properties: Clonidine is well absorbed from the GI tract. Peak plasma concentrations are observed 3-5 hours after administration, declining with a half life up to about 23 hours. Clonidine is metabolised in the liver. About 65% is excreted in the urine, partly as unchanged clonidine and about 20% is excreted in the faeces.

Pharmaceutical particulars

List of excipients: Lactose; calcium hydrogen phosphate; maize starch; colloidal silica; polyvinylpyrrolidone; soluble starch; stearic acid.

Incompatibilities: None stated.

Shelf life: 5 years

Special precautions for storage: Store in a dry place below 30°C. Protect from light.

Nature and contents of container: Catapres Tablets 100 micrograms and 300 micrograms are currently marketed in PVC blister packs of 100 tablets.

Instructions for use/handling: None stated.

Marketing authorisation numbers

Catapres Tablets 100 micrograms	0015/5009R
Catapres Tablets 300 micrograms	0015/5041R

Date of first authorisation/renewal of authorisation

Catapres Tablets 100 micrograms	22.08.90
Catapres Tablets 300 micrograms	25.08.95

Date of approval/revision of SPC October 1995

Legal category POM

CATAPRES* PL PERLONGETS*

Qualitative and quantitative composition Red/yellow size 2 gelatin capsules. Each Perlonget contains 5 mini tablets constituting 250 micrograms clonidine hydrochloride in a sustained release form.

Pharmaceutical form Sustained release capsule for oral administration.

Clinical particulars

Therapeutic indications: All degrees of hypertension excluding hypertensive crisis.

Posology and method of administration: Most patients will be satisfactorily controlled on one perlonget daily (usually given in the evening). This dosage can be increased if necessary up to 2 or 3 perlongets daily (one in the morning and one or two at night).

Catapres PL may be added to an existing antihypertensive regimen where blood pressure control has not been satisfactorily achieved. If side effects with existing therapy are troublesome the concomitant use of Catapres PL may allow a lower dose of the established regimen to be employed.

Patients changing treatment should have their existing therapy reduced gradually whilst Catapres is added to their regime.

Contra-indications: There are no absolute contra-indications to the use of Catapres PL.

Special warnings and special precautions for use: Sudden withdrawal of Catapres PL, particularly in those patients receiving high doses may result in rebound hypertension. Termination of long-term therapy with Catapres PL for any reason should therefore be performed gradually. With Catapres PL this may be achieved by increasing progressively the interval between doses. If a hypertensive episode should nevertheless occur conventional oral or intravenous Catapres should reverse any such effect.

Patients with a known history of depression should be carefully supervised while under long-term treatment with Catapres PL as there have been occasional reports of further depressive episodes during oral treatment in such patients.

Caution should be exercised in patients with Raynaud's disease or other peripheral vascular occlusive disease. As with all drugs used in hypertension, Catapres PL should be used with caution in patients with cerebrovascular, coronary or renal insufficiency.

There is as yet insufficient experience to enable Catapres PL to be recommended in children.

Interaction with other medicaments and other forms of interaction: Concomitant use of diuretics or other antihypertensive agents will usually result in an increased hypotensive effect.

Concomitant administration of tricyclic antidepressants may reduce the hypotensive effect of Catapres PL.

Alpha-adrenergic blocking drugs antagonise the acute effects of Catapres PL.

No adverse reaction has been reported following the concurrent administration of clonidine hydrochloride with digoxin, aminophylline, anticonvulsants, or anti-arrhythmic preparations. Monitoring of haematological and hepatic status in large numbers of patients has revealed no drug-related adverse effects. Renal blood flow and glomerular filtration rates are maintained and there is no deterioration in renal function. There is evidence that plasma renin levels are reduced. Clonidine hydrochloride does not affect the estimation of VMA levels.

Pregnancy and lactation: This product should only be used in pregnancy or lactating women if considered essential by the physician.

Effects on ability to drive and use machines: This product may cause drowsiness. Patients who are affected should not drive or operate machinery. Sedation due to the drug may be increased by the concomitant use of other central nervous depressants.

Undesirable effects: Initially, sedation or dry mouth are encountered in a few patients on treatment with Catapres PL. These effects usually subside as treatment continues. Other drug-related side effects from clonidine hydrochloride which have been reported include: constipation, nausea and vomiting, headache, malaise, impotence, decreased libido, gynaecomastia, orthostatic hypotension and associated dizziness, paraesthesia of the extremities, Raynaud's phenomenon, pain in the parotid gland, drying out of the nasal mucosa and reduced lachrymal flow (caution: contact lens wearers) skin reactions with symptoms such as rash, urticaria, pruritus and alopecia. Nocturnal unrest, nightmares, depression, perceptual disorders, hallucinations, confusion, disturbance of accommodation and also agitation on withdrawal of long-term therapy may occur.

There are occasional reports of fluid retention during initial stages of oral treatment with clonidine hydrochloride. This is usually transitory and can be corrected by the addition of a diuretic.

In very rare cases, pseudo-obstruction of the large bowel has been observed.

Clonidine may cause or potentiate bradyarrhythmic conditions such as sinus bradycardia or AV-block.

Occasional reports of abnormal liver function tests and two cases of hepatitis have been reported.

Acute administration of clonidine hydrochloride in animals or in man has occasionally induced a transient elevation of blood sugar. This is believed to be due to the initial pharmacological effect of alpha-adrenergic stimulation. Investigators agree that this has no clinical significance. The inclusion of diabetic patients in many clonidine hydrochloride investigations has confirmed its suitability as an antihypertensive agent for such patients.

Overdose: Accidental overdosage may cause hypotension, bradycardia, sedation and coma. Transient hypertension may be seen if the total dose is over 10 mg.

Gastric lavage should be performed. In most cases all that is required are general supportive measures. Forced diuresis has been employed. Where bradycardia is severe atropine will increase the heart rate. If hypotension is giving rise to concern the administration of an alpha-adrenergic blocking drug such as phentolamine may help.

Pharmacological properties

Pharmacodynamic properties: Catapres PL has been shown to have both central and peripheral sites of action. With long-term treatment Catapres PL reduces the responsiveness of peripheral vessels to vasoconstrictor and vasodilator substances and to synthetic nerve stimulation. Early in treatment, however, blood pressure reduction is associated with a central reduction of sympathetic outflow and increased vagal tone.

Clinically, there may be reduced venous return and slight bradycardia resulting in reduced cardiac output. Although initially peripheral resistance may be unchanged, it tends to be reduced as treatment continues. There is no interference with myocardial contractility. Studies have shown that cardiovascular reflexes, as shown by the lack of postural hypotension and exercise hypotension, are preserved.

Pharmacokinetic properties: Catapres PL contains clonidine hydrochloride in a sustained release formulation. Clonidine is well absorbed from the GI tract. Peak plasma concentrations are observed 3–5 hours after administration, declining with a half-life up to about 23 hours. Clonidine is metabolised in the liver. About 65% is excreted in the urine, partly as unchanged clonidine and about 20% is excreted in the faeces.

Pharmaceutical particulars

List of excipients:
Lactose
Red-brown pigment (E172 and E171)
Magnesium stearate
Povidone
Hydroxypropyl methylcellulose
Poly (0-ethyl) cellulose
Macrogol 6000
Titanium dioxide
Brown pigment (E172)
Lebensmittelblau (E132).

Incompatibilities: None stated.

Shelf life: 3 years.

Special precautions for storage: Store below 25°C in a dry place. Protect from light.

Nature and contents of container: PVC/PVDC blister packs of 56.

Instructions for use/handling: None stated.

Marketing authorisation number PL 0015/0072

Date of renewal of authorisation 21.08.95

Date of revision of the text July 1998

Legal category POM

COMBIVENT* METERED AEROSOL

Qualitative and quantitative composition Combivent Metered Aerosol is a combination of ipratropium bromide monohydrate and salbutamol sulphate. Each valve activation delivers 21 micrograms of ipratropium bromide monohydrate (corresponds to 20 micrograms ipratropium bromide anhydrous) and 120 micrograms of salbutamol sulphate.

Pharmaceutical form Combivent is a metered dose aerosol for inhalation.

Clinical particulars

Therapeutic indications: Combivent is indicated as a bronchodilator for the treatment of bronchospasm associated with chronic obstructive pulmonary disease in patients who require regular treatment with both ipratropium and salbutamol.

Posology and method of administration:
Adults (including elderly patients): Two inhalations four times a day.

Children: There is no experience of the use of Combivent in children below the age of 12 years.

Contra-indications: Combivent is contra-indicated in patients with a history of hypersensitivity to any of its components, or to atropine or its derivatives.

Special warnings and special precautions for use:
Ocular complications

There have been rare reports of ocular complications (i.e. mydriasis, blurring of vision, eye pain) when the contents of metered aerosols containing ipratropium bromide have been sprayed inadvertently into the eye. Care must be taken to prevent Combivent from entering the eye. Should patients develop effects in the eye they should be warned to seek medical advice.

Patients must be instructed in the correct administration of Combivent metered aerosol.

In the following conditions Combivent should only be used after careful risk/benefit assessment: Hypertrophic obstructive cardiomyopathy, tachyarrhythmia, insufficiently controlled diabetes mellitus, recent myocardial infarction and/or severe organic heart or vascular disorders, hyperthyroidism.

The patient should be instructed to consult a doctor immediately in the event of acute, rapidly worsening dyspnoea. In addition, the patient should be warned to seek medical advice should a reduced response become apparent.

Potentially serious hypokalemia may result from $beta_2$-agonist therapy. Particular caution is advised in severe asthma, as this effect may be potentiated by concomitant treatment with xanthine derivatives, steroids and diuretics. Additionally, hypoxia may aggravate the effects of hypokalemia on cardiac rhythm. It is recommended that serum potassium levels are monitored in such situations.

Interaction with other medicaments and other forms of interaction: Beta-adrenergics, xanthine derivatives and corticosteroids may enhance the effect of Combivent. The concurrent administration of other betamimetics, systemically absorbed anticholinergics and xanthine derivatives may increase the side effects.

A potentially serious reduction in effect may occur during concurrent administration of beta-blockers.

Anticholinergic effects of other drugs can be enhanced.

Pregnancy and lactation: Ipratropium bromide has been in general use for several years and there is no definite evidence of ill-consequence during pregnancy; animal studies have shown no hazard.

Salbutamol has been in widespread use for many years without apparent ill-consequence during pregnancy. There is inadequate published evidence of safety in the early stages of human pregnancy but in animal studies there has been evidence of some harmful effects on the foetus at very high dose levels.

As with all medicines, Combivent should not be used in pregnancy, especially the first trimester, unless the expected benefit is thought to outweigh any possible risk to the foetus. Similarly, Combivent should not be administered to breast-feeding mothers unless the expected benefit is thought to outweigh any possible risk to the neonate.

Effects on ability to drive and use machines: None stated.

Undesirable effects: In common with other beta-agonists more frequent undesirable effects of Combivent are fine tremor of skeletal muscles and nervousness, less frequent are tachycardia, dizziness, palpitations or headache, especially in hypersensitive patients.

Potentially serious hypokalemia may result from $beta_2$-agonist therapy.

In isolated cases there may be local reactions such as dryness of the mouth, throat irritation, or allergic reactions.

As with other bronchodilators, in some cases cough, in very rare instances paradoxical bronchoconstrictions have been observed.

Use of anticholinergic agents (e.g. ipratropium bromide) may precipitate urinary retention, in particular in patients with pre-existing outflow tract obstruction.

Overdose: The effects of overdosage are expected to be primarily related to salbutamol because acute overdosage with ipratropium bromide is unlikely as it is not well absorbed systemically after inhalation or oral administration.

Manifestations of overdosage with salbutamol may include anginal pain, hypertension, hypokalaemia and tachycardia. The preferred antidote for overdosage with salbutamol is a cardioselective beta-blocking agent but due care and attention should be used in administering these drugs in patients with a history of bronchospasm.

Pharmacological properties

Pharmacodynamic properties: Ipratropium bromide is an anticholinergic agent which inhibits vagally mediated reflexes by antagonising the action of acetylcholine, the transmitter agent released from the vagus nerve. The bronchodilation following inhalation of ipratropium bromide is primarily local and site specific to the lung and not systemic in nature.

Salbutamol sulphate is a $beta_2$-adrenergic agent which acts on airway smooth muscle resulting in relaxation. Salbutamol relaxes all smooth muscle from the trachea to the terminal bronchioles and protects against all bronchoconstrictor challenges.

Combivent metered aerosol provides the simultaneous release of ipratropium bromide and salbutamol sulphate allowing the synergetic efficacy on the muscarinic and $beta_2$-adrenergic receptors in the lung to cause bronchodilation.

Pharmacokinetic properties: Ipratropium bromide is not readily absorbed into the systemic circulation either from the surface of the lung or from the gastrointestinal tract as compared by blood level and renal excretion studies. The half-life elimination is about 3–4 hours after inhalation or intravenous administration. Ipratropium bromide does not penetrate the blood brain barrier.

Salbutamol sulphate is rapidly and completely absorbed following oral adminstration either by the inhaled or gastric route. Peak plasma salbutamol concentrations are seen within three hours of administration and the drug is excreted unchanged in the urine after 24 hours. Intravenous salbutamol will cross the blood brain barrier reaching concentrations amounting to about five percent of the plasma concentrations.

From a pharmacokinetic perspective, the additive activity of Combivent is due to the local effect of the fixed dose of the active components (ipratropium bromide and salbutamol sulphate) on the muscarinic and $beta_2$-adrenergic receptors in the lung.

Preclinical safety data: The individual active ingredients ipratropium bromide and salbutamol sulphate have been extensively investigated in animal models and the safety concerns are not clinically significant when Combivent is used as metered aerosol at the recommended dosage levels to patients.

Pharmaceutical particulars

List of excipients: Dichlorodifluoromethane; dichlorotetrafluoroethane; trichloromonofluoromethane; soya lecithin.

Incompatibilities: None known.

Shelf life: 3 years

Special precautions for storage: Store below 25°C. Protect from direct sunlight and frost.

Nature and contents of container: Combivent Metered Aerosol is a creamy-white suspension of micronised substances in halogenated propellants filled in metal canisters with a metering valve.

Instructions for use/handling: The correct operation of the metered aerosol apparatus is essential for successful therapy.

The aerosol should be shaken and the valve depressed once or twice before the apparatus is initially used.

Before each use the following rules should be observed:

1. Remove protective cap.
2. Shake the metered aerosol well before each use.
3. Breathe out deeply.
4. Hold the metered aerosol and close lips over the mouthpiece. The arrow and the base of the container should be pointing upwards.
5. Breathe in as deeply as possible, pressing the base of the container firmly at the same time, this releases one metered dose. Hold the breath for a few seconds, then remove the mouthpiece from the mouth and breathe out.
6. Replace the protective cap after use.

The container is under pressure and should on no account be opened by force or exposed to temperatures exceeding 50°C. As the container is not transparent it is not possible to see when the contents are used up, but if on shaking the container seems to be empty, it probably still contains a further 10 effective inhalations.

The mouthpiece should always be kept clean and can be washed with warm water. If soap or detergent is used, the mouthpiece should be thoroughly rinsed in clear water.

Marketing authorisation number 0015/0191

Date of approval/revision of SPC September 1996

Legal category POM

COMBIVENT* UDVs*

Qualitative and quantitative composition Each 2.5 ml single dose unit contains 500 micrograms ipratropium bromide and 3 mg salbutamol sulphate (corresponds to 2.5 mg salbutamol base).

Pharmaceutical form Solution for inhalation.

Clinical particulars

Therapeutic indications: Combivent UDVs are indicated for the management of bronchospasm in patients suffering from chronic obstructive pulmonary disease who require regular treatment with both ipratropium and salbutamol.

Posology and method of administration: Combivent UDVs may be administered from a suitable nebuliser or an intermittent positive pressure ventilator.

The recommended dose is:
Adults (including elderly patients and children over 12 years): 1 vial three or four times daily.

Children under 12 years: There is no experience of the use of Combivent UDVs in children under 12 years.

Contra-indications: Combivent UDVs are contra-indicated in patients with a history of hypersensitivity to ipratropium bromide, salbutamol sulphate or to atropine or its derivatives.

Special warnings and special precautions for use: Patients must be instructed in the correct use of Combivent UDVs and warned not to allow the solution or mist to enter the eyes. Acute angle glaucoma has been reported rarely when nebulised solutions of ipratropium bromide have been used in conjunction with $beta_2$-agonist bronchodilators. Protection of the eyes appears to prevent any increase in intra-ocular pressure and patients who may be susceptible to glaucoma should be warned specifically on the need for ocular protection.

In the following conditions Combivent UDVs should only be used after careful risk/benefit assessment: hypertrophic obstructive cardiomyopathy, tachyarrhythmia, inadequately controlled diabetes mellitus, recent myocardial infarction and/or severe organic heart or vascular disorders, hyperthyroidism.

The patient should be instructed to consult a doctor immediately in the event of acute, rapidly worsening dyspnoea. In addition, the patient should be warned to seek medical advice should a reduced response become apparent.

Potentially serious hypokalaemia may result from $beta_2$-agonist therapy. Particular caution is advised in severe airway obstruction, as this effect may be potentiated by concomitant treatment with xanthine derivatives, steroids and diuretics. Additionally, hypoxia may aggravate the effects of hypokalaemia on cardiac rhythm. It is recommended that serum potassium levels are monitored in such situations.

Interaction with other medicaments and other forms of interaction: The use of additional beta-agonists, xanthine derivatives and corticosteroids may enhance the effect of Combivent UDVs. The concurrent administration of other beta-mimetics, systemically absorbed anticholinergics and xanthine derivatives may increase the severity of side effects. A potentially serious reduction in effect may occur during concurrent administration of beta-blockers.

Pregnancy and lactation: Ipratropium bromide has been in general use for several years and there is no definite evidence of ill-consequence during pregnancy; animal studies have shown no hazard.

Salbutamol has been in widespread use for many years without apparent ill-consequence during pregnancy. There is inadequate published evidence of safety in the early stages of human pregnancy but in animal studies there has been evidence of some harmful effects on the foetus at very high dose levels.

As with all medicines, Combivent should not be used in pregnancy, especially the first trimester, unless the expected benefit is thought to outweigh any possible risk to the foetus. Similarly, Combivent should not be administered to breast-feeding mothers unless the expected benefit is thought to outweigh any possible risk to the neonate.

Effects on ability to drive and use machines: None stated.

Undesirable effects: Nebulisation-induced bronchospasm, dyspnoea and cough have been reported infrequently following the use of Combivent UDVs.

In common with other beta-agonist bronchodilators the undesirable effects of Combivent UDVs include fine tremor of skeletal muscles and nervousness and less frequently, tachycardia, dizziness, palpitations or headache, especially in hypersensitive patients.

Potentially serious hypokalaemia may result from $beta_2$-agonist therapy.

Use of anticholinergic agents (e.g. ipratropium bromide) may precipitate urinary retention, in particular in patients with pre-existing obstruction of the urinary tract. Dry mouth has occasionally been reported.

Overdose: Acute effects of overdosage with ipratropium bromide are unlikely due to its poor systemic absorption after either inhalation or oral administration. Any effects of overdosage are therefore likely to be related to the salbutamol component.

Manifestations of overdosage with salbutamol may include anginal pain, hypertension, hypokalaemia and tachycardia. The preferred antidote for overdosage with salbutamol is a cardioselective beta-blocking agent but caution should be used in administering these drugs in patients with a history of bronchospasm.

Pharmacological properties
Pharmacodynamic properties: Ipratropium bromide is an anticholinergic agent which inhibits vagally-mediated reflexes by antagonising the action of acetylcholine, the transmitter agent released from the vagus nerve. The bronchodilation following inhalation of ipratropium bromide is primarily local and site specific to the lung and not systemic in nature.

Salbutamol is a $beta_2$-adrenergic agent which acts on airway smooth muscle resulting in relaxation. Salbutamol relaxes all smooth muscle from the trachea to the terminal bronchioles and protects against bronchoconstrictor challenges.

Combivent UDVs provide the simultaneous delivery of ipratropium bromide and salbutamol sulphate allowing effects on both muscarinic and $beta_2$-adrenergic receptors in the lung leading to increased bronchodilation over that provided by each agent singly.

Pharmacokinetic properties: Ipratropium bromide is not readily absorbed into the systemic circulation either from the surface of the lung or from the gastrointestinal tract as assessed by blood level and renal excretion studies. The elimination half-life is about 1.5 hours after inhalation or intravenous administration. Ipratropium bromide does not cross the blood-brain barrier.

Salbutamol is rapidly and completely absorbed following oral administration either by the inhaled or the gastric route. Peak plasma salbutamol concentrations are seen within three hours of administration and the drug is excreted unchanged in the urine after 24 hours. The elimination half-life is 4 hours. Salbutamol will cross the blood brain barrier reaching concentrations amounting to about five percent of the plasma concentrations.

It has been shown that co-nebulisation of ipratropium bromide and salbutamol sulphate does not potentiate the systemic absorption of either component and that therefore the additive activity of Combivent UDVs is due to the combined local effect on the lung following inhalation.

Preclinical safety data: The individual active ingredients, ipratropium bromide and salbutamol sulphate, have been extensively investigated in animal models and there are no clinically relevant safety issues when Combivent UDVs are used at the recommended doses by patients.

Pharmaceutical particulars
List of excipients:
Sodium chloride
Hydrochloric acid
Purified water

Incompatibilities: None known.

Shelf life: 24 months.

Special precautions for storage: Store below 25°C. Protect from light. Do not freeze. Do not use if solution is discoloured.

Nature and contents of container: Low density polyethylene vials containing 2.5 ml of solution, formed into strips of 10 and packed into cartons containing 10 (sample pack) or 60 vials.

Instructions for use/handling:
i) Prepare the nebuliser by following the manufacturer's instructions and the advice of your doctor.
ii) Carefully separate a new vial from the strip. NEVER use one that has been opened already.
iii) Open the vial by simply twisting off the top, always taking care to hold it in an upright position.
iv) Unless otherwise instructed by your doctor squeeze all the contents of the plastic vial into the nebuliser chamber.
v) Assemble the nebuliser and use it as directed by your doctor.
vi) After nebulisation clean the nebuliser according to the manufacturer's instructions.

Marketing authorisation number PL 0015/0197

Date of first authorisation 07.06.95

Date of revision of the text May 1997

Legal category POM

DEXA-RHINASPRAY* DUO

Qualitative and quantitative composition Tramazoline hydrochloride (INN) 120 micrograms/metered dose as tramazoline hydrochloride monohydrate 128.59 micrograms/metered dose equivalent to tramazoline (base) 111.22 micrograms/metered dose and dexamethasone 21-isonicotinate 20 micrograms/metered dose.

Pharmaceutical form Nasal spray.

Clinical particulars
Therapeutic indications: Treatment of allergic rhinitis.

Posology and method of administration
Adults (including the elderly): 1 metered dose into each nostril up to six times in 24 hours, although 2 or 3 applications a day are usually sufficient.

Children 5–12 years: 1 metered dose into each nostril up to twice daily.

Children under 5 years: Not recommended.

Each course of treatment should not exceed 14 days.

No specific information on the use of this product in the elderly is available. No adverse reactions specific to this age group have been reported with tramazoline and dexamethasone.

Contra-indications: The use of Dexa-Rhinaspray Duo is contra-indicated in patients hypersensitive to any of the components and in infants and nursing mothers.

Special warnings and special precautions for use: Care should be used to avoid contact with the eyes as conjunctival irritation may occur. The use of Dexa-Rhinaspray Duo for prolonged periods is not recommended. The possibility of side-effects from the systemic absorption of dexamethasone should be borne in mind.

Interaction with other medicaments and other forms of interaction: None stated.

Pregnancy and lactation: There is inadequate evidence of safety in human pregnancy. Topical administration of corticosteroids to pregnant animals can cause abnormalities of foetal development including cleft palate and intra-uterine growth retardation. There may therefore be a very small risk of such effects in the human foetus. Dexa-Rhinaspray Duo should not be used by nursing mothers.

Effects on ability to drive and use machines: None stated.

Undesirable effects: A slight burning sensation in the nose, with sneezing, has been reported when using tramazoline hydrochloride alone. Rebound congestion of the nasal mucosa has been reported following prolonged use of nasal decongestants.

Overdose: Absorption of tramazoline may produce pallor, sweating, tachycardia and anxiety. These should be treated symptomatically if necessary.

Pharmacological properties
Pharmacodynamic properties: Tramazoline hydrochloride is a sympathomimetic with local vasoconstrictor activity. It has a quick-acting, long-lasting decongestant effect on the nasal mucosa.

Dexamethasone 21-isonicotinate is a corticosteroid with marked anti-inflammatory and anti-allergic properties.

Pharmacokinetic properties: Although Dexa-Rhinaspray Duo is intended for topical administration, the possibility of systemic absorption, particularly of the steroid component, should be borne in mind.

Pharmaceutical precautions
List of excipients:
Benzalkonium chloride
Sodium chloride
Polyoxyethylene-sorbitan monooleate (Polysorbate 80)
Glycerol 85%
Purified water
0.1N Sodium hydroxide is used for pH adjustment

Incompatibilities: None stated.

Shelf life: 2 years.

After opening use within 6 months after which discard any remaining product.

Special precautions for storage: Store below 25°C.

Nature and contents of container: Amber-coloured glass (Type I) bottle fitted with a 0.07 ml metering pump and white nasal adaptor and a protective cap. Nominal contents 10 ml equivalent to not less than 125 doses.

Instructions for use/handling:
1. Shake the bottle each time before use.
2. Remove the dust cap.
3. Blow your nose to clear your nostrils, if necessary.
4. The nasal pump spray must be primed before Dexa-Rhinaspray Duo is used for the first time. To prime the pump, hold the bottle with your thumb at the base and your index and middle fingers on the white shoulder area. Make sure the bottle points upwards and away from your eyes. Press your thumb firmly and quickly against the bottle seven times. The pump is now primed and can be used. Your pump should be reprimed if you have not used the medication for more than 24 hours; repriming the pump will only require one or two sprays.
5. Close one nostril by gently placing your finger against the side of your nose. Tilt your head slightly forward and, keeping the bottle upright, insert the nasal tip into the other nostril. Point the tip toward the back and outer side of the nose.

   Press firmly and quickly upwards with the thumb at the base while holding the white shoulder portion of the pump between your index and middle fingers. Following each spray, sniff and breathe out through your mouth.

   After spraying the nostril and removing the unit,

tilt your head backwards for a few seconds to let the spray spread over the back of the nose.
6. Repeat step 5 in the other nostril.
7. Replace the cap.

Avoid spraying Dexa-Rhinaspray Duo in or around your eye. Should this occur, immediately flush your eye with cold tap water for several minutes.

If the nasal tip becomes clogged, remove the clear plastic dust cap. Hold the nasal tip under running warm tap water for about a minute. Dry the nasal tip, reprime the nasal pump spray and replace the plastic dust cap.

Marketing authorisation number PL 0015/0213

Date of first authorisation 22 December 1997

Date of revision of the SPC October 1997

Legal category POM.

DIXARIT* TABLETS

Qualitative and quantitative composition Blue, biconvex, sugar-coated tablets. Each tablet contains clonidine hydrochloride 25 micrograms.

Pharmaceutical form Sugar-coated tablets for oral administration.

Clinical particulars
Therapeutic indications:
(a) The prophylactic management of migraine or recurrent vascular headache.
(b) The management of vasomotor conditions commonly associated with the menopause and characterised by flushing.

Posology and method of administration:
Adults: Initially 2 tablets twice daily. If after two weeks there has been no remission, increase to 3 tablets twice daily.

The duration of treatment depends upon the severity of the condition.

Children: Not generally recommended for administration to children under 12 years.

Elderly: No specific information on the use of this product in the elderly is available.

Clinical trials have included patients over 65 years and no adverse reactions specific to this age group have been reported.

Contra-indications: Dixarit should not be used in patients with sick-sinus syndrome or with known hypersensitivity to the active ingredient, clonidine.

Special warnings and special precautions for use: Dixarit should be used with caution in patients with cerebrovascular disease, coronary insufficiency, occlusive peripheral vascular disorders, such as Raynaud's disease, or those with a history of depression.

At doses higher than those recommended above, clonidine is an effective antihypertensive agent. Caution should therefore be observed where antihypertensive agents are being used, as potentiation of the hypotensive effect may occur. Provided the recommended Dixarit dosage regimen is followed, no difficulty with hypotension should arise during the routine management of patients with either migraine or menopausal flushing.

Depending on the dose given, Dixarit can cause bradycardia. In patients with pre-existing cardiac conduction abnormalities, arrhythmias have been observed after high doses of Dixarit.

Patients with renal failure require extreme care.

Clonidine is available for the management of hypertension as Catapres Tablets (100 micrograms and 300 micrograms), Perlongets (250 micrograms) and Ampoules (150 micrograms in 1 ml). Where Catapres is already being used Dixarit therapy is obviously not indicated.

Interaction with other medicaments and other forms of interaction: Concurrent administration of antihypertensive agents, vasodilators or diuretics, may lead to an increased hypotensive effect.

Concomitant use of beta-blockers and/or cardiac glycosides can cause bradycardia or dysrhythmia (AV-block) in isolated cases.

If during combined treatment with a beta-blocker there is need to interrupt or discontinue antihypertensive therapy, the beta-blocker must always be discontinued slowly first (reducing the dose gradually to avoid sympathetic hyperactivity) and then the Dixarit, which should also be reduced gradually over several days if previously given in high doses.

As the effects of clonidine can be antagonised by tricyclic anti-depressants, it may be necessary to adjust the dosage of Dixarit, if these agents are administered concurrently. Although there is no experience from clinical trials, the effect of tranquillisers, hypnotics or alcohol could theoretically be potentiated by Dixarit.

Pregnancy and lactation: Clonidine has been in wide general use for many years and has shown no evidence of untoward effects when taken during human pregnancy. However, as with all medicines, Dixarit should not be used in pregnancy, especially the first trimester, unless the expected benefit is thought to outweigh any possible risk to the foetus.

In animal studies involving doses higher than the equivalent maximum therapeutic dose in man, effects on foetal development were only seen in one species. Foetal malformations did not occur.

The drug enters breast milk, but is not likely to affect the infant when therapeutic doses are used.

Effects on ability to drive and use machines: Because of different individual reactions including drowsiness, the ability to drive or operate machinery may be impaired, particularly in the initial phase of treatment with Dixarit.

Undesirable effects: There may be some initial sedation or dry mouth in some patients when Dixarit therapy is started. Dizziness, nausea and nocturnal unrest have been reported. Orthostatic hypotension has been reported, but only following the first administration of high doses.

Rare cases of constipation, impotence and disturbances in peripheral blood flow have been observed.

Very rarely, and only after very high doses of clonidine, have there been reports of hypersensitivity reactions, skin rash, perceptual disorders, nightmares, gynaecomastia, pain in the parotid gland, depressive moods, drying of nasal mucosa and reduced lachrymal flow.

In the management of hypertension a single case of toxic hepatitis has been reported with clonidine. However, the role of clonidine in hepatotoxicity in this patient remains questionable. Monitoring of haematological, renal and hepatic status in large numbers of patients has revealed no drug-related adverse effects.

Overdose: Symptoms: Sedation to somnolence, hypotension, orthostatic hypotension, bradycardia, occasionally vomiting, very occasionally hypertension, dryness of the mouth.

Treatment: Gastric lavage and/or administration of activated charcoal should be performed where appropriate. In most cases all that is required are general supportive measures.

Pharmacological properties
Pharmacodynamic properties: Clonidine is an antihypertensive agent which acts centrally by stimulating alpha$_2$-adrenergic receptors and producing a reduction in sympathetic tone, resulting in a fall in diastolic and systolic blood pressure and a reduction in heart rate.

Treatment with Dixarit diminishes the responsiveness of peripheral vessels to constrictor and dilator stimuli, thereby preventing the vascular changes associated with migraine. The same direct action on peripheral vessels moderates the vascular changes associated with menopausal flushing.

Pharmacokinetic properties: Clonidine is well absorbed from the gastro-intestinal tract. Peak plasma concentrations are observed 3 to 5 hours post administration, decreasing with a half life of up to approximately 23 hours. Clonidine is metabolised in the liver. About 65% is excreted in the urine, partly as unchanged clonidine and about 20% is excreted in the faeces.

Pharmaceutical particulars
List of excipients: Tablet core: Calcium hydrogen phosphate; lactose; maize starch; colloidal silica; polyvinylpyrrolidone; soluble starch; colouring E132; magnesium stearate.

Tablet coating: Polyvinylpyrrolidone; sucrose; talc; gum arabic; titanium dioxide; colouring E132; polyethylene glycol; carnauba wax; white wax.

Incompatibilities: None stated.

Shelf life: 5 years.

Special precautions for storage: Protect from light.

Nature and contents of container: PVC/aluminium blister packs of 84, 100 & 112. Currently the 112 pack is the only marketed pack.

Instructions for use/handling: None stated.

Marketing authorisation number 0015/5014R

Date of approval/revision of SPC July 1996

Legal category POM

DUOVENT* INHALER

Qualitative and quantitative composition Cream coloured suspension. Each metered dose contains fenoterol hydrobromide 100 micrograms and ipratropium bromide 40 micrograms.

Pharmaceutical form Pressurised metered dose aerosol.

Clinical particulars
Therapeutic indications: For the treatment of reversible airways obstruction in bronchial asthma and chronic obstructive pulmonary disease.

Posology and method of administration
For inhalational use only
Adults: The recommended dose of Duovent Inhaler is one to two puffs given as a single dose. This may be given 3–4 times daily. Dosing should not exceed two puffs every six hours (i.e. the maximum dose is 800 micrograms of fenoterol plus 320 micrograms of ipratropium).

Children over 6 years: Children aged 6–12 years will normally require one puff. This may be given 3 times daily. Dosing should not exceed two puffs every six hours (i.e. the maximum dose is 800 micrograms of fenoterol plus 320 micrograms of ipratropium).

Elderly: No specific information on the use of this product in the elderly is available. Clinical trials have included patients over 65 years and no adverse reactions specific to this age group have been reported.

Some patients may find it beneficial to use the metered dose inhaler with an extension tube.

Contra-indications: Known sensitivity to atropine.

Special warnings and special precautions for use: Potentially serious hypokalaemia may result from beta$_2$-agonist therapy.

Caution should be observed should it be necessary to administer Duovent to patients with thyrotoxicosis, myocardial insufficiency, angina, cardiac dysrhythmias, hypertension or hypertrophic subvalvular aortic stenosis. Generally, caution is advocated in the use of anticholinergic agents in patients with glaucoma and prostatic hypertrophy. However, specific studies with ipratropium in patients with these conditions showed no adverse effects.

Patients must be instructed in the correct use of a metered dose inhaler and warned against the accidental release of the contents into the eye. If relief is not obtained after correct administration of the prescribed dose, then patients should contact their doctor for advice.

Interactions with other medicaments and other forms of interaction: In view of the possible interaction between sympathomimetic amines and monoamine oxidase inhibitors or tricyclic anti-depressants, care should be taken if it is proposed to administer these compounds concurrently with Duovent. Duovent should be used with caution in patients already receiving other sympathomimetic agents as cardiovascular effects may be additive.

Beta-adrenergic blocking agents may antagonise fenoterol hydrobromide and reduce its bronchodilator effect if administered concurrently.

Potentially serious hypokalaemia may result from beta$_2$-agonist therapy. Particular caution is advised in severe asthma as this effect may be potentiated by concomitant treatment with xanthine derivatives, steroids, diuretics and by hypoxia. It is recommended that serum potassium levels are monitored in such situations.

Pregnancy and lactation: Although both fenoterol hydrobromide and ipratropium bromide have been in general use for several years, there is no definite evidence of ill-consequence during human pregnancy; animal studies have shown no hazard.

Beta-adrenergic agents have been shown to prolong pregnancy and inhibit labour, although the amount in the prescribed dose of Duovent is probably insufficient to do so.

Medicines should not be used in pregnancy, especially the first trimester, unless the expected benefit is thought to outweigh any possible risk to the foetus.

Effects on ability to drive and use machines: None stated.

Undesirable effects: See *Special warnings and special precautions for use.*

Overdose: Accidental overdosage may give rise to tachycardia, palpitations and tremor. It is suggested that the patient should be treated symptomatically. Should the administration of beta-adrenergic blocking agents be considered necessary to counteract the effects of overdosage, its use in a patient liable to bronchospasm should be carefully monitored. Very high doses (30 mg) of ipratropium bromide by mouth have been reported to cause anticholinergic side-effects but these were not severe and did not require specific reversal.

Pharmacological properties
Pharmacodynamic properties: The bronchospasmolytic effect of Duovent was demonstrated in dogs; the individual agents of the combination when tested together had an additive effect when administered by inhalation.

In guinea pigs, the ingredients given intravenously, both separately and together, demonstrated a synergistic dose-related bronchospasmolytic action. A tachycardic effect was also noted with the combination: as ipratropium had no tachycardic effect alone, this represented a potentiation of action.

Dose response studies in man using the inhaled drug showed a bronchospasmolytic effect as judged by improvement in lung function (total airway resistance).

Pulse rates did not vary significantly between the individual components and the combination. No significant change in blood pressure was noted. The time of onset of action on lung function with the combination was the same for fenoterol alone but more prolonged.

Pharmacokinetic properties: Ipratropium bromide is a quaternary ammonium compound which is poorly absorbed from the gastro-intestinal tract and is slow to cross mucous membranes and the blood brain barrier. Following inhalation, uptake into the plasma is minimal, a peak blood concentration is attained 1½ to 3 hours after inhalation (and similarly for oral administration). Excretion is chiefly via the kidneys.

Fenoterol hydrobromide in man is very rapidly distributed through the tissues following intravenous administration. The kidneys excrete up to 65% mainly in the form of acidic conjugates. Following oral administration, the plasma levels reach their maximum 2 hours after ingestion and then drop exponentially. The renal excretion is 39% following peroral administration and over 98% of the renal excretory products consist of acidic conjugates. The half life for total excretion is 7.2 hours and absorption was calculated to be 60%.

The duration of action following the use of a metered dose aerosol is considerably longer and can be explained by the dose independent absorption in the upper bronchial tree. The concentration-independent absorption at this site, from the depot produced by the metered aerosol is maintained for several hours.

Pharmaceutical particulars

List of excipients:

Sorbitan trioleate
Monofluorotrichloromethane
Difluorodichloromethane
Tetrafluorodichloroethane

Incompatibilities: None stated.

Shelf life: 3 years.

Special precautions for storage: Protect from heat, including the sun. The vials should not be punctured or incinerated even when apparently empty. Protect from frost.

Nature and contents of container: 10 ml vial (200 metered doses) (OP) complete with mouthpiece.

Instructions for use/handling: None stated.

Marketing authorisation number PL 00015/0091

Date of renewal of the authorisation 5 April 1992

Date of revision of the text April 1998

Legal category POM

DUOVENT* AUTOHALER*

Qualitative and quantitative composition Cream coloured suspension. Each metered dose contains 42 micrograms of ipratropium bromide monohydrate EP (equivalent to 40 micrograms of ipratropium bromide) and 100 micrograms fenoterol hydrobromide BP.

Pharmaceutical form Breath actuated pressurised metered aerosol.

Clinical particulars

Therapeutic indications: For the treatment of reversible airways obstruction in bronchial asthma and chronic obstructive pulmonary disease.

Posology and method of administration

By inhalation:

Adults: The recommended dose of Duovent Autohaler is one to two puffs given as a single dose. This may be given 3–4 times daily. Dosing should not exceed two puffs every six hours (i.e. the maximum dose is 800 micrograms of fenoterol plus 320 micrograms of ipratropium).

Children: Children aged 6–12 years will normally require one puff. This may be given 3 times daily. Dosing should not exceed two puffs every six hours (i.e. the maximum dose is 800 micrograms of fenoterol plus 320 micrograms of ipratropium).

Elderly: No specific information on the use of this product in the elderly is available. Clinical trials have included patients over 65 years and no adverse reactions specific to this age group have been reported.

Some patients may find it beneficial to use the metered dose inhaler with an extension tube.

Contra-indications: Known sensitivity to atropine.

Special warnings and special precautions for use: Potentially serious hypokalaemia may result from $beta_2$-agonist therapy.

Caution should be observed should it be necessary to administer Duovent to patients with thyrotoxicosis, myocardial insufficiency, angina, cardiac dysrhythmias, hypertension or hypertrophic subvalvular aortic stenosis. Generally, caution is advocated in the use of anticholinergic agents in patients with glaucoma and prostatic hypertrophy. However, specific studies with ipratropium in patients with these conditions showed no adverse effects.

Patients must be instructed in the correct use of the Autohaler device. If relief is not obtained after correct administration of the prescribed dose, the patients should contact their doctor for advice.

Interaction with other medicaments and other forms of interaction: In view of the possible interaction between sympathomimetic amines and monoamine oxidase inhibitors or tricyclic anti-depressants, care should be taken if it is proposed to administer these compounds concurrently with Duovent. Duovent should be used with caution in patients already receiving other sympathomimetic agents as cardiovascular effects may be additive.

Beta-adrenergic blocking agents may antagonise fenoterol hydrobromide and reduce its bronchodilator effect if administered concurrently.

Potentially serious hypokalaemia may result from $beta_2$-agonist therapy. Particular caution is advised in severe asthma as this effect may be potentiated by concomitant treatment with xanthine derivatives, steroids, diuretics and by hypoxia. It is recommended that serum potassium levels are monitored in such situations.

Pregnancy and lactation: Although both fenoterol hydrobromide and ipratropium bromide have been in general use for several years, there is no definite evidence of ill-consequence during human pregnancy; animal studies have shown no hazard.

Beta-adrenergic agents have been shown to prolong pregnancy and inhibit labour, although the amount in the prescribed dose of Duovent is probably insufficient to do so.

Medicines should not be used in pregnancy, especially the first trimester, unless the expected benefit is thought to outweigh any possible risk to the foetus.

Effects on ability to drive and use machines: None stated.

Undesirable effects: See *Special warnings and special precautions for use.*

Overdose: Accidental overdosage may give rise to tachycardia, palpitation and tremor. It is suggested that the patient should be treated symptomatically. Should the administration of beta-adrenergic blocking agents be considered necessary to counteract the effects of overdosage, its use in a patient liable to bronchospasm should be carefully monitored. Very high doses (30 mg) of ipratropium bromide by mouth have been reported to cause anticholinergic side-effects but these were not severe and did not require specific reversal.

Pharmacological properties

Pharmacodynamic properties: The bronchospasmolytic effect of Duovent was demonstrated in dogs; the individual agents of the combination when tested together had an additive effect when administered by inhalation.

In guinea pigs, the ingredients given intravenously, both separately and together, demonstrated a synergistic dose-related bronchospasmolytic action. A tachycardic effect was also noted with the combination: as ipratropium had no tachycardic effect when administered alone, this effect may represent a potentiation of action.

Dose-response studies in man using the inhaled drug combination showed a significant bronchospasmolytic effect as judged by improvement in lung function (total airway resistance), following administration of 1, 2, 4 and 6 puffs of Duovent (100:40, 200:80, 400:160, 600:240 mcg fenoterol hydrobromide: ipratropium bromide).

Pulse rates did not vary significantly between patients administered therapeutic doses of the individual components or the combination. No significant change in blood pressure was noted. The time to onset of bronchodilatation with the combination was the same as for fenoterol alone but of longer duration.

Pharmacokinetic properties: Ipratropium bromide is a quaternary ammonium antimuscarinic compound which is poorly absorbed from the gastro-intestinal tract and is slow to cross mucous membranes and the blood-brain barrier. Following inhalation, uptake into the plasma is minimal, a peak blood concentration is attained 1½ to 3 hours after inhalation (and similarly for oral administration). Excretion is chiefly via the kidneys.

Fenoterol hydrobromide is a beta-adrenergic sympathomimetic agent. Following inhalation of fenoterol hydrobromide, bronchodilatation occurs within a few minutes. The duration of action is about 3–5 hours.

Inhaled fenoterol acts topically on the airway by binding the $beta_2$-receptors on airway smooth muscle. Fenoterol concentrations in the circulation do not reflect those at the site of action.

The pharmacokinetics of fenoterol are therefore not related to the pharmacodynamics of the bronchodilatation it produces.

Orally administered fenoterol undergoes extensive first-pass metabolism.

Fenoterol hydrobromide can pass through the placenta and also into human milk.

Preclinical safety data: None stated.

Pharmaceutical particulars

List of excipients:

Sorbitan trioleate
Monofluorotrichloromethane
Difluorodichloromethane
Tetrafluorodichloroethane

Incompatibilities: None stated.

Shelf life: 3 years.

Special precautions for storage: Protect from heat, including the sun. Protect from frost. The vials should not be opened, punctured or incinerated even when apparently empty.

Nature and contents of container: 10 ml vial (200 metered doses) complete with Autohaler device.

Instructions for use/handling:

1. To remove the mouthpiece cover, pull down on the lip at the back.
2. Hold the Autohaler device upright. Push the lever up so that it stays up.
3. With the lever still up, shake the Autohaler device.
4. Continue to hold the Autohaler device upright, making sure that your hand is not blocking the air vents at the bottom.

   Breathe out normally and close your lips firmly around the mouthpiece.
5. Breathe in through the mouthpiece. When you hear the slight click, continue to breathe in.

   This click lets you know you have received your puff of medication.

   Hold your breath for 10 seconds, or as long as is comfortable, and then breathe out normally.
6. The lever must be lowered after each puff. If your doctor has prescribed more than one puff, wait one minute before repeating steps 2–6. Replace the mouthpiece cover after use.

Marketing authorisation number PL 00015/0162

Date of first authorisation 09/09/91

Date of revision of SPC January 1998

Legal category POM

DUOVENT* UDVs*

Qualitative and quantitative composition Each single dose unit contains fenoterol hydrobromide 1.25 mg and ipratropium bromide 0.5 mg.

Pharmaceutical form Nebuliser solution for inhalation.

Clinical particulars

Therapeutic indications: The management of acute severe asthma or acute exacerbation of chronic asthma presenting as an emergency requiring treatment by nebuliser.

Posology and method of administration: Duovent UDVs may be administered from an intermittent positive pressure ventilator or from a properly maintained and functioning nebuliser.

The recommended dose for adults and children over 14 years is one vial (4 ml) to be nebulised immediately upon presentation. Each dose should be inhaled to dryness from the nebuliser. Repeat dosing may be given at the discretion of the treating physician, up to a maximum of 4 vials in 24 hours.

In acute severe asthma additional doses may be necessary depending on clinical response. Nebuliser treatment of acute severe asthma should be replaced by standard inhaler devices 24–48 hours before discharge unless the patient requires a nebuliser at home.

Clinical trials have included patients over 65 years. No adverse reactions specific to this age group have been reported.

Contra-indications: Known hypersensitivity to atropine, ipratropium or fenoterol.

Special warnings and special precautions for use: As with other beta-agonists, caution should be observed when using Duovent UDVs in patients with thyrotoxicosis, myocardial insufficiency, angina, cardiac dysrhythmias, hypertension, hypertrophic subvalvular aortic stenosis or hypertrophic obstructive cardiomyopathy.

The administration of nebuliser solutions has occasionally been associated with cases of paradoxical bronchoconstriction.

Patients must be instructed in the correct use of a

nebuliser and warned not to exceed the prescribed dose. The patient must be instructed to seek medical advice in the event of Duovent failing to provide relief of bronchospasm.

Care should be taken to prevent the solution or mist from entering the eyes. Acute angle-closure glaucoma has been reported rarely when nebulised ipratropium bromide has been used in conjunction with nebulised beta$_2$-agonist bronchodilators. Protection of the eyes appears to prevent any increase in intra-ocular pressure and patients who may be susceptible to glaucoma should be warned specifically on the need for ocular protection. Inhaled doses of ipratropium bromide nebuliser solution up to 1 mg have not been associated with elevation of intra-ocular pressure.

Caution is advocated in the use of anticholinergic agents in patients with prostatic hypertrophy.

Interaction with other medicaments and other forms of interaction: In view of a possible interaction between sympathomimetic amines and monoamine oxidase inhibitors or tricyclic antidepressants, care should be exercised if it is proposed to administer these compounds concurrently with Duovent UDVs.

Duovent UDVs should be used with caution in patients already receiving other sympathomimetic agents as cardiovascular effects may be additive.

Potentially serious hypokalaemia may result from beta$_2$-agonist therapy. Particular caution is advised in severe asthma as this effect may be potentiated by concomitant treatment with xanthine derivatives, steroids, diuretics and by hypoxia. It is recommended that serum potassium levels are monitored on such occasions.

Beta-adrenergic blocking agents may antagonise fenoterol hydrobromide and reduce its bronchodilator effect if administered concurrently.

Pregnancy and lactation: Ipratropium bromide and fenoterol hydrobromide have been in wide general use for several years and there is no definite evidence of ill-consequence during pregnancy; animal studies have shown no hazard. Medicines should, however, not be used in pregnancy, especially during the first trimester, unless the expected benefit is thought to outweigh any possible risk to the foetus.

Beta-adrenergic agents have been shown to prolong pregnancy and inhibit labour although the amount in the recommended dose of Duovent UDVs is probably insufficient to do so.

Effects on ability to drive and use machines: None stated.

Undesirable effects: Anticholinergic side-effects are unlikely at therapeutic doses, but some patients may complain of a dry mouth.

As with other beta-adrenergic agonists transient sympathomimetic side-effects such as tremor, palpitations, tachycardia and headache may occur but are uncommon with administration by inhalation.

Potentially serious hypokalaemia may result from beta$_2$-agonist therapy.

Overdose: Inhaled doses of 5 mg ipratropium produce an increase in heart rate and palpitation but single doses of 2 mg have been given to adults and 1 mg to children without causing side-effects. Single doses of ipratropium bromide 30 mg by mouth cause anticholinergic side-effects but these are not severe and do not require specific reversal.

Accidental overdose with fenoterol may give rise to tachycardia, palpitation, flushing, nausea, restlessness, dizziness, headache and tremor. It is suggested that the patient should be treated symptomatically. Beta$_1$-selective beta-adrenergic blocking agents should be chosen and blood pressure should be monitored. Should the administration of a beta-adrenergic blocking agent be considered necessary to counteract the effects of overdosage, its use in a patient liable to bronchospasm should be carefully monitored.

Pharmacological properties

Pharmacodynamic properties:

Fenoterol hydrobromide is a direct acting sympathomimetic agent where the catechol nucleus of isoprenaline has been replaced by a resorcinol nucleus, and the substituent moiety on the amino group is larger. This substitution has the effect of depressing the affinity of the molecule to the beta-1 (cardiac and lipolytic) adrenergic receptors and enhancing the affinity towards the beta-2 (bronchial, vascular and intestinal) adrenergic receptors.

Ipratropium bromide affects airway function primarily through its neural effect on the parasympathetic nervous system. Ipratropium bromide blocks the acetylcholine receptors on smooth muscle in the lung. Stimulation of these receptors normally produces contraction and, depending on the degree of actuation, bronchoconstriction. Thus, even in normal subjects, ipratropium bromide will cause bronchodilatation.

Pharmacokinetic properties:

Fenoterol hydrobromide: In man fenoterol is very rapidly distributed through the tissues following intravenous administration. The kidneys excrete up to 65% mainly in the form of acidic conjugates. Following oral administration, the plasma levels reach their maximum 2 hours after ingestion and then drop exponentially. Renal excretion is 39% following peroral administration and over 98% of the renal excretory products consist of acidic conjugates. The half life for total excretion is 7.2 hours and absorption was calculated to be 60%.

The duration of action following use of a metered dose aerosol is considerably larger and can be explained by the dose independent absorption in the upper bronchial tree. The concentration-independent absorption at this site, from the depot produced by the metered dose aerosol is maintained for several hours.

Ipratropium bromide: It is a quaternary ammonium compound which is poorly absorbed from the gastro-intestinal tract and is slow to cross mucous membranes and the blood brain barrier. Following inhalation, uptake into the plasma is minimal, a peak blood concentration is attained 1½ to 3 hours after inhalation (and similarly for oral administration). Excretion is chiefly via the kidneys.

Pharmaceutical particulars

List of excipients:

Sodium chloride
Hydrochloric acid
Purified water

Incompatibilities: None stated.

Shelf life: 3 years

Special precautions for storage: Store below 25°C. Protect from heat and light.

Nature and contents of container: Low density polyethylene (LDPE) vials formed in strips of 10 packed into cartons containing 20 or 60 vials. Each vial contains 4 ml of solution.

Instructions for use/handling: None stated.

Marketing authorisation number PL 0015/0164

Date of first authorisation 09/06/93

Date of revision of the text May 1997

Legal category POM

MOBIC* 7.5 mg TABLETS ▼

Qualitative and quantitative composition Meloxicam 7.5 mg.

Pharmaceutical form Tablet.

Clinical particulars

Therapeutic indications: Short-term symptomatic treatment of acute exacerbations of osteoarthrosis.

Long-term symptomatic treatment of rheumatoid arthritis (chronic polyarthritis).

Symptomatic treatment of ankylosing spondylitis.

Posology and method of administration:

Acute exacerbations of osteoarthrosis: 7.5 mg/day (one tablet). If necessary, in the absence of improvement, the dose may be increased to 15 mg/day (two tablets).

Rheumatoid arthritis: 15 mg/day (two tablets). In elderly patients the recommended dose for long term treatment is 7.5 mg per day. Patients with increased risks for adverse reactions should start treatment with 7.5 mg per day.

Ankylosing spondylitis: 15 mg/day (two 7.5 mg tablets).

DO NOT EXCEED THE DOSE OF 15 mg/day.

In dialysis patients with severe renal failure the dose should not exceed 7.5 mg per day.

The total daily amount should be taken as a single dose, with water or another liquid, during a meal.

Contra-indications: Hypersensitivity to meloxicam or to one of the excipients. The possibility exists of crossover sensitivity with aspirin and other non-steroidal anti-inflammatory drugs (NSAIDs). Mobic should not be given to patients who have developed signs of asthma, nasal polyps, angioneurotic oedema or urticaria following the administration of aspirin or NSAIDs.

- Active peptic ulcer during the last six months or a history of recurrent peptic ulcer disease.
- Severe hepatic failure.
- Non-dialysed severe renal failure.
- Children aged under 15.
- Pregnancy (see *Pregnancy and lactation*).
- Lactation.
- Gastrointestinal bleeding, cerebrovascular bleeding or other bleeding disorders.

Special warnings and special precautions for use:

Warnings: As with all NSAIDs, any history of oesophagitis, gastritis and/or peptic ulcer must be sought in order to ensure their total cure before starting treatment with meloxicam. Attention should routinely be paid to the possible onset of a recurrence in patients treated with meloxicam and with a past history of this type.

Patients with gastrointestinal symptoms or history of gastrointestinal disease should be monitored for digestive disturbances, especially for gastrointestinal bleeding.

Gastrointestinal bleeding or ulceration/perforation, have in general more serious consequences in the elderly. They can occur at any time during treatment, with or without warning symptoms or a previous history of serious gastrointestinal events.

In the rare instance where gastrointestinal bleeding or ulceration occurs in patients receiving meloxicam, the drug should be withdrawn.

Withdrawal of treatment with meloxicam must be envisaged in case of onset of cutaneo-mucosal adverse events. The possible occurrence of severe skin reactions and serious life threatening hypersensitivity reactions is known to occur with NSAIDs including oxicams.

In rare instances, NSAIDs may be the cause of interstitial nephritis, glomerulonephritis, renal medullary necrosis or nephrotic syndrome.

As with most NSAIDs, occasional increases in serum transaminase levels, increases in serum bilirubin or other liver function parameters as well as increases in serum creatinine and blood urea nitrogen as well as other laboratory disturbances have been reported. The majority of these instances involved transitory and slight abnormalities. Should any such abnormality prove significant or persistent, the administration of meloxicam should be stopped and appropriate investigations prescribed.

Induction of sodium, potassium and water retention and interference with the natriuretic effects of diuretics and consequently possible exacerbations of the condition of patients with cardiac insufficiency or hypertension may occur with NSAIDs.

Precautions: NSAIDs inhibit the synthesis of renal prostaglandins involved in the maintenance of renal perfusion in patients with decreased renal blood flow and blood volume. Administration of NSAIDs in such situations may result in the decompensation of latent renal failure. However renal function returns to its initial status when treatment is withdrawn. This risk concerns all elderly individuals, patients with congestive cardiac failure, cirrhosis of the liver, nephrotic syndrome or renal failure as well as patients on diuretics or having undergone major surgery leading to hypovolaemia. Careful monitoring of urine output and renal function during treatment is necessary in such patients.

Adverse reactions are often less well tolerated in elderly, fragile or weakened individuals, who therefore require careful surveillance. As with other NSAIDs, particular caution is required in the elderly, in whom renal, hepatic and cardiac functions are frequently impaired.

The recommended maximum daily dose should not be exceeded in case of insufficient therapeutic effect nor should an additional NSAID be added to the therapy because this may increase the toxicity while therapeutic advantage has not been proven.

Interaction with other medicaments and other forms of interaction:

Inadvisable combinations: Other NSAIDs, including high doses of salicylates: administration of several NSAIDs together may increase the risk of ulcers and of gastrointestinal bleeding, via a synergistic effect.

Oral anticoagulants, heparin and ticlopidine: increased risk of bleeding via inhibition of platelet function and damage to the gastroduodenal mucosa. Careful monitoring of the effects of anticoagulants is thus essential if it proves impossible to avoid such combined prescription.

Lithium: NSAIDs increase blood lithium levels, which may then reach toxic values (decreased renal excretion of lithium). This parameter therefore requires monitoring during the initiation, adjustment and withdrawal of treatment with meloxicam.

Methotrexate: NSAIDs may accentuate the haematologic toxicity of methotrexate. A case of agranulocytosis with meloxicam has been reported in a patient who was also taking methotrexate. The direct causality of meloxicam was not confirmed, but caution is required before prescribing such a combination. Strict monitoring of blood cell count is recommended in this situation.

Intrauterine contraceptive devices: NSAIDs appear to decrease the efficacy of intrauterine contraceptive devices.

Combinations requiring precautions: Diuretics: treatment with NSAIDs is associated with a risk of acute renal failure in dehydrated patients (decreased glomerular filtration via decreased renal prostaglandin synthesis). In case of combined prescription of meloxicam and a diuretic, it is essential to ensure that the patient is adequately hydrated and to monitor renal function at the start of treatment.

Nephrotoxicity of cyclosporin may be enhanced by NSAIDs via renal prostaglandin mediated effects.

During combined treatment renal function is to be measured.

Associations needing to be taken into consideration: Antihypertensive drugs [beta-blockers, angiotensin converting enzyme (ACE) inhibitors, diuretics]: treatment with a NSAID may decrease their antihypertensive effect via inhibition of vasodilator prostaglandin synthesis.

Thrombolytics: increased risk of haemorrhage.

Concomitant administration of antacids, cimetidine, β-acetyl digoxin and frusemide has not given rise to any notable pharmacokinetic interactions with meloxicam. Cholestyramine accelerates the elimination of meloxicam via binding in the digestive tract.

Interactions with oral anti-diabetics cannot be excluded.

Pregnancy and lactation:
Pregnancy: In animals, lethal effects on the embryo have been reported at doses far higher than those used clinically.

It is advisable to avoid the administration of meloxicam during pregnancy.

During the final three months, all prostaglandin synthesis inhibitors may expose the foetus to cardiopulmonary (pulmonary hypertension with premature closure of the ductus arteriosus) and renal toxicity or inhibit the contraction of the uterus. This effect on the uterus has been associated with an increase in the incidence of dystocia and delayed parturition in animals. Thus all NSAIDs are absolutely contraindicated during the final three months.

Lactation: It is unknown whether meloxicam passes into mothers milk. Meloxicam should not be given to nursing mothers.

Effects on ability to drive and use machines: There are no specific studies about such effects. However, when adverse effects such as vertigo or drowsiness occur it is advisable to refrain from these activities.

Undesirable effects: Digestive system: dyspepsia, nausea, vomiting, abdominal pain, constipation, flatulence, diarrhoea. More rarely, peptic ulcers, perforation or gastrointestinal bleeding, which may be severe, may occur.

Haematologic adverse events: disturbances of blood count, including differential white cell count: anaemia, leukopenia, thrombocytopenia have been described in patients taking meloxicam. Certain cases have been attributed to treatment. Concomitant administration of a potentially myelotoxic drug, in particular methotrexate, appears to be a predisposing factor to the onset of a cytopenia. In particular, a case of agranulocytosis has been described in a patient treated with meloxicam and also taking methotrexate.

Cutaneo-mucosal reactions: stomatitis, oesophagitis, pruritus, skin rash, urticaria, photosensitisation have been reported. Very rare cases of bullous reactions such as erythema multiforme, Stevens-Johnson Syndrome and toxic epidermal necrolysis may develop.

Respiratory system: onset of an asthma attack has been reported in certain individuals allergic to aspirin or to other NSAIDs.

Central nervous system: possibility of lightheadedness, headache, vertigo, tinnitus, drowsiness.

Cardiovascular system: oedema, oedema of the lower limbs, palpitations, flushes may occur during treatment.

Genitourinary system: possibility of disturbances of laboratory tests investigating renal function (e.g. raised serum creatinine or urea).

Transitory disturbances of liver function tests (e.g. raised transaminases or bilirubin).

Overdose: Appropriate measures are required in case of overdose since there is no known antidote. Evidence was found in one clinical trial of acceleration of the elimination of meloxicam by cholestyramine. Severe gastrointestinal lesions may be treated with antacids and H_2 receptor antagonists.

Pharmacological properties
Pharmacodynamic properties: NON-STEROIDAL ANTI-INFLAMMATORY AGENT (M: locomotor system).

Meloxicam is a non-steroidal anti-inflammatory drug (NSAID) of the oxicam family, with anti-inflammatory, analgesic and antipyretic properties.

The anti-inflammatory activity of meloxicam has been proven in classical models of inflammation. As with other NSAIDs, its precise mechanism of action remains unknown. However there is at least one common mode of action shared by all NSAIDs (including meloxicam): inhibition of the biosynthesis of prostaglandins, known inflammation mediators.

Pharmacokinetic properties: The bioavailability of meloxicam following oral administration is on the average 89%.

With the doses of 7.5 and 15 mg, plasma concentrations are proportional to dose: 0.4 to 1.0 mg/l for 7.5 mg and 0.8 to 2.0 mg/l for 15 mg, on average (C_{min} and C_{max} at steady state).

Meloxicam is very strongly bound to plasma proteins, essentially albumin (99%).

Meloxicam is extensively metabolised, chiefly by oxidation of the methyl radical attached to the thiazolyl ring. Elimination in unchanged form accounts for 3% of the dose. Half of the substance is eliminated in urine and the other half in faeces.

The mean elimination half-life is of the order of 20 hours.

Steady state is reached in 5 days.

In terminal renal failure, the volume of distribution is increased and a daily dose of 7.5 mg must not be exceeded.

Plasma clearance is on average 8 ml/min. Clearance is decreased in the elderly. Volume of distribution is low, on average 11 l. Inter-individual variation is the order of 30–40%.

Preclinical safety data: The toxicological profile of meloxicam has been found in preclinical studies to be identical to that of NSAIDs: gastrointestinal ulcers and erosions, renal papillary necrosis at high doses during chronic administration in two animal species. Non toxic doses were 3 to 10 times higher than clinically used doses, according to animal species used.

Reproduction studies have reported lethal effects on the embryo at doses far higher than those used clinically. Fetotoxic effects at the end of gestation, shared by all prostaglandin synthesis inhibitors, have been described. No evidence has been found of any mutagenic effect, either in vitro or in vivo. No carcinogenic risk has been found in the rat and mouse at doses far higher than those used clinically.

Pharmaceutical particulars
List of excipients:
Sodium citrate dihydrate
Lactose monohydrate
Microcrystalline cellulose (AVICEL PH 102)
Polyvidone (KOLLIDON 25)
Anhydrous colloidal silica (AEROSIL 200)
Crospolyvidone (KOLLIDON CL)
Magnesium stearate.

Incompatibilities: None stated.

Shelf life: Five years when stored below 25°C for the packaging in blister cards. Five years for packaging in glass bottle and polypropylene tube.

Special precautions for storage: Should be stored away from dampness (in the case of blister cards).

Nature and contents of container: Glass bottle or polypropylene tube with polyethylene cap. PVC/PVDC-aluminium blister cards.

Instructions for use/handling: None stated.

Marketing authorisation holder Boehringer Ingelheim International GmbH, D-55216 Ingelheim am Rhein, Germany.

Marketing authorisation number PL 14598/0002

Date of first authorisation 21 February 1996

Date of approval/revision of SPC June 1998

Legal category POM

MOBIC* 15 mg TABLETS ▼

Qualitative and quantitative composition Meloxicam 15.0 mg.

Pharmaceutical form Tablet with breakline.

Clinical particulars
Therapeutic indications: Short-term symptomatic treatment of acute exacerbations of osteoarthrosis.

Long-term symptomatic treatment of rheumatoid arthritis (chronic polyarthritis).

Symptomatic treatment of ankylosing spondylitis.

Posology and method of administration:
Acute exacerbations of osteoarthrosis: 7.5 mg/day (half a tablet). If necessary, in the absence of improvement, the dose may be increased to 15 mg/day (one tablet).

Rheumatoid arthritis: 15 mg/day (one tablet). In elderly patients the recommended dose for long term treatment is 7.5 mg per day. Patients with increased risks for adverse reactions should start treatment with 7.5 mg per day.

Ankylosing spondylitis: 15 mg/day.

DO NOT EXCEED THE DOSE OF 15 mg/day.

In dialysis patients with severe renal failure the dose should not exceed 7.5 mg per day.

The total daily amount should be taken as a single dose, with water or another liquid, during a meal.

Contra-indications: Hypersensitivity to meloxicam or to one of the excipients. The possibility exists of crossover sensitivity with aspirin and other non-steroidal anti-inflammatory drugs (NSAIDs). Mobic should not be given to patients who have developed signs of asthma, nasal polyps, angioneurotic oedema or urticaria following the administration of aspirin or NSAIDs.

- Active peptic ulcer during the last six months or a history of recurrent peptic ulcer disease.
- Severe hepatic failure.
- Non-dialysed severe renal failure.
- Children aged under 15.
- Pregnancy (see *Pregnancy and lactation*).
- Lactation.
- Gastrointestinal bleeding, cerebrovascular bleeding or other bleeding disorders.

Special warnings and special precautions for use:
Warnings: As with all NSAIDs, any history of oesophagitis, gastritis and/or peptic ulcer must be sought in order to ensure their total cure before starting treatment with meloxicam. Attention should routinely be paid to the possible onset of a recurrence in patients treated with meloxicam and with a past history of this type.

Patients with gastrointestinal symptoms or history of gastrointestinal disease should be monitored for digestive disturbances, especially for gastrointestinal bleeding.

Gastrointestinal bleeding or ulceration/perforation, have in general more serious consequences in the elderly. They can occur at any time during treatment, with or without warning symptoms or a previous history of serious gastrointestinal events.

In the rare instance where gastrointestinal bleeding or ulceration occurs in patients receiving meloxicam, the drug should be withdrawn.

Withdrawal of treatment with meloxicam must be envisaged in case of onset of cutaneo-mucosal adverse events. The possible occurrence of severe skin reactions and serious life threatening hypersensitivity reactions is known to occur with NSAIDs including oxicams.

In rare instances, NSAIDs may be the cause of interstitial nephritis, glomerulonephritis, renal medullary necrosis or nephrotic syndrome.

As with most NSAIDs, occasional increases in serum transaminase levels, increases in serum bilirubin or other liver function parameters as well as increases in serum creatinine and blood urea nitrogen as well as other laboratory disturbances have been reported. The majority of these instances involved transitory and slight abnormalities. Should any such abnormality prove significant or persistent, the administration of meloxicam should be stopped and appropriate investigations prescribed.

Induction of sodium, potassium and water retention and interference with the natriuretic effects of diuretics and consequently possible exacerbations of the condition of patients with cardiac insufficiency or hypertension may occur with NSAIDs.

Precautions: NSAIDs inhibit the synthesis of renal prostaglandins involved in the maintenance of renal perfusion in patients with decreased renal blood flow and blood volume. Administration of NSAIDs in such situations may result in the decompensation of latent renal failure. However renal function returns to its initial status when treatment is withdrawn. This risk concerns all elderly individuals, patients with congestive cardiac failure, cirrhosis of the liver, nephrotic syndrome or renal failure as well as patients on diuretics or having undergone major surgery leading to hypovolaemia. Careful monitoring of urine output and renal function during treatment is necessary in such patients.

Adverse reactions are often less well tolerated in elderly, fragile or weakened individuals, who therefore require careful surveillance. As with other NSAIDs, particular caution is required in the elderly, in whom renal, hepatic and cardiac functions are frequently impaired.

The recommended maximum daily dose should not be exceeded in case of insufficient therapeutic effect nor should an additional NSAID be added to the therapy because this may increase the toxicity while therapeutic advantage has not been proven.

Interaction with other medicaments and other forms of interaction:
Inadvisable combinations: Other NSAIDs, including high doses of salicylates: administration of several NSAIDs together may increase the risk of ulcers and of gastrointestinal bleeding, via a synergistic effect.

Oral anticoagulants, heparin and ticlopidine: increased risk of bleeding via inhibition of platelet function and damage to the gastroduodenal mucosa. Careful monitoring of the effects of anticoagulants is thus essential if it proves impossible to avoid such combined prescription.

Lithium: NSAIDs increase blood lithium levels, which may then reach toxic values (decreased renal excretion of lithium). This parameter therefore requires monitoring during the initiation, adjustment and withdrawal of treatment with meloxicam.

Methotrexate: NSAIDs may accentuate the haematologic toxicity of methotrexate. A case of agranulocytosis with meloxicam has been reported in a patient who was also taking methotrexate. The direct causality of meloxicam was not confirmed, but caution is required before prescribing such a combination. Strict monitoring of blood cell count is recommended in this situation.

Intrauterine contraceptive devices: NSAIDs appear to decrease the efficacy of intrauterine contraceptive devices.

Combinations requiring precautions: Diuretics: treatment with NSAIDs is associated with a risk of acute renal failure in dehydrated patients (decreased glomerular filtration via decreased renal prostaglandin synthesis). In case of combined prescription of meloxicam and a diuretic, it is essential to ensure that the patient is adequately hydrated and to monitor renal function at the start of treatment.

Nephrotoxicity of cyclosporin may be enhanced by NSAIDs via renal prostaglandin mediated effects. During combined treatment renal function is to be measured.

Associations needing to be taken into consideration: Antihypertensive drugs [beta-blockers, angiotensin converting enzyme (ACE) inhibitors, diuretics]: treatment with a NSAID may decrease their antihypertensive effect via inhibition of vasodilator prostaglandin synthesis.

Thrombolytics: increased risk of haemorrhage.

Concomitant administration of antacids, cimetidine, β-acetyl digoxin and frusemide has not given rise to any notable pharmacokinetic interactions with meloxicam. Cholestyramine accelerates the elimination of meloxicam via binding in the digestive tract.

Interactions with oral anti-diabetics cannot be excluded.

Pregnancy and lactation:
Pregnancy: In animals, lethal effects on the embryo have been reported at doses far higher than those used clinically.

It is advisable to avoid the administration of meloxicam during pregnancy.

During the final three months, all prostaglandin synthesis inhibitors may expose the foetus to cardiopulmonary (pulmonary hypertension with premature closure of the ductus arteriosus) and renal toxicity or inhibit the contraction of the uterus. This effect on the uterus has been associated with an increase in the incidence of dystocia and delayed parturition in animals.

Thus all NSAIDs are absolutely contra-indicated during the final three months.

Lactation: It is unknown whether meloxicam passes into mothers milk. Meloxicam should not be given to nursing mothers.

Effects on ability to drive and use machines: There are no specific studies about such effects. However, when adverse effects such as vertigo or drowsiness occur it is advisable to refrain from these activities.

Undesirable effects: Digestive system: dyspepsia, nausea, vomiting, abdominal pain, constipation, flatulence, diarrhoea. More rarely, peptic ulcers, perforation or gastrointestinal bleeding, which may be severe, may occur.

Haematologic adverse events: disturbances of blood count, including differential white cell count: anaemia, leukopenia, thrombocytopenia have been described in patients taking meloxicam. Certain cases have been attributed to treatment. Concomitant administration of a potentially myelotoxic drug, in particular methotrexate, appears to be a predisposing factor to the onset of a cytopenia. In particular, a case of agranulocytosis has been described in a patient treated with meloxicam and also taking methotrexate.

Cutaneo-mucosal reactions: stomatitis, oesophagitis, pruritus, skin rash, urticaria, photosensitisation have been reported. Very rare cases of bullous reactions such as erythema multiforme, Stevens-Johnson Syndrome and toxic epidermal necrolysis may develop.

Respiratory system: onset of an asthma attack has been reported in certain individuals allergic to aspirin or to other NSAIDs.

Central nervous system: possibility of lightheadedness, headache, vertigo, tinnitus, drowsiness.

Cardiovascular system: oedema, oedema of the lower limbs, palpitations, flushes may occur during treatment.

Genitourinary system: possibility of disturbances of laboratory tests investigating renal function (e.g. raised serum creatinine or urea).

Transitory disturbances of liver function tests (e.g. raised transaminases or bilirubin).

Overdose: Appropriate measures are required in case of overdose since there is no known antidote. Evidence was found in one clinical trial of acceleration of the elimination of meloxicam by cholestyramine. Severe gastrointestinal lesions may be treated with antacids and H_2 receptor antagonists.

Pharmacological properties
Pharmacodynamic properties: NON-STEROIDAL ANTI-INFLAMMATORY AGENT (M: locomotor system).

Meloxicam is a non-steroidal anti-inflammatory drug (NSAID) of the oxicam family, with anti-inflammatory, analgesic and antipyretic properties.

The anti-inflammatory activity of meloxicam has been proven in classical models of inflammation. As with other NSAIDs, its precise mechanism of action remains unknown. However there is at least one common mode of action shared by all NSAIDs (including meloxicam): inhibition of the biosynthesis of prostaglandins, known inflammation mediators.

Pharmacokinetic properties: The bioavailability of meloxicam following oral administration is on the average 89%.

With the doses of 7.5 and 15 mg, plasma concentrations are proportional to dose: 0.4 to 1.0 mg/l for 7.5 mg and 0.8 to 2.0 mg/l for 15 mg, on average (C_{min} and C_{max} at steady state).

Meloxicam is very strongly bound to plasma proteins, essentially albumin (99%).

Meloxicam is extensively metabolised, chiefly by oxidation of the methyl radical attached to the thiazolyl ring. Elimination in unchanged form accounts for 3% of the dose. Half of the substance is eliminated in urine and the other half in faeces.

The mean elimination half-life is of the order of 20 hours.

Steady state is reached in 5 days.

In terminal renal failure, the volume of distribution is increased and a daily dose of 7.5 mg must not be exceeded.

Plasma clearance is on average 8 ml/min. Clearance is decreased in the elderly. Volume of distribution is low, on average 11 l. Interindividual variation is the order of 30–40%.

Preclinical safety data: The toxicological profile of meloxicam has been found in preclinical studies to be identical to that of NSAIDs: gastrointestinal ulcers and erosions, renal papillary necrosis at high doses during chronic administration in two animal species. Non toxic doses were 3 to 10 times higher than clinically used doses, according to animal species used.

Reproduction studies have reported lethal effects on the embryo at doses far higher than those used clinically. Fetotoxic effects at the end of gestation, shared by all prostaglandin synthesis inhibitors, have been described. No evidence has been found of any mutagenic effect, either in vitro or in vivo. No carcinogenic risk has been found in the rat and mouse at doses far higher than those used clinically.

Pharmaceutical particulars
List of excipients:
Sodium citrate dihydrate
Lactose monohydrate
Microcrystalline cellulose (AVICEL PH 102)
Polyvidone (KOLLIDON 25)
Anhydrous colloidal silica (AEROSIL 200)
Crospolyvidone (KOLLIDON CL)
Magnesium stearate

Incompatibilities: None stated.

Shelf life: Five years when stored below 25°C for the packaging in blister cards. Five years for packaging in glass bottle and polypropylene tube.

Special precautions for storage: Should be stored away from dampness (in the case of blister cards).

Nature and contents of container: Glass bottle or polypropylene tube with polyethylene cap. PVC/PVDC-aluminium blister cards.

Instructions for use/handling: None stated.

Marketing authorisation holder Boehringer Ingelheim International GmbH, D-55216 Ingelheim am Rhein, Germany.

Marketing authorisation number PL 14598/0003

Date of first authorisation 21 February 1996

Date of approval/revision of SPC June 1998

Legal category POM

MOBIC* 7.5 mg SUPPOSITORIES ▼

Qualitative and quantitative composition Meloxicam 7.50 mg per suppository.

Pharmaceutical form Suppository.

Clinical particulars
Therapeutic indications: Short term symptomatic treatment of acute exacerbations of osteoarthrosis; long term symptomatic treatment of rheumatoid arthritis.

Posology and method of administration:
Osteoarthrosis: 7.5 mg/day, i.e. one 7.5 mg suppository. If necessary, in the absence of improvement, the dosage can be increased to 15 mg/day, i.e. one 15 mg suppository.

Rheumatoid arthritis: 15 mg a day, i.e. one 15 mg suppository. In elderly patients with rheumatoid arthritis, the recommended dose for long term treatment is 7.5 mg per day.

DO NOT EXCEED THE DOSE OF 15 mg/day.

Patients with increased risks for adverse reactions should start with 7.5 mg per day. In dialysis patients with severe renal failure, the dose should not exceed 7.5 mg per day.

Rectal administration should be used for the shortest time possible, in view of the risk of local toxicity added to the risks of oral administration.

Contra-indications: This medicinal product is contra-indicated in the following situations:
- pregnancy and lactation (see *Pregnancy and lactation*);
- hypersensitivity to meloxicam or to one of the excipients, or hypersensitivity to substances with a similar action, e.g. NSAIDs, aspirin;
- active peptic ulcer or history of recurrent peptic ulcer;
- severely impaired liver function;
- non-dialysed severe renal failure;
- past history of proctitis or rectal bleeding;
- children aged under 15;
- gastrointestinal bleeding, cerebrovascular bleeding or other bleeding disorders.

This medicinal product is generally inadvisable in combination with other NSAIDs, oral anticoagulants, heparin by injection, lithium, high doses of methotrexate, high doses of salicylates, ticlopidine (see *Interaction with other medicinal products and other forms of interaction*).

Special warnings and special precautions for use
Warnings: As with all NSAIDs, any history of oesophagitis, gastritis and/or peptic ulcer must be sought in order to ensure their total cure before starting treatment with meloxicam. Attention should routinely be paid to the possible onset of a recurrence in patients treated with meloxicam and with a past history of this type.

Patients with gastrointestinal symptoms or history of gastrointestinal disease should be monitored for digestive disturbances, especially for gastrointestinal bleeding.

Gastrointestinal bleeding or ulceration/perforation, have in general more serious consequences in the elderly. They can occur at any time during treatment, with or without warning symptoms or a previous history of serious gastrointestinal events.

In the rare instance where gastrointestinal bleeding or ulceration occurs in patients receiving meloxicam, the drug should be withdrawn.

Mobic should not be given to patients who have developed signs of asthma, nasal polyps angioneurotic oedema or urticaria following the administration of aspirin or other NSAIDs.

Withdrawal of treatment with meloxicam must be envisaged in case of onset of cutaneo-mucosal adverse events. The possible onset of severe skin reactions and serious life threatening hypersensitivity reactions is known to occur with NSAIDs including oxicams.

In rare instances, NSAIDs may be the cause of interstitial nephritis, glomerulonephritis, renal medullary necrosis or nephrotic syndrome.

As with most NSAIDs, occasional increases in serum transaminase level, increases in serum bilirubin or other liver function parameters, as well as increases in serum creatinine and blood urea nitrogen as well as other laboratory disturbances, have been reported. The majority of these instances involved transitory and slight abnormalities. Should any such abnormality prove significant or persistent, the administration of meloxicam should be stopped and appropriate investigations prescribed.

Induction of sodium, potassium and water retention and interference with the natriuretic effects of diuretics and consequently possible exacerbations of the condition of patients with cardiac failure or hypertension may occur with NSAIDs.

Precautions: This medicinal product exists in other dosages, which may be more appropriate.

The onset of asthma attacks in certain patients may be linked to allergy to aspirin or to NSAIDs. The medicinal product is contra-indicated in this situation.

NSAIDs inhibit the synthesis of renal prostaglandins involved in the maintenance of renal perfusion, in patients with decreased renal blood flow and blood volume. Administration of NSAIDs in such situations may result in the decompensation of latent renal failure. However, renal function returns to its initial status when treatment is withdrawn. This risk concerns all elderly individuals, patients with congestive cardiac failure, cirrhosis of the liver, nephrotic syndrome or renal failure as well as patients on diuretics or having undergone major surgery leading to hypovolaemia. Careful monitoring of urine output and renal function during treatment is necessary in such patients.

Adverse reactions are often less well tolerated in elderly, fragile or weakened individuals, who therefore require careful monitoring. As with other NSAIDs, particular caution is required in the elderly, in whom renal, hepatic and cardiac functions are frequently impaired.

The recommended maximum daily dose should not be exceeded in case of insufficient therapeutic effect, nor should an additional NSAID be added to the therapy because this may increase the toxicity while therapeutic advantage has not been proven.

Interaction with other medicaments and other forms of interaction: Simultaneous administration of meloxicam with the following substances requires careful monitoring of the patient's clinical and laboratory status.

Inadvisable combinations:

Oral anticoagulants, parenteral heparin and ticlopidine: increased risk of bleeding, via inhibition of platelet function and damage to the gastroduodenal mucosa. Careful monitoring of the effects of anticoagulants is thus essential if it proves impossible to avoid such combined prescription.

Other NSAIDs, including high doses of salicylates: administration of several NSAIDs together may increase the risk of gastrointestinal ulcers and bleeding, via a synergistic effect.

Lithium (described with several NSAIDs): NSAIDs increase blood lithium levels, which may reach toxic values (decreased renal excretion of lithium). This parameter therefore requires monitoring during the initiation, adjustment and withdrawal of treatment with meloxicam.

Methotrexate, used at high doses of 15 mg/week or more: increased haematological toxicity of methotrexate via a decrease in its renal clearance by anti-inflammatory agents in general.

A case of agranulocytosis with meloxicam has been reported in a patient also treated with methotrexate. The direct causality of meloxicam was not confirmed, but caution is required before prescribing such a combination. Strict monitoring of blood cell count is recommended in this situation.

Combinations requiring precautions:

Cyclosporin: Nephrotoxicity of cyclosporin may be enhanced by NSAIDs via renal prostaglandin mediated effects. During combined treatment, renal function is to be measured.

Diuretics: treatment with NSAIDs is associated with a risk of acute renal failure in dehydrated patients (decreased glomerular filtration via decreased renal prostaglandin synthesis). In case of combined prescription of meloxicam and a diuretic, it is essential to ensure that the patient is adequately hydrated and to monitor renal function at the start of the treatment.

Methotrexate, used at low doses, less than 15 mg/week: increased hematological toxicity of methotrexate via a decrease in its renal clearance by anti-inflammatory agents in general. Weekly monitoring of blood count during the first weeks of the combination.

Increased surveillance in the presence of even mildly impaired renal function, as well as in the elderly.

Pentoxifylline: increased risk of bleeding. Increase clinical monitoring and check bleeding time more often.

Zidovudine: risk of increased red cell line toxicity via action on reticulocytes, with severe anaemia occurring one week after the NSAID is started. Check CBC and reticulocyte count one to two weeks after starting treatment with the NSAID.

Associations needing to be taken into account:

Antihypertensive agents, e.g. beta-blockers, angiotensin converting enzyme inhibitors, diuretics (by extrapolation from indomethacin): treatment with a NSAID may decrease their antihypertensive effect via inhibition of prostaglandin synthesis.

IUD: controversial risk of impaired efficacy.

Thrombolytics: increased risk of bleeding.

Others: Concomitant administration of antacids, cimetidine, beta-acetyl digoxin and frusemide has not given rise to any notable pharmacokinetic interactions with meloxicam. Cholestyramine accelerates the elimination of meloxicam via binding in the digestive tract.

Interaction with oral anti-diabetics cannot be excluded.

Pregnancy and lactation:

Pregnancy: In animals, lethal effects on the embryo have been reported at doses far higher than those used clinically.

It is advisable to avoid the administration of meloxicam during pregnancy.

During the final three months, all prostaglandin synthesis inhibitors may expose the foetus to cardio-pulmonary (pulmonary hypertension with premature closure of the ductus arteriosus) and renal toxicity or inhibit the contraction of the uterus. This effect on the uterus has been associated with an increase in the incidence of dystocia and delayed parturition in animals. Thus all NSAIDs are absolutely contra-indicated during the final three months.

Lactation: NSAIDs pass into mothers milk. Administration should therefore be avoided, as a precautionary measure, in women who are breast feeding.

Effects on ability to drive and use machines: There have been no specific studies. However, when adverse effects such as vertigo and drowsiness occur, it is advisable to refrain from these activities.

Undesirable effects:

Digestive system: dyspepsia, nausea, vomiting, abdominal pain, constipation, flatulence, diarrhoea. More rarely, peptic ulcers, perforation or gastrointestinal bleeding, which may be severe, may occur.

Haematological system: disturbances of blood count: anaemia, leucocytopenia, thrombocytopenia have been reported in patients on meloxicam. Some cases have been atrributed to treatment. Concomitant administration of a potentially myelotoxic drug (methotrexate in particular) appears to be a predisposing factor to the onset of a cytopenia. In particular, a case of agranulocytosis has been reported in a patient treated with meloxicam and also taking methotrexate.

Cutaneo-mucosal reactions: stomatitis, oesophagitis, pruritus, skin rash, urticaria, photosensitivity reactions. Very rare cases of bullous reaction such as erythema multiforme, Stevens-Johnson Syndrome and toxic epidermal necrolysis may develop.

Respiratory system: onset of asthma attacks have been reported in certain individuals allergic to aspirin or other NSAIDs.

Central nervous system: possibility of lightheadedness, headache, vertigo, tinnitus, drowsiness.

Cardiovascular system: oedema, oedema of the lower limbs, palpitations, flushes may occur during treatment.

Genitourinary system: possibility of disturbances of laboratory tests investigating renal function (e.g. raised creatinine or urea).

Transitory disturbances of liver function tests (e.g. raised transaminases or bilirubin).

Adverse effects related to route of administration: risk of local toxicity all the more frequent and severe when treatment is for a long period and the number of daily doses and dosage are high.

Overdose: Appropriate measures are required in case of overdosage since there is no known antidote. Evidence was found in one clinical trial of accleration of the elimination of meloxicam by cholestyramine. Severe gastrointestinal lesions may be treated with antacids and H_2 receptor antagonists.

Pharmacological properties

Pharmacodynamic properties: NON-STEROIDAL ANTI-INFLAMMATORY DRUG (M: locomotor system).

Meloxicam is a non-steriodal anti-inflammatory drug (NSAID) of the oxicam group, with anti-inflammatory, analgesic and antipyretic properties.

The anti-inflammatory activity of meloxicam has been proven in classical models of inflammation. As with other NSAIDs, its precise mechanism of action remains unknown.

However, there is at least one common mode of action shared by all NSAIDs (including meloxicam): inhibition of the biosynthesis of prostaglandins, known inflammation mediators.

Pharmacokinetic properties: The bioavailability of meloxicam following oral administration is on the average 89%.

Meloxicam 7.5 mg suppositories have a bioavailability of 88% in comparison to capsules and mean drug concentrations fluctuate in steady state between 0.40±0.16 μg/ml and 0.96±0.24 μg/ml.

This corresponds to an absolute bioavailability of 85%.

With the doses of 7.5 and 15 mg, plasma concentrations are proportional to dose: 0.4 to 1.0 mg/l for 7.5 mg and 0.8 to 2.0 mg/l for 15 mg, on average (C_{min} and C_{max} at steady state).

Meloxicam is very strongly bound to proteins, essentially albumin (99%).

Meloxicam is extensively metabolised, chiefly by oxidation of the methyl radical attached to the thiazolyl ring. Elimination in unchanged form accounts for 3% of the dose. Half of the substance is eliminated in urine and the other half in faeces.

The mean elimination half-life is of the order of 20 hours.

Steady state is reached in 5 days.

Plasma clearance is on average 8 ml/min. Clearance is decreased in the elderly. Volume of distribution is low, on average 11 l. Interindividual variation is the order of 30–40%.

In terminal renal failure, the volume of distribution is increased, and a daily dose of 7.5 mg must not be exceeded.

Preclinical safety data: The toxicological profile of meloxicam has been found in preclinical studies to be identical to that of NSAIDs: gastrointestinal ulcers and erosions, renal papillary necrosis at high doses during chronic administration in two animal species. Non toxic doses were 3 to 10 times higher than clinically used doses according to animal species used.

Reproduction studies have reported lethal effects on the embryo at doses far higher than those used clinically. Fetotoxic effects at the end of gestation, shared by all prostaglandin synthesis inhibitors, have been described. No evidence has been found of any mutagenic effect, either *in vitro* or *in vivo*. No carcinogenic risk has been found in the rat and mouse at doses far higher than those used clinically.

Pharmaceutical particulars

List of excipients: Hard fat (Type SU BP), Polyoxyethylenated hydrogenated castor oil 40.

Incompatibilities: None stated.

Shelf life: 3 years.

Special precautions for storage: Should be stored at a temperature not exceeding 30°C.

Nature and contents of container:

Cartons containing 6 suppositories in aluminium blister sheets.
Cartons containing 7 suppositories in aluminium blister sheets.
Cartons containing 10 suppositories in aluminium blister sheets.
Cartons containing 12 suppositories in aluminium blister sheets.
Cartons containing 20 suppositories in aluminium blister sheets.
Cartons containing 30 suppositories in aluminium blister sheets.
Cartons containing 50 suppositories in aluminium blister sheets.
Cartons containing 60 suppositories in aluminium blister sheets.
Cartons containing 120 suppositories in aluminium blister sheets.
Cartons containing 10×50 suppositories in aluminium blister sheets.

Instructions for use/handling: None stated.

Marketing authorisation holder Boehringer Ingelheim International GmbH, D-55216 Ingelheim am Rhein, Germany.

Marketing authorisation number PL 14598/0007

Date of authorisation/renewal of authorisation 31 July 1997

Date of revision of the text June 1998

Legal category POM

MOBIC* 15 mg SUPPOSITORIES 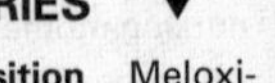

Qualitative and quantitative composition Meloxicam 15.0 mg.

Pharmaceutical form Suppository.

Clinical particulars

Therapeutic indications: Long-term symptomatic treatment of rheumatoid arthritis (chronic polyarthritis).

Symptomatic treatment of ankylosing spondylitis.

Posology and method of administration:

Rheumatoid arthritis: 15 mg/day (one suppository). In elderly patients the recommended dose for long term treatment is 7.5 mg per day. Patients with increased risks for adverse reactions should start treatment with 7.5 mg per day. Mobic suppositories are not suitable for the initiation of treatment.

Ankylosing spondylitis: 15 mg/day (one suppository).

DO NOT EXCEED THE DOSE OF 15 mg/day.

In dialysis patients with severe renal failure the dose should not exceed 7.5 mg per day.

Contra-indications: Hypersensitivity to meloxicam or to one of the excipients. The possibility exists of crossover sensitivity with aspirin and other non-steroidal anti-inflammatory drugs (NSAIDs). Meloxicam should not be given to patients who have developed signs of asthma, nasal polyps, angioneurotic oedema or urticaria following the administration of aspirin or NSAIDs.

- Active peptic ulcer during the last six months or a history of recurrent peptic ulcer disease.
- Severe hepatic failure.
- Non-dialysed severe renal failure.
- Children aged under 15.
- Past history of proctitis or of rectal bleeding.
- Pregnancy (see *Pregnancy and lactation*).
- Lactation.
- Gastrointestinal bleeding, cerebrovascular bleeding or other bleeding disorders.

Special warnings and special precautions for use:

Warnings: As with all NSAIDs, any history of oesophagitis, gastritis and/or peptic ulcer must be sought in order to ensure their total cure before starting treatment with meloxicam. Attention should routinely be paid to the possible onset of a recurrence in patients treated with meloxicam and with a past history of this type.

Patients with gastrointestinal symptoms or history of gastrointestinal disease should be monitored for digestive disturbances, especially for gastrointestinal bleeding.

Gastrointestinal bleeding or ulceration/perforation, have in general more serious consequences in the elderly. They can occur at any time during treatment, with or without warning symptoms or a previous history of serious gastrointestinal events.

In the rare instance where gastrointestinal bleeding or ulceration occurs in patients receiving meloxicam, the drug should be withdrawn.

Withdrawal of treatment with meloxicam must be envisaged in case of onset of cutaneo-mucosal adverse events. The possible occurrence of severe skin reactions and serious life threatening hypersensitivity reactions is known to occur with NSAIDs including oxicams.

In rare instances, NSAIDs may be the cause of interstitial nephritis, glomerulonephritis, renal medullary necrosis or nephrotic syndrome.

As with most NSAIDs, occasional increases in serum transaminase levels, increases in serum bilirubin or other liver function parameters, as well as increases in serum creatinine and blood urea nitrogen as well as other laboratory disturbances, have been reported. The majority of these instances involved transitory and slight abnormalities. Should any such abnormality prove significant or persistent, the administration of meloxicam should be stopped and appropriate investigations prescribed.

Induction of sodium, potassium and water retention and interference with the natriuretic effects of diuretics and consequently possible exacerbations of the condition of patients with cardiac insufficiency or hypertension may occur with NSAIDs.

Precautions: NSAIDs inhibit the synthesis of renal prostaglandins involved in the maintenance of renal perfusion in patients with decreased renal blood flow and blood volume. Administration of NSAIDs in such situations may result in the decompensation of latent renal failure. However renal function returns to its initial status when treatment is withdrawn. This risk concerns all elderly individuals, patients with congestive cardiac failure, cirrhosis of the liver, nephrotic syndrome or renal failure as well as patients on diuretics or having undergone major surgery leading to hypovolaemia. Careful monitoring of urine output and renal function during treatment is necessary in such patients.

Adverse reactions are often less well tolerated in elderly, fragile or weakened individuals, who therefore require careful surveillance. As with other NSAIDs, particular caution is required in the elderly, in whom renal hepatic and cardiac functions are frequently impaired.

The recommended maximum daily dose should not be exceeded in case of insufficient therapeutic effect nor should an additional NSAID be added to the therapy because this may increase the toxicity while therapeutic advantage has not been proven.

Interaction with other medicaments and other forms of interaction:

Inadvisable combinations: Other NSAIDs, including high doses of salicylates: administration of several NSAIDs together may increase the risk of ulcers and of gastrointestinal bleeding, via a synergistic effect.

Oral anticoagulants, heparin and ticlopidine: increased risk of bleeding via inhibition of platelet function and damage to the gastroduodenal mucosa. Careful monitoring of the effects of anticoagulants is thus essential if it proves impossible to avoid such combined prescription.

Lithium: NSAIDs increase blood lithium levels, which may then reach toxic values (decreased renal excretion of lithium). This parameter therefore requires monitoring during the initiation, adjustment and withdrawal of treatment with meloxicam.

Methotrexate: NSAIDs may accentuate the haematologic toxicity of methotrexate. A case of agranulocytosis with meloxicam has been reported in a patient who was also taking methotrexate. The direct causality of meloxicam was not confirmed, but caution is required before prescribing such a combination. Strict monitoring of blood cell count is recommended in this situation.

Intrauterine contraceptive devices: NSAIDs appear to decrease the efficacy of intrauterine contraceptive devices.

Combinations requiring precautions: Diuretics: treatment with NSAIDs is associated with a risk of acute renal failure in dehydrated patients (decreased glomerular filtration via decreased renal prostaglandin synthesis). In case of combined prescription of meloxicam and a diuretic, it is essential to ensure that the patient is adequately hydrated and to monitor renal function at the start of treatment.

Nephrotoxicity of cyclosporin may be enhanced by NSAIDs via renal prostaglandin mediated effects. During combined treatment renal function is to be measured.

Associations needing to be taken into consideration: Antihypertensive drugs [beta-blockers, angiotensin converting enzyme (ACE) inhibitors, diuretics]: treatment with a NSAID may decrease their antihypertensive effect via inhibition of vasodilator prostaglandin synthesis.

Thrombolytics: increased risk of haemorrhage.

Concomitant administration of antacids, cimetidine, β-acetyl digoxin and frusemide has not given rise to any notable pharmacokinetic interactions with meloxicam. Cholestyramine accelerates the elimination of meloxicam via binding in the digestive tract.

Interactions with oral anti-diabetics cannot be excluded.

Pregnancy and lactation:

Pregnancy: In animals, lethal effects on the embryo have been reported at doses far higher than those used clinically.

It is advisable to avoid the administration of meloxicam during pregnancy.

During the final three months, all prostaglandin synthesis inhibitors may expose the foetus to cardiopulmonary (pulmonary hypertension with premature closure of the ductus arteriosus) and renal toxicity or inhibit the contraction of the uterus. This effect on the uterus has been associated with an increase in the incidence of dystocia and delayed parturition in animals.

Thus all NSAIDs are absolutely contra-indicated during the final three months.

Lactation: It is unknown whether meloxicam passes into mothers' milk. Meloxicam should not be given to nursing mothers.

Effects on ability to drive and use machines: There are no specific studies about such effects. However when adverse effects such as vertigo or drowsiness occur it is advisable to refrain from these activities.

Undesirable effects: Digestive system: dyspepsia, nausea, vomiting, abdominal pain, constipation, flatulence, diarrhoea. More rarely, peptic ulcers, perforation or gastrointestinal bleeding, which may be severe, may occur.

Haematologic adverse events: disturbances of blood count, including differential white cell count: anaemia, leukopenia, thrombocytopenia have been described in patients taking meloxicam. Certain cases have been attributed to treatment. Concomitant administration of a potentially myelotoxic drug, in particular methotrexate, appears to be a predisposing factor to the onset of a cytopenia. In particular, a case of agranulocytosis has been described in a patient treated with meloxicam and also taking methotrexate.

Cutaneo-mucosal reactions: stomatitis, oesophagitis, pruritus, skin rash, urticaria, photosensitisation have been reported. Very rare cases of bullous reactions such as erythema multiforme, Stevens-Johnson Syndrome and toxic epidermal necrolysis may develop.

Respiratory system: onset of an asthma attack has been reported in certain individuals allergic to aspirin or to other NSAIDs.

Central nervous system: possibility of lightheadedness, headache, vertigo, tinnitus, drowsiness.

Cardiovascular system: oedema, oedema of the lower limbs, palpitations, flushes may occur during treatment.

Genitourinary system: possibility of disturbances of laboratory tests investigating renal function (e.g. raised serum creatinine or urea).

Transitory disturbances of liver function tests (e.g. raised transaminases or bilirubin).

Overdose: Appropriate measures are required in case of overdose since there is no known antidote. Evidence was found in one clinical trial of acceleration of the elimination of meloxicam by cholestyramine. Severe gastrointestinal lesions may be treated with antacids and H_2 receptor antagonists.

Pharmacological properties

Pharmacodynamic properties: NON-STEROIDAL ANTI-INFLAMMATORY AGENT (M: locomotor system).

Meloxicam is a non-steroidal anti-inflammatory drug (NSAID) of the oxicam family, with anti-inflammatory, analgesic and antipyretic properties.

The anti-inflammatory activity of meloxicam has been proven in classical models of inflammation. As with other NSAIDs, its precise mechanism of action remains unknown. However there is at least one common mode of action shared by all NSAIDs (including meloxicam): inhibition of the biosynthesis of prostaglandins, known inflammation mediators.

Pharmacokinetic properties: Pharmacokinetic studies have involved use of the oral formulation of meloxicam.

Meloxicam suppositories have been shown to be bioequivalent to oral formulations.

The bioavailability of meloxicam following oral administration is on the average 89%.

With the doses of 7.5 and 15 mg plasma concentrations are proportional to dose: 0.4 to 1.0 mg/l for 7.5 mg and 0.8 to 2.0 mg/l for 15 mg, on average (C_{min} and C_{max} at steady state).

Meloxicam is very strongly bound to plasma proteins, essentially albumin (99%).

Meloxicam is extensively metabolised, chiefly by oxidation of the methyl radical attached to the thiazolyl ring. Elimination in unchanged form accounts for 3% of the dose. Half of the substance is eliminated in urine and the other half in faeces.

The mean elimination half-life is of the order of 20 hours.

Steady state is reached in 5 days.

In terminal renal failure, the volume of distribution is increased and a daily dose of 7.5 mg must not be exceeded.

Plasma clearance is on average 8 ml/min. Clearance is decreased in the elderly. Volume of distribution is low, on average 11 l. Interindividual variation is the order of 30–40%.

Preclinical safety data: The toxicological profile of meloxicam has been found in preclinical studies to be identical to that of NSAIDs: gastrointestinal ulcers and erosions, renal papillary necrosis at high doses during chronic administration in two animal species. Non toxic doses were 3 to 10 times higher than clinically used doses, according to animal species used.

Reproduction studies have reported lethal effects on the embryo at doses far higher than those used clinically. Fetotoxic effects at the end of gestation, shared by all prostaglandin synthesis inhibitors, have been described. No evidence has been found of any mutagenic effect, either in vitro or in vivo. No carcinogenic risk has been found in the rat and mouse at doses far higher than those used clinically.

Pharmaceutical particulars

List of excipients: Hard fat (SUPPOCIRE BP); Polyoxyethylenated hydrogenated castor oil (CREMOPHOR RH 40)

Incompatibilities: None stated.

Shelf life: Three years.

Special precautions for storage: Should be stored at a temperature of below 30°C.

Nature and contents of container:

Cartons containing 6 suppositories in aluminium blister sheets.

Cartons containing 7 suppositories in aluminium blister sheets.

Cartons containing 10 suppositories in aluminium blister sheets.

Cartons containing 12 suppositories in aluminium blister sheets.

Cartons containing 20 suppositories in aluminium blister sheets.

Cartons containing 30 suppositories in aluminium blister sheets.

Cartons containing 50 suppositories in aluminium blister sheets.

Cartons containing 60 suppositories in aluminium blister sheets.

Cartons containing 120 suppositories in aluminium blister sheets.

Cartons containing 10×50 suppositories in aluminium blister sheets.

Instructions for use/handling: None stated.

Marketing authorisation holder Boehringer Ingelheim International GmbH, D-55216 Ingelheim am Rhein, Germany.

Marketing authorisation number PL 14598/0001

Date of first authorisation 21 February 1996

Date of revision of the SPC June 1998

Legal category POM

MOTENS* TABLETS 2 mg

Qualitative and quantitative composition Tablets containing lacidipine 2 mg.

Pharmaceutical form Film coated tablets.

Clinical particulars

Therapeutic indications: Motens is indicated for the treatment of hypertension either alone or in combination with other antihypertensive agents, including β-adrenoceptor antagonists, diuretics, and ACE-inhibitors.

Posology and method of administration:

Adults: The treatment of hypertension should be adapted to the severity of the condition, and according to the individual response.

The recommended initial dose is 2 mg once daily. The dose may be increased to 4 mg (and then, if necessary, to 6 mg) after adequate time has been allowed for the full pharmacological effect to occur. In practice, this should not be less than 3 to 4 weeks. Daily doses above 6 mg have not been shown to be significantly more effective.

Motens should be taken at the same time each day, preferably in the morning.

Treatment with Motens may be continued indefinitely.

Patients with kidney disease: As Motens is not cleared by the kidneys, the dose does not require modification in patients with kidney disease.

Use in children: No experience has been gained with Motens in children.

Contra-indications: Motens tablets are contra-indicated in patients with known hypersensitivity to any ingredient of the preparation. Motens should only be used with great care in patients with a previous allergic reaction to another dihydropyridine because there is a theoretical risk of cross-reactivity.

In healthy volunteers, patients and pre-clinical studies, Motens did not inhibit myocardial contractility. As with other calcium antagonists, Motens should be discontinued in patients who develop cardiogenic shock. In addition, dihydropyridines have been shown to reduce coronary arterial blood-flow in patients with aortic stenosis and in such patients Motens is contra-indicated.

Motens should not be used during or within one month of a myocardial infarction.

Special warnings and precautions for use: In specialised studies Motens has been shown neither to affect the spontaneous function of the sinoatrial (SA) node nor to cause prolonged conduction within the atrioventricular (AV) node. However, the theoretical potential for a calcium antagonist to affect the activity of the SA and AV nodes should be noted, and care should be taken in patients with pre-existing abnormalities.

There is no evidence that Motens is useful for secondary prevention of myocardial infarction.

Motens should be used with caution in patients with poor cardiac reserve.

The efficacy and safety of Motens in the treatment of malignant hypertension has not been established.

Caution should be exercised in patients with hepatic impairment because the antihypertensive effect may be increased.

There is no evidence that Motens impairs glucose tolerance or alters diabetic control.

Interaction with other medicaments and other forms of interaction: Concomitant administration of Motens with other antihypertensive agents e.g. diuretics, β-adrenoceptor antagonists or ACE-inhibitors may have an additive hypotensive effect.

The plasma concentration of Motens may be increased by simultaneous administration of cimetidine.

As with other dihydropyridines, Motens should not be taken with grapefruit juice as bioavailability may be altered.

Motens is highly protein-bound (>95%) to albumin and α_1-acid glycoprotein. No specific pharmacodynamic interaction problems have been identified in studies with common antihypertensive agents e.g. β-adrenoceptor antagonists and diuretics, or with digoxin, tolbutamide or warfarin.

Pregnancy and lactation: Although some dihydropyridine compounds have been found to be teratogenic in animals, data in the rat and rabbit for Motens provide no evidence of a teratogenic effect. Using doses far above the therapeutic range, in animals Motens shows evidence of maternal toxicity resulting in increased pre- and post-implantation losses and possibly delayed ossification. There is, however, no clinical experience of Motens in pregnancy and lactation. Accordingly, Motens should not be used during pregnancy or lactation.

Effects on ability to drive and use machines: None reported.

Undesirable effects: Motens is generally well tolerated. Some individuals may experience minor side effects which are related to its known pharmacological action of peripheral vasodilation. The most common of these are headache, flushing, oedema, dizziness and palpitations. Such effects are usually transient and usually disappear with continued administration of Motens at the same dosage.

Asthenia, skin rash (including erythema and itching), gastric upset, nausea, gingival hyperplasia, polyuria muscle cramps and disturbances of mood have also been reported rarely.

As with other dihydropyridines aggravation of underlying angina has been reported in a small number of individuals, especially after the start of treatment. This is more likely to happen in patients with symptomatic ischaemic heart disease. Motens should be discontinued under medical supervision in patients who develop unstable angina.

Transient and reversible increases in alkaline phosphatase have been noted on rare occasions.

Overdose

Symptoms: There have been no recorded cases of Motens overdosage. The expected symptoms could comprise prolonged peripheral vasodilation associated with hypotension and tachycardia. Bradycardia or prolonged AV conduction could occur.

Therapy: Symptomatic treatment is warranted. There is no specific antidote.

Pharmacological properties

Pharmacodynamic properties: Motens is a specific and potent calcium antagonist with a predominant selectivity for calcium channels in the vascular smooth muscle. Its main action is to dilate peripheral arterioles, reducing peripheral vascular resistance and lowering blood pressure.

In a study of ten patients with a renal transplant, Motens has been shown to prevent an acute decrease in renal plasma flow and glomerular filtration rate about six hours after administering oral cyclosporin. During the trough phase of cyclosporin treatment, there was no difference in renal plasma flow and glomerular filtration rate between patients with or without Motens.

Pharmacokinetic properties: Motens is a highly lipophilic compound; it is rapidly absorbed from the gastrointestinal tract following oral dosing. Absolute bioavailability averages about 10% due to extensive first-pass metabolism in the liver.

Peak plasma concentrations are reached between 30 and 150 minutes. The drug is eliminated primarily by hepatic metabolism. There is no evidence that Motens causes either induction or inhibition of hepatic enzymes.

The principal metabolites possess little, if any, pharmacodynamic activity.

Approximately 70% of the administered dose is eliminated as metabolites in the faeces and the remainder as metabolites in the urine.

The average terminal half-life of Motens ranges from between 13 and 19 hours at steady state.

Preclinical safety data: In acute toxicity studies, Motens has shown a wide safety margin.

In repeated dose toxicological studies, findings in animals, related to the safety profile of Motens in man, were reversible and reflected the pharmacodynamic effect of Motens.

No data of clinical relevance have been gained from *in vivo* and *in vitro* studies on reproduction toxicity, genetic toxicity or oncogenicity.

Pharmaceutical particulars

List of excipients

Tablet core: Lactose (monohydrate); lactose (spray-dried); povidone K30; magnesium stearate.

Film coating: Titanium dioxide (E171), methylhydroxypropylcellulose.

Incompatibilities: None known.

Shelf life: 24 months.

Special precautions for storage: Store below 30°C. Motens is light sensitive. Motens tablets should, therefore, be protected from light and should not be removed from their foil pack until required for administration.

Keep out of the reach of children.

Nature and contents of container: Cartons containing 7, 14 and 28 tablets packed in blister strips.

[The 7 tablet pack is not currently marketed.]

Instructions for use/handling: Do not remove from foil pack until required for administration.

Marketing authorisation number PL 0015/0188

Date of first authorisation 29 April 1993

Date of revision of the text January 1998

Legal category POM

MOTENS* TABLETS 4 mg

Qualitative and quantitative composition Tablets containing lacidipine 4 mg.

Pharmaceutical form Film coated tablets.

Clinical particulars

Therapeutic indications: Motens is indicated for the treatment of hypertension either alone or in combination with other antihypertensive agents, including β-adrenoceptor antagonists, diuretics, and ACE-inhibitors.

Posology and method of administration:

Adults: The treatment of hypertension should be adapted to the severity of the condition, and according to the individual response.

The recommended initial dose is 2 mg once daily. The dose may be increased to 4 mg (and then, if necessary, to 6 mg) after adequate time has been allowed for the full pharmacological effect to occur. In practice, this should not be less than 3 to 4 weeks. Daily doses above 6 mg have not been shown to be significantly more effective.

Motens should be taken at the same time each day, preferably in the morning.

Treatment with Motens may be continued indefinitely.

Patients with kidney disease: As Motens is not cleared by the kidneys, the dose does not require modification in patients with kidney disease.

Use in children: No experience has been gained with Motens in children.

Contra-indications: Motens tablets are contra-indicated in patients with known hypersensitivity to any ingredient of the preparation. Motens should only be used with great care in patients with a previous allergic reaction to another dihydropyridine because there is a theoretical risk of cross-reactivity.

In healthy volunteers, patients and pre-clinical studies, Motens did not inhibit myocardial contractility. As with other calcium antagonists, Motens should be discontinued in patients who develop cardiogenic shock. In addition, dihydropyridines have been shown to reduce coronary arterial blood-flow in patients with aortic stenosis and in such patients Motens is contra-indicated.

Motens should not be used during or within one month of a myocardial infarction.

Special warnings and precautions for use: In specialised studies Motens has been shown neither to affect the spontaneous function of the sinoatrial (SA) node nor to cause prolonged conduction within the atrioventricular (AV) node. However, the theoretical potential for a calcium antagonist to affect the activity of the SA and AV nodes should be noted, and care should be taken in patients with pre-existing abnormalities.

There is no evidence that Motens is useful for secondary prevention of myocardial infarction.

Motens should be used with caution in patients with poor cardiac reserve.

The efficacy and safety of Motens in the treatment of malignant hypertension has not been established.

Caution should be exercised in patients with hepatic impairment because the antihypertensive effect may be increased.

There is no evidence that Motens impairs glucose tolerance or alters diabetic control.

Interaction with other medicaments and other forms of interaction: Concomitant administration of Motens with other antihypertensive agents e.g. diuretics, β-adrenoceptor antagonists or ACE-inhibitors may have an additive hypotensive effect.

The plasma concentration of Motens may be increased by simultaneous administration of cimetidine.

As with other dihydropyridines, Motens should not be taken with grapefruit juice as bioavailability may be altered.

Motens is highly protein-bound (>95%) to albumin and α_1-acid glycoprotein. No specific pharmacodynamic interaction problems have been identified in studies with common antihypertensive agents e.g. β-adrenoceptor antagonists and diuretics, or with digoxin, tolbutamide or warfarin.

Pregnancy and lactation: Although some dihydropyridine compounds have been found to be teratogenic in animals, data in the rat and rabbit for Motens provide no evidence of a teratogenic effect. Using doses far above the therapeutic range, in animals Motens shows evidence of maternal toxicity resulting in increased pre- and post-implantation losses and possibly delayed ossification. There is, however, no clinical experience of Motens in pregnancy and lactation. Accordingly, Motens should not be used during pregnancy or lactation.

Effects on ability to drive and use machines: None reported.

Undesirable effects: Motens is generally well tolerated. Some individuals may experience minor side effects which are related to its known pharmacological action of peripheral vasodilation. The most common of these are headache, flushing, oedema, dizziness and palpitations. Such effects are usually transient and usually disappear with continued administration of Motens at the same dosage.

Asthenia, skin rash (including erythema and itching), gastric upset, nausea, gingival hyperplasia, polyuria, muscle cramps and disturbances of mood have also been reported rarely.

As with other dihydropyridines aggravation of underlying angina has been reported in a small number of individuals, especially after the start of treatment. This is more likely to happen in patients with symptomatic ischaemic heart disease. Motens should be discontinued under medical supervision in patients who develop unstable angina.

Transient and reversible increases in alkaline phosphatase have been noted on rare occasions.

Overdose

Symptoms: There have been no recorded cases of Motens overdosage. The expected symptoms could comprise prolonged peripheral vasodilation associated with hypotension and tachycardia. Bradycardia or prolonged AV conduction could occur.

Therapy: Symptomatic treatment is warranted. There is no specific antidote.

Pharmacological properties

Pharmacodynamic properties: Motens is a specific and potent calcium antagonist with a predominant selectivity for calcium channels in the vascular smooth muscle. Its main action is to dilate peripheral arterioles, reducing peripheral vascular resistance and lowering blood pressure.

In a study of ten patients with a renal transplant, Motens has been shown to prevent an acute decrease in renal plasma flow and glomerular filtration rate about six hours after administering oral cyclosporin. During the trough phase of cyclosporin treatment, there was no difference in renal plasma flow and glomerular filtration rate between patients with or without Motens.

Pharmacokinetic properties: Motens is a highly lipophilic compound; it is rapidly absorbed from the gastrointestinal tract following oral dosing. Absolute bioavailability averages about 10% due to extensive first-pass metabolism in the liver.

Peak plasma concentrations are reached between 30 and 150 minutes. The drug is eliminated primarily by hepatic metabolism. There is no evidence that Motens causes either induction or inhibition of hepatic enzymes.

The principal metabolites possess little, if any, pharmacodynamic activity.

Approximately 70% of the administered dose is eliminated as metabolites in the faeces and the remainder as metabolites in the urine.

The average terminal half-life of Motens ranges from between 13 and 19 hours at steady state.

Preclinical safety data: In acute toxicity studies, Motens has shown a wide safety margin.

In repeated dose toxicological studies, findings in animals, related to the safety profile of Motens in man, were reversible and reflected the pharmacodynamic effect of Motens.

No data of clinical relevance have been gained from *in vivo* and *in vitro* studies on reproduction toxicity, genetic toxicity or oncogenicity.

Pharmaceutical particulars

List of excipients

Tablet core: Lactose (monohydrate); lactose (spray-dried); povidone K30; magnesium stearate.

Film coating: Titanium dioxide (E171), methylhydroxypropylcellulose.

Incompatibilities: None known.

Shelf life: 24 months.

Special precautions for storage: Store below 30°C. Motens is light sensitive. Motens tablets should, therefore, be protected from light and should not be removed from their foil pack until required for administration.

Keep out of the reach of children.

Nature and contents of container: Cartons containing 7, 14 and 28 tablets packed in blister strips.

[The 7 tablet pack is not currently marketed.]

Instructions for use/handling: Do not remove from foil pack until required for administration.

Marketing authorisation number PL 0015/0189

Date of first authorisation 29 April 1993

Date of revision of the text January 1998

Legal category POM

OXIVENT* INHALER

Qualitative and quantitative composition Each actuation delivers 100 micrograms of oxitropium bromide.

Pharmaceutical form Pressurised metered aerosol.

Clinical particulars

Therapeutic indications: For the management of airways obstruction in patients suffering from chronic stable asthma and chronic obstructive pulmonary disease.

Posology and method of administration: For administration by inhalation only.

Adults: Two puffs, two or three times daily.

Children: Oxivent has not been evaluated in children.

Elderly patients: There are no special dosage requirements for the elderly.

All patients should be instructed in the correct use of a metered dose inhaler.

Contra-indications: Oxivent Inhaler is contraindicated in patients with a history of hypersensitivity to soya lecithin or related food products such as soya beans or peanuts.

Oxivent Inhaler should not be taken by patients who have known hypersensitivity to atropine or its derivatives, or to any other component of the product.

Special warnings and special precautions for use: Symptoms of aerosol-induced bronchospasm including wheeze, cough and chest tightness, have been reported following the use of Oxivent. If patients report respiratory symptoms associated with the use of the inhaler, treatment should be discontinued.

The patient should be warned to seek medical advice should a reduced response become apparent. In the case of acute or rapidly worsening dyspnoea (difficulty in breathing) a doctor should be consulted immediately.

Oxivent should be prevented from coming into contact with the eye. Accidental release of Oxivent into the eye should be avoided, as there have been isolated reports of ocular complications (such as mydriasis, increased intraocular pressure, narrow-angle glaucoma and eye pain) following unintended exposure of the eye to anticholinergics.

Eye pain or discomfort, blurred vision, visual halos or coloured images in association with red eyes from conjunctival and corneal congestion may be signs of acute narrow-angle glaucoma. Should any combination of these symptoms develop, treatment with miotic drops should be initiated and specialist advice sought immediately.

Patients therefore should be instructed in the correct administration of Oxivent Inhaler. Antiglaucoma therapy is also effective in the prevention of acute narrow-angle glaucoma in susceptible individuals.

As patients with cystic fibrosis may be prone to gastro-intestinal motility disturbances, Oxivent as with other anticholinergics should be used with caution in these patients.

Caution is advocated in patients with narrow-angle glaucoma or those with prostatic hypertrophy.

Interaction with other medicaments and other forms of interaction: Oxivent has been administered in conjunction with sympathomimetic bronchodilators, xanthines, steroids and sodium cromoglycate with no evidence of adverse interaction. There is evidence that the administration of Oxivent with beta$_2$-agonist drugs and xanthine preparations may intensify the bronchodilator effect of Oxivent.

Oxivent has been shown to prevent and reverse propranolol-induced bronchoconstriction in patients with reversible airways obstruction.

Pregnancy and lactation: The safety of this product for use in human pregnancy has not been established. Animal studies have shown reproductive toxicity with high doses of oxitropium.

Oxivent should not therefore be used during pregnancy, particularly the first trimester, unless the expected benefit is thought to outweigh any risk to the foetus.

Animal studies have shown that oxitropium bromide can be secreted in mother's milk. It is unlikely that the drug would reach the infant to any great extent, but caution should be exercised by nursing mothers.

Effects on ability to drive and use machines: None known.

Undesirable effects: The most frequent non-respiratory adverse reactions reported in clinical trials were headache, nausea and dryness of the mouth.

Anticholinergic side effects such as tachycardia, palpitations, visual accommodation disturbances, gastro-intestinal motility disturbances and urinary retention have been reported. The risk of urinary retention may be increased in patients with pre-existing urinary outflow obstruction.

Ocular side effects have been reported (see: *Special warnings and special precautions for use*).

As with other inhaled bronchodilator therapy, cough and paradoxical bronchoconstriction may occur. Cases of unpleasant taste have been reported. Local irritation of the oropharynx may occur.

Allergic type reactions cannot be excluded.

Overdose: No symptoms specific to overdosage have been encountered. The poor absorption of Oxivent, and limited experience of the outcome of overdose with the product in clinical use, suggest that serious anticholinergic symptoms are unlikely. As seen with other anticholinergics, dry mouth, visual accommodation disturbances, tachycardia and urinary retention may occur.

Pharmacological properties

Pharmacodynamic properties: Oxitropium bromide is an anticholinergic bronchodilator that competitively antagonises the effects of acetylcholine at muscarinic receptors. When administered by inhalation, it produces only local effects on the lung due to its poor absorption through the lungs and gastrointestinal tract.

Pharmacokinetic properties: Studies in man have shown that, following oral administration (20 mg), peak plasma levels were not reached for 3 hours (36.5 ng/ml). At 96 hours, 12.6% was excreted by the kidneys and 77% in the faeces. The decline of the plasma level showed a biphasic course. Absorption after oral administration was calculated to be 16.2%. Following inhalation 10.4% was eliminated by the kidneys and 87.9% in the faeces. The absorption after inhalation was 15.4% of the dose.

Pharmaceutical particulars

List of excipients:

- Soya lecithin
- Monofluorotrichloromethane
- Difluorodichloromethane
- Tetrafluorodichloroethane

Incompatibilities: None stated.

Shelf life: 3 years.

Special precautions for storage: Protect from heat, including the sun. The vials should not be punctured or incinerated even when apparently empty. Protect from frost.

Nature and contents of container: A one piece aluminium vial fitted with a 50 microlitre metering valve and containing 10 ml (200 doses) of a cream-coloured suspension, complete with mouth piece.

Instructions for use/handling:

To make sure that your inhaler is working, test fire it twice into the air before using it for the first time and whenever your inhaler has not been used for a week or more.

1. Remove the dustcap from the mouthpiece and **shake the inhaler vigorously.**
2. Holding the inhaler as shown, breathe out gently and then immediately . . .
3. . . . place the mouthpiece in the mouth and close your lips around it. After starting to breathe in slowly and deeply, through your mouth, press the inhaler firmly as shown to release the Oxivent. *Continue to breathe in as deeply as you can.*
4. Hold your breath for 10 seconds, or as long as is comfortable, before breathing out slowly.
5. If you are to take more than one puff you should wait at least one minute before shaking the inhaler again and repeating steps 2, 3 and 4.
6. After use, replace the dustcap on the mouthpiece.
7. Follow the instructions for how to clean and care for the inhaler.

As the container is not transparent it is not possible to see when the contents are used up, but shaking the container will show is there is any remaining fluid.

Marketing authorisation number PL 0015/0142

Date of renewal of authorisation 09.01.96

Date of revision of the text May 1998

Legal category POM.

OXIVENT* AUTOHALER*

Qualitative and quantitative composition Each actuation delivers 100 micrograms of oxitropium bromide.

Pharmaceutical form A breath-actuated pressurised metered aerosol for inhalation therapy.

Clinical particulars

Therapeutic indications: For the management of airways obstruction in patients suffering from chronic stable asthma and chronic obstructive pulmonary disease.

Posology and method of administration: For administration by inhalation only.

Adults: Two puffs, two or three times daily.

Children: Oxivent has not been evaluated in children.

Elderly patients: There are no special dosage requirements for the elderly.

All patients should be instructed in the correct use of the Autohaler device.

Contra-indications: Oxivent Autohaler is contraindicated in patients with a history of hypersensitivity to soya lecithin or related food products such as soya beans or peanuts.

Oxivent Autohaler should not be taken by patients who have known hypersensitivity to atropine or its derivatives, or to any other component of the product.

Special warnings and special precautions for use: Symptoms of aerosol-induced bronchospasm including wheeze, cough and chest tightness, have been reported following the use of Oxivent. If patients report respiratory symptoms associated with the use of the inhaler, treatment should be discontinued.

The patient should be warned to seek medical advice should a reduced response become apparent. In the case of acute or rapidly worsening dyspnoea (difficulty in breathing) a doctor should be consulted immediately.

Oxivent should be prevented from coming into

contact with the eye. It is unlikely that correct use of the Oxivent Autohaler would result in accidental release of Oxivent into the eye, however, there have been isolated reports of ocular complications (such as mydriasis, increased intraocular pressure, narrow-angle glaucoma and eye pain) following unintended exposure of the eye to anticholinergics.

Eye pain or discomfort, blurred vision, visual halos or coloured images in association with red eyes from conjunctival and corneal congestion may be signs of acute narrow-angle glaucoma.Should any combination of these symptoms develop, treatment with miotic drops should be initated and specialist advice sought immediately.

Patients therefore should be instructed in the correct administration of Oxivent Autohaler. Antiglaucoma therapy is also effective in the prevention of acute narrow-angle glaucoma in susceptible individuals.

As patients with cystic fibrosis may be prone to gastro-intestinal motility disturbances, Oxivent as with other anticholinergics should be used with caution in these patients.

Caution is advocated in patients with narrow-angle glaucoma or those with prostatic hypertrophy.

Interaction with other medicaments and other forms of interaction: Oxivent had been administered in conjunction with sympathomimetic bronchodilators, xanthines, steroids and sodium cromoglycate with no evidence of adverse interaction. There is evidence that the administration of Oxivent with beta$_2$-agonist drugs and xanthine preparations may intensify the bronchodilator effect of Oxivent.

Oxivent has been shown to prevent and reverse propranolol-induced bronchoconstriction in patients with reversible airways obstruction.

Pregnancy and lactation: The safety of this product for use in human pregnancy has not been established. Animal studies have shown reproductive toxicity with high doses of oxitropium. Oxivent should not therefore be used during pregnancy, particularly the first trimester, unless the expected benefit is thought to outweigh any risk to the foetus.

Animal studies have shown that oxitropium bromide can be secreted in mother's milk. It is unlikely that the drug would reach the infant to any great extent, but caution should be exercised by nursing mothers.

Effects on ability to drive and use machines: None known.

Undesirable effects: The most frequent non-respiratory adverse reactions reported in clinical trials were headache, nausea and dryness of the mouth.

Anticholinergic side effects such as tachycardia, palpitations, visual accommodation disturbances, gastro-intestinal motility disturbances and urinary retention have been reported. The risk of urinary retention may be increased in patients with pre-existing urinary outflow obstruction.

Ocular side effects have been reported (see *Special warnings and special precautions for use*).

As with other inhaled bronchodilator therapy, cough and paradoxical bronchoconstriction may occur. Cases of unpleasant taste have been reported. Local irritation of the oropharynx may occur.

Allergic type reactions cannot be excluded.

Overdose: No symptoms specific to overdosage have been encountered. The poor absorption of Oxivent, and limited experience of the outcome of overdose with the product in clinical use, suggest that serious anticholinergic symptoms are unlikely.

As seen with other anticholinergics, dry mouth, visual accommodation disturbances, tachycardia and urinary retention may occur.

Pharmacological properties
Pharmacodynamic properties: Oxitropium bromide is an anticholinergic bronchodilator that competitively antagonises the effects of acetylcholine at muscarinic receptors. When administered by inhalation, it produces only local effects on the lung due to its poor absorption through the lungs and gastrointestinal tract.

Pharmacokinetic properties: Studies in man have shown that, following oral administration (20 mg), peak plasma levels were not reached for 3 hours (36.5 ng/ml). At 96 hours, 12.6% was excreted by the kidneys and 77% in the faeces. The decline of the plasma level showed a biphasic course. Absorption after oral administration was calculated to be 16.2%. Following inhalation 10.4% was eliminated by the kidneys and 87.9% in the faeces. The absorption after inhalation was 15.4% of the dose.

Pharmaceutical particulars
List of excipients:
- Soya lecithin
- Monofluorotrichloromethane
- Difluorodichloromethane
- Tetrafluorodichloroethane

Incompatibilities: None stated.

Shelf life: 3 years.

Special precautions for storage: Protect from heat, including the sun. The vials should not be punctured or incinerated even when apparently empty. Protect from frost.

Nature and contents of container: A one piece aluminium vial fitted with a 50 mcl metering valve and containing 10 ml (200 doses) of a cream-coloured suspension, in a breath-actuated device.

Instructions for use/handling:
1. To remove the mouthpiece cover, pull down on the lip at the back.
2. Hold the Autohaler device upright as shown. Push the lever up so that it stays up.
3. With the lever still up, shake the Autohaler device.
4. Continue to hold the Autohaler device upright, making sure that your hand is not blocking the air vents at the bottom. Breathe out normally and close your lips firmly around the mouthpiece.
5. Breathe in through the mouthpiece. When you hear the slight click, continue to breathe in.

This click lets you know you have received your puff of medication. Hold your breath for 10 seconds, or as long as is comfortable, and then breathe out normally.

6. The lever must be lowered after each puff. If your doctor has prescribed more than one puff, wait one minute before repeating steps 2–6. Replace the mouthpiece cover after use.
7. Follow the instructions for how to clean and care for the Autohaler device.

As the container is not transparent it is not possible to see when the contents are used up, but shaking the container will show if there is any remaining fluid.

Marketing authorisation number 0015/0163

Date of authorisation/renewal of authorisation 30.08.91

Date of revision of SPC May 1998

Legal category POM

PAVACOL-D*

Qualitative and quantitative composition Dark brown liquid containing 5 mg of Pholcodine BP in each 5 ml.

Pharmaceutical form Liquid for oral administration.

Clinical particulars
Therapeutic indications: For the symptomatic treatment of dry troublesome coughs.

Posology and method of administration:
Adults: One or two 5 ml spoonfuls as required. The dose may be increased to three 5 ml spoonfuls if necessary. No more than 60 ml should be taken in 24 hours.

Children:
6 to 12 years: One 5 ml spoonful four or five times daily.
3 to 5 years: One 5 ml spoonful three times daily.
1 to 2 years: Half a 5 ml spoonful three or four times daily.

Pavacol-D may be diluted with Sorbitol Solution BPC.

No specific information on the use of this product in the elderly is available. Clinical trials have included patients over 65 years and no adverse reactions specific to this age group have been reported.

Contra-indications: Hypersensitivity to any of the ingredients, or liver disease.

Special warnings and special precautions for use: Cough suppressants may cause sputum retention and this may be harmful in patients with chronic bronchitis and bronchiectasis. If symptoms persist longer than 5 days a physician should be consulted.

Interaction with other medicaments and other forms of interaction: Alcohol or other CNS depressants may lead to greater drowsiness and sedation.

Pregnancy and lactation: Although Pavacol-D has been in general use for many years, there is no evidence of ill-consequence during human pregnancy.

Medicines should not be used in pregnancy, especially the first trimester, unless the expected benefit is thought to outweigh any possible risk to the foetus.

Effect on ability to drive and use machines: Drowsiness occurs occasionally after taking pholcodine.

Undesirable effects: Nausea, sputum retention and constipation occur occasionally after taking pholcodine.

Overdose: Symptoms of overdosage include nausea, drowsiness, restlessness, excitement, ataxia and respiratory depression.

Treatment consists of emptying the stomach by aspiration and lavage. In case of severe poisoning the specific narcotic antagonist nalaxone may be used. Otherwise, treatment is supportive and symptomatic.

Pharmacological properties
Pharmacodynamic properties: Pholcodine is a specific anti-tussive lacking the unwanted side-effects of opium and its derivatives. The specificity of action suggests that pholcodine acts via a distinct subset of opioid receptors.

Pharmacokinetic properties: In a study of male volunteers receiving 15, 30 and 60 mg doses of pholcodine at 7 day intervals, pharmacokinetics were found to be independent of dose. The elimination of pholcodine is described by a two-compartment model with an elimination half-life of 37±4.2 hours. Pholcodine undergoes little conjugation and is not transformed to morphine.

Pharmaceutical particulars
List of excipients: Tolu balsam solution; N.I. special flavour; ethanol 96%; anise oil; clove oil; peppermint oil; capsicum tincture; strong ginger tincture; sorbitol solution; saccharin sodium; hydroxyethylcellulose; treacle flavour; caramel; L-menthol; methyl paraben; propyl paraben; deionised water.

Incompatibilities: None stated.

Shelf life: The shelf life expiry date for Pavacol-D is 3 years from the date of its manufacture.

When Pavacol-D is diluted an in-use shelf life of 14 days is recommended.

Special precautions for storage: Store below 25°C. Protect from light.

Nature and contents of container: 300 ml round amber glass bottle (Type III glass) with an aluminium roll-on pilfer proof cap.

Instructions for use/handling: None stated.

Marketing authorisation number 00015/0207

Date of renewal of authorisation 29 April 1996

Date of approval/revision of SPC February 1996

Legal category P

PERSANTIN*

Presentation Persantin Tablets 25 mg: orange sugar-coated tablets containing dipyridamole 25 mg.

Persantin Tablets 100 mg: white sugar-coated tablets containing dipyridamole 100 mg.

Uses
Action: Dipyridamole has an antithrombotic action based on its ability to modify various aspects of platelet function, such as platelet aggregation, adhesion and survival, which have been shown to be factors associated with the initiation of thrombus formation.

Indications: An adjunct to oral anticoagulation for prophylaxis of thromboembolism associated with prosthetic heart valves.

Dosage and administration
Adults: 300-600 mg daily in three or four doses.

Children: The normal total oral daily dose is 5 mg/kg in divided doses.

Persantin should usually be taken before meals.

Contra-indications, warnings, etc
Contra-indications: There are no absolute contra-indications to the administration of Persantin.

Precautions: Persantin is a potent vasodilator and should therefore be used with caution in patients with rapidly worsening angina, subvalvular aortic stenosis or haemodynamic instability associated with a recently sustained myocardial infarction.

There is inadequate evidence of safety in human pregnancy but Persantin has been used for many years without apparent ill-consequence. Animal studies have shown no hazards. Medicines should not be used in pregnancy, especially the first trimester, unless the expected benefit is thought to outweigh any possible risk to the foetus.

The concurrent administration of antacids may reduce the efficacy of Persantin.

It is possible that Persantin may enhance the effects of oral anticoagulants.

Persantin should be used with caution in patients with coagulation disorders.

Side-effects: If these occur it is usually during the early part of treatment and they are often dose-related. The vasodilating properties of Persantin may occasionally produce a vascular headache which normally disappears with dosage reduction. Dizziness, faintness, dyspepsia, mild diarrhoea and rash have also been reported occasionally.

Overdosage: Overdosage may lead to headache, gastro-intestinal symptoms and hypotension. Coronary vasodilatation may cause chest pain in patients with ischaemic heart disease. General supportive measures should be employed. Coronary vasodilatation may be reversed by administering aminophylline by slow IV injection, whilst monitoring the ECG.

Pharmaceutical precautions Protect from heat, light and moisture.

Legal category POM.

Package quantities Blister packs of 84 (OP)

Further information There is evidence that the effects of aspirin and dipyridamole on platelet behaviour are synergistic.

Product licence numbers
Persantin Tablets 25 mg 0015/0052R
Persantin Tablets 100 mg 0015/5016R

PERSANTIN* AMPOULES

Qualitative and quantitative composition 2 ml ampoules containing a clear, yellow coloured, sterile solution. Each ampoule contains 10 mg of Dipyridamole BP in 2 ml.

Pharmaceutical form Injection for slow intravenous infusion.

Clinical particulars
Therapeutic indications: As an alternative to exercise stress in thallium-201 myocardial imaging, particularly in patients unable to exercise or in those for whom exercise may be contra-indicated.

Posology and method of administration: 0.56 mg/kg injected intravenously over 4 minutes. The injection of thallium-201 should be given from 1–2 minutes after completion of the dipyridamole injection.

Contra-indications: Known hypersensitivity to dipyridamole. Subvalvular aortic stenosis, aortic disease, hypotension associated with a recently sustained myocardial infarction, significant valvular disease, or uncompensated congestive heart failure. Patients with known cardiac conduction defects or dysrhythmias.

Special warnings and special precautions for use: The product should be administered with care in unstable angina. As with exercise stress, dipyridamole-thallium scanning should be performed with continuous monitoring of the patients ECG.

Interaction with other medicaments and other forms of interaction: Concurrent administration of other vasodilators may cause a severe hypotensive effect.

Pregnancy and lactation: There is inadequate evidence of safety in human pregnancy, but dipyridamole has been used for many years without apparent ill-consequence.

Effect on ability to drive and use machines: None stated.

Undesirable effects: Some patients may experience chest pain or a worsening of their angina. Transient headache, dizziness, facial flushing, faintness and nausea are common side-effects. A bitter taste has been experienced after i.v. injection.

Overdose: Adverse effects may usually be reversed with intravenous aminophylline.

Pharmacological properties
Pharmacodynamic properties: Dipyridamole has two main actions:
1. Coronary vasodilator.
2. Inhibitor of platelet aggregation and adhesion.

Pharmacokinetic properties
Distribution: Does not cross blood brain barrier; very small placental transfer; $\frac{1}{17}$ of plasma concentration detectable in breast milk.
Protein binding: 97–99% Protein bound mainly to alpha 1-acid glycoprotein.
Metabolism: Mainly in liver to a monoglucuronide.
Excretion: 95% of i.v. injection excreted via bile into faeces.

Pharmaceutical particulars
List of excipients: Tartaric acid, Polyethylene glycol 600, Hydrochloric acid, Water for injections.

Incompatibilities: None stated.

Shelf life: 3 years.

Special precautions for storage: Protect from light.

Nature and contents of container: Cartons containing 5×2 ml clear glass (Type I) ampoules.

Instructions for use/handling: None stated.

Marketing authorisation number PL 0015/0119

Date of first authorisation/renewal of authorisation 23.04.92.

Date of (partial) revision of the text December 1997.

Legal category POM.

PERSANTIN* RETARD 200 mg

Qualitative and quantitative composition Each modified release capsule contains dipyridamole 200 mg.

Pharmaceutical form Modified release capsule.

Clinical particulars
Therepeutic indications: Secondary prevention of ischaemic stroke and transient ischaemic attacks either alone or in conjunction with aspirin.

An adjunct to oral anti-coagulation for prophylaxis of thromboembolism associated with prosthetic heart valves.

Posology and method of administration: For oral administration.

Adults, including the elderly: The recommended dose is one capsule twice daily, usually one in the morning and one in the evening preferably with meals.

The capsules should be swallowed whole without chewing.

Children: Persantin Retard 200 mg is not recommended for children.

Contra-indications: Hypersensitivity to any component of the product.

Special warnings and special precautions for use: Among other properties dipyridamole acts as a potent vasodilator. It should therefore be used in caution in patients with severe coronary artery disease (e.g. unstable angina or recently sustained myocardial infarction), subvalvular aortic stenosis or haemodynamic instability (e.g. decompensated heart failure).

In patients with myasthenia gravis readjustment of therapy may be necessary after changes in dipyridamole dosage (see *Interactions*).

Persantin should be used in caution in patients with coagulation disorders.

Interaction with other medicaments and other forms of interaction: Dipyridamole increases the plasma levels and cardiovascular effects of adenosine. Adjustment of adenosine dosage should therefore be considered if use with dipyridamole is unavoidable.

There is evidence that the effects of aspirin and dipyridamole on platelet behaviour are additive.

When dipyridamole is used in combination with anticoagulants and aspirin, the statements on intolerance and risks for these preparations must be observed. Addition of dipyridamole to aspirin does not increase the incidence of bleeding events. When dipyridamole was administered concomitantly with warfarin, bleeding was no greater in frequency or severity than that observed when warfarin was administered alone.

Dipyridamole may increase the hypotensive effect of blood pressure lowering drugs and may counteract the anticholinesterase effect of cholinesterase inhibitors thereby potentially aggravating myasthenia gravis.

Pregnancy and lactation: There is inadequate evidence of safety in human pregnancy, but dipyridamole has been used for many years without apparent ill-consequence. Animal studies have shown no hazard. Nevertheless, medicines should not be used in pregnancy, especially the first trimester unless the expected benefit is thought to outweigh the possible risk to the foetus.

Persantin Retard 200 mg should only be used during lactation if considered essential by the physician.

Effects on ability to drive and use machines: None stated.

Undesirable effects: Adverse reactions at therapeutic doses are usually mild. Vomiting, diarrhoea and symptoms such as dizziness, nausea, dyspepsia, headache and myalgia have been observed. These tend to occur early after initiating treatment and may disappear with continued treatment. As side effects may be dose related dose reduction may need to be considered.

As a result of its vasodilating properties, Persantin Retard 200 mg may cause hypotension, hot flushes and tachycardia. In rare cases, worsening of the symptoms of coronary heart disease has been observed.

Hypersensitivity reactions such as rash and urticaria have been reported. In very rare cases, increased bleeding during or after surgery has been observed.

Overdose: Due to the low number of observations, experience with dipyridamole overdose is limited. Symptoms such as feeling warm, flushes, sweating, accelerated pulse, restlessness, feeling of weakness, dizziness, drop in blood pressure and anginal complaints can be expected.

Symptomatic therapy is recommended. Administration of xanthine derivatives (e.g. aminophylline) may reverse the haemodynamic effects of dipyridamole overdose. ECG monitoring is advised in such a situation. Due to its wide distribution to tissues and its predominantly hepatic elimination, dipyridamole is not likely to be accessible to enhanced removal procedures.

Pharmacological properties
Pharmacodynamic properties: The antithrombotic action of dipyridamole is based on its ability to modify various aspects of platelet function such as inhibition of platelet adhesion and aggregation, which have been shown to be factors associated with the initiation of thrombus formation, as well as lengthening shortened platelet survival time.

Pharmacokinetic properties: Persantin Retard 200 mg given twice daily has been shown to be bioequivalent to the same total daily dose of Persantin Tablets given in four divided doses.

Peak plasma concentrations are reached 2–3 hours after administration. Steady state conditions are reached within 3 days.

Metabolism of dipyridamole occurs in the liver predominantly by conjugation with glururonic acid to form a monoglucuronide. In plasma about 70–80% of the total amount is present as parent compound and 20–30% as the monoglucuronide.

Renal excretion is very low (1–5%).

Preclinical safety data: Dipyridamole has been extensively investigated in animal models and no clinically significant findings have been observed at doses equivalent to therapeutic doses in humans.

Pharmaceutical particulars
List of excipients: Tartaric acid; povidone; Eudragit S 100; talc; acacia; methylhydroxypropylcellulose phthalate; methylhydroxypropylcellulose; triacetin; dimethicone 300; stearic acid; and in the capsule shells – gelatin; erythrosine (E127); titanium dioxide (E171); red and yellow iron oxides (E172).

Incompatibilities: None stated.

Shelf life: 3 years.

Special precautions for storage: Store below 25°C. Discard any capsules remaining 6 weeks after first opening.

Nature and contents of container: White polypropylene tubes with low-density polyethylene Air-sec stoppers filled with dessicating agent (90% white silicon gel/10% molecular sieves).

Packs contain 30, 60 or 100 capsules. Packs of 60 are marketed.

Instructions for use/handling: None stated.

Marketing authorisation number 0015/0206

Date of approval/revision of SPC April 1997

Legal category POM

RINATEC* NASAL SPRAY 0.03%

Qualitative and quantitative composition Rinatec* Nasal Spray 0.03% is an aqueous formulation (adjusted to pH 4.0–5.0) available as a 15 ml (180 metered doses) and 30 ml (380 metered doses) pump spray. Each valve actuation delivers 70 µl of solution containing 21 micrograms of ipratropium bromide.

Pharmaceutical form Aqueous Nasal Spray.

Clinical particulars
Therapeutic indications: Rinatec* Nasal Spray 0.03% is indicated for the symptomatic relief of rhinorrhoea in allergic and non-allergic rhinitis.

Posology and method of administration:
Adults: Two sprays (42 mcg) in each nostril administered 2–3 times a day.

Children: The use of Rinatec* Nasal Spray 0.03% has not been evaluated in children, and therefore is not recommended for use in patients below the age of 12 years.

Contra-indications: Rinatec* Nasal Spray 0.03% is contra-indicated in patients known to be hypersensitive to atropine-like substances or inactive ingredients of the product.

Special warnings and special precautions for use: There have been isolated reports of ocular complications (i.e. mydriasis, increased intraocular pressure, angle-closure glaucoma, eye pain) when nebulised ipratropium bromide either alone or in combination with an adrenergic beta$_2$-agonist, was sprayed into the eyes. Thus patients must be instructed in the correct administration of Rinatec* Nasal Spray 0.03%.

Eye pain or discomfort, blurred vision, visual halos or coloured images in association with red eyes from conjunctival and corneal congestion may be signs of acute angle-closure glaucoma. Should any combination of these symptoms develop, treatment with miotic drops should be initiated and specialist advice sought immediately.

Interaction with other medicaments and other forms of interaction: The concomitant use of Rinatec* Nasal Spray 0.03% with other drugs commonly prescribed for perennial rhinitis i.e. antihistamines, decongesttants or nasal steroids does not increase the incidence of nasal or non-nasal side effects.

Anticholinergic adverse events with chronic use of Rinatec* Nasal Spray 0.03% are rare, limited to local adverse events of dryness of nose and mouth and are not increased by concomitant use of drugs with anticholinergic properties.

Pregnancy and lactation: No adequate or well controlled studies have been conducted in pregnant women. Oral reproduction studies performed in mice, rats and rabbits [at doses approximately 2,000, 200,000 and 25,000 times the maximum recommended human daily dose of Rinatec* Nasal Spray 0.03% in perennial rhinitis (252 mcg/day), respectively] and inhalation reproduction studies in rats and rabbits (at doses approximately 305 and 357 times the maximum recommended human daily dose, respectively) have demonstrated no evidence of teratogenic effects as a result of administration of ipratropium bromide. Fertility of male or female rats at oral doses up to approximately 10,000 times the maximum recommended human daily dose was unaffected by ipratropium bromide administration. At doses above 18,000 times the maximum recommended human daily dose, increased resorption and decreased conception rates were observed. Because animal studies are not always predictive of human response, Rinatec* Nasal Spray 0.03% should be used during pregnancy only if the potential benefit outweighs the potential risk.

It is not known whether ipratropium bromide is excreted in human milk. Although lipid-insoluble quaternary bases pass into breast milk, it is unlikely that ipratropium bromide would reach the infant to an important extent, especially when taken intranasally. However, because many drugs are excreted in human milk, caution should be exercised when Rinatec* Nasal Spray 0.03% is administered to a nursing woman.

Effects on ability to drive and use machines: None known, however see *Overdose*.

Undesirable effects: Local reactions can cause nasal drying in 10% of patients and epistaxis in 6% of patients. These effects may necessitate reduced frequency of administration.

Blurring of vision, precipitation or worsening of narrow angle glaucoma or eye pain may result if Rinatec* Nasal Spray 0.03% comes into direct contact with the eyes. Patients should read and follow the Patient's *Instructions for use* carefully.

Overdose: Acute overdosage by intranasal administration is unlikely since ipratropium bromide is not well absorbed systemically after intranasal or oral administration. The oral LD_{50} of ipratropium bromide ranged between 1001 and 2010 mg/kg in mice; between 1667 and more than 4000 mg/kg in rats; and between 400 and 1300 mg/kg in dogs.

Pharmacological properties

Pharmacodynamic properties: Ipratropium bromide is an anticholinergic drug. As such it directly reduces mucous secretions from the nasal serous and seromucous glands especially in cases where secretion is raised.

Pharmacokinetic properties: The active ingredient is adsorbed to the local muscarinic receptor very quickly after both nasal and oral inhalation. Following intranasal administration of an ipratropium bromide solution, plasma ipratropium concentration above 0.1 mcg/ml are not observed. The systemic bioavailability following intranasal administration or after inhalation is estimated to be less than 10.

The basic pharmacokinetic parameters were calculated from the plasma level data after i.v. administration. The active ingredient was eliminated from the plasma with a terminal half-life of 1.6 h. The half-life of the active ingredient and the metabolites was 3.6 h. The three metabolites whose structure has been determined bind poorly to the muscarinic receptor. The total clearance of the active ingredient is 2300 ml/min. Approx. 40% of clearance is renal (872 ml/min) and 60% non-renal i.e. mainly hepato-metabolic. The volume of distribution in the steady state (Vss) is 176 l (corresponding to approx. 2.4 l/kg) and the volume of distribution in the terminal phase (Vz) is 338 l (approx. 4.6 l/kg).

Renal excretion of the active ingredient is given as 46.3% of the dose after intravenous administration, 3.1% of the dose after inhalation, and 3.7% of the dose after intranasal administration.

The plasma protein binding is minimal (0–9%). It was not observed that the blood brain barrier was penetrated consistent with the quaternary amino structure of the molecule.

Preclinical safety data: The toxicity of ipratropium bromide has been investigated extensively in the following types of studies: acute, subchronic and chronic toxicity, carcinogenicity, reproductive toxicity and mutagenicity via oral, intravenous, subcutaneous, intranasal and/or inhalation routes. Based on these toxicity studies, the probability of systemic anticholinergic side effects decreases in the following order: intravenous > subcutaneous > oral > inhalation > intranasal.

Pre-clinically, ipratropium bromide was found to be well-tolerated. Two-year carcinogenicity studies in rats and mice have revealed no carcinogenic activity at doses up to approximately 1200 times the maximum recommended human daily dose for Rinatec* Nasal Spray 0.03%. Results of various mutagenicity tests were negative.

Pharmaceutical particulars

List of excipients: Sodium chloride; benzalkonium chloride; disodium edetate dihydrate; purified water. Hydrochloric acid and sodium hydroxide are used for pH adjustment.

Incompatibilities: None known.

Shelf life: 2 years.

Special precautions for storage: Store below 25°C. Avoid excessive heat.

Nature and contents of container: Rinatec* Nasal Spray 0.03% is a clear colourless aqueous solution adjusted to the optimum pH 4.0–5.0. The solution is filled into either 15 ml or 30 ml amber glass bottles (Type I glass) fitted with 70 μL manually activated nasal pump/closures.

Instructions for use/handling: To obtain the best results from your nasal spray follow the simple instructions given below. If you are unclear about how to use the nasal spray ask your doctor or pharmacist to explain.

1. Remove the dust cap.
2. The nasal spray pump must be primed before Rinatec Nasal Spray is used for the first time. To prime the pump, hold the bottle with your thumb at the base and your index and middle fingers on the white shoulder area. Make sure the bottle points upright and away from your eyes. Press your thumb firmly and quickly against the bottle seven times. The pump is now primed and can be used. Your pump will hold its prime for up to 24 hours. If you have not used your pump for more than 24 hours, you will need to prime it again before use. Reprime the pump as before, but this time only two sprays are required. If you have not used your pump for more than 7 days reprime using 7 sprays.
3. Blow your nose to clear your nostrils if necessary.
4. Close one nostril by gently placing your finger against the side of your nose. Tilt your head slightly forward and, keeping the bottle upright, insert the nasal tip into the other nostril. Point the tip toward the back and outer side of the nose.

Press firmly and quickly upwards with the thumb at the base while holding the white shoulder portion of the pump between your index and middle fingers. Following each spray, sniff deeply and breathe out through your mouth.

After spraying the nostril and removing the unit, tilt your head backwards for a few seconds to let the spray spread over the back of the nose.

5. Repeat step 4 in the other nostril.
6. Replace the cap.

Avoid spraying Rinatec Nasal Spray in or around your eye. Should this occur, immediately flush your eye with cold tap water for several minutes. If you accidentally spray Rinatec Nasal Spray in your eyes, you may experience a temporary blurring of vision and increased sensitivity to light, which may last a few hours. Follow your doctor's instructions about when and how to take your medicine and always read the label.

If the nasal tip becomes clogged, remove the clear plastic dust cap. Hold the nasal tip under running warm tap water for about a minute. Dry the nasal tip, reprime the nasal spray pump and replace the plastic dust cap.

Marketing authorisation number PL 0015/0196

Date of first authorisation 20 March 1996

Date of revision of the text April 1998

Legal category POM

TRANXENE* CAPSULES 7.5 mg

Qualitative and quantitative composition Maroon/grey hard gelatin capsules imprinted with the product name, 7.5 mg and the Company symbol. Each capsule contains dipotassium clorazepate 7.5 mg.

Pharmaceutical form Capsules for oral administration.

Clinical particulars

Therapeutic indications: Anxiety. Benzodiazepines are only indicated when the disorder is severe, disabling or subjecting the individual to extreme distress.

Posology and method of administration: Anxiety: Treatment should be as short as possible (2–4 weeks). The patient should be reassessed regularly and the need for continued treatment should be evaluated, especially in case the patient is symptom free.

Treatment should be started with the lowest recommended dose. The maximum dose should not be exceeded.

Adults: One capsule up to 3 times daily.

Children: Not generally recommended for children under 16 years.

Elderly: Half the normal dose may be sufficient for a therapeutic response in the elderly.

The lowest dose which can control symptoms should be used, it should not be continued beyond 4 weeks.

Long-term chronic use is not recommended.

Treatment should always be tapered off gradually.

Patients who have taken benzodiazepines for a long time may require a longer period during which doses are reduced.

Contra-indications: Myasthenia gravis, hypersensitivity to benzodiazepines, severe respiratory insufficiency, sleep apnoea syndrome, severe hepatic insufficiency.

Special warnings and special precautions for use:

Tolerance: Some loss of efficacy to the hypnotic effects of benzodiazepines may develop after repeated use for a few weeks.

Dependence: Use of benzodiazepines may lead to the development of physical and psychic dependence upon these products. The risk of dependence increases with dose and duration of treatment; it is also greater in patients with a history of alcholol or drug abuse.

Once physical dependence has developed, abrupt termination of treatment will be accompanied by withdrawal symptoms. These may consist of headaches, muscle pain, extreme anxiety, tension, restlessness, confusion and irritability. In severe cases the following symptoms may occur: derealisation, depersonalisation, hyperacusis, numbness and tingling of the extremities, hypersensitivity to light, noise and physical contact, hallucinations or epileptic seizures.

Rebound insomnia and anxiety: a transient syndrome whereby the symptoms that led to treatment with a benzodiazepine recur in an enhanced form, may occur on withdrawal of treatment. It may be accompanied by other reactions including mood changes, anxiety or sleep disturbances and restlessness. Since the risk of withdrawal phenomena/rebound phenomena is greater after abrupt discontinuation of treatment, it is recommended that the dosage is decreased gradually.

Duration of treatment: The duration of treatment should be as short as possible (see *Posology*) depending on the indication, but should not exceed 4 weeks. Extension beyond these periods should not take place without re-evaluation of the situation.

It may be useful to inform the patient when treatment is started that it will be of limited duration and to explain precisely how the dosage will be progressively decreased. Moreover it is important that the patient should be aware of the possibility of rebound phenomena, thereby minimising anxiety over such symptoms should they occur while the medicinal product is being discontinued.

There are indications that, in the case of benzodiazepines with a short duration of action, withdrawal phenomena can become manifest within the dosage interval, especially when the dosage is high. When benzodiazepines with a long duration of action are being used it is important to warn against changing to a benzodiazepine with a short duration of action, as withdrawal symptoms may develop.

Amnesia: Benzodiazepines may induce anterograde amnesia. The condition occurs most often several hours after ingesting the product and therefore to reduce the risk patients should ensure that they will be able to have an uninterrupted sleep of 7–8 hours (see also *Undesirable effects*).

Psychiatric and 'paradoxical' reactions: Reactions like restlessness, agitation, irritability, aggressiveness, delusion, rages, nightmares, hallucinations, psychoses, inappropriate behaviour and other adverse behavioural effects are known to occur when using benzodiazepines. Should this occur, use of the drug should be discontinued.

They are more likely to occur in children and the elderly.

Specific patient groups: Benzodiazepines should not be given to children without careful assessment of the need to do so; the duration of treatment must be kept to a minimum.

Elderly should be given a reduced dose (see *Posology*). A lower dose is also recommended for patients with chronic respiratory insufficiency due to the risk of respiratory depression. Benzodiazepines are not indicated to treat patients with severe hepatic insufficiency as they may precipitate encephalopathy.

Benzodiazepines are not recommended for the primary treatment of psychotic illness.

Benzodiazepines should not be used alone to treat depression or anxiety associated with depression (suicide may be precipitated in such patients).

Benzodiazepines should be used with extreme caution in patients with a history of alcohol or drug abuse.

Interaction with other medicaments and other forms of interaction

Not recommended: Concomitant intake with alcohol.

The sedative effect may be enhanced when the product is used in combination with alcohol. This affects the ability to drive or use machines.

Take into account: Combination with CNS depressants.

Enhancement of the central depressive effect may occur in cases of concomitant use with antipsychotics (neuroleptics), hypnotics, anxiolytics/sedatives, antidepressant agents, narcotic analgesics, anti-epileptic drugs, anaesthetics and sedative antihistamines.

In the case of narcotic analgesics enhancement of the euphoria may also occur leading to an increase in psychic dependence.

Compounds which inhibit certain hepatic enzymes (particularly cytochrome P450) may enhance the activity of benzodiazepines. To a lesser degree this also applies to benzodiazepines that are metabolised only by conjugation.

Pregnancy and lactation: There is no evidence as to drug safety in human pregnancy nor is there evidence from animal work that it is free from hazard. Do not use during pregnancy, especially during the first and last trimesters, unless there are compelling reasons.

If the product is prescribed to a woman of child bearing potential, she should be warned to contact her physician regarding discontinuance of the product if she intends to become or suspects she is pregnant. If, for compelling medical reasons, the product is administered during the late phase of pregnancy, or during labour at high doses, effects on the neonate such as hypothermia, hypotonia and moderate respiratory depression, can be expected, due to the pharmacological action of the compound.

Moreover, infants born to mothers who took benzodiazepines chronically during the latter stages of pregnancy may have developed physical dependence and may be at some risk for developing withdrawal symptoms in the postnatal period.

Tranxene and its metabolites are excreted in human milk in minimal quantities and therefore use during lactation should be avoided if possible.

Effects on ability to drive and use machines: Sedation, amnesia, impaired concentration and impaired muscular function may adversely affect the ability to drive or to use machines. If insufficient sleep duration occurs, the likelihood of impaired alertness may be increased (see also *Interactions*).

Undesirable effects: Drowsiness, numbed emotions, reduced alertness, confusion, fatigue, headache, dizziness, muscle weakness, ataxia or double vision. These phenomena occur predominantly at the start of therapy and usually disappear with repeated administration.

Other side effects like gastrointestinal disturbances, changes in libido or skin reactions have been reported occasionally.

Amnesia: Anterograde amnesia may occur using therapeutic dosages, the risk increasing at higher dosages. Amnesic effects may be associated with inappropriate behaviour (see *Special warnings and special precautions for use*).

Depression: Pre-existing depression may be unmasked during benzodiazepine use.

Psychiatric and 'paradoxical' reactions: Reactions like restlessness, agitation, irritability, aggressiveness, delusion, rages, nightmares, hallucinations, psychoses, inappropriate behaviour and other adverse behavioural effects are known to occur when using benzodiazepines or benzodiazepine-like agents. They may be quite severe with this product. They are more likely to occur in children and the elderly.

Dependence: Use (even at therapeutic doses) may lead to the development of physical dependence: discontinuation of the therapy may result in withdrawal or rebound phenomena (see *Special warnings and special precautions for use*). Psychic dependence may occur. Abuse of benzodiazepines has been reported.

Overdose: As with other benzodiazepines, overdose should not present a threat to life unless combined with other CNS depressants (including alcohol).

In the management of overdose with any medical product, it should be borne in mind that multiple agents have been taken.

Following overdose with any medicinal product, vomiting should be induced (within one hour) if the patient is conscious or gastric lavage undertaken with the airway protected if the patient is unconscious. If there is no advantage in emptying the stomach, activated charcoal should be given to reduce absorption. Special attention should be paid to respiratory and cardiovascular functions in intensive care.

Overdose of benzodiazepines usually manifested by degrees of central nervous system depression ranging from drowsiness to coma. In mild cases, symptoms include drowsiness, mental confusion and lethargy, in more serious cases, symptoms may include ataxia, hypotonia, hypotension, respiratory depression, rarely coma and very rarely death.

Flumazenil may be useful as an antidote.

Pharmacological properties

Pharmacodynamic properties: Tranxene is a tranquilliser exhibiting many characteristics of the benzodiazepine group of preparations. Particular features which distinguish Tranxene from other members of this group are the rapid appearance in the blood of the anxiolytic compound, nordiazepam, the maintenance of satisfactory therapeutic effect in most patients with once daily administration, and little sedation. In common with other benzodiazepines, Tranxene has a central muscle relaxant effect and synergism with peripherally acting muscle relaxants is a theoretical possibility.

Pharmacokinetic properties: After oral administration of Tranxene, there is essentially no circulating parent drug. Nordiazepam, its primary metabolite quickly appears in the blood stream. The serum half life is about 2 days. Tranxene is metabolised in the liver. In 2 volunteers given 15 mg (50 μC) of 14C-Tranxene, about 80% was recovered in the urine and faeces within 10 days. Excretion was primarily in the urine with about 1% excreted per day on day 10.

Pharmaceutical particulars

List of excipients

Ingredients: Potassium carbonate, Talc.

Capsule shell ingredients: Erythrosine (E127), Indigo carmine (E132), Iron oxide black (E172), Iron oxide red (E172), Titanium dioxide (E171), Gelatin.

Incompatibilities: None stated.

Shelf life: 5 years.

Special precautions for storage: Tranxene Capsules should be stored in a dry place below 25°C. Protect from light.

Nature and contents of container:

Registered packs: (1) Aluminium foil strips
(2) Tropical blister packs

Registered pack sizes: 20, 28 and 100.

The current marketed packs for Tranxene Capsules 7.5 mg are tropical blister packs of 20 and 100.

Instructions for use/handling: None stated.

Marketing authorisation number PL 0015/0045R

Date of first authorisation 30.11.82

Date of revision of the text November 1997

Legal category POM

TRANXENE* CAPSULES 15 mg

Qualitative and quantitative composition Pink/grey hard gelatin capsules imprinted with the notation 15 mg and the Company symbol. Each capsule contains dipotassium clorazepate 15 mg.

Pharmaceutical form Capsules for oral administration.

Clinical particulars

Therapeutic indications: Anxiety. Benzodiazepines are only indicated when the disorder is severe, disabling or subjecting the individual to extreme distress.

Posology and method of administration: Anxiety: Treatment should be as short as possible (2–4 weeks). The patient should be reassessed regularly and the need for continued treatment should be evaluated, especially in case the patient is symptom free.

Treatment should be started with the lowest recommended dose. The maximum dose should not be exceeded.

Adults: One capsule daily, usually administered at night.

Children: Not generally recommended for children under 16 years.

Elderly: Half the normal dose may be sufficient for a therapeutic response in the elderly.

The lowest dose which can control symptoms should be used, it should not be continued beyond 4 weeks.

Long-term chronic use is not recommended.

Treatment should always be tapered off gradually.

Patients who have taken benzodiazepines for a long time may require a longer period during which doses are reduced.

Contra-indications: Myasthenia gravis, hypersensitivity to benzodiazepines, severe respiratory insufficiency, sleep apnoea syndrome, severe hepatic insufficiency.

Special warnings and special precautions for use:

Tolerance: Some loss of efficacy to the hypnotic effects of benzodiazepines may develop after repeated use for a few weeks.

Dependence: Use of benzodiazepines may lead to the development of physical and psychic dependence upon these products. The risk of dependence increases with dose and duration of treatment; it is also greater in patients with a history of alcohol or drug abuse.

Once physical dependence has developed, abrupt termination of treatment will be accompanied by withdrawal symptoms. These may consist of headaches, muscle pain, extreme anxiety, tension, restlessness, confusion and irritability. In severe cases the following symptoms may occur: derealisation, depersonalisation, hyperacusis, numbness and tingling of the extremities, hypersensitivity to light, noise and physical contact, hallucinations or epileptic seizures.

Rebound insomnia and anxiety: a transient syndrome whereby the symptoms that led to treatment with a benzodiazepine recur in an enhanced form, may occur on withdrawal of treatment. It may be accompanied by other reactions including mood changes, anxiety or sleep disturbances and restlessness. Since the risk of withdrawal phenomena/rebound phenomena is greater after abrupt discontinuation of treatment, it is recommended that the dosage is decreased gradually.

Duration of treatment: The duration of treatment should be as short as possible (see *Posology*) depending on the indication, but should not exceed 4 weeks. Extension beyond these periods should not take place without re-evaluation of the situation.

It may be useful to inform the patient when treatment is started that it will be of limited duration and to explain precisely how the dosage will be progressively decreased. Moreover it is important that the patient should be aware of the possibility of rebound phenomena, thereby minimising anxiety over such symptoms should they occur while the medicinal product is being discontinued.

There are indications that, in the case of benzodiazepines with a short duration of action, withdrawal phenomena can become manifest within the dosage interval, especially when the dosage is high. When benzodiazepines with a long duration of action are being used it is important to warn against changing to a benzodiazepine with a short duration of action, as withdrawal symptoms may develop.

Amnesia: Benzodiazepines may induce anterograde amnesia. The condition occurs most often several hours after ingesting the product and therefore to reduce the risk patients should ensure that they will be able to have an uninterrupted sleep of 7–8 hours (see also *Undesirable effects*).

Psychiatric and 'paradoxical' reactions: Reactions like restlessness, agitation, irritability, aggressiveness, delusion, rages, nightmares, hallucinations, psychoses, inappropriate behaviour and other adverse behavioural effects are known to occur when using benzodiazepines. Should this occur, use of the drug should be discontinued.

They are more likely to occur in children and the elderly.

Specific patient groups: Benzodiazepines should not be given to children without careful assessment of the need to do so; the duration of treatment must be kept to a minimum.

Elderly should be given a reduced dose (see *Posology*). A lower dose is also recommended for patients with chronic respiratory insufficiency due to the risk of respiratory depression. Benzodiazepines are not indicated to treat patients with severe hepatic insufficiency as they may precipitate encephalopathy.

Benzodiazepines are not recommended for the primary treatment of psychotic illness.

Benzodiazepines should not be used alone to treat depression or anxiety associated with depression (suicide may be precipitated in such patients).

Benzodiazepines should be used with extreme caution in patients with a history of alcohol or drug abuse.

Interaction with other medicaments and other forms of interaction

Not recommended: Concomitant intake with alcohol.

The sedative effect may be enhanced when the product is used in combination with alcohol. This affects the ability to drive or use machines.

Take into account: Combination with CNS depressants.

Enhancement of the central depressive effect may occur in cases of concomitant use with antipsychotics (neuroleptics), hypnotics, anxiolytics/sedatives, antidepressant agents, narcotic analgesics, anti-epileptic drugs, anaesthetics and sedative antihistamines.

In the case of narcotic analgesics enhancement of the euphoria may also occur leading to an increase in psychic dependence.

Compounds which inhibit certain hepatic enzymes

(particularly cytochrome P450) may enhance the activity of benzodiazepines. To a lesser degree this also applies to benzodiazepines that are metabolised only by conjugation.

Pregnancy and lactation: There is no evidence as to drug safety in human pregnancy nor is there evidence from animal work that it is free from hazard. Do not use during pregnancy, especially during the first and last trimesters, unless there are compelling reasons.

If the product is prescribed to a woman of child bearing potential, she should be warned to contact her physician regarding discontinuance of the product if she intends to become or suspects she is pregnant. If, for compelling medical reasons, the product is administered during the late phase of pregnancy, or during labour at high doses, effects on the neonate such as hypothermia, hypotonia and moderate respiratory depression, can be expected, due to the pharmacological action of the compound.

Moreover, infants born to mothers who took benzodiazepines chronically during the latter stages of pregnancy may have developed physical dependence and may be at some risk for developing withdrawal symptoms in the postnatal period.

Tranxene and its metabolites are excreted in human milk in minimal quantities and therefore use during lactation should be avoided if possible.

Effects on ability to drive and use machines: Sedation, amnesia, impaired concentration and impaired muscular function may adversely affect the ability to drive or to use machines. If insufficient sleep duration occurs, the likelihood of impaired alertness may be increased (see also *Interactions*).

Undesirable effects: Drowsiness, numbed emotions, reduced alertness, confusion, fatigue, headache, dizziness, muscle weakness, ataxia or double vision. These phenomena occur predominantly at the start of therapy and usually disappear with repeated administration.

Other side effects like gastrointestinal disturbances, changes in libido or skin reactions have been reported occasionally.

Amnesia: Anterograde amnesia may occur using therapeutic dosages, the risk increasing at higher dosages. Amnesic effects may be associated with inappropriate behaviour (see *Special warnings and special precautions for use*).

Depression: Pre-existing depression may be unmasked during benzodiazepine use.

Psychiatric and 'paradoxical' reactions: Reactions like restlessness, agitation, irritability, aggressiveness, delusion, rages, nightmares, hallucinations, psychoses, inappropriate behaviour and other adverse behavioural effects are known to occur when using benzodiazepines or benzodiazepine-like agents. They may be quite severe with this product. They are more likely to occur in children and the elderly.

Dependence: Use (even at therapeutic doses) may lead to the development of physical dependence: discontinuation of the therapy may result in withdrawal or rebound phenomena (see *Special warnings and special precautions for use*). Psychic dependence may occur. Abuse of benzodiazepines has been reported.

Overdose: As with other benzodiazepines, overdose should not present a threat to life unless combined with other CNS depressants (including alcohol).

In the management of overdose with any medical product, it should be borne in mind that multiple agents have been taken.

Following overdose with any medicinal product, vomiting should be induced (within one hour) if the patient is conscious or gastric lavage undertaken with the airway protected if the patient is unconscious. If there is no advantage in emptying the stomach, activated charcoal should be given to reduce absorption. Special attention should be paid to respiratory and cardiovascular functions in intensive care.

Overdose of benzodiazepines usually manifested by degrees of central nervous system depression ranging from drowsiness to coma. In mild cases, symptoms include drowsiness, mental confusion and lethargy, in more serious cases, symptoms may include ataxia, hypotonia, hypotension, respiratory depression, rarely coma and very rarely death.

Flumazenil may be useful as an antidote.

Pharmacological properties

Pharmacodynamic properties: Tranxene is a tranquilliser exhibiting many characteristics of the benzodiazepine group of preparations. Particular features which distinguish Tranxene from other members of this group are the rapid appearance in the blood of the anxiolytic compound, nordiazepam, the maintenance of satisfactory therapeutic effect in most patients with once daily administration, and little sedation. In common with other benzodiazepines, Tranxene has a central muscle relaxant effect and synergism with peripherally acting muscle relaxants is a theoretical possibility.

Pharmacokinetic properties: After oral administration of Tranxene, there is essentially no circulating parent drug. Nordiazepam, its primary metabolite quickly appears in the blood stream. The serum half life is about 2 days. Tranxene is metabolised in the liver. In 2 volunteers given 15 mg (50 μC) of 14C-Tranxene, about 80% was recovered in the urine and faeces within 10 days. Excretion was primarily in the urine with about 1% excreted per day on day 10.

Pharmaceutical particulars

List of excipients

Ingredients: Potassium carbonate, Talc.

Capsule shell ingredients: Erythrosine (E127), Indigo carmine (E132), Iron oxide black (E172), Titanium dioxide (E171), Gelatin.

Incompatibilities: None stated.

Shelf life: 5 years.

Special precautions for storage: Tranxene Capsules should be stored in a dry place below 25°C. Protect from light.

Nature and contents of container:

Registered packs: (1) Aluminium foil strips
(2) Tropical blister packs

Registered pack sizes: 20, 28 and 100.

The current marketed packs for Tranxene Capsules 15 mg are tropical blister packs of 20 and 100.

Instructions for use/handling: None stated.

Marketing authorisation number PL 0015/0057R

Date of first authorisation 30.11.82

Date of revision of the text November 1997

Legal category POM.

**Trade Mark*

Boehringer Ingelheim Limited–Hospital Division

Ellesfield Avenue
Bracknell
Berkshire RG12 8YS

☎ 01344 424600 📠 01344 741157

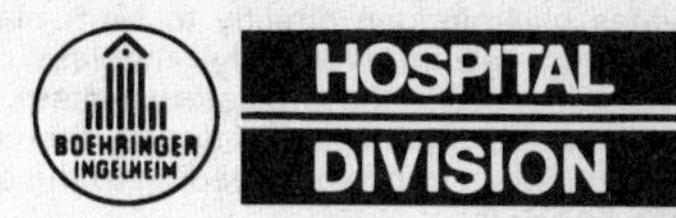

ACTILYSE*

Qualitative and quantitative composition

10 mg/vial: Actilyse 10 mg contains 10 mg (equivalent to 5.8 million International Units) alteplase (recombinant human tissue-type plasminogen activator) per vial.

20 mg/vial: Actilyse 20 mg contains 20 mg (equivalent to 11.6 million International Units) alteplase (recombinant human tissue-type plasminogen activator) per vial.

50 mg/vial: Actilyse 50 mg contains 50 mg (equivalent to 29 million International Units) alteplase (recombinant human tissue-type plasminogen activator) per vial.

The specific activity of alteplase in-house reference material is 580,000 International Units/mg. This has been confirmed by comparison with the second international WHO Standard for t-PA. The specification for the specific activity of alteplase batches is 522.000 to 696.000 International Units/mg.

Following reconstitution with the appropriate volume of Water for Injections, the pH of the resulting solution is 7.3±0.5.

Pharmaceutical form Vial with freeze–dried product, to be reconstituted with Water for Injection (PhEur), for intravenous administration.

Clinical particulars

Therapeutic indications: Thrombolytic treatment in acute myocardial infarction

- 90 minutes (accelerated) dose regimen (see posology and method of administration): for patients in whom treatment can be started within 6 hours after symptom onset

- 3 hour dose regimen (see posology and method of administration): for patients in whom treatment can be started between 6-12 hours after symptom onset provided that the above-mentioned indication is clear.

Actilyse has proven to reduce 30-day-mortality in patients with acute myocardial infarction.

Thrombolytic treatment in acute massive pulmonary embolism with haemodynamic instability. The diagnosis should be confirmed whenever possible by objective means such as pulmonary angiography or non-invasive procedures such as lung scanning.

There is no evidence for positive effects on mortality and late morbidity related to pulmonary embolism.

Posology and method of administration: Actilyse should be given as soon as possible after symptom onset.

Under aseptic conditions the contents of an injection vial of Actilyse (10 or 20 or 50 mg) dry substance is dissolved with water for injection (10 or 20 or 50 ml depending on the size of the rt–PA vial) to a concentration of 1 mg Actilyse/ml and is then administered intravenously. The reconstituted solution may be diluted further with sterile physiological saline solution (0.9 %) up to a minimal concentration of 0.2 mg/ml.

1) Myocardial infarction

a) 90 minutes (accelerated) dose regimen for patients with myocardial infarction, in whom treatment can be started within 6 hours after symptom onset:

15 mg as an intravenous bolus,

50 mg as an infusion over the first 30 minutes,

followed by an infusion of 35 mg over 60 minutes, up to the maximum dose of 100 mg.

In patients with a body weight below 65 kg the dose should be weight adjusted with 15 mg as an intravenous bolus, and 0.75 mg/kg body weight over 30 minutes (maximum 50 mg), followed by an infusion of 0.5 mg/kg over 60 minutes (maximum 35 mg).

b) 3 hour dose regimen for patients, in whom treatment can be started between 6 and 12 hours after symptom onset:

10 mg as an intravenous bolus,

50 mg as an intravenous infusion over the first hour, followed by infusions of 10 mg over 30 minutes, up to the maximum dose of 100 mg over 3 hours.

In patients with a body weight below 65 kg the total dose should not exceed 1.5 mg/kg.

The maximum acceptable dose of Actilyse is 100 mg.

Adjunctive therapy: Aspirin should be initiated as soon as possible after symptom onset and continued for several months after myocardial infarction. The recommended dose is 160 - 300 mg/day.

Heparin should be administered concomitantly for at least 24 hours (at least 48 hours with the accelerated dose regimen). An initial intravenous bolus of 5,000 Units prior to thrombolytic therapy is recommended, followed by an infusion of 1,000 Units/hour. The dose of heparin should be adjusted according to repeated measurements of aPTT values of 1.5 to 2.5 fold of the initial value.

2) Pulmonary embolism

A total dose of 100 mg should be administered in 2 hours. The most experience available is with the following dose regimen:

10 mg as an intravenous bolus over 1-2 minutes, 90 mg as an intravenous infusion over 2 hours.

The total dose should not exceed 1.5 mg/kg in patients with a body weight below 65 kg.

Adjunctive therapy: After treatment with Actilyse heparin therapy should be initiated (or resumed) when aPTT values are less than twice the upper limit of normal. The infusion should be adjusted according to aPTT values of 1.5 to 2.5 fold of the initial value.

Contra–indications: Like all thrombolytic agents, Actilyse should not be used in cases where there is a high risk of haemorrhage such as:

–known haemorrhagic diathesis

–patients receiving oral anticoagulants, e.g. warfarin sodium

–manifest or recent severe or dangerous bleeding

–any history of stroke or central nervous system damage (i.e. neoplasm, aneurysm, intracranial or spinal surgery)

–haemorrhagic retinopathy, e.g. in diabetes (vision disturbances may indicate haemorrhagic retinopathy)

–recent (less than 10 days) traumatic external heart massage, obstetrical delivery, recent puncture of a non-compressible blood–vessel (e.g. subclavian or jugular vein puncture)

–severe uncontrolled arterial hypertension

–bacterial endocarditis, pericarditis

–acute pancreatitis

–documented ulcerative gastrointestinal disease during the last 3 months, oesophageal varices, arterial aneurismus, arterial/venous malformations

–neoplasm with increased bleeding risk

–severe liver disease, including hepatic failure, cirrhosis, portal hypertension (oesophageal varices) and active hepatitis

–major surgery or significant trauma in past 3 months

Special warnings and special precautions for use: Actilyse should be used by physicians experienced in the use of thrombolytic treatment and with the facilities to monitor that use.

The risk of intracerebral haemorrhage is increased in elderly patients. As the therapeutic benefit is also increased in elderly patients, the risk–benefit–evaluation should be carried out carefully.

As yet, there is only limited experience with the use of Actilyse in children.

As with all thrombolytics, the expected therapeutic benefit should be weighed up particularly carefully against the possible risk, especially in patients with

-smaller recent traumas, such as biopsies, puncture of major vessels, intramuscular injections, cardiac massage for resuscitation

-conditions with an increased risk of haemorrhage which are not mentioned in the *Contra-indications* section.

A dose exceeding 100 mg of alteplase should not be given because it has been associated with an additional increase in intracranial bleeding.

There is limited experience with readministration of Actilyse. Actilyse is not suspected to cause anaphylactic reactions. If an anaphylactoid reaction occurs, the infusion should be discontinued and appropriate treatment initiated.

The use of rigid catheters should be avoided.

Interaction with other medicaments and other forms of interaction: The risk of haemorrhage can be increased with the use of coumarine derivatives, platelet aggregation inhibitors, heparin and other agents influencing coagulation.

Pregnancy and lactation: There is very limited experience with the use of Actilyse during pregnancy and lactation. In cases of an acute life–threatening disease the benefit has to be evaluated against the potential risk.

In pregnant animals no teratogenic effects were observed after iv. infusion of pharmacologically effective doses. In rabbits embryotoxicity (embryolethality, growth retardation) was induced by more than 3 mg/kg/day. No effects on peri–postnatal development or on fertility parameters were observed in rats with doses up to 10 mg/kg/day.

Effects on ability to drive and use machines: Not applicable.

Undesirable effects: The most frequent adverse reaction associated with Actilyse is bleeding resulting in a fall in haematocrit and/or haemoglobin values. The type of bleeds associated with thrombolytic therapy can be divided into two broad categories:

-superficial bleeding, normally from punctures or damaged blood vessels,

- internal bleedings into the gastro–intestinal or uro–genital tract, retro–peritoneum or CNS or bleeding of parenchymatous organs.

In clinical studies with Actilyse significant blood–loss was observed occasionally from gastro–intestinal, uro–genital or retro–peritoneal bleeding. Ecchymosis, epistaxis and gingival bleeding are observed rather frequently but usually do not require any specific action. In studies, where patients were treated according to clinical routine, i.e. without acute left–heart catheterisation, a blood transfusion was only occasionally necessary. Intracranial haemorrhage has been reported rarely (less than 1%).

If a potentially dangerous haemorrhage occurs, in particular cerebral haemorrhage, the fibrinolytic therapy must be discontinued. In general, however, it is not necessary to replace the coagulation factors because of the short half–life and the minimal effect on the systemic coagulation factors. Most patients who have bleeding can be managed by interruption of thrombolytic and anticoagulant therapy, volume replacement, and manual pressure applied to an incompetent vessel. Protamine should be considered if heparin has been administered within 4 hours of the onset of bleeding. In the few patients who fail to respond to these conservative measures, judicious use of transfusion products may be indicated. Transfusion of cryoprecipitate, fresh frozen plasma, and platelets should be considered with clinical and laboratory reassessment after each administration. A target fibrinogen level of 1 gram/litre is desirable with cryoprecipitate infusion. Antifibrinolytic agents are available as a last alternative.

Actilyse therapy may lead to cholesterol crystal embolisation or thrombotic embolisation in rare cases. The clinical consequences depend on the organ involved (e.g. renal failure in the case of renal involvement).

In patients receiving Actilyse for myocardial infarction successful reperfusion is often accompanied by arrythmias. These may require the use of conventional antiarrhythmic therapies.

In rare cases nausea, vomiting, hypotension and fever have been reported. These reactions can also occur as concomitant symptoms of myocardial infarction.

In rare cases, anaphylactoid reactions (urticaria, bronchospasm, hypotension) have been reported. A causal relationship could not be established. Clinical relevant antibody formation after alteplase administration has not been observed. No definite allergic reactions with Actilyse are known.

Overdose: The relative fibrin specificity notwithstanding, a clinically significant reduction in fibrinogen and other blood coagulation components may occur after overdosage. In most cases, it is sufficient to await the physiological regeneration of these factors after the Actilyse therapy has been terminated. If, however, severe bleeding results, the infusion of fresh frozen plasma or fresh blood is recommended and if necessary, synthetic antifibrinolytics may be administered.

Pharmacological properties

Pharmacodynamic properties: The active ingredient of Actilyse (alteplase) is a glycoprotein, which activates plasminogen directly to form plasmin. When administered intravenously, alteplase remains relatively inactive in the circulatory system. Once bound to fibrin, it is activated, inducing the conversion of plasminogen to plasmin leading to the dissolution of the fibrin clot.

In a study including more than 40,000 patients with an acute myocardial infarction (Global Utilization of Streptokinase and t-PA for Occluded Coronary Arteries Study–GUSTO) the administration of 100 mg alteplase over 90 minutes, with concomitant iv heparin infusion, led to a lower mortality after 30 days (6.3 %) as compared to the administration of streptokinase, 1.5 million Units over 60 minutes, with sc or iv heparin (7.3%). Actilyse-treated patients showed higher infarct related vessel patency rates at 90 minutes after thrombolysis than the streptokinase-treated patients. No differences in patency rates were noted at 180 minutes or longer.

30-day-mortality is reduced as compared to patients not undergoing thrombolytic therapy (Anglo-Scandinavian Study of Early Thrombolysis–ASSET).

The release of alpha-hydroxybutyrate-dehydrogenase (HBDH) is reduced. Global ventricular function as well as regional wall motion is less impaired as compared to patients receiving no thrombolytic therapy.

A placebo controlled trial with 100 mg Actilyse over 3 hours (Late Assessment of Thrombolytic Efficacy Study–LATE) showed a reduction of 30-day-mortality compared to placebo for patients treated within 6-12 hours after symptom onset. In cases in which clear signs of myocardial infarction are present, treatment initiated up to 24 hours after symptom onset may still be beneficial.

In patients with acute massive pulmonary embolism with haemodynamic instability thrombolytic treatment with Actilyse leads to a fast reduction of the thrombus size and a reduction of pulmonary artery pressure. Mortality data are not available.

Due to its relative fibrin-specificity Actilyse at a dose of 100 mg leads to a modest decrease of the circulating fibrinogen levels to about 60% at 4 hours, which generally reverts to more than 80% after 24 hours. Plasminogen and alpha-2-antiplasmin decrease to about 20% and 35% respectively after 4 hours and increase again to more than 80% at 24 hours. A marked and prolonged decrease of the circulating fibrinogen level is only seen in a few patients.

Actilyse is not suspected to be antigenic.

Pharmacokinetic properties: Actilyse is cleared rapidly from the circulating blood and metabolized mainly by the liver (plasma clearance 550 – 680 ml/min.). The relevant plasma half-life $t_{\frac{1}{2}}$alpha is 4-5 minutes. This means that after 20 minutes less than 10% of the initial value is present in the plasma. For the residual amount remaining in a deep compartment, a beta-half-life of about 40 minutes was measured.

Preclinical safety data: In subchronic toxicity studies in rats and marmosets no unexpected side effects were found.

No indications of a mutagenic potential were found in mutagenic tests.

Pharmaceutical particulars

List of excipients: L-Arginine, phosphoric acid and polysorbate 80.

Incompatibilities: The reconstituted solution may be diluted further with sterile physiological saline solution (0.9 %) up to 1:5.

It may not, however, be diluted further with water for injection or carbohydrate infusion solutions, e. g. dextrose.

Actilyse must not be mixed with other drugs, neither in the same infusion-vial nor via the same catheter (not even with heparin).

Shelf life: 36 months under controlled room temperature storage conditions (not exceeding 25°C, PhEur).

The prepared solution may be stored under refrigeration up to 24 hours and up to 8 hours at a temperature not exceeding 25°C.

Special precautions for storage: Protect the lyophilized substance from light.

Nature and contents of container: 10, 20 or 50 ml sterilized glass vials, which are stoppered with sterile siliconized grey butyl–lyophilization–type stoppers with aluminium/plastic flip–off caps.

The water for injection is filled into either 10, 20 or 50 ml vials, depending on the size of the rt–PA–vials. The water for injection vials are stoppered with appropriate rubber stoppers and aluminium/plastic flip–off type caps.

Instructions for use/handling: Not applicable

Marketing authorisation number 0015/0120

Date of approval/revision of SPC October 1995.

Legal category POM

BONEFOS* CAPSULES

Qualitative and quantitative composition Pale yellow, hard gelatin capsules, printed 'BONEFOS' in black and containing 500 mg sodium clodronate tetrahydrate, equivalent to 400 mg anhydrous sodium clodronate.

Pharmaceutical form Capsules for oral administration.

Clinical particulars

Therapeutic indications: Bonefos Capsules are indicated for the management of osteolytic lesions, hypercalcaemia and bone pain associated with skeletal metastases in patients with carcinoma of the breast or multiple myeloma.

Bonefos Capsules are also indicated for the maintenance of clinically acceptable serum calcium levels in patients with hypercalcaemia of malignancy initially treated with an intravenous infusion of Bonefos concentrate.

Posology and method of administration: Adequate fluid intake should be maintained during treatment.

Adults: The recommended daily dose of Bonefos is 1600 mg sodium clodronate taken as a single dose or in two divided doses (800 mg bd). The capsules should be taken with a little fluid, but not milk, at least 1 hour before or 1 hour after food. If necessary, the dose may be increased but should not exceed a maximum of 3200 mg sodium clodronate daily.

The oral bioavailability of bisphosphonates is poor. Bioequivalence studies have shown appreciable differences in bioavailability between different oral formulations of sodium clodronate, as well as marked inter- and intra-patient variability. Dose adjustment may be required if the formulation is changed.

Dose adjustment is not recommended when switching between Bonefos capsule and tablet formulations (please refer to *Pharmacokinetic properties* below for additional information).

Renal impairment: In patients with moderate renal impairment (creatinine clearance between 10 and 30 ml/min), the daily dose should be reduced to half the adult dose, i.e. 800 mg sodium clodronate. Sodium clodronate is contra-indicated in patients with creatinine clearance below 10 ml/min.

Children: Bonefos has not been evaluated in children.

Elderly: There are no special dosage recommendations in the elderly. Clinical trials have included patients over 65 years and no adverse reactions specific to this age group have been reported.

Contra-indications: Bonefos Capsules are contra-indicated in patients with known hypersensitivity to bisphosphonates, in patients with moderate to severe renal failure (serum creatinine greater than 440 micromol/l or creatinine clearance below 10 ml/min), in children, in pregnant and lactating women, and in patients receiving other bisphosphonates.

Special warnings and special precautions for use: Bonefos Capsules should be administered with care to patients with renal insufficiency. It is recommended that appropriate monitoring of renal function with serum creatinine measurement be carried out during treatment. Serum calcium should be monitored periodically.

Interaction with other medicaments and other forms of interaction: Patients receiving NSAIDs in addition to sodium clodronate have developed renal dysfunction. However, a synergistic action has not been established. As aminoglycosides can cause hypocalcaemia, concomitant clodronate should be administered with caution. There is no evidence from clinical experience that sodium clodronate interacts with other medication such as steroids, diuretics, analgesics or chemotherapeutic agents.

Bonefos forms complexes with divalent metal ions, and therefore simultaneous administration with food, antacids and mineral supplements may impair absorption.

Pregnancy and lactation: There are insufficient data either from animal or human studies on the effects of sodium clodronate on the foetus and on reproduction. No studies have been conducted on secretion in breast milk. Bonefos Capsules are therefore contra-indicated in pregnancy and lactation and should not be given to women of childbearing age unless they are taking adequate contraceptive precautions. Sodium clodronate is likely to adversely affect bone formation both in the foetus and in young children.

Effect on ability to drive and use machines: None known.

Undesirable effects: Side-effects include gastro-intestinal disturbances, for example, nausea, vomiting and diarrhoea may occur during oral treatment, but these are usually mild. If these symptoms occur, use of the divided dose regimen rather than a single daily dose may improve gastro-intestinal tolerance. Hypersensitivity reactions have been mainly confined to the skin: pruritus, urticaria, exfoliative dermatitis. Bronchospasm has been precipitated rarely in patients with and without a previous history of asthma. Renal dysfunction, including failure, has been reported.

Reversible elevations of serum creatinine, parathyroid hormone, lactic acid dehydrogenase, transaminase and alkaline phosphatase have been reported. Asymptomatic hypocalcaemia has been noted infrequently, symptomatic hypocalcaemia is rare.

Overdose: No reports of overt poisoning with sodium clodronate have been received. It is theoretically possible that hypocalcaemia may develop up to 2 or 3 days following the overdose. Serum calcium should be monitored and oral or parenteral calcium supplementation may be needed.

Pharmacological properties

Pharmacodynamic properties: Clodronate is a bisphosphonate (formerly diphosphonates), a group of analogues of pyrophosphate which have been shown, *in vitro*, to inhibit the formation and dissolution of calcium phosphate (hydroxyapatite). *In vivo*, they have been shown to inhibit bone resorption to a greater or lesser extent, depending on the compound, and clodronate is one of the most effective in this respect.

Pharmacokinetic properties: Clodronate is eliminated mainly via the kidneys, and after intravenous doses, 60–80% will be found in urine within 48 hours. Distribution studies in animals suggest that the remainder is retained in bone tissue. Total systemic clearance is, on average, 110 ml/min and the renal clearance 90 ml/min. Clodronate is not metabolised. The half life for elimination from plasma is 2 hours but a second phase with a half life of 13 hours has been identified although less than 10% of total urinary excretion takes place during this phase. The substance which is bound to bone will be excreted more slowly at a rate corresponding to bone turnover. The binding of clodronate to serum proteins is low.

Due to low uptake from gastrointestinal tract, the bioavailability of oral doses is 1–4%. The kinetics of clodronate are linear after both iv and oral doses.

Data from a bioequivalence study show that, based on serum clodronate concentrations, the relative bioavailability of the tablet formulation is 113% (90% confidence interval 91–141%) of that of the capsule formulation. Urinary excretion of clodronate from one Bonefos 800 mg tablet is 95% (90% confidence interval 83–109%) of that of two Bonefos 400 mg capsules.

Preclinical safety data: No further information relevant to clinical practice is available from preclinical studies.

Pharmaceutical particulars

List of excipients: Calcium stearate, colloidal silica, lactose and talc. The capsule shell contains gelatin, titanium dioxide (E171), erythrosine (E127) and yellow iron oxide (E172).

Incompatibilities: None stated.

Shelf life: The shelf life expiry date for this product shall not exceed 5 years from the date of its manufacture.

Special precautions for storage: Bonefos Capsules should be stored below 25°C.

Nature and contents of container:

(i) *Registered packing:* HDPE containers, Clear PVC/aluminium blister packs.

(ii) *Registered pack sizes:* 28, 30, 100, 112 and 120.

(iii) *Current marketed pack:* PVC/aluminium blister packs of 30 and 120 capsules.

Instructions for use/handling: None stated.

Marketing authorisation number PL 0015/0136

Date of first authorisation/renewal of the authorisation 05.04.91

Date of (partial) revision of the text July 1998

Legal category POM.

BONEFOS* CONCENTRATE

Qualitative and quantitative composition Colourless 5 ml ampoules containing 60 mg/ml sodium clodronate. One 5 ml ampoule contains 300 mg sodium clodronate.

Pharmaceutical form Concentrate for intravenous infusion.

Clinical particulars

Therapeutic indications: The treatment of hypercalcaemia of malignancy.

Posology and method of administration: Patients must be kept adequately hydrated before, during and after the administration of Bonefos Concentrate.

Adults: Bonefos Concentrate may be administered to adults as follows:

Single infusion: 1500 mg (five 5 ml ampoules) Bonefos Concentrate in 500 ml of either 0.9% w/v saline or 5% glucose solution administered as an intravenous infusion over a period of four hours. Serum calcium levels should start to decrease 24–48 hours after the infusion.

Multiple infusions: As an alternative, 300 mg (one 5 ml ampoule) Bonefos Concentrate in 500 ml of either 0.9% w/v saline or 5% glucose solution administered as an intravenous infusion over a period of at least two hours on successive days until normocalcaemia is achieved or to a maximum of 7 days.

Response: Whichever method of infusion is employed, most patients will achieve normocalcaemia within 5 days. For those who do not achieve a clinically acceptable serum calcium level, the infusion with Bonefos Concentrate may be repeated.

Further treatment: The length of time that a clinically acceptable serum calcium level is maintained after infusion of Bonefos Concentrate varies considerably from patient to patient. The infusion can be repeated as necessary to control the serum calcium level or, alternatively, treatment with oral Bonefos Capsules at a dose of 1600–3200 mg daily may be appropriate.

Renal function and serum calcium levels should be monitored during therapy. Dose reduction is recommended if deterioration in renal function becomes apparent (see below). Treatment should be stopped if hypocalcaemia develops, and serum calcium levels monitored to determine whether further treatment is required.

Renal impairment: There are no published data at present on which to base recommendations for dose reduction in renal impairment when considering the option of a single 1500 mg infusion in hypercalcaemia.

The dose of clodronate should be reduced in renal impairment according to creatinine clearance when using divided intravenous doses of 300 mg. Thus in mild renal impairment with creatinine clearance of 50–80 ml/minute a 25% reduction in dose is recommended, in moderate renal impairment (10–50 ml/minute) a 25–50% reduction in dose is recommended. Sodium clodoronate is contra-indicated in patients with creatinine clearance below 10 ml/minute.

Children: Bonefos has not been evaluated in children.

Elderly: There are no special dosage recommendations in the elderly. Clinical trials have included patients over 65 years and no adverse reactions specific to this age group have been reported.

Contra-indications: Bonefos Concentrate is contra-indicated in patients with known hypersensitivity to bisphosphonates, in patients with moderate to severe renal failure (serum creatinine greater than 440 micromol/l or creatinine clearance below 10 ml/minute), in children, in pregnant and lactating women, and in patients receiving other bisphosphonates.

Special warnings and precautions for use: Bonefos Concentrate should be administered with care to patients with renal insufficiency. It is recommended that appropriate monitoring of renal function with serum creatinine measurement be carried out during treatment.

Interaction with other medicaments and other forms of interaction: Patients receiving NSAIDs in addition to sodium clodronate have developed renal dysfunction. However, a synergistic action has not been established. As aminoglycosides can cause hypocalcaemia concomitant clodronate should be administered with caution. There is no evidence from clinical experience that sodium clodronate interacts with other medication such as steroids, diuretics, analgesics or chemotherapeutic agents.

Pregnancy and lactation: There are insufficient data either from animal or human studies on the effects of sodium clodronate on the foetus and on reproduction. No studies have been conducted on secretion in breast milk. Bonefos Concentrate is, therefore, contra-indicated in pregnancy and lactation and should not be given to women of childbearing age unless they are taking adequate contraceptive precautions. Sodium clodronate is likely to adversely affect bone formation both in the foetus and in young children.

Effects on ability to drive and use machines: There is no indication to suggest any effects of Bonefos on a patient's ability to drive or use machinery.

Undesirable effects: Hypersensitivity reactions have been mainly confined to the skin: pruritus, urticaria, exfoliative dermatitis. Bronchospasm has been precipitated rarely in patients with and without a previous history of asthma. Renal dysfunction, including failure, has been reported.

Transient proteinuria has been noted immediately after intravenous infusion.

Reversible elevations of serum creatinine, parathyroid hormone, lactic acid dehydrogenase transaminase and alkaline phosphatase have been reported. Asymptomatic hypocalcaemia has been noted infrequently; symptomatic hypocalcaemia is rare.

Overdosage: No reports of overt poisoning with clodronate have been received.

One patient developed fatal renal failure after receiving extremely high doses of intravenous clodronate. Transient increases in serum creatinine have been observed in two studies, suggesting that overdosage of intravenous clodronate may lead to reduced renal function.

It is theoretically possible that hypocalcaemia may develop up to 2 or 3 days following the overdose. Serum calcium should be monitored and oral or parenteral calcium supplementation may be needed.

Pharmacological properties

Pharmacodynamic properties: Clodronate is a bisphosphonate (formerly diphosphonate), a group of analogues of pyrophosphate which have been shown, *in vitro*, to inhibit the formation and dissolution of calcium phosphate (hydroxyapatite). *In vivo*, they have been shown to inhibit bone resorption to a greater or lesser extent, depending on the compound, and clodronate is one of the most effective in this respect.

Pharmacokinetic properties: Clodronate is eliminated mainly via the kidneys, and after intravenous doses, 60–80% will be found in urine within 48 hours. Distribution studies in animals suggest that the remainder is retained in bone tissue. Total systemic clearance is, on average, 110 ml/min and the renal clearance 90 ml/min. Clodronate is not metabolised. The half life for elimination from plasma is 2 hours but a second phase with a half life of 13 hours has been identified although less than 10% of total urinary excretion takes place during this phase. The substance which is bound to bone will be excreted more slowly at a rate corresponding to bone turnover. The binding of clodronate to serum proteins is low.

Due to low uptake from gastrointestinal tract, the bioavailability of oral doses is 1–4%. The kinetics of clodronate are linear after both iv and oral doses.

Preclinical safety data: No further information relevant to clinical practice is available from preclinical studies.

Pharmaceutical particulars

List of excipients: Sodium hydroxide, water for injections.

Incompatibilities: None stated.

Shelf life: The shelf life expiry date for this product shall not exceed 2 years from the date of its manufacture.

Special precautions for storage: The ampoules should be stored below 25°C. Diluted solution must be used within 12 hours.

Nature and contents of container: Bonefos Concentrate is available in 5 ml colourless ampoules of Type I glass, packed into cartons containing 5 or 10 ampoules.

Instructions for use/handling: None stated.

Marketing authorisation number PL 0015/0134

Date of first authorisation/renewal of authorisation
Approved 5 April 1991
Renewed 17 July 1996

Date of (partial) revision of the text December 1997

Legal category POM

BONEFOS* TABLETS

Qualitative and quantitative composition Each tablet contains 1000 mg of disodium clodronate tetrahydrate, equivalent to 800 mg of anhydrous disodium clodronate.

Pharmaceutical form Pale white, oval-shaped, film-coated tablets for oral use.

Clinical particulars

Therapeutic indications: Bonefos tablets are indicated in the management of osteolytic lesions, hypercalcaemia and bone pain associated with skeletal metastases in patients with carcinoma of the breast or multiple myeloma.

Bonefos tablets are also indicated for the maintenance of clinically acceptable serum calcium levels in patients with hypercalcaemia of malignancy initially treated with an intravenous infusion of Bonefos concentrate.

Posology and method of administration

Adults: The recommended daily dose of Bonefos tablets is 1600 mg sodium clodronate taken as a single dose or in two divided doses (800 mg bd). The tablets should be taken with a little fluid, but not milk, at least 1 hour before or 1 hour after food.

If necessary, the dose may be increased but should not exceed a maximum of 3200 mg daily.

The oral bioavailability of bisphosphonates is poor. Bioequivalence studies have shown appreciable differences in bioavailability between different oral formulations of sodium clodronate, as well as marked inter- and intra-patient variability. Dose adjustment may be required if the formulation is changed.

Dose adjustment is not recommended when switching between Bonefos capsule and tablet formulations (please refer to *Pharmacokinetic properties* below for additional information).

Children: Bonefos has not been evaluated in children.

Elderly: There are no special dosage recommendations in the elderly. Clinical trials have included patients over 65 years and no adverse reactions specific to this age group have been reported.

Renal impairment: In patients with moderate renal impairment (creatinine clearance between 10 and 30 ml/min), the daily dose should be reduced to half the adult dose, i.e. 800 mg sodium clodronate. Sodium clodronate is contra-indicated in patients with creatinine clearance below 10 ml/min.

Contra-indications: Bonefos tablets are contra-indicated in patients with known hypersensitivity to bisphosphonates, in patients with moderate to severe renal failure (serum creatinine greater than 440 micromol/l or creatinine clearance less than 10 ml/min), in children, in pregnant and lactating women, and in patients receiving other bisphosphonates.

Special warnings and precautions for use: Adequate fluid intake should be maintained during treatment.

Bonefos tablets should be administered with care to patients with renal insufficiency. It is recommended that appropriate monitoring of hydration status and of renal function with serum creatinine measurement should be carried out during treatment. Serum calcium should be monitored periodically.

Interaction with other medicaments and other forms of interaction: Concomitant use with other bisphosphonates is contra-indicated. Patients receiving non-steroidal anti-inflammatory drugs in addition to sodium clodronate have been reported to develop renal dysfunction. However, a synergistic action has not been established. As aminoglycosides can cause hypocalcaemia, concomitant clodronate should be administered with caution. There is no evidence from clinical experience that sodium clodronate interacts with other medication such as steroids, diuretics, analgesics or chemotherapeutic agents.

Bonefos forms complexes with divalent ions and, therefore, simultaneous administration with food, antacids and mineral supplements may impair absorption.

Pregnancy and lactation: There are insufficient data either from animal or human studies on the effects of sodium clodronate on the foetus and on reproduction. No studies have been conducted on secretion in breast milk. Bonefos tablets are therefore contra-indicated in pregnancy and lactation and should not be given to women of childbearing age unless they are taking adequate contraceptive precautions. Sodium clodronate is likely to adversely affect bone formation both in the foetus and in young children.

Effects on ability to drive and use machines: None known.

Undesirable effects: Gastro-intestinal disturbance, including nausea, vomiting and diarrhoea, may occur during oral treatment, but these are usually mild. If these symptoms occur, use of the divided dose regimen rather than a single daily dose may improve gastro-intestinal tolerance.

Hypersensitivity reactions have been mainly confined to the skin: pruritus, urticaria and exfoliative dermatitis. Bronchospasm has been precipitated rarely in patients with and without a previous history of asthma. Renal dysfunction, including failure, has been reported.

Reversible elevations of serum parathyroid hormone, creatinine, lactic acid dehydrogenase, transaminase and alkaline phosphatase have been reported. Asymptomatic hypocalcaemia has been noted infrequently; symptomatic hypocalcaemia is rare.

Overdose: No reports of overt poisoning with sodium clodronate have been received. It is theoretically possible that hypocalcaemia may develop up to 2 or 3 days following the overdose. Serum calcium should be monitored and oral or parenteral calcium supplementation may be needed.

Pharmacological properties

Pharmacodynamic properties: Clodronate is a bisphosphonate (formerly diphosphonates), a group of analogues of pyrophosphate, which have been shown, *in vitro*, to inhibit the formation and dissolution of calcium phosphate (hydroxyapatite). *In vivo*, they have been shown to inhibit bone resorption to a greater or lesser extent, depending on the compound, and clodronate is one of the most effective in this respect.

Pharmacokinetic properties: Clodronate is eliminated mainly via the kidneys and, after intravenous doses, 60–80% will be found in urine within 48 hours. Distribution studies in animals suggest that the remainder is retained in bone tissue. Total systemic clearance is, on average, 110 ml/min and the renal clearance is 90 ml/min. Clodronate is not metabolised.

The half-life for elimination from plasma is 2 hours but a second phase with a half-life of 13 hours has been identified although less than 10% of total urinary excretion takes place during this phase. The substance, which is bound to bone, will be excreted more slowly at a rate corresponding to bone turnover. The binding of clodronate to serum proteins is low.

Due to low uptake from gastrointestinal tract, the bioavailability of oral doses is 1–4%. The kinetics of clodronate are linear after both intravenous and oral doses.

Data from a bioequivalence study show that, based on serum clodronate concentrations, the relative bioavailability of the tablet formulation is 113% (90% confidence interval 91–141%) of that of the capsule formulation. Urinary excretion of clodronate from one Bonefos 800 mg tablet is 95% (90% confidence interval 83–109%) of that of two Bonefos 400 mg capsules.

Preclinical safety data: No further information relevant to clinical practice is available from preclinical studies.

Pharmaceutical particulars

List of excipients: Croscarmellose sodium, microcrystalline cellulose, magnesium stearate, stearic acid, and Opadry Y-1-7000 [coating substance contains methocel, titanium dioxide (E171) and polyethylene glycol 400].

Incompatibilities: None stated.

Shelf life: The shelf life of Bonefos 800 mg tablets is three years.

Special precautions for storage: Bonefos tablets are stored below 25°C.

Nature and contents of container: Bonefos tablets are supplied in clear, colourless PVC/aluminium blister packs of 10 and 60 tablets.

Instructions for use/handling: None stated.

Marketing authorisation number PL 0015/0199

Date of first authorisation/renewal of authorisation 3rd February, 1995

Date of (partial) revision of the text December 1997

Legal category POM.

IMMUKIN*

Presentation Vials containing an isotonic solution (pH5.0±0.5) for subcutaneous injection. Each vial contains 100 micrograms recombinant human interferon gamma-1b (equivalent to 3 x 10^6 Units) per 0.5 ml.

When compared with native human interferon gamma which is a mixture of clipped forms of a heterogeneously glycosylated protein with two allelic forms (position 137: arginine or glutamine, respectively) of different polypeptide chain lengths, interferon gamma-1b is a recombinant homogeneous 140 amino acid long non-glycosylated (position 137: arginine) containing a N-terminal methionine.

Uses

Properties: Interferons are a family of functionally related proteins synthesised by eukaryotic cells in response to viruses and a variety of natural and synthetic stimuli. While alpha, beta and gamma interferons share certain properties, IFN-gamma has potent phagocyte-activating effects not seen with other interferon preparations.

In a placebo-controlled clinical trial in patients with chronic granulomatous disease (CGD), Immukin was shown to reduce the frequency of serious infections during the trial period of 12 months. The overwhelming majority of these patients were also receiving prophylactic antimicrobial therapy.

Pharmacokinetics: Immukin is rapidly cleared after intravenous administration and slowly and well absorbed after intramuscular or subcutaneous administration. Clearance is via the liver and kidney.

The mean elimination half-lives were 38 minutes, 2.9 hours and 5.9 hours after administration of a single 100 micrograms/m² injection by intravenous, intramuscular and subcutaneous routes. Peak plasma concentrations occurred approximately 4 hours after i.m. dosing and 7 hours after s.c. dosing. Multiple-dose subcutaneous pharmacokinetic studies were conducted in healthy male subjects. There was no accumulation of Immukin after 12 consecutive daily injections of 100 micrograms/m².

No pharmacokinetic studies have been performed with the recommended dosage regimen.

Indications: Immukin is indicated as an adjunct therapy to antibiotics to reduce the frequency of serious infections in patients with chronic granulomatous disease (CGD).

Dosage and administration The recommended dose is 50 micrograms/m² or 1.5 micrograms/kg/dose for patients whose body surface area is 0.5 m² or less, to be given by subcutaneous injection three times a week.

The volume withdrawn from the vial should be controlled according to the required dosage before administration. Although the optimum dose of Immukin is not yet known, the recommended dose should not be exceeded. If severe reactions occur, the dosage should be modified (50% reduction) or therapy should be discontinued until the adverse reaction has subsided.

Safety and efficacy in children under the age of 6 months has not been established.

Clinical experience in the elderly is limited.

Contra-indications, warnings etc

Contra-indications: Immukin is contra-indicated in patients who develop or have known acute hypersensitivity to interferon gamma or known hypersensitivity to closely related interferons.

Interaction with other medicaments and other forms of interactions: Immukin does not reduce the efficacy of antibiotics or glucocorticoids in CGD patients.

Immukin can potentially alter the half-lives of simultaneously administered drugs which are metabolised by the cytochrome P-450 system.

It is theoretically possible that hepatotoxic and/or nephrotoxic drugs might have effects on the clearance of Immukin.

Concurrent use of drugs having neurotoxic (including effects on the central nervous system), haemotoxic or cardiotoxic effects may increase the toxicity of interferons in these systems.

The effects of anti-inflammatory drugs, NSAIDs, theophylline, immunosuppressive and cytostatic drugs on the acute cellular effects of Immukin and its therapeutic effects in CGD patients when such drugs are used concomitantly in chronic conditions are not known.

Theoretically, concomitant administration of heterologous serum protein preparations or immunological preparations (e.g. vaccines) might increase the immunogenicity of Immukin.

Immukin should not be mixed with other drugs in the same syringe.

Effects on ability to drive and use machines: Immukin may impair the ability to drive or operate machinery. Patients should be warned of this, and that the effect may be enhanced by alcohol.

Undesirable effects: The clinical and laboratory toxicity associated with multiple-dose Immukin therapy is dose-, route- and schedule-dependent.

Serious adverse reactions have not been observed in patients receiving the recommended dose of Immukin.

The most common adverse experiences are fever, headache, chills, myalgia or fatigue which may decrease in severity as treatment continues. Vomiting, nausea, arthralgia and injection site tenderness have been reported in some patients.

Acute serious hypersensitivity reactions have not been observed in patients receiving Immukin. However, transient cutaneous rashes, e.g. dermatitis, maculopapular rash, pustular and vesicular eruptions and erythema at injection site have occurred in some patients following injection but have rarely necessitated interruption of treatment.

Pregnancy and lactation: There is insufficient information about use during pregnancy in the human to assess possible risk. Immukin should be used during pregnancy only if the potential benefit justifies the potential risk to the foetus. There is no indication of maternal toxicity, embryotoxicity, foetotoxicity or teratogenicity in animal studies.

It is not known whether Immukin is excreted in human milk. Because of unknown risk to the infant breast feeding is inadvisable.

Other special warnings and precautions: Patients with serious liver disease and patients with severe renal insufficiency should be treated with caution because of the possibility of interferon gamma-1b accumulation.

Caution should be exercised when treating patients with known seizure disorders and/or compromised central nervous system function.

Although no direct cardiotoxic effects have been demonstrated Immukin should be used with caution in patients with pre-existing cardiac disease, including symptoms of ischaemia, congestive heart failure or arrhythmia.

Simultaneous administration of interferon gamma-1b with other heterologous serum protein preparations or immunological preparations (e.g. vaccines,) should be avoided because of the risk of unexpected amplified immune response.

In addition to tests normally required for monitoring patients with CGD, patients should undergo the following tests before beginning Immukin therapy and at appropriate periods during treatment: haematologic tests, including full blood counts, differential wbc and platelet counts; blood chemistry, including renal and liver function tests; urinalysis.

Although antibodies to interferon gamma-1b have not been detected in several hundred patients, it would be prudent to monitor patients periodically for the presence of antibodies to Immukin.

Parenteral drug products should be inspected visually for particulate matter and discolouration prior to administration.

Overdose: Experience of doses in excess of 50 micrograms/m² has been confined to patients with conditions other than CGD.

Central nervous system adverse reactions including decreased mental status, gait disturbance and dizziness have been observed, particularly in cancer patients receiving doses greater than 100 micrograms/m²/day. These abnormalities were reversible within a few days upon dose reduction or discontinuation of therapy.

Reversible neutropenia and elevation of hepatic enzymes have been observed at doses equal to or above 250 micrograms/m²/day. Thrombocytopenia and proteinuria have also been seen rarely.

It is possible that at very high doses (250 micrograms/m²/day or higher), acute, self-limiting constitutional toxicities such as arrhythmia, pulmonary and renal insufficiency, confusion and seizure may exacerbate pre-existing cardiac conditions.

Pharmaceutical precautions Store in a refrigerator (2-8°C). Do not freeze. Do not shake vigorously.

The formulation does not contain a preservative. Once opened, the contents of a vial should be used immediately. The unused portion of any vial should be discarded. Immukin is for single use only.

Legal category POM.

Package quantities Immukin is available in packs containing 6 vials.

Further information Immukin also contains mannitol, disodium succinate hexahydrate, succinic acid, polysorbate 20 and water for injection.

Product licence number 0015/0154.

MEXITIL* AMPOULES

Qualitative and quantitative composition Colourless, glass, ampoules contains 250 mg mexiletine hydrochloride (equivalnt to 207.7 mg of mexiletine) in 10 ml of solution.

Pharmaceutical form Ampoules for intravenous injection.

Clinical particulars

Therapeutic indications: For the treatment of ventricular arrhythmias which are considered as serious and/or life-threatening by the physician.

i.v. mexiletine has been used successfully in the treatment of ventricular arrhythmias induced by digitalis or other drugs; mexiletine has also been proven to be of some benefit in idiopathic and other arrhythmic states. Mexiletine is often effective in patients with good left ventricular function, in suppressing ventricular arrhythmias refractory to other treatment. Mexiletine is not of proven value in arrhythmias in pre-excitation syndromes.

Posology and method of administration:

Intravenous mexitil: Mexitil should never be injected in bolus form.

(a) Loading dose: i.v. injection of 4–10 ml (100–250 mg) Mexitil given at a suggested rate of 1 ml per minute (25 mg per minute).

THEN

Add 500 mg (2 ampoules) Mexitil to 500 ml of a suitable infusion solution. Administer the first 250 ml by i.v. infusion over 1 hour (4 ml per minute).

THEN

Administer the second 250 ml by i.v. infusion over 2 hours (2 ml per minute).

(b) Maintenance dose: Add 250 mg (1 ampoule) Mexitil to 500 ml of a suitable infusion solution. Administer by i.v. infusion at a suggested rate of 1 ml per minute (0.5 mg per minute), according to patient response. Continue for as long as required or until oral maintenance therapy is commenced.

2. *Alternative loading dose regimes:*

(a) Combination i.v. Mexitil and Oral Mexitil Loading Dose: i.v. injection of 8 ml (200 mg) Mexitil given at a suggested rate of 1 ml per minute. On completion of injection or infusion give 400 mg Mexitil orally.

(b) Maintenance dose: As in 1(b) above.

3. *Change over from i.v. to oral Mexitil maintenance:* On discontinuing the i.v. infusion commence the maintenance dose. The first capsule should be taken at, or shortly before, the end of the infusion (an oral loading dose should not be given).

Notes:

1. The loading dose regime is designed to compensate for the rapid phase of tissue distribution which occurs especially with i.v. loading.

2. Side effects are more likely to be encountered during the initial tissue loading phase in which case the rate of infusion should be reduced.

3. If the optimum therapeutic effect is not achieved the rate of infusion or oral dosage may be increased, side-effects permitting.

4. When mexiletine therapy is commenced, patients should be monitored closely (ECG and blood pressure, routine laboratory tests) over a period of at least 24 hours, particularly in the following situations: sinus node dysfunction, conduction defects, bradycardia, hypotension or cardiac, renal or hepatic failure. There may be potentiation of tremor in patients with Parkinsonism.

Regular monitoring of cardiac function throughout treatment is advisable.

The duration of treatment required in any patient is of necessity variable, and although no precise guide can be given withdrawal of treatment may be attempted after a suitable period of free arrhythmia. Gradual withdrawal, i.e. over 1–2 weeks, is preferable as arrhythmias which have been satisfactorily controlled may recur.

No specific information on the use of this product in the elderly is available. Clinical trials have included patients over 65 years and no adverse reactions specific to this age group have been reported.

Instructions for dilution: Mexitil solution for injection is known to be compatible with the following infusion solutions: sodium chloride 0.9%; sodium chloride 0.9% with potassium chloride 0.3% or 0.6%; dextrose 5%; sodium bicarbonate 1.4%; sodium lactate (M/6). Diluted Mexitil should not be stored for longer than 8 hours.

Contra-indications: Hypersensitivity to mexiletine or local anaesthetics, cardiogenic shock and high degree A-V block unless a pacemaker is *in situ*.

Mexitil should not be used in the first three months following myocardial infarction or where cardiac output is limited (left ventricular stroke work <35% except in patients with life-threatening ventricular arrhythmias.

Warnings: When using Mexitil, it should be noted that the long-term use of anti-arrhythmic agents has not been shown to prolong life.

Special warnings and special precautions for use: Myocardial infarction results in prolonged absorption half-life of mexiletine. Plasma elimination half-life may be prolonged in moderate to severe hepatic disease, and in patients with creatinine clearance of less than 10 ml/min: individual dose titration is advised in these conditions.

Interaction with other medicaments and other forms of interaction:

(i) Drugs which delay the rate of absorption (narcotic analgesics, some antacids) may reduce peak plasma concentration of mexiletine.

(ii) Drugs which induce the hepatic mixed function oxidase system (e.g. rifampicin, phenytoin and phenobarbitone) can influence the metabolism and hence lower plasma levels of mexiletine. Conversely, drugs which inhibit hepatic function may increase mexiletine levels in the plasma.

(iii) Drugs which acidify or alkalinise urine will enhance or reduce (respectively) the rate of drug elimination.

(iv) Concurrent administration of mexiletine may increase plasma levels of theophylline and caffeine.

(v) No interactions have been observed with warfarin, diazepam or nitrazepam.

(vi) Mexitil may be used concurrently with the cardiovascular drugs digoxin, amiodarone, quinidine and beta-adrenergic blocking agents. Concomitant i.v. therapy with other local anaesthetic-type agents such as lignocaine or procainamide is not recommended. However, no problems have been encountered when oral mexiletine has been given in conjunction with these drugs.

Pregnancy and lactation: Although Mexitil has been in general use for several years, there is no definite evidence of safety during human pregnancy. Mexiletine freely crosses the placenta: however, animal studies have shown no hazard.

As with all medicines, mexiletine should not be used in pregnancy, especially the first trimester, unless the expected benefit is thought to outweigh any possible risk to the foetus.

Mexiletine is secreted in breast milk (at concentrations on average slightly higher than maternal blood), but has not been detected in the plasma of the suckling infant. Nevertheless caution should be exercised, particularly when nursing a premature infant.

Effect on ability to drive and use machines: Mexitil may impair the ability to drive or operate machinery, especially when taken in combination with alcohol.

Indesirable effects: Side-effects are mainly related to blood concentration and may therefore be seen during the initial phases of both i.v. and oral treatment when fluctuation may occur before the blood and tissue concentrations reach equilibrium. Reducing the rate of injection of infusion or delaying the next oral dose allows the blood concentration to fall and usually reduces side-effects.

Generally side-effects are of the following types:

Gastrointestinal – nausea, vomiting, indigestion, constipation, diarrhoea, dry mouth, unpleasant taste, hiccoughs. Oesophageal ulceration may occur if oral Mexitil is swallowed without adequate liquid and is lodged in the oesophagus.

Central nervous system – light-headedness, drowsiness, confusion, dizziness, unco-ordination, diplopia, blurred vision, nystagmus, dysarthria, ataxia, tremor, paraesthesiae, convulsion, psychiatric disorders, insomnia. Animals studies using toxic doses have shown that benzodiazepines reduce the CNS effects.

Cardiovascular – hypotension, sinus bradycardia, atrial fibrillation, palpitation, conduction defects, exacerbation of arrhythmias and torsade de pointes. When hypotension has occurred this has tended to be in patients with severe illness who have already been given a variety of anti-arrhythmic or other preparations and, if associated with bradycardia, may be reduced by the use of atropine. Pulmonary fibrosis has been observed in isolated cases.

Haematological – rash, jaundice, arthralgia, fever, thrombocytopenia and appearance of positive but symptomless antinuclear factor titres. Leucopernia has been observed rarely. Rare cases of Stevens-Johnson Syndrome, some with liver involvement, have been reported in Japan.

Hepatic – liver damage has been observed following Mexitil administration.

Overdose: The minimum fatal dose is unknown but 4.40 g proved fatal in a healthy young adult.

The clinical features include nausea, vomiting, drowsiness, confusion, ataxia and convulsions. Blurred vision and paraesthesiae have also been reported. Hypotension, sinus bradycardia, atrial fibrillation and cardiac arrest are more specific effects. Arrhythmias should be treated as appropriate and diazepam may be useful to control convulsions.

Acidification of the urine enhances the rate of drug elimiation and so may be useful.

Pharmacological properties

Pharmacodynamic properties: Mexitil is an anti-arrhythmic agent which depresses the maximum rate of depolarisation with little or no modification of resting potentials or the duration of action potentials.

Pharmacokinetic properties: Mexiletine is metabolised in the liver to a number of metabolites. It is excreted in the urine, mainly in the form of its metabolites with a small proportion of unchanged mexiletine; the clearance of mexiletine is increased in acid urine. Mexiletine is widely distributed throughout the body and is about 60–70% bound to plasma proteins. It has a plasma half life of 10 hours in healthy subjects but this may be prolonged in patients with heart disease.

Pharmaceutical particulars

List of excipients: Sodium chloride; water for injections.

Incompatibilities: None stated.

Shelf life: The ampoules have a shelf life expiry date of 5 years from date of manufacture. Diluted Mexitil should be discarded after 8 hours.

Special precautions for storage: Store below 25°C. Protect from light.

Nature and contents of container: Cartons containing 5×10 ml colourless glass ampoules.

Instructions for use/handling: None stated.

Marketing authorisation number 0015/0065R.

Date of approval/revision of SPC January 1996.

Legal category POM.

MEXITIL* CAPSULES

Qualitative and quantitative composition

Mexitil Capsules 50 mg: Red/purple hard gelatin capsules imprinted with the notation 50 mg and the Company symbol. Each capsule contains mexiletine hydrochloride 50 mg, equivalent to 41.5 mg of mexiletine base.

Mexitil Capsules 200 mg: Red/red hard gelatin capsules imprinted with the notation 200 mg and the Company symbol. Each capsule contains mexiletine hydrochloride 200 mg, equivalent to 166.2 mg of mexiletine base.

Pharmaceutical form Capsules for oral administration.

Clinical particulars

Therapeutic indications: For the treatment of ventricular arrhythmias which are considered as serious and/or life-threatening by the physician.

i.v. mexiletine has been used successfully in the treatment of ventricular arrhythmias induced by digitalis or other drugs; mexiletine has also been proven to be of some benefit in idiopathic and other arrhythmic states. Mexiletine is often effective in patients with good left ventricular function, in suppressing ventricular arrhythmias refractory to other treatment. Mexiletine is not of proven value in arrhythmias in pre-excitation syndromes.

Posology and method of administration: Capsules should be swallowed whole with ample liquid, preferably with the patient in an upright position. It is advisable to take Mexitil after food.

(i) Loading dose: Give 400 mg Mexitil.

(ii) Maintenance dose: Give 200–250 mg Mexitil three to four times daily commencing 2 hours after the loading dose. The usual daily dose is between 600–800 mg in divided doses; optimal doses range from 300–1200 mg daily in divided doses.

Note: Mexitil is absorbed in the upper part of the small intestine. In acute myocardial infarction and particularly when opiates have been given, *rate* of absorption *but not bioavailability* may be delayed and therefore a larger loading dose e.g. 600 mg may be preferable.

Alternative loading dose regimes

(a) *Combination i.v. Mexitil and oral mexitil loading dose:* i.v. injection of 8 ml (200 mg) Mexitil given at a suggested rate of 1 ml per minute. On completion of injection or infusion give 400 mg Mexitil orally. Maintenance dose as in (ii).

(b) *Combination i.v. Lignocaine and oral Mexitil loading dose:* Give i.v. lignocaine according to manufacturer's instructions. On completion of injection give 400 mg Mexitil orally. Maintenance dose as in (ii).

Change over from i.v. to oral maintenance: On discontinuing the i.v. infusion commence the maintenance dose. The first capsule should be taken at, or shortly before, the end of the infusion (an oral loading dose should not be given). Give 200–250 mg Mexitil orally three or four times a day.

Notes:

1. The loading dose regime is designed to compensate for the rapid phase of tissue distribution which occurs especially with i.v. loading.

2. Side-effects are more likely to be encountered during the initial tissue loading phase in which case the rate of infusion should be reduced.

3. If the optimum therapeutic effect is not achieved the rate of infusion or oral dosage may be increased, side-effects permitting.

4. Gastric emptying time may be delayed in patients with myocardial infarction and/or to whom opiates have been given and thus, it may be necessary to titrate the dose against therapeutic effects and side-effects.

5. The 50 mg capsule is available in order that a more precise dose titration may be undertaken should this be required. Small increments will also reduce the incidence of side effects.

6. When mexiletine therapy is commenced, patients should be monitored closely (ECG and blood pressure, routine laboratory tests) over a period of at least 24 hours, particularly in the following situations: sinus node dysfunction, conduction defect, bradycardia, hypotension or cardiac, renal or hepatic failure. There may be potentiation of tremor in patients with Parkinsonism.

Regular monitoring of cardiac function throughout treatment is advisable.

The duration of treatment required in any patient is of necessity variable, and although no precise guide can be given, withdrawal of treatment may be attempted after a suitable period free of arrhythmia. Gradual withdrawal, i.e. over 1–2 weeks, is preferable as arrhythmias which have been satisfactorily controlled may recur.

No specific information on the use of this product in the elderly is available. Clinical trials have included patients over 65 years and no adverse reactions specific to this age group have been reported.

Contra-indications: Hypersensitivity to mexiletine or local anaesthetics, cardiogenic shock and high degree A-V block unless a pacemaker is *in situ*.

Mexitil should not be used in the first three months following myocardial infarction or where cardiac output is limited (left ventricular stoke work <35%) except in patients with life-threatening ventricular arrhythmias.

Warnings: When using Mexitil, it should be noted that the long-term use of anti-arrhythmic agents has not been shown to prolong life.

Special warnings and special precautions for use: Myocardial infarction results in prolonged absorption half-life of mexiletine. Plasma elimination half-life may be prolonged in moderate to severe hepatic disease, and in patients with creatinine clearance of less than 10 ml/min: individual dose titration is advised in these conditions.

Interactions with other medicaments and other forms of interaction:

(i) Drugs which delay the rate of absorption (narcotic analgesics, some antacids) may reduce peak plasma concentration of mexiletine.

(ii) Drugs which induce the hepatic mixed function oxidase system (e.g. rifampicin, phenytoin and phenobarbitone) can influence the metabolism and hence lower plasma levels of mexiletine. Conversely, drugs which inhibit hepatic function may increase mexiletine levels in the plasma.

(iii) Drugs which acidify or alkalinise urine will enhance or reduce (respectively) the rate of drug elimination.

(iv) Concurrent administration of mexiletine may increase plasma levels of theophylline and caffeine.

(v) No interactions have been observed with warfarin, diazepam or nitrazepam.

(vi) Mexitil may be used concurrently with the cardiovascular drugs digoxin, amiodarone, quinidine and beta-adrenergic blocking agents. Concomitant I.V. therapy with other local anaesthetic-type agents such as lignocaine or procainamide is not recommended. However no problems have been encountered when oral mexiletine has been given in conjunction with these drugs.

Pregnancy and lactation: Although Mexitil has been in general use for several years, there is no definite evidence of safety during human pregnancy. Mexiletine freely crosses the placenta: however, animal studies have shown no hazard. As with all medicines, mexiletine should not be used in pregnancy, especially the first trimester, unless the expected benefit is thought to outweigh any possible risk to the foetus. Mexiletine is secreted in breast milk (at concentrations on average slightly higher than maternal blood), but has not been detected in the plasma of the suckling infant. Nevertheless caution should be exercised, particularly when nursing a premature infant.

Effect on ability to drive and use machines: Mexitil may impair the ability to drive or operate machinery, especially when taken in combination with alcohol.

Undesirable effects: Side-effects are mainly related to blood concentration and may, therefore be seen during the initial phases of both i.v. and oral treatment when fluctuation may occur before the blood and tissue concentrations reach equilibrium. Reducing the rate of injection of infusion or delaying the next oral dose allows the blood concentration to fall and usually reduces side-effects.

Generally side-effects are of the following types:

Gastrointestinal – nausea, vomiting, indigestion, constipation, diarrhoea, dry mouth, unpleasant taste, hiccoughs. Oesophageal ulceration may occur if oral Mexitil is swallowed without adequate liquid and is lodged in the oesophagus.

Central nervous system – light-headedness, drowsiness, confusion, dizziness, unco-ordination, diplopia, blurred vision, nystagmus, dysarthria, ataxia, tremor, paraesthesiae, convulsion, psychiatric disorders, insomnia. Animal studies using toxic doses have shown that benzodiazepines reduce the CNS effects.

Cardiovascular – hypotension, sinus bradycardia, atrial fibrillation, palpitation, conduction defects, exacerbation of arrhythmias and torsade de pointes. When hypotension has occurred this has tended to be in patients with severe illness who have already been given a variety of anti-arrhythmic or other preparations and, if associated with bradycardia, may be reduced by the use of atropine. Pulmonary fibrosis has been observed in isolated cases.

Haematological – rash, jaundice, arthralgia, fever, thrombocytopenia and appearance of positive but symptomless antinuclear factor titres. Leucopenia has been observed rarely. Rare cases of Stevens-Johnson Syndrome, some with liver involvement, have been reported in Japan.

Hepatic – Liver damage has been observed following Mexitil administration.

Overdose: The minimum fatal dose is unknown but 4.40 g proved fatal in a healthy young adult.

The clinical features include nausea, vomiting, drowsiness, confusion, ataxia and convulsions. Blurred vision and paraesthesiae have also been reported. Hypotension, sinus bradycardia, atrial fibrillation and cardiac arrest are more specific effects.

Gastric lavage should be performed where appropriate and the patient should be transferred to an intensive/coronary care unit for possible cardiopulmonary support.

Arrhythmias should be treated as appropriate and diazepam may be useful to control convulsions.

Acidification of the urine enhances the rate of drug elimination and so may be useful.

Pharmacological properties

Pharmacodynamic properties: The basic cellular electrophysiological effect of mexiletine is a slowing of the maximal rate of depolarisation of the action potential. Mexiletine blocks sodium channels with a rapid rate of onset and recovery. Mexiletine may have a vagolytic activity.

In patients, mexiletine increases the functional refractory period of the atrio-ventricular node and atrio-ventricular conduction time, and shifts the Wenckebach point to a lower rate. Mexiletine increases the relative and effective refractory periods of his-purkinje system. (Reference: Campbell, RNF, *NEJ Medicine* **316** 29–34 (1987)).

Pharmacokinetic properties: Mexiletine is primarily absorbed in the upper portion of the small intestine. Peak plasma levels are reached 1.5 hours after administration to normal subjects; absorption is slower after myocardial infarction. Mexiletine shows a fast distribution phase, a slow distribution phase, and a slow elimination phase. Tissue up-take is substantial. Mexiletine undergoes less than 10% first-pass hepatic metabolism. Bioavailability is about 90%. Renal clearance varies with urine pH but this is unlikely to have clinical significance. In patients the elimination half-life is 10–15 hours. (Reference: Campbell, RNF, *NEJ Medicine* **316** 29–34 (1987)).

Pharmaceutical particulars

List of excipients: Dried maize starch, colloidal silica, magnesium stearate, hard gelatin capsules.

Incompatibilities: None stated.

Shelf life: The capsules have a shelf life expiry of 5 years from date of manufacture.

Special precautions for storage: Store below 25°C.

Nature and contents of container: PVC blister packs (backed with PVC-lacquered aluminium) of 100.

Instructions for use/handling: None stated.

Marketing authorisation numbers

Mexitil Capsules 50 mg 0015/0062R
Mexitil Capsules 200 mg 0015/0064R

Date of approval/revision of SPC January 1996.

Legal category POM.

MEXITIL* PL PERLONGETS*

Qualitative and quantitative composition Mexitil PL Perlongets are sustained release hard gelatin capsules consisting of a scarlet opaque cap and a turquoise opaque body and containing five round, biconvex, beige-yellow film-coated tablets wth a dull sheen. Each capsule contains 360 mg of mexiletine hydrochloride (equivalent to 299.1 mg mexiletine).

Pharmaceutical form Sustained release capsules for oral administration.

Clinical particulars

Therapeutic indications: For the treatment of ventricular arrhythmias which are considered as serious and/or life-threatening by the physician. Mexiletine has also been proven to be of some benefit in idiopathic and other arrhythmic states. Mexiletine is often effective in patients with good left ventricular function, in suppressing ventricular arrhythmias refractory to other treatment. Mexiletine is not of proven value in arrhythmias in pre-excitation syndromes.

Posology and method of administration: Capsules should be swallowed whole with ample liquid, preferably with the patient in an upright position. It is advisable to take Mexitil after food.

One Mexitil PL capsule twice daily (twelve hourly) will maintain therapeutic blood levels of mexiletine. If this regimen is used initially in new patients, therapeutic blood levels of mexiletine will be achieved after about 36 hours. If a more rapid effect is required, one of the following loading doses may be used:

(a) Two Mexitil PL capsules. This will give therapeutic blood levels of mexiletine within 6 hours.

(b) One Mexitil PL Capsule together with 250 mg Mexitil as conventional capsules. This will give therapeutic blood levels of mexiletine within 2½ hours.

(c) Intravenous loading dose. See Mexitil Capsules and Ampoules SPCs for details. This will give therapeutic blood levels of mexiletine within 5 minutes.

Change over from i.v. to Mexitil PL Capsules: Commence oral maintenance therapy 1–2 hours before the end of the infusion (an oral loading dose should not be given).

Change over from Mexitil Capsules to Mexitil PL Capsules: The first Perlonget should be given in the evening, in place of the capsule. Alternatively, the first Perlonget may be given in the morning together with the last capsule.

Where individually adjusted dosage is necessary, titration of dosage may be accomplished with lower-dosed Mexitil capsules, where appropriate.

Notes: Gastric emptying time may be delayed in patients with myocardial infarction and/or to whom opiates have been given and thus it may be necessary to titrate the dose against therapeutic effects and side-effects. When mexiletine therapy is commenced, patients should be monitored closely (ECG and blood pressure, routine laboratory tests) over a period of at least 24 hours, particularly in the following situations:

Sinus node dysfunction, conduction defect, bradycardia, hypotension or cardiac, renal or hepatic failure. There may be potentiation of tremor in patients with Parkinsonism.

Regular monitoring of cardiac function throughout treatment is advisable.

The duration of treatment required in any patient is of necessity variable, and although no precise guide can be given, withdrawal of treatment may be attempted after a suitable period free of arrhythmia. Gradual withdrawal, i.e. over 1–2 weeks, is preferable as arrhythmias which have been satisfactorily controlled may recur.

No specific information on the use of this product in the elderly is available. Clinical trials have included patients over 65 years and no adverse reactions specific to this age group have been reported.

Contra-indications: Hypersensitivity to mexiletine or local anaesthetics, cardiogenic shock and high degree A-V block unless a pacemaker is *in situ*.

Mexitil should not be used in the first three months following myocardial infarction or where cardiac output is limited (left ventricular stroke work <35%) except in patients with life-threatening ventricular arrhythmias.

When using Mexitil, it should be noted that the long-term use of antiarrhythmic agents has not been shown to prolong life.

Special warnings and special precautions for use: Myocardial infarction results in prolonged absorption half-life of mexiletine. Plasma elimination half-life may be prolonged in moderate to severe hepatic disease, and in patients with creatinine clearance of less than 10 ml/min: individual dose titration is advised in these conditions.

Interactions with other medicaments and other forms of interaction:

(i) Drugs which delay the rate of absorption (narcotic analgesics, some antacids) may reduce peak plasma concentration of mexiletine.

(ii) Drugs which induce the hepatic mixed function oxidase system (e.g. rifampicin, phenytoin and phenobarbitone) can influence the metabolism and hence lower plasma levels of mexiletine. Conversely, drugs which inhibit hepatic function may increase mexiletine levels in the plasma.

(iii) Drugs which acidify or alkalinise urine will enhance or reduce (respectively) the rate of drug elimination.

(iv) Concurrent administration of mexiletine may increase plasma levels of theophylline and caffeine.

(v) No interactions have been observed with warfarin, diazepam or nitrazepam.

(vi) Mexitil may be used concurrently with the cardiovascular drugs digoxin, amiodarone, quinidine and beta-adrenergic blocking agents. Concomitant i.v. therapy with other local anaesthetic-type agents such as lignocaine or procainamide is not recommended. However no problems have been encountered when oral mexiletine has been given in conjunction with these drugs.

Pregnancy and lactation: Although Mexitil has been in general use for several years, there is no definite evidence of safety during human pregnancy. Mexiletine freely crosses the placenta; however animal studies have shown no hazard. As with all medicines, mexiletine should not be used in pregnancy, especially the first trimester, unless the expected benefit is thought to outweigh any possible risk to the foetus. Mexiletine is secreted in breast milk (at concentrations on average slightly higher than maternal blood), but has not been detected in the plasma of the suckling infant. Neverthelss caution should be exercised, particularly when nursing a premature infant.

Effect on ability to drive and use machines: Mexitil may impair the ability to drive or operate machines, especially when taken in combination with alcohol.

Undesirable effects: Side-effects are mainly related to blood concentration and may therefore be seen during the initial phases of both i.v. and oral treatment when fluctuation may occur before the blood and tissue concentrations reach equilibrium. Reducing the rate of injection or infusion or delaying the next oral dose allows the blood concentration to fall and usually reduces side-effects. Generally side-effects are of five types:

Gastro-intestinal – Nausea, vomiting, indigestion, constipation, diarrhoea, dry mouth, unpleasant taste, hiccoughs. Oesophageal ulceration may occur if oral Mexitil is swallowed without adequate liquid and is lodged in the oesophagus.

Central nervous system – Light headedness, drowsiness, confusion, dizziness, unco-ordination, diplopia, blurred vision, nystagmus, dysarthria, ataxia, tremor, paraesthesiae, convulsion, psychiatric disorders, insomnia. Animal studies using toxic doses have shown that benzodiazepines reduce the CNS effects.

Cardiovascular – Hypotension, sinus bradycardia, atrial fibrillation, palpitation, conduction defects, exacerbation of arrhythmias and torsade de pointes.

When hypotension has occurred this has tended to be in patients with severe illness who have already been given a variety of anti-arrhythmic or other preparations and, if associated with bradycardia, may be reduced by the use of atropine. Pulmonary fibrosis has occurred in isolated cases.

Haematological – rash, jaundice, arthralgia, fever, thrombocytopenia and appearance of positive but symptomless antinuclear factor titres. Leucopenia has been observed rarely. Rare cases of Stevens-Johnson syndrome, some with liver involvement, have been reported in Japan.

Hepatic – Liver damage has been observed following Mexitil administration.

Overdose: The minimum fatal dose is unknown but 4.40 g proved fatal in a healthy young adult. The clinical features include: nausea, vomiting, drowsiness, confusion, ataxia and convulsions. Blurred vision and paraesthesiae have also been reported. Hypotension, sinus bradycardia, atrial fibrillation and cardiac arrest are more specific effects.

Gastric lavage should be performed where appropriate and the patient should be transferred to an intensive/coronary care unit for possible cardio-pulmonary support. Arrhythmias should be treated as appropriate and diazepam may be useful to control convulsions. Acidification of the urine enhances the rate of drug elimination and so may be useful.

Pharmacological properties

Pharmacodynamic properties: Mexitil is an anti-arrhythmic agent which depresses the maximum rate of depolarisation with little or no modification of resting potentials or the duration of action potentials.

Pharmacokinetic properties: Mexiletine is readily and almost completely absorbed from the gastrointestinal tract, peak plasma concentrations being obtained 2–4 hours after oral administration.

Pharmaceutical particulars

List of excipients: Tablet core: Lactose; povidone; yellow iron oxide; magnesium stearate. *Tablet coating:* Ethylcellulose; polyethylene glycol 6000. *Capsule shell:* Gelatin; erythrosine; indigo carmine; titanium dioxide; yellow iron oxide; black iron oxide.

Incompatibilities: None stated.

Shelf Life: 5 years.

Special precautions for storage: Store below 25°C.

Nature and content of container: Mexitil PL Perlongets are packed into blister packs of 56 and 60 consisting of aluminium foil coated with a heat seal lacquer (PVC/PVDC combination) and a PVC/PVDC film is used as the sealing surface.

Instructions for use/handling: None stated.

Marketing authorisation number 0015/0084.

Date of approval/revision of SPC November 1996.

Legal category POM.

MYDRILATE* 0.5% W/V EYE DROPS
MYDRILATE* 1.0% W/V EYE DROPS

Qualitative and quantitative composition Solutions containing Cyclopentolate Hydrochloride BP 0.5% w/v and 1.0% w/v.

Pharmaceutical form Eye drops.

Clinical particulars

Therapeutic indications:

(i) Diagnostic purposes for fundoscopy and cycloplegic refraction.
(ii) Dilating the pupil in inflammatory conditions of the iris and uveal tract.

Posology and method of administration

(i) Refraction/Fundoscopy

Adults (and the elderly): One drop of 0.5% w/v solution instilled into the eye, repeated after 15 minutes if necessary, approximately 40 minutes before examination. Deeply pigmented eyes may require the use of a 1% w/v solution.

N.B.: Maximum effect is reached after 30–60 minutes.

Children 6–16 years: One drop of 1% w/v solution instilled into the eye, repeated after 15 minutes if necessary, approximately 40 minutes before examination.

Children under 6 years: One or two drops of 1% w/v solution instilled into the eye, repeated after 15 minutes if necessary, approximately 40 minutes before examination.

(ii) For Uveitis, Iritis and Iridocyclitis

Adults and the elderly: One or two drops of 0.5% w/v solution instilled into the eye up to 4 times daily or as required. Deeply pigmented eyes may require the use of a 1% w/v solution.

Children: At the discretion of the physician.

Do not use during the first three months of life due to possible association between the cycloplegia produced and the development of amblyopia and also the increased risks of systemic toxicity in neonates.

Cycloplegia following administration is quick in onset and short-lived. Maximal cycloplegia is achieved within 15–45 minutes of instillation and lasts on average about 20 minutes. Recovery normally takes place in about 4 hours, but very occasionally some effect persists for up to 24 hours.

Mydriasis is produced very rapidly and an average pupil diameter of 7 mm is usually reached 15–30 minutes after instillation of one drop of 0.5% w/v solution. Complete recovery from the mydriatic effect generally occurs spontaneously in not more than 20 hours.

No specific information on the use of this product in the elderly is available. Clinical trials have included patients over 65 years and no adverse reactions specific to this group have been reported.

Contra-indications:

(i) Use in narrow-angle glaucoma or those with a tendency towards glaucoma e.g. patients with a shallow anterior chamber.
(ii) Hypersensitivity to cyclopentolate hydrochloride, benzalkonium chloride or any other components of the formulation.
(iii) This preparation contains benzalkonium chloride and should not be used whilst soft contact lenses are being worn.
(iv) Use in patients with paralytic ileus.
(v) Use in children with organic brain syndromes, including congenital or neuro-developmental abnormalities, particularly those predisposing to epileptic seizures.

Special warnings and special precautions for use: Because of the risk of precipitating angle-closure glaucoma in the elderly and others prone to raised intraocular pressure, an estimate of the depth of the anterior chamber should be made before use, particularly if therapy is likely to be intense or protracted.

Caution should be observed when drugs of this group are administered to patients with prostatic enlargement, coronary insufficiency or cardiac failure, or ataxia. Atropine-like effects have been reported as side-effects.

Extreme caution is advised for use in children and individuals susceptible to belladonna alkaloids because of the increased risk of systemic toxicity.

Patients should be warned of the oral toxicity of this preparation, and advised to wash their hands after use. If accidentally swallowed, patients should be advised to seek medical attention.

Use with caution in an inflamed eye as the hyperaemia greatly increases the rate of systemic absorption through the conjunctiva.

To reduce systemic absorption the lacrimal sac should be compressed at the medial canthus by digital pressure for at least two minutes after instillation of the drops.

Interaction with other medicaments and other forms of interaction: The effects of anti-muscarinic agents may be enhanced by the concomitant administration of other drugs with anti-muscarinic properties such as some antihistamines, butyrophenones, phenothiazines, tricyclic antidepressants and amantadine.

Pregnancy and lactation: There is insufficient evidence as to drug safety in pregnancy and lactation. This product should not be used during pregnancy unless it is considered essential by a physician.

Effects on ability to drive and to use machines: May cause blurred vision, difficulty in focusing and sensitivity to light. Patients should be warned not to drive or engage in other hazardous activities (including climbing ladders and scaffolding) unless vision is clear. Complete recovery from the effects of Mydrilate Eye Drops may take up to 24 hours.

Undesirable effects

Local: Increased intraocular pressure, transient stinging, and sensitivity to light secondary to pupillary dilation. Prolonged administration may lead to local irritation, hyperaemia, oedema and conjunctivitis.

Systemic: Systemic anticholinergic toxicity is manifested by dryness of the mouth, flushing, dryness of the skin, bradycardia followed by tachycardia with palpitations and arrhythmias, urinary urgency, difficulty and retention, reduction in the tone and motility of the gastrointestinal tract leading to constipation.

Vomiting, giddiness and staggering may occur, a rash may be present in children, abdominal distension in infants. Psychotic reactions, behavioural disturbances and cardio-respiratory collapse may occur in children.

Overdose: Systemic toxicity may occur following topical use, particularly in children. It is manifested by flushing and dryness of the skin (a rash may be present in children), blurred vision, a rapid and irregular pulse, fever, abdominal distension in infants, convulsions and hallucinations and the loss of neuromuscular co-ordination.

Treatment is supportive (there is no evidence that physostigmine is superior to supportive management). In infants and small children the body surface must be kept moist. If accidentally ingested, induce emesis or perform gastric lavage.

Pharmacological properties Cyclopentolate is an anti-muscarinic agent used topically in the eye as a mydriatic and cycloplegic. The effects are similar to those of atropine, but with a more rapid onset and a shorter duration of action.

Pharmaceutical particulars

List of excipients: Boric acid, potassium chloride, benzalkonium chloride solution, purified water.

Incompatibilities: None stated.

Shelf life: 2 years.

Special precautions for storage: Store at 2–8°C. Refrigerate, do not freeze. Protect from light. Do not dilute or dispense from any container other than the original bottle. Discard one month after opening.

Nature and contents of container: 5 ml dropper bottles of 0.5% w/v and 1.0% w/v.

Bottle:	BASF Lupolen 1810E (LDPE) Natural colour
Dropper	BASF Lupolen 1800H (LDPE)
Insert:	Natural colour
Cap and Tamper Evident Closure:	Hostalen GC 7260 (HDPE) White colour
Collar:	LDPE Red colour

Instructions for use/handling: When using the product for the first time, remove both the cap and collar. Replace the cap and screw down firmly to pierce the seal at the tip of the plastic nozzle.

Marketing authorisation numbers

Mydrilate 0.5% w/v Eye Drops	PL 1416/5030
Mydrilate 1.0% w/v Eye Drops	PL 1416/5031

Date of first authorisation/renewal of authorisation 12 February 1990

Date of (partial) revision of the text May 1996

Legal category POM.

ORAMORPH* ORAL SOLUTION

Qualitative and quantitative composition Each 5 ml contains 10 mg of Morphine Sulphate BP.

Pharmaceutical form A clear, colourless solution for oral administration.

Clinical particulars

Therapeutic indications: For the relief of severe pain.

Posology and method of administration

Adults: Usual dose 10–20 mg (5–10 ml) every 4 hours.

Children 6–12 years: Maximum dose 5–10 mg (2.5–5 ml) every 4 hours.

Children 1–5 years: Maximum dose 5 mg (2.5 ml) every 4 hours.

Children under 1 year: Not recommended.

Dosage can be increased under medical supervision according to the severity of the pain and the patient's previous history of analgesic requirements. Reductions in dosage may be appropriate in the elderly.

Morphine sulphate is readily absorbed from the gastro-intestinal tract following oral administration. However, when Oramorph Oral Solution is used in place of parenteral morphine, a 50% to 100% increase in dosage is usually required in order to achieve the same level of analgesia.

Contra-indications: Respiratory depression, obstructive airways disease, known morphine sensitivity, acute hepatic disease, acute alcoholism, head injuries, coma, convulsive disorders and where the intracranial pressure is raised. Concurrent administration of monoamine oxidase inhibitors or within two weeks of discontinuation of their use.

Special warnings and special precautions for use: Care should be exercised if morphine sulphate is given in the first 24 hours post-operatively, in hypothyroidism, and where there is reduced respiratory reserve, such as kyphoscoliosis, emphysema and severe obesity.

Morphine sulphate should not be given if paralytic ileus is likely to occur. If constipation occurs, this may be treated with appropriate laxatives.

It is wise to reduce dosage in chronic hepatic and renal disease, myxoedema, adrenocortical insufficiency, prostatic hypertrophy or shock.

Tolerance and dependence may occur.

Interaction with other medicaments and other forms of interaction: Phenothiazine antiemetics may be given with morphine, but it should be noted that morphine potentiates the effects of tranquillisers, anaesthetics, hypnotics, sedatives and alcohol.

Pregnancy and lactation: Although morphine sulphate has been in general use for many years, there is inadequate evidence of safety in human pregnancy and lactation.

Morphine is known to cross the placenta and is excreted in breast milk, and may thus cause respiratory depression in the newborn infant.

Medicines should not be used in pregnancy, especially the first trimester unless the expected benefit is thought to outweigh any possible risk to the foetus.

Effects on ability to drive and use machines: Morphine sulphate is likely to impair ability to drive and to use machinery.

Undesirable effects: Nausea, vomiting and confusion may be troublesome. If constipation occurs, this may be treated with appropriate laxatives. Morphine may cause dry mouth, sweating, facial flushing, vertigo, bradycardia, palpitations, orthostatic hypotension, hypothermia, restlessness, changes of mood and miosis. Micturition may be difficult and there may be ureteric or biliary spasm. There is also an antidiuretic effect. These effects are more common in ambulant patients than in those who are bedridden. Raised intracranial pressure occurs in some patients.

Overdose

Symptoms: Signs of morphine toxicity and overdosage are likely to consist of pin-point pupils, respiratory depression and hypotension. Circulatory failure and deepening coma may occur in more severe cases. Convulsions may occur in infants and children. Death may occur from respiratory failure.

Treatment of morphine overdose: Administer 400 microgram of naloxone intravenously. Repeat at 2–3 minute intervals as necessary, or by an infusion of 2 mg in 500 ml of normal saline or 5% dextrose (4 microgram/ml). Empty the stomach. A 0.02% aqueous solution of potassium permanganate may be used for lavage. Assist respiration if necessary. Maintain fluid and electrolyte levels.

Pharmacological properties

Pharmacodynamic properties: Morphine binds to opiate receptors, which are located on the cell surfaces of the brain and nervous tissue. This action results in alteration of neurotransmitter release and calcium uptake. It has been postulated that this is the basis of the modulation of sensory input from afferent nerves sensitive to pain.

Pharmacokinetic properties: Morphine N-methyl ^{14}C sulphate administered orally to humans reaches a peak plasma level after around 15 minutes: levels of plasma-conjugated morphine peak at about 3 hours, and slowly decrease over the following 24 hours. After the first hour no significant differences in total plasma levels of radioactivity are seen whether administration is by intravenous, intramuscular, subcutaneous or oral route.

Morphine is a basic amine, and rapidly leaves the plasma and concentrates in the tissues. In animals it has been shown that a relatively small amount of free morphine crosses the blood-brain barrier. Morphine is metabolised in the liver and probably also in the mucosal cells of the small intestine. The metabolites recovered in the urine, in addition to free morphine, are morphine-3-glucuronide and morphine ethereal sulphate. These account for over 65% of administered radioactivity; further radioactivity can be recovered as exhaled $^{14}CO_2$.

Preclinical safety data: No further relevant preclinical data are available.

Pharmaceutical particulars

List of excipients: Alcohol, corn syrup, sucrose, methyl hydroxybenzoate, propyl hydroxybenzoate and purified water.

Incompatibilities: None stated.

Shelf life: 3 years. Discard Oramorph Oral Solution 90 days after first opening.

Special precautions for storage: Store below 25°C. Protect from light.

Nature and contents of container

Registered packs: Amber glass bottles with a tamper-evident, child resistant closure with an outer cap of HDPE and expanded PE liner are available in packs of 100 ml, 250 ml or 300 ml.

Amber glass bottle with a tamper-evident closure available in packs of 500 ml.

Marketed packs: Oramorph Oral Solution is available in 100 ml and 300 ml amber glass bottles with a tamper-evident, child resitant closure with an outer cap of HDPE and expanded PE liner.

Amber glass bottle with a tamper-evident closure available in packs of 500 ml.

Instructions for use/handling: None stated.

Marketing authorisation number PL 0015/0122

Date of first authorisation/renewal of the authorisation 08.03.88/08.03.93

Date of (partial) revision of the text June 1998

Legal category POM

ORAMORPH CONCENTRATED ORAL SOLUTION

Presentation A clear, red solution of Morphine Sulphate BP 20 mg/ml.

Uses For the relief of severe pain.

Dosage and administration

Adults: Usual dose 10–20 mg every 4 hours.

Children 6–12 years: Maximum dose 5–10 mg every 4 hours.

Children 1–5 years: Maximum dose 5 mg every 4 hours.

Children under 1 year: Not recommended.

Dosage can be increased under medical supervision according to the severity of the pain and the patient's previous history of analgesic requirement. Reductions in dosage may be appropriate in the elderly and in debilitated patients.

When patients are transferred from other morphine preparations to Oramorph Oral preparations dosage titration may be appropriate.

Morphine Sulphate BP is readily absorbed from the gastro-intestinal tract following oral administration. However, when oral Oramorph preparations are used in place of parenteral morphine, a 50% to 100% increase in dosage is usually required in order to achieve the same lever of analgesia.

A calibrated dropper is supplied with this dosage form for accurate and convenient dose adjustment. The required dose may be added to a soft drink immediately prior to administration.

Contra-indications, warnings, etc

Contra-indications: Respiratory depression, obstructive airways disease, known morphine sensitivity, acute hepatic disease, acute alcoholism, head injuries, coma, convulsive disorders and where intracranial pressure is raised. Concurrent administration of monoamine oxidase inhibitors or within two weeks of discontinuation of their use.

Warnings and precautions: Care should be exercised if morphine sulphate is given in the first 24 hours post-operatively, in hyperthyroidism or hypothyroidism, and where there is reduced respiratory reserve, such as kyphoscoliosis, emphysema and severe obesity. Morphine sulphate should not be given if paralytic ileus is likely to occur. It is wise to reduce dosage in chronic hepatic and renal disease, myxoedema, adrenocortical insufficiency, prostatic hypertrophy or shock. Tolerance and dependence may occur.

Interactions: The depressant effects of morphine are enhanced by depressants of the central and peripheral nervous system such as alcohol, anaesthetics, muscle relaxants, hypnotics and sedatives, tricyclic antidepressants and phenothiazines.

Side effects: In normal doses, the commonest side effects of morphine sulphate are nausea, vomiting, constipation, drowsiness and confusion. If constipation occurs, this may be treated with appropriate laxatives. Micturition may be difficult and there may be ureteric or biliary spasm. There is also an antidiuretic effect. Dry mouth, sweating, facial flushing, vertigo, bradycardia, palpitations, orthostatic hypotension, hypothermia, restlessness, changes of mood and miosis can also occur. These effects are more common in ambulant patients than in those who are bedridden. Raised intracranial pressure occurs in some patients. As a consequence of histamine release, urticaria and or pruritis may occur in some individuals.

Use in pregnancy and lactation: Although morphine sulphate has been in general use for many years, there is inadequate evidence of safety in human pregnancy and lactation. Morphine is known to cross the placenta and is excreted in breast milk, and may thus cause respiratory depression in the newborn infant.

Medicines should not be used in pregnancy, especially in the first trimester, unless the expected benefit outweighs any possible risk to the foetus.

Effects on ability to drive and use machinery: Patients should be warned not to drive or operate dangerous machinery after taking Oramorph.

Overdosage:

Signs of morphine toxicity and overdosage: These are likely to consist of pin-point pupils, respiratory depression and hypotension. Circulatory failure and deepening coma may occur in more severe cases. Convulsions may occur in infants and children. Death may occur from respiratory failure.

Treatment of morphine overdosage: Managed with intravenous naloxone therapy at an initial dose of 400 micrograms (10 micrograms per kilogram body weight in children). If the desired degree of counteraction and improvement is not observed within 2–3 minutes repeat dosing or establish an infusion of 2 mg in 500 ml of normal saline or 5% dextrose to provide a concentration of 4 micrograms/mL. Empty the stomach. A 0.02% aqueous solution of potassium permanganate may be used for lavage. Assist respiration if necessary. Maintain fluid and electrolyte levels.

Pharmaceutical precautions Store at below 25°C. Protect from light. Discard 120 days after opening.

Legal category
UK: POM CD (Sch. 2).

Package quantities Bottles of 30 ml and 120 ml with calibrated dropper.

Further information Contains preservatives.

Product licence and authorisation data:
Product licence number: PL 0015/0125

Data sheet reference: This data sheet was written in September 1998.

ORAMORPH SR TABLETS

Qualititative and quantitative composition

Oramorph SR Tablets 10 mg: each tablet contains 10 mg Morphine Sulphate BP, equivalent to 7.5 mg anhydrous morphine.

Oramorph SR Tablets 30 mg: each tablet contains 30 mg Morphine Sulphate BP, equivalent to 22.5 mg anhydrous morphine.

Oramorph SR Tablets 60 mg: each tablet contains 60 mg Morphine Sulphate BP, equivalent to 45.0 mg anhydrous morphine.

Oramorph SR Tablets 100 mg: each tablet contains 100 mg Morphine Sulphate BP, equivalent to 75.0 mg anhydrous morphine.

Pharmaceutical form Slow release morphine tablet.

Clinical particulars

Therapeutic indication: For the prolonged relief of severe pain.

Posology and method of administration: Oramorph SR tablets must be swallowed whole and not chewed.

The dosage of Oramorph SR tablets is dependent upon the severity of the pain and the patient's previous history of analgesic requirements. Oramorph SR should normally be administered twice daily at 12 hourly intervals.

One Oramorph SR 30 mg tablet twice daily is the recommended starting dose if Oramorph is taken to replace a weaker opioid analgesic (such as co-proxamol).

One or two Oramorph SR 10 mg tablets twice daily is the recommended starting dosage for a patient presenting with severe pain who has not been previously treated with a weaker opioid analgesic. With increasing severity of pain it is recommended that the dosage of morphine be increased to achieve the desired relief. The dosage may be varied by choosing combinations of the available strengths (10, 30, 60 and 100 mg) or by using higher strength tablets alone.

Alternatively, the effective dose of Oramorph SR Tablets can be found by giving Oramorph liquid every 4 hours in increasing doses until the pain has been controlled and then transferring the patient to the same total 24 hour dose of Oramorph SR, divided into 2 portions taken 12-hourly. The first dose of Oramorph SR should be given 4 hours after the last dose of the oral solution.

It is recommended that a patient transferred from another oral morphine preparation, having similar bioavailability to oral morphine liquid, should receive the same total morphine dose in one twenty-four hour period, divided between the morning and evening dose.

If it is necessary to transfer a patient from another modified release preparation to Oramorph SR it is recommended that the patient receives the same total dose in one 24 hour period, divided into two portions for 12-hourly administration. The first dose of Oramorph SR should not be administered before the dosing interval of the previous morphine preparation has been completed. The patient should be monitored initially and the dose of Oramorph SR adjusted if necessary.

Where a patient had previously received parenteral morphine prior to being transferred to Oramorph SR tablets, a higher total dosage of Oramorph SR may be required. Individual dosage adjustment will be necessary to compensate for any reduction in analgesic effect associated with oral administration.

Oramorph SR tablets should be used with caution post-operatively (as with all morphine preparations) but especially in cases of 'acute abdomen' and following abdominal surgery. Gastric motility should have returned and be maintained.

When Oramorph SR is to be given for the relief of post-operative pain, it is not advisable to administer it during the first 24 hours. Following this initial period, the dosage should be at the physician's discretion.

As with all modified release morphine preparations, breakthrough pain may occur. An immediate release form of morphine should, therefore, be available to the patient as rescue medication. Careful attention should be paid to the total daily morphine dosage. The prolonged effects of morphine in the Oramorph SR formulation should also be borne in mind.

Oramorph SR is not recommended for use in children.

Contra-indications: Respiratory depression, obstructive airways disease, known morphine sensitivity, acute hepatic disease, acute abdomen, paralytic ileus, acute alcoholism, head injuries and where the intracranial pressure is raised. Concurrent administration of monoamine oxidase inhibitors or within two weeks of discontinuation of their use. Oramorph SR Tablets should not be given during an attack of bronchial asthma nor in heart failure secondary to chronic lung disease.

Special warnings and special precautions for use: *Precautions:* Nausea, vomiting and confusion may be troublesome. Care should be exercised in hypothyroidism, and where there is reduced respiratory reserve, such as kyphoscoliosis, emphysema and severe obesity. If constipation occurs, this may be treated with appropriate laxatives.

It is wise to reduce dosage in chronic hepatic and renal disease, myxoedema, adrenocortical insufficiency, prostatic hypertrophy or shock. It should be used with caution in patients with either obstructive bowel disorders, convulsive disorders or myasthenia gravis. Tolerance and dependence may occur.

Interaction with other medicaments and other forms of interaction: Phenothiazine anti-emetics may be given with morphine, but it should be noted that morphine potentiates the effects of tranquillisers, anaesthetics, hypnotics, sedatives and alcohol. Morphine's gastrointestinal effects may also delay the absorption of certain drugs, e.g. mexiletine, or be counteractive, as with metoclopramide.

Pregnancy and lactation: Although morphine sulphate has been in general use for many years, there is inadequate evidence of safety in human pregnancy and lactation. Morphine is known to cross the placenta and is excreted in breast milk, and may thus cause respiratory depression in the newborn infant.

Medicines should not be used in pregnancy, especially the first trimester, unless the expected benefit outweighs any possible risk to the foetus.

Effects on ability to drive and use machines: Patients taking Oramorph SR tablets should not operate dangerous machinery. Patients should be warned that Oramorph may affect their ability to drive.

Undesirable effects: Morphine may cause dry mouth, sweating, facial flushing, vertigo, bradycardia, palpitations, orthostatic hypotension, hypothermia, restlessness, changes of mood and miosis. Micturition may be difficult and there may be ureteric or biliary spasm. There is also an antidiuretic effect. These effects are more common in ambulant patients than in those who are bedridden. Raised intracranial pressure occurs in some patients.

Overdose:

Signs of morphine toxicity and overdosage: These are likely to consist of pin-point pupils, respiratory depression and hypotension. Circulatory failure and deepening coma may occur in more severe cases. Convulsions may occur in infants and children. Death may occur from respiratory failure.

Treatment of morphine overdosage: Administer naloxone 400 micrograms intravenously. Repeat at 2–3 minute intervals as necessary, or by an infusion of 2 mg in 500 ml of normal saline or 5% dextrose (4 micrograms/ml). Empty the stomach. A 0.02% aqueous solution of potassium permanganate may be used for lavage. Assist respiration if necessary. Maintain fluid and electrolyte levels.

Pharmacological properties

Pharmacodynamic properties: Morphine is an opioid analgesic. It acts mainly on the central nervous system and thus on smooth muscle. Although morphine is predominantly a central nervous system depressant it has some central stimulant actions which result in nausea and vomiting and miosis. Morphine generally increases smooth muscle tone, especially the sphincters of the gastro-intestinal tract.

Morphine and related analgesics may produce both physical and psychological dependence and should therefore be used with discrimination. Tolerance may also develop.

Morphine is an alagesic used for the symptomatic relief of moderate to severe pain, especially that associated with neoplastic disease, myocardial infarction and surgery. When pain is likely to be of short duration, a short-acting analgesic is usually preferred. In addition to relieving pain, morphine also alleviates the anxiety associated with severe pain. It is useful as a hypnotic where sleeplessness is due to pain and may also relieve the pain of biliary or renal colic, although an antispasmodic may also be required since morphine may increase smooth muscle tone.

Morphine reduces motility and is used in the symptomatic treatment of diarrhoea. It also relieves the dyspnoea of left ventricular failure and of pulmonary oedema. It is effective for the suppression of cough, but codeine is usually preferred as there is less risk of dependence. Morphine has been used preoperatively as an adjunct to anaesthesia for pain relief and to allay anxiety. It has also been used in high doses as a general anaesthetic in specialised procedures. Morphine is usually administered as the sulphate, although the hydrochloride and the tartrate are used in simular doses; the acetate has also been used. Routes of administration include the oral, subcutaneous, intramuscular, intravenous, intraspinal and rectal routes. Parenteral doses may be intermittent injections or continuous or intermittent infusions adjusted according to individual analgesic requirements.

Pharmacokinetic properties: Morphine has a plasma half-life of about 2 to 3 hours and if given I.V. must be administered frequently. Oramorph SR on the other hand, being a sustained release preparation of morphine, has the advantage that it is only administered twice daily.

A summary of the morphine pharmacokinetic parameters is given below:

(a) Half-life; Plasma half-life; about 2–3 hours
(b) Volume of Distribution; about 3–5 litres/kg
(c) Clearance; Plasma clearance; about 15 to 20 ml/min/kg
(d) Protein Binding; in plasma 20–35%

Pharmacokinetic parameters pertinent to Oramorph SR are summarised in the following table:

Parameters	*Oramorph SR Fasting (A)*	*Oramorph SR Food (B)*
AUC_{0-t} (NG.HR/ML)	46.02±18.85	59.88±20.52
C_{max} (NG/ML)	9.2±3.6	13.6±4.6
T_{max} (Hours)	2.5±1.7	3.9±1.6

Preclinical safety data: No preclinical safety data are available which are additional to the experience gained in man over many years.

Pharmaceutical particulars

List of excipients: Lactose, hydroxyethylcellulose, hypromellose, polyvinylpyrrolidone, talc, magnesium stearate, Opadry buff OY-3607 (10 mg tablet), Opadry violet OY-6708 (30 mg tablet), Opadry orange OY-3533 (60 mg tablet), and Opadry grey OY-8238 (100 mg tablet). The coating agents contain the following constituents:

Opadry Buff OY-3607: Hypromellose; polyethylene glycol 400; titanium dioxide (E171); iron oxide yellow (E172); iron oxide red (E172).

Opadry Orange OY-3533: Hypromellose; polyethylene glycol 400; titanium dioxide (E171); sunset yellow FCF aluminium lake (E110).

Opadry Violet OY-6708: Hypromellose; polyethylene glycol 400; titanium dioxide (E171); erythrosine aluminium lake (E121); indigo carmine aluminium lake (E132); sunset yellow FCF aluminium lake (E110).

Opadry Grey OY-8238: Hypromellose; polyethylene glycol 400; titanium dioxide (E171); iron oxide black (E172).

Incompatibilities: None known.

Shelf life: 3 years below 25°C.

Special precautions for storage: Store below 25°C in a dry place and protect from light.

Nature and contents of container: Polypropylene securitainers with low density polyethylene caps, containing 10 or 60 tablets; or blister packs of a hard-tempered aluminium foil (20 microns), coated outside with nitrocellulose lacquer and inside with a heat-seal lacquer bonded to clear PVC (250 microns) containing 10 or 60 tablets.

Instructions for use/handling: No special handling instructions are required.

Marketing authorisation numbers

Oramorph SR Tablets 10 mg 0015/0208
Oramorph SR Tablets 30 mg 0015/0209
Oramorph SR Tablets 60 mg 0015/0210
Oramorph SR Tablets 100 mg 0015/0211

Date of approval/revision of SPC October 1995.

Legal category CD (Sch 2), POM.

ORAMORPH* UNIT DOSE VIALS

Presentation Clear, colourless solution in 5 ml polyethylene Unit Dose Vials containing 10 mg/5 ml, 30 mg/5 ml, 100 mg/5 ml Morphine Sulphate.

Uses Oramorph Unit Dose Vials are indicated for the relief of severe pain.

Dosage and administration For oral use only.
Adults: The usual starting dose is 10-20 mg (5-10 ml) or Oramorph 10 mg/5 ml Unit Dose Vials every 4 hours.

The dosage can be increased under medical supervision according to the severity of the pain and the patients previous history of analgesic requirements, using Oramorph 30 mg/5 ml Unit Dose Vials or Oramorph 100 mg/5 ml Unit Dose Vials.

Children under 5 years: Not recommended.

6-12 years: Maximum dose 10 mg (5 ml of Oramorph 10 mg/5 ml Unit Dose Vial) every 4 hours.

Reductions in dosage may be appropriate in the elderly or in debilitated patients or where sedation is undesirable.

The required dose may be added to a soft drink immediately prior to administration.

When patients are transferred from other morphine preparations to Oramorph Unit Dose Vials, dosage titration may be appropriate. Morphine sulphate BP is readily absorbed from the gastro-intestinal tract following oral administration. However, when Oramorph Unit Dose Vials are used in place of parenteral morphine, a 50% to 100% increase in dosage is usually required to achieve the same level of analgesia.

Contra-indications, warnings, etc: Respiratory depression, obstructive airways disease, known morphine sensitivity, acute hepatic disease, acute alcoholism, head injuries, coma, convulsive disorders and where the intracranial pressure is raised. Concurrent administration of monoamine oxidase inhibitors or within 10 days of discontinuation of their use.

Precautions: Nausea, vomiting and constipation may be troublesome. Phenothiazine anti-emetics may be given with morphine, but it should be noted that morphine potentiates the effects of tranquillisers, anaesthetics, hypnotics, sedatives and alcohol.

Care should be exercised if morphine sulphate is given in the first 24 hours post-operatively, in hyperthyroidism, and where there is reduced respiratory reserve, such as kyphoscoliosis, emphysema and severe obesity. Morphine sulphate should not be given if paralytic ileus is likely to occur. If constipation occurs, this may be treated with appropriate laxatives.

It is wise to reduce dosage in chronic hepatic and renal disease, myxoedema, adrenocortical insufficiency, prostatic hypertrophy or shock. Tolerance and dependence may occur.

Side effects: In routine clinical practice, the commonest side effects of morphine sulphate are nausea, vomiting, constipation, drowsiness and confusion. If constipation occurs, this may be treated with appropriate laxatives. Micturition may be difficult and there may be ureteric or biliary spasm. There is also an antidiuretic effect. Dry mouth, sweating, facial flushing, vertigo, bradycardia, palpitations, orthostatic hypotension, hypothermia, restlessness, changes of moods and miosis can also occur. These effects are more common in ambulant patients than in those who are bedridden. Raised intracranial pressure occurs in some patients. As a consequence of histamine release, urticaria and/or pruritus may occur in some individuals.

Use in pregnancy and lactation: Although morphine sulphate has been in general use for many years, there is inadequate evidence of safety in human pregnancy and lactation. Morphine is known to cross the placenta and is excreted in the breast milk, and may thus cause respiratory depression in the new born infant.

Medicines should not be used in pregnancy, especially the first trimester, unless the expected benefit outweighs any possible risk to the foetus.

Effects on ability to drive and use machinery: Morphine may cause drowsiness and confusion. Patients should be warned not to drive or operate dangerous machinery after taking Oramorph.

Overdosage: Signs of morphine toxicity and overdosage: These are likely to consist of pin-point pupils, respiratory depression and hypotension. Circulatory failure and deepening coma may occur in more severe cases. Convulsions may occur in infants and children. Death may occur from respiratory failure.

Treatment of morphine overdosage: Administer 400 micrograms naloxone intravenously.

Thereafter repeat at 2-3 minute intervals as necessary, or by an infusion of 2 mg in 500 ml of normal saline or 5% dextrose (4 micrograms/ml). Empty the stomach. A 0.02% aqueous solution of potassium permanganate may be used for lavage. Assist respiration if necessary. Maintain fluid and electrolyte levels.

Pharmaceutical precautions Store below 25°C. Protect from light. Discard unused solution after administration.

Legal category
10 mg/5 ml UDV POM
30 mg/5 ml UDV POM, CD
100 mg/5 ml UDV POM, CD

Package quantities Packs containing 25 vials.

Further information Oramorph UDVs do not contain preservatives

Oramorph is also available as Oramorph Oral Solution (10 mg/5 ml), Oramorph Concentrated Oral Solution (20 mg/5 ml) and Oramorph SR Tablets.

Product licence numbers
10 mg/5 ml UDV 0015/0157
30 mg/5 ml UDV 0015/0158
100 mg/5 ml UDV 0015/0159

POSIJECT*

Presentation Posiject (dobutamine hydrochloride for injection): ampoules containing 5 ml of a colourless to pale yellow sterile solution for intravenous use only. Each ml contains 50 mg dobutamine, 1 mg ascorbic acid and water for injections.

Uses
Actions: The primary action of dobutamine is to augment cardiac contractility by stimulating the $\beta 1$ receptors of the heart. It is a direct-acting agent.

Indications: Posiject is indicated for adults who require inotropic support in the treatment of low output cardiac failure associated with myocardial infarction, open heart surgery, cardiomyopathies, septic shock and cardiogenic shock. Posiject can also increase or maintain cardiac output during positive end expiratory pressure (PEEP) ventilation.

Posiject may also be used for cardiac stress testing as an alternative to exercise in patients for whom routine exercise testing cannot be satisfactorily performed. This use of dobutamine should only be undertaken in units which already perform exercise stress testing and all normal care and precautions required for such testing are also required when using dobutamine for this purpose.

Dosage and administration For intravenous administration only.

Posiject Solution must be diluted to at least 50 ml with either: Sodium Chloride Intravenous Infusion BP or 5% Dextrose Intravenous Infusion BP.

Dilution to 250 ml or 500 ml, will give the following concentrations:

250 ml contains 1,000 micrograms/ml of dobutamine.

500 ml contains 500 micrograms/ml of dobutamine.

The final volume administered should be determined by the fluid requirements of the patient. Concentrations as high as 5,000 micrograms/ml have been used in patients on a restricted fluid intake. High concentrations of dobutamine should only be given with an infusion pump, to ensure accurate dosage.

The diluted solution may be stored for up to 24 hours in a refrigerator.

Administration: Due to its short half life, Posiject must be administered as a continuous intravenous infusion. After dilution, Posiject should be administered intravenously through an intravenous needle or catheter. An i.v. drip chamber or other suitable metering device is essential for controlling the rate of flow in drops per minute.

Recommended dosage for adults and the elderly:
Cardiac stress testing: When used as an alternative to exercise for cardiac stress testing the content of one ampoule (250 mg) should be diluted to 250 ml with Sodium Chloride Intravenous Infusion BP or 5% Dextrose Intravenous Infusion BP to give a final concentration of 1,000 micrograms/ml. The diluted solution should be administered with an infusion pump to ensure accurate delivery. The recommended dose is an incremental increase of 5 micrograms/kg/minute from 5 up to 20 micrograms/kg/minute, each dose being infused for 8 minutes. Continuous ECG monitoring is essential and the infusion should be terminated in the event of > 3 mm ST segment depression or any ventricular arrhythmia. The infusion should also be terminated if heart rate reaches the age/sex maximum, systolic blood pressure rises above 220 mm Hg or any side-effects occur – see 'Side-effects'.

Other uses: Most patients will respond satisfactorily to doses ranging from 2.5 to 10 micrograms/kg/minute. Occasionally, however, a dose as low as 0.5 micrograms/kg/minute will elicit a response.

The rate of administration and the duration of therapy should be adjusted according to the individual patient's response.

Rather than abruptly discontinuing therapy with Posiject, it is advisable to decrease the dosage gradually.

Side-effects, which are dose-related, are infrequent when Posiject is administered at rates below 10 micrograms/kg/minute. Rates as high as 40 micrograms/kg/minute have been used occasionally without significant adverse effects.

Paediatric use: The safety and efficacy of dobutamine for use in children have not been established.

Contra-indications, warnings, etc
Contra-indications: Previous hypersensitivity to dobutamine. Patients with hypovolaemia.

Warnings: If an undue increase in heart rate or systolic blood pressure occurs or if an arrythmia is precipated the dose of dobutamine should be reduced or the drug should be discontinued temporarily.

Dobutamine may precipitate or exacerbate ventricular ectopic activity: rarely it has caused ventricular tachycardia or fibrillation. Because dobutamine facilitates atrioventricular conduction, patients with atrial flutter or fibrillation may develop rapid ventricular responses.

Particular care should be exercised when dobutamine is used in patients with acute myocardial infarction because any significant increase in heart rate or excessive increases in arterial pressure that occur may intensify ischaemia and cause anginal pain and ST segment elevation.

Inotropic agents, including dobutamine, do not improve haemodynamics in most patients with mechanical obstruction that hinders either ventricular filling or outflow, or both. Inotropic response may be inadequate in patients with markedly reduced ventricular compliance. Such conditions are present in cardiac tamponade, valvular aortic stenosis, and idiopathic hypertrophic subaortic stenosis.

Minimal vasoconstriction has occasionally been observed, most notably in patients recently treated with a β-blocking drug. As the inotropic effect of dobutamine stems from stimulation of cardiac β_1 receptors, this effect is prevented by β-blocking drugs. However, dobutamine has been shown to counteract the cardiodepressive effects of β-blocking drugs. Conversely, α-adrenergic blockade may make the β_1 and β_2 effects apparent, resulting in tachycardia and vasodilatation.

The use of dobutamine as an alternative to exercise for cardiac stress testing is not recommended for patients with unstable angina, bundle branch block, valvular heart disease, aortic outflow obstruction or any cardiac condition that could make them unsuitable for exercise stress testing.

Usage in pregnancy: Reproduction studies performed in rats and rabbits have revealed no evidence of impaired fertility, harm to the foetus, or teratogenic effects due to dobutamine. As there are no adequate and well-controlled studies in pregnant women, and as animal reproduction studies are not always predictive of human response, dobutamine should not be used during pregnancy unless the potential benefits outweigh the potential risks to the foetus.

Precautions: During the administration of dobutamine, as with any parenteral catecholamine, heart rate and rhythm, arterial blood pressure, and infusion rate should be monitored closely. When initiating therapy, electrocardiographic monitoring is advisable until a stable response is achieved. Dobutamine should only be used in specialist units in which adequate facilities are available for patient surveillance and the monitoring of responses.

Precipitous decreases in blood pressure have occasionally been described in association with dobutamine therapy. Decreasing the dose or discontinuing the infusion typically results in rapid return of blood pressure to base line values, but rarely intervention may be required and reversibility may not be immediate. Dobutamine should be used with caution in the presence of severe hypotension complicating cardiogenic shock (mean arterial pressure less than 70 mm Hg).

Hypovolaemia should be corrected when necessary with whole blood or plasma before dobutamine is administered.

If arterial blood pressure remains low or decreases progressively during administration of dobutamine despite adequate ventricular filling pressure and cardiac output, consideration may be given to the concomitant use of a peripheral vasoconstrictor agent, such as dopamine or noradrenaline.

Side-effects: For cardiovascular effects, see *Warnings* and *Precautions*.

The following side-effects have been reported rarely: nausea, headache, anginal pain, non-specific chest pain, palpitations, shortness of breath, and reactions suggestive of hypersensitivity, including rash, fever, eosinophilia and bronchospasm.

As with other catecholamines, decreases in serum potassium concentrations have occurred, rarely to hypokalaemic values.

Reactions at site of intravenous infusion: Phlebitis has occasionally been reported. Local inflammatory changes have been described following inadvertent infiltration.

Long-term safety: Infusions for up to 72 hours have revealed no adverse effects other than those seen with shorter infusions. There is evidence that partial tolerance develops with continuous infusions of dobutamine for 72 hours or more; therefore, higher doses may be required to maintain the same effects.

Overdosage: Overdoses of dobutamine have been reported rarely. The symptoms of toxicity may include anorexia, nausea, vomiting, tremor, anxiety, palpitations, headache, shortness of breath and anginal and non-specific chest pain. The positive inotropic and chronotropic effects of dobutamine may cause hypertension, tachyarrhythmias, myocardial ischaemia and ventricular fibrillation. Hypotension may result from vasodilatation.

The duration of action of dobutamine hydrochloride is generally short (half-life approximately 2 minutes).

Temporarily discontinue dobutamine until the patient's condition stabilises. The patient should be monitored and any appropriate resuscitative measures initiated promptly.

Forced diuresis, peritoneal dialysis, or charcoal haemoperfusion have not been established as beneficial.

If the product is ingested, unpredictable absorption may occur from the mouth and gastrointestinal tract.

Pharmaceutical precautions Store undiluted ampoules of Posiject below 25°C and protect from light. If solid particles are evident, do not use.

Prior to administration, Posiject Concentrate must be further diluted to at least 50 ml with either: Sodium Chloride Intravenous Infusion BP or 5% Dextrose Intravenous Infusion BP.

The diluted solution may be stored for up to 24 hours in a refrigerator.

No other intravenous preparation should be administered in the same solution as Posiject.

Posiject should not be mixed with alkaline solutions.

Discard any unused contents of the ampoule.

Legal category POM.

Package quantities Packs containing 5×5 ml ampoules.

Further information Nil.

Product licence number 0015/0180.

VIRAMUNE 200 mg TABLETS ▼

Qualitative and quantitative composition Tablets each containing 200 mg of nevirapine anhydrate (active substance).

Pharmaceutical form Tablets.

Clinical particualrs
Therapeutic indications: Nevirapine is indicated as part of combination therapy for the antiviral treatment of HIV-1 infected adult patients with advanced or progressive immunodeficiency.

Most of the experience with nevirapine is in combination with nucleoside reverse transcriptase inhibitors. There is at present insufficient data on the efficacy of subsequent use of triple combination including protease inhibitors after nevirapine therapy. Refer to *Pharmacodynamic properties.*

Posology and method of administration: The recommended dose for nevirapine is one 200 mg tablet daily for the first 14 days (this lead-in period should be used because it has been found to lessen the frequency of rash), followed by one 200 mg tablet twice daily, in combination with at least two additional antiretroviral agents to which the patient has not been previously exposed. Resistant virus emerges rapidly and uniformly when nevirapine is administered as monotherapy; therefore nevirapine should always be administered in combination therapy. For concomitantly administered antiretroviral therapy, the recommended dosage and monitoring should be followed.

Clinical chemistry tests, which include liver function tests, should be performed prior to initiating nevirapine therapy and at appropriate intervals during therapy.

Nevirapine should be discontinued if patients experience severe rash or a rash accompanied by constitutional findings such as fever, blistering, oral lesions, conjunctivitis, swelling, muscle or joint aches, or general malaise. Patients experiencing rash during the 14-day lead-in period of 200 mg/day should not have their nevirapine dose increased until the rash has resolved. Refer to *Special warnings and special precautions for use.*

Nevirapine administration should be interrupted in

patients experiencing moderate or severe liver function test abnormalities (excluding GGT), until the liver function tests return to baseline values. Nevirapine may then be restarted at 200 mg per day. Increasing the daily dose to 200 mg twice daily should be done with caution, after extended observation. Nevirapine should be permanently discontinued if moderate or severe liver function test abnormalities recur.

Patients who interrupt nevirapine dosing for more than 7 days should restart the recommended lead-in dosing, using one 200 mg tablet daily for the first 14 days followed by one 200 mg tablet twice daily.

No data are available to recommend a dosage of nevirapine in patients with hepatic dysfunction, renal insufficiency, or undergoing dialysis.

Safety and effectiveness of nevirapine in paediatric patients under the age of 16 have not been established.

Nevirapine should be administered by physicians who are experienced in the treatment of HIV infection.

Contra-indications: Nevirapine is contra-indicated in patients with clinically significant hypersensitivity to the active substance or to any of the excipients of the medicinal product.

Special warnings and special precautions for use: On the basis of pharmacodynamic data (see *Pharmacodynamic properties*), nevirapine should only be used with at least two other antiretroviral agents.

Severe and life-threatening skin reactions have occurred in patients treated with nevirapine, including Stevens-Johnson syndrome (SJS) and rarely, toxic epidermal necrolysis (TEN). Fatal cases of TEN have been reported. Nevirapine must be discontinued in patients developing a severe rash or a rash accompanied by constitutional symptoms such as fever, blistering, oral lesions, conjunctivitis, swelling, muscle or joint aches, or general malaise.

While nevirapine is extensively metabolised by the liver and nevirapine metabolites are extensively eliminated by the kidney, the pharmacokinetics of nevirapine have not been evaluated in patients with either hepatic or renal dysfunction. Therefore, nevirapine should not be used in patients with hepatic or renal failure.

Abnormal liver function tests have been reported with nevirapine, some in the first few weeks of therapy, including cases of hepatitis which have resulted in at least one fatal outcome. Nevirapine administration should be interrupted in patients experiencing moderate or severe liver function test abnormalities (except for isolated, asymptomatic GGT elevations) until liver function tests return to baseline values. Nevirapine may then be restarted at 200 mg per day. Increasing the daily dose to 200 mg twice daily should be done with caution, after extended observation. Nevirapine should be permanently discontinued if moderate or severe liver function abnormalities recur. Because clinical hepatitis has occasionally been reported in nevirapine treated patients, some in the first few weeks after initiation of therapy, monitoring of ALT (SGPT) and AST (SGOT) is strongly recommended, especially during the first 6 months of nevirapine treatment.

Nevirapine is not a cure for HIV-1 infection; patients may continue to experience illnesses associated with advanced HIV-1 infection, including opportunistic infections.

The long-term effects of nevirapine are unknown at this time. Nevirapine therapy has not been shown to reduce the risk of transmission of HIV-1 to others through sexual contact or blood contamination.

Patients should be instructed that the major toxicity of nevirapine is rash. They should be advised to promptly notify their physician of any rash. The majority of rashes associated with nevirapine occur within the first 6 weeks of initiation of therapy. Therefore, patients should be monitored carefully for the appearance of rash during this period. Patients should be instructed that dose escalation is not to occur if any rash occurs during the two-week lead-in dosing period, until the rash resolves. Any patient experiencing severe rash or a rash accompanied by constitutional symptoms such as fever, blistering, oral lesions, conjunctivitis, swelling, muscle or joint aches, or general malaise should discontinue medication and consult a physician.

Nevirapine may interact with some medicinal products; therefore, patients should be advised to report to their doctor the use of any other medications.

Oral contraceptives and other hormonal methods of birth control should not be used as the sole method of contraception in women taking nevirapine, since nevirapine might lower the plasma concentrations of these medications. For this reason, and to reduce the risk of HIV transmission, barrier contraception (e.g., condoms) is recommended. Additionally, when oral contraceptives are used for hormonal regulation during administration of nevirapine therapeutic effect should be monitored.

Interaction with other medicinal products and other forms of interaction

Nucleoside analogues: No dosage adjustments are required when nevirapine is taken in combination with zidovudine, didanosine, or zalcitabine. When the zidovudine data were pooled from two studies (n=33) in which HIV-1-infected patients received nevirapine 400 mg/day either alone or in combination with 200–300 mg/day didanosine or 0.375 to 0.75 mg/day zalcitabine on a background of zidovudine therapy, nevirapine produced a non-significant decline of 13% in zidovudine area under the curve (AUC) and a non-significant increase of 5.8% in zidovudine C_{max}. In a subset of patients (n=6) who were administered nevirapine 400 mg/day and didanosine on a background of zidovudine therapy, nevirapine produced a significant decline of 32% in zidovudine AUC and a non-significant decline of 27% in zidovudine C_{max}. Paired data suggest that zidovudine had no effect on the pharmacokinetics of nevirapine. In one crossover study, nevirapine had no effect on the steady-state pharmacokinetics of either didanosine (n=18) or zalcitabine (n=6).

Protease inhibitors: Nevirapine is a mild to moderate inducer of the hepatic enzyme CYP3A; therefore, it is possible that co-administration with protease inhibitors (also metabolised by CYP3A) may result in an alteration in the plasma concentration of either agent.

Results from a clinical trial (n=31) with HIV infected patients administered nevirapine and saquinavir (hard gelatin capsules; 600 mg t.i.d.) indicated that their co-administration leads to a mean reduction of 27% (p=0.03) in saquinavir AUC and no significant change in nevirapine plasma levels. The reduction in saquinavir levels due to this interaction may further reduce the marginal plasma levels of saquinavir which are achieved with the hard gelatin capsule formulation.

Results from a clinical trial (n=25) with HIV infected patients administered nevirapine and indinavir (800 mg q8h) indicated that their co-administration leads to a 28% mean decrease (p<0.01) in indinavir AUC and no significant change in nevirapine plasma levels. No definitive clinical conclusions have been reached regarding the potential impact of co-administration of nevirapine and indinavir. A dose increase of indinavir to 1000 mg q8h should be considered when indinavir is given with nevirapine 200 mg b.i.d.; however, there are no data currently available to establish that the short term or long term antiviral activity of indinavir 1000 mg q8h with nevirapine 200 mg b.i.d. will differ from that of indinavir 800 mg q8h with nevirapine 200 mg b.i.d.

Results from a clinical trial (n=25) with HIV infected patients administered nevirapine and ritonavir (600 mg b.i.d. [using a gradual dose escalation regimen]) indicated that their co-administration leads to no significant change in ritonavir or nevirapine plasma levels. There were no increased safety concerns noted with the co-administration of nevirapine with any of these three protease inhibitors when used in combination.

Ketoconazole: In one study, administration of nevirapine 200 mg b.i.d. with ketoconazole 400 mg q.d. resulted in a significant reduction (63% median reduction in ketoconazole AUC and a 40% median reduction in ketoconazole C_{max}). In the same study, ketoconazole administration resulted in a 15–28% increase in the plasma levels of nevirapine compared to historical controls. Ketoconazole and nevirapine should not be given concomitantly. The effects of nevirapine on itraconazole are not known. Although interaction studies have not been performed, antifungal medicinal products which are eliminated renally (e.g., fluconazole) might be substituted for ketoconazole.

Oral contraceptives: There are no clinical data on the effects of nevirapine on the pharmacokinetics of oral contraceptives. Nevirapine might decrease the plasma concentrations of oral contraceptives (also other hormonal contraceptives); therefore, oral contraceptives should not be used as the sole method of birth control in patients being treated with nevirapine. For other therapeutic uses requiring hormonal regulation, the therapeutic effect in patients being treated with nevirapine should be monitored.

Other medicinal products metabolised by CYP3A: Nevirapine is an inducer of CYP3A and potentially CYP2B6, with maximal induction occurring within 2–4 weeks of initiating multiple-dose therapy. Other compounds that are substrates of these isoforms may have decreased plasma concentrations when co-administered with nevirapine. Therefore, careful monitoring of the therapeutic effectiveness of P450 metabolised medicinal products is recommended when taken in combination with nevirapine.

Other information: Monitoring of steady-state nevirapine trough plasma concentrations in patients who received long-term nevirapine treatment revealed that nevirapine trough concentrations were elevated in patients who received cimetidine (+21%, n=11) and macrolides (+12%, n=24), known inhibitors of CYP3A. Steady-state nevirapine trough concentrations were reduced in patients who received rifabutin (–16%, n=19) and rifampicin (–37%, n=3), known inducers of CYP3A.

There are insufficient data to assess whether dose adjustments are necessary when nevirapine and rifampicin or rifabutin are co-administered. Therefore, these medicinal products should only be used in combination if clearly indicated and with careful monitoring.

Studies using human liver microsomes indicated that the formation of nevirapine hydroxylated metabolites was not affected by the presence of dapsone, rifabutin, rifampicin, and trimethoprim/sulfamethoxazole. Ketoconazole and erythromycin significantly inhibited the formation of nevirapine hydroxylated metabolites.

Use during pregnancy and lactation: No observable teratogenicity was detected in reproductive studies performed in pregnant rats and rabbits. There are no adequate and well-controlled studies in pregnant women.

Preliminary results from an ongoing pharmacokinetic study (ACTG 250) of 10 HIV-1-infected pregnant women who were administered a single oral dose of 100 or 200 mg nevirapine at a median of 5.8 hours before delivery, indicate that nevirapine readily crosses the placenta and is found in breast milk. It is recommended that HIV-infected mothers do not breast-feed their infants to avoid risking postnatal transmission of HIV and that mothers should discontinue nursing if they are receiving nevirapine.

Nevirapine cannot be recommended for pregnant or lactating women at this time.

Effects on ability to drive and use machines: Somnolence has been reported in association with nevirapine therapy.

Undesirable effects: The most frequently reported adverse events related to nevirapine therapy, across all clinical trials, were rash, nausea, fatigue, fever, headache, somnolence and abnormal liver function tests.

The major clinical toxicity of nevirapine is rash, with nevirapine attributable rash occurring in 16% of patients in combination regimens in Phase II/III controlled studies. In these clinical trials 35% of patients treated with nevirapine experienced rash compared with 19% of patients treated in control groups of either zidovudine+didanosine or zidovudine alone. Severe or life-threatening skin reactions occurred in 6.6% of nevirapine-treated patients compared with 1.3% of patients treated in the control groups. Overall, 7% of patients discontinued nevirapine due to rash.

Rashes are usually mild to moderate, maculopapular erythematous cutaneous eruptions, with or without pruritus, located on the trunk, face and extremities. Severe and life-threatening skin reactions have occurred in patients treated with nevirapine, including Stevens-Johnson syndrome (SJS) and, rarely, toxic epidermal necrolysis (TEN). Fatal cases of TEN have been reported. The majority of severe rashes occurred within the first 28 days of treatment and some required hospitalisation, with one patient requiring surgical intervention.

Liver function test abnormalities have occurred in patients treated with nevirapine, some in the first few weeks of therapy, including cases of hepatitis which have resulted in at least one fatal outcome.

Overdose: There is no known antidote for nevirapine overdosage. No acute toxicities or sequelae were reported for one patient who ingested 800 mg of nevirapine in one day.

Pharmacological properties

Pharmacodynamic properties: Pharmacotherapeutic group: antiviral agent, ATC code J05AX04.

Mechanism of action: Nevirapine is a non-nucleoside reverse transcriptase inhibitor (NNRTI) of HIV-1. Nevirapine binds directly to reverse transcriptase and blocks the RNA-dependent and DNA-dependent DNA polymerase activities by causing a disruption of the enzyme's catalytic site. The activity of nevirapine does not compete with template or nucleoside triphosphates. HIV-2 reverse transcriptase and eukaryotic DNA polymerases (such as human DNA polymerases α, β, γ, or δ) are not inhibited by nevirapine.

Resistance: HIV isolates with reduced susceptibility (100 to 250-fold) to nevirapine emerge *in vitro*. Phenotypic and genotypic changes occur in HIV isolates from patients treated with nevirapine or nevirapine+zidovudine over one to 12 weeks. By week 8 of nevirapine monotherapy, 100% of the patients tested had HIV isolates with a >100-fold decrease in susceptibility to nevirapine, regardless of dose. Nevirapine+zidovudine combination therapy did not alter the emergence rate of nevirapine-resistant virus. In a trial with nevirapine+zidovudine+didanosine in previously untreated patients, after 6 months of therapy, decreased phenotypic nevirapine susceptibility emerged in 21% (5/24) patients who had plasma submitted for testing. Virus was suppressed in the other 19 plasma specimens. The clinical relevance of phenotypic and genotypic changes associated with nevirapine therapy has not been established.

Cross-resistance: Rapid emergence of HIV strains

which are cross-resistant to NNRTIs has been observed *in vitro*. Data on cross-resistance between the NNRTI nevirapine and nucleoside analogue reverse transcriptase inhibitors are very limited. In four patients, zidovudine-resistant isolates tested *in vitro* retained susceptibility to nevirapine and in six patients, nevirapine-resistant isolates were susceptible to zidovudine and didanosine. Cross-resistance between nevirapine and HIV protease inhibitors is unlikely because the enzyme targets involved are different.

Pharmacodynamic effects: Nevirapine has been evaluated in both treatment naive and treatment experienced patients. Results from a trial (ACTG 241) evaluated triple therapy with nevirapine, zidovudine and didanosine compared to zidovudine+didanosine, in 398 HIV-1-infected patients (mean baseline 153 CD4+cells/mm^3; plasma HIV-1 RNA 4.59 $\log_{10}$ copies/ml), who had received at least 6 months of nucleoside analogue therapy prior to enrolment (median 115 weeks). These heavily experienced patients demonstrated a significant improvement of the triple therapy group over the double therapy group for one year in both viral RNA and CD4+ cell counts.

A durable response for at least one year was documented in a trial (INCAS) for the triple therapy arm with nevirapine, zidovudine and didanosine compared to zidovudine+didanosine or nevirapine+zidovudine in 151 HIV-1 infected, treatment naive patients with CD4+ cell counts of 200–600 cells/mm^3 (mean 376 cells/mm^3) and a mean baseline plasma HIV-1 RNA concentration of 4.41 $\log_{10}$ copies/ml (25,704 copies/ml). Treatment doses were nevirapine, 200 mg daily for two weeks, followed by 200 mg twice daily, or placebo; zidovudine, 200 mg three times daily; didanosine, 125 or 200 mg twice daily (depending on the weight).

The two largest controlled trials of nevirapine described above have both evaluated nevirapine in combination with zidovudine and didanosine; there is currently limited information on long term safety and activity with combinations of other antiretroviral medicinal products. Nevirapine has also been studied in combination with other antiretroviral agents, e.g., zalcitabine, indinavir, ritonavir, and saquinavir. Ongoing trials are examining nevirapine in combinations with nelfinavir, lamivudine, and stavudine. No new and overt safety problems have been reported for these combinations, but clinical experience is still somewhat limited.

Studies are on-going to evaluate the efficacy and safety of combination therapies with nevirapine in patients failing protease inhibitor therapy. Data will be collected on the efficacy and safety of protease inhibitor therapy following failure with nevirapine combination.

Pharmacokinetic properties: Nevirapine is readily absorbed (>90%) after oral administration in healthy volunteers and in adults with HIV-1 infection. Absolute bioavailability in 12 healthy adults following single-dose administration was 93±9% (mean SD) for a 50 mg tablet and 91±8% for an oral solution. Peak plasma nevirapine concentrations of 2 0.4 mcg/ml (7.5 μM) were attained by 4 hours following a single 200 mg dose. Following multiple doses, nevirapine peak concentrations appear to increase linearly in the dose range of 200 to 400 mg/day. Steady state trough nevirapine concentrations of 4.5 1.9 mcg/ml (17±7 μM), (n=242) were attained at 400 mg/day.

The absorption of nevirapine is not affected by food, antacids or medicinal products which are formulated with an alkaline buffering agent (e.g., didanosine).

Nevirapine is lipophilic and is essentially non-ionised at physiologic pH. Following intravenous administration to healthy adults, the volume of distribution (Vdss) of nevirapine was 1.21±0.09 L/kg, suggesting that nevirapine is widely distributed in humans. Nevirapine readily crosses the placenta and is found in breast milk. Nevirapine is about 60% bound to plasma proteins in the plasma concentration range of 1–10 mcg/ml. Nevirapine concentrations in human cerebrospinal fluid (n=6) were 45% (5%) of the concentrations in plasma; this ratio is approximately equal to the fraction not bound to plasma protein.

In vivo studies in humans *in vitro* studies with human liver microsomes have shown that nevirapine is extensively biotransformed via cytochrome P450 (oxidative) metabolism to several hydroxylated metabolites. *In vitro* studies with human liver microsomes suggest that oxidative metabolism of nevirapine is mediated primarily by cytochrome P450 isozymes from the CYP3A family, although other isozymes may have a secondary role. In a mass balance/excretion study in eight healthy male volunteers dosed to steady state with nevirapine 200 mg given twice daily followed by a single 50 mg dose of 14C-nevirapine, approximately 91.4±10.5% of the radiolabeled dose was recovered, with urine (81.3±11.1%) representing the primary route of excretion compared to faeces (10.1±1.5%). Greater than 80% of the radioactivity in urine was made up of glucuronide conjugates of hydroxylated metabolites. Thus cytochrome P450 metabolism, glucuronide conjugation, and urinary excretion of glucuronidated metabolites represent the primary route of nevirapine biotransformation and elimination in humans. Only a small fraction (<5%) of the radioactivity in urine (representing <3% of the total dose) was made up of parent compound; therefore, renal excretion plays a minor role in elimination of the parent compound.

Nevirapine has been shown to be an inducer of hepatic cytochrome P450 metabolic enzymes. The pharmacokinetics of autoinduction are characterised by an approximately 1.5 to 2 fold increase in the apparent oral clearance of nevirapine as treatment continues from a single dose to two-to-four weeks of dosing with 200–400 mg/day. Autoinduction also results in a corresponding decrease in the terminal phase half-life of nevirapine in plasma from approximately 45 hours (single dose) to approximately 25–30 hours following multiple dosing with 200–400 mg/day.

The pharmacokinetics of nevirapine have not been evaluated in patients with either renal of hepatic dysfunction.

Although a slightly higher weight adjusted volume of distribution of nevirapine was found in female subjects compared to males, no significant gender differences in nevirapine plasma concentrations following single or multiple dose administrations were seen. Nevirapine pharmacokinetics in HIV-1 infected adults do not appear to change with age (range 19–68 years) or race (Black, Hispanic, or Caucasian). Nevirapine has not been specifically investigated in patients over the age of 65.

Preclinical safety data: Preclinical data revealed no special hazard for humans other than those observed in clinical studies based on conventional studies of safety, pharmacology, repeated dose toxicity, and genotoxicity. Long-term carcinogenicity studies of nevirapine in animals are currently under progress. In reproductive toxicology studies, evidence of impaired fertility was seen in rats.

Pharmaceutical particulars

List of excipients: Microcrystalline cellulose, lactose monohydrate, polyvidone K26/28 or K/25, sodium starch glycolate, colloidal silicon dioxide and magnesium stearate.

Incompatibilities: None reported.

Shelf life: 2 years.

Special precautions for storage: There are no special storage precautions.

Nature and content of container: Polyvinyl chloride (PVC)/aluminium foil push-through blister units (blister card of 10 tablets, 6 blister cards per carton).

Marketing authorisation holder Boehringer Ingelheim International GmbH, Binger Strasse 173, 55216 Ingelheim am Rhein, Germany.

Marketing authorisation number EU/1/97/055/001

Date of first authorisation/renewal of the authorisation 5 February 1998

Date of (partial) revision of the text February 1998

Legal category POM.

***Trade Mark**

Boehringer Ingelheim Limited Self-Medication Division
Ellesfield Avenue
Bracknell
Berkshire RG12 8YS

☎ 01344 424600 🖷 01344 741399

DULCO-LAX*

Qualitative and quantitative composition
Dulco-lax: Circular, biconvex, yellow, sugar-coated and enteric-coated tablets each containing 5 mg of bisacodyl.

Dulco-lax Suppositories for Children 5 mg: Smooth white torpedo shaped suppositories, each containing 5 mg of bisacodyl.

Dulco-lax Suppositories 10 mg: Smooth white torpedo shaped suppositories, each containing 10 mg of bisacodyl.

Pharmaceutical form
Tablets for oral administration.
Suppositories for rectal administration.

Clinical particulars
Therapeutic indications: Constipation, either chronic or of recent onset, whenever a stimulant laxative is required.

Bowel clearance before surgery or radiological investigation. Replacement of the evacuant enema in all its indications.

Posology and method of administration Dulco-lax is suitable for routine use in adults of all ages, and in children over 10 years of age. Children under 10 years should not take Dulco-lax without medical advice. Unless otherwise prescribed by the doctor, the following dosages are recommended:

1. For constipation
Sugar-coated tablets (5 mg)
Adults and children over 10 years: One to two tablets at night (5–10 mg).

Children under 10 years should not take Dulco-lax without medical advice.

Children aged 4 to 10 years: One tablet (5 mg) at night.

Children under 4 years: Paediatric suppositories (5 mg) are recommended.

Sugar-coated tablets should be taken at night to produce evacuation the following morning. The tablets have a special coating and should, therefore, not be taken together with milk or antacids. The tablets should be swallowed whole with adequate fluid.

Suppositories (5 & 10 mg)
Adults and children over 10 years: One 10 mg suppository to be administered in the morning.

Children under 10 years: One 5 mg suppository to be administered under medical supervision only.

Suppositories are usually effective in about 30 minutes. A suppository should be unwrapped and inserted into the rectum pointed end first.

2. For preparation for diagnostic procedures and preoperatively
When using Dulco-lax to prepare the patient for radiographic examination of the abdomen or employing it preoperatively, tablets should be combined with suppositories in order to achieve complete evacuation of the intestine.

Adults and children over 10 years: Two to four tablets the night before and insert one 10 mg suppository the following morning.

Children aged 4–10 years: One tablet the night before and insert one 5 mg suppository the following morning.

No specific information on the use of this product in the elderly is available. Clinical trials have included patients over 65 years and no adverse reactions specific to this age group have been reported.

Contra-indications: Dulco-lax must not be used in patients with ileus, intestinal obstruction, acute surgical abdominal conditions such as acute appendicitis, acute inflammatory bowel diseases, and in severe dehydration.

Dulco-lax suppositories should not be used when anal fissures or ulcerative proctitis with mucosal damage are present.

Special warnings and special precautions for use: As with all laxatives, Dulco-lax should not be used on a continuous daily basis for long periods.

If laxatives are needed every day, the cause of constipation should be investigated. Prolonged excessive use may lead to electrolyte imbalance and hypokalaemia, and may precipitate the onset of rebound constipation.

The use of suppositories may lead to painful sensations and local irritation, especially in anal fissures and ulcerative proctitis.

Children under 10 years should not take Dulco-lax without medical advice.

Interaction with other medicaments and other forms of interaction: The concomitant use of antacids and milk products may reduce the resistance of the coating of the tablets and result in dyspepsia and gastric irritation.

The concomitant use of diuretics or adreno-corticosteroids may increase the risk of electrolyte imbalance. However, this situation only arises if excessive doses of Dulco-lax are taken (see *Overdose* section).

Pregnancy and lactation: There are no reports of undesirable or damaging effects during pregnancy or to the foetus attributable to the use of Dulco-lax. Nevertheless, medicines should not be used in pregnancy, especially the first trimester, unless the expected benefit is thought to outweigh any possible risk to the foetus.

Although the active ingredient of Dulco-lax is not known to be excreted in breast milk, its use during breast feeding is not recommended.

Effects on ability to drive and use machines: Dulco-lax has no effect on ability to drive and use machinery.

Undesirable effects: Abdominal discomfort and diarrhoea may occasionally occur. Local irritation has been reported when the suppository formulation has been administered.

Overdose: Symptoms: If high doses are taken diarrhoea, abdominal cramps and a clinically significant loss of potassium and other electrolytes can occur. This may also lead to increased sensitivity to cardiac glycosides.

Therapy: Within a short time after ingestion of oral forms of Dulco-lax, absorption can be minimised or prevented by inducing vomiting. Otherwise, gastric lavage should be performed. Replacement of fluids and correction of electrolyte imbalance (particularly hypokalaemia) may be required. This is especially important in the elderly and the young. Administration of antispasmodics may be of some value.

Pharmacological properties
Pharmacodynamic properties: Bisacodyl is a locally acting laxative from the triarylmethane group, which after bacterial cleavage in the colon, has the dual-action of stimulating the mucosa of both the large intestine causing peristalsis and of the rectum causing increased motility and a feeling of rectal fullness. The rectal effect may help to restore the 'call to stool' although its clinical relevance remains to be established.

Pharmacokinetic properties: Hydrolysis of bisacodyl by enzymes of the enteric mucosa forms desacetylbisacodyl which is absorbed and excreted partly via urine and bile as glucuronide. By bacterial cleavage the active form, the free diphenol, is formed in the colon. Formulations of bisacodyl which are resistant to gastric and small intestinal juice, like Dulco-lax sugar-coated tablets, reach the colon without any appreciable absorption and therefore avoid enterohepatic circulation. Consequently, these oral forms have an onset of action between 6–12 hours after administration.

Suppository formulations of bisacodyl have an onset of action within 15–30 minutes, although in some cases it may be prolonged to 15–60 minutes. The onset of action is determined by the release of the active substance from the preparation.

After administration, only small amounts of the drug are systemically available. Urinary excretion reflects low systemic burden after oral and rectal administraiton.

There is no relationship between the laxative effect and plasma levels of the active diphenol.

Preclinical safety data: There are no preclinical data of relevance to the prescriber which are additional to that already included in other sections of the SPC.

Pharmaceutical particulars
List of excipients: Tablets: Lactose, maize starch (dried), soluble maize starch, glycerol (85%), magnesium stearate, sucrose, talc, acacia (powered), titanium dioxide, eudragit L, eudragit S, dibutyl phthalate, macrogol 6000, yellow iron oxide, white beeswax, carnauba wax and shellac.
Suppositories: Hard fat (Adeps solidus).
Incompatibilities: None stated.
Shelf life: 5 years.
Special precautions for storage: Store below 25°C. Protect from light.
Nature and contents of container: Dulco-lax Tablets are presented in aluminium foil blister strips coated with PVC film or combination lacquer.

Dulco-lax Suppositories and Dulco-lax Suppositories for Children are presented in aluminium foil blister strips coated with polyethylene.

Dulco-lax Tablets are available in packs of 10, 20 and 60 (Packs of 10 are available for general sale in the UK). Dulco-lax Suppositories are available in packs of 10 and 20, and Dulco-lax Suppositories for Children are available in packs of 5.
Instructions for use/handling: None stated.

Marketing authorisation numbers

Dulco-lax Tablets	6772/0007
Dulco-lax Suppositories	6772/0009
Dulco-lax Suppositories for Children	6772/0008

Date of approval/revision of SPC March 1998
Legal category P.

LAXOBERAL* LIQUID
DULCO-LAX* LIQUID

Qualitative and quantitative composition A golden orange coloured liquid, with a fruit-like odour and taste containing 5 mg of sodium picosulphate in each 5 ml.

Pharmaceutical form Oral solution.

Clinical particulars
Therapeutic indications: Constipation of any aetiology and bowel clearance before surgery, childbirth or radiological investigations.
Posology and method of administration: For oral administration.

Unless otherwise prescribed by the doctor, the following dosages are recommended:

Adults and children over 10 years: One to two 5 ml spoonfuls (5–10 mg) at night.

Children under 10 years: Not to be taken by children under 10 years without medical advice.

Children (4–10 years): Half to one 5 ml spoonful (2.5–5 mg) at night.

Children under 4 years: The recommended dosage is 250 micrograms per kilogram body weight.

Diluent: Can be diluted with purified water.
Contra-indications: Not to be used in patients with ileus, intestinal obstruction, acute surgical abdominal conditions like acute appendicitis, acute inflammatory bowel diseases, and in severe dehydration.
Special warnings and special precautions for use: As with all laxatives, this product should not be taken on a continuous daily basis for long periods.

If laxatives are needed every day, the cause of constipation should be investigated.

Prolonged excessive use may lead to electrolyte imbalance and hypokalaemia, and may precipitate onset of rebound constipation.

Not to be taken by children under 10 years without medical advice.
Interaction with other medicaments and other forms of interaction: The concomitant use of diuretics or adreno-corticosteroids may increase the risk of electrolyte imbalance. However, this situation only arises if excessive doses are taken (see *Overdose*).

Concurrent administration of broad spectrum antibiotics may reduce the laxative action of this product.
Pregnancy and lactation: There are no reports of undesirable or damaging effects during pregnancy or to the foetus attributable to the use of this product. Nevertheless, medicines should not be used in pregnancy, especially the first trimester, unless the expected benefit is thought to outweigh any possible risk to the foetus.

Although the active ingredient is not known to be excreted in breast milk, use of this product during breast feeding is not recommended.

Effects on ability to drive and use machines: None stated.

Undesirable effects: Abdominal discomfort and diarrhoea may occasionally occur.

Overdose

Symptoms: If high doses are taken diarrhoea, abdominal cramps and a clinically significant loss of potassium and other electrolytes can occur. This may also lead to increased sensitivity to cardiac glycosides.

Therapy: Within a short time of ingestion, absorption can be minimised or prevented by inducing vomiting or by gastric lavage. Replacement of fluids and correction of electrolyte imbalance may be required. This is especially important in the elderly and the young.

Administration of antispasmodics may be of some value.

Pharmacological properties

Pharmacodynamic properties: Sodium picosulphate is a locally acting laxative from the triarylmethane group, which after bacterial cleavage in the colon, has the dual-action of stimulating the mucosa of both the large intestine causing peristalsis and of the rectum causing increased motility and a feeling of rectal fullness. The rectal effect may help to restore the 'call to stool' although its clinical relevance remains to be established.

Pharmacokinetic properties: After oral ingestion, sodium picosulphate reaches the colon without any appreciable absorption. Therefore, enterohepatic circulation is avoided. By bacterial cleavage the active form, the free diphenol, is formed in the colon. Consequently, there is an onset of action between 6–12 hours, which is determined by the release of the active substance from the preparation.

After administration, only small amounts of the drug are systemically available. Urinary excretion reflects low systemic burden after oral administration.

There is no relationship between the laxative effect and plasma levels of the active diphenol.

Preclinical safety data: There are no pre-clinical data of relevance to the prescriber which are additional to that already included in other sections of the SPC.

Pharmaceutical particulars

List of excipients: Sodium Carboxymethylcellulose; Methyl p-Hydroxybenzoate; Propyl p-Hydroxybenzoate; Glycerine; Aroma Tutti Frutti (flavouring); Saccharin Sodium; FD & C Yellow 6 (E110) (colouring); Alcohol 96%; 0.1 M Sodium Hydroxide; Purified Water.

Incompatibilities: None stated.

Shelf life: 5 years.

Special precautions for storage: Store at room temperature. Protect from light.

Nature and contents of container: Pack sizes of 30, 40, 50, 60, 90, 100, 300 and 500 ml are registered.

100 ml and 300 ml amber glass bottles with aluminium ROPP caps are marketed under the trade name of Laxoberal.

100 ml amber glass bottles with aluminium ROPP caps underfilled to 90 ml are marketed under the trade name of Dulco-Lax liquid.

Instructions for use/handling: Not applicable.

Marketing authorisation holder: Windsor Healthcare Limited, Ellesfield Avenue, Bracknell, Berkshire RG12 8YS.

Marketing authorisation number PL 6772/0011

Date of revision of the text March 1998

Legal category
90, 100, 300, 500 ml: P
30, 40, 50, 60 ml: GSL

PHARMATON* CAPSULES

Qualitative and quantitative composition Each capsule contains:

Active ingredients	*Declaration per capsule*
Standardised Panax ginseng extract	40.0 mg
G115 Pharmaton	41.0
Vitamin A Palmitate	(Vit.A) 2667 IU
Cholecalciferol	(Vit.D3) 200 IU
D,L-α-Tocopherol acetate	(Vit.E) 10 mg
Thiamine mononitrate	(Vit.B1) 1.4 mg
Riboflavine	(Vit.B2) 1.6 mg
Pyridoxine hydrochloride	(Vit.B6) 2.0 mg
Cyanocobalamine	(Vit.B12) 1.0 mcg
Biotin	150.0 mcg
Nicotinamide	18.0 mg
Ascorbic acid	60.0 mg
Folic acid	0.1 mg
Copper(II) sulphate dried	(Cu: 2.0 mg) 5.6 mg
Sodium selenite, dried	(Se: 50.0 mcg) 111.0 mcg
Manganese(II) sulphate monohydrate	(Mn: 2.5 mg) 7.75 mg
Magnesium sulphate, dried	(Mg: 10.0 mg) 71.0 mg
Iron(II) sulphate, dried	(Fe: 10.0 mg) 33.0 mg
Zinc sulphate, monohydrate	(Zn: 1.0 mg) 2.75 mg
Dibasic calcium phosphate, anhydrous	(Ca: 100.0 mg) 340.0 mg
Lecithin	100.0 mg

Pharmaceutical form Soft gelatin capsules for oral use.

Clinical particulars

Therapeutic indications: Pharmaton Capsules contain vitamins, minerals and standardised Ginseng Extract G115 in amounts which suit the body's daily requirements. The capsules are indicated for:

States of exhaustion (eg caused by stress), tiredness, feeling of weakness, vitality deficiency.

Prevention and treatment of symptoms caused by ill-balanced or deficient nutrition.

Posology and method of administration:

Adults: The recommended daily dosage is one to two capsules per day. The first capsule should preferably be taken with breakfast and the second with lunch.

Children: Not recommended for use in children.

Elderly: There no special dosage recommendations for the elderly.

Contra-indications: Hypersensitivity to any of the ingredients. Hypercalcaemia and/or hypercalciuria, haemochromatosis, iron overload syndrome, hypervitaminosis A or D, concomitant retinoid (eg against acne) or vitamin D therapy, renal insufficiency, pregnancy.

Other special warnings and precautions: An allowance should be made for vitamins or minerals obtained from other sources.

Interaction with other medicaments and other forms of interaction: There is no evidence from clinical experience that Pharmaton Capsules interacts with other medications.

Pregnancy and lactation: Reproduction studies with animals using the standardised Panax ginseng extract G115 Pharmaton showed no adverse effects on fertility, nor any teratogenic effects. However, controlled studies with pregnant women are not available.

Controlled studies with women using multivitamin-mineral preparations at the usual dosage during the course of the first trimester resulted in no fetal risks. There are no signs indicating a risk if this type of preparation is taken during the second and third trimesters, and probability of injuring the fetus appears to be very low.

Large doses of vitamin A (10,000 IU per day) have been found to be teratogenic if administered during the first trimester of pregnancy. Vitamin D given during the last trimester of pregnancy may cause hypercalcaemia in infants. As with many other medicines an assessment of benefits versus risks should be made before this product is administered during this period.

WARNING: Do not take Vitamin A supplements if you are pregnant or likely to become pregnant except on the advice of a doctor or ante-natal clinic.

Effects on ability to drive and use machines: None known.

Undesirable effects: Gastrointestinal reactions (eg abdominal pain, nausea) have been reported rarely.

Overdose: Nervousness may occur following an overdose of the product.

The toxicity of the product in large overdoses is caused by the toxicity of the liposoluble vitamins A and D. A *safe dose* for both vitamins is considered to be 5-10 x RDA (each capsule contains the EU %RDA for vitamins A and D).

Prolonged supply of larger amounts (40-55 x RDA for Vitamin A; 10-25 x RDA for Vitamin D) can cause symptoms of chronic toxicity. Acute toxic symptoms are only seen at even higher doses.

Iron: Severe acute toxicity in man has been reported from doses of iron ranging from 12-1500 x RDA (each capsule contains the UK %RDA for iron). Most incidents of acute iron toxicity have resulted from accidental oral ingestion of iron pills by children. Longer-term doses of iron up to 6-7 x RDA have been reported to have no toxic effect.

Symptoms: Initial symptoms include nausea, vomiting, diarrhoea, abdominal pain, haematemesis, rectal bleeding, lethargy and circulatory collapse. Hyperglycaemia and metabolic acidosis may also occur.

Treatment: To minimise or prevent further absorption of the medication, as follows:

– Induce vomiting eg by administration of an emetic

– Gastric lavage with desferrioxamine solution (2 g/l). Then desferrioxamine (5–10 g in 50-100 ml water) should be introduced into the stomach to be retained.

– Severe poisoning: Shock and/or coma with high iron levels (serum iron >90 μmol/l in children, >142 μmol/l in adults); immediate supportive measures plus i.v. infusion of desferrioxamine should be instituted.

– Less severe poisoning: i.m. desferrioxamine is recommended (1 g 4-6 hourly in children; 50 mg/kg up to a maximum dose of 4 g in adults).

Pharmacological properties

Pharmacodynamic properties: Pharmaton Capsules exert a stimulant effect at physical and psychological levels through the combined action of various substances on the basic metabolic processes.

The standardised ginseng extract G115 raises the general level of cellular activity, which is expressed by a pronounced increase in the physical and mental capacity.

In animal experiments, it caused a reduction of lactic acid concentration in muscles during exercise. An increase in the dopamine and noradrenaline content and a reduction in the serotonin content in the brain stem could be observed.

Vitamins, minerals and trace elements correct and prevent impairment of the cell metabolism in situations with increased demands. Low supply of vitamins, minerals, and trace elements may cause disturbances, such as debility, tiredness, decrease in vitality, reduced force of resistance, and decelerated convalescence. The composition and dosages of the preparation were chosen according to the European RDA-requirements for food supplements.

Choline, inositol, linoleic acid and linolenic acid, in the form of lecithin, improve energy output and lipid metabolism.

Pharmacokinetic properties: Pharmacokinetic studies of Pharmaton Capsules have not been carried out, because of the complex composition of the product and the small quantities of the active ingredients contained. Moreover, these substances are well known.

Pharmacokinetic studies of the standardised ginseng extract G115 are not possible, because it is a complex extract. In the ginseng root more than 200 substances have been identified to date. Pharmacokinetic studies of individual purified ginsenosides have been carried out in various animal species:

Using radioactively labelled (^{14}C) Ginsenoside Rgl, originated from the standarised Panax ginseng extract G115 Pharmaton, a bioavailability of 30% was determined in mice.

With intraperitoneal application, depending on the tested animal species and the Ginsenoside type, a half-life of between 27 minutes and 14.5 hours was measured.

Preclinical safety data

Acute toxicity: The oral LD_{50} of the standardized Panax ginseng extract G115 Pharmaton is more than 5 g/kg of body weight in the mouse and the rat, and more than 2 g/kg in the mini-pig.

Reproduction toxicity: The effect of standardised Panax ginseng extract G115 Pharmaton on reproductive performance was studied in two generations of Sprague-Dawley rats. Animals of both sexes were fed either control diet or diet supplemented with the standardised Panax ginseng extract G115 Pharmaton at dose levels of 1.5, 5 or 15 mg/kg body weight/day. Parameters of reproduction and lactation in the treated groups were comparable to those of the controls for two generations of dams and pups. No treatment-related effects were seen in weekly body weights and food consumption, haematological and blood chemistry parameters, and ophthalmic, macroscopic and histopathological examinations.

Fetal toxicity: The standardised Panax ginseng extract G115 Pharmaton, administered to pregnant Wistar rats and pregnant New Zealand rabbits, caused no abnormality in the foetal development.

The rats were treated with 40 mg/kg/day from the 1st to the 15th day after mating.

The rabbits were treated with 20 mg/kg/day from the 7th to the 16th day after mating.

The fetuses were removed by caesarean section on the 21st day in the rats and on the 27th day in the rabbits.

Pharmaceutical particulars

List of excipients:

Capsule: Rape oil; hard fat; ethyl vanillin; arachis oil; triglycerides, medium chain; gelatin powder.

Capsule shell: Gelatin; glycerol 85%; iron oxide red (E172); iron oxide black (E172).

Incompatibilities: None stated.

Shelf-life: Two years

Special precautions for storage: Pharmaton Capsules should be kept tightly closed in a dry place below 25°C.

Nature and contents of container: Registered packs: Brown glass bottles (hydrolytical class III, PhEur) with

pilfer proof aluminium caps (with rubber inserts) containing either 30, 60, 90 or 100 capsules.
or
Aluminium foil/polyvinylchloride/polyvinylidenchloride blister packs of 4, 30, 60, 90 and 100 capsules.
Current marketed packs: Brown glass bottles (hydrolytical class III, PhEur) with pilfer proof aluminium caps (with rubber inserts) containing either 30, 60 or 100 capsules.

Instructions for use/handling: None stated.

Marketing authorisation number 00015/0250

Date of approval/revision of SPC January 1999.

Legal category P.

**Trade Mark*

Borg Medicare
Dornstauden 15
91233 Neunkirchen-Rollhofen
Germany

☎ 9153 923983 🗋 9153 923983

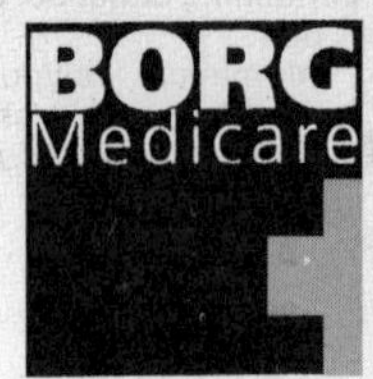

LASIKAL* TABLETS

Presentation Lasikal Tablets each contain 20 mg Frusemide BP and 750 mg (10 mmol K^+) slow-release potassium chloride. They are presented as film-coated, biconvex, twin-layered tablets, 12.5 mm in diameter, marked 'LK' on one side. The frusemide layer is white and the slow-release potassium chloride layer is yellow.

Excipients include lactose and Sunset Yellow.

Uses Lasikal contains a short-acting diuretic and a slow-release potassium supplement. It is intended for the treatment of oedema in patients who require potassium supplementation.

Dosage and administration The recommended initial adult dose is 2 tablets (40 mg frusemide and 20 mmol K^+) to be taken each morning. This may be increased to four tablets daily, to be taken as 2 tablets each morning and evening, or may be decreased to 1 tablet each morning, according to clinical response.

Lasikal tablets must be swallowed whole.

Children: Lasikal tablets cannot be sub-divided and are unsuitable for paediatric use.

Elderly: Frusemide and potassium may both be excreted more slowly in the elderly.

Contra-indications, warnings, etc
Contra-indications: Lasikal is contra-indicated in anuria, hyperkalaemia, precomatose states associated with liver cirrhosis, Addison's disease and in patients taking potassium-sparing diuretics. Hypersensitivity to frusemide or sulphonamides is also a contra-indication.

Warnings: Patients with prostatic hypertrophy or impairment of micturition have an increased risk of developing acute retention.

Where indicated, steps should be taken to correct hypotension or hypovolaemia before commencing therapy.

The dosage of concurrently administered cardiac glycosides or antihypertensive agents may require adjustment.

ACE inhibitors should not be used in combination with Lasikal as serum potassium levels may be increased.

The toxic effects of nephrotoxic antibiotics may be increased by concomitant administration of potent diuretics such as frusemide.

Latent diabetes may become manifest or the insulin requirements of diabetic patients may increase.

Care should be exercised when treating patients with renal insufficiency because of the risk of hyperkalaemia.

In common with other diuretics, serum lithium levels may be increased when lithium is given concomitantly with frusemide, necessitating adjustment of the lithium dosage.

Certain non-steroidal anti-inflammatory agents have been shown to antagonise the action of diuretics such as frusemide and may cause renal failure in cases of pre-existing hypovolaemia.

Frusemide may sometimes attenuate the effects of other drugs (e.g. the effects of antidiabetics and of pressor amines) and sometimes potentiate them (e.g. the effects of salicylates, theophylline, lithium and curare-type muscle relaxants).

Interactions have also been reported with ototoxic antibiotics. In cases of concomitant glucocorticoid therapy or abuse of laxatives, the risk of an increased potassium loss should be borne in mind.

Precautions: Results of animal work, in general, show no hazardous effect of frusemide in pregnancy. There is clinical evidence of safety of the drug in the third trimester of human pregnancy; however, frusemide should be used in pregnancy only if strictly indicated and for short term treatment.

Nursing mothers: As frusemide may inhibit lactation or pass into breast milk, it should be used with caution in nursing mothers.

Overdosage: In cases of overdose there is a danger of dehydration and electrolyte depletion due to excessive diuresis. Treatment should therefore be aimed at fluid replacement and correction of the electrolyte imbalance.

Side-effects: Lasikal is generally well tolerated. Side-effects of a minor nature such as nausea, malaise or gastric upset may occur but are not usually severe enough to necessitate withdrawal of treatment.

As with other diuretics, electrolytes and water balance may be disturbed as a result of diuresis after prolonged therapy. This may cause symptoms such as headache, hypotension or muscle cramps.

Serum calcium levels may be reduced; in very rare cases tetany has been observed. Nephrocalcinosis has been reported in premature infants.

Isolated cases of acute pancreatitis have been reported after long-term diuretic (including frusemide) treatment. Disorders of hearing after frusemide are rare and, in most cases reversible. They may occur if frusemide is injected too rapidly, particularly in patients with renal insufficiency.

As with other diuretics a transient rise in creatinine and urea levels has also been reported with frusemide.

The incidence of allergic reactions, such as skin rash, photosensitivity, vasculitis, fever or interstitial nephritis, is very low, but when these occur treatment should be withdrawn.

In common with other sulphonamide-based diuretics, hyperuricaemia may occur and, in rare cases, clinical gout may be precipitated.

Serum cholesterol and triglyceride levels may rise during frusemide treatment. During long term therapy they will usually return to normal within six months.

Bone marrow depression has been reported as a rare complication and necessitates withdrawal of treatment.

Pre-existing metabolic alkalosis (e.g. in decompensated cirrhosis of the liver) may be aggravated by frusemide treatment.

Reduced mental alertness may impair ability to drive or operate dangerous machinery.

Pharmaceutical precautions Lasikal should be stored below 25°C in a dry place, protected from light, in the original container or in containers similar to those of the manufacturer. Lasikal tablets should be dispensed in moisture-tight containers which offer protection from light.

Legal category POM.

Package quantities Lasikal is available in containers of 100 tablets.

Further information Frusemide produces a prompt and effective diuresis which lasts for approximately four hours following oral administration. The potassium chloride in Lasikal tablets is contained in an inert matrix which allows slow release of potassium ions, thereby helping to avoid high local K^+ion concentrations in the intestine.

Ghost tablets may appear in the patient's faeces.

Product licence number 13402/0032.

Product licence holder: Hoechst Marion Roussel Ltd., Broadwater Park, Denham, Uxbridge, Middlesex UB9 5HP.

LASILACTONE* CAPSULES

Presentation Lasilactone Capsules each contain 20 mg of Frusemide BP and 50 mg Spironolactone BP (micronised). They are presented as hard gelatin capsules with a light blue opaque cap and white opaque body. Excipients include lactose.

Uses Lasilactone contains a short-acting diuretic and a long-acting aldosterone antagonist. It is indicated in the treatment of resistant oedema where this is associated with secondary hyperaldosteronism; conditions include chronic congestive cardiac failure and hepatic cirrhosis.

Treatment with Lasilactone should be reserved for cases refractory to a diuretic alone at conventional dosage.

This fixed ratio combination should only be used if titration with the component drugs separately indicates that this product is appropriate.

The use of Lasilactone in the management of essential hypertension should be restricted to patients with demonstrated hyperaldosteronism. It is recommended that in these patients also, this combination should only be used if titration with the component drugs separately indicates that this product is appropriate.

Dosage and administration In accordance with the recommendations on usage given above the dosage of Lasilactone will normally be in the range of 1 to 4 capsules daily (20–80 mg Lasix and 50–200 mg spironolactone).

Children: The product is not suitable for use in children.

Elderly: Frusemide and spironolactone may both be excreted more slowly in the elderly.

Contra-indications, warnings, etc
Contra-indications: Lasilactone should not be given in acute renal failure, renal insufficiency (creatinine clearance <30 ml/minute ≡ serum creatinine of about 1.8–2.0 mg/100 ml), anuric states, hyperkalaemia, Addison's disease or in patients hypersensitive to frusemide, spironolactone or sulphonamides.

Warnings: Patients with prostatic hypertrophy or impairment of micturition have an increased risk of developing acute retention. Caution should also be exercised in the presence of liver disease as hepatic coma may be precipitated in susceptible cases. Administration of Lasilactone should be avoided in the presence of hyperkalaemia and hyponatraemia. Concomitant administration of triamterene, amiloride or potassium supplements or non-steroidal anti-inflammatory drugs is not recommended as hyperkalaemia may result. Where indicated, steps should be taken to correct hypotension, hypovolaemia and severe hypokalaemia before starting therapy.

The dosage of concurrently administered cardiac glycosides or hypotensive agents may require adjustment.

ACE inhibitors should not be used in combination with Lasilactone as serum potassium levels may be increased.

The toxic effects of nephrotoxic antibiotics may be potentiated by concurrent administration of potent diuretics such as frusemide.

Latent diabetes may become manifest or the insulin requirements of diabetic patients may increase.

In common with other diuretics, serum lithium levels may be increased when lithium is given concomitantly with frusemide, necessitating adjustment of the lithium dosage.

Certain non-steroidal anti-inflammatory agents have been shown to antagonise the action of diuretics such as frusemide and may cause renal failure in cases of pre-existing hypovolaemia. Frusemide may sometimes attenuate the effects of other drugs (e.g. the effects of antidiabetics and of pressor amines) and sometimes potentiate them (e.g. the effects of salicylates, theophylline, lithium and curare-type muscle relaxants). Salicylates may attenuate the effect of spironolactone. Concomitant glucocorticoid medication or abuse of laxatives may lead to potassium deficiency. In the presence of potassium deficiency the effect of cardiac glycosides may be enhanced.

Interactions have also been reported with carbenoxolone and with ototoxic antibiotics.

Concurrent administration of Lasilactone and sucralfate should be avoided as sucralfate decreases the absorption of frusemide.

Carcinogenicity: Spironolactone has been shown to produce tumours in rats when administered at high doses over a long period of time. The significance of these findings with respect to clinical use is not certain. However, the long-term use of spironolactone in young patients requires careful consideration of the benefits and the potential hazard involved.

Precautions: Caution should be observed in patients liable to electrolyte deficiency.

Results of animal work, in general, show no hazardous effect of frusemide in pregnancy. There is clinical evidence of the safety of the drug in the third trimester of human pregnancy; however, frusemide should be used in pregnancy only if strictly indicated and for short term treatment.

Spironolactone or its metabolites may cross the placental barrier.

Nursing mothers: Lasilactone is contra-indicated in nursing mothers because canrenone, a metabolite of the spironolactone component of this preparation, appears in breast milk. (Frusemide may inhibit lactation or pass into breast milk).

Overdosage: In cases of overdosage with Lasilactone there is a danger of severe electrolyte disturbance and dehydration due to excessive diuresis. Signs of overdosage may include drowsiness, mental confusion, nausea, vomiting, dizziness or diarrhoea. Electrolyte disturbances such as hyperkalaemia and hyponatraemia may be induced. Hyperkalaemia may be manifested clinically by paraesthesia, weakness, flaccid paralysis or muscle spasm and may be difficult to distinguish from hypokalaemia. Electrocardiographic changes may be the earliest signs of potassium disturbances.

Treatment should be aimed at the replacement of fluid and the correction of any electrolyte imbalance.

Side-effects: Frusemide is generally well tolerated. Side-effects of a minor nature such as nausea, malaise or gastric upset may occur but are not usually severe enough to necessitate withdrawal of treatment.

As with other diuretics, electrolytes and water balance may be disturbed as a result of diuresis after prolonged therapy. This may cause symptoms such as headache, hypotension or muscle cramps.

Calcium depletion may occur. Nephrocalcinosis has been reported in premature infants treated with frusemide.

The incidence of allergic reactions, such as skin rashes (including photosensitivity reactions), vasculitis, fever or interstitial nephritis, is very low, but when these occur treatment should be withdrawn.

Auditory disorders and acute pancreatitis have been reported with high dose parenteral frusemide.

A transient rise in creatinine and urea levels has also been reported. In common with other sulphonamide-based diuretics, the administration of frusemide may induce a rise in serum uric acid; in rare cases, clinical gout may be precipitated.

Serum cholesterol and triglyceride levels may rise during frusemide treatment. During long term therapy they will usually return to normal within six months.

Bone marrow depression has been reported as a rare complication of Lasix therapy and necessitates withdrawal of treatment.

Spironolactone has been reported to induce gastrointestinal intolerance. Stomach ulcers (sometimes with bleeding) have been reported rarely. Eosinophilia may occur occasionally. Spironolactone may also cause drowsiness, headache, ataxia, lethargy and mental confusion. Dose-dependent mastodynia and reversible gynaecomastia may occur in both sexes. Urticaria may occur occasionally. Maculopapular or erythematous cutaneous eruptions have been reported rarely. In women, dose dependent menstrual irregularities and hirsuitism may be seen and in men impairment of potency. Spironolactone may cause vocal changes in the form of hoarseness and deepening of the voice in women and increase in the pitch in men. These vocal changes in both sexes may be irreversible. Therefore, this risk should be carefully considered for patients whose voice is of professional importance e.g. singers, teachers, actors.

Reduced mental alertness may impair the ability to drive or operate dangerous machinery.

Pharmaceutical precautions Lasilactone should be stored at ambient temperature, protected from light, in the original container or in containers similar to those of the manufacturer.

Legal category POM.

Package quantities Lasilactone is available in blister (calendar) packs of 28 capsules (original packs).

Further information Frusemide is an effective short-acting diuretic; diuresis usually commences within one hour and lasts for four to six hours.

Spironolactone is a competitive inhibitor of aldosterone and thus increases sodium excretion whilst reducing potassium loss at the distal renal tubule. It has a slow and prolonged action, maximum response being usually attained after 2–3 days' treatment.

Product licence number PL 13402/0033.

Product licence holder: Hoechst Marion Roussel Ltd., Broadwater Park, Denham, Uxbridge, Middlesex UB9 5HP United Kingdom.

LASIX* INJECTION 20 mg/2 ml

Qualitative and quantitative composition Lasix injection 20 mg/2 ml contains 20 mg frusemide BP in 2 ml aqueous solution.

Pharmaceutical form Solution for injection.

Clinical particulars

Therapeutic indications: Lasix is a diuretic indicated for use when a prompt and effective diuresis is required. The intravenous formulation is appropriate for use in emergencies or when oral therapy is precluded. Indications include cardiac, pulmonary, hepatic and renal oedema.

Posology and method of administration: Route of administration: intramuscular or intravenous.

Adults: Lasix injection must always be given slowly. The diuretic effect is proportional to the dose. An infusion rate of 4 mg/minute should not be exceeded.

Doses of 20 mg to 50 mg intramuscularly or intravenously may be given initially. If larger doses are required, they should be given by slow infusion and titrated according to the response. In such cases the use of Lasix 250 mg ampoules should be considered.

Elderly: The dose recommendation for adults applies.

In the elderly frusemide is generally eliminated more slowly. Dosage should be titrated until the required response is achieved.

Children: Parenteral doses for children range from 0.5 to 1.5 mg/kg body weight daily up to a maximum total daily dose of 20 mg.

Contra-indications: Lasix is contra-indicated in: electrolyte deficiency and pre-comatose states associated with liver cirrhosis. Hypersensitivity to sulphonamides. Anuria.

Special warnings and special precautions for use: Latent diabetes may become manifest or the insulin requirements of diabetic patients may increase.

Patients with prostatic hypertrophy or impairment of micturition have an increased risk of developing acute retention.

Where indicated, steps should be taken to correct hypotension or hypovolaemia before commencing therapy.

Caution should be observed in patients liable to electrolyte deficiency.

Interaction with other medicaments and other forms of interaction: The dosage of concurrently administered cardiac glycosides or antihypertensive agents may require adjustment.

The toxic effects of nephrotoxic antibiotics may be increased by concomitant administration of potent diuretics such as frusemide.

As with other diuretics, serum lithium levels may be increased when lithium is given concomitantly, necessitating adjustment of lithium dosage.

Certain non-steroidal anti-inflammatory agents have been shown to antagonise the action of diuretics such as frusemide and may cause renal failure in cases of pre-existing hypovolaemia.

Interactions have been reported with ototoxic antibiotics and parenteral cisplatin.

Corticosteroids administered concurrently may cause sodium retention and exacerbate potassium loss.

A marked fall in blood pressure may be seen when ACE inhibitors are added to frusemide therapy. The dose of frusemide should be reduced, or the drug stopped, before initiating the ACE inhibitor.

Frusemide may sometimes attenuate the effects of other drugs (e.g. antidiabetics and pressor amines) and sometimes potentiate them (e.g. salicylates, theophylline, lithium and curare-type muscle relaxants).

Pregnancy and lactation: Results of animal work, in general, show no hazardous effect of Lasix in pregnancy. There is clinical evidence of safety of the drug in the third trimester of human pregnancy. However, Lasix should be used in pregnancy only if strictly indicated and for short term treatment.

As Lasix may inhibit lactation or may pass into breast milk, it should be used with caution in nursing mothers.

Effects on ability to drive and use machines: Reduced mental alertness may impair ability to drive or operate dangerous machinery.

Undesirable effects: Lasix is generally well tolerated. Nausea, malaise or gastric upset may occur but are not usually severe enough to necessitate withdrawal of treatment.

As with other diuretics, electrolytes and water balance may be disturbed as a result of diuresis after prolonged therapy. This may cause symptoms such as headache, hypotension or muscle cramps.

Calcium depletion may occur. Nephrocalcinosis has been reported in premature infants.

The incidence of allergic reactions, such as skin rashes, or interstitial nephritis or shock, is very low but treatment should be withdrawn when these occur. Standard measures for the treatment of shock should be taken.

Auditory disorders and acute pancreatitis have been reported with high dose parenteral frusemide.

A transient rise in creatinine and urea levels has been reported with frusemide, as with other diuretics.

In common with other sulphonamide-based diuretics, hyperuricaemia may occur and, in rare cases, clinical gout has been precipitated.

Bone marrow depression has been reported as a rare complication and necessitates withdrawal of treatment.

There may be aggravation of metabolic alkalosis.

Serum cholesterol and triglyceride levels may rise during frusemide treatment but will usually return to normal within 6 months.

Overdose: In case of overdose there is a danger of dehydration and electrolyte depletion due to excessive diuresis. Treatment should therefore be aimed at fluid replacement and correction of the electrolyte imbalance.

Pharmacological properties

Pharmacodynamic properties: The evidence from many experimental studies suggests that frusemide acts along the entire nephron with the exception of the distal exchange site. The main effect is on the ascending limb of the loop of Henle with a complex effect on renal circulation. Blood-flow is diverted from the juxta-medullary region to the outer cortex. The principle renal action of frusemide is to inhibit active chloride transport in the thick ascending limb. Re-absorption of sodium chloride from the nephron is reduced and a hypotonic or isotonic urine produced. It has been established that prostaglandin (PG) biosynthesis and the renin-angiotensin system are affected by frusemide administration and that frusemide alters the renal permeability of the glomerulus to serum proteins.

Pharmacokinetic properties: Frusemide is a weak carboxylic acid which exists mainly in the dissociated form in the gastrointestinal tract. Frusemide is rapidly but incompletely absorbed (60–70%) on oral administration and its effect is largely over within 4 hours. The optimal absorption site is the upper duodenum at pH 5.0. Regardless of route of administration 69–97% of activity from a radio-labelled dose is excreted in the first 4 hours after the drug is given. Frusemide is bound to plasma albumin and little biotransformation takes place. Frusemide is mainly eliminated via the kidneys (80–90%); a small fraction of the dose undergoes biliary elimination and 10–15% of the activity can be recovered from the faeces.

In renal/ hepatic impairment: Where liver disease is present, biliary elimination is reduced up to 50%. Renal impairment has little effect on the elimination rate of Lasix, but less than 20% residual renal function increases the elimination time.

The elderly: The elimination of frusemide is delayed in the elderly where a certain degree of renal impairment is present.

New born: A sustained diuretic effect is seen in the newborn, possibly due to immature tubular function.

Pre-clinical safety data: Not applicable

Pharmaceutical particulars

List of excipients: Sodium hydroxide BP, Sodium chloride BP, Water for Injection BP.

Incompatibilities: Frusemide may precipitate out of solution in fluids of low pH (e.g. dextrose solutions).

Shelf life: 60 months.

Special precautions for storage: Lasix injection should be stored protected from light.

Nature and contents of container: Each pack contains 5×2 ml Lasix Injection in amber glass ampoules.

Instruction for use/handling: Lasix injection solution should not be mixed with any other drugs in the injection bottle.

Marketing authorisation holder: Hoechst Marion Roussel Ltd, Broadwater Park, Denham, Uxbridge, Middlesex, UB9 5HP.

Marketing authorisation number PL 13402/0035.

Date of approval/revision of SPC September 1998.

Legal category POM.

LASIX* TABLETS 20 mg

Qualitative and quantitative composition Lasix Tablets 20 mg each contain 20 mg Frusemide BP.

Pharmaceutical form Uncoated tablets.

Clinical particulars

Therapeutic indications: Lasix is a diuretic recommended for use in all indications when a prompt and effective diuresis is required.

Lasix Tablets 20 mg are indicated for the maintenance therapy of mild oedema of any origin.

Posology and method of administration: Lasix has an exceptionally wide therapeutic range, the effect being proportional to the dosage. Lasix is best given as a single dose either daily or on alternate days.

The usual initial daily dose is 40 mg. This may require adjustment until the effective dose is achieved. In mild cases, 20 mg daily or 40 mg on alternate days may be sufficient, whereas in cases of resistant oedema, daily doses of 80 mg and above may be used.

Children: Oral doses for children range from 1 to 3 mg/kg body weight daily up to a maximum total dose of 40 mg/day.

Elderly: In the elderly, frusemide is generally eliminated more slowly. Dosage should be titrated until the required response is achieved.

Contra-indications: Lasix is contra-indicated in anuria, electrolyte deficiency and pre-comatose states associated with liver cirrhosis. Hypersensitivity to frusemide or sulphonamides.

Special warnings and special precautions for use: Patients with prostatic hypertrophy or impairment of micturition have an increased risk of developing acute retention.

Where indicated, steps should be taken to correct hypotension or hypovolaemia before commencing therapy.

Latent diabetes may become manifest or the insulin requirements of diabetic patients may increase.

Caution should be observed in patients liable to electrolyte deficiency.

Interaction with other medicaments and other forms of interaction: The dosage of concurrently administered cardiac glycosides or anti-hypertensive agents may require adjustment.

A marked fall in blood pressure may be seen when ACE inhibitors are added to frusemide therapy. The dose of frusemide should be reduced, or the drug stopped, before initiating the ACE inhibitor.

The toxic effects of nephrotoxic antibiotics may be increased by concomitant administration of potent diuretics such as frusemide.

In common with other diuretics, serum lithium levels may be increased when lithium is given concomitantly with frusemide, necessitating adjustment of the lithium dosage.

Certain non-steroidal anti-inflammatory agents (e.g. indomethacin, acetylsalicylic acid) may attenuate the action of frusemide and may cause renal failure in cases of pre-existing hypovolaemia. Frusemide may sometimes attenuate the effects of other drugs (e.g. the effects of antidiabetics and of pressor amines) and sometimes potentiate them (e.g. the effects of salicylates, theophylline, lithium and curare-type muscle relaxants).

Interactions have also been reported with ototoxic antibiotics. In cases of concomitant gluco-corticoid therapy or abuse of laxatives, the risk of an increased potassium loss should be borne in mind.

Pregnancy and lactation: Results of animal work, in general, show no hazardous effect of Lasix in pregnancy.

There is clinical evidence of safety of the drug in the third trimester of human pregnancy; however, Lasix should be used in pregnancy only if strictly indicated and for short term treatment.

As Lasix may inhibit lactation or may pass into the breast milk it should be used with caution in nursing mothers.

Effects on ability to drive and use machines: Reduced mental alertness may impair ability to drive or operate dangerous machinery.

Undesirable effects: Lasix is generally well tolerated. Side-effects of a minor nature such as nausea, malaise or gastric upset may occur but are not usually severe enough to necessitate withdrawal of treatment.

As with other diuretics, electrolytes and water balance may be disturbed as a result of diuresis after prolonged therapy. This may cause symptoms such as headache, hypotension or muscle cramps.

Serum calcium levels may be reduced; in very rare cases tetany has been observed. Nephrocalcinosis has been reported in premature infants.

Isolated cases of acute pancreatitis have been reported after long-term diuretic (including frusemide) treatment. Disorders of hearing after frusemide are rare and, in most cases reversible. They may occur if frusemide is injected too rapidly, particularly in patients with renal insufficiency.

As with other diuretics a transient rise in creatinine and urea levels has also been reported with frusemide.

The incidence of allergic reactions, such as skin rashes, photosensitivity, vasculitis, fever or interstitial nephritis, is very low, but when these occur treatment should be withdrawn.

In common with other sulphonamide-based diuretics, hyperuricaemia may occur and, in rare cases, clinical gout may be precipitated.

Serum cholesterol and triglyceride levels may rise during frusemide treatment. During long term therapy they will usually return to normal within six months.

Bone marrow depression has been reported as a rare complication and necessitates withdrawal of treatment.

Pre-existing metabolic alkalosis (e.g. in decompensated cirrhosis of the liver) may be aggravated by frusemide treatment.

Overdose: In cases of overdose there is a danger of dehydration and electrolyte depletion due to excessive diuresis. Treatment should therefore be aimed at fluid replacement and correction of the electrolyte imbalance.

Pharmacological properties

Pharmacodynamic properties: The evidence from many experimental studies suggests that frusemide acts along the entire nephron with the exception of the distal exchange site. The main effect is on the ascending limb of the loop of henle with a complex effect on renal circulation. Blood-flow is diverted from the juxta-medullary region to the outer cortex the principal renal action of frusemide is to inhibit active chloride transport in the thick ascending limb. Reabsorption of sodium chloride from the nephron is reduced and a hypotonic or isotonic urine produced.

It has been established that prostaglandin (PG) biosynthesis and the renin-angiotensin system are affected by frusemide administration and that frusemide alters the renal permeability of the glomerulus to serum proteins.

Pharmacokinetic properties: Frusemide is a weak carboxylic acid which exists mainly in the dissociated form in the gastro-intestinal tract. Frusemide is rapidly but incompletely absorbed (60–70%) on oral administration and its effect is largely over within four hours. The optimal absorption site is the upper duodenum at pH 5.0. Regardless of route of administration, 69–97% of activity from a radio-labelled dose is excreted in the first 4 hours after the drug is given. Frusemide is bound to plasma albumin and little biotransformation takes place. Frusemide is mainly eliminated via the kidneys (80–90%); a small fraction of the dose undergoes biliary elimination and 10–15% of the activity can be recovered from the faeces.

(a) In renal/hepatic impairment: Where liver disease is present, biliary elimination is reduced. Up to 50% renal impairment has little effect on the elimination rate of Lasix, but less than 20% residual renal function increases the elimination time.

(b) The elderly: The elimination of frusemide is delayed in the elderly where a certain degree of renal impairment is present.

(c) New-born: A sustained diuretic effect is seen, possibly due to immature tubular function.

Preclinical safety data: None applicable.

Pharmaceutical particulars

List of excipients: Lactose, maize starch, talc, magnesium stearate and colloidal silicon dioxide.

Incompatibilities: None.

Shelf life: Five years.

Special precautions for storage: Store protected from light in the manufacturers containers or similar.

Nature and contents of container: Lasix Tablets 20 mg are available in blister packs of 28.

Instructions for use/handling: None.

Marketing authorisation holder: Hoechst Marion Roussel Ltd, Broadwater Park, Denham, Uxbridge, Middlesex, UB9 5HP.

Marketing authorisation number PL 13402/0037.

Date of approval/revision of SPC December 1997.

Legal category POM.

LASIX TABLETS 40 mg*

Presentation Lasix Tablets 40 mg each contain 40 mg Frusemide BP. They are presented as flat white tablets with bevelled edges, 8 mm in diameter, one face bearing the Hoechst logo, the other face with a break line, each half marked DLI.

Excipients include lactose.

Uses Lasix is a diuretic recommended for use in all indications when a prompt and effective diuresis is required. Indications for Lasix Tablets 40 mg include cardiac, pulmonary, hepatic and renal oedema, peripheral oedema due to mechanical obstruction or venous insufficiency and hypertension.

Dosage and administration Lasix has an exceptionally wide therapeutic range, the effect being proportional to the dosage. Lasix is best given as a single dose either daily or on alternate days.

The usual initial daily dose is 40 mg. This may require adjustment until the effective dose is achieved. In mild cases, 20 mg daily or 40 mg on alternate days may be sufficient, whereas in cases of resistant oedema, daily doses of 80 mg and above may be used.

Children: Oral doses for children range from 1 to 3 mg/kg body weight daily up to a maximum total dose of 40 mg/day.

Elderly: In the elderly, frusemide is generally eliminated more slowly. Dosage should be titrated until the required response is achieved.

Contra-indications, warnings, etc

Contra-indications: Lasix is contra-indicated in anuria, electrolyte deficiency and pre-comatose states associated with liver cirrhosis. Hypersensitivity to frusemide or sulphonamides.

Warnings: Patients with prostatic hypertrophy or impairment of micturition have an increased risk of developing acute retention.

Where indicated, steps should be taken to correct hypotension or hypovolaemia before commencing therapy.

The dosage of concurrently administered cardiac glycosides or anti-hypertensive agents may require adjustment. A marked fall in blood pressure may be seen when ACE inhibitors are added to frusemide therapy. The dose of frusemide should be reduced, or the drug stopped, before initiating the ACE inhibitor.

The toxic effects of nephrotoxic antibiotics may be increased by concomitant administration of potent diuretics such as frusemide.

Latent diabetes may become manifest or the insulin requirements of diabetic patients may increase.

In common with other diuretics, serum lithium levels may be increased when lithium is given concomitantly with frusemide, necessitating adjustment of the lithium dosage.

Certain non-steroidal anti-inflammatory agents (e.g. indomethacin, acetylsalicylic acid) may attenuate the action of frusemide and may cause renal failure in cases of pre-existing hypovolaemia. Frusemide may sometimes attenuate the effects of other drugs (e.g. the effects of antidiabetics and of pressor amines) and sometimes potentiate them (e.g. the effects of salicylates, theophylline, lithium and curare-type muscle relaxants).

Interactions have also been reported with ototoxic antibiotics. In cases of concomitant glucocorticoid therapy or abuse of laxatives, the risk of an increased potassium loss should be borne in mind.

Precautions: Caution should be observed in patients liable to electrolyte deficiency.

Results of animal work, in general, show no hazardous effect of Lasix in pregnancy. There is clinical evidence of safety of the drug in the third trimester of human pregnancy; however, Lasix should be used in pregnancy only if strictly indicated and for short term treatment.

Nursing mothers: As Lasix may inhibit lactation or may pass into the breast milk it should be used with caution in nursing mothers.

Overdosage: In cases of overdose there is a danger of dehydration and electrolyte depletion due to excessive diuresis. Treatment should therefore be aimed at fluid replacement and correction of the electrolyte imbalance.

Side-effects: Lasix is generally well tolerated. Side-effects of a minor nature such as nausea, malaise or gastric upset may occur but are not usually severe enough to necessitate withdrawal of treatment.

As with other diuretics, electrolytes and water balance may be disturbed as a result of diuresis after prolonged therapy. This may cause symptoms such as headache, hypotension or muscle cramps.

Serum calcium levels may be reduced; in very rare cases tetany has been observed. Nephrocalcinosis has been reported in premature infants.

Isolated cases of acute pancreatitis have been reported after long-term diuretic (including frusemide) treatment. Disorders of hearing after frusemide are rare and, in most cases reversible. They may occur if frusemide is injected too rapidly, particularly in patients with renal insufficiency.

As with other diuretics a transient rise in creatinine and urea levels has also been reported with frusemide.

The incidence of allergic reactions, such as skin rashes, photosensitivity, vasculitis, fever or interstitial nephritis, is very low, but when these occur treatment should be withdrawn.

In common with other sulphonamide-based diuretics, hyperuricaemia may occur and, in rare cases, clinical gout may be precipitated.

Serum cholesterol and triglyceride levels may rise during frusemide treatment. During long term therapy they will usually return to normal within six months.

Bone marrow depression has been reported as a rare complication and necessitates withdrawal of treatment.

Pre-existing metabolic alkalosis (e.g. in decompensated cirrhosis of the liver) may be aggravated by frusemide treatment.

Reduced mental alertness may impair ability to drive or operate dangerous machinery.

Pharmaceutical precautions Lasix tablets should be stored protected from light, in the manufacturer's containers or similar.

Legal category POM.

Package quantities Lasix Tablets 40 mg are available in packs of 28 and 250 (The pack size of 28 is an original pack).

Further information Lasix produces a prompt and effective diuresis which lasts for approximately four hours following oral administration. Therefore the time of administration can be adjusted to suit the patient's requirements.

Product licence number 13402/0038.

Product licence holder: Hoechst Marion Roussel Ltd, Broadwater Park, Denham, Uxbridge, Middlesex, UB9 5HP.

LASIX PAEDIATRIC LIQUID*

Qualitative and quantitative composition Lasix contains Frusemide BP as active ingredient. When reconstituted, Lasix Paediatric Liquid contains 1 mg Frusemide BP in 1 ml of liquid.

Pharmaceutical form Granules for reconstitution to oral solution.

Clinical particulars

Therapeutic indications: Lasix Paediatric Liquid is a diuretic for treatment of oedema in children or in patients unable to take solid oral dosage forms of Lasix.

Posology and method of administration:

Children: Dosage 1–3 mg/kg body weight daily. (1–3 ml/kg as reconstituted liquid).

Adults: Substitution for oral tablet therapy, dosage 20–80 mg (20–80 ml) daily.

Lasix Paediatric Liquid contains sorbitol and may cause flatulence, abdominal distension or diarrhoea if given in large quantities to adults who are unable to take solid oral dose forms of Lasix. (see *Special warnings and special precautions for use*).

Elderly: The dose range for adults applies but in the elderly, frusemide is generally eliminated more slowly. Dosage should be titrated until the required response is achieved.

Contra-indications: Electrolyte deficiency and pre-comatose states associated with liver cirrhosis. Hypersensitivity to frusemide or sulphonamides.

Special warnings and special precautions for use: Lasix Paediatric Liquid contains sorbitol and may cause flatulence, abdominal distension or diarrhoea if given in large quantities to adults who are unable to take solid oral dosage forms of Lasix.

Patients with prostatic hypertrophy or impairment of micturition have an increased risk of developing acute retention.

Where indicated steps should be taken to correct hypotension or hypovolaemia before commencing therapy.

Latent diabetes may become manifest or the insulin requirements of diabetic patients may increase.

Caution should be observed in patients liable to electrolyte deficiency.

Interaction with other medicaments and other forms of interaction: The dosage of concurrently administered cardiac glycosides or antihypertensive agents may require adjustment. A marked fall in blood pressure may be seen when ACE inhibitors are added to frusemide therapy. The dose of frusemide should be reduced or the drug stopped, before initiating the ACE inhibitor.

The toxic effects of nephrotoxic antibiotics may be increased by concomitant administration of potent diuretics such as frusemide.

In common with other diuretics, serum lithium levels may be increased when lithium is given concomitantly with frusemide, necessitating adjustment of the lithium dosage.

Certain non-steroidal anti-inflammatory agents have been shown to antagonise the action of diuretics such as frusemide and may cause renal failure in cases of pre-existing hypovolaemia.

Interactions have also been reported with ototoxic antibiotics and parenteral cisplatin. In cases of concomitant glucocorticoid therapy or abuse of laxatives, the risk of an increased potassium loss should be borne in mind.

Frusemide may sometimes attenuate the effects of other drugs (e.g. the effects of antidiabetics and pressor amines) and some times potentiate them (e.g. the effects of salicylates, theophylline and curare-type muscle relaxants.

Pregnancy and lactation: Results of animal work in general show no hazardous effect of Lasix in pregnancy. There is clinical evidence of the safety of the drug in the third trimester of pregnancy in humans. However, Lasix should be used in pregnancy only if strictly indicated and for short-term treatment.

As Lasix may inhibit lactation, it should be used with caution in nursing mothers.

Effects on ability to drive and use machines: Reduced mental alertness may impair ability to drive or operate dangerous machinery.

Undesirable effects: Lasix is generally well-tolerated. Nausea, malaise or gastric upset may occur but are not usually severe enough to necessitate withdrawal of treatment.

As with other diuretics, electrolytes and water balance may be disturbed as a result of diuresis after prolonged therapy. This may cause symptoms such as headache, hypotension or muscle cramps.

Flatulence, abdominal distension or diarrhoea may occur following the ingestion of large quantities of Lasix Paediatric Liquid, due to its sorbitol content.

Serum calcium levels may be reduced; in very rare cases tetany has been observed. Nephrocalcinosis has been reported in premature infants.

The incidence of allergic reactions, such as skin rashes, photosensitivity, vasculitis, fever or interstitial nephritis, is very low but treatment should be withdrawn when these occur.

Isolated cases of acute pancreatitis have been reported after long term diuretic (including frusemide) treatment. Disorders of hearing after frusemide are rare, and in most cases reversible. They may occur if frusemide is injected too rapidly, particularly in patients with renal insufficiency.

A transient rise in creatinine and urea levels has been reported with frusemide, as with other diuretics.

In common with other sulphonamide-based diuretics, hyperuricaemia may occur and in rare cases, clinical gout be precipitated.

Bone marrow depression has been reported as a rare complication and necessitates withdrawal of treatment.

Pre-existing metabolic alkalosis (e.g in decompensated cirrhosis of the liver) may be aggravated by frusemide treatment.

Serum cholesterol and triglyceride levels may rise during frusemide treatment. During long term therapy they will usually return to normal levels within six months.

Overdose: In cases of overdose there is a danger of dehydration and electrolyte depletion due to excessive diuresis. Treatment should be aimed at fluid replacement and correction of the electrolyte imbalance.

Pharmacological properties

Pharmacodynamic properties: The evidence from many experimental studies suggests that frusemide acts along the entire nephron with the exception of the distal exchange site. The main effect is on the ascending limb of the loop of henle with a complex effect on renal circulation. Blood-flow is diverted from the juxta-medullary region to the outer cortex. The principle renal action of frusemide is to inhibit active chloride transport in the thick ascending limb. Re-absorption of sodium chloride from the nephron is reduced and a hypotonic or isotonic urine produced. It has been established that prostaglandin (PG) biosynthesis and the renin-angiotensin system are affected by frusemide administration and that frusemide alters the renal permeability of the glomerulus to serum proteins.

Pharmacokinetic properties: Frusemide is a weak carboxylic acid which exists mainly in the dissociated form in the gastrointestinal tract. Frusemide is rapidly but incompletely absorbed (60–70%) on oral administration and its effect is largely over within 4 hours. The optimal absorption site is the upper duodenum at pH 5.0. Regardless of route of administration 69–97% of activity from a radio-labelled dose is excreted in the first 4 hours after the drug is given. Frusemide is bound to plasma albumin and little biotransformation takes place. Frusemide is mainly eliminated via the kidneys (80–90%); a small fraction of the dose undergoes biliary elimination and 10–15% of the activity can be recovered from the faeces.

In renal/hepatic impairment: Where liver disease is present, biliary elimination is reduced up to 50%, renal impairment has little effect on the elimination rate of Lasix. But less than 20% residual renal function increases the elimination time.

The elderly: The elimination of frusemide is delayed in the elderly where a certain degree of renal impairment is present.

Newborn: A sustained diuretic effect is seen in the newborn, possibly due to immature tubular function.

Preclinical safety data: Not applicable.

Pharmaceutical particulars

List of excipients: Sorbitol, disodium hydrogen orthophosphate, sodium sulphite, disodium edetate, sodium hydroxide, nipasept sodium, vanilla flavour and saccharin sodium distilled water (not detected in finished product).

Incompatibilities: Frusemide should not be mixed with fluids of low pH.

Shelf life: Three years unopened, 30 days after reconstitution.

Special precautions for storage: Store in a dry place at ambient temperature, protected from light in the original container.

Reconstituted liquid should be stored in a cool place e.g. in a refrigerator at 5°C, protected from light.

Nature and contents of container: Lasix Paediatric Liquid is available in amber glass bottles, which on reconsitutution of the product contain 150 ml.

Instructions for use/handling: The granulate should only be reconstituted with 142 ml of distilled water. The use of sterile distilled water is recommended when the product is intended for administration to neonates.

Marketing authorisation holder: Hoechst Marion Roussel Ltd, Broadwater Park, Denham, Uxbridge, UB9 5HP.

Marketing authorisation number PL 13402/0036.

Date of approval/revision of SPC December 1997.

Legal category POM.

LASORIDE* (co-amilofruse 5/40)

Qualitative and quantitative composition Each tablet contains, as active ingredients, 40 mg frusemide and 5 mg amiloride hydrochloride.

Pharmaceutical form Oblong, biconvex yellow tablets.

Clinical particulars

Therapeutic indications: Where a prompt diuresis is required and where potassium conservation is important.

Posology and method of administration: The adult dose is one to two tablets, to be taken in the morning.

Elderly: The elderly are more likely to experience hyperkalaemia since renal reserve may be reduced. The dosage should be adjusted according to renal function, blood electrolytes and diuretic response.

Children: Not recommended for use in children (see *Contra-indications*).

Contra-indications: Hyperkalaemia (serum potassium >5.3 mmol/litre), Addison's disease, acute renal failure, anuria, severe progressive renal disease, electrolyte imbalance, precomatose states associated with cirrhosis, concomitant potassium supplements, spironolactone or triamterene, known sensitivity to frusemide or amiloride.

Lasoride is contra-indicated in children as safety in this age group has not been established.

Special warnings and special precautions for use: *Warnings:* Hyperkalaemia has been observed in patients receiving amiloride hydrochloride.

Frusemide may cause latent diabetes to become manifest. It may be necessary to increase the dose of hypoglycaemic agents in diabetic patients.

Lasoride should be discontinued before a glucose tolerance test.

Patients with prostatic hypertrophy or impairment of micturition have an increased risk of developing acute urinary retention during diuretic therapy.

Serum uric acid levels may rise during treatment with Lasoride and acute attacks of gout may be precipitated.

Precautions: Patients who are being treated with the preparation require regular supervision, with monitoring of fluid and electrolyte states to avoid excessive loss of fluid.

Lasoride should be used with particular caution in elderly patients or those with potential obstruction in the urinary tract or disorders rendering electrolyte balance precarious.

Hyponatraemia, hypochloraemia and raised blood urea nitrogen may occur during vigorous diuresis, especially in seriously ill patients or the elderly. Careful monitoring of serum electrolytes and urea should therefore be undertaken in these patients.

Interaction with other medicaments and other forms of interaction: The dosage of concurrently administered cardiac glycosides or antihypertensive agents may require adjustment.

The toxic effects of nephrotoxic antibiotics may be increased by concomitant administration of potent diuretics such as Lasoride.

In common with other diuretics, serum lithium levels may be increased when lithium is given concomitantly with frusemide, necessitating adjustment of the lithium dosage.

ACE inhibitors should not be used in combination with Lasoride as serum potassium levels may be increased.

Certain non-steroidal anti-inflammatory agents (e.g. indomethacin, acetylsalicylic acid) may attenuate the action of diuretics such as frusemide and may cause renal failure in cases of pre-existing hypovolaemia. Frusemide may sometimes attenuate the effects of other drugs (e.g. the effect of antidiabetics and of pressor amines) and sometimes potentiate them (e.g.

the effects of salicylates, theophylline, lithium and curare-type muscle relaxants).

Interactions have also been reported with ototoxic antibiotics. In cases of concomitant corticosteroid therapy or abuse of laxatives, the risk of an increased potassium loss should be borne in mind.

Pregnancy and lactation: The safety of Lasoride use during pregnancy and lactation has not been established.

Effects on ability to drive and use machines: Reduced mental alertness may impair ability to drive or operate dangerous machinery.

Undesirable effects: Malaise, gastric upset, nausea, vomiting, diarrhoea, and constipation may occur.

If skin rashes or pruritus occur, treatment should be withdrawn.

Serum calcium levels may be reduced; in very rare cases tetany has been observed.

Serum cholesterol and triglyceride levels may rise during frusemide treatment but will usually return to normal within six months.

Rare complications may include minor psychiatric disturbances and disturbances in liver function tests. Isolated cases of acute pancreatitis have been reported after long-term diuretic (including frusemide) treatment.

Disorders of hearing after frusemide are rare and, in most cases reversible. They may occur if frusemide is injected too rapidly, particularly in patients with renal insufficiency.

Bone marrow depression occasionally complicates treatment, necessitating withdrawal of the product. The haematopoietic state should be regularly monitored during treatment.

Overdose: Treatment of overdosage should be aimed at reversing dehydration and correcting electrolyte imbalance, particularly hyperkalaemia. Emesis should be induced or gastric lavage performed. Treatment is symptomatic and supportive. If hyperkalaemia is seen, appropriate measures to reduce serum potassium must be instituted.

Pharmacological properties

Pharmacodynamic properties: Frusemide: Frusemide is a potent diuretic acting on the loop of Henle to inhibit electrolyte re-absorption, excretion of sodium, potassium and chloride ions is increased and water excretion enhanced.

Amiloride: Amiloride is a mild diuretic acting mainly on distal renal tubules. It increases excretion of sodium and chloride and reduces excretionof potassium. It is mainly used as an adjunct to the thiazides, frusemide and similar diuretics

Pharmacokinetic properties: Frusemide: Frusemide is rapidly absorbed from the gastrointestinal tract after oral administration. It has a biphasic half-life in the plasma with a terminal elimination of about 1.5 hours.

It is up to 99% bound to plasma proteins..

Amiloride: Amiloride is relatively well absorbed from the gastro-intestinal tract after oral administration.

Peak serum concentration are attained 3 to 4 hours after administration. It is estimated to have a serum half-life of about 9–10 hours.

Preclinical safety data: None stated.

Pharmaceutical particulars

List of excipients: Lactose, maize starch, talc, colloidal silicon dioxide, magnesiun stearate and colouring agent E104 (dispersed quinoline yellow).

Incompatibilities: Not applicable.

Shelf life: 3 years.

Special precautions for storage: Protect from light.

Nature and contents of container: Amber glass bottles of 50 and 100 tablets and securitainers of 50, 100 and 1000 tablets.

Also blister pack of 28 tablets in a calendar pack.

Instructions for use/handling: Not applicable.

Marketing authorisation holder: Hoechst Marion Roussel Ltd, Broadwater Park, Denham, Uxbridge, Middlesex, UB9 5HP.

Marketing authorisation number PL 13402/0040.

Date of approval/revision of SPC December 1997.

Legal category POM.

METENIX* 5 TABLETS

Qualitative and quantitative composition Metolazone 5 mg.

Pharmaceutical form Tablet.

Clinical particulars

Therapeutic indications: Metenix 5 is a diuretic for use in the treatment of mild and moderate hypertension. Metenix 5 may be used in conjunction with non-diuretic antihypertensive agents and, in these circumstances, it is usually possible to achieve satisfactory control of blood pressure with a reduced dose of the non-diuretic agent. Patients who have become resistant to therapy with these agents may respond to the addition of Metenix 5 to their antihypertensive regimen.

Metenix 5 may also be used for the treatment of cardiac, renal and hepatic oedema, ascites or toxaemia of pregnancy.

Posology and method of administration: Route of administration:oral.

Hypertension: The recommended initial dose in mild and moderate hypertension is 5 mg daily. After three to four weeks, the dose may be reduced if necessary to 5 mg on alternate days as maintenance therapy.

Oedema: In oedematous conditions, the normal recommended dose is 5–10 mg daily, given as a single dose. In resistant conditions, this may be increased to 20 mg daily or above. However, no more than 80 mg should be given in any 24–hour period.

Children: There is insufficient knowledge of the effects of Metenix 5 in children for any dosage recommendations to be made.

Elderly: Metolazone may be excreted more slowly in the elderly.

Contra-indications: Metenix 5 is contra-indicated in electrolyte deficiency states, anuria, coma or pre-comatose states associated with liver cirrhosis; also in patients with known allergy or hypersensitivity to metolazone.

Special warnings and special precautions for use: Because of the antihypertensive effects of metolazone the dosage of concurrently administered non-diuretic antihypertensive agents may need to be reduced.

Caution should be exercised during Metenix 5 therapy in patients liable to electrolyte deficiency.

Chloride deficit, hyponatraemia and a low salt syndrome may also occur, particularly when the patient is also on a diet with restricted salt intake. Hypomagnesaemia has been reported as a consequence of prolonged diuretic therapy.

Prolonged therapy with Metenix 5 may result in hypokalaemia. Serum potassium levels should be determined at regular intervals and, if necessary, potassium supplementation should be instituted.

Fluid and electrolyte balance should be carefully monitored during therapy especially if Metenix 5 is used concurrently with other diuretics. In particular, Metenix 5 may potentiate the diuresis produced by frusemide and, if the two agents are used concurrently, patients should be carefully monitored.

Interaction with other medicaments and other forms of interaction: The dosage of concurrently administered cardiac glycosides may require adjustment. Metenix 5 may aggravate the increased potassium excretion associated with steroid therapy or diseases such as cirrhosis or severe ischaemic heart disease. Latent diabetes may become manifest or the insulin requirements of diabetic patients may increase.

Non steroidal anti-inflammatory drugs (e.g. Indomethacin, Sulindac) may attenuate the action of Metolazone.

Prolongation of bleeding time has been reported during concomitant administration of Metenix and warfarin.

Pregnancy and lactation: There is little evidence of safety of the drug in human pregnancy, but it has been in wide, general use for many years without apparent ill consequence, animal studies having shown no hazard.

If Metenix 5 is given to nursing mothers, metolazone may be present in the breast milk.

Effects on ability to drive and use machines: None known.

Undesirable effects: Metenix 5 is generally well tolerated. There have been occasional reports of headache, anorexia, vomiting, abdominal discomfort, muscle cramps and dizziness. There have been isolated reports of urticaria, leucopenia, tachycardia, chills and chest pain.

Hyperuricaemia or azotaemia may occur during treatment with Metenix 5, particularly in patients with impaired renal function. On rare occasions, clinical gout has been reported.

Overdose: In cases of overdose there is a danger of dehydration and electrolyte depletion. Treatment should therefore be aimed at fluid replacement and correction of the electrolyte imbalance.

Pharmacological properties

Pharmacodynamic properties: Metolazone is a substituted quinazolinone diuretic.

Pharmacokinetic properties: Diuresis and saluresis begin within one hour of administration of Metenix 5 tablets, reaching a maximum in two hours and continuing for 12–24 hours according to dosage.

Preclinical safety data: None applicable.

Pharmaceutical particulars

List of excipients: Microcrystalline cellulose, magnesium stearate, F and D C blue no 2 lake (E132).

Incompatibilities: None.

Shelf life: 5 years.

Special precautions for storage: Metenix 5 tablets should be stored in a cool dry place, protected from light, in the original container or in containers similar to those of the manufacturer.

Nature and contents of container: Blister pack of 30 or 100 tablets.

Instruction for use/handling: None.

Marketing authorisation holder: Hoechst Marion Roussel Ltd., Broadwater Park, Denham, Uxbridge, Middlesex, UB9 5HP.

Marketing authorisation number PL 13402/0041.

Date of first approval/revision of SPC December 1997.

Legal category POM.

RYTHMODAN CAPSULES 100 mg*

Qualitative and quantitative composition Capsules containing Disopyramide BP 100 mg.

Pharmaceutical form Capsules.

Clinical particulars

Therapeutic indications:

Rythmodan is used in the treatment of cardiac arrhythmias as follows:–

1. The prevention and treatment of arrhythmias occurring after myocardial infarction.
2. Maintenance of normal rhythm following electro-conversion eg atrial fibrillation, atrial flutter.
3. Persistent ventricular extrasystoles.
4. Control of arrhythmias following the use of digitalis or similar glycosides.
5. Suppression of arrhythmias during surgical procedures eg cardiac catheterisation.
6. The prevention of paroxysmal supraventricular tachycardia.
7. Other types of arrhythmias e.g. atrial extrasystoles, Wolff-Parkinson-White Syndrome.

Posology and method of administration: Route of administration: Oral.

300 mg to 800 mg daily in divided doses.

Children: Not recommended as insufficient data available.

Contra-indications: Disopyramide is contra-indicated in un-paced second or third degree atrioventricular block; bundle-branch block associated with first degree atrioventricular block; un-paced bifasicular block; pre-existing long QT syndromes; severe sinus node dysfunction; severe heart failure, unless secondary to cardiac arrhythmia; and hypersensitivity to disopyramide. It is also contra-indicated in concomitant admistration with other anti-arrhythmics or other drugs liable to provoke ventricular arrythmias, especially Torsade de Pointes (see *Interaction with other medicaments and other forms of interaction*). The sustained release formulation is contra-indicated in patients with renal or hepatic impairment.

Special warnings and special precautions for use: In view of the serious nature of many of the conditions being treated it is suggested that Rythmodan Injection should only be used when facilities exist for cardiac monitoring or defibrillation, should the need arise.

Antiarrhythmic drugs belonging to the class 1c (Vaughan Williams Classification) were included in the Cardiac Arrhythmia Suppression Trial (CAST), a long term multicentre randomised, double blind study in patients with asymptomatic non life–threatening ventricular arrhythmia who had a myocardial infarction more than six days but less than two years previously. A significant increase in mortality and non-fatal cardiac arrest rate was seen in patients treated with class 1c antiarrhythmic drugs when compared with a matched placebo group. The applicability of the CAST results to other antiarrhythmics and other populations (e.g. those without recent infarction) is uncertain. At present, it is best to assume that the risk extends to other antiarrhythmic agents for patients with structural heart disease.

There is no evidence that prolonged suppression of ventricular premature contractions with antiarrhythmic drugs prevents sudden death.

All antiarrhythmic drugs can produce unwanted effects when they are used to treat symptomatic but not life threatening arrhythmia; the expected benefit should be balanced against their risks.

In patients with structural heart disease, proarrhythmia and cardiac decompensation are special risks associated with antiarrhythmic drugs. Special caution should be exercised when prescribing in this taken context.

Disopyramide should not be used in patients with uncompensated congestive heart failure, unless this heart failure is secondary to cardiac arrhythmia. If disopyramide is to be given under these circumstances, special care and monitoring are essential.

Haemodynamically significant arrhythmias are difficult to treat and affected patients have a high mortality risk. Treatment of these arrhythmias, by whatever modality, must be initiated in hospital.

Owing to its negative inotropic effect, disopyramide should be used with caution in patients suffering from significant cardiac failure. This group may be specially sensitive to the negative inotropic properties of disopyramide. Such patients should be fully digitalised or controlled with other therapy before treatment with disopyramide is commenced.

Aggravation of existing arrhythmia, or emergence of a new type of arrhythmia, demands urgent review disopyramide treatment.

Similarly, if an atrioventricular block or a bifasicular block occurs during treatment, the use of disopyramide should be reviewed.

There have been reports of ventricular tachycardia, ventricular fibrillation and Torsade de Pointes in patients receiving disopyramide. These have usually, but not always, been associated with significant widening of the QRS complex or prolonged QT interval. The QT interval and QRS duration must be monitored and disopyramide should be stopped if these are increased by more than 25%. If these changes or arrhythmias develop the drug should be discontinued. Disopyramide should be used only with caution in patients with atrial flutter or atrial tachycardia with block as conversion of a partial AV block to a 1:1 response may occur, leading to a potentially more serious tachyarrhythmia.

The occurrence of hypotension following disopyramide administration, requires prompt discontinuation of the drug. This has been observed especiallyin patients with cardiomyopathy or uncompensated congestive heart failure. Any resumption of therapy should be at a lower dose with close patient monitoring. Disopyramide should be used with caution in the treatment of digitalis intoxication.

Potassium imbalance: Antiarrhythmic drugs may be hazardous in patients with potassium imbalance, as potassium abnormalities can induce arrhythmias.

During treatment with disopyramide, potassium levels should be checked regularly. Patients treated with diuretics or stimulant laxatives are at particular risk of hypokalaemia.

Renal insufficiency: In renal insufficiency, the dosage of disopyramide should be reduced by adjusting the interval between administrations.

Hepatic insufficiency: Hepatic impairment causes an increase in the plasma half-life of Rythmodan and a reduced dosage may be required.

Hypoglycaemia: Hypoglycaemia has been reported in association with disopyramide administration. Patients at particular risk are the elderly, the malnourished, or diabetics. The risk of hypoglycaemia occurring is increased with impaired renal function or cardiac failure. Blood glucose should be monitored in all patients. Strict adherence to the dosing recommendations is advised. If hypoglycaemia occurs then treatment with disopyramide should be stopped.

Atropine-like effects: There is a risk of:
- ocular hypertension in patients with narrow-angle glaucoma,
- acute urinary retention in patients with prostatic enlargement,
- aggravation of myasthenia gravis.

Interaction with other medicaments and other forms of interaction:

Combination with other antiarrhythmic drugs: Combinations of antiarrhythmic drugs are not well researched and their effect may be unpredictable. Thus, antiarrhythmic combination should be avoided except under certain circumstances, e.g. Beta-blockers for angina pectoris; digoxin with beta-blocker and/or verapamil for the control of atrial fibrillation, when defined as effective for an individual.

Interaction with drugs associated with risk of Torsade de Pointes, such as:
- tricyclic and tetracyclic antidepressants
- intravenous erythromycin
- astemizole; cisapride; pentamidine; pimozide; sparfloxacin; terfenadine

The concomitant use of these medications whilst undergoing treatment with disopyramide increases the chance of cardiac arrhythmia.

There is some evidence that disopyramide is metabolised by hepatic CYP3A. Concomitant administration of significant inhibitors of this isozyme (e.g. certain macrolide or azole antifungal antibiotics) may therefore increase the serum levels of disopyramide. On the other hand, inducers of CYP3A (e.g. rifampicin, certain anticonvulsants) may reduce disopyramide and increase MN-disopyramide serum levels. Since the magnitude of such potential effects is not foreseeable, such drug combinations are not recommended.

When prescribing a drug metabolised by CYP3A [such as theophylline, HIV protease inhibitors (e.g. ritonavir, indinavir, saquinavir), cyclosporin A, warfarin] it should be kept in mind that disopyramide is probably also a substrate of this isozyme and thus competitive inhibition of metabolism might occur, possibly increasing serum levels of these drugs.

Interactions with hypokalaemia inducing drugs: Concomitant use with drugs that can induce hypokalaemia such as: diuretics, amphotericin B, tetracosactrin (corticotrophin analogue), gluco and mineralocorticoids may reduce the action of the drug, or potentiate proarrhythmic effects. Stimulant laxatives are not recommended to be given concomitantly, due to their potassium lowering potential.

Other drug interactions: Atropine and other anticholinergic drugs, including phenothiazines, may potentiate the atropine-like effects of disopyramide.

Pregnancy and lactation:

Pregnancy: Although Rythmodan has undergone animal tests for teratogenicity without evidence of any effect on the developing foetus, its safety in human pregnancy has not been established. Rythmodan has been reported to stimulate contractions of the pregnant uterus. The drug should only be used during pregnancy if benefits clearly outweigh the possible risks to the mother and foetus.

Lactation: No data for Rythmodan Injection, but studies have shown that oral disopyramide is secreted in breast milk, although no adverse effects to the infant have been noted. However, clinical experience is limited and disopyramide should only be used in lactation if, in the clinician's judgement, it is essential for the welfare of the patient. The infant should be closely supervised, particularly for anticholinergic effects and drug levels determined if necessary. Ideally, if the drug is considered essential, an alternative method of feeding should be used.

Effects on ability to drive and use machines: Some adverse reactions may impair the patients' ability to concentrate and react, and hence the ability to drive or operate machinery (see *Undesirable effects*).

Undesirable effects:

Cardiac: It is accepted that the arrhythmogenic potential of disopyramide is weak. However, as with all antiarrhythmic drugs, disopyramide may worsen or provoke arrhythmias. This proarrhythmic effect is more likely to occur in the presence of hypokalaemia with the associated use of antiarrhythmic drugs, in patients with severe structural heart disease or prolongation of the QT interval.

Intra-cardiac conduction abnormalities may occur: QT interval prolongation, widening of the QRS complex, atrioventricular block and bundle-branch block.

Other types of arrhythmia have been reported: Bradycardia, sinus block.

Episodes of severe heart failure or even cardiogenic shock have also been described particularlyin patients with severe structural heart disease. The resulting low cardiac output can cause hypotension, renal insufficiency and/or acute hepatic ischemia.

Other adverse reactions include: Atropine like: Urinary (dysuria; acute urinary retention); ocular (disorders of accommodation; diplopia); gastrointestinal – (dry mouth; abdominal pain; nausea, vomiting, anorexia, diarrhoea, constipation); impotence; psychiatric disorders.

Skin reactions: Very rarely, rashes; isolated reports of anaphylactic-type reactions possibly culminating in shock (only reported in association with the injectable formulation).

Rarely: Hypoglycaemia.

Very rarely: cholestatic jaundice, headache, dizzy sensation, neutropenia.

Rapid infusion may cause profuse sweating.

Overdose: There is no specific antidote for disopyramide. Prostigmine derivatives can be used to treat anticholinergic effects. Symptomatic supportive measures may include: early gastric lavage; administration of a cathartic followed by activated charcoal by mouth or stomach tube; IV administration of isoprenaline, other vasopressors and/or positive inotropic agents; if needed – infusion of lactate and/or magnesium, electro-systolic assistance, cardioversion, insertion of an intra-aortic balloon for counterpulsion and mechanically assisted ventilation. Haemodialysis, haemofiltration or haemoperfusion with activated charcoal has been employed to lower the serum concentration of the drug.

Pharmacological properties

Pharmacodynamic properties: Class 1 anti-arrhythmic agent.

It decreases membrane responsiveness, prolongs the effective refractory period (ERP) and slows automaticity in cells with augmented automaticity. Effective refractory period of the atrium is lengthened, ERP of the A-V node is shortened and conduction in accessory pathways is prolonged.

Disopyramide is a myocardial depressant and has anti-cholinergic effects.

Pharmacokinetic properties:

Elimination phase of plasma t1/2: 5–8 hours. Increased in hepatic impairment, cardiac and hepatic disease.

Protein binding: 50–60%. Saturable and concentration dependent.

Volume of distribution: Variable according to method of determination.

Metabolism: Approximately 25% of a dose metabolised to a mono-N-dealkylated derivative. Additional 10% as other metabolites.

Excretion: 75% unchanged drug via urine, remainder in faeces mono-N-dealkylated metabolite 25% in urine, 64% via faeces.

Preclinical safety data: Not applicable.

Pharmaceutical particulars

List of excipients: The capsules contain maize starch, magnesium stearate, STA-RX 1500 and talc.

The capsule shell consists of an opaque green body (indigo carmine, iron oxide and titanium dioxide) and an opaque beige body (iron oxide and titanium dioxide).

Incompatibilities: Not known.

Shelf life: Glass bottle: 5 years. PVC Blister: 5 years.

Special precautions for storage: None.

Nature and contents of container: Glass Bottle containing 100 capsules. PVC Blister containing 84 capsules.

Instructions for use/handling: None.

Marketing authorisation holder: Hoechst Marion Roussel Ltd., Broadwater Park, Denham, Uxbridge, Middlesex UB9 5HP, UK.

Marketing authorisation number PL 13402/0113.

Date of approval/revision of SPC June 1998.

Legal category POM.

RYTHMODAN INJECTION*

Qualitative and quantitative composition Each glass ampoule contains 12.88 mg disopyramide phosphate (equivalent to 10 mg of disopyramide) per 1 ml of solution.

Pharmaceutical form Intravenous.

Clinical particulars

Therapeutic indications: Conversion of ventricular and supraventricular arrythmias after myocardial infarction, including patients not responding to lignocaine or other intravenous treatment.

Control of ventricular and atrial extrasystoles, supraventricular tachycardia, and Wolff-Parkinson-White syndrome.

Control of arrhythmias following digitalis or similar glycosides when Rythmodan cannot be given orally.

Posology and method of administration: Route of Administration: Rythmodan Injection is intended for intravenous use only.

Adults including the elderly: The recommended dosage can be given by two different regimes:–

1. An initial direct intravenous injection of 2 mg/kg (but not exceeding 150 mg (15 ml) irrespective of body weight) should be given slowly over not less than five minutes, ie, the rate of injection must not exceed 30 mg (3 ml) per minute in order to reduce or avoid unwanted haemodynamic effects. If conversion occurs during this time the injection should be stopped. If the arrhythmia is to respond to Rythmodan it will usually do so within 10–15 minutes after completion of the injection.

If conversion is achieved by intravenous Rythmodan but the arrhythmia subsequently recurs, a further slow direct intravenous injection over not less than five minutes may be administered cautiously and preferably under ECG control. The total administration by the intravenous route should not exceed 4 mg/kg (maximum 300 mg) in the first hour, nor should the combined administration by the intravenous and oral routes exceed 800 mg in 24 hours.

2. An initial direct intravenous injection as above, ie over not less than five minutes, maintained by intravenous infusion by drip of 20–30 mg/hour (or 0.4 mg/kg/hour) up to a maximum of 800 mg daily. This regime should be employed if the patient is unable to take oral medication or in particularly serious arrhythmias being treated in coronary care units.

Children: Not applicable. Rythmodan Injection is not intended for use in children.

Contra-indications: Disopyramide is contra-indicated in un-paced second or third degree atrioventricular block; bundle-branch block associated with first degree atrioventricular block; un-paced bifasicular block; pre-existing long QT syndromes; severe sinus node dysfunction; severe heart failure, unless secondary to cardiac arrhythmia; and hypersensitivity to disopyramide. It is also contra-indicated in concomitant admistration with other anti-arrhythmics or other drugs liable to provoke ventricular arrythmias, especially Torsade de Pointes (see *Interactions with other medicaments and other forms of interaction*). The sustained release formulation is contra-indicated in patients with renal or hepatic impairment.

Special warnings and special precautions for use: In view of the serious nature of many of the conditions being treated it is suggested that Rythmodan Injection should only be used when facilities exist for cardiac monitoring or defibrillation, should the need arise.

Antiarrhythmic drugs belonging to the class 1c (Vaughan Williams Classification) were included in the Cardiac Arrhythmia Suppression Trial (CAST), a long term multicentre randomised, double blind study in patients with asymptomatic non life-threatening ventricular arrhythmia who had a myocardial infarction more than six days but less than two years previously. A significant increase in mortality and non-fatal cardiac arrest rate was seen in patients treated with class 1c antiarrhythmic drugs when compared with a matched placebo group. The applicability of the CAST results to other antiarrhythmics and other populations (e.g. those without recent infarction) is uncertain. At present, it is best to assume that the risk extends to other antiarrhythmic agents for patients with structural heart disease.

There is no evidence that prolonged suppression of ventricular premature contractions with antiarrhythmic drugs prevents sudden death.

All antiarrhythmic drugs can produce unwanted effects when they are used to treat symptomatic but not life threatening arrhythmia; the expected benefit should be balanced against their risks.

In patients with structural heart disease, proarrhythmia and cardiac decompensation are special risks associated with antiarrhythmic drugs. Special caution should be exercised when prescribing in this taken context.

Disopyramide should not be used in patients with uncompensated congestive heart failure, unless this heart failure is secondary to cardiac arrhythmia. If disopyramide is to be given under these circumstances, special care and monitoring are essential.

Haemodynamically significant arrhythmias are difficult to treat and affected patients have a high mortality risk. Treatment of these arrhythmias, by whatever modality, must be initiated in hospital.

Owing to its negative inotropic effect, disopyramide should be used with caution in patients suffering from significant cardiac failure. This group may be specially sensitive to the negative inotropic properties of disopyramide. Such patients should be fully digitalised or controlled with other therapy before treatment with disopyramide is commenced.

Aggravation of existing arrhythmia, or emergence of a new type of arrhythmia, demands urgent review of disopyramide treatment.

Similarly, if an atrioventricular block or a bifasicular block occurs during treatment, the use of disopyramide should be reviewed.

There have been reports of ventricular tachycardia, ventricular fibrillation and Torsade de Pointes in patients receiving disopyramide. These have usually, but not always, been associated with significant widening of the QRS complex or prolonged QT interval. The QT interval and QRS duration must be monitored and disopyramide should be stopped if these are increased by more than 25%. If these changes or arrhythmias develop the drug should be discontinued. Disopyramide should be used with caution in patients with atrial flutter or atrial tachycardia with block as conversion of a partial AV block to a 1:1 response may occur, leading to a potentially more serious tachyarrhythmia.

The occurrence of hypotension following disopyramide administration, requires prompt discontinuation of the drug. This has been observed especially in patients with cardiomyopathy or uncompensated congestive heart failure. Any resumption of therapy should be at a lower dose with close patient monitoring. Disopyramide should be used with caution in the treatment of digitalis intoxication.

Potassium imbalance: Antiarrhythmic drugs may be hazardous in patients with potassium imbalance, as potassium abnormalities can induce arrhythmias.

During treatment with disopyramide, potassium levels should be checked regularly. Patients treated with diuretics or stimulant laxatives are at particular risk of hypokalaemia.

Renal insufficiency: In renal insufficiency, the dosage of disopyramide should be reduced by adjusting the interval between administrations.

Hepatic insufficiency: Hepatic impairment causes an increase in the plasma half-life of Rythmodan and a reduced dosage may be required.

Hypoglycaemia: Hypoglycaemia has been reported in association with disopyramide administration. Patients at particular risk are the elderly, the malnourished, or diabetics. The risk of hypoglycaemia occurring is increased with impaired renal function or cardiac failure. Blood glucose should be monitored in all patients. Strict adherence to the dosing recommendations is advised. If hypoglycaemia ocurs then treatment with disopyramide should be stopped.

Atropine-like effects: There is a risk of:

– ocular hypertension in patients with narrow-angle glaucoma,

– acute urinary retention in patients with prostatic enlargement,

– aggravation of myasthenia gravis.

Interaction with other medicaments and other forms of interaction:

Combination with other antiarrhythmic drugs: Combinations of antiarrhythmic drugs are not well researched and their effect may be unpredictable. Thus, antiarrhythmic combination should be avoided except under certain circumstances, e.g. Beta-blockers for angina pectoris; digoxin with beta-blocker and/or verapamil for the control of atrial fibrillation, when defined as effective for an individual.

Interaction with drugs associated with risk of Torsade de Pointes, such as

– tricyclic and tetracyclic antidepressants

– intravenous erythromycin

– astemizole; cisapride; pentamidine; pimozide; sparfloxacin; terfenadine

The concomitant use of these medications whilst undergoing treatment with disopyramide increases the chance of cardiac arrhythmia.

There is some evidence that disopyramide is metabolised by hepatic CYP3A. Concomitant administration of significant inhibitors of this isozyme (e.g. certain macrolide or azole antifungal antibiotics) may therefore increase the serum levels of disopyramide. On the other hand, inducers of CYP3A (e.g. rifampicin, certain anticonvulsants) may reduce disopyramide and increase MN-disopyramide serum levels. Since the magnitude of such potential effects is not foreseeable, such drug combinations are not recommended.

When prescribing a drug metabolised by CYP3A [such as theophylline, HIV protease inhibitors (e.g. ritonavir, indinavir, saquinavir), cyclosporin A, warfarin] it should be kept in mind that disopyramide is probably also a substrate of this isozyme and thus competitive inhibition of metabolism might occur, possibly increasing serum levels of these drugs.

Interactions with hypokalaemia inducing drugs: Concomitant use with drugs that can induce hypokalaemia such as: diuretics, amphotericin B, tetracosactrin (corticotrophin analogue), gluco and mineralocorticoids may reduce the action of the drug, or potentiate proarrhythmic effects. Stimulant laxatives are not recommended to be given concomitantly, due to their potassium lowering potential.

Other drug interactions: Atropine and other anticholinergic drugs, including phenothiazines, may potentiate the atropine-like effects of disopyramide.

Pregnancy and lactation:

Pregnancy: Although Rythmodan has undergone animal tests for teratogenicity without evidence of any effect on the developing foetus, its safety in human pregnancy has not been established. Rythmodan has been reported to stimulate contractions of the pregnant uterus. The drug should only be used during pregnancy if benefits clearly outweigh the possible risks to the mother and foetus.

Lactation: No data for Rythmodan Injection, but studies have shown that oral disopyramide is secreted in breast milk, although no adverse effects to the infant have been noted. However, clinical experience is limited and disopyramide should only be used in lactation if, in the clinician's judgement, it is essential for the welfare of the patient. The infant should be closely supervised, particularly for anticholinergic effects and drug levels determined if necessary. Ideally, if the drug is considered essential, an alternative method of feeding should be used.

Effects on ability to drive and use machines: Some adverse reactions may impair the patients' ability to concentrate and react, and hence the ability to drive or operate machinery (see *Undesirable effects*).

Undesirable effects:

Cardiac: It is accepted that the arrhythmogenic potential of disopyramide is weak. However, as with all antiarrhythmic drugs, disopyramide may worsen or provoke arrhythmias. This proarrhythmic effect is more likely to occur in the presence of hypokalaemia with the associated use of antiarrhythmic drugs, in patients with severe structural heart disease or prolongation of the QT interval.

Intra-cardiac conduction abnormalities may occur: QT interval prolongation, widening of the QRS complex, atrioventricular block and bundle-branch block.

Other types of arrhythmia have been reported: Bradycardia, sinus block.

Episodes of severe heart failure or even cardiogenic shock have also been described particularly in patients with severe structural heart disease. The resulting low cardiac output can cause hypotension, renal insufficiency and/or acute hepatic ischemia.

Other adverse reactions include: Atropine like: Urinary (dysuria; acute urinary retention); ocular (disorders of accommodation; diplopia); gastrointestinal – (dry mouth; abdominal pain; nausea, vomiting, anorexia, diarrhoea, constipation); impotence; psychiatric disorders.

Skin reactions: Very rarely, rashes; isolated reports of anaphylactic-type reactions possibly culminating in shock (only reported in association with the injectable formulation).

Rarely: Hypoglycaemia.

Very rarely: cholestatic jaundice, headache, dizzy sensation, neutropenia.

Rapid infusion may cause profuse sweating.

Overdose: There is no specific antidote for disopyramide. Prostigmine derivatives can be used to treat anticholinergic effects. Symptomatic supportive measures may include: early gastric lavage; administration of a cathartic followed by activated charcoal by mouth or stomach tube; IV administration of isoprenaline, other vasopressors and/or positive inotropic agents; if needed – infusion of lactate and/or magnesium, electro-systolic assistance, cardioversion, insertion of an intra-aortic balloon for counterpulsion and mechanically assisted ventilation. Haemodialysis, haemofiltration or haemoperfusion with activated charcoal has been employed to lower the serum concentration of the drug.

Pharmacological properties

Pharmacodynamic properties: Class 1 antiarrhythmic agent.

Pharmacokinetic properties: Following intravenous administration, disopyramide is rapidly distributed. Doses of 1.5–2 mg/kg produce plasma levels of about 10 microg/ml, declining rapidly to 3.8–4.2 microg/ml at 5 minutes and to less than 3 microg/ml at 15 minutes.

In multidose studies, direct slow intravenous injection of 2 mg/kg followed by an infusion of 20 mg/hr, maintained plasma levels of disopyramide between 2.5 and 2.8 microg/ml from the first hour onwards.

Distribution T1/2: 2–4 minutes in healthy volunteers. Longer (15 minutes) in patients with acute myocardial infarct.

Elimination phase of plasma T1/2: 5–8 hours. Increased in renal impairment, cardiac and hepatic disease.

Protein binding: 50–60%. Saturable and concentration dependent.

Volume of distribution: Variable according to method of determination

Metabolism: Approximately 25% of a dose is metabolised to a mono-n-dealkylated derivative. Additional 10% as other metabolites.

Excretion: 75% unchanged drug via urine, remainder in faeces. Mono-n-dealkylated metabolite 25% in urine, 64% via faeces.

Preclinical safety data: Not applicable.

Pharmaceutical particulars

List of excipients: Benzyl Alcohol, Sorbitol and Water for Injection.

Incompatibilities: Not applicable.

Shelf life: 60 Months.

Special precautions for storage: Store below 25°C.

Nature and contents of container: Colourless neutral glass ampoules are available as 5 ml, 10 ml or 15 ml.

Instructions for use/handling: Not applicable.

Marketing authorisation holder: Hoechst Marion Roussel Ltd., Broadwater Park, Denham, Uxbridge, Middlesex UB9 5HP UK.

Marketing authorisation number PL 13402/0112.

Date of approval/revision of SPC June 1998.

Legal category POM.

RYTHMODAN 150 mg CAPSULES*

Presentation

Rythmodan

Capsules containing a white powder. The cap and body are opaque white. The capsules are printed 'RY' on one part and '150' on the other, in black.

Uses Rythmodan is used in the treatment of cardiac arrhythmias as follows:

1. The prevention and treatment of arrhythmias occurring after myocardial infarction.
2. Maintenance of normal rhythm following electro-conversion e.g. atrial fibrillation, atrial flutter.
3. Persistent ventricular extrasystoles.
4. Control of arrhythmias following the use of digitalis or similar glycosides.
5. Suppression of arrhythmias during surgical procedures e.g. cardiac catheterisation.
6. The prevention of paroxysmal supraventricular tachycardia.

7. Other types of arrhythmias e.g. atrial extrasystoles, Wolff-Parkinson-White Syndrome.

Dosage and administration
Route of administration: Oral
300 mg to 800 mg daily in divided doses.

Children: Not recommended as insufficient data available.

Contra-indications, warnings, etc
Contra-indications: Disopyramide is contra-indicated in un-paced second or third degree atrioventricular block; bundle-branch block associated with first-degree atrioventricular block; unpaced bifasicular block; pre-existing long QT syndromes; severe sinus node dysfunction; severe heart failure, unless secondary to cardiac arrhythmia; hypersensitivity to disopyramide. It is also contra-indicated in concomitant administration with other anti-arrhythmics or other drugs liable to provoke ventricular arrythmias, especially Torsade de Pointes (see *Drug interactions*). The sustained release formulation is contra-indicated in patients with renal or hepatic impairment.

Warnings and precautions: In view of the serious nature of many of the conditions being treated it is suggested that Rythmodan Injection should only be used when facilities exist for cardiac monitoring or defibrillation, should the need arise.

Antiarrhythmic drugs belonging to the class 1c (Vaughan Williams Classification) were included in the Cardiac Arrhythmia Suppression Trial (CAST), a long term multicentre randomised, double blind study in patients with asymptomatic non life-threatening ventricular arrhythmia who have had a myocardial infarction more than six days but less than two years previously. A significant increase in mortality and non-fatal cardiac arrest rate was seen in patients treated with class 1c antiarrhythmic drugs when compared with a matched placebo group. The applicability of the CAST results to other antiarrhythmics and other populations (e.g. those without recent infarction) is uncertain. At present, it is best to assume that the risk extends to other antiarrhythmic agents for patients with structural heart disease.

There is no evidence that prolonged suppression of ventricular premature contractions with antiarrhythmic drugs prevents sudden death.

All antiarrhythmic drugs can produce unwanted effects when they are used to treat symptomatic but not life threatening arrhythmia ; the expected benefits should be balanced against their risks.

In patients with structural heart disease, proarrhythmia and cardiac decompensation are special risks associated with antiarrhythmic drugs. Special caution should be exercised when prescribing in this context.

Disopyramide should not be used in patients with uncompensated congestive heart failure, unless this heart failure is secondary to cardiac arrhythmia. If disopyramide is to be given under these circumstances, special care and monitoring are essential.

Haemodynamically significant arrhythmias are difficult to treat and affected patients have a high mortality risk. Treatment of these arrhythmias, by whatever modality, must be initiated in hospital.

Owing to its negative inotropic effect, disopyramide should be used with caution in patients suffering from significant cardiac failure.This group may be specially sensitive to the negative inotropic properties of disopyramide. Such patients should be fully digitalised or controlled with other therapy before treatment with disopyramide is commenced.

Aggravation of existing arrhythmia, or emergence of a new type of arrhythmia, demands urgent review of disopyramide treatment.

Similarly, if an atrioventricular block or a bifasicular block occurs during treatment, the use of disopyramide should be reviewed.

There have been reports of ventricular tachycardia, ventricular fibrillation and Torsade de Pointes in patients receiving disopyramide. These have usually, but not always, been associated with significant widening of the QRS complex or prolonged QT interval. The QT interval and QRS duration must be monitored and disopyramide should be stopped if these are increased by more than 25%. If these changes or arrhythmias develop the drug should be discontinued. Disopyramide should be used only with caution in patients with atrial flutter or atrial tachycardia with block as conversion of a partial AV block to a 1:1 response may occur, leading to a potentially more serious tachyarrhythmia.

The occurrence of hypotension following disopyramide administration requires prompt discontinuation of the drug. This has been observed especially in patients with cardiomyopathy or uncompensated congestive heart failure. Any resumption of therapy should be at a lower dose with close patient monitoring. Disopyramide should be used with caution in the treatment of digitalis intoxication.

Potassium imbalance: Antiarrhythmic drugs may be hazardous in patients with potassium imbalance, as potassium abnormalities can induce arrhythmias.

During treatment with disopyramide, potassium levels should be checked regularly. Patients treated with diuretics or stimulant laxatives are at particular risk of hypokalaemia.

Renal insufficiency: In renal insufficiency, the dosage of disopyramide should be reduced by adjusting the interval between administrations.

Hepatic insufficiency: Hepatic impairment causes an increase in the plasma half-life of Rythmodan and a reduced dosage may be required.

Hypoglycaemia: Hypoglycaemia has been reported in association with disopyramide administration. Patients at particular risk are the elderly, the malnourished, or diabetics. The risk of hypoglycaemia occurring is increased with impaired renal function or cardiac failure. Blood glucose should be monitored in all patients. Strict adherence to the dosing recommendations is advised. If hypoglycaemia occurs then treatment with disopyramide should be stopped.

Atropine-like effects: There is a risk of:
– ocular hypertension in patients with narrow-angle glaucoma,
– acute urinary retention in patients with prostatic enlargement,
– aggravation of myasthenia gravis.

Drug interactions:
Combination with other antiarrhythmic drugs: Combinations of antiarrhythmic drugs are not well researched and their effect may be unpredictable. Thus, antiarrhythmic combination should be avoided except under certain circumstances, e.g. beta-blockers for angina pectoris; digoxin with beta-blocker and/or verapamil for the control of atrial fibrillation, when defined as effective for an individual.

Interaction with drugs associated with risk of Torsade de Pointes, such as
– tricyclic and tetracyclic antidepressants
– intravenous erythromycin
– astemizole; cisapride; pentamidine; pimozide; sparfloxacin; terfenadine

The concomitant use of these medications whilst undergoing treatment with disopyramide increases the chance of cardiac arrhythmia.

There is some evidence that disopyramide is metabolised by hepatic CYP3A. Concomitant administration of significant inhibitors of this isozyme (e.g. certain macrolide or azole antifungal antibiotics) may therefore increase the serum levels of disopyramide. On the other hand, inducers of CYP3A (e.g. rifampicin, certain anticonvulsants) may reduce disopyramide and increase MN-disopyramide serum levels. Since the magnitude of such potential effects is not foreseeable, such drug combinations are not recommended.

When prescribing a drug metabolised by CYP3A [such as theophylline, HIV protease inhibitors (e.g. ritonavir, indinavir, saquinavir), cyclosporin A, warfarin] it should be kept in mind that disopyramide is probably also a substrate of this isozyme and thus competitive inhibition of metabolism might occur, possibly increasing serum levels of these drugs.

Interactions with hypokalaemia inducing drugs: Concomitant use with drugs that can induce hypokalaemia such as: diuretics, amphotericin B, tetracosactrin (corticotrophin analogue), gluco and mineralocorticoids may reduce the action of the drug, or potentiate proarrhythmic effects.

Stimulant laxatives are not recommended to be given concomitantly, due to their potassium lowering potential.

Other drug interactions: Atropine and other anticholinergic drugs, including phenothiazines, may potentiate the atropine-like effects of disopyramide.

Pregnancy: Although Rythmodan has undergone animal tests for teratogenicity without evidence of any effect on the developing foetus, its safety in human pregnancy has not been established. Disopyramide has been reported to stimulate contractions of the pregnant uterus. The drugs should only be used during pregnancy if benefits clearly outweigh the possible risks to the mother and foetus.

Lactation: Studies have shown that oral disopyramide is secreted in breast milk although no adverse effects to the infant have been noted. However, clinical experience is limited and Rythmodan should only be used in lactation if, in the clinicians judgement, it is essential for the welfare of the patient. The infant should be closely supervised, particularly for anticholinergic effects and drug levels determined if necessary. Ideally, if the drug is considered essential an alternative method of feeding should be used.

Effects on ability to drive and use machines: Some adverse reactions may impair the patient's ability to concentrate and react, and hence the ability to drive or operate machinery.

Side-effects:
Cardiac: It is accepted that the arrhythmogenic potential of disopyramide is weak. However, as with all antiarrhythmic drugs, disopyramide may worsen or provoke arrhythmias. This proarrhythmic effect is more likely to occur in the presence of hypokalaemia, with the associated use of antiarrhythmic drugs, in patients with severe structural heart disease with prolongation of the QT interval.

Intra-cardiac conduction abnormalities may occur: QT interval prolongation, widening of the QRS complex, atrioventricular block and bundle-branch block.

Other types of arrhythmia have been reported: bradycardia, sinus block.

Episodes of severe heart failure or even cardiogenic shock have also been described particularly in patients with severe structural heart disease. The resulting low cardiac output can cause hypotension, renal insufficiency and/or acute hepatic ischemia.

Other adverse reactions include: Atropine like: Urinary (dysuria; acute urinary retention); ocular (disorders of accommodation; diplopia); gastrointestinal – (dry mouth, abdominal pain, nausea; vomiting, anorexia, diarrhoea, constipation); impotence; psychiatric disorders.

Skin reactions: very rarely, rashes ; isolated reports of anaphylactic-type reactions possibly culminating in shock (only reported in association with the injectable formulation).

Rarely: hypoglycaemia.

Very rarely: cholestatic jaundice, headache, dizzy sensation, neutropenia.

Rapid infusion may cause profuse sweating.

Overdose: There is no specific antidote for disopyramide. Prostigmine derivatives can be used to treat anticholinergic effects. Symptomatic supportive measures may include: early gastric lavage; administration of a cathartic followed by activated charcoal by mouth or stomach tube; IV administration of isoprenaline, other vasopressors and/or positive inotropic agents; if needed – infusion of lactate and/or magnesium, electro-systolic assistance, cardioversion, insertion of an intra-aortic balloon for counterpulsion and mechanically assisted ventilation. Haemodialysis, haemofiltration or haemoperfusion with activated charcoal has been employed to lower the serum concentrations of the drug.

Pharmaceutical precautions Shelf life: 5 years.

Legal category POM.

Package quantities
Amber glass bottle with jaycap closure containing 100 capsules. PVC/PVdC blister strips in cardboard cartons containing 84 capsules.

Further information
Class 1 anti-arrhythmic agent.

It decreases membrane responsiveness, prolongs the effective refractory period (ERP) and slows automaticity in cells with augmented automaticity. Effective refractory period of the atrium is lengthened, ERP of the A-V node is shortened and conduction in accessory pathways is prolonged.

Disopyramide is a myocardial depressant and has anti-cholinergic effects.

Elimination phase of plasma t1/2: 5–8 hours. Increased in hepatic impairment, cardiac and hepatic disease.

Protein binding: 50–60%. Saturable and concentration dependent.

Volume of distribution: Variable according to method of determination.

Metabolism: Approximately 25% of a dose metabolised to a mono-N-dealkylated derivative. Additional 10% as other metabolites.

Excretion: 75% unchanged drug via urine, remainder in faeces mono-N-dealkylated metabolite 25% in urine, 64% via faeces.

Product licence number 13402/0114.

Product licence holder: Hoechst Marion Roussel Ltd., Broadwater Park, Denham, Uxbridge, Middlesex UB9 5HP.

Date of revision June 1998

RYTHMODAN RETARD*

Qualitative and quantitative composition Tablets containing Disopyramide Phosphate 322.5 mg (equivalent to 250 mg base).

Pharmaceutical form Tablet.

Clinical particulars
Therapeutic indications:
Properties: Prevention and control of a wide variety of cardiac arrhythmias, probably by slowing conduction in the his-Purkinje system and by increasing the effective refractory period of the atria and ventricles.

Indications:
1. Maintenance of normal rhythm following conversion by Rythmodan injection, other parenteral drugs or electroconversion.
2. Prevention of arrhythmias after myocardial infarction.
3. Treatment of persistent ventricular and atrial extrasystoles, paroxysmal supra ventricular tachycardia, Wolff-Parkinson-White syndrome.

4. Suppression of arrhythmias during surgical procedures.

5. Control of arrhythmias following the use of digitalis or similar glycosides.

Posology and method of administration: Route of administration: Oral.

Recommended dose for stabilised patients or those receiving Rythmodan for the first time is one to one and a half tablets (250–375 mg) twice daily. Patients being transferred from intravenous therapy with Rythmodan should be stabilised on standard Rythmodan capsules for the first 24 hours. Tablets should be swallowed and not crushed or chewed.

Children: There are insufficient data to recommend the use of Rythmodan in children.

Elderly: No special dosage recommendations.

Contra-indications: Disopyramide is contra-indicated in un-paced second or third degree atrioventricular block; bundle-branch block associated with first degree atrioventricular block; un-paced bifasicular block; pre-existing long QT syndromes; severe sinus node dysfunction; severe heart failure, unless secondary to cardiac arrhythmia; and hypersensitivity to disopyramide. It is also contra-indicated in concomitant administration with other anti-arrhythmics or other drugs liable to provoke ventricular arrythmias, especially Torsade de Pointes (see *Interaction with other medicaments and other forms of interaction*). The sustained release formulation is contra-indicated in patients with renal or hepatic impairment.

Special warnings and special precautions for use: In view of the serious nature of many of the conditions being treated it is suggested that Rythmodan Injection should only be used when facilities exist for cardiac monitoring or defibrillation, should the need arise.

Antiarrhythmic drugs belonging to the class 1c (Vaughan Williams Classification) were included in the Cardiac Arrhythmia Suppression Trial (CAST), a long term multicentre randomised, double blind study in patients with asymptomatic non life-threatening ventricular arrhythmia who had a myocardial infarction more than six days but less than two years previously. A significant increase in mortality and non-fatal cardiac arrest rate was seen in patients treated with class 1c antiarrhythmic drugs when compared with a matched placebo group. The applicability of the CAST results to other antiarrhythmics and other populations (e.g. those without recent infarction) is uncertain. At present, it is best to assume that the risk extends to other antiarrhythmic agents for patients with structural heart disease.

There is no evidence that prolonged suppression of ventricular premature contractions with antiarrhythmic drugs prevents sudden death.

All antiarrhythmic drugs can produce unwanted effects when they are used to treat symptomatic but not life threatening arrhythmia; the expected benefit should be balanced against their risks.

In patients with structural heart disease, proarrhythmia and cardiac decompensation are special risks associated with antiarrhythmic drugs. Special caution should be exercised when prescribing in this taken context.

Disopyramide should not be used in patients with uncompensated congestive heart failure, unless this heart failure is secondary to cardiac arrhythmia. If disopyramide is to be given under these circumstances, special care and monitoring are essential.

Haemodynamically significant arrhythmias are difficult to treat and affected patients have a high mortality risk. Treatment of these arrhythmias, by whatever modality, must be initiated in hospital.

Owing to its negative inotropic effect, disopyramide should be used with caution in patients suffering from significant cardiac failure. This group may be specially sensitive to the negative inotropic properties of disopyramide. Such patients should be fully digitalised or controlled with other therapy before treatment with disopyramide is commenced.

Aggravation of existing arrhythmia, or emergence of a new type of arrhythmia, demands urgent review disopyramide treatment.

Similarly, if an atrioventricular block or a bifasicular block occurs during treatment, the use of disopyramide should be reviewed.

There have been reports of ventricular tachycardia, ventricular fibrillation and Torsade de Pointes in patients receiving disopyramide. These have usually, but not always, been associated with significant widening of the QRS complex or prolonged QT interval. The QT interval and QRS duration must be monitored and disopyramide should be stopped if these are increased by more than 25%. If these changes or arrhythmias develop the drug should be discontinued. Disopyramide should be used with caution in patients with atrial flutter or atrial tachycardia with block as conversion of a partial AV block to a 1:1 response may occur, leading to a potentially more serious tachyarrhythmia.

The occurrence of hypotension following disopyramide administration, requires prompt discontinuation of the drug. This has been observed especially in patients with cardiomyopathy or uncompensated congestive heart failure. Any resumption of therapy should be at a lower dose with close patient monitoring. Disopyramide should be used with caution in the treatment of digitalis intoxication.

Potassium imbalance: Antiarrhythmic drugs may be hazardous in patients with potassium imbalance, as potassium abnormalities can induce arrhythmias.

During treatment with disopyramide, potassium levels should be checked regularly. Patients treated with diuretics or stimulant laxatives are at particular risk of hypokalaemia.

Renal insufficiency: In renal insufficiency, the dosage of disopyramide should be reduced by adjusting the interval between administrations.

Hepatic insufficiency: Hepatic impairment causes an increase in the plasma half-life of Rythmodan and a reduced dosage may be required.

Hypoglycaemia: Hypoglycaemia has been reported in association with disopyramide administration. Patients at particular risk are the elderly, the malnourished, or diabetics. The risk of hypoglycaemia occurring is increased with impaired renal function or cardiac failure. Blood glucose should be monitored in all patients. Strict adherence to the dosing recommendations is advised. If hypoglycaemia occurs then treatment with disopyramide should be stopped.

Atropine-like effects: There is a risk of:

– ocular hypertension in patients with narrow-angle glaucoma,

– acute urinary retention in patients with prostatic enlargement,

– aggravation of myasthenia gravis.

Interaction with other medicaments and other forms of interaction:

Combination with other antiarrhythmic drugs: Combinations of antiarrhythmic drugs are not well researched and their effect may be unpredictable. Thus, antiarrhythmic combination should be avoided except under certain circumstances, e.g. Beta-blockers for angina pectoris; digoxin with beta-blocker and/or verapamil for the control of atrial fibrillation, when defined as effective for an individual.

Interaction with drugs associated with risk of Torsade de Pointes, such as:

– tricyclic and tetracyclic antidepressants

– intravenous erythromycin

– astemizole; cisapride; pentamidine; pimozide; sparfloxacin; terfenadine

The concomitant use of these medications whilst undergoing treatment with disopyramide increases the chance of cardiac arrhythmia.

There is some evidence that disopyramide is metabolised by hepatic CYP3A. Concomitant administration of significant inhibitors of this isozyme (e.g. certain macrolide or azole antifungal antibiotics) may therefore increase the serum levels of disopyramide. On the other hand, inducers of CYP3A (e.g. rifampicin, certain anticonvulsants) may reduce disopyramide and increase MN-disopyramide serum levels. Since the magnitude of such potential effects is not foreseeable, such drug combinations are not recommended.

When prescribing a drug metabolised by CYP3A [such as theophylline, HIV protease inhibitors (e.g. ritonavir, indinavir, saquinavir), cyclosporin A, warfarin] it should be kept in mind that disopyramide is probably also a substrate of this isozyme and thus competitive inhibition of metabolism might occur, possibly increasing serum levels of these drugs.

Interactions with hypokalaemia inducing drugs: Concomitant use with drugs that can induce hypokalaemia such as: diuretics, amphotericin B, tetracosactrin (corticotrophin analogue), gluco and mineralocorticoids may reduce the action of the drug, or potentiate proarrhythmic effects. Stimulant laxatives are not recommended to be given concomitantly, due to their potassium lowering potential.

Other drug interactions: Atropine and other anticholinergic drugs, including phenothiazines, may potentiate the atropine-like effects of disopyramide.

Pregnancy and lactation:

Pregnancy: Although Rythmodan has undergone animal tests for teratogenicity without evidence of any effect on the developing foetus, its safety in human pregnancy has not been established. Rythmodan has been reported to stimulate contractions of the pregnant uterus. The drug should only be used during pregnancy if benefits clearly outweigh the possible risks to the mother and foetus.

Lactation: No data for Rythmodan Injection, but studies have shown that oral disopyramide is secreted in breast milk, although no adverse effects to the infant have been noted. However, clinical experience is limited and disopyramide should only be used in lactation if, in the clinician's judgement, it is essential for the welfare of the patient. The infant should be closely supervised, particularly for anticholinergic effects and drug levels determined if necessary. Ideally, if the drug is considered essential, an alternative method of feeding should be used.

Effects on ability to drive and use machines: Some adverse reactions may impair the patients' ability to concentrate and react, and hence the ability to drive or operate machinery (see *Undesirable effects*).

Undesirable effects:

Cardiac: It is accepted that the arrhythmogenic potential of disopyramide is weak. However, as with all antiarrhythmic drugs, disopyramide may worsen or provide arrhythmias. This proarrhythmic effect is more likely to occur in the presence of hypokalaemia with the associated use of antiarrhythmic drugs, in patients with severe structural heart disease or prolongation of the QT interval.

Intra-cardiac conduction abnormalities may occur: QT interval prolongation, widening of the QRS complex, atrioventricular block and bundle-branch block.

Other types of arrhythmia have been reported: Bradycardia, sinus block.

Episodes of severe heart failure or even cardiogenic shock have also been described particularly in patients with severe structural heart disease. The resulting low cardiac output can cause hypotension, renal insufficiency and/or acute hepatic ischemia.

Other adverse reactions include: Atropine like: Urinary (dysuria; acute urinary retention); ocular (disorders of accommodation; diplopia); gastrointestinal – (dry mouth; abdominal pain; nausea, vomiting, anorexia, diarrhoea, constipation); impotence; psychiatric disorders.

Skin reactions: Very rarely, rashes; isolated reports of anaphylactic-type reactions possibly culminating in shock (only reported in association with the injectable formulation).

Rarely: Hypoglycaemia.

Very rarely: cholestatic jaundice, headache, dizzy sensation, neutropenia.

Rapid infusion may cause profuse sweating.

Overdose: There is no specific antidote for disopyramide. Prostigmine derivatives can be used to treat anticholinergic effects. Symptomatic supportive measures may include: early gastric lavage; administration of a cathartic followed by activated charcoal by mouth or stomach tube; IV administration of isoprenaline, other vasopressors and/or positive inotropic agents; if needed – infusion of lactate and/or magnesium, electro-systolic assistance, cardioversion, insertion of an intra-aortic balloon for counterpulsion and mechanically assisted ventilation. Haemodialysis, haemofiltration or haemoperfusion with activated charcoal has been employed to lower the serum concentration of the drug.

Pharmacological properties

Pharmacodynamic properties: Disopyramide is a Class 1 antiarrhythmic agent with a depressant action on the heart similar to that of quinidine and is used for the prevention and treatment of a wide variety of cardiac arrhythmias.

Pharmacokinetic properties: The dissolution characteristics of Rythmodan Retard are designed to release 250 mg disopyramide over 12 hours. The dissolution profile is matched to the drug half life of 6–8 hours with good therapeutic levels followed by steady release of disopyramide to sustain therapeutic effect. The sustained release mechanism is based on the matrix principle, adapted for disopyramide. Reliable release is achieved by strict control of particle size.

Preclinical safety data: Not applicable.

Pharmaceutical particulars

List of excipients: The tablets contain glyceryl monostearate, castor sugar, povidone and magnesium stearate.

The film coating consists of hydroxypropyl methylcellulose, propylene glycol, sorbitan monolaurate and titanium dioxide E171.

Incompatibilities: Not known.

Shelf life: Glass bottle: 5 years. PVC Blister: 5 years.

Special precautions for storage:

Glass Bottle: Store below 30°C.

PVC Blister: Store below 30°C.

Nature and contents of container: Glass Bottle containing 100 tablets. PVC Blister containing 56 or 100 tablets.

Instructions for use/handling: Not applicable.

Marketing authorisation holder: Hoechst Marion Roussel Ltd., Broadwater Park, Denham, Uxbridge, Middlesex UB9 5HP, UK.

Marketing authorisation number PL 13402/0115.

Date of approval/revision of SPC June 1998.

Legal category POM.

TRENTAL 400

Qualitative and quantitative composition Oxpentifylline 400 mg.

Pharmaceutical form Slow release sugar coated tablet.

Clinical particulars
Therapeutic indications: Trental 400 is indicated in the treatment of peripheral vascular disease, including intermittent claudication and rest pain.

Posology and method of administration: The recommended initial dose is 1 tablet (400 mg) three times daily; two tablets daily may prove sufficient in some patients, particularly for maintenance therapy. Tablets should be taken with or immediately after meals, and swallowed whole with plenty of water.

Elderly: No special dosage requirements.

Children: Trental 400 is not suitable for use in children.

Special cases: In patients with impairment of renal function (creatinine clearance below 30 ml/min) a dose reduction by approximately 30% to 50% may be necessary guided by individual tolerance.

Contra-indications: Trental 400 is contra-indicated in cases where there is known hypersensitivity to the active constituent, oxpentifylline other methyl xanthines or any of the excipients. Also in patients with cerebral haemorrhage, extensive retinal haemorrhage, acute myocardial infarction and severe cardiac arrhythmias.

Special warnings and special precautions for use: In patients with hypotension or severe coronary artery disease, Trental 400 should be used with caution, as a transient hypotensive effect is possible and, in isolated cases, might result in a reduction in coronary artery perfusion.

Particularly careful monitoring is required in patients with impaired renal function. In patients with a creatinine clearance of less than 30 ml/min it may be necessary to reduce the daily dose of Trental 400 to one or two tablets to avoid accumulation. In patients with severely impaired liver function the dosage may need to be reduced.

Interaction with other medicaments and other forms of interaction: High doses of Trental injection have been shown, in rare cases, to intensify the hypoglycaemic action of insulin and oral hypoglycaemic agents. However, no effect on insulin release has been observed with Trental following oral administration.

Trental 400 may potentiate the effect of anti-hypertensive agents and the dosage of the latter may need to be reduced.

Trental 400 should not be given concomitantly with ketorolac as there is increased risk of bleeding and/or prolongation of prothrombin time.

Concomitant administration of oxpentifylline and theophylline may increase theophylline levels in some patients. Therefore there may be an increase in and intensification of adverse effects of theophylline.

Pregnancy and lactation: There is no information on the use of Trental in pregnancy but no untoward effects have been found in animal studies. Trental 400 should not be administered during pregnancy.

Oxpentifylline passes into breast milk in minute quantities. Because insufficient experience has been gained, the possible risks and benefits must be weighed before administration of Trental 400 to breast feeding mothers.

Effects on ability to drive and use machines: No effect known.

Undesirable effects: Gastrointestinal side-effects (e.g. nausea, vomiting, diarrhoea), may occur which, in individual cases, could necessitate discontinuation of treatment. Headache, dizziness, agitation and sleep disorders may occasionally occur as well as, in isolated cases intrahepatic cholestasis and transaminase elevation.

There have been reports of flushing, occasionally tachycardia and rarely angina pectoris and hypotension, particularly if using high doses of oxpentifylline. In such cases a discontinuation of the medication or a reduction of the daily dosage is required.

Hypersensitivity reactions such as pruritus, rash, urticaria, anaphylactic or anaphylactoid reactions with angioneurotic edema or bronchospasm may occur in isolated cases and usually disappear rapidly after discontinuation of the drug treatment.

A few very rare events of bleeding (e.g. skin, mucosa) have been reported in patients treated with Trental with and without anticoagulants or platelet aggregation inhibitors. The serious cases are predominantly concentrated in the gastrointestinal, genitourinary, multiple site and surgical wound areas and are associated with bleeding risk factors. A causal relationship between Trental therapy and bleeding has not been established. Thrombocytopenia has occurred in isolated cases.

Overdose: The treatment of overdosage should be symptomatic with particular attention to supporting the cardiovascular system.

Pharmacological properties
Pharmacodynamic properties: Leukocyte properties of haemorrheologic importance have been modified in animal and in vitro human studies. Oxpentifylline has been shown to increase leukocyte deformability and to inhibit neutrophil adhesion and activation.

Pharmacokinetic properties: The half life of absorption of Trental 400 is 4–6 hours. Oxpentifylline is extensively metabolised, mainly in the liver. Sixty percent of a single dose of Trental 400 is eliminated via the kidney over 24 hours.

Preclinical safety data: Nothing of clinical relevance.

Pharmaceutical particulars
List of excipients: Hydroxyethyl cellulose, polyvinylpyrrolidone, talc, magnesium stearate, sucrose, gum arabic, polyethylene glycol 6000, erythrosine (E127). titanium dioxide (E171).

Incompatibilities: None known.

Shelf life: 5 years.

Special precautions for storage: Store below 25°C in a dry place.

Nature and contents of container: Blister Pack (Alu/PVC) of 10 or 90 tablets, amber glass bottles of 100 or 250 tablets, plastic pots of 100 or 250 tablets.

Instruction for use/handling: None.

Marketing authorisation holder: Hoechst Marion Roussel Ltd., Broadwater Park, Denham, Uxbridge, Middlesex, UB9 5HP.

Marketing authorisation number PL 13402/0055.

Date of approval/revision of SPC December 1997.

Legal Category POM.

**Trade Mark*

Bristol-Myers Pharmaceuticals

Bristol-Myers Squibb House
Staines Road
Hounslow TW3 3JA

☎ 0181 572 7422 🗋 0181 754 3789

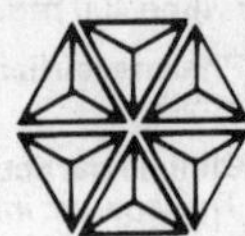

ALPHA KERI* BATH OIL

Qualitative and quantitative composition Bath oil containing Mineral oil 91.7% and Lanolin oil 3%.

Pharmaceutical form Bath oil.

Clinical particulars
Therapeutic indications: Alpha Keri effective deposits a thin uniform emulisified film of oil over the skin, and this retards evaporation of moisture, helps to relieve itching, lubricates and softens the skin. Alpha Keri is valuable as an aid in the management of dry pruritic skin, especilly in senile pruritus, ichthyosis and other dermotases wher dermal hydration is an important part of the therapy (as in the prevention of decubitus ulcer).

Posology and method of administration
Adults: Bath: Add 10-20 ml to the bath water. Soak for 10-20 minutes.

Sponge bath: Add 10-20 ml to basin of warm water. Apply over the entire body with a sponge or flannel.

Skin cleansing: Rub a small amount onto wet skin, rinse and pat dry.

Infant bath: Add 5 ml to bath water.

Shower: Pour a small amount onto a wet sponge or flannel and rub onto wet skin, rinse and pat dry.

Contra-indications: As Alpha Keri deposits a film of oil over the skin, special care should be taken to guard against slipping, especially in the bath or shower.

Alpha Keri contains lanolin oil and is there contra-indicated in thos patients allergic to this ingredient.

Special warnings and special precautions for use: None known.

Interactions with other medicinal products and other forms of interaction: Do not use Alpha Keri bath oil if you are allergic to lanolin oil or any of the other ingredients. Go back to your doctor as soon as possible to discuss your concerns and follow the advice given.

Pregnancy and lactation: Alpha Keri oil works on the suface of the skin and is unlikely to be absorbed

Effects on ability to drive and use machines: None known.

Undesirable effects: Alpha Keri deposits a film of oil over the skin, special care should be taken to guard against slipping, especailly in the bath or shower.

Overdose: If swallowed, Alpha Keri bath oil will not enter the bloodstream but may cause a stomach upset.

Pharmacological properties
Pharmacodynamic properties: Mineral and lanolin oils have emollient properties. The product deposits a thin uniform emulsified film of oil over the skin and thus retards the evaporation of moisture, helping to relieve itching, lubricates and softens the skin.

Pharmacokinetic properties: Not applicable for this type of product.

Preclinical safety data: No further relevant information.

Pharmaceutical particulars
List of excipients: Oxybenzone, perfume, PEG-4-dilaurate.

Incompatibilities: None known.

Shelf life: 36 months.

Special precautions for storage: Store Alpha Keri bath oil at room temperature.

Nature and contents of container: Clear PVC Bottles, closures are polypropylene with pulp/SA-66 liners or linerless polypropylene dispenser closure with hinge (flip-top closure) in pack sizes of 240 or 480 ml.

Instructions for use/handling: None known.

Marketing authorisation number 0125/0141.

Date of first authorisation/renewal of authorisation 24 March 1982/23 June 1992.

Date of (partial) revision of the text May 1997

AMIKIN* INJECTION

Qualitative and quantitative composition Each vial contains in 2 ml amikacin sulphate equivalent to amikacin activity 100 mg (100,000 international units).

Each vial contains in 2 ml amikacin sulphate equivalent to amikacin activity 500 mg (500,000 international units)

Pharmaceutical form Solution for administration to human beings by injection.

Clinical particulars
Therapeutic indications: Amikacin sulphate is an aminoglycoside antibiotic which is active against a broad spectrum of gram-negative organisms, including *Pseudomonas* spp., *Escherichia coli*, indole-positive and indole-negative *Proteus* spp. *Klebsiella-Enterobacter-Serratia* spp, *Salmonella*, *Shigella*, *Minea-Herellae*, *Citrobacter freundii* and *Providencia* spp.

Many strains of these gram-negative organisms resistant to gentamicin and tobramycin may show sensitivity to amikacin *in vitro*. The principal gram-positive organism sensitive to amikacin is *Staphylococcus aureus*, including methicillin-resistant strains. Amikacin has some activity against other gram-positive organisms including certain strains of *Streptococcus pyogenes*, Enterococci and *Diplococcus pneumoniae*.

Amikin is indicated in the short-term treatment of serious infections due to susceptible strains of gram-negative bacteria. It may also be indicated for the treatment of known or suspected staphylococcal disease.

Posology and method of administration: For most infections the intramsucular route is preferred, but in life-threatening infections, or in patients in whom intramuscular injection is not feasible the intravenous route may be used.

Intramuscular and intravenous administration: At the recommended dosage level, uncomplicated infections due to sensitive organisms should respond to therapy within 24 to 48 hours.

If clinical response does not occur within three to five days consideration should be given to alternative therapy.

Adults and children: 15 mg/kg/day in two equally divided doses (equivalent to 500 mg b.i.d. in adults): use of the 100 mg/2 ml strength is recommended for children for the accurate measurement of the appropriate dose.

Neonates and premature infants: An initial loading dose of 10 mg/kg followed by 15 mg/kg/day in two equally divided doses.

Elderly: Amikacin is excreted by the renal route, renal function should be assessed whenever possible and dosage adjusted as described under impaired renal function.

Life-threatening infections and/or those caused by pseudomonas: The adult dose may be increased to 500 mg every eight hours but should neither exceed 1.5 g/day nor be administered for a period longer than 10 days. A maximum total adult dose of 15 g should not be exceeded.

Urinary tract infections: (other than pseudomonal infections): 7.5 mg/kg/day in two equally divided doses (equivalent to 250 mg b.i.d. in adults). As the activity of amikacin is enhanced by increasing the pH, a urinary alkalising agent may be administered concurrently.

Serum Creatinine Concentration (mg/100 ml)		*Interval between AMIKACIN doses of 7.5 mg/kg/IM (hours)*
1.5		13.5
2.0		18
2.5		22.5
3.0		27
3.5	X9 =	31.5
4.0		36
4.5		40.5
5.0		45
5.5		49.5
6.0		54

Impaired renal function: In patients with impaired renal function, the daily dose should be reduced and/or the intervals between doses increased to avoid accumulation of the drug. A suggested method for estimating dosage in patients with known or suspected diminished renal function is to multiply the serum creatinine concentration (in mg/100 ml) by 9 and use the resulting figure as the interval in hours between doses.

As renal function may alter appreciably during therapy, the serum creatinine should be checked frequently and the dosage regimen modified as necessary.

Intraperitoneal use: Following exploration for established peritonitis, or after peritoneal contamination due to faecal spill during surgery, Amikin may be used as an irrigant after recovery from anaesthesia in concentrations of 0.25% (2.5 mg/ml). If instillation is desired in adults, a single dose of 500 mg is diluted in 20 ml of sterile distilled water and may be instilled through a polyethylene catheter sutured into the wound at closure. If possible, instillation should be postponed until the patient has fully recovered from the effects of anaesthesia and muscle-relaxing drugs.

Other routes of administration: Amikin in concentrations of 0.25% may be used satisfactorily as an irrigating solution in abscess cavities, the pleural space, the peritoneum and the cerebral ventricles

Contra-indications: None.

Special warnings and special precautions for use: Patients should be well hydrated during amikacin therapy.

In patients with impaired renal function or diminished glomerular filtration, amikacin should be used cautiously. In such patients, renal function should be assessed by the usual methods prior to therapy and periodically during therapy. Daily doses should be reduced and/or the interval between doses lengthened in accordance with serum creatinine concentrations to avoid accumulation of abnormally high blood levels and to minimise the risk of ototoxicity.

As with other aminoglycosides, ototoxicity and/or nephrotoxicity can result from the use of amikacin; precautions on dosage and adequate hydration should be observed.

If signs of renal irritation appear (such as albumin, casts, red or white blood cells), hydration should be increased and a reduction in dosage may be desirable. These findings usually disappear when treatment is completed. However, if azotaemia or a progressive decrease in urine output occurs, treatment should be stopped.

The use of amikacin in patients with a history of allergy to aminoglycosides or in patients who may have subclinical renal or eighth nerve damage induced by prior administration of nephrotoxic and/or ototoxic agents such as streptomycin, dihydrostreptomycin, gentamicin, tobramycin, kanamycin, bekanamycin, neomycin, polymyxin B, colistin, cephaloridine, or viomycin should be considered with caution, as toxicity may be additive.

In these patients amikacin should be used only if, in the opinion of the physician, therapeutic advantages outweigh the potential risks.

The intraperitoneal use of amikacin is not recommend in young children.

Interactions with other medicinal products and other forms of interaction: The risk of ototoxicity is increased when amikacin is used in conjunction with rapidly acting diuretic drugs, particularly when the diuretic is administered intravenously. Such agents include frusemide and ethacrynic acid. Irreversible deafness may result.

The intraperitoneal use of amikacin is not recommended in patients under the influence of anaesthetics or muscle-relaxing drugs (including ether, halothane, d-tubocurarine, succinylcholine and decamethonium) as neuromuscular blockade and consequent respiratory depression may occur.

Pregnancy and lactation: The safety of Amikin in pregnancy has not yet been established.

Effects on ability to drive and use machines: None stated.

Undesirable effects: When the recommended precautions and dosages are followed the incidence of toxic reactions, such as tinnitus, vertigo, and partial reversible or irreversible deafness, skin rash, drug fever, headache, paraesthesia, nausea and vomiting is low. Urinary signs of renal irritation (albumin, casts, and red or white blood cells), azotaemia and oliguria have been reported.

Overdose: In the event of overdosage or toxic reaction, peritoneal dialysis or haemodialysis will aid in the removal of amikacin from the blood.

Pharmacological properties

Pharmacodynamic properties: Amikacin sulphate is an aminoglycoside antibiotic which is active against a broad spectrum of gram-negative organisms, including *Pseudomonas* spp, *Escherichia coli*, indole-positive and indole-negative *Proteus* spp. *Klebsiella-Enterobacter-Serratia* spp, *Salmonella, Shigella, Minea-Herellae, Citrobacter Freundii* and *Providencia* spp.

Many strains of these gram-negative organisms resistant to gentamicin and tobramycin may show sensitivity to amikacin *in vitro*. The principal gram-positive organism sensitive to amikacin is *Staphylococcus aureus*, including methicillin-resistant strains. Amikacin has some activity against other gram-positive organisms including certain strains of *Streptococcus pyogenes*, Enterococci and *Diplococcus pneumoniae*.

Pharmacokinetic properties: Amikin is rapidly absorbed after intramuscular injection. Peak serum levels of approximately 11 mg/l and 23 mg/l are reached one hour after i.m. doses of 250 mg and 500 mg respectively. Levels 10 hours after injection are of the order of 0.3 mg/l and 2.1 mg/l respectively.

Twenty per cent or less is bound to serum protein and serum concentrations remain in the bactericidal range for sensitive organisms for 10 to 12 hours.

Pharmacokinetic properties: Amikin diffuses readily through extracellular fluids and is excreted in the urine unchanged, primarily by glomerular filtration. Half-life in individuals with normal renal functions is two to three hours.

Following intramuscular administration of a 250 mg dose, about 65% is excreted in six hours and 91% within 24 hours. The urinary concentrations average 563 mg/l in the first 6 hours and 163 mg/l over 6 to 12 hours. Mean urine concentrations after a 500 mg i.m. dose average 832 mg/l in the first six hours.

Single doses of 500 mg administered to normal adults as an intravenous infusion over a period of 30 minutes produce a mean peak serum concentration of 38 mg/l at the end of the infusion. Repeated infusions do not produce drug accumulation.

Amikin has been found in cerebrospinal fluid, pleural fluid, amniotic fluid and in the peritoneal cavity following parenteral administration.

Preclinical safety data: No further relevant information.

Pharmaceutical particulars

List of excipients: Sodium Citrate, Sodium Bisulphite, Sulphuric Acid, Water for Injection.

Incompatibilities: None.

Shelf life: 36 months.

Special precautions for storage: Store below 25°C.

Nature and contents of container: 2 ml flint glass Type 1 vial with butyl rubber stopper and aluminium seal.

Instructions for use/handling: None stated.

Marketing authorisation numbers
100 mg/2 ml 0125/0090R
500 mg/2 ml 0215/0092R

Date of approval/revision of SPC October 1995

Legal category POM

ANGETTES* 75

Qualitative and quantitative composition Each tablet contains: Aspirin BP 75 mg

Pharmaceutical form Oral tablet.

Clincial particulars

Therapeutic indications: As a platelet antiaggregatory agent for the prevention of secondary myocardial infarction and in patients suffering from unstable angina.

Posology and method of administration

Adults: Following myocardial infarction; two tablets to be taken once daily. Treatment should commence as soon as possible. Patients suffering from unstable angina: four tablets once daily.

Elderly: The risk/benefit ratios in the elderly have not been fully established.

Children: Children (under 12 years) not recommended except under medical supervision for use for example in juvenile rheumatoid arthritis.

Contra-indications: Active peptic ulceration, haemophilia and other bleeding disorders, hypersensitivity to aspirin.

Special warnings and special precautions for use: Aspirin may induce gastro-intestinal haemorrhage, occasionally major. Patients with hypertension should be carefully monitored.

There is a possible association between Aspirin and Reye's Syndrome when administered to children with a fever. For this reason it should not normally be given to children under 12 years of age except on medical advice.

Interactions with other medicinal products and other forms of interaction: Aspirin may enhance the effects of anticoagulants and may inhibit the action of uricosurics.

Pregnancy and lactation: There is clinical and epidemiological evidence of safety in human pregnancy. Aspirin may prolong labour and contribute to maternal and neonatal bleeding, and should be avoided at term.

Effects on ability to drive and use machines: None known.

Undesirable effects: Aspirin may enhance the effects of anticoagulants and may inhibit the action of uricosurics. Aspirin may precipitate bronchospasm and may induce attacks of asthma in susceptible subjects.

Overdose: Overdosage is unlikely due to the low level of aspirin in Angettes. If necessary gastric lavage, forced alkaline diuresis and supportive therapy may be employed. Restoration of acid/base balance may be required.

Pharmacological properties

Pharmacodynamic properties: Aspirin has antiplatelet, analgesic, antipyretic and anti-inflammatory properties.

Pharmacokinetic properties: After a single oral dose of a salicylate, the plasma concentration becomes appreciable within 30 minutes, reaches a peak in about 2 hours and then slowly declines.

The highest concentrations occur in plasma, kidney, liver, heart and lung.

From 50-80% of salicylic acid in plasma is bound to plasma proteins, mainly albumin.

Salicylate is metabolised chiefly in the smooth endoplasmic reticulum of liver cells.

Preclinical safety data: There are no preclinical safety data of relevance to the prescriber which are additional to that already included in other sections of the SPC.

Pharmaceutical particulars

List of excipients: Lactose, maize starch, sodium saccharin.

Incompatibilities: None.

Shelf life: 36 months.

Special precautions for storage: Store below 30°C.

Nature and contents of container: HDPE bottle with white opaque polypropylene CR cap.

2 x 7 blister pack of PVC/PVDC with 20 micron lacquered hard temper aluminium foil.

Instructions for use/handling: None.

Marketing authorisation number 0125/5020R

Date of first authorisation/renewal of authorisation
6th June 1990

Date of (partial) revision of the text January 1998

BAXAN*

Presentation *Baxan Capsules:* white capsules imprinted with the number 7244 containing cefadroxil monohydrate equivalent to 500 mg cefadroxil activity.

Other ingredients: Colloidal silicon dioxide, lactose, magnesium stearate; gelatin capsules contain titanium dioxide.

Baxan Suspension: supplied as a bottle containing powder for reconstitution to provide 125 mg, 250 mg or 500 mg per 5 ml.

Other ingredients: Flavours, polysorbate 40, sodium benzoate, sucrose, titanium dioxide, xanthan gum.

Uses Baxan is a cephalosporin antibiotic bactericidal *in vitro* against a wide range of Gram-positive and Gram-negative micro-organisms. Sensitive Gram-positive organisms include: penicillinase and non-penicillinase-producing *staphylococci*, beta-haemolytic *streptococci, Streptococcus pneumoniae* and *Streptococcus pyogenes*. Sensitive Gram-negative organisms include *Escherichia coli*, Klebsiella species, *Proteus mirabilis, Moraxella [Branhamella] catarrhalis* and *Bacteroides spp.* (excluding *Bacteroides fragilis*) and some strains of *Haemophilus influenzae*.

Baxan is indicated in the treatment of the following infections when due to susceptible micro-organisms.

Respiratory tract infections: Tonsillitis, pharyngitis, lobar and bronchopneumonia, acute and chronic bronchitis, pulmonary abscess, empyema, pleurisy, sinusitis, laryngitis, otitis media.

Skin and soft-tissue infections: Lymphadenitis, abscesses, cellulitis, decubitus ulcers, mastitis, furunculosis, erysipelas.

Genitourinary tract infections: Pyelonephritis, cystitis, urethritis, gynaecological infections.

Other infections: Osteomyelitis, septic arthritis.

Dosage and administration

Adults and children weighing more than 40 kg (88 lbs): 500 mg to 1 g twice a day, depending upon the severity of infection.

Alternatively, in skin and soft tissue and uncomplicated urinary tract infections, 1 g once a day.

In the treatment of beta-haemolytic streptococcal infections, Baxan should be administered for at least 10 days.

Children weighing less than 40 kg (88 lbs):
Under 1 year: 25 mg/kg daily in divided doses, e.g. 2.5 ml of the 125 mg per 5 ml suspension twice a day for a 6 month old infant weighing 5 kg, or 5 ml of the 125 mg per 5 ml suspension twice a day for a 1 year old infant weighing 10 kg.
1–6 years: 250 mg twice a day
Over 6 years: 500 mg twice a day.

Elderly: No specific dosage recommendations or precautions for use in the elderly except to monitor those patients with impaired renal function.

The bioavailability and consequent chemotherapeutic effects of cefadroxil are unaffected by food. It may, therefore, be taken with meals or on an empty stomach.

Renal Impairment Dosage: In patients with renal impairment, the dosage should be adjusted according to creatinine clearance rates to prevent drug accumulation and serum levels should be monitored. A modified dosage schedule is unnecessary in patients with creatinine clearance rates of greater than 50 ml/min. In those patients with creatinine clearance rates of 50 ml/min or less, the following reduced dosage schedule is recommended as a guideline, based upon the creatinine clearance rate (ml/min/1.73m²).

Patients with renal insufficiency may be treated with an initial dose of 500 mg to 1000 mg of Baxan. Subsequent doses may be administered according to the following table:

Creatinine clearance	*Dose*	*Dose Interval*
0–10 ml/min/1.73m²	500–1000 mg	36 hrs
11–25 ml/min/1.73m²	500–1000 mg	24 hrs
26–50 ml/min/1.73m²	500–1000 mg	12 hrs

Baxan can be removed from the body by haemodialysis.

Contra-indications, warnings, etc Baxan is contra-indicated in patients with a history of hypersensitivity to any of the ingredients.

Use in pregnancy and lactation: Although animal studies and clinical experience have not shown any evidence of teratogenicity the safe use of Baxan during pregnancy has not been established. Baxan is excreted in breast milk and should be used with caution in lactating mothers.

Precautions: In patients with a history of penicillin allergy, Baxan should be used with caution. There is evidence of partial cross-allergenicity between the penicillins and the cephalosporins. Should an allergic reaction to Baxan occur, the drug should be discontinued and the patient treated with the usual agents (pressor amines, corticosteroids and/or antihistamines), depending on the severity of the reaction.

As experience in premature infants and neonates is limited, the use of Baxan in these patients should only be undertaken with caution.

As with all antibiotics, prolonged use may result in over-growth of non-susceptible organisms.

As with other broad spectrum antibiotics, pseudomembranous colitis has been reported. It is important to consider its diagnosis in patients who develop diarrhoea in association with Baxan therapy.

Adverse reactions: The most commonly reported side-effects are gastrointestinal disturbances and hypersensitivity phenomena. Rash, pruritus, urticaria, angioneurotic oedema have been observed infrequently. Serum sickness, erythema multiforme and anaphylaxis have been reported rarely. Side effects, including nausea, vomiting, diarrhoea, dyspepsia, abdominal discomfort, fever, dizziness, headache, arthralgia and genital candidiasis may also occur. Reversible neutropenia may occur rarely, as may leucopenia, thrombocytopenia, agranulocytosis and minor elevations in serum transaminase and Stevens-Johnson Syndrome. Colitis, including rare instances of pseudo-membraneous colitis, has been reported.

Overdosage: Ingestion of <250 mg/kg in children under six years of age was not associated with significant outcomes. The patient should be observed and treated symptomatically. For amounts >250 mg/kg gastric lavage or stimulation of vomiting is appropriate.

Drug interactions: There are not sufficient data available to indicate whether the concurrent use of Baxan and potential nephrotoxic agents such as aminoglycosides causes any alteration in their nephrotoxic effects.

A false-positive Coombs' reaction may occur in some patients receiving Baxan.

Urine from patients treated with Baxan may give a false-positive glycosuria reaction when tested with Benedict's or Fehling's solutions. This does not occur with enzyme based tests.

Pharmaceutical precautions Store below 30°C in a dry place.

Legal category POM.

Package quantities Capsules – Containers of 100. Suspension – Bottles containing 60 ml

Further information Nil.

Product licence numbers

Baxan 500 mg capsules	0125/0107
Baxan 125 mg/5 ml suspension	0125/0110
Baxan 250 mg/5 ml suspension	0125/0111
Baxan 500 mg/5 ml suspension	0125/0112

BiCNU*

Presentation *BiCNU Injection:* each package contains a 30 ml vial containing 100 mg carmustine and a 5 ml vial containing 3 ml sterile ethanol diluent.

Uses BiCNU is indicated as palliative therapy as a single agent or in established combination therapy with other approved chemotherapeutic agents in the following:

1. Brain tumours – Glioblastoma, brainstem glioma, medulloblastoma, astrocytoma, ependymoma, and metastatic brain tumours.
2. Multiple myeloma – In combination with prednisone.
3. Hodgkin's Disease – As secondary therapy in combination with other approved drugs in patients who relapse while being treated with primary therapy, or who fail to respond to primary therapy.
4. Non-Hodgkin's lymphomas – As secondary therapy in combination with other approved drugs in patients who relapse while being treated with primary therapy, or who fail to respond to primary therapy.

Dosage and administration

Intravenous administration: The recommended dose of BiCNU as single agent in previously untreated patients is 200 mg/m² intravenously every six weeks. This may be given as a single dose or divided into daily injections such as 100 mg/m² on two successive days.

When BiCNU is used in combination with other myelosuppressive drugs or in patients in whom bone marrow reserve is depleted the doses should be adjusted accordingly.

A repeat course of BiCNU should not be given until circulating blood elements have returned to acceptable levels (platelets above 100,000/mm³; leucocytes above 4,000/mm³) and this is usually in six weeks. Blood counts should be monitored frequently and repeat courses should not be given before six weeks because of delayed toxicity.

Doses subsequent to the initial dose should be adjusted according to the haematological response of the patient to the preceding dose. The following schedule is suggested as a guide to dosage adjustment.

Nadir after Prior Dose		*Percentage of prior dose to be given*
Leucocytes (/mm³)	*Platelets (/mm³)*	
> 4000	> 100,000	100
3000–3999	75,000–99,999	100
2000–2999	25,000–74,999	70
< 2000	< 25,000	50

Children: BiCNU should be used with extreme caution in children due to the high risk of pulmonary toxicity (see *Warnings*).

Elderly: No dosage adjustment is required on the grounds of age.

Contra-indications, warnings, etc *Contra-indications:* BiCNU should not be given to individuals who have demonstrated a previous hypersensitivity to it.

BiCNU should not be given to individuals with decreased circulating platelets, leucocytes, or erythrocytes either from previous chemotherapy or other causes.

Warnings and precautions: Pulmonary toxicity characterised by pulmonary infiltrates and/or fibrosis has been reported to occur with a frequency ranging up to 30%. This may occur within 3 years of therapy and appears to be dose related with total cumulative doses of 1200–1500 mg/m² being associated with increased likelihood of lung fibrosis. Risk factors include smoking, the presence of a respiratory condition, pre-existing radiographic abnormalities, sequential or concomitant thoracic irradiation and association with other agents that cause lung damage.

Cases of late pulmonary fibrosis, occurring up to 17 years after treatment, have also been reported. In a long-term follow-up of 17 patients who survived childhood brain tumours eight (47%) died of lung fibrosis. Of these eight deaths, two occurred within 3 years of treatment and 6 occurred 8–13 years after treatment. Of the patients who died, the median age at treatment was 2.5 years (range 1–12); the median age of the long-term survivors was 10 years (5–16 years at treatment). All five patients treated under the age of 5 years have died of pulmonary fibrosis. In this study, the dose of BiCNU did not influence fatal outcome nor did co-administration of vincristine or spinal irradiation. Of the remaining survivors available for follow-up, evidence of lung fibrosis was detected in all patients. The risks and benefits of BiCNU therapy must be carefully considered especially in young patients, due to extremely high risk of pulmonary toxicity.

BiCNU should be administered by individuals experienced in antineoplastic therapy. Bone marrow toxicity is a common and severe toxic effect of BiCNU. Complete blood counts should be monitored frequently for at least six weeks after a dose. Repeat doses of BiCNU should not be given more frequently than every six weeks. The bone marrow toxicity of BiCNU is cumulative and therefore dosage adjustment must be considered on the basis of nadir blood counts from prior dose (see Dosage Adjustment Table under Dosage).

It is recommended that liver function, kidney function and pulmonary function also be monitored.

Pregnancy and lactation: BiCNU should not normally be administered to patients who are pregnant or mothers who are breast-feeding. Male patients should be advised to use adequate contraceptive measures.

Safe use in pregnancy has not been established and therefore the benefit to risk of toxicity must be carefully weighed. BiCNU is embryotoxic and teratogenic in rats and embryotoxic in rabbits at dose levels equivalent to the human dose. BiCNU also affects fertility in male rats at doses somewhat higher than the human dose.

BiCNU is carcinogenic in rats and mice, producing a marked increase in tumour incidence in doses approximating those employed clinically.

Adverse reactions: Haematological: Delayed myelosuppression is a frequent and serious adverse event associated with BiCNU administration. It usually occurs four to six weeks after drug administration and is dose-related. Platelet nadirs occur at four to five weeks; leucocyte nadirs occur at five to six weeks post therapy. Thrombocytopenia is generally more severe than leucopenia. However both may be dose limiting toxicities. Anaemia also occurs, but is generally less severe. The occurrence of acute leukaemia and bone marrow dysplasias have been reported in patients following long term nitrosourea therapy.

Gastro-intestinal: Nausea and vomiting after i.v. administration of BiCNU are noted frequently. This reaction appears within two hours of dosing, usually lasting four to six hours and is dose-related. Prior administration of anti-emetics is effective in diminishing and sometimes preventing this side-effect.

Hepatic: When high doses of BiCNU have been employed, a reversible type of hepatic toxicity, manifested by increased transaminase, alkaline phosphatase and bilirubin levels, has been reported in a small percentage of patients.

Pulmonary: See *Warnings and Precautions.*

Renal: Renal abnormalities consisting of decrease in kidney size, progressive azotaemia and renal failure have been reported in patients who receive large cumulative doses after prolonged therapy with BiCNU and related nitrosoureas. Kidney damage has also been reported in patients receiving lower total doses.

Cardiovascular: Hypotension, tachycardia have been reported.

Local: Burning at the site of injection is common but true thrombosis is rare.

Other: Rapid i.v. infusion of BiCNU may produce intense flushing of the skin and suffusion of the conjunctiva within two hours, lasting about four hours. Neuroretinitis, chest pain, headache, allergic reactions have been reported.

Pharmaceutical precautions **IMPORTANT NOTE:** The lyophilised dosage formulation contains no preservatives and is not intended as multiple dose vial. Reconstitutions and further dilutions should be carried out under aseptic conditions.

Unopened vials of the dry powder must be stored in a refrigerator (2–8°C).

Once reconstituted as recommended, resulting solutions, undiluted or further diluted (with 500 ml of sodium chloride for injection or 500 ml of 5% glucose for injection) may be stored up to a total of 24 hours when stored at 2–8°C and protected from light.

Compatibility/incompatibility with containers: The intravenous solution is suitable for infusion in polythene or glass containers. Studies have shown carmustine to be incompatible with PVC containers as it is readily absorbed on plastic.

Preparation of intravenous solution: Dissolve BiCNU with 3 ml of the supplied sterile diluent (absolute ethanol) and then aseptically add 27 ml of sterile water for injection to the alcohol solution. Each ml of the resulting solution will contain 3.3 mg of BiCNU in 10% ethanol and has a pH of 5.6 to 6.0.

Reconstitution as recommended results in a clear colourless solution which may be further diluted with sodium chloride for injection, or 5% glucose for injection.

The reconstituted solution must be given intravenously and should be administered by i.v. drip over a one- to two-hour period. Injection of BiCNU over shorter periods of time may produce intense pain and burning at the site of injection.

IMPORTANT NOTE: BiCNU has a low melting point (approximately 30·5–32·0°C or 86·9–89·6°F). Exposure of the drug to this temperature or above will cause the drug to liquefy and appear as an oil film in the bottom of the vials. This is a sign of decomposition and vials should be discarded.

Guidelines for the safe handling of antineoplastic agents:

1. Trained personnel should reconstitute the drug.
2. This should be performed in a designated area.
3. Adequate protective gloves should be worn.
4. Precautions should be taken to avoid the drug accidentally coming into contact with the eyes. In the event of contact with the eyes, flush with copious amounts of water and/or saline.
5. The cytotoxic preparation should not be handled by pregnant staff.
6. Adequate care and precaution should be taken in the disposal of items (syringes, needles etc) used to reconstitute cytotoxic drugs. Excess material and body waste may be disposed of by placing in double sealed polythene bags and incinerating at a temperature of 1,000°C. Liquid waste may be flushed with copious amounts of water.
7. The work surface should be covered with disposable plastic-backed absorbent paper.
8. Use Luer-Lock fittings on all syringes and sets. Large bore needles are recommended to minimise pressure and the possible formation of aerosols. The latter may also be reduced by the use of a venting needle.

Legal category POM.

Package quantities BiCNU Injection packed in cartons of 10 units, each unit consisting of one vial of carmustine 100 mg and one vial of sterile absolute alcohol 3 ml.

Further information BiCNU alkylates DNA and RNA and has also been shown to inhibit several enzymes by carbamoylation of amino acids in proteins.

Intravenously administered BiCNU is rapidly degraded, with no intact drug detectable after 15 minutes. However, in studies with C_{14} labelled drug, prolonged levels of the isotope were observed in the plasma and tissue, probably representing radioactive fragments of the parent compound.

It is thought that the antineoplastic and toxic activities of BiCNU may be due to metabolites. Approximately 60 to 70% of a total dose is excreted in the urine in 96 hours and about 10% as respiratory CO_2. The fate of the remainder is undetermined.

Because of the high lipid solubility and the relative lack of ionisation at a physiological pH, BiCNU crosses the blood brain barrier.

Levels of radioactivity in the CSF are at least 50% higher than those measured concurrently in plasma.

Product licence number 0125/0108.

BUSPAR* TABLETS

Qualitative and quantitative composition Each tablet contains: buspirone hydrochloride 5 mg or 10 mg.

Pharmaceutical form Oral tablet.

Clincal particulars
Therapeutic indications: Buspar is indicated for the short-term management of anxiety disorders and the relief of symptoms of anxiety with or without accompanying depression.

Posology and method of administration
Adults: Dosage should be adjusted according to response for maximum effect. The recommended initial dose is 5 mg two to three times daily and this may be increased every two to three days. The usual therapeutic dose is 15 to 30 mg daily in divided doses with a maximum recommended dose of 45 mg daily in divided doses.

Elderly: Dosage should be adjusted according to response for maximum effect. The recommended initial dose is 5 mg two to three times daily and this may be increased as required. The usual therapeutic dose is 15 to 30 mg daily in divided doses with a maximum recommended dose of 45 mg daily in divided doses.

Children: Use in children has not been established.

Contra-indications: Buspar should not be used in patients hypertensive to buspirone hydrochloride. Buspar should not be used in patients with epilepsy. In patients with a history of renal or hepatic impairment, Buspar should be used with caution. Buspar should not be used in patients with severe renal impairment, defined as creatinine clearance of 20 ml/minute or below, or a plasma creatinine above 200 micromoles/litre. Buspar should not be used in patients with severe hepatic disease.

Special warnings and special precautions for use: In controlled studies in healthy volunteers, Buspar in single doses up to 20 mg caused no significant impairment of cognitive or psychomotor functions, unlike the benzodiazepines, diazepam or lorazepam. In studies in healthy volunteers, Buspar did not potentiate the psychomotor impairment produced by alcohol, in contrast to a comparative benzodiazepine. However, no data are available on concomitant use of alcohol and Buspar at single doses greater than 20 mg. It is prudent therefore to avoid alcohol while taking Buspar.

As Buspar does not exhibit cross-tolerance with benzodiazepines and other common sedative/hypnotic agents, it will not block the withdrawal syndrome often seen with cessation of therapy with these compounds. Before starting therapy with Buspar, it is advisable to withdraw patients gradually from prior chronic treatment with these agents.

Interactions with other medicinal products and other forms of interaction: The occurrence of elevated blood pressure in patients receiving both buspirone and monoamine oxidase inhibitors (phenelzine and tranylcypromine) has been reported. It is therefore recommended that Buspar should not be used concomitantly with a monoamine oxidase inhibitor (MAOI).

In vitro studies have shown that buspirone does not displace warfarin, digoxin, phenytoin or propranolol from plasma proteins.

In a study in normal volunteers, no interaction with amitriptyline was seen. A similar study with diazepam showed a slight increase in metabolite (nordiazepam) levels.

Pregnancy and lactation: In some studies, administration of high doses of buspirone to pregnant animals produced effects on survival, birth and weanling weights, although there was no effect on foetal development. Since the relevance of this finding in humans has not been established, Buspar is contraindicated in pregnancy and in lactation.

Effects on ability to drive and use machines: See *Undesirable effects.*

Undesirable effects: Buspar is generally well tolerated. If side-effects occur they are normally observed at the beginning of treatment and usually subside with continued use and/or decreased dosage.

In controlled trials, the only side-effects that occurred with significantly greater frequency with buspirone treatment than with placebo were dizziness, headache, nervousness, light-headedness, excitement and nausea. Tachycardia, palpitations, chest pain, drowsiness, confusion, dry mouth, fatigue and sweating/clamminess have also been reported rarely.

Overdose: There is no specific antidote to Buspar. Buspar is not removed by haemodialysis. The stomach should be emptied as quickly as possible. Treatment should be symptomatic and supportive. The ingestion of multiple agents should be suspected.

Death by deliberate or accidental overdose has not been observed. A dose of 375 mg per day in healthy volunteers produced no significant adverse effects. As maximum dose levels are reached symptoms most commonly observed are: nausea, vomiting, dizziness, drowsiness and miosis.

Pharmacological properties
Pharmacodynamic properties: Buspar is an azaspirodecanedione. The exact mechanism of Buspar anxioselective action is not fully known. It does not act on benzodiazepine receptor sites and lacks sedative, anticonvulsant and muscle relaxant properties. From animal studies it is known to interact with serotonin, noradrenaline, acetylcholine and dopamine systems of the brain. Buspar enhances the activity of specific noradrenergic and dopaminergic pathways, whereas the activity of serotonin and acetylcholine are reduced.

Pharmacokinetic properties: Buspar is rapidly absorbed when given orally. It is then subject to considerable first-pass metabolism. Peak plasma levels occur 60-90 minutes after dosing. Plasma concentration is linearly related to dose. Following multiple dosing steady state plasma concentrations are achieved within 2 days. Buspar is 95% protein bound. Buspar is eliminated primarily by liver metabolism. In pharmacokinetic studies mean plasma half-lives varied from 2 to 11 hours.

Preclinical safety data: No further relevant information.

Pharmaceutical particulars
List of excipients: Lactose anhydrous, sodium carboxymethyl starch, microcrystalline cellulose, silicon dioxide colloidal, magnesium stearate.

Incompatibilities: None known.

Shelf life: 24 months.

Special precautions for storage: Store below 25°C

Nature and contents of container: The tablets are packed in bottles containing 100 tablets. Buspar 5 mg is also available in a blister pack containing 126 tablets.

Instructions for use/handling: None

Marketing authorisation numbers
Buspar 5 mg 0125/0162
Buspar 10 mg 0125/0163

Date of revision of SPC October 1997.

KERI* THERAPEUTIC LOTION

Qualitative and quantitative composition Mineral Oil 16%.

Pharmaceutical form Lotion.

Clincial particulars
Therapeutic indications: Keri Therapeutic Lotion has emollient properties. It is indicated for the symptomatic treatment of dermatitis, eczema, ichthyosis, nappy rash, protection of raw and abraded skin areas, pruritus and related conditions where dry scaly skin is a problem It is also indicated as an emollient before bathing for dry/eczematous skin, to alleviate drying effects.

Posology and method of administration: Topical Administration.

Adults: Keri Therapeutic Lotion should be gently massaged into the skin three times daily or as often as required.

Elderly: No dosage adjustment is necessary.

Contra-indications: Keri Therapeutic Lotion contains lanolin oil and is therefore contraindicated in those patients allergic to this ingredient.

Special warnings and special precautions for use: None known.

Interactions with other medicinal products and other forms of interaction: None known.

Pregnancy and lactation: No special precautions.

Effects on ability to drive and use machines: Not applicable

Undesirable effects: None known.

Overdose: Not applicable.

Pharmacological properties
Pharmacodynamic properties: Mineral oil has emollient properties. Keri lotion lubrication helps hydrate the skin. It relieves itching, helps maintain a normal moisture balance and supplements the protective action of skin lipids.

Pharmacokinetic properties: Not applicable for this type of product.

Preclinical safety data: Nothing of relevance to the prescriber.

Pharmaceutical particulars
List of excipients: Carbomer 934, glycerol monostearate, lanolin oil, laureth 4, methyl hydroxybenzoate, perfume, PEG-4 dilaurate, polyethylene glycol 40 stearate, propyl hydroxybenzoate, propylene glycol, quaternium 15, sodium dioctyl sulphosuccinate, triethanolamine, water.

Incompatibilities: None known.

Shelf life: 36 months.

Special precautions for storage: Store at room temperature (below 25°C)

Nature and contents of container: HDPE opaque white bottle with either a polypropylene pump or a polypropylene disc cap closure (Pack sizes of 190 or 380 ml).

Instructions for use/handling: Not applicable to this product.

Marketing authorisation number 0125/0152

Date of first authorisation/renewal of authorisation 18th October 1992

Date of (partial) revision of the text August 1997

MEGACE* TABLETS

Qualitative and quantitative composition Each tablet contains Megestrol Acetate BP 40 or 160 mg.

Pharmaceutical form Oral tablets.

Clinical particulars
Therapeutic indications: Megace is a progestational agent, indicated for the treatment of certain hormone dependent neoplasms, such as a endometrial or breast cancer.

Posology and method of administration:
Breast cancer: 160 mg/day (40 mg qid or 160 mg taken once daily).

Endometrial cancer: 40–320 mg/day in divided doses (40–80 mg one to four times daily or one to two 160 mg tablets daily).

At least two months of continuous treatment is considered an adequate period for determining the efficacy of Megace.

Children: Megace is not recommended for use in children.

Elderly: No dosage adjustments is necessary.

Contra-indications: Megace is contra-indicated in patients who have demonstrated hypersensitivity to the drug.

Special warnings and special precautions for use:
Precautions: Megace should be used with caution in patients with a history of thrombophlebitis and in patients with severe impaired liver function.

Interactions with other medicinal products and other forms of interaction: None stated.

Pregnancy and lactation: Megace should not normally be administered to women who are pregnant or to mothers who are breast feeding.

Fertility and reproduction studies with high doses of megestrol acetate have shown a reversible feminising effect on some male rat foetuses.

Several reports suggest an association between intrauterine exposure to progestational drugs in the first trimester of pregnancy and genital abnormalities in male and female foetuses. The risk of hypospadias in male foetuses may be approximately doubled with the exposure to progestational drugs. There are insufficient data to quantify the risk to exposed female foetuses, however some of these drugs induce mild virilisation of the external genitalia of the female foetuses.

If a patient is exposed to Megace during the first four months of pregnancy or if she becomes pregnant whilst taking Megace, she should be apprised of the potential risks to the foetus.

Women of child bearing potential should be advised to avoid becoming pregnant.

Because of the potential for adverse effects, nursing should be discontinued during treatment with Megace.

Effects on the ability to drive and use machines: None stated.

Undesirable effects: The major side-effect experienced by patients while taking megestrol acetate, particularly at high doses, is weight gain, which is usually not associated with water retention, but which is secondary to an increased appetite and food intake. Other occasionally noted side effects are nausea, vomiting, oedema and breakthrough uterine bleeding. Rare reports have been received of patients developing dyspnoea, heart failure, hypertension, hot flushes, mood changes, cushingoid faces, tumour flare (with or without hypercalcaemia), hyperglycaemia, alopecia and carpal tunnel syndrome while taking megestrol acetate. Thromboembolic phenomena including thrombophlebitis and pulmonary embolism (in some cases fatal) have been reported. A rarely encountered side effect of prolonged administration of megestrol acetate is urticaria, presumably an idiosyncratic reaction to the drug. The drug is devoid of the myelosuppressive activity characteristic of many cytotoxic drugs and it causes no significant changes in haematology, blood chemistry or urinalysis.

Pituitary adrenal axis abnormalities including glucose intolerance, and Cushing's syndrome have been reported with the use of megestrol acetate. Clinically apparent adrenal insufficiency has been rarely reported in patients shortly after discontinuing megestrol acetate. The possibility of adrenal suppression should be considered in all patients taking or withdrawing from chronic megestrol acetate therapy. Replacement stress doses of glucocorticoids may be indicated.

Overdose: No serious side-effects have resulted from studies involving Megace (megestrol acetate) administered in dosages as high as 1600 mg/day.

There is no specific antidote to overdosage and treatment should therefore be symptomatic.

Pharmacological properties

Pharmacodynamic properties: Megace (megestrol acetate) possesses pharmacological properties similar to those of natural progesterone. Its progestational activity is slightly greater than that of medroxyprogesterone acetate, norethindrone, norethindrone acetate and norethynodrel; slightly less than that of chlormadinone acetate; and substantially less than that of norgestrel.

Megestrol acetate is a potent progestogen that exerts significant anti-oestrogenic effects. It has no androgenic or oestrogenic properties. It has anti-gonadotropic, anti-uterotropic and anti-androgenic/anti-myotropic actions. It has a slight but significant glucocorticoid effect and a very slight mineralocorticoid effect.

The progestational activity of megestrol acetate has been assessed in a number of standard tests, including clauberg-mcphail, mcginty, uterotropic and carbonic anhydrase tests in rabbits; pregnancy maintenance and delay-of-implantation tests in rats; endometrial response in rhesus monkeys; conversion of an oestrogen-primed endometrium to a secretory one in normal women and in those with secondary amenorrhea with resultant withdrawal bleeding; induction of pseudopregnancy for treatment of endometriosis; and the delay-of-menses and thermogenic tests. In all these tests, progestational activity was high.

It has been demonstrated that megestrol acetate blocks oestrogen effects in the uteri of rats and mice in human cervical mucus and vaginal mucosa. Anti-gondotropic activity has been demonstrated in rats of both sexes.

Pharmacokinetic properties:

Animal: Peak plasma levels occur four to six hours after oral administration of radioactively labelled megestrol acetate to female rats. High concentrations are found in the liver, fat, adrenal glands, ovaries and kidneys. Radioactivity is almost wholly cleared within a week, chiefly by biliary excretion to the faeces.

In dogs, megestrol acetate metabolite are excreted primarily in the faeces. In rabbits, the principal route of metabolic excretion is urinary and the major metabolites are the 2-alpha-hydroxy-6-hydroxymethyl and 6-hydroxymethyl derivatives.

Human: Peak plasma levels of tritiated megestrol acetate and metabolites occur one to three hours after oral administration. When 4 to 91 mg of c-labelled megestrol acetate were administered orally to women, the major route of drug elimination was in the urine. The urinary and fecal recovery of total radioactivity within 10 days ranged from 56.6% to 78.4% (mean 66.4%) and 7.7% to 30.3% (mean 19.8%), respectively. The total recovered radioactivity varied between 83.1% and 94.7% (mean 86.2%). Megestrol acetate metabolites, which were identified in the urine as glucuronide conjugates, were 17-alpha-acetoxy-2-alpha hydroxy-6-methylpregna-4,6-diene-3,20-dione; 17-alpha-acetoxy-6-hydroxymethylpregna-4,6-diene-3, 20-dione; and 17-alpha-acetoxy-2-alpha-hydroxy-6-hydromethylpregna-4, 6-diene-3, 20-dione; these identified metabolites accounted for only 5-8% of the administered dose.

Serum concentrations were measured after the administration of single and multiple oral doses of megestrol acetate. Adult male and post-menopausal female volunteers, no more than 65 years of age participated in the study.

Megestrol acetate is readily absorbed following oral administration of 20, 40, 80 and 200 mg doses. Megestrol serum concentrations increase with increasing doses, the relationship between increasing dosage and increasing serum levels not being arithmetically proportional. Average peak serum concentrations for the four doses tested were 89, 190, 209 and 465 ng/ml.

Mean peak serum concentrations are found three hours after single-dose administration for all dosage levels studied. The serum concentration curve appears biphasic, and the beta-phase half-life is 15 to 20 hours long.

After multiple doses over a three-day period, serum levels increase each day and are estimated to reach 80% to 90% predicted steady-state levels on the third day.

Preclinical safety data: No further relevant data.

Pharmaceutical particulars

List of excipients: 40 mg Tablets: Acacia, calcium hydrogen phosphate, lactose, magnesium stearate, maize starch, silicon dioxide.

160 mg Tablets: Colloidal silicon dioxide, lactose monohydrate, magnesium stearate, microcrystalline cellulose, povidone, sodium starch glycollate.

Incompatibilities: None stated.

Shelf life: 36 months.

Special precautions for storage: Megace tablets should be stored below 25°C.

Nature and contents of container:
40 mg tablet – blister packs of 100 tablets.
160 mg tablet – blister packs of 30 tablets.

Instructions for use handling: None.

Marketing authorisation numbers
Megace 40 mg 0125/0144
Megace 160 mg 0125/0173

Date of approval/revison of SPC 12 October 1998.

Legal Category POM.

PARAPLATIN* SOLUTION

Qualitative and quantitative composition Paraplatin Solution contains carboplatin (cis-diammine (1,1-cyclobutane-dicarboxylato) platinum) as a 10 mg/ml solution in water for injection.

Pharmaceutical form Solution for intravenous injection.

Clinical particulars

Therapeutic indications: Paraplatin is indicated for the treatment of:

1. advanced ovarian carcinoma of epithelial origin in:
   a. first line therapy
   b. second line therapy, after other treatments have failed.
2. small cell carcinoma of the lung.

Posology and method of administration: Paraplatin should be used by the intravenous route only. The recommended dosage of Paraplatin in previously untreated adult patients with normal kidney function is 400 mg/m² as a single i.v. dose administered by a 15 to 60 minutes infusion. Alternatively, see Calvert formula below. Therapy should not be repeated until four weeks after the previous Paraplatin course and/or until the neutrophil count is at least 2,000 cells/mm³ and the platelet count is at least 100,000 cells/mm³.

Reduction of the initial dosage by 20-25% is recommended for those patients who present with risk factors such as prior myelosuppressive treatment and low performance status (ECOG-Zubrod 2-4 or Karnofsky below 80).

Determination of the haematological nadir by weekly blood counts during the initial courses of treatment with Paraplatin is recommended for future dosage adjustment.

Impaired Renal Function: The optimal use of Paraplatin in patients presenting with impaired renal function requires adequate dosage adjustments and frequent monitoring of both haematological nadirs and renal function.

Dosage (mg) = target AUC (mg/ml x min) x [GFR ml/min + 25]

Note: With the Calvert formula, the total dose of carboplatin is calculated in mg, not mg/m².

Target AUC	*Planned Chemotherapy*	*Patient treatment status*
5-7 mg/ ml.min	single agent carboplatin	Previously untreated
4-6 mg/ ml.min	single agent carboplatin	Previously treated
4-6 mg/ ml.min	carboplatin plus cyclophosphamide	Previously untreated

Combination therapy: The optimal use of Paraplatin in combination with other myelosuppressive agents requires dosage adjustments according to the regimen and schedule to be adopted.

Paediatrics: Sufficient usage of Paraplatin in paediatrics has not occurred to allow specific dosage recommendations to be made.

Elderly: Dosage adjustment, initially or subsequently, may be necessary, dependent on the physical condition of the patient.

Dilution and reconstitution: See *Instructions for use/handling.*

Contra-indications: Paraplatin should not be used in patients with severe pre-existing renal impairment (creatinine clearance at or below 20 ml/minute).

It should not be employed in severely myelosuppressed patients. It is also contra-indicated in patients with a history of several allergic reactions to Paraplatin or other platinum containing compounds.

Special warnings and special precautions for use

Warnings: Paraplatin should be administered by individuals experienced in the use of anti-neoplastic therapy.

Paraplatin myelosuppression is closely related to its renal clearance. Patients with abnormal kidney function or receiving concomitant therapy with other drugs with nephrotoxic potential are likely to experience more severe and prolonged myelotoxicity. Renal function parameters should therefore be carefully assessed before and during therapy. Paraplatin courses should not be repeated more frequently than monthly under normal circumstances. Thrombocytopenia, leukopenia and anaemia occur after administration of Paraplatin. Frequent monitoring of peripheral blood counts is recommended throughout and following therapy with Paraplatin. Paraplatin combination therapy with other myelosuppressive compounds must be planned very carefully with respect to dosages and timing in order to minimise additive effects. Supportive transfusional therapy may be required in patients who suffer severe myelosuppression.

Paraplatin can cause nausea and vomiting. Premedication with anti-emetics has been reported to be useful in reducing the incidence and intensity of these effects.

Renal and hepatic function impairment may be encountered with Paraplatin. Very high doses of Paraplatin (>5 times single agent recommended dose) have resulted in severe abnormalities in hepatic and renal function. Although no clinical evidence on compounding nephrotoxicity has been accumulated, it is recommended not to combine Paraplatin with aminoglycosides or other nephrotoxic compounds.

Infrequent allergic reactions to Paraplatin have been reported, i.e. skin reactions usually designated as a rash. Rarely anaphylaxis, angio-oedema and anaphylactoid reactions including bronchospasm, urticaria and facial oedema have occurred. These reactions are similar to those observed after administration of other platinum containing compounds and may occur within minutes. Patients should be observed carefully for possible allergic reactions and managed with appropriate supportive therapy.

The carcinogenic potential of Paraplatin has not been studied but compounds with similar mechanisms of action and mutagenicity have been reported to be carcinogenic.

Precautions: Peripheral blood counts and renal and hepatic function tests should be monitored closely. Blood counts at the beginning of the therapy and weekly to assess haematological nadir for subsequent dose adjustment are recommended. Neurological evaluations should also be performed on a regular basis.

Interactions with other medicinal products and other forms of interaction: The use of Paraplatin with nephrotoxic compounds is not recommended.

Pregnancy and lactation: The safe use of Paraplatin during pregnancy has not been established: Paraplatin has been shown to be an embryotoxin and teratogen in rats. If Paraplatin is used during pregnancy the patient should be apprised of the potential hazard to the foetus. Women of child-bearing potential should be advised to avoid becoming pregnant.

Carboplatin has been shown to be mutagenic *in vivo* and *in vitro.*

Nursing mothers: It is not known whether Paraplatin is excreted in human milk.

Effects on ability to drive and use machines: None reported.

Undesirable effects: Incidences of adverse reactions reported hereunder are based on cumulative data obtained in a large group of patients with various pretreatment prognostic features.

Haematological toxicity: Myelosuppression is the dose-limiting toxicity of Paraplatin. At maximum tolerated dosages of Paraplatin administered as a single agent, thrombocytopenia, with nadir platelet counts of less than 50 x 10⁹/L, occurs in about a quarter of the patients.

The nadir usually occurs between days 14 and 21, with recovery within 35 days from the start of therapy. Leukopenia has also occurred in approximately 14% of patients but its recovery from the day of nadir (day 14-28) may be slower and usually occurs within 42 days from the start of therapy. Neutropenia with granulocyte counts below 1 x 10⁹/L occurs in approximately one fifth of patients. Anaemia with haemoglobin values below 11 g/dL has been observed in more than two-thirds of patients with normal baseline values.

Myelosuppression may be more severe and prolonged in patients with impaired renal function, extensive prior treatment, poor performance status and age above 65. Myelosuppression is also worsened by therapy combining Paraplatin with other compounds that are myelosuppressive.

Myelosuppression is usually reversible and not cumulative when Paraplatin is used as a single agent and at the recommended dosages and frequencies of administration.

Infectious complications have occasionally been reported. Haemorrhagic complications, usually minor, have also been reported.

Nephrotoxicity: Renal toxicity is usually not dose-limiting in patients receiving Paraplatin, nor does it require preventive measures such as high volume fluid hydration or forced diuresis. Nevertheless, increasing blood urea or serum creatinine levels can occur. Renal function impairment, as defined by a decrease in the creatinine clearance below 60 ml/min, may also be observed. The incidence and severity of nephrotoxicity may increase in patients who have impaired kidney function before Paraplatin treatment. It is not clear whether an appropriate hydration programme might overcome such an effect, but dosage reduction or discontinuation of therapy is required in the presence of severe alteration of renal function tests.

Decreases in serum electrolytes (sodium, magnesium, potassium and calcium) have been reported after treatment with Paraplatin but have not been reported to be severe enough to cause the appearance of clinical signs or symptoms.

Cases of hyponatraemia have been reported. Haemolytic uraemic syndrome has been reported rarely.

Gastrointestinal toxicity: Nausea without vomiting occurs in about 15% of patients receiving Paraplatin; vomiting has been reported in over half of the patients and about one-fifth of these suffer severe emesis. Nausea and vomiting usually disappear within 24 hours after treatment and are usually responsive to (and may be prevented by) anti-emetic medication. A fifth of patients experience no nausea or vomiting.

Cases of anorexia have been reported.

Allergic reactions: Infrequent allergic reactions to Paraplatin have been reported. These reactions are similar to those observed after administration of other platinum-containing compounds, i.e. erythematous rash, fever with no apparent cause and pruritus.

Ototoxicity: Subclinical decrease in hearing acuity, consisting of high-frequency (4000-8000 Hz) hearing loss determined by audiogram, has been reported in 15% of the patients treated with Paraplatin. However, only 1% of patients present with clinical symptoms, manifested in the majority of cases by tinnitus. In patients who have been previously treated with cisplatin and have developed hearing loss related to such treatment, the hearing impairment may persist or worsen.

At higher than recommended doses in combination with other ototoxic agents, clinically significant hearing loss has been reported to occur in paediatric patients when Paraplatin Solution was administered.

Neurotoxicity: The incidence of peripheral neuropathies after treatment with Paraplatin is 4%. In the majority of the patients neurotoxicity is limited to paraesthesia and decreased deep tendon reflexes. The frequency and intensity of this side effect increases in elderly patients and those previously treated with cisplatin.

Paraesthesia present before commencing Paraplatin therapy, particularly if related to prior cisplatin treatment, may persist or worsen during treatment with Paraplatin.

Ocular toxicity: Transient visual disturbances, sometimes including transient sight loss, have been reported rarely with platinum therapy. This is usually associated with high dose therapy in renally impaired patients.

Other: Abnormalities of liver function tests (usually mild to moderate) have been reported with Paraplatin in about one-third of the patients with normal baseline values. The alkaline phosphatase level is increased more frequently than SGOT, SGPT or total bilirubin. The majority of these abnormalities regress spontaneously during the course of treatment.

Infrequent events consisting of taste alteration, asthenia, alopecia, fever and chills without evidence of infection have occurred.

Overdose: There is no known antidote for Paraplatin overdosage. The anticipated complications of overdosage would be related to myelosuppression as well as impairment of hepatic and renal function.

Pharmacological properties

Pharmacodynamic properties: Carboplatin is an antineoplastic agent. Its activity has been demonstrated against several murine and human cell lines.

Carboplatin exhibited comparable activity to cisplatin against a wide range of tumours regardless of implant site.

Alkaline elution techniques and DNA binding studies have demonstrated the qualitatively similar modes of action of carboplatin and cisplatin. Carboplatin, like cisplatin, induces changes in the superhelical conformation of DNA which is consistent with a "DNA shortening effect".

Pharmacokinetic properties: Paraplatin has biochemical properties similar to that of cisplatin, thus producing predominantly interstrand and intrastrand DNA crosslinks. Following administration of Paraplatin in man, linear relationships exist between dose and plasma concentrations of total and free ultrafilterable platinum. The area under the plasma concentration versus time curve for total platinum also shows a linear relationship with the dose when creatinine clearance ≥60 ml/min.

Repeated dosing during four consecutive days did not produce an accumulation of platinum in plasma. Following the administration of Paraplatin reported values for the terminal elimination of half-lives of free ultrafilterable platinum and Paraplatin in man are approximately 6 hours and 1.5 hours respectively. During the initial phase, most of the free ultrafilterable platinum is present as Paraplatin. The terminal half-life for total plasma platinum is 24 hours. Approximately 87% of plasma platinum is protein bound within 24 hours following administration. Paraplatin is excreted primarily in the urine, with recovery of approximately 70% of the administered platinum within 24 hours. Most of the drug is excreted in the first 6 hours. Total body and renal clearances of free ultrafilterable platinum correlate with the rate of glomerular filtration but not tubular secretion.

Preclinical safety data: Paraplatin has been shown to be embryotoxic and teratogenic in rats. (See *Pregnancy and lactation.*) It is mutagenic in vivo and in vitro and although the carcinogenic potential of Paraplatin has not been studied, compounds with similar mechanisms of action and mutagenicity have been reported to be carcinogenic.

Pharmaceutical particulars

List of excipients: Water for Injections.

Incompatibilities: Needles or intravenous sets containing aluminium parts that may come into contact with Paraplatin should not be used for preparation or administration of Paraplatin.

Shelf life: Unopened product: 18 months. After dilution: 8 hours at room temperature (15–25°C), or 24 hours under refrigeration (2–8°C)

Special precautions for storage: Paraplatin should be stored at room temperature (15–25°C) and protected from light. When diluted as directed, it is recommended that any Paraplatin Solution be discarded after 8 hours from dilution if stored at room temperature (15–25°C) or after 24 hours if stored refrigerated (2–8°C).

Nature and contents of container: Cardboard carton containing a flint glass vial with a rubber or Daikyo compound Teflon coated stopper and aluminium closure with polypropylene top, containing either 50 mg, 150 mg or 450 mg carboplatin as a 10 mg/ml solution.

Instructions for use/handling: This product is for single dose use only.

Reconstitution: The product may be diluted with 5% Glucose for Injection BP, or 0.9% Sodium Chloride for Injection BP, to concentrations as low as 0.5 mg/ml (500 micrograms / ml).

When diluted as directed, Paraplatin solutions are stable for eight hours stored at room temperature or 24 hours stored under refrigeration. Since no antibacterial preservatives are contained in the formulation, it is recommended that any Paraplatin solution be discarded after eight hours from dilution if stored at room temperature or after 24 hours if stored refrigerated. This product is for single dose use only.

Guidelines for the safe handling of anti-neoplastic agents:

1. Trained personnel should reconstitute the drug.
2. This should be performed in a designated area.
3. Adequate protective gloves should be worn.
4. Precautions should be taken to avoid the drug accidentally coming into contact with the eyes. In the event of contact with the eyes, wash with water and/or saline.
5. The cytotoxic preparation should not be handled by pregnant staff.
6. Adequate care and precautions should be taken in the disposal of items (syringes, needles, etc.) used to reconstitute cytotoxic drugs. Excess material and body waste may be disposed of by placing in double sealed polythene bags and incinerating at a temperature of 1,000 degrees C. Liquid waste may be flushed with copious amounts of water.

Reconstitution:

7. The work surface should be covered with disposable plastic-backed absorbent paper.
8. Use Luer-Lock fittings on all syringes and sets. Large bore needles are recommended to minimise pressure and the possible formation of aerosols. The latter may also be reduced by the use of a venting needle.

Marketing authorisation number 0125/0201

Date of approval/revision of SPC July 1997

Legal category POM

QUESTRAN*
QUESTRAN LIGHT*

Qualitative and quantitative composition Each sachet contains 4 g anhydrous cholestyramine (a basic anion-exchange resin).

Pharmaceutical form Each sachet contains 9 g orange-flavoured powder which produces a pale orange-coloured oral suspension when reconstituted with water.

Clinical particulars

Therapeutic indications: Questran is used for:

1. Primary prevention of coronary heart disease in men between 35 and 59 years of age and with primary hypercholesterolaemia who have not responded to diet and other appropriate measures.
2. Reduction of plasma cholesterol in hypercholesterolaemia, particularly in those patients who have been diagnosed as Fredrickson's Type II (high plasma cholesterol with normal or slightly elevated triglycerides).
3. Relief of pruritus associated with partial biliary obstruction and primary biliary cirrhosis.
4. Relief of diarrhoea associated with ileal resection, Crohn's disease, vagotomy and diabetic vagal neuropathy.
5. Management of radiation-induced diarrhoea.

Posology and method of administration

Adults: As a precautionary measure, where concurrent drug therapy exists then such drugs should be administered at least one hour before or 4-6 hours after Questran.

Questran should not be taken in its dry form.

Questran should be administered mixed with water or a suitable liquid, such as fruit juice, and stirred to a uniform consistency.

Questran may also be mixed with skimmed milk, thin soups, pulpy fruits with high moisture content, e.g. apple sauce, etc..

1. For primary prevention of coronary heart disease and to reduce cholesterol: After initial introduction over a three to four week period, 3 to 6 Questran sachets per day, administered either as a single daily dose or in divided doses up to four times daily, according to dosage requirements and patient acceptability. Dosage may be modified according to response and can be increased to 9 sachets per day if necessary.

Occasional slight gastro-intestinal upsets, e.g. constipation, may occur when starting Questran. These usually pass with continued usage of Questran and are minimised by starting therapy gradually.

Final dose required	*Sachets per day*			
	Week 1	*Week 2*	*Week 3*	*Week 4*
3	1	2	3	3
4	1	2	3	4
6	1	2	3	6

2. To relieve pruritus: One or two sachets daily are usually sufficient.

3. To relieve diarrhoea: As for reduction of cholesterol but it may be possible to reduce this dosage. In all patients presenting with diarrhoea induced by bile acid malabsorption, if a response is not seen within 3 days, then alternative therapy should be initiated.

Children: Children 6–12 years: The initial dose is determined by the following formula:

$$\frac{\textit{Child's Weight in Kg} \times \textit{Adult Dose}}{70}$$

Subsequent dosage adjustment may be necessary where clinically indicated.

Children under 6 years: The dose has not been established in infants and children under 6 years.

Elderly: No dosage adjustment is necessary.

Contra-indications: Questran is contra-indicated in patients who have shown hypersensitivity to any of the product ingredients.

In patients with complete biliary obstruction, since

Questran cannot be effective where bile is not secreted into the intestine.

Special warnings and special precautions for use: Reduction of serum folate concentrations has been reported in children with familial hypercholesterolaemia. Supplementation with folic acid should be considered in these cases.

Questran Light contains aspartame, a source of phenylalanine.

Interactions with other medicinal products and other forms of interaction: Questran may delay or reduce the absorption of certain drugs (such as digitalis, tetracycline, chlorothiazide, warfarin and thyroxine). The response to concomitant medication should be closely monitored and appropriate adjustments made if necessary.

Questran may interfere with the pharmacokinetics of drugs that undergo enterohepatic recirculation.

Patients should take other drugs at least one hour before or 4-6 hours after Questran to minimise possible interference with their absorption.

Pregnancy and lactation: The safety of cholestyramine in pregnancy and lactation has not been established and the possibility of interference with absorption of fat soluble vitamins should be considered.

Effects on ability to drive and use machines: None.

Undesirable effects: Since Questran may interfere with the absorption of fat soluble vitamins, the diet may require supplementation with Vitamins A, D and K during prolonged high dose administration.

Chronic use of Questran may be associated with increased bleeding tendency due to hyperprothrombinaemia associated with Vitamin K deficiency. This will usually respond promptly to parenteral Vitamin K administration; recurrences can be prevented by oral administration of Vitamin K.

Hyperchloraemic acidosis has occasionally been reported following the prolonged use of anion exchange resins.

Gastro-intestinal side effects are those most frequently reported. The principal complaint is constipation which may be controlled with the usual remedies, and frequently disappears on continued usage of Questran. Large doses of Questran can cause diarrhoea.

Taste disturbance and skin irritation have been reported rarely but causal relationship to cholestyramine remains undetermined.

Overdose: One case of medication error experienced heartburn and nausea after taking cholestyramine 27 g t.i.d. for a week. The potential problem in overdosage would be obstruction of the gastro-intestinal tract.

Pharmacological properties

Pharmacodynamic properties: Cholesterol is a major, if not the sole precursor of bile acids. During normal digestion, bile acids are secreted via the bile from the liver and gall bladder into the small intestine. Bile acids emulsify the fat and lipid materials present in foods, thus facilitating absorption. A major portion of the bile acids secreted are reabsorbed from the ileum and returned via the portal vein to the liver, thus completing the enterohepatic cycle. Only very small amounts of bile acids are found in normal serum.

Cholestyramine resin absorbs and combines with the bile acids in the intestine to form an insoluble complex which is excreted in the faeces. This results in a continuous, though partial, removal of bile acids from the enterohepatic circulation by preventing their reabsorption. The increased faecal loss of bile acids leads to an increased oxidation of cholesterol to bile acids and a decrease in serum cholesterol levels and low density lipoprotein serum levels. Cholestyramine is hydrophilic but it is not soluble in water, nor is it hydrolysed by digestive enzymes.

In patients with partial biliary obstruction, the reduction of serum bile acid levels reduces excess bile acids deposited in the dermal tissue with resultant decrease in pruritus.

Pharmacokinetic properties: The cholestyramine resin in Questran and Questran Light is not absorbed from the digestive tract.

Preclinical safety data: No further significant information.

Pharmaceutical particulars

List of excipients

Questran: Acacia, citric acid anhydrous, orange juice flavour, polysorbate 80, propylene glycol alginate, sucrose, sunset yellow.

Questran Light: Aspartame, citric acid anhydrous, colloidal anhydrous silica, orange juice flavour, propylene glycol alginate, quinoline yellow, sucrose, xanthan gum.

Incompatibilities: None known.

Shelf life:

Questran: 48 months.

Questran Light: 36 months

Special precautions for storage: Store in a dry place.

Nature and contents of container: Original packs containing 60 laminate sachets composed of paper, polyethylene and aluminium.

Instructions for use/handling: No special instructions.

Marketing authorisation number

Questran 0125/5009R.
Questran Light 0125/0192.

Date of first authorisation/renewal of authorisation

Questran 22 January 1987
Questran Light 25th July 1988

Date of (partial) revision of the text

January 1998

SOTACOR* TABLETS

Qualitative and quantitative composition

White, circular, tablets engraved 'SOTACOR 80MG' on one face, each tablet containing 80 mg sotalol hydrochloride.

White, circular, tablets engraved 'SOTACOR 160' on one face, each tablet containing 160 mg sotalol hydrochloride.

Pharmaceutical form Oral tablets.

Clincal particulars

Therapeutic indications:

SOTACOR tablets are indicated for:

Ventricular arrhythmias:

Treatment of life-threatening ventricular tachyarrhythmias;

Treatment of symptomatic non-sustained ventricular tachyarrhythmias;

Supraventricular arrhythmias:

Prophylaxis of paroxysmal atrial tachycardia, paroxysmal atrial fibrillation, paroxysmal A-V nodal re-entrant tachycardia, paroxysmal A-V re-entrant tachycardia using accessory pathways, and paroxysmal supraventricular tachycardia after cardiac surgery;

Maintenance of normal sinus rhythm following conversion of atrial fibrillation or atrial flutter.

Posology and method of administration: The initiation of treatment or changes in dosage with SOTACOR should follow an appropriate medical evaluation including ECG control with measurement of the corrected QT interval, and assessment of renal function, electrolyte balance, and concomitant medications (see *Special warnings and special precautions for use*).

As with other antiarrhythmic agents, it is recommended that SOTACOR be initiated and doses increased in a facility capable of monitoring and assessing cardiac rhythm. The dosage must be individualized and based on the patient's response. Proarrhythmic events can occur not only at initiation of therapy, but also with each upward dosage adjustment.

In view of its -adrenergic blocking properties, treatment with SOTACOR should not be discontinued suddenly, especially in patients with ischaemic heart disease (angina pectoris, prior acute myocardial infarction) or hypertension, to prevent exacerbation of the disease (see *Special warnings and special precautions for use*).

The following dosing schedule can be recommended:

The initial dose is 80 mg, administered either singly or as two divided doses.

Oral dosage of SOTACOR should be adjusted gradually allowing 2-3 days between dosing increments in order to attain steady-state, and to allow monitoring of QT intervals. Most patients respond to a daily dose of 160 to 320 mg administered in two divided doses at approximately 12 hour intervals. Some patients with life-threatening refractory ventricular arrhythmias may require doses as high as 480–640 mg/day. These doses should be used under specialist supervision and should only be prescribed when the potential benefit outweighs the increased risk of adverse events, particularly proarrhythmias (see *Special warnings and special precautions for use*).

Children: SOTACOR is not intended for administration to children.

Dosage in renally impaired patients: Because SOTACOR is excreted mainly in urine, the dosage should be reduced when the creatinine clearance is less than 60 ml/min according to the following table:

Creatinine clearance (ml/min)	*Adjusted doses*
> 60	Recommended SOTACOR Dose
30-60	½ recommended SOTACOR Dose
10-30	¼ recommended SOTACOR Dose
< 10	Avoid

The creatinine clearance can be estimated from serum creatinine by the Cockroft and Gault formula:

Men:

$$\frac{(140-\text{age})\times\text{weight (kg)}}{72\times\text{serum creatinine (mg/dl)}}$$

Women: idem×0.85

When serum creatinine is given in μmol/l, divide the value by 88.4 (1 mg/dl = 88.4 μmol/l).

Dosage in hepatically impaired patients: No dosage adjustment is required in hepatically impaired patients.

Contra-indications: SOTACOR should not be used where there is evidence of sick sinus syndrome; second and third degree AV heart block unless a functioning pacemaker is present; congenital or acquired long QT syndromes; torsades de pointes; symptomatic sinus bradycardia; uncontrolled congestive heart failure; cardiogenic shock; anaesthesia that produces myocardial depression; untreated phaeochromocytoma; hypotension (except due to arrhythmia); Raynaud's phenomenon and severe peripheral circulatory disturbances; history of chronic obstructive airway disease or bronchial asthma (a warning will appear on the label); hypersensitivity to any of the components of the formulation; metabolic acidosis; renal failure (creatinine clearance < 10 ml/min).

Special warnings and special precautions for use:

Abrupt withdrawal: Hypersensitivity to catecholamines is observed in patients withdrawn from beta-blocker therapy. Occasional cases of exacerbation of angina pectoris, arrhythmias, and in some cases, myocardial infarction have been reported after abrupt discontinuation of therapy. Patients should be carefully monitored when discontinuing chronically administered SOTACOR, particularly those with ischaemic heart disease. If possible the dosage should be gradually reduced over a period of one to two weeks, if necessary at the same time initiating replacement therapy. Abrupt discontinuation may unmask latent coronary insufficiency. In addition, hypertension may develop.

Proarrhythmias: The most dangerous adverse effect of Class I and Class III antiarrhythmic drugs (such as sotalol) is the aggravation of pre-existing arrhythmias or the provocation of new arrhythmias. Drugs that prolong the QT-interval may cause torsades de pointes, a polymorphic ventricular tachycardia associated with prolongation of the QT-interval. Experience to date indicates that the risk of torsades de pointes is associated with the prolongation of the QT-interval, reduction of the heart rate, reduction in serum potassium and magnesium, high plasma sotalol concentrations and with the concomitant use of sotalol and other medications which have been associated with torsades de pointes (see *Interactions with other medicinal products and other forms of interation*). Females may be at increased risk of developing torsades de pointes.

The incidence of torsades de pointes is dose dependent. Torsades de pointes usually occurs early after initiating therapy or escalation of the dose and can progress to ventricular fibrillation.

In clinical trials of patients with sustained VT/VF the incidence of severe proarrhythmia (torsades de pointes or new sustained VT/VF) was <2% at doses up to 320 mg. The incidence more than doubled at higher doses.

Other risk factors for torsades de pointes were excessive prolongation of the QT_C and history of cardiomegaly or congestive heart failure. Patients with sustained ventricular tachycardia and a history of congestive heart failure have the highest risk of serious proarrhythmia (7%). Proarrhythmic events must be anticipated not only on initiating therapy but with every upward dose adjustment. Initiating therapy at 80 mg with gradual upward dose titration thereafter reduces the risk of proarrhythmia. In patients already receiving SOTACOR caution should be used if the QT_C exceeds 500 msec whilst on therapy, and serious consideration should be given to reducing the dose or discontinuing therapy when the QT_C-interval exceeds 550 msec. Due to the multiple risk factors associated with torsades de pointes, however, caution should be exercised regardless of the QT_C-interval.

Electrolyte disturbances: SOTACOR should not be used in patients with hypokalaemia or hypomagnesaemia prior to correction of imbalance; these conditions can exaggerate the degree of QT prolongation, and increase the potential for torsades de pointes. Special attention should be given to electrolyte and acid-base balance in patients experiencing severe or prolonged diarrhoea or patients receiving concomitant magnesium- and/or potassium-depleting drugs.

Congestive heart failure: Beta-blockade may further depress myocardial contractility and precipitate more severe heart failure. Caution is advised when initiating therapy in patients with left ventricular dysfunction controlled by therapy (i.e. ACE Inhibitors, diuretics, digitalis, etc); a low initial dose and careful dose titration is appropriate.

Recent MI: In post-infarction patients with impaired left ventricular function, the risk versus benefit of sotalol administration must be considered. Careful monitoring and dose titration are critical during initiation and follow-up of therapy. SOTACOR should be avoided in patients with left ventricular ejection fractions ≤40% without serious ventricular arrhythmias.

Electrocardiographic changes: Excessive prolongation of the QT-interval can be a sign of toxicity and should be avoided (see *Proarrhythmias* above). Bradycardia increases the risk of torsades de pointes.

Anaphylaxis: Patients with a history of anaphylactic reaction to a variety of allergens may have a more severe reaction on repeated challenge while taking beta-blockers. Such patients may be unresponsive to the usual doses of adrenaline used to treat the allergic reaction.

Anaesthesia: As with other beta-blocking agents, SOTACOR should be used with caution in patients undergoing surgery and in association with anaesthetics that cause myocardial depression, such as cyclopropane or trichloroethylene.

Diabetes mellitus: SOTACOR should be used with caution in patients with diabetes (especially labile diabetes) or with a history of episodes of spontaneous hypoglycaemia, since beta-blockade may mask some important signs of the onset of acute hypoglycaemia, e.g. tachycardia.

Thyrotoxicosis: Beta-blockade may mask certain clinical signs of hyperthyroidism (e.g., tachycardia). Patients suspected of developing thyrotoxicosis should be managed carefully to avoid abrupt withdrawal of beta-blockade which might be followed by an exacerbation of symptoms of hyperthyroidism, including thyroid storm.

Renal impairment: As sotalol is mainly eliminated via the kidneys the dose should be adjusted in patients with renal impairment (see *Dosage*).

Psoriasis: Beta-blocking drugs have been reported rarely to exacerbate the symptoms of psoriasis vulgaris.

Interactions with other medicinal products and other forms of interaction:

Antiarrhythmics: Class 1a antiarrhythmic drugs, such as disopyramide, quinidine and procainamide and other antiarrhythmic drugs such as amiodarone and bepridil are not recommended as concomitant therapy with SOTACOR, because of their potential to prolong refractoriness (see *Special warnings and special precautions for use*). The concomitant use of other beta-blocking agents with SOTACOR may result in additive Class II effects.

Other drugs prolonging the QT-interval: SOTACOR should be given with extreme caution in conjunction with other drugs known to prolong the QT-interval such as phenothiazines, tricyclic antidepressants, terfenadine and astemizole. Other drugs that have been associated with an increased risk for torsades de pointes include vincamine, fénoxedil, erythromycin IV, halofantrine, pentamidine, sultopride.

Floctafenine: Beta-adrenergic blocking agents may impede the compensatory cardiovascular reactions associated with hypotension or shock that may be induced by Floctafenine.

Calcium channel blocking drugs: Concurrent administration of beta-blocking agents and calcium channel blockers has resulted in hypotension, bradycardia, conduction defects, and cardiac failure. Beta-blockers should be avoided in combination with cardiodepressant calcium-channel blockers such as verapamil and diltiazem because of the additive effects on atrioventricular conduction, and ventricular function.

Potassium-depleting diuretics: Hypokalaemia or hypomagnesaemia may occur, increasing the potential for torsade de pointes (see *Special warnings and special precautions for use*).

Other potassium-depleting drugs: Amphotericin B (IV route), corticosteroids (systemic administration), and some laxatives may also be associated with hypokalemia; Potassium levels should be monitored and corrected appropriately during concommitant administration with SOTACOR.

Clonidine: Beta-blocking drugs may potentiate the rebound hypertension sometimes observed after discontinuation of clonidine; therefore, the beta-blocker should be discontinued slowly several days before the gradual withdrawal of clonidine.

Digitalis glycosides: Single and multiple doses of SOTACOR do not significantly affect serum digoxin levels. Proarrhythmic events were more common in sotalol treated patients also receiving digitalis glycosides; however, this may be related to the presence of CHF, a known risk factor for proarrhythmia, in patients receiving digitalis glycosides. Association of digitalis glycosides with beta-blockers may increase auriculo-ventricular conduction time.

Catecholamine-depleting agents: Concomitant use of catecholamine-depleting drugs, such as reserpine, guanethidine, or alpha methyldopa, with a beta-blocker may produce an excessive reduction of resting sympathetic nervous tone. Patients should be closely monitored for evidence of hypotension and/or marked bradycardia which may produce syncope.

Insulin and oral hypoglycaemics: Hyperglycaemia may occur, and the dosage of antidiabetic drugs may require adjustment. Symptoms of hypoglycaemia (tachycardia) may be masked by beta-blocking agents.

Neuromuscular blocking agents like Tubocurarine: The neuromuscular blockade is prolonged by beta-blocking agents.

Beta-2-receptor stimulants: Patients in need of beta-agonists should not normally receive SOTACOR. However, if concomitant therapy is necessary beta-agonists may have to be administered in increased dosages.

Drug/laboratory interaction: The presence of sotalol in the urine may result in falsely elevated levels of urinary metanephrine when measured by photometric methods. Patients suspected of having phaeochromocytoma and who are treated with sotalol should have their urine screened utilizing the HPLC assay with solid phase extraction.

Pregnancy and lactation:

Pregnancy: Animal studies with sotalol hydrochloride have shown no evidence of teratogenicity or other harmful effects on the foetus. Although there are no adequate and well-controlled studies in pregnant women, sotalol hydrochloride has been shown to cross the placenta and is found in amniotic fluid. Beta-blockers reduce placental perfusion, which may result in intrauterine foetal death, immature and premature deliveries. In addition, adverse effects (especially hypoglycaemia and bradycardia) may occur in foetus and neonate. There is an increased risk of cardiac and pulmonary complications in the neonate in the postnatal period. Therefore, SOTACOR should be used in pregnancy only if the potential benefits outweigh the possible risk to the foetus. The neonate should be monitored very carefully for 48–72 hours after delivery if it was not possible to interrupt maternal therapy with SOTACOR 2-3 days before the birthdate.

Most beta-blockers, particularly lipophilic compounds, will pass into breast milk although to a variable extent. Breast feeding is therefore not recommended during administration of these compounds.

Effect on ability to drive and use machines: There are no data available, but the occasional occurrence of side-effects such as dizziness and fatigue should be taken into account (see *Undesirable effects*).

Undesirable effects: The most frequent adverse effects of sotalol arise from its beta-blockade properties. Adverse effects are usually transient in nature and rarely necessitate interruption of, or withdrawal from treatment. If they do occur, they usually disappear when the dosage is reduced. The most significant adverse effects, however, are those due to proarrhythmia, including torsades de pointes (see *Special warnings and special precautions for use*).

The following are adverse events considered related to therapy, occuring in 1% or more of patients treated with SOTACOR.

Cardiovascular: Bradycardia, dyspnoea, chest pain, palpitations, oedema, ECG abnormalities, hypotension, proarrhythmia, syncope, heart failure, presyncope.

Dermatologic: Rash.

Gastro-intestinal: Nausea/vomiting, diarrhoea, dyspepsia, abdominal pain, flatulence.

Musculoskeletal: Cramps.

Nervous/psychiatric: Fatigue, dizziness, asthenia, lightheadedness, headache, sleep disturbances, depression, paresthesia, mood changes, anxiety.

Urogenital: Sexual dysfunction.

Special senses: Visual disturbances, taste abnormalities, hearing disturbances.

Body as a whole: Fever.

In trials of patients with cardiac arrhythmia, the most common adverse events leading to discontinuation of SOTACOR were fatigue 4%, bradycardia (<50 bpm) 3%, dyspnoea 3%, proarrhythmia 2%, asthenia 2%, and dizziness 2%.

Overdose: Intentional or accidental overdosage with SOTACOR has rarely resulted in death. Haemodialysis results in a large reduction of plasma levels of sotalol.

Symptoms and treatment of overdosage: The most yycommon signs to be expected are bradycardia, congestive heart failure, hypotension, bronchospasm and hypoglycaemia. In cases of massive intentional overdosage (2-16 g) of SOTACOR the following clinical findings were seen: hypotension, bradycardia, prolongation of QT-interval, premature ventricular complexes, ventricular tachycardia, torsades de pointes.

If overdosage occurs, therapy with SOTACOR should be discontinued and the patient observed closely. In addition, if required, the following therapeutic measures are suggested:

Bradycardia: Atropine (0.5 to 2 mg IV), another anticholinergic drug, a beta-adrenergic agonist (isoprenaline, 5 microgram per minute, up to 25 microgram, by slow IV injection) or transvenous cardiac pacing.

Heart block (second and third degree): Transvenous cardiac pacing.

Hypotension: Adrenaline rather than isoprenaline or noradrenaline may be useful, depending on associated factors.

Bronchospasm: Aminophylline or aerosol beta-2-receptor stimulant.

Torsades de pointes: DC cardioversion, transvenous cardiac pacing, adrenaline, and/or magnesium sulphate.

Pharmacological properties

Pharmacodynamic properties: D,l-sotalol is a non-selective hydrophilic -adrenergic receptor blocking agent, devoid of intrinsic sympathomimetic activity or membrane stabilizing activity.

SOTACOR has both beta-adrenoreceptor blocking (Vaughan Williams Class II) and cardiac action potential duration prolongation (Vaughan Williams Class III) antiarrhythmic properties. Sotalol has no known effect on the upstroke velocity and therefore no effect on the depolarisation phase.

Sotalol uniformly prolongs the action potential duration in cardiac tissues by delaying the repolarisation phase. Its major effects are prolongation of the atrial, ventricular and accessory pathway effective refractory periods.

The Class II and III properties may be reflected on the surface electrocardiogram by a lengthening of the PR, QT and QT_c (QT corrected for heart rate) intervals with no significant alteration in the QRS duration.

The d- and l-isomers of sotalol have similar Class III antiarrhythmic effects while the l-isomer is responsible for virtually all of the beta-blocking activity. Although significant beta-blockade may occur at oral doses as low as 25 mg, Class III effects are usually seen at daily doses of greater than 160 mg.

Its -adrenergic blocking activity causes a reduction in heart rate (negative chronotropic effect) and a limited reduction in the force of contraction (negative inotropic effect). These cardiac changes reduce myocardial oxygen consumption and cardiac work. Like other -blockers, sotalol inhibits renin release. The renin-suppressive effect of sotalol is significant both at rest and during exercise. Like other beta adrenergic blocking agents, SOTACOR produces a gradual but significant reduction in both systolic and diastolic blood pressures in hypertensive patients. Twenty-four-hour control of blood pressure is maintained both in the supine and upright positions with a single daily dose.

Pharmacokinetic properties: The bioavailability of oral sotalol is essentially complete (greater than 90%). After oral administration, peak levels are reached in 2.5 to 4 hours, and steady-state plasma levels are attained within 2-3 days. The absorption is reduced by approximately 20% when administered with a standard meal, in comparison to fasting conditions. Over the dosage range 40-640 mg/day SOTACOR displays dose proportionality with respect to plasma levels. Distribution occurs to a central (plasma) and a peripheral compartment, with an elimination half-life of 10-20 hours. Sotalol does not bind to plasma proteins and is not metabolised. There is very little inter-subject variability in plasma levels. Sotalol crosses the blood brain barrier poorly, with cerebrospinal fluid concentrations only 10% of those in plasma. The primary route of elimination is renal excretion. Approximately 80 to 90% of a dose is excreted unchanged in the urine, while the remainder is excreted in the faeces. Lower doses are necessary in conditions of renal impairment (see *Dosage and Administration in patients with renal dysfunction*). Age does not significantly alter the pharmacokinetics, although impaired renal function in geriatric patients can decrease the excretion rate, resulting in increased drug accumulation.

Preclinical safety data: No further particulars.

Pharmaceutical particulars

List of excipients: 80 mg Tablets: Lactose, magnesium stearate, maize starch, talc.

160 mg Tablets: Magnesium stearate, maize starch, microcrystalline cellulose, pregelatinised starch.

Incompatibilities: There are no known incompatibilities.

Shelf-life: Three years.

Special precautions for storage: Sotacor 80 mg: Store below 30°C. Protect from light.

Sotacor 160 mg: Store below 30°C in a dry place. Protect from light.

Nature and contents of container: Polypropylene securitainers of 100 or 300.

Original packs of 28–blister strips of 14 tablets with 2 strips toa carton.

Polypropylene securitainers of 50 or 300 tablets.

Original packs of 28 or 56–blister strips of 14 tablets with 2 or 4 strips to a carton.

Instructions for use/handling: None.

Marketing authorisation numbers

80 mg Tablets:	0125/0076
160 mg Tablets:	0125/0093

Date of first authorisation/renewal of authorisation

80 mg Tablets:	9th August 1989
160 mg Tablets:	11th February 1992

Date of (partial) revision of the text

80 mg Tablets:	May 1997
160 mg Tablets:	June 1997

SOTACOR* INJECTION

Qualitative and quantitative composition

Ampoules containing sotalol hydrochloride 40 mg in each 4 ml of solution.

Pharmaceutical form(s): Intravenous injection

Clinical particulars

Therapeutic indications: Termination of acute and life-threatening arrhythmias, including life-threatening ventricular tachyarrhythmias, symptomatic non-sustained ventricular achyarrhythmias;

Testing of drug efficacy during programmed electrical stimulation in patients with inducible ventricular and supraventricular tachyarrhythmias;

Transitory substitution for oral SOTACOR in patients temporarily unable to take oral medications.

Posology and method of administration: The initiation of treatment or changes in dosage with SOTACOR should follow an appropriate medical evaluation including ECG control with measurement of the corrected QT interval, and assessment of renal function, electrolyte balance, and concomitant medications (see *Special warnings and special precautions for use*).

As with other antiarrhythmic agents, it is recommended that SOTACOR be initiated and doses increased in a facility capable of monitoring and assessing cardiac rhythm. The dosage must be individualized and based on the patient's response. Proarrhythmic events can occur not only at initiation of therapy, but also with each upward dosage adjustment.

In view of its β-adrenergic blocking properties, treatment with SOTACOR should not be discontinued suddenly, especially in patients with ischaemic heart disease (angina pectoris, prior acute myocardial infarction) or hypertension, to prevent exacerbation of the disease (see *Special warnings and special precautions for use*).

The following dosing schedule can be recommended:

For the management of acute arrhythmias, dosage range is from 20-120 mg intravenously (0.5 mg to 1.5 mg/kg). The total calculated dose has been safely administered over a 10-minute period and can be repeated at 6-hour intervals if necessary. For high risk patients with acute myocardial infarction and/or congestive heart failure, careful monitoring for hemodynamic or electrocardiographic changes is recommended.

For programmed electrical stimulation, an initial bolus of 1.5 mg/kg should be given over 10 to 20 minutes, followed by maintenance infusion at a rate of between 0.2 and 0.5 mg/kg/hour.

For substitution in place of oral therapy, infusion of between 0.2 and 0.5 mg/kg/hour should be used with the total daily dose not exceeding 640 mg.

Children: SOTACOR is not intended for administration to children.

Dosage in renally impaired patients: Because SOTACOR is excreted mainly in urine, the dosage should be reduced when the creatinine clearance is less than 60 ml/min according to the following table:

Creatinine clearance (ml/min)	*Adjusted doses*
> 60	Recommended SOTACOR Dose
30-6 0	½ recommended SOTACOR Dose
10-30	¼ recommended SOTACOR Dose
< 10	Avoid

The creatinine clearance can be estimated from serum creatinine by the Cockroft and Gault formula:

Men:

$$\frac{(140-\text{age})\times\text{weight (kg)}}{72\times\text{serum creatinine (mg/dl)}}$$

Women: idem×0.85

When serum creatinine is given in μmol/l, divide the value by 88.4 (1 mg/dl = 88.4 mol/l).

Dosage in hepatically impaired patients: No dosage adjustment is required in hepatically impaired patients.

Contra-indications: SOTACOR should not be used where there is evidence of sick sinus syndrome; second and third degree AV heart block unless a functioning pacemaker is present; congenital or acquired long QT syndromes; torsades de pointes; symptomatic sinus bradycardia; uncontrolled congestive heart failure; cardiogenic shock; anaesthesia that produces myocardial depression; untreated phaeochromocytoma; hypotension (except due to arrhythmia); Raynaud's phenomenon and severe peripheral circulatory disturbances; history of chronic obstructive airway disease or bronchial asthma; hypersensitivity to any of the components of the formulation; metabolic acidosis; renal failure (creatinine clearance < 10 ml/min).

Special warnings and special precautions for use:

Abrupt withdrawal: Hypersensitivity to catecholamines is observed in patients withdrawn from beta-blocker therapy. Occasional cases of exacerbation of angina pectoris, arrhythmias, and in some cases, myocardial infarction have been reported after abrupt discontinuation of therapy. Patients should be carefully monitored when discontinuing chronically administered SOTACOR, particularly those with ischaemic heart disease. If possible the dosage should be gradually reduced over a period of one to two weeks, if necessary at the same time initiating replacement therapy. Abrupt discontinuation may unmask latent coronary insufficiency. In addition, hypertension may develop.

Proarrhythmias: The most dangerous adverse effect of Class I and Class III antiarrhythmic drugs (such as sotalol) is the aggravation of pre-existing arrhythmias or the provocation of new arrhythmias. Drugs that prolong the QT-interval may cause torsades de pointes, a polymorphic ventricular tachycardia associated with prolongation of the QT-interval. Experience to date indicates that the risk of torsades de pointes is associated with the prolongation of the QT-interval, reduction of the heart rate, reduction in serum potassium and magnesium, high plasma sotalol concentrations and with the concomitant use of sotalol and other medications which have been associated with torsades de pointes (see *Interactions with other medicinal products and other forms of interaction*). Females may be at increased risk of developing torsades de pointes.

The incidence of torsades de pointes is dose dependent. Torsades de pointes usually occurs early after initiating therapy or escalation of the dose and can progress to ventricular fibrillation.

In clinical trials of patients with sustained VT/VF the incidence of severe proarrhythmia (torsades de pointes or new sustained VT/VF) was <2% at doses up to 320 mg. The incidence more than doubled at higher doses.

Other risk factors for torsades de pointes were excessive prolongation of the QT_C and history of cardiomegaly or congestive heart failure. Patients with sustained ventricular tachycardia and a history of congestive heart failure have the highest risk of serious proarrhythmia (7%). Proarrhythmic events must be anticipated not only on initiating therapy but with every upward dose adjustment. Initiating therapy at 80 mg with gradual upward dose titration thereafter reduces the risk of proarrhythmia. In patients already receiving SOTACOR caution should be used if the QT_C exceeds 500 msec whilst on therapy, and serious consideration should be given to reducing the dose or discontinuing therapy when the QT_C-interval exceeds 550 msec. Due to the multiple risk factors associated with torsades de pointes, however, caution should be exercised regardless of the QT_C-interval.

Electrolyte disturbances: SOTACOR should not be used in patients with hypokalaemia or hypomagnesaemia prior to correction of imbalance; these conditions can exaggerate the degree of QT prolongation, and increase the potential for torsades de pointes. Special attention should be given to electrolyte and acid-base balance in patients experiencing severe or prolonged diarrhoea or patients receiving concomitant magnesium- and/or potassium-depleting drugs.

Congestive heart failure: Beta-blockade may further depress myocardial contractility and precipitate more severe heart failure. Caution is advised when initiating therapy in patients with left ventricular dysfunction controlled by therapy (i.e. ACE Inhibitors, diuretics, digitalis, etc); a low initial dose and careful dose titration is appropriate.

Recent MI: In post-infarction patients with impaired left ventricular function, the risk versus benefit of sotalol administration must be considered. Careful monitoring and dose titration are critical during initiation and follow-up of therapy. SOTACOR should be avoided in patients with left ventricular ejection fractions ≤40% without serious ventricular arrhythmias.

Electrocardiographic changes: Excessive prolongation of the QT-interval can be a sign of toxicity and should be avoided (see *Proarrhythmias* above). Bradycardia increases the risk of torsades de pointes.

Anaphylaxis: Patients with a history of anaphylactic reaction to a variety of allergens may have a more severe reaction on repeated challenge while taking beta-blockers. Such patients may be unresponsive to the usual doses of adrenaline used to treat the allergic reaction.

Anaesthesia: As with other beta-blocking agents, SOTACOR should be used with caution in patients undergoing surgery and in association with anaesthetics that cause myocardial depression, such as cyclopropane or trichloroethylene.

Diabetes mellitus: SOTACOR should be used with caution in patients with diabetes (especially labile diabetes) or with a history of episodes of spontaneous hypoglycaemia, since beta-blockade may mask some important signs of the onset of acute hypoglycaemia, e.g. tachycardia.

Thyrotoxicosis: Beta-blockade may mask certain clinical signs of hyperthyroidism (e.g., tachycardia). Patients suspected of developing thyrotoxicosis should be managed carefully to avoid abrupt withdrawal of beta-blockade which might be followed by an exacerbation of symptoms of hyperthyroidism, including thyroid storm.

Renal impairment: As sotalol is mainly eliminated via the kidneys the dose should be adjusted in patients with renal impairment (see *Posology and method of administration*).

Psoriasis: Beta-blocking drugs have been reported rarely to exacerbate the symptoms of psoriasis vulgaris.

Interactions with other medicinal products and other forms of interaction:

Antiarrhythmias: Class 1a antiarrhythmic drugs, such as disopyramide, quinidine and procainamide and other antiarrhythmic drugs such as amiodarone and bepridil are not recommended as concomitant therapy with SOTACOR, because of their potential to prolong refractoriness (see *Special warnings and special precautions for use*). The concomitant use of other beta-blocking agents with SOTACOR may result in additive Class II effects.

Other drugs prolonging the QT-interval: SOTACOR should be given with extreme caution in conjunction with other drugs known to prolong the QT-interval such as phenothiazines, tricyclic antidepressants, terfenadine and astemizole. Other drugs that have been associated with an increased risk for torsades de pointes include vincamine, fénoxedil, erythromycin IV, halofantrine, pentamidine, sultopride.

Floctafenine: beta-adrenergic blocking agents may impede the compensatory cardiovascular reactions associated with hypotension or shock that may be induced by Floctafenine.

Calcium channel blocking drugs: Concurrent administration of beta-blocking agents and calcium channel blockers has resulted in hypotension, bradycardia, conduction defects, and cardiac failure. Beta-blockers should be avoided in combination with cardiodepressant calcium-channel blockers such as verapamil and diltiazem because of the additive effects on atrioventricular conduction, and ventricular function.

Potassium-depleting diuretics: Hypokalaemia or hypomagnesaemia may occur, increasing the potential for torsade de pointes (see *Special warnings and special precautions for use*).

Other potassium-depleting drugs: Amphotericin B (IV route), corticosteroids (systemic administration), and some laxatives may also be associated with hypokalemia; Potassium levels should be monitored and corrected appropriately during concommitant administration with SOTACOR.

Clonidine: Beta-blocking drugs may potentiate the rebound hypertension sometimes observed after discontinuation of clonidine; therefore, the beta-blocker should be discontinued slowly several days before the gradual withdrawal of clonidine.

Digitalis glycosides: Single and multiple doses of SOTACOR do not significantly affect serum digoxin levels. Proarrhythmic events were more common in sotalol treated patients also receiving digitalis glycosides; however, this may be related to the presence of CHF, a known risk factor for proarrhythmia, in patients receiving digitalis glycosides. Association of digitalis glycosides with beta-blockers may increase auriculo-ventricular conduction time.

Catecholamine-depleting agents: Concomitant use of catecholamine-depleting drugs, such as reserpine, guanethidine, or alpha methyldopa, with a beta-blocker may produce an excessive reduction of resting sympathetic nervous tone. Patients should be closely monitored for evidence of hypotension and/or marked bradycardia which may produce syncope.

Insulin and oral hypoglycaemics: Hyperglycaemia may occur, and the dosage of antidiabetic drugs may require adjustment. Symptoms of hypoglycaemia (tachycardia) may be masked by beta-blocking agents.

Neuromuscular blocking agents like Tubocurarine: The neuromuscular blockade is prolonged by beta-blocking agents.

Beta-2-receptor stimulants: Patients in need of beta-agonists should not normally receive SOTACOR. However, if concomitant therapy is necessary beta-agonists may have to be administered in increased dosages.

Drug/laboratory interaction: The presence of sotalol in the urine may result in falsely elevated levels of urinary metanephrine when measured by photometric methods. Patients suspected of having phaeochromocytoma and who are treated with sotalol should have their urine screened utilizing the HPLC assay with solid phase extraction.

Pregnancy and lactation:

Pregnancy: Animal studies with sotalol hydrochloride have shown no evidence of teratogenicity or other harmful effects on the foetus. Although there are no adequate and well-controlled studies in pregnant women, sotalol hydrochloride has been shown to cross the placenta and is found in amniotic fluid. Beta-blockers reduce placental perfusion, which may result in intrauterine foetal death, immature and premature deliveries. In addition, adverse effects (especially hypoglycaemia and bradycardia) may occur in foetus and neonate. There is an increased risk of cardiac and pulmonary complications in the neonate in the postnatal period. Therefore, SOTACOR should be used in pregnancy only if the potential benefits outweigh the possible risk to the foetus. The neonate should be monitored very carefully for 48–72 hours after delivery if it was not possible to interrupt maternal therapy with SOTACOR 2-3 days before the birthdate.

Most beta-blockers, particularly lipophilic compounds, will pass into breast milk although to a variable extent. Breast feeding is therefore not recommended during administration of these compounds.

Effect on ability to drive and use machines: There are no data available, but the occasional occurrence of side-effects such as dizziness and fatigue should be taken into account (see *Undesirable effects*).

Undesirable effects: The most frequent adverse effects of sotalol arise from its beta-blockade properties. Adverse effects are usually transient in nature and rarely necessitate interruption of, or withdrawal from treatment. If they do occur, they usually disappear when the dosage is reduced. The most significant adverse effects, however, are those due to proarrhythmia, including torsades de pointes (see *Special warnings and special precautions for use*).

The following are adverse events considered related to therapy, occuring in 1% or more of patients treated with SOTACOR.

Cardiovascular: Bradycardia, dyspnoea, chest pain, palpitations, oedema, ECG abnormalities, hypotension, proarrhythmia, syncope, heart failure, presyncope.

Dermatologic: Rash.

Gastro-intestinal: Nausea/vomiting, diarrhoea, dyspepsia, abdominal pain, flatulence.

Musculoskeletal: Cramps.

Nervous/psychiatric: Fatigue, dizziness, asthenia, lightheadedness, headache, sleep disturbances, depression, paresthesia, mood changes, anxiety.

Urogenital: Sexual dysfunction.

Special senses: Visual disturbances, taste abnormalities, hearing disturbances.

Body as a whole: Fever.

In trials of patients with cardiac arrhythmia, the most common adverse events leading to discontinuation of SOTACOR were fatigue 4%, bradycardia (<50 bpm) 3%, dyspnoea 3%, proarrhythmia 2%, asthenia 2%, and dizziness 2%.

Overdose: Intentional or accidental overdosage with SOTACOR has rarely resulted in death. Haemodialysis results in a large reduction of plasma levels of sotalol.

Symptoms and treatment of overdosage: The most common signs to be expected are bradycardia, congestive heart failure, hypotension, bronchospasm and hypoglycaemia. In cases of massive intentional overdosage (2-16 g) of SOTACOR the following clinical findings were seen: hypotension, bradycardia, prolongation of QT-interval, premature ventricular complexes, ventricular tachycardia, torsades de pointes.

If overdosage occurs, therapy with SOTACOR should be discontinued and the patient observed closely. In addition, if required, the following therapeutic measures are suggested:

Bradycardia: Atropine (0.5 to 2 mg IV), another anticholinergic drug, a beta-adrenergic agonist (isoprenaline, 5 microgram per minute, up to 25 microgram, by slow IV injection) or transvenous cardiac pacing.

Heart block (second and third degree): Transvenous cardiac pacing.

Hypotension: Adrenaline rather than isoprenaline or noradrenaline may be useful, depending on associated factors.

Bronchospasm: Aminophylline or aerosol beta-2-receptor stimulant.

Torsades de pointes: DC cardioversion, transvenous cardiac pacing, adrenaline, and/or magnesium sulphate.

Pharmacological properties

Pharmacodynamic properties: D,l-sotalol is a non-selective hydrophilic -adrenergic receptor blocking agent, devoid of intrinsic sympathomimetic activity or membrane stabilizing activity.

SOTACOR has both beta-adrenoreceptor blocking (Vaughan Williams Class II) and cardiac action potential duration prolongation (Vaughan Williams Class III) antiarrhythmic properties. Sotalol has no known effect on the upstroke velocity and therefore no effect on the depolarisation phase.

Sotalol uniformly prolongs the action potential duration in cardiac tissues by delaying the repolarisation phase. Its major effects are prolongation of the atrial, ventricular and accessory pathway effective refractory periods.

The Class II and III properties may be reflected on the surface electrocardiogram by a lengthening of the PR, QT and QT^c (QT corrected for heart rate) intervals with no significant alteration in the QRS duration.

The d- and l-isomers of sotalol have similar Class III antiarrhythmic effects while the l-isomer is responsible for virtually all of the beta-blocking activity. Although significant beta-blockade may occur at oral doses as low as 25 mg, Class III effects are usually seen at daily doses of greater than 160 mg.

Its β-adrenergic blocking activity causes a reduction in heart rate (negative chronotropic effect) and a limited reduction in the force of contraction (negative inotropic effect). These cardiac changes reduce myocardial oxygen consumption and cardiac work. Like other -blockers, sotalol inhibits renin release. The renin-suppressive effect of sotalol is significant both at rest and during exercise. Like other beta adrenergic blocking agents, SOTACOR produces a gradual but significant reduction in both systolic and diastolic blood pressures in hypertensive patients. Twenty-four-hour control of blood pressure is maintained both in the supine and upright positions with a single daily dose.

Pharmacokinetic properties: The bioavailability of oral sotalol is essentially complete (greater than 90%). After oral administration, peak levels are reached in 2.5 to 4 hours, and steady-state plasma levels are attained within 2-3 days. The absorption is reduced by approximately 20% when administered with a standard meal, in comparison to fasting conditions. Over the dosage range 40-640 mg/day SOTACOR displays dose proportionality with respect to plasma levels. Distribution occurs to a central (plasma) and a peripheral compartment, with an elimination half-life of 10-20 hours. Sotalol does not bind to plasma proteins and is not metabolised. There is very little inter-subject variability in plasma levels. Sotalol crosses the blood brain barrier poorly, with cerebrospinal fluid concentrations only 10% of those in plasma. The primary route of elimination is renal excretion. Approximately 80 to 90% of a dose is excreted unchanged in the urine, while the remainder is excreted in the faeces. Lower doses are necessary in conditions of renal impairment (see *Dosage and administration in patients with renal dysfunction*). Age does not significantly alter the pharmacokinetics, although impaired renal function in geriatric patients can decrease the excretion rate, resulting in increased drug accumulation.

Preclinical safety data: No further particulars.

Pharmaceutical particulars

List of excipients: Glacial acetic acid, sodium chloride, sodium hydroxide, water.

Incompatibilities: There are no known incompatibilities.

Shelf-life: Three years.

Special precautions for storage: Store between 15 and 30°C in a dry place, protected from light.

Nature and contents of container: SOTACOR injection is supplied as 40 mg sotalol hydrochloride in 4 ml ampoules, with 5 ampoules per box.

Instructions for use/handling: SOTACOR injection fluid can be administered as an intravenous infusion with 5% glucose intravenous infusion or 0.9% sodium chloride intravenous infusion. The final concentration should be between 0.01-2 mg/ml.

In concentrations of 0.01-2 mg/ml, dilution of SOTACOR injection fluid with 5% glucose intravenous infusion or 0.9% sodium chloride intravenous infusion, is chemically and physically stable during at least 4 days at room temperature (15-25°C) and 3 weeks under refrigeration (2-8°C).

As the formulation does not contain a preservative, the solutions of SOTACOR should be prepared in an aseptic manner. Prompt use of the solution is recommended.

Marketing authorisation number 0125/0123

Date of first authorisation/renewal of authorisation 25 January 1990

Date of (partial) revision of the text March 1996

VEPESID* CAPSULES 100 mg

Qualitative and quantitative composition Pale pink, soft gelatin capsules containing 100 mg etoposide.

Pharmaceutical form Oral capsules

Clinical particulars

Therapeutic indications: Vepesid is an anti-neoplastic drug for intravenous or oral use, which can be used alone or in combination with other oncolytic drugs. Present data indicate that Vepesid is applicable in the therapy of: small cell lung cancer, resistant non-seminomatous testicular carcinoma.

Posology and method of administration: The recommended course of Vepesid capsules is 120-240 mg/m2 orally daily, for five consecutive days. The dose of Vepesid capsules is based on the recommended i.v. dose with consideration given to the bioavailability of Vepesid capsules appearing to be dependent upon the dose administered. The bioavailability also varies from patient to patient following any oral dose. This should be taken into consideration when prescribing this medication. In view of significant intra-patient variability, dose adjustments may be required in order to achieve the desired therapeutic effect. As Vepesid produces myelosuppression, courses may not be repeated more frequently than at 21 day intervals. In any case, a repeat course of Vepesid should not be given until the blood picture has been checked for evidence of myelosuppression and found to be satisfactory.

The capsules should be taken on an empty stomach.

Elderly: No dosage adjustment is necessary.

Paediatric use: Safety and effectiveness in children have not been established.

Contra-indications: Vepesid is contra-indicated in patients with severe hepatic dysfunction or in those patients who have demonstrated hypersensitivity to the drug.

Special warnings and special precautions for use: Vepesid should be administered by individuals experienced in the use of anti-neoplastic therapy.

When Vepesid is administered intravenously care should be taken to avoid extravasation.

If radiotherapy and/or chemotherapy has been given prior to starting Vepesid treatment, an adequate interval should be allowed to enable the bone marrow to recover. If the leucocyte count falls below 2,000 mm^3, treatment should be suspended until the circulating blood elements have returned to acceptable levels (platelets above 100,000 mm^3, leucocytes above 4,000/mm^3), this is usually within 10 days.

Peripheral blood counts and liver function should be monitored. (See *Undesirable effects*).

Bacterial infections should be brought under control before treatment with Vepesid commences.

The occurrence of acute leukaemia, which can occur with or without a preleukaemic phase has been reported rarely in patients treated with etoposide in association with other anti-neoplastic drugs.

Interactions with other medicinal products and other forms of interaction: None stated.

Pregnancy and lactation: Vepesid is teratogenic in rats and mice at dose levels equivalent to those employed clinically. There are no adequate and well-controlled studies in pregnant women.

Vepesid should not normally be administered to patients who are pregnant or to mothers who are breast feeding. Women of childbearing potential should be advised to avoid becoming pregnant.

The influence of Vepesid on human reproduction has not been determined.

In-vitro tests indicate that Vepesid is mutagenic.

Effects on ability to drive and use machines: None stated.

Undesirable effects:

Haematological: The dose limiting toxicity of Vepesid is myelosuppression, predominantly leucopenia and thrombocytopenia. Anaemia occurs infrequently.

The leucocyte count nadir occurs approximately 21 days after treatment.

Alopecia: Alopecia occurs in approximately two-thirds of patients and is reversible on cessation of therapy.

Gastrointestinal: Nausea and vomiting are the major gastrointestinal toxicities and occur in over one-third of patients. Anti-emetics are useful in controlling these side effects. Abdominal pain, anorexia, diarrhoea, oesophagitis and stomatitis occur infrequently.

Other toxicities: Hypotension may occur following an excessively rapid infusion and may be reversed by slowing the infusion rate.

Anaphylactoid reactions have been reported following administration of Vepesid. Higher rates of anaphylactoid reactions have been reported in children who received infusions at concentrations higher than those recommended. The role that concentration of infusion (or rate of infusion) plays in the development of anaphylactoid reactions is uncertain. These reactions have usually responded to cessation of therapy and administration of pressor agents, corticosteroids, antihistamines or volume expanders as appropriate.

Apnoea with spontaneous resumption of breathing following discontinuation of etoposide injection has been reported. Sudden fatal reactions associated with bronchospasm have been reported. Hypertension and/or flushing have also been reported. Blood pressure usually returns to normal within a few hours after cessation of the infusion.

The use of etoposide has been reported infrequently to cause peripheral neuropathy.

Vepesid has been shown to reach high concentrations in the liver and kidney, thus presenting a potential for accumulation in cases of functional impairment.

Somnolence, fatigue, aftertaste, fever, rash, pigmentation, pruritus, urticaria, dysphagia, transient cortical blindness and a single case of radiation recall dermatitis have also been reported following the administration of Vepesid.

Overdose: No proven antidotes have been established for Vepesid overdosage. Treatment should be symptomatic and supportive.

Total doses of 2.4 to 3.5 g/m² administered i.v. over three days have resulted in severe mucositis and myelotoxicity. Metabolic acidosis and cases of severe hepatic toxicity have been reported in patients receiving higher than recommended doses of etoposide.

Pharmacological properties

Pharmacodynamic properties: Etoposide is a semi-synthetic derivative of podophyllotoxin.

Experimental data indicate that etoposide arrests the cell cycle in the G^2 phase. Etoposide differs from the vinca alkaloids in that it does not cause an accumulation of cells in metaphase, but prevents cells from entering mitosis or destroys cells in the G^2 phase. The incorporation of thymidine into DNA is inhibited in vitro by etoposide. Etoposide does not interfere with microtubule assembly.

Pharmacokinetic properties: Etoposide is approximately 94% protein-bound in human serum. Plasma decay kinetics follow a bi-exponential curve and correspond to a two compartmental model. The mean volume of distribution is approximately 32% of body weight. Etoposide demonstrates relatively poor penetration into the cerebrospinal fluid. Urinary excretion is approximately 45% of an administered dose, 29% being excreted unchanged in 72 hours.

Preclinical safety data: No further relevant data.

Pharmaceutical particulars

List of excipients

Other ingredients: Citric acid, glycerol, polyethylene glycol 400, water. Gelatin capsules containing glycerol, iron oxide, sodium hydroxybenzoic acid ethyl ester, sodium propylhydroxybenzoate, titanium dioxide, water.

Incompatibilities: None stated.

Shelf life: 36 months

Special precautions for storage: Vepesid capsules should be stored between 10-25°C. Do not open any blister in which there is evidence of capsule leakage.

Nature and contents of container: Vepesid 100 mg capsules are packed in blister packs of 10 capsules, each capsule containing 100 mg etoposide.

Instructions for use/handling: Vepsid should be administered by individuals experienced in the use of anti-neoplastic therapy.

Marketing authorisation number

Vepesid Capsules 100 mg PL 0125/0124

Date of first authorisation/renewal of authorisation

03 July 1981 / 03 July 1991

Date of (partial) revision of the text

December 1997

VEPESID* CAPSULES 50 mg VEPESID* INJECTION

Presentation Vepesid Injection-vials containing 100 mg etoposide in 5 ml.

Other ingredients: Benzyl alcohol, citric acid anhydrous, dehydrated ethanol, polyethylene glycol, polysorbate 80.

Vepesid Capsules-soft gelatin, pale pink capsules containing 50 mg etoposide.

Other ingredients: citric acid, glycerol, polyethylene glycol 400, water; gelatin capsules containing glycerol, iron oxide, sodium hydroxybenzoic acid, ethyl ester, sodium propyl hydroxybenzoate, titanium dioxide, water.

Uses Vepesid is an anti-neoplastic drug for intravenous or oral use, which can be used alone or in combination with other oncolytic drugs.

Present data indicate that Vepesid is applicable in the therapy of: small cell lung cancer, resistant non-sèminomatous testicular carcinoma.

Dosage and administration The recommended course of Vepesid Injection is 60–120 mg/m², i.v., daily for five consecutive days. As Vepesid produces myelosuppression, courses may not be repeated more frequently than at 21 day intervals. In any case, repeat courses of Vepesid should not be given until the blood picture has been checked for evidence of myelosuppression and found to be satisfactory

Immediately before administration, the required dose of Vepesid Injection must be diluted with 0.9% saline solution for injection to give a solution concentration of not more than 0.25 mg/ml of etoposide; it should then be given by intravenous infusion over a period of not less than 30 minutes.

Care should be taken to avoid extravasation.

If oral dosing is preferred, 120–240 mg/m² should be given daily, for five consecutive days. The dose of Vepesid capsules is based on the recommended i.v. dose with consideration given to the bioavailability of Vepesid capsules appearing to be dependent upon the dose administered. The bioavailability also varies from patient to patient following any oral dose. This should be taken into consideration when prescribing this medication. In view of significant intra-patient variability, dose adjustments may be required in order to achieve the desired therapeutic effect. As Vepesid produces myelosuppression, courses may not be repeated more frequently than at 21 day intervals. In any case, a repeat course of Vepesid should not be given until the blood picture has been checked for evidence of myelosuppression and found to be satisfactory.

The capsules should be taken on an empty stomach.

Elderly: No dosage adjustment is necessary.

Paediatric use: Safety and effectiveness in children have not been established.

Contra-indications, warnings, etc Vepesid is contra-indicated in patients with severe hepatic dysfunction or in those patients who have demonstrated hypersensitivity to the drug.

Vepesid must not be given by intra-cavitary injection.

Warnings

Use in pregnancy: Vepesid is teratogenic in rats and mice at dose levels equivalent to those employed clinically. There are no adequate and well-controlled studies in pregnant women.

Vepesid should not normally be administered to patients who are pregnant or to mothers who are breast feeding. Women of childbearing potential should be advised to avoid becoming pregnant.

The influence of Vepesid on human reproduction has not been determined.

In-vitro tests indicate that Vepesid is mutagenic.

Precautions: Vepesid should be administered by individuals experienced in the use of antineoplastic therapy.

When Vepesid is administered intravenously care should be taken to avoid extravasation.

If radiotherapy and/or chemotherapy has been given prior to starting Vepesid treatment, an adequate interval should be allowed to enable the bone marrow to recover. If the leucocyte count falls below 2,000/mm³, treatment should be suspended until the circulating blood elements have returned to acceptable levels (platelets above 100,000mm³, leucocytes above 4,000/mm³), this is usually within 10 days.

Peripheral blood counts and liver function should be monitored. (See Adverse Reactions.)

Bacterial infections should be brought under control before treatment with Vepesid commences.

The occurrence of acute leukaemia, which can occur with or without a preleukaemic phase has been reported rarely in patients treated with etoposide in association with other anti-neoplastic drugs.

Adverse reactions: Haematological: The dose limiting toxicity of Vepesid is myelosuppression, predominantly leucopenia and thrombocytopenia. Anaemia occurs infrequently.

The leucocyte count nadir occurs approximately 21 days after treatment.

Alopecia: Alopecia occurs in approximately two-thirds of patients and is reversible on cessation of therapy.

Gastrointestinal: Nausea and vomiting are the major gastrointestinal toxicities and occur in over one-third of patients. Anti-emetics are useful in controlling these side effects. Abdominal pain, anorexia, diarrhoea, oesophagitis and stomatitis occur infrequently.

Other Toxicities: Hypotension may occur following an excessively rapid infusion and may be reversed by slowing the infusion rate.

Anaphylactoid reactions have been reported following administration of Vepesid. Higher rates of anaphylactoid reactions have been reported in children who received infusions at concentrations higher than those recommended. The role that concentration of infusion (or rate of infusion) plays in the development of anaphylactoid reactions is uncertain. These reactions have usually responded to cessation of therapy and administration of pressor agents, corticosteroids, antihistamines or volume expanders as appropriate.

Apnoea with spontaneous resumption of breathing following discontinuation of etoposide injection has been reported. Sudden fatal reactions associated with bronchospasm have been reported. Hypertension and/or flushing have also been reported. Blood pressure usually returns to normal within a few hours after cessation of the infusion.

The use of etoposide has been reported infrequently to cause peripheral neuropathy.

Vepesid has been shown to reach high concentrations in the liver and kidney, thus presenting a potential for accumulation in cases of functional impairment.

Somnolence, fatigue, aftertaste, fever, rash, pigmentation, pruritus, urticaria, dysphagia, transient cortical blindness and a single case of radiation recall dermatitis have also been reported following the administration of Vepesid.

Overdosage: No proven antidotes have been established for Vepesid overdosage. Treatment should be symptomatic and supportive.

Total doses of 2.4 to 3.5 g/m² administered i.v. over three days have resulted in severe mucositis and myelotoxicity. Metabolic acidosis and cases of severe hepatic toxicity have been reported in patients receiving higher than recommended doses of etoposide.

Pharmaceutical precautions Vepesid injection should be stored at room temperature. The injection should be protected from light.

Vepesid capsules should be stored between 10–25°C. Do not open any blister in which there is evidence of capsule leakage.

Preparation of intravenous solution: Immediately before administration the required dose of Vepesid Injection must be diluted with 0.9% sodium chloride for injection to give a solution concentration of not more than 0.25 mg/ml of etoposide; it should then be given by intravenous infusion over a period of not less than 30 minutes. The infusion solution should be kept at room temperature and should be used within six hours of preparation. Solutions of concentration greater than 0.25 mg/ml may show signs of precipitation, and are therefore not recommended. Any solutions showing signs of precipitation should be discarded.

The intravenous solution is suitable for infusion in glass or PVC containers.

Hard plastic devices made of acrylic or ABS (a polymer composed of acrylonitrile, butadiene and styrene) have been reported to crack and leak when used with undiluted Vepesid Injection. This effect has not been reported with diluted Vepesid Injection.

Vepesid should not be physically mixed with any other drug.

Guidelines for the safe handling of antineoplastic agents:

1. Trained personnel should reconstitute the drug.
2. This should be performed in a designated area.
3. Adequate protective gloves should be worn.
4. Precautions should be taken to avoid the drug accidentally coming into contact with the eyes. In the event of contact with the eyes, irrigate with large amounts of water and/or saline.
5. The cytotoxic preparation should not be handled by pregnant staff.
6. Adequate care and precautions should be taken in the disposal of items (syringes, needles etc) used to reconstitute cytotoxic drugs. Excess material and body waste may be disposed of by placing in double sealed polythene bags and incinerating at a temperature of 1,000°C. Liquid waste may be flushed with copious amounts of water.
7. The work surface should be covered with disposable plastic-backed absorbent paper.
8. Use Luer-Lock fittings on all syringes and sets. Large bore needles are recommended to minimise pressure and the possible formation of aerosols. The latter may also be reduced by the use of a venting needle.

Legal category POM.

Package quantities Vepesid injection is packed in cartons of 10 vials, each vial containing 100 mg etoposide in 5 ml of solution.

Vepesid 50 mg capsules are packed in blister packs of 20 capsules, each capsule containing 50 mg etoposide.

Further information Etoposide is a semisynthetic derivative of podophyllotoxin.

Experimental data indicate that etoposide arrests the cell cycle in the G_2 phase. Etoposide differs from the vinca alkaloids in that it does not cause an accumulation of cells in metaphase, but prevents cells from entering mitosis or destroys cells in the G_2 phase. The incorporation of thymidine into DNA is inhibited in-vitro by etoposide. Etoposide does not interfere with microtubule assembly. Etoposide is approximately 94% protein-bound in human serum. Plasma decay kinetics follow a bi-exponential curve and correspond to a two compartmental model. The mean volume of distribution is approximately 32% of body weight. Etoposide demonstrates relatively poor penetration into the cerebrospinal fluid. Urinary excretion is approximately 45% of an administered dose, 29% being excreted unchanged in 72 hours.

An information sheet on the storage, preparation and handling of the product is available

Product licence numbers

Vepesid 50 mg Capsules	0125/0153
Vepesid Injection	0125/0184

**Trade Mark*

Bristol-Myers Squibb Pharmaceuticals Ltd

Bristol-Myers Squibb House
Staines Road
Hounslow TW3 3JA

☎ 0181 572 7422 🗋 0181 754 3789

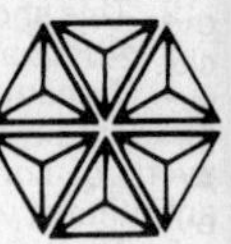

APROVEL* ▼

Qualitative and quantitative composition Each tablet contains 75 mg, 150 mg or 300 mg irbesartan.

Pharmaceutical form Tablet.

White to off-white, biconvex, and oval-shaped with a heart debossed on one side and the number 2771 (75 mg), 2772 (150 mg) or 2773 (300 mg) engraved on the other side.

Clinical particulars

Therapeutic indication: Treatment of essential hypertension.

Posology and method of administration: The usual recommended initial and maintenance dose is 150 mg once daily, with or without food. Aprovel at a dose of 150 mg once daily generally provides a better 24 hour blood pressure control than 75 mg. However, initiation of therapy with 75 mg could be considered, particularly in haemodialysed patients and in the elderly over 75 years.

In patients insufficiently controlled with 150 mg once daily, the dose of Aprovel can be increased to 300 mg, or other anti-hypertensive agents can be added. In particular, the addition of a diuretic such as hydrochlorothiazide has been shown to have an additive effect with Aprovel. (See *Interactions with other medicinal products and other forms of interaction*)

Renal impairment: No dosage adjustment is necessary in patients with impaired renal function. A lower starting dose (75 mg) should be considered for patients undergoing haemodialysis.

Intravascular volume depletion: Volume and/or sodium depletion should be corrected prior to administration of Aprovel.

Hepatic impairment: No dosage adjustment is necessary in patients with mild to moderate hepatic impairment. There is no clinical experience in patients with severe hepatic impairment.

Elderly patients: Although consideration should be given to initiating therapy with 75 mg in patients over 75 years of age, dosage adjustment is not usually necessary for the elderly.

Children: Safety and efficacy of Aprovel have not been established in children.

Contra-indications: Hypersensitivity to any component of the product (see *List of excipients*)

Pregnancy and lactation: (see *Use during pregnancy and lactation*).

Special warnings and special precautions for use:

Intravascular volume depletion: Symptomatic hypotension, especially after the first dose, may occur in patients who are volume and/or sodium depleted by vigorous diuretic therapy, dietary salt restriction, diarrhoea or vomiting. Such conditions should be corrected before the administration of Aprovel.

Renovascular hypertension: There is an increased risk of severe hypotension and renal insufficiency when patients with bilateral renal artery stenosis or stenosis of the artery to a single functioning kidney are treated with drugs that affect the renin-angiotensin-aldosterone system. While this is not documented with Aprovel, a similar effect should be anticipated with angiotensin II receptor antagonists.

Renal impairment and kidney transplantation: When Aprovel is used in patients with impaired renal function, a periodic monitoring of potassium and creatinine serum levels is recommended. There is no experience regarding the administration of Aprovel in patients with a recent kidney transplantation.

Hyperkalemia: During treatment with other drugs that affect the renin-angiotensin-aldosterone system hyperkalemia may occur, especially in the presence of renal impairment and/or heart failure. While this is not documented with Aprovel, adequate monitoring of serum potassium in patients at risk is recommended (see *Interactions with other medicinal products and other forms of interaction*).

Aortic and mitral valve stenosis, obstructive hypertrophic cardiomyopathy: As with other vasodilators, special caution is indicated in patients suffering from aortic or mitral stenosis, or obstructive hypertrophic cardiomyopathy.

Primary aldosteronism: Patients with primary aldosteronism generally will not respond to anti-hypertensive drugs acting through inhibition of the renin-angiotensin system. Therefore, the use of Aprovel is not recommended.

General: In patients whose vascular tone and renal function depend predominantly on the activity of the renin-angiotensin-aldosterone system (e.g. patients with severe congestive heart failure or underlying renal disease, including renal artery stenosis), treatment with other drugs that affect this system has been associated with acute hypotension, azotaemia, oliguria, or rarely acute renal failure. Although the possibility of similar effects cannot be excluded with angiotensin II receptor antagonists, these effects are not documented with Aprovel. As with any antihypertensive agent, excessive blood pressure decrease in patients with ischemic cardiopathy or ischemic cardiovascular disease could result in a myocardial infarction or stroke.

Interactions with other medicinal products and other forms of interaction:

Diuretics and other antihypertensive agents: Other antihypertensive agents may increase the hypotensive effects of irbesartan; however Aprovel has been safely administered with other antihypertensive agents, such as beta-blockers, long-acting calcium channel blockers, and thiazide diuretics. Prior treatment with high dose diuretics may result in volume depletion and a risk of hypotension when initiating therapy with Aprovel (see *Special warnings and special precautions for use*).

Potassium supplements and potassium-sparing diuretics: Based on experience with the use of other drugs that affect the renin-angiotensin system, concomitant use of potassium-sparing diruetics, potassium supplements, salt substitutes containing potassium or other drugs that may increase serum potassium levels (e.g. heparin) may lead to increases in serum potassium (see *Special warnings and special precautions for use*)

Lithium: Reversible increases in serum lithium concentrations and toxicity have been reported during concomitant administration of lithium with angiotensin converting enzyme inhibitors. While this is not documented with Aprovel, the possibility of a similar effect can not be excluded and careful monitoring of serum lithium levels is recommended during concomitant use.

Additional information on drug interactions: The pharmacokinetics of digoxin were not altered by co-administration of a 150 mg dose of irbesartan in healthy male volunteers. The pharmacokinetics of irbesartan are not affected by co-administration of hydrochlorothiazide. Irbesartan is mainly metabolised by CYP2C9 and to a lesser extent by glucuronidation. Inhibition of the glucuronyl transferase pathway is unlikely to result in clinically significant interactions. In-vitro interactions were observed between irbesartan and warfarin, tolbutamide (CYP2C9 substrates) and nifedipine (CYP2C9 inhibitor). However, no significant pharmacokinetic or pharmacodynamic interactions were observed when irbesartan was co-administered with warfarin in healthy male volunteers. The pharmacokinetics of irbesartan are not affected by co-administration of nifedipine. The effects of CYP2C9 inducers such as rifampicin on the pharmacokinetics of irbesartan were not evaluated. Based on *in-vitro* data, no interaction would be expected to occur with drugs whose metabolism is dependent upon cytochrome P450 isoenzymes CYP1A1, CYP1A2, CYP2A6, CYP2B6, CYP2D6, CYP2E1 or CYP3A4.

Use during pregnancy and lactation:

Pregnancy: Aprovel is contraindicated during pregnancy. Although there is no experience with Aprovel in pregnant women, *in utero* exposure to ACE inhibitors given to pregnant women during the second and third trimesters has been reported to cause injury and death to the developing foetus.

As for any drug that also acts directly on the renin-angiotensin-aldosterone system, Aprovel, should not be used during pregnancy. If pregnancy is detected during therapy, Aprovel should be discontinued as soon as possible (see *Contra-indications*).

Lactation: Aprovel is contraindicated during lactation. It is not known whether irbesartan is excreted in human milk. Irbesartan is excreted in the milk of lactating rats (see *Contra-indications*).

Effects on ability to drive and use machines: The effect of irbesartan on ability to drive and use machines has not been studied, but based on its pharmacodynamic properties, irbesartan is unlikely to affect this ability. When driving vehicles or operating machines, it should be taken into account that occasionally dizziness or weariness may occur during treatment of hypertension.

Undesirable effects: Undesirable effects in patients receiving Aprovel are generally mild and transient. In placebo-controlled trials in patients with hypertension, the overall incidence of adverse events did not differ between the irbesartan and the placebo groups. Discontinuation due to any clinical or laboratory adverse event was less frequent for irbesartan-treated patients than for placebo-treated patients. The incidence of adverse events was not related to dose (in the recommended dose range), gender, age, race, or duration of treatment.

Clinical adverse events, regardless of whether attributed to therapy, occurring in 1% or more of hypertensive patients with Aprovel in placebo-controlled trials are presented in the following table:

	% of Patients	
Adverse Event	*Irbesartan Monotherapy N=1965*	*Placebo N=641*
respiratory infection[a]	18.4	18.6
headache	12.3	16.7*
musculoskeletal pain[b]	7.3	8.4
dizziness	4.9	5.0
fatigue	4.3	3.7
diarrhoea	3.1	2.2
cough	2.8	2.7
nausea/vomiting	2.1	2.8
musculoskeletal trauma	1.9*	0.5
chest pain	1.8	1.7
dyspepsia/heartburn	1.7	1.1
oedema	1.5	2.3
abdominal pain	1.4	2.0
rash	1.3	2.0
tachycardia	1.2	0.9
anxiety/nervousness	1.1	0.9
UTI	1.1	1.4

[a] Includes upper respiratory infection, sinus abnormality, influenza, pharyngitis, and rhinitis.

[b] Includes musculoskeletal pain, musculoskeletal ache, and myalgia.

* Indicates a statistically significant difference between groups ($p < 0.05$).

Adverse events occurred with similar frequency in placebo and irbesartan-treated patients, with the exception of headache, musculoskeletal trauma, and flushing. Headache occurred significantly more often in the placebo group. Musculoskeletal trauma of differing types and causes occurred with a significantly higher incidence in the irbesartan group; all reports of musculoskeletal trauma were considered unrelated to irbesartan by the investigators. Flushing occurred in 0.6% of irbesartan patients and in no placebo patients. The occurrence of flushing was not related to dose, was not accompanied by other clinical events, and the relationship with irbesartan therapy is unknown. In over 5500 subjects exposed to irbesartan in clinical trials, there has been no report of angioedema.

No clinically significant changes in laboratory test parameters occurred in controlled clinical trials. Although significant increases in plasma creatine kinase occurred more frequently in irbesartan-treated subjects (1.7% vs 0.7% in placebo-treated subjects), none of these increases were classified as serious, resulted in drug discontinuation, or were associated with identifiable clinical musculoskeletal events. No special monitoring of laboratory parameters is necessary for patients with essential hypertension receiving therapy with Aprovel, when the renal function is normal (see *Special warnings and special precautions for use*).

Overdose: Experience in adults exposed to doses of up to 900 mg/day for 8 weeks revealed no toxicity. The most likely manifestations of overdosage are expected to be hypotension and tachycardia; bradycardia might also occur from overdose. No specific information is available on the treatment of overdosage with Aprovel. The patient should be closely monitored, and the treatment should be symptomatic and supportive. Suggested measures include induction of emesis and/or gastric lavage. Activated charcoal may be useful in the treatment of overdosage. Irbesartan is not removed by haemodialysis.

Pharmacological properties

Pharmacodynamic properties:

Pharmaco-therapeutic group: Angiotensin II antagonists, ATC code C09C A: Irbesartan is a potent, orally active, selective angiotensin II receptor (type AT_1) antagonist. It is expected to block all actions of angiotensin II mediated by the AT_1 receptor, regardless of the source or route of synthesis of angiotensin II. The selective antagonism of the angiotensin II (AT_1) receptors results in increases in plasma renin levels and angiotensin II levels, and a decrease in plasma aldosterone concentration. Serum potassium levels are not significantly affected by irbesartan alone at the recommended doses. Irbesartan does not inhibit ACE (kininase II), an enzyme which generates angiotensin II and also degrades bradykinin into inactive metabolites. Irbesartan does not require metabolic activation for its activity.

Irbesartan lowers blood pressure with minimal change in heart rate. The decrease in blood pressure is dose-related for once a day doses with a tendency towards plateau at doses above 300 mg. Doses of 150-300 mg once daily lower supine or seated blood pressures at trough (i.e., 24 hours after dosing) by an average of 8-13/5-8 mm Hg (systolic/diastolic) greater than those associated with placebo.

Peak reduction of blood pressure is achieved within 3-6 hours after administration and the blood pressure lowering effect is maintained for at least 24 hours. At 24 hours the reduction of blood pressure was 60-70% of the corresponding peak diastolic and systolic responses at the recommended doses. Once daily dosing with 150 mg produced trough and mean 24 hour responses similar to twice daily dosing on the same total dose.

The blood pressure lowering effect of Aprovel is evident within 1-2 weeks, with the maximal effect occurring by 4-6 weeks after start of therapy. The antihypertensive effects are maintained during long term therapy. After withdrawal of therapy, blood pressure gradually returns toward baseline. Rebound hypertension has not been observed.

The blood pressure lowering effects of irbesartan and thiazide-type diuretics are additive. In patients not adequately controlled by irbesartan alone, the addition of a low dose of hydrochlorothiazide (12.5 mg) to irbesartan once daily results in a further placebo-adjusted blood pressure reduction at trough of 7-10/3-6 mm Hg (systolic/diastolic).

The efficacy of Aprovel is not influenced by age or gender. As is the case with other drugs that affect the renin-angiotensin system, black hypertensive patients have notably less response to irbesartan monotherapy. When irbesartan is administered concomitantly with a low dose of hydrochlorothiazide (e.g., 12.5 mg daily), the antihypertensive response in black patients approaches that of white patients.

There is no clinically important effect on serum uric acid or urinary uric acid secretion.

Pharmacokinetic properties: After oral administration, irbesartan is well absorbed: studies of absolute bioavailability gave values of approximately 60-80%. Concomitant food intake does not significantly influence the bioavailability of irbesartan.

Plasma protein binding is approximately 90%, with negligible binding to cellular blood components. The volume of distribution is 53-93 litres.

Following oral or intravenous administration of ^{14}C irbesartan, 80-85% of the circulating plasma radioactivity is attributable to unchanged irbesartan. Irbesartan is metabolised by the liver via glucuronide conjugation and oxidation. The major circulating metabolite is irbesartan glucuronide (approximately 6%). *In vitro* studies indicate that irbesartan is primarily oxidised by the cytochrome P450 enzyme CYP2C9; isoenzyme CYP3A4 has negligible effect.

Irbesartan exhibits linear and dose proportional pharmacokinetics over the dose range of 10 to 600 mg. A less than proportional increase in oral absorption at doses beyond 600 mg (twice the maximal recommended dose) was observed; the mechanism for this is unknown. Peak plasma concentrations are attained at 1.5-2 hours after oral administration. The total body and renal clearance are 157-176 and 3-3.5 ml/min, respectively. The terminal elimination half-life of irbesartan is 11-15 hours. Steady-state plasma concentrations are attained within 3 days after initiation of a once-daily dosing regimen. Limited accumulation of irbesartan (<20%) is observed in plasma upon repeated once-daily dosing. In a study, somewhat higher plasma concentrations of irbesartan were observed in female hypertensive patients. However, there was no difference in the half-life and accumulation of irbesartan. No dosage adjustment is necessary in female patients. Irbesartan AUC and C_{max} values were also somewhat greater in elderly subjects (≥65 years) than those of young subjects (18-40 years). However the terminal half-life was not significantly altered. No dosage adjustment is necessary in elderly patients.

Irbesartan and its metabolites are eliminated by both biliary and renal pathways. After either oral or IV administration of ^{14}C irbesartan, about 20% of the radioactivity is recovered in the urine, and the remainder in the faeces. Less than 2% of the dose is excreted in the urine as unchanged irbesartan.

Renal impairment: In patients with renal impairment or those undergoing haemodialysis, the pharmacokinetic parameters of irbesartan are not significantly altered. Irbesartan is not removed by haemodialysis.

Hepatic impairment: In patients with mild to moderate cirrhosis, the pharmacokinetic parameters of irbesartan are not significantly altered. Studies have not been performed in patients with severe hepatic impairment.

Preclinical safety data: There was no evidence of abnormal systemic or target organ toxicity at clinically relevant doses. In preclinical safety studies, high doses of irbesartan (≥250 mg/kg/day in rats and ≥100 mg/kg/day in macaques) caused a reduction of red blood cell parameters (erythrocytes, haemoglobin, haematocrit). At very high doses (≥500 mg/kg/day), degenerative changes in the kidney (such as interstitial nephritis, tubular distension, basophilic tubules, increased plasma concentrations of urea and creatinine) were induced by irbesartan in the rat and the macaque and are considered secondary to the hypotensive effects of the drug which led to decreased renal perfusion. Furthermore, irbesartan induced hyperplasia/hypertrophy of the juxtaglomerular cells (in rats at ≥250 mg/kg/day, in macaques at ≥10 mg/kg/day). All of these changes were considered to be caused by the pharmacological action of irbesartan. For therapeutic doses of irbesartan in humans, the hyperplasia/hypertrophy of the renal juxtaglomerular cells does not appear to have any relevance.

There was no evidence of mutagenicity, clastogenicity or carcinogenicity.

Animal studies with irbesartan showed transient toxic effects (increased renal pelvic cavitation, hydroureter or subcutaneous oedema) in rat foetuses, which were resolved after birth. In rabbits, abortion or early resorption were noted at doses causing significant maternal toxicity, including mortality. No teratogenic effects were observed in the rat or rabbit.

Pharmaceutical particulars

List of excipients: Microcrystalline cellulose, croscarmellose sodium, lactose monohydrate, magnesium stearate, colloidal hydrated silica, pregelatinised maize starch, and poloxamer 188.

Incompatibilities: None

Shelf-life: 24 months

Special precautions for storage: Store in a dry place below 30°C.

Nature and content of container: Aprovel tablets are packaged in blister packs containing 28 tablets in PVC/PVDC/Aluminium strips.

Instructions for use, handling and disposal (if appropriate): None.

Marketing authorisation holder: Sanofi Pharma Bristol-Myers Squibb SNC, 174 Avenue de France, F-75013, Paris, France.

Numbers in the community register of medicinal products

Aprovel 75 mg	EU/1/97/046/001
Aprovel 150 mg	EU/1/97/046/004
Aprovel 300 mg	EU/1/97/046/007

Date of first authorisation/renewal of the authorisation 27 August 1997

Date of revision of the text Not applicable

Legal category: POM

DUTONIN*

Qualitative and quantitative composition Nefazodone is a phenylpiperazine antidepressant, available as tablets containing 50, 100 and 200 mg of nefazodone HCl.

Nefazodone tablets contain the following inactive ingredients: microcrystalline cellulose, povidone, sodium starch glycollate, colloidal silicon dioxide, magnesium stearate and iron oxides.

Pharmaceutical form Nefazodone is supplied as flat faced, bevelled edged, hexagonal shaped tablets containing 50 mg, 100 mg or 200 mg of nefazodone HCl. Tablets are imprinted with the product strength on one side. The 100 and 200 mg tablets are bisect scored. Tablet colours are pink (50 mg), white (100 mg) and light yellow (200 mg).

Clinical particulars

Therapeutic indications: Nefazodone is indicated for the symptomatic treatment of all types of depressive illness, including depressive syndromes accompanied by anxiety or sleep disturbances.

Posology and method of administration:

Adults: The usual therapeutic dose is 200 mg twice daily. The recommended starting dose is 50-100 mg twice daily which should be increased to 200 mg twice daily after 5-7 days. Depending on the clinical response, the daily dose can be increased gradually to a maximum of 300 mg twice daily.

In patients being transferred from another CNS medication, treatment should be initiated at a dose of 50 mg twice daily before being titrated at weekly intervals to the usual therapeutic dose.

While benefit is seen during the first week of treatment, as with all antidepressants, up to 4 weeks' treatment may be required to obtain the full antidepressant effect in some patients. It is recommended that treatment should continue for a sufficient period which may be several months. Patients treated with nefazodone for up to one year have shown continued beneficial response.

Elderly: The effects of the starting dose (50 mg twice daily) and the rate of subsequent dose titration should be carefully assessed, since increased plasma concentrations have been seen to occur in the elderly, especially females. Maximum therapeutic benefit is usually achieved at doses of 100-200 mg twice daily.

Renal impairment: No significant relationship between pharmacokinetic parameters and degree of renal impairment has been observed. However, with chronic administration, accumulation of nefazodone or its metabolites may occur in patients with severely impaired renal function, and use of the lower end of the dose range is advised.

Hepatic impairment: The elimination half-life of nefazodone in patients with cirrhosis was significantly prolonged. This suggests that if nefazodone is administered to patients with liver disease, dosage should be restricted to the lower end of the dose range.

Children: The use of nefazodone in children is not recommended, as safety and effectiveness in children below the age of 18 years have not yet been established.

Contra-indications: Nefazodone is contra-indicated in patients with known hypersensitivity to nefazodone hydrochloride, any of the inactive ingredients, or other phenylpiperazine antidepressants.

Special warnings and special precautions for use:

Hepatic or renal impairment: see section *Posology and Method of administration.*

Electro-convulsive therapy: There are no clinical studies involving the combined use of ECT and nefazodone.

Epilepsy: As with other antidepressants, nefazodone should be used with caution in patients with epilepsy.

History of mania/hypomania: Nefazodone should be used with caution in these patients as rare occurrences of activation of mania / hypomania have been reported.

Cardiovascular: Patients with a recent history of myocardial infarction or unstable heart disease should be treated with caution.

Sexual function: Unlike other antidepressants, nefazodone has not been associated with impotence and abnormal ejaculation in men or inability to achieve orgasm in women. Priapism has been reported with another phenylpiperazine compound and, should this occur during nefazodone treatment, the patient should be advised to discontinue therapy immediately and seek medical attention.

Suicide: The possibility of suicide attempt in seriously depressed patients is inherent to the illness and may persist even during apparent improvement of symptoms. Close supervision of high risk patients is advised.

Interactions with other medicinal products and other forms of interaction:

Centrally active medication: As with all centrally acting drugs, caution is advised when drugs are used in combination. Concurrent or immediate pretreatment with fluoxetine increases the AUC of the nefazodone metabolite m-chlorophenylpiperazine (mCPP). Such patients may experience transient increased side effects which can be minimised by reducing the dose of nefazodone or allowing an adequate washout period.

Benzodiazepines: In healthy volunteers, the half-life of triazolam, a short-acting sedative hypnotic, was significantly increased (from 2.3 to 7 h) when co-administered with nefazodone. The pharmacokinetics of nefazodone were not altered. When alprazolam and nefazodone were co-administered the half life of alprazolam was doubled and, although the nefazodone concentration was unaffected, the concentration of its metabolite, mCPP, was increased. A reduction in the alprazolam dosage is recommended. The co-administration of lorazepam and nefazodone resulted in minimal changes in the pharmacokinetic parameters of either drug. No dosage adjustment is required. Caution should be exercised when using nefazodone and other benzodiazepines concomitantly.

Protein binding: Nefazodone is extensively (>99%) bound to plasma proteins in man. The effect of nefazodone on the plasma protein binding of co-administered drugs should be considered. The protein binding of chlorpromazine, desipramine, diazepam, phenytoin, lidocaine, prazosin, propranolol, verapamil or warfarin was not affected by nefazodone *in vitro*.

Warfarin: No significant clinical or pharmacokinetic interactions between nefazodone and warfarin were observed in a multidose study using healthy male subjects.

Terfenadine/astemizole/cisapride: Nefazodone has been shown *in vitro* to be an inhibitor of cytochrome P_{450} III A4. Therefore, the concomitant use of nefazodone with terfenadine, astemizole or cisapride, which are all metabolised by this isoenzyme, is not recommended.

Other drugs metabolised by cytochrome $P_{450}III_{A4}$: As their clearance may be affected, caution is indicated in the combined use of nefazodone with other drugs metabolised by this isoenzyme.

Lithium: Co-administration of nefazodone with lithium did not cause any untoward effects (e.g. tremor, hyperthermia) associated with serotonin syndrome. However, caution should be exercised when using nefazodone and lithium concomitantly.

Carbamazepine: Monitoring of carbamazepine plasma concentrations is recommended when co-administered with nefazodone as a 23% increase of both C_{max} and AUC for carbamazepine was observed in a multidose volunteer study. No adjustment in the initial dose of nefazodone is necessary when administered with carbamazepine but, based on clinical effect, subsequent dose adjustments may be required due to marked decreases in nefazodone plasma concentrations.

Haloperidol: In a multi-dose study involving healthy volunteers, the AUC of haloperidol was increased by 35% with no significant increase in the C_{max} or T_{max} when co-administered with nefazodone. Slight protein binding displacement of haloperidol was also noted. Caution should be exercised when using nefazodone and haloperidol concomitantly.

Monoamine oxidase inhibitors: As with other antidepressants, nefazodone should not be used in combination with an MAOI or within two weeks of discontinuing treatment with an MAOI. Conversely, at least one week should be allowed after stopping nefazodone before starting an MAOI.

Cimetidine: No significant clinical or pharmacokinetic interactions between nefazodone and cimetidine were observed in a multiple dose clinical trial involving healthy volunteers.

Cardiovascular: Although nefazodone is not a potent alpha-adrenergic blocking agent, there have been reports of orthostatic hypotension and syncope occurring in nefazodone-treated patients. Concomitant administration of antihypertensive therapy, e.g. propranolol, and nefazodone may require an adjustment in the dose of the antihypertensive drug. Caution is advised with co-administration of nefazodone and digoxin as serum concentrations of digoxin have been shown to increase by as much as 30%. Other cardiovascular agents have not been formally studied but the potential for interaction exists.

Theophylline: There was no effect on FEV_1 values, nor any change in the pharmacokinetics of either nefazodone or theophylline when co-administered to patients with chronic obstructive pulmonary disease.

General anaesthetics: Concomitant use of nefazodone with general anaesthetics has not been formally evaluated but the potential for interaction exists; therefore, prior to elective surgery, nefazodone should be discontinued for as long as clinically feasible.

Alcohol: Whilst in a controlled trial with young normal volunteers, nefazodone did not alter the psychomotor or cognitive impairment caused by alcohol, it is prudent to avoid concomitant use of alcohol and nefazodone.

Pregnancy and lactation: The safety of nefazodone for use in human pregnancy has not been established. An evaluation of experimental animal studies does not indicate direct or indirect harmful effects with respect to development of the embryo: however, both maternal and foetal / neonatal toxicities occurred. Findings consisted of non-specific delay in foetal development and increased mortality and decreased body weight in the neonates. Because animal reproductive studies are not always predictive of human response, this drug should be used during pregnancy only if clearly needed.

It is not known whether nefazodone or its metabolites are excreted in human milk. Hence use in nursing mothers is not recommended.

Effects on ability to drive and use machines: In healthy volunteers nefazodone caused a modest decrease in some psychomotor function tests but no impairment of cognitive function. However, any psychoactive drug may impair judgement, cognitive or motor skills, and patients should be cautioned about operating hazardous machinery, including automobiles.

Undesirable effects: Nefazodone is generally well tolerated. If side effects occur, they are normally observed at the beginning of treatment and usually subside with decreased dosage. In controlled clinical trials, certain side effects occurred with significantly greater frequency than placebo: the most frequent were asthenia, dry mouth, nausea, constipation, somnolence, dizziness and lightheadedness; side effects which sometimes occurred were chills, fever, postural hypotension, vasodilation, abnormal dreams, paraesthesia, arthralgia, memory impairment, confusion, ataxia, amblyopia and other minor visual disturbances; a side effect which rarely occurred was syncope.

Over a six week trial period, there was evidence of progressive adaptation with continued therapy to the following adverse experiences: asthenia, visual disturbances, constipation, dizziness, dry mouth, lightheadedness, nausea and somnolence.

Overdose: There have been rare reported cases of overdose with nefazodone (up to 11.2 g). No death has occurred. The reactions most frequently reported from overdose have been drowsiness and vomiting. Overdosage may cause an increase in incidence or severity of any of the reported adverse reactions (see *Undesirable effects*).

Any patient suspected of having taken an overdose should have the stomach emptied by gastric lavage. Treatment should be symptomatic and supportive in the case of hypotension or excessive sedation. There is no specific antidote for nefazodone.

Pharmacological properties

Pharmacodynamic properties: Nefazodone blocks serotonin type 2 ($5HT_2$) receptors and inhibits serotonin uptake. It lacks anticholinergic and antihistamine effects, has little $alpha_1$-adrenergic blocking activity and does not potentiate the sedative effects of alcohol in man or pentobarbital in animal studies.

In elderly volunteers, nefazodone caused a small fall in mean supine blood pressure and pulse rate; however, no significant orthostatic blood pressure or ECG changes were observed.

Nefazodone has positive effects on sleep architecture. It slightly decreased (20%) the time between sleep initiation and the first REM episode, increased total REM sleep time, and did not affect the number or timing of REM episodes through the night. There were no changes in detumescence time for nocturnal erections associated with REM episodes. Additionally, Dutonin decreased the number of arousals and wakefulness during sleep in patients with major depression.

Pharmacokinetic properties: Nefazodone is rapidly and completely absorbed with peak plasma concentrations 1-3 hours after oral administration. It undergoes extensive presystemic metabolism and is highly protein bound (>99%). The estimated systemic bioavailability of nefazodone is 15-23%. The plasma elimination half-life is 2-4 hours for nefazodone, with elimination primarily by liver metabolism. Steady state is reached within 3-4 days after initiating treatment or making a dose adjustment. Pharmacokinetic parameters are non-linear with relatively higher peak serum levels and greater AUCs occurring as doses are increased through the recommended dosage range. Nefazodone is eliminated within 24 hours of discontinuing treatment.

Effect of age, gender and phenotype: In repeat dose studies, plasma levels of nefazodone and its major metabolite were higher in elderly than in young females. In male subjects, no significant effect of age was observed. The pharmacokinetics of nefazodone and its metabolites were unchanged in slow metabolisers of dextromethorphan, except that the clearance of the metabolite, m-chlorophenylpiperazine (mCPP), is reduced in this phenotype.

Effect of food: Food delays the absorption of nefazodone and decreases the systemic exposure to nefazodone (AUC) on average by approximately 20%. These effects are not considered to be clinically significant.

Preclinical safety data: There is no evidence of carcinogenic, mutagenic or genotoxic effects with nefazodone. There were no specific organ toxicities noted in animal studies.

Pharmaceutical particulars

List of excipients: Microcrystalline Cellulose; Povidone; Sodium Starch Glycollate; Colloidal Silicon Dioxide; Magnesium Stearate; Red Ferric Oxide; Yellow Ferric Oxide.

Incompatibilities: Not applicable.

Shelf life: PVC, PVDC blisters on foil flexible packaging: 24 months

Special precautions for storage: Storage should be below 30°C, in a dry place.

Nature and contents of container: Polyvinyl chloride (PVC) or polyvinylidene chloride (PVDC) blister packs on foil flexible packaging, containing 14 or 56 tablets per carton. Treatment initiation pack containing blisters of 14 pink 50 mg, 14 white 100 mg and 28 light yellow 200 mg tablets.

Instructions for use/handling: No special handling instructions.

Marketing authorisation numbers

Dutonin Tablets 50 mg	11184/0027
Dutonin Tablets 100 mg	11184/0028
Dutonin Tablets 200 mg	11184/0029

Date of approval/revision of SPC January 1997

Legal category POM

ETOPOPHOS* INJECTION (ETOPOSIDE PHOSPHATE)

Qualitative and quantitative composition Each vial contains 113.6 mg etoposide phosphate (equivalent to 100 mg etoposide).

Pharmaceutical form Lyophilised powder for injection.

Clincial particulars

Therapeutic indications: Etopophos is an anti-neoplastic drug for intravenous use, which can be used alone or in combination with other cytotoxic drugs.

Present data indicate that Etopophos is applicable in the therapy of: small cell lung cancer, resistant non-seminomatous testicular carcinoma.

Posology and method of administration: Etopophos should be administered by individuals experienced in the use of anti-neoplastic therapy.

The recommended course of Etopophos Injection is 60-120 mg/m², (etoposide equivalent) i.v daily for five consecutive days. As Etopophos produces myelosuppression, courses should not be repeated more frequently than at 21 day intervals. In any case, repeat courses of Etopophos should not be given until the blood picture has been checked for evidence of myelosuppression and found to be satisfactory.

When used as part of combination therapy, the dosage should be reduced toward the lower end of the dosage range to take into account the myelosuppressive effects of radiation therapy or chemotherapy which may have compromised bone marrow reserve.

Immediately prior to administration, the content of each vial must be reconstituted with either 5 ml or 10 ml Water for Injections B.P., 5% Glucose Intravenous Infusion B.P. or 0.9% Sodium Chloride Intravenous Infusion B.P. to a concentration equivalent to 20 mg/ml or 10 mg/ml etoposide (22.7 mg/ml or 11.4 mg/ml etoposide phosphate) respectively. Following reconstitution the solution may be administered without further dilution or it can be further diluted to concentrations as low as 0.1 mg/ml etoposide (0.14 mg/ml etoposide phosphate) with either 5% Glucose Intravenous Infusion B.P. or 0.9% Sodium Chloride Intravenous Infusion B.P.

Etopophos solutions may be infused over 5 minutes to 3.5 hours.

Care should be taken to avoid extravasation. Occasionally following extravasation of etoposide, soft tissue irritation and inflammation has occurred, ulceration was generally not seen.

Elderly: No dosage adjustment is necessary.

Paediatric use: Safety and effectiveness in children have not been established. Until further data are available, Etopophos should not be given to children under 12 years of age.

Contra-indications: Etopophos is contra-indicated in patients with severe hepatic dysfunction or in those patients who have demonstrated hypersensitivity to etoposide, etoposide phosphate or any other component of the formulation.

Special warnings and special precautions for use: Since etoposide phosphate is rapidly and completely converted to etoposide, the WARNINGS and PRECAUTIONS that are considered when prescribing etoposide should be considered when prescribing Etopophos.

When Etopophos is administered intravenously care should be taken to avoid extravasation.

Etopophos should not be given by intracavitary injection.

If radiotherapy and/or chemotherapy has been given prior to starting Etopophos treatment, an adequate interval should be allowed to enable the bone marrow to recover. If the leucocyte count falls below 2,000/mm^3, treatment should be suspended until the circulating blood elements have returned to acceptable levels (platelets above 100,000/mm^3, leucocytes above 4,000/mm^3), this is usually within 10 days.

Peripheral blood counts and liver function should be monitored. (See *Adverse reactions.*)

Bacterial infections should be brought under control before treatment with Etopophos commences.

No data are available on the use of Etopophos in patients with renal and hepatic impairment.

The occurrence of acute leukaemia, which can occur with or without myelodysplasia has been reported rarely in patients treated with etoposide containing regimens.

Interactions with other medicinal products and other forms of interaction: There are no data on administering Etopophos with drugs that are known to inhibit phosphatase activities (e.g. levamisole hydrochloride). Increased frequency of monitoring of haematological indices will ensure adequate chemotherapeutic effect when Etopophos is used with such agents.

Pregnancy and lactation: Etoposide is teratogenic in rats and mice at dose levels equivalent to those employed clinically and it is therefore assumed that Etopophos is also teratogenic. There are no adequate and well-controlled studies in pregnant women.

Etopophos should not be administered to patients who are pregnant or to mothers who are breast feeding. It is not known whether Etopophos is excreted in human milk. Women of childbearing potential should be advised to avoid becoming pregnant.

The influence of etoposide on human reproduction has not been determined.

In-vitro tests indicate that etoposide is mutagenic and Etopophos is expected to have similar mutagenic effects.

Effects on ability to drive and use machines: None.

Undesirable effects: In clinical studies with Etopophos the most frequent clinically significant adverse experiences were leucopenia and neutropenia which occurred in almost all patients. The leucopenia was severe in approximately 20% of the patients, with neutropenia severe in about one third. Thrombocytopenia was reported in about a quarter of the patients and was severe in about 10% of the cases. Anaemia was observed in about three quarters of the patients and was severe in about 20%. Gastrointestinal adverse events were usually mild to moderate. Nausea and/or vomiting was seen in about a third of the patients. Anorexia and mucositis was reported by 10-20% of the patients and constipation, abdominal pain, diarrhoea and taste alteration was seen in between 5 to 10%. Asthenia or malaise affected about a third of the patients. Alopecia was also observed in a third of the patients. Chills and/or fever were reported in a quarter of the patients, dizziness and extravasation/ phlebitis in about 5% of the patients. No cardiovascular symptoms including hypotension, have been observed during administration of 5 minute infusions of Etopophos.

Since etoposide phosphate is converted to etoposide, the adverse experiences reported below that are associated with etoposide may occur with Etopophos.

The following data on adverse reactions are based on both oral and intravenous administration of etoposide.

Haematological: The dose limiting toxicity of etoposide is myelosuppression, predominantly leucopenia and thrombocytopenia. Anaemia occurs infrequently.

The leucocyte count nadir occurs approximately 21 days after treatment.

Alopecia: Alopecia occurs in approximately two-thirds of patients and is reversible on cessation of therapy.

Gastrointestinal: Nausea and vomiting are the major gastrointestinal toxicities and occur in over one-third of patients. Anti-emetics are useful in controlling these side effects. Abdominal pain, anorexia, diarrhoea, oesophagitis and stomatitis occur infrequently.

Other Toxicities: Hypotension may occur following an excessively rapid infusion of etoposide and may be reversed by slowing the infusion rate. Symptomatic hypotension has not been seen with Etopophos.

Anaphylactoid reactions have been reported following administration of etoposide. Higher rates of anaphylactoid reactions have been reported in children who received infusions at concentrations higher than those recommended. The role that concentration of infusion (or rate of infusion) plays in the development of anaphylactoid reactions is uncertain. These reactions have usually responded to cessation of therapy and administration of pressor agents, cortico-steroids, antihistamines or volume expanders as appropriate.

Apnoea with spontaneous resumption of breathing following discontinuation of etoposide injection has been reported. Sudden fatal reactions associated with bronchospasm have been reported. Hypertension and/or flushing have also been reported. Blood pressure usually returns to normal within a few hours after cessation of the infusion.

The use of etoposide has been reported infrequently to cause peripheral neuropathy.

Etoposide has been shown to reach high concentrations in the liver and kidney, thus presenting a potential for accumulation in cases of functional impairment.

Somnolence, fatigue, aftertaste, fever, rash, pigmentation, pruritus, urticaria, dysphagia, transient cortical blindness and a single case of radiation recall dermatitis have also been reported following the administration of etoposide.

Overdose: High doses of etoposide or etoposide phosphate may result in bone marrow suppression or mucositis. Total etoposide doses of 2.4 to 3.5 g/m^2 administered intravenously over three days have resulted in severe mucositis and myelotoxicity. Metabolic acidosis and cases of severe hepatic toxicity have been reported in patients receiving higher than recommended doses of etoposide.

No proven antidotes have been established for Etopophos overdosage. Treatment should therefore be symptomatic and supportive.

Pharmacological properties

Pharmacodynamic properties: Etoposide phosphate is converted *in vivo* to the active moiety, etoposide, by dephosphorylation. The mechanism of action of etoposide phosphate is believed to be the same as that of etoposide.

Etoposide is a semi-synthetic derivative of podophyllotoxin. Experimental data indicate that etoposide arrests the cell cycle in the G^2 phase. Etoposide differs from the vinca alkaloids in that it does not cause an accumulation of cells in metaphase, but prevents cells from entering mitosis or destroys cells in the G^2 phase. The incorporation of thymidine into DNA is inhibited in vitro by etoposide.

Pharmacokinetic properties: Following intravenous administration of Etopophos, etoposide phosphate is rapidly and completely converted to etoposide in plasma. A direct comparison of the pharmacokinetic parameters (AUC and CMAX) of etoposide following intravenous administration of molar equivalent doses of Etopophos and etoposide was made in two randomised cross-over studies in patients. Results from both studies demonstrated no statistically significant differences in the AUC and CMAX for etoposide when administered as Etopophos or etoposide. In addition, there were no statistically significant differences in the pharmacodynamic parameters (haematologic toxicity) after administration of Etopophos or etoposide. Because of the pharmacokinetic and pharmaco-dynamic bioequeivalence of Etopophos to etoposide, the following information on etoposide should be considered.

Etoposide is approximately 94% protein-bound in human serum. Plasma decay kinetics follow a bi-exponential curve and correspond to a two compartmental model. The mean volume of distribution is approximately 32% of body weight. Etoposide demonstrates relatively poor penetration into the cerebrospinal fluid. Urinary excretion is approximately 45% of an administered dose, 29% being excreted unchanged in 72 hours. There is a significant negative correlation between the plasma clearance of etoposide and serum creatinine. This finding is consistent with the significant role that renal clearance plays in the elimination of etoposide as 30-50% of an intravenous dose is excreted unchanged in the urine.

Preclinical safety data: The carcinogenic potential of Etopophos has not been studied. However, based upon its pharmacodynamic mechanism of action, Etopophos is a potential carcinogenic and genotoxic agent. Etoposide has been shown to be mutagenic in mammalian cells and Etopophos is expected to have similar mutagenic effects.

Pharmaceutical particulars

List of excipients: Dextran 40, sodium citrate dihydrate.

Incompatibilities: Etopophos should not be physically mixed with any other drug.

Shelf life: 18 months.

Special precautions for storage: Store between 2-8°C. Protect from light.

Nature and contents of container: 20 ml flint glass type I vial with a butyl rubber stopper and flip-off aluminium seal.

Instructions for use/handling: Immediately prior to administration, the content of each vial must be reconstituted with either 5 ml or 10 ml Water for Injection BP, 5% Glucose Intravenous Infusion BP or 0.9% Sodium Chloride Intravenous Infusion BP to a concentration equivalent to 20 mg/ml or 10 mg/ml etoposide (22.7 mg/ml or 11.4 mg/ml etoposide phosphate), respectively. Following reconstitution the solution may be administered without further dilution or it can be further diluted to concentrations as low as 0.1 mg/mL etoposide (0.14 mg/ml etoposide phosphate) with either 5% Glucose Intravenous Infusion BP or 0.9% Sodium Chloride Intravenous Infusion BP.

When reconstituted and/or diluted as directed Etopophos solutions are chemically and physically stable for 48 hours at 37°C, 96 hours at 25°C and 7 days under refrigeration (2-8°C) under normal room fluorescent light in both glass and plastic containers. For microbiological reasons, the product should be stored for not more than 8 hours at room temperature or 24 hours in a refrigerator. Solutions of Etopophos should be prepared in an aseptic manner.

Etopophos should not be physically mixed with any other drug.

Instructions for use/handling:

Guidelines for the safe handling of anti-neoplastic agents:

1. Trained personnel should reconstitute the drug.
2. This should be performed in a designated area.
3. Adequate protective gloves should be worn.
4. Precautions should be taken to avoid the drug accidentally coming into contact with the eyes. In the event of contact with the eyes, irrigate with large amounts of water and/or saline.
5. The cytotoxic preparation should not be handled by pregnant staff.
6. Adequate care and precautions should be taken in the disposal of items (syringes, needles etc) used to reconstitute cytotoxic drugs. Excess material and body waste may be disposed of by placing in double sealed polythene bags and incinerating at a temperature of 1,000°C. Liquid waste may be flushed with copious amounts of water.
7. The work surface should be covered with disposable plastic backed absorbent paper.
8. Use Luer-Lock fittings on all syringes and sets. Large bore needles are recommended to minimise pressure and the possible formation of aerosols. The latter may also be reduced by the use of a venting needle.

Instruction for disposal: As *Instructions for use/ handling* section.

Marketing authorisation number PL 11184/0052

Date of first authorisation/renewal of authorisation 23rd May 1996

Date of (partial) revision of the text May 1996.

LIPOSTAT* TABLETS

Qualitative and quantitative composition

Lipostat tablets 10 mg: Yellow capsule shaped biconvex tablet each containing pravastatin sodium 10 mg. Each tablet is engraved '10' on one side, with a breakline.

Lipostat tablets 20 mg: Yellow capsule shaped biconvex tablet each containing pravastatin sodium 20 mg. Each tablet is engraved '20' on one side, with a breakline.

Lipostat tablets 40 mg: Yellow capsule shaped biconvex tablet each containing pravastatin sodium 40 mg. Each tablet is engraved '40' on one side.

Pharmaceutical form Uncoated tablet

Clinical particulars

Therapeutic indications:

Post-myocardial infarction: Lipostat is indicated to reduce the risk of recurrent myocardial infarction, need for myocardial revascularisation procedure, and to reduce the risk of stroke in patients with previous myocardial infarction and a total serum cholesterol level in excess of 4.8 mmol/L or a LDL-cholesterol in excess of 3.2 mmol/L.

Coronary heart disease: As an adjunct to diet to slow the progressive course of coronary atherosclerosis and reduce the incidence of clinical cardiac events in patients with hypercholesterolaemia and documented atherosclerotic coronary artery disease.

Prevention of coronary heart disease: As an adjunct to diet in hypercholesterolaemic patients without clinically evident coronary heart disease to:

- reduce the risk of fatal and non-fatal myocardial infarction;
- reduce the need to undergo myocardial revascularisation procedures;
- improve survival by reducing cardiovascular deaths.

Hypercholesterolaemia: The reduction of elevated total and LDL cholesterol levels in patients with primary hypercholesterolaemia who have not responded adequately to dietary measures.

Posology and method of administration: Prior to initiating Lipostat, secondary causes of hypercholesterolaemia should be excluded and patients should be placed on a standard cholesterol-lowering diet which should be continued during treatment. In addition, physicians are recommended to consult guidelines issued by consensus groups such as the European Atherosclerosis Society.

Adults: The usual dosage range is 10-40 mg administered once a day at bedtime.

The maximal effect of a given dose occurs within four weeks, therefore periodic lipid determinations should be performed and the dosage adjusted accordingly.

Elderly patients and patients with hepatic or renal impairment: There is no clinical evidence to suggest the dose range needs to be different in these patients. In common with other treatments, treatment should be initiated at the lower end of the dosage range.

Children: There are insufficient clinical data to recommend use in individuals less than 18 years old.

Concomitant therapy: The effects of Lipostat on lowering total and LDL cholesterol are enhanced when combined with a bile acid-binding resin. When administering a bile acid-binding resin (e.g. cholestyramine, colestipol) Lipostat should be given either one hour or more before or at least four hours after the resin. The bioavailability of pravastatin is not altered by concurrent administration with nicotinic acid, probucol and gemfibrozil (see *Precautions, Skeletal Muscle*).

Patients taking immunosuppressive drugs such as cyclosporin (see *Precautions, Skeletal Muscle*) concomitantly with pravastatin, should begin treatment with 10 mg of pravastatin once daily and be titrated to higher doses with caution.

Contra-indications: Hypersensitivity to any component of this medication.

Active liver disease or unexplained persistent elevations in liver function tests.

Pregnancy and lactation: (see *Pregnancy and lactation* section).

Special warnings and special precautions for use: Lipostat should not be used when hypercholesterolaemia is due to elevated HDL-C or in patients with homozygotic familial hypercholesterolaemia.

Liver function: As with other lipid-lowering agents, liver function tests should be performed periodically. Special attention should be given to patients who develop increased transaminase levels and therapy should be discontinued if increases in alanine aminotransferase (ALT) and aspartate aminotransferase (AST) exceed three times the upper limit of normal and persist.

In clinical trials 0.5% of patients treated with pravastatin had marked persistent increases (greater than 3 times the upper limit of normal) in serum transaminases. These elevations were not associated with clinical signs and symptoms of liver disease and usually declined to pre-treatment levels upon discontinuation of therapy.

Caution should be exercised when pravastatin is administered to patients with a history of liver disease or heavy alcohol ingestion.

Skeletal muscle: As with other HMG-CoA reductase inhibitors, sporadic elevations of creatine phosphokinase levels (CPK [MM fraction]) have been observed. If a markedly elevated (greater than 10 times upper limit of normal) serum CPK develops, or if myopathy is suspected, discontinuation of pravastatin therapy is recommended. There have been rare reports of rhabdomyolysis with renal dysfunction secondary to myoglobinuria. An increase in the incidence of myositis and myopathy has been seen in patients receiving HMG-CoA reductase inhibitors, especially those being treated concomitantly with cyclosporin (see *Drug interactions*), fibric acid derivatives and nicotinic acid.

In clinical trials involving small numbers of patients who were treated concurrently with pravastatin and nicotinic acid, there were no reports of myopathy. However, such combinations should continue to be used with caution.

The combined use of pravastatin and fibric acid derivatives may be useful in selected patients requiring further lipid level reductions. However, since the occurrence of myopathy cannot be excluded, concomitant use of pravastatin and fibric acid derivatives should generally be avoided.

Interactions with other medicinal products and other forms of interaction: No clinically significant effects were seen in a range of interaction studies.

Cholestyramine/Colestipol: There was no clinically significant decrease in bioavailability or therapeutic effect when pravastatin was administered one hour before or four hours after cholestyramine or one hour before colestipol and a standard meal. Concomitant administration resulted in approximately 40 to 50% decrease in the bioavailability of pravastatin.

Cyclosporin: Some investigators have measured cyclosporin plasma levels in patients receiving pravastatin and cyclosporin concomitantly and to date these results indicate no clinically meaningful elevations in cyclosporin levels. In one single-dose study, pravastatin plasma levels were found to be increased in cardiac transplant patients receiving cyclosporin.

Warfarin: Bioavailability parameters at steady state for pravastatin were not altered following administration with warfarin. Chronic dosing of the two drugs did not produce any changes in the anticoagulant action of warfarin.

In interaction studies with aspirin, antacids (one hour prior to Lipostat) cimetidine, gemfibrozil, nicotinic acid or probucol, no statistically significant differences in bioavailability were seen.

Other drugs: During clinical trials, no noticeable drug interactions were reported when Lipostat was added to: diuretics, antihypertensives, digitalis, converting-enzyme inhibitors, calcium channel blocker, beta-blockers, or nitroglycerins.

Pregnancy and lactation: There have been no teratogenic effects seen in animal studies. The safety of pravastatin therapy during pregnancy has not been established. Lipostat should only be used in women of child-bearing potential who are protected by effective contraception. As cholesterol and other products of cholesterol synthesis are essential components for foetal development, HMG-CoA reductase inhibitors are contra-indicated during pregnancy.

A small amount of pravastatin is excreted in human milk. Breastfeeding should be discontinued during pravastatin therapy.

Effects on ability to drive and use machines: None.

Undesirable effects: Lipostat is generally well tolerated. Adverse events, both clinical and laboratory are usually mild and transient.

In two long-term placebo-controlled trials West of Scotland Study (WOSCOPS) and Cholesterol and Recurrent Events study (CARE) involving a total of 10,754 patients treated with pravastatin 40 mg, (N=5383) or placebo (N=5371), the safety and tolerability profile in the pravastatin group was comparable to that of the placebo group over a media of 4.8–4.9 years of follow-up.

In smaller placebo controlled studies, the following events showed a small increase in incidence over placebo: those occurring with a frequency >1% were rash, myalgia, headache, non-cardiac chest pain; those occurring with a frequency >0.1% were nausea/vomiting, diarrhoea, fatigue.

Pravastatin was not associated with cataract formation in patients treated for up to a year or more in clinical studies nor in long-term animal studies.

Pravastatin has been administered concurrently with cholestyramine, colestipol, nicotinic acid and probucol. No adverse reactions unique to the combination or in addition to those previously reported for each drug alone have been reported.

Overdose: To date there have been only two reported cases of overdose, both of which were asymptomatic and did not give rise to abnormal laboratory tests. In the event of accidental overdose patients should be treated symptomatically.

Pharmacological properties

Pharmacodynamic properties: Pravastatin sodium is a competitive inhibitor of 3-hydroxy-3-methylglutaryl-coenzyme A (HMG-CoA) reductase, the enzyme catalysing the early rate-limiting step in cholesterol biosynthesis, and produces its lipid-lowering effect in two ways. First, it effects modest reductions in intracellular pools of cholesterol which results in an increased number of LDL-receptors on cell surfaces, enhanced receptor-mediated catabolism and clearance of circulating low density lipoprotein cholesterol (LDL-C). Second, pravastatin inhibits LDL-C production by inhibiting hepatic synthesis of very low density lipoprotein (VLDL-C), the LDL-C precursor. These effects result in a reduction of total cholesterol (Total-C), LDL-C, VLDL-C, apolipoprotein B and triglycerides, whilst increasing high density, lipoprotein cholesterol (HDL-C) and apolipoprotein A. Unlike other HMG-CoA reductase inhibitors, Lipostat has little effect on cholesterol synthesis in other tissues (e.g. lens, adrenal glands). *In vitro* studies demonstrated that pravastatin is transported into hepatocytes with substantially less uptake into other cells.

In controlled clinical trials, pravastatin was shown to reduce the progression of atherosclerosis and cardiovascular events (e.g. fatal and non-fatal M.I.) or death, in patients with moderate hypercholesterolaemia with or without atherosclerotic cardiovascular disease.

In the Cholesterol and Recurrent Events (CARE) study, Lipostat was effective in reducing the risk of fatal coronary events (fatal myocardial infarction and sudden death) plus non-fatal myocardial infarction, and frequency of stroke in patients with previous myocardial infarction and a total serum cholesterol level in excess of 4.8 mmol/L or a LDL-cholesterol in excess of 3.2 mmol/L.

Pharmacokinetic properties: Pravastatin is administered orally in the active form and is rapidly absorbed, with peak plasma levels occurring 1 to 1.5 hours after dosing. Whilst the presence of food reduces the systemic biovailability, the lipid-lowering effect is unaffected. Pravastatin undergoes extensive first-pass extraction in the liver which is its primary site of action and the primary site of cholesterol synthesis and of LDL-C clearance. Plasma levels are of limited value in predicting lipid-lowering efficacy. Approximately 50% of the circulating drug is bound to plasma proteins. The plasma elimination half life of pravastatin is between 1.5 and 2 hours. After oral dosing approximately 20% of the dose is excreted in the urine and 70% in the faeces. Although there are dual routes of elimination, and the potential exists for compensatory excretion by the alternate route, accumulation of drug and/or metabolites may occur in patients with renal or hepatic insufficiency. The major metabolite of pravastatin has one-tenth to one-fortieth of the activity of the parent compound.

Preclinical safety data: Pravastatin has not demonstrated any carcinogenic potential in mice. However, in a 2 year study in male rats given 125 times the maximum human dose of pravastatin, a statistically significant increase in the incidence of hepatocellular carcinomas was observed. This change was not seen in male rats given less than or equal to 50 times the recommended human dose, or in female rats at any dose level.

In vitro toxicology studies have shown no evidence of mutagenic potential.

Pharmaceutical particulars

List of excipients: Croscarmellose sodium, lactose, magnesium stearate, magnesium oxide, microcrystalline cellulose, polyvidone, yellow ferric oxide E172.

Incompatibilities: Not applicable.

Shelf life: 36 months

Special precautions for storage: Store below 30°C. Protect from light and moisture.

Nature and contents of container: PVC blister or aluminium foil packs of 28 tablets.

Instructions for use/handling: Not applicable.

Marketing authorisation numbers

Lipostat 10 mg	11184/0055
Lipostat 20 mg	11184/0056
Lipostat 40 mg	11184/0057

Date of approval/revision of SPC 24 July 1998

Legal category POM

PLAVIX* ▼

Qualitative and quantitative compostion Clopidogrel hydrogen sulphate 97.875 mg (molar equivalent of 75 mg of clopidogrel base)

Pharmaceutical form Film-coated tablet.

Plavix 75 mg film-coated tablets are pink, round, biconvex, film-coated and engraved with « 75 » on one side.

Clinical particulars

Therapeutic indications: Reduction of atherosclerotic events (myocardial infarction, stroke, death due to vascular causes) in patients with a history of symptomatic atherosclerotic disease defined by ischaemic stroke (from 7 days until less than 6 months), myocardial infarction (from a few days until less than 35 days) or established peripheral arterial disease.

This indication is based on the results of the CAPRIE study comparing clopidogrel with acetyl salicylic acid (ASA). The slight but statistically significant difference of clopidogrel over ASA was mainly related to patients enrolled due to peripheral arterial disease.

For further information please refer to *Special warnings and special precautions for use* and *Pharmacodynamic properties.*

Posology and method of administration:

Adults and elderly: Clopidogrel should be given as a single daily dose of 75 mg with or without food.

Children and adolescents: Safety and efficacy in

subjects below the age of 18 have not been established.

Contra-indications: Hypersensitivity to the active substance or any component of the medicinal product.

Severe liver impairment.

Active pathological bleeding such as peptic ulcer or intracranial haemorrhage.

Breast-feeding (see *Use during pregnancy and lactation*).

Special warnings and special precautions for use: In patients with acute myocardial infarction, clopidogrel therapy should not be initiated within the first few days following myocardial infarction.

In view of the lack of data, clopidogrel can not be recommended in unstable angina, PTCA (stenting), CABG and acute ischaemic stroke (less than 7 days).

As with other anti-platelet agents, clopidogrel should be used with caution in patients who may be at risk of increased bleeding from trauma, surgery or other pathological conditions. If a patient is to undergo elective surgery and an antiplatelet effect is not desired, clopidogrel should be discontinued 7 days prior to surgery.

Clopidogrel prolongs bleeding time and should be used with caution in patients who have lesions with a propensity to bleed (particularly gastrointestinal and intraocular).

Patients should be told that it may take longer than usual to stop bleeding when they take clopidogrel, and that they should report any unusual bleeding to their physician. Patients should inform physicians and dentists that they are taking clopidogrel before any surgery is scheduled and before any new drug is taken.

Therapeutic experience with clopidogrel is limited in patients with renal impairment. Therefore clopidogrel should be used with caution in these patients.

Experience is limited in patients with moderate hepatic disease who may have bleeding diatheses. Clopidogrel should therefore be used with caution in this population.

The concomitant administration of clopidogrel with warfarin is not recommended since it may increase the intensity of bleedings.

In view of the possible increased risk of bleeding, the concomitant administration of clopidogrel with ASA, heparin, or thrombolytics should be undertaken with caution (see *Interaction with other medicinal products and other forms of interaction*).

Drugs that might induce gastrointestinal lesions (such as Non-Steroidal Anti-Inflammatory Drugs) should be used with caution in patients taking clopidogrel (see *Interaction with other medicinal products and other forms of interaction*).

Interaction with other medicinal products and other forms of interaction:

Warfarin: See *Special warnings and special precautions for use.*

Acetylsalicylic acid (ASA): ASA did not modify the clopidogrel-mediated inhibition of ADP-induced platelet aggregation, but clopidogrel potentiated the effect of ASA on collagen-induced platelet aggregation. However, concomitant administration of 500 mg of ASA twice a day for one day did not significantly increase the prolongation of bleeding time induced by clopidogrel intake. The safety of the chronic concomitant administration of ASA and clopidogrel has not been established (see *Special warnings and special precautions for use*).

Heparin: In a clinical study conducted in healthy subjects, clopidogrel did not necessitate modification of the heparin dose or alter the effect of heparin on coagulation. Co-administration of heparin had no effect on the inhibition of platelet aggregation induced by clopidogrel. However, the safety of this combination has not been established and concomitant use should be undertaken with caution (see *Special warnings and special precautions for use*).

Thrombolytics: The safety of the concomitant administration of clopidogrel, rt-PA and heparin was assessed in patients with recent myocardial infarction. The incidence of clinically significant bleeding was similar to that observed when rt-PA and heparin are co-administered with ASA. The safety of the concomitant administration of clopidogrel with other thrombolytic agents has not been established and should be undertaken with caution (see *Special warnings and special precautions for use*).

Non-Steroidal Anti-Inflammatory Drugs (NSAIDs): In a clinical study conducted in healthy volunteers, the concomitant administration of clopidogrel and naproxen increased occult gastrointestinal blood loss. However, due to the lack of interaction studies with other NSAIDs it is presently unclear whether there is an increased risk of gastrointestinal bleeding with all NSAIDs. Consequently, NSAIDs and clopidogrel should be co-administered with caution (see *Special warnings and special precautions for use*).

Other concomitant therapy: A number of other clinical studies have been conducted with clopidogrel and other concomitant medications to investigate the potential for pharmacodynamic and pharmacokinetic interactions. No clinically significant pharmacodynamic interactions were observed when clopidogrel was co-administered with atenolol, nifedipine, or both atenolol and nifedipine. Furthermore, the pharmacodynamic activity of clopidogrel was not significantly influenced by the co-administration of phenobarbital, cimetidine, or oestrogen.

The pharmacokinetics of digoxin or theophylline were not modified by the co-administration of clopidogrel. Antacids did not modify the extent of clopidogrel absorption.

Data from studies with human liver microsomes indicated that the carboxylic acid metabolite of clopidogrel could inhibit the activity of Cytochrome P_{450} 2C9. This could potentially lead to increased plasma levels of drugs such as phenytoin and tolbutamide and the NSAIDs which are metabolised by Cytochrome P_{450} 2C9. Data from the CAPRIE study indicate that phenytoin and tolbutamide can be safely co-administered with clopidogrel.

Use during pregnancy and lactation:

Pregnancy: Reproduction studies performed in rats and in rabbits revealed no evidence of impaired fertility or harm to the foetus due to clopidogrel. There are, however, no adequate and well-controlled studies in pregnant women. In view of the lack of data, clopidogrel is not recommended during pregnancy.

Lactation: Studies in rats have shown that clopidogrel and/or its metabolites are excreted in the milk. It is not known whether this medicinal product is excreted in human milk (see *Contra-indications*).

Effects on ability to drive and use machines: No impairment of driving or psychometric performance was observed following clopidogrel administration.

Undesirable effects: Clopidogrel has been evaluated for safety in more than 11,300 patients, including over 7,000 patients treated for 1 year or more. Clopidogrel 75 mg/day was well tolerated compared to ASA 325 mg/day in a large controlled clinical trial (CAPRIE). The overall tolerability of clopidogrel in this study was similar to ASA, regardless of age, gender and race. The clinically relevant adverse effects observed in CAPRIE are discussed below.

Haemorrhagic disorders: in patients treated with either clopidogrel or ASA, the overall incidence of any bleeding was 9.3%. The incidence of severe cases was 1.4% for clopidogrel and 1.6% for ASA.

In patients that received clopidogrel, gastro-intestinal bleeding occurred at a rate of 2.0%, and required hospitalisation in 0.7%. In patients that received ASA, the corresponding rates were 2.7% and 1.1%, respectively.

The incidence of other bleeding was higher in patients that received clopidogrel compared to ASA (7.3% vs. 6.5%). However, the incidence of severe events was similar in both treatment groups (0.6% vs. 0.4%). The most frequently reported events in both treatment groups were: purpura/bruising/haematoma, and epistaxis. Other less frequently reported events were haematoma, haematuria, and eye bleeding (mainly conjunctival).

The incidence of intracranial bleeding was 0.4% in patients that received clopidogrel and 0.5% for patients that received ASA.

Haematological: Severe neutropaenia ($<0.45 \times 10^9$/l) was observed in 4 patients (0.04%) that received clopidogrel and 2 patients (0.02%) that received ASA. Two of the 9599 patients who received clopidogrel and none of the 9586 patients who received ASA had neutrophil counts of zero. One case of aplastic anaemia occurred on clopidogrel treatment.

The incidence of severe thrombocytopaenia ($<80 \times 10^9$/l) was 0.2% on clopidogrel and 0.1% on ASA.

Gastrointestinal: The overall, incidence of gastro-intestinal events (e.g. abdominal pain, dyspepsia, gastritis and constipation) was significantly lower in patients treated with clopidogrel compared to ASA (27.1% vs. 29.8%). In addition, the number of events resulting in early permanent discontinuation was lower in the clopidogrel group compared to ASA (3.2% vs. 4.0%). However, the incidence of adverse events judged as clinically severe were not statistically different in the groups (3.0% vs. 3.6%). The most frequently reported events in both treatment groups were: abdominal pain, dyspepsia, diarrhoea, and nausea. Other less frequently reported events were constipation, tooth disorder, vomiting, flatulence and gastritis.

Cases of diarrhoea were reported at a significantly higher frequency in patients taking clopidogrel compared to ASA (4.5% vs. 3.4%). The incidence of severe diarrhoea was similar in both treatment groups (0.2% vs. 0.1%). The incidence of peptic, gastric or duodenal ulcers was 0.7% for clopidogrel and 1.2% for ASA.

Skin and appendage disorders: The overall incidence of skin and appendage disorders in patients taking clopidogrel was significantly higher (15.8%) compared to ASA (13.1%). The incidence of severe events was similar in both treatment groups (0.7% vs.0.5%).

There were significantly more patients with rash in the clopidogrel group compared to the ASA group (4.2% vs. 3.5%). More patients reported pruritus in the clopidogrel group compared to ASA (3.3% vs. 1.6%).

Central and peripheral nervous system disorders: The overall incidence of central and peripheral nervous system disorders (e.g. headache, dizziness, vertigo and paraesthesia) was significantly lower in patients taking clopidogrel compared to ASA (22.3% vs. 23.8%).

Hepatic and biliary disorders: The overall incidence of hepatic and biliary disorders was similar in patients treated with clopidogrel compared to ASA (3.5% vs. 3.4%).

Overdose: One case of deliberate overdosage with clopidogrel has been reported. A 34 year old woman took a single 1,050 mg dose of clopidogrel (equivalent to 14 standard 75 mg tablets). There were no associated undesirable effects. No special therapy was instituted and she recovered without sequelae.

No adverse events were reported after single oral administration of 600 mg (equivalent to 8 standard 75 mg tablets) of clopidogrel to healthy subjects. The bleeding time was prolonged by a factor of 1.7 which is similar to that typically observed with the therapeutic dose of 75 mg per day.

No antidote to the pharmacological activity of clopidogrel has been found. If prompt correction of prolonged bleeding time is required, platelet transfusion may reverse the effects of clopidogrel.

Pharmacological properties

Pharmacodynamic properties: Pharmacotherapeutical group: platelet aggregation inhibitors excl. Heparin, ATC Code: BO1AC/04.

Clopidogrel selectively inhibits the binding of adenosine diphosphate (ADP) to its platelet receptor, and the subsequent ADP-mediated activation of the GPIIb/IIIa complex, thereby inhibiting platelet aggregation. Biotransformation of clopidogrel is necessary to produce inhibition of platelet aggregation. Clopidogrel also inhibits platelet aggregation induced by other agonists by blocking the amplification of platelet activation by released ADP. Clopidogrel acts by irreversibly modifying the platelet ADP receptor. Consequently, platelets exposed to clopidogrel are affected for the remainder of their lifespan and recovery of normal platelet function occurs at a rate consistent with platelet turnover.

Repeated doses of 75 mg per day produced substantial inhibition of ADP-induced platelet aggregation from the first day; this increased progressively and reached steady state between Day 3 and Day 7. At steady state, the average inhibition level observed with a dose of 75 mg per day was between 40% and 60%. Platelet aggregation and bleeding time gradually returned to baseline values, generally within 5 days after treatment was discontinued.

The safety and efficacy of clopidogrel in preventing vascular ischaemic events have been evaluated in a blinded comparison with ASA (CAPRIE, Clopidogrel versus ASA in Patients at Risk of Ischaemic Events). This study included 19,185 patients with atherothrombosis as manifested by recent myocardial infarction (<35 days), recent ischaemic stroke (between 7 days and 6 months) or established peripheral arterial disease (PAD). Patients were randomised to clopidogrel 75 mg/day or ASA 325 mg/day, and were followed for 1 to 3 years. In the myocardial infarction subgroup, most of the patients received ASA for the first few days following the acute myocardial infarction.

Clopidogrel significantly reduced the incidence of new ischaemic events (combined end point of myocardial infarction, ischaemic stroke and vascular death) when compared to ASA. In the intention to treat analysis, 939 events were observed in the clopidogrel group and 1,020 events with ASA (relative risk reduction (RRR) 8.7%, [95% CI: 0.2 to 16.4]; p = 0.045), which corresponds, for every 1000 patients treated for 2 years, to 10 [CI: 0 to 20] additional patients being prevented from experiencing a new ischaemic event. Analysis of total mortality as a secondary endpoint did not show any significant difference between clopidogrel (5.8%) and ASA (6.0%).

In a subgroup analysis by qualifying condition (myocardial infarction, ischaemic stroke, and PAD) the benefit appeared to be strongest (achieving statistical significance at p=0.003) in patients enrolled due to PAD (especially those who also had a history of myocardial infarction) (RRR=23.7%; CI: 8.9 to 36.2) and weaker (not significantly different from ASA) in stroke patients (RRR=7.3%; CI: -5.7 to 18.7). In patients who were enrolled in the trial on the sole basis of a recent myocardial infarction, clopidogrel was numerically inferior, but not statistically different from ASA (RRR=-4.0%; CI: -22.5 to 11.7). In addition, a subgroup analysis by age suggested that the benefit of clopidogrel in patients over 75 years was less than that observed in patients ≤75 years

Since the CAPRIE trial was not powered to evaluate efficacy of individual subgroups, it is not clear whether the differences in relative risk reduction across qualifying conditions are real, or a result of chance.

Pharmacokinetic properties: After repeated oral doses of 75 mg per day, clopidogrel is rapidly absorbed. However, plasma concentrations of the parent compound are very low and below the quantification limit (0.00025 mg/l) beyond 2 hours. Absorption is at least 50%, based on urinary excretion of clopidogrel metabolites.

Clopidogrel is extensively metabolised by the liver and the main metabolite, which is inactive, is the carboxylic acid derivative which represents about 85% of the circulating compound in plasma. Peak plasma levels of this metabolite (approx. 3 mg/l after repeated 75 mg oral doses) occurred approximately 1 hour after dosing.

Clopidogrel is a prodrug. The active metabolite, a thiol derivative, is formed by oxidation of clopidogrel to 2-oxo-clopidogrel and subsequent hydrolysis. The oxidative step is regulated primarily by Cytochrome P_{450} isoenzymes 2B6 and 3A4 and to a lesser extent by 1A1, 1A2 and 2C19. The active thiol metabolite, which has been isolated *in vitro*, binds rapidly and irreversibly to platelet receptors, thus inhibiting platelet aggregation. This metabolite has not been detected in plasma.

The kinetics of the main circulating metabolite were linear (plasma concentrations increased in proportion to dose) in the dose range of 50 to 150 mg of clopidogrel.

Clopidogrel and the main circulating metabolite bind reversibly *in vitro* to human plasma proteins (98% and 94% respectively). The binding is non-saturable *in vitro* over a wide concentration range.

Following an oral dose of ^{14}C-labelled clopidogrel in man, approximately 50% was excreted in the urine and approximately 46% in the faeces in the 120 hour interval after dosing. The elimination half-life of the main circulating metabolite was 8 hours after single and repeated administration.

After repeated doses of 75 mg clopidogrel per day, plasma levels of the main circulating metabolite were lower in subjects with severe renal disease (creatinine clearance from 5 to 15 ml/min) compared to subjects with moderate renal disease (creatinine clearance from 30 to 60 ml/min) and to levels observed in other studies with healthy subjects. Although inhibition of ADP-induced platelet aggregation was lower (25%) than that observed in healthy subjects, the prolongation of bleeding was similar to that seen in healthy subjects receiving 75 mg of clopidogrel per day. In addition, clinical tolerance was good in all patients.

The pharmacokinetics and pharmacodynamics of clopidogrel were assessed in a single and multiple dose study in both healthy subjects and those with cirrhosis (Child-Pugh class A or B). Daily dosing for 10 days with clopidogrel 75 mg/day was safe and well tolerated. Clopidogrel C_{max} for both single dose and steady state for cirrhotics was many fold higher than in normal subjects. However, plasma levels of the main circulating metabolite together with the effect of clopidogrel on ADP-induced platelet aggregation and bleeding time were comparable between these groups.

Preclinical safety data: During preclinical studies in rat and baboon, the most frequently observed effects were liver changes. These occurred at doses representing at least 25 times the exposure seen in humans receiving the clinical dose of 75 mg/day and were a consequence of an effect on hepatic metabolising enzymes. No effect on hepatic metabolising enzymes were observed in humans receiving clopidogrel at the therapeutic dose.

At very high doses, a poor gastric tolerability (gastritis, gastric erosions and/or vomiting) of clopidogrel was also reported in rat and baboon.

There was no evidence of carcinogenic effect when clopidogrel was administered for 78 weeks to mice and 104 weeks to rats when given at doses up to 77 mg/kg per day (representing at least 25 times the exposure seen in humans receiving the clinical dose of 75 mg/day).

Clopidogrel has been tested in a range of *in vitro* and *in vivo* genotoxicity studies, and showed no genotoxic activity.

Clopidogrel was found to have no effect on the fertility of male and female rats and was not teratogenic in either rats or rabbits. When given to lactating rats, clopidogrel caused a slight delay in the development of the offspring. Specific pharmacokinetic studies performed with radiolabelled clopidogrel have shown that the parent compound or its metabolites are excreted in the milk. Consequently, a direct effect (slight toxicity), or an indirect effect (low palatability) cannot be excluded.

Pharmaceutical particulars

List of excipients:

Core: Anhydrous lactose, Modified maize starch, Macrogol 6000, Microcrystalline cellulose, Hydrogenated castor oil

Coating: Hypromellose, Macrogol 6000, Titanium dioxide (E171), Red iron oxide (E172), Carnauba wax

Incompatibilities: Not applicable

Shelf-life: Three years

Special precautions for storage: No special precautions for storage

Nature and content of container: 28, 50, and 84, tablets packed in blisters in cardboard cartons.

Instruction for use and handling, and disposal (if appropriate): Not applicable

Marketing authorisation holder: Sanofi Pharma Bristol-Myers Squibb SNC, 174 Avenue de France, F-75013, Paris, France.

Number(s) in the community register of medicinal products

EU/1/98/069/001–Cartons of 28 tablets
EU/1/98/069/002–Cartons of 50 tablets
EU/1/98/069/003–Cartons of 84 tablets

Date of first authorisation/renewal of the authorisation 15.07.98

Date of revision of the text Not applicable

Legal category POM

SULPAREX* TABLETS 200 MG

Presentation Plain white round tablets with BMS 1510 on one side and a break bar on the other, each containing 200 mg sulpiride.

Other ingredients: magnesium stearate, maize starch, microcrystalline cellulose and polyvidone.

Uses For the treatment of acute and chronic schizophrenia.

Sulparex is a highly selective dopamine antagonist with bi-modal dose-dependant antidepressant and antipsychotic activity. Florid schizophrenic symptoms respond to high doses of Sulparex, whereas administration of lower doses results in mood elevation and alerting effect. Schizophrenia characterised by lack of social contact can benefit strikingly from treatment. Improvement of both florid and negative symptoms occurs, often within the first few days of treatment. The sedation and blunted effect characteristically associated with classical neuroleptics of the phenothiazine or butyrophenone type are not features of Sulparex therapy.

Dosage and administration *Adults:* The initial dose depends on the nature of the symptoms.

Predominantly positive symptoms (formal thought disorder, hallucinations, delusions, incongruity of effect) respond to higher doses, and a starting dose of at least 400 mg twice daily is recommended, increasing if necessary up to a suggested maximum of 1200 mg twice daily. Increasing the dose beyond this level has not been shown to produce further improvement.

Predominantly negative symptoms (flattening of effect, poverty of speech, anergia, apathy), as well as depression, usually respond best to a total of 200 mg to 400 mg daily, given in divided doses.

Patients with mixed positive and negative symptoms, with neither predominating, will normally respond to dosage of 200 mg to 600 mg twice daily.

Elderly: The same dose ranges may be required in the elderly but, as a general rule with the use of psychotropics in elderly patients, starting doses should be lower and increased gradually, particularly in those with renal impairment.

Children: Clinical experience in children under 14 years of age is insufficient to permit specific recommendations.

Contra-indications, warnings, etc

Contra-indications: Hypersensitivity to any of the ingredients of Sulparex. Phaeochromocytoma. Severe hepatic, renal or haematological disease. Alcoholic intoxication or other disorders which depress CNS function.

Warnings: Increased motor agitation has been reported at low dosage in a small number of patients. Low doses of Sulparex may aggravate symptoms in aggressive, agitated, or excited phases of the disease process. Consequently, low doses are not recommended when hypomania is present. Insomnia may occur in a small percentage of patients.

Extra-pyramidal reactions, including akathisia, have been reported in a small number of cases. If warranted, reduction in dosage or anti-parkinsonian medication may be necessary.

Tardive dyskinesia has occurred rarely.

As with all neuroleptic drugs, the presence of unexplained hyperthermia could indicate the neuroleptic malignant syndrome (NMS). In this event Sulparex and any associated neuroleptic treatment should be discontinued until the origin of the fever has been determined.

Hormonal effects of neuroleptic drugs include hyperprolactinaemia, which may cause galactorrhoea, gynaecomastia and oligomenorrhoea/amenorrhoea. Sexual function may be increased or decreased. These side-effects are reversible on cessation of treatment. In long term animal studies with neuroleptic compounds, including sulpiride, an increase of various endocrine tumours (a small proportion of which were malignant) have been seen in some but not all strains of rats and mice studied. The significance of these findings to man is not known; there is no evidence of an association between Sulparex use and tumour risk in man. However, when prescribing neuroleptics to patients with existing mammary neoplasia or a personal history of this disease, possible risk should be weighed against benefits of therapy.

Precautions: As with all drugs for which the kidney is the major elimination pathway, caution should be exercised when administering Sulparex to patients with impairment of renal function. Dose levels and/or the frequency of administration may need to be amended.

Although Sulparex is less prone to produce drowsiness than conventional neuroleptic compounds, patients receiving high doses of medication should be warned about the hazards of driving or operating machinery until the compound has been shown not to interfere with their physical or mental ability.

Patients should be warned against taking alcohol with sulpiride as reaction capacity may be impaired.

Patients with epilepsy: Although Sulparex produces only slight modifications to the EEG, anti-convulsant medication should be continued unchanged in epileptics. Patients with unstable epilepsy should be monitored frequently.

Drug interactions: As with other psychotropic compounds, sulpiride may increase the effect of antihypertensives and CNS depressants (including alcohol) or stimulants.

Use in pregnancy and lactation: Despite the negative results of teratogenicity studies in animals and the lack of teratogenic effects during widespread clinical use, Sulparex should not be considered an exception to the general principle of avoiding drug treatment during pregnancy, particularly during the first 16 weeks, with potential benefits being weighed against possible hazards.

Passage of sulpiride into breast milk has been reported.

Side-effects: Hepatic reactions, including jaundice and hepatitis, have been reported.

Cases of convulsions, sometimes in patients with no previous history, have been reported.

Toxicity and treatment of overdose: Overdoses have been reported ranging from 1 g to 16 g but no death has occurred even at the 16 g dose. Doses of 1 g to 3 g have been reported to produce restlessness and clouding of consciousness and (rarely) extrapyramidal symptoms. Doses of 3 g to 7 g may produce a degree of agitation, confusion, low blood pressure and extra-pyramidal symptoms. In cases where coma has occurred, Sulparex has been administered in conjunction with other psychotropic medication. The duration of intoxication is generally short, the symptoms disappearing within a few hours. There are no specific complications from overdose. In particular no haematological or hepatic toxicity has been reported.

Overdose may be treated with alkaline osmotic diuresis and, if necessary, anti-parkinsonian drugs. Emetic drugs are unlikely to be effective. Coma needs appropriate nursing.

Pharmaceutical precautions Store below 30°C.

Legal category POM.

Package quantities Cardboard cartons containing blister strips of 100 tablets.

Further information Sulparex is a member of the group of substituted benzamides, which are structurally distinct from the phenothiazines, butyrophenones and thioxanthenes. Current evidence suggests that the actions of Sulparex hint at an important distinction between different types of dopamine receptors or receptor mechanisms in the brain. Behaviourally and biochemically, Sulparex shares with these conventional neuroleptics a number of properties indicative of cerebral dopamine receptor antagonism. Essential and intriguing differences include lack of catalepsy at doses active in other behavioural tests, lack of effect in the dopamine sensitive adenylate cyclase systems, lack of effect upon noradrenaline or 5HT turnover, negligible anticholinesterase activity, no effect on muscarinic or GABA receptor binding, and a radical difference in the binding of tritiated sulpiride to striatal preparations *in-vitro*, compared to ^{3}H-spiperone or ^{3}H-haloperidol. These findings indicate a major differentiation between Sulparex and conventional neuroleptics which lack such specificity.

Sulparex is slowly absorbed after oral dosing.

Peak sulpiride serum levels are reached 2–6 hours after an oral dose. The majority of studies have shown that the elimination half-life in plasma is 6–8 hours. Approximately 40% sulpiride is bound to plasma proteins. The mean concentration of sulpiride in the cerebrospinal fluid is 13% of its serum concentration. 95% of the compound is excreted in the urine and faeces as unchanged sulpiride.

Sulparex has no significant cardiovascular or anticholinergic activity.

Product licence number 11184/0032.

TAXOL*
TAXOL*-100

Qualitative and quantitative composition Taxol vials contain 30 mg or 100 mg paclitaxel per vial as a 6 mg/ml solution.

Pharmaceutical form Concentrate for solution for infusion

Clinical particulars
Therapeutic indications:
Ovarian carcinoma: The primary treatment of carcinoma of the ovary, in combination with cisplatin, in patients with advanced disease or residual disease (>1cm) after initial laparotomy.

The secondary treatment of metastatic carcinoma of the ovary after failure of standard platinum containing therapy.

Breast carcinoma: The treatment of metastatic carcinoma of the breast in patients who have failed, or are not candidates for, standard anthracycline containing therapy.

Non-small cell lung carcinoma: The treatment of non-small cell lung carcinoma (NSCLC) in combination with cisplatin in patients who are not candidates for potentially curative surgery and/or radiation therapy.

Limited efficacy data supports this indication, a summary of the relevant studies is shown in *Pharmacodynamic properties*.

Posology and method of administration:
Primary treatment of ovarian carcinoma: although other dosage regimens are under investigation, a combination regimen is recommended consisting of Taxol 135 mg/m² administered over 24 hours, followed by cisplatin 75 mg/m², with a 3 week interval between courses (see *Interactions with other medicinal products and other forms of interaction*).

Secondary treatment of ovarian and breast carcinoma: the recommended dose of Taxol is 175 mg/m² administered over a period of 3 hours, with a 3 week interval between courses.

Treatment of advanced NSCLC: the recommended dose of Taxol is 175 mg/m² administered over a period of 3 hours, followed by cisplatin 80 mg/m², with a 3 week interval between courses.

Subsequent doses of Taxol should be administered according to individual patient tolerance.

Taxol should not be readministered until the neutrophil count is ≥1.5x10⁹/L and the platelet count is ≥100x10⁹/L. Patients who experience severe neutropenia (neutrophil count <0.5x10⁹/L for ≥7 days) or severe peripheral neuropathy should receive a dose reduction of 20% for subsequent courses (see *Special warnings and special precautions for use*).

All patients must be premedicated with corticosteroids, antihistamines, and H_2 antagonists prior to Taxol, eg.

Drug	*Dose*	*Administration prior to Taxol*
dexamethasone	20 mg oral	approximately 12 and 6 hours
diphenhydramine	50 mg IV	30 to 60 minutes
or chlorpheniramine	10 mg IV	
cimetidine	300 mg IV	30 to 60 minutes
or ranitidine	50 mg IV	

Taxol should be administered through an in-line filter with a microporous membrane ≤0.22µm (see *Instructions for use/handling*).

Contra-indications: Taxol is contra-indicated in patients with severe hypersensitivity reactions to paclitaxel or any other component of the formulation, especially polyethoxylated castor oil.

Taxol is contraindicated during pregnancy and lactation.

Taxol should not be used in patients with baseline neutrophils <1.5x10⁹/L

Special warnings and special precautions for use: Taxol should be administered under the supervision of a physician experienced in the use of cancer chemotherapeutic agents. Since significant hypersensitivity reactions may occur, appropriate supportive equipment should be available.

Patients must be pretreated with corticosteroids, antihistamines and H_2 antagonists (see *Posology and method of administration*).

Taxol should be given *before* cisplatin when used in combination (see *Interactions with other medicinal products and other forms of interaction*).

Significant hypersensitivity reactions: Characterized by dyspnea and hypotension requiring treatment, angioedema and generalized urticaria have occurred in <1% of patients receiving Taxol after adequate premedication. These reactions are probably histamine-mediated. In the case of severe hypersensitivity reactions, Taxol infusion should be discontinued immediately, symptomatic therapy should be initiated and the patient should not be rechallenged with the drug.

Bone marrow suppression: (Primarily neutropenia) is the dose-limiting toxicity. Frequent monitoring of blood counts should be instituted. Patients should not be retreated until neutrophils recover to a level ≥1.5x10⁹/L and platelets recover to a level ≥100x10⁹/L.

Severe cardiac conduction abnormalities: Have been reported rarely. If patients develop significant conduction abnormalities during Taxol administration, appropriate therapy should be administered and continuous cardiac monitoring should be performed during subsequent therapy with Taxol. Hypotension, hypertension, and bradycardia have been observed during Taxol administration; patients are usually asymptomatic and generally do not require treatment. Frequent vital sign monitoring, particularly during the first hour of Taxol infusion, is recommended. Severe cardiovascular events were observed more frequently in patients with NSCLC than in those with breast- or ovarian carcinoma.

Although the occurrence of **peripheral neuropathy** is frequent, the development of severe symptoms is unusual. In severe cases, a dose reduction of 20% is recommended for all subsequent courses of Taxol. In NSCLC patients, the administration of Taxol in combination with cisplatin, resulted in a greater incidence of severe neurotoxicity than single agent Taxol.

There is no evidence that the toxicity of Taxol is increased when given as a 3-hour infusion to patients with mildly abnormal liver function. No data are available for patients with severe baseline cholestasis. When Taxol is given as a longer infusion, increased myelosuppression may be seen in patients with moderate to severe hepatic impairment.

Taxol is not recommended in patients with **severely impaired hepatic function.**

Since Taxol contains dehydrated alcohol (396 mg/mL), consideration should be given to possible CNS and other effects.

Special care should be taken to avoid intra-arterial administration of Taxol. In animal studies investigating local tolerance, severe tissue reactions occurred following intra-arterial administration.

Interactions with other medicinal products and other forms of interaction: Paclitaxel clearance is not affected by cimetidine premedication.

The recommended regimen of Taxol administration for the primary treatment of ovarian carcinoma is for Taxol to be given *before* cisplatin. When Taxol is given *before* cisplatin, the safety profile of Taxol is consistent with that reported for single-agent use. When Taxol was given *after* cisplatin, patients showed a more profound myelosuppression and an approximately 20% decrease in paclitaxel clearance.

The metabolism of paclitaxel is catalyzed, in part, by cytochrome P450 isoenzymes CYP2C8 and 3A4 (see *Pharmacokinetic properties*). Clinical studies have demonstrated that CYP2C8-mediated metabolism of paclitaxel, to 6a-hydroxypaclitaxel, is the major metabolic pathway in humans. Based on current knowledge, clinically relevant interactions between paclitaxel and other CYP2C8 substrates are not anti-cipated. Concurrent administration of ketoconazole, a known potent inhibitor of CYP3A4, does not inhibit the elimination of paclitaxel in patients; thus, both medicinal products may be administered together without dosage adjustment. Further data on the potential of drug interactions between paclitaxel and other CYP3A4 substrates/inhibitors are limited. Therefore, caution shoud be exercised when administering paclitaxel concomitantly with known substrates or inhibitors of CYP3A4.

Pregnancy and lactation: Taxol has been shown to be embryotoxic and fetotoxic in rabbits, and to decrease fertility in rats.

There is no information on the use of Taxol in pregnant women. As with other cytotoxic drugs, Taxol may cause fetal harm, and is therefore contraindicated during pregnancy. Women should be advised to avoid becoming pregnant during therapy with Taxol, and to inform the treating physician immediately should this occur.

It is not known whether paclitaxel is excreted in human milk. Taxol is contraindicated during lactation. Breastfeeding should be discontinued for the duration of Taxol therapy.

Effect on ability to drive and use machines: Taxol has not been demonstrated to interfere with this ability. However, it should be noted that the formulation contains alcohol (see *Special warnings and special precautions for use* and *List of excipients*).

Undesirable effects: The frequency and severity of adverse events are generally similar between patients receiving Taxol for the treatment of ovarian carcinoma, breast carcinoma or NSCLC. None of the observed toxicities was clearly influenced by age.

The following safety data relate to 95 patients with ovarian cancer and 289 patients with breast cancer treated with 175 mg/m² single agent Taxol over a 3 hour infusion in phase III clinical trials.

Safety of the Taxol/platinum combination has been evaluated in a large randomised trial in ovarian carcinoma (24-hr infusion, GOG-III) and in major phase III trials in NSCLC (3-hr infusion) (see *Pharmacodynamic properties*). Unless otherwise mentioned, the combination of Taxol with platinum agents, or the infusion of Taxol over 24 hours, did not result in any clinically relevant changes to the safety profile of single agent Taxol.

The most frequent significant undesirable effect of Taxol was **bone marrow suppression**. Severe neutropenia (<0.5x10⁹/L) occurred in 28% of patients, but was not associated with febrile episodes. Only 1% of patients experienced severe neutropenia for 7 days or more.

Twenty-four percent of patients had an **infectious episode.** In the phase III clinical trials, 2 fatal infections were seen at the recommended dose and infusion schedule.

Thrombocytopenia: Was reported in 11% of patients. Three percent of patients had a platelet count nadir <50x10⁹/L at least once while on study.

Anemia: Was observed in 64% of patients, but was severe (Hb<8 g/dL) in only 6% of patients. Incidence and severity of anemia is related to baseline hemoglobin status.

One case each of **acute myeloid leukemia and myelodysplastic syndrome** has been reported outside the phase III trials.

Myelosuppression: Is less frequent and less severe with a 3-hour infusion than with a 24-hour infusion schedule. The recommended Taxol/cisplatin regimen for the primary treatment of ovarian cancer caused more severe myelosuppression than single dose Taxol using the recommended schedule of 175 mg/m² over 3 hour infusion. However, there was no increase in clinical sequelae.

A **significant hypersensitivity reaction** with possible fatal outcome (defined as hypotension requiring therapy, angioedema, respiratory distress requiring bronchodilator therapy, or generalized urticaria) occurred in 2 (<1%) patients. Thirty-four percent of patients (17% of all courses) experienced minor hypersensitivity reactions. These minor reactions, mainly flushing and rash, did not require therapeutic intervention nor did they prevent continuation of Taxol therapy.

Hypotension and bradycardia: Were experienced by 22% and 5% of patients, respectively. The degree of change was usually mild and did not require therapeutic intervention.

Seventeen percent of patients had an **abnormal ECG** during clinical trials. In most cases, no clear relationship between Taxol and ECG alterations could be defined and these alterations were of little or no clinical relevance.

One (<1%) patient experienced **hypertension** during Taxol therapy. In addition, 2 (<1%) patients presented **severe thrombotic events** (upper extremity thrombosis and thrombophlebitis). One patient each (<1%) experienced the following **significant cardiovascular events**: hypotension associated with septic shock, cardiomyopathy and tachycardia associated with fever. In early clinical studies, conducted with varying dosages and infusion schedules, 2% patients experienced severe cardiovascular events possibly related to Taxol which included asymptomatic ventricular tachycardia, tachycardia with bigeminy, AV block and syncope. These occur more frequently in patients with NSCLC (see *Special warnings and special precautions for use*).

Cases of myocardial infarction have been reported rarely. Congestive heart failure has been reported typically in patients who have received other chemotherapy, notably anthracyclines.

Peripheral neuropathy: Mainly manifested by paresthesia, affected 66% of patients, but was severe in only 5% of patients. In NSCLC patients, the incidence of severe peripheral neuropathy is slightly greater (6%). Peripheral neuropathy can occur following the first course and can worsen with increasing exposure to Taxol. Peripheral neuropathy was the cause of Taxol discontinuation in 3 cases. Sensory symptoms have usually improved or resolved within several months of Taxol discontinuation. Pre-existing neuropathies resulting from prior therapies are not a contraindication for Taxol therapy. Among patients treated with Taxol outside these randomized trials, grand mal seizures, encephalopathy, motor neuropathy with resultant minor distal weakness, autonomic neuropathy resulting in paralytic ileus, and orthostatic hypotension have been reported. Optic nerve and/or visual disturbances (scintillating scotomata) have also been reported, particularly in patients who have received higher doses than recommended. These effects generally have been reversible.

Arthralgia or myalgia: Affected 60% of patients and was severe in 13% of patients.

Alopecia: Was observed in almost all patients.

Transient and mild nail and skin changes: Have been observed. Rare reports of skin abnormalities related to radiation recall have been received outside the phase III trials.

Gastrointestinal side effects: Were usually mild to moderate: nausea/vomiting, diarrhea and mucositis were reported by 43%, 28% and 18% of patients, respectively. Other gastrointestinal events reported outside these randomized trials included bowel obstruction/perforation, and (mesenteric thrombosis including ischemic) colitis.

Severe elevations: (> 5 x normal values) **in AST (SGOT), alkaline phosphatase or bilirubin** were seen in 5%, 4%, and <1% of patients, respectively. Hepatic necrosis and hepatic encephalopathy have been reported in patients treated with Taxol outside the phase III trials.

Injection site reactions: During intravenous administration may lead to localized edema, pain, erythema, and induration; on occasion, extravasation can result in cellulitis. Skin discoloration may also occur. Recurrence of skin reactions at a site of previous extravasation following administration of Taxol at a different site, ie. "recall", has been reported rarely. A specific treatment for extravasation reactions is unknown at this time.

Radiation pneumonitis has been reported in patients receiving concurrent radiotherapy.

Overdose: There is no known antidote for Taxol overdosage. The primary anticipated complications of overdosage would consist of bone marrow suppression, peripheral neurotoxicity and mucositis.

Pharmacological properties

Pharmacodynamic properties: Pharmacotherapeutic group/ATC code: cystostatic agent, L01C D01. Paclitaxel is a novel antimicrotubule agent that promotes the assembly of microtubules from tubulin dimers and stabilizes microtubules by preventing depolymerization. This stability results in the inhibition of the normal dynamic reorganization of the microtubule network that is essential for vital interphase and mitotic cellular functions. In addition, paclitaxel induces abnormal arrays or bundles of microtubules throughout the cell cycle and multiple asters of microtubules during mitosis.

The safety and efficacy of Taxol (135 mg/m² over 24 hr) followed by cisplatin (75 mg/m²) was evaluated in a major randomized, controlled clinical trial (GOG-111). Patients in the control group received cyclophosphamide 750 mg/m² + cisplatin 75 mg/m². The trial involved over 400 patients with stage III/IV primary ovarian cancer with a >1 cm residual disease after staging laparotomy or with distant metastases. There were statistically significant gains in median time to progression (>3.5 months) and overall median survival (>11 months) for the Taxol arm. The level of serious toxicity was comparable between the two groups.

Taxol 175 mg/m² followed by cisplatin 80 mg/m² has been evaluated in two phase III trials of advanced NSCLC (367 patients on Taxol containing regimens). Both were randomised trials, one compared to treatment with cisplatin 100 mg/m², the other used teniposide 100 mg/m² followed by cisplatin 80 mg/m² as comparator (367 patients on comparator). Results in each trial were similar. For the primary outcome of mortality, there was no significant difference between the Taxol containing regimen and the comparator (median survival times 8.1 and 9.5 months on Taxol containing regimens, 8.6 and 9.9 months on comparators). Similarly, for progression-free survival there was no significant difference between treatments. There was a significant benefit in terms of clinical response rate. Quality of life results are suggestive of a benefit on Taxol containing regimens in terms of appetite loss and provide clear evidence of the inferiority of Taxol containing regimens in terms of peripheral neuropathy ($p<0.008$).

Pharmacokinetic properties: Following intravenous administration, paclitaxel exhibits a biphasic decline in plasma concentrations.

The pharmacokinetics of paclitaxel were determined following 3 and 24 hour infusions at doses of 135 and 175 mg/m². Mean terminal half-life estimates ranged from 3.0 to 52.7 hours, and mean, non-compartmentally derived, values for total body clearance ranged from 11.6 to 24.0 L/hr/m²; total body clearance appeared to decrease with higher plasma concentrations of paclitaxel. Mean steady-state volume of distribution ranged from 198 to 688 L/m², indicating extensive extravascular distribution and/or tissue binding. With the 3-hour infusion, increasing doses result in non-linear pharmacokinetics. For the 30% increase in dose from 135 mg/m² to 175 mg/m², the C_{MAX} and $AUC_{0-\infty}$ values increased 75% and 81%, respectively.

Intrapatient variability in systemic paclitaxel exposure was minimal. There was no evidence of accumulation of paclitaxel with multiple treatment courses.

In vitro studies of binding to human serum proteins indicate that 89-98% of drug is bound. The presence of cimetidine, ranitidine, dexamethasone or diphenhydramine did not affect protein binding of paclitaxel.

The disposition of paclitaxel has not been fully elucidated in humans. Mean values for cumulative urinary recovery of unchanged drug have ranged from 1.3 to 12.6% of the dose, indicating extensive non-renal clearance. Hepatic metabolism and biliary clearance may be the principal mechanism for disposition of paclitaxel. Paclitaxel appears to be metabolized primarily by cytochrome P450 enzymes. Following administration of a radiolabeled paclitaxel, an average of 26, 2, and 6% of the radioactivity was excreted in the faeces as 6a-hydroxypaclitaxel, 3'-p-hydroxypaclitaxel, and 6a-3'-p-dihydroxy-paclitaxel, respectively. The formation of these hydroxylated metabolites is catalyzed by CYP2C8, -3A4, and both -2C8 and -3A4 respectively. The effect of renal or hepatic dysfunction on the disposition of paclitaxel following a 3-hour infusion has not been investigated formally. Pharmacokinetic parameters obtained from one patient undergoing hemodialysis who received a 3-hour infusion of Taxol 135 mg/m² were within the range of those defined in non-dialysis patients.

Preclinical safety data: The carcinogenic potential of Taxol has not been studied. However, paclitaxel is a potential carcinogenic and genotoxic agent, based upon its pharmacodynamic mechanism of action. Taxol has been shown to be mutagenic in both *in vitro* and *in vivo* mammalian test systems.

Pharmaceutical particulars

List of excipients: Dehydrated alcohol (396 mg/mL), cleaned polyethoxylated castor oil.

Incompatibilities: Polyethoxylated castor oil can result in DEHP [di-(2-ethylhexyl)phthalate] leaching from plasticized polyvinyl chloride (PVC) containers, at levels which increase with time and concentration. Consequently, the preparation, storage and administration of diluted Taxol should be carried out using non-PVC-containing equipment.

Shelf life: Unopened vials are stable until the date indicated on the package (24 months), when stored at room temperature (15-25°C) in the original carton.

If unopened vials are refrigerated, a precipitate may form that redissolves with little or no agitation upon reaching room temperature. Product quality is not affected. If the solution remains cloudy or if an insoluble precipitate is noted, the vial should be discarded. Freezing does not adversely affect the product.

Taxol-100

After first use, any unused concentrate may be stored at room temperature (15-25°C) and under normal room lighting conditions for up to 28 days. Other in-use storage times and conditions are the responsibility of the user.

Special precautions for storage: Store the unopened vials at room temperature (15-25°C) in the original cartons to protect from light.

Taxol-100

After first use, any unused concentrate may be stored at room temperature (15-25°C) and under normal room lighting conditions (see *Shelf life*). Other in-use storage times and conditions are the responsibility of the user.

Nature and contents of container: Glass vials with butyl rubber stoppers containing 30 mg or 100 mg of paclitaxel as a 6 mg/ml solution. The 100 mg presentation may be used as a multidose vial. The vials are available individually packed in a carton or in a shelf pack of 10 cartons.

Instructions for use/handling:

Handling: As with all antineoplastic agents, caution should be exercised when handling Taxol. Dilution should be carried out under aseptic conditions by trained personnel in a designated area. Adequate protective gloves should be worn. Precautions should be taken to avoid contact with the skin and mucous membranes. In the event of contact with the skin, the area should be washed with soap and water. Following topical exposure, tingling, burning and redness have been observed. In the event of contact with the mucous membranes, these should be flushed thoroughly with water. Upon inhalation, dyspnea, chest pain, burning throat and nausea have been reported.

The Chemo-Dispensing Pin device or similar devices with spikes should not be used since they can cause the vial stopper to collapse, resulting in loss of sterile integrity.

Preparation for IV administration: Prior to infusion, Taxol must be diluted, using aseptic techniques, in 0.9% Sodium Chloride Injection, or 5% Dextrose Injection, or 5% Dextrose and 0.9% Sodium Chloride Injection, or 5% Dextrose in Ringer's Injection, to a final concentration of 0.3 to 1.2 mg/mL. The prepared solutions are physically and chemically stable for up to 27 hours (including preparation and administration) at ambient temperature (approximately 25°C) and room lighting conditions. Diluted solutions should not be refrigerated.

Upon preparation, solutions may show haziness, which is attributed to the formulation vehicle, and is not removed by filtration. Taxol should be administered through an in-line filter with a microporous membrane ≤0.22μm. No significant losses in potency have been noted following simulated delivery of the solution through IV tubing containing an in-line filter.

To minimize patient exposure to DEHP, which may be leached from plasticized PVC infusion bags, sets, or other medical instruments, diluted Taxol solutions should be stored in non-PVC bottles (glass, polypropylene) or plastic bags (polypropylene, polyolefin) and administered through polyethylene-lined administration sets. Use of filter devices (eg. IVEX-2®) which incorporate short inlet and/or outlet plasticized PVC tubing has not resulted in significant leaching of DEHP.

There have been rare reports of precipitation during Taxol infusions, usually towards the end of a 24 hour infusion period. Although the cause of this precipitation has not been elucidated, it is probably linked to the supersaturation of the diluted solution. To reduce the precipitation risk, Taxol should be used as soon as possible after dilution and excessive agitation, vibration or shaking should be avoided. The infusion sets should be flushed thoroughly before use. During infusion the appearance of the solution should be inspected regularly and the infusion should be stopped if precipitation is present.

Disposal: All items used for preparation, administration or otherwise coming into contact with Taxol should undergo disposal according to local guidelines for the handling of cytotoxic compounds.

Marketing authorisation number(s)

PL 11184/0026 TAXOL
PL 11184/0058 TAXOL-100

Date of first authorisation/renewal of the authorisation

TAXOL 18 November 1993/20 September 1998
TAXOL-100 15 November 1996

Date of (partial) revision of text September 1998

VIDEX* TABLETS

Qualitative and quantitative composition Chewable/dispersible buffered tablets containing didanosine 25 mg, 100 mg and 150 mg.

Pharmaceutical form Tablets.

Clinical particulars

Therapeutic indications: Videx is indicated as part of a combination therapy for antiviral treatment of HIV infected patients.

Clinical benefit of Videx was demonstrated in several important clinical trials (see *Pharmacodynamic properties*).

Posology and method of administration: Because of reduced absorption in the presence of food, it is recommended that Videx be administered at least 30 minutes before a meal (see *Pharmacokinetic properties*). Although the optimal dose of Videx has not been finally established, the following recommendations can be made:

Dosage

Adults: The recommended starting dose is dependent

on weight; the dosing interval should be approximately 12 hours (BID). Doses up to 750 mg/day (sachet) or 600 mg/day (tablet) have been used in clinical trials. The recommended average starting doses are outlined in the table below.

ADULT DOSING GUIDELINES

Patient Baseline Weight	Videx tablets (*)
≥60 kg	200 mg BID
<60 kg	125 mg BID

(*) To ensure that patients receive a sufficient amount of antacid, each dose must be given as 2 tablets (eg 200 mg BID, or a total daily dose of 400 mg should be given as 2 doses of 2x100 mg tablets with approximately 12 hours between each dose).

Children: The recommended starting dose, based on body surface area, is 240 mg/m²/day (180 mg/m²/day in combination with ZDV). The recommended dosing interval is 12 hours.

Insufficient clinical experience exists to recommend a dosing regimen in infants under 3 months of age.

Dose adjustment: Significant elevations of serum amylase should prompt discontinuation of therapy and careful evaluation of the possibility of pancreatitis, even in the absence of symptoms of pancreatitis. Fractionation of amylase may help distinguish amylase of salivary origin. Only after pancreatitis has been ruled out or after clinical and biological parameters have returned to normal, should dosing be resumed, and then only if treatment is considered essential. Treatment should be re-initiated with low doses and increased slowly, if appropriate.

Many patients who present with symptoms of neuropathy and who experience resolution of symptoms upon drug discontinuation will tolerate a reduced dose of Videx.

Renal impairment: The following dosages are recommended:

Videx dose adjustment in renal impairment

Patient Weight	≥60 kg		<60 kg
Creatinine Clearance (mL/min)	*Tablet(*)*	*Tablet(*)*	*Dosing Frequency*
≥60	200 mg	125 mg	BID
30-59	100 mg	75 mg	BID
10-29	150 mg	100 mg	once daily
<10	100 mg	75 mg	once daily

(*) to ensure that patients receive a sufficient amount of antacid, each dose must be given as 2 tablets (eg. 200 mg BID, or a total daily dose of 400 mg should be given as 2 doses of 2 x 100 mg tablets with approximately 12 hours between each dose).

The dose should preferably be administered after dialysis (see *Special warnings and special precautions for use*). However, it is not necessary to administer a supplemental dose of Videx following haemodialysis.

Children: Since urinary excretion is also a major route of elimination of didanosine in children, the clearance of didanosine may be altered in children with renal impairment. Although there are insufficient data to recommend a specific dosage adjustment of Videx in this patient population, a reduction in the dose and/or an increase in the interval between doses should be considered.

Hepatic impairment: There are insufficient data to recommend a specific dose adjustment of Videx in patients with hepatic impairment, but an adjustment in the dose in these patients should also be considered (see *Special warnings and special precautions for use*).

Contra-indications: Videx is contraindicated in patients with hypersensitivity to any of the components of the formulations.

Special warnings and special precautions for use:
Pancreatitis: Is a known serious complication among HIV-infected patients. It has also been associated with Videx therapy and has been fatal in some cases. Videx should be used only with extreme caution in patients with a history of pancreatitis. Positive relationships have been found between the risk of pancreatitis and daily dose.

Whenever warranted by clinical conditions, Videx dosing should be suspended until the diagnosis of pancreatitis is excluded by appropriate laboratory and imaging techniques. Similarly, when treatment with other drugs known to cause pancreatic toxicity is required (e.g. i.v. pentamidine), didanosine should be suspended during therapy wherever possible. If concomitant therapy is unavoidable there should be close observation. Dose suspension should also be considered when biochemical markers of pancreatitis have increased to a clinically significant degree above the upper limit of normal, even in the absence of symptoms. Significant elevations of triglycerides are a known cause of pancreatitis and warrant close observation.

Peripheral neuropathy: Patients on Videx may develop toxic peripheral neuropathy, usually characterized by bilateral symmetrical distal numbness, tingling, and pain in feet and, less frequently, hands. Whenever warranted by clinical conditions, Videx therapy should be suspended until resolution of symptoms. Many patients tolerate a reduced dose after resolution of symptoms.

Hyperuricaemia: Videx has been associated with hyperuricaemia. Treatment should be suspended if significant elevations in uric acid levels occur during treatment.

Liver failure of unknown etiology: Has occurred rarely in patients on Videx. Patients should be observed for liver enzyme elevations and Videx should be suspended if enzymes rise to a clinically significant level above the upper limit of normal. Rechallenge should be considered only if the potential benefits of Videx treatment clearly outweigh the potential risks for the individual patient

Paediatric patients on Videx therapy have demonstrated **retinal or optic nerve changes** on rare occasions, particularly at doses above those recommended. There have been reports of retinal depigmentation in adult patients. Especially for children, periodic dilated retinal examinations (every 6 months), or if a change in vision occurs, should be considered.

Lactic acidosis: Occurrences of lactic acidosis (in the absence of hypoxia), usually associated with severe hepatomegaly and hepatic steatosis have been reported with the use of nucleoside analogues. Treatment with nucleoside analogues should be discontinued in the setting of rapidly elevating aminotransferase levels, progressive hepatomegaly or metabolic/lactic acidosis of unknown etiology. Caution should be exercised when administering nucleoside analogues to any patient (particularly obese women) with hepatomegaly, hepatitis or other known risk factors for liver disease. These patients should be followed closely.

Insufficient clinical experience exists to recommend a dosing regimen in infants under 3 months of age.

Patients receiving Videx or any antiretroviral therapy may continue to develop opportunistic infections and other complications of HIV infection or therapy. They therefore should remain under close clinical observation by physicians experienced in the treatment of patients with HIV associated diseases. To carry out the treatment in an appropriate way, one needs access to appropriate equipment, e.g., the possibility to carry out special laboratory tests including the necessary controls of T4-lymphocytes and biochemical markers of pancreatitis.

Renal impairment: The half-life of didanosine after oral administration increased from an average of 1.4 hours in subjects with normal renal function to 4.1 hours in subjects with severe renal impairment requiring dialysis. After an oral dose, didanosine was not detectable in peritoneal dialysis fluid; recovery in hemodialysate ranged from 0.6 to 7.4% of the dose over a 3-4 hour dialysis period. Patients with a creatinine clearance <60 mL/min may be at greater risk of Videx toxicity due to decreased drug clearance. A dose reduction is recommended for these patients (see *Posology and method of administration*). Further, the magnesium content of each Videx tablet is 8.7 mEq which may represent an excessive load of magnesium to patients with significant renal impairment.

Hepatic impairment: No significant changes in the pharmacokinetics of didanosine were observed among hemophiliac patients with chronic, persistent elevations in liver function enzymes, which may be indicative of impaired hepatic function; hemophiliac patients with normal or less severe increases in liver function enzymes; and non-hemophiliac patients with normal enzyme levels following a single IV or oral dose. The metabolism of didanosine may, however, be altered in patients with more severe or other forms of hepatic impairment; an adjustment of the dose should also be considered (see *Posology and method of administration*).

Phenylketonurics: Videx tablets contain 36.5 mg phenylalanine (from the aspartame). Therefore, the use of Videx in phenylketonuria patients should be considered only if clearly indicated.

Patients on sodium-restricted diets: Videx tablets do not contain Sodium

Interaction with other medicinal products and other forms of interaction: Combination studies of Videx (up to 500 mg/day) and zidovudine (ZDV) (up to 600 mg/day) have not revealed any unexpected toxicities.

Specific drug interaction studies have been conducted with zidovudine, stavudine, ranitidine, loperamide, metoclopramide, foscarnet, trimethoprim, sulfamethoxazole, dapsone and rifabutin without evidence of interaction. Based upon the results from a study with ketoconazole, it is recommended that drugs which can be affected by stomach acidity (eg. oral azoles such as ketoconazole and itraconazole), be given at least 2 hours prior to dosing with Videx.

Administration of Videx 2 hours prior to, or concurrent with, ganciclovir was associated with a mean increase of 111% in the steady state AUC for didanosine. A minor decrease (21%) in the steady state AUC of ganciclovir was seen when Videx was given 2 hours prior to ganciclovir, but not when both drugs were given simultaneously. There were no changes in renal clearance for either drug. It is not known whether these changes are associated with alterations in either the safety of Videx or the efficacy of ganciclovir. There is no evidence that Videx potentiates the myelosuppressive effects of ganciclovir or zidovudine.

Coadministration of Videx with drugs that are known to cause peripheral neuropathy or pancreatitis may increase the risk of these toxicities. Patients who receive these drugs should be carefully observed.

As with other products containing aluminum and/or magnesium antacid components, Videx tablets should not be taken with any tetracycline antibiotic. Likewise, plasma concentrations of some quinolone antibiotics (eg. ciprofloxacin) are decreased by administration with antacids contained in or adminstered with Videx. It is recommended that drugs that may interact with antacids should not be administered within 2 hours of taking Videx tablets.

Ingestion of Videx with food reduces the amount of didanosine absorbed by approximately 50% (see *Pharmacokinetic properties*)

Pregnancy and lactation
Pregnancy: There are no adequate and well-controlled studies in pregnant women and it is not known whether didanosine can cause foetal harm or affect reproductive capacity when administered during pregnancy. Therefore, the use of Videx during pregnancy should be considered only if clearly indicated, and only when the potential benefit outweighs the possible risk.

Teratology studies in rats and rabbits did not produce evidence of embryotoxic, foetotoxic, or teratogenic effects. A study in rats showed that didanosine and/or its metabolites are transferred to the foetus through the placenta.

Lactation: It is not known whether didanosine is excreted in human milk. It is recommended that women taking Videx do not breast-feed because of the potential for serious adverse reactions from didanosine in nursing infants.

At the 1000 mg/kg/day dose levels in rats, didanosine was slightly toxic to females and pups during mid and late lactation (reduced food intake and body weight gains), but the physical and functional development of the subsequent offsprings were not impaired. A further study showed that, following oral administration, didanosine and/or its metabolites were excreted into the milk of lactating rats.

Reproduction: In rats, didanosine did not impair the reproduction ability of male or female parents following treatment prior to and during mating, gestation and lactation at daily didanosine doses up to 1000 mg/kg/day. In a perinatal and postnatal reproduction study in rats, didanosine did not induce toxic effects.

Effects on ability to drive and use machines: At present, no data are known regarding these effects.

Undesirable effects
Adults: Most of the serious adverse events observed have generally reflected the recognized clinical course of AIDS and HIV infection. Concurrent dosing with a variety of drugs was allowed in the studies. Therefore, it is difficult to distinguish which events are related to Videx, to the disease itself, or to other therapy-related events.

Clinically significant undesirable effects reported in controlled clinical studies which may be possibly related to treatment with Videx at the recommended dose include pancreatitis and elevations in serum amylase and lipase levels. Pancreatitis, which may be fatal in some cases, was more frequent in patients who were treated with doses above those recommended; patients with advanced HIV disease or a history of pancreatitis may also be at increased risk of developing pancreatitis. Peripheral neuropathy has been associated with Videx therapy. Abnormal liver function tests, with rare reports of liver failure and death have also been reported. Events of less clinical importance which may possibly be associated with Videx treatment include diarrhoea, nausea/vomiting, allergic reactions, diabetes mellitus, dry mouth and elevated uric acid levels. Retinal or optic nerve changes have been reported rarely. Leukopenia, thrombocytopenia, anaemia were reported at significantly lower incidence than with ZDV, and the relationship with Videx treatment has not been established.

Cases of lactic acidosis (in the absence of hypoxemia), usually associated with severe hepatomegaly and hepatic steatosis have been reported with the use of nucleoside analogues.

Children: Undesirable effects were generally similar to those seen in adults. A higher incidence of haematotoxicity has been reported in patients treated with the combination with ZDV compared with Videx monotherapy. Retinal or optic nerve changes have been reported in a small number of paediatric patients usually at doses above those recommended. It is recommended that children on Videx treatment undergo dilated retinal examination every 6 months or if a change in vision occurs.

Overdose: There is no known antidote for didanosine overdosage. Experience in early studies, in which didanosine was initially administered at doses ten times the recommended doses indicates that the anticipated complications of overdosage would be secondary to hyperuricaemia or, possibly, to hepatic dysfunction.

Didanosine is not dialyzable by peritoneal dialysis, although there is some clearance by hemodialysis. (The fractional removal of didanosine during an average hemodialysis session of 3 to 4 hours was approximately 20-35% of the dose present in the body at the start of dialysis.)

Pharmacological properties

Pharmacodynamic properties: Didanosine (2′,3′-dideoxyinosine) is an inhibitor of the *in vitro* replication of HIV in cultured human cells and cell lines. After didanosine enters the cell, it is enzymatically converted to dideoxyadenosine-triphosphate (ddATP), its active metabolite. In viral nucleic acid replication, incorporation of this 2′-3′-dideoxynucleoside prevents chain extension, and thereby inhibits viral replication.

In addition, ddATP inhibits HIV-reverse transcriptase by competing with dATP for binding to the enzyme's active site, preventing proviral DNA synthesis.

The relationship between *in vitro* susceptibility of HIV to didanosine, and clinical response to therapy has not been established. Likewise, *in vitro* sensitivity results vary greatly and methods to establish virologic responses have not been proven.

The effect of Videx, alone or in combination with ZDV (zidovudine), was evaluated in several major randomized, controlled clinical trials (ACTG 175, ACTG 152, DELTA, CPCRA 007). These trials confirmed the reduced risk of HIV disease progression or death with Videx therapy, alone or in combination with ZDV, as compared with ZDV monotherapy in HIV-infected individuals, including symptomatic and asymptomatic adults with CD4 counts < 500 cells/mm³ and children with evidence of immunosuppression. The clinical benefits of initial Videx therapy were demonstrated in adults with CD4 counts 200-500 cells/mm³, as well as in children. The ACTG 175 trial showed that eight weeks of treatment with ZDV, Videx, or Videx plus ZDV decreased mean plasma HIV RNA by 0.26, 0.65 and 0.93 $\log_{10}$ copies /mL, respectively.

Pharmacokinetic properties

Adults: Didanosine is rapidly degraded at an acidic pH. Therefore, all oral formulations must contain buffering agents designed to increase gastric pH. The administration of didanosine with a meal results in a significant decrease in bioavailability. This decrease is about 50 % with the tablet. All Videx formulations should be administered at least 30 minutes before a meal. A study in 10 asymptomatic HIV seropositive patients demonstrated that administration of Videx tablets 30 min to 1 hr before a meal did not result in any significant changes in the bioavailability of didanosine compared to administration under fasting conditions. Administration of the tablets 1 to 2 hr after a meal was associated with a 55% decrease in CMAX and AUC values, which was comparable to the decrease observed when the formulation was given immediately after a meal.

The volume of distribution at steady state averages 54 L, suggesting that there is some uptake of didanosine by body tissues.

The level of didanosine in the cerebrospinal fluid (CSF), one hour after infusion, averages 21% of that of the simultaneous plasma level.

The average elimination half-life after intravenous administration of didanosine is approximately 1.4 hours. Renal clearance represents 50% of total body clearance (800 mL/min), indicating that active tubular secretion, in addition to glomerular filtration, is responsible for the renal elimination of didanosine.

Urinary recovery of didanosine is approximately 20% of the dose after oral treatment. There is no evidence of didanosine accumulation after the administration of oral doses for 4 weeks.

Children: Variability in the amount of didanosine (non-buffered Videx powder reconstituted with water and antacid) absorbed in children is greater than in adults. The absolute bioavailability of didanosine administered orally was approximately 36% after the first dose and 47% at steady state.

The CSF didanosine level averages 46% of that of the simultaneous plasma level after intravenous administration of doses of 60 or 90 mg/m² and equivalent oral doses of 120 or 180 mg/m². Measurable concentrations of didanosine in the CSF were detectable for up to 3.5 hours after dosing.

The average elimination half-life after intravenous didanosine administration is approximately 0.8 hours. Renal clearance represents approximately 59% of the total body clearance (315 mL/min/m²), indicating that both renal and nonrenal pathways are involved in the elimination.

Urinary recovery of didanosine is approximately 17% of dose after oral treatment.

There is no evidence of didanosine accumulation after oral administration for an average of 26 days. The metabolism of didanosine in man has not been evaluated. However, based on animal studies, it is presumed that it follows the same pathways responsible for the elimination of endogenous purines.

In vitro human plasma protein binding is less than 5% with didanosine, indicating that drug interactions involving binding site displacement are not anticipated.

There are currently incomplete data concerning the effect of impaired renal or hepatic function on the pharmacokinetics of didanosine.

Preclinical safety data: The lowest dose to cause death in acute toxicity studies in the mouse, rat and dog was greater than 2000 mg/kg which is equivalent to approximately 300 times the maximum recommended human dose of the tablet formulation. Repeat-dose oral toxicity studies revealed evidence of a dose-limiting skeletal muscle toxicity in rodents (but not in dogs) following long-term (> 90 days) dosing with didanosine at doses that were approximately 1.2–12 times the estimated human dose. Additionally, in repeat dose studies, leucopenia was observed in dogs and rats, and gastrointestinal disturbances (soft stool, diarrhoea) were seen in dogs at doses approximately 5–14 times the maximum human dose. In the carcinogenicity studies, non-neoplastic alterations have been observed including skeletal muscle myopathy, hepatic alterations and an exacerbation of spontaneous age-related cardiomyopathy. Results from the genotoxicity studies suggest that didanosine is not mutagenic at biologically and pharmacologically relevant doses. At significantly elevated concentrations *in vitro*, the genotoxic effects of didanosine are similar in magnitude to those seen with natural DNA nucleosides. Lifetime dietary carcinogenicity studies were conducted in mice and rats for 22 or 24 months, respectively. No drug-related neoplasms were observed in any didanosine-treated groups of mice during, or at the end of, the dosing period. In rats, statistically significant increased incidences of granulosa cell tumors in females receiving the high dose, of subcutaneous fibrosarcomas and histiocytic sarcomas in males receiving the high dose and of hemangiomas in males receiving the high and intermediate dose of didanosine were noted. The drug-relationship and clinical relevance of these statistical findings were not clear.

Pharmaceutical particulars

List of excipients: Aspartame, calcium carbonate, crospovidone, magnesium hydroxide, magnesium stearate, mandarin orange flavour, microcrystalline cellulose, sorbitol.

Incompatibilities: None.

Shelf life: 24 months at room temperature (15°-30°C). If dispersed in water, the dose may be held for up to 1 hour at 15°-30°C.

Special precautions for storage: Store in tightly closed bottles at 15°-30°C.

Nature and contents of container: High-density polyethylene bottle with child-resistant cap (60 tablets per bottle).

Instructions for use/handling:

Method of preparation:

Adults: Patients should take two tablets in each dose, to provide sufficient antacid against acid degradation of didanosine. The tablets should be thoroughly chewed, or crushed, or dispersed in at least 30 mL of water prior to consumption. To disperse tablets, stir until a uniform dispersion forms, and drink the entire dispersion immediately. If additional flavouring is desired, the dispersion may be diluted with 30 mL of clear apple juice.

Stir the further dispersion just prior to consumption. The dispersion with clear apple juice is stable at room temperature for up to one hour.

Children: Children older than 1 year of age should receive a 2-tablet dose, children under 1 year should receive a 1-tablet dose. Tablets should be chewed, or crushed, or dispersed in water prior to consumption, as described in the preceding Adult Dosing Method of Preparation. When a one tablet dose is required, the volume of water for dispersion should be 15 mL. Fifteen mL of clear apple juice may be added to the dispersion as a flavouring.

Marketing authorisation numbers

25 mg: PL 11184/0008
100 mg: PL 11184/0010
150 mg: PL 11184/0011

Date of first authorisation/renewal of authorisation 17th February 1994

Date of (partial) revision of text 7th January 1998

ZERIT* ▼

Qualitative and quantitative composition Capsules each containing stavudine 15 mg, 20 mg, 30 mg or 40 mg.

Pharaceutical form Capsules.

Clinical particulars

Therapeutic indications: Treatment of HIV-infected adults and children with progressive or advanced immunodeficiency (for combination use, see *Pharmacodynamic properties*).

Posology and method of administration:

Adults: the recommended starting dosage is:

Patient weight	*Zerit dosage*
<60 kg	30 mg twice daily (every 12 hours)
≥60 kg	40 mg twice daily

Children over the age of 3 months: The recommended starting dosage is:

Patient weight	*Zerit dosage*
<30 kg	1 mg/kg twice daily (every 12 hours)
≥30 kg	adult dosing

For optimal absorption, Zerit should be taken on an empty stomach (i.e. at least 1 hour prior to meals) but, if this is not possible, it may be taken with a light meal. Zerit may also be administered by carefully opening the capsule and mixing the contents with food (see *Pharmacokinetic properties*).

The therapy should be initiated by a doctor experienced in the management of HIV infection.

Dose adjustments

Peripheral neuropathy: Is usually characterised by persistent numbness, tingling, or pain in the feet and/or hands. If these symptoms develop, Zerit therapy should be interrupted. Stavudine-related peripheral neuropathy should resolve if therapy is withdrawn promptly although some patients may experience a temporary worsening of symptoms following discontinuation. If symptoms resolve satisfactorily, resumption of treatment with Zerit at 50% of the previous dosage may be considered.

Clinically significant elevations of hepatic transaminase: (ALT/AST, > 5 x upper limit of normal, ULN) should be managed in the same way as peripheral neuropathy.

Hepatic impairment: No initial dosage adjustment is necessary.

Renal impairment: The following dosages are recommended:

Patient weight	*Zerit dosage (according to creatinine clearance)*	
	26-50 mL/min	≤25 mL/min (including dialysis dependence*)
<60 kg	15 mg twice daily	15 mg every 24 hours
≥60 kg	20 mg twice daily	20 mg every 24 hours

* Patients on haemodialysis should take Zerit after the completion of haemodialysis, and at the same time on non-dialysis days.

Contra-indications: Zerit is contraindicated in patients with hypersensitivity to stavudine or to any of the excipients (see *List of excipients*).

Special warnings and special precautions for use: Patients with a history of peripheral neuropathy are at increased risk for development of neuropathy. If Zerit must be administered in this setting, careful monitoring is essential.

Patients with a history of pancreatitis had an incidence of approximately 5% on Zerit, as compared to approximately 2% in patients without such a history. Patients with a high risk of pancreatitis or those receiving products known to be associated with pancreatitis should be closely followed for symptoms of this condition.

Clinically significant elevations of ALT and AST may require dose modifications (see *Posology and method of administration*).

Lactic acidosis: Occurrences of lactic acidosis (in the absence of hypoxemia), usually associated with severe hepatomegaly and hepatic steatosis have been reported with the use of nucleoside analogues.

Treatment with nucleoside analogues should be discontinued in the setting of rapidly elevating aminotransferase levels, progressive hepatomegaly or metabolic/lactic acidosis of unknown etiology.

Caution should be exercised when administering nucleoside analogues to any patient (particularly obese women) with hepatomegaly, hepatitis or other known risk factors for liver disease. These patients should be followed closely.

Elderly: Zerit has not been specifically investigated in patients over the age of 65.

Children under the age of 3 months: There is insufficient documentation on the use of Zerit in children under the age of 3 months.

Lactose intolerance: The capsules contain lactose;
120 mg in the 15 mg strength
182 mg in the 20 mg and 30 mg strength
238 in the 40 mg strength

These quantities are probably not sufficient to induce specific symptoms of intolerance.

***Pneumocystis carinii* pneumonia (PCP) prophylaxis:** in the main clinical trial, the incidence of PCP among patients not receiving sulfamethoxazole-trimethoprim prophylaxis was greater in the stavudine group than in the zidovudine group. For patients on stavudine therapy, sulfamethoxazole-trimethoprim is the agent of choice when PCP-prophylaxis is warranted.

Interaction with other medicinal products and other forms of interaction: Since stavudine is actively secreted by the renal tubules, interactions with other actively secreted drugs are possible.

Zidovudine may inhibit the intracellular phosphorylation of stavudine. Zidovudine is therefore not recommended to be used in combination with stavudine. The activation of stavudine has also been shown to be inhibited by doxorubicin, but not by other drugs used in HIV-infection and which are similarly phosphorylated, eg. didanosine, zalcitabine, ganciclovir and foscarnet.

Use during pregnancy and lactation: Embryo-foetal toxicities were seen only at high exposure levels in animals. Clinical experience in pregnant women is lacking. Until additional data become available, Zerit should be given during pregnancy only after special consideration.

An *ex vivo* study using a term human placenta model demonstrated that stavudine reaches the foetal circulation by simple diffusion. A rat study also showed placental transfer of stavudine, with the foetal tissue concentration approximately 50% of the maternal plasma concentration.

The data available on stavudine excretion into human breast milk are insufficient to assess the risk to the child. Studies in lactating rats showed that stavudine is excreted in breast milk. Therefore, mothers should be instructed to discontinue breast feeding prior to receiving Zerit. Some health experts recommend that HIV-infected women should not breast feed their infants under any circumstances in order to avoid transmission of HIV.

Effects on ability to drive and use machines: There is no indication that Zerit affects this ability.

Undesirable effects
Adults: Many of the serious undesirable effects reported in clinical trials with Zerit are consistent with the course of HIV-infection, or with the side effects of concomitant therapies.

The major clinical toxicity is dose-related peripheral neuropathy requiring dose modification (see *Posology and method of administration*). The yearly rate of neuropathy in an expanded access programme of approximately 12,000 patients with advanced HIV disease (median CD4: 44 cells/mm³) and prolonged prior treatment with other antiretroviral nucleosides was 24% and 19% for patients receiving 40 or 20 mg twice daily, respectively. The intensity of this complaint was usually mild and patients usually experienced resolution of symptoms after dose reduction or interruption. The 24-week rates of therapy discontinuation due to neuropathy in this population were 13% and 10% for the two doses, respectively.

In a comparative trial involving patients with less advanced HIV-infection (median CD4: 250 cells/mm³), after a median duration of 79 weeks on Zerit treatment versus 53 weeks on zidovudine, asymptomatic elevations of AST and ALT (≤ 5 times ULN) were observed while receiving Zerit. Yearly rates of peripheral neuropathy in this comparative trial were 12% for Zerit and 4% for zidovudine.

Cases of lactic acidosis, usually associated with severe hepatomegaly and hepatic steatosis, have been reported with the use of nucleoside analogues.

Pancreatitis, occasionally fatal, has been reported in up to 2-3% of patients enrolled in the clinical studies.

Other undesirable effects reported from >5% of patients in the zidovudine-comparative trial which are considered potential adverse reactions included: headache, chills/fever, malaise, diarrhoea, constipation, dyspepsia, asthenia, anorexia, nausea/ vomiting, pneumonia, pain, chest-, abdominal-, and back-pain, myalgia, arthralgia, insomnia, depression, anxiety, flu syndrome, sweating, dizziness, dyspnoea, allergic reaction, rash, maculopapular rash, pruritus, benign skin neoplasms, peripheral neurologic symptoms, neuropathy, lymphadenopathy, and neoplasms.

Abnormalities of laboratory tests in the same trial were infrequent. Clinically significant elevations of ALT and AST were reported in 13% and 11% of Zerit recipients, respectively, and in 11% and 10% of zidovudine recipients, respectively. Alkaline phosphatase >5 times ULN, and bilirubin >2.5 times ULN each were reported in 1% of Zerit recipients and in 0% and 3% of zidovudine recipients, respectively. Neutropenia (<750 cells/mm³) was reported in 5% and 9%, thrombocytopenia (platelets <50,000/mm³) in 3% of Zerit and zidovudine recipients, amylase (>1.0 times ULN) in 23% and 22% of Zerit and zidovudine recipients, respectively.

Children: Undesirable effects and serious laboratory abnormalities were generally similar in type and frequency to those seen in adults. However, clinically significant peripheral neuropathy is less frequent.

Overdose: Experience in adults treated with up to 12 times the recommended daily dosage revealed no acute toxicity. Complications of chronic overdosage could include peripheral neuropathy and hepatic dysfunction. The mean haemodialysis clearance of stavudine is 120 mL/min. The contribution of this to the total elimination in an overdose situation is unknown. It is not known whether stavudine is removed by peritoneal dialysis.

Pharmacological properties
Pharmacodynamic properties: Pharmaco-therapeutic group: antiviral agent, ATC code J05AX04.

Stavudine, a thymidine analog, is an antiviral agent with *in vitro* activity against HIV in human cells. It is phosphorylated by cellular kinases to stavudine triphosphate which inhibits HIV reverse transcriptase by competing with the natural substrate, thymidine triphosphate. It also inhibits viral DNA synthesis by causing DNA chain termination.

HIV-1 strains with reduced sensitivity to stavudine have been isolated following *in vitro* passage, and in some post-treatment patient isolates. However, few data are available addressing the development of HIV-resistance to stavudine *in vivo*, or the development of cross-resistance to other nucleoside analogues.

Efficacy of stavudine monotherapy in terms of reduced incidence of AIDS defining events and death has been demonstrated in adult patients after prolonged zidovudine monotherapy. In children, the safety profile of stavudine monotherapy is adequately documented in treatment-naive subjects. The safe use in previously treated children is supported by non-comparative data indicating acceptable tolerance. Stavudine has been studied in combination with other antiretroviral agents, eg. didanosine, lamivudine, ritonavir, indinavir, saquinavir and nelfinavir. No new or overt safety problems have been reported for these combinations, but clinical experience is still rather limited. Zidovudine is not recommended to be used in combination with stavudine (see *Interactions with other medicinal products and other forms of interaction*).

Pharmacokinetic properties
Adults: The absolute bioavailability is 86±18%. After multiple oral administration of 0.5–0.67 mg/kg doses, a Cmax value of 810±175 ng/mL was obtained. Cmax and AUC increased proportionally with dose in the dose ranges, i.v. 0.0625–0.75 mg/kg, and oral 0.033–4.0 mg/kg.

A study in asymptomatic patients demonstrated that systemic exposure is similar while Cmax is lower and Tmax is prolonged when stavudine is administered with a standardised, high-fat meal compared with fasting conditions. The clinical significance of this is unknown.

The apparent volume of distribution at steady state is 46±15 L. Cerebrospinal fluid (CSF) levels of stavudine were not possible to detect until at least 2 hours after oral administration. Four hours after administration the CSF/plasma ratio was 0.39±0.06. No significant accumulation of stavudine is observed with repeated administration every 6, 8, or 12 hours.

The terminal elimination half-life is 1.3±0.2 hours after a single dose, and 1.4±0.2 hours after multiple doses, and is independent of dose. *In vitro*, stavudine triphosphate has an intracellular half-life of 3.5 hours in CEM T-cells (a human T-lymphoblastoid cell line) and peripheral blood mononuclear cells, supporting twice daily dosing.

Total clearance of stavudine is 600±90 mL/min, and renal clearance is 240±50 mL/min, indicating active tubular secretion in addition to glomerular filtration. After i.v. administration, 42±7% of dose is excreted unchanged in the urine. The corresponding values after oral single and multiple dose administration are 34±5% and 40±12%, respectively. The remaining 60% of the drug is presumably eliminated by endogenous pathways.

The metabolism of stavudine has not been elucidated in humans. Studies in monkeys indicate that the majority of the dose that is not excreted unchanged in the urine (approximately 50%) is hydrolysed to thymine and sugar.

The pharmacokinetics of stavudine was independent of time, since the ratio between AUC(ss) at steady state and the AUC(0-t) after the first dose was approximately 1. Intra- and interindividual variation in pharmacokinetic characteristics of stavudine is low, approximately 15% and 25%, respectively, after oral administration.

Children: stavudine pharmacokinetics in children are comparable to those in adults. Stavudine clearance is related to both body surface area and body weight. Total exposure to stavudine was comparable between children receiving the 2 mg/kg/day dose and adults receiving 1 mg/kg/day. Two to 3 hours post-dose, CSF/plasma ratios of stavudine ranged from 16% to 125% (mean of 59%±35%).

Renal impairment: The clearance of stavudine decreases as creatinine clearance decreases; therefore, it is recommended that the dosage of Zerit be adjusted in patients with reduced renal function (see *Posology and method of administration*).

Hepatic impairment: Stavudine pharmacokinetics in patients with hepatic impairment were similar to those in patients with normal hepatic function.

Preclinical safety data: Animal data showed embryo-foetal toxicity at very high exposure levels. Stavudine was genotoxic in *in vitro* tests in human lymphocytes possessing triphosphorylating activity (in which no no-effect level was established), in mouse fibroblasts, and in an *in vivo* test for chromosomal aberrations. Similar effects have been observed with other nucleoside analogues.

Stavudine was carcinogenic in mice (liver tumours) and rats (liver tumours: cholangiocellular, hepatocellular, mixed hepatocholangiocellular, and/ or vascular; and urinary bladder carcinomas) at very high exposure levels. No carcinogenicity was noted at doses of 400 mg/kg/day in mice and 600 mg/kg/day in rats, corresponding to exposures ~39 and 168 times the expected human exposure, respectively, suggesting an insignificant carcinogenic potential of stavudine in clinical therapy.

Pharmaceutical particulars
List of excipients: Lactose, magnesium stearate, microcrystalline cellulose and sodium starch glycolate. The capsule shell is composed of gelatin, iron oxide colorant (E172), silicon dioxide, sodium lauryl sulphate and titanium dioxide colorant (E171). The capsules are marked using edible printing ink.

Incompatibilities: None.

Shelf-life: 24 months between 15°C and 30°C.

Special precautions for storage: Store at 15°C to 30°C.

Nature and content of container: Aclar/aluminum blisters with 14 capsules per card and 4 cards (56 capsules) per carton.

Marketing authorisation holder: Bristol-Myers Squibb Pharma EEIG, Swakeleys House, Milton Road, Ickenham UB10 8PU, United Kingdom

Numbers in the community register of medicinal products

Capsule 15 mg	Blister pack of 56	EU/1/96/009/002
Capsule 20 mg	Blister pack of 56	EU/1/96/009/004
Capsule 30 mg	Blister pack of 56	EU/1/96/009/006
Capsule 40 mg	Blister pack of 56	EU/1/96/009/008

Date of first authorisation/renewal of the authorisation 8 MAY 1996

Date of revision of text 21 November 1997

ZERIT* POWDER FOR ORAL SOLUTION ▼

Qualitative and quantitative composition Powder for oral solution containing 1 mg of stavudine per mL of constituted solution (200 mL per bottle).

Pharmaceutical form: Powder for oral solution.

Clincial particulars
Therapeutic indications: Treatment of HIV-infected adults and children with progressive or advanced immunodeficiency (for combination use, see *Pharmacodynamic properties*).

Posology and method of administration
Adults: the recommended starting dosage is:

Patient weight	*Zerit dosage*
<60 kg	30 mg twice daily (every 12 hours)
≥60 kg	40 mg twice daily

Children over the age of 3 months: the recommended starting dosage is:

Patient weight	*Zerit dosage*
<30 kg	1 mg/kg twice daily (every 12 hours)
≥30 kg	adult dosing

For optimal absorption, Zerit should be taken on an empty stomach (i.e. at least 1 hour prior to meals) but, if this is not possible, it may be taken with a light meal (see *Pharmacokinetic properties*).

The therapy should be initiated by a doctor experienced in the management of HIV infection.

Dose adjustments
Peripheral neuropathy: Is usually characterized by persistent numbness, tingling, or pain in the feet and/or hands. If these symptoms develop, Zerit therapy should be interrupted. Stavudine-related peripheral neuropathy should resolve if therapy is withdrawn promptly although some patients may experience a temporary worsening of symptoms following discontinuation. If symptoms resolve satisfactorily, resumption of treatment with Zerit® at 50% of the previous dosage may be considered.

Clinically significant elevations of hepatic transaminase: (ALT/AST, > 5 x upper limit of normal, ULN) should be managed in the same way as peripheral neuropathy.

Hepatic impairment: No initial dosage adjustment is necessary.

Renal impairment: The following dosages are recommended:

Patient weight	*Zerit dosage (according to creatinine clearance)* 26-50 mL/min	≤25 mL/min (including dialysis dependence*)
<60 kg	15 mg twice daily	15 mg every 24 hours
≥60 kg	20 mg twice daily	20 mg every 24 hours

* Patients on haemodialysis should take Zerit after the completion of haemodialysis, and at the same time on non-dialysis days.

Contra-indications: Zerit is contraindicated in patients with hypersensitivity to stavudine or to any of the excipients (see *List of excipients*).

Special warnings and special precautions for use: Patients with a history of peripheral neuropathy are at increased risk for development of neuropathy. If Zerit must be administered in this setting, careful monitoring is essential.

Patients with a history of pancreatitis had an incidence of approximately 5% on Zerit, as compared to approximately 2% in patients without such a history. Patients with a high risk of pancreatitis or those receiving products known to be associated with pancreatitis should be closely followed for symptoms of this condition.

Clinically significant elevations of ALT and AST may require dose modifications (see *Posology and method of administration*).

Lactic acidosis: Occurrences of lactic acidosis (in the absence of hypoxemia), usually associated with severe hepatomegaly and hepatic steatosis have been reported with the use of nucleoside analogues.

Treatment with nucleoside analogues should be discontinued in the setting of rapidly elevating aminotransferase levels, progressive hepatomegaly or metabolic/lactic acidosis of unknown etiology.

Caution should be exercised when administering nucleoside analogues to any patient (particularly obese women) with hepatomegaly, hepatitis or other known risk factors for liver disease. These patients should be followed closely.

Elderly: Zerit has not been specifically investigated in patients over the age of 65.

Children under the age of 3 months: There is insufficient documentation on the use of Zerit in children under the age of 3 months.

Diabetic patients: The constituted powder for oral solution contains 50 mg sucrose per mL of constituted solution.

***Pneumocystis carinii* pneumonia (PCP) prophylaxis:** In the main clinical trial, the incidence of PCP among patients not receiving sulfamethoxazole-trimethoprim prophylaxis was greater in the stavudine group than in the zidovudine group. For patients on stavudine therapy, sulfamethoxazole-trimethoprim is the agent of choice when PCP-prophylaxis is warranted.

Interaction with other medicinal products and other forms of interaction: Since stavudine is actively secreted by the renal tubules, interactions with other actively secreted drugs are possible.

Zidovudine may inhibit the intracellular phosphorylation of stavudine. Zidovudine is therefore not recommended to be used in combination with stavudine. The activation of stavudine has also been shown to be inhibited by doxorubicin, but not by other drugs used in HIV-infection and which are similarly phosphorylated, eg. didanosine, zalcitabine, ganciclovir and foscarnet.

Use during pregnancy and lactation: Embryo-foetal toxicities were seen only at high exposure levels in animals. Clinical experience in pregnant women is lacking. Until additional data become available, Zerit should be given during pregnancy only after special consideration.

An *ex vivo* study using a term human placenta model demonstrated that stavudine reaches the foetal circulation by simple diffusion. A rat study also showed placental transfer of stavudine, with the foetal tissue concentration approximately 50% of the maternal plasma concentration.

The data available on stavudine excretion into human breast milk are insufficient to assess the risk to the child. Studies in lactating rats showed that stavudine is excreted in breast milk. Therefore, mothers should be instructed to discontinue breast feeding prior to receiving Zerit. Some health experts recommend that HIV-infected women should not breast feed their infants under any circumstances in order to avoid transmission of HIV.

Effects on ability to drive and use machines: There is no indication that Zerit affects this ability.

Undesirable effects
Adults: Many of the serious undesirable effects reported in clinical trials with Zerit are consistent with the course of HIV-infection, or with the side effects of concomitant therapies.

The major clinical toxicity is dose-related peripheral neuropathy requiring dose modification (see *Posology and method of administration*). The yearly rate of neuropathy in an expanded access programme of approximately 12,000 patients with advanced HIV disease (median CD4: 44 cells/mm³) and prolonged prior treatment with other antiretroviral nucleosides was 24% and 19% for patients receiving 40 or 20 mg twice daily, respectively. The intensity of this complaint was usually mild and patients usually experienced resolution of symptoms after dose reduction or interruption. The 24-week rates of therapy discontinuation due to neuropathy in this population were 13% and 10% for the two doses, respectively.

In a comparative trial involving patients with less advanced HIV-infection (median CD4: 250 cells/mm³), after a median duration of 79 weeks on Zerit treatment versus 53 weeks on zidovudine, asymptomatic elevations of AST and ALT (≤5 times ULN) were observed while receiving Zerit Yearly rates of peripheral neuropathy in this comparative trial were 12% for Zerit and 4% for zidovudine.

Cases of lactic acidosis, usually associated with severe hepatomegaly and hepatic steatosis, have been reported with the use of nucleoside analogues.

Pancreatitis, occasionally fatal, has been reported in up to 2-3% of patients enrolled in the clinical studies. Other undesirable effects reported from >5% of patients in the zidovudine-comparative trial which are considered potential adverse reactions included: headache, chills/fever, malaise, diarrhoea, constipation, dyspepsia, asthenia, anorexia, nausea/vomiting, pneumonia, pain, chest-, abdominal-, and back-pain, myalgia, arthralgia, insomnia, depression, anxiety, flu syndrome, sweating, dizziness, dyspnoea, allergic reaction, rash, maculopapular rash, pruritus, benign skin neoplasms, peripheral neurologic symptoms, neuropathy, lymphadenopathy, and neoplasms.

Abnormalities of laboratory tests in the same trial were infrequent. Clinically significant elevations of ALT and AST were reported in 13% and 11% of Zerit recipients, respectively, and in 11% and 10% of zidovudine recipients, respectively. Alkaline phosphatase > 5 times ULN, and bilirubin >2.5 times ULN each were reported in 1% of Zerit recipients and in 0% and 3% of zidovudine recipients, respectively. Neutropenia (<750 cells/mm³) was reported in 5% and 9%, thrombocytopenia (platelets <50,000/mm³) in 3% of Zerit and zidovudine recipients, amylase (>1.0 times ULN) in 23% and 22% of Zerit and zidovudine recipients, respectively.

Children: Undesirable effects and serious laboratory abnormalities were generally similar in type and frequency to those seen in adults. However, clinically significant peripheral neuropathy is less frequent.

Overdose: Experience in adults treated with up to 12 times the recommended daily dosage revealed no acute toxicity. Complications of chronic overdosage could include peripheral neuropathy and hepatic dysfunction. The mean haemodialysis clearance of stavudine is 120 mL/min. The contribution of this to the total elimination in an overdose situation is unknown. It is not known whether stavudine is removed by peritoneal dialysis.

Pharmacological properties
Pharmacodynamic properties: Pharmacotherapeutic group: antiviral agent, ATC code J05AX04.

Stavudine, a thymidine analog, is an antiviral agent with *in vitro* activity against HIV in human cells. It is phosphorylated by cellular kinases to stavudine triphosphate which inhibits HIV reverse transcriptase by competing with the natural substrate, thymidine triphosphate. It also inhibits viral DNA synthesis by causing DNA chain termination.

HIV-1 strains with reduced sensitivity to stavudine have been isolated following *in vitro* passage, and in some post-treatment patient isolates. However, few data are available addressing the development of HIV-resistance to stavudine *in vivo*, or the development of cross-resistance to other nucleoside analogues.

Efficacy of stavudine monotherapy in terms of reduced incidence of AIDS defining events and death has been demonstrated in adult patients after prolonged zidovudine monotherapy. In children, the safety profile of stavudine monotherapy is adequately documented in treatment-naive subjects. The safe use in previously treated children is supported by non-comparative data indicating acceptable tolerance. Stavudine has been studied in combination with other antiretroviral agents, eg. didanosine, lamivudine, ritonavir, indinavir, saquinavir and nelfinavir. No new or overt safety problems have been reported for these combinations, but clinical experience is still rather limited. Zidovudine is not recommended to be used in combination with stavudine (see *Interaction with other medicinal products and other forms of interaction*).

Pharmacokinetic properties
Adults: The absolute bioavailability is 86 ± 18%. After multiple oral administration of 0.5–0.67 mg/kg doses, a Cmax value of 810±175 ng/mL was obtained. Cmax and AUC increased proportionally with dose in the dose ranges, i.v. 0.0625–0.75 mg/kg, and oral 0.033–4.0 mg/kg.

A study in asymptomatic patients demonstrated that systemic exposure is similar while Cmax is lower and Tmax is prolonged when stavudine is administered with a standardised, high-fat meal compared with fasting conditions. The clinical significance of this is unknown.

The apparent volume of distribution at steady state is 46±15 L. Cerebrospinal fluid (CSF) levels of stavudine were not possible to detect until at least 2 hours after oral administration. Four hours after administration the CSF/plasma ratio was 0.39±0.06. No significant accumulation of stavudine is observed with repeated administration every 6, 8, or 12 hours.

The terminal elimination half-life is 1.3±0.2 hours after a single dose, and 1.4±0.2 hours after multiple doses, and is independent of dose. *In vitro*, stavudine triphosphate has an intracellular half-life of 3.5 hours in CEM T-cells (a human T-lymphoblastoid cell line) and peripheral blood mononuclear cells, supporting twice daily dosing.

Total clearance of stavudine is 600±90 mL/min, and renal clearance is 240±50 mL/min, indicating active tubular secretion in addition to glomerular filtration. After i.v. administration, 42±7% of dose is excreted unchanged in the urine. The corresponding values after oral single and multiple dose administration are 34±5% and 40±12%, respectively. The remaining 60% of the drug is presumably eliminated by endogenous pathways.

The metabolism of stavudine has not been elucidated in humans. Studies in monkeys indicate that the majority of the dose that is not excreted unchanged in the urine (approximately 50%) is hydrolysed to thymine and sugar.

The pharmacokinetics of stavudine was independent of time, since the ratio between AUC(ss) at steady state and the AUC(0-t) after the first dose was approximately 1. Intra- and interindividual variation in pharmacokinetic characteristics of stavudine is low, approximately 15% and 25%, respectively, after oral administration.

Children: stavudine pharmacokinetics in children are comparable to those in adults. Stavudine clearance is related to both body surface area and body weight. Total exposure to stavudine was comparable between children receiving the 2 mg/kg/day dose and adults receiving 1 mg/kg/day. Two to 3 hours post-dose, CSF/plasma ratios of stavudine ranged from 16% to 125% (mean of 59%±35%).

Renal impairment: The clearance of stavudine decreases as creatinine clearance decreases; therefore, it is recommended that the dosage of Zerit be adjusted in patients with reduced renal function (see *Posology and method of administration*).

Hepatic impairment: Stavudine pharmacokinetics in patients with hepatic impairment were similar to those in patients with normal hepatic function.

Preclinical safety data: Animal data showed embryo-foetal toxicity at very high exposure levels. Stavudine was genotoxic in *in vitro* tests in human lymphocytes possessing triphosphorylating activity (in which no no-effect level was established), in mouse fibroblasts, and in an *in vivo* test for chromosomal aberrations. Similar effects have been observed with other nucleoside analogues.

Stavudine was carcinogenic in mice (liver tumours) and rats (liver tumours: cholangiocellular, hepatocellular, mixed hepatocholangiocellular, and/or vascular; and urinary bladder carcinomas) at very high exposure levels. No carcinogenicity was noted at doses of 400 mg/kg/day in mice and 600 mg/kg/day in rats, corresponding to exposures ~39 and 168 times the expected human exposure, respectively, suggesting an insignificant carcinogenic potential of stavudine in clinical therapy.

Pharmaceutical particulars

List of excipients: Cherry flavour, methylparaben, propylparaben, silicon dioxide, simethicone, sodium carboxymethylcellulose, sorbic acid, stearate emulsifiers and sucrose.

Incompatibilities: None.

Shelf-life: 24 months between 15°C and 30°C.

After constitution, the solution may be stored for up to 30 days under refrigeration (2°C to 8°C) (see *Special precautions for storage*).

Special precautions for storage: Store and protect from excessive moisture in tightly closed bottles at 15°C to 30°C. After constitution, store the solution in tightly closed bottles under refrigeration (2°C to 8°C).

Nature and content of container: Powder for oral solution: HDPE bottle with child resistant screw cap, fill mark (200 mL of solution after constitution) and measuring cup.

Instructions for use/handling: Constitute with water to a 200 mL deliverable volume solution (stavudine concentration of 1 mg/mL):

Add 202 mL of water to the original bottle (when the patient makes up the solution, they should be instructed to fill to the mark). Replace the cap.

Shake the bottle well until the powder dissolves completely. The solution may remain slightly hazy.

Dispense the solution with the measuring cup provided. The patient should be instructed to shake the bottle well prior to measuring each dose.

Marketing authorisation holder: Bristol-Myers Squibb Pharma EEIG, Swakeleys House, Milton Road, Ickenham UB10 8PU, United Kingdom

Number in the community register of medicinal products EU/1/96/009/009

Date of first authorisation/renewal of the authorisation 8 May 1996

Date of revision of the text 21st November 1997

**Trade Mark*

Britannia Pharmaceuticals Limited

41–51 Brighton Road
Redhill
Surrey RH1 6YS

☎ +44 01737 773741 🗋 +44 01737 762672

ALEC*

Presentation ALEC is presented as a vial of white, sterile, freeze-dried powder stored under nitrogen together with a 5 ml syringe, catheter, and 2 ml ampoule of sterile sodium chloride 0.9% w/v.

Each vial of ALEC contains 100 mg pumactant for reconstitution with 1.2 ml of cold, sterile sodium chloride solution 0.9% w/v. ALEC is for intratracheal administration.

When reconstituted the product appears as a white, creamy suspension. The reconstituted product contains 0.18 mmol (10.8 mg) of sodium.

Uses ALEC treatment reduces neonatal mortality in newborn babies of an estimated gestational age of 25–29 weeks, and who are intubated and undergoing mechanical ventilation because they are at risk of developing, or have developed Respiratory Distress Syndrome (RDS).

Dosage and administration ALEC must be reconstituted with 1.2 ml of cold, sterile sodium chloride solution 0.9% w/v before administration.

Dosage: Adults and older children—Not applicable.

Neonates: The reconstituted contents of one vial (i.e. 100 mg pumactant) should be given via the endotracheal tube as soon as possible after the baby is intubated. If the baby remains intubated, a second dose should be given 1 hour later. A third dose should be given at 24 hours from the time of intubation, but only if the baby is still undergoing mechanical ventilation.

Infants should not be intubated solely for the purpose of administering ALEC.

Reconstitution: ALEC should be reconstituted immediately before use as it contains no antimicrobial preservatives. The reconstituted product should be used within 8 hours.

The phospholipids in reconstituted ALEC will undergo a physical transition when warmed to body temperature to give molecular lamellar structures. This change involves a rapid spreading of the phospholipids, and it is essential that this occurs only after ALEC has been instilled into the endotracheal tube. Therefore, care should be taken to ensure that ALEC is kept cool up to the time of administration. ALEC (powder, syringe, catheter and the sterile sodium chloride solution 0.9% w/v) must be stored in the refrigerator (below 8°C) before use, BOTH as the packaged product AND as the reconstituted suspension ready for use. Do not freeze.

ONLY preservative-free sodium chloride solution 0.9% w/v for injection should be used for reconstitution, which should be performed as follows:

1. Remove the centre of the metal cover on the pumactant vial. Tap the vial to loosen the powder which may have settled on storage.
2. Draw 1.2 ml of cold, sterile sodium chloride solution 0.9% w/v into the 5 ml syringe. Push the syringe needle through the stopper of the pumactant vial and inject the sodium chloride solution. Withdraw the syringe with needle still attached.
3. Shake the vial gently, just enough to ensure dispersal of the pumactant; the contents of the vial should appear as a creamy suspension with a few lumps. (Any lumps of pumactant remaining in the vial will be disrupted in drawing up the reconstituted ALEC or will melt on warming to body temperature after administration).

Vigorous shaking will cause the suspension to form a foam, and should be avoided.

4. Draw 2 ml of air into the syringe and push the syringe needle through the rubber stopper of the pumactant vial. Inject the air to create a positive pressure.
5. Invert the vial and carefully draw as much of the suspension as possible into the syringe, followed by about 1 ml of air. Withdraw the syringe with needle still attached.
6. Hold the syringe with the needle pointing upwards and expel air so that the final volume reading on the syringe is 1.2 ml. Remove the needle from the syringe.
7. Attach the catheter supplied in the pack of ALEC to the syringe.

Administration: ALEC should be administered only by those trained and experienced in the care and resuscitation of preterm infants.

ALEC is administered rapidly from the syringe through the catheter which has been passed to the end of the endotracheal tube. It is necessary to disconnect the ventilator from the neonate temporarily during administration, although the time taken to deliver a whole single dose of ALEC should not generally be more than a few seconds.

The administration of ALEC should be performed as follows:

1. Prepare the ALEC as described under *Reconstitution* above, and have it ready to use before proceeding to the following steps.
2. Disconnect the ventilator (or the resuscitation bag in the event of the baby being hand-ventilated) from the endotracheal tube. Proceed quickly through the next five steps.
3. Suction the baby's airway to clear any mucous immediately before ALEC is administered. This will not be appropriate if the dose is being given immediately after the baby has been intubated and it is known that the endotracheal tube is essentially clear from any obstruction.
4. Having noted the length of the endotracheal tube, pass the catheter on the syringe containing ALEC down it so that the lower end is just at the end of the endotracheal tube.
5. Instill ALEC by quickly injecting the suspension and air from the syringe into the trachea; it should not take more than two seconds.
6. With the catheter still in the endotracheal tube, quickly disconnect the syringe from the catheter. Draw 3 ml of air into the syringe and reconnect to the catheter. Rapidly inject all the air down the endotracheal tube into the neonate; this empties the syringe and catheter of any residual ALEC suspension.
7. Withdraw the catheter from the endotracheal tube and reconnect the ventilator (or the resuscitation bag) to the endotracheal tube.

Some 'milky' surfactant suspension will be seen in the endotracheal tube. This should NOT be aspirated; it will melt on warming from body heat and spread slowly into the baby's lungs.

8. Ensure that satisfactory ventilation has been re-established. Arterial oxygen monitors may record a more than transitory depression of arterial oxygen suggestive of a blockage of the endotracheal tube. If there is any concern that the airways have been obstructed by surfactant the first action should be hand ventilation with oxygen and resuscitation bag. If this is unsuccessful the endotracheal tube should be aspirated. If this does not remedy the problem, the baby should be re-intubated.

Care should be taken to avoid prolonged disconnection from the ventilator.

Contra-indications, warnings, etc
Contra-indications: There are no known contra-indications to the use of ALEC.

Precautions: ALEC should only be administered where there are adequate facilities for ventilation and monitoring of neonates with, or at risk from, RDS.

Preterm birth is hazardous. Surfactant administration can be expected to diminish the severity of RDS and hence to diminish the complications of intensive care, especially the ventilatory support required for the treatment of RDS, but cannot be expected to eliminate entirely the mortality and morbidity associated with preterm delivery. Infants who, but for the administration of surfactant, might have died from RDS may be exposed to other complications of their immaturity.

As a consequence of the surfactant properties of ALEC, chest expansion may improve rapidly after dosing, necessitating rapid reduction in peak ventilator inspiratory pressure.

The improvement in lung mechanics resulting from ALEC administration may result in rapid improvement in arterial oxygen concentration. After any appropriate reduction in ventilator pressure, rapid reduction in inspired oxygen concentration may be needed to avoid hyperoxia.

ALEC was non-mutagenic in Chinese Hamster Ovaries cells. No long-term studies have been performed in animals to determine whether ALEC has carcinogenic potential. The only constituents of pumactant are synthetic phospholipids which are also naturally occurring in human lung surfactant. These are not known to be carcinogenic.

The effects of ALEC on fertility have not been studied.

Side-effects: In rare instances (less than 1% of cases) ALEC administration has been associated with obstruction of the endotracheal tube. In infants in whom endotracheal tube obstruction is suspected this should be treated, according to normal practice, by hand-ventilation with oxygen and a resuscitation bag, followed by suction of the tube, or by replacement of the tube if this is unsuccessful.

Pregnancy and lactation: Not applicable.

Interactions: No drug interactions have been reported with ALEC.

Treatment of overdosage: ALEC contains only phospholipids which are naturally occurring in human lung surfactant. There have been no reports of overdosage with ALEC.

In case of a severe accidental overdosage, as much as possible of the surfactant should be aspirated and the baby should then be managed with supportive treatment.

Pharmaceutical precautions ALEC (powder, syringe, catheter and 2 ml ampoule of sterile sodium chloride 0.9% w/v) must be stored in the refrigerator (below 8°C) before use, BOTH as the packaged product AND as the reconstituted product ready for use.

Do not freeze packs of ALEC or the reconstituted product.

ALEC should be used within 8 hours from reconstitution.

Legal category POM.

Package quantities ALEC contains one vial of pumactant, packaged with a 5 ml syringe, catheter and 2 ml ampoule of sterile sodium chloride 0.9% w/v.

Further information ALEC contains pumactant which is a 7:3 mixture (by weight) of dipalmitoylphosphatidylcholine (DPPC) and unsaturated phosphatidylglycerol (PG). Both of these phospholipids are naturally occurring in human lung surfactant. ALEC contains no protein, alcohol or other artificial surface-active agents.

Neonates with RDS have a deficiency in lung surfactant, and what surfactant is present has an abnormal composition compared to that of healthy full-term babies. ALEC mimics closely the properties of natural lung surfactant and can improve lung compliance. In a multicentre clinical trial, ALEC was able to reduce neonatal mortality from 27% to 14% in babies of less than 30 weeks gestation.

Product licence number 04483/0040.

BRITAJECT*

Presentation Britaject Pen 10 mg/ml is a disposable multiple dose pen injector system incorporating a clear glass cartridge containing apomorphine hydrochloride 10 mg/ml in aqueous solution for subcutaneous injection. It contains sodium bisulphite 0.093% w/v as an antioxidant.

Britaject Injection 10 mg/ml is presented as ampoules each containing apomorphine hydrochloride 10 mg/ml in aqueous solution for subcutaneous injection. It contains sodium metabisulphite 0.1% w/v as an antioxidant.

Britaject Pen 10 mg/ml contains 3 ml of solution and Britaject Injection 10 mg/ml is available in ampoules of 2 ml and 5 ml.

Uses
Indication: Britaject is indicated for the management of refractory motor fluctuations in Parkinson's disease; i.e. patients with disabling fluctuations in motor performance ('off' episodes) which are inadequately controlled by levodopa or other dopamine agonists (e.g. bromocriptine, lisuride, pergolide, etc.).

Properties: Apomorphine HCl is a potent dopamine agonist with antiparkinsonian activity. Other pharmacological effects include induction of emesis, nausea, retching, sedation, and yawning.

Apomorphine HCl is recommended for use in parkinsonian patients who have reached a stage of the disease at which they are exhibiting frequent 'on-off' disabling fluctuations in motor performance which are inadequately controlled by conventional antiparkinsonian medication.

Benefits are best seen in those Parkinson's disease patients who have good quality motor performance with levodopa, but in whom the duration of 'on' time is frequently unsatisfactory and is associated with unpredictable, disabling motor fluctuations.

Apomorphine HCl has an onset of action of between 5–10 minutes with a duration of action of about one hour, and, when administered by subcutaneous injection, may prevent an 'off' episode.

Dosage and administration The following general guidance applies to initiation and maintenance of apomorphine HCl therapy. It is administered as a subcutaneous injection. The optimal dosage of apomorphine HCl has to be determined on an individual patient basis. Hospital admission under appropriate specialist supervision is advised when establishing a patient's therapeutic regime.

It is essential that the patient is established on the antiemetic domperidone for at least 3 days prior to initiation of therapy.

Patient selection: Apomorphine HCl injections are only considered to be suitable for Parkinson's disease patients capable of recognising and anticipating 'off' episodes in motor performance. Patients must be capable and motivated for apomorphine HCl to be used effectively. Adult patients through all age ranges have been successfully managed with apomorphine HCl injections. Apomorphine HCl is contra-indicated in children and adolescents up to 18 years of age.

Elderly patients, in appropriate circumstances, can be successfully managed with apomorphine HCl.

The practical steps described below should be followed when commencing a patient on treatment;

- Pre-treat with domperidone.
- Discontinue all existing antiparkinsonian medication to provoke an 'off' episode in motor performance.
- Determine the threshold dose response to apomorphine HCl that produces an unequivocal motor response.
- Re-establish other antiparkinsonian agents.
- Determine effective treatment regimen for apomorphine HCl.
- Teach patient and/or carer how and when to administer.
- Discharge from hospital.
- Monitor frequently and adjust dosage regimen as appropriate.

Full details are given below:

Pre-treatment: Patient admission to hospital at least 3 days before initiation of apomorphine HCl treatment is recommended. On admission treatment with domperidone should be commenced (see *Use of domperidone with apomorphine HCl*, below). Over the following 3 days a clinical assessment must be made of the fluctuations in the patient's motor performance and response to conventional antiparkinsonian drug therapy.

Provoking and assessing an 'off' state: After at least 3 days of hospitalisation all anti-parkinsonian therapy is withheld overnight to provoke an 'off'-state in motor performance and to undertake a baseline motor assessment as follows:

(a) Alternate, unilateral hand-tapping for 30 seconds on mounted digital counters (preferably 20 cm apart) (Ref. Hughes, AJ et al., Lancet, 1990; *336*: 32–34).
(b) Time taken to walk 12 metres.
(c) Clinical assessment of tremor and dyskinesia according to a four point scale (0=nil, 1=mild, 2=moderate, 3=severe).
(d) Scoring on a modified Webster disability scale to assess 12 features of parkinsonism (maximum disability score of 36) (Ref. Kempster, PA et al., J Neurol Neurosurg Psychiatry, 1989; *52*: 718–23).

Determination of the threshold dose: Following baseline motor assessment the patient is challenged for apomorphine responsiveness according to the following schedule;

- 1.5 mg apomorphine HCl (0.15 ml) is injected subcutaneously and the patient is observed over 30 minutes for motor responsiveness.
- if no or poor response is obtained, a second dose of 3 mg apomorphine HCl (0.3 ml) is given 40 minutes after the first dose, and the patient observed for a further 30 minutes.
- The dosage is increased in an incremental fashion every 40 minutes and the patient observed carefully for an unequivocal motor response. The third dose is 5 mg s.c., and the fourth dose is 7 mg s.c. If the patient shows no response to the 7 mg dose then the patient must be classified as a non-responder to apomorphine HCl and no further attempts to provoke a motor response should be made. If the patient shows only a mild response to the 7 mg dose, a maximum dose of 10 mg can be used to see if an unequivocal motor response is possible.
- The lowest dose producing an unequivocal motor response is called the 'threshold dose'. For the majority of patients the threshold dose is less than 7 mg apomorphine HCl (0.7 ml), although very occasionally it can be up to 10 mg apomorphine HCl (1.0 ml).

Since Britaject Pen 10 mg/ml can only be administered in unit increments of 1 mg of apomorphine hydrochloride, it is recommended that the determination of the threshold dose is carried out with Britaject Injection 10 mg/ml.

Motor responsiveness is judged to be positive if 2 or more of the following are seen:

(a) More than 15% increase in tapping score.
(b) More than 25% improvement in walking time.
(c) An improvement of at least 2 points of tremor score.
(d) An improvement of Webster's score of 3 or more.

Initiation of treatment: Following establishment of an acceptable threshold dose of apomorphine HCl injection, the patient should be restarted on conventional antiparkinsonian therapy.

A subcutaneous injection of the established threshold dose may then be given into the lower abdomen or outer thigh at the first signs of an 'off' episode. The patient should then be observed over the following hour and the quality of their 'on' period noted. It may be appropriate to modify the dose of apomorphine HCl according to the patient's response.

Close monitoring of therapeutic benefits and side-effects under specialist supervision is required after initiation of treatment. The daily dose can vary between patients and will typically be in the range of 3 mg up to 30 mg per day in divided doses. The frequency of injection will also vary between patients and may be between 1 to 10 per day but in rare cases may be up to 12 times per day.

Patients who have shown a good 'on' period response during the initiation stage, but whose overall control remains unsatisfactory using intermittent injections, or who require many and frequent injections (more than 10 per day), may be commenced on or transferred to continuous subcutaneous infusion by minipump as follows;

Continuous infusion is started at a rate of 1 mg apomorphine HCl (0.1 ml) per hour then increased according to the individual response. Increases in the infusion rate should not exceed 0.5 mg per hour at intervals of not less than 4 hours. Hourly infusion rates may range between 1 mg and 4 mg (0.1 ml and 0.4 ml), equivalent to 0.015–0.06 mg/kg/hour. Infusions should run for waking hours only. Unless the patient is experiencing severe night-time problems, 24-hour infusions are not advised. In any event, the infusion site should be changed every 12 hours.

Patients normally need to supplement their continuous infusion with intermittent bolus boosts via the pump system as necessary. Patients who experience severe dyskinesias should only use bolus doses when absolutely necessary.

It is recommended that the total daily dose of apomorphine HCl should not exceed 100 mg and that individual bolus injections should not exceed 10 mg.

Transferring patients established on intermittent apomorphine injections using standard syringes to Britaject Pen 10 mg/ml: Britaject Pen 10 mg/ml is a convenient delivery system for administering frequent intermitttent injections. Patients already receiving apomorphine injections may be transferred to Britaject Pen 10 mg/ml but should be given a clear explanation by suitably trained medical staff on the use of the new delivery system. Some patients may require re-training in the administration technique. Full instructions for use are given in the leaflet enclosed with each pack.

Patients who are injecting apomorphine HCl in mg doses corresponding to whole digits may transfer directly to the corresponding mg dose on Britaject Pen 10 mg/ml.

However, since the dose dial increments on Britaject Pen 10 mg/ml are in single whole digits, patients who receive doses in between (e.g. 3.5 mg) will need to retitrate their dose on transferring to the Pen.

The appropriate dose (either up or down to the single, whole digit) should be selected according to the requirements of the individual patient. This can be established by instructing the patient to use the lower dose at the first sign of an off-episode. If the response is considered to be sub-optimal, a higher dose may be used for subsequent off-episodes.

In cases where over or under-dosing is achieved with Britaject Pen 10 mg/ml, it may be necessary to revert back to the original dose using their previous delivery system, or alternatively, the patient may be referred to their hospital specialist physician to determine whether he or she may be successfully transferred to Britaject Pen 10 mg/ml.

Monitoring treatment: Long-term specialist supervision of patients is advised.

There is a high probability of adverse effects to apomorphine HCl therapy (see *Side-effects*, below). The frequency and severity of adverse events should be monitored carefully at regular intervals and a reassessment of the patient carried out if appropriate. Adjustments to the dosage or discontinuation may be necessary.

Use of domperidone with apomorphine HCl: Domperidone maleate is a peripherally acting dopamine receptor antagonist and is recommended for the treatment of drug-induced nausea and vomiting in Parkinson's disease. Pre-treatment with domperidone is necessary during the initiation of therapy to control apomorphine's emetic actions.

The typical pre-treatment dose of domperidone used in specialist centres during the clinical development of Britaject, was 20 mg three times a day. However, the appropriate pre-treatment and maintenance doses of domperidone should be established on an individual patient basis. Domperidone treatment can normally be withdrawn gradually over several weeks to 6 months, according to the degree of nausea being experienced by the patient, although occasionally it has to be continued indefinitely. Where nausea and vomiting occur during treatment it is usually as a result of omission or sub-therapeutic dosing of domperidone.

Contra-indications, warnings, etc

Contra-indications: Apomorphine HCl is contra-indicated in patients with respiratory or central nervous system depression. Apomorphine HCl should not be administered to patients who are sensitive to morphine or its derivatives.

Apomorphine HCl can lead to neuropsychiatric disturbances and should not be administered to patients with pre-existing neuropsychiatric problems or dementias due to other pathological processes, e.g. dementia of the Alzheimer's type or multiinfarct dementia.

Apomorphine HCl treatment is not suitable for patients who have an 'on' response to levodopa which is marred by severe dyskinesia, hypotonia or psychotoxicity.

Use in pregnancy and lactation: Animal reproduction studies have not been conducted with apomorphine HCl. It is not known whether apomorphine can damage the foetus or affect the mother's reproductive capacity. Therefore, apomorphine HCl is not recommended for use in women of child bearing potential.

It is not known whether apomorphine is excreted in breast milk. However, breast-feeding is not recommended where a nursing mother is on apomorphine HCl therapy.

Precautions: Apomorphine HCl should be given with caution to patients with endocrine, renal, pulmonary or cardiovascular disease and persons prone to nausea and vomiting.

Extra caution is recommended during initiation of therapy in elderly and/or debilitated patients. Periodic evaluation of hepatic, haemopoietic, renal and cardiovascular functions is advised.

If the patient has a history of postural hypotension, particularly if associated with other dopamine agonists, extra caution is recommended during the initiation stages of therapy with lying and standing blood pressure monitored before and after apomorphine test doses.

Patients selected for treatment with apomorphine HCl are almost certain to be taking concomitant medications for their Parkinson's disease. In the initial stages of apomorphine HCl therapy the patient should be monitored for unusual side-effects or signs of potentiation of effect.

Drugs which interfere with central amine mechanisms such as reserpine, tetrabenazine, metoclopramide, antipsychotic dopamine-blocking agents (such as phenothiazines, thioxanthines, and butyrophenones), amphetamines and papaverine should be avoided if possible. If, however, their administration is considered essential, extreme care should be taken and the patient monitored for signs of potentiation, antagonism or other interactions and for any unusual side-effects.

Side-effects: Local induration and nodules often develop at subcutaneous sites of injection. In patients on high doses of apomorphine HCl these may persist and give rise to areas of erythema, tenderness and induration. Panniculitis has been reported from those patients where a skin biopsy has been undertaken. These local subcutaneous effects can sometimes be reduced by rotation of injection sites, dilution of the solution with Sodium Chloride 0.9% injection, and possibly the use of ultrasound to areas of nodularity and induration. Care should be taken to ensure that areas of ulceration do not become infected. Rarely, cutaneous ulceration has led to cessation of apomorphine HCl therapy.

Drug-induced dyskinesias during 'on' periods can be severe, and in a few patients may result in cessation of therapy. Postural instability, falls, increasing cognitive impairment, personality change and disabling dyskinesias during the 'on' phase can mar the therapeutic response in some patients. Motor deficits in skilled tasks can still be detectable during 'on' periods, and impaired speech and balance may not improve with apomorphine HCl therapy.

Nausea and vomiting may occur, usually as a result of the omission of domperidone (*see Use of Domperidone*, above).

Neuropsychiatric disturbances are common in parkinsonian patients. Apomorphine HCl can lead to neuropsychiatric disturbances and should not be given to patients with pre-existing neuropsychiatric problems or dementias due to other pathological processes, e.g. dementia of the Alzheimer's type or multiinfarct dementia. Transient mild confusion and visual hallucinations have occurred during apomorphine HCl therapy, most commonly in patients reporting previous levodopa-induced neuropsychiatric complications. In the event of the continued development of confusion or hallucinations during treatment with apomorphine HCl an attempt should be made to identify the contributing factor under the direct supervision of a hospital specialist. The dose of apomorphine HCl should be reduced gradually and the effects on the patient's motor and psychiatric states closely observed.

Transient sedation with each dose of apomorphine HCl at the start of therapy is common; this usually resolves over the first few weeks. Postural hypotension is seen infrequently and is usually transient.

Euphoria, light-headedness, restlessness and tremors have also been reported.

The use of apomorphine HCl in conjunction with levodopa treatment may cause Coombs' positive haemolytic anaemia. An initial screen prior to commencement of treatment and at 6 monthly intervals is recommended. In the event of the development of a haemolytic anaemia, a haematological specialist should be consulted. The dose of apomorphine HCl and/or levodopa should be reduced, with careful monitoring of the patient's motor state. It may be necessary to discontinue treatment with levodopa and/or apomorphine HCl in the event that it is not possible to control the anaemia satisfactorily.

Eosinophilia has occurred in only a few patients during treatment with apomorphine HCl.

Treatment of overdosage: In a few cases hypotension and bradycardic episodes have occurred during test doses with apomorphine HCl. These are usually transient. If necessary, measures should be taken to increase the blood pressure, e.g. raising the foot of the bed. There is no clearly established pharmacological antidote to excessive doses of apomorphine HCl. However, treatment with an opioid antagonist such as naloxone has been reported to reduce yawning, sleepiness, nausea, retching, and vomiting when administered prior to a dose of apomorphine HCl. (Ref. Bonuccelli, U et al., Clin Neuropharmacol 1991, *14*: 442–449) and may be considered in severe cases where excessive doses of apomorphine HCl have been given.

Domperidone maleate is a recognised peripherally acting dopamine antagonist and is used to counter the emetic actions of apomorphine. Its use may be considered in cases of overdose.

Antipsychotic (neuroleptic) drugs, which interfere with dopaminergic transmission in the brain by blocking dopamine receptors, may be considered in the treatment of overdosage with apomorphine HCl.

Pharmaceutical precautions
Britaject Pen 10 mg/ml: Store in a cool dry place (below 25°C) but not in a refrigerator. Do not store in direct heat or sunlight. Do not use if the solution turns green. Discard each pen no later than 48 hours from first use.

Britaject Injection 10 mg/ml ampoules: Protect from light and store at a temperature not exceeding 25°C. Do not use if the solution turns green. Britaject ampoules do not contain an antimicrobial preservative, so solutions should be used within 24 hours of opening.

Legal category POM.

Package quantities
Britaject Pen 10 mg/ml: Each pen contains apomorphine hydrochloride 10 mg/ml in 3 ml solution. The pens are supplied in cartons of 5.

Britaject Injection 10 mg/ml is presented as ampoules containing apomorphine hydrochloride 10 mg/ml:

20 mg apomorphine hydrochloride in 2 ml of solution.

50 mg apomorphine hydrochloride in 5 ml of solution.

The ampoules are supplied in cartons of 5.

Further information Nil.

Product licence numbers
Britaject Pen 10 mg/ml 4483/0042.
Britaject Injection 10 mg/ml 2 ml and 5 ml ampoules 4483/0038.

BRITLOFEX* TABLETS 0.2 mg

Presentation Round, peach, film coated tablets; 6.5 mm diameter containing 0.2 mg lofexidine hydrochloride.

Uses To relieve symptoms in patients undergoing opiate detoxification.

Dosage and administration Initial dosage should be one 0.2 mg tablet twice daily. The dose may be increased by increments of 0.2–0.4 mg per day up to a maximum of 2.4 mg (12 tablets) per day, according to the patient's response. In cases where no opiate use occurs during detoxification a duration of treatment of 7–10 days is recommended. In some cases a longer treatment period may be warranted.

At the end of treatment dosage should be reduced gradually over a period of at least 2–4 days (see under Precautions).

Contra-indications, warnings, etc
Contra-indications: Lofexidine is contra-indicated in cases of sensitivity to other Imidazoline derivatives.

Interactions: Lofexidine may enhance the CNS depressive effects of alcohol, barbiturates and other sedatives, although concurrent medication to aid sleeping has frequently been used in withdrawal studies. Concomitant use of tricyclic antidepressants may reduce the efficacy of lofexidine.

Pregnancy: The safety of lofexidine in pregnant women has not been established and it should only be administered during pregnancy if the benefit outweighs the potential risk to mother and foetus. It is not known whether lofexidine is excreted in human milk and caution should be exercised when it is administered to nursing mothers.

Precautions: Lofexidine may have a mild sedative effect. If affected, patients should be advised not to drive or operate machinery.

Lofexidine does not normally produce any clinically significant effects on blood pressure, but since lofexidine possesses mild hypotensive properties it should be used with caution in patients with severe coronary insufficiency, recent myocardial infarction, cerebrovascular disease or chronic renal failure. Lofexidine should not be discontinued abruptly, but withdrawn gradually over 2–4 days, or longer, to minimise any risk of blood pressure elevation and associated signs and symptoms. It should also be used with caution in patients with marked bradycardia (55 beats per minute); pulse rate should be assessed frequently. Patients with a history of depression should be carefully observed during long term therapy with lofexidine.

Side-effects: The side-effects of lofexidine are primarily related to its central alpha-adrenergic effects and comprise drowsiness and related symptoms and dryness of mucous membranes especially mouth, throat and nose. Hypotension and bradycardia may occur.

Treatment of overdosage: Overdosage may cause hypotension, bradycardia, sedation and coma. Gastric lavage should be carried out where appropriate. In most cases all that is required are general supportive measures.

Pharmaceutical precautions Protect from heat, moisture and light.

Legal category POM.

Package quantities 60 tablets.

Further information Nil.

Product licence number 4483/0036.

CRYSTAPEN* INJECTION

Qualitative and quantitative composition Benzylpenicillin sodium BP available as 600 mg and 1,200 mg vials.

Pharmaceutical form White crystalline, water-soluble sterile powder for injection

Clinical particulars
Therapeutic indications: Crystapen has bactericidal activity in infections due to penicillin-sensitive organisms, particularly streptococci, pneumococci (Streptococcus Pneumoniae), meningococci, gonococci and staphylococci (excluding penicillinase-producing strains). Crystapen is indicated for most wound infections, pyogenic infections of the skin, soft tissue infections and infections of the nose, throat, nasal sinuses, respiratory tract and middle ear, etc.

Generalised infections, septicaemia and pyaemia from susceptible bacteria. Acute and chronic osteomyelitis, sub-acute bacterial endocarditis and meningitis caused by susceptible organisms. Gonorrhoea. Suspected meningococcal disease.

Posology and method of administration:
Route of administration: Intramuscular, intravenous.

For other routes of administration, please contact Britannia Pharmaceuticals.

Preparation of solutions: Pharmaceutical preparation: Only freshly prepared solutions should be used. Reconstituted solutions of benzylpenicillin sodium BP are intended for immediate administration but may be stored for up to 24 hours at 2–8°C if necessary.

600 mg vial: Intramuscular injection: 600 mg (1 mega unit) is usually dissolved in 1.6 to 2.0 ml of Water for Injections BP.

600 mg and 1,200 mg vials: Intravenous injection: A suitable concentration is 600 mg (1 mega unit) dissolved in 4 to 10 ml of Water for Injections BP or Sodium Chloride Injection and 1,200 mg (2 mega units) dissolved in at least 8 ml of Sodium Chloride Injection BP.

Intravenous infusion: It is recommended that 600 mg (1 mega unit) should be dissolved in at least 10 ml of Sodium Chloride Injection or other infusion solution and 1,200 mg (2 mega units) should be dissolved in at least 20 ml of Sodium Chloride Injection or other infusion solution.

Dosage and administration The following dosages apply to both intramuscular and intravenous injection.

Adults: Usually 600 to 1,200 mg (1 to 2 mega units) daily, divided into 2 to 4 doses. Higher doses (up to 14.4 g/day (24 mega units) in divided doses) may be given in adult meningitis by the intravenous route.

In bacterial endocarditis, 4.8 g (8 mega units) or more may be given daily in divided doses by the intravenous route, often by infusion.

Intravenous doses in excess of 1.2 g (2 mega units) should be given slowly taking at least one minute for each 300 mg (0.5 mega unit) to avoid high levels causing irritation of the central nervous system.

High dosage of benzylpenicillin sodium may result in hypernatraemia and hypokalaemia unless the sodium content is taken into account.

Children aged 1 month to 12 years: 100 mg/kg/day in 4 divided doses; not exceeding 4 g/day.

Infants 1–4 weeks: 75 mg/kg/day in 3 divided doses.

Newborn infants: 50 mg/kg/day in 2 divided doses.

Meningitis in infants and children:

Children 1 month to 12 years	180–300 mg/kg/day in 4–6 divided doses, not exceeding 12 g/day.
Infants 1–4 weeks	150 mg/kg/day in 3 divided doses.
Newborn infants	100 mg/kg/day in 2 divided doses.

Suspected meningococcal disease:

Adults and children over 10 years	1,200 mg iv (or im)
Children 1–9 years	600 mg iv (or im)
Children under 1 year	300 mg iv (or im)

Contra-indications: Allergy to penicillins. Hypersensitivity to any ingredient of the preparation.

Special warnings and special precautions for use: Massive doses of Benzylpenicillin Sodium BP can cause hypokalaemia and sometimes hypernatraemia. Use of a potassium-sparing diuretic may be helpful. In the presence of impaired renal function, large doses of penicillin can cause cerebral irritation, convulsions and coma. Skin sensitisation may occur in persons handling the antibiotic and care should be taken to avoid contact with the substance. It should be recognised that any patient with a history of allergy, especially to drugs, is more likely to develop a hypersensitivity reaction to penicillin.

Interaction with other medicaments and other forms of interaction: None known.

Pregnancy and lactation: Benzylpenicillin has been taken by a large number of pregnant women and women of childbearing age without an increase in malformations or other direct or indirect harmful effects on the foetus having been observed.

Effects on ability to drive and use machines: None known.

Undesirable effects: Occasionally hypersensitivity to penicillin in the form of urticarial rash, may occur; it may be treated with antihistamine drugs. More rarely, anaphylactic reactions have been reported. Haemolytic anaemia and granulocytopenia have been reported in patients receiving prolonged high dosage of Benzylpenicillin Sodium BP (e.g. Subacute bacterial endocarditis).

Overdose: Excessive blood levels of Benzylpenicillin Sodium BP can be corrected by haemodialysis.

Pharmacological properties
Pharmacodynamic properties: Benzylpenicillin So-

dium BP has bacteriostatic and bactericidal actions, depending on its concentration, against most Gram-negative coli.

Pharmacokinetic properties: Benzylpenicillin Sodium BP rapidly appears in the blood following intramuscular injection of water soluble salts and maximum concentrations are usually reached in 15–30 minutes. Peak plasma concentrations of about 12 mcg/ml have been reported after doses of 600 mg with therapeutic plasma concentrations for most susceptible organisms detectable for about 5 hours.

The plasma half life is about 30 minutes.

Preclinical safety data: There are no pre-clinical data of relevance to the prescriber which are additional to that already included in other sections of the SmPC.

Pharmaceutical particulars

List of excipients: None.

Incompatibilities: None known.

Shelf life: Unopened 36 months. Opened 24 hours.

Special precautions for storage: Store below 25°C.

Nature and contents of container: Tubular type III glass vials sealed with bromobutyl rubber plugs with aluminium overseals or plastic 'flip-top' caps. This product is supplied in vials containing 600 mg and 1.2 g of powder in boxes containing 25 vials, and 'GP pack' containing 2 vials of 600 mg.

Instructions for use/handling: After contact with skin, wash immediately with water. In case of contact with eyes, rinse immediately with plenty of water and seek medical advice if discomfort persists.

Marketing authorisation number PL 04483/0039.

Date of first authorisation December 1992.

Renewal of authorisation March 1998.

Date of (partial) revision of the text November 1998.

**Trade Mark*

Cambridge Healthcare Supplies Ltd
Francis House
112 Hills Rd
Cambridge CB2 1PH
☎ 01202 734100 🗋 01202 735100

CAM* MIXTURE

Presentation CAM is a clear colourless liquid. Each 5 ml contains: Ephedrine Hydrochloride PhEur 4 mg. Contains parabens in a sugar free base.

Uses CAM is indicated in the symptomatic treatment of bronchospasm in children and adults with bronchitis.

Dosage and administration
Children 6 months to 2 years: 2.5 ml 3 times daily.
2 to 4 years: 5 ml 3 times daily.
Over 4 years: 10 mls 3 times daily.

Adults and elderly: 20 mls 3 to 4 times daily.

Contra-indications, warnings, etc
Contra-indications: CAM should be avoided in patients with most types of cardiovascular disorders, hypertension, hyperthyroidism, hyperexcitability, phaeochromocytoma and closed-angle glaucoma. In patients with prostatic enlargement it may increase difficulty with micturition. It should not be given to patients taking monoamine oxidase inhibitors or within 14 days of stopping such treatment.

Precautions: Care should be taken in patients with any of the following conditions; diabetes mellitus, ischaemic heart disease and renal impairment.

Interactions: When possible CAM should be discontinued prior to giving chloroform, cyclopropane, halothane or other halogenated anaesthetics. The effects of ephedrine are diminished by guanethidine, reserpine and probably methyldope and may be diminished or enhanced by tricyclic antidepressants. It may also diminish the effects of guanethidine and β blockers and may increase the possibility of arrhythmias in digitalised patients.

Side-effects: Although not reported for CAM, the following effects are possible based on experience with other ephedrine containing products: tachycardia, anxiety, restlessness, insomnia, tremor, arrhythmias, dry mouth and cold extremities.

Use in pregnancy and lactations: While no evidence of ill-consequences have been reported, as with most drugs, administration should be avoided especially during the first and third trimesters.

Overdosage: The effects of overdosage include CNS stimulation, hallucinations and hypertension. Management involves supportive and symptomatic treatment. In severe overdosage the stomach should be emptied by aspiration and lavage. If within 4 hours of ingestion, Diazepam may be given to control CNS stimulation and convulsions. For marked excitement or hallucinations chlorpromazine may be necessary. Severe hypertension may call for administration of an alpha-receptor blocking agent such as phentolamine.

Pharmaceutical precautions Store below 25°C. Once opened, use within 4 weeks.

Legal category P

Package quantities CAM is available in bottles of 200 ml and 1 litre.

Further information Does not contain colouring agents or sucrose. Contains parabens.

Product licence number 0237/5014R

CLINITAR* CREAM 1%

Qualitative and quantitative composition Stantar 1% w/w (a coal tar extract).

Pharmaceutical form Cream.

Clinical particulars
Therapeutic indications: Subacute and chronic psoriasis and eczema. For use alone or with UVB irradiation.

Posology and method of administration: For topical administration. Apply to the affected area(s) once or twice daily. In combined treatment with UVB irradiation, Clinitar should be removed before exposure to light. Suitable for all ages.

Contra-indications: Allergy to the ingredients. Contraindicated in generalised pustular psoriasis and infections of the skin.

Special warnings and precautions for use: The patient should be warned against exposing skin areas treated with Clinitar Cream to the sun or any artificial light source unless otherwise prescribed by the doctor.

Interaction with other medicaments and other forms of interaction: Senaltises the skin to UV light, which may lead to an unintended sunburn.

Pregnancy and lactation: Clinitar has not been tested in classical animal reproduction studies. There are insufficient human data to rule out the possibility of adverse effects in pregnancy and lactation, therefore it is recommended that Clinitar should not be used during pregnancy or lactation.

Effects on ability to drive and use machinery: None known.

Undesirable effects: Primary irritation and folliculitis. Phototoxic dermatitis has been seen in a few cases.

Overdose: Not applicable.

Pharmacological properties
Pharmacodynamic properties: The toxicology and the pharmacology of coal tar is well-known, coal tar having been used for topical treatment in therapeutic medicine since antiquity. The first clinical reports, however, only date back to the 1920's. Today, preparations containing coal tar are used world-wide in large quantities.

Pharmacokinetic properties: Percutaneous absorption of coal tar is assumed to be negligiible. There is, however, a risk of absorption of phenols, of which coal tar contains up to 3–4%. Systemic toxicity after human use of coal tar has only been seen very rarely and only in patients who were seriously weakened by immunological and systemic diseases. It is therefore recommended not to apply coal tar to more than 25% of the body surface.

Pharmaceutical particulars
List of excipients: 1,2 propylene glycol, cetostearyl alcohol, glyceryl stearate, isopropylpalmitate, purified water.

Incompatibilities: None known.

Shelf life: 3 years.

Special storage precautions: No special precautions.

Nature and contents of container: 100 g aluminium tubes.

Instructions for use/handling: No special conditions.

Market authorisation number 8557/0024

Date of approval/revision of SPC 3 June 1996

Legal category P

CLINITAR* SHAMPOO 2%

Qualitative and quantitative composition Stantar 2% w/w (a coal tar extract).

Pharmaceutical form Shampoo.

Clinical particulars
Therapeutic indications: Indicated for the treatment of pityriasis simplex capitis (dandruff). Seborrhoeic dermatitis of the scalp, and psoriasis of the scalp.

Posology and method of administration: For topical administration.

Moisten hair and rub a little shampoo into the hair and scalp. Rinse and repeat the treatment, this time producing a heavy lather. Leave in the hair for 5 minutes after the second treatment and then rinse carefully.

Use 1–3 times a week.
Suitable for all ages.

Contra-indications: Contains coal tar, therefore should not be used on coal tar sensitive skin, or where there is sensitivity to any of the other ingredients. Do not use in contact dermatitis.

Special warnings and precautions for use: If undue irritation occurs, the patient should be advised to discontinue use and see their doctor. Avoid getting shampoo into the eyes.

Interaction with other medicaments and other forms of interaction: None stated.

Pregnancy and lactation: Clinitar Shampoo has not been tested in classical animal reproduction studies. There are insufficient human data to rule out the possibility of adverse effects in pregnancy and lactation. It is therefore recommended that Clinitar should not be used.

Effects on ability to drive and use machinery: None known.

Undesirable effects: Coal tar may cause primary irritation and folliculitis.

Overdose: None stated.

Pharmacological properties
Pharmacological properties: Coal tar has been used in medicine for thousands of years. The use of tar preparations in the treatment of eczema, psoriasis and dandruff of the scalp can be considered well established. Tar reduces excess production of skin lipids (seborrhoea) especially from the sebaceous glands. Excessive production of skin surface lipids very often leads to a very troublesome seborrhoea capillitil with greasy hair, dandruff and seborrhoeic dermatitis.

Pharmacokinetic properties: Not much is known about the pharmacokinetics of coal tar. Knoth, Herrman and Meyhofer (1959) found that the distribution of tar in the skin showed the highest concentration in the hair follicles and the sebaceous glands, suggesting that these may make up an important route of penetration for the coal tar into the skin.

Pharmaceutical particulars
List of excipients: Sodium laurylethylsulphate, triethanolamine laurylsulphate, polyoxyethylene glycerolmonostearate, polysorbate 80, cocamidopropyl amine oxide, cocamide DEA, cocamidopropyl betain, perfume mixture and purified water.

Incompatibilities: None known.

Shelf life: 5 years.

Special storage precautions: No special precautions.

Nature and contents of container: 100 g polypropylene tubes.

Instructions for use/handling: No special conditions.

Marketing authorisation number 8557/0025

Date of approval/revison of SPC 3 June 1996

Legal category P

IONAMIN 15

Qualitative and quantitative composition
Active constituent:
Phentermine (as a resin complex) 15 mg

Pharmaceutical form Modified release capsule.

Clinical particulars
Therapeutic indications: Ionamin is an anorectic agent intended as an adjunctive therapy to diet in patients with obesity and a body mass index (BMI) of 30 kg/m² or higher, who have not responded to an appropriate weight reducing regimen alone.

Note: Short term efficacy only has been demonstrated with regard to weight reduction. No significant data on changes in morbidity or mortality are yet available.

Posology and method of administration:
Oral administration:
Adults: 15 mg or 30 mg daily at breakfast time. Evening dosing should be avoided as Ionamin may induce nervousness and insomnia.

It is recommended that treatment should be conducted under the care of physicians experienced in the treament of obesity.

Secondary organic causes of obesity must be excluded by diagnosis before prescribing Ionamin.

The recommended dose should not be exceeded in an attempt to increase the anorectic effect, and the drug should be discontinued in non-responsive cases.

The management of obesity should be undertaken using a overall approach which should include dietary, medical and pschotherapeutic methods.

The duration of treatment is four to six weeks and should not exceed three months. An intermittent dosage regimen consisting of treatment for up to four weeks, followed by a similar period without medication may be as effective as continuous treatment.

Children (below 12 years) and the elderly: Ionamin is not recommended for use.

Contra-indications: Pulmonary artery hypertension; severe arterial hypertension. Thyrotoxicosis, glaucoma, epilepsy. Hypersensitivity to sympathomimetic amines. Current or past medical history of cardio-vascular or cerebro-vascular disease or psychiatric disorders including anorexia nervosa and depression. Propensity towards drug abuse, known alcoholism. Ionamin should not be administered to children under 12 years of age.

Combination drug therapy: Concurrent use with any other centrally acting anorectic agent is contra-indicated due to the increased risk of potentially fatal pulmonary artery hypertension. Concurrent or recent use of monoamine oxidase inhibitors (MAOI's) also contra-indicates the use of Iomamin.

Special warnings and precautions for use:
Special warnings: Cases of severe, often fatal, pulmonary artery hypertension, have been reported in patients who have received anorectics of the type in this product. An epidemiological study has shown that anorectic intake is a risk factor involved in the development of pulmonary artery hypertension and that the use of anorectics is strongly associated with an increased risk for this adverse drug reaction. In view of this rare but serious risk, it must be emphasised that:

- careful compliance with the indication and the duration of treatment is required,
- duration of treatment greater than 3 months and a BMI ≥ 30 kg/m^2 increase the risk of pulmonary artery hypertension.
- the onset or aggravation of exertional dyspnoea suggests the possibility of occurrence of pulmonary artery hypertension. Under these circumstances, treatment should be immediately discontinued and the patient referred to a specialist unit for investigation.

Special precautions for use:
- Prolonged treatment may give rise to pharmacological tolerance and drug dependence, and more rarely to severe psychotic disorders in predisposed patients.
- Rarely, cases of cardiac and cerebro-vascular accidents have been reported, often following rapid weight loss. Special care should be taken to ensure gradual and controlled weight loss in obese patients, who are subject to a risk of vascular disease. Ionamin should not be prescribed in patients with current or a past medical history of cardio-vascular or cerebro-vascular disease.
- Ionamin should be used with caution in epileptic patients.

Interaction with other medicaments and other forms of interaction: Phentermine may enhance the response to alcohol and, in combination with dieting, may alter the insulin requirements of diabetics. Caution should be exercised when Ionamin is administered with anti-hypertensive, psychotropic and sympathomimetic drugs.

Pregnancy and lactation:
Pregnancy: There is inadequate evidence of safety of Ionamin in human pregnancy. There is evidence of harmful effects in animals with amphetamines. Treatment with Ionamin should cease during pregnancy.

Lactation: No information is available.

Effects on ability to drive and use machines: Phentermine may produce mild CNS excitation and there is a theoretical risk of sedation on withdrawal of the drug. If the patient is affectd, his ability to drive or operate machinery may be impaired.

Undesirable effects:
Pulmonary artery hypertension:
- An epedemiological study has shown that anorectic intake is a risk factor involved in the development of pulmonary artery hypertension and that the use of anorectics is strongly associated with an increased risk for this adverse drug reaction. Cases of pulmonary artery hypertension have been reported in patients with phentermine. Pulmonary artery hypertension is a severe and often fatal disease. The occurrence or aggravation of exertional dyspnoea is usually the first clinical sign and requires treatment discontinuation and investigation in a specialised unit (see *Special warnings*).

CNS effects:
- The prolonged use of this agent associated with a risk of pharmacological tolerance, dependence and withdrawal syndrome.
- The most common adverse reactions which have been described are: psychotic reactions or psychosis, depression, nervousness, agitation, sleep disorders and vertigo.
- Convulsions, dry mouth and headache have also been reported.

Cardio-vascular effects:
- The most common reported reactions are tachycardia, palpitations, hypertension, precordial pain.
- Rarely, cases of cardiovascular or cerebro-vascular accidents have been described in patients treated with anorectic agents. In particular stroke, angina, myocardial infarction, cardiac failure and cardiac arrest have been reported.

Other effects:
- Constipation, nausea, vomiting and rashes have been reported.

Overdose:
Signs and symptoms: CNS stimulation such as restlessness, agitation and hallucinations may occur, usually followed by fatigue and depression. Cardiovascular effects include arrhythmias, hypertension and circulatory collapse. Gastrointestinal effects include nausea, vomiting, diarrhoea and abdominal cramps. Since Ionamin is a sustained release product, effects may be slow in onset and prolonged.

Treatment: Management includes emesis or gastric lavage (depending on the clinical state of the patient) and activated charcoal. The patient should be kept quiet and chlorpromazine used if necessary for sedation. Cardiovascular function should be monitored and treated symptomatically. In serious cases, forced acid diuresis my be indicated but only after discussion with a poisons centre.

Pharmacological properties
Pharmacodynamic properties: Phentermine is a sympathomimetic amine with CNS stimulant activity. It has not been established whether its anorectic action is primarily one of appetite suppression or whether other central nervous or metabolic effects may be involved.

Pharmacokinetic propeties: After ingestion, phenermine is gradually released from the ion exchange resin complex providing smooth and maintained plasma concentrations.

Preclinical safety data: No remarks.

Pharmaceutical particulars
List of excipients: Amberlite Resin*, Calcium Hydrogen Phosphate BP, Lactose BP, Magnesium Stearate BP, Purified Water BP, Titanium Dioxide (E171), Sunset Yellow (E110), Quinoline Yellow (E104), Gelatin USP, Black Iron Oxide (E172) and Black Ink.

* Sulphonated styrene – divinyl benzene copolymer.

Incompatibilities: None known.

Shelf life: Three years.

Special precautions for storage: Store below 25°C in a dry place.

Nature and contents of container: Tablet container with screw cap (100 capsules) or strips (4 or 28 capsules).

Instructions for use/handling: No special instructions are necessary.

Marketing authorisation holder: Cambridge Healthcare Supplies Ltd, 57/58 King Street, Great Yarmouth, Norfolk, NR30 2PW.

Marketing authorisation number PL 16794/0001

Date of first authorisation/renewal of authorisation 30 April 1998

Date of (partial) revision of the text January 1997

IONAMIN 30

Qualitative and quantitative composition
Active constituent:
Phentermine (as a resin complex) 30 mg

Pharmaceutical form Modified release capsule.

Clinical particulars
Therapeutic indications: Ionamin is an anorectic agent intended as an adjunctive therapy to diet in patients with obesity and a body mass index (BMI) of 30 kg/m^2 or higher, who have not responded to an appropriate weight reducing regimen alone.

Note: Short term efficacy only has been demonstrated with regard to weight reduction. No significant data on changes in morbidity or mortality are yet available.

Posology and method of administration:
Oral administration:
Adults: 15 mg or 30 mg daily at breakfast time. Evening dosing should be avoided as Ionamin may induce nervousness and insomnia.

It is recommended that treatment should be conducted under the care of physicians experienced in the treament of obesity.

Secondary organic causes of obesity must be excluded by diagnosis before prescribing Ionamin.

The recommended dose should not be exceeded in an attempt to increase the anorectic effect, and the drug should be discontinued in non-responsive cases.

The management of obesity should be undertaken using a overall approach which should include dietary, medical and psychotherapeutic methods.

The duration of treatment is four to six weeks and should not exceed three months. An intermittent dosage regimen consisting of treatment for up to four weeks, followed by a similar period without medication may be as effective as continuous treatment.

Children (below 12 years) and the elderly: Ionamin is not recommended for use.

Contra-indications: Pulmonary artery hypertension; severe arterial hypertension. Thyrotoxicosis, glaucoma, epilepsy. Hypersensitivity to sympathomimetic amines. Current or past medical history of cardio-vascular or cerebro-vascular disease or psychiatric disorders including anorexia nervosa and depression. Propensity towards drug abuse, known alcoholism. Ionamin should not be administered to children under 12 years of age.

Combination drug therapy: Concurrent use with any other centrally acting anorectic agent is contra-indicated due to the increased risk of potentially fatal pulmonary artery hypertension. Concurrent or recent use of monoamine oxidase inhibitors (MAOI's) also contra-indicates the use of Iomamin.

Special warnings and precautions for use:
Special warnings: Cases of severe, often fatal, pulmonary artery hypertension, have been reported in patients who have received anorectics of the type in this product. An epidemiological study has shown that anorectic intake is a risk factor involved in the development of pulmonary artery hypertension and that the use of anorectics is strongly associated with an increased risk for this adverse drug reaction. In view of this rare but serious risk, it must be emphasised that:

- careful compliance with the indication and the duration of treatment is required,
- duration of treatment greater than 3 months and a BMI ≥ 30 kg/m^2 increase the risk of pulmonary artery hypertension.
- the onset or aggravation of exertional dyspnoea suggests the possibility of occurrence of pulmonary artery hypertension. Under these circumstances, treatment should be immediately discontinued and the patient referred to a specialist unit for investigation.

Special precautions for use:
- Prolonged treatment may give rise to pharmacological tolerance and drug dependence, and more rarely to severe psychotic disorders in predisposed patients.
- Rarely, cases of cardiac and cerebro-vascular accidents have been reported, often following rapid weight loss. Special care should be taken to ensure gradual and controlled weight loss in obese patients, who are subject to a risk of vascular disease. Ionamin should not be prescribed in patients with current or a past medical history of cardio-vascular or cerebro-vascular disease.
- Ionamin should be used with caution in epileptic patients.

Interaction with other medicaments and other forms of interaction: Phentermine may enhance the response to alcohol and, in combination with dieting, may alter the insulin requirements of diabetics. Caution should be exercised when Ionamin is administered with anti-hypertensive, psychotropic and sympathomimetic drugs.

Pregnancy and lactation:
Pregnancy: There is inadequate evidence of safety of Ionamin in human pregnancy. There is evidence of harmful effects in animals with amphetamines. Treatment with Ionamin should cease during pregnancy.

Lactation: No information is available.

Effects on ability to drive and use machines: Phentermine may produce mild CNS excitation and there is a theoretical risk of sedation on withdrawal of the drug. If the patient is affectd, his ability to drive or operate machinery may be impaired.

Undesirable effects:
Pulmonary artery hypertension:
- An epedemiological study has shown that anorectic intake is a risk factor involved in the development of pulmonary artery hypertension and that the use of anorectics is strongly associated with an increased risk for this adverse drug reaction. Cases of pulmonary artery hypertension have been reported in patients with phentermine. Pulmonary artery hypertension is a severe and often fatal disease. The occurrence or aggravation of exertional dyspnoea is usually the first clinical sign and requires treatment discontinuation and investigation in a specialised unit (see *Special warnings*).

CNS effects:
- the prolonged use of this agent associated with a risk of pharmacological tolerance, dependence and withdrawal syndrome.

- The most common adverse reactions which have been described are: psychotic reactions or psychosis, depression, nervousness, agitation, sleep disorders and vertigo.
- Convulsions, dry mouth and headache have also been reported.

Cardio-vascular effects:

- The most common reported reactions are tachycardia, palpitations, hypertension, precordial pain.
- Rarely, cases of cardiovascular or cerebro-vascular accidents have been described in patients treated with anorectic agents. In particular stroke, engine, myocardial infarction, cardiac failure and cardiac arrest have been reported.

Other effects:

- Constipation, nausea, vomiting and rashes have been reported.

Overdose:

Signs and symptoms: CNS stimulation such as restlessness, agitation and hallucinations may occur, usually followed by fatigue and depression. Cardiovascular effects include arrhythmias, hypertension and circulatory collapse. Gastrointestinal effects include nausea, vomiting, diarrhoea and abdominal cramps. Since Ionamin is a sustained release product, effects may be slow in onset and prolonged.

Treatment: Management includes emesis or gastric lavage (depending on the clinical state of the patient) and activated charcoal. The patient should be kept quiet and chlorpromazine used if necessary for sedation. Cardiovascular function should be monitored and treated symptomatically. In serious cases, forced acid diuresis my be indicated but only after discussion with a poisons centre.

Pharmacological properties

Pharmacodynamic properties: Phentermine is a sympathomimetic amine with CNS stimulant activity. It has not been established whether its anorectic action is primarily one of appetite suppression or whether other central nervous or metabolic effects may be involved.

Pharmacokinetic propeties: After ingestion, phenermine is gradually released from the ion exchange resin complex providing smooth and maintained plasma concentrations.

Preclinical safety data: No remarks.

Pharmaceutical particulars

List of excipients: Amberlite Resin*, Calcium Hydrogen Phosphate BP, Lactose BP, Magnesium Stearate BP, Purified Water BP, Titanium Dioxide (E171), Sunset Yellow (E110), Quinoline Yellow (E104), Gelatin USP, Black Iron Oxide (E172) and Black Ink.

* Sulphonated styrene – divinyl benzene copolymer.

Incompatibilities: None known.

Shelf life: Three years.

Special precautions for storage: Store below 25°C in a dry place.

Nature and contents of container: Tablet container with screw cap (100 capsules) or strips (4 or 28 capsules).

Instructions for use/handling: No special instructions are necessary.

Marketing authorisation holder: Cambridge Healthcare Supplies Ltd, 57/58 King Street, Great Yarmouth, Norfolk, NR30 2PW.

Marketing authorisation number PL 16794/0002

Date of first authorisation/renewal of authorisation 30 April 1998

Date of (partial) revision of the text January 1997

**Trade Mark*

Cambridge Laboratories
Richmond House
Old Brewery Court
Sandyford Road
Newcastle upon Tyne NE2 1XG
☎ 0191 2615950 ▯ 0191 2221006

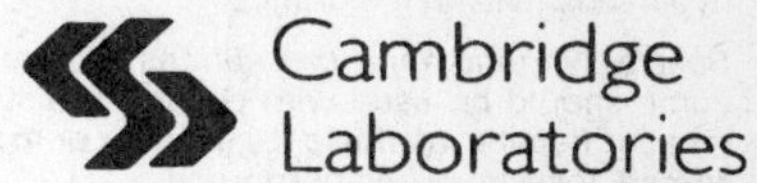

ACTIDOSE-AQUA*

Qualitative and quantitative composition Actidose-Aqua contains 1.040 g of activated charcoal/5 ml.

Pharmaceutical form Suspension for oral administration.

Clinical particulars
Therapeutic indications: For the emergency treatment of acute poisoning and drug overdosage where substances such as those listed below have been ingested. The list is not exhaustive and Actidose-Aqua may be of benefit following ingestion of many other toxins.

Also indicated for a limited number of systemic poisonings resulting from parenteral overdosage or when the ingested toxin has been totally absorbed. This usually involves repeated doses of Actidose-Aqua to remove compounds which undergo enterohepatic recycling or which can diffuse into the gastrointestinal tract along a concentration gradient. Under these circumstances, multiple doses of Actidose-Aqua adsorb the toxin, thereby preventing its reabsorbtion and increasing the concentration gradient in favour of further diffusion of the toxin into the gastrointestinal tract. Compounds most effectively transferred by this mechanism are lipophilic, uncharged and not excessively protein-bound. Examples of compounds which can be eliminated more rapidly by 'gastrointestinal dialysis' in this way are phenobarbitone and theophylline.

Posology and method of administration: The container should be shaken thoroughly prior to administration. If the dose of poison that has been ingested is known, a ratio of 10:1 (activated charcoal:toxin) may be used to determine the optimal dose of activated charcoal, subject to the limits of practicality. In the absence of any information regarding the amount of poison ingested, the following doses are recommended:

Adults (including the elderly) and children over 12 years of age: For single dose therapy, 50–100 grams of activated charcoal (240–480 ml) taken as soon as possible after ingestion of the poison.

For multiple dose therapy, 25–50 grams of activated charcoal (120–240 ml) every 4–6 hours.

Children aged 1–12 years: For single dose therapy, 25–50 grams of activated charcoal (120–240 ml) taken as soon as possible after ingestion of the poison. For multiple dose therapy, the dose may be repeated every 4–6 hours.

Children under 1 year: For single dose therapy, 1 g or 5 ml per kg bodyweight taken as soon as possible after ingestion of the poison. For multiple dose therapy, the dose may be repeated every 4–6 hours.

When syrup of ipecac is used to produce emesis, administration of Actidose-Aqua should be delayed until 30–60 minutes after vomiting has ceased. If gastric lavage is being used to facilitate stomach evacuation, a single dose of Actidose-Aqua may be administered early in the procedure. This has the advantage of prompt administration of activated charcoal, but the gastric lavage returns will be black which may make it difficult to evaluate what the patient ingested by visual examination.

Actidose-Aqua may be effective even when several hours have elapsed after ingestion of the poison if gastrointestinal motility is reduced by the toxin or if the drug is subject to enterohepatic or enteroenteric recycling.

Contra-indications: Use of Actidose-Aqua is contra-indicated in persons who are not fully conscious.

Special warnings and precautions for use: Actidose-Aqua is not recommended for patients who have ingested corrosive agents such as strong acids or alkalis since the activated charcoal may obscure endoscopic visualisation of oesophageal and gastric lesions produced by the toxin. Actidose-Aqua is of little or no value in the treatment of poisoning with cyanides, alcohols, iron salts, malathion and DDT.

Actidose-Aqua is an adjunct in the management of poisoning emergencies. Prior to its use, proper basic life support measures must be implemented where required, as well as the appropriate gastric emptying technique if indicated.

Actidose-Aqua should be used with caution in patients who have been exposed to toxins which interfere with gastrointestinal motility (e.g. anticholinergics, opioids). Bowel sounds should be monitored frequently to assess peristaltic action, especially in patients undergoing multiple dose activated charcoal therapy.

Interactions with other medicaments and other forms of interaction: Actidose-Aqua will adsorb most medicaments and many other chemical substances. If a specific antidote is to be administered, the likelihood of its adsorption by activated charcoal should be borne in mind and a parenteral route of administration used if possible. Thus, in the case of paracetamol, Actidose-Aqua should not be given as well as oral methionine but may be used alone or in conjunction with intravenous N-acetylcysteine.

Other concurrent medications to counteract shock or associated infection should also be given parenterally since orally administered drugs may be bound to the activated charcoal in the gut.

Pregnancy and lactation: The safety of this medicinal product for use in human pregnancy has not been established. Experimental animal studies are insufficient to assess the safety with respect to the development of the embryo or foetus, the course of gestation and peri- and postnatal development.

Activated charcoal is, however, essentially inert pharmacologically and is not absorbed from the gastrointestinal tract. No hazard is therefore anticipated from its use during pregnancy or lactation.

Effects on ability to drive and use machines: None known.

Undesirable effects: Both the patient and health care professionals should be aware that Actidose-Aqua will produce black stools. A laxative may be given concurrently to accelerate the removal of the activated charcoal-toxin complex, but should be used with caution and only intermittently during multiple dose activated charcoal therapy since profuse and protracted diarrhoea may lead to fluid and electrolyte imbalance.

Aspiration of activated charcoal has been reported to produce airways obstruction and appropriate precautions should be taken. Gastrointestinal obstruction associated with the use of multiple dose activated charcoal therapy has been reported rarely.

Overdose: Actidose-Aqua is well tolerated and due to its lack of toxicity, overdosage requiring treatment is unlikely. A laxative may be administered to enhance elimination of the product.

Pharmacological properties
Pharmacodynamic properties: Activated charcoal has a high adsorptive capacity for a wide range of compounds, including many of those which are most commonly encountered in deliberate and accidental poisoning. Substances adsorbed include the following:

Aspirin and other salicylates
Barbiturates
Benzodiazepines
Chlormethiazole
Chloroquine
Chlorpromazine and related phenothiazines
Clonidine
Cocaine and other stimulants
Digoxin and digitoxin
Ibuprofen
Mefenamic Acid
Mianserin
Nicotine
Paracetamol
Paraquat
Phenelzine and other monoamine oxidase inhibitors
Phenytoin
Propranolol and other beta-blockers
Quinine
Theophylline
Zidovudine

Pharmacokinetic properties: Activated charcoal is not absorbed from the gastrointestinal tract or subject to any metabolic processes. It is eliminated in the faeces.

Preclinical safety data: Activated charcoal is essentially inert pharmacologically and it would therefore be expected to be virtually devoid of toxicity, other than any ill-effects arising from mechanical obstruction of the gut or, if inhaled, the lungs.

The excipients in the product are all well known and widely used in medicinal products and should not give rise to any toxicological problems.

Pharmaceutical particulars
List of excipients: Methylparaben, propylparaben, butylparaben, potassium sorbate, sucrose, propylene glycol, glycerine, citric acid, purified water.

Incompatibilities: None known.

Shelf life: Two years.

Special precautions for storage: Store at 15–30°C. Do not refrigerate.

Nature and contents of container:
1. Low density polyethylene bottles containing 120 ml
2. Low density polyethylene bottles containing 240 ml
3. Low density polyethylene tubes containing 120 ml.

Instructions for use/handling: Shake well before use.

Marketing authorisation number 12070/0011.

Date of approval/revision of SPC March 1996.

Legal category P.

DEBRISOQUINE TABLETS

Qualitative and quantitative composition Each tablet contains 12.8 mg Debrisoquine Sulphate, equivalent to 10.0 mg Debrisoquine.

Pharmaceutical form Tablets.

Clinical particulars
Therapeutic indications: Debrisoquine is indicated for the treatment of all grades of hypertension. It can be given either alone or together with other antihypertensive drugs or diuretics.

Posology and method of administration: Debrisoquine Tablets are for oral administration.

Adults: Mild to moderate hypertension: 10 mg once or twice daily. This dose can be increased by 10 mg at 3-day intervals. The total dose usually falls within the range 20–60 mg daily.

Adults: Severe hypertension: 20 mg once or twice daily. This dose can be increased, depending on response, by 10–20 mg every 3 or 4 days provided a close check is kept on the blood pressure.

When initially treating severe hypertension with Debrisoquine, the diastolic pressure should not be reduced below 110 mm Hg as impaired autoregulatory mechanisms may lead to impaired perfusion of vital organs.

The total dose usually falls within the range 40–120 mg but in cases of severe hypertension 300 mg or more daily may be given. Although some tolerance to the drug may occur during long term therapy, requiring increased dosage, this has usually been moderate and has not posed special problems.

Should postural hypotension occur with a dosage that controls the blood pressure, the total daily dose should be adjusted to give a small dose in the morning, a relatively large dose at midday and a moderate evening dose.

Adequate control of blood pressure is frequently obtained with Debrisoquine alone but, if necessary, its effects can be enhanced by the addition of therapy with a diuretic or another antihypertensive drug (e.g. a beta-adrenergic blocking agent).

Use in the elderly: There is inadequate evidence of the safety of Debrisoquine in the elderly, although it has been in wide use for many years without apparent ill consequence specifically relating to elderly populations. However, as with other potent hypotensive agents, including α-adrenergic blockers, the possibility of postural hypotension occurring should be borne in mind.

Children: There is inadequate evidence of the safety of Debrisoquine in children, although it has been in wide use for many years without apparent ill consequence specifically relating to childhood.

Contra-indications: Debrisoquine should not be given to patients with a phaeochromocytoma or with a recent history of cerebral or myocardial infarction. It is contra-indicated in patients who have shown hypersensitivity to the drug.

Special warnings and precautions for use: Debrisoquine should be used with caution in patients with renal or hepatic insufficiency; smaller or more widely spread doses may be appropriate.

Debrisoquine may give rise to exertional and postural hypotension. Caution should therefore be exercised in patients with coronary or cerebral insufficiency. As with other potent hypotensive agents, including α-adrenergic blockers, the possibility of postural hypotension occurring in the elderly should be borne in mind.

Patients on antihypertensive drugs often have a lower blood pressure in warm weather, therefore in hot climates their dose of Debrisoquine may need to be reduced.

If anaesthesia for surgery or dentistry is necessary, the anaesthetist should be informed that the patient is being treated with Debrisoquine.

Abrupt cessation of Debrisoquine should be avoided as this may lead to rebound hypertension.

The metabolism of Debrisoquine is subject to genetic polymorphism such that non-metabolisers may show a marked response (e.g. orthostatic hypotension) to doses that have little effect in metabolisers.

New patients should be carefully monitored during the initial treatment to determine possible non-metabolisers (approximately 8 per cent of Caucasian populations).

Interactions with other medicaments and other forms of interaction: The possibility of an enhanced hypotensive effect should be borne in mind when any drug with a tendency to lower blood pressure is given concomitantly with Debrisoquine.

Evidence from both animal experiments and clinical observation suggests that the hypotensive action of adrenergic neurone-blocking drugs such as Debrisoquine may be inhibited by simultaneous treatment with tricyclic antidepressants, monoamine oxidase inhibitors and fenfluramine. Extra care should be taken when prescribing antihypertensive drugs in patients being treated with levodopa. Patients taking Debrisoquine are sensitive to sympathomimetic drugs.

Pregnancy and lactation: There is inadequate evidence of safety of Debrisoquine in human pregnancy but it has been in wide use for many years without apparent ill-consequence, animal studies having shown no hazard.

Effects on ability to drive and use machines: Not known.

Undesirable effects: Debrisoquine is well tolerated. Overdosage causes postural hypotension, most noticeable in the early morning or with long standing and associated with weakness, giddiness, fatigue and very rarely syncope. The patient should be warned of the possibility of these symptoms occurring. This can be minimised by reducing the dose. Other reported side-effects include malaise, nausea, headache, sweating, oedema, muscle weakness, failure of ejaculation in the male, and sometimes disturbances of micturition and nocturia. Diarrhoea, common with some other anti-hypertensive agents, is seen only very rarely. Aggravation of angina pectoris has been reported in a few cases.

Overdose: Excessive fall in blood pressure will be shown by orthostatic collapse. This will usually respond rapidly to placing the patient in a recumbent position. Patients receiving Debrisoquine are particularly sensitive to the effects of catecholamines. Sympathomimetic agents should therefore be administered only with great caution.

Pharmacological properties
Pharmacodynamic properties: Debrisoquine lowers blood pressure markedly and promptly in the hypertensive patient. It does this by blocking the transmission of sympathetic nerve impulses at the nerve terminals, thereby decreasing peripheral vascular resistance. Reduction in post-ganglionic sympathetic transmission is achieved by interfering with the physiological release of noradrenaline, without depleting major catecholamine stores in cardiovascular tissues and without impairing the cardiac contractile mechanism. The action, as with other alpha-adrenergic blocking agents, is most marked in the standing position.

Pharmacokinetic properties: Debrisoquine is rapidly absorbed from the gastrointestinal tract. The major metabolite is 4-hydroxydebrisoquine; metabolism is subject to polymorphism.

Preclinical safety data: The oral LD_{50} of Debrisoquine in rats has been reported to be 88±18 mg/kg (neonates) and 1580±163 mg/kg (adults). There is no evidence that Debrisoquine has teratogenic, mutagenic or carcinogenic actions.

Pharmaceutical particulars
List of excipients: Lactose, Starch, Purified talc, Magnesium stearate.

Incompatibilities: None known.

Shelf life: Five years.

Special precautions for storage: None.

Nature and contents of container: White HDPE bottles.

Instruction for use/handling: None.

Marketing authorisation holder: Lifehealth Limited, Richmond House, Old Brewery Court, Sandyford Road, Newcastle upon Tyne NE2 1XG.

Marketing authorisation number 14576/0001.

Date of first authorisation/renewal of authorisation 17 October 1995.

Date of (partial) revision of the text Not applicable.

DICOBALT EDETATE INJECTION 300 mg

Qualitative and quantitative composition Each ampoule contains 300 mg Dicobalt Edetate INN (15mg/ml).

Pharmaceutical form Solution for injection.

Clinical particulars
Therapeutic indications: Dicobalt Edetate Injection is a specific antidote for acute cyanide poisoning. In view of the difficulty of certain diagnosis in emergency situations, it is recommended that Dicobalt Edetate Injection only be given when the patient is tending to lose or has lost consciousness. The product should not be used as a precautionary measure.

Posology and method of administration: Cyanide poisoning must be treated as quickly as possible and intensive supportive measures must be instituted: clear airways and adequate ventilation are essential. 100% oxygen should be administered concurrently with Dicobalt Edetate Injection.

Expert advice on the treatment of poisoning is available at the local poisons centre.

Adults: One 300 mg ampoule intravenously over approximately one minute. If the patient shows inadequate response, a second ampoule may be given. If there is no response after a further five minutes, a third ampoule may be administered.

Each ampoule of Dicobalt Edetate Injection may be followed immediately by 50 ml Glucose intravenous infusion BP 500 g/l.

When the patient's condition is less severe but in the physician's judgement still warrants the use of Dicobalt Edetate Injection, the period over which the injection is given should be extended to 5 minutes.

Children: There is no clinical experience of the use of Dicobalt Edetate Injection in children. As with adults the dose required will be related to the quantity of cyanide ingested.

The elderly: There is no clinical evidence of the use of Dicobalt Edetate Injection in the elderly, but there is no reason to believe that the dosage schedule should be different from that for adults.

Contra-indications: None.

Special warnings and precautions for use: There is a reciprocal antidote action between cyanide and cobalt. Thus in the absence of cyanide, Dicobalt Edetate Injection itself is toxic. It is therefore essential that the product only be used in cases of cyanide poisoning. When the patient is fully conscious, it is unlikely that the extent of poisoning warrants the use of Dicobalt Edetate Injection.

Interactions with other medicaments and other forms of interaction: No information is available.

Pregnancy and lactation: No information is available.

Effects on ability to drive and use machines: Not applicable.

Undesirable effects: The initial effects of Dicobalt Edetate Injection are vomiting, a fall in blood pressure and compensatory tachycardia. After this the patient should recover.

Overdose: Signs and symptoms – these may be due to cobalt toxicity or to an anaphylactic type reaction, which may be dramatic. Oedema (particularly of the face and neck), vomiting, chest pain, sweating, hypotension, cardiac irregularities and rashes may occur.

Treatment – intensive supportive therapy is required.

Pharmacological properties
Pharmacodynamic properties: Cyanide blocks intracellular respiration by binding to cytochrome oxidase. Dicobalt Edetate Injection forms a stable complex with the cyanide thereby acting as an antidote.

Pharmacokinetic properties: Only very limited data are available.

Intravenous infusion of Dicobalt Edetate Injection is likely to result in rapid distribution in the extracellular fluid compartment.

Excretion is entirely via the kidneys within 24 hours and it is not metabolised.

Preclinical safety data: There are no preclinical data of relevance to the prescriber which are additional to that already included in other sections of the SPC.

Pharmaceutical particulars
List of excipients: Dextrose Monohydrate, Water for Injections.

Incompatibilities: Not applicable.

Shelf life: Three years.

Special precautions for storage: Store below 25°C away from light.

Nature and contents of container: Packs of six PhEur Type I glass ampoules containing 20 ml of a rose-violet coloured sterile pyrogen free solution.

Instruction for use/handling: None.

Marketing authorisation holder: L'Arguenon Limited, Richmond House, Old Brewery Court, Sandyford Road, Newcastle upon Tyne NE2 1XG.

Marketing authorisation number PL 14945/0001.

Date of first authorisation/renewal of authorisation 31 May 1996.

Date of (partial) revision of the text December 1997.

EDROPHONIUM INJECTION BP 10 mg/1 ml

Qualitative and quantitative composition Each ampoule contains 10 mg Edrophonium Chloride BP in 1 ml of solution.

Pharmaceutical form Ampoules.

Clinical particulars
Therapeutic indications: Myasthenia gravis, as a diagnostic test; to distinguish between overdosage and underdosage of cholinergic drugs in myasthenic patients; diagnosis of suspected 'dual block'; antagonist to non-depolarising neuromuscular blockade.

Posology and method of administration: Edrophonium Injection BP is for intramuscular or intravenous injection. In view of the possibility of provoking a cholinergic crisis it is recommended that facilities for resuscitation should be available whenever Edrophonium Injection BP is administered.

Adults: Test for myasthenia gravis
A syringe is filled with the contents of 1 ampoule (10 mg) and 2 mg is given intravenously, the needle and syringe being left in situ. If no response occurs within 30 seconds, the remaining 8 mg is injected. In adults with unsuitable veins, 10 mg is given by intramuscular injection.

To differentiate between 'myasthenic' and 'cholinergic' crises: In a myasthenic patient who is suffering from marked muscle weakness, in spite of taking large doses of Mestinon or Prostigmin, a test dose of 2 mg Edrophonium Injection BP is given intravenously one hour after the last dose of the cholinergic compound. If therapy has been inadequate, there is a rapid, transient increase in muscle strength; if the patient has been overtreated, Edrophonium Injection BP causes a transient increase of muscle weakness.

Diagnosis of suspected 'dual block': Edrophonium Injection BP 10 mg intravenously. If the block is due to depolarisation, it is briefly potentiated, whereas in a 'dual block', it is reversed.

Children: Diagnostic tests: A total dose of 100 micrograms/kg body-weight may be given intravenously. One fifth of this dose should be injected initially; if no reaction occurs, the remainder of the dose is administered 30 seconds later.

Antagonist to non-depolarising neuromuscular blockade: Generally, reversal of neuromuscular block with Edrophonium Injection BP should not be attempted until there is evidence of spontaneous recovery from paralysis. It is recommended that the patient be well ventilated and a patent airway maintained until complete recovery of normal respiration is assured.

Adults and children: Edrophonium Injection BP 500–700 micrograms/kg body-weight and atropine 7 micrograms/kg body-weight, by slow intravenous injection over several minutes, is usually adequate for reversal of non-depolarising muscle relaxants within 5–15 minutes. The two drugs are usually given simultaneously, but in patients who show bradycardia the pulse rate should be increased to about 80/minute with atropine before administering Edrophonium Injection BP.

The speed of recovery from neuromuscular blockade is primarily determined by the intensity of the block at the time of antagonism but it is also subject to other factors, including the presence of drugs (e.g. anaesthetic agents, antibiotics, antiarrhythmic drugs) and physiological changes (electrolyte and acid-base imbalance, renal impairment). These factors may prevent successful reversal with Edrophonium Injection BP or lead to recurarisation after apparently successful reversal. Therefore it is imperative that patients should not be left unattended until these possibilities have been excluded.

Elderly: There are no specific dosage recommendations for Edrophonium Injection BP in elderly patients.

Contra-indications: Edrophonium Injection BP should not be given to patients with mechanical intestinal or urinary obstruction.

Edrophonium Injection BP is contra-indicated in patients with known hypersensitivity to the drug.

Special warnings and precautions for use: Extreme caution is required when administering Edrophonium Injection BP to patients with bronchial asthma.

Care should also be taken in patients with bradycardia, recent coronary occlusion, vagotonia, hypotension, peptic ulcer, epilepsy or Parkinsonism.

In diagnostic uses of Edrophonium Injection BP, a syringe containing 1 mg of atropine should be kept at hand to counteract severe cholinergic reactions, should they occur. In view of the possibility of provoking a cholinergic crisis it is recommended that facilities for resuscitation should always be available.

When Edrophonium Injection BP is used as an antagonist to neuromuscular blockade bradycardia may occur, to a possibly dangerous level, unless atropine is given simultaneously. In this indication, Edrophonium Injection BP should not be given during cyclopropane or halothane anaesthesia; however, it may be used after withdrawal of these agents.

There is no evidence to suggest that Edrophonium Injection BP has any special effects in the elderly. However, elderly patients may be more susceptible to dysrhythmias than younger adults.

Interactions with other medicaments and other forms of interaction: With doses above 10 mg, especially the higher dosage employed to antagonise neuromuscular blockade, Edrophonium Injection BP should not be used in conjunction with depolarising muscle relaxants such as suxamethonium as neuromuscular blockade may be potentiated and prolonged apnoea may result.

Pregnancy and lactation: The safety of Edrophonium Injection BP during pregnancy or lactation has not been established. Although the possible hazards to mother and child must be weighed against the potential benefits in every case, experience with Edrophonium Injection BP in pregnant patients with myasthenia gravis has revealed no untoward effect of the drug on the course of pregnancy.

There is no information on the excretion of Edrophonium Injection BP into breast milk. Although only negligible amounts would be expected to be present, due regard should be paid to possible effects on the breast-feeding infant.

Effects on ability to drive and use machines: None.

Undesirable effects: These may include nausea and vomiting, increased salivation, diarrhoea and abdominal cramps.

Overdose: Edrophonium Injection BP overdosage may given rise to bradycardia, arrhythmias, hypotension and bronchiolar spasm. Perspiration, gastro-intestinal hypermotility and visual disturbances may also occur.

Artificial ventilation should be instituted if respiration is severely depressed. Atropine sulphate 1–2 mg intravenously is an antidote to the muscarinic effects.

Pharmacological properties

Pharmacodynamic properties: Edrophonium Injection BP is an antagonist to cholinesterase, the enzyme which normally destroys acetylcholine. The action of Edrophonium Injection BP can briefly be described, therefore, as the potentiation of naturally occurring acetylcholine. It differs from Prostigmin (neostigmine) and Mestinon (pyridostigmine) in the rapidity and brevity of its action.

Pharmacokinetic properties: Following intravenous injection of Edrophonium Injection BP an initial rapid phase of elimination (0.5–2 minutes) precedes a much slower decline (24–45 minutes). It is suggested that the rapid fall in plasma concentration of edrophonium is not primarily due to metabolism and excretion but to the rapid uptake of the drug by other tissues.

Preclinical safety data: There are no pre-clinical data of relevance to the prescriber which are additional to that already included in other sections of the SPC.

Pharmaceutical particulars

List of excipients: Sodium Sulphite anhydrous, Sodium Citrate BP, Citric Acid BP, Water for Injections BP.

Incompatibilities: None known.

Shelf life: Five years.

Special precautions for storge: Protect from light.

Nature and contents of container: Colourless glass ampoules each containing 1 ml of solution, in packs of 10 ampoules. The ampoule solution is almost colourless.

Instruction for use/handling: None.

Marketing authorisation holder: Cambridge Selfcare Diagnostics Limited, t/a Cambridge Laboratories, Richmond House, Old Brewery Court, Sandyford Road, Newcastle upon Tyne NE2 1XG.

Marketing authorisation number 12070/0008.

Date of first authorisation/renewal of authorisation 24 April 1992.

Date of (partial) revision of the text November 1996.

FLUOROURACIL

Presentation Ampoules containing 250 mg of fluorouracil in the form of the sodium salt in 10 ml Water for Injections BP. The ampoule solution is colourless to slightly yellow.

Capsules with powder opaque cap and orange opaque body with ROCHE printed in black along both cap and body, containing 250 mg fluorouracil.

Uses

Properties: Fluorouracil, a cytostatic agent, is a fluorinated pyrimidine belonging to the category of antimetabolites. It inhibits cell division by interfering with the synthesis of deoxyribonucleic acid (DNA) and to a lesser extent of ribonucleic acid (RNA).

Indications: The palliative treatment of carcinoma.

Dosage and administration Various techniques are employed when using Fluorouracil in the treatment of carcinoma. The following examples are given for guidance.

Adults by the intravenous route: Fluorouracil may be administered by intravenous infusion or by intravenous injection. Dosages are generally based on the patient's body weight. If the patient is obese or there has been a spurious gain due to oedema, ascites or other forms of fluid retention, the patient's ideal weight should be used in calculating the dosage. The initial dose given below should be reduced by one-third to a half if the following conditions are present: poor nutritional state; after major surgery (within the previous 30 days); poor bone-marrow function (anaemia, leucopenia, thrombocytopenia); impaired hepatic or renal function.

Initial treatment: This may be in the form of an infusion or injection, the former usually being preferred because of lesser toxicity.

Infusion: A daily dose of 15 mg/kg, but not more than 1 g per infusion, is diluted in 500 ml 5% dextrose solution or 500 ml 0.9% sodium chloride solution and given by intravenous infusion at the rate of 40 drops per minute over 4 hours. Alternatively, the daily dose may be infused over 30–60 minutes, or given as a continuous infusion over 24 hours. This daily dose is given on successive days until toxicity occurs or until 12 to 15 g has been given. This sequence of injections constitutes a 'course' of therapy. Some patients have received up to 30 g at a maximum rate of 1 g daily. The daily dose should never exceed 1 g. An interval of four to six weeks should be allowed between any two 'courses' of Fluorouracil.

Injection: A dose of 12 mg/kg i.v. daily on three consecutive days. If there are no signs of toxicity the patient receives 6 mg/kg on the 5th, 7th and 9th days. If toxicity occurs the signs should be allowed to regress before further doses are administered.

Maintenance therapy consists of 5 to 15 mg/kg i.v. once weekly.

A more recent alternative method is to give 15 mg/kg i.v. once a week throughout the course of treatment. This obviates the need for an initial period of daily administration.

Regional perfusion intra-arterially: Continuous infusion of Fluorouracil into an artery supplying a localised growth has been shown to produce a better result in some tumours than would have been expected from systemic administration by the intravenous route, together with a decrease in toxicity. The usual dose is 5 to 7.5 mg/kg daily.

In combination with radiotherapy: Irradiation combined with Fluorouracil has been found to be useful in the treatment of certain types of metastatic lesions in the lungs and for relief of pain caused by recurrent, inoperable growth. The standard dose of Fluorouracil is used.

By the oral route: Fluorouracil may be administered orally using either the capsule or the ampoule solution. Oral administration is not recommended when Fluorouracil is being used initially as the sole agent in palliative treatment of carcinoma.

Oral administration may be useful in: palliative therapy employing a combination of drugs; long-term maintenance or post-operative prophylactic therapy in weekly doses; and where therapy with Fluorouracil is indicated, but it is impractical to administer the drug parenterally.

The usual dosage for maintenance treatment is 15 mg/kg once weekly. For palliative therapy a more rapid onset of therapeutic effect may be obtained by giving a daily dose of 15 mg/kg on six successive days. This is followed by maintenance therapy of 15 mg/kg once weekly. The daily dose should not exceed 1 g. The capsules should be taken with water after a meal.

The solution may be mixed with fruit juice or other similar beverages immediately before oral ingestion to mask its rather bitter taste. Multi-dose preparations must not be made up.

Elderly: Fluorouracil should be used in the elderly with similar consideration as in younger adults, notwithstanding that incidence of concomitant medical illness is higher in the former group.

Children: No dosage recommendations are made for the administration of Fluorouracil to children.

Fluorouracil Ampoules are for intra-arterial, intravenous or oral administration.

Fluorouracil Capsules are for oral administration.

Contra-indications, warnings, etc

Contra-indication: Fluorouracil should not be used in the management of non-malignant disease.

Use in pregnancy: Fluorouracil has been shown to be teratogenic. It therefore should not normally be administered to patients who are pregnant. Fluorouracil should also be regarded as contra-indicated in mothers who are breast-feeding.

Precautions: It is recommended that Fluorouracil be given only by or under the supervision of a physician who is experienced in cancer chemotherapy and who is well versed in the use of potent antimetabolites. Because of the possibility of severe toxic reactions, all patients should be admitted to hospital for initial treatment. Fluorouracil should be used with great care in debilitated patients.

The margin between the effective and toxic doses of Fluorouracil is narrow and a therapeutic response is unlikely without some evidence of toxicity. Even with meticulous selection of patients and careful adjustment of dosage, there may be severe haematological toxicity and gastro-intestinal haemorrhage. Severe toxicity is more likely in poor-risk patients.

Treatment should be discontinued promptly whenever one of the following signs of toxicity appears: Leucopenia (WBC under 3,500 per mm^3). Thrombocytopenia (platelets under 100,000 per mm^3). Stomatitis (the first small ulceration at the inner margin of the lips is a signal for stopping treatment. Severe diarrhoea (frequent bowel movements and watery stools). Gastro-intestinal ulceration and bleeding. Haemorrhage at any site.

Isolated cases of angina, ECG abnormalities and, rarely, myocardial infarction have been reported following Fluorouracil administration. Caution should therefore be exercised in treating patients who experience chest pain during courses of therapy, or patients with a history of heart disease.

The carcinogenic potential of Fluorouracil has not been evaluated but, as with all cytostatic drugs, this possibility should be borne in mind when designing long-term management of patients.

Side-effects: During treatment, diarrhoea, nausea and vomiting commonly occur, but may be controlled by the use of appropriate drugs.

Leucopenia usually follows an adequate course of treatment with Fluorouracil. The lowest white cell count commonly occurs between the seventh and fourteenth days after the first dose, but it may be delayed for as long as the twentieth day. By the thirtieth day, the count has usually returned to the normal range. Because of the importance of leucopenia, the white cell count should be checked frequently throughout the course. If it falls, it is advisable to obtain differential counts. If the total is less than 2,000 per mm^3, and especially if there is granulocytopenia, it is recommended that the patient be placed in protective isolation in the hospital and treated with appropriate measures for the prevention of systemic infection.

Alopecia and dermatitis may occur in a substantial proportion of cases. Female patients particularly should be warned as to the possibility of alopecia. Since the alopecia appears to be reversible, special measures do not seem to be indicated.

Treatment of overdosage: Signs and symptoms are qualitatively similar to the side-effects, and similar measures should be taken to treat them.

Handling precautions: Fluorouracil is irritant, contact with skin and mucous membranes should be avoided.

Handling guidelines:

Ampoules: Fluorouracil Ampoules should only be opened by trained staff and as with all cytotoxic agents, precautions should be taken to avoid exposing staff during pregnancy. Preparation of solution for administration should be carried out in a designated handling area and working over a washable tray or disposable plastic-backed absorbent paper.

Suitable eye protection, disposable gloves, face mask and disposable apron should be worn. Syringes and infusion sets should be assembled carefully to avoid leakage (use of Luer lock fittings is recommended).

On completion, any exposed surface should be thoroughly cleaned and hands and face washed.

Capsules: Undamaged capsules present minimal risk of contamination but in accordance with good hygiene requirements, direct handling should be avoided. As with all cytotoxic agents, precautions should be taken to avoid exposing staff during pregnancy.

Disposal guidelines: All sharps should be placed in an appropriate container and all other disposable items in a sealed plastic bag which should be incinerated with other clinical waste.

Waste material may be disposed of by incineration. Waste ampoule solution may first be absorbed on to cotton wool and double wrapped in sealed polythene bags.

First aid: Eye contact: Irrigate immediately with water and seek medical advice.

Skin contact: Wash thoroughly with soap and water and remove contaminated clothing.

Inhalation, ingestion: Seek immediate medical attention.

Pharmaceutical precautions

Storage: Fluorouracil Ampoule solution should be stored between 15°C and 25°C. Fluorouracil Capsules in blister packings should be stored in a dry place; the recommended maximum storage temperature is 25°C.

Additives: Fluorouracil Ampoule solution may be diluted with dextrose injection, sodium chloride injection or Water for Injections BP immediately before parenteral use.

Fluorouracil Ampoule solution may be diluted with fruit juice or other similar beverages immediately before use to facilitate ingestion by the oral route. Fluorouracil Ampoule solution must not be made up into multidose preparations.

Legal category POM

Package quantities Fluorouracil Ampoules in packings of 10.

Fluorouracil Capsules in blister packings of 30.

Further information *Availability:* Fluorouracil Ampoules are available through hospital pharmacies for use in hospitals and hospital clinics and can be supplied to retail chemists for dispensing prescriptions for patients whose treatment has been initiated in hospital practice.

Product licence numbers

Ampoules 14576/0002
Capsules 14576/0003

GESTRONOL HEXANOATE AMPOULES

Qualitative and quantitative composition 1 ml of solution contains 100 mg of gestronol hexanoate.

Pharmaceutical form Solution for injection.

Clinical particulars

Therapeutic indications: For the treatment of endometrial carcinoma and benign prostatic hyperplasia in adults.

Posology and method of administration: To be administered by slow intramuscular injection.

Endometrial carcinoma, before hysterectomy and for advanced disease: Gestronol hexanoate is a well-tolerated adjunct to other therapy. To inhibit metastatic spread before and after operation, 200–400 mg intramuscularly every 5–7 days, starting immediately following diagnosis and continuing for a minimum of 12 weeks.

For treating existing metastases: 200–400 mg can be administered intramuscularly every 5–7 days. If the metastases are hormone-responsive, improvement will be observed within 8–12 weeks of therapy. Treatment should than be continued for as long as it appears beneficial.

Benign prostatic hyperplasia: Where (a) the patient is an operation risk; (b) symptoms are mild; (c) there is a waiting list for operation, the following standard dosage applies: 200 mg weekly by intramuscular injection. In view of Gestronol hexanoate's good tolerance, this dosage can confidently be increased. In trials, 300 mg and 400 mg weekly have been used. The full benefit of treatment is unlikely to be established in a shorter period than three months, and trial results suggest that improvement can continue during substantially longer periods.

Contra-indications: Pregnancy. History of herpes gestationis. Previous or existing liver tumours (in progressive endometrial carcinoma only if these are not due to metastases).

Special warnings and precautions for use: Patients suffering from bronchial asthma, diabetes, epilepsy or migraine should be supervised closely.

In patients with chronic liver damage it is advisable to check liver function at intervals during long-term treatment or repeated courses of Gestronol hexanoate. Transient moderate rises in bromsulphthalein retention and serum transaminases have occasionally been observed but have always proved harmless.

In rare cases benign and, in even rarer cases malignant liver tumours leading in isolated cases to life-threatening intra-abdominal haemorrhage, have been observed after the use of hormonal substances such as Gestronol hexanoate. If severe upper abdominal complaints, liver enlargement or signs of intra-abdominal haemorrhage occur, a liver tumour should be considered in the differential diagnosis.

During treatment of prostatic adenoma, supervision of bladder and renal function is necessary.

Interactions with other medicaments and other forms of interaction: The requirement for oral antidiabetic agents or insulin can change.

Pregnancy and lactation: Gestronol hexanoate is contra-indicated in pregnancy.

Effects on ability to drive and use machines: None stated.

Undesirable effects: Rarely, local reactions may occur at the site of injection. Exacerbation of bronchial asthma, diabetes, epilepsy and migraine may sometimes occur. Side-effects are infrequent.

In males, a reversible depression of libido and gynaecomastia with discomfort have been reported by a few patients. Spermatogenesis is temporarily inhibited.

In rare cases, coughing, dyspnoea and circulatory irregularities may develop during, or immediately after, the injection.

Experience has shown that these reactions can be avoided by injecting very slowly.

Should severe or repeated symptomatology occur despite this injection technique, withdrawal of therapy will have to be considered.

Overdose: Overdose with injectable drugs is unlikely to occur, but if it does arise, treatment should be symptomatic.

Pharmacological properties

Pharmacodynamic properties: Gestronol hexanoate is 25 times more potent than its parent substance progesterone. In the female, the action of Gestronol hexanoate is concentrated on the endometrium. This action is direct and does not involve suppression via the pituitary. Except in some highly anaplastic tumours, Gestronol hexanoate has a strong antimitotic effect, with regression or arrest of primary endometrial carcinoma and of soft-tissue metastases.

In the male, Gestronol hexanoate has been shown to reduce prostatic weight significantly. It may effect an objective improvement in peak urine flow rates and residual urine and in subjective symptoms such as nocturia.

Pharmacokinetic properties: Gestronol hexanoate is administered intramuscularly as an oily solution. Therapeutic effects are dependent upon the release of gestronol hexanoate from its intramuscular depot which is retarded but complete. Liberation of active ingredient from the depot, however, is slower than its elimination from the plasma. This is why the disposition half-lives from plasma reflect the liberation process from the oily depot. About 3 days after administration, peak plasma levels reach about 420 ng/ml. Plasma levels decrease with a half-life of about 7.5 days.

The unchanged drug substance is probably responsible for the therapeutic effects observed. Its fraction of the whole sum of metabolites in plasma may not exceed 5%, however. The predominant part of the main metabolite is rapidly conjugated. There is virtually no free gestronol hexanoate.

Gestronol hexanoate is excreted mainly in the faeces (72%) and also in the urine (25%). The recovery was 48% of the administered dose within 14 days and 85% within 37 days. The observed half-lives of renal (3.2 days; with urine) and biliary (3.7 days; with faeces) excretion reflect the release of drug substance from its oily depot.

Gestronol hexanoate is completely bioavailable.

Preclinical safety data: There are no preclinical safety data which could be of relevance to the prescriber and which are not already included in other relevant sections of the SPC.

Pharmaceutical particulars

List of excipients: Benzyl benzoate; castor oil for injection.

Imcompatibilities: None known.

Shelf life: 5 years.

Special precautions for storage: Store below 25°C. Protect from light.

Nature and contents of container: 2 ml amber glass ampoules in packs of 5 ampoules.

Instruction for use/handling: Keep out of the reach of children.

Marketing authorisation holder: Cambridge Selfcare Diagnostics Limited, Newcastle upon Tyne NE2 1XG.

Marketing authorisation number 12070/0014.

Date of approval/revision of SPC March 1996.

Legal category POM.

ISOCARBOXAZID TABLETS 10 mg

Qualitative and quantitative composition Each tablet contains 10 mg Isocarboxazid.

Pharmaceutical form Tablets.

Clinical particulars

Therapeutic indications: For the treatment of the symptoms of depressive illness.

Posology and method of administration: Isocarboxazid Tablets are for oral administration.

Adults: A daily dose of 30 mg, in single or divided doses, should be given until improvement is obtained. The maximal effect is only observed after a period varying from 1–4 weeks. If no improvement has been seen by 4 weeks, doses up to 60 mg may be tried, according to the patient's tolerance, for no longer than 4–6 weeks, provided the patient is closely monitored because of the increased risk of adverse reactions occurring.

Once the optimal effect is achieved, the dose should be reduced to the lowest possible amount sufficient to maintain the improvement. Clinical experience has shown this to be usually 10–20 mg daily but up to 40 mg daily may be required in some cases.

The elderly: The elderly are more likely to experience adverse reactions such as agitation, confusion and postural hypotension. Half the normal maintenance dose may be sufficient to produce a satisfactory clinical response.

Children: Isocarboxazid Tablets are not indicated for paediatric use.

Contra-indications: Isocarboxazid is contra-indicated in patients with any impairment of hepatic function, cerebrovascular disorders or severe cardiovascular disease, and in those with actual or suspected phaeochromocytoma.

Special warnings and precautions for use: Some monoamine oxidase inhibitors have occasionally caused hepatic complications and jaundice in patients, therefore regular monitoring of liver function should be carried out during Isocarboxazid therapy. If there is any evidence of a hepatotoxic reaction, the drug should be withdrawn immediately.

The drug should be used cautiously in patients with impaired renal function, to prevent accumulation taking place, and also in the elderly or debilitated and those with cardiovascular disease, diabetes or blood dyscrasias.

In restless or agitated patients, Isocarboxazid may precipitate states of excessive excitement. Isocarboxazid appears to have varying effects in epileptic patients; while some have a decrease in frequency of seizures, others have more seizures.

Interactions with other medicaments and other forms of interaction: Like other monoamine oxidase inhibitors, Isocarboxazid potentiates the action of a number of drugs and foods. Patients being treated with a monoamine oxidase inhibitor should not receive indirectly-acting sympathomimetic agents such as amphetamines, metaraminol, fenfluramine or similar anorectic agents, ephedrine or phenylpropanolamine (contained in many proprietary 'cold-cure' medications), dopamine or levodopa. Patients should also be warned to avoid foodstuffs and beverages with a high tyramine content: mature cheeses (including processed cheeses), hydrolysed yeast or meat extracts, alcoholic beverages, particularly heavy red wines such as Chianti, non-alcoholic beers, lagers and wines, and other foods which are not fresh and are fermented, pickled, 'hung', 'matured' or otherwise subject to protein degradation before consumption. Broad bean pods (which contain levodopa) and banana skins may also present a hazard. In extreme cases interactions may result in severe hypertensive episodes. Isocarboxazid should therefore be discontinued immediately upon the occurrence of palpitations or frequent headaches.

Pethidine should not be given to patients receiving

monoamine oxidase inhibitors as serious, potentially fatal reactions, including central excitation, muscle rigidity, hyperpyrexia, circulatory collapse, respiratory depression and coma, can result. Such reactions are less likely with morphine, but experience of the interaction of Isocarboxazid with narcotic analgesics other than pethidine is limited and extreme caution is therefore necessary when administering morphine to patients undergoing therapy with Isocarboxazid.

Isocarboxazid should not be administered together with other monoamine oxidase inhibitors or most tricyclic antidepressants (clomipramine, desipramine, imipramine, butriptyline, nortriptyline or protriptyline). Although there is no proof that combined therapy will be effective, refractory cases of depression may be treated with Isocarboxazid in combination with amitriptyline or trimipramine, provided appropriate care is taken. Hypotensive and other adverse reactions are likely to be increased.

An interval of 1–2 weeks should be allowed after treatment with Isocarboxazid before the administration of antidepressants with a different mode of action or any other drug which may interact. A similar interval is recommended before administration of Isocarboxazid when another antidepressant has been used; in the case of drugs with a very long half-life (such as fluoxetine), it may be advisable to extend this interval.

Isocarboxazid should be discontinued for at least 2 weeks prior to elective surgery requiring general anaesthesia. The anaesthetist should be warned that a patient is being treated with Isocarboxazid, in the event of emergency surgery being necessary. Concurrent administration of Isocarboxazid with other central nervous system depressants (especially barbiturates and phenothiazines), stimulants, local anaesthetics, ganglion-blocking agents and other hypotensives (including methyl-dopa and reserpine), diuretics, vasopressors, anticholinergic drugs and hypoglycaemic agents may lead to potentiation of their effects. This should be borne in mind if dentistry, surgery or a change in treatment of a patient becomes necessary during treatment with Isocarboxazid.

All patients taking Isocarboxazid should be warned against self-medication with proprietary 'cold-cure' preparations and nasal decongestants and advised of the dietary restrictions listed under 'warnings'.

With Isocarboxazid, as with other drugs acting on the central nervous system, patients should be instructed to avoid alcohol while under treatment, since the individual response cannot be foreseen.

Pregnancy and lactation: Do not use in pregnancy, especially during the first and last trimesters, unless there are compelling reasons. There is no evidence as to drug safety in human pregnancy, nor is there evidence from animal work that it is free from hazard. In addition, the effect of psychotropic drugs on the fine brain structure of the foetus is unknown. Since there is no information on the secretion of the drug into breast milk, Isocarboxazid is contra-indicated during lactation.

Effects on ability to drive and use machines: Like all medicaments of this type, Isocarboxazid may modify patients' reactions (driving ability, operation of machinery etc.) to a varying extent, depending on dosage and individual susceptibility.

Undesirable effects: In general, Isocarboxazid is well tolerated by the majority of patients. Side-effects, if they occur, are those common to the group of monoamine oxidase inhibitors.

The most frequently reported have been orthostatic hypotension, associated in some patients with disturbances in cardiac rhythm, peripheral oedema, complaints of dizziness, dryness of the mouth, nausea and vomiting, constipation, blurred vision, insomnia, drowsiness, weakness and fatigue. These side-effects can usually be controlled by dosage reduction.

There have been infrequent reports of mild headaches, sweating, paraesthesiae, peripheral neuritis, hyperreflexia, agitation, overactivity, muscle tremor, confusion and other behavioural changes, difficulty in micturition, impairment of erection and ejaculation, and skin rashes. Although rare, blood dyscrasias (purpura, granulocytopenia) have been reported. Response to Isocarboxazid may be accompanied by increased appetite and weight gain.

Overdose: The primary symptoms of overdosage include dizziness, ataxia and irritability. In acute cases, hypotension or hypertension, tachycardia, pyrexia, psychotic manifestations, convulsions, respiratory depression and coma may occur and continue for 8–14 days before recovery.

Gastric lavage should be performed soon after ingestion and intensive supportive therapy carried out. Sympathomimetic agents should not be given to treat hypotension but plasma expanders may be used in severe cases. Hypertensive crises may be treated by pentoliniurn or phentolamine, severe shock with hydrocortisone. Diazepam may be used to control convulsions or severe excitement. Dialysis is of value in eliminating the drug in severe cases.

Pharmacological properties

Pharmacodynamic properties: Isocarboxazid is a monoamine oxidase inhibitor, effective in small doses. Its antidepressant action is thought to be related to its effect on physiological amines such as serotonin and noradrenaline, and this effect is cumulative and persistent.

Pharmacokinetic properties: Isocarboxazid is readily absorbed after oral administration. Most of the drug-related material is excreted as metabolites in the urine.

Preclinical safety data: There are no pre-clinical data of relevance to the prescriber which are additional to that already included in other sections of the SPC.

Pharmaceutical particulars

List of excipients: Lactose, Starch, Talc, Magnesium stearate, Gelatin, Iron oxide yellow E172, Iron Oxide red E172.

Incompatibilities: None known.

Shelf life: Three years.

Special precautions for storage: The recommended maximum storage temperature is 25°C.

Isocarboxazid Tablets should be stored in well-closed containers.

Nature and contents of container: HDPE bottles with snap closures, containing 56 tablets.

Instruction for use/handling: None.

Marketing authorisation holder: Cambridge Selfcare Diagnostics Limited, t/a Cambridge Laboratories, Richmond House, Old Brewery Court, Sandyford Road, Newcastle upon Tyne NE2 1XG.

Marketing authorisation number PL 12070/0003.

Date of first authorisation/renewal of authorisation 21 April 1992.

Date of (partial) revision of the text November 1996.

ISONIAZID AMPOULES 50 mg/2 ml

Qualitative and quantitative composition Each ampoule contains 50 mg Isoniazid BP in 2 ml of solution.

Pharmaceutical form Ampoules.

Clinical particulars

Therapeutic indications: For all forms of pulmonary and extra-pulmonary tuberculosis.

Posology and method of administration: Isoniazid ampoules are for intramuscular, intravenous, intrapleural, or intrathecal injection.

Adults and children: The usual intramuscular or intravenous dose for adults is 200 to 300 mg as a single daily dose, for children 100 to 300 mg daily (10–20 mg/kg), but doses much larger than these are sometimes given, especially in conditions such as tuberculous meningitis. It is recommended to give an intravenous dose slowly as an undiluted bolus injection, although other methods may be employed.

Neonates: The recommended intravenous or intramuscular dose for neonates is 3–5 mg/kg with a maximum of 10 mg/kg daily. Isoniazid may be present in the milk of lactating mothers.

The elderly: No dosage reduction is necessary in the elderly.

Intrapleural use: 50 to 250 mg may be instilled intrapleurally after aspiration of pus, the dosage of oral isoniazid on that day being correspondingly reduced. The ampoule solution is also used for the local treatment of tuberculous ulcers, for irrigation of fistulae, etc.

Intrathecal use: It should be noted that CSF concentrations of isoniazid are approximately 90% of plasma concentrations. Where intrathecal use is required, 25–50 mg daily has been given to adults and 10–20 mg daily for children, according to age.

It is usual to give Isoniazid together with other antituberculous therapy, as determined by current practice and/or sensitivity testing.

It is recommended that pyridoxine 10–50 mg daily be given during Isoniazid therapy to minimise adverse reactions, especially in malnourished patients and those predisposed to neuropathy (e.g. diabetics and alcoholics).

Contra-indications: Isoniazid should not be given to patients with a history of sensitivity to isoniazid.

Special warnings and precautions for use: Use in renal and hepatic impairment: no dosage reduction of Isoniazid is necessary when given to patients with mild renal failure. Patients with severe renal failure (glomerular filtration rate of less than 10 ml/minute) and slow acetylator status might require a dose reduction of about 100 mg to maintain trough plasma levels at less than 1 mcg/ml. The possible risks of administration of Isoniazid to patients with pre-existing non-tuberculous hepatic disease should be balanced against the benefits expected from treating tuberculosis. Care is also required in chronic alcoholism and when prescribing isoniazid for patients with pre-existing hepatitis. Convulsions and psychotic reactions have occurred, especially in patients with a previous history of these conditions. These manifestations usually subside rapidly when the drug is withdrawn. Isoniazid should therefore be given with caution to patients with convulsive disorders and should be avoided in those with manic or hypomanic psychoses.

Isoniazid is metabolised by acetylation, which is subject to genetic variation. The 'slow acetylators' may be more susceptible to drug-induced peripheral neuropathy. However, dose adjustment is not normally required.

Interactions with other medicaments and other forms of interaction: Isoniazid may inhibit the metabolism of phenytoin, primidone and carbamazepine. Plasma levels of these drugs should be monitored if concurrent therapy with Isoniazid is necessary. See also statement under *Undesirable effects* regarding Rifampicin.

Pregnancy and lactation: While Isoniazid is generally regarded to be safe in pregnancy, there is a possibility of an increased risk of foetal malformations occurring when Isoniazid is given in early pregnancy. If pregnancy cannot be excluded possible risks should be balanced against therapeutic benefits. Isoniazid is excreted in breast milk at concentrations equivalent to those found in maternal plasma, i.e. 6–12 mcg/ml. This could result in an infant ingesting up to 2 mg/kg/day.

Effects on ability to drive and use machines: None known.

Undesirable effects: Isoniazid is generally well tolerated. Side-effects have been reported mainly in association with high doses or in slow acetylators who develop higher blood levels of the drug. Fever, peripheral neuropathy (preventable with pyridoxine), optic neuritis and atrophy, allergic skin conditions (including erythema multiforme), and rarely lupoid syndrome, pellagra, purpura and haematological reactions have occurred during isoniazid therapy. Hyperglycaemia and gynaeco-mastia have been reported with isoniazid treatment. Isoniazid, especially if given with rifampicin, may induce abnormalities in liver function, particularly in patients with pre-existing liver disorders, in the elderly, the very young and the malnourished. Monthly review is suggested to detect and limit the severity of this side-effect by stopping treatment if plasma transaminases exceed three times the upper limit of normal. There is conflicting opinion as to the relationship of this side-effect to acetylator status.

Overdose: In severe poisoning the main risk is of epileptiform convulsions. In addition any of the side-effects listed above may occur together with metabolic acidosis and hyperglycaemia. Treatment should be directed to the control of convulsions and large doses of pyridoxine may limit the occurrence of other adverse effects. Metabolic acidosis may require sodium bicarbonate infusion. The drug is removed by dialysis.

Pharmacological properties

Pharmacodynamic properties: Isoniazid is a highly active tuberculostatic drug, and at high concentrations it is bactericidal to mycobacterium tuberculosis, possibly acting by interference with the synthesis of mycolic acid (a constituent of the bacterial cell wall).

Phamacokinetic properties: Isoniazid is not appreciably protein-bound and diffuses readily throughout the body. It affects intracellular as well as extracellular bacilli. The primary metabolic route involves acetylation the rate of which is determined genetically.

Preclinical safety data: There are no pre-clinical data of relevance to the prescriber which are additional to that already included in other sections of the SPC.

Pharmaceutical particulars

List of excipients: Hydrochloric Acid, Water for Injections BP.

Incompatibilities: None known.

Shelf life: Three years.

Special precautions for storage: The recommended maximum storage temperature is 25°C. Protect from light.

Nature and contents of container: 10 Colourless glass ampoules, each containing 2 ml of solution.

Instruction for use/handling: None.

Marketing authorisation holder: Cambridge Selfcare Diagnostics Limited, t/a Cambridge Laboratories,

Richmond House, Old Brewery Court, Sandyford Road, Newcastle upon Tyne NE2 1XG.

Marketing authorisation number PL 12070/0005.

Date of first authorisation/renewal of authorisation 21 April 1992.

Date of (partial) revision of the text July 1997.

LEVODOPA TABLETS 500 mg

Qualitative and quantitative composition Each tablet contains 500 mg Levodopa PhEur.

Pharmaceutical form Tablets.

Clinical particulars

Therapeutic indications: For the treatment of Parkinsonism – idiopathic, post-encephalitic, arteriosclerotic. Previous neurosurgery is not a contra-indication to levodopa.

Posology and method of administration: Lovodopa Tablets are for oral administration.

Dosage and administration are variable and no more than a guide can be given.

Adults: Hospitalised patients: Initially 0.25 to 1 g daily in up to 5 divided doses immediately after food. Dosage should be increased by 0.5 to 1g every three to four days until adequate improvement results or intolerable side-effects appear. If severe side-effects appear, the dosage should be gradually decreased to the maximum tolerated. The majority of patients will tolerate the rapid dose increase outlined above, but occasionally intolerance may prevent patients from reaching effective dosage levels. When patients discontinue therapy due to intolerance they should be restarted on 0.25 to 0.5 g daily in small divided doses, increasing by 0.125 to 0.5 g at weekly intervals.

Adults: General practice patients and out-patients: Initially 0.125 g twice daily immediately after food. After one week, the dose may be increased to 0.125 g four or five times daily. Thereafter dosage should be increased at weekly intervals by 0.375 g daily, the total daily dose being given in four or five divided doses. The response of individual patients varies and some patients may tolerate a more rapid rate of increase, e.g. by 0.25 to 0.5 g daily at intervals of three to four days.

Improvement is usually seen in two to three weeks with the normal dosage range being 2.5 to 8 g daily, but further improvement may occur up to six months or even longer.

When the optimum daily dosage for any particular patient has been reached, it may need to be redistributed throughout the day to meet fluctuations in the individual's requirements. Most patients find a four or five times daily dosage scheme satisfactory; some obtain a smoother effect with two-hourly administration; others, who develop akinetic crises at particular times of the day, learn by experience the daily dosage scheme most suited to their needs.

After a period at the maximum tolerated dosage level, side-effects may slowly develop, usually in the form of involuntary movements. These generally regress without loss of therapeutic effect if the dosage is slightly reduced.

Anticholinergic drugs should be continued during levodopa therapy. As treatment with levodopa proceeds and the therepeutic effect is found, the dosage of the anticholinergic drugs may need to be changed.

Children: No dosage recommendations are made for the administration of levodopa to children.

Contra-indications: Levodopa is contra-indicated in narrow-angle glaucoma (it may be used in wide-angle glaucoma provided that the intra-ocular pressure remains under control); severe psychoneuroses or psychoses; severe endocrine, renal, hepatic or cardiac disorders. It should not be given in conjunction with monoamine oxidase (MAO) inhibitors except selective MAO-B inhibitors, or within two weeks of their withdrawal. It should not be given to patients under 25 years of age.

Suspicion has arisen that levodopa may activate a malignant melanoma. Therefore levodopa should not be used in persons who have a history of, or who may be suffering from, a malignant melanoma.

Special warnings and precautions for use: Pyridoxine (vitamin B6), which is often included in multi-vitamin preparations, is known to block the effect of levodopa. When other drugs must be given in conjunction with levodopa, the patient should be carefully observed for unusual side-effects or potentiating effects. In the event of general anaesthesia being required, levodopa therapy may be continued as long as the patient is able to take fluid and medication by mouth.

If therapy is temporarily interrupted, the usual daily dosage may be administered as soon as the patient is able to take oral medication. Whenever therapy has been interrupted for longer periods, dosage should again be adjusted gradually, however, in many cases the patient can rapidly be returned to his previous therapeutic dosage.

There have been occasional reports of a neuroleptic malignant-like syndrome, involving hyperthermia, on abrupt withdrawal of levodopa preparations. Sudden discontinuation of levodopa, without close supervision, or 'drug holidays' should therefore be avoided. Care should be taken when using levodopa in the following circumstances: in endocrine, renal, pulmonary or cardiovascular disease; particularly where there is a history of myocardial infarction or arrhythmia; psychiatric disturbances; hepatic disorder; peptic ulcer; osteomalacia; where sympathomimetic, drugs may be required (e.g. bronchial asthma), due to possible potentiation of the cardiovascular effects of levodopa; where anti-hypertensive drugs are being used due to possible increased hypotensive action.

Periodic evaluation of hepatic, haemopoietic, renal and cardiovascular functions is advised. Patients who improve on levodopa therapy should be advised to resume normal activities gradually as rapid mobilisation may increase the risk of injury.

Interactions with other medicaments and other forms of interaction: Drugs which interfere with central amine mechanisms, such as rauwolfia alkaloids (reserpine), tetrabenazine, metoclopramide, phenothiazines, thioxanthenes, butyrophenones, amphetamines and papaverine, should be avoided where possible. If, however, their administration is considered essential, extreme care should be exercised and a close watch kept for any signs of potentiation, antagonism or other interactions and for unusual side-effects.

Pregnancy and lactation: There is no, or inadequate evidence of safety of the drug in human pregnancy; it has been in wide use for many years without apparent ill-consequence; there is evidence of harmful effects in pregnancy in animals. Levodopa therapy may interfere with lactation; this should be borne in mind if treatment is required in breast-feeding mothers.

Effects on ability to drive and use machines: Not applicable.

Undesirable effects: Tolerance to levodopa varies widely between patients and is often related to the rate of dosage increase. Post-encephalitic Parkinsonian patients tolerate the drug less well. Side-effects, usually dose-related, occur at some time in most patients. During the initiation of therapy nausea and vomiting, anorexia, weakness and hypotension, which is usually postural (but a little hypertension may rarely be seen), are most frequent. Nausea and vomiting may be minimised by administering levodopa immediately after food; an anti-emetic, e.g. cyclizine hydrochloride 50 mg three times daily, may also be helpful.

Psychiatric disturbances are common in Parkinsonian patients, including those being treated with levodopa. They include mild elation, anxiety, agitation, insomnia, depression, aggression, delusions, hallucinations and 'unmasking' of psychoses.

Although there have been rare reports of possible antagonism of levodopa by diazepam, in general diazepam and nitrazepam have been found to be useful in the treatment of anxiety and insomnia, respectively, occurring in Parkinsonism. Depression may be treated with tricyclic antidepressants although isolated cases of hypertensive crises have been reported with the concomitant use of tricyclic drugs. ECT may be administered if appropriate. MAO inhibitors, except selective MAO-B inhibitors, must not be used.

Involuntary movements, commonly in the form of oral dyskinesias, often accompanied by 'paddling' foot movements, or of the choreo-athetoid type, are common, particularly on long-term administration. These are usually dose-dependent and may disappear or become tolerable after dose adjustment. With long-term administration, fluctuations in the therapeutic response may be encountered. They include 'freezing' episodes, end-of-dose deterioration and the so called 'on-off' effect. Patients may be helped by dosage reduction or by giving smaller and more frequent doses.

Other side-effects which have occasionally been reported with levodopa therapy include gastrointestinal bleeding, flushing, sweating and drowsiness. On some occasions the urine passed during levodopa treatment may be altered in colour; usually red-tinged, this will turn dark on standing. These changes are due to metabolites and are no cause for concern. Transient rises in SGOT, SGPT and alkaline phosphatase values have been noted: serum uric acid and blood urea nitrogen levels are occasionally increased. In rare instances, haemolytic anaemia, mild transient leucopenia and thrombocytopenia have been reported.

Also, in rare instances, headache and peripheral neuropathy have been reported.

Overdose: Symptoms of overdosage are qualitatively similar to the side-effects but may be of greater magnitude. Treatment should include gastric lavage, general supportive measures, intravenous fluids and the maintenance of an adequate airway. Electrocardiographic monitoring should be instituted and the patient carefully observed for the possible development of arrhythmias. If necessary, anti-arrhythmic therapy should be given and other symptoms treated as they arise.

Pharmacological properties

Pharmacodynamic properties: Levodopa is an anti-parkinsonian agent. Levodopa is the metabolic precursor of dopamine. The latter is severely depleted in the striatum, pallidum and substantia nigra of parkinsonian patients and it is considered that administration of levodopa raises the level of available dopamine in these centres.

Treatment with levodopa gives worthwhile sustained relief in about two-thirds of these patients. Akinesia usually responds first, then rigidity, and then tremor. Amelioration may be seen in other symptoms, including oculogyric crises. It may take six months or more before maximal improvement is achieved.

Pharmacokinetic properties: Although there may be considerable inter-individual variation in the systemic absorption of levodopa following oral administration, peak plasma levels are generally achieved within two hours.

Estimates of the elimination half-life for levodopa are usually within the range 30–60 minutes.

Preclinical safety data: There are no pre-clinical data of relevance to the prescriber which are additional to that already included in other sections of the SPC.

Pharmaceutical particulars

List of excipients: Starch, Purified talc, Citric acid, anhydrous, Magnesium stearate, Microcrystalline cellulose.

Incompatibilities: Levodopa may interfere chemically with several diagnostic laboratory tests including those for glucose, ketone bodies, or catecholamines in urine and for glucose or uric acid in blood. Levodopa therapy has been reported to inhibit the response to protirelin in tests of thyroid function.

Shelf life: Five years.

Special precautions for storage: Protect from light.

Nature and contents of container: Amber glass bottles with screw cap or HDPE bottles with polyethylene caps, containing 200 tablets.

Instruction for use/handling: None.

Marketing authorisation holder: Cambridge Selfcare Diagnostics Limited, t/a Cambridge Laboratories, Richmond House, Old Brewery Court, Sandyford Road, Newcastle upon Tyne NE2 1XG.

Marketing authorisation number PL 12070/0002.

Date of first authorisation/renewal of authorisation 21 April 1992.

Date of (partial) revision of the text November 1996.

LISURIDE TABLETS 200 mcg

Qualitative and quantitative composition Each tablet contains 200 micrograms Lisuride Maleate (equivalent to 149 micrograms Lisuride).

Pharmaceutical form Tablet.

Clinical particulars Lisuride is a selective dopamine agonist. Parkinson's disease, which is characterised by a deficiency of dopamine in the nigro-striatal pathway, responds to Lisuride, which can be used either alone or in combination with levodopa, for the management of previously untreated patients and those exhibiting 'on-off' phenomena. It is suitable for patients who cannot tolerate levodopa or whose response to levodopa is declining.

Therapeutic indications: For the treatment of Parkinson's disease.

Posology and method of administration: The following general rules apply: Lisuride should always be taken with food. The initial dose should preferably be taken at bedtime. Dosage should be low initially, increasing gradually to the appropriate final level, as determined by the efficacy and tolerance of the drug.

Adults and elderly patients: Initially, one tablet at bedtime. After one week, the dosage may be increased to 200 micrograms at bedtime and 200 micrograms at midday. After a further week, an additional 200 micrograms may be added in the morning. The dosage should continue to be increased by 200 micrograms per week (beginning each sequence of three increases with the bedtime dose) until the optimum dosage is achieved.

The maximum daily dosage should not normally exceed 5 mg (25 tablets).

Children: Lisuride is not recommended in children.

Contra-indications: Severe disturbances of peripheral circulation, coronary insufficiency.

Special warnings and precautions for use: Lisuride

should be given with extreme caution to a patient who has, or has had treated, a pituitary tumour. Enlargement can occur, particularly during pregnancy, which may result in early visual field defects.

Psychiatric reactions have been seen with the use of Lisuride and this is more likely with high dosage and in patients who have a history of psychotic disturbance.

Interactions with other medicaments and other forms of interaction: The effects of some psychotropic drugs may possibly be impaired by the simultaneous use of Lisuride. Dopamine antagonists (e.g. haloperidol, sulpiride and metoclopramide) can weaken the effects and side-effects of Lisuride.

Pregnancy and lactation: Although many foetuses have been exposed to Lisuride, without evidence of teratogenicity in women of child bearing potential, the potential risks of use must be weighed against the benefits of treatment.

Lactation is unlikely to be inhibited if suckling or a breast pump is used.

Effects on ability to drive and use machines: The possibility of hypotensive reactions demands particular care in activities such as driving or operating machinery.

Undesirable effects: Nausea and vomiting are the most common side-effects experienced in patients with Parkinson's disease. In these patients domperidone can be freely used, since although it is an antidopaminergic drug it does not pass the blood brain barrier and therefore does not antagonise the anti-Parkinsonian effects of Lisuride. A sudden severe fall in blood pressure has been observed in isolated cases. Tolerance is rapidly acquired, and side-effects are most likely during the first few days of treatment. Dizziness, headache, lethargy, malaise and slight drowsiness are possible. There are occasional transient slightly itchy exanthemata. Abdominal pains and constipation occur rarely. Raynaud's phenomenon has been reported in one case so far.

Overdose: Expected symptoms of overdosage include severe nausea and vomiting, confusion, hallucinations and postural hypotension. Treatment should include the use of a specific dopamine antagonist as well as general supportive measures and maintenance of the blood pressure. Gastric lavage should be employed if overdosage is discovered soon enough.

Pharmacological properties

Pharmacodynamic properties: Numerous pharmacological experiments have shown Lisuride to be a potent direct dopamine agonist. It has been shown to interact with peripheral 5-HT systems as an antagonist and with central 5-HT systems as an agonist. At higher doses, it also has alpha-adrenolytic and even beta-receptor-blocking activity.

Biochemical investigations have confirmed that it is one of the most potent dopamine-receptor agonists known, displaying very high affinity for both D_1 and D_2 receptors.

Pharmacokinetic properties

Absorption: In man, Lisuride is completely absorbed after oral administration with an absorption half-life of 1.2±0.3 h. Lisuride maleate is a semi-synthetic ergot derivative with a high affinity for central dopamine receptors. Lisuride maleate is subject to a high first-pass metabolism.

Drug level/metabolic clearance: In man, following an intravenous bolus injection, the plasma concentration of Lisuride falls in three phases with half-lives of 3–5 minutes, 20 mins and 2–3 hours. Values found in younger and older healthy volunteers were almost identical. The basic pharmacokinetic data for Lisuride were unchanged in Parkinson patients. Metabolic clearance was 13 ml/kg/min in young healthy volunteers, 16 ml/kg/min in elderly volunteers and 11±12.7 ml/kg/min in patients.

Bioavailability: Bioavailability is low in man and all animal species tested because of the high level of first-pass metabolism.

Elimination: In man, only 1.8% of the IV dose and 0.1% of the oral dose are recovered in the urine as unchanged metabolite. The metabolites of Lisuride are eliminated in almost equal portions via the kidney and liver.

Preclinical safety data: There are no pre-clinical data of relevance to the prescriber which are additional to that already included in other sections of the SPC.

Pharmaceutical particulars

List of excipients: Tartaric acid, lactose, magnesium stearate, calcium disodium edetate, microcrystalline cellulose.

Incompatibilities: None known.

Shelf life: 18 months.

Special precautions for storage: Recommended maximum storage temperature for Lisuride tablets is 25°C. Lisuride tablets should be stored in a dry place.

Nature and contents of container: Amber glass bottle with white polyethylene snap-in stopper, containing 100 tablets.

Instruction for use/handling: No special requirements.

Marketing authorisation holder: Cambridge Selfcare Diagnostics Limited, t/a Cambridge Laboratories, Richmond House, Old Brewery Court, Sandyford Road, Newcastle upon Tyne NE2 1XG.

Marketing authorisation number 12070/0021.

Date of first authorisation/renewal of authorisation 16 June 1997.

Date of (partial) revision of the text 30 January 1998.

MENADIOL SODIUM DIPHOSPHATE TABLETS 10 mg

Qualitative and quantitative composition Each tablet contains 10 mg Menadiol Sodium Diphosphate USP.

Pharmaceutical form Tablets.

Clinical particulars

Therapeutic indications: For the treatment of haemorrhage or threatened haemorrhage associated with a low blood level of prothrombin or factor vii. The main indication is obstructive jaundice (before and after surgery).

Posology and method of administration: Menadiol Sodium Diphosphate Tablets are for oral administration.

Adults: Usual therapeutic dose: 10–40 mg daily.

Children: If, on the recommendation of a physician, a children's dosage is required, it is suggested that 5–20 mg daily be given.

The elderly: Recommendations for use in the elderly do not differ from those for other adults.

Contra-indications: Administration to neonates, infants or to mothers in the pre- and post-natal periods.

Special warnings and precautions for use: None.

Interactions with other medicaments and other forms of interaction: Large doses of menadiol sodium diphosphate may decrease patient sensitivity to anti-coagulants.

Pregnancy and lactation: There is evidence of hazard if menadiol sodium diphosphate is used in human pregnancy. It is known to be associated with a small risk of haemolytic anaemia, hyperbilirubinaemia and kernicterus in the infant if administered to the mother in late pregnancy or during labour. Menadiol sodium diphosphate is therefore contra-indicated during late pregnancy.

Effects on ability to drive and use machines: None known.

Undesirable effects: Menadiol sodium diphosphate may induce haemolysis (especially in the newborn infant) in the presence of erythrocyte glucose-6-phosphate dehydrogenase deficiency or low concentrations of alpha-tocopherol in the blood.

Overdose: No information is available.

Pharmacological properties

Pharmacodynamic properties: Menadiol sodium diphosphate is a water-soluble vitamin K analogue. The presence of vitamin K is essential for the formation within the body of prothrombin, factor VII, factor IX and factor X. Lack of vitamin K leads to increased tendency to haemorrhage.

Pharmacokinetic properties: Menadione is absorbed from the gastro-intestinal tract without being dependent upon the presence of bile salts. Vitamin K is rapidly metabolised and excreted by the body.

Preclinical safety data: There are no pre-clinical data of relevance to the prescriber which are additional to that already included in other sections of the SPC.

Pharmaceutical particulars

List of excipients: Lactose, Maize starch, Talc, Magnesium stearate.

Incompatibilities: No information is available.

Shelf life: Three years.

Special precautions for storage: Recommended maximum storage temperature 30°C. Protect from light.

Nature and contents of container: White HDPE bottles containing 100 tablets.

Instruction for use/handling: None.

Marketing authorisation holder: Cambridge Selfcare Diagnostics Limited, t/a Cambridge Laboratories, Richmond House, Old Brewery Court, Sandyford Road, Newcastle upon Tyne NE2 1XG.

Marketing authorisation number PL 12070/0007.

Date of first authorisation/renewal of authorisation 30 April 1992.

Date of (partial) revision of the text November 1996.

NABILONE CAPSULES

Qualitative and quantitative composition Nabilone Capsules contain 1.0 mg nabilone per capsule.

Pharmaceutical form Capsules.

Clinical particulars

Therapeutic indications: Nabilone is indicated for the control of nausea and vomiting, caused by chemotherapeutic agents used in the treatment of cancer, in patients who have failed to respond adequately to conventional antiemetic treatments.

Posology and method of administration: Nabilone is for administration to adults only. It is not recommended for use in children younger than 18 years of age as safety and efficacy have not been established.

The usual adult doage is 1 mg or 2 mg twice a day. To minimise side-effects, it is recommended that the lower starting dose is used and that the dose is increased as necessary. The first dose should be administered the night before initiation of chemotherapy, and the second dose should be given one to three hours before the first dose of the oncolytic agent is administered.

The maximum daily dose should not exceed 6 mg, given in three divided doses.

Nabilone may be administered throughout each cycle of chemotherapy and, if necessary, for 48 hours after the last dose of each cycle. Data on the chronic use of nabilone are not available.

The elderly: as for adults (see 'precautions').

Treatment for respiratory depression and comatose state consists of symptomatic and supportive therapy. Attention should be paid to the occurrence of hypothermia. Consider fluids, inotropes and/or vasopressors for hypotension.

Pharmacological properties

Pharmacodynamic properties: Nabilone is a synthetic cannabinoid which has been shown to have significant anti-emetic activity in patients undergoing chemotherapy for malignant neoplasms. The mode of action of nabilone has been studied in cats and dogs. Although its anti-emetic action is not yet fully understood, it is apparent that there are a number of points in the control systems of the body at which nabilone could block the emetic mechanism.

Pharmacokinetic properties

Absorption: Two fasted subjects were given an oral dose of 2 mg ^{14}C-nabilone. Nabilone was readily absorbed from the gastrointestinal tract. Pharmacokinetic comparison between the oral and intravenous routes of administration suggested that most of the drug was available after oral dosage. Similarly, the percentages of radioactivity in the faeces and urine were approximately sixty per cent and twenty-four per cent respectively whichever route was employed, supporting the view that most of the oral dose was absorbed.

Half life: The plasma half-life of unchanged nabilone in these volunteers was approximately two hours. The estimated half-life of the carbinol metabolite was somewhat longer at between five and ten hours. Total radioactivity had a half-life of approximately thirty-five hours.

Transport: The rapid disappearance of absorbed drug from the plasma has been related to extensive tissue distribution and to rapid metabolism and excretion.

Metabolism: Two metabolic pathways have been suggested. The major pathway probably involves the direct oxidation of nabilone to produce hydroxylic and carboxylic analogues. These compounds are thought to account for the remaining plasma radioactivity when carbinol metabolites have been extracted.

Excretion: When 2 mg of ^{14}C-nabilone was administered orally, over sixty per cent of the total radioactivity was eliminated in the faeces and about twenty five per cent in the urine. The discrepancy is probably due to additive analytical errors, since respiratory $^{14}C\ CO_2$ did not account for the remaining fifteen per cent. Comparison with intravenous administration indicated no significant differences in the excretion pattern suggesting the biliary system to be the major excretory pathway.

Preclinical safety data: Monkeys treated with nabilone at doses as high as 2 mg/kg/day for a year experienced no significant adverse events. This result contrasts with the finding in a planned 1-year dog study that was prematurely terminated because of deaths associated with convulsions in dogs receiving as little as 0.5 mg/kg/day. The earliest deaths, however, occurred at 56 days in dogs receiving 2 mg/kg/day. The unusual vulnerability of the dog is not understood; it is hypothesised, however, that the explanation lies in the fact that the dog differs markedly from other species (including humans) in its metabolism of nabilone.

Carcinogenesis, mutagenesis, impairment of fertility: Carcinogenicity studies have not been performed with nabilone. The influence on fertility and reproduction at doses of 150 and 40 times the maximum recommended human dose was evaluated in rats and rabbits, respectively. In these studies there was no evidence of teratogenicity due to nabilone. In high dose groups, however, nabilone produced a slight decrease in mean litter size, although the number of implantations was unaffected by treatment.

Pharmaceutical particulars

List of excipients: Povidone, Starch flowable, Indigo carmine, Red iron oxide, Titanium dioxide, Gelatin, Edible black ink.

Incompatibilities: None known.

Shelf life: Three years.

Special precautions for storage: Bottles: Keep tightly closed. Store at 15°–25°C. Blisters: Store at 15°–25°C.

Nature and contents of container: High density polyethylene bottles with screw caps or blister packs, each containing 20 capsules.

Instructions for use/handling: None.

Marketing authorisation holder: Cambridge Selfcare Diagnostics Limited, Richmond House, Old Brewery Court, Sandyford Road, Newcastle upon Tyne NE2 1XG.

Marketing authorisation number 12070/0013.

Date of first authorisation/renewal of authorisation Not applicable.

Date of (partial) revision of the text Not applicable.

NEOSTIGMINE BROMIDE TABLETS

Qualitative and quantitative composition Each tablet contains 15 mg Neostigmine Bromide PhEur.

Pharmaceutical form Tablets.

Clinical particulars

Therapeutic indications: Myasthenia gravis, antagonist to non-depolarising neuromuscular blockade; paralytic ileus; post-operative urinary retention.

Posology and method of administration: Neostigmine bromide has a slower onset of effect when given orally than when given parenterally, but the duration of action is longer and the intensity of action more uniform.

To facilitate change of treatment from one route of administration to another, the following doses are approximately equivalent in effect: 0.5 mg intravenously = 1–1.5 mg intramuscularly or subcutaneously = 15 mg orally.

Myasthenia gravis

Adults: Doses of 15 to 30 mg by mouth are given at intervals throughout the day when maximum strength is needed (for example, on rising and before mealtimes). The usual duration of action of a dose is two to four hours.

The total daily dose is usually in the range of 5–20 tablets but doses higher than these may be needed by some patients.

Newborn infants: Neostigmine bromide (Prostigmin) ampoules are recommended.

Older children: Children under 6 years old should receive an initial dose of half a tablet (7.5 mg) of Neostigmine Bromide; children 6–12 years old should receive one tablet (15 mg). Dosage requirements should be adjusted according to the response but are usually in the range of 15–90 mg orally per day.

The requirement for Neostigmine Bromide is usually markedly decreased after thymectomy, or when additional therapy (steroids, immunosuppressant drugs) is given.

When relatively large doses of Neostigmine Bromide are taken by myasthenic patients, it may be necessary to give atropine or other anticholinergic drugs to counteract the muscarinic effects. It should be noted that the slower gastro-intestinal motility caused by these drugs may affect the absorption of oral Neostigmine Bromide.

In all patients the possibility of 'cholinergic crisis', due to overdosage of Neostigmine Bromide, and its differentiation from 'myasthenic crisis', due to increased severity of disease, must be borne in mind. Both types of crisis are manifested by increased muscle weakness, but whereas myasthenic crisis may require more intensive anticholinesterase treatment, cholinergic crisis calls for immediate discontinuation of this treatment and institution of appropriate supportive measures, including respiratory assistance.

Antagonist to non-depolarising neuromuscular blockade: Neostigmine bromide (Prostigmin) ampoules are recommended.

Other indications

Adults: The usual dose is 1 to 2 tablets orally.

Children: 2.5–15 mg orally. The frequency of these doses may be varied according to the needs of the patient.

The elderly: There are no specific dosage recommendations for Neostigmine Bromide in elderly patients.

Contra-indications: Neostigmine Bromide should not be given to patients with mechanical gastro-intestinal or urinary obstruction.

Neostigmine Bromide is contra-indicated in patients with known hypersensitivity to the drug and to bromides.

Neostigmine Bromide should not be used in conjunction with depolarising muscle relaxants such as suxamethonium as neuromuscular blockade may be potentiated and prolonged apnoea may result.

Special warnings and special precautions for use: Extreme caution is required when administering Neostigmine Bromide to patients with bronchial asthma.

Care should also be taken in patients with bradycardia, recent coronary occlusion, hypotension, peptic ulcer, vagotonia, epilepsy or Parkinsonism.

Interaction with other medicaments and other forms of interaction: Neostigmine Bromide should not be given during cyclopropane or halothane anaesthesia; however, it may be used after withdrawal of these agents.

Pregnancy and lactation: The safety of Neostigmine Bromide during pregnancy or lactation has not been established. Although the possible hazards to mother and child must therefore be weighed against the potential benefits in every case, experience with Neostigmine Bromide in pregnant patients with myasthenia gravis has revealed no untoward effect of the drug on the course of pregnancy.

As the severity of myasthenia gravis often fluctuates considerably, particular care is required to avoid cholinergic crisis, due to overdosage of the drug, but otherwise management is no different from that in non-pregnant patients.

Observations indicate that only negligible amounts of Neostigmine Bromide are excreted in breast milk; nevertheless due regard should be paid to possible effects on the breast-feeding infant.

Effects on ability to drive and use machines: Not known.

Undesirable effects: There is no evidence to suggest that Neostigmine Bromide has any special effects in the elderly. However, elderly patients may be more susceptible to dysrhythmias than the younger adult.

Side-effects and adverse reactions may include nausea and vomiting, increased salivation, diarrhoea and abdominal cramps.

Overdose: Signs of overdose due to muscarinic effects may include abdominal cramps, increased peristalsis, diarrhoea, nausea and vomiting, increased bronchial secretions, salivation, diaphoresis and miosis. Nicotinic effects consist of muscular cramps, fasciculations and general weakness. Bradycardia and hypotension may also occur.

Artificial ventilation should be instituted if respiration is severely depressed. Atropine sulphate 1 to 2 mg intravenously is an antidote to the muscarinic effects.

Pharmacological properties

Pharmacodynamic properties: Neostigmine Bromide is an antagonist to cholinesterase, the enzyme which normally destroys acetylcholine. The action of Neostigmine Bromide can briefly be described, therefore, as the potentiation of naturally occurring acetylcholine.

Pharmacokinetic properties: Neostigmine Bromide is a quaternary ammonium compound and is poorly absorbed from the gastro-intestinal tract. Following parenteral administration as the methylsulphate, neostigmine is rapidly eliminated with a plasma half-life of 50–90 minutes and is excreted in the urine both as unchanged drug and metabolites. It is metabolised partly by hydrolysis of the ester linkage.

Preclinical safety data: Neostigmine has not been reported to have mutagenic or carcinogenic potential. In rats, acute and chronic exposure causes changes in the fine structure at the end-plate region of muscle.

Pharmaceutical particulars

List of excipients: Lactose, Maize starch, Talc, Magnesium stearate.

Incompatibilities: None known.

Shelf life: Five years.

Special precautions for storage: The recommended maximum storage temperature is 30°C. The tablets should be protected from light.

Nature and contents of container: White pigmented HDPE bottles with plastic snap-on caps, each containing 140 tablets.

Instructions for use/handling: None.

Marketing authorisation holder: Lifehealth Limited, Richmond House, Old Brewery Court, Sandyford Road, Newcastle upon Tyne NE2 1XG.

Marketing authorisation number 14576/0004.

Date of first authorisation/renewal of authorisation 23 October 1995.

Date of (partial) revision of the text Not applicable.

PENTAGASTRIN INJECTION BP

Qualitative and quantitative composition Pentagastrin BP 0.025 w/v.

Pharmaceutical form Solution for injection.

Clinical particulars

Therapeutic indications: Pentagastrin Injection BP is used for the diagnostic testing of gastric secretion.

Posology and method of administration: For administration either subcutaneously or by continuous intravenous infusion.

Adults (including the elderly) and children: The following procedure is adopted for testing gastric secretion with Pentagastrin Injection BP.

The patient receives no medication (e.g. antacids, etc.) that might affect the results of the test for 24 hours and no food for 12 hours before the test. On the morning of the test a radio-opaque tube (Leven No. 7 or Ryle's 12-16Fr.) is passed into the patient's stomach by way of the nose. Radiological observation is used to ensure that the tube is correctly positioned in the lower part of the body of the stomach.

The tube is securely fastened to the patient's nose and forehead with adhesive tape to ensure that it is not displaced. The patient lies on his left side.

The gastric juices are then collected by applying continuous suction (at 30–50 mm Hg below atmospheric pressure) to this tube, supplemented by manual suction. The patient takes occasional deep breaths to improve collection. The basal secretion is obtained by collecting samples at 15 minute intervals over an hour.

Pentagastrin Injection BP is then given, either at a dose of:

(a) 6 micrograms/kg/body weight subcutaneously, or

(b) 0.6 micrograms/kg/hour as a continuous intravenous infusion. A Tuberculin syringe is used to give a dose correct to 0.01 ml.

If dilution is required normal saline may be used.

Specimens of the gastric juices are again collected over periods of 10 or 15 minutes. The volume of the sample is measured and it is immediately filtered through gauze into a bottle. The acidity at each sample is determined by titration.

Contra-indications: When the patient has previously shown a severe idiosyncratic response to the drug, Pentagastrin Injection BP should not be administered.

Special warnings and special precautions for use: As pentagastrin stimulates gastric acid secretion it should be used with caution in patients with acute or bleeding peptic ulcer disease, though there is no clinical evidence to contra-indicate use.

Interactions with other medicaments and forms of interaction: None known.

Pregnancy and lactation: Pregnancy: Pentagastrin Injection BP should not be administered during pregnancy.

Lactation: No special precautions are required.

Effects on ability to drive and use machines: No precautions are required.

Undesirable effects: At the recommended dosage the incidence of side-effects is extremely small, although very occasionally an individual may respond with hypotension and associated dizziness and faintness. Other unwanted effects reported are mild abdominal discomfort, abdominal cramps, nausea, vomiting, flushing, sweating, headaches, drowsiness or exhaustion, heaviness or weakness of the legs, allergic reactions, bradycardia, tachycardia. These effects disappear once administration of Pentagastrin Injection BP has ceased.

Overdosage: The form of presentation makes it unlikely that overdosage will occur, and no such occurrence has been reported. As maximal secretory response is produced by the normal dosage, increased dosage would be expected to have no sequel other than an accentuation of the known side-effects.

Pharmacological properties

Pharmacodynamic properties: Pentagastrin is a synthetic pentapeptide containing the carboxyl terminal tetrapeptide responsible for the actions of natural gastrins. The most prominent action of pentagastrin is to stimulate the secretion of gastric acid, pepsin and intrinsic factor. Additionally, it stimulates pancreatic secretion, inhibits absorption of water and electrolytes from the ileum, contracts the smooth muscle of the lower oesophageal sphincter and stomach (but delays gastric emptying time), relaxes the sphincter of Oddi and increases blood flow in the gastric mucosa.

Pharmacokinetic properties: Pentagastrin stimulates gastric acid secretion approximately ten minutes after subcutaneous injection, with peak response occurring in most cases twenty to thirty minutes after administration. Duration of activity is usually between sixty and eighty minutes.

Pentagastrin is rapidly absorbed after administration. Pentagastrin has a short half-life (10 minutes or less) in the circulation. It is metabolised primarily in the liver and excretion is mainly by the kidneys.

Preclinical safety data: Pentagastrin is a drug on which extensive clinical experience has been obtained. All relevant information for the prescriber is provided elsewhere in the Summary of Product Characteristics.

Pharmaceutical particulars
List of excipients: Sodium chloride, ammonium chloride, water.

Incompatibilities: None known.

Shelf life: 24 months.

Special precautions for storage: Store away from light, below 4°C but above freezing.

Nature and contents of container: 2 ml glass ampoules in boxes of 5.

Instructions for use/handling: If dilution is required Sodium Chloride Injection BP may be used. This solution should be prepared immediately before it is required for use.

Marketing authorisation holder: Cambridge Selfcare Diagnostics Limited, Richmond House, Old Brewery Court, Sandyford Road, Newcastle upon Tyne NE2 1XG.

Marketing authorisation number 12070/0020.

Date of first authorisation/renewal of authorisation First authorisation 9/2/73.
Renewal 15/10/95.

Date of (partial) revision of text December 1997.

PROCARBAZINE CAPSULES 50 mg

Qualitative and quantitative composition Each capsule contains 58.3 mg procarbazine hydrochloride (equivalent to 50 mg of procarbazine).

Pharmaceutical form Capsules with opaque ivory cap and body.

Clinical particulars
Therapeutic indications: The main indication is Hodgkin's disease (lymphadenoma).

Procarbazine may also be useful in other advanced lymphomata and a variety of solid tumours which have proved resistant to other forms of therapy.

Posology and method of administration
In combination chemotherapeutic regimens: Procarbazine is usually administered concomitantly with other appropriate cytostatic drugs in repeated four- to six-weekly cycles. In most such combination chemotherapy regimens currently in use (e.g. the so-called MOPP schedule with mustine, vincristine and prednisone) Procarbazine is given daily on the first 10–14 days of each cycle in a dosage of 100 mg per m² of body surface (to nearest 50 mg).

As sole therapeutic agent:
Adults: Treatment should begin with small doses which are increased gradually up to a maximum daily dose of 250 or 300 mg divided as evenly as possible throughout the day.

Initial dosage scheme:

1st day:	50 mg	4th day:	200 mg
2nd day:	100 mg	5th day:	250 mg
3rd day:	150 mg	6th day et seq:	250–300 mg

Further procedure: Treatment should be continued with 250 or 300 mg daily until the greatest possible remission has been obtained, after which a maintenance dose is given.

Maintenance dose: 50–150 mg daily. Treatment should be continued until a total dose of at least 6 g has been given. Otherwise, a negative result is not significant.

Elderly: Procarbazine should be used with caution in the elderly. Patients in this group should be observed very closely for signs of early failure or intolerance of treatment.

Children: If, on the recommendation of a physician, a children's dosage is required, 50 mg daily should be given for the first week. Daily dosage should then be maintained at 100 mg per m² of body surface (to nearest 50 mg) until leucopenia or thrombocytopenia occurs or maximum response is obtained.

Procarbazine capsules are for oral administration.

Contra-indications: Pre-existing severe leucopenia or thrombocytopenia from any cause; severe hepatic or renal damage.

Procarbazine should not be used in the management of non-malignant disease.

Special warnings and precautions for use: Procarbazine should be given only under the supervision of a physician who is experienced in cancer chemotherapy and having facilities for regular monitoring of clinical and haematological effects during and after administration.

Introduction of therapy should only be effected under hospital conditions.

Caution is advisable in patients with hepatic or renal dysfunction, cardiovascular or cerebrovascular disease, phaeochromocytoma, or epilepsy.

Regular blood counts are of great importance. If during the initial treatment the total white cell count falls to 3000 per mm³ or the platelet count to 80,000 per mm³, treatment should be suspended temporarily until the leucocyte and/or platelet levels recover, when therapy with the maintenance dose may be resumed.

Treatment should be interrupted on the appearance of allergic skin reactions.

Procarbazine has been shown to be carcinogenic in animals. The increased risk of carcinogenicity in man should be borne in mind when long-term management of patients is proposed.

Interactions with other medicaments and other forms of interaction: Procarbazine is a weak MAO inhibitor and therefore interactions with certain foodstuffs and drugs, although very rare, must be borne in mind. Thus, owing to possible potentiation of the effect of barbiturates, narcotic analgesics (especially pethidine), drugs with anticholinergic effects (including phenothiazine derivatives and tricyclic antidepressants), other central nervous system depressants (including anaesthetic agents) and anti-hypertensive agents, these drugs should be given concurrently with caution and in low doses. Intolerance to alcohol (disulfiram-like reaction) may occur.

Pregnancy and lactation: Procarbazine is teratogenic in animals. Isolated human foetal malformations have been reported following MOPP combination therapy. Therefore Procarbazine should not be administered to patients who are pregnant unless considered absolutely essential by the physician. Procarbazine should not be given to breast feeding mothers.

Effects on ability to drive and use machines: None known.

Undesirable effects: Loss of appetite and nausea occur in most cases, sometimes with vomiting. These symptoms are usually confined to the first few days of treatment and then tend to disappear.

Procarbazine causes leucopenia and thrombocytopenia. These haematological changes are almost always reversible and seldom require complete cessation of therapy.

Overdose: Signs of overdosage include severe nausea and vomiting, dizziness, hallucinations, depression and convulsions; hypotension or tachycardia may occur.

Gastric lavage and general supportive treatment should be performed, with prophylactic treatment against possible infection, and frequent blood counts.

Pharmacological properties
Pharmacodynamic properties: Procarbazine, a methylhydrazine derivative, is a cytostatic agent with weak MAO inhibitor properties. Its exact mode of action on tumour cells is unknown. It may be effective in patients who have become resistant to radiation therapy and other cytostatic agents.

Pharmacokinetic properties: Procarbazine is readily absorbed from the gastrointestinal tract. It is rapidly metabolised, the primary circulating metabolite is the azo derivative while the major urinary metabolite has been shown to be N-isopropyl-terephthalamic acid.

Preclinical safety data: There are no pre-clinical data of relevance to the prescriber which are additional to that already included in other sections of the SPC.

Pharmaceutical particulars
List of excipents: Mannitol, Maize starch, Talc, Magnesium stearate.

Capsule shell components: Gelatin, Yellow iron oxide E172, Titanium dioxide E171.

Incompatibilities: None known.

Shelf life: Three years.

Special precautions for storage: Procarbazine capsules should be stored in a dry place; the recommended maximum storage temperature is 25°C.

Nature and contents of container: Blister packs of 50 capsules.

Instruction for use/handling: Handling guidelines: Undamaged capsules present minimal risk of contamination, but in accordance with good hygiene requirements, direct handling should be avoided. As with all cytotoxics, precautions should be taken to avoid exposing staff during pregnancy.

Waste material may be disposed of by incineration.

Marketing authorisation holder: Cambridge Selfcare Diagnostics Limited, t/a Cambridge Laboratories, Richmond House, Old Brewery Court, Sandyford Road, Newcastle upon Tyne NE2 1XG.

Marketing authorisation number PL 12070/0004.

Date of first authorisation/renewal of authorisation 10 November 1992.

Date of (partial) revision of the text May 1997.

PROTIRELIN AMPOULES

Qualitative and quantitative composition Each ampoule contains 200 micrograms of Protirelin (Thyrotrophin-releasing hormone, TRH) in 2 ml of solution.

Pharmaceutical form Solution for injection.

Clinical particulars
Therapeutic indications: The administration of Protirelin provides a means of assessing thyroid function and the reserve of TSH in the pituitary gland and is recommended as a test procedure where such assessment is indicated.

It is particularly useful as a diagnostic test for:
1. Mild hyperthyroidism.
2. Ophthalmic Graves' disease.
3. Mild or preclinical hypothyroidism.
4. Hypopituitarism.
5. Hypothalamic disease.

It may also be used in place of the T_3 suppression test.

Posology and method of administration: Protirelin ampoules are for intravenous injection.

Intravenous injection: Tests employing intravenous Protirelin are based on the serum TSH response to a standard dose. They provide a means of both quantitative and qualitative assessment of thyroid function. It is essential for each laboratory to establish its own normal range of values for serum TSH before attempting quantitative assessment of Protirelin responses by this means.

Intravenous Protirelin test
(a) Blood sample taken for control TSH assay.
(b) Protirelin 200 µg given as a single bolus injection.
(c) Blood sample taken 20 minutes after injection for peak TSH assay.
(d) If necessary, a further blood sample may be taken 60 minutes after injection to detect a delayed TSH response.

The ampoule solution should not be diluted.

The elderly: The use of Protirelin in the elderly has been well documented. Dosage requirements and the side-effects are similar to those of younger adults. The response may be decreased in elderly subjects, but this does not interfere with the interpretation of the test results.

Children up to the age of 12: The procedures for administering Protirelin to children are identical to those outlined above. An intravenous dose of 1 µg/kg bodyweight may be used.

Interpretation of results: Interpretation of the responses to Protirelin is based on the increase in TSH and/or PBI, T_3 or T_4 levels from the basal values. In normal subjects, there is a prompt rise in serum levels of TSH. The changes observed in various conditions are briefly outlined below:

1. Hyperthyroidism – no rise in serum TSH or thyroid hormone levels.
2. Ophthalmic Graves' disease – often no rise in serum TSH or thyroid hormone levels.
3. Primary hypothyroidism – exaggerated and prolonged rise in serum TSH but no change in thyroid hormone levels.
4. Hypopituitarism – absent or impaired TSH or thyroid hormone response implies diminished TSH reserve.
5. Hypothalamic disease – a rise in serum TSH or thyroid hormone levels can occur in the presence of hypothyroidism; delayed responses are common.

The Protirelin test provides, in most instances, information similar to that obtained from a T_3 suppression test in that an absent or impaired response usually correlates with an absent or impaired response to T_3 suppression.

Contra-indications: There are no absolute contra-indications to Protirelin.

Special warnings and special precautions for use: In view of the postulated effect of bolus injections of Protirelin on smooth muscle, patients with bronchial asthma or other types of obstructive airways disease should be closely monitored. Caution should always be observed in patients with myocardial ischaemia and severe hypopituitarism.

Interactions with other medicaments and other forms of interaction: The secretion of thyrotrophin appears to be modulated by dopaminergic and noradrenergic pathways. The TSH response to Protirelin may be reduced by thyroid hormones, levodopa, phenothiazines, salicylates, bromocriptine, carbamazepine, lithium and by pharmacological doses of corticosteroids.

An increased response may be seen in subjects taking metoclopramide, amiodarone or theophyllines and in men taking oestrogens. Over-treatment with antithyroid drugs may also cause an enhanced response.

Pregnancy and lactation: Animal studies and clinical experience have shown no evidence of hazard in human pregnancy at the recommended dosage. Nevertheless, the established medical principle of not administering drugs during early pregnancy should be observed.

Breast enlargement and leaking of milk have been reported following the administration of protirelin to lactating women.

Effects on ability to drive and use machines: None known.

Undesirable effects: Protirelin is well tolerated. Following rapid intravenous injection, side-effects of a mild and transient nature may be experienced. These comprise nausea, a desire to micturate, a feeling of flushing, slight dizziness and a peculiar taste, and have been attributed to a local action of the bolus of Protirelin on the muscle of the gastro-intestinal and genito-urinary tracts. A transient increase in pulse rate and blood pressure may also be noted.

Overdose: No symptoms of overdosage have been noted in patients receiving up to 1 mg i.v.

Pharmacological properties

Pharmacodynamic properties: Pharmacotherapeutic group: H01AB.

Protirelin stimulates the secretion of thyroid stimulating hormone (TSH). Intravenous injection results in a prompt rise in serum TSH levels in normal subjects, peak levels being observed about twenty minutes after administration. There is a concomitant rise in serum levels of prolactin.

Pharmacokinetic properties: TSH rapidly disappears from the plasma after intravenous injection. Over 90% is removed within 20 minutes with a half life of about 5.3 minutes. About 5.5% of the dose is excreted in the urine, mostly within 30 minutes.

Preclinical safety data: There are no pre-clinical data of relevance to the prescriber which are additional to that already included in other sections of the SPC.

Pharmaceutical particulars

List of excipients: Mannitol PhEur; Glacial acetic acid PhEur; Water for injections PhEur.

Incompatibilities: None known.

Shelf life: Three years.

Special precautions for storage: The recommended maximum storage temperature is 30°C.

Nature and contents of container: Clear glass ampoules each containing 2 ml of solution, in packs of 10 ampoules.

Instruction for use/handling: None.

Marketing authorisation holder: Cambridge Selfcare Diagnostics Limited, t/a Cambridge Laboratories, Richmond House, Old Brewery Court, Sandyford Road, Newcastle upon Tyne NE2 1XG.

Marketing authorisation number 12070/0009.

Date of first authorisation/renewal of authorisation 9 July 1992
Renewed 9 July 1997.

Date of (partial) revision of the text July 1998.

RAZOXANE TABLETS 125 mg

Qualitative and quantitative composition Razoxane Tablets contain 125.00 mg Razoxane (BAN) per tablet. Razoxane is described chemically as (±)-4,4'-propylenebis(piperazine-2,6-dione).

Pharmaceutical form Tablets.

Clinical particulars

Therapeutic indications: In contrast to most anti-cancer agents Razoxane interferes with cell division at the G_2M phase of the cycle.

Razoxane in combination with radiotherapy may be used for all forms of soft-tissue, chondro- and osteo-sarcomas. In comparison with radiotherapy alone, this combination may increase the response rate and reduce recurrence. Razoxane can produce remissions in previous radio-resistant lesions.

Razoxane may be useful alone or in combination with other antimitotic agents in the treatment of malignant lymphomas, including mycosis fungoides, acute leukaemias, especially the acute blast cell-crisis of chronic myeloid leukaemia, and Kaposi's sarcoma. Experience to date has been in open studies which indicate that the product is of value in patients in whom previous therapies have been unsuccessful.

Note: Because of an association between administration of Razoxane and the development of acute myeloid leukaemia or skin epitheliomata, the drug should only be used in the above malignant conditions and then when its administration is essential such as when other treatments have failed.

Posology and method of administration

Adults and children: Razoxane is administered orally. The following guidelines are based on the regimens with which responses have been obtained. In all regimens, if unacceptable degrees of leucopenia, thrombocytopenia or gastrointestinal disturbance occur, the dosage of Razoxane should be reduced or temporarily withdrawn to allow recovery.

Soft-tissue, osteo- and chondro-sarcomata: 125 mg (1 tablet) twice daily 3 days before the start of radiotherapy, continued throughout that therapy. On days when radiation is given, 1 tablet of Razoxane should be taken 1–4 hours before radiotherapy; the other tablet in the evening. The dosage of radiation should be selected and administered using normal criteria.

Malignant lymphomas (including mycosis fungoides): 0.5–1.5 g/m²/week should be administered orally as long as a remission is maintained. For example the dosage can be given as:

(a) 125 mg (1 tablet) twice daily on 3–5 days/week

or

(b) three doses of 375 mg (3 tablets) given eight hours apart and repeated weekly.

If an inadequate response is obtained the dosage may be increased, provided that the white cell count permits.

Acute leukaemias (including blast cell crisis of chronic myeloid leukaemia): 150–500 mg/m²/day for 3–5 days. Treatment should be repeated at 14–28 day intervals, depending on the peripheral blood count. Allopurinol may also be given to prevent uric acid deposition.

Kaposi's sarcoma: 333 mg/m² three times daily for 3 days every 3 weeks, and adjusted as necessary according to peripheral blood count.

Elderly patients: There are no special dosage recommendations for the elderly, but it may be advisable to monitor elderly patients so that optimum dosage can be individually determined.

Contra-indications

Razoxane is contra-indicated in the treatment of non-malignant conditions such as psoriasis.

Razoxane is contra-indicated in pregnancy because of its action on cell division. Animal studies have revealed abnormalities of foetal development. It should not normally be administered to mothers who are breast feeding.

Special warnings and precautions for use: It is recommended that adequate protective gloves be worn when handling Razoxane Tablets and that Razoxane tablets should not be handled by pregnant staff.

Interactions with other medicaments and other forms of interaction: None.

Pregnancy and lactation: Razoxane is contra-indicated in pregnancy because of its action on cell division. Animal studies have revealed abnormalities of foetal development. It should not normally be administered to mothers who are breast feeding.

Effects on ability to drive and use machines: There is no evidence that Razoxane results in impairment of these activities.

Undesirable effects: The principal reported side-effects include leucopenia, thrombocytopenia, nausea, vomiting, diarrhoea, skin reactions and alopecia. Early skin reactions in patients receiving Razoxane plus radiotherapy may be more marked than those expected from radiotherapy alone. Severe late subcutaneous fibrosis has been reported in some patients receiving the combined therapy. There appears to be an increased likelihood of oesophagitis and pneumonitis in patients who require radiotherapy for thoracic lesions.

Overdose: In cases of overdosage, signs and symptoms are likely to be qualitatively similar to side-effects; there is no specific antidote and treatment must be symptomatic.

Pharmacological properties

Pharmacodynamic properties: In contrast to most anti-cancer agents Razoxane interferes with cell division at the G_2M phase of the cell cycle and in multiple-drug chemotherapy regimes it is logical to combine Razoxane with agents acting at the other phases in the cell cycle.

Pharmacokinetic properties: Absorption of Razoxane after oral dosing is slow and incomplete, followed by rapid urinary excretion.

Preclinical safety data: Mice and rats developed tumours following long term intraperitoneal administration of Razoxane. Animal studies have revealed abnormalities of foetal development when the drug was administered to pregnant females.

Pharmaceutical particulars

List of excipients: Alginic acid; Povidone; Microcrystalline cellulose; Magnesium stearate.

Incompatibilities: None stated.

Shelf life: Two years.

Special precautions for storage: Store below 25°C, protect from light and moisture.

Nature and contents of container: Aluminium tubes fitted with aluminium screw caps with flowed-in PVC gaskets, each containing 30 tablets.

Instruction for use/handling: It is recommended that adequate protective gloves be worn when handling Razoxane Tablets and that Razoxane Tablets should not be handled by pregnant staff.

Marketing authorisation holder: Cambridge Selfcare Diagnostics Limited, t/a Cambridge Laboratories, Richmond House, Old Brewery Court, Sandyford Road, Newcastle upon Tyne NE2 1XG.

Marketing authorisation number 12070/0012.

Date of first authorised/renewal of authorisation 15 May 1995.

Date of (partial) revision of the text 24 January 1996.

RHEOMACRODEX* IN DEXTROSE

Qualitative and quantitative composition Dextran 40. 10 g in 100 mls.

Pharmaceutical form Colourless, clear, slightly viscous sterile solution 500 ml.

Clinical particulars

Therapeutic indications: Rheomacrodex is used for the early fluid replacement or for plasma volume expansion in the adjunctive treatment of certain types of shock or in impending shock including those resulting from burns, surgery, haemorrhage or trauma in which circulatory volume deficit is present.

Rheomacrodex is not a substitute for whole blood or blood products where these are clearly indicated.

Rheomacrodex may be used in embolic episodes and for prophylaxis of venous thrombosis and pulmonary embolism in patients at moderate or high risk of thromboembolism.

Rheomacrodex is also used as a priming fluid during extracorporeal circulation.

Rheomacrodex is used in conditions where improvement of microcirculatory flow is required.

Posology and method of administration: Rheomacrodex is for intravenous administration only.

The recommended dosage is dependent upon the age, weight and clinical condition of the patient.

The solution is hyperoncotic and draws extravascular fluid into the vascular space such that 500 ml infused rapidly into a normally hydrated patient may produce an expansion of almost one litre. This expansion is short lived due to excretion of smaller molecules, and by 3 hours expansion will have declined to about 520 ml, by 6 hours 430 ml and 12 hours 360 ml. Such expansion rapidly fills circulation deficit, reduces haematocrit and concentration of clotting factors, and may produce oozing from recent surgical incisions due to increase in capillary flow.

Dehydration must be corrected before giving the drug.

In shock: The suggested total adult dose for the first 24 hours should not exceed 20 ml per kg body weight. The first 10 ml per kg may be infused as rapidly as necessary to effect improvement. Monitoring central venous pressure; strongly recommended as guide to infusion. Daily doses after the first 24 hours should not exceed 10 ml per kg and therapy should not be continued beyond 5 days.

For the treatment of thromboembolism: Initially 500–1000 ml over 4–6 hours on the first day followed by 500 ml over 4–6 hours the next day. Then, the treatment may be continued with 500 ml over 4–6 hours on alternate days for a maximum of 10 days.

For the prophylaxis of thromboembolism: Infuse 500 ml over 4–6 hours during or at the end of surgery followed by 500 ml over 4–6 hours the next day. In high-risk patients, the treatment may be continued with 500 ml over 4–6 hours on alternate days for a maximum of 10 days.

In extracorporeal perfusion: The dose of Rheomacrodex will depend upon the volume needed to prime the pump oxygenator. Usually, a total dose of 10–20 ml per kg of body weight is added to the perfusion circuit. The total dose should not exceed 2 g per kg of body weight and this can be limited and controlled by adding other priming fluids.

In improvement of microcirculatory flow: Infuse 500–1000 ml in the first 24 hours. 500 ml is given the next day and then alternate days to a maximum of two weeks.

Infants: up to 5 ml per kg of body weight.

Children: up to 10 ml per kg of body weight.

Elderly: as per adults, but take extra care regarding dehydration, overloading and renal function.

Contra-indications: Rheomacrodex is contra-indicated in the presence of thrombocytopenia, hypofibrinogenaemia, severe congestive heart failure, renal disease with severe oliguria or anuria and where there is known intolerance to dextran.

Rheomacrodex in sodium chloride should not be administered to patients in whom sodium restriction is indicated. Rheomacrodex in 5% dextrose is available.

Special warnings and special precautions for use: *Warnings:* Because Rheomacrodex is a colloidal solution it withdraws water from the extravascular space and the resultant fluid shifts may become critical in poorly hydrated patients. The renal excretion of dextran is associated with elevations of the specific gravity of the urine and these may become significant in patients with reduced renal function. It is therefore, essential that the patient's state of hydration is assessed before Rheomacrodex is administered. If signs of dehydration are present, appropriate parenteral fluids should be administered and the infusion of Rheomacrodex limited to 500 ml per hour. An osmotic diuretic like mannitol may be used to maintain urine excretion following adequate hydration. Urine flow should be kept above 250 ml/6 hours and the s.g. below 1.065.

Recommended dosage of Rheomacrodex effects only minor and transient changes in the coagulation of the blood. Excessive dosage may induce a prolonged bleeding time. Therefore, the physician should be aware of the possibility of a slight increase in blood loss.

It is strongly recommended that central venous pressure is frequently monitored during the initial infusion of Rheomacrodex. With monitoring, the first 500 ml may be administered rapidly, but should be immediately discontinued if there is a steep rise in central venous pressure. Without monitoring, the intravenous infusion should be slower and the patient carefully observed for signs of circulatory overloading.

Following the administration of Rheomacrodex, an increase in urinary output usually occurs in oliguric patients. If no increase is observed after the administration of 500 ml, the infusion should be discontinued until adequate diuresis develops spontaneously or can be provoked by other means.

The amount of Rheomacrodex given should not cause a depression of the haemoglobin concentration below 9 g% for more than a short time. Care should be taken to prevent a depression of the haematocrit below 30% volume.

Precautions: Although dextrans of higher molecular weight produce erythrocyte aggregation which may interfere with blood-typing and cross-matching, no such interference occurs with Rheomacrodex. Blood sugar determinations that employ high concentrations of acid may result in hydrolysis of dextran, yielding falsely elevated glucose assay results. This has been observed both with sulphuric acid and with acetic acid. In other laboratory tests, the presence of dextran in the blood may result in the development of turbidity, which can interfere with the assay. This has been observed in bilirubin assays in which alcohol is employed and in total protein assays employing biuret reagent. Thus consideration should be given to withdrawal of blood for chemical laboratory tests prior to initiation of therapy.

Patients should be closely observed for signs of anaphylaxis during the first few minutes and resuscitative measures should be readily available. Large doses may result in pulmonary oedema. Caution is advised in patients with poor cardiac function.

In patients in whom restriction of sodium is indicated Rheomacrodex in glucose should be used, and conversely, in patients in whom dextrose restriction is indicated, Rheomacrodex in saline should be used.

Interaction with other medicaments and other forms of interaction: Rheomacrodex crystallises occasionally due to swings of temperature causing expansion changes of meniscus level. Seed crystals form on the meniscus line which may grow into full crystals. Storage should therefore, be at a constant temperature not exceeding 25°C. If flakes of dextran appear, these can be redissolved by heating for a short time at a low temperature not to exceed 100°C. The solution should then be cooled to 37°C before infusion.

As with all parenterals, compatibilities should be checked when additives are used.

Thorough and careful mixing of any additives is mandatory.

Avoid storage of solution so prepared.

Pregnancy and lactation: Although anaphylactic reactions to Rheomacrodex are rare, the product should only be used during pregnancy when strictly indicated, since anaphylactic reactions in the mother have been reported to cause anoxic brain damage which has resulted in death of the foetus in a number of cases.

Effects on ability to drive and use machines: Not applicable.

Undesirable effects: Mild urticarial reactions, rarely severe anaphylactoid reactions, increase in viscosity and specific gravity of urine, reversible tubular vacuolisation, and occasionally transient acidosis due to improved tissue perfusion. Rarely renal failure has been reported.

Overdose: In the event of an accidental over infusion, treatment should temporarily be either discontinued or rate of infusion decreased significantly, depending on extent of over infusion. The patient should be observed for symptoms and signs of cardiorespiratory decompensation and hepatic and renal functions, and fluid and electrolyte balance should be carefully monitored together with any evidence of bleeding diathesis, other symptomatic and supportive measures should be provided.

Pharmacological properties

Pharmacodynamic properties: Dextran 40 has a mean molecular weight of 40,000. Dextran of this weight binds about 20 ml of water per gram of dextran when in the circulation and the dextran 40 is known to have disaggregative effects on erythrocytes. This effect combined with the volume expansion and haemodilution produced by the infusion serves to improve microcirculatory flow. Inhibition of platelet adhesiveness combined with haemodilution, improved flow due to reduced viscosity and dilution of clotting factors serve to inhibit post surgical thrombo embolic disease without altering normal haemostasis. Thrombi formed in the presence of dextran have a structure more readily attacked by body lytic processes.

The solution is hyperoncotic and draws extravascular fluid into the vascular space such that 500 ml infused rapidly into a normal hydrated patient may produce an expansion of almost one litre. This expansion is short lived due to excretion of smaller molecules and by 3 hours expansion will have declined to about 520 ml, by 6 hours 430 ml and 12 hours 360 ml. Such expansion rapidly fills circulatory deficit, reduces haematocrit and concentration of clotting factors and may produce oozing from recent surgical incisions due to increase in capillary flow.

Dehydration must be corrected before giving the drug.

Pharmacokinetic properties: Following intravenous infusion the dextran 40 remains largely in the vasculature, producing the volume changes outlined above. Molecules below a mw of about 50,000 are rapidly excreted through the kidneys, about 60% of the dextran in the first 6 hours. The large molecules are metabolised at about 70–100 mg/kg/body weight/day by the reticulo endothelial system (mainly the liver) to glucose, which joins the body pool. This slower mode of elimination means that by 24 hours only 70% of the dextran has gone.

Preclinical safety data: None stated.

Pharmaceutical particulars

List of excipients: Dextrose Monohydrate PhEur; water for injections.

Incompatibilities: The slight acid pH of Rheomacrodex despite negligible buffering capacity (<2mEq/L) may precipitate salts of weak acids such as the various penicillins, unless they are buffered. Aminocaproic acid, dihydrallazine mesylate, warfarin sodium (dextrose vehicle only). 95% ethanol, dexamethasone sodium phosphate, isoxaprin hydrochloride and propantheline bromide have been reported incompatible.

Shelf life: 5 years.

Special precautions for storage: Store at steady temperature not exceeding 30°C. Do not freeze.

Nature and contents of container: Type II. Glass infusion bottle complying with EP and DIN 58363, bromo chlorbutyl rubber stoppers to DIN 58363 and EP. Aluminium seal.

Instructions for use/handling: None stated.

Marketing authorisation holder: Medisan Pharmaceuticals AB, AR4, S-741 74 Uppsala, Sweden.

Marketing authorisation number 15135/0001.

Date of approval/revision of SPC 15 March 1996.

Legal category POM.

RHEOMACRODEX* IN NORMAL SALINE

Qualitative and quantitative composition Dextran 40. 10 g in 100 mls.

Pharmaceutical form Colourless, clear, slightly viscous sterile solution 500 ml.

Clinical particulars

Therapeutic indications: Rheomacrodex is used for the early fluid replacement or for plasma volume expansion in the adjunctive treatment of certain types of shock or in impending shock including those resulting from burns, surgery, haemorrhage or trauma in which circulatory volume deficit is present.

Rheomacrodex is not a substitute for whole blood or blood products where these are clearly indicated.

Rheomacrodex may be used in embolic episodes and for prophylaxis of venous thrombosis and pulmonary embolism in patients at moderate or high risk of thromboembolism.

Rheomacrodex is also used as a priming fluid during extracorporeal circulation.

Rheomacrodex is used in conditions where improvement of microcirculatory flow is required.

Posology and method of administration: Rheomacrodex is for intravenous administration only.

The recommended dosage is dependent upon the age, weight and clinical condition of the patient.

The solution is hyperoncotic and draws extravascular fluid into the vascular space such that 500 ml infused rapidly into a normal hydrated patient may produce an expansion of almost one litre. The expansion is short lived due to excretion of smaller molecules, and by 3 hours expansion will have declined to about 520 ml, by 6 hours 430 ml and 12 hours 360 ml. Such expansion rapidly fills circulation deficit, reduces haematocrit and concentration of clotting factors, and may produce oozing from recent surgical incisions due to increase in capillary flow.

Dehydration must be corrected before giving the drug.

In shock: The suggested total dose for the first 24 hours should not exceed 20 ml per kg body weight. The first 10 ml per kg may be infused as rapidly as necessary to effect improvement. Monitoring central venous pressure; strongly recommended as guide to infusion. Daily doses after the first 24 hours should not exceed 10 ml per kg and therapy should not be continued beyond 5 days.

For the treatment of thromboembolism: Initially 500–1000 ml over 4–6 hours on the first day followed by 500 ml over 4–6 hours the next day. Then, the treatment may be continued with 500 ml over 4–6 hours on alternate days for a maximum of 10 days.

For the prophylaxis of thromboembolism: Infuse 500 ml over 4–6 hours during or at the end of the surgery followed by 500 ml over 4–6 hours the next day. In high-risk patients, the treatment may be continued with 500 ml over 4–6 hours on alternate days for a maximum of 10 days.

In extracorporeal perfusion: The dose of Rheomacrodex will depend upon the volume needed to prime the pump oxygenator. Usually, a total dose of 10–20 ml per kg of body weight is added to the perfusion circuit. The total dose should not exceed 2 g per kg of body weight and this can be limited and controlled by adding other priming fluids.

In improvement of microcirculatory flow: Infuse 500–1000 ml in the first 24 hours. 500 ml is given the next day and then alternate days to a maximum of two weeks.

Infants: Up to 5 ml per kg of body weight.

Children: Up to 10 ml/kg of body weight.

Elderly: As per adults, but take extra care regarding dehydration, overloading and renal function.

Contra-indications: Rheomacrodex is contra-indicated in the presence of thrombocytopenia, hypofibrinogenaemia, severe congestive heart failure, renal disease with severe oliguria or anuria and where there is known intolerance to dextran.

Rheomacrodex in sodium chloride should not be administered to patients in whom sodium restriction is indicated. Rheomacrodex in 5% dextrose is available.

Special warnings and special precautions for use: *Warnings:* Because Rheomacrodex is a colloidal solution it withdraws water from the extravascular space and the resultant fluid shifts may become critical in poorly hydrated patients. The renal excretion of dextran is associated with elevations of the specific gravity of the urine and these may become significant in patients with reduced renal function. It is therefore, essential that the patient's state of hydration is assessed before Rheomacrodex is administered. If signs of dehydration are present, appropriate parenteral fluids should be administered and the infusion of Rheomacrodex limited to 500 ml per hour. An osmotic diuretic like mannitol may be used to maintain urine excretion following adquate hydration. Urine flow should be kept above 250 ml/6 hours and the s.g. below 1.065.

Recommended dosage of Rheomacrodex effects only minor and transient changes in the coagulation of the blood. Excessive dosage may induce a prolonged bleeding time. Therefore, the physician should be aware of the possibility of a slight increase in blood loss.

It is strongly recommended that central venous pressure is frequently monitored during the initial infusion of Rheomacrodex. With monitoring, the first 500 ml may be administered rapidly, but should be immediately discontinued if there is a steep rise in central venous pressure. Without monitoring, the intravenous infusion should be slower and the patient carefully observed for signs of circulatory overloading.

Following the administration of Rheomacrodex, an increase in urinary output usually occurs in oliguric patients. If no increase is observed after the administration of 500 ml, the infusion should be discontinued until adequate diuresis develops spontaneously or can be provoked by other means.

The amount of Rheomacrodex given should not cause a depression of the haemoglobin concentration below 9 g% for more than a short time. Care should be taken to prevent a depression of the haematocrit below 30% volume.

Precautions: Although dextrans of higher molecular weight produce erythrocyte aggregation which may interfere with blood-typing and cross-matching, no such interference occurs with Rheomacrodex. Blood sugar determinations that employ high concentration of acid may result in hydrolysis of dextran, yielding falsely elevated glucose assay results. This has been observed both with sulphuric acid and with acetic acid. In other laboratory tests, the presence of dextran in the blood may result in the development of turbidity, which can interfere with the assay. This has been observed in bilirubin assays in which alcohol is employed and in total protein assays employing biuret reagent. Thus consideration should be given to withdrawal of blood for chemical laboratory tests prior to initiation of therapy.

Patients should be closely observed for signs of anaphylaxis during the first few minutes and resuscitative measures should be readily available. Large doses may result in pulmonary oedema. Caution is advised in patients with poor cardiac function.

In patients in whom restriction of sodium is indicated Rheomacrodex in glucose should be used, and conversely, in patients in whom dextrose restriction is indicated, Rheomacrodex in saline should be used.

Interaction with other medicaments and other forms of interaction: Rheomacrodex crystallises occasionally due to swings of temperature causing expansion changes of meniscus level. Seed crystals form on the meniscus line which may grow into full crystals. Storage should therefore, be at a constant temperature not exceeding 25°C. If flakes of dextran appear, these can be redissolved by heating for a short time at a low temperature not to exceed 100°C. The solution should then be cooled to 37°C before infusion.

As with all parenterals, compatibilities should be checked when additives are used.

Thorough and careful mixing of any additives is mandatory.

Avoid storage of solution so prepared.

Pregnancy and lactation: Although anaphylactic reactions to Rheomacrodex are rare, the product should only be used during pregnancy when strictly indicated, since anaphylactic reactions in the mother have been reported to cause anoxic brain damage which has resulted in death of the foetus in a number of cases.

Effects on ability to drive and use machines: Not applicable.

Undesirable effects: Mild urticarial reactions, rarely severe anaphylactoid reactions, increase in viscosity and specific gravity of urine, reversible tubular vacuolisation and occasionally transient acidosis due to improved tissue perfusion. Rarely renal failure has been reported.

Overdose: In the event of an accidental over infusion, treatment should temporarily be either discontinued or rate of infusion decreased significantly, depending on extent of over infusion. The patient should be observed for symptoms and signs of cardiorespiratory decompensation and hepatic and renal functions, and fluid and electrolyte balance should be carefully monitored together with any evidence of bleeding diathesis, other symptomatic and supportive measures should be provided.

Pharmacological properties

Pharmacodynamic properties: Dextran 40 has a mean molecular weight of 40,000. Dextran of this weight binds about 20 ml of water per gram of dextran when in the circulation and the dextran 40 is known to have disaggregative effects on erythrocytes. This effect combined with the volume expansion and haemodilution produced by the infusion serve to improve microcirculatory flow. Inhibition of platelet adhesiveness combined with haemodilution, improved flow due to reduced viscosity and dilution of clotting factors serves to inhibit post surgical thrombo embolic disease without altering normal haemostasis. Thrombi formed in the presence of dextran have a structure more readily attached by body lytic processes.

The solution is hyperoncotic and draws extravascular fluid into the vascular space such that 500 ml infused rapidly into a normal hydrated patient may produce an expansion of almost one litre. This expansion is short lived due to excretion of smaller molecules and by 3 hours expansion will have declined to about 520 ml, by 6 hours 430 ml and 12 hours 360 ml. Such expansion rapidly fills circulatory deficit, reduces haematocrit and concentration of clotting factors and may produce oozing from recent surgical incisions due to increase in capillary flow.

Dehydration must be corrected before giving the drug.

Pharmacokinetic properties: Following intravenous infusion the dextran 40 remains largely in the vasculature, producing the volume changes outlined above. Molecules below a mw of about 50,000 are rapidly excreted through the kidneys, about 60% of the dextran in the first 6 hours. The large molecules are metabolised at about 70–100 mg/kg/body weight/day by the reticulo endothelial system (mainly the liver) to glucose, which joins the body pool. This slower mode of elimination means that by 24 hours only 70% of the dextran has gone.

Preclinical safety data: None stated.

Pharmaceutical particulars

List of excipients: Sodium chloride; water for injections.

Incompatibilities: The slight acid pH of Rheomacrodex despite negligible buffering capacity (<2mEq/L) may precipitate salts of weak acids such as the various penicillins, unless they are buffered. Aminocaproic acid, dihydrallazine mesylate, warfarin sodium (dextrose vehicle only), 95% ethanol, dexamethasone sodium phosphate, isoxaprin hydrochloride and propantheline bromide have been reported incompatible.

Shelf life: 5 years.

Special precautions for storage: Store at steady temperature not exceeding 25°C. Do not freeze.

Nature and contents of container: Type II. Glass infusion bottle complying with EP and DIN 58363, bromo or chlorbutyl rubber stoppers to DIN 58363 and EP. Aluminium seal.

Instructions for use/handling: None stated.

Marketing authorisation holder: Medisan Pharmaceuticals AB, AR4, S-741 74 Uppsala, Sweden.

Marketing authorisation number 15135/0002.

Date of approval/revision of SPC 24 May 1996.

Legal cateogry POM.

TESTOSTERONE ENANTHATE AMPOULES

Qualitative and quantitative composition Each ampoule contains 250 mg Testosterone Enanthate PhEur in oily solution.

Pharmaceutical form Solution for injection.

Clinical particulars

Therapeutic indications: Mammary carcinoma in the female. Androgen deficiency in the male.

Posology and method of administration:

Females – mammary carcinoma: 250 mg every two weeks by intramuscular injection.

Males – Hypogonadism: To stimulate development of underdeveloped androgen-dependent organs and for initial treatment of deficiency symptoms, 250 mg Testosterone Enanthate intramuscularly every two to three weeks.

For maintenance treatment: 250 mg Testosterone Enanthate intramuscularly every three to six weeks, according to individual requirement.

Contra-indications: Prostatic carcinoma, mammary carcinoma in males and pregnancy. Previous or existing liver tumours (in advanced mammary carcinoma in females only) if these are not due to metastases.

Special warnings and precautions for use: Androgens should not be used for enhancing muscular development in healthy individuals or for increasing physical ability.

High dose or long-term administration of testosterone occasionally increases the tendency to water retention and oedema. Caution should therefore be exercised in patients predisposed to oedema.

In rare cases benign and in even rarer cases malignant liver tumours leading in isolated cases to life-threatening intra-abdominal haemorrhage have been observed after the use of hormonal substances such as testosterone enanthate. If severe upper abdominal complaints, liver enlargement or signs of intra-abdominal haemorrhage occur, a liver tumour should be included in the differential diagnosis and, if necessary, the preparation should be withdrawn. Regular examination of the prostate is advisable for men receiving androgen therapy.

If, in individual cases, frequent or persistent erections occur, the dose should be reduced or the treatment discontinued in order to avoid injury to the penis.

In women: If hypercalcaemia develops, therapy must be discontinued.

Interactions with other medicaments and other forms of interaction: Phenobarbitone increases the breakdown of steroid hormones in the liver (possible impairment of efficacy).

The clotting status should be monitored particularly closely when testosterone enanthate is administered together with coumarin derivatives.

Pregnancy and lactation: Contra-indicated in pregnancy.

Effects on ability to drive and use machines: None known.

Undesirable effects: Women treated with Testosterone Enanthate may develop signs of virilisation, (e.g. acne, hirsutism, voice changes). Particular care is therefore necessary in women whose occupations involve singing or speaking.

Spermatogenesis is inhibited by long-term and high-dose treatment with testosterone enanthate.

In rare cases, coughing, dyspnoea and circulatory irregularities may occur during or immediately after the injection. Experience has shown that these reactions can be avoided by injecting very slowly.

Overdose: Acute toxicity data show that Testosterone Enanthate can be classified as non-toxic following a single intake. Even in the case of an inadvertent administration of a multiple of the dose required for therapy, no acute toxicity risk is expected.

Pharmacological properties

Pharmacodynamic properties: Testosterone enanthate is an ester of the natural male sex hormone testosterone and exhibits all the pharmacological effects of the natural hormone. It differs in that it has a depot effect, due to the fact that testosterone enanthate is only slowly degraded to testosterone in the body.

Pharmacokinetic properties: Following intramuscular administration of 200 mg of testosterone enanthate to 6 hypogonadal males:

– Peak serum testosterone levels of 1233±484 ng/ml were achieved at 24 hours.

– Physiological levels of testosterone (approx. 500 ng/ml) were maintained for 11 days.

Half-life in blood was 2–3 days (healthy male volunteers).

Preclinical safety data: Studies in animals showed that the formulation has minimal potential for causing sensitisation or local irritation following intramuscular injection. Long-term systemic studies showed no evidence of testicular toxicity although a temporary inhibition of spermatogenesis may occur. No fertility studies with testosterone enanthate have been carried out. Administration of Testosterone Enanthate is contraindicated during pregnancy due to the possibility of virilisation of the female foetus. However, investigations into embryotoxic, in particular teratogenic, effects gave no indication that further impairment of organ development may occur.

In vitro investigations of mutagenicity gave negative results.

Pharmaceutical particulars

List of excipients: Benzyl benzoate; castor oil for injection.

Incompatibilities: None so far known.

Shelf life: 5 years.

Special precautions for storage: Protect from light.

Nature and contents of container: Clear glass ampoules of 1 ml in packs of 3.

Instruction for use/handling: Not applicable.

Marketing authorisation holder: Cambridge Selfcare Diagnostics Limited, Newcastle upon Tyne NE2 1XG.

Marketing authorisation number 12070/0015.

Date of approval/revision of SPC April 1996.

Legal category POM.

TETRABENAZINE TABLETS 25 mg

Qualitative and quantitative composition Each tablet contains 25 mg tetrabenazine.

Pharmaceutical form Tablets.

Clinical particulars

Therapeutic indications: Movement disorders associated with organic central nervous system conditions, e.g. Huntington's chorea, hemiballismus and senile chorea.

Posology and method of administration: The tablets are for oral administration.

Adults: Dosage and administration are variable and only a guide is given. An initial starting dose of 25 mg three times a day is recommended. This can be increased by 25 mg a day every three or four days until 200 mg a day is being given or the limit of tolerance, as dictated by unwanted effects, is reached, whichever is the lower dose.

If there is no improvement at the maximum dose in seven days, it is unlikely that the compound will be of benefit to the patient, either by increasing the dose or by extending the duration of treatment.

The elderly: No specific studies have been performed in the elderly, but Tetrabenazine has been administered to elderly patients in standard dosage without apparent ill effect.

Children: No specific dosage recommendations are made for the administration of Tetrabenazine to children, although it has been used without ill effect.

Contra-indications: Tetrabenazine blocks the action of reserpine.

Special warnings and precautions for use: None.

Interaction with other medicaments and other forms of interaction: Levodopa should be administered with caution in the presence of Tetrabenazine.

Pregnancy and lactation: There is inadequate evidence of safety of the drug in human pregnancy and no evidence from animal work, but it has been in wide use for many years without apparent ill consequence. Tetrabenazine should be avoided in breast-feeding mothers.

Effects on ability to drive and use machines: Patients should be advised that Tetrabenazine may cause drowsiness and therefore may modify their performance at skilled tasks (driving ability, operation of machinery, etc.) to a varying degree, depending on dose and individual susceptibility.

Undesirable effects: Side-effects are usually mild with little hypotensive action and few digestive disorders. The main unwanted effect reported to date has been drowsiness, which occurs with higher doses. If depression occurs, it can be controlled by reducing the dose or by giving antidepressant drugs such as the monoamine oxidase inhibitors. However, Tetrabenazine should not be given immediately after a course of any of the monoamine oxidase inhibitors as such treatment may lead to a state of restlessness, disorientation and confusion. In man, a Parkinsonian-like syndrome has been reported on rare occasions, usually in doses above 200 mg per day, but this disappears on reducing the dose.

Overdose: Signs and symptoms of overdosage may include drowsiness, sweating, hypotension and hypothermia. Treatment is symptomatic.

Pharmacological properties

Pharmacodynamic properties: The central effects of Tetrabenazine closely resemble those of reserpine, but it differs from the latter in having less peripheral activity and being much shorter-acting.

Pharmacokinetic properties: Tetrabenazine has a low and erratic bioavailability. It appears to be extensively metabolised by first-pass metabolism. The major metabolite, hydroxytetrabenazine, is formed by reduction. Little unchanged tetrabenazine can be detected in the urine. Since hydroxybenazine is reported to be as active as tetrabenazine in depleting brain amines, it is likely that this is the major therapeutic agent.

Preclinical safety data: It is known from animal experiments that Tetrabenazine intervenes in the metabolism of biogenic amines, such as serotonin and noradrenaline, and that this activity is mainly limited to the brain. It is thought that the effect of Tetrabenazine on brain amines explains its clinical effects in man.

Pharmaceutical particulars

List of excipients:

Starch	BP	33.30 mg
Lactose	BP	64.0 mg
Talc	BP	2.0 mg
Magnesium stearate	BP	0.8 mg
Iron oxide yellow	E172	0.2 mg

Incompatibilities: None known.

Shelf life: 5 years.

Special precautions for storage: The recommended maximum storage temperature is 30°C.

Nature and contents of container: White HDPE bottle, pack size 112 tablets.

Instructions for use/handling: None.

Marketing authorisation holder: Lifehealth Limited, Richmond House, Old Brewery Court, Sandyford Road, Newcastle upon Tyne NE2 1XG.

Marketing authorisation number 14576/0005

Date of first authorisation/renewal of authorisation 23 October 1995.

Date of (partial) revision of the text September 1997.

TRIMETAPHAN CAMSYLATE AMPOULES

Qualitative and quantitative composition Each ampoule contains 250 mg trimetaphan camsylate in 5 ml of solution.

Pharmaceutical form Ampoules.

Clinical particulars

Therapeutic indications: Trimetaphan camsylate is used to induce controlled hypotension during certain surgical procedures. These may include: neurosurgery; vascular surgery; prostatectomy; chest surgery; thyroidectomy; bone and joint surgery.

Posology and method of administration: Trimetaphan Camsylate ampoules are for administration by intravenous drip and intermittent intravenous injection.

Adults and children:

(a) Dilution to 250 ml with normal saline or dextrose-saline gives a 0.1% solution (1 mg per ml) which is the strength usually used for an intravenous drip. The trimetaphan camsylate drip is started at an average of 60 drops (approximately 3 to 4 mg) per minute and, having ascertained the patient's response, the rate of administration is then adjusted to maintain the desired level of hypotension. Since there is marked variation in individual response, continuous blood pressure monitoring is essential to maintain proper control.

(b) If a weaker solution is preferred, a 0.05% solution can be prepared by diluting the 5% ampoule solution to 500 ml.

(c) It may be necessary to use a more concentrated solution in operations in which intravenous fluid should be restricted. For such patients a solution containing 0.25% trimetaphan camsylate should be prepared by diluting the original 5% solution to 100 ml with normal saline or dextrose-saline. The rate at which the drip is given should be correspondingly reduced.

(d) The undiluted solution has also been used by intermittent intravenous injection.

As with other hypotensive drugs, trimetaphan camsylate should be stopped before wound closure to allow the blood pressure to rise.

Trimetaphan camsylate ampoule solution may be diluted with water for injections, normal saline or dextrose-saline immediately before use.

The elderly: See *Special warnings and precautions for use.*

Contra-indications: Trimetaphan camsylate should not be used for hypotensive surgery in patients with severe arteriosclerosis, severe cardiac disease, or pyloric stenosis.

Special warnings and precautions for use: Trimetaphan camsylate should be used with caution in the elderly, in patients with cerebral or coronary vascular insufficiency, diabetes mellitus, hepatic or renal insufficiency and in adrenal insufficiency. Care should also be taken in patients receiving neuromuscular blocking drugs (especially suxamethonium), other anti-hypertensive agents, myocardial depressants or systemic corticosteroids.

Use in the elderly: No specific data are available on the use of trimetaphan camsylate in the elderly. Whilst there is no indication that this is accompanied by particular problems, it is known that the elderly may be more sensitive to hypotensive drugs. Trimetaphan camsylate should be used with particular caution in patients with coronary artery disease, prostatic hypertrophy or glaucoma (cf. pupillary dilatation effect).

Use in other special groups: Extreme caution should also be exercised when using trimetaphan camsylate in patients with degenerative disease of the central nervous system, Addison's disease and diabetes. Owing to its histamine-releasing effects, trimetaphan camsylate should be used with caution in subjects with a history of allergy.

Interactions with other medicaments and other forms of interaction: Since the effect of trimetaphan camsylate is neutralised by vasopressor drugs such as adrenaline, noradrenaline and ephedrine, local adrenaline infiltration at the site of incision is contra-indicated. Trimetaphan camsylate may sensitise patients to the cardiovascular effects of sympathomimetic agents.

Pregnancy and lactation: Use of trimetaphan camsylate in pregnancy should be avoided due to the risk of producing paralytic ileus or meconium ileus in the newborn.

Effects on ability to drive and use machines: Not applicable.

Undesirable effects: Ganglionic blockade due to trimetaphan camsylate may reduce gastro-intestinal motility and bladder function and affect visual accommodation. Constipation, mydriasis, increased intra-ocular pressure, decreased oral and nasal secretion, respiratory arrest (on rapid infusion of greater than 5 mg/minute), hypoglycaemia and hypokalaemia may also rarely occur.

Overdose: The major effect will be a marked fall in blood pressure below the desired level of hypotension. Tachycardia and respiratory depression may result, particularly if trimetaphan camsylate is used concomitantly with a muscle relaxant. Vasopressor agents such as phenylephrine, ephedrine or noradrenaline are antidotes and may be used to effect a rapid return to normotensive level.

Pharmacological properties

Pharmacodynamic properties: Trimetaphan camsylate is a ganglion-blocking agent which also has a direct dilator effect on peripheral vessels. It has a rapid, short and readily reversible action, which permits minute-to-minute control of the blood pressure.

Pharmacokinetic properties: Trimetaphan crosses the placenta. Further pharmacokinetic data are unavailable as there is no acceptable assay procedure for the determination of trimetaphan in biological specimens, however most of a parenteral dose is excreted unchanged by the kidney.

Preclinical safety data: There are no pre-clinical data of relevance to the prescriber which are additional to that already included in other sections of the SPC.

Pharmaceutical particulars

List of excipients: Sodium acetate; Hydrochloric acid; Water for injections.

Incompatibilities: It is inadvisable to use the trimetaphan camsylate drip as a vehicle for administering other drugs. Trimetaphan camsylate is known to be incompatible with thiopentone, gallamine triethiodide, strongly alkaline solutions, iodides and bromides.

Shelf life: Three years.

Special precautions for storage: The recommended maximum storage temperature is 6°C; avoid freezing.

Nature and contents of container: Colourless neutral glass ampoules each containing 5 ml of solution. 10 ampoules packed in a carton.

Instruction for use/handling: None.

Marketing authorisation holder: Cambridge Selfcare Diagnostics Limited, t/a Cambridge Laboratories, Richmond House, Old Brewery Court, Sandyford Road, Newcastle upon Tyne NE2 1XG.

Marketing authorisation number PL 12070/0001.

Date of first authorisation/renewal of authorisation 10 July 1992.

Date of (partial) revision of the text November 1996.

VITAMIN A PALMITATE AMPOULES 100,000 IU/2 ml

Qualitative and quantitative composition Each ampoule containing 100,000 IU Vitamin A, equivalent to 30 mg retinol.

Pharmaceutical form Ampoules containing a sterile solution.

Clinical particulars

Therapeutic indications: For the treatment and prevention of Vitamin A deficiency symptoms when oral therapy is inappropriate.

Posology and method of administration: Vitamin A Palmitate Ampoules 100,000 IU/2 ml are for deep intramuscular injection.

Adults: A maintenance dose of 100,000 i.u. by deep intramuscular injection once monthly is usually sufficient.

In acute deficiency states 100,000 i.u. may be given once weekly. However, if patients are receiving high doses continuously for a prolonged period, it is recommended that Vitamin A Palmitate be given in courses of no longer than six weeks separated by treatment-free intervals of two weeks in order to minimise the risk of hypervitaminosis A.

In patients with liver disease, a dose of 100,000 i.u. once every two to four months by deep intramuscular injection is recommended subject to a regular check of Vitamin A status.

Children: For children, and infants under one year of age, a dose of 50,000 i.u. by deep intramuscular injection once monthly is recommended.

The elderly: No specific studies of vitamin A have

been performed in elderly patients but Vitamin A Palmitate has been widely used for many years in the dosages recommended for younger adults without apparent ill consequence.

Contra-indications: Use in patients with a known hypersensitivity to any of the constituents.

Special warnings and precautions for use: Vitamin A Palmitate ampoules contain a polyethoxylated castor oil as solubiliser. In animal studies, polyethoxylated castor oil can produce severe anaphylactoid reactions associated with histamine release. There is strong circumstantial evidence that similar reactions occurring in patients may have been caused by polyethoxylated castor oil. If such a reaction should occur the usual measures should be taken (e.g. administration of glucocorticoids and/or antihistamines).

Local injection site reactions have been reported following co-administration of Vitamin A Palmitate ampoules with oil-based formulations. Vitamin A Palmitate should not, therefore, be mixed with oil-based formulations.

Massive doses of vitamin A are required to produce toxicity and therefore it is extremely unlikely that even exceptionally large single doses would cause hypervitaminosis A, except possibly in children, and in patients with underlying liver disease where enhanced susceptibility to vitamin A toxicity should be anticipated.

Small children are sometimes sensitive to single doses of 100,000 i.u. vitamin A. While children are taking Vitamin A Palmitate no other vitamin supplement containing vitamin A should be taken, unless under medical supervision.

If ampoules show signs of flocculation (as may be the case after unsuitable storage) they must not be used.

Interactions with other medicaments and other forms of interaction: None known.

Pregnancy and lactation: High doses of vitamin A can be teratogenic. Vitamin A Palmitate is therefore contra-indicated during pregnancy.

Effects on ability to drive and use machines: None known.

Undesirable effects: Yellowing of the skin is one of the signs of toxicity associated with high doses.

Overdose: Manifestations of acute overdosage in children include severe headache, nausea or vomiting, drowsiness, irritability and pruritus.

In chronic overdosage in children the following have been noted after periods of 2.5 to 15 months: hydrocephaly, alopecia, painful swellings over the long bones, with bone and joint pains, hyperostosis and deep, hard, tender swellings in the extremities. Adults are likely to complain of bone and joint pain. The vitamin should be discontinued. Symptoms of acute overdosage subside within 72 hours and of chronic overdosage over a period of several months, without further treatment.

Pharmacological properties

Pharmacodynamic properties: Vitamin A Palmitate is a synthetic vitamin A preparation. Vitamin A may be considered to act chiefly as a regulator of the growth and activity of epithelial tissues. It plays an essential role in the visual cycle through its participation in the synthesis of rhodopsin by the retina.

The cardinal signs and symptoms of vitamin A deficiency are those affecting the eyes, such as xerosis, swelling and destruction of the cornea and night-blindness. Hyperkeratosis of the skin and keratinising and metaplastic changes in the mucous membranes of the respiratory, digestive and urinary tracts have been reported.

Pharmacokinetic properties: After a single injection of 100,000 i.u. of Vitamin A Palmitate in a water miscible preparation the following results were obtained.

Plasma levels of Vitamin A Palmitate of up to 6000 µg/l were obtained at 10 to 20 hours after administration.

Baseline levels of 10 to 50 µg/l were reached after approximately 150 hours. Elimination from plasma appears to be governed by non-linear kinetics.

The bioavailability of this water miscible preparation is approximately 50%.

Preclinical safety data: There are no pre-clinical data of relevance to the prescriber which are additional to that already included in other sections of the SPC.

Pharmaceutical particulars

List of excipients: Polyoxyl 40 hydrogenated castor oil; DL-α-tocopherol; Sodium benzoate; Hydrochloric Acid; Purified Water.

Incompatibilities: Vitamin A Palmitate ampoule solution should not be diluted or mixed with other agents before injection. In particular, mixing of the water miscible Vitamin A Palmitate ampoule solution with oil-based formulations (e.g. Calciferol Injection BP) may be expected to result in emulsification.

Shelf life: Three years.

Special precautions for storage: Store below 15°C. Protect from light.

Nature and contents of container: Amber neutral type I glass ampoules each containing 10×2 ml of solution.

Instruction for use/handling: None.

Marketing authorisation holder: Cambridge Selfcare Diagnostics Limited, t/a Cambridge Laboratories, Richmond House, Old Brewery Court, Sandyford Road, Newcastle upon Tyne NE2 1XG.

Marketing authorisation number PL 12070/0006.

Date of first authorisation/renewal of authorisation 21 April 1992.

Date of (partial) revision of the text August 1997.

VITAMIN E SUSPENSION 100 mg/ml

Qualitative and quantitative composition Each 5 ml of suspension contains 500 mg of DL-alpha-tocopheryl acetate.

Pharmaceutical form Oral suspension.

Clinical particulars

Therapeutic indications: For the correction of Vitamin E deficiency occurring in malabsorption disorders i.e. cystic fibrosis, chronic cholestasis and abetalipoproteinaemia.

Posology and method of administration

Route of administration: For oral use.

Adults (including the elderly): For the treatment of malabsorption disorders the following doses should be administered:

Cystic fibrosis	100–200 mg/day
Abetalipoproteinaemia	50–100 mg/kg/day

Children: For the treatment of cystic fibrosis a dose of 50 mg/day should be given to children less than 1 year and 100 mg/day to children 1 year and over.

The adult dosage should be used for the treatment of abetalipoproteinaemia (50–100 mg/kg/day).

Infants with vitamin E deficiency which is secondary to chronic cholestasis may be treated with doses of 150–200 mg/kg/day.

Contra-indications: Use in patients with a known hypersensitivity to Vitamin E.

Special warnings and precautions for use: Vitamin E has been reported to increase the risk of thrombosis in patients predisposed to this condition, including patients taking oestrogens. This finding has not been confirmed but should be borne in mind when selecting patients for treatment, in particular women taking oral contraceptives containing oestrogens.

A higher incidence of necrotising enterocolitis has been noted in lower weight premature infants (less than 1.5 kg) treated with vitamin E.

Interactions with other medicaments and other forms of interaction: Vitamin E may increase the risk of thrombosis in patients taking oestrogens (see *Special warnings and precautions for use*).

Pregnancy and lactation: There is no evidence of the safety of high doses of vitamin E in pregnancy nor is there evidence from animal work that it is free from hazard, therefore do not use in pregnancy especially in the first trimester. No information is available on excretion in breast milk, therefore it is advisable not to use during lactation.

Effects on ability to drive and use machines: None known.

Undesirable effects: Diarrhoea and abdominal pain may occur with doses greater than 1 g daily.

Overdose: Transient gastro-intestinal disturbances have been reported with doses greater than 1 g daily and where necessary, general supportive measures should be employed.

Pharmacological properties

Pharmacodynamic properties: The exact role of Vitamin E in the animal organism has not yet been established. Vitamin E is known to exert an important physiological function as an antioxidant for fats, with a sparing action on vitamin A, carotenoids and on unsaturated fatty acids. Other work has demonstrated that vitamin E is connected with the maintenance of certain factors essential for the normal metabolic cycle.

Pharmacokinetic properties: Vitamin E is absorbed from the gastro-intestinal tract. Most of the vitamin appears in the lymph and is then widely distributed to all tissues. Most of the dose is slowly excreted in the bile and the remainder is eliminated in the urine as glucuronides of tocopheronic acid or other metabolites.

Preclinical safety data: There are no preclinical data of relevance to the prescriber which are additional to that already included in other sections of the SPC.

Pharmaceutical particulars

List of excipients: Castor oil polyethylene glycol ether; Benzoic acid; Sorbic acid; Glycerol; Syrup; Flavour raspberry; Purified water.

Incompatibilities: None.

Shelf life:

Unopened:	Two years.
After first opening:	One month (The product will be stable after opening for the normal duration of treatment providing the cap is replaced after use and the recommended storage conditions on the label are observed).

Special precautions for storage: Store below 25°C.

Nature and contents of container: 100 ml Amber glass bottles with aluminium screw caps or Vistop tamper-evident caps.

Instruction for use/handling: Vitamin E Suspension may be diluted with Syrup BP but should be used immediately and not stored.

Marketing authorisation holder: Cambridge Selfcare Diagnostics Limited, t/a Cambridge Laboratories, Richmond House, Old Brewery Court, Sandyford Road, Newcastle upon Tyne NE2 1XG.

Marketing authorisation number PL 12070/0010.

Date of first authorisation/renewal of authorisation 8 March 1993.

Date of (partial) revision of the text October 1997.

**Trade Mark*

Castlemead Healthcare Limited
20 Clanwilliam Terrace
Dublin 2
Ireland

☎ 278 0755   278 0763

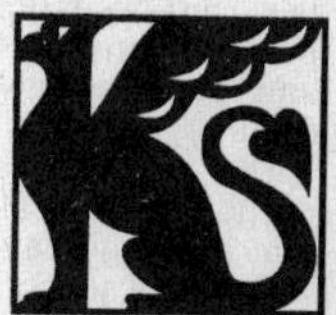

AEROCROM* INHALER AND SYNCRONER

Qualitative and quantitative composition

Ingredients	*mg per actuation*
Sodium cromoglycate, micronised	1.00
Salbutamol sulphate, micronised (equivalent to 0.10 mg salbutamol base).	0.1205

Pharmaceutical form Aerocrom Inhaler is presented as a metered dose pressurised aerosol containing sodium cromoglycate and salbutamol sulphate as a suspension in chlorofluorocarbon propellants, for inhalation.

Clinical particulars
Therapeutic indications: Aerocrom is indicated for patients who have been shown to require regular doses of sodium cromoglycate and salbutamol for the treatment of asthma. Aerocrom is not intended for first line maintenance treatment but is only for use once the need for regular combination therapy has been established.

Posology and method of administration: Adults (including the elderly): Two inhalations (2 mg Sodium cromoglycate and 200 micrograms salbutamol) four times daily. This is the maximum recommended dose for regular treatment with salbutamol.

In patients who experience exercise-induced asthma, one of the scheduled doses may be administered a few minutes prior to exercise. In the event of isolated episodes of breakthrough wheezing an additional dose of two inhalations may be administered. If the patient experiences breakthrough symptoms regularly or notices the effectiveness of the inhaler in relieving bronchospasm is diminishing they should be advised to seek medical advice.

Children: Aerocrom is not recommended for use in children.

Contra-indications, warnings, etc:
Contra-indications: Aerocrom is contra-indicated in patients with a history of hypersensitivity to any of the ingredients. Not for use in children.

Special warnings and special precautions for use: Patients who experience breakthrough wheezing regularly should be advised to obtain medical advice. Aerocrom Inhaler is not for use in acute attacks but for regular maintenance treatment. If the patient notices that the effectiveness of the inhaler in relieving bronchospasm or symptoms is diminishing they should be advised to seek further medical advice.

Aerocrom should be administered with caution to patients suffering from thyrotoxicosis. Potentially serious hypokalaemia may result from beta$_2$-agonist therapy.

If it is necessary to withdraw this treatment, it should normally be done progressively over a period of one week. Symptoms of asthma may recur.

Interactions with other medicaments and other forms of interaction: Potentially serious hypokalaemia may result from beta$_2$-agonist therapy. Particular caution is advised in severe asthma as this effect may be potentiated by concomitant treatment with xanthine derivatives, steroids, diuretics and by hypoxia. It is recommended that serum potassium levels are monitored in such situations. Non-selective beta-blockers such as propranolol should not usually be prescribed with Aerocrom.

Use during pregnancy and lactation: As with all medicines, administration during pregnancy should only be considered if the expected benefit to the mother is greater than any possible risk to the foetus. Particular caution must be exercised during the first trimester of pregnancy.

Both sodium cromoglycate and salbutamol have been in widespread use for many years without apparent effects on foetal development. However, there is little published evidence concerning safety in early human pregnancy. Animal studies with salbutamol are reported as showing evidence of some harmful effects on the foetus at high dose levels.

It is not known whether sodium cromoglycate is excreted in breast milk. On the basis of animal studies this is unlikely. There is no information to suggest that the use of sodium cromoglycate by nursing mothers has any undesirable effects on the nursing infant. However, as salbutamol is reported as probably being excreted in breast milk the use of Aerocrom in nursing mothers needs to be carefully considered. The effect of salbutamol on neonates is not known. The use of Aerocrom should be limited to cases where the expected benefit to the mother outweighs any potential risk to the neonate.

Effects on ability to drive and use machines: Aerocrom has no known effects on ability to drive or operate machinery.

Undesirable effects: Some patients may experience mild tremor, throat irritation, coughing, headache, transient muscle cramps, bronchospasm or rash particularly when treatment is first started.

Very rarely following administration of sodium cromoglycate or salbutamol by inhalation, severe bronchospasm associated with a marked fall in pulmonary function has been reported. Hypersensitivity reactions such as angioedema, urticaria, hypotension and collapse have been reported very rarely in association with the use of salbutamol. In such cases Aerocrom should be stopped immediately and not be reintroduced. Medical advice should be sought. Consideration should be given to the introduction of other anti-inflammatory asthma therapy.

Overdose: Overdosage with Aerocrom leading to signs of excessive beta-stimulation may be managed by the administration of a cardioselective beta-blocking agent, but such drugs should be used with caution in patients with a history of bronchospasm. No action other than medical observation should be necessary for overdosage with sodium cromoglycate.

Pharmacological properties
Pharmacodynamic properties: Sodium cromoglycate is believed to act by inhibiting the release of chemical mediators from sensitised mast cells, thereby preventing the allergic reaction in the lung. This inhibition prevents the asthmatic response. Salbutamol is a direct-acting sympathomimetic agent with predominantly beta-adrenergic activity and a selective action on beta$_2$-receptors. When applied topically to the lungs this action is seen as a sustained bronchodilation.

Pharmacokinetic properties: Sodium cromoglycate: Following inhalation as a fine powder, about 8% of the dose is reported to be deposited in the lungs, from where it is rapidly absorbed and excreted unchanged in the urine and bile. The majority of an inhaled dose is swallowed and excreted unchanged via the alimentary canal.

Salbutamol: As with sodium cromoglycate much of the inhaled dose is swallowed. Oral salbutamol is well absorbed from the gut giving peak plasma concentrations about 3 hours after administration. Salbutamol is subject to extensive first pass metabolism; 50% is excreted in the urine as an inactive sulphate conjugate. The remainder is excreted unchanged. Absorption from the lung is slower giving peak plasma concentrations about 3–5 hours after administration. The half life is similarly prolonged.

Preclinical safety data: Animal studies have shown that sodium cromoglycate has a very low order of local or systemic toxicity. The safety of salbutamol has been established during more than 20 years of worldwide clinical use.

Pharmaceutical particulars
List of excipients: Sorbitan trioleate; propellant mixture 12:114 (dichlorodifluoromethane and dichlorotetrafluoroethane, 60:40% w/w).

Incompatibilities: None known.

Shelf life: 36 months.

Special precautions for storage: Store below 25°C. The aerosol canister is pressurised and should be protected from direct sunlight, heat and frost and must not be punctured or burnt even when empty. As with most other inhaled medications in aerosol canisters, the therapeutic effect of Aerocrom may decrease when the canister is cold.

Nature and contents of container:
Aerocrom Inhaler: A pressurised aerosol containing sodium cromoglycate and salbutamol sulphate as a suspension in compressed, liquefied propellant gas mixture. The aluminium can is fitted with a metering valve (delivering 200 actuations) and a plastic valve cover.

Aerocrom Syncroner: The cartoned pack contains an aerosol canister, a moulded polyethylene mouthpiece with a spacer device fitted with a dustcap and instructions for use.

Marketing authorisation number PL 16946/0001

Date of approval/revision of SPC July 1998.

Legal category POM.

STEMETIL Eff*

Qualitative and quantitative composition The active component of Stemetil Eff is prochlorperazine mesylate BP 5 mg equivalent to 3.3 mg prochlorperazine base.

Pharmaceutical form White effervescent granular powder which dissolves in water to give a lemon flavoured effervescent solution.

Clinical Particulars:
Therapeutic indications: Prevention of nausea and vomiting. Treatment of nausea and vomiting. Treatment of vertigo and Meniere's syndrome. Adjunct in the short-term management of anxiety.

Posology and method of administration: For oral administration.

Adults

Indication	*Dosage*
Prevention of nausea and vomiting	5 to 10 mg b.d. or t.d.s.
Treatment of nausea and vomiting	20 mg stat, followed if necessary by 10 mg two hours later.
Vertigo and Meniere's syndrome	5 mg t.d.s increasing if necessary to a total of 30 mg daily. After several weeks dosage may be reduced gradually to 5–10 mg daily.
Adjunct in the short-term management of anxiety	15–20 mg daily in divided doses initially but this may be increased if necessary to maximum of 40 mg daily in divided doses.

Children: Not recommended.

Elderly: A lower initial dose is recommended. Please see *Special warnings and special precautions for use* section.

Contra-indications: None stated.

Special warnings and special precautions for use: Stemetil should be avoided in patients with liver or renal dysfunction, epilepsy, Parkinson's disease, hypothyroidism, phaeochromocytoma, myasthenia gravis, prostate hypertrophy. It should be avoided in patients known to be hypersensitive to phenothiazines or with a history of narrow angle glaucoma. It should be used with caution in the elderly, particularly during very hot or very cold weather (risk of hyper-, hypothermia).

The elderly are particularly susceptible to postural hypotension.

Stemetil should be used cautiously in the elderly owing to their susceptibility to drugs acting centrally on the nervous system and a lower initial dosage is recommended. There is an increased risk of drug-induced Parkinsonism in the elderly, particularly after prolonged use. Care should also be taken not to confuse the adverse effects of Stemetil e.g. orthostatic hypotension, with effects due to the underlying disorder.

Due to its aspartame content, Stemetil Eff should not be given to patients with phenylketonuria.

Children: Stemetil has been associated with dystonic reactions particularly after a cumulative dosage of 0.5 mg/kg. It should therefore be used cautiously in children.

Interaction with other medicaments and other forms of interaction: Interactions of phenothiazine neuroleptics: The CNS depressant actions of neuroleptic agents may be intensified (additively) by alcohol, barbiturates and other sedatives. Respiratory depression may occur.

The hypotensive effect of most antihypertensive drugs especially alpha adrenoceptor blocking agents may be exaggerated by neuroleptics.

The mild anticholinergic effect of neuroleptics may be enhanced by other anticholinergic drugs possibly leading to constipation, heat stroke, etc.

The action of some drugs may be opposed by phenothiazine neuroleptics; these include amphetamine, levodopa, clonidine, guanethidine, adrenaline.

Anticholinergic agents may reduce the antipsychotic effect of neuroleptics.

Some drugs interfere with absorption of neuroleptic agents: antacids, anti-Parkinson, lithium. Increases or decreases in the plasma concentrations of a number of drugs, e.g. propranolol, phenobarbitone have been observed but were not of clinical significance.

High doses of neuroleptics reduce the response to hypoglycaemic agents the dosage of which might have to be raised.

Adrenaline must *not* be used in patients overdosed with Stemetil. Most of the above interactions are of a theoretical nature and not dangerous.

Simultaneous administration of desferrioxamine and prochlorperazine has been observed to induce a transient metabolic encephalopathy characterised by loss of consciousness for 48–72 hours.

Pregnancy and lactation: Stemetil is contraindicated in pregnancy. There is inadequate evidence of the safety of Stemetil in human pregnancy but it has been widely used for many years without apparent ill consequence. There is evidence of harmful effects in animals. Like other drugs it should be avoided in pregnancy unless the physician considers it essential. Neuroleptics may occasionally prolong labour and at such a time should be withheld until the cervix is dilated 3–4 cm. Possible adverse effects on the neonate include lethargy or paradoxical hyperexcitability, tremor and low Apgar score. Phenothiazines may be excreted in milk, breastfeeding should be suspended during treatment.

Effects on ability to drive and use machines: Patients should be warned about drowsiness during the early days of treatment, and advised not to drive or operate machinery.

Undesirable effects: Minor side-effects of neuroleptics are nasal stuffiness, dry mouth, insomnia, agitation. Adverse effects of neuroleptics: *Liver function:* Jaundice, usually transient, occurs in a very small percentage of patients taking neuroleptics. A premonitory sign may be a sudden onset of fever after one to three weeks of treatment followed by the development of jaundice. Neuroleptic jaundice has the biochemical and other characteristics of obstructive jaundice and is associated with obstruction of the canaliculi by bile thrombi; the frequent presence of an accompanying eosinophilia indicates the allergic nature of this phenomenon. Treatment should be withheld on the development of jaundice. *Cardiorespiratory:* Hypotension, usually postural, commonly occurs. Elderly or volume depleted subjects are particularly susceptible, it is more likely after intramuscular injection. Cardiac arrhythmias, including atrial arrhythmia, A-V block, ventricular tachycardia and fibrillation have been reported during neuroleptic therapy, possibly related to dosage. Pre-existing cardiac disease, old age, hypokalaemia and concurrent tricyclic antidepressants may pre-dispose. ECG changes, usually benign, include widened QT interval, ST depression, U-waves and T-wave changes. *Respiratory depression* is possible in susceptible patients. *Blood picture:* A mild leucopenia occurs in up to 30% of patients on prolonged high dosage. Agranulocytosis may occur rarely; it is not dose related. The occurrence of unexplained infections or fever requires immediate haematological investigation. *Extrapyramidal:* Acute dystonias or dyskinesias, usually transitory, are more common in children and young adults, and usually occur within the first 4 days of treatment or after dosage increases. Akathisia characteristically occurs after large initial doses. Parkinsonism is more common in adults and the elderly. It usually develops after weeks or months of treatment. One or more of the following may be seen: tremor, rigidity, akinesia or other features of Parkinsonism, commonly just tremor. *Tardive dyskinesia:* If this occurs it is usually, but not necessarily, after prolonged or high dosage. It can even occur after treatment has been stopped. Dosage should therefore be kept low whenever possible. *Skin and eyes:* Contact skin sensitisation is a serious but rare complication in those frequently handling preparations of certain phenothiazines; the greatest care must be taken to avoid contact of the drug with the skin. Skin rashes of various kinds may also be seen in patients treated with the drug. Patients on high dosage should be warned that they may develop photosensitivity in sunny weather and should avoid exposure to direct sunlight. Ocular changes and the development of a metallic greyish-mauve coloration of exposed skin have been noted in some individuals mainly females, who have received chlorpromazine continuously for long periods (four to eight years). This could possibly happen with Stemetil. *Endocrine:* Hyperprolactinaemia which may result in galactorrhoea, gynaecomastia, amenorrhoea and impotence. Neuroleptic malignant syndrome (hyperthermia, rigidity, autonomic dysfunction and altered consciousness) may occur with any neuroleptic.

Overdose: Symptoms of phenothiazine overdosage include drowsiness or loss of consciousness, hypotension, tachycardia, ECG changes, ventricular arrhythmias and hypothermia. Severe extra-pyramidal dyskinesias may occur.

If the patient is seen sufficiently soon (up to 6 hours) after ingestion of a toxic dose, gastric lavage may be attempted. Pharmacological induction of emesis is unlikely to be of any use. Activated charcoal should be given. There is no specific antidote. Treatment is supportive.

Generalised vasodilatation may result in circulatory collapse; raising the patient's legs may suffice. In severe cases, volume expansion by intravenous fluids may be needed; infusion fluids should be warmed before administration in order not to aggravate hypothermia.

Positive inotropic agents such as dopamine may be tried if fluid replacement is insufficient to correct the circulatory collapse. Peripheral vasoconstrictor agents are not generally recommended; avoid the use of adrenaline.

Ventricular or supraventricular tachy-arrhythmias usually respond to restoration of normal body temperature and correction of circulatory or metabolic disturbances. If persistent or life threatening, appropriate anti-arrhythmic therapy may be considered. Avoid lignocaine and, as far as possible, long acting anti-arrhythmic drugs.

Pronounced central nervous system depression requires airway maintenance or, in extreme circumstances, assisted respiration. Severe dystonic reactions usually respond to procyclidine (5–10 mg) or orphenadrine (20–40 mg) administered intramuscularly or intravenously. Convulsions should be treated with intravenous diazepam.

Neuroleptic malignant syndrome should be treated with cooling. Dantrolene sodium may be tried.

Pharmacological properties

Pharmacodynamic properties: Prochlorperazine (PCP) is a dopamine and histamine antagonist. The mechanism of the anti-emetic is due predominantly to blockade of the histamine H_1 and dopamine D_2 neurotransmitter receptors in the chemoreceptor trigger zone and vomiting centre. It also has weak anticholinergic effect and prevents acid reflux by increasing the tone of the lower oesphangeal sphincter.

Pharmacokinetic properties: Peak prochlorperazine (PCP) concentrations of approximately 1.1ng/ml were reached at 2.8 hours after oral administration of an aqueous solution of prochlorperazine mesylate (Stemetil syrup) to healthy volunteers.

PCP was rapidly metabolised to the S-oxide due to a first pass effect during absorption, thus producing peak metabolite concentrations of 17ng/ml at 0.5 hour. The AUC values for the S-oxide indicate that PCP is well absorbed orally, compared with i.m. injection. Plasma concentrations of PCP and S-oxide fell with half-lives of 6.2 and 8.5 hours, respectively.

PCP is widely distributed throughout the body and diffuses rapidly across the placenta. It is excreted in the urine and faeces mainly as metabolites.

Preclinical safety data: There is no pre-clinical data of relevance to the prescriber which are additional to that already included in other sections of the SPC.

Pharmaceutical particulars

List of excipients: Tartaric acid BP (E334), Povidone K30 BP, sodium bicarbonate BP (E500), fresh lemon juice (Flav-O-Lok 610406E), citric acid anhydrous BP (E330), ascorbic acid BP (E300), sodium carbonate dried 1968 BPC (E500), aspartame (E951).

Incompatibilities: None stated.

Shelf life: 36 months.

Special precautions for storage: Store below 25°C.

Nature and content of container: Stemetil Eff is available in sealed sachets consisting of paper/foil/polyethylene laminate in cartons of 21.

Instructions for use/handling: None stated.

Marketing authorisation number PL 16946/0002

Date of approval/partial revision of SPC July 1998

Legal category POM.

STEMETIL* INJECTION

Qualitative and quantitative composition Each 1 ml of Stemetil Injection contains 12.5 mg prochlorperazine mesylate BP.

Pharmaceutical form Colourless sterile solution.

Clinical Particulars

Therapeutic indications: Stemetil is a potent phenothiazine neuroleptic. Uses: The treatment of nausea and vomiting and in schizophrenia (particularly the chronic stage) and acute mania.

Posology and method of administration: For deep intramuscular injection.

Adults

Indication	*Dosage*
Treatment of nausea and vomiting	12.5 mg by deep i.m. injection followed by oral therapy medication 6 hours later if necessary.
Schizophrenia and other psychotic disorders	12.5 mg to 25 mg b.i.d. or t.d.s. by deep intramuscular injection until oral treatment becomes possible

Children: Intramuscular Stemetil should not be given to children.

Elderly: A lower dose is recommended. Please see *Special warnings and special precautions for use* section.

Contra-indications: The use of Stemetil injection is contraindicated in children as it has been associated with dystonic reactions after the cumulative dose of 0.5 mg/kg.

Special warnings and special precautions for use: Stemetil should be avoided in patients with liver or renal dysfunction, epilepsy, Parkinson's disease, hypothyroidism, phaeochromocytoma, myasthenia gravis, prostate hypertrophy. It should be avoided in patients known to be hypersensitive to phenothiazines or with a history of narrow angle glaucoma. It should be used with caution in the elderly, particularly during very hot or very cold weather (risk of hyper-, hypothermia).

Postural hypotension with tachycardia as well as local pain or nodule formation may occur after i.m. administration.

The elderly are particularly susceptible to postural hypotension.

Stemetil should be used cautiously in the elderly owing to their susceptibility to drugs acting centrally on the nervous system and a lower initial dosage is recommended. There is an increased risk of drug-induced Parkinsonism in the elderly particularly after prolonged use. Care should also be taken not to confuse the adverse effects of Stemetil e.g. orthostatic hypotension with effects due to the underlying disorder.

Interaction with other medicaments and other forms of interaction: Interactions of phenothiazine neuroleptics: The CNS depressant actions of neuroleptic agents may be intensified (additively) by alcohol, barbiturates and other sedatives. Respiratory depression may occur.

The hypotensive effect of most antihypertensive drugs especially alpha adrenoceptor blocking agents may be exaggerated by neuroleptics.

The mild anticholinergic effect of neuroleptics may be enhanced by other anticholinergic drugs possibly leading to constipation, heat stroke, etc.

The action of some drugs may be opposed by phenothiazine neuroleptics; these include amphetamine, levodopa, clonidine, guanethidine, adrenaline.

Anticholinergic agents may reduce the antipsychotic effect of neuroleptics.

Some drugs interfere with absorption of neuroleptic agents: antacids, anti-Parkinson, lithium. Increases or decreases in the plasma concentrations of a number of drugs, e.g. propranolol, phenobarbitone have been observed but were not of clinical significance.

High doses of neuroleptics reduce the response to hypoglycaemic agents the dosage of which might have to be raised.

Adrenaline must *not* be used in patients overdosed with Stemetil. Most of the above interactions are of a theoretical nature and not dangerous.

Simultaneous administration of desferrioxamine and prochlorperazine has been observed to induce a transient metabolic encephalopathy characterised by loss of consciousness for 48–72 hours.

Pregnancy and lactation: Stemetil is contraindicated in pregnancy. There is inadequate evidence of the safety of Stemetil in human pregnancy but it has been widely used for many years without apparent ill consequence. There is evidence of harmful effects in animals. Like other drugs it should be avoided in pregnancy unless the physician considers it essential. Neuroleptics may occasionally prolong labour and at such a time should be withheld until the cervix is dilated 3–4 cm. Possible adverse effects on the neonate include lethargy or paradoxical hyperexcitability, tremor and low Apgar score. Phenothiazines may be excreted in milk, breastfeeding should be suspended during treatment.

Effects on ability to drive and use machines: Patients should be warned about drowsiness during the early days of treatment, and advised not to drive or operate machinery.

Undesirable effects: Minor side-effects of neuroleptics are nasal stuffiness, dry mouth, insomnia, agitation. Adverse effects of neuroleptics: *Liver function*: Jaundice, usually transient, occurs in a very small percentage of patients taking neuroleptics. A premonitory sign may be a sudden onset of fever after one to three weeks of treatment followed by the development of jaundice. Neuroleptic jaundice has the biochemical and other characteristics of obstructive jaundice and is associated with obstruction of the canaliculi by bile thrombi; the frequent presence of an accompanying eosinophilia indicates the allergic nature of this phenomenon. Treatment should be withheld on the development of jaundice. *Cardiorespiratory:* Hypotension, usually postural, commonly occurs. Elderly or volume depleted subjects are particularly susceptible, it is more likely to occur after intramuscular injection. Cardiac arrhythmias, including atrial arrhythmia, A-V block, ventricular tachycardia and fibrillation have been reported during neuroleptic therapy, possibly related to dosage. Pre-existing cardiac disease, old age, hypokalaemia and concurrent tricyclic antidepressants may predispose. ECG changes, usually benign, include widened QT interval, ST depression, U-waves and T-wave changes. Respiratory depression is possible in susceptible patients. *Blood picture:* A mild leucopenia occurs in up to 30% of patients on prolonged high dosage. Agranulocytosis may occur rarely; it is not dose related. The occurrence of unexplained infections or fever requires immediate haematological investigation. *Extrapyramidal:* Acute dystonias or dyskinesias, usually transitory, are more common in children and young adults, and usually occur within the first 4 days of treatment or after dosage increases. Akathisia characteristically occurs after large initial doses. Parkinsonism is more common in adults and the elderly. It usually develops after weeks or months of treatment. One or more of the following may be seen: tremor, rigidity, akinesia or other features of Parkinsonism. Commonly just tremor. *Tardive dyskinesia:* If this occurs it is usually, but not necessarily, after prolonged or high dosage. It can even occur after treatment has been stopped. Dosage should therefore be kept low whenever possible. *Skin and eyes:* Contact skin sensitisation is a serious but rare complication in those frequently handling preparations of certain phenothiazines; the greatest care must be taken to avoid contact of the drug with the skin. Skin rashes of various kinds may also be seen in patients treated with the drug. Patients on high dosage should be warned that they may develop photosensitivity in sunny weather and should avoid exposure to direct sunlight. Ocular changes and the development of a metallic greyish-mauve coloration of exposed skin have been noted in some individuals mainly females, who have received chlorpromazine continuously for long periods (four to eight years). This could possibly happen with Stemetil. *Endocrine:* Hyperprolactinaemia which may result in galactorrhoea, gynaecomastia, amenorrhoea; impotence. Neuroleptic malignant syndrome (hyperthermia, rigidity, autonomic dysfunction and altered consciousness) may occur with any neuroleptic.

Overdose: Symptoms of phenothiazine overdosage include drowsiness or loss of consciousness, hypotension, tachycardia, ECG changes, ventricular arrhythmias and hypothermia. Severe extra-pyramidal dyskinesias may occur.

If the patient is seen sufficiently soon (up to 6 hours) after ingestion of a toxic dose, gastric lavage may be attempted. Pharmacological induction of emesis is unlikely to be of any use. Activated charcoal should be given. There is no specific antidote. Treatment is supportive.

Generalised vasodilatation may result in circulatory collapse; raising the patient's legs may suffice. In severe cases, volume expansion by intravenous fluids may be needed; infusion fluids should be warmed before administration in order not to aggravate hypothermia.

Positive inotropic agents such as dopamine may be tried if fluid replacement is insufficient to correct the circulatory collapse. Peripheral vasoconstrictor agents are not generally recommended; avoid the use of adrenaline.

Ventricular or supraventricular tachy-arrhythmias usually respond to restoration of normal body temperature and correction of circulatory or metabolic disturbances. If persistent or life threatening, appropriate anti-arrhythmic therapy may be considered. Avoid lignocaine and, as far as possible, long acting anti-arrhythmic drugs.

Pronounced central nervous system depression requires airway maintenance or, in extreme circumstances, assisted respiration. Severe dystonic reactions usually respond to procyclidine (5–10 mg) or orphenadrine (20–40 mg) administered intramuscularly or intravenously. Convulsions should be treated with intravenous diazepam.

Neuroleptic malignant syndrome should be treated with cooling. Dantrolene sodium may be tried.

Pharmacological properties

Pharmacodynamic properties: Stemetil is a potent phenothiazine neuroleptic. It is used in vertigo due to Meniere's syndrome, labryrinthitis and other causes, and for nausea and vomiting from whatever cause including that associated with migraine. It may also be used for schizophrenia (particularly the chronic stage), acute mania and as an adjunct to the short term management of anxiety.

Pharmacokinetic properties: There is little information about blood levels, distribution and excretion in humans. The rate of metabolism and excretion of phenothiazines decreases in old age.

Preclinical safety data: There is no pre-clinical data of relevance to the prescriber which are additional to that already included in other sections of the SPC.

Pharmaceutical particulars

List of excipients: Sodium sulphite anhydrous BP (E221), sodium metabisulphite powder BP (E223), sodium chloride Ph Eur, ethanolamine BP and water for injections (non-sterilised) BP.

Incompatibilities: None stated.

Shelf life: 60 months.

Special precautions for storage: Protect from light. Discoloured solutions should not be used.

Nature and content of container: Stemetil injection is supplied in colourless glass ampoules in packs of 10 x 1 ml.

Instructions for use/handling: None.

Marketing Authorisation number PL 16946/0003

Date of approval/revision of SPC July 1998

Legal category POM.

STEMETIL* SUPPOSITORIES

Qualitative and quantitative composition Each Stemetil 5 mg suppository contains 0.32% w/w prochlorperazine base, equivalent to 5 mg prochlorperazine maleate. Each Stemetil 25 mg suppository contains 0.78% w/w prochlorperazine base, equivalent to 25 mg prochlorperazine maleate

Pharmaceutical form Cream, smooth, torpedo-shaped suppositories.

Clinical Particulars

Therapeutic indications: Stemetil is a potent phenothiazine neuroleptic. Uses: The treatment of nausea and vomiting, the prevention of post-operative vomiting. The management of nausea and vomiting and in schizophrenia (particularly the chronic stage) and acute mania.

Posology and method of administration: Route of administration: Rectal

Adults

Indication	*Dosage*
Treatment of nausea and vomiting	25 mg followed by oral medication 6 hours later if necessary.
For the management of nausea and vomiting due to migraine	One 5 mg suppository three times a day. In acute cases an intramuscular injection may be administered followed by the use of suppositories.
Prevention of post-operative vomiting	Two 5 mg suppositories before operation followed by two every 5 hours for up to 20 hours thereafter.
Schizophrenia and other psychotic disorders	25 mg b.d. or t.d.s. until oral treatment becomes possible.

Children: Stemetil suppositories should not be given to children.

Elderly: A lower dose is recommended. Please see *Special warnings and special precautions for use* section.

Contra-indications: Pregnancy.

Special warnings and special precautions for use: Stemetil should be avoided in patients with liver or renal dysfunction, epilepsy, Parkinson's disease, hypothyroidism, phaeochromocytoma, myasthenia gravis, prostate hypertrophy. It should be avoided in patients known to be hypersensitive to phenothiazines or with a history of narrow angle glaucoma. It should be used with caution in the elderly, particularly during very hot or very cold weather (risk of hyper-, hypothermia).

The elderly are particularly susceptible to postural hypotension.

Stemetil should be used cautiously in the elderly owing to their susceptibility to drugs acting centrally on the nervous system and a lower initial dosage is recommended. There is an increased risk of drug-induced Parkinsonism in the elderly particularly after prolonged use. Care should also be taken not to confuse the adverse effects of Stemetil e.g. orthostatic hypotension with effects due to the underlying disorder.

Interaction with other medicaments and other forms of interaction: Interactions of phenothiazine neuroleptics: The CNS depressant actions of neuroleptic agents may be intensified (additively) by alcohol, barbiturates and other sedatives. Respiratory depression may occur.

The hypotensive effect of most antihypertensive drugs especially alpha adrenoceptor blocking agents may be exaggerated by neuroleptics.

The mild anticholinergic effect of neuroleptics may be enhanced by other anticholinergic drugs possibly leading to constipation, heat stroke, etc.

The action of some drugs may be opposed by phenothiazine neuroleptics; these include amphetamine, levodopa, clonidine, guanethidine, adrenaline.

Anticholinergic agents may reduce the antipsychotic effect of neuroleptics.

Some drugs interfere with absorption of neuroleptic agents: antacids, anti-Parkinson, lithium. Increases or decreases in the plasma concentrations of a number of drugs, e.g. propranolol, phenobarbitone have been observed but were not of clinical significance.

High doses of neuroleptics reduce the response to hypoglycaemic agents the dosage of which might have to be raised.

Adrenaline must *not* be used in patients overdosed with Stemetil. Most of the above interactions are of a theoretical nature and not dangerous.

Simultaneous administration of desferrioxamine and prochlorperazine has been observed to induce a transient metabolic encephalopathy characterised by loss of consciousness for 48–72 hours.

Pregnancy and lactation: Stemetil is contraindicated in pregnancy. There is inadequate evidence of the safety of Stemetil in human pregnancy but it has been widely used for many years without apparent ill consequence. There is evidence of harmful effects in animals. Like other drugs it should be avoided in pregnancy unless the physician considers it essential. Neuroleptics may occasionally prolong labour and at such a time should be withheld until the cervix is dilated 3–4 cm. Possible adverse effects on the neonate include lethargy or paradoxical hyperexcitability, tremor and low Apgar score. Phenothiazines may be excreted in milk, breastfeeding should be suspended during treatment.

Effects on ability to drive and use machines: Patients should be warned about drowsiness during the early days of treatment, and advised not to drive or operate machinery.

Undesirable effects: Minor side-effects of neuroleptics are nasal stuffiness, dry mouth, insomnia, agitation. Adverse effects of neuroleptics: *Liver function:* Jaundice, usually transient, occurs in a very small percentage of patients taking neuroleptics. A premonitory sign may be a sudden onset of fever after one to three weeks of treatment followed by the development of jaundice. Neuroleptic jaundice has the biochemical and other characteristics of obstructive jaundice and is associated with obstruction of the canaliculi by bile thrombi; the frequent presence of an accompanying eosinophilia indicates the allergic nature of this phenomenon. Treatment should be withheld on the development of jaundice. *Cardiorespiratory:* Hypotension, usually postural, commonly occurs. Elderly or volume depleted subjects are particularly susceptible, it is more likely to occur after intramuscular injection. Cardiac arrhythmias, including atrial arrhythmia, A-V block, ventricular tachycardia and fibrillation have been reported during neuroleptic therapy, possibly related to dosage. Pre-existing cardiac disease, old age, hypokalaemia and concurrent tricyclic antidepressants may predispose. ECG changes, usually benign, include widened QT interval, ST depression, U-waves and T-wave changes. Respiratory depression is possible in susceptible patients. *Blood picture:* A mild leucopenia occurs in up to 30% of patients on prolonged high dosage. Agranulocytosis may occur rarely; it is not dose related. The occurrence of unexplained infections or fever requires immediate haematological investigation. *Extrapyramidal:* Acute dystonias or dyskinesias, usually transitory, are more common in children and young adults, and usually occur within the first 4 days of treatment or after dosage increases. Akathisia characteristically occurs after large initial doses. Parkinsonism is more common in adults and the elderly. It usually develops after weeks or months of treatment. One or more of the following may be seen: tremor, rigidity, akinesia or other features of Parkinsonism. Commonly just tremor. *Tardive dyskinesia:* If this occurs it is usually, but not necessarily, after prolonged or high dosage. It can even occur after treatment has been stopped. Dosage should therefore be kept low whenever possible. *Skin and eyes:* Contact skin sensitisation is a serious but rare complication in those frequently handling preparations of certain phenothiazines; the greatest care must be taken to avoid contact of the drug with the skin. Skin rashes of various kinds may also be seen in patients treated with the drug. Patients on high dosage should be warned that they may develop photosensitivity in sunny weather and should avoid exposure to direct sunlight. Ocular changes and the development of a metallic greyish-mauve coloration of exposed skin have been noted in some individuals mainly females, who have received chlorpromazine continuously for long periods (four to eight years). This could possibly happen with Stemetil. *Endocrine:* hyperprolactinaemia which may result in galactorrhoea, gynaecomastia, amenorrhoea; impotence. Neuroleptic malignant syndrome (hypothermia, rigidity, autonomic dysfunction and altered consciousness) may occur with any neuroleptic.

Overdose: Symptoms of phenothiazine overdosage include drowsiness or loss of consciousness, hypotension, tachycardia, ECG changes, ventricular arrhythmias and hypothermia. Severe extra-pyramidal dyskinesias may occur.

If the patient is seen sufficiently soon (up to 6 hours) after ingestion of a toxic dose, gastric lavage may be attempted. Pharmacological induction of emesis is unlikely to be of any use. Activated charcoal should be given. There is no specific antidote. Treatment is supportive.

Generalised vasodilatation may result in circulatory collapse; raising the patient's legs may suffice. In severe cases, volume expansion by intravenous fluids may be needed; infusion fluids should be warmed before administration in order not to aggravate hypothermia.

Positive inotropic agents such as dopamine may be tried if fluid replacement is insufficient to correct the circulatory collapse. Peripheral vasoconstrictor agents are not generally recommended; avoid the use of adrenaline.

Ventricular or supraventricular tachy-arrhythmias usually respond to restoration of normal body temperature and correction of circulatory or metabolic disturbances. If persistent or life threatening, appropriate anti-arrhythmic therapy may be considered. Avoid lignocaine and, as far as possible, long acting anti-arrhythmic drugs.

Pronounced central nervous system depression requires airway maintenance or, in extreme circumstances, assisted respiration. Severe dystonic reactions usually respond to procyclidine (5–10 mg) or orphenadrine (20–40 mg) administered intramuscularly or intravenously. Convulsions should be treated with intravenous diazepam.

Neuroleptic malignant syndrome should be treated with cooling. Dantrolene sodium may be tried.

Pharmacological properties

Pharmacodynamic properties: Stemetil is a potent phenothiazine neuroleptic.

Pharmacokinetic properties: There is little information about blood levels, distribution and excretion in humans. The rate of metabolism and excretion of phenothiazines decreases in old age.

Preclinical safety data: There is no pre-clinical data of relevance to the prescriber which are additional to that already included in other sections of the SPC.

Pharmaceutical particulars

List of excipients: Suppository base E75 and suppository base W35.

Incompatibilities: None stated.

Shelf life: 36 months.

Special precautions for storage: Store below 25°C. Protect from light.

Nature and content of container: Suppositories enclosed automatically during filling in preformed strips of PVC and polyethylene being the inner surface in contact with the product. Sealing of bandolier effected by the action of heat and pressure. Stemetil suppositories are available in packs of 10.

Instructions for use/handling: None.

Marketing authorisation numbers

Suppositories 5 mg 16946/0004
Suppositories 25 mg 16946/0005

Date of approval/revision of SPC July 1998

Legal category POM.

STEMETIL* TABLETS AND SYRUP

Qualitative and quantitative composition The active component of the Stemetil tablets 5 mg is prochlorperazine maleate BP 5 mg. The active component of the Stemetil tablets 25 mg is prochlorperazine maleate BP 25 mg. The active component of the Stemetil syrup is prochlorperazine mesylate BP 5 mg per 5 ml.

Pharmaceutical form Stemetil tablets 5 mg: Off-white to pale cream coloured circular tablets for oral use. The tablets are marked on one face 'STEMETIL' around a centrally impressed '5', reverse face plain. Stemetil tablets 25 mg: Off-white to pale cream coloured tablets for oral use. The tablets are marked 'STEMETIL' around a centrally impressed '25', a breakline on the reverse. Stemetil syrup: A dark straw coloured syrup.

Clinical Particulars

Therapeutic indications: Vertigo due to Meniere's Syndrome, labyrinthis and other causes, and for nausea and vomiting from whatever cause including that associated with migraine. It may also be used for schizophrenia (particularly in the chronic stage), acute mania and as an adjunct to the short-term management of anxiety.

Posology and method of administration: For oral administration.

Adults

Indication	*Dosage*
Prevention of nausea and vomiting	5 to 10 mg b.d. or t.d.s.
Treatment of nausea and vomiting	20 mg stat, followed if necessary by 10 mg two hours later.
Vertigo and Meniere's syndrome	5 mg t.d.s. increasing if necessary to a total of 30 mg daily. After several weeks dosage may be reduced gradually to 5-10 mg daily.
Adjunct in the short term management of anxiety	15-20 mg daily in divided doses initially but this may be increased if necessary to a maximum of 40 mg daily in divided doses.
Schizophrenia and other psychotic disorders	Usual effective daily oral dosage is in the order of 75-100 mg daily. Patients very widely in response. The following schedule is suggested: Initially 12.5 mg twice daily for 7 days, the daily amount being subsequently increased 12.5 mg at 4 to 7 days interval until a satisfactory response is obtained. After some weeks at the effective dosage, an attempt should be made reduce this dosage. Total daily amounts as small as 50 mg or even 25 mg have sometimes been found to be effective.

Children:

Indication	*Dosage*
Prevention and treatment of nausea and vomiting	If it is considered unavoidable to use Stemetil for a child, the dosage is 0.25 mg/kg bodyweight two or three times a day. Stemetil is not recommended for children weighing less than 10 Kg or below 1 year of age.

Elderly: A lower dose is recommended. Please see *Special warnings and special precautions for use* section.

Contra-indications: Pregnancy.

Special warnings and special precautions for use: Stemetil should be avoided in patients with liver or renal dysfunction, epilepsy, Parkinson's disease, hypothyroidism, phaeochromocytoma, myasthenia gravis, prostate hypertrophy. It should be avoided in patients known to be hypersensitive to phenothiazines or with a history of narrow angle glaucoma. It should be used with caution in the elderly, particularly during very hot or very cold weather (risk of hyper-, hypothermia).

The elderly are particularly susceptible to postural hypotension.

Stemetil should be used cautiously in the elderly owing to their susceptibility to drugs acting centrally on the nervous system and a lower initial dosage is recommended. There is an increased risk of drug-induced Parkinsonism in the elderly particularly after prolonged use. Care should also be taken not to confuse the adverse effects of Stemetil e.g. orthostatic hypotension with effects due to the underlying disorder.

Children: Stemetil has been associated with dystonic reactions particularly after a cumulative dosage of 0.5 mg/kg. It should therefore be used cautiously in children.

Interaction with other medicaments and other forms of interaction: Interactions of phenothiazine neuroleptics: The CNS depressant actions of neuroleptic agents may be intensified (additively) by alcohol, barbiturates and other sedatives. Respiratory depression may occur.

The hypotensive effect of most antihypertensive drugs especially alpha adrenoceptor blocking agents may be exaggerated by neuroleptics.

The mild anticholinergic effect of neuroleptics may be enhanced by other anticholinergic drugs possibly leading to constipation, heat stroke, etc.

The action of some drugs may be opposed by phenothiazine neuroleptics; these include amphetamine, levodopa, clonidine, guanethidine, adrenaline.

Anticholinergic agents may reduce the antipsychotic effect of neuroleptics.

Some drugs interfere with absorption of neuroleptic agents: antacids, anti-Parkinson, lithium. Increases or decreases in the plasma concentrations of a number of drugs, e.g. propranolol, phenobarbitone have been observed but were not of clinical significance.

High doses of neuroleptics reduce the response to hypoglycaemic agents the dosage of which might have to be raised.

Adrenaline must *not* be used in patients overdosed with Stemetil. Most of the above interactions are of a theoretical nature and not dangerous.

Simultaneous administration of desferrioxamine and prochlorperazine has been observed to induce a transient metabolic encephalopathy characterised by loss of consciousness for 48–72 hours.

Pregnancy and lactation: Stemetil is contraindicated in pregnancy. There is inadequate evidence of the safety of Stemetil in human pregnancy but it has been widely used for many years without apparent ill consequence. There is evidence of harmful effects in animals. Like other drugs it should be avoided in pregnancy unless the physician considers it essential. Neuroleptics may occasionally prolong labour and at such a time should be withheld until the cervix is dilated 3–4 cm. Possible adverse effects on the neonate include lethargy or paradoxical hyperexcitability, tremor and low Apgar score. Phenothiazines may be excreted in milk, breastfeeding should be suspended during treatment.

Effects on ability to drive and use machines: Patients should be warned about drowsiness during the early days of treatment, and advised not to drive or operate machinery.

Undesirable effects: Minor side-effects of neuroleptics are nasal stuffiness, dry mouth, insomnia, agitation. Adverse effects of neuroleptics: *Liver function:* Jaundice, usually transient, occurs in a very small percentage of patients taking neuroleptics. A premonitory sign may be a sudden onset of fever after one to three weeks of treatment followed by the development of jaundice. Neuroleptic jaundice has the biochemical and other characteristics of obstructive jaundice and is associated with obstruction of the canaliculi by bile thrombi; the frequent presence of an accompanying eosinophilia indicates the allergic nature of this phenomenon. Treatment should be withheld on the development of jaundice. *Cardiorespiratory:* Hypotension, usually postural, commonly occurs. Elderly or volume depleted subjects are particularly susceptible, it is more likely to occur after intramuscular injection. Cardiac arrhythmias, including atrial arrhythmia, A-V block, ventricular tachycardia and fibrillation have been reported during neuroleptic therapy, possibly related to dosage. Pre-existing cardiac disease, old age, hypokalaemia and concurrent tricyclic antidepressants may predispose. ECG changes, usually benign, include widened QT interval, ST depression, U-waves and T-wave changes. Respiratory depression is possible in susceptible patients. *Blood picture:* A mild leucopenia occurs in up to 30% of patients on prolonged high dosage. Agranulocytosis may occur rarely; it is not dose related. The occurrence of unexplained infections or fever requires immediate haematological investigation. *Extrapyramidal:* Acute dystonias or dyskinesias, usually transitory, are more common in children and young adults, and usually occur within the first 4 days of treatment or after dosage increases. Akathisia characteristically occurs after large initial doses. Parkinsonism is more common in adults and the elderly. It usually develops after weeks or months of treatment. One or more of the following may be seen: tremor, rigidity, akinesia or other features of Parkinsonism. Commonly just tremor. *Tardive dyskinesia:* If this occurs it is usually, but not necessarily, after prolonged or high dosage. It can even occur after treatment has been stopped.

Dosage should therefore be kept low whenever possible. *Skin and eyes:* Contact skin sensitisation is a serious but rare complication in those frequently handling preparations of certain phenothiazines; the greatest care must be taken to avoid contact of the drug with the skin. Skin rashes of various kinds may also be seen in patients treated with the drug. Patients on high dosage should be warned that they may develop photosensitivity in sunny weather and should avoid exposure to direct sunlight. Ocular changes and the development of a metallic greyish-mauve coloration of exposed skin have been noted in some individuals mainly females, who have received chlorpromazine continuously for long periods (four to eight years). This could possibly happen with Stemetil. *Endocrine:* Hyperprolactinaemia which may result in galactorrhoea, gynaecomastia, amenorrhoea; impotence. Neuroleptic malignant syndrome (hyperthermia, rigidity, autonomic dysfunction and altered consciousness) may occur with any neuroleptic.

Overdose: Symptoms of phenothiazine overdosage include drowsiness or loss of consciousness, hypotension, tachycardia, ECG changes, ventricular arrhythmias and hypothermia. Severe extra-pyramidal dyskinesias may occur.

If the patient is seen sufficiently soon (up to 6 hours) after ingestion of a toxic dose, gastric lavage may be attempted. Pharmacological induction of emesis is unlikely to be of any use. Activated charcoal should be given. There is no specific antidote. Treatment is supportive.

Generalised vasodilatation may result in circulatory collapse; raising the patient's legs may suffice. In severe cases, volume expansion by intravenous fluids may be needed; infusion fluids should be warmed before administration in order not to aggravate hypothermia.

Positive inotropic agents such as dopamine may be tried if fluid replacement is insufficient to correct the circulatory collapse. Peripheral vasoconstrictor agents are not generally recommended; avoid the use of adrenaline.

Ventricular or supraventricular tachy-arrhythmias usually respond to restoration of normal body temperature and correction of circulatory or metabolic disturbances. If persistent or life threatening, appropriate anti-arrhythmic therapy may be considered. Avoid lignocaine and, as far as possible, long acting anti-arrhythmic drugs.

Pronounced central nervous system depression requires airway maintenance or, in extreme circumstances, assisted respiration. Severe dystonic reactions usually respond to procyclidine (5–10 mg) or orphenadrine (20–40 mg) administered intramuscularly or intravenously. Convulsions should be treated with intravenous diazepam.

Neuroleptic malignant syndrome should be treated with cooling. Dantrolene sodium may be tried.

Pharmacological properties
Pharmacodynamic properties: Stemetil is a potent phenothiazine neuroleptic.

Pharmacokinetic properties: There is little information about blood levels, distribution and excretion in humans. The rate of metabolism and excretion of phenothiazines decreases in old age.

Preclinical safety data: There is no pre-clinical data of relevance to the prescriber which are additional to that already included in other sections of the SPC.

Pharmaceutical particulars
List of excipients: Stemetil tablets: lactose BP, starch maize BP, aerosil (E551) and magnesium stearate BP. *Stemetil syrup:* liquid sugar gran. liquors, Tween 80 Ph Eur. (E433), Zimm banana 504, caramel HT (E150a), citric acid anhydrous BP (E330), sodium citrate gran. BP (E331), sodium benzoate BP (E211), sodium sulphite anhydrous BP (E221), sodium metabisulphite powder BP (E223), ascorbic acid L(+) BP (E300) and demineralised water BP.

Incompatibilities: None stated.

Shelf life: Tablets: 60 months. *Syrup:* 36 months.

Special precautions for storage: Store protected from light.

Nature and content of container: Stemetil tablets 5 mg are available in PVDC coated UPVC/aluminium foil blisters containing 84 tablets. Stemetil tablets 25 mg are available in PVDC coated UPVC/aluminium foil blisters containing 56 tablets. Stemetil syrup is available in amber glass bottles containing 100 ml.

Instructions for use/handling: None.

Marketing authorisation numbers

Tablets 5 mg	PL 16946/0006
Tablets 25 mg	PL 16946/0007
Syrup	PL 16946/0008

Date of approval/revision of SPC July 1998

Legal category POM.

VALLERGAN* TABLETS, SYRUP AND FORTE SYRUP

Qualitative and quantitative composition *Tablets:* Trimeprazine Tartrate BP (alimemazine tartrate (rINN)) 10 mg.

Syrup: Trimeprazine tartrate 0.15w/v (7.5 mg Trimeprazine Tartrate BP (alimemazine tartrate (rINN))/ 5 ml).

Forte Syrup: Trimeprazine tartrate 0.6w/v (30 mg Trimeprazine Tartrate BP (alimemazine tartrate (rINN))/5 ml).

Pharmaceutical form *Tablet:* Circular, film coated biconvex tablet with bevelled edge, dark blue in colour, one face impressed V/10. The reverse side is plain.

Syrup and Forte Syrup: Syrup.

Clinical Particulars
Therapeutic Indications: Vallergan is used in the management of urticaria and pruritus and in premedication for anaesthesia in children.

Posology and method of administration: The product is administered orally. Not recommended for infants less than 2 years old.

Vallergan Forte Syrup may be diluted if required, using simple syrup (without preservative)

The Syrup and Forte Syrup may be diluted up to 3:2 in syrup BP to provide convenient dosing quantity

Urticaria and pruritus: Adults: 10 mg two or three times daily; up to 100 mg per day have been used in intractable cases. Elderly: Dosage should be reduced to 10 mg once or twice daily. Children over 2 years of age: 2.5–5 mg three or four times daily.

Pre-anaesthetic medication: The dosage for children is best achieved by use of Vallergan Syrup or Vallergan Forte Syrup. (Children aged 2-7 years:) the maximum dosage recommended is 2 mg per kg bodyweight 1–2 hours before the operation.

Contra-indications: Vallergan should be avoided in patients with hepatic or renal dysfunction, epilepsy, Parkinson's disease, hypothyroidism, phaeochromocytoma, myasthenia gravis, prostatic hypertrophy. It should be avoided in patients known to be hypersensitive to phenothiazines or with history of narrow angle glaucoma.

Special warnings and special precautions for use: Vallergan should be used with caution in the elderly, particularly in very hot or very cold weather (risk of hyper-hypothermia). The elderly are particularly susceptible to postural hypotension.

Interaction with other medicaments and other forms of interaction: The CNS depressant actions of phenothiazines may be intensified (additively) by alcohol, barbiturates and other sedatives. Respiratory depression may occur.

The hypotensive effect of most antihypertensive drugs especially alpha adrenoreceptor blocking agents may be exaggerated by phenothiazines.

The mild anticholinergic effect of phenothiazines may be enhanced by other anticholinergic drugs possibly leading to constipation, heat stroke, etc

The action of some drugs may be opposed by phenothiazines; these include amphetamine, levodopa, clonidine, guanethidine, adrenaline.

Anticholinergic agents may reduce the antipsychotic effect of phenothiazines.

Some drugs interfere with absorption of phenothiazines: antacids, anti-Parkinson, lithium. Increases or decreases in the plasma concentrations of a number of drugs, eg propranolol, phenobarbitone have been observed but were not of clinical significance.

High doses of phenothiazines reduce the response to hypoglycaemic agents, the dosage of which may have to be raised. Adrenaline must not be used in patients overdosed with phenothiazines.

Most of the above interactions are of a theoretical nature and not dangerous

Pregnancy and lactation: There is inadequate evidence of the safety of Vallergan in human pregnancy, but it has been widely used for many years without apparent ill consequence. Some phenothiazines have shown evidence of harmful effects in animals. Vallergan, like other drugs, should be avoided in pregnancy unless the physician considers it essential. Neuroleptics may occasionally prolong labour and at such a time should be withheld until the cervix is dilated 3-4cm. Possible adverse effects on the neonate include lethargy or paradoxical hyperexcitability, tremor and low Apgar score. Phenothiazines may be excreted in milk: breast feeding should be suspended during treatment.

Effects on ability to drive and use machines: Patients should be warned about drowsiness during the early days of treatment, and advised not to drive or operate machinery.

Undesirable effects: Minor side-effects of phenothiazines are nasal stuffiness, dry mouth, insomnia, agitation. *Liver function:* Jaundice, usually transient, occurs in a very small percentage of patients taking phenothiazines. A premonitory sign may be a sudden onset of fever after one to three weeks of treatment followed by the development of jaundice. Neuroleptic jaundice has the biochemical and other characteristics of obstructive jaundice and is associated with obstructions of the canaliculi by bile thrombi; the frequent presence of an accompanying eosinophilia indicates the allergic nature of this phenomenon. Treatment should be withheld on the development of jaundice. *Cardiorespiratory:* hypotension, or pallor may occur in children. Elderly or volume depleted subjects are particularly susceptible to postural hypotension. Cardiac arrhythmias, including atrial arrhythmia. A-V block, ventricular tachycardia and fibrillation have been reported during phenothiazine therapy, possibly related to dosage. Pre-existing cardiac disease, old age, hypokalaemia and concurrent tricyclic antidepressants may predispose. ECG changes, usually benign, include widened QT interval, ST depression, U-waves and T-wave changes. Respiratory depression is possible in susceptible patients. *Blood picture:* A mild leukopenia occurs in up to 30% of patients on prolonged high dosage of phenothiazines. Agranulocytosis may occur rarely; it is not dose related. The occurrence of unexplained infections or fever requires immediate haematological investigation. *Extrapyramidal:* Acute dystonias or dyskinesias, usually transitory are commoner in children and young adults and usually occur within the first 4 days of treatment or after dosage increases. Akathisia characteristically occurs after large doses. Parkinsonism is commoner in adults and the elderly. It usually develops after weeks or months of treatment. One or more of the following may be seen: tremor, rigidity, akinesia or other features of Parkinsonism. Commonly just tremor. *Tardive dyskinesia:* If this occurs it is usually, but not necessarily, after prolonged or high dosage. It can even occur after treatment has been stopped. Dosage should therefore be kept low whenever possible. *Skin and eyes:* Contact skin sensitisation is a serious but rare complication in those frequently handling preparations of phenothiazines: Care must be taken to avoid contact of the drug with the skin. Skin rashes of various kinds may also be seen in patients treated with the drug. Patients on high dosage should be warned that they may develop photosensitivity in sunny weather and should avoid exposure to direct sunlight. Ocular changes and the development of a metallic greyish-mauve coloration of exposed skin have been noted in some individuals, mainly females, who have received chlorpromazine continuously for long periods (four to eight years). *Endocrine:* Hyperprolactinaemia which may result in galactorrhoea, gynaecomastia, amenorrhoea: impotence. Neuroleptic malignant syndrome (hyperthermia, rigidity, autonomic dysfunction and altered consciousness) may occur with any phenothiazine

Overdose: Symptoms of phenothiazine overdosage include drowsiness or loss of consciousness, hypotension, tachycardia, ECG changes, ventricular arrhythmias and hypothermia. Severe extra-pyramidal dyskinesias may occur. If the patient is seen sufficiently soon (up to 6 hours) after ingestion of a toxic dose, gastric lavage may be attempted. Pharmacological induction of emesis is unlikely to be of any use. Activated charcoal should be given. There is no specific antidote. Treatment is supportive. Generalised vasodilatation may result in circulatory collapse; Raising the patient's legs may suffice, in severe cases, volume expansion by intravenous fluids may be needed; infusion fluids should be warmed before administration in order not to aggravate hypothermia. Positive inotropic agents such as dopamine may be tried if fluid replacement is insufficient to correct the circulatory collapse. Peripheral vasoconstrictor agents are not generally recommended; avoid the use of adrenaline. Ventricular or supraventricular tachyarrhythmias usually respond to restoration of normal body temperature and correction of circulatory or metabolic disturbances. If persistent or life-threatening, appropriate anti-arrhythmic therapy may be considered. Avoid lignocaine and, as far as possible, long acting anti-arrhythmic drugs.

Pronounced central nervous system depression requires airway maintenance or, in extreme circumstances, assisted respiration. Severe dystonic reactions, usually respond to procyclidine (5–10 mg) or orphenadrine (20–40 mg) administered intramuscularly or intravenously. Convulsions should be treated with intravenous diazepam. Neuroleptic malignant syndrome should be treated with cooling. Dantrolene sodium may be tried.

Pharmacological properties
Pharmacodynamic properties: Trimeprazine has a central sedative effect, comparable to that of chlorpromazine, but largely devoid of the latter's anti-adrenaline action. It has powerful antihistamine and anti-emetic actions.

Pharmacokinetic properties: There is little information

about blood levels, distribution and excretion in humans. The rate of metabolism and excretion of phenothiazines decreases in old age.

Pharmaceutical particulars

List of excipients: Tablet: Microcrystalline Cellulose BP, Lactose Spray Dried BP, Colloidal Silicone Dioxide, Magnesium Stearate BP, Sodium Starch Glycollate BP, Hydroxypropyl Methylcellulose, Polyethylene glycol 200, Blue opaspray M-1-4229 (purified water EP, Indigo Carmine, Titanium Dioxide EP, Industrial Methylated Spirits 74 OP BP, Hydroxypropyl methylcellulose USP/EP), Demineralised Water BP.

Syrup and Forte Syrup: Liquid sugar gran.liquors HSE, Apricot Flavour no. 1 NS HSE

Ethanol 96% v/v BP, Caramel HT HSE, Citric Acid Anhydrous BP, Sodium Citrate gran BP, Sodium Benzoate BP, Sodium Sulphite Anhydrous BP, Sodium metabisulphite powder, L(+) Ascorbic Acid BP, Demineralised Water BP.

Incompatibilities: None stated.

Shelf life: Tablet: 36 months.

Syrup and Forte Syrup: 36 months unopened, 1 month opened. Diluted product shelf life 28 days.

Special precautions for storage: Protect from light. *Tablet:* Store below 30°C.

Syrup and Forte Syrup: Store below 25°C.

Nature and contents of container: Tablet: Blister pack containing 28 tablets.

Syrup and Forte Syrup: Glass bottle 100 ml. Rolled on pilfer proof aluminium cap and a PVDC emulsion coated wad.

or HDPE polypropylene child resistant cap with a tamper evident band.

Instructions for use/handling: None stated.

Marketing authorisation numbers

Tablet	PL 16946/0009
Syrup	PL 16946/0010
Forte Syrup	PL 16946/0011

Date of Approval/Revision of SPC July 1998

Legal Category POM

***Trade Mark**

Centeon Limited
Centeon House
Market Place
Haywards Heath
West Sussex RH16 1DB
☎ 01444 447400 🗋 01444 447401

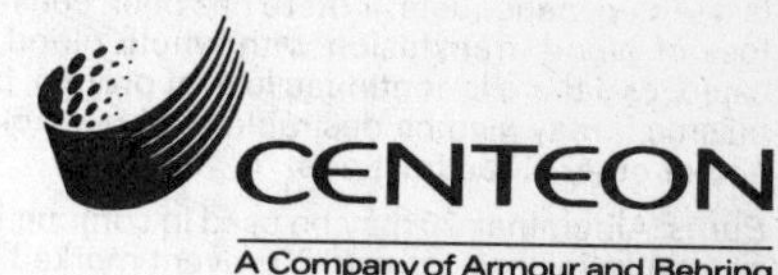

ALBUMINAR*-5

Presentation Albuminar-5 is a sterile aqueous solution of Human Albumin 5% obtained from large pools of adult human venous plasma. Each 100 ml of Albuminar-5 contains 5 g of human albumin which is osmotically equivalent to normal human plasma.

The product conforms to the monograph for Human Albumin Solution PhEur.

Other ingredients are: Sodium acetyltryptophanate, sodium caprylate, sodium chloride, sodium bicarbonate, sodium hydroxide, glacial acetic acid, water for injection.

Indications Albuminar-5 is indicated in: The emergency treatment of shock and in other conditions where the restoration of blood volume is urgent.

Serious burns to prevent haemoconcentration and to combat fluid and sodium losses.

Clinical situations associated with low plasma protein (hypoproteinaemia) with or without oedema, provided that sodium restriction is not imperative.

Therapeutic Plasma Exchange as a replacement fluid for apheresed plasma.

Dosage and administration (a) *Administration:* Albuminar-5 is for intravenous infusion.

Albuminar-5 may be given intravenously without further dilution; 5% solution is approximately isotonic and isosmotic with citrated plasma.

When albumin solution is administered to patients with normal blood volume, particular attention should be given to the rate of infusion so that the plasma volume is not expanded too rapidly.

(b) *Standard dose: Urgent restoration of blood volume:* In the emergency treatment of shock, the amount of albumin and duration of therapy must be based on the responsiveness of the patient as indicated by blood pressure, central venous pressure, degree of pulmonary congestion and haematocrit. The initial dose may be followed by additional albumin within 15–30 minutes if the response is deemed inadequate. If there has been considerable loss of blood, transfusion with whole blood is indicated, or if there is continued loss of protein, blood or plasma it may also be desirable to give whole blood and/or other blood fractions.

Burns: Albuminar-5 may be used to prevent marked haemoconcentration and to maintain appropriate electrolyte balance. An optimal regimen involving the use of albumin, crystalloids and water has not been established. Suggested therapy in the treatment of burns includes administration of large volumes of crystalloid solution during the first 24 hours to maintain an adequate plasma volume, even when albumin is infused. Continuation of therapy beyond 24 hours usually requires more albumin and less crystalloid solution. Duration of treatment varies depending on the extent of protein loss through renal excretion, denuded areas of skin and decreased albumin synthesis. Attempts to raise the albumin level above 40 g/litre may only result in an increased rate of catabolism.

Conditions associated with hypoproteinaemia: In these conditions, 1,000 to 1,500 ml of Albuminar-5 may be required to reduce oedema and to bring serum protein values to normal. Since such patients usually have approximately normal blood volume, doses of more than 500 ml of Albuminar-5 should not be given faster than 500 ml in 30–45 minutes for acute replacement of protein lost in hypoproteinaemic conditions, with careful monitoring of cardiovascular status. Further therapy should be guided by clinical response, blood pressure and assessments of serum protein levels and degree of anaemia. If slower administration is desired, e.g. in patients with hypertension or cardiac insufficiency, 1,000 ml of Albuminar-5 may be administered by continuous drip at a rate of 100 ml of this solution per hour. Unless the pathological condition responsible for the hypoproteinaemia can be corrected, albumin in any form can afford only symptomatic or supportive relief. The 5% solution should not be administered in situations where sodium restriction is imperative.

Therapeutic plasma exchange: In plasma exchange procedures the volume of plasma removed may be replaced with an equivalent volume of Albuminar-5.

(c) *Children:* The amount of albumin given and the duration of therapy must be determined by the child's condition, response and other parameters, as stated under '*Standard Dose*'. However, when treating children, their body weight should also be taken into account.

Pharmacology: Action: Albuminar-5 is active osmotically and is therefore important in regulating the volume of circulating blood. When the circulating blood volume has been depleted, the haemodilution following albumin administration persists for many hours. In individuals with normal blood volumes, it usually lasts only a few hours.

Contra-indications, warnings, etc *Contra-indications:* Albuminar-5 may be contra-indicated in patients with severe anaemia or cardiac failure or with known hypersensitivity to human albumin.

Precautions: If dehydration is present additional fluids must accompany or follow the administration of Albuminar-5.

The rise in blood pressure which may follow rapid administration of albumin necessitates careful observation of the injured patient to detect bleeding points which failed to bleed at the lower blood pressure; otherwise new haemorrhage and shock may occur.

Albuminar-5 should be administered with caution to patients with low cardiac reserve or with no albumin deficiency, because a rapid increase in plasma volume may cause circulatory embarrassment or pulmonary oedema. In cases of hypertension or cardiac insufficiency, a slower rate of administration is desirable, at a rate of 5 g of albumin (100 ml) per hour. A careful watch must be kept for the possible development of pulmonary oedema. Should pulmonary oedema occur, the infusion must be stopped immediately.

Use in pregnancy: There is some experience of albumin being used in the treatment of pre-eclampsia and eclampsia. However, there is very little experience of the use of albumin in the early stages of pregnancy. There is no evidence either in human pregnancy or in animal work that administration of albumin is free from hazard.

Warnings and adverse effects: Do not use if the solution is turbid or contains a deposit. Since the solution contains no preservative, it should be used within 3 hours after entering the vial.

The incidence of adverse reactions to human albumin 5% is low, although nausea, vomiting, increased salivation, urticaria and febrile reactions may occasionally occur. Anaphylactic reactions may rarely occur, in which cases the infusion should be stopped and appropriate treatment initiated.

When medical products prepared from human blood or plasma are administered, infectious diseases due to the transmission of infective agents cannot be totally excluded. This applies also to pathogens of hitherto unknown nature. See also 'Further information'.

Toxicity and treatment of overdosage: Administration of large quantities of albumin should be supplemented with red cell concentrates or replaced by whole blood to combat the relative anaemia which would follow such use. If circulatory embarrassment or pulmonary oedema should develop, the infusion must be stopped immediately and specific treatment given.

Pharmaceutical precautions
(a) *Presentation and composition:* Albuminar-5 is a sterile, clear, yellowish, slightly viscous aqueous solution of human serum albumin. It is stabilised with 0.004 M sodium acetyltryptophanate and 0.004 M sodium caprylate and the pH of the solution is adjusted with sodium bicarbonate or acetic acid. The solution contains approximately 145 mmol/l of sodium and not more than 200 micrograms/l of aluminium. The solution contains no preservative.

(b) *Incompatibilities:* Albuminar-5 should not be mixed with protein hydrolysates, amino acid mixtures or solutions containing alcohol.

(c) *Storage:* Albuminar-5 should be stored at a temperature between 2° and 25°C. Freezing will not harm the solution, but might damage the container and allow contamination of the contents.

Protect solution from light.

When stored as directed Albuminar-5 has a shelf-life of 3 years.

Legal category POM.

Package quantities
Albuminar-5 is supplied as a 5% solution in:
250 ml glass vials containing 12.5 grams of albumin
500 ml glass vials containing 25.0 grams of albumin
1,000 ml glass vials containing 50.0 grams of albumin.

Further information The source plasma or blood from which Albuminar-5 is prepared has been tested and found non-reactive for hepatitis B surface antigen (HBsAg), negative for antibody to hepatitis C and negative for antibody to human immunodeficiency viruses (Anti-HIV-1-and Anti-HIV-2). In addition, Albuminar-5 is pasteurized at 60°C for 10 hours, a procedure designed to reduce the risks of viral transmission. So prepared, Albuminar-5, unlike whole blood or plasma, has not been associated with homologous serum hepatitis or AIDS transmission.

Albuminar-5 may be given in conjunction with other parenteral fluids, such as whole blood, plasma, saline, dextrose, or sodium lactate. It is convenient to use, since no cross-matching is required and the absence of cellular elements removes the danger of sensitisation with repeated infusions.

Albuminar-5 contains none of the recognised components of the clotting mechanism of normal blood or plasma. It does not interfere with the normal clotting of blood.

Product licence number 0231/0056.

ALBUMINAR-20

Presentation Albuminar-20 is a sterile aqueous solution of Human Albumin 20% obtained from large pools of adult human venous plasma. Each 100 ml of Albuminar-20 contains 20 g of human serum albumin which is osmotically equivalent to 400 ml of normal human plasma.

Other ingredients are: Sodium acetyltryptophanate, sodium caprylate, sodium chloride, sodium bicarbonate, sodium hydroxide, glacial acetic acid, water for injection.

The product conforms to the monograph for Human Albumin Solution Ph Eur.

Indications Albuminar-20 is indicated in: The emergency treatment of shock and in other conditions where the restoration of blood volume is urgent.

Serious burns to prevent haemoconcentration and to combat fluid and sodium losses.

Clinical situations associated with low plasma protein (hypoproteinaemia) with or without oedema.

As an adjunct to exchange transfusion for the treatment of hyperbilirubinaemia in haemolytic disease of the newborn.

In priming heart lung machines for cardiopulmonary by-pass surgery.

Dosage and administration
(a) *Administration:* Albuminar-20 is for intravenous infusion.

Albuminar-20 may be given intravenously without dilution or it may be diluted with normal saline or 5% dextrose before administration, 250 ml per litre gives a solution which is approximately isotonic and isosmotic with citrated plasma.

When undiluted albumin solution is administered to patients with normal blood volume, particular attention should be given to the rate of infusion so that the plasma volume is not expanded too rapidly.

(b) *Standard dose: Urgent restoration of blood volume:* In these conditions the effectiveness of Albuminar-20 depends on its ability to draw tissue fluid into the blood stream, when such fluid is available. Therefore, if dehydration is present, other fluids must be administered by any available route, either with albumin or following it. In the emergency treatment of shock, the amount of albumin and duration of therapy must be based on the responsiveness of the patient as indicated by blood pressure, central venous pressure, degree of pulmonary congestion and haematocrit. The initial dose may be followed by additional albumin within 15–30 minutes if the response is deemed inadequate. If there has been considerable loss of blood, transfusion with whole blood is indicated, or if there is continued loss of protein, blood or plasma it may also be desirable to give whole blood and/or other blood fractions.

Burns: Albuminar-20 may be used in conjunction with normal saline or dextrose to prevent marked haemoconcentration and to maintain appropriate electrolyte balance. An optimal regimen involving the use of albumin, crystalloids and water has not been established. Suggested therapy in the treatment of burns includes administration of large volumes of crystalloid solution during the first 24 hours to maintain an adequate plasma volume, even when albumin is infused. Continuation of therapy beyond 24 hours usually requires more albumin and less crystalloid solution. Duration of treatment varies depending on the extent of protein loss through renal excretion, denuded areas of skin and decreased albumin synthesis. Attempts to raise the albumin level above 40 g/litre may only result in an increased rate of catabolism.

Conditions associated with hypoproteinaemia: In these conditions, 200 to 300 ml of Albuminar-20 may be required to reduce oedema and to bring serum protein values to normal. Since such patients usually have approximately normal blood volume, doses of more than 100 ml of Albuminar-20 should not be given faster than 100 ml in 30–45 minutes for acute replacement of protein lost in hypoproteinaemic conditions, with careful monitoring of cardiovascular status. Further therapy should be guided by clinical response, blood pressure and assessments of serum protein levels and degree of anaemia. If slower administration is desired, e.g. in patients with hypertension or cardiac insufficiency, 250 ml of Albuminar-20 may be mixed with 250 ml of 10% dextrose solution and administered by continuous drip at a rate of 100 ml of this dextrose solution per hour. Unless the pathological condition responsible for the hypoproteinaemia can be corrected, albumin in any form can afford only symptomatic or supportive relief.

Hyperbilirubinaemia in haemolytic disease of the newborn: In neonates, with serum bilirubin levels above 20 mg per 100 ml severe cerebral damage can develop due to kernicterus. In hypoalbuminaemia the reserve binding capacity for bilirubin is decreased and consequently bilirubin toxicity increases and with it the risk of cerebral damage. The risk of cerebral damage can be reduced by correction of the bilirubin binding capacity with Albuminar-20.

If immediate protection of the patient is required an intravenous injection of 1.0–1.5 g/kg albumin (5–7 ml Albuminar-20/kg bodyweight) can be given. Following this injection the exchange transfusion procedure should be instituted within 6 hours.

If albumin is intended for increasing the removal of bilirubin during exchange transfusion, it is suggested that 1.5–2.5 g albumin (7–12 ml Albuminar-20) is added to each 100 ml donor blood during exchange transfusion.

In priming heart lung machines for cardiopulmonary by-pass surgery: Pre-operative dilution of the blood by use of a pump prime consisting of only albumin and crystalloid has been shown to be well tolerated during clinical studies. An albumin concentration of 5 g per cent has been widely used. A commonly employed programme is an albumin and crystalloid pump prime adjusted so as to achieve a haematocrit reading of 20 per cent and a plasma albumin level of 2.5 g/100 ml in the patient.

(c) *Children:* The amount of albumin given and the duration of therapy must be determined by the child's condition, response and other parameters, as stated under '*Standard Dose*'. However, when treating children, their body weight should also be taken into account.

Pharmacology: Action: Albuminar-20 is active osmotically and is therefore important in regulating the volume of circulating blood. When injected intravenously, 50 ml of Albuminar-20 draws approximately 3 volumes of additional fluid into the circulation within 15 minutes, except in the presence of marked dehydration. This extra fluid reduces haematocrit and blood viscosity. The degree of volume expansion is dependent on the initial blood volume. When circulating blood volume has been depleted, the haemodilution following albumin administration persists for many hours. In individuals with normal blood volume, it usually lasts only a few hours.

Contra-indications, warnings, etc
Contra-indications: Albuminar-20 may be contra-indicated in patients with severe anaemia or cardiac failure or with known hypersensitivity to human albumin.

Precautions: If dehydration is present additional fluids must accompany or follow the administration of Albuminar-20.

The rise in blood pressure which may follow rapid administration of albumin necessitates careful observation of the injured patient to detect bleeding points which failed to bleed at the lower blood pressure; otherwise new haemorrhage and shock may occur.

Albuminar-20 should be administered with caution to patients with low cardiac reserve or with no albumin deficiency, because a rapid increase in plasma volume may cause circulatory embarrassment or pulmonary oedema. In cases of hypertension or cardiac insufficiency, a slower rate of administration is desirable: 250 ml of Albuminar-20 may be mixed with 250 ml of 10% dextrose solution and administered at a rate of 10 g of albumin (100 ml) per hour. A careful watch must be kept for the possible development of pulmonary oedema. Should pulmonary oedema occur, the infusion must be stopped immediately.

Use in pregnancy: There is some experience of albumin being used in the treatment of pre-eclampsia and eclampsia. However, there is very little experience of the use of albumin in the early stages of pregnancy. There is no evidence either in human pregnancy or in animal work that administration of albumin is free from hazard.

Warnings and adverse effects: Do not use if the solution is turbid or contains a deposit. Since the solution contains no preservative, it should be used within 3 hours after entering the vial.

The incidence of adverse reactions to human albumin 20% is low, although nausea, vomiting, increased salivation, urticaria and febrile reactions may occasionally occur. Anaphylactic reactions may rarely occur, in which cases the infusion should be stopped and appropriate treatment initiated.

When medical products prepared from human blood or plasma are administered, infectious diseases due to the transmission of infective agents cannot be totally excluded. This applies also to pathogens of hitherto unknown nature. See also 'Further information'.

Toxicity and treatment of overdosage: Administration of large quantities of albumin should be supplemented with red cell concentrates or replaced by whole blood to combat the relative anaemia which would follow such use.

If circulatory embarrassment or pulmonary oedema should develop, the infusion must be stopped immediately and specific treatment given.

Pharmaceutical precautions
(a) *Presentation and composition:* Albuminar-20 is a sterile, clear, brownish, slightly viscous aqueous solution of human albumin. It is stabilised with 0.016 M sodium acetyltryptophanate and 0.016 M sodium caprylate and the pH of the solution is adjusted with sodium bicarbonate or acetic acid. The solution contains approximately 145 mmol/l of sodium and not more than 200 micrograms/l of aluminium. The solution contains no preservative.

(b) *Incompatibilities:* Albuminar-20 should not be mixed with protein hydrolysates, amino acid mixtures or solutions containing alcohol.

(c) *Storage:* Albuminar-20 should be stored at a temperature between 2° and 25°C. Freezing will not harm the solution, but might damage the container and allow contamination of the contents. Protect solution from light.

When stored as directed, Albuminar-20 has a shelf-life of 3 years.

Legal category POM.

Package quantities Albuminar-20 is supplied as a 20% solution in:
50 ml vials containing 10.0 grams of albumin;
100 ml vials containing 20.0 grams of albumin.

Further information The source plasma or blood from which Albuminar-20 is prepared has been tested with licensed reagents and found non-reactive for hepatitis B surface antigen (HBsAg), negative for antibody to hepatitis C and negative for antibody to human immunodeficiency viruses (Anti-HIV-1 and Anti-HIV-2). In addition, Albuminar-20 is pasteurized at 60°C for 10 hours, a procedure designed to reduce the risks of viral transmission. So prepared, Albuminar-20, unlike whole blood or plasma, has not been associated with homologous serum hepatitis of AIDS transmission.

Albuminar-20 may be given in conjunction with other parenteral fluids, such as whole blood, plasma, saline, dextrose, or sodium lactate. It is convenient to use, since no cross-matching is required and the absence of cellular elements removes the danger of sensitisation with repeated infusions.

Albuminar-20 contains none of the recognised components of the clotting mechanism of normal blood or plasma. It does not interfere with the normal clotting of blood.

Product licence number 0231/0057

ALBUMINAR-25

Presentation Albuminar-25 is a sterile aqueous solution of Human Albumin 25% obtained from large pools of adult human venous plasma. Each 100 ml of Albuminar-25 contains 25 g of human serum albumin which is osmotically equivalent to 500 ml of normal human plasma.

Other ingredients are: Sodium acetyltryptophanate, sodium caprylate, sodium chloride, sodium bicarbonate, sodium hydroxide, glacial acetic acid, water for injection.

The product conforms to the monograph for Human Albumin Solution PhEur.

Indications Albuminar-25 is indicated in: The emergency treatment of shock and in other conditions where the restoration of blood volume is urgent.

Serious burns to prevent haemoconcentration and to combat fluid and sodium losses.

Clinical situations associated with low plasma protein (hypoproteinaemia) with or without oedema.

As an adjunct to exchange transfusion for the treatment of hyperbilirubinaemia in haemolytic disease of the newborn.

In priming heart-lung machines for cardiopulmonary by-pass surgery.

Dosage and administration
(a) *Administration:* Albuminar-25 is for intravenous infusion.

Albuminar-25 may be given intravenously without dilution or it may be diluted with normal saline or 5% dextrose before administration; 200 ml per litre gives a solution which is approximately isotonic and isosmotic with citrated plasma.

When undiluted albumin solution is administered to patients with normal blood volume, particular attention should be given to the rate of infusion so that it is slow enough to prevent too rapid expansion of plasma volume.

(b) *Standard dose: Urgent restoration of blood volume:* In these conditions the effectiveness of Albuminar-25 depends on its ability to draw tissue fluid into the blood stream, when such fluid is available. Therefore, if dehydration is present, other fluids must be administered by any available route, either with albumin or following it. In the emergency treatment of shock, the amount of albumin and duration of therapy must be based on the responsiveness of the patient as indicated by blood pressure, central venous pressure, degree of pulmonary congestion and haematocrit. The initial dose may be followed by additional albumin within 15–30 minutes if the response is deemed inadequate. If there has been considerable loss of blood, transfusion with whole blood is indicated, or if there is continued loss of protein, blood or plasma it may also be desirable to give whole blood and/or other blood fractions.

Burns: Albuminar-25 may be used in conjunction with normal saline or dextrose to prevent marked haemoconcentration and to maintain appropriate electrolyte balance. An optimal regimen involving the use of albumin, crystalloids and water has not been established. Suggested therapy in the treatment of burns includes administration of large volumes of crystalloid solution during the first 24 hours to maintain an adequate plasma volume, even when albumin is infused. Continuation of therapy beyond 24 hours usually requires more albumin and less crystalloid solution. Duration of treatment varies depending on the extent of protein loss through renal excretion, denuded areas of skin and decreased albumin synthesis. Attempts to raise the albumin level above 40 g/litre may only result in an increased rate of catabolism.

Conditions associated with hypoproteinaemia: In these conditions, 200 to 300 ml of Albuminar-25 may be required to reduce oedema and to bring serum protein values to normal. Since such patients usually have approximately normal blood volume, doses of more than 100 ml of Albuminar-25 should not be given faster than 100 ml in 30–45 minutes for acute replacement of protein lost in hypoproteinaemic conditions, with careful monitoring of cardiovascular status. Further therapy should be guided by clinical response, blood pressure and assessments of serum protein levels and degree of anaemia. If slower administration is desired, e.g. in patients with hypertension or cardiac insufficiency, 200 ml of Albuminar-25 may be mixed with 300 ml of 10% dextrose solution and administered by continuous drip at a rate of 100 ml of this dextrose solution per hour. Unless the pathological condition responsible for the hypoproteinaemia can be corrected, albumin in any form can afford only symptomatic or supportive relief.

Hyperbilirubinaemia in haemolytic disease of the newborn: In neonates with serum bilirubin levels above 20 mg per 100 ml severe cerebral damage can develop due to kernicterus. In hypoalbuminaemia the reserve binding capacity for bilirubin is decreased and consequently bilirubin toxicity increases and with it the risk of cerebral damage. The risk of cerebral damage can be reduced by correction of the bilirubin binding capacity with Albuminar-25.

If immediate protection of the patient is required an intravenous injection of 1.0–1.5 g/kg albumin (4–6 ml Albuminar-25/kg bodyweight) can be given. Following this injection the exchange transfusion procedure should be instituted within 6 hours.

If albumin is intended for increasing the removal of bilirubin during exchange transfusion, it is suggested that 1.5–2.5 g albumin (6–10 ml Albuminar-25) is added to each 100 ml donor blood during exchange transfusion.

In priming heart lung machines for cardiopulmonary by-pass surgery: Pre-operative dilution of the blood by use of a pump prime consisting of only albumin and crystalloid has been shown to be well tolerated during clinical studies. An albumin concentration of 5 g per cent has been widely used. A commonly employed programme is an albumin and crystalloid pump prime adjusted so as to achieve a haematocrit reading of 20 per cent and a plasma albumin level of 2.5 g/100 ml in the patient.

(c) *Children:* The amount of albumin given and the duration of therapy must be determined by the child's condition, response and other parameters, as stated under '*Standard Dose*'. However, when treating children, their body weight should also be taken into account.

Pharmacology: Action: Albuminar-25 is active osmotically and is therefore important in regulating the volume of circulating blood. When injected intravenously, 50 ml of Albuminar-25 draws approximately 175 ml of additional fluid into the circulation within 15 minutes, except in the presence of marked dehydration. This extra fluid reduces haematocrit and blood viscosity. The degree of volume expansion is dependent on the initial blood volume. When circulating blood volume has been depleted, the haemodilution following albumin administration persists for many hours. In individuals with normal blood volume, it usually lasts only a few hours.

Contra-indications, warnings, etc

Contra-indications: Albuminar-25 may be contra-indicated in patients with severe anaemia or cardiac failure or with known hypersensitivity to human albumin.

Precautions: If dehydration is present additional fluids must accompany or follow the administration of Albuminar-25.

The rise in blood pressure which may follow rapid administration of albumin necessitates careful observation of the injured patient to detect bleeding points which failed to bleed at the lower blood pressure; otherwise new haemorrhage and shock may occur.

Albuminar-25 should be administered with caution to patients with low cardiac reserve or with no albumin deficiency, because a rapid increase in plasma volume may cause circulatory embarrassment or pulmonary oedema. In cases of hypertension or cardiac insufficiency, a slower rate of administration is desirable: 200 ml of Albuminar-25 may be mixed with 300 ml of 10% dextrose solution and administered at a rate of 10 g of albumin (100 ml) per hour. A careful watch must be kept for the possible development of pulmonary oedema. Should pulmonary oedema occur, the infusion must be stopped immediately.

Use in pregnancy: There is some experience of albumin being used in the treatment of pre-eclampsia and eclampsia. However, there is very little experience of the use of albumin in the early stages of pregnancy. There is no evidence either in human pregnancy or in animal work that administration of albumin is free from hazard.

Warnings and adverse effects: Do not use if the solution is turbid or contains a deposit. Since the solution contains no preservative, it should be used within 3 hours after entering the vial.

The incidence of adverse reactions to human albumin 25% is low, although nausea, vomiting, increased salivation, urticaria and febrile reactions may occasionally occur. Anaphylactic reactions may rarely occur, in which case the infusion should be stopped and appropriate treatment initiated.

When medicinal products prepared from human blood or plasma are administered, infectious diseases due to the transmission of infective agents cannot be totally excluded. This applies also to pathogens of hitherto unknown nature.

Toxicity and treatment of overdosage: Administration of large quantities of albumin should be supplemented with red cell concentrates or replaced by whole blood to combat the relative anaemia which would follow such use.

If circulatory embarrassment or pulmonary oedema should develop, the infusion must be stopped immediately and specific treatment given.

Pharmaceutical precautions

(a) *Presentation and composition:* Albuminar-25 is a sterile, clear, brownish, slightly viscous aqueous solution of human albumin. It is stabilised with 0.02 M sodium acetyltryptophanate and 0.02 M sodium caprylate and the pH of the solution is adjusted with sodium bicarbonate or acetic acid. The solution contains approximately 145 mmol/l of sodium and not more than 200 micrograms/l of aluminium. The solution contains no preservative.

(b) *Incompatibilities:* Albuminar-25 should not be mixed with protein hydrolysates, amino acid mixtures or solutions containing alcohol.

(c) *Storage:* Albuminar-25 should be stored at a temperature between 2° and 25°C. Freezing will not harm the solution, but might damage the container and allow contamination of the contents. Protect solution from light.

When stored as directed, Albuminar-25 has a shelf-life of 3 years.

Legal category POM.

Package quantities Albuminar-25 is supplied as a 25% solution in:

50 ml vials containing 12.5 grams of albumin;
100 ml vials containing 25.0 grams of albumin.

Further information The source plasma or blood from which Albuminar-25 is prepared has been tested with licensed reagents and found non-reactive for hepatitis B surface antigen (HBsAg), negative for antibody to hepatitis C and negative for antibody to human immunodeficiency viruses (Anti-HIV-1 and Anti-HIV-2). In addition, Albuminar-25 is pasteurized at 60°C for 10 hours, a procedure designed to reduce the risks of viral transmission. So prepared, Albuminar-25, unlike whole blood or plasma, has not been associated with homologous serum hepatitis or AIDS transmission.

Albuminar-25 may be given in conjunction with other parenteral fluids, such as whole blood, plasma, saline, dextrose, or sodium lactate. It is convenient to use, since no cross-matching is required and the absence of cellular elements removes the danger of sensitisation with repeated infusions.

Albuminar-25 contains none of the recognised components of the clotting mechanism of normal blood or plasma. It does not interfere with the normal clotting of blood.

Product licence number 0231/0045.

FIBROGAMMIN P ▼

Qualitative and quantitative composition Human plasma coagulation factor XIII.

Fibrogammin P 250 U 1250 U
dried substance 68–135 mg 340–673 mg.
coagulation factor XIII 250 U* 1250 U*.
total protein 24–64 mg 120–320 mg.

* 1 Unit (U) is equivalent to the factor-XIII-activity of 1 ml fresh citrated plasma (pooled plasma) of healthy donors.

Pharmaceutical form Powder for intravenous injection or infusion.

Clinical particulars

Therapeutic indications: Congenital deficiency of Factor XIII and resultant haemorrhagic syndroms, haemorrhages and disturbances in wound healing.

Posology and method of administration:

Posology: 1 ml is equivalent to 62.5 U or 100 U are equivalent to 1.6 ml.

Prophylaxis:

– of haemorrhages:

Approx. 10 U/kg body weight at intervals of 4 weeks. The interval is to be shortened if spontaneous haemorrhages develop;

– before surgical operations:

Adults are to receive up to 35 U/kg body weight immediately before the operation, and approx. 10 U/kg body weight on each of the following 5 days or until the wound has healed completely.

Therapy: In the case of severe haemorrhages and extensive haematomas, administer 10-20 U/kg body weight daily until the bleeding has stopped.

Due to the different pathogenesis of factor-XIII-deficiency half-lives differ considerably. Thus, it is recommended to monitor the increase in factor-XIII-activity with a factor-XIII-assay (e.g. with Berichrom(R) Factor XIII). In the case of major operations and severe haemorrhages the aim is to obtain normal values.

Important: The amount to be administered and the frequency of administration should always be orientated towards clinical efficacy in the individual case.

Method of administration: Reconstitute the preparation as described under 6.6 and inject or infuse slowly intravenously.

Contra-indications: No absolute contraindications are known. In cases of recent thrombosis caution should be exercised on account of the fibrin-stabilizing effect of factor XIII.

Special warnings and special precautions for use: Caution is advised in patients with a known allergic reaction to constituents of the product.

In the case of patients known to have a tendency towards allergies, antihistaminics and corticosteroids should be administered prophylactically.

If allergic or anaphylactic reactions occur the injection/ infusion should be stopped immediately. The current specific guidelines of shock therapy should be followed.

Interactions with other medicinal products and other forms of interaction: No interactions of Fibrogammin P with other medicinal products are known so far.

Pregnancy and lactation: Experimental animal studies are not suitable to assess the safety with respect to reproduction, development of the embryo or foetus, the course of gestation and peri- and postnatal development.

The safety of Fibrogammin P for use in human pregnancy has not been established in controlled clinical trials.

The clinical use of Fibrogammin P in pregnancy did not show any negative effects on the course of gestation and the peri- or postnatal development. The efficacy of Fibrogammin P in pregnant women with congenital factor-XIII-deficiency has been described.

Therefore, Fibrogammin P should only be used if clearly needed during pregnancy and lactation.

Effects on ability to drive and use machines: There are no indications that Fibrogammin P may impair the ability to drive or to operate machines.

Undesirable effects:

- In rare cases allergic reactions and rise in temperature are observed. The treatment required depends on the nature and severity of the side-effect.
- In very rare cases the development of inhibitors to Factor XIII may occur.
- In case of existing thrombosis a stabilization of the thrombus might occur, consecutively resulting in a favourization of vessel occlusions.
- When medicinal products prepared from human blood or plasma are administered it is not totally improbable that infectious diseases might be transmitted due to the transmission of infective agents– this also applies to pathogens of hitherto unknown nature.

To reduce the risk of transmission of infective agents, selection of donors and donations by suitable measures is performed and removal and/or inactivation procedures are included in the production process (see also 5.4, viral safety).

Overdose: No symptoms of overdosage with Fibrogammin P are known so far.

Pharmacological properties

Pharmacodynamic properties: Biochemically factor XIII acts as transglutaminase. Physiologically, this corresponds to cross-linking of fibrin-monomers representing the final steps of blood coagulation. Fibrin cross-linking and stabilization promote penetration of fibroblasts. Thus, factor XIII is essentially involved in the principal steps of wound healing and tissue repair.

Pharmacokinetic properties: In congenital factor-XIII-deficiency the biological half-life of Fibrogammin P was determined to be 9.2 days (median).

Fibrogammin P is metabolized in the same way as is the endogenous coagulation factor XIII.

Preclinical safety data:

Toxicological properties: Concentrate of human factor XIII as a normal constituent of the human plasma acts like the physiological factor XIII. Single dose toxicity testing revealed no adverse findings in different species even at dose levels several times higher than the recommended human dose.

Repeated dose toxicity testing is impracticable due to the development of antibodies in animal models.

To date, Fibrogammin P has not been reported to be associated with embryo-fetal toxicity, oncogenic or mutagenic potential.

Viral safety: Fibrogammin P is derived from the plasma of healthy donors which is negative for HBsAg, anti-HCV, anti-HIV-1 and anti-HIV-2. The levels of ALT (GPT) in the plasma are also determined and donations are rejected if the values found are above double the upper limit of the normal range specified in the test.

Important steps of the production procedure, including the heat-treatment in aqueous solution at 60 °C for 10 hours (pasteurization), were validated with regard to the inactivation and/or removal of enveloped viruses (e.g. HIV, herpes simplex) and non-enveloped viruses (e.g. poliomyelitis).* High cumulative virus inactivation and/or removal rates were demonstrated.

On the basis of the current state of scientific knowledge it is safe to assume that Fibrogammin P

does not transmit HIV-induced AIDS as AIDS-inducing viruses such as HIV-1 and HIV-2 are inactivated by the special production process.
Due to production procedures, the risk of transmission of hepatitis B and hepatitis C is very small, as has been shown by experience with other pasteurized preparations.
* with reference to the CPMP Note for Guidance 'Validation of Virus Removal and Inactivation Procedures'

Pharmaceutical particulars
List of excipients: Fibrogammin P 250 U 1250 U
human albumin 24–40 mg 120–200 mg
glucose 16–24 mg 80–120 mg
sodium chloride 28–44 mg 140–220 mg
Supplied diluent Water for injections 4 ml 20 ml.

Incompatibilities: Fibrogammin P should not be mixed with other medicinal products.

Shelf-life: Fibrogammin P has a shelf-life of 24 months.

Special precautions for storage: Fibrogammin P should be stored at +2 to +8°C.
Do not freeze.

Nature and contents of container:
Containers:
–250 U: 6 ml injection vial of colourless tube glass, Type I (Ph.Eur.) - 1250 U: 30 ml injection vial of colourless blow moulded glass, Type II (Ph.Eur.) Vials are sealed with a rubber stopper, a plastic disc and an aluminium cap.
Presentations: Pack with 250 U
1 vial with dried substance
1 ampoule with 4 ml water for injections
Pack with 1250 U
1 vial with dried substance
1 vial with 20 ml water for injections
1 transfer spike.

Instructions for use/handling: Completely dissolve the dried substance with the supplied solvent prewarmed to body temperature within 10 minutes. Reconstitute under sterile conditions. Inject or infuse slowly intravenously.
Usually the solution is slightly opalescent. Do not use solutions which are cloudy or contain particles.
The reconstituted preparation is to be used within 8 hours, sterile conditions provided, and stored at +2 to +8 °C.
Do not use after the expiry date given on the pack and container.
Any unused solution must be discarded appropriately.

Marketing authorisation holder: Centeon Pharma GmbH, Emil-von-Behring-Str. 76, P.O. Box 1230, D-35002 Marburg, Germany.

Marketing authorisation number PL 15036/0006.

Date of (partial) revision of the text February 1998.

Date of last revision February 1998.
[based on the Core-SmPC Human Plasma Coagulation Factor XIII, Guideline III/3560/92-EN, effective December 1992.]

HAEMATE P*

Presentation Haemate P (Factor VIII HS, heat treated) is presented in clear glass vials containing 250 or 500 units of Factor VIII as a lyophilised concentrate. When reconstituted with the vial of solvent provided, the solution will contain 25 IU Factor VIII per ml.

Uses Prophylaxis and therapy of haemorrhages in Hemophilia A and other diseases with Factor VIII deficiency.

Dosage and administration Unless prescribed otherwise the dosage should depend on the degree of Factor VIII deficiency and the extent and location of the bleeding. The amount of Factor VIII required can be estimated as follows: On administration of 1 IU/kg body-weight a rise in Factor VIII activity by about 1% of the normal is to be expected.
In the case of the following haemorrhagic events, the Factor VIII activity should not fall below the given level (in per cent of normal) in the corresponding period:

Haemorrhagic event	*Therapeutically necessary blood level of Factor VIII*	*Period during which it is necessary to maintain the therapeutic blood level*
1. Haemorrhages into joints; Gastro-intestinal haemorrhages; Bite injuries in the oral cavity; Slighter injuries (where local therapy is unsuccessful)	10–20%	2–3 days
2. Haemorrhages into muscles; Larger injuries; Minor operations; (Teeth extractions)	20–30%	3–4 days
3. Intracranial, intra-abdominal or intrathoracic haemorrhages; Medium operations; Fractures	30–50%	4–14 days or until wound completely healed.
4. Major operations	over 50%	14–21 days or until wound completely healed

The amount to be administered should always be oriented to the clinical effectiveness in the individual case. Under certain circumstances larger amounts than those calculated can be required, especially in the case of the initial dose.
In the case of major surgical interventions in particular, a precise monitoring of the substitution therapy by means of coagulation analyses is indispensable.

Administration: The contents of one vial should be dissolved, by slow swirling of the vial, in the appropriate amount of water for injection previously brought to 20°-37°C. The material will dissolve in less than 10 minutes to give a clear to slightly opalescent solution.

Injection: Using a filter needle, withdraw solution from the vial into a syringe. Inject the solution slowly (maximum 4 ml per minute) intravenously. Administration may be effected with the infusion set or with a suitable injection needle. Do not use the filter needle for injection.

Infusion: Dissolve the preparation as described and infuse slowly by means of a disposable transfusion set (with filter inset).

Contra-indications, warnings, etc
Contra-indications: None known.

Warnings: In the case of patients with known allergic diathesis, antihistamines and corticosteroids should be administered as prophylaxis. Caution should be observed in cases of impaired liver or kidney function.
In the case of massive therapy, symptoms of hypervolaemia and–in rare cases–haemolytic reactions through blood-group isoagglutinins should be watched for.
The therapeutic effect may not be achieved if the blood of the patient contains a high level of inhibitors for Factor VIII ('inhibitor hemophilia'). In such cases an attempt must be made to override the inhibitors by administration of large amounts of Factor VIII.
This concentrate has been prepared from large pools of human plasma non-reactive for hepatitis B surface antigen (HbsAg). However, such plasma may contain one or more causative agents of viral hepatitis. Haemate P is heated to 60°C for 10 hours in solution form. However, no procedure has been shown to be totally effective in removing hepatitis infectivity from Antihemophilic Factor (Human).

Side-effects: Haemate P is usually tolerated without reaction. Rare cases of allergic reactions and rise in temperature have been observed. Therapeutic countermeasures depend on nature and severity of the side-effect. In the case of slight reactions, corticosteroids and antihistamines may be used.
In the case of severe reactions (anaphylactic shock), immediate discontinuation of the preparation and injection of adrenalin slowly iv supplemented by high doses of corticosteroids slowly iv.

Pharmaceutical precautions Haemate P should be stored in a refrigerator at +2°C to +8°C and used on or before the expiry date given on the pack. The dissolved preparation should be used within 3 hours of reconstitution.

Legal category POM.

Package quantities The product is supplied as a single vial with an ampoule containing Water for Injections.

Further information Haemate P is a specific hemostatic agent for intravenous application in hemophilia A. The lyophilised preparation is sterile and pyrogen-free and does not contain any preservative. No fibrinogen can be detected by the Clauss method.
Haemate P is obtained from HBsAg-negative and anti HIV-negative plasma of healthy donors. In addition the ALT in the plasma is determined and donations with pathological values are rejected. The pasteurisation process, heating to 60°C for 10 hours in solution form, has been shown to inactivate several DNA viruses (Epstein Barr, cytomegalovirus, herpes simplex and hepatitis B) and RNA viruses (rubella, mumps, measles, poliomyelitis and HIV), and the pathogens of hepatitis non-A/non-B (Hutchison Pool).
Haemate P prepared from cryoprecipitate experimentally infected with Hepatitis B virus was given to chimpanzees. After 6 and 9 months follow-up the test animals remained serologically negative.

Product licence number 15036/0001.

Product licence holder: Centeon Pharma GmbH, PO Box 1230, 35002 Marburg, Germany.

MONOCLATE-P*

Presentation Sterile vials containing nominally 250, 500 or 1000iu Freeze Dried Human Coagulation Factor VIII Ph Eur, highly purified by affinity chromatography using a murine antibody to von Willebrand's Factor. Supplied with Water for Injection for reconstitution prior to intravenous administration.
The concentrate as formulated contains pasteurised Human Albumin Solution as a stabiliser, resulting in a concentrate with a specific activity between 5 and 10 units/mg of total protein. In the absence of this pasteurised Human Albumin stabiliser, specific activity has been determined to exceed 3000 units/mg of protein.
The lyophilised vials also contain sodium chloride, histidine, calcium chloride and mannitol.
The product has been pasteurised in aqueous solution at 60°C for 10 hours during manufacture to further reduce the risk of viral transmission.

Uses Monoclate-P is indicated for the treatment of classical haemophilia (Haemophilia A). Affected individuals frequently require therapy following minor accidents. Surgery, when required in such individuals, must be preceded by temporary correction of the clotting abnormality. Pre-surgical correction of severe Factor VIII (AHF) deficiency can be accomplished with a small volume of Monoclate-P.
Monoclate-P is not effective in controlling the bleeding of patients with von Willebrand's disease.

Dosage and administration Freeze-Dried Human Coagulation Factor VIII, Monoclate-P, Factor VIII: C Pasteurised is for intravenous administration only. As a general rule one unit of Factor VIII activity per kg will increase the circulating Factor VIII by 2%. The following formula provides a guide for dosage calculations:

$$\text{Number of Factor VIII IU Required} = \frac{\text{Body weight}}{\text{(in kg)}} \times \frac{\text{desired Factor VIII}}{\text{increase (\% normal)}} \times 0.5$$

Although dosage must be individualised according to the needs of the patient (weight, severity of haemorrhage, presence of inhibitors), the following general dosages are suggested.

Mild haemorrhages: Minor haemorrhagic episodes will generally subside with a single infusion if a level of 30% of normal or more is attained.

Moderate haemorrhage and minor surgery: For more serious haemorrhages and minor surgical procedures, the patient's Factor VIII level should be raised to 30–50% of normal, which usually requires an initial dose of 15–25 IU per kg. If further therapy is required a maintenance dose is 10–15 IU per kg every 8–12 hours.

Severe haemorrhage: In haemorrhages near vital organs (neck, throat, subperitoneal) it may be desirable to raise the Factor VIII level to 80–100% of normal which can be achieved with an initial dose of 40–50 IU per kg and a maintenance dose of 20–25 IU per kg every 8–12 hours.

Major surgery: For surgical procedures a dose of Factor VIII sufficient to achieve a level 80–100% of normal should be given an hour prior to surgery. A second dose, half the size of the priming dose, should be given five hours after the first dose. Factor VIII levels should be maintained at a daily minimum of at least 30% of normal for a period of 10–14 days post-operatively. Close laboratory control to maintain Factor VIII plasma levels deemed appropriate to maintain haemostasis is recommended.

Reconstitution and administration: Specific instructions for reconstitution and administration are included on the package insert and patient instruction leaflet.
Monoclate-P is for intravenous injection only. Plastic disposable syringes are recommended with Mono-

clate-P solution. The ground glass surfaces of all-glass syringes tend to stick with solutions of this type.

A winged infusion needle with microbore tubing is supplied with each pack. Use of other winged needles without microbore tubing, although compatible with the concentrate, will result in a larger retention of solution within the infusion set.

Contra-indications, warnings, etc
Contra-indications: None known.

Warnings: Monoclate-P is prepared from pooled units of human plasma which may contain the causative agents of hepatitis B, non-A non-B hepatitis (hepatitis C), acquired immune deficiency syndrome (AIDS) and other viral diseases. Each unit of plasma used in the production of Monoclate-P has been tested and found nonreactive for hepatitis B surface antigen (HB_sAg), negative for antibody to human immunodeficiency viruses (Anti-HIV-1 and Anti-HIV-2) and negative for antibody to hepatitis C virus by FDA approved tests, and has been shown to have ALT levels not exceeding two times the upper limit of normal. Additional screening procedures used to eliminate high risk plasma donors, and the purification techniques and pasteurisation step used in the manufacturing process, are all designed to reduce the risk of transmitting viral infection. However, testing methods presently available are not sensitive enough to detect all units of potentially infectious plasma, and treatment methods have not been shown to be totally effective in eliminating any of the aforementioned viral diseases from this concentrate. Accordingly, the benefits and risks of treatment with this concentrate should be carefully assessed prior to use.

Individuals who have not received multiple infusions of blood or plasma products are likely to develop signs and/or symptoms of some viral infections, especially non-A non-B hepatitis as shown by recent data, when treated with coagulant factor concentrates. However, a group of such patients treated with Monoclate, Heat-Treated, did not demonstrate signs or symptoms of a non-A, non-B hepatitis over observation periods ranging from 6 months to 36 months.

Precautions: Patients should be informed of the early signs of hypersensitivity reactions including hives, generalised urticaria, tightness of the chest, wheezing, hypotension and anaphylaxis, and should be advised to discontinue use of the concentrate and contact their physician if these symptoms occur.

Adverse reactions: Products of this type are known to cause allergic reactions, mild chills, nausea or stinging at the infusion site.

Pharmaceutical precautions Monoclate-P should not be mixed with other drugs before injection.

Storage: When stored at refrigerator temperature, 2°–8°C (36°–46°F), Monoclate-P, is stable for the period indicated by the expiration date on its label. Within this period, Monoclate-P may be stored at room temperature not to exceed 30°C (86°F), for up to six months. Avoid freezing which may damage the container for the diluent.

Legal category POM.

Package quantities Monoclate-P is supplied in a single dose vial. IU activity is stated on the label of each vial. Nominal strengths available are 250, 500 and 1000 IU. A patient user kit is supplied with each vial of Monoclate-P. The kit includes a vial of sterile Water for Injections, sterile 10 ml plastic syringe, sterile vented filter spike, sterile winged infusion set, sterile double ended transfer needle, sterile plaster dressing, disposable alcohol swabs and plastic disposal bag.

Further information Upon reconstitution, a clear, colourless solution is obtained, containing 50 to 150 times as much Factor VIII: C as does an equivalent volume of plasma.

Each vial contains the labelled amount of Factor VIII: C activity as expressed in terms of International Units of Factor VIII: C activity. One unit of antihaemophilic activity is equivalent to that quantity of Factor VIII: C present in one ml of normal human plasma. When reconstituted as recommended, the resulting solution contains approximately 300 to 450 millimoles of sodium ions per litre and has 2–3 times the tonicity of saline. It contains approximately 2–5 millimoles of calcium per litre, contributed as calcium chloride, approximately 1–2% pasteurised Human Albumin Solution, 0.8% mannitol, and 1.2 mM histidine. The pH is adjusted with hydrochloric acid and/or sodium hydroxide. Monoclate-P also contains trace amounts (less than 50 ng per 100 IU Factor VIII) of mouse protein.

The half-life of the second elimination phase in haemophiliacs is 17.5±4.8 hours and recovery 1.9 units/dl increase per unit per kg BW (95%) which is comparable to other commercially available Factor VIII products.

The pasteurisation process used in the manufacture of this concentrate has demonstrated in vitro inactivation of 10.5 logs of Human Immunodeficiency Virus (HIV-1) and 7.8 logs of murine encephalomyocarditis (EMC), a non-lipid encapsulated model virus were inactivated to undetectable levels.

The purification and preparative steps used in the production of Monoclate-P are capable of providing a non-specific viral reduction of approximately 5–6 logs independent of the pasteurisation process.

Product licence numbers

250 IU/vial	0231/0090
500 IU/vial	0231/0091
1,000 IU/vial	0231/0092
Diluent	0231/0107

MONONINE*

Presentation Mononine (Freeze Dried Human Coagulation Factor IX PhEur) is supplied as a sterile freeze dried concentrate in single dose vials of nominally 250, 500 or 1000 International Units (iu) with diluent for intravenous administration. Other ingredients include histidine (approximately) 10 mM), sodium chloride (approximately 66 mM) and mannitol (approximately 165 mM).

Unlike lower purity concentrates of Factor IX which are typically complexes of Factor IX with other vitamin K-dependent clotting factors, this product is further purified by a process which includes affinity chromatography using a murine antibody.

Uses Mononine is indicated for the prevention and control of bleeding in Factor IX deficiency, also known as Haemophilia B or Christmas disease.

Mononine is not indicated in the treatment or prophylaxis of Haemophilia A patients with inhibitors to Factor VIII. It contains non-detectable levels of Factors II, VII and X and is, therefore, not indicated for replacement therapy of these clotting factors. Mononine is also not indicated in the treatment or reversal of coumarin-induced anticoagulation or in a haemorrhagic state caused by hepatitis-induced lack of production of liver dependent coagulation factors.

Dosage and administration Mononine is intended for intravenous administration only. It should be reconstituted with the volume of Water for Injections PhEur supplied with the batch, and administered within three hours of reconstitution. Do not refrigerate after reconstitution. After administration, any unused solution and the administration equipment should be discarded.

As a general rule, one unit of Factor IX activity per kg can be expected to increase the circulating level of Factor IX by 1% of normal. The following formula provides a guide for dosage calculations:

$$\text{Number of Factor IX iu required} = \text{Body weight (in kg)} \times \text{Desired Factor IX increase (\% normal)} \times 1.0\,\text{iu/kg}$$

The amount of Mononine to be infused, as well as the frequency of infusions, will vary with each patient and with the clinical situation.

As a general rule, the level of Factor IX required for treatment of different conditions is as follows:

	Minor spontaneous haemorrhage, prophylaxis	*Major trauma or surgery*
Desired levels of Factor IX for haemostasis	15–25%	25–50%
Initial loading dose to achieve desired level	up to 20–30 iu/kg	up to 75 iu/kg
Frequency of dosing	once; repeated in 24 hours if necessary	every 18–30 hours, depending on $T_{1/2}$ and measured Factor IX levels
Duration of treatment	once; repeated if necessary	up to 10 days, depending upon nature of insult

Recovery of the loading dose varies from patient to patient. Doses administered should be titrated to the patient's response.

In the presence of an inhibitor to Factor IX, higher doses of Mononine might be necessary to overcome the inhibitor. No data on the treatment of patients with inhibitors to Factor IX with Mononine are available.

Reconstitution and administration: Specific instructions for reconstitution and administration are included on the package insert and patient instruction leaflet.

Plastic disposable syringes are recommended with Mononine solution. The ground glass surfaces of all-glass syringes tend to stick with solutions of this type.

A winged infusion needle with microbore tubing is supplied with each pack. Use of other winged needles without microbore tubing, although compatible with the concentrate, will result in a larger retention of solution within the winged infusion set.

Rate of administration: The rate of administration should be determined by the response and comfort of the patient; intravenous dosage administration rates of up to 225 units/minute have been regularly tolerated without incident. When reconstituted as directed, i.e. to approximately 100 units/ml, Mononine should be administered at a rate of approximately 2.0 ml per minute.

Contra-indications, warnings, etc
Contra-indications: Known hypersensitivity to mouse protein.

Warnings: This product is prepared from pooled human plasma which may contain the causative agents of hepatitis, AIDS and other viral diseases. Prescribed manufacturing procedures utilised at the plasma collection centres, plasma testing laboratories, and the fractionation facilities are designed to reduce the risk of transmitting viral infection. However, the risk of viral infectivity from this product cannot be totally eliminated. Accordingly, the benefits and risks of treatment with this concentrate should be carefully assessed prior to use.

Individuals who receive infusions of blood or plasma products may develop signs and/or symptoms of some viral infections, particularly nonA nonB hepatitis.

Since the use of Factor IX Complex concentrates has historically been associated with the development of thromboembolic complications, the use of Factor IX containing products may be potentially hazardous in patients with signs of fibrinolysis and in patients with disseminated intravascular coagulation (DIC).

Precautions: The administration of Factor IX Complex concentrates, containing Factors II, VII, IX and X, has been associated with the development of thromboembolic complications. Although Mononine contains highly purified Factor IX, the potential risk of thrombosis or disseminated intravascular coagulation observed with the use of other products containing Factor IX should be recognised. Patients should be given Mononine under specialist direction with appropriate facilities for clinical and laboratory monitoring and observed closely for signs or symptoms of intravascular coagulation or thrombosis. Because of the potential risk of thromboembolic complications, caution should be exercised when administering this concentrate to patients with liver disease, to patients post-operatively, to neonates, or to patients at risk of thromboembolic phenomena or disseminated intravascular coagulation. In each of these situations, the potential benefit of treatment with Mononine should be weighed against the risk of these complications.

The product should be administered intravenously at a rate that wil permit observation of the patient for any immediate reaction. Rates of infusion of up to 225 units per minute have been regularly tolerated with no adverse reactions. If any reaction takes place that is thought to be related to the administration of Mononine, the rate of infusion should be decreased or the infusion stopped, as dictated by the response of the patient.

During the course of treatment, determination of daily Factor IX levels is advised to guide the dose to be administered and the frequency of repeated infusions. Individual patients may vary in their response to Mononine, achieving different levels of in vivo recovery and demonstrating different half-lives.

The use of high doses of Factor IX Complex concentrates has been reported to be associated with instances of myocardial infarction, disseminated intravascular coagulation, venous thrombosis and pulmonary embolism. Generally a Factor IX level of 25% to 50% is considered adequate for haemostasis, including major haemorrhages and surgery. Attempting to maintain Factor IX levels of >75% to 100% during treatment is not recommended. To achieve Factor IX levels that will remain above 25% between once-a-day administrations, each daily dose should attempt to raise the level to 50–60% (see 'Dosage and administration').

No data are available regarding the use of ε-amino caproic acid following an initial infusion of Mononine for the prevention or treatment of oral bleeding following trauma or dental procedures such as extractions.

Formation of antibodies to mouse protein: Although no hypersensitivity reactions have been observed, because Mononine contains trace amounts of mouse protein (<50 ng per 100 Factor IX activity units), the possibility exists that patients treated with Mononine may develop hypersensitivity to the mouse protein.

Information for patients: Patients shouuld be informed of the early signs of hypersensitivity reactions including hives, generalised urticaria, tightness of the chest, wheezing, hypotension and anaphylaxis, and should be advised to discontinue use of the concentrate and contact their physician if these symptoms occur.

Use in pregnancy: Animal reproduction studies have not been conducted with Mononine. It is also not known whether it can cause foetal harm when administered to a pregnant woman or can affect reproduction capacity. Mononine should therefore be given to a pregnant woman only if clearly needed.

Adverse reactions: In clinical trials there were occasional reports of sinusitis, pruritus, rash, fatigue and bitter taste. As with the administration of any product intravenously, the following reactions may be observed following administration: headache, fever, chills, flushing, nausea, vomiting, tingling, lethargy, hives; stinging or burning at the infusion site or other manifestations of allergic reactions.

There is a potential risk of thromboembolic episodes following the administration of Mononine (see *Warnings and Precautions*).

Overdosage: See *Precautions.*

Pharmaceutical precautions Mononine should be administered by a separate infusion line without mixing with other drugs or medication.

Storage: Mononine should be stored at 2°–8°C. Mononine does not contain a preservative. Upon reconstitution, it is advisable that Mononine be administered immediately; in any case it should be administered within three hours in order to assure sterility.

Stability data for Mononine stored under room temperature conditions support the stability of the product for a period of up to one month at a temperature of ≤30°C. These data would supoort a one-time-only storage of Mononine at room temperature in cases where refrigeration is not available and such storage is unavoidable. Precautions should be followed to monitor the time and temperature conditions to assure that they do not exceed one month and 30°C, respectively.

Avoid freezing which may damage the diluent container.

Legal category POM

Package quantities Mononine is supplied in a single dose vial with diluent, double-end needle for reconstitution, vented filter spike for withdrawal, winged infusion set, sterile 10 ml plastic syringe, alcohol swabs, sterile plaster dressing and plastic disposal bag. Factor IX activity in International Units (iu) is stated on the label of each vial which contains nominally 250, 500 or 1000 iu.

One iu represents the activity of Factor IX present in 1 ml of normal, pooled plasma.

Further information Infusion of Freeze-Dried Human Coagulation Factor IX, Mononine into ten patients with severe or moderate Haemophilia B has shown a mean recovery of 67% and a mean half-life of 22.6 hours. Determinations of half-life and recovery six months later in nine of the same ten patients showed a mean recovery of 68% and a mean half-life of 25.3 hours. This pharmacokinetic profile compares favourably to published results for prothrombin complex concentrates.

This concentrate has been processed by monoclonal antibody immunoaffinity chromatography during its manufacture which has been shown to be capable of reducing the risk of viral transmission. Additionally, a chemical treatment protocol and two ultrafiltration steps used in its manufacture have been shown to be capable of significant viral reductions. However, no procedure has been shown to be totally effective in removing viral infectivity from coagulation factor concentrates.

Product licence numbers

250 iu/vial	0231/0097
500 iu/vial	0231/0098
1,000 iu/vial	0231/0099
Diluent	0231/0100

**Trade Mark*

Cephalon UK Limited
11/13 Frederick Sanger Road
Surrey Research Park
Guildford GU2 5YD
☎ 01483 453360 📠 01483 453324

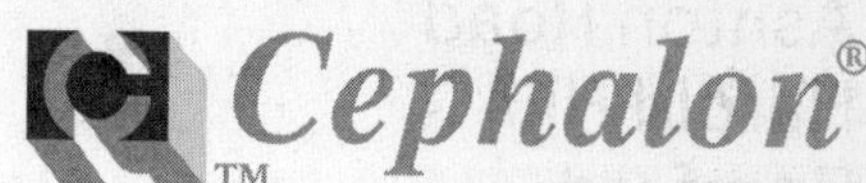

PROVIGIL* ▼

Qualitative and quantitative composition Modafinil 100 mg per tablet.

Pharmaceutical form Tablets.

Clinical particulars

Therapeutic indications: Narcolepsy.

Posology and Method of Administration:
Adults: The recommended daily dose is 200-400 mg. PROVIGIL may be taken as two divided doses in the morning and at noon, or as a single dose in the morning according to physician assessment of the patient and the patient's response.

Elderly: There are limited data available on the use of PROVIGIL in elderly patients. In view of lower clearance and increased AUC, it is recommended that patients over 65 years of age should commence therapy at 100 mg daily. The maximum dose of 400 mg per day should only be used in the absence of renal or hepatic impairment.

Hepatic and renal failure: The dose in patients with severe hepatic or renal failure should be reduced by half (100-200 mg/day).

Children: See *Contra-indications*.

Contra-indications: PROVIGIL is contra-indicated for use during pregnancy and lactation, in children, moderate to severe hypertension, and arrhythmia. Known hypersensitivity to PROVIGIL or any component of the preparation.

Special warnings and special precautions for use: Patients with major anxiety should only receive treatment with PROVIGIL in a specialist unit.
Sexually active women of child-bearing potential should be established on a contraceptive programme before taking PROVIGIL.
Blood pressure and heart rate should be monitored in hypertensive patients.

It is recommended that PROVIGIL tablets not be used in patients with a history of left ventricular hypertrophy or ischaemic ECG changes, chest pain, arrhythmia or other clinically significant manifestations of mitral valve prolapse in association with CNS stimulant use.

Whilst studies with modafinil have demonstrated a low potential for dependence, as with other psychoactive agents, the possibility of dependence with long term use cannot be entirely excluded.

Interactions with other medicaments and other forms of interaction:

Oral contraceptives: The effectiveness of oral contraceptives may be impaired due to enzyme induction activity of PROVIGIL. When oral contraceptives are used, a product containing 50 micrograms or more of ethinyl oestradiol should be taken. Adequate contraception will require continuation of the oral contraceptive for two cycles after stopping PROVIGIL.

Tricyclic antidepressants: In a single dose pharmacokinetic interaction study of PROVIGIL (200 mg) and clomipramine (50 mg), no clinically important alterations in the pharmacokinetic profile of PROVIGIL or clomipramine were noted, however, patients receiving such medication should be carefully monitored.

Anti-convulsant therapy: In view of the enzyme inducing potential of PROVIGIL, care should be observed with co-administration of these drugs.

Pregnancy and lactation: Modafinil has been shown to be non-teratogenic in preclinical reproductive toxicology investigations at doses greater than the maximum clinical dose. However, blood levels in preclinical safety studies, due to metabolic autoinduction, were less than or similar to that expected in patients. As there have been no adequate or well controlled studies of modafinil in pregnant women, PROVIGIL should be contra-indicated for use in pregnancy and lactation.

Effects on ability to drive and use machines: There is no information available concerning the effects of PROVIGIL on vehicle driving and/or the ability to use machinery.

Undesirable effects: Episodes of feelings of nervousness, excitation, aggressive tendencies, insomnia, personality disorder, anorexia, headache, CNS stimulation, euphoria, abdominal pain, dry mouth, palpitation, tachycardia, hypertension, and tremor have been reported.

Gastrointestinal disturbances (nausea, gastric discomfort) have been reported in clinical trials, usually regressing when tablets are taken during meals. There have also been reports of pruritic skin rashes and, very rarely, cases of buccofacial dyskinesia.

A dose related increase in alkaline phosphatase has been observed.

The safety of PROVIGIL has not been studied beyond 40 weeks of continuous use.

Overdose: The chief symptom following massive ingestion is insomnia.

Management: Induced emesis or gastric lavage should be considered. Hospitalisation and surveillance of psychomotor status; cardiovascular monitoring or surveillance until the patient's symptoms have resolved.

Pharmacological properties

Pharmacodynamic properties: Modafinil promotes wakefulness in a variety of species, including man. The precise mechanism(s) through which modafinil promotes wakefulness is unknown, although the wake-promoting effects of modafinil can be attenuated by alpha-adrenergic antagonists.

Modafinil in man restores and/or improves the level of wakefulness and daytime alertness in relation to the dose administered. Starting from the dose of 100 mg in the morning, changes are found in electrophysiological parameters reflecting alertness (ratio of power of α rhythm to power of θ rhythm). Starting from 200 mg in the morning, an increase is seen in latency periods in the multiple sleep latency test. It opposes the impairment of cognitive (memory in particular), psychomotor and neurosensorial performances induced by sleep deprivation. This activity is obtained in the absence of any modifications concerning behaviour, appetite and habituation.

Morning administration of 200 mg does not appear to affect nocturnal sleep. Administration of 100 mg morning and noon may prolong the subjective time taken to fall asleep. Evening administration may disturb sleep. This pharmacodynamic activity does not appear to affect the autonomic nervous system.

Pharmacokinetic properties: The pharmacokinetics of modafinil are linear and independent of the dose administered. Absorption of modafinil following oral administration is good but slow. Peak plasma concentration is reached two to three hours after ingestion. Amounts absorbed increase in proportion to doses administered.

Modafinil is moderately bound to plasma proteins (62%), essentially to albumin. This degree of protein binding is such that the risk of interaction with strongly bound drugs is unlikely.

Modafinil is metabolised by the liver. The chief metabolite (40-50% of the dose), acid modafinil, has no pharmacological activity. The excretion of modafinil and its metabolites is chiefly renal, with a small proportion being eliminated unchanged (< 10%).
The elimination half-life of modafinil is long (10-12 hours) and enables a treatment regimen based upon one or two doses/day.

Preclinical safety data: Toxicology studies by single and repeated dosing have revealed no particular toxic action in animals.

Reproduction function studies have revealed no effect on fertility, nor any teratogenic effect, nor any effect on viability, growth or development of the offspring.

This drug is not considered to be mutagenic or carcinogenic.

Animal exposure to modafinil, based on actual blood levels in the general toxicology, reproductive and carcinogenicity studies, was less than or similar to that expected in humans. This circumstance is the result of metabolic auto-induction noted in the preclinical studies. However, animal exposure on a mg/kg dose basis to modafinil in the general toxicology, reproductive and carcinogenicity studies was greater than the expected exposure, calculated on a similar basis, in humans.

Pharmaceutical particulars

List of excipients: Lactose monohydrate, corn starch, magnesium silicate, croscarmellose sodium, povidone K90, talc and magnesium stearate.

Incompatibilities: None known

Shelf life: Three years

Special precautions for storage: Store at less than 25°C in a dry place. Protect from direct heat and sunlight.

Nature and contents of container: 30 tablets in PVC/PE/Aclar/Aluminium blister
60 tablets in PVC/PE/Aclar/Aluminium blister
90 tablets in PVC/PE/Aclar/Aluminium blister

Instructions for use/handling: Not applicable.

Marketing authorisation number PL 16260/0001

Date of first authorisation/renewal of authorisation 14 October 1997

Date of (partial) revision of text 22 June 1998

**Trade Mark*

Chauvin Pharmaceuticals Ltd

Ashton Road
Harold Hill
Romford
Essex RM3 8SL

☎ 01708 383838 🖷 01708 371316

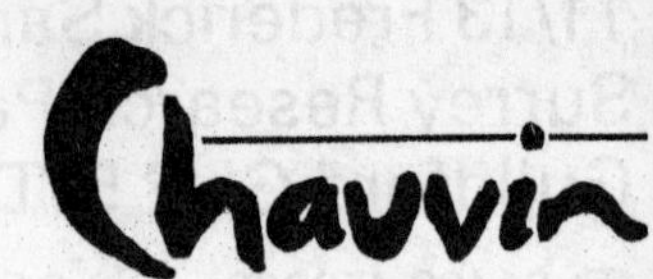

EPPY*

Qualitative and quantitative composition Colourless to pale yellow solution containing Adrenaline BP 1% w/v in a buffered solution preserved with benzalkonium chloride 0.01% w/v.

Pharmaceutical form Multidose, seterile eye drops.

Clinical particulars

Therapeutic indications: Indicated for the treatment of elevated intraocular pressure in open-angle (chronic simple) glaucoma.

It may be used in combination with miotics, beta-adrenergic blocking agents or carbonic anhydrase inhibitors where indicated.

Posology and method of administration:

Adults (including the elderly) and children: One or two drops to each eye, usually once or twice daily. May be given as infrequently as once every three days. Determine the frequency of instillation by tonometry.

When used in conjunction with miotics, instil this drug five or ten minutes after the miotic drops.

Children: As directed by a physician. Safety and efficacy of use in children has not been established.

Contra-indications: Closed-angle glaucoma (unless previously treated with iridectomy).

Patients with a narrow angle prone to angle block precipitated by mydriatics.

Hypersensitivity to adrenaline or any other component of the preparation.

This product contains benzalkonium chloride and should not be used when soft contact lenses are worn.

Special warnings and precautions for use: Do not use until the diagnosis of glaucoma has been verified and the nature of the glaucoma has been confirmed (as the use of adrenaline is contraindicated in narrow-angle glaucoma).

To reduce the risk of precipitating an attack of narrow-angle glaucoma, evaluate the anterior chamber angle by gonioscopy before initiating therapy.

Adrenaline eye drops should be used with caution by patients with hypertension, cardiac disease, aneurysms, arrhythmias or tachycardia, hyperthyroidism, cerebral arteriosclerosis and diabetes mellitus.

Maculopathy with a central scotoma may occur following use in aphakic patients. Discontinue use in such patients if visual acuity deteriorates.

Systemic absorption of adrenaline from eye drops may be reduced by compressing the lacrimal sac at the medial canthus for a minute during and following the instillation of the drops. (This blocks the passage of the drops via the naso-lacrimal duct to the wide absorptive area of the nasal and pharyngeal mucosa. It is especially advisable in children.)

Interaction with other medicaments and other forms of intereaction: Monoamine oxidase inhibitors: There is an increased risk of adrenergic reactions when used simultaneously with or up to three weeks after the administration of MAOIs.

Tricyclic antidepressants: The pressor response to adrenergic agents and the risk of cardiac arrhythmia may be potentiated in patients receiving tricyclic antidepressants (or within several days of their discontinuation).

Halothane: Because of the increased risk of ventricular fibrillation adrenaline should not be given during general anaesthesia with anaesthetic agents which sensitise the myocardium to sympathomimetics.

There has been work that has suggested that as adrenaline probably exerts its effect on increasing outflow via Beta 2 receptors, additive effects on reducing IOP may be expected if a Beta 1 selective beta-blocker is used, but not if a non-selective beta-blocker is used.

Preganancy and lactation: Safety for use in pregnancy and lactation has not been established. This product should not be used during pregnancy unless it is considered essential by the physician.

Effects on the ability to drive and use machines: May cause temporarily blurred vision. Warn patients not to drive or operate hazardous machinery unless vision is clear.

Undesirable effects: Local: Severe smarting on instillation, blurred vision, photophobia, eye pain, conjunctival hyperaemia (resulting in a red eye as a frequent response). Conjunctival sensitisation and allergy and local skin reactions occur occasionally. Pigmentary deposits in the conjunctiva, cornea or eyelids may occur after prolonged use.

CNS: Headache or browache are also common but usually diminish as treatment is continued.

Systemic: Systemic adverse reactions are rare following topical use at normal dosage, however, palpitations, tachycardia, raised blood pressure, extrasystoles, cardiac arrhythmias, faintness, sweating, pallor, trembling and perspiration may occur.

Overdose: Systemic reactions to topical adrenaline are unlikely at normal doses. Greater caution is necessary in children and the elderly and those patients predisposed to such reactions e.g. hypertensive cardiac disease or thyrotoxicosis. A severe reaction to adrenaline is of rapid onset and short duration. The treatment of a severe toxic reaction is an immediate intravenous injection of a quick-acting alpha-adrenoceptor blocking agent (such as 2 mg to 5 mg of phentolamine) followed by a beta-adrenoceptor blocking agent (such as 1 mg of propranolol injected over 1 minute and repeated, if necessary, at 2 minute intervals up to a maximum of 10 mg (5 mg in anaesthesia)). Adrenaline is almost totally inactive when given by mouth as a result of enzymic degradation in the gut and first pass metabolism in the liver.

Pharmacological properties

Pharmacodynamic properties: Adrenaline is a sympathomimetic drug which acts as an agonist on both alpha and beta type receptors. In the eye, this sympathomimetic action initiates a contraction of the radial muscle of the iris, which leads to a mydriatic effect on the pupil. Adrenaline is also capable of causing local vasoconstriction in the conjunctiva and increased uveal vascular resistance. Except where angle block is produced in eyes with a narrow angle, the intraocular pressure is reduced via actions on both the production and drainage of aqueous humour.

Pharmacokinetic properties: There are no data on the pharmacokinetics of Eppy.

Preclinical safety data: Adrenaline is a naturally occurring molecule; its use in ophthalmology is well established. Little toxicology work has been carried out, however, the breadth of clinical experience confirms its suitability as a topical ophthalmic agent.

Pharmaceutical particulars

List of excipients: N-Actyl-L-Cysteine; Amonium Lactate Syrup; Benzalkonium Chloride; Ammonium Hydroxide; Purified Water.

Incompatibilities: None known.

Shelf life; Unopened: 24 months.
Opened: 28 days.

Special precautions for storage: Store below 25°C. Do not freeze. Protect from light.

Nature and contents of container: 7.5 ml of Eppy is supplied in a polyethylene dropper bottle fitted with a pilfer proof cap. Each bottle is enclosed in a nitrogen filled sealed pouch inside a carton.

Instructions for use/handling: Eppy should not be used if the solution has become dark amber.

Discard any remaining solution 28 days after first opening the container.

Avoid contact between the dropper nozzle and other surfaces.

Marketing authorisation number PL 0033/5022R

Date of approval/revision of SPC November 1998

Legal category POM

FLUORETS*

Qualitative and quantitative composition Paper strips each impregnated with approximately 1 mg Fluorescein Sodium BP.

Pharmaceutical form Sterile, individually wrapped paper strips.

Clinical particulars

Therapeutic indications: Fluorescein is a corneal stain and can be used in diagnostic examinations of the eye including Goldmann tonometry and the fitting of contact lenses.

Posology and method of administration:

Adults (including the elderly) and children: One Fluoret moistened with tear fluid, sterile water or sterile ophthalmic solution applied topically to the eye should be sufficient to provide adequate corneal staining.

Contra-indications: Not for use in patients with known hypersensitivity to fluorescein. Not to be used with soft contact lenses.

Special warnings and precautions for use: Care should be taken to handle the strip by the non-impregnated end. The applicator should be used once and discarded.

Interaction with other medicaments and other forms of interaction: None known.

Pregnancy and lactation: Safety for use in pregnancy and lactation has not been established, therefore, use only when considered essential by a physician.

Effects on ability to drive and use machines: May cause transient blurring of vision when applied. Warn patients not to drive or operate hazardous machinery unless vision is clear.

Undesirable effects: None.

Overdose: Not applicable.

Pharmacological properties

Pharmacodynamic properties: Fluorescein sodium acts as a diagnostic stain.

Pharmacokinetic properties: Fluorescein will resist penetration of a normal cornea and most excess solution will, therefore, be carried with the tear film away from the conjunctival sac. The majority will be lost through the naso-lacrimal ducts and absorbed via the gastro-intestinal tract from where it is converted rapidly to its glucuronide and excreted via the urine.

If fluorescein crosses the cornea it will enter the Bowman's membrane, stroma and possibly the anterior chamber. Aqueous flow and diffusion into the blood in the anterior chamber finally removes fluorescein from the eye and it is excreted unchanged in the urine.

Preclinical safety data: There are no preclinical data of relevance to the prescriber which are additional to that already included in other sections of this SPC.

Pharmaceutical particulars

List of excipients: None.

Incompatibilities: None.

Shelf life: 5 years.

Special precautions for storage: Store below 25°C.

Nature and contents of container: Individually wrapped sterile paper strips, supplied in cartons containing 100 Fluorets.

Instructions for use/handling: Each Fluoret should be handled by the non-impregnated end. Fluorets should be used once and discarded.

Marketing authorisation holder: Chauvin Pharmaceuticals Ltd, Ashton Road, Harold Hill, Romford, Essex RM3 8SL.

Marketing authorisation number PL 0033/5095R.

Date of approval/revision of SPC January 1998.

Legal category P

GANDA*

Qualitative and quantitative composition Clear, viscous, colourless to almost colourless liquid containing Guanethidine Monosulphate BP + Epinephrine (Adrenaline) BP. Two strengths are available: 1% w/v Guanethidine Monosulphate + 0.2% w/v Epinephrine (Adrenaline) and 3% w/v Guanethidine Monosulphate + 0.5% w/v Epinephrine (Adrenaline).

Pharmaceutical form Multidose sterile eye drops.

Clinical particulars

Therapeutic indications: For the reduction of intraocular pressure in primary open angle or secondary glaucoma. It may be used alone or in conjunction with miotics or carbonic anhydrase inhibitor therapy.

Posology and method of administration:

Adults (including the elderly): One drop to be instilled into the eye once or twice daily or at the discretion of the physician.

Children: As instructed by the practitioner.

Light pressure may be applied for a few minutes to the inner canthus to reduce systemic absorption via the naso-lacrimal duct.

When used in conjunction with miotics, Ganda 3+0.5 should follow the miotic after an interval of 5–10 minutes.

Contra-indications: Ganda should not be used in narrow angle glaucoma or in the case of a narrow angle between the iris and cornea as pupillary dilation may precipitate angle closure.

Special warnings and special precautions for use: After prolonged treatment with Ganda (more than 9–12 months) cicatrising changes of the conjunctiva and cornea leading to corneal ulceration and scarring have been reported in some patients. If the initial changes are detected on slit lamp examination, treatment with Ganda should be stopped. These cicatrising changes develop slowly and six-monthly examination of the conjunctiva and cornea will enable Ganda to be withdrawn in any patients who are starting to show conjunctival damage.

A paradoxical increase in intraocular pressure has been reported in a small number of cases.

Some degree of ptosis may represent an adverse effect in glaucoma but will usually respond to a reduction in dosage or in the frequency of administration.

At prolonged high dosage a tendency to superficial punctate keratitis has been reported, responding either to a reduction in dosage or termination of treatment.

Interaction with other medicaments and other forms of interaction: Miotics and other forms of glaucoma treatment produce an enhancement of the therapeutic effect of Ganda.

Monoamine oxidase inhibitors: There is an increased risk of adrenergic reactions when used simultaneously with or up to three weeks after the administration of MAOIs.

Tricyclic antidepressants: The pressor response to adrenergic agents and the risk of cardiac arrhythmia may be potentiated in patients receiving tricyclic antidepressants (or within several days of their discontinuation).

Halothane: Because of the increased risk of ventricular fibrillation adrenaline should not be given during general anaesthesia with anaesthetic agents which sensitise the myocardium to sympathomimetics.

Pregnancy and lactation: No data are available on the use of Ganda in pregnancy and lactation therefore Ganda cannot be recommended in pregnancy or during lactation unless the therapeutic benefit exceeds the potential risk and there is no safer alternative.

Effects on ability to drive and use machines: May cause temporarily blurred vision. Warn patients not to drive or operate hazardous machinery unless vision is clear.

Undesirable effects:

Local: Occasionally a patient may complain of orbital discomfort or red eye. Rarely, headache, irritation and local skin reactions may occur. As with other adrenaline preparations, melanosis may occasionally occur, but this has no pathological significance. Topical adrenaline has been shown to occasionally cause macular oedema in aphakic eyes and thus the use of adrenaline-containing eye drops in aphakic patients is not recommended.

Systemic: Systemic side effects are rare but can include tachycardia, extrasystoles, and elevation of blood pressure. Although no reports of such reactions to Ganda have been received, caution is recommended in patients with thyrotoxicosis, hypertension or cardiovascular problems including tachycardia and arrhythmias.

Systemic absorption of adrenaline from eye drops may be minimised by compressing the lacrimal sac at the medial canthus for a minute during and following the instillation of the drops. (This blocks the passage of the drops via the naso-lacrimal duct to the wide absorptive area of the nasal and pharyngeal mucosa. It is especially advisable in children.)

Overdose: Overdose is unlikely to occur at normal doses, however, caution is necessary in children, the elderly and patients with predisposing conditions e.g. hypertensive cardiac disease or thyrotoxicosis. A severe reaction to adrenaline is of rapid onset and short duration. The treatment of a severe toxic reaction is an immediate intravenous injection of a quick-acting alpha-adrenoceptor blocking agent (such as 2 mg to 5 mg of phentolamine) followed by a beta-adrenoceptor blocking agent, such as 1 mg of propranolol injected over 1 minute and repeated, if necessary at 2 minute intervals up to a maximum of 10 mg (5 mg in anaesthesia). Adrenaline is almost totally inactive when given by mouth as a result of enzymic degradation in the gut and first pass metabolism in the liver.

Pharmacological properties

Pharmacodynamic properties: Guanethidine is a post-ganglionic adrenergic neurone blocker which acts by displacing noradrenaline from the sympathetic nerve terminals. In the eye, this causes mydriasis and a transitory increase of facility of aqueous outflow. Stores of noradrenaline are then depleted, resulting in reduced production of aqueous humour. Both these effects contribute to a lowering of the intraocular pressure.

Adrenaline is a sympathomimetic alpha and beta receptor agonist. Topical ocular adrenaline reduces the intraocular pressure by decreasing aqueous humour production and increasing aqueous outflow.

The presence of guanethidine results in potentiation of the effect of adrenaline due to the prevention of noradrenaline re-uptake at the sympathetic nerve terminals.

Pharmacokinetic properties: Extensive pharmacokinetic data are available for oral guanethidine. 50–60% of the dose is absorbed and this is believed to be widely distributed in the tissues. Less than 10% of the drug is bound to plasma protein. The plasma half life is in the range 2–8 days. Specific information on the ocular pharmacokinetics of guanethidine following topical application is not available.

Adrenaline is rapidly distributed into the heart, spleen, endocrine system and adrenergic nerves following intramuscular or subcutaneous injection. Oral administration leads to rapid oxidation and pharmacologically active concentrations are not achieved. Plasma protein binding is around 50% and metabolism is rapid. The plasma half life is therefore in the range 3–10 minutes. Once again, specific ocular pharmacokinetic data is not available.

Preclinical safety data: Ames tests have shown guanethidine to be non-mutagenic. It is also non-teratogenic. Repeated high intraperitoneal doses in rats have been shown to cause structural changes in sympathetic ganglia which are only partly reversible. However, neuronal destruction by guanethidine has not been described in man and there are no reports of irreversible sympathetic inhibition following prolonged use.

Systemic oral daily therapeutic doses of guanethidine are frequently in the 50–60 mg range, but doses of 200–300 mg per day have been used without untoward adverse reactions. The average daily topical ocular dose of guanethidine is likely to be in the range of ≅ 0–2 mg. Systemic toxicity is therefore unlikely to be a feature.

Adrenaline is a naturally occurring molecule whose use in ophthalmology is well established. Little specific toxicology work has been carried out, however, the breadth of clinical experience confirms its suitability as a topical ophthalmic agent.

Pharmaceutical particulars

List of excipients: N-Acetyl-L-cysteine; Ammonium dihydrogen phosphate; Hydroxyethylcellulose; Benzalkonium chloride; Strong solution of ammonia; Purified water.

Incompatibilities: Not applicable.

Shelf life: The shelf life expiry date for this product shall not exceed two years from the date of its manufacture when stored below 25°C and protected from light.

The bottle should be discarded one month after the pouch has been opened.

Special precautions for storage: The product should be transported and stored in the original packaging. It should be stored below 25°C and protected from light.

Nature and contents of container: Multidose polyethylene bottles fitted with a polyethylene dropper nozzle and a polystyrene or polyethylene pilfer proof cap. The bottle is contained in a nitrogen filled pouch and packed into cartons. Each bottle contains 7.5 ml of solution.

Marketing authorisation numbers
Ganda 1+0.2 0033/0075
Ganda 3+0.5 0033/0071

Date of approval/revision of SPC Ganda 1+0.2 July 98, Ganda 3+0.5 February 98.

Legal category POM.

GELTEARS

Qualitative and quantitative composition Clear, colourless gel containing 0.2% w/w Carbomer 940.

Pharmaceutical form Sterile eye gel.

Clinical particulars

Therapeutic indications: Substitution of tear fluid in the management of dry eye conditions, including keratoconjunctivitis sicca and unstable tear film.

Posology and method of administration:

Adults (including the elderly) and children: One drop to be instilled into the conjunctival fold of each affected eye 3–4 times daily or as required, depending on the degree of discomfort.

Contra-indications: Use in patients with a known hypersensitivity to any component of the preparation.

Special warnings and precautions for use: Blurred vision can occur if too much gel is instilled at one time, or if the gel is used too frequently. This effect can last for up to an hour. Recovery can be aided by blinking vigorously for a few seconds. If this fails, the lower eyelid should be manipulated until the gel returns to the lower fornix and normal vision is restored.

Contact lenses should be removed during treatment with GelTears.

Interaction with other medicaments and other forms of interaction: No significant interactions have been reported.

Pregnancy and lactation: Safety for use in pregnancy and lactation has not been established, therefore, GelTears should not be used in these circumstances.

Effects on ability to drive and use machines: As with other ophthalmic preparations, transient blurring of vision may occur on instillation. If affected, the patient should be advised not to drive or operate hazardous machinery until normal vision is restored.

Undesirable effects: Corneal irritation due to benzalkonium chloride could possibly occur with prolonged use.

Overdose: Not applicable.

Pharmacological properties

Pharmacodynamic properties: GelTears contains Carbomer 940, a hydrophilic, high molecular weight polymer of carboxyvinylic acid. The gel forms a transparent lubricating and moistening film on the surface of the eye. The preparation has a pH similar to that found in the normal tear film and is slightly hypotonic with respect to tears. GelTears relieves the symptoms of irritation linked with dry eye syndromes and protects the cornea against drying out.

The use of vital stains has provided objective evidence that the corneal and conjunctival epithelial lesions associated with dry eye syndromes show improvement on treatment with GelTears. The gel remains on the surface of the eye for longer than low viscosity artificial tears and hence, less frequent application is required.

Pharmacokinetic properties: No human pharmacokinetic studies are available, however, absorption or accumulation in ocular tissues is likely to be negligible due to the high molecular weight of the active ingredient.

Preclinical safety data: No adverse safety issues were detected during the development of this formulation. The ingredients are well established in clinical ophthalmology.

Pharmaceutical particulars

List of excipients: Benzalkonium chloride 0.01% w/w (as a preservative); purified water; sorbitol; sodium hydroxide.

Incompatibilities: None known.

Shelf life: The shelf life expiry date shall not exceed 3 years from the date of its manufacture when stored below 25°C. Any remaining gel should be discarded 28 days after first opening the tube.

Special precautions for storage: The product should be transported in the original packaging. It should be stored below 25°C.

Nature and contents of container: Sterile ophthalmic gel presented in 5 g and 10 g plasticised, lacquered aluminium tubes, closed with a tamper evident polyethylene cap. Each tube is individually cartonned with a patient information leaflet.

Marketing authorisation number 0033/0149

Date of approval/revision of SPC January 1996

Legal category P

MINIMS* AMETHOCAINE HYDROCHLORIDE

Quantitative and qualitative composition Single-use, clear, colourless, sterile eye drops containing amethocaine (tetracaine) hydrochloride PhEur solution. There are two strengths 0.5% w/v amethocaine (tetracaine) hydrochloride and 1.0% w/v amethocaine (tetracaine) hydrochloride.

Pharmaceutical form Single-use, sterile eye drops.

Clinical particulars
Therapeutic indications: Ocular anaesthetic for topical instillation into the conjunctival sac.

Posology and method of administration:
Adults (including the elderly) and children: One drop or as required.

Contra-indications: Not to be used in patients with a known hypersensitivity to the product.

Amethocaine is hydrolysed in the body to p-aminobenzoic acid and should not therefore be used in patients being treated with sulphonamides.

In view of the immaturity of the enzyme system which metabolises the ester type local anaesthetics in premature babies, amethocaine should be avoided in these patients.

Special warnings and precautions for use: The anaesthetised eye should be protected from dust and bacterial contamination.

Amethocaine may give rise to dermatitis in hypersensitive patients.

On instillation an initial burning sensation may be experienced. This may last for up to 30 seconds.

The cornea may be damaged by prolonged application of anaesthetic eye drops.

Systemic absorption may be reduced by compressing the lacrimal sac at the medial canthus for a minute during and following the instillation of the drops. (This blocks the passage of the drops via the naso lacrimal duct to the wide absorptive area of the nasal and pharyngeal mucosa. It is especially advisable in children.)

Interaction with other medicaments and other forms of interaction: Amethocaine should not be used in patients being treated with sulphonamides (see *Contra-indications*).

Pregnancy and lactation: Safety for use in pregnancy and lactation has not been established, therefore, use only when considered essential by the physician.

Effects on ability to drive and use machines: May cause transient blurring of vision on instillation. Warn patients not to drive or operate hazardous machinery unless vision is clear.

Undesirable effects: Not applicable.

Overdose: Not expected.

Pharmacological properties
Pharmacodynamic properties: Amethocaine hydrochloride is used as a local anaesthetic which acts by reversibly blocking the propagation and conduction of nerve impulses along nerve axons. Amethocaine stabilises the nerve membrane, preventing the increase in sodium permeability necessary for the production of an action potential.

Pharmacokinetic properties: Amethocaine is a weak base (pK_a 8.5), therefore, significant changes in the rate of ionised lipid soluble drug uptake may occur with changes in the acid base balance.

In vitro studies have shown that amethocaine has a high affinity for melanin, therefore, differences in duration of action may be expected between deeply pigmented eyes and less pigmented eyes.

The primary site of metabolism for amethocaine is the plasma. Pseudocholinesterases in the plasma hydrolyse amethocaine to 4-aminobenzoic acid. Unmetabolised drug is excreted in the urine.

Preclinical safety data: No adverse safety issues were detected during the development of this formulation. The active ingredient is well established in clinical ophthalmology.

Pharmaceutical particulars
List of excipients: Hydrochloric acid; Purified water.

Incompatibilities: None known.

Shelf life: Unopened: 15 months.

Special precautions for storage: Store below 25°C. Do not freeze. Protect from light.

Nature and contents of container: A sealed conical shaped polypropylene container fitted with a twist and pull off cap. Overwrapped in an individual polypropylene/paper pouch. Each container holds approximately 0.5 ml of solution.

Instructions for use/handling: Each Minims unit should be discarded after a single use.

Marketing authorisation number Minims Amethocaine 0.5% PL 0033/5000R, Minims Amethocaine 1.0% PL 0033/5001R

Date of approval/revision of the SPC Minims Amethocaine 0.5% December 1997, Minims Amethocaine 1.0% December 1997

Legal category POM

MINIMS* ARTIFICIAL TEARS

Qualitative and quantitative composition Clear, colourless, sterile eye drops containing Hydroxyethylcellulose 0.44% w/w BP and Sodium Chloride PhEur 0.35% w/w.

Pharmaceutical form Sterile single-use eye drop.

Clinical particulars
Therapeutic indications: For the relief of dry eye syndromes associated with deficient tear secretion.

Posology and method of administration: One or two drops instilled into the affected eye three or four times daily, or as often as is required.

Contra-indications: None known.

Special warnings and precautions for use: If irritation persists or worsens or continued redness occurs, discontinue use and consult a physician or ophthalmologist.

Interaction with other medicaments and other forms of interaction: None known.

Pregnancy and lactation: There is no evidence of safety of the drug in human pregnancy but it has been in wide use for many years without apparent ill consequence. If drug therapy is needed in pregnancy this preparation can be used if recommended by a physician and it is considered that the benefits outweigh the possible risks.

Effects on ability to drive and use machines: May cause transient blurring of vision on instillation. Do not drive or operate hazardous machinery unless vision is clear.

Undesirable effects: May cause transient mild stinging or temporarily blurred vision.

Overdose: Overdose would not be expected to produce symptoms.

Pharmacological properties
Pharmacodynamic properties: The viscolising properties of hydroxyethylcellulose combined with sodium chloride have been shown to increase the tear breakup time in animal models, whilst also acting as a lubricating agent for dry eyes.

Pharmacokinetic properties: Not applicable.

Preclinical safety data: No adverse safety issues were detected during the development of this formulation. The active ingredients are well-established in clinical ophthalmology.

Pharmaceutical particulars
List of excipients: Purified water; borax; boric acid.

Incompatibilities: None known.

Shelf life: 15 months.

Special precautions for storage: Store below 25°C. Do not freeze. Protect from light.

Nature and contents of container: A sealed conical shaped polypropylene container fitted with a twist and pull off cap. Each Minims unit is overwrapped in an individual polypropylene/paper pouch.

Instructions for use/handling: Do not use if solution is more than pale yellow in colour. Each Minims unit should be discarded after a single use.

Marketing authorisation number 0033/0137

Date of approval/revision of SPC December 1996

Legal category P

MINIMS* ATROPINE SULPHATE

Quantitative and qualitative composition Single-use, clear, colourless, sterile eye drops containing Atropine Sulphate PhEur 1% w/v.

Pharmaceutical form Single-use, sterile eye drops.

Clinical particulars
Therapeutic indications: As a topical mydriatic and cycloplegic.

Posology and method of administration:
Adults (including the elderly): One drop to be instilled into the eye, or as required.

Contra-indications: Hypersensitivity to any component of the preparation.

Due to the risk of precipitating an acute attack, do not use in cases of confirmed narrow-angle glaucoma or where latent narrow angle glaucoma is suspected. If in doubt it is recommended that an alternative preparation is used.

Special warnings and precautions for use: The protracted mydriasis which is difficult to reverse, may be a disadvantage.

Systemic absorption may be reduced by compressing the lacrimal sac at the medial canthus for a minute during and following the instillation of the drops. (This blocks the passage of the drops via the naso-lacrimal duct to the wide absorptive area of the nasal and pharyngeal mucosa. It is especially advisable in children.)

Interaction with other medicaments and other forms of interaction: None known.

Pregnancy and lactation: The safety for use in pregnancy and lactation has not been established, therefore, use only when directed by a physician.

Effects on ability to drive and use machines: May cause transient blurring of vision on instillation. Warn patients not to drive or operate hazardous machinery unless vision is clear.

Undesirable effects: Side effects rarely occur but include anticholinergic effects such as dry mouth and skin, flushing, increased body temperature, urinary symptoms, gastrointestinal symptoms and tachycardia. These effects are more likely to occur in infants and children.

Overdose: Systemic reactions to topical atropine are unlikely at normal doses. Symptoms which can occur following an overdose, however, include anticholinergic effects (as listed in the undesirable effects section above), cardiovascular changes (tachycardia, atrial arrhythmias, atrio-ventricular dissociation) and central nervous system effects (confusion, ataxia, restlessness, hallucination, convulsions). Treatment is supportive.

Pharmacological properties
Pharmacodynamic properties: Atropine sulphate is a competitive antagonist of acetylcholine at postganglionic cholinergic (parasympathetic) nerve endings.

Atropine does not discriminate between the recently discovered muscarinic receptor sub types M1 (in parasympathetic ganglia of the submucous plexus, with high affinity for selecting antimuscarinic pirenzepine) and M2 (low affinity for pirenzepine and occurring predominantly in heart and smooth muscle).

Pharmacokinetic properties: Atropine is well absorbed from the small bowel and not at all from the stomach. Thus the effects of oral dosing are much slower in onset than after parenteral dosing. Atropine is also absorbed by mucous membranes but less readily from the eye and skin, although significant toxicity can sometimes occur through absorption of excessive eye drops.

Atropine has a volume of distribution of 1–6 L/kg. Protein binding is moderate, with approximately 50% of the drug bound in plasma. Its plasma clearance is 8 ml/min/kg.

Only traces of atropine are found in breast milk. The drug readily crosses the blood-brain barrier and may cause confusion and delirium post-operatively. It crosses the placenta readily.

Atropine is metabolised by hepatic oxidation and conjugation to inactive metabolites, with about 2% undergoing hydrolysis to tropine and tropic acid. About 30% of the dose is excreted unchanged in the urine. Only trace amounts of the dose are eliminated in the faeces.

There is some evidence of prolonged elimination in elderly subjects.

Preclinical safety data: There are no preclinical data of relevance to the prescriber which are additional to that already included in other sections of the SPC.

Pharmaceutical particulars
List of excipients: Hydrochloric acid; Purified water.

Incompatibilities: None known.

Shelf life: 15 months.

Special precautions for storage: Store below 25°C. do not freeze. Protect from light.

Nature and contents of container: A sealed conical shaped polypropylene container fitted with a twist and pull off cap. Overwrapped in an individual polypropylene/paper pouch. Each container holds approximately 0.5 ml of solution.

Instructions for use/handling: Each Minims unit should be discarded after a single use.

Marketing authorisation number 0033/5002R

Date of approval/revision of the SPC August 1997

Legal category POM

MINIMS* BENOXINATE (OXYBUPROCAINE) HYDROCHLORIDE

Quantitative and qualitative composition Single-use, clear, colourless, sterile eye drops, available as a 0.4% w/v solution of Benoxinate (Oxybuprocaine) Hydrochloride USP.

Pharmaceutical form Single-use, sterile eye drops.

Clinical particulars
Therapeutic indications: As a topical ocular anaesthetic.

Posology and method of administration:
Adults (including the elderly) and children: One drop is sufficient when dropped into the conjunctival sac to anaesthetise the surface of the eye to allow tonometry after one minute. A further drop after 90 seconds provides adequate anaesthesia for the fitting of contact lenses. Three drops at 90 second intervals provides sufficient anaesthesia for a foreign body to be removed from the corneal epithelium or for incision of a meibomian cyst through the conjunctiva. Corneal sensitivity is normal again after about one hour.

Instil dropwise into the eye according to the recommended dosage.

Each Minims unit should be discarded after use.

Contra-indications: Not to be used in patients with a known hypersensitivity to the product.

Special warnings and precautions for use: Transient stinging and blurring of vision may occur on instillation.

The anaesthetised eye should be protected from dust and bacterial contamination.

When applied to the conjunctiva, benoxinate is less irritant than amethocaine in normal concentrations.

The cornea may be damaged by prolonged application of anaesthetic eye drops.

Systemic absorption may be reduced by compressing the lacrimal sac at the medial canthus for a minute during and following the instillation of the drops. (This blocks the passage of the drops via the naso-lacrimal duct to the wide absorptive area of the nasal and pharyngeal mucosa. It is especially advisable in children.)

Interaction with other medicaments and other forms of interaction: None stated.

Pregnancy and lactation: This product should not be used in pregnancy or lactation, unless considered essential by the physician.

Effects on ability to drive and use machines: Patients should be advised not to drive or operate hazardous machinery until normal vision is restored.

Undesirable effects: See *Special warnings and precautions for use.*

Overdose: Overdose following the recommended use is unlikely.

Pharmacological properties
Pharmacodynamic properties: Benoxinate hydrochloride is used as a local anaesthetic as it reversibly blocks the propagation and conduction of nerve impulses along nerve axons.

Pharmacokinetic properties: The rate of loss of local anaesthetics through tearflow is very high as they induce an initial stinging reaction which stimulates reflex lacrimation and leads to dilution of the drugs. It is thought that this is responsible for the very short duration of maximum effect of local anaesthetics. The non-ionised base of benoxinate is rapidly absorbed from the pre-corneal tear film by the lipophilic corneal epithelium. The drug then passes into the corneal stroma and from there into the anterior chamber where it is carried away by the aqueous flow and diffuses into the blood circulation in the anterior uvea. As with other ester type local anaesthetics, benoxinate is probably rapidly metabolised by plasma cholinesterases (and also by esterases in the liver).

Preclinical safety data: No adverse safety issues were detected during the development of this formulation. The active ingredient is well established in clinical ophthalmology.

Pharmaceutical particulars
List of excipients: Hydrochloric acid; Purified water.

Incompatibilities: None known.

Shelf life: Unopened: 15 months.

Special precautions for storage: Store below 25°C. Do not freeze. Protect from light.

Nature and contents of container: A sealed conical shaped polypropylene container fitted with a twist and pull off cap. Overwrapped in an individual polypropylene/paper pouch. Each container holds approximately 0.5 ml of solution.

Instructions for use/handling: Each Minims unit should be discarded after a single use.

Marketing authorisation number 0033/5004R

Date of approval/revision of the SPC December 1997

Legal category POM

MINIMS* CHLORAMPHENICOL

Quantitative and qualitative composition Clear, colourless, sterile eye drops containing Chloramphenicol PhEur 0.5% w/v.

Pharmaceutical form Sterile single use eye drop.

Clinical particulars
Therapeutic indications: Chloramphenicol is a broad spectrum bacteriostatic antibiotic. It is active against a wide variety of gram-negative and gram-positive organisms as well as rickettsiae and spirochaetes. It is indicated for use as a topical antibacterial in the treatment of superficial ocular infections.

Posology and method of administration:
Adults (including the elderly) and children: One to two drops applied topically to each affected eye up to six times daily or more frequently if required. (Severe infections may require one to two drops every fifteen to twenty minutes initially, reducing the frequency of instillation gradually as the infection is controlled.)

Contra-indications: Hypersensitivity to chloramphenicol or any component of the preparation.

Special warnings and precautions for use: In severe infections topical use of chloramphenicol should be supplemented with appropriate systemic treatment.

Aplastic anaemia has, rarely, followed topical use of chloramphenicol eye drops and, whilst this hazard is an uncommon one, it should be borne in mind when the benefits of the use of chloramphenicol are assessed.

Prolonged use should be avoided as it may increase the likelihood of sensitisation and the emergence of resistant organisms.

Contact lenses should be removed during the period of treatment.

Systemic absorption may be reduced by compressing the lacrimal sac at the medial canthus for a minute during and following the instillation of the drops. (This blocks the passage of the drops via the naso-lacrimal duct to the wide absorptive area of the nasal and pharyngeal mucosa. It is especially advisable in children.)

Interaction with other medicaments and other forms of interaction: Chymotrypsin will be inhibited if given simultaneously with chloramphenicol.

Pregnancy and lactation: Safety for use in pregnancy and lactation has not been established, therefore, use only when considered essential by the physician.

Effects on ability to drive and use machines: May cause transient blurring of vision on instillation. Warn patients not to drive or operate hazardous machinery unless vision is clear.

Undesirable effects: Local: Sensitivity reactions such as transient irritation, burning, stinging, itching and dermatitis, may occur.

Systemic: Rarely, cases of major adverse haematological events (bone marrow depression, aplastic anaemia and death) have been reported following ocular use of chloramphenicol.

Overdose: Not applicable.

Pharmacological properties
Pharmacodynamic properties: Chloramphenicol is an antibiotic which is mainly bacteriostatic in action, but exerts a bactericidal effect against some strains of gram-positive cocci and against *Haemophilus influenzae* and *Neisseria.* It has a broad spectrum of action against both gram-positive and gram-negative bacteria, rickettsiae and chlamydia.

Pharmacokinetic properties: Chloramphenicol is rapidly absorbed after oral administration. In the liver, chloramphenicol is inactivated by conjugation with glucuronic acid or by reduction to inactive aryl amines. Excretion is mainly renal, though some bile excretion occurs following oral administration.

Preclinical safety data: There are no preclinical data of relevance to the prescriber which are additional to that already included in other sections of the SPC.

Pharmaceutical particulars
List of excipients: Borax; Boric acid; Purified water.

Incompatibilities: None known.

Shelf life: 30 months.

Special precautions for storage: Store between 2° and 8°C. Do not freeze. Protect from light.

Nature and contents of container: A sealed conical shaped polypropylene container fitted with a twist and pull off cap. Each Minims Chloramphenicol unit is overwrapped in an individual polyethylene sachet. 20 units each containing 0.5 ml are packed into a suitable carton.

Instructions for use/handling: Each Minims unit should be discarded after a single use.

Marketing authorisation number 0033/0055R.

Date of approval/revision of the SPC April 1997.

Legal catgegory POM.

MINIMS* CYCLOPENTOLATE HYDROCHLORIDE

Quantitative and qualitative composition Clear, colourless, sterile eye drops containing cyclopentolate hydrochloride BP. Two strengths are available: Cyclopentolate Hydrochloride BP 0.5% and 1% w/v solutions.

Pharmaceutical form Sterile single use eye drop.

Clinical particulars
Therapeutic indications: As a topical mydriatic and cycloplegic.

Posology and method of administration:
Adults (including the elderly): Instil dropwise into eye according to the recommended dosage.

One or two drops as required. Maximum effect is induced 30–60 minutes after instillation.

For refraction and examination of the back of the eye: 1 drop of solution, which may be repeated after five minutes, is usually sufficient.

For anterior and posterior uveitis (if associated with signs of anterior uveitis) and for the breakdown of posterior synechiae: 1–2 drops are instilled every 6–8 hours.

Resistance to cycloplegia can occur in young children, in patients with dark skin and/or patients with dark irides, therefore, the strength of cyclopentolate used should be adjusted accordingly.

Children: <3 months: Not recommended.

3 months–12 years: 1 drop of a 1% solution to each eye.

12 years–adult: 1 drop of 0.5% solution to each eye repeated after 10 minutes if necessary.

Children should be observed for 45 minutes after instillation.

Contra-indications: Do not use in patients with a known hypersensitivity to any component of the preparation.

Should not be used in neonates except where, on expert evaluation, the need is considered to be compelling.

Do not use in patients with confirmed or suspected narrow-angle glaucoma as an acute attack may be precipitated.

Special warnings and precautions for use: Recovery of accommodation occurs within 24 hours.

Use with caution in very young children and other patients at special risk, such as debilitated or aged patients.

Caution is also advised in hyperaemia as increased systemic absorption may occur.

Systemic absorption may be reduced by compressing the lacrimal sac at the medial canthus for a minute during and following the instillation of the drops. (This blocks the passage of the drops via the naso-lacrimal duct to the wide absorptive area of the nasal and pharyngeal mucosa. It is especially advisable in children.)

Interaction with other medicaments and other forms of interaction: None known.

Pregnancy and lactation: The safety for use in pregnancy and lactation has not been established, therefore, use only when considered essential by the physician.

Effects on ability to drive and use machines: May cause transient blurring of vision on instillation. Warn patients not to drive or operate hazardous machinery unless vision is clear.

Undesirable effects:
Local: Local irritation may result following the use of this product. The frequency of this effect occurring is dependant on the concentration instilled.

Increased intraocular pressure may occur in predisposed patients.

Allergic reactions may rarely occur, manifesting as diffusely red eyes with lacrimation and stringy white mucus discharge.

Systemic: Systemic cyclopentolate toxicity is dose-related and is uncommon following administration of 1% solution and would not be expected to occur following instillation of 0.5% solution. Children are, however, more susceptible to such reactions than adults. Toxicity is usually transient and is manifest mainly by CNS disturbances. Any CNS disturbances are characterised by signs and symptoms of cerebellar dysfunction and visual and tactile hallucinations.

Peripheral effects typical of anti-cholinergics, such as flushing or dryness of the skin and mucous membranes, have not been observed with topical cyclopentolate in children or adults. Temperature, pulse and blood pressure are not normally affected.

Overdose: Overdose is rare but symptoms can include those mentioned in the section above. Treatment is supportive.

Pharmacological properties
Pharmacodynamic properties: Cyclopentolate hydrochloride is a synthetic tertiary amine, antimuscarinic compound with actions similar to atropine.

Pharmacokinetic properties: As a group, the synthetic tertiary amine antimuscarinic compounds are well absorbed following oral administration. Cyclopentolate may be absorbed systemically either by transcorneal absorption, direct topical absorption through the skin or by absorption from the nasal or naso lacrimal system.

Preclinical safety data: There are no preclinical data of relevance to the prescriber which are additional to that already included in other sections of the SPC.

Pharmaceutical particulars
List of excipients: Hydrochloric acid; Purified water.

Incompatibilities: None known.

Shelf life: 15 months.

Special precautions for storage: Store below 25°C. Do not freeze. Protect from light.

Nature and contents of container: A sealed, conical shaped container fitted with a twist and pull-off cap. Each Minims unit is overwrapped in an individual polypropylene/paper pouch. Each container holds approximately 0.5 ml of solution.

Instructions for use/handling: Each Minims unit should be discarded after a single use.

Marketing authorisation numbers
Cyclopentolate Hydrochloride 0.5% 0033/5005R
Cyclopentolate Hydrochloride 1% 0033/5006R

Date of approval/revision of the SPC
Cyclopentolate Hydrochloride 0.5% July 1997.
Cyclopentolate Hydrochloride 1% July 1997.

Legal category POM

MINIMS* DEXAMETHASONE

Quantitative and qualitative composition Clear, colourless, sterile eye drops containing dexamethasone sodium phosphate BP 0.1% w/v.

Pharmaceutical form Single-use, sterile eye drops.

Clinical particulars
Therapeutic indications: Non-infected, steroid responsive, inflammatory conditions of the eye.

Posology and method of administration:
Adults (including the elderly): One or two drops should be applied topically to the eye up to six times a day. Note: In severe conditions the treatment may be initiated with 1 or 2 drops every hour, the dosage should then be gradually reduced as the inflammation subsides.

Children: At the discretion of the physician.

Contra-indications: Use is contra-indicated in herpes simplex and other viral diseases of the cornea and conjunctiva, fungal disease, ocular tuberculosis, untreated purulent infections and hypersensitivity to any component of the preparation.

In children, long-term, continuous corticosteroid therapy should be avoided due to possible adrenal suppression.

Special warnings and precautions for use: Care should be taken to ensure that the eye is not infected before Minims Dexamethasone is used.

These drops should be used cautiously in patients with glaucoma and should be considered carefully in patients with a family history of this disease.

Topical corticosteroids should not be used for longer than one week except under ophthalmic supervision, as prolonged application to the eye of preparations containing corticosteroids has caused increased intraocular pressure. The dose of anti-glaucoma medication may need to be adjusted in these patients. Prolonged use may also increase the hazard of secondary ocular infections.

Contact lenses should not be worn during treatment with corticosteroid eye drops due to increased risk of infection.

Systemic absorption may be reduced by compressing the lacrimal sac at the medial canthus for a minute during and following the instillation of the drops. (This blocks the passage of drops via the naso-lacrimal duct to the wide absorptive area of the nasal and pharyngeal mucosa. It is especially advisable in children.)

Interaction with other medicaments and other forms of interaction: The risk of increased intraocular pressure associated with prolonged corticosteroid therapy may be more likely to occur with concomitant use of anticholinergics, especially atropine and related compounds, in patients predisposed to acute angle closure.

The following drug interactions are possible, but are unlikely to be of clinical significance, following the use of Minims Dexamethasone in the eye:

The therapeutic efficacy of dexamethasone may be reduced by phenytoin, phenobarbitone, ephedrine and rifampicin.

Glucocorticoids may increase the need for salicylates as plasma salicylate clearance is increased.

Pregnancy and lactation: Topically applied steroids can be absorbed systemically and have been shown to cause abnormalities of foetal development in pregnant animals. Although the relevance of this finding to human beings has not been established, the use of Minims Dexamethasone during pregnancy should be avoided.

Topically applied dexamethasone is not recommended in breastfeeding mothers, as it is possible that traces of dexamethasone may enter the breast milk.

Effects on ability to drive and use machines: Instillation of this eye drop may cause transient blurring of vision. Warn patients not to drive or operate hazardous machinery until vision is clear.

Undesirable effects: Administration of dexamethasone to the eye may rarely cause stinging, burning, redness or watering of the eyes.

Prolonged treatment with corticosteroids in high dosage is, rarely, associated with subcapsular cataract. In diseases which cause thinning of the cornea or sclera, perforations of the globe have been known to occur. In addition, optic nerve damage and visual acuity and field defects may arise following long term use of this product.

The systemic effects of corticosteroids are possible with excessive use of steroid eye drops.

Overdose: As Minims are single-dose units, overdose is unlikely to occur.

Pharmacological properties
Pharmacodynamic properties: Dexamethasone is a highly potent and long-acting glucocorticoid. It has an approximately 7 times greater anti-inflammatory potency than prednisolone, another commonly prescribed corticosteroid.

The actions of corticosteroids are mediated by the binding of the corticosteroid molecules to receptor molecules located within sensitive cells. Corticosteroid receptors are present in human trabecular meshwork cells and in rabbit iris ciliary body tissue.

Corticosteroids will inhibit phospholipase A2 thereby preventing the generation of substances which mediate inflammation, for example, prostaglandins. Corticosteroids also produce a marked, though transient, lymphocytopenia. This depletion is due to redistribution of the cells, the T lymphocytes being affected to a greater degree than the B lymphocytes. Lymphokine production is reduced, as is the sensitivity of macrophages to activation by lymphokines. Corticosteroids also retard epithelial regeneration, diminish post-inflammatory neo-vascularisation and reduce towards normal levels the excessive permeability of inflamed capillaries.

The actions of corticosteroids described above are exhibited by dexamethasone and they all contribute to its anti-inflammatory effect.

Pharmacokinetic properties: When given topically to the eye, dexamethasone is absorbed into the aqueous humour, cornea, iris, choroid, ciliary body and retina. Systemic absorption occurs but may be significant only at higher dosages or in extended paediatric therapy.

Up to 90% of dexamethasone is absorbed when given by mouth; peak plasma levels are reached between 1 and 2 hours after ingestion and show wide individual variations. Dexamethasone sodium phosphate is rapidly converted to dexamethasone within the circulation. Up to 77% of dexamethasone is bound to plasma proteins, mainly albumin. This percentage, unlike cortisol, remains practically unchanged with increasing steroid concentrations. The mean plasma half life of dexamethasone is 3.6±0.9 h.

Tissue distribution studies in animals show a high uptake of dexamethasone by the liver, kidney and adrenal glands; a volume of distribution has been quoted as 0.58 l/kg. In man, over 60% of circulating steroids are excreted in the urine within 24 hours, largely as unconjugated steroid.

Dexamethasone also appears to be cleared more rapidly from the circulation of the foetus and neonate than in the mother; plasma dexamethasone levels in the foetus and the mother have been found in the ratio of 0.32:1.

Preclinical safety data: The use of corticosteroids, including dexamethasone and its derivatives, is well established in ophthalmology. Little relevant toxicology has been reported, however, the breadth of clinical experience confirms its suitability as a topical ophthalmic agent.

Pharmaceutical particulars
List of excipients: Anhydrous disodium hydrogen phosphate; Sodium dihydrogen phosphate ($2H_2O$); Disodium edetate; Purified water.

Incompatibilities: None known.

Shelf life: 15 months.

Special precautions for storage: Store below 25°C. Do not freeze. Protect from light.

Nature and contents of container: A sealed conical shaped polypropylene container fitted with a twist and pull-off cap. Each Minims unit contains approximately 0.5 ml of solution. Each unit is overwrapped in a sachet. 20 units are packed into a suitable carton.

Instructions for use/handling: Each Minims unit should be discarded after a single use.

Marketing authorisation number PL 0033/0153

Date of approval/revision of SPC November 1997

Legal category POM

MINIMS* FLUORESCEIN SODIUM

Quantitative and qualitative composition Solution of Fluorescein Sodium BP. Two strengths are available: Fluorescein Sodium BP 1% and 2% w/v.

Pharmaceutical form Single-use, sterile eye drops.

Clinical particulars
Therapeutic indications: As a diagnostic stain.

Fluorescein does not stain a normal cornea but conjunctival abrasions are stained yellow or orange, corneal abrasions or ulcers are stained a bright green and foreign bodies are surrounded by a green ring.

Fluorescein can be used in diagnostic examinations including Goldmann tonometry and in the fitting of hard contact lenses.

Posology and method of administration:
Adults (including the elderly) and children: Instil dropwise into the eye.

Sufficient solution should be applied to stain the damaged areas. Excess may be washed away with sterile saline solution.

Contra-indications: Not to be used with soft contact lenses.

Special warnings and precautions for use: Special care should be taken to avoid microbial contamination. *Pseudomonas aeruginosa* grows well in fluorescein solutions, therefore, a single dose solution is preferred. Each Minims unit should be discarded after a single use.

Interaction with other medicaments and other forms of interaction: None known.

Pregnancy and lactation: Safety for use in pregnancy and lactation has not been established, therefore, use only when considered essential by the physician.

Effects on ability to drive and use machines: May cause transient blurring of vision on instillation. Warn patients not to drive or operate hazardous machinery unless vision is clear.

Undesirable effects: None.

Overdose: Overdose following the recommended use is unlikely.

Pharmacological properties
Pharmacodynamic properties: Fluorescein acts as a diagnostic stain.

Pharmacokinetic properties: Fluorescein will resist penetration of a normal cornea and most excess solution will, therefore, be carried with the tear film away from the conjunctival sac. The majority will be lost through the naso-lacrimal ducts and absorbed via the gastro-intestinal tract from where it is converted rapidly to its glucuronide and excreted via the urine.

If fluorescein crosses the cornea it will enter the Bowman's membrane, stroma and possibly the anterior chamber. Aqueous flow and diffusion into the blood in the anterior chamber finally removes fluorescein from the eye and it is excreted unchanged in the urine.

Preclinical safety data: There are no preclinical data of relevance to the prescriber which are additional to that already included in other sections of this SPC.

Pharmaceutical particulars
List of excipients: Purified water.

Incompatibilities: None known.

Shelf life: Unopened 15 months.

Special precautions for storage: Store below 25°C. Do not freeze. Protect from light.

Nature and contents of container: A sealed conical shaped polypropylene container fitted with a twist and pull off cap. Each Minims unit contains approximately 0.5 ml of solution. Each unit is overwrapped in a polypropylene/paper pouch. 20 units are packed into a suitable carton.

Instructions for use/handling: Each Minims unit should be discarded after a single use.

Marketing authorisation numbers
Fluorescein Sodium 1% PL 0033/0079
Fluorescein Sodium 2% PL 0033/5008R

Date of approval/revision of the SPC Fluorescein Sodium 1% October 1997, Fluorescein Sodium 2% July 1997

Legal category P.

MINIMS* GENTAMICIN SULPHATE

Presentation Single-use, clear, colourless sterile eye drops containing Gentamicin Sulphate BP equivalent to 0.3% w/v gentamicin base. The other ingredients are purified water, sodium chloride, borax and sodium hydroxide. No preservatives are included in the formulation.

Uses As a broad-spectrum bactericidal antibiotic, for the treatment of ocular infections caused by both Gram-positive and Gram-negative organisms.

Dosage and administration
Adults (including the elderly): One drop as required.

Children: At the discretion of the physician.

Each Minims unit should be discarded after a single use.

Contra-indications, warnings, etc Gentamicin should not be used in patients with hypersensitivity to gentamicin and/or other aminoglycosides.

Gentamicin has been used topically without any evidence of significant absorption of the drug causing systemic reactions. Gentamicin is well tolerated when applied topically to the eye.

The use of sulphacetamide with gentamicin in the treatment of eye infections is not recommended. Concomitant administration of frusemide and gentamicin may reduce the renal clearance of gentamicin but this is unlikely to be of significance with topical use.

Gentamicin is incompatible with amphotericin, cephalosporins, erythromycin, heparin, penicillins, sodium bicarbonate and sulphadiazine sodium. This is unlikely to be relevant regarding topical use.

The use of gentamicin during pregnancy is not recommended.

Gentamicin should not be the first choice antibiotic for minor infections, in order to minimise the possibility of bacterial resistance.

Systemic absorption may be reduced by compressing the lacrimal sac at the medial canthus for a minute during and following the instillation of the drops. (This blocks the passage of the drops via the naso-lacrimal duct to the wide absorptive area of the nasal and pharyngeal mucosa. It is especially advisable in children.)

Pharmaceutical precautions Minims Gentamicin Sulphate should be stored below 25°C and should not be exposed to strong light. Do not freeze.

Legal category POM

Package quantities Cartons of 20 units, each unit containing approximately 0.5 ml. OP.

Further information Nil.

Product licence number 0033/0094

MINIMS* HOMATROPINE HYDROBROMIDE

Quantitative and qualitative composition Clear, colourless, sterile eye drops containing Homatropine Hydrobromide PhEur 2% w/v.

Pharmaceutical form Sterile single use eye drop.

Clinical particulars
Therapeutic indications: Mydriatic and cycloplegic.

Posology and method of administration:
Adults and children: One drop applied topically to the eye, as required.

Instil dropwise into the eye according to the recommended dose.

Homatropine hydrobromide has properties similar to those of atropine and is often used in preference to the latter because its action is more rapid in onset and it has a less prolonged mydriatic action.

Contra-indications: All mydriatics and cycloplegics are contra-indicated in eyes where the filtration angle is narrow, as an acute attack of angle closure glaucoma may be precipitated.

Minims Homatropine Hydrobromide should not be used in patients who are hypersensitive to atropine, patients with myasthenia gravis or patients with tachycardia secondary to cardiac insufficiency or thyrotoxicosis.

Special warnings and precautions for use: Use with caution in patients with fever or in those who may be exposed to elevated environmental temperatures, as there is a risk of heat prostration and hyperthermia.

Minims Homatropine Hydrobromide should not be used during the first three months of life. The safety and efficacy of homatropine in children has not been established. Children with blond hair and blue eyes are more susceptible to the effects of homatropine.

Systemic absorption may be reduced by compressing the lacrimal sac at the medial canthus for a minute during and following the instillation of the drops. (This blocks the passage of the drops via the naso-lacrimal duct to the wide absorptive area of the nasal and pharyngeal mucosa. It is especially advisable in children.)

Interaction with other medicaments and other forms of interaction: None stated.

Pregnancy and lactation: The safety for use in pregnancy and lactation has not been established, therefore, use only when considered essential by the physician.

Effects on ability to drive and use machines: May cause transient blurring of vision on instillation. Warn patients not to drive or operate hazardous machinery unless vision is clear.

Undesirable effects: None known.

Overdose: Not applicable.

Pharmacological properties
Pharmacodynamic properties: Homatropine is an anticholinergic agent which, like atropine, blocks the effects of the acetylcholine at post ganglionic parasympathetic receptor sites. Its effect on receptor sites in the smooth muscle of the ciliary body and sphincter pupillae result in paralysis of accommodation and mydriasis.

Pharmacokinetic properties: Since homatropine is a tertiary ammonium compound like atropine, it is likely to be readily absorbed from the conjunctival mucosa and rapidly distributed throughout the body. At physiological pH only 0.32% of homatropine is in the non-ionised form, which limits its corneal penetration. Very little is known about the distribution, metabolism and elimination of homatropine.

Preclinical safety data: There are no preclinical data of relevance to the prescriber which are additional to that already included in other sections of the SPC.

Pharmaceutical particulars
List of excipients: Hydrochloric acid; Purified water.

Incompatibilities: None known.

Shelf life: 15 months.

Special precautions for storage: Store below 25°C. Do not freeze. Protect from light.

Nature and contents of container: A sealed, conical shaped container fitted with a twist and pull-off cap. Each Minims unit is overwrapped in an individual polypropylene/paper pouch. Each container holds approximately 0.5 ml of solution.

Instructions for use/handling: Each Minims unit should be discarded after a single use.

Marketing authorisation number 0033/5010R

Date of approval/revision of the SPC July 1997

Legal category POM

MINIMS* LIGNOCAINE AND FLUORESCEIN

Presentation Single-use, clear, yellow, sterile eye drops containing Lignocaine (Lidocaine) Hydrochloride PhEur 4.0% w/v and Fluorescein Sodium BP 0.25% w/v. The other ingredients are purified water, polyvinyl pyrrolidone and hydrochloric acid. No preservatives are included in the formulation.

Uses As a diagnostic stain and topical anaesthetic combined. Minims Lignocaine and Fluorescein units are used in the measurement of intraocular pressure by Goldmann tonometry.

Dosage and administration
Adults: One or more drops as required.

Children: At the discretion of the physician.

Each Minims unit should be discarded after a single use.

Contra-indications, warnings etc Known hypersensitivity to lignocaine and other local anaesthetics.

Special care should be taken to protect the anaesthetised eye from foreign body contamination, particularly in elderly patients in whom the duration of anaesthesia may exceed 30 minutes.

This combination has been in use during pregnancy and lactation for a number of years without apparent ill consequence.

Overdose is not expected to cause adverse effects. However, overuse of local anaesthetics can cause keratitis, with loss of corneal epithelium and stromal opacity.

Pharmaceutical precautions Minims Lignocaine and Fluorescein should be stored below 25°C and should not be exposed to strong light. Do not freeze.

Legal category POM

Package quantities Cartons of 20 units, each unit containing approximately 0.5 ml. OP.

Further information Nil.

Product licence number 0033/0073

MINIMS* METIPRANOLOL

Presentation Single-use, clear, colourless, sterile eye drops. Two strengths are available: 0.1% w/v and 0.3% w/v Metipranolol. The other ingredients are purified water, sodium chloride, hydrochloric acid and sodium hydroxide. No preservatives are included in the formulation.

Uses Metipranolol is a non-selective beta-adrenoceptor blocking agent.

Minims Metipranolol is indicated for the treatment of raised intraocular pressure. It is particularly suitable for the control of post-operative intraocular pressure and for the treatment of chronic open-angle glaucoma in patients who are allergic to preservatives.

The use of Minims Metipranolol in patients with chronic glaucoma should be restricted only to those patients who are allergic to the preservatives commonly used in multidose preparations, or those patients wearing soft contact lenses in whom benzalkonium chloride should be avoided.

Dosage and administration
Adults (including the elderly): The recommended dose is one drop instilled into the affected eye twice daily. Newly diagnosed patients should be treated in the first instance with the 0.1% w/v strength, changing to a higher strength if adequate control is not achieved or maintained.

In the treatment of post-operative rises in intraocular pressure, the dosage and frequency should be at the discretion of the physician.

Children: At the discretion of the physician. No clinical trials in children have been carried out.

Each Minims unit should be discarded after a single use.

Contra-indications, warnings, etc
Contra-indications: Bronchial asthma, history of bronchial asthma, chronic obstructive airways disease, sinus bradycardia, second or third degree atrioventricular block, cardiac failure, cardiogenic shock, hypersensitivity to any of the components of the preparation.

Precautions and warnings: As with other topically applied beta-blockers, systemic absorption may occur giving adverse reactions similar to those of orally administered beta-blockers.

Cardiac and respiratory reactions have been reported with topically applied beta-blockers including, rarely, death due to bronchospasm or cardiac failure.

Congestive cardiac failure should be adequately controlled before starting therapy with Minims Metipranolol. If the patient has a history of cardiac disease, pulse rate should be monitored.

Diabetic control should be monitored during Minims Metipranolol therapy in patients with labile diabetes.

Granulomatous anterior uveitis has been reported in association with the use of the multidose preparation of metipranolol in patients with chronic glaucoma. In any case where a patient shows symptoms or signs suggestive of anterior uveitis, Minims Metipranolol should be withdrawn and an alternative ocular hypotensive agent substituted.

Systemic absorption may be reduced by compressing the lacrimal sac at the medial canthus for a minute during and following the instillation of the drops. (This blocks the passage of the drops via the naso-lacrimal duct to the wide absorptive area of the nasal and pharyngeal mucosa. It is especially advisable in children.)

Use in pregnancy: Although there is no evidence to suggest that metipranolol has teratogenic properties, its use during pregnancy should be avoided unless the potential benefits are considered to outweigh the possible hazards.

Use in lactation: As beta-blockers can pass into breast milk, consideration should be given to stopping breast-feeding if Minims Metipranolol is considered necessary.

Side-effects:
Ocular: Transient burning or stinging on instillation, blurred vision, superficial punctate keratitis, blepharoconjunctivitis and anterior uveitis have been reported.

Cardiovascular: Bradycardia and hypotension can occasionally occur following the systemic absorption of topically applied beta-blockers.

Respiratory: Bronchospasm can occur, predominantly in patients with a history of reversible obstructive airways disease. Dyspnoea and respiratory failure have also been reported with topically applied beta-blockers.

CNS: Headache, ataxia, weakness and lethargy can occur.

Dermatological: Local manifestations of contact sensitivity. Reactions around the eyes can involve skin rashes on the lower lids and cheeks and periorbital oedema.

Drug interactions: Caution should be exercised if used in conjunction with oral beta-blockers as additive effects on systemic beta-blockade may occur. In particular, care should be taken in patients with sinus bradycardia and greater than first-degree heart block.

Beta-blockers should not be given with verapamil and neither drug should be administered within several days of discontinuing the other.

Pharmaceutical precautions Minims should be stored below 25°C and should not be exposed to strong light. Do not freeze.

Legal category POM

Package quantities Cartons of 20 units, each unit containing approximately 0.5 ml solution. OP.

Further information Metipranolol has little or no effect on pupil size or accommodation. Metipranolol is generally well tolerated but some patients may experience slight transient stinging. Transient headaches have been reported.

Product licence numbers
Metipranolol 0.1% 0033/0121
Metipranolol 0.3% 0033/0122

MINIMS* NEOMYCIN SULPHATE

Qualitative and quantitative composition Clear, colourless, sterile eye drops, available as a 0.5% w/v solution of Neomycin Sulphate PhEur.

Pharmaceutical form Sterile single-use eye drop.

Clinical particulars
Therapeutic indications: For the topical treatment of superficial ocular infections caused by sensitive pathogens.

Posology and method of administration: One or two drops applied to each affected eye up to six times daily or more frequently if required. (Severe infections may require one or two drops every fifteen to twenty minutes initially, reducing the frequency of instillation gradually as the infection is controlled.)

Contra-indications: Hypersensitivity to neomycin or to any component of the preparation. (Cross-sensitivity with other aminoglycoside antibiotics may occur.)

Special warnings and special precautions for use:
(a) In severe infections topical use of neomycin should be supplemented with appropriate systemic treatment.
(b) Prolonged use should be avoided as it may lead to skin sensitisation and the emergence of resistant organisms.
(c) Neomycin may cause irreversible, partial or total deafness when given systemically or when applied topically to open wounds or damaged skin. This effect is dose-related and is enhanced by renal or hepatic impairment. Although this effect has not been reported following topical ocular use, the possibility should be considered when high dose topical treatment is given to small children or infants.
(d) Contact lenses should be removed during the period of treatment.
(e) Systemic absorption may be reduced by compressing the lacrimal sac at the medial canthus for a minute during and following the instillation of the drops. (This blocks the passage of the drops via the naso lacrimal duct to the wide absorptive area of the nasal and pharyngeal mucosa. It is especially advisable in children.)

Interaction with other medicaments and other forms of interaction: None relevant to topical use.

Pregnancy and lactation: Safety for use in pregnancy and lactation has not been established therefore use only when considered essential by the physician.

Effects on ability to drive and use machines: May cause transient blurring of vision on instillation. Warn patients not to drive or operate hazardous machinery until vision is clear.

Undesirable effects: Hypersensitivity reactions, usually of the delayed type, occur frequently with local treatment with neomycin. Irritation, burning, stinging, itching and dermatitis may occur.

Overdose: Please see *'Special warnings and special precautions for use'* above.

Pharmacological properties
Pharmacodynamic properties: Neomycin is a broad spectrum antibiotic effective against a wide range of Gram-positive and Gram-negative micro-organisms. It has no activity against viruses or fungi.

Pharmacokinetic properties: No specific human topical ocular pharmacokinetic data are available.

Preclinical safety data: No unexpected safety issues were identified during the development of this product.

Pharmaceutical particulars
List of excipients: Purified water; sodium dihydrogen phosphate; disodium edetate.

Incompatibilities: None applicable.

Shelf life: 15 months.

Special precautions for storage: Store below 25°C. Do not freeze. Protect from light.

Nature and contents of container: A sealed conical shaped polypropylene container fitted with a twist and pull off cap. Each Minims unit is overwrapped in an individual polypropylene/paper pouch.

Instructions for use/handling: Each Minims unit should be discarded after a single use.

Marketing authorisation number 0033/5012R

Date of approval/revision of SPC July 1996

Legal category POM

MINIMS* PHENYLEPHRINE HYDROCHLORIDE

Quantitative and qualitative composition

Pharmaceutical form Single-use, clear, colourless, sterile eye drops. Two strengths are available: Phenylephrine Hydrochloride BP 2.5% and 10% w/v solutions. No preservatives are included in the formulation.

Clinical particulars
Therapeutic indications: Phenylephrine is a directly acting sympathomimetic agent used topically in the eye as a mydriatic. It may be indicated to dilate the pupil in diagnostic or therapeutic procedures.

Posology and method of administration:
Adults: Apply one drop to each eye. If necessary, this dose may be repeated once only, at least one hour after the first drop.

N.B. The use of a drop of topical anaesthetic a few minutes before instillation of phenylephrine is recommended to prevent stinging.

Children and the elderly: The use of phenylephrine 10% solution is contra-indicated in these groups because of the increased risks of systemic toxicity.

Contra-indications: Patients with cardiac disease, hypertension, aneurysms, thyrotoxicosis, long-standing insulin dependent diabetes mellitus and tachycardia.

Patients on monoamine oxidase inhibitors, tricyclic antidepressants and anti-hypertensive agents (including beta-blockers).

Patients with closed angle glaucoma (unless previously treated with iridectomy) and patients with a narrow angle prone to glaucoma precipitated by mydriatics.

Hypersensitivity to phenylephrine or any component of the preparation.

Special warnings and precautions for use: Use with caution in the presence of diabetes, cerebral arteriosclerosis or long standing bronchial asthma.

To reduce the risk of precipitating an attack of narrow angle glaucoma evaluate the anterior chamber angle before use.

Corneal clouding may occur if phenylephrine 10% is instilled when the corneal epithelium has been denuded or damaged.

Systemic absorption may be minimised by compressing the lacrimal sac at the medial canthus for one minute during and after the instillation of the drops. This blocks the passage of the drops via the naso-lacrimal duct to the wide absorptive area of the nasal and pharyngeal mucosa.

Interaction with other medicaments and other forms of interaction:
Anti-hypertensive agents: Topical phenylephrine should not be used as it may reverse the action of many anti-hypertensive agents with possibly fatal consequences.

Monoamine oxidase inhibitors: There is an increased risk of adrenergic reactions when used simultaneously with, or up to three weeks after, the administration of MAOIs.

Tricyclic Antidepressants: The pressor response to adrenergic agents and the risk of cardiac arrhythmia may be potentiated in patients receiving tricyclic antidepressants (or within several days of their discontinuation).

Halothane: Because of the increased risk of ventricular fibrillation, phenylephrine should be used with caution during general anaesthesia with anaesthetic agents which sensitise the myocardium to sympathomimetics.

Cardiac glycosides or quinidine: There is an increased risk of arrhythmias.

Pregnancy and lactation: Safety for use in pregnancy and lactation has not been established. This product should only be used during pregnancy if it is considered by the physician to be essential.

Effects on ability to drive and use machines: May cause stinging and temporarily blurred vision. Warn patients not to drive or operate hazardous machinery until vision is clear.

Undesirable effects:
Local: Eye pain and stinging on instillation (use of a drop of topical anaesthetic a few minutes before the instillation of phenylephrine is recommended), temporarily blurred vision and photophobia, conjunctival sensitisation and allergy may occur.

Systemic: Palpitations, tachycardia, extrasystoles, cardiac arrhythmias and hypertension.

Serious cardiovascular reactions including coronary artery spasm, ventricular arrhythmias and myocardial infarctions have occurred following topical use of 10% phenylephrine. These sometimes fatal reactions have usually occurred in patients with pre-existing cardiovascular disease.

Overdose: Because a severe toxic reactions to phenylephrine is of rapid onset and short duration, treatment is primarily supportive. Prompt injection of a rapidly acting alpha-adrenergic blocking agent such as phentolamine (dose 2 to 5 mg iv) has been recommended.

Pharmacological properties
Pharmacodynamic properties: Phenylephrine is a direct acting sympathomimetic agent. It causes mydriasis via the stimulation of alpha receptors. There is almost no cycloplegic effect.

Maximal mydriasis occurs in 60- 90 minutes with recovery after 5–7 hours.

The mydriatic effects of phenylephrine can be reversed with thymoxamine.

Pharmacokinetic properties: Phenylephrine is a weak base at physiological pH. The extent of ocular penetration is determined by the condition of the cornea. A healthy cornea presents a physical barrier, in addition to which, some metabolic activity may occur. Where the corneal epithelium is damaged, the effect of the barrier and the extent of metabolism are reduced, leading to greater absorption.

Preclinical safety data: The use of phenylephrine in ophthalmology has been well-established for many years. No unexpected adverse safety issues were identified during the development of the Minims format.

Pharmaceutical particulars
List of excipients: Purified water; sodium metabisulphite; disodium edetate.

Incompatibilities: None relevant.

Shelf life: 15 months.

Special precautions for storage: Store below 25°C. Do not freeze. Protect from light.

Nature and contents of container: A sealed conical shaped polypropylene container fitted with a twist and pull off cap. Overwrapped in an individual polypropylene/paper pouch. Each container holds approximately 0.5 ml of solution.

Instructions for use/handling: Each Minims unit should be discarded after a single use.

Marketing authorisation numbers
Minims Phenylephrine 2.5% 0033/0117
Minims Phenylephrine 10% 0033/5021R

Date of approval/revision of SPC
Minims Phenylephrine 2.5% September 1996
Minims Phenylephrine 10% January 1997

Legal category P

MINIMS* PILOCARPINE NITRATE

Quantitative and qualitative composition Three strengths are available: Pilocarpine Nitrate PhEur 1%, 2% and 4% w/v solutions. No preservatives are included in the formulation.

Pharmaceutical form Single-use, clear, colourless, sterile eye drops.

Clinical particulars
Therapeutic indications: Pilocarpine is used as a miotic for reversing the action of weaker mydriatics and in the emergency treatment of glaucoma.

Posology and method of administration:

Adults (including the elderly) and children: Instil dropwise into the eye according to the recommended dosage.

To induce miosis, one or two drops should be used.

In cases of emergency treatment of acute narrow-angle glaucoma, one drop should be used every five minutes until miosis is achieved.

Contra-indications: Conditions where pupillary constriction is undesirable e.g. acute iritis, anterior uveitis and some forms of secondary glaucoma.

Hypersensitivity to any component of the preparation.

Patients with soft contact lenses should not use this preparation.

Special warnings and precautions for use: Systemic reactions rarely occur when treating chronic simple glaucoma at normal doses. However, in the treatment of acute closed-angle glaucoma the possibility of systemic reactions must be considered because of the higher doses given. Caution is particularly advised in patients with acute heart failure, bronchial asthma, peptic ulceration, hypertension, urinary tract obstruction, Parkinson's disease and corneal abrasions.

Retinal detachments have been caused in susceptible individuals and those with pre-existing retinal disease, therefore, fundus examination is advised in all patients prior to the initiation of therapy.

Patients with chronic glaucoma on long-term pilocarpine therapy should have regular monitoring of intraocular pressure and visual fields.

Systemic absorption may be minimised by compressing the lacrimal sac at the medial canthus for one minute during and after the instillation of the drops. This blocks the passage of the drops via the naso-lacrimal duct to the wide absorptive area of the nasal and pharyngeal mucosa.

Interaction with other medicaments and other forms of interaction: Although clinically not proven, the miotic effects of pilocarpine may be antagonised by long-term topical or systemic corticosteroid therapy, systemic anticholinergics, antihistamines, pethidine, sympathomimetics or tricyclic antidepressants.

Concomitant administration of two miotics is not recommended because of inter-drug antagonism and the risk that unresponsiveness may develop to both drugs.

Pregnancy and lactation: Safety for use in pregnancy and lactation has not been established. This product should only be used during pregnancy if it is considered by the physician to be essential.

Effects on ability to drive and use machines: Causes difficulty with dark adaptation, therefore, caution is necessary when night driving and when hazardous tasks are undertaken in poor illumination. May cause accommodation spasm. Patients should be advised not to drive or use machinery if vision is not clear.

Undesirable effects:
Local: Burning, itching, smarting, blurring of vision, ciliary spasm, conjunctival vascular congestion, induced myopia, sensitisation of the lids and conjunctiva, reduced visual acuity in poor illumination, lens changes with chronic use, increased pupillary block, retinal detachments and vitreous haemorrhages.

CNS: Browache and headache (especially in younger patients who have recently started therapy).

Systemic: Systemic reactions rarely occur in the treatment of chronic simple glaucoma but they may include hypertension, tachycardia, bronchial spasm, pulmonary oedema, salivation, sweating, nausea, vomiting, diarrhoea and lacrimation.

Overdose: If accidentally ingested, induce emesis or perform gastric lavage. Observe for signs of toxicity (salivation, lacrimation, sweating, bronchial spasm, cyanosis, nausea, vomiting and diarrhoea).

Pharmacological properties
Pharmacodynamic properties: Pilocarpine is a direct acting parasympathomimetic drug. It duplicates the muscarinic effect of acetyl choline, but not its nicotinic effects. Consequently, pilocarpine stimulates the smooth muscle and secretary glands but does not affect the striated muscle.

Pharmacokinetic properties: Pilocarpine has a low ocular bioavailability when topically applied and this has been attributed to extensive pre-corneal drug loss in conjunction with the resistance to normal corneal penetration. Further, pilocarpine appears to bind to the eye pigments from which it is gradually released to the muscles.

Inactivation of pilocarpine in the eye is thought to occur by a hydrolysing enzyme. The amount of this enzyme is not changed by the prolonged use of pilocarpine by glaucoma patients, nor is it changed in patients poorly controlled by glaucoma therapy.

Preclinical safety data: There are no preclinical data of relevance to the prescriber which are additional to that already included in other sections of the SPC.

Pharmaceutical particulars
List of excipients: Purified water.

Incompatibilities: None known.

Shelf life: 15 months.

Special precautions for storage: Store below 25°C. Do not freeze. Protect from light.

Nature and contents of container: A sealed conical shaped polypropylene container fitted with a twist and pull off cap. Overwrapped in an individual polypropylene/paper pouch. Each container holds approximately 0.5 ml of solution.

Instructions for use/handling: Each Minims unit should be discarded after a single use.

Marketing authorisation numbers
Minims Pilocarpine 1% 0033/5013R
Minims Pilocarpine 2% 0033/5014R
Minims Pilocarpine 4% 0033/5016R

Date of approval/revision of SPC February 1997

Legal category POM

MINIMS* PREDNISOLONE SODIUM PHOSPHATE

Quantitative and qualitative composition Clear, colourless, sterile eye drops containing Prednisolone Sodium Phosphate BP 0.5% w/v.

Pharmaceutical form Single-use, sterile eye drops.

Clinical particulars
Therapeutic indications: Non-infected inflammatory conditions of the eye.

Posology and method of administration:
Adults (including the elderly): One or two drops applied topically to the eye as required.
Children: At the discretion of the physician.

Contra-indications: Use is contra-indicated in viral, fungal, tuberculous and other bacterial infections.

Prolonged application to the eye of preparations containing corticosteroids has caused increased intraocular pressure and therefore the drops should not be used in patients with glaucoma.

In children, long-term, continuous topical corticosteroid therapy should be avoided due to possible adrenal suppression.

Special warnings and precautions for use: Care should be taken to ensure that the eye is not infected before Minims Prednisolone is used.

Systemic absorption may be reduced by compressing the lacrimal sac at the medial canthus for a minute during and following the instillation of the drops. (This blocks the passage of drops via the naso-lacrimal duct to the wide absorptive area of the nasal and pharyngeal mucosa. It is especially advisable in children.)

Interaction with other medicaments and other forms of interaction: Corticosteroids are known to increase the effects of barbiturates, sedative hypnotics and tricyclic antidepressants.

They will, however, decrease the effects of anticholinesterases, antiviral eye preparations and salicylates.

Pregnancy and lactation: Topical administration of corticosteroids to pregnant animals can cause abnormalities of foetal development and although the relevance of this finding to human beings has not been established, the use of Minims Prednisolone during pregnancy should be avoided.

Effects on ability to drive and use machines: None known.

Undesirable effects: Prolonged treatment with corticosteroids in high dosage is occasionally associated with cataract.

The systemic effects of steroids are possible following the use of Minims Prednisolone, but are, however, unlikely due to the reduced absorption of topical eye drops.

Overdose: As Minims are single dose units, overdose is unlikely to occur.

Pharmacological properties
Pharmacodynamic properties: The actions of corticosteroids are mediated by the binding of the corticosteroid molecules to receptor molecules located within sensitive cells. Corticosteroid receptors are present in human trabecular meshwork cells and in rabbit iris ciliary body tissue.

Prednisolone, in common with other corticosteroids, will inhibit phospholipase A2 and thus decrease prostaglandin formation.

The activation and migration of leucocytes will be affected by prednisolone. A 1% solution of prednisolone has been demonstrated to cause a 5.1% reduction in polymorphonuclear leucocyte mobilisation to an inflamed cornea. Corticosteroids will also lyse and destroy lymphocytes. These actions of prednisolone all contribute to its anti-inflammatory effect.

Pharmacokinetic properties: The oral availability, distribution and excretion of prednisolone is well documented. A figure of 82 ± 13% has been quoted as the oral availability and 1.4 ± 0.3 ml/min/kg as the clearance rate. A half life of 2.1–4.0 hours has been calculated.

With regard to ocular pharmacokinetics, prednisolone sodium phosphate is a highly water soluble compound and is almost lipid insoluble. Therefore, theoretically it should not penetrate the intact corneal epithelium. Nevertheless, 30 minutes after instillation of a drop of 1% drug, corneal concentrations of 10μg/g and aqueous levels of 0.5μg/g have been attained. When a 0.5% solution was instilled in rabbit eyes every 15 minutes for an hour, an aqueous concentration of 2.5μg/ml was measured. Considerable variance exists in the intraocular penetration of prednisolone depending on whether the cornea is normal or abraded.

It can be seen that only low levels of prednisolone will be absorbed systemically, particularly where the cornea is intact.

Any prednisolone which is absorbed will be highly protein-bound in common with other corticosteroids.

Preclinical safety data: The use of prednisolone in ophthalmology is well-established. Little specific toxicology work has been reported, however, the breadth of clinical experience confirms its suitability as a topical ophthalmic agent.

Pharmaceutical particulars
List of excipients: Disodium edetate; disodium dihydrogen phosphate; sodium chloride; sodium hydroxide for pH adjustment; purified water.

Incompatibilities: None known.

Shelf life 15 months.

Special precautions for storage: Store below 25°C. Do not freeze. Protect from light.

Nature and contents of container: A sealed conical shaped polypropylene container fitted with a twist and pull off cap. Overwrapped in an individual polypropylene/paper pouch. Each container holds approximately 0.5 ml of solution.

Instructions for use/handling: Each Minims unit should be discarded after a single use.

Marketing authorisation number 0033/0091

Date of approval/revision of SPC December 1996

Legal category POM

MINIMS* PROXYMETACAINE

Quantitative and qualitative composition Clear, colourless to pale yellow 0.5% w/v solution of Proxymetacaine Hydrochloride BP.

Pharmaceutical form Single-use, sterile eye drops.

Clinical particulars
Therapeutic indications: To be used as a topical ocular anaesthetic.

Posology and method of administration:
Adults (including the elderly) and children:
Deep anaesthesia: Instil 1 drop every 5–10 minutes for 5–7 applications.

Removal of sutures: Instil 1 or 2 drops 2–3 minutes before removal of sutures.

Removal of foreign bodies: Instil 1 or 2 drops prior to operating.

Tonometry: Instil 1 or 2 drops immediately before measurement.

Contra-indications: Use in patients with a known hypersensitivity to proxymetacaine.

In view of the immaturity of the enzyme system which metabolises the ester-type local anaesthetics in premature babies, this product should be avoided in these patients.

Special warnings and precautions for use: This product should be used cautiously and sparingly in patients with known allergies, cardiac disease or hyperthyroidism because of the increased risk of sensitivity reactions.

Minims Proxymetacaine is not miscible with fluorescein, however, fluorescein can be added to the eye after it has been anaesthetised with Minims Proxymetacaine.

This product is not intended for long term use. Regular and prolonged use of topical ocular anaesthetics e.g. in conjunction with contact lens insertion, may cause softening and erosion of the corneal epithelium, which could produce corneal opacification with accompanying loss of vision.

Protection of the eye from rubbing, irritating chemicals and foreign bodies during the period of anaesthesia is very important. Patients should be advised to avoid touching the eye until the anaesthesia has worn off.

Tonometers soaked in sterilising or detergent solutions should be thoroughly rinsed with sterile distilled water prior to use.

Systemic absorption may be reduced by compressing the lacrimal sac at the medial canthus for a minute during and following the instillation of the drops. (This blocks the passage of the drops via the naso lacrimal duct to the wide absorptive area of the nasal and pharyngeal mucosa. It is especially advisable in children.)

Interaction with other medicaments and other forms of interaction: None stated.

Pregnancy and lactation: Safety for use in pregnancy and lactation has not been established, therefore, use only when considered essential by the physician.

Effects on ability to drive and use machines: May

cause transient blurring of vision on instillation. Warn patients not to drive or operate hazardous machinery unless vision is clear.

Undesirable effects: Pupillary dilatation or cycloplegic effects have rarely been observed with proxymetacaine preparations. Irritation of the conjunctiva or other toxic reactions have occurred only rarely. A severe, immediate-type apparently hyperallergic corneal reaction may rarely occur. This includes acute, intense and diffuse epithelial keratitis, a grey groundglass appearance, sloughing of large areas of necrotic epithelium, corneal filaments and sometimes, iritis with descemetitis.

Overdose: Not applicable.

Pharmacological properties
Pharmacodynamic properties: Proxymetacaine, in common with other local anaesthetics, reversibly blocks the initiation and conduction of nerve impulses by decreasing the permeability of the neuronal membrane to sodium ions.

The delay to onset of effect, duration of effect and potency of proxymetacaine are similar to those of amethocaine.

Pharmacokinetic properties: Proxymetacaine is readily absorbed into the systemic circulation where, in common with other ester-type local anaesthetics, it is hydrolysed by plasma esterases. Proxymetacaine is also subject to hepatic metabolism.

Preclinical safety data: No adverse safety issues were identified during the development of this formulation. The ingredients are well established in clinical ophthalmology.

Pharmaceutical particulars
List of excipients: Purified water; hydrochloric acid; sodium hydroxide

Incompatibilities: None known.

Shelf life: 2 years.

Special precautions for storage: The product should be transported in the original packaging. It should be stored at 2–8°C. Do not freeze.

Nature and contents of container: A sealed conical shaped polypropylene container fitted with a twist and pull off cap. Each Minims unit contains approximately 0.5 ml of solution. Each unit is overwrapped in a polyethylene sachet. 20 units are packed into a suitable carton.

Instructions for use/handling: Do not use if solution is more than pale yellow in colour.

Each Minims unit should be discarded after a single use.

Marketing authorisation number 0033/0151

Date of approval/revision of SPC March 1996

Legal category POM

MINIMS* PROXYMETACAINE AND FLUORESCEIN

Quantitative and qualitative composition Clear, yellow solution containing 0.5% w/v Proxymetacaine Hydrochloride BP and 0.25% w/v Fluorescein Sodium BP.

Pharmaceutical form Single-use, sterile eye drops.

Clinical particulars
Therapeutic indications: As a combined topical ocular anaesthetic and diagnostic stain. Uses include tonometry, removal of corneal foreign bodies and other corneal or conjunctival procedures of short duration.

Posology and method of administration:
Adults (including the elderly) and children: Instil one or two drops into the conjunctival sac prior to the procedure.

Each Minims unit should be discarded after a single use to avoid risk of cross infection.

Contra-indications: Do not use in patients with a known hypersensitivity to any component of the preparation. In view of the immaturity of the enzyme system which metabolises the ester type local anaesthetics in premature babies, this product should be avoided in these patients.

Special warnings and precautions for use: This product should be used cautiously and sparingly in patients with known allergies, cardiac disease or hyperthyroidism because of the increased risk of sensitivity reactions.

This product is not intended for long term use. Regular and prolonged use of topical ocular anaesthetics e.g. in conjunction with contact lens insertion, may cause softening and erosion of the corneal epithelium, which could produce corneal opacification with accompanying loss of vision.

Protection of the eye from rubbing, irritating chemicals and foreign bodies during the period of anaesthesia is very important. Patients should be advised to avoid touching the eye until the anaesthesia has worn off.

Tonometers soaked in sterilising or detergent solutions should be thoroughly rinsed with sterile distilled water prior to use.

Systemic absorption may be reduced by compressing the lacrimal sac at the medial canthus for a minute during and following instillation of the drops. (This blocks the passage of the drops via the naso-lacrimal duct to the wide absorptive area of the nasal and pharyngeal mucosa. It is especially advisable in children.)

Interaction with other medicaments and other forms of interaction: None stated.

Pregnancy and lactation: Safety for use in pregnancy and lactation has not been established, therefore, use only when considered essential by the doctor or eye specialist.

Effects on ability to drive and use machines: May cause transient blurring of vision on instillation. Warn patients not to drive or operate hazardous machinery unless vision is clear.

Undesirable effects: Transient mild stinging or blurring of vision may occur immediately following the use of this product.

Pupillary dilatation or cycloplegic effects have been observed infrequently with proxymetacaine preparations. Irritation of the conjunctiva or other toxic reactions have occurred only rarely. A severe, immediate-type apparently hyperallergic corneal reaction may rarely occur. This includes acute, intense and diffuse epithelial keratitis; a grey ground-glass appearance; sloughing of large areas of necrotic epithelium; corneal filaments and sometimes, iritis with descemetitis.

Overdose: Not applicable.

Pharmacological properties
Pharmacodynamic properties: Proxymetacaine, in common with other local anaesthetics, reversibly blocks the initiation and conduction of nerve impulses by decreasing the permeability of the neuronal membrane to sodium ions.

The time to onset of effect, duration of effect and potency of proxymetacaine are similar to those of amethocaine.

Fluorescein does not stain a normal cornea but conjunctival abrasions are stained yellow or orange, corneal abrasions are stained a bright green and foreign bodies are surrounded by a green ring.

Pharmacokinetic properties: Proxymetacaine is readily absorbed into the systemic circulation where, in common with other ester-type local anaesthetics, it is hydrolysed by plasma esterases. Proxymetacaine is also subject to hepatic metabolism.

Fluorescein will resist penetration of a normal cornea and most will therefore be carried with the tear film away from the conjunctival sac. The majority will be lost through the naso-lacrimal ducts and absorbed via the gastro-intestinal tract from where it is converted rapidly to glucuronide and excreted via the urine.

If fluorescein crosses the cornea it will enter the Bowman's membrane, stroma and possibly the anterior chamber. Aqueous flow and diffusion into the blood in the anterior area finally remove fluorescein from the eye and it is excreted unchanged in the urine.

Preclinical safety data: No adverse safety issues were identified during the development of this formulation. The ingredients are well established in clinical ophthalmology.

Pharmaceutical particulars
List of excipients: Purified water; Povidone K30; hydrochloric acid; sodium hydroxide.

Incompatibilities: None known.

Shelf life: 18 months.

Special precautions for storage: The product should be transported in the original packaging. It should be stored at 2–8°C and prevented from freezing.

Nature and contents of container: A sealed conical shaped polypropylene container fitted with a twist and pull off cap. Each Minims unit contains approximately 0.5 ml of solution. Each unit is overwrapped in a polyethylene sachet. 20 units are packed into a suitable carton.

Instructions for use/handling: Each Minims unit should be discarded after a single use. Excess solution may be washed away with sterile saline solution.

Marketing authorisation number 0033/0152

Date of approval/revision of SPC February 1997

Legal category POM

MINIMS* ROSE BENGAL

Quantitative and qualitative composition 1% w/v solution of Rose Bengal.

Pharmaceutical form Single-use, sterile eye drops.

Clinical particulars
Therapeutic indications: As a diagnostic stain.

Rose Bengal solution stains degenerated conjunctival and corneal epithelial cells. It is particularly useful in demonstrating these changes in Sjögren's syndrome, where lack of tears has caused damage.

Posology and method of administration:
Adults (including the elderly) and children: One or two drops to be instilled topically into the eye, as required.

Contra-indications: Rose Bengal can produce severe stinging in dry eyes, where it should be used with care.

Special warnings and precautions for use: Rose Bengal should not be instilled into the eye when the patient is wearing contact lenses.

Interaction with other medicaments and other forms of interaction: None known.

Pregnancy and lactation: The use of Rose Bengal over the last 15 years has not shown any adverse effects. In the absence of any teratology studies, however, Rose Bengal is not recommended in pregnancy unless the therapeutic benefit exceeds the potential risk.

Effects on ability to drive and use machines: May cause transient blurring of vision on instillation. Warn patients not to drive or operate hazardous machinery unless vision is clear.

Undesirable effects: Rose Bengal may discolour the eye lids and/or conjunctiva.

Overdose: As Minims are single-dose units, overdose is unlikely to occur.

Pharmacological properties
Pharmacodynamic properties: Not applicable.

Pharmacokinetic properties: Rose Bengal stains degenerated conjunctival and corneal epithelial cells. It will resist penetration through a normal cornea as it is virtually unable to pass through the membrane of live cells. Therefore, the majority of solution will be carried with the tear film away from the conjunctiva and lost via the naso-lacrimal ducts. In rabbits, this has been demonstrated to occur within a few minutes, but in humans with a normal function, this would seem to occur within 15–30 minutes. Rose Bengal remains in the stained structure and does not diffuse further nor penetrate into the aqueous humour from a mucosal defect. Thus, the stain will remain in the damaged corneal cells and be removed together with these cells. Therefore, the concentration of Rose Bengal absorbed systemically is likely to be negligible.

Preclinical safety data: There are no preclinical data of relevance to the prescriber which are additional to that already included in other sections of this SPC.

Pharmaceutical particulars
List of excipients: Sodium hydroxide; Purified water.

Incompatibilities: None known.

Shelf life: 15 months.

Special precautions for storage: Store below 25°C. Do not freeze. Protect from light.

Nature and contents of container: A sealed conical shaped polypropylene container fitted with a twist and pull off cap. Each Minims unit contains approximately 0.5 ml of solution. Each unit is overwrapped in a polypropylene/paper pouch. 20 units are packed into a suitable carton.

Instructions for use/handling: Each Minims unit should be discarded after a single use.

Marketing authorisation numbers 0033/0048R

Date of approval/revision of the SPC July 1997

Legal category P

MINIMS* SALINE

Quantitative and qualitative composition A clear, colourless liquid containing Sodium Chloride PhEur 0.9% w/v.

Pharmaceutical form Single-use, sterile eye drops.

Clinical particulars
Therapeutic indications: As a topical ocular irrigating solution.

Posology and method of administration:
Adults (including the elderly) and children: Adequate solution should be used to irrigate the eye.

Contra-indications: None.

Special warnings and precautions for use: None.

Interaction with other medicaments and other forms of interaction: None known.

Pregnancy and lactation: Not applicable.

Effects on ability to drive and use machines: None known.

Undesirable effects: None known.

Overdose: Not applicable.

Pharmacological properties
Pharmacodynamic properties: Minims Saline is an isotonic solution of sodium chloride used for irrigation of the eye. There are no pharmacodynamic properties of relevance for this product.

Pharmacokinetic properties: There are no pharmacokinetic properties which are applicable for this product.

Preclinical safety data: There are no preclinical data of relevance to the prescriber which are additional to that already included in other sections of the SPC.

Pharmaceutical particulars
List of excipients: Purified water.

Incompatibilities: None known.

Shelf life: 15 months.

Special precautions for storage: Store below 25°C. Do not freeze. Protect from light.

Nature and contents of container: A sealed conical shaped container fitted with a twist and pull off cap overwrapped in an individual polypropylene/paper pouch. Each Minims unit contains approximately 0.5 ml of solution.

Instructions for use/handling: Discard each unit after a single use.

Marketing authorisation number PL 0033/5017R

Date of approval/revision of SPC June 1997

Legal catgegory P

MINIMS* TROPICAMIDE

Presentation Single-use, clear, colourless, sterile eye drops. Two strengths are available: Tropicamide BP 0.5% and 1% w/v solutions. The other ingredients are purified water, hydrochloric acid and sodium hydroxide. No preservatives are included in the formulation.

Uses As a mydriatic and cycloplegic.

Dosage and administration
Adults: 2 drops at five minute intervals, with a further 1 or 2 drops after 30 minutes if required.

Children: At the discretion of the physician.

Each Minims unit should be discarded after a single use.

Contra-indications, warnings, etc All mydriatics and cycloplegics are contra-indicated in eyes where the filtration angle is narrow, as an acute attack of angle closure glaucoma may be precipitated.

Patients who receive a mydriatic may suffer from photophobia and this may impair their ability to drive under certain circumstances.

There is no evidence as to the drug's safety in human pregnancy nor is there evidence from animal work that it is free from hazard. This product should only be used during pregnancy if considered essential by the physician.

Systemic effects from Minims Tropicamide are not expected. Absorption, however, may be reduced by compressing the lacrimal sac at the medial canthus for a minute during and following the instillation of the drops. (This blocks the passage of the drops via the naso-lacrimal duct to the wide absorptive area of the nasal and pharyngeal mucosa. It is especially advisable in children.)

Should an overdosage occur causing local effects eg. sustained mydriasis, physostigmine 0.25% w/v should be applied.

Pharmaceutical precautions Minims Tropicamide should be stored below 25°C and should not be exposed to strong light. Do not freeze.

Legal category POM

Package quantities Cartons of 20 units, each unit containing approximately 0.5 ml. OP.

Further information The 0.5% solution in particular may be expected to cause little or no cycloplegia.

Product licence numbers
Minims Tropicamide 0.5% 0033/0077
Minims Tropicamide 1% 0033/0078

SIMPLENE*

Qualitative and quantitative composition Clear, viscous, colourless to almost colourless liquid containing Adrenaline BP. Two strengths are available: 0.5% and 1.0% w/v Adrenaline BP in a buffered solution preserved with benzalkonium chloride 0.01% w/v.

Pharmaceutical form Multidose eye drops.

Clinical particulars
Therapeutic indications: Indicated for the treatment of elevated intraocular pressure in open-angle (chronic simple) glaucoma. It may be used in combination with miotics, beta-adrenergic blocking agents or carbonic anhydrase inhibitors where indicated.

Posology and method of administration:
Adults (including the elderly): One or two drops to each eye, usually once or twice daily. (May be given as infrequently as every three days.) Determine the frequency of instillation by tonometry.

When used in conjunction with miotics, instil this drug 5 to 10 minutes after the miotic drops.

Children: As directed by a physician. Safety and efficacy of use in children has not been established.

Contra-indications: Closed-angle glaucoma (unless previously treated with iridectomy). Patients with a narrow angle prone to angle block precipitated by mydriatics. Hypersensitivity to adrenaline or any other component of the preparation. This product contains benzalkonium chloride and should not be used when soft contact lenses are worn.

Special warnings and special precautions for use: Do not use until the diagnosis of glaucoma has been verified and the nature of the glaucoma has been confirmed (as the use of adrenaline is contra-indicated in narrow-angle glaucoma).

To reduce the risk of precipitating an attack of narrow-angle glaucoma, evaluate the anterior chamber angle by gonioscopy before initiating therapy.

Adrenaline eye drops should be used with caution by patients with hypertension, cardiac disease, aneurysms, arrhythmia or tachycardia, hyperthyroidism, cerebral arteriosclerosis and diabetes mellitus.

Maculopathy with a central scotoma may occur following use in aphakic patients. Discontinue use in such patients if visual acuity deteriorates.

Systemic absorption of adrenaline from eye drops may be minimised by compressing the lacrimal sac at the medial canthus for a minute during and following the instillation of the drops. (This blocks the passage of the drops via the naso-lacrimal duct to the wide absorptive area of the nasal and pharyngeal mucosa. It is especially advisable in children.)

Interaction with other medicaments and other forms of interaction:
Monoamine oxidase inhibitors: There is an increased risk of adrenergic reactions when used simultaneously with or up to three weeks after the administration of MAOIs.

Tricyclic antidepressants: The pressor response to adrenergic agents and the risk of cardiac arrhythmia may be potentiated in patients receiving tricyclic antidepressants (or within several days of their discontinuation).

Halothane: Because of the increased risk of ventricular fibrillation, adrenaline should not be given during general anaesthesia with anaesthetic agents which sensitise the myocardium to sympathomimetics.

Pregnancy and lactation: Safety for use in pregnancy and lactation has not been established. This product should not be used during pregnancy unless it is considered essential by the physician.

Effects on ability to drive and use machines: May cause temporarily blurred vision. Warn patients not to drive or operate hazardous machinery unless vision is clear.

Undesirable effects:
Local: Severe smarting on instillation, blurred vision, photophobia, eye pain, conjunctival hyperaemia (resulting in a red eye as a frequent response). Conjunctival sensitisation and allergy and local skin reactions occur occasionally. Pigmentary deposits in the conjunctiva, cornea or eyelids may occur after prolonged use.

CNS: Headache or browache are also common but usually diminish as treatment is continued.

Systemic: Systemic adverse reactions are rare following topical use at normal dosage. However, palpitations, tachycardia, raised blood pressure, extrasystoles, cardiac arrhythmias, faintness, sweating, pallor, trembling and perspiration may occur.

Overdose: Systemic reactions to topical adrenaline are unlikely at normal doses. Greater caution is necessary in children and the elderly and those patients predisposed to such reactions e.g. hypertensive cardiac disease or thyrotoxicosis. A severe reaction to adrenaline is of rapid onset and short duration. The treatment of severe toxic reaction is an immediate intravenous injection of a quick-acting alpha-adrenoceptor blocking agent (such as 2 mg to 5 mg of phentolamine) followed by a beta-adrenoceptor blocking agent (such as 1 mg of propranolol injected over 1 minute and repeated, if necessary at 2 minute intervals up to a maximum of 10 mg (5 mg in anaesthesia)). Adrenaline is almost totally inactive when given by mouth as a result of enzymic degradation in the gut and first pass metabolism in the liver.

Pharmacological properties
Pharmacodynamic properties: Adrenaline is a sympathomimetic drug which acts as an agonist on both alpha and beta type receptors. In the eye, this sympathomimetic action initiates a contraction of the radial muscle of the iris, which leads to a mydriatic effect on the pupil. Adrenaline is also capable of causing local vasoconstriction in the conjunctiva and increased uveal vascular resistance. Except where angle block is produced in eyes with a narrow angle, the intraocular pressure is reduced via actions on both the production and drainage of aqueous humour.

Pharmacokinetic properties: There are no data on the pharmacokinetics of topical Simplene.

Caution should be exercised when treating patients with cardiovascular disease and thyrotoxicosis.

No reports have been received which would indicate that clinically significant systemic reactions have occurred following the use of Simplene.

Preclinical safety data: Adrenaline is a naturally occurring molecule; its use in ophthalmology is well established. Little specific toxicology work has been carried out, however, the breadth of clinical experience confirms its suitability as a topical ophthalmic agent.

Pharmaceutical particulars
List of excipients: Benzalkonium chloride 50% solution (as preservative); purified water; ammonium lactate (as 60% syrup); N-acetyl-L-cysteine; hydroxyethylcellulose; 0.880 ammonium hydroxide.

Incompatibilities: Not known.

Shelf life: Unopened: 24 months. Opened: 28 days.

Special precautions for storage: Store below 25°C. Protect from light.

Nature and contents of container: 7.5 ml of Simplene is supplied in a dropper bottle fitted with a polystyrene or polyethylene pilfer proof cap. Each bottle is enclosed in a nitrogen filled sealed pouch inside a carton. Simplene has a shelf life of 2 years provided the pouch remains unopened.

Instructions for use/handling: Contact between the dropper nozzle and other surfaces should be avoided.

Discard any remaining solution 28 days after first opening the container.

Marketing authorisation numbers
Simplene 0.5% 0033/0072
Simplene 1% 0033/0057R

Date of approval/revision of SPC
Simplene 0.5% May 1997
Simplene 1% October 1995

Legal category POM

SNO* PHENICOL

Qualitative and quantitative composition Multidose, colourless to pale straw coloured eye drops containing Chloramphenicol BP 0.5% w/v.

Pharmaceutical form Multidose sterile eye drops.

Clinical particulars
Therapeutic indications: Chloramphenicol is a broad spectrum bacteriostatic antibiotic. It is active against a wide variety of gram-negative and gram-positive organisms as well as *rickettsiae* and *spirochaetes*. It is indicated for use as a topical antibacterial in the treatment of superficial ocular infections caused by sensitive organisms.

Posology and method of administration:

Adults (including the elderly): One to two drops applied to each affected eye up to six times daily or more frequently if required. (Severe infections may require one to two drops every fifteen to twenty minutes initially, reducing the frequency of instillation gradually as the infection is controlled.)

Children: One drop as required.

Contra-indications: This product is not intended as a long term treatment for dry eye syndromes. Hypersensitivity to chloramphenicol or to any component of the formulation.

Special warnings and special precautions for use: In severe infections topical use of chloramphenicol should be supplemented with appropriate systemic treatment.

Aplastic anaemia has followed topical use of chloramphenicol eye drops and, whilst this hazard is a rare one, it should be considered when the benefits of the use of chloramphenicol are assessed.

Prolonged use should be avoided as it may increase the likelihood of sensitisation and the emergence of resistant organisms.

Contact lenses should be removed during the period of treatment.

Systemic absorption may be reduced by compressing the lacrimal sac at the medial canthus for a minute during and following instillation of the drops. (This blocks the passage of the drops via the naso-lacrimal duct to the wide absorptive area of the nasal and pharyngeal mucosa. This procedure is especially advisable in children).

Interaction with other medicaments and other forms of interaction: Chymotrypsin will be inhibited if given simultaneously with chloramphenicol.

Pregnancy and lactation: Safety for use in pregnancy and lactation has not been established. Therefore, use only when considered essential by the physician.

Effects on ability to drive and use machines: May cause transient blurring of vision on instillation. Warn patients not to drive or operate hazardous machinery unless vision is clear.

Undesirable effects:
Local: Sensitivity reactions such as transient irritation, burning, stinging, itching and dermatitis.
Systemic: Several cases of major adverse haematological events (bone marrow depression, aplastic anaemia and death) have been reported following ocular use of chloramphenicol.

Overdose: Not applicable.

Pharmacological properties
Pharmacodynamic properties: Chloramphenicol binds to the 50S subunit of 70S ribosomes. This prevents the translation of mRNA into protein by inhibiting peptide bond synthesis.

Pharmacokinetic properties: Systemically absorbed chloramphenicol is widely distributed throughout the body. Approximately 53% of the absorbed dose is bound to plasma protein. Plasma half life has a mean of around 5 hours. Excretion is mainly in the form of the glucuronide.

Preclinical safety data: There are no preclinical data of relevance to the prescriber which are additional to that already included in other sections of the SPC.

Pharmaceutical particulars
List of excipients: Chlorhexidine acetate 0.01% w/v as a preservative; purified water; polyvinyl alcohol; disodium citrate; citric acid.

Incompatibilities: None known.

Shelf life: Unopened: 18 months. After opening: 28 days.

Special precautions for storage: Store between 2°C and 8°C. Do not freeze.

Nature and contents of container: Sno phenicol is supplied as a sterile ophthalmic solution in a 10 ml polyethylene bottle with a polyethylene dropper and a polyethylene or polystyrene cap.

Instructions for use/handling: Contact between the dropper nozzle and other surfaces should be avoided.
Discard any remaining solution 28 days after first opening the container.

Marketing authorisation number 0033/0076

Date of approval/revision of SPC April 1996

Legal category POM

SNO* PILO

Quantitative and qualitative composition Three strengths are available: Pilocarpine Hydrochloride PhEur 1.0% w/v, 2.0% w/v and 4.0% w/v.

Pharmaceutical form Multidose eye drops.

Clinical particulars
Therapeutic indications: Sno pilo is a directly-acting miotic used for the treatment of glaucoma. It is indicated for: (1) Chronic simple glaucoma. (2) Acute (closed-angle) glaucoma. Pilocarpine may be used alone or in conjunction with other agents to decrease intraocular pressure prior to surgical treatment. (3) Miosis: To counter the effects of cycloplegic and mydriatic eye drops.

Posology and method of administration:
Adults (including the elderly): One or two drops up to four times daily or as prescribed. The frequency of instillation and concentration of drops used are determined by the severity of the glaucoma and the response to treatment.
Children: At the discretion of the physician. Safety and efficacy of use in children has not been established.

Contra-indications: Conditions where pupillary constriction is undesirable, e.g. acute iritis, anterior uveitis and some forms of secondary glaucoma.
Hypersensitivity to any component of the preparation.
Patients with soft contact lenses should not use this preparation.

Special warnings and precautions for use: Systemic reactions rarely occur in the treatment of chronic simple glaucoma with the usual doses used.

In the treatment of acute closed-angle glaucoma the possibility of systemic reactions must be considered because of the higher doses given. Caution is particularly advised in patients with acute heart failure, bronchial asthma, peptic ulceration, hypertension, urinary tract obstruction, Parkinson's disease and corneal abrasions.

Retinal detachments have been caused in susceptible individuals and those with pre-existing retinal disease, therefore, fundus examination is advised in all patients prior to the initiation of therapy.

Patients with chronic simple glaucoma on long-term pilocarpine therapy should have regular monitoring of intraocular pressure and visual fields.

Interaction with other medicaments and other forms of interaction: Although clinically not proven, the miotic effects of pilocarpine may be antagonised by long-term topical or systemic corticosteroid therapy, systemic anticholinergics, antihistamines, pethidine, sympathomimetics or tricyclic antidepressants. Concomitant administration of two miotics is not recommended because of interdrug antagonism, and unresponsiveness may develop to both drugs.

Pregnancy and lactation: Safety for use in pregnancy and lactation has not been established, therefore, use only when clearly indicated.

Effects on ability to drive and use machines: Causes difficulty with dark adaptation, therefore, caution is necessary with night driving and when hazardous tasks are undertaken in poor illumination. May cause accommodation spasm. Patients should be advised not to drive or use machinery if vision is affected.

Undesirable effects: Local: Burning, itching, smarting, blurring of vision, ciliary spasm, conjunctival vascular congestion, induced myopia, sensitisation of the lids and conjunctiva, reduced visual acuity in poor illumination, lens changes with chronic use, increased pupillary block, retinal detachments and vitreous haemorrhages.
CNS: Browache and headache (especially in younger patients who have recently started therapy).
Systemic: Systemic reactions rarely occur in the treatment of chronic simple glaucoma but they may include hypertension, tachycardia, bronchial spasm, pulmonary oedema, salivation, sweating, nausea, vomiting, diarrhoea and lacrimation.

Overdose: If accidentally ingested, induce emesis or perform gastric lavage. Observe for signs of toxicity (salivation, lacrimation, sweating, bronchial spasm, cyanosis, nausea, vomiting and diarrhoea).

Pharmacological properties
Pharmacodynamic properties: Pilocarpine is a direct-acting parasympathomimetic agent. Its primary action is the stimulation (or inhibition) of autonomic effector cells in a similar manner to that accomplished by the acetylcholine released by stimulation of post-ganglionic parasympathetic nerves i.e. it exhibits a muscarinic action. There is also some nicotinic action.

In the eye, pilocarpine causes a constriction of the ciliary muscle which opens up the trabecular spaces and increases the facility of outflow of the aqueous humour. This together with the diminution of the blood supply to the anterior portion of the uvea, resulting from a constriction of the anterior ciliary arteries as they travel through the belly of the muscle and an opening up of the choroidal veins by traction by the muscle from its origin, assumes a primary importance in lowering the intraocular pressure when the drainage channels are pathologically obstructed in simple glaucoma.

Similarly in closed-angle glaucoma the iris is pulled away from the angle of the anterior chamber, re-establishing filtration in favourable cases when this has been obstructed. The lacrimal secretion is considerably increased. The action of the drug on the blood vessels is important and is effective independently of the mioisis. Although it acts as a vasoconstrictor to the splanchnic areas, it is a dilator to the vessels in the head, a fact seen both in the conjunctival and intraocular vessels. A secondary action of considerable importance in simple glaucoma is its vasodilatory effect which, quite apart from the hypotensive action of the drug, helps to maintain an adequate circulation in the visual state of vasosclerosis which characterises long standing cases of this malady.

Pharmacokinetic properties: Pilocarpine being a tertiary amine, is lipophilic and traverses the cornea well, after topical application. After instillation of two drops of a 2% solution in man, an aqueous humour concentration of 0.2% is achieved at 20 minutes post-instillation.

Small amounts of pilocarpine may be excreted in breast milk. It is not known if it crosses the placenta. Given the normal dosage of pilocarpine by an ocular application, the possible effects of old age, renal and hepatic disease or the kinetics of the drug are unlikely to be of any consequence.

Preclinical safety data: There are no preclinical data of relevance to the prescriber which are additional to that already included in other sections of the SPC.

Pharmaceutical particulars
List of excipients: Sodium acetate; Acetic acid; Polyvinyl alcohol; Benzalkonium chloride; Purified water.

Incompatibilities: None known.

Shelf life: Unopened: 15 months; Opened: 1 month.

Special precautions for storage: Store below 25°C. Do not freeze.

Nature and contents of container: A 10 ml polyethylene bottle fitted with a polyethylene plug and a tamper evident polystyrene or polyethylene pilfer proof cap.

Instructions for use/handling: Discard the remaining solution 1 month after first opening the container.

Marketing authorisation numbers

Sno Pilo 1%	PL 0033/0065R
Sno Pilo 2%	PL 0033/0066R
Sno Pilo 4%	PL 0033/0068R

Date of approval/revision of SPC Sno Pilo 1% September 1997, Sno Pilo 2% September 1997, Sno Pilo 4% September 1997

Legal category POM.

SNO* TEARS

Quantitative and qualitative composition Polyvinyl Alcohol 1.4% w/v.

Pharmaceutical form Multidose eye drops.

Clinical particulars
Therapeutic indications: Sno Tears is used topically to provide tear-like lubrication for the symptomatic relief of dry eyes and eye irritation associated with deficient tear production (usually in cases of keratoconjunctivitis sicca and xerophthalmia).
Sno Tears is also used as an ocular lubricant for artificial eyes.

Posology and method of administration:
Adults (including the elderly) and children: The dose depends on the need for lubrication. Usually one or more drops should be used as required, or as prescribed.

Contra-indications: Hypersensitivity to any component of the preparation.
This product contains benzalkonium chloride, therefore, soft contact lenses should be removed during treatment with Sno tears.

Special warnings and precautions for use: If irritation persists or worsens, or headache, eye pain, vision changes or continued redness occurs, discontinue use and consult a physician.

Interaction with other medicaments and other forms of interaction: None known.

Pregnancy and lactation: There is no evidence of safety of the drug in human pregnancy, but it has been in widespread use for many years without apparent ill-consequence. If any therapy is needed in pregnancy, this preparation can be used if recommended by a physician.

Effects on ability to drive and use machines: May cause transient blurring of vision on instillation. Do not drive or operate hazardous machinery unless vision is clear.

Undesirable effects: May cause transient, mild stinging or temporarily blurred vision.

Overdose: Not applicable.

Pharmacological properties
Pharmacodynamic properties: Polyvinyl alcohol is a wetting agent and as such enables the formation of a tear film to relieve the symptoms of dry eye.

Pharmacokinetic properties: There are not expected to be any systemic reactions occurring following the use of Sno tears.

Preclinical safety data: There are no preclinical data of relevance to the prescriber which are additional to that already included in other sections of the SPC.

Pharmaceutical particulars
List of excipients: Benzalkonium chloride; Disodium edetate; Hydroxyethylcellulose; Sodium chloride; Sodium hydroxide; Purified water.

Incompatibilities: None known.

Shelf life: Unopened: 36 months; Opened: 1 month.

Special precautions for storage: Store below 25°C.

Nature and contents of container: A 10 ml polyethylene bottle fitted with a polyethylene plug and a tamper evident polystyrene or polyethylene pilfer proof cap.

Instructions for use/handling: Discard any remaining solution 1 month after first opening the container.

Marketing authorisation number PL 0033/0097

Date of approval/revision of SPC October 1997

Legal category P

*Trade Mark

Chugai Pharma UK Limited
Mulliner House,
Flanders Road,
Turnham Green,
London W4 1NN

☎ 0181 9875600 🗋 0181 9875660

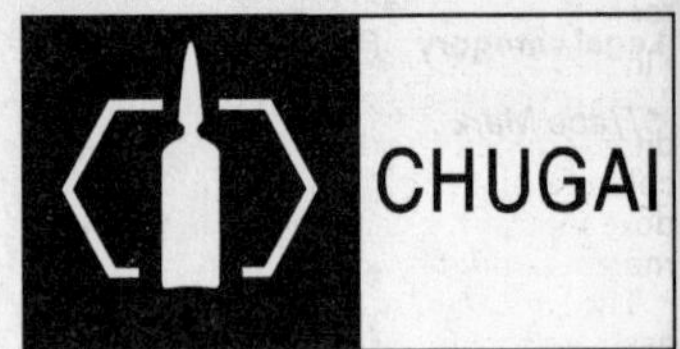

GRANOCYTE* 13, GRANOCYTE* 34 ▼

Qualitative and quantitative composition
Granocyte contains lenograstim, a recombinant glycoprotein (rHuG-CSF) equivalent to the Human Granulocyte Colony Stimulating Factor isolated from CHU-2, a human cell line.

Lenograstim is expressed and glycosylated in a mammalian host cell system, Chinese hamster ovary (CHO) cells.

Composition of the lyophilisate:

	Granocyte 13	Granocyte 34
rHuG-CSF	13.4 MIU*	33.6 MIU*
(lenograstim)	(105 micrograms)	(263 micrograms)

*as measured by the GNFS-60 in vitro bioassay in comparison with the WHO International Standard for human G-CSF.

Composition of the solvent:
Water for Injections 1 ml

Both the product and the solvent are 5% overfilled. The extractable volume of the solvent is therefore 1.05 ml to be used for reconstitution of the lyophilisate in order finally to extract up to 1 ml of Granocyte for use.

Granocyte 13 contains 13.4 Million International Units rHuG-CSF (105 µg) in 1 ml of reconstituted product.

Granocyte 34 contains 33.6 Million International Units rHuG-CSF (263 µg) in 1 ml of reconstituted product.

The reconstituted product is formulated as an aqueous phosphate buffer at pH 6.5 containing 5% mannitol, 0.1% Human Albumin and 0.01% Polysorbate 200.01%.

Pharmaceutical form Powder and solvent for solution for injection or infusion.

Clinical particulars
Therapeutic indications:
Reduction in the duration of neutropenia in patients (with non myeloid malignancy) undergoing myeloablative therapy followed by bone marrow transplantation (BMT) in patients considered to be at increased risk of prolonged severe neutropenia.

Reduction of duration of severe neutropenia and its associated complications in patients with non myeloid malignancy undergoing established cytotoxic chemotherapy associated with a significant incidence of febrile neutropenia.

Mobilisation of peripheral blood progenitor cells (PBPCs).

Note: The safety of the use of Granocyte with antineoplastic agents characterized by cumulative or predominant myelotoxicity vis-à-vis the platelet lineage (nitrosourea, mitomycin) has not been established. Administration of Granocyte might even enhance the toxicities of these agents, particularly vis-à-vis platelets.

Posology and method of administration: The recommended dose of Granocyte 13 is 150 µg (19.2 MIU) per m² per day, therapeutically equivalent to 5 µg (0.64 MIU) per kg per day for: bone marrow transplantation, established cytotoxic chemotherapy, PBPC mobilisation after chemotherapy,
Granocyte 13.4 MIU/vial can be used in patients with body surface area up to 0.7 m²
Granocyte 33.6 MIU/vial can be used in patients with body surface area up to 1.8 m²

For PBPC mobilisation with Granocyte alone, the recommended dose is 10 µg (1.28 MIU) per kg per day

Adults: In bone marrow transplantation: Granocyte should be administered daily at the recommended dose of 150 µg (19.2 MIU) per m² per day as a 30-minute intravenous infusion diluted in isotonic saline solution or as a subcutaneous injection, starting the day following transplantation (see below section on instructions for use). Dosing should continue until the expected nadir has passed and the neutrophil count returns to a stable level compatible with treatment discontinuation, with, if necessary, a maximum of 28 consecutive days of treatment.

It is anticipated that by day 14 following bone marrow transplantation, 50% of patients will achieve neutrophil recovery.

In established cytotoxic chemotherapy: Granocyte should be administered daily at the recommended dose of 150 µg (19.2 MIU) per m² per day as a subcutaneous injection starting on the day following completion of chemotherapy (see below section on instructions for use). Daily administration of Granocyte should continue until the expected nadir has passed and the neutrophil count returns to a stable level compatible with treatment discontinuation, with, if necessary, a maximum of 28 consecutive days of treatment.

A transient increase in neutrophil count may occur within the first 2 days of treatment, however Granocyte treatment should not be stopped, since the subsequent nadir usually occurs earlier and recovers more quickly if treatment continues.

In peripheral blood progenitor cell (PBPC) mobilisation: After chemotherapy, Granocyte should be administered daily, at the recommended dose of 150 µg (19.2 MIU) per m² per day as a subcutaneous injection starting on the day after completion of chemotherapy until the expected nadir has passed and neutrophil count returns to a normal range compatible with treatment discontinuation.

Leucapheresis should be performed when the post nadir leucocyte count is rising or after assessment of CD34⁺ cells in blood with a validated method. For patients who have not had extensive chemotherapy, one leucapheresis if often sufficient to obtain the acceptable minimum yield (≥ 2.0 x 10^6 CD34⁺ cells per kg).

In PBPC mobilisation with Granocyte alone, Granocyte should be administered daily at the recommended dose of 10 µg (1.28 MIU) per kg per day as a subcutaneous injection for 4 to 6 days. Leucapheresis should be performed between day 5 and 7.

In patients who have not had extensive chemotherapy one leucapheresis is often sufficient to obtain the acceptable minimum yield (≥ 2.0 x 10^6 CD34⁺ cells per kg).

In healthy donors, a 10µg/kg daily dose administered subcutaneously for 5-6 days allows a CD34+ cells collection ≥ 3 x 10^6 /kg body weight with a single leukapheresis in 83% of subjects and with 2 leukaphereses in 97%.

Therapy should only be given in collaboration with an experienced oncology and/or hematology centre.

Elderly: Clinical trials with Granocyte have included a small number of patients up to the age of 70 years but special studies have not been performed in the elderly and therefore specific dosage recommendations cannot be made.

Children: The safety and efficacy of Granocyte have been established in patients older than 2 years in BMT.

Contraindications: Granocyte should not be administered to patients or subjects with known hypersensitivity to the product or its constituents.

Granocyte should not be used to increase the dose intensity of cytotoxic chemotherapy beyond established doses and dosage regimens since the drug could reduce myelo-toxicity but not overall toxicity of cytotoxic drugs.

Granocyte should not be administered concurrently with cytotoxic chemotherapy.

Granocyte should not be administered to patients with myeloid malignancy.

Special warning and special precautions for use:
• Malignant Cell Growth

Granulocyte colony stimulating factor can promote growth of myeloid cells in vitro and similar effects may be seen on some non-myeloid cells in vitro.

The safety and efficacy of Granocyte administration in patients with myelodysplasia, acute myelogenous leukemia, or chronic myelogenous leukemia have not been established. Therefore, because of the possibility of tumour growth, Granocyte should not be used in any myeloid malignancy.

Clinical trials have not established whether Granocyte influences the progression of myelodysplastic syndrome to acute myeloid leukemia. Caution should be exercised in using Granocyte in any pre-malignant myeloid condition. As some tumours with non-specific characteristics can exceptionally express a G-CSF receptor, caution should be exerted in the event of unexpected tumour regrowth concomitantly observed with rHuG-CSF therapy.

• Leucocytosis

A leucocyte count greater than 50 x 10^9/l has not been observed in any of the 174 clinical trials patients treated with 5 µg/kg/day (0.64 million units/kg/day) following bone marrow transplantation. White blood cell counts of 70 x 10^9/l or greater have been observed in less than 5% of patients who received cytotoxic chemotherapy and were treated with Granocyte at 5 µg/kg/day (0.64 million units/kg/day). No adverse events directly attribuable to this degree of leucocytosis have been reported. In view of the potential risks associated with severe leucocytosis, a white blood cell count should, however, be performed at regular intervals during Granocyte therapy. If leucocyte counts exceed 50 x 10^9/l after the expected nadir, Granocyte should be discontinued immediately.

During PBPC mobilisation, Granocyte should be discontinued if the leucocyte count rises to > 70 x 10^9/l.

• Pulmonary adverse effect

The onset of pulmonary signs, such as cough, fever and dyspnoea, in association with radiological signs of pulmonary infiltrates and deterioration in pulmonary function may be preliminary signs of adult respiratory distress syndrome (ARDS).

Granocyte should be discontinued and appropriate treatment given.

• In Bone Marrow Transplantation

The effect of Granocyte on the incidence and severity of acute and chronic graft- versus- host disease has not been accurately determined.

• Risks Associated with Increased Doses of Chemotherapy

The safety and efficacy of Granocyte have yet to be established in the context of intensified chemotherapy. Granocyte should not be used to decrease, beyond the established limits, intervals between chemotherapy courses and/or to increase the doses of chemotherapy. Non-myeloid toxicities were limiting factors in a phase II chemotherapy intensification trial with Granocyte

• Special precautions in Peripheral Blood Progenitor Cell mobilisation

Choice of the mobilisation method.

Clinical trials carried out among the same patient population have shown that PBPC mobilisation, as assessed within the same laboratory, was higher when Granocyte was used after chemotherapy than when used alone. Nevertheless the choice between the two mobilisation methods should be considered in relation to the overall objectives of treatment for an individual patient.

Prior exposure to radiotherapy and/or cytotoxic agents.

Patients who have undergone extensive prior myelosuppressive therapy and/or radiotherapy, may not show sufficient PBPC mobilisation to achieve the acceptable minimum yield (≥ 2 x10^6 CD34⁺ /kg) and therefore adequate haematological reconstitution.

A PBPC transplantation program should be defined early in the treatment course of the patient and particular attention should be paid to the number of PBPCs mobilised before the administration of high-dose chemotherapy. If yields are low, the PBPC transplantation program should be replaced by other forms of treatment.

Assessment of progenitor cell yields

Particular attention should be paid to the method of quantification of progenitor cell yields as the results of flow cytometric analysis of CD34⁺ cell number vary among laboratories.

The minimum yield of CD34⁺ cells is not well defined. The recommendation of a minimum yield of ≥ 2.0 x 10^6 CD34⁺ cells/kg is based on published experience in order to achieve adequate haematological reconstitution. Yields higher than ≥ 2.0 x 10^6 CD34⁺

cells/kg are associated with more rapid recovery, including platelets, while lower yields result in slower recovery.

• In healthy donors

The PBPC mobilisation which is a procedure without direct benefit for healthy people should only be considered in accord through a clear selection procedure in accordance with local regulations as for bone marrow donation when applicable.

The efficacy and safety of Granocyte has not been assessed in donors aged over 60 years, therefore the procedure cannot be recommended. Based on some local regulations and lack of studies, minor donors should not be considered.

PBPC mobilisation procedure should be considered for donors who fit usual clinical and laboratory eligibility criteria for bone marrow donation especially normal haematological values.

Marked leucocytosis (WBC ≥ 50 x 10^9/l) was observed in 24% of subjects studied.

Apheresis-related thrombocytopenia (platelets < 100 x 10^9/l) was observed in 42% of subjects studied and values < 50 x 10^9/l were occasionally noted following leukapheresis without related clinical adverse events, all recovered.

Therefore leukapheresis should not be performed in donors who are anticoagulated or who have known defects in hemostasis. If more than one leukapheresis is required particular attention should be paid to donors with platelets < 100 x 10^9/l prior to apheresis; in general apheresis should not be performed if platelets < 75 x 10^9/l.

Insertion of a central venous catheter should be avoided if possible with consideration given to venous access in selection of donors.

Data on long term follow-up of donors are available on a small number of subjects. Up to six years, no emerging long term sequelae have been reported. Nevertheless, a risk of promotion of a malignant myeloid clone is possible.Therefore, it is recommended that systematic record and tracking of the stem-cell donors be made by the apheresis centers.

• In recipients of allogeneic peripheral blood stem-cells mobilized with Granocyte

Allogeneic stem-cell grafting may be associated with an increased risk for chronic GVH (Graft Versus Host Disease), and long-term data of graft functioning are sparse.

• Other Special Precautions

In patients with severe impairment of hepatic or renal function, the safety and efficacy of Granocyte have not been established.

In patients with substantially reduced myeloid progenitor cells (e.g. due to prior intensive radiotherapy/chemotherapy), neutrophil response is sometimes diminished and the safety of Granocyte has not been established.

Interaction with other medications and other forms of interaction: In view of the sensitivity of rapidly dividing myeloid cells to cytotoxic chemotherapy, the use of Granocyte is not recommended from 24 hours before until 24 hours after chemotherapy ends. Possible interactions with other hematopoietic growth factors and cytokines have yet to be investigated in clinical trials.

Pregnancy and lactation: The safety of Granocyte has not been established in pregnant women.

There is no evidence from studies in rats and rabbits that Granocyte is teratogenic. An increased incidence of embryo-loss has been observed in rabbits, but no malformation has been seen. In pregnancy, the possible risk to the foetus for Granocyte use must be weighed against the expected therapeutic benefit.

Granocyte is not recommended for use in nursing women, as it is not known whether Granocyte is excreted in human breast milk.

Effects on ability to drive and use machines: None.

Undesirable Effects:

In Bone Marrow Transplantation

Special attention should be paid to platelet recovery since in double-blind placebo-controlled trials the mean platelet count was lower in patients treated with Granocyte as compared with placebo. However, this did not result in an increase in incidence of adverse events related to blood loss and the median number of days following BMT to last platelet infusion was similar in both groups.

In placebo-controlled trials, the most frequently reported adverse events (15% in at least one treatment group) occurred with equal frequency in patients treated with Granocyte or placebo. These adverse events were those usually encountered with conditioning regimens and were apparently unrelated to Granocyte which did not prevent them. The events consisted of infection/inflammatory disorder of the buccal cavity, fever, diarrhea, rash, abdominal pain, vomiting, alopecia, sepsis and infection.

In Chemotherapy-Induced Neutropenia

The safety of Granocyte use with antineoplastic agents with cumulative bone marrow toxicity or predominant toxicity to the platelet lineage (nitrosourea, mitomycin) has not been established. Granocyte use may even result in enhanced toxicity particularly vis-à-vis platelets.

In trials, the most frequently reported adverse events were the same in patients treated with either Granocyte or placebo. The most commonly reported adverse events were alopecia, nausea, vomiting, fever and headache, similar to those observed in cancer patients treated with chemotherapy.

A slightly higher incidence of bone pain (approximately 10% higher) and injection site reaction (approximately 5% higher) were reported in Granocyte-treated patients.

Other undesirable effects

Pulmonary infiltrates have been reported in some cases with an outcome of respiratory failure or adult respiratory distress syndrome (ARDS), which may be fatal.

In peripheral blood progenitor cell mobilisation

When Granocyte is administered to healthy subjects, the most commonly reported clinical adverse events were headache in 30%, bone pain in 23%, back pain in 17.5%, asthenia in 11%, abdominal pain in 6% and pain in 6% of subjects. The risk of occurrence of pain is increased in subjects with high peak WBC values, especially when WBC ≥ 50 x 10^9/l. Leukocytosis ≥ 50 x 10^9/l was reported in 24% of donors and thrombocytopenia (platelets < 100 x 10^9/l) apheresis-related in 42%.

Transient increase of ASAT and/or ALAT was observed in 12% of subjects and alkaline phosphatase in 16%.

Overdosage: In animals, acute toxicity studies (up to 1000 µg/kg/day in mice) and subacute toxicity studies (up to 100 µg/kg/day in monkey) showed the effects of overdose were restricted to an exaggerated and reversible pharmacological effect.

The effects of Granocyte overdosage have not been established. Discontinuation of Granocyte therapy usually results in a 50% decrease in circulating neutrophils within 1 to 2 days, with a return to normal levels in 1 to 7 days. A white blood cell count of approximately 50 x 10^9/l was observed in one patient out of three receiving the highest Granocyte dose of 40 µg/kg/day (5.12 MIU/kg/day) on the 5th day of treatment

In humans, doses up to 40 µg/kg/day were not associated with toxic side effects except musculoskeletal pain.

Pharmacological properties

Pharmacodynamic properties: Granocyte (rHuG-CSF) listed in the therapeutic classification as L03 A A10, belongs to the cytokine group of biologically active proteins which regulate cell differentiation and cell growth.

rHuG-CSF is a factor that stimulates neutrophil precursor cells as demonstrated by the CFU-S and CFU-GM cell count which increases in peripheral blood.

Granocyte induces a marked increase in peripheral blood neutrophil counts within 24 hours of administration.

Elevations of neutrophil count are dose-dependent over the 1–10 µg/kg/day range. At the recommended dose, repeated doses induce an enhancement of the neutrophil response. Neutrophils produced in response to Granocyte show normal chemotactic and phagocytic functions.

Granulocyte colony stimulating factors displayed angiogenic properties in several experimental systems in vitro.

Use of Granocyte in patients who underwent Bone Marrow Transplantation or who are treated with cytotoxic chemotherapy leads to significant reductions in duration of neutropenia and its associated complications.

Use of Granocyte, either alone or after chemotherapy mobilises haematopoietic progenitor cells into the peripheral blood. These autologous Peripheral Blood Progenitor Cells (PBPCs) can be harvested and infused after high dose cytotoxic chemotherapy, either in place of, or in addition to bone marrow transplantation.

Reinfused PBPCs, as obtained following mobilisation with Granocyte, have been shown to reconstitute haemopoiesis and reduce the time to engraftment, leading to a marked decrease of the days to platelet independance when compared to autologous bone marrow transplantation.

Pharmacokinetic properties: The pharmacokinetics of Granocyte are dose and time dependent.

During repeated dosing (iv and sc routes), peak serum concentration (immediately after iv infusion or after sc injection) are proportional to the injected dose. Repeated dosing with Granocyte by the two administration routes showed no evidence of drug accumulation.

At the recommended dose, the absolute bioavailability of Granocyte is 30%. The apparent volume of distribution (Vd) is approximatively 1 l/kg body weight and the mean residence time close to 7 h following subcutaneous dosing.

The apparent serum elimination half-life of Granocyte (sc route) is approximatively 3–4 h, at steady state (repeated dosing) and is shorter (1–1.5 h) following repeated iv infusion.

Plasma clearance of rHuG-CSF increased 3-fold (from 50 up to 150 ml/min) during repeated sc dosing. Less than 1% of Granocyte is excreted in urine unchanged and Granocyte is considered to be metabolized to peptides. During multiple sc dosing, peak serum concentrations of Granocyte are close to 100 pg/ml/kg body weight at the recommended dosage. There is a positive correlation between the dose and the serum concentration of Granocyte and between the neutrophil response and the total amount of Granocyte recovered in serum.

Pharmaceutical particulars

List of excipients: Human albumin, Mannitol, Polysorbate 20, Disodium phosphate, Sodium dihydrogen phosphate, Sodium chloride.

Incompatibilities: Dilution of Granocyte 13 (13.4 MIU/vial) to a final concentration of less than 0.26 Million International Units/ml (2 µg/ml) is not recommended.

Dilution of Granocyte 34 (33.6 MIU/vial) to a final concentration of less than 0.32 Million International Units/ml (2 µg/ml) is not recommended.

Shelf life: The shelf life of Granocyte is 2 years when stored in a refrigerator at between +2°C and +8°C.

Special precautions for storage: Granocyte should be stored in a refrigerator at between +2°C and +8°C.

Short exposure of the vials to elevated temperatures (up to 2 weeks at +30°C) does not affect the product stability.

No decrease in activity was observed after dilution to a final concentration of not less than 0.26 MIU/ml (2µg/ml) for Granocyte 13 (13.4 MIU/vial) or not less than 0.32 MIU/ml (2µg/ml) for Granocyte 34 (33.6 MIU/vial) when the dilution was stored at +5°C or at +25°C for 24 hours.

Granocyte should not be reconstituted and/or diluted more than 24 hours before administration and solutions should be stored refrigerated at +2–+8°C.

Unused reconstitued or diluted solution should be discarded.

Nature and contents of container: Lyophilisate (white lyophilised powder) in vial (glass) + 1 ml of solvent (Water for Injections) in pre-filled syringe (glass) + 2 needles (19 G for reconstitution and 26 G for administration) or lyophilisate (white lyophilised powder) in vial (glass) + 1 ml of solvent (Water for Injections) in ampoule (glass) for reconstitution and administration

Presentations of Granocyte 13:

1 pack of 5 x 1 [13.4 MIU (105 µg)] vial + 5 x 1 (1 ml) prefilled syringe with solvent

1 pack of 1 x 1 [13.4 MIU (105 µg)] vial + 1 x 1 (1 ml) ampoule with solvent

Presentations of Granocyte 34:

1 pack of 5 x 1 [33.6 MIU (263 µg)] vial + 5 x 1 (1 ml) prefilled syringe with solvent

1 pack of 5 x 1 [33.6 MIU (263 µg)] vial + 5 x 1 (1 ml) ampoule with solvent

Instructions for use: Granocyte vials are for single-dose use only.

Preparation of subcutaneous injection solution: Aseptically add the extractable contents of one ampoule or of one prefilled syringe of solvent (Water for Injection) to the Granocyte vial :

1.05 ml for Granocyte

Agitate gently until complete dissolution (about 5 seconds). Do not shake vigorously.

Withdraw the required volume from the vial.

Administer immediately by SC injection.

Preparation of infusion: Aseptically add the extractable contents of one ampoule or of one prefilled syringe of solvent (Water for Injection) to the Granocyte vial :

1.05 ml for Granocyte

Agitate gently until complete dissolution (about 5 seconds). Do not shake vigorously.

Withdraw the required volume from the vial.

Dilute the resulting solution in 0.9% sodium chloride solution.

Administer by IV route.

Dilution of Granocyte 13 (13.4 MIU/vial) to a final concentration of less than 0.26 Million International Units/ml (2 µg/ml) is not recommended.

(i.e. One vial of reconstituted Granocyte 13 should be diluted in 0.9% sodium chloride solution to give a total volume of no more than 50 ml).

Dilution of Granocyte 34 (33.6 MIU/vial) to a final concentration of less than 0.32 Million International Units/ml (2.5 μg/ml) is not recommended.

(i.e. One vial of reconstituted Granocyte 34 should be diluted in 0.9% sodium chloride solution to give a total volume of no more than 100 ml).

When diluted in a 0.9% saline solution Granocyte is compatible with the commonly used giving-sets for injection (polyvinyl chloride).

Marketing authorisation holder: Chugai Pharma UK Ltd, Mulliner House, Flanders Road, Turnham Green, London W4 1NN.

Marketing authorisation number
PL 12185/0002
PL 12185/0005 (water for injection in prefilled syringe)

Date of first authorisation November 1993

Date of revision of the text November 1998

**Trade Mark*

CIBA Vision
Flanders Road
Hedge End
Southampton
Hampshire SO30 2LG

☎ 01489 775534 🗋 01489 798074

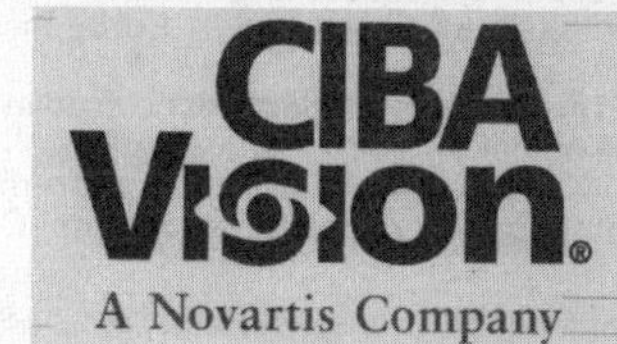

HYPOTEARS*

Presentation A sterile colourless, hypotonic aqueous solution, containing 1.0% w/v polyvinyl alcohol. It also contains disodium edetate, benzalkonium chloride (preservative), polyethylene glycol and purified water.

Uses An ocular lubricant for the treatment and symptomatic relief of physiological dry eye conditions and associated irritation.

Dosage and administration
Adults: One or two drops in the affected eye(s) as required.

Elderly and children: No dosage amendment is necessary in the elderly or in children.

Contra-indications, warnings, etc
Contra-indications: Patients with known hypersensitivity to benzalkonium chloride.

Due to the presence of benzalkonium chloride this product should not be prescribed for patients who wear soft contact lenses.

Precautions: Discontinue use if allergy develops to any component of the preparation. To avoid contamination of the solution, do not touch dropper tip to any surface, particularly the eyelids or surrounding area. For topical use only. Discard any remainder 28 days after opening. If eye irritation persists discontinue use and seek medical advice.

Pregnancy: There is no experience regarding the safety of Hypotears in human pregnancy or lactation.

Side-effects: As with other lubricating artificial tear solutions, transient stinging and/or burning has been reported.

Overdosage: Not applicable.

Effect on ability to drive or use machines: Hypotears does not have any sedative effect and so will not affect ability to drive and to use machines.

Pharmaceutical precautions Store below 30°C

Legal category P

Package quantities 15 ml

Further information Hypotears is an ocular lubricant which relieves irritation or dryness of eyes due to physiological dry eye conditions. Hypotears normalises the pre-corneal tear film by balancing tear film osmolarity and stabilises the mucin and aqueous tear layers. The polyvinyl alcohol contained in Hypotears has mucomimetic properties to soothe and lubricate the dry eye and enhance tear film stability. Polyvinyl alcohol also reduces the surface tension of the tears to increase the wetting of the cornea by the tear film.

There are no pharmacologically active constituents in Hypotears. The action of polyvinyl alcohol in the eye is based on its demulcent and lubricating properties rather than chemical or pharmacological actions.

Product licence number 8685/0012

LIVOSTIN* EYE DROPS ▼

Presentation White sterile ophthalmic microsuspension (pH6-8) containing levocabastine hydrochloride equivalent to 0.5 mg/ml levocabastine. Livostin eye drops also contain benzalkonium chloride, disodium edetate, propylene glycol, polysorbate 80, disodium phosphate, monosodium phosphate, hypromellose and water.

Uses Levocabastine is a selective histamine H_1 antagonist.

Livostin eye drops are indicated for the symptomatic treatment of seasonal allergic conjunctivitis.

Dosage and administration As Livostin eye drops are a microsuspension, the bottle should be shaken before each application.

Adults, the elderly and children 9 years and over: The usual dose is 1 drop of Livostin eye drops per eye, twice a day. The dose may be increased to 1 drop per eye 3 to 4 times daily, if necessary. Treatment should not be continued beyond 4 weeks. Exposure to the product is limited to a total of 4 weeks in any one year.

It is not useful to continue treatment for more than 3 days if no improvement is seen.

Use in children: Livostin eye drops are not recommended for use in children less than 9 years.

Contra-indications, warnings, etc
Contra-indications: Hypersensitivity to any of the ingredients.

Precautions: As with all ophthalmic preparations containing benzalkonium chloride patients are advised not to wear soft (hydrophilic) contact lenses whilst being treated with Livostin eye drops.

Use in pregnancy and lactation: In mice, rats and rabbits, Livostin, at oral doses up to 8,300 times the recommended ocular clinical dose, did not reveal any embryotoxic or teratogenic effect. In rodents, at 16,500 times this dose and higher, teratogenicity and/or increased embryonal resorption were observed.

There are no adequate data on the use of Livostin eye drops in pregnant women, therefore Livostin eye drops should not be used during pregnancy, unless the potential benefit justifies the potential risk to the foetus.

Based on determinations of levocabastine concentrations in saliva and breast milk in a nursing woman, it was calculated that the daily dose of levocabastine in the infant would not exceed 0.5µg after ophthalmic treatment of the mother. Therefore levocabastine eye drops can be given to nursing mothers.

Effects on ability to drive or use machines: Sedation has rarely been reported during concomitant use of the eye drops and nasal spray. This should be borne in mind when special alertness is necessary eg in connection with driving or in performance of skilled tasks.

Side-effects: Effects such as local irritation, blurring of vision, eye oedema, urticaria, dyspnoea and headache have been reported after instillation of Livostin Eye Drops. If effects are severe it may be necessary to discontinue treatment.

Overdosage: Overdosage is unlikely following topical use. In the event of accidental oral ingestion, supportive measures should be taken.

Pharmaceutical precautions Store below 25°C. Use within one month of opening the bottle. Shake well before use

Legal category POM

Package quantities White plastic bottles containing 4 ml microsuspension.

Further information Nil

Product licence number 0242/0151

LIVOSTIN* NASAL SPRAY ▼

Presentation White sterile microsuspension (pH6-8) containing levocabastine hydrochloride equivalent to 0.5 mg/ml levocabastine. Livostin nasal spray also contains benzalkonium chloride, disodium edetate, propylene glycol, polysorbate 80, disodium phosphate, monosodium phosphate, hypromellose and water.

Uses Levocabastine is a selective histamine H_1 antagonist.

Livostin nasal spray is indicated for the symptomatic treatment of seasonal allergic rhinitis.

Dosage and administration As Livostin nasal spray is a microsuspension, the bottle should be shaken before each application.

Adults and children 9 years and over: The usual dose is 2 sprays per nostril of Livostin nasal spray, twice daily. The dose may be increased to 2 sprays per nostril 3 to 4 times daily, if necessary. Treatment should not be continued for more than 4 weeks.

Patients should be instructed to clean the nasal passages prior to administering the spray and to inhale gently through the nose during spraying. Before using the pump delivery system for the first time the pump reservoir should be filled up by squeezing the bottle once or twice until a fine spray is delivered.

Use in the elderly: As for adults

Use in children: Livostin nasal spray is not recommended for use in children less than 9 years of age.

Contra-indications, warnings, etc
Contra-indications: Hypersensitivity to any of the ingredients.

The main route of excretion of levocabastine is via the kidneys. In patients with renal impairment elimination of levocabastine was found to be prolonged. Use of Livostin nasal spray in patients with significant renal impairment is therefore contraindicated.

Use in pregnancy and lactation: In mice, rats and rabbits, levocabastine, at oral doses up to 1,250 times the recommended nasal clinical dose, did not reveal any embryotoxic or teratogenic effect. In rodents, at 2,500 times this dose and higher, teratogenicity and/or increased embryonal resorption were observed.

There are no adequate data on the use of Livostin nasal spray in pregnant women. Livostin nasal spray should therefore not be used during pregnancy, unless the potential benefit justifies the potential risk to the foetus.

Based on determination of levocabastine concentrations in saliva and the breast milk in a nursing woman, it was calculated that the daily dose of levocabastine in the infant would not exceed 3.5µg after nasal treatment of the mother. Livostin nasal spray can therefore be given to nursing mothers.

Interactions: No interaction with alcohol or with any other drugs was reported during clinical trials. In specially designed psychoperformance studies, no interaction with diazepam or alcohol was observed.

Treatment with Livostin nasal spray may cause sedation in some patients. This should be borne in mind when special alertness is necessary, eg in connection with driving or the performance of skilled tasks. Excess alcohol should be avoided.

Side-effects: Symptoms of local irritation (eg nasal stinging and burning), have been reported following the application of Livostin nasal spray.

Headache, fatigue and somnolence have also been reported. Conclusive evidence of the causation of these effects has not been demonstrated.

Overdosage: Overdosing with Livostin nasal spray is unlikely. In the event of accidental oral ingestion, supportive measures should be taken.

Pharmaceutical precautions Store at room temperature, not greater than 30°C. Shake well before use.

Legal category POM

Package quantities White plastic bottles with a spray pump containing 10 ml microsuspension.

Further information Nil

Product licence number 0242/0152
Product licence holder: Janssen-Cilag Ltd

OTRIVINE-ANTISTIN* STERILE EYE DROPS

Presentation A clear colourless odourless solution containing Xylometazoline Hydrochloride BP 0.05% w/v and antazoline sulphate 0.5% w/v with Benzalkonium Chloride Ph Eur 0.01% w/v as a preservative.

Also contains: boric acid, disodium edetate, sodium tetraborate and water.

Uses Otrivine-Antistin is a combination of a long acting vasoconstrictor and an antihistamine. The eye drops are for temporary relief of redness and itching of the eye due to seasonal and perennial allergies such as hay fever, or allergy due to house dust.

Dosage and administration Otrivine-Antistin Eye Drops are intended for local administration to the eye.

Adults: 1 or 2 drops instilled 2-3 times per day into the conjunctival sac.

Children 5–12 years and the elderly: No specific studies have been performed in these patients. Due to possible systemic effects caution must be exercised and the dosage reduced to 1 drop instilled 2-3 times per day.

The eye drops should not be used in children under the age of 5 years.

When necessary, mydriatics or miotics may be administered simultaneously with Otrivine-Antistin Eye Drops.

Contra-indications, warnings, etc
Contra-indications: Hypersensitivity to any of the components of the formulation. Presence of narrow angle glaucoma. The use of monoamine oxidase inhibitors within the last 14 days. Otrivine-Antistin is not recommended in patients who wear contact lenses of any type.

Precautions: In patients who are receiving medication for hypertension, cardiac irregularities, hyperthyroidism or diabetes mellitus particular caution should be exercised. Caution should be observed in patients with relevant previous eye disease or surgery. Otrivine-Antistin is not suitable for patients suffering from dry eyes without first seeking medical advice. Rebound congestion may follow continued use. Inflammation arising from infection should receive appropriate antibacterial therapy.

Use in pregnancy and lactation: In line with common practice, the use of medication during pregnancy is not recommended unless considered essential.

Drug interactions: No interactions with other drugs have been reported. There is a theoretical potential for interaction with clonidine.

Side-effects: Otrivine-Antistin Eye Drops are well tolerated in the eye and for the majority of the patients will be non-irritant, but in a few cases, slight transient local stinging may occur. Other side effects which have been reported very occasionally are blurred vision, headache and drowsiness.

Overdosage: There is no experience of overdosage.

Pharmaceutical precautions Protect from heat. The drops should not be used later than one month after first breaking the seal.

Legal category P

Package quantities Otrivine-Antistin Sterile Eye drops 10 ml (OP)

Further information Nil

Product licence number 8685/0002

TEOPTIC* EYE-DROPS

Presentation A clear colourless odourless sterile solution containing carteolol hydrochloride 1% or 2% w/v with Benzalkonium Chloride PhEur 0.005% w/v as a preservative.

Also contains: sodium chloride, dibasic sodium phosphate, monobasic sodium phosphate and water.

Uses Teoptic is a beta-adrenergic-receptor-blocking agent possessing intrinsic sympathomimetic activity. Teoptic Eye-Drops are a topical treatment for the reduction of intra-ocular pressure, eg in ocular hypertension, chronic open angle glaucoma, some secondary glaucomas.

Dosage and administration Teoptic Eye-Drops are for local administration to the eye. Initially, the recommended adult dose is one drop of Teoptic 1% Eye-Drops instilled twice daily in each affected eye. If the clinical response is not adequate, the dosage may be altered to one drop of Teoptic 2% Eye-Drops instilled twice daily in each affected eye.

Teoptic Eye-Drops may, if necessary, be used in association with pilocarpine, adrenaline, carbachol and carbonic anhydrase inhibitors.

Children: Teoptic Eye-Drops have not been studied in children. Their use in these patients is, therefore, not recommended.

Use in the elderly: In clinical trials, the efficacy and tolerability profiles of Teoptic Eye-Drops were similar in elderly patients and in the general adult patient population. The usual recommended adult dose may, therefore, be considered suitable for elderly patients.

Contra-indications, warnings, etc
Contra-indications: Unsatisfactorily controlled cardiac insufficiency; bronchospasm, including bronchial asthma, or chronic obstructive pulmonary disease; pregnancy; hypersensitivity to any of the components of the formulation.

Precautions: As with other topically applied ophthalmic preparations, Teoptic may be absorbed systemically. Teoptic Eye-Drops should, therefore, be used with caution in patients receiving systemic beta-adrenergic-receptor-blocking therapy and in patients with known contra-indications to systemic beta-blockers, eg sinus bradycardia, second and third degree atrioventricular block, cardiogenic shock, right ventricular insufficiency due to pulmonary hypertension and congestive heart failure, unsatisfactorily controlled diabetes mellitus.

As with all ophthalmic preparations containing benzalkonium chloride, soft contact lenses (hydrophilic lenses) should not be worn during treatment with Teoptic Eye-Drops.

Side-effects: Local ocular reactions such as irritation, burning, itching and pain, blurred vision, photophobia, xerosis, conjunctival hyperaemia, conjunctival discharge and corneal disorders such as diffuse superficial keratitis may occasionally develop. As with all beta-blocking agents, bradycardia, bronchospasm, rashes, dyspnoea, headache, lassitude and vertigo have occasionally been reported.

Use in pregnancy and lactation: Teoptic Eye-Drops have not been studied in human pregnancy and lactation. Use during pregnancy is, therefore, contra-indicated. In animal studies, orally administered carteolol has been shown to penetrate the breast milk and the use of Teoptic Eye-Drops in lactating mothers should, therefore, be at the discretion of the physician.

Overdosage: There is no experience of overdosage with Teoptic Eye-Drops. However, potential symptoms (typical of beta-blocking agents) which may occur after accidental oral ingestion include bradycardia, severe hypotension, acute cardiac failure, bronchospasm, hypoglycaemia, delirium and unconsciousness. Initially, treatment should be by removal of any unabsorbed drug (eg gastric lavage) and general supportive measures, ie marked bradycardia should be treated in the first instance by intravenous atropine sulphate at a dose of 500 micrograms-2.0 mg depending on severity; intravenous glucagon and cardiac pacemakers may be required in more severe cases; bronchospasm should be treated with appropriate bronchodilators, including B_2-agonists and aminophylline where necessary. Patients should be monitored for several days as the beta-blocking effects of Teoptic may exceed its plasma half life.

Pharmaceutical precautions Protect from heat. Teoptic Eye-Drops are sterile until the seal is broken. The container should not be accepted for initial use if the seal is damaged. The drops should not be used later than one month after first breaking the seal.

Legal category POM

Package quantities 1%: 1 X 5 ml dropper-bottle, 3 X 5 ml dropper-bottle; 2%: 1 X 5 ml dropper-bottle; 3 X 5 ml dropper-bottle

Further information Unlike miotics, Teoptic Eye-Drops reduce intra-ocular pressure without altering accommodation or pupil diameter. A slight increase in pupil diameter may be noted, however, if patients are transferred from miotic therapy to Teoptic Eye-Drops.

Product licence numbers
1% Eye-Drops: 8685/0005
2% Eye-Drops: 8685/0006

VISCOTEARS* LIQUID GEL

Presentation Sterile, colourless and translucent liquid gel, containing 2.0 mg/g Carbomer 940 (polyacrylic acid). It also contains cetrimide (0.1 mg/g), sorbitol, disodium edetate, sodium hydroxide and water.

Uses Substitute of tear fluid for management of dry eye conditions including keratoconjunctivitis sicca, and for unstable tear film.

Dosage and administration
Adults: 1 drop 3–4 times daily or as required, depending upon the severity of the disease

Elderly: No dosage amendment is necessary in the elderly

Children: No specific studies with Viscotears have been performed in children. Use in these patients, is therefore, at the responsibility of the physician.

Hold the tube vertically. This results in the formation of a small drop which readily becomes detached from the tube opening. This drop is instilled into the conjunctival sac.

Contra-indications,warnings, etc
Contra-indications: Patients with known hypersensitivity to one of the components of the gel.

Precautions: Contact lenses should not be worn during instillation of the drug. After instillation there should be an interval of at least 30 minutes before reinsertion.

Pregnancy and lactation: There is no experience regarding the safety of Viscotears Liquid Gel in human pregnancy or lactation. Administration during pregnancy and lactation is therefore not recommended, except for compelling reasons.

Drug interactions: In case of any additional local ocular treatment (eg glaucoma therapy) there should be an application interval of at least 5 minutes between the two medications, Viscotears Liquid Gel always should be the last medication instilled.

Side-effects: In clinical studies with Viscotears Liquid Gel the following adverse events have been occasionally reported: mild, transient burning sensation; sticky eyelid; blurred vision after instillation of the gel.

Overdosage: Not applicable

Effects on ability to drive or use machines: Viscotears Liquid Gel may temporarily influence the visual acuity. Patients with blurred vision driving a vehicle or operating machines should be alerted to the possibility of impaired reactions.

Pharmaceutical precautions Store below 30°C.

Legal category P

Package quantities Viscotears Liquid Gel 10 g (OP)

Further information Viscotears Liquid Gel is a stable, well preserved liquid gel containing Carbomer 940. After local instillation it spreads rapidly over the conjunctiva and cornea and forms a lubricating film with prolonged contact time.

The retention times of Viscotears Liquid Gel and a conventional tear substitute based on polyvinylalcohol were studied in 30 healthy volunteers with fluorescein staining. The retention time of Viscotears Liquid Gel was approximately 16 minutes compared with approximately 2 minutes for the conventional artificial tears eye drops.

Tear film stability was maintained for a period of up to 6 hours. Data of clinical studies on healthy volunteers, patients with dry eye and patients in intensive care or during operation suggest evidence that Viscotears Liquid Gel improves tear film stability and prolongs tear break-up time (BUT).

There are no controlled animal or human pharmacokinetic studies available. However, absorption or accumulation in eye tissues can presumably be excluded due to the high molecular weight of polyacrylic acid (4 mio D).

Product licence number 8685/0009

VOLTAROL* OPHTHA

Presentation A clear, slightly yellow, sterile eye drop solution presented in single dose units, containing 0.1% (w/v) diclofenac sodium in a preservative free formulation.

Also contains boric acid, polyoxyl 35 castor oil, tromethamine and water.

Uses Inhibition of peroperative miosis during cataract surgery. Voltarol Ophtha does not have intrinsic mydriatic properties and does not replace standard mydriatic agents. Voltarol Ophtha is also indicated for the treatment of post-operative inflammation in cataract surgery, and the control of ocular pain and discomfort associated with corneal epithelial defects after excimer PRK (photorefractive keratectomy) surgery or accidental trauma.

Dosage and administration
Adults: For the prophylaxis of peroperative miosis: apply 1 drop four times during the 2 hours prior to surgery.

For the control of post-operative inflammation: apply 1 drop four times daily for up to 28 days.

For the control of post-PRK pain and discomfort: apply 1 drop 2 times in the hour prior to surgery, one drop 2 times five minutes apart immediately after PRK surgery and then post-operatively 1 drop every 2–5 hours while awake for up to 24 hours.

Control of ocular pain associated with corneal epithelial defects after accidental trauma: apply 1 drop 4 times daily for up to 2 days.

Elderly patients: No dosage amendment is necessary in the elderly.

Children: Safety and efficacy in children have not been established.

Note: Each Voltarol Ophtha single dose unit should be used for a single dose only. Discard the single dose unit immediately after use. Do not save unused contents.

Contra-indications, warnings,etc
Contra-indications: Patients with known hypersensitivity to any of the ingredients of the formulation.

Like other non-steroidal anti-inflammatory agents, Voltarol Ophtha is also contraindicated in patients in whom attacks of asthma, urticaria, or acute rhinitis are precipitated by acetylsalicylic acid or by other drugs with prostaglandin synthetase inhibiting activity. Intraocular use during surgical procedure is also contraindicated

Special precautions and warnings: In the presence of infection, or if there is a risk of infection, appropriate therapy (eg antibiotic) should be given concurrently with Voltarol Ophtha.

Although there have been no reported adverse events, there is a theoretical possibility that patients receiving other medications which may prolong bleeding time, or with known haemostatic defects may experience exacerbation with Voltarol Ophtha.

Adverse reactions: The following adverse events have been reported:

Frequent: a mild to moderate burning sensation

Rare: blurred vision immediately after instillation of the eye drops, hypersensitivity reactions with itching and reddening, photosensitivity, keratitis punctata, corneal epithelial discontinuity.

Use during pregnancy and lactation: There is no experience concerning the safety of Voltarol Ophtha in human pregnancy. Administration during pregnancy and lactation is therefore not recommended except for compelling reasons.

Overdosage: There is practically no risk of adverse effects due to accidental oral ingestion, since the eye drop solution in a block of ten units contains only 3 mg of diclofenac sodium, corresponding to about 1.8% of the recommended maximum daily adult dose of Voltarol after oral administration. By way of comparison, the maximum oral daily dose for diclofenac sodium recommended in children is 2 mg/kg body weight.

Drug interactions: None reported to date. Clinical findings have shown that Voltarol Ophtha can, if necessary, be combined with steroid containing eye drops.

To prevent the active substances from being washed out when additional ophthalmic medication is used, an interval of at least 5 minutes between each application should be adhered to.

Ability to drive and operate machinery: Patients with blurred vision should refrain from driving a vehicle or operating machinery.

Pharmaceutical precautions Store below 15°C until the pack is dispensed. The pack is then stable for 28 days when stored below 25°C. The single dose units should not be used more than 28 days after dispensing. Discard each single dose unit after single dose use.

Legal category POM

Package quantities Voltarol Ophtha is available in packs of 5 and 40 single dose units.

Further information Voltarol Ophtha solution contains diclofenac sodium, a non-steroidal compound with pronounced anti-inflammatory and analgesic properties. Inhibition of prostaglandin biosynthesis, which has been demonstrated experimentally, is regarded as having an important bearing on its mechanism of action.

Prostaglandins play a major role in miosis which occurs during ocular surgery through the constriction of the iris sphincter and in the causation of inflammation and pain.

In clinical trials Voltarol Ophtha has been found to inhibit miosis during cataract surgery, to reduce inflammation following surgical interventions and to reduce ocular pain and discomfort associated with corneal epithelial defects after excimer PRK surgery.

Penetration of diclofenac into the anterior chamber has been confirmed in humans. No measurable plasma levels of diclofenac could be found in humans after ocular application of diclofenac eye drops.

Product licence number 00101/0478

***Trade Mark*

Cortecs Healthcare Limited

Abbey Road
Wrexham Industrial Estate
Wrexham
LL13 9PW

☎ 01244 288888 🗋 01244 280299

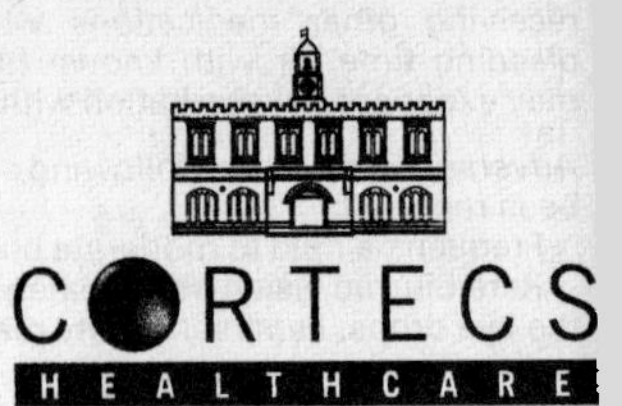

BIOPLEX* MOUTHWASH

Qualitative and quantitative composition Carbenoxolone Sodium BP 1% m/m. USAN, INNM: Carbenoxolone disodium. INN: Carbenoxolone sodium.

Pharmaceutical form Granules.

Clinical particulars
Therapeutic indications: The treatment of mouth ulcers.

Posology and method of administration: To be used topically in the mouth. Adults, children and elderly: 2 g of the granules to be dissolved in 30 to 50 ml warm water and used as a mouthwash 3 times a day and once at night until the ulcers have healed. The mouthwash is to be spat out and not swallowed.

Contra-indications: None known.

Special warnings and special precautions for use: No special warnings or precautions are necessary for the small dose of carbenoxolone in Bioplex Mouthwash.

Interactions with other medicaments and other forms of interaction: Spironoloactone and amiloride inhibit the healing of gastric ulcers by carbenoxolone but their effect on Bioplex Mouthwash is unknown.

Pregnancy and lactation: No teratogenic effects have been reported with carbenoxolone but, in common with other drugs, Bioplex Mouthwash should be used with caution in patients who may become pregnant.

Effects on ability to drive and use machines: None known.

Undesirable effects: Undesirable effects of carbenoxolone are exceedingly rare with the low local dose applied as Bioplex Mouthwash. When given by mouth in larger doses (80 to 300 mg/day) carbenoxolone can produce a mineralocorticoid-like hypernatræmia with hypokalæmia and occasional hypertension with oedema.

Overdose: Unlikely, even if the total daily dose were ingested.

Pharmacological properties
Pharmacodynamic properties: Carbenoxolone Sodium BP is an ulcer healing agent whose exact mechanism of action is unknown. In the stomach carbenoxolone is cytoprotective and associated with increased mucus production.

Pharmacokinetic properties:
(a) General characteristics: Carbenoxolone is readily absorbed from the gastric mucosa (and presumably from other mucosae). The carbenoxolone circulates reversibly bound to plasma proteins, is conjugated in the liver to mono- and diglucuronides and excreted via the bile. Enterohepatic recirculation may occur.
(b) Characteristics in patients: Absorption of carbenoxolone from Bioplex Mouthwash is low.

Preclinical safety data: No additional data are available for Carbenoxolone Sodium BP.

Pharmaceutical particulars
List of excipients: Inactive ingredients in Bioplex Mouthwash are; Sodium Citrate BP, Lactose BP, Disodium Edetate BP and Peppermint Oil BP.

Incompatibilities: None known.

Shelf life: Three years.

Special precautions for storage: Store in a dry place.

Nature and contents of container: Paper 44 gsm/polythene 10–12 gsm/aluminium foil 0.008 mm/polythene 23–25 gsm.

Instructions for handling: None.

Marketing authorisation holder: Biorex Laboratories Limited, 2 Crossfield Chambers, Gladbeck Way, Enfield, Middlesex, EN2 7HT.

Marketing authorisation number 0181/0029

Date of approval/revision of SPC August 1996

Legal category POM

CALCEOS*

Qualitative and quantitative composition Each tablet contains 1250 mg calcium carbonate PhEur (equivalent to 500 mg elemental calcium) plus 400 IU vitamin D_3 PhEur (10 mcg colecalciferol).

Pharmaceutical form Greyish white square chewable tablets, with a lemon flavour.

Clinical particulars
Therapeutic indications: Vitamin D and calcium deficiency correction in the elderly. Vitamin and calcium supplement as an adjunct to specific therapy for osteoporosis.

Posology and method of administration: For adults only. One tablet, twice per day. Chew the tablets and take with a glass of water.

Contra-indications: Hypersensitivity to one of the constituents. Hypercalcaemia as a result of hyperparathyroidism (primary or secondary). Hypercalciuria, calcium lithiasis, tissue calcification (nephrocalcinosis). Vitamin D overdose. Myeloma and bone metastases. Renal insufficiency (creatinin clearance less than 20 ml/min). Calceos is also contra-indicated in patients where prolonged immobilisation is accompanied by hypercalcaemia and/or hypercalciuria. In these cases, treatment should only be resumed when the patient becomes mobile.

Special warnings and special precautions for use: Calculate the total vitamin D intake in case of treatment with another drug containing this vitamin.

Plasma and urinary calcium levels should be monitored regularly.

In the elderly, renal function must be monitored regularly.

In patients with renal failure, dosage has to be adapted according to the creatinine clearance.

In case of long term treatment, the urinary calcium excretion must be monitored and treatment must be reduced or suspended if urinary calcium exceeds 7.5 to 9 mmol/24 h (300 to 360 mg/24 h).

Interaction with other medicaments and other forms of interaction:
- In case of treatment with digitalis glycosides: risk of cardiac arrhythmias. Clinical surveillance is required and possibly electrocardiographic and serum calcium monitoring are recommended.
- Associations to be taken into account in the case of treatment with thiazide diuretics: Risk of hypercalcaemia by decreasing urinary calcium excretion.
- Calcium may impair the absorption of tetracyclines, etidronate, iron or fluoride. At least 3 hours should intervene between taking Calceos and these agents.

Pregnancy and lactation: Normal requirements for calcium and vitamin D are raised during pregnancy and lactation. If supplementation is necessary, it should be given at a different time to iron supplements. Calcium is excreted in breast milk but not sufficiently to produce an adverse effect in the infant.

Effects on ability to drive and use machines: None known.

The following side effects have been observed:
- Hypercalciuria in cases of prolonged treatment at high doses, exceptionally hypercalcaemia.
- Hypophosphataemia.
- Nausea.
- Mild gastro-intestinal disturbances such as constipation can occur but are infrequent.

Overdose: Clinical signs: anorexia, intense thirst, nausea, vomiting, polyuria, polydipsia, dehydration, hypertension, vasomotor disorders, constipation.

Laboratory signs: hypercalcaemia, hypercalciuria, impaired renal function tests.

Emergency treatment: Calcium and vitamin D treatment must be stopped. Rehydration and, according to the severity, isolated or combined use of diuretics, corticosteriods, calcitonin. Peritoneal dialysis may be necessary in severe cases.

Pharmacological properties
Pharmacodynamic properties: Calceos is a fixed combination of calcium and vitamin D. The high calcium and vitamin D concentration in each dose unit facilitates absorption of a sufficient quantity of calcium, with a limited number of doses. Vitamin D is involved in calcium-phosphorus metabolism. It allows active absorption of calcium and phosphorus from the intestine and their uptake by bone.

Pharmacokinetic properties:
Calcium carbonate: Absorption: In the stomach, calcium carbonate releases calcium ions as a function of pH. Calcium is essentially absorbed in the proximal part of the small intestine. The rate of absorption of calcium in the gastrointestinal tract is of the order of 30% of the dose ingested.

Elimination: Calcium is eliminated in sweat and gastrointestinal secretions. The urinary calcium excretion depends on the glomerular filtration and rate of tubular resorption of calcium.

Vitamin D_3: Vitamin D_3 is absorbed from the intestine and transported by protein binding in the blood to the liver (first hydroxylation) and to the kidney (2nd hydroxylation).

Non-hydroxylated vitamin D_3 is stored in reserve compartments such as muscle and adipose tissues.

Its plasma half-life is of the order of several days; it is eliminated in faeces and urine.

Pharmaceutical particulars
List of excipients: Xylitol, Sorbitol, Polyvinylpyrrolidone, Lemon flavouring*, Magnesium stearate.

*Composition of the lemon flavouring: essential oils of lemon, orange, litsea cubeba, maltodextrin, acacia gum, sodium citrate.

Incompatibilities: None known.

Shelf life: 36 months.

Special precautions of storage: None.

Nature and contents of container: Polypropylene tubes containing 15 chewable tablets. Cartons of 1, 2 or 4 tubes are available.

Instructions for use/handling: None.

Marketing authorisation holder: Laboratoire Innothera, 10 av. Paul Vaillant-Couturier, BP 35–94111 Arcueil Cedex, France.

Marketing authorisation number 5856/0001

Date of approval/revision of SPC November 1996.

Legal category P.

CLOTAM* RAPID

Qualitative and quantitative composition Tolfenamic acid 200 mg.

Pharmaceutical form Tablets.

Clinical particulars
Therapeutic indications: Acute migraine.

Posology and method of administration:
Adults: Migraine – acute attacks: 200 mg when the first symptoms of migraine appear. The treatment can be repeated once after 1–2 hours if a satisfactory response is not obtained.

Children: A paediatric dosage regimen has not yet been established.

Elderly: Normal adult dose.

Contra-indications: Active peptic ulceration. Significantly impaired kidney or liver function. Tolfenamic acid is contraindicated in patients in whom attacks of asthma, urticaria or acute rhinitis are precipitated by aspirin or other non-steroidal anti-inflammatory agents.

Special warnings and precautions for use: As is the case with other NSAIDs, tolfenamic acid should be used with caution in patients with a history of gastrointestinal ulceration, or impaired liver or kidney function.

Interaction with other medicaments and other forms of interaction: Anticoagulants: In patients treated with anticoagulants, close monitoring of blood coagulation is recommended.

Diuretics: The effect of loop diuretics may be reduced.

Lithium: The effect of lithium may be increased.

Pregnancy and lactation: Pregnancy: Reproduction studies in animals have not shown any signs of foetal damage. Controlled studies in pregnant women are not available. As is the case with the use of other NSAIDs, tolfenamic acid should not be given in the last trimester, due to risks of premature closure of the ductus arteriosus and prolonged parturition.

Lactation: Tolfenamic acid is excreted to such a very small extent in mothers' milk that it should be without risk to the breast-fed baby.

Effects on ability to drive and use machines: None.

Undesirable effects: Tolfenamic acid is well tolerated at the recommended dosage. The following side effects have been observed:

Gastrointestinal tract: Diarrhoea, nausea, epigastric pain, vomiting, dyspepsia. Isolated reports of gastric ulcertation.

Allergic skin reactions: Drug exanthema, erythema, pruritus, urticaria.

Urinary tract: Harmless dysuria in the form of smarting during urination may occur occasionally, most commonly in males. The occurrence is correlated with the concentration of a metabolite and is most probably due to local irritation of the urethra. Increased consumption of liquid or reduction of the dose diminishes the risk of smarting. The urine may, due to coloured metabolites, become a little more lemon-coloured.

As is the case with the use of other NSAIDs, the side effects listed below have occasionally been observed:

Central nervous system: Headache, vertigo, tremor, euphoria, fatigue.

Respiratory tract: Isolated cases of dyspnoea, pulmonary infiltration, bronchospasm and asthma attack.

Haematology: Isolated cases of thrombocytopenia, anaemia and leucopenia.

Liver: Isolated cases of reversible liver function disturbances and toxic hepatitis.

Overdose: No symptoms of overdosage are known in man. In cases where treatment is required, this should be symptomatic. There is no specific antidote to tolfenamic acid.

Pharmacological properties

Pharmacodynamic properties: NSAID with anti-inflammatory, analgesic and antipyretic effects. Tolfenamic acid is a prostaglandin synthesis inhibitor and a leukotriene synthesis inhibitor.

Pharmacokinetic properties: Tolfenamic acid is absorbed quickly and almost completely after oral administration. Hepatic first pass metabolism is as low as 15% (bioavailability 85%). Maximum plasma concentrations are reached after about 1–1½ hours. The half-life in plasma is about 2 hours. Tolfenamic acid is extensively bound to plasma proteins (99%). It is metabolised in the liver and tolfenamic acid, as well as the metabolites are conjugated with glucuronic acid. About 90% of a given dose of tolfenamic acid is excreted in the urine as glucuronic acid conjugates, and about 10% is excreted in the faeces. Enterohepatic circulation exists.

Preclinical safety data: The therapeutic index for tolfenamic acid is high, and gastrointestinal ulceration and kidney changes have only been seen with oral doses approximately 6–10 times the maximum therapeutic dose recommended for tolfenamic acid. In human volunteers, tolfenamic acid did not affect renal function.

Pharmaceutical particulars

List of excipients: Maize starch; Sodium starch glycollate (Type A); Macrogol 6000; Alginic acid; Cellulose, microcrystalline; Croscarmellose sodium; Silica, colloidal anhydrous; Sodium stearyl fumarate.

Incompatibilities: None known.

Shelf-life: Three years.

Special precautions for storage: Store below 25°C.

Nature and contents of container: Al/PVC blister. HDPE tablet container with LDPE closure. Pack sizes: 3, 10 and 30 capsules.

Instructions for use/handling: None.

Marketing authorisation holder: A/S GEA Farmaceutisk Fabrik, Holger Danskes Vej 89, DK-2000 Frederiksberg, Denmark.

Marketing authorisation number 4012/0043.

Date of approval/revision of SPC April 1997.

Legal category POM

SALOFALK* SUPPOSITORIES 500 mg
SALOFALK* ENEMA 2 g

Qualitative and quantitative composition Each suppository contains Mesalazine 500 mg. Each enema contains Mesalazine 2 g in 59 ml of suspension.

Pharmaceutical form Suppository/Enema.

Clinical particulars

Therapeutic indications: Suppositories: Management of mild and moderate attacks of ulcerative colitis, especially in the rectum and sigmoid colon and also in the descencing colon.

Enemas: Therapeutic and prophylaxis of acute attacks of mild ulcerative colitis, especially in the rectum and sigmoid colon and also in the descending colon.

Posology and method of administration:

Method of administration: Rectal.

Adults and the elderly: Suppositories: 1 to 2 suppositories.

Enema: 1 enema once a day at bedtime. The action of Salofalk is enhanced if the patient lies on the left side when introducing the enema. The dosage should be adjusted to suit the progress of the condition. Do not discontinue treatment suddenly.

Children: There is no recommended dose for children. Mesalazine should not be used in babies and infants.

Contra-indications: Severe renal and hepatic function disturbances. Active gastrointestinal ulcers. Hypersensitivity to salicylates.

Special warnings and special precautions for use: The drug should not be prescribed for infants or young children. Serious blood dyscrasias have been reported very rarely with mesalazine. Haematological investigations should be performed if the patient develops unexplained bleeding, bruising, purpura, anaemia, fever or sore throat. Treatment should be stopped if there is suspicion or evidence of blood dyscrasia.

Interactions with other medicaments and other forms of interactions: Although the following interactions are theoretically possible, owing to the low degree of absorption of the rectally administered mesalazine, the risk of their onset is extremely low: mesalazine may potentiate the actions of sulphonylureas. Interactions with coumarin, methotrexate, probenicid, sulphinpyrazone, spironolactone, frusemide and rifampicin cannot be excluded. Mesalazine can theoretically potentiate the side effects of glucocorticoids on the stomach.

Use during pregnancy and lactation: Animal experiments on mesalazine have produced no evidence of embryonic effects. No untoward effects were seen in a reproductive and fertility study with mesalazine in breast-fed rat pups. Mesalazine is acetylated in the body and passes in this form into breast milk. Limited use of mesalazine in pregnancy has shown no untoward effect on the foetus: however, it should be used with caution during pregnancy and only if the potential benefits outweigh the potential risk.

Effects on ability to drive and use machines: Salofalk Enema is not expected to affect ability to drive and use machines.

Undesirable effects: Salofalk may cause hypersensitivity reactions. These are unrelated to dose. Mesalazine may be associated with an exacerbation of the symptoms of colitis in those patients who have previously had such problems with sulphasalazine. There have been rare reports of leucopenia, neutropenia, agranulocytosis, aplastic anaemia and thrombocytopenia, pancreatitis, hepatitis, allergic lung reactions, lupus erythematosus-like reactions and rash (including urticaria), interstitial nephritis and nephrotic syndrome with oral mesalazine treatment, usually reversible on withdrawal. Renal failure has been reported. Mesalazine-induced nephrotoxicity should be suspected in patients developing renal dysfunction during treatment. Increased methaemaglobin levels may occur. Headache and digestive disturbances such as nausea and diarrhoea may occur. Isolated cases of hair loss have been reported.

Overdose: Symptoms of renal disturbances have been reported in the course of studies on animals at dosages considerably higher than those used in human medicine (a factor in the order of magnitude of 28).

Pharmacological properties

Pharmacodynamic properties: Mesalazine is the biologically active metabolite of salicylazosulphapyridine that is used in the treatment of certain chronic inflammatory conditions of the intestine.

Pharmacokinetic particulars: Following rectal administration the major fraction is recovered from the faeces, a small percentage (approximately 15%) is absorbed; the absorbed mesalazine is excreted mainly in the urine; biliary excretion is secondary. The acetylated and the non-acetylated forms of mesalazine bind slightly to plasma proteins.

Pharmaceutical particulars

List of excipients: Salofalk Suppositories contain the following excipients: Hard fat, docusate sodium, cetyl alcohol.

Salofalk Enemas contain the following excipients: Carbomer, disodium edetate, potassium acetate, potassium metabisulphite, purified water, sodium benzoate, xanthan gum.

Incompatibilities: None known.

Shelf-life: Suppositories: 36 months.
Enema: 24 months.

Special precautions for storage: Store at room temperature (15-25°C) and protect from light.

Nature and contents of container: Suppositories: Carton of 10 or 30 suppositories in white, opaque PVC/PE moulded strips. Each strip contains 5 suppositories.

Enema: Low density concertina shaped polythene bottle with a low density polythene application nozzle packed in cartons containing seven individually blister packed bottles.

Instructions for use/handling: None.

Marketing authorisation number
Suppositories: 14568/0003.
Enema: 14568/0002.

Date of approval/revision of SPC August 1997.

Legal category POM

SALOFALK TABLETS

Qualitative and quantitative composition Mesalazine 250 mg.

Pharmaceutical form Enteric coated tablet.

Therapeutic indications: Treatment of mild to moderate acute exacerbations of ulcerative colitis and for the maintenance of remission of ulcerative colitis.

Posology and method of administration: Method of administration: Oral.

Adults: Acute treatment: six tablets daily in three divided doses.

Maintenance treatment: three to six tablets daily in divided doses.

Elderly: As for adults.

Contra-indications: Patients with an active peptic ulcer, blood clotting abnormalities, severe hepatic or renal disease or where there is a pathological propensity to bleeding.

Salofalk should not be used in babies and young children.

Special warnings and precautions for use: Serious blood dyscrasias have been reported very rarely with mesalazine. Haematological investigations should be performed if the patient develops unexplained bleeding, bruising, purpura, anaemia, fever or sore throat. Treatment should be stopped if there is suspicion or evidence of blood dyscrasia.

Interactions with other medicaments and other forms of interaction: The hypoglycaemic action of sulphonureas can be intensified, as can gastro-intestinal haemorrhage caused by coumarins. The toxicity of methotrexate can be increased. The uricosuric action of probenecid and sulphinpyrazone can be decreased, as can the diuretic action of frusemide and the action of spironolactone. The antituberculosis action of rifampicin can also be diminished.

Pregnancy and lactation: Animal experiments on mesalazine have produced no evidence of embryonic effects. All competent authors recommend to continue treatment with sulphasalazine, the parent drug of mesalazine, during pregnancy. Up to now, they didn't see any untoward effect on its course or on the foetus. Therefore there is no reason to prohibit Salofalk treatment during pregnancy. No untoward effects were seen in a reproductive and fertility study with mesalazine in breast-fed rat pups. But up to now there is a limited experience in using mesalazine/sulphasalazine during the lactation period in man. Therefore, it should be stated that the experience with Salofalk 250 during lactation up to now is not sufficient. The acetylated form of mesalazine is found in the breast milk in slight amounts.

Effects on ability to drive and use machines: Salofalk is not expected to affect ability to drive and use machines.

Undesirable effects: Salofalk may cause hypersensitivity reactions. These are unrelated to dose.

Mesalazine may be associated with an exacerbation of the symptoms of colitis in those patients who have previously had such problems with sulphasalazine. There have been rare reports of leucopenia, neutropenia, agranulocytosis, aplastic anaemia and thrombocytopenia, pancreatitis, hepatitis, allergic lung reactions, lupus erythematosus-like reactions and rash (including urticaria), interstitial nephritis and nephrotic syndrome with oral mesalazine treatment, usually reversible on withdrawal. Renal failure has been reported. Mesalazine-induced nephrotoxicity should be suspected in patients developing renal dysfunction during treatment.

Increased metahaemoglobin levels may occur.

Overdose: Due to the enteric nature of the formulation of Salofalk tablets and the particular pharmacokinetic properties of mesalazine, only small amounts of the drug are available for systemic action. Consequently signs of intoxication are unlikely even after large doses. However, in principle, symptoms consistent with salicylate intoxication may occur (management of which is shown in brackets).

- Mixed Acidosis-Alkalosis (reinstatement of the acid-base balance to match the situation and electrolytic substitutions).
- Hyperventilation
- Pulmonary Oedema
- Dehydration from perspiration and vomiting (fluid intake)
- Hypoglycaemia (glucose intake)

There is no specific antidote to mesalazine but in many cases of overdose, gastric lavage and intravenous transfusion of electrolytes to promote diuresis should be implemented.

Pharmacodynamic properties: The main site of action of mesalazine is the inflamed mucosa in the terminal ileum and colon. The pH dependent enteric coating applied to Salofalk tablets (Eudragit L) disintegrates above pH 6.0 ensuring that the drug is released at the site of action, where it is absorbed to a certain degree. The absorbed portion is acetylated and excreted predominantly in the acetylated form via the kidneys. A small portion (about 5% of the absorbed quantity) is excreted in the bile. In faeces, mesalazine is found particularly in unchanged form and partially in acetylated form.

Pharmacokinetic properties: The elimination half-lives are 0.7–2.4 hours (mean 1.4±0.6 hours). The plasma protein binding of mesalazie is 43% and of acetylated mesalazine 78%. The rapid acetylation is not reversible and, in contrast to sulphapyridine, there is no differentiation between slow and rapid acetylation.

List of excipients: Sodium carbonate, glycine, polyvidone, microcrystalline cellulose (E460), colloidal anhydrous silica, calcium stearate, hydroxypropylmethylcellulose (E464), methacrylic acid copolymer (Eudragit L), dibutyl phthalate, talc, titanium dioxide (E171), iron oxide (E172), polyethylene glycol.

Incompatibilities: None stated.

Shelf life: 3 years.

Special precautions for storage: None.

Nature and contents of container: Orange PVC/Al blister strips packed in cartons 10†, 100 or 300† tablets.

† not currently marketed.

Instructions for use/handling: Salofalk tablets should be swallowed whole and not chewed.

Marketing authorisation holder Interfalk UK Ltd, Thames House, Wellington Street, London SE18 6NZ.

Marketing authorisation number PL 10341/0004.

Date of first authorisation/renewal of authorisation First authorised: September 1991, renewal pending.

Date of (partial) revision of the text April 1997.

Legal category POM

SOLVAZINC*

Qualitative and quantitative composition Each Solvazinc tablet contains the following active ingredient: Zinc sulphate monohydrate: 125 mg (equivalent to 45 mg elemental zinc).

Pharmaceutical form Effervescent tablet.

Clinical particulars

Therapeutic indications: Zinc sulphate is a source of zinc which is an essential trace element and involved in a number of body enzyme systems.

Indications: For the treatment of zinc deficiency.

Posology and method of administration: Method of administration: oral after dissolution in water.

Adults: One tablet, dissolved in water, once to three times daily after meals.

Children: More than 30 kg: One tablet, dissolved in water, once to three times daily after meals.

10-30 kg: ½ tablet, dissolved in water, once to three times daily after meals.

Less than 10 kg: ½ tablet, dissolved in water, once daily after meals.

Contra-indications: None.

Special warnings and precautions for use: Accumulation of zinc may occur in cases of renal failure.

Interactions with other medicaments and other forms of interaction: Zinc may inhibit the absorption of concurrently administered tetracyclines; when both are being given an interval of at least 3 hours should be allowed.

Pregnancy and lactation: The safety of this product in human pregnancy has not been established. Zinc crosses the placenta and is present in breast milk.

Effects on ability to drive and use machines: Solvazinc is not expected to affect ability to drive and use machines.

Undesirable effects: Zinc salts may cause abdominal pain and dyspepsia.

Overdose: Zinc sulphate is corrosive in overdosage. Symptoms are corrosion and inflammation of the mucous membrane of the mouth and stomach; ulceration of the stomach followed by perforation may occur. Gastric lavage and emesis should be avoided. Demulcents such as milk should be given. Chelating agents such as sodium edetate may be useful.

Pharmacological properties

Pharmacodynamic properties: Zinc is an essential trace element involved in many enzyme systems. Severe deficiency causes skin lesion, alopecia, diarrhoea, increased susceptibility to infections and failure to thrive in children. Symtoms of less severe deficiency include distorted or absent perceptions of taste and smell and poor wound healing.

Pharmacokinetic properties: Zinc is absorbed from the gastrointestinal tract and distributed throughout the body. The highest concentrations occur in hair, eyes, male reproductive organs and bone. Lower levels are present in liver, kidney and muscle.

In blood 80% is found in erythrocytes. Plasma zinc levels range from 70 to 110 μg per dl and about 50% of this is loosely bound to albumin. About 7% is amino-acid bound and the rest is tightly bound to alpha 2-macroglobulins and other proteins.

Pharmaceutical particulars

List of excipients: Solvazinc contains the following excipients: Sorbitol, polyethylene glycol, sodium hydrogen carbonate, citric acid, saccharin sodium, liquid paraffin.

Incompatibilities: None.

Shelf-life: 3 years.

Special precautions for storage: Store below 25°C, protect from moisture.

Nature and contents of container: Aluminium tubes with polythene caps containing a desiccant capsule and packed in cardboard cartons. Each carton contains 3 tubes of 30 tablets.

Instruction for use/handling: None.

Marketing authorisation number 14568/0004

Date of approval/revision of SPC September 1998

Legal category P

URSOFALK*

Qualitative and quantitative composition Each capsule of Ursofalk contains the following active ingredient: ursodeoxycholic acid 250 mg.

Pharmaceutical form White, opaque, hard gelatin capsules.

Clinical particulars

Therapeutic indications: Ursofalk is indicated in the treatment of primary biliary cirrhosis (PBC) and for the dissolution of radiolucent gallstones in patients with a functioning gall bladder.

Posology and method of administration: Method of administration: Oral.

Primary biliary cirrhosis

Adults and the elderly: 10–15 mg ursodeoxycholic acid (UDCA) per kg per day in two to four divided doses. The following dosage regimen is recommended:

Body Weight (kg)	*Capsules daily (in 2–4 divided doses)*	*mg (UDCA)/kg/day*
50–62	2–4	10.0–16.1
63–85	3–5	11.9–14.7
86–120	4–7	11.6–14.6

Children: Dosage should be related to bodyweight.

Dissolution of gallstones

Adults: 8–12 mg ursodeoxycholic acid (UDCA) per kg per day in two divided doses. The following dosage regime is recommended:

Body weight (kg)	*Capsules daily (in 2 divided doses)*	*mg (UDCA)/kg/day*
50–62	2	8.1–10.0
63–85	3	8.8–11.9
86–120	4	8.3–11.6

If doses are unequal the larger dose should be taken in late evening to counteract the rise in biliary cholesterol saturation which occurs in the early morning. The late evening dose may usefully be taken with food to help maintain bile flow overnight.

The time required for dissolution of gallstones is likely to range from 6 to 24 months depending on stone size and composition. Follow-up cholecystograms or ultrasound investigation may be useful at 6 month intervals until the gallstones have disappeared.

Treatment should be continued until 2 successive cholecystograms and/or ultrasound investigations 4–12 weeks apart have failed to demonstrate gallstones. This is because these techniques do not permit reliable visualisation of stones less than 2 mm in diameter.

The likelihood of recurrence of gallstones after dissolution by bile acid treatment has been estimated as up to 50% at 5 years.

The efficiency of Ursofalk in treating radio-opaque or partially radio-opaque gallstones has not been tested but these are generally thought to be less soluble than radiolucent stones.

Non-cholesterol stones account for 10–15% of radiolucent stones and may not be dissolved by bile acids.

Elderly: There is no evidence to suggest that any alteration in the adult dose is needed but the relevant precautions should be taken into account.

Children: Cholesterol rich gallstones are rare in children but when they occur, dosage should be related to bodyweight.

Contra-indications: Ursofalk is not suitable for the dissolution of radio-opaque gallstones and should not be used in patients with non-functioning gall bladder.

Special warnings and precautions for use: A product of this class has been found to be carcinogenic in animals. The relevance of these findings to the clinical use of Ursofalk has not been established.

Interactions with other medicaments and other forms of interaction: Some drugs, such as cholestyramine, charcoal, colestipol and certain antacids (e.g. aluminium hydroxide) bind bile acids *in vitro* and may interfere with the absorption of Ursofalk.

Drugs which increase cholesterol elimination in bile, such as oestrogenic hormones, oestrogen-rich contraceptive agents and certain blood cholesterol lowering agents, such as clofibrate, should not be taken with Ursofalk.

UDCA may increase the absorption of cyclosporin in transplantation patients.

Pregnancy and lactation: Ursofalk should not be used in pregnancy. When treating women of childbearing potential, non-hormonal or low oestrogen oral contraceptive measures are recommended.

Effects on ability to drive and use machines: Ursofalk is not expected to affect ability to drive and use machines.

Undesirable effects: Diarrhoea may occur rarely.

Overdose: Serious adverse effects are unlikely to occur in overdosage, however, liver function should be monitored. If necessary, ion-exchange resins may be used to bind bile acids in the intestines.

Pharmacological properties

Pharmacodynamic properties: UDCA is a bile acid which effects a reduction in cholesterol in biliary fluid primarily by dispersing the cholesterol and forming a liquid-crystal phase.

UDCA affects the enterohepatic circulation of bile salts by reducing the ileal reabsorption of endogenous more hydrophobic and potentially toxic salts such as cholic and chenodeoxycholic acids.

In-vitro studies show that UDCA has a direct hepatoprotective effect and reduces the hepatoxicity of hydrophobic bile salts. Immunological effects have also been demonstrated with a reduction in abnormal expression of HLA Class I antigens on hepatocytes as well as suppression of cytokine and interleukin production.

Pharmacokinetic properties: Ursodeoxycholic acid occurs naturally in the body. When given orally it is rapidly and completely absorbed. It is 96–98% bound to plasma proteins and efficiently extracted by the liver and excreted in the bile as glycine and taurine conjugates. In the intestine some of the conjugates are deconjugated and reabsorbed. The conjugates may also be dehydroxylated to lithocholic acid, part of which is absorbed, sulphated by the liver and excreted via the biliary tract.

Pharmaceutical particulars

List of excipients: Ursofalk contains the following excipients: Maize starch, colloidal anhydrous silica, magnesium stearate, gelatin, titanium dioxide.

Incompatibilities: None known.

Shelf-life: 36 months.

Special precautions for storage: None.

Nature and contents of container: Clear PVC blister strips with aluminium foil backing packed in cardboard cartons. Each carton contains six blister strips of ten capsules.

Instructions for handling: None.

Marketing authorisation number 14658/0001

Date of approval/revision of SPC September 1998

Legal category POM

**Trade Mark*

Cox Pharmaceuticals

A. H. Cox & Co. Limited
Whiddon Valley
Barnstaple
North Devon EX32 8NS

☎ 01271 311200 📠 01271 346106

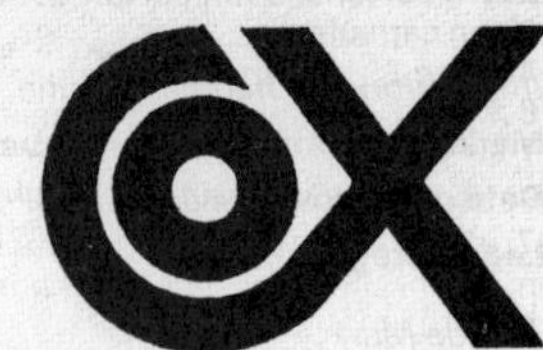

ASPAV*

Presentation White, circular, flat bevelled-edge uncoated tablets impressed with the identifying letters 'AP' on one face; or as an alternative, plain tablets devoid of surface markings; each containing 500 mg Aspirin PhEur, 7.71 mg Papaveretum BP (equivalent to 5 mg anhydrous morphine).

Uses (1) For the relief of moderate to severe pain in post-operative states and in the relief of chronic pain associated with inoperable carcinoma.

Dosage and administration *Adults:* One or two tablets to be dispersed in water every 4–6 hours. Not more than eight tablets in any 24 hour period.

Children under 12 years: Not recommended.

Contra-indications, warnings, etc

Contra-indications: Aspav should not be taken by patients with the following conditions:

- Known hypersensitivity to aspirin, papaveretum, other ingredients in the product, other opioids, other salicylates or non-steroidal anti-inflammatory drugs (a patient may have developed anaphylaxis, angioedema, asthma, rhinitis or urticaria induced by aspirin or other NSAIDs).
- Nasal polyps associated with asthma (high risk of severe sensitivity reactions).
- Active peptic ulceration or a past history of ulceration or dyspepsia.
- Haemophilia or other haemorrhagic disorder (including thrombocytopenia) as there is an increased risk of bleeding.
- Concurrent anticoagulant therapy should be avoided.
- Diarrhoea caused by poisoning until the toxic material has been eliminated, or diarrhoea associated with pseudomembraneous colitis.
- Respiratory depression.
- Obstructive airways disease.

Interactions: The following drug interactions should be considered when prescribing Aspav:

- Alcohol – may enhance gastro-intestinal side effect of aspirin.
- Analgesics – avoid concomitant administration of other salicylates or other NSAIDs (including topical formulations) as increased risk of side effects.
- Alkalisers of urine (eg carbonic anhydrase inhibitors, antacids, citrates) – increased excretion of aspirin.
- Anticoagulants or platelet aggregation inhibitors – increased risk of bleeding.
- Antiepileptic drugs (eg phenytoin, sodium valproate) – increased effect.
- Corticosteroids – increased risk of gastro-intestinal bleeding or ulceration.
- Dipyridamole – increase in peak concentration.
- Diuretics – frusemide and acetazolamide (risk of toxic effects), spironolactone (antagonised diuretic action).
- Hypoglycaemics – enhanced activity.
- Methotrexate – increased toxicity.
- Metoclopramide and domperidone – increased rate of absorption of aspirin.
- Mifepristone – avoid aspirin until 8–12 days after mifepristone.
- Ototoxic medicine (eg vancomycin) – potential for ototoxicity increased. Hearing loss may occur and may progress to deafness even after discontinuation of the medication. Effects may be reversible but are usually permanent.
- Uricosurics (eg probenecid, sulphinpyrazone) – effects of uricosurics reduced.
- Laboratory investigations – aspirin may interfere with some laboratory tests such as urine 5-hydroxyindoleactic acid determinations and copper sulphate urine sugar tests.
- CNS depressants – enhanced sedative and/or hypotensive effect with alcohol, anaesthetics, hypnotics, anxiolytics, antipsychotics, hydroxyzine, tricyclic antidepressants.
- Antibacterials, eg ciprofloxacin – avoid premedication with opioids as reduced plasma ciprofloxacin concentration.
- MAOIs – use only with extreme caution.
- Cyclizine.
- Mexiletine – delayed absorption.
- Metoclopramide and domperidone – antagonise GI effects.
- Cisapride – possible antagonism of GI effects.
- Dopaminergics (eg selegiline) – possible risk of hyperpyrexia and CNS toxicity. This risk is greater with pethidine but with other opioids the risk is uncertain.
- Ulcer healing drugs – cimetidine inhibits the metabolism of opioid analgesics.
- Anticholinergics (eg atropine) – risk of severe constipation which may lead to paralytic illness, and/or urinary retention.
- Antidiarrhoeal drugs (eg loperamide, kaolin) – increased risk of severe constipation.
- Antihypertensive drugs (eg guanethidine, diuretics) – enhanced hypotensive effect.
- Opioid antagonists (eg buprenorphine, naltrexone, naloxone).
- Neuromuscular blocking agents – additive respiratory depressant effects.

Effects on ability to drive and use machines: Opioid analgesics can impair mental function and can cause blurred vision and dizziness. Patients should make sure they are not affected before driving or operating machinery.

Other undesirable effects: Adverse effects of aspirin treatment which have been reported include:

- Allergic reactions – rhinitis, urticaria, angioneurotic oedema and worsening of asthma.
- Effects on GI system – gastro-intestinal bleeding or ulceration which can occasionally be major (may develop bloody or black tarry stools, severe stomach pain and vomiting blood), gastro-intestinal irritation (mild stomach pain, heartburn and nausea) and hepatitis (particularly in patients with SLE or connective tissue disease).
- Effects on blood – anaemia, haemolytic anaemia, hypoprothrombinaemia, thrombocytopenia, aplastic anaemia, pancytopenia.
- Effects on sensory system – tinnitus.
- Salicylism – mild chronic salicylate intoxication may occur after repeated administration of large doses, symptoms include dizziness, tinnitus, deafness, sweating, nausea, vomiting, headache and mental confusion, and may be controlled by reducing the dose.
- Effects in children – aspirin may be associated with the development of Reye's Syndrome (encephalopathy and hepatic failure) in children presenting with an acute febrile illness.

Adverse effects of opioid treatment which have been reported include:

- Allergic reactions (may be caused by histamine release) – including rash, urticaria, difficulty breathing, increased sweating, redness or flushed face.
- Effects on CNS – confusion, drowsiness, vertigo, dizziness, changes in mood, hallucinations, CNS excitation (restlessness/excitement), convulsions, mental depression, headache, trouble sleeping, or nightmares, raised intracranial pressure, tolerance or dependence.
- Effects on GI system – constipation, GI irritation, biliary spasm, nausea, vomiting, loss of appetite, dry mouth, paralytic ileius or toxic megacolon.
- Effects on CVS – bradycardia, palpitations, hypotension.
- Effects on sensory system – blurred or double vision.
- Effects on GU system – ureteral spasm, antidiuretic effect.
- Other effects – trembling, unusual tiredness or weakness, malaise, miosis, hypothermia.
- Effects of withdrawal – abrupt withdrawal precipitates a withdrawal syndrome. Symptoms may include tremor, insomnia, nausea, vomiting, sweating and increase in heart rate, respiratory rate and blood pressure. NOTE – tolerance diminishes rapidly after withdrawal so a previously tolerated dose may prove fatal.

Use in pregnancy and lactation: Controlled trials in humans using aspirin have not shown evidence of teratogenic effects. However, studies in animals have shown that salicylates can cause birth defects including fissure of the spine and skull, facial clefts and malformations of the CNS, viscera and skeleton. Ingestion of aspirin during the last two weeks of pregnancy may increase the risk of fetal or neonatal haemorrhage. Regular or high dose use of salicylates late in pregnancy may result in constriction or premature closing of the fetal ductus arteriosus, increased risk of still birth or neonatal death, decreased birth weight, prolonged labour, complicated deliveries and increased risk of maternal or fetal haemorrhage and possibly persistent pulmonary hypertension of newborn or kernicterus in jaundiced neonates. Pregnant women should be advised not to take aspirin in the last three months of pregnancy unless under medical supervision.

Risk benefit must be considered because opioid analgesics cross the placenta. Studies in animals have shown opioids to cause delayed ossification in mice and increased resorption in rats.

Regular use during pregnancy may cause physical dependence in the fetus, leading to withdrawal symptoms in the neonate. During labour opioids enter the fetal circulation and may cause respiratory depression in the neonate. Administration should be avoided during the late stages of labour and during the delivery of a premature infant.

Aspirin is distributed in breast milk. Aspirin should be avoided while breast feeding.

Papaveretum is distributed in breast milk in small amounts. It is advisable to avoid administration opioids in a breast feeding woman.

Other special warnings and precautions: Aspav should be used with caution in patients with:

- Allergic disease.
- Anaemia (may be exacerbated by GI blood loss).
- Asthma (increased risk of bronchospastic sensitivity reactions).
- Cardiac failure (conditions which predispose to fluid retention).
- Children under 12 – there is possible association between aspirin and Reye's Syndrome when administered to children with a fever. For this reason it should not normally be given to children under 12 years of age except on medical advice.
- Dehydration.
- Glucose-6-phosphate dehydrogenase deficiency (aspirin rarely causes haemolytic anaemia).
- Gout (serum urate may be increased).
- Hepatic function impairment (avoid if severe).
- Renal function impairment.
- Surgery. Aspirin should be discontinued several days before scheduled surgery (including dental extractions).
- Systemic lupus erythematosus and other connective tissue disorders (hepatic and renal function may be impaired in these conditions).
- Thyrotoxicosis (may be exacerbated by large doses of salicylates).
- Hypothyroidism (risk of depression and prolonged CNS depression is increased).
- Inflammatory bowel disease – risk of toxic megacolon.
- Opioids should not be administered during an asthma attack.
- Convulsions – may be induced or exacerbated.
- Drug abuse, dependence (including alcoholism), enhanced instability, suicidal ideation or attempts – predisposed to drug abuse.
- Head injuries or conditions where intracranial pressure is raised.
- Gall bladder disease or gall stones – opioids may cause biliary contraction.
- Gastro-intestinal surgery – use with caution after recent GI surgery as opioids may alter GI motility.
- Prostatic hypertrophy or recent urinary tract surgery.
- Adrenocortical insufficiency, eg Addison's Disease.
- Hypotension and shock.
- Myasthenia gravis.
- Phaeochromocytoma – opioids may stimulate catecholamine release by inducing the release of endogenous histamine.

Overdosage: Salicylates:
Symptoms of overdose depend upon plasma salicylate concentration. Concentration greater than 300 mg/l⁻¹ – tinnitus and vertigo; concentration approx 400 mg/l⁻¹ – hyperventilation; concentration above 600 mg/l⁻¹ – metabolic acidosis; concentration range 700–900 mg/l⁻¹ – coma, fever, hypothrombinaemia, cardiovascular collapse, renal failure.

Treatment: Aspirin may remain in the stomach for many hours after ingestion and should be removed by gastric lavage.

Plasma salicylate, pH and electrolytes should be measured. Fluid losses replaced and forced alkaline diuresis (eg with sodium bicarbonate) should be considered when the plasma salicylate concentration is greater than 500 mg/l⁻¹; (3.6 mmol/l⁻¹) in adults or 300 mg/l⁻¹ (2.2 mmol/l⁻¹) in children. In very severe cases of poisoning haemodialysis may be needed.

Opioids:
Symptoms: cold clammy skin, confusion, convulsions, severe drowsiness, tiredness, low blood pressure, pinpoint pupils of eyes, slow heart beat and respiratory rate coma.

Treatment: Treat respiratory depression or other life-threatening adverse effects first. Empty the stomach via gastric lavage or induction of emesis.

The opioid antagonist naloxone (0.4–2 mg subcutaneous) can be given and repeated at 2–3 minute intervals to a maximum of 10 mg. Naloxone may also be given by intramuscular injection or intravenous infusion. The patient should be monitored as the duration of opioid analgesic may exceed that of the antagonist.

Pharmaceutical precautions Keep tightly closed and store below 25°C in a dry place. Protect from light.

Legal category POM.

Package quantities Aspav is available in packs of 100 tablets.

Further information Aspav has advantages over morphine combinations, as papaveretum has intrinsic spasmolytic activity in addition to its analgesic properties. Aspav is not subject to the prescribing regultions of the Misuse of Drugs Act. Each tablet contains 1607.29 mg Lactose BP.

Product licence number 0142/5597R.

COBADEX*

Presentation Cobadex Cream is a white cream containing 1% w/w Hydrocortisone PhEur and 20% w/w Dimethicone 350 PhEur.

Uses Cobadex Cream is formulated to include volatile and skin-penetrating solvents. This enables the hydrocortisone to be carried into the skin by the organic solvent vehicle, and at the same time evaporation of water will take place from the external surface of the cream, leaving a water-repellent silicone film in contact with the air. Cobadex is indicated, therefore, in all steroid responsive dermatoses wherever water, soap, chemicals, etc. cause irritation, e.g. contact dermatitis (especially of hands and body).

Dosage and administration A thin layer of cream should be applied to the affected area two or three times daily.

Contra-indications, warnings, etc
Contra-indications: Bacterial (impetigo), viral (herpes simplex) or fungal (candida or dermatophyte) infections. The cream should not be used on raw, weeping surfaces because it tends to hold back any exudate. The area of skin around the eye should be avoided.

Use in pregnancy and lactation: There is inadequate evidence of safety in human pregnancy. Topical administration of corticosteroids to pregnant animals can cause abnormalities of foetal development including cleft palate and intra-uterine growth retardation. There may therefore be a very small risk of such effects in the human foetus.

Other undesirable effects: Discontinue treatment should sensitisation occur.

Other special warnings and precautions: Steroid therapy in infants should not exceed seven days, since adrenal suppression may occur, even without occlusion.

Pharmaceutical precautions Cobadex should be stored below 25°C. Do not freeze.

Legal category POM.

Package quantities Cobadex is available in 20 g tubes.

Further information Cobadex Cream also contains propylene glycol, cetostearyl alcohol, paraffin, isopropyl myristate, cetomacrogol, polysorbate, methyl and propyl hydroxy benzoates, isobornyl acetate and disodium edetate.

Product licence number 0142/0201.

KLOREF*

Presentation White, effervescent, lemon and lime flavoured tablets impressed 'Kloref' on one face; each tablet contains Potassium Bicarbonate BPC, Potassium Chloride BP, potassium benzoate and Betaine Hydrochloride BPC 1949, which provides 6.7 mmol potassium (K^+) and 6.7 mmol chloride (Cl^-) (equivalent to 500 mg potassium chloride) when dissolved in water.

Uses Kloref is indicated in all cases of potassium depletion resulting from prolonged or intensive diuretic therapy, an inadequate dietary potassium intake, and those receiving digitalis – here the elderly population are a special risk. A lack of cellular potassium in the latter can increase the toxic effect of digitalis.

Other indications are corticosteroid therapy, use of carbenoxolone sodium, advanced hepatic cirrhosis, chronic renal disease, Cushing's syndrome, diabetic ketosis, patients on a low-salt diet and in conditions requiring potassium supplementation due to prolonged or chronic diarrhoea or vomiting.

Dosage and administration Each tablet should be fully dissolved in at least 100 ml of cold or refrigerated water before drinking. The tablets themselves should not be swallowed.

Adults: In most cases 1–2 tablets three times daily (20–40 mmol K^+ and Cl^-). A few patients may need considerably bigger doses.

Children and pregnant women: Treatment should only be initiated under close medical supervision in hospital, with frequent monitoring of serum electrolytes.

Elderly: The elderly also require monitoring of serum electrolytes.

Contra-indications, warnings, etc
Contra-indications: Hyperchloraemia; renal tubular or metabolic acidosis.

Use in pregnancy and lactation: Potassium may be indicated as replacement therapy for pregnant women with low potassium levels such as those receiving diuretics. Serum levels should be closely monitored.

Administration of potassium during lactation is considered to be safe providing that maternal serum levels are maintained in the physiological range.

Other special warnings and precautions: Cautious administration is required in cases of chronic renal disease.

Overdosage: Hyperkalaemia. Poisoning is usually minimal below 6.5 mmol/l, moderate between 6.5 and 8 mmol/l and severe above that level. The absolute toxicity is governed by both pH and associated sodium levels.

Hyperkalaemic symptoms and particularly the ECG effects, may be transiently controlled by calcium gluconate, administration of glucose or glucose and insulin, sodium bicarbonate or hypertonic sodium infusions, cation exchange resins or by haemodialysis and peritoneal dialysis. Caution should be exercised in patients who are digitalised and who may experience acute digitalis intoxication in the course of potassium removal.

Pharmaceutical precautions Kloref Tablets should be dispensed in a moisture proof container and stored below 25°C in a dry place. Securely fasten lid immediately after use.

Legal category P.

Package quantities Kloref is available in packs of 50 tablets.

Further information The addition of each tablet to water brings about a reaction between the betaine hydrochloride and potassium bicarbonate; effervescence results from the liberation of carbon dioxide.

Betaine is a naturally occurring substance found in beet, and is metabolised by the body.

Kloref also contains citric acid, povidone, macrogol, saccharin calcium and dioctyl sodium sulphosuccinate.

Product licence number 0142/0275.

KLOREF-S*

Presentation Lemon and lime flavoured effervescent granules in individual sachets; each sachet contains Potassium Bicarbonate BPC, Potassium Chloride BP and Betaine Hydrochloride BPC 1949, which provide 20 mmol potassium (K^+) and 20 mmol chloride (Cl^-) (equivalent to 1.5 g potassium chloride) when dissolved in water.

Uses Kloref-S is indicated in all cases of potassium depletion resulting from intensive or prolonged diuretic therapy, an inadequate potassium dietary intake, and those receiving digitalis – here the elderly population are a special risk. A lack of cellular potassium in the latter can increase the toxic effect of digitalis.

Other indications are corticosteroid therapy, use of carbenoxolone sodium, advanced hepatic cirrhosis, chronic renal disease, Cushing's syndrome, diabetic ketosis, patients on a low-salt diet and in conditions requiring potassium supplementation due to prolonged or chronic diarrhoea or vomiting.

Dosage and administration *Adults:* In most cases 1 or 2 sachets daily (20–40 mmol K^+ and Cl^-) preferably after meals. A few patients may need considerably bigger doses. Each sachet should be dissolved in at least 200 ml of cold water.

Children and pregnant women: Treatment should only be initiated under close medical observation in hospital, with frequent monitoring of serum electrolytes.

Elderly: The elderly also require monitoring of serum electrolytes.

Contra-indications, warnings, etc
Contra-indications: Contra-indicated in hyperchloraemia, renal tubular or metabolic acidosis.

Interactions with other medicaments and other forms of interaction: Combined treatment with the following increase the risk of hyperkalaemia: Angiotensin-converting enzyme inhibitors, cyclosporin, NSAIDs, beta-blockers, heparin, digoxin, potassium sparing diuretics.

Other undesirable effects: Abdominal discomfort, diarrhoea, nausea and vomiting may occur. If there are any signs of gastric irritancy, Kloref-S should be given with or after food.

Use in pregnancy and lactation: Potassium may be indicated as replacement therapy for pregnant women with low potassium levels such as those receiving diuretics. Serum levels should be closely monitored.

Administration of potassium during lactation is considered to be safe providing that maternal serum levels are maintained in the physiological range.

Other special warnings and precautions: Cautious administration is required in cases of chronic renal disease.

Periodic evaluation of the patient's clinical status, serum electrolytes and the ECG should be carried out when replacement therapy is undertaken. This is particularly important in patients with cardiac disease and in those receiving digitalis.

The following warnings appear on the product labelling: 'To be taken only under medical supervision. Keep out of the reach of children'.

Overdosage: Hyperkalaemia. Poisoning is usually minimal below 6.5 mmol/l, moderate between 6.5 and 8 mmol/l and severe above that level. The absolute toxicity is governed by both pH and associated sodium levels.

Hyperkalaemic symptoms and particularly the ECG effects, may be transiently controlled by calcium gluconate, administration of glucose or glucose and insulin, sodium bicarbonate or hypertonic sodium infusions, cation exchange resins or by haemodialysis and peritoneal dialysis. Caution should be exercised in patients who are digitalised and who may experience acute digitalis intoxication in the course of potassium removal.

Pharmaceutical precautions Kloref-S should be stored below 25°C in a dry place.

Legal category P.

Package quantities Kloref-S is available in boxes of 30 sachets.

Further information The addition of each sachet to water brings about a reaction between the betaine hydrochloride and potassium bicarbonate; effervescence results from the liberation of carbon dioxide.

Betaine is a naturally occurring substance found in beet, and is metabolised by the body.

Kloref-S also contains citric acid, povidone, macrogol, saccharin calcium and dioctyl sodium sulphosuccinate.

Product licence number 0142/0367.

**Trade Mark*

CP Pharmaceuticals Limited

Ash Road North
Wrexham Industrial Estate
Wrexham
LL13 9UF

☎ +44 01978 6611261 📠 +44 01978 660130

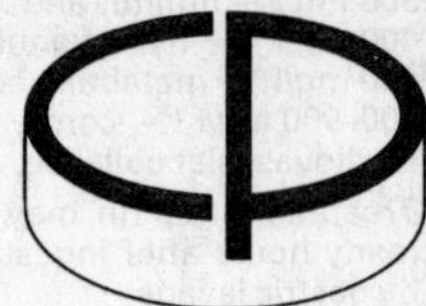

CANUSAL*

Presentation A sterile, pyrogen-free, clear, colourless solution of porcine mucosal Heparin Sodium BP in Sodium Chloride Injection BP adjusted to pH 5 to 8. The solution is preservative free. Each 2 ml ampoule contains 200 iu heparin sodium (100 iu per ml).

Uses Heparin is an anticoagulant. It acts by potentiating the naturally occurring inhibitors of thrombin and factor X (Xa).

Canusal is indicated in any clinical circumstances in which it is desired to maintain the patency of indwelling intravascular catheters/cannulae, attendant lines or heparin locks.

Canusal is not recommended for systemic use.

Dosage and administration

Adults: Flush with 2 ml (200 iu) every 4 hours or as required.

Children/elderly: As for adults.

Contra-indications, warnings, etc.

Contra-indications: Established hypersensitivity to heparin which occurs only rarely.

Precautions: When used as directed, it is extremely unlikely that the low levels of heparin reaching the blood will have any systemic effect.

Rigorous aseptic technique should be observed at all times in its use.

Use in pregnancy: The safety of Canusal in pregnancy is not established but the dose of heparin involved would not be expected to constitute a hazard.

Heparin does not appear in breast milk.

Pharmaceutical precautions Heparin may be incompatible with solutions of certain other drugs, e.g. some antibiotics, opioid analgesics and antihistamines. Canusal should be stored below 25°C. It should not be frozen and should be stored protected from light.

Legal category POM

Package quantities Box of 10 ampoules

Further information Nil

Product licence number 4543/0322

DIAMORPHINE HYDROCHLORIDE FOR INJECTION BP

Quantitative and qualitative composition Each ampoule contains 5 mg, 10 mg, 30 mg, 100 mg, 250 mg or 500 mg of Diamorphine Hydrochloride BP.

Pharmaceutical form A white to off-white, sterile, freeze dried powder of Diamorphine Hydrochloride BP for reconstitution for injection.

Clinical particulars

Therapeutic indications: Diamorphine may be used in the treatment of severe pain associated with surgical procedures, myocardial infarction or pain in the terminally ill and for the relief of dyspnoea in acute pulmonary oedema.

Posology and method of administration: Diamorphine may be given by the intramuscular, intravenous or subcutaneous routes. Glucose intravenous infusion is the preferred diluent, particularly when the drug is administered by a continuous infusion pump over 24 to 48 hours, although it is also compatible with sodium chloride intravenous infusion.

The dose should be suited to the individual patient.

Adults:

Acute pain, 5 mg repeated every four hours if necessary (up to 10 mg for heavier, well muscled patients) by subcutaneous or intramuscular injection. By slow intravenous injection, one quarter to one half the corresponding intramuscular dose.

Chronic pain, 5-10 mg regularly every four hours by subcutaneous or intramuscular injection. The dose may be increased according to individual needs.

Myocardial infarction, 5 mg by slow intravenous injection (1 mg/minute) followed by a further 2.5 mg to 5 mg if necessary.

Acute pulmonary oedema, 2.5 mg to 5 mg by slow intravenous injection (1 mg/minute).

Children and elderly: As diamorphine has a respiratory depressant effect, care should be taken when giving the drug to the very young and the elderly and a lower starting dose than normal is recommended.

Contra-indications: Respiratory depression and obstructive airways disease.

Phaeochromocytoma (endogenous release of histamine may stimulate catecholamine release).

Raised intracranial pressure.

Concurrent use of monoamine oxidase inhibitors or within two weeks of their discontinuation.

Special warnings and special precautions for use: Diamorphine should be administered with care to patients with head injuries as there is an increased risk of respiratory depression which may lead to elevation of CSF pressure. The sedation and pupillary changes produced may interfere with accurate monitoring of the patient.

Repeated administration of diamorphine may lead to dependence and tolerance developing. Abrupt withdrawal in patients who have developed dependence may precipitate a withdrawal syndrome. Great caution should be exercised in patients with a known tendency or history of drug abuse.

Use with caution in patients with toxic psychosis, CNS depression, myxoedema, prostatic hypertrophy or urethral stricture, kyphoscoliosis, acute alcoholism, delirium tremens, severe inflammatory or obstructive bowel disorders, adrenal insufficiency or severe diarrhoea. Care should be exercised in treating the elderly or debilitated patients and those with hepatic or renal impairment.

Interaction with other medicaments and other forms of interaction: The depressant effects of diamorphine may be exaggerated and prolonged by phenothiazines, monoamine oxidase inhibitors, tricyclic antidepressants, anxiolytics and hypnotics. There may be antagonism of the gastrointestinal effects of cisapride, domperidone and metoclopramide. The risk of severe constipation and/or urinary retention is increased by administration of antimuscarinic drugs (e.g. atropine). There may be increased risk of toxicity with 4-quinolone antibacterials.

Alcohol may enhance the sedative and hypotensive effects of diamorphine.

Cimetidine inhibits metabolism of opioid analgesics.

Hyperpyrexia and CNS toxicity have been reported when opioid analgesics are used with selegiline.

Pregnancy and lactation: Safety has not been established in pregnancy.

Administration during labour may cause respiratory depression in the neonate and gastric stasis during labour, increasing the risk of inhalation pneumonia.

Diamorphine should not be given to women who are breast-feeding as there is limited information available on diamorphine in breast milk.

Effects on ability to drive and to use machinery: Diamorphine causes drowsiness and mental clouding. If affected patients should not drive or use machines.

Undesirable effects: The most serious hazard of therapy is respiratory depression although circulatory depression is also possible. The most common side effects are sedation, nausea and vomiting, constipation and sweating. Other side effects include dizziness, miosis, confusion, urinary retention, biliary spasm, orthostatic hypotension, facial flushing, vertigo, palpitations, mood changes, dry mouth, dependence, urticaria, pruritus and raised intracranial pressure.

Overdose: Symptoms: Respiratory depression, pulmonary oedema, muscle flaccidity, coma or stupor, constricted pupils, cold, clammy skin and occasionally bradycardia and hypotension.

Treatment: Respiration and circulation should be maintained and naloxone is indicated if coma or bradypnoea are present. A dose of 0.4 to 2 mg repeated at intervals of two to three minutes (up to 10 mg) may be given by subcutaneous, intramuscular or intravenous injection. The usual initial dosage for children is 10 micrograms per kg body weight. Naloxone may also be given by continuous intravenous infusion, 2 mg diluted in 500 ml, at a rate adjusted to the patient's response. Oxygen and assisted ventilation should be administered if necessary.

Pharmacological properties

Pharmacodynamic properties: Diamorphine is a narcotic analgesic which acts primarily on the central nervous system and smooth muscle. It is predominantly a central nervous system depressant but it has stimulant actions resulting in nausea, vomiting and miosis.

Pharmacokinetic properties: Diamorphine is a potent opiate analgesic which has a more rapid onset of activity than morphine as the first metabolite, monoacetylmorphine, more readily crosses the blood brain barrier. In man, diamorphine has a half life of two to three minutes. Its first metabolite, monoacetylmorphine, is more slowly hydrolysed in the blood to be concentrated mainly in skeletal muscle, kidney, lung, liver and spleen. Monoacetylmorphine is metabolised to morphine. Morphine forms conjugates with glucuronic acid. The majority of the drug is excreted via the kidney as glucuronides and to a much lesser extent as morphine. About 7-10% is eliminated via the biliary system into the faeces.

Diamorphine does not bind to protein. However, morphine is about 35% bound to human plasma proteins, mainly to albumin. The analgesic effect lasts approximately three to four hours.

Preclinical safety data: There are no additional preclinical data of relevance to the prescriber.

Pharmaceutical particulars

List of excipients: Water for Injections BP* Not detectable in the finished product.

Incompatibilities: Physical incompatibility has been reported with mineral acids and alkalis.

Shelf life: Three years from date of manufacture

Special precautions for storage: Store below 25°C, protect from light

Nature and contents of container: 5 mg, 10 mg, 30 mg: 2 ml Neutral glass ampoules, PhEur. Type 1. Ampoules are packed into cartons of 5, 10 or 50.

Nature and contents of container: 100 mg, 250 mg, 500 mg: 5 ml Neutral glass ampoules, PhEur. Type 1. Ampoules are packed into cartons of 5, 10 or 50.

Instruction for use/handling: The solution should be used immediately after preparation.

Marketing authorisation numbers

Diamorphine Hydrochloride for Injection BP:

5 mg	4543/0303
10 mg	4543/0304
30 mg	4543/0305
100 mg	4543/0306
250 mg	4543/0307
500 mg	4543/0308

Date of approval/revision of SPC March 1998

Legal category CD (Sch 2), POM

DIAZEPAM INJECTION BP

Qualitative and quantitative composition Diazepam BP 5.0 mg/ml

Pharmaceutical form Solution for Injection.

Clinical Particulars

Therapeutic indications: Diazepam injection may be used in severe or disabling anxiety and agitation; for the control of status epilepticus, epileptic and febrile convulsions; to relieve muscle spasm; as a sedative in minor surgical and dental procedures; or other circumstances in which a rapid effect is required.

Posology and method of administration: Dosage depends on individual response, age and weight.

Adults:

In severe anxiety or acute muscle spasm, diazepam 10 mg may be given intravenously or intramuscularly and repeated after 4 hours.

In tetanus, 0.1 to 0.3 mg per kg bodyweight may be given intravenously and repeated every 1-4 hours; alternatively, a continuous infusion of 3 to 10 mg per kg every 24 hours may be used or similar doses may be given by nasoduodenal tube.

In status epilepticus or epileptic convulsions, 0.15-0.25 mg per kg (usually 10-20 mg) is given by intravenous injection. If no effect is seen after 5 minutes, the dose can be repeated, up to a maximum of 30 mg. Once the patient is controlled, recurrence of seizures may be prevented by a slow infusion (maximum total dose 3 mg per kg over 24 hours).

In minor surgical procedures and dentistry, 0.1-0.2 mg per kg by injection (usually 10-20 mg) adjusted to the patient's requirements.

Elderly: Elderly or debilitated patients should be given not more than half of the usual dose.

Hepatic/renal impairment: Dosage reduction may also be required in patients with liver or kidney dysfunction.

Children:

In status epilepticus, epileptic or febrile convulsions: 0.2-0.3 mg per kg (or 1 mg per year of life) is given by intravenous injection. If no effect is seen after 5 minutes, the dose can be repeated.

Sedation or muscle relaxation: up to 0.2 mg per kg may be given parenterally.

Neonates: Not recommended; dosage has not been established.

IMPORTANT: In order to reduce the likelihood of adverse effects during intravenous administration the injection should be given slowly (1.0 ml solution per minute). It is advisable to keep the patient supine for at least an hour after administration. Except in emergencies, a second person should always be present during intravenous use and facilities for resuscitation should always be available.

It is recommended that patients should remain under medical supervision until at least one hour has elapsed from the time of injection. They should always be accompanied home by a responsible adult, with a warning not to drive or operate machinery for 24 hours.

Intravenous injection may be associated with local reactions and thrombophlebitis and venous thrombosis may occur. In order to minimise the likelihood of these effects, intravenous injections of diazepam should be given into a large vein of the antecubital fossa.

Where continuous intravenous infusion is necessary it is suggested that 2 ml Diazepam Injection is mixed with at least 200 ml of infusion fluid such as Sodium Chloride Injection or Dextrose Injection and that such solutions should be used immediately. There is evidence that diazepam is adsorbed onto plastic infusion bags and giving sets. It is therefore recommended that glass bottles should be used for the administration of diazepam by intravenous infusion.

Contra-indications: Known sensitivity to benzodiazepines or any of the ingredients, Myasthenia gravis, Severe respiratory insufficiency

Diazepam injection should not be used in phobic or obsessional states nor be used alone in the treatment of depression or anxiety associated with depression due to the risk of suicide being precipitated in this patient group. Diazepam Injection should not be used in the treatment of chronic psychosis. In common with other benzodiazepines the use of diazepam may be associated with amnesia and Diazepam Injection should not be used in cases of loss or bereavement as psychological adjustment may be inhibited.

Special warnings and precautions for use: Diazepam injection should be used with caution in patients with renal or hepatic dysfunction, chronic pulmonary insufficiency, closed angle glaucoma or organic brain changes, particularly arteriosclerosis.

Diazepam may enhance the effects of other CNS depressants; their concurrent use should be avoided.

The dependence potential of diazepam is low when limited to short term use. Withdrawal symptoms may occur with benzodiazepines following normal use of therapeutic doses for only short periods and may be associated with physiological and psychological sequelae, including depression. This should be considered when treating patients for more than a few days.

As with other benzodiazepines extreme caution should be used if prescribing diazepam for patients with personality disorders. The disinhibiting effects of benzodiazepines may be manifested as the precipitation of suicide in patients who are depressed or show aggressive behaviour towards self and others.

Interactions with other medicaments and other forms of interaction: Enhanced sedation or respiratory and cardiovascular depression may occur if diazepam is given with other drugs that have CNS depressant properties (e.g. antipsychotics, anxiolytics, sedatives, antidepressants, hypnotics, narcotic analgesics, anaesthetics, antiepileptics).

If such centrally acting depressant drugs are given parenterally in conjunction with intravenous diazepam, severe respiratory and cardiovascular depression may occur. When intravenous diazepam is to be administered concurrently with a narcotic analgesic agent (e.g. in dentistry), it is recommended that diazepam be given after the analgesic and that the dose be carefully titrated to meet the patient's needs.

Agents that interfere with metabolism by hepatic enzymes (e.g. isoniazid, disulfiram, cimetidine, omeprazole, oral contraceptives) have been shown to reduce the clearance of benzodiazepines and may potentiate their actions, whilst known inducers of hepatic enzymes, for example, rifampicin, may increase the clearance of benzodiazepines.

Diazepam metabolism is accelerated by theophylline and smoking.

Diazepam may interact with other hepatically metabolised drugs, causing inhibition (levodopa) or potentiation (phenytoin, muscle relaxants).

Pregnancy and lactation: There is no evidence regarding the safety of diazepam in pregnancy. It should not be used, especially in the first and third trimesters, unless the benefit is considered to outweigh the risk.

If the product is prescribed to a woman of childbearing potential she should be warned to contact her physician regarding the discontinuance of the product if she intends to become or suspects that she is pregnant.

If for compelling medical reasons, the product is administered during the late phase of pregnancy, or during labour at high doses, effects on the neonate, such as hypothermia, hypotonia and moderate respiratory depression, can be expected, due to the pharmacological action of the compound.

Since benzodiazepines are found in the breast milk, benzodiazepines should not be given to breast feeding mothers.

Effects on ability to drive and to use machines: Patients treated with Diazepam Injection should not drive or use machinery.

Undesirable effects: High dosage or parenteral administration can produce respiratory depression and hypotension.

The side effects of diazepam are usually mild and infrequent. The most common side effects are sedation, drowsiness, headaches, muscle weakness, dizziness (with risk of falls in the elderly), ataxia, confusion, slurred speech, tremor, numbed emotions, reduced alertness, fatigue, double vision, anterograde amnesia and a hangover effect. Elderly or debilitated patients are particularly susceptible to side effects and may require lower doses. Other effects which may occur rarely are dry mouth, increased appetite, gastrointestinal and visual disturbances, jaundice, urinary retention, hypotension, bradycardia, changes in libido, menstrual disturbances, skin reactions, blood dyscrasias, laryngeal spasm, chest pain, respiratory depression and apnoea.

In susceptible patients, an unnoticed depression may become evident. Paradoxical reactions (restlessness, agitation, instability, rages, hallucinations) are known to occur with benzodiazepines and are more likely in children and the elderly.

Overdose: Symptoms: The symptoms of mild overdose may include confusion, somnolence, ataxia, dysarthria, hypotension, muscular weakness. In severe overdose, depression of vital functions may occur, particularly the respiratory centre. As drug levels fall severe agitation may develop.

Treatment: Treatment is symptomatic. Respiration, heart rate, blood pressure and body temperature should be monitored and supportive measures taken to maintain cardiovascular and respiratory function. Flumazenil is indicated to counteract the central depressive effect of benzodiazepines.

Pharmacological properties

Pharmacodynamic properties: Diazepam is a psychotropic substance from the class of 1,4-benzodiazepines with marked properties of suppression of tension, agitation and anxiety as well as sedative and hypnotic effects. In addition, diazepam demonstrates muscle relaxant and anticonvulsive properties. It is used in the short-term treatment of anxiety and tension states, as a sedative and premedicant, in the control of muscle spasm and in the management of alcohol withdrawal symptoms.

Diazepam binds to specific receptors in the central nervous system and particular peripheral organs. The benzodiazepine receptors in the CNS have a close functional connection with receptors of the GABA-ergic transmitter system. After binding to the benzodiazepine receptor, diazepam augments the inhibitory effect of GABA-ergic transmission.

Pharmacokinetic properties: Diazepam is highly lipid soluble and crosses the blood brain barrier. These properties qualify it for intravenous use in short term anaesthetic procedures since it acts promptly on the brain, and its initial effects decrease rapidly as it is distributed into fat deposits and tissues. Following the administration of an adequate intravenous dose of diazepam, effective plasma concentrations are usually reached within 5 minutes (ca. 150-400 ng/ml).

Absorption is erratic following intramuscular administration and lower peak plasma concentrations may be obtained than those following oral administration.

Diazepam is extensively protein bound (95-99%). The volume of distribution is between 0.95 and 2 l/kg depending on age. Diazepam and its main metabolite, N-desmethyldiazepam, cross the placenta and are secreted in breast milk.

Diazepam is metabolised predominantly in the liver. Its metabolites, N-desmethyldiazepam (nordiazepam), temazepam and oxazepam, which appear in the urine as glucuronides, are also pharmacologically active substances. Only 20% of the metabolites are detected in the urine in the first 72 hours.

Diazepam has a biphasic half life with an initial rapid distribution phase followed by a prolonged terminal elimination phase of 1-2 days. For the active metabolites N-desmethyldiazepam, temazepam and oxazepam, the half lives are 30-100 hours, 10-20 hours and 5-15 hours, respectively.

Excretion is mainly renal and also partly biliary. It is dependent on age as well as hepatic and renal function.

Metabolism and elimination in the neonate are markedly slower than in children and adults. In the elderly, elimination is prolonged by a factor of 2 to 4. In patients with impaired renal function, elimination is also prolonged. In patients with hepatic disorders (liver cirrhosis, hepatitis), elimination is prolonged by a factor of 2.

Pre-clinical safety data: Chronic toxicity studies have demonstrated no evidence of drug induced changes. There are no long term animal studies to investigate the carcinogenic potential of diazepam. Several investigations pointed to a weakly mutagenic potential at doses far above the human therapeutic dose.

Local tolerability has been studied following single and repeat dose applications into the conjunctival sac of rabbits and the rectum of dogs. Only minimal irritation was observed. There were no systemic changes.

In humans it would appear that the risk of congenital abnormalities from the ingestion of therapeutic doses of benzodiazepines is slight, although a few epidemiological studies have pointed to an increased risk of cleft palate. There are case reports of congenital abnormalities and mental retardation in prenatally exposed children following overdosage and intoxication with benzodiazepines.

Pharmaceutical particulars

List of excipients: Benzoic acid; ethanol; propylene glycol; sodium benzoate; benzyl alcohol; water for injections

Incompatibilities: Diazepam Injection should not be mixed with other drugs in the same infusion solution or the same syringe.

Shelf life: Three years

Special precautions for storage: Store protected from light. Store below 25°C

Nature and contents of container: Amber glass ampoules (2 ml or 4 ml) packed in 10s in an outer printed carton.

Instructions for use/handling: None

Marketing authorisation number 4543/0179

Date of approval /revision of SPC November 1997

Legal category CD (Sch 4), POM

DIAZEPAM RECTUBES*

Qualitative and quantitative composition

Diazepam Ph Eur 2.5 mg in 1.25 ml (2 mg/ml)
Diazepam Ph Eur 5 mg in 2.5 ml (2 mg/ml)
Diazepam Ph Eur 10 mg in 2.5 ml (4 mg/ml)
Diazepam Ph Eur 20 mg in 5.0 ml (4 mg/ml)

Pharmaceutical form Solution in rectal tube–rectal use

Clinical particulars

Therapeutic indications: Diazepam rectal tubes may be used in severe or disabling anxiety and agitation; epileptic and febrile convulsions; to relieve muscle spasm caused by tetanus; as a sedative in minor surgical and dental procedures, or other circumstances in which a rapid effect is required but where intravenous injection is impracticable or undesirable.

Diazepam rectal tubes may be of particular value for the immediate treatment of convulsions in children.

Posology and method of administration: Dosage depends on age and weight.

Children: 0.5 mg/kg (not recommended in infants under 10 kg)

Adults: 0.5 mg/kg

If convulsions are not controlled other anticonvulsive measures should be instituted. The dose can be repeated every 12 hours.

Elderly and debilitated patients should be given not more than one half the appropriate adult dose.

Dosage reduction may also be required in patients with liver or kidney dysfunction.

Contra-indications: Known hypersensitivity to benzodiazepines or any of the ingredients. Myasthenia gravis. Severe respiratory insufficiency.

Diazepam should not be used in phobic or obsessional states, nor be used alone in the treatment of depression or anxiety associated with depression due to the risk of suicide being precipitated in this patient group. Diazepam should not be used in the treatment of chronic psychosis. In common with other benzodiazepines the use of diazepam may be associated with amnesia and diazepam should not be used in cases of loss or bereavement as psychological adjustments may be inhibited.

Special warnings and special precautions for use: Diazepam should be used with caution in patients with renal or hepatic dysfunction, chronic pulmonary insufficiency, closed angle glaucoma or organic brain changes, particularly arteriosclerosis.

Diazepam may enhance the effects of other CNS depressants, their concurrent use should be avoided.

The dependence potential of diazepam is low when limited to short-term use. Withdrawal symptoms may occur with benzodiazepines following normal use of therapeutic doses for only short periods and may be associated with physiological and psychological sequelae, including depression. This should be considered when treating patients for more than a few days.

As with other benzodiazepines extreme caution should be used if prescribing diazepam for patients with personality disorders. The disinhibiting effects of benzodiazepines may be manifested as the precipitation of suicide in patients who are depressed or show aggressive behaviour towards self and others.

Interaction with other medicaments and other forms of interactions: Enhanced sedation or respiratory and cardiovascular depression may occur if diazepam is given with other drugs that have CNS depressant properties (e.g. antipsychotics, anxiolytics, sedatives, antidepressants, hypnotics, narcotic analgesics, anaesthetics, antiepileptics) or with agents that interfere with its metabolism by hepatic enzymes (e.g. isoniazid, disulfiram, cimetidine, omeprazole, oral contraceptives). Cimetidine and omeprazole have been shown to reduce the clearance of benzodiazepines and may potentiate their action whilst known inducers of hepatic enzymes e.g. rifampicin, may increase the clearance of benzodiazepines.

Diazepam metabolism is accelerated by theophylline and smoking.

Diazepam may interact with other hepatically metabolised drugs, causing inhibition (levodopa) or potentiation (phenytoin, muscle relaxants).

Pregnancy and lactation: There is no evidence regarding the safety of diazepam in pregnancy. It should not be used especially in the first and third trimesters, unless the benefit is considered to outweigh the risk.

In labour, high single doses or repeated low doses have been reported to produce hypothermia, hypotonia, respiratory depression and poor suckling (floppy infant syndrome) in the neonate and irregularities in the foetal heart.

Diazepam is excreted in the breast milk and therefore its use during lactation should be avoided.

Effects on ability to drive and use machines: Patients treated with Diazepam Rectal Tubes should not drive or operate machines.

Undesirable effects: The side effects of diazepam are usually mild and infrequent. The most common side effects are sedation, drowsiness, headaches, muscle weakness, dizziness (with risk of falls in the elderly), ataxia, confusion, slurred speech, tremor, numbed emotions, reduced alertness, fatigue, double vision, anterograde amnesia and a hangover effect. Elderly or debilitated patients are particularly susceptible to side effects and may require lower doses. Other effects which may occur rarely are dry mouth, increased appetite, gastrointestinal and visual disturbances, jaundice, urinary retention, hypotension, bradycardia, changes in libido, menstrual disturbances, skin reactions, blood dyscrasias, laryngeal spasm, chest pain, respiratory depression and apnoea.

In susceptible patients, an unnoticed depression may become evident. Paradoxical reactions (restlessness, agitation, instability, rages, hallucinations) are known to occur with benzodiazepines and are more likely in children and the elderly.

Overdose: Symptoms: The symptoms of mild overdose may include confusion, somnolence, ataxia, dysarthria, hypotension, muscular weakness. In severe overdose, depression of vital functions may occur, particularly the respiratory centre. As drug levels fall severe agitation may develop.

Treatment: Treatment is symptomatic. Respiration, heart rate, blood pressure and body temperature should be monitored and supportive measures taken to maintain cardiovascular and respiratory function. Flumazenil is indicated to counteract the central depressive effect of benzodiazepines.

Pharmacological properties

Pharmacodynamic properties: Diazepam is a psychotropic substance from the class of 1,4-benzodiazepines with marked properties of suppression of tension, agitation and anxiety as well as sedative and hypnotic effects. In addition, diazepam demonstrates muscle relaxant and anticonvulsive properties. It is used in the short-term treatment of anxiety and tension states, as a sedative and premedicant, in the control of muscle spasm and in the management of alcohol withdrawal symptoms.

Diazepam binds to specific receptors in the central nervous system and particular peripheral organs. The benzodiazepine receptors in the CNS have a close functional connection with receptors of the GABA-ergic transmitter system. After binding to the benzodiazepine receptor, diazepam augments the inhibitory effect of GABA-ergic transmission.

Pharmacokinetic properties: After rectal administration of the solution, diazepam is absorbed rapidly and almost completely from the rectum.

The onset of the therapeutic effect occurs within a few minutes of rectal administration. The rapidity of the rise in the serum level following rectal administration corresponds approximately to that following an intravenous dose but peak plasma concentrations are lower after rectal tubes than after intravenous administration. In adults maximal plasma concentrations following the administration of 10 mg diazepam in rectal solution are reached after about 10–30 minutes (ca. 150–400 ng/ml).

Diazepam is extensively protein bound (95-99%). The volume of distribution is between 0.95 and 2 l/kg depending on age. Diazepam is lipophilic and rapidly enters the cerebrospinal fluid. Diazepam and its main metabolite, N-desmethyldiazepam, cross the placenta and are secreted in breast milk.

Diazepam is metabolised predominantly in the liver. Its metabolites, N-desmethyldiazepam (nordiazepam), temazepam and oxazepam, which appear in the urine as glucuronides, are also pharmacologically active substances. Only 20% of the metabolites are detected in the urine in the first 72 hours.

Diazepam has a biphasic half life with an initial rapid distribution phase followed by a prolonged terminal elimination phase of 1-2 days. For the active metabolites N-desmethyldiazepam, temazepam and oxazepam, the half lives are 30-100 hours, 10-20 hours and 5-15 hours, respectively.

Excretion is mainly renal and also partly biliary. It is dependent on age as well as hepatic and renal function.

Metabolism and elimination in the neonate are markedly slower than in children and adults. In the elderly, elimination is prolonged by a factor of 2 to 4. In patients with impaired renal function, elimination is also prolonged. In patients with hepatic disorders (liver cirrhosis, hepatitis), elimination is prolonged by a factor of 2.

Preclinical safety data: Chronic toxicity studies in animals have demonstrated no evidence of drug-induced changes. There are no long-term animal studies to investigate the carcinogenic potential of diazepam. Several investigations pointed to a weakly mutagenic potential at doses far above the human therapeutic dose.

Local tolerability has been studied following single and repeat dose applications into the conjunctival sac of rabbits and the rectum of dogs. Only minimal irritation was observed. There were no systemic changes.

In humans it would appear that the risk of congenital abnormalities from the ingestion of therapeutic doses of benzodiazepines is slight, although a few epidemiological studies have pointed to an increased risk of cleft palate. There are case reports of congenital abnormalities and mental retardation in prenatally exposed children following overdosage and intoxication with benzodiazepines.

Pharmaceutical particulars

List of excipients: Benzyl alcohol; Alcohol; Propylene glycol; Benzoic acid; Sodium benzoate; Purified Water

Incompatibilities: None known.

Shelf life: Three years in alufoil pack.

Special precautions for storage: Store below 25°C. Short-term exposure to higher temperatures (eg in emergencies), is of no consequence.

Nature and contents of container:

2.5 mg: Packs of 5 rectal tubes each containing 1.25 ml of solution

5 mg: Packs of 5 rectal tubes each containing 2.5 ml of solution

10 mg: Packs of 5 rectal tubes each containing 2.5 ml of solution

20 mg: Packs of 5 rectal tubes each containing 5 ml of solution

The tubes are made of low density polyethylene.

Instructions for use/handling: The solution is administered rectally. Adults should be in the lateral position; children should be in the prone or lateral position.

a) Tear open the foil pack. Remove the cap.

b) Insert the tube nozzle completely into the rectum. For children under 15 kg, insert only half way. Hold the tube with the spout downwards. The contents of the tube should be completely emptied by using firm pressure with the index finger and thumb.

c) To avoid suction, maintain pressure on the tube until it is withdrawn from the rectum. Press together the patient's buttocks for a short time.

Marketing authorisation numbers

2.5 mg	4543/0364
5 mg	4543/0340
10 mg	4543/0341
20 mg	4543/0363

Date of approval/revision of SPC August 1996

Legal Category CD (Sch 4), POM

HEPSAL* 10 iu/ml

Qualitative and quantitative composition Heparin Sodium (Mucous) BP 10iu per ml.

Pharmaceutical form Injection

Clinical particulars

Therapeutic indications: Heparin is an anticoagulant and acts by potentiating the naturally occurring inhibitors of thrombin and factor X (Xa).

Hepsal is indicated in any clinical circumstances in which it is desired to maintain the patency of indwelling catheters/cannulae, attendant lines or heparin locks.

Hepsal is not recommended for systemic use.

Posology and method of administration: Route of administration: For cleaning indwelling cannulae. Material to be used as a cannula flush (5 ml; 50 units) every 4 hours or as required.

Contra-indications: The very rare occurrence of established hypersensitivity to heparin is the only contra-indication to Hepsal.

Special warnings and precautions for use: Rigorous aseptic technique should be observed at all times in its use.

Interaction with other medicaments: None stated.

Pregnancy and lactation: None stated.

Effects on ability to drive and to use machinery: None stated.

Undesirable effects: Used as directed, it is extremely unlikely that the low levels of heparin reaching the blood will have any systemic effect.

Overdose: None stated

Pharmacological properties

Pharmacodynamic properties: Hepsal, containing only 50 iu of sodium heparin per ampoule (5 ml), is to be used as directed for flushing indwelling cannulae. This is unlikely to produce blood levels of heparin having any systemic effect.

Pharmacokinetic properties: None stated

Pre-clinical safety data: There are no pre-clinical data of relevance to the prescriber which are additional to that already included in other sections.

Pharmaceutical particulars

List of excipients: Sodium Chloride BP; Water for Injection BP; Hydrochloric Acid 3M; Sodium Hydroxide 3M

Incompatibilities: None stated

Shelf life: 36 months in glass ampoules; 24 months in polypropylene ampoules

Special precautions for storage: Store below 25°C. Do not freeze

Nature and contents of container: 5 ml clear glass ampoules. Carton contains 10 ampoules. 5 ml polypropylene ampoules. Carton contains 20 ampoules.

Instructions for use/handling: Not applicable

Marketing authorisation number

Glass ampoules	4543/0228
Polypropylene ampoules	4543/0358

Date of approval/revision of SPC July 1996

Legal category POM

HYPURIN* BOVINE NEUTRAL CARTRIDGES
HYPURIN* BOVINE ISOPHANE CARTRIDGES

Qualitative and quantitative formula Highly Purified Crystalline Bovine Insulin Ph Eur 100 international units/ml.

Pharmaceutical form
Neutral: Sterile injection for subcutaneous, intramuscular or intravenous injection.
Isophane: Sterile injection for subcutaneous or intramuscular injection.

Clinical particulars
Therapeutic indications: The treatment of insulin dependent diabetes mellitus.

Hypurin Bovine Neutral: May be used for diabetics who require an insulin of prompt onset and short duration. It is a suitable preparation for admixture with longer acting insulins. It is particularly useful where intermittent, short term or emergency therapy is required, during initial stabilisation and in the treatment of labile diabetes.

Hypurin Bovine Isophane: May be used for diabetics requiring a depot insulin of medium duration. Where a more rapid, intense onset is desirable it may be mixed with Hypurin Neutral.

Posology and method of administration: To be determined by the physician according to the needs of the patient.

Hypurin Bovine Neutral: Usually administered subcutaneously but where necessary it may be given intramuscularly or intravenously. After subcutaneous injection onset of action occurs within 30-60 minutes with an overall duration of 6-8 hours. Maximum effect is exerted over the mid-range.

Hypurin Bovine Isophane: Usually administered subcutaneously but where necessary it may be given intramuscularly in which case onset is more rapid and overall duration shorter. It should not be given intravenously. Onset of action occurs within 2 hours after subcutaneous injection with an overall duration of 18-24 hours. Maximum effect is exerted between 6-12 hours.

Contra-indications: Hypoglycaemia.

Special warnings and precautions: In no circumstances must Hypurin Bovine Isophane be given intravenously.

Blood or urinary glucose concentrations should be monitored and the urine tested for ketones by patients on insulin therapy.

Patients transferred to Hypurin Bovine insulins from other commercially available preparations may require dosage adjustments. Patients whose blood glucose control is greatly improved, e.g. by intensified insulin therapy, may lose some or all of the warning symptoms of hypoglycaemia and should be advised accordingly.

Interactions with other medicaments and other forms of interaction: Insulin requirements may increase during illness, puberty or emotional upset or during concurrent administration of drugs associated with hyperglycaemic activity e.g.oral contraceptives, chlorpromazine, thyroid hormone replacement therapy, thiazide diuretics and sympathomimetic agents.

Insulin requirements may decrease with liver or kidney disease, disease of the adrenal, pituitary or thyroid glands or during concomitant use of drugs with hypoglycaemic activity, e.g salicylates, anabolic steroids, monoamine oxidase inhibitors, NSAIDS. Drugs which may decrease or increase insulin requirements include alcohol, cyclophosphamide, isoniazid and beta blockers (which may also mask some of the warning signs of insulin-induced hypoglycaemia).

Insulin requirements are usually reduced but occasionally increased during periods of increased activity.

Pregnancy and lactation: A decreased requirement for insulin may be observed in the early stages of pregnancy. However, in the second and third trimesters, insulin requirements may increase. Diabetic patients who are breast feeding may require adjustments in their insulin dose.

Effects on ability to drive and to use machinery: The patient's ability to concentrate and react may be impaired as a result of hypoglycaemia. This may constitute a risk in situations where these abilities are of special importance (e.g. driving a car or operating machinery).

Patients should be advised to take precautions to avoid hypoglycaemia whilst driving, this is particularly important in those who have reduced or absent awareness of the warning signs of hypoglycaemia or have frequent episodes of hypoglycaemia. The advisability of driving should be considered in these circumstances.

Undesirable effects: Lipodystrophy (atrophy or hypertrophy of the fat tissue) or oedema may occur at the injection site. Insulin hypersensitivity can occur with animal insulins , but appears less likely with purified insulins and there is minimal evidence that such effects occur with Hypurin® Bovine insulins.

Intolerability reactions to phenol and m-cresol contained as preservative may occur.

Overdosage: Symptoms: Overdosage causes hypoglycaemia. Symptoms include weakness, sweating, trembling, nervousness, excitement and irritability which, if untreated, will lead to collapse and coma.

Treatment: Mild hypoglycaemia will respond to oral administration of glucose or sugar and rest.

Moderately severe hypoglycaemia can be treated by intramuscular or subcutaneous injection of glucagon followed by oral carbohydrate when the patient is sufficiently recovered.

For patients who are comatose or who have failed to respond to glucagon injection an intravenous injection of Strong Dextrose Injection BP should be given.

Pharmacological particulars
Pharmacodynamic properties: Insulin output from the pancreas of a healthy person is about 50 units per day, which is sufficient to maintain the fasting blood sugar concentration in the range 0.8±0.2 mg/ml. In diabetes mellitus, the blood sugar rises in an uncontrolled manner. Parenterally administered insulin causes a fall in blood sugar concentration and increased storage of glycogen in the liver. In the diabetic it raises the respiratory quotient after a carbohydrate meal and prevents the formation of ketone bodies. The rise in blood sugar concentration caused by adrenaline and corticosteroids, glucagon and posterior pituitary extract is reversed by insulin.

Pharmacokinetic properties: Insulin is rapidly absorbed from subcutaneous tissue or muscle following injection.

Insulin is metabolised mainly in the liver and a small amount is excreted in the urine.

The plasma half life is 4 to 5 minutes. The half life after subcutaneous injection is about 4 hours and after intramuscular injection about 2 hours.

Pre-clinical safety data: There are no preclinical data of relevance to the prescriber which are additional to that already included in other sections.

Pharmaceutical particulars
List of excipients

Neutral: m-cresol, Phenol Ph Eur, Sodium Phosphate Ph Eur, Glycerol Ph Eur, Water for Injections Ph Eur.

Isophane: Protamine Sulphate Ph Eur, Zinc Chloride Ph Eur, m-cresol, Phenol Ph Eur, Sodium Phosphate Ph Eur, Glycerol Ph Eur, Water for Injections Ph Eur.

Incompatibilities: None

Shelf life: 36 months.

Following injection of the first dose the product should be used within 28 days. Discard any unused material after this time.

Special precautions for storage: Store between 2°C and 8°C. Do not freeze.

Cartridges in use must not be stored in a refrigerator. They may be kept at room temperature (maximum 25°C) for four weeks.

Nature and contents of container: 1.5 ml neutral glass cartridge sealed with a rubber bung and metal closure.

Instruction for use/handling: Prior to use the cartridge of Hypurin® Bovine Isophane should be inverted at least ten times. The injection should then be made immediately.

The cartridge must not be used if the contents have been frozen or it contains lumps that do not disperse on mixing.

Marketing authorisation numbers

Hypurin Bovine Neutral cartridge	PL 4543/0366
Hypurin Bovine Isophane cartridge	PL 4543/0367

Date of approval/revision of SPC April 1998.

Legal Category POM

HYPURIN* BOVINE NEUTRAL VIALS
HYPURIN* BOVINE ISOPHANE VIALS
HYPURIN* BOVINE LENTE VIALS
HYPURIN* BOVINE PROTAMINE ZINC VIALS

Qualitative and quantitative composition Highly Purified Crystalline Bovine Insulin Ph Eur 100 international units/ml.

Pharmaceutical form
Neutral: Sterile injection for subcutaneous, intramuscular or intravenous injection.

Isophane: Sterile injection for subcutaneous or intramuscular injection.

Lente: Sterile suspension for subcutaneous injection.

Protamine Zinc: Sterile suspension for subcutaneous injection.

Clinical particulars
Therapeutic indications: The treatment of insulin dependent diabetes mellitus.

Hypurin Bovine Neutral: May be used for diabetics who require an insulin of prompt onset and short duration. It is a suitable preparation for admixture with longer acting insulins. It is particularly useful where intermittent, short term or emergency therapy is required, during initial stabilisation and in the treatment of labile diabetes.

Hypurin Bovine Isophane: May be used for diabetics requiring a depot insulin of medium duration. Where a more rapid, intense onset is desirable it may be mixed with Hypurin Neutral.

Hypurin Bovine Lente: May be used for diabetics requiring a depot insulin of medium to extended duration.

Hypurin Bovine Protamine Zinc: May be used for diabetics requiring a depot insulin of extended duration. It is characteristically slow in onset and is commonly used in conjunction with Hypurin Neutral.

Posology and method of administration: To be determined by the physician according to the needs of the patient.

Hypurin Bovine Neutral: Usually administered subcutaneously but where necessary it may be given intramuscularly or intravenously. After subcutaneous injection onset of action occurs within 30-60 minutes with an overall duration of 6-8 hours. Maximum effect is exerted over the mid-range.

Hypurin Bovine Isophane: Usually administered subcutaneously but where necessary it may be given intramuscularly in which case onset is more rapid and overall duration shorter. It should not be given intravenously. Onset of action occurs within 2 hours after subcutaneous injection with an overall duration of 18-24 hours. Maximum effect is exerted between 6-12 hours.

Hypurin Bovine Lente: Administered subcutaneously. It is not recommended for intramuscular use and should not be given intravenously. Onset of action occurs approximately 2 hours after subcutaneous injection with an overall duration extending up to 30 hours. Maximum effect is exerted between 8-12 hours.

Hypurin Bovine Protamine Zinc: Administered subcutaneously. It is not recommended for intramuscular use and should not be given intravenously. Onset of action occurs after 4-6 hours with an overall duration of 24-36 hours. Maximum effect is exerted between 10-20 hours.

Contra-indications: Hypoglycaemia.

Special warnings and precautions for use: In no circumstances must Hypurin Bovine Isophane, Hypurin Bovine Lente or Hypurin Bovine Protamine Zinc be given intravenously.

Blood or urinary glucose concentrations should be monitored and the urine tested for ketones by patients on insulin therapy.

Patients transferred to Hypurin Bovine insulins from other commercially available preparations may require dosage adjustments. Patients whose blood glucose control is greatly improved, e.g. by intensified insulin therapy, may lose some or all of the warning symptoms of hypoglycaemia and should be advised accordingly.

Interactions with other medicaments and other forms of interaction: Insulin requirements may increase during illness, puberty or emotional upset or during concurrent administration of drugs associated with hyperglycaemic activity e.g. oral contraceptives, chlorpromazine, thyroid hormone replacement therapy, thiazide diuretics and sympathomimetic agents.

Insulin requirements may decrease with liver or kidney disease, disease of the adrenal, pituitary or thyroid glands or during concomitant use of drugs with hypoglycaemic activity, e.g salicylates, anabolic steroids, monoamine oxidase inhibitors, NSAIDS. Drugs which may decrease or increase insulin requirements include alcohol, cyclophosphamide, isoniazid and beta blockers (which may also mask some of the warning signs of insulin-induced hypoglycaemia).

Insulin requirements are usually reduced but occasionally increased during periods of increased activity.

Pregnancy and lactation: A decreased requirement for insulin may be observed in the early stages of pregnancy. However, in the second and third trimesters, insulin requirements may increase. Diabetic patients who are breast-feeding may require adjustments in their insulin dose.

Effects on ability to drive and to use machinery: The patient's ability to concentrate and react may be impaired as a result of hypoglycaemia. This may constitute a risk in situations where these abilities are of special importance (e.g. driving a car or operating machinery).

Patients should be advised to take precautions to avoid hypoglycaemia whilst driving, this is particularly important in those who have reduced or absent awareness of the warning signs of hypoglycaemia or have frequent episodes of hypoglycaemia. The advisability of driving should be considered in these circumstances.

Undesirable effects: Lipodystrophy (atrophy or hypertrophy of the fat tissue) or oedema may occur at the injection site. Insulin hypersensitivity can occur with animal insulins, but appears less likely with purified insulins and there is minimal evidence that such effects occur with Hypurin Bovine insulins.

Intolerability reactions to phenol and m-cresol contained as preservative may occur.

Overdosage: Symptoms: Overdosage causes hypoglycaemia. Symptoms include weakness, sweating, trembling, nervousness, excitement and irritability which, if untreated, will lead to collapse and coma.

Treatment: Mild hypoglycaemia will respond to oral administration of glucose or sugar and rest.

Moderately severe hypoglycaemia can be treated by intramuscular or subcutaneous injection of glucagon followed by oral carbohydrate when the patient is sufficiently recovered.

For patients who are comatose or who have failed to respond to glucagon injection, 50% glucose intravenous infusion should be given.

Pharmacological particulars

Pharmacodynamic properties: Insulin output from the pancreas of a healthy person is about 50 units per day, which is sufficient to maintain the fasting blood sugar concentration in the range 0.8±0.2 mg/ml. In diabetes mellitus, the blood sugar rises in an uncontrolled manner. Parenterally administered insulin causes a fall in blood sugar concentration and increased storage of glycogen in the liver. In the diabetic it raises the respiratory quotient after a carbohydrate meal and prevents the formation of ketone bodies. The rise in blood sugar concentration caused by adrenaline and corticosteroids, glucagon and posterior pituitary extract is reversed by insulin.

Pharmacokinetic properties: Insulin is rapidly absorbed from subcutaneous tissue or muscle following injection.

Insulin is metabolised mainly in the liver and a small amount is excreted in the urine.

The plasma half life is 4 to 5 minutes. The half life after subcutaneous injection is about 4 hours and after intramuscular injection about 2 hours.

Pre-clinical safety data: There are no preclinical data of relevance to the prescriber which are additional to those already included in other sections.

Pharmaceutical particulars

List of excipients:

Neutral: m-cresol, Phenol Ph Eur, Sodium Phosphate Ph Eur, Glycerol Ph Eur, Water for Injections Ph Eur.

Isophane: Protamine Sulphate Ph Eur, Zinc Chloride Ph Eur, m-cresol, Phenol Ph Eur, Sodium Phosphate Ph Eur, Glycerol Ph Eur, Water for Injections Ph Eur.

Lente: Sodium Chloride Ph Eur, Sodium Acetate Ph Eur, Methylparahydroxybenzoate Ph Eur, Zinc Chloride Ph Eur, Water for Injections Ph Eur.

Protamine Zinc: Protamine Sulphate Ph Eur, Zinc Chloride Ph Eur, Glycerol Ph Eur, Sodium Phosphate Ph Eur, Phenol Ph Eur, Water for Injections Ph Eur.

Incompatibilities: None

Shelf life: 36 months.

Following injection of the first dose the product should be used within 28 days. Discard any unused material after this time.

Special precautions for storage: Store between 2°C and 8°C. Do not freeze.

Vials in use may be kept at room temperature (maximum 25°C) for four weeks.

Nature and contents of container: 10 ml neutral glass vial sealed with a rubber bung and metal closure.

Instruction for use/handling: The vial must not be used if the contents have been frozen or it contains lumps that do not disperse on mixing.

Prior to use the vial of Hypurin Bovine Isophane or Hypurin Bovine Lente or Hypurin Bovine Protamine Zinc should be rolled gently between the palms or inverted several times.

Hypurin Bovine Isophane and Hypurin Bovine Lente may be mixed with Hypurin Bovine Neutral in the syringe, in which case Hypurin Bovine Neutral should be the first dose to be withdrawn.

The injection should then be made immediately upon withdrawal of the contents.

Hypurin Bovine Neutral and Hypurin Bovine Protamine Zinc should not be mixed together.

Marketing authorisation numbers

Hypurin Bovine Neutral	PL 4543/0203
Hypurin Bovine Isophane	PL 4543/0196
Hypurin Bovine Lente	PL 4543/0214
Hypurin Bovine Protamine Zinc	PL 4543/0199

Date of approval/revision of SPC April 1998

Legal category POM

HYPURIN* PORCINE NEUTRAL CARTRIDGES
HYPURIN* PORCINE ISOPHANE CARTRIDGES
HYPURIN* PORCINE 30/70 MIX CARTRIDGES

Qualitative and quantitative formula Highly Purified Crystalline Porcine Insulin PhEur 100 international units/ml.

Pharmaceutical form

Neutral: Sterile injection for subcutaneous, intramuscular or intravenous injection.

Isophane and 30/70 Mix: Sterile injection for subcutaneous or intramuscular injection.

Clinical particulars

Therapeutic indications: The treatment of insulin dependent diabetes mellitus.

Hypurin Porcine Neutral: May be used for diabetics who require an insulin of prompt onset and short duration. It is a suitable preparation for admixture with longer acting insulins. It is particularly useful where intermittent, short term or emergency therapy is required, during initial stabilisation and in the treatment of labile diabetes.

Hypurin Porcine Isophane: May be used for diabetics requiring a depot insulin of medium duration. Where a more rapid, intense onset is desirable it may be mixed with Hypurin Porcine Neutral.

Hypurin Porcine 30/70 Mix: May be used for diabetics requiring a depot insulin of intermediate duration.

Posology and method of administration: To be determined by the physician according to the needs of the patient.

Hypurin Porcine Neutral: Usually administered subcutaneously but where necessary it may be given intramuscularly or intravenously. After subcutaneous injection onset of action occurs within 30-60 minutes with an overall duration of 6-8 hours. Maximum effect is exerted over the mid-range.

Hypurin Porcine Isophane: Usually administered subcutaneously but where necessary it may be given intramuscularly in which case onset is more rapid and overall duration shorter. It should not be given intravenously. Onset of action occurs within 2 hours after subcutaneous injection with an overall duration of 18-24 hours. Maximum effect is exerted between 6-12 hours.

Hypurin Porcine 30/70 Mix: Usually administered subcutaneously but where necessary it may be given intramuscularly in which case onset is more rapid and overall duration shorter. It should not be given intravenously. Onset of action occurs within 2 hours after subcutaneous injection with an overall duration up to 24 hours. Maximum effect is exerted between 4-12 hours.

Contra-indications: Hypoglycaemia.

Special warnings and precautions for use: In no circumstances must Hypurin Porcine Isophane or Hypurin Porcine 30/70 Mix be given intravenously.

Blood or urinary glucose concentrations should be monitored and the urine tested for ketones by patients on insulin therapy.

Patients transferred to Hypurin Porcine insulins from other commercially available preparations may require dosage adjustments. Patients whose blood glucose control is greatly improved, e.g. by intensified insulin therapy, may lose some or all of the warning symptoms of hypoglycaemia and should be advised accordingly.

Interactions with other medicaments and other forms of interaction: Insulin requirements may increase during illness, puberty or emotional upset or during concurrent administration of drugs associated with hyperglycaemic activity e.g. oral contraceptives, chloropromazine, thyroid hormone replacement therapy, thiazide diuretics and sympathomimetic agents.

Insulin requirements may decrease with liver or kidney disease, disease of the adrenal, pituitary or thyroid glands or during concomitant use of drugs with hypoglycaemic activity, e.g. salicylates, anabolic steroids, monoamine oxidase inhibitors, NSAIDs. Drugs that may decrease or increase insulin requirements include alcohol, cyclophosphamide, isoniazid and beta-blockers (which may also mask some of the warning signs of insulin-induced hypoglycaemia).

Insulin requirements are usually reduced but occasionally increased during periods of increased activity.

Pregnancy and lactation: A decreased requirement for insulin may be observed in the early stages of pregnancy. However, in the second and third trimesters, insulin requirements may increase. Diabetic patients who are breast-feeding may require adjustments in their insulin dose.

Effects on ability to drive and to use machinery: The patient's ability to concentrate and react may be impaired as a result of hypoglycaemia. This may constitute a risk in situations where these abilities are of special importance (e.g. driving a car or operating machinery).

Patients should be advised to take precautions to avoid hypoglycaemia whilst driving, this is particularly important in those who have reduced or absent awareness of the warning signs of hypoglycaemia or have frequent episodes of hypoglycaemia. The advisability of driving should be considered in these circumstances.

Undesirable effects: Lipodystrophy (atrophy or hypertrophy of the fat tissue) or oedema may occur at the injection site. Insulin hypersensitivity can occur with animal insulins, but appears less likely with purified insulins.

Intolerability reactions to phenol and m-cresol contained as preservative may occur.

Overdosage: Symptoms: Overdosage causes hypoglycaemia. Symptoms include weakness, sweating, trembling, nervousness, excitement and irritability which, if untreated, will lead to collapse and coma.

Treatment: Mild hypoglycaemia will respond to oral administration of glucose or sugar and rest.

Moderately severe hypoglycaemia can be treated by intramuscular or subcutaneous injection of glucagon followed by oral carbohydrate when the patient is sufficiently recovered.

For patients who are comatose or who have failed to respond to glucagon injection an intravenous injection of strong Dextrose Injection BP should be given.

Pharmacological particulars

Pharmacodynamic properties: Insulin output from the pancreas of a healthy person is about 50 units per day, which is sufficient to maintain the fasting blood sugar concentration in the range 0.8±0.2 mg/ml. In diabetes mellitus, the blood sugar rises in an uncontrolled manner. Parenterally administered insulin causes a fall in blood sugar concentration and increased storage of glycogen in the liver. In the diabetic it raises the respiratory quotient after a carbohydrate meal and prevents the formation of ketone bodies. The rise in blood sugar concentration caused by adrenaline and corticosteroids, glucagon and posterior pituitary extract is reversed by insulin.

Pharmacokinetic properties: Insulin is rapidly absorbed from subcutaneous tissue or muscle following injection.

Insulin is metabolised mainly in the liver and a small amount is excreted in the urine.

The plasma half-life is four to five minutes. The half-life after subcutaneous injection is about four hours and after intramuscular injection about two hours.

Pre-clinical safety data: There are no preclinical data of relevance to the prescriber that are additional to that already included in other sections.

Pharmaceutical particulars

List of excipients

Neutral: m-cresol, Phenol Ph Eur, Sodium Phosphate Ph Eur, Glycerol Ph Eur, Water for Injections Ph Eur.

Isophane: Protamine Sulphate Ph Eur, Zinc Chloride Ph Eur, m-cresol, Phenol Ph Eur, Sodium Phosphate Ph Eur, Glycerol Ph Eur, Water for Injections Ph Eur.

30/70 Mix: Protamine Sulphate Ph Eur, Zinc Chloride Ph Eur, m-cresol, Phenol Ph Eur, Sodium Phosphate Ph Eur, Glycerol Ph Eur, Water for Injections Ph Eur.

Incompatibilities: None

Shelf life: 36 months (except Hypurin® Porcine 30/70 mix which is 24 months).

Following injection of the first dose the product should be used within 28 days. Discard any unused material after this time.

Special precautions for storage: Store between 2°C and 8°C. Do not freeze.

Cartridges in use should not be stored in a refrigerator. They may be kept at room temperature (maximum 25°C) for four weeks.

Nature and contents of container: 1.5 ml neutral glass cartridge sealed with a rubber bung and metal closure.

Instruction for use/handling: Prior to use the cartridge of Hypurin Porcine Isophane or Hypurin Porcine 30/70 Mix should inverted at least ten times. The injection should then be made immediately.

The cartridge must not be used if the contents have been frozen or it contains lumps that do not disperse on mixing.

Marketing authorisation numbers

Hypurin Porcine Neutral cartridge PL 4543/0373

Hypurin Porcine Isophane cartridge PL 4543/0374
Hypurin Porcine 30/70 Mix cartridge PL 4543/0375

Date of approval/revision of SPC April 1998

Legal category POM

HYPURIN* PORCINE NEUTRAL VIALS HYPURIN* PORCINE ISOPHANE VIALS HYPURIN* PORCINE 30/70 MIX VIALS

Qualitative and quantitative formula Highly Purified Crystalline Porcine Insulin Ph Eur 100 international units/ml.

Pharmaceutical form
Neutral: Sterile injection for subcutaneous, intramuscular or intravenous injection.

Isophane and 30/70 Mix: Sterile injection for subcutaneous or intramuscular injection.

Clinical particulars
Therapeutic indications: The treatment of insulin dependent diabetes mellitus.

Hypurin Porcine Neutral: May be used for diabetics who require an insulin of prompt onset and short duration. It is a suitable preparation for admixture with longer acting insulins. It is particularly useful where intermittent, short term or emergency therapy is required, during initial stabilisation and in the treatment of labile diabetes.

Hypurin Porcine Isophane: May be used for diabetics requiring a depot insulin of medium duration. Where a more rapid, intense onset is desirable it may be mixed with Hypurin Neutral.

Hypurin Porcine 30/70 Mix: May be used for diabetics requiring a depot insulin of intermediate duration.

Posology and method of administration: To be determined by the physician according to the needs if the patient.

Hypurin Porcine Neutral: Usually administered subcutaneously but where necessary it may be given intramuscularly or intravenously. After subcutaneous injection onset of action occurs within 30-60 minutes with an overall duration of 6-8 hours. Maximum effect is exerted over the mid-range.

Hypurin Porcine Isophane: Usually administered subcutaneously but where necessary it may be given intramuscularly in which case onset is more rapid and overall duration shorter. It should not be given intravenously. Onset of action occurs within 2 hours after subcutaneous injection with an overall duration of 18-24 hours. Maximum effect is exerted between 6-12 hours.

Hypurin Porcine 30/70 Mix: Usually administered subcutaneously but where necessary it may be given intramuscularly in which case onset is more rapid and overall duration shorter. It should not be given intravenously. Onset of action occurs within 2 hours after subcutaneous injection with an overall duration up to 24 hours. Maximum effect is exerted between 4-12 hours.

Contra-indications: Hypoglycaemia.

Special warnings and precautions: In no circumstances must Hypurin Porcine Isophane or Hypurin Porcine 30/70 Mix be given intravenously.

Blood or urinary glucose concentrations should be monitored and the urine tested for ketones by patients on insulin therapy.

Patients transferred to Hypurin Porcine insulins from other commercially available preparations may require dosage adjustments. Patients whose blood glucose control is greatly improved, e.g. by intensified insulin therapy, may lose some or all of the warning symptoms of hypoglycaemia and should be advised accordingly.

Interactions with other medicaments and other forms of interaction: Insulin requirements may increase during illness, puberty or emotional upset or during concurrent administration of drugs associated with hyperglycaemic activity e.g. oral contraceptives, chloropromazine, thyroid hormone replacement therapy, thiazide diuretics and sympathomimetic agents.

Insulin requirements may decrease with liver or kidney disease, disease of the adrenal, pituitary or thyroid glands or during concomitant use of drugs with hypoglycaemic activity, e.g salicylates, anabolic steroids, monoamine oxidase inhibitors, NSAIDS. Drugs which may decrease or increase insulin requirements include alcohol, cyclophosphamide, isoniazid and beta blockers (which may also mask some of the warning signs of insulin-induced hypoglycaemia).

Insulin requirements are usually reduced but occasionally increased during periods of increased activity.

Pregnancy and lactation: A decreased requirement for insulin may be observed in the early stages of pregnancy. However, in the second and third trimesters, insulin requirements may increase. Diabetic patients who are breast-feeding may require adjustments in their insulin dose.

Affects on ability to drive and to use machinery: The patient's ability to concentrate and react may be impaired as a result of hypoglycaemia. This may constitute a risk in situations where these abilities are of special importance (e.g. driving a car or operating machinery).

Patients should be advised to take precautions to avoid hypoglycaemia whilst driving, this is particularly important in those who have reduced or absent awareness of the warning signs of hypoglycaemia or have frequent episodes of hypoglycaemia. The advisability of driving should be considered in these circumstances.

Undesirable effects: Lipodystrophy (atrophy or hypertrophy of the fat tissue) or oedema may occur at the injection site. Insulin hypersensitivity can occur with animal insulins, but appears less likely with purified insulins and there is minimal evidence that such effects occur with Hypurin insulins.

Intolerability reactions to phenol and m-cresol contained as preservative may occur.

Overdosage: Symptoms: Overdosage causes hypoglycaemia. Symptoms include weakness, sweating, trembling, nervousness, excitement and irritability which, if untreated, will lead to collapse and coma.

Treatment: Mild hypoglycaemia will respond to oral administration of glucose or sugar and rest.

Moderately severe hypoglycaemia can be treated by intramuscular or subcutaneous injection of glucagon followed by oral carbohydrate when the patient is sufficiently recovered.

For patients who are comatose or who have failed to respond to glucagon injection an intravenous injection of strong Dextrose Injection BP should be given.

Pharmacological particulars
Pharmacodynamic properties: Insulin output from the pancreas of a healthy person is about 50 units per day, which is sufficient to maintain the fasting blood sugar concentration in the range 0.8±0.2 mg/ml. In diabetes mellitus, the blood sugar rises in an uncontrolled manner. Parenterally administered insulin causes a fall in blood sugar concentration and increased storage of glycogen in the liver. In the diabetic it raises the respiratory quotient after a carbohydrate meal and prevents the formation of ketone bodies. The rise in blood sugar concentration caused by adrenaline and corticosteroids, glucagon and posterior pituitary extract is reversed by insulin.

Pharmacokinetic properties: Insulin is rapidly absorbed from subcutaneous tissue or muscle following injection.

Insulin is metabolised mainly in the liver and a small amount is excreted in the urine.

The plasma half-life is 4 to 5 minutes. The half-life after subcutaneous injection is about 4 hours and after intramuscular injection about 2 hours.

Pre-clinical safety data: There are no preclinical data of relevance to the prescriber that are additional to that already included in other sections.

Pharmaceutical particulars
List of excipients
Neutral: m-cresol, Phenol Ph Eur, Sodium Phosphate Ph Eur, Glycerol Ph Eur, Water for Injections BP.

Isophane: Protamine Sulphate Ph Eur, Zinc Chloride Ph Eur, m-cresol, Phenol Ph Eur, Sodium Phosphate Ph Eur, Glycerol Ph Eur, Water for Injections BP.

30/70 Mix: Protamine Sulphate Ph Eur, Zinc Chloride Ph Eur, m-cresol, Phenol Ph Eur, Sodium Phosphate Ph Eur, Glycerol Ph Eur, Water for Injections BP.

Incompatibilities: None

Shelf life: 36 months.

Following withdrawal of the first dose the product should be used within 28 days. Discard any unused material.

Special precautions for storage: Store between 2°C and 8°C. Do not freeze.

Vials in use may be kept at room temperature (maximum 25°C) for four weeks.

Nature and contents of container: 10 ml neutral glass vial sealed with a rubber bung and metal closure.

Instruction for use/handling: Prior to use the vial of Hypurin Porcine Isophane or Hypurin Porcine 30/70 Mix should be gently rolled between the palms or inverted several times.

The vial must not be used if the contents have been frozen or it contains lumps that do not disperse on mixing.

The injections should be made immediately upon withdrawal of the contents.

Marketing authorisation numbers
Hypurin Porcine Neutral vials PL 4543/0370
Hypurin Porcine Isophane vials PL 4543/0371
Hypurin Porcine 30/70 Mix vials PL 4543/0372

Date of approval/revision of SPC April 1998

Legal category POM

MONOPARIN*

Qualitative and quantitative composition
Monoparin 1,000 iu/ml: Heparin Sodium (Mucous) BP 1,000 iu/ml

Monoparin 5,000 iu/ml: Heparin Sodium (Mucous) BP 5,000 iu/ml

Monoparin 10,000 iu/ml: Heparin Sodium (Mucous) BP 10,000 iu/ml

Monoparin 25,000 iu/ml: Heparin Sodium (Mucous) BP 25,000 iu/ml

Pharmaceutical form
Monoparin 1,000 iu/ml: Intravenous Injection

Monoparin 5,000 iu/ml, Monoparin 10,000 and Monoparin 25,000 iu/ml: Intravenous or subcutaneous injection

Clinical particulars
Therapeutic indications:

Monoparin 1,000 iu/ml, 5000 iu/ml, 10,000 iu/ml and 25,000 iu/ml: Treatment of deep vein thrombosis, pulmonary embolism, unstable angina pectoris and acute peripheral arterial occlusion.

In extracorporeal circulation and haemodialysis.

Monoparin 5,000 iu/ml, 10,000 iu/ml and 25,000 iu/ml: Prophylaxis of deep vein thrombosis and pulmonary embolism. Prophylaxis of mural thrombosis following myocardial infarction.

Posology and method of administration:
Route of administration: Monoparin 5,000 iu/ml, 10,000 iu/ml and 25,000 iu/ml: By continuous intravenous infusion in 5% glucose or 0.9% sodium chloride or by intermittent intravenous injection, or by subcutaneous injection.

As the effects of heparin are short-lived, administration by intravenous infusion or subcutaneous injection is preferable to intermittent intravenous injections.

Monoparin 1,000 iu/ml: By continuous intravenous infusion in 5% glucose or 0.9% sodium chloride or by intermittent intravenous injection.

As the effects of heparin are short-lived, administration by intravenous infusion is preferable to intermittent intravenous injections.

Recommended dosage:
Prophylaxis of deep vein thrombosis and pulmonary embolism (Monoparin 5,000 iu/ml, 10,000 iu/ml and 25,000 iu/ml only)

Adults: 2 hours pre-operatively: 5,000 units subcutaneously followed by: 5,000 units subcutaneously every 8-12 hours, for 7-10 days or until the patient is fully ambulant.

No laboratory monitoring should be necessary during low dose heparin prophylaxis. If monitoring is considered desirable, anti-Xa assays should be used as the activated partial thromboplastin time (APTT) is not significantly prolonged.

During pregnancy: 5,000–10,000 units every 12 hours, subcutaneously, adjusted according to APTT or anti-Xa assay.

Elderly: Dosage reduction and monitoring of APTT may be advisable.

Children: No dosage recommendations.

Treatment of deep vein thrombosis, pulmonary embolism, unstable angina pectoris, acute peripheral arterial occlusion (Monoparin 1,000 iu/ml, 5,000 iu/ml, 10,000 iu/ml, 25,000 iu/ml):

Adults: Loading dose: 5,000 units intravenously (10,000 units may be required in severe pulmonary embolism)

Maintenance: 1,000-2,000 units/hour by intravenous infusion,

or 5,000-10,000 units 4-hourly by intravenous injection

or (except Monoparin 1,000 iu/ml) 10,000-20,000 units 12 hourly subcutaneously,

Elderly: Dosage reduction may be advisable.

Children and small adults:
Loading dose: 50 units/kg intravenously

Maintenance: 15-25 units/kg/hour by intravenous infusion,

or 100 units/kg 4-hourly by intravenous injection

or (except Monoparin 1,000 iu/ml) 250 units/kg 12 hourly subcutaneously

Daily laboratory monitoring (ideally at the same time each day, starting 4-6 hours after initiation of treatment) is essential during full-dose heparin treatment, with adjustment of dosage to maintain an APTT value 1.5-2.5 x midpoint of normal range or control value.

Prophylaxis of mural thrombosis following myocardial infarction (Monoparin 5,000 iu/ml, 10,000 iu/ml and 25,000 iu/ml only)

Adults: 12,500 units 12 hourly subcutaneously for at least 10 days.

Elderly: Dosage reduction may be advisable

In extracorporeal circulation and haemodialysis (Monoparin 1,000 iu/ml, 5,000 iu/ml, 10,000 iu/ml25,000 iu/ml)

Adults: Cardiopulmonary bypass: Initially 300 units/kg intravenously, adjusted thereafter to maintain the activated clotting time (ACT) in the range 400-500 seconds.

Haemodialysis and haemofiltration: Initially 1-5,000 units, Maintenance: 1-2,000 units/hour, adjusted to maintain clotting time >40 minutes.

Contra-indications: Patients who consume large amounts of alcohol, who are sensitive to the drug, who are actively bleeding or who have haemophilia, purpura, severe hypertension, active tuberculosis or increased capillary permeability.

Patients with present or previous thrombocytopenia. The rare occurrence of skin necrosis in patients receiving heparin contra-indicates the further use of heparin either by subcutaneous or intravenous routes because of the risk of thrombocytopenia. Because of the special hazard of post-operative haemorrhage heparin is contra-indicated during surgery of the brain, spinal cord and eye, and in patients undergoing lumbar puncture or regional anaesthetic block.

The relative risks and benefits of heparin should be carefully assessed in patients with a bleeding tendency or those patients with an actual or potential bleeding site eg. hiatus hernia, peptic ulcer, neoplasm, bacterial endocarditis, retinopathy, bleeding haemorrhoids, suspected intracranial haemorrhage, cerebral thrombosis or threatened abortion.

Menstruation is not a contra-indication.

Special warnings and special precautions for use: Platelet counts should be measured in patients receiving heparin treatment for longer than 5 days and the treatment should be stopped immediately in those who develop thrombocytopenia.

In patients with advanced renal or hepatic disease, a reduction in dosage may be necessary.

Although heparin hypersensitivity is rare, it is advisable to give a trial dose of 1,000 iu in patients with a history of allergy.

In most patients, the recommended low-dose regimen produces no alteration in clotting time. However, patients show an individual response to heparin, and it is therefore essential that the effect of therapy on coagulation time should be monitored in patients undergoing major surgery.

Heparin can suppress adrenal secretion of aldosterone leading to hyperkalemia, particularly in patients such as those with diabetes mellitus, chronic renal failure, pre-existing metabolic acidosis, a raised plasma potassium, or taking potassium sparing drugs. The risk of hyperkalemia appears to increase with duration of therapy but is usually reversible. Plasma potassium should be measured in patients at risk before starting heparin therapy and in all patients treated for more than 7 days.

Interactions with other medicaments: Drugs that interfere with platelet aggregation eg. aspirin, dextran solutions, dipyridamole or any other drug which may interfere with coagulation, should be used with care.

Pregnancy and lactation: Heparin is not contraindicated in pregnancy. Heparin does not cross the placenta or appear in breast milk. The decision to use heparin in pregnancy should be taken after evaluation of the risk/benefit in any particular circumstances.

Effects on ability to drive and to use machinery: None stated.

Undesirable effects: Haemorrhage (see *Overdosage*).

Thrombocytopenia has been observed occasionally (see *Warnings*).

There is some evidence that prolonged dosing with heparin (ie. over many months) may cause alopecia and osteoporosis. Significant bone demineralisation has been reported in women taking more than 10,000 iu per day of heparin for at least 6 months.

Heparin products can cause hypoaldosteronism which may result in an increase in plasma potassium. Rarely, clinically significant hyperkalemia may occur particularly in patients with chronic renal failure and diabetes mellitus (see *Warnings and Precautions*).

Hypersensitivity reactions, local irritation and skin necrosis may occur but are rare.

Overdose: A potential hazard of heparin therapy is haemorrhage, but this is usually due to overdosage and the risk is minimised by strict laboratory control. Slight haemorrhage can usually be treated by withdrawing the drug. If bleeding is more severe, clotting time and platelet count should be determined. Prolonged clotting time will indicate the presence of an excessive anticoagulant effect requiring neutralisation by intravenous protamine sulphate, at a dosage of 1 mg for every 100 iu of heparin to be neutralised. The bolus dose of protamine sulphate should be given slowly over about 10 minutes and not exceed 50 mg. If more than 15 minutes have elapsed since the injection of heparin, lower doses of protamine will be necessary.

Pharmacological properties

Pharmacodynamic properties: Heparin is an anticoagulant and acts by inhibiting thrombin and by potentiating the naturally occurring inhibitors of activated Factor X (Xa).

Pharmacokinetic particulars: As heparin is not absorbed from the gastrointestinal tract and sublingual sites it is administered by injection. After injection heparin extensively binds to plasma proteins.

Heparin is metabolised in the liver and the inactive metabolic products are excreted in the urine.

The half life of heparin is dependent on the dose.

Pre-clinical safety data: There are no pre-clinical data of relevance to the prescriber which are additional to that already included in other sections.

Pharmaceutical particulars

List of excipients: Water for Injections BP, sodium hydroxide solution 3M, hydrochloric acid 3M

Incompatibilities: Heparin is incompatible with many injectable preparations e.g. some antibiotics, opioid analgesics and antihistamines.

Shelf life: 36 months

Special precautions for storage: Monoparin should be stored below 25°C.

Nature and contents of container:
Monoparin 1,000 iu/ml: Neutral glass ampoules (Type I Ph Eur) of 1 ml, 5 ml, 10 ml and 20 ml capacity containing 1 ml, 5 ml, 10 ml and 20 ml of solution respectively. Cartons contain 10 ampoules.

Monoparin 5,000 iu/ml: Neutral glass ampoules (Type I Ph Eur) of 1 ml and 5 ml capacity containing 1 ml and 5 ml of solution respectively. Cartons contain 10 ampoules.

Monoparin 10,000 iu/ml: Neutral glass ampoules (Type I Ph Eur) of 1 ml capacity containing 1 ml of solution. Cartons contain 10 ampoules.

Monoparin 25,000 iu/ml: Neutral glass ampoules (Type I Ph Eur) of 1 ml capacity containing 0.2 ml, 0.5 ml and 1 ml of solution respectively and 5 ml ampoules containing 5 ml of solution. Cartons contain 10, 15 or 50 ampoules.

Instructions for use/handling: Not applicable

Marketing authorisation numbers

Monoparin 1,000 iu/ml	PL 4543/0221
Monoparin 5,000 iu/ml	PL 4543/0208
Monoparin 10,000 iu/ml	PL 4543/0209
Monoparin 25,000 iu/ml	PL 4543/0210

Date of approval/revision of SmPC: June 1998

Legal category POM

MONOPARIN CA*

Qualitative and quantitative composition

Monoparin Ca 1,000 iu/ml: Heparin Calcium (Mucous) BP 1,000 iu/ml

Monoparin Ca 5,000 iu/ml: Heparin Calcium (Mucous) BP 5,000 iu/ml

Monoparin Ca 25,000 iu/ml: Heparin Calcium (Mucous) BP 25,000 iu/ml

Pharmaceutical form

Monoparin Ca 1,000 iu/ml: Intravenous Injection
Monoparin Ca 5,000 iu/ml and Monoparin Ca 25,000 iu/ml: Intravenous or subcutaneous injection

Clinical particulars

Therapeutic indications: Monoparin Ca 1,000 iu/ml, 5000iu/ml and 25,000 iu/ml: Treatment of deep vein thrombosis, pulmonary embolism, unstable angina pectoris and acute peripheral arterial occlusion.

In extracorporeal circulation and haemodialysis.

Monoparin Ca 5,000iu/ml and 25,000 iu/ml: Prophylaxis of deep vein thrombosis and pulmonary embolism. Prophylaxis of mural thrombosis following myocardial infarction.

Posology and method of administration:
Route of administration: Monoparin Ca 5,000 iu/ml and 25,000 iu/ml: By continuous intravenous infusion in 5% glucose or 0.9% sodium chloride or by intermittent intravenous injection, or by subcutaneous injection.

As the effects of heparin are short-lived, administration by intravenous infusion or subcutaneous injection is preferable to intermittent intravenous injections.

Monoparin Ca 1,000 iu/ml: By continuous intravenous infusion in 5% glucose or 0.9% sodium chloride or by intermittent intravenous injection.

As the effects of heparin are short-lived, administration by intravenous infusion is preferable to intermittent intravenous injections.

Recommended dosage:
Prophylaxis of deep vein thrombosis and pulmonary embolism (Monoparin Ca 5,000 iu/ml and 25,000 iu/ml only)

Adults: 2 hours pre-operatively: 5,000 units subcutaneously followed by: 5,000 units subcutaneously every 8-12 hours, for 7-10 days or until the patient is fully ambulant.

No laboratory monitoring should be necessary during low dose heparin prophylaxis. If monitoring is considered desirable, anti-Xa assays should be used as the activated partial thromboplastin time (APTT) is not significantly prolonged.

During pregnancy: 5,000–10,000 units every 12 hours, subcutaneously, adjusted according to APTT or anti-Xa assay.

Elderly: Dosage reduction and monitoring of APTT may be advisable.

Children: No dosage recommendations.

Treatment of deep vein thrombosis, pulmonary embolism, unstable angina pectoris, acute peripheral arterial occlusion (Monoparin Ca 1,000 iu/ml, 5,000 iu/ml, 25,000 iu/ml):

Adults: Loading dose: 5,000 units intravenously (10,000 units may be required in severe pulmonary embolism)

Maintenance: 1,000-2,000 units/hour by intravenous infusion,

or 5,000-10,000 units 4-hourly by intravenous injection

or (except Monoparin 1,000 iu/ml) 10,000-20,000 units 12 hourly subcutaneously,

Elderly: Dosage reduction may be advisable.

Children and small adults:
Loading dose: 50 units/kg intravenously

Maintenance: 15-25 units/kg/hour by intravenous infusion,

or 100 units/kg 4-hourly by intravenous injection

or (except Monoparin Ca 1,000 iu/ml) 250 units/kg 12 hourly subcutaneously

Daily laboratory monitoring (ideally at the same time each day, starting 4-6 hours after initiation of treatment) is essential during full-dose heparin treatment, with adjustment of dosage to maintain an APTT value 1.5-2.5 x midpoint of normal range or control value.

Prophylaxis of mural thrombosis following myocardial infarction (Monoparin Ca 5,000 iu/ml and 25,000 iu/ml only)

Adults: 12,500 units 12 hourly subcutaneously for at least 10 days.

Elderly: Dosage reduction may be advisable

In extracorporeal circulation and haemodialysis (Monoparin Ca 1,000 iu/ml, 5,000 iu/ml, 25,000 iu/ml)
Adults:

Cardiopulmonary bypass: Initially 300 units/kg intravenously, adjusted thereafter to maintain the activated clotting time (ACT) in the range 400-500 seconds.

Haemodialysis and haemofiltration: Initially 1-5,000 units, Maintenance: 1-2,000 units/hour, adjusted to maintain clotting time >40 minutes.

Contra-indications: Patients who consume large amounts of alcohol, who are sensitive to the drug, who are actively bleeding or who have haemophilia, purpura, severe hypertension, active tuberculosis or increased capillary permeability.

Patients with present or previous thrombocytopenia. The rare occurrence of skin necrosis in patients receiving heparin contra-indicates the further use of heparin either by subcutaneous or intravenous routes because of the risk of thrombocytopenia. Because of the special hazard of post-operative haemorrhage heparin is contra-indicated during surgery of the brain, spinal cord and eye, and in patients undergoing lumbar puncture or regional anaesthetic block.

The relative risks and benefits of heparin should be carefully assessed in patients with a bleeding tendency or those patients with an actual or potential bleeding site eg. hiatus hernia, peptic ulcer, neoplasm, bacterial endocarditis, retinopathy, bleeding haemorrhoids, suspected intracranial haemorrhage, cerebral thrombosis or threatened abortion.

Menstruation is not a contra-indication.

Special warnings and special precautions for use: Platelet counts should be measured in patients receiving heparin treatment for longer than 5 days and the treatment should be stopped immediately in those who develop thrombocytopenia.

In patients with advanced renal or hepatic disease, a reduction in dosage may be necessary.

Although heparin hypersensitivity is rare, it is advisable to give a trial dose of 1,000 iu in patients with a history of allergy.

In most patients, the recommended low-dose regimen produces no alteration in clotting time. However, patients show an individual response to heparin, and it is therefore essential that the effect of therapy on coagulation time should be monitored in patients undergoing major surgery.

Heparin can suppress adrenal secretion of aldosterone leading to hyperkalemia, particularly in patients such as those with diabetes mellitus, chronic renal failure, pre-existing metabolic acidosis, a raised plasma potassium, or taking potassium sparing drugs. The risk of hyperkalemia appears to increase with duration of therapy but is usually reversible. Plasma potassium should be measured in patients at risk before starting heparin therapy and in all patients treated for more than 7 days.

Interactions with other medicaments: Drugs that interfere with platelet aggregation eg. aspirin, dextran solutions, dipyridamole or any other drug which may interfere with coagulation, should be used with care.

Pregnancy and lactation: Heparin is not contra-indicated in pregnancy. Heparin does not cross the placenta or appear in breast milk. The decision to use heparin in pregnancy should be taken after evaluation of the risk/benefit in any particular circumstances.

Effects on ability to drive and to use machinery: None stated.

Undesirable effects: Haemorrhage (see *Overdosage*).

Thrombocytopenia has been observed occasionally (see *Warnings and precautions*).

There is some evidence that prolonged dosing with heparin (ie. over many months) may cause alopecia and osteoporosis. Significant bone demineralisation has been reported in women taking more than 10,000 iu per day of heparin for at least 6 months.

Heparin products can cause hypoaldosteronism which may result in an increase in plasma potassium. Rarely, clinically significant hyperkalemia may occur particularly in patients with chronic renal failure and diabetes mellitus (see *Warnings and precautions*).

Hypersensitivity reactions, local irritation and skin necrosis may occur but are rare.

Overdose: A potential hazard of heparin therapy is haemorrhage, but this is usually due to overdosage and the risk is minimised by strict laboratory control. Slight haemorrhage can usually be treated by withdrawing the drug. If bleeding is more severe, clotting time and platelet count should be determined. Prolonged clotting time will indicate the presence of an excessive anticoagulant effect requiring neutralisation by intravenous protamine sulphate, at a dosage of 1 mg for every 100 iu of heparin to be neutralised. The bolus dose of protamine sulphate should be given slowly over about 10 minutes and not exceed 50 mg. If more than 15 minutes have elapsed since the injection of heparin, lower doses of protamine will be necessary.

Pharmacological properties

Pharmacodynamic properties: Heparin is an anticoagulant and acts by inhibiting thrombin and by potentiating the naturally occurring inhibitors of activated Factor X (Xa).

Pharmacokinetic particulars: As heparin is not absorbed from the gastrointestinal tract and sublingual sites it is administered by injection. After injection heparin extensively binds to plasma proteins.

Heparin is metabolised in the liver and the inactive metabolic products are excreted in the urine.

The half life of heparin is dependent on the dose.

Pre-clinical safety data: There are no pre-clinical data of relevance to the prescriber which are additional to that already included in other sections.

Pharmaceutical particulars

List of excipients: Water for Injections BP, calcium hydroxide solution 3M, hydrochloric acid 3M

Incompatibilities: Heparin is incompatible with many injectable preparations e.g. some antibiotics, opioid analgesics and antihistamines.

Shelf life: 36 months

Special precautions for storage: Monoparin Ca should be stored below 25°C.

Nature and contents of container:

Monoparin Ca 1,000 iu/ml and 5,000 iu/ml: Neutral glass ampoule (Type I Ph Eur) of 1 ml and 5 ml capacity containing 1 ml and 5 ml of solution respectively. Cartons contain 10 ampoules.

Monoparin Ca 25,000 iu/ml: Neutral glass ampoules (Type I Ph Eur) of 1 ml capacity containing 0.2 ml of solution. Cartons contain 10 ampoules.

Instructions for use/handling: Not applicable

Marketing authorisation numbers

Monoparin Ca 1,000 iu/ml	PL 4543/0211
Monoparin Ca 5,000 iu/ml	PL 4543/0212
Monoparin Ca 25,000 iu/ml	PL 4543/0213

Date of approval/revision of SmPC September 1998

Legal category POM

MULTIPARIN*

Qualitative and quantitative composition

Multiparin 1,000 iu/ml: Heparin Sodium (Mucous) BP 1,000 iu/ml

Multiparin 5,000 iu/ml: Heparin Sodium (Mucous) BP 5,000 iu/ml

Multiparin 25,000 iu/ml: Heparin Sodium (Mucous) BP 25,000 iu/ml

Pharmaceutical form

Multiparin 1,000 iu/ml: Intravenous Injection

Multiparin 5,000 iu/ml and Multiparin 25,000 iu/ml: Intravenous or subcutaneous injection

Clinical particulars

Therapeutic indications:

Multiparin 1,000 iu/ml, 5000iu/ml and 25,000 iu/ml: Treatment of deep vein thrombosis, pulmonary embolism, unstable angina pectoris and acute peripheral arterial occlusion.

In extracorporeal circulation and haemodialysis.

Multiparin 5,000iu/ml and 25,000 iu/ml: Prophylaxis of deep vein thrombosis and pulmonary embolism. Prophylaxis of mural thrombosis following myocardial infarction.

Posology and method of administration:

Route of administration: Multiparin 5,000 iu/ml and 25,000 iu/ml: By continuous intravenous infusion in 5% glucose or 0.9% sodium chloride or by intermittent intravenous injection, or by subcutaneous injection.

The intravenous injection volume of Multiparin should not exceed 15 ml.

As the effects of heparin are short-lived, administration by intravenous infusion or subcutaneous injection is preferable to intermittent intravenous injections.

Multiparin 1,000 iu/ml: By continuous intravenous infusion in 5% glucose or 0.9% sodium chloride or by intermittent intravenous injection.

The intravenous injection volume of Multiparin should not exceed 15 ml.

As the effects of heparin are short-lived, administration by intravenous infusion is preferable to intermittent intravenous injections.

Recommended dosage:

Prophylaxis of deep vein thrombosis and pulmonary embolism (Multiparin 5,000 iu/ml and 25,000 iu/ml only)

Adults: 2 hours pre-operatively: 5,000 units subcutaneously followed by: 5,000 units subcutaneously every 8-12 hours, for 7-10 days or until the patient is fully ambulant.

No laboratory monitoring should be necessary during low dose heparin prophylaxis. If monitoring is considered desirable, anti-Xa assays should be used as the activated partial thromboplastin time (APTT) is not significantly prolonged.

During pregnancy: 5,000–10,000 units every 12 hours, subcutaneously, adjusted according to APTT or anti-Xa assay.

Elderly: Dosage reduction and monitoring of APTT may be advisable.

Children: No dosage recommendations.

Treatment of deep vein thrombosis, pulmonary embolism, unstable angina pectoris, acute peripheral arterial occlusion (Multiparin 1,000 iu/ml, 5,000 iu/ml, 25,000 iu/ml):

Adults:

Loading dose: 5,000 units intravenously (10,000 units may be required in severe pulmonary embolism)

Maintenance: 1,000-2,000 units/hour by intravenous infusion,

or 5,000-10,000 units 4-hourly by intravenous injection

or (except Multiparin 1,000 iu/ml) 10,000-20,000 units 12 hourly subcutaneously,

Elderly: Dosage reduction may be advisable.

Children and small adults:

Loading dose: 50 units/kg intravenously

Maintenance: 15-25 units/kg/hour by intravenous infusion,

or 100 units/kg 4-hourly by intravenous injection

or (except Multiparin 1,000 iu/ml) 250 units/kg 12 hourly subcutaneously

Daily laboratory monitoring (ideally at the same time each day, starting 4-6 hours after initiation of treatment) is essential during full-dose heparin treatment, with adjustment of dosage to maintain an APTT value 1.5-2.5 x midpoint of normal range or control value.

Prophylaxis of mural thrombosis following myocardial infarction (Multiparin 5,000 iu/ml and 25,000 iu/ml only)

Adults: 12,500 units 12 hourly subcutaneously for at least 10 days.

Elderly: Dosage reduction may be advisable

In extracorporeal circulation and haemodialysis (Multiparin 1,000 iu/ml, 5,000 iu/ml, 25,000 iu/ml)

Adults:

Cardiopulmonary bypass: Initially 300 units/kg intravenously, adjusted thereafter to maintain the activated clotting time (ACT) in the range 400-500 seconds.

Haemodialysis and haemofiltration: Initially 1-5,000 units, Maintenance: 1-2,000 units/hour, adjusted to maintain clotting time >40 minutes.

Contra-indications: Patients who consume large amounts of alcohol, who are sensitive to the drug, who are actively bleeding or who have haemophilia, purpura, severe hypertension, active tuberculosis or increased capillary permeability.

Patients with present or previous thrombocytopenia. The rare occurrence of skin necrosis in patients receiving heparin contra-indicates the further use of heparin either by subcutaneous or intravenous routes because of the risk of thrombocytopenia. Because of the special hazard of post-operative haemorrhage heparin is contra-indicated during surgery of the brain, spinal cord and eye, and in patients undergoing lumbar puncture or regional anaesthetic block.

The relative risks and benefits of heparin should be carefully assessed in patients with a bleeding tendency or those patients with an actual or potential bleeding site eg. hiatus hernia, peptic ulcer, neoplasm, bacterial endocarditis, retinopathy, bleeding haemorrhoids, suspected intracranial haemorrhage, cerebral thrombosis or threatened abortion.

Menstruation is not a contra-indication.

Special warnings and special precautions for use: Platelet counts should be measured in patients receiving heparin treatment for longer than 5 days and the treatment should be stopped immediately in those who develop thrombocytopenia.

In patients with advanced renal or hepatic disease, a reduction in dosage may be necessary.

Although heparin hypersensitivity is rare, it is advisable to give a trial dose of 1,000 iu in patients with a history of allergy.

In most patients, the recommended low-dose regimen produces no alteration in clotting time. However, patients show an individual response to heparin, and it is therefore essential that the effect of therapy on coagulation time should be monitored in patients undergoing major surgery.

Heparin can suppress adrenal secretion of aldosterone leading to hyperkalemia, particularly in patients such as those with diabetes mellitus, chronic renal failure, pre-existing metabolic acidosis, a raised plasma potassium, or taking potassium sparing drugs. The risk of hyperkalemia appears to increase with duration of therapy but is usually reversible. Plasma potassium should be measured in patients at risk before starting heparin therapy and in all patients treated for more than 7 days.

Interactions with other medicaments: Drugs that interfere with platelet aggregation eg. aspirin, dextran solutions, dipyridamole or any other drug which may interfere with coagulation, should be used with care.

Pregnancy and lactation: Heparin is not contraindicated in pregnancy. Heparin does not cross the placenta or appear in breast milk. The decision to use heparin in pregnancy should be taken after evaluation of the risk/benefit in any particular circumstances.

Effects on ability to drive and to use machinery: None stated.

Undesirable effects: Haemorrhage (see *Overdosage*).

Thrombocytopenia has been observed occasionally (see *Warnings and precautions*).

There is some evidence that prolonged dosing with heparin (ie. over many months) may cause alopecia and osteoporosis. Significant bone demineralisation has been reported in women taking more than 10,000 iu per day of heparin for at least 6 months.

Heparin products can cause hypoaldosteronism which may result in an increase in plasma potassium. Rarely, clinically significant hyperkalemia may occur particularly in patients with chronic renal failure and diabetes mellitus (see *Warnings and precautions*).

Hypersensitivity reactions, local irritation and skin necrosis may occur but are rare.

Overdose: A potential hazard of heparin therapy is haemorrhage, but this is usually due to overdosage and the risk is minimised by strict laboratory control. Slight haemorrhage can usually be treated by withdrawing the drug. If bleeding is more severe, clotting time and platelet count should be determined. Prolonged clotting time will indicate the presence of an excessive anticoagulant effect requiring neutralisation by intravenous protamine sulphate, at a dosage of 1 mg for every 100 iu of heparin to be neutralised. The bolus dose of protamine sulphate should be given slowly over about 10 minutes and not exceed 50 mg. If more than 15 minutes have elapsed since the injection of heparin, lower doses of protamine will be necessary.

Pharmacological properties

Pharmacodynamic properties: Heparin is an anticoagulant and acts by inhibiting thrombin and by potentiating the naturally occurring inhibitors of activated Factor X (Xa).

Pharmacokinetic particulars: As heparin is not absorbed from the gastrointestinal tract and sublingual sites it is administered by injection. After injection heparin extensively binds to plasma proteins.

Heparin is metabolised in the liver and the inactive metabolic products are excreted in the urine.

The half life of heparin is dependent on the dose.

Pre-clinical safety data: There are no pre-clinical data of relevance to the prescriber which are additional to that already included in other sections.

Pharmaceutical particulars

List of excipients: Water for Injections BP, 0.15% chlorocresol, sodium hydroxide solution 3M, hydrochloric acid 3M

Incompatibilities: Heparin is incompatible with many injectable preparations e.g. some antibiotics, opioid analgesics and antihistamines.

Shelf life: 36 months

Special precautions for storage: Multiparin should be stored below 25°C.

Nature and contents of container: 5 ml multidose neutral glass (Type I, Ph Eur) vial. Cartons contain 10 vials.

Instructions for use/handling: Not applicable

Marketing authorisation numbers

Multiparin 1,000 iu/ml	PL 4543/0218
Multiparin 5,000 iu/ml	PL 4543/0219
Multiparin 25,000 iu/ml	PL 4543/0220

Date of approval/revision of SmPC June 1998

Legal category POM

ORLEPT* TABLETS
ORLEPT* (SF) LIQUID

Qualitative and quantitative composition

Orlept Tablets: Sodium Valproate Ph Eur 200 mg or 500 mg

Orlept Liquid: Sodium Valproate Ph Eur 200 mg in 5 ml

Pharmaceutical form

Orlept Tablets: Enteric coated tablet for oral administration.

Orlept Liquid: Oral liquid.

Clinical particulars

Therapeutic indications: Sodium valproate is used in the treatment of all forms of epilepsy.

Posology and method of administration: Dosage requirements vary according to age and body weight and should be adjusted individually to achieve adequate seizure control. The tablets or liquid may be given in divided doses.

Monotherapy: usual requirements are as follows:

Adults: Dosage should start at 600 mg daily increasing by 200 mg at three day intervals until control is achieved. This is generally within the dosage range 1000 mg to 2000 mg per day i.e. 20-30 mg/kg body weight daily. Where adequate control is not achieved within this range the dose may be further increased to a maximum of 2500 mg per day.

Children over 20 kg: Initial dosage should be 400 mg/day increasing until control is achieved. This is usually within the range 20-30 mg/kg body weight per day.

Children under 20 kg: 20 mg/kg of body weight per day; in severe cases this may be increased up to 40 mg/kg/day.

Use in the elderly: Care should be taken when adjusting dosage in the elderly since the pharmacokinetics of sodium valproate are modified. Dosage should be determined by seizure control.

Combined therapy: In certain cases it may be necessary to raise the dose by 5 to 10 mg/kg/day when used in combination with liver enzyme inducing drugs such as phenytoin, phenobarbitone and carbamazepine.

Contra-indications: Liver disease. Hypersensitivity to valproate

Special warnings and precautions for use: Clinical symptoms are a more sensitive indicator in the early stages of hepatic failure than laboratory investigations. The onset of an acute illness, especially within the first six months, which may include symptoms of vomiting, lethargy or weakness, drowsiness, anorexia, jaundice or loss of seizure control is an indication for immediate withdrawal of the drug.

Patients should be instructed to report any such signs to the clinician should they occur.

Routine measurement of liver function should be undertaken in those at risk before and during the first six months of therapy including children under three years, especially those with mental retardation, organic brain damage or metabolic disorder.

The drug should be discontinued if signs of liver damage occur or if serum amylase levels are elevated.

Valproic acid inhibits the second stage of platelet aggregation. If spontaneous bruising or bleeding occurs medication should be withdrawn. It is recommended that patients receiving sodium valproate be monitored for platelet function and clotting time before major surgery.

Withdrawal of sodium valproate or transition to another antiepileptic should be made gradually to avoid precipitation of an increase in seizure frequency.

Sodium valproate may give false positives for ketone bodies in the urine testing of diabetics.

Interactions with other medicaments and other forms of interaction: Concomitant use of hepatic enzyme inducers (e.g. barbiturates, carbamazepine, phenytoin) may enhance metabolism of valproic acid, while cimetidine has been reported to decrease clearance. Valproic acid has been reported to have variable effects on blood levels of other hepatically metabolised or highly protein bound agents. Caution is recommended when administering with other drugs affecting clotting (e.g. warfarin, aspirin). Other hepatotoxic drugs should be avoided. Antidepressants and antipsychotics may lower the threshold for convulsions and higher doses of sodium valproate may be needed.

Pregnancy and lactation: There is an increased incidence of congenital abnormalities in offspring born to mothers with epilepsy, both untreated and treated.

The benefits of anti-epileptic therapy in pregnancy should be evaluated against the possible risks. There have been reports of foetal abnormalities including neural tube defects in women receiving valproate during the first trimester. This incidence has been estimated to be in the region of 1%. Women should be informed of the possible risk and carefully screened by alpha foetoprotein measurement and ultra sound, and if indicated, amniocentesis.

The concentration of valproate in breast milk is very low, between 1% and 10% of total maternal plasma levels, and at this level appears not to have harmful effects on the nursing child.

Effects on ability to drive and to operate machinery: Sodium valproate in appropriate doses may not impair driving skills but driving should be restricted to patients whose seizures are adequately controlled. Administration of the drug may occasionally induce drowsiness.

Undesirable effects: Most frequently, gastrointestinal disturbances, particularly on initiation of therapy. Less commonly, increased appetite and weight gain, tremor, drowsiness, ataxia, confusion, headache, reversible prolongation of bleeding time, thrombocytopenia, leucopenia and bone marrow depression have been reported. Occasionally rashes, transient alopecia with regrowth of curly hair. Transient elevation of liver enzyme levels is common and dose related. Liver dysplasia and hepatic failure (rarely fatal) occurs occasionally, usually in the first few months, necessitating withdrawal. Hyperammonaemia without liver failure, hyperglycinaemia and pancreatitis have been reported.

Congenital malformations have been reported in women receiving anti-epileptic agents including sodium valproate during pregnancy.

Overdosage: Treatment includes induced vomiting, gastric lavage, assisted ventilation and forced diuresis.

Pharmacological properties

Pharmacodynamic properties: The mode of action of valproic acid in epilepsy is not fully understood but may involve an elevation of gamma-amino butyric acid levels in the brain.

Pharmacokinetic properties: Sodium valproate is rapidly and completely absorbed after oral administration; the rate of absorption is delayed by administration as enteric coated tablets.

Sodium valproate is extensively metabolised in the liver, it is excreted in the urine almost entirely in the form of its metabolites.

Sodium valproate is extensively bound to plasma protein. Peak plasma levels are attained 1-4 hours after oral dosing and the half life is of the order of 8-22 hours.

Sodium valproate crosses the blood brain barrier and small amounts are excreted in milk. Data from animal studies indicate that sodium valproate crosses the placenta.

Preclinical safety data: There are no additional preclinical data of relevance to the prescriber which have not been included in the main body of the text.

Pharmaceutical particulars

List of excipients:

200 mg & 500 mg Tablets: Microcrystalline cellulose anhydrous Ph Eur; Methylated colloidal anhydrous silica HSE; Enzymatically hydrolysed gelatin HSE; Calcium behenate DAB; Talc Ph Eur.

Coating: Methacrylic acid copolymer USP; Talc Ph Eur; Triacetin USP; Titanium Dioxide Ph Eur; Polyethylene Glycol 6000 Ph Eur.

Oral liquid: Maltilol Solution (Syrup); Nipasept; Cherry flavour black NA D3923; 3M Hydrochloric acid; 3M Sodium hydroxide; Purified water

Incompatibilities: None known

Shelf life:

Tablets: 24 months in polypropylene or polyethylene container or glass bottles.

24 months in blister strips of PVC/PVDC and aluminium foil.

Oral liquid: 24 months

Special precautions for storage:

Tablets: Store below 25°C in a dry place.

Oral liquid: Store below 25°C and protect from light

Nature and contents of container:

Tablets: Polypropylene or polyethylene containers or glass botles containing 100 tablets.

Blister strips of rigid PVC/PVDC film and aluminium foil of 10 tablets used in multiples of 5, 6 or 10 giving pack sizes of 10, 50, 60 or 100 tablets.

Oral liquid: 100 ml opaque HDPE bottles with polypropylene caps.

500 ml, 300 ml and 2000 ml amber glass bottles with black bakelite screw-on caps.

Instructions for use/handling: None.

Marketing authorisation numbers

Orlept Tablets 200 mg	PL 4543/0283
Orlept Tablets 500 mg	PL 4543/0284
Orlept (SF) Liquid	PL 4543/0323

Date of approval/revision of SPC April 1997

Legal category POM

PROSULF*

Qualitative and quantitative composition Protamine Sulphate PhEur 1% (50 mg in 5 ml)

Pharmaceutical form Solution for injections

Clinical particulars

Therapeutic indications: Protamine sulphate is used to counteract the anticoagulant effect of heparin: before surgery; after renal dialysis; after open-heart surgery; if excessive bleeding occurs and when an overdose has inadvertently been given.

Posology and method of administration:

Adults: Prosulf should be administered by slow intravenous injection over a period of about 10 minutes. No more than 50 mg of protamine sulphate should be given in any one dose.

The dose is dependent on the amount and type of heparin to be neutralised, its route of administration and the time elapsed since it was last given, since heparin is continuously being excreted. Ideally, the dose required to neutralise the action of heparin should be guided by blood coagulation studies or calculated from a protamine neutralisation test.

Patients should be carefully monitored using either the activated partial thromboplastin time or the activated coagulation time, carried out 5-15 minutes after protamine sulphate administration. Further doses may be needed because protamine is cleared from the blood more rapidly than heparin, especially low molecular weight heparin.

In gross excess, protamine itself acts as an anticoagulant.

Neutralisation of unfractionated (UF) heparins: 1 mg of protamine sulphate will usually neutralise at least 100 international units of mucous heparin or 80 units of lung heparin. The dose of protamine sulphate should be reduced if more than 15 minutes have elapsed since intravenous injection.

For example, if 30-60 minutes have elapsed since heparin was injected intravenously, 0.5-0.75 mg protamine sulphate per 100 units of mucous heparin is recommended. If two hours or more have elapsed, 0.25-0.375 mg per 100 units of mucous heparin should be administered.

If the patient is receiving an intravenous infusion of heparin, the infusion should be stopped and 25-50 mg of protamine sulphate given by slow intravenous injection.

If heparin was administered subcutaneously, 1 mg protamine sulphate should be given per 100 units of mucous heparin–25-50 mg by slow intravenous injection and the balance by intravenous infusion over 8-16 hours.

In the reversal of UF heparin following cardiopulmonary bypass, either a standard dose of protamine may be given, as above, or the dose may be titrated according to the activated clotting time.

Neutralisation of low molecular weight (LMW) heparins: A dose of 1 mg per 100 units is usually recommended but the manufacturer's own guidelines should be consulted.

The anti-Xa activity of LMW heparins may not be completely reversible with protamine sulphate and may persist for up to 24 hours after administration.

The longer half-life of LMW heparins (approximately twice that of UF heparin) should also be borne in mind when estimating the dose of protamine sulphate required in relation to the time which has elapsed since the last heparin dose.

Theoretically, the dose of protamine sulphate should be halved when one half-life has elapsed since the last LMW heparin dose. Intermittent injections or continuous infusion of protamine sulphate have been recommended for the neutralisation of LMW heparin following subcutaneous administration, as there may be continuing absorption from the subcutaneous depot.

Elderly: There is no current evidence for alteration of the recommended dose.

Children: Safety and efficacy in children have not been established. Not recommended.

Contra-indications: None known.

Special warnings and precautions for use: Too rapid administration of protamine sulphate may cause severe hypotension and anaphylactoid reactions. Facilities for resuscitation and treatment of shock should be available.

Protamine sulphate is not suitable for reversing the effects of oral anticoagulants. Caution should be observed when administering protamine sulphate to patients who may be at increased risk of allergic reaction to protamine. These patients include those who have previously undergone procedures such as coronary angioplasty or cardio-pulmonary by-pass which may include use of protamine, diabetics who have been treated with protamine insulin, patients allergic to fish and men who have had a vasectomy or are infertile and may have antibodies to protamine.

Patients undergoing prolonged procedures involving repeated doses of protamine should be subject to careful monitoring of clotting parameters. A rebound bleeding effect may occur up to 18 hours post-operatively which responds to further doses of protamine.

Interaction with other medicaments: None known.

Pregnancy and lactation: As with most drugs, to be used only if clearly indicated in pregnancy and with caution during lactation.

Effects on ability to drive and to use machinery: None.

Undesirable effects: When used at doses in excess of that required to neutralise the anticoagulant effect of heparin, protamine sulphate exerts its own anticoagulant effect. Following injection of protamine sulphate the following effects have been observed; a sudden fall in blood pressure, bradycardia, pulmonary and systemic hypertension, dyspnoea, transitory flushing and a feeling of warmth, back pain, nausea and vomiting, lassitude. Hypersensitivity reactions and fatal anaphylaxis have been reported.

Overdose: Symptoms: Overdosage may cause hypotension, bradycardia and dyspnoea with a sensation of warmth, nausea, vomiting, lassitude and transitory flushing.

Treatment: Includes monitoring of coagulation tests, respiratory ventilation and symptomatic treatment. If bleeding is a problem, fresh frozen plasma or fresh whole blood should be given.

Pharmacological properties
Pharmacodynamic properties: Although protamine is a potent antidote for heparin, its precise mechanism of action is unknown. However, when the strongly basic protamine combines with the strongly acid heparin, a stable salt is formed lacking in anticoagulant activity. One mg of protamine sulphate neutralises between 80 and 120 units of heparin. However, methods of standardisation and the use of heparin from different sources (mucosal, lung) may produce different responses to protamine.

Pharmacokinetic properties: The onset of action of protamine occurs within five minutes following intravenous administration. The fate of the protamine-heparin complex is unknown, but it may be partially degraded, thus freeing heparin.

Pre-clinical safety data: No data are available.

Pharmaceutical particulars
List of excipients: Sodium Chloride; Hydrochloric Acid 3M; Sodium Hydroxide 3M; Water for Injections

Incompatibilities: Protamine sulphate is incompatible with certain antibiotics, including several cephalosporins and penicillin.

Shelf life: 48 months in glass ampoules, 24 months in polypropylene ampoules.

Special precautions for storage: Store between 15°C and 25°C.

Nature and contents of container: 5 ml and 10 ml neutral type 1 hydrolytic glass ampoules in pack sizes of 10 ampoules in cartons. 5 ml polypropylene ampoules

Instructions for use/handling: Not applicable.

Marketing authorisation numbers
Glass ampoules PL 4543/0234
Polypropylene ampoules PL 4543//0359

Date of approval/revision of text October 1997

Legal category POM

URDOX* TABLETS 300 mg.

Qualitative and quantitative composition Ursodeoxycholic acid 300 mg.

Pharmaceutical form Tablet for oral use.

Clinical particulars
Therapeutic indications: Urdox tablets are indicated for the dissolution of small to medium sized radiolucent, cholesterol-rich gall-stones in functioning gall bladders.

Cholesterol stones coated with calcium or stones composed of bile pigments are not dissolved by ursodeoxycholic acid. Urdox has a particular place in the treatment of patients in whom surgery is contra-indicated or who are anxious to avoid surgery.

Posology and method of administration: Urdox tablets are for oral administration. To be taken with a drink of water.

Adults and elderly: The usual dose is 6–12 mg/kg/day either as a single night time dose or in divided doses. This may be increased to 15 mg/kg/day in obese patients, if necessary.

The duration of treatment may be up to two years, depending on the size of the stone(s), and should be continued for three months after the apparent dissolution of the stone(s).

Children: Not recommended.

Contra-indications: Use in patients with radio-opaque calcified gall-stones, or in those with non-functioning gall bladders.

Use in women who may become pregnant.

Use in patients with chronic liver disease, peptic ulcers or in those with inflammatory diseases of the small intestine and colon.

Special warnings and precautions for use: None known

Interaction with other medicaments and other forms of interaction: Urdox tablets should not be administered with oral contraceptives, oestrogenic hormones and other drugs which reduce the blood cholesterol level and increase the bile cholesterol level. Antacids bind bile acids in the gut. Drugs such as charcoal, colestipol and cholestyramine bind bile acids *in vitro*. All the above should be avoided during bile acid therapy as they may limit the effectiveness of therapy.

Pregnancy and lactation: This product should not be used during pregnancy or lactation. Measures should be taken to prevent pregnancy if given to women of childbearing age. A non-hormonal contraceptive should be used. Treatment should be discontinued immediately if pregnancy occurs and medical advice sought.

Effects on ability to drive and to use machinery: None known.

Undesirable effects: Urdox may give rise to nausea, vomiting, diarrhoea and pruritus. A calcified layer may develop on the surface of the stone making it unable to be dissolved by bile acid therapy, resulting in surgery for some patients.

Overdose: Bile acids are removed in the faeces either unchanged or as bacterial metabolites. It is unlikely therefore that serious toxicity would occur following overdose. The most likely result is diarrhoea which should be treated symptomatically and supportively.

Pharmacological properties
Pharmacodynamic properties: When given by mouth, ursodeoxycholic acid reduces the ratio of cholesterol to bile salts plus phospholipids in bile, causing desaturation of cholesterol saturated bile. The exact mechanism of action has not been fully elucidated.

Pharmacokinetic properties: Ursodeoxycholic acid is absorbed from the gastro-intestinal tract and undergoes first pass metabolism and enterohepatic recycling. It is partially conjugated in the liver before being excreted into bile and undergoing 7-α-dehydroxylation to lithocholic acid, some of which is excreted directly in the faeces. The rest is absorbed and mainly conjugated and sulphated by the liver before excretion in the faeces.

Pre-clinical safety data: There are no pre-clinical data of relevance to the prescriber which are additional to those already included in other sections.

Pharmaceutical particulars
List of excipients: Lactose PhEur; Maize Starch PhEur; Povidone PhEur; Sodium Starch Glycollate PhEur; Magnesium Stearate PhEur; Purified Water PhEur

Tablet Coating: Hydroxypropylmethylcellulose (E464) PhEur; Titanium dioxide (E171) PhEur; Polyethylene glycol PhEur

Incompatibilities: None known.

Shelf life: Three years.

Special precautions for storage: Store below 25°C. Protect from light.

Nature and contents of container: Polypropylene or polyethylene tablet container with tamper evident closure of 60, 100 or 500 tablets.

Strips of 60 tablets in white opaque 250 micron UPVC with 20 micron hard tempered foil.

Instructions for use/handling: None.

Marketing authorisation number 4543/0318

Date of approval/revision of SPC May 1997

Legal Category POM

**Trade Mark*

Dermal Laboratories Limited

Tatmore Place
Gosmore, Hitchin
Herts, SG4 7QR

☎ 01462 458866 📄 01462 420565

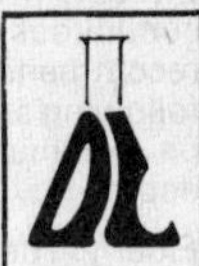

ANHYDROL* FORTE

Qualitative and quantitative composition Aluminium Chloride Hexahydrate 20.0% w/v.

Pharmaceutical form Clear, colourless evaporative topical solution.

Clinical particulars
Therapeutic indications: For the topical treatment of hyperhidrosis specifically involving axillae, hands or feet.

Posology and method of administration: For adults, children and the elderly. Apply to the affected sites at night, as required, and allow to dry. Wash off in the morning.

Contra-indications: Not to be used in cases of sensitivity to any of the ingredients.

Special warnings and special precautions for use: Care should be taken to restrict the application to the affected sites only. Keep away from the eyes and mucous membranes. Care should be taken to avoid Anhydrol Forte coming into direct contact with clothing, polished surfaces, jewellery or metal. Replace cap tightly after use. For external use only.

Interaction with other medicaments and other forms of interaction: Do not bathe immediately before use and, if the axillae are treated, do not shave or use depilatories on this area within 12 hours before or after use.

Pregnancy and lactation: No special precautions.

Effects on ability to drive and use machines: None known.

Undesirable effects: If applied too frequently, Anhydrol Forte may cause irritation which should be treated with a mild topical hydrocortisone cream.

Overdose: See section above (*Undesirable effects*).

Pharmacological properties
Pharmacodynamic properties: Aluminium chloride is believed to denature the protein content of sweat issuing from eccrine glands, and to combine with the intraductal keratin fibrils, producing a functional closure. The antibacterial action of the aluminium ion also precludes the development of miliaria. Accordingly, there is no secondary inflammation. The intraluminal pressure rises to the point where it acts as a feedback system, shutting off acinar secretion.

The formulation of Anhydrol Forte has been tested in widespread clinical practice, and has been shown to be effective when used in accordance with the recommended instructions.

Pharmacokinetic properties: As the active ingredient is applied in an alcoholic solution of low surface tension, it therefore penetrates into the terminal pores of the sweat ducts, when applied, as recommended, to dry skin. The alcohol then evaporates off, leaving the salt deposited in close contact with the lining of the duct. The use of the preparation is restricted to small areas of skin, namely the axillae, hands or feet, to ensure that there are no detrimental effects from widespread obstruction of sweating.

Preclinical safety data: No special information.

Pharmaceutical particulars
List of excipients: IMS BP.

Incompatibilities: None known.

Shelf life: 36 months.

Special precautions for storage: Highly flammable. Store at room temperature (not exceeding 25°C). Store upright and away from flames.

Nature and contents of container: 60 ml plastic bottle with roll-on applicator and screwcap. This is supplied as an original pack (OP).

Instructions for use/handling: Not applicable.

Marketing authorisation number 0173/0030.

Date of approval/revision of SPC February 1995.

Legal category P.

BETACAP* SCALP APPLICATION

Presentation Transparent, slightly gelled emollient scalp application containing 0.1% w/w betamethasone as valerate. The vehicle also contains isopropyl alcohol, which has antiseptic activity.

Ingredients: Betamethasone Valerate BP; PEG-7 Glyceryl Cocoate (a water-dispersible derivative of coconut oil); Isopropyl Alcohol BP; Carbomer; Sodium Hydroxide BP; Purified Water BP.

Uses For the treatment of dermatoses of the scalp, such as psoriasis and seborrhoeic dermatitis unresponsive to less potent corticosteroids.

Dosage and administration
For adults, including the elderly, and children over the age of one year: Betacap Scalp Application should be applied sparingly to the scalp night and morning until improvement is noticeable. It may then be possible to sustain improvement by applying once a day, or less frequently. For the treatment of seborrhoeic dermatitis in children, this product should not be used for longer than 5 to 7 days.

Contra-indications, warnings, etc
Contra-indications: Do not use in cases of bacterial, fungal and/or viral infection of the scalp or where there is a known sensitivity to any of the ingredients. Do not use on children under the age of one year.

Precautions: Care must be taken to keep the preparation away from the eyes. As it is highly flammable, do not use the product near a fire or naked flame. Allow treated scalp to dry naturally.

Continuous long-term treatment should be avoided, particularly in children, as systemic side-effects can occur even without occlusion.

Complications sometimes associated with topical corticosteroids in psoriasis include the possibility of rebound relapses, development of tolerance, risk of generalised pustular psoriasis and development of local or systemic toxicity due to impaired barrier function of the skin. If used in psoriasis careful patient supervision is therefore important.

Development of secondary infection requires withdrawal of topical corticosteroid therapy and commencement of appropriate systemic antimicrobial treatment.

Use in pregnancy and lactation: There is inadequate evidence of safety in human pregnancy. Topical administration of corticosteroids to pregnant animals can cause abnormalities of foetal development, including cleft palate and intra-uterine growth retardation. There may therefore be a very small risk of such effects in the human foetus. The risk/benefit needs to be carefully assessed, therefore, before prescribing this medicine.

Side-effects: Betamethasone preparations are usually well tolerated, but if signs of hypersensitivity appear, application should be stopped immediately.

As with other topical corticosteroids, prolonged use of large amounts, or treatment of extensive areas, can result in sufficient systemic absorption to produce the features of hypercorticism and suppression of the HPA axis. These effects are more likely to occur in infants and children, and if occlusive dressings are used. Local atrophy may occur after prolonged treatment, particularly under occlusion.

In rare instances, treatment of psoriasis with corticosteroids (or its withdrawal) is thought to have provoked the pustular form of the disease.

Overdosage: Acute overdosage is very unlikely to occur. In the case of chronic overdosage or misuse, the features of hypercorticism may appear and in this situation treatment with Betacap Scalp Application should be discontinued.

Pharmaceutical precautions Store upright at room temperature (not exceeding 25°C), with the cap replaced. Return bottle to carton between use. Protect from light. Avoid spillage.

Legal category POM.

Package quantity Betacap Scalp Application is supplied in a plastic squeeze bottle with integral nozzle applicator, containing 100 ml. This is supplied as an original pack (OP).

Further information Betacap Scalp Application is specially formulated to include a coconut-oil related emollient ingredient designed to reduce the drying effect that a standard alcoholic vehicle may otherwise have on the scalp. The viscosity of the preparation has been adjusted so that it spreads easily without being too fluid. The squeeze bottle and nozzle also allow easy application direct to the scalp through the hair.

Marketing authorisation number 0173/0149.

CAPASAL* THERAPEUTIC SHAMPOO

Qualitative and quantitative composition Salicylic Acid BP 0.5% w/w; Coconut Oil BP 1.0% w/w; Distilled Coal Tar 1.0% w/w.

Pharmaceutical form Golden brown therapeutic shampoo.

Clinical particulars
Therapeutic indications: For use as a shampoo in the treatment of dry, scaly scalp conditions such as seborrhoeic eczema, seborrhoeic dermatitis, pityriasis capitis, psoriasis, and cradle cap in children. It may also be used to remove previous scalp applications.

Posology and method of administration: For adults, children and the elderly. Use as a shampoo, daily if necessary. Wet the hair thoroughly. Massage a small amount of the shampoo into the scalp, leaving on for a few minutes before washing out. Repeat, producing a rich lather. Rinse hair well and dry.

Contra-indications: Not to be used in cases of sensitivity to any of the ingredients.

Special warnings and special precautions for use: Keep away from the eyes. Keep out of the reach of children. In case of irritation, discontinue treatment. For external use only.

Interaction with other medicaments and other forms of interaction: None known.

Pregnancy and lactation: No known side-effects.

Effects on ability to drive and use machines: None known.

Undesirable effects: None known.

Overdose: There are no known toxic effects resulting from excessive use of Capasal Therapeutic Shampoo.

Pharmacological properties
Pharmacodynamic properties: The preparation has been designed for use in the treatment of dry, scaly scalp conditions by incorporating into a convenient shampoo formulation three well known ingredients which have been established as safe and effective, for example, in Coconut Oil Compound Ointment (Ung Cocois Co), for use in these indications. They are as follows:

- 0.5% salicylic acid – mild keratolytic
- 1.0% coconut oil – emollient, softening agent and lubricant
- 1.0% distilled coal tar – anti-pruritic, keratoplastic

The preparation may also be used conveniently to remove any previous topical application.

Pharmacokinetic properties: The active ingredients of the formulation are readily available for intimate contact with the skin, as the shampoo is massaged into the scalp and left on for a few minutes before washing out. This is then repeated in order to produce a rich lather. The detergent effect of the shampoo will also remove any previous application to the scalp.

Preclinical safety data: No special information.

Pharmaceutical particulars
List of excipients: Lauric Acid Diethanolamide; Coco Amido Propyl Dimethyl Betaine; Triethanolamine Lauryl Sulphate; Phenoxyethanol BP; Water.

Incompatibilities: None known.

Shelf life: 36 months.

Special precautions for storage: Store at room temperature (not exceeding 25°C) and away from direct sunlight.

Nature and contents of container: Plastic 'flip top' bottle containing 250 ml. This is supplied as an original pack (OP).

Instructions for use/handling: Not applicable.

Marketing authorisation number 0173/0048.

Date of approval/revision of SPC January 1996.

Legal category P.

DERMOL* 200 SHOWER EMOLLIENT

Presentation White, non-greasy shower emollient containing 0.1% w/w Benzalkonium Chloride BP, 0.1% w/w Chlorhexidine Hydrochloride BP, 2.5% w/w Liquid Paraffin BP, 2.5% w/w Isopropyl Myristate BP.

Ingredients: Benzalkonium Chloride BP; Chlorhexidine Hydrochloride BP; Liquid Paraffin BP; Isopropyl Myristate BP; Cetostearyl Alcohol BP; Cetomacrogol 1000 BP; Phenoxyethanol BP; Purified Water BP.

Uses An antimicrobial shower emollient for the management of dry and pruritic skin conditions, especially eczema and dermatitis. Dermol 200 Shower Emollient is for direct application onto the skin and is suitable for use as a soap substitute in the shower.

Dosage and administration
For adults, children and the elderly. For application to the skin (eg after showering): Apply to the affected areas as required and massage into the skin until absorbed. For use as a soap substitute in the shower: As required, use the shower emollient instead of an ordinary shower gel or soap. Pat dry.

Contra-indications, warnings, etc Do not use in cases of known sensitivity to any of the ingredients. Take care to avoid contact with the eyes, especially when used on the face. Take care to avoid slipping in the shower or bath. Although the shower emollient has been especially formulated for use on dry or problem skin, in the unlikely event of a reaction, discontinue treatment.

Pharmaceutical precautions Store at room temperature (not exceeding 25°C).

Legal category P.

Package quantity Dermol 200 Shower Emollient is supplied in a plastic 200 ml bottle with a hooked overcap. This is supplied as an original pack (OP).

Further information Bacteria (especially *Staphylococcus aureus*) are implicated in the pathogenesis of inflammatory dry skin conditions such as atopic eczema or dermatitis.

Dermol 200 Shower Emollient contains 5% of emollient oils in a non-greasy aqueous system which also contains the well-known antiseptics benzalkonium chloride and chlorhexidine hydrochloride. Its antimicrobial properties assist in overcoming infection, whether from *Staph. aureus*, the pathogen which often complicates eczema and associated pruritus, or secondary infection caused by scratching.

The emollients, liquid paraffin and isopropyl myristate, permit rehydration of dry skin by forming an occlusive barrier within the skin surface, thus reducing drying from evaporation of water that diffuses from the underlying layers.

Marketing authorisation number 0173/0156.

DERMOL* 500 LOTION

Qualitative and quantitative composition Benzalkonium Chloride BP 0.1% w/w; Chlorhexidine Hydrochloride BP 0.1% w/w; Liquid Paraffin BP 2.5% w/w; Isopropyl Myristate BP 2.5% w/w.

Pharmaceutical form White, non-greasy aqueous lotion.

Clinical particulars
Therapeutic indications: An antimicrobial emollient for the management of dry and pruritic skin conditions, especially eczema and dermatitis. The lotion is suitable for direct application, and for use as a soap substitute.

Posology and method of administration: For adults, children and the elderly. For application to the skin*:* apply the lotion to the affected areas as required. Massage well into the skin, until absorbed. For periodic use as a soap substitute*:* as required, use the lotion in the bath or shower, or for other toiletry purposes, instead of ordinary soap or shower gel.

Contra-indications: Do not use in cases of known sensitivity to any of the ingredients.

Special warnings and special precautions for use: Avoid contact with the eyes.

Interaction with other medicaments and other forms of interaction: None known.

Pregnancy and lactation: No special precautions.

Effects on ability to drive and use machines: None known.

Undesirable effects: Although the lotion has been specially formulated for use on dry or problem skin, in the unlikely event of a reaction discontinue treatment.

Overdose: Not applicable.

Pharmacological properties
Pharmacodynamic properties: Bacteria (especially *Staphylococcus aureus*) are implicated in the pathogenesis of inflammatory dry skin conditions such as atopic eczema or dermatitis. Dermol 500 Lotion contains 5% of emollient oils in a non-greasy aqueous lotion which also contains the well-known and effective antiseptics benzalkonium chloride and chlorhexidine hydrochloride. Its antimicrobial properties assist in overcoming infection, whether from *Staph. aureus*, the pathogen which often complicates eczema and associated pruritus, or secondary infection caused by scratching.

Massaged into the skin, the emollients, liquid paraffin and isopropyl myristate, permit rehydration of dry skin by forming an occlusive barrier within the skin surface, thus reducing drying from evaporation of water that diffuses from the underlying layers.

Pharmacokinetic properties: The active ingredients are presented in an aqueous lotion and so are readily absorbed into the stratum corneum when the product is gently massaged over the areas of dry skin. The antiseptic ingredients are in intimate contact with the skin, and as they are in solution, their availability is optimal.

Preclinical safety data: No special information.

Pharmaceutical particulars
List of excipients: Cetostearyl Alcohol BP; Cetomacrogol 1000 BP; Phenoxyethanol BP; Purified Water BP.

Incompatibilities: None known.

Shelf life: 30 months in unopened container. Use within 18 months of first opening.

Special precautions for storage: Store at room temperature (not exceeding 25°C).

Nature and contents of container: Plastic 500 ml bottle with a white polypropylene pump dispenser. Supplied as an original pack (OP).

Instructions for use/handling: Not applicable.

Marketing authorisation number 0173/0051.

Date of approval/revision of SPC October 1996.

Legal category P.

DIODERM*

Qualitative and quantitative composition Hydrocortisone BP 0.1% w/w.

Pharmaceutical form Smooth white aqueous cream.

Clinical particulars
Therapeutic indications: For the topical treatment of eczema and dermatitis.

Posology and method of administration: For adults, children and the elderly. Apply to the affected areas twice daily. For infants, the treatment period should not normally exceed 7 days.

Contra-indications: As with all topical steroids, Dioderm is not to be used where there is bacterial, viral or fungal infection.

Not be used on open wounds, ulcers or broken skin.

Not to be used in cases of sensitivity to any of the ingredients.

Special warnings and special precautions for use: Although generally regarded as safe, even for long-term administration in adults, there is a potential for overdosage in infancy. Extreme caution is required in dermatoses in infancy, including napkin eruption. In such patients, courses of treatment should not normally exceed 7 days.

Prolonged or extensive uninterrupted application should be avoided, particularly if used on the face or with occlusive dressings.

Topical corticosteroids may complicate psoriasis for a number of reasons including rebound relapses following development of tolerance, risk of generalised pustular psoriasis and local and systemic toxicity due to impaired barrier function of the skin. In such patients, careful patient supervision is important.

Keep away from the eyes.

For external use only.

Interaction with other medicaments and other forms of interaction: None known.

Pregnancy and lactation: There is inadequate evidence of safety in human pregnancy. Topical administration of corticosteroids to pregnant animals can cause abnormalities of foetal development including cleft palate and intra-uterine growth retardation. There may therefore be a very small risk of such effects in the human foetus.

Effects on ability to drive and use machines: None known.

Undesirable effects: None known.

Overdose: Under exceptional circumstances, if Dioderm is used excessively, particularly in young children, it is theoretically possible that adrenal suppression and skin thinning may occur. The symptoms are normally reversible on cessation of treatment.

Pharmacological properties
Pharmacodynamic properties: Corticosteroids are used in pharmacological doses for their anti-inflammatory and immunosuppressive glucocorticoid properties which suppress the clinical manifestations of a wide range of diseases. Although many synthetic derivatives have been developed, hydrocortisone is still used widely in topical formulations for inflammatory dermatoses. It has the advantage over its synthetic derivatives that it is metabolised in the skin and therefore cannot accumulate to form a depot which may result in local side effects.

Pharmacokinetic properties: The cream formulation of Dioderm was developed in order to optimise the release and partition of its active ingredient, hydrocortisone, into the skin. The hydrocortisone is presented as a saturated or near saturated solution in aqueous propylene glycol, which represents the continuous phase of the emulsion system. It has been shown, by the vasoconstrictor assay on normal skin, that, in this environment, a 0.1% concentration of the hydrocortisone is equivalent to the 1.0% concentration of the official cream formulations appearing in the British Pharmacopoeia where the drug substance is in suspension. Clinical studies have confirmed that 0.1% Dioderm is equivalent to 1.0% Hydrocortisone Cream BP whilst the reduced strength of Dioderm increases the margin of safety.

Preclinical safety data: No special information.

Pharmaceutical particulars
List of excipients: Citric Acid BP; Emulsifying Ointment BP; Propylene Glycol BP; Purified Water BP.

Incompatibilities: None known.

Shelf life: 30 months.

Special precautions for storage: Store at room temperature (not exceeding 25°C). Replace cap tightly after use.

Nature and contents of container: 30 g collapsible tube. This is supplied as an original pack (OP).

Instructions for use/handling: Not applicable.

Marketing authorisation number 0173/0047.

Date of approval/revision of SPC February 1998.

Legal category POM.

DITHROCREAM*

Qualitative and quantitative composition Dithranol BP 0.1%, 0.25%, 0.5%, 1.0% or 2.0% w/w.

Pharmaceutical form Yellow aqueous cream.

Clinical particulars
Therapeutic indications: For the topical treatment of subacute and chronic psoriasis including psoriasis of the scalp.

Posology and method of administration: Dithranol therapy customarily involves titrating the concentration applied to the skin to suit individual patient's circumstances. Dithrocream is, therefore, available in five strengths. The different packs are colour coded as follows:

0.1%	pale blue
0.25%	red
0.5%	purple
1.0%	brown
2.0%	yellow

For adults and the elderly: It is important to determine each patient's optimal treatment strength, as too high a strength may induce a burning sensation. Where the response to Dithrocream has not previously been established, always commence with Dithrocream 0.1%, continuing for at least one week and then, if necessary, increase to the 0.25% followed by the 0.5%, the 1.0% and finally the 2.0% strength. The aim should be to build up gradually over approximately 4 weeks to the highest tolerated strength to produce the optimum therapeutic effect. This optimum concentration will depend upon such factors as the thickness and location of the psoriatic plaques, as well as the variation between individual patients in their reaction to dithranol.

Dithrocream should be applied sparingly, and only to the affected areas, once every 24 hours, at any convenient time of the day or evening. Rub the cream gently and carefully into the skin until completely absorbed. For use on the scalp, first comb the hair to remove scalar debris and, after suitably parting, rub the cream well into the affected areas. Remove by washing off the skin or scalp, usually no more than one hour after application (Short Contact Therapy). Alternatively, it may be applied at night before retiring and washed off in the morning.

Treatment should be continued until the skin is entirely clear, i.e. when there is nothing to feel with the fingers and the texture is normal. By gradually increasing the strength of cream applied, it should be possible to clear psoriasis patches within 4 to 6 weeks.

For children: No additional special precautions necessary. However, use cautiously as described above for adults and the elderly, with regular supervision.

Contra-indications: Not to be used on the face, or for acute or pustular psoriasis. Not to be used in cases of sensitivity to any of the ingredients.

Special warnings and special precautions for use: Dithrocream 0.5%, Dithrocream 1.0% and Dithocream 2.0% should only be used for those patients who have failed to respond to lower strengths of dithranol. Dithrocream 1.0% and 2.0% should normally only be applied for 'short contact' periods.

Dithrocream 0.5%, Dithrocream 1.0% and Dithrocream 2.0% should always be used under medical supervision.

It is most important to avoid applying an excessive amount of the cream, which may cause unnecessary soiling and staining of clothing and/or bed linen. After each period of treatment, a bath/shower should be taken to remove any residual cream. To prevent the possibility of discolouration, particularly where Dithrocream 1.0% or 2.0% has been used, always rinse the bath/shower with hot water immediately after washing/showering and then use a suitable cleanser to remove any deposit on the surface of the bath/shower.

After use on the scalp, a shampoo may be used to remove the Dithrocream residue. Great care must be taken when washing out the shampoo (which may contain some Dithrocream residue), to ensure that it does not get into the eyes or on the face. This is particularly important when the high strengths of Dithrocream have been used.

Although a feeling of warmth at the application site is normal, if this amounts to a burning sensation, or if the lesions spread, treatment should be stopped at once, and the dosage re-evaluated by a doctor.

Dithrocream is not normally recommended for use on areas of folded skin such as the groin and beneath the breasts. Do not use high strengths on these sites.

Keep away from the eyes and mucous membranes. Always wash the hands after use.

As long term use of topical corticosteroids is known to destabilise psoriasis, and withdrawal may give rise to a rebound phenomenon, an interval of at least one week should be allowed between the discontinuance of such steroids and the commencement of Dithrocream therapy. A suitably bland emollient may usefully be applied in the intervening period.

Contact with fabrics, plastics and other materials may cause permanent staining and should be avoided.

Interaction with other medicaments and other forms of interaction: None known.

Pregnancy and lactation: Although there is no experimental evidence to support the safety of the drug in pregnancy or during lactation, no adverse effects have been reported.

Effects on ability to drive and use machines: None known.

Undesirable effects: Some skin irritation and/or a feeling of warmth at the site of application is normally associated with dithranol therapy. Dithrocream applied at too high a strength or left in contact with the skin for too long may induce a burning sensation. Dithrocream may cause temporary staining of the skin and/or hair.

Overdose: Dithranol is a cathartic (laxative) and if accidentally swallowed, it should be removed by gastric lavage.

Pharmacological properties
Pharmacodynamic properties: Dithranol has been used in the treatment of sub-acute and chronic psoriasis for over 70 years and, during that time, it has become established as a safe and effective form of therapy. Its precise mode of action is still to be confirmed, although it has been shown to inhibit DNA replication, cellular respiration and key cellular enzymes eg glucose-6-phosphate dehydrogenase.

Because dithranol causes staining and irritation, it is now widely used in short contact therapy where the preparation is washed off the skin after periods of one hour or less. For this purpose, Dithrocream is particularly suitable, as it is convenient to apply and washes off easily with ordinary soap and warm water in a bath or shower.

Pharmocokinetic properties: The traditional formulations of dithranol are based on soft paraffin from which it is effectively released into the skin. In Dithrocream, during manufacture, the oily paraffin phase of the cream is heated until the dithranol entirely dissolves so that, on cooling, it is retained solely within the paraffin phase and does not spread into the aqueous phase. After application of Dithrocream to the skin, the water is lost through absorption and evaporation, leaving the oily phase which then acts in the same way as a dithranol ointment. However, since the cream may be rubbed into the skin more effectively than the ointment, it is convenient to apply and, owing to the presence of the emulsifying components, is easier to wash off. The availability of the dithranol has now been confirmed in numerous publications detailing the results of clinical trials.

Preclinical safety data: No special information.

Pharmaceutical particulars
List of excipients: White Soft Paraffin BP; Cetostearyl Alcohol BP; Salicylic Acid BP; Ascorbic Acid BP; Sodium Lauryl Sulphate BP; Chlorocresol BP; Purified Water BP. Dithrocream 2.0% also contains Liquid Paraffin BP.

Incompatibilities: None known.

Shelf life: 36 months.

Special precautions for storage: Store at room temperature (not exceeding 25°C). Replace cap tightly after use.

Nature and contents of container: All strengths of Dithrocream are supplied in collapsible tubes containing 50 g. These are supplied as original packs (OP).

Instructions for use/handling: Not applicable.

Marketing authorisation numbers

Dithrocream 0.1%	0173/0029
Dithrocream 0.25%	0173/0028
Dithrocream 0.5%	0173/0027
Dithrocream 1.0%	0173/0039
Dithrocream 2.0%	0173/0045

Date of approval/revision of SPC October 1997.

Legal category P except for Dithrocream 2.0% (POM).

EMULSIDERM* EMOLLIENT

Presentation Pale blue/green liquid emulsion containing Benzalkonium Chloride BP 0.5% w/w, Liquid Paraffin BP 25.0% w/w and Isopropyl Myristate BP 25.0% w/w.

Ingredients: Benzalkonium Chloride BP; Liquid Paraffin BP; Isopropyl Myristate BP; Sorbitan Monostearate BP; Polysorbate 60 BP; Methylene Blue; IMS BP; Purified Water BP.

Uses For the treatment of dry skin conditions, including those associated with dermatitis and psoriasis. It permits re-hydration of the keratin by replacing lost lipids, and its antibacterial properties assist in overcoming *Staph. aureus*, the pathogen which often complicates atopic eczema and associated pruritus.

Dosage and administration
Adults, children and the elderly: Shake bottle before use.

Add 7 to 30 ml to a bath of warm water (more or less according to the size of the bath and individual patient requirements). Soak for 5 to 10 minutes. Pat dry.

For application to the skin: rub a small amount of undiluted emollient into the dry areas of skin until absorbed.

Contra-indications, warnings, etc Keep away from the eyes. Take care to avoid slipping in the bath.

Do not use if sensitive to any of the ingredients.

Pharmaceutical precautions Store at room temperature (not exceeding 25°C). Replace cap after use.

Legal category P.

Package quantities Emulsiderm is supplied in plastic bottles; a 300 ml with a measuring cap, and a 1 litre with a measuring cup. These are supplied as original packs (OP).

Further information Bacteria (especially *Staph. aureus*) have been implicated in the pathogenesis of inflammatory dry skin conditions such as atopic eczema or dermatitis. Dual action bactericidal and emollient Emulsiderm is specially formulated in a unique emulsion system optimised for convenient application to the skin, either directly or via the patient's bath water.

Marketing authorisation number 0173/0036.

EXTEROL*

Qualitative and quantitative composition Urea Hydrogen Peroxide 5.0% w/w.

Pharmaceutical form Clear, straw-coloured, viscous ear drops.

Clinical particulars
Therapeutic indications: As an aid in the removal of hardened ear wax.

Posology and method of administration: For adults, children and the elderly. Instil up to 5 drops into the ear. Retain drops in ear for several minutes by keeping the head tilted and then wipe away any surplus. Repeat once or twice daily for at least 3 to 4 days, or as required.

Contra-indications: Do not use if the eardrum is known or suspected to be damaged, in cases of dizziness, or if there is, or has been, any other ear disorder (such as pain, discharge, inflammation, infection or tinnitus). Do not use after ill-advised attempts to dislodge wax using fingernails, cotton buds or similar implements, as such mechanical efforts can cause the ear's delicate inner lining to become damaged, inflamed or infected, whereupon the use of ear drops can be painful. For similar reasons, it is inadvisable to use Exterol within 2 to 3 days of syringing. Do not use where there is a history of ear problems, unless under close medical supervision. Do not use if sensitive to any of the ingredients.

Special warnings and special precautions for use: Keep Exterol away from the eyes. For external use only.

Interaction with other medicaments and other forms of interaction: Exterol should not be used at the same time as anything else in the ear.

Pregnancy and lactation: No known side-effects.

Effects on ability to drive and use machines: None known.

Undesirable effects: Due to the release of oxygen, patients may experience a mild, temporary effervescence in the ear. Stop usage if irritation or pain occurs. Instillation of ear drops can aggravate the painful symptoms of excessive ear wax, including some loss of hearing, dizziness and tinnitus. Very rarely, unpleasant taste has been reported. If patients encounter any of these problems, or if their symptoms persist or worsen, they should discontinue treatment and consult a doctor.

Overdose: No adverse effects.

Pharmacological properties
Pharmacodynamic properties: After insertion of the drops into the ear, the urea hydrogen peroxide complex liberates oxygen which acts to break up the hardened wax. The hydrogen peroxide component is also an antiseptic, especially in sites with relative anaerobiosis. The glycerol assists in softening the wax, so that it may more easily be removed from the ear, either with or without syringing. The urea acts as a mild keratolytic, helping to reduce the keratin-load in the wax debris, thereby assisting penetration of the other components.

Pharmacokinetic properties: Exterol is intended only for the treatment of impacted wax in the *external* auditory canal. The ingredients of the formulation are therefore readily available for intimate contact with the affected area, as the drops are instilled into the ear and retained therein for several minutes by tilting the head.

Preclinical safety data: No special information.

Pharmaceutical particulars
List of excipients: 8-Hydroxyquinoline; Glycerol BP.

Incompatibilities: None known.

Shelf life: 30 months.

Special precautions for storage: Store at room temperature (not exceeding 25°C). Replace cap after use, and return bottle to carton.

Nature and contents of container: 8 ml easy squeeze plastic dropper bottle with screw cap. This is supplied as an original pack (OP).

Instructions for use/handling: Not applicable.

Marketing authorisation number 0173/0037.

Date of approval/revision of SPC January 1997.

Legal category P.

GLUTAROL*

Qualitative and quantitative composition Glutaraldehyde 10.0% w/v.

Pharmaceutical form Colourless, evaporative wart paint.

Clinical particulars
Therapeutic indications: For the topical treatment of warts, especially plantar warts.

Posology and method of administration: For adults, children and the elderly.

1. Gently rub the surface of the wart with a piece of pumice stone or manicure emery board, or pare down any hard skin.
2. Using the applicator provided, carefully apply a few drops of the paint to the wart, taking care to localise the application to the affected area. Allow each drop to dry before the next is applied.
3. Repeat twice daily.
4. On subsequent days, repeat steps 1 to 3.

It is not necessary to cover the treated wart(s) with an adhesive plaster.

Contra-indications: Not to be used in cases of sensitivity to any of the ingredients. Not to be used on the face, anal or perineal region. Not to be used on moles or on any other skin lesion for which it is not indicated.

Special warnings and special precautions for use: Keep away from the eyes and mucous membranes. Avoid spreading onto surrounding uninvolved skin. Avoid spillage. Avoid inhaling vapour. Replace cap tightly after use. For external use only.

Interaction with other medicaments and other forms of interaction: None known.

Pregnancy and lactation: No special precautions.

Effects on ability to drive and use machines: None known.

Undesirable effects: Undesirable effects occur very occasionally and mostly involve mild local skin rashes and irritation. Very rarely, a severe reaction may occur particularly on the hands or when the product is used excessively and allowed to spread onto surrounding normal skin. If mild irritation should occur, apply a reduced amount (taking special care to avoid spreading beyond the wart or verruca) and apply less often. If the irritation is severe, patients should stop treatment immediately and seek medical advice.

Overdose: Accidental oral ingestion should be treated immediately by gastric lavage with 2 to 5% aqueous sodium bicarbonate solution. Fluid and electrolyte balance should be monitored and appropriate supportive measures should be provided. Symptoms include headache, nausea, vomiting, diarrhoea and respiratory depression.

Pharmacological properties
Pharmacodynamic properties: Glutaraldehyde is virucidal and thus inactivates the wart virus. On the skin, it also acts as an anhidrotic, drying the warts and surrounding skin, thus reducing the spread of lesions and simplifying the removal of persistent warts by curettage.

As glutaraldehyde stains the outer layer of the skin brown, treatment can be seen to be carried out. This stain soon disappears after cessation of treatment.

Pharmacokinetic properties: Addition of ethanol to the formulation stabilises the glutaraldehyde against irreversible polymerisation during storage but at the same time diminishes its activity. However, when the aqueous ethanolic solution is applied to the skin, the alcohol rapidly evaporates leaving a concentrated aqueous solution of glutaraldehyde which is highly reactive and attacks the wart before it has time to polymerise. Thus, the ethanolic formulation is stable in storage, as confirmed by stability tests, but is immediately activated when applied to the skin and the alcohol is allowed to evaporate.

Preclinical safety data: No special information.

Pharmaceutical particulars
List of excipients: Bitrex; IMS BP; Purified Water BP.

Incompatibilities: None known.

Shelf life: 36 months.

Special precautions for storage: Flammable. Keep away from flames. Store upright at room temperature (not exceeding 25°C).

Nature and contents of container: 10 ml amber glass bottle incorporating a specially designed spatula for ease of application. This is supplied as an original pack (OP).

Instructions for use/handling: Not applicable.

Marketing authorisation number 0173/0022.

Date of approval/revision of SPC April 1996.

Legal category P.

IBUGEL*

Qualitative and quantitative composition Ibuprofen BP 5.0% w/w.

Pharmaceutical form Non-greasy, fragrance-free, clear, colourless aqueous-alcoholic gel.

Clinical particulars
Therapeutic indications: For the topical treatment of backache, rheumatic and muscular pain, sprains, strains and neuralgia. Ibugel is also indicated for symptomatic relief of pain due to non-serious arthritic conditions.

Posology and method of administration: Apply the gel to the affected areas, up to three times daily, or as directed by the physician. On each occasion apply only enough gel to thinly cover the affected area, and gently massage well into the skin, until completely absorbed. Do not use excessively. Hands should be washed after use (unless treating them). Therapy should be reviewed after a few weeks, particularly if symptoms worsen or persist.

The same dosage and dosage schedule applies to all age groups, although Ibugel is not normally recommended for use on children under the age of 12 years, unless instructed by their doctor.

Contra-indications: Not to be used in cases of sensitivity to any of the ingredients, particularly if asthmatic or suffering from rhinitis or urticaria and have previously shown hypersensitivity to aspirin, ibuprofen or related painkillers. Not to be used on broken skin.

Special warnings and special precautions for use: Seek medical advice if symptoms worsen or persist. Oral NSAIDs, including ibuprofen, can sometimes be associated with renal impairment, aggravation of active peptic ulcers, and can induce allergic bronchial reactions in susceptible asthmatic patients. Although the systemic absorption of topically applied ibuprofen is less than for oral dosage forms, these complications can occur in rare cases. For these reasons, patients with an active peptic ulcer, a history of kidney problems, asthma or intolerance to aspirin or ibuprofen taken orally should seek medical advice before using Ibugel. Keep Ibugel away from the eyes and mucous membranes. For external use only.

Interaction with other medicaments and other forms of interaction: Non-steroidal anti-inflammatory drugs may interact with blood pressure lowering drugs, although the chance of this occurring with a topically administered preparation is extremely remote.

Pregnancy and lactation: Do not use during pregnancy or lactation.

Effects on ability to drive and use machines: None known.

Undesirable effects: Local side-effects do not normally occur. In rare instances, skin rashes may occur, in which case the application of Ibugel should be stopped.

Overdose: Not applicable. Any overdose with a topical presentation of ibuprofen is extremely unlikely.

Pharmacological properties
Pharmacodynamic properties: Ibugel is a topical preparation which has anti-inflammatory and analgesic properties. It contains the active ingredient, ibuprofen, which exerts its effects directly in inflamed tissues underlying the site of application, mainly by inhibiting prostaglandin biosynthesis.

Because it is formulated in an aqueous/alcoholic gel, Ibugel also exerts a soothing and cooling effect when applied to the affected area.

Pharmacokinetic properties: Specially formulated for external application, the active ingredient penetrates through the skin rapidly and extensively, achieving high, therapeutically relevant local concentrations in underlying soft tissues, joints and synovial fluid, whilst producing plasma levels that are unlikely to be sufficient to cause any systemic side-effects, other than in rare individuals who are hypersensitive to ibuprofen.

Furthermore, there do not appear to be any appreciable differences between the oral and topical routes of administration regarding metabolism or excretion of ibuprofen.

Preclinical safety data: Published information on subchronic toxicity studies confirms that topically applied ibuprofen is well tolerated both locally and by the gastro-intestinal tract. Any local erythema is only mild and no signs of mucosal lesions or ulcerogenic effects have been determined in the gastro-intestinal tract.

In the course of assessing mucosal tolerance, topical ibuprofen has been found to cause acute, but reversible, irritant reactions in the eyes and mucous membranes.

Pharmaceutical particulars
List of excipients: IMS BP; Carbomer; Propylene Glycol BP; Diethylamine; Purified Water BP.

Incompatibilities: None known.

Shelf life: 36 months.

Special precautions for storage: Store at room temperature (not exceeding 25°C).

Nature and contents of container: 100 g collapsible aluminium tube, fitted with a screw cap. This is supplied as an original pack (OP).

Instructions for use/handling: Not applicable.

Marketing authorisation number 0173/0050.

Date of approval/revision of SPC September 1997.

Legal category P.

IBUMOUSSE*

Qualitative and quantitative composition Ibuprofen BP 5.0% w/w.

Pharmaceutical form Non-greasy, fragrance-free, white aqueous cutaneous foam.

Clinical Particulars
Therapeutic indications: For backache, rheumatic and muscular pain, and neuralgia. Ibumousse is also indicated for symptomatic relief of pain due to non-serious arthritic conditions.

Posology and method of administration: Shake container before use. Hold container upright, then press nozzle to dispense the mousse into the palm of your hand. Gently massage the mousse into and around the affected areas until absorbed. The exact amount to be applied will vary, depending on the extent and severity of the condition, but it should normally be sufficient to apply 1 to 2 g (1 to 2 golf-ball sized quantities of mousse dispensed into the palm of the hand). This amount may be repeated 3 to 4 times daily, unless otherwise directed by the doctor.

Treatment should not normally continue for more than a few weeks, unless recommended by a doctor.

The same dosage and dosage schedule applies to all age groups, although the mousse is not normally recommended for children under 12 years, unless instructed by their doctor.

Contra-indications: Not to be used if allergic to any of the ingredients, or in cases of hypersensitivity to aspirin, ibuprofen or related painkillers (including when taken by mouth), especially where associated with a history of asthma, rhinitis or urticaria.

Not to be used on broken or damaged skin, or where there is infection or other skin disease.

Special warnings and special precautions for use: This product is flammable. Do not spray near flames, burning cigarettes, electric heaters or similar objects.

Keep away from the eyes and mucous membranes.

Oral NSAIDs, including ibuprofen, can sometimes be associated with renal impairment or aggravation of active peptic ulcers, and they can induce allergic bronchial reactions in susceptible asthmatic patients. Although systemic absorption of topically applied ibuprofen is much less than for oral dosage forms, these complications can still occur in rare cases. For these reasons, patients with asthma, an active peptic ulcer or a history of kidney problems, should seek medical advice before using the mousse, as should patients already taking other painkillers.

Patients should seek medical advice if symptoms worsen or persist. For external use only. Wash hands after use unless treating them. Do not use excessively.

The label will include statements to the following effect:

Do not exceed the stated dose. Not recommended for children under 12 years without medical advice. For external use only. Not to be used during pregnancy or breastfeeding. Do not use if you are allergic to any of the ingredients or have experienced problems with aspirin, ibuprofen or related painkillers (including when taken by mouth). If symptoms persist consult your doctor or pharmacist. Patients with asthma, an active peptic ulcer or a history of kidney problems should consult their doctor before use, as should patients already taking aspirin or other painkillers.

Interaction with other medicaments and other forms of interaction: Non-steroidal anti-inflammatory drugs may interact with blood pressure lowering drugs, although the chance of this occurring with a topically administered preparation is extremely remote. Concurrent aspirin or other NSAIDs may result in an increased incidence of undesirable effects.

Pregnancy and lactation: Not to be used during pregnancy or lactation. Although no teratogenic effects have been demonstrated, ibuprofen should be avoided during pregnancy. The onset of labour may be delayed, and the duration of labour increased. Ibuprofen appears in breast milk in very low concentrations, but is unlikely to affect breast-fed infants adversely.

Effects on ability to drive and use machines: None known.

Undesirable effects: The cooling effect of the mousse may result in a temporary paling of the skin.

Undesirable effects occur very occasionally, in which case treatment should be discontinued. Mostly these involve application site skin rashes, pruritus or urticaria.

Very rarely, the following side-effects may also occur in susceptible patients. Bronchospasm can be precipitated in patients suffering from, or with a history of, asthma or allergic disease. Renal impairment can occur in patients with a history of kidney problems. Additionally, gastro-intestinal side-effects, such as abdominal pain and dyspepsia, are possible in rare cases.

Overdose: Any overdose with a topical presentation of ibuprofen is extremely unlikely. Symptoms of severe ibuprofen overdosage (eg following accidental oral ingestion) include headache, vomiting, drowsiness and hypotension. Correction of severe electrolyte abnormalities should be considered.

Pharmacological properties
Pharmacodynamic properties: The mousse is for topical application. Ibuprofen is a phenylpropionic acid derivative with analgesic and anti-inflammatory properties. It exerts its effects directly in inflamed tissues underlying the site of application, mainly by inhibiting prostaglandin biosynthesis.

Because it is formulated in an aqueous mousse, the preparation also exerts a soothing and cooling effect when applied to the affected area.

Pharmacokinetic properties: Ibumousse has been designed for external application. The formulation delivers the active ingredient through the skin rapidly and extensively, achieving high, therapeutically relevant local concentrations in underlying soft tissues, joints and the synovial fluid, whilst producing plasma levels that are unlikely to be sufficient to cause any systemic side-effects, other than in rare individuals who are hypersensitive to ibuprofen. There do not appear to be any appreciable differences between the oral and topical routes of administration regarding metabolism or excretion of ibuprofen.

Preclinical safety data: No relevant information additional to that contained elsewhere in the SPC.

Pharmaceutical particulars
List of excipients: Propylene Glycol BP; Carbomer; Phenoxyethanol BP; Diethylamine; Butane 40; Purified Water BP.

(The ozone-friendly aerosol propellent is a blend of C_2-H_5 hydrocarbons consisting primarily of propane, iso-butane and n-butane).

Incompatibilities: None known.

Shelf life: 36 months.

Special precautions for storage: Store upright at room temperature (not exceeding 25°C), and away from direct heat or sunlight. Do not expose pressurised container to temperatures higher than 50°C. Do not pierce or burn container, even when empty.

Nature and contents of container: Aluminium pressurised container incorporating a spray valve and cap containing 125 g of product. This is supplied as an original pack (OP).

Instructions for use/handling: Not applicable.

Marketing authorisation number 0173/0169.

Date of approval/revision of SPC September 1998.

Legal category P.

IBUSPRAY*

Qualitative and quantitative composition Ibuprofen BP 5.0% w/w.

Pharmaceutical form Clear, colourless, fragrance-free, aqueous-alcoholic topical spray.

Clinical particulars
Therapeutic indications: For the topical treatment of backache, rheumatic and muscular pain, sprains, strains and neuralgia. Ibuspray is also indicated for symptomatic relief of pain due to non-serious arthritic conditions.

Posology and method of administration: Holding the bottle upright or upside down, spray approximately 4 inches to 6 inches away from the skin. After every 2 to 3 sprays, gently massage the preparation into the skin, spreading the product over a wide area around the affected site. The exact amount to be applied will vary, depending on the extent and severity of the condition, but it should normally be sufficient to apply 5 to 10 sprays (1 to 2 ml). This amount may be repeated three to four times daily, or more often if required.

Therapy should be reviewed after a few weeks, particularly if symptoms worsen or persist.

The same dosage and dosage schedule applies to all age groups, although Ibuspray is not normally recommended for use on children under the age of 12 years, unless instructed by their doctor.

Contra-indications: Not to be used in cases of sensitivity to any of the ingredients, particularly if asthmatic and have previously shown hypersensitivity to aspirin or ibuprofen. Not to be used on broken skin.

Special warnings and special precautions for use: This product is flammable. Do not spray near flames, electric heaters or similar objects. Patients should seek medical advice if symptoms worsen or persist. Oral NSAIDs, including ibuprofen, can sometimes be associated with renal impairment, aggravation of active peptic ulcers, and can induce allergic bronchial reactions in susceptible asthmatic patients. Although the systemic absorption of topically applied ibuprofen is less than for oral dosage forms, these complications can occur in rare cases. For these reasons, patients with an active peptic ulcer, a history of kidney problems, asthma or intolerance to aspirin or ibuprofen taken orally should seek medical advice before using Ibuspray. Keep away from the eyes and mucous membranes. For external use only.

Interaction with other medicaments and other forms of interaction: Non-steroidal anti-inflammatory drugs may interact with blood pressure lowering drugs, although the chance of this occurring with a topically administered preparation is extremely remote.

Pregnancy and lactation: Do not use during pregnancy or lactation.

Effects on ability to drive and use machines: None known.

Undesirable effects: The side-effects known to occur with oral ibuprofen are theoretically possible, although much less likely with topical application. In rare instances, skin rashes may occur, in which case the application of Ibuspray should be stopped.

Overdose: Not applicable. Any overdose with a topical presentation of ibuprofen is extremely unlikely.

Pharmacological properties
Pharmacodynamic properties: Ibuspray is a topical preparation which has anti-inflammatory and analgesic properties. It contains the active ingredient, ibuprofen, which exerts its effects directly in inflamed tissues underlying the site of application, mainly by inhibiting prostaglandin biosynthesis. Because it is formulated in an evaporative aqueous/alcoholic solution, Ibuspray also exerts a soothing and cooling effect when applied to the affected area.

Pharmacokinetic properties: Specially formulated for external application, the active ingredient penetrates through the skin rapidly and extensively, achieving high, therapeutically relevant local concentrations in underlying soft tissues, joints and synovial fluid, whilst producing plasma levels that are unlikely to be sufficient to cause any systemic side-effects, other than in rare individuals who are hypersensitive to ibuprofen. Furthermore, there do not appear to be any appreciable differences between the oral and topical routes of administration regarding metabolism or excretion of ibuprofen.

Preclinical safety data: Published information on subchronic toxicity studies confirms that topically applied ibuprofen is well tolerated both locally and by the gastro-intestinal tract. Any local erythema is only mild and no signs of mucosal lesions or ulcerogenic effects have been determined in the gastro-intestinal tract.

In the course of assessing mucosal tolerance, topical ibuprofen has been found to cause acute, but reversible, irritant reactions in the eyes and mucous membranes.

Pharmaceutical particulars
List of excipients: IMS BP; Polyethylene Glycol 300 BP; Cetomacrogol 1000 BP; Purified Water BP.

Incompatibilities: None known.

Shelf life: 30 months.

Special precautions for storage: Store at room temperature (not exceeding 25°C).

Nature and contents of container: 100 ml plastic bottle incorporating a controlled metered-dose spray pump dispenser and overcap. This is supplied as an original pack (OP). Ibuspray is not an aerosol, does not contain potentially irritant propellants and is ozone-friendly.

Instructions for use/handling: Not applicable.

Marketing authorisation number 0173/0150.

Date of approval/revision of SPC May 1998.

Legal category P.

PERINAL* SPRAY

Qualitative and quantitative composition Hydrocortisone BP 0.2% w/w; Lignocaine Hydrochloride BP 1.0% w/w.

Pharmaceutical form Colourless to pale yellow aqueous cutaneous spray solution.

Clinical particulars
Therapeutic indications: For the symptomatic relief of anal and perianal itch, irritation and pain, such as associated with haemorrhoids.

Posology and method of administration: The same dosage schedule applies to all age groups, although the spray is not normally recommended for children under 14 years unless on medical advice:

Spray twice over the affected area up to three times daily, depending on the severity of the condition.

Contra-indications: Not to be used if sensitive to lignocaine or any of the other ingredients. Not to be used on broken or infected skin. Not to used internally (inside the anus), or anywhere other than the anal area.

Special warnings and special precautions for use: Perinal Spray is intended for use for limited periods and so should not be used continuously for longer than 7 days without medical advice. Patients should be instructed to seek medical advice if they experience persistent pain or bleeding from the anus, especially when associated with a change in bowel habit, if the stomach is distended or if they are losing weight. Prompt medical treatment may be very important under such circumstances. Perinal Spray should be kept away from the eyes, nose and mouth.

The label will state:

Perinal Spray should not be used during pregnancy, while breast feeding or by children under the age of 14 without medical advice. Keep spray away from the eyes, nose and mouth, and do not apply to broken or infected skin, or to any part of the body except the anal area. Prime pump before initial use by depressing its top once or twice. Wash hands, and replace cap after use. Consult your doctor if the condition does not improve, or if rectal bleeding occurs. Do not use continuously for more than 7 days, unless recommended by your doctor. Do not use if sensitive to any of the ingredients. For external use only.

Interaction with other medicaments and other forms of interaction: No known interactions. Medical supervision is required if used in conjunction with other medicines containing steroids, owing to possible additive effects.

Pregnancy and lactation: There is inadequate evidence of safety in human pregnancy. Topical administration of corticosteroids to pregnant animals can cause abnormalies of foetal development including cleft palate and intra-uterine growth retardation. There may therefore be a very small risk of such effects in the human foetus. The risk/benefit needs to be carefully assessed, therefore, before prescribing this medicine.

Effects on ability to drive and use machines: None known.

Undesirable effects: A temporary tingling sensation may be experienced locally after initial application. Hypersensitivity to lignocaine has rarely been reported.

Overdose: Under exceptional circumstances, if Perinal Spray is used excessively, particularly in young children, it is theoretically possible that adrenal suppression and skin thinning may occur. The symptoms are normally reversible on cessation of treatment.

Pharmacological properties
Pharmacodynamic properties: The preparation combines the well-known local anti-inflammatory and anti-pruritic properties of hydrocortisone and the analgesic effect of lignocaine in an aqueous spray formulation. On application, finger contact with the affected area can be avoided which makes for improved hygiene, and lessens the risk of infection.

Pharmacokinetic properties: The active ingredients of the formulation are readily available for intimate contact with the skin and mucous membranes, as the preparation is sprayed in small droplets which dry after application to leave the active ingredients in close contact with the affected area.

Because the preparation is a clear solution, it is entirely homogeneous, and the availability of the active ingredient is optimal.

Preclinical safety data: No special information.

Pharmaceutical particulars
List of excipients: Cetomacrogol 1000 BP; Citric Acid Monohydrate BP; Sodium Citrate BP; Propyl Gallate BP; Phenoxyethanol BP; Purified Water BP.

Incompatibilities: None known.

Shelf life: 30 months.

Special precautions for storage: Store at room temperature (not exceeding 25°C).

Nature and contents of container: 30 ml collapsible laminate tube with metering-dose spray pump and cap, which is ozone-friendly.

The spray operates when held in any direction. It is

not an aerosol and does *not* contain any potentially irritant propellants.

This is supplied as an original pack (OP).

Instructions for use/handling: Not applicable.

Marketing authorisation number 0173/0049.

Date of approval/revision of SPC February 1998.

Legal category P.

PSORIDERM* BATH EMULSION

Qualitative and quantitative composition Distilled Coal Tar 40.0% w/v.

Pharmaceutical form Buff coloured liquid emulsion.

Clinical particulars The use of coal tar has long been advocated as a therapeutic agent in the management of psoriasis. Psoriderm Bath Emulsion conveniently provides a coal tar bath which may be used alone, or as part of a more extensive treatment regime.

Therapeutic indications: For use topically as an aid in the treatment of sub-acute and chronic psoriasis.

Posology and method of administration: For adults, children and the elderly. Add 30 ml of the emulsion to a standard bath of warm water. Soak for 5 minutes, pat dry.

Contra-indications: Not to be used in cases of sensitivity to any of the ingredients.

Special warnings and special precautions for use: Do not use product undiluted. Keep away from the eyes and broken or inflamed skin. Replace cap after use. Avoid spillage. For external use only.

Interaction with other medicaments and other forms of interaction: None known.

Pregnancy and lactation: No special precautions.

Effects on ability to drive and use machines: None known.

Undesirable effects: Local side-effects do not normally occur. In rare cases of skin irritation, discontinue treatment.

Overdose: There are no known toxic effects resulting from excessive use of Psoriderm Bath Emulsion. In case of accidental ingestion, patients should contact a doctor or hospital immediately.

Pharmacological properties
Pharmacodynamic properties: Coal tar has been used dermatologically for hundreds of years and has been shown to be safe and effective in the treatment of scaly skin conditions such as psoriasis. The British Pharmacopoeia contains monographs on coal tar and coal tar solution, and many formulations of coal tar are used in hospitals throughout the country. The coal tar used in Psoriderm Bath Emulsion has been specially distilled and is based on a neutral fraction which has been shown to be effective in the treatment of psoriasis.

The precise mechanism of action of coal tar is not understood, largely as a result of it comprising up to 10,000 components. There is evidence that topical application of coal tar improves psoriasis by reducing the excessive rate of mitotic epidermal cell division.

Pharmacokinetic properties: Dry scales, which are a common feature of psoriasis, generally reduce the effectiveness of topically applied treatments by reducing absorption of the active ingredient. An established means of overcoming this problem is to add a mild softening agent such as lecithin. In the case of Psoriderm Bath Emulsion, however, no such softening agent is included because the dosage and administration regime involves prolonged soaking (5 minutes) in a warm water emulsion which achieves a similar effect.

Preclinical safety data: No special information.

Pharmaceutical particulars
List of excipients: Polysorbate 20 BP; Triethanolamine BP; Phenoxyethanol BP; Water.

Incompatibilities: None known.

Shelf life: 36 months.

Special precautions for storage: Store at room temperature (not exceeding 25°C).

Nature and contents of container: Amber glass bottle containing 200 ml. This is supplied as an original pack (OP).

Instructions for use/handling: Not applicable.

Marketing authorisation number 0173/5003R.

Date of approval/revision of SPC March 1995.

Legal category P.

PSORIDERM* CREAM

Qualitative and quantitative composition Distilled Coal Tar 6.0% w/w; Lecithin 0.4% w/w.

Pharmaceutical form Buff coloured cream.

Clinical particulars The use of coal tar has long been advocated as a therapeutic agent in the management of psoriasis. Psoriderm Cream may be used alone, or as part of a more extensive treatment regime, and is particularly suitable for treating the hair bearing parts of the body and the flexures.

Therapeutic indications: For the topical treatment of sub-acute and chronic psoriasis, including psoriasis of the scalp and flexures.

Posology and method of administration: For adults, children and the elderly. Apply to the affected area once or twice daily, or as recommended by the physician. Wash hands after use.

Contra-indications: Not to be used for acute psoriasis. Not to be used in cases of sensitivity to any of the ingredients.

Special warnings and special precautions for use: Keep away from the eyes and mucous membranes. Replace cap after use. Avoid spillage. For external use only.

Interaction with other medicaments and other forms of interaction: None known.

Pregnancy and lactation: No special precautions.

Effects on ability to drive and use machines: None known.

Undesirable effects: Local side-effects do not normally occur. In rare cases of skin irritation, discontinue treatment.

Overdose: There are no known toxic effects resulting from excessive use of Psoriderm Cream.

Pharmacological properties
Pharmacodynamic properties: Coal tar has been used dermatologically for hundreds of years and has been shown to be safe and effective in the treatment of scaly skin conditions such as psoriasis. The British Pharmacopoeia contains monographs on coal tar and coal tar solution, and many formulations of coal tar are used in hospitals throughout the country. The coal tar used in Psoriderm Cream has been specially distilled and is based on a neutral fraction which has been shown to be effective in the treatment of psoriasis.

The precise mechanism of action of coal tar is not understood, largely as a result of it comprising up to 10,000 components. There is evidence that topical application of coal tar improves psoriasis by reducing the excessive rate of mitotic epidermal cell division.

Lecithin is a well known phospholipid which is present in foodstuffs. It is added to Psoriderm Cream to soften psoriasis scales and thereby enhance the absorption of the coal tar.

Pharmacokinetic properties: Not applicable.

Preclinical safety data: No special information.

Pharmaceutical particulars
List of excipients: Stearic Acid BP; Isopropyl Palmitate; Propylene Glycol BP; Triethanolamine BP; Phenoxyethanol BP; Purified Water BP.

Incompatibilities: None known.

Shelf life: 36 months.

Special precautions for storage: Store in a cool, dark place.

Nature and contents of container: Amber glass jar containing 225 ml. This is supplied as an original pack (OP).

Instructions for use/handling: Not applicable.

Marketing authorisation number 0173/5000R.

Date of approval/revision of SPC September 1995.

Legal category P.

PSORIDERM* SCALP LOTION

Qualitative and quantitative composition Distilled Coal Tar 2.5% w/v; Lecithin 0.3% w/v.

Pharmaceutical form Golden brown coloured foaming therapeutic shampoo.

Clinical particulars The use of coal tar has long been advocated as a therapeutic agent in the management of psoriasis. Psoriderm Scalp Lotion may be used alone as a coal tar shampoo, or as part of a more extensive treatment regime.

Therapeutic indications: For the topical treatment of psoriasis of the scalp.

Posology and method of administration: For adults, children and the elderly. Wet the hair thoroughly. Apply a small amount of the shampoo to the scalp, and massage gently until a rich lather has been generated. Retain on the scalp for a few minutes. Remove excess lather with the hands before rinsing with warm water. Repeat the above procedure.

Contra-indications: Not to be used for acute psoriasis. Not to be used in cases of sensitivity to any of the ingredients.

Special warnings and special precautions for use: Keep away from the eyes and mucous membranes. Replace cap after use. Avoid spillage. For external use only.

Interaction with other medicaments and other forms of interaction: None known.

Pregnancy and lactation: No special precautions.

Effects on ability to drive and use machines: None known.

Undesirable effects: Local side-effects do not normally occur. In rare cases of skin irritation, discontinue treatment.

Overdose: There are no known toxic effects resulting from excessive use of Psoriderm Scalp Lotion.

Pharmacological properties
Pharmacodynamic properties: Coal tar has been used dermatologically for hundreds of years and has been shown to be safe and effective in the treatment of scaly scalp conditions such as psoriasis. The British Pharmacopoeia contains monographs on coal tar and coal tar solution, and many formulations of coal tar are used in hospitals throughout the country. The coal tar used in Psoriderm Scalp Lotion has been specially distilled and is based on a neutral fraction which has been shown to be effective in the treatment of psoriasis.

The precise mechanism of action of coal tar is not understood, largely as a result of it comprising up to 10,000 components. There is evidence that topical application of coal tar improves psoriasis by reducing the excessive rate of mitotic epidermal cell division.

Lecithin is a well known phospholipid which is present in foodstuffs. It is added to Psoriderm Scalp Lotion to soften psoriasis scales and thereby enhance the absorption of the coal tar.

Pharmacokinetic properties: Not applicable.

Preclinical safety data: No special information.

Pharmaceutical particulars
List of excipients: Triethanolamine Lauryl Sulphate; Lauric Acid Diethanolamide; Disodium Edetate BP; Sodium Chloride BP; Phenoxyethanol BP; Purified Water BP.

Incompatibilities: None known.

Shelf life: 36 months.

Special precautions for storage: Store in a cool, dark place.

Nature and contents of container: White plastic bottle containing 250 ml. This is supplied as an original pack (OP).

Instructions for use/handling: Not applicable.

Marketing authorisation number 0173/5001R.

Date of approval/revision of SPC April 1995.

Legal category P.

SALACTOL*

Qualitative and quantitative composition Salicylic Acid BP 16.7% w/w; Lactic Acid BP 16.7% w/w.

Pharmaceutical form Colourless or pale yellow/brown evaporative wart paint.

Clinical particulars
Therapeutic indications: For the topical treatment of warts, verrucas, corns and calluses.

Posology and method of administration: For adults, children and the elderly. Soak the affected site in warm water and pat dry. Gently rub the surface of the wart, verruca, corn or callus with a pumice stone or manicure emery board to remove any hard skin. Using the applicator provided, carefully apply a few drops of Salactol to the lesion, taking care to localise the application to the affected area. Plantar warts should be covered with an adhesive plaster. Leave for 24 hours. Repeat the procedure daily, removing old collodion on each occasion.

Contra-indications: Not to be used on or near the face, intertriginous or anogenital regions. Not to be used by diabetics or individuals with impaired peripheral blood circulation. Not to be used in cases of sensitivity to any of the ingredients. Not to be used on moles, birthmarks, hairy warts or on any other skin lesions for which Salactol is not indicated.

Special warnings and special precautions for use: Keep away from the eyes and mucous membranes. Avoid spreading onto surrounding normal skin. If the treated area becomes inflamed or painful, treatment should be suspended until the inflammation resolves. Extremely flammable. Avoid spillage. Avoid inhaling vapour. Replace cap tightly after use. For external use only.

Interaction with other medicaments and other forms of interaction: None known.

Pregnancy and lactation: No special precautions.

Effects on ability to drive and use machines: None known.

Undesirable effects: Salactol may be irritant on the skin in certain patients.

Overdose: Any excessive use of Salactol could cause irritation of the skin. If this occurs, Salactol should be used more sparingly or applied less frequently. Accidental oral ingestion should be treated immediately by gastric lavage with a 2 to 5% aqueous sodium bicarbonate solution. Fluid and electrolyte balance should be monitored and appropriate supportive measures should be provided. Symptoms include headache, nausea, vomiting, diarrhoea and respiratory depression.

Pharmacological properties

Pharmacodynamic properties: The combination of salicylic acid and lactic acid in flexible collodion has been shown to be particularly efficacious in treating warts, verrucas, corns and calluses.

Salicylic acid has bacteriostatic and fungicidal actions as well as keratolytic properties. Its effectiveness for topical treatment of hyperkeratotic skin lesions is based on mild keratolytic action which produces slow and painless destruction of the epithelium. In the treatment of warts, a mild irritant reaction, which may render the virus more prone to immunologic stimulation or response, may add to the mechanical removal of infected cells. Apart from its antiseptic and caustic properties, lactic acid enhances the availability of salicylic acid from the dried collodion.

Pharmacokinetic properties: Salactol contains 16.7% salicylic acid and 16.7% lactic acid in flexible collodion. The bioavailability of salicylic acid is reduced as the collodion film dries on the skin due to entrapment of the drug which inhibits release. The addition of lactic acid to salicylic acid collodion provides more efficient release of the salicylic acid, since the non-volatile lactic acid remains in the film, thus permitting continued release of the keratolytic which may otherwise be entrapped within the dried collodion film. Systemic absorption of salicylic acid or lactic acid after application to small circumscribed areas is exceedingly unlikely.

Preclinical safety data: No special information.

Pharmaceutical particulars

List of excipients: Pyroxylin BP; Colophony BP; Castor Oil BP; IMS BP; Solvent Ether BP.

Incompatibilities: None known.

Shelf life: 36 months in unopened container. 3 months in opened container.

Special precautions for storage: Store at room temperature (not exceeding 25°C).

Nature and contents of container: Amber glass bottle containing 10 ml, incorporating a specially designed spatula for ease of application. This is supplied as an original pack (OP).

Instructions for use/handling: Not applicable.

Marketing authorisation number 0173/5006R.

Date of approval/revision of SPC October 1996.

Legal category P.

SALATAC* GEL

Qualitative and quantitative composition Salicylic Acid BP 12.0% w/w; Lactic Acid BP 4.0% w/w.

Pharmaceutical form Clear, colourless, collodion-like wart gel.

Clinical particulars

Therapeutic indications: For the topical treatment of warts, verrucas, corns and calluses.

Posology and method of administration: For adults, children and the elderly. Salatac Gel should be applied once daily. The gel should be applied once every night. Treatment can take up to twelve (12) weeks for resistant lesions to disappear, and it is necessary to persevere with treatment.

1. Every night, soak the affected site in warm water for 2 to 3 minutes.
2. Dry thoroughly with the patient's own towel.
3. Carefully apply one or two drops of the gel to the lesion and allow to dry over its surface. Take care to avoid spreading on to surrounding normal skin. No adhesive plaster is necessary.
4. The following evening, carefully remove and discard the elastic film formed from the previous application, and reapply the gel. Occasionally, if removal of the elastic film proves difficult, carefully reapply the gel over it and allow to dry. This should help thicken the film to assist removal. If necessary, such re-application may be made on two or three successive days.
5. Once a week, gently rub away the treated surface using an emery board, as provided, or pumice stone used only for this purpose, before re-applying the gel.
6. The wart, verruca, corn or callus may take up to twelve (12) weeks to disappear and it is important to persevere with the treatment.
7. At the end of treatment, if the elastic film is difficult to remove, it may be allowed to remain on the skin until it sheds.

Contra-indications: Not to be used on or near the face, intertriginous or anogenital regions, or by diabetics or individuals with impaired peripheral blood circulation. Not to be used on moles or on any other skin lesions for which the gel is not indicated. Not to be used in cases of sensitivity to any of the ingredients.

Special warnings and special precautions for use: Keep away from the eyes, mucous membranes and from cuts and grazes. Apply only to warts, verrucas, corns and calluses, avoiding surrounding normal skin. Do not use excessively. Some mild, transient irritation may be expected, but in cases of more severe inflammation, treatment should be suspended. Avoid inhaling vapour, and keep cap firmly closed when not in use. Contact with clothing, fabrics, plastics and other materials may cause damage, and should be avoided. For external use only.

Interaction with other medicaments and other forms of interaction: None known.

Pregnancy and lactation: No special precautions.

Effects on ability to drive and use machines: None known.

Undesirable effects: Salatac Gel may be irritant on the skin in certain patients.

Overdose: Any excessive use of Salatac Gel could cause irritation of the skin. If this occurs, Salatac Gel should be used more sparingly or applied less frequently.

Pharmacological properties

Pharmacodynamic properties: The active ingredients, salicylic acid and lactic acid, are well-established pharmacopoeial substances. In combination, they are routinely used in the treatment of verrucas, warts, corns and calluses for their keratolytic properties.

When applied topically, and in high enough concentrations, salicylic acid acts by achieving a slow, painless destruction of the thickened stratum corneum. It softens and destroys the stratum corneum of the affected tissue by reducing the adhesiveness of the corneocytes while causing the cornified epithelium to swell, soften, macerate and finally desquamate. In the treatment of warts, a mild irritant reaction, which may render the virus more prone to immunologic stimulation or response, may add to the mechanical removal of infected cells. The other active ingredient, lactic acid, enhances the availability of the salicylic acid from the dried collodion, in addition to having antiseptic and caustic properties.

Pharmacokinetic properties: Salatac Gel contains 12% salicylic acid and 4% lactic acid in an evaporative collodion-like gel which forms a cohesive and adhesive film on the skin.

The formulation is presented in a collapsible aluminium tube fitted with a special applicator nozzle allowing the formulation to be dispensed precisely to the affected areas only. This minimises the spread of the preparation onto the surrounding healthy skin.

The gel quickly forms a surface film, well before it dries completely, thereby prolonging the period during which the keratolytic solution can properly infiltrate and achieve intimate contact with the surface layers of the thickened stratum corneum.

Furthermore, even when the film appears to have dried completely, the inclusion of the non-evaporative lactic acid ensures that a proportion of the salicylic acid remains in solution within the vehicle, thus permitting continued release of the keratolytic, which may otherwise be entrapped within the collodion-like film.

Systemic absorption of salicylic acid or lactic acid after application of the recommended daily dose of one or two drops of the preparation to small, circumscribed areas is exceedingly unlikely.

Preclinical safety data: No special information.

Pharmaceutical particulars

List of excipients: Camphor BP; Pyroxylin BP; Ethanol (96%) BP; Ethyl Acetate.

Incompatibilities: None known.

Shelf life: 36 months.

Special precautions for storage: Highly flammable – keep away from flames. Store at room temperature (not exceeding 25°C).

Nature and contents of container: Collapsible tube containing 8 g, complete with special applicator, emery board and instructions. This is supplied as an original pack (OP).

Instructions for use/handling: Not applicable.

Marketing authorisation number 0173/0046.

Date of approval/revision of SPC August 1997.

Legal category P.

**Trade Mark*

DermaPharm Limited
The Old Coach House
34 Elm Road
Chessington
Surrey KT9 1AW

☎ 0181 9742266 🗋 0181 9742005

≈DermaPharm Limited

ACNISAL*

Qualitative and quantitative composition Salicylic acid BP 2.0% w/w.

Pharmaceutical form Lotion for topical administration.

Clinical particulars
Therapeutic indications: Acnisal is for the management of acne. It helps prevent new comedones (blackheads and whiteheads) papules and pustules (acne pimples).

Posology and method of administration: For topical administration.

Adults: Acnisal is used to wash the affected area 2 to 3 times daily. Lather with warm water, massage into skin, rinse and dry.
Children: As for adults.
Elderly: As for adults.

Contra-indications: Acnisal is contra-indicated in persons with a sensitivity to salicylic acid.

Special warnings and precautions for use: For external use only. Avoid contact with the mouth, eyes and other mucous membranes to avoid irritation.

As with other topical preparations containing salicylic acid, excessive prolonged use may result in symptoms of salicylism.

Interactions with other medicaments and other forms of interaction: None known.

Pregnancy and lactation: No limitations to the use of Acnisal during pregnancy or lactation are known.

Effects on ability to drive and use machines: None known.

Undesirable effects: Salicylic acid is a mild irritant and may cause skin irritation. If undue skin irritation develops or increases adjust the usage schedule or consult your physician.

Overdose: Not applicable.

Pharmacological properties
Pharmacodynamic properties: Human comedones, naturally or coal tar induced, are fiirmly anchored and are dislodged with great difficulty. Most classic 'peeling' agents are ineffective: they are merely irritants which cause scaling, creating the illusion of comedolysis. While salicylic acid is an irritant its efficacy is dependent on specific pharmacological effects. It seems to detach horny cells from each other by weakening the intercellular cement. As a result, the comedones tend to undergo disorganisation. The effect is probably a good deal more complex. Salicylic acid penetrates skin readily and increases turnover which also favours exfoliation of the comedo. In concentrations of 0.5 to 2% it significantly reduces the formation of micromedones, which are the precursors of all other acne lesions.

Pharmacokinetic properties: There is no evidence of any systemic absorption from the use of Acnisal.

Preclinical safety data: None presented.

Pharmaceutical particulars
List of excipients: Purified water; Benzyl alcohol; Sodium chloride; Sodium C14–C16 olefin sulphonate; Lauramide DEA (monoamide 716); PEG-7 glycerol cocoate; Lytron 614.

Incompatibilities: None known.

Shelf life: 36 months.

Special precautions for storage: Store below 30°C.

Nature and cotents of container: Acnisal is supplied in a white HDPE bottle with a white polypropylene screw cap. Each bottle contains either 30 ml or 177 ml of Acnisal.

Instructions for use/handling: For external use only. Keep out of reach of children.

Marketing authorisation number PL 16874/0003.

Date of first authorisation/renewal of authorisation 11 September 1998.

Date of (partial) revision of the text January 1997.

METED* SHAMPOO

Qualitative and quantitative composition

Salicylic acid	USP 3.0%
Colloidal sulphur	HSE 6.25% (equivalent to sulphur 5.0%).

Pharmaceutical form Shampoo.

Clinical particulars
Therapeutic indications: For the relief of itching, irritation, redness, flaking and/or scaling due to dandruff, seborrhoeic dermatitis, or psoriasis of the scalp.

Posology and method of administration: For topical administration.

Adults: The hair should be thoroughly wetted and sufficient Meted shampoo applied to produce an abundant lather. The hair should be rinsed and the procedure repeated.

Use at least twice weekly or as directed by a physician.
Children: As for adults.
Elderly: As for adults.

Contra-indications: Meted Shampoo is contra-indicated in persons with a sensitivity to any of the ingredients.

Special warnings and precautions: Avoid contact with the eyes. If shampoo gets into the eyes rinse thoroughly with water.

If the condition worsens or does not improve after regular use of the product as directed, consult a physician.

Interaction with other medicaments and other forms of interaction: None known.

Pregnancy and lactation: No limitations to the use of Meted Shampoo during pregnancy or lactation are known.

Effects on ability to drive and use machinery: None known.

Undesirable effects: There have been no reports of adverse effects following the use of Meted Shampoo. However, salicylic acid is a mild irritant and may cause dermatitis.

Overdose: There is no evidence of systemic absorption following the use this shampoo. There are no reports available of its ingestion.

Pharmacological properties
Pharmacodynamic properties: Sulphur is a keratolytic and mild antiseptic. Salicylic acid has keratolytic and fungicidal properties.

Pharmacokinetic properties: There is no evidence of systemic absoprtion of sulphur or salicylic acid following use of Meted Shampoo.

Preclinical safety data: None presented.

Pharmaceutical particulars
List of excipients: Magnesium aluminium silicate; Hydroxypropyl methyl cellulose; Panthenol; Sodium laureth sulphate; Sodium cocoyl sarcosinate; Cocamido propyl betaine; Fragrance—Firmenich 430 018; Purified water.

Incompatibilities: None known.

Shelf life: 36 months.

Special precautions for storage: No special precautions—store at room temperature.

Nature and contents of container: Meted Shampoo is supplied in a white HDPE bottle with a white polypropylene screw cap. Each bottle contains either 30 ml or 120 ml of Meted Shampoo.

Instructions for use/handling: For exernal use only. Keep out of reach of children.

Marketing authorisation holder Euroderma Limited, The Old Coach House, 34 Elm Road, Chessington, Surrey KT9 1AW.

Marketing authorisation number PL 10670/0001.

Date of first authorisation/renewal of authorisation 17 September 1996.

Date of (partial) revision of the text 22 March 1996.

OCCLUSAL*

Qualitative and quantitative composition Salicylic Acid BP 26% w/w.

Pharmaceutical form Solution for topical application.

Clinical particulars
Therapeutic indications: Occlusal is indicated for the treatment and removal of common warts and plantar warts.

Posology and method of administration: For topical application.

Prior to application soak wart in warm water for five minutes. Remove loose tissue with a brush, washcloth or emery board. Dry thoroughly with a towel not used by others to avoid contagion. Carefully apply Occusal twice to the wart using the brush applicator allowing the first application to dry before applying the second. Thereafter repeat treatment once daily or as directed by physician. Do not apply to surrounding healthy skin. Clinically visible improvement should occur in one to two weeks but maximum effect may be expected after four to six weeks.

There are no differences in dosage for children, adults or the elderly.

Contra-indications: Occlusal should not be used by diabetics or patients with impaired blood circulation. Do not use on moles, birthmarks, unusual warts with hair growth, on facial warts, or in the anal or perineal region.

Special warnings and precautions for use: Occlusal is for external use only. Do not permit contact with eyes or mucous membranes. If contact occurs flush with water for 15 minutes. Do not allow contact with normal skin around wart. Avoid using on areas of broken or damaged skin. Discontinue treatment if excessive irritation occurs.

Interactions with other medicaments and other forms of interaction: None known.

Pregnancy and lactation: The chronic use of this product during pregnancy and lactation, particularly when large areas of skin are involved, should be avoided.

Effects on ability to drive and use machines: None known.

Undesirable effects: A localised irritant reaction may occur if Occlusal is applied to normal skin surrounding the wart. This may normally be controlled by temporarily discontinuing the use of Occlusal and by being careful to apply the solution only to the wart itself when treatment is resumed.

Overdose: Salicylism can occur following large doses of salicylic acid or prolonged use of topical salicylic acid preparations, or in the unlikely event of accidental consumption.

Pharmacological properties
Pharmacodynamic properties: Salicylic acid has bacteriostatic and fungicidal actions, but it is its keratolytic properties which are important for this medicinal product. When applied externally it produces slow and painless destruction of the epithelium. Salicylic acid is usually applied in the form of a paint in a collodian base (10 to 17%) or as a plaster (20 to 50%) to destroy warts or corns.

Pharmacokinetic properties: Not applicable.

Preclinical safety data: None presented.

Pharmaceutical particulars
List of excipients: Polyvinyl butyral; Dibutyl phthalate; Isopropyl alcohol; Butyl acetate; Acrylates copolymer.

Incompatibilities: None known.

Shelf life: 2 years.

Special precautions for storage: Store below 25°C.

Nature and contents of container: The product is presented in a 10 ml amber glass with cap brush assembly. The cap brush assembly comprises of a black cap and a white polythene wand nylon brush with a stainless steel staple.

Instructions for use/handling: Occlusal is flammable and should be kept away from flame or fire. Keep the bottle tightly capped when not in use. Do not allow the solution to drip from the brush onto the bottle neck thread, otherwise subsequent opening of the bottle may be difficult.

Marketing authorisation number PL 16874/0001.

Date of first authorisaiton/renewal of authorisation 7 September 1998.

Date of (partial) revision of the text April 1998.

PENTRAX* SHAMPOO

Qualitative and quantitative composition
Fractar 5 HSE 7.71%
(equivalent to coal tar 4.3%).

Pharmaceutical form Shampoo.

Clinical particulars
Therapeutic indications: For the relief of itching, irritation, redness, flaking and/or scaling due to dandruff, seborrhoeic dermatitis, or psoriasis of the scalp.

Posology and method of administration: For topical administration.

Adults: Pentrax Shampoo should be massaged into wet hair and scalp to produce a lather. The hair should be rinsed and the procedure repeated applying a liberal amount of Pentrax and allowing the lather to remain on the hair for up to 10 minutes. The hair should be rinsed thoroughly.

Use at least twice weekly or as otherwise directed by a physician.

Children: As for adults.

Elderly: As for adults.

Contra-indications: Pentrax shampoo is contra-indicated in persons with a sensitivity to any of the ingredients.

Special warnings and precautions for use: Avoid contact with the eyes. If shampoo gets into the eyes rinse thoroughly with water.

If the condition worsens or does not improve after regular use of the product as directed, consult a physician.

Interaction with other medicaments and other forms of interaction: None known.

Pregnancy and lactation: No limitations to the use of Pentrax shampoo during pregnancy or lactation are known.

Effects on ability to drive and use machinery: None known.

Undesirable effects: There have been no reports of adverse effects following the use of Pentrax Shampoo. However, coal tar may cause irritation to the skin, and hypersensitivity to coal tar has been reported.

Overdose: There is no evidence of systemic absorption following the use of this shampoo. There are no reports available of its ingestion.

Pharmacological properties
Pharmacodynamic properties: Coal tar is an antipruritic, keratolytic and a weak antiseptic.

Pharmacokinetic properties: There is no evidence of systemic absorption following the use of Pentrax Shampoo.

Preclinical safety data: None presented.

Pharmaceutical particulars
List of excipients: Dioctyl sodium sulphosuccinate; Laureth 23; Polyethylene glycol 8; Sodium lauryl sulphate; Cocamide DEA; Lauramine oxide.

Incompatibilities: None known.

Shelf life: 48 months.

Special precautions for storage: None.

Nature and contents of container: Pentrax Shampoo is supplied in a polyvinylchloride bottle with a polypropylene screw cap with triseal. Each bottle contains either 30 ml, 120 ml or 240 ml of Pentrax Shampoo.

Instructions for use/handling: For external use only. Keep out of reach of children.

Marketing authorisation holder Euroderma Limited, The Old Coach House, 34 Elm Road, Chessington, Surrey KT9 1AW.

Marketing authorisation number PL 10670/0002.

Date of first authorisation/renewal of authorisation 24 September 1996.

Date of (partial) revision of the text 22 March 1996.

**Trade Mark*

E. C. De Witt & Company Limited
Tudor Road, Manor Park
Runcorn, Cheshire WA7 1SZ

☎ 01928 579029 🗋 01928 579712

FLEET* MICRO-ENEMA

Presentation A disposable polyethylene tube with a pre-lubricated pliable nozzle and integral finger guard, which delivers 5 ml of a smooth white, opaque solution comprising 450 mg Sodium Citrate Dihydrate and 45 mg Sodium Lauryl Sulphoacetate.

Excipients: Glycerin, Sorbitol, Propylene Glycol, Carbomer.

Nozzle Lubricant: White Soft Paraffin.

Uses Fleet Micro-enema is indicated for the occasional treatment of constipation in bedridden patients, geriatrics, paediatrics and obstetrics.

Dosage and administration

Dosage: Adults and children aged 3 years and over: Administer the contents of one Fleet Micro-enema rectally and expect a bowel movement within 15 minutes.

FOR RECTAL USE ONLY.

Directions for use: Lie on left side with both knees bent, arms at rest. (Fig. 1)

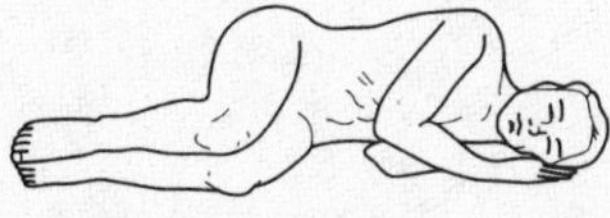

Fig. 1

Remove orange protective shield. Pull shield gently while grasping grooved cap underneath finger guard. (Fig. 2)

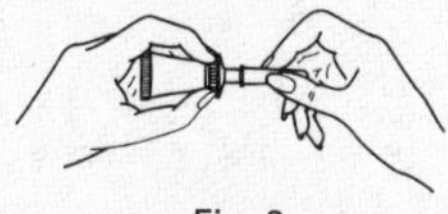

Fig. 2

With steady pressure, gently insert enema full length into the rectum with tip pointing towards navel. Squeeze tube until contents are expelled.

Discontinue use if resistance is encountered. Forcing an enema can result in injury.

Contra-indications, warnings, etc

Contra-indications: Do not administer to children under 3 years of age.

It is advisable to avoid the use of Fleet Micro-enema in cases of haemorrhoid eruptions and in patients with inflammatory bowel disease.

Warnings: Excessive use may cause diarrhoea and fluid loss, which should be treated symptomatically. Propylene glycol can cause local irritancy and hypersensitivity. Frequent or prolonged use of a laxative for more than one week may result in dependence.

Rectal bleeding or failure to have a bowel movement after use of a laxative may indicate a serious problem. In such cases Fleet Micro-enema should not be administered further and a doctor's advice sought.

Use in pregnancy and lactation: There is no data on toxicity in animals and man, therefore should only be used under medical supervision.

Effects on ability to drive and use machines: Not applicable.

Undesirable effects: Not applicable.

Overdose: In case of accidental ingestion, seek medical advice.

Pharmaceutical precautions Store below 25°C.

Legal category P.

Package quantities 5 ml tubes packed in 12s.

Further information The laxative action is due to the combined action of sodium citrate and sodium lauryl sulphoacetate. Sodium citrate acts by retaining fluid in the bowel by osmosis and by changing the pattern of water distribution in the faeces, while sodium lauryl sulphoacetate is a wetting agent.

Product licence number 0083/0045.

FLEET* PHOSPHO-SODA*

Presentation Two polyethylene bottles, each containing 45 ml of a clear, colourless, ginger-lemon flavoured solution for oral use, with the equivalent of 24.4 g Sodium Dihydrogen Phosphate Dihydrate and 10.8 g Disodium Phosphate Dodecahydrate per 45 ml. Sodium content is 5.0 g per 45 ml. Excipients: Glycerol, Sodium Saccharin, Sodium Benzoate (E211), Ginger-Lemon Flavour, Purified Water.

Uses As a bowel cleanser in preparing the patient for colon surgery or for preparing the colon for x-ray or endoscopic examination.

Dosage and administration

Adults only: The taking of Fleet Phospho-soda should be started the day before the hospital appointment. If the hospital appointment is before 12 noon the dosage instructions for morning appointments should be followed and for appointments after 12 noon the dosage instructions for an afternoon appointment should be followed. 'Clear liquids' include water, clear soup, strained fruit juices without pulp (not red or purple coloured), black tea or black coffee and clear fizzy/non fizzy soft drinks, e.g. lemonade.

Morning apppointment

Day before appointment: 7am – In place of breakfast drink at least one full glass of 'clear liquid' or water, more if desired.

1st dose – Straight after breakfast. Dilute the contents of one bottle (45 ml) in half a glass (120 ml) of cold water. Drink this solution followed by one full glass (240 ml) of cold water, more if desired.

1pm lunch – In place of lunch drink at least three full glasses (720 ml) of 'clear liquid' or water, more if desired.

7pm supper – In place of supper drink at least one full glass of 'clear liquid' or water, more if desired.

2nd dose – Straight after supper. Dilute the contents of the second bottle (45 ml) in half a glass (120 ml) of cold water. Drink this solution followed by one full glass (240 ml) of cold water, more if desired. Additional water or 'clear liquids' may be taken up until midnight if necessary.

Afternoon appointment

Day before appointment: 1pm lunch– A light snack may be taken. After lunch no more solid food must be taken until after the hospital appointment.

7pm supper – In place of supper drink at least one full glass of 'clear liquid' or water, more if desired.

1st dose – Straight after supper. Dilute the contents of one bottle (45 ml) in half a glass (120 ml) of cold water. Drink this solution followed by one full glass (240 ml) of cold water, more if desired.

During the evening drink at least three full glasses of water or 'clear liquid' before going to bed.

Day of appointment: 7am breakfast – In place of breakfast drink at least one full glass of 'clear liquid' or water, more if desired.

2nd dose – Straight after breakfast. Dilute the contents of the second bottle (45 ml) in half a glass (120 ml) of cold water. Drink this solution followed by one full glass (240 ml) of cold water. More water or 'clear liquid' may be taken up until 8am.

Contra-indications, warnings, etc

Contra-indications: Do not use in children and in patients with known or suspected gastrointestinal obstruction or ileus, congestive heart failure, megacolon (congenital or acquired), renal failure or inflammatory bowel disease. Do not use when nausea, vomiting or abdominal pain are present.

Warnings: Use with caution in patients with impaired renal function, heart disease, colostomy or on a low salt diet as hyperphosphataemia, hypocalcaemia, hypernatraemic dehydration and acidosis may occur.

This product normally produces a bowel movement in ½ to 6 hours.

Patients should be warned to expect frequent, liquid stools.

Interactions: Use with caution in patients taking calcium channel blockers, diuretics, lithium treatment or other medications that might affect electrolyte levels as hyperphosphataemia, hypocalcaemia, hypernatraemic dehydration and acidosis may occur. The absorption of regularly taken oral drugs (e.g. oral contraceptives, antiepileptic drugs, antidiabetics, antibiotics) may be delayed or completely prevented.

Use in pregnancy and lactation: Due to there being no relevant data available to evaluate a potential malformative or foetotoxic effect when administered during pregnancy, this product should only be used under medical supervision.

Effect on ability to drive and use machines: Not applicable.

Undesirable effects: As with other bowel cleansing regimens treatment with Fleet Phospho-soda may cause vomiting, fatigue (sickness), nausea, abdominal bloating, gastrointestinal cramping and diarrhoea. Isolated cases of allergic reactions with/without rash have also been reported. Transient hyperphosphataemia, without accompanying hypocalcaemia, has been noted in clinical trials. All such patients have remained asymptomatic and plasma phosphate levels have returned to intial pre-treatment levels within 24 hours.

Overdose: Recovery from the toxic effects of accidental excess ingestion can normally be achieved by re-hydration, though the intravenous administration of 10% calcium gluconate may be necessary.

Pharmaceutical precautions Store below 25°C. Do not refrigerate.

Legal category P.

Package quantities Two single-dose disposable bottles, each containing 45 ml of solution in a single carton.

Further information Fleet Phospho-soda is a saline laxative which acts by osmotic processes to increase fluid retention in the lumen of the small intestine. Fluid accumulation in the ileum produces distension, in turn promoting peristalsis and evacuation.

Product licence number 0083/0044.

FLEET* READY-TO-USE ENEMA

Presentation A disposable LDPE bottle with a prelubricated pliable nozzle, which delivers a single dose equivalent to Sodium Acid Phosphate 21.4 g (18.1% w/v) and Sodium Phosphate 9.4 g (8.0% w/v) per 118 ml. Sodium content is 4.4 g per 118 ml. Excipients: Benzalkonium Chloride, Disodium Edetate, Purified Water. Nozzle lubricant: White Soft Paraffin.

Uses Fleet Ready-to-use enema is for use in the relief of occasional constipation, pre- and post-operative bowel cleansing, obstetrics and prior to proctoscopy, sigmoidoscopy and x-ray examination.

Dosage and administration

Adults and childen 12 years and over: 1 enema (118 ml delivered dose), no more than once daily or as directed by a physician.

Children 3 years to under 12: as directed by physician.

Do not administer to children under 3 years of age.

FOR RECTAL USE ONLY.

Directions for use: Lie on left side with both knees bent, arms at rest. (Fig. 1)

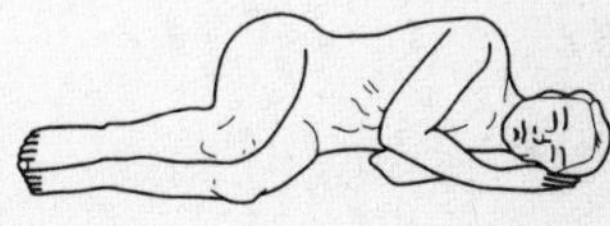

Fig. 1

Remove orange protective shield. Pull shield gently while holding bottle upright and grasping grooved bottle cap with fingers. (Fig. 2)

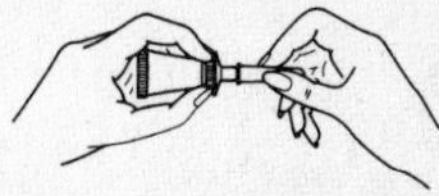

Fig. 2

With steady pressure, gently insert enema into the rectum with tip pointing towards navel. Squeeze bottle until nearly all liquid is expelled. **Discontinue use if resistance is encountered. Forcing the enema can result in injury.** Return enema to carton for disposal.

Contra-indications, warnings, etc
Contra-indications: Do not use in patients with congenital megacolon, Hirschsprung's Disease, imperforate anus or congestive heart failure. Do not use when nausea, vomiting or abdominal pain is present unless directed by a physician.

Warnings: Use with caution in patients with impaired renal function, heart disease, colostomy, or pre-existing electrolyte disturbances as hyperphosphataemia, hypocalcaemia, hypernatraemia and acidosis may occur. Prolonged repeated use is not recommended and may lead to dependence, Unless directed by a physician, Fleet Ready-to-use enema should not be used for more than two weeks.

Interactions: Use with caution in patients taking calcium channel blockers, diuretics or other medications which may affect electrolyte levels as hypocalcaemia, hyperphosphataemia, hypernatraemia and acidosis may occur.

Use in pregnancy and lactation: For use only under medical supervision.

Effect on ability to drive and use machines: Not applicable.

Undesirable effects: Rectal bleeding or failure to have bowel movement after use of a laxative may indicate a serious condition. Use should be discontinued and medical advice sought.

Overdose: In case of accidental ingestion or overdose seek medical advice.

Pharmaceutical precautions Store below 25°C. Do not refrigerate.

Legal category P.

Package quantities A LDPE bottle containing 133 ml of solution in a single carton.

Further information Phosphates act as a mild saline laxative when administered by the rectal route. They stimulate peristalsis, leading to an approximately normal bowel movement, in that only the rectum, sigmoid colon and part or all of the descending colon are evacuated.

Product licence number 0083/0043.

**Trade Mark*

Dista Products Limited
Kingsclere Road,
Basingstoke,
Hants. RG21 6XA

☎ 01256 52011 🖷 01256 315858

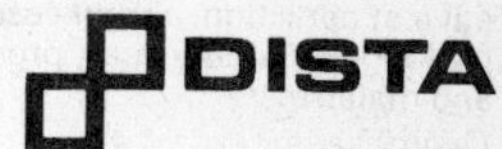

ALLEGRON*

Presentation Tablets each containing Nortriptyline Hydrochloride BP equivalent to 25 mg nortriptyline. The tablets are orange, scored and have a diameter of 8 mm. They are marked 'DISTA'.

Tablets each containing Nortriptyline Hydrochloride BP equivalent to 10 mg nortriptyline. The tablets are white, unscored and have a diameter of 5.5 mm. They are marked 'DISTA'.

Uses Allegron is indicated for the relief of symptoms of depression. It may also be used for the treatment of some cases of nocturnal enuresis.

Dosage and administration For oral administration.

Adults: The usual adult dose is 25 mg three or four times daily. Dosage should begin at a low level and be increased as required. Alternatively, the total daily dose may be given once a day. When doses above 100 mg daily are administered, plasma levels of nortriptyline should be monitored and maintained in the optimum range of 50 to 150 ng/ml. Doses above 150 mg per day are not recommended.

Lower than usual dosages are recommended for elderly patients and adolescents. Lower dosages are also recommended for outpatients than for hospitalised patients who will be under close supervision. The physician should initiate dosage at a low level and increase it gradually, noting carefully the clinical response and any evidence of intolerance. Following remission, maintenance medication may be required for a longer period of time at the lowest dose that will maintain remission.

If a patient develops minor side-effects, the dosage should be reduced. The drug should be discontinued promptly if adverse effects of a serious nature or allergic manifestations occur.

The elderly: 30 to 50 mg/day in divided doses.

Adolescent patients: 30 to 50 mg/day in divided doses.

Plasma levels: Optimal responses to nortriptyline have been associated with plasma concentrations of 50 to 150 ng/ml. Higher concentrations may be associated with more adverse experiences. Plasma concentrations are difficult to measure, and physicians should consult the laboratory professional staff.

Many antidepressants (tricyclic antidepressants, including nortriptyline, selective serotonin re-uptake inhibitors and others) are metabolised by the hepatic cytochrome P450 isoenzyme P450IID6. Three to ten per cent of the population have reduced isoenzyme activity ('poor metabolisers') and may have higher than expected plasma concentrations at usual doses. The percentage of 'poor metabolisers' in a population is also affected by its ethnic origin.

Older patients have been reported to have higher plasma concentrations of the active nortriptyline metabolite 10-hydroxynortriptyline. In one case, this was associated with apparent cardiotoxicity, despite the fact that nortriptyline concentrations were within the 'therapeutic range'. Clinical findings should predominate over plasma concentrations as primary determinants of dosage changes.

Children: (for nocturnal enuresis only).

Age (years)	*Weight*		*Dose (mg)*
	kg	*lb*	
6-7	20-25	44-55	10
8-11	25-35	55-77	10-20
>11	35-54	77-119	25-35

The dose should be administered thirty minutes before bedtime.

The maximum period of treatment should not exceed three months. A further course of treatment should not be started until a full physical examination, including an ECG, has been made.

Contra-indications, warnings, etc

Contra-indications: Hypersensitivity to nortriptyline.

Recent myocardial infarction, any degree of heart block or other cardiac arrhythmias.

Severe liver disease. Mania.

Nortriptyline is contra-indicated for the nursing mother and for children under the age of six years.

Please also refer to 'Drug interactions' section.

Warnings: As improvement may not occur during the initial weeks of therapy, patients, especially those posing a high suicidal risk, should be closely monitored during this period.

Withdrawal symptoms, including insomnia, irritability and excessive perspiration, may occur on abrupt cessation of therapy.

The use of nortriptyline in schizophrenic patients may result in an exacerbation of the psychosis or may activate latent schizophrenic symptoms. If administered to overactive or agitated patients, increased anxiety and agitation may occur. In manic-depressive patients, nortriptyline may cause symptoms of the manic phase to emerge.

Cross sensitivity between nortriptyline and other tricyclic antidepressants is a possibility.

Patients with cardiovascular disease should be given nortriptyline only under close supervision because of the tendency of the drug to produce sinus tachycardia and to prolong the conduction time. Myocardial infarction, arrhythmia and strokes have occurred. Great care is necessary if nortriptyline is administered to hyperthyroid patients or to those receiving thyroid medication, since cardiac arrhythmias may develop.

The use of nortriptyline should be avoided, if possible, in patients with a history of epilepsy. If it is used, however, the patients should be observed carefully at the beginning of treatment, for nortriptyline is known to lower the convulsive threshold.

Nortriptyline may impair the mental and/or physical abilities required for the performance of hazardous tasks, such as operating machinery or driving a car; therefore the patient should be warned accordingly.

Drug interactions: Under no circumstances should nortriptyline be given concurrently with, or within two weeks of cessation of, therapy with monoamine oxidase inhibitors. Hyperpyretic crises, severe convulsions and fatalities have occurred when similar tricyclic antidepressants were used in such combinations.

Nortriptyline should not be given with sympathomimetic agents such as adrenaline, ephedrine, isoprenaline, noradrenaline, phenylephrine and phenylpropanolamine.

Nortriptyline may decrease the antihypertensive effect of guanethidine, debrisoquine, bethanidine and possibly clonidine. Concurrent administration of reserpine has been shown to produce a 'stimulating' effect in some depressed patients. It would be advisable to review all antihypertensive therapy during treatment with tricyclic antidepressants.

Barbiturates may increase the rate of metabolism of nortriptyline.

Anaesthetics given during tricyclic antidepressant therapy may increase the risk of arrhythmias and hypotension. If surgery is necessary, the drug should be discontinued, if possible, for several days prior to the procedure, or the anaesthetist should be informed if the patient is still receiving therapy.

Tricyclic antidepressants may potentiate the CNS depressant effect of alcohol.

The potentiating effect of excessive consumption of alcohol may lead to increased suicidal attempts or overdosage, especially in patients with histories of emotional disturbances or suicidal ideation.

Steady-state serum concentrations of the tricyclic antidepressants are reported to fluctuate significantly as cimetidine is either added to or deleted from the drug regimen. Higher than expected steady-state serum concentrations of the tricyclic antidepressant have been observed when therapy is initiated in patients already taking cimetidine. A decrease may occur when cimetidine therapy is discontinued.

Because nortriptyline's metabolism (like other tricyclic and SSRI antidepressants) involves the hepatic cytochrome P450IID6 isoenzyme system, concomitant therapy with drugs also metabolised by this system may lead to drug interactions. Lower doses than are usually prescribed for either the tricyclic antidepressant or the other drug may therefore be required.

Greater than two-fold increases in previously stable plasma levels of nortriptyline have occurred when fluoxetine was administered concomitantly. Fluoxetine and its active metabolite, norfluoxetine, have long half-lives (4–16 days for norfluoxetine).

Concomitant therapy with other drugs that are metabolised by this isoenzyme, including other antidepressants, phenothiazines, carbamazepine, propafenone, flecainide and encainide, or that inhibit this enzyme (e.g. quinidine), should be approached with caution.

Supervision and adjustment of dosage may be required when nortriptyline is used with other anticholinergic drugs.

Usage in pregnancy: The safety of nortriptyline for use during pregnancy has not been established, nor is there evidence from animal studies that it is free from hazard; therefore the drug should not be administered to pregnant patients or women of childbearing age unless the potential benefits clearly outweigh any potential risk.

Usage in nursing mothers: See *Contra-indications.*

Precautions: The elderly are particularly liable to experience adverse reactions, especially agitation, confusion and postural hypotension.

Troublesome hostility in a patient may be aroused by the use of nortriptyline.

Behavioural changes may occur in children receiving therapy for nocturnal enuresis.

If possible, the use of nortriptyline should be avoided in patients with narrow angle glaucoma or symptoms suggestive of prostatic hypertrophy.

The possibility of a suicide attempt by a depressed patient remains after the initiation of treatment. This possibility should be considered in relation to the quantity of drug dispensed at any one time.

When it is essential, nortriptyline may be administered with electroconvulsive therapy, although the hazards may be increased.

Both elevation and lowering of blood sugar levels have been reported. Significant hypoglycaemia was reported in a Type II diabetic patient maintained on chlorpropamide (250 mg/day), after the addition of nortriptyline (125 mg/day).

Side-effects: Included in the following list are a few adverse reactions that have not been reported with this specific drug. However, the pharmacological similarities among the tricyclic antidepressant drugs require that each of the reactions be considered when nortriptyline is administered.

Cardiovascular: Hypotension, hypertension, tachycardia, palpitation, myocardial infarction, arrhythmias, heart block, stroke.

Psychiatric: Confusional states (especially in the elderly) with hallucinations, disorientation, delusions; anxiety, restlessness, agitation; insomnia, panic, nightmares; hypomania; exacerbation of psychosis.

Neurological: Numbness, tingling, paraesthesia of extremities; inco-ordination, ataxia, tremors; peripheral neuropathy; extrapyramidal symptoms; seizures, alteration of EEG patterns; tinnitus.

Anticholinergic: Dry mouth and, rarely, associated sublingual adenitis or gingivitis; blurred vision, disturbance of accommodation, mydriasis; constipation, paralytic ileus; urinary retention, delayed micturition, dilation of the urinary tract.

Allergic: Rash, petechiae, urticaria, itching, photosensitisation (avoid excessive exposure to sunlight); oedema (general or of face and tongue), drug fever, cross-sensitivity with other tricyclic drugs.

Haematological: Bone-marrow depression, including agranulocytosis; aplastic anaemia; eosinophilia; purpura; thrombocytopenia.

Gastro-intestinal: Nausea and vomiting, anorexia, epigastric distress, diarrhoea; peculiar taste, stomatitis, abdominal cramps, black tongue, constipation, paralytic ileus.

Endocrine: Gynaecomastia in the male; breast enlargement and galactorrhoea in the female; increased or decreased libido, impotence; testicular swelling; elevation or depression of blood sugar levels; syndrome of inappropriate secretion of antidiuretic hormone.

Other: Jaundice (simulating obstructive); altered liver function, hepatitis and liver necrosis; weight gain or loss; sweating; flushing; urinary frequency, nocturia; drowsiness, dizziness, weakness, fatigue; headache; parotid swelling; alopecia.

Withdrawal symptoms: Though these are not indicative of addiction, abrupt cessation of treatment after prolonged therapy may produce nausea, headache and malaise.

Overdosage

Signs and symptoms: 50 mg of a tricyclic antidepressant can be an overdose in a child. Of patients who are alive at presentation, mortality of 0-15% has been reported. Symptoms may begin within several hours and may include blurred vision, confusion, restlessness, dizziness, hypothermia, hyperthermia, agitation, vomiting, hyperactive reflexes, dilated pupils, fever, rapid heart rate, decreased bowel sounds, dry mouth, inability to void, myoclonic jerks, seizures, respiratory depression, myoglobinuric renal failure, nystagmus, ataxia, dysarthria, choreoathetosis, coma, hypotension and cardiac arrhythmias. Cardiac conduction may be slowed, with prolongation of QRS complex and QT intervals, right bundle branch and AV block, ventricular tachyarrhythmias (including Torsade de pointes and fibrillation) and death. Prolongation of QRS duration to more than 100 msec is predictive of more severe toxicity. The absence of sinus tachycardia does not ensure a benign course. Hypotension may be caused by vasodilatation, central and peripheral alpha-adrenergic blockade and cardiac depression. In a healthy young person, prolonged resuscitation may be effective; one patient survived 5 hours of cardiac massage.

Treatment: Symptomatic and supportive therapy is recommended. Activated charcoal may be more effective than emesis or lavage to reduce absorption.

Ventricular arrhythmias, especially when accompanied by lengthened QRS intervals, may respond to alkalinisation by hyperventilation or administration of sodium bicarbonate. Serum electrolytes should be monitored and managed. Refractory arrhythmias may respond to propranolol, bretylium or lignocaine. Quinidine and procainamide usually should not be used because they may exacerbate arrhythmias and conduction already slowed by the overdose.

Seizures may respond to diazepam. Phenytoin may treat seizures and cardiac rhythm disturbances. Physostigmine may antagonise atrial tachycardia, gut immotility, myoclonic jerks and somnolence. The effects of physostigmine may be short-lived.

Diuresis and dialysis have little effect. Haemoperfusion is unproven. Monitoring should continue, at least until the QRS duration is normal.

Pharmaceutical precautions Store below 25°C.

Legal category POM.

Package quantities

Tablets 25 mg: Bottles of 100
Tablets 10 mg: Bottles of 100

Further information Nil.

Product licence numbers

Tablets 25 mg: 0006/5003
Tablets 10 mg: 0006/5002

CAPASTAT*

Presentation Capreomycin sulphate as sterile white powder for intramuscular injection only, in sealed vials each containing 1,000,000 units (approximately equivalent to 1 g capreomycin base).

Uses

Actions: Capreomycin is active against human strains of *Mycobacterium tuberculosis.*

Frequent cross-resistance occurs between capreomycin and viomycin. Varying degrees of cross-resistance between capreomycin and kanamycin and neomycin have been reported. No cross-resistance has been observed between capreomycin and isoniazid, aminosalicylic acid, cycloserine, streptomycin, ethionamide or ethambutol.

Indications: Capastat should be used concomitantly with other appropriate antituberculous agents for the treatment of pulmonary infections caused by capreomycin-susceptible strains of *Mycobacterium tuberculosis* when the primary agents (isoniazid, rifampicin, streptomycin and ethambutol) have been ineffective or cannot be used because of toxicity or the presence of resistant tubercle bacilli.

Dosage and administration The usual dose is 1 g daily (but 20 mg/kg/day should not be exceeded) given by deep intramuscular injection only for 60 to 120 days, followed by 1 g intramuscularly two or three times a week. Capastat is always administered in combination with at least one other antituberculous agent to which the patient's strain of tubercle bacillus is susceptible.

Capastat should be dissolved in 2 ml of 0.9% Sodium Chloride Intravenous Infusion BP or Water for Injections PhEur. Two to three minutes should be allowed for complete solution.

For administration of a 1 g dose, the entire contents of the vial should be given. For dosages of less than 1 g the following dilution table may be used:

Diluent to be added (ml)	*Approximate volume of Capastat solution (ml)*	*Approximate average concentration (mg/ml) in terms of mg of capreomycin activity*
2.15	2.85	350
2.63	3.33	300
3.3	4.0	250
4.3	5.0	200

The elderly: As for adults. Reduce dosage if renal function is impaired.

Patients with reduced renal function: A reduced dosage should be given based on creatinine clearance using the guidance given in the following table. These dosages are designed to achieve a mean steady-state capreomycin level of 10 micrograms/ml, at various levels of renal function:

Creatinine clearance (ml/min)	*Capreomycin clearance ($l/kg/h \times 10^{-2}$)*	*Half-life (hours)*	*Dose for these dosing intervals (mg/kg)*		
			24 h	*48 h*	*72 h*
0	0.54	55.5	1.29	2.58	3.87
10	1.01	29.4	2.43	4.87	7.30
20	1.49	20.0	3.58	7.16	10.70
30	1.97	15.1	4.72	9.45	14.20
40	2.45	12.2	5.87	11.70	
50	2.92	10.2	7.01	14.00	
60	3.40	8.8	8.16		
80	4.35	6.8	10.40		
100	5.31	5.6	12.70		
110	5.78	5.2	13.90		

Infants and children: Not for paediatric use, since the safety of capreomycin for use in infants and children has not been established.

Contra-indications, warnings, etc

Contra-indication: Hypersensitivity to capreomycin.

Warnings: The use of capreomycin in patients with renal insufficiency or pre-existing auditory impairment must be undertaken with great caution, and the risk of additional eighth cranial nerve impairment or renal injury should be weighed against the benefits to be derived from treatment.

Simultaneous administration of other antituberculous drugs which also have ototoxic and nephrotoxic potential (e.g. streptomycin, viomycin) is not recommended. Also, use with other drugs that are not given for the treatment of tuberculosis but have ototoxic or nephrotoxic potential (e.g. polymyxin, colistin sulphate, amikacin, gentamicin, tobramycin, vancomycin, kanamycin and neomycin) should also be undertaken only with great caution.

Pregnancy: The safety of capreomycin for use during pregnancy has not been established. Capreomycin has been shown to be teratogenic in rats when given at 3.5 times the human dose. There are no adequate and well controlled studies in pregnant women. Capastat should be used during pregnancy only if the potential benefit justifies the potential risk to the foetus.

Studies have not been performed to determine potential for carcinogenicity, mutagenicity, or impairment of fertility.

Nursing mothers: It is not known whether capreomycin is excreted in human milk. Caution should be exercised when administering to a nursing woman.

Precautions: As capreomycin is potentially ototoxic, audiometry and assessment of vestibular function should be performed before starting treatment and at regular intervals during treatment.

Regular tests of renal function should be made throughout the period of treatment, and reduced dosage should be used in patients with known, or suspected, renal impairment (see 'Dosage and administration').

Since hypokalaemia may occur during capreomycin therapy, serum potassium levels should be determined frequently.

A partial neuromuscular block can occur after large doses of capreomycin.

Capreomycin should be administered cautiously to patients with a history of allergy, particularly to drugs.

Side-effects

Renal: Elevation of serum creatinine or blood urea and abnormal urine sediment have been observed. Toxic nephritis was reported in one patient with tuberculosis and portal cirrhosis who was treated with capreomycin (1 g) and aminosalicylic acid daily for one month. This patient developed renal insufficiency and oliguria and died. The post-mortem showed subsiding acute tubular necrosis.

Electrolyte disturbances resembling Bartter's syndrome have been reported in one patient.

Hepatic: A decrease in bromsulphthalein excretion without change in serum enzymes has been noted in the presence of pre-existing liver disease. Abnormal results in liver function tests have occurred in many patients receiving capreomycin in combination with other antituberculous agents which are also known to cause changes in hepatic function. Periodic determinations of liver function are recommended.

Haematological: Leucocytosis and leucopenia have been observed. Rare cases of thrombocytopenia have been reported. Most patients receiving daily capreomycin have had eosinophilia exceeding 5%, but this has subsided with the reduction of capreomycin dosage to two or three times weekly.

Hypersensitivity: Urticaria and maculopapular rashes associated in some cases with febrile reactions have been reported when capreomycin and other antituberculous drugs were given concomitantly.

Otic: Clinical and subclinical auditory loss has been noted. Some audiometric changes have proved reversible and others with permanent loss have not been progressive following withdrawal of capreomycin. Tinnitus and vertigo have occurred.

Injection site reactions: Pain and induration at injection sites have been observed. Excessive bleeding and sterile abscesses have also been reported at these sites.

Overdosage

Signs and symptoms: Hypokalaemia, hypocalcaemia, hypomagnesaemia and an electrolyte disturbance resembling Bartter's syndrome have been reported to occur in patients with capreomycin toxicity. Nephrotoxicity, including acute tubular necrosis; and ototoxicity, including dizziness, tinnitus, vertigo and loss of high-tone acuity (see 'Warnings' and 'Precautions'). Neuromuscular blockage or respiratory paralysis may occur following rapid intravenous administration.

If capreomycin is ingested, toxicity is unlikely because less than 1% is absorbed from an intact gastro-intestinal system.

Treatment: Symptomatic and supportive therapy is recommended. Activated charcoal may be more effective than emesis or lavage in reducing absorption.

Patients who have received an overdose of capreomycin and have normal renal function should be hydrated to maintain a urine output of 3-5 ml/kg/hr. Fluid balance electrolytes and creatinine clearance should be monitored.

Haemodialysis is effective in patients with significant renal disease.

Pharmaceutical precautions Store below 25°C. The reconstituted product should be used within 24 hours.

The solution may acquire a pale straw colour and darken with time, but this is not associated with loss of potency or the development of toxicity.

Legal category POM.

Package quantities Vials of 1,000,000 units (1 g base approximately): Pack of 5 vials.

Further information Capastat must be used only in conjunction with adequate doses of other antituberculous drugs. The use of Capastat alone allows the rapid development of strains resistant to it.

Product licence number 0006/5005.

DISTACLOR*

Presentation Capsules (violet and grey, printed Lilly 3062) containing 500 mg cefaclor.

Granules (pink) for suspension containing 125 mg cefaclor/5 ml.

Granules (pink) for suspension containing 250 mg cefaclor/5 ml.

Uses Distaclor is indicated for the treatment of the following infections due to susceptible micro-organisms:

Respiratory tract infections, including pneumonia, bronchitis, exacerbations of chronic bronchitis, pharyngitis and tonsillitis, and as part of the management of sinusitis
Otitis media
Skin and soft tissue infections
Urinary tract infections, including pyelonephritis and cystitis
Distaclor has been found to be effective in both acute and chronic urinary tract infections.

Cefaclor is active against the following organisms *in vitro:*

Alpha- and beta-haemolytic streptococci
Staphylococci; including coagulase-positive, coagulase-negative and penicillinase-producing strains
Streptococcus pneumoniae
Streptococcus pyogenes (group A beta-haemolytic streptococci)
Branhamella catarrhalis
Escherichia coli
Proteus mirabilis
Klebsiella species
Haemophilus influenzae, including ampicillin-resistant strains.

Cefaclor has no activity against *Pseudomonas* species or *Acinetobacter* species. Methicillin-resistant staphylococci and most strains of enterococci (e.g. *Str. faecalis*) are resistant to cefaclor. Cefaclor is not active against most strains of *Enterobacter* spp, *Serratia* spp, *Morganella morganii, Proteus vulgaris* and *Providencia rettgeri*.

Cefaclor is generally effective in the eradication of streptococci from the nasopharynx, however, data establishing efficacy in the subsequent prevention of either rheumatic fever or bacterial endocarditis are not available.

Dosage and administration Distaclor is administered orally.

Adults: The usual adult dosage is 250 mg every eight hours. For more severe infections or those caused by less susceptible organisms, doses may be doubled. Doses of 4 g per day have been administered safely to normal subjects for 28 days, but the total daily dosage should not exceed this amount.

Please see the separate Distaclor MR data sheet for extended release tablets of cefaclor, equivalent to 375 mg cefaclor.

Distaclor may be administered in the presence of impaired renal function. Under such conditions dosage is usually unchanged (see *Precautions*).

Patients undergoing haemodialysis: Haemodialysis shortens serum half-life by 25–30%. In patients undergoing regular haemodialysis, a loading dose of 250 mg–1 g administered prior to dialysis and a therapeutic dose of 250–500 mg every six to eight hours maintained during interdialytic periods is recommended.

The elderly: As for adults.

Children: The usual recommended daily dosage for children is 20 mg/kg/day in divided doses every eight hours, as indicated. For bronchitis and pneumonia, the dosage is 20 mg/kg/day in divided doses administered 3 times daily. For otitis media and pharyngitis, the total daily dosage may be divided and administered every 12 hours. Safety and efficacy have not been established for use in infants aged less than one month.

Distaclor Suspension

	125 mg/5 ml	*250 mg/5 ml*
<1 year (9 kg)	*2.5 ml t.i.d.*	
1–5 years (9–18 kg)	*5.0 ml t.i.d.*	
Over 5 years		*5.0 ml t.i.d.*

In more serious infections, otitis media, sinusitis and infections caused by less susceptible organisms, 40 mg/kg/day in divided doses is recommended, up to a daily maximum of 1 g.

In the treatment of beta-haemolytic streptococcal infections, therapy should be continued for at least 10 days.

Contra-indications, warnings, etc

Contra-indication: Hypersensitivity to cephalosporins.

Warnings: Before instituting therapy with cefaclor, every effort should be made to determine whether the patient has had previous hypersensitivity reactions to cefaclor, cephalosporins, penicillins or other drugs. Cefaclor should be given cautiously to penicillin-sensitive patients, because cross-hypersensitivity, including anaphylaxis, among beta-lactam antibiotics has been clearly documented.

If an allergic reaction to cefaclor occurs, the drug should be discontinued and the patient treated with the appropriate agents.

Pseudomembranous colitis has been reported with virtually all broad-spectrum antibiotics, including macrolides, semi-synthetic penicillins and cephalosporins. It is important, therefore, to consider its diagnosis in patients who develop diarrhoea in association with the use of antibiotics. Such colitis may range in severity from mild to life-threatening. Mild cases usually respond to drug discontinuance alone. In moderate to severe cases, appropriate measures should be taken.

Usage in pregnancy: Animal studies have shown no evidence of impaired fertility or teratogenicity. However, since there are no adequate or well-controlled studies in pregnant women, caution should be exercised when prescribing for the pregnant patient.

Usage in nursing mothers: Small amounts of cefaclor have been detected in breast milk following administration of single 500 mg doses. Average levels of about 0.2 micrograms/ml or less were detected up to 5 hours later. Trace amounts were detected at one hour. As the effect on nursing infants is not known, caution should be exercised when cefaclor is administered to a nursing woman.

Precautions: Cefaclor should be administered with caution in the presence of markedly impaired renal function. Since the half-life of cefaclor in anuric patients is 2.3 to 2.8 hours (compared to 0.6–0.9 hours in normal subjects), dosage adjustments for patients with moderate or severe renal impairment are not usually required. Clinical experience with cefaclor under such conditions is limited; therefore, careful clinical observation and laboratory studies should be made.

Broad-spectrum antibiotics should be prescribed with caution in individuals with a history of gastro-intestinal disease, particularly colitis.

Prolonged use of cefaclor may result in the overgrowth of non-susceptible organisms. If superinfection occurs during therapy, appropriate measures should be taken.

Positive direct Coombs' tests have been reported during treatment with the cephalosporin antibiotics. In haematological studies or in transfusion cross-matching procedures, when anti-globulin tests are performed on the minor side, or in Coombs' testing of newborns whose mothers have received cephalosporin antibiotics before parturition, it should be recognised that a positive Coombs' test may be due to the drug.

A false-positive reaction for glucose in the urine may occur with Benedict's or Fehling's solutions or with copper sulphate test tablets.

Drug interactions: There have been rare reports of increased prothrombin time, with or without clinical bleeding, in patients receiving cefaclor and warfarin concomitantly. It is recommended that in such patients, regular monitoring of prothrombin time should be considered, with adjustment of dosage if necessary.

The renal excretion of cefaclor is inhibited by probenecid.

Side-effects

Gastro-intestinal: The most frequent side-effect has been diarrhoea. It is rarely severe enough to warrant cessation of therapy. Colitis, including rare instances of pseudomembranous colitis, has been reported. Nausea and vomiting have also occurred.

Hypersensitivity: Allergic reactions such as morbilliform eruptions, pruritus and urticaria have been observed. These reactions usually subside upon discontinuation of therapy. Serum sickness-like reactions (erythema multiforme minor, rashes or other skin manifestations accompanied by arthritis/arthralgia, with or without fever) have been reported. Lymphadenopathy and proteinuria are infrequent, there are no circulating immune complexes and no evidence of sequelae. Occasionally, solitary symptoms may occur, but do not represent a serum sickness-like reaction. Serum sickness-like reactions are apparently due to hypersensitivity and have usually occurred during or following a second (or subsequent) course of therapy with cefaclor. Such reactions have been reported more frequently in children than in adults. Signs and symptoms usually occur a few days after initiation of therapy and usually subside within a few days of cessation of therapy. Antihistamines and corticosteroids appear to enhance resolution of the syndrome. No serious sequelae have been reported.

There are rare reports of erythema multiforme major (Stevens-Johnson syndrome), toxic epidermal necrolysis, and anaphylaxis. Anaphylaxis may be more common in patients with a history of penicillin allergy. Anaphylactoid events may present as solitary symptoms, including angioedema, asthenia, oedema (including face and limbs), dyspnoea, paraesthesias, syncope, or vasodilatation.

Rarely, hypersensitivity symptoms may persist for several months.

Haematological: Eosinophilia, positive Coombs' tests and, rarely, thrombocytopenia. Transient lymphocytosis, leucopenia and, rarely, haemolytic anaemia, aplastic anaemia, agranulocytosis and reversible neutropenia of possible clinical significance. See 'Drug interactions'.

Hepatic: Transient hepatitis and cholestatic jaundice have been reported rarely, slight elevations in AST, ALT or alkaline phosphatase values.

Renal: Reversible interstitial nephritis has occurred rarely, also slight elevations in blood urea or serum creatinine or abnormal urinalysis.

Central Nervous System: Reversible hyperactivity, agitation, nervousness, insomnia, confusion, hypertonia, dizziness, hallucinations and somnolence have been reported rarely.

Miscellaneous: Genital pruritus, vaginitis and vaginal moniliasis.

Overdosage: Symptoms of nausea, vomiting, epigastric distress and diarrhoea would be anticipated.

Treatment: Unless 5 times the normal total daily dose has been ingested, gastro-intestinal decontamination will not be necessary.

General management may consist of supportive therapy.

Pharmaceutical precautions Store below 25°C. Keep containers tightly closed and protect from light.

After reconstitution, the 125 mg/5 ml and 250 mg/5 ml suspensions should be stored in a refrigerator (2°-8°C) and be used within 14 days. When dilution is unavoidable, Syrup BP should be used after the suspension has been prepared according to the manufacturer's instructions.

Legal category POM.

Package quantities

Capsules 500 mg:	Bottles of 50
Suspension 125 mg/5 ml:	Bottles of 100 ml
Suspension 250 mg/5 ml:	Bottles of 100 ml

Further information Nil.

Product licence numbers

Capsules 500 mg:	0006/0119
Suspension 125 mg/5 ml:	0006/0120
Suspension 250 mg/5 ml:	0006/0121

DISTACLOR MR*

Presentation Extended release tablets of cefaclor 'Modified Release' (blue, printed 'TA 4220'), equivalent to 375 mg cefaclor.

Cefaclor 'Modified Release' differs from cefaclor in its rate of dissolution, producing a lower peak serum concentration, but retaining sustained measurable serum concentrations, which provides the advantage of twice daily dosing.

Uses Distaclor MR is indicated in the treatment of the following infections when caused by susceptible strains of the designated organisms:

Acute bronchitis and acute exacerbations of chronic bronchitis caused by *Streptococcus pneumoniae, Haemophilus influenzae* (including beta-lactamase producing strains), *Haemophilus parainfluenzae, Moraxella catarrhalis* (including beta-lactamase producing strains) and *Staphylococcus aureus.*

Pharyngitis and tonsillitis caused by *Streptococcus pyogenes* (group A streptococci).

Pneumonia caused by *S. pneumoniae, H. influenzae* (including beta-lactamase producing strains) and *M. catarrhalis* (including beta-lactamase producing strains).

Uncomplicated lower urinary tract infections, including cystitis and asymptomatic bacteriuria, caused by *Escherichia coli, Klebsiella pneumoniae, Proteus mirabilis* and *Staphylococcus saprophyticus.*

Skin and skin structure infections caused by *S. pyogenes* (group A streptococci), *S. aureus* (including beta-lactamase producing strains) and *Staphylococcus epidermidis* (including beta-lactamase producing strains).

Bacteriological studies, to determine the causative organism and its susceptibility to cefaclor, should be performed. Therapy may be started while awaiting the results of these studies. Once these results become available, antimicrobial therapy should be adjusted accordingly.

Note: Distaclor MR is generally effective in the eradication of streptococci from the oropharynx. However, data establishing the efficacy of this antibiotic in the subsequent prevention of rheumatic fever are not available.

Distaclor MR has been shown to be active *in vitro* against most strains of the following organisms, although clinical efficacy has not been established:

Gram-negative organisms:

Citrobacter diversus
Neisseria gonorrhoeae

Anaerobic organisms:

Propionibacterium acnes
Bacteroides species (excluding *Bacteroides fragilis*)
Peptococci
Peptostreptococci

Note: *Pseudomonas* sp, *Acinetobacter calcoaceticus*, most strains of enterococci, *Enterobacter* sp, indole-positive *Proteus* and *Serratia* sp are resistant to cefaclor. Cefaclor is inactive against methicillin-resistant staphylococci.

Cefaclor is a semi-synthetic cephalosporin antibiotic.

Dosage and administration Distaclor MR is administered orally.

Adults and the elderly: Pharyngitis, bronchitis, tonsillitis, skin and skin structure infections: 375 mg twice daily.

Lower urinary tract infections: 375 mg twice daily.

Pneumonia: 750 mg twice daily.

In clinical trials, doses of 1.5 g/day of Distaclor MR have been administered safely for 14 days. Doses of 4 g/day of cefaclor have been administered safely, to normal subjects, for 28 days.

Elderly subjects with normal renal function do not require dosage adjustment.

Children: The safety and effectiveness of Distaclor MR have not been established. Cefaclor suspensions are available (see Distaclor data sheet for dosages).

In the treatment of infections caused by *S. pyogenes* (group A streptococci), a therapeutic dosage should be administered for at least 10 days.

Distaclor MR is well absorbed from the gastro-intestinal tract. Since absorption is enhanced by administration with food, Distaclor MR should be taken with meals.

The tablets should not be cut, crushed or chewed.

There is no evidence of metabolism in humans.

Contra-indications, warnings, etc

Contra-indication: Hypersensitivity to cefaclor and other cephalosporins.

Warnings: Before instituting therapy with cefaclor, every effort should be made to determine whether the patient has had previous hypersensitivity reactions to the cephalosporins, penicillins or other drugs. Cefaclor should be given cautiously to penicillin-sensitive patients and to any patient who has demonstrated some form of allergy, particularly to drugs.

If an allergic reaction to cefaclor occurs, the drug should be discontinued and the patient treated with the appropriate agents.

Pseudomembranous colitis has been reported with virtually all broad-spectrum antibiotics, including macrolides, semi-synthetic penicillins and cephalosporins. It is important, therefore, to consider its diagnosis in patients who develop diarrhoea in association with the use of antibiotics. Such colitis may range in severity from mild to life-threatening. Mild cases usually respond to drug discontinuance alone. In moderate to severe cases, appropriate measures should be taken.

Usage in pregnancy: Although animal studies have shown no evidence of impaired fertility or harm to the foetus due to cefaclor, there are no adequate and well-controlled studies in pregnant women. Distaclor MR should be used during pregnancy only if clearly needed.

Usage in nursing mothers: Small amounts of cefaclor have been detected in breast milk following administration of single 500 mg doses. Average levels of about 0.2 micrograms/ml or less were detected up to 5 hours later. Trace amounts were detected at one hour. As the effect on nursing infants is not known, caution should be exercised when cefaclor is administered to a nursing woman. No studies have been done with Distaclor MR.

Usage during labour and delivery: Treatment should be given only if clearly needed.

Precautions: Prolonged use of cefaclor may result in the overgrowth of non-susceptible organisms. If superinfection occurs during therapy, appropriate measures should be taken.

A false-positive reaction for glucose in the urine may occur with Benedict's or Fehling's solutions or with copper sulphate test tablets.

Drug interactions: The extent of absorption of Distaclor MR is diminished if magnesium hydroxide or aluminium hydroxide containing antacids are taken within 1 hour of administration. H_2 blockers do not alter either the rate or extent of absorption.

The renal excretion of cefaclor is inhibited by probenecid.

Adverse reactions: The majority of adverse reactions observed in clinical trials of Distaclor MR were mild and transient. Drug-related adverse reactions requiring discontinuation of therapy occurred in 1.7% of patients. The following adverse reactions were reported in clinical trials. Incidence rates were less than 1 in 100 (less than 1%), except as stated:

Gastro-intestinal: Diarrhoea (3.4%), nausea (2.5%), vomiting and dyspepsia.

Hypersensitivity: Rash, urticaria or pruritus occurred in approximately 1.7% of patients. One serum sickness-like reaction (0.03%) was reported among the 3,272 patients treated with Distaclor MR during the controlled clinical trials.

Serum sickness-like reactions (erythema multiforme minor, rashes or other skin manifestations accompanied by arthritis/arthralgia, with or without fever) have been reported with cefaclor. Lymphadenopathy and proteinuria are infrequent, there are no circulating immune complexes and no evidence of sequelae. Occasionally, solitary symptoms may occur, but do not represent a serum sickness-like reaction. Serum sickness-like reactions are apparently due to hypersensitivity and have usually occurred during or following a second (or subsequent) course of therapy with cefaclor. Such reactions have been reported more frequently in children than in adults. Signs and symptoms usually occur a few days after initiation of therapy and usually subside within a few days of cessation of therapy. Antihistamines and corticosteroids appear to enhance resolution of the syndrome. No serious sequelae have been reported.

Haematological and lymphatic systems: Eosinophilia.

Genitourinary: Vaginal moniliasis (2.5%) and vaginitis (1.7%).

The following adverse effects have been reported, but causal relationship is uncertain:

Central nervous system: Headache, dizziness and somnolence.

Hepatic: Transient elevations in AST, ALT and alkaline phosphatase.

Renal: Transient increase in BUN or creatinine.

Laboratory tests: Transient thrombocytopenia, leucopenia, lymphocytosis, neutropenia and abnormal urinalysis.

In addition to the adverse reactions listed above that have been observed in patients taking Distaclor MR, the following have been reported in patients treated with cefaclor:

Erythema multiforme, fever, anaphylaxis (may be more common in patients with a history of penicillin allergy), Stevens–Johnson syndrome, positive direct Coombs' test and genital pruritus. Symptoms of pseudomembranous colitis may appear either during or after antibiotic treatment. Anaphylactoid events may present as solitary symptoms, including angio-edema, asthenia, oedema (including face and limbs), dyspnoea, paraesthesias, syncope, or vasodilatation.

Rarely, hypersensitivity symptoms may persist for several months.

The following reactions have been reported rarely in patients treated with cefaclor:

Toxic epidermal necrolysis, reversible interstitial nephritis, hepatic dysfunction, including cholestasis, increased prothrombin time in patients receiving cefaclor and warfarin concomitantly, reversible hyperactivity, agitation, nervousness, insomnia, confusion, hallucinations, hypertonia, aplastic anaemia, agranulocytosis and haemolytic anaemia.

The following adverse reactions have been reported in patients treated with other beta-lactam antibiotics:

Colitis, renal dysfunction and toxic nephropathy.

Several beta-lactam antibiotics have been implicated in triggering seizures, particularly in patients with renal impairment when the dosage was not reduced. If seizures associated with drug therapy should occur, the drug should be discontinued. Anticonvulsant therapy can be given if clinically indicated.

Overdosage: Symptoms of nausea, vomiting, epigastric distress and diarrhoea would be anticipated.

General management consists of supportive therapy. Consider activated charcoal instead of, or in addition to, gastric emptying.

Forced diuresis, peritoneal dialysis, haemodialysis or charcoal haemoperfusion have not been established as beneficial.

Pharmaceutical precautions Store at room temperature (15°–25°C). Protect from light.

Legal category POM

Package quantity Blister packs of 14 tablets.

Product licence number 0006/0274

DISTALGESIC*
Approved name: Co-proxamol Tablets

Qualitative and quantitative composition Each tablet contains 32.5 mg Dextropropoxyphene Hydrochloride BP (equivalent to approximately 30 mg dextropropoxyphene base) with 325 mg Paracetamol PhEur.

Pharmaceutical form White, pillow-shaped, film coated tablets, 14 mm in length and marked 'DG'.

Clinical particulars

Therapeutic indications:

Actions: Dextropropoxyphene is a mild narcotic analgesic structurally related to methadone.

Indication: For the management of mild to moderate pain.

Posology and method of administration: For oral administration to adults only. The usual dose is 2 tablets three or four times daily and should not normally be exceeded.

Consideration should be given to a reduced total daily dosage in patients with hepatic or renal impairment.

The elderly: There is evidence of prolonged half-life in the elderly, so reduction in dosage should be considered.

Children: Distalgesic is not recommended for use in children.

Contra-indications: Hypersensitivity to dextropropoxyphene or paracetamol.

Use in patients who are suicidal or addiction-prone.

Special warnings and special precautions for use:

Warnings: PATIENTS SHOULD BE ADVISED NOT TO EXCEED THE RECOMMENDED DOSE AND TO AVOID ALCOHOL.

Dextropropoxyphene products in excessive doses, either alone or in combination with other CNS depressants, including alcohol, are a major cause of drug-related deaths. Fatalities within the first hour of overdosage are not uncommon and can occur within 15 minutes. Some deaths have occurred as a consequence of the accidental ingestion of excessive quantities of Distalgesic alone, or in combination with other drugs.

Distalgesic should not be taken with any other paracetamol-containing products.

Overdosage may damage the liver, due predominantly to the accumulation of intermediate metabolites of paracetamol which cause hepatic necrosis. Immediate medical advice should be sought in the event of an overdose, even if the patient feels well, because of the risk of delayed, serious liver damage.

Distalgesic should be prescribed with caution for those patients whose medical condition requires the concomitant administration of sedatives, tranquillisers, muscle relaxants, antidepressants or other CNS-depressant drugs; patients should be advised of the additive depressant effects of these combinations. Distalgesic should also be prescribed with caution in patients who use alcohol in excess.

Drug dependence: Dextropropoxyphene, when taken in higher than recommended doses over long periods of time, can produce drug dependence.

Precautions: Distalgesic should be administered with caution to patients with hepatic or renal impairment, since higher serum concentrations or delayed elimination may occur.

Interaction with other medicaments and other forms of interaction:

Drug interactions: The CNS-depressant effect of dextropropoxyphene is additive with that of other CNS depressants, including alcohol.

Dextropropoxyphene may interfere with the metabolism of antidepressants, anticonvulsants and warfarin-like drugs. Severe neurological signs, including coma, have occurred with concomitant use of carbamazepine.

Pregnancy and lactation:

Pregnancy: Safety in pregnancy has not been established relative to possible adverse effects on fetal development. Withdrawal symptoms in neonates have been reported following use during pregnancy. Therefore, Distalgesic should not be used in pregnant women unless, in the judgment of the physician, the potential benefits outweigh the possible hazards.

Nursing mothers: Low levels of dextropropoxyphene have been detected in human milk. In postpartum studies involving nursing mothers who were given dextropropoxyphene, no adverse effects were noted in the infants.

Effects on ability to drive and use machines:

Ambulatory patients: Dextropropoxyphene may impair abilities required for tasks such as driving a car or operating machinery. The patient should be cautioned accordingly.

Undesirable effects: The most frequently reported have been dizziness, sedation, nausea and vomiting. Some of these side-effects may be alleviated if the patient lies down.

Other side-effects include constipation, abdominal pain, rashes, light-headedness, headache, weakness, euphoria, dysphoria, hallucinations and minor visual disturbances.

Dextropropoxyphene therapy has been associated with abnormal liver function tests and, more rarely, with instances of reversible jaundice (including cholestatic jaundice).

Hepatic necrosis may result from acute overdose of paracetamol. In chronic alcohol abusers, this has been reported rarely with short-term use of paracetamol dosages of 2.5 to 10 g/day. Fatalities have occurred.

Renal papillary necrosis may result from chronic paracetamol use, particularly when the dosage is greater than recommended and when combined with aspirin.

Subacute painful myopathy has occurred following chronic dextropropoxyphene overdosage.

Chronic ingestion of dextropropoxyphene in doses exceeding 720 mg per day has caused toxic psychoses and convulsions.

Overdose: Initial consideration should be given to the management of the CNS effects of dextropropoxyphene overdosage. Resuscitative measures should be initiated promptly.

Dextropropoxyphene: In the acute phase dextropropoxyphene produces symptoms typical of narcosis, with somnolence or coma and respiratory depression, sometimes with convulsions. Blood pressure falls and cardiac performance deteriorates. Cardiac arrhythmias and conduction delay may be present. A combined respiratory-metabolic acidosis occurs, which may be severe if large amounts of salicylates have also been ingested. Death may occur.

Naloxone will reduce the respiratory depression

and 0.4-2 mg IV should be administered promptly. (This may be repeated at 2-3 minute intervals, but if there is no response after 10 mg of naloxone the diagnosis should be questioned.) The duration of antagonism may be brief and need repeating for up to 24 hours. Mechanical ventilation, with oxygen may be required, and PEEP ventilation is desirable if pulmonary oedema is present.

Blood gases, pH and electrolytes should be monitored and electrocardiographic monitoring is essential. Ventricular fibrillation or cardiac arrest may occur. Respiratory acidosis rapidly subsides as ventilation is restored and hypercapnoea eliminated, but lactic acidosis may require IV bicarbonate for prompt correction. In addition to the use of a narcotic antagonist, the patient may require titration with an anti-convulsant to control convulsions. Gastric lavage may be useful and activated charcoal can absorb a significant amount of ingested dextropropoxyphene.

Treatment of dextropropoxyphene overdose in children: See general comments above. Naloxone at 0.01 mg/kg body weight IV should be administered promptly. If there is no response a dose of 0.1 mg/kg IV may be used.

Paracetamol: Overdose symptoms may not become apparent until later but early measurement of paracetamol levels is essential. N-acetylcysteine given as early as possible is effective in reducing the toxic effects of paracetamol. Treatment should be instituted within 16 hours of ingestion. Initial symptoms may be anorexia, nausea, vomiting, profuse sweating, malaise and abdominal pain, but the patient may have no symptoms. Subsequent evidence of liver dysfunction may be apparent up to 72 hours after ingestion, and if severe lead to irreversible hepatic necrosis and death within 3-7 days.

In adults, hepatic toxicity has rarely been reported with acute overdoses of less than 10 g and fatalities with less than 15 g.

Acute renal failure may accompany the hepatic dysfunction and can occur without signs of fulminant hepatic failure. Typically renal impairment is more apparent 6-9 days after overdose.

Pharmacological properties

Pharmacodynamic properties: The product is a compound analgesic containing the non-narcotic drug (paracetamol) for the relief of pain of musculoskeletal conditions and a narcotic drug (dextropropoxyphene) for the relief of pain of visceral origin.

Pharmacokinetic properties: Single dose studies have shown peak plasma levels of 0.06 mg/l two hours after administration of 65 mg of dextropropoxyphene HCl. Variation of plasma levels between subjects may be due to individual differences in drug absorption and metabolism.

Multiple dose studies have shown that differences in plasma levels obtained with the hydrochloride salt or the napsylate salt have little therapeutic significance and that a 65 mg dextropropoxyphene HCl dose administered six hourly will achieve steady state plasma levels in the 0.13-0.19 mg/l range after 48 hours. The minimum lethal dose of dextropropoxyphene has been reported to be 500-800 mg and could result in blood concentrations of 0.45-0.74 mg/l. Mean half-lives of 11.8 hours for dextropropoxyphene and 36.6 hours for norpropoxyphene have been demonstrated.

Preclinical safety data: There are no preclinical data of relevance to the prescriber in addition to that summarised in other sections of the summary of product characteristics.

Pharmaceutical particulars

List of excipients: Maize Starch; Pregelatinised Maize Starch; Magnesium Stearate; Methylhydroxypropylcellulose 15; Glycerol; Titanium Dioxide.

Incompatibilities: Not applicable.

Shelf-life: 3 years.

Special precautions for storage: None.

Nature and contents of container: Blister packs containing 100 white, pillow-shaped, film coated tablets, 14 mm in length and marked 'DG' (10 strips of 10 tablets).

Instructions for use/handling: None.

Marketing authorisation number PL 0006/5000

Date of approval/revision of SPC January 1998

Legal category CD (Sch 5), POM

DISTAMINE*

Presentation Tablets each containing 125 mg or 250 mg D-penicillamine base. The 125 mg tablets are white, coated and have a diameter of 8 mm. They are marked 'DS' on one face and '125' on the other. The 250 mg tablets are white, coated and have a diameter of 10 mm. They are marked 'DM' on one face and '250' on the other.

Uses

(a) Severe active rheumatoid arthritis, including juvenile forms.

(b) Wilson's disease (hepatolenticular degeneration).

(c) Cystinuria—dissolution and prevention of cystine stones.

(d) Lead poisoning.

(e) Chronic active hepatitis.

Dosage and administration For oral administration.

(a) Rheumatoid arthritis: Adults: 125–250 mg daily for the first month. Increase by the same amount every 4 to 12 weeks until remission occurs. The minimum maintenance dose to achieve suppression of symptoms should be used and treatment should be discontinued if no benefit is obtained within twelve months. Improvement may not occur for some months.

The usual maintenance dose is 500–750 mg daily. Up to 1.5 g daily may be required. If possible, penicillamine should be taken at least half an hour before meals, or on retiring.

If remission is established and has been sustained for six months, gradual reduction by 125–250 mg amounts every 12 weeks may be attempted.

The elderly: Increased toxicity has been observed in this patient population regardless of renal function. Initial dose should not exceed 125 mg daily for the first month, increasing by a similar increment every 4 to 12 weeks until the minimum maintenance dose to suppress symptoms is reached. Daily dosage should not exceed 1 g.

Children: 15-20 mg/kg/day is considered appropriate in the majority of cases. The initial dose should be 2.5–5.0 mg/kg/day and increased at four-weekly intervals over a period of three to six months. Please note that as the smallest available tablet is 125 mg, this may not be suitable for children under 8 years.

(b) Wilson's disease: Adults: 1.5-2 g daily in divided doses 30 minutes before food. Dose may be reduced to 750 mg-1 g daily when control of the disease is achieved. Patients must be maintained in negative copper balance and the minimum dosage of penicillamine required to achieve this should be given.

It is advisable that a dose of 2 g/day should not be continued for more than a year.

The elderly: 20 mg/kg/day in divided doses. Adjust dosage to control disease and maintain negative copper balance.

Children: Up to 20 mg/kg/day in divided doses before food. Minimum dose 500 mg/day.

(c) Cystinuria: Ideally, establish the lowest effective dose by quantitative amino acid chromatography of urine.

(i) *Dissolution of cystine stones: Adults:* 1-3 g daily in divided doses 30 minutes before food, where possible.

Urine cystine levels of not more than 200 mg/l should be maintained.

(ii) *Prevention of cystine stones: Adults:* 500 mg-1 g on retiring. Fluid intake should be not less than 3 litres/day.

Urine cystine levels of not more than 300 mg/l should be maintained.

The elderly: Use the minimum dose to maintain urinary cystine levels below 200 mg/l.

Children: No dose range established, but urinary cystine levels must be kept below 200 mg/l. The minimum dose of penicillamine required to achieve this should be given.

(d) Lead poisoning: Adults: 1-1.5 g daily in divided doses before food until urinary lead is stabilised at less than 0.5 mg/day.

The elderly: 20 mg/kg/day in divided doses until urinary lead is stabilised at less than 0.5 mg/day.

Children: 20 mg/kg/day.

(e) Chronic active hepatitis: Adults: For maintenance treatment after the disease process has been brought under control with corticosteroids. The initial dosage of 500 mg daily, in divided doses, should be increased gradually over three months to a maintenance dose of 1.25 g daily. During this period, the dosage of corticosteroids should be phased out. Throughout therapy, liver function tests should be carried out periodically to assess the disease status.

The elderly: Not recommended.

(f) Desensitisation: No fixed dose regimen. An initial dose of 25 mg daily is suggested, this to be gradually increased in accordance with the response of the patient. Higher initial doses have been employed in cystinuric patients.

Contra-indications, warnings, etc

Contra-indications: Hypersensitivity to penicillamine, except in a life-threatening situation, when desensitisation should be attempted (see 'Dosage and Administration').

Agranulocytosis or severe thrombocytopenia due to penicillamine.

Lupus erythematosus.

Warnings

Usage in pregnancy: The safety of penicillamine for use during pregnancy has not been established. It has been shown to be teratogenic in rats when given in doses several times higher than those recommended for human use.

Wilson's disease: There has been one case reported of reversible cutis laxa in an infant born to a mother taking 1.5 g penicillamine daily throughout pregnancy. Although there have been no controlled studies on the use of penicillamine during pregnancy, two retrospective studies have reported the successful delivery of 43 normal infants to 28 women receiving between 0.5 g and 2 g of penicillamine daily.

Cystinuria: There have been reports of patients delivered of normal infants, and one report of a severe connective tissue abnormality in the infant of a mother who received 2 g penicillamine daily throughout pregnancy. Whenever possible, penicillamine should be withheld during pregnancy, but if stones continue to form, the benefit of resuming treatment must be weighed against the possible risk to the foetus.

Rheumatoid arthritis or chronic active hepatitis: Penicillamine should not be administered to patients who are pregnant, and therapy should be stopped when pregnancy is diagnosed or suspected, unless considered to be absolutely essential by the physician.

Precautions: Full blood and platelet counts should be performed and renal function should be assessed prior to treatment with penicillamine. Monitoring of blood and platelet counts should be carried out at appropriate intervals, together with urinalysis for detection of haematuria and proteinuria.

If concomitant oral iron therapy is indicated, this should not be given within two hours of taking penicillamine.

Caution should be observed when anti-inflammatory or other drugs with known propensity for causing marrow injury are taken concurrently with penicillamine.

Care should be exercised in patients with renal insufficiency; modification of dosage may be necessary.

Side-effects: NB: The incidence and severity of some of the adverse reactions, noted below, varies according to the dosage and nature of the disease under treatment.

Nausea, anorexia, fever and rash may occur early in therapy, especially when full doses are given from the start. Antihistamines, steroid cover, or temporary reduction of dose will control urticarial reactions.

Reversible loss of taste may occur. Mineral supplements to overcome this are not recommended. Rarely, mouth ulceration/stomatitis has occurred.

Thrombocytopenia occurs commonly and neutropenia less often. These reactions may occur at any time during treatment and are usually reversible. Deaths from agranulocytosis and aplastic anaemia have occurred. Full blood counts should be carried out weekly or fortnightly during the first eight weeks of therapy, in the week after any increase in dose, and otherwise monthly thereafter. In cystinuria or Wilson's disease, longer intervals may be adequate.

Withdrawal of treatment should be considered if platelets fall below 120,000 or white blood cells below 2,500/mm^3, or if three successive falls are noted within the normal range. Treatment may be restarted at a reduced dosage when counts return to normal, but should be permanently withdrawn on recurrence of neutropenia or thrombocytopenia.

Proteinuria occurs in up to 30 per cent of patients and is partially dose-related. Urine should be tested weekly at first and after each increase in dose, then monthly, though again longer intervals may be adequate with cystinuria and Wilson's disease. Increasing proteinuria may necessitate withdrawal of treatment.

Haematuria is rare, but if it occurs in the absence of renal stones or other known cause, treatment should be stopped immediately.

Other rare adverse reactions are as follows: alopecia and inflammatory conditions of the respiratory system, such as bronchiolitis and pneumonitis.

Other complications have included haemolytic anaemia, nephrotic syndrome, drug induced lupus erythematosus, and conditions closely resembling myasthenia gravis, polymyositis (with rare cardiac involvement), dermatomyositis, pemphigus, Goodpasture's syndrome, Stevens-Johnson syndrome and rheumatoid arthritis.

A late rash, described as acquired epidermolysis

bullosa and penicillamine dermopathy, may occur after several months or years of therapy. This may necessitate a reduction in dosage. Pseudoxanthoma elasticum and skin laxity have been reported rarely.

Overdosage: No instances of adverse reactions to an overdose of penicillamine have been recorded and no specific measures are indicated.

Further information Nil.

Pharmaceutical precautions Store in a dry place below 25°C. Keep containers tightly closed.

Legal category POM.

Package quantities
Tablets 125 mg: Bottles of 100
Tablets 250 mg: Bottles of 100

Product licence numbers
Tablets 125 mg: 0006/0090
Tablets 250 mg: 0006/5008

ILOSONE*

Qualitative and quantitative composition Erythromycin Estolate.

Equivalent to base 250 mg (pulvules) or base 500 mg (tablets).

Pharmaceutical form The capsules are ivory/red, marked DISTA, and are 2.1cm long.

The tablets are pink, para-capsule shaped, 1.9cm long, and coded DISTA DI.

Clinical particulars

Therapeutic indications: Antibiotic. Erythromycin is indicated in the treatment of the following infections when due to susceptible organisms:

Upper and lower respiratory tract infections
Otitis media
Skin and soft-issue infections, including erythrasma and acne
Dental infections
Genito-urinary infections, including gonorrhoea, syphilis, and chlamydial infections
Intestinal amoebiasis (extra-enteric amoebiasis requires treatment with other agents)

Erythromycin is also indicated for the following:

Endocarditis: Continuous or short-term prophylaxis against bacterial endocarditis, especially prior to dental or other operative procedures, in patients with a history of rheumatic fever or congenital heart disease and who are hypersensitive to penicillin. Erythromycin is not suitable for prophylaxis prior to genito-urinary or gastro-intestinal tract surgery.

Diphtheria: As an adjunct to antitoxin, to prevent establishment of carriers, and to eradicate the organism in carriers.

Whooping cough: When given early after exposure, erythromycin may reduce the risk of development of classical symptoms.

Legionnaires' disease: Limited clinical experience would suggest that erythromycin may be effective in treating Legionnaires' disease.

Erythromycin is active against the following organisms *in vitro: Streptococcus pyogenes; Str. pneumoniae;* Alpha-haemolytic streptococci (viridans group); *Staphylococcus aureus; Haemophilus influenzae; Mycoplasma pneumoniae; Corynebacterium* spp.; *Listeria monocytogenes; Bordetella pertussis; Legionella pneumophila; Helicobacter* spp.; *Neisseria gonorrhoeae; Treponema pallidum; Chlamydia trachomatis;* Anaerobic bacteria, including *Bacteroides* spp., *Clostridium* spp. and *Propionibacterium acnes; Entamoeba histolytica.*

Posology and method of administration: For oral administration.

Adults: The usual dose is 250 mg every six hours. This may be increased up to 4 g per day according to the severity of the infection. Dosage should be limited to a maximum of 1.5 g daily in patients with severe renal impairment.

The elderly: As for adults.

Children: Age, weight and severity of the infection are important factors in determining the correct dosage. The usual range is 20-50 mg/kg/day in divided doses.

If administration on a twice daily schedule is desirable, one-half of the total daily dose may be given every 12 hours. Twice daily dosing is not recommended when doses larger than 1 g daily are administered.

Streptococcal infections: For streptococcal pharyngitis and tonsillitis, the usual dosage range is 20-50 mg/kg/day in divided doses. In the treatment of group A beta-haemolytic streptococcal infections, a therapeutic dosage of erythromycin should be administered for at least 10 days. In continuous prophylaxis of streptococcal infections in persons with a history of rheumatic heart disease, the dosage is 250 mg twice daily.

When Ilosone is used prior to surgery to prevent endocarditis caused by alpha-haemolytic streptococci (viridans group), a recommended schedule for adults is 1 g pre-operatively (20 mg/kg for children) and 500 mg (10 mg/kg for children) 6 hours later.

Pertussis: Doses of erythromycin estolate utilised in reported clinical studies were 40-50 mg/kg/day, given in divided doses for five to 14 days.

Gonorrhoea: For disseminated infection, 500 mg four times daily for 7 days.

Syphilis: A regimen of 20 g of erythromycin estolate in divided doses over a period of 10 days has been shown to be effective.

Amoebic dysentery: Dosage for adults is 250 mg four times daily for 10 to 14 days; for children, 30-50 mg/kg/day in divided doses for 10 to 14 days.

Legionnaires' disease: Although optimum regimens have not been established, 1-4 g daily in divided doses has been utilised in reported clinical studies.

Urogenital infections during pregnancy due to C. trachomatis: 500 mg four times a day for at least seven days. For women who cannot tolerate this regimen, a decreased dose of 250 mg four times a day should be used for at least fourteen days.

For adults with uncomplicated urethral, endocervical, or rectal infections caused by C. trachomatis in whom tetracyclines are contra-indicated or not tolerated: 500 mg four times a day for at least seven days.

Contra-indications: Hypersensitivity to erythromycin.

Patients who have previously developed jaundice or who have pre-existing liver disease or dysfunction.

Patients taking terfenadine or astemizole.

Special warnings and special precautions for use: The administration of erythromycin estolate has been associated with the infrequent occurrence of reversible cholestatic hepatitis. Hepatic dysfunction with or without jaundice has occurred, chiefly in adults. It may be accompanied by malaise, nausea, vomiting, abdominal colic and fever. In some instances severe abdominal pain may simulate the pain of biliary colic, pancreatitis, perforated ulcer, or an acute abdominal surgical problem. In other instances, clinical symptoms and results of liver function tests have resembled findings in extrahepatic obstructive jaundice. Laboratory findings have been characterised by abnormal hepatic function test values, peripheral eosinophilia and leucocytosis. If the above findings occur, discontinue Ilosone promptly.

Initial symptoms have developed in some cases after a few days of treatment, but generally have followed one or two weeks of continuous therapy. Symptoms re-appear promptly, usually within 48 hours, after the drug is re-administered to sensitive patients. The syndrome seems to result from a form of sensitisation, occurs chiefly in adults, and has been reversible when medication is discontinued.

The diagnosis of pseudomembranous colitis should be considered should diarrhoea develop. Mild cases usually respond to drug discontinuation alone. Additional measures will be required in more severe cases, which may be life-threatening.

The antibacterial activity of erythromycin is markedly greater in alkaline than in neutral or acid media. Urinary alkalinisation should be considered when treating urinary infections.

Laboratory tests: Erythromycin interferes with some clinical laboratory tests, for example, high SGOT values may be artefacts and may not necessarily reflect changes in liver function.

During prolonged or repeated therapy, there is a possibility of overgrowth of non-susceptible bacteria or fungi. If such infections arise, the drug should be discontinued and appropriate therapy instituted.

Interaction with other medicaments and other forms of interaction:

Drug interactions: Erythromycin significantly alters the metabolism of terfenadine or astemizole when taken concomitantly. Rare cases of serious cardiovascular events, including death, cardiac arrest, torsade de pointes and other ventricular arrhythmias, have been observed (see *Contra-indications*).

Since probenecid inhibits tubular re-absorption of erythromycin in animals, it prolongs maintenance of plasma levels.

Erythromycin and lincomycin or clindamycin may, under some conditions, be antagonistic. Lincomycin or clindamycin therapy should be avoided in treatment of infections due to erythromycin-resistant organisms.

The use of erythromycin in patients who are receiving concomitant high doses of theophylline may be associated with an increase in serum theophylline levels and potential theophylline toxicity. If symptoms of toxicity or elevated serum theophylline levels develop, the dose of theophylline should be reduced.

Concomitant administration of erythromycin and digoxin has been reported to result in elevated digoxin serum levels.

There have been reports of increased anticoagulant effects when erythromycin and oral anticoagulants were used concomitantly. Increased anticoagulation effects due to this drug interaction may be more pronounced in the elderly.

Concurrent use of erythromycin and ergotamine or dihydroergotamine has been associated in some patients with acute ergot toxicity characterised by severe peripheral vasospasm and dysaesthesia.

Erythromycin has been reported to decrease the clearance of triazolam and midazolam, and thus may increase the pharmacological effect of these benzodiazepines.

The use of erythromycin in patients concurrently taking drugs metabolised by the cytochrome P450 system may be associated with elevation in serum levels of these other drugs. Elevated serum concentrations of the following drugs have been reported when administered concurrently with erythromycin: carbamazepine, cyclosporin, hexobarbitone, phenytoin, alfentanil, disopyramide, lovastatin and bromocriptine. Serum concentrations of such drugs should be monitored closely in patients concurrently receiving erythromycin.

Pregnancy and lactation:

Usage in pregnancy: Reproduction studies in rats, mice and rabbits, with doses several times the usual human dose, have revealed no evidence of impaired fertility or foetal harm related to erythromycin. There are no adequate studies in pregnant women. Because animal reproductive studies are not always predictive of human response, this drug should be used during pregnancy only if clearly needed.

Usage in nursing mothers: Erythromycin is excreted in breast milk. Caution should be exercised when it is administered to a nursing woman.

Effects on ability to drive and use machines: Not applicable.

Undesirable effects: The most frequent side-effects of erythromycin preparations are gastro-intestinal (eg, abdominal cramping and discomfort) and are dose-related. Nausea, vomiting and diarrhoea occur infrequently with usual oral doses.

Mild allergic reactions, such as urticaria and other skin rashes, have occurred. Serious allergic reactions, including anaphylaxis, have been reported.

There have been isolated reports of hearing loss and/or tinnitus occurring chiefly in patients with renal or hepatic insufficiency and in patients receiving high doses of erythromycin. Ototoxic effects are usually reversible upon discontinuation, but in rare instances, involving intravenous administration, the ototoxic effect has been irreversible.

Rarely, erythromycin has been associated with ventricular arrhythmias, including ventricular tachycardia and torsade de pointes, in individuals with prolonged QT intervals.

Overdose:

Symptoms: Nausea, vomiting and dose-related epigastric distress and diarrhoea. Reversible mild acute pancreatitis has been reported. Hearing loss, with or without tinnitus and vertigo, may occur (see *Undesirable effects*).

Treatment: Unless 5 times the normal single dose has been ingested, gastro-intestinal decontamination should not be necessary. Consider activated charcoal instead of, or in addition to, gastric emptying.

Forced diuresis, peritoneal dialysis, haemodialysis, or charcoal haemoperfusion have not been established as beneficial.

Pharmacological properties

Pharmacodynamic properties: Erythromycin acts by interfering with bacterial protein synthesis and is bacteriostatic or bactericidal, depending on the concentration of the drugs and the type of organism.

Pharmacokinetic properties: Erythromycin estolate is stable to acid, and is not affected by food to the same extent as other erythromycins. It is rapidly absorbed, with peak serum levels being achieved within 4 hours in adults. Serum concentrations are significantly higher than those obtained with the base or other esters.

Preclinical safety data: Reproduction studies in rats, mice and rabbits, with doses several times the usual human dose, have revealed no evidence of impaired fertility or foetal harm related to erythromycin.

Pharmaceutical particulars

List of excipients:

Capsules: Talc; Silica Gel Powder; Magnesium Stearate; Liquid Paraffin; Erythrosine (E127); Titanium Dioxide (E171); Quinoline Yellow (E104); Red Iron Oxide (E172); Yellow Iron Oxide (E172); Gelatin.

Tablets: Magnesium Stearate; Starch; Amaranth Aluminium Lake (E123); Erythrosine Aluminium Lake (E127); Sunset Yellow Aluminium Lake (E110).

Incompatibilities: Not applicable.

Shelf-life: 5 years.

Special precautions for storage:

Capsules: Store below 25°C.

Tablets: Store in a cool, dry place (6-15°C). Keep tightly closed.

Nature and contents of container: High density polyethylene bottle.

Package quantities
Capsules 250 mg: Bottles of 100.
Tablets 500 mg: Bottles of 12.

Instructions for use/handling: Not applicable.

Marketing authorisation numbers
Capsules: PL 0006/5022R
Tablets: PL 0006/5015R

Date of approval/revision of SPC September 1996

Legal category POM

KEFADOL*

Presentation 10 ml vials containing cefamandole nafate for injection equivalent to 1 g cefamandole.

The vials also contain 63 mg Sodium Carbonate USP per gram of cefamandole. The total sodium content is approximately 77 mg per gram of cefamandole activity.

Uses Cefamandole is indicated in the treatment of infections of the lower respiratory tract, genito-urinary tract, bones and joints, bloodstream (septicaemia), skin and soft tissue, gall bladder and peritoneum, and pelvic inflammatory disease in women, when due to susceptible micro-organisms.

Prophylactic use: Perioperative administration of cefamandole may reduce the incidence of postoperative infections in patients undergoing contaminated or potentially contaminated surgical procedures associated with a high risk of infection, or where the occurrence of a postoperative infection could be especially serious.

Cefamandole is usually active against the following organisms *in vitro* and in clinical infections:

Gram-positive:

Staphylococci, including coagulase-positive, coagulase-negative (e.g. *Staphylococcus epidermidis*) and penicillinase-producing strains

Beta-haemolytic and other streptococci (most strains of enterococci, e.g. *Enterococcus faecalis*, are resistant)

Streptococcus pneumoniae

Gram-negative:

Escherichia coli

Klebsiella spp.

Enterobacter spp. (initially susceptible organisms occasionally may become resistant during therapy)

Haemophilus influenzae

Proteus mirabilis

Providencia rettgeri

Morganella morganii

Proteus vulgaris (some strains of *P. vulgaris* have been shown by *in vitro* tests to be resistant to cefamandole and certain other cephalosporins)

Anaerobic organisms:

Gram-positive and gram-negative cocci (including *Peptococcus* and *Peptostreptococcus* spp.)

Gram-positive bacilli (including *Clostridium* spp.)

Gram-negative bacilli (including *Bacteroides*)

Most strains of *Bacteroides fragilis* are resistant.

Pseudomonas, Acinetobacter calcoaceticus and most *Serratia* strains are resistant to cefamandole and certain other cephalosporins. Cefamandole is resistant to degradation by β-lactamases from certain members of the *Enterobacteriaceae*.

Dosage and administration Cefamandole nafate may be given intravenously or by deep intramuscular injection into a large muscle mass to minimise pain.

Adults and the elderly: The dosage range for cefamandole is 500 mg to 2 g every four to eight hours, depending on the severity and site of infection.

Impaired renal function: When renal function is impaired, a reduced dosage must be employed and serum concentrations should be monitored when feasible. After an initial dose of 1 to 2 g (depending on the severity of infection), a maintenance dosage schedule should be followed (see table). Continued dosage should be determined by degree of renal impairment, severity of infection and susceptibility of the causative organism.

Maintenance dosage of cefamandole in patients with impaired renal function

Creatinine clearance ml/min/1.73 m²	*Life-threatening infections*	*Severe infections*	*Less severe infections*
80-50	2 g q 6 h	1.5 g q 6 h	0.75 g q 6 h
50-25	2 g q 8 h	1.5 g q 8 h	0.75 g q 8 h
25-10	1.25 g q 8 h	1.0 g q 8 h	0.5 g q 8 h
10-2	1 g q 12 h	0.75 g q 12 h	0.5 g q 12 h
<2	0.75 g q 12 h	0.5 g q 12 h	0.25 g q 12 h

Intramuscular administration: Each gram of cefamandole should be reconstituted with 3 ml of Water for Injections PhEur or Sodium Chloride Intravenous Infusion BP. Shake well until dissolved.

Intravenous administration: Intravenous route may be preferable for bacterial septicaemia, localised parenchymal abscesses, peritonitis, or other severe or life-threatening infections.

1. *For direct intermittent intravenous administration,* each gram of cefamandole should be reconstituted with 10 ml of Water for Injections PhEur, 5% Dextrose Intravenous Infusion BP, or Sodium Chloride Intravenous Infusion BP. Slowly inject directly into the vein over a period of three to five minutes or give through the tubing of an administration set while the patient is also receiving one of the following intravenous fluids:

Sodium Chloride Intravenous Infusion BP
5% Dextrose Intravenous Infusion BP
10% Dextrose Intravenous Infusion BP
5% Dextrose and 0.9% Sodium Chloride Intravenous Infusion BP
5% Dextrose and 0.45% Sodium Chloride Intravenous Infusion BP
Sodium Lactate Intravenous Infusion BP

2. *Intermittent intravenous infusion with a Y-type administration set or volume control set* can also be accomplished while any of the above mentioned intravenous fluids are being infused. However, during infusion of the solution containing cefamandole, it is desirable to discontinue the other solution. When this technique is employed, careful attention should be paid to the volume of the solution containing cefamandole so that the calculated dose will be infused. When a Y-tube connection is used, 100 ml of an appropriate diluent should be added to 2 g cefamandole. If Water for Injections PhEur is used as the diluent, reconstitute with approximately 20 ml per g to avoid a hypotonic solution.

3. *For continuous intravenous infusion,* each gram of cefamandole should be diluted with 10 ml of Water for Injections PhEur. An appropriate quantity of the resulting solution may be added to an i.v. bottle containing one of the previously mentioned intravenous fluids.

If combination therapy with cefamandole and an aminoglycoside is indicated, each of these should be administered at separate sites.

Infants and children: Administration of 50 to 100 mg/kg/day in equally divided doses every four to eight hours has been effective for most infections susceptible to cefamandole. This may be increased to a total daily dose of 150 mg/kg (not to exceed the maximum adult dose) for serious infections.

Infants: Cefamandole has been effectively used in this age group, but all laboratory parameters have not been extensively studied in infants between 1 and 6 months of age. Safety of this product has not been established in prematures and infants under 1 month of age; therefore, if cefamandole is to be administered to infants, the physician should determine whether the potential benefits outweigh the possible risks involved. Accumulation of cephalosporins (with resulting prolongation of drug half-life) has been reported in neonates.

Prophylactic use: The following schedules are recommended for perioperative use:

Adults and the elderly: 1 or 2 g intravenously or intramuscularly one-half to one hour prior to surgical incision, followed by 1 or 2 g every six hours for 24 to 48 hours.

For patients undergoing procedures involving implantation of prosthetic devices, administration for up to 72 hours is recommended.

Children (more than three months of age): 50–100 mg/kg/day in equally divided doses by the same routes and schedule designated for adults.

If signs of infection occur, cultures should be obtained and appropriate therapy instituted.

Kefadol should be continued for a minimum of 48 to 72 hours after the patient becomes asymptomatic or bacterial eradication has occurred. A minimum of 10 days treatment is recommended in infections caused by group A beta-haemolytic streptococci. In chronic urinary tract infection, frequent bacteriological and clinical appraisal is necessary during therapy and possibly for several months after completion. Persistent infections may require treatment for several weeks.

Contra-indications, warnings, etc

Contra-indication: Cefamandole is contra-indicated in patients with known allergy to the cephalosporin group of antibiotics.

Warnings: Before cefamandole therapy is instituted, careful enquiry should be made concerning previous hypersensitivity reactions to cephalosporins, penicillins or other drugs. Kefadol should be given cautiously to penicillin-sensitive patients.

There is some clinical and laboratory evidence of partial cross-allergenicity of the penicillins and the cephalosporins. Patients have been reported to have had severe reactions (including anaphylaxis) to both drugs.

Antibiotics should be administered with caution to any patient who has demonstrated some form of allergy, particularly to drugs.

Pseudomembranous colitis has been reported with most broad-spectrum antibiotics. Its diagnosis should be considered in patients who develop diarrhoea with antibiotics. Such colitis may range from mild to life-threatening.

Usage in pregnancy: Reproduction studies in rats given doses of 500 or 1000 mg/kg/day (approximately 5 times the maximum clinical dose) revealed no evidence of impaired fertility or harm to the foetus due to cefamandole nafate. There are, however, no adequate and well-controlled studies in pregnant women. Because animal studies are not always predictive of human response, this drug should be used during pregnancy only if clearly needed.

Nursing mothers: Caution should be exercised.

Precautions: Although cefamandole rarely produces alteration in kidney function, evaluation of renal status is recommended, especially in seriously ill patients receiving maximum doses. Patients with impaired renal function should be placed on the dosage schedule recommended under 'Dosage and administration'. Usual doses in such individuals may result in excessive serum concentrations.

Nephrotoxicity has been reported following concomitant administration of aminoglycoside antibiotics and cephalosporins.

The results of experimental studies in animals suggest that the concurrent use of potent diuretics such as frusemide or ethacrynic acid may also increase the risk of renal toxicity with cephalosporin antibiotics.

As with other broad-spectrum antibiotics, hypoprothrombinaemia with or without bleeding has been reported rarely, but it has been promptly reversed by administration of vitamin K. Such episodes have usually occurred in elderly, debilitated or otherwise compromised patients with deficient stores of vitamin K. Prophylactic administration of vitamin K may be indicated in such patients, especially when intestinal sterilisation and surgical procedures are performed.

In a few patients receiving cefamandole, nausea, vomiting and vasomotor instability with hypotension and peripheral vasodilatation, has occurred following the ingestion of alcohol. Cefamandole inhibits the enzyme acetaldehyde dehydrogenase in laboratory animals. This causes accumulation of acetaldehyde when ethanol is administered concurrently.

Broad-spectrum antibiotics should be prescribed with caution in individuals with a history of gastro-intestinal disease, particularly colitis.

Prolonged use of cefamandole may result in the overgrowth of non-susceptible organisms. Careful observation of the patient is essential. If superinfection occurs during therapy, appropriate measures should be taken.

A false positive reaction for glucose in the urine may occur with Benedict's or Fehling's solutions or with Clinitest tablets. A false positive test for proteinuria may occur with acid and denaturisation precipitation tests.

Impairment of fertility: Very high doses of cefamandole (equivalent to approximately 5 times the maximum clinical dose) have been found to delay maturation of the testicular germinal epithelium in rats. This effect was seen only when cefamandole was given to neonatal rats during initial spermatogenic development. The clinical significance of this finding is unknown due to differences in the time of initiation of spermatogenesis, rate of spermatogenic development and duration of puberty.

Side-effects

Hypersensitivity: Anaphylaxis, maculopapular rash, urticaria, eosinophilia and drug fever have been reported. These reactions are more likely to occur in patients with a history of allergy, particularly to penicillin.

Haematological: Thrombocytopenia has been reported rarely. Neutropenia has been reported, especially in long courses of treatment. Some individuals have developed positive direct Coombs' tests during treatment with the cephalosporin antibiotics.

Gastro-intestinal: Nausea and vomiting occur rarely. Colitis, including rare instances of pseudomembranous colitis, has been reported.

Liver: Transient rise in AST, ALT and ALP levels have been noted. Transient hepatitis and cholestatic jaundice have been reported rarely.

Kidney: Decreased creatinine clearance has been reported in patients with prior renal impairment. As with some other cephalosporins, transitory elevations of blood urea have occasionally been observed; their frequency increases in patients over 50 years of age. In some of these cases, there was also a mild increase in serum creatinine.

Local reactions: Pain on intramuscular injection is infrequent. Thrombophlebitis occurs rarely.

Overdosage: The administration of inappropriately large doses of parenteral cephalosporins may cause seizures, particularly in patients with renal impairment. Dosage reduction is necessary when renal function is impaired (see 'Dosage and administration'). If seizures occur, the drug should be promptly discontinued; anticonvulsant therapy may be administered if clinically indicated.

In the event of serious overdosage, general supportive care is recommended, with monitoring of haematological, renal and hepatic functions, and coagulation status, until the patient is stable. Haemodialysis may be considered in cases of overwhelming overdosage.

Pharmaceutical precautions *Unreconstituted vials:* Store below 25°C. Protect from light.

It is good practice to reconstitute immediately before use. If this is not feasible, reconstituted solutions may be stored in a refrigerator (2°-8°C) and used within 96 hours. If kept below 25°C, use within 24 hours. During storage at room temperature, carbon dioxide develops inside the vial after reconstitution. This pressure may be dissipated prior to withdrawal of the vial contents, or it may be used to aid withdrawal if the vial is inverted over the syringe needle and the contents are allowed to flow into the syringe.

The pH of freshly reconstituted solutions usually ranges from 6.0 to 8.5.

Do not mix an aminoglycoside with cefamandole in the same intravenous fluid container.

Legal category POM.

Package quantities Vials 1 g: Individual vials in packs of 10.

Further information Solutions of cefamandole range from light yellow to amber, depending upon a variety of factors, including concentration and the diluent used.

Product licence number 0006/0111.

PROZAC*

Presentation Capsules (green and yellow, marked 'Prozac 20 mg') each containing 20 mg fluoxetine, as the hydrochloride.

Capsules (yellow, coded 3109) each containing 60 mg fluoxetine, as the hydrochloride.

Liquid (clear, colourless, mint odoured) containing 20 mg fluoxetine, as the hydrochloride, per 5 ml syrup.

Uses

Depression: Prozac is indicated for the treatment of the symptoms of depressive illness, with or without associated anxiety symptoms, especially where sedation is not required.

Obsessive-compulsive disorder.

Bulimia nervosa: Prozac is indicated for the reduction of binge-eating and purging activity.

Dosage and administration For oral administration to adults only.

Depression, with or without associated anxiety symptoms – adults and the elderly: A dose of 20 mg/day is recommended.

Obsessive-compulsive disorder: 20 mg/day to 60 mg/day. A dose of 20 mg/day is recommended as the initial dose. Although there may be an increased potential for side-effects at higher doses, a dose increase may be considered after several weeks if there is no response.

Bulimia nervosa – adults and the elderly: A dose of 60 mg/day is recommended.

Fluoxetine has a half-life of 1 to 3 days after acute administration. The half-life may be prolonged to 4 to 6 days after chronic administration. The active metabolite, norfluoxetine, has a mean half-life of 9.3 days after multiple dosing (range 4 to 16 days). Steady state plasma concentrations are only achieved after continuous dosing for weeks.

When dosing is stopped, active drug substances will persist in the body for weeks. This should be borne in mind when starting or stopping treatment.

Plasma concentrations do not appear to increase without limit because, in addition to metabolism by the hepatic cytochrome P450IID6 isoenzyme system, there are non-saturable pathways. Patients receiving fluoxetine for as long as 3 years exhibited average plasma concentrations, similar to those seen among patients treated for 4 or 5 weeks.

The capsule and liquid dosage forms are bioequivalent.

Children: The use of Prozac in children is not recommended, as safety and efficacy have not been established.

Patients with renal and/or hepatic dysfunction: See 'Contra-indications' and 'Precautions' sections.

Contra-indications, warnings, etc

Contra-indications: Hypersensitivity to fluoxetine.

Fluoxetine should not be administered to patients with severe renal failure (GFR <10 ml/min) because accumulation may occur in these patients during chronic treatment.

Usage in nursing mothers: Prozac should not be prescribed to nursing mothers. In one breast milk sample the concentration of fluoxetine, plus norfluoxetine, was 70.4 ng/ml, compared to 295.0 ng/ml in the mother's plasma. No adverse effects on the infant were noted. In another infant the plasma level of fluoxetine was 340 ng/ml and 208 ng/ml of norfluoxetine on the second day of breast feeding from a mother on Prozac. This infant developed crying, sleep disturbance, vomiting and watery stools.

Monoamine oxidase inhibitors: At least 14 days should elapse between discontinuation of an MAOI and initiation of treatment with Prozac. At least five weeks (longest if fluoxetine has been prescribed chronically and/or at higher doses) should elapse between discontinuation of Prozac and initiation of therapy with an MAOI.

Serious, sometimes fatal reactions (including hyperthermia, rigidity, myoclonus, autonomic instability with possible rapid fluctuations of vital signs, and mental status changes that include extreme agitation progressing to delirium and coma) have been reported with concomitant use or when fluoxetine had been recently discontinued and an MAOI started. Some cases presented with features resembling neuroleptic malignant syndrome. Cyproheptadine or dantrolene may benefit patients experiencing such reactions.

Warnings

Rash and allergic reactions: Angioneurotic oedema, urticaria and other allergic reactions have been reported. Upon the appearance of rash or of other allergic phenomena for which an alternative aetiology cannot be identified, Prozac should be discontinued.

Pregnancy: The safety of fluoxetine in human pregnancy has not been established; accordingly, the drug should be avoided in pregnancy unless there is no safer alternative. There was no evidence of teratogenicity from animal studies but full testing was limited by maternal toxicity.

Lactation: See 'Contra-indications'.

Precautions: Prozac should be discontinued in any patient who develops seizures. Prozac should be avoided in patients with unstable epilepsy; patients with controlled epilepsy should be carefully monitored. There have been rare reports of prolonged seizures in patients on fluoxetine receiving ECT treatment.

Fluoxetine is extensively metabolised by the liver and excreted by the kidneys. A lower dose, e.g., alternate day dosing, is recommended in patients with significant hepatic dysfunction or mild to moderate renal failure (GFR 10–50 ml/min).

Clinical experience in acute cardiac disease is limited, therefore caution is advisable. However, the ECG of 312 patients who received fluoxetine in double-blind trials were retrospectively evaluated; no conduction abnormalities that resulted in heart block were observed.

Prozac may cause weight loss which may be undesirable in underweight depressed patients. Only rarely have depressed or bulimic patients been discontinued for weight loss when treated with fluoxetine.

In patients with diabetes, fluoxetine may alter glycaemic control. Hypoglycaemia has occurred during therapy with fluoxetine and hyperglycaemia has developed following discontinuation. Insulin and/or oral hypoglycaemic dosage may need to be adjusted.

There have been reports of abnormal bleeding in several patients, but causal relationship to fluoxetine and clinical importance are unclear.

Although fluoxetine has been shown not to affect psychomotor performance in healthy volunteers, any psychoactive drug may impair judgement or skills. Therefore, patients should be cautioned that their ability to perform potentially hazardous tasks (e.g., driving, operating machinery) may be impaired.

As improvement may not occur during the first two or more weeks of treatment, patients should be closely monitored during this period. The possibility of a suicide attempt is inherent in depression and may persist until significant remission occurs.

Drug interactions: Monoamine oxidase inhibitors: (see 'Contra-indications').

Caution is advised if the concomitant administration of Prozac and CNS active drugs, including lithium, is required. There have been reports of both increased and decreased lithium levels when used concomitantly with fluoxetine. Cases of lithium toxicity have been reported. Lithium levels should be monitored.

Because fluoxetine's metabolism (like tricyclic antidepressants and other selective serotonin antidepressants) involves the hepatic cytochrome P450IID6 isoenzyme system, concomitant therapy with drugs also metabolised by this enzyme system may lead to drug interactions.

Concomitant therapy with drugs predominantly metabolised by this isoenzyme, and which have a narrow therapeutic index (such as flecainide, encainide, vinblastine, carbamazepine and tricyclic antidepressants), should be initiated at or adjusted to the low end of their dose range. This will also apply if fluoxetine has been taken in the previous 5 weeks.

Greater than two-fold increases of previously stable plasma levels of cyclic antidepressants have been observed when Prozac has been administered in combination.

Agitation, restlessness and gastro-intestinal symptoms have been reported in a small number of patients receiving fluoxetine in combination with tryptophan.

Patients on stable doses of phenytoin have developed elevated plasma phenytoin concentrations and clinical phenytoin toxicity following initiation of concomitant fluoxetine treatment.

The long elimination half-lives should be borne in mind (see 'Dosage and administration') when considering pharmacodynamic or pharmacokinetic drug interactions.

Fluoxetine is bound to plasma protein and concurrent administration may alter plasma concentrations of other plasma protein bound drugs or conversely fluoxetine. In formal testing, no drug interaction of clinical significance has been observed between fluoxetine and chlorothiazide, ethanol, secobarbital and tolbutamide.

In formal testing, no drug interaction of clinical significance has been observed between fluoxetine and warfarin. Possible interactions have been reported rarely.

Fluoxetine does not appear to potentiate the effects of alcohol.

Adverse effects

Body as a whole: Asthenia, fever.

Digestive system: Nausea, diarrhoea, dry mouth, appetite loss, dyspepsia, vomiting. Abnormal liver function tests have been reported rarely.

Nervous system: Headache, nervousness, insomnia, drowsiness, anxiety, tremor, dizziness, fatigue, decreased libido, seizures (see 'Precautions'). Hypomania or mania occurred in approximately one per cent of fluoxetine treated trial patients. Dyskinesia (including, for example, a case of buccal-lingual-masticatory syndrome, which resolved following drug discontinuation), movement disorders developing in patients with risk factors (including drugs associated with such events) and worsening of pre-existing movement disorders, and neuroleptic malignant syndrome-like events have been reported.

Respiratory system: Pharyngitis, dyspnoea. Pulmonary events (including inflammatory processes of varying histopathology and/or fibrosis) have been reported rarely. Dyspnoea may be the only preceding symptom.

Skin and appendages: A small percentage of patients developed rash and/or urticaria (see 'Warnings'). Serious systemic reactions, possibly related to vasculitis, have developed in patients with rash, and rarely death has been reported. Excessive sweating, arthralgia, myalgia, serum sickness and anaphylactoid reactions have also been reported. Hair loss, usually reversible, has been reported.

Urinogenital system: Sexual dysfunction (delayed or inhibited orgasm).

Hyponatraemia (including serum sodium below 110 mmol/l) has been rarely reported and appeared to be reversible when Prozac was discontinued. Some cases were possibly due to the syndrome of inappropriate antidiuretic hormone secretion. The majority of reports were associated with older patients, and patients taking diuretics or otherwise volume depleted.

The following have been reported in association with fluoxetine but no causal relationship has been established: aplastic anaemia, cerebral vascular accident, confusion, ecchymoses, eosinophilic pneumonia, gastro-intestinal haemorrhage, hyperprolactinaemia, immune-related haemolytic anaemia, pancreatitis, pancytopenia, suicidal ideation, thrombocytopenia, thrombocytopenic purpura, vaginal bleeding after drug withdrawal and violent behaviour.

Overdosage: On the evidence available, fluoxetine has a wide margin of safety in overdose. Since introduction, reports of death attributed to overdosage of fluoxetine alone have been extremely rare.

One patient who reportedly took 3000 mg of fluoxetine experienced 2 grand mal seizures that remitted spontaneously. Nausea and vomiting were prominent in overdoses involving higher fluoxetine doses. Agitation, restlessness, hypomania and other signs of CNS excitation were also observed.

Management: No specific antidote is known.

An airway should be established. Cardiac and vital signs monitoring is recommended, along with general symptomatic and supportive measures.

An extended time for close medical observation may be needed in patients who have taken excessive quantities of a tricyclic antidepressant if they are also taking, or have recently taken, fluoxetine. Accumulation of the parent tricyclic or an active metabolite may increase the possibility of clinically relevant sequelae.

Based on experience with animals, fluoxetine-induced seizures which fail to remit spontaneously may respond to diazepam. Due to the large volume of distribution of fluoxetine, forced diuresis, dialysis, haemoperfusion and exchange transfusion are unlikely to be of benefit. Activated charcoal, which may be used with sorbitol, may be as or more effective than emesis or lavage.

Pharmaceutical precautions Store at room temperature (15°–25°C).

Legal category POM.

Package quantities
20 mg: Calendar packs of 30 capsules (2 strips of 15 capsules).
20 mg: Packs of 98 capsules (14 strips of 7 capsules).
60 mg: Packs of 30 capsules (3 strips of 10 capsules).
Bottles of 70 ml liquid.

Further information Fluoxetine is chemically unrelated to tricyclic and tetracyclic antidepressant agents. It is a specific serotonin (5-hydroxytryptamine, 5-HT) reuptake inhibitor, whose specificity is unaltered by its major metabolite. Fluoxetine is a 50:50 mixture of two isomers which have equivalent pharmacological activity in animals. Individuals with reduced P450IID6 isoenzyme activity (3–10% of the normal human population – 'poor metabolisers') were compared to normal metabolisers. The total sum at steady state of the two isomers and their active norfluoxetine metabolites was similar. Thus, net pharmacodynamic activities were essentially the same.

Product licence numbers

20 mg capsules:	0006/0195
60 mg capsules:	0006/0198
Liquid:	0006/0272

**Trade Mark*

Dominion Pharma Ltd
Dominion House
Lion Lane
Haslemere
Surrey GU27 1JL

☎ 01428 661078   🖷 01428 661075

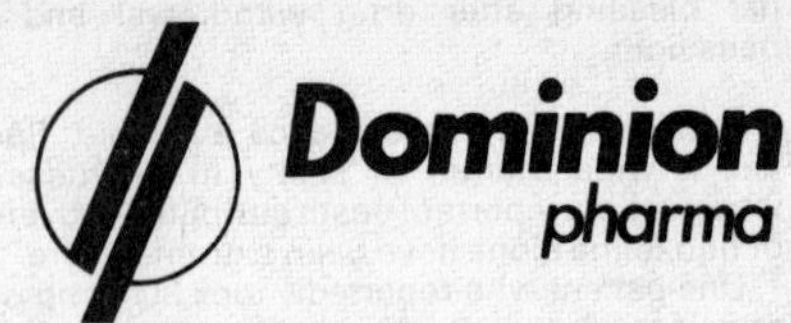

CLOBURATE* EYE DROPS

Qualitative and quantitative composition Clobetasone butyrate 0.1% w/v.

Pharmaceutical form Sterile suspension.

Clinical particulars
Therapeutic indications: For short-term treatment of steroid responsive inflammatory conditions of the eye after clinical exclusion of bacterial, viral and fungal infections. Cloburate eye drops have less effect on intra-ocular pressure than hydrocortisone (1%), betamethasone sodium phosphate (0.1%), prednisolone sodium phosphate (0.5%) or dexamethasone (0.1%) eye drops.

Posology and method of administration:
Adult: The drops are instilled into the eye. Usual dosage: One or two drops four times a day.
For severe inflammatory conditions: One or two drops every one or two hours until signs of improvement are apparent when the frequency may be reduced.
Elderly: As Adults above.
Children: As Adults above.

Contraindications: Bacterial, viral, fungal, tuberculous or purulent conditions of the eye. Use is contra-indicated if glaucoma is present or herpetic keratitis (e.g. dendritic ulcer) is considered a possibility. Use of topical steroids in the latter condition can lead to extension of the ulcer and marked visual deterioration.
Hypersensitivity to any ingredient in the preparation.

Special warnings and precautions: Topical corticosteroids should never be given for an undiagnosed red eye as inappropriate use is potentially blinding. Prolonged use may lead to the risk of adrenal suppression in infants. Although Cloburate eye drops have been shown to have little adverse effect on intra-ocular pressure in most patients, ophthalmological treatment with corticosteroid preparations should not be repeated or prolonged without regular review to exclude raised intra-ocular pressure, cataract formation or unsuspected infections.

Interactions with other medicaments and other forms of interaction: Cloburate eye drops contain benzalkonium chloride as a preservative and therefore should not be used to treat patients who wear soft contact lenses.

Pregnancy and lactation: Safety for use in pregnancy and lactation has not been established. There is inadequate evidence of safety in human pregnancy. Topical administration of corticosteroids to pregnant animals can cause abnormalities of foetal development including cleft palate and intrauterine growth retardation. There may therefore be a very small risk of such effects in the human foetus.

Effects on ability to drive and use machines: May cause transient blurring of vision on instillation. Warn patients not to drive or operate hazardous machinery unless vision is clear.

Undesirable effects: Hypersensitivity reactions, usually of the delayed type, may occur leading to irritation, burning, stinging, itching and dermatitis.
Topical corticosteroid use may result in increased intra-ocular pressure leading to optic nerve damage, reduced visual acuity and visual field defects.
Rises in intra-ocular pressure have been reported in susceptible patients, but these are generally much less than with other corticosteroid eye preparations, including hydrocortisone.
Intensive or prolonged use of topical corticosteroids may lead to formation of posterior subcapsular cataracts.
In those diseases causing thinning of the cornea or sclera, corticosteroid therapy may result in thinning of the globe leading to perforation.

Overdosage: Long-term intensive topical use may lead to systemic effects.
Oral ingestion of the contents of one bottle (up to 10ml) of drops is unlikely to lead to any serious adverse effects.

Pharmacological properties
Pharmacodynamic properties: Clobetasone butyrate is a topically active corticosteroid which provides an exceptional combination of activity and safety.
When used in the treatment of eye conditions it has been shown to be as active as Betamethasone sodium phosphate, but has less adverse effects on intra-ocular pressure.
It has been shown to have little effect on hypothalamic-pituitary-adrenal function when used in the treatment of inflammatory skin conditions.
Pharmacokinetic properties: Not applicable for this use of clobetasone butyrate.

Preclinical safety data: No further relevant data.

Pharmaceutical particulars
List of excipients: Polyethylene glycol 300, Benzalkonium chloride, Sodium citrate, Citric acid monohydrate, Purified water.

Incompatibilities: None known.

Shelf life: Opened: 4 weeks. Unopened: 24 months.

Special precautions for storage: Store at a temperature not exceeding 25°C. Store upright. Replace in carton to protect from light.

Nature and contents of container: Bottle with nozzle insert moulded in natural low density polyethylene closed with a tamper evident high density polyethylene cap. Bottles containing 5 ml and 10 ml.

Instructions for use/handling: No special instructions are required.

Marketing authorisation number PL 10622/0014

Date of approval/revision of SPC November 1997

Legal Category POM

KALSPARE*

Qualitative and quantitative composition Chlorthalidone BP 50 mg, Triamterene BP 50 mg.

Pharmaceutical form Coated tablets.

Clinical particulars
Therapeutic indications: Management of mild to moderate hypertension. Oedema associated with congestive cardiac failure, nephrosis, corticosteroid or oestrogen therapy. Ascites associated with hepatic cirrhosis.

Posology and method of administration: Hypertension: Usually one tablet daily taken after breakfast. If necessary the dose may be increased to two tablets taken once daily. Oedema: The usual dose is one tablet daily taken after breakfast. If oedema persists after seven to ten days the dose may be increased to two tablets daily.
Dosage in children has not been established and Kalspare is recommended for the treatment of adults only.
The elderly may require a lower dosage schedule.

Contra-indications: Hypersensitivity to the individual components or to other sulphonamide-derived drugs. Progressive renal failure. Concomitant lithium therapy. Kalspare should not be used in the presence of hyperkalaemia (plasma potassium above 5.0 mmol/litre) or in patients receiving other potassium-sparing agents such as spironolactone or amiloride.

Special warnings and precautions: Caution should be exercised in patients with severe kidney disease, impaired liver function or progressive liver disease.
As with thiazide diuretics and chlorthalidone, treatment with Kalspare may result in hyperuricaemia or the precipitation of acute gout in certain patients.
Potassium supplements should not be given with Kalspare except in the presence of hypokalaemia.
Chlorthalidone has, in common with other sulphonamide diuretics, occasionally aggravated or precipitated diabetes mellitus. The effect is usually reversible on cessation of therapy.
Chlorthalidone and related drugs may decrease serum protein bound iodine levels without signs of thyroid disturbance.
Triamterene may cause a decreasing alkali reserve, with the possibility of metabolic acidosis.
Although no clinically significant hyperkalaemia has occurred in studies with Kalspare, all potassium conserving diuretic combinations can cause an abnormal elevation of plasma potassium. It is recommended that measurements of potassium are made at the time of dosage adjustments and at appropriate intervals during therapy, particularly in elderly or diabetic patients with confirmed or suspected renal insufficiency.
Signs or symptoms of hyperkalaemia include paresthesia, muscular weakness, fatigue, flaccid paralysis of the extremities, bradycardia, shock and ECG abnormalities. If hyperkalaemia occurs in patients taking Kalspare the drug should be withdrawn, a diuretic substituted and potassium intake restricted. If the plasma potassium level exceeds 6.5 mmol per litre, active measures should be taken to reduce it. Such measures include the intravenous administration of sodium bicarbonate solution or oral or parenteral glucose with a rapid-acting insulin preparation.
If progressive renal impairment becomes evident, Kalspare therapy should be withdrawn and alternative therapy instituted if necessary.

Interactions with other medicaments and other forms of interaction: Kalspare may add to or potentiate the action of other antihypertensive drugs. Any tendency to orthostatic hypotension on Kalspare treatment may be aggravated by concomitant alcohol, barbiturates or narcotics. Chlorthalidone and related drugs may increase the responsiveness to tubocurarine.

Pregnancy and lactation: Thiazide diuretics have been shown to cross the placenta and also to appear in breast milk. In rare instances, thrombocytopenia, pancreatitis or hypokalaemia have been reported in newborn infants of mothers treated with thiazide diuretics. The use of Kalspare in pregnant or nursing mothers should therefore be avoided unless essential.

Effects on ability to drive and use machines: None

Undesirable effects: Side effects are similar to those that have been associated with thiazide therapy and include nausea, dry mouth, constipation, leg cramp, headaches, dizziness and fatigue. Rare cases of megaloblastic anaemia have been reported in association with triamterene.

Overdosage: The stomach contents should be emptied immediately. Treatment should be symptomatic and supportive with correction of electrolyte imbalance and fluid depletion. No specific antidote exists for Kalspare.

Pharmacological properties
Pharmacodynamic properties: Kalspare is a long acting potassium sparing diuretic and antihypertensive of particular value in conditions where potassium conservation is important.
Chlorthalidone blocks the reabsorption of sodium and chloride in the cortical diluting segment of the nephron thereby increasing both the quantity of sodium delivered to the distal tubule and the volume of water excreted. However, a portion of the additional sodium reaching the distal tubule is exchanged at this site for potassium and hydrogen.
Triamterene is a weak diuretic found to spare potassium. It acts on the membrane of the lumen in the collecting duct of the kidney to inhibit the reabsorption of sodium and decrease the passive forces influencing the secretion of potassium and hydrogen.

Pharmacokinetic properties: Triamterene is incompletely but fairly rapidly absorbed from the gastrointestinal tract. It is extensively metabolised and mainly excreted in the urine as metabolites with some unchanged triamterene.
Chlorthalidone is also incompletely absorbed from the gastro-intestinal tract and is mainly excreted unchanged in the urine.
From a bioequivalence single dose study
Serum triamterene levels:
C max (ng/ml) mean: 67.05
T max (h) median: 1
Auc to 24 hours mean: 257.75

Urinary chlorthalidone levels:
Peak urinary excretion rate (mg/h) mean: 0.804
Time to peak urinary excretion rate (h) median: 3
Total amount excreted by 120 hours (mg) mean: 15.856
Auc to 120 hours mean: 15.85

Preclinical safety data: There are no pre-clinical data of relevance to the prescriber which are additional to that in other sections of the SPC.

Pharmaceutical particulars
List of excipients: Lactose BP, Starch BP, STA RX 1500 starch, Microcrystalline cellulose BP, Sodium starch glycollate BP, Magnesium stearate BP, Hypromellose, Polyethylene glycol 4000, Polyethylene glycol 400, Antifoam, Sodium propyl hydroxybenzoate BP, Carnauba wax BP, Titanium dioxide E171, Sunset Yellow E110.

Incompatibilities: None known

Shelf life: 36 months

Special precautions for storage: Store in a dry place, below 25°C.

Nature and contents of container: PVC/aluminium blister strips containing 4 or 14 tablets.
4 or 28 tablets (2 strips) are packed into cardboard cartons.

Instructions for use/handling: None stated.

Marketing authorisation number 10622/0019

Date of approval/revision of SPC January 1997

Legal category POM

LOMEXIN* PESSARY

Qualitative and quantitative composition Fenticonazole nitrate 200 mg or 600 mg.

Pharmaceutical form Pessary.

Clinical particulars
Therapeutic indications: Vulvovaginal candidiasis.

Contra-indications: Ascertained hypersensitivity to the product and other imidazole derivatives.

Side-effects: After intravaginal administration slight transient burning–which usually disappears rapidly–may occasionally occur.

Precautions: In the event of hypersensitivity reactions or development of resistant organisms, treatment should be discontinued and the physician consulted.

Use during pregnancy and lactation: Oral administration of fenticonazole in rats has been reported to produce prolonged gestation and embryotoxic effects after doses above 40 mg/kg/day. Fenticonazole does not interfere with the function of male and female gonads and does not modify the first phases of reproduction.
Fenticonazole has shown no teratogenic effects in rats and rabbits.
Fenticonazole or its metabolites cross the placental barrier in pregnant rats and rabbits after vaginal application and are excreted in milk of lactating rats.
Since there is no experience of use during pregnancy and lactation Lomexin should not be used unless the physician considers it essential to the welfare of the patient.

Interactions with other medicaments: Not yet investigated. Since fenticonazole systemic absorption after vaginal application is low, interactions with other drugs are unlikely to occur.

Dosage and administration: Adults: One 200 mg pessary at bedtime for 3 days, or one 600 mg pessary once only, at bedtime. The pessary must be introduced deep into the vagina.
Children: The use of Lomexin in children is not recommended.
Lomexin is not greasy, does not soil and can easily be removed with water.

Overdosage: Because of the low systemic absorption after vaginal application, overdosage is unlikely. In case of a suspected oral accidental ingestion emesis should be induced or gastric lavage may be attempted. Irrespective of success in inducing emesis make patient drink water or lemonade with active charcoal and a laxative. Symptomatic therapy may be administered if indicated.

Special warnings: Prolonged topical application may cause sensitisation reactions. The product should not be used in conjunction with barrier contraceptives.

Effects on driving ability and control of machinery: None

Pharmacological properties
Pharmacodynamic properties: Lomexin is a broad-spectrum antimycotic agent.
In vitro: high fungistatic and fungicidal activity against *Candida albicans.*
In vivo: healing of vaginal mycoses due to candida within 5 days in mice.

Pharmacokinetic properties: Pharmacokinetic studies in humans have shown that systemic absorption of fenticonazole nitrate after vaginal administration is minimal.

Preclinical safety data: In mice, rats and dogs, the oral LD_{50} values were 3000 mg/kg, 3000 mg/kg and 1000 mg/kg, respectively.
Long term oral administration to rats and dogs at and above 60 mg/kg/day has been reported to produce morphological and functional modifications of the liver, while cutaneous and ocular reactions were noticed in dogs only.
Fenticonazole has no mutagenic potential.
Satisfactory results were obtained in tolerability tests performed in rabbit, dog, guinea pig and mini-pig.
Fenticonazole has shown no evidence of phototoxicity and photoallergy.

Pharmaceutical particulars
List of excipients: Lomexin 200 mg: Triglycerides of saturated fatty acids, colloidal silicon dioxide, gelatin, glycerin, titanium dioxide, sodium ethyl hydroxybenzoate, sodium propyl hydroxybenzoate.
Lomexin 600 mg: Liquid paraffin, white soft paraffin, soya lecithin, gelatin, titanium dioxide, sodium ethyl hydroxybenzoate, sodium propyl hydroxybenzoate.

Incompatibilities: None

Shelf life: in integral package: 36 months.

Special precautions for storage: No special storage conditions are required.

Nature and contents of container:
200 mg Pessary: PVC/PVDC/aluminium foil blisters in packs of 3 pessaries
600 mg Pessary: PVC/PVDC/aluminium foil blisters in packs of 1 pessary

Marketing authorisation numbers
200 mg Pessary PL 10622/0024
600 mg Pessary PL 10622/0025

Date of approval/revision of SPC 9 March 1995

Legal category POM

LOTRIDERM* CREAM

Qualitative and quantitative composition Betamethasone Dipropionate USP 0.064% w/w, Clotrimazole USP 1.0% w/w.

Pharmaceutical form Cream.

Clinical particulars
Therapeutic indications: Short-term topical treatment of tinea infections due to *Trichophyton rubrum; T. mentagrophytes; Epidermophyton floccusum* and *Microsporum canis;* candidiasis due to *Candida albicans.*

Posology and method of administration:

Adults and children over the age of 12 years: Topical administration twice daily for two weeks (tinea cruris, tinea corporis and candidiasis) or for four weeks (tinea pedis).
Lotriderm cream is not recommended for children under the age of twelve years.

Contraindications: Lotriderm is contraindicated in those patients with a history of sensitivity to any of its components or to other corticosteroids or imidazoles.
If irritation or sensitisation develops with the use of Lotriderm cream, treatment should be discontinued and appropriate therapy instituted.
Lotriderm is contraindicated in facial rosacea, acne vulgaris, perioral dermatitis, napkin eruptions and bacterial or viral infections.

Special warnings and precautions: Local and systemic toxicity is common especially following long continued use on large areas of damaged skin and in flexures. If used in children or on the face, courses should be limited to 5 days. Long term continuous therapy should be avoided in all children irrespective of age. Lotriderm cream should not be used with adhesive dressing.
The safety and effectiveness of Lotriderm cream has not been established in children below the age of 12.
Lotriderm cream should not be used with occlusive dressing.
Topical corticosteroids may be hazardous in psoriasis for a number of reasons including rebound relapses following the development of tolerance, risk of generalised pustular psoriasis and local and systemic toxicity due to impaired barrier function of the skin.
Lotriderm Cream is not intended for ophthalmic use.

Interactions with other medicaments and other forms of interaction: There are no known interactions.

Pregnancy and lactation: There is inadequate evidence of safety in pregnancy. Clotrimazole has shown no teratogenic effect in animals but is foetotoxic at high oral doses.
Topical administration of corticosteroids to pregnant animals can cause abnormalities of foetal development including cleft palate and intra-uterine growth retardation. There may therefore be a very small risk of such effects in the human foetus. Hence Lotriderm Cream should only be used in pregnancy if the benefit justifies the potential risk to the foetus and such use should not be extensive i.e. in large amounts or for long periods.
It is not known whether the components of Lotriderm are excreted in human milk and therefore caution should be exercised when treating nursing mothers.

Effects on ability to drive and use machines: None known.

Undesirable effects: Adverse reactions reported for Lotriderm include: burning and stinging, maculopapular rash, oedema and secondary infection.
Reported reactions to clotrimazole include erythema, stinging, blistering, peeling, oedema, pruritus, urticaria and general irritation of the skin.
Reactions to betamethasone dipropionate include: burning, itching, irritation, dryness, folliculitis, hypertrichosis, acneiform eruptions, hyperpigmentation, perioral dermatitis, allergic contact dermatitis, maceration of the skin, secondary infection, skin atrophy, striae and miliaria.

Overdosage: Acute overdosage with topical application of Lotriderm Cream is unlikely and would not be expected to lead to a life-threatening situation; however topically applied corticosteroids can be absorbed in sufficient amounts to produce systemic effects.
Toxic effects are unlikely to occur following accidental ingestion of Lotriderm Cream. Signs of toxicity appearing after such accidental ingestion should be treated symptomatically.

Pharmacological properties
Pharmacodynamic properties: Lotriderm Cream contains the dipropionate ester of betamethasone, a glucocorticoid exhibiting the general properties of corticosteroids, and clotrimazole which is an imidazole antifungal agent.
Topical corticosteroids are effective in the treatment of a range of dermatoses because of their anti-inflammatory anti-pruritic and vasoconstrictive actions.
Clotrimazole is a broad-spectrum antifungal agent with activity against Trichomones, Staphylococci and Bacteroides.

Pharmacokinetic properties: Lotriderm is intended for treatment of skin conditions and is applied topically. Thus there are minimal pharmacokinetic aspects related to bioavailability at the site of action.
Clotrimazole penetrates the epidermis after topical administration but there is little, if any, systemic absorption.
The extent of percutaneous absorption of topical corticosteroids is determined by many factors including vehicle, integrity of skin and use of occlusion.
Systemically absorbed topical corticosteroids are bound to plasma proteins, metabolised in the liver and excreted by the kidneys. Some corticosteroids and their metabolites are also excreted in the bile.

Preclinical safety data: There are no pre-clinical data of relevance to the prescriber which are additional to that already included in other sections of this SmPC.

Pharmaceutical particulars
List of excipients: Liquid paraffin, white petroleum jelly, cetostearyl alcohol, cetomacrogol 1000, benzyl alcohol, sodium phosphate monobasic, phosphoric acid, sodium hydroxide, propylene glycol and purified water.

Incompatibilities: None known.

Shelf life: 48 months.

Special precautions for storage: Store at or below 25°C.

Nature and contents of container: The product is marketed in standard epoxy-lined aluminium tubes with low density polyethylene caps. Tubes contain 15 g.

Instructions for use/handling: There are no special instructions for use.

Marketing authorisation number PL 0201/0081

Date of approval/revision of SPC August 1997

Legal Category POM.

Product licence holder: Schering-Plough Ltd., Welwyn Garden City

MASNODERM* CREAM

Qualitative and quantitative composition Clotrimazole B.P. 1% w/w

Pharmaceutical form Topical cream

Clinical particulars
Therapeutic indications: For the treatment of skin infections due to dermatophytes (e.g. trycophyton species), yeasts (e.g. candida species), moulds and other fungi. These include ringworm (tinea) infections, athlete's foot, paronychia, pityriasis versicolor, erythrasma and intertrigo, as well as fungal nappy rash, candidal vaginitis and candidal balanitis.

Posology and method of administration:

Dosage: Adult, children and elderly: Apply to the affected area two or three times daily.

Dermatophyte infections: treat for at least one month

Candida infections: treat for at least two weeks.

Route of administration: Directly applied to the affected area.

Contraindications: Known hypersensitivity to any of the components.

Special warnings and precautions: None.

Interactions with other medicaments and other forms of interaction: None known.

Pregnancy and lactation: Use is not recommended during pregnancy and lactation.

Effects on ability to drive and use machines: None known.

Undesirable effects: Rarely patients may experience burning or irritation immediately after applying the cream. Rarely hypersensitivity reactions.

Overdosage: Accidental oral ingestion: in case of accidental oral ingestion, routine supportive measures such as gastric lavage should be performed as soon as possible.

Pharmacological properties
Pharmacodynamic properties: Clotrimazole is a broad spectrum imidazole antifungal agent which interferes with ergosterol synthesis and therefore alters the permeability of the cell membrane of sensitive fungi.

Pharmacokinetic properties: Not applicable.

Preclinical safety data: Not applicable.

Pharmaceutical particulars
List of excipients: Sorbitan monostearate, Polysorbate 60, Cetyl Esters Wax, Stearyl Alcohol, Cetyl Alcohol, 2-Octyldodecanol, Benzyl Alcohol, Purified Water.

Incompatibilities: None known.

Shelf life: 36 months.

Special precautions for storage: None.

Nature and contents of container: Aluminium tube with polypropylene screw-on cap containing 20 g of cream.

Instructions for use/handling: None.

Marketing authorisation number PL 10622/0004

Date of approval/revision of SPC January 1998

Legal category P

MODRASONE* CREAM
MODRASONE* OINTMENT

Qualitative and quantitative composition Alclometasone dipropionate 0.05% w/w.

Pharmaceutical form Cream/Ointment for topical use.

Clinical particulars
Therapeutic indications: Alclometasone dipropionate is a non-fluorinated topically active synthetic corticosteroid. Modrasone is indicated for the treatment of inflammatory and pruritic manifestations of corticosteroid responsive dermatoses.

Posology and method of administration:
Adult and children: A thin film of Modrasone should be applied to the affected area two or three times daily or as directed by the physician. Massage gently into the skin until the medication disappears.

Contra-indications: Hypersensitivity to any of the ingredients; rosacea; acne and perioral dermatitis; tuberculous and viral lesions of the skin, particularly Herpes Simplex; vaccinia; varicella.

Modrasone should not be used in fungal or bacterial skin infections.

Special warnings and precautions: As with all topical steroids, long term continuous therapy should be avoided where possible, particularly in infants and children as adrenal suppression may occur even without occlusion. In infants the napkin may act as an occlusive dressing and thus increase absorption.

Interactions with other medicaments and other forms of interaction: None known.

Pregnancy and lactation: Topical administration of corticosteroids to pregnant animals can cause abnormalities in foetal development. The relevance of this finding to human beings has not been established; however, topical steroids should not be used extensively in pregnancy i.e. in large amounts or for long periods.

It is not known whether topical administration of corticosteroids could result in sufficient systemic absorption to produce detectable quantities in breast milk. Modrasone should be administered to nursing mothers only after careful consideration of the benefit/risk relationship.

Effects on ability to drive and use machines: Not applicable.

Undesirable effects: Excessive prolonged use may result in local atrophy of the skin, striae and superficial vascular dilation, particularly on the face.

Overdosage: Excessive prolonged use of topical corticosteroids can suppress pituitary-adrenal function resulting in secondary adrenal insufficiency which is usually reversible. In such cases appropriate symptomatic treatment is indicated. In cases of chronic toxicity, corticosteroids should be withdrawn.

The steroid content is so low as to have little or no effect in the unlikely event of accidental oral ingestion.

Pharmacological properties
Pharmacodynamic properties: Alclometasone dipropionate is a non-fluorinated, topically active synthetic corticosteroid. Alclometasone dipropionate suppresses local inflammation at doses producing minimal systemic effects. Studies have shown alclometasone dipropionate to be approximately 2/3 as potent as betamethasone valerate and 60 x as potent as hydrocortisone.

Pharmacokinetic properties: Not applicable in view of topical action and application.

Preclinical safety data: Modrasone appears to be a relatively non-toxic and non-irritating drug product that produces no unusual or unexpected teratologic effects in laboratory animals. A wide margin of safety was demonstrated in all species studied. Acute oral and intraperitoneal doses more than 3,000 times the proposed topical human dose were without any toxicologically significant effects.

Pharmaceutical particulars
List of excipients: Cream: Propylene Glycol PhEur, White Soft Paraffin BP, Cetostearyl Alcohol BP, Glyceryl stearate PEG 100 stearate, Polyoxyethylene (20) cetyl ether, Sodium dihydrogenium phosphate dihydrate, 4-Chloro-M-Cresol BP, Phosphoric Acid Ph Eur, Purified Water PhEur.

Ointment: Hexylene glycol, Propylene glycol monostearate, White Beeswax BP, White Soft Paraffin BP.

Incompatibilities: None known

Shelf life: Cream and Ointment: 60 months

Special precautions for storage: Store below 25°C.

Nature and contents of container: Cream and Ointment: Aluminium tubes with white LDPE caps. Pack size: 50 g.

Instructions for use/handling: Not applicable.

Marketing authorisation numbers
Cream: PL 0201/0060
Ointment: PL 0201/0061

Date of approval/revision of SPC March 1996

Legal category POM

Product licence holder: Schering-Plough Ltd., Welwyn Garden City.

NEO-CORTEF* EYE/EAR DROPS
NEO-CORTEF* EYE/EAR OINTMENT

Qualitative and quantitative composition
Eye/Ear Drops: Hydrocortisone acetate 15 mg and neomycin sulphate 5 mg (equivalent to neomycin 3.5 mg) per ml.

Eye/Ear Ointment: Hydrocortisone acetate 15 mg and neomycin sulphate 5 mg (equivalent to neomycin 3.5 mg) per g.

Pharmaceutical form
Eye/Ear Drops
Eye/Ear Ointment

Clinical particulars
Therapeutic indications:
Eye: Short-term treatment of steroid responsive conditions of the eye when prophylactic antibiotic treatment is also required, after excluding the presence of fungal and viral disease.
Eyelid: Blepharitis
Ear: Otitis externa caused by susceptible organisms

Posology and method of administration:
Adults and children:
DROPS:
Eye: One or two drops to be applied to each eye up to six times daily or more frequently if required.

Ear: Two or three drops to be instilled into the ear three to four times daily.
OINTMENT:
Eye: Apply sparingly two or three times daily, or at night if drop treatment is given during the day.

Ear: Apply once or twice daily.

Elderly patients: There is no information to suggest that a change in dosage is warranted in the elderly, however care should be taken when the drops/ointment are administered in this group (see Special warnings and special precautions for use).

Do not exceed the recommended dose.

Contra-indications: Viral, fungal, tuberculous or purulent conditions of the eye. Use is contra-indicated if glaucoma is present or herpetic keratitis (eg dendritic ulcer) is considered a possibility.

Use of topical steroids in the latter condition can lead to extension of the ulcer and marked visual deterioration.

Otitis externa should not be treated when the eardrum is perforated because of the risk of ototoxicity.

Hypersensitivity to any of the ingredients of the preparation.

Special warnings and precautions: Topical corticosteroids should never be given for an undiagnosed red eye as inappropriate use is potentially blinding.

Treatment with corticosteroid/antibiotic combinations should not be continued for more than 7 days in the absence of any clinical improvement, since prolonged use may lead to occult extension of infection due to the masking effect of the steroid. Prolonged use may also lead to skin sensitisation and the emergence of resistant organisms.

Prolonged use may lead to the risk of adrenal suppression in infants.

Treatment with corticosteroid preparations should not be repeated or prolonged without regular review to exclude raised intra-ocular pressure, cataract formation or unsuspected infections.

Aminoglycoside antibiotics may cause irreversible, partial or total deafness when given systemically or when applied topically to open wounds or damaged skin. This effect is dose related and is enhanced by renal or hepatic impairment. Although this effect has not been reported following topical ocular use, the possibility should be considered when high dose topical treatment is given to small children or infants and patients suffering from renal impairment.

Care should also be taken when the drops/ointment are administered to the elderly and those with existing hearing loss.

Interactions with other medicaments and other forms of interaction: None relevant to ocular/aural use.

Pregnancy and lactation: Safety for use in pregnancy and lactation has not been established. There is inadequate evidence of safety in human pregnancy. Topical administration of corticosteroids to pregnant animals can cause abnormalities of foetal development including cleft palate and intra-uterine growth retardation. There may therefore be a very small risk of such effects in the human foetus. There is a risk of foetal ototoxicity if aminoglycoside antibiotic preparations are administered during pregnancy.

Effects on ability to drive and use machines: Transient blurring of vision on instillation or application. Warn patients not to drive or operate hazardous machinery unless vision is clear.

Undesirable effects: Hypersensitivity reactions, usually of the delayed type, may occur leading to irritation, burning, stinging, itching and dermatitis.

Topical steroid use may result in increased intraocular pressure leading to optic nerve damage, reduced visual acuity, and visual field defects.

In those diseases causing thinning of the cornea or sclera, corticosteroid therapy may result in thinning of the globe leading to perforation.

Overdosage: Long-term intensive topical use may lead to systemic effects.

Oral ingestion of the contents of one bottle is unlikely to lead to any serious adverse effects.

Pharmacological properties
Pharmacodynamic properties: Neomycin is an aminoglycoside antibiotic. It has activity against many Gram-negative bacteria (not *Pseudomonas* spp), and *Staphylococcus aureus*.

Hydrocortisone is a mild corticosteroid.

Pharmacokinetic properties: Activity is intended to be restricted locally to the eye/ear.

Preclinical safety data: There are no pre-clinical data of relevance to the prescriber which are additional to that in other sections of the SPC.

Pharmaceutical particulars
List of excipients:
Eye/Ear Drops: Sodium citrate, polyethylene glycol, myristyl gamma-picolinium chloride, povidone, water.
Eye/Ear Ointment: White soft paraffin, wool fat, liquid paraffin.

Incompatibilities: None known

Shelf life:
Eye/Ear Drops: 36 months
Eye/Ear Ointment: 48 months

Special precautions for storage:
Eye/Ear Drops: Store at room temperature below 25°C. Protect from freezing.
Eye/Ear Ointment: Store at room temperature below 25°C.

Nature and contents of container:
Eye/Ear Drops: Polyethylene squeeze bottle with applicator tip, containing 10 ml of sterile suspension.
Eye/Ear Ointment: Collapsible, internally lacquered tubes, containing 3.9 g ointment.

Instructions for use/handling:
Eye/Ear Drops: The contents are sterile whilst the bottle seal is intact. Discard one month after opening.
Eye/Ear Ointment: Discard one month after opening.

Marketing authorisation numbers
Eye/Ear Drops: PL 0032/5026
Eye/Ear Ointment: PL 0032/5027

Date of approval/revision of SPC December 1996

Legal category POM

Product licence holder: Pharmacia & Upjohn Limited, Milton Keynes

NEOSPORIN* EYE DROPS

Presentation A colourless to very pale yellow, slightly hazy solution. Each ml contains:

Polymyxin B Sulphate BP	5,000 units
Neomycin Sulphate BP	1,700 units
Gramicidin USP	25 units

Also contains Thiomersal BP (0.001%) as a preservative.

Uses Topical antibacterial agent. For the prophylaxis and treatment of external bacterial infections of the eye. Prophylactically, it is useful following removal of foreign bodies, and before and after ophthalmic surgery, to help provide and maintain a sterile field.

Dosage and administration *Adults and children:* 1 or 2 drops in the affected eye, two to four times daily or more frequently as required. In severe infections, therapy should be started with 1 or 2 drops every 15 to 30 minutes, reducing the frequency of instillation gradually as the infection is controlled.

Use in the elderly: No special comment.

Contra-indications, warnings, etc
Contra-indications: Hypersensitivity to polymyxins, gramicidin or neomycin group of antibiotics.

Precautions: Neomycin is ototoxic and nephrotoxic if absorbed from open surfaces. Polymyxin B and gramicidin are also nephrotoxic. However, these effects are unlikely with ocular administration.
Neosporin Eye Drops should not be used during surgical procedures nor before surgery in circumstances where access of the product to intra-ocular fluids could occur.

Side- and adverse effects: Allergic reactions following the topical application of neomycin have been reported in the literature, but such reactions following the application of polymyxin B and gramicidin are rare events.
As with all antibacterial preparations prolonged use may result in the overgrowth of non-susceptible organisms including fungi.

Use in pregnancy and lactation: Neosporin Eye Drops have been in use for many years. There has been no evidence of untoward effects in pregnancy. However, caution should be exercised by balancing the potential benefits of treatment against any possible hazard.
No information is available regarding the excretion of the active ingredients or their metabolites in human breast milk.

Toxicity and treatment of overdosage: Not applicable.

Pharmaceutical precautions Store below 15°C. Keep dry. Protect from light. Not suitable for injection. Discard four weeks after opening.

Legal category POM

Package quantities Special dropper bottle of 5 ml (OP).

Further information Neosporin is a non-irritating isotonic solution and is well tolerated by the sensitive structures of the eye.

Product licence number 0003/5108R

Product licence holder: The Wellcome Foundation Limited, Greenford, Middlesex.

OCUSERT*

Qualitative and quantitative composition
Ocusert Pilo 20: Pilocarpine USP 5.0 mg per unit.
Ocusert Pilo 40: Pilocarpine USP 11.0 mg per unit.

Pharmaceutical form Ocular inserts. Elliptically shaped units designed to release pilocarpine continuously following placement into the upper or lower conjunctival sac.
The systems consist of a core reservoir of pilocarpine surrounded by a membrane which controls the drug's diffusion from the system into the tear fluid. Two systems are available, Ocusert Pilo 20 and Ocusert Pilo 40, which release 20 and 40 micrograms per hour, respectively, for one week. The Ocusert Pilo 20 system is 5.7 x 13.4 mm across its axis, 0.3 mm thick and contains 5 mg pilocarpine: the Ocusert Pilo 40 system is 5.5 x 13 mm across its axis, 0.5 mm thick, and contains 11 mg pilocarpine. Except for the opaque white margin, the systems are clear.

Clinical particulars
Therapeutic indications: The Ocusert pilocarpine system is indicated for control of elevated intra-ocular pressure in glaucoma, in pilocarpine-responsive patients.

Posology and method of administration:
Route of administration: Placement in the conjunctival sac. Suitable for use with contact lenses.
Recommended doses and dosage schedules:
Adults and elderly: Initiation of therapy: The Ocusert Pilo 20 system will usually control a patient previously controlled by 1 per cent or 2 per cent pilocarpine eye drops; a patient who has used higher strengths of pilocarpine eye drops may require the Ocusert Pilo 40. However, there is no direct correlation between the two strengths of Ocusert and the strength of pilocarpine eye drops necessary to achieve the required reduction of pressure. The Ocusert systems reduce the amount of pilocarpine necessary to achieve adequate reduction of intra-ocular pressure; therapy may be started therefore with the Ocusert Pilo 20 system irrespective of the strength of pilocarpine eye drops used previously by the patient. If the pressure is satisfactorily reduced with the Ocusert Pilo 20 system the patient should continue with its use, replacing each unit every 7 days; if greater reduction of intra-ocular pressure is required, the patient should be transferred to the Ocusert Pilo 40 system. Depending on the patient's age, family history, and disease status, the ophthalmologist may elect to begin therapy with the Ocusert Pilo 40 system.
Concomitant therapy: Where necessary, adrenaline or timolol eye drops or a diuretic of the carbonic anhydrase inhibitor type may be used concurrently with Ocusert systems. The release rate of pilocarpine from the Ocusert system is not influenced by the beta adrenoceptor antagonists, carbonic anhydrase inhibitors, adrenaline eye drops, fluorescein or local anaesthetics, antibiotics or anti-inflammatory steroid eye drops.
Placement and removal of the Ocusert systems: Patient instructions for the replacement of the Ocusert systems in the eye and their removal are included in each package. It is strongly recommended that the patient's ability to manage the placement and removal of the system be reviewed at the first patient visit after initiation of therapy.
Since pilocarpine-induced myopia from the Ocusert system may occur during the first few hours of therapy, the patient should be advised to place the system into the conjunctival sac at bedtime. By morning the induced myopia is at a stable level.
Handling precautions: Patients should be instructed to wash their hands thoroughly with soap and water before touching or manipulating the Ocusert systems. If a displaced unit contacts unclean surfaces, rinsing with cool tap water before replacing is advisable. Bacteriologically contaminated units should be discarded and replaced with fresh ones.
Retention in the eye: During the initial adaptation period, the Ocusert unit may slip out of the conjunctival sac to the cheek. The patient is usually aware of such movement and can replace the unit without difficulty. In those patients in whom retention of the Ocusert is a problem, placement in the upper conjunctival sac may be more acceptable. The Ocusert unit can be manipulated from the lower to the upper conjunctival sac by a gentle digital massage through the lid, a technique readily learned by the patient. For best retention, the unit should be moved before sleep to the upper conjunctival sac. Should the unit slip out of the conjunctival sac during sleep, its ocular hypotensive effect continues for a period of time comparable to that following instillation of eye drops. The patient should be instructed to check for the presence of the Ocusert unit before sleep and on rising.
Children: Not recommended.

Contra-indications: Ocusert systems are contra-indicated where pupillary constriction is undesirable, such as glaucomas associated with acute inflammatory disease of the anterior segment of the eye, and glaucomas occurring or persisting after extra-capsular cataract extraction where posterior synechiae may occur.

Special warnings and precautions: Ocusert systems should not be used in patients with acute infectious conjunctivitis or keratitis except on specialist advice. Damaged or deformed systems should not be placed or retained in the eye. Systems believed to be associated with an unexpected increase in drug action should be removed and replaced with new systems.
The safety of Ocusert systems in patients with retinal detachment or with filtration blebs has not been established.
Although withdrawal of the peripheral iris from the anterior chamber angle by miosis may reduce the tendency for narrow angle closure, miotics can occasionally precipitate angle closure by increasing the resistance to aqueous flow from posterior to anterior chamber. Miotic agents may also cause retinal detachment; thus, care should be exercised with all miotic therapy especially in young myopic patients.
The use of pilocarpine eye drops should be considered when intense miosis is desired in certain ocular conditions.

Interaction with other medicaments and other forms of interaction: Although eye drops have been used effectively in conjunction with the Ocusert systems, systemic reactions consistent with an increased rate of absorption from the eye of an automotive drug, such as adrenaline, have been observed. In rare instances, reactions of this type can be severe. The conjunctival erythema and oedema associated with adrenaline eye drops are not substantially altered by concomitant use of an Ocusert system.

Pregnancy and lactation: Pilocarpine has no known effect on pregnancy and lactation.

Effect on the ability to drive and use machines: The effect of Pilocarpine on visual accommodation may affect the patient's ability to drive and use machinery.

Undesirable effects: Ciliary spasm is encountered with Pilocarpine usage but is not a contra-indication to continued therapy unless the induced myopia is debilitating to the patient. Irritation from Pilocarpine has been infrequently encountered and may require cessation of therapy depending on judgement of the doctor. True allergic reactions are uncommon, but require discontinuation of therapy if they occur.
Some patients may notice signs of conjunctival irritation including mild erythema with or without a slight increase in mucous secretion when they first use Ocusert systems. These signs tend to lessen or disappear after the first week of therapy. In rare instances a sudden increase in pilocarpine effect has been reported.

Overdose: Patients are unlikely to experience pilocarpine overdosage with the use of the Ocusert system.

Pharmacological properties
Pharmacodynamic properties: Pilocarpine is released from the Ocusert system as soon as it is placed in contact with the conjunctival surfaces. Pilocarpine is a direct acting parasympathomimetic drug which produces pupillary constriction, stimulates the ciliary muscle and increased aqueous humour outflow facility.

Pharmacokinetic properties: The ocular hypotensive effect of both the Ocusert Pilo 20 and Ocusert Pilo 40 systems is fully developed within 1½ to 2 hours after placement in the conjunctival sac and is maintained for 24 hours a day for seven days.

Preclinical safety data: Not applicable.

Pharmaceutical particulars
List of excipients: Alginic acid, Ethylene vinyl acetate, Titanium dioxide. Ocusert Pilo 40 also contains Di (2-Ethylhexyl) phthalate.

Incompatibilities: None known.

Shelf life: 36 months.

Special precautions for storage: Ocusert Pilo 20/40 should be stored in a refrigerator at 2–8°C.

Nature and contents of container: Containers of 1, 2, 4 or 8 inserts (sterile units).

Instructions for use/handling: None.

Marketing authorisation numbers
Ocusert Pilo 20 10622/0012
Ocusert Pilo 40 10622/0013

Date of approval/revision of SPC 25 April 1997

Legal category POM

PERCUTOL*

Qualitative and quantitative composition The active ingredient of Percutol is glyceryl trinitrate 2% w/w.

Pharmaceutical form A homogeneous cream coloured ointment.

Clinical particulars
Therapeutic indications: Prophylaxis of angina pectoris.

Posology and method of administration: Topical application.
Adults (including elderly): The usual dose is 1 to 2 inches squeezed from the tube, although some patients may require more. This dose may be repeated every 3 to 4 hours as required.

The dose may be titrated to individual patients' needs by finding the dose that causes headache and then reducing this dose by half an inch. Half an inch of ointment should be applied on the first day, one inch on the second, etc. increasing by half an inch per day until headache occurs and then reducing by half an inch. If several applications per day are required the dose may need to be reduced.

The ointment may be conveniently measured and applied using the paper "Applirules" enclosed in the carton. After squeezing the required length of ointment onto the "Applirule" it should be pressed on to any convenient area of skin (e.g. chest, thigh, or arm) until the ointment is spread in a thin layer under the paper. The ointment should not be rubbed in. The "Applirule" may be secured in place with surgical tape.

Children: The safety and efficacy of Percutol in children has not been established.

Contra-indications: May be contra-indicated in patients with marked anaemia, or raised intra cranial pressure. Should not be employed in patients with known idiosyncrasies to nitrates.

Special warnings and precautions: In the elderly the development of postural hypotension may be more pronounced especially on sudden rising. Caution should be exercised in patients with cerebrovascular disease. As with other vasodilators chronic therapy should not be discontinued abruptly. The frequency of application and the dosage should gradually be reduced (over a period of 4 to 6 weeks).

Interactions with other medicaments and other forms of interaction: Some effects of glyceryl trinitrate are enhanced by alcohol.

Pregnancy and lactation: The safety of Percutol in pregnancy is not established. The product should therefore be given during pregnancy, only if clearly needed. It is not known whether glyceryl trinitrate is excreted in human milk, therefore caution should be exercised when administered to a nursing mother.

Effects on ability to drive and use machines: Glyceryl trinitrate may cause dizziness. In consequence until the effect of treatment is known, patients should be warned not to take charge of vehicles or machinery.

Undesirable effects: Headache, flushing, dizziness or postural hypotension.

Overdosage: A hypotensive headache is a sign of overdosage. High doses of glyceryl trinitrate may cause marked hypotension and collapse, however topical application reduces the likelihood of overdosage and the effect can be quickly terminated by washing the ointment off the skin.

Pharmacological properties
Pharmacodynamic properties: The active ingredient relaxes smooth muscle and reduces blood pressure. Its use as a vasodilator in the prophylaxis and treatment of angina pectoris is well established.

Pharmacokinetic properties: In human volunteers the mean absorption of glyceryl trinitrate from 1 inch of ointment was 0.8 mg/hour.

Preclinical safety data: There are no preclinical data of relevance to the prescriber which are additional to that already included in other sections of the SPC.

Pharmaceutical particulars
List of excipients: Percutol also contains lanolin anhydrous USP, purified water USP, white petroleum USP, and lactose anhydrous USP.

Incompatibilities: None stated.

Shelf life: 36 months.

Special precautions for storage: Store below 25°C.

Nature and contents of container: Collapsible aluminium tube containing 60 g.

Instructions for use/handling: None stated.

Marketing authorisation number PL 10622/0046

Date of approval/revision of SPC July 1998

Legal category P

POLYFAX* OINTMENT

Presentation Polyfax Ointment contains 10,000 units of Polymyxin B Sulphate BP and 500 units of Zinc Bacitracin BP per gram, in a stable petrolatum base. The translucent ointment is off-white in colour.

Uses Topical antibacterial agent. Polyfax Ointment is indicated for the treatment of infected wounds, burns, skin grafts, ulcers, pyoderma, sycosis barbae, impetigo, and in secondarily infected skin lesions of scabies, pediculosis, tinea pedis and contact and allergic dermatitis.

Dosage and administration
Adults: Polyfax Ointment should be applied thinly over the affected area, which is best left exposed. Two or more applications a day may be necessary, depending on the severity of the condition.

Children: As for adults.

Use in the elderly: No specific studies have been carried out in the elderly, however it may be advisable to monitor renal function in these patients and if there is any impairment then caution should be exercised.

Contra-indications, warnings, etc
Contra-indications: Hypersensitivity to bacitracin, polymyxins or cross-sensitising substances.

Precautions: The following statements take into account the possibility that the constituent drugs of Polyfax Ointment may be absorbed to a significant degree after topical application. However, the normal use of Polyfax is unlikely to present any risk of systemic toxicity unless the application were excessive eg more than 200 g per day in adults or proportionately less in children and in patients with compromised renal function.

Nephrotoxicity may result from the absorption of bacitracin, and nephrotoxicity and neurotoxicity from polymyxin B.

As with all antibacterial preparations prolonged use may result in the overgrowth of non-susceptible organisms including fungi.

Side- and adverse effects: Allergic reactions following topical application of polymyxin B and zinc bacitracin have rarely been reported.

Anaphylactic reactions have been reported, as rare events, following topical application of zinc bacitracin. Following significant systemic absorption, polymyxin B can intensify and prolong the respiratory depressant effects of neuromuscular blocking agents.

Use in pregnancy and lactation: Due to a lack of detailed information, the use of Polyfax Ointment during pregnancy and lactation cannot be recommended in circumstances where significant systemic absorption of the active ingredients may occur.

No information is available regarding the excretion of the active ingredients or their metabolites in human milk.

Toxicity and treatment of overdosage: In the unlikely event of significant systemic absorption of the active ingredients of Polyfax Ointment occurring, signs of neurotoxicity and nephrotoxicity may be noted. In such an event, the patient's general status and renal function should be monitored and blood levels of polymyxin B and zinc bacitracin determined.

Pharmaceutical precautions Store below 25°C.

Legal category POM

Package quantities Tube of 20 g (OP)

Further information Nil

Product licence number 0003/5230

Product licence holder: The Wellcome Foundation Limited, Greenford, Middlesex.

POLYFAX* OPHTHALMIC OINTMENT

Qualitative and quantitative compositions 10K IU Polymyxin B Sulphate EP, 500 IU Bacitracin Zinc EP

Pharmaceutical form Ointment

Clinical particulars
Therapeutic indications: Polyfax Ophthalmic Ointment is indicated for the treatment of bacterial infections of the eye and its adnexa, including conjunctivitis, keratitis, corneal ulceration and ulcerative blepharitis.

Polyfax Ophthalmic Ointment may be applied both pre- and post-operatively to prevent ocular infection following surgical procedures, including the removal of foreign bodies from the eye.

The use of Polyfax does not exclude concomitant systemic therapy or other forms of local therapy where appropriate.

Posology and method of administration:
Adults: A thin film of ointment should be applied to the affected part or inside of the lower eyelid two or more times a day depending on the severity of the condition.

Treatment should be continued until at least two days after the eye has apparently recovered.

Children: As for adults.

Use in the elderly: No special comment.

Contra-indications: Hypersensitivity to bacitracin, polymyxin B sulphate or cross-sensitising substances.

Special warnings and special precautions for use: Ocular administration of Polyfax Ophthalmic Ointment is extremely unlikely to lead to significant absorption of the constituents and therefore present no risk of systemic toxicity.

Interaction with other medicaments and other forms of interaction: None known.

Pregnancy and lactation: Polyfax has been used for several years without any untoward effect in pregnancy. The clinical benefit of the treatment to the patient must be balanced against any possible but unknown hazards to the developing foetus. No information is available regarding the excretion of the active ingredients or their metabolites in human milk.

Undesirable effects: Allergic reactions following topical (dermatological) application of polymyxin B and bacitracin zinc is rare but has been reported.

As with other antibacterial preparations, prolonged use may result in the overgrowth of non-susceptible organisms, including fungi.

Overdose: Not applicable

Pharmacological properties
Pharmacodynamic properties: Polymyxin B sulphate and bacitracin zinc are both bactericidal antibiotics. The former exerts its action by binding with the cellular membrane and the latter by inhibiting bacterial cell wall development.

It has been shown in animal studies that both polymyxin B sulphate and bacitracin zinc may be absorbed into the aqueous humour following topical application to the eye, especially in circumstances where the cornea is either abraded or inflamed.

In vitro activity: Gram positive: Species of staphylococcus; streptococcus, including
S. Pyogenes (B haemolytic streptococcus) and *S. Pneumoniae* (Pneumococcus); and corynebacterium.
Gram negative: Species of pseudomonas (including *P. Aeruginosa*), haemophilus, klebsiella. enterobacter, escherichia and neisseria.

Pharmaceutical particulars
List of excipients: White Petrolatum USP.

Incompatibilities: None known.

Shelf life: 5 years.

Special precautions for storage: Store below 25°C.

Nature and contents of container: Pack size 4 g. Laminate ophthalmic ointment tubes with polyolefin screw caps.

Instructions for use/handling: No special instructions.

Marketing authorisation number PL 0003/5229R

Date of approval/revision of SPC April 1996

Legal category POM

Product licence holder: The Wellcome Foundation Limited, Greenford, Middlesex.

POLYTRIM* EYE DROPS

Presentation A clear, colourless, sterile, aqueous solution containing in each ml Trimethoprim BP 1 mg and Polymyxin B Sulphate BP 10,000 units. Thiomersal BP (0.05 mg per ml) is included as a preservative.

Uses Antibacterial agent. For the treatment and prophylaxis of external bacterial infections of the eye including conjunctivitis, keratitis, corneal ulceration, ulcerative blepharitis with associated conjunctivitis, and chronic dacryocystitis. Prophylactically, it is useful following removal of foreign bodies, and before and after ophthalmic surgery to help provide and maintain a sterile field. Use of Polytrim does not exclude concomitant systemic therapy or other forms of local therapy, where appropriate.

Dosage and administration
Adults and children: 1 drop in affected eye four times daily. More frequent administration may be required, depending on the severity of the condition. Treatment should normally be continued for at least forty-eight hours after the eye has apparently returned to normal.

Use in the elderly: No special precautions.

Contra-indications, warnings, etc
Contra-indications: Contra-indicated in individuals who have a history of hypersensitivity to trimethoprim, polymyxins, or cross-sensitising substances, such as the polypeptide group of antibiotics.

Precautions: As with all antibacterial preparations, prolonged use may result in the overgrowth of non-susceptible organisms including fungi.

Side- and adverse effects: Polytrim is isotonic with tear fluid and is well tolerated in the eye. No local adverse effects are to be expected except, rarely, a hypersensitivity reaction. If one is suspected during treatment, administration should be discontinued.

Use in pregnancy and lactation: The active ingredients of Polytrim Eye Drops have been used for several years without any evidence of untoward effect in pregnancy, however the clinical benefit of treatment to the patient must be balanced against any possible hazard to the developing foetus.

No information is available regarding the excretion of polymyxin B sulphate or its metabolites in human breast milk.

Trimethoprim is excreted in breast milk following *systemic* administration but this presents a negligible risk to the suckling infant. No information, however, is available on the excretion of trimethoprim or its metabolites in human breast milk following topical application.

Toxicity and treatment of overdosage: Not applicable.

Pharmaceutical precautions Do not use if the container seal has been broken. Use within one month of opening container. Store below 25°C, and protect from light. Not suitable for injection.

Legal category POM

Package quantities Screw-capped plastic dropper bottle containing 5 ml (OP).

Further information The combination is effective against a wide variety of Gram-positive and Gram-negative bacterial ocular pathogens, including *Pseudomonas aeruginosa.*

Product licence number 0003/0153

Product licence holder: The Wellcome Foundation Limited, Greenford, Middlesex.

POLYTRIM* OPHTHALMIC OINTMENT

Presentation A white to off-white sterile ointment containing Trimethoprim BP 0.5% w/w and Polymyxin B Sulphate BP 10,000 units per gram in a sterile, anhydrous, soft paraffin base.

Uses An antibacterial agent for the treatment and prophylaxis of external bacterial infections of the eye and surrounding tissues including conjunctivitis, keratitis, corneal ulceration, ulcerative blepharitis with associated conjunctivitis, and chronic dacryocystitis. Prophylactically, it can be used following removal of foreign bodies, and before and after ophthalmic surgery to help provide and maintain a sterile field.

Dosage and administration
Dosage in adults: Apply a thin film of ointment either directly to the affected part or inside the lower conjunctival sac 3 to 4 times a day depending on the severity of the condition.

Dosage in children: As for adults. Suitable for use in subjects of all ages including infants.

Treatment should normally be continued until at least forty-eight hours after the eye has apparently returned to normal. Debris such as crusts or pus should be removed prior to application of the ointment.

Use in the elderly: No special studies have been carried out in the elderly, although no special precautions are expected to be applied to this group.

Contra-indications, warnings, etc
Contra-indications: Contra-indicated in individuals who have a history of hypersensitivity to trimethoprim or to polymyxins.

Precautions: As with all antibacterial preparations prolonged use may result in the overgrowth of non-susceptible organisms including fungi.

Side- and adverse effects: Rarely, hypersensitivity reactions may occur. If one is suspected during treatment, administration should be discontinued.

Use in pregnancy and lactation: There is no evidence of safety of Polytrim Ophthalmic Ointment in human pregnancy, however the active ingredients have been in use for many years without apparent ill consequence. In high systemic dosage (40 times the human systemic dose), trimethoprim had been shown to be teratogenic in rats. Although topical application is unlikely to be associated with risk, the clinical benefit of treatment to the patient must be balanced against any possible but unknown hazards to the developing foetus.

No information is available on the excretion of polymyxin in breast milk.

Excretion of trimethoprim into breast milk has been noted after oral administration to lactating women, but this represents a negligible risk to the suckling infant.

Toxicity and treatment of overdosage: Not applicable.

Pharmaceutical precautions Do not use if the container seal has been broken. Use within one month of opening container. Store below 25°C.

Legal category POM

Package quantities Tubes of 4 g (OP).

Further information The combination is effective against a wide variety of Gram-positive and Gram-negative bacterial ocular pathogens, including *Pseudomonas aeruginosa,* but not *Neisseria gonorrhoeae.*

Product licence number 0003/0223

Product licence holder: The Wellcome Foundation Limited, Greenford, Middlesex.

**Trade Mark*

Dumex Limited
at Cox Pharmaceuticals
Whiddon Valley
Barnstaple
North Devon EX32 8NS

☎ 01271 311200 ▯ 01271 346106

DUMEX

ANTABUSE*

Presentation White scored tablet marked DUMEX 110L. Each tablet contains 200 mg Disulfiram BP. Inactive ingredients include lactose.

Uses Alcoholic deterrent compound. Antabuse is indicated as an adjuvant in the treatment of carefully selected and co-operative patients with drinking problems. Its use should be supported by appropriate supportive treatment.

Dosage and administration

Adults and the elderly: It is recommended that treatment with Antabuse should be initiated only in a hospital or specialised clinic and by physicians experienced in its use.

On the first day of treatment: 4 tablets as a single dose. The second day: 3 tablets, followed on the third day by 2 tablets and on each of the fourth and fifth days by 1 tablet. Subsequently, 1 or half a tablet daily for the duration of the treatment. Treatment should not be continued for longer than six months without review.

In the routine management of the alcoholic an alcoholic challenge test is not recommended. If it is considered that this test is necessary for the success of the therapy, this should be carried out in a specialised unit by physicians acquainted with the procedure since severe reactions can occur. Full resuscitation facilities should be immediately available.

Children: Not applicable.

Contra-indications, warnings, etc

Contra-indications: Antabuse is contra-indicated in the presence of cardiac failure, coronary artery disease, previous history of CVA, hypertension, severe personality disorder, suicidal risk or psychosis.

Warnings/precautions: Caution should be exercised in the presence of renal failure, hepatic or respiratory disease, diabetes mellitus and epilepsy.

Before initiating treatment it is advised that appropriate examinations should be carried out to establish the suitability of the patient for treatment. Patients must not have taken alcohol for at least 24 hours prior to initiation of Antabuse therapy, during treatment or for 1 week after cessation of treatment with Antabuse. Patients should be warned of the unpredictable and potentially severe nature of an Antabuse-alcohol reaction as in rare cases deaths have been reported following the drinking of alcohol by patients receiving Antabuse. Personnel involved in administration of therapy should be made aware that disulfiram should not be given during a drinking episode. Adequate social and family support to avoid ingestion of alcohol should be available.

Liquid medicines, remedies, tonics and foods may contain sufficient alcohol to elicit an Antabuse-alcohol reaction and patients should be made aware of this.

Use in pregnancy and lactation: The use of disulfiram in the first trimester of pregnancy is not advised. The risk/benefit ratio in assessing adverse effects of alcoholism in pregnancy should be taken into account when considering the use of disulfiram in pregnancy.

There have been rare reports of congenital abnormalities in infants whose mothers have received disulfiram in conjunction with other medicines.

No information is available on whether disulfiram is excreted in breastmilk. Its use during breast feeding is not advised.

Drug interactions: Antabuse may potentiate the toxic effects of warfarin, antipyrine, phenytoin, chlordiazepoxide and diazepam by inhibiting their metabolism. The intensity of the Antabuse-alcohol reaction may be increased by amitriptyline and decreased by diazepam. Chlorpromazine, while decreasing certain components of the Antabuse-alcohol reaction, may increase the overall intensity. Disulfiram inhibits the oxidation and renal excretion of rifampicin. Animal studies have indicated similar inhibition of metabolism of pethidine, morphine and amphetamines. A few case reports of increased confusion and changes in affective behaviour have been noted with the concurrent administration of metronidazole, isoniazid or paraldehyde. Potentiation of organic brain syndrome with amitriptyline and choreoathetosis following pimozide have occurred very rarely.

Side-effects: During initial treatment, drowsiness and fatigue may occur. Nausea, vomiting, halitosis and reduction in libido have been reported. If side-effects are marked the dosage may be reduced. Psychotic reactions, including depression, paranoia, schizophrenia and mania occur rarely in patients receiving Antabuse. There are occasional reports of allergic dermatitis, peripheral neuritis and hepatic cell damage.

Treatment of Antabuse-alcohol reaction: Antabuse interferes with the metabolism of alcohol and leads to an accumulation of acetaldehyde in the bloodstream. The Antabuse-alcohol reaction can occur within 10 minutes of ingestion of alcohol and may last several hours. It is characterised by violent flushing, dyspnoea, headache, palpitations, tachycardia, nausea and vomiting.

Intensive supportive therapy should be available in the event of severe reaction to alcohol. Oxygen should be available and supportive measures may be necessary to counteract hypotension.

Severe vomiting may occur which may require administration of intravenous fluids.

Overdosage and treatment of overdose: Antabuse has low toxicity. Ingestion of quantities of up to 25 g have resulted in central and peripheral neurological symptoms which have resolved without sequelae. Treatment should be symptomatic; gastric lavage and observation are recommended.

Pharmaceutical precautions Keep tightly closed, protect from light.

Legal category POM.

Package quantities Pack of 50 tablets.

Further information Antabuse is rapidly absorbed from the gastro-intestinal tract but is very slowly eliminated and may be detected in body fluids up to seven days after cessation of administration.

Product licence number 4938/0011.

DIAZEMULS*

Presentation Ampoules of a white, opaque emulsion containing Diazepam BP 10 mg in 2 ml.

Uses *Action:* Diazepam is a potent anxiolytic, anticonvulsant and central muscle relaxant mediating its effects mainly via the limbic system as well as the polysynaptic spinal reflexes. The formulation of diazepam in an oil-in-water emulsion similar to Intralipid reduces the incidence of local pain and thrombophlebitis after injection.

Indications:

1. Sedation prior to procedures such as endoscopy, dentistry, cardiac catheterisation and cardioversion.
2. Premedication prior to anaesthesia.
3. Control of acute muscle spasm due to tetanus or poisoning.
4. Control of convulsions; status epilepticus.
5. Management of severe acute anxiety or agitation including delirium tremens.

Dosage and administration Diazemuls may be administered by slow intravenous injection (1 ml per min), or by continuous infusion. Diazemuls should be drawn up into the syringe immediately prior to administration.

1. *Sedation:* 0.1–0.2 mg diazepam/kg body weight by iv injection. The normal adult dose is 10–20 mg, but dosage should be titrated to the patient's response.

2. *Premedication:* 0.1–0.2 mg diazepam/kg body weight by iv injection. Dosage should be titrated to the patient's response. In this indication, prior treatment with diazepam leads to a reduction in fasciculations and postoperative myalgia associated with the use of suxamethonium.

3. *Tetanus:* 0.1–0.3 mg diazepam/kg body weight by iv injection repeated every 1–4 hours as required. Alternatively, a continuous infusion (see below) of 3–10 mg/kg body weight every 24 hours may be used.

4. *Status epilepticus:* An initial dose of 0.15–0.25 mg/kg body weight by iv injection repeated in 30 to 60 minutes if required, and followed if necessary by infusion (see below) of up to 3 mg/kg body weight over 24 hours.

5. *Anxiety and tension, acute muscle spasm, acute states of excitation, delirium tremens:* The usual dose is 10 mg repeated at intervals of 4 hours, or as required.

Elderly or debilitated patients: Elderly or debilitated patients are particularly sensitive to benzodiazepines. Dosage should initially be reduced to one half of the normal recommendations.

If a continuous infusion is required Diazemuls may be added to 5% or 10% dextrose solution to achieve a final diazepam concentration within the range 0.1–0.4 mg/ml (i.e. 2–8 ml Diazemuls per 100 ml dextrose solution). A dextrose solution containing added Diazemuls should be used within 6 hours of the admixture. Diazemuls can be mixed in all proportions with Intralipid 10% or 20% but not with saline solutions. It can be injected into the infusion tube during an ongoing infusion of isotonic saline or dextrose solution 5% or 10%. As with other diazepam injections, adsorption may occur to plastic infusion equipment. This adsorption occurs at a lesser degree with Diazemuls than with aqueous diazepam injection preparations when mixed with dextrose solutions.

Contra-indications, warnings, etc As with other benzodiazepine preparations:

1. Should not be used in phobic or obsessional states since there is inadequate evidence of efficacy and safety.
2. Should not be used in the treatment of chronic psychosis.

Warnings and precautions:

1. Treatment with diazepam may cause drowsiness and increase the patient's reaction time. This should be considered in situations where alertness is required, e.g. driving a car.
2. Use with caution in patients with impairment of renal or hepatic function and in patients with pulmonary insufficiency or myasthenia gravis.
3. Should not be used alone to treat depression or anxiety associated with depression.
4. Amnesia may occur. In cases of loss or bereavement psychological adjustment may be inhibited by benzodiazepines.
5. Disinhibiting effects may be manifested in various ways. Suicide may be precipitated in patients who are depressed and aggressive behaviour toward self and others may be precipitated. Extreme caution should therefore be used in prescribing benzodiazepines in patients with personality disorders.
6. Physiological and psychological symptoms of withdrawal including depression may be associated with discontinuation of benzodiazepines even after normal therapeutic doses for short periods of time.

Interactions with other medicaments: Concomitant use of central nervous system depressants, e.g. alcohol, general anaesthetics, narcotic analgesics, or antidepressants, including MAOI's will result in accentuation of their sedative effects. When Diazemuls is combined with centrally depressant drugs administered parenterally, severe respiratory and cardiovascular depression may occur. It is recommended that Diazemuls is administered following the analgesic, and that the dose should be carefully titrated to the patient's response. Diazepam clearance is increased by concomitant administration of phenobarbitone, and is decreased by administration of cimetidine.

Use in pregnancy: Diazepam crosses the placenta and should not be used during pregnancy. Maternal doses administered during delivery may produce clinical effects in the newborn, for example hypotonia and hypothermia.

Lactation: Diazepam can be transmitted in breast milk and clinical effects may occur in the breast-fed infant.

Diazemuls should be administered during lactation only if considered essential.

Side-effects: This formulation may rarely cause local pain or thrombophlebitis in the vein used for administration.

Rare instances have been reported of a local painless erythematous rash around the site of injection, which has resolved in 1–2 days. Urticaria and, rarely, anaphylaxis have been reported following the injection of Diazemuls.

Overdosage: CNS depression and coma. Treatment symptomatic.

Pharmaceutical precautions For full information on admixture see dosage and administration. Diazemuls should only be mixed in the same container or syringe with dextrose solution 5% or 10% or Intralipid 10% or 20%. The contents of the ampoule should not be mixed with any drugs other than the infusion solutions mentioned above. Store at room temperature. Do not freeze.

Legal category CD (Sch 4), POM.

Package quantities Boxes of 10×2 ml ampoules.

Further information During prolonged administration, for example in the treatment of tetanus, the plasma concentration of desmethyldiazepam, the main (and similarly potent) active metabolite of diazepam, may exceed that of the parent compound. Accordingly, there is a risk of accumulation and prolonged CNS depression if the dosage is not reduced following continuous administration for 5–7 days.

The clinician should be aware that intravenous sedation is associated with a significant incidence of anterograde and retrograde amnesia.

Product licence number 10183/0001.

DUMICOAT* DENTURE LACQUER

Presentation Dumicoat denture lacquer contains miconazole 50 mg/g. Each bottle contains 1 g of denture lacquer. After application to the upper surface of the upper denture, the lacquer forms a film, which slowly releases miconazole during the course of a week.

Uses Dumicoat denture lacquer is to be used in the treatment of Candida-associated denture stomatitis. Miconazole is an imidazole antifungal active against Candida spp., e.g. C. albicans, dermatophytes, Aspergillus spp., and Pityrosporon spp.

Kinetics: Miconazole is incompletely absorbed from the gastrointestinal tract after oral ingestion, the bioavailability being about 25–30%.

The apparent volume of distribution is about 1400 L. More than 90% of the drug is bound to plasma proteins. Miconazole is metabolised in the liver to inactive metabolites, with less than 1% excreted unchanged in the urine. About 50% of an oral dose may be recovered, mainly unchanged in the faeces. The elimination half-life is 20–25 hours.

Dosage and administration

Adults: One gram of denture lacquer (content of one bottle) is applied to the upper surface of the upper denture 3 times with weekly intervals. It may be necessary to repeat the treatment after a time.

Before each application, the denture must be cleaned thoroughly, as described in the directions for use. The lacquer is applied with a brush to the upper surface of the denture down to the rim of the teeth. When the lacquer is dry, the denture may be replaced in the mouth. It should be noted that the lacquer is not suitable for use with soft linings, nor to be used with poorly fitting dentures.

Use in the elderly: As for adults.

Contra-indications, warnings, etc

Contra-indications: There are no known contra-indications to the use of miconazole denture lacquer.

Warnings and precautions: Miconazole may potentiate the effect of oral anticoagulants, anti-epileptics, and hypoglycaemic drugs.

Side-effects: Transient smarting has been reported in a few cases immediately after the lacquered denture was placed in the mouth.

Use in pregnancy: Miconazole has shown no teratogenic effects in animals. No information is available regarding secretion into human breast milk. Dumicoat denture lacquer is considered to be safe for use during pregnancy, owing to the small amount of miconazole administered.

Pharmaceutical precautions Nil.

Legal category POM.

Package quantities Three glass bottles, each containing 1 g of Dumicoat denture lacquer, 3 brushes, and 4 cleaning tissues to a carton.

Further information Nil.

Product licence number 10183/0007.

ELYZOL* 25% DENTAL GEL

Presentation Elyzol dental gel is an off-white semi-solid suspension containing metronidazole benzoate corresponding to 250 mg metronidazole per g.

The dental gel is designed for application into gingival pockets. After application the gel assumes greater flowability and fills the pockets. On contact with the gingival fluid it forms a highly viscous gel. This is slowly broken down and metronidazole is released gradually from the gel.

Uses Elyzol dental gel is to be used in the treatment of chronic periodontal disease as an adjunct to conventional therapy.

Metronidazole is an antibiotic active against most of the organisms that are predominant in the subgingival flora in adult periodontitis. Metronidazole has a bactericidal effect against *Bacteroides spp., Fusobacterium, Selemonas, Wolinella, Spirochetes* and other obligate anaerobic organisms, but does not affect aerobic bacteria. Also some facultatively anaerobic bacteria, such as *Actinobacillus actinomycetemcomitans* are sensitive to the concentrations of metronidazole obtained after local application of Elyzol 25% dental gel. Development of resistance against metronidazole is seldom reported, and only with high doses after long-term use. Metronidazole does not affect the commensal flora.

Kinetics: After application of Elyzol 25% dental gel, metronidazole concentrations of above 100 μg/ml are measurable locally in the crevicular fluid for at least 8 hours. At 36 hours, concentrations above 1 μg/ml are still measurable. Metronidazole is released slowly from the dental gel with a bioavailability of about 70%. The maximal plasma concentration is found after about four hours. Systemic concentrations above 1.3 μg/ml have not been found.

Metronidazole is metabolised by means of hydroxylation and oxidation, and it conjugates with glucuronic acid. Metronidazole is mainly excreted with urine, in which 15–20% is found unchanged, and the rest as metabolites. A certain amount is excreted in the bile.

Dosage and administration Elyzol 25% dental gel is administered into the periodontal pocket twice with a one week interval. Dosage is individual, dependent upon the number of teeth to be treated.

Treatment should not normally be repeated within six months of initial therapy.

Contra-indications, warnings, etc

Contra-indications: Known hypersensitivity to metronidazole.

Precautions: In some patients metronidazole may have an effect similar to that of disulfiram on the metabolism of alcohol, resulting in intolerance symptoms.

Side-effects: Because of the low plasma concentrations after local application of the dental gel, the risk of systemic side-effects is low. The most frequent side-effects are local and occur directly in connection with the application, such as bitter taste and temporary local tenderness. Headache has been reported.

Interactions: Some potentiation of anticoagulant therapy has been reported when metronidazole has been used with warfarin type oral anticoagulants. Metronidazole and disulfiram taken concurrently may cause a confusional condition.

Use in pregnancy: Metronidazole should not be given during the first trimester of pregnancy unless it is considered essential.

Lactation: Metronidazole is excreted in milk but the risk of affecting the child seems unlikely with therapeutic doses.

Pharmaceutical precautions Use each applicator on one patient during one session of treatment only. If only part is used the remainder should be discarded.

Legal category POM.

Package quantities Disposable applicator containing 1 g dental gel. Cartons of 2×1 g.

Further information Nil.

Product licence number 4938/0007.

LITAREX*

Presentation Oval, white, biconvex, scored, controlled release tablets marked 160I on one side. Each tablet contains lithium citrate 564 mg equivalent to 6 mmol lithium.

Uses Litarex is a source of lithium ions in a controlled release dosage form. Lithium may act by competing with sodium ions at various sites in the body. It changes the electrolyte composition of body fluids and increases the intracellular and total body water volume. The mechanism of action in affective disorders is not known. For the prophylaxis and treatment of mania. For the prophylaxis of manic depression and depression.

Dosage and administration Tablets should be swallowed whole and not chewed and taken in single or divided doses as necessary.

Adults – Prophylactic long term treatment: Start with a low dosage and then increase step-wise over a period of several weeks. Treatment is managed by monitoring clinical symptoms and by measuring plasma lithium concentration. Plasma concentrations should initially be taken after 48 hours then, following any required adjustments to the dosage, at weekly intervals for a period of one month and thereafter at monthly intervals for the duration of treatment.

The initial dose is one tablet (6 mmol Li^+) each morning and evening. The dosage should be adjusted to produce a concentration of about 0.80 mmol/litre. In some patients effective plasma lithium may be within the range 0.4 to 1.0 mmol/litre. Toxic symptoms are usually associated with plasma lithium exceeding 1.2 mmol/litre. During prophylactic treatment, blood samples for estimation of lithium should be taken 12 hours after the evening dose.

Adults – Treatment of acute mania: Initiate in hospital. There is considerable biological variation in renal lithium clearance and thus the number of Litarex tablets required by individual patients to reach their particular effective plasma concentration is variable. The initial dose required for the acute treatment of mania may be high, for example 48 mmol lithium daily. Close monitoring of plasma lithium is necessary to maintain the plasma lithium concentration within the optimum range. The dose of Litarex may need to be reduced as soon as the acute phase has passed and restabilisation of plasma lithium levels may be required. Lithium concentrations should not exceed 1.2 mmol/litre.

Use in elderly: Elderly patients, or patients below 50 kg in weight, may require smaller doses of Litarex. Elderly patients may be more sensitive to the undesirable effects of lithium. Plasma lithium levels should be adjusted to the lower end of the recommended range and not exceeding 1.0 mmol/litre.

Contra-indications, warnings, etc

Use in children: Not recommended.

Contra-indications: Renal disease, sodium depletion, cardiovascular disease or Addison's disease and in women who are breast feeding.

Precautions: Lithium therapy should not be initiated unless adequate facilities for monitoring serum concentrations are available.

The use of lithium for long-term prophylactic treatment requires careful supervision. Plasma lithium concentration should be monitored regularly and determined from a blood sample drawn 12 hours after the last dose. More frequent monitoring is advisable after a change in dose; during an intercurrent illness provoking fluid loss; after starting a slimming diet; in the treatment of elderly patients; if signs of lithium toxicity on mania or depressive relapse occur.

As bioavailability varies from product to product, a change of product should be regarded as initiation of new treatment. Blood levels should therefore be monitored weekly until restabilisation is achieved.

ECG, renal function and thyroid function should be determined prior to treatment. Patients should be euthyroid before starting treatment.

Renal function should be routinely monitored in patients with polyuria and polydypsia. Clear instructions regarding the symptoms of impending toxicity should be given by the doctor to all patients receiving long-term lithium therapy. Patients should also be warned to report the development of polyuria or polydypsia. Episodes of nausea and vomiting or other conditions leading to salt/water depletion should also be reported. Patients should be advised to maintain their usual salt and fluid intake.

Use in pregnancy: The lithium ion crosses the placenta. It is therefore, advisable that a pregnancy test should be carried out prior to treatment, that women treated with lithium should adopt adequate contraceptive methods, and that treatment should be withdrawn for the first trimester of pregnancy. Treatment with lithium throughout pregnancy is associated with an incidence of congenital abnormality greater than that for the general population. Lithium dosage requirements may vary during pregnancy and after delivery; serum lithium concentrations should be monitored closely. Lithium is excreted in breast milk, and therefore lithium-treated patients should not breast feed.

Drug interactions: ACE inhibitors and NSAIDs reduce excretion of lithium, possibility of toxicity. Antacids and adsorbents, e.g. sodium bicarbonate increases excretion of lithium (reduced plasma lithium concentration). Lithium toxicity has been reported with metronidazole and spectinomycin. Serum lithium concentrations may increase during concomitant therapy with tetracycline.

Antidepressants, e.g. fluoxetine, fluvoxamine, paroxetine and sertraline increases the risk of CNS toxicity. Symptoms of nephrogenic diabetes are particularly prevalent in patients receiving concurrent treatment with tri/tetracyclic anti-depressants.

Antidiabetics: Lithium may occasionally impair glucose tolerance.

Antiepileptics: Neurotoxicity may occur with carbamazepine and phenytoin without increase in plasma-lithium concentration.

Antihypertensives: Neurotoxicity may occur with methyldopa without increased plasma-lithium concentration.

Antipsychotics: Increased risk of extrapyramidal effects and possibility of neurotoxicity (notably with haloperidol). Symptoms of nephrogenic diabetes insipidus are particularly prevalent in patients receiving concurrent treatment with tri/tetracyclic antidepressants.

Calcium-channel blockers: Neurotoxicity may occur with diltiazem and verapamil without increased plasma-lithium concentration.

Cholinergics: Lithium antagonises the effect of neostigmine and pyridostigmine.

Diuretics: Lithium excretion is reduced by loop diuretics and thiazide (increased plasma-lithium concentration and risk of toxicity; loop diuretics are safer than thiazides); lithium excretion is increased by acetazolamide.

Domperidone and metoclopramide: Increased risk of extrapyramidal effects and possibility of neurotoxicity with metoclopramide.

Muscle relaxants: Muscle relaxant effect enhanced by lithium; baclofen possibly aggravates hyperkinesis.

Sumatriptan: Risk of CNS toxicity.

Theophylline: Lithium excretion increased (reduced plasma lithium concentration).

Other interactions: Lithium treatment may lead to aggravation of myasthenia gravis. Lithium intake should be stopped 2 days before major surgery. A low sodium intake facilitates lithium re-absorption in the renal tubule and may lead to lithium accumulation. Raised plasma levels of ADH may occur during treatment.

Side-effects: Thirst and polyuria, fine tremor of the hands, muscular weakness, nausea and loose stools are the commonest side-effects during the first days or weeks of treatment. These often subside as treatment progresses.

During maintenance therapy fine hand tremor, weight gain, oedema, polyuria, hypothyroidism and goitre may occur.

More serious side-effects which may signal imminent lithium toxicity include loss of appetite, slurred speech, drowsiness, coarse hand tremor, vomiting, diarrhoea, fasciculation, vertigo and confusion. Mild cognitive impairment may occur during long-term use.

Hypercalcaemia, hypermagnesaemia, hyperparathyroidism and an increase in antinuclear antibodies have also been reported. Exacerbation of psoriasis may occur.

Long-term treatment with lithium may result in permanent changes in the kidney and impairment of renal function. High serum concentrations of lithium, including episodes of acute lithium toxicity may enhance these changes. The minimum clinically effective dose of lithium should always be used. Patients should be maintained on lithium after 3–5 years only if benefit persists.

Overdosage: Early signs of toxicity (see side effects) may respond to a reduction in, or cessation of, lithium therapy.

Symptoms of severe lithium poisoning include hyper-reflexia, attacks of hyper-extension of the limbs, epileptic seizures, toxic psychosis, syncope, oliguria, circulatory failure and coma. Deaths have been reported.

Treatment consists of the induction of vomiting and/or gastric lavage together with appropriate supportive and symptomatic measures. It is essential that fluid and electrolyte balance and adequate renal function are maintained. In cases of gross overdosage (plasma concentrations greater than 3 mmol per litre) lithium clearance can be enhanced by haemodialysis or peritoneal dialysis.

Since Litarex is a controlled-release preparation, clinicians should be aware of the possibility of lithium release continuing over a period of time. Following overdose, plasma lithium levels should be monitored for at least 24 hours and subsequently as considered necessary.

Pharmaceutical precautions No special requirements.

Legal category POM.

Package quantities Containers of 100.

Further information The lithium citrate in Litarex tablets is distributed in a plastic/lipid matrix from which the lithium salt is released over a period of four to five hours during passage through the gastro-intestinal tract. The tablets are formulated in such a way as to give absorption which is slow and even, so that rapid increases and high peak levels in serum lithium concentrations are avoided.

Product licence number 4938/0012.

METRONIDAZOLE TABLETS 500 mg

Qualitative and quantitative composition Each tablet contains metronidazole 500 mg.

Pharmaceutical form Tablets.

Clinical particulars

Therapeutic indications: Metronidazole is active against infections caused by *Trichomonas vaginalis, Gardnerella vaginalis, Giardia lamblia,* and *Entamoeba histolytica.* It is also active against a broad spectrum of obligate anaerobic bacteria, including Bacteroides, Fusobacterium, Clostridium and various anaerobic cocci. The action is trichomonacidal, amoebacidal and bactericidal.

Metronidazole tablets may be used in the treatment of *Trichomonas vaginalis* infestations in men and women; *Gardnerella vaginalis;* giardiasis (lambliasis); amoebiasis; and infections in which anaerobic bacteria have been identified or are suspected as pathogens.

Metronidazole tablets may be used in combination with other recommended agents in the treatment of *Helicobacter pylori* infection associated with peptic ulcer.

Metronidazole tablets may be used in the prevention of postoperative infections caused by anaerobic bacteria, particularly following gynaecological and gastrointestinal surgery.

Metronidazole tablets may be used in acute ulcerative gingivitis (Vincent's Infection).

Posology and method of administration: As given below under the specific indications.

The dose should be reduced in the presence of severe liver insufficiency.

Trichomoniasis: 2 g (4 tablets) in a single dose or 250 mg (½ tablet) each morning and evening for 6 days. In severe cases 500 mg each morning and evening for 6 days. Both the patient and partner should be treated simultaneously.

Gardnerella vaginalis: 500 mg (1 tablet) each morning and evening for 7 days.

Amoebiasis – acute intestinal amoebiasis: 2 to 2.5 g (4 to 5 tablets) in a single dose for 2 to 3 days or 750 mg three times daily for 5 to 10 days.

Hepatic amoebiasis: 1.5 to 2.5 g (3 to 5 tablets) in a single dose for 2 to 3 days or 500 mg three times daily for 5 days.

Eradication of cysts in symptomless carriers: Adults: 500 to 750 mg three times daily for 5 to 10 days.

Children: Half the adult dose.

Infants: 50 mg/kg body weight daily.

Giardiasis: Adults: 2 g (4 tablets) in 3 single dose for 3 days or 500 mg (1 tablet) twice daily for 1 to 10 days.

Children: 250 mg (½ tablet) once daily for 10 days.

Infants: 25 mg/kg body weight for 10 days.

Eradication of Helicobacter pylori in infected patients: Generally, metronidazole treatment should be given for at least 7 days in triple combination with other agents recommended for use in the treatment of Helicobacter pylori infection.

Adults: 500 mg two to three daily for 7–14 days.

There are no specific recommendations for use in children.

Acute ulcerative gingivitis: Adults: 250 mg (½ tablet) three times daily for 3 days.

Treatment of anaerobic infections: Generally metronidazole treatment should be given for at least 7 days.

Adults and children over 12 years of age: 500 mg every 8 hours.

Children under 12 years: 7 mg/kg body weight every 8 hours.

Prevention of anaerobic infections: Generally metronidazole prophylaxis should be given for 3 to 7 days.

Elective surgery: e.g. hysterectomy and colonic surgery.

Preoperatively: Adults and children over 12 years of age: 24 hours before surgery 1 g (2 tablets) followed by 500 mg by mouth every 8 hours until preoperative starvation.

Children under 12 years: 7 mg/kg body weight every 8 hours.

Postoperative periods: Adults and children over 12 years of age: 500 mg (1 tablet) every 8 hours once oral medication is possible.

Children under 12 years: 7 mg/kg body weight every 8 hours once oral medication is possible.

Acute surgery: e.g. appendectomy, gastrointestinal perforation.

Adults and children over 12 years of age: 500 mg (1 tablet) every 8 hours postoperatively, once oral medication is possible.

Children under 12 years: 7 mg/kg body weight every 8 hours postoperatively, once oral medication is possible.

Contra-indications: A history of known allergy to metronidazole.

Special warnings and precautions for use: Metronidazole tablets should not be used in patients with blood dyscrasias or with active non-infectious disease of the central nervous system. High doses of metronidazole may mask the presence of syphilis.

The dose should be prescribed with caution in patients with renal or hepatic impairment.

Regular clinical and biological surveillance are advised if administration of metronidazole tablets for more than 10 days is considered necessary.

Interaction with other medicaments and other forms of interaction: Metronidazole may provoke a disulfiram-like reaction with alcohol. Concurrent ingestion of disulfiram may cause conditions of acute confusion.

Metronidazole enhances the activity of warfarin. Anticoagulant therapy should be closely monitored in patients receiving metronidazole concurrently.

Cimetidine decreases the plasma clearance of metronidazole by 30%. This is not thought to have major clinical significance.

Metronidazole has exhibited synergism with several agents active against anaerobes, for instance clindamycin, erythromycin, nifampicin and nalidixic acid. Phenobarbitone increases the metabolism of metronidazole, reducing the half-life to about three hours.

Pregnancy and lactation: Should not be used unless the physician considers it essential.

Effect on ability to drive and use machines: None.

Undesirable effects: Serious adverse reactions occur rarely. Side effects of metronidazole are usually mild and may include gastrointestinal disturbances, nausea, unpleasant taste in the mouth, coated tongue, headache and skin rashes. There have been occasional reports of erythema multiforme, urticaria and angioedema, which may be reversed on drug withdrawal. Anaphylaxis may occur rarely. Drowsiness, dizziness, depression and darkening of the urine have been reported.

Abnormal liver function tests, cholestatic hepatitis and jaundice, which may be reversed upon drug withdrawal have been reported. During intensive and/or prolonged metronidazole therapy, peripheral neuropathy, transient epileptiform seizures and paraesthesia i.e. tingling, have been reported.

There have been reports of bone marrow depression disorders, such as agranulocytosis, neutropenia, thrombocytopenia and pancytopenia, which may be reversed on drug withdrawal, although fatalities have been reported.

Overdose: There is no specific treatment for gross overdosage of metronidazole.

Pharmacological properties

Pharmacodynamic properties: Metronidazole is active against obligate anaerobic bacteria, *Gardnerella vaginalis, Trichomonas vaginalis, Giardia lamblia* and *Entamoeba histolytica.*

Pharmacokinetic properties: Metronidazole is absorbed readily and almost completely from the gastrointestinal tract. Maximum concentrations occur after about 1 hour. Metronidazole penetrates well into body tissues and fluids. About 10% of the drug is bound to plasma proteins.

At least half the dose is excreted in the urine as metronidazole and its metabolites, including an acid oxidation product, a hydroxy derivative and a glucuronide. The elimination half-life of metronidazole is about 8.5 hours.

Preclinical data: None.

Pharmacological particulars

List of excipients: Lactose, maize starch, povidone, magnesium stearate ac-di-sol, microcrystalline cellulose, purified water, ethanol, methocel E5, propylene glycol, dimethicone, titanium dioxide (E-171).

Incompatibilities: None.

Shelf life: 3 years.

Special precautions for storage: Store below 25°C. Protect from light.

Nature and contents of container: Amber glass bottle (500 tablets). Blister packs (21 tablets).

Instruction for use/handling: Not applicable.

Marketing authorisation holder: A/S Dumex (Dumex Ltd), Prags Boulevard 37, DK-2300 Copenhagen S.

Marketing authorisation number 4938/0014.

Date of approval/revision of SPC 16 July 1996.

Legal category POM.

STESOLID* RECTAL TUBES

Presentation Transparent, yellow, polyethylene Rectal Tubes containing a clear, colourless to slightly yellowish solution of 2 mg/ml or 4 mg/ml diazepam. The formulation also includes the following inactive ingredients: benzoic acid, benzyl alcohol, ethanol, propylene glycol and sodium benzoate. Approximately 2.5 ml can be squeezed from each tube, giving an individual dose of 5 mg or 10 mg diazepam. The small amount left in the tube will not affect the correct dose.

Uses Diazepam has anti-convulsant, sedative and muscle relaxant properties. It is used in the treatment of severe anxiety and tension states, as a sedative and premedicant in the control of muscle spasm and in the management of alcohol withdrawal symptoms.

Stesolid Rectal Tubes may be used in acute severe anxiety and agitation, epileptic and febrile convulsions, tetanus, as a sedative in minor surgical and dental procedures or other circumstances in which a rapid effect is required but where intravenous injection is impracticable or undesirable. Stesolid Rectal Tubes may be of particular value for the immediate treatment of convulsions in children. (1 year and over).

Dosage and administration Sensitivity to diazepam varies with age.

Children: 1 to 3 years of age – one 5 mg tube. Insert tube half way to mark on nozzle. Over 3 years of age – one 10 mg tube. Note: these recommendations assume normal frame size for age. In particularly small children the depth of insertion should be reduced accordingly.

Adults: One 10 mg tube.

Elderly patients: One 5 mg tube.

If no effect is seen after five minutes, one further tube (5 mg or 10 mg) diazepam respectively can be administered. Further doses of Stesolid Rectal Tubes should be administered only after consultation with a physician. If convulsions are still not controlled, then other anti-convulsive measures should be instituted.

Contra-indications, warnings, etc

Contra-indications: Known sensitivity to any of the ingredients. Acute pulmonary insufficiency, respiratory depression.

Use in pregnancy and lactation: There is no evidence as to the safety of diazepam in human pregnancy. It should not be used, especially during the first and last trimesters, unless the benefit is considered to outweigh the potential risk.

In labour, high single doses or repeated low doses have been reported to produce hypotonia, poor suckling and hypothermia in the neonate and irregularities in the foetal heart.

Diazepam is excreted in breast milk and therefore its use during lactation should be avoided.

Warnings: Stesolid Rectal Tubes should not be used in phobic or obsessional states as there is insufficient evidence of efficacy and safety in this situation, nor should they be used alone in the treatment of depression or anxiety associated with depression due to the risk of suicide being precipitated in this patient group. Stesolid Rectal Tubes should not be used in the treatment of chronic psychosis. In common with other benzodiazepines the use of diazepam may be associated with amnesia and Stesolid Rectal Tubes should not be used in cases of loss or bereavement as psychological adjustment may be inhibited.

As with other benzodiazepines extreme caution should be used if prescribing Stesolid Rectal Tubes for patients with personality disorders. The disinhibiting effects of benzodiazepines may be manifested as the precipitation of suicide in patients who are depressed and aggressive behaviour towards self and others.

Withdrawal symptoms occur with benzodiazepines following normal therapeutic doses given for short periods of time and may be associated with physiological and psychological sequelae including depression.

Precautions: Stesolid Rectal Tubes should be used with caution in patients with renal or hepatic dysfunction, chronic pulmonary insufficiency or close-angle glaucoma.

Elderly or debilitated patients are particularly susceptible to side-effects and may require lower doses.

Alertness and performance at skilled tasks may be impaired. Patients should be warned not to drive or operate machinery. Alcohol may potentiate these effects.

Drug interactions: Diazepam may enhance the effects of other CNS depressants. Their concurrent use should be avoided. Diazepam may potentiate the effect of phenytoin when taken concurrently. Sodium valproate displaces protein bound diazepam and inhibits its metabolism. Occasionally, diazepam has been reported to antagonise the effect of levodopa.

Cimetidine may potentiate the effect of diazepam because of decreased hepatic metabolism.

Alcohol may alter the response to diazepam.

Side-effects: The side-effects of diazepam are usually mild and infrequent. The most common side-effects are drowsiness, light-headedness, unsteadiness and ataxia.

Elderly and debilitated patients are particularly susceptible to these effects and may require lower doses. Other rare side-effects include hypotension, apnoea, respiratory depression, gastro-intestinal and visual disturbances, skin rashes, urinary retention, headache, confusion, vertigo, changes in libido, blood dyscrasias and jaundice.

Paradoxical reactions to benzodiazepines have been reported, provoking excitement instead of sedation.

Treatment of overdosage: The symptoms of overdose are hypnosis, hypotension, respiratory depression and coma. Treatment is symptomatic, with airway maintenance. Intravenous fluids may be administered. Flumazenil is a specific I.V. antidote for use in emergency situations. Patients requiring such intervention should be monitored closely in hospital.

Pharmaceutical precautions Stesolid Rectal Tubes should be stored at a temperature below 25°C. Do not open the foil before use.

Legal category CD (Sch 4), POM.

Package quantities Single-packed Rectal Tubes, 5 tubes to a carton.

Further information Shelf life of two and a half years from date of manufacture.

Product licence numbers
5 mg Rectal Tube 10183/0003
10 mg Rectal Tube 10183/0004

VANCOMYCIN CAPSULES

Qualitative and quantitative composition Vancomycin 125 mg (125,000 IU) per capsule and 250 mg (250,000 IU) per capsule as vancomycin hydrochloride.

Pharmaceutical form Capsules.

Clinical particulars

Therapeutic indications: Staphylococcal enterocolitis and pseudomembraneous colitis due to *Clostridium difficile.*

Vancomycin is not significantly absorbed from the normal gastro-intestinal tract and is therefore not effective by the oral route for other types of infection.

Posology and method of administration:
Adults and the elderly: The usual daily dose is 500 mg in 4 divided doses for 7 to 10 days. In severe cases up to 2 g daily in 3 or 4 divided doses. The total daily dose should not exceed 2 g.

Children: 40 mg/kg daily in 3 or 4 divided doses for 7 to 10 days. The total daily dosage should not exceed 2 g.

Contra-indications: Hypersensitivity to vancomycin.

Special warnings and precautions for use: Although in general very little vancomycin is absorbed from the gastro-intestinal tract following oral administration, absorption may be enhanced in patients with inflammatory disorders of the intestinal mucosa. These patients may be at risk for the development of adverse reactions. The risk is greater in patients with renal impairment. The greater the renal impairment, the greater the risk of developing the adverse reactions associated with the parental administration of vancomycin.

Monitoring of serum concentrations of these patients should therefore be performed. It should be noted that the total systemic and renal clearances of vancomycin are reduced in the elderly.

Nephrotoxicity: Nephrotoxicity has occurred in patients receiving vancomycin. It has been reported mostly in patients who have been given excessive intravenous doses, have a pre-existing kidney dysfunction, or are receiving concomitant treatment with aminoglycoside.

In order to minimise the risk of nephrotoxicity when treating patients with underlying renal dysfunction or patients receiving concomitant therapy with an aminoglycoside, serial monitoring at renal function should be performed.

Ototoxicity: Ototoxicity has occurred in patients receiving vancomycin. It may be transient or permanent. It has been reported mostly in patients who have been given excessive intravenous doses, have a pre-existing hearing loss, or are receiving concomitant treatment with an ototoxic drug. Serial tests of auditory function may be helpful in order to minimise the risk of ototoxicity.

Haematological: Haematological problems have occurred in patients receiving vancomycin. Most of the conditions are reversible.

Interaction with other medicaments and other forms of interaction: None known.

Pregnancy and lactation: Teratology studies have been performed at 5 times the human dose in rats and 3 times the human dose in rabbits, and have revealed no evidence of harm to the foetus due to vancomycin. In a controlled clinical study, the potential ototoxic and nephrotoxic effects of vancomycin hydrochloride on infants were evaluated when the drug was administered to pregnant women for serious staphylococcal infections complicating intravenous drug abuse. Vancomycin hydrochloride was found in cord blood. No sensorineural hearing loss or nephrotoxocity attributable to vancomycin was noted. One infant, whose mother received vancomycin in the third trimester, experienced conductive hearing loss that was not attributable to vancomycin. Because vancomycin was administered only in the second and third trimesters. It is not known whether it causes foetal harm, Vancomycin should therefore, only be given to pregnant women if clearly needed.

Vancomycin hydrochloride is excreted in human milk. Caution should be exercised when vancomycin is administered to a nursing woman.

Effect on ability to drive and use machines: Not applicable.

Undesirable effects: Since vancomycin is not usually significantly absorbed from the gastro-intestinal tract, the adverse reactions encountered with parental therapy is unlikely to occur after oral administration.

Nephrotoxicity: Rarely, renal failure, principally manifested by increased serum creatinine or blood urea concentrations, have been observed, especially in patients given large doses of intravenously administered vancomycin. Rare cases of interstitial nephritis have been reported. Most occurred in patients who were given aminoglycosides concomitantly or who had pre-existing kidney dysfunction.

Ototoxicity: Hearing loss associated with intravenously administered vancomycin has been reported. Most of those patients had kidney dysfunction, pre-existing hearing loss, or concomitant treatment with an ototoxic drug. Vertigo, dizziness, and tinnitus have been reported rarely.

Haematological: Reversible neutropenia, usually starting one week or more after onset of intravenous therapy or after a total dose of more than 25 g. Neutropenia appears to be promptly reversible when vancomycin is discontinued. Thrombocytopenia and reversible agranulocytosis (granulo-cyte count less than 500/mm^3) have been reported rarely.

Miscellaneous: Anaphylaxis, chills, drug fever, eosinophilia, hypotension, wheezing, dyspnoea, urticaria, pruritus, flushing of the upper body, pain, muscle spasm of the chest and back, nausea and rashes, including exfoliative dematitis, Stevens-Johnson syndrome and rare cases of vasculitis.

Overdose: Symptoms: See *Undesirable effects.*

Treatment: Supportive care is advised, with maintenance of glomeruler filtration. Vancomycin is poorly removed by dialysis. Haemofiltration and haemoperfusion with Amberlite resin XAD-4 have been reported to be of limited benefit.

Pharmacological properties

Pharmacodynamic properties: Vancomycin is a narrow spectrum antibiotic. The mechanism of action is an inhibition of the enzyme glycopeptide synthetase which is reponsible for condensation of the glycopeptide backbone of the cell wall.

Vancomycin has a bactericidal effect against gram-positive bacteria, especially Staphylococcus aureus. Staphylococcus epidermis, streptococcus faecalis, and Clostridium difficile. All gram negative organisms are resistant.

Resistance is not readily acquired *in vitro* and it has not been observed during the use of vancomycin *in vivo.* There is no cross resistance with other known antibiotics.

Pharmacokinetic properties: Vancomycin is not normally absorbed from the gastro-intestinal tract, but in patients with inflammatory disorders of the intestinal mucosa some systemic absorption may occur. The orally administered drug is active only locally within the gut lumen, making it useful in enterocolitis. An oral dose is excreted exclusively in the faeces.

Preclinical safety data: None.

Pharmacological particulars

List of excipients: Polyethylene glycol 6000.

Capsule 125 mg: Black iron oxide E-172, titanium-dioxide E-171, yellow iron oxide E-172, gelatin.

Capsule 250 mg: Black iron oxide E-172, titanium-dioxide E-171, yellow iron oxide E-172, indigo carmine E-132, gelatin.

Incompatibilities: Not applicable.

Shelf life: 2 years.

Special precautions for storage: Room temperature (15–25°C). Protect from moisture.

Nature and contents of container: Unit dose blister

packs of PVC/PVdC (250/35 μm) on aluminium foil (20 μm). Pack sizes: 28 capsules.

Instructions for use/handling: Not applicable.

Marketing authorisation holder: Dumex-Alphama A/S, Dalslandsgrade 11, DK-23000 Copenhagen S, Denmark.

Marketing authorisation numbers

125 mg Capsules	4938/0015
250 mg Capsules	4938/0016

Date of approval/revision of SPC 28 May 1996

Legal category POM

VANCOMYCIN POWDER for INFUSION

Qualitative and quantitative composition *Vancomycin Powder for Infusion 1 g:* Vancomycin 1 g (equivalent to 1,000,000 IU) as vancomycin hydrochloride.

Vancomycin Powder for Infusion 500 mg: Vancomycin 500 mg (equivalent to 500,000 IU) as vancomycin hydrochloride.

Pharmaceutical form Powder for infusion.

Clinical particulars

Therapeutic indications: Severe infections caused by bacteria that are susceptible to vancomycin and resistant to other antibiotics; when therapy fails; and in the presence of allergy to penicillin. For instance, sepsis and/or endocarditis, peritonitis in dialysis patients which is caused by Staphlococcus aureus or Staphylococcus epidermidis.

Posology and method of administration:

Adults: 500 mg every six hours or 1 g every twelve hours by slow intravenous infusion.

Children: 40 mg/kg body weight every 24 hours divided into 2 doses given by slow intravenous infusion.

The rate of infusion should not exceed 10 mg/min, corresponding to a rate of 2 ml/min with a concentration of vancomycin of 5 mg/ml.

The dose must be reduced in the presence of decreased renal function. The initial dose is at least 15 mg/kg. The following tables give a guideline for use in patients with decreased renal function.

Creatinine clearance ml/min	*Dose Vancomycin mg/24 hours*
>100	2000–1500
100–70	1500–1000
70–30	1000–50
20	300
10	150

Contra-indications: None.

Special warnings and precautions for use: The serum concentation must be determined daily and the dose regulated accordingly. Two hours after completion of infusion serum concentrations are in the region of 18–26 mg/litre. Serum concentrations measured immediately prior to the next dose should be in the 5–10 mg/litre range.

Care must be exercised in administration to patients with decreased kidney function and in elderly patients.

Concomitant treatment with potentially ototoxic or nephrotoxic medication should be avoided.

Interactions with other medicaments and other forms of interaction: None.

Pregnancy and lactation:

Pregnancy: Reproduction studies of animals have been faulty or non-existent. The data available gives no reason to suspect an increased frequency in foetal damage or other serious effects on the reproductive process. Should not be given in pregnancy, except when the clinical suituation is sufficiently serious to outweigh potential foetal risks.

Lactation: Vancomycin is secreted into breast milk. Information on the levels of vancomycin in breast milk is insufficient to judge the risk to the infant. During lactation avoid breast feeding.

Effects on ability to drive and use machines: None.

Undesirable effects: Commonest are phlebitis and pseudo-allergic reactions occurring when the information is given too quickly.

Frequent (>1/100):

General: Anaphylactoid reactions including hypotension, wheezing, dyspnoea, urticaria, pruritus, and flushing of the upper body (red man effect), pain and muscle spasm of the chest and back.

Circulation: Thrombophlebitis.

Urogenital: Elevated serum creatinine and serum urea, indicating nephrotoxicity.

Less frequent:

Skin: Rash.

Ears: Reduced hearing.

Rare:

Miscellaneous: Anaphylaxis, fever, chills, dizziness.

Haematological: Thromobocytopenia, neutropenia.

Skin: Exfoliative dermatitis.

Ears: Tinnitus.

Reversible agranulocystosis and pseudomembranous colitis have been reported in a few cases. Ototoxicity may be reversible or permanent, and has been reported mainly in patients given an overdose, in patients with a history of reduced hearing, and with concomitant therapy with other ototoxoc drugs, such as aminoglycosides.

Overdose: Symptoms: see *Undesirble effects.*

Treatment: Symptomatic. Cannot be removed by haemodialysis.

Pharmacological properties

Pharmacodynamic properties: Vancomycin inhibits the construction of the cellular wall of gram-positive bacteria. It has a rapid bacterial action on bacteria in the growth phase. Vancomycin is active against gram-positive cocci, especially Staphylococcus aureus, Staph. epidermidis, Streptococcus faecalis, and gram-positive rods, particularly Clostridium difficile. Other micro-organisms are resistant.

Pharmacokinetic properties: Intravenous administration of 2 g over 24 hours produces a mean serum concentration of 10–20 micg/ml. Protein binding is 55%. Vancomycin is distributed rapidly to most tissue and body fluids after intravenous infusion. It penetrates the intact blood-brain barrier only to a low degree. Elimination occurs via kidneys and more than 95% of the dose administered is recovered in the urine. The plasma half-life in adults is 4–6 hours, in children 2–3 hours, and 6–10 hours in the newborn.

Preclinical safety data: LD_{50} values after intravenous administration: 489 mg/kg (mice), 319 mg/kg (rats). Teratogenic and mutagenic effects have not been demonstrated in animal studies.

Pharmaceutical particulars

List of excipients: Nitrogen, Water for Injections.

Incompatibilities: After reconstitution in sterile water, the pH value is 2.8–4.5. Should only be dissolved in or mixed with the infusion fluids described under *Instruction for use/handling.* The prepared infusion fluid should not be mixed with other drugs.

Shelf life: Powder for infusion: 2 years at a temperature below 25°C.

Dissolved powder for infusion: 24 hours in a refrigerator at 2–8°C.

Special precautions for storage: Temperature below 25°C.

Nature and contents of container:

Nature: Vials, closed with stoppers of chlorobutyl type 1 coated with silicone, sealed with a grey flip-off capsule of aluminium with polypropylene tops, and packaged into a carton.

Contents of container:

Vancomycin Powder for Infusion 1 g: 1 vial containing 1 g vancomycin packaged into a carton.

Vancomycin Powder for Infusion 500 mg: 1 vial containing 500 mg vancomycin packaged into a carton.

Instruction for use/handling:

Vancomycin Powder for Infusion 1 g: Dissolve the powder for infusion in and dilute to a strength of 50 mg/ml with 20 ml of sterile water. Dilute this stock solution with at least 200 ml of sodium chloride infusion fluid 9 mg/ml or glucose infusion fluid 50 mg/ml.

Vancomycin Powder for Infusion 500 mg: Dissolve the powder for infusion in and dilute to a strength of 50 mg/ml with 10 ml of sterile water. Dilute this stock solution with at least 100 ml of sodium chloride infusion fluid 9 mg/ml or glucose infusion fluid 50 mg/ml.

Marketing authorisation holder: Dumex-Alpharma A/S, Dalslandsgade 11, DK-2300 Copenhagen S.

Marketing authorisation number 0438/0018

Date of approval/revision of SPC 2 April 1997

Date of (partial) revision of the text 22 January 1997

**Trade Mark*

DuPont Pharmaceuticals Limited
Wedgwood Way
Stevenage
Hertfordshire SG1 4QN

☎ 01438 842530   🗋 01438 842533

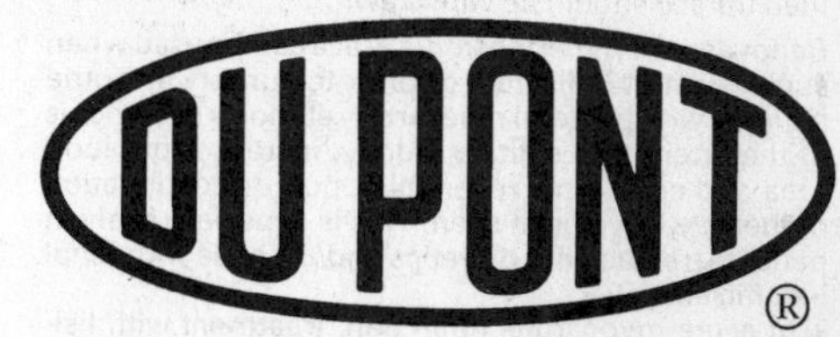

CARACE

Presentation Blue, oval tablets, marked 'MSD 15', containing 2.5 mg lisinopril.

White, half-scored, oval tablets, marked 'CARACE' and '5', containing 5 mg lisinopril.

Yellow, half-scored, oval tablets, marked 'CARACE' and '10', containing 10 mg lisinopril.

Orange, half-scored, oval tablets, marked 'CARACE' and '20', containing 20 mg lisinopril.

Uses

Indications

Hypertension: All grades of essential hypertension and renovascular hypertension. Carace may be used alone or with other antihypertensive agents.

Heart failure: In heart failure, Carace should be used as an adjunctive therapy with non-potassium-sparing diuretics and, where appropriate, digitalis.

Severe heart failure: Treatment with Carace should always be initiated in hospital under close medical supervision.

Mild to moderate heart failure: Treatment with Carace should always be initiated under close medical supervision.

Acute myocardial infarction: Carace is indicated for the treatment of haemodynamically stable patients, defined as patients not in cardiogenic shock and who have a systolic blood pressure greater than 100 mmHg. Carace may be initiated within 24 hours of acute myocardial infarction to prevent the subsequent development of left ventricular dysfunction or heart failure and to improve survival. Patients should receive, as appropriate, the standard recommended treatments such as thrombolytics, aspirin and beta-blocker.

Action: Lisinopril is a peptidyl dipeptidase inhibitor. It inhibits the angiotensin converting enzyme (ACE) that catalyses the conversion of Angiotensin I to the vasoconstrictor peptide, Angiotensin II. Angiotensin II also stimulates aldosterone secretion by the adrenal cortex. Inhibition of ACE results in decreased concentrations of Angiotensin II which results in decreased vasopressor activity and reduced aldosterone secretion. The latter decrease may result in a small increase in serum potassium concentration.

While the mechanism through which lisinopril lowers blood pressure is believed to be primarily suppression of the renin-angiotensin-aldosterone system, lisinopril is antihypertensive even in patients with low-renin hypertension. ACE is identical to kinanase II, an enzyme that degrades bradykinin. Whether increased levels of bradykinin, a potent vasodilatory peptide, play a role in the therapeutic effects of lisinopril remains to be elucidated.

The disposition of lisinopril in patients with renal insufficiency was similar to that in patients with normal renal function until the glomerular filtration rate reached 30 ml/min or less. Older patients have higher blood levels and higher values for the area under the plasma concentration time curve than younger patients. Lisinopril can be removed by dialysis.

Following oral administration of lisinopril, peak serum concentrations occur within about 7 hours. On multiple dosing lisinopril has an effective half life of accumulation of 12.6 hours.

Declining serum concentrations exhibited a prolonged terminal phase which did not contribute to drug accumulation. This terminal phase probably represents saturable binding to ACE and was not proportional to dose. Lisinopril did not appear to be bound to other plasma proteins.

Based on urinary recovery, the mean extent of absorption of lisinopril is approximately 25%, with interpatient variability (6–60%) at all doses tested (5–80 mg).

Lisinopril does not undergo metabolism and absorbed drug is excreted unchanged entirely in the urine. Lisinopril absorption is not affected by the presence of food in the gastrointestinal tract.

Studies in rats indicate that lisinopril crosses the blood-brain barrier poorly.

Dosage and administration The absorption of Carace is not affected by food.

Hypertension: The need for dosage titration should be determined by measurement of the blood pressure just before the next dose.

Essential and renovascular hypertension: Treatment should be started with 2.5 mg once daily, and titrated upwards to achieve optimal blood pressure control. A 2.5 mg dose seldom achieves a therapeutic response.

The usual effective dose range is 10–20 mg once daily.

The maximum recommended dose is 40 mg daily.

Diuretic-treated patients: If possible, the diuretic should be discontinued or the dose reduced, two to three days before beginning therapy with Carace (see 'Precautions') and may be resumed later if required.

Use in the elderly: Age alone does not appear to affect the efficacy or safety profile of Carace. Thus, elderly patients should start treatment with Carace as directed above.

Congestive heart failure: Carace may be used as adjunctive therapy with non-potassium-sparing diuretics with or without digitalis.

Initial dosage: Therapy with Carace should be initiated under close medical supervision (in hospital for severe heart failure) with a recommended starting dose of 2.5 mg once daily. If possible, the dose of diuretic should be reduced before beginning treatment.

Blood pressure and renal function should be monitored closely both before and during treatment because severe hypotension and, more rarely, consequent renal failure have been reported with angiotensin-converting enzyme (ACE) inhibitors (see 'Precautions').

The appearance of hypotension after the initial dose of Carace does not preclude subsequent careful dose adjustment with the drug, following effective treatment of the hypotension.

Some patients, other than those with severe heart failure, are considered to be at higher risk when started on an ACE inhibitor and are recommended for initiation of therapy in hospital. Research data have shown such patients to be: those on multiple or high-dose diuretics (e.g., >80 mg frusemide); patients with hypovolaemia; hyponatraemia (serum sodium <130 mEq/l); pre-existing hypotension (systolic blood pressure <90 mm Hg); patients with unstable cardiac failure; renal impairment (serum creatinine >150 micromol/l); those on high-dose vasodilator therapy; patients aged 70 years or over.

Maintenance dosage: The dose should be gradually increased, depending on the patient's response, to the usual maintenance dose (5–20 mg). This dose adjustment may be performed over a two- to four-week period, or more rapidly if clinically indicated.

Acute myocardial infarction: Treatment with Carace may be started within 24 hours of the onset of symptoms. The first dose of Carace is 5 mg given orally, followed by 5 mg after 24 hours, 10 mg after 48 hours and then 10 mg once daily thereafter. Patients with a low systolic blood pressure (120 mmHg or less) should be given a lower dose – 2.5 mg orally (see precautions). If hypotension occurs (systolic blood pressure less than or equal to 100 mmHg) a daily maintenance dose of 5 mg may be given with temporary reductions to 2.5 mg if needed. If prolonged hypotension occurs (systolic blood pressure less than 90 mmHg for more than 1 hour) Carace should be withdrawn.

Dosing for patients with acute myocardial infarction should continue for six weeks. The benefit appears to be greatest in patients with large myocardial infarctions and evidence of impaired left ventricular function. For patients who develop symptoms of heart failure, see Dosage and administration, Congestive heart failure.

Carace is compatible with intravenous or transdermal glyceryl trinitrate.

Impaired renal function: Carace is excreted by the kidney, and should be used with caution in patients with renal insufficiency.

Carace is dialysable. Dialysis patients may be given the usual dose of 'Carace' on dialysis days. On the days when patients are not on dialysis the dosage should be tailored to the blood pressure response.

Paediatric use: Carace has not been studied for use in children.

Contra-indications, warnings, etc

Contra-indications

Pregnancy: The use of Carace during pregnancy is not recommended. When pregnancy is determined Carace should be discontinued as soon as possible unless it is considered life-saving for the mother (see Precautions).

Hypersensitivity to Carace, and in patients with a history of angioneurotic oedema relating to previous treatment with an ACE inhibitor.

Precautions:

Assessment of renal function: Evaluation of the patient should include assessment of renal function prior to initiation of therapy, and during treatment.

Impaired renal function: Carace should be used with caution in patients with renal insufficiency, as they may require reduced or less frequent doses (see 'Dosage'). Close monitoring of renal function during therapy should be performed as deemed appropriate in those with renal insufficiency. In the majority, renal function will not alter, or may improve.

Renal failure has been reported in association with ACE inhibitors and has been mainly in patients with severe congestive heart failure or underlying renal disease, including renal artery stenosis. If recognised promptly and treated appropriately, renal failure is usually reversible.

Some hypertensive patients, with no apparent pre-existing renal disease, have developed increases in blood urea and creatinine when Carace has been given concurrently with a diuretic. Dosage reduction of Carace and/or discontinuation of the diuretic may be required. This situation should raise the possibility of underlying renal artery stenosis (see 'Renovascular hypertension').

Symptomatic hypotension was seen rarely in uncomplicated hypertensive patients. It is more likely to occur in patients who have been volume-depleted by diuretic therapy, dietary salt restriction, dialysis, diarrhoea, or vomiting. In these patients, by discontinuing diuretic therapy or significantly reducing the diuretic dose for two to three days prior to initiating Carace, the possibility of this occurrence is reduced.

Similar caution and close supervision may apply also to patients with ischaemic heart or cerebrovascular disease in whom severe hypotension could result in a myocardial infarct or cerebrovascular accident.

Severe hypotension has been reported with ACE inhibitors, mainly in patients with severe heart failure. Many of these patients were on high doses of loop diuretics, and some had hyponatraemia or functional renal impairment. If hypotension develops, the patient should be placed in a supine position. Volume repletion with oral fluids or intravenous normal saline may be required. Intravenous atropine may be necessary if there is associated bradycardia. Treatment with Carace may be restarted with careful dose titration following restoration of effective blood volume and pressure.

In some patients with congestive heart failure who have normal or low blood pressure, additional lowering of systemic blood pressure may occur with Carace. If such hypotension becomes symptomatic, a reduction of dose or discontinuation of Carace may become necessary.

The appearance of hypotension after the initial dose of Carace does not preclude subsequent careful dose titration with the drug after effective management of hypotension.

Hypotension in acute myocardial infarction: Treatment with lisinopril must not be initiated in acute myocardial infarction patients who are at risk of further serious haemodynamic deterioration after treatment with a vasodilator. These are patients with systolic blood pressure of 100 mmHg or lower or cardiogenic shock. During the first 3 days following the infarction, the dose should be reduced if the systolic blood pressure is 120 mmHg or lower. Maintenance doses should be reduced to 5 mg or temporarily to 2.5 mg if systolic blood pressure is 100 mmHg or lower. If hypotension persists (systolic blood pressure less than 90 mmHg for more than 1 hour) then Carace should be withdrawn.

Renovascular hypertension: Carace can be used when surgery is not indicated, or prior to surgery. In some patients with bilateral renal artery stenosis or stenosis of the artery to a solitary kidney, increases of blood urea and creatinine, reversible upon discontinuation of therapy, have been seen. This is especially likely in patients treated with diuretics and/or those with renal insufficiency.

In acute myocardial infarction, treatment with lisinopril should not be initiated in patients with evidence of renal dysfunction, defined as serum creatinine concentration exceeding 177 micromol/l and/or proteinuria exceeding 500 mg/24 h. If renal dysfunction develops during treatment with Carace (serum creatinine concentration exceeding 265 micromol/l or a doubling from the pre-treatment value) then the physician should consider withdrawal of Carace.

Angioneurotic oedema: It has been reported with angiotensin-converting enzyme inhibitors, including Carace. This may occur at any time during treatment. In such cases, Carace should be discontinued promptly and appropriate monitoring should be instituted to ensure complete resolution of symptoms prior to dismissing the patient. Where swelling is confined to the face, lips and mouth, the condition will usually resolve without further treatment although antihistamines may be useful in relieving symptoms. These patients should be followed carefully until the swelling has resolved. However, where there is involvement of the tongue, glottis or larynx likely to cause airways obstruction, appropriate therapy such as subcutaneous adrenaline (0.5 ml 1:1,000) should be administered promptly.

Patients with a history of angioedema unrelated to ACE-inhibitor therapy may be at an increased risk of angioedema while receiving an ACE inhibitor (see also 'Contra-indications').

Other hypersensitivity reactions have been reported.

Anaphylactoid reactions during hymenoptera desensitisation: Rarely, patients receiving ACE inhibitors during desensitisation with hymenoptera venom have experienced life-threatening anaphylactoid reactions. These reactions were avoided by temporarily withholding ACE inhibitor therapy prior to each desensitisation.

Haemodialysis patients: Anaphylactoid reactions have been reported in patients dialysed with high-flux membrances (e.g. AN 69®) and treated concomitantly with an ACE inhibitor. In these patients consideration should be given to using a different type of dialysis membrane or a different class of antihypertensive agent.

Cough: Cough has been reported with the use of ACE-inhibitors. Characteristically, the cough is non-productive, persistent, and resolves after discontinuation of therapy. ACE-inhibitor-induced cough should be considered as part of the differential diagnosis of cough.

Surgery/anaesthesia: In patients undergoing major surgery or during anaesthesia with agents that produce hypotension, Carace blocks angiotensin II formation secondary to compensatory renin release. This may lead to hypotension which can be corrected by volume expansion.

General: Carace should not be used in patients with aortic stenosis, cor pulmonale or outflow tract obstruction.

Where Carace is used as a single agent in hypertension, Afro-Caribbean patients may show a reduced therapeutic response.

Drug interactions: When Carace is combined with other antihypertensive agents such as beta-blockers and diuretics the antihypertensive effect is usually additive.

Carace minimises the development of thiazide-induced hypokalaemia and hyperuricaemia.

Carace has been used with nitrates without significant clinical interaction.

Indomethacin may reduce the antihypertensive efficacy of Carace.

As Carace may reduce the elimination of lithium, serum levels of lithium should be monitored if lithium salts are administered.

Plasma potassium usually remains within normal limits, although a few cases of hyperkalaemia have occurred. If Carace is given with a diuretic, the likelihood of diuretic-induced hypokalaemia may be lessened. Carace may elevate plasma potassium levels in patients with renal failure. Potassium supplements, potassium-sparing diuretics and potassium-containing salt substitutes are not recommended.

Use in pregnancy and lactation: The use of Carace during pregnancy is not recommended. When pregnancy is detected Carace should be discontinued as soon as possible, unless it is considered life-saving for the mother.

ACE inhibitors can cause foetal and neonatal morbidity and mortality when administered to pregnant women during the second and third trimesters. Use of ACE inhibitors during this period has been associated with foetal and neonatal injury including hypotension, renal failure, hyperkalaemia, and/or skull hypoplasia in the newborn. Maternal oligohydramnios, presumably representing decreased foetal renal function, has occurred and may result in limb contractures, craniofacial deformations and hypoplastic lung development. If Carace is used, the patient should be appraised of the potential hazard to the foetus.

These adverse effects to the embryo and foetus do not appear to have resulted from intrauterine ACE-inhibitor exposure limited to the first trimester.

In those rare cases where ACE inhibitor use during pregnancy is deemed essential, serial ultrasound examinations should be performed to assess the intraamniotic environment. If oligohydramnios is detected, Carace should be discontinued unless it is considered life-saving to the mother. Patients and physicians should be aware, however, that oligohydramnios may not appear until after the foetus has sustained irreversible injury.

Infants whose mothers have taken Carace should be closely observed for hypotension, oliguria and hyperkalaemia. Lisinopril, which crossed the placenta, has been removed from the neonatal circulation by peritoneal dialysis with some clinical benefit, and theoretically may be removed by exchange transfusion.

Nursing mothers: It is not known whether Carace is excreted in human milk. Because many drugs are secreted in human milk, caution should be exercised if Carace is given to a nursing mother.

Side-effects: Hypotension has occurred in association with therapy with Carace. This appears to occur in certain specific sub-groups (see 'Precautions').

Hypersensitivity/angioneurotic oedema: Angioneurotic oedema of the face, extremities, lips, tongue, glottis and/or larynx has been reported rarely (see 'Precautions').

Other adverse reactions: Dizziness, headache, diarrhoea, fatigue, cough, and nausea are the most frequent. Other less frequent side effects include: orthostatic effects (including hypotension), rash, and asthenia.

Rare side-effects include myocardial infarction or cerebrovascular accident possibly secondary to excessive hypotension in high-risk patients (see 'Precautions'), palpitation, tachycardia, pancreatitis, abdominal pain, dry mouth, hepatitis (hepatocellular or cholestatic), mood alterations, mental confusion, bronchospasm, paraesthesia, urticaria, pruritus, diaphoresis, alopecia, uraemia, oliguria/anuria, renal dysfunction, acute renal failure, impotence.

There have been reports of haemolytic anaemia in patients taking lisinopril, although no causal relationship has been established.

A symptom complex has been reported which may include fever, vasculitis, myalgia, arthralgia/arthritis, a positive ANA, elevated erythrocyte sedimentation rate, eosinophilia, and leucocytosis. Rash, photosensitivity, or other dermatological manifestations may occur.

Laboratory test findings: Increases in blood urea and creatinine, reversible on discontinuation of Carace, are most likely in the presence of bilateral renal artery stenosis, especially in patients with renal insufficiency (see 'Precautions'). However, increases in blood urea and creatinine may occur without evidence of pre-existing renal impairment, especially in patients taking diuretics. In this event, undiagnosed renal artery stenosis should be suspected. Dosage reduction of Carace and/or discontinuation of the diuretic should be considered. Rare cases of neutropenia have been reported, although no causal relationship has been shown.

Increases in liver enzymes and serum bilirubin have occurred which are usually reversible on discontinuation of Carace.

Decreases in haemoglobin and haematocrit have been reported in a few patients but were rarely of clinical importance unless another cause of anaemia was present.

Hyperkalaemia and hyponatraemia have occurred occasionally (see also 'Plasma potassium').

Thrombocytopenia and leukopenia have been reported: a causal relationship to therapy with Carace cannot be excluded.

Overdosage: There are no data on overdosage in humans. The most likely manifestation of overdosage would be hypotension, which can be treated, if necessary, by intravenous infusion of normal saline solution. Carace can be removed by haemodialysis.

Pharmaceutical precautions Store in a dry place below 25°C.

Legal category POM.

Package quantities
Tablets 20 mg: Calendar packs of 28 tablets.
Tablets 10 mg: Calendar packs of 28 tablets.
Tablets 5 mg: Calendar packs of 28 tablets.
Tablets 2.5 mg: Calendar packs of 28 tablets.

Further information Nil.

Product licence numbers

2.5 mg tablet	11173/0027
5 mg tablet	11173/0028
10 mg tablet	11173/0029
20 mg tablet	11173/0030

Product licence holder: DuPont Pharmaceuticals Limited, Wedgwood Way, Stevenage, Herts SG1 4QN

CARACE* 10 PLUS and CARACE 20* PLUS

Presentation Carace 10 Plus: Blue, hexagonal, biconvex tablet with the product code 145 on one side. Each tablet contains 10 mg lisinopril and 12.5 mg hydrochlorothiazide.

Carace 20 Plus: Hexagonal, yellow tablets marked MSD 140 on one side and scored. Each tablet contains 20 mg lisinopril and 12.5 mg hydrochlorothiazide.

Uses For the management of mild to moderate hypertension in patients who have been stabilised on the individual components given in the same proportions.

Action: Carace 10 Plus and Carace 20 Plus are fixed combinations of an angiotensin-converting enzyme inhibitor (lisinopril) and a diuretic (hydrochlorothiazide). Carace 10 Plus and Carace 20 Plus are highly effective in the treatment of hypertension. Hydrochlorothiazide stimulates the renin-angiotensin-aldosterone system which produces an additive effect with lisinopril.

Lisinopril is an inhibitor of the angiotensin-converting enzyme (ACE). Inhibition of the formation of angiotensin II results in vasodilation and a fall in blood pressure.

Hydrochlorothiazide is a diuretic and antihypertensive agent. Use of this agent alone results in increased renin secretion. Although lisinopril alone is antihypertensive, even in patients with low renin hypertension, concomitant administration with hydrochlorothiazide results in a greater reduction in blood pressure. Lisinopril attenuates the potassium loss associated with hydrochlorothiazide.

Dosage and administration
Adults:

Essential hypertension: The usual dosage of Carace 10 Plus or Carace 20 Plus is 1 tablet, administered once daily. If necessary, the dosage may be increased to 2 tablets, administered once daily.

Dosage in renal insufficiency: Thiazides may not be appropriate diuretics for use in patients with renal impairment and are ineffective at creatinine clearance values of 30 ml/min or below (i.e. moderate or severe renal insufficiency).

Carace 10 Plus or Carace 20 Plus are not to be used as initial therapy in any patient with renal insufficiency.

In patients with creatinine clearance of >30 and <80 ml/min, Carace 10 Plus or Carace 20 Plus may be used, but only after titration of the individual components.

Prior diuretic therapy: Symptomatic hypotension may occur following the initial dose of Carace 10 Plus or Carace 20 Plus: this is more likely in patients who are volume and/or salt depleted as a result of prior diuretic therapy. If possible, the diuretic therapy should be discontinued for 2–3 days prior to initiation of therapy with lisinopril alone, in a 2.5 mg dose.

Use in the elderly: Lisinopril was equally effective in elderly (65 years or older) and non-elderly hypertensive patients. In elderly hypertensive patients, monotherapy with lisinopril was as effective in reducing diastolic blood pressure as monotherapy with either hydrochlorothiazide or atenolol. In clinical studies, age did not affect the tolerability of lisinopril.

In clinical studies the efficacy and tolerability of lisinopril and hydrochlorothiazide, administered concomitantly, were similar in both elderly and younger hypertensive patients.

Paediatric use: Safety and effectiveness in children have not been established.

Contra-indications, warnings, etc
Contra-indications: Carace 10 Plus or Carace 20 Plus are contra-indicated in patients with anuria or aortic stenosis or hyperkalaemia.

Carace 10 Plus or Carace 20 Plus are contra-indicated in patients who are hypersensitive to any component of the product and in patients with a history of angioneurotic oedema relating to previous treatment with an angiotensin-converting-enzyme inhibitor.

Carace 10 Plus and Carace 20 Plus are contra-indicated in patients who are hypersensitive to other sulphonamide-derived drugs.

The use of Carace 10 Plus or Carace 20 Plus during

pregnancy is not recommended. When pregnancy is detected Carace 10 Plus or Carace 20 Plus should be discontinued as soon as possible, unless it is considered life-saving for the mother.

ACE inhibitors can cause foetal and neonatal morbidity and mortality when administered to pregnant women during the second and third trimesters. Use of ACE inhibitors during this period has been associated with foetal and neonatal injury including hypotension, renal failure, hyperkalaemia, and/or skull hypoplasia in the newborn. Maternal oligohydramnios, presumably representing decreased foetal renal function, has occurred and may result in limb contractures, craniofacial deformations and hypoplastic lung development.

These adverse effects to the embryo and foetus do not appear to have resulted from intrauterine ACE inhibitor exposure limited to the first trimester.

The routine use of diuretics in otherwise healthy pregnant women is not recommended and exposes mother and foetus to unnecessary hazard including foetal or neonatal jaundice, thrombocytopenia and possibly other adverse reactions which have occurred in the adult.

If Carace 10 Plus or Carace 20 Plus are used during pregnancy, the patient should be apprised of the potential hazard to the foetus. In those rare cases where use during pregnancy is deemed essential, serial ultrasound examinations should be performed to assess the intraamniotic environment. If oligohydramnios is detected, Carace 10 Plus or Carace 20 Plus should be discontinued unless it is considered life-saving for the mother. Patients and physicians should be aware, however, that oligohydramnios may not appear until after the foetus has sustained irreversible injury.

Infants whose mothers have taken Carace 10 Plus or Carace 20 Plus should be closely observed for hypotension, oliguria and hyperkalaemia. Lisinopril, which crosses the placenta, has been removed from the neonatal circulation by peritoneal dialysis with some clinical benefit, and theoretically may be removed by exchange transfusion. There is no experience with the removal of hydrochlorothiazide, which also crosses the placenta, from the neonatal circulation.

Carace 10 Plus or Carace 20 Plus are contra-indicated in lactating women who are breast-feeding infants. It is not known whether lisinopril is excreted in human milk. Thiazides do appear in human milk.

See also 'Breast-feeding mothers' under 'Precautions'.

Precautions:

Hypotension and electrolyte/fluid imbalance: As with all antihypertensive therapy, symptomatic hypotension may occur in some patients. This was rarely seen in uncomplicated hypertensive patients but is more likely in the presence of fluid or electrolyte imbalance, e.g. volume depletion, hyponatraemia, hypochloraemic alkalosis, hypomagnesaemia or hypokalaemia which may occur from prior diuretic therapy, dietary salt restriction, dialysis, or during intercurrent diarrhoea or vomiting. Periodic determination of serum electrolytes should be performed at appropriate intervals in such patients.

Particular consideration should be given when therapy is administered to patients with ischaemic heart or cerebrovascular disease, because an excessive fall in blood pressure could result in myocardial infarction or cerebrovascular accident.

If hypotension occurs, the patient should be placed in the supine position and, if necessary, should receive an intravenous infusion of normal saline. A transient hypotensive response is not a contra-indication to further doses. Following restoration of effective blood volume and pressure, reinstitution of therapy at reduced dosage may be possible; or either of the components may be used appropriately alone.

Renal function impairment: Thiazides may not be appropriate diuretics for use in patients with renal impairment and are ineffective at creatinine clearance values of 30 ml/min or below (i.e. moderate or severe renal insufficiency). Carace 10 Plus or Carace 20 Plus should not be administered to patients with renal insufficiency (creatinine clearance <80 ml/min) until titration of the individual components has shown the need for the doses present in the combination tablet.

Some hypertensive patients, with no apparent preexisting renal disease, have developed usually minor and transient increases in blood urea and serum creatinine when lisinopril has been given concomitantly with a diuretic. If this occurs during therapy with Carace 10 Plus or Carace 20 Plus the combination should be discontinued. Reinstitution of therapy at reduced dosage may be possible, or either of the components may be used appropriately alone.

In some patients, with bilateral renal artery stenosis or stenosis of the single artery to a solitary kidney, increases in blood urea and serum creatinine, reversible upon discontinuation of therapy, have been seen with angiotensin-converting enzyme (ACE) inhibitors.

Haemodialysis patients: The use of Carace 10 Plus or Carace 20 Plus are not indicated in patients requiring dialysis for renal failure. A high incidence of anaphylactoid reactions have been reported in patients dialysed with high-flux membranes (e.g. AN 69®) and treated concomitantly with an ACE inhibitor. These combinations should therefore be avoided.

Hepatic disease: Thiazides should be used with caution in patients with impaired hepatic function or progressive liver disease, since minor alterations of fluid and electrolyte balance may precipitate hepatic coma.

Surgery/anaesthesia: In patients undergoing major surgery or during anaesthesia with agents that produce hypotension, lisinopril may block angiotensin II formation secondary to compensatory renin release. If hypotension occurs and is considered to be due to this mechanism, it can be corrected by volume expansion.

Metabolic and endocrine effects: Thiazide therapy may impair glucose tolerance. Dosage adjustment of antidiabetic agents, including insulin, may be required.

Thiazides may decrease urinary calcium excretion and may cause intermittent and slight elevation of serum calcium. Marked hypercalcaemia may be evidence of hidden hyperparathyroidism. Thiazides should be discontinued before carrying out tests for parathyroid function.

Increases in cholesterol and triglyceride levels may be associated with thiazide diuretic therapy.

Thiazide therapy may precipitate hyperuricaemia and/or gout in certain patients. However, lisinopril may increase urinary uric acid and thus may attenuate the hyperuricaemic effect of hydrochlorothiazide.

Hypersensitivity/angioneurotic oedema: Angioneurotic oedema of the face, extremities, lips, tongue, glottis, and/or larynx has been reported rarely in patients treated with angiotensin-converting enzyme inhibitors, including lisinopril. This may occur at anytime during treatment. In such cases, Carace 10 Plus or Carace 20 Plus should be discontinued promptly, and appropriate monitoring should be instituted to ensure complete resolution of symptoms prior to dismissing the patient.

In those instances where swelling has been confined to the face and lips, the condition generally resolved without treatment, although antihistamines have been useful in relieving symptoms. Angioneurotic oedema associated with laryngeal oedema may be fatal. Where there is involvement of the tongue, glottis or larynx, likely to cause airway obstruction, appropriate therapy such as subcutaneous adrenaline solution 1:1,000 (0.3 ml to 0.5 ml) should be administered promptly. Patients with a history of angioedema unrelated to ACE-inhibitor therapy may be at increased risk of angioedema while receiving an ACE inhibitor. (See also 'Contra-indications').

In patients receiving thiazides, sensitivity reactions may occur with or without a history of allergy or bronchial asthma. Exacerbation or activation of systemic lupus erythematosus has been reported with the use of thiazides.

Anaphylactoid reactions during hymenoptera desensitization: Rarely, patients receiving ACE inhibitors during desensitization with hymenoptera venom have experienced life-threatening anaphylactoid reactions. These reactions were avoided by temporarily withholding ACE inhibitor therapy prior to each desensitisation.

Cough: Cough has been reported with the use of ACE inhibitors. Characteristically, the cough is non-productive, persistent, and resolves after discontinuation of therapy. ACE inhibitor-induced cough should be considered as part of the differential diagnosis of cough.

Breast-feeding mothers: It is not known whether lisinopril is secreted in human milk; however, thiazides do appear in human milk. Because of the potential for serious reactions in nursing infants, a decision should be made whether to discontinue breast-feeding or to discontinue Carace 10 Plus or Carace 20 Plus, taking into account the importance of the drug to the mother.

Drug interactions:

Serum potassium: The potassium-losing effect of thiazide diuretics is usually attenuated by the potassium-conserving effect of lisinopril.

The use of potassium supplements, potassium-sparing agents or potassium-containing salt substitutes, particularly in patients with impaired renal function, may lead to a significant increase in serum potassium. If concomitant use of Carace 10 Plus or Carace 20 Plus and any of these agents is deemed appropriate, they should be used with caution and with frequent monitoring of serum potassium.

Lithium: Lithium generally should not be given with diuretics or ACE inhibitors. Diuretic agents and ACE inhibitors reduce the renal clearance of lithium and add a high risk of lithium toxicity. Refer to prescribing information for lithium preparations before use of such preparations.

Other agents: Indomethacin may diminish the antihypertensive effect of concomitantly administered Carace 10 Plus or Carace 20 Plus. The antihypertensive effect of Carace 10 Plus or Carace 20 Plus may be potentiated when given concomitantly with other agents likely to cause postural hypotension.

Thiazides may increase the responsiveness to tubocurarine.

Side-effects: Carace 10 Plus or Carace 20 Plus are usually well tolerated. In clinical studies, side effects have usually been mild and transient, and in most instances have not required interruption of therapy. The side-effects that have been observed have been limited to those reported previously with lisinopril or hydrochlorothiazide.

One of the most common clinical side-effects was dizziness, which generally responded to dosage reduction and seldom required discontinuation of therapy.

Other, less frequent side-effects were headache, dry cough, fatigue, and hypotension including orthostatic hypotension.

Still less common were diarrhoea, nausea, vomiting, dry mouth, rash, gout, palpitation, chest discomfort, muscle cramps and weakness, paraesthesia, asthenia, and impotence.

Pancreatitis has been reported rarely with lisinopril and with hydrochlorothiazide and therefore is a potential side-effect of Carace 10 Plus and Carace 20 Plus.

Hypersensitivity/angioneurotic oedema: Angioneurotic oedema of the face, extremities, lips, tongue, glottis and/or larynx has been reported rarely (see 'Precautions').

A symptom complex has been reported which may include fever, vasculitis, myalgia, arthralgia/arthritis, a positive ANA, elevated ESR, eosinophilia, and leucocytosis. Rash photosensitivity, or other dermatological manifestations may occur.

Laboratory test findings: Laboratory side-effects have rarely been of clinical importance. Occasional hyperglycaemia, hyperuricaemia and hyperkalaemia or hypokalaemia have been noted. Usually minor and transient increases in blood urea nitrogen and serum creatinine have been seen in patients without evidence of pre-existing renal impairment. If such increases persist, they are usually reversible upon discontinuation of Carace 10 Plus or Carace 20 Plus. Small decreases in haemoglobin and haematocrit have been reported frequently in hypertensive patients treated with Carace 10 Plus or Carace 20 Plus but were rarely of clinical importance unless another cause of anaemia co-existed. Rarely, elevation of liver enzymes and/or serum bilirubin have occurred, but a causal relationship to Carace 10 Plus or Carace 20 Plus has not been established.

Other side-effects reported with the individual components alone, and which may be potential side-effects with Carace 10 Plus or Carace 20 Plus, are:

Lisinopril: Myocardial infarction or cerebrovascular accident possibly secondary to excessive hypotension in high-risk patients (see 'Precautions'), tachycardia, abdominal pain, hepatitis – either hepatocellular or cholestatic jaundice, mood alterations, mental confusion, bronchospasm, urticaria, pruritus, diaphoresis, alopecia, uraemia, oliguria/anuria, renal dysfunction, acute renal failure, thrombocytopenia, leukopenia, hyponatraemia. Rare cases of neutropenia have been reported, although no causal relationship has been established. There have been reports of haemolytic anaemia in patients taking lisinopril, although no causal relationship has been established.

Hydrochlorothiazide: Anorexia, gastric irritation, constipation, jaundice (intrahepatic cholestatic jaundice), sialoadenitis, vertigo, xanthopsia, leucopenia, agranulocytosis, thrombocytopenia, aplastic anaemia, haemolytic anaemia, purpura, photosensitivity, urticaria, necrotising angiitis (vasculitis, cutaneous vasculitis), fever, respiratory distress including pneumonitis and pulmonary oedema, anaphylactic reactions, hyperglycaemia, glycosuria, hyperuricaemia, electrolyte imbalance including hyponatraemia, muscle spasm, restlessness, transient blurred vision, renal failure, renal dysfunction, and interstitial nephritis.

Overdosage: No specific information is available on the treatment of overdosage with Carace 10 Plus or Carace 20 Plus. Treatment is symptomatic and supportive. Therapy with Carace 10 Plus or Carace 20 Plus should be discontinued and the patient observed closely. Suggested measures include induction of emesis and/or gastric lavage, if ingestion is recent, and correction of dehydration, electrolyte imbalance and hypotension by established procedures.

Lisinopril: The most likely features of overdosage would be hypotension, for which the usual treatment would be intravenous infusion of normal saline solution.

Lisinopril may be removed from the general circulation by haemodialysis. (See *Precautions*).

Hydrochlorothiazide: The most common signs and symptoms observed are those caused by electrolyte depletion (hypokalaemia, hypochloraemia, hyponatraemia) and dehydration resulting from excessive diuresis. If digitalis has also been administered, hypokalaemia may accentuate cardiac arrhythmias.

Pharmaceutical precautions Store in a dry place below 25°C.

Legal category POM.

Package quantities Calendar packs of 28 tablets.

Further information Nil.

Product licence numbers
Carace 10 Plus 11173/0036.
Carace 20 Plus 11173/0033

Product licence holder: DuPont Pharmaceuticals Limited, Wedgwood Way, Stevenage, Herts SG1 4QN.

CARDIOLITE*

Name of the medicinal product CARDIOLITE, Kit for the preparation of Technetium Tc-99m Sestamibi.

Qualitative and quantitative composition
Active ingredients/1 vial contains: Tetrakis (2-methoxy isobutyl isonitrile) Copper (I)
Tetrafluoroborate 1.0 mg
Stannous chloride dihydrate 0.075 mg
L-Cysteine hydrochloride monohydrate 1.0 mg.

Pharmaceutical form Powder for injection.

Clinical particulars
Therapeutic indications: For intravenous injection after reconstitution with Sodium Pertechnetate [^{99m}Tc] solution and may be used for:

Adjunct for diagnosis of ischaemic heart disease.

Adjunct for diagnosis and localisation of myocardial infarction.

Assessment of global ventricular function (first pass technique for determination of ejection fraction and/or regional wall motion).

A second line diagnostic aid in the investigation of patients with suspected breast cancer when the results of mammography are unsatisfactory or equivocal, particularly in patients with dense breasts.

Posology and method of administration: The vial is reconstituted with a maximum of 5.55 GBq (150 mCi) of oxidant-free Sodium Pertechnetate Tc-99m Injection PhEur in 1–3 ml. Radiochemical purity should be checked prior to patient administration (see *Instructions for use/handling*).

The suggested dose range for intravenous administration to a patient of average (70 kg) is:

Diagnosis of reduced coronary perfusion and myocardial infarction: 185–740 MBq

Assessment of global ventricular function: 600–800 MBq injected as a bolus.

For diagnosis of ischaemic heart disease two injections (stress and rest) are required in order to differentiate transiently from persistently reduced myocardial uptake. Not more than a total of 925 MBq should be administered by these two injections which should be done at least six hours apart but may be performed in either order. After the stress injection, exercise should be encouraged for an additional one minute (if possible).

For diagnosis of myocardial infarction one injection at rest may be sufficient.

For breast imaging: 740–925 MBq injected as a bolus.

(The dose used should in every case be as low as reasonably practical).

Cardiac imaging: If possible, patients should fast for *at least* four hours prior to the study. It is recommended that patients eat a light fatty meal or drink a glass or two of milk after each injection, prior to imaging. This will promote rapid hepatobiliary clearance of Technetium Tc-99m Sestamibi resulting in less liver activity in the image.

The heart to background ratio will increase with time but the ideal imaging time, reflecting the best compromise between heart count rate and contrast, is approximately 1–2 hours after rest injection and stress injection. There is no evidence for significant changes in myocardial tracer concentration or redistribution, therefore imaging for up to 6 hours post injection is possible.

Either planar or tomographic imaging can be performed for diagnosis of ischaemic heart disease and myocardial infarction. Both may be performed ECG gated.

For planar imaging the standard three view (anterior, LAO 45°, LAO 70° or LL) planar projections should be used (e.g. 5–10 minutes each).

For tomographic imaging each projection should be acquired for approximately 20–40 seconds depending on injected dose.

For assessment of *global ventricular function* the same standard techniques and projections can be used, as established for Tc-99m first pass ejection studies; data should be acquired in list or fast frame mode in a computer using a high count rate scintillation camera. Gated Blood Pool Imaging protocols may be used for assessment of regional wall motion, however, must only be evaluated visually.

Breast imaging is optimally initiated 5 to 10 minutes post injection with the patient in the prone position with breast freely pendant. A 10 minute lateral image of the breast suspected of containing cancer should be obtained with the camera face as close to the breast as practical.

The patient should then be repositioned so that the contralateral breast is pendant and a lateral image of it should be obtained. An anterior supine image may then be obtained with the patient's arms behind her head.

Contra-indications: Pregnancy.

Special warnings and special precautions for use: Radiopharmaceutical agents should be used only by qualified personnel with the appropriate government authorisation for use and manipulation of radionuclides.

This radiopharmaceutical may be received, used and administered only by authorised persons in designated clinical settings. Its receipt, storage, use, transfer and disposal are subject to the regulations and/or appropriate licences of the local competent official organisation.

Radiopharmaceuticals should be prepared by the user in a manner which satisfies both radiation safety and pharmaceutical quality requirements. Appropriate aseptic precautions should be taken, complying with the requirements of Good Manufacturing Practice for pharmaceuticals.

Contents of the vial are intended only for use in the preparation of Technetium Tc-99m Sestamibi and are not to be administered directly to the patient without first undergoing the preparative procedure.

Safety and efficacy in children below the age of 18 years have not been established.

PROPER HYDRATION AND FREQUENT URINATION ARE NECESSARY TO REDUCE BLADDER IRRADIATION.

IN CASE OF KIDNEY FAILURE, EXPOSURE TO IONISING RADIATION CAN BE INCREASED. THIS MUST BE TAKEN INTO ACCOUNT WHEN CALCULATING THE ACTIVITY TO BE ADMINISTERED.

Interaction with other medications and other forms of interaction: No drug interactions have been described to date.

Pregnancy and lactation: When it is necessary to administer radioactive products to women of childbearing potential, information should be sought about pregnancy. Any woman who has missed a period should be assumed to be pregnant until proven otherwise. Where uncertainty exists it is important that radiation exposure should be the minimum consistent with obtaining the desired clincial information. Alternative techniques which do not involve ionising radiation should be considered.

The anticipated dose to the uterus from a 740 MBq rest injection would be 5.8 mGy. A radiation dose above 0.5 mGy (approximately equivalent to that exposure from annual background radiation) could potentially result in risk to the foetus. It is therefore contra-indicated in women known to be pregnant.

Before administering a radioactive medicinal product to a mother who is breast feeding consideration should be given as to whether the investigation could be reasonably delayed until after the mother has ceased breast feeding and as to whether the most appropriate choice of radiopharmaceutical has been made, bearing in mind the secretion of activity in breast milk.

If the administration is considered necessary, breast feeding should be interrupted for 24 hours and the expressed feeds discarded. It is usual to advise that breastfeeding can be restarted when the level in the milk will not result in a radiation dose to the child greater than 1 mSv.

Effects on ability to drive and use machines: Effects on the ability to drive and use machines have not been described.

Undesirable effects: Immediately after injection of Technetium Tc-99m Sestamibi, a small percentage of patients experienced a metallic or bitter taste, transient headache, flushing and a non-itching rash. A few cases of transient headache, flushing, oedema, injection site inflammation, dyspepsia, nausea, vomiting, pruritus, rash, urticaria, dry mouth, fever, dizziness, fatigue, dyspnoea and hypotension have been attributed to administration of the agent.

For each patient, exposure to ionising radiation must be justified on the basis of likely benefit. The activity administered must be such that the resulting radiation dose is as low as reasonably achievable bearing in mind the need to obtain the intended diagnostic or therapeutic result.

Exposure to ionising radiation is linked with cancer induction and a potential for development of hereditary defects. For diagnostic nuclear medicine investigations the current evidence suggests that these adverse effects will occur with low frequency because of the low radiation doses incurred.

For most diagnostic investigations using a nuclear medicine procedure the radiation dose delivered (effective dose/EDE) is less than 20 mSv. Higher doses may be justified in some clinical circumstances.

Overdose: In the event of administration of a radiation overdose with Technetium Tc-99m Sestamibi the absorbed dose to the patient should be reduced where possible by increasing the elimination of the radionuclide from the body by frequent micturation and defaecation.

Pharmacological properties
Pharmacodynamic properties: Pharmacodynamic effects are not expected after administration of Cardiolite.

Pharmacokinetics: After reconstitution with Sodium Pertechnetate Tc-99m Injection, PhEur solution, the following complex forms (Technetium Tc-99m Sestamibi):

Tc-99m $(MIBI)_6^+$ Where: MIBI=2-methoxyisobutylisonitrile

Like Thallous Chloride T1 201, this cationic complex accumulates in the viable myocardial tissue proportional to the circulation. Scintigraphic pictures which where obtained after i.v. injection of Technetium Tc-99m Sestamibi to animals and man are comparable with those obtained with Thallous Chloride T1 201. This correlation applies to normal as well as infarcted and ischaemic cardiac tissue.

Technetium Tc-99m Sestamibi from the blood is rapidly distributed into the tissue: 5 minutes after injection only about 8% of the injected dose is still in circulation.

Animal experiments have shown that uptake is not dependent on the functional capability of the sodium-potassium pump.

Elimination: The major metabolic pathway for clearance of Technetium Tc-99m Sestamibi is the hepatobiliary system. Activity from the gallbladder appears in the intestine within one hour of injection. About twenty-seven percent of the injected dose is cleared through renal elimination after 24 hours and approximately thirty-three percent of the injected dose is cleared through the faeces in 48 hours. At five minutes post injection about 8% of the injected dose remains in circulation.

Half-life: The biological myocardial $T_{\frac{1}{2}}$ is approximately seven (7) hours at rest and stress. The effective $T_{\frac{1}{2}}$ (which includes biological and physical half-lives) is approximately three (3) hours.

Myocardial uptake: Myocardial uptake which is coronary flow dependent is 1.5% of the injected dose at stress and 1.2% of the injected dose at rest.

Preclinical: In acute intravenous toxicity studies in mice, rats and dogs, the lowest dose of the reconstituted Cardiolite kit that resulted in any deaths was 7 mg/kg (expressed as Cu $(MIBI)_4$ BF_4 content) in female rats. This corresponds to 500 times the maximal human dose (MHD) of 0.014 mg/kg for adults (70 kg). Neither rats nor dogs exhibited treatment related effects at reconstituted Cardiolite kit doses of 0.42 mg/kg (30 times MHD) and 0.07 mg/kg (5 times MHD) respectively for 28 days. Studies on reproductive toxicity have not been conducted. Cu $(MIBI)_4$ BF_4 showed no genotoxic activity in the Ames, CHO/HPRT and sister chromatid exchange tests. At cytoxic concentrations, an increase in chromosome aberration was observed in the *in-vitro* human lymphocyte assay. No genotoxic activity was observed in the *in-vivo* mouse micronucleus test at 9 mg/kg. Studies to assess the carcinogenic potential of Cardiolite have not been conducted.

Radiation dosimetry: The projected radiation doses to organs and tissues of a patient of average weight (70 kg) after intravenous injection of Technetium Tc-99m Sestamibi are given below:

Absorbed dose per unit administered activity (mGy/MBq) for adults

Organ	*At rest*	*Stress*
Pancreas	7.7E-03	6.9E-03
Uterus	7.8E-03	7.2E-03
Adrenals	7.5E-03	6.6E-03
Bladder wall	1.1E-02	9.8E-03
Breast	3.8E-03	3.4E-03
Bone surface	8.2E-03	7.8E-03
Gall bladder wall	3.9E-02	3.3E-02
Heart	6.3E-03	7.2E-03
Brains	5.2E-03	4.4E-03
Skin	3.1E-03	2.9E-03
Liver	1.1E-02	9.2E-03
Lungs	4.6E-03	4.4E-03
GI-tract		
Stomach	6.5E-03	5.9E-03
Small intestine	1.5E-02	1.2E-02
Upper large intestine	2.7E-02	2.2E-02
Lower large intestine	1.9E-02	1.6E-02

Organ	At rest	Stress
Spleen	6.5E-03	5.8E-03
Kidneys	3.6E-02	2.6E-02
Ovaries	9.1E-03	8.1E-03
Red marrow	5.5E-03	5.0E-03
Thyroid	5.3E-03	4.4E-03
Esophagus	4.1E-03	4.0E-03
Salivary glands	1.4E-02	9.2E-03
Muscle	2.9E-03	3.2E-03
Testes	3.8E-03	3.7E-03
Thymus	4.1E-03	4.0E-03
Other organs	3.1E-03	3.3E-03
ED (mSv/MBq)	8.5E-03	7.5E-03

Data adopted from ICRP-publication nr. 62 (Volume 22. nr. 3. 1993): 'Radiological Protection in Biomedical Research.'

The effective dose resulting from an administered amount of 925 MBq in the adult is 7.9 mSv at rest and 6.9 mSv at stress.

Pharmaceutical particulars

List of excipients

Sodium citrate dihydrate

Mannitol

Incompatibilities: The Technetium labelling reactions involved depend on maintaining the stannous level in the reduced state. Hence, Sodium Pertechnetate Tc-99m Injection, PhEur, containing oxidants should not be employed.

Shelf-life: Of the finished drug in an unopened container: 24 months.

After preparation of the ready-to-use formulation: 6 hours.

Special precautions for storage: Before and after preparation, the drug should be stored at 15–25°C and protected from light. The contents of the vial are not radioactive. However, after labelling with Sodium Pertechnetate Tc-99m Injection PhEur the contents are radioactive and the currently valid protection and safety regulations must be be complied with.

Nature and contents of container: 5 ml glass vials, type 1 borosilicate glass (PhEur) sealed with a halobutyl rubber stopper.

Instructions for use/handling: The contents of the kit before preparation are not radioactive. However, after Sodium Pertechnetate Tc-99m Injection, PhEur is added, adequate shielding of the final preparation must be maintained.

The administration of radiopharmaceuticals create risks for other persons from external radiation or contamination from spill of urine, vomiting etc. Radiation protection precautions in accordance with national regulations must therefore be taken.

The preparation contains no bacteriostatic preservative.

Technetium Tc-99m Sestamibi is to be used within six (6) hours of reconstitution.

Reconstitute with oxidant-free Sodium Pertechnetate Tc-99m Injection, PhEur.

As with any pharmaceutical product, if at any time in the preparation of this product the integrity of this vial is compromised it should not be used.

Instructions for preparation of Technetium Tc-99m Sestamibi

A. Boiling procedure:

Preparation of Technetium Tc-99m Sestamibi from the Cardiolite Kit is to be done according to the following aseptic procedure:

1 Waterproof gloves should be worn during the preparation procedure. Remove the plastic disc from the Cardiolite Kit vial and swab the top of the vial closure with alcohol to disinfect the surface.
2 Place the vial in a suitable radiation shield appropriately labelled with date, time of preparation, volume and activity.
3 With a sterile shielded syringe, aseptically obtain additive-free, sterile, non-pyrogenic Sodium Pertechnetate Tc-99m solution (max 5.55 GBq–150 mCi) in approximately 1 to 3 ml.
4 Aseptically add the Sodium Pertechnetate Tc-99m solution to the vial in the lead shield. Without withdrawing the needle, remove an equal volume of headspace to maintain atmospheric pressure within the vial.
5 Swirl the contents of the vial for a few seconds.
6 Remove the vial from the lead shield and place **upright** in a boiling water bath, such that the vial is suspended above the bottom of the bath, and boil for 10 minutes. The bath must be shielded. Timing for the 10 minutes commences as soon as the water **begins to boil** again.
Note: The vial **must** remain upright during the boiling step. Use a water bath where the stopper will be above the level of the water.
7 Remove the shielded vial from the water bath and allow to cool for fifteen minutes.
8 Inspect visually for the absence of particulate matter and discoloration prior to administration.
9 Aseptically withdraw material using a sterile shielded syringe. Use within six (6) hours of preparation.
10 Radiochemical purity should be checked prior to patient administration according to the Radio TLC Method as detailed below.

B. Thermal Cycler procedure:

Preparation of Technetium Tc-99m Sestamibi from the Cardiolite Kit is to be done according to the following aseptic procedure:

1 Waterproof gloves should be worn during the preparation procedure. Remove the plastic disc from the Cardiolite Kit vial and swab the top of the vial closure with alcohol to disinfect the surface.
2 Place the vial in a suitable radiation shield appropriately labelled with date, time of preparation, volume and activity.
3 With a sterile shielded syringe, aseptically obtain additive-free, sterile, non-pyrogenic Sodium Pertechnetate Tc-99m solution (max 5.55 GBq–150 mCi-) in approximately 1 to 3 ml.
4 Aseptically add the Sodium Pertechnetate Tc-99m solution to the vial in the lead shield. Without withdrawing the needle, remove an equal volume of headspace to maintain atmospheric pressure within the vial.
5 Shake vigorously, about 5 to 10 quick upward-downward motions.
6 Place Shield in the sample block. While slightly pressing downwards, give the shield a quarter turn to make certain there is a firm fit between the shield and the sample block.
7 Press the proceed button to initiate the program (the thermal cycler automatically heats and cools the vial and contents). Please see the Recon-o-stat Instruction Manual for further details.
8 Inspect visually for the absence of particulate matter and discoloration prior to administration.
9 Aseptically withdraw material using a sterile shielded syringe. Use within six (6) hours of preparation.
10 Radiochemical purity should be checked prior to patient administration according to the Radio TLC Method as detailed below.

Radio-TLC Method for the Quantification of Technetium Tc-99m Sestamibi

A. Materials

1 Baker-Flex-Aluminium Oxide plate, # 1 B-F, pre-cut to 2.5 cm×7.5 cm.
2 Ethanol, >95%.
3 Capintec, or equivalent instrument for measuring radioactivity in the 0.74–11.12 GBq (20–300 mCi) range.
4 1 ml syringe with a 22–26 gauge needle.
5 Small developing tank with cover (100 ml beaker covered with Parafilm[R] is sufficient).

B. Procedure

1 Pour enough ethanol into the developing tank (beaker) to have a depth of 3–4 mm of solvent. Cover the tank (beaker) with Parafilm[R] and allow it to equilibrate for approximately 10 minutes.
2 Apply 1 drop of ethanol, using a 1 ml syringe with a 22–26 gauge needle on to the Aluminium Oxide TLC plate, 1.5 cm from the bottom. **Do not allow the spot to dry.**
3 Apply 1 drop of the kit solution on top of the ethanol spot. Dry the spot. **Do not heat!**
4 Develop the plate a distance of 5.0 cm from the spot.
5 Cut the strip 4.0 cm from the bottom, and measure each piece in your dose calibrator.
6 Calculate the % Radiochemical purity as:
% Tc-99m Sestamibi= (Activity top portion)/(Activity both pieces)×100.
7 % Tc-99m Sestamibi should >90%; otherwise the preparation should be discarded.

Note: Do not use material if the radiochemical purity is less than 90%.

The potential for cracking and significant contamination exists whenever vials containing radioactive material are heated. After reconstitution the container and any unused contents should be disposed of in accordance with local requirements for radioactive materials.

Marketing authorisation holder
DuPont Pharmaceuticals Limited, Wedgwood Way, Stevenage, Hertfordshire SG1 4QN, United Kingdom.

Marketing authorisation number PL 11173/0021.

Date of first authorisation/renewal of authorisation
8 October 1998.

Date of (partial) revision of text October 1998.

Legal category POM.

MODURET* 25

Presentation Moduret 25 is available as off-white, diamond-shaped tablets, with a break line and marked '923', containing Amiloride Hydrochloride BP equivalent to 2.5 mg anhydrous amiloride hydrochloride and 25 mg Hydrochlorothiazide BP.

Uses Potassium-conserving diuretic and antihypertensive.

Moduret 25 is indicated alone or as an adjunct to other antihypertensive agents in: hypertension, congestive heart failure, hepatic cirrhosis with ascites and oedema.

Moduret 25 is intended for the treatment of patients in whom potassium depletion might be suspected or anticipated. The presence of amiloride hydrochloride minimises the likelihood of potassium loss during vigorous diuresis for long term maintenance therapy. The combination is thus indicated especially in conditions where potassium balance is particularly important.

Dosage and administration

Hypertension: Usually two or four Moduret 25 tablets given once a day or in divided doses. Some patients may require only one Moduret 25 Tablet a day. The dosage may be increased if necessary, but must not exceed eight Moduret 25 tablets a day.

Congestive heart failure: Initially two or four tablets of Moduret 25 a day, subsequently adjusted if required, but not exceeding eight Moduret 25 tablets a day. Optimal dosage is determined by the diuretic response and the plasma potassium level. Once an initial diuresis has been achieved, reduction in dosage may be attempted for maintenance therapy. Maintenance therapy may be on an intermittent basis.

Hepatic cirrhosis with ascites: Initiate therapy with a low dose. A single daily dose of two Moduret 25 tablets may be increased gradually until there is an effective diuresis. Dosage should not exceed eight Moduret 25 tablets a day. Maintenance dosages may be lower than those required to initiate diuresis; dosage reduction should therefore be attempted when the patient's weight is stabilised. A gradual weight reduction is especially desirable in cirrhotic patients to reduce the likelihood of untoward reactions associated with diuretic therapy.

Paediatric use: Moduret 25 is not recommended for children (see 'Contra-indications').

Use in the elderly: Particular caution is needed in the elderly because of their susceptibility to electrolyte imbalance; the dosage should be carefully adjusted to renal function and clinical response.

Contra-indications, warnings, etc

Contra-indications: Hyperkalaemia (plasma potassium over 5.5 mmol/l); other potassium-conserving diuretics. Potassium supplements or potassium-rich food (except in severe and/or refractory cases of hypokalaemia under careful monitoring); concomitant use with spironolactone or triamterene; anuria; acute renal failure, severe progressive renal disease, severe hepatic failure, precoma associated with hepatic cirrhosis, Addison's disease, hypercalcaemia, concurrent lithium therapy, diabetic nephropathy; patients with blood urea over 10 mmol/l, patients with diabetes mellitus, or those with serum creatinine over 130 umol/l in whom serum electrolyte and blood urea levels cannot be monitored carefully and frequently. Prior hypersensitivity to amiloride hydrochloride, hydrochlorothiazide or other sulphonamide derived drugs. Because the safety of amiloride hydrochloride for use in children has not been established, Moduret 25 is not recommended for children. For 'Use in pregnancy' and 'Use in breast-feeding mothers', see 'Precautions'.

Precautions: Hyperkalaemia has been observed in patients receiving amiloride hydrochloride, either alone or with other diuretics, particularly in the aged or in hospital patients with hepatic cirrhosis or congestive heart failure with renal involvement, who were seriously ill, or were undergoing vigorous diuretic therapy. Such patients should be carefully observed for clinical, laboratory, and ECG evidence of hyperkalaemia (not always associated with an abnormal ECG).

Neither potassium supplements nor a potassium-rich diet should be used with Moduret 25 except under careful monitoring in severe and/or refractory cases of hypokalaemia.

Some deaths have been reported in this group of patients.

Treatment of hyperkalaemia: Should hyperkalaemia develop, discontinue treatment immediately and, if necessary, take active measures to reduce the plasma potassium to normal.

Impaired renal function: Renal function should be monitored because the use of Moduret 25 in impaired renal function may result in the rapid development of hyperkalaemia. Thiazide diuretics become ineffective when creatinine levels fall below 30 ml/min.

Electrolyte imbalance: Although the likelihood of electrolyte imbalance is reduced by Moduret 25, careful check should be kept for such signs of fluid and electrolyte imbalance as hyponatraemia, hypochloraemic alkalosis, hypokalaemia and hypomagnesaemia. It is particularly important to make serum and urine electrolyte determinations when the patient is vomiting excessively or receiving parenteral fluids. Warning signs or symptoms of fluid or electrolyte imbalance include: dryness of the mouth, weakness, lethargy, drowsiness, restlessness, seizures, muscle pains or cramps, muscular fatigue, hypotension, oliguria, tachycardia, and gastro-intestinal disturbances such as nausea and vomiting.

Hypokalaemia may develop, especially as a result of brisk diuresis, after prolonged therapy or when severe cirrhosis is present. Hypokalaemia can sensitise or exaggerate the response of the heart to the toxic effects of digitalis (e.g. increased ventricular irritability).

Diuretic-induced hyponatraemia is usually mild and asymptomatic. It may become severe and symptomatic in a few patients who will then require immediate attention and appropriate treatment.

Thiazides may decrease urinary calcium excretion. Thiazides may cause intermittent and slight elevation of serum calcium in the absence of known disorders of calcium metabolism. Therapy should be discontinued before carrying out tests for parathyroid function.

Azotaemia may be precipitated or increased by hydrochlorothiazide. Cumulative effects of the drug may develop in patients with impaired renal function. If increasing azotaemia and oliguria develop during treatment of renal disease, Moduret 25 should be discontinued.

Hepatic disease: Thiazides should be used with caution in patients with impaired hepatic function or progressive liver disease (see 'Contra-indications'), since minor alterations of fluid and electrolyte balance may precipitate hepatic coma.

Metabolic: Hyperuricaemia may occur, or gout may be precipitated or aggravated, in certain patients receiving thiazides. Thiazides may impair glucose tolerance. Diabetes mellitus may be precipitated or aggravated by therapy with Moduret 25 (see 'Contra-indications'). Dosage adjustment of antidiabetic agents, including insulin, may be required.

Increases in cholesterol and triglyceride levels may be associated with thiazide diuretic therapy.

To minimise the risk of hyperkalaemia in diabetic or suspected diabetic patients, the status of renal function should be determined before initiating therapy with Moduret 25. Therapy should be discontinued at least three days before giving a glucose tolerance test. Potassium-conserving therapy should be initiated only with caution in severely ill patients in whom metabolic or respiratory acidosis may occur, e.g. patients with cardiopulmonary disease or patients with inadequately controlled diabetes.

Shifts in acid-base balance alter the balance of extracellular/intracellular potassium, and the development of acidosis may be associated with rapid increases in plasma potassium.

Sensitivity reactions: The possibility that thiazides may activate or exacerbate systemic lupus erythematosus has been reported.

Ability to drive and to use machines: Infrequently, patients may experience weakness, fatigue, dizziness, stupor and vertigo. Should any of these occur, the patient should be cautioned not to drive or operate machinery.

Use in pregnancy: The routine use of diuretics in otherwise healthy pregnant women with or without mild oedema is not indicated, because they may be associated with hypovolaemia, increased blood viscosity, and decreased placental perfusion. Diuretics do not prevent the development of toxaemia of pregnancy and there is no satisfactory evidence that they are useful for its treatment.

Since thiazides cross the placental barrier and appear in cord blood, use where pregnancy is present or suspected requires that the benefits of the drug be weighed against possible hazards to the fetus. These hazards include fetal or neonatal jaundice, thrombocytopenia, bone marrow depression and possibly other side effects that have occurred in the adult.

Use in breast-feeding mothers: Although it is not known whether amiloride hydrochloride is excreted in human milk, it is known that thiazides do appear in breast milk. If use of the drug combination is deemed essential, the patient should stop breast-feeding.

Drug interactions: When amiloride hydrochloride is administered concomitantly with an ACE inhibitor, the risk of hyperkalaemia may be increased. Therefore, if concomitant use of these agents is indicated because of demonstrated hypokalaemia, they should be used with caution and with frequent monitoring of serum potassium.

When given concurrently, the following drugs may interact with thiazide diuretics:

Alcohol, barbiturates or narcotics: Co-administration may potentiate orthostatic hypotension. Oral and parenteral antidiabetic drugs may require adjustment of dosage with concurrent use. Other antihypertensive drugs may have an additive effect. Therefore the dosage of these agents, especially adrenergic-blockers, may need to be reduced when Moduret 25 is added to the regimen. Diuretic therapy should be discontinued for 2–3 days prior to initiation of therapy with an ACE inhibitor to reduce the likelihood of first dose hypotension. Corticosteroids or ACTH may intensify any thiazide-induced electrolyte depletion, particularly hypokalaemia. Pressor amines such as adrenaline may show decreased arterial responsiveness when used with Moduret 25 but this reaction is not enough to preclude their therapeutic usefulness. Non-depolarising muscle relaxants such as tubocurarine may possibly interact with Moduret 25 to increase muscle relaxation. Lithium may accumulate as a result of reduced renal clearance. Non-steroidal anti-inflammatory drugs may attenuate the diuretic, natriuretic and antihypertensive effects of diuretics. Chlorpropamide: Moduret 25 can act synergistically with chlorpropramide to increase the risk of hyponatraemia. Drug/laboratory tests: Because thiazides may affect calcium metabolism, Moduret 25 may interfere with tests for parathyroid function.

Side-effects: Although minor side effects are relatively common, significant side effects are infrequent.

Reported side effects are generally associated with diuresis, thiazide therapy, or with the underlying disease.

No increase in the risk of adverse reactions has been seen over those of the individual components.

The reported adverse reactions of the combination:

Body as a whole: headache, weakness, fatigue, malaise, chest pain, back pain, syncope.

Cardiovascular: arrhythmias, tachycardia, digitalis toxicity, orthostatic hypotension, angina pectoris.

Digestive: anorexia, nausea, vomiting, diarrhoea, constipation, abdominal pain, GI bleeding, appetite changes, abdominal fullness, flatulence, thirst, hiccups.

Metabolic: elevated plasma potassium levels (above 5.5 mmol/l), electrolyte imbalance, hyponatraemia, gout, dehydration, symptomatic hyponatraemia.

Integumentary: rash, pruritus, flushing, diaphoresis.

Musculoskeletal: leg ache, muscle cramps, joint pain.

Nervous: dizziness, vertigo, paraesthesiae, stupor.

Psychiatric: insomnia, nervousness, mental confusion, depression, sleepiness.

Respiratory: dyspnoea.

Special senses: bad taste, visual disturbance, nasal congestion.

Urogenital: impotence, dysuria, nocturia, incontinence, renal dysfunction including renal failure.

The reported adverse reactions of amiloride:

Body as a whole: neck/shoulder ache, pain in extremities.

Digestive: abnormal liver function, activation of probable pre-existing peptic ulcer, dyspepsia, jaundice.

Integumentary: dry mouth, alopecia, diaphoresis.

Nervous: tremors, encephalopathy.

Haematological: aplastic anaemia, neutropenia.

Cardiovascular: one patient with partial heart block developed complete heart block, palpitation.

Psychiatric: decreased libido, somnolence.

Respiratory: cough.

Special senses: tinnitus, increased intra-ocular pressure.

Urogenital: polyuria, urinary frequency, bladder spasm.

The reported adverse reactions of hydrochlorothiazide:

Body as a whole: anaphylactic reaction, fever.

Cardiovascular: necrotising angiitis (vasculitis, cutaneous vasculitis).

Digestive: jaundice (intrahepatic cholestatic jaundice), pancreatitis, cramping, gastric irritation.

Endocrine/Metabolic: glycosuria, hyperglycaemia, hyperuricaemia.

Integumentary: photosensitivity, sialadenitis, urticaria.

Haematological: agranulocytosis, aplastic anaemia, haemolytic anaemia, leucopenia, purpura, thrombocytopenia.

Psychiatric: restlessness.

Renal: interstitial nephritis.

Respiratory: respiratory distress, including pneumonitis, pulmonary oedema.

Special senses: transient blurred vision, xanthopsia.

Overdosage: No specific data are available on overdosage with Moduret 25. No specific antidote is available, and it is not known whether the drug is dialysable.

Treatment should be symptomatic and supportive. Therapy should be discontinued and the patient watched closely. Emesis should be induced and/or gastric lavage performed. The most common signs and symptoms of overdosage with amiloride hydrochloride are dehydration and electrolyte imbalance. Blood pressure should be monitored and corrected where necessary. If hyperkalaemia occurs, active measures should be taken to reduce the plasma potassium levels.

Electrolyte depletion (hypokalaemia, hypochloraemia, hyponatraemia) and dehydration are the most common signs and symptoms of hydrochlorothiazide overdosage. If digitalis has been administered, hypokalaemia may accentuate cardiac arrhythmias.

The plasma half-life of hydrochlorothiazide is 5.6 hours with a subsequent longer terminal half-life: the plasma half-life of amiloride is about six hours.

Pharmaceutical precautions Store in a dry place below 25°C, protected from light.

Legal category POM.

Package quantities Calendar packs of 28 tablets.

Further information The combination of amiloride with hydrochlorothiazide has been shown to cause less magnesium excretion than either the thiazides or the loop diuretics when used alone.

Onset of diuretic action begins within two hours after administration, and reaches a peak at about the fourth hour; there is detectable activity for about 24 hours.

Product licence number 0025/0178.

Product licence holder: Merck Sharp & Dohme Limited, Hertford Road, Hoddesdon, Hertfordshire, EN11 9BU.

MODURETIC*

Presentation Moduretic is available as peach-coloured, half-scored, diamond shaped tablets, marked 'MSD 917', containing amiloride hydrochloride BP, equivalent to 5 mg anhydrous amiloride hydrochloride and 50 mg hydrochlorothiazide BP.

Uses Potassium-conserving diuretic and antihypertensive.

Moduretic is indicated in patients with: hypertension, congestive heart failure, hepatic cirrhosis with ascites and oedema. In hypertension, Moduretic may be used alone or in conjunction with other antihypertensive agents.

Moduretic is intended for the treatment of patients in whom potassium depletion might be suspected or anticipated. The presence of amiloride hydrochloride minimises the likelihood of potassium loss during vigorous diuresis for long term maintenance therapy. The combination is thus indicated especially in conditions where potassium balance is particularly important.

Dosage and administration

Hypertension: Usually one or two Moduretic tablets given once a day or in divided doses. Some patients may require only half a Moduretic tablet a day. The dosage may be increased if necessary, but must not exceed four Moduretic tablets a day.

Congestive heart failure: Initially one or two tablets of Moduretic a day, subsequently adjusted if required, but not exceeding four Moduretic tablets a day. Optimal dosage is determined by the diuretic response and the plasma potassium level. Once an initial diuresis has been achieved, reduction in dosage may be attempted for maintenance therapy. Maintenance therapy may be on an intermittent basis.

Hepatic cirrhosis with ascites: Initiate therapy with a low dose. A single daily dose of one Moduretic tablet or equivalent may be increased gradually until there is an effective diuresis. Dosage should not exceed four Moduretic tablets a day. Maintenance dosages may be lower than those required to initiate diuresis; dosage reduction should therefore be attempted when the patient's weight is stabilised. A gradual weight reduction is especially desirable in cirrhotic patients to reduce the likelihood of untoward reactions associated with diuretic therapy.

Paediatric use: Moduretic is not recommended for children (see 'Contra-indications').

Use in the elderly: Particular caution is needed in the elderly because of their susceptibility to electrolyte imbalance; the dosage should be carefully adjusted to renal function and clinical response.

Contra-indications, warnings, etc

Contra-indications: Hyperkalaemia (plasma potassium over 5.5 mmol/l); other potassium-conserving diuretics. Potassium supplements or potassium-rich food (except in severe and/or refractory cases of hypokalaemia under careful monitoring); concomitant use with spironolactone or triamterene; anuria; acute renal failure, severe progressive renal disease, severe hepatic failure, precoma associated with hepatic cirrhosis, Addison's disease, hypercalcaemia, concurrent lithium therapy, diabetic nephropathy; patients with blood urea over 10 mmol/l, patients with diabetes mellitus, or those with serum creatinine over 130 umol/l in whom serum electrolyte and blood urea levels cannot be monitored carefully and frequently. Prior hypersensitivity to amiloride hydrochloride, hydrochlorothiazide or other sulphonamide derived drugs. Because the safety of amiloride hydrochloride for use in children has not been established, Moduretic is not recommended for children. For 'Use in pregnancy' and 'Use in breast-feeding mothers', see 'Precautions'.

Precautions: Hyperkalaemia has been observed in patients receiving amiloride hydrochloride, either alone or with other diuretics, particularly in the aged or in hospital patients with hepatic cirrhosis or congestive heart failure with renal involvement, who were seriously ill, or were undergoing vigorous diuretic therapy. Such patients should be carefully observed for clinical, laboratory, and ECG evidence of hyperkalaemia (not always associated with an abnormal ECG).

Neither potassium supplements nor a potassium-rich diet should be used with Moduretic except under careful monitoring in severe and/or refractory cases of hypokalaemia.

Some deaths have been reported in this group of patients.

Treatment of hyperkalaemia: Should hyperkalaemia develop, discontinue treatment immediately and, if necessary, take active measures to reduce the plasma potassium to normal.

Impaired renal function: Renal function should be monitored because the use of Moduretic in impaired renal function may result in the rapid development of hyperkalaemia. Thiazide diuretics become ineffective when creatinine levels fall below 30 ml/min.

Electrolyte imbalance: Although the likelihood of electrolyte imbalance is reduced by Moduretic, careful check should be kept for such signs of fluid and electrolyte imbalance as hyponatraemia, hypochloraemic alkalosis, hypokalaemia and hypomagnesaemia. It is particularly important to make serum and urine electrolyte determinations when the patient is vomiting excessively or receiving parenteral fluids. Warning signs or symptoms of fluid or electrolyte imbalance include: dryness of the mouth, weakness, lethargy, drowsiness, restlessness, seizures, muscle pains or cramps, muscular fatigue, hypotension, oliguria, tachycardia, and gastro-intestinal disturbances such as nausea and vomiting.

Hypokalaemia may develop, especially as a result of brisk diuresis, after prolonged therapy or when severe cirrhosis is present. Hypokalaemia can sensitise or exaggerate the response of the heart to the toxic effects of digitalis (e.g. increased ventricular irritability).

Diuretic-induced hyponatraemia is usually mild and asymptomatic. It may become severe and symptomatic in a few patients who will then require immediate attention and appropriate treatment.

Thiazides may decrease urinary calcium excretion. Thiazides may cause intermittent and slight elevation of serum calcium in the absence of known disorders of calcium metabolism. Therapy should be discontinued before carrying out tests for parathyroid function.

Azotaemia may be precipitated or increased by hydrochlorothiazide. Cumulative effects of the drug may develop in patients with impaired renal function. If increasing azotaemia and oliguria develop during treatment of renal disease, Moduretic should be discontinued.

Hepatic disease: Thiazides should be used with caution in patients with impaired hepatic function or progressive liver disease (see 'Contra-indications'), since minor alterations of fluid and electrolyte balance may precipitate hepatic coma.

Metabolic: Hyperuricaemia may occur, or gout may be precipitated or aggravated, in certain patients receiving thiazides. Thiazides may impair glucose tolerance. Diabetes mellitus may be precipitated or aggravated by therapy with Moduretic (see 'Contra-indications'). Dosage adjustment of antidiabetic agents, including insulin, may be required.

Increases in cholesterol and triglyceride levels may be associated with thiazide diuretic therapy.

To minimise the risk of hyperkalaemia in diabetic or suspected diabetic patients, the status of renal function should be determined before initiating therapy with Moduretic. Therapy should be discontinued at least three days before giving a glucose tolerance test. Potassium-conserving therapy should be initiated only with caution in severely ill patients in whom metabolic or respiratory acidosis may occur, e.g. patients with cardiopulmonary disease or patients with inadequately controlled diabetes.

Shifts in acid-base balance alter the balance of extracellular/intracellular potassium, and the development of acidosis may be associated with rapid increases in plasma potassium.

Sensitivity reactions: The possibility that thiazides may activate or exacerbate systemic lupus erythematosus has been reported.

Ability to drive and to use machines: Infrequently, patients may experience weakness, fatigue, dizziness, stupor and vertigo. Should any of these occur, the patient should be cautioned not to drive or operate machinery.

Use in pregnancy: The routine use of diuretics in otherwise healthy pregnant women with or without mild oedema is not indicated, because they may be associated with hypovolaemia, increased blood viscosity, and decreased placental perfusion. Diuretics do not prevent the development of toxaemia of pregnancy and there is no satisfactory evidence that they are useful for its treatment.

Since thiazides cross the placental barrier and appear in cord blood, use where pregnancy is present or suspected requires that the benefits of the drug be weighed against possible hazards to the foetus. These hazards include foetal or neonatal jaundice, thrombocytopenia, bone marrow depression and possibly other side effects that have occurred in the adult.

Use in breast-feeding mothers: Although it is not known whether amiloride hydrochloride is excreted in human milk, it is known that thiazides do appear in breast milk. If use of the drug combination is deemed essential, the patient should stop breast-feeding.

Drug interactions: When amiloride hydrochloride is administered concomitantly with an ACE inhibitor, the risk of hyperkalaemia may be increased. Therefore, if concomitant use of these agents is indicated because of demonstrated hypokalaemia, they should be used with caution and with frequent monitoring of serum potassium.

When given concurrently, the following drugs may interact with thiazide diuretics:

Alcohol, barbiturates or narcotics: Co-administration may potentiate orthostatic hypotension. Oral and parenteral antidiabetic drugs may require adjustment of dosage with concurrent use. Other antihypertensive drugs may have an additive effect. Therefore the dosage of these agents, especially adrenergic-blockers, may need to be reduced when Moduretic is added to the regimen. Diuretic therapy should be discontinued for 2–3 days prior to initiation of therapy with an ACE inhibitor to reduce the likelihood of first dose hypotension. Corticosteroids or ACTH may intensify any thiazide-induced electrolyte depletion, particularly hypokalaemia. Pressor amines such as adrenaline may show decreased arterial responsiveness when used with Moduretic but this reaction is not enough to preclude their therapeutic usefulness. Non-depolarising muscle relaxants such as tubocurarine may possibly interact with Moduretic to increase muscle relaxation. Lithium may accumulate as a result of reduced renal clearance. Non-steroidal anti-inflammatory drugs may attenuate the diuretic, natriuretic and antihypertensive effects of diuretics. Chlorpropamide: Moduretic can act synergistically with chlorpropamide to increase the risk of hyponatraemia. Drug/laboratory tests: Because thiazides may affect calcium metabolism, Moduretic may interfere with tests for parathyroid function.

Side-effects: Although minor side effects are relatively common, significant side effects are infrequent.

Reported side effects are generally associated with diuresis, thiazide therapy, or with the underlying disease.

No increase in the risk of adverse reactions has been seen over those of the individual components.

The reported adverse reactions of the combination:

Body as a whole: headache, weakness, fatigue, malaise, chest pain, back pain, syncope.

Cardiovascular: arrhythmias, tachycardia, digitalis toxicity, orthostatic hypotension, angina pectoris.

Digestive: anorexia, nausea, vomiting, diarrhoea, constipation, abdominal pain, GI bleeding, appetite changes, abdominal fullness, flatulence, thirst, hiccups.

Metabolic: elevated plasma potassium levels (above 5.5 mmol/l), electrolyte imbalance, hyponatraemia, gout, dehydration, symptomatic hyponatraemia.

Integumentary: rash, pruritus, flushing, diaphoresis.

Musculoskeletal: leg ache, muscle cramps, joint pain.

Nervous: dizziness, vertigo, paraesthesiae, stupor.

Psychiatric: insomnia, nervousness, mental confusion, depression, sleepiness.

Respiratory: dyspnoea.

Special senses: bad taste, visual disturbance, nasal congestion.

Urogenital: impotence, dysuria, nocturia, incontinence, renal dysfunction including renal failure.

The reported adverse reactions of amiloride:

Body as a whole: neck/shoulder ache, pain in extremities.

Digestive: abnormal liver function, activation of probable pre-existing peptic ulcer, dyspepsia, jaundice.

Integumentary: dry mouth, alopecia, diaphoresis.

Nervous: tremors, encephalopathy.

Haematological: aplastic anaemia, neutropenia.

Cardiovascular: one patient with partial heart block developed complete heart block, palpitation.

Psychiatric: decreased libido, somnolence.

Respiratory: cough.

Special senses: tinnitus, increased intra-ocular pressure.

Urogenital: polyuria, urinary frequency, bladder spasm.

The reported adverse reactions of hydrochlorothiazide:

Body as a whole: anaphylactic reaction, fever.

Cardiovascular: necrotising angiitis (vasculitis, cutaneous vasculitis).

Digestive: jaundice (intrahepatic cholestatic jaundice), pancreatitis, cramping, gastric irritation.

Endocrine/Metabolic: glycosuria, hyperglycaemia, hyperuricaemia.

Integumentary: photosensitivity, sialadenitis, urticaria.

Haematological: agranulocytosis, aplastic anaemia, haemolytic anaemia, leucopenia, purpura, thrombocytopenia.

Psychiatric: restlessness.

Renal: interstitial nephritis.

Respiratory: respiratory distress, including pneumonitis, pulmonary oedema.

Special senses: transient blurred vision, xanthopsia.

Overdosage: No specific data are available on overdosage with Moduretic. No specific antidote is available, and it is not known whether the drug is dialysable.

Treatment should be symptomatic and supportive. Therapy should be discontinued and the patient watched closely. Emesis should be induced and/or gastric lavage performed. The most common signs and symptoms of overdosage with amiloride hydrochloride are dehydration and electrolyte imbalance. Blood pressure should be monitored and corrected where necessary. If hyperkalaemia occurs, active measures should be taken to reduce the plasma potassium levels.

Electrolyte depletion (hypokalaemia, hypochloraemia, hyponatraemia) and dehydration are the most common signs and symptoms of hydrochlorothiazide overdosage. If digitalis has been administered, hypokalaemia may accentuate cardiac arrhythmias.

The plasma half-life of hydrochlorothiazide is 5.6 hours with a subsequent longer terminal half-life: the plasma half-life of amiloride is about six hours.

Pharmaceutical precautions Keep container tightly closed. Store in a dry place below 25°C, protected from light.

Legal category POM.

Package quantities Calendar packs of 28 tablets.

Further information The combination of amiloride with hydrochlorothiazide has been shown to cause less magnesium excretion than either the thiazides or the loop diuretics when used alone.

Onset of diuretic action begins within two hours after administration, and reaches a peak at about the fourth hour; there is detectable activity for about 24 hours.

Product licence numbers
Moduretic Tablets 0025/5016.

Product licence holder: Merck Sharp & Dohme Limited, Hertford Road, Hoddesdon, Hertfordshire, EN11 9BU.

NALOREX*

Presentation Pale yellow, film coated capsule-shaped tablet, debossed on one side with 'DuPont' and scored and debossed with '11' on the other side, containing naltrexone hydrochloride 50 mg.

Uses Nalorex is indicated as an adjunctive prophylactic therapy in the maintenance of detoxified, formerly opioid-dependent patients.

Dosage and administration Nalorex treatment should be initiated in a drug addiction centre and supervised by suitably qualified physicians.

Nalorex is an opioid antagonist with only minimal agonist activity under ordinary conditions. It is extensively metabolised in the liver. One of its metabolites, 6-Beta-Naltrexol, may also have activity as an opioid antagonist. It is excreted mainly in urine.

The initial dose of Nalorex should be 25 mg (half a tablet) followed by 50 mg (one tablet) daily.

A three-times a week dosing schedule may be considered if it is likely to result in better compliance, e.g. 100 mg on Monday, 100 mg on Wednesday and 150 mg on Friday.

Treatment with Nalorex should be considered only in patients who have remained opioid-free for a minimum of 7–10 days.

Narcan* (Naloxone hydrochloride) challenge is recommended to minimise the chance of a prolonged withdrawal syndrome precipitated by Nalorex (see also 'Warnings').

As Nalorex is a prophylactic agent and full recovery from opioid dependence is variable, no standard duration of therapy can be recommended; an initial period of three months should be considered. However, prolonged administration may be necessary.

Contra-indications, warnings, etc
Contra-indications: Nalorex should not be given to patients currently dependent on opioids since an acute withdrawal syndrome may ensue.

Nalorex should not be used in conjunction with an opioid-containing medication.

Nalorex should not be given to patients who are hypersensitive to it.

Nalorex should not be given to patients with acute hepatitis or liver failure.

Warnings: It is not uncommon for opioid abusing individuals to have impaired liver function. Liver function test abnormalities have been reported in obese and elderly patients taking naltrexone who have no history of drug abuse. Liver function tests should be carried out both before and during treatment.

A withdrawal syndrome may be precipitated by Nalorex* in opioid dependent patients; signs and symptoms may develop within 5 minutes and last up to 48 hours.

Treatment should be symptomatic and may include opioid administration.

Narcan (Naloxone hydrochloride) challenge is recommended to screen for presence of opioid use; a withdrawal syndrome precipitated by Narcan* will be of shorter duration than one precipitated by Nalorex*.

The recommended procedure is as follows:
- i.v. injection of 0.2 mg Narcan
- if after 30 seconds no adverse reactions occur, a further i.v. injection of 0.6 mg Narcan may be administered.
- continue to observe the patient for withdrawal effects for a further 30 minutes.

If doubt exists that the patient is opioid-free, the challenge may be repeated with a Narcan dose of 1.6 mg.

If there is no evidence of a reaction, Nalorex administration may be initiated with 25 mg by mouth (half a tablet).

Drug interactions: Concomitant administration of Nalorex with an opioid containing medication should be avoided. Patients should be warned that attempts to overcome the blockade may result in acute opioid intoxication which may be life threatening. In an emergency requiring opioid analgesia an increased dose of opioid may be required to control pain. The patient should be closely monitored for evidence of respiratory depression or other adverse symptoms and signs.

Use in pregnancy: Animal studies do not suggest a teratogenic effect.

Because of absence of documented clinical experience Nalorex should only be given to pregnant or breast-feeding women when, in the judgement of the attending physician, the potential benefits outweigh the possible risks.

Use in children: Safe use in children has not been established.

Use in elderly: There is no experience of use in the elderly.

Effects on ability to drive and use machines: Nalorex may impair the mental and/or physical abilities for performance of potentially hazardous tasks such as driving a car or operating machinery.

Precautions: Since Nalorex* is extensively metabolised by the liver and excreted predominantly in the urine, caution should be observed in administering the drug to patients with impaired hepatic or renal function.

Adverse effects: The following adverse reactions have been reported before and during naltrexone medication: an incidence of more than 10% in detoxified opioid abusers; difficulty in sleeping, anxiety, nervousness, abdominal pain/cramps, nausea and/or vomiting, low energy, joint and muscle pain, and headache: an incidence of less than 10%; loss of appetite, diarrhoea, constipation, increased thirst, increased energy, feeling down, irritability, dizziness, skin rash, delayed ejaculation, decreased potency, chills, chest pain, increased sweating, and increased lacrimation. Occasional liver function abnormalities have also been reported. One case of reversible idiopathic thrombocytopenic purpura has occurred in a patient taking Nalorex*.

Overdose: There is no clinical experience with Nalorex* overdose in patients. There was no evidence of toxicity in volunteers receiving 800 mg/day for seven days, however, in case of overdose, patients should be monitored and treated symptomatically in a closely supervised environment.

Pharmaceutical precautions Store below 30°C. Protect from light.

Legal category POM.

Package quantities Calendar pack of 28 tablets.

Further information The development of tolerance and dependence have not been observed with Nalorex.

Product licence number 11173/0026.

Product licence holder: DuPont Pharmaceuticals Limited, Wedgwood Way, Stevenage, Herts SG1 4QN.

NARCAN* INJECTION 400 mcg/ml

Qualitative and quantitative composition
NARCAN (1 ml ampoules) – each 1 ml of solution contains 400 micrograms naloxone hydrochloride.

Pharmaceutical form Solution for injection.

Clinical particulars
Therapeutic indications: Narcan may be used for the complete or partial reversal of opioid depression, including mild to severe respiratory depression induced by natural and synthetic opioids, the agonist/antagonist nalbuphine and pentazocine, or dextropropoxyphene. It may also be used for the diagnosis of suspected acute opioid overdosage. Narcan Neonatal may be used to counteract respiratory and other CNS depression in the newborn resulting from the administration of analgesics to the mother during childbirth.

Posology and method of administration: Narcan is for intravenous, intramuscular or subcutaneous injection or intravenous infusion.

Intravenous infusion: Narcan may be diluted for intravenous infusion in normal saline (0.9%) or 5% dextrose in water or saline: the addition of 2 mg (5 ml of 400 mcg/ml concentration) of Narcan in 500 ml of either solution provides a concentration of 4 micrograms/ml. Mixtures should be used within 12 hours. After 12 hours the remaining unused solution must be discarded. The rate of administration should be titrated in accordance with the patient's response to both the Narcan infusion and to any previous bolus doses administered.

Parenteral drug products should be inspected visually for particulate matter and discoloration prior to administration whenever solution and container permit.

Adults: Opioid overdosage (known or suspected): An initial dose of 400–2000 micrograms of Narcan may be administered intravenously. If the desired degree of counteraction and improvement in respiratory function is not obtained it may be repeated at 2 to 3 minute intervals. If no response is observed after 10 mg of Narcan have been administered the diagnosis of opioid induced or partial opioid induced toxicity should be questioned. Intramuscular or subcutaneous administration may be necessary if dosing by the intravenous route is not feasible.

NB The duration of action of certain opioids can outlast that of an i.v. bolus of Narcan, e.g. dextropropoxyphene (present in commonly prescribed analgesics which in over-dosage have been associated with suicide), dihydrocodeine and methadone. In situations where one of these opioids is known or suspected it is recommended that an infusion of Narcan (see above) be used to produce sustained antagonism to the opioid without repeated injection.

Post-operative use: When Narcan is used post-operatively, the dose should be titrated for each patient in order to obtain optimum respiratory response while maintaining adequate analgesia. Intravenous doses of 100–200 micrograms (approximately 1.5–3 micrograms/kg body weight) are usually sufficient, but a full two minutes should be allowed between each 100 microgram increment of Narcan administered. Further intramuscular doses may be needed within one to two hours, depending on the interval since the last opioid administration and the amount and type (i.e. long or short-acting) of drug used. Alternatively Narcan may be administered as an intravenous infusion (see above).

Children: The usual initial dose in children is 10 micrograms/kg body weight given i.v. If this dose does not result in the desired degree of clinical improvement, a subsequent dose of 100 micrograms/kg of body weight may be administered. Narcan may be required by infusion as described above. If an i.v. route of administration is not feasible, Narcan my be administered i.m. or s.c. in divided doses.

Neonatal use: An adequate airway should be established in the apnoeic infant before Narcan is administered. The usual dose for opioid-induced depression is 10 micrograms/kg body weight administered i.v., i.m., or s.c. If the desired degree of counteraction and improvement in respiratory function is not obtained it may be repeated at 2 to 3 minute intervals. Alternatively, a single dose of 200 micrograms, approximately 60 micrograms/kg body weight may be given intramuscularly at birth.

It should, however, be noted that onset of action is slower following i.m. injection. In neonates needing infusion of Narcan in saline care should be taken to avoid excessive sodium intake.

Elderly: There have been no specific studies of use in the elderly.

Contra-indications: Narcan should not be given to patients who are known to be hypersensitive to it.

Special warnings and special precautions for use: It should be administered cautiously to patients who have received large doses of opioids or to those physically dependent on opioids since too rapid reversal of opioid effects by Narcan may precipitate an acute withdrawal syndrome in such patients. The same caution is needed when giving Narcan to neonates delivered of such patients.

Patients who have responded satisfactorily to Narcan should be kept under observation. Repeated doses of Narcan may be necessary since the duration of action of some opioids may exceed that of Narcan.

Narcan is not effective against respiratory depression caused by non-opioid drugs. Reversal of buprenorphine-induced respiratory depression may be incomplete. If an incomplete response occurs, respiration should be mechanically assisted.

Several instances of hypotension, hypertension, ventricular tachycardia and fibrillation, and pulmonary oedema have been reported. These have occurred in postoperative patients, most of whom had pre-existing cardiovascular disorders or received other drugs which may have similar adverse cardiovascular effects. Although a direct cause and effect relationship has not been established, Narcan should be used with caution in patients with pre-existing cardiac disease or patients who have received potentially cardiotoxic drugs.

In addition to Narcan, other resuscitative measures such as maintenance of a free airway, artificial ventilation, cardiac massage and vasopressor agents should be available and employed when necessary to counteract acute poisoning.

Interaction with other medications and other forms of interaction: Narcan should be administered cautiously to persons including newborns of mothers who are known or suspected to be physically dependent on opioids. In such cases an abrupt and complete reversal of narcotic effects may precipitate an acute abstinence syndrome.

Pregnancy and lactation: The safety of this medicinal product for use in human pregnancy has not been established. Evaluation of experimental animal studies does not indicate direct or indirect harmful effects with respect to the development of the embryo or foetus, the course of gestation and peri- and postnatal development. Narcan should, like all drugs, be used with caution during pregnancy. Narcan may be administered to mothers during the second stage of labour to correct respiratory depression caused by opioids used to provide obstetrical analgesia.

It is not known whether Narcan is excreted in human milk. Because many drugs are excreted in human milk caution should be exercised when Narcan is administered to a nursing mother.

Effects on ability to drive and use machines: Not applicable.

Undesirable effects: Abrupt reversal of narcotic depression may result in nausea, vomiting, sweating, tachycardia, increased blood pressure, tremulousness, seizures and cardiac arrest. In post operative patients, larger than necessary dosage of Narcan may result in significant reversal of analgesia and excitement. Hypotension, hypertension, ventricular tachycardia and fibrillation, and pulmonary oedema have been associated with the use of Narcan post-operatively.

Overdose: There have been no reports of acute overdosage with Narcan. Single doses of 10 mg intravenously and subcutaneous doses of 15 mg every four hours for two weeks have been administered without producing either respiratory depression or psychotomimetic effects.

Pharmacological properties
Pharmacodynamic properties: Naloxone is N-allyl-nor-oxymorphone, an opioid antagonist which is devoid of the agonist or morphine-like properties characteristic of other opioid antagonists. In the absence of opioids or agonistic effects of other antagonists it exhibits essentially no pharmacologic activity.

Pharmacokinetic properties: Narcan usually acts within two minutes of intravenous administration and the onset of action is only slightly less rapid following intramuscular or subcutaneous injection. The duration of action is dependent upon the dose, route of administration, intramuscular injection producing a more prolonged effect than intravenous doses. However, the need for repeat doses of Narcan also depends on the amount, type and route of administration of the opioid being antagonised.

The rate of administration should be titrated in accordance with the patient's response to both the Narcan infusion and to any previous bolus dose.

Preclinical safety data: Narcan is well established in medical use. Preclinical data is broadly consistent with clinical experience. For reproductive toxicity, see *Pregnancy and lactation.*

Pharmaceutical particulars

List of excipients: Sodium Chloride, Hydrochloric Acid, Water for Injection, Nitrogen.

Incompatibilities: Narcan should not be mixed with preparations containing bisulphite, metabisulphite, long-chain or high molecular weight anions or any solution having an alkaline pH: no drug or chemical agent should be added to Narcan unless its effect on the chemical and physical stability of the solution has first been established.

Shelf-life: 36 months.

Special precautions for storage: Protect from light.

Nature and contents of container: Narcan ampoules each containing 1 ml (equivalent to 400 micrograms naloxone hydrochloride) are supplied in boxes of three and ten ampoules.

Instructions for use/handling: Not applicable.

Marketing authorisation holder
DuPont Pharmaceuticals Limited, Wedgwood Way, Stevenage, Hertfordshire SG1 4QN.

Marketing authorisation numbers PL 11173/0009.

Date of first authorisation/renewal of authorisation 27 August 1991.

Date of (partial) revision of text Date of preparation of text: September 1998.

Legal category POM.

NARCAN* NEONATAL 20 mcg/ml

Qualitative and quantitative composition NARCAN NEONATAL (2 ml ampoules) - each 1 ml of solution contains 20 micrograms naloxone hydrochloride.

Pharmaceutical form Solution for injection.

Clinical particulars

Therapeutic indications: Narcan Neonatal is indicated for the complete or partial reversal of opioid-induced depression and other CNS depression in the newborn resulting from the administration of analgesics to the mother during childbirth.

Posology and method of administration: Narcan Neonatal is for intravenous, intramuscular or subcutaneous injection or intravenous infusion.

Intravenous infusion: Narcan 0.4 mg/ml, may be diluted for intravenous infusion in normal saline (0.9%) or 5% dextrose in water or saline: the addition of 2 mg (5 ml of 0.4 mg/ml concentration) of Narcan in 500 ml of either solution provides a concentration of 4 micrograms/ml. Mixtures should be used within 12 hours. After 12 hours the remaining unused solution must be discarded. The rate of administration should be titrated in accordance with the patient's response to both the Narcan infusion and to any previous bolus doses administered.

Parenteral drug products should be inspected visually for particulate matter and discoloration prior to administration whenever solution and container permit.

An adequate airway should be established in the apnoeic infant before naloxone hydrochloride is administered. The usual dose for opioid-induced depression is 10 micrograms/kg body weight administered i.v., i.m., or s.c. If the desired degree of counteraction and improvement in respiratory function is not obtained it may be repeated at 2 to 3 minute intervals. Alternatively, a single dose of 200 micrograms, approximately 60 micrograms/kg body weight may be given intramuscularly at birth.

It should, however, be noted that onset of action is slower following i.m. injection. In neonates needing infusion of naloxone hydrochloride in saline care should be taken to avoid excessive sodium intake.

Contra-indications: Naloxone hydrochloride should not be given to patients who are known to be hypersensitive to it.

Special warnings and special precautions for use: It should be administered cautiously to new-borns of mothers who have received large doses of opioids or to those physically dependent on opioids since too rapid reversal of opioid effects by naloxone hydrochloride may precipitate an acute withdrawal syndrome.

New-borns who have responded satisfactorily to naloxone hydrochloride should be kept under observation. Repeated doses of naloxone hydrochloride may be necessary since the duration of action of some opioids may exceed that of naloxone hydrochloride.

Naloxone hydrochloride is not effective against respiratory depression caused by non-opioid drugs. Reversal of buprenorphine-induced respiratory depression may be incomplete. If an incomplete response occurs, respiration should be mechanically assisted.

Several instances of hypotension, hypertension, ventricular tachycardia and fibrillation, and pulmonary oedema have been reported. These have occurred in postoperative adult patients, most of whom had pre-existing cardiovascular effects. Although a direct cause and effect relationship has not been established, naloxone hydrochloride should be used with caution in patients with pre-existing cardiac disease or patients who have received potentially cardiotoxic drugs.

In addition to naloxone hydrochloride, other resuscitative measures such as maintenance of a free airway, artificial ventilation, cardiac massage and vasopressor agents should be available and employed when necessary to counteract acute poisoning.

Interaction with other medications and other forms of interaction: Naloxone hydrochloride should be administered cautiously to new-borns of mothers who are known or suspected to be physically dependent on opioids. In such cases an abrupt and complete reversal of narcotic effects may precipitate an acute abstinence syndrome.

Pregnancy and lactation: Not relevant.

Effects on ability to drive and use machines: Not applicable.

Undesirable effects: Abrupt reversal of narcotic depression may result in nausea, vomiting, sweating, tachycardia, increased blood pressure, tremulousness, seizures and cardiac arrest.

In postoperative patients, larger than necessary dosage of naloxone hydrochloride may result in significant reversal of analgesia and excitement. Hypotension, hypertension, ventricular tachycardia and fibrillation, and pulmonary oedema have been associated with the use of naloxone hydrochloride postoperatively.

Overdose: There have been no reports of acute overdosage with naloxone hydrochloride in the newborn. Single doses of 10 mg intravenously and subcutaneous doses of 15 mg every four hours for two weeks have been administered to adults without producing either respiratory depression or psychotomimetic effects.

Pharmacological properties

Pharmacodynamic properties: Naloxone is N-allyl-noroxymorphone, an opioid antagonist which is devoid of the agonist or morphine-like properties characteristic of other opioid antagonists. In the absence of opioids or the agonist/antagonist it shows essentially no pharmacological activity.

Pharmacokinetic properties: Naloxone hydrochloride usually acts within two minutes of intravenous administration and the onset of action is only slightly less rapid following intramuscular or subcutaneous injection. The duration of action is dependent upon the dose, route of administration, intramuscular injection producing a more prolonged effect than intravenous doses. However, the need for repeat doses of naloxone hydrochloride also depends on the amount, type and route of administration of the opioid being antagonised.

The rate of administration should be titrated in accordance with the patient's response to both the naloxone hydrochloride infusion and to any previous bolus dose.

Preclinical safety data: Naloxone hydrochloride is well established in medical use. Preclinical data is broadly consistent with clinical experience. For reproductive toxicity, see *Pregnancy and lactation.*

Pharmaceutical particulars

List of excipients: Sodium Chloride, Hydrochloric Acid, Water for Injection, Nitrogen.

Incompatibilities: Narcan should not be mixed with preparations containing bisulphite, metabisulphite, long-chain or high molecular weight anions or any solution having an alkaline pH: no drug or chemical agent should be added to Narcan unless its effect on the chemical and physical stability of the solution has first been established.

Shelf-life: 24 months.

Special precautions for storage: Protect from light.

Nature and contents of container: Narcan Neonatal ampoules each containing 2 ml (equivalent to 40 micrograms naloxone hydrochloride) are supplied in boxes of ten ampoules.

Instructions for use/handling: Not applicable.

Marketing authorisation Holder
DuPont Pharmaceuticals Limited, Wedgwood Way, Stevenage, Hertfordshire SG1 4QN.

Marketing authorisation numbers PL 11173/0012.

Date of first authorisation/renewal of authorisation 23 January 1992.

Date of (partial) revision of text Date of preparation of text: September 1998.

Legal category POM.

NUBAIN*

Qualitative and quantitative composition Each 1 ml of solution contains 10 mg nalbuphine hydrochloride.

Pharmaceutical form Solution for injection.

Clinical particulars

Therapeutic indications: Nubain injection is indicated for the relief of moderate to severe pain. It can also be used as a premedication, for pre- and post-operative analgesia, and as a component of balanced anaesthesia. It can also be used in the management of pain due to suspected myocardial infarction. It can also be used to treat moderate to severe pain in children.

Posology and method of administration: Nubain injection may be administered subcutaneously, intramuscularly or intravenously. It may also be administered by patient-controlled on demand intravenous infusion, using a delivery system which is appropriately calibrated and does not interact with the drug.

Nubain is compatible with 0.9% Sodium Chloride, 5% Dextrose, 4.3% Dextrose/0.18% Saline and Hartmann's solution used in glass, PVC and Polyethylene Infusion containers.

Use in adults: The usual recommended dosage is 10 mg–20 mg for a 70 kg individual. The dosage should be adjusted according to the severity of pain, physical status of the patient and other medications the patient may be receiving.

Balanced anaesthesia:

Induction: 0.3 mg/kg to 1 mg/kg i.v. over a 10–15 minute period.

Maintenance: 0.25–0.5 mg/kg at 30 minute intervals.

Premedication: 0.1–0.2 mg/kg.

Suspected myocardial infarction: Usual dose 20 mg by slow intravenous injection. Some patients may be successfully managed on 10 mg while others may need to have the dose increased to 30 mg. In the absence of pain relief a repeat dose of 20 mg may be given within 30 minutes.

Use in children: An initial dose of up to 0.3 mg/kg i.v., i.m. or s.c. which may be repeated once or twice as necessary.

Contra-indications: Nubain should not be administered to patients who are hypersensitive to it.

Special warnings and special precautions for use: Drug dependence: Nubain has low abuse potential. However, caution should be observed in prescribing it for emotionally unstable patients or for patients with a history of opioid abuse.

When Nubain is selected for the control of chronic pain, its suggested prolonged activity may delay the need for larger or more frequent doses.

Abrupt discontinuation of Nubain following prolonged use has been followed by symptoms of opioid withdrawal.

Nubain should only be considered essential and only used with extreme caution to provide analgesia in patients with head injury and increased intracranial pressure.

Nubain used as a premedication causes some respiratory depression. Caution should therefore be observed in administering the drug to patients with impaired respiration, or with other medications which produce respiratory depression.

During evaluation of Nubain in anaesthesia, a higher incidence of bradycardia has been reported in patients not administered pre-operative atropine.

In the presence of bronchial asthma, uraemia, severe infection, cyanosis or respiratory obstruction, Nubain should be administered with caution and in reduced doses.

Nubain should be used with caution and administered in reduced amounts in patients with impaired renal or hepatic function.

Interaction with other medicaments and other forms of interaction: Patients receiving an opioid analgesic, general anaesthetic, phenothiazine or other tranquilliser, sedative, hypnotic or other CNS depressant (including alcohol) concomitantly with Nubain may exhibit an additive effect. When such combined therapy is contemplated, the dose of one or both agents should be reduced.

Pregnancy and lactation: Safe use of Nubain in pregnancy (including labour) has not been established. A few cases of severe foetal respiratory depression and bradycardia have been reported when Nubain has been used during labour.

Although animal studies have not revealed teratogenic or embryotoxic effects, nalbuphine should only be administered to pregnant women when, in the judgement of the physician, the potential benefits outweigh the possible hazards.

It is not known whether Nubain is excreted in human milk. Because many drugs are excreted in human milk, caution should be exercised when Nubain is administered to a nursing woman.

Effects on ability to drive and use machines: Nubain may impair the mental or physical abilities required for the performance of potentially dangerous tasks such as driving a car or operating machinery. Therefore, Nubain should be administered with caution to ambulatory patients who should be warned to avoid such hazards.

Undesirable effects: The most frequently seen reaction to Nubain is sedation. Less frequent are sweating, nausea, vomiting, dizziness, dry mouth, vertigo and headache. Rarely seen are CNS effects such as nervousness, depression, confusion and dysphoria. Also reported have been hyper- and hypotension, bradycardia, tachycardia, urticaria, speech difficulty, blurred vision and flushing.

Overdose: The immediate intravenous administration of Narcan* (naloxone hydrochloride) is a specific antidote. Oxygen, intravenous fluids, vasopressors and other supportive measures should be used as indicated.

Pharmacological properties

Pharmacodynamic properties: Nubain (nalbuphine hydrochloride) is a potent semi-synthetic agonist/antagonist analgesic of the phenanthrene series. It is primarily a kappa-agonist/mu-antagonist analgesic. Analgesic tolerance is uncommon and nalbuphine has low abuse potential.

Unlike morphine, there is a ceiling effect to the respiratory depressant effect of nalbuphine.

Nalbuphine causes minimal haemodynamic effects and minimal inhibition of gastrointestinal motility.

Pharmacokinetic properties: The onset of action occurs within 2–3 minutes after i.v. injection and within 15 minutes after i.m. or s.c. administration. The duration of effect is 3–5 hours. The elimination half-life ($t_{\frac{1}{2}}$) of Nubain is approximately 2.5 hours following i.v., i.m. or s.c. administration.

Nalbuphine hydrochloride is extensively metabolised and excreted predominantly (approximately 70 percent) in the urine. About five percent of nalbuphine is excreted as unchanged drug.

Preclinical safety data: Nubain is well established in medical use. Preclinical data is broadly consistent with clinical experience. For reproductive toxicity, see *Pregnancy and lactation.*

Pharmaceutical particulars

List of excipients:

Citric Acid, Anhydrous	PhEur/USP
Sodium Citrate, Dihydrate	PhEur/USP
Sodium Chloride	PhEur
Hydrochloric Acid	PhEur
Water for Injection	PhEur

Incompatibilities: None known.

Shelf life: 36 months.

Special precautions for storage: Protect from light. Store at room temperature.

Nature and contents of container: Nubain 20 mg ampoules are supplied in boxes of 10. Nubain 10 mg ampoules are supplied in boxes of 10.

Instructions for use/handling: Not applicable.

Marketing authorisation number

Nubain 10 mg/ml – Ampoule: PL 11173/0013.

Date of first authorisation/renewal of authorisation 14 November 1991.

Date of (partial) revision of text September 1998.

Legal category POM.

SINEMET*

Presentation

Sinemet-LS is available as yellow, half-scored, oval tablets, marked 'SINEMET LS', containing 12.5 mg carbidopa (as carbidopa monohydrate) and 50 mg levodopa.

Sinemet-110 is available as dapple-blue, half-scored, oval tablets, marked 'MSD 647' containing 10 mg carbidopa (as carbidopa monohydrate) and 100 mg levodopa.

Sinemet-Plus is available as yellow, half-scored, oval tablets, marked 'SINEMET PLUS', containing 25 mg carbidopa (as carbidopa monohydrate) and 100 mg levodopa.

Sinemet-275 is available as dapple-blue, half-scored, oval tablets, marked 'MSD 654', containing 25 mg carbidopa (as carbidopa monohydrate) and 250 mg levodopa.

Uses Antiparkinsonian agent.

For treatment of Parkinson's disease and syndrome. Sinemet is useful in relieving many of the symptoms of parkinsonism, particularly rigidity and bradykinesia. It is frequently helpful in the management of tremor, dysphagia, sialorrhoea, and postural instability associated with Parkinson's disease and syndrome.

When response to levodopa alone is irregular, and signs and symptoms of Parkinson's disease are not controlled evenly throughout the day, substitution of Sinemet usually reduces fluctuations in response. By reducing some of the adverse reactions produced by levodopa alone, Sinemet permits more patients to obtain adequate relief of the symptoms of Parkinson's disease.

Sinemet may be given to patients with Parkinson's disease and syndrome who are taking vitamin preparations that contain pyridoxine hydrochloride (Vitamin B6).

Dosage and administration The optimum daily dosage of Sinemet must be determined by careful titration for each patient.

Sinemet Tablets are available in a ratio of 1:4 or 1:10 of carbidopa to levodopa to provide facility for fine dosage titration for each patient.

General considerations: Studies show that the peripheral enzyme dopa-decarboxylase is fully inhibited (saturated) by carbidopa at doses between 70 and 100 mg a day. Patients receiving less than this amount of carbidopa are more likely to experience nausea and vomiting.

Standard anti-parkinsonism drugs other than levodopa alone, may be continued while 'Sinemet' is being administered, although their dosage may have to be adjusted.

Because both therapeutic and adverse effects are seen more rapidly with Sinemet than with levodopa, patients should be carefully monitored during the dosage adjustment period. Involuntary movements, particularly blepharospasm, are a useful early sign of excess dosage in some patients.

If general anaesthesia is required, therapy with Sinemet may be continued for as long as the patient is permitted to take fluids and medicines by mouth. If therapy has to be stopped temporarily, Sinemet may be restarted as soon as oral medication can be taken at the same daily dosage as before.

Patients not receiving levodopa: Dosage may be best initiated with one tablet of Sinemet-Plus three times a day. This dosage schedule provides 75 mg of carbidopa per day. Dosage may be increased by one tablet of Sinemet-LS or Sinemet-Plus every day or every other day, as necessary, until a dosage equivalent of eight tablets of Sinemet-Plus a day is reached.

If Sinemet-110 or Sinemet-LS is used, dosage may be initiated with one tablet three or four times a day. Titration upward may be required in some patients to achieve optimum dosage of carbidopa. The dosage may be increased by one tablet every day or every other day until a total of eight tablets (two tablets q.d.s.) is reached. For patients starting with Sinemet-275, the initial dose is one-half tablet taken once or twice daily. However, this may not provide the optimal amount of carbidopa needed by many patients. If necessary, add one-half tablet every day or every other day until optimal response is reached.

Response has been observed in one day, and sometimes after one dose. Fully effective doses usually are reached within seven days as compared to weeks or months with levodopa alone.

Sinemet-LS or Sinemet-110 may be used to facilitate dosage titration according to the needs of the individual patient.

Patients receiving levodopa: Discontinue levodopa at least 12 hours (24 hours for slow-release preparations) before starting therapy with Sinemet. The easiest way to do this is to give Sinemet as the first morning dose after a night without any levodopa. The dose of Sinemet should be approximately 20% of the previous daily dosage of levodopa.

Patients taking less than 1,500 mg levodopa a day should be started on one tablet of Sinemet-Plus three or four times a day dependent on patient need. The suggested starting dose for most patients taking more than 1,500 mg levodopa a day is one tablet of Sinemet-275 three or four times a day.

Maintenance: Therapy with Sinemet should be individualised and adjusted gradually according to response. When a greater proportion of carbidopa is required, each tablet of Sinemet-110 may be replaced with a tablet of Sinemet-Plus or Sinemet-LS.

When more levodopa is required, Sinemet-275 should be substituted at a dosage of one tablet three or four times a day. If necessary, the dosage of Sinemet-275 may be increased by half to one tablet every other day to a maximum of eight tablets a day. Experience with a total daily dosage greater than 200 mg carbidopa is limited.

Patients receiving other antiparkinsonian agents: The combination of Sinemet with MAO-B inhibitors (e.g. selegiline) has been reported to improve the efficacy of Sinemet in controlling episodes of akinesia and/or dyskinesia.

Use in children: The safety of Sinemet in patients under 18 years of age has not been established.

Use in the elderly: There is wide experience in the use of this product in elderly patients. The recommendations set out above reflect the clinical data derived from this experience.

Contra-indications, warnings, etc

Contra-indications: MAO-inhibitors (except low doses of selective MAO-B inhibitors) and Sinemet should not be given concomitantly (these must be discontinued at least two weeks before starting Sinemet); narrow-angle glaucoma; known hypersensitivity to any component of this medication. Because levodopa may activate a malignant melanoma, it should not be used in patients with suspicious undiagnosed skin lesions or a history of melanoma. See also 'Pregnancy and lactation', under 'Precautions'.

Precautions: Sinemet is not recommended for the treatment of drug-induced extrapyramidal reactions.

Sinemet should be administered cautiously to patients with severe cardiovascular or pulmonary disease, bronchial asthma, renal, hepatic or endocrine disease; or a history of peptic ulcer disease (because of the possibility of upper gastrointestinal haemorrhage).

Care should be exercised when Sinemet is administered to patients with a history of myocardial infarction who have atrial, nodal, or ventricular arrhythmias. Cardiac function should be monitored with particular care in such patients during the period of initial dosage adjustment.

All patients should be monitored carefully for the development of mental changes, depression with suicidal tendencies, and other serious antisocial behaviour. Patients with current psychoses should be treated with caution.

Dyskinesias may occur in patients previously treated with levodopa alone, because carbidopa permits more levodopa to reach the brain and, thus, more dopamine to be formed. The occurence of dyskinesias may require dosage reduction.

As with levodopa, Sinemet may cause involuntary movements and mental disturbances. Patients with a history of severe involuntary movements or psychotic episodes when treated with levodopa alone should be observed carefully when Sinemet is substituted. These reactions are thought to be due to increased brain dopamine following administration of levodopa, and use of Sinemet may cause a recurrence. A syndrome resembling the neuroleptic malignant syndrome including muscular rigidity, elevated body temperature, mental changes and increased serum creatine phosphokinase has been reported with the abrupt withdrawal of antiparkinsonian agents. Therefore, any abrupt dosage reduction or withdrawal of Sinemet should be carefully observed, particularly in patients who are also receiving neuroleptics.

Concomitant administration of psycho-active drugs such as phenothiazines or butyrophenones should be carried out with caution, and the patients carefully observed for loss of antiparkinsonian effect. Patients with a history of convulsions should be treated with caution.

As with levodopa, periodic evaluations of hepatic haematopoietic, cardiovascular and renal functions are recommended during extended therapy.

Patients with chronic wide-angle glaucoma may be treated cautiously with Sinemet, provided the intra-ocular pressure is well controlled and the patient monitored carefully for changes in intra-ocular pressure during therapy.

Laboratory tests: Commonly, levels of blood urea, creatinine and uric acid are lower during administration of Sinemet than with levodopa. Transient abnormalities include elevated levels of blood urea, AST (SGOT), ALT (SGPT), LDH, bilirubin, alkaline phosphatase, and protein-bound iodine.

Decreased haemoglobin, haematocrit, elevated serum glucose, and white blood cells, bacteria and blood in the urine have been reported.

Positive Coombs tests have been reported, both with Sinemet and levodopa alone, but haemolytic anaemia is extremely rare.

Sinemet may cause a false positive result when a dipstick is used to test for urinary ketone; and this reaction is not altered by boiling the urine. The use of glucose oxidase methods may give false negative results for glycosuria.

Drug interactions: Caution should be exercised when the following drugs are administered concomitantly with Sinemet:

Antihypertensive agents: Postural hypotension can occur when Sinemet is added to the treatment of patients already receiving antihypertensive drugs. Dosage adjustments of the antihypertensive agent may be required.

Antidepressants: Rarely, reactions including hypertension and dyskinesia have been reported with the concomitant use of tricyclic antidepressants. (See the Contra-indications for patients receiving MAOIs.)

Other drugs: Phenothiazines, butyrophenones, phenytoin and papaverine may reduce the therapeutic effect of levodopa. Patients taking these drugs with Sinemet should be carefully observed for loss of therapeutic response.

Since levodopa competes with certain amino acids, the absorption of Sinemet may be impaired in some patients on a high protein diet.

Pregnancy: Although the effects of Sinemet on human pregnancy are unknown, both levodopa and combinations of carbidopa and levodopa have caused visceral and skeletal malformations in rabbits. Therefore, use of Sinemet in women of childbearing potential requires that the anticipated benefits of the drug be weighed against possible hazards should pregnancy occur.

Breast-feeding mothers: It is not known whether carbidopa or levodopa is excreted in human milk. Because many drugs are excreted in human milk and because of the potential for serious adverse reactions in infants, a decision should be made whether to discontinue breast-feeding or to discontinue the use of Sinemet taking into account the importance of the drug to the mother.

Side-effects: Side-effects that occur frequently with Sinemet are those due to the central neuropharmacological activity of dopamine. These reactions can usually be diminished by dosage reduction. The most common are dyskinesias including choreiform, dystonic, and other involuntary movements. Muscle twitching and blepharospasm may be taken as early signs to consider dosage reduction.

Other serious side-effects are mental changes, including paranoid ideation and psychotic episodes; depression, with or without development of suicidal tendencies; and dementia. A common but less serious side effect is nausea.

Less frequent side-effects are cardiac irregularities and/or palpitations, orthostatic hypotensive episodes, bradykinetic episodes (the 'on-off' phenomenon), anorexia, vomiting, dizziness, and somnolence.

Gastro-intestinal bleeding, development of duodenal ulcer, hypertension, phlebitis, leucopenia, haemolytic and non-haemolytic anaemia, thrombocytopenia, agranulocytosis, chest pain, dyspnoea and paraesthesia have occurred rarely.

Other side-effects that have been reported with levodopa and may be potential side effects with Sinemet include:

Neurological: ataxia, numbness, increased hand tremor, muscle twitching, muscle cramp, trismus, activation of latent Horner's syndrome.

Psychiatric: confusion, insomnia, nightmares, hallucinations, delusions, agitation, anxiety, euphoria.

Gastro-intestinal: dry mouth, bitter taste, sialorrhoea, dysphagia, bruxism, hiccups, abdominal pain and distress, constipation, diarrhoea, flatulence, burning sensation of the tongue.

Metabolic: weight gain or loss, oedema.

Integumentary: flushing, increased sweating, dark sweat, rash, hair loss.

Genito-urinary: urinary retention, urinary incontinence, dark urine, priapism.

Special senses: diplopia, blurred vision, dilated pupils, oculogyric crises.

Miscellaneous: weakness, faintness, fatigue, headache, hoarseness, malaise, hot flushes, sense of stimulation, bizarre breathing patterns, neuroleptic malignant syndrome, malignant melanoma (see 'Contra-indications').

Other side-effects that have been reported with Sinemet CR and may be potential side-effects with Sinemet include:

Neurological: Falling, gait abnormalities.

Overdosage: Management of acute overdosage with Sinemet is basically the same as management of acute overdosage with levodopa; however, pyridoxine is not effective in reversing the actions of Sinemet. ECG monitoring should be instituted, and the patient carefully observed for the possible development of arrhythmias; if required, appropriate anti-arrhythmic therapy should be given.

The possibility that the patient may have taken other drugs as well as Sinemet should be taken into consideration. To date, no experience has been reported with dialysis, and hence its value in the treatment of overdosage is not known.

The terminal half-life of levodopa is about two hours in the presence of carbidopa.

Pharmaceutical precautions Keep container tightly closed; store in a cool place, protected from light.

Legal category POM.

Package quantities
Sinemet-LS in bottles of 84.
Sinemet-110 in bottles of 100.
Sinemet-Plus in bottles of 100.
Sinemet-275 in bottles of 100.

Further information Levodopa relieves the symptoms of Parkinson's disease presumably by being decarboxylated to dopamine in the brain. Carbidopa, which does not cross the blood-brain barrier, inhibits only the extra-cerebral decarboxylation of levodopa, making more levodopa available for transport to the brain and subsequent conversion to dopamine. This obviates the need for large doses of levodopa at frequent intervals. The lower dosage reduces or eliminates many adverse reactions, some of which are attributed to dopamine being formed in extra-cerebral tissues.

Product licence numbers

Sinemet-LS	0025/0226
Sinemet-110	0025/0084
Sinemet-Plus	0025/0150
Sinemet-275	0025/0085

Product licence holder: Merck, Sharp & Dohme Limited, Hertford Road, Hoddesdon, Hertfordshire EN11 9BU.

SINEMET* CR HALF SINEMET CR

Qualitative and quantitative composition Each tablet of Sinemet CR (code 'DPP' and '521') contains carbidopa PhEur (equivalent to 50 mg of anhydrous carbidopa) and 200 mg levodopa PhEur.

Each tablet of Half Sinemet CR (code 'DPP' and '601') contains carbidopa PhEur (equivalent to 25 mg of anhydrous carbidopa) and 100 mg levodopa PhEur.

Pharmaceutical form Tablets.

Clinical particulars

Therapeutic indications: Antiparkinson agent.

Idiopathic Parkinson's disease, in particular to reduce off-period in patients who previously have been treated with levodopa/decarboxylase inhibitors, or with levodopa alone and who have experienced motor fluctuations. The experience is limited with Sinemet CR and Half Sinemet CR in patients who have not been treated with levodopa before.

Posology and method of administration: Sinemet CR and Half Sinemet CR tablets contain a 1:4 ratio of carbidopa to levodopa (Sinemet CR: carbidopa 50 mg/levodopa 200 mg, Half Sinemet CR 25 mg/100 mg per tablet). The daily dosage of Sinemet CR must be determined by careful titration. Patients should be monitored closely during the dose adjustment period, particularly with regard to appearance or worsening of nausea or abnormal involuntary movements, including dyskinesias, chorea and dystonia.

Route of administration: oral: Sinemet CR and Half Sinemet CR may only be administered as whole tablets. So that the controlled release properties of the product can be maintained, tablets should not be chewed, crushed, or halved.

Standard antiparkinson drugs, other than levodopa alone, may be continued while Sinemet CR or Half Sinemet CR are being administered, although their dosage may have to be adjusted.

Since carbidopa prevents the reversal of levodopa effects caused by pyridoxine, Sinemet CR or Half Sinemet CR can be given to patients receiving supplemental pyridoxine (vitamin B_6).

Initial dose

Patients currently treated with conventional levodopa/decarboxylase inhibitor combinations: Dosage with Sinemet CR should be substituted initially at an amount that provides no more than approximately 10% more levodopa per day when higher dosages are given (more than 900 mg per day). The dosing interval between doses should be prolonged by 30 to 50% at intervals ranging from 4 to 12 hours. It is recommended to give the smaller dose, if divided doses are not equal, at the end of the day. The dose needs to be titrated further depending on clinical response, as indicated below under *Titration.* Dosages that provide up to 30% more levodopa per day may be necessary.

A guide for substitution of Sinemet CR treatment for conventional levodopa/decarboxylase inhibitor combinations is shown in the table below:

Guideline for conversion from Sinemet to Sinemet CR

Sinemet	*Sinemet CR*	
Daily dosage Levodopa (mg)	*Daily dosage Levodopa (mg)*	*Dosage regimen*
300– 400	400	1 2×daily
500– 600	600	1 3×daily
700– 800	800	4 Tablets in 3 or more divided doses
900–1000	1000	5 Tablets in 3 or more divided doses
1100–1200	1200	6 Tablets in 3 or more divided doses
1300–1400	1400	7 Tablets in 3 or more divided doses
1500–1600	1600	8 Tablets in 3 or more divided doses

Half Sinemet CR is available to facilitate titration when 100 mg steps are required.

Patients currently treated with levodopa alone: Levodopa must be discontinued at least eight hours before therapy with Sinemet CR is started. In patients with mild to moderate disease, the initial recommended dose is one tablet of Sinemet CR twice daily.

Patients not receiving levodopa: In patients with mild to moderate disease, the initial recommended dose is one tablet of Sinemet CR twice daily. Initial dosages should not exceed 600 mg per day of levodopa, nor be given at intervals of less than six hours.

Titration: Following initiation of therapy, doses and dosing intervals may be increased or decreased, depending upon therapeutic response. Most patients have been adequately treated with two to eight tablets per day of Sinemet CR administered as divided doses at intervals ranging from four to twelve hours during the waking day. Higher doses (up to 12 tablets) and shorter intervals (less than 4 hours) have been used, but are not usually recommended.

When doses of Sinemet CR are given at intervals of less than 4 hours, or if the divided doses are not equal, it is recommended that the smaller doses be given at the end of the day. In some patients the onset of effect of the first morning dose may be delayed for up to one hour compared with the response usually obtained from the first morning dose of Sinemet.

An interval of at least three days between dosage adjustments is recommended.

Maintenance: Because Parkinson's disease is progressive, periodic clinical evaluations are recommended and adjustment of the dosage regimen of Sinemet CR or Half Sinemet CR may be required.

Addition of other antiparkinson medication: Anticholinergic agents, dopamine agonists and amantadine can be given with Sinemet CR or Half Sinemet CR. Dosage adjustment of Sinemet CR or Half Sinemet CR may be necessary when these agents are added to an existing treatment regimen for Sinemet CR or Half Sinemet CR.

Interruption of therapy: Patients should be observed carefully if abrupt reduction or discontinuation of Sinemet CR or Half Sinemet CR is required, especially if the patient is receiving antipsychotics (see *Special warnings and special precautions for use*).

If general anaesthesia is required, Sinemet CR or Half Sinemet CR may be continued as long as the patient is permitted to take oral medication. If therapy is interrupted temporarily, the usual dosage should be administered as soon as the patient is able to take oral medicine.

Use in children: Safety and effectiveness of Sinemet CR or Half Sinemet CR in infants and children have not been established, and its use in patients below the age of 18 is not recommended.

Contra-indications: Sinemet CR or Half Sinemet CR should not be given when administration of a sympathomimetic amine is contra-indicated.

Monoamine oxidase inhibitors (except low doses of selective MAO-B inhibitors) and Sinemet CR or Half Sinemet CR should not be given concomitantly. These inhibitors must be discontinued at least two weeks prior to initiating therapy with Sinemet CR or Half Sinemet CR.

Sinemet CR or Half Sinemet CR is contra-indicated in patients with known hypersensitivity to any component of this medication, and in patients with narrow-angle glaucoma.

Because levodopa may activate a malignant melanoma, Sinemet CR or Half Sinemet CR should not be used in patients with suspicious undiagnosed skin lesions or a history of melanoma.

Use in patients with severe psychoses.

Special warnings and special precautions for use: When patients are receiving levodopa monotherapy, levodopa must be discontinued at least eight hours before therapy with Sinemet CR or Half Sinemet CR is started (at least 12 hours if slow-release levodopa has been administered).

Dyskinesias may occur in patients previously treated with levodopa alone because carbidopa permits more levodopa to reach the brain and, thus, more dopamine to be formed. The occurrence of dyskinesias may require dosage reduction.

Sinemet CR and Half Sinemet CR are not recommended for the treatment of drug-induced extrapyramidal reactions or for the treatment of Huntington's chorea.

Based on the pharmacokinetic profile of Sinemet CR the onset of effect in patients with early morning dyskinesias may be slower than with conventional Sinemet. The incidence of dyskinesias is slightly higher during treatment with Sinemet CR than with conventional Sinemet (16.5% vs 12.2%) in advanced patients with motor fluctuations.

Sinemet CR or Half Sinemet CR should be administered cautiously to patients with severe cardiovascular or pulmonary disease, bronchial asthma, renal, hepatic or endocrine disease, or with a history of peptic ulcer disease or of convulsions.

Care should be exercised in administering Sinemet CR or Half Sinemet CR to patients with a history of recent myocardial infarction who have residual atrial, nodal, or ventricular arrhythmia. In such patients, cardiac function should be monitored with particular care during the period of initial dosage administration and titration.

As with levodopa, Sinemet CR or Half Sinemet CR may cause involuntary movements and mental disturbances. Patients with a history of severe involuntary movements or psychotic episodes when treated with levodopa alone or levodopa/decarboxylase inhibitor combination should be observed carefully when Sinemet CR or Half Sinemet CR is substituted. These reactions are thought to be due to increased brain dopamine following administration of levodopa and use of Sinemet CR or Half Sinemet CR may cause recurrence. Dosage reduction may be required. All patients should be observed carefully for the development of depression with concomitant suicidal tendencies. Patients with past or current psychoses should be treated with caution.

A symptom complex resembling the neuroleptic malignant syndrome including muscular rigidity, elevated body temperature, mental changes, and increased serum creatine phosphokinase has been reported when antiparkinsonian agents were withdrawn abruptly. Therefore, patients should be observed carefully when the dosage of carbidopa-levodopa combinations is reduced abruptly or discontinued, especially if the patient is receiving antipsychotics.

Patients with chronic wide-angle glaucoma may be treated cautiously with Sinemet CR or Half Sinemet CR, provided the intraocular pressure is well controlled and the patient monitored carefully for changes in intraocular pressure during therapy.

Periodic evaluations of hepatic, haematopoietic, cardiovascular and renal function are recommended during extended therapy.

Laboratory tests: Abnormalities in various laboratory tests have occurred with carbidopa-levodopa preparations and may occur with Sinemet CR or Half Sinemet CR. These include elevations of liver function tests such as alkaline phosphatase, SGOT (AST), SGPT (ALT), LDH, bilirubin, blood urea nitrogen and positive Coombs' test.

Carbidopa-levodopa preparations may cause a false-positive reaction for urinary ketone bodies when a test tape is used for determination of ketonuria. This reaction will not be altered by boiling the urine specimen. False-negative tests may result with the use of glucose-oxidase methods of testing for glycosuria.

Decreased haemoglobin and haematocrit, elevated serum glucose and white blood cells, bacteria and blood in the urine have been reported with standard Sinemet.

Interaction with other medications and other forms of interaction: Caution should be exercised when the following drugs are administered concomitantly with Sinemet CR or Half Sinemet CR:

Antihypertensive agents: Symptomatic postural hypotension has occurred when levodopa/decarboxylase inhibitor combinations were added to the treatment of patients receiving some antihypertensive drugs. Therefore when therapy with Sinemet CR or Half Sinemet CR is started, dosage adjustment of the antihypertensive drug may be required.

Antidepressants: There have been rare reports of adverse reactions, including hypertension and dyskinesia, resulting from the concomitant use of tricyclic antidepressants and carbidopa-levodopa preparations. (For patients receiving monomine oxidase inhibitors, see *Contra-indications*).

Anticholinergics: Anticholinergics may affect the absorption and thus the patient's response.

Other drugs: Antipsychotics may reduce the therapeutic effects of levodopa. The beneficial effects of levodopa in Parkinson's disease have been reported to be reversed by phenytoin and papaverine. Patients taking these drugs with Sinemet CR or Half Sinemet CR should be observed carefully for loss of therapeutic response.

Since levodopa competes with certain amino acids, the absorption of levodopa may be impaired in some patients on a high protein diet.

The effect of simultaneous administration of antacids with Sinemet CR or Half Sinemet CR on the bioavailability of levodopa has not been studied.

Pregnancy and lactation: There are insufficient data to evaluate the possible harmfulness of this substance when used in human pregnancy. (See *Preclinical safety data*). It is not known whether carbidopa or levodopa is excreted in human milk. Sinemet CR or Half Sinemet CR should not be given during pregnancy and to nursing mothers.

Effects on ability to drive and use machines: No data are known about the effect of this product on the ability to drive. If they occur, side-effects such as dizziness or somnolence may affect the ability to drive or to operate machinery.

Undesirable effects: In controlled clinical trials in patients with moderate to severe motor fluctuations Sinemet CR did not produce side-effects which were unique to the controlled-release formulation.

The side-effect reported most frequently was dysksinesia (a form of abnormal involuntary movements). A greater incidence of dyskinesias was seen with Sinemet CR than with Sinemet.

Other side-effects that also were reported frequently (above 2%) were: nausea, hallucinations, confusion, dizziness, chorea and dry mouth.

Side-effects occurring less frequently (1–2%) were: dream abnormalities, dystonia, somnolence, insomnia, depression, asthenia, vomiting and anorexia.

Side-effects observed rarely (0.5%–1%) were: headache, on-off phenomenon, constipation, disorientation, paraesthesia, dyspnoea, fatigue, orthostatic effects, palpitation, dyspepsia, intestinal pain, muscle cramps, decreased mental acuity, chest pain, diarrhoea, weight loss, agitation, anxiety, falling, gait abnormalities and blurred vision.

Other side-effects that have been reported with levodopa or levodopa/carbidopa combinations and may be potential side-effects with Sinemet CR are listed below:

Nervous system: Ataxia, numbness, increased hand tremor, muscle twitching, blepharospasm, trismus, activation of latent Horner's syndrome.

Psychiatric: Euphoria, paranoid ideation and psychotic episodes, and dementia.

Gastrointestinal: Bitter taste, sialorrhoea, dysphagia, bruxism, hiccups, gastrointestinal bleeding, flatulence, burning sensation of tongue, development of duodenal ulcer.

Cardiovascular: Cardiac irregularities, hypertension, phlebitis.

Integumentary: Flushing, increased sweating, dark sweat, rash, hair loss.

Genitourinary: Urinary retention, urinary incontinence, dark urine, priapism.

Special senses: Diplopia, dilated pupils, oculogyric crises.

Haematologic: Leukopenia, haemolytic and non-haemolytic anaemia, thrombocytopenia, agranulocytosis.

Miscellaneous: Weakness, faintness, hoarseness, malaise, hot flushes, sense of stimulation, bizarre breathing patterns, neuroleptic malignant syndrome, malignant melanoma (see *Contra-indications*). Convulsions have occurred; however, a causal relationship with levodopa or levodopa/carbidopa combinations has not been established.

Overdose: Management of acute overdosage with Sinemet CR or Half Sinemet CR is basically the same as management of acute overdosage with levodopa; however, pyridoxine is not effective in reversing the actions of Sinemet CR or Half Sinemet CR.

Electrocardiographic monitoring should be instituted and the patient observed carefully for the development of arrhythmias; if required, appropriate antiarrhythmic therapy should be given. The possibility that the patient may have taken other drugs as well as Sinemet CR or Half Sinemet CR should be taken into consideration. To date, no experience has been reported with dialysis; hence, its value in overdosage is not known.

Pharmacological properties

Pharmacodynamic properties: Sinemet CR and Half Sinemet CR are a combination of carbidopa, an aromatic amino acid decarboxylase inhibitor, and levodopa, the metabolic precursor of dopamine, in a polymer-based controlled-release tablet formulation, for use in the treatment of Parkinson's disease. Sinemet CR and Half Sinemet CR are particularly useful to reduce 'off' time in patients treated previously with a conventional levodopa/decarboxylase inhibitor combination who have had dyskinesias and motor fluctuations.

Patients with Parkinson's disease treated with preparations containing levodopa may develop motor fluctuations characterised by end-of-dose failure, peak dose dyskinesia, and akinesia. The advanced form of motor fluctuations ('on-off' phenomenon) is characterised by unpredictable swings from mobility to immobility. Although the causes of the motor fluctuations are not completely understood, it has been demonstrated that they can be attenuated by treatment regimens that produce steady plasma levels of levodopa.

Levodopa relieves the symptoms of Parkinson's disease by being decarboxylated to dopamine in the brain. Carbidopa, which does not cross the blood-brain barrier, inhibits only the extracerebral decarboxylation of levodopa, making more levodopa available for transport to the brain and subsequent conversion to dopamine. This normally obviates the necessity for large doses of levodopa at frequent intervals. The lower dosage reduces or may help eliminate gastrointestinal and cardiovascular side-effects, especially those which are attributed to dopamine being formed in extracerebral tissues.

Sinemet CR and Half Sinemet CR are designed to release their active ingredients over a four–six hour period. With this formulation there is less variation in plasma levodopa levels and the peak plasma level is 60% lower than with conventional Sinemet, as established in healthy volunteers.

In clinical trials, patients with motor fluctuations experienced reduced 'off'-time with Sinemet CR when compared with Sinemet. The reduction of the 'off'-time is rather small (about 10%) and the incidence of dyskinesias increases slightly after administration of Sinemet CR compared to standard Sinemet. Global ratings of improvement and activities of daily living in the 'on' and 'off' state, as assessed by both patient and physician, were better during therapy with Sinemet CR than with Sinemet. Patients considered Sinemet CR to be more helpful for their clinical fluctuations, and preferred it over Sinemet. In patients without motor fluctuations, Sinemet CR under controlled conditions, provided the same therapeutic benefit with less frequent dosing than with Sinemet. Generally, there was no further improvement of other symptoms of Parkinson's disease.

Pharmacokinetic properties: The pharmacokinetics of levodopa following administration of Sinemet CR were studied in young and elderly healthy volunteers. The mean time to peak plasma levodopa level after Sinemet CR was approximately two hours compared to 0.75 hours with Sinemet. The mean peak plasma levodopa levels were 60 percent lower with Sinemet CR than with Sinemet. The in vivo absorption of levodopa following administration of Sinemet CR was continuous for 4 to 6 hours. In these studies, as with patients, plasma levodopa concentrations fluctuated in a narrower range than with Sinemet. Because the bioavailability of levodopa from Sinemet CR relative to Sinemet is approximately 70 percent, the daily dosage of levodopa in the controlled release formulation will usually be higher than with conventional formulations. There was no evidence that Sinemet CR released its ingredients in a rapid or uncontrolled fashion.

The pharmacokinetics of levodopa following administration of Half Sinemet CR were studied in patients with Parkinson's disease. Chronic three month, open-label, twice daily dosing with Half Sinemet CR (range: 50 mg carbidopa, 200 mg levodopa up to 150 mg carbidopa, 600 mg levodopa per day) did not result in accumulation of plasma levodopa. The dose-adjusted bioavailability for one Half Sinemet CR tablet was equivalent to that for one Sinemet CR tablet. The mean peak concentration of levodopa following administration of one Half Sinemet CR tablet was greater than 50% of that following one Sinemet CR tablet. Mean time-to-peak plasma levels may be slightly less for Half Sinemet CR than for Sinemet CR.

It is not known whether or not or to what extent the absorption is influenced by a protein rich diet. The bioavailability may be influenced by drugs which affect the gastrointestinal propulsion.

Preclinical safety data: The medicine has appeared harmful in animal trials (visceral and skeletal malformations in rabbits). For reproductive toxicity, see *Pregnancy and lactation*.

Pharmaceutical particulars

List of excipients: Hydroxypropylcellulose PhEur, Magnesium Stearate PhEur, Poly (Vinyl Acetate-Crotonic Acid) Copolymer, Quinoline Yellow 10 Aluminium Lake E104 (Sinemet CR only), Red Iron Oxide E172.

Incompatibilities: Not applicable.

Shelf life: 36 months.

Special precautions for storage: Avoid storage above 30°C.

Nature and contents of container: All aluminium blister pack of 60 tablets.

Instructions for use/handling: Not applicable.

Marketing authorisation holder: Merck Sharp & Dohme Limited, Hertford Road, Hoddesdon, Hertfordshire, EN11 9BU.

Marketing authorisation numbers

Sinemet CR PL 0025/0269

Half Sinemet CR PL 0025/0287

Date of first authorisation/renewal of authorisation
Sinemet CR 5 September 1991
Half Sinemet CR 7 October 1992

Date of (partial) revision of text November 1998

Legal category POM

VIAZEM* XL

Qualitative and quantitative composition Diltiazem hydrochloride : 120-180-240-300-360 mg per capsule. Each capsule of Viazem XL is composed of coated pellets.

	120 mg	180 mg	240 mg	300 mg	360 mg
Size:	3	2	1	0	0

Pharmaceutical form Prolonged release capsule. For oral administration.

Clinical particulars

Therapeutic indications: Viazem XL is indicated for the management of angina pectoris and the treatment of mild to moderate hypertension.

Posology and method of administration: Dosage requirements may differ between patients with angina and patients with hypertension. In addition, individual patients responses may vary, necessitating careful titration. This range of strengths facilitates titration to the optimal dose.

One capsule per day is to be taken, before or during a meal. The capsules should be swallowed whole and not chewed.

Adults: For hypertensive patients; the usual daily dose is 300 mg, to be adapted according to the patient's response.

For angina patients; the usual starting dose is one 240 mg capsule daily.

Elderly and patients with impaired hepatic or renal function: The usual starting dose is one 120 mg capsule daily. If necessary, the dose may be gradually increased, but careful monitoring of this group of patients is advised.

Children: Viazem XL capsules are not recommended for children.

Safety and efficacy in children have not been established.

Contra-indications: Diltiazem is contra-indicated in pregnancy and in women of child-bearing potential. Diltiazem is excreted in breast milk in concentrations similar to those in serum. If use of diltiazem is considered essential during lactation, an alternative method of infant feeding should be instituted.

Diltiazem depresses atrioventricular node conduction and is therefore contra-indicated in patients with marked bradycardia, sick sinus syndrome, left ventricular failure with stasis, or second or third degree AV block except in the presence of a functioning pacemaker.

Special warnings and precautions for use: Diltiazem should be used with caution in patients with reduced left ventricular function. Patients with mild bradycardia, first degree AV block or prolonged PR interval should be observed closely.

No special precautions are necessary in cases of isolated branch block. In cases of general anaesthesia, the anaesthetist should be informed that the drug is being taken.

Diltiazem may be used without risk in patients with chronic respiratory diseases.

Interaction with other medicaments and other forms of interaction: Combinations contra-indicated as a safety measure:

In animals, fatal ventricular fibrillations are constantly seen during administration of verapamil and dantrolene via the i.v. route. The combination of a calcium antagonist and dantrolene is therefore potentially dangerous.

Combinations requiring safety precautions:

In common with other calcium antagonists, when diltiazem is used with drugs which may induce bradycardia or with antiarrhythmic or other antihypertensive drugs the possibility of an additive effect should be borne in mind.

Diltiazem has been used safely in combination with beta-blockers, diuretics, ACE-inhibitors and other antihypertensive agents. It is recommended that patients receiving these combinations should be regularly monitored. Concomitant use of diltiazem with alphablockers such as prazosin should be strictly monitored because of the possible synergistic hypotensive effect of this combination.

Case reports have suggested that blood levels of carbamazepine, cyclosporin and theophylline may be increased when given concurrently with diltiazem. Care should be exercised in patients taking these drugs. In common with other calcium antagonists diltiazem may cause small increases in plasma levels of digoxin.

In patients taking H_2-antagonists concurrently with diltiazem there may be increased levels of diltiazem.

Magnification of the hypotensive and lipothymic effects (summation of vasodilator properties) of nitrate derivatives can occur. In patients on calcium inhibitors, prescription of nitrate derivatives should be made at progressively increasing doses. Diltiazem treatment has been continued without problem during anaesthesia, but the anaesthetist should be informed that the patient is receiving a calcium antagonist.

Pregnancy and lactation:
Pregnancy: Diltiazem is teratogenic in some animal species. In the absence of adequate evidence of safety in human pregnancy, Viazem XL should not be used in pregnancy or in women of childbearing potential.

Lactation: Diltiazem is excreted in breast milk in concentrations similar to those in serum. If the use of diltiazem is considered essential, an alternative method of infant feeding should be instituted.

Effects on ability to drive and use machines: None of note at the recommended dosage.

Undesirable effects: Certain undesirable effects may lead to suspension of treatment : sinus bradycardia, sinoatrial heart block, 2nd and 3rd degree atrioventricular heart block, skin rash, oedema of the lower limbs.

In hypertensive patients, adverse effects are generally mild and transient and are most commonly vasodilatory related events

The following have been described in decreasing order of frequency : lower limb oedema, headache, hot flushes/flushing, asthenia/fatigue, palpitations, malaise, minor gastro-intestinal disorders (dyspepsia, abdominal pain, dry mouth) and skin rash. Vasodilatory related events (in particular, oedema) are dose-dependent and appear to be more frequent in elderly subjects.

Rare cases of symptomatic bradycardia and exceptionally sino-atrial block and atrioventricular block were also recorded.

Experience with use in other indications and with other formulations, has shown that skin rashes are usually localised and are limited to cases of erythema, urticaria or occasionally desquamative erythema, with or without fever, which regress when treatment is discontinued.

Isolated cases of moderate and transient elevation of liver transaminases have been observed at the start of treatment. Isolated cases of clinical hepatitis have been reported which resolved on cessation of therapy.

Overdose: The clinical consequences of overdose can be severe hypotension leading to collapse, and sinus bradycardia which may be accompanied by isorhythmic dissociation and atrioventricular conduction disturbances. Observation in a coronary care unit is advisable. Vasopressors such as adrenaline may be indicated in patients exhibiting profound hypotension. Calcium gluconate may help reverse the effects of calcium entry blockade. Atropine administration and temporary cardiac pacing may be required to manage bradycardia and/or conduction disturbances.

Glucagon can be used in cases of established hypoglycaemia.

Diltiazem and its metabolites are very poorly dialysable.

Pharmacological properties

Pharmacodynamic properties: Diltiazem hydrochloride is a calcium antagonist. It selectively reduces calcium entry through voltage-dependent calcium-n channels into vascular smooth muscle cells and myocardial cells. This lowers the concentration of intracellular calcium which is available to activate contractile proteins. This action of diltiazem results in dilation of coronary arteries causing an increase in myocardial oxygen supply. It reduces cardiac work by moderating the heart rate and by reducing systemic vascular resistance thus reducing oxygen demand.

Pharmacokinetic properties: The kinetics of diltiazem are linear and non-saturable. In the healthy volunteer, following a single oral administration, diltiazem is well absorbed (90%).

Viazem XL formulations allow a prolonged absorption of the active element. In most cases, the 300 mg capsule translates into therapeutic levels (50-200 ng/ml) over 24 hours following chronic administration. In other cases the therapeutic level is obtained with lower or higher dosages.

Diltiazem is bound to plasma proteins in proportions of 80 to 85%. It is metabolised by the liver.

After chronic administration, the unchanged substance is found in the urine at levels of 1 to 3%.

Deacetyldiltiazem, the active metabolite, represents 15% of circulating levels of diltiazem. Food does not significantly alter the kinetics of diltiazem when administered as the Viazem XL formulation.

Diltiazem and its metabolites are very poorly dialysable.

The apparent half-life of elimination is from 5 to 7 hours.

Preclinical safety data:
Toxicity: Toxicity by single ingestion: The LD_{50} for rats and mice are 560 mg/kg/day and 508 mg/kg/day respectively by the oral route. By the intravenous route, the LD_{50} are 38 mg/kg/day (males) and 39 mg/kg/day (females) in rats, and 61 mg/kg/day (males) and 58 mg/kg/day (females) in mice. It has been estimated that the smallest lethal dose in dogs is 40 mg/kg/day.

Subacute toxicity: In rats, 500 mg/kg/day for 30 days via the oral route or 25 mg/kg/day via the intraperitoneal route constitute lethal doses. In dogs, the lethal dose is 50 mg/kg/day.

Chronic toxicity: In studies carried out in rats for 6 months, a 60% mortality rate was noted at a dose of 125 mg/kg/day. In dogs after the same period, a sole death took place with a dose of 40 mg/kg/day.

Fertility and general capacity for reproduction: The effects of diltiazem on fertility and reproductive function were studied in rats. Toxic effects were revealed at an oral dose of 100 mg/kg/day and via the intraperitoneal route at a dose of 80 mg/kg/day. Via the intravenous route, a dose of 18 mg/kg/day produced toxic effects.

Embryotoxicity–Teratogenicity: In mice, a teratogenic effect is evidenced via the oral route from doses of 50 mg/kg/day. In rats, oral administration of diltiazem from the 9th to the 14th days of gestation at high doses (200 to 400 mg/kg/day) induce toxic effects.

In rabbits, doses from 18 to 70 mg/kg/day exert a teratogenic effect, which becomes lethal to the embryo at doses of 35 mg/kg/day.

Peri- and post natal toxicity: In rats, oral doses (from 100 mg/kg/day) produce maternal toxicity. A teratogenic effect has been observed in the retina and in the tongue upwards of 30 mg/kg/day. Toxic effects become evident at a dose of 130 mg/kg/day via the intravenous route on the neonatal survival rate and on the average growth rate.

Mutagenesis–Carcinogenesis: Diltiazem has no known carcinogenic potential.

Toxicity in man: The lethal dose in man is not known.

Pharmaceutical particulars

List of excipients: Saccharose stearate; Microcrystalline cellulose; Polyvidone; Magnesium stearate; Talc; Methylhydroxypropylcellulose; Polysorbate 80; Polyacrylate dispersion 30% (dry); Simethicone emulsion, gelatin capsule.

Gelatin capsule colours

	Capsule body	Capsule cap
120 mg	Lavender opaque (1)	Lavender opaque (1)
180 mg	White opaque (2)	Blue green opaque (3)
240 mg	Blue green opaque (3)	Lavender opaque (1)
300 mg	White opaque (2)	Lavender opaque (1)
360 mg	Blue green opaque (3)	Blue green opaque (3)

(1) Colour is composed of Azorubine E122, Indigotine E132, and Titanium Dioxide E171.
(2) Colour is composed of Titanium Dioxide E171.
(3) Colour is composed of Quinoline Yellow E104, Indigotine E132 and Titanium Dioxide E171.

Gelatin capsule markings (printed radially):

	Capsule body	*Capsule cap*
120 mg	Viazem XL 120 (white ink EEC approved)	Viazem XL 120 (white ink EEC approved)
180 mg	Viazem XL 180 (black ink EEC approved)	Viazem XL 180 (black ink EEC approved)
240 mg	Viazem XL 240 (white ink EEC approved)	Viazem XL 240 (white ink EEC approved)
300 mg	Viazem XL 300 (black ink EEC approved)	Viazem XL 300 (black ink EEC approved)
360 mg	Viazem XL 360 (white ink EEC approved)	Viazem XL 360 (white ink EEC approved)

Incompatibilities: Not applicable.

Shelf life: 3 years.

Special precautions for storage: At room temperature (at or below 25°C), avoiding excessive humidity.

Nature and contents of container: The capsules are packed in PVC/aluminium blisters.

Instructions for use/handling: Swallow capsules whole, do not chew.

Marketing authorisation holder: Biovail (UK) Ltd, Thames House, Wellington Street, London SE18 6NZ.

Marketing authorisation numbers

Viazem XL 120 mg 15136/0006
Viazem XL 180 mg 15136/0007
Viazem XL 240 mg 15136/0008
Viazem XL 300 mg 15136/0009
Viazem XL 360 mg 15136/0010

Date of first authorisation 2 April 1997.

Date of (partial) revision of the text September 1998.

Legal category POM.

**Trade Mark*

Eisai Ltd

Hammersmith International Centre
3 Shortlands
London W6 8EE

☎ 0181 600 1400  0181 600 1401

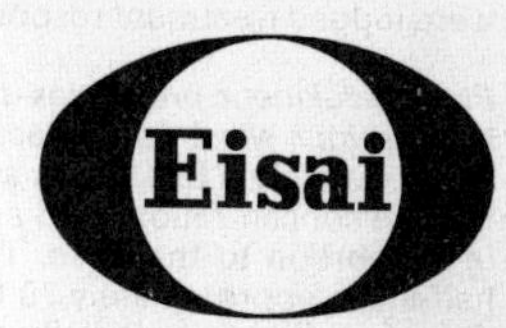

ARICEPT* 5 mg, 10 mg ▼

Qualitative and quantitative composition 5 mg donepezil hydrochloride tablets each containing 4.56 mg donepezil free base. 10 mg donepezil hydrochloride tablets each containing 9.12 mg donepezil free base.

Pharmaceutical form Film-Coated tablets.

Clinical particulars

Therapeutic indications: Aricept tablets are indicated for the symptomatic treatment of mild to moderately severe Alzheimer's dementia.

Special warnings and precautions for use in this indication may be found in *Special warnings and special precautions for use.*

Posology and method of administration:

Adults/elderly: Treatment is initiated at 5 mg/day (once-a-day dosing). Aricept should be taken orally, in the evening, just prior to retiring. The 5 mg/day dose should be maintained for at least one month in order to allow the earliest clinical responses to treatment to be assessed and to allow steady-state concentrations of donepezil hydrochloride to be achieved. Following a one-month clinical assessment of treatment at 5 mg/day, the dose of Aricept can be increased to 10 mg/day (once-a-day dosing). The maximum recommended daily dose is 10 mg. Doses greater than 10 mg/day have not been studied in clinical trials.

Duration of treatment has not been investigated in placebo-controlled trials beyond 6 months. Upon discontinuation of treatment, a gradual abatement of the beneficial effects of Aricept is seen. There is no evidence of a rebound effect after abrupt discontinuation of therapy.

Renal and hepatic impairment: A similar dose schedule can be followed for patients with renal or mild to moderate hepatic impairment as clearance of donepezil hydrochloride is not affected by these conditions.

Children: Aricept is not recommended for use in children.

Contra-indications: Aricept is contra-indicated in patients with a known hypersensitivity to donepezil hydrochloride, piperidine derivatives, or to any excipients used in the formulation. Aricept is contra-indicated in pregnancy.

Special warnings and special precautions for use: Treatment should be initiated and supervised by a physician experienced in the diagnosis and treatment of Alzheimer's dementia. Diagnosis should be made according to accepted guidelines (e.g. DSM IV, ICD 10). Therapy with donepezil should only be started if a caregiver is available who will regularly monitor drug intake for the patient. Maintenance treatmemt can be continued for as long as a therapeutic benefit for the patient exists. Therefore, the clinical benefit of donepezil should be reassessed on a regular basis. Discontinuation should be considered when evidence of a therapeutic effect is no longer present. Individual response to donepezil cannot be predicted. The use of Aricept in patients with severe Alzheimer's dementia, other types of dementia or other types of memory impairment (e.g. age-related cognitive decline), has not been investigated.

Anaesthesia: Aricept, as a cholinesterase inhibitor is likely to exaggerate succinylcholine-type muscle relaxation during anaesthesia.

Cardiovascular conditions: Because of their pharmacological action, cholinesterase inhibitors may have vagotonic effects on heart rate (e.g. bradycardia). The potential for this action may be particularly important to patients with "sick sinus syndrome" or other supraventricular cardiac conduction conditions, such as sinoatrial or atrioventricular block.

Gastro-intestinal conditions: Patients at increased risk for developing ulcers, e.g. those with a history of ulcer disease or those receiving concurrent nonsteroidal anti-inflammatory drugs (NSAIDs), should be monitored for symptoms. However, the clinical studies with Aricept showed no increase, relative to placebo, in the incidence of either peptic ulcer disease or gastrointestinal bleeding.

Genito-urinary: Although not observed in clinical trials of Aricept, cholinomimetics may cause bladder outflow obstruction.

Neurological conditions: Seizures: Cholinomimetics are believed to have some potential to cause generalised convulsions. However, seizure activity may also be a manifestation of Alzheimer's Disease.

Pulmonary conditions: Because of their cholinomimetic actions, cholinesterase inhibitors should be prescribed with care to patients with a history of asthma or obstructive pulmonary disease.

The administration of Aricept concimitantly with other inhibitors of acetylcholinesterase, agonists or antagonists of the cholinergic system should be avoided.

Interaction with other medicaments and other forms of interaction: The clinical experience with donepezil is presently limited. For this reason, it may be that all possible interactions have not been recorded. The prescribing physician should be aware of the possibility of new, as yet unknown interactions with donepezil.

Donepezil hydrochloride and/or any of its metabolites does not inhibit the metabolism of theophylline, warfarin, cimetidine or digoxin in humans. The metabolism of donepezil hydrochloride is not affected by concurrent administration of digoxin or cimetidine. *In vitro* studies have shown that the cytochrome P450 isoenzymes 3A4 and to a minor extent 2D6 are involved in the metabolism of donepezil. Drug interaction studies performed *in vitro* show that ketaconazole and quinidine, inhibitors of CYP3A4 and 2D6 respectively, inhibit donepezil metabolism. Therefore these and other CYP3A4 inhibitors, such as itraconazole and erythromycin, and CYP2D6 inhibitors, such as fluoxetine could inhibit the metabolism of donepezil. In a study in healthy volunteers, ketoconazole increased mean donepezil concentrations by about 30%. Enzyme inducers, such as rifampicin, phenytoin, carbamazepine and alcohol may reduce the levels of donepezil. Since the magnitude of an inhibiting or inducing effect is unknown, such drug combinations should be used with care. Donepezil hydrochloride has the potential to interfere with medications having anticholinergic activity. There is also the potential for synergistic activity with concomitant treatment involving medications such as succinylcholine, other neuromuscular blocking agents or cholinergic agonists or beta blocking agents which have effects on cardiac conduction.

Pregnancy and lactation:

Pregnancy: Teratology studies conducted in pregnant rats at doses up to approximately 80 times the human dose and in pregnant rabbits at doses up to approximately 50 times the human dose did not disclose any evidence for a teratogenic potential. However, in a study in which pregnant rats were given approximately 50 times the human dose from day 17 of gestation through day 20 postpartum, there was a slight increase in stillbirths and a slight decrease in pup survival through day 4 postpartum. No effect was observed at the next lower dose tested, approximately 15 times the human dose. Aricept should not be used during pregnancy.

Lactation: It is not known whether donepezil hydrochloride is excreted in human breast milk and there are no studies in lactating women. Therefore, women on donepezil should not breast feed.

Effects on ability to drive and use machines: Alzheimer's Dementia may cause impairment of driving performance or compromise the ability to use machinery. Furthermore, donepezil can induce fatigue, dizziness and muscle cramps, mainly when initiating or increasing the dose. The ability of Alzheimer patients on donepezil to continue driving or operating complex machines should be routinely evaluated by the treating physician.

Undesirable effects: The most common adverse events (incidence ≥ 5% and twice the frequency of placebo) were diarrhoea, muscle cramps, fatigue nausea, vomiting and insomnia. Other common adverse events (incidence ≥ 5% and ≥ placebo) were headache, pain, accident, common cold, abdominal disturbance and dizziness.

Rare cases of syncope, bradycardia, sinoatrial block and atrioventricular block were observed.

There have been reports of psychiatric disturbances, including hallucinations, agitation and aggressive behaviour which were resolved on dose reduction or discontinuation of treatment.

No notable abnormalities in laboratory values were observed, except for minor increases in serum concentrations of muscle creatine kinase.

Overdose: The estimated median lethal dose of donepezil hydrochloride following administration of a single oral dose in mice and rats is 45 and 32 mg/kg, respectively, or approximately 225 and 160 times the maximum recommended human dose of 10 mg per day. Dose-related signs of cholinergic stimulation were observed in animals and included reduced spontaneous movement, prone position, staggering gait, lacrimation, clonic convulsions, depressed respiration, salivation, miosis, fasciculation and lower body surface temperature.

Overdosage with cholinesterase inhibitors can result in cholinergic crisis characterised by severe nausea, vomiting, salivation, sweating, bradycardia, hypotension, respiratory depression, collapse and convulsions. Increasing muscle weakness is a possibility and may result in death if respiratory muscles are involved.

As in any case of overdose, general supportive measures should be utilised. Tertiary anticholinergics such as atropine may be used as an antidote for Aricept overdosage. Intravenous atropine sulphate titrated to effect is recommended: an initial dose of 1.0 to 2.0 mg IV with subsequent doses based upon clinical response. Atypical responses in blood pressure and heart rate have been reported with other cholinomimetics when co-administered with quaternary anticholinergics such as glycopyrrolate. It is not known whether donepezil hydrochloride and/or its metabolites can be removed by dialysis (hemodialysis, peritoneal dialysis, or hemofiltration).

Pharmacological properties

Pharmacodynamic properties: Donepezil hydrochloride is a specific and reversible inhibitor of acetylcholinesterase, the predominant cholinesterase in the brain. Donepezil hydrochloride is *in vitro* over 1000 times more potent an inhibitor of this enzyme than of butyrylcholinesterase, an enzyme which is present mainly outside the central nervous system.

In patients with Alzheimer's Dementia participating in clinical trials, administration of single daily doses of 5 mg or 10 mg of Aricept produced steady-state inhibition of acetylcholinesterase activity (measured in erythrocyte membranes) of 63.3% and 77.3%, respectively when measured post dose. The inhibition of acetylcholinesterase (AChE) in red blood cells by donepezil hydrochloride has been shown to correlate to changes in ADAS-cog, a sensitive scale which examines selected aspects of cognition. The potential for donepezil hydrochloride to alter the course of the underlying neuropathology has not been studied. Thus Aricept can not be considered to have any effect on the pregress of the disease.

In the clinical trials, an analysis was done at the conclusion of 6 months of donepezil treatment using a combination of three efficacy criteria: the ADAS-cog (a measure of cognitive performance), the Clinician Interview Based Impression of Change with Caregiver Input (a measure of global function) and the Activities of Daily Living Subscale of the Clinical Dementia Rating Scale (a measure of capabilities in community affairs, home and hobbies and personal care).

Patients who fulfilled the criteria listed below were considered treatment responders.

Response = Improvement of ADAS-cog of at least 4 points
No deterioration of CIBIC
No deterioration of Activities of Daily Living Subscale of the Clinical Dementia Rating Scale

	% Response	
	Intent to Treat Population n = 365	*Evaluable Population n = 352*
Placebo group	10%	10%
Aricept 5 mg group	18%*	18%*
Aricept 10 mg group	21%*	22%**

* P < 0.05 **P < 0.01

Aricept produced a dose-dependent statistically significant increase in the percentage of patients who were judged treatment responders.

Pharmacokinetic properties–General characteristics: Absorption: Maximum plasma levels are reached approximately 3 to 4 hours after oral administration. Plasma concentrations and area under the curve rise in proportion to the dose. The terminal disposition half-life is approximately 70 hours, thus, administration of multiple single-daily doses results in gradual approach to steady-state. Approximate steady-state is achieved within 3 weeks after initiation of therapy. Once at steady-state, plasma donepezil hydrochloride concentrations and the related pharmacodynamic activity show little variability over the course of the day.

Food did not affect the absorption of donepezil hydrochloride.

Distribution: Donepezil hydrochloride is approximately 95% bound to human plasma proteins. The plasma protein binding of the active metabolite 6-O-desmethyl donepezil is not known. The distribution of donepezil hydrochloride in various body tissues has not been definitively studied. However, in a mass balance study conducted in healthy male volunteers, 240 hours after the administration of a single 5 mg dose of ^{14}C-labelled donepezil hydrochloride, approximately 28% of the label remained unrecovered. This suggests that donepezil hydrochloride and/or its metabolites may persist in the body for more than 10 days.

Metabolism/excretion: Donepezil hydrochloride is both excreted in the urine intact and metabolised by the cytochrome P450 system to multiple metabolites, not all of which have been identified. Following administration of a single 5 mg dose of ^{14}C-labelled donepezil hydrochloride, plasma radioactivity, expressed as a percent of the administered dose, was present primarily as intact donepezil hydrochloride (30%), 6-O-desmethyl donepezil (11%–only metabolite that exhibits activity similar to donepezil hydrochloride), donepezil-cis-N-oxide (9%), 5-O-desmethyl donepezil (7%) and the glucuronide conjugate of 5-O-desmethyl donepezil (3%). Approximately 57% of the total administered radioactivity was recovered from the urine (17% as unchanged donepezil), and 14.5% was recovered from the faeces, suggesting biotransformation and urinary excretion as the primary routes of elimination. There is no evidence to suggest enterohepatic recirculation of donepezil hydrochloride and/or any of its metabolites.

Plasma donepezil concentrations decline with a half-life of approximately 70 hours.

Sex, race and smoking history have no clinically significant influence on plasma concentrations of donepezil hydrochloride. The pharmacokinetics of donepezil have not been formerly studied in healthy elderly subjects or in Alzheimer's patients. However mean plasma levels in patients closely agreed with those of young healthy volunteers.

Preclinical safety data: Extensive testing in experimental animals has demonstrated that this compound causes few effects other than the intended pharmacological effects consistent with its action as a cholinergic stimulator (see *Overdose* above). Donepezil is not mutagenic in bacterial and mammalian cell mutation assays. Some clastogenic effects were observed *in vitro* at concentrations overtly toxic to the cells and more than 3000 times the steady-state plasma concentrations. No clastogenic or other genotoxic effects were observed in the mouse micronucleus model *in vivo*. Data regarding carcinogenic potential are not yet available.

Donepezil hydrochloride had no effect on fertility in rats, and was not teratogenic in rats or rabbits, but had a slight effect on still births and early pup survival when administered to pregnant rats at 50 times the human dose (see *Pregnancy and lactation* above).

Pharmaceutical particulars

List of excipients: Inactive ingredients are lactose monohydrate, maize starch, microcrystalline cellulose, hydroxypropyl cellulose, and magnesium stearate. The film coating contains talc, polyethylene glycol, hypromellose and titanium dioxide. Additionally, the 10 mg tablet contains yellow iron oxide (synthetic) as a colouring agent.

Incompatibilities: None.

Shelf life: 36 months.

Special precautions for storage: Store below 30°C.

Nature and contents of container: 5 mg tablets: Unit Dose blister strips (PVC/foil, calendar marked) of 14. Two strips of 14 per carton.

10 mg tablets: Unit Dose blister strips (PVC/foil, calendar marked) of 14. Two strips of 14 per carton.

Instructions for use/handling: No special instructions.

Marketing authorisation holder Eisai Ltd., Hammersmith International Centre, 3 Shortlands, London W6 8EE.

Marketing authorisation numbers
PL 10555/0006 (5 mg)
PL 10555/0007 (10 mg)

Date of first authorisation /renewal of the authorisation 14 February 1997

Date of (partial) revision of the text May 1998

**Trade Mark*

Elan Pharma Ltd
1 Meadway Court
Rutherford Close
Stevenage
Herts SG1 2EF

☎ 01438 730200 🖷 01438 741452

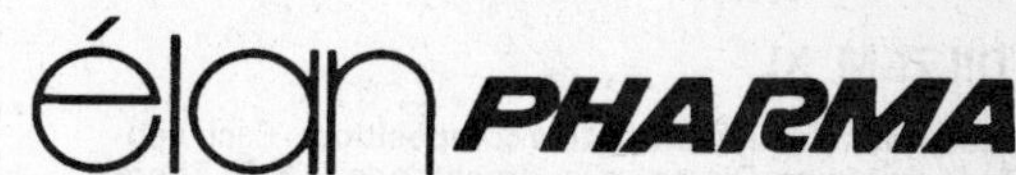

DILZEM SR

Presentation Dilzem SR 60, Dilzem SR 90, Dilzem SR120. Each sustained release capsule contains Diltiazem hydrochloride U.S.P. 60 mg, 90 mg and 120 mg respectively. The capsules are beige in colour and overprinted with the product strength.

Uses *Action:* Diltiazem has pharmacologic actions similar to those of other calcium channel blocking agents such as nifedipine or verapamil. The principal physiologic action of diltiazem is to inhibit the transmembrane influx of extracellular calcium ions across the membranes of myocardial cells and vascular smooth muscle cells.

Calcium plays important roles in the excitation-contraction coupling processes of the heart and vascular smooth muscle cells and in the electrical discharge of the specialised conduction cells of the heart. The membranes of these cells contain numerous channels that carry a slow inward current and that are selective for calcium.

By inhibiting calcium influx, diltiazem inhibits the contractile processes of cardiac and vascular smooth muscle, thereby dilating the main coronary and systemic arteries. Dilation of systemic arteries by diltiazem results in a decrease in total peripheral resistance, a decrease in systemic blood pressure and a decrease in the afterload of the heart. The reduction in afterload, seen at rest and with exercise and its resultant decrease in myocardial oxygen consumption are thought to be responsible for the beneficial effects of diltiazem in patients with chronic stable angina pectoris. In patients with Prinzmetal variant angina, inhibition of spontaneous and ergonovine-induced coronary artery spasm by diltiazem results in increased myocardial oxygen delivery.

Indications
Dilzem SR: Treatment of angina pectoris including Prinzmetal's angina and treatment of mild to moderate hypertension.

Dosage and administration
Route of administration: Oral.

Adults
Hypertension: The usual initial dose is one Dilzem SR 90 capsule twice daily (corresponding to 180 mg of diltiazem hydrochloride). Depending upon clinical response the dosage may be increased to 180 mg twice daily if required.

Angina pectoris: The usual initial dose is one Dilzem SR 90 capsule twice daily (corresponding to 180 mg of diltiazem hydrochloride). Depending upon clinical response, the patient's dosage may be increased to 180 mg twice daily if required.

Elderly patients and those with renal or hepatic impairment: Dosage should commence at the lower level of either Dilzem SR 60 twice daily and be increased slowly. Do not increase the dose if the heart rate falls below 50 beats per minute.

Children: This product is not recommended for use in children.

Contra-indications, warnings, etc
Contra-indications
(1) Use in women of child-bearing potential.
(2) Concomitant administration of dantrolene infusion due to the risk of ventricular fibrillation.
(3) Shock
(4) Acute cardiac infarct with complications (bradycardia, severe hypotension, left heart insufficiency).
(5) Bradycardia (pulse rate, at rest, of less than 50 beats per minute), hypotension (less than 90 mm Hg systole), second or third degree heart block, or sick sinus syndrome except in the presence of a functioning ventricular pacemaker.
(6) Atrial fibrillation / flutter and simultaneous presence of a WPW (Wolff-Parkinson-White) syndrome (increased risk of triggering a ventricular tachycardia).
(7) Manifest myocardial insufficiency.
(8) Left ventricular failure with stasis.
(9) Hypersensitivity to diltiazem or any of the excipients.

Use in pregnancy and lactation: Diltiazem must not be taken during pregnancy as experimental studies have shown indications of teratogenicity. There is no experience of its effects in humans. As diltiazem is known to enter the breast milk and there is no experience of possible effects in infants, infants should be weaned if treatment of the mother with diltiazem is necessary.

Adverse effects: In studies carried out to date, serious adverse reactions with diltiazem have been rare; however, it should be recognised that patients with impaired ventricular function and cardiac conduction abnormalities have usually been excluded from these studies.

In 900 patients with hypertension, the most common adverse effects were oedema (9%), headache (8%), dizziness (6%), asthenia (5%), sinus bradycardia (3%), flushing (3%) and first degree AV block (3%). Only oedema and perhaps bradycardia were dose related.

The most common adverse events (>1%) observed in clinical studies of over 2100 angina and hypertensive patients receiving diltiazem were oedema (5.4%), headache (4.5%), dizziness (3.4%), asthenia (2.8%), first degree AV block (1.8%), flushing (1.7%), nausea (1.6%), bradycardia (1.5%) and rash (1.5%).

Less common adverse events have included the following:

Cardiovascular: angina, arrhythmia, AV block (second or third degree), congestive heart failure, hypotension, palpitations, syncope.

Nervous system: amnesia, depression, gait abnormality, hallucinations, insomnia, nervousness, paraesthesia, personality change, somnolence, tinnitus, tremor.

Gastro-intestinal: anorexia, constipation, diarrhoea, dyspepsia, mild elevations of alkaline phosphatase, SGOT, SGPT and LDH (see *special warnings and precautions)*, vomiting, weight increase, gingivitis.

Dermatologic: Petechiae, pruritus, photosensitivity, urticaria. Allergic skin reactions including erythema multiforme, vasculitis, lymphadenopathy and eosinophilia have been observed in isolated cases. Dermatological events may be transient and may disappear despite continued use of diltiazem. Should a dermatologic reaction persist, the drug should be discontinued.

Other: amblyopia, CK elevation, dyspnoea, epistaxis, eye irritation, hyperglycaemia, nasal congestion, nocturia, osteoarticular pain, polyuria, sexual difficulties.

Precautions and warnings: Capsules should not be sucked or chewed.
The use of diltiazem hydrochloride in diabetic patients may require adjustment of their control.

The product should be used with caution in patients with hepatic dysfunction. Abnormalities of liver function may occur during therapy. Very occasional reports of abnormal liver function have been received, these reactions have been reversible upon discontinuation of therapy.

First degree AV block or prolonged PR interval. Dilzem prolongs AV node refractory periods without significantly prolonging sinus node recovery time, except in patients with sick sinus syndrome. This effect may rarely result in abnormally slow heart rates (particularly in patients with sick sinus syndrome) or second- or third- degree AV block (see Interactions section for information concerning beta-blockers and digitalis).

Mild bradycardia.
Patients with reduced left ventricular function.
Renally impaired patients.

As with any drug given over prolonged periods, laboratory parameters should be monitored at regular intervals.

Interactions: Diltiazem undergoes biotransformation by cytochrome P-450 mixed function oxidase. Co-administration with other agents which follow the same route of biotransformation may result in competitive inhibition of metabolism.

Diltiazem hydrochloride should only be administered with great care to patients receiving concurrent treatment with antihypertensives or other hypotensive agents including halogenated anaesthetics or drugs with moderate protein binding.

Diltiazem hydrochloride will not protect against the effects of withdrawal of beta-adrenoceptor blocking agents, nor the rebound effects seen with various antihypertensives. Combination with beta-adrenoceptor blockers having a significant 'first pass' loss, e.g. propanolol may require a decrease in their dose and may lead to bradycardia. There may be an additive effect when used with drugs which may induce bradycardia or with other antihypertensives.

Concomitant H_2 antagonist therapy may increase diltiazem blood levels.

Diltiazem may affect the blood levels of concomitant carbamazepine, theophylline, cyclosporin and digoxin. Careful attention should therefore be given to signs of overdosage. If necessary, the levels should be determined and the dose of carbamazepine, theophylline, cyclosporin or digoxin reduced if necessary. Patients receiving beta-blockers, diuretics, ACE inhibitors or other antihypertensive agents should be strictly monitored. Use with alpha blockers should be strictly monitored.

The simultaneous administration of diltiazem with drugs such as beta-blockers, antiarrythmics or heart glycosides may cause a greater degree of AV blocking, reduce the heart rate or induce a hypotensive effect.

Intravenous administration of beta-blockers should be discontinued during therapy with diltiazem.

Anaesthetists should be warned that a patient is on a calcium antagonist. The depression of cardiac contractility, conductivity and automaticity as well as the vascular dilation associated with anaesthetics may be potentiated by calcium channel blockers. When used concomitantly, anaesthetics and calcium channel blockers should be titrated carefully.

There have been reports in the literature of diltiazem interactions with warfarin, rifampicin and lithium.

Overdosage: Experience of overdosage in man is limited but cases of spontaneous recovery have been reported. However, it is recommended that patients with suspected overdose, should be placed under observation in a coronary care unit with facilities available for treatment of any possible hypotension and conduction disturbances that may occur.

Most patients suffering from overdosage of diltiazem become hypotensive within 8 hours of ingestion. With bradycardia and first to third degree atrioventricular block also developing cardiac arrest may ensue. Hyperglycaemia is also a recognised complication. The elimination half-life of diltiazem after overdosage is estimated to be about 5.5-10.2 hours. If a patient presents early after overdose, gastric lavage should be performed and activated charcoal administered to reduce diltiazem absorption.

Hypotension should be corrected with plasma expanders, intravenous calcium gluconate and inotropic agents (dopamine, dobutamine or isoprenaline), symptomatic bradycardia and high grade AV block may respond to atropine, isoprenaline or occasionally cardiac pacing which may be useful if cardiac standstill occurs.

Pharmaceutical precautions Store in a dry place at a temperature not exceeding 25°C.

Legal category POM

Package quantities
Dilzem SR 60: Blister pack containing 56 capsules
Dilzem SR 90: Blister pack containing 56 capsules
Dilzem SR 120: Blister pack containing 56 capsules

Further information None

Product licence numbers

Dilzem SR 60	10038/0024
Dilzem SR 90	10038/0025
Dilzem SR 120	10038/0026

Product licence holder: Elan Pharma Ltd, Monksland, Athlone, Co. Westmeath, Ireland.

Trading as: Elan Pharma, 1 Meadway Court, Rutherford Close, Stevenage, Hertfordshire SG1 2EF, UK.

Date of revision April 1998

DILZEM XL

Qualitative and quantitative composition Each capsule contains Diltiazem hydrochloride U.S.P. There are three strengths of Dilzem XL capsule containing 120 mg, 180 mg and 240 mg respectively.

Pharmaceutical form The product consists of hard gelatin capsules containing roughly spherical beads.

Clinical particulars

Therapeutic indications: Prophylaxis and treatment of angina pectoris.

Treatment of mild to moderate hypertension.

Posology and method of administration

Adults: Hypertension: The usual initial dose is one 180 mg capsule per day (corresponding to 180 mg of diltiazem hydrochloride once daily). Depending upon the clinical response the dosage may be increased stepwise to 360 mg/day if required.

Angina pectoris: The usual initial dose is one 180 mg capsule per day (corresponding to 180 mg of diltiazem hydrochloride once daily). Depending upon the clinical response the dosage may be increased stepwise to 360 mg/day if required.

Elderly patients and those with renal or hepatic impairment: Dosage should commence at the lower level of 120 mg once daily and be increased slowly. Do not increase the dose if the heart rate falls below 50 beats per minute.

Children: Not recommended.

Contra-indications

1. Use in women of child-bearing potential.
2. Concomitant administration of dantrolene infusion due to the risk of ventricular fibrillation.
3. Shock.
4. Acute cardiac infarct with complications (bradycardia, severe hypotension, left heart insufficiency).
5. Bradycardia (pulse rate, at rest, of less than 50 bpm), hypotension (less than 90 mm Hg systole), second or third degree heart block or sick sinus syndrome except in the presence of a functioning ventricular pacemaker.
6. Atrial fibrillation/flutter and simultaneous presence of a WPW (Wolff-Parkinson-White) syndrome (increased risk of triggering a ventricular tachycardia).
7. Manifest myocardial insufficiency.
8. Left ventricular failure with stasis
9. Hypersensitivity to diltiazem or any of the excipients

Special warnings and special precautions for use: Capsules should not be sucked or chewed.

The use of diltiazem hydrochloride in diabetic patients may require adjustment of their control.

The product should be used with caution in patients with hepatic dysfunction. Abnormalities of liver function may occur during therapy. Very occasional reports of abnormal liver function have been received, these reactions have been reversible upon discontinuation of therapy.

First degree atrio-ventricular block or prolonged PR interval. Dilzem prolongs AV node refractory periods without significantly prolonging sinus node recovery time, except in patients with sick sinus syndrome. This effect may rarely result in abnormally slow heart rates (particularly in patients with sick sinus syndrome) or second- or third- degree AV block (see interactions section for information concerning beta-blockers and digitalis).

Mild bradycardia. Patients with reduced left ventricular function and renally impaired patients

As with any drug given over prolonged periods, laboratory parameters should be monitored at regular intervals.

Interaction with other medicaments and other forms of interaction

1. Diltiazem undergoes biotransformation by cytochrome P-450 mixed function oxidase. Coadministration with other agents which follow the same route of biotransformation may result in competitive inhibition of metabolism.
2. Diltiazem hydrochloride should be administered with great care to patients receiving concurrent treatment with antihypertensives or other hypotensive agents including halogenated anaesthetics or drugs with moderate protein binding.
3. Diltiazem hydrochloride will not protect against effects of withdrawal of β-adrenoceptor blocking agents, nor the rebound effects seen with various antihypertensives. Combination with β-adrenoceptor blockers having a significant "first pass" loss, eg. propanolol may require a decrease in their dose and may lead to bradycardia.
4. There may be an additive effect when used with drugs which may induce bradycardia or with other antihypertensives. Concomitant H_2 antagonist therapy may increase diltiazem blood levels.
5. Diltiazem may affect the blood levels of concomitant carbamazepine, theophylline, cyclosporin and digoxin. Careful attention should therefore be given to signs of overdosage, if necessary, the levels should be determined and the dose of carbamazepine, theophylline, cyclosporin, or digoxin reduced if necessary.
6. Patients receiving β-blockers, diuretics, ACE inhibitors or other antihypertensive agents should be regularly monitored. Use with alpha blockers should be strictly monitored. The simultaneous administration of diltiazem with drugs such as β-blockers, antiarrythmics or heart glycosides may cause a greater degree of AV blocking, reduce the heart rate or induce a hypotensive effect. Intravenous administration of β-blockers should be discontinued during therapy with diltiazem.
7. Anaesthetists should be warned that a patient is on a calcium antagonist. The depression of cardiac contractility, conductivity, and automaticity as well as the vascular dilation associated with anaesthetics may be potentiated by calcium channel blockers. When used concomitantly, anaesthetics and calcium channel blockers should be titrated carefully.

There have been reports in the literature of diltiazem interactions with warfarin, rifampacin, and lithium.

Pregnancy and lactation: Diltiazem must not be taken during pregnancy as experimental studies have shown indications of teratogenicity. There is no experience of its effects in humans. As diltiazem is known to enter the breast milk and there is no experience of possible effects in infants, infants should be weaned if treatment of the mother with diltiazem is necessary.

Effects on ability to drive and use machines: Diltiazem is not known to have any effect on ability to drive or operate machinery.

Undesirable effects: In studies carried out to date, serious adverse reactions with diltiazem have been rare; however, it should be recognised that patients with impaired ventricular function and cardiac conduction abnormalities have usually been excluded from these studies.

In 900 patients with hypertension, the most common adverse events were oedema (9%), headache (8%), dizziness (6%), asthenia (5%), sinus bradycardia (3%), flushing (3%), and first degree AV block (3%). Only oedema and perhaps bradycardia were dose related. The most common adverse events (>1%) observed in clinical studies of over 2100 angina and hypertensive patients receiving diltiazem were: oedema (5.4%), headache (4.5%), dizziness (3.4%), asthenia (2.8%), first-degree AV block (1.8%), flushing (1.7%), nausea (1.6%), bradycardia (1.5%) and rash (1.5%).

Less common adverse events have included the following:

Cardiovascular: angina, arrhythmia, AV block (second or third degree), congestive heart failure, hypotension, palpitations, syncope.

Nervous system: amnesia, depression, gait abnormality, hallucinations, insomnia, nervousness, paraesthesia, personality change, somnolence, tinnitus, tremor.

Gastrointestinal: anorexia, constipation, diarrhoea, dyspepsia, mild elevations of alkaline phosphatase, SGOT, SGPT and LDH (see Special Warnings and Precautions), vomiting, weight increase, gingivitis.

Dermatologic: petechiae, pruritus, photosensitivity, urticaria. Allergic skin reactions including erythema multiforme, vasculitis, lymphadenopathy and eosinophilia have been observed in isolated cases. Dermatological events may be transient and may disappear despite continued use of diltiazem. Should a dermatologic reaction persist, the drug should be discontinued.

Other: amblyopia, CK elevation, dyspnoea, epistaxis, eye irritation, hyperglycaemia, nasal congestion, nocturia, osteoarticular pain, polyuria, sexual difficulties.

Overdose: Experience of overdosage in man is limited but cases of spontaneous recovery have been reported. However, it is recommended that patients with suspected overdose, should be placed under observation in a coronary care unit with facilities available for treatment of any possible hypotension and conduction disturbances that may occur.

Most patients suffering from overdosage of diltiazem become hypotensive within 8 hours of ingestion. With bradycardia and first to third degree atrioventricular block also developing cardiac arrest may ensue. Hyperglycaemia is also a recognised complication. The elimination half-life of diltiazem after overdosage is estimated to be about 5.5-10.2 hours. If a patient presents early after overdose, gastric lavage should be performed and activated charcoal administered to reduce diltiazem absorption.

Hypotension should be corrected with plasma expanders, intravenous calcium gluconate and inotropic agents (dopamine, dobutamine, isoprenaline), symptomatic bradycardia and high grade AV block may respond to atropine, isoprenaline or occasionally cardiac pacing which may be useful if cardiac standstill occurs.

Pharmacological properties

Pharmacodynamic properties: Diltiazem has pharmacologic actions similar to those of other calcium channel blocking agents such as nifedipine or verapamil. The principal physiologic action of diltiazem is to inhibit the transmembrane influx of extracellular calcium ions across the membranes of myocardial cells and vascular smooth muscle cells.

Calcium plays important roles in the excitation-contraction coupling processes of the heart and vascular smooth muscle cells and in the electrical discharge of the specialised conduction cells of the heart. The membranes of these cells contain numerous channels that carry a slow inward current and that are selective for calcium.

By inhibiting calcium influx, diltiazem inhibits the contractile processes of cardiac and vascular smooth muscle, thereby dilating the main coronary and systemic arteries. Dilation of systemic arteries by diltiazem results in a decrease in total peripheral resistance, a decrease in systemic blood pressure and a decrease in the afterload of the heart. The reduction in afterload, seen at rest and with exercise, and its resultant decrease in myocardial oxygen consumption are thought to be responsible for the beneficial effects of diltiazem in patients with chronic stable angina pectoris. In patients with prinzmetal variant angina, inhibition of spontaneous and ergonovine-induced coronary artery spasm by diltiazem results in increased myocardial oxygen delivery.

Pharmacokinetic properties: (a) General Characteristics

Absorption: Capsules seem to have a similar bioavailability to tablets (30-40%), with peak concentrations for the sustained release product after 8-11 hours compared to 1-2 hours after the conventional release product. The relatively low bioavailability is due to first pass metabolism in the liver to an active metabolite.

Distribution: Diltiazem hydrochloride is lipophilic and has a high volume of distribution. Typical study results are in the range of 3-8 litres per kilogramme. Protein binding is about 80% and is not concentration-dependent at levels likely to be found clinically. Protein binding does not appear to be influenced by phenylbutazone, warfarin, propanolol, salicylic acid or digoxin.

Metabolism: Diltiazem hydrochloride is extensively metabolised in the liver. N-monodesmethyl diltiazem is the predominant metabolite followed quantitatively by the desacetyl metabolite, which has some pharmacological activity. The efficacy of the metabolites, desacetyl diltiazem and N-monodesmethyl diltiazem is 25-50% and about 20% respectively of that of diltiazem. In liver function disorders delayed metabolism in the liver is likely. These metabolites are converted to conjugates, generally the glucuronide or the sulphate.

Elimination: Diltiazem is excreted in the form of its metabolites (about 35%) and in the non-metabolised form (about 2-4%) via the kidneys whilst about 60% is excreted via the faeces. The average elimination half life period for diltiazem is 6-8 hours but may vary between 2 and 11 hours. Although the elimination half life is not changed after repeated oral administration, diltiazem and also the desacetyl metabolite show a slight accumulation in the plasma.

(b) Characteristics in Patients

Decreased first-pass metabolism in the elderly tends to result in increased plasma concentrations of calcium antagonists but no major changes have been found with diltiazem. Renal impairment did not cause significant changes in diltiazem pharmacokinetics. Plasma concentrations of diltiazem also tend to be higher in hepatic cirrhosis due to impaired oxidative metabolism.

Preclinical safety data: Chronic toxicity studies in rats revealed no remarkable changes at oral doses up to 125 mg/kg/day although there was a 60% mortality at this dose. In dogs chronically treated with oral doses of 20 mg/kg/day, transient rises in SGPT were observed. Embryotoxicity has been reported in mice, rats and rabbits following i.p. administration of diltiazem. Main types of malformations included limb and tail defects with a small number of vertebral and rib deformities also noted.

Pharmaceutical particulars

List of excipients:

Fumaric Acid – NF
Talc – Ph.Eur
Povidone – BP/EP
Non-Pareil Seeds – USP
Poly (ethylacrylate, methylacrylate, trimethylam-

monio-ethylmethacrylate chloride (1:2:0.1) (Eudragit RS 12.5%), Poly (ethylacrylate, methylacrylate, trimethylammonio-ethylmethacrylate chloride (1:2:0.2) (Eudragit RL 12.5%)

Incompatibilities: Not applicable.

Shelf life: Two years from the date of manufacture.

Special precautions for storage: Store in a dry place at a temperature not exceeding 25°C.

Nature and contents of the container: Jaysquare container, containing 7, 20, 30, 50, 60 and 100 capsules.

PVC/PVDC blister pack containing 4, 28 and 30 capsules

Instructions for use/handling: Not applicable.

Name and address of marketing authorisation holder: Elan Pharma Ltd, Monksland, Athlone, Co. Westmeath, Ireland.

Trading as: Elan Pharma, 1 Meadway Court, Rutherford Close, Stevenage, Herts, SG1 2EF, UK.

Marketing authorisation numbers
PL 10038/0027 Dilzem XL capsules 120
PL 10038/0028 Dilzem XL capsules 180
PL 10038/0029 Dilzem XL capsules 240

Date of first authorisation/renewal of authorisation 30 April 1998

Date of (partial) revision of the text December 1996

ERYMAX CAPSULES

Qualitative and quantitative composition Each capsule contains 250 mg of Erythromycin Ph Eur.

Pharmaceutical form Capsules containing enteric-coated pellets of erythromycin base.

Clinical particulars

Therapeutic indications: Erythromycin is an antibiotic effective in the treatment of bacterial disease caused by susceptible organisms.

Examples of its use are in the treatment of upper and lower respiratory tract infections of mild to moderate severity; skin and soft tissue infections including pustular acne.

Erythromycin is usually active against the following organisms in vitro and in clinical infection: Streptococcus pyogenes; Alpha haemolytic streptococci; Staphylococcus aureus; Streptococcus pneumoniae; Haemophilus influenzae; Mycoplasma pneumoniae; Treponema pallidum; Corynebacterium diphtheriae; Corynebacterium minutissimum; Entamoeba histolytica; Listeria monocytogenes; Neisseria gonorrhoeae; Bordetella pertussis; Legionella pneumophila; Chlamydia trachomatis; Propionibacterium acnes.

Posology and method of administration: Oral administration.

Adults and elderly: 250 mg every six hours- before or with meals. 500 mg every twelve hours–may be given if desired; b.i.d. dosage should not be used if dosage exceeds one gram.

Children: The usual dose is 30-50 mg/kg/day erythromycin, in divided doses given twice daily or every six hours. In severe infections, this dose may be doubled; elevated doses should be given every six hours. The drug should be given before or with meals.

Note: Erymax Capsules may be given to children of any age who can swallow the capsules whole.

The capsules should be swallowed whole either before or with food; they should not be chewed.

Streptococcal infections: For active infection–a full therapeutic dose is given for at least ten days.

For continuous prophylaxis against recurrences of streptococcal infections in patients with evidence of rheumatic fever or heart disease, the dose is 250 mg b.i.d.

For the prevention of bacterial endocarditis in patients with valvular disease scheduled for dental or surgical procedures of the upper respiratory tract, the adult dose is 1 gram (children 20 mg/kg) 2 hours before surgery. Following surgery, the dose is 500 mg for adults (children 10 mg/kg) orally every six hours for 8 doses.

Primary syphilis: 30-40 grams given in divided doses over a period of 10-15 days.

Intestinal amoebiasis: 250 mg four times daily for 10 to 14 days for adults: 30 to 50 mg/kg/day in divided doses for 10 to 14 days for children.

Legionnaires' disease: 1-4 g daily until clinical signs and symptoms indicate a clinical cure. Treatment may be prolonged.

Pertussis: 30-50 mg/kg/day given in divided doses for 5–14 days, depending upon eradication of a positive culture.

Acne: initially, 250 mg twice daily, which may be reduced to a maintenance dose of 250 mg once daily after one month according to response.

Contra-indications: Use in patients hypersensitive to erythromycin, and in patients taking either astemizole or terfenadine.

Special warnings and special precautions for use: In patients with impaired hepatic function, liver function should be monitored, since a few reports of hepatic dysfunction have been received in patients taking erythromycin as the estolate, base or stearate. Extended administration requires regular evaluation particularly of liver function. Therapy should be discontinued if significant hepatic dysfunction occurs.

Prolonged use of erythromycin has caused overgrowth of nonsusceptible bacteria or fungi; this is a rare occurrence.

Interaction with other medicaments and other forms of interaction: Concomitant administration of erythromycin and digoxin has been reported to result in elevated digoxin serum levels.

The use of erythromycin in patients taking concurrent drugs which are metabolised by the cytochrome P450 system may be associated with elevated serum levels of these other drugs.

Concomitant use of erythromycin with terfenadine or astemizole is likely to result in an enhanced risk of cardiotoxicity with these drugs. The concomitant use of erythromycin with either of these drugs is therefore contraindicated.

There have been reports of interactions of erythromycin with cyclosporin, hexobarbital and phenytoin.

In a few patients receiving high doses of theophylline, concomitant use of erythromycin has caused increase of serum theophylline levels and signs of toxicity.

Erythromycin administration in patients receiving carbamazepine has been reported to cause increased serum levels of carbamazepine with subsequent development of signs of carbamazepine toxicity.

There have been reports of increased anticoagulant effects when erythromycin and oral anticoagulants were used concomitantly.

There are reports that ischaemic reactions may occur when erythromycin is given concurrently with ergotamine containing drugs.

Erythromycin should be used with caution if administered concomitantly with lincomycin, clindamycin or chloramphenicol, as competitive inhibition may occur.

The concomitant use of erythromycin with alfentanil can significantly inhibit the clearance of alfentanil and may increase the risk of prolonged or delayed respiratory depression.

Patients receiving concomitant lovastatin and erythromycin should be carefully monitored as cases of rhabdomyolysis have been reported in seriously ill patients.

Pregnancy and lactation: Like all drugs erythromycin should be used in pregnancy only when clearly indicated. Erythromycin crosses the placental barrier.

Nursing mothers: erythromycin is excreted in human milk and should be used in lactating women only if clearly needed.

Effects on ability to drive and use machines: None known.

Undesirable effects: Serious allergic reaction, including anaphylaxis, has been reported.

Nausea and abdominal discomfort can occur at elevated doses; diarrhoea and vomiting are less common.

Hepatotoxicity: There have been reports of hepatic dysfunction, with or without jaundice, occurring in patients receiving erythromycin products and due to combined cholestatic and hepatocellular injury although less commonly than with erythromycin estolate.

Superinfections including pseudomembranous colitis have been occasionally reported to occur in association with erythromycin therapy.

Transient hearing disturbances and deafness have been reported with doses of erythromycin usually greater than 4 g daily, and usually given intravenously.

There have been isolated reports of transient central nervous system side effects including confusion, hallucinations, seizures, and vertigo; however, a cause and effect relationship has not been established.

Overdose: Nausea, vomiting and diarrhoea have been reported.

Treatment: Gastric lavage and general supportive therapy. Erythromycin is not removed by peritoneal dialysis or haemodialysis.

Pharmacological properties

Pharmacodynamic properties: Erythromycin base and its salts are readily absorbed in the microbiologically active form. Erythromycin is largely bound to plasma proteins and after absorption erythromycin diffuses readily into most body fluids.

Erythromycin acts by inhibition of protein synthesis by binding 50s ribosomal subunits of susceptible organisms. It does not affect nucleic acid synthesis.

Pharmacokinetic properties: After administration of a single dose of Erymax 250 mg, peak serum levels are attained in approximately 3 hours.

In the presence of normal hepatic function, erythromycin is concentrated in the liver and is excreted in the bile. After oral administration, less than 5% of the administered dose can be recovered in the active form in the urine.

Preclinical safety data: Pre-clinical safety data does not add anything of further significance to the prescriber.

Pharmaceutical particulars

List of excipients: Cellulose acetate phthalate, lactose, potassium phosphate monobasic, povidone, diethyl phthalate, purified water, sunset yellow, titanium dioxide, gelatin, erythrosine, quinoline yellow.

Incompatibilities: None known.

Shelf life: 36 months.

Special precautions for storage: Store below 25°C. Protect from moisture and light.

Nature and contents of containers: Polypropylene Securitainers containing 100 capsules

HDPE Tampertainers containing 28, 100 capsules

Blister packs containing 4, 8, 28, 30 and 100 capsules.

Instructions for use/handling: No special requirements.

Name and address of marketing authorisation holder: Elan Pharma Ltd, Monksland, Athlone, Co. Westmeath, Ireland.

Trading as: Elan Pharma, 1 Meadway Court, Rutherford Close, Stevenage, Hertfordshire, SG1 2EF, UK.

Marketing authorisation number PL 10038/0030

Date of first authorisation/renewal of authorisation 3/10/97

Date of (partial) revision of the text July 1998

PONSTAN CAPSULES

Qualitative and quantitative composition Mefenamic acid BP 250 mg

Pharmaceutical form A practically white to greyish or creamy-white powder in a No 1 hard gelatin capsule having an ivory opaque body and powder blue opaque cap and imprinted "PONSTAN 250".

Clinical particulars

Therapeutic indications: Mefenamic acid is a non-steroidal anti-inflammatory agent with analgesic properties, and a demonstrable antipyretic effect. It has been shown to inhibit prostaglandin activity.

Indications:
1. As an anti-inflammatory analgesic for the symptomatic relief of rheumatoid arthritis (including Still's Disease), osteoarthritis, and pain including muscular, traumatic and dental pain, headaches of most aetiology, post-operative and post-partum pain; pyrexia in children.
2. Primary dysmenorrhoea.
3. Menorrhagia due to dysfunctional causes and presence of an IUD when other pelvic pathology has been ruled out.

Posology and method of administration
Adults: 2 capsules (500 mg) three times daily.

In menorrhagia to be administered on the first day of excessive bleeding and continued according to the judgement of the physician.

In dysmenorrhoea to be administered at the onset of menstrual pain and continued according to the judgement of the physician.

Elderly (over 65 years): As for adults.

Whilst no pharmacokinetic or clinical studies specific to the elderly have been undertaken with Ponstan, it has been used at normal dosage in trials which included many elderly patients. Ponstan should be used with caution in elderly patients suffering from dehydration and renal disease.

Non-oliguric renal failure and proctocolitis have been reported mainly in elderly patients who have not discontinued Ponstan after the development of diarrhoea.

Children: It is recommended that children under 12 years of age should be given Ponstan Paediatric Suspension (50mg/5ml).

Do not exceed the stated dose.

Contra-indications: Patients hypersensitive to mefenamic acid.

Mefenamic acid is contra-indicated in inflammatory bowel disease and in patients suffering from peptic and/or intestinal ulceration, and in patients with renal or hepatic impairment.

Because the potential exists for cross-sensitivity to aspirin or other non-steroidal anti-inflammatory drugs, mefenamic acid should not be given to patients in whom these drugs induce symptoms of bronchospasm, allergic rhinitis, or urticaria.

Special warnings and special precautions for use: Precaution should be taken in patients suffering from dehydration and renal disease, particularly the elderly.

In dysmenorrhoea and menorrhagia lack of response should alert the physician to investigate other causes.

Caution should be exercised when treating patients suffering from epilepsy.

Interaction with other medicaments and other forms of interaction: Concurrent therapy with other plasma protein binding drugs may necessitate a modification in dosage. In the case of anticoagulants the dose of the anticoagulant may need to be reduced. Concurrent administration of mefenamic acid with oral anticoagulant drugs requires careful prothrombin time monitoring.

The following interactions have been reported with NSAIDS but have not necessarily been associated with Ponstan Capsules:

Antihypertensives and diuretics: a reduction in antihypertensive and diuretic effect has been observed.

Cardiac glycosides: NSAIDs may exacerbate cardiac failure and increases in plasma cardiac glycoside levels may occur when renal function is affected.

Lithium and methotrexate: Elimination of these drugs can be reduced.

Cyclosporin: The risk of nephrotoxicity of cyclosporin may be increased with NSAIDs.

Mifepristone: NSAIDs should not be taken for 8 -12 days after mifepristone administration, NSAIDs can reduce the effects of mifepristone.

Corticosteroids: Concomitant use may increase the risk of gastrointestinal bleeding.

Quinolone antibiotics: Animal data indicates that NSAIDs can increase the risk of convulsions associated with quinolone antibiotics. Patients taking NSAIDs and quinolones may have an increased risk of developing convulsions.

Other analgesics: Concomitant use of two or more NSAIDs should be avoided.

Pregnancy and lactation: Safety in pregnancy has not been established and because of the effects of drugs in this class on the foetal cardiovascular system, the use of mefenamic acid in pregnant women is not recommended.

Trace amounts of mefenamic acid may be present in breast milk and transmitted to the nursing infant.

Therefore, mefenamic acid should not be taken by nursing mothers.

Effects on ability to drive and use machines: Drowsiness and dizziness have rarely been reported.

Undesirable effects: Diarrhoea occasionally occurs following the use of mefenamic acid. Although this may occur soon after starting treatment, it may also occur after several months of continuous use. The diarrhoea has been investigated in some patients who have continued this drug in spite of its continued presence. These patients were found to have associated proctocolitis. If diarrhoea does develop the drug should be withdrawn immediately and this patient should not receive mefenamic acid again.

Skin rashes have been observed following the administration of mefenamic acid and the occurrence of a rash is a definite indication to withdraw medication. There have been rare reports of Stevens-Johnson syndrome, Lyell's syndrome (toxic epidermal necrolysis) and erythema multiforme.

Serious gastrointestinal toxicity such as bleeding, ulceration, and perforation can occur at any time with or without warning symptoms, in patients treated chronically with NSAID therapy. GI bleeding has been associated with a previous history of peptic ulcer, smoking and alcohol use.

Elderly or debilitated patients seem to tolerate ulceration or bleeding less well than other individuals and most spontaneous reports of fatal GI events are in this population.

As with other prostaglandin inhibitors allergic glomerulonephritis has occurred occasionally. There have also been reports of acute interstitial nephritis with haematuria and proteinuria and occasionally nephrotic syndrome. Non-oliguric renal failure has been reported on a few occasions in elderly patients with dehydration usually from diarrhoea. Toxicity has been seen in patients with pre-renal conditions leading to a reduction in renal blood flow or blood volume. Patients at greatest risk of this reaction are those with impaired renal function, heart failure, liver dysfunction, those taking diuretics and the elderly. The drug should not be administered to patients with significantly impaired renal function. It has been suggested that the recovery is more rapid and complete than with other forms of analgesic induced renal impairment, with discontinuation of NSAID therapy being typically followed by recovery to the pre-treatment state.

Thrombocytopenic purpura has been reported with mefenamic acid. In some cases reversible haemolytic anaemia has occurred. Temporary lowering of the white blood cell count which may have been due to mefenamic acid has been reported. Rarely eosinophilia, agranulocytosis, pancytopenia and aplastic anaemia have been reported. Blood studies should therefore be carried out during long term administration and the appearance of any dyscrasia is an indication to discontinue therapy.

Bronchospasm and/or urticaria may be precipitated in patients suffering from, or with a previous history of, bronchial asthma or allergic disease.

Borderline elevations of one or more liver function tests may occur in some patients receiving mefenamic acid therapy. A patient with symptoms and/or signs suggesting liver dysfunction, or in whom an abnormal liver test has occurred, should have their therapy discontinued. Patients on prolonged therapy should be kept under surveillance with particular attention to liver dysfunction. Pancreatitis and cholestatic jaundice have also been reported.

Other adverse reactions: Nausea, vomiting, abdominal pain, headache, facial oedema, laryngeal oedema and anaphylaxis. Drowsiness, dizziness, abnormal vision, palpitations, glucose intolerance in diabetic patients and hypotension have rarely been reported.

NOTE: A positive reaction in certain tests for bile in the urine of patients receiving mefenamic acid has been demonstrated to be due to the presence of the drug and its metabolites and not to the presence of bile.

Overdose: Gastric lavage in the conscious patient and intensive supportive therapy where necessary. Vital functions should be monitored and supported. Activated charcoal has been shown to be a powerful adsorbent for mefenamic acid and its metabolites. Studies in experimental animals and human volunteers have shown that a 5 to 1 ratio of charcoal to mefenamic acid results in considerable suppression of absorption of the drug. Haemodialysis is of little value since mefenamic acid and its metabolites are firmly bound to plasma proteins. Overdose has led to fatalities.

Mefenamic acid has a tendency to induce tonic-clonic (grand mal) convulsions in overdose. Acute renal failure and coma have been reported with mefenamic acid overdose. It is important that the recommended dose is not exceeded and the regime adhered to since some reports have involved daily dosages under 3g.

Pharmacological properties

Pharmacodynamic properties: ANIMAL MODELS

Mefenamic acid is a non-steroidal anti-inflammatory drug (NSAID) and anti-inflammatory, analgesic and antipyretic properties.

Its anti-inflammatory effect was first established in the UV erythema model of inflammation. Further studies included inhibition of granulation tissue growth into subcutaneous cotton pellets in rats and carrageenin induced rat paw oedema tests.

Antipyretic activity was demonstrated in yeast-induced pyresis in rats. In this model its antipyretic activity was roughly equal to that of phenylbutazone and flufenamic acid, but less than that of indomethacin.

Analgesic activity was demonstrated in tests involving pain sensitivity of rats paws inflamed by brewers yeast. Mefenamic acid was less potent than flufenamic acid in this model.

Prostaglandins are implicated in a number of disease processes including inflammation, modulation of the pain response, dysmenorrhoea, menorrhagia and pyrexia.

In common with most NSAID's mefenamic acid inhibits the action of prostaglandin synthetase (cyclo oxygenase). This results in a reduction in the rate of prostaglandin synthesis and reduced prostaglandin levels.

The anti-inflammatory activity of NSAID's in the rat paw oedema test has been correlated with their ability to inhibit prostaglandin synthetase. When mefenamic acid is ranked in both these tests it falls between indomethacin and phenylbutazone and it is probable that inhibition of prostaglandin synthesis contributes to the pharmacological activity and clinical efficacy of mefenamic acid.

There is also considerable evidence that the fenamates inhibit the action of prostaglandins after they have been formed. They therefore both inhibit the synthesis and response to prostaglandins. This double blockade may well be important in their mode of action.

Pharmacokinetic properties: ABSORPTION AND DISTRIBUTION

Mefenamic acid is absorbed from the gastrointestinal tract. Peak levels of 10 mg/l occur two hours after the administration of a 1g oral dose to adults.

METABOLISM: Mefenamic acid is extensively metabolised, first to A3 hydroxymethyl derivative (metabolite I) and then A3 carboxyl derivative (metabolite II). Both metabolites undergo secondary conjugation to form glucuronides.

ELIMINATION: Fifty two percent of a dose is recovered from the urine, 6% as mefenamic acid, 25% as metabolite I and 21% as metabolite II. Assay of stools over a 3 day period accounted for 10-20% of the dose chiefly as unconjugated metabolite II.

The plasma levels of unconjugated mefenamic acid decline with a half life of approximately two hours.

Preclinical safety data: Preclinical safety data does not add anything of further significance to the prescriber.

Pharmaceutical particulars

List of excipients: Lactose, gelatin, sodium lauryl sulphate, potable water*, titanium dioxide (E171), patent blue (E131), quinoline yellow (E104), erythrosine (E127).

* not detectable

Incompatibilities: None known

Shelf life: 36 months

Special precautions for storage: Store at a temperature not exceeding 30°C.

Nature and contents of container:

(a) Securitainer (polypropylene body and polyethylene cap). Pack size : 500.

(b) High density polyethylene (HDPE) bottle fitted with a white low density polyethylene (LDPE) tamper evident "J" cap. Pack size : 100 and 500.

(c) Polyvinylchloride/aluminium foil blister pack. Pack size : 6, 10, 12, 20, 30, 50, 100 and 168.

Instructions for use/handling: Not applicable

Marketing authorisation holder: Elan Pharma Ltd, Monksland, Athlone, Co. Westmeath, Ireland

Trading as: Elan Pharma, 1 Meadway Court, Rutherford Close, Stevenage, Hertfordshire SG1 2EF, UK.

Marketing authorisation number PL 10038/0021

Date of first authorisation/renewal of authorisation 8 September 1997

Date of (partial) revision of the text June 1998

PONSTAN PAEDIATRIC SUSPENSION 50 mg/5 ml

Qualitative and quantitative composition Mefenamic acid BP 50 mg

Pharmaceutical form An off-white suspension with typical aroma and taste.

Clinical particulars

Therapeutic indications: Mefenamic acid is a non-steroidal anti-inflammatory agent with analgesic properties, and a demonstrable antipyretic effect. It has been shown to inhibit prostaglandin activity.

Indications:

1. As an anti-inflammatory analgesic for the symptomatic relief of rheumatoid arthritis (including Still's Disease), osteoarthritis, and pain including muscular, traumatic and dental pain, headaches of most aetiology, post-operative and post-partum pain; pyrexia in children.
2. Primary dysmenorrhoea in older children.

Posology and method of administration:

Children: It is recommended that children under 12 years of age should be given Ponstan Paediatric Suspension (50 mg/5ml) in the following dosage regime:

Infants over 6 months – 25 mg/kg of bodyweight daily in divided doses, or,

6 months to under 2 years - one 5ml spoonful
2 years to under 5 years - two 5ml spoonfuls
5 years to under 9 years - three 5ml spoonfuls
9 years to 12 years - four 5ml spoonfuls

Dose may be repeated as necessary, up to three times daily.

Apart from the treatment of Still's Disease, therapy should not be continued for longer than 7 days in children.

Do not exceed the stated dose.

Contra-indications: Patients hypersensitive to mefenamic acid.

Mefenamic acid is contra-indicated in inflammatory bowel disease and in patients suffering from peptic and/or intestinal ulceration, and in patients with renal or hepatic impairment.

Because the potential exists for cross-sensitivity to aspirin or other non-steroidal anti-inflammatory drugs, mefenamic acid should not be given to patients in whom these drugs induce symptoms of bronchospasm, allergic rhinitis, or urticaria.

Special warnings and special precautions for use: Patients suffering from dehydration and renal disease, particularly the elderly, when Ponstan Paediatric Suspension has been considered appropriate in this age group.

In dysmenorrhoea lack of response should alert the physician to investigate other causes.

Caution should be exercised when treating patients suffering from epilepsy.

Interaction with other medicaments and other forms of interaction: Concurrent therapy with other plasma protein binding drugs may necessitate a modification in dosage. In the case of anticoagulants the dose of the anticoagulant may need to be reduced. Concurrent administration of mefenamic acid with oral anticoagulant drugs requires careful prothrombin time monitoring.

The following interactions have been reported with NSAIDS but have not necessarily been associated with Ponstan Paediatric Suspension:

Antihypertensives and diuretics: a reduction in antihypertensive and diuretic effect has been observed.

Cardiac glycosides: NSAIDs may exacerbate cardiac failure and increases in plasma cardiac glycoside levels may occur when renal function is affected.

Lithium and methotrexate: Elimination of these drugs can be reduced.

Cyclosporin: The risk of nephrotoxicity of cyclosporin may be increased with NSAIDs.

Mifepristone: NSAIDs should not be taken for 8-12 days after mifepristone administration, NSAIDs can reduce the effects of mifepristone.

Corticosteroids: Concomitant use may increase the risk of gastrointestinal bleeding.

Quinolone antibiotics: Animal data indicates that NSAIDs can increase the risk of convulsions associated with quinolone antibiotics. Patients taking NSAIDs and quinolones may have an increased risk of developing convulsions.

Other analgesics: Concomitant use of two or more NSAIDs should be avoided.

Pregnancy and lactation: In the event of Ponstan Paediatric Suspension being used in older children and women of child bearing potential, the following should be noted:

Safety in pregnancy has not been established and because of the effects of drugs in this class on the foetal cardiovascular system, the use of mefenamic acid in pregnant women is not recommended.

Trace amounts of mefenamic acid may be present in breast milk and transmitted to the nursing infant. Therefore, mefenamic acid should not be taken by nursing mothers.

Effects on ability to drive and use machines: Drowsiness and dizziness have rarely been reported.

Undesirable effects: Diarrhoea occasionally occurs following the use of mefenamic acid. Although this may occur soon after starting treatment, it may also occur after several months of continuous use. The diarrhoea has been investigated in some patients who have continued this drug in spite of its continued presence. These patients were found to have associated proctocolitis. If diarrhoea does develop the drug should be withdrawn immediately and this patient should not receive mefenamic acid again.

Skin rashes have been observed following the administration of mefenamic acid and the occurrence of a rash is a definite indication to withdraw medication. There have been rare reports of Stevens-Johnson syndrome, Lyell's syndrome (toxic epidermal necrolysis) and erythema multiforme.

Serious gastrointestinal toxicity such as bleeding, ulceration, and perforation can occur at any time with or without warning symptoms, in patients treated chronically with NSAID therapy. GI bleeding has been associated with a previous history of peptic ulcer, smoking and alcohol use.

Although Ponstan Paediatric Suspension is not usually taken by the elderly; elderly or debilitated patients seem to tolerate ulceration or bleeding less well than other individuals and most spontaneous reports of fatal GI events are in this population.

As with other prostaglandin inhibitors allergic glomerulonephritis has occurred occasionally. There have also been reports of acute interstitial nephritis with haematuria and proteinuria and occasionally nephrotic syndrome. Non-oliguric renal failure has been reported on a few occasions, although these have been in elderly patients with dehydration, usually from diarrhoea. Toxicity has been seen in patients with pre-renal conditions leading to a reduction in renal blood flow or blood volume. Patients at greatest risk of this reaction are those with impaired renal function, heart failure, liver dysfunction, those taking diuretics and the elderly. The drug should not be administered to patients with significantly impaired renal function. It has been suggested that the recovery is more rapid and complete than with other forms of analgesic induced renal impairment, with discontinuation of NSAID therapy being typically followed by recovery to the pre-treatment state.

Thrombocytopenic purpura has been reported with mefenamic acid. In some cases reversible haemolytic anaemia has occurred. Temporary lowering of the white blood cell count which may have been due to mefenamic acid has been reported. Rarely eosinophilia, agranulocytosis, pancytopenia and aplastic anaemia have been reported. Blood studies should therefore be carried out during long term administration and the appearance of any dyscrasia is an indication to discontinue therapy.

Bronchospasm and/or urticaria may be precipitated in patients suffering from, or with a previous history of, bronchial asthma or allergic disease.

Borderline elevations of one or more liver function tests may occur in some patients receiving mefenamic acid therapy. A patient with symptoms and/or signs suggesting liver dysfunction, or in whom an abnormal liver test has occurred, should have their therapy discontinued. Patients on prolonged therapy should be kept under surveillance with particular attention to liver dysfunction. Pancreatitis and cholestatic jaundice have also been reported.

Other adverse reactions: Nausea, vomiting, abdominal pain, headache, facial oedema, laryngeal oedema and anaphylaxis. Drowsiness, dizziness, abnormal vision, palpitations, glucose intolerance in diabetic patients and hypotension have rarely been reported.

NOTE: A positive reaction in certain tests for bile in the urine of patients receiving mefenamic acid has been demonstrated to be due to the presence of the drug and its metabolites and not to the presence of bile.

Overdose: Gastric lavage in the conscious patient and intensive supportive therapy where necessary. Vital functions should be monitored and supported. Activated charcoal has been shown to be a powerful adsorbent for mefenamic acid and its metabolites. Studies in experimental animals and human volunteers have shown that a 5 to 1 ratio of charcoal to mefenamic acid results in considerable suppression of absorption of the drug. Haemodialysis is of little value since mefenamic acid and its metabolites are firmly bound to plasma proteins. Overdose has led to fatalities.

Mefenamic acid has a tendency to induce tonic-clonic (grand mal) convulsions in overdose. Acute renal failure and coma have been reported with mefenamic acid overdose. It is important that the recommended dose is not exceeded and the regime adhered to since some reports have involved daily dosages under 3g.

Pharmacological properties

Pharmacodynamic properties: ANIMAL MODELS

Mefenamic acid is a non-steroid anti-inflammatory drug (NSAID) and anti-inflammatory, analgesic and antipyretic properties.

Its anti-inflammatory effect was first established in the UV erythema model of inflammation. Further studies included inhibition of granulation tissue growth into subcutaneous cotton pellets in rats and carrageenin induced rat paw oedema tests.

Antipyretic activity was demonstrated in yeast-induced pyresis in rats. In this model its antipyretic activity was roughly equal to that of phenylbutazone and flufenamic acid, but less than that of indomethacin.

Analgesic activity was demonstrated in tests involving pain sensitivity of rats paws inflamed by brewers yeast. Mefenamic acid was less potent than flufenamic acid in this model.

Prostaglandins are implicated in a number of disease processes including inflammation, modulation of the pain response, dysmenorrhoea, menorrhagia and pyrexia.

In common with most NSAID's mefenamic acid inhibits the action of prostaglandin synthetase (cyclo oxygenase). This results in a reduction in the rate of prostaglandin synthesis and reduced prostaglandin levels.

The anti-inflammatory activity of NSAID's in the rat paw oedema test has been correlated with their ability to inhibit prostaglandin synthetase. When mefenamic acid is ranked in both these tests it falls between indomethacin and phenylbutazone and it is probable that inhibition of prostaglandin synthesis contributes to the pharmacological activity and clinical efficacy of mefenamic acid.

There is also considerable evidence that the fenamates inhibit the action of prostaglandins after they have been formed. They therefore both inhibit the synthesis and response to prostaglandins. This double blockade may well be important in their mode of action.

Pharmacokinetic properties: ABSORPTION AND DISTRIBUTION

Mefenamic acid is absorbed from the gastrointestinal tract. Peak levels of 10 mg/l occur two hours after the administration of a 1g oral dose to adults.

METABOLISM: Mefenamic acid is extensively metabolised, first to A3 hydroxymethyl derivative (metabolite I) and then A3 carboxyl derivative (metabolite II). Both metabolites undergo secondary conjugation to form glucuronides.

ELIMINATION: Fifty two percent of a dose is recovered from the urine, 6% as mefenamic acid, 25% as metabolite I and 21% as metabolite II. Assay of stools over a 3 day period accounted for 10-20% of the dose chiefly as unconjugated metabolite II.

The plasma levels of unconjugated mefenamic acid decline with a half life of approximately two hours.

Preclinical safety data: Preclinical safety data does not add anything of further significance to the prescriber.

Pharmaceutical particulars

List of excipients:

SUSPENSION: Sorbitol solution, aluminium magnesium silicate, sodium carboxymethylcellulose, ethanol 96%, sodium benzoate, hydrochloric acid, saccharin sodium, sodium hydroxide, glucono delta lactone, Purified water Ph. Eur, polyvidone 25, sugar mineral water, banana flavour (510120E), imitation chocolate flavour IFF, pure anise mint 108 IFF.

Incompatibilities: None known

Shelf life: 36 months

Special precautions for storage: Store at a temperature not exceeding 30° C.

Nature and contents of container: Clear amber glass bottle (Type III glass) with metal roll-on-pilfer-proof cap. Pack sizes: 30 & 125ml.

Instructions for use/handling: Not applicable

Marketing authorisation holder: Elan Pharma Ltd, Monksland, Athlone, County Westmeath, Ireland.

Trading as: Elan Pharma, 1 Meadway Court, Rutherford Close, Stevenage, Herts SG1 2EF, UK.

Marketing authorisation number PL 10038/0022

Date of first authorisation/renewal of authorisation
8 September 1997

Date of revision June 1998

PONSTAN FORTE TABLETS

Qualitative and quantitative composition Mefenamic acid BP 500mg

Pharmaceutical form Yellow film coated tablet, inscribed 'Ponstan' on one side

Clinical particulars

Therapeutic indications: Mefenamic acid is a non-steroidal anti-inflammatory agent with analgesic properties, and a demonstrable antipyretic effect. It has been shown to inhibit prostaglandin activity.

Indications:

1. As an anti-inflammatory analgesic for the symptomatic relief of rheumatoid arthritis (including Still's Disease), osteoarthritis, and pain including muscular, traumatic and dental pain, headaches of most aetiology, post-operative and post-partum pain.
2. Primary dysmenorrhoea.
3. Menorrhagia due to dysfunctional causes and presence of an IUD when other pelvic pathology has been ruled out.

Posology and method of administration: Adults: 1 tablet (500 mg) three times daily.

In menorrhagia to be administered on the first day of excessive bleeding and continued according to the judgement of the physician.

In dysmenorrhoea to be administered at the onset of menstrual pain and continued according to the judgement of the physician.

Elderly (over 65 years): As for adults.

Whilst no pharmacokinetic or clinical studies specific to the elderly have been undertaken with Ponstan, it has been used at normal dosage in trials which included many elderly patients.

Ponstan should be used with caution in elderly patients suffering from dehydration and renal disease. Non-oliguric renal failure and proctocolitis have been reported mainly in elderly patients who have not discontinued Ponstan after the development of diarrhoea.

Children: It is recommended that children under 12 years of age should be given Ponstan Paediatric Suspension (50 mg/5 ml).

Do not exceed the stated dose.

Contra-indications: Patients hypersensitive to mefenamic acid. Mefenamic acid is contra-indicated in inflammatory bowel disease and in patients suffering from peptic and/or intestinal ulceration, and in patients with renal or hepatic impairment.

Because the potential exists for cross-sensitivity to aspirin or other non-steroidal anti-inflammatory drugs, mefenamic acid should not be given to patients in whom these drugs induce symptoms of bronchopsasm allergic rhinitis, or urticaria.

Special warnings and special precautions for use: Precaution should be taken in patients suffering from dehydration and renal disease, particularly the elderly.

In dysmenorrhoea and menorrhagia lack of response should alert the physician to investigate other causes.

Caution should be exercised when treating patients suffering from epilepsy.

Interaction with other medicaments and other forms of interaction: Concurrent therapy with other plasma protein binding may necessitate a modification in dosage. In the case of anticoagulants the dose of the anticoagulant may need to be reduced. Concurrent administration of mefenamic acid with oral anticoagulant drugs requires careful prothrombin time monitoring.

The following interactions have been reported with NSAIDS but have not necessarily been associated with Ponstan Tablets:

Antihypertensives and diuretics: a reduction in antihypertensive and diuretic effect has been observed.

Cardiac glycosides: NSAIDS may exacerbate cardiac failure and increase in plasma cardiac glycoside levels may occur when renal function is affected.

Lithium and methotrexate: Elimination of these drugs can be reduced.

Cyclosporin: The risk of nephrotoxicity of cyclosporin may be increase with NSAIDs.

Mifepristone: NSAIDs should not be taken for 8-12 days after mifepristone administration. NSAIDs can reduce the effects of mifepristone.

Corticosteroids: Concomitant use may increase the risk of gastrointestinal bleeding.

Quinolone antibiotics: Animal data indicates that NSAIDs can increase the risk of convulsions associated with quinolone antibiotics. Patients taking NSAIDs and quinolone may have an increased risk of developing convulsions.

Other analgesics: Concomitant use of two or more NSAIDs should be avoided.

Pregnancy and lactation: Safety in pregnancy has not been established and because of the effects of drugs in this class on the foetal cardiovascular system, the use of mefenamic acid in pregnant women is not recommended.

Trace amounts of mefenamic acid may be present in breast milk and transmitted to the nursing infant. Therefore, mefenamic acid should not be taken by nursing mothers.

Effects on ability to drive and use machines: Drowsiness and dizziness have rarely been reported.

Undesirable effects: Diarrhoea occasionally occurs following the use of mefenamic acid. Although this may occur soon after starting treatment, it may also occur after several months of continuous use. The diarrhoea has been investigated in some patients who have continued this drug in spite of its continued presence. These patients were found to have associated proctocolitis. If diarrhoea does develop the drug should be withdrawn immediately and this patient should not receive mefenamic acid again.

Skin rashes have been observed following the administration of mefenamic acid and the occurrence of a rash is a definite indication to withdraw medication. There have been rare reports of Steven-Johnson syndrome, Lyell's syndrome (toxic epidermal necrolysis) and erythema multiforme.

Serious gastrointestinal toxicity such as bleeding, ulceration, and perforation can occur at any time with or without warning symptoms, in patients treated chronically with NSAID therapy. GI bleeding has been associated with a previous history of peptic ulcer, smoking and alcohol use.

Elderly or debilitated patients seem to tolerate ulceration or bleeding less well than other individuals and most spontaneous reports of fatal GI events are in this population.

As with other prostaglandin inhibitors allergic glomerulonephritis has occurred occasionally. There have also been reports if acute intestinal nephritis with haematuria and proteinuria and occasionally nephrotic syndrome. Non-oliguric renal failure has been reported on a few occasions in elderly patients with dehydration usually from diarrhoea. Toxicity has been seen in patients with pre-renal conditions leading to a reduction in renal blood flow or blood volume. Patients at greatest risk of this reaction are those with impaired renal function, heart failure, liver dysfunction, those taking diuretics and the elderly. The drug should not be administered to patients with significantly impaired renal function. It has been suggested that the recovery is more rapid and complete than with other forms of analgesic induced renal impairment, with discontinuation of NSAID therapy being typically followed by recovery to the pre-treatment state.

Thrombocytopenic purpura has been reported with mefenamic acid. In some cases reversible haemolytic anaemia has occurred. Temporary lowering of the white blood cell count which may have been due to mefenamic acid has been reported. Rarely eosinophilia, agranulocytosis, pancytopenia and aplastic anaemia have been reported. Blood studies should therefore be carried out during long term administration and the appearance of any dyscrasia is an indication to discontinue therapy.

Bronchospasm and/or urticaria may be precipitated in patients suffering from, or with a previous history of, bronchial asthma or allergic disease.

Borderline elevations of one or more liver function tests may occur in some patients receiving mefenamic acid therapy. A patient with symptoms and/or signs suggesting liver dysfunction, or in whom an abnormal liver test has occurred, should have their therapy discontinued. Patients on prolonged therapy should be kept under surveillance with particular attention to liver dysfunction. Pancreatitis and cholestatic jaundice have also been reported.

Other adverse reactions: Nausea, vomiting, abdominal pain, headache, facial oedema, laryngeal oedema and anaphylaxis. Drowsiness, dizziness, abnormal vision, palpitations, glucose intolerance in diabetic patients and hypotension have rarely been reported.

NOTE: A positive reaction in certain tests for bile in the urine of patients receiving mefenamic acid has been demonstrated to be due to the presence of the drug and its metabolites and not to the presence of bile.

Overdose: Gastric lavage in the conscious patient and intensive supportive therapy where necessary. Vital functions should be monitored and supported. Activated charcoal has been shown to be a powerful absorbent for mefenamic acid and its metabolites. Studies in experimental animals and human volunteers have shown that a 5 to 1 ratio of charcoal to mefenamic acid results in considerable suppression of absorption of the drug. Haemodialysis is of little value since mefenamic acid and its metabolites are firmly bound to plasma proteins. Overdose has led to fatalities.

Mefenamic acid has a tendency to induce tonic-clonic (grand mal) convulsions in overdose. Acute renal failure and coma have been reported with mefenamic acid overdose. It is important that the recommended failure and coma have been reported with mefenamic acid overdose. It is important that the recommended dose is not exceeded and the regime adhered to since some reports have involved daily dosages under 3g.

Pharmacological properties

Pharmacodynamic properties: Mefenamic acid is non-steroidal anti-inflammatory drug (NSAID) and anti-inflammatory, analgesic and antipyretic properties.

Its anti-inflammatory effect was first established in the UV erythema model of inflammation. Further studies included inhibition of granulation tissue growth into subcutaneous cotton pellets in rats and carrageenin induced rat paw oedema tests.

Antipyretic activity was demonstrated in yeast-induced pyresis in rats. In this model its antipyretic activity was roughly equal to that of phenylbutazone and flufenamic acid, but less that that of indomethacin.

Analgesic activity was demonstrated in tests involving pain sensitivity of rats paws inflamed by brewers yeast. Mefenamic acid was less potent than flufenamic acid in this model.

Prostaglandins are implicated in a number of disease processes including inflammation, modulation of the pain response, dysmenorrhoea, menorrhagia and pyrexia.

In common with most NSAIDs mefenamic acid inhibits the action of prostaglandin synthetase (cyclo oxygenase). This results in a reduction in the rate of prostaglandin synthesis and reduced prostaglandin levels.

The anti-inflammatory activity of NSAIDs in the rat paw oedema test has been correlated with their ability to inhibit prostaglandin synthetase. When mefenamic acid is ranked in both these tests it falls between indomethacin and phenylbutazone and it is probable that inhibition of prostaglandin synthesis contributes to the pharmacological activity and clinical efficacy of mefenamic acid.

There is also considerable evidence that the fenamates inhibit the action of prostaglandins after they have been formed. They therefore both inhibit the synthesis and response to prostaglandins. This double blockade may well be important in their mode of action.

Pharmacokinetic properties: ABSORPTION AND DISTRIBUTION

Mefenamic acid is absorbed from the gastrointestinal tract. Peak levels of 10mg/1 occur two hours after the administration of a 1g oral dose to adults.

METABOLISM: Mefenamic acid is extremely metabolised, first to A3 hydroxymethyl derivative (metabolite I) and then A3 carboxyl derivative (metabolite II). Both metabolites undergo secondary conjugation to form glucuronides.

ELIMINATION: Fifty two percent of a dose is recovered from the urine, 6% as mefenamic acid, 25% as metabolite I and 21% as metabolite II. Assay of stools over a 3 day period accounted for 10-20% of the dose chiefly as unconjugated metabolite II.

The plasma levels of unconjugated mefenamic acid decline with a half life of approximately two hours.

Preclinical safety data: Preclinical safety data does not add anything of further significance to the prescriber.

Pharmaceutical particulars

List of excipients

EACH TABLET CONTAINS: Lactose, pregelatinised starch, maize starch, polyvidone, silicon dioxide, talc, magnesium stearate, croscarmellose sodium type A, sodium lauryl sulphate, purified water*, Opadry OY-LS-22808 (H.P.M.C.2910 15cP, lactose, polyethylene glycol 4000, vanillin, E104, E110, E171), Opaglos AG7350 (purified water, beeswax white, carnauba wax yellow, polysorbate 20, sorbic acid).

*not detectable

Incompatibilities: None Known

Shelf life: 36 months for amber polystyrene bottle

48 months for blister and HDPE DUMA and polypropylene container

Special precautions for storage: Store below 30°C.

Nature and contents of container:

(a) Aluminium foil/pvc blister pack in cardboard carton. Pack sizes: 100

(b) HDPE duma and polypropylene container. Pack sizes: 100 and 500

(c) Amber polystyrene bottle with a high density polyethene anti-arthritic closure. Pack sizes: 6, 12, 84, 100 and 500.

Instructions for use/handling: Not applicable

Marketing authorisation holder: Elan Pharma Ltd, Monksland, Athlone, Co. Westmeath, Ireland

Trading as: Elan Pharma, 1 Meadway Court, Rutherford Close, Stevenage, Hertfordshire SG1 2EF, UK.

Marketing authorisation number PL 10038/0020

Date of first authorisation/renewal of authorisation
8 September 1997

Date of (partial) revision of the text June 1998

UNIVER CAPSULES

Qualitative and quantitative composition Univer capsules containing 120mg, 180mg or 240mg of verapamil hydrochloride BP.

Pharmaceutical form Hard gelatin capsules containing slow release beads.

Clinical particulars

Therapeutic indications: Mild to moderate hypertension. Angina pectoris.

Posology and method of administration:

Adults: Hypertension: Initial dose in patients new to verapamil therapy should be 120mg od. This can be increased to 240mg od which is the normal maintenance dosage. The dose may be further increased to a maximum of 480mg od if required.

Angina: The usual dose is 360mg od. Dosage may be increased to a maximum of 480mg daily if required.

Elderly: Elderly patients show enhanced bioavailability of verapamil and therapeutic control may be achieved with lower doses in this patient population.

Children: Univer is not recommended in children as no studies have been undertaken.

Univer is for oral administration.

Contra-indications: Significant bradycardia (less than 50 bpm), second or third degree heart block, sick sinus syndrome or uncontrolled heart failure. Verapamil should not be used when atrial flutter/fibrillation complicates Wolfe-Parkinson-White syndrome. Porphyria.

Concomitant ingestion of grapefruit juice.

Special warnings and special precautions for use: Special care should be taken in hypotension, especially in acute myocardial infarction as this is a condition where atrioventricular conduction defects may develop and contractility may be impaired.

Elderly: Elderly subjects show enhanced bioavailability of verapamil and therapeutic control may be achieved with lower doses in this population.

Interaction with other medicaments and other forms of interaction: Since beta-blocking agents may tend to interfere with conduction and decrease contractility, this product should be used with caution in combination with beta-blocking agents, and a period between stopping beta-blocking therapy and starting therapy with this product may be advisable. Verapamil is extensively metabolised in the liver and special care should be taken in cases where liver damage exists, as plasma levels of verapamil may be increased. Caution is required when verapamil is given with digoxin, theophylline and carbamazepine as plasma levels of these drugs may rise. With phenytoin and phenobarbital, plasma levels of verapamil may be reduced, whilst with cimetidine, plasma verapamil levels may be increased. Increased plasma levels of lithium have been noted when given with verapamil; because lithium alone can enhance neuromuscular block during anaesthesia, this pharmacodynamic effect could be increased in the presence of verapamil.

Grapefruit juice – an increase in verapamil serum level has been reported.

Pregnancy and lactation: Although there is no evidence of teratogenicity for verapamil its use in pregnancy, particularly in the first trimester, should be avoided if at all possible.

Effects on ability to drive and use machines: None stated.

Undesirable effects: Verapamil alters conduction in the heart and caution should be exercised in first degree heart block. It also has an effect that reduces the contractility of the myocardium and this may aggravate or occasionally precipitate heart failure in borderline cases. In cases of pre-existing poor ventricular function it is prudent to treat this condition before initiating Univer therapy. Constipation may occur and flushing has been reported. Headaches are uncommon. Very infrequently nausea, vomiting and allergic reactions have been observed.

Overdose: Normal resuscitation procedures should be initiated in the event of cardiovascular collapse, ie if atrioventricular conduction defects such as second or third degree block develop these should be treated in the usual way using atropine, isoprenaline or the temporary insertion of a pacemaker, as required. Hypotension may be observed and, if persistent, and in the absence of a conduction defect, treatment with systemic dopaminergic agents, eg dopamine, dobutamine or noradrenaline should be started.

Pharmacological properties

Pharmacodynamic properties: Verapamil hydrochloride is a well established calcium antagonist agent.

Pharmacokinetic properties: The pharmacokinetics of verapamil are widely published and well known. The relevant parameters for this sustained release product, verapamil od are:

SINGLE DOSE KINETICS	*MULTIDOSE KINETICS* (7 AVS)
(W=22, male volunteers are 18-39 years, mean 27 years – both studies)	
Dose 240 mg	*Dose 240 mg once daily*
C_{max}: 83.8 ng/ml	117.6 ng/ml
T_{max}: 7.6 hrs	7.7 hrs
AUC_{24} 1128.5 ng x hr/ml	1573.0 ng x hr/ml
Elimination Rate: 0.08 hr	0.08 hr

Preclinical safety data: No further information is available.

Pharmaceutical particulars

List of excipients

Excipient	Pharmacopoeial Specification
Fumaric Acid	USP
Non-Pareil Seeds (0.40-0.50 mm)	
Talc (Blend)	BP
Talc (Dusting)	BP
Polyvinylpyrrolidone	BP
Shellac	USP
Hard Gelatin Capsules	BP

Incompatibilities: None stated

Shelf life: 3 years

Special precautions for storage: Store in a dry place below 25°C

Nature and contents of container: The capsules are available in plastic bottles containing 500 or 100 capsules and in blister packs containing 4, 8, 28 or 56 capsules

Instructions for use/handling: None

Marketing authorisation holder: Elan Pharma Ltd, Monksland, Athlone, Co Westmeath, Ireland
Trading as: Elan Pharma, 1 Meadway Court, Rutherford Close, Stevenage, Hertfordshire SG1 2EF UK.

Marketing authorisation number

120mg capsules	PL 10038/0033
180mg capsules	PL 10038/0034
240mg capsules	PL 10038/0035

Date of first authorisation/renewal of authorisation
12 April, 1995

Date of (partial) revision of the text February, 1998

Ethical Generics Ltd

West Point
46–48 West Street
Newbury
Berkshire RG14 1BD
☎ 01635 568400 🖷 01635 568401

TENSIPINE* MR 10 and 20

Qualitative and quantitative composition
Tensipine MR 20 tablets: Pink-grey lacquered modified release tablets each containing 20 mg nifedipine, one side marked TMR and the reverse side marked 20.

Tensipine MR 10 tablets: Pink-grey lacquered modified release tablets each containing 10 mg nifedipine, one side marked TMR and the reverse side marked 10.

Pharmaceutical form Modified release tablets for oral administration.

Clinical particulars
Therapeutic indications: For the prophylaxis of chronic stable angina pectoris and the treatment of hypertension.

Posology and method of administration:
Adults: The recommended starting dose of Tensipine MR is 10 mg every 12 hours swallowed with water with subsequent titration of dosage according to response. The dose may be adjusted to 40 mg every 12 hours.

Tensipine MR 10 permits titration of initial dosage. The recommended dose is one Tensipine MR 10 tablet (10 mg) every 12 hours.

Nifedipine is metabolised primarily by the liver therefore patients with liver dysfunction should be carefully monitored.

Patients with renal impairment should not require adjustment of dosage.

Elderly patients: The pharmacokinetics of nifedipine are altered in the elderly so that lower maintenance doses of nifedipine may be required compared to younger patients.

Children: Nifedipine is not recommended for use in children.

Treatment may be continued indefinitely.

Contra-indications: Tensipine MR should not be administered to patients with known hypersensitivity to nifedipine or other dihydropyridines because of the theoretical risk of cross-reaction, to women capable of child-bearing or to nursing mothers.

Tensipine MR should not be used in cardiogenic shock, clinically significant aortic stenosis, unstable angina, or during or within one month of a myocardial infarction.

Tensipine MR should not be used for the treatment of acute attacks of angina.

The safety of Tensipine MR in malignant hypertension has not been established.

Tensipine MR should not be used for secondary prevention of myocardial infarction.

Tensipine MR should not be administered concomitantly with rifampicin since effective plasma levels of nifedipine may not be achieved owing to enzyme induction.

Special warnings and precautions for use: Tensipine MR is not a beta-blocker and therefore gives no protection against the dangers of abrupt beta-blocker withdrawal; any such withdrawal should be by gradual reduction of the dose of beta-blocker preferably over 8–10 days.

Tensipine MR may be used in combination with beta-blocking drugs and other antihypertensive agents but the possibility of an additive effect resulting in postural hypotension should be borne in mind. Tensipine MR will not prevent possible rebound effects after cessation of other antihypertensive therapy.

Tensipine MR should be used with caution in patients whose cardiac reserve is poor. Deterioration of heart failure has occasionally been observed with nifedipine.

Caution should be exercised in patients with severe hypotension.

Diabetic patients taking Tensipine MR may require adjustment of their control.

In dialysis patients with malignant hypertension and hypovolaemia, a marked decrease in blood pressure can occur.

Interactions with other medicaments and other forms of interaction: The antihypertensive effect of Tensipine MR may be potentiated by simultaneous administration of cimetidine.

When used in combination with nifedipine, serum quinidine levels have been shown to be suppressed regardless of dosage of quinidine.

The simultaneous administration of nifedipine and digoxin may lead to reduced digoxin clearance and hence an increase in the plasma digoxin level. Plasma digoxin levels should be monitored and, if necessary, the digoxin dose reduced.

Diltiazem decreases the clearance of nifedipine and hence increases plasma nifedipine levels. Therefore, caution should be taken when both drugs are used in combination and a reduction of the nifedipine dose may be necessary.

Nifedipine may increase the spectrophotometric values of urinary vanillylmandelic acid falsely. However, HPLC measurements are unaffected.

Rifampicin interacts with nifedipine (see Contra-indications).

As with other dihydropyridines, nifedipine should not be taken with grapefruit juice because bioavailability is increased.

Pregnancy and lactation: Tensipine MR is contra-indicated in women capable of child-bearing and nursing mothers.

Effects on ability to drive and use machines: None known.

Undesirable effects: Ischaemic pain has been reported in a small proportion of patients within one to four hours of the introduction of Tensipine MR therapy. Although a 'steal' effect has not been demonstrated, patients experiencing this effect should discontinue Tensipine MR.

Most side-effects are consequences of the vasodilatory effects of nifedipine. Headache, flushing, tachycardia and palpitations may occur, most commonly in the early stages of treatment with nifedipine. Gravitational oedema not associated with heart failure or weight gain may also occur.

Paraesthesia, dizziness, lethargy and gastro-intestinal symptoms such as nausea and altered bowel habit occur occasionally.

There are reports of skin reactions such as rash, pruritus and urticaria.

Other less frequently reported side-effects include myalgia, tremor and visual disturbances.

Impotence may occur rarely.

Increased frequency of micturition may occur.

There are reports of gingival hyperplasia and, in older men on long-term therapy, gynaecomastia, which usually regress upon withdrawl of therapy.

Mood changes may occur rarely.

Side-effects which may occur in isolated cases are photosensitivity, exfoliative dermatitis, systemic allergic reactions and purpura. Usually, these regress after discontinuation of the drug.

Rare cases of hypersensitivity-type jaundice have been reported. In addition, disturbances of liver function such as intra-hepatic cholestasis may occur. These regress after discontinuation of therapy.

As with other sustained release dihydropyridines, exacerbation of angina pectoris may occur rarely at the start of treatment. The occurrence of myocardial infarction has been described although it is not possible to distinguish such as an event from the natural course of ischaemic heart disease.

Overdose:
Clincial effects: Reports of nifedipine overdosage are limited and symptoms are not necessarily dose-related.

Severe hypotension due to vasodilatation, and tachycardia or bradycardia are the most likely manifestations of overdose.

Metabolic disturbances include hyperglycaemia, metabolic acidosis and hypo- or hyperkalaemia.

Cardiac effects may include heart block, AV dissociation and asystole, and cardiogenic shock with pulmonary oedema.

Other toxic effects include nausea, vomiting, drowsiness, dizziness, confusion, lethargy, flushing, hypoxia and unconsciousness to the point of coma.

Treatment: As far as treatment is concerned, elimination of nifedipine and the restoration of stable cardiovascular conditions have priority.

After oral ingestion, gastric lavage is indicated, if necessary in combination with irrigation of the small intestine. Ipecacuanha should be given to children.

Elimination must be as complete as possible, including the small intestine, to prevent the otherwise inevitable subsequent absorption of the active substance. Activated charcoal should be given in 4-hourly doses of 25 g for adults, 10 g for children.

Blood pressure, ECG, central arterial pressure, pulmonary wedge pressure, urea and electrolytes should be monitored.

Hypotension as a result of cardiogenic shock and arterial vasodilatation should be treated with elevation of the feet and plasma expanders. If these measures are ineffective, hypotension may be treated with 10% calcium gluconate 10–20 ml intravenously over 5–10 minutes. If the effects are inadequate, the treatment can be continued, with ECG monitoring. In addition, beta-sympathomimetics may be given, e.g. isoprenaline 0.2 mg slowly i.v. or as a continuous infusion of 5 μg/min. If an insufficient increase in blood pressure is achieved with calcium and isoprenaline, vasoconstricting sympathomimetics such as dopamine or noradrenaline should be administered. The dosage of these drugs should be determined by the patient's response.

Bradycardia may be treated with atropine, beta-sympathomimetics or a temporary cardiac pacemaker, as required.

Additional fluids should be administered with caution to avoid cardiac overload.

Pharmacological properties
Pharmacodynamic properties
Mode of action: Nifedipine is a specific and potent calcium antagonist. In hypertension, the main action of Tensipine MR is to cause peripheral vasodilatation and thus reduce peripheral resistance.

In angina, Tensipine MR reduces peripheral and coronary vascular resistance, leading to an increase in coronary blood flow, cardiac output and stroke volume, whilst decreasing after-load.

Additionally, nifedipine dilates submaximally both clear and atherosclerotic coronary arteries, thus protecting the heart against coronary artery spasm and improving perfusion to the ischaemic myocardium.

Nifedipine reduces the frequency of painful attacks and the ischaemic ECG changes irrespective of the relative contribution from coronary artery spasm or atherosclerosis.

Tensipine MR administered twice-daily provides 24-hour control of raised blood pressure. Tensipine MR causes reduction in blood pressure such that the percentage lowering is directly related to its initial level. In normotensive individuals, Tensipine MR has little or no effect on blood pressure.

Pharmacokinetic properties: Nifedipine is absorbed almost completely from the gastro-intestinal tract regardless of the oral formulation used and undergoes extensive metabolism in the liver to inactive metabolites, with less than 1% of the parent drug appearing unchanged in the urine. The rate of absorption determines the drug's apparent elimination. The terminal elimination half-life of the modified release formulation is 6–11 hours.

After enteral or intravenous doses, 70–80% of activity is eliminated (primarily as metabolites) via the urine. Remaining excretion is via the faeces.

After 24 hours, 90% of the administered dose is eliminated.

Protein binding of nifedipine exceeds 90% in human serum.

Pre-clinical safety data
Reproduction toxicology: Nifedipine administration has been associated with a variety of embryotoxic, placentotoxic and fetotoxic effects in rats, mice and rabbits. All of the doses associated with the teratogenic, embryotoxic or fetotoxic effects in animals were maternally toxic and several times the recommended maximum dose for humans.

Pharmaceutical particulars
List of excipients: Tensipine MR tablets contain the following excipients:

Microcrystalline cellulose, maize starch, lactose, polysorbate 80, magnesium stearate, hydroxypropyl methylcellulose, polyethylene glycol 4000, iron oxide red and titanium dioxide.

Incompatibilities: Not applicable.

Shelf life: PVC blister strips: 48 months. PP blister strips: 30 months.

Special precautions for storage: The tablets should be protected from strong light and stored in the manufacturer's original container.

Nature and contents of container: Tensipine MR 10 tablets: blister strips of 14 tablets in a cardboard outer container, packs of 56 tablets.

Tensipine MR 20 tablets: blister strips of 14 tablets in a cardboard outer container, packs of 56 tablets.

Blister strips are composed of red polypropylene foil (0.3 mm) with aluminium backing foil (0.02 mm) or red PVC foil (0.3 mm) with aluminium backing foil (0.02 mm).

Instructions for use/handling: No additional information.

Marketing authorisation numbers
Tensipine MR 10 tablets 6831/0048
Tensipine MR 20 tablets 6831/0049

Date of approval/revision of SPC November 1996.

Legal category POM.

UNIPINE* XL

Qualitative and quantitative composition Circular, biconvex, red, film-coated tablets marked 'UXL 30' on one side and blank on the other side containing 30 mg Nifedipine Ph.Eur.

Pharmaceutical form Nifedipine (30 mg) in tablet form for oral administration. It is a sustained release preparation.

Clinical particulars
Therapeutic indications: Unipine XL is indicated for the treatment of hypertension.

Posology and method of administration: Adults and elderly: The recommended starting dose of nifedipine is 30 mg every 24 hours swallowed with water with subsequent titration of dosage according to response. The dose may be adjusted to 60 mg every 24 hours.

Nifedipine should be taken with a little water. Tablets should be swallowed whole. Do not chew. *Not* to be taken with or immediately after food.

The pharmacokinetics of nifedipine are altered in the elderly so that lower maintenance doses of nifedipine may be required compared to younger patients.

Nifedipine is metabolised primarily by the liver and therefore patients with liver dysfunction should be carefully monitored. Patients with renal impairment should not require adjustment of dosage.

Children: Nifedipine is not recommended for use in children.

Contra-indications: Hypersensitivity to nifedipine or other dihydropyridines because of the theoretical risk of cross reactivity.

Nifedipine should not be used in clinically significant aortic stenosis, unstable angina, or during or within one month of a myocardial infarction.

Nifedipine should not be used for the treatment of acute attacks of angina.

The safety of nifedipine in malignant hypertension has not been established.

Nifedipine should not be used for secondary prevention of myocardial infarction.

Nifedipine should not be administered concomitantly with rifampicin since effective plasma levels of nifedipine may not be achieved owing to enzyme induction.

Special warnings and precautions for use: Unipine XL should be used with caution in patients whose cardiac reserve is poor and in patients with hepatic impairment. A marked decrease in blood pressure may occur in dialysis patients with malignant hypertension and hypovolaemia.

Unipine XL should be discontinued in patients who experience ischaemic pain following its administration.

Interactions with other medicaments and other forms of interaction: When Unipine XL is used in combination with beta-blocking drugs and other antihypertensive drugs, there is the possibility of an additive effect resulting in postural hypotension.

Decreased plasma quinidine and increased plasma phenytoin and theophylline concentrations have been reported when nifedipine is administered concomitantly.

Adjustment of hypoglycaemic medication may be required in diabetic patients.

There may be potentiation of the antihypertensive action of nifedipine when administered simultaneously with cimetidine.

Unipine XL is not a beta-blocker and therefore gives no protection against the dangers of abrupt beta-blocker withdrawal. Any such withdrawal should be by gradual reduction of the dose of beta-blocker preferably over 8 to 10 days. Unipine XL will not prevent possible rebound effects after cessation of antihypertensive therapy.

The simultaneous administration of nifedipine and digoxin may lead to reduced digoxin clearance and hence an increase in the plasma digoxin. Digoxin levels should be monitored and, if necessary the digoxin dose reduced.

Nifedipine should not be administered concomitantly with rifampicin since effective plasma levels of nifedipine may not be achieved owing to enzyme induction (see *Contra-indications*).

As with other dihydropyridines, nifedipine should not be taken with grapefruit juice because bioavailability is increased.

Pregnancy and lactation: Unipine XL should not be administered to women who are pregnant, women of child-bearing potential or to nursing mothers.

Effects on ability to drive and use machines: Not applicable.

Undesirable effects: Side-effects, mainly associated with the vasodilatory action of nifedipine include headache, dizziness, flushing and gravitational oedema. These effects usually disappear with continued treatment. Common side-effects include rash, nausea, lethargy, increased frequency of micturition, hypersensitivity type jaundice and gingival hyperplasia.

As with other sustained release dihydropyridines, exacerbation of angina pectoris may occur rarely at the start of treatment with sustained release formulations of nifedipine. The occurrence of myocardial infarction has been described although it is not possible to distinguish such an event from the natural course of ischaemic heart disease.

Overdose: Following overdosage, the stomach should be emptied by aspiration and lavage and charcoal instillation. Standard measures such as atropine and noradrenaline may be used for resultant bradycardia and hypotension. Intravenous calcium gluconate may be of benefit combined with metaraminol.

Pharmacological properties
Pharmacodynamic properties: Nifedipine is a potent and specific Class II calcium antagonist. The main action is to reduce contraction of vascular smooth muscle in both the coronary and peripheral circulation resulting in a reduction in blood pressure.

Pharmacokinetic properties: Nifedipine is absorbed over the whole length of the gastrointestinal tract the majority of an oral dose being absorbed in the jejunum. There is however considerable inter-individual variation in the rate and extent to which nifedipine is absorbed. It undergoes extensive yet variable first pass metabolism. The absorption of nifedipine from Nifedipine (30 mg) SR Tablets occurs over several hours which is typical of a sustained release preparation. At steady state C_{max} was approximately 20 ng/ml with T_{max} of 7 hours. At 24 hours the mean plasma concentration was approximately 8 ng/ml supporting once daily administration. In a single dose study the mean elimination half life was shown to be 10 hours (range 3.5–16.5 hours) in the fasting state.

Pre-clinical safety data: The LD_{50} of oral nifedipine has been found to be 494 mg/kg in mice and 1022 mg/kg in rats. Reproductive studies have shown reduced fertility in male and female rats dosed 100 mg/kg/day nifedipine for 10 weeks. Pregnant rats and rabbits receiving 30 mg/kg/day nifedipine showed increased rates of resorption and abortion. In pregnant mice dosed at 24 mg/kg/day nifedipine caused a low incidence of embryo lethality and a dosage-related reduction in foetal weight.

Nifedipine showed no mutagenic activity in the dominant lethal or micronucleus tests in mice, or in an *in vivo* cytogenic study in hamsters. Nor was it carcinogenic in rats.

The widespread clinical usage of nifedipine in accordance with the data sheet has established its safety and efficacy in man in the treatment of hypertension.

Pharmaceutical particulars
List of excipients: Povidone, Ammoniomethacrylate copolymer, Lactose, Hydrogentated castor oil, Talc, Colours E110, E171, E120, E132.

Incompatibilities: Unipine XL should not be taken with cimetidine as this causes potentiation of the antihypertensive action of nifedipine.

Shelf life: 2 years.

Special precautions for storage: Unipine XL should be protected from light and stored below 25°C, in a dry place in the manufacturer's original container.

Nature and contents of container: Unipine XL is available in blister packs each containing 28 tablets.

Instructions for use/handling: No special instructions.

Marketing authorisation number 6831/0047.

Date of approval/revision of SPC February 1997.

Legal category POM.

**Trade Mark*

Exelgyn Laboratoires

6 Rue Christophe Colomb
75008 Paris
France

☎ 0800 7316120 📠 0800 7316120

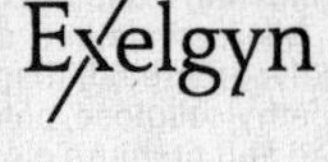

MIFEGYNE*
(Mifepristone)

Special note: The treatment procedures detailed below, must be fully explained to and completely understood by the patient. A patient information leaflet for each of the indications listed below, is available in the tablet carton. Prior to administration of Mifegyne the appropriate leaflet should be given to the patient to read.

Presentation Mifegyne tablets contain 200 mg of mifepristone. The tablets are light yellow, cylindrical, bi-convex, 11 mm in diameter with an identification code 167B engraved on one face.

Indication:

1. Medical alternative to surgical termination of intra-uterine pregnancy of up to 63 days gestation based on the first day of the last menstrual period and/or ultrasound scan.
2. Softening and dilatation of the cervix uteri prior to mechanical cervical dilatation for pregnancy termination.
3. For use in combination with gemeprost for termination of pregnancy of between 13 and 20 weeks gestation.

Mifepristone must not be administered if there is doubt as to the existence and age of the pregnancy. The prescribing doctor should in this case perform an ultrasound scan and/or measure hCG before administration.

Dosage and administration

1. Therapeutic termination of pregnancy of up to 63 days gestation.

600 mg of mifepristone (3×200 mg tablets) is taken by mouth in a single dose, in the presence of the doctor. The dosage is independent of body weight.

The patient should be observed for at least 2 hours following administration. In the absence of any effect at this time the patient may leave the treatment centre.

Unless abortion has already been completed, gemeprost 1 mg p.v. must be given 36–48 hours later in the treatment centre. The use of mifepristone must be followed, 36 to 48 hours later, by a prostaglandin analogue, unless abortion is already completed as mifepristone alone is effective in less than 80% of cases.

In the majority of cases abortion will occur within 4 hours following prostaglandin administration. There is a risk of profound hypotension, related to the administration of prostaglandin, occurring during this period. Hence, the patient must be observed in the treatment centre for at least 6 hours or until any bleeding or pain has diminished to an acceptable level, whichever is the longer. It is imperative that suitably experienced medical personnel and resuscitation equipment are available during this period.

If abortion has not occurred by this time and if the patient leaves the treatment centre, she must be informed specifically whom she should contact at the treatment centre and where to go in the event of any problems emerging, particularly in the case of very heavy vaginal bleeding. It should be noted that in pregnancies of 8 to 9 weeks gestation, blood loss may be heavier than that seen at earlier gestations.

A follow-up visit must always take place within a period of 8 to 12 days after administration of mifepristone to verify by the appropriate means (clinical examination, ultrasound scan, etc) that expulsion has been completed and that vaginal bleeding has stopped or has substantially reduced. The patient must be informed that vaginal bleeding occurs in almost all cases and is not in any way a proof of complete expulsion and that, for this reason, a follow-up visit is absolutely necessary.

Persistence of moderate vaginal bleeding at this point or later could signify incomplete abortion and appropriate investigation/treatment should be considered.

Mifepristone may only be administered for pregnancy termination in accordance with the Abortion Act 1967 as amended by the Human Fertilisation and Embryology Act 1990.

The administration of mifepristone must be supervised by a registered medical practitioner; follow-up of patients after administration of mifepristone may be carried out by registered medical practitioners only. Both administration of mifepristone and follow-up must take place in an NHS hospital or place approved by the Secretary of State under Section 1(3) of the Abortion Act 1967 and which has received DOH approval to undertake medical terminations with mifepristone.

2. Softening and dilatation of the cervix.

600 mg mifepristone (3×200 mg tablets) is taken by mouth 36–48 hours prior to the planned operative procedure. Softening and dilatation has been shown to be detectable from 24 hours after administration of mifepristone and increases to a maximum at approximately 36–48 hours after administration. Administration more than 48 hours before surgery increases the risk of bleeding and abortion prior to surgery, particularly with pregnancies of earlier gestations (less than nine weeks).

Mifepristone may only be administered for pregnancy termination in accordance with the Abortion Act 1967 as amended by the Human Fertilisation and Embryology Act 1990.

The administration of mifepristone must be supervised by a registered medical practitioner; any treatment necessary to effect complete termination of the pregnancy may be carried out by registered medical pratitioners only. Administration of mifepristone and any treatment necessary to effect complete termination of the pregnancy must take place in an NHS hospital or place approved by the Secretary of State under Section 1(3) of the Abortion Act 1967.

3. For use in combination with gemeprost for termination of pregnancy between 13 and 20 weeks gestation.

600 mg mifepristone (3×200 mg tablets) is taken by mouth 36–48 hours prior to scheduled prostaglandin termination of pregnancy. The patient should remain in the treatment centre for 2 hours following administration of the mifepristone to ensure that she does not vomit. In the absence of any effect at this time the patient may leave the treatment centre.

The patient must return to the treatment centre 36–48 hours later, the recommended procedure for therapeutic termination of pregnancy with gemeprost **must** then be followed. Gemeprost 1 mg p.v. should be given at 3 hourly intervals, up to a maximum of 5 pessaries. If abortion does not occur, a further course of pessaries may be instituted 24 hours after commencement of treatment. If abortion does not occur after a total of 10 pessaries, an alternative procedure to effect uterine emptying should be employed. It is not necessary to perform a dilation and curettage procedure if it is clear that a complete abortion has occurred. (NB pre-treatment with mifepristone has been shown to reduce the total dose of gemeprost required to cause expulsion of the fetus and to reduce the interval between initiation of prostaglandin treatment and abortion).

A follow-up visit is recommended at an appropriate interval after delivery of the fetus to verify that vaginal bleeding has stopped or has substantially reduced. Persistence of vaginal bleeding could signify incomplete abortion and appropriate investigation/treatment should be considered.

Mifepristone may only be administered for pregnancy termination in accordance with the Abortion Act 1967 as amended by the Human Fertilisation and Embryology Act 1990.

The administration of mifepristone must be supervised by a registered medical practitioner; any treatment necessary to effect complete termination of the pregnancy may be carried out by registered medical practitioners only. The administration of mifepristone and any treatment necessary to effect complete termination of the pregnancy must take place in an NHS hospital or place approved by the Secretary of State under Section 1(3) of the Abortion Act 1967 and which has received DOH approval to undertake medical terminations with mifepristone.

The administation of the treatment for the above indications must be carried out in an NHS hospital or place approved by the Secretary of State under Section 1(3) of the Abortion Act 1967, and which has immediate access to suitably experienced medical practitioners and adequate resuscitation equipment.

Pregnancy may occur between fetal expulsion and the resumption of mensus: it is, therefore, recommended that contraceptive advice be given prior to discharge from hospital after prostaglandin administration and/or surgery.

If appropriate, contraception can be initiated, according to normal clinical practice, within the period of 3 to 9 days after taking the mifepristone tablets.

Contra-indications, warnings, etc

Contra-indications: Suspected ectopic pregnancy, chronic adrenal failure, long-term corticosteroid therapy, known allergy to mifepristone, haemorrhagic disorders and tretment with anti-coagulants.

In addition to the above contra-indications, mifepristone is contra-indicated in smokers over 35 years of age when used in association with gemeprost for therapeutic termination of pregnancy up to 63 days gestation, and between 13 and 20 weeks gestation.

Precautions: As they could affect the efficacy of the treatment, NSAIDs including aspirin, should be avoided until pregnancy termination is complete. For termination of pregnancy of up to 63 days gestation, NSAIDs should not be given at least until the follow-up visit 8–12 days after mifepristone administration.

When mifepristone is used, special consideration must be given to patients in the following high risk categories: Asthmatics and other patients with COAD, patients with cardiovascular disease or risk factors.

It is not recommended to use this treatment for patients with the following conditions: Renal or hepatic failure; patients with prosthetic heart valves or who have had one previous episode of infective endocarditis should receive chemoprophylaxis according to the current UK recommendations.

Drug interactions and other interactions: **In view of the single dose administration, no specific interactions have been studied. However, there could be interactions with drugs which modulate or inhibit prostaglandin synthesis and metabolism. See *Precautions* above).**

Side effects:

A Relating to the treatment procedure:

1. Therapeutic termination of pregnancy of up to 63 days gestation:

i) Bleeding: 48 hours after administration of the mifepristone tablets, approximately 55% of patients have started to bleed. During this time, in up to 9% of patients, the bleeding has been described as 'heavy'.

By 4 hours after the prostaglandin administration, bleeding is observed in over 96% of patients, with 9% of patients experiencing heavy bleeding.

In approximately 0.7% of patients, transfusion and curettage has been necessary.

The blood loss associated with this procedure is considered acceptable, in that it will not cause significant anaemia and is comparable to that observed during surgical termination. The duration of bleeding, following the treatment procedure, is approximately 12 days.

ii) Pain: Up to 48 hours after administration of the mifepristone tablets, very few patients have experienced any pain. During the first few hours after prostaglandin administration, uterine pain is often experienced, with about 40% of patients requiring no analgesic support, 30% requiring simple analgesia, e.g. paracetamol, and 30% requiring parenteral or oral narcotic analgesia, e.g. pethidine or dihydrocodeine.

Nulliparous women and those with a history of dysmenorrhoea are more likely to require narcotic analgesia.

iii) Other complications: In a small number of patients, other complications such as uterine and urinary tract infections, have been experienced. These should be treated according to normal clinical practice.

2. Softening and dilatation of the cervix:

i) Bleeding: Uterine bleeding may commence between administration of mifepristone and surgery especially in pregnancies of less than 9 weeks gestation. In a very small number of cases abortion may occur prior to surgery.

ii) Pain: Uterine cramps may be experienced between administration of mifepristone and surgery.

3. For use in combination with gemeprost for termination of pregnancy between 13 and 20 weeks gestation:

i) Bleeding: Bleeding has rarely been observed in the interval between administration of mifepristone tablets and initiation of gemeprost. After the initiation of gemeprost, vaginal bleeding may commence within one to two hours.

ii) Pain: Uterine cramps may be experienced between administration of mifepristone and initiation of gemeprost therapy.

iii) Other complications: Uterine rupture has been reported in association with prostaglandin induction of second trimester termination of pregnancy, the risk of this may be increased in patients with a caesarean section scar.

B Drug related:
i) Mifepristone: Malaise, faintness, headache, nausea and vomiting, and skin rashes have been reported in a minority of patients.

ii) Prostaglandin: Diarrhoea, nausea, vomiting, and vagal symptoms (hot flushes, dizziness, chills and headaches) have been reported and hyperthermia in a few patients.

Cardiovascular incidents have been rarely reported, probably due to coronary spasm, induced by the prostaglandin analogue administration.

Warning: Patients must be informed that in the event of the failure or interruption of the method, the pregnancy is liable to continue to develop. The foetus may then be exposed to a risk of malformation, as suggested by studies with mifepristone in rabbits, although not confirmed in rats and mice. Similarly there is a foreseeable effect of certain synthetic prostaglandin analogues on the foetus. It is essential that termination of pregnancy by another method be undertaken at a follow-up visit in the event of such failure.

Although no data on mifepristone in human breast milk exists, it is recommended that breast feeding is interrupted for 14 days after mifepristone is administered. This time is based on the clearance of mifepristone from the circulation.

Special notes: The use of mifepristone requires the prevention of rhesus allo-immunisation and other general measures taken during an abortion.

The precautions for synthetic prostaglandin analogues must be observed viz:

1. The patient should be lying down and blood pressure measurements made every 30 minutes, for several hours after the administration of the prostaglandin. This should be carried out, under medical supervision, in the treatment centre which must be fitted with the appropriate cardiovascular monitoring and resuscitation equipment.
2. Parenteral and sublingual forms of medication for the treatment of coronary spasm, such as nitrate derivatives and calcium antagonists, must be readily available.
3. An electrocardiogram should be performed, in cases of chest pain, suspected arrhythmias or severe arterial hypotension.
4. Patients should not smoke or take alcohol, on the 2 days prior to and the day of the prostaglandin administration.

Overdosage: Tolerance studies have shown that administration of doses of mifepristone of up to 2 g caused no unwanted reactions. Nevertheless, in the event of massive ingestion signs of adrenal failure might occur. Any suggestion of acute intoxication, therefore, requires treatment in a specialist environment.

Pharmaceutical precautions No special storage conditions are necessary.

Legal category POM.

This product can only be supplied to NHS hospitals and premises approved under the Abortion Act 1967.

Package quantities Blister pack of three tablets.

Further information After oral administration of a single 600 mg dose, the peak plasma level is obtained after 1.30 hours, (mean of 10 subjects). The absolute bioavailability is 69% and the active drug is 98% bound to plasma proteins.

Following the distribution phase, elimination is slow at first with the plasma concentration decreasing by 50% between 12 and 72 hours, and then more rapidly giving an elimination half-life of 18 hours.

Mifepristone is a synthetic steroid with an anti-progestational action. The sequential use of mifepristone with a synthetic prostaglandin analogue, 36–48 hours later, has a success rate of about 95% for aborting pregnancies of up to 63 days gestation.

Administration of mifepristone, 36 to 48 hours prior to prostaglandin induction of termination of pregnancy between 13 and 20 weeks gestation, significantly shortens the interval between the beginning of treatment with prostaglandin and foetal expulsion and reduces the dose of prostaglandin necessary for expulsion.

Product licence holder: Exelgyn, 6 rue Christophe Colomb, 75008 Paris, France.

Product licence number PL 16152/0001

Date of issue September 1997.

**Trade Mark*

Fauldling Pharmaceuticals Plc
Queensway
Royal Leamington Spa
Warwickshire CV31 3RW
☎ 01926 820820 🗋 01926 821041

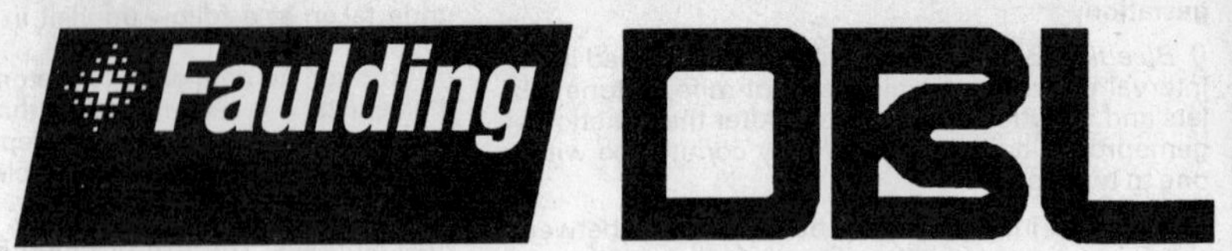

ACICLOVIR I.V. FOR INTRAVENOUS INFUSION

Qualitative and quantitative composition

	250 mg/ 10 mL	*500 mg/ 20 mL*	*1 g/40 mL*
Active constituent			
Aciclovir PhEur	250 mg	500 mg	1 gram
Other constituents			
Sodium hydroxide PhEur	46.45 mg	92.9 mg	185.8 mg
Water for injections PhEur	to10 ml	to 20 ml	to 40 ml

Pharmaceutical form Aciclovir iv is a clear colourless or almost colourless sterile solution containing the equivalent of 25 mg/ml Aciclovir I.V. in water for injections PhEur; the aciclovir is present as aciclovir sodium. It is available in the following concentrations 250 mg/10 ml, 500 mg/20 ml, 1 g/40 ml.

Clinical particulars

Therapeutic indications: Aciclovir i.v. is indicated for the treatment of *Herpes simplex* infections in immunocompromised patients.

Aciclovir I.V. is indicated for the prophylaxis of *Herpes simplex* infections in Immunocompromised patients.

Aciclovir I.V. is indicated for the treatment of *Varicella zoster* infections.

Aciclovir I.V. is indicated for the treatment of herpes encephalitis.

Aciclovir I.V. is indicated for the treatment of *Herpes simplex* infections in the neonate and infant up to 3 months of age.

Posology and method of administration: A course of treatment with Aciclovir I.V. usually lasts 5 days, but this may be adjusted according to the patient's condition and response to therapy. Treatment for herpes encephalitis and neonatal *Herpes simplex* infections usually lasts 10 days.

The duration of prophylactic administration of Aciclovir I.V. is determined by the duration of the period at risk.

Dosage in adults: Patients with *Herpes simplex* (except herpes encephalitis) or *Varicella zoster* infections should be given Aciclovir I.V. in doses of 5 mg/kg bodyweight every 8 hours.

Immunocompromised patients with *Varicella zoster* infections or patients with herpes encephalitis should be given Aciclovir I.V. in doses of 10 mg/kg bodyweight every 8 hours provided renal function is not impaired. (see dosage in renal impairment).

Dosage in children: the dose of Aciclovir I.V. for children aged between 3 months and 12 years is calculated on the basis of body surface area.

Children with *Herpes simplex* (except herpes encephalitis) or *Varicella zoster* infections should be given Aciclovir I.V. in doses of 250 mg per square metre of body surface area every 8 hours.

In immunocompromised children with *Varicella zoster* infections or children with herpes encephalitis, Aciclovir I.V. should be given in doses of 500 mg per square metre body surface area every 8 hours if renal function is not impaired.

Children with impaired renal function require an appropriately modified dose, according to the degree of impairment.

The dosage of Aciclovir I.V. in neonates and infants up to 3 months of age is calculated on the basis of bodyweight.

Neonates and infants up to 3 months of age with *Herpes simplex* infections should be given Aciclovir I.V. in doses of 10 mg/kg bodyweight every 8 hours. Treatment for neonatal *Herpes simplex* infections usually lasts 10 days.

Dosage in the elderly: in the elderly, total aciclovir body clearance declines in parallel with creatinine clearance. Special attention should be given to dosage reduction in elderly patients with impaired creatinine clearance. It is recommended that the state of hydration and the creatinine clearance should be evaluated before the administration of high dosages of aciclovir, especially in elderly patients, who may have reduced renal function despite a normal serum creatinine concentration.

Dosage in renal impairment: caution is advised when administering Aciclovir I.V. to patients with impaired renal function since the drug is excreted through the kidneys. The following adjustments in dosage are suggested:

Creatinine clearance	*Dosage*
25 to 50 ml/min	the dose recommended above (5 or 10 mg/kg bodyweight or 500 mg/m²) should be given every 12 hours.
10 to 25 ml/min	the dose recommended above (5 or 10 mg/kg bodyweight or 500 mg/m²) should be given every 24 hours.
0(anuric) to 10 ml/min	in patients receiving continuous ambulatory peritoneal dialysis (CAPD) the dose recommended above (5 or 10 mg/kg bodyweight or 500 mg/m²) should be halved and administered every 24 hours. In patients receiving haemodialysis the dose recommended above (5 or 10 mg/kg bodyweight or 500 mg/m²) should be halved and administered every 24 hours and after dialysis.

Administration: the required dose of Aciclovir I.V. should be administered by slow intravenous infusion over a one-hour period.

Aciclovir I.V. may be administered by a controlled-rate infusion pump.

For adults, it is recommended that infusion bags containing 100 ml of infusion fluid are used, even when this would give an aciclovir concentration substantially below 0.5% w/v. Thus one 100 ml infusion bag may be used for any dose between 250 mg and 500 mg aciclovir but a second bag must be used for doses between 500 and 1000 mg. Aciclovir injection should not be diluted to a concentration greater than 5 mg/ml (0.5%w/v) for administration by infusion. After addition of Aciclovir I.V. to an infusion solution the mixture should be shaken to ensure through mixing.

For children and neonates, where it is advisable to keep the volume of infusion fluid to a minimum, it is recommended that dilution is on the basis of 4 ml of solution, (100 mg aciclovir), added to 20 ml of infusion fluid.

When diluted in accordance with the recommended schedules, Aciclovir I.V. is known to be compatible with the following infusion fluids and stable for up to 24 hours at room temperature, below 25°C:

Sodium chloride intravenous infusion BP 0.9% w/v;
Sodium chloride (0.18% w/v) and glucose (4% w/v) intravenous infusion BP;
Sodium chloride (0.9% w/v) and glucose (5% w/v) intravenous infusion BP;
Compound sodium lactate intravenous infusion BP (hartmann's solution).

Aciclovir I.V. when diluted in accordance with the above schedule will give an aciclovir concentration not greater that 0.5% w/v.

Aciclovir I.V. contains no preservative. Dilution should therefore be carried out immediately before use and any unused solution should be discarded.

Should any visible turbidity or crystallisation appear in the solution before or during infusion, the preparation should be discarded.

The solution should not be refrigerated as this causes precipitation of crystals.

Contra-indications: Aciclovir I.V. is contra-indicated in patients known to be previously hypersensitive to aciclovir.

Special warnings and special precautions for use: Aciclovir I.V. is intended for intravenous infusion only and should not be used by any other route.

Special warnings and special precautions for use: The dose of Aciclovir I.V. must be adjusted in patients with impaired renal function in order to avoid accumulation of aciclovir in the body. Infusions of aciclovir must be given over a period of at least one hour in order to avoid renal tubular damage. (see dosage in renal impairment).

Although the aqueous solubility of aciclovir exceeds 100 mg/ml, precipitation of aciclovir crystals in renal tubules and the consequent renal tubular damage can occur if the maximum solubility of free aciclovir (2.5 mg/ml at 37°C in water) is exceeded. Aciclovir infusions must be accompanied by adequate hydration. Since maximum urine concentration occurs within the first few hours following infusion particular attention should be given to establish sufficient urine flow during that period. Concomitant use of other nephrotoxic drugs, pre-existing renal disease and dehydration increase the risk of further renal impairment by aciclovir.

In patients receiving Aciclovir I.V. at higher doses (e.g. For herpes encephalitis), specific care regarding renal function should be taken, particularly when patients are dehydrated or have any renal impairment.

Aciclovir I.V. has a pH of approximately 11.0 and should not be administered by mouth.

Interaction with other medicaments and other forms of interaction: Probenecid increases the aciclovir mean half-life and area under the plasma concentration-time curve. Other drugs affecting renal physiology could potentially influence the pharmacokinetics of aciclovir. However, clinical experience has not identified other drug interactions with aciclovir.

Pregnancy and lactation: Limited data are available on the use of aciclovir during pregnancy. Aciclovir should not be used during pregnancy unless the potential benefits to the patient outweigh the potential risk to the foetus.

Limited human data show that aciclovir is excreted in human breast milk. Aciclovir should only be administered to nursing mothers if the benefits to the mother outweigh the potential risks to the baby.

Effects on ability to drive and use machines: Not applicable.

Undesirable effects: Renal: Rapid increases in blood urea and creatinine levels may occasionally occur in patients given Aciclovir I.V. These are usually reversible but progression to acute renal failure can occur in rare cases. The rapid increases in blood urea and creatinine levels are believed to be related to peak plasma levels and the state of hydration of the patient. To avoid this effect the drug should not be given as an intravenous bolus injection but by slow infusion over a one hour period. Adequate hydration of the patient should be maintained.

The risk of renal damage is increased by concomitant use of other nephrotoxic drugs and pre-existing renal disease.

Renal impairment developing during treatment with Aciclovir I.V. usually responds rapidly to rehydration of the patient and/or dosage reduction or withdrawal of the drug. Progression to acute renal failure, however, can occur in exceptional cases.

Skin: Severe local inflammatory reactions or phlebitis have occurred at the injection site sometimes leading to breakdown of the skin. Rashes and hives may occur.

Local necrosis and inflammation have occurred when Aciclovir I.V. has been inadvertently infused into extravascular tissues.

Neurological: Reversible neurological reactions such as confusion, lethargy, hallucinations, agitation, tremors, somnolence, psychosis, convulsions and coma have been associated with Aciclovir I.V. therapy, usually in medically complicated cases.

Therefore aciclovir should be used with caution in patients with underlying neurological abnormalities. It should also be used with caution in patients who have manifested neurological reactions to cytotoxic drugs or are receiving concomitant interferon or intrathecal methotrexate.

Other: Other events reported in patients receiving Aciclovir I.V. include increases in liver-related enzymes, fever and decreases in haematological indices (anaemia, thrombocytopenia, leucopoenia).

Aciclovir should be used with caution in patients with significant hypoxia or serious hepatic or electrolyte abnormalities.

Other less frequent adverse effects reported in patients receiving therapy with Aciclovir I.V. include, diaphoresis, haematuria, hypotension, reversible psychiatric effects and headache, nausea and vomiting.

Overdose: Toxicity and treatment of overdosage: There is little experience concerning overdosage with aciclovir however single doses of Aciclovir I.V. up to 80 mg/kg bodyweight have been inadvertently administered without adverse effects. Effects of overdosage may be expected to be similar in nature to those described under adverse reactions. Adequate hydration is essential to reduce the possibility of crystal formation in the urine. Aciclovir can be removed from the circulation by haemodialysis.

Pharmacological properties

Pharmacodynamic properties: Mode of action: Aciclovir is a synthetic acyclic purine nucleoside analogue with in vitro and in vivo inhibitory activity against human herpes viruses, including Herpes simplex virus (HSV) types 1 and 2 and Varicella Zoster virus (VZV), Epstein Barr virus (EBV) and Cytomegalovirus (CMV). In cell culture aciclovir has the greatest antiviral activity against HSV-1, followed (in decreasing order of potency) by HSV-2, VZV, EBV, and CMV.

The inhibitory activity of aciclovir for HSV-1, HSV-2, VZV and EBV is highly selective. The enzyme thymidine kinase (TK) of normal, uninfected cells does not use aciclovir effectively as a substrate, hence toxicity to mammalian host cells is low; however, TK encoded by HSV, VZV and EBV converts aciclovir to aciclovir monophosphate, a nucleoside analogue, which is further converted to the diphosphate and finally to the triphosphate by cellular enzymes. Aciclovir needs to be phosphorylated to the active compound aciclovir triphosphate, in order to become active against the virus. Aciclovir triphosphate acts as an inhibitor of, and a substrate for, the herpes specified DNA polymerase preventing further viral DNA synthesis.

Animal studies indicate that at high does aciclovir is cytotoxic.

Pharmacokinetic properties: Pharmacokinetics: in adults, the terminal plasma half-life of aciclovir after the administration of Aciclovir I.V. is about 2.9 hours. Approximately 60% of the drug is excreted unchanged by the kidney. Renal clearance of aciclovir is substantially greater than creatinine clearance, indicating that tubular secretion, in addition to glomerular filtration, contributes to the renal elimination of the drug.

When aciclovir is given one hour after 1 gram of probenecid the terminal half-life and the area under the plasma concentration time curve, are extended by 18% and 40% respectively. 9-carboxymethoxymethylguanine is the major significant metabolite of aciclovir and accounts for 10 to 15% of the dose excreted in the urine.

In adults, mean steady state peak plasma concentrations (c^{ss}max) following a one-hour infusion of 2.5 mg/kg, 5 mg/kg, 10 mg/kg and 15 mg/kg were 22.7 micromolar (5.1 microgram/ml), 43.6 micromolar (9.8 microgram/ml), 92 micromolar (20.7 microgram/ml) and 105 micromolar (23.6 microgram/ml) respectively. The corresponding trough levels (c^{ss}min) 7 hours later were 2.2 micromolar (0.5 microgram/ml), 3.1 micromolar (0.7 microgram/ml) 10.2 micromolar (2.3 microgram/ml), and 8.8 micromolar (2.0 microgram/ml), respectively. In children over 1 year of age similar mean peak (c^{ss}max) and trough (c^{ss}min) levels were observed when a dose of 250 mg/m^2 was substituted for 5 mg/kg and a dose of 500 mg/m^2 was substituted for 10 mg/kg. Ir. Neonates (0 to 3 months of age) treated with doses of 10 mg/kg administered by infusion over a one-hour period every 8 hours the c^{ss}max was found to be 61.2 micromolar (13.8 microgram/ml) and the c^{ss}min. To be 10.1 micromolar (2.3 microgram/ml).

The terminal plasma half-life in these patients was 3.8 hours. In the elderly, total body clearance falls with increasing age and is associated with decreases in creatinine clearance although there is little change in the terminal plasma half-life.

In patients with chronic renal failure the mean terminal half-life was found to be 19.5 hours. The mean aciclovir half-life during haemodialysis was 5.7 hours. Plasma aciclovir levels dropped approximately 60% during dialysis.

Cerebrospinal fluid levels are approximately 50% of corresponding plasma levels.

Plasma protein binding is relatively low (9 to 33%) and drug interactions involving binding site displacement are not anticipated.

Preclinical safety data: The results of a wide range of mutagenicity test *in vitro* and *in vivo* indicate that aciclovir is unlikely to pose a genetic risk to man.

Aciclovir was not found to be carcinogenic in long-term studies in the rat and the mouse.

Systemic administration of aciclovir in internationally accepted standard tests did not produce embryotoxic or teratogenic effects in rabbits, rats or mice.

In a non-standard test in rats, foetal abnormalities were observed but only following such high subcutaneous doses that maternal toxicity was produced. The clinical relevance of these findings is uncertain.

Largely reversible adverse effects on spermatogenesis in association with overall toxicity in rats and dogs have been reported only at doses of aciclovir greatly in excess of those employed therapeutically. Two-generation studies in mice did not reveal any effect of (orally administered) aciclovir on fertility.

There is no experience of the effect of Aciclovir I.V. on human fertility. Aciclovir tablets have shown to have no definitive effect upon sperm count, morphology or motility in man.

Pharmaceutical particulars

List of excipients:

	250 mg/ 10 mL	*500 mg/ 20 mL*	*1 g/40 mL*
Sodium hydroxide PhEur	46.45 mg	92.9 mg	185.8 mg
Water for injections PhEur	to10 ml	to 20 ml	to 40 ml

Incompatibilities: Aciclovir sodium is reported to be incompatible with solutions of dobutamine hydrochloride, dopamine hydrochloride, amsacrine, fludarabine phosphate, foscarnet sodium, idarubicin hydrochloride, ondansetron hydrochloride, and piperacillin sodium–tazobactam sodium. Diltiazem hydrochloride 5 mg/ml, pethidine hydrochloride 10 mg/ml and morphine sulphate 1 mg/ml cause precipitation, although solutions containing lower concentrations of these drugs are compatible with aciclovir.

Biologic or colloidal fluids (e.g. blood products, protein containing solutions) are incompatible with aciclovir sodium.

Shelf life: 24 months.

Special precautions for storage: Store below 25°C. Do not refrigerate. Refrigeration is not recommended as precipitation may occur. Such a precipitate will redissolve at room temperature without affecting potency however.

Instructions for use/handling: Aciclovir I.V. contains no preservative. Dilution should therefore be carried out immediately before use and any unused solution should be discarded.

Diluted solutions should not be refrigerated.

Marketing authorisation number 4515/0098.

Date of approval/revision of SPC May 1997

Legal category POM

AMIKACIN SULPHATE INJECTION

Qualitative and quantitative composition

Amikacin (as Amikacin Sulphate USP)	500.0 mg
Sodium Citrate BP	50.0 mg
Sodium Metabisulphite BP	4.8 mg
Water for Injections BP	2.0 ml

Pharmaceutical form Each vial contains in 2 ml, Amikacin sulphate equivalent to Amikacin activity 500 mg.

Clinical particulars

Therapeutic indications: Amikacin Sulphate Injection is a semi-synthetic, aminoglycoside antibiotic which is active against a broad spectrum of Gram-negative organisms, including pseudomonas and some Gram-positive organisms.

Sensitive Gram-negative organisms include; *Pseudomonas aeruginosa, Escherichia coli,* indole-positive and indole-negative Proteus spp, Klebsiella, Enterobacter and Serratia spp, *Citrobacter freundii,* Salmonella, Shigella, Acinetobacter and Providencia spp.

Many strains of these Gram-negative organisms resistant to gentamicin and tobramycin show sensitivity to Amikacin in vitro.

The principal Gram-positive organism sensitive to Amikacin is *Staphylococcus aureus,* including some methicillin-resistant strains.

Amikacin is indicated in the short-term treatment of serious infections due to susceptible strains of Gram-negative bacteria, including Pseudomonas species. Although Amikacin is not the drug of choice for infections due to staphylococci, at times it may be indicated for the treatment of known or suspected staphylococcal disease. These situations include: the initiation of therapy for severe infections when the organisms suspected are either Gram-negative or staphylococci, patients allergic to other antibiotics, and mixed staphylococcal/Gram-negative infections.

Therapy with Amikacin may be instituted prior to obtaining the results of sensitivity testing. Surgical procedures should be performed where indicated.

Posology and method of administration: At the recommended dosage level, uncomplicated infections due to sensitive organisms should respond to therapy within 24 to 48 hours.

If clinical response does not occur within two to three days, consideration should be given to alternative therapy.

Amikacin Sulphate Injection can be administered by intramuscular injection or the intravenous route, when either a slow bolus (two to three minutes) or an infusion (0.25% over 30 minutes) maybe used. The dosage is identical for either route of administration and should be based on an estimate of ideal body weight.

If required, suitable diluents for intravenous use are: Normal saline, 5% dextrose in water. Once the product has been diluted the solution must be used as soon as possible and NOT STORED.

Adults and children: 15 mg/kg/day in two equally divided doses (equivalent to 500 mg b.i.d.in adults).

Neonates and premature infants: In neonates an initial loading dose of 10 mg/kg followed by 15 mg/kg/day in two equally divided doses.

Sufficient extensive clinical use has not been achieved to enable firm dosage guidelines to be given in premature infants.

Use in elderly: Amikacin is excreted by the renal route, renal function should be assessed whenever possible and dosage adjusted as described under impaired renal function.

Life-threatening infections and/or those caused by pseudomonas: The adult dose may be increased to 500 mg every eight hours but should never exceed 1.5 g/day nor be administered for a period longer than 10 days. A maximum total adult dose of 15 g should not be exceeded.

Urinary tract infections: (other than pseudomonas infections): 7.5 mg/kg/day in two equally divided doses (equivalent to 250 mg b.i.d. in adults). As the activity of Amikacin is enhanced by increasing the pH, a urinary alkalinising agent may be administered concurrently.

Impaired renal function: In patients with impaired renal function, the daily dose should be reduced and/or the intervals between doses increased to avoid accumulation of the drug. A suggested method for estimating dosage in patients with known or suspected diminished renal function is to multiply the serum creatinine concentration (in mg/100 ml) by 9 and use the resulting figure as the interval in hours between doses.

Serum creatinine concentration (mg/100 ml)		*Interval between Amikacin doses of 7.5 mg/kg/IM (hours)*
1.5	x 9 =	13.5
2.0		18.0
2.5		22.5
3.0		27.0
3.5		31.5
4.0		36.0
4.5		40.5
5.0		45.0
5.5		49.5
6.0		54.0

As renal function may alter appreciably during therapy, the serum creatinine should be checked frequently and the dosage regimen modified as necessary.

Intraperitoneal use: Following exploration for established peritonitis, or after peritoneal contamination due to faecal spill during surgery, Amikacin may be used as an irrigant after recovery from anaesthesia in concentrations of 0.25% (2.5 mg/ml).

Other routes of administration: Amikacin in concentrations 0.25% (2.5 mg/ml) may be used satisfactorily as an irrigating solution in abscess cavities, the pleural space, the peritoneum and the cerebral ventricles.

Contra-indications: Patients should be well hydrated during Amikacin therapy. In patients with impaired renal function or diminished glomerular filtration Amikacin should be used with caution.

If therapy is expected to last seven days or more in patients with renal impairment, or 10 days in other patients, a pre-treatment audiogram should be obtained and repeated during therapy. Amikacin therapy should be stopped if tinnitus or subjective hearing loss develops, or if follow-up audiograms show significant loss of high frequency response.

As with other aminoglycosides, ototoxicity and/or nephrotoxicity can result from the use of Amikacin; precautions on dosage and adequate hydration should be observed.

If signs of renal irritation appear (such as albumin, casts, red or white blood cells), hydration should be increased and a reduction in dosage may be desirable. These findings usually disappear when treatment is completed. However, if azotaemia or a progressive decrease in urine output occurs, treatment should be stopped.

The use of Amikacin in patients with a history of allergy to aminoglycosides or in patients who may have subclinical renal or eighth cranial nerve damage induced by prior administration of nephrotoxic and/or ototoxic agents such as streptomycin, gentamicin, tobramycin, kanamycin, neomycin, polymyxin B, colistin, cephaloridine, should be considered with caution, as toxicity may be additive. In these patients Amikacin should be used only if, in the opinion of the physician, therapeutic advantages outweigh the potential risks.

The risk of ototoxicity is increased when Amikacin is used in conjunction with rapidly acting diuretic drugs, particularly when the diuretic is administered intravenously. Such agents include frusemide and ethacrynic acid. Irreversible deafness may result.

The intraperitoneal use of Amikacin is not recommended in young children or in patients under the influence of anaesthetics or muscle-relaxing drugs (including ether, halothane, d-tubocurarine, succinylcholine and decamethonium) as neuromuscular blockade and consequent respiratory depression may occur.

Special warnings and special precautions for use: In such patients, renal function should be assessed by the usual methods prior to therapy and periodically during therapy. Daily doses should be reduced and/or the interval between doses lengthened in accordance with serum creatinine concentrations to avoid accumulation of abnormally high blood levels and tominimise the risk of ototoxicity. Regular monitoring of serum drug concentration and of renal function is particularly important in elderly patients, who may have reduced renal function that may not be evident in the results of routine screening tests ie. blood urea and serum creatinine.

If signs of renal irritation appear (such as albumin, casts, red or white blood cells), hydration should be increased and a reduction in dosage may be desirable. These findings usually disappear when treatment is completed. However, if azotaemia or a progressive decrease in urine output occurs, treatment should be stopped.

Interaction with other medicaments and other forms of interaction: Amikacin sulphate is incompatible with some penicillins and cephalosporins, amphotericin, chlorothiazide sodium, erythromycin gluceptate, heparin, nitrofurantoin sodium, phenytoin sodium, thiopentone sodium and warfarin sodium, and depending on the composition and strength of the vehicle, tetracyclines, vitamins of the B group with vitamin C, and potassium chloride.

Pregnancy and lactation: The safety of Amikacin in pregnancy has not yet been established

Effects on ability to drive and use machines: Not applicable.

Undesirable effects: When the recommended precautions and dosages are followed the incidence of toxic reactions, such as tinnitis, vertigo, and partial reversible deafness, skin rash, drug fever, headache, paraesthesia, nausea and vomiting is low. Urinary signs of renal irritation (albumen, casts, and red or white cells), azotaemia and oliguria have been reported.

Overdose: In the event of overdosage or toxic reaction, peritoneal dialysis or haemodialysis will aid in the removal of Amikacin from the blood.

Pharmacological properties

Pharmacodynamic properties: Amikacin is a semi-synthetic aminoglycoside antibiotic derived from Kanamycin A. It is active against a broad spectrum of Gram-negative organisms, including pseudomonas, *Escherichia coli* and some Gram-positive organisms, e.g. *Staphylococcus aureus*.

Aminoglycoside antibiotics are bactericidal in action. Although the exact mechanism of action has not been fully elucidated, the drugs appear to inhibit protein synthesis in susceptible bacteria by irreversibly binding to 30S ribosomal subunits.

Pharmacokinetic properties: Amikacin is rapidly absorbed after intramuscular injection. Peak plasma concentrations equivalent to about 20 mcg/ml are achieved one hour after I.M. doses of 500 mg, reducing to about 2 mcg/ml 10 hours after injections.

Single doses of 500 mg administered as an intravenous infusion over a period of 30 minutes produce a mean peak serum concentration of 38 mcg/ml. Repeated infusions do not produce drug accumulation in adults with normal renal function. However, decreased renal function will lead to accumulation

In adults with normal renal function the plasma elimination half-life of Amikacin is usually 2–3 hours. 94–98% of a single I.M. or I.V. dose of Amikacin is excreted unchanged by glomerular filtration within 24 hours. Urine concentrations of Amikacin average 563 mcg/ml for 6 hours following a single 250-mg I.M. dose and 832 mcg/ml following a single 500-mg I.M. dose in adults with normal renal function.

Amikacin diffuses readily through extracellular fluids. It has been found in pleural fluid, amniotic fluid and in the peritoneal cavity following parenteral administration.

Preclinical safety data: There are no pre-clinical data of relevance to the prescriber which are additional to that already included in other sections of the SPC.

Pharmaceutical particulars

List of excipients:

Sodium Citrate BP	50.0 mg
Sodium metabisulphite BP	4.8 mg
Water for Injections BP	2.0 ml

Incompatibilities: Amikacin sulphate is incompatible with some penicillins and cephalosporins, amphotericin chlorothiazide sodium, erythromycin gluceptate, heparin, nitrofurantoin sodium, phenytoin sodium, thiopentone sodium and warfarin sodium, and depending on the composition and strength of the vehicle, tetracyclines, vitamins of the B group with vitamin C, and potassium chloride.

Shelf life: 36 months shelf life in the medicinal product as packaged for sale.

Special precautions for storage: At times, Amikacin may be indicated as concurrent therapy with other antibacterial agents in mixed or superinfections. In such instances, Amikacin should not be physically mixed with other antibacterial agents in syringes, infusion bottles or any other equipment. Each agent should be administered separately.

Store below 25°C. The solution may darken from colourless to a pale yellow but this does not indicate a loss of potency

Marketing authorisation number 4515/0075

Date of approval/revision of SPC March 1998

Legal category POM

ATRACURIUM BESILATE INJECTION

Qualitative and quantitative composition Atracurium besilate 10 mg/ml.

Pharmaceutical form Solution for injection.

Clinical particulars

Therapeutic indications: Atracurium Besilate Injection is indicated as an adjunct to general anaesthesia during surgery to relax skeletal muscles, and to facilitate endotracheal intubation and mechanical ventilation. It is also indicated to facilitate mechanical ventilation in intensive care unit (ICU) patients.

Posology and method of administration:

Use as an adjunct to general anaesthia: Atracurium Besilate Injection should only be administered by intravenous injection. **Do not give Atracurium Besilate Injection intramuscularly** since this may result in tissue irritation and there are no clinical data to support this route of administration.

To avoid distress to the patient, Atracurium Besilate Injection should not be administered before unconsciousness has been induced. Atracurium Besilate Injection should not be mixed in the same syringe, or administered simultaneously through the same needle, with alkaline solutions (e.g. barbiturate solutions).

In common with all neuromuscular blocking agents, monitoring of neuromuscular function is recommended during the use of Atracurium Besilate Injection in order to individualise dosage requirements.

Initial bolus doses for intubation: An initial atracurium besilate dose of 0.3 to 0.6 mg/kg (depending on the duration of full block required), given as an intravenous bolus injection, is recommended. This will provide adequate relaxation for about 15 to 35 minutes.

Endotracheal intubation can usually be accomplished within 90 to 120 seconds of the intravenous injection of 0.5 to 0.6 mg/kg. Maximum neuromuscular blockade is generally achieved approximately 3 to 5 minutes after administration. Spontaneous recovery from the end of full block occurs in about 35 minutes as measured by the restoration of the tetanic response to 95% of normal neuromuscular function.

Although atracurium is potentiated by (approximately 35%) isoflurane or enflurane anaesthesia, the same initial atracurium besilate dose (0.3 to 0.6 mg/kg) may be used for intubation if given prior to the administration of these inhalation agents. However if the initial atracurium dose is administered after steady state anaesthesia with isoflurane or enflurane has been achieved, the dose of atracurium should be reduced by approximately one-third. Smaller dosage reductions may be considered with concomitant halothane anaesthesia since it has only a marginal (approximately 20%) potentiating effect on atracurium.

Maintenance doses:

Intermittent IV injection: During prolonged surgical procedures neuromuscular blockade may be maintained with atracurium besilate maintenance doses of 0.1 to 0.2 mg/kg. Generally, under balanced anaesthia, using maintenance doses of 0.1 mg/kg, the first maintenance dose is required within 20 to 45 minutes of the initial bolus dose, then typically at 15 to 25 minute intervals, however, the need for maintenance doses should be determined by the individual patient's requirements and response. Successive supplementary dosing does not give rise to accumulation of neuromuscular blocking effect.

Use as an infusion: After the initial atracurium bolus dose, neuromuscular blockade may be maintained during prolonged surgical procedures by administering atracurium besilate as a continuous intravenous infusion at a rate of 0.3 to 0.6 mg/kg/hour. The infusion should not be commenced until early spontaneous recovery from the initial atracurium bolus dose is evident.

Atracurium besilate infusion solutions may be prepared by admixing Atracurium Besilate Injection with an appropriate diluent (see below) to give an atracurium besilate concentration of 0.5 mg/ml to 5 mg/ml.

Atracurium Besilate Injection can be administered by infusion during cardiopulmonary bypass surgery at the recommended infusion rates. Induced hypothermia to a body temperature of 25 to 26°C reduces the rate of inactivation of atracurium, and therefore full neuromuscular block may be maintained with approximately half the original infusion rate at these temperatures.

Compatibility with infusion solutions: Atracurium Besilate Injection diluted to 0.5 mg/ml with the following infusion solutions, and stored at 30°C protected from light, was shown to be stable for the times stated below.

Infusion Solution	*Period of stability*
Sodium Chloride 0.9% Intravenous Infusion	24 hours
Glucose 5% Intravenous Infusion	24 hours
Glucose 4% and Sodium Chloride 0.18% Intravenous Infusion	24 hours
Ringer's Injection USP	24 hours
Compound Sodium Lactate Intravenous Infusion (Hartmann's Solution for Injection)	4 hours

Atracurium Besilate Injection diluted to 5 mg/ml with the following infusion solutions, and stored at 30°C protected from light in 50 ml plastic syringes, was shown to be stable for the times stated below.

Infusion Solution	*Period of stability*
Sodium Chloride 0.9% Intravenous Infusion	24 hours
Glucose 5% Intravenous Infusion	24 hours
Glucose 4% and Sodium Chloride 0.18% Intravenous Infusion	24 hours
Ringer's Injection USP	24 hours
Compound Sodium Lactate Intravenous Infusion (Hartmann's Solution for Injection)	8 hours

Reversal of neuromuscular blockade: The neuromuscular blockade induced by atracurium can be reversed with an anticholinesterase agent such as neostigmine or pyridostigmine, usually in conjunction with an anticholinergic agent such as atropine or glycopyronium to prevent the adverse muscarinic effects of the anticholinesterase. Under balanced anaesthesia, reversal can usually be attempted approximately 20 to 35 minutes after the initial atracurium dose, or approximately 10 to 30 minutes after the last atracurium maintenance dose, when recovery of muscle twitch has started. Complete reversal of neuromuscular blockade is usually achieved within 8 to 10 minutes after administration of the reversing agents.

Rare instances of breathing difficulties, possibly related to incomplete reversal, have been reported following attempted pharmacological antagonism of atracurium induced neuromuscular blockade. As with other agents in this class, the tendency for residual neuromuscular block is increased if reversal is attempted at deep levels of blockade or if inadequate doses of reversal agents are employed.

Facilitation of mechanical ventilation in intensive care unit (ICU) patients: After an optional initial bolus of 0.3 to 0.6 mg/kg, neuromuscular block may be maintained by administering a continuous atracurium besilate infusion at rates of between 11 and 13 microgram/kg/min (0.65 to 0.78 mg/kg/hr). There may be wide inter-patient variability in dosage requirements and these may increase of decrease with time. Infusion rates as low as 4.5 microgram/kg/min (0.27 mg/kg/hr) or as high as 29.5 microgram/kg/min (1.77 mg/kg/hr) are required in some patients.

The rate of spontaneous recovery from neuromuscular block after infusion of atracurium besilate in ICU patients is independent of the duration of administration.

Spontaneous recovery to a train-of-four ratio >0.75 (the ratio of the height of the fourth to the first twitch in a train-of-four) can be expected to occur in approximately 60 minutes. A range of 32 to 108 minutes has been observed in clinical trials.

Dosage considerations
Use in children: The dosage in children over the age of 1 month is similar to that in adults on a body weight basis, however, large individual variability in the neuromuscular response in paediatric patients indicates that neuromuscular monitoring is essential.

Use in neonates: There are insufficient data to recommend a dose in neonates, however, this patient group is known to have increased sensitivity to non-depolarising muscle relaxants.

Use in the elderly: The standard dose of atracurium may be used in elderly patients, however, it is recommended that it be administered slowly.

Use in patients with reduced renal and/or hepatic function: Standard dosages may be used at all levels of renal or hepatic function, including endstage failure.

Use in patients with cardiovascular disease: In patients with significant cardiovascular disease the initial dose of atracurium should be administered over a period of at least 60 seconds.

See also *Special warnings and special precautions for use.*

Contra-indications: Known or suspected hypersensitivity to the product.

Special warnings and special precautions for use: Atracurium Besilate Injection should be used only by those skilled in the management of artificial respiration and only when facilities are immediately available for endotracheal intubation and for providing adequate ventilation support, including the administration of oxygen under positive pressure and the elimination of carbon dioxide. The clinician must be prepared to assist or control ventilation, and anticholinesterase agents should be immediately available for reversal of neuromuscular blockade.

Atracurium has no known effect on consciousness, pain threshold, or cerebration. In surgery, it should be used only with adequate general anaesthesia.

In common with other neuromuscular blocking agents, the potential for histamine release exists in susceptible patients during administration of atracurium besilate. Caution should be exercised in patients with a history suggestive of an increased sensitivity to the effects of histamine.

Do not give Atracurium Besilate Injection by intramuscular administration.

Atracurium Besilate Injection has an acid pH and therefore should not be mixed with alkaline solutions (e.g. barbiturate solutions) in the same syringe or administered simultaneously during intravenous infusion through the same needle. Depending on the resultant pH of such mixtures, Atracurium Besilate Injection may be inactivated and a free acid may be precipitated.

When a small vein is selected as the injection site, Atracurium Besilate Injection should be flushed through the vein with physiological saline after injection. When other anaesthetic drugs are administered through the same indwelling needle or cannula as Atracurium Besilate Injection, it is important that each drug is flushed through with an adequate volume of physiological saline.

Atracurium may have profound effects in patients with myasthenia gravis, Eaton-Lambert syndrome, or other neuromuscular diseases in which potentiation of non-depolarising agents has been noted. A reduced dosage of atracurium and the use of a peripheral nerve stimulator for assessing neuromuscular blockade is especially important in these patients. Similar precautions should be taken in patients with severe electrolyte disorders.

Atracurium does not have significant vagal or ganglion blocking properties in the recommended dosage range. Consequently, atracurium will not counteract the bradycardia produced by many anaesthetic agents or by vagal stimulation during surgery. Therefore, bradycardia during anaesthesia may be more common with atracurium than with other muscle relaxants.

As with other non-depolarising neuromuscular blocking agents, resistance to atracurium may develop in patients suffering from burns. Such patients may require increased doses of atracurium depending on the time elapsed since the burn injury and the extent of the burn.

Atracurium Besilate Injection should be administered over a period of at least 60 seconds to patients who may be unusually sensitive to falls in arterial blood pressure, for example those who are hypovolaemic.

Atracurium Besilate Injection is hypotonic and must not be applied into the infusion line of a blood transfusion.

Interaction with other medicinal products and other forms of interaction: As with other non-depolarising neuromuscular blocking agents, the magnitude and/or duration of atracurium's effects may be increased as a result of an interaction with the following agents.

Inhalation anaesthetics: atracurium is potentiated by isoflurane and enflurane anaesthesia, and only marginally potentiated by halothane anaesthesia.

Antibiotics: including the aminoglycosides, polymyxins, spectinomycin, tetracyclines, lincomycin, clindamycin and vancomycin.

Antiarrhythmic drugs: lignocaine, procainamide, quinidine.

Beta-blockers: propranolol.

Calcium channel blockers: diltiazem, nicardipine, nifedipine, verapamil.

Diuretics: frusemide, thiazides, acetazolamide and possibly mannitol.

Ganglion blocking agents: trimetaphan, hexamethonium.

Others: dantrolene, parenteral magnesium sulphate, ketamine, lithium salts and quinine.

The administration of combinations of non-depolarising neuromuscular blocking agents in conjunction with atracurium may produce a degree of neuromuscular blockade in excess of that which might be expected were an equipotent total dose of atracurium administered. Any synergistic effect may vary between different drug combinations.

A depolarising muscle relaxant such as suxamethonium chloride should not be administered to prolong the neuromuscular blocking effects of non-depolarising blocking agents such as atracurium, as this may result in a prolonged and complex block which can be difficult to reverse with anticholinesterase drugs.

The prior use of suxamethonium reduces the onset (to maximum blockade) by approximately 2 to 3 minutes and may increase the depth of neuromusculare blockade induced by the atricurium. Therefore, the initial atracurium dose should be reduced and the reduced dose should not be administered until the patient has recovered from the neuromuscular blocking effects of suxamethonium.

Rarely, certain drugs may aggravate or unmask latent myasthenia gravis or actually induce a myasthenic syndrome. Such drugs include various antibiotics, beta-blockers (propranolol, oxprenolol), antiarrhythmic drugs (procainamide, quinidine), antirheumatic drugs (chloroquine, d-penicillamine), trimetaphan, chlorpromazine, steroids, phenytoin and lithium. In these situations a consequent increased sensitivity to atracurium would be expected.

The use of corticosteroids with neuromuscular blocking agents has been reported to antagonise neuromuscular blockades. In addition, prolonged coadminstration of these agents may increase the risk and/or severity of myopathy resulting in prolonged flaccid paralysis following discontinuation of the neuromuscular blocking agent.

The onset of neuromuscular blockade is likely to be lengthened and the duration of blockade shortened in patients receiving chronic anticonvulsant therapy (e.g. carbamazepine, phenytoin).

In principle, maintaining neuromuscular monitoring until complete reversal of neuromuscular monitoring should permit detection of most interactions. Nevertheless, recurrence of neuromuscular blockade may occur, for example, upon treatment with post surgical antibiotics.

Use during pregnancy and lactation: Atracurium crosses the placenta, but, there have been no demonstrated adverse effects in the foetus or newborn infant. Animal studies have indicated that atracurium has no adverse effects on foetal development. Nevertheless, as with all neuromuscular blocking agents, atracurium should be used during pregnancy only if the potential benefit to the mother outweighs any potential risk to the foetus and use in the first 3 months of pregnancy should be avoided.

It is not known whether muscle relaxants administered during vaginal delivery have immediate or delayed effects on the foetus or increase the likelihood that resuscitation of the newborn infant will be necessary. The possibility that a forceps delivery will be necessary may increase.

Atricurium Besilate Injection is suitable for maintenance of muscle relaxation during Caesarean section as it does not cross the placenta in clinically significant amounts following the recommended doses. In an open study, atracurium besilate (0.3 mg/kg) was administered to 26 pregnant women during delivery by caesarean section. No harmful effects were attributable to atracurium in any of the newborn infants, although small amounts of atracurium were shown to cross the placental barrier. The possibility of respiratory depression in the newborn infant should always be considered following caesarean section during which a neuromuscular blocking agent has been administered. In patients receiving magnesium sulphate, the reversal of neuromuscular blockade may be unsatisfactory and the atracurium dose should be lowered as indicated.

It is not known whether atracurium is excreted in human milk. After administration of Atracurium Besilate Injection breast feeding should be stopped for 24 hours.

Effects on ability to drive and use machines: As atracurium is indicated for use with general anaesthetics consideration of the effects of atracurium on the ability to drive and use machines is irrelevant.

Undesirable effects: As with most neuromuscular blocking agents, the potential exists for adverse reactions suggestive of histamine release in susceptible patients. In clinical trials involving 875 patients, reports of skin flushing ranged from 1% at doses up to 0.3 mg/kg, to 29% at doses of 0.6 mg/kg or greater. The incidence of transient hypotension ranged from 1 to 14% respectively for the corresponding dosages. Other undesirable effects reported included bronchospasm, tachycardia and rarely anaphylactoid reactions.

In large scale atracurium surveillance studies, undesirable effects considered possibly or probably related to atracurium were observed in approximately 10% of patients. Localised skin reactions, generalised flushing and hypotension each occurred in approximately 2 to 3% of patients. Hypertension, tachycardia and bradycardia were observed in approximately 1% of patients. Bronchospasm was reported in approximately 0.2% of patients.

The following undesirable effects have been reported for atracurium:

General: Allergic reactions (i.e. anaphylactic or anaphylactoid responses) which in rare instances were severe (e.g. shock, cardiac failure, cardiac arrest), angioneurotic oedema.

Musculoskeletal: Inadequate block, prolonged block.

Cardiovascular: Hypotension, hypertension, vasodilatation (flushing), tachycardia, bradycardia, hypoxaemia.

Respiratory: Dyspnoea, bronchospasm, laryngospasm, wheezing.

Dermatological: Rash, urticaria, generalised erythema, skin flushing, reaction at injection site.

After prolonged administration of atracurium besilate in severely ill patients under intensive care, some incidences of muscle weakness and/or myopathy occurred. Most patients were concomitantly treated with cortiscosteroids. A causal relationship with atricurium therapy has not been established.

There have been rare reports of seizures in ICU patients who have been receiving atracurium concurrently with several other agents. These patients usually had one or more medical conditions predisposing to seizures (e.g. cranial trauma, cerebral oedoma, viral encephalitis, hypoxic encephalopathy, uraemia). In clinical trials, there appears to be not correlation between plasma laudanosine concentration and the occurrence of seizures.

Overdose: Prolonged muscle paralysis and its consequences are the main signs of overdose.

There is limited experience with atracurium overdosage following parenteral administration. The possibility of iatrogenic overdosage can be minimised by carefully monitoring muscle twitch response to peripheral nerve stimulation. Excessive doses of atracurium are likely to produce symptoms consistent with extensions of the usual pharmacological effects. Overdosage may increase the risk of histamine release and adverse cardiovascular effects, especially hypotension. If cardiovascular support is necessary, this should include proper positioning, fluid administration, and the use of vasopressor agents if necessary. It is essential to maintain a patent airway with assisted positive pressure ventilation until spontaneous respiration is adequate. Full sedation will be required since consciousness is not impaired. The duration of neuromuscular blockade may be prolonged and a peripheral nerve stimulator should be used to monitor recovery. Recovery may be hastened by the administration of an anticholinesterase agent such as neostigmine or pyridostigmine in conjunction with an anticholinergic agent such as atropine, once evidence of spontaneous recovery is present.

Pharmacodological properties

Pharmacodynamic properties: Atracurium besilate is a non-depolarising neuromuscular blocking agent

(ATC code M03A C04) with an intermediate duration of action, administered intravenously to produce skeletal muscle relaxation.

Non-depolarising neuromuscular blocking agents antagonise the action of the neurotransmitter acetylcholine by competitively binding with cholinergic receptor sites on the motor endplate of the myoneural junction. These effects may be inhibited or reversed by the administration of anticholinesterases such as neostigmine or pyridostigmine.

As with other non-depolarising neuromuscular blocking agents, the time to onset or paralysis is reduced, and the duration of maximum effect prolonged, with increasing atracurium doses.

Once recovery from atracurium's neuromuscular blocking effect begins, it proceeds more rapidly than recovery from tubocurarine, alcuronium, and pancuronium. Regardless of the atracurium dose, the time from start of recovery (from complete block) to complete recovery (as measured by restoration of the tetanic response to 95% of normal) is approximately 30 minutes under balanced anaesthesia, and approximately 40 minutes under halothane, enflurane or isoflurane anaesthesia. Repeated doses have no cumulative effect on recovery state.

With initial atracurium besilate doses up to 0.5 mg/kg, plasma histamine levels were shown to increase by 15% in a dose dependant way, but haemodynamic changes were minor within this dose range. Following the administration of 0.6 mg/kg of atracurium besilate, histamine levels were shown to increase by 92%, and were shown to correlate with a transient (5 minutes) decrease in blood pressure and a brief (2 to 3 minutes) episode of skin flushing. While these effects are of little clinical significance in most patients, the possibility of substantial histamine release at recommended doses must be considered in sensitive individuals, or in patients in whom substantial histamine release would be especially hazardous (e.g. patients with significant respiratory or cardiovascular disease).

Studies in malignant hyperthermia-susceptible pigs indicated that atracurium besilate does not trigger this syndrome. Clinical studies in patients with a history of malignant hyperthermia revealed the same results.

Atricurium besilate does not appear to affect intraocular pressure, therefore, it is not a suitable agents for ophthalmic surgery.

Pharmacokinetic properties: The pharmacokinetics of atracurium besilate in humans are essentially linear within the dose range of 0.3 to 0.6 mg/kg. The elimination half-life is approximately 20 minutes. The protein binding of atracurium is approximately 82%. The volume of distribution of atracurium is 0.16 l/kg. Some placental transfer occurs in humans.

The duration of neuromuscular blockade produced by atracurium does not correlate with plasma pseudocholinesterase levels and is not altered by the absence of renal function. This is is consistent with the results of *in vitro* studies which have shown that atracurium is inactivated in plasma via two non-oxidative pathways: ester hydrolysis, catalysed by non-specific esterases; and Hofmann elimination, a non-enzymatic chemical process which occurs at physiological pH and body temperature. The rate of Hofmann elimination, which is the principal route of elimination for atracurium, is increased at a higher pH or at higher temperatures, and reduced at a lower pH or lower temperatures.

Limited clinical experience on long term administration of atracurium besilate show only minimal effects of haemofiltration or haemodialysis on plasma levels of atracurium and its metabolites. The effects of haemoperfusion on plasma levels of atracurium and it metabolites are not known.

Preclinical safety data:
Carcinogenicity/mutagenicity: Carcinogenicity studies have not been performed. Atracurium yielded negative results for gene mutation in bacteria, and chromosomal damage in bone marrow of rats. A positive response in the mouse lymphoma assay was observed only at highly cytotoxic concentrations. This single positive response is not considered to be of clinical relevance.

Reproductive toxicity: Studies on fertility and post-natal growth, development and function of offspring have not been performed.

Pharmaceutical particulars

List of excipients: Benzenesulphonic acid and water for injections.

Incompatibilities: Atracurium Besilate Injection has an acid pH and therefore should not be mixed with alkaline solutions (e.g. barbiturate solutions) in the same syringe or administered simultaneously during intravenous infusion through the same needle.

Shelf life: 18 months

Special precautions for storage: Store at 2 to 8°C. Protect from light. Do not freeze.

Nature and contents of container: Box of 5×3 ml Type I glass ampoules (each ampoule contains atracurium besilate 25 mg/2.5 ml).

Box of 5×5 ml Type I glass ampoules (each ampoule contains atracurium besilate 50 mg/5 ml).

Box of 1×30 ml Type I glass vial with rubber closure (the vial contains atracurium besilate 250 mg/25 ml).

Instructions for use/handling: Contains no preservative. Discard residue immediately after use.

Marketing authorisation holder
Fauldling Pharmaceuticals plc, trading as David Bull Laboratories, Spartan Close, Tachbrook Park, Warwick CV34 6RS, United Kingdom.

Marketing authorisation number PL 4515/0099

Date of first authorisation/renewal of authorisation
15 October 1996

Date of (partial) revision of the text 8 April 1998

CALCIUM LEUCOVORIN INJECTION

Qualitative and quantitative composition

	3 mg/mL	*7.5 mg/mL*	*10 mg/mL presentations*
Active Constituent			
Leucovorin Calcium USP	3.24 mg	8.1 mg	10.8 mg
Equivalent to Leucovorin USP	3.0 mg	7.5 mg	10.0 mg
Other Constituents			
Sodium Chloride BP	8.6 mg	8.1 mg	8.5 mg
Water for Injections BP	to 1.0 ml	to 1.0 ml	to 1.0 ml

There is no overage included in the formulation.

Pharmaceutical form Sterile solution for injection.

Clinical particulars

Therapeutic indications: Calcium Leucovorin is indicated in:

a. Neutralising the immediate toxic effects of folic acid antagonists, e.g. Methotrexate.
b. Calcium Leucovorin Rescue–a treatment technique using Calcium Leucovorin in conjunction with folic acid antagonists, e.g. methotrexate, to minimise systemic toxicity.
c. The treatment of megaloblastic anaemias due to sprue, nutritional deficiency, pregnancy, infancy, liver disease and malabsorption syndrome.

Posology and method of administration:
Adults and children: Calcium Leucovorin may be given parenterally by intramuscular injection, intravenous injection or intravenous infusion. When required for intravenous infusion, it may be diluted with 5% glucose injection or 0.9% sodium chloride injection. Such solutions are stable for 24 hours when stored below 25°C.

Treatment of Overdosage of Folic Acid Antagonists: In cases of overdosage of folic acid antagonists, Calcium Leucovorin maybe administered by intravenous infusion in doses of up to 75 mg within 12 hours, followed by 12 mg intramuscularly every 6 hours for 4 doses.

In general, where overdosage is suspected, the dose of Calcium Leucovorin should be equal to or greater than the offending dose of the folic acid antagonist administered, and should be given as soon as possible; preferably within the first hour and certainly within 4 hours after which it may not be effective.

Calcium Leucovorin Rescue: Calcium Leucovorin may be used in conjunction with folic acid antagonists, e.g. methotrexate, to reduce their systemic toxicity. It is given 12 to 24 hours after the antineoplastic drug. Doses of up to 120 mg may be given over 12 to 24 hours by intramuscular injection or intravenous injection or infusion, followed by 12 to 15 mg intramuscularly, or 15 mg orally, every 6 hours for the next 48 hours. With lower doses of methotrexate, leucovorin 15 mg orally every 6 hours for 48 to 72 hours may be sufficient.

Treatment of Megaloblastic Anaemia: The dose should not exceed 1 mg daily given intramuscularly. When given orally, the recommended dosage is one Calcium Leucovorin Tablet (15 mg) daily. Children up to 12 years: 0.25 mg/kg/day. Normal adult dosage: 10-20 mg daily.

Contra-indications: Calcium Leucovorin Injection is contra-indicated in the treatment of pernicious anaemia or other megaloblastic anaemias where vitamin B_{12} is deficient. Its use can lead to an apparent response of the haematopoietic system, but neurological damage may occur or progress if already present.

Special warnings and special precautions for use:
Warnings: In the treatment of inadvertent overdosage of a folic acid antagonist, leucovorin should be administered as soon as possible; if a period exceeding 4 hours intervenes, the treatment may not be effective.

Precautions: In general, Calcium Leucovorin should not be given simultaneously with folic acid antagonists, e.g. methotrexate, to abort clinical toxicity as the therapeutic effect of the antagonist may be nullified. However, Calcium Leucovorin given concurrently with folate antagonists, such as pyrimethamine and trimethoprim does not inhibit their antibacterial activity.

Parenteral administration of leucovorin is preferable to oral dosing following chemotherapy with folic acid antagonists if there is a possibility that the patient may vomit and not absorb the leucovorin.

Calcium Leucovorin Injection should be given with haematological control.

Interaction with other medicaments and other forms of interaction: Not applicable.

Pregnancy and lactation: Animal reproduction studies have not been performed with Leucovorin. It is also not known whether Leucovorin can cause foetal harm, when administered to pregnant women. Leucovorin should be used during pregnancy only when clearly needed.

Since it is not known if Leucovorin is distributed into milk, the drug should be used with caution in nursing women.

Effects on ability to drive and use machines: Not applicable.

Undesirable effects: Adverse reactions are rare but occasional allergic reactions have been reported; pyrexia has occurred after parenteral administration.

Overdose: Not applicable.

Pharmacological properties

Pharmacodynamic properties: Leucovorin is a derivative of tetrahydrofolic acid, the reduced form of folic acid, which is involved as a cofactor for 1-carbon transfer reactions in the biosynthesis of purine and pyrimidines of nucleic acids.

Impairment of thymidylate synthesis in patients with folic acid deficiency is thought to account for the defective DNA synthesis that leads to megaloblast formation and megaloblastic and macrocytic anaemias. Because of its ready conversion to other tetrahydrofolic acid derivatives, Leucovorin is a potent antidote for both hematopoietic and reticuloendothelial toxic effects of folic acid antagonists, (e.g. Methotrexate, Pyrimethamine, Trimethoprim). It is postulated that in some cancers, Leucovorin enters and 'rescues' normal cells from the toxic effects of folic acid antagonists, in preference to tumour cells, because of a difference in membrane transport mechanisms; this principle is the basis of high-dose Methotrexate therapy with 'Leucovorin rescue'.

Pharmacokinetic properties: Absorption and distribution: In vivo, Leucovorin Calcium is rapidly and extensively converted to other tetrahydrofolic acid derivatives including 5-methyl tetrahydrofolate, which is the major transport and storage form of folate in the body.

Normal total serum folate concentrations have been reported to range from 0.005-0.015 mcg/mL. Folate is actively concentrated in CSF, and normal CSF concentrations are reported to be about 0.016-0.021 mcg/mL. Normal erythrocyte folate concentrations range from 0.175-0.316 mcg/mL.

In general, serum folate concentrations less than 0.005 mcg/mL indicate folate deficiency and concentrations less than 0.002 mcg/mL usually result in megaloblastic anaemia. Following i.m. administration of a 15 mg (7.5 mg/m^2) dose in healthy men, mean peak serum folate concentrations of 0.241 mcg/mL occur within about 40 minutes. Following oral administration of a 15 mg (7.5 mg/m^2) dose in healthy men, mean peak serum folate concentrations of 0.268 mcg/mL occur within about 1.72 hours. Areas under the serum folate concentration-time curves (AUCs) are reported to be about 8% less following i.m. injection in the gluteal region than in the deltoid region and about 12% less following i.m. injection in the gluteal region than following i.v. or oral administration.

Tetrahydrofolic acid and its derivatives are distributed to all body tissues; the liver contains about one-half of total body folate stores. In a small number of patients, biliary concentration of folates was about 4.5 times the plasma folate concentration after oral administration of a 2 mg dose of Leucovorin; this is believed to represent the hepatic folate pool rather than excretion of the administered dose.

Elimination: Leucovorin is excreted in urine, mainly as 10-formyl tetrahydrofolate and 5, 10-methenyl tetrahydrofolate. There is some evidence that 5-methyltetrahydrofolate may be conserved by the kidneys in preference to 5-formyltetrahydrofolate

(Leucovorin). Loss of folate in the urine becomes approximately logarithmic as the amount of Leucovorin administered exceeds 1 mg.

Pharmaceutical particulars
List of excipients:

	3 mg/mL	*7.5 mg/mL*	*10 mg/mL*
Sodium Chloride BP	8.6 mg	8.1 mg	8.5 mg
Water for Injections BP	to 1.0 mL	to 1.0 mL	to 1.0 mL

There is no overage included in the formulation.

Incompatibilities: Immediate precipitation results when combined with Droperidol in syringe.

Shelf life: 24 months.

Special precautions for storage: Store 2°C-8°C. Protect from light.

Ampoules and Vials of Calcium Leucovorin do not contain a preservative. They should be used once and discarded.

Instructions for use/handling: Not applicable.

Marketing authorisation number 4515/0032.

Date of approval/revision of SPC March 1998

Legal category POM

CARBOPLATIN INJECTION SOLUTION 10MG PER ML

Qualitative and quantitative composition

	per unit dose		*per vial*	
Carboplatin	10 mg	50 mg	150 mg	450 mg
Water for Injection BP	1.0 mL	5.0 mL	15.0 mL	45.0 mL

Pharmaceutical form Aqueous solution for injection.

Clinical particulars
Therapeutic indications: Antineoplastic agent indicated in the treatment of ovarian carcinoma of epithelial origin or in the treatment of small cell lung carcinoma.

Posology and method of administration: The recommended dose of Carboplatin in previously untreated adults with normal renal function is 400 mg/m2 given as a single short term intravenous infusion over 15 to 60 minutes. Therapy should not be repeated until 4 weeks after the previous Carboplatin course.

Initial dosage should be reduced by 20-25% in patients with risk factors such as previous myelosuppressive therapy and/or poor performance status.

Determination of haematologic nadir by weekly blood counts during initial courses is recommended for future dosage adjustment and scheduling of Carboplatin.

Impaired renal function: In patients with impaired renal function dosage of Carboplatin should be reduced and haematological nadirs and renal function monitored.

A suggested dosage schedule based on creatinine clearance is as follows:

Creatinine Clearance (ml/min)	*Dosage of Carboplatin*
40 ml per minute	400 mg per square metre
20–39 ml per minute	250 mg per square metre

Elderly: Dosage adjustment may be necessary in elderly patients and also in patients receiving combination chemotherapy.

Children: Specific dosage recommendations for use in children and infants cannot be made due to insufficient use in paediatrics at this time.

Contra-indications: Carboplatin is contra-indicated in patients with severe myelosuppression, preexisting severe renal impairment (with creatinine clearance of less than 20 ml per minute) and a history of severe allergic reaction to Carboplatin, other platinum containing compounds or Mannitol. Dosage adjustment may allow use in the presence of mild renal impairment (See *Posology and method of administration*).

Special warnings and special precautions for use:
Warnings: Myelosuppression as a result of Carboplatin treatment is closely related to the renal clearance of the drug. Therefore, in patients with abnormal renal function, or who are receiving concomitant therapy with nephrotoxic drugs, myelosuppression, especially thrombocytopenia, may be more severe and prolonged.

The occurrence, severity and protraction of toxicity is likely to be greater in patients who have received extensive prior treatment for their disease, have poor performance status and are advanced in years. Renal function parameters should be assessed prior to, during, and after Carboplatin therapy. Peripheral blood counts (including platelets, white blood cells and haemoglobin) should be followed during and after therapy. Combination therapy with other myelosuppressive drugs may require modification of dosage/timing of schedules in order to minimize additive effects.

Carboplatin courses should not, in general, be repeated more frequently than every 4 weeks in order to ensure that the nadir in blood counts has occurred and there has been recovery to a satisfactory level.

Precautions:
Carboplatin should only be administered under the supervision of a qualified physician who is experienced in the use of chemotherapeutic agents. Diagnostic and treatment facilities should be readily available for management of therapy and possible complications.

Peripheral blood counts and renal function tests should be monitored closely. Blood counts should be performed prior to commencement of Carboplatin therapy, and at weekly intervals thereafter. This will monitor toxicity and help determine the nadir and recovery of haematological parameters, and assist in subsequent dosage adjustments. Lowest levels of platelets are generally seen between days 14 and 21 of initial therapy. A greater reduction is seen in patients who previously received extensive myelosuppressive chemotherapy. Lowest Levels of white cells occur generally between days 14 and 28 of initial therapy. If levels fall below 2000 cells/mm³ or platelets less than 50,000 cells/mm³ then postponement of Carboplatin therapy until bone marrow recovery is evident, should be considered. This recovery usually takes 5 to 6 weeks. Transfusions may be necessary and dosage reductions recommended for subsequent treatment.

Renal toxicity is not usually dose limiting. Pretreatment and post-treatment hydration is not necessary. However, about 25% of patients show a decrease in creatinine clearance and, less frequently, a rise in serum creatinine and blood urea nitrogen. Impairment of renal function is more likely in patients who have previously experienced nephrotoxicity as a result of Cisplatin therapy.

Neurological evaluation and an assessment of hearing should be performed on a regular basis. Neurotoxicity, such as parasthesia, decreased deep tendon reflexes, and ototoxicity are more likely seen in patients previously treated with Cisplatin.

Aluminium containing equipment should not be used during preparation and administration of Carboplatin (see *Interactions*).

Interaction with other medicaments and other forms of interaction: Carboplatin may interact with aluminium to form a black precipitate. Needles, syringes, catheters or IV administration sets that contain aluminium parts which may come into contact with Carboplatin should not be used for the preparation or administration of the drug.

Concurrent therapy with nephrotoxic drugs may increase or exacerbate toxicity due to Carboplatin induced changes in renal clearance.

Combination therapy with other myelosuppressive agents may require dose changes or rescheduling of doses in order to minimise the additive myelosuppressive effects.

Pregnancy and lactation: Safe use of Carboplatin in pregnancy has not been established and its use is not recommended during pregnancy. It is not known whether Carboplatin is excreted in breast milk. To avoid possible harmful effects in the infant, breast feeding is not advised during Carboplatin therapy.

Effects on ability to drive and use machines: None known.

Undesirable effects:
Adverse reactions: Myelosuppression is the dose limiting toxic reaction of Carboplatin. It is generally reversible and not cumulative when Carboplatin is used as a single agent at recommended frequencies of administration. Adverse reactions which have occurred in studies to date can be grouped under the following systems:

Haemopoietic System: Leucopenia (55%), thrombocytopenia (32%) and anaemia (59%) of patients. Transfusion support has been required in about 20% of patients.

Gastrointestinal System: Nausea and vomiting (53%), nausea only in 25%. Nausea and vomiting are generally delayed until 6 to 12 hours after administration of Carboplatin, are readily controlled or prevented with antiemetics and disappear within 24 hours. Diarrhoea occurred in 6% and constipation in 3% of patients.

Renal System: Creatinine clearance decreased in 25% of patients. Increases in uric acid (25%), blood urea nitrogen (16%) and serum creatinine (7%).

Biochemistry: Decreased serum levels of magnesium (37% patients), potassium (16% patients) and calcium (5% patients) have occurred although not severe enough to cause clinical symptoms.

Neurotoxicity: Mild peripheral neuropathy occurred in 6% of patients and dysgeusia in less than 1% of patients. Parasthesias present prior to treatment, especially if caused by Cisplatin, may persist or worsen during Carboplatin therapy. (See Precautions).

Ototoxicity: A subclinical decrease in hearing acuity in the high frequency range (4000-8000 Hz), determined by audiogram, occurred in 15% of patients. Clinical ototoxicity also manifested itself as tinnitus (1% of patients). Hearing loss as a result of Cisplatin therapy may give rise to persistent or worsening symptoms.

Hepatic System: Transient increases in liver enzymes have been reported in some patients. Alkaline phosphatase was increased in 30% of patients, with aspartate aminotransferase (15% patients) and elevated serum bilirubin (4% patients) occurring less frequently.

Allergic Reactions: Erythematous rash, fever and pruritis have been observed in less than 2% of patients treated. These were reactions similar to those seen after Cisplatin therapy but in a few cases no cross-reactivity was present.

Other Reactions: Rare events have included alopecia (2%), a flu-like syndrome (1%) and reaction at the injection site (<1%).

Overdose: No overdosage occurred during clinical trials. If necessary, however, the patient may need supportive treatment relating to myelosuppression, renal and hepatic impairment. Reports of doses up to 1600 mg/m2 indicate patients feeling extremely ill with diarrhoea and alopecia developing.

Pharmacological properties
Pharmacodynamic properties: Carboplatin, like Cisplatin, interferes with DNA intrastrand and interstrand crosslinks in cells exposed to the drug. DNA reactivity has been correlated with cytotoxicity.

Pharmacokinetic properties: After a 1 hour infusion (20-520 mg/m²) plasma levels of total platinum and free (ultrafilterable) platinum decay biphasically following first order kinetics. For free platinum the initial phase (t alpha) half life is approximately 90 minutes, and the later phase (t beta) half life approximately 6 hours. All free platinum is in the form of Carboplatin in the first 4 hours after administration.

Carboplatin is excreted primarily by glomerular filtration in urine, with recovery of 65% of a dose within 24 hours. Most of the drug is excreted within the first 6 hours. Approximately 32% of a given dose of Carboplatin is excreted unchanged.

Protein binding of Carboplatin reaches 85-89% within 24 hours of administration although during the first 4 hours only up to 29% of the dose is protein bound. Patients with poor renal function may require dosage adjustments due to altered pharmacokinetics of Carboplatin.

Pharmaceutical particulars
List of excipients: Water for Injection BP

Incompatibilities: Aluminium-containing equipment should not be used (see *Interactions*).

Shelf life: A shelf life of 24 months when stored below 25°C and protected from light.

Special precautions for storage: Store below 25°C. Protect from light.

Carboplatin Injection Solution may be further diluted in Glucose 5% or Sodium Chloride 0.9% BP and administered as an intravenous infusion. This infusion solution is chemically stable for 24 hours when stored at room temperature.

Instructions for use/handling:
Handling: Carboplatin should be prepared for administration only by professionals who have been trained in the safe use of chemotherapeutic agents.

Transfer to syringes and infusion containers should be carried out only in the designated area. Personnel carrying out these procedures should be adequately protected with clothing, gloves, and an eye shield.

Pregnant personnel are advised not to handle chemotherapeutic agents.

Contamination: In the event of contact of Carboplatin with eyes or skin, wash the affected area with copious amounts of water or Normal Saline. A bland cream may be used to treat transient stinging of skin. Medical advice should be sought if the eyes are affected.

In the event of spillage, two operators should put on gloves and mop up the spilled material with a sponge kept for that purpose. Rinse the area twice with water. Put all solutions and sponges in a plastic bag, seal and label with the words 'CYTOTOXIC WASTE' and incinerate.

Disposal: Syringes, containers, absorbent materials, solutions and any other material which has come into contact with Carboplatin should be placed in a thick plastic bag or other impervious container and incinerated at 1000°C.

Marketing authorisation number 4515/0050

Date of approval/revision of SPC June 1995

Legal category POM

CISPLATIN INJECTION SOLUTION

Qualitative and quantitative composition

	10 mg	*50 mg*	*100 mg*
Active Constituent			
Cis-Diammine Dicloroplatinum (II) HSE	10.0 mg	50.0 mg	100.0 mg
Other Constituents			
Mannitol BP	10.0 mg	50.0 mg	100.0 mg
Sodium Chloride BP	90.0 mg	450.0 mg	900.0 mg
Dilute Hydrochloric Acid BP	QS	QS	QS
Water for Injections BP to:	10.0 ml	50.0 ml	100.0 ml

There is no overage included in the above formulations.

Pharmaceutical form A sterile, clear, colourless to pale yellow preservative-free solution free from visible particulates.

Clinical particulars

Therapeutic indications: Cisplatin is indicated in metastatic, non-seminomatous germ cell carcinoma, advanced stage and refractory ovarian carcinoma, advanced stages and refractory bladder carcinoma and squamous cell carcinoma of head and neck.

Cisplatin is indicated in combination with other antineoplastic agents for the treatment of metastatic testicular tumours. The combination of Cisplatin, Vinblastine and Bleomycin is reported to be highly effective.

Posology and method of administration:

Adults and children: Cisplatin should be administered by I.V. infusion over a 6-8 hour period. The recommended dose of Cisplatin in adults and children is 50 to 100 mg/m² as a single I.V. dose every 3 to 4 weeks, or 15 to 20 mg/m² intravenously daily for 5 days every 3 to 4 weeks.

Interaction with aluminium:

Cisplatin may interact with metal aluminium to form a black precipitate of platinum. All aluminium-containing I.V. sets, needles, catheters and syringes should be avoided.

1. Pretreatment Hydration: Pretreatment hydration is required to induce diuresis during (and after) Cisplatin administration. This hydration is achieved by giving 2 litres of either 0.9% Sodium Chloride or Dextrose 4% in one-fifth Normal Saline (0.18%) over a 2-hour period. During the last 30 minutes of the pre-treatment hydration or after the hydration, administer by side arm drip 37.5 g of Mannitol (i.e., 375 ml of Mannitol 10% Injection).
2. Preparation of Cisplatin Infusion: Cisplatin Injection Solution 1 mg/mL may be diluted in 2 litres of 0.9% Sodium Chloride Injection. Do not refrigerate solutions.
3. Treatment: Following prehydration, administer the Cisplatin infusion over 1 to 2 hours. It has been proposed that a longer infusion time of 6 to 8 hours may decrease the gastrointestinal and renal toxicities. The container should be covered to exclude light. Discard remaining contents after use.
4. Post Treatment Hydration: Continue I.V. hydration with the aim of administering another 2 litres of Sodium Chloride 0.9% Injection, or Dextrose 4% in Sodium Chloride 0.18% Injection, over a period of 6 to 12 hours.

Contra-indications: Cisplatin may give allergic reactions in some patients. Use is contraindicated in those patients with a history of allergic reaction to Cisplatin or other platinum containing compounds. Cisplatin induces nephrotoxicity which is cumulative. It is therefore contraindicated in patients with renal impairment. The serum creatinine, BUN, and creatinine clearance should be measured prior to initiating therapy and monitored throughout treatment with Cisplatin. To reduce nephrotoxicity of Cisplatin treatment pretreatment hydration procedures, together with maintenance of hydration and urinary output during the 24 hours following administration are necessary.

Cisplatin has been shown to be cumulatively ototoxic and should not be given to patients with hearing impairment. It is recommended that hearing function should be monitored prior to and during treatment with Cisplatin. Cisplatin is also contraindicated in myelosuppressed patients.

Special warnings and precautions for use:

Warnings and precautions: Cisplatin must only be used by physicians experienced in cytotoxic chemotherapy.

Cisplatin reacts with metallic aluminium to form a black precipitate of platinum. All aluminium containing I.V. sets, needles, catheters and syringes should be avoided.

The solution for infusion should not be mixed with other drugs or additives.

Interactions with other medicaments and other forms of interaction: Cisplatin and antihypertensive therapy with Frusemide, Hydralazine Diazoxide and Propanolol have been reported to cause nephrotoxicity.

Cisplatin may interact with aluminium. See *Dosage and Administration.*

Pregnancy and lactation:

Use in pregnancy: The safe use of Cisplatin in human pregnancy has not been established. Cisplatin has been shown to be mutagenic in bacteria. It produces chromosome aberrations in tissue-cultures of animal cells and is teratogenic and embryotoxic in mice.

Use in lactation: Cisplatin should not normally be administered to mothers who are breastfeeding.

Effects on ability to drive and use machines: Not applicable.

Undesirable effects:

1. Nephrotoxicity: Renal toxicity has been shown in 28-38% of patients treated with a single dose of Cisplatin 50 mg/m². Renal toxicity becomes more prolonged and severe with repeated courses of the drug. Renal function must be restored before additional Cisplatin therapy is used.
2. Ototoxicity: Ototoxicity has occurred in up to 31% of patients treated with a single dose of Cisplatin 50 mg/m². Ototoxicity may be more severe in children and more frequent and severe with repeated doses.
3. Haemotoxicity: Myelosuppression is observed in about 30% of patients treated with Cisplatin. Leucopenia and thrombocytopenia are more pronounced at higher doses.
4. Myelosuppression: This may occur in patients treated with Cisplatin. The nadirs in circulating platelets and leucocytes generally occur between days 18-32 (range 7.3 to 45) with most patients recovering by day 39 (range 13 to 62). Leucopenia and thrombocytopenia are more pronounced at doses greater than 50 mg/m². Anaemia (decreases of greater than 2 g% haemoglobin) occurs at approximately the same frequency, but generally with a later onset than leucopenia and thrombocytopenia. Subsequent courses of Cisplatin should not be instituted until platelets are present at levels greater than 100.000/mm³ and white cells greater than 4.000/mm³. A high incidence of severe anaemia requiring transfusion of packed red cells has been observed in patients receiving combination chemotherapy including Cisplatin.
5. Anaphylaxis: Reactions possibly secondary to Cisplatin therapy have been occasionally reported in patients who were previously exposed to Cisplatin. Patients who are particularly at risk are those with a prior history or family history of atopy. Facial oedema, wheezing, tachycardia, hypotension and skin rashes of urticarial non-specific maculopapular type can occur within a few minutes of administration. Serious reactions seem to be controlled by I.V. adrenaline, corticosteroids or antihistamines.
6. Hypomagnesaemia and Hypocalcaemia: Hypomagnesaemia occurs quite frequently with Cisplatin administration, while hypocalcaemia occurs less frequently. The loss of magnesium seems to be associated with renal tubular damage which prevents resorption of this cation. Where both electrolytes are deficient, tetany may result. It does not appear to be dose related. Monitoring of electrolytes is necessary.
7. Neurotoxicity and Seizures: Peripheral neuropathy, postural hypotension and seizures may occur with Cisplatin administration. This appears to be common after Cisplatin administration. The development of clinically significant symptoms should generally contra-indicate further Cisplatin usage.

Overdose: Overdosage can be expected to cause the toxic effects described above, but to an exaggerated degree. Adequate hydration and osmotic diuresis may help reduce the toxicity of Cisplatin if administered promptly following overdosage.

Convulsions may be treated with appropriate anticonvulsants. Renal function, cardiovascular function and blood counts should be monitored daily in order to assess the potential toxicity to these systems. Serum magnesium and calcium levels should be carefully monitored as should symptoms and signs of voluntary muscle irritability. If symptomatic tetany develops, electrolyte supplements should be administered. Serum liver enzymes and uric acid should also be monitored daily after an acute overdose.

If fever develops during prolonged myelosuppression, appropriate presumptive antibiotic coverage should be instilled after cultures have been obtained.

Pharmacological properties

Pharmacodynamic properties: Cisplatin has biochemical properties similar to those of bifunctional alkylating agents. The drug inhibits DNA synthesis by producing intrastrand and interstrand cross links in DNA. Protein and RNA synthesis are also inhibited to a lesser extent.

Although the principal mechanism of action of Cisplatin appears to be inhibition of DNA synthesis, other mechanisms, including enhancement of tumour immunogenicity, may be involved in its antineoplastic activity. Cisplatin also has immunosuppressive, radiosensitising, and antimicrobial properties.

Cisplatin does not appear to be cell cycle specific.

Pharmacokinetic properties: There is good uptake of Cisplatin by the kidneys, liver and intestine. More than 90% of platinum containing species remaining in the blood are bound (possibly irreversibly) to plasma proteins.

Penetration into the CSF is poor although significant amounts of Cisplatin can be detected in intracerebral tumours.

The clearance of total platinum from plasma is rapid during the first four hours after intravenous administration, but then proceeds more slowly because of covalent binding to serum proteins. Levels of unbound platinum fall with a half-life of 20 minutes to 1 hour depending on the rate of drug infusion.

The elimination of intact drug and various platinum-containing biotransformation products is via the urine. About 15-25% of administered platinum is rapidly excreted in the first 2-4 hours after administration of Cisplatin. This early excretion is mostly of intact Cisplatin. In the first 24 hours after administration, 20-80% is excreted, the remainder representing drug bound to tissues or plasma protein.

Preclinical safety data: There are no pre-clinical data of relevance to the prescriber which are additional to that already included in other sections of the SPC.

Pharmaceutical particulars

List of excipients:

	10 mg	*50 mg*	*100 mg*
Mannitol BP	10.0 mg	50.0 mg	100.0 mg
Sodium Chloride BP	90.0 mg	450.0 mg	900.0 mg
Dilute Hydrochloric Acid BP	QS	QS	QS
Water for Injections BP to:	10.0 ml	50.0 ml	100.0 ml

There is no overage included in the above formulations.

Incompatibilities: There is a total loss of Cisplatin in 30 minutes at room temperature when mixed with Metoclopramide and Sodium Metabisulphite in concentrations equivalent to those that would be found on mixing with a commercial formulation of Metoclopramide.

Cisplatin and Sodium Bisulphite have been known to react chemically. Such antioxidants might inactivate Cisplatin before administration if they are present in intravenous fluids.

Shelf life: 48 months.

Special precautions for storage: All preparations and reconstituted solutions must be stored between 15°C and 25°C. Do not store in refrigerator. Protect from light.

Instruction for use/handling: Not applicable.

Marketing authorisation number 4515/0026

Date of approval/revision of SPC 12 March 1996

Legal category POM

STERILE CO-TRIMOXAZOLE CONCENTRATE BP

Qualitative and quantitative composition

	480 mg/ 5 ml	*960 mg/ 10 ml*	*1920 mg/ 20 ml*
Active Constituent			
Trimethoprim BP	80 mg	160 mg	320 mg
Sulphamethoxazole BP	400 mg	800 mg	1600 mg

	480 mg/ 5 ml	960 mg/ 10 ml	1920 mg/ 20 ml
Other Constituents			
Diethanolamine HSE	0.015 mL	0.030 mL	0.06 mL
Propylene Glycol BP	2.0 mL	4.0 mL	8.0 mL
Ethanol BP	0.5 mL	1.0 mL	2.0 mL
Sodium Metabisulphite BP	5.0 mg	10 mg	20 mg
Sodium Hydroxide BP	62.5 mg	125 mg	250 mg
Water for Injections BP to:	5.0 mL	10 mL	20 mL

There is no overage included in the above formulations.

Pharmaceutical form Strong sterile solution.

Clinical particulars

Therapeutic indications: Co-trimoxazole is an antibacterial combination product. It is bactericidal at concentrations at which the components are usually bacteriostatic, and is frequently active against organisms which are resistant to one of the components.

Treatment and prophylaxis (primary and secondary) of Pneumocystis carinii pneumonitis in adults and children.

Treatment and prophylaxis of toxoplasmosis, treatment of nocardia.

Treatment of urinary tract infections and acute exacerbations of chronic bronchitis, where there is bacterial evidence of sensitivity to Cotrimoxazole and good reason to prefer this combination to a single antibiotic.

Treatment of acute otitis media in children, where there is a good reason to prefer cotrimoxazole to a single antibiotic.

Parenteral administration of Co-trimoxazole is indicated where oral dosage is not desirable or practical, e.g. pre- and post-operative infections associated with surgery, trauma and gynaecology.

Posology and method of administration: Sterile Co-trimoxazole Concentrate BP MUST BE DILUTED prior to administration.

It should be administered intravenously only in the form of an infusion solution, and may not be injected undiluted either intravenously or directly into infusion tube.

The prepared infusion should be shaken well to ensure thorough mixing. Should visible turbidity or crystallisation appear in the solution at any time before or during infusion, the mixture should be discarded and replaced by a freshly prepared solution.

It is recommended that infusion of co-trimoxazole be commenced within half an hour of preparation and the duration of infusion should not exceed one and a half hours. However, this should be balanced against the fluid requirements of the patient.

Sterile Co-trimoxazole Concentrate BP may be mixed only with the following infusion solutions:

Glucose Injection BP 5% or 10%
Laevulose Injection BP 5%
Sodium Chloride Injection BP 0.45% or 0.9%
Sodium Chloride Injection BP 0.45% in Glucose 2.5%
Sodium Chloride Injection BP 0.18% in Glucose 4%
Dextran 40 Injection BP
Dextran 70 Injection BP
Dextran Injection BP 6% or 10% in Glucose 5%
Dextran Injection BP 6% or 10% in normal saline
Ringer's Injection USP

No other agent should be added to or mixed with the infusion.

It is important to adhere to the following dilution scheme:

Add 5 mL Sterile Co-trimoxazole Concentrate BP to 125 mL infusion solution

10 mL Sterile Co-trimoxazole Concentrate BP to 250 mL infusion solution

15 mL to 500 mL infusion solution or an equivalent dilution

In addition, dilutions of the following for the treatment of patients with PCP can be used:

2 x 5 mL amps in 125 mL of 5% dextrose, normal saline or saline/dextrose.

or

4 x 5 mL amps in 125 mL of normal saline injection solution

Dosage for adults and children over 12 years: Standard dose: 10 ml diluted and infused twice daily.

For severe infections: 15 ml diluted and infused twice daily.

Dosage for children up to 12 years: The recommended dosage is approximately 6 mg trimethoprim and 30 mg sulphamethoxazole per kg bodyweight per day, divided into two equal doses, morning and evening.

As a guide, the following doses of Sterile Co-trimoxazole Concentrate BP may be used:

6 weeks to 5 months: 1.25 mL diluted to 30 mL and infused twice daily.

6 months to 5 years: 2.5 mL diluted to 60 mL and infused twice daily.

6 years to 12 years: 5 mL diluted to 120 mL and infused twice daily.

In severe infections the paediatric dosage may be increased by 50%.

Table 1: Co-trimoxazole dosages in impaired renal function

Criteria of kidney function		*Recommended dosage regimens*
Creatinine Clearance (ml/min.)	Serum Creatinine (μmol/l) (a)	One standard dose for adults. 160 mg trimethoprim and 800 mg sulphamethoxazole.
Above 30	Men <260 Women < 170	Dosage as for patients with normal kidney function.
30-15	Men 260-600 Women 170-400	One standard dose every 12 hours for 3 days; thereafter one standard dose every 24 hours as long as allowed by control analyses (b).
Below 15	Men >600 Women >400	Until further experience is gained, the combination should be given only if patients can undergo haemodialysis when necessary (c); under this condition one standard dose may be administered every 24 hours as long as allowed by control analyses (b).

a. Serum creatinine levels can be used as the basis of dosing only in cases of stable chronic renal impairment, but not acute or subacute kidney failure.

b. The concentration of total sulphamethoxazole should be measured in plasma samples obtained 12 hours after every third day of treatment.

Treatment must be interrupted if at any time the determined plasma level of total sulphamethoxazole exceeds 150 microgram/ml. As soon as the value of total sulphamethoxazole drops again below 120 microgram/ml (e.g. in patients undergoing haemodialysis), treatment can be continued as recommended.

c. Both trimethoprim and sulphamethoxazole are readily dialysable, leading to a significantly shortened half-life for each drug during dialysis. It is suggested that patients undergoing haemodialysis receive a dose just before and at the end of the procedure.

No data are available relating to dosage in children with renal failure.

The recommended dosage for patients with documented Pneumocystis carinii pneumonitis is 20 mg/kg trimethoprim and 100mg/kg sulphamethoxazole per 24 hours given in equally divided doses every 6 hours for 14 days.

Duration of treatment: Sterile Co-trimoxazole Concentrate BP should be used ONLY during such periods as the patient is unable to accept oral therapy. In general, administration is unlikely to be required for more than a few days.

Dosage in impaired renal function: In patients with impaired renal function, the dosage and/or frequency of administration of co-trimoxazole needs to be modified. Dosages are suggested in Table 1.

Contra-indications: Co-trimoxazole should not be given to patients with known hypersensitivity or with documented megaloblastic anaemia secondary to folate deficiency.

It is contraindicated in patients showing marked liver parenchymal damage, blood dyscrasias and severe renal insufficiency where repeated measurements of the plasma concentrations cannot be performed.

Infants under 6 weeks of age except in the management of PCP where this may be from 4 weeks of age should not be given co-trimoxazole because sulphamethoxazole may interfere with the serum albumin binding of bilirubin and produce kernicterus.

Special warnings and special precautions for use: *Warnings:* Prolonged parenteral administration of preparations containing propylene glycol can lead to lactic acidosis.

A number of serious side effects; aplastic anaemia, pancytopenia and thrombocytopenia are reported as occurring more frequently in the elderly. Accordingly, co-trimoxazole should not be prescribed in elderly patients unless the benefits are felt to exceed the increased risk of these serious side effects.

Fatalities may occur in severe skin, hepatic and blood disorders and pulmonary hypersensitivity; discontinue immediately with skin rashes; haemolysis in patients with G6PD deficiency; avoid in patients at risk of acute porphyria; do not use in Group A beta-haemolytic streptococci; can be used in patients with phenylketonuria on special diet.

Precautions: Care should be taken when giving Co-trimoxazole, to patients with liver damage, renal damage, urinary obstruction, blood dyscrasias, allergies or bronchial asthma.

In renal impairment reduced or less frequent dosage is recommended in order to avoid accumulation of trimethoprim in the blood. For such patients serum assays are necessary and adequate fluid intake must be maintained in order to avoid crystalluria and stone formation (see Table 1).

Because of the possible interference with folate metabolism, regular blood counts are advisable in patients on long-term therapy; in those who are predisposed to folate deficiency (i.e. the elderly, chronic alcoholics and rheumatoid arthritics), in malabsorption syndromes, malnutrition states or during the treatment of epilepsy with anticonvulsant drugs such as phenytoin, primidone and barbiturates.

Finally, the possibility of super-infection with a non-sensitive organism should be born in mind.

Interaction with other medicaments and other forms of interaction: Sulphamethoxazole may displace methotrexate from protein binding sites.

PABA or its derivatives may antagonise the antibacterial effects of sulphamethoxazole, while rifampicin may decrease trimethoprim concentrations. Increased sulphamethoxazole blood levels may occur in patients who are also receiving urinary acidifiers, oral anticoagulants, phenylbutazone, oxyphenbutazone and indomethacin.

As co-trimoxazole possesses anti-folate properties, the drug increases the incidence of folate deficiencies induced by other drugs such as phenytoin and pyrimethamine when used concomitantly.

Cross sensitisation may exist between Co-trimoxazole and some antithyroid agents, diuretics (acetazolamide), cyclosporin and oral hypoglycaemic drugs.

Care should be taken in patients receiving warfarin and sulphonylurea hypoglycaemic agents and cations at physiological pH, e.g. procainamide, amantadine and digoxin since their action could be increased.

Pregnancy and lactation

Use in pregnancy: Since trimethoprim is a folate antagonist, it might be expected to cause teratogenic effects. Foetal malformations commonly associated with lack of folic acid have occurred in several animal species when trimethoprim was administered to the pregnant female. The teratogenic effects were prevented by concurrent administration of dietary folates. No teratogenic effects have yet been reported in women. Nevertheless, since folate levels are probably marginal in pregnant women, the combination of trimethoprim and sulphamethoxazole is generally contraindicated, or should only be used with the full knowledge of the potential danger during pregnancy.

Furthermore, sulphamethoxazole should not be administered in late pregnancy because of the risk of kernicterus.

Use in lactation: Both trimethoprim and sulphamethoxazole are excreted in breast milk at concentrations comparable or somewhat lower than that in the blood. Although the quantity of Co-trimoxazole ingested by a breast-feeding infant is small, it is recommended that the possible risks be balanced against the therapeutic benefits.

Effects on ability to drive and use machines: Not applicable.

Undesirable effects: At the recommended dose Co-trimoxazole is well tolerated, but may occasionally give rise to local side effects in the form of mild to moderate venous pain and phlebitis.

In general, the adverse reactions (5-7%) correspond to those of a sulphonamide of moderately low toxicity.

During the administration of Co-trimoxazole, the possibility of blood dyscrasias should be taken into account.

Nausea and vomiting are the most frequent gastro-intestinal reactions to Cotrimoxazole, but glossitis, stomatitis, abdominal pain, pancreatitis, diarrhoea, anorexia, raised hepatic transaminases, rarely cholestatic jaundice and hepatic necrosis have been reported.

Haematological changes have been observed in some patients, particularly the elderly. The great majority of these changes were mild, asymptomatic and proved reversible on withdrawal of the drug. The reported changes consist primarily of neutropenia and thrombocytopenia. Leucopenia, aplastic and haemolytic anaemia, purpura, agranulocytosis and bone marrow depression rare. Reports have also been noted of megaloblastic anaemia, methaemoglobinaemia, haemolysis in patients with G6PD deficiency; reactions may be worse in patients with poor hepatic or renal function and poor folate status.

A number of serious side effects; aplastic anaemia, pancytopenia and thrombocytopenia are reported as occurring more frequently in the elderly. Accordingly, Co-trimoxazole should not be prescribed in elderly patients the benefits are felt to exceed the increased risk of these serious side effects.

Pseudomembranous colitis has been reported as well as several cases of Stevens-Johnson and Lyell's syndrome. Jaundice rarely occurs and has usually been mild and transient, frequently occurring in patients with a past history of infectious hepatitis.

Skin reactions which have been noted include rashes, photosensitivity, exfoliative dermatitis and erythema multiforme.

Allergic reactions which have been noted include serum sickness, anaphylaxis, allergic myocarditis, angiodema, drug fever, peri-arteritis nodosa and SLE.

Neurological reactions which have been noted include aseptic meningitis (reversible on withdrawal), convulsions, peripheral neuritis, ataxia, vertigo, tinnitus, headache, depression, dizziness and hallucinations.

Genitourinary reactions include impaired renal function and rarely interstitial nephritis.

Reported respiratory reactions include cough, dyspnoea, pulmonary infiltration and indicative of hypersensitivity.

Reported metabolic reactions include hyperkalaemia and hyponatraemia, which may be worse in the elderly and with high doses.

Musculoskeletal reactions which have been noted include arthralgia and myalgia.

It should be noted that adverse reactions may be more severe in the management of PCP.

Overdose: Stop therapy. Force fluids orally or parenterally if renal function is normal.

In excessive overdosage in patients with impaired renal function, consider dialysis, since both drugs are readily dialysable.

Calcium leucovorin may be used as an effective antidote for adverse effects in the haemopoietic system caused by trimethoprim.

Pharmacological properties

Pharmacodynamic properties: Co-trimoxazole usually is bactericidal. Of its components, sulphamethoxazole is bacteriostatic and trimethoprim usually is bactericidal. Co-trimoxazole acts by sequentially inhibiting enzymes of the folic acid pathway; sulphamethoxazole inhibits the formation of dihydrofolic acid from p-aminobenzoic acid and, by inhibiting dihydrofolate reductase, trimethoprim inhibits the formation of tetrahydrofolic acid from dihydrofolic acid.

By inhibiting synthesis of tetrahydrofolic acid, the metabolically active form of folic acid, co-trimoxazole inhibits bacterial thymidine synthesis.

Sequential inhibition by co-trimoxazole of two steps in the folic acid pathway appears to be responsible for the antibacterial synergism of the trimethoprim-sulphamethoxazole combination. For most organisms optimum synergistic antibacterial action occurs in vitro at a trimethoprim : sulphamethoxazole ratio about 1 : 20, which is also the approximate peak serum concentration ratio of 2 drugs achieved following oral or I.V. administration of co-trimoxazole. Synergistic activity also has been observed in vitro at trimethoprim : sulphamethoxazole ratios of 1:1 - 1:40.

Susceptibility of organisms to trimethoprim usually is more critical to the efficacy of co-trimoxazole than is susceptibility to sulphamethoxazole.

Many organisms that are resistant to sulphamethoxazole but susceptible to trimethoprim will show synergistic antibacterial response to co-trimoxazole. However, for Neisseria gonorrhoeae, susceptibility to sulphamethoxazole is required for antibacterial response to co-trimoxazole.

Pharmacokinetic properties: Co-trimoxazole is rapidly and well absorbed from the G.I. tract. Peak serum concentrations of 1-2 mg/ml of trimethoprim and 40-60 mg/ml of unbound sulphamethoxazole are reached 1-4 hours after a single oral dose of co-trimoxazole containing 160 mg trimethoprim and 800 mg of sulphamethoxazole.

Co-trimoxazole is widely distributed into body tissues and fluids including sputum, aqueous humour, middle ear fluid, prostatic fluid, vaginal fluid, bile and CSF. Trimethoprim is approximately 44% and sulphamethoxazole is approximately 70% bound to plasma proteins. Co-trimoxazole readily crosses the placenta and is distributed into breast milk. High concentrations of co-trimoxazole are achieved in the urine.

Sulphamethoxazole and trimethoprim are both excreted unchanged and as metabolites mainly by the kidneys. Both compounds have elimination half-lives of approximately 12 hours.

Renal Impairment: Because both compounds are cleared largely via the kidneys, their half-lives are significantly increased in patients with creatinine clearance less than 30 ml per minute. This reduction of dosage is required when patients with renal impairment are treated with co-trimoxazole.

Pharmaceutical particulars

List of excipients:

	480 mg/ 5 ml	*960 mg/ 10 ml*	*1920 mg/ 20 ml*
Diethanolamine HSE	0.015 mL	0.030 mL	0.06 mL
Propylene Glycol BP	2.0 mL	4.0 mL	8.0 mL
Ethanol BP	0.5 mL	1.0 mL	2.0 mL
Sodium Metabisulphite BP	5.0 mg	10 mg	20 mg
Sodium Hydroxide BP	62.5 mg	125 mg	250 mg
Water for Injections BP to:	5.0 mL	10 mL	20 mL

There is no overage included in the above formulations.

Incompatibilities: No other agent should be added to or mixed with the infusion.

Shelf life: 36 months.

Special precautions for storage: Store below 30°C. Do not refrigerate. Protect from light. If stored at low temperatures, precipitation may occur, and solutions in which precipitation has occurred could be discarded.

Instructions for use/handling: Not applicable.

Marketing authorisation number 4515/0023.

Date of approval/revision of SPC 5 February 1996

Legal category POM

CYTARABINE INJECTION SOLUTION 20MG/ML

Qualitative and quantitative composition

Active Constituent	
Cytarabine BP	2.0% w/v
Other Constituents	
Sodium Chloride BP	6.8 mg
Water for Injections BP	to 1.0 mL

There is no overage in the formulation.

Pharmaceutical form Aqueous, sterile isotonic solution for injection.

Clinical particulars

Therapeutic indications: Cytarabine may be used alone or in combination with other antineoplastic agents. It is indicated alone or in combination for induction of remission and/or maintainance in patients with acute myeloid leukaemia, acute non-lymphoblastic leukaemias, acute lymphoblastic leukaemias, acute lymphocytic leukaemia, erythroleukaemia, blast crises of chronic myeloid leukaemia, diffuse histiocytic lymphomas (non-hodgkin's lymphomas of high malignancy), meningeal leukaemia and meningeal neoplasms. Clinicians should refer to the current literature on combination therapy before initiating treatment.

Posology and method of administration: Cytarabine Injection Solution is a ready to use solution with a concentration of 20 mg/mL. The 20 mg/mL presentation is suitable for intravenous, subcutaneous and intrathecal use.

Cytarabine Injection Solution can be diluted with Sterile Water for Injection BP, Glucose 5% Injection BP or Sodium Chloride 0.9% Injection BP. Prepared infusions, in the recommended diluents should be used immediately. Alternatively, the diluted infusion fluids may be stored at 2-8°C, protected from light, but portions remaining unused after 24 hours must be discarded.

Remission induction: Adults

Continuous dosing: The usual dose in leukaemia, is 2 mg/kg by rapid intravenous injection daily for ten days. If after ten days neither therapeutic response not toxicity has been observed, the dose may be increased to 4 mg per kg until a therapeutic response or toxicity is evident. Daily blood counts should be taken. Almost all patients can be carried to toxicity with these doses.

Alternatively, 0.5 to 1 mg/kg may be infused daily in 1-24 hours for ten days, and then at a rate of 2 mg/kg/day until toxicity is observed. Continue to toxicity or until remission occurs. Results from one hour infusions have been satisfactory in the majority of patients.

Intermittent dosing: Cytarabine may be given as intermittent IV doses of 3-5 mg/kg daily, for five consecutive days This course of treatment can be repeated after an interval of 2 to 9 days, and repeated until the therapeutic response or toxicity is exhibited.

Evidence of bone marrow improvement has been reported to occur 7-64 days after the beginning of therapy.

In general, if a patient shows neither remission or toxicity after a trial period, then cautiously administered higher doses can be administered. Generally patients tolerate higher doses given by rapid intravenous injection rather than slow infusion.

As a single agent for induction of remissions in patients with acute leukaemia, Cytarabine has been given in doses of 200 mg/m² by continuous IV infusion for five days at approximately 2 week intervals.

Maintainance therapy: To maintain remission, doses of 1-1.5 mg/kg may be given intravenously or subcutaneously, once or twice weekly.

Leukaemic meningitis: Therapy for established meningitis employs a wide variety of dose regimens but a recommended total daily dose not exceeding 100 mg, alternating with Methotrexate (given either systemically or intrathecally) is recommended. Cytarabine Injection has been given intrathecally at doses of 10-30 mg per m² three times a week until CSF findings return to normal.

Myelosuppression, anaemia and thrombocytopenia occur in almost all patients given daily infusions or injections. Myelosuppression is biphasic and nadirs at 7-9 and 15-24 days. Evidence of bone marrow improvement may be expected 7-64 (mean 28) days after the beginning of treatment.

Children: Children appear to tolerate higher doses of Cytarabine than adults, and where the range of doses is given, children should receive the higher dose.

Elderly: No data is available to suggest that a change in dose is necessary in the elderly. However, the elderly patient is more susceptable to toxic reactions and therefore particular attention should be paid to drug induced leucopenia, thrombocytopenia and anaemia.

Contra-indications: Cytarabine is contra-indicated in patients with known hypersensitivity to the drug. Therapy with Cytarabine should not be considered in patients with pre-existing drug-induced bone marrow suppression, unless in the opinion of the physician the potential benefits outweigh the hazards. Cytarabine should not be used in the management of non-malignant disease, except for immunosuppression.

Special warnings and special precautions for use: Cytarabine is a potent bone marrow suppressant. Patients receiving the drug should be kept under close medical supervision. Leucocyte and platelet counts should be performed frequently and daily during induction. One case of anaphylaxis that resulted in cardiopulmonary arrest and necessitated resuscitation has been reported. This occurred immediately after intravenous Cytarabine was administered.

Severe and at times fatal CNS, GI and pulmonary toxicity (different from that seen with conventional therapy regimens of dosage schedules). These reactions include reversible corneal toxicity; cerebral and cerebellar dysfunction, usually reversible; severe gastrointestinal ulceration including pneumatosis cysteroides intestinalis, leading to peritonitis; sepsis and liver abscess; and pulmonary oedema.

Cytarabine has been shown to be mutagenic and carcinogenic in animals.

Cytarabine should only be used under the constant supervision of physicians experienced in therapy with cytotoxic agents. Hyperuricaemia secondary to lysis of neoplastic cells may occur in patients receiving Cytarabine; serum uric acid concentrations should be monitored.

Periodic determinations of renal and hepatic functions and bone marrow should also be performed and the drug should be used with caution in patients with impaired hepatic function.

However, dosage reduction does not appear to be necessary in patients with impaired renal function. The human liver apparently detoxifies a substantial fraction of the administered dose. The drug should be used with caution and at a reduced dose when liver function is poor. Frequent platelet and leucocyte counts are manditory. Therapy should be suspended or modified when drug-induced bone marrow depression results in a platelet count of less than 50,000 or a polymorphonuclear count of under 1000 per cubic mm. Counts may continue to fall after the therapy has been discontinued and may reach lowest values after five to seven days. Therapy may be restarted when the bone marrow appears to be recovering on successive bone marrow studies. Therapy should not wait until the normal blood values are obtained to be re-initiated.

When intravenous doses are given quickly, patients may become nauseated and may vomit for several hours afterwards. The problem tends to be less severe when infused.

When given intrathecally, as with any other intrathecal drug, care must be taken with radiotherapy given either during or after treatment; it is well recognised that this can exacerbate the toxicity of radiotherapy.

The safety of the drug has not been established in infants.

Interaction with other medicaments and other forms of interaction

(i) *Cardiac glycosides:* G.I. absorption of oral digoxin tablets may be substantially reduced in patients receiving combination chemotherapy regimens (including regimens containing cytarabine), possibly as a result of temporary damage to intestinal mucosa caused by the cytotoxic agents. Limited data suggest that the extent of G.I. absorption of digitoxin is not substantially affected by concomitant administration of combination chemotherapy regimens known to decrease absorption of digoxin.

(ii) *Anti-infective agents:* One in vitro study indicates that cytarabine may antagonise the activity of gentamicin against *Klebsiella pneumoniae*. Limited data may suggest that cytarabine may antagonise the anti-infective activity of flucytosine, possibly by competitive inhibition of the anti-infective uptake by fungi.

Pregnancy and lactation: Cytarabine is teratogenic in some animal species. It should not be used in pregnant women (especially during the first trimester) or in those who may become pregnant, unless the possible benefits outweigh the potential risks. Women who are, or become, pregnant during treatment with Cytarabine should be informed of the risks.

It is not known if Cytarabine or its metabolite is distributed into breast milk, and it should not be used.

Effects on ability to drive and use machines: No documented effect on ability to drive or operate machinery.

Undesirable effects:

Central nervous system: Rarely, neurological effects such a quadriplegia and paralysis have been reported with cytosine arabinoside and have predominantly been associated with intrathecal administration. Isolated cases have also been reported with high intravenous doses during combination chemotherapeutic regimens.

Haematological effects: The major adverse effect of Cytarabine is the haematological toxicity. Myelosuppression is manifested by megaloblastosis, reticulocytopenia, thrombocytopenia and anaemia.

These appear to be more evident after high doses and continuous infusions; the severity depends on the dose of the drug and schedule of administration.

GI effects: Nausea and vomiting occur and are generally more frequent following rapid IV administration than with continuous IV infusion of the drug.

Diarrhoea, anorexia, oral and anal inflammation or ulceration and less frequently abdominal pain, sore throat, oesphagitis, oesophageal ulceration and gastrointestinal haemorrhage may also occur.

Other reported adverse effects of Cytarabine include fever, rash, alopecia, skin ulceration, conjunctivitis, chest pain, urinary retention, dizziness, neuritis or neural toxicity and pain, cellulitis or thrombophlebitis at the site of injection. Cytarabine has also been associated with renal dysfunction, hepatic dysfunction and jaundice in some patients. It has also been associated with sepsis, irritation or sepsis at the injection site, neuritis or neurotoxicity rash, freckling, skin and mucosal bleeding, chest pain, joint pain and reduction in reticulocytes.

A Cytarabine reaction is characterised by fever, myalgia, bone pain, occasionally chest pain, maculopapular rash, conjunctivitis and malaise. It usually occurs 6-12 hours after administration. Corticosteroids have been shown to be beneficial in treating or preventing this syndrome. If the symptoms of the syndrome are serious enough to warrant treatment, corticosteroids should be contemplated as well as continuation of Cytarabine therapy.

Overdose: Cessation of therapy followed by management of ensuing bone marrow depression including whole blood or platelet transfusion and antibiotics as required.

Pharmacological properties

Pharmacodynamic properties: Cytarabine (ARA-C) is metabolised in vivo to ARA-CTP phosphorylated compound. This competitively inhibits DNA polymerase and may also inhibit certain acid kinase enzymes. Primarily the drug acts as a false nucleoside and competes for enzymes involved in the conversion of Cytidine nucleotide to deoxycytidine nucleotide and also incorporation into the DNA.

Cytarabine has no effect on non proliferating cells nor on proliferating cells unless in the S phase. It is a cell cycle specific antineoplastic drug.

Pharmacokinetic properties: Oral administration is ineffective due to rapid deamination in the gut. Cytidine deaminase is concentrated in the liver and intravenous doses show biphasic elimination with half lifes of approximately 10 minutes and 1-3 hours.

After 24 hours 80% of a dose has been eliminated either as the inactive metabolite or as the unchanged Cytarabine, mostly in urine but some in bile.

CSF levels of 50% of plasma levels are achieved with IV infusion. Intrathecal dosing results in slower elimination (T1/2 2-11 hours).

Cytarabine is rapidly and widely distributed into tissues, crosses the blood brain barrier and also the placenta.

Preclinical safety data: Not applicable.

Pharmaceutical particulars

List of excipients:

Sodium Chloride BP	6.8 mg
Water for Injections BP	to 1.0 mL

There is no overage in the formulation.

Incompatibilities: Solutions of Cytarabine have been reported to be incompatible with various drugs, i.e. Carbenicillin Sodium, Cephalothin Sodium, Fluorouracil, Gentamicin Sulphate, Heparin Sodium, Hydrocortisone Sodium Succinate, Insulin-regular, Methylprednisolone Sodium Succinate, Nafacillin Sodium, Oxacillin Sodium, Penicillin G Sodium. However, the incompatibility depends on several factors (e.g. concentrations of the drug, specific diluents used, resulting pH, temperature). Specialised references should be consulted for specific compatibility information.

Shelf life: 36 months.

Special precautions for storage: Store below 25°C. Protect from light.

In diluted infusion fluids store at 2-8°C and protect from light for a maximum of 24 hours.

Instructions for use/handling: Not applicable.

Marketing authorisation number 4515/0040.

Date of approval/revision of SPC March 1996

Legal category POM

CYTARABINE INJECTION SOLUTION 100 mg/mL

Qualitative and quantitative composition

Active constituent

Cytarabine BP	10.0 % w/v

Other constituents

Water for Injections BP to	1.0 mL

There is no overage in the formulation.

Pharmaceutical form Aqueous, sterile hypertonic solution for injection.

Clinical particulars

Therapeutic indications: Cytarabine may be used alone or in combination with other antineoplastic agents. It is indicated alone or in combination for induction of remission and/or maintainance in patients with acute myeloid leukaemia, acute non-lymphoblastic leukaemias, acute lymphoblastic leukaemias, acute lymphocytic leukaemia, erythroleukaemia, blast crises of chronic myeloid leukaemia, diffuse histiocytic lymphomas (non-hodgkin's lymphomas of high malignancy), meningeal leukaemia and meningeal neoplasms. Clinicians should refer to the current literature on combination therapy before initiating treatment.

Posology and method of administration: Cytarabine Injection Solution is a ready to use solution with a concentration of 100 mg/mL.

Cytarabine Injection Solution 100 mg/mL can be administered by the intravenous and subcutaneous routes. **Cytarabine Injection Solution 100 mg/mL should not be administered by the intrathecal route due to the slight hypertonicity of this formulation.**

Cytarabine Injection Solution can be diluted with Sterile Water for Injection BP, Glucose Injection BP or Sodium Chloride 0.9% Injection BP. Prepared infusions, in the recommended diluents should be used immediately. Alternatively, the diluted infusion fluids may be stored at 2–8°C, protected from light, but portions remaining unused after 24 hours must be discarded.

Remission induction: Adults.

Continuous dosing: The usual dose in leukaemia, is 2 mg/kg by rapid intravenous injection daily for ten days. If after ten days neither therapeutic response nor toxicity has been observed, the dose may be increased to 4 mg per kg until a therapeutic response or toxicity is evident. Daily blood counts should be taken. Almost all patients can be carried to toxicity with these doses.

Alternatively, 0.5 to 1 mg/kg may be infused daily in 1–24 hours for ten days, and then at a rate of 2 mg/kg/day until toxicity is observed. Continue to toxicity or until remission occurs. Results from one hour infusions have been satisfactory in the majority of patients.

Intermittent dosing: Cytarabine may be given as intermittent IV doses of 3–5 mg/kg daily, for five consecutive days This course of treatment can be repeated after an interval of 2 to 9 days, and repeated until the therapeutic response or toxicity is exhibited.

Evidence of bone marrow inprovement has been reported to occur 7–64 days after the beginning of therapy.

In general, if a patient shows neither remission or toxicity after a trial period, then cautiously administered higher doses can be administered. Generally patients tolerate higher doses given by rapid intravenous injection rather than slow infusion.

As a single agent for induction of remissions in patients with acute leukaemia, Cytarabine has been given in doses of 200 mg/m² by continuous IV Infusion for five days at approximately 2 week intervals.

Maintainance therapy: To maintain remission, doses of 1–1.5 mg/kg may be given intravenously or subcutaneously, once or twice weekly.

Leukaemic meningitis: Therapy for established meningitis employs a wide variety of dose regimens but a recommended total daily dose not exceeding 100 mg, alternating with Methotrexate (given either systemically or intrathecally) is recommended. Cytarabine Injection has been given intrathecally at doses of 10–30 mg per m² three times a week until CSF findings return to normal. **Cytarabine Injection Solution 100 mg/mL should not be administered by the intrathecal route due to the slight hypertonicity of this formulation.**

Myelosuppression, anaemia and thrombocytopenia occur almost to all patients given daily infusions or injections. Myelosuppression is biphasic and nadirs at 7–9 and 15–24 days. Evidence of bone marrow improvement may be expected 7–64 (mean 28) days after the beginning of treatment.

Children: Children appear to tolerate higher doses of Cytarabine than adults, and where the range of doses is given, children should receive the higher dose.

Elderly: No data is available to suggest that a change in dose is necessary in the elderly. However, the elderly patient is more susceptable to toxic reactions and therefore particular attention should be paid to drug induced leucopenia, thrombocytopenia and anaemia.

Contra-indications: Cytarabine is contraindicated in patients with known hypersensitivity to the drug. Therapy with Cytarabine should not be considered in patients with pre-existing drug-induced bone marrow suppression, unless in the opinion of the physician the potential benefits outweigh the hazards. Cytarabine should not be used in the management of non-malignant disease, except for immunosuppression.

Special warnings and special precautions for use: Cytarabine is a potent bone marrow suppressant. Patients receiving the drug should be kept under close medical supervision. Leucocyte and platelet counts should be performed frequently and daily during induction. One case of anaphylaxis that resulted in cardiopulmonary arrest and necessitated resuscitation has been reported. This occurred immediately after intravenous Cytarabine was administered.

Severe and at times fatal CNS, GI and pulmonary toxicity (different from that seen with conventional therapy regimens of dosage schedules). These reactions include reversible corneal toxicity; cerebral and cerebellar dysfunction, usually reversible; severe gastrointestinal ulceration including pneumatosis cysteroides intestinalis, leading to peritonitis; sepsis and liver abscess; and pulmonary oedema.

Cytarabine has been shown to be mutagenic and carcinogenic in animals.

Cytarabine should only be used under the constant supervision of physicians experienced in therapy with cytotoxic agents. Hyperuricaemia secondary to lysis of neoplastic cells may occur in patients receiving Cytarabine; serum uric acid concentrations should be monitored.

Periodic determinations of renal and hepatic functions and bone marrow should also be performed and the drug should be used with caution in patients with impaired hepatic function.

However, dosage reduction does not appear to be necessary in patients with impaired renal function. The human liver apparently detoxifies a substantial fraction of the administered dose. The drug should be used with caution and at a reduced dose when liver function is poor. Frequent platelet and leucocyte counts are manditory. Therapy should be suspended or modified when drug-induced bone marrow depression results in a platelet count of less than 50,000 or a polymorphonuclear count of under 1000 per cubic mm. Counts may continue to fall after the therapy has been discontinued and may reach lowest values after five to seven days. Therapy may be restarted when the bone marrow appears to be recovering on successive bone marrow studies. Therapy should not wait until the normal blood values are obtained to be re-initiated.

When intravenous doses are given quickly, patients may become nauseated and may vomit for several hours afterwards. The problem tends to be less severe when infused.

The safety of the drug has not been established in infants.

Interaction with other medicaments and other forms of interaction:

(i) *Cardiac glycosides:* G.I. absorption of oral digoxin tablets may be substantially reduced in patients receiving combination chemotherapy regimens (including regimens containing cytarabine), possibly as a result of temporary damage to intestinal mucosa caused by the cytotoxic agents. Limited data suggest that the extent of G.I. absorption of digitoxin is not substantially affected by concomitant administration of combination chemotherapy regimens known to decrease absorption of digoxin.

(ii) *Anti-infective agents:* One *in vitro* study indicates that cytarabine may antagonise the activity of gentamicin against *Klebsiella pneumoniae.* Limited data may suggest that cytarabine may antagonise the anti-infective activity of flucytosine, possibly by competitive inhibition of the anti-infective uptake by fungi.

Pregnancy and lactation: Cytarabine is teratogenic in some animal species. It should not be used in pregnant women (especially during the first trimester) or in those who may become pregnant, unless the possible benefits outweigh the potential risks. Women who are, or become, pregnant during treatment with Cytarabine should be informed of the risks.

It is not known if Cytarabine or its metabolite is distributed into breast milk, and it should not be used.

Effects on ability to drive and use machines: No documented effect on ability to drive or operate machinery.

Undesirable effects:
Haematological effects: The major adverse effect of Cytarabine is the haematological toxicity. Myelosuppression is manifested by megaloblastosis, reticulocytopenia, thrombocytopenia and anaemia.

These appear to be more evident after high doses and continuous infusions; the severity depends on the dose of the drug and schedule of administration.

GI effects: Nausea and vomiting occur and are generally more frequent following rapid IV administration than with continuous IV infusion of the drug.

Diarrhoea, anorexia, oral and anal inflammation or ulceration and less frequently abdominal pain, sore throat, oesphagitis, oesophageal ulceration and gastrointestinal haemorrhage may also occur.

Other reported adverse effects of Cytarabine include fever, rash, alopecia, skin ulceration, conjunctivitis, chest pain, urinary retention, dizziness, neuritis or neural toxicity and pain, cellulitis or thrombophlebitis at the site of injection. Cytarabine has also been associated with renal dysfunction, hepatic dysfunction and jaundice in some patients. It has also been associated with sepsis, irritation or sepsis at the injection site, neuritis or neurotoxicity rash, freckling, skin and mucosal bleeding, chest pain, joint pain and reduction in reticulocytes.

A Cytarabine reaction is characterised by fever, myalgia, bone pain, occasionally chest pain, maculopapular rash, conjunctivitis and malaise. It usually occurs 6–12 hours after administration. Corticosteroids have been shown to be beneficial in treating or preventing this syndrome. If the symptoms of the syndrome are serious enough to warrant treatment, corticosteroids should be contemplated as well as continuation of Cytarabine therapy.

Overdose: Cessation of therapy followed by management of ensuing bone marrow depression including whole blood or platelet transfusion and antibiotics as required.

Pharmacological properties

Pharmacodynamic properties: Cytarabine (ARA-C) is metabolised *in vivo* to ARA-CTP phosphorylated compound. This competitively inhibits DNA polymerase and may also inhibit certain acid kinase enzymes. Primarily the drug acts as a false nucleoside and competes for enzymes involved in the conversion of Cytidine nucleotide to deoxycytidine nucleotide and also incorporation into the DNA.

Cytarabine has no effect on non proliferating cells nor on proliferating cells unless in the S phase. It is a cell cycle specific antineoplastic drug.

Pharmacokinetic properties: Oral administration is ineffective due to rapid deamination in the gut. Cytidine deaminase is concentrated in the liver and intravenous doses show biphasic elimination with half lifes of approximately 10 minutes and 1–3 hours.

After 24 hours 80% of a dose has been eliminated either as the inactive metabolite or as the unchanged Cytarabine, mostly in urine but some in bile.

CSF levels of 50% of plasma levels are achieved with IV infusion. Intrathecal dosing results in slower elimination ($T_{\frac{1}{2}}$ 2–11 hours).

Cytarabine is rapidly and widely distributed into tissues, crosses the blood brain barrier and also the placenta.

Preclinical safety data: Not applicable.

Pharmaceutical particulars

List of excipients: Water for Injections BP to 1.0 mL.
There is no overage in the formulation.

Incompatibilities: Solutions of Cytarabine have been reported to be incompatible with various drugs, i.e. Carbenicillin Sodium, Cephalothin Sodium, Fluorouracil, Gentamicin Sulphate, Heparin Sodium, Hydrocortisone Sodium Succinate, Insulin-regular, Methylprednisolone Sodium Succinate, Nafacillin Sodium, Oxacillin Sodium, Penicillin G Sodium. However, the incompatibility depends on several factors (e.g. concentrations of the drug, specific diluents used, resulting pH, temperature). Specialised references should be consulted for specific compatibility information.

Shelf life:
Conventional Glass Vials and Onco-Tain Vials:* 36 months.
Shell Glass Vials: 24 months

Special precautions for storage:
Conventional Glass Vials and Onco-Tain Vials:* Store below 25°C. Protect from light.

In diluted infusion fluids store at 2–8°C and protect from light for a maximum of 24 hours.

Shell Glass Vials: Store below 25°C. Protect from light.

Unused portions of opened vials or prepared infusions if not used immediately must be stored at 2–8°C for no longer than 24 hours from the time of opening or preparation.

Nature and contents of container:
Conventional Glass Vials: Clear Type I Glass Vials, 13 mm West 1816 Style Rubber Stopper in 1 ml and 5 ml.

Clear Type I Glass Vials, 20 mm West 1816 Style Rubber Stopper in 10 ml and 20 ml.

Onco-Tain Vials:* Clear Type I Onco-Tain* Vials, 13 mm West 1816 Style Rubber Stopper in 1 ml and 5 ml.

Clear Type Onco-Tain* Glass Vials, 20 mm West 1816 Style Rubber Stopper in 10 ml and 20 ml.

Shell Glass Vials: Clear Type I 3 mL Shell Glass Vials, 10 mm West Type 4405/50 Style Rubber Stopper.

Clear Type I 10 mL Shell Glass Vials, 15 mm West Type 4405/50 Style Rubber Stopper.

Clear Type I 30 mL Shell Glass Vials, 27 mm West Type 4405/50 Style Rubber Stopper.

Clear Type I 50 mL Shell Glass Vials, 27 mm West Type 4405/50 Style Rubber Stopper.

Instructions for use/handling: Not applicable.

Marketing authorisation number 4515/0057

Date of first authorisation/renewal of authorisation
Date of first authorisation: 7/7/92 – (Conv. Glass Vials 1 ml & 10 ml).
Date of first authorisation: 18/1/94 – (Conv. Glass Vials 5 ml & 20 ml).
Date of first authorisation: 14/9/94 – (Onco-Tain* Vials).
Date of first authorisation: 27/4/95 – (Shell Glass Vials).

Date of (partial) revision of the text 11 March 1998

Legal category POM

DACARBAZINE FOR INJECTION

Qualitative and quantitative composition Dacarbazine for Injection BP is a cytotoxic agent presented as vials containing 100 mg and 200 mg of sterile dacarbazine as a white/pale yellow powder or plug which is to be reconstituted with Water for Injections BP.

When reconstituted as directed each ml of the solution of the 100 mg vial contains dacarbazine 10 mg, citric acid 10 mg, mannitol 5 mg, and sodium hydroxide 1N has been used to adjust the pH. Each ml of the 200 mg vial contains dacarbazine 20 mg, citric acid 20 mg, mannitol 7.5 mg, and sodium hydroxide 1N has been used to adjust the pH.

Pharmaceutical form Freeze dried powder for injection.

Clinical particulars

Therapeutic indications:

1. Metastatic malignant melanoma
2. Sarcoma
3. Hodgkin's disease.

In addition, dacarbazine has been shown, when used in combination with other cytotoxic agents, to be of use in the treatment of other malignant diseases including: carcinoma of the colon, ovary, breast, lung, testicular teratoma, and solid tumours in children.

Posology and method of administration:
Dosage: Standard dose. The following dosage schedules are recommended:

1. 2.0-4.5 mg/kg/day for 10 days, which may be repeated at 4 week intervals.
2. 250 mg/m²/day for five days, which may be repeated at 3 week intervals.
3. A further alternative is to administer the total schedule dose on the first day.

Other schedules may be used at the discretion of the prescribing physician.

Children: The dosage for children is calculated on a mg/kg or mg/m² basis as per the standard dosage. There is no indication that children require a different dosage range or metabolise or react differently to the drug.

Geriatric: As for paediatric use.

With impaired hepatic function: As the drug partly undergoes metabolism in the liver, impairment of liver function is likely to necessitate a variation in dosage.

With impaired renal function: As the drug is excreted 50% unchanged in the urine by tubular secretion, impairment of renal function is likely to necessitate a change in dosage.

Administration: Administration is by the IV route only.

Dacarbazine 100 mg and 200 mg vials should be reconstituted with 9.9 ml and 19.7 ml respectively, with Water for Injections BP. The resulting solutions contain the equivalent of 10 mg/ml of dacarbazine and have a pH of 3 to 4. The resultant solution should be injected intravenously over one to two minutes.

If desired the reconstituted solution can be further diluted with 125-250 ml of Dextrose Injection BP 5% or Sodium Chloride Injection BP 0.9% and administered by intravenous infusion over 15-30 minutes.

Contra-indications: Dacarbazine is contra-indicated in patients who have demonstrated a hypersensitivity to Dacarbazine in the past.

Dacarbazine should not be administered to patients who are pregnant or may become pregnant or breast feeding mothers.

Patients who have previously had severe myelosuppression.

Special warnings and special precautions for use:
Warnings: Haemopoietic depression is the most common toxic side-effect of dacarbazine and involves primarily the leucocytes and platelets, although mild anaemia may sometimes occur. Leucopenia and thrombocytopenia may be severe enough to cause death. Possible bone marrow depression requires careful monitoring of white blood cells, red blood cells and platelet levels. Such toxicity may necessitate temporary suspension or cessation of therapy.

Hepatic toxicity, accompanied by hepatic vein thrombosis and hepatocellular necrosis resulting in death, have been reported. The incidence of such reactions has been low. This toxicity has been observed mostly when dacarbazine has been adminstered concommitantly with other anti-neoplastic drugs; however, it has also been reported in some patients treated with dacarbazine alone.

Precautions: The drug can produce severe and possibly fatal, haematologic or hepatic toxicity and severe GI reactions and should be administered to patients preferably within the hospital setting, where they can be observed frequently during and after therapy, particularly with regards to the haemopoietic toxicity.

It is recommended that dacarbazine be administered by physicians experienced in the use of cytotoxic therapy. Laboratory facilities should be available for blood monitoring.

Restriction of food intake for 4-6 hours prior to treatment may reduce the severity of the nausea and vomiting which occurs in most patients particularly during the first two days of treatment. Administration of an anti-emetic may also reduce the severity of these effects.

Impairment of renal and liver function: See dosage in impaired renal and liver function

Care must be taken to avoid extravasation during intravenous administration as this may cause tissue damage and severe pain.

Care should be taken to avoid contact with the skin and eyes when reconstituting or administering dacarbazine.

Interaction with other medicaments and other forms of interaction: Microsomal liver enzyme inducers e.g. barbiturates, rifampicin, phenytoin may theoretically hasten the activation of dacarbazine to aminoimidazole-carboxamide.

Mercaptopurine, azathioprine, allopurinol: dacarbazine inhibits xanthine oxidase and may theoretically potentiate the activity of these drugs.

Patients receiving Dacarbazine should not receive immunisation with live vaccines. Dacarbazine may impair the immunological response to the vaccine with the development of a generalised vaccinia.

Pregnancy and lactation: Studies have demonstrated that this agent is carcinogenic and teratogenic when administered to animals. Dacarbazine therefore should not be administered to pregnant or lactating women unless the benefit clearly justifies the potential risk to the foetus.

Effects on ability to drive and use machines: Dacarbazine in appropriate doses should not impair the ability to drive. However, rare adverse reactions affecting the nervous system may cause blurred vision, seizures, headache, confusion, malaise and lethargy. Patients affected by these adverse effects should not drive or operate machinery.

Undesirable effects:
Common reactions: Symptoms of anorexia, nausea, and vomiting are the most frequent side-effects. Vomiting may last for 1-12 hours and is incompletely and unpredictably palliated with prochlorperazine. Diarrhoea is a rarer side-effect of Dacarbazine therapy. Rarely have intractable nausea and vomiting have necessitated discontinuation of therapy.

It is suggested that restriction fo the patients oral fluid intake and food 4-6 hours prior to treatment may be helpful. The rapid toleration of these symptoms suggests a central nervous system mechanism, and usually these symptoms subside after the first 1-2 days.

Haematological:Bone marrow depression, leucocytopenia, thrombocytopenia.

Haemopoietic toxicity may warrant temporary suspension or cessation of Dacarbazine therapy.

Less common reactions:
Cardiovascular: Facial flushing
Dermatological: Transient rash, alopecia

General : Infrequently some patients have experienced an influenza type syndrome of fever, myalgias and malaise. This syndrome usually occurs after large single doses and approximately seven days after treatment with dacarbazine and lasts 7-21 days, and may reoccur with successive treatments.

Hepatic: Increases in transaminases (AST, ALT), alkaline phosphatase, LDH. Levels usually return to normal within two weeks; hepatic toxicity accompanied by hepatic vein thrombosis and hepatocellular necrosis,(Budd-Chiari Syndrome) resulting in death.

Nervous System: Blurred vision, seizures, headache, facial paraesthesia, confusion, malaise, lethargy.

Anaphylaxis can occur very rarely following administration of Dacarbazine.

Photosensitivity reactions may occur rarely.

Overdose: Signs and Symptoms: Severe bone marrow depression and gastrointestinal effects such as nausea, vomiting and diarrhoea may be expected.

Treatment: Cease dacarbazine administration and institute supportive measures, e.g. appropriate transfusions for bone marrow suppression.

Pharmacological properties

Pharmacodynamic properties: Dacarbazine is an imidazole dimethyltriazene with reproducible activity in patients with metastatic melanoma. The structure of Dacarbazine bears a striking resemblance to the metabolite 5-aminoimidazole-4-carboxamide (AIC) which is converted to inosinic acid by enzymes involved in purine synthesis.

It was therefore initially thought to act as an antimetabolite, by inhibiting purine metabolism and nucleic acid synthesis. However the similarity of structure is of little relevance since Dacarbazine is extensively metabolised by the cytochrome P450 system in the liver by N-demethylation reaction. The monomethyl derivative then spontaneously cleaves to yield AIC and an intermediate compound, probably diazomethane, which decomposes to produce the methyl carbonium ion. This ion attached to nucleophilic groups on nucleic acids and other macromolecules, thus acting as an alkylating agent. The 7-position of guanine on DNA is especially susceptible to alkylation.

Dacarbazine is thought to act as an alkylating agent in man. It interferes with the synthesis of DNA, RNA and proteins but its cytotoxicity is not specific for any phase of the cell cycle. In general, it is most effective in inhibiting synthesis of RNA. Dacarbazine kills cells slowly and no immunosuppressive action has been shown in man. There are no systemic studies of dose-response effects but one anecdotal report has suggested that there may be an increased chance of response as the dose increases.

Dacarbazine undergoes spontaneous photodegradation in light, decomposing into 5-diazoimidazole-4-carboxamide and dimethylamine. 5-Diazoimidazole-4-carboxamide can attack nucleophilic groups of DNA and also undergoes structural rearrangement to form 2-azahypoxanthine. However, the products of photodegradation of dacarbazine probably do not contribute greatly to its cytotoxicity, although they may be implicated in the local burning pain on intravenous injection and systemic problems associated with the drug.

Pharmacokinetic properties: The volume of distribution of dacarbazine exceeds body water content, suggesting localisation in some body tissues, probably the liver. Dacarbazine is only slightly (approximately 5%) bound to plasma proteins. Its plasma half-life after intravenous administration is approximately 35 minutes. In animal studies, approximately 46% of radio-labelled dose was recovered from the urine after 6 hours. Of this 46%, almost half, was unchanged dacarbazine and a similar quantity was amino-imidazole carboxamide, a metabolite. Dacarbazine is subject to renal tubular secretion rather than glomerular filtration.

Dacarbazine crosses the blood-brain barrier to a limited extent; CSF concentrations are reported to be about 14% of plasma concentrations. It is not known if dacarbazine crosses the placenta or distributes into milk.

Preclinical safety data: Not applicable.

Pharmaceutical particulars

List of excipients: Citric Acid BP; Mannitol BP; Sodium Hydroxide 1.0N.

Incompatibilities: Dacarbazine is incompatible with hydrocortisone sodium succinate in solution, forming an inmediate precipitate.

It has been reported to be incompatible with heparin, although only with concentrated solutions (25 mg/ml).

Shelf life: 3 years.

Special precautions for storage: Store between 2-8°C. Protect from light.

After reconstitution the vial should be stored, protected from light, at 2-8°C and the contents used within 24 hours. If the reconstituted solution is further diluted in 5% Dextrose Injection BP or Sodium Chloride 0.9% BP the resulting solution should be stored protected from light, at 2-8°C and used within 24 hours.

Instructions for use/handling: Dacarbazine for Injection should only be prepared for administration by professionals who have been trained in the safe use of the preparation. In the event of spillage, operators should put on gloves and mop up the spilled material with a sponge kept in the area for that purpose, and transfer the sponge to a plastic bag. The procedure should be repeated and the area rinsed with water and absorbed solution placed in the plastic bag, which is then sealed. Repeat if necessary. The plastic container should then be incinerated and the gloves destroyed.

Marketing authorisation numbers
100 mg 4515/0091
200 mg 4515/0092

Date of approval/revision of SPC November 1995

Legal category POM

DEXAMETHASONE SODIUM PHOSPHATE INJECTION

Qualitative and quantitative composition 4 mg/1 mL, 8 mg/2 mL, 120 mg/5 mL.

Pharmaceutical form Sterile solution for injection.

Clinical particulars

Therapeutic indications: Dexamethasone Injection is indicated in acute conditions in which oral glucocorticoid therapy is not feasible such as:

Shock: of haemorrhagic, traumatic, surgical or septic origin; Cerebral oedema associated with cerebral neoplasm; Inflammatory diseases of joints and soft tissue such as rheumatoid arthritis

Short term management of acute self-limited allergic conditions such as angioneurotic oedema or acute exacerbations of chronic allergic disorders such as bronchial asthma or serum sickness.

High doses of Dexamethasone are intended for the adjunctive treatment of shock where massive doses of corticosteroids are needed. There is a lack of evidence that use of corticosteriods in septic shock affects mortality in the long term. Use must be accompanied by the appropriate concomitant systemic antibiotic treatment and supportive measures which the patient's condition may require.

Posology and method of administration: Dosage of Dexamethasone Sodium Phosphate is usually expressed in terms of Dexamethasone Phosphate.

The lowest effective dose should be used for the minimum period and this should be reviewed frequently to appropriately titrate the dose against disease activity. (See Warnings Section).

Dexamethasone Sodium Phosphate Injection 4 mg/ml may be administered by intramuscular, intra-articular or direct intravenous injection, intravenous infusion or soft tissue infiltration.

Dexamethasone Sodium Phosphate Injection 24 mg/ml is for intravenous administration only.

Intravenous and intramuscular administration: I.M. or I.V. dosage of Dexamethasone Phosphate is variable, depending on the condition being treated. It usually ranges from 0.5-24 mg daily. The duration of therapy is dependent on the clinical response of the patient and as soon as improvement is indicated, the dosage should be adjusted to the minimum required to maintain the desired clinical response. Withdrawal of the drug on completion of therapy should be gradual.

Shock: A single I.V. injection of 2 to 6 mg/kg bodyweight which may be repeated in 2-6 hours if shock persists. High-dose therapy should be continued only until the patient's condition has stabilised and usually for no longer than 48-72 hours. This bolus injection can then be followed by continuous I.V. infusion of 3 mg/kg bodyweight per 24 hours. Dexamethasone Sodium Phosphate Injection can be diluted with Sodium Chloride Injection BP or Glucose Injection BP

Cerebral oedema associated with neoplasm: An initial dose of 10 mg I.V. followed by 4 mg I.M. every 6 hours until the symptoms of oedema subside (usually after 12 to 24 hours). After 2 to 4 days the dosage should be reduced and gradually stopped over a period of 5 to 7 days. In patients with recurrent or inoperable neoplasms, maintenance therapy may be effective at doses of 2 mg I.M. or I.V. 2-3 times daily.

Life-Threatening Cerebral Oedema:

High Dose Schedule:

	Adults	*Children > 35 kg*	*Children <35 kg*
Initial dose	50 mg IV	25 mg IV	20 mg IV
1st day	8 mg IV every 2 hrs	4 mg IV every 2 hrs	4 mg IV every 3 hrs
2nd day	8 mg IV every 2 hrs	4 mg IV every 2 hrs	4 mg IV every 3 hrs
3rd day	8 mg IV every 2 hrs	4 mg IV every 2 hrs	4 mg IV every 3 hrs
4th day	4 mg IV every 2 hrs	4 mg IV every 4 hrs	4 mg IV every 6 hrs
5th-8th day	4 mg IV every 4 hrs	4 mg IV every 6 hrs	4 mg IV every 6 hrs
After 8 days	decrease by 4 mg daily	decrease by 2 mg daily	decrease by 1 mg daily

Note: The intravenous and intramuscular routes of administration of Dexamethasone Sodium Phosphate should only be used where acute illness or life-threatening situations exist. Oral therapy should be substituted as soon as possible.

Intra-articular and soft tissue injections: Dosage varies with the degree of inflammation and the size and location of the affected area. Injections may be repeated from once every 3-5 days (e.g. for bursae) to once every 2-3 weeks (for joints).

Site of injection	*Dosage*
Large Joint	2 mg to 4 mg
Small Joints	800 microgram to 1 mg
Bursae	2 mg to 3 mg
Tendon Sheaths	400 microgram to 1 mg
Soft Tissue Infiltration	2 mg to 6 mg
Ganglia	1 mg to 2 mg

Children: Dosage requirements are variable and may have to be changed according to individual need. Usually 200 micrograms/kg to 400 micrograms/kg of body weight daily.

Corticosteroids cause growth retardation in infancy, childhood and adolescence, which may be irreversible. Treatment should be limited to the minimum dosage for the shortest possible time. In order to minimise suppression of the hypothalamopituitary-adrenal axis and growth retardation, treatment should be limited, where possible, to a single dose on alternative days.

Growth and development of infants and children on prolonged corticosteriod therapy should be carefully monitored.

Elderly: Treatment of elderly patients, particularly long-term, should be planned, bearing in mind the more serious consequences in old age. Such effects include osteoporosis, hypertension, hypokalaemia, diabetes, susceptibility to infection, thinning and fragility of the skin. Close clinical supervision is required to avoid life-threatening reactions.

Contra-indications: Unless considered to be life-saving systemic administration of corticosteroids are generally contraindicated in patients with systemic infections, (unless specific anti-infective therapy is employed). Hypersensitivity to any components of the injection.

Special warnings and special precautions for use:
Warnings: A Patient Information Leaflet should be supplied with this product.

The lowest effective dose of corticosteroid should

be used to control the condition under treatment for the minimum period. Frequent patient review is required to appropriately titrate the dose against disease activity (see dosage section). When dose reduction is possible, it should occur gradually. Too rapid a reduction of dexamethasone dosage following prolonged treatment can lead to acute adrenal insufficiency, hypotension and death.

A 'withdrawal syndrome' may also occur including fever, myalgia, arthralgia, rhinitis, conjunctivitis, painful itchy skin nodules and loss of weight.

Adrenal suppression: Adrenal cortical atrophy develops during prolonged therapy and may persist for years after stopping treatment. Withdrawal of corticosteroids after prolonged therapy must, therefore, be gradual to avoid acute adrenal insufficiency, being tapered off over weeks or months according to the dose and duration of treatment. During prolonged therapy any intercurrent illness, trauma or surgical procedure will require a temporary increase in dosage; if corticosteroids have been stopped following prolonged therapy they may need to be temporarily reintroduced.

Patients should carry 'steroid treatment' cards which give clear guidance on the precautions to be taken to minimise risk and which provide details of prescriber, drug, dosage and the duration of treatment.

There is lack of evidence to support the prolonged use of corticosteroids in septic shock. Although they may be of value in the early treatment, the overall survival may not be influenced.

Severe anaphylactoid reactions have occurred after administration of parenteral corticosteroids, particularly in patients with history of allergy. Appropriate precautions should be taken prior to administration.

The slower rate of absorption after intramuscular injection should be noted.

Intra-articular corticosteroids are associated with a substantially increased risk of an inflammatory response in the joint, particularly a bacterial infection introduced with the injection. Great care is required and all intra-articular corticosteroid injections should be undertaken in an aseptic environment. Charcot like arthropathies have been reported particularly after repeated injections.

Prior to intra-articular injection the joint fluid should be examined to exclude a septic process. A marked increase in pain, accompanied by local swelling, further restriction of joint motion, fever and malaise are suggestive of septic arthritis. If this complication occurs and sepsis is confirmed, appropriate antimicrobial therapy should be commenced.

Patients should be impressed strongly with the importance of not overusing joints in which symptomatic benefit has been obtained, but the inflammatory process remains active.

Suppression of the inflammatory response and the immune function increases the susceptibility to infections and their severity. The clinical presentation may be atypical and serious infections, such as septicaemia and tuberculosis, may be masked and may reach an advanced stage before being recognised.

Chickenpox is of particular concern since this normally minor illness may be fatal in immunosuppressed patients. Patients (or parents of children) without a definite history of chickenpox should be advised to avoid close personal contact with chickenpox or herpes zoster and if exposed they should seek urgent medical attention. Passive immunisation with varicella/zoster immunoglobulin (VZIG) is needed by exposed non-immune patients who are receiving systemic dexamethasone or who have received it during the previous 3 months; this should be given within 10 days of exposure to chicken pox. If a diagnosis of chickenpox is confirmed, the illness warrants specialist care and urgent treatment. Dexamethasone should not be stopped and the dose may need to be increased.

Live vaccines should not be given to individuals with impaired immune responsiveness. The antibody response to other vaccines may be diminished.

False negative results may occur with the nitroblue tetrazolium test for bacterial infection.

Extreme caution should be exercised in the treatment of patients with the following conditions and frequent patient monitoring is necessary:

Liver failure, chronic renal failure, congestive heart failure, hypertension, epilepsy, migraine.

Osteoporosis, since corticosteriods increase calcium excretion. Post-menopausal women are at particular risk.

Latent tuberculosis, as corticosteroids can cause reactivation.

Hypothyroidism or cirrhosis, because such patients often show an exaggerated response to corticosteroids.

Latent amoebiasis, as corticosteroids may cause reactivation. Prior to treatment, amoebiasis should be ruled out in any patient with unexplained diarrhoea or who has recently spent time in the tropics.

Ocular herpes simplex, because corticosteroids may cause corneal perforation.

Corticosteroids should also be used with caution in patients with diabetes mellitus (or a family history of diabetes), affective disorders (especially previous steroid psychosis), glaucoma (or a family history of glaucoma), peptic ulceration or previous corticosteroid-induced myopathy.

Interaction with other medicaments and other forms of interaction: Liver enzyme inducing drugs such as barbiturates, ephedrine, rifampicin, rifabutin, carbamazepine, phenytoin, primidone and aminoglutethimide may enhance the metabolism of corticosteroids, resulting in a decrease in pharmacological action, and a need for dosage adjustment.

The efficacy of coumarin anticoagulants may be enhanced by concurrent corticosteroid therapy and close monitoring of prothombin time or INR is required to avoid spontaneous bleeding. Corticosterioids may affect glucose tolerance and increase the dosage requirement for hypoglycaemic drugs (including insulin).

The incidence of gastro-intestinal ulceration is increased in patients receiving concomitant nonsteroidal anti-inflammatory drugs and corticosteroids.

The renal clearance of salicylates is increased by corticosteroids and steroid withdrawal may result in salicylate intoxication.

Diuretics are antagonised by corticosteroids and the hypokalaemic effects of acetozolamide, loop diuretics, thiazide diuretics and carbenoxolone are enhanced. Patients receiving corticosterioids and potassium depleting diuretics and/or cardiac glycosides, should be monitored for hypokalaemia. This is of particular importance in patients receiving cardiac glycosides, since hypokalamia increases the toxicity of these drugs. The effects of anti-hypertensive drugs are also antagonised by corticosteroids.

Pregnancy and lactation:

Use in pregnancy: The ability of corticosteroids to cross the placenta varies between individual drugs, however, methylpredisolone does cross the placenta.

Administration of corticosteroids to pregnant animals can cause abnormalities of foetal development including cleft palate, intra-uterine growth retardation and affects on brain growth and development. There is no evidence that corticosteroids result in an increased incidence of congenital abnormalities, such as cleft palate/lip in man. However, when administered for prolonged periods or repeatedly during pregnancy, corticosteroids may increase the risk of intrauterine growth retardation. Hypoadrenalism may, in theory, occur in the neonate following prenatal exposure to the corticosteroids but usually resolves spontaneously following birth and is rarely clinically important. As with all drugs, corticosteroids should only be prescribed when the benefits to the mother and child outweigh the risks. When corticosteroids are essential however, patients with normal pregnancies may be treated as though they were in the nongravid state.

There may be a very small risk of cleft palate and intrauterine growth retardation in the foetus. There is evidence of harmful effects on pregnancy in animals. Infants born to mothers who have received substantial doses of corticosteroids during the pregnancy should be carefully observed, for signs of adrenal insufficiency.

When corticosteroids are essential however, patients with normal pregnancies may be treated as though they were in the non-gravid state. Patients with pre-eclampsia or fluid retention require close monitoring.

Use in lactation: Corticosteroids are excreted in small amounts in breast milk. However, doses of up to 40 mg daily of methylprednisolone are unlikely to cause systemic effects in the infant. Infants of mothers taking higher doses than this may gave a degree of adrenal suppression but the benefits of breast feeding are likely to outweigh any theoretical risk.

Suppression of growth or other adverse effects may occur. Infants of mothers taking pharmacological doses of steroids should be monitored carefully for signs of adrenal suppression.

Effects on ability to drive and use machines: Not applicable.

Undesirable effects:

Adverse reactions: The incidence of predictable undesirable effects, including hypothalamic-pituitary-adrenal suppression correlates with the relative potency of the drug, dosage, timing of administration and the duration of treatment (see *Other Special Warnings and Precautions*).

High doses of Dexamethasone Sodium Phosphate are intended for short term therapy and therefore adverse reactions are uncommon. However, peptic ulceration and bronchospasm may occur.

Except for hypersensitivity, the following adverse effects have been associated with prolonged systemic corticosteroid therapy.

Endocrine and metabolic disturbances: Suppression of the hypothalamic-pituitary adrenal axis; Cushing-like syndrome, hirsuitism and weight gain; suppression of growth in infants, children and adolescents; secondary adrenocortical unresponsiveness, particularly in times of stress, as in surgery or trauma; menstrual irregularities and amenorrhoea; impaired glucose tolerance with increased requirement for antidiabetic therapy; hyperglycaemia; negative protein/nitrogen and calcium balance; increased appetite.

Metabolic: Electrolyte imbalance (retention of sodium and water with oedema and hypertension); nitrogen depletion; hyperglycaemia; hypokalaemic alkalosis; increased calcium and potassium excretion and hypertension.

Anti-inflammatory and Immunosupressive effects: Increased susceptibility to and severity of infection with supression of clinical symptoms and signs; opportunistic infections; recurrence of dormant tuberculosis. (See Warnings Section).

Musculoskeletal: Muscular atrophy, proximal myopathy, premature epiphyseal closure, osteoporosis, avascular osteonecrosis, muscle weakness, tendon rupture, vertebral compression and long bone fractures.

Gastro-intestinal: Dyspepsia, peptic ulceration with perforation and haemorrhage, oesophageal ulcerations, acute pancreatitis and candidiasis.

Dermatological: Impaired wound healing; skin atrophy; bruising; telangiectasia and striae; petechiae and ecchymoses; erythema; increased sweating; possible suppression of skin tests; burning or tingling; bruising; allergic dermatitis; urticaria, candidiasis, acne.

Neurological: Mental disturbances, psychological dependence, euphoria, depression, insomnia, headache, convulsions, vertigo. Aggravation of epilepsy and schizoprenia. Increased intra-cranial pressure with papilloedema in children (pseudotumour cerebri), usually after treatment withdrawal.

Ophthalmic: Posterior sub-capsular cataracts or increased intraocular pressure may result in glaucoma or occasionally damage to the optic nerve; exophthalmos papilloedema; corneal or scleral thinning; exacerbation of ophthalmic viral or fungal diseases.

Other: Hypersensitivity including anaphylaxis, has been reported; blindness associated with intralesional therapy around the face and neck; hyperpigmentation; hypopigmentation; subcutaneous and cutaneous atrophy; sterile abscess; post injection flare (following intra-articular injection): Charcot-like arthropathy. Leucocytosis. Thromboembolism.

Withdrawal symptoms and signs: In patients who have received more than physiological doses of systemic corticosteroids (approximately 6 mg methylprednisolone) for greater than 3 weeks, withdrawal should not be abrupt. How dose reduction should be carried out depends largely on whether the disease is likely to relapse as the dose of systemic corticosteroids is reduced. Clinical assessment of disease activity may be needed during withdrawal. If the disease is unlikely to relapse on withdrawal of systemic corticosteroids but there is uncertainty about HPA suppression, the dose of systemic corticosteroid *may* be reduced rapidly to physiological doses. Once a daily dose of 6 mg methylprednisolone is reached, dose reduction should be slower to allow the HPA-axis to recover.

Abrupt withdrawal of systemic corticosteroid treatment, which has continued up to 3 weeks is appropriate if it is considered that the disease is unlikely to relapse. Abrupt withdrawal of doses up to 32 mg of dexamethasone for 3 weeks is unlikely to lead to clinically relevant HPA-axis suppression, in the majority of patients. In the following patient groups, gradual withdrawal of systemic corticosteroid therapy should be considered even after courses lasting 3 weeks or less:

- Patients who have had repeated courses of systemic corticosteroid, particularly if taken for greater than 3 weeks,
- When a short course has been prescribed within one year of cessation of long-term therapy (months or years),
- Patients who may have other reasons for adrenocortical insufficiency other than exogenous corticosteroid therapy
- Patients receiving doses of systemic corticosteroid greater than 32 mg daily of methylprednisolone.
- Patients repeatedly taking doses in the evening.

Overdose: Treat anaphylaxis with adrenaline and positive pressure ventilation. Other supportive measures aimed to maintain the patient unstressed.

Pharmacological properties

Pharmacodynamic properties: Pharmacology of the corticosteroids is complex and the drugs affect almost all body systems. Maximum pharmacologic activity lags behind peak blood concentrations, suggesting that most effects of the drugs result from modification of enzyme activity rather than from direct actions by the drugs.

Pharmacokinetic properties: Intramuscular injections of Dexamethasone Phosphate gives maximum plasma concentrations of Dexamethasone at 1 hour. Dexamethasone is readily absorbed from the gastro-intestinal tract. Its biological half-life in plasma is about 190 minutes. Binding of Dexamethasone to plasma proteins is less than for most other corticosteroids. Dexamethasone penetrates into tissue fluids and cerebrospinal fluids. Metabolism of the drug takes place in the kidneys and liver and excretion is via the urine.

Preclinical safety data: Not applicable.

Pharmaceutical particulars

List of excipients:

	4 mg	*8 mg*	*120 mg*
Dexamethasone Sodium Phosphate BP, equivalent to Dexamethasone Phosphate:	4.0 mg	8.0 mg	120.0 mg
Creatinine	8.0 mg	16.0 mg	40.0 mg
Disodium Edetate BP			2.5 mg
Sodium Citrate BP	10.0 mg	20.0 mg	50.0 mg
Water for Injection BP to	1.0 mL	2.0 mL	5.0 mL

Incompatibilities: Dexamethasone Sodium Phosphate is physically incompatible with Daunorubicin, Doxorubicin and Vancomycin and should not be admixed with solutions containing these drugs. Also incompatible with Doxapram HCl and glycopyrrolate in syringe.

Shelf life: 3 years.

Special precautions for storage: Store below 25°C and protect from freezing and from light. Do not use heat to sterilise the exterior of vials. Any unused portion should be discarded immediately after use.

When Dexamethasone Sodium Phosphate is given by intravenous infusion, only Sodium Chloride Injection BP or Glucose Injection BP should be used as diluents. The exact concentration of Dexamethasone Sodium Phosphate per infusion container should be determined by the desired dose, patient fluid intake and drip rate required. Dilutions should be used within 24 hours and discarded after use.

Instructions for use/handling: Not applicable.

Marketing authorisation numbers

120 mg/5 ml	4515/0018
4 mg/1 ml	4515/0019
8 mg/2 ml	4515/0020

Date of approval/revision of SPC July 1995

Legal category POM

STERILE DOBUTAMINE HYDROCHLORIDE CONCENTRATE.

Qualitative and quantitative composition

	per vial	*per mL*
Dobutamine Hydrochloride USP	280.2 mg*	14.01 mg
(equivalent to Dobutamine)	(250.0 mg)	(12.50 mg)
Sodium Metabisulphite BP	4.4 mg	0.22 mg
Water for Injections BP to	20.0 mL	1.0 mL

* No overage is required in the formulation.

Pharmaceutical form Aqueous solution for injection.

Clinical particulars

Therapeutic indications: Dobutamine Hydrochloride is a sympathomimetic agent which acts by stimulating the ß1 adrenergic receptors of the heart promoting a prominent inotropic action on the heart, increasing cardiac contractility and stroke volume It is a direct acting agent.

Dobutamine is indicated for adults who require inotropic support in the treatment of low output cardiac failure associated with organic heart disease, myocardial infarction, open heart surgery, cardiomyopathies, septic shock and cardiogenic shock. Dobutamine can increase or maintain cardiac output during positive end expiratory pressure (PEEP) ventilation.

Posology and method of administration: Dobutamine Hydrochloride should be administered by IV infusion only using an infusion pump or other apparatus to control the flow rate.

Dobutamine Hydrochloride must be diluted to a final volume of at least 50 mL with the following IV infusion solutions:

Sodium Chloride Intravenous Infusion BP
5% Dextrose Intravenous Infusion BP

If diluting to 250 mL or 500 mL, dilution will give a concentration for administration as follows:

250 mL contains 1,000 micrograms/ml of Dobutamine

500 mL contains 500 micrograms/ml of Dobutamine
1000 mL contains 250 micrograms/ml of Dobutamine

Diluted solution should be used within 24 hours, when aseptically prepared and stored in the refrigerator.

Administration: The concentration of Dobutamine administered depends upon the dosage and fluid requirements of the individual patient. Concentrations of 5000 microgram/ml have been used in fluid restricted patients but this concentration should not be exceeded. High concentrations of Dobutamine should only be given with an infusion pump to ensure accurate dosage. Due to it's short half-life Dobutamine should be administered as a continuous intravenous infusion. Dobutamine should be administered intravenously through an intravenous needle or catheter. An intravenous pump or other suitable apparatus should be used to control the flow rate in drops per minute.

Dosage:
Adults: The usual rate is 2.5 to 10 mcg per kg bodyweight per minute,which should be adjusted according to the patients heart rate, blood pressure, cardiac output and urine output. Up to 40 micrograms per kg per minute may occasionally be required but this is rare. Dobutamine infusions have been given for up to 72 hours without a decrease in effectiveness. It is recommended that treatment with Dobutamine should be discontinued gradually.

Side-effects which are dose related, are infrequent when Dobutamine is administered at rates below 10 microgram/kg/min. Rates as high as 40 microgram/kg/min have been used occasionally without significant adverse effects.

Children: The safety and efficacy of Dobutamine has not been established in children.

Contra-indications: Patients with known or suspected hypersensitivity to dobutamine or sulphites. Patients with marked mechanical obstruction affecting ventricular filling or outflow, or both such as cardiac tamponade, valvular aortic stenosis or idiopathic hypertrophic subaortic stenosis. Patients with hypovolaemia unless it has been corrected by volume replacement.

Special warnings and special precautions for use:
Warnings: If an undue increase in heart rate or systolic blood pressure occurs or if an arrythmia is precipitated the dose of Dobutamine should be reduced or the drug should be discontinued temporarily.

Dobutamine may precipitate or exacerbate ventricular ectopic activity, rarely has it caused ventricular tachycardia or fibrillation. Because Dobutamine increases atrioventricular conduction, patients with atrial flutter or fibrillation may develop a rapid ventricular response, and therefore should be digitalised prior to administration of Dobutamine.

Experience with the use of Dobutamine following acute myocardial infarction is limited. However there is a possibility that Dobutamine can cause a significant increase in heart rate or excessive increase in arterial pressure which may intensify or extend myocardial ischaemia, cause anginal pain and elevate ST segment, therefore care should be exercised following myocardial infarction.

Dobutamine will not improve haemodynamics in most patients with mechanical obstruction affecting ventricular filling or outflow, or both. Inotropic response may be inadequate in patients with markedly reduced ventricular compliance, e.g. with cardiac tamponade, valvular aortic stenosis, and idiopathic hypertrophic subaortic stenosis (see *Contra-indications*).

Minor vasoconstriction has been observed in patients treated with beta blocking drugs. This may occur due to the inotropic effect of Dobutamine which stimulates cardiac ß1 receptors and which is blocked by ß blockers. Conversely alpha adrenergic blockade may make the ß1 and ß2 effects apparent, resulting in tachycardia and vasodilatation.

Precautions: Before administration of Dobutamine, hypovolaemia should be corrected with an appropriate plasma volume expander. The ECG, blood pressure and when possible, cardiac output and pulmonary wedge pressure should be monitored.

Like other drugs with ß2 agonist activity, Dobutamine may produce slight reductions in serum potassium concentrations and hypokalaemia may occur occasionally. Consideration should be given to monitoring serum potassium during Dobutamine therapy.

During administration of Dobutamine heart rate and rhythm, arterial blood pressure, and infusion rate should be monitored closely. When starting therapy, electrocardiographic monitoring is recommended until a stable response is obtained.

Interaction with other medicaments and other forms of interaction: ß-Adrenergic blocking agents: In animals the cardiac effects of Dobutamine are antagonised by ß-adrenergic blocking agents such as propranolol and metoprolol, resulting in predominance of alpha-adrenergic blocking agents and increased peripheral resistance.

General anaesthetics: Ventricular arrythymias have been reported in animals receiving usual doses of Dobutamine during Halothane or Cyclopropane anaesthesia; therefore, caution should be exercised when administering Dobutamine to patients receiving these anaesthetics.

Pregnancy and lactation: Safe use of Dobutamine during pregnancy has not been established. Reproductive studies in rats and rabbits have not revealed any evidence of impaired fertility, evidence of harm to the foetus or teratogenic effects. Dobutamine should not be used in pregnant women unless the possible benefits outweigh the potential risks.

It is not known if Dobutamine crosses the placenta or is distributed into milk.

Effects on ability to drive and use machines: Not applicable.

Undesirable effects:
Adverse effects: Principal adverse effects are ectopic heart beats, increased heart rate, angina, chest pain, palpitation and elevations in blood pressure. All of these cardiovascular effects are usually dose related, and dosage should be reduced or temporarily discontinued if they occur. Rarely Dobutamine has caused ventricular tachycardia.

Other less frequent adverse effects include nausea, vomiting, tingling sensation, parasthesia, dyspnoea, headache and mild leg cramps; pruritis of the scalp during IV infusion of Dobutamine has been reported as with other reactions indicative of hypersensitivity, including rash, fever, eosinophilia and bronchospasm.

Phlebitis at the site of the IV infusion has been reported occasionally. Inadvertant subcutaneous infiltration of Dobutamine has caused local inflammatory changes and local pain without local ischaemia, however rarely dermal necrosis has been reported.

As with other catecholamines, decreases in serum potassium concentrations have occurred, rarely to hypokalaemic values.

Infusions for up to 72 hours have revealed no adverse effects other than those seen with shorter infusions. There is evidence that partial tolerance develops with continuous infusions of Dobutamine for 72 hours or more; therefore higher doses may be required to maintain the same effects.

Overdose: Overdosage have been reported rarely. The symptoms of toxicity may include anorexia, nausea, vomiting, tremor, anxiety, palpitations, headache, shortness of breath, fatigue and anginal and specific chest pain. The positive inotropic and chronotropic effects of Dobutamine may cause hypertension, tachyarrythmias, myocardial ischaemia and ventricular fibrillation. Hypotension may result from vasodilatation. The duration of action of Dobutamine Hydrochloride is generally short (half-life, approximately 2 minutes).

Temporarily discontinue Dobutamine until the patient's condition stabilises. The patient should be monitored and any appropriate resusitative measures started immediately.

Forced diuresis, peritoneal dialysis, haemodialysis or charcoal haemoperfusion have not been established as beneficial.

If the product is ingested, unpredictable absorption may occur from the mouth and gastrointestinal tract.

Dobutamine should be used with caution in severe hypotension complicating cardiogenic shock (mean arterial pressure less than 70 mm Hg). If the blood pressure drops quickly decreasing the dose or stopping the infusion typically results in a return to baseline blood pressure values. Occasionally intervention may be required and reversibility may not be immediate.

If arterial blood pressure remains low or decreases progressively during administration of Dobutamine despite adequate ventricular filling pressure and cardiac output consideration may be given to the use of a peripheral vasoconstrictor agent e.g. Noradrenaline or Dopamine.

DBL Dobutamine Hydrochloride contains sodium metabisulphite in the formulation. This may cause allergic type reactions including anaphylaxis and life-threatening or less severe asthmatic episodes, in certain susceptable individuals. The overall prevalence of sulphite sensitivity in the general population is unknown but probably low; such sensitivity seems to occur more frequently in asthmatic patients.

Pharmacological properties

Pharmacodynamic properties: Dobutamine is a selective ß-adrenergic agonist whose mechanism of action is complex.

It is believed that the ß-adrenergic effects result from stimulation of adenyl cyclase activity. In therapeutic doses, Dobutamine also has mild ß2- and a1-

adrenergic receptor agonist effects, which are relatively balanced and result in minimal net direct effect on systemic vasculature. Dobutamine does not cause release of endogenous norepinephrine. The main effect of therapeutic doses of Dobutamine is cardiac stimulation. While the positive inotropic effect of the drug on the myocardium appears to be mediated principally via ß1-adrenergic stimulation, experimental evidence suggests that a1-adrenergic stimulation may also be involved and that the a1-adrenergic activity results mainly from the (-)-stereoisomer of the drug.

The ß1-adrenergic effects of Dobutamine exert a positive inotropic effect on the myocardium and result in an increase in cardiac output due to increased myocardial contractility and stroke volume. Increased left ventricular filling pressure decreases in patients with congestive heart failure. In therapeutic doses, Dobutamine causes a decrease in peripheral resistance; however, systolic blood pressure and pulse pressure may remain unchanged or be increased because of augmented cardiac output. With usual doses, heart rate is usually not substantially changed. Coronary blood flow and myocardial oxygen consumption are usually increased because of increased myocardial contractility.

Dobutamine facilitates atrioventricular conduction and shortens or causes no important change in intraventricular conduction. The tendency of Dobutamine to induce cardiac arrhythmias may be slightly less than that of dopamine and is considerably less than that of isoproterenol or other catecholamines. Pulmonary vascular resistance may decrease if it is elevated initially and mean pulmonary artery pressure may decrease or remain unchanged. Dobutamine does not seem to affect dopaminergic receptors and causes no renal or mesenteric vasodilation; however, urine flow may increase because of increased cardiac output.

Pharmacokinetic properties:

Absorption: Orally administered Dobutamine is rapidly metabolized in the GI tract. Following IV administration, the onset of action of Dobutamine occurs within 2 minutes. Peak plasma concentrations of the drug and peak effects occur within 10 minutes after initiation of an IV infusion. The effects of the drug cease shortly after discontinuing an infusion.

Distribution: It is not known if Dobutamine crosses the placenta or is distributed into milk.

Elimination: The plasma half-life of Dobutamine is about 2 minutes. Dobutamine is metabolized in the liver and other tissues by catechol-O-methyltransferase to an inactive compound, 3-O-methyldobutamine, and by conjugation with glucuronic acid. Conjugates of Dobutamine and 3-O-methyldobutamine are excreted mainly in urine and to a minor extent in faeces.

Pharmaceutical particulars

List of excipients:

Sodium Metabisulphite BP	0.22 mg
Water for Injections BP	to 1.0 mL.

Incompatibilities: Dobutamine Hydrochloride has been reported to be incompatible with alkaline solutions and should not be mixed with sodium bicarbonate 5%, or other strong alkaline solutions ie. aminophylline, frusemide. Precipitation has occured with bumetanide, calcium gluconate, insulin, diazepam and phenytoin Because of the potential physical incompatibilities, it is recommended that Dobutamine Hydrochloride not be mixed with other drugs in the same solution.

Dobutamine should not be used with drugs or diluents containing bisulphites or ethanol.

Shelf life: 24 months

Special precautions for storage: Undiluted vials of Dobutamine Hydrochloride should be stored below 25°C.

Prepared intravenous solutions are stable for 24 hours, when aseptically prepared and stored in the refrigerator.

Solutions of Dobutamine Hydrochloride may have a pink discolouration. This discolouration, which will increase with time, results from a slight oxidation of the drug. However, there is no significant loss of drug potency within the recommended storage times for solutions of the drug.

Instructions for use/handling: Not applicable.

Marketing authorisation number 4515/0077.

Date of approval/revision of SPC September 1995

Legal category POM

STERILE DOPAMINE CONCENTRATE 200 mg/5 ml

Qualitative and quantitative composition

Active constituent

Dopamine Hydrochloride HSE	200.0 mg

Other constituents

Sodium Metabisulphite BP	50.0 mg
Water for Injections BP	5.0 mL

There is no overage included in the formulation.

Pharmaceutical form Concentrated solution for intravenous infusion.

Clinical particulars

Therapeutic indications: Dopamine is indicated for the correction of haemodynamic imbalance present in:

(a) Acute hypotension or shock associated with myocardial infarction, endotoxic septicaemia, trauma and renal failure.
(b) As an adjunct after open heart surgery, where there is persistent hypotension after correction of hypovolaemia.
(c) In chronic cardiac decompensation as in congestive failure.

Posology and method of administration: To be administered by intravenous infusion only after dilution with the appropriate diluents.

Adults: The rate of administration and duration of therapy should be carefully adjusted accoriding to the patient's response. Dopamine infusion is usually begun at a rate of 1–5 mcg/kg per minute. Increases of 1 to 4 mcg/kg/min at 10- to 30-minute intervals may be made until the optimal response is attained. Such low doses dilate the renal and mesenteric vascular bed by acting on 'dopaminergic' receptors, causing increases in glomerular filtration rate, renal blood flow, sodium excretion, and urine output.

In severely ill patients, the infusion should be initiated at a rate of 5 mcg/kg/min gradually increased by increments of 5–10 mcg/kg/min, until the optimum dose for the patient is achieved as judged by increases in blood pressure, urine flow and perfusion generally. Infusion rates greater than 50 mcg/kg/min have been safely used although urine output should be checked frequently and should it fall, the lowest effective dosage should be used.

Children: The safety and efficacy of Dopamine in paediatric patients has not been established.

Geriatric: No variation in dosage is suggested for geriatric patients. However, close monitoring is suggested for blood pressure, urine flow and peripheral tissue perfusion.

Contra-indications: Dopamine should not be used in patients with:

(i) Phaeochromocytoma
(ii) Arterial or ventricular tachyarrhythmias
(iii) Hyperthroidism
(iv) Avoid Cyclopropane and halogenated anaesthetics.

Special warnings and special precautions for use: Dopamine should not be used in the presence of uncorrected tachyarrhythmias or ventricular fibrillation. Nor should it be used in patients with phaeochromocytoma or hyperthyroidism. Cyclopropane and halogenated hydrocarbon anaesthetics should be avoided.

Patients who have been treated with MAO inhibitors prior to Dopamine should be given reduced doses; the starting dose should be one tenth (1/10th) of the usual dose.

Hypovolaemia should be corrected where necessary prior to Dopamine infusion. Low doses should be used in shock due to acute myocardial infarction.

Interaction with other medicaments and other forms of interaction:

(i) *Anaesthetics:* The myocardium is sensitised by the effect of Dopamine, Cyclopropane or halogenated hydrocarbon anaesthetics, and these should be avoided. This interaction applies both to pressor activity and cardiac beta adrenergic stimulation.

(ii) *Monoamine Oxidase (MAO) Inhibitors:* MAO inhibitors potentiate the effect of Dopamine and its duration of action. Patients who have been treated with monoamine oxidase (MAO) inhibitors prior to administration of dopamine will therefore require a substantially reduced dosage. (The starting dose should be reduced to at least one tenth (1/10th) of the usual dose.)

(iii) *Alpha and Beta Blockers:* The cardiac effects of Dopamine are antagonised by β-adrenergic blocking agents such as Propanolol and Metroprolol, and the peripheral vasoconstriction caused by high doses of Dopamine is antagonised by a-adrenergic blocking agents. Dopamine-induced renal and mesenteric vasodilation is not antagonised by either a β-adrenergic blocking agents, but, in animals, is antagonised by Haloperidol or other butyrophenes, phenothiazines, and opiates.

(iv) *Phenytoin:* Administration of I.V. Phenytoin to patients receiving Dopamine has resulted in hypotension and bradycardia; some clinicians recommend that Phenytoin be used with extreme caution, if at all, in patients receiving Dopamine.

Pregnancy and lactation:

Use in pregnancy: The effect of Dopamine on the human foetus is not known; therefore, the drug should be used in pregnant women only when the possible benefits outweight the potential risks.

Use in lactation: It is not known if Dopamine is excreted in breast milk, nor is the effect on the infant known.

Effects on ability to drive and use machines: Not applicable.

Undesirable effects: Adverse reactions to dopamine are related to its pharmacological action.

More common reactions include:

Cardiovascular: Ectopic beats, tachycardia, anginal pain, palpitation, hypotension, vasoconstriction.
Gastrointestinal: Nausea, vomiting.
Nervous System:Headache.
Respiratory: Dyspnoea.

Less common reactions include:

Biochemical Abnormalities: Azotaemia.
Cardiovasular: Aberrant conduction, bradycardia, widened QRS complex, hypertension, gangrene.
Nervous system: Piloerection.

Serious or life-threatening reactions: Gangrene of the feet has occurred following doses of 10–14 mcg/kg/min and higher in a few patients with pre-existing vascular disease.

Overdose: Excessive elevation of blood pressure and vasoconstriction can occur due to the alpha adrenergic actions of dopamine, especially in patients with a history of occlusive vascular disease. If desired, this condition can be rapidly reversed by dose reduction or discontinuing the infusion, since dopamine has a half-life of less than 2 minutes in the body.

Should these measures fail, an infusion of an alpha adrenergic blocking agent e.g., phentolamine mesylate should be considered.

Dopamine at the infusion site can cause local vasoconstriction, hence the desirability of infusing into a large vein. The resulting ischaemia can be reversed by infiltration of the affected area with 10–15 ml of saline containing 5 mg to 10 mg phentolamine mesylate. A syringe with a fine hypodermic needle should be used to liberally infiltrate the ischaemic area as soon as extravasation is noted.

Accidental overdosage: Accidental overdosage as evidenced by excessive blood pressure elevation can be controlled by dose reduction or discontinuing the dopamine infusion for a short period, since the duration of action of dopamine is short.

Should these measures fail, an infusion of phentolamine mesylate should be considered.

Pharmacological properties

Pharmacodynamic properties: Dopamine stimulates adrenergic receptors of the sympathetic nervous system. The drug has principally a direct stimulatory effect on β1-adrenergic receptors, but also appears to have an indirect effect by releasing norepinephrine from its storage sites. Dopamine also appears to act on specific dopaminergic receptors in the renal, mesenteric, coronary, and intracerebral vascular beds to cause vasodilation. The drug has little or no effect on β2-adrenergic receptors.

In I.V. doses of 0.5–2 mcg/kg per minute, the drug acts predominantly on dopaminergic receptors; in I.V. doses of 2–10 mcg/kg per minute, the drug also stimulates β1-adrenergic receptors. In higher therapeutic doses, a-adrenergic receptors are stimulated and the net effect of the drug is the result of a-adrenergic, β1-adrenergic, and dopaminergic stimulation. The main effects of Dopamine depend on the dose administered. In low doses, cardiac stimulation and renal vascular dilation occur and in larger doses vasoconstriction occurs. It is believed that a-adrenergic effects result from inhibition of the production of cyclic adenosine -31, 51-monophosphate (cAMP) by inhibition of the enzyme adenyl cyclase, whereas β-adrenergic effects result from stimulation of adenyl cyclase activity.

Pharmacokinetic properties:

Absorption: Orally administered Dopamine is rapidly metabolised in the G.I. tract. Following I.V. administration, the onset of action of Dopamine occurs within 5 minutes, and the drug has a duration of action of less than 10 minutes.

Distribution: The drug is widely distributed in the body but does not cross the blood-brain barrier to a substantial extent. It is not known if Dopamine crosses the placenta.

Elimination: Dopamine has a plasma half-life of about 2 minutes. Dopamine is metabolised in the liver, kidneys, and plasma by monoamine oxidase (MAO) and catechol-0-methyltransferase to the inactive compounds homovanillic acid (HVA) and 3,4-dihydroxyphenylacetic acid. In patients receiving MAO inhibitors, the duration of action of Dopamine may be as long as 1 hour. About 25% of a dose of Dopamine is metabolised to norepinephrine within the adrenergic nerve terminals.

Dopamine is excreted in urine principally as HVA and its sulphate and glucuronide conjugates and as

3,4-dihydroxyphenylacetic acid. A very small fraction of a dose is excreted unchanged. Following administration of radio labelled Dopamine, approximately 80% of the radioactivity reportedly is excreted in urine within 24 hours.

Pharmaceutical particulars

List of excipients:

Sodium Metabisulphite BP	50.0 mg
Water for Injections BP	5.0 mL

There is no overage included in the formulation.

Incompatibilities: Sterile Dopamine Concentrate should not be added to any alkaline intravenous solutions, i.e. Sodium Bicarbonate. Any solution which exhibits physical or chemical incompatibility through a colour change or precipitate should not be administered.

It is suggested that admixtures containing Gentamicin Sulphate, Cephalothin Sodium, Cephalothin Sodium Neutral or Oxacillin Sodium should be avoided unless all other viable alternatives have been exhausted.

Admixtures of Ampicillin and Dopamine in 5% Glucose Solution are alkaline and incompatible and result in decomposition of both drugs. They should not be admixed.

Admixtures of Dopamine, Amphotericin B in 5% Glucose Solution are incompatible as a precipitate forms immediately on mixing.

Shelf life: 36 months.

Special precautions for storage: Store below 30°C. Protect from light.

Nature and contents of container: Clear, 5 ml Type I Glass Ampoules in a pack of 5.

Instructions for use/handling: Not applicable.

Marketing authorisation number PL 4515/0011

Date of first authorisation/renewal of authorisation

Date of First Authorisation: 10/9/85
First Renewal of Authorisation: 12/1/93

Date of (partial) revision of the text 16/3/98

STERILE DOPAMINE CONCENTRATE 800 mg/5 ml

Qualitative and quantitative composition

Active constituent

Dopamine Hydrochloride HSE 800.0 mg

Other constituents

Sodium Metabisulphite BP 50.0 mg
Water for Injections BP 5.0 mL

There is no overage included in the formulation.

Pharmaceutical form Concentrated solution for intravenous infusion.

Clinical particulars

Therapeutic indications: Dopamine is indicated for the correction of haemodynamic imbalance present in:

(a) Acute hypotension or shock associated with myocardial infarction, endotoxic septicaemia, trauma and renal failure.
(b) As an adjunct after open heart surgery, where there is persistent hypotension after correction of hypovolaemia.
(c) In chronic cardiac decompensation as in congestive failure.

Posology and method of administration: Dopamine is a potent drug; it must be diluted before administration.

Adults: Where appropriate, the circulating blood volume must be restored with a suitable plasma expander or whole blood, prior to administration of dopamine hydrochloride.

Begin infusion of dopamine hydrochloride solution at doses of 2.5 mcg/kg/min in patients who are likely to respond to modest increments of heart force and renal perfusion.

In more severe cases, administration may be initiated at a rate of 5 mcg/kg/min and increased gradually in 5 to 10 mcg/kg/min increments up to 20 to 50 mcg/kg/min as needed. If doses in excess of 50 mcg/kg/min are required, it is advisable to check urine output frequently.

Should urinary flow begin to decrease in the absence of hypotension, reduction of dopamine dosage should be considered. It has been found that more than 50% of patients have been satisfactorily maintained on doses less than 20 mcg/kg/min.

In patients who do not respond to these doses, additional increments of dopamine may be given in an effort to achieve adequate blood pressure, urine flow and perfusion generally.

Treatment of all patients requires constant evaluation of therapy in terms of blood volume, augmentation of cardiac contractility, and distribution of peripheral perfusion and urinary output.

Dosage of dopamine should be adjusted according to the patient's response, with particular attention to diminution of established urine flow rate, increasing tachycardia or development of new dysrhythmias as indications for decreasing or temporarily suspending the dosage.

Preparation of infusion solutions:

Suggested dilution: Aseptically transfer Sterile Dopamine Concentrate into the I.V. solution as shown in the following table:

Strength	*Volume (ml)*	*I.V. solution volume (ml)*	*Final concentration (microgram/ml)*
200 mg/5 ml	5	500	400
200 mg/5 ml	5	250	800
200 mg/5 ml	10	250	1600
200 mg/5 ml	20	500	1600
800 mg/5 ml	5	500	1600
800 mg/5 ml	5	250	3200

Dopamine Hydrochloride can be diluted with:
0.9% Sodium Chloride Injection
5% Dextrose, 0.45% Sodium Chloride Solution
Compound Sodium Lactate (Hartmann's) Solution

Dilution in these fluids retain at least 95% of the original potency for 48 hours at room temperature under normal fluorescent light. Dilutions should be discarded immediately after use.

Children: The safety and efficacy of Dopamine in paediatric patients has not been established.

Geriatric: No variation in dosage is suggested for geriatric patients. However, close monitoring is suggested for blood pressure, urine flow and peripheral tissue perfusion.

Contra-indications: Dopamine should not be used in patients with phaeochromocytoma or hyperthyroidism.

Dopamine should not be used in the presence of uncorrected arterial or ventricular tachyarrhythmias or ventricular fibrillation.

Cyclopropane and halogenated hydrocarbon anaesthetics should be avoided.

Special warnings and special precautions for use:

Warnings: Dopamine should not be used in the presence of uncorrected tachyarrhythmias or ventricular fibrillation. Nor should it be used in patients with phaeochromocytoma or hyperthyroidism. Cyclopropane and halogenated hydrocarbon anaesthetics should be avoided.

Patients who have been treated with MAO inhibitors prior to Dopamine should be given reduced doses; the starting dose should be one tenth (1/10th) of the usual dose.

Excess administration of potassium-free solutions may result in significant hypokalaemia.

The intravenous administration of these solutions can cause fluid and/or solute overloading resulting in dilution of serum electrolyte concentrations, overhydration, congested states or pulmonary oedema.

Precautions: Hypovolaemia should be corrected where necessary prior to Dopamine infusion. Low doses should be used in shock due to acute myocardial infarction.

If a disproportionate rise in diastolic pressure (i.e. a marked decrease in pulse pressure) is observed, the infusion rate should be decreased and the patients observed carefully for further evidence of predominant vasoconstriction activity, unless such an effect is desired.

Patients with a history of peripheral vascular disease should be closely monitored for any changes in colour or temperature of the skin of the extremities. If a change of skin colour or temperature occurs and is thought to be the result of compromised circulation to the extremities, the benefits of continued dopamine infusion should be weighed against the risk of possible necrosis. These changes may be reversed by decreasing the rate or discontinuing the infusion.

Dopamine hydrochloride in 5% dextrose injection should be infused into a large vein whenever possible to prevent the possibility of infiltration of perivascular tissue adjacent to the infusion site. Extravasation may cause necrosis and sloughing of the surrounding tissue. Ischaemia can be reversed by infiltration of the affected area with 10–15 ml of saline containing 5 to 10 mg phentolamine mesylate. A syringe with a fine hypodermic needle should be used to liberally infiltrate the ischaemic area as soon as extravasation is noted.

Dopamine should be used with extreme caution in patients inhaling cyclopropane or halogenated hydrocarbon anaesthetics due to the arterial arrhythmogenic potential.

Dextrose solutions should be used with caution in patients with known subclinical or overt diabetes mellitus.

Interaction with other medicaments and other forms of interaction:

Anaesthetics: The myocardium is sensitised by the effect of Dopamine, Cyclopropane or halogenated hydrocarbon anaesthetics, and these should be avoided. This interaction applies both to pressor activity and cardiac beta adrenergic stimulation.

Alpha and beta blockers: The cardiac effects of Dopamine are antagonised by β-adrenergic blocking agents such as Propanolol and Metoprolol, and the peripheral vasoconstriction caused by high doses of Dopamine is antagonised by a-adrenergic blocking agents. Dopamine-induced renal and mesenteric vasodilation is not antagonised by either a or β-adrenergic blocking agents, but, in animals, is antagonised by Haloperidol or other butyrophenones, phenothiazines, and opiates.

Monoamine Oxidase (MAO): MAO inhibitors potentiate the effect of Dopamine and its duration of action. Patients who have been treated with monoamine oxidase (MAO) inhibitors prior to dopamine should be given reduced doses; the starting dose should be one tenth (1/10th) of the usual dose.

Phenytoin: Administration of I.V. Phenytoin to patients receiving Dopamine has resulted in hypotension and bradycardia; some clinicians recommend that Phenytoin be used with extreme caution, if at all, in patients receiving Dopamine.

Pregnancy and lactation:

Use in pregnancy: Animal studies have shown no evidence of teratogenic effects with dopamine. However, the effect of Dopamine on the human foetus is unknown therefore the drug should be used in pregnant women only when the expected benefits outweight the potential risk to the foetus.

Use in lactation: It is not known if Dopamine is excreted in breast milk nor if there is any effect on the infant.

Effects on ability to drive and use machines: Not applicable.

Undesirable effects: Adverse reactions to dopamine are related to its pharmacological action.

More common reactions:

Cardiovascular: Ectopic beats, tachycardia, anginal pain, palpitation, hypotension, vasoconstriction.
Gastrointestinal: Nausea, vomiting.
Nervous System: Headache.
Respiratory: Dyspnoea.

Less common reactions:

Biochemical Abnormalities: Azotaemia.
Cardiovasular: Aberrant conduction, bradycardia, widened QRS complex, hypertension, gangrene.
Nervous system: Piloerection.

Serious or life-threatening reactions: Gangrene of the feet has occurred following doses of 10–14 mcg/kg/min and higher in a few patients with pre-existing vascular disease.

Overdose: Excessive elevation of blood pressure and vasoconstriction can occur due to the alpha adrenergic actions of dopamine, especially in patients with a history of occlusive vascular disease. If desired, this condition can be rapidly reversed by dose reduction or discontinuing the infusion, since dopamine has a half-life of less than 2 minutes in the body. Should these measures fail, an infusion of an alpha adrenergic blocking agent e.g., phentolamine mesylate should be considered. Dopamine at the infusion site can cause local vasoconstriction, hence the desirability of infusing into a large vein. The resulting ischaemia can be reversed by infiltration of the effected area with 10–15 ml of saline containing 5 to 10 mg phentolamine mesylate. A syringe with a fine hypodermic needle should be used to liberally infiltrate the ischaemic area as soon as extravasation is noted.

Accidental overdosage: Accidental overdosage as evidenced by excessive blood pressure elevation can be controlled by dose reduction or discontinuing the dopamine infusion for a short period, since the duration of action of dopamine is short.

Should these measures fail, an infusion of phentolamine mesylate should be considered.

Pharmacological properties

Pharmacodynamic properties: Dopamine stimulates adrenergic receptors of the sympathetic nervous system. The drug has principally a direct stimulatory effect on β1-adrenergic receptors, but also appears to have an indirect effect by releasing norepinephrine from its storage sites. Dopamine also appears to act on specific dopaminergic receptors in the renal, mesenteric, coronary, and intracerebral vascular beds to cause vasodilation. The drug has little or no effect on β2-adrenergic receptors.

In I.V. doses of 0.5–2 mcg/kg per minute, the drug acts predominantly on dopaminergic receptors; in I.V. doses of 2–10 mcg/kg per minute, the drug also stimulates β1-adrenergic receptors. In higher therapeutic doses, a-adrenergic receptors are stimulated and the net effect of the drug is the result of a-adrenergic, β1-adrenergic, and dopaminergic stimulation. The main effects of Dopamine depend on the dose administered. In low doses, cardiac stimulation and renal vascular dilation occur and in larger doses vasoconstriction occurs. It is believed that a-adrenergic effects result from inhibition of the production of cyclic adenosine -31, 51-monophosphate (cAMP) by inhibition of the enzyme adenyl cyclase, whereas β-adrenergic effects result from stimulation of adenyl cyclase activity.

Pharmacokinetic properties:
Absorption: Orally administered Dopamine is rapidly metabolised in the G.I. tract. Following I.V. administration, the onset of action of Dopamine occurs within 5 minutes, and the drug has a duration of action of less than 10 minutes.

Distribution: The drug is widely distributed in the body but does not cross the blood-brain barrier to a substantial extent. It is not known if Dopamine crosses the placenta.

Elimination: Dopamine has a plasma half-life of about 2 minutes. Dopamine is metabolised in the liver, kidneys, and plasma by monoamine oxidase (MAO) and catechol-0-methyltransferase to the inactive compounds homovanillic acid (HVA) and 3,4-dihydroxyphenylacetic acid. In patients receiving MAO inhibitors, the duration of action of Dopamine may be as long as 1 hour. About 25% of a dose of Dopamine is metabolised to norepinephrine within the adrenergic nerve terminals.

Dopamine is excreted in urine principally as HVA and its sulphate and glucuronide conjugates and as 3,4-dihydroxyphenylacetic acid. A very small fraction of a dose is excreted unchanged. Following administration of radio labelled Dopamine, approximately 80% of the radioactivity reportedly is excreted in urine within 24 hours.

Pharmaceutical particulars

List of excipients:

Sodium Metabisulphite BP	50.0 mg
Water for Injections BP	5.0 mL

There is no overage included in the formulation.

Incompatibilities: Sterile Dopamine Concentrate should not be added to any alkaline intravenous solutions, i.e. Sodium Bicarbonate. Any solution which exhibits physical or chemical incompatibility through a colour change or precipitate should not be administered.

It is suggested that admixtures containing Gentamicin Sulphate, Cephalothin Sodium, Cephalothin Sodium Neutral or Oxacillin Sodium should be avoided unless all other viable alternatives have been exhausted.

Admixtures of Ampicillin and Dopamine in 5% Glucose Solution are alkaline and incompatible and result in decomposition of both drugs. They should not be admixed.

Admixtures of Dopamine, Amphotericin B in 5% Glucose Solution are incompatible as a precipitate forms immediately on mixing.

Shelf life: 36 months.

Special precautions for storage: Store below 30°C. Protect from light.

Do not add dopamine to 5% sodium bicarbonate or other alkaline solutions, since the drug is inactivated. Store below 30°C, protect from light, do not use if discoloured. Any solution which exhibits physical or chemical incompatibility through a colour change or precipitate should not be administered.

Nature and contents of container: Clear, 5 ml Type I Glass Ampoules in a pack of 5.

Instructions for use/handling: Not applicable.

Marketing authorisation number PL 4515/0022

Date of first authorisation/renewal of authorisation
Date of First Authorisation: 2/9/85
First Renewal of Authorisation: 17/10/90

Date of (partial) revision of the text
Amended 29/5/97 SF/vg
Amended 16/3/98 DM

DOXORUBICIN HYDROCHLORIDE FOR INJECTION

Qualitative and quantitative composition

Active constituent	*10 mg*	*50 mg*
Doxorubicin USP	10.0 mg	50.0 mg

Pharmaceutical form Sterile freeze dried powder for injection.

Clinical particulars

Therapeutic indications: Doxorubicin has been used successfully in the treatment of neoplastic conditions such as acute leukaemia, soft tissue and osteogenic sarcomas, breast carcinoma, lymphomas , bronchogenic (lung) carcinoma. It has also been used in the treatment of paediatric malignancy. Doxorubicin is frequently used in combination chemotherapy regimen involving other cytotoxic drugs. Doxorubicin can be used in the treatment of non-metastatic transitional cell carcinoma, carcinoma in situ and papillary tumours of the bladder, by intravesical administration.

Posology and method of administration: When used as a single agent, the recommended dosage schedule is 60- 75 mg/m² body surface area, as a single intravenous injection administered at 21 day intervals. If using body weight to calculate the dose, then dosages of 1.2–2.4 mg/kg are recommended.

It has been shown that giving doxorubicin as a single dose every three weeks greatly reduces the distressing toxic effect, mucositis. However, there are some regimens which divide the dose over three successive days (20-25 mg/m² or 0.4-0.8 mg/kg). It is thought that this regimen has greater effectiveness although at a cost of higher toxicity

Administration of doxorubicin in a weekly regimen has been shown to be as effective as the three weekly regimen. The recommended dosage is 20 mg/m² once a week although objective responses have been seen at 6-12 mg/m². This regimen of weekly dosing also reduces the incidence of cardiotoxicity.

It is particularly important to reduce the dose of doxorubicin if it is used in combination with other drugs with a similar toxicity profile. The recommended lifetime cumulative dose limit is 450-550 mg doxorubicin hydrochloride/m² body surface area.

It is recommended that doxorubicin be slowly administered into the tubing of a freely running intravenous infusion of Sodium Chloride Injection 0.9% or 5% Dextrose Injection. The tubing should be attached to a Butterfly needle inserted preferably into a large vein. The rate of administration is dependent on the size of the vein and the dosage. However the dose should be administered in not less than 3 to 5 minutes. This technique minimises the risk of thrombosis or perivenous extravasation which can lead to severe cellulitis and vesication.

Intravenous infusion is not advised due to the tissue damage that may occur if the infusion infiltrates the tissues. If a central vein catheter is used then infusion of Doxorubicin in Sodium Chloride 0.9% Injection is advised.

Local erythematous streaking along the vein as well as facial flushing may be indicative of too rapid administration. A burning or stinging sensation may be indicative of perivenous infiltration and the infusion should be immediately terminated and restarted in another vein. Doxorubicin should not be mixed with heparin since it has been reported that these drugs are incompatible to the extent that a precipitate may form. Until specific compatibility data are available, it is not recommended that doxorubicin be mixed with other drugs.

Intravesical administration: This technique may be used for the treatment of transitional cell carcinoma, papillary bladder tumours and carcinoma in situ. It should not be used for invasive tumours of the bladder which have penetrated the bladder wall.

Many regimens are in use, making interpretation difficult, but the following procedure may be a helpful guide:

1. Patient should be instructed not to drink fluids for 12 hours prior to the examination.
2. Dissolve 50 mg of doxorubicin in 50 mL of normal saline and instil via the catheter into the bladder.
3. The catheter should be removed and the patient instructed to be on one side. At 15 minute intervals the patient should make a quarter turn over a 1 hour period. At the end of this period, the patient may void.
4. The procedure may be repeated at monthly intervals.

Intra-arterial administration: Doxorubicin Hydrochloride has been administered as an intra-arterial infusion in an attempt to produce local intense activity and reduce systemic toxicity. However it must be recognised that this route of administration is potentially extremely hazardous and can lead to widespread necrosis of perfused tissue unless careful precautions are taken. Intraarterial administration should be undertaken only by experienced professionals.

Paediatric: Adult dosage regimens may be suitable for paediatric cases, but may need to be reduced.

Geriatric: It is recommended that the total cumulative dose of doxorubicin for adults aged 70 or older be restricted to 450 mg/m² body surface area. Adult doses may be suitable for geriatric patients, but may need to be reduced.

Impaired hepatic function: Doxorubicin is metabolised by the liver and excreted in bile. Impairment of liver function results in slower excretion of the drug and consequently increased retention and accumulation in the plasma and tissues, resulting in enhanced clinical toxicity.

Doxorubicin dosage must be reduced if hepatic function is impaired according to the following table:

Serum bilirubin levels	*BSP retention*	*Recommended dose*
1.2–3.0 mg/100 mL	9–15%	50% normal dose
over 3.0 mg/100 mL	over 15%	25% normal dose

Impaired renal function: Doxorubicin and metabolites are excreted in the urine to a minor degree and there are no clear indications that the pharmacokinetics or toxicity of doxorubicin are altered in patients with impaired renal function.

Contra-indications: Dosage should not be repeated in cases of bone marrow depression or buccal ulceration or buccal burning sensation, which can precede ulceration.

Experienced Physician: Doxorubicin should be administered only under the supervision of a physician who is experienced in the use of cancer chemotherapeutic agents.

Special warnings and special precautions for use:
Warnings: Cardiac toxicity: Special attention must be given to the cardiac toxicity exhibited by doxorubicin. This may present as tachycardia or ECG changes including supraventricular tachycardia. Severe cardiac failure may occur suddenly, without premonitory ECG changes.

It is recommended that the cumulative total lifetime dose of doxorubicin (including related drugs such as daunorubicin) should not exceed 450–550 mg/sq m body surface area. Above this dosage, the risk of irreversible congestive cardiac failure increases greatly. Total dose should also take account of any previous or concomitant mediastinal irradiation, other anthracycline chemotherapy or concurrent high dose cyclophosphamide, which may also exhibit cardiotoxic effects.

Congestive heart failure and/or cardiomyopathy may be encountered several weeks after discontinuation of doxorubicin therapy and for this reason extreme care should be taken in patients with existing associated heart disease.

Cardiac failure is often not favourably affected by presently known medical or physical therapy for cardiac support. Early clinical diagnosis of drug induced heart failure appears to be essential for successful treatment with digitalis, diuretics, low salt diet and bed rest. Severe cardiac toxicity may occur precipitously without antecedent ECG changes. Base line ECG and periodic follow up ECG during and immediately after active drug therapy is an advisable precaution. Transient ECG changes, such as T-wave flattening, S-T depression and arrhythmias are not considered indications for suspension of doxorubicin therapy. A persistent reduction in the voltage of the QRS wave is presently considered more specifically predictive for cardiac toxicity. If this occurs, the benefit of continued therapy must be carefully evaluated against the risk of producing irreversible cardiac damage.

Bone marrow depression: There is a high incidence of bone marrow depression, primarily of leucocytes, requiring careful haematological monitoring. With the recommended dosage schedule, leucopenia is usually transient, reaching its nadir at 10–14 days after treatment, with recovery usually occurring by the 21st day. White blood cell counts as low as 1000/cubic mm are to be expected during treatment with appropriate doses of doxorubicin. Red blood cell and platelet levels should also be monitored, since they may also be depressed.

Haematologic toxicity may require dose reduction or suspension or delay of doxorubicin therapy.

Immunosuppression: Doxorubicin is a powerful but temporary immunosuppressant agent. Appropriate measures should be taken to prevent secondary infection.

Severe myelosuppression: Persistent severe myelosuppression may result in superinfection or haemorrhage.

Enhanced toxicity: It has been reported that doxorubicin may enhance the severity of the toxicity of anticancer therapies, such as cyclophosphamide induced haemorrhagic cystitis, mucositis induced by radiotherapy and hepatotoxicity of 6-mercaptopurine.

Infertility: Doxorubicin may cause infertility during the time of drug administration. Although ovulation and menstruation appear to return after termination of therapy, there is no information about the restoration of male fertility.

Hepatic impairment: Toxicity to recommended doses of doxorubicin is enhanced by hepatic impairment. It is recommended that an evaluation of hepatic function be carried out prior to individual dosing, using conventional clinical laboratory tests such as AST, ALT, alkaline phosphatase, bilirubin and BSP. If required, dosage schedules should be reduced accordingly (see Dosage and administration).

Extravasation: On intravenous administration of doxorubicin, a stinging or burning sensation signifies extravasation and, even if blood return from aspiration of the infusion needle is good, the injection or infusion should be immediately terminated and restarted in another vein.

Should extravasation occur, stop the infusion immediately and apply ice packs to the injection site. Local injection of dexamethasone or hydrocortisone may be used to minimise local tissue necrosis. Hydrocortisone cream 1% may also be applied locally.

Precautions: Initial treatment with doxorubicin requires close observation of the patient and extensive laboratory monitoring.

It is strongly recommended therefore, that patients be hospitalised at least during the first phase of treatment. Blood count and liver function tests should be carried out prior to each doxorubicin treatment.

Interaction with other medicaments and other forms of interaction: Not applicable.

Pregnancy and lactation:

Use In pregnancy: The drug is embryotoxic and teratogenic in rats and embryotoxic and abortifacient in rabbits, and trace amounts of the drug have been found in mouse foetuses and in one aborted human foetus. Although there is no conclusive evidence, there is data which suggests that doxorubicin may harm the foetus. It is therefore recommended that doxorubicin is not administered to women who are pregnant.

Use In lactation: Doxorubicin is distributed into milk. Experimental data suggests that doxorubicin may harm the infant and should therefore not be administered to mothers who are breast feeding.

Use In intravesical administration: Urine cytologies and blood counts should be monitored monthly, and cytoscopic examinations should be performed at regular intervals.

Effects on ability to drive and use machines: Not known.

Undesirable effects:

Adverse reactions–more common reactions:

Cardiovascular: Cardiotoxicity i.e. cardiomyopathy, congestive heart failure, supraventricular tachycardia.

Dermatological: Doxorubicin extravasation, skin necrosis, cellulitis, vesication, phlebitis, reversible alopecia, erythematous streaking along the vein proximal to the site of injection, phlebosclerosis. Hair growth returns to normal after cessation of treatment.

Gastrointestinal: Nausea and vomiting, mucositis (stomatitis and oesophagitis), diarrhoea. Mucositis is a frequent and painful complication of doxorubicin treatment. Mucositis most commonly develops 5 to 10 days after treatment, and typically begins as a burning sensation in the mouth and pharynx. It may involve the vagina, rectum and oesophagus, and progress to ulceration with risk of secondary infection and usually subsides in 10 days. Retrospective comparison of the incidence of mucositis suggests that it is less frequent as the intervals between doses increase. Mucositis may be severe in patients who have had previous irradiation to the mucosae.

General: Dehydration, facial flushing (if an injection has been given too rapidly). Administration of Doxorubicin may cause red colouration of the urine. Patients should be advised that this is no cause for alarm.

Haematological: Myelosuppression, leucopenia.

Less common reactions:

Dermatological: Urticarial rash, hyperpigmentation of nailbeds and dermal increases (primarily in children in a few cases), recall of skin reaction due to prior radiotherapy.

General: Chills and fever, anorexia, anaphylaxis.

Haematological: Leucopenia, thrombocytopenia, anaemia. Myelosuppression is more common in patients who have had extensive radiotherapy, bone infiltration by tumour, impaired liver function (when appropriate dosage reduction has not been adopted. See DOSAGE: WITH IMPAIRED HEPATIC FUNCTION) and simultaneous treatment with other myelosuppressive agents. The nadir (time from treatment to peripheral blood evidence of maximal myelosuppression) of leucopenia and thrombocytopenia is 10 to 15 days after treatment, and counts return to normal before day 21.

Nervous System: Drowsiness.

Ocular: Conjunctivitis.

Renal: Renal damage.

Overdose: Clinical features: The symptoms of overdosage are likely to be an extension of doxorubicin's pharmacological action. Single doses of 250 mg and 500 mg of doxorubicin have proved fatal. Such doses may cause acute myocardial degeneration within 24 hours, and severe myelosuppression, the greatest effects of which are seen between 10 and 15 days after administration.

Delayed cardiac failure may occur up to six months after the overdose. Patients should be monitored carefully and if symptoms appear, conventional treatment started.

Management: Symptomatic supportive measures should be instituted. Particular attention should be given to prevention and treatment of possible severe haemorrhage or infections secondary to severe, persistent bone marrow depression. Blood transfusion and reverse barrier nursing may be considered.

Pharmacological properties

Pharmacodynamic properties: Doxorubicin hydrochloride is a cytotoxic anthracycline antibiotic.

Although not completely elucidated, the mechanism of action of doxorubicin is related to its ability to bind to DNA and inhibit nucleic acid synthesis. Cell culture studies have demonstrated rapid cell penetration and perinucleolar chromatin binding, rapid inhibition of mitotic activity and nucleic acid synthesis, mutagenesis and chromosomal aberrations.

The specificity of doxorubicin toxicity appears to be related primarily to proliferative activity of normal tissue. Thus, bone marrow, gastro-intestinal tract and gonads are the main normal tissues damaged.

Doxorubicin is not suitable for oral administration as less than 5% of the drug is absorbed.

Pharmacokinetic properties: Pharmacokinetic studies show the intravenous administration of normal or radiolabelled doxorubicin for injection is followed by rapid plasma clearance and significant tissue binding. No information on plasma-protein binding of doxorubicin is available.

The metabolism and disposition of doxorubicin is still to be defined. The drug is metabolised predominantly by the liver to doxorubicinol and several aglycone metabolites. It should be noted that several of the metabolites are cytotoxic. However, it is not certain whether any are more cytotoxic than the parent compound. High levels of metabolites appear rapidly in plasma and undergo a distribution phase with a measurable short initial half-life. Metabolism may be impaired in patients with abnormal liver function.

The disappearance of doxorubicin and its metabolites from the plasma follows a triphasic pharmacokinetic pattern with a mean half-life of the first phase of 12 minutes, of a second phase of 3.3 hours and a prolonged third phase of 29.6 hours.

Urinary excretion of doxorubicin hydrochloride and its metabolites is prolonged and accounts for only 5% of the drug excreted during the first 5 days. Approximately 50% of an administered dose is excreted in bile.

Impairment of liver function results in slower excretion, and consequently, increased retention and accumulation in plasma and tissues. Doxorubicin does not cross the blood brain barrier. However it is known to cross the placenta barrier.

Pharmaceutical particulars

List of excipients:

Doxorubicin content	*10 mg*	*50 mg*
Lactose monohydrate BP	52.6 mg	263.1 mg

There is no overage included in the above formulations.

Incompatibilities: Doxorubicin should not be mixed with heparin since it has been reported that these drugs are incompatible to the extent that a precipitate may form. Until specific compatibility data are available, it is not recommended that doxorubicin be mixed with other drugs.

Shelf life: 36 months.

Special precautions for storage: Store below 25°C and protect from light.

Instructions for use/handling: Doxorubicin is a potent cytotoxic agent which should only be prescribed, prepared and administered by professionals who have been trained in the safe use of the preparation. The following guidelines should be followed when handling, preparing and disposing of Doxorubicin.

Preparation:

1. Reconstitution of powder, transfer to syringes or infusion bags should be carried out in designated areas, preferably a laminar flow station.

2. Personnel must be adequately protected with suitable clothing, gloves, mask and eye shield.

3. Pregnant women should be excluded from handling cytotoxic agents.

Contamination:

1. In the event of contact with the skin or eyes, the affected area should be washed with copious amounts of water or Normal saline. A bland cream may be used to treat transient stinging of skin. Medical advice should be sought if the eyes are affected.

2. In the event of spillage treat with 1% Sodium Hypochlorite solution using a cloth/sponge kept in the designate area. Rinse twice with water. Put all cloths into a plastic bag and seal for incineration.

Disposal: All items used during preparation or administration including syringes,containers, absorbent materials, residual solutions should all be placed in a thick plastic bag and incinerated at 700oC.

Preparation of the injection: The contents of the vial should be reconstituted with Water for Injection BP, Sodium Chloride 0.9%, or Dextrose 5% Injection to a solution concentration of 2 mg per ml.

The reconstituted solution is stable at room temperature, in the vial or in a polypropylene (Terumo) syringe, in the presence or absence of light, for a period of 48 hours. However, it is recommended that the solution be stored at 2-8°C in a refrigerator, and used within 24 hours, in line with good pharmaceutical practice.

Marketing authorisation number 4515/0072-73

Date of approval/revision of SPC May 1996

Legal category POM

ERYTHROMYCIN LACTOBIONATE FOR I.V. INJECTION.

Qualitative and quantitative composition

Erythromycin BP	1000.0 mg
Lactobionic Acid H.S.E.	448.0 mg

Pharmaceutical form Freeze dried powder for injection in a vial.

Clinical particulars

Therapeutic indications:

1. Upper respiratory tract infections (tonsillitis, pharyngitis, sinusitis, secondary bacterial infections).
2. Lower respiratory tract infections (pneumonia, bronchitis, primary atypical pneumonia, Legionnaire's disease).
3. Skin and soft tissue infections (furunculosis, erysipelas).
4. Other infections – diphtheria carriers and cases as an adjunct to antitoxin, syphilis and gonorrhoea (in cases of penicillin allergy), subacute bacterial endocarditis, otitis media.

Posology and method of administration: Intravenous injection by:

1. Continuous I.V. infusion.
2. Intermittent I.V infusion.
   (Small volume I.V. infusion, minimum volume 100 ml, is the preferred method so as to minimise venous irritation).
3. Slow intravenous injection should be made over a period of 3–5 minutes.

Dosage and administration: Intravenous administration of erythromycin is suitable to patients who are unable to tolerate oral medication or when it is necessary to produce a high blood concentration to control severe infections. Oral administration should replace parenteral administration as soon as practicable.

Due to the local irritant effects of erythromycin as well as reports of QT interval prolongation and ventricular arrhythmias (some of which have been fatal) being associated with elevated serum concentrations of erythromycin, the drug must not be administered rapidly by direct intravenous injection (IV push).

Erythromycin lactobionate vials labelled as containing 1 gram of Erythromycin should be initially reconstituted by adding 20 ml of Sterile Water for Injections BP without preservative, to provide a solution containing 50 mg per ml. No other diluent should be used to prepare this initial solution. It is important to ensure that the product is completely dissolved by vigorous shaking before transferring to infusion containers. Prior to administration the concentrated solution should be further diluted in glass or flexible plastic containers of 0.9% Sodium Chloride Injection. If, for clinical reasons, 0.9% saline is not suitable, then neutralised Glucose Intravenous Infusion BP 5% w/v may be used. Neutralised glucose solution is prepared by the addition of 5 ml of sterile 8.4% w/v sodium bicarbonate solution to each litre of Glucose Intravenous Injection BP 5% w/v.

It is necessary to buffer the glucose solution in this way because the stability of Erythromycin Lactobionate is adversely affected below pH 5.5.

To ensure potency, all solutions for administration should be used within 8 hours of preparation.

It is recommended that a clarifying filter is used to minimise the particulate levels in resultant infusions.

For continuous I.V. infusion the concentrated solution should be diluted to a concentration of 1 mg per ml. If required, solution strengths up to 5 mg/ml (0.5% solution) may be used, but should not be exceeded. Higher concentrations may result in pain along the vein. Bolus injection is not recommended.

For intermittent I.V. infusion the appropriate daily dose can be given as 4 doses once every 6 hours. The erythromycin concentration should not exceed 5 mg per ml and the infusion should be administered over 60 minutes, as a rapid infusion is more likely to be associated with arrhythmias or hypotension. A longer period of infusion should be used in patients with risk factors or previous evidence of arrhythmias. Not less than 100 ml of diluent should be used for preparing intermittent I.V. solutions.

Intravenous therapy should be replaced by oral administration at the appropriate time.

Adults: The usual adult dose is the equivalent of 25–50 mg/kg per day in divided doses of erythromycin, by intravenous infusion every 6 hours, or the equivalent of 1 to 2 g of erythromycin daily by intermittent intravenous infusion over 20 to 60 minutes every 6 hours or by infusion over 24 hours. The equivalent of 4 gram daily has been recommended for severe infections.

Small volume I.V. infusion, minimum volume 100 ml, is the preferred method so as to minimise venous irritation.

Children: 25–50 mg per kg by intravenous injection, daily in divided doses.

Elderly: Use adult dosage with care, taking into consideration any impairments in liver or biliary functions.

Patients with impaired hepatic function: In the presence of normal hepatic function, erythromycin is concentrated in the liver and excreted in the bile. Although the effect of hepatic dysfunction on the excretion of erythromycin and its half-life in such patients is not known, caution should be exercised in administering the antibiotic in such cases.

Patients with impaired renal function: The low proportion of renal excretion would suggest that dosage modification in patients with impaired renal function may not be necessary. In severely impaired patients however, toxicity has been reported and dosage adjustment in these cases may be warranted.

Contra-indications: Patients with known hypersensitivity to erythromycin.

Erythromycin is contraindicated with either astemizole, terfenadine, cisapride or pimozide. The concurrent administration of these drugs with erythromycin has been associated with the increased blood levels of astemizole, terfenadine, cisapride or pimozide, with an increased risk of life threatening cardiac arrhythmias.

Prolongation of the QT interval and development of ventricular arrhythmias (some of which have been fatal), including atypical ventricular tachycardia (torsades de pointes) have been reported with the intravenous administration of erythromycin. Limited data suggest that these adverse effects may be associated with abnormally elevated serum erythromycin concentrations following rapid administration. Erythromycin therefore must not be administered rapidly by direct intravenous injection (IV push).

Special warnings and precautions for use: Allergic reactions ranging from urticaria to anaphylaxis have been reported with intravenous erythromycin.

Superinfection may occur with prolonged use, giving rise to overgrowth of non susceptible organisms.

Erythromycin is excreted principally via the liver and caution should be exercised when using erythromycin in patients with a degree of hepatic impairment.

In severe renal impairment the half life may be prolonged to 4–7 hours requiring a dose modification.

Interactions with other medicaments and other forms of interaction: Penicillin: Erythromycin, in low bacteriostatic concentrations, may inhibit the actions of bactericidal drugs. In high concentrations, erythromycin may act synergistically with penicillin.

Use of erythromycin in patients receiving digoxin, warfarin, carbemazepine or high doses of theophylline may result in potentiation of the effects due to impairment of excretion. A possible interaction between Erythromycin and Vinblastine has been reported in which patients receiving the two agents concurrently may experience myalgia, neutropenia and fever. It is recommended that patients should avoid receiving Erythromycin and Vinblastine at the same time.

Increased plasma levels of cyclosporin may occur in patients on erythromycin.

Ergotism has been reported in patients receiving erythromycin in combination with ergot.

Concomitant use of erythromycin with astemizole, terfenadine, cisapride, or pimozide is likely to result in an enhanced risk of cardiotoxicity with these drugs, and is therefore contraindicated (see *Contra-indications*).

Laboratory tests used for measurement of urinary catecholamines, SGOT and 17-hydroxycorticosteroids, may be affected if a colorimetric test is used. This interference may complicate interpretation of liver function tests. Suppression of growth of *Lactobacillus casei* by erythromycin, may interfere with serum folate measurements.

Pregnancy and lactation:

Use in pregnancy and lactation: Erythromycin crosses the placenta and gives rise to foetal plasma levels which are approximately 5–20% of maternal levels. However the risks associated with this phenomenon have not been clearly established. Erythromycin should not be administered to pregnant women unless the benefits outweigh the potential risks.

In lactating women, erythromycin is secreted into breast milk in quantities of between 0.5 and 6.2 micrograms/ml. These quantities are not known to be harmful. Erythromycin is not recommended for nursing mothers unless the expected benefits outweigh the potential risks.

Effects on ability to drive and use machines: Not applicable.

Undesirable effects:

Hepatic: Administration may be followed, in up to 10% of cases, by increases in AST and ALT enzymes, which sometimes recur on challenge.

Cardiovascular: Thrombophlebitis, venous irritation. Irritation can be reduced by either slow I.V. injection, or preferably a small volume I.V. infusion.

Prolongation of the QT interval and development of ventricular arrhythmias (some of which have been fatal), including atypical ventricular tachycardia (torsades de pointes), have been reported with the intravenous administration of erythromycin. Limited data suggest that these adverse effects may be associated with abnormally elevated serum erythromycin concentrations following rapid administration.

Auditory/vestibular: In very high doses, erythromycin may cause transient perceptive deafness.

Dermatological: Mild allergic reactions, urticaria, skin eruptions, rashes with fever, and reports of erythema multiforme reaction have been noted.

Overdose: The toxicity is low. Overdosage may be associated with ototoxicity. No specific treatment has been proposed other than general supportive measures.

Pharmacological properties

Pharmacodynamic properties: Erythromycin binds to the ribosomes of bacteria and affects protein synthesis without affecting nucleic acid synthesis. Erythromycin does not bind to cytoplasmic membranes of the host cells. This is a possible explanation of its low toxicity and safety record.

Erythromycin is bacteriostatic and bactericidal depending on its concentration and the type of organism. It inhibits protein synthesis by binding to ribosomal subunits, inhibiting translocation of aminocyl transfer RNA and inhibiting polypeptide synthesis without causing any alteration in the nucleic acid cycle.

Pharmacokinetic properties:

Distribution: The apparent volume of distribution of erythromycin is around 45% of body weight in normal subjects. This large distribution volume is consistent with the extensive tissue penetration of erythromycin.

Erythromycin diffuses readily into most body fluids, except the cerebrospinal fluid. However, in cases of meningeal inflammation, higher concentrations are apparent.

Metabolism: In studies using rabbit microsomes it has been shown that erythromycin is demethylated to des-N-methyl erythromycin and formaldehyde.

Excretion: In the presence of normal hepatic function, erythromycin is concentrated in the liver and excreted in the bile; the effect of hepatic dysfunction on excretion of erythromycin by the liver is not known.

From 12% to 15% of intravenously administered erythromycin is excreted in active form in the urine.

The drug is also excreted in the faeces.

Half-life: The plasma elimination half-life in patients with normal renal function is about 2 hours. In severe renal impairment the half-life may be prolonged to between 4 and 7 hours.

Preclinical safety data: There are no preclinical data of relevance to the prescriber which are additional to that already included in other sections of the SPC.

Pharmaceutical particulars

List of excipients: None.

Incompatibilities: Erythromycin should not be reconstituted with inorganic salt solutions. Use only Water for Injections.

Subsequent dilution into infusion fluids should be made prior to administration. Recommended fluids are Sodium Chloride Injection BP 0.9%, or Dextrose 5% Injection BP.

The stability of solutions of Erythromycin Lactobionate is adversely affected below pH 5.5. 5 ml of sterile 8.4% sodium bicarbonate solution will neutralise 1 litre of Glucose Injection BP 5% and should be added to the bag prior to addition of Erythromycin Lactobionate.

Shelf life: 24 months.

Special precautions for storage: Store below 25°C. Diluted solutions should be used within 8 hours of preparation.

Nature and contents of container: 30 mL clear Type I glass vials in single and packs of 10.

Instruction for use/handling: Not applicable.

Marketing authorisation number PL 4515/0054

Date of first authorisation/renewal of authorisation Date of first authorisation: 18/10/91.

Date of (partial) revision of the text R/LC/vg 7/96, V/MJ/8/98.

FENTANYL CITRATE INJECTION

Qualitative and quantitative composition

Fentanyl Citrate Injection 100 micrograms in 2 mL:

	per unit dose	*per mL*
Fentanyl (as Fentanyl Citrate BP)	100 micrograms (157 micrograms)	50 micrograms (78.5 micrograms/mL)
Water for Injections BP to	2 mL	1 mL

Fentanyl Citrate Injection 500 micrograms in 10 mL:

	per unit dose	*per mL*
Fentanyl (as Fentanyl Citrate BP)	500 micrograms (785 micrograms)	50 micrograms (78.5 micrograms/mL)
Water for Injections BP to	10 mL	1 mL

Pharmaceutical form Aqueous injection solution.

Clinical particulars

Therapeutic indications: Fentanyl is a narcotic analgesic indicated for short term analgesia during short surgical procedures. Alternatively, in higher doses, it may be used in ventilated patients as an analgesic and respiratory depressant. In combination with a neuroleptic agent, Fentanyl may be used in the technique of neuroleptanalgesia.

Posology and method of administration: Fentanyl Citrate Injection is for administration by the intravenous or intramuscular routes. When administered as an analgesic to patients with spontaneous respiration, adult doses should be as follows:

Initial dose: 50–200 micrograms. Supplemental: 50 micrograms

Doses in excess of 200 micrograms are for general anaesthesia only. Patients on assisted ventilation may be given the following intravenous doses of Fentanyl Citrate:

Initial dose: 300–3500 micrograms. Supplemental: 100-200 micrograms

Fentanyl may also be given intramuscularly, 30–60 minutes before induction of anaesthesia, in doses of 50–100 micrograms.

Dosage in children: In children, Fentanyl Citrate is given on a bodyweight basis according to the following schedule:

Spontaneous respiration: Initially 3–5 micrograms per kg, followed by 1 microgram per kg.

Assisted ventilation: Initially 15 micrograms per kg, followed by 1–3 micrograms per kg.

Safe use of Fentanyl has not been established in children under 2 years of age, and it should not be administered to such patients.

Dosage in the elderly: Because of the adverse reactions associated with Fentanyl, particularly those affecting the respiratory and cardiovascular systems, it is wise to use reduced doses in treatment of the elderly.

Fentanyl Citrate has a short duration of action and a single dose may be expected to provide analgesia for 10–20 minutes in an unpremedicated adult patient. Larger doses provide analgesia for up to 4 hours when doses of 50 micrograms per kg are used. It is important to assess the degree of stimulation, effect of other drugs and the duration of the surgical procedure when calculating the dosage.

Contra-indications: Fentanyl citrate is contraindicated in patients with a known hypersensitivity to the drug, or in patients who have received monoamine oxidase inhibitor (MAOI) drugs within the previous 2 weeks. In addition, patients with obstructive airway disease or respiratory depression should not be treated with Fentanyl Citrate.

Special warnings and special precautions for use:

Warnings: At high doses (more than 200 micrograms), respiratory depression occurs, which can be reversed by administration of Naloxone 100–200 micrograms in adult patients, or 10–20 micrograms in children.

A transient fall in blood pressure may occur after intravenous administration. Bradycardia, which can be reversed by atropine, may also occur.

Muscular rigidity may occur which can affect respiration, particularly in myasthenia gravis patients. The effects can be minimised by a slow intravenous injection, or alternatively muscle relaxants can be used to treat the rigidity.

In combination with other narcotic analgesics, Fentanyl may cause additive effects on CNS depression and respiration. Resuscitative measures should be available at all times, and the patient kept under close medical supervision. As Fentanyl is a narcotic drug, tolerance and dependence may occur. Nausea and vomiting may also be a problem although the incidence is lower than with other opiates.

As with all potent opioids, profound analgesia is accompanied by marked respiratory depression, which may persist into or recur in the early postoperative period. Care should be taken after large doses or infusions of fentanyl to ensure that adequate spontaneous breathing has been established and maintained before disharging the patient from the recovery area. Hyperventilation during anaethesia may alter the patient's response to CO_2, thus affecting respiration postoperatively. Use of opioid premedication may enhance or prolong the respiratory depressant effects of fentanyl.

Where early discharge is envisaged patients should be advised not to drive or operate machinery. Fentanyl is for single use only. Use once and any unused product must be discarded.

Precautions: Fentanyl should only be administered by experienced clinicians to patients under close medical supervision. It should be administered with caution to patients in the following cases:

(a) Severe, chronic liver or renal impairment
(b) Severe impairment of pulmonary function
(c) Myasthenia gravis
(d) Hypothyroidism

When used in conjunction with neuroleptics, the different duration of action should be taken into account.

Interaction with other medicaments and other forms of interaction: Used in combination with CNS depressants, Fentanyl may have additive or potentiating effects. MAO inhibitors are known to interact with narcotic analgesics, and the safe use of Fentanyl Citrate has not been established in this situation.

Pregnancy and lactation:

Use in pregnancy: Administration in labour may induce respiratory depression in the newborn. Safe use has not been established during pregnancy and it should not be used unless the benefits to the mother outweigh the potential risks to mother and child.

Use in lactation: Safe use of Fentanyl Citrate has not been established in mothers who are breast feeding their children. However, because of the nature of the drug and its indications it is unlikely that Fentanyl would be administered to a lactating mother.

Effects on ability to drive and use machines: Where early discharge is envisaged patients should be advised not to drive or operate machinery.

Undesirable effects: As with all opiates, profound analgesia is accompanied by respiratory depression which may persist longer than the analgesic effect, through into the immediate post-operative period.

Respiratory depression can be immediately reversed with a narcotic agonist and is more likely to occur following too rapid intravenous administration.

Muscular rigidity can be reversed by intravenous administration of a relaxant such as suxamethonium, in combination with assisted ventilation.

Bradycardia may occur, but is less likely if atropine is included in the premedication regimen.

Other reported adverse effects include hypertension, hypotension, blurred vision, dizziness, nausea, vomiting, laryngospasm, sweating, itching and spasm of the sphincter of Oddi.

Overdose: The symptoms of overdosage are extensions of the pharmacological effects. Respiratory depression may be reversed using naloxone in combination with other supportive measures.

If respiratory depression is associated with muscular rigidity, then use of suxamethonium has been successful in reversing the effects. Bradycardia may be treated with atropine sulphate.

Pharmacological properties

Pharmacodynamic properties: Fentanyl is a potent narcotic analgesic, chemically related to pethidine and estimated to be about 80 times as potent as morphine as an analgesic. Fentanyl is a centrally acting opiate analgesic which produces profound analgesia of short duration, which is reversed by narcotic antagonists such as naloxone. Its primary indication is for analgesia during short term surgical procedures, or at higher doses, for analgesia in ventilated patients.

Pharmacokinetic properties: Following IV administration, the onset of action is within a few minutes, with analgesia lasting for 30-60 minutes following one dose of 100 micrograms. Following IM administration, onset of action occurs with 7-15 minutes, and duration is 1-2 hours.

Fentanyl is rapidly metabolised and excreted in the urine. The short duration of action is primarily due to redistribution. Up to 70% of a dose may be protein bound. The drug also crosses the placental barrier.

Pharmaceutical particulars

List of excipients: Water for Injections BP qs.

Incompatibilities: Fentanyl is stated to be chemically incompatible with Thiopentone Sodium, Methohexitone and Phenobarbitone.

Shelf life: The medicinal product as packaged for sale has a 2 year shelf life.

Special precautions for storage: Storage is recommended below 25°C. Protect from light. Store as specified in Misuse of Drugs Act in respect of Schedule 2 drugs.

Instructions for use/handling: Not applicable.

Marketing authorisation numbers

100 micrograms in 2 ml	4515/0046
500 micrograms in 10 ml	4515/0046

Date of approval/revision of SPC 26 July 1995

Legal category CD(Sch 2), POM

FLUOROURACIL INJECTION BP 25MG/ML

Qualitative and quantitative composition

	250mg in 10ml	*500mg in 20ml*	*2.5gm in 100ml*
Active Ingredient			
Fluorouracil BP	250mg	500mg	2.5gram
Other Ingredients			
Sodium Hydroxide BP	69.7mg	139.4mg	697mg
Water for Injections BP	to 10ml	to 20ml	to 100ml

No overage is required in the formulation.

Pharmaceutical form Aqueous solution for injection.

Clinical particulars

Therapeutic indications: Fluorouracil may be used alone or in combination, for its palliative action in the management of common malignancies particularly cancer of the colon and breast.

Posology and method of administration:

Routes of administration: Fluorouracil Injection BP can be given by intravenous injection or intravenous or intra-arterial infusion.

Adults: Selection of an appropriate dose and treatment regime depends upon the condition of the patient, the type of carcinoma being treated and whether fluorouracil is to be administered alone or in combination with other therapy. Initial treatment should be given in hospital and the *total daily dose should not exceed 0.8–1 gram.* It is customary to calculate the dose in accordance with the patient's actual bodyweight unless there is obesity, oedema or some form of abnormal fluid retention such as ascites. Ideal weight is used as the basis for calculation in such cases.

The initial dose should be reduced by one-third to one half in patients with any of the following:

1. Cachexia.
2. Major surgery within preceding 30 days.
3. Reduced bone marrow function.
4. Impaired hepatic or renal function.

The following regimen have been recommended for use as a single agent:

Initial Treatment: This may be in the form of an infusion or an injection, the former usually being preferred because of lesser toxicity.

Intravenous infusion: 15 mg/kg bodyweight but not more than 1 g per infusion, diluted in 300–500 ml of 5% glucose or 9% NaCl injection and given over 4 hours. Alternatively the daily dose may be infused over 30–60 minutes or may be given as a continuous infusion over 24 hours. The infusion may be repeated daily until there is evidence of toxicity or a total dose of 12–15 g has been reached.

Intravenous Injection: 12 mg/kg bodyweight may be given daily for 3 days and then, if there is no evidence of toxicity, 6 mg/kg on alternate days for 3 further doses.

An alternative regimen is 15 mg/kg as a single intravenous injection once a week throughout the course.

Intra-arterial infusion: 5/7.5 mg/kg bodyweight daily may be given by 24 hour continuous intra-arterial infusion.

Maintenance therapy: An initial intensive course may be followed by maintenance therapy providing there are no significant toxic effects.

In all instances, toxic side effects must disappear before maintenance therapy is started.

The initial course of fluorouracil can be repeated after an interval of 4 to 6 weeks from the last dose or, alternatively, treatment can be continued with intravenous injections of 5-15 mg/kg bodyweight at weekly intervals. This sequence constitutes a course of therapy. Some patients have received up to 30 g at a maximum rate of 1 g daily.

A more recent alternative method is to give 15 mg/kg IV once a week throughout the course of treatment. This obviates the need for an initial period of daily administration.

In combination with Irradiation

Irradiation combined with 5-FU has been found to be useful in the treatment of certain types of metastatic lesions in the lungs and for the relief of pain caused by recurrent, inoperable growth. The standard dose of 5FU should be used.

Children: No recommendations are made regarding the use of fluorouracil in children.

Elderly: Fluorouracil should be used in the elderly with similar considerations as in younger adults, notwithstanding that incidence of concomitant medical illness is higher in the former group.

Contra-indications: Fluorouracil is contra-indicated in seriously debilitated patients or those with bone marrow depression after radiotherapy or treatment with other antineoplastic agents.

Fluorouracil is strictly contra-indicated in pregnant or breast feeding women.

Fluorouracil should not be used in the management of non-malignant disease.

Special warnings and special precautions for use

Precautions

It is recommended that fluorouracil be given only by, or under the strict supervision of, a qualified physician who is conversant with the use of potent antimetabolites.

All patients should be admitted to hospital for initial treatment.

Adequate treatment with fluorouracil is usually followed by leucopoenia, the lowest white blood cell (W.B.C.) count commonly being observed between the 7th and 14th day of the first course, but occasionally being delayed for as long as 20 days.

The count usually returns to normal by the 30th day. Daily monitoring of platelet and W.B.C. count is recommended and treatment should be stopped if platelets fall below 100,000 per mm^3 or the W.B.C. count falls below 3,500 per mm^3. If the total count is less than 2000 per mm^3, and especially if there is granulocytopenia, it is recommended that the patient be placed in protective isolation in the hospital and treated with appropriate measures to prevent systemic infection.

Treatment should also be stopped at the first sign of oral ulceration or if there is evidence of gastrointestinal side effects such as stomatitis, diarrhoea, bleeding from the G.I. tract or haemorrage at any site. The ratio between effective and toxic dose is small and therapeutic response is unlikely without some degree of toxicity. Care must be taken, therefore, in the selection of patients and adjustment of dosage.

Fluorouracil should be used with caution in patients with reduced renal or liver function or jaundice. Isolated cases of angina, ECG abnormalities and rarely, myocardial infarction have been reported following administration of Fluorouracil. Caution should therefore be exercised in treating patients who experience chest pain during courses of treatment, or patients with a history of heart disease.

Interaction with other medicaments and other forms of interaction: Various agents have been reported to biochemically modulate the antitumour efficacy or toxicity of Fluorouracil, common drugs include Methotrexate, Metronidazole, Leucovorin as well as Allopurinol and Cimetidine which can affect the availability of the active drug.

Pregnancy and lactation: Fluorouracil is strictly contra-indicated in pregnant or breast feeding women.

Effects on ability to drive and use machines: Not applicable.

Undesirable effects: Diarrhoea, nausea and vomiting are observed quite commonly during therapy and may be treated symptomatically. An antiemetic may be given for nausea and vomiting. Alopecia may be seen in a substantial number of cases, particularly in females, but is reversible. Other side effects include dermatitis, pigmentation, changes in the nails, ataxia and fever.

There have been reports of chest pain, tachycardia, breathlessness and ECG changes after administration of fluorouracil. Special attention is therefore advisable in treating patients with a history of heart disease or those who develop chest pain during treatment.

Leucopoenia is common and the precautions described above should be followed.

Systemic fluorouracil treatment has been associated with various types of ocular toxicity.

Additionally several other reports have been noted including:

Incidences of excessive lacrimation, dacryostenosis, visual changes and photophobia.

A transient reversible cerebellar syndrome can occur after the use of 5-fluorouracil. Rarely, a reversible confusional state may occur. Both neurological conditions usually respond to withdrawal of 5-fluorouracil.

Palmar-Plantar Erythrodysesthesia Syndrome has been reported as an unusual complication of high dose bolus or protracted continuous therapy with fluorouracil.

Thrombophlebitis/vein tracking.

Overdose: The symptoms and signs of overdosage are qualitatively similar to the adverse reactions and should be managed as indicated under *Precautions* and *Adverse Reactions.*

Pharmacological properties

Pharmacodynamic properties: Fluorouracil is an analogue of uracil, a component of ribonucleic acid. The drug is believed to function as an antimetabolite. After intracellular conversion to the active deoxynucleotide, it interferes with the synthesis of DNA by blocking the conversion of deoxyuridylic acid to thymidylic acid by the cellular enzyme thymidylate synthetase. Fluorouracil may also interfere with RNA synthesis.

Pharmacokinetic properties: After intravenous administration, Fluorouracil is distributed through the body water and disappears from the blood within 3 hours. It is preferentially taken up by actively dividing tissues and tumours after conversion to its nucleotide. Fluorouracil ready enters the C.S.F and brain tissue.

Following IV administration, the plasma elimination half-life averages about 16 minutes and is dose dependant. Following a single IV dose of Fluorouracil approximately 15% of the dose is excreted unchanged in the urine within 6 hours; over 90% of this is excreted in the first hour. The remainder is mostly metabolised in the liver by the usual body mechanisms for uracil.

Pharmaceutical particulars

List of excipients:

	250 mg in 10 ml	*500 mg in 20 ml*	*2.5 gm in 100 ml*
Sodium Hydroxide BP	69.7 mg	139.4 mg	697 mg
Water for Injections BP	to 10 ml	to 20 ml	to 100 ml

No overage is required in the formulation.

Incompatibilities: 5-Fluorouracil is incompatible with Carboplatin, Cisplatin, Cytarabine, Diazepam, Doxorubicin, other Anthracyclines and possibly Methotrexate.

Formulated solutions are alkaline and it is recommended that admixture with acidic drugs or preparations should be avoided.

Shelf life: 24 months.

Special precautions for storage: Fluorouracil Injection BP should be stored between 15°C and 25°C and should be protected from light. The pH of Fluorouracil Injection BP is 8.9 and the drug has maximal stability over the pH range 8.6 to 9.0.

If a precipitate has formed as a result of exposure to low temperatures, redissolve by heating to 60°C accompanied by vigorous shaking. Allow to cool to body temperature prior to use.

Instructions for use/handling: Fluorouracil is an irritant, contact with skin and mucous membranes should be avoided. Please refer to company for COSHH hazard datasheets.

Diluents: Fluorouracil Injection BP may be diluted with Glucose or Sodium Chloride Injection BP or Water for Injections BP immediately before parenteral use. The remainder of solutions should be discarded after use: do not make up into multidose preparations. Fluorouracil Injection should only be prepared for administration by professionals who have been trained in the safe use of the preparation. Preparation should only be carried out in a designated area.

First aid: Eye contact: Irrigate immediately with water and seek medical advice.

Skin contact: Wash thorughly with soap and water and remove contaminated clothing.

Inhalation, Ingestion: Seek medical advice.

Marketing authorisation number 4515/0024.

Date of approval/revision of SPC 22 July 1996

FLUOROURACIL INJECTION BP 50MG/ML

Qualitative and quantitative composition Fluorouracil Injection BP 50 mg/ml is available in the following presentations:- 250 mg/5 ml, 500 mg/10 ml and 2.5 g/50 ml conventional glass vials and Onco-Tain* vials

Pharmaceutical form Sterile solution for injection.

Clinical particulars

Therapeutic indications: Fluorouracil may be used alone, or in combination for its palliative action in the management of common malignancies particularly cancer of the colon and breast, either as a single agent or in combination with other cytotoxic agents.

Posology and method of administration: Selection of an appropriate dose and treatment regime will depend upon the condition of the patient, the type of carcinoma being treated and whether Fluorouracil is to be administered alone or in combination with other therapy. Initial treatment should be given in hospital and the total daily dose should not exceed 1 gram. It is customary to calculate the dose in accordance with the patient's actual weight unless there is obesity, oedema or some other form of abnormal fluid retention such as ascites. In this case, ideal weight should be used as the basis for the calculation. Reduction of the dose is advisable in patients with any of the following:

(1) Cachexia
(2) Major surgery within preceding 30 days
(3) Reduced bone marrow function
(4) Impaired hepatic or renal function

Fluorouracil injection can be given by intravenous injection or, intravenous or intra-arterial infusion.

Adult dose: The following regimes have been recommended for use as a single agent:

Initial treatment: This may be in the form of an infusion or an injection, the former usually being preferred because of lesser toxicity.

Intravenous infusion: 15 mg/kg bodyweight but not more than 1 g per infusion, diluted in 500 ml of 5% glucose or 0.9% NaCl injection and given by intravenous infusion at a rate of 40 drops per minute over 4 hours. Alternatively the daily dose may be infused over 30–60 minutes or may be given as a continuous infusion over 24 hours. The infusion may be repeated daily until there is evidence of toxicity or a total dose of 12–15 g has been reached.

Intravenous injection: 12 mg/kg bodyweight may be given daily for 3 days and then if there is no evidence of toxicity 6 mg/kg on alternate days for 3 further doses. An alternative regime is 15 mg/kg as a single intravenous injection once a week throughout the course.

Intra-arterial infusion: 5-7.5 mg/kg may be given by 24 hour continuous intra-arterial infusion.

Maintenance therapy: An initial intensive course may be followed by maintenance therapy providing there are no significant toxic effects. In all instances, toxic side effects must disappear before maintainance therapy is started.

The initial course of Fluorouracil can be repeated after an interval of 4 to 6 weeks from the last dose, or alternatively, treatment can be continued with intravenous injections of 5-15 mg/kg at weekly intervals. This sequence constitutes a course of therapy. Some patients have received up to 30 g at a maximum rate of 1 g daily. A more recent alternative method is to give 15 mg/kg IV Once a week throughout the course of treatment. This obviates the need for an initial period of daily administration.

In combination with irradiation: Irradiation combined with 5-FU has been found to be useful in the treatment of certain types of metastatic lesions in the lungs and for the relief of pain caused by recurrent, inoperable growth. The standard dose of 5-FU should be used.

Children: No recommendations are made regarding the use of Fluorouracil in children.

Elderly: Fluorouracil should be used in the elderly with similar considerations as with normal adult dosages.

Contra-indications: Fluorouracil is contra-indicated in seriously debilitated patients or those with bone marrow depression after radiotherapy or treatment with other antineoplastic agents.

Fluorouracil is strictly contra-indicated in pregnant or breast feeding women.

Fluorouracil should not be used in the management of non-malignant disease.

Special warnings and special precautions for use: It is recommended that Fluorouracil be given only by, or under the strict supervision of,a qualified physician who is conversant with the use of potent antimetabolites.

All patients should be admitted to hospital for initial treatment.

Adequate treatment with Fluorouracil is usually followed by leucopenia, the lowest white blood cell (W.B.C.) count comonly being observed between the 7th and 14th day of the first course, but occasionally being delayed for as long as 20 days.

The count usually returns to normal by the 30th day. Daily monitoring of platelet and W.B.C. count is recommended and treatment should be stopped if platelets fall below 100,000 per mm3 or the W.B.C. count falls below 3,500 per mm^3. If the total count is less than 2000 mm^3, and especially if there is granulocytopenia, it is recommended that the patient be placed in protective isolation in the hospital and treated with appropriate measures to prevent systemic infection.

Treatment should also be stopped at the first sign of oral ulceration or if there is evidence of gastrointestnal side effects such as stomatitis, diarrhoea, bleeding from the G.I. tract ot haemorrage at any site. The ratio between effective and toxic dose is small and therapeutic response is unlikely without some degree of toxicity. Care must be taken therefore, in the selection of patients and adjustment of dosage.

Fluorouracil should be used with caution in patients with reduced renal or liver function or jaundice. Isolated cases of angina, ECG abnormalities and rarely, myocardial infarction have been reported following administration of Fluorouracil. Care should therefore be exercised in treating patients who experience chest pain during courses of treatment, or patients with a history of heart disease.

Interaction with other medicaments and other forms of interaction

Drug interactions: Various agents have been reported to biochemically modulate the antitumour efficacy or toxicity of Fluorouracil, common drugs include Methotrexate, Metronidazole, Leucovorin as well as Allopurinol and Cimetidine which can affect the availability of the active drug.

Pregnancy and lactation: Fluorouracil is strictly contra-indicated in pregnant and breast feeding women.

Effects on ability to drive and use machines: Not applicable.

Undesirable effects: Diarrhoea, nausea and vomiting are observed quite commonly during therapy and may be treated symptomatically. An anti-emetic may be given for nausea and vomiting.

Alopecia may be seen in a substantial number of cases, partcularly females, but is reversible. Other side effects include dermatitis, pigmentation, changes in the nails, ataxia and fever.

There have been reports of chest pain, tachycardia, breathlessness and E.C.G. changes after administration of Fluorouracil. Special attention is advisable in treating patients with a history of heart disease or those who develop chest pain during treatment.

Leucopenia is common and the precautions described above should be followed.

Systemic Fluorouracil treatment has been associated with various types of ocular toxicity.

A transient reversible cerebellar syndrome can occur after the use of 5-fluorouracil. Rarely, a reversible confusional state may occur. Both neurological conditions usually respond to withdrawal of 5-fluorouracil.

Additionally several other reports have been noted including:

Incidences of excessive lacrimation, dacryostenosis, visual changes and photophobia.

Palmar-Plantar Erythrodysesthesia Syndrome has been reported as an unusual complication of high dose bolus or protracted continuous therapy with fluorouracil.

Thrombophlebitis/ Vein Tracking

Overdose: The symptoms and signs of overdosage are qualitatively similar to the adverse reactions and should be managed as indicated under *Other Undesirable Effects* and *Special Warnings and Precautions.*

Pharmacological properties

Pharmacodynamic properties: Fluorouracil is an analogue of uracil, a component of ribonucleic acid. The drug is believed to function as an antimetabolite. After intracellular conversion to the active deoxynucleotide, it interferes with the synthesis of DNA by blocking the conversion of deoxyuridylic acid to thymidylic acid by the cellular enzyme thymidylate synthetase. Fluorouracil may also interfere with RNA synthesis.

Pharmacokinetic properties: After intravenous administration, Fluorouracil is distributed through the body water and disappears from the blood within 3 hours. It is preferentially taken up by actively dividing tissues and tumours after conversion to its nucleotide. Fluorouracil ready enters the C.S.F and brain tissue.

Following IV administration, the plasma elimination half-life averages about 16 minutes and is dose dependant. Following a single IV dose of Fluorouracil approximately 15% of the dose is excreted unchanged in the urine within 6 hours; over 90% of this is excreted in the first hour. The remainder is mostly metabolised in the liver by the usual body mechanisms for uracil.

Preclinical safety data: Not applicable.

Pharmaceutical particulars

List of excipients: Sodium Hydroxide BP; Water for Injections BP.

Incompatibilities: Fluorouracil is incompatible with Carboplatin, Cisplatin, Cytarabine, Diazepam, Doxorubicin, other Anthracyclines and possibly Methotrexate.

Formulated solutions are alkaline and it is recommended that admixture with acidic drugs or preparations should be avoided.

Shelf life: 24 months.

Special precautions for storage: Storage: Fluorouracil Injection BP should be stored between 15°C and 25°C and should be protected from light. Do not refrigerate. Unused portions of opened vials or prepared infusions if not used immediately must be stored at 2-8°C for no longer than 24 hours from the time of opening or preparation.

The pH of Fluorouracil Injection BP is 8.9 and the drug has maximal stability over the pH range 8.6 to 9.0.

If a precipitate has formed as a result of exposure

to low temperatures, redissolve by heating to 60°C accompanied by vigorous shaking. Allow to cool to body temperature prior to use.

The product should be discarded if it appears brown or dark yellow in solution.

Instructions for use/handling: Cytotoxic Handling Guidelines: Should be administered only by or under the direct supervision of a qualified physician who is experienced in the use of cancer chemotherapeutic agents.

Fluorouracil Injection should only be prepared for administration by professionals who have been trained in the safe use of the preparation. Preparation should only be carried out in a designated area.

In the event of spillage, operators should put on gloves, face mask, eye protection and disposible apron and mop up the spilled material with a absorbant material kept in the area for that purpose. The area should then be cleaned and all contaminated material transferred to a cytotoxic spillage bag or bin and sealed for incineration.

Contamination: Fluorouracil is an irritant, contact with skin and mucous membranes should be avoided.

In the event of contact with the skin or eyes, the affected area should be washed with copious amounts of water or normal saline. A bland cream may be used to treat the transient stinging of the skin. Medical advice should be sought if the eyes are affected or if the preparation is inhaled or ingested.

Please refer to company for COSHH hazard datasheets.

Preparation guidelines:

a. Chemotherapeutic agents should be prepared for administration only by professionals who have been trained in the safe use of the preparation.
b. Operations such as reconstitution of powder and transfer to syringes should be carried out only in the designated area.
c. The personnel carrying out these procedures should be adequately protected with clothing, gloves and eye shield.
d. Pregnant personnel are advised not to handle chemotherapeutic agents.

Disposal: Syringes containing remaining solution, absorbent materials, and any other contaminated material should be placed in a thick plastic bag or other impervious container and incinerated at 700°C.

Diluents: Fluorouracil Injection BP may be diluted with Glucose or Sodium Chloride Injection BP or Water for Injections BP immediately before parenteral use.

Marketing authorisation number 4515/0088

Date of approval/revision of SPC 22 July 1996

Legal category POM

FLUPHENAZINE DECANOATE INJECTION BP 25 mg/mL

Qualitative and quantitative composition

Fluphenazine Decanoate Injection BP

	per ml	*per unit dose*	*per unit dose*	*per unit dose*
Fluphenazine Decanoate	25 mg	12.5mg	25 mg	50 mg
Sesame Oil	to 1mL	to 0.5mL	to 1 ml	in 2 ml

Pharmaceutical form Oily injection solution.

Clinical particulars

Therapeutic indications: The management of schizophrenic patients and those with paranoid psychoses. Fluphenazine is also particularly useful in the managment of patients who are unreliable at taking oral medication and of those who do not absorb their oral phenothiazines in adequate amounts.

Posology and method of administration: Fluphenazine Decanoate is given by deep intramuscular injection into the gluteal muscle region, using a needle of at least 21 gauge size. Dosage will depend on any previous exposure to Fluphenazine or other phenothiazines prior to treatment.

Adults: In patients with no previous treatment, initially 12.5 mg to 25 mg should be given. Onset of action will normally occur between 24 and 72 hours after injection with an antipsychotic effect being noticed within 2 to 4 days. Subsequent dosages schedules must be determined with the individual patient response. Maintenance therapy can be effected using a single injection for as long as four to six weeks, although most patients symptoms can be contolled on 12.5–100 mg given at two to five week intervals.

Dosage would not normally exceed 100 mg. If doses in excess of 50 mg are required then increments of 12.5 mg should be implemented.

Fluphenazine Decanoate Injection 100 mg per ml is indicated for those patients requiring high doses as part of maintenance therapy and where a small injection volume is required. When transferring from Fluphenazine Decanoate 25 mg/ml to Fluphenazine Decanoate 100 mg/ml Injection the dose volume should be divided by four to obtain equivalent milligram dosage.

Children: Fluphenazine Decanoate and Fluphenazine Decanoate 100 mg/ml Injection are not recommended for use in children under the age of twelve.

Elderly: Reduced maintenance doses may be needed in patients showing extra-pyramidal symptoms, following initial dosing as above.

Initial dose–0.25 ml (25 mg)

Patients not previously treated with a depot fluphenazine formulation, and over sixty years of age, should receive a lower initial dose.

Contra-indications: Fluphenazine Decanoate is contra-indicated in comatose patients or those under the influence of central nervous system depressants. The presence of liver damage, history of jaundice and renal insufficiency preclude use of Fluphenazine Decanoate. Cerebral atherosclerosis, phaeochromocytoma, severely depressed states and severe cardiac insufficiency are also contra-indications for Fluphenazine Decanoate therapy.

Special warnings and special precautions for use:
Warnings: Sudden, unexplained deaths have been reported in hospitalised psychotic patients receiving phenothiazines. Autopsy findings have revealed acute, fulminating pneumonia, aspiration of gastric contents or intramyocardial lesions. Some patients exhibited acute exacerbations of psychotic behaviour shortly prior to their death.

Fluphenazine Decanoate may impair the mental and physical abilities required for driving or operating machinery. Potentiation of the central nervous system depressant effects of alcohol may occur.

The drug should be administered under the direction of a physician experienced in the use of psychotropic drugs. Hepatic and renal function should be monitored periodically as well as haematological monitoring.

Precautions: Fluphenazine Decanoate should be used with caution in patients with cardiovascular or respiratory disease.

The drug may cause cross sensitivity with other phenothiazines, so caution is necessary in patients with a known history of hypersensitivity to phenothiazines.

On prolonged therapy patients may show symptoms of liver damage, pigmentary retinopathy, corneal deposits and irreversible dyskinesia.

The preparation should be used with caution in patients with a history of convulsive disorders, and grand mal seizures have been reported in patients on Fluphenazine.

Psychotic patients on high doses who will be undergoing surgery may be at risk to hypotension, and may additionally require reduced amounts of anaesthetic agents or central nervous system depressants. Body temperature control mechanisms may be affected giving rise to hypothermia or hyperpyrexia in patients on high doses of Fluphenazine Decanoate. In addition elderly patients or those subjected to extremes of temperature and humidity may be affected.

The anticholinergic effects of atropine may be potentiated. Antiparkinsonian drug effects may be diminished in patients on Fluphenazine therapy.

Interaction with other medicaments and other forms of interaction: Fluphenazine Decanoate may interact additionally with CNS depressants (alcohol, barbiturates, hypnotics, sedatives and strong analgesics) to enhance their depressant effects. Guanethidine and levodopa efficacy may be impaired. Plasma levels of Fluphenazine may be increased by high doses of tricyclic antidepressants, and lowered by barbiturates.

Adrenaline action may be reversed and the antihypertensive properties of adrenergic blocking drugs may be antagonised. The antiparkinsonian effect of Levodopa may be impaired as well as the effects of anticonvulsants.

Pregnancy and lactation:
Use in pregnancy: The safety of this drug during pregnancy has not been established. The possible hazards should be weighed against the benefits when administering the drug to pregnant patients.

Use in lactation: Fluphenazine Decanoate may possibly be excreted in breast milk, as other phenothiazines are. Breast feeding is therefore not recommended during treatment.

Effects on ability to drive and use machines: Use may impair mental and physical abilities to drive or operate heavy machinery.

Undesirable effects:
Adverse reactions: Extrapyramidal disturbances: Extrapyramidal side effects occur with Fluphenazine Decanoate including pseudo-parkinsonism, dystonia, dyskinesia, akathisia, oculogyric crises, opisthotonos and hyperreflexia.

Dystonic reactions such as acute spasm of facial, neck and back muscles may occur within 24 hours of an injection and require immediate administration of an anticholinergic such as benztropine, benzhexol oir procyclidine. This may need to be continued orally for a few days to prevent recurrence. Young male patients seem most at risk from dystonic reactions.

Parkinsonism effects occur frequently, particularly in elderly patients, usually within 2-5 days after an injection. Early detection is important so that the patients neurological system can be examined regularly. Extrapyramidal symptoms are persistent but usually reversible.

Tardive dyskinesia: As with all antipsychotic agents, tardive dyskinesia may occur in patients on long-term therapy or after drug treatment has been discontinued. The risk seems greatest in elderly female patients on high doses. Symptoms are persistent and may be irreversible. The disorder consists of repetitive involuntary movements of the tongue, face, and muscles of mastication. The trunk and limbs are less frequently involved. Fine vermicular movements of the tongue may be an early sign of the syndrome, and if medication is stopped at this stage, the syndrome may not develop.

There is no known effective treatment for tardive dyskinesia. Increasing the dose of medication may result in temporary suppression but with subsequent deterioration. Anticholinergic drugs may exacerbate the problem. All antipsychotic agents may be withdrawn if these symptoms appear. Subsequently symptoms of dyskinesia may be masked if a different antipsychotic agent is used, or if the dose of Fluphenazine Decanoate is increased.

Other central nervous system effects: Drowsiness, lethargy may necessitate a reduction in dosage. Phenothiazine derivatives have been known to cause restlessness, excitement or bizarre dreams.

Autonomic nervous system: Hypotension is infrequently found except in patients with pre-existing cerebrovascular disease or cardiac insufficiency such as mitral valve disease. Such patients should be closely monitored when the drug is administered. In acute hypotension, supportive measures including the use of intravenous vasopressor drugs is recommended, but excluding the use of adrenaline which has been found to further lower blood pressure through drug interaction with Fluphenazine Decanoate.

Nausea, and loss of appetite, salivation, polyuria, perspiration, dry mouth, headache and constipation may occur. These can usually be controlled by a dosage reduction or temporary discontinuation of treatment. Blurred vision, glaucoma, constipation, urinary incontinence and epileptiform attacks are also occasionally seen.

Allergic reactions: Skin disorders such as itching, erythema, urticaria, and dermatitis have been reported occasionally. SLE and skin pigmentation have rarely been reported.

Haemopoietic system: Blood dyscrasias including transient leucopenia, thrombocytopenia and agranulocytosis have been reported. Accordingly, if patients show signs of sore throat, gums or mouth, then regular blood counts should be instituted and if symptoms persist, the treatment be discontinued until the haematological system has recovered.

Hepatic system: Cholestatic jaundice may occur during the first three months of treatment, and if so therapy should be stopped. Alterations in liver function tests have been reported in the absence of jaundice.

Metabolic and endocrine system: Weight changes, peripheral oedema, gynacomastia, alterations in lactation, menstrual irregularities and impotence have been reported. Blood glucose levels may also be erratic causing problems in diabetic patients.

Cardiovascular system: Phenothiazines may cause changes in ECG patterns which are dose related. Moderate to high dosages can cause prolongation of QT interval and alteration in T waves. Rarely these effects precede serious arrhythmias including ventricular tachycardia and fibrillation.

Overdose: Supportive and symptomatic treatment should be used. Oral or parenteral procyclidine or benztropine will control extrapyramidal symptoms. In severe hypotension, management of circulatory failure should be instituted including vasoconstrictors and intravenous fluids.

N.B. Avoid the use of adrenaline as this may exacerbate the hypotension due to interaction with Fluphenazine.

Pharmacological properties

Pharmacodynamic properties: Fluphenazine is a piperazine phenothiazine used widely in the treatment of schizophrenia. The action is thought to be through dopamine receptor blockade in the mesolimbic system. Fluphenazine has weak anticholinergic effects, sedative effects, antiadrenal effects and neuroendocrine effects. Side effects from extrapyramidal symptoms are common.

In an oil vehicle as the decanoate, fluphenazine ester slowly diffuses into the circulation. After hydrolysis, the drug passes the blood brain barrier as free drug.

Pharmacokinetic properties: Esterification of fluphenazine slows the rate of release from fat and thus prolongs the duration of action. Further delay is achieved by formulation in an oily solvent. Onset of action is within 48-72 hours, duration may be 1-6 weeks with an average of 2 weeks.

Distribution and metabolism are not fully described. Plasma half life has been shown to be 6-9 days following intramuscular administration of the decanoate.

Pharmaceutical particulars

List of excipients:

Fluphenazine Decanoate Injection BP 25 mg in 1 mL

	per unit dose	per mL
Sesame Oil	to 1 mL	to 1 mL

Incompatibilities: Not applicable. An oily injection for intramuscular use only.

Shelf life: The medicinal product as packaged for sale has a 24 month shelf life.

Special precautions for storage: Storage: store between 15°C–25°C. Protect from light. Do not refrigerate.

Instructions for use/handling: Not applicable.

Marketing authorisation number 4515/0048

Date of approval/revision of SPC 21 July 1997

Legal category POM

FLUPHENAZINE DECANOATE INJECTION BP 100 mg/mL

Qualitative and quantitative composition

Fluphenazine Decanoate Injection BP

	per ml	*per unit dose*	*per unit dose*
Fluphenazine Decanoate	100mg	50mg	100mg
Sesame Oil	to 1 mL	to 0.5mL	to 1 ml

Pharmaceutical form Oily injection solution.

Clinical particulars

Therapeutic indications: The management of schizophrenic patients and those with paranoid psychoses. Fluphenazine is also particularly useful in the management of patients who are unreliable at taking oral medication and of those who do not absorb their oral phenothiazines in adequate amounts.

Posology and method of administration:

Adults: Suitable where a reduced injection volume is desirable and therefore most suitable for patients on high dose maintenance therapy.

Not previously treated: Initially 0.5 ml by deep intramuscular injection into the gluteal region given at 2-5 week intervals, depending on patient response. Most patients are maintained on dose range of 0.5–4 ml.

If doses in excess of 100 mg are needed, increments of 12.5 mg (0.125 ml) should be implemented.

Previously treated:

(i) Oral: Dosage must be titrated as for new patients.

(ii) Depot: Restart on same dose as previously, possibly required at shorter dose intervals in the early weeks of treatment.

Children: Not recommended for patients under 12 years of age.

Elderly: Reduced maintenance doses may be needed in patients showing extrapyramidal symptoms, following initial dosing as above.

Initial dose–0.25 ml (25 mg).

N.B. Dose should not be increased without close supervision. Patients will respond in varying degrees to the drug. The response may be delayed. Symptoms may not recur for several weeks after discontinuation of treatment.

Contra-indications: Comatose patients, hepatic damage, jaundice, renal insufficiency, marked cerebral atherosclerosis, phaeochromocytoma, cardiac insufficiency and severely depressed states.

Special warnings and special precautions for use

Sudden, unexplained death has been reported in patients on phenothiazines, revealing at autopsy an acute, fulminating pneumonia with aspiration.

The drug should be administered under the direction of an experienced clinician. Renal and hepatic function should be monitored periodically during treatment.

Use with caution in patients with cardiovascular disease, known hypersensitivity to other phenothiazines, convulsive disorders. Patients undergoing surgery may be at risk to hypotension. Body temperature controls may become altered particularly at high doses. Atropinic effects may be potentiated.

Interaction with other medicaments and other forms of interaction:

CNS depressants: (alcohol, barbiturates, hypnotics, sedatives, strong analgesics all may show increased depressant effects).

May impair:
Antiparkinson effect of levodopa
Effect of anticonvulsants
Metabolism of tricyclic antidepressants
Control of diabetes
Action of adrenalin and other sympathomimetics.
May interact with lithium.
May enhance:
Cardiac depressant effect of quinidine
Absorption of corticosteroids
Absorption of digoxin
Absorption of neuromuscular blocking agents
Effect of anticoagulants.

Pregnancy and lactation:

Use in pregnancy: The safety of this drug during pregnancy has not been established. The possible hazards should be weighed against the benefits when administering the drug to pregnant patients.

Use in Lactation: Fluphenazine Decanoate may possibly be excreted in breast milk, as other phenothiazines are. Breast feeding is therefore not recommended during treatment.

Effects on ability to drive and use machines

Use may impair mental and physical abilities to drive or operate heavy machinery.

Undesirable effects:

Adverse reactions: Acute dystonic reactions occur frequently, usually within 24-48 hours. In susceptible individuals they may occur after small doses. Reaction may include oculogyric crises and opisthotonos. Rapidly relived by intravenous antiparkinsonian agent such as procyclidine.

Parkinsonian-like state may occur particularly between second and fifth day after injection. Can be reduced by using smaller doses more frequently or concomitant use of benzhexol, benztropine or procyclidine. Antiparkinson drugs should not be prescribed routinely because of the risk of aggravating antiucholinergic side effects or precipitating toxic confusion states or impairing therapeutic response. Careful monitoring will minimise use of antiparkinsonian drugs.

Tardive dyskinesia may appear on long term therapy or after drug has been discontinued. Elderly female patients on high doses seem to be most at risk. Symptoms are persistent and in some cases irreversible. The syndrome is characterised by rhythmical, involuntary movement of the tongue, face, mouth or jaw. Sometimes accompanied by involuntary movements of limbs. There is no known effective treatment. Antiparkinson drugs do not usually alleviate symptoms. It is suggested that antipsychotic agents be discontinued if such symptoms occur. It is reported that fine vermicular movements of the tongue may be an early sign of the syndrome, and cessation of treatment at this stage may prevent development of the full syndrome.

Drowsiness, lethargy, blurred vision, dryness of the mouth, constipation, urinary hesitancy or incontinence, mild hypotension, impairment of judgement and mental skills, epileptic form attacks are all occasionally seen.

Blood dyscrasias are rarely reported. Blood counts should be performed if persistent infection develops. Transient leucopenia and thrombocytopenia have been reported. Antinuclear antibodies and SLE are very rarely reported.

Jaundice and transient abnormalities of liver function are rarely reported.

Long term high dose phenothiazine use may result occasionally in abnormal skin pigmentation and lens opacity.

Skin rashes have been rarely reported.

Elderly patients may be more susceptible to sedative or hypertensive effects.

Cardiovascular effects of phenothiazines are dose related. ECG changes, including prolongation of QT interval and T wave changes have been reported commonly in patients treated with moderate to high dose therapy. The effects are reversible on reducing the dose. Rarely the effects may precipitate arrhythmias including ventricular tachycardia and fibrillation. These effects may also occur on overdosage.

Sudden, unexplained death has also been reported in hospitalised psychotic patients receiving phenothiazines.

Phenothiazines may impair body temperature regulation. Severe hypothermia or hyperpyrexia have been reported in association with moderate or high doses. Elderly patients may be particularly susceptible to hypothermia. Hyperpyrexia may be increased by hot or humid weather or by antiparkinsonian drugs which impair sweating.

Neuroleptic malignant syndrome (NMS) is rarely reported. The syndrome is characterised by hyperthermia, together with some or all of the following: muscular rigidity, autonomic instability, akinesia, altered consciousness, sometimes progressing to coma or stupor. Leucocytoses, elevated CPK, liver function abnormalities and acute renal failure. Neuroleptic drug therapy should be discontinued immediately. The syndrome is potentially fatal, and must be treated with vigorous symptomatic treatment.

Hormonal effects of phenothiazines include hyperprolactinaemia, which may cause galactorrhoea, gynacomastia and oligo or ammenorrhoea. Sexual function may be impaired.

Overdose: Supportive measures and symptomatic treatment. Extrapyramidal symptoms can be controlled with procyclidine or benztropine. Hypotension can be treated with vasoconstrictors and fluid replacement–but avoid using adrenalin.

Pharmacological properties

Pharmacodynamic properties: Fluphenazine is a piperazine phenothiazine used widely in the treatment of schizophrenia. The action is thought to be through dopamine receptor blockade in the mesolimbic system. Fluphenazine has weak anticholinergic effects, sedative effects, antiadrenal effects and neuroendocrine effects. Side effects from extrapyramidal symptoms are common.

In an oil vehicle as the decanoate, fluphenazine ester slowly diffuses into the circulation. After hydrolysis, the drug passes the blood brain barrier as free drug.

Pharmacokinetic properties: Esterification of fluphenazine slows the rate of release from fat and thus prolongs the duration of action. Further delay is achieved by formulation in an oily solvent. Onset of action is within 48-72 hours, duration may be 1-6 weeks with an average of 2 weeks.

Distribution and metabolism are not fully described. Plasma half life has been shown to be 6-9 days following intramuscular administration of the decanoate.

Pharmaceutical particulars

List of excipients:

Fluphenazine Decanoate Injection BP 50 mg in 0.5 mL

	per unit dose	per mL
Sesame Oil BP	to 0.5 mL	to 1 mL

Fluphenazine Decanoate Injection BP 100 mg in 1 mL

	per unit dose	per mL
Sesame Oil	to 1 mL	to 1 mL

Incompatibilities: Not applicable. An oily injection for intramuscular use only.

Shelf life: The medicinal product as packaged for sale has an 24 month shelf life.

Special precautions for storage: Store between 15°C–25°C. Protect from light.

Instructions for use/handling: Not applicable.

Marketing authorisation numbers

50 mg in 0.5 ml	4515/0056.
100 mg in 1 ml	4515/0056.

Date of approval/revision of SPC 20 February 1996

Legal category POM

GENTAMICIN INJECTION BP

Qualitative and quantitative composition Active constituent: Gentamicin Sulphate BP, equivalent to Gentamicin Base: 40 mg/mL solutions, presented as 1 mL and 2 mL ampoules and 2 mL vials. 3.5% overage included in formulation.

Pharmaceutical form Sterile solution of Gentamicin Sulphate BP in Water for Injections BP

Clinical particulars

Therapeutic indications: Gentamicin is bactericidal and is active against many strains of Gram-positive and Gram-negative pathogens including species of *Escherichia, Enterobacter, Klebsiella, Salmonella, Serratia, Shigella, Staphylococcus aureus,* some *Proteus* and against *Pseudomonas aeruginosa.* Gentamicin is often effective against strains of these organisms which are resistant to other antibiotics such as streptomycin, kanamycin and neomycin. Gentamicin is effective against penicillin-resistant *Staphylococci*, but rarely effective against *Streptococci*.

Gentamicin is indicated in the treatment of the following infections when caused by susceptible organisms:

Severe Gram-negative Infections
Upper and lower urinary tract infections
Burn and wound infections
Septicaemia, bacteraemia
Abscesses
Subacute bacterial endocarditis
Respiratory tract infections (bronchopneumonia)
Neonatal infections
Gynaecological infections
Gram-positive Infections:
Bacteraemia
Abscesses
Accidental and operative trauma
Burns and serious skin lesions

Posology and method of administration: Gentamicin is normally given by the intramuscular route, but can be given intravenously when intramuscular administration is not feasible.

Gentamicin is normally given by the intramuscular route, but can be given intravenously when intramuscular administration is not feasible, e.g. in shocked or severely burned patients. When given intravenously, the prescribed dose should be administered slowly over 2 to 3 minutes directly into a vein or into the rubber tubing of a giving set. Rapid, direct intravenous administration may give rise, initially, to potentially neurotoxic concentrations and it is essential that the prescribed dose is administered over the recommended period of time. Alternatively the prescribed dose should be dissolved in up to 100 ml of normal saline or 5% glucose in water, but not solutions containing bicarbonate (see *Incompatibilities*), and the solution infused over a period of 20 to 30 minutes.

The same dosage schedule is recommended for intramuscular and intravenous dosing. Dosage is related to the severity of infection, the age of the patient and the patient's renal function.

Dosage in Patients with Normal Renal Function:

Adult dosage:

Type of infection	*Dosage*	*Time interval between doses*	*Duration of therapy*
Systemic and urinary tract infections	3 mg/kg/day up to 80 mg	8 hours	7-10 days
Life threatening infections	5 mg/kg/day initially then 3 mg/kg/day as soon as improvement is indicated	6-8 hours	7-10 days (Longer therapy may be required. If so, auditory renal and vestibular functions should be monitored).

Paediatric dosage:

Infection	*Age*	*Dose/Route*	*Frequency*
Systemic	0–7 days	5 mg/kg/day IM	12 hours
	1 week–1 yr	6 mg/kg/day IM	12 hours
	1 yr–12 yrs	4.5 mg/kg/ day IM	8 hours
Urinary tract infections	-	3 mg/kg/day IM	8 hours–12 hours
Life threatening infections	0–7 days	5 mg/kg/day	12 hours
	1 week–1 yr	7.5 mg/kg/ day	8 hours
	1 yr–12 yrs	6 mg/kg/day	8 hours

Doses in patients with impaired renal function: Dosage is adjusted for patients with renal impairment to minimise the risk of toxicity. The first dose should be as normal–after this, doses should be given less frequently, the interval being determined by results of renal function tests as below:

Renal function tests:

Dose	*Creatinine clearance (ml/mn)*	*Serum creatinine (mmol/l)*	*BUN (mmol/l)*	*Interval between doses*
80 mg	over 70	less than 0.12	less than 6.5	8 hours
	35-70	0.12-0.17	6.5-10	12 hours
	24-34	0.18-0.25	11-14	18 hours
	16-23	0.26-0.33	15-18	24 hours
	10-15	0.34-0.47	19-26	36 hours
	5-9	0.48-0.64	27-36	48 hours

Serum levels should be monitored daily.

Peak levels in infants and young children: Peak serum levels are reached in 1 hour and dosage should be adjusted to achieve levels of more than 4 micrograms/ml, but not exceed 10 micrograms/ml.

Contra-indications: Patients being treated with Gentamicin should be under close clinical observation because of its potential toxicity. There are no absolute contraindications other than a history of hypersensitivity to Gentamicin. Gentamicin should be used with caution in premature infants because of their renal immaturity, in elderly people and generally in patients with impaired renal function. Diabetes, auditory vestibular dysfunctions, otitis media, a history of otitis media, previous use of ototoxic drugs and a genetically determined high sensitivity to aminoglycoside induced ototoxicity, are other main factors which may pre-dispose the patient to toxicity.

Special warnings and precautions for use: As with other aminoglycosides toxicity is related to serum concentration. At serum levels more than 10 micrograms/ml the vestibular mechanism may be affected. Toxicity can be minimised by monitoring serum concentrations and it is advisable to check serum levels to confirm that peak levels (one hour) do not exceed 10 micrograms/ml and that trough levels (one hour before next injection) do not exceed 2 micrograms/ml. Evidence of toxicity requires adjustment of dosage or withdrawal of the drug.

Concurrent use of other neurotoxic and/or nephrotoxic drugs can increase the possibility of Gentamicin toxicity. Co-administration with the following agents should be avoided:

Neuromuscular blocking agents such as succinylcholine and tubocurarine.

Other potentially nephrotoxic or ototoxic drugs such as cephalosporins and methicillin.

Potent diuretics such as ethacrynic acid and frusemide.

Other aminoglycosides.

Interactions with other Medicaments and other forms of Interaction:

(i) Antibacterials: increased risk of nephrotoxicity with *cephalosporins notably cephalothin*.
(ii) Gentamicin has been known to potentiate anticoagulants such as warfarin and phenindione.
(iii) Antifungals: increased risk of nephrotoxicity with *amphotericin*.
(iv) Cholinergics: antagonism of effect of *neostigmine and pyridostigmine*.
(v) Cyclosporin: increased risk of nephrotoxicity.
(vi) Cytotoxics: increased risk of nephrotoxicity and possible risk of ototoxicity with *cisplatin*.
(vii) Diuretics: increased risk of ototoxicity with *loop diuretics*.
(viii) Muscle relaxants: effect of non-depolarising muscle relaxants such as *tubocurarine* enhanced.

Pregnancy and lactation:

Use in pregnancy: Although no teratogenic effects have been observed, Gentamicin is known to cross the placenta. Ototoxicity in the foetus is also a potential hazard. The benefits should, therefore, be weighed against such hazards to the foetus before using Gentamicin during pregnancy.

Use in lactation: Small amounts of Gentamicin have been reported in breast milk. Because of the potential for serious adverse reactions to an aminoglycoside in nursing infants, a decision should be made whether to discontinue nursing or the drug, taking into account the importance of the drug to the woman.

Effects on ability to drive and use machines: Not applicable.

Undesirable effects: Ototoxicity and nephrotoxicity are the most common side effects associated with Gentamicin therapy. Both effects are related to renal impairment and hence the dosage in such patients should be altered as suggested.

Other adverse reactions associated with Gentamicin therapy include nausea, vomiting, urticaria, reversible granulocytopenia, allergic contact sensitization and neuromuscular blockade.

Overdose: As in the case of other aminoglycosides, toxicity is associated with serum levels above a critical value. In patients with normal renal function it is unlikely that toxic serum levels (in excess of 10 micrograms/ml) will be reached after administration of recommended doses. Where higher levels occur because of renal impairment, dosage should be reduced. In the event of an overdose or toxic reaction, peritoneal dialysis or haemodialysis will lower serum Gentamicin levels.

Pharmacological properties

Pharmacodynamic properties: Gentamicin is usually bactericidal in action. Although the exact mechanism of action has not been fully elucidated, the drug appears to inhibit protein synthesis in susceptible bacteria by irreversibly binding to 30S ribosomal subunits.

In general, Gentamicin is active against many aerobic gram-negative bacteria and some aerobic gram-positive bacteria. Gentamicin is inactive against fungi, viruses, and most anaerobic bacteria.

In vitro, Gentamicin concentrations of 1-8 mcg/mL inhibit most susceptible strains of *Escherichia coli, Haemophilus influenzae, Moraxella lacunata, Neisseria*, indole positive and indole negative *Proteus, Pseudomonas* (including most strains of *Ps. aeruginosa*), *Staphylococcus aureus, S. epidermidis, and Serratia*. However, different species and different strains of the same species may exhibit wide variations in susceptibility *in vitro*. In addition, *in vitro* susceptibility does not always correlate with *in vivo* activity. Gentamicin is only minimally active against *Streptococci*.

Natural and acquired resistance to Gentamicin has been demonstrated in both gram-negative and gram-positive bacteria. Gentamicin resistance may be due to decreased permeability of the bacterial cell wall, alteration in the ribosomal binding site, or the presence of a plasmid-mediated resistance factor which is acquired by conjugation. Plasmid-mediated resistance enables the resistant bacteria to enzymatically modify the drug by acetylation, phosphorylation, or adenylylation and can be transferred between organisms of the same or different species. Resistance to other aminoglycosides and several other anti-infectives (e.g. chloramphenicol, sulphonamides, tetracycline) may be transferred on the same plasmid.

There is partial cross-resistance between Gentamicin and other aminoglycosides.

Pharmacokinetic properties: Gentamicin and other aminoglycosides are poorly absorbed from the gastro-intestinal tract but are rapidly absorbed after intramuscular injection. Average peak plasma concentrations of about 4 mcg per mL have been obtained 30 to 60 minutes after intramuscular administration of a dose equivalent to 1 mg of Gentamicin per kg bodyweight although there may be considerable individual variation and higher concentrations in patients with renal failure. Similar concentrations are obtained after intravenous administration. Several doses are required before equilibrium concentrations are obtained in the plasma and this may represent the saturation of binding sites in body tissues such as the kidney. Binding of Gentamicin to plasma proteins is usually low.

Following parenteral administration Gentamicin and other aminoglycosides diffuse mainly into extracellular fluids and factors which affect the volume of distribution will also affect plasma concentrations. However, there is little diffusion into the cerebrospinal fluid and even when the meninges are inflamed effective concentrations may not be achieved; diffusion into the eye is also poor. Aminoglycosides diffuse readily into the perilymph of the inner ear. Gentamicin crosses the placenta but only small amounts have been reported in breast milk.

Systemic absorption of Gentamicin and other aminoglycosides has been reported after topical use on denuded skin and burns and following instillation into and irrigation of wounds, body-cavities, and joints.

Preclinical safety data: There are no preclinical data of relevance to the prescriber which are additional to that already included in other sections of the SPC.

Pharmaceutical particulars

List of excipient:

Sodium Metabisulphite BP	6.4 mg
Disodium Edetate BP	0.2 mg
Water for Injections BP	2.0 ml
Sulphuric Acid (2.5N) BP	Q.S.
Sodium Hydroxide (2.5N) BP	Q.S.
(In presentations with bactericide only):	
Methyl Hydroxybenzoate BP	3.6 mg
Propyl Hydroxybenzoate BP	0.4 mg

Incompatibilities: Gentamicin Injection should not be mixed with other drugs before injection and where co-administration of penicillins, cephalosporins, erythromycin, sulphadiazine, frusemide and betalactam antibiotics and heparin is necessary, the drugs should be administered separately, either as bolus injections into the tubing of the giving set or at separate sites. Addition of Gentamicin to solutions containing bicarbonate may lead to the release of carbon dioxide.

Shelf life: 36 months.

Special precautions for storage: Store below 25°C.

Instruction for use/handling: Not applicable.

Marketing authorisation numbers

Ampoules	4515/0028
80 mg/2 mL vial	4515/0037

Date of approval/revision of SPC 24 January 1997

Legal category POM

GLYCERYL TRINITRATE FOR INJECTION 5MG/1ML.

Qualitative and quantitative composition

Active Constituent	
Glyceryl Trinitrate HSE	5.0 mg.
Other Constituents	
Ethanol BP	30.0% v/v
Propylene Glycol BP	30.0% v/v
Water for Injections BP	to 1.0 mL.

There is no overage included in the formulation.

Pharmaceutical form A sterile, non-pyrogenic, clear, practically colourless solution.

Clinical particulars

Therapeutic indications: Surgery: Glyceryl Trinitrate is indicated for the prompt control of hypertension during cardiac surgery.

It may also be used for the production and maintenance of controlled hypotension during surgical procedures.

Glyceryl Trinitrate may be given for the control of myocardial ischaemia both during and following cardiovascular surgery.

Unresponsive congestive cardiac failure secondary to acute myocardial infarction: Glyceryl Trinitrate may be used in patients presenting with unresponsive congestive heart failure secondary to acute myocardial infarction.

Unstable angina: Glyceryl Trinitrate Infusion may be used to reduce myocardial oxygen demand in proportion to the reduction in pre- and after-load. It may be indicated for the control of anginal episodes in patients with unstable angina who do not respond to standard treatment and/or beta-blockers.

It is recommended that blood pressure and pulse rate are regularly monitored during infusion of Glyceryl Trinitrate.

Posology and method of administration: Glyceryl Trinitrate for Injection is a concentrated, potent drug which must be diluted in Dextrose (5%) Injection BP or Sodium Chloride (0.9%) Injection BP prior to its infusion.

The dosage range for most patients is 10-20mcg/min. However, doses up to 400 mcg/min may be required during surgical procedures.

Compatibility: Glyceryl Trinitrate for Injection is compatible with glass infusion bottles and some rigid infusion packs made of polyethylene. Examples of such suitable infusion packs are: Boots polyfusor and the bottle pack distributed by Dylade, Cheshire UK (bottlepak, flatpak) or Antigen Ltd. Roscrea, Eire (Braun).

Glyceryl Trinitrate for Injection may also be administered using a syringe pump or rigid plastic syringe (Gillette Sabre syringe, Brunswick Disposable, Plastipak syringe or Monojet disposable syringe).

Suitable giving sets are Types A261 or A2001 available from David Bull Laboratories or Avon Medicals. Lectrocath tubing (Vygon UK Ltd) is also known to be compatible with the preparation.

The method of choice of administration should ensure that the drug is given at a constant infusion rate.

Incompatibility: Glyceryl Trinitrate for Injection is incompatible with polyvinyl chloride (PVC) since 40-80% of the total amount thereof in the final diluted solution for infusion is absorbed by the PVC tubing of the intravenous administration sets.

Dosage: The recommended dose range is 10-200 mcg/min, although larger doses than this have been used. During some surgical procedures, doses of up to 400 mcg/min may be required. In order to maintain the appropriate infusion rate, clinical assessment and regular blood pressure monitoring are necessary. Measurement of pulmonary capillary wedge pressure and cardiac out-put may also be used to titrate dosage to response.

Surgery: For the control of hypertensive episodes the recommended starting dose is 25 mcg/min increasing in steps to 25 mcg/min at 5 minute intervals until the desired drop in blood pressure is achieved. Although most patients respond to doses between 10-200 mcg/min, doses up to 400 mcg/min have been required during some surgical procedures. In the treatment of perioperative myocardial ischaemia, the recommended starting dose is 15-20 mcg/min increasing in steps of 10-15 mcg/min until the desired effect is achieved.

Unresponsive congestive cardiac failure secondary to acute myocardial infarction: The recommended starting dose is 20-25 mcg/min which can be decreased to 10 mcg/min or increased in steps of 20-25 mcg/min at 15-30 minute intervals until the desired effect is achieved.

Unstable angina: The recommended starting dose is 10 mcg/min increasing in steps of 5-10 mcg/min at approximately 30 minute intervals.

Children and the elderly: The use of Glyceryl Trinitrate in children and elderly patients is not recommended, as the safety and effectiveness of Glyceryl Trinitrate in children and elderly patients have not been established.

Contra-indications: To those who have or are:

1. Hypersensitive to Glyceryl Trinitrate
2. Hypotensive or hypovolaemic
3. Increased intracranial pressure
4. Constrictive pericarditis and pericardial tamponade
5. Severe anaemia and arterial hypoxaemia.

Special warnings and special precautions for use: *Warnings:* DBL Glyceryl Trinitrate for Injection contains propylene glycol which can lead to lactic acidosis. It is recommended that the use of this preparation be restricted to not more than three successive days.

Precautions: Glyceryl Trinitrate for Injection should not be administered to patients known to be hypersensitive to organic nitrates, nor should it be given to patients with uncorrected hypovolaemia, severe anaemia or cerebral haemorrhage or hypotension.

Glyceryl Trinitrate should be used with caution in patients presenting with malnutrition, hypothyroidism, severe hypothermia, or severe impairment of hepatic and/or renal function.

Evidence is not available to demonstrate the safety of Glyceryl Trinitrate for intracoronary injection.

Glyceryl Trinitrate for Injection should be used with caution in patients predisposed to closed angle glaucoma.

Interaction with other medicaments and other forms of interaction:

Anti-arrhythmics: disopyramide may reduce effect of sublingual nitrates (owing to dry mouth)

Anti-depressants: tricyclics may reduce effects of sublingual nitrates (owing to dry mouth)

Antimuscarinics: antimuscarinics such as atropine and propantheline may reduce effect of sublingual nitrates (owing to dry mouth).

Pregnancy and lactation: The safety of Glyceryl Trinitrate during pregnancy and lactation has not been demonstrated and therefore it should not be used in these situations unless considered essential by the physician.

Effects on ability to drive and use machines: Not applicable.

Undesirable effects: Adverse reactions to organic nitrates which have been reported include hypotension, tachycardia, nausea, retching, diaphoresis, apprehension, headache, restlessness, muscle twitching, retrosternal discomfort, palpitations, dizziness, and abdominal pain, paradoxical bradycardia has rarely been observed.

Overdose: Overdosage usually results in hypotension and tachycardia and can be reversed by elevating the legs or decreasing or terminating the infusion. In severe cases of overdosage, intravenous administration of methoxamine or phenylephrine is recommended.

Pharmacological properties

Pharmacodynamic properties: Glyceryl Trinitrate, an organic nitrate, is a vasodilator. The principal pharmacological action of Glyceryl Trinitrate is the relaxation of vascular smooth muscle. Glyceryl Trinitrate produces, in a dose-related manner, dilation of both arterial and venous beds. Dilatation of the post-capillary vessels, including large veins, promotes peripheral pooling of blood and decreases venous return to the heart, reducing left ventricular end-diastolic pressure (pre-load).

Arteriolar relaxation reduces systemic vascular resistance and arterial pressure (after-load). Myocardial oxygen consumption or demand (as measured by the pressure-rate product, tension time index and stroke work index) is decreased by both arterial and venous effects of Glyceryl Trinitrate, and a more favourable supply demand ratio can be achieved.

Therapeutic doses of intravenous Glyceryl Trinitrate reduce systolic, diastolic and mean arterial blood pressure. Effective coronary perfusion pressure is usually maintained, but can be compromised if blood pressure falls excessively or increased heart rate decreases diastolic filling time.

Glyceryl Trinitrate reduces elevated central venous and pulmonary capillary wedge pressures, pulmonary vascular resistance and systemic vascular resistance. Heart rate is usually slightly increased, presumably a reflex response to the fall in blood pressure. Cardiac index may be increased, decreased or unchanged.

Patients with elevated left ventricular filling pressure and systemic vascular resistance values in conjunction with a depressed cardiac index are likely to experience an improvement in cardiac index. Alternatively, when filling pressures and cardiac index are normal, cardiac index may be slightly reduced by intravenous Glyceryl Trinitrate.

Pharmacokinetic properties: Glyceryl Trinitrate is widely distributed in the body with an apparent volume of distribution of 200 L in adult male subjects, and is rapidly metabolised to dinitrates and mononitrates, with a short half-life estimated at 1-4 minutes. This results in a low plasma concentration after intravenous infusion. Glyceryl Trinitrate is also well absorbed from the gastro-intestinal tract, but it is not known if it is distributed into milk.

At plasma concentrations of between 50 and 500ng/ml, the binding of Glyceryl Trinitrate to plasma proteins is approximately 60% and 30% respectively. The plasma half-life of Glyceryl Trinitrate is about 1-4 minutes. Glyceryl mononitrate which is inactive, is the principal metabolite.

Preclinical safety data: Not applicable.

Pharmaceutical particulars

List of excipients:	
Ethanol BP	30.0% v/v
Propylene Glycol BP	30.0% v/v
Water for Injections BP	to 1.0 mL.

There is no overage included in the formulation.

Incompatibilities: The manufacturers of Glyceryl Trinitrate for Injection recommend that this concentrated and potent drug must be diluted in Dextrose (5%) Injection BP or Sodium Chloride (0.9%) Injection BP prior to its infusion. They also state that no other drug should be admixed with it.

Shelf life: 36 months.

Special precautions for storage: Store below 25°C. Protect from light.

Open ampoules of Glyceryl Trinitrate should be used immediately and any unused portion discarded.

Dilutions of Glyceryl Trinitrate for Injection in Sodium Chloride Injection or Dextrose Injection are stable for 40 hours at room temperature when stored in glass containers or recommended plastic containers. Similar dilutions are stable for 7 days at 2°C-8°C.

Solutions containing 1 mg or 4 mg per Glyceryl Trinitrate, diluted in Dextrose 5% Injection BP are stable for up to 72 hours, at room temperature protected from light, using either polycarbonate (Plastipak) or polypropylene syringes.

Glyceryl Trinitrate is rapidly lost from solutions stored in polyvinylchloride (PVC) containers, and the use of such infusion packs should therefore be avoided.

Glyceryl Trinitrate should be administered in the recommended plastic containers (see under compatibility).

Glyceryl Trinitrate should be protected from strong light.

Do not use if the solution is discoloured.

Instructions for use/handling: Not applicable.

Marketing authorisation number 4515/0006

Date of approval/revision of SPC August 1995

Legal category POM

METHOTREXATE INJECTION

Qualitative and quantitative composition

2.5 mg/mL presentations

Presentation	*5 mg/2 mL*	
Active Constituent	*per unit dose*	*per mL*
Methotrexate BP	5.0 mg*	2.5 mg

*There is a 5% manufacturing overage included in the formulation.

25 mg/mL presentations

Presentation	*50 mg/2 mL*		*500 mg/20 mL*	
Active Constituent	*per unit dose*	*per mL*	*per unit dose*	*per mL*
Methotrexate BP	50.0 mg*	25.0 mg	500.0 mg*	25.0 mg.

*There is a 5% manufacturing overage included in the formulation.

100 mg/mL presentations

Presentation	*1 g/10 mL*		*5 g/50 mL*	
Active Constituent	*per unit dose*	*per mL*	*per unit dose*	*per mL*
Methotrexate BP	1000.0 mg*	100.0 mg	5000.0 mg*	100.0 mg.

*There is a 5% manufacturing overage included in the formulation.

Pharmaceutical form Sterile solution of Methotrexate in Water for Injections.

Clinical particulars

Therapeutic indications: Methotrexate is indicated in the treatment of neoplastic disease, such as trophoblastic neoplasms and leukaemia, and the symptomatic treatment of severe recalcitrant disabling psoriasis which is not adequately responsive to other forms of treatment.

Methotrexate Injection BP may be given by the intramuscular, intravenous, intra-arterial, intrathecal routes.

NOTE: Methotrexate Injection BP 1 g in 10 ml and 5 g in 50 ml are hypertonic and therefore are not suitable for intrathecal use. The 500 mg in 20 ml should not be administered by the intrathecal route.

Posology and method of administration:
Adults and children: Antineoplastic chemotherapy: Methotrexate is active orally and parenterally. Methotrexate Injection BP may be given by the intramuscular, intravenous, intra-arterial or intrathecal routes. Dosage is related to the patient's body weight or surface area. Methotrexate has been used with beneficial effect in a wide variety of neoplastic diseases, alone and in combination with other cytotoxic agents. Note: Methotrexate Injection BP 1 g in 10 ml and 5 g in 50 ml are hypertonic and thus are not recommended for intrathecal use.

Choriocarcinoma and Similar Trophoblastic Diseases: Methotrexate is administered orally or intramuscularly in doses of 15-30 mg daily for a 5 day course. Such courses may be repeated for 3-5 times as required, with rest periods of one or more weeks interposed between courses until any manifesting toxic symptoms subside.

The effectiveness of therapy can be evaluated by 24 hours quantitative analysis of urinary chorionic gonadotrophin hormone (HCG). Alternation of Methotrexate, and combination therapy with other cytotoxic drugs, has also been reported as useful.

Hydatidiform mole may precede or be followed by choriocarcinoma, and Methotrexate has been used in similar doses for the treatment of hydatidiform mole and chorioadenoma destruens.

Breast Carcinoma: Prolonged cyclic combination with Cyclophosphamide, Methotrexate and Fluorouracil has given good results when used as adjuvant treatment to radical mastectomy in primary breast cancer with positive axillary lymph nodes. Methotrexate dosage was 40 mg/m2 intravenously on the first and eight days.

Leukaemia: Acute granulocytic leukaemia is rare in children but common in adults and this form of leukaemia responds poorly to chemotherapy.

Methotrexate is not generally a drug of choice for induction of remission of lymphoblastic leukaemia. Oral Methotrexate dosage of 3.3 mg/m2 daily, and Prednisolone 40-60 mg/m2 daily for 4-6 weeks has been used. After a remission is attained, Methotrexate in a maintenance dosage of 20-30 mg/m2 orally or by I.M. injection has been administered twice weekly. Twice weekly doses appear to be more effective than daily drug administration. Alternatively, 2.5 mg/kg has been administered I.V. every 14 days.

Meningeal Leukaemia: Some patients with leukaemia are subject to leukaemic invasions of the central nervous system and the CSF should be examined in all leukaemia patients.

Passage of Methotrexate from blood to the cerebrospinal fluid is minimal and for adequate therapy the drug should be administered intrathecally. Methotrexate may be given in a prophylactic regimen in all cases of lymphocytic leukaemia. Methotrexate is administered by intrathecal injection in doses of 200-500 micrograms/kg body weight. The administration is at intervals of 2 to 5 days and is usually repeated until the cell count of cerebrospinal fluid returns to normal. At this point one additional dose is advised. Alternatively, Methotrexate 12 mg/m2 can be given once weekly for 2 weeks, and then once monthly. Large doses may cause convulsions and untoward side effects may occur as with any intrathecal injection, and are commonly neurological in character.

NOTE: Methotrexate Injection BP 1 g in 10 ml, 5 g in 50 ml and 500 mg in 20 ml are not recommended for intrathecal use.

Lymphomas: In Burkitt's Tumour, stages 1-2, Methotrexate has prolonged remissions in some cases. Recommended dosage is 10-25 mg per day orally for 4 to 8 days. In stage 3, Methotrexate is commonly given concomitantly with other antitumour agents. Treatment in all stages usually consists of several courses of the drug interposed with 7 to 10 day rest periods, and in stage 3 they respond to combined drug therapy with Methotrexate given in doses of 0.625 mg to 2.5 mg/kg daily. Hodgkin's Disease responds poorly to Methotrexate and to most types of chemotherapy.

Mycosis Fungoides: Therapy with Methotrexate appears to produce clinical remissions in one half of the cases treated. Recommended dosage is usually 2.5 to 10 mg daily by mouth for weeks or months and dosage should be adjusted according to the patient's response and haematological monitoring. Methotrexate has also been given intramuscularly in doses of 50 mg once weekly or 25 mg twice weekly.

Psoriasis Chemotherapy: Cases of severe uncontrolled psoriasis, unresponsive to conventional therapy, have responded to weekly single, oral, I.M. or I.V. doses of 10-25 mg per week, and adjusted according to the patient's response. An initial test dose one week prior to initiation of therapy is recommended to detect any idiosyncrasy. A suggested dose range is 5-10 mg parenterally.

An alternative dosage schedule consists of 2.5 to 5 mg of Methotrexate administered orally at 12 hour intervals for 3 doses each week or at 8-hour intervals for 4 doses each week; weekly dosages should not exceed 30 mg.

A daily oral dosage schedule of 2 to 5 mg administered orally for 5 days followed by a rest period of at least 2 days may also be used. The daily dose should not exceed 6.25 mg.

The patient should be fully informed of the risks involved and the clinician should pay particular attention to the appearance of the liver toxicity by carrying out liver function tests before starting Methotrexate treatment, and repeating these at 2 to 4 month intervals during therapy. The aim of therapy should be to reduce the dose to the lowest possible level with the longest possible rest period. The use of Methotrexate may permit the return to conventional topical therapy which should be encouraged.

Contra-indications: Impaired renal or hepatic function.

Pre-existing blood dyscrasias, such as marrow hypoplasia, leukopenia, thromocytopenia or anaemia.

Pregnancy and lactation: Methotrexate is contraindicated in pregnancy. Because of the potential for serious adverse reactions from methotrexate in breast fed infants, breast feeding is contra-indicated in women taking methotrexate. Patients with a known allergic hypersensitivity to methotrexate should not receive methotrexate.

Special warnings and special precautions for use:
Warnings: Methotrexate must be used only by physicians experienced in antimetabolic chemotherapy.

Because of the possibility of fatal or severe toxic reactions, the patient should be fully informed by the physician of the risks involved and be under his constant supervision.

Deaths have been reported with the use of Methotrexate in the treatment of psoriasis.

In the treatment of psoriasis, Methotrexate should be restricted to severe recalcitrant, disabling psoriasis which is not adequately responsive to other forms of therapy, but only when the diagnosis has been established as by biopsy and/or after dermatological consultation.

1. Methotrexate may produce marked depression of bone marrow, anaemia, leukopenia, thrombocytopenia and bleeding.

2. Methotrexate may be hepatotoxic, particularly at high dosage or with prolonged therapy. Liver atrophy, necrosis, cirrhosis, fatty changes, and periportal fibrosis have been reported. Since changes may occur without previous signs of gastrointestinal or haematological toxicity, it is imperative that hepatic function be determined prior to initiation of treatment and monitored regularly throughout therapy. Special caution is indicated in the presence of pre-existing liver damage of impaired hepatic function. Concomitant use of other drugs with hepatotoxic potential (including alcohol) should be avoided.

3. Methotrexate has been shown to be teratogenic; it has caused foetal death and/or congenital anomalies. Therefore it is not recommended in women of childbearing potential unless there is appropriate medical evidence that the benefits can be expected to outweigh the considered risks. Pregnant psoriatic patients should not receive Methotrexate.

4. Impaired renal function is usually a contraindication.

5. Diarrhoea and ulcerative stomatitis are frequent toxic effects and require interruption of therapy, otherwise haemorrhagic enteritis and death from intestinal perforation may occur.

6. Methotrexate affects gametogenesis during the period of its administration and may result in decreased fertility which is thought to be reversible on discontinuation of therapy. Conception should be avoided during the period of Methotrexate administration and for at least 6 months thereafter. Patients and their partners should be advised to this effect.

7. Methotrexate has some immunosuppressive activity and immunological responses to concurrent vaccination may be decreased. The immunosuppressive effect of Methotrexate should be taken into account when immune responses of patients are important or essential.

8. Patients with pleural effusions or ascites should have these drained if appropriate before treatment or treatment should be withdrawn.

9. Deaths have been reported with the use of methotrexate. Serious adverse reactions including deaths have been reported with concomitant administration of methotrexate (usually in high doses) along with some non-steroidal anti-inflammatory drugs (NSAIDs).

10. Concomitant administration of folate antagonists such as trimethoprim/sulphamethoxazole has been reported to cause an acute megaloblastic pancytopenia in rare instances.

Precautions: Methotrexate has a high potential toxicity, usually dose related, and should be used only by physicians experienced in antimetabolite chemotherapy, in patients under their constant supervision. The physician should be familiar with the various characteristics of the drug and its established clinical usage.

Before beginning methotrexate therapy or reinstituting methotrexate after a rest period, assessment of renal function, liver function and blood elements should be made by history, physical examination and laboratory tests.

It should be noted that intrathecal doses are transported into the cardiovascular system and may give rise to systemic toxicity. Systemic toxicity of methotrexate may also be enhanced in patients with renal dysfunction, ascites, or other effusions due to prolongation of serum half-life.

High doses may cause the precipitation of methotrexate or its metabolites in the renal tubules. A high fluid throughout and alkalinisation of the urine to pH 6.5-7.0 by oral or intravenous administration of sodium bicarbonate (5 x 625 mg tablets every three hours) or acetazolamide (500 mg orally four times a day) is recommended as a preventative measure.

Carcinogenesis, mutagenesis, and impairment of fertility: Animal carcinogencity studies have demonstrated methotrexate to be free of carcinogenic potential. Although methotrexate has been reported to cause chromosomal damage to animal somatic cells and bone marrow cells in humans, these effects are transient and reversible. In patients treated with methotrexate, evidence is insufficient to permit conclusive evaluation of any increased risk of neoplasia.

Methotrexate has been reported to cause impairment of fertility, oligospermia, menstrual dysfunction and amenorrhoea in humans, during and for a short period after cessation of therapy. In addition, methotrexate causes, embryotoxicity, abortion and foetal defects in humans. Therefore the possible risks of effects on reproduction should be discussed with patients of childbearing potential (see 'Warnings').

Patients undergoing therapy should be subject to appropriate supervision so that signs or symptoms of possible toxic effects or adverse reactions may be detected and evaluated with minimal delay. Pretreatment and periodic haematological studies are essential to the use of Methotrexate in chemotherapy because of its common effect of haematopoietic suppression. This may occur abruptly and on apparent safe dosage, and any profound drop in blood cell count indicates immediate stopping of the drug and appropriate therapy. In patients with malignant disease who have pre-existing bone marrow aplasia, leukopenia, thrombocytopenia or anaemia, the drug should be used with caution, if at all.

Methotrexate is excreted primarily by the kidneys. Its use in the presence of impaired renal function may result in accumulation of toxic amounts or even additional renal damage. The patient's renal status should be determined prior to or during Methotrexate therapy and proper caution exercised, should significant renal impairment be disclosed.

Drug dosage should be reduced or discontinued until renal function is improved or restored.

In general, the following laboratory tests are recommended as part of essential clinical evaluation and appropriate monitoring of patients chosen for or receiving Methotrexate therapy: complete haemogram; haematocrit; urinalysis; renal function tests; and liver function tests.

A chest X-ray is also recommended. The purpose is to determine any existing organ dysfunction or system impairment. The tests should be performed prior to therapy, at appropriate periods during therapy and after termination of therapy. It may be useful or important to perform liver biopsy or bone marrow aspiration studies where high dose or long term therapy is being followed.

Methotrexate is bound in part to serum albumin after absorption, and toxicity may be increased because of displacement by certain drugs such as salicylates, sulphonamides, phenytoin, and some antibacterials such as tetracycline, chloramphenicol and para-aminobenzoic acid. These drugs, especially salicylates and sulphonamides, whether antibacterial, hypoglycaemic or diuretic, should not be given concurrently until the significance of these findings is established.

Vitamin preparations containing folic acid or its derivatives may alter response to Methotrexate.

Methotrexate should be used with extreme caution in the presence of infection, peptic ulcer, ulcerative colitis, debility, and in extreme youth and old age. If profound leukopenia occurs during therapy, bacterial infection may occur or become a threat. Cessation of the drug and appropriate antibiotic therapy is usually indicated. In severe bone marrow depression, blood or platelet transfusions may be necessary.

Since it is reported that Methotrexate may have an immunosuppressive action, this factor must be taken into consideration in evaluating the use of the drug where immune responses in a patient may be important or essential.

In all instances where the use of Methotrexate is considered for chemotherapy, the physician must evaluate the need and usefulness of the drug against the risks of toxic effects or adverse reactions. Most such adverse reactions are reversible if detected early. When such effects or reactions do occur, the drug should be reduced in dosage or discontinued and appropriate corrective measures should be taken according to the clinical judgement of the physician. Reinstitution of Methotrexate therapy should be carried out with caution, with adequate consideration of further need for the drug and alertness as to the possible recurrence of toxicity.

Interaction with other medicaments and other forms of interaction: Methotrexate is extensively protein bound and may be displaced by certain drugs such as salicylates, hypoglycaemics, diuretics, sulphonamides, diphenylhydantoins, tetracyclines, chloramphenicol and p-aminobenzoic acid, and the acidic anti-inflammatory agents, so causing a potential for increased toxicity when used concurrently. Concomitant use of other drugs with nephrotoxic or hepatotoxic potential (including alcohol) should be avoided. Vitamin preparations containing folic acid or its derivatives may decrease the effectiveness of methotrexate.

Caution should be used when NSAIDs and salicylates are administered concomitantly with methotrexate. These drugs have been reported to reduce the tubular secretion of methotrexate in an animal model and thereby may enhance its toxicity. Renal tubular transport is also diminished by probenecid; use of methotrexate with this drug should be carefully monitored.

Patients using constant dosage regimens of NSAIDs have received concurrent doses of methotrexate problems. Therefore, until more is known about the NSAIDs/methotrexate interaction, it is recommended that methotrexate dosage be carefully controlled during treatment with NSAIDs.

Methotrexate should be used with caution in patients taking drugs known to have an antifolate potential.

Pregnancy and lactation: Abortion, foetal death, and/or congenital anomalies have occurred in pregnant women receiving Methotrexate, especially during the first trimester of pregnancy. Methotrexate is contra-indicated in the management of psoriasis or rheumatoid arthritis in pregnant women. Women of childbearing potential should not receive Methotrexate until pregnancy is excluded. For the management of psoriasis or rheumatoid arthritis, Methotrexate therapy in women should be started immediately following a menstrual period and appropriate measures should be taken in men or women to avoid conception during and for at least 12 weeks following Methotrexate therapy.

Both men and women receiving Methotrexate should be informed of the potential risk of adverse effects on reproduction. Women of childbearing potential should be fully informed of the potential hazard to the foetus should they become pregnant during Methotrexate therapy. In cancer chemotherapy, Methotrexate should not be used in pregnant women or women of childbearing potential who might become pregnant unless the potential benefits to the mother outweigh the possible risks to the foetus.

Defective oogenesis or spermatogenesis, transient oligospermia, menstrual dysfunction, and infertility have been reported in patients receiving Methotrexate.

Methotrexate is distributed into breast milk. Because of the potential for serious adverse reactions to Methotrexate in nursing infants, a decision should be made whether to discontinue nursing or the drug, taking into account the importance of the drug to the woman.

Effects on ability to drive and use machines: Not applicable.

Undesirable effects: The most common adverse reactions include ulcerative stomatitis, leukopenia, nausea and abdominal distress. Although very rare, anaphylactic reactions to methotrexate have occurred. Others reported are malaise, undue fatigue, chills and fever, dizziness and decreased resistance to infection. In general, the incidence and severity of side effects are considered to be dose-related. Adverse reactions as reported for the various systems are as follows:

Skin: Erythematous rashes, pruritus, urticaria, photosensitivity, depigmentation, alopecia, ecchymosis, telangiectasia, acne, furunculosis. Lesions of psoriasis may be aggravated by concomitant exposure to ultraviolet radiation. Skin ulceration has been reported in psoriatic patients. The recall phenomenon has been reported in both radiation and solar damaged skin.

Blood: Bone marrow depression, leukopenia, thrombocytopenia, anaemia, hypogammaglobulinaemia, haemorrhage from various sites, septicaemia.

Alimentary System: Gingivitis, pharyngitis, stomatitis, anorexia, vomiting, diarrhoea, haematemesis, melena, gastrointestinal ulceration and bleeding, enteritis, hepatic toxicity resulting in active liver atrophy, necrosis, fatty metamorphosis, periportal fibrosis, or hepatic cirrhosis. In rare cases the effect of methotrexate on the intestinal mucosa has led to malabsorption or toxic megacolon.

Hepatic: Hepatic toxicity resulting in significant elevations of liver enzymes, acute liver atrophy, necrosis, fatty metamorphosis, periportal fibrosis or cirrhosis or death may occur, usually following chronic administration.

Urogenital System: Renal failure, azotaemia, cystitis, haematuria, defective oogenesis or spermatogenesis, transient oligospermia, menstrual dysfunction, infertility, abortion, foetal defects, severe nephropathy. Vaginitis, vaginal ulcers, cystitis, haematuria and nephropathy have also been reported.

Pulmonary System: Infrequently an acute or chronic interstitial pneumonitis, often associated with blood eosinophilia, may occur and deaths have been reported. Acute pulmonary oedema has also been reported after oral and intrathecal use. Pulmonary fibrosis is rare. A syndrome consisting of pleuritic pain and pleural thickening has been reported following high doses.

Central Nervous System: Headaches, drowsiness, blurred vision, aphasia, hemiparesis and convulsions have occurred possibly related to haemorrhage or to complications from intra-arterial catheterization. Convulsion, paresis, Guillain-Barre syndrome and increased cerebrospinal fluid pressure have followed intrathecal administration.

Other reactions related to, or attributed to the use of Methotrexate such as pneumonitis, metabolic changes, precipitation of diabetes, osteoporotic effects, abdominal changes in tissue cells and even sudden death have been reported.

There have been reports of leukoencephalopathy following intravenous methotrexate in high doses, or low doses following cranial-spinal radiation.

Adverse reactions following intrathecal methotrexate are generally classified into three groups, acute, subacute, and chronic. The acute form is a chemical arachnoiditis manifested by headache, back or shoulder pain, nuchal rigidity, and fever. The subacute form may include paresis, usually transient, paraplegia, nerve palsies, and cerebellar dysfunction. The chronic form is a leukoencephalopathy manifested by irritability, confusion, ataxia, spasticity, occasionally convulsions, dementia, somnolence, coma, and rarely, death. There is evidence that the combined use of cranial radiation and intrathecal methotrexate increases the incidence of leukoencephalopathy.

Additional reactions related to or attributed to the use of methotrexate such as osteoporosis, abnormal (usually 'megaloblastic') red cell morphology, precipitation of diabetes, other metabolic changes, and sudden death have been reported.

Overdose: Calcium Folinate (Calcium Leucovorin) is a potent agent for neutralizing the immediate toxic effects of Methotrexate on the haematopoietic system. Where large doses or overdoses are given, Calcium Folinate may be administered by intravenous infusion in doses up to 75 mg within 12 hours, followed by 12 mg intramuscularly every 6 hours for 4 doses. Where average doses of Methotrexate appear to have an adverse effect 6-12 mg of Calcium Folinate may be given intramuscularly every 6 hours for 4 doses. In general, where overdosage is suspected, the dose of Calcium Folinate should be equal to or higher than, the offending dose of Methotrexate and should be administered as soon as possible; preferably within the first hour and certainly within 4 hours after which it may not be effective. Other supporting therapy such as blood transfusion and renal dialysis may be required.

Pharmacological properties

Pharmacodynamic properties

Methotrexate is an antimetabolite which acts principally by competitively inhibiting the enzyme, dihydrofolate reductase. In the process of DNA synthesis and cellular replication, folic acid must be reduced to tetrahydrofolic acid by thisenzyme, and inhibition by Methotrexate interfers with tissue cell reproductions. Actively proliferating tissues such as malignant cells are generally more sensitive to this effect of Methotrexate. It also inhibits antibody synthesis.

Methotrexate also has immunosuppressive activity, in part possibly as a result of inhibition of lymphocyte multiplication. The mechanism(s) of action in the management of rheumatoid arthritis of the drug is not known, although suggested mechanisms have included immunosuppressive and/or anti-inflammatory effect.

Pharmacokinetic properties

In doses of 0.1 mg (of Methotrexate) per kg, Methotrexate is completely absorbed from the G.I. tract; larger oral doses may be incompletely absorbed. Peak serum concentrations are achieved with 0.5–2 hours following I.V., I.M. or intra-arterial administration. Serum concentrations following oral administration of Methotrexate may be slightly lower than those following I.V. injection.

Methotrexate is actively transported across cell membranes. The drug is widely distributed into body tissues with highest concentrations in the kidneys, gall bladder, spleen, liver and skin. Methotrexate is retained for several weeks in the kidneys and for months in the liver. Sustained serum concentrations and tissue accumulation may result from repeated daily doses. Methotrexate crosses the placental barrier and is distributed into breast milk. Approximately 50% of the drug in the blood is bound to serum proteins.

In one study, Methotrexate had a serum half-life of 2-4 hours following I.M. administration. Following oral doses of 0.06 mg/kg or more, the drug had a serum half-life of 2-4 hours, but the serum half-life was reported to be increased to 8-10 hours when oral doses of 0.037 mg/kg were given.

Methotrexate does not appear to be appreciably metabolised. The drug is excreted primarily by the kidneys via glomerular filtration and active transport. Small amounts are excreted in the faeces, probably via the bile. Methotrexate has a biphasic excretion pattern. If Methotrexate excretion is impaired accumulation will occur more rapidly in patients with impaired renal function. In addition, simultaneous administration of other weak organic acids such as salicylates may suppress Methotrexate clearance.

Pharmaceutical particulars

List of excipients:

2.5 mg/mL presentations

Presentation	*5 mg/2 mL per unit dose*	*per mL*
Sodium Chloride BP	17.2 mg	8.6 mg
Sodium Hydroxide BP	qs	qs
Water for Injections BP	to 2.0 mL	to 1.0 mL

25 mg/mL presentations

Presentation	*50 mg/2 mL per unit dose*	*per mL*	*500 mg/20 mL per unit dose*	*per mL*
Sodium Chloride BP	9.8 mg	4.90 mg	98 mg	4.90 mg
Sodium Hydroxide BP	qs	qs	qs	qs
Water for Injections BP	to 2.0 mL	to 1.0 mL	to 20 mL	to 1.0 mL

There is a 5% manufacturing overage included in the formulation.

100 mg/mL presentations

Presentation	*1 g/10 mL per unit dose*	*per mL*	*5 g/50 mL per unit dose*	*per mL*
Sodium Hydroxide BP	qs	qs	qs	qs
Water for Injections BP	to 10.0 mL	to 1.0 mL	to 50.0 mL	to 1.0 mL

Incompatibilities: Immediate precipitation or turbidity results when combined with certain concentrations of Droperidol, Heparin Sodium, Metoclopramide Hydrochloride, Ranitidine Hydrochloride in syringe.

Shelf life: 24 months.

Special precautions for storage: Store below 25°C. Protect from light and freezing.

Unused portions of opened vials or prepared infusions if not used immediately must be stored at 2-8°C for no longer than 24 hours from the time of opening or preparation.

Instructions for use/handling: Not applicable.

Marketing authorisation numbers

2.5 mg/mL	4515/0013
25 mg/mL	4515/0015
100 mg/mL	4515/0038

Date of approval/revision of SPC June 1994

Legal category POM

METHOTREXATE TABLETS BP

Qualitative and quantitative composition *Active constituent:* Methotrexate PhEur 2.5 mg and 10.0 mg. There is no overage included in the formulation.

Pharmaceutical form Tablet for oral administration.

Clinical particulars

Therapeutic indications: Methotrexate is indicated in the treatment of neoplastic disease, such as trophoblastic neoplasms and leukaemia and in the control of severe recalcitrant psoriasis which is not responsive to other forms of therapy.

Posology and method of administration:
Adults and children:

Antineoplastic chemotherapy: Methotrexate is active orally and parenterally. Methotrexate Injection BP may be given by the intramuscular, intravenous, intra-arterial or intrathecal routes. Dosage is related to the patient's body weight or surface area. Methotrexate has been used with beneficial effect in a wide variety of neoplastic *diseases, alone and in combination with other cytotoxic agents.*

Choriocarcinoma and similar trophoblastic diseases: Methotrexate is administered orally or intramuscularly in doses of 15-30 mg daily for a 5 day course. Such courses may be repeated for 3-5 times as required, with rest periods of one or more weeks interposed between courses until any manifesting toxic symptoms subside.

The effectiveness of therapy can be evaluated by 24 hours quantitative analysis of urinary chorionic gonadotrophin hormone (HCG). Alternation of Methotrexate, and combination therapy with other cytotoxic drugs, has also been reported as useful.

Hydatidiform mole may precede or be followed by choriocarcinoma, and Methotrexate has been used in similar doses for the treatment of hydatidiform mole and chorioadenoma destruens.

Breast Carcinoma: Prolonged cyclic combination with Cyclophosphamide, Methotrexate and Fluorouracil has given good results when used as adjuvant treatment to radical mastectomy in primary breast cancer with positive axillary lymph nodes. Methotrexate dosage was 40 mg/m2 intravenously on the first and eight days.

Leukaemia: Acute granulocytic leukaemia is rare in children but common in adults and this form of leukaemia responds poorly to chemotherapy.

Methotrexate is not generally a drug of choice for induction of remission of lymphoblastic leukaemia. Oral Methotrexate dosage of 3.3 mg/m2 daily, and Prednisolone 40-60 mg/m2 daily for 4-6 weeks has been used. After a remission is attained, Methotrexate in a maintenance dosage of 20-30 mg/m2 orally or by I.M. injection has been administered twice weekly. Twice weekly doses appear to be more effective than daily drug administration. Alternatively, 2.5 mg/kg has been administered I.V. every 14 days.

Meningeal Leukaemia: Some patients with leukaemia are subject to leukaemic invasions of the central nervous system and the CSF should be examined in all leukaemia patients.

Passage of Methotrexate from blood to the cerebrospinal fluid is minimal and for adequate therapy the drug should be administered intrathecally. Methotrexate may be given in a prophylactic regimen in all cases of lymphocytic leukaemia. Methotrexate is administered by intrathecal injection in doses of 200-500 micrograms/kg body weight. The administration is at intervals of 2 to 5 days and is usually repeated until the cell count of cerebrospinal fluid returns to normal. At this point one additional dose is advised. Alternatively, Methotrexate 12 mg/m2 can be given once weekly for 2 weeks, and then once monthly. Large doses may cause convulsions and untoward side effects may occur as with any intrathecal injection, and are commonly neurological in character.

Lymphomas: In Burkitt's Tumour, stages 1-2, Methotrexate has prolonged remissions in some cases. Recommended dosage is 10-25 mg per day orally for 4 to 8 days. In stage 3, Methotrexate is commonly given concomitantly with other antitumour agents. Treatment in all stages usually consists of several courses of the drug interposed with 7 to 10 day rest periods, and in stage 3 they respond to combined drug therapy with Methotrexate given in doses of 0.625 mg to 2.5 mg/kg daily. Hodgkin's Disease responds poorly to Methotrexate and to most types of chemotherapy.

Mycosis Fungoides: Therapy with Methotrexate appears to produce clinical remissions in one half of the cases treated. Recommended dosage is usually 2.5 to 10 mg daily by mouth for weeks or months and dosage should be adjusted according to the patient's response and haematological monitoring. Methotrexate has also been given intramuscularly in doses of 50 mg once weekly or 25 mg twice weekly.

Psoriasis Chemotherapy: Cases of severe uncontrolled psoriasis, unresponsive to conventional therapy, have responded to weekly single, oral, I.M. or I.V. doses of 10-25 mg per week, and adjusted according to the patient's response. An initial test dose one week prior to initiation of therapy is recommended to detect any idiosyncrasy. A suggested dose range is 5-10 mg parenterally.

An alternative dosage schedule consists of 2.5 to 5 mg of Methotrexate administered orally at 12 hour intervals for 3 doses each week or at 8-hour intervals for 4 doses each week; weekly dosages should not exceed 30 mg.

A daily oral dosage schedule of 2 to 5 mg administered orally for 5 days followed by a rest period of at least 2 days may also be used. The daily dose should not exceed 6.25 mg.

The patient should be fully informed of the risks involved and the clinician should pay particular attention to the appearance of the liver toxicity by carrying out liver function tests before starting Methotrexate treatment, and repeating these at 2 to 4 month intervals during therapy. The aim of therapy should be to reduce the dose to the lowest possible level with the longest possible rest period. The use of Methotrexate may permit the return to conventional topical therapy which should be encouraged.

Contra-indications: Impaired renal or hepatic function. Pre-existing blood dyscrasias, such as marrow hypoplasia, leukopenia, thromocytopenia or anaemia. Methotrexate is contraindicated in pregnancy.

Methotrexate is contra-indicated in pregnant patients. Because of the potential for serious adverse reactions from methotrexate in breast fed infants, breast feeding is contra-indicated in women taking methotrexate. Patients with a known allergic hypersensitivity to methotrexate should not receive methotrexate.

Special warnings and special precautions for use:
Warnings: Methotrexate must be used only by physicians experienced in antimetabolic chemotherapy.

Because of the possibility of fatal or severe toxic reactions, the patient should be fully informed by the physician of the risks involved and be under his constant supervision.

Deaths have been reported with the use of Methotrexate in the treatment of psoriasis.

In the treatment of psoriasis, Methotrexate should be restricted to severe recalcitrant, disabling psoriasis which is not adequately responsive to other forms of therapy, but only when the diagnosis has been established as by biopsy and/or after dermatological consultation.

1. Methotrexate may produce marked depression of bone marrow, anaemia, leukopenia, thrombocytopenia and bleeding.

2. Methotrexate may be hepatotoxic, particularly at high dosage or with prolonged therapy. Liver atrophy, necrosis, cirrhosis, fatty changes, and periportal fibrosis have been reported. Since changes may occur without previous signs of gastrointestinal or haematological toxicity, it is imperative that hepatic function be determined prior to initiation of treatment and monitored regularly throughout therapy. Special caution is indicated in the presence of pre-existing liver damage of impaired hepatic function. Concomitant use of other drugs with hepatotoxic potential (including alcohol) should be avoided.

3. Methotrexate has been shown to be teratogenic; it has caused foetal death and/or congenital anomalies. Therefore it is not recommended in women of childbearing potential unless there is appropriate medical evidence that the benefits can be expected to outweigh the considered risks. Pregnant psoriatic patients should not receive Methotrexate.

4. Impaired renal function is usually a contraindication.

5. Diarrhoea and ulcerative stomatitis are frequent toxic effects and require interruption of therapy, otherwise haemorrhagic enteritis and death from intestinal perforation may occur.

6. Methotrexate affects gametogenesis during the period of its administration and may result in decreased fertility which is thought to be reversible on discontinuation of therapy. Conception should be avoided during the period of Methotrexate administration and for at least 6 months thereafter. Patients and their partners should be advised to this effect.

7. Methotrexate has some immunosuppressive activity and immunological responses to concurrent vaccination may be decreased. The immunosuppressive effect of Methotrexate should be taken into account when immune responses of patients are important or essential.

8. Patients with pleural effusions or ascites should have these drained if appropriate before treatment or treatment should be withdrawn.

9. Deaths have been reported with the use of methotrexate. Serious adverse reactions including deaths have been reported with concomitant administration of methotrexate (usually in high doses) along with some non-steroidal anti-inflammatory drugs (NSAIDs).

10. Concomitant administration of folate antagonists such as trimethoprim/sulphamethoxazole has been reported to cause an acute megaloblastic pancytopenia in rare instances.

Precautions: Methotrexate has a high potential toxicity, usually dose related, and should be used only by physicians experienced in antimetabolite chemotherapy, in patients under their constant supervision. The physician should be familiar with the various characteristics of the drug and its established clinical usage.

Before beginning methotrexate therapy or reinstituting methotrexate after a rest period, assessment of renal function, liver function and blood elements should be made by history, physical examination and laboratory tests.

It should be noted that intrathecal doses are transported into the cardiovascular system and may give rise to systemic toxicity. Systemic toxicity of methotrexate may also be enhanced in patients with renal dysfunction, ascites, or other effusions due to prolongation of serum half-life.

High doses may cause the precipitation of methotrexate or its metabolites in the renal tubules. A high fluid throughout and alkalinisation of the urine to pH 6.5-7.0 by oral or intravenous administration of sodium bicarbonate (5 x 625 mg tablets every three hours) or acetazolamide (500 mg orally four times a day) is recommended as a preventative measure.

Carcinogenesis, mutagenesis, and impairment of fertility: Animal carcinogencity studies have demonstrated methotrexate to be free of carcinogenic potential. Although methotrexate has been reported to cause chromosomal damage to animal somatic cells and bone marrow cells in humans, these effects are transient and reversible. In patients treated with methotrexate, evidence is insufficient to permit conclusive evaluation of any increased risk of neoplasia.

Methotrexate has been reported to cause impairment of fertility, oligospermia, menstrual dysfunction and amenorrhoea in humans, during and for a short period after cessation of therapy. In addition, methotrexate causes, embryotoxicity, abortion and foetal defects in humans. Therefore the possible risks of effects on reproduction should be discussed with patients of childbearing potential (see 'Warnings').

Patients undergoing therapy should be subject to appropriate supervision so that signs or symptoms of possible toxic effects or adverse reactions may be detected and evaluated with minimal delay. Pretreatment and periodic haematological studies are essential to the use of Methotrexate in chemotherapy because of its common effect of haematopoietic suppression. This may occur abruptly and on apparent safe dosage, and any profound drop in blood cell count indicates immediate stopping of the drug and appropriate therapy. In patients with malignant disease who have pre-existing bone marrow aplasia, leukopenia, thrombocytopenia or anaemia, the drug should be used with caution, if at all.

Methotrexate is excreted primarily by the kidneys. Its use in the presence of impaired renal function may result in accumulation of toxic amounts or even additional renal damage. The patient's renal status should be determined prior to or during Methotrexate therapy and proper caution exercised, should significant renal impairment be disclosed.

Drug dosage should be reduced or discontinued until renal function is improved or restored.

In general, the following laboratory tests are recommended as part of essential clinical evaluation and appropriate monitoring of patients chosen for or receiving Methotrexate therapy: complete haemogram; haematocrit; urinalysis; renal function tests; and liver function tests.

A chest X-ray is also recommended. The purpose is to determine any existing organ dysfunction or system impairment. The tests should be performed prior to therapy, at appropriate periods during therapy and after termination of therapy. It may be useful or important to perform liver biopsy or bone marrow aspiration studies where high dose or long term therapy is being followed.

Methotrexate is bound in part to serum albumin after absorption, and toxicity may be increased because of displacement by certain drugs such as salicylates, sulphonamides, phenytoin, and some antibacterials such as tetracycline, chloramphenicol and para-aminobenzoic acid. These drugs, especially salicylates and sulphonamides, whether antibacterial, hypoglycaemic or diuretic, should not be given concurrently until the significance of these findings is established.

Vitamin preparations containing folic acid or its derivatives may alter response to Methotrexate.

Methotrexate should be used with extreme caution in the presence of infection, peptic ulcer, ulcerative colitis, debility, and in extreme youth and old age. If profound leukopenia occurs during therapy, bacterial infection may occur or become a threat. Cessation of the drug and appropriate antibiotic therapy is usually indicated. In severe bone marrow depression, blood or platelet transfusions may be necessary.

Since it is reported that Methotrexate may have an immunosuppressive action, this factor must be taken into consideration in evaluating the use of the drug where immune responses in a patient may be important or essential.

In all instances where the use of Methotrexate is considered for chemotherapy, the physician must evaluate the need and usefulness of the drug against the risks of toxic effects or adverse reactions. Most such adverse reactions are reversible if detected early. When such effects or reactions do occur, the drug should be reduced in dosage or discontinued and appropriate corrective measures should be taken according to the clinical judgement of the physician. Reinstitution of Methotrexate therapy should be carried out with caution, with adequate consideration of further need for the drug and alertness as to the possible recurrence of toxicity.

Interaction with other medicaments and other forms of interaction: Methotrexate is extensively protein bound and may be displaced by certain drugs such as salicylates, hypoglycaemics, diuretics, sulphonamides, diphenylhydantoins, tetracyclines, chloramphenicol and p-aminobenzoic acid, and the acidic anti-inflammatory agents, so causing a potential for increased toxicity when used concurrently. Concomitant use of other drugs with nephrotoxic or hepatotoxic potential (including alcohol) should be avoided. Vitamin preparations containing folic acid or its derivatives may decrease the effectiveness of methotrexate.

Caution should be used when NSAIDs and salicylates are administered concomitantly with methotrexate. These drugs have been reported to reduce the tubular secretion of methotrexate in an animal model and thereby may enhance its toxicity. Renal tubular transport is also diminished by probenecid; use of methotrexate with this drug should be carefully monitored.

Patients using constant dosage regimens of NSAIDs have received concurrent doses of methotrexate problems. Therefore, until more is known about the NSAIDs/methotrexate interaction, it is recommended that methotrexate dosage be carefully controlled during treatment with NSAIDs.

Methotrexate should be used with caution in patients taking drugs known to have an antifolate potential.

Pregnancy and lactation: Abortion, foetal death, and/or congenital anomalies have occurred in pregnant women receiving Methotrexate, especially during the first trimester of pregnancy. Methotrexate is contraindicated in the management of psoriasis or rheumatoid arthritis in pregnant women. Women of childbearing potential should not receive Methotrexate until pregnancy is excluded. For the management of psoriasis or rheumatoid arthritis, Methotrexate therapy in women should be started immediately following a menstrual period and appropriate measures should be taken in men or women to avoid conception during and for at least 12 weeks following Methotrexate therapy.

Both men and women receiving Methotrexate should be informed of the potential risk of adverse effects on reproduction. Women of childbearing potential should be fully informed of the potential hazard to the foetus should they become pregnant during Methotrexate therapy. In cancer chemotherapy, Methotrexate should not be used in pregnant women or women of childbearing potential who might become pregnant unless the potential benefits to the mother outweigh the possible risks to the foetus.

Defective oogenesis or spermatogenesis, transient oligospermia, menstrual dysfunction, and infertility have been reported in patients receiving Methotrexate.

Methotrexate is distributed into breast milk. Because of the potential for serious adverse reactions to Methotrexate in nursing infants, a decision should be made whether to discontinue nursing or the drug, taking into account the importance of the drug to the woman.

Effects on ability to drive and use machines: Not applicable.

Undesirable effects: The most common adverse reactions include ulcerative stomatitis, leukopenia, nausea and abdominal distress. Although very rare, anaphylactic reactions to methotrexate have occurred. Others reported are malaise, undue fatigue, chills and fever, dizziness and decreased resistance to infection. In general, the incidence and severity of side effects are considered to be dose-related. Adverse reactions as reported for the various systems are as follows:

Skin: Erythematous rashes, pruritus, urticaria, photosensitivity, depigmentation, alopecia, ecchymosis, telangiectasia, acne, furunculosis. Lesions of psoriasis may be aggravated by concomitant exposure to ultraviolet radiation. Skin ulceration has been reported in psoriatic patients. The recall phenomenon has been reported in both radiation and solar damaged skin.

Blood: Bone marrow depression, leukopenia, thrombocytopenia, anaemia, hypogammaglobulinaemia, haemorrhage from various sites, septicaemia.

Alimentary System: Gingivitis, pharyngitis, stomatitis, anorexia, vomiting, diarrhoea, haematemesis, melena, gastrointestinal ulceration and bleeding, enteritis, hepatic toxicity resulting in active liver atrophy, necrosis, fatty metamorphosis, periportal fibrosis, or hepatic cirrhosis. In rare cases the effect of methotrexate on the intestinal mucosa has led to malabsorption or toxic megacolon.

Hepatic: Hepatic toxicity resulting in significant elevations of liver enzymes, acute liver atrophy, necrosis, fatty metamorphosis, periportal fibrosis or cirrhosis or death may occur, usually following chronic administration.

Urogenital System: Renal failure, azotaemia, cystitis, haematuria, defective oogenesis or spermatogenesis, transient oligospermia, menstrual dysfunction, infertility, abortion, foetal defects, severe nephropathy. Vaginitis, vaginal ulcers, cystitis, haematuria and nephropathy have also been reported.

Pulmonary System: Infrequently an acute or chronic interstitial pneumonitis, often associated with blood eosinophilia, may occur and deaths have been reported. Acute pulmonary oedema has also been reported after oral and intrathecal use. Pulmonary fibrosis is rare. A syndrome consisting of pleuritic pain and pleural thickening has been reported following high doses.

Central Nervous System: Headaches, drowsiness, blurred vision, aphasia, hemiparesis and convulsions have occurred possibly related to haemorrhage or to complications from intra-arterial catheterization. Convulsion, paresis, Guillain-Barre syndrome and increased cerebrospinal fluid pressure have followed intrathecal administration.

Other reactions related to, or attributed to the use of Methotrexate such as pneumonitis, metabolic changes, precipitation of diabetes, osteoporotic effects, abdominal changes in tissue cells and even sudden death have been reported.

There have been reports of leukoencephalopathy following intravenous methotrexate in high doses, or low doses following cranial-spinal radiation.

Adverse reactions following intrathecal methotrexate are generally classified into three groups, acute, subacute, and chronic. The acute form is a chemical arachnoiditis manifested by headache, back or shoulder pain, nuchal rigidity, and fever. The subacute form may include paresis, usually transient, paraplegia, nerve palsies, and cerebellar dysfunction. The chronic form is a leukoencephalopathy manifested by irritability, confusion, ataxia, spasticity, occasionally convulsions, dementia, somnolence, coma, and rarely, death. There is evidence that the combined use of cranial radiation and intrathecal methotrexate increases the incidence of leukoencephalopathy.

Additional reactions related to or attributed to the use of methotrexate such as osteoporosis, abnormal (usually 'megaloblastic') red cell morphology, precipitation of diabetes, other metabolic changes, and sudden death have been reported.

Overdose: Calcium Folinate (Calcium Leucovorin) is a potent agent for neutralizing the immediate toxic effects of Methotrexate on the haematopoietic system. Where large doses or overdoses are given, Calcium Folinate may be administered by intravenous infusion in doses up to 75 mg within 12 hours, followed by 12 mg intramuscularly every 6 hours for 4 doses. Where average doses of Methotrexate appear to have an adverse effect 6-12 mg of Calcium Folinate may be given intramuscularly every 6 hours for 4 doses. In general, where overdosage is suspected, the dose of Calcium Folinate should be equal to or higher than, the offending dose of Methotrexate and should be administered as soon as possible; preferably within the first hour and certainly within 4 hours after which it may not be effective.

Other supporting therapy such as blood transfusion and renal dialysis may be required.

Pharmacological properties

Pharmacodynamic properties: Methotrexate is an antimetabolite which acts principally by competitively inhibiting the enzyme, dihydrofolate reductase. In the process of DNA synthesis and cellular replication, folic acid must be reduced to tetrahydrofolic acid by this enzyme, and inhibition by Methotrexate interfers with tissue cell reproductions. Actively proliferating tissues such as malignant cells are generally more sensitive to this effect of Methotrexate. It also inhibits antibody synthesis.

Methotrexate also has immunosuppressive activity, in part possibly as a result of inhibition of lymphocyte multiplication. The mechanism(s) of action in the management of rheumatoid arthritis of the drug is not known, although suggested mechanisms have included immunosuppressive and/or anti-inflammatory effect.

Pharmacokinetic properties: In doses of 0.1 mg (of Methotrexate) per kg, Methotrexate is completely absorbed from the G.I. tract; larger oral doses may be incompletely absorbed. Peak serum concentrations are achieved with 0.5–2 hours following I.V., I.M. or intra-arterial administration. Serum concentrations following oral administration of Methotrexate may be slightly lower than those following I.V. injection.

Methotrexate is actively transported across cell membranes. The drug is widely distributed into body tissues with highest concentrations in the kidneys, gall bladder, spleen, liver and skin. Methotrexate is retained for several weeks in the kidneys and for months in the liver. Sustained serum concentrations and tissue accumulation may result from repeated daily doses. Methotrexate crosses the placental barrier and is distributed into breast milk. Approximately 50% of the drug in the blood is bound to serum proteins.

In one study, Methotrexate had a serum half-life of 2-4 hours following I.M. administration. Following oral doses of 0.06 mg/kg or more, the drug had a serum half-life of 2-4 hours, but the serum half-life was reported to be increased to 8-10 hours when oral doses of 0.037 mg/kg were given.

Methotrexate does not appear to be appreciably metabolised. The drug is excreted primarily by the kidneys via glomerular filtration and active transport. Small amounts are excreted in the faeces, probably via the bile. Methotrexate has a biphasic excretion pattern. If Methotrexate excretion is impaired accumulation will occur more rapidly in patients with impaired renal function. In addition, simultaneous administration of other weak organic acids such as salicylates may suppress Methotrexate clearance.

Pharmaceutical particulars

List of excipients:	*2.5 mg tablets*	*10 mg tablets*
Maize Starch PhEur	30.0 mg	27.6 mg
Lactose PhEur	41.8 mg	38.5 mg
Pre gelatinized Starch (Prejel PA5) USNF	2.5 mg	2.5 mg
Polysorbate 80 PhEur	0.2 mg	0.2 mg
Microcrystalline Cellulose (AVICEL 101) USNF	20.0 mg	18.2 mg
Magnesium Stearate PhEur	3.0 mg	3.0 mg

There is no overage included in the formulation.

Incompatibilities: Immediate precipitation or turbidity results when combined with certain concentrations of Droperidol, Heparin Sodium, Metaclopramide Hydrochloride, Ranitidine Hydrochloride in syringe.

Shelf life: 60 months.

Special precautions for storage: There are no specific storage requirements.

Instructions for use/handling: Not applicable.

Marketing authorisation numbers

10 mg tabs	4515/0005
2.5 mg tabs	4515/0004

Date of approval/revision of SPC May 1996

Legal category POM

METHYLENE BLUE INJECTION USP

Presentation Methylene Blue Injection USP is presented as a clear, blue coloured sterile solution containing in each 5.0 mL ampoule; Methylene Blue Trihydrate USP 50.0 mg, approximately a 1% solution. The pH of the solution ranges between 3.0 and 4.5.

Uses Methylene blue is primarily used in the treatment of drug-induced and genetic methaemoglobinaemia that are not due to a structural abnormality of haemoglobin.

Dosage and administration Methylene blue may be administered orally or by intravenous (IV) injection. In the treatment of acute methaemoglobinaemia, the IV route of administration is usually preferred because it provides a more rapid onset of effect. However, in large doses, methylene blue can itself produce methaemoglobinaemia and the methaemoglobin concentration should therefore be closely monitored during treatment. The usual IV dose of methylene blue for adults and children is as a 1% solution in doses of 1 to 2 mg/kg body weight injected over a period of several minutes. A repeat dose may be given after one hour if required.

When treatment is less urgent, and for chronic dosing of genetic methaemoglobinaemias, methylene blue 3-6 mg/kg (generally 300 mg daily in adults) is given orally in divided doses over 24 hours with ascorbic acid 500 mg daily. A suitable dilution for oral dosing would be 5-10 mL of the 1% solution diluted to 100-200 mL with water for injection. The high volume is suggested to reduce the degree of gastro-intestinal disturbance and dysuria.

The dosage of methylene blue should be calculated on the basis of lean body weight.

Contra-indications, warnings, etc

Contra-indications: Use of methylene blue in pregnancy and lactation is contraindicated as its safe use during pregnancy has not yet been established

Methylene blue is contra-indicated in patients with severe renal impairment or a known hypersensitivity to the drug.

Methylene blue should not be used for the treatment of methaemoglobinaemia due to chlorate poisoning as it may convert the chlorate to hypochlorite which is an even more toxic compound.

Methylene blue may cause haemolytic anaemia in patients with glucose-6-phosphate dehydrogenase deficiency.

Intrathecal injection of methylene blue can result in neural damage and is therefore contraindicated.

Warnings/precautions: Long-term administration of methylene blue may result in marked anaemia due to accelerated destruction of erythrocytes; haemoglobin concentrations should be checked frequently. If methylene blue is injected subcutaneously or if extravasation occurs, necrotic abscesses may result.

Use in pregnancy: Safe use of methylene blue during pregnancy has not been established. Therefore, the drug should be used in pregnant women only if clearly indicated.

Although intra-amniotic injection of methylene blue has been used to diagnose premature rupture of foetal membranes or to identify separate amniotic sacs in twin pregnancies, there have been several reports of haemolytic anaemia and hyperbilirubinaemia in neonates exposed to methylene blue in the amniotic activity.

Use in lactation: There is no information on whether or not the drug passes into the breast milk. Consequently, the potential hazard to the infant must be considered prior to administration of the drug to nursing mothers.

Drug interactions: No information available.

Adverse reactions: After intravenous administration, methylene blue may cause nausea, vomiting, abdominal and chest pain, headache, dizziness, mental confusion, profuse sweating and hypotension; with very high doses methaemoglobinaemia and haemolysis may occur. Infants and patients with glucose-6-phosphate dehydrogenase deficiency are particularly susceptible to haemolysis from treatment with methylene blue.

Oral administration may cause gastrointestinal disturbances (nausea, vomiting and diarrhoea) and dysuria.

High doses, if not adequately diluted, could cause thrombophlebitis. Not more than 350 mg of methylene blue should be diluted in each 500 mL of infusion fluid.

Methylene blue imparts a blue colour to the saliva, urine and faeces.

Overdosage: No specific information is available. However, in high concentrations, methylene blue can oxidize haemoglobin to methaemoglobinemia, thus increasing methaemoglobinemia. Nonspecific side effects seen with high doses included precordial pain, dyspnea, restlessness, apprehension, tremors, and a sense of oppression. Large doses are irritant to the urinary tract. In addition, it can produce a mild haemolysis with moderate hyper bilrubinemia, reticulosis and slight anaemia. Rarely, however, a severe haemolytic anaemia with Heinz body formation has resulted. Methylene blue in large doses could cause a blue discolouration to the skin after methaemoglobin levels had returned to normal.

Treatment of overdosage: General supportive care and removal of the toxin should be carried out. Depending on the severity of the poisoning and the etiologic agent, this may include removal of contaminated clothing, rinsing the skin with water, ipecac-induced emesis or gastric lavage, charcoal, cathartics, and even haemodialysis.

There is no specific antidotal therapy. Although in severe and refractory cases of methaemoglobinemia, blood transfusions and even exchange transfusions, and (possibly) hyperbaric oxygen therapy maybe the only alternative available. Ascorbic acid works slowly and is probably no benefit in the acute situation. Removal of the toxic compound and supportive therapy are essential.

Pharmaceutical precautions

Incompatibilities: Methylene blue is reported to be incompatible with caustic alkalis, iodides and dichromates and oxidising and reducing substances.

Storage: Methylene Blue Injection USP is to be stored below 25°C and protected from light.

Legal category POM

Package quantities 1% solution: 5×5 ml ampoules.

Further information Nil

Product licence number 4515/0079

METHYLPREDNISOLONE SODIUM SUCCINATE FOR INJECTION

Qualitative and quantitative composition

Active Constituents	500 mg	1 gram
Methylprednisolone HSE (as Sodium Succinate)	500.0 mg	1.0 gm
Prepared in situ from:		
Methylprednisolone Hemisuccinate USP	633.6 mg	1.267 gm
Other Constituents		
Sodium Hydroxide BP	53.4 mg	106.8 mg
Disodium Hydrogen Phosphate HSE	69.8 mg	139.6 mg
Sodium Dihydrogen Phosphate HSE	6.4 mg	12.8 mg
Sodium Hydroxide BP	QS	QS
Hydrochloric Acid BP	QS	QS
Water for Injections BP	removed on lyophilisation	removed on lyophilisation

There is no overage in these formulations.

Pharmaceutical form Sterile freeze dried powder for injection.

Clinical particulars

Therapeutic indications: Parenteral, short term treatment of:

1. Acute anaphylactic and severe allergic reactions such as bronchial asthma, severe seasonal and perennial allergic rhinitis or angioneurotic oedema.
2. Gastrointestinal disease such as Crohns disease or ulcerative colitis.
3. Severe dermatological disease such as erythema multiforme.
4. Aspiration of gastric contents, with appropriate supportive treatment.
5. Tuberculosis, in combination with appropriate anti tubercular chemotherapy, for example TB meningitis or fulminating disseminated tuberculosis.
6. Cerebral oedema secondary to neoplasm.
7. Organ transplant rejection as part of a treatment regimen.

Posology and method of administration: Intravenous injection.

Intravenous infusion in the recommended diluents. Injection.

High doses should be administered as an intermittent infusion over at least 30 minutes.

The product should be reconstituted with Water for Injections BP.

The drug may be safely diluted in either Sodium Chloride 0.9% or Dextrose 5% Infusion fluids before administration.

The normal adult dose is 10-500 mg repeated up to 4 hourly. In severe shock, doses of 100 mg-250 mg four hourly may be used or up to 30 mg/kg every four hours have been used for limited periods.

Intramuscular doses are the same as for intravenous administration.

Intravenous infusion of Methylprednisolone Sodium Succinate may be administered by diluting the reconstituted solution in either Dextrose 5%, Sodium Chloride 0.9% or Dextrose 5% in Sodium Chloride 0.9%.

In the treatment of organ transplant rejection and also in autoimmune disorders, intermittent infusion of 1 gram in 100 ml Sodium Chloride 0.9% has been used. This regimen may be given daily or on alternate days, depending on the indication.

In an acute situation or medical crisis, direct intravenous injection should be administered over at least five minutes.

When treating patients with organ transplant rejection, three daily doses of Methylprednisolone Sodium Succinate 1 gram diluted in 100 ml infusion fluid is given over 30 minutes for maximum period of 72 hours.

In the management of autoimmune disorders a number of different regimens have been used including three doses of 1 gram diluted in 100 ml infusion fluid, given on alternate days. This course may be repeated at intervals where necessary.

In anaphylactic reactions, adrenaline or noradrenaline should be administered before methylprednisolone, in order to acheive the required haemoodynamic effect.

In allergic reactions, the effect can commence within 1–2 hours. Status asthmaticus patients are given 40 mg IV repeated as necessary.

Cerebral oedema treated with corticosteroids must have a tapering dosage programme to avoid rebound increases in intracranial pressure. The following are recommended schedules:

A:	*Dose*	*Route*	*Interval*	*Duration*
Preoperative	20 mg	IM	3-6 hours	
During surgery	20-40mg	IV	hourly	
Post operative	20 mg	IM	3 hourly	Day 1
	16 mg	IM	3 hourly	Day 2
	12 mg	IM	3 hourly	Day 3
	8 mg	IM	3 hourly	Day 4
	4 mg	IM	3 hourly	Day 5
	4 mg	IM	6 hourly	Day 6
	4 mg	IM	12 hourly	Day 7
B:				
Preoperative	40 mg	IM	6 hourly	2-3 days
Post operative	40 mg	IM	6 hourly	3-5 days
	20 mg	oral	6 hourly	24 hours
	12 mg	oral	6 hourly	24 hours
	8 mg	oral	8 hourly	24 hours
	4 mg	oral	12hourly	24 hours
	4 mg	oral	24 hours	24 hours

Children: Dosage may be determined by disease state and response but should be not more than 1 gram per day. Normal doses are 30 mg/kg/day for the treatment of haemotological, rheumatic, renal or dermatological conditions. Doses may be repeated either daily or on alternate days, for three days.

10-20 mg/kg/day for organ transplant rejection reactions. Repeated for up to three days, to a maximum of 1 gram per day.

1-4 mg/kg/day for treatment of status asthmaticus, repeated for up; to three days.

N.B. Corticosteroids cause dose-related growth retardation in infancy, childhood and adolescence which may be irreversible (see *Warnings* section).

Elderly: There is no indication that dosage adjustment is necessary in elderly patients although the detailed warnings and precautions should be considered when treatment is considered.

Contra-indications: Severe infections and septic shock do not appear to respond to Methylprednisolone and this drug should preferably not be used in this situation.

Methylprednisolone is contraindicated when there is hypersensitivity to the drug or its excipients.

Various local or systemic infections are contraindications for use of corticosteroid therapy unless specific anti-infective therapy is employed.

Special warnings and precautions for use:

Warnings: A patient information leaflet should be supplied with this product.

Short term administration of corticosteroids and short courses of high dose intermittent Methylprednisolone are unlikely to produce harmful effects provided the drug is given at the recommended rate of administration. However if used for longer than 48-72 hours continuously, severe endocrinological and cardiovascular side effects can occur. Secondary adrenocortical insufficiency leading to adrenal atrophy and generalised protein depletion have been reported. Antibiotic therapy should be initiated in patients treated for long periods of time.

Adrenal cortical atrophy develops during prolonged therapy and may persist for years after treatment has ceased. Withdrawal of corticosteroids after prolonged therapy must therefore be gradual to avoid acute adrenal insufficiency, being tapered off over weeks or months according to the dose and duration of treatment, (see *Dosage and Administration* section). During prolonged therapy any intercurrent illness, trauma or surgical procedure will require a temporary increase in dosage, if corticosteroids have been stopped following prolonged therapy they may need to be temporarily re-introduced.

Undesirable effects may be minimised by using the lowest effective dose for the minimum period. Frequent patient review is required to appropriately titrate the dose against disease activity (see *Dosage and Administration* section).

Patients should carry 'steroid treatment' cards which give clear guidance on the precautions to be taken to minimise the risk and which provide details of prescriber, drug, dosage and duration of treatment.

If used to treat adrenal insufficiency a mineralocorticoid drug will also be necessary as Methylprednisolone has only minimal mineralocorticoid action.

Intramuscular injection repeated at the same site may cause subcutaneous atrophy and should be avoided. Deep injection into the gluteal muscle is recommended.

Use in children may cause growth retardation in infancy, childhood and adolescence. Minimise the suppression of hypothalamic-pituitary-adrenal axis by administering the drug as a single dose on alternate days, where possible (see *Dosage* section).

Use in the elderly: The common adverse effects of systemic corticosteroids may be associated with more serious consequences in old age, especially osteoporosis, hypertension, hypokalaemia, diabetes, susceptibility to infection and thinning of the skin. Close clinical supervision is required to avoid life-threatening reactions.

High dose intravenous injection must be administered in diluted form and given slowly over at least 30 minutes to avoid the possibility of cardiovascular toxicity. Occasional reports of cardiac arrhythmia, congestive heart failure, circulatory collapse or cardiac arrest have been reported following high doses given over a very short period of time. Monitoring facilities should be available at all times when high dose intravenous therapy is used.

Suppression of the anti-inflammatory response increases the susceptibility to infections and their severity. The clinical presentation may often be atypical and serious infections such as septicaemia and tuberculosis may be masked and may reach an advanced stage before being recognised.

Use in the treatment of tuberculosis should be confined to fulminating disseminated tuberculosis, or TB meningitis. If use in latent disease, a reactivation of the disease may occur. During prolonged treatment these patients should receive chemotherapy prophylactically.

Chickenpox is of particular concern since this normally minor illness may be fatal in immunosuppressed patients. Patients (or parents of children) without a definite history of chickenpox should be advised to avoid close personal contact with chickenpox of herpes zoster and if exposed they should seek urgent medical attention. Passive immunisation with varicella/zoster immunoglobulin (VZIG) is needed by exposed non-immune patients who are receiving systemic corticosteroids or who have had them within the previous 3 months; this should be given within 10 days of exposure of chickenpox. If a diagnosis of chickenpox is confirmed, the illness warrants specialist care and urgent treatement. Corticosteroids should not be stopped and the dose may need to be increased.

Live vaccines should not be given to individuals with impaired immune responsiveness. The antibody response to other vaccines may be diminished.

Precautions: Gastric irritation may occur in patients with cerebral oedema induced by trauma, and prophylactic antacids may be advisable.

Special precautions: Particular care is required when considering the use of systemic corticosteroids in patients with the following conditions and frequent patient monitoring is necessary.

a. Osteoporosis (post-menopausal females are particularly at risk).
b. Hypertension or congestive heart failure.
c. Existing or previous history of severe affective disorders (especially previous steroid psychosis).
d. Diabetes mellitus (or a family history of diabetes).
e. History of tuberculosis.
f. Glaucoma (or a family history of glaucoma).
g. Previous corticosteroid-induced myopathy.
h. Liver failure.
i. Renal insufficiency.
j. Epilepsy.
k. Peptic ulceration.
l. Myasthenia gravis.
m. Ulcerative colitis, if there is a probability of impending perforation, abscess or other infection.
n. Fresh anastomoses.
o. Diverticulosis.
p. Herpes simplex keratitis.
q. Cushing's syndrome.
r. Cerebral oedema in malaria.

Interactions with other medicaments and other forms of interaction: Non steroidal anti-inflammatory drugs may increase the risk of gastrointestinal ulceration.

Vaccinations are not recommended during treatment due to the inhibitory effect on antibody responses.

Concurrent use of non-steroidal anti-inflammatory drugs may increase the risk of gastrointestinal ulceration.

Rifampicin, rifabutin, carbamazepine, phenobarbitone, phenytoin, primidone and aminoglutethimide enhance the metabolism of corticosteroids and its therapeutic effects may be reduced.

The desired effects of hypoglycaemic agents (including insulin), anti-hypertensives and diuretics are antagonised by corticosteroids, and the hypokalaemic effects of acetazolamide, loop diuretics, thiazide diuretics and carbenoxolone are enhanced. Potassium depleting diuretics may enhance the potassium wasting effects of glucocorticoids. Serum potassium levels should be closely monitored during treatment.

The efficacy of coumarin anticoagulants may be enhanced by concurrent corticosteroid therapy and close monitoring of the INR or prothrombin time is required to avoid spontaneous bleeding.

The renal clearance of salicylates is increased by corticosteroids and steroid withdrawal may result in salicylate intoxication.

Pregnancy and lactation:
Use in pregnancy: The ability of corticosteroids to cross the placenta varies between individual drugs, however, methylpredisolone does cross the placenta.

Administration of corticosteroids to pregnant animals can cause abnormalities of foetal development including cleft palate, intra-uterine growth retardation and affects of brain growth and development. There is no evidence that corticosteroids result in an increased incidence of congenital abnormalities, such as cleft palate/lip in man. However, when administered for prolonged periods or repeatedly during pregnancy, corticosteroids may increase the risk of intrauterine growth retardation. Hypoadrenalism may, in theory, occur in the neonate following prenatal exposure to the corticosteroids but usually resolves spontaneously following birth and is rarely clinically important. As with all drugs, corticosteroids should only be prescribed when the benefits to the mother and child outweigh the risks. When corticosteroids are essential however, patients with normal pregnancies may be treated as though they were in the non-gravid state.

There may be a small risk of cleft palate and intrauterine growth retardation. There is evidence of harmful effects on pregnancy in animals. Hypoadrenalism may also occur in the neonate. When corticosteroids are essential however, patients with normal pregnancies may be treated as though they were in a non-gravid state. Patients with pre-eclampsia or fluid retention require close monitoring.

Use in lactation: Corticosteroids are excreted in small amounts in breast milk. However, doses of up to 40 mg daily of methylprednisolone are unlikely to cause systemic effects in the infant. Infants of mothers taking higher doses than this may have a degree of adrenal suppression but the benefits of breast feeding are likely to outweigh any theoretical risk.

Corticosteroids may be distributed into breast milk and could suppress growth or cause adverse effects in nursing infants. Infants or mother taking pharmacological doses of steroids should be monitored carefully for signs of adrenal suppression.

Effects on ability to drive and use machines: Not applicable.

Undesirable effects:
Side effects: The incidence of predictable undesirable effects, including hypothalamic-pituatary-adrenal suppression correlates with the relative potency of the drug, dosage, timing and administration and duration of treatment (see *Warnings* section).

Gastrointestinal: Dyspepsia, peptic ulceration with perforation and haemorrhage. Abdominal distention, oesophageal ulceration or candidiasis, acute pancreatitis, liver failure. Nausea, vomiting and bad taste may occur with repeated administration.

Musculoskeletal: Proximal myopathy, osteoporosis, long bone or vertebral fracture, avascular osteonecrosis, tendon rupture.

Sodium and water retention, hypertension, potassium loss, hypokalaemic alkalosis.

Dermatological: Impaired wound healing, skin atrophy, bruising, striae, telangiectasia, acne.

Endocrine: Suppression of the hypothalamic-pituitary-adrenal axis, growth suppression in infancy, childhood and adolescence, menstrual irregularity and amenorrhoea, Cushinoid face, hirsutism, weight gain, diabetes mellitus, a family history of diabetes or impaired carbohydrate tolerance with increased requirement for antidiabetic therapy, negative protein and calcium balance and increased appetite.

Neuropsychiatric: Existing or previous history of severe affective disorders, euphoria, psychological dependence, depression, insomnia, intracranial hypertension with papilloema in children (pseudotumour cerebri), usually after treatment, withdrawal, aggravation of schizophrenia and epilepsy.

Ophthalmic: Increased intraocular pressure, glaucoma or family history of glaucoma, papilloedema, posterior subcapsular cataracts, corneal or scleral thinning, exacerbation of opthalmic viral or fungal disease.

Anti-inflammatory and Immunosuppressive effects: Increased susceptibility and severity of infections with suppression of clinical symptoms and signs, opportunistic infections, recurrence of dormant tuberculosis (see *Warnings* and *Precautions*).

General: Hypersensitivity including anaphylaxis, has been reported. Leucocytosis, thromboembolism.

Withdrawal: In patients who have received more than physiological doses of systemic corticosteroids (approximately 6 mg methylprednisolone) for greater than 3 weeks, withdrawal should not be abrupt. How dose reduction should be carried out depends largely on whether the disease is likely to relapse as the dose of systemic corticosteroids is reduced. Clinical assessment of disease activity may be needed during withdrawal. If the disease is unlikely to relapse on withdrawal of systemic corticosteroids but there is uncertainty about HPA suppression, the dose of systemic corticosteroid *may* be reduced rapidly to physiological doses. Once a daily dose of 6 mg methylprednisolone is reached, dose reduction should be slower to allow the HPA-axis to recover.

Abrupt withdrawal of systemic corticosteroid treatment, which has continued up to 3 weeks is appropriate if it is considered that the disease is unlikely to relapse. Abrupt withdrawal of doses up to 32 mg of dexamethasone for 3 weeks is unlikely to lead to clinically relevant HPA-axis suppression, in the majority of patients. In the following patient groups, gradual withdrawal of systemic corticosteroid therapy should be considered even after courses lasting 3 weeks or less:

- Patients who have had repeated courses of systemic corticosteroid, particularly if taken for greater than 3 weeks,
- When a short course has been prescribed within one year of cessation of long-term therapy (months or years),
- Patients who may have other reasons for adrenocortical insufficiency other than exogenous corticosteroid therapy
- Patients receiving doses of systemic corticosteroid greater than 32 mg daily of methylprednisolone.
- Patients repeatedly taking doses in the evening-

Overdose: Adrenal suppression may occur and appropriate measures should be taken during the withdrawal period. There is no known antidote to Methylprednisolone sodium succinate.

Pharmacological properties

Pharmacodynamic properties: A potent anti-inflammatory corticosteriod with predominantly glucocorticoid activity.

Methylprednisolone Sodium Succinate is primarily used in the acute treatment of shock, as part of post transplant rejection regimens, in severe rheumatoid arthritis, collagen vascular disease and in severe anaphylaxis or allergic reactions.

Methylprednisolone may cause profound metabolic effects and modify the body's immune response. Use of the parenteral form should therefore be confined to short term treatment.

Methylprednisolone stabilises leucocyte lysosomal membranes, preventing release of destructive acid hydrolases, inhibiting macrophage accumulation, reducing leucocyte adhesion, reducing capilliary wall permeability and antagonising histamine activity.

The immune system is suppressed by reducing the activity and volume of the lymphatic system, decreasing immunoglobulin and complement and decreasing the passage of immune complexes through membranes.

Pharmacokinetic properties: Methylprednisolone is rapidly removed from the plasma and widely distributed. The drug is extensively bound to plasma proteins. The drug may also cross the placenta and be distributed into milk.

Metabolism is primarily by reduction in the liver to biologically inactive compounds and subsequent excretion through the kidney.

Preclinical safety data: There are no pre-clinical data of relevance to the prescriber which are additional to that already included in other sections of the SPC.

Pharmaceutical particulars

List of excipients:

	500 mg	*1 gram*
Disodium Hydrogen Phosphate HSE	69.8 mg	139.6 mg
Sodium Dihydrogen Phosphate HSE	6.4 mg	12.8 mg
Sodium Hydroxide BP	QS	QS
Hydrochloric Acid BP	QS	QS
Water for Injections BP	removed on lyophilisation	removed on lyophilisation

There is no overage in these formulations.

Incompatibilities: Infusion solutions of methylprednisolone sodium succinate in the recommended diluents are stable for 24 hours at room temperature exposed to light. Only clear solutions should be used and any solutions developing a haze after preparation should be discarded. Methylprednisolone has approximately five times the glucocorticoid potency of hydrocortisone. Each gram of Methylprednisolone Sodium Succinate contains 2 mmol of Sodium.

Shelf life: 24 months.

Special precautions for storage: Methylprednisolone sodium succinate for Injection should be stored below 25°C and protected from light. Do not freeze, reconstituted solutions using the recommended diluent should be stored at 2-8°C and used within 24 hours of preparation.

Instruction for use/handling: Not applicable.

Marketing authorisation number 4515/0042

Date of approval/revision of SPC July 1995

Legal category POM

MITOMYCIN FOR INJECTION

Qualitative and quantitative composition

Active Constituent	10 mg/vial	20 mg/vial
Mitomycin USP	10.0 mg	20.0 mg

Pharmaceutical form Mitomycin for Injection is a sterile, lyophilised product intended for intravenous administration upon reconstitution with Water for Injections.

Clinical particulars

Therapeutic indications: Antimitotic and Cytotoxic: Mitomycin for Injection is recommended for certain types of cancer, either in combination with other drugs or after primary therapy has failed. In particular, Mitomycin for Injection has been successfully used to improve subjective and objective symptoms in a wide range of neoplastic conditions:

It has been used as a single agent in the treatment of superficial bladder cancer. In addition it has been shown that post-operative instillations of Mitomycin for Injection can reduce recurrence rates in newly diagnosed patients with superficial bladder cancer.

As a single agent and in combination with other drugs in metastatic breast cancer.

In combination with other agents in advanced squamous cell carcinoma of the uterine cervix.

It shows a degree of activity as part of combination therapy in carcinoma of the stomach, pancreas and lung (particularly non-small cell).

It shows a degree of activity as a single agent and in combination in liver cancer when given by the intra-arterial route.

It has a possible role in combination with other cytotoxic drugs in colorectal cancer.

It shows a degree of activity as a single agent or part of combination therapy in cancer of the head and neck.

It shows a degree of activity as a single agent in cancer of the prostate.

It has a possible role in skin cancer.

It has a degree of activity in leukaemia and non solid tumours.

It has a possible role in sarcomas.

It has been successfully used in combination with surgery, preoperatively (oesophageal, squamous cell carcinoma) and post-operatively (gastric cancer).

It has been shown to be effective when used in combination with radiotherapy.

Posology and method of administration: Reconstitution and Administration: Mitomycin for Injection is administered via a functioning I.V. catheter, *care should be taken to avoid extravasation of the drug,* and it is recommended that the reconstituted solution be administered through the tubing of an I.V. infusion. (If extravasation occurs, cellulitis, ulceration, and tissue sloughing may result).

Mitomycin for Injection is reconstituted by adding 10 or 20 mL of sterile water for injection to a vial labelled as containing 10 or 20 mg of mitomycin respectively, to provide a solution containing approximately 1 mg/ml. The vial should be shaken to enhance dissolution; if the powder for injection does not dissolve immediately, allow to stand at room temperature until complete dissolution occurs.

Dosage: For systemic administration, Mitomycin for Injection should be given intravenously using great care to avoid extravasation. The usual initial dosage is in the range 10-20 mg per m^2 body-surface given as a single dose through a running intravenous infusion and repeated every 6-8 weeks. Alternatively it may be given intravenously in divided doses of 2 mg per m^2 daily for 5 days, repeated after 2 days. Subsequent doses are adjusted according to the effect on bone marrow and treatment should not be repeated until leucocyte count is above 3000/mm^3, and the platelet count above at least 75,000/mm^3.

Dosage of Mitomycin subsequent to the initial dose maybe adjusted according to the following suggested schedule:

Nadir after prior dose (cells/mm^3)		*Percentage of prior dose to be given*
Leucocytes	Platelets	
>4000	>100,000	100%
3000-3999	75,000-99,999	100%
2000-2999	25,000-74,999	70%
<2000	<25,000	Nil

Dosage may be reduced when used in combination with other antineoplastics. However, when disease continues to progress after 2 courses of Mitomycin therapy, the drug should be discontinued since the likelihood of response is minimal.

For administration to specific tissues, Mitomycin for Injection can be given by the intra-arterial route in the treatment of liver tumours.

Because of cumulative myelosuppression and/or thrombocytopenia patients should be fully re-evaluated after each course of Mitomycin for Injection and the dose reduced if the patient has experienced any toxic effects. Doses greater than 20 mg/m^2 increase the risk of toxicity and have not been shown to be more effective than lower doses.

Treatment of superficial urinary bladder tumours: In the prevention of recurrent bladder tumours the usual dose is the equivalent of 4-10 mg potency of Mitomycin for Injection instilled into the bladder through a urethral catheter once or three times a week. In the treatment of bladder tumours, the usual dose is the equivalent of 10-40 mg potency of Mitomycin for Injection instilled into the bladder either weekly or three times a week for a total of 20 doses. In either case, it should be dissolved in 10 ml–40 ml of water for injections before use. The dose should be adjusted in accordance with the age and condition of the patient.

Topical use has rarely been reported to cause fibrosis of the bladder, leading to decreased bladder capacity, manifesting as urinary frequency, urgency, dysuria, and also to cause palmer rash, which is thought to be secondary to contact dermatitis. After continued use, renal failure has been reported to develop. Accordingly, maintenance therapy of Mitomycin is not recommended, unless the physician considers that such administration will provide benefits which outweigh the risks incurred.

Contra-indications: Mitomycin is contra-indicated in patients with platelet counts of less than 75,000/mm^3, white cell counts of less than 2,500/mm$^{3\ or\ 8}$ serum creatinine concentration greater than 1.7 mg/dL.

Mitomycin is contraindicated in patients who have substantial prolongation of prothrombin time or bleed time, coagulation disorders, increased bleeding due to other causes, or potentially serious infections.

Mitomycin is contraindicated in patients who have demonstrated a hypersensitive or idiosyncratic reaction to it in the past.

Special warnings and special precautions for use: Mitomycin for Injection should not be administered orally, intrathecally, into tissues (such as intramuscularly or subcutaneously). Mitomycin is a highly toxic drug with a low therapeutic index. The drug should be used only under the supervision of a physician experienced in cytotoxic cancer chemotherapy. Patients should be monitored closely during each course of treatment, paying particular attention to peripheral blood count including platelet count.

The principal toxicity of Mitomycin for Injection is bone marrow suppression, particularly thrombocytopenia and leucopenia. The nadir is usually around four weeks after treatment and toxicity is cumulative, with increasing risk after each course of treatment.

No repeat dosage should be given until the bone marrow nadir has passed. If disease progression continues after two courses of treatment, the drug should be stopped since the chances of response are then minimal.

Severe renal toxicity has occasionally been reported after treatment and renal function should be monitored before starting treatment and again after each course. The incidence of this is reduced considerably if the total cumulative dose does not exceed 120 mg; this may of course temporize the therapeutic response. Nausea and vomiting are sometimes experienced immediately after treatment but these are usually mild and of short duration. Local ulceration and cellulitis may be caused by tissue extravasation during intravenous injection and utmost care should be taken in administration. In the event of extravasation following an intravenous injection of Mitomycin for Injection, it is recommended that 5 ml of Sodium Bicarbonate 8.4% solution is immediately infiltrated into the area where extravasation has occurred followed by an injection of 4 mg of Dexamethasone. In addition, a systemic injection of 200 mg Vitamin B6 may be of some value in promoting the regrowth of tissues that have been damaged.

Following the intravesicle use of mitomycin, cases of bladder wall fibrosis have been reported, some of which may have led to renal failure.

The person administering the injection of Mitomycin for Injection should not allow the solution to come into contact with his or her skin.

Treatment of skin or eye contact: Any Mitomycin for Injection substance or solution in contact with the skin should be washed several times with 8.4% sodium bicarbonate solution, followed by washing with soap and water. Use of handcreams or other emollient preparations is inappropriate as this may assist the penetration of any traces of Mitomycin for Injection into the epidermal tissue.

Contact with the eye: The eye should be rinsed several times with sodium bicarbonate eye lotion and the eye examined for several days after contact for evidence of corneal damage. If this occurs, appropriate treatment should be instituted.

Interaction with other medicaments and other forms of interaction:

Potentially hazardous interactions:: As free radical generation is noted with this drug, there may be some synergistic cardiotoxicity with adriamycin. The possible enhancement of lung damage by nitrosoureas and doxorubicin has been reported.

Microsomal enzyme inducers such as barbiturates or liver enzyme inhibitors such as cimetidine may alter activity by an effect on host and tumour metabolism.

Potentially useful interactions: Mitomycin may show synergy with 5-Fluorouracil.

Mitomycin may enhance cell kill induced by radiation therapy, particularly under hypoxic conditions.

Pregnancy and lactation: Mitomycin for Injection should not normally be administered to patients who are pregnant or to mothers who are breast feeding. Teratological changes have been noted in animal studies. The effect of Mitomycin for Injection on fertility is unknown.

Effects on ability to drive and use machines: None known.

Undesirable effects:

Adverse reactions: Potentially life-threatening effects: A microangiopathic haemolytic anaemia (renal failure syndrome with anaemia, thrombocytopenia, haematuria, proteinuria. hypertension and neurological abnormalities) has been reported and is frequently fatal. It usually occurs after 6 months treatment, but has been reported earlier. In small series where renal histopathology has been studied, fibrin deposition in the glomeruli has been noted, but the precise mechanism is not known. Hepatic veno-occlusive disease has been reported in one high-dose study.

Severe or irreversible adverse effects: The dose-limiting toxicity is myelosuppression, which may be delayed with a nadir at 4-8 weeks. The effect is cumulative and affects both leucocytes and platelets. Diffuse pulmonary infiltration has also been recorded and exposure to oxygen in high concentration may be contributory. This side effect is thought to be related to generation of free radicals following activation of the drug.

Symptomatic adverse effects: Nausea and vomiting of moderate severity are seen in about 25% of patients and alopecia, stomatitis and diarrhoea are also observed. Local tissue necrosis is observed if the solution is extravasated from a vein or artery.

Overdose: No specific antidote for mitomycin is known. Management of overdose should include general supportive measures to sustain the patient through any period of oxicity that might occur.

Pharmacological properties

Pharmacodynamic properties: Mitomycin for Injection is an antitumour antibiotic that is activated in the tissues to an alkylating agent which disrupts deoxyribonucleic acid (DNA) in cancer cells by forming a complex with DNA and also acts by inhibiting division of cancer cells by interfering with the biosynthesis of DNA. In high concentrations, the drug may also inhibit RNA and protein synthesis.

Pharmacokinetic properties: In vivo, Mitomycin for Injection is rapidly cleared from the serum after intravenous administration. The time required to reduce the serum concentration by 50% after a 30 mg bolus injection is 17 minutes. After injection of 30 mg, 20 mg, or 10 mg intravenously, the maximal serum concentrations were 2.4 mcg/ml, 1.7 mcg/ml and 0.52 mcg/ml respectively. Clearance is effected primarily by metabolism in the liver but metabolism occurs in other tissues as well. The rate of clearance is inversely proportional to the maximal serum concentration because, it is thought, of saturation of the degradative pathways. Approximately 10% of a dose of Mitomycin for Injection is excreted unchanged in the urine. Since metabolic pathways are saturated at relatively low doses, the percentage dose excreted in the urine increases with increasing dose. In children, excretion of intravenously administered Mitomycin for Injection is similar to that in adults.

In animals, highest mitomycin concentration are found in the kidneys followed by muscles, eyes, lungs, intestines and stomach. The drug is not detectable in the liver, spleen or brain which rapidly inactivate mitomycin. Higher concentrations of the drug are generally present in cancer tissues than in normal tissues.

Pharmaceutical particulars

List of excipients:

	per 10mg vial	*per 20mg vial*	*per mL*	*Function*	*Reference to Standards*
Mannitol	20mg	40mg	2.0mg	Bulking agent	BP
Water for Injections*	qs 10ml	qs 20ml	qs 1.00ml	Solvent*	BP/USP

*Removed during the lyophilisation process.

Incompatibilities: Concentrations of Mitomycin for Injection of 10 mg and 50 mg/L in sodium chloride 0.9% resulted in a 20% and 54% loss respectively in bleomycin activity when added to a 20-30 units/L solution of bleomycin.

Shelf life:

(1) 3 years shelf life in the medicinal product as packaged for sale.

(2) The reconstituted product should be used immediately and any unused portion discarded.

Special precautions for storage: Unreconstituted Mitomycin for Injection remains stable for three years from the date of manufacture when stored below 25°C. Reconstitution, as directed, should be accomplished using aseptic technique and the resulting solutions should be used immediately. Any unused portion should be discarded. When reconstituted solution is added to infusion fluids, especially where these contain dextrose, the resulting solution should be used immediately, and any unused portion discarded.

Instructions for use/handling: There is limited but increasing concern that personnel involved in preparation and administration of parenteral antineoplastics may be at some risk because of the potential mutagenicity, teratogenicity, and/or carcinogenicity of these agents, although the actual risk is unknown. Cautious handling both in preparation and disposal of antineoplastic agents is recommended.

Precautions that have been suggested include:

Use of a biological containment cabinet during reconstitution and dilution of parenteral medications and wearing of disposable surgical gloves and masks.

Use of proper technique to prevent contamination of the medication, work area, and operator during transfer between containers (including proper training of personnel in this technique.

Cautious and proper disposal of needles, syringes, vials, ampoules and unused medication.

Marketing authorisation numbers

Mitomycin for Injection 10 mg Vial 4515/0093
Mitomycin for Injection 20 mg Vial 4515/0094

Date of approval/revision of SPC 26 June 1996

Legal category POM

MORPHINE SULPHATE INJECTION BP

Qualitative and quantitative composition Morphine Sulphate Injection BP is a clear colourless to slightly yellow sterile solution of morphine sulphate in Water for Injections. Morphine Sulphate Injection BP is available in two presentations as a prefilled Pharma-Ject* syringe in the following strengths: 50 mg/50 ml and 100 mg/50 ml.

Morphine Sulphate Injection BP available in a prefilled Pharma-Ject* syringe is a sterile solution of morphine sulphate BP with sodium chloride BP, in water for injections BP/USP.

Pharmaceutical form Pre-filled Pharma-Ject* syringe containing a sterile solution of Morphine Sulphate Injection BP.

Clinical particulars

Therapeutic indications: Morphine Sulphate Injection BP in a prefilled (Pharma-Ject*) syringe is specifically indicated for continuous intravenous infusion in patients with severe pain not responsive to non-narcotic analgesics.

In addition, the product is suitable for use with controlled rate infusion pumps in accordance with appropriate protocols for patient controlled analgesia (PCA).

Posology and method of administration:
Continuous Intravenous Infusion

Adults: Morphine Pharma-Ject* may be administered for severe pain not responsive to non-narcotic analgesics by slow continuous intravenous infusion. The dosage should respond to $\frac{1}{4}$ to $\frac{1}{2}$ of the intramuscular dose typically prescribed or in accordance with the individual patient's needs.

The dosage of morphine administered should be titrated according to the patient's requirements. However, most adult patients with no previous history of narcotic intake, can initially tolerate a morphine dosage 0.5 to 1.0 mg/hour. Higher doses generally result in an increased incidence of adverse effects.

Elderly: As with other narcotics, a reduction in dosage may be advisable in the elderly.

Children: In children, an infusion dose of 10 to 50 mcg/kg/hour morphine is recommended. A maximum intravenous dose of 4 mg/hour should be exceeded with caution.

It is recommended that an opioid antagonist and equipment for artificial ventilation be available.

Patient-controlled analgesia: Patient-controlled analgesia allows patients to assess their own level of pain and consequently titrate the amount of morphine they require for adequate pain control against sedation and other side effects.

The dosage and time intervals are preset into a microprocessor-controlled infusion pump. When the patient experiences pain, a button is depressed by the patient and a dose of morphine is administered intravenously. If the patient should depress the button before the preset time interval (lockout interval) has elapsed, no extra drug is administered.

Adults: Prescribers are advised to refer to the practices and procedures of the hospital, hospice, or clinic concerned for the appropriate dose and dose schedules when using Morphine Pharma-Ject* for patient controlled analgesia.

For adults, demand doses of 0.05 to 1.5 mg morphine have been given via PCA using a lockout interval of 6 to 10 minutes. Along with the self-administered dose of morphine, some devices also deliver a background continuous infusion of morphine at a basal rate. If a background infusion is adopted, a dose of 1 mg/hour is often used in adults.

Patient controlled analgesia should be supervised by hospitals and healthcare professionals familiar with the technique.

Elderly: As with other narcotics, a reduction in dosage may be advisable in the elderly.

Children: There is limited clinical experience of the use of patient-controlled analgesia in children. However, a demand dose of 0.01 to 0.025 mg/kg morphine has been used successfully in children and adolescents between the ages of 7 and 19. If a background infusion is employed, an infusion dose of 0.015 mg/kg/hour morphine may be used in children.

The demand dosage and lockout interval should be determined according to the patient's analgesic requirements. Patients receiving a background infusion of morphine should generally receive a smaller demand dose relative to equivalent patients utilising a demand dose only.

Contra-indications: Morphine sulphate is contraindicated in patients with known hypersensitivity to morphine; with acute or severe bronchial asthma; respiratory insufficiency or depression; obstructive airways disease; severe CNS depression; following biliary tract surgery or surgical anastomosis, biliary colic, acute hepatic disease gastrointestinal obstruction, delayed gastric emptying, paralytic ileus; in patients who are taking or who have taken MAO inhibitors within the previous fourteen days; cardiac arrythmias; heart failure secondary to pulmonary disease; acute alcoholism; head injuries; brain tumour; raised intracranial or cerebrospinal pressure and in convulsive states such as status epilepticus, tetanus or strychnine poisoning.

The administration of morphine via patient-controlled analgesia in young children and adults with poor cognitive function is contraindicated.

The continuous intravenous infusion of morphine in patients with hepatic disease is contraindicated.

Special warnings and special precautions for use:
Warnings

Drug dependence and tolerance: Morphine can produce drug dependence and therefore has the potential for being abused. Psychic dependence, physical dependence, and tolerance may develop upon repeated administration of morphine. However it should be noted that clinically significant respiratory depression, addiction, rapid tolerance and euphoria rarely develop when doses of morphine are carefully titrated against the pain in patients with terminal disease and severe pain.

Drug dependence does not develop if morphine is administered regularly at individually optimised doses to the cancer patient with moderate to severe pain. While a certain degree of physical dependence occurs, a psychological dependence does not occur. If a cancer patient no longer requires a narcotic for pain control, a gradual reduction in dose will prevent any withdrawal symptoms, although these are usually mild or absent even after abrupt discontinuance.

Clincally significant tolerance to morphine is unusual in the cancer patient being treated for severe pain. In most cases, a plateauing of dose requirements is seen as a need to increase morphine dose means an increase in pain and not tolerance.

Morphine should be used with caution and in reduced dosage in patients who are concurrently receiving other narcotic analgesics, general anaesthetics, pheniothiazines, other tranquilisers, sedative-hypnotics, tricyclic antidepressants, and other CNS depressants (including alcohol). Respiratory depression, hypotension and profound sedation or coma may result.

Impaired respiration: The respiratory depressant effects of morphine and its capacity to elevate cerebrospinal fluid pressure may be markedly exaggerated in the presence of head injury, other intracranial lesions, or a pre-existing increase in intracranial pressure. Furthermore, narcotics produce adverse reactions which may obscure the clinical course of patients with head injuries.

Morphine should be used with extreme caution in patients having an acute asthmatic attack, patients with chronic obstructive pulmonary disease or cor pulmonale, patients having a substantially decreased respiratory reserve, and patients with pre-existing respiratory depression, hypoxia or hypercapnia. In such patients, even usual therapeutic doses of narcotics may decrease respiratory drive while simultaneously increasing airway resistance to the point of apnoea. Resuscitative equipment and a narcotic antagonist must be readily available.

Hypotensive effect: The administration of morphine may result in severe hypotension in the post-operative patient or any individual whose ability to maintain blood pressure has been compromised by a depleted blood volume, shock, or the administration of such drugs as the phenothiazines or certain anaesthetics.

Morphine may produce orthostatic hypotension in ambulatory patients.

Precautions

Supreventricular tachycardias: Because of possible vagolytic action that may produce a significant increase in the ventricular response rate, morphine should be used with caution in patients with atrial flutter and other supreventricular tachycardias.

Acute abdominal condition: The administration of morphine or other narcotics may obscure the diagnosis or clinical course in patients with acute abdominal conditions.

Convulsions: Morphine may aggravate pre-existing convulsions in patients with convulsive disorders. If dosage is escalated substantially above recommened levels becuase of tolerance development, convulsions may occur in individuals without a history of convulsive disorders.

Other special risk patients: Morphine should be given with caution to certain patients, such as the elderly or debilitated and those with severe impairment or hepatic or renal function, hypothyroidism, Addison's disease, and prostatic hypertrophy or urethral stricture. Morphine should be used with extreme caution in patients with disorders characterised by hypoxia, since even usual therapeutic doses of narcotics may decrease respiratory drive to the point of apnoea while simultaneously increasing airway resistance.

Renal or hepatic disease: Morphine may have a prolonged duration and cumulative effect in patients with kidney or liver dysfunction. In these patients, analgesia may last for 6, 8 or even up to 24 hours following a standard dose. Continuous infusions are contraindicated in these patients. (See *Contra-indications.*)

Shock patients: In patients with shock, impaired perfusion may prevent complete absorption following subcutaneous or intramuscular injection of morphine. Repeated administration may result in overdosage due to an excessive amount of morphine suddenly being absorbed when circulation is restored.

Paediatrics: Safety and efficacy of morphine in neonates and children have not been established.

Interaction with other medicaments and other forms of interaction:

CNS depressants: Morphine should be used with great caution and in reduced dosage in patients concurrently receiving other central nervous system depressants including sedatives, hypnotics, general anaesthetics, phenothiazines, other tranquilisers and alcohol because of the risk of respiratory depression, depression, hypotension and profound sedation or coma. When such combined therapy is contemplated, the dose of one or both agents should be reduced.

Muscle relaxants: Morphine may enhance the neuromuscular blocking action of skeletal relaxants and produce an increase degree of respiratory depression.

Mixed agonist/antagonist opioid analgesics: From a theoretical perspective, mixed agonist/antagonist opioid analgesics (e.g. pentazocine, and buprenorphine) should NOT be administerd to a patient who has received or is receiving a course of therapy with a pure opioid agonist analgesic. In these patients, mixed agonist/antagonist analgesics may reduce the analgesic effect or may precipitate withdrawal symptoms.

Monoamine oxidase inhibitors (MAOIs): MAOIs

intensify the effects of morphine and other opioid drugs which can cause anxiety, confusion and significant depression of respiration, sometimes leading to coma. Morphine should not be given to patients taking MAOIs or within 14 days of stopping such treatment.

Cimetidine: There is a report of confusion and severe respiratory depression when a haemodialysis patient was administered morphine and cimetidine.

Diuretics: Morphine reduces the efficacy of diuretics by inducing the release of antidiuretic hormone. Morphine may also lead to acute retention of urine by causing spasm of the sphincter of the bladder, particularly in men with prostatism.

Pregnancy and lactation
Use in pregnancy: Animal reproduction studies have not been performed using morphine. It is not known whether morphine can cause foetal damage when administered throughout pregnancy or if it can effect reproductive capacity in humans. Pregnant patients should only be given morphine when the benefits clearly outweigh potential risk to the foetus.

Use in lactation: Morphine is excreted in human milk and breast-feeding is not recommended while a patient is receiving morphine. Withdrawal symptoms have been observed in breast-fed infants when maternal administration of morphine sulphate is stopped.

Use in labour/delivery: Morphine is not recommended for use in women during and immediately before labour. The effects of opioid analgesics are unpredictable. They may prolong labour by temporarily reducing the strength, duration and frequency of uterine contractions, or conversely they may tend to shorten labour by increasing the rate of cervical dilatation. Infants born to mothers receiving opioid analgesics during labour should be observed closely for signs of respiratory depression. In such infants a specific opioid antagonist, naxolone hydrochloride, should be available for reversal of narcotic-induced respiratory depression.

Effects on ability to drive and use machines: Morphine may impair the mental and/or physical abilities required for the performance of potentially hazardous tasks, such as driving a car or operating machinery. Morphine in combination with other narcotic analgesics, phenothiazines, sedative-hypnotics, and alcohol have additive depressant effects. Patients should be cautioned accordingly.

Undesirable efects
Adverse reactions: The adverse reactions caused by morphine are essentially the same as those observed with other opioid analgesics. They include the following major hazards: respiratory depression, apnoea and to a lesser degree circulatory depression, respiratory arrest, shock and cardiac arrest.

Most common adverse effects: Constipation, lightheadedness, dizziness, sedation, nausea, vomiting, sweating, dysphoria and euphoria.

Sedation: Most patients receiving morphine will experience initial drowsiness. This usually disappears in three to five days and is not a cause for concern unless it is excessive, or accompanied by unsteadiness or confusion. Excessive or persistent sedation should be investigated. Factors to be considered should include: concurrent sedative medications, the presence of hepatic or renal insufficiency, exacerbated respiratory failure, tolerance to the dose used especially in older patients, disease severity and the patient's general condition. If the dose of morphine has been reduced and pain is not adequately controlled, the dose may be carefully increased again after a few days.

Dizziness and unsteadiness may be associated with morphine-induced postural hypotension, particularly in elderly or debilitated patients. The dosage should be adjusted according to individual needs but, because of reduced clearance, dosage may be lower in patients over 50 years of age.

Nausea and vomiting: Nausea and vomiting is common after single doses of morphine or as an early undesirable effect of regular opioid therapy. The prescription of a suitable antiemetic should be considered. The frequency of nausea and vomiting usually decreases within a week or so but may persist due to opioid-induced gastric stasis. Metoclopramide is often useful in such patients.

Constipation: Virtually all patients suffer from constipation while taking opioids on a chronic basis. Some patients, particularly elderly, debilitated or bedridden patients may become impacted. Patients must be cautioned accordingly and laxatives, softeners and other appropriate treatments should be initiated at the beginning of opioid therapy.

Other adverse reactions include
Cardiovascular: Flushing of the face, chills, tachycardia, bradycardia, palpitations, faintness, vertigo, syncope, hypothermia, hypotension, orthostatic hypotension, and hypertension.

Central nervous system: Euphoria, dysphoria, weakness, headache, agitation, tremor, uncoordinated muscle movements, insomnia, dizziness, confusional symptoms and occasionally hallucinations.

Gastrointestinal: Dry mouth, anorexia, constipation, laryngospasm, colic, taste alterations and biliary colic.

Genitourinary: Urinary retention or hesitancy, reduced libido or potency.

Endocrine: A syndrome of inappropriate antidiuretic hormone secretion characterised by hyponatraemia secondary to decreased free-water excretion may occur (monitoring of electrolytes may be necessary).

Visual disturbances: Blurred vision, nystagmus, diplopia and miosis.

Allergic: Pruritus, urticaria, other skin rashes and oedema.

Withdrawal (abstinence) syndrome: Chronic use of opioid analgesics may be associated with the development of physcial dependence. An abstinence syndrome may be precipitated when opioid administration is suddenly discontinued or opioid antagonists administered.

Other: Pain at injection site; local tissue irritation and induration following subcutaneous injection, particularly when repeated.

Withdrawal symptoms that may be observed after discontinuation of opioid use include: body aches, diarrhoea, piloerection, anorexia, lacrimation, mydriasis, nervousness, insomnia, or restlessness, rhinorrhoea, sneezing, tremors or shivering, abdominal colic, abdominal and muscle cramps, bone pain, nausea, vomiting or loss of weight, sleep disturbance, unusual increase in sweating and yawning, weakness, dehydration, increased respiratory rate, blood pressure, vagomotor disturbances, tachycardia and unexplained fever. With appropriate dose adjustments and gradual withdrawal these symptoms are usually mild.

Overdose: Overdosage with morphine is characterised by respiratory depression (a decrease in respiratory rate and/or tidal volume, Cheynes-Stokes respiration, cyanosis), pinpoint pupils, extreme somnolence progressing to stupor and coma, skeletal muscle flaccidity, cold and clammy skin and sometimes bradycardia and hypotension. In severe overdosage, apnoea, circulatory collapse, cardiac arrest and death may occur.

Treatment: Immediate attention should be given to the re-establishment of adequate respiratory exchange through provision of a patent airway and institution of assisted or controlled ventilation.

Oxygen, IV fluids, vasopressors and other supportive measures should be employed as indicated.

The narcotic antagonist, naloxone, is a specific antidote against respiratory depression which may result from overdosage or unusual sensitivity to narcotics. The recommeneded adult dose of naloxone is 0.4 to 2 mg IV every 2 to 3 minutes as necessary, simultaneously with assisted respiration.

For children, the initial recommended dose is 0.01 mg/kg naloxone. A response should be seen after 2–3 doses.

Note the duration of action of naloxone is usually shorter than that of morphine and thus the patient should be carefully monitored for signs of CNS depression returning.

If the response to naloxone is suboptimal or not sustained, additional naloxone may be administered as needed, or given by continuous intravenous infusion to maintain alertness and respiratory function. There is no additional information available about the cumulative dose of naloxone that may be safely administered.

Naloxone should not be administered in the absence of clinically significant respiratory or circulatory depression secondary to morphine overdosage.

Naloxone should be administered cautiously to persons who are known or suspected to be physically dependent on morphine. In such cases, an abrupt or complete reversal of opioid effects may precipitate an acute withdrawal syndrome. The severity of the withdrawl syndrome produced will depend on the degree of physical dependence and the dose of the antagonist administered. If it is necessary to treat serious respiratory depression in the physically dependent patient, the antagonist should be administered with extreme care and by titration with smaller than usual doses of the antagonist.

Morphine toxicity may be a result of overdosage but because of the large inter-individual variation in sensitivity to opioids it is difficult to assess the exact dose of any opioid that is toxic or lethal. The toxic effects of morphine tend to be overshadowed by the presence of pain or tolerance. Patients having chronic morphine therapy have been known to take in excess of 3000 mg/day with no apparent toxic effects being present.

Pharmacological properties
Pharmacodynamic properties: Morphine is the principal alkaloid of opium. Morphine acts as an agonist, binding to receptors in the brain, spinal cord and other tissues. These sites have been classified as mu receptors and are widely distributed throughout the cental nervous system being present in highest concentration in the limbic system.

Morphine exerts its primary effects in the central nervous system and organs containing smooth muscle.

Morphine produces many effects including analgesia, decreased gastrointestinal motility, respiratory depression, drowsiness, changes in mood and alterations of the endocrine and autonomic nervous system. Nausea and vomiting may occur through direct stimulation of the chemoreceptor trigger zone (CTZ).

Urinary retention may occur due to increased bladder sphincter tone.

Pharmacokinetic properties: Absorption of morphine sulphate after intramuscular and subcutaneous injection is fairly rapid with peak analgesia occurring 30–60 minutes and 5–90 minutes after injection via the respective routes. Morphine is distributed throughout the body, but particularly to paranchymatous tissue such as kidney, lung, liver and spleen. Lower concentrations are found in skeletal muscle and brain tissue. Morphine diffuses across the placenta and trace amounts are found in sweat and breast milk. About 35% is protein bound, mainly to albumin. Morphine is metabolised principally in the liver by conjugation with glucuronic acid at the 3-hydroxyl group, and to much lesser extent to 3,6-diglucuronide. Elimination half-life is approximately 1.5 to 2 hours in healthy subjects and 90% of the dose is recovered in urine within 24 hours.

Approximately 7 to 10% of the dose is recovered in faeces, the majority after conjugation and excretion via bile.

Preclinical safety data: None.

Pharmaceutical particulars
List of excipients:

	Dosage strength ***50 mg/50 ml***	*Function*	*Reference to standards*
Active constituent			
Morphine Sulphate	50.0 mg	Active	BP
Other constituents			
Sodium Chloride	442.0 mg	Isotonicity	BP
Water for Injections	50.0 ml	Solvent	BP/USP

	Dosage strength ***100 mg/50 ml***	*Function*	*Reference to standards*
Active constituent			
Morphine Sulphate	100.0 mg	Active	BP
Other constituents			
Sodium Chloride	434.0 mg	Isotonicity	BP
Water for Injections	50.0 ml	Solvent	BP/USP

Incompatibilities: As with all parenteral drug products, intravenous admixtures should be inspected visually for clarity, particulate matter, precipitate and leakage prior to administration, whenever solution and container permit. Solutions showing haziness, particulate matter, precipitate or leakage should not be used.

Morphine Sulphate has been reported to be physically or chemically incompatible with solutions containing aminophylline, amobarbital sodium, chlorothiazide sodium, phenytoin sodium, heparin sodium, meperidine hydrochloride, methicillin sodium, nitrofurantoin sodium, pentobarbital sodium, phenobarbital sodium, sodium bicarbonate, sodium iodide, and thiopental sodium. Specialised references should be consulted for specific compatibility information.

Shelf life: 12 months.

Special precautions for storage: Store below 25°C. Protect from light. Morphine Sulphate Injection BP should be used within 24 hours of opening, in order to avoid the risk of microbial contamination.

Nature and contents of container:
Container: 50 ml clear, Type I glass, Shell glass vial.
Closure: 27 mm West Type 4405/50 SGV rubber stopper.
Seal: SGV 27 mm End Cap.

Carton: Cardboard containing 1 vial of Morphine Sulphate BP 50 mg/50 ml with an insert leaflet plus cardboard containing 1 Pharma-Ject* adaptor.

OR

Carton: Cardboard containing 1 vial of Morphine Sulphate BP 100 mg/50 ml with an insert leaflet plus cardboard containing 1 Pharma-Ject* adaptor.

Instructions fo use/handling: Morphine Sulphate Injection BP in a prefilled (Pharma-Ject*) syringe is specifically indicated for either continuous intravenous infusion or for use in patient-controlled analgesia (PCA) in patients with severe pain of medium to long duration (i.e. postoperative pain, cancer patients, burns patients etc.). The use of Pharma-Ject* is explained in the diagrams below.

Directions for use of Pharma-Ject prefilled syringe.*
Remove protective sheath from vial before use.

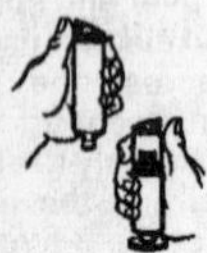

Remove protective caps from vial and injector.

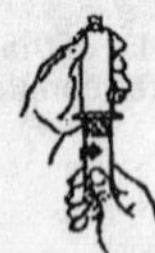

Insert vial into injector. Rotate vial three times in a clockwise direction until some resistance occurs. Then rotate vial another half turn. The needle will then be in contact with the morphine solution.

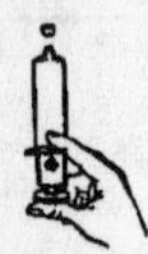

Remove the needle cap and expel air. The Pharma-Ject* is now ready for use.

Marketing authorisation number

50 mg/50 ml	UK PL 4515/0089	IR PA 437/39/1
100 mg/50 ml	UK PL 4515/0090	IR PA 437/39/2

Date of first authorisation/renewal of authorisation Not applicable.

Date of (partial) revision of the text
July 1995
December 1995
November 1996
25/2/97 SF/vg
4/3/97 SF/vg
18/3/98 DM

NALOXONE HYDROCHLORIDE INJECTION

Qualitative and quantitative composition

Active Constituents	
Naloxone Hydrochloride USP	400 mcg
Other Constituents	
Sodium Chloride BP	9.0 mg
Water for Injections BP to	1.0 mL

There is no overage in this formulation.

Pharmaceutical form Aqueous solution for injection.

Clinical particulars

Therapeutic indications:

1. Treatment of respiratory depression induced by synthetic and natural opiates.
2. Treatment of respiratory depression induced by partial opiate agonists.
3. Diagnosis of suspected acute opiate overdosage.

Posology and method of administration: Intravenous, intramuscular and subcutaneous injection.

Adults: Overdosage of narcotics–known or suspected: 400-2000 micrograms intravenously repeated at 2-3 minute intervals up to 10 mg. Dosage is similar if intramuscular or subcutaneous routes are used.

Postoperative Respiratory Depression: 100-200 micrograms intravenously at 2-3 minute intervals, to the required degree of reversal.

Children: This presentation of Naloxone is not recommended for use in children.

Elderly: No dosage adjustment is necessary for use in elderly patients.

Naloxone Hydrochloride is compatible with either Sodium Chloride 0.9% Infusion BP or Dextrose 5% Infusion BP for a period of 24 hours when stored at room temperature in fluorescent light.

Contra-indications: Naloxone is contra-indicated in patients with known hypersensitivity to the drug.

Special warnings and precautions for use: Naloxone should be given with caution to patients known or suspected to be physically dependent on opiates (including neonates born to women who are opiate dependent), because the drug may precipitate severe withdrawal symptoms.

Patients who have satisfactorily responded to naloxone should be carefully monitored since the duration of action of some opiates may exceed that of naloxone. Repeated doses of naloxone should be administered when necessary.

Naloxone is not effective against respiratory depression not due to opioid drugs.

When naloxone is used in the management of acute opioid overdosage, other resuscitative measures such as maintenance of a free airway, artificial ventilation, cardiac massage and vasopressor agents should be readily available and used when necessary.

Naloxone should be used with caution in patients with pre-existing cardi-vascular disease or in those receiving potentially cardiotoxic drugs, since serious adverse cardiovascular effects (e.g. ventricular tachycardia and fibrillation) have occurred in postoperative patients following naloxone administration.

Excessive dosage of naloxone following the use of opiates in surgery should be avoided because it may result in excitement, increased blood pressure and clinically important reversal of analgesia. Too rapid reversal of opiate effects may induce nausea, vomiting, sweating or tachycardia.

Interactions with other medicaments and other forms of interaction Not known.

Pregnancy and lactation: Reproduction studies in mice and rats using naloxone hydrochloride in doses up to 1000 times the usual human dosage revealed no evidence of impaired fertility or harm to the foetus. There are no adequate and controlled studies to date in pregnant women. Naloxone should be administered to pregnant patients only when, in the judgement of the physician, the potential benefits outweigh the possible hazards.

It is not known whether naloxone is excreted in human milk. Therefore, naloxone should be used with caution in nursing women.

Effects on ability to drive and use machines: Not applicable.

Undesirable effects: Abrupt reversal of narcotic depression has been reported to result in nausea, vomiting, sweating, tachycardia, tremor and hyperventilation. In postoperative patients excessive dosage of naloxone may result in excitement, increased blood pressure and significant reversal of analgesia.

Hypertension, pulmonary oedema, atrial and ventricular arrhythmias and cardiac-arrest have been reported in certain patients, particularly those with pre-existing cardiac abnormalities.

Seizures have occurred rarely following administration of naloxone, however, a causal relationship has not been established.

Overdose: No documented reports of acute overdosage are available.

Pharmacological properties

Pharmacodynamic properties: Naloxone hydrochloride is essentially a pure opiate antagonist, it has little or no agonistic activity. Naloxone is thought to act as a competitive antagonist at μ-, k- and σ- opioid receptors in the CNS. Small doses (0.4 mg to 0.8 mg) of naloxone given intramuscularly or intravenously prevent or promptly reverse the effects of opioids. In patients with respiratory depression, there is an increase in respiratory rate within 1 or 2 minutes. Sedative effects are reversed and blood pressure, if depressed, returns to normal. Naloxone also reverses the psychotomimetic and dysphoric effects of agonist-antagonists such as pentazocine, but higher doses (10-15 mg) are required. One milligram of naloxone intravenously completely blocks the effects of 25 mg of diacetylmorphine.

When administered in usual doses to patients who have not recently received opiates, naloxone exerts little or no pharmacological effect. Even extremely high doses (10 times the usual therapeutic dose) produce insignificant analgesia, only slight drowsiness, and no respiratory depression, psychotomimetic effects, circulatory changes, or miosis.

Naloxone does not produce tolerance or physical or psychological dependence.

Parenteral administration (S.C., I.M. or I.V.) of naloxone will produce withdrawal symptoms in patients physically dependent on opiates or pentazocine.

Pharmacokinetic properties: Naloxone has an onset of action within 1-2 minutes following I.V. administration and within 2-5 minutes following subcutaneous or intramuscular administration. The duration of action depends on the dose and route of administration and is more prolonged following I.M. administration than after I.V. administration. Duration of action is reported up to several hours but practical duration probably 1 hour or less.

Following parenteral administration, naloxone is rapidly distributed into body tissues and fluids. It is rapidly metabolised in the liver, principally by conjugation with glucuronic acid, and is excreted in the urine. The plasma half-life of naloxone has been reported to be 60-90 minutes in adults and about 3 hours in neonates.

Preclinical safety data: There are no pre-clinical data of relevance to the prescriber which are additional to that already included in other sections of the SPC.

Pharmaceutical particulars

List of excipients:	
Sodium Chloride BP	9.0 mg
Water for Injections BP	to 1.0 mL

There is no overage in this formulation.

Incompatibilities: None known.

Shelf life: 24 months.

Special precautions for storage: Store below 25°C. Protect from light.

Instruction for use/handling: Not applicable.

Marketing authorisation number 4515/0052

Date of approval/revision of SPC 12 March 1996

Legal category POM

PANCURONIUM BROMIDE INJECTION BP

Qualitative and quantitative composition *Active constituent:* Pancuronium Bromide BP 2 mg per mL. There is no overage in this formulation.

Pharmaceutical form Aqueous solution for injection.

Clinical particulars

Therapeutic indications: The active substance of Pancuronium Bromide is an amino steroid which effectively blocks transmission of motor nerve impulses to the striated muscle receptors. It is a non-depolarising neuromuscular blocking agent with a medium duration of action and is used in the following indications:

1. As an adjuvant in surgical anaesthesia to obtain relaxation of skeletal muscles in a wide range of surgical procedures.
2. Use in intensive care as a non-depolarising neuromuscular blocker for the treatment of various pathologies e.g. intractable status asthmaticus and tetanus.

Posology and method of administration: Pancuronium should be administered intravenously.

It is not recommended to be given by infusion.

The dosage should be individualised as there is a wide variation in individual response to muscle relaxants. When determining the dose, the method of anaesthesia, expected duration of surgery, potential interaction with other drugs that are administered before and during anaesthesia and the condition of the patient should be taken into account.

The use of a peripheral nerve stimulator is recommended for monitoring the neuromuscular block and recovery.

Adult: Initial dosage range 80-100 micrograms/kg body weight depending on the surgical procedure and for intubation. Incremental doses10-20 micrograms/kg.

For endotracheal intubation when Pancuronium is given in the dosage range of 80-100 micrograms/kg conditions satisfactory for intubation are usually present within 1-2 minutes.

Paediatric: 60-80 micrograms/kg initially I/V by increments increased by increments of 10-20 micrograms/kg thereafter.

Neonates: Doses of Pancuronium in neonates up to one month of age must be carefully individualised since neonates are particularly sensitive to non-depolarising neuromuscular blocking agents.

Dosage 30-40 micrograms/kg initially I/V followed by 10-20 micrograms/kg thereafter.

Elderly: The neuromuscular blocing activity of Pancuronium is prolonged in the elderly and lower doses may be necessary.

Obesity: In heavy obese patients doses of Pancuronium based on a mg/kg basis may lead to overdosage. Dosage must be adjusted according to response.

Intensive care: Pancuronium is longer acting in the

intensive care patient, and an intravenous dose of 60 micrograms/kg every one to one and a half hours, or even less frequently is usually adequate.

Impaired liver and renal function: Care must be exercised in patients with impaired liver or renal function as mentioned in the special warnings and precautions section.

Hyperdiuresis may result in a decreased neuromuscular blocking effect.

In the control of tetanus, duration of Pancuronium relaxation probably depends upon the severity of the spasm, therefore duration of effect can be variable.

The duration of action depends upon the clinical condition of the patient and the dose administered, but in normal subjects receiving perioperative muscle relaxant doses the duration of action is usually 45-60 minutes.

Pancuronium should not be mixed with other agents in the same syringe, or with solutions for intravenous infusions as a change in pH may cause precipitation.

Discard any unused solution.

Contra-indications: Patients with a known hypersensitivity to Pancuronium or the Bromide ion Concurrent use of a depolarising neuromuscular blocking agent e.g. Suxamethonium.

Special warnings and precautions for use:
Renal failure: As Pancuronium Bromide is excreted mainly in the renal system, the elimination half-life is prolonged in renal failure, resulting in a reduction in plasma clearance and prolonged duration of action.

Impaired hepatic/biliary tract disease: The duration of action may be prolonged in these conditions and resistance to neuromuscular blocking action of Pancuronium Bromide may occur because of the increased volume of distribution of the drug.

In such conditions, the drug has a slower onset and coupled with the increased total dosage requirements, there may be a prolongation of blockade and recovering time in these patients.

As with other non-depolarising muscle relaxants Pancuronium should be used with care in patients with pre-existing pulmonary, hepatic or renal disease and with particular care in patients with muscular dystrophies, myasthenia gravis and myasthenic syndrome unless it is intended to administer prolonged post-operative respiratory assistance. Before administration of Pancuronium conditions such as electrolyte disturbance, altered pH, and dehydration should be corrected if possible. Pancuronium should be used cautiously in patients with a tendancy to hypertension.

Pancuronium can cause a reduction in the partial prothromboplastin time and prothrombin time. Conditions associated with slower circulation times e.g. cardiovascular disease, oedema, old age result in an increased volume of distribution which may lead to an increased onset time.

Pancuronium should be used with particular care in neo-nates, in ill or cachetic patients, in the presence of liver disease or obstructive jaundice (resistant to the effects of drugs) in states with altered plasma protein levels or when there is diminished renal blood flow or renal disease. In operations employing the hypothermic techniques the neuromuscular blocking effect of non-depolarising drugs is decreased and increased by warming the patient.

Pancuronium should be administered in carefully adjusted dosage or under the supervision of a qualified anaesthetist and only when facilities for controlled ventilation, insufflation with oxygen and endotracheal intubation are available for immediate use.

Interactions with other medicaments and other forms of interaction:

1. Suxamethonium. Used prior to Pancuronium (for endotracheal intubation) enhances the relaxation effect of the Pancuronium and the duration of action. Therefore administration of Pancuronium should be delayed until Suxamethonium shows signs of wearing off.
2. Anaesthetics. The following anaesthetics may potentiate the neuromuscular blocking activity of Pancuronium, Halothane, Ether, Enflurane, Isoflurane, Methoxyflurane, Cyclopropane, Thiopentone, Methohexitone.
3. The following drugs may influence the duration of action of Pancuronium and the intensity of neuromuscular block.

Potentiation: Other muscle relaxants, antibiotics of the polypeptide and aminoglycoside groups, diazepam, propranolol, thiamine (high dose), MAO inhibiting agents, quinidine, magnesium sulphate, protamine, nitroglycerin, narcotic analgesics, diuretics, phenytoin, alpha adrenergic blocking agents, imidazoles, metronidazole, noradrenaline and adrenaline.

Decreased effect: Neostigmine, edrophonium, corticosteriods (high dose), adrenaline, potassium chloride, calcium chloride, sodium chloride, heparin (temporary decrease), azathioprine, theophylline, pyridostigmine.

Pancuronium should be given with caution to patients receiving chronic tricyclic antidepressant therapy who are anaesthetised with Halothane or any inhalation anaesthetic since this enhances the predisposition to the development of cardiac arrythmias associated with tricyclic antidepressants.

Pregnancy and lactation: The use of Pancuronium in pregnant or breast feeding women with respect to safety has not been established. Therefore the drug should only be administered to pregnant women when the attending physician decides that the potential benefits outweigh the risks.

Pancuronium may be used for caesarian section but the reversal of Pancuronium may be unsatisfactory in patients receiving Magnesium sulphate for toxaemia of pregnancy because magnesium salts enhance neuromuscular blockade.

Effects on ability to drive and use machines: Not applicable.

Undesirable effects: High doses of a depolarising drug may cause end-plate desensitisation and prolong post-operative apnoea.

Cardiovascular: Increased pulse rate and cardiac output. Blood pressure may rise. Arrhythmias may occur occasionally.

Gastrointestinal: Salivation is sometimes noted during anaesthesia.

Hypersensitivity: Occasional transient rash has been noted.

Injection Site Reactions: Pain or local skin reactions noted at the site of injection.

Respiratory: Bronchospasm has rarely been reported. Patients with carcinomatosis especially associated with bronchial carcinoma may exhibit a marked sensitivity to this agent, and the neuromuscular block produced may respond poorly to Neostigmine.

Serious or life threatening reactions: Severe anaphylactoid reactions have been reported uncommonly.

Overdose: Clinical features: The symptoms are those of prolonged apnoea, respiratory depression and/or muscle weakness. Death may follow acute respiratory failure.

Management: Neostigmine at a dose of 2.5 mg and Atropine at a dose of 1.2 mg can be administered to reverse the neuromuscular block whilst ventilation is continued. When administration of the cholinesterase inhibiting agent fails to reverse the neuromuscular blocking effects of Pancuronium ventilation must continue until spontaneous breathing is restored.

Pharmacological properties

Pharmacodynamic properties: Pancuronium bromide produces pharmacologic effects similar to those other non-depolarising neuromuscular blocking agents. The drug may produce an increase in heart rate which appears to result from a direct blocking effect on the acetylcholine receptors of the heart. The increase in heart rate appears to be dose related and is minimal with usual doses. Pancuronium causes little or no histamine release and no ganglionic blockade and therefore does not cause hypotension or bronchospasm. Despite its steroidal structure, the drug exhibits no hormonal activity.

Pharmacokinetic properties: Following I/V administration of Pancuronium Bromide 0.06 mg/kg, muscle relaxation reaches a level suitable for endotracheal intubation within 2-3 minutes, slightly more rapidly than with tubocurarine. The onset and duration of paralysis are dose related. After a dose of 0.06 mg/kg, the effects of the drug begin to subside in about 35-45 minutes. Supplemental doses may increase the magnitude and duration of the neuromuscular blockade. The duration of action depends upon the clinical condition of the patient and the dose administered, but in normal subjects receiving perioperative muscle relaxant doses the duration of action is usually 45-60 minutes.

Protein binding of Pancuronium does not appear to be substantial. The activity of the drug is not greatly affected by plasma carbon dioxide concentrations or pH. Redistribution is responsible for the termination of activity following single doses. Pancuronium crosses the placenta in small amounts.

Plasma concentrations appear to decline in a triphasic manner. In adults with normal renal and hepatic function, the half-life in the terminal phase is about 2 hours. The elimination half-life may be prolonged in patients with impaired renal and/or hepatic function. The drug is eliminated mainly unchanged by the kidneys, although small amounts may be metabolised and some of the drug may be eliminated in the bile.

Preclinical safety data: There are no pre-clinical data of relevance to the prescriber which are additional to that already included in other sections of the SPC.

Pharmaceutical particulars

List of excipients

Sodium Chloride BP	8.0 mg
Sodium Acetate BP	2.0 mg
Acetic Acid 6N BP	Q.S.
Sodium Hydroxide 1N BP	Q.S.
Nitrogen BP	Q.S.
Water for Injections BP	to 1.0 ml

There is no overage in this formulation.

Incompatibilities: Do not mix other solutions in the same syringe as a change in pH can cause precipitation.

Pancuronium should be stored at 2-8°C.

Shelf life: 24 months.

Special precautions for storage: Store between 2-8°C. Protect from light. Do not freeze.

Instruction for use/handling: Not applicable.

Marketing authorisation number 4515/0062

Date of approval/revision of SPC June 1997

Legal category POM

PARALDEHYDE INJECTION BP

Qualitative and quantitative composition Paraldehyde BP.

Pharmaceutical form Sterile liquid intended for parenteral use.

Clinical particulars

Therapeutic indications: Status Epilepticus.

Posology and method of administration: Deep intramuscular injection or rectal administration.

Adults: 5–10 ml administered by deep intramuscular injection. The usual maximum is 20 ml daily with not more than 5 ml at any one site. 15 to 30 ml suitably diluted can be administered rectally (usually 10% paraldehyde in isotonic sodium chloride solution).

Children: Reduced doses are necessary in children with suggested daily as follows:

Up to 3 months	0.5 ml
3–6 months	1.0 ml
6–12 months	1.5 ml
1–2 years	2.0 ml
3–5 years	3–4 ml
6–12 years	5–6 ml

Elderly: No special recommendations.

Contra-indications: Paraldehyde should not be administered to patients with gastric disorders or patients receiving disulfiram. Paraldehyde should not be administered rectally in patients with colitis.

Special warnings and precautions for use: Paraldehyde should be used with extreme caution in patients with bronchopulmonary disease or hepatic impairment. The injection is painful and care should be taken to avoid the neighbourhood or nerve trunks which could be damaged by paraldehyde. Prolonged use of paraldehyde may lead to dependence particularly in alcoholics. When administered intramuscularly not more than 5 ml should be injected into any one site to minimise the possibility of sterile abscess formation.

Paraldehyde decomposes on storage particularly after opening. Administration of partly decomposed paraldehyde is dangerous and the product should not be used if it has a brownish colour or sharp penetrating odour of acetic acid. After injection, any unused contents should be discarded.

Interactions with other medicaments and other forms of interaction: Effects of paraldehyde are enhanced by the simultaneous administration of CNS depressants.

Pregnancy and lactation: Paraldehyde readily crosses the placental barrier and appears in the foetal circulation and is also found in breast milk. Safety in human pregnancy and during breast feeding has not been established and therefore, as with all drugs, paraldehyde should not be administered during pregnancy or breast feeding unless considered essential.

Effects on ability to drive and use machines: Paraldehyde causes drowsiness and patients should not be allowed to drive or operate machinery.

Undesirable effects: Paraldehyde may cause occasional allergic skin rashes. Intramuscular injection is painful and associated with tissue necrosis, sterile abscesses and nerve damage.

Overdose: Symptoms – rapid laboured breathing owing to damage in the lungs and to acidosis. Hepatic and renal damage may occur.

Treatment – intensive symptomatic and supportive therapy, in particular, the maintenance of cardiovascular, respiratory and renal functions, and maintenance of electrolyte balance. Intravenous hydrocortisone may be given to reduce hepatic and renal damage.

Pharmacological properties

Pharmacodynamic properties: Paraldehyde is a rapidly acting hypnotic and sedative with anticonvulsant effects.

Pharmacokinetic properties: Paraldehyde is readily absorbed after intrasmuscular injection and is distributed throughout the body tissue. About 80% of a dose is metabolised in the liver. Unmetabolised drug is largely excreted unchanged through the lungs. Small amounts are excreted in urine. Paraldehyde crosses the placental barrier.

Preclinical safety data: There is no pre-clinical data of relevance to the prescriber which are additional to that already included in other sections of the SPC.

Pharmaceutical particulars

List of excipients: Hydroquinone USP 0.5 mg.

Incompatibilities: Paraldehyde should not be administered in plastic syringes or be placed in contact with rubber components. Paraldehyde should always be administered in glass syringes.

Shelf life: 24 months.

Special precautions for storage: Store between 15°C to 20°C in complete darkness.

Nature and contents of container: Neutral Glass (Type 1) 5 ml ampoules. In packs of 5.

Instruction for use/handling. Not applicable.

Marketing authorisation number PL 4515/0104

Date of first authorisation/renewal of authorisation 30 June 1997

Date of (partial) revision of the text July 1998

PHENYTOIN INJECTION BP

Qualitative and quantitative composition Phenytoin Sodium BP 250 mg in 5 mL

Pharmaceutical form Sterile Solution for Injection

Clinical particulars

Therapeutic indications: Control of status epilepticus and the prevention of seizures occurring during or following neurosurgery. Treatment of certain cardiac dysrhythmias, particularly those unresponsive to conventional antidysrhythmic agents or to cardioversion.

Posology and method of administration: Phenytoin Injection BP solution is suitable for use as long as it remains free of haziness and precipitate. A precipitate might form if the product has been kept in a refrigerator or freezer. This precipitate will dissolve if allowed to stand at room temperature. The product will then be suitable for use.

Phenytoin Injection BP should be injected slowly and directly into a large vein through a large-gauge needle or intravenous catheter. It must be administered slowly. Intravenous administration should not exceed 50 mg/minute in adults. In neonates the drug should be administered at a rate not exceeding 1 to 3 mg/kg/min. Each injection should be followed by an injection of 0.9% sodium chloride through the same needle or catheter to avoid local venous irritation due to the alkalinity of the solution.

For infusion administration the parenteral phenytoin should be diluted in 50–100 ml of normal saline, with the final concentration of phenytoin in the solution not exceeding 10 mg/ml. Administration should commence immediately after the mixture has been prepared and must be completed within one hour (the infusion mixture should not be refrigerated). An in-line filter (0.22–0.50 microns) should be used. The diluted form is suitable for use as long as it remains free of haziness and precipitate.

Continuous monitoring of the electrocardiogram and blood pressure is essential. Cardiac resuscitative equipment should be available. The patient should be observed for signs of respiratory depression. If administration of intravenous Phenytoin Injection does not terminate seizures, the use of other measures, including general anaesthesia, should be considered.

For the control of status epilepticus, 150 to 250 mg should be given by slow intravenous injection at a rate not exceeding 50 mg/minute to avoid hypotension. This dose can be repeated if necessary after 30 minutes. A previously untreated adult may require 10-15 mg/kg. The loading dose is then followed by a maintenance dose of 100 mg given orally or intravenously every 6-8h. In geriatric patients with heart disease, it has been recommended that the drug be given at a rate of 50 mg over 2-3 minutes. Dosage for children is usually determined according to weight. Paediatric dosage may also be calculated on the basis of 250 mg/m^2 of body surface area or 15-20 mg/kg administered in 2 or 3 equally divided doses. Subsequent dosage should be adjusted carefully and slowly according to the patients requirements. Maintenance dosage for children usually ranges from 4-8 mg/kg daily.

Determination of phenytoin serum levels is advised when using Phenytoin Injection BP in the management of status epilepticus and in the subsequent establishing of maintenance dosage. The clinically effective level is usually 10-20 mg/l although some cases of tonic-clonic seizures may be controlled with lower serum levels of phenytoin.

In a patient who has not previously received the drug, Phenytoin Injection, 100 mg-200 mg (2-4 ml), maybe given intramuscularly at approximately 4 hourly intervals prophylactically during neurosurgery and continued during the postoperative period for 48-72 hours. The dosage should then be reduced to a maintenance dose of 300 mg and adjusted according to serum level estimations.

When given by intramuscular injection, phenytoin precipitates out at the injection site and is absorbed slowly and erratically. This route is not, therefore, recommended for treating status epilepticus. If phenytoin is administered by intramuscular injection to patients unable to take the drug orally, the dose should be increased by 50% over the previously established oral dose. To avoid drug accumulation resulting from eventual absorption from intramuscular injection sites, it is recommended that for the first week back on oral therapy the dose is reduced to one-half the original dose. Monitoring of serum concentrations is also recommended. Intramuscular therapy should generally be limited to I week.

Phenytoin sodium can be useful in ventricular arrhythmias, particularly those due to digitalis. The recommended dosage is one intravenous injection of Phenytoin Injection BP of 3 to 5 mg/kg bodyweight initially, repeating if necessary.

Contra-indications: In patients with a known hypersensitivity to phenytoin or other hydantoins.

In patients with sinus bradycardia, sino-atrial block, second and third degree AV block or Adams-Stokes syndrome.

Intra-arterial administration must be avoided in view of the high pH of the preparation.

Special warnings and special precautions for use:
Warnings: This drug must be administered slowly, at a rate not exceeding 50 mg/minute in adults. In neonates, the drug should be administered at a rate not exceeding 1-3 mg/kg/min. The response to phenytoin may be significantly altered by the concomitant use of other drugs (see Interactions with other Drugs).

Rapid administration may result in hypotension. In patients with cardiovascular disease, parenteral administration may result in atrial and ventricular conduction depression, ventricular fibrillation or reduced cardiac output. Severe complications are most commonly encountered in elderly or gravely ill patients. In these patients, the drug should be administered at a rate not exceeding 25 mg/minute, and if necessary, at a slow rate of 5 to 10 mg/minute.

Serum levels of phenytoin sustained above the optimal range may produce encephalopathy, or confusional states (delirium psychosis), or rarely irreversible cerebellar dysfunction. Plasma level determinations are recommended at the first signs of acute toxicity. If plasma levels are excessive, then dosage reduction is indicated. Termination is recommended if symptoms persist.

Abrupt withdrawal of phenytoin in epileptic patients may precipitate status epilepticus. When it is necessary to reduce the dose of phenytoin, this should be done gradually. In hypersensitivity reactions, where rapid substitution of therapy is warranted, the alternative drug should be one not belonging to the hydantoin class of compounds.

Subcutaneous or perivascular injection should be avoided because of the highly alkaline nature of the solution. Such injection may cause irritation of the tissues varying from slight tenderness to extensive necrosis, sloughing and in rare instances has led to amputation.

The intramuscular route is not recommended for the treatment of status epilepticus because of slow absorption. Serum levels of phenytoin in the therapeutic range cannot be rapidly achieved by this method.

Precautions: The liver is the principal site of biotransformation of phenytoin; patients with impaired liver function, elderly patients, or those who are gravely ill may show early signs of toxicity.

Patients with renal function impairment should also be carefully observed when prescribing phenytoin, as excretion and protein binding may be altered.

A small percentage of individuals who have been treated with phenytoin have been shown to metabolize the drug slowly. Slow metabolism appears to be due to limited enzyme availability and lack of induction, which may be genetically determined.

Phenytoin should be used with caution in diabetic patients as hyperglycaemia may be potentiated.

Measurement of serum phenytoin levels is recommended when using phenytoin in the management of status epilepticus and in establishing a maintenance dose. The usually accepted therapeutic level is 10-20 mg/L, although some patients with tonic-clonic seizures can be controlled with lower serum levels.

Phenytoin is not effective for petit mal seizures. Therefore, combined therapy is required if both grand mal and petit mal seizures are present.

Interaction with other medicaments and other forms of interaction: Drugs which may increase serum levels of phenytoin include: chloramphenicol, coumarin anticoagulants, disulfiram, phenylbutazone, isoniazid, salicylates, chlordiazepoxide, phenothiazines, diazepam, oestrogens, ethosuximide, sulthiame, halothane, methylphenidate, trimethadione, mephenytoin, sulphonamides, cimetidine, trazodone, ranitidine, fluconazole, ketoconazole, miconazole.

Drugs which may decrease serum levels of phenytoin include: carbamazepine, reserpine, bleomycin, carboplatin, carmustine, cisplatin, methotrexate, vinblastine, folic acid, calcium folinate, rifampicin.

Drugs which may either increase or decrease serum levels of phenytoin and vice versa include: barbiturates, valproic acid and sodium valproate, primidone.

Acute alcoholic intake may increase serum levels of phenytoin while chronic alcoholic use may decrease them.

Tricyclic antidepressants, haloperidol, monoamine oxidase inhibitors and thioxanthenes may precipitate seizures in susceptible patients and phenytoin dosage may need to be adjusted.

Phenytoin impairs the efficacy of several drugs, including:

anticonvulsants, corticosteroids, coumarin anticoagulants, cyclosporine, dacarbazine, vitamin D, digoxin, disopyramide, doxycycline, frusemide, L-dopa, mexiletine, oestrogens, oral contraceptives, quinidine, succinimide and xanthines.

Caution is advised when nifedipine or verapamil are used concurrently with phenytoin. All are highly protein bound medications and therefore changes in serum concentrations of the free, unbound medications may occur.

Phenytoin may increase serum glucose levels and therefore dosage adjustments for Insulin or oral antidiabetic agents may be necessary.

Concurrent use of phenytoin and oral diazoxide may decrease the efficacy of phenytoin and the hyperglycaemic effect of diazoxide and is not recommended.

Use of intravenous phenytoin in patients maintained on dopamine may produce sudden hypotension and bradycardia. This appears to be dose-dependent. If anticonvulsant therapy is necessary during administration of dopamine, an alternative to phenytoin should be considered.

Concurrent use of intravenous phenytoin with lignocaine or beta-blockers may produce additive cardiac depressant effects. Phenytoin may also increase the metabolism of lignocaine.

Pregnancy and lactation:

Use in pregnancy: Adverse effects on the foetus of status epilepticus, specifically hypoxia, make it imperative to control the condition. However, Phenytoin readily crosses the placenta about 10% of exposed fetuses have been noted to show minor craniofacial and digital abnormalities–the so-called fetal hydantoin syndrome. Common features include broad lower nasal bridge, epicanthic folds, hypertelorism, malformed ears, wide mouth and hypoplasia of the distal phalanges and nails. A few of these babies have microencephaly and are retarded. Facial clefts and congenital heart disease are also seen more commonly than might be expected. Overall, however, the risk of having an abnormal child as a result of medication is far outweighed by the dangers to the mother and foetus of uncontrolled epilepsy.

The adverse effects on the foetus of status epilepticus, specifically hypoxia, make it imperative to control the condition in the shortest possible time.

The pharmacokinetics of phenytoin are altered in pregnancy. A fall in plasma albumin together with more efficient hepatic metabolism act to a reduce total and unbound plasma phenytoin concentrations. Neonatal coagulation defects have been reported within the first 24 hours in babies born to epileptic mothers receiving phenytoin. Vitamin K has been shown to prevent or correct this defect and may be given to the mother before delivery and to the neonate after birth.

Use in lactation: Phenytoin concentrations in breast milk are 20 to 25% of simultaneous maternal plasma levels. If maternal plasma levels are within the therapeutic range, and considering the daily volume of milk taken by the infant, it is unlikely that the infant will be exposed to clinically significant phenytoin concentrations. Breast feeding is not, therefore, contraindicated.

Effects on ability to drive and use machines: Phenytoin in appropriate doses may as such impair driving skills but epilepsy itself dictates the practice of driving. Patients affected by drowsiness should not drive or operate machinery.

Undesirable effects: The most notable signs of toxicity are cardiovascular collapse and/or depression of the central nervous system. Hypotension can occur when the drug is administered rapidly by intravenous injection. Toxicity should be minimised by following the appropriate directions (see *Dosage and Administration*).

Cardiovascular: Severe cardiotoxic reactions and fatalities have been reported, most commonly in gravely ill patients or the elderly (see *Warnings)*.

Central Nervous System: There are the most common reactions encountered with phenytoin and include nystagmus, ataxia, slurred speech, decreased coordination and mental confusion. Cases of dizziness, insomnia, transient nervousness, motor twitchings and headaches have also been reported. These side effects are usually dose related.

There have also been rare reports of phenytoin induced dyskinesias, including chorea, dystonia, tremor and asterixis, similar to those induced by phenothiazine and other neuroleptic drugs. These may be due to sudden intravenous administration for status epilepticus. The effect usually lasts 24-48h after discontinuation.

A predominantly sensory peripheral polyneuropathy has been reported for patients on long-term phenytoin therapy.

Gastrointestinal: Nausea, vomiting and constipation.

Dermatological: A measle-like rash is the most common dermatological manifestation. Rashes are sometimes accompanied by fever, and are generally more common in children and young adults. Other types of rashes are more rare, and more serious forms which may be fatal include bullous, exfoliative or purpuric dermatitis, lupus erythematosus, Stevens-Johnson syndrome and toxic epidermal necrolysis. Phenytoin should be discontinued if a skin rash appears. If the rash is exfoliative, purpuric, or bullous or if lupus erythematosus, Stevens-Johnson syndrome or toxic epidermal necrolysis is suspected, phenytoin should not be resumed. If the rash is mild (measles-like or scarlatiniform), therapy may be resumed when the rash has completely disappeared. However, in the case of the rash recurring upon reinstitution of therapy, further phenytoin medication is contraindicated.

Haemopoietic: Some fatal haemopoietic complications have occasionally been reported in association with the use of phenytoin. These have included thrombocytopenia, leukopaenia, granulocytopaenia, agranulocytosis, and pancytopaenia with or without bone marrow suppression. Although macrocytosis and megaloblastic anaemia have occurred, these conditions usually respond to folic acid therapy. There have been a number of reports suggesting a relationship between phenytoin and the development of local or generalised lymphadenopathy, including benign lymph node hyperplasia, lymphoma, pseudolymphoma and Hodgkin's Disease. Although a cause and effect relationship has not been established, the occurrence of lymphadenopathy indicates the need to differentiate such a condition from other types of lymph node pathology. Lymph node involvement may occur with or without symptoms resembling serum sickness e.g. rash, fever and liver involvement. In all cases of lymphadenopathy, seizure control should be sought using alternative antiepileptic drugs and observation of patients for an extended period is recommended.

Injection Site: Local irritation, inflammation and tenderness. Necrosis and sloughing have been reported after subcutaneous or perivascular injection. Subcutaneous or perivascular injection should be avoided. Soft tissue irritation and inflammation have occurred at the site of injection with or without extravasation of intravenous phenytoin.

Others: Gingival hyperplasia is common with long-term therapy. Its incidence may be reduced by maintaining good oral hygiene such as frequent brushing, gum massage and appropriate dental care.

Coarsening of the facial features, enlargement of the lips, hypertrichosis, Peyronies Disease, systemic lupus erythematosus, periarteritis nodosa, toxic hepatitis, liver damage, and immunoglobulin abnormalities may occur.

Rare reports of pulmonary infiltrates or fibrosis, with symptoms including fever, troubled or quick, shallow breathing, unusual tiredness or weakness, loss of appetite and weight and chest discomfort, have also occurred.

Overdose:

Symptoms: The lethal dose in adults is considered to be 2 to 5 grams. The lethal dose in children is not known. The initial symptoms are nystagmus, ataxia, and dysarthria. Other signs are tremor, hyperflexia, lethargy, slurred speech, nausea and vomiting. The patient may become comatose and hypotensive. Death is due to respiratory and circulatory depression.

Treatment: Treatment is nonspecific since there is no known antidote. (If ingestion has taken place, the stomach should be emptied). If the gag reflex is absent, the airway should be supported. Oxygen and assisted ventilation may be necessary for central nervous system, respiratory and cardiovascular depression. Haemodialysis can be considered since phenytoin is not completely bound to plasma proteins. Total exchange transfusion has been utilised in the treatment of severe intoxication in children.

Pharmacological properties

Pharmacodynamic properties: Phenytoin sodium inhibits the spread of seizure activity in the motor cortex. It appears that by promoting sodium efflux from neurons, phenytoin sodium tends to stabilise the threshold against hyperexcitability caused by environmental changes or excessive stimulation capable of reducing membrane sodium gradient. This includes the reduction of post tetanic potentiation of synapses. Loss of post tetanic potentiation prevents cortical seizure foci from detonating adjacent cortical areas. Phenytoin thereby reduces the over-activity of brain stem centres responsible for the tonic phase of grand mal seizures.

Phenytoin sodium antiarrhythmic action may be attributed to the normalization of influx of sodium and calcium to cardiac Purkinje fibres. Abnormal ventricular automaticity and membrane responsiveness are decreased. It also shortens the refractory period, and therefore shortens the QT interval and the duration of the action potential.

Hydantoins induce production of liver microsomal enzymes, thereby accelerating the metabolism of concomitantly administered drugs.

Pharmacokinetic properties: The onset of action after an intravenous dose is 30 to 60 minutes and the effect persists up to 24 hours. Phenytoin is about 90% protein bound. Protein binding may be lower in neonates and hyperbilirubinemic infants; also altered in patients with hypoalbuminaemia, uraemia or acute trauma, and in pregnancy. Optimum control without clinical signs of toxicity occurs most often with serum levels between 10 and 20 mcg/mL. In renal failure or hypoalbuminaemia, 5 to 12 mcg/mL or even less may be therapeutic.

Phenytoin is metabolised in the liver, the major inactive metabolite is 5-(p-hydroxyphenyl)-5-phenylhydantoin (HPPH). The rate of metabolism is increased in younger children, pregnant women, in women during menses and in patients with acute trauma. The rate decreases with advancing age. Phenytoin may be metabolised slowly in a small number of individuals due to genetic factors, which may cause limited enzyme availability and lack of induction.

The plasma half-life is normally from 10 to 15 hours. Because phenytoin exhibits saturable or dose-dependent pharmacokinetics, the apparent half-life of phenytoin changes with dose and serum concentration. At therapeutic concentrations of the drug, the enzyme system responsible for metabolising phenytoin becomes saturated. Thus a constant amount of drug is metabolised, and small increases in dose may cause disproportionately large increases in serum concentrations and apparent half-life, possibly causing unexpected toxicity.

Pharmaceutical particulars

List of excipients

Propylene Glycol BP	2.0 ml
Absolute Alcohol BP	0.5 ml
Water for Injection BP	to 5.0 ml

Incompatibilities: Incompatible with amikacin sulphate, cephapirin sodium clindamycin phosphate, and many other drugs. It is recommended that phenytoin sodium not be mixed with other drugs or with any infusion solution other than sodium chloride 0.9%.

Shelf life: 24 months.

Special precautions for storage: Phenytoin Injection BP should be stored below 25°C and protected from light. The product should be visually inspected for particulate matter and discolouration prior to administration.

Instructions for use/handling: See under *Posology and Method of Administration.*

Marketing authorisation number 4515/0083

Date of approval/revision of SPC May 1996

Legal category POM

SODIUM NITROPRUSSIDE FOR INJECTION BP 50MG

Qualitative and quantitative composition Active constituent: Sodium Nitroprusside Dihydrate BP 50.0 mg. There is no overage included in the formulation.

Pharmaceutical form Lyophilised powder for reconstitution with Glucose Injection BP

Clinical particulars

Therapeutic indications: Sodium Nitroprusside is indicated for the immediate reduction of blood pressure in patients in hypertensive crises.

The drug is effective in the management of hypertensive emergencies, irrespective of aetiology, and may be useful when other drugs have failed.

Sodium nitroprusside may also be used to produce controlled hypotension during anaesthesia in order to reduce bleeding in surgical procedures when surgeon and anaesthetist deem it appropriate.

Nitroprusside has also been used in the treatment of heart failure and other cardiac disorders where it is necessary to quickly reduce left ventricular outflow (afterload) and lower raised ventricular pressure (preload).

Posology and method of administration: Sodium Nitroprusside is to be administered only by intravenous infusion using a controlled infusion device, infusion pump, drip regulator, micro-drip regulator or similar device that will allow precise measurements of flow rate. Care should be taken to avoid extravasation.

Reconstitution of Sodium Nitroprusside for Injection BP to produce the Intravenous Infusion

Reconstitution can only be carried out using Glucose Injection BP A concentrated solution of sodium nitroprusside may be prepared by dissolving 50 mg of the drug in 2-3 ml of glucose Injection BP The concentrated solution should be further diluted in 250, 500, or 1000 ml of Glucose Injection BP to provide solutions containing 200, 100 or 50 micrograms per ml respectively. Nitroprusside solutions should be protected from light by promptly wrapping the containers in aluminium foil or other opaque material. Both the concentrated solution and the infusion solution should be freshly prepared and any unused portion discarded after 24 hours. The freshly prepared infusion solution has a very faint brownish tint; if it is highly coloured it should be discarded.

Administration should be carried out at all times under close supervision. No other drug should be added to the infusion fluid for simultaneous administration with sodium nitroprusside and in hypotensive patients receiving concomitant antihypertensive medication, smaller doses of sodium nitroprusside might be required.

It is recommended that the blood pressure should not be allowed to drop rapidly and that systolic pressure should not be lowered below 60 mmHg. This can be achieved by increasing the dose slowly which should also prevent any physiological compensatory reactions resulting from the release of catecholamines and renins into the blood, which would lead to tachycardia.

The rate of administration should be adjusted to maintain the desired hypotensive effect, as determined by continous blood pressure monitoring.

In order to avoid excessive levels of cyanide and thiocyanate and lessen the possibility of a precipitous drop in blood pressure, infusion rates greater than 10 micrograms per kilogram per minute should not be used. If, at this rate, an adequate reduction of blood pressure is not obtained within 10 minutes, the administration of sodium nitroprusside should be stopped.

The intravenous infusion should not be stopped suddenly as this might lead to an excessive rebound rise in blood pressure, but rather over a period of 15 to 30 minutes. In hypertensive emergencies sodium nitroprusside infusion may be continued until an alternative oral therapy can be safely introduced.

Intravenous infusion of sodium nitroprusside may be continued for several days but care must be taken to ensure that the blood cyanide concentration does not exceed 100 micrograms per 100 ml and that the serum cyanide concentration does not exceed 8 micrograms per 100 ml. If infusion is carried out for a period in excess of three days then the blood thiocyanate concentration should be checked and not exceed 100 micrograms per ml.

Dosage in adults:

Hypertensive crisis: Dosage varies considerably between patients, hence the need for individual titration. In adults not receiving other hypotensive agents, the average dosage of sodium nitroprusside is 3 micrograms per kilogram per minute.The initial dose is normally within the range of 0.5-1.5 micrograms per kilogram per minute, but can then be adjusted in a stepwise fashion, e.g. in increments of 0.5 micrograms per kilogram per minute every 5 minutes, to fall between 0.5–8 micrograms per kilogram per minute.To maintain the blood pressure at 30 to 40 % lower than the pretreatment diastolic blood pressure levels an average of 200 micrograms/minute (range of 20 to 400 micrograms/minute) is usually sufficient. In hypertensive patients receiving concomitant antihypertensive medication, smaller doses might be required.

Heart failure: The initial dose should be between 10-15 micrograms per minute increased every 5-10 minutes in increments of 10 to 15 micrograms per minute as necessary to the normal range of 10-200 microgram per minute to obtain the desired response.In some patients the additive effects of a vasodilator and a potent inotropic agent may be used to advantage. If a vasodilator is used haemodynamic monitoring should be used to guide its administration.If during treatment signs of hypotension, hypoperfusion or any other adverse effects are observed the infusion rate should be reduced or administration stopped.The infusion may be continued until an alternative oral therapy can be safely introduced. The infusion therapy should not normally exceed 3 days.

In controlled hypotension during general anaesthesia: For the induction of hypotension during anaesthesia a maximum dose of 1.5 microgram per kilogram bodyweight per minute is recommended. The intrinsic hypotensive effect of many anaesthetic agents must be remembered and all normal procedures for hypotensive techniques should be carried out.

Geriatric Patients: Commence therapy with low doses since geriatric patients appear to be more sensitive to the hypotensive effects of the drug. Therefore the drug should be administered with caution in this age group.

Children: Dosage recommendations have not been established.

Contra-indications:

1. Treatment of compensatory hypertension, e.g. arteriovenous shunt or coarctation of the aorta.
2. Inadequate cerebral circulation
3. Cyanide and thiocyanate are metabolites of nitroprusside and may interfere with the metabolism of cyanocobalamin. Nitroprusside is therefore contra-indicated in patients suffering from severe vitamin B12 deficiency, hepatic failure and Leber's optic atrophy.

Special warnings and special precautions for use:
Precautions: Thiocyanate may accumulate in the blood of patients receiving sodium nitroprusside therapy, especially those with impaired renal function or hyponatraemia. Since thiocyanate inhibits both uptake and binding of iodine, symptoms of hypothyroidism may occur.

Sodium nitroprusside should be administered only when adequate facilities are available to frequently monitor blood pressure, since the hypotensive effect is rapid. When I.V. infusion of sodium nitroprusside is decreased or discontinued, blood pressure usually begins to increase immediately and returns to pretreatment levels within 1-10 minutes.

Because sodium nitroprusside may interfere with vitamin B12 distribution and metabolism, the drug should be used with caution in patients with low plasma vitamin B12 concentrations.

The drug should be used with extreme caution if the patient is hypothermic.

Interaction with other medicaments and other forms of interaction: e hypotensive effects of Sodium Nitroprusside are additive when used concomitantly with ganglionic blocking agents, general anaesthetics (e.g. halothane, enflurane), and with most other circulatory depressants.

Pregnancy and lactation:

Use in pegnancy: Adequate reproduction studies have not been performed with sodium nitroprusside, and its its use in pregnancy or women of child bearing potential requires that the potential benefits be weighed against possible hazards to the mother and child or foetus.

Use in lctation: It is not known if sodium nitroprusside is distributed into milk, therefore the drug should be used with caution in nursing mothers.

Effects on ability to drive and use machines: Not applicable.

Undesirable effects: Nausea,retching, diaphoresis, apprehension, headache, restlessness, muscle twitching, retrosternal discomfort, palpitations, drowsiness, dizziness, paraesthesial warmth and abdominal pain have been noted when the reduction in blood pressure is too rapid, but these symptoms quickly disappear when the rate of infusion is decreased or the infusion is temporarily discontinued and do not reappear with continued slower rate of administration.

Tachycardia and postural hypotension have also been reported. Irritation and reddening of the skin may occur at the injection site.

Overdose: Overdosage will result in a fall in blood pressure below the desired level. Discontinuation of administration or a reduction in the rate of administration are usually sufficient measures for managing an overdose of sodium nitroprusside.

Infusion rates exceeding 10 micrograms per kilogram per minute may result in cyanide intoxication. This is best managed by the intravenous injection of sodium nitrate in conjunction with sodium thiosulphate.

Pharmacological properties

Pharmacodynamic properties: When Sodium Nitroprusside is administered by IV infusion to hypertensive or normotensive patients, a marked lowering of arterial blood pressure is produced. Venous pressure is also lowered and a moderate reduction in total peripheral resistance occurs. The effects of the drug on blood pressure are more pronounced in hypertensive than in normotensive patients.

The hypotensive action of Sodium Nitroprusside results from peripheral vasodilation caused by a direct action on vascular smooth muscle. Animal tests performed in situ have demonstrated no relaxation of other smooth muscle tissue, such as the uterus or duodenum, by Sodium Nitroprusside. The drug has no direct effect on vasomotor centres, sympathetic nerves, or adrenergic receptors. The hypotensive effect of Sodium Nitroprusside is augmented by concomitant use of other hypotensive agents and is not blocked by adrenergic blocking agents or vagotomy. Pressor agents such as epinephrine which stimulate the myocardium directly are the only drugs that cause an increase in blood pressure during Sodium Nitroprusside therapy. Resistance to the drug's hypotensive effects and tachyphylaxis are very rare.

The effects of Sodium Nitroprusside on cardiac performance appear to depend on preexisting performance. Changes in cardiac performance are attributed mainly to a reduction in left ventricular afterload resulting from vasodilation but may also be related to reduction in venous return to the heart resulting from peripheral vascular pooling of blood, decreased arteriolar resistance, and increased diastolic compliance. The drug has no direct effect on the myocardium, but it may exert a direct coronary vasodilator effect. When Sodium Nitroprusside is administered to hypertensive patients, a slight increase in heart rate usually occurs and cardiac output is usually decreased slightly. Decreases in cardiac index and stroke index are common; however, these decreases do not occur consistently and increases have occurred in some patients. When Sodium Nitroprusside is administered to patients with refractory heart failure and/or acute myocardial infarction, substantial improvement in left ventricular performance results with cardiac output, cardiac index, and stroke volume being increased and left ventricular filling pressure being decreased. In patients with congestive heart failure, a slight but clinically important slowing of the heart rate results, as well as reduction or cessation of arrhythmias.

A reduction in myocardial oxygen consumption during Sodium Nitroprusside use has been noted which could prove beneficial when infarcted areas of the heart are already short of oxygen. In patients with congestive heart failure, improvement in cardiac performance is accompanied by prompt diuresis, with urine volume and sodium excretion both being increased.

Moderate doses of Sodium Nitroprusside in hypertensive patients produce renal vasodilation without an appreciable increase in renal blood flow or a decrease in glomerular filtration. Mean renal arterial pressure and renal vascular resistance are slightly decreased. The acute reduction in mean arterial pressure is accompanied by an increase in renin activity of renal venous plasma.

Pharmacokinetic properties:

Absorption: IV infusion of Sodium Nitroprusside produces an almost immediate reduction in blood pressure. Blood pressure begins to rise immediately when the infusion is slowed or stopped and returns to pretreatment levels within 1-10 minutes.

Distribution: Distribution of Nitroprusside in the body as well as passage across the placenta into milk, or across the blood-brain barrier has not been studied.

Elimination: Sodium Nitroprusside is rapidly metabolised, probably by interaction with sulphhydryl groups in the erythrocytes and tissues. Cyanogen (cyanide radical) is produced which is converted to thiocyanate in the liver by the enzyme rhodanase. A thiocyanate oxidase present in the erythrocytes may oxidise small quantities of thiocyanate back to cyanogen. Toxic symptoms begin to appear at plasma thiocyanate concentrations of 50-100 mcg/ml; fatalities have been reported at concentrations of 200 mcg/ml.

Sodium Nitroprusside is excreted entirely as metabolites, principally thiocyanate. In animals, Sodium Nitroprusside metabolites are excreted mainly in urine, exhaled air, and probably in faeces. The elimination half-life of thiocyanate is 2.7-7 days when renal function is normal but is longer in patients with impaired renal function or hyponatraemia.

Pharmaceutical particulars

List of excipients: Not applicable. There is no overage included in the formulation.

Incompatibilities: Nitroprusside forms highly coloured reaction products with a wide variety of therapeutic agents, and admixture should be avoided.

Shelf life: 36 months.

Special precautions for storage: Sodium nitroprusside vials and infusion solution should be protected from light; heat and moisture. Reconstituted intravenous infusion should be protected from light by covering with aluminium foil or other opaque material as quickly as possible.

Sodium Nitroprusside when reconstituted should be discarded after 24 hours. If the reconstituted solution is highly coloured, the solution should be discarded.

No preparation other than Glucose Injection BP should be added to the sodium nitroprusside vial or mixed with the infusion solution.

Instructions for use/handling: Not applicable.

Marketing authoristion number 4515/0016

Date of approval/revision of SPC 31 January 1997

Legal category POM

TOBRAMYCIN INJECTION BP

Presentation Tobramycin Injection BP is a sterile, colourless solution. It contains tobramycin 40 mg per ml or 10 mg per ml (paediatric formulation only). The solution also contains in each ml; 0.1 mg disodium edetate BP, and 2.4 mg metabisulphite presented in clear glass vials.

Uses Tobramycin is an aminoglycoside antibiotic obtained from cultures of Streptomyces tenebrarius. Tobramycin Injection BP is indicated in the treatment of the following serious infections caused by susceptible micro-organisms:

1. central nervous system infections including meningitis, septicaemia and neonatalsepsis;
2. gastro-intestinal infections including peritonitis;
3. complicated and recurrent urinary tract infections such as pyelonephritis and cystitis;
4. lower respiratory tract infections, including pneumonia, bronchopneumonia and acutebronchitis;
5. skin, bone and soft tissue infections including burns.

Tobramycin may be considered in serious staphylococcal infections for which penicillin or other less potentially toxic drugs are contra-indicated and when bacterial susceptibility testing and clinical judgement indicate its use.

Tobramycin is usually active against most strains of the following organisms:

Pseudomonas aeruginosa

Proteus species (indole-positive and indole-negative), including *Pr. mirabilis, Pr. rettgeri* and *Pr. vulgaris; Morganella morganii, Escherichia coli,* Klebsiella-Enterobacter-Serratia species, Citrobacter species, Providencia species, Staphylococci including *Staphylococcus aureus* (coagulase-positive and coagulase-negative).

Most strains of enterococci demonstrate resistance although some strains of group D streptococci are susceptible in vivo. The combination of tobramycin and carbenicillin is synergistic in vitro against most strains of *Ps. aeruginosa.* Other Gram-negative organisms may be affected synergistically by the combination of tobramycin and a cephalosporin.

Prior to initiation of tobramycin therapy, appropriate specimens should be collected for identification of the causative organism and in vitro susceptibility tests. Tobramycin may be started pending results of susceptibility tests but should be discontinued if the causative organism is shown to be resistant to the drug. The decision to continue tobramycin therapy should be based upon the results of susceptibility studies, severity of the infection, and the important additional concepts discussed under 'Warnings'.

Dosage and administration Tobramycin may be given intramuscularly or intravenously and the dosage is the same for either route of administration. To calculate the correct dosage, the patients pretreatment bodyweight should be obtained.

Patients with normal renal funtion:
Adults: For adults with serious infections the usual recommended dosage is 3 mg/kg/day, administered in three equal doses every eight hours (see Table 1)

Patients with life-threatening infections, dosages up to 5 mg/kg/day may be administered in three or four equal dosages. The dosage should be reduced to 3 mg/kg/day as soon as clinically indicated. Dosage should not exceed 5 mg/kg/day, unless serum levels are monitored in order to prevent increased toxicity due to excessive blood levels (See *Warnings and Precautions*).

It may be necessary to administer up to 8 to 10 mg/kg/day in equally divided doses, to achieve therapeutic serum levels for patients with cystic fibrosis. Serum levels should be monitored because serum concentrations of tobramycin vary from patient to patient.

In adults with normal renal function, mild to moderate infections of the urinary tract have responded to a dosage of 2-3 mg/kg/day administered as a single intramuscular injection.

Table 1: Dosage schedule for adults with normal renal function

(Dosage at 8-hour intervals)

Patient Weight	*Usual dose for Serious Infections 1 mg/kg q 8h. (Total 3 mg/kg/day)*		*Maximum dose for Life-threatening Infections (Reduce as soon as possible) 1.66 mg/kg q 8h (Total 5 mg/kg/day-unless monitored)*	
kg	*mg/dose*	*ml/dose**	*mg/dose*	*ml/dose**
120	120	3.0	200	5.0
100	100	2.5	166	4.0
80	80	2.0	133	3.0
60	60	1.5	100	2.5
40	40	1.0	66	1.6

* Applicable to 40 mg/ml product forms.

Elderly: As for adults, but see recommendations for patients with impaired renal function.

Children: The recommended dosage is 6-7.5 mg/kg/day, administered in 3 or 4 equally divided doses. It may be necessary to administer higher doses in some patients.

Premature or full-term neonates: Dosages of up to 4 mg/kg/day may be administered in two equal doses every 12 hours, for children between 1.5 and 2.5 kg body weight.

The usual length of treatment is seven to ten days. However, in difficult and complicated infections, a longer course of therapy may be necessary. In such cases monitoring of renal, auditory and vestibular functions is advised because neurotoxicity is more likely to occur when treatment is extended longer than ten days.

To ensure the correct dosage is given, it is recommended that blood levels should be determined whenever possible. Blood levels should always be determined in patients with chronic infections such as cystic fibrosis, or where longer duration of treatment may be necessary, or in patients with decreased renal function.

Patients with impaired renal function: Following a loading dose of 1 mg/kg, subsequent dosage must be adjusted, either with lower doses administered at 8hr intervals or with normal doses at prolonged intervals, (see Table 2). Both these regimens are suggested as guides to be used when serum levels of tobramycin can not be measured directly. They are based on either the creatinine clearance or the serum creatinine of the patient, because these values correlate with the half-life of tobramycin. Neither regimen should be used when dialysis is being performed.

Regimen I-Reduced dosage at 8-hour intervals: An appropriate reduced dosage range can be found in the accompanying table, (Table 2) for any patient for whom the creatinine clearance or serum creatinine values are known. The choice of dose within the indicated range should be based on the severity of the infection, the sensitivity of the pathogen, and individual patient considerations, especially renal function. Another rough guide for determining reduced dosage at 8-hour intervals, e.g. for patients whose steady-state serum creatinine values are known is to divide the normally recommended dose by the patient's serum creatinine value (mg/100 ml).

Regimen II - Normal dosage at prolonged intervals: Table 2 illustrates the recommended intervals between doses. As a general rule, the dosage frequency in hours can be determined by multiplying the patient's serum creatinine level (expressed as mg/100 ml) by six.

The dosage schedules derived from either method should be used in conjunction with careful clinical and laboratory observations of the patient and should be modified as necessary (see *Warnings*).

Intramuscular administration: Tobramycin may be administered by withdrawing the appropriate dose directly from the vial.

Intravenous administration: Tobramycin Injection BP may be given by intravenous infusion or by direct intravenous injection. When given by infusion, tobramycin may be diluted (with 0.9% Sodium Chloride Intravenous Infusion BP or 5% Dextrose Intravenous Infusion BP) to volumes of 50-100 ml for adult doses. For children, the volume of diluent should be proportionately less than for adults. The diluted solution should be infused over a period of 20-60 minutes avoiding admixture with any other drug. Tobramycin may be administered by direct intravenous injection or into the tubing of a drip set. When given in this way, serum levels may exceed 12 mg/L for a short time (See *Contra-indications, warnings, etc*).

It is recommended that both peak and trough serum levels should be determined whenever possible to ensure the correct dosage is given.

Following IM administration of a single dose of tobramycin of 1 mg/kg in adults with normal renal function, peak plasma tobramycin concentrations averaging 4-6 mcg/mL are attained within 30-90 minutes; plasma concentrations of the drug are 1 mcg/mL or less at 8 hours. Following intravenous infusion of the same dose over 30-60 minutes, similar plasma concentrations of the drug are obtained. In neonates, average peak plasma tobramycin concentrations of about 5 mcg/mL are attained 30-60 minutes after a single IM dose of 2 mg/kg; plasma concentrations average 1-2 mcg/mL at 12 hours.

Contra-indications, warnings, etc

Contra-indications: Intrathecal administration. Because of the known cross-allergenicity of drugs in this class, hypersensitivity to any aminoglycoside is a contraindication to the use of tobramycin.

Warnings: Tobramycin contains sodium metabisulphite which may cause allergic-type reactions, including anaphylactic symptoms and life-threatening or less severe asthmatic episodes, in certain susceptible people. The overall prevalence of sulphite sensitivity in the general population is unknown and probably low, but it occurs more frequently in asthmatic patients.

Cross-allergenicity among aminoglycosides has been known to occur. Patients treated with aminoglycoside antibiotics such as tobramycin should be under close clinical observation because these drugs have an inherent potential for causing nephrotoxicity and ototoxicity.

Both vestibular and auditory ototoxicity can occur. Eighth nerve impairment may develop in patients with pre-existing renal damage, and if tobramycin is administered for longer periods or in higher doses than those recommended. Other manifestations of neurotoxicity may include numbness, skin tingling, muscle twitching and convulsions. The risk of aminoglycoside-induced hearing loss increases with the degree of exposure to either high peak or high trough serum concentrations. Patients who develop cochlear damage may not have symptoms during therapy to warn of eighth-nerve toxicity, and partial or total irreversible bilateral deafness may continue to develop after the drug has been discontinued. Rarely, nephrotoxicity may not become manifest until the first few days after cessation of therapy. Aminoglycoside-induced nephrotoxicity is usually reversible. Therefore, renal and eighth cranial nerve function should be closely monitored in patients with known or suspected renal impairment and also in those whose renal function is initially normal but who develop signs of renal dysfunction during therapy.

*Table 2: Two maintenance regimens based on renal function and body weight following a loading dose of 1 mg/kg**

Renal Function°			*Regimen I*		*or Regimen II*
			Adjusted doses at 8-hour intervals		*Normal dosage at prolonged intervals*
Serum Creatinine		*Creatinine Clearance*	*Weight*		*Weight/Dose 50-60 kg : 60 mg 60-80 kg : 80 mg*
mg/100 ml	*mmol/L*	*ml/min*	*50-60 kg*	*60-80 kg*	
< 1.3	< 114.9	> 70	60 mg	80 mg	q. 8h
1.4–1.9	123.8–168	69–40	30–60 mg	50–80 mg	q. 12h
2.0–3.3	176.8–291.7	39–20	20–25 mg	30–45 mg	q. 18h
3.4–5.3	300.6–468.5	19–10	10–18 mg	15–24 mg	q. 24h
5.3–7.5	477.4–663	9–5	5–9 mg	7–12 mg	q. 36h
> 7.6	> 671.8	< 4	2.5–4.5 mg	3.5–6 mg	q. 48h†

* For life-threatening infections, dosages 50% above those normally recommended may be used. The dosages should be reduced as soon as possible when improvement is noted.

° If used to estimate degree of renal impairment, serum creatinine concentrations should reflect a steady state of renal azotaemia.

† When dialysis is not being performed.

Evidence of impairment in renal, vestibular and/or auditory function requires discontinuation of the drug or dosage adjustment.

In elderly patients, it is particularly important to monitor renal function, when reduced renal function may not be evident in the results of routine screening tests, such as blood urea or serum creatinine. A creatinine clearance determination may be more useful.

Serum concentrations should be monitored when possible, and prolonged concentrations above 12 mg/L should be avoided. A useful guideline would be to perform serum level assays after 2 or 3 doses and also at 3 or 4 day intervals during therapy, so that the dosage could be adjusted if necessary. In the event of changing renal function, more frequent serum levels should be obtained and the dosage or dosage intervals adjusted according to the guidelines provided in the 'Dosage and Administration' section. In order to measure the peak level, a serum sample should be drawn about 30 minutes following intravenous infusion or at one hour after intramuscular injection. Trough levels are measured by obtaining serum samples at 8 hours or just prior to the next dose of tobramycin.

Urine should be examined for increased excretion of protein, cells and casts. Serum creatinine or creatinine clearance (preferred over blood urea) should be measured periodically. When possible, it is recommended that serial audiograms be obtained in patients old enough to be tested, particularly high-risk patients.

In patients with normal renal function who do not receive tobramycin in higher doses or for longer periods of time than those recommended, the risk of toxic reactions is low. However, patients with reduced renal function are prone to the potential ototoxic and nephrotoxic effects of this drug, so dosage should be adjusted carefully on the basis of regular monitoring of serum drug concentrations and of renal function.

Concurrent and sequential use of other nephrotic, neurotoxic or ototoxic drugs, particularly streptomycin, neomycin, kanamycin, gentamicin, cephaloridine, paromomycin, viomycin, polymyxin B, colistin, cisplatin, vancomycin and amikacin, should be avoided. Advanced age and dehydration may also increase patient risk.

Tobramycin should not be given concurrently with potent diuretics. Some diuretics themselves cause ototoxicity, and diuretics administered intravenously enhance aminoglycoside toxicity by altering antibiotic concentrations in serum and tissue.

Use in pregnancy and lactation:

Use in pregnancy: Aminoglycosides can cause foetal harm when administered to a pregnant woman. Aminoglycosides such as tobramycin cross the placenta. Serious side-effects to mother, foetus, or newborn have not been reported in the treatment of pregnant women with other aminoglycosides, but tobramycin should not be administered to the pregnant patient unless the potential benefits clearly outweigh any potential risk. If tobramycin is used during pregnancy or if the patient becomes pregnant whilst taking tobramycin, she should be informed of the potential hazard to the foetus.

Use in lactation: Tobramycin is excreted in the breast milk and should be avoided in nursing women.

Precautions:

Use in neonates: Tobramycin should be used with caution and in reduced dosage in premature and full term neonate infants younger than 6 weeks of age because of their renal immaturity and the resulting prolongation of serum half-life of the drug.

General: It is desirable to measure both peak and trough serum concentrations as high doses of drug may be associated with a greater risk of toxicity.

Serum calcium, magnesium and sodium should be monitored. It is particularly important to monitor serum levels closely in patients with known renal impairment.

In patients with extensive burns, altered pharmacokinetics may result in reduced serum drug levels. Dosage must be based on measured serum levels in these patients.

Aminoglycosides may be absorbed in significant quantities from body surfaces for local irrigation or application and may cause neurotoxicity and nephrotoxicity.

Aminoglycosides should be used with caution in patients with muscular disorders, such as myasthenia gravis or parkinsonism, since these drugs may aggravate muscle weakness because of their potential curare-like effect on neuromuscular function.

The possibility of prolonged secondary apnoea should be considered if tobramycin is administered to anaesthetised patients who are also receiving neuromuscular blocking agents such as succinylcholine, tubocurarine or decamethonium, or to patients receiving massive transfusions of citrated blood. If neuromuscular blockade occurs, it may be reversed by the administration of calcium salts.

The inactivation of tobramycin by beta-lactam-type antibiotics (penicillins or cephalosporins) has been demonstrated in vitro and in patients with severe renal impairment. Such inactiviation has not been found in patients with normal renal function if the drugs are administered by separate routes.

If overgrowth of non-susceptible organisms occurs appropriate therapy should be initiated.

Side-effects: Renal function changes such as rising blood urea and serum creatinine and by oliguria, cylindruria and increased proteinuria, have been reported, especially in patients with a history of renal impairment who are treated for longer periods or with higher doses than these recommended. These changes can occur in patients with initially normal renal function.

In patients receiving high doses or prolonged therapy, side effects on both vestibular and auditory branches of the eighth cranial nerve have been reported. Similar effects have been noted in those given previous courses of therapy with an ototoxin, and in cases of dehydration. Symptoms include dizziness, vertigo, tinnitus, roaring in the ears and hearing loss. Hearing loss is usually irreversible and is manifested initially by diminution of high tone acuity.

Other side effects attributed to tobramycin have been reported such as increased AST, ALT, and serum bilirubin; decreased serum calcium, magnesium, sodium, potassium; anaemia, granulocytopenia, thrombocytopenia, leucopenia, leucocytosis and eosinophilia; and fever, rash, itching, urticaria, nausea, vomiting, headache, lethargy, pain at injection site, mental confusion and disorientation.

Overdose: Severity of the manifestations of a tobramycin overdose depend on the dose, the patient's renal function, state of hydration, age and whether concurrent medication with similar toxicities is being given.

Nephrotoxicity following the parenteral administration of an aminoglycoside is most closely related to the AUC of serum concentrations versus time. Nephrotoxicity is more likely if trough levels fail to fall below 2 mcg/mL and is also proportional to the average blood concentration. Patients who are elderly, have renal impairment, are receiving other nephrotoxic or ototoxic drugs, or are volume depleted, are at greater risk for developing acute tubular necrosis or auditory and vestibular toxicity. These patients often experience dizziness, tinnitus, vertigo and a loss of high-tone acuity. Neuromuscular blockade or respiratory failure may occur following rapid intravenous administration of many aminoglycosides. These reactions and prolonged respiratory paralysis may occur more commonly in patients with myasthenia gravis or Parkinson's disease, or those receiving decamethonium, tubocurarine or succinylcholine.

Toxicity from ingested tobramycin is unlikely because aminoglycosides are poorly absorbed from an intact gastro-intestinal tract.

Treatment of overdose: Haemodialysis or peritoneal dialysis will help remove tobramycin from the blood in the event of overdosage or toxic reactions. Depending on the duration and type of dialysis employed, approximately 25-70% of the administered dose may be removed. Haemodialysis is the more effective method. Calcium salts given intravenously have been used to counter neuromuscular blockade, the effectiveness of neostigmine has been variable.

Pharmaceutical precautions

Incompatibilities: Incompatibility or loss of activity has been reported between tobramycin sulphate and some cephalosporins and penicillins and also heparin sodium. Solutions with clindamycin phosphate in glucose injection are reported to be unstable.

Tobramycin Injection BP should not be physically premixed with other drugs but should be administered separately according to the recommended dose and route.

Storage: Store below 25°C and protect from light.

Legal category POM

Package quantities All presentations are available in packs of 5.

Further information Nil.

Product licence numbers

40 mg/ml	4515/0066
80 mg/2 ml	4515/0066
20 mg/2 ml	4515/0067

VANCOMYCIN HYDROCHLORIDE FOR INJECTION BP

Qualitative and quantitative composition Vancomycin BP 500 mg and 1 gram.

Pharmaceutical form Freeze dried powder in clear glass vial for reconstitution before injection.

Clinical particulars

Therapeutic indications: Vancomycin is an amphoteric glycopeptide antimicrobial substance produced by the growth of certain strains of *Nocardia orientalis* (formerly known as *Streptomyces orientalis*). It is bactericidal against many gram-positive organisms. Vancomycin is not chemically related to any of the presently used antimicrobial agents.

Vancomycin is indicated in potentially life-threatening infections due to susceptible gram-positive organisms which cannot be treated by other effective, less toxic antimicrobial drugs, such as the penicillins and cephalosporins. As Vancomycin is the only currently available antibiotic to which nearly all strains of Staphylococcus remain susceptible, it should be reserved for those cases where there is a specific indication, to minimise the chance of resistance emerging. Vancomycin is one of the agents of choice in treating methicillin resistant Staphylococcal infection.

Staphylococcal infections: Vancomycin is useful in therapy of severe Staphylococcal infections in patients who cannot receive or who have failed to respond to the penicillins and cephalosporins or who have infections with Staphylococci that are resistant to other antibiotics, including methicillin. Vancomycin has been used successfully alone in the treatment of staphylococcal endocarditis. Its efficacy has been documented in other infections due to staphylococci, including osteomyelitis, pneumonia, septicaemia and soft tissue infections.

Pseudomembranous colitis:

Oral Vancomycin is indicated for severe cases of antibiotic-associated pseudomembranous colitis (usually involving *Clostridium difficile*). Vancomycin is not absorbed from the gastrointestinal tract and faecal levels are many times higher than the M.I.C.'s needed. The incidence of relapse is approximately 14% and usually occurs 4 to 21 days after Vancomycin is discontinued. Patients appear to respond to a second course of oral Vancomycin. (Note: Intravenous Vancomycin is ineffective in treating pseudomembranous colitis.)

Posology and method of administration: The usual adult intravenous dose is 500 mg every six hours or 1 g every twelve hours. Staphylococcal infections normally respond within 48 to 72 hours. Duration of therapy depends on type and severity of infections and patient response. For bacterial endocarditis, the generally accepted regimen is 500 mg Vancomycin intravenously every six hours for a minimum of three weeks either alone or in combination with other antibiotics.

Therapeutic range of serum levels: During chronic therapy peak concentration should be kept within the range 10-20 micrograms/ml.

Pseudomembranous colitis: The recommended dose is 250 mg taken orally every six hours for 5 to 10 days. Even doses of 125 mg six hourly, produce faecal levels of Vancomycin well above those needed to kill most strains of C. difficile. Relapse rate is about 14% and may appear within 1 to 3 weeks of stopping therapy but responds to a further course of Vancomycin.

Preparation of solution: At the time of use, add 10 ml of sterile Water for Injections BP to a 500 mg vial of Vancomycin powder for Injection. Similarly, add 20 ml of sterile Water for Injections BP to a 1 gram vial of Vancomycin powder for Injection. Vials reconstituted in this manner will give a solution of 50 mg/ml. Further dilution is required depending on method of administration.

Intravenous: Intermittent infusion (the preferred method of administration): Reconstituted solutions containing 500 mg Vancomycin must be diluted with at least 100 ml diluent. Reconstituted solutions containing 1 g vancomycin must be diluted with at least 200 ml diluent. Sodium Chloride Intravenous infusion BP or 5% Dextrose Intravenous Infusion BP are suitable diluents. The desired dose should be given by intravenous infusion over a period of at least 60 minutes. If administered over a shorter period of time or in higher concentrations there is the possibility of inducing marked hypotension in addition to thrombophlebitis. Rapid administration may also produce flushing and a transient rash over the neck and shoulders.

Continuous infusion (should only be used when intermittent infusion not feasible): 1 g or 2 g of Vancomycin may be added to a sufficiently large volume of Sodium Chloride 0.9% Injection or Glucose 5% in Water for Injection to permit the desired dose to be infused over twenty-four hours.

Oral: After initial reconstitution of the vial, the selected dose 250 mg (5 ml) or 125 mg (2.5 ml) may be diluted in 30 ml of water and given to the patient to drink or the diluted material may be given down a nasogastric tube. Vancomycin is not effective orally for conditions other than pseudomembranous colitis.

Paediatric: Intravenous: The usual intravenous dosage is 10 mg/kg per dose given every 6 hours (total daily dosage 40 mg/kg of body weight). Each dose should be administered over a period of at least 60 minutes. In neonates and young infants, the total daily dosage may be lower. An initial dose of 15 mg/kg is suggested, followed by 10 mg/kg every 12 hours in the first week of life and every 8 hours thereafter until one month of age. Each dose should be administered over 60 minutes. Close monitoring of serum vancomycin concentrations may be warranted in these patients.

Oral: Can be administered using 40 mg per kg body weight in three or four divided doses for 7–10 days. The total daily dose of Vancomycin is normally 125 mg every six hours for a period of 7-14 days for the treatment of antibiotic associated diarrhoea caused by *Clostridium difficile*.

Geriatric: Because of its ototoxicity and nephrotoxicity, Vancomycin should be used with caution in patients with renal insufficiency or previous hearing loss. The elderly are particularly at risk. Doses should be titrated on the basis of serum levels. The elderly are particularly susceptible to auditory damage and should be given serial tests for auditory function if over the age of 60. Concurrent or sequential use of other neurotoxic substances should be avoided.

With impaired renal function: In patients with impaired renal function, dosage regimen of Vancomycin must be modified in response to degree of renal impairment, severity of infection, susceptibility of causative organism and serum concentrations of the drug. A suggested starting dose in patients with impaired renal function is 15 mg/kg with subsequent doses based mainly on renal function and serum concentrations of the drug.

In patients on haemodialysis, the drug is not significantly removed by haemodialysis. A dose of 1 g of Vancomycin every seven days produces effective blood levels. Serum levels should be monitored to avoid drug accumulation and resultant toxicity. The serum half-life ranges from 120 to 216 hours.

In patients undergoing peritoneal dialysis, the half-life of Vancomycin has been reported at around 18 hours. To prevent undue lowering of serum levels during peritoneal dialysis, an additional amount of Vancomycin could be added to the dialysate in a concentration of 25 microgram per ml.

Contra-indications: Vancomycin is contra-indicated in patients with known hypersensitivity to this drug.

Special warnings and special precautions for use:
Warnings: Because of its toxicity and nephrotoxicity, Vancomycin should be used with care in patients with renal impairment. The risk of toxicity is increased by high blood concentrations or prolonged therapy. Therefore, blood levels should be monitored and dosage adjusted if it is necessary to use Vancomycin in such patients.

The concurrent or sequential use of other nephrotoxic drugs requires careful monitoring and should be avoided if possible.

Vancomycin should, if possible, be avoided in patients with previous hearing loss. If used it is very important that the dose be adjusted by monitoring the blood concentrations of the drug. Deafness may be preceded by tinnitus. The elderly are more susceptible to auditory damage. Experience with other antibiotics suggests that deafness may be progressive despite cessation of treatment.

Precautions: Vancomycin is very irritating to tissue and causes necrosis if injected intramuscularly. Pain and thrombophlebitis occur in many patients receiving Vancomycin and are occasionally severe. The frequency and severity of thrombophlebitis can be minimised if the drug is administered in a volume of at least 200 ml of glucose or saline solution and if the sites of injection are changed regularly. Complications of occasional severe hypotension, histamine like responses and maculopapular or erythematous rash ('red man's syndrome' or 'red neck syndrome') are thought to be related to the rate of the infusion and can be avoided by administration of the recommended dilute solutions over at least 20 to 30 minutes. One gram doses should be given over at least one hour and slow infusions over one hour are recommended for infants and children.

All patients receiving Vancomycin should have periodic haematological studies, urine analysis, liver and renal function tests.

Anaesthetic induced myocardial depression may be enhanced by Vancomycin. During anaesthesia, doses must be well diluted and administered slowly with close cardiac monitoring. Position changes should be delayed until the infusion is completed to allow for postural adjustment.

Patients taking oral Vancomycin should be warned of its offensive taste.

Interaction with other medicaments and other forms of interaction: Concurrent administration with other neurotoxic or nephrotoxic antibiotics, e.g. streptomycin, neomycin, gentamicin, kanamycin, amikacin, tobramycin, polymyxin B and colistin requires careful monitoring.

Diuretics such as ethacrynic acid and frusemide may aggravate ototoxicity.

Cholestyramine has been shown to bind Vancomycin in-vitro. Therefore, if oral Vancomycin is used with cholestyramine, the two drugs should be administered several hours apart.

Pregnancy and lactation:

Use in pregnancy: As there is little information on the use of Vancomycin in pregnancy, the drug should not be used in pregnant women or those likely to become pregnant unless the expected benefits outweigh any potential risk.

Use in lactation: Vancomycin is excreted in breast milk but it is not known whether it is harmful to the newborn. Therefore, it is not recommended for nursing mothers unless the expected benefits outweigh any potential risk.

Effects on ability to drive and use machines: Not applicable.

Undesirable effects:

Adverse reactions: Auditory and vestibular: Sensorineural deafness which may be accompanied by tinnitus has occurred but the incidence is low. Permanent deafness is more likely to occur in patients with compromised auditory or renal function but reversible deafness has been reported in normal patients.

Cardiovascular: Hypotension, palpitations, substernal pressure, tachycardia. (All effects due to excessively rapid infusion or insufficient dilution of drug.)

Dermatological: Pruritus at injection site, generalised flushing, erythematous macular rash with intense pruritus over face, neck and upper body have occurred after too rapid injection of the drug. Tissue irritation and necrosis occurs after I.M. injection or extravasation from I.V. site.

Gastrointestinal: Oral doses are extremely unpalatable. In leukaemic patients, oral dosing regimens are associated with frequent nausea, diarrhoea and occasional vomiting.

General: The use of Vancomycin may result in overgrowth of non-susceptible organisms resulting in new bacterial or fungal infections.

Genitourinary: Transient elevations of urea and granular casts in the urine occasionally occur. Nephrotoxicity in the presence of normal renal function at therapeutic serum levels is rare.

Haematological: Eosinophilia and neutropenia have been reported.

Immunological: Histamine release with chills, nausea, urticaria, macular rash, fever and rigors, even at normal doses but usually following rapid drug administration. Anaphylactoid reactions have been reported.

Ocular: Subconjunctival injections have infrequently been used in the treatment of bacterial corneal ulcers but may cause severe inflammation or sloughing.

Overdose: No information available except for that given under *Adverse Reactions* above.

Pharmacological properties

Pharmacodynamic properties: Vancomycin is a biological material, described as a tricyclic glycopeptide obtained from cultures of *Nocardia orientalis (Streptomyces orientalis)*. It is structurally unrelated to other antibiotics and is presented as the hydrochloride salt for parenteral administration. The drug is not absorbed from the gastrointestinal tract, and an aqueous solution of the product can be administered orally in the treatment of Pseudomembranous colitis.

Vancomycin is a bactericidal antibiotic and appears to bind to the bacterial cell wall causing blocckage of glycopeptide polymerisation. This effect produces immediate inhibition of cell wall synthesis and secondary damage to the cytoplasmic membrane. It is active against may gram positive organisms including staphylococci, group A beta haemolytic streptococci, streptococcus pneumoniae, enterococci, corynebacterium and clostridium species. It does not demonstrate clinical efficacy against gram negative bacteria, fungi or yewasts, and hence the product literature only indicates use in severe infections caused by gram positive organisms.

Pharmacokinetic properties: Vancomycin is poorly absorbed by mouth. An intravenous dose of 1 g produces serum levels averaging 25 microgram per ml after two hours in patients with normal renal function. Serum levels are higher in patients with renal impairment and toxicity may result. Vancomycin is excreted unchanged in the urine, at least 80% is excreted in the first 24 hours. It has a half-life of about 6 hours in patients with normal renal function.

Vancomycin readily diffuses into pleural, pericardial, ascitic and synovial fluids. It does not diffuse into cerebrospinal fluid with normal meninges, but therapeutic concentrations may be reached in patients with acute meningitis. Vancomycin is active against many gram-positive organisms including staphylococci, streptococci, corynebacterium and clostridium, including Clostridium difficile. Gram-negative bacteria, mycobacteria and fungi are highly resistant. Many strains of gram-positive bacteria are sensitive in-vitro toVancomycin concentrations of 0.5 to 5 microgram/ml, but a few Staph. aureus strains require 10-20 microgram/ml for inhibition.

Using the Bauer-Kirby method of disc susceptibility testing, a 30 microgram Vancomycin disc should produce a zone of more than 11 mm when tested against a Vancomycin sensitive strain.

Vancomycin appears to act by inhibiting the production of bacterial cell wall mucopeptide. This effect occurs at a site different from that affected by penicillins and produces immediate inhibition of cell wall synthesis and secondary damage to the cytoplasmic membrane.

Preclinical safety data: Not applicable.

Pharmaceutical particulars

List of excipients: Water for Injections BP removed during lyophilisation.

Incompatibilities: Chemically incompatible with Dexamethasone sodium phosphate, Heparin sodium, Methicillin sodium, phenobarbitone sodium, sodium bicarbonate.

Shelf life: 18 months.

Special precautions for storage: Store below 25°C and protect from light.

When aseptically prepared, the product may be stored for up to 24 hours at 2°C to 8°C. The product does not contain an antimicrobial preservative. Therefore if aseptic preparation cannot be ensured, the product should be prepared immediately before use and any unused portion discarded.

Instructions for use/handling: Vancomycin is very irritating to tissue and causes necrosis if injected intramuscularly. Pain and thrombophlebitis occur in many patients receiving vancomycin and are occasionally severe. The frequency and severity of thrombophlebitis can be minimised if the drug is administered in a volume of at least 200 ml of glucose or saline solution and if the sites of injection are changed regularly.

Complications of occasional severe hypotension, histamine like responses and maculopapular or erythematous rash ('red man's syndrome' or 'red neck syndrome') are thought to be related to the rate of the infusion and can be avoided by administration of the recommended dilute solutions over at least 20 to 30 minutes. One gram doses should be given over at least one hour and slow infusions over one hour are recommended for infants and children.

All patients receiving vancomycin should have periodic haematological studies, urine analysis, liver and renal function tests.

Anaesthetic induced myocardial depression may be enhanced by vancomycin. During anaesthesia, doses must be well diluted and administered slowly with close cardiac monitoring. Position changes should be delayed until the infusion is completed to allow for postural adjustment.

Patients taking oral vancomycin should be warned of its offensive taste.

Marketing authorisation number 4515/0053

Date of approval/revision of SPC 12 February 1997

Legal category POM

VINBLASTINE SULPHATE INJECTION SOLUTION 10MG/10ML

Qualitative and quantitative composition

	per unit dose	*per mL*
Vinblastine Sulphate	10 mg	1 mg
Sodium Chloride	90 mg	9 mg
Water for Injection	to 10 mL	to 1 mL

1N Sodium Hydroxide or 1N Sulphuric Acid is added to adjust the pH to be approximately 4.5

Pharmaceutical form Vinblastine Sulphate Injection Solution is a clear, colourless, sterile solution of Vinblastine Sulphate BP in Water for Injection BP It is presented in conventional glass vials and Onco-Tain* vials containing 10 ml of a 1 mg/ml solution of Vinblastine Sulphate BP and 9 mg/ml Sodium Chloride BP The solution does not contain any preservatives.

Clinical particulars

Therapeutic indications: Vinblastine Sulphate is a cytotoxic drug that arrests cell growth at the metaphase. Its actions are more pronounced on the rapidly dividing cell than on the normal cell. It appears to act, like Vincristine, by binding to the microtubular proteins of the mitotic spindle, preventing polymerisation.

Vinblastine Sulphate is effective as a single agent, but its therapeutic effect is enhanced when used in combination with other antineoplastic drugs. Vinblastine Sulphate has been used in the treatment of Hodgkin's Disease (Stages III and IV); lymphocytic lymphoma (nodular and diffuse, poorly and well differentiated); histiocytic lymphoma; advanced stages of mycosis fungoides; advanced carcinoma of the testis; Kaposi's sarcoma and Letterer-Siwe disease (histocytosis X). Vinblastine Sulphate may be used in the treatment of choriocarcinoma resistant to other chemotherapeutic agents; carcinoma of the breast, unresponsive to appropriate endocrine surgery and hormonal therapy.

Posology and method of administration: The solution may be injected either directly into the vein or into the injection site of a running intravenous infusion. Injection of Vinblastine Sulphate may be completed in about one minute.

This preparation is for intravenous use only. Intrathecal administration usually results in death. (See warnings).

Syringes containing this product should be overlabelled with the intrathecal warning label provided –'NOT FOR INTRATHECAL USE'.

Dosage: Vinblastine Sulphate is given intravenously at weekly intervals according to the needs of the patient. Therapy is initiated by a single intravenous dose in accordance with the following dosage table, and white blood cell counts should be made to determine the sensitivity of the patient to Vinblastine. Dosage should not be increased after that dose which reduces the white cell count to approximately 3000 cells/mm³.

	Adults *mg/m² bsa*	*Children* *mg/m² bsa*
First Dose	3.7	2.5
Second Dose	5.5	3.75
Third Dose	7.4	5.0
Fourth Dose	9.25	6.25
Fifth Dose	11.1	7.5

Dosage increase may be continued but must not exceed 18.5 mg/m² for adults or 12.5 mg/m² for children.

Patients should be maintained on the maximum weekly dose that does not cause the above degree of leucopenia.

For most adult patients this dosage will be 5.5 mg/m²–7.4 mg/m², however, leucopenia can be produced at 3.7 mg/m², other patients may require 11.1 mg/m² and, very rarely, 18.5 mg/m².

A FURTHER DOSE OF VINBLASTINE SHOULD NOT BE GIVEN UNTIL THE WHITE CELL COUNT HAS RETURNED TO AT LEAST 4000/mm³, EVEN THOUGH 7 DAYS MAY HAVE ELAPSED.

In some cases, oncolytic activity may be encountered before the leucopenic effect and, when this occurs, there is no necessity to increase subsequent doses.

Duration of maintenance therapy is dependent upon the disease state and the antineoplastic agent combination.

Differing clinical opinions are held for the appropriate duration of maintenance therapy in Hodgkin's Disease. Prolonged chemotherapy for maintaining remissions involves several risks such as life-threatening infections, sterility and possibly the appearance of other cancers through suppression of immune response.

Vinblastine should not be given intramuscularly, subcutaneously or intrathecally.

Contra-indications: This preparation is for intravenous use only. Intrathecal administration usually results in death (see *Warnings*).

Vinblastine Sulphate is contra-indicated in patients who are leucopenic. It should not be used in the presence of bacterial infection. Such infections should be brought under control with antiseptics or antibiotics before the initiation of therapy with Vinblastine Sulphate.

Special warnings and special precautions for use:

Warnings: Vinblastine Sulphate must be used only by physicians experienced in cytotoxic chemotherapy.

Syringes containing this product should be overlabelled with the intrathecal warning label provided –'NOT FOR INTRATHECAL USE'.

The following treatment successfully arrested progresive paralysis in a single patient mistakenly given the related vincristine sulphate, intrathecally. This treatment should be initiated immediately:

1. Removal of as much CSF as is safely possible.
2. Flushing with Lactated Ringer's solution by continuous infusion at 150 ml/h, through a catheter in a cerebral lateral ventricle and removed through lumbar access, until fresh plasma becomes available.
3. Fresh frozen plasma, 25 ml, diluted with 1 L of Lactated Ringer's was then infused similarly at 75 ml/h. The rate of infusion should be adjusted to maintain a spinal fluid protein level of 150 mg/dl.
4. Glutamic acid, 10 gm, was given iv over 24 hours, followed by 500 mg tds by mouth for 1 month. Glutamic acid may not be essential.

Vinblastine SHOULD NOT BE GIVEN intramuscularly, subcutaneously or intrathecally.

Caution is necessary with the use of Vinblastine Sulphate during pregnancy. There is insufficient information to assess Vinblastine Sulphate's effect on fertility in men and women. However, aspermia has been reported in man.

Animal studies suggest that teratogenic effects may occur. The drug should not be used in pregnant women unless the expected benefit outweighs the potential risk.

As with other antineoplastic agents, vinblastine may cause a severe local reaction on extravasation. If leakage into the surrounding tissue should occur during intravenous administration of Vinblastine Sulphate, the injection should be discontinued immediately and any remaining portion of the dose should be introduced into another vein. Local injection of hyaluronidase with the application of heat has been used to disperse the drug in order to minimise discomfort and the possibility of tissue damage.

Liver disease may alter the elimination of vinblastine in the bile, markedly increasing toxicity to peripheral nerves and necessitating a dosage modification in affected patients.

Precautions: Patients should be carefully monitored for infection until the white cell count has returned to normal levels, if leucopenia with less than 2000 white blood cells per mm3 occurs following a dose of Vinblastine Sulphate.

When cachexia or ulcerated areas of the skin are present, a more profound leucopenic response may be produced by vinblastine. Therefore, its use should be avoided in older persons suffering from either of these conditions.

Leucocyte and platelet counts have sometimes fallen precipitously after moderate doses of Vinblastine Sulphate in patients with malignant cell infiltration of the bone marrow.

Further use of the drug in such patients is inadvisable. Avoid contamination of the eye with Vinblastine Sulphate injection. If accidental contamination occurs, severe irritation or corneal ulceration may result. The affected eye should be thoroughly irrigated with water immediately.

Interaction with other medicaments and other forms of interaction:

(i) Vinblastine used as part of a combination regimen with mitomycin may result in acute respiratory distress and pulmonary infiltration.

(ii) Cases of respiratory distress with interstitial pulmonary infiltrates have been reported in patients given a regimen comprising vinblastine, mitomycin, and progesterone (MVP).

Pregnancy and lactation: Although information on the use of vinblastine during pregnancy is limited, the drug may cause foetal toxicity when administered to pregnant women. The drug causes resorption of foetuses in animals and produces gross foetal abnormalities in surviving offspring. There are no adequate and controlled studies to date using vinblastine in pregnant women, and the drug should be used during pregnancy only in life-threatening situations or severe disease for which safer drugs cannot be used or are ineffective. Women of childbearing potential should be advised to avoid becoming pregnant while receiving the drug. When vinblastine is administered during pregnancy or the patient becomes pregnant while receiving the drug, the patient should be informed of the potential hazard to the foetus.

The effect of vinblastine on fertility in humans is not fully known. Aspermia has occurred in some individuals during vinblastine therapy.

It is not known whether vinblastine is excreted in human milk. Because of the potential for serious adverse reactions due to vinblastine in nursing infants, a decision should be made whether to discontinue nursing or the drug, taking into account the importance of the drug to the mother.

Effects on ability to drive and use machines: Not applicable.

Undesirable effects: The incidence of side effects with Vinblastine Sulphate appears to be dose related and most do not persist longer than 24 hours. Neurological effects are uncommon but can occur and may last longer than 24 hours.

Leucopenia is the most common side effect and dose limiting factor.

The following side effects have been reported:

Gastrointestinal: nausea, vomiting, constipation, vesiculation of the mouth, diarrhoea, anorexia, abdominal pain, rectal bleeding, pharyngitis, haemorrhagic enterocolitis, bleeding for an old peptic ulcer.

Neurological: numbness, paraesthesias, peripheral neuritis, mental depression, loss of deep tendon reflexes, headache, convulsions.

Miscellaneous: malaise, weakness, dizziness, pain in tumour site, vesiculation of the skin, alopecia.

Antiemetics may be used to control nausea and vomiting. Alopecia is usually not total and in some cases the hair regrows during maintenance therapy.

Extravasation during intravenous injection may result in cellulitis and phlebitis. In extreme instances sloughing may occur.

Overdose: Side-effects following the use of vinblastine are dose related. Therefore, following administration of more than the recommended dose, patients can be expected to experience these effects in an exaggerated fashion.

In addition, neurotoxicity similar to that seen with vincristine sulphate may be observed.

Treatment: Supportive care should include: (1) prevention of the side effects that result from the syndrome of inappropriate secretion of antidiuretic hormone. This includes restriction of fluid intake and perhaps the use of a diuretic acting on the loop of Henle and distal tubule function; (2) administration of an anticonvulsant; (3) prevention and treatment of ileus; (4) monitoring the patient's cardiovascular system; and (5) daily blood counts for guidance in transfusion requirement.

The major effect of excessive doses of vinblastine will be on granulocytopoeisis, and this may be life-threatening.

Pharmacological properties

Pharmacodynamic properties: Although the mechanism of action has not been definitely established, vinblastine appears to bind to or crystallize critical microtubular proteins of the mitotic spindle, thus preventing their proper polymerization and causing metaphase arrest. In high concentrations, vinblastine also exerts complex effects on nucleic acid and protein synthesis. Vinblastine reportedly also interferes with amino acid metabolism by blocking cellular utilization of glutamic acid and thus inhibits purine synthesis, the citric acid cycle, and the formation of urea. Vinblastine exerts some immunosuppressive activity.

Pharmacokinetic properties: Vinblastine sulphate is unpredictably absorbed from the GI tract. Following intravenous administration, the drug is rapidly cleared from the blood and distributed into body tissues.

Vinblastine crosses the blood-brain barrier poorly and does not appear in the CSF in therapeutic concentrations. Vinblastine is reported to be extensively metabolized, primarily in the liver, to desacetylvinblastine, which is more active than the parent compound on a weight basis. The drug is excreted slowly in urine and in faeces via the bile.

Pharmaceutical particulars

List of excipients:

Sodium Chloride BP	9.0 mg
Water for Injection BP	to 10.0 mL.

Incompatibilities: Vinblastine Sulphate is incompatible with furosemide, when injected sequentially into Y-site with no flush between or when mixed in syringe. Immediate precipitation results.

Shelf life: 24 months.

Special precautions for storage: The product must be stored between 2°C and 8°C and protected from light.

Instructions for use/handling:
Cytotoxic Handling Guidelines:

Administration: Should be administered only by or under the direct supervision of a qualified physician who is experienced in the use of cancer chemotherapeutic agents.

Preparation (Guidelines)

(a) Chemotherapeutic agents should be prepared for administration only by professionals who have been trained in the safe use of the preparation.

(b) Operations such as reconstitution of powder and transfer to syringes should be carried out only in the designated area.

(c) The personnel carrying out these procedures should be adequately protected with clothing, gloves and eye shield.

(d) Pregnant personnel are advised not to handle chemotherapeutic agents.

Contamination

(a) In the event of contact with the skin or eyes, the affected area should be washed with copious amounts of water or normal saline. A bland cream may be used to treat the transient stinging of skin. Medical advice should be sought if the eyes are affected.

(b) In the event of spillage, operators should put on gloves and mop up the spilled material with a sponge kept in the area for that purpose. Rinse the area twice with water. Put all solutions and sponges into a plastic bag and seal it.

Disposal: Syringes, containers, absorbent materials, solution and any other contaminated material should be placed in a thick plastic bag or other impervious container and incinerated.

Marketing authorisation number 4515/0051

Date of approval/revision of SPC 9 August 1996

Legal category POM

VINCRISTINE SULPHATE INJECTION SOLUTION

Qualitative and quantitative composition

Active Constituent	
Vincristine Sulphate BP	1.0 mg.
Other Constituents	
Mannitol BP	100.0 mg
Water for Injections BP	to 1.0 mL.

There is no overage in this formulation.

Pharmaceutical form A sterile, colourless solution.

Clinical particulars

Therapeutic indications: Vincristine Sulphate is used primarily as a component of various chemotherapeutic regimens for the treatment of acute leukaemias. It has also been used in conjunction with other oncolytic drugs in the treatment of Hodgkin's Disease, all forms of lymphoma, Wilm's tumour, sarcomas and tumours of the breast, brain and lung.

Posology and method of administration: This preparation is for intravenous use only. Intrathecal administration usually results in death (see *Warnings* for treatment).

Vincristine Sulphate is administered by intravenous injection at weekly intervals, the precise dose being determined by body weight.

Great care should be exercised in calculating the dose as overdosage may be extremely serious or even fatal. The dose should not be increased beyond the level which produces therapeutic benefit. In general, individual doses should not exceed 2 mg; and white cell counts should be carried out before and after giving each dose.

Vincristine Sulphate for Injection BP after reconstitution as directed (see below) or Vincristine Sulphate Injection Solution may be injected into the tubing or side arm of a free-flowing I.V. infusion or directly into a vein over a one-minute period. For safety reasons when administering Vincristine Injection into a side arm of a fast running infusion, please ensure that pressure is maintained on the syringe plunger during administration, to avoid back pressure from the infusion forcing the plunger out of the syringe barrel. Care should be taken to avoid extravasation as this may cause local ulceration.

Because of the narrow range between therapeutic and toxic levels and variations in response, the dosage must always be adjusted to the individual.

The following dosage regimens have been used:

Acute leukaemia:

Adults: The suggested dose is 25-75 micrograms/kg body weight (1.4 mg/m2 body surface area) by weekly intravenous injection.

Children: Weekly intravenous injections starting with 50 micrograms/kg body weight (1.5-2 mg/m2 body surface area) increasing by weekly increments of 25 micrograms/kg body weight to a maximum of 150 micrograms/kg body weight. The dose should not be increased after a response has been obtained and it may be possible to maintain remission with a reduced dose.

Elderly: The normal adult dose is still appropriate in the elderly.

Other tumours: 25 micrograms/kg body weight by weekly intravenous injection until a response is observed and 5-10 micrograms/kg body weight thereafter for maintenance.

Contra-indications: Intrathecal administration of Vincristine Sulphate is usually fatal. Although there are no other known contraindications to the use of Vincristine Sulphate, careful notice should be given to those conditions listed under *Warnings* and *Precautions.*

Breast feeding during treatment.

Special warnings and special precautions for use:
Warnings: Syringes containing this product should be labelled 'VINCRISTINE FOR INTRAVENOUS USE ONLY'.

After intrathecal administration, removal of cerebrospinal fluid, and flushing with Lactated Ringer's and other solutions, has not prevented ascending paralysis leading to death. In one adult paralysis was arrested, with some recovery, by the following treatment initiated immediately:-

1. Removal of as much CSF as is safely possible.
2. Flushing with Lactated Ringer's solution by continuous infusion at 150 ml/h, through a catheter in a cerebral lateral ventricle and removed through lumbar access, until fresh frozen plasma became available.
3. Fresh frozen plasma, 25 ml, diluted with 1l of Lactated Ringer's was then infused similarly at 75 ml/h. The rate of infusion was adjusted to maintain a spinal fluid protein level of 150 mg/dl.
4. Glutamic acid, 10 gm, was given iv over 24 hours, followed by 500 mg tds by mouth for 1 month. Glutamic acid may not be essential.

Vincristine Sulphate should only be administered by physicians experienced in cytotoxic chemotherapy.

Vincristine Sulphate should not be given by intrathecal, intramuscular or subcutaneous injection.

Vincristine Sulphate is a vesicant and may cause a severe local reaction or extravasation. If leakage into the surrounding tissue should occur during I.V. administration of Vincristine Sulphate, the injection should be discontinued immediately and any remaining portion of the dose should be introduced into another vein. Local injection of hyaluronidase with the application of heat has been used to disperse the drug in order to minimise discomfort and the possibility of tissue damage.

Precautions: Leucopenia is less likely following therapy with Vincristine Sulphate than is the case with other oncolytic agents. However, because of its possibility both physician and patient should remain alert for signs of any complicating infection. If leucopenia or a complicating infection is present, then administration of the next dose of Vincristine Sulphate warrants careful consideration.

Acute uric acid nephropathy, which may occur after administration of oncolytic agents, has also been reported with Vincristine Sulphate.

As Vincristine Sulphate penetrates the blood-brain barrier poorly, additional agents and routes of administration may be required for central nervous system leukaemias.

The neurotoxic effect of Vincristine Sulphate may be additive with other neurotoxic agents or increased by spinal cord irradiation and neurological disease. Elderly patients may be more susceptible to the neurotoxic effects of Vincristine Sulphate.

The elimination of Vincristine Sulphate may be reduced in the presence of impaired hepatic or biliary function and the dose must be decreased accordingly.

Care should be exercised to avoid accidental contamination of the eyes as Vincristine Sulphate is highly irritant and can cause corneal ulceration.

Interaction with other medicaments and other forms of interaction: Allopurinol, pyridoxine and isoniazid may increase the incidence of cytotoxic induced bone marrow depression. The mechanism for this potentiation has not been fully classified.

The neurotoxicity of Vincristine Sulphate may be additive with that of other drugs acting on the peripheral nervous system.

Vincristine Sulphate appears to increase the cellular uptake of Methotrexate by malignant cells and this principle has been applied in high-dose Methotrexate therapy.

Pregnancy and lactation: Safe use of Vincristine Sulphate during pregnancy has not been established. The drug should not be used in women who are or who may become pregnant, unless the expected benefit outweighs the potential risk. Women being treated with Vincristine should take appropriate contraceptive measures during therapy. Vinca alkaloids may effect fertility and have been shown to be embryocidal.

Vincristine Sulphate should not be used in women who are breastfeeding, unless the expected benefit outweighs the potential risk.

Effects on ability to drive and use machines: Not applicable.

Undesirable effects: Vincristine is a vesicant and may cause a severe local reaction on extravasation. It should only be administered by physicians experienced in cytotoxic chemotherapy.

Vincristine may cause granulocytopenia and users should be alert to signs of infection. Preexisting granulocytopenia does not preclude treatment, but care should be taken in such patients.

Daily administration of small doses of Vincristine Sulphate may result in the prolongation of side-effects which would otherwise be of short duration.

Side-effects of Vincristine Sulphate appear to be dose-related and, particularly in the case of neurotoxicity, related to the total accumulated dose given.

Neuropathies are the most common side effect in all age groups and are often dose-limiting. The neuropathy may occur as neuritic pain, paraesthesia, sensory loss and peroneal weakness resulting in foot drop and impaired gait. Headache and jaw pain are associated with cranial nerve involvement. No reversal agent for the neuromuscular effects has been reported as yet.

Gastrointestinal side-effects such as constipation, abdominal cramps, paralytic ileus, vomiting and diarrhoea may be encountered. The prophylactic use of stool softeners and mild cathartics is recommended to avoid impaction as a result of constipation.

Bladder neuropathies are uncommon but have been reported.

Reversible alopecia occurs in approximately 20% of all cases treated with Vincristine Sulphate and patients should be warned of this possibility. Other side effects reported in a small number of patients are weight loss, polyuria, dysuria and fever.

Overdose: Symptoms are those associated with acute neurotoxicity, seizures, fluid retention, paralytic ileus.

Side effects of Vincristine Sulphate are dose related and are exaggerated by overdosage. There is, as yet, no antidote for Vincristine Sulphate.

Support therapy should be directed to the prevention of the side effects resulting from hypersecretion of antidiuretic hormone by restriction of fluid intake and possibly the use of an appropriate diuretic. Anticonvulsants, e.g. phenobarbitone may be necessary for control of seizure and cathartics administered to prevent ileus.

Routine cardiovascular monitoring is recommended together with daily haematology as an indicator for transfusion requirements.

Folinic Acid has been used for the treatment of overdosage. An intravenous injection of 15 mg Folinic Acid may be given every 3 hours for 24 hours, then every 6 hours for at least 48 hours.

Pharmacological properties

Pharmacodynamic properties: Although the mechanism of action has not been definitely established, Vincristine appears to bind to or crystallize critical microtubular proteins of the mitotic spindle, thus preventing their proper polymerization and causing metaphase arrest. In high concentrations, the drug also exerts complex effects on nucleic acid and protein synthesis. Vincristine exerts some immuno-suppressive activity.

Pharmacokinetic properties: Vincristine is not reliably absorbed from the gastro-intestinal tract. After intravenous injection it disappears rapidly from the blood. It is extensively protein bound and it is reported to be concentrated in blood platelets. It is metabolised in the liver and excreted primarily in the bile–about 70% of a dose is found in faeces, as unchanged drug and metabolites, over 72 hours. Some also appears in the urine. Vincristine does not appear to cross the blood-brain barrier in significant amounts.

Following rapid I.V. injection of Vincristine, serum concentrations of the drug appear to decline in a triphasic manner. The terminal elimination half-life of Vincristine has ranged from 10.5-15.5 hours.

Pharmaceutical particulars

List of excipients:

Mannitol BP	100.0 mg
Water for Injections BP	to 1.0 mL.

There is no overage in this formulation.

Incompatibilities: It is not recommended that Vincristine Sulphate should be mixed with any other drug and should not be diluted in solutions that raise or lower the pH outside the range 3.5 to 5.5. Frusemide both in syringe and injected sequentially into Y-site with no flush between, results in immediate precipitation.

Shelf life: 24 months.

Special precautions for storage: Store between 2°C and 8°C. Protect from light.

Marketing authorisation number 4515/0008

Date of approval/revision of SPC August 1996

Legal category POM

**Trade Mark*

Ferring Pharmaceuticals Ltd
The Courtyard
Waterside Drive
Langley
Berkshire SL3 6EZ

☎ 01753 214800 🖷 01753 214801

FERRING
PHARMACEUTICALS

APROTININ INJECTION BP

Presentation A sterile, pyrogen-free, clear, colourless solution of Aprotinin 5.56 BP/EP Units per ml/ 10,000 KIU (Kallikrein Inactivator Units) per ml in 0.9% sodium chloride solution presented in 50 ml vials containing 70 mg aprotinin (500,000 KIU) and 5 ml ampoules containing 7 mg aprotinin (50,000 KIU).

Uses Aprotinin is a polyvalent protease inhibitor, isolated from animal tissue. It is active against certain proteolytic enzymes such as kallikrein, kinin, trypsin, chymotrypsin, plasmin, plasmin-activator, fibrin enzymes and tissue proteases. Aprotinin may be used therapeutically or prophylactically when these enzyme systems fail.

Aprotinin is a haemostatic. High doses offer major reductions in peri-operative blood loss and the need for donor blood transfusions. It is indicated for the treatment of life-threatening haemorrhage due to hyperplasminaemia.

Dosage and administration Intravenously by slow injection or infusion.

Dosage in adults: 500,000 to 1,000,000 KIU (277.8–555.6 EP Units) given by slow IV infusion (maximum rate 5 ml/min), followed by 200,000 KIU (111.1 EP Units) hourly until bleeding stops.

Dosage in the elderly: The dosage given above applies to persons of average bodyweight. Reductions of these doses should be considered in patients of below average weight.

Dosage in children: It is recommended that a dose proportional to the adult dose is calculated.

Contra-indications, warnings, etc
Contra-indications: Known hypersensitivity to aprotinin.

Interactions: None known.

Effects on ability to drive/use machines: None known; unlikely to be applicable as indications are for hospitalised patients.

Side-effects: Aprotinin is usually well tolerated but local thrombophlebitis, nausea and vomiting, diarrhoea, muscle pains, and blood-pressure changes can occur.

Allergic reactions such as erythema, urticaria, and bronchospasm have occasionally been reported and can occur on first administration. On repeated dosage, a reddening may occur at the point of injection, but this disappears after 1 or 2 hours. Anaphylaxis, tachycardia, pallor or cyanosis and dyspnoea have also occurred.

Use in pregnancy/lactation: There is no evidence that aprotinin has teratogenic or embryotoxic effects in animals. Experience in human pregnancy and lactation is limited and inadequate to assess safety. As the use of aprotinin is in life-threatening situations it may be used in pregnancy and lactation when the benefit is considered to outweigh the risk.

Warnings/precautions: Rapid IV injection of large doses should be avoided for the high basicity of aprotinin may cause liberation of histamine and lead to an anaphylactic reaction. Aprotinin should be administered slowly (maximum 5 ml/min) with the patient lying down. Care should be taken in treating patients intermittently and in those who have received Aprotinin previously. If hypersensitivity reactions are observed, the injection/infusion must be stopped immediately and the appropriate therapeutic measures initiated (administration of adrenaline, antihistamines, intravenous corticosteroids). Intra-ocular or intra-dermal testing may be useful for detecting allergic patients.

Overdose: There is no specific antidote and symptomatic treatment is advised. The use of more than 6×10^6 KIU (equivalent to 12×50 ml vials) per day is not recommended.

Incompatibilities: Antibiotics which react with proteins, corticosteroid and nutrient solutions containing amino-acids or fat emulsions.

Pharmaceutical precautions Store at a temperature not exceeding 25°C and protect from light. Both 5 ml ampoules and 50 ml vials should be considered as single dose containers and any contents not used in a single administration should be discarded.

Legal category POM.

Package quantities 5 ml ampoules each containing 50,000 KIU in boxes of 10 ampoules; 50 ml vials containing 500,000 KIU.

Product licence numbers

5 ml ampoule	0051/0027
50 ml vial	0051/0028

CHORAGON* 5000 U and CHORAGON SOLVENT

Presentation Choragon 5000 U is presented in ampoules containing a white, sterile, freeze-dried plug of 5000 Units of Chorionic Gonadotrophin PhEur (HCG) in the inactive carrier mannitol, for injection. It is supplied with a 1 ml ampoule of solvent for reconstitution of the powder.

Uses Human chorionic gonadotrophin (HCG) is obtained from the urine of pregnant women. The action of HCG is predominantly that of the pituitary luteinising hormone.

In the female: In the management of anovulatory infertility, Choragon can be given to induce ovulation after follicular development has been stimulated with follicle stimulating hormone.

In the male: HCG stimulates the interstitial cells to secrete testosterone. Choragon can therefore be used in the management of delayed puberty, undescended testes and oligospermia.

Dosage and administration Choragon is given by intramuscular injection. Treatment should only commence after expert assessment.

In the female: Induction of ovulation: 10,000 units mid-cycle if plasma oestrogen levels are favourable following follicular stimulation.

In the male: Delayed puberty: Dose should be titrated against plasma testosterone, starting with 500 units twice weekly. Treatment should be continued for 4–6 weeks.

Undescended testes: Treatment should begin before puberty, the optimum age range being 7–10 years. 500 units three times weekly is a suitable starting dose, but this may be increased up to 4000 units thrice weekly if necessary. Treatment should continue for 6–10 weeks. In males over 17 years of age a commencing dose of 1000 units twice weekly can be given. Treatment should be continued for one or two months after testicular descent.

Oligospermia: Dose should be titrated against seminal analysis starting with 500 units two or three times weekly. Treatment should be continued for 16 weeks.

Contra-indications, warnings, etc
Contra-indications: HCG should not be given to patients with disorders that might be exacerbated by androgen release.

Warnings: HCG should be given with care to patients in whom fluid retention might be a hazard, as in asthma, epilepsy, migraine, or cardiac or renal disorders.

Allergic reactions may occur and patients thought to be susceptible should be given skin tests before treatment.

HCG preparations should only be used under the supervision of a specialist having available adequate facilities for appropriate laboratory monitoring.

In the female: Use in induction of ovulation may result in ovarian enlargement or cysts, acute abdominal pain, superovulation, or multiple pregnancies, particularly if endocrine monitoring is inadequate.

In the male: Treatment for undescended testes may produce precocious puberty; use should cease immediately. Gynaecomastia has been reported. A growth spurt may also be associated with use and this should be kept in mind particularly where epiphyseal growth is still potentially active.

Side-effects: Headache, tiredness and mood changes have been described.

Pharmaceutical precautions In the dry state, in sealed ampoules, Choragon will remain stable if protected from light and stored at a temperature not exceeding 20°C. Solutions are unstable and should be freshly prepared.

Legal category POM.

Package quantities Cartons containing 3 ampoules of Choragon 5000 U and solvent for reconstitution of the powder.

Further information The solvent contains 0.9% Sodium Chloride in Water for Injection PhEur.

Product licence number 03194/0065

DDAVP* TABLETS

Presentation Uncoated, white, flat, round tablets of 8 mm diameter, scored on one side and marked '0.1' on the other side, each containing desmopressin acetate 0.1 mg.

Uncoated, white, flat, round tablets of 8 mm diameter, scored one side and marked "0.2" on the other side, each containing desmopressin acetate 0.2 mg.

Uses DDAVP Tablets are indicated for the treatment of vasopressin-sensitive cranial diabetes insipidus or in the treatment of post-hypophysectomy polyuria/ polydipsia.

DDAVP Tablets are also indicated for the treatment of primary nocturnal enuresis.

Dosage and administration
Treatment of diabetes insipidus: Dosage is individual but clinical experience has shown that the total daily dose normally lies in the range of 0.2 to 1.2 mg. A suitable starting dose in adults and children is 0.1 mg three times daily. This dosage regimen should then be adjusted in accordance with the patient's response. For the majority of patients, the maintenance dose is 0.1 mg to 0.2 mg three times daily.

Post-hypophysectomy polyuria/polydipsia: The dose of DDAVP Tablets should be controlled by measurement of urine osmolality.

Primary nocturnal enuresis: Children (from 5 years of age) and adults (up to 65 years of age) with normal urine concentrating ability who have primary nocturnal enuresis should take 0.2 mg at bedtime and only if needed should the dose be increased to 0.4 mg.

The need for continued treatment should be reassessed after 3 months by means of a period of at least 1 week without DDAVP Tablets.

During the treatment of enuresis the fluid intake should be limited to a minimum and only to satisfy thirst for 8 hours following administration.

Contra-indications, warnings, etc
Contra-indications: DDAVP Tablets are contraindicated in cases of cardiac insufficiency and other conditions requiring treatment with diuretic agents. When used to control primary nocturnal enuresis DDAVP Tablets should only be used in patients with normal blood pressure.

Before prescribing DDAVP Tablets the diagnoses of psychogenic polydipsia and alcohol abuse should be excluded.

Desmopressin should not be prescribed to patients over the age of 65 for the treatment of primary nocturnal enuresis.

Use in pregnancy: DDAVP Tablets should be given with caution to pregnant patients, although the oxytocic effect of desmopressin is very low.

Reproduction studies performed in rats and rabbits with doses of more than 100 times the human dose have revealed no evidence of a harmful action of desmopressin on the fetus. There have been rare reports of malformations in children born to mothers treated for diabetes insipidus during pregnancy. However, a review of available data suggests no increase in the rate of malformations in children exposed to desmopressin throughout pregnancy.

Use in lactation: Results from analyses of milk from nursing mothers receiving high dose desmopressin (300 micrograms intranasally) indicate that the amounts of desmopressin that may be transferred to the child are considerably less than the amounts required to influence diuresis.

Precautions: Care should be taken with patients who have reduced renal function and/or cardiovascular disease or cystic fibrosis. In chronic renal disease the antidiuretic effect of DDAVP Tablets would be less than normal.

Patients being treated for primary nocturnal enuresis should be warned to avoid ingesting water while swimming and to discontinue DDAVP Tablets during an episode of vomiting and/or diarrhoea until their fluid balance is once again normal.

Special precautions for use: Precautions to prevent fluid overload must be taken in:
- conditions characterised by fluid and/or electrolyte imbalance
- patients at risk for increased intracranial pressure

Side-effects: Occasional side-effects include headache, stomach pain and nausea. Treatment with desmopressin without concomitant reduction of fluid intake may lead to fluid retention, hyponatraemia and in more serious cases, convulsions.

Interactions: Indomethacin may augment the magnitude but not the duration of response to desmopressin.

Substances which are known to release antidiuretic hormone e.g. tricyclic antidepressants, chlorpromazine and carbamazepine, may cause an additive antidiuretic effect and increase the risk of water retention.

Overdose: An overdose of DDAVP Tablets can lead to hyponatraemia and convulsions.

Treatment of overdose: Overdosage increases the risk of fluid retention and hyponatraemia. If hyponatraemia occurs desmopressin treatment should immediately be discontinued and fluid intake restricted until serum sodium is normalised.

Pharmaceutical precautions DDAVP Tablets should be stored at room temperature.

Legal category POM.

Package quantities Cartons containing 90 tablets in blister strip packing.

Further information Oral administration of desmopressin acetate results in an antidiuretic effect lasting about eight hours.

The antidiuretic effect of DDAVP Tablets is not influenced by concomitant food intake.

Product licence numbers
DDAVP Tablets 0.1 mg 3194/0040
DDAVP Tablets 0.2 mg 3194/0041.

DDAVP*/DESMOPRESSIN INJECTION

Presentation Ampoules containing a clear colourless solution of 4 micrograms desmopressin acetate in 1 ml normal saline.

Uses DDAVP/Desmopressin Injection is indicated as follows:
1. Diagnosis and treatment of cranial diabetes insipidus.
2. To increase Factor VIII:C and Factor VIII:Ag in patients with mild to moderate haemophilia or von Willebrand's disease undergoing surgery or following trauma.
3. To establish renal concentration capacity.
4. To treat headache resulting from a lumbar puncture.
5. To test for fibrinolytic response.

Dosage and administration
Diabetes insipidus: By subcutaneous, intramuscular or intravenous injection.

Adults: The usual dose is 1 to 4 micrograms given once daily.

Children and infants: Doses from 0.4 micrograms (0.1 ml) may be used.

The diagnostic dose in adults and children is 2 micrograms given by subcutaneous or intramuscular injection. Failure to elaborate a concentrated urine after water deprivation, followed by the ability to do so after the administration of Desmopressin confirms a diagnosis of cranial diabetes insipidus. Failure to concentrate after the administration suggests nephrogenic diabetes insipidus.

When used for diagnostic purposes the fluid intake must be limited and not exceed 0.5 litres from 1 hour before until 8 hours after administration.

Mild to moderate haemophilia and von Willebrand's Disease: By intravenous administration.

The dose for adults, children and infants is 0.4 micrograms per kilogram body weight.

The dose should be diluted in 50 ml of 0.9% sodium chloride for injection and given by infusion over 20 minutes immediately prior to surgery. During administration of intravenous desmopressin, vasodilation may occur resulting in decreased blood pressure and tachycardia with facial flushing in some patients.

Increase of Factor VIII levels are dependent on basal levels and are normally between 2 and 5 times the pre-treatment levels. If results from a previous administration of desmopressin are not available then blood should be taken pre-dose and 20 minutes post-dose for assay of Factor VIII levels in order to monitor response.

Further doses may be administered at 12 hourly intervals so long as cover is required. As some patients have shown a diminishing response to successive doses, Factor VIII levels should continue to be monitored.

Unless contra-indicated, when surgery is undertaken tranexamic acid may be given orally at the recommended dose from 24 hours beforehand until healing is complete.

Renal function testing: By subcutaneous or intramuscular injection.

Adults and children can be expected to achieve urine concentrations above 700 mOsm/kg in the period of 5 to 9 hours following a dose of 2 micrograms DDAVP/Desmopressin injection. It is recommended that the bladder should be emptied at the time of administration.

When used for diagnostic purposes the fluid intake must be limited and not exceed 0.5 litres from 1 hour before until 8 hours after administration.

In normal infants, a urine concentration of 600 mOsm/kg should be achieved in the five hour period following a dose of 0.4 micrograms DDAVP/Desmopressin Injection. The fluid intake at the two meals following the administration should be restricted to 50% of the ordinary intake to avoid water overload.

Post lumbar puncture headache: By subcutaneous or intramuscular injection.

Where a headache is thought to be due to a lumbar puncture, an adult patient can be given a dose of 4 micrograms DDAVP/Desmopressin Injection which may be repeated 24 hours later if necessary.

Alternatively, a prophylactic dose of 4 micrograms can be given immediately prior to the lumbar puncture and repeated 24 hours later.

Fibrinolytic response testing: By intravenous administration.

The dose for adults and children is 0.4 micrograms per kilogram body weight. The dose should be diluted in 50 ml of 0.9% sodium chloride for injection and given by infusion over 20 minutes.

A sample of venous blood should be taken 20 minutes after the infusion. In patients with a normal response the sample should show fibrinolytic activity of euglobulin clot precipitate on fibrin plates of at least 240 mm².

Contra-indications, warnings, etc
Contra-indications: DDAVP/Desmopressin Injection is contra-indicated in cases of:

General: habitual and psychogenic polydipsia.

Renal function testing, treatment of lumbar puncture headache or fibrinolytic response testing: Should not be carried out in patients with hypertension, heart disease, cardiac insufficiency and other conditions requiring treatment with diuretic agents.

For haemostatic use:
- unstable angina pectoris
- decompensated cardiac insufficiency
- von Willebrand's Disease Type IIB where the administration of desmopressin may result in pseudothrombocytopenia due to the release of clotting factors which cause platelet aggregation.

Use in pregnancy: DDAVP/Desmopressin Injection should be given with caution to pregnant patients, although the oxytocic effect of desmopressin is very low.

Reproduction studies performed in rats and rabbits with doses of more than 100 times the human dose have revealed no evidence of a harmful action of desmopressin on the fetus. There have been rare reports of malformations in children born to mothers treated for diabetes insipidus during pregnancy. However, a review of available data suggests no increase in the rate of malformations in children exposed to desmopressin throughout pregnancy.

Use in lactation: Results from analyses of milk from nursing mothers receiving high dose desmopressin (300 micrograms intranasally) indicate that the amounts of desmopressin that may be transferred to the child are considerably less than the amounts required to influence diuresis or haemostasis.

Precautions:
General: Precautions to prevent fluid overload must be taken in:
- conditions characterised by fluid and/or electrolyte imbalance
- patients at risk for increased intracranial pressure.

Care should be taken with patients who have reduced renal function and/or cardiovascular disease or cystic fibrosis.

For renal concentration capacity testing: Testing in children below the age of 1 year should only be performed under carefully supervised conditions in hospital.

For haemostatic use: When repeated doses are used to control bleeding in haemophilia or von Willebrand's disease, care should be taken to prevent fluid overload. Fluid should not be forced, orally or parenterally, and patients should only take as much fluid as they require to satisfy thirst. Intravenous infusions should not be left up as a routine after surgery. Fluid accumulation can be readily monitored by weighing the patient or by determining plasma sodium or osmolality.

Measures to prevent fluid overload must be taken in patients with conditions requiring treatment with diuretic agents.

Special warnings: Special attention must be paid to the risk of water retention. The fluid intake should be restricted to the least possible and the body weight should be checked regularly.

If there is a gradual increase of the body weight, decrease of serum sodium to below 130 mmol/l or plasma osmolality to below 270 mOsm/kg, the fluid intake must be reduced drastically and the administration of DDAVP/Desmopressin Injection interrupted.

During infusion of DDAVP/Desmopressin Injection for haemostatic use, it is recommended that the patient's blood pressure is monitored continuously.

DDAVP/Desmopressin Injection does not reduce prolonged bleeding time in thrombocytopenia.

Side-effects: Occasional side-effects include headache, stomach pain, and nausea. Treatment with desmopressin without concomitant reduction of fluid intake may lead to fluid retention, hyponatraemia and in more severe cases, convulsions.

During infusion of DDAVP/Desmopressin Injection for haemostatic indications, vasodilation may occur, resulting in decreased blood pressure and tachycardia with facial flushing. This side effect is normally avoided by infusing the product over 20 minutes.

Interactions: Indomethacin may augment the magnitude but not the duration of the antidiuretic response to desmopressin.

Substances which are known to release antidiuretic hormone e.g. tricyclic antidepressants, chlorpromazine and carbamazepine, may cause an additive antidiuretic effect and increase the risk of water retention.

Overdose: An overdose of DDAVP/Desmopressin Injection can lead to hyponatraemia and convulsions.

Treatment of overdose: Overdosage increases the risk of fluid retention and hyponatraemia. If hyponatraemia occurs, desmopressin treatment should immediately be discontinued and fluid intake restricted until serum sodium is normalised.

Pharmaceutical precautions DDAVP/Desmopressin injection should be stored in the refrigerator at 4 to 8°C and must be protected from light. Doses of less than 4 micrograms (1 ml) should be measured using a suitable syringe because dilution may result in the loss of desmopressin by adsorption onto glass or plastic surfaces.

Legal category POM.

Package quantities Cartons containing 10 × 1 ml ampoules.

Further information Desmopressin is a structural analogue of vasopressin in which the antidiuretic activity has been increased and the duration of action prolonged. Desmopressin also retains the ability of vasopressin to increase the levels of clotting factors, Factor VIII:C, Factor VIIIR:Ag, Factor VIII:Rcof and Plasminogen Activator. Pressor activity is reduced to less than 0.01% of vasopressin as a result of which side-effects are rarely seen.

Product licence number 3194/0002.

DDAVP*/DESMOPRESSIN INTRANASAL SOLUTION

Presentation 2.5 ml dropper bottle containing a clear solution of desmopressin acetate 100 micrograms per ml. DDAVP/Desmopressin Intranasal Solution contains chlorbutol 0.5% as a preservative.

Uses DDAVP/Desmopressin Intranasal Solution is indicated for:
1. The diagnosis and treatment of vasopressin-sensitive cranial diabetes insipidus.
2. The treatment of primary nocturnal enuresis.
3. The treatment of nocturia associated with multiple sclerosis where other treatments have failed.
4. Establishing renal concentration capacity.

Dosage and administration
Treatment of diabetes insipidus: Dosage is individual but clinical experience has shown that the average maintenance doses are as follows:

Adults: 10 to 20 micrograms once or twice daily.

Children: 5 to 20 micrograms daily, (a lower dose may be required for infants).

Diagnosis of diabetes insipidus: The diagnostic dose in adults and children is 20 micrograms. Failure to elaborate a concentrated urine after water deprivation, followed by the ability to do so after the administration of desmopressin confirms the diagnosis of cranial diabetes insipidus. Failure to concentrate after the administration suggests nephrogenic diabetes insipidus.

When used for diagnostic purposes the fluid intake must be limited and not exceed 0.5 litres from 1 hour before until 8 hours after administration.

Primary nocturnal enuresis: The starting dose for children (from 5 years of age) and adults (up to 65 years of age) with normal urine concentrating ability who have primary nocturnal enuresis is 20 micrograms at bedtime and only if needed should the dose be increased up to 40 micrograms.

The need for continued treatment should be reassessed after 3 months by means of a period of at least one week without DDAVP/Desmopressin Intranasal.

During the treatment of enuresis the fluid intake should be limited to a minimum and only to satisfy thirst for 8 hours following administration.

Treatment of nocturia: For multiple sclerosis patients up to 65 years of age with normal renal function suffering from nocturia the dose is 10 to 20 micrograms at bedtime. Not more than one dose should be used in any 24 hour period.

During the treatment of nocturia the fluid intake should be limited to a minimum and only to satisfy thirst for 8 hours following adminstration.

Renal function testing: Recommended doses for the renal concentration capacity test:

Adults: 40 micrograms.
Children (1–15 years): 20 micrograms.
Infants (to 1 year): 10 micrograms.

Adults and children with normal renal function can be expected to achieve concentrations above 700 mOsm/kg in the period of 5–9 hours following administration of DDAVP/Desmopressin Intranasal. It is recommended that the bladder should be emptied at the time of administration.

When used for diagnostic purposes the fluid intake must be limited and not exceed 0.5 litres from 1 hour before until 8 hours after administration.

In normal infants a urine concentration of 600 mOsm/kg should be achieved in the 5 hour period following the administration of DDAVP/Desmopressin Intranasal. The fluid intake at the two meals following the administration should be restricted to 50% of the ordinary intake in order to avoid water overload.

Contra-indications, warnings, etc
Contra-indications: DDAVP/Desmopressin Intranasal is contra-indicated in cases of:
- cardiac insufficiency and other conditions requiring treatment with diuretic agents
- hypersensitivity to the preservative

When used to control primary nocturnal enuresis DDAVP/Desmopressin Intranasal should only be used in patients with normal blood pressure.

Before prescribing DDAVP/Desmopressin Intranasal the diagnoses of psychogenic polydipsia and alcohol abuse should be excluded.

When used to control nocturia in patients with multiple sclerosis, desmopressin should not be used in patients with hypertension or cardiovascular disease.

Desmopressin should not be prescribed to patients over the age of 65 for the treatment of primary nocturnal enuresis or nocturia associated with multiple sclerosis.

Use in pregnancy: DDAVP/Desmopressin Intranasal should be given with caution to pregnant patients, although the oxytocic effect of desmopressin is very low.

Reproduction studies performed in rats and rabbits with doses of more than 100 times the human dose have revealed no evidence of a harmful action of desmopressin on the fetus. There have been rare reports of malformations in children born to mothers treated for diabetes insipidus during pregnancy. However, a review of available data suggests no increase in the rate of malformations in children exposed to desmopressin throughout pregnancy.

Use in lactation: Results from analyses of milk from nursing mothers receiving high dose desmopressin (300 micrograms intranasally) indicate that the amounts of desmopressin that may be transferred to the child are considerably less than the amounts required to influence diuresis.

Precautions: Care should be taken with patients who have reduced renal function and/or cardiovascular disease or cystic fibrosis.

Patients being treated for primary nocturnal enuresis should be warned to avoid ingesting water while swimming and to discontinue DDAVP/Desmopressin Intranasal during an episode of vomiting and/or diarrhoea until their fluid balance is once again normal.

When DDAVP/Desmopressin Intranasal is used in the treatment of nocturia, periodic assessments should be made of blood pressure and weight to monitor the possibility of fluid overload.

Following diagnostic testing for diabetes insipidus or renal concentration capacity, care should be taken to prevent fluid overload. Fluid should not be forced, orally or parenterally, and patients should only take as much fluid as they require to satisfy thirst.

Special precautions for use: Precautions to prevent fluid overload must be taken in:
- conditions characterised by fluid and/or electrolyte imbalance
- patients at risk for increased intracranial pressure

Additional precautions for using the renal concentration capacity test: Renal concentration capacity test in children below the age of 1 year should only be performed under carefully supervised conditions in hospital.

Side-effects: Occasional side-effects include headache, stomach pain, nausea, nasal congestion, rhinitis and epistaxis. Allergic reactions to the preservative have been reported rarely. Treatment with desmopressin without concomitant reduction of fluid intake may lead to fluid retention, hyponatraemia and in more serious cases, convulsions.

Interactions: Indomethacin may augment the magnitude but not the duration of response to desmopressin.

Substances which are known to release antidiuretic hormone e.g. tricyclic antidepressants, chlorpromazine and carbamazepine, may cause an additive antidiuretic effect and increase the risk of water retention.

Overdose: An overdose of DDAVP/Desmopressin Intranasal can lead to hyponatraemia and convulsions.

Treatment of overdose: Overdosage increases the risk of fluid retention and hyponatraemia. If hyponatraemia occurs, desmopressin treatment should immediately be discontinued and fluid intake restricted until serum sodium is normalised.

Pharmaceutical precautions DDAVP/Desmopressin Intranasal should be stored in the refrigerator at 2 to 8°C and must be protected from light.

Legal category POM.

Package quantities 2.5 ml bottle.

Further information Patients sensitive to chlorbutol should use DDAVP* Tablets or Desmotabs*.

Product licence number 3194/0001.

DESMOSPRAY*

Presentation Metered-dose, pre-compression atomiser delivering 60 doses of 10 micrograms desmopressin acetate per spray.

Desmospray contains benzalkonium chloride as a preservative.

Uses Desmospray is indicated for:
1. The treatment of primary nocturnal enuresis.
2. The treatment of nocturia associated with multiple sclerosis where other treatments have failed.
3. The diagnosis and treatment of vasopressin-sensitive cranial diabetes insipidus.
4. Establishing renal concentration capacity.

Dosage and administration
Primary nocturnal enuresis: The starting dose for children (from 5 years of age) and adults (up to 65 years of age) with normal urine concentrating ability who have primary nocturnal enuresis is one spray (10 micrograms) into each nostril (a total of 20 micrograms) at bedtime and only if needed should the dose be increased up to two sprays (20 micrograms) into each nostril (a total of 40 micrograms).

The need for continued treatment should be reassessed after 3 months by means of a period of at least 1 week without Desmospray.

During the treatment of enuresis the fluid intake should be limited to a minimum and only to satisfy thirst for 8 hours following administration.

Treatment of nocturia: For multiple sclerosis patients up to 65 years of age with normal renal function suffering from nocturia the dose is one or two sprays intranasally (10 to 20 micrograms) at bedtime. Not more than one dose should be used in any 24 hour period. If a dose of two sprays is required, this should be as one spray into each nostril.

During the treatment of nocturia the fluid intake should be limited to a minimum and only to satisfy thirst for 8 hours following administration.

Treatment of diabetes insipidus: Dosage is individual but clinical experience has shown that the average maintenance dose in adults and children is one or two sprays (10 to 20 micrograms) once or twice daily. If a dose of two sprays is required, this should be as one spray into each nostril.

Diagnosis of diabetes insipidus: The diagnostic dose in adults and children is two sprays (20 micrograms).

Failure to elaborate a concentrated urine after water deprivation, followed by the ability to do so after the administration of Desmospray confirms the diagnosis of cranial diabetes insipidus. Failure to concentrate after the administration suggests nephrogenic diabetes insipidus.

When used for diagnostic purposes the fluid intake must be limited and not exceed 0.5 litres from 1 hour before until 8 hours after administration.

Renal function testing: Recommended doses for the renal concentration capacity test:
Adults: Two sprays into each nostril (a total of 40 micrograms).
Children (1–15 years): One spray into each nostril (a total of 20 micrograms).
Infants (to 1 year): One spray (10 micrograms).

Adults and children with normal renal function can be expected to achieve concentrations above 700 mOsm/kg in the period of 5 to 9 hours following administration of Desmospray. It is recommended that the bladder should be emptied at the time of administration.

When used for diagnostic purposes the fluid intake must be limited and not exceed 0.5 litres from 1 hour before until 8 hours after administration.

In normal infants a urine concentration of 600 mOsm/kg should be achieved in the 5 hour period following administration of Desmospray. The fluid intake at the two meals following the administration should be restricted to 50% of the ordinary intake in order to avoid water overload.

Contra-indications, warnings, etc
Contra-indications: Desmospray is contraindicated in cases of:
- cardiac insufficiency and other conditions requiring treatment with diuretic agents
- hypersensitivity to the preservative

When used to control primary nocturnal enuresis Desmospray should only be used in patients with normal blood pressure.

Before prescribing Desmospray the diagnoses of psychogenic polydipsia and alcohol abuse should be excluded.

When used to control nocturia in patients with multiple sclerosis, desmopressin should not be used in patients with hypertension or cardiovascular disease.

Desmopressin should not be prescribed to patients over the age of 65 for the treatment of primary nocturnal enuresis or nocturia associated with multiple sclerosis.

Use in pregnancy: Desmospray should be given with caution to pregnant patients, although the oxytocic effect of desmopressin is very low.

Reproduction studies performed in rats and rabbits with doses of more than 100 times the human dose have revealed no evidence of a harmful action of desmopressin on the fetus. There have been rare reports of malformations in children born to mothers treated for diabetes insipidus during pregnancy. However, a review of available data suggests no increase in the rate of malformations in children exposed to desmopressin throughout pregnancy.

Use in lactation: Results from analyses of milk from nursing mothers receiving high dose desmopressin (300 micrograms intranasally) indicate that the amounts of desmopressin that may be transferred to the child are considerably less than the amounts required to influence diuresis.

Precautions: Care should be taken with patients who have reduced renal function and/or cardiovascular disease or cystic fibrosis.

Patients being treated for primary nocturnal enuresis should be warned to avoid ingesting water while swimming and to discontinue Desmospray during an episode of vomiting and/or diarrhoea until their fluid balance is once again normal.

When Desmospray is used in the treatment of nocturia, periodic assessments should be made of blood pressure and weight to monitor the possibility of fluid overload.

Following diagnostic testing for diabetes insipidus or renal concentration capacity, care should be taken to prevent fluid overload. Fluid should not be forced, orally or parenterally, and patients should only take as much fluid as they require to satisfy thirst.

Special precautions for use: Precautions to prevent fluid overload must be taken in:

– conditions characterised by fluid and/or electrolyte imbalance
– patients at risk for increased intracranial pressure

Additional precautions for using the renal concentration capacity test: Renal concentration capacity test in children below the age of 1 year should only be performed under carefully supervised conditions in hospital.

Side-effects: Occasional side-effects include headache, stomach pain, nausea, nasal congestion, rhinitis and epistaxis. Allergic reactions to the preservative have been reported rarely. Treatment with desmopressin without concomitant reduction of fluid intake may lead to fluid retention, hyponatraemia and in more serious cases, convulsions.

Interactions: Indomethacin may augment the magnitude but not the duration of response to desmopressin.

Substances which are known to release antidiuretic hormone e.g. tricyclic antidepressants, chlorpromazine and carbamazepine, may cause an additive antidiuretic effect and increase the risk of water retention.

Overdose: An overdose of Desmospray can lead to hyponatraemia and convulsions.

Treatment of overdose: Overdosage increases the risk of fluid retention and hyponatraemia. If hyponatraemia occurs, desmopressin treatment should immediately be discontinued and fluid intake restricted until serum sodium is normalised.

Pharmaceutical precautions Desmospray should be stored at room temperature (up to 25°C) and must be protected from light.

Legal category POM.

Package quantities 6 ml bottle (60 doses of 10 micrograms desmopressin acetate per spray).

Further information Children requiring doses of less than 10 micrograms should use DDAVP Tablets, Desmotabs 0.2 mg or DDAVP/Desmopressin Intranasal solution which employs a small plastic calibrated catheter to administer doses of 5 to 20 micrograms. Patients sensitive to benzalkonium chloride should use DDAVP* Tablets or Desmotabs* 0.2 mg.

Product licence number 3194/0024.

DESMOTABS* 0.2 mg

Presentation Uncoated, white, flat, round tablets of 8 mm diameter, scored one side and marked '0.2' on the other side, each containing desmopressin acetate 0.2 mg.

Uses Desmotabs are indicated for the treatment of primary nocturnal enuresis.

Dosage and administration

Primary nocturnal enuresis: Children (from 5 years of age) and adults (up to 65 years of age) with normal urine concentrating ability who have primary nocturnal enuresis should take 0.2 mg at bedtime and only if needed should the dose be increased to 0.4 mg.

The need for continued treatment should be reassessed after 3 months by means of a period of at least 1 week without Desmotabs.

During the treatment of enuresis the fluid intake should be limited to a minimum and only to satisfy thirst for 8 hours following administration.

Contra-indications, warnings, etc

Contra-indications: Desmotabs are contra-indicated in cases of cardiac insufficiency and other conditions requiring treatment with diuretic agents. Desmotabs should only be used in patients with normal blood pressure.

Before prescribing Desmotabs the diagnoses of psychogenic polydipsia and alcohol abuse should be excluded.

Desmopressin should not be prescribed to patients over the age of 65 for the treatment of primary nocturnal enuresis.

Use in pregnancy: Desmotabs should be given with caution to pregnant patients, although the oxytocic effect of desmopressin is very low.

Reproduction studies performed in rats and rabbits with doses of more than 100 times the human dose have revealed no evidence of a harmful action of desmopressin on the fetus. There have been rare reports of malformations in children born to mothers treated for diabetes insipidus during pregnancy. However, a review of available data suggests no increase in the rate of malformations in children exposed to desmopressin throughout pregnancy.

Use in lactation: Results from analyses of milk from nursing mothers receiving high dose desmopressin (300 micrograms intranasally) indicate that the amounts of desmopressin that may be transferred to the child are considerably less than the amounts required to influence diuresis.

Precautions: Care should be taken with patients who have cystic fibrosis.

Patients being treated for primary nocturnal enuresis should be warned to avoid ingesting water while swimming and to discontinue Desmotabs during an episode of vomiting and/or diarrhoea until their fluid balance is once again normal.

Special precautions for use: Precautions to prevent fluid overload must be taken in:
– conditions characterised by fluid and/or electrolyte imbalance;
– patients at risk for increased intracranial pressure.

Side-effects: Occasional side-effects include headache, stomach pain and nausea. Treatment with desmopressin without concomitant reduction of fluid intake may lead to fluid retention, hyponatraemia and in more serious cases, convulsions.

Interactions: Indomethacin may augment the magnitude but not the duration of response to desmopressin.

Substances which are known to release antidiuretic hormone e.g. tricyclic antidepressants, chlorpromazine and carbamazepine, may cause an additive antidiuretic effect and increase the risk of water retention.

Overdose: An overdose of Desmotabs can lead to hyponatraemia and convulsions.

Treatment of overdose: Overdosage increases the risk of fluid retention and hyponatraemia. If hyponatraemia occurs, desmopressin treatment should immediately be discontinued and fluid intake restricted until serum sodium is normalised.

Pharmaceutical precautions Desmotabs should be stored at room temperature (maximum 25°C).

Legal category POM.

Package quantities Cartons containing 28 tablets in blister strip packing.

Further information Oral administration of Desmopressin acetate results in an antidiuretic effect lasting about eight hours.

The antidiuretic effect of Desmotabs is not influenced by concomitant food intake.

Product licence number 3194/0046.

GESTONE*

Presentation Ampoules of a sterile straw-coloured solution of Progesterone BP 25 or 50 mg per ml in ethyl oleate for injection containing 10% v/v benzyl alcohol.

Uses Gestone is indicated for the treatment of dysfunctional uterine bleeding.

It is also indicated for the maintenance of early pregnancy in cases of documented history of repeated miscarriages due to luteal phase defect and in selected cases as an adjunct to successful treatment of infertility with techniques such as in-vitro fertilisation (IVF) or gamete intra-fallopian transfer (GIFT) in order to facilitate uterine implantation of the fertilised ovum.

Dosage and administration Gestone is given by intramuscular injection. It should be injected deep into the buttock, rather than the thigh or deltoid, using a 1.5 inch (3.8 cm) needle. This site has ample fat cells where a depot of progesterone can be formed for slow release.

Dysfunctional uterine bleeding: 5–10 mg daily for 5–10 days until 2 days before anticipated onset of menstruation.

Maintenance of pregnancy: Twice weekly or more frequent (maximum: daily) injections of 25–100 mg from approximately day 15, or day of transfer of embryo or gametes usually until 8–16 weeks of pregnancy when secretion of progesterone from the placenta should be established.

Daily dosage can be increased to 200 mg at the discretion of the physician.

As the indications for Gestone are restricted to women of child-bearing age, dosage recommendations for children and the elderly are not appropriate.

Contra-indications, warnings, etc

Contra-indications: Hypersensitivity to progestins, undiagnosed vaginal bleeding, missed or incomplete abortion, mammary or genital tract carcinoma, thrombophlebitis, cerebral haemorrhage, marked hepatic dysfunction. Contraindicated as a diagnostic test for pregnancy.

Interactions: Gestone may interfere with the effects of bromocriptine. Gestone may affect the results of laboratory tests of hepatic and/or endocrine functions. Gestone may raise the plasma concentration of cyclosporin.

Effects on ability to drive and use machinery: No known effect.

Other undesirable effects: Breakthrough bleeding, change in menstrual flow, amenorrhoea, changes in cervical erosion and secretions, breast changes, oedema, weight gain, catabolism, cholestatic jaundice, allergic reactions and rashes, acne, chloasma, mental depression, pyrexia, insomnia, somnolence, nausea, alopecia, hirsutism, local reactions at site of injection.

Use in pregnancy and lactation: Gestone may be used to maintain pregnancy where there is deficient production of endogenous progesterone from the corpus luteum. It should not be necessary to administer Gestone once there is adequate secretion of placental progesterone. Gestone contains progesterone itself, the same as the naturally secreted hormone, and is not associated with masculinization of a female foetus as are synthetic progestins.

Detectable amounts of progesterone enter the breast milk. As the effect on the suckling infant has not been determined, the use of Gestone during lactation is not recommended.

Other special warnings and precautions: Gestone should be used cautiously in patients with conditions that might be aggravated by fluid retention (e.g. hypertension, cardiac disease, renal disease, epilepsy), with a history of mental depression, diabetes, mild to moderate hepatic dysfunction, acute intermittent porphyria, migraine or photosensitivity.

If unexplained, sudden or gradual, partial or complete loss of vision, proptosis or diplopia, papilloedema, retinal vascular lesions or migraine occur during therapy, the drug should be discontinued and appropriate diagnostic and therapeutic measures instituted.

Overdosage: This is unlikely and is not expected to produce any adverse effects. Treatment is observation and, if necessary, symptomatic and supportive measures should be provided.

Pharmaceutical precautions Store at room temperature (15–25°C) and protect from light. On storage, solid matter may separate and this should be redissolved by warming before use.

Legal category POM.

Package quantities Ampoules containing: 25 mg in 1 ml; 50 mg in 1 ml; 100 mg in 2 ml. Boxes of 10.

Further information Nil.

Product licence numbers
25 mg/ml 3194/0061
50 mg/ml 3194/0062
100 mg/2 ml 3194/0063.

GHRH FERRING

Presentation Freeze dried powder for injection containing 50 micrograms Somatorelin (as the acetate), per ampoule. Supplied with a 1 ml ampoule of sterile diluent.

Uses GHRH Ferring is applied to determine the somatotropic function of the anterior pituitary gland in cases of suspected growth hormone deficiency. The test distinguishes between hypophysic and hypothalamic disorders but is not suitable as a screening test for growth hormone deficiencies.

Dosage and administration The recommended dosage for adult patients of standard weight is the content of one ampoule of GHRH Ferring (50 micrograms Somatorelin as the acetate) dissolved in 1 ml of the supplied solvent. The solution is administered intravenously as a bolus injection.

In cases of highly overweight adults and in children, a dosage of 1 microgram per kilogram body weight is indicated. The application is intended as a single test.

GHRH test: After withdrawal of approximately 2 ml of venous blood from the fasted patient, the increase of basal growth hormone levels in plasma or serum after a single intravenous injection of the product is measured. For this procedure, the content of one ampoule is dissolved in 1 ml of the solvent (0.9% NaCl), or a volume corresponding to 1 microgram per kilogram body weight if appropriate, is administered intravenously to the fasted patient as a bolus injection (within 30 seconds).

To evaluate the growth hormone increment in plasma or serum, a second blood sample is taken 30 minutes after the injection. Peak growth hormone values may occasionally occur sooner or later. Therefore, additional blood samples may be taken 15, 45, 60 and 90 minutes after the GHRH Ferring injection for better assessment of growth hormone release.

Contra-indications, warnings, etc Hypersensitivity to growth hormone releasing hormone.

Interactions: The concomitant administration of substances which influence the release of growth hormone, such as growth hormone itself, somatostatin or its analogues, atropine, levodopa, dopamine, clonidine, arginine, ornithine, glycine, glucagon, insulin, oral glucose, anti-thyroid drugs and propranolol should be avoided. High levels of glucocorticoids as well as somatostatin may inhibit the growth hormone response.

Use in pregnancy and lactation: GHRH Ferring is not indicated during pregnancy and lactation.

Warnings and precautions: Because of the possible inhibitory influence of human growth hormone on the somatotropic function of the pituitary gland, the GHRH Ferring test should not be carried out earlier than one week after discontinuation of treatment with human growth hormone. The test results may be affected in conditions such as:
- untreated hyperthyroidism
- obesity, hyperglycaemia, elevated plasma fatty acid levels
- high levels of somatostatin.

Although no hypersensitivity reactions have yet been reported, the possibility of this kind of adverse event cannot be completely ruled out because of the peptide nature of the product and the intravenous route of administration. It is recommended that emergency facilities should be available to treat such a reaction if it occurs.

Side-effects: Occasionally a mild sensation of warmth may appear in the head, neck and upper part of the body, and there may be mild disturbances of taste and smell. These side effects are short lasting and will fade rapidly. In combination with 'hot flush', a slight increase or decrease in blood pressure may occasionally occur in conjunction with the corresponding alterations in heart rate.

The described side effects are insignificant when the suggested dose is applied and they do not need any special treatment.

Incompatibilities: GHRH Ferring should not be administered together with other preparations for parenteral use (e.g. mixed injections or infusion solutions).

Overdose: In cases of higher dosage, the known side effects may occur. The undesirable effects fade rapidly and do not need any special treatment.

Pharmaceutical precautions Freeze dried powder and diluent may be stored at room temperature. The powder should be reconstituted with 1 ml of the diluent supplied and used immediately.

Legal category POM.

Package quantity Cartons containing one ampoule of GHRH Ferring 50 micrograms and one diluent ampoule of sterile isotonic saline solution 1 ml.

Product licence numbers
GHRH Ferring: PL 03194/0050
Diluent for dissolution of GHRH Ferring: PL 03194/0051.

GLYPRESSIN* INJECTION

Presentation Glypressin is presented in vials containing a white, freeze dried powder of Terlipressin acetate 1 mg. The powder also contains the inactive carrier mannitol. For reconstitution of the powder, each vial is supplied with an ampoule containing 5 ml of sterile isotonic saline 0.9% w/v, and hydrochloric acid to adjust pH.

Uses Glypressin is indicated in the treatment of bleeding oesophageal varices.

Glypressin (triglycyl-lysine-vasopressin) is a hormonogen. When injected into the blood the glycyl residues of the molecule are slowly cleaved off by enzymatic action generating the release of vasopressin. Glypressin may thus be regarded as a circulating depot, releasing lysine vasopressin at a constant rate.

Dosage and administration In acute variceal bleeding, 2 mg Glypressin should be administered by intravenous bolus injection followed by 1 or 2 mg every 4 to 6 hours until bleeding is controlled, up to a maximum of 72 hours.

Contra-indications, warnings, etc
Contra-indications: Due to its effect on smooth muscle Glypressin is contra-indicated in pregnancy.

Warnings and precautions: The pressor and antidiuretic effects of Glypressin are reduced (compared with lysine or arginine vasopressin) but the product should still be used with great caution in patients with hypertension, advanced atherosclerosis, cardiac dysrhythmias or coronary insufficiency. Constant monitoring of blood pressure, serum sodium, potassium and fluid balance are essential. The possibility of immunological sensitisation cannot be excluded.

Side-effects: Because the severity of pressor and antidiuretic activities are reduced, few side-effects have been recorded. Infrequent effects include: abdominal cramps, headache, transient blanching, increase in arterial blood pressure.

Drug interactions: Glypressin is intended for the short term treatment of acute bleeding oesophageal varices. No interactions are known with other products likely to be used concurrently.

Treatment of overdose: Increase in blood pressure following the use of Glypressin in patients with known hypertension has been controlled with clonidine 150 micrograms intravenously.

Pharmaceutical precautions Freeze-dried powder and the diluent may be stored at room temperature, protected from direct sunlight. Each 1 mg vial of Glypressin should be reconstituted with 5 ml diluent supplied and used immediately.

Legal category POM.

Package quantity Glypressin Terlipressin 1 mg freeze dried powder: Single use vial. Diluent 5 ml ampoule supplied with each vial. Cartons of five vials and ampoules.

Further information Extensive tests in animals and humans have shown that Glypressin in itself is without hormonal activity. Appropriate doses of Glypressin however, lead to a reduction of portal vein pressure, but arterial blood pressure changes are far less marked than after vasopressin and Glypressin does not increase the fibrinolytic activity of the blood.

Product licence number 3194/0018.

MENOGON*

Presentation Menogon is a sterile freeze-dried powder for injection, containing menotrophin BP 75 IU providing 75 IU FSH and 75 IU LH. The powder also contains the inactive carrier, lactose and sodium hydroxide to adjust the pH. Each ampoule is supplied with a diluent ampoule of sodium chloride solution for injections 0.9% w/v.

Uses Treatment of female and male infertility in the following groups of patients:

In the female:
Anovulatory women: Menogon can be used to stimulate follicle development in amenorrhoeic patients who are unresponsive to clomiphene citrate or a similar ovulation induction agent.

Women undergoing superovulation within a medically assisted fertilisation programme: Menogon can be used to induce multiple follicular development in women undergoing an assisted conception technique such as in-vitro fertilisation (IVF).

In the male
Hypogonadotrophic hypogonadism in men: Menogon may be given in combination with hCG (e.g. Choragon) for the stimulation of spermatogenesis. Patients with primary testicular failure are usually unresponsive.

Dosage and administration Menogon should be reconstituted immediately prior to use and any remaining solution discarded. The product is administered by intramuscular injection.

In the female
Anovulatory women: Menogon is administered to induce follicular maturation and is followed by treatment with hCG to stimulate ovulation and corpus luteum formation.

The dosage and schedule of treatment must be determined according to the needs of each patient. Response is monitored by studying the patient's urinary oestrogen excretion or by ultrasound visualisation of follicles. Menogon may be given daily by intramuscular injection to provide a dose of 75 to 150 IU menotrophin, and gradually adjusted if necessary until an adequate response is achieved, followed after 1 or 2 days by hCG. In menstruating patients treatment should be started within the first 7 days of the menstrual cycle. The treatment course should be abandoned if no response is seen in 3 weeks. It may be repeated at least twice more if necessary. Alternatively, three equal doses of Menogon, each providing 225 to 375 IU may be given on alternate days followed by hCG one week after the first dose.

In the daily therapy schedule, the dose is gradually increased until oestrogen levels start to rise. The effective dose is then maintained until adequate preovulatory oestrogen levels are reached. If oestrogen levels rise too rapidly, the dose should be decreased.

As a measure of follicle maturity the following values can be taken:
- total urinary oestrogen: 75–150 microgram (270–540 nmol)/24 hours
- plasma 17 β-oestradiol: 400–800 picogram/ml (1500–3000 pmol/L).

When adequate pre-ovulatory oestrogen levels have been reached, administration of Menogon is stopped, and ovulation induced by administration of hCG at a dose of 5000–10000 IU.

Women undergoing superovulation within a medically assisted fertilisation programme: In in-vitro fertilisation procedures or other assisted conception techniques menotrophin is used in conjunction with hCG and sometimes also clomiphene citrate or a gonadorelin agonist. Stimulation of follicular growth is produced by Menogon in a daily dose of 75 to 300 IU. Treatment is continued until an adequate response is obtained. It is recommended there should be at least 3 follicles greater than 17 mm in diameter with 17 β-oestradiol levels of at least 3500 pmol/L (920 picogram/ml). Egg maturation occurs by administration of hCG in a dose of 5000–10000 IU, 30–40 hours after the last Menogon injection.

hCG should not be administered if these criteria have not been met. Egg retrieval is carried out 32–36 hours after the hCG injection.

In the male
Spermatogenesis is stimulated with hCG (1000–2000 IU two to three times a week) and then menotrophin is given in a dose of 75 or 150 IU two or three times weekly. Treatment should be continued for at least 3 or 4 months.

Contra-indications, warnings, etc
Contra-indications: Pregnancy, enlargement of the ovaries or cysts not caused by polycystic ovarian syndrome, gynaecological bleeding of unknown cause, tumours in the uterus, ovaries, breasts, or testes, carcinoma of the prostate, structural abnormalities in which a satsifactory outcome cannot be expected, for example, tubal occlusion (unless superovulation is to be induced for IVF), ovarian dysgenesis, absent uterus or premature menopause.

Other undesirable effects: Treatment with menotrophin can often lead to ovarian hyperstimulation. This, however, mostly becomes clinically relevant only after hCG has been administered to induce ovulation. This can lead to the formation of large ovarian cysts that tend to rupture and can cause intra-abdominal bleeding. In addition, ascites, hydrothorax, oliguria, hypotension, and thromboembolic phenomena can occur. Treatment should be immediately discontinued when the first signs of hyperstimulation can be detected by ultrasound or physically (abdominal pain and distension). With pregnancy, these side effects can intensify, continue over a long period of time, and become life threatening.

Occasional adverse effects of menotrophin treatment are nausea and vomiting.

There is an increased risk of miscarriage and also multiple pregnancies with menotrophin therapy.

Rarely reported side effects are fever and joint pain, hypersensitivity reactions (skin rash) and local reactions at the site of injection.

In very rare cases, long term use of menotrophin can lead to the formation of antibodies making treatment ineffectual.

Use in pregnancy and lactation: Menogon should not be given during pregnancy or to lactating mothers.

Warnings and precautions: The following conditions should be properly treated and excluded as the cause of infertility before menotrophin therapy is initiated: dysfunction of the thyroid gland and cortex of the suprarenal gland, hyperprolactinaemia, tumours in the pituitary or hypothalamic glands.

In the treatment of female infertility, ovarian activity should be checked (by ultrasound and plasma 17β-oestradiol measurement) prior to Menogon administration. During treatment, these tests and urinary oestrogen measurement should be carried out at regular intervals, until stimulation occurs. Close supervision is imperative during treatment. If urinary oestrogen levels exceed 540 nmol (150 micrograms)/24 hours, or if plasma 17β-oestradiol levels exceed 3000 pmol/L (800 picograms/ml), or if there is any steep rise in values, there is an increased risk of hyperstimulation and Menogon treatment should be immediately discontinued and hCG withheld. Ultrasound will reveal any excessive follicular development and unintentional hyperstimulation. In the event of hyperstimulation, the patient should refrain from sexual intercourse until they are no longer at risk.

If during ultrasound, several mature follicles are visualised, hCG should not be given as there is a risk of multiple ovulation and the occurrence of hyperstimulation syndrome.

Patients undergoing superovulation may be at an increased risk of developing hyperstimulation in view of the excessive oestrogen response and multiple follicular development. Aspiration of all follicles, prior to ovulation, may reduce the incidence of hyperstimulation syndrome.

The severe form of hyperstimulation syndrome may be life threatening and is characterised by large ovarian cysts which are prone to rupture, acute abdominal pain, ascites, very often hydrothorax and occasionally thromboembolic phenomena.

Prior to treatment with Menogon, primary ovarian failure should be excluded by the determination of gonadotrophin levels.

Overdose: The acute toxicity of menotrophin has been shown to be very low. However, too high a dosage for more than one day may lead to hyperstimulation, which is categorised as mild, moderate or severe. Symptoms of overdosage usually appear 3–6 days after treatment with hCG.

Mild hyperstimulation – Symptoms include some abdominal swelling and pain, ovaries enlarged to about 5 cm diameter. Therapy is rest, careful observation and symptomatic relief. Ovarian enlargement declines rapidly.

Moderate hyperstimulation – Symptoms include more pronounced abdominal distension and pain, nausea, vomiting, occasional diarrhoea, ovaries enlarged up to 12 cm diameter. Therapy is bed rest, close observation especially in the case of conception occurring, to detect any progression to severe hyperstimulation.

Pelvic examination of enlarged ovaries should be gentle in order to avoid rupture of the cysts. Symptoms subside spontaneously over 2–3 weeks.

Severe hyperstimulation – This is a rare but serious complication – symptoms include pronounced abdominal distension and pain, ascites, pleural effusion, decreased blood volume, reduced urine output, electrolyte imbalance and sometimes shock, ovaries enlarge to in excess of 12 cm diameter. Therapy is hospitalisation; treatment should be conservative and concentrate on restoring blood volume and preventing shock. Acute symptoms subside over several days and ovaries return to normal over 20–40 days if conception does not occur – symptoms may be prolonged if conception occurs.

Pharmaceutical precautions Protect from light. Store at a temperature not exceeding 25°C.

Legal category POM.

Package quantities Each carton contains 10 ampoules of Menogon and 10 ampoules of sodium chloride solution for injections 0.9% w/v, for reconstitution of the dry powder.

Further information 75 IU menotrophin contains 75 IU FSH and 75 IU LH and is obtained from the urine of post menopausal women.

Product licence numbers
Menogon: PL 03194/0059
Sodium chloride solution for injections 0.9% w/v: PL 03194/0060.

PENTASA* MESALAZINE ENEMA

Presentation Individually foil-wrapped unit dose polythene enema bottles with protective sleeve. Each bottle contains 100 ml of a colourless to pale yellow aqueous suspension containing 1 g mesalazine.

Uses Pentasa Mesalazine Enema is indicated for the treatment of ulcerative colitis affecting the distal colon and rectum.

Dosage and administration *Adults:* The recommended dosage is one enema at bedtime.
Children: Not recommended.

Contra-indications, warnings, etc
Contra indications: Pentasa is contraindicated in:
- Patients with known sensitivity to salicylates
- Patients with severe liver and/or renal impairment
- Patients allergic to any of the ingredients

Use during pregnancy and lactation: Pentasa should be used with caution during pregnancy and lactation and only if the potential benefit outweighs the possible hazards in the opinion of the physician.

Mesalazine is known to cross the placental barrier, but the limited data available on its use in pregnant women do not allow assessment of possible adverse effects. No teratogenic effects have been observed in animal studies.

Mesalazine is excreted in breast milk. The concentration is lower than in maternal blood, whereas the metabolite, acetyl mesalazine appears in similar or increased concentrations. No adverse effects in suckling babies of mothers treated with Pentasa have been reported, but the data are very limited.

Precautions and warnings: Serious blood dyscrasias have been reported rarely with mesalazine. Haematological investigations should be performed if the patient develops unexplained bleeding, bruising, purpura, anaemia, fever or sore throat. Treatment should be stopped if there is suspicion or evidence of blood dyscrasia.

Most patients who are intolerant or hypersensitive to sulphasalazine are able to take Pentasa without risk of similar reactions. However, caution is recommended when treating patients allergic to sulphasalazine (risk of allergy to salicylates). Caution is recommended in patients with impaired liver function.

The drug is not recommended for use in patients with renal impairment. Renal function should be monitored regularly (e.g. serum creatinine), especially during the initial phase of treatment.

Mesalazine induced cardiac hypersensitivity reactions (myocarditis and pericarditis) have been reported rarely. Treatment should be discontinued on suspicion or evidence of these reactions.

Side effects: Minor side effects which may occur include headache, nausea, vomiting, diarrhoea, abdominal pain and rash (including urticaria and exanthema). Mesalazine may be associated with an exacerbation of the symptoms of colitis in those patients who have previously had such problems with sulphasalazine. There have been rare reports of leucopenia, neutropenia, agranulocytosis, aplastic anaemia and thrombocytopenia, pancreatitis, hepatitis, allergic lung reactions, lupus erythematosus-like reactions, nephropathy including interstitial nephritis and nephrotic syndrome with oral mesalazine treatment, usually reversible on withdrawal. Rarely, myocarditis, pericarditis and increased amylase have also been reported. Reversible alopecia, increased liver enzymes, myalgia and arthralgia have been reported very rarely. The mechanism of mesalazine induced myocarditis, pericarditis, pancreatitis, nephritis and hepatitis is unknown, but it might be of allergic origin. Renal failure has been reported. Mesalazine-induced nephrotoxocity should be suspected in patients developing renal dysfunction during treatment.

Following rectal administration local reactions such as pruritus, rectal discomfort and urge may occur.

Interactions: There are no data on interactions between Pentasa and other drugs.

Treatment of overdose

Acute experience in animals: Single oral doses of mesalazine of up to 5 g/kg in pigs or a single intravenous dose of mesalazine at 920 mg/kg in rats were not lethal.

Human experience: No cases of overdose have been reported.

Management of overdose in man: Symptomatic treatment at hospital. Close monitoring of renal function. Intravenous infusion of electrolytes may be used to promote diuresis.

Pharmaceutical precautions Pentasa Enema should be stored at room temperature (15°C–25°C). Protect from light. Use immediately after opening individual foil pack.

Legal category POM.

Package quantities Cartons containing seven individually foil-wrapped 100 ml enemas.

Further information A plastic sleeve bearing administration instructions is provided for each enema bottle. The sleeve also facilitates hygienic application of the enema and disposal after use.

Product licence number 3194/0027.

PENTASA* SLOW RELEASE TABLETS

Presentation Pentasa Slow Release Tablets 250 mg: White to light grey, specked, round tablets, scored and marked '250' on one side and 'PENTASA' on the reverse side. Each tablet contains 250 mg mesalazine in a slow release presentation.

Pentasa Slow Release Tablets 500 mg: White to light grey, specked, round tablets, scored and marked '500 mg' on one side and 'PENTASA' on the reverse side. Each tablet contains 500 mg mesalazine in a slow release presentation.

Uses Pentasa Slow Release Tablets are indicated for the treatment of mild to moderate acute exacerbations of ulcerative colitis.

For the maintenance of remission of ulcerative colitis.

Dosage and administration The tablets may be dispersed in water to facilitate swallowing but they should not be chewed.

Adults:
Acute treatment: Individual dosage up to 4 g mesalazine daily in 2 or 3 divided doses.

Maintenance treatment: Individual dosage. Recommended starting dose is 1500 mg mesalazine daily in 2 or 3 divided doses.

Children: Not recommended.

Elderly patients: The usual adult dose applies.

Contra-indications, warnings, etc
Contra-indications: Pentasa is contraindicated in:
- Patients with known sensitivity to salicylates
- Children under the age of 15 years
- Patients with severe liver and/or renal impairment
- Patients allergic to any of the ingredients

Use during pregnancy and lactation: Pentasa should be used with caution during pregnancy and lactation and only if the potential benefit outweighs the possible hazards in the opinion of the physician.

Mesalazine is known to cross the placental barrier, but the limited data available on its use in pregnant women do not allow assessment of possible adverse effects. No teratogenic effects have been observed in animal studies.

Mesalazine is excreted in breast milk. The concentration is lower than in maternal blood, whereas the metabolite, acetyl mesalazine appears in similar or increased concentrations. No adverse effects in suckling babies of mothers treated with Pentasa have been reported, but the data are very limited.

Precautions and warnings: Serious blood dyscrasias have been reported rarely with mesalazine. Haematological investigations should be performed if the patient develops unexplained bleeding, bruising, purpura, anaemia, fever or sore throat. Treatment should be stopped if there is suspicion or evidence of blood dyscrasia.

Most patients who are intolerant or hypersensitive to sulphasalazine are able to take Pentasa without risk of similar reactions. However, caution is recommended when treating patients allergic to sulphasalazine (risk of allergy to salicylates). Caution is recommended in patients with impaired liver function.

The drug is not recommended for use in patients with renal impairment. Renal function should be monitored regularly (e.g. serum creatinine), especially during the initial phase of treatment.

Mesalazine induced cardiac hypersensitivity reactions (myocarditis and pericarditis) have been reported rarely. Treatment should be discontinued on suspicion or evidence of these reactions.

Side effects: Minor side effects which may occur include headache, nausea, vomiting, diarrhoea, abdominal pain and rash (including urticaria and exanthema). Mesalazine may be associated with an exacerbation of the symptoms of colitis in those patients who have previously had such problems with sulphasalazine. There have been rare reports of leucopenia, neutropenia, agranulocytosis, aplastic anaemia and thrombocytopenia, pancreatitis, hepatitis, allergic lung reactions, lupus erythematosus-like reactions, nephropathy including interstitial nephritis and nephrotic syndrome with oral mesalazine treatment, usually reversible on withdrawal. Rarely, myocarditis, pericarditis and increased amylase have also been reported. Reversible alopecia, increased liver enzymes, myalgia and arthralgia have been reported very rarely. The mechanism of mesalazine induced myocarditis, pericarditis, pancreatitis, nephritis and hepatitis is unknown, but it might be of allergic origin. Renal failure has been reported. Mesalazine-induced nephrotoxocity should be suspected in patients developing renal dysfunction during treatment.

Interactions: There are no data on interactions between Pentasa and other drugs.

Treatment of overdose

Acute experience in animals: Single oral doses of mesalazine of up to 5 g/kg in pigs or a single intravenous dose of mesalazine at 920 mg/kg in rats were not lethal.

Human experience: No cases of overdose have been reported.

Management of overdose in man: Symptomatic treatment at hospital. Close monitoring of renal function. Intravenous infusion of electrolytes may be used to promote diuresis.

Pharmaceutical precautions Pentasa Slow Release Tablets should be stored at room temperature (15°C–25°C).

Legal category POM.

Package quantities Amber glass screw-top bottles each containing 200×250 mg tablets. Cartons containing 100×500 mg tablets in double aluminium foil blister packs.

Further information Pentasa Slow Release Tablets disintegrate in the stomach to yield coated slow release granules which are conveyed into the intestinal tract. The release of mesalazine from the granulation takes place at all physiological pH values but is slower in the acidic conditions found in the upper gastrointestinal tract. This approach ensures that mesalazine is available in the lumen of the intestine for topical activity in ulcerative colitis. Plasma levels of mesalazine and its metabolites are similar to those observed during therapy with sulphasalazine.

Product licence numbers
Pentasa Slow Release Tablets 250 mg 3194/0043.
Pentasa Slow Release Tablets 500 mg 3194/0044.

PENTASA* SUPPOSITORIES 1 g

Presentation Oblong, compressed white to light tan, specked suppositories each containing 1 g mesalazine in a macrogol 6000 base.

Uses Pentasa Suppositories are indicated for the treatment of ulcerative proctitis.

Dosage and administration
Adults:
Acute treatment: The recommended dosage is one suppository daily for two to four weeks.
Maintenance Treatment: One suppository daily.
Children: Not recommended.
Elderly patients: The usual adult dose applies.

Contra-indications, warnings, etc
Contra-indications: Pentasa is contraindicated in:
- Patients with known sensitivity to salicylates
- Children under the age of 15 years
- Patients with severe liver and/or renal impairment
- Patients allergic to any of the ingredients

Use during pregnancy and lactation: Pentasa should be used with caution during pregnancy and lactation and only if the potential benefit outweighs the possible hazards in the opinion of the physician.

Mesalazine is known to cross the placental barrier, but the limited data available on its use in pregnant women do not allow assessment of possible adverse effects. No teratogenic effects have been observed in animal studies.

Mesalazine is excreted in breast milk. The concentration is lower than in maternal blood, whereas the metabolite, acetyl mesalazine appears in similar or increased concentrations. No adverse effects in suckling babies of mothers treated with Pentasa have been reported, but the data are very limited.

Precautions and warnings: Serious blood dyscrasias have been reported rarely with mesalazine. Haematological investigations should be performed if the patient develops unexplained bleeding, bruising, purpura, anaemia, fever or sore throat. Treatment should be stopped if there is suspicion or evidence of blood dyscrasia.

Most patients who are intolerant or hypersensitive to sulphasalazine are able to take Pentasa without risk of similar reactions. However, caution is recommended when treating patients allergic to sulphasalazine (risk of allergy to salicylates). Caution is recommended in patients with impaired liver function.

The drug is not recommended for use in patients with renal impairment. Renal function should be monitored regularly (e.g. serum creatinine), especially during the initial phase of treatment.

Mesalazine induced cardiac hypersensitivity reactions (myocarditis and pericarditis) have been reported rarely. Treatment should be discontinued on suspicion or evidence of these reactions.

Adverse reactions: Minor side effects which may occur include headache, nausea, vomiting, diarrhoea, abdominal pain and rash (including urticaria and exanthema). Mesalazine may be associated with an exacerbation of the symptoms of colitis in those patients who have previously had such problems with sulphasalazine. There have been rare reports of leucopenia, neutropenia, agranulocytosis, aplastic anaemia and thrombocytopenia, pancreatitis, hepatitis, allergic lung reactions, lupus erythematosus-like reactions, nephropathy including interstitial nephritis and nephrotic syndrome with oral mesalazine treatment, usually reversible on withdrawal. Rarely, myocarditis, pericarditis and increased amylase have also been reported. Reversible alopecia, increased liver enzymes, myalgia and arthralgia have been reported very rarely. The mechanism of mesalazine induced myocarditis, pericarditis, pancreatitis, nephritis and hepatitis is unknown, but it might be of allergic origin. Renal failure has been reported. Mesalazine-induced nephrotoxocity should be suspected in patients developing renal dysfunction during treatment.

Following rectal administration local reactions such as pruritus, rectal discomfort and urge may occur.

Interactions: There are no data on interactions between Pentasa and other drugs.

Treatment of overdose

Acute experience in animals: Single oral doses of mesalazine of up to 5 g/kg in pigs or a single intravenous dose of mesalazine at 920 mg/kg in rats were not lethal.

Human experience: No cases of overdose have been reported.

Management of overdose in man: Symptomatic treatment at hospital. Close monitoring of renal function. Intravenous infusion of electrolytes may be used to promote diuresis.

Pharmaceutical precautions Pentasa Suppositories should be stored at room temperature (15°C–25°C).

Legal category POM.

Package quantities Each suppository is individually packed in double aluminium foil presented in cartons of 28 suppositories.

Further information Each pack contains administration instructions for patients and rubber finger-protectors to facilitate hygenic insertion. The release profile for Pentasa Suppositories is comparable to Pentasa Enemas.

Product licence number 3194/0045.

PICOLAX*

Presentation Sachets each containing 16.1 g of powder for oral administration. Active ingredients: Sodium picosulphate 10 mg with magnesium citrate formed in solution.

Uses For clearance of the bowel prior to examination by radiography, endoscopy or surgery.

Dosage and administration
Adults: The contents of one sachet are reconstituted in a cup of water. Stir for 2–3 minutes and drink the mixture. If it becomes hot, wait until it cools sufficiently to drink.
1st dose – 1 sachet before 8 am on the day prior to examination.
2nd dose – 1 sachet between 2 and 4 pm on the day prior to examination.

Children: Timings as above.
1–2 years: ¼ sachet morning, ¼ sachet afternoon.
2–4 years: ½ sachet morning, ½ sachet afternoon.
4–9 years: 1 sachet morning, ½ sachet afternoon.
9 and above: adult dose.

Elderly patients: As for adults.

A low residue diet is recommended for 2 days prior to examination, and a liberal intake of clear fluids. Patients should drink as much as is required to satisfy thirst. A suggested diet plan is given in the Patient Information Leaflet.

Patients should be warned to expect frequent, loose bowel movements. Some authorities recommend a high fluid intake but no food at all during the 24 hours prior to examination.

Contra-indications, warnings, etc The usual general contraindications to purgatives apply. In patients with severely reduced renal function, accumulation of magnesium in plasma may occur. Another preparation should be used in such cases.

Picolax should not be used in suspected toxic dilatation of the colon. Picolax is also contraindicated in patients with clinical evidence of bowel obstruction.

Use in pregnancy and lactation: Reproduction studies with sodium picosulphate performed in animals have revealed no evidence of a harmful action on the fetus. However, clinical experience of the use of Picolax during pregnancy is limited and caution should be observed, particularly during the first trimester.

Neither sodium picosulphate nor magnesium citrate have been shown to be excreted in breast milk.

Warnings and precautions: Picolax should not be used in patients with undiagnosed abdominal symptoms. Care should also be taken in patients with inflammatory bowel disease and in patients with suspected bowel obstruction.

A suboptimal oral intake of water and electrolytes could create clinically significant deficiencies in less fit patients. In this regard, elderly, debilitated and patients at risk of hypokalaemia may need particular attention.

The period of bowel cleansing should not exceed 24 hours because longer preparation may increase the risk of water and electrolyte imbalance.

Side effects: As with other bowel cleansing regimens, treatment with Picolax may cause headache, tiredness, nausea, griping and anal pain. Isolated cases have been reported of allergic reactions including anaphylaxis or of vomiting and severe diarrhoea leading to hyponatraemia and convulsions in the absence of adequate salt replacement.

Interactions: As a purgative, Picolax increases gastrointestinal transit rate. Absorption of other orally administered medicines may therefore be modified during the treatment period. The efficacy of Picolax is lowered by bulk-forming laxatives.

Care should be taken with patients already receiving drugs which may be associated with hypokalaemia (such as diuretics or corticosteroids, or drugs where hypokalaemia is a particular risk i.e. cardiac glycosides).

Treatment of overdose: Overdosage would lead to profuse diarrhoea. Treatment is by general supportive measures and maintenance of fluid intake.

Pharmaceutical precautions Store at room temperature, in a cool dry place.

Legal category P.

Package quantity Treatment units of two sachets in cartons of 25×2 sachets.

Product licence number 3194/0014

PROPESS*

Presentation Propess is presented as a thin, flat, semi-opaque polymeric pessary which is rectangular in shape with radiused corners contained within a knitted polyester retrieval system.

Each pessary consists of a non-biodegradable polymeric drug delivery device containing dinoprostone (PGE_2) dispersed throughout its matrix, and releasing approximately 5 mg PGE_2 over 12 hours. The reservoir of 10 mg dinoprostone serves to maintain constant release.

The retrieval system, within which each pessary is supplied, consists of a one-piece knitted polyester pouch and withdrawal tape. This ensures easy and reliable removal of the pessary when the patient's requirement for PGE_2 has been fulfilled or an obstetric event makes it necessary to stop further drug administration.

Uses Propess is indicated for the initiation and/or continuation of cervical ripening in patients at term (from 38 weeks gestation) when there is a singleton cephalic presentation. The ripeness of the cervix should be assessed by a Bishop's Score or modification thereof. Propess is indicated for induction of labour when the score is 6 or less by the original Bishop's Score (Bishop, E.H., (1964) Obstetrics & Gynecology, *24* (2), 266–268). There should be no fetal or maternal contra-indications.

Dosage and administration
Dosage: One pessary. This is usually sufficient to achieve cervical ripening.

If there has been insufficient cervical ripening in 8–12 hours, the pessary should be removed. It may be replaced by a second pessary. This should also be removed not more than 12 hours later. Not more than 2 consecutive pessaries should be used in the course of therapy.

Administration: Do not remove the pessary from the retrieval system in which it is supplied.

The pessary should be inserted high into the posterior vaginal fornix using only small amounts of water soluble lubricants to aid insertion. After the pessary has been inserted, the withdrawal tape may be cut with scissors always ensuring there is sufficient tape outside the vagina to allow removal. No attempt should be made to tuck the end of the tape into the vagina as this may make retrieval more difficult.

The patient should be recumbent for 20 mins–30 mins after insertion. As PGE_2 will be released continuously over a period of 12 hours, it is important to monitor uterine contractions and fetal condition at frequent regular intervals.

Retrieval: It is necessary to remove the pessary to terminate drug administration when cervical ripening is judged to be complete or for any of the reasons listed below.

The pessary can be removed quickly and easily by gentle traction on the retrieval tape.

The pessary should be removed immediately under any of the following circumstances:

1. Onset of labour. For the purpose of induction of labour with Propess, the onset of labour is defined as the presence of regular painful uterine contractions occurring every 3 minutes irrespective of any cervical change. There are two important points to note:

(i) Once regular, painful contractions have been established with Propess they will not reduce in frequency or intensity as long as Propess remains *in situ* because PGE_2 is still being administered.

(ii) Patients, particularly multigravidae, may develop regular painful contractions without any apparent cervical change. Effacement and dilatation of the cervix may not occur until uterine activity is established. Because of this, once regular painful uterine activity is established with Propess *in situ*, the pessary should be removed irrespective of cervical state to avoid the possibility of uterine hyperstimulation.

2. Spontaneous rupture of the membranes and at artificial rupture of membranes.
3. Any suggestion of uterine hyperstimulation or hypertonic uterine contractions.
4. Evidence of fetal distress.
5. Evidence of maternal systemic adverse PGE_2 effects such as nausea, vomiting, hypotension or tachycardia.
6. Prior to starting an intravenous infusion of oxytocin.

Contra-indications, warnings, etc
Contra-indications: Propess should not be used or left in place:
1. When labour has started.
2. When the membranes have ruptured.
3. When oxytocic drugs are being given.
4. When strong prolonged uterine contraction would be inappropriate such as in patients:
   a. who have had previous major uterine surgery.
   b. who have had previous surgery to the cervix of the uterus.

c. with a major degree of cephalopelvic disproportion.
d. with fetal malpresentation.
e. with suspicion or evidence of fetal distress.
f. with a history of difficult or traumatic deliveries.
g. who have had more than three full term deliveries.

5. When there is a history of, or current pelvic inflammatory disease, unless adequate prior treatment has been instituted.
6. When there is reason to believe there may be hypersensitivity to PGE_2.
7. When there is a multiple pregnancy.

Precautions and warnings: The suitability of the patient and the condition of the cervix should be assessed carefully before Propess is used. After insertion, uterine activity and fetal condition must be monitored regularly. If there is any suggestion of maternal or fetal complications or adverse effects, PGE_2 delivery should be stopped by removing the pessary from the vagina.

Propess should be used with caution in patients with a previous history of uterine hypertony, glaucoma, or asthma.

Medication with non-steroidal anti-inflammatory drugs, including aspirin, should be stopped before administration of PGE_2.

If uterine contractions are prolonged and excessive, there is a possibility of uterine hypertonus or rupture and the pessary should be removed immediately.

It would be prudent to remove the Propess pessary should epidural anaesthesia be given in anticipation of labour before membrane rupture.

High doses of Prostaglandin of the E and F series have been shown to induce bone proliferation in animals at high doses. Similar effects have been observed in neonates exposed to prostaglandins for long periods but no such changes have been seen with the short term administration of Propess for cervical ripening.

Side-effects: The occasional effects seen have been those normally associated with intravaginal PGE_2 administration.

CTG changes and unspecified fetal distress have been reported during and after administration of intravaginal PGE_2. Increased uterine activity with hypertonic contractions with or without fetal distress has been reported and immediate removal of the pessary is recommended. There is a much greater risk of hyperstimulation if the PGE_2 source is not removed before administration of oxytocin because prostaglandins are known to potentiate the uterotonic effects of oxytocic drugs.

Gastrointestinal effects such as nausea, vomiting and diarrhoea have been reported.

PGE_2 is known to be responsible for the patency of the ductus arteriosus in pregnancy but there have been no reports of 'blue babies' in the neonatal period after the use of Propess. In a 3 year follow up of 121 babies after labour induction with PGE_2, 51 of whom received Propess, there were no adverse effects on physical development or psychomotor evolution in the infants.

Overdose: Overdosage or hypersensitivity may lead to hyperstimulation of the uterine muscle or fetal distress. The Propess pessary should be removed immediately and the patient should be managed in accordance with local protocol.

Pharmaceutical precautions Propess should be stored unopened, in the foil pack in a freezer (−10 to −20°C) until immediately before use.

The opening on one side of the retrieval device is present only to allow the manufacturer to enclose the pessary into the retrieval device during manufacture.

The pessary should NEVER be removed from the retrieval device. On removal of the product, the pessary will have swollen to 2–3 times its original size and be pliable. The whole product should be disposed as clinical waste.

Legal category POM.

Package quantities Propess is presented in cartons of one individual, sealed aluminium foil/polyethylene laminate sachet.

Further information Propess is not approved nor intended for use as an abortifacient.

Drug delivery system information: The vaginal pessary is a product designed around the Controlled Therapeutics Delivery System. It is a patented hydrophilic hydrogel polymer which controls the delivery of PGE_2 at a near constant rate as it swells in vaginal fluid. In this process the pessary slowly becomes softer and rubbery in consistency, but maintains its physical integrity.

The retrieval system which encloses the pessary is a knitted product made from a polyester which is also used in the manufacture of long-term, vascular implants.

The nature of the device and its retrieval system allow easy and reliable removal of the product when required.

Product licence number 8731/0003.

Product licence holder: Controlled Therapeutics (Scotland) Limited, East Kilbride G74 5PB.

VIRORMONE*

Presentation Ampoules of 100 mg of Testosterone Propionate BP in ethyl oleate for intramuscular injection.

Uses Testosterone is the androgenic hormone of male testis. It is used as replacement therapy in castrated adults and in those who are hypogonadal due to either pituitary or testicular disease.

May also be used for control of carcinoma of the breast in post-menopausal women.

Dosage and administration
In the male: Hypogonadism (adults), delayed puberty, cryptorchidism.

In the female: Carcinoma of the breast in post-menopausal women.

Hypogonadism	50 mg 2–3 times weekly
Delayed puberty cryptorchidism	50 mg weekly
Carcinoma of the breast	100 mg 2–3 times weekly

Contra-indications, warnings, etc

Contra-indications: Breast cancer in men, prostatic carcinoma, pregnancy, breast feeding and nephrosis.

Interactions: None stated.

Effects on ability to drive and use machines: None stated.

Other undesirable effects: None stated.

Use in pregnancy and lactation: Contra-indicated.

Warning: Tumours of the liver have been reported occasionally in patients subjected to prolonged treatment with androgenic-anabolic steroids. The possibility that these compounds may induce or enhance the development of hepatic tumours cannot at present be excluded and this should be considered when the use of this product is proposed, especially in young people who are not suffering with life threatening disorders.

Precautions: Do not use before puberty in males, unless for treatment of delayed puberty. In any case caution is advised since the fusion of the epiphyses is hastened and may lead to short stature.

Use with care in patients with cardiac, renal or hepatic impairment, circulatory failure, hypertension or epilepsy. A reduced dosage may be advisable in elderly male patients since hyperstimulation can occur.

Virilism may occur in female patients on high doses.

Overdose: None stated.

Incompatibilities: None stated.

Pharmaceutical precautions Protect from light.

Legal category POM.

Package quantities 100 mg in 2 ml ampoules. Boxes of 10.

Further information Nil.

Product licence number 3194/0064.

ZOMACTON* INJECTION-12 iu (Somatropin)

Presentation Zomacton Injection-12 iu is presented as a sterile lyophilised powder in a glass vial, with a potency of 3.0 iu per mg. Each vial is supplied with a diluent ampoule of sterile isotonic saline for injection 0.9% w/v (with benzyl alcohol 0.9% w/v preservative).

Uses Zomacton Injection is indicated for the long-term treatment of children who have growth failure due to inadequate secretion of growth hormone.

Dosage and administration
Children only: The dosage and schedule of administration of Zomacton Injection should be individualised for each patient.

The product should be reconstituted using only the diluent supplied. To prevent foaming of the solution, the stream of diluent should be aimed against the side of the vial. The vial must then be swirled with a gentle rotary motion until the contents are completely dissolved and a clear, colourless solution is produced. Since Zomacton Injection is a protein, shaking or vigorous mixing is not recommended. If, after the mixing, the solution is cloudy or contains particulate matter, the contents must be discarded. In the case of cloudiness after refrigeration, the product should be allowed to warm to room temperature. If cloudiness persists, discard the vial and its contents.

Generally a dose of 0.5–0.7 iu/kg bodyweight (corresponding to 0.17 mg/kg–0.23 mg/kg bodyweight or 14.8 iu/m²–20.7 iu/m² body surface area) per week divided into 6–7 subcutaneous injections is recommended (corresponding to a daily injection of 0.07–0.1 iu/kg bodyweight equivalent to 0.023 mg/kg–0.033 mg/kg bodyweight or 2.1–3.0 iu/m² body surface area). The total weekly dose of 0.81 iu/kg bodyweight corresponding to 0.27 mg/kg or 24 iu/m² body surface area should not be exceeded (corresponding to daily injections of up to 0.116 iu/kg equivalent to 0.039 mg/kg). The duration of treatment, usually a period of several years, will depend on maximum achievable therapeutic benefit.

Contra-indications, warnings, etc
Contra-indications: Zomacton Injection should not be used in children with closed epiphyses.

Patients with evidence of progression of an underlying intracranial lesion or other tumour should not receive Zomacton Injection, since the possibility of a tumour growth promoting effect cannot be excluded. Prior to the initiation of therapy with Zomacton Injection, intracranial tumours must be inactive and anti-tumour therapy completed.

Patients with a known sensitivity to benzyl alcohol should not be treated with Zomacton Injection-12 iu.

Use in pregnancy and lactation: Zomacton should not be used during pregnancy or lactation. There is no evidence from either human or animal studies of the safety of growth hormone treatment during pregnancy. Also, no information is available as to whether peptide hormones pass into breast milk.

Special warnings and precautions for use: Zomacton Injection therapy should be used only under the supervision of a qualified physician, experienced in the management of patients with growth hormone deficiency.

Patients should be observed for evidence of glucose intolerance because growth hormone may induce a state of insulin resistance. Zomacton Injection should be used with caution in patients with diabetes mellitus or a familial predisposition to the disease. Strict monitoring of urine and blood glucose is necessary in these patients. In childen with diabetes mellitus, the dose of insulin may need to be increased to maintain glucose control during Zomacton Injection therapy.

Children with hypopituitarism sometimes experience fasting hypoglycaemia which is improved by therapy with growth hormone. There have been reports that some of these children, when treated with growth hormone injections three times weekly, experience hypoglycaemia on non-treatment days. Thus, in children who have fasting hypoglycaemia associated with hypopituitarism, daily growth hormone administration is recommended.

In patients with growth hormone deficiency secondary to an intracranial lesion, frequent monitoring for progression or recurrence of the underlying disease process is advised. Discontinue Zomacton Injection therapy if progression or recurrence of the lesion occurs.

Fundoscopic examination for papilloedema is recommended at the initiation and periodically during the course of growth hormone treatment, especially if the patients report recurrent headache, visual problems, nausea and/or vomiting which may indicate intracranial hypertension.

Hypothyroidism may develop during treatment with growth hormone. Inadequate treatment of hypothyroidism may prevent optimal response to Zomacton Injection. Therefore, patients should have periodic thyroid function tests and be treated with thyroid hormone when indicated.

Leukaemia has been reported in a small number of growth hormone deficient patients treated with Somatropin as well as in untreated patients. Based on current evidence, experts cannot conclude that Somatropin is responsible for this. If there is any increase in risk to an individual patient it is small.

Slipped capital femoral epiphysis may occur more frequently in patients with endocrine disorders. A patient treated with Zomacton Injection who develops a limp or complains of hip or knee pain should be evaluated by a physician.

Side-effects: The subcutaneous administration of growth hormone may lead to the loss or increase of adipose tissue at the injection site. Therefore, injection sites should be changed frequently. Rarely, pain and an itchy rash may develop at the injection site.

Transient headache has been reported. Infrequently, a slight transient oedema may occur during treatment.

Formation of antibodies against Somatropin or *E. coli* has not yet been observed.

In individual cases, especially during the first weeks of growth hormone therapy, a benign intracranial hypertension has been reported. Symptoms usually are headache, nausea and/or vomiting and visual problems requiring fundoscopic examination for papilloedema. In most cases the symptoms resolved without discontinuation of therapy; in severe cases the dose should be reduced or treatment interrupted.

Interactions: Glucocorticoid therapy may inhibit the growth promoting effect of Zomacton Injection. Patients with co-existing ACTH deficiency should have their glucocorticoid replacement dose carefully adjusted to avoid impairment of the growth promoting effect of Zomacton Injection.

High doses of androgens, oestrogens or anabolic steroids can accelerate bone maturation and inhibit an increase in growth.

Because human growth hormone can induce a state of insulin resistance, insulin dose may have to be adjusted in the patient receiving concomitant Zomacton Injection.

Overdose: The recommended dose of Zomacton Injection should not be exceeded. Acute overdosage may result in an initial hypoglycaemia followed by a subsequent hyperglycaemia.

The effects of long term, repeated use of Zomacton Injection in doses exceeding those recommended, are unknown. However, it is possible that such use might produce signs and symptoms consistent with the known effects of excess human growth hormone (e.g. acromegaly).

Pharmaceutical precautions Zomacton Injection should be stored in the refrigerator at 2°C to 8°C and protected from light. After reconstitution with sterile isotonic saline 0.9% w/v (containing benzyl alcohol preservative 0.9% w/v), Zomacton Injection is stable for 14 days when stored in the refrigerator at 2°C to 8°C and protected from light. Discard any solution left in the vial at the end of this period.

Legal category POM.

Package quantities Each carton contains one vial of Zomacton Injection-12 iu and one diluent ampoule of sterile isotonic saline solution 0.9% w/v 3.5 ml (containing benzyl alcohol preservative 0.9% w/v).

Further information Zomacton Injection contains human growth hormone (Somatropin) produced in a genetically modified Escherichia Coli strain using a recombinant DNA technique. It is chemically identical and biologically equivalent to pituitary-derived Somatropin. It does not contain a terminal methionine residue. The lyophilised powder contains the inactive ingredient mannitol.

Product licence numbers

Zomacton Injection	3194/0052
Diluent	3194/0054.

**Trade Mark*

Florizel Ltd
15 Kritis Street
10451 Athens
Greece

Florizel Ltd

DIMETRIOSE*

Qualitative and quantitative composition Gestrinone capsules 2.5 mg.

Pharmaceutical form Hard white, size no. 4 gelatin capsules containing a white to slightly yellow powder. The capsule will be printed "Roussel" and logo.

Clinical particulars
Therapeutic indications: Therapeutic treatment of endometriosis.

Posology and method of administration:
Adults: Gestrinone is for oral administration to adult females only. The dose is one capsule twice a week. To ensure that pregnant patients are not treated, it is essential that **the first dose is taken on the first day of the menstrual cycle.**

The second dose should be taken three days later. Thereafter, Gestrinone capsules should be taken on the same two days of the week (preferably at the same time) every week for the duration of the treatment, which will normally be six months.

Should one dose be missed, then a capsule should be taken as soon as possible and the original sequence maintained.

Should two or more doses be missed, treatment should be discontinued and therapy re-started on the first day of the new cycle, following a negative pregnancy test and according to the usual dosage schedule.

Children & elderly adults: Treatment with Gestrinone is not appropriate.

Contra-indications: Pregnancy. Lactation. Severe cardiac, renal or hepatic insufficiency. Metabolic and/or vascular disorders during previous oestrogen and/or progestogen therapy.

Special warnings and special precautions for use: The possibility of pregnancy must be ruled out before starting treatment, especially in the case of pre-existing amenorrhoea.

Gestrinone, at the recommended dose, may inhibit ovulation in some women but, pregnancies can occur with this treatment and gestrinone must **not** be relied on for contraception.

As concurrent administration of oral contraceptives may modify the action of gestrinone, it is, therefore, essential that barrier methods are used throughout treatment as the use of gestrinone is totally contra-indicated in pregnancy.

Because gestrinone may occasionally cause some degree of fluid retention, patients with cardiac or renal dysfunction require close monitoring.

Monitor ALAT, ASAT, cholesterol fractions in hyperlipidaemic subjects and blood sugar levels in diabetics.

Gestrinone will cause a decrease in the concentration of thyroid-binding globulin. Hence there will be a decrease in serum total thyroxine levels. This is without clinical significance as free thyroxine levels remain within the reference range as do thyroid-stimulating hormone levels.

Interactions with other medicaments and other forms of interaction: Concomitant administration of anti-epileptic drugs or rifampicin may result in accelerated metabolism of gestrinone.

Use in pregnancy and lactation: Gestrinone is specifically contraindicated in pregnancy and lactation.

Administration should be discontinued if a patient is found to be pregnant as animal studies have shown embryotoxicity in some species, albeit at doses well in excess of those used clinically.

Effects on ability to drive and to use machines: None stated.

Undesirable effects (frequency and seriousness): Spotting has been reported in some patients both during the first few weeks and throughout treatment.

Acne, oily skin, fluid retention, weight gain, hirsutism, voice change and other androgen-type effects have been reported by some patients.

Other unwanted reactions recorded during gestrinone therapy include transient increases in liver transaminases, headache, gastro-intestinal disturbance, change in libido, hot flushes, decrease in breast size, nervousness and depression, cramp and change in appetite.

Overdose: Acute toxicity studies in animals indicate that serious reactions are unlikely as an immediate result of a single excessive dose.

In the case of acute overdosage, the drug should be removed by emesis or gastric lavage if ingestion is recent and the patient kept under observation in case of delayed reaction.

Pharmacological properties
Pharmacodynamic properties: Gestrinone, a synthetic steroid hormone, is an antiprogestin: it is not an oestrogen-progestogen combination. Gestrinone has an inhibitory effect on endometrial tissue. It is believed to act by direct inhibition of the synthesis-release mechanisms of pituitary gonadotrophins and a direct antagonist action on endometrial tissues.

Pharmacokinetic properties: Gestrinone shows linear pharmacokinetics after oral administration of 1.25 mg, 2.5 or 5 mg. The peak concentration appears between 2.8 and 3.1 hours after administration.

The plasma half life is about 24 hours.

Three days after administration blood levels are only 5% of the maximum plasma concentration. The steady state is reached since the second administration, which is three days after the initial dose, therefore there is virtually no risk of accumulation under normal conditions of use.

Investigation of the absolute bioavailability in a subject after gestrinone administration demonstrates that after oral administration, absorption is virtually complete and the first pass metabolism is negligible.

Gestrinone undergoes important hepatic metabolism, essentially through hydroxylation processes, resulting in the formation of conjugated metabolites.

Pharmaceutical particulars
List of excipients: The product contains Colloidal Silicon Dioxide, Maize Starch, Microcrystalline Cellulose, Lactose, Magnesium Stearate, and Talc.

The white opaque capsule shell contains Titanium Dioxide and Gelatin.

Incompatibilities: None stated.

Shelf life: 60 months.

Special precautions for storage: Store below 25°C protected from light.

Nature and contents of container: Dimetriose capsules are supplied in blister packs of 8 capsules.

Instructions for use/handling: None.

Marketing authorisation holder: Roussel Laboratories Ltd., Broadwater Park, Denham, Uxbridge, Middlesex UB9 5HP, UK

Marketing authorisation number 0109/0207

Date of revision/approval of SPC May 1997

Legal category POM

MERBENTYL* 20

Qualitative and quantitative composition Dicyclomine hydrochloride BP 20 mg

Pharmaceutical form Tablets.

Clinical particulars
Therapeutic indications: Smooth muscle antispasmodic primarily indicated for treatment of functional conditions involving smooth muscle spasm of the gastrointestinal tract.

Posology and method of administration: Route of administration: Oral

Adults and children over 12 years: 1 tablet three times a day before or after meals.

Contra-indications: Known idiosyncrasy to dicyclomine hydrochloride.

Special warnings and special precautions for use: Products containing dicyclomine hydrochloride should be used with caution in any patient with or suspected of having glaucoma or prostatic hypertrophy. Use with care In patients with hiatus hernia associated with reflux oesophagitis because anticholinergic drugs may aggravate the condition.

Interaction with other medicaments and other forms of interaction: None stated.

Pregnancy and lactation: Epidemiological studies in pregnant women with products containing dicyclomine hydrochloride (at doses up to 40 mg/day) have not shown that dicyclomine hydrochloride increases the risk of foetal abnormalities if administered during the first trimester of pregnancy. Reproduction studies have been performed in rats and rabbits at doses of up to 100 times the maximum recommended dose (based on 60 mg per day for an adult person) and have revealed no evidence of impaired fertility or harm to the foetus due to dicyclomine. Since the risk of teratogenicity cannot be excluded with absolute certainty for any product, the drug should be used during pregnancy only if clearly needed.

It is not known whether dicyclomine is secreted in human milk. Because many drugs are excreted in human milk, caution should be exercised when dicyclomine is administered to a nursing woman.

Effects on ability to drive and use machines: None stated.

Undesirable effects: Side-effects seldom occur with Merbentyl tablets. However, in susceptible individuals, dry mouth, thirst and dizziness may occur. On rare occasions, fatigue, sedation, blurred vision, rash, constipation, anorexia, nausea and vomiting, headache and dysuria have also been reported.

Overdose: Symptoms of Merbentyl overdosage are headache, dizziness, nausea, dry mouth, difficulty in swallowing, dilated pupils and hot dry skin. Treatment may include emetics, gastric lavage and symptomatic therapy if indicated.

Pharmacological properties
Pharmacodynamic properties: Dicyclomine hydrochloride relieves smooth muscle spasm of the gastrointestinal tract.

Animal studies indicate that this action is achieved via a dual mechanism: (1) a specific anticholinergic effect (antimuscarinic at the ACh-receptor sites) and (2) a direct effect upon smooth muscle (musculotropic).

Pharmacokinetic properties: After a single oral 20 mg dose of dicyclomine hydrochloride in volunteers, peak plasma concentration reached a mean value of 58 ng/ml in 1 to 1.5 hours. ^{14}C labelled studies demonstrated comparable bioavailability from oral and intravenous administration. The principal route of elimination is via the urine.

Preclinical safety data: None stated.

Pharmaceutical particulars
List of excipients: The product contains Lactose, Calcium Hydrogen Phosphate, Icing Sugar (mixture of Sucrose 97%, Starch 3%), Maize Starch, Glucose Liquid, Magnesium Stearate and Purified Water.

Incompatibilities: None stated.

Shelf life: 5 years.

Special precautions for storage: None stated.

Nature and contents of container: Container: Opaque blue 250 micron PVC blisters with aluminium foil 20 micron. Pack Size: 84 tablets.

Instructions for use/handling: None stated.

Marketing authorisation holder: Marion Merrell Ltd, Broadwater Park, Denham, Uxbridge, Middlesex, UB9 5HP

Marketing authorisation number PL 4425/0081

Date of approval/revision of SPC February 1996

Legal category POM

MERBENTYL* SYRUP

Presentation Merbentyl Syrup is colourless, and raspberry flavoured. Each 5 ml contains 10 mg Dicyclomine Hydrochloride BP.

Uses Merbentyl is a smooth muscle antispasmodic primarily indicated for the treatment of functional conditions involving smooth muscle spasm of the gastro-intestinal tract. The commonest of these is irritable colon (mucous colitis, spastic colon).

Dosage and administration *Adults:* One to two 5 ml spoonfuls (10–20 mg) three times daily before or after meals.

Children (2–12 years): One 5 ml spoonful (10 mg) three times daily.

Children (6 months–2 years): 5–10 mg three or four times daily, 15 minutes before feeds. Do not exceed a daily dose of 40 mg. If it is necessary to dilute Merbentyl syrup this may be done using Syrup BP or, if diluted immediately prior to use, with water.

Contra-indications, warnings, etc
Contra-indications: Known idiosyncrasy to dicyclomine hydrochloride. Infants under 6 months of age.

Precautions: Products containing dicyclomine hydrochloride should be used with caution in any patient with, or suspected of having, glaucoma or prostatic hypertrophy. Use with care in patients with hiatus hernia associated with reflux oesophagitis because anticholinergic drugs may aggravate the condition.

There are rare reports of infants, 3 months of age and under, administered dicyclomine hydrochloride syrup, who have evidenced respiratory symptoms (breathing difficulty, shortness of breath, breathlessness, respiratory collapse, apnoea), as well as seizures, syncope, asphyxia, pulse rate fluctuations, muscular hypotonia and coma. The above symptoms have occurred within minutes of ingestion and lasted 20–30 minutes. The symptoms were reported in association with dicyclomine hydrochloride syrup therapy but the cause and effect relationship has neither been disproved nor proved. The timing and nature of the reactions suggest that they were a consequence of local irritation and/or aspiration, rather than to a direct pharmacological effect. Although no causal relationship between these effects, observed in infants, and dicyclomine administration has been established, dicyclomine hydrochloride is contra-indicated in infants under 6 months of age. See *Contra-indications* above.

Use in pregnancy and lactation: Epidemiological studies in pregnant women with products containing dicyclomine hydrochloride (at doses up to 40 mg/day) have not shown that dicyclomine hydrochloride increases the risk of foetal abnormalities if administered during the first trimester of pregnancy. Reproduction studies have been performed in rats and rabbits at doses of up to 100 times the maximum recommended dose (based on 60 mg per day for an adult person) and have revealed no evidence of impaired fertility or harm to the foetus due to dicyclomine.

Since the risk of teratogenicity cannot be excluded with absolute certainty for any product, the drug should be used during pregnancy only if clearly needed.

It is not known whether dicyclomine is secreted in human milk. Because many drugs are excreted in human milk, caution should be exercised when dicyclomine is administered to a nursing woman.

Side-effects: Side-effects seldom occur with Merbentyl. However, in susceptible individuals, dry mouth, thirst and dizziness may occur. On rare occasions, fatigue, sedation, blurred vision, rash, constipation, anorexia, nausea and vomiting, headache and dysuria have also been reported.

Overdosage: Symptoms of Merbentyl overdosage are headache, dizziness, nausea, dry mouth, difficulty in swallowing, dilated pupils and hot dry skin. Treatment may include emetics, gastric lavage and symptomatic therapy if indicated.

Pharmaceutical precautions Should be stored and dispensed in amber glass bottles.

Legal category POM

P – Preparations of Dicyclomine Hydrochloride for internal use with a maximum dose of 10 mg and a maximum daily dose of 60 mg.

Package quantities Amber glass bottle of 500 ml.

Further information Nil.

Product licence number PL 4425/0047

Product licence holder: Marion Merrell Ltd., Broadwater Park, Denham, Uxbridge, Middlesex UB9 5HP

MERBENTYL* TABLETS

Presentation
Merbentyl Tablets: White, round, plain biconvex tablets, stamped 'M' in two concentric circles, containing Dicyclomine Hydrochloride BP 10 mg.

Uses Merbentyl is a smooth muscle antispasmodic primarily indicated for the treatment of functional conditions involving smooth muscle spasm of the gastro-intestinal tract.

Dosage and administration *Adults:* 10–20 mg three times daily before or after meals.

Children: (2–12 years): 10 mg three times daily.

Contra-indications, warnings, etc
Contra-indications: Known idiosyncrasy to dicyclomine hydrochloride.

Precautions: Products containing dicyclomine hydrochloride should be used with caution in any patient with, or suspected of having glaucoma or prostatic hypertrophy. Use with care in patients with hiatus hernia associated with reflux oesophagitis because anticholinergic drugs may aggravate the condition.

Use in pregnancy and lactation: Epidemiological studies in pregnant women with products containing dicyclomine hydrochloride (at doses up to 40 mg/day) have not shown that dicyclomine hydrochloride increases the risk of foetal abnormalities if administered during the first trimester of pregnancy. Reproduction studies have been performed in rats and rabbits at doses of up to 100 times the maximum recommended dose (based on 60 mg per day for an adult person) and have revealed no evidence of impaired fertility or harm to the foetus due to dicyclomine.

Since the risk of teratogenicity cannot be excluded with absolute certainty for any product, the drug should be used during pregnancy only if clearly needed.

It is not known whether dicyclomine is secreted in human milk. Because many drugs are excreted in human milk, caution should be exercised when dicyclomine is administered to a nursing woman.

Side-effects: Side-effects seldom occur with Merbentyl. However, in susceptible individuals, dry mouth, thirst and dizziness may occur. On rare occasions, fatigue, sedation, blurred vision, rash, constipation, anorexia, nausea and vomiting, headache and dysuria have also been reported.

Overdosage: Symptoms of Merbentyl overdosage are headache, dizziness, nausea, dry mouth, difficulty in swallowing, dilated pupils and hot dry skin. Treatment may include emetics, gastric lavage and symptomatic therapy if indicated.

Pharmaceutical precautions None.

Legal category POM.

P – Preparations of Dicyclomine Hydrochloride for internal use with a maximum dose of 10 mg and a maximum daily dose of 60 mg.

Package quantities Blister pack of 100 tablets.

Further information Nil.

Product licence numbers
Merbentyl Tablets PL 4425/0035

Product licence holder: Marion Merrell Ltd., Broadwater Park, Denham, Uxbridge, Middlesex UB9 5HP

SOFRADEX* EAR/EYE DROPS
SOFRADEX* EAR/EYE OINTMENT

Qualitative and quantitative composition
Sofradex ear/eye drops: Each bottles contains 0.525% w/v of Framycetin Sulphate (includes a 5% overage), Dexamethasone Sodium Metasulphobenzoate (equivalent to 0.050% w/v of Dexamethasone) and 0.005% w/v of Gramicidin.

Sofradex ear/eye ointment: Ear/eye ointment containing 0.5% w/w Framycetin Sulphate, 0.05% w/w Dexamethasone and 0.005% w/w Gramicidin USP.

Pharmaceutical form
Sofradex ear/eye drops: Sterile clear colourless ear/eye drops.

Sofradex ear/eye ointment: Ear/eye ointment.

Clinical particulars
Therapeutic indications:
In the eye: For the short-term treatment of steroid responsive conditions of the eye when prophylactic antibiotic treatment is also required, after excluding the presence of fungal and viral disease.

In the ear: Otitis externa.

Application to the eyelid: Blepharitis. (Sofradex Ear/Eye ointment only)

Posology and method of administration: Route of Administration: Auricular and ocular use.

Sofradex Ear/Eye Drops: Adults (and the elderly) and children: In the Eye: One or two drops applied to each affected eye up to six times daily or more frequently if required. In the Ear: Two or three drops instilled into the ear three or four times daily

Sofradex Ear/Eye Ointment: Adults (and the elderly) and children: In the eye: Apply sparingly two or three times daily, or at night if drop treatment is given during the day. In the ear: Apply once or twice daily.

Contra-indications: Viral, fungal, tuberculous or purulent conditions of the eye. Use is contraindicated if glaucoma is present or herpetic keratitis (e.g. dendritic ulcer) is considered a possibility. Use of topical steroids in the latter condition can lead to extension of the ulcer and marked visual deterioration.

Otitis externa should not be treated when the eardrum is perforated because of the risk of ototoxicity.

Hypersensitivity to the preparation.

Special warnings and special precautions for use: Topical corticosteroids should never be given for an undiagnosed red eye as inappropriate use is potentially blinding.

Treatment with corticosteroid/antibiotic combinations should not be continued for more than 7 days in the absence of any clinical improvement, since prolonged use may lead to occult extension of infection due to the masking effect of the steroid. Prolonged use may also lead to skin sensitisation and the emergence of resistant organisms.

Prolonged use may lead to the risk of adrenal suppression in infants.

Treatment with corticosteroid preparations should not be repeated or prolonged without regular review to exclude raised intraocular, pressure, cataract formation or unsuspected infections.

Aminoglycoside antibiotics may cause irreversible, partial or total deafness when given systemically or when applied topically to open wounds or damaged skin. This effect is dose related and is enhanced by renal or hepatic impairment. Although this effect has not been reported following topical ocular use, the possibility should be considered when high dose topical treatment is given to small children or infants.

Interactions with other medicaments and other forms of interaction: Non relevant to topical use.

Use in pregnancy and lactation: Safety for use in pregnancy and lactation has not been established. There is inadequate evidence of safety in human pregnancy. Topical administration of corticosteroids to pregnant animals can cause abnormalities of foetal development including cleft palate and intrauterine growth retardation. There may therefore be a very small risk of such effects in the human foetus. There is a risk of foetal ototoxicity if aminoglycoside antibiotic preparations are administered during pregnancy.

Effects on ability to drive and to use machines: May cause blurring of vision on application. Warn patients not to drive or operate hazardous machinery unless vision is clear.

Undesirable effects: Hypersensitivity reactions, usually of the delayed type, may occur leading to irritation, burning, stinging, itching and dermatitis.

Topical steroid use may result in increased intraocular pressure leading to optic nerve damage, reduced visual acuity and visual field defects.

Intensive or prolonged use of topical corticosteroids may lead to formation of posterior subcapsular cataracts.

In those diseases causing thinning of the cornea or sclera, corticosteroid therapy may result in the thinning of the globe leading to perforation.

Overdosage: Long-term intensive topical use may lead to systemic effects.

Oral ingestion of the contents of one bottle (up to 10 ml) of the eye drops, is unlikely to lead to any serious adverse effects.

Pharmacological properties
Pharmacodynamic properties: Framycetin sulphate is an aminoglycoside antibiotic with a spectrum of activity similar to that of neomycin, this includes *Staphylococcus aureus* and most clinically significant gram negative organisms.

Gramicidin is an antimicrobial cyclic polypeptide active in vitro against many gram positive bacteria. It is used for the local treatment and susceptible infections, sometimes in combination with other antimicrobial agents and frequently with a corticosteroid.

Dexamethasone is a synthetic glucocorticoid and has the same general properties as other corticosteroids.

Pharmacokinetic properties: Framycetin sulphate absorption occurs from inflamed skin and wounds. Once absorbed it is rapidly excreted by the kidneys in active form. It has been reported to have a half life of 2-3 hours.

Gramicidin has properties similar to those of tyrothricin and is too toxic to be administered systemically.

Dexamethasone is readily absorbed from the gastro-intestinal tract. It has a biological half-life in plasma of about 190 minutes.

Preclinical safety data: Not applicable.

Pharmaceutical particulars
List of excipients: The ointment contains Plastibase 30w. The drops contain citric acid, sodium citrate, lithium chloride, phenylethyl alcohol, industrial methylated spirit, polysorbate 80, purified water.

Incompatibilities: None known.

Shelf life: Sofradex Ear/Eye Drops: 24 Months. Discard contents 28 days after opening. Sofradex Ear/Eye Ointment: 5 years. Discard contents 28 days after opening.

Special precautions for storage: Store below 25°C, do not refrigerate.

Nature and contents of container: Sofradex Ear/ Eye Drops: Glass bottle fitted with a special dropper attachment. Pack sizes of 8 or 10 ml. Plastic dropper bottle: Pack sizes of 5, 8 or 10 ml.

Sofradex Ear/Eye Ointment: 5 g white pigment plasticised PVC tube with tamper evident seal or white pigment multilaminated tube (Aluminium Foil Barrier/ Inner Coating HDPE) with tamper evident seal.

Instructions for use/handling: None.

Marketing authorisation holder: Roussel Laboratories Ltd., Broadwater Park, Denham, Uxbridge, Middlesex UB9 5HP

Marketing authorisation numbers
Sofradex Ear/Eye Drops PL 0109/0030R
Sofradex Ear/Eye Ointment PL 0109/0031R

Date of approval/revision of SPC Sofradex ear/eye drops: July 1997. Sofradex ear/eye ointment September 1997

Legal category POM

SOFRAMYCIN* EYE OINTMENT SOFRAMYCIN* EYE DROPS

Qualitative and quantitative composition Soframycin Eye Ointment and Soframycin Eye Drops contain 0.5% w/w Framycetin Sulphate BP.

Pharmaceutical form Eye ointment. Eye Drops.

Clinical particulars
Therapeutic indications: The topical treatment of bacterial infections such as blepharitis, conjunctivitis, styes, infected corneal abrasions and burns of the eye caused by sensitive organisms.

It may also be used prophylactically in patients undergoing removal of occular foreign bodies.

It may also be indicated for corneal ulcers.

Posology and method of administration: Route of Administration: Ocular.

Soframycin Eye Ointment: Adults (& Elderly) & Children: For continued effect, Soframycin Ointment should be applied, to each affected eye two or three times daily, or before retiring if drops have been used during the day.

Soframycin Eye Drops: Adults (& Elderly) & Children: For rapid effect, preferably during the daytime, one or two drops should be applied to each affected eye every one or two hours or more frequently if required.

Severe infections may require one or two drops every 15-20 minutes initially, reducing the frequency of instillation gradually as the infection is controlled.

Contra-indications: Known hypersensitivity to framycetin or chemically related antibiotics or any of the other components in the preparation.

Special warnings and precautions for use:

1. Prolonged use of an anti-infective may result in the development of superinfection due to microorganisms, including fungi, resistant to that anti-infective.
2. Contact lenses should be removed during the period of treatment.
3. Aminoglycosides have been reported to cause irreversible partial or total deafness when given systemically, topically to open wounds or broken skin, or intraperitoneally. These effects have not been reported with topical ocular administration of framycetin. However, the possibility should be considered when using high dose topical treatment in the elderly, small children, or those patients with renal or hepatic impairment.
4. In cases of severe infections the topical use of framycetin should be supplemented with appropriate systemic treatment.

Interactions with other medicaments and other forms of interaction: None relevant to topical use.

Pregnancy and lactation: There is inadequate evidence for the safety of framycetin in pregnancy and lactation, however, it has been used for many years with no direct evidence for ill consequences. Use should be only when considered essential by the physician.

Effects on ability to drive and use machines:

Soframycin Eye Ointment: Eye ointment preparations when applied topically will cause blurring of vision. Patients should be warned not to drive or operate hazardous machinery unless vision is clear.

Soframycin Eye Drops: Topical eye drop preparations may cause transient blurring of vision on instillation. Patients should be warned not to drive or operate hazardous machinery unless vision is clear.

Undesirable effects: Hypersensitivity reactions, usually of the delayed type, may occur with local treatment with framycetin (cross-sensitivity with other aminoglycoside antibiotics may occur). Irritation, stinging or burning, itching and dermatitis may sometimes occur.

Overdose: Not applicable.

Pharmacological properties
Pharmacodynamic properties: Framycetin is an aminoglycoside antibiotic with a spectrum of activity similar to that of neomycin, this includes *Staph. aureus* and most clinically significant gram negative organisms.

It is not active against *Pseudomonas aeruginosa* and resistant strains of gram-negative bacteria which are more common than with gentamicin.

Pharmacokinetic properties: Absorption occurs from inflamed skin and wounds. Once absorbed it is rapidly excreted by the kidneys in active form. It has been reported to have a half life of 2-3 hours.

Preclinical safety data: Not applicable.

Pharmaceutical particulars
List of excipients:

Soframycin Eye Ointment: The eye ointment contains Plastibase 30W.

Soframycin Eye Drops: The product contains citric acid, sodium citrate, sodium chloride, benzalkonium chloride solution, purified water, sodium hydroxide and hydrochloric acid.

Incompatibilities: No major incompatibilities *in vivo* are known.

Shelf-life:

Soframycin Eye Ointment: 3 years. Discard 28 days after opening.

Soframycin Eye Drops: Finished Product: 36 months. After first opening the container: discard contents 4 weeks after opening.

Special precautions for storage:

Soframycin Eye Ointment: Store below 25°C.

Soframycin Eye Drops: Store below 25°C. Protect from light. Avoid contamination during use.

Nature and contents of container:

Soframycin Eye Ointment: 5 g PVC tube fitted with ophthalmic nozzle.

Soframycin Eye Drops: Polypropylene dropper bottle fitted with a plug and cap: Pack size of 5 ml or 10 ml.

Instructions for use/handling: None/not applicable.

Marketing authorisation holder: Roussel Laboratories Ltd., Broadwater Park, Denham, Uxbridge, Middlesex UB9 5HP

Marketing authorisation numbers
Soframycin Eye Ointment: PL 0109/5041R
Soframycin Eye Drops: PL 0109/0140

Date of approval/revision of SPC
Soframycin Eye Ointment: November 1997
Soframycin Eye Drops: June 1997

Legal category POM

SURGAM TABLETS 200 mg* SURGAM TABLETS 300 mg* Surgam SA CAPSULES*

Qualitative and quantitative composition
Surgam Tablets 200 mg: contain 200 mg Tiaprofenic Acid.

Surgam Tablets 300 mg: contain 300 mg Tiaprofenic Acid.

Surgam SA Capsules: contain 300 mg Tiaprofenic Acid.

Pharmaceutical form Tablets. Capsules containing a pellet formulation providing sustained release.

Clinical particulars
Therapeutic indications: Rheumatoid arthritis, osteoarthritis, ankylosing spondylitis, low back pain, musculo-skeletal disorders such as fibrositis, capsulitis, epicondylitis and other soft-tissue inflammatory conditions, sprains and strains, post-operative inflammation and pain and other soft tissue injuries.

Posology and method of administration: For oral administration.

Tablets to be swallowed whole.

Capsules to be swallowed whole.

Adults: *Surgam Tablets 200 mg and 300 mg:* 600 mg Tiaprofenic acid daily.

Surgam SA Capsules: Two capsules (600 mg tiaprofenic acid) once daily.

Elderly: As for adults (see Section on Special warnings and precautions). NSAIDs should be used with particular caution in older patients who generally are more prone to adverse reactions.

In cases of renal, cardiac or hepatic impairment, the dosage should be kept as low as possible. It is suggested that in such cases, the dosage be reduced to 200 mg twice daily.

Children: There are insufficient data to recommend use of Surgam in children.

Contra-indications:

- Active gastroduodenal ulceration or history of gastroduodenal ulceration.
- Active bladder or prostatic disease or symptoms.
- History of recurrent urinary tract disorders.
- Hypersensitivity to tiaprofenic acid or to any of the ingredients in the drug.
- History of asthma, rhinitis or urticaria whether or not induced by aspirin and other NSAIDs.
- Pregnancy (see Section on Pregnancy and lactation)
- Severe renal or hepatic insufficiency.

Special warnings and precautions for use: As with other NSAIDs, Surgam should be used with care in the elderly and in patients with renal, cardiac or hepatic insufficiency as the use of these drugs may result in the deterioration of renal function. The dose should be kept as low as possible and renal function should be monitored. Renal function should also be monitored in patients on diuretics. Tiaprofenic acid should be used with caution in patients with arterial hypertension.

Tiaprofenic acid can cause cystitis which may become severe if the treatment is continued after the onset of urinary symptoms. If urinary symptoms such as frequency, urgency, dysuria, nocturia or haematuria occur, tiaprofenic acid should be stopped immediately and urinalysis and urine culture performed. Patients should be warned about the onset of urinary symptoms which may suggest cystitis and are advised to stop taking the drug and seek medical advice if these occur.

Because of the risk of serious gastrointestinal side effects, especially in patients on anticoagulant treatment, special attention should be paid to the appearance of any gastrointestinal symptoms; treatment should be stopped immediately in the event of gastrointestinal haemorrhage.

There is a risk of cross-sensitivity among aspirin and NSAIDs, including the group to which tiaprofenic acid belongs. These pseudo-allergic reactions may include rash, urticaria and angioedema or more potentially severe manifestations (e.g. laryngeal oedema, bronchoconstriction and shock). The risk of pseudo-allergic reactions is greater in patients with recurrent rhino-sinusitis, nasal polyposis or chronic urticaria. Asthmatic patients are particularly at risk of dangerous reactions. Therefore tiaprofenic acid must not be administered to patients with a history of asthma.

Interactions with other medicaments and other forms of interaction: Since Surgam is highly protein-bound, it is not recommended for co-administration with other highly protein-bound drugs such as heparin. Modification of the dosage may be necessary with hypoglycaemic agents, phenytoin and diuretics.

Concomitant use of Surgam with corticosteroids and other NSAIDs including high-dose salicylates and high dose methotrexate should be avoided. Caution should be exercised when administered with cardiac glycosides, low dose methotrexate and sulphonamides. As with other NSAIDs, careful patient monitoring is suggested if Surgam and an oral anticoagulant are administered together.

NSAIDs have been reported to increase steady state plasma levels of lithium and it is therefore recommended that these levels are monitored in patients receiving Surgam therapy.

The use of aspirin and other NSAIDs should be avoided for at least 8-12 days after taking mifepristone.

NSAIDs may cause sodium and fluid retention and may interfere with the natriuretic action of diuretic agents, thus reducing the effects of these. NSAIDs also interact with antihypertensive drugs (e.g. beta-blockers, ACE inhibitors and anti-angiotensin II receptor antagonists) and cause an increased risk of renal impairment and an increased risk of hyperkalaemia. This should be borne in mind in patients with incipient or actual congestive heart failure and/or hypertension.

The risk of nephrotoxicity may be increased if NSAIDs are given with cyclosporins. Convulsions may occur due to an interaction with quinolone antibiotics.

Pregnancy and lactation: Pregnancy: Tiaprofenic acid crosses the placental barrier. Although animal studies have not revealed evidence of teratogenicity, safety in human pregnancy and lactation cannot be assumed and, in common with other NSAIDs, administration during the first trimester should be avoided.

Lactation: The level of Surgam in mother's milk has been studied and the total daily exposure is very small; approximately 0.2% of the administered dose and is unlikely to be of pharmacological significance. Breast feeding or treatment of the mother should be stopped as necessary.

Effects on ability to drive and use machines: None known.

Undesirable effects:

Gastrointestinal tract: Reported reactions include dyspepsia, nausea, vomiting, abdominal pain, anorexia, indigestion, heartburn, constipation, gastritis, flatulence and diarrhoea. In common with other NSAIDs, gastroduodenal ulcers, perforation and overt or occult gastrointestinal haemorrhage resulting in anaemia have occasionally been reported and in exceptional cases may have been associated with fatalities.

Muco-cutaneous: Rash, urticaria, pruritus, purpura, alopecia and very rarely erythema multiforme and bullous eruptions (Stevens Johnson Syndrome or, exceptionally, toxic epidermal necrolysis) have been reported. Very rarely photosensitivity reactions and aphthous stomatitis.

Hypersensitivity reactions: Asthmatic attacks, especially in subjects allergic to aspirin and other NSAIDs. Angio-oedema. Anaphylactic shock has also been reported.

Haematological: Thrombocytopenia , prolongation of bleeding time may occur.

Nervous system: Headaches, dizziness, tinnitus and drowsiness.

Urinary system: Bladder pain, dysuria, frequency and cystitis have been reported with tiaprofenic acid and other NSAIDs. On the basis of spontaneous reports, tiaprofenic acid appears to have a greater propensity than other NSAIDs to cause urinary disorders. Although generally reversible, in some cases where tiaprofenic acid has continued after the onset of urinary symptoms and an association with tiaprofenic acid not recognised, serious consequences requiring surgical intervention have resulted. Therefore, treatment with tiaprofenic acid should be discontinued immediately if urinary disorders develop.

Renal: Sodium and water retention (see Section on Special warnings and precautions).

NSAIDs have been reported to cause nephrotoxicity in various forms. As with other NSAIDs, isolated cases of acute interstitial nephritis, nephrotic syndrome and renal failure have also been reported with tiaprofenic acid.

Hepatic: Liver test abnormalities

Overdose: In the event of overdosage with Surgam, supportive and symptomatic therapy is indicated.

Pharmacological properties

Pharmacodynamic properties: Surgam Tablets 200 mg and 300 mg: Non-steroidal anti-inflammatory drug.

Surgam SA capsules: Tiaprofenic acid is a propionic acid derivative having anti-inflammatory and analgesic properties.

Pharmacokinetic properties:

Surgam Tablets 200 mg and 300 mg:

Single dose studies: Following oral administration (max. at 90 mins). Plasma level zero at 24 hours. $t_{\frac{1}{2}}$ = 1.5 to 2 hours.

Repeated dose studies: Surgam is rapidly eliminated and there is no accumulation after repeated doses of 600 mg/day in divided doses. Steady state after first day. No impairment of absorption in patients with RA undergoing long term therapy. There is no evidence of different pharmacokinetics in the elderly.

Protein binding = 97–98%

Plasma clearance = 6 litres/hour

Elimination = 60% of urine remainder in bile

Metabolites = there are two main metabolites which account for about 10% of urinary excretion and have low pharmacological activity. The parent compound is excreted mostly in the form of acylglucuronide.

Surgam SA Capsules: Surgam SA (600 mg) gives a Cmax of 28.1 mg/l which is not significantly different from 300 mg conventional Surgam (37.3 mg/l).

The plasma concentration remains above 10 mg/l for 6-8 hours, against 2 to 3 hours with the conventional tablet.

Despite these differences in profile, there was no significant difference in the amount of Tiaprofenic acid absorbed as measured by areas under the plasma concentration curve and quantities eliminated in the urine.

Preclinical safety data: Not applicable

Pharmaceutical particulars

List of excipients: Surgam Tablets 200 mg and 300 mg: Maize starch, pluronic F68, magnesium stearate and talc.

Surgam SA Capsules: Pellets: Glyceryl monostearate; Microcrystalline Cellulose; Purified Talc

Capsule Shell – CAP: Erythrosine E127; Titanium Dioxide E171; Indigo carmine E132

Capsule Shell – BODY: Erythrosine E127; Indigo carmine E132; Gelatin

Incompatibilities: None known

Shelf life: 60 Months

Special precautions for storage: *Surgam Tablets 200 mg and 300 mg:* Store below 25°C. Protect from light.

Surgam SA capsules: Store below 25°C in a dry place and protect from light.

Nature and contents of container: Polyethylene bottles with screw cap, amber glass bottles with polyethylene caps or blister packs sealed with aluminium foil in a cardboard carton in packs of 10, 20, 21, 30, 42, 84 or 100.

Surgam Tablets 300 mg: Polyethylene bottles with screw cap, amber glass bottles with polyethylene caps or blister packs sealed with aluminium foil in a cardboard carton in packs of 10, 12, 14, 20, 28, 30, 56 or 60.

Surgam SA Capsules: Blister packs of 8, 20 or 56 capsules manufactured from 250 µm PVC/20 µm aluminium foil.

Polyethylene bottle with screw-neck fitted with a polyethylene cap. Contains a pack size of 60 capsules.

Instructions for use/handling: Not applicable.

Marketing authorisation holder: Roussel Laboratories Ltd., Broadwater Park, Denham, Uxbridge, Middlesex UB9 5HP UK

Marketing authorisation numbers

Surgam tablets 200 mg	PL 0109/0108
Surgam tablets 300 mg	PL 0109/0109
Surgam SA Capsules	PL 0109/0167

Date of approval/revision of SPC March 1998

Legal category POM

**Trade Mark*

Forley Ltd
4 Priory Hall
Stillorgan Road
Stillorgan
Co Dublin
Eire

☎ 00353 1 2836665 　 🗋 00353 1 2836603

DIBENYLINE* CAPSULES

Presentation Opaque white capsules with clear ruby-red caps, each containing 10 mg phenoxybenzamine hydrochloride as a white powder.

Uses Dibenyline is a non-competitive long-acting α-adrenergic receptor antagonist.

It is indicated in the short-term management of severe hypertensive episodes associated with phaeochromocytoma. Dibenyline should only be used after careful consideration of the likely benefit of treatment compared with the mutagenic and carcinogenic risk (see *Precautions* below).

Dosage and administration
Adults: The usual starting dose is 10 mg daily. This may be increased by 10 mg daily until control of hypertensive episodes is achieved or postural hypotension occurs. Usually the dosage required is 1 to 2 mg/kg body weight daily in two doses. Concomitant β-adrenergic blockade may be necessary to control tachycardia and arrhythmias notably when tumours are secreting an appreciable amount of adrenaline as well as noradrenaline.

Elderly: Use with caution (see *Contra-indications* and *Precautions* below).

Children: There is little experience in children, but doses of 1 to 2 mg/kg daily have been used successfully.

Contra-indications, warnings, etc
Contra-indications: Do not use in patients who have had a cerebrovascular accident; or in the recovery period (usually 3 to 4 weeks) after acute myocardial infarction.

Precautions: Use with great caution in patients in whom a fall in blood pressure and/or tachycardia may be undesirable, such as the elderly, or those with severe heart disease, congestive heart failure, cerebrovascular disease or renal damage. The mode of action should be borne in mind if used concurrently with α-sympathomimetics or myocardial depressants.

Phenoxybenzamine is carcinogenic in the rat and has shown mutagenic activity in the bacterial Ames test and the mouse lymphoma assay. It should, therefore, be used only after very careful consideration of the risks, in patients in whom alternative treatment is inappropriate.

Use in pregnancy: There is little evidence as to the safety of Dibenyline in pregnancy and it should not be used in pregnancy unless essential.

Adverse reactions: Side-effects are generally mild and transient, but may include postural hypotension with dizziness and compensatory tachycardia, nasal congestion, inhibition of ejaculation, miosis and lassitude. Gastro-intestinal upset has also been reported.

Overdosage: The main effect of overdosage is profound hypotension, which may last several hours, tachycardia and collapse. Treatment consists of the induction of vomiting and/or gastric lavage together with appropriate symptomatic and supportive measures. Treat hypotension with plasma expanders and the 'head down' position. Noradrenaline is of little value when α-adrenergic receptors are blocked. Adrenaline should not be used since stimulation of β-adrenergic receptors will further decrease blood pressure.

Pharmaceutical precautions Store in a dry place and protect from light.

Legal category POM.

Package quantities Opaque blister packs (OP) of 30 (2×15) capsules.

Further information Treatment should be started as soon as possible after diagnosis and time allowed for stabilisation of the condition before invasive investigations or operations are carried out. Operative cover with intravenous phenoxybenzamine may be given.

In a few inoperable cases, long-term treatment with Dibenyline has been used.

Inactive ingredients include lactose.

Product licence number 12300/0007.

DIBENYLINE* INJECTION

Presentation Clear colourless ampoules, each containing 100 mg phenoxybenzamine hydrochloride in 2 ml clear colourless to mid-straw coloured solution.

This solution contains absolute ethyl alcohol, hydrochloric acid and propylene glycol.

Uses Phenoxybenzamine is a long-acting, non-competitive, alpha-adrenergic receptor antagonist. By intravenous infusion it is used as part of the investigational, pre-operative and operative management of phaeochromocytoma, and as an adjunct to the treatment of severe shock, not responding to conventional therapy, in the presence of an adequate circulating blood volume.

Dibenyline should only be used after careful consideration of the likely benefit of treatment compared with the mutagenic and carcinogenic risk. See *Precautions* below.

Dosage and administration Dibenyline Injection Concentrate *must be diluted* before use. The dose selected should be added aseptically to 200–500 ml 0.9 per cent sodium chloride immediately before use.

The intravenous route only must be used, preferably through a large vein. Not more than one dose should be given in 24 hours, infused over at least two hours. It is suggested that one-third of the dose is given over the first hour, and the remaining two-thirds over the second hour if no precipitous fall in blood pressure has occurred. Any solution remaining four hours after dilution should be discarded because of reduced potency.

Adults:
Phaeochromocytoma: Where alpha-blockade is required as a preparation for investigation or operation in cases of phaeochromocytoma, a daily dose of 1 mg/kg body weight intravenously in 200 ml of physiological saline over two hours has been used, for several days preceding and during the procedure. This dose is a guide and it is often necessary to titrate the dose on a daily basis according to individual response, concomitant beta-receptor blockade may be necessary.

Shock: 1 mg/kg body weight in 200 to 500 ml of 0.9 per cent Sodium chloride given over not less than two hours.

Children: Dosage in children has not been established.

Precautions in use: The patient should be recumbent. Blood pressure must be determined every few minutes during the administration. Facilities for rapid infusion of intravenous fluid should be available. The Dibenyline infusion should be slowed or stopped if there is a precipitous fall in blood pressure. This usually indicates an inadequate circulating blood volume, but occasionally may occur in the presence of an adequate blood volume in hypertensives or in patients with carbon dioxide retention, and in these cases is relatively unresponsive to the administration of intravenous fluids. Nevertheless, if severe hypotension does occur, treatment can be attempted with plasma expanders and the 'head down' position. Noradrenaline may be of little value when alpha-adrenergic receptors are blocked. Adrenaline should not be used since stimulation of beta-adrenergic receptors will further decrease blood pressure. If blood pressure has been stabilised by the administration of appropriate fluids, the Dibenyline infusion may be restarted under close supervision. The blockade produced is often still exerting an effect 24 hours after administration and, even in patients with a favourable response, close attention to their cardiovascular status should be maintained for at least this period. Little can be accomplished by a second administration of Dibenyline within 24 hours and the drug should not be given more than twice during a 48-hour period.

Care should be taken to avoid extravasation, as the diluted solution is irritant to muscle tissue.

Avoid contamination of the hands with Dibenyline as reactions may occur in sensitive skins.

Contra-indications, warnings, etc
Contra-indications: Do not use in patients who have had a cerebrovascular accident; or in the recovery period (usually 3 to 4 weeks) after acute myocardial infarction. Do not use in the presence of hypovolaemia in patients with severe shock.

Precautions: Use with great caution in patients in whom a fall in blood pressure and/or tachycardia may be undesirable, such as the elderly or those with severe ischaemic heart disease, congestive heart failure, extensive arteriosclerosis, cerebrovascular disease or renal damage. The adrenergic blocking effect may aggravate symptoms of respiratory infections. Alpha-sympathomimetics may be ineffective if used concomitantly with phenoxybenzamine. Care should be taken if phenoxybenzamine is used concomitantly with myocardial depressants, e.g. beta-blockers and anti-arrhythmics.

Phenoxybenzamine is carcinogenic in the rat and has shown mutagenic activity in the bacterial Ames test and the mouse lymphoma assay. It should therefore be used only after very careful consideration of the risks, in patients in whom alternative treatment is inappropriate.

Use in pregnancy: There is no available evidence as to the safety of Dibenyline in pregnancy and it should not be used in pregnancy or lactation unless essential.

Adverse reactions: Dibenyline given intravenously has a sedative effect and patients may become more drowsy or less responsive during the infusion. This may occur in spite of an excellent cardiovascular response and should not be confused with the decreased responsiveness associated with worsening of the shock syndrome.

Other side-effects include orthostatic hypotension with dizziness and compensatory tachycardia, miosis, dry mouth, nasal congestion, decreased sweating and gastrointestinal upset. Convulsions have been reported after rapid infusion.

Some fall in blood pressure is a normal response but an idiosyncratic profound hypotensive effect can occur, usually within five minutes of starting the infusion.

The effect of one dose of Dibenyline on sympathetic motor responses may last 48 hours or more.

Overdosage: As described in *Precautions in use*, there may be a precipitous fall in blood pressure even at the recommended dosage. Facilities for rapid infusion of intravenous fluid should therefore be available and in the event of such a severe hypotensive episode, the Dibenyline infusion should be slowed or stopped. Treatment can be attempted with plasma expanders and the 'head down' position. Noradrenaline may be of little value when alpha-adrenergic receptors are blocked and adrenaline is contra-indicated.

Pharmaceutical precautions Protect the ampoules from light. Dibenyline solutions should be made up immediately before administration. Any that remains four hours after dilution should be discarded because of reduced potency. A transient clouding of the solution, due to low aqueous solubility of Dibenyline near neutral pH, is unimportant. If markedly discoloured in the ampoule, the preparation should be discarded.

Legal category POM.

Package quantities Ampoules: 100 mg phenoxybenzamine hydrochloride/2 ml in boxes of 3.

Further information Nil.

Product licence number 12300/0008.

**Trade Mark*

Fournier Pharmaceuticals Limited

22–23 Progress Business Centre
Whittle Parkway
Slough SL1 6DG

☎ 01753 740400   🗋 01753 74044

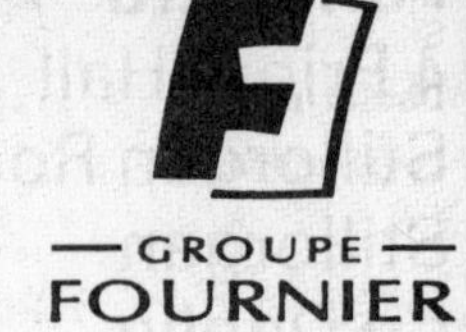

LIPANTIL* Micro 67

Qualitative and quantitative composition Each LIPANTIL Micro 67 capsule contains 67 mg of micronised fenofibrate (INN).

Pharmaceutical form Yellow, hard gelatin capsule.

Clinical particulars

Therapeutic indications: LIPANTIL Micro 67 reduces elevated serum cholesterol and triglycerides and is of benefit in the treatment of severe dyslipidaemia in patients in whom dietary measures alone have failed to produce an adequate response. LIPANTIL Micro 67 is indicated in appropriate cases of dyslipidaemia (Fredrickson classification types IIa, IIb, III, IV and V).

Type	*Major lipid elevated*	*Lipoproteins elevated*
IIa	Cholesterol	LDL
IIb	Cholesterol, triglycerides	LDL, VLDL
III (rare)	Cholesterol, triglycerides	LDL and chylomicron remnants
IV	Triglycerides	VLDL
V (rare)	Triglycerides	Chylomicrons, VLDL

LIPANTIL Micro 67 should only be used in patients in whom a full investigation has been performed to define their abnormality. Other risk factors, such as hypertension and smoking, may also require management.

Posology and method of administration:

Adults: In adults, the recommended initial dose is 3 capsules taken daily in divided doses. LIPANTIL Micro 67 should always be taken with food, because it is less well absorbed from an empty stomach. Dietary measures instituted before therapy should be continued.

The response to therapy should be monitored by determination of serum lipid values and the dosage may be altered within the range 2-4 capsules of LIPANTIL Micro 67 daily.

Children: In children, the recommended dose is one capsule (67 mg) micronised fenofibrate / day / 20 kg body weight.

Elderly: In elderly patients without renal impairment, the normal adult dose is recommended.

Renal impairment: In renal dysfunction, the dosage may need to be reduced depending on the rate of creatinine clearance, for example:

Creatinine clearance (ml/min)	*Dosage*
<60	Two 67 mg capsules
<20	One 67 mg capsule

Contra-indications: LIPANTIL Micro 67 is contra-indicated in patients with severe liver or renal dysfunction, existing gallbladder disease and in patients hypersensitive to fenofibrate.

See also section 4.6.

Special warnings and special precautions for use:

In renal impairment: In renal dysfunction the dose of fenofibrate may need to be reduced, depending on the rate of creatinine clearance, (see section 4.2). Dose reduction should be considered in elderly patients with impaired renal function.

Transaminases: Moderately elevated levels of serum transaminases may be found in some patients but rarely interfere with treatment. However, it is recommended that serum transaminases should be monitored every three months during the first twelve months of treatment. Treatment should be interrupted in the event of ALT (SGPT) or ASAT (SGOT) elevations to more than one hundred international units.

Myopathy: There have been reports of elevations (sometimes marked) of creatine phosphokinase (CPK), myositis and myopathy associated with fibrates as well as other systemically absorbed lipid modifying drugs. Rhabdomyolysis has also been reported rarely. Patients at risk of developing, or who show signs of muscle toxicity should be monitored closely and CPK levels checked.

Treatment with fenofibrate should be stopped if myopathy is suspected or if CPK rises to ≥10 times the upper limit of normal. The risk of serious muscle toxicity is increased if fenofibrate is used concomitantly with HMG-CoA reductase inhibitors or other fibrates. Such combination therapy should be used with caution and patients monitored closely for signs of muscle toxicity.

In children: Only an hereditary disease (familial hyperlipidaemia) justifies early treatment, and the precise nature of the hyperlipidaemia must be determined by genetic and laboratory investigations. It is recommended to begin treatment with controlled dietary restrictions for a period of at least 3 months. Proceeding to medicinal treatment should only be considered after specialist advice and only in severe forms with clinical signs of atherosclerosis and/or xanthomata and/or in cases where patients suffer from atherosclerotic cardiovascular disease before the age of 40.

Interactions with other medicaments and other forms of interaction:

Oral anticoagulants: In patients receiving anticoagulant therapy, the dose of anticoagulant should be reduced by about one-third at the commencement of treatment and then gradually adjusted if necessary.

Oral hypoglycaemic agents: Possible interactions with oral hypoglycaemic agents should also be considered, but there are no adequately documented cases of this.

HMG-CoA reductase inhibitors: The risk of serious muscle toxicity is increased if fenofibrate is used concomitantly with HMG-CoA reductase inhibitors or other fibrates. Such combination therapy should be used with caution and patients monitored closely for signs of muscle toxicity.

Other: No proven clinical interactions of fenofibrate with other drugs have been reported, although in vitro interaction studies suggest displacement of phenylbutazone from plasma protein binding sites. In common with other fibrates, fenofibrate induces microsomal mixed-function oxidases involved in fatty acid metabolism in rodents and may interact with drugs metabolised by these enzymes.

Pregnancy and lactation: Fenofibrate has not been shown to be teratogenic in animals. However, signs of embryotoxicity have been seen in animals and it is therefore recommended that LIPANTIL Micro 67 should not be administered to women who are pregnant or are breast feeding.

Effects on ability to drive and use machines: No effect noted to date.

Undesirable effects: Fenofibrate is generally well tolerated. Adverse reactions observed during fenofibrate treatment are not very frequent; they are generally minor, transient and do not interfere with treatment. Most commonly reported are mild gastro-intestinal disturbances, skin reactions, headache, fatigue and vertigo. Sexual asthenia has been reported less frequently. Gallstones have occasionally been reported during fenofibrate treatment but any causal relationship remains inconclusive.

Photosensitivity reactions have been reported rarely.

Hepatic effects: Moderately elevated levels of serum transaminases may be found in some patients but rarely interfere with treatment (see also section 4.4). Episodes of hepatitis have been reported rarely.

Muscle effects: As with other systemically absorbed lipid modifying drugs, there have been reports of elevated levels of CPK (sometimes marked), myalgia and myopathy, including rare cases of rhabdomyolysis. Patients at risk of developing muscle toxicity should be monitored (see also section 4.4).

Overdose: No reports of ill effects from overdosage have been reported. There are no specific antidotes and treatment of acute overdosage should be symptomatic. Gastric lavage and appropriate supportive care may be instituted if necessary.

Pharmacological properties

Pharmacodynamic properties: LIPANTIL Micro 67 is a formulation containing 67 mg of micronised fenofibrate.

The lipid-lowering properties of fenofibrate seen in clinical practice have been explained *in vivo* in transgenic mice and in human hepatocyte cultures by activation of Peroxisome Proliferator Activated Receptor type α (PPARα). Through this mechanism, fenofibrate increases lipolysis and elimination of triglyceride rich particles from plasma by activating lipoprotein lipase and reducing production of Apoprotein C-III. Activation of PPARα also induces an increase in the synthesis of Apoproteins A-I, A-II and of HDL cholesterol.

Epidemiological studies have demonstrated a positive correlation between increased serum lipid levels and an increased risk of coronary heart disease. The control of such dyslipidaemias forms the rationale for treatment with fenofibrate. However, the possible beneficial and adverse long-term consequences of drugs used in the hyperlipidaemias are still the subject of scientific discussion. Therefore the presumptive beneficial effect of LIPANTIL Micro 67 on cardiovascular morbidity and mortality is as yet unproven.

Studies with fenofibrate consistently show decreases in levels of LDL-cholesterol. HDL-cholesterol levels are frequently increased. Triglyceride levels are also reduced. This results in a decrease in the ratio of low and very low density lipoproteins to high density lipoproteins, which has been correlated with a decrease in atherogenic risk in epidemiological studies. Apolipoprotein-A and apolipoprotein-B levels are altered in parallel with HDL and LDL and VLDL levels respectively.

Regression of xanthomata has been observed during fenofibrate therapy.

Plasma uric acid levels are increased in approximately 20% of hyperlipidaemic patients, particularly in those with type IV phenotype. LIPANTIL Micro 67 has a uricosuric effect and is therefore of additional benefit in such patients.

Patients with raised levels of fibrinogen and Lp(a) have shown significant reductions in these measurements during clinical trials with fenofibrate.

Pharmacokinetic properties: Absorption: The unchanged compound is not recovered in the plasma. Fenofibric acid is the major plasma metabolite. Peak plasma concentration occurs after a mean period of 5 hours following dosing.

Mean plasma concentration is 15μg/ml for a daily dosage of 200 mg of micronised fenofibrate, equivalent to 3 capsules of LIPANTIL Micro 67.

Steady state levels are observed throughout continuous treatments.

Fenofibric acid is highly bound to plasma albumin: it can displace antivitamin K compounds from the protein binding sites and potentiate their anticoagulant effect.

Plasma half-life: The plasma half-life of elimination of fenofibric acid is approximately 20 hours.

Metabolism and excretion: The product is mainly excreted in the urine: 70% in 24 hours and 88% in 6 days, at which time total excretion in urine and faeces reaches 93%. Fenofibrate is mainly excreted as fenofibric acid and its derived glucuroconjugate.

Kinetic studies after administration of repeated doses show the absence of accumulation of the product.

Fenofibric acid is not eliminated during haemodialysis.

Preclinical safety data: None stated.

Pharmaceutical particulars

List of excipients: Excipients: lactose, magnesium stearate, pregelatinised starch, sodium lauryl sulphate, crospovidone.

Composition of the capsule shell: gelatin, titanium dioxide (E171), quinoline yellow (E104) and erythrosine (E127).

Incompatibilities: No effect noted to date.

Shelf life: 3 years.

Special precautions for storage: Store below 25°C in a dry place.

Protect from light.

Nature and contents of container: LIPANTIL Micro 67 is available in a pack containing 9 strips of 10 capsules per blister.

Instructions for use/handling: Capsules should be swallowed whole with water.

Marketing authorisation number PL 12509/0004.

Date of first authorisation/renewal of authorisation September 1997.

Date of (partial) revision of the text September 1998.

Legal category POM.

LIPANTIL* Micro 200

Qualitative and quantitative composition Each LIPANTIL Micro 200 capsule contains 200 mg of micronised fenofibrate (INN).

Pharmaceutical form Orange, hard gelatin capsule

Clinical particulars

Therapeutic indications: LIPANTIL Micro 200 reduces elevated serum cholesterol and triglyceride and is of benefit in the treatment of severe dyslipidaemia in patients in whom dietary measures alone have failed to produce an adequate response. LIPANTIL Micro 200 is therefore indicated in appropriate cases of hyperlipidaemia (Fredrickson classification types IIa, IIb, III, IV and V).

Type	Major Lipid elevated	Lipoproteins elevated
IIa	Cholesterol	LDL
IIb	Cholesterol, triglyceride	LDL, VLDL
III (rare)	Cholesterol, triglyceride	LDL and Chylomicron Remnants
IV	Triglyceride	VLDL
V (rare)	Triglyceride	Chylomicrons, VLDL

LIPANTIL Micro 200 should only be used in patients whose disease is unresponsive to dietary control and in whom a full investigation has been performed to define their abnormality, and where long-term risks associated with their condition warrant treatment. Other risk factors, such as hypertension and smoking may also require management.

Posology and method of administration:

Adults: The recommended initial dose is one capsule taken daily during a main meal. In elderly patients without renal impairment, the normal adult dose is recommended. Since it is less well absorbed from an empty stomach, LIPANTIL Micro 200 should always be taken with food. Dietary restrictions instituted before therapy should be continued.

Response to therapy should be monitored by determination of serum lipid values. Rapid reduction of serum lipid levels usually follows LIPANTIL Micro 200 treatment, but treatment should be discontinued if an adequate response has not been achieved within three months.

Contra-indications: LIPANTIL Micro 200 is contra-indicated in children, in patients with severe liver dysfunction, existing gallbladder disease, severe renal disorders and in patients hypersensitive to fenofibrate.

Special warnings and special precautions for use:

Renal impairment: In renal dysfunction the dose of fenofibrate may need to be reduced, depending on the rate of creatinine clearance. In this case, LIPANTIL Micro 67 (micronised fenofibrate) should be used, eg. 2 capsules of LIPANTIL Micro 67 daily for creatinine clearance levels of <60 ml/min and 1 capsule of LIPANTIL Micro 67 daily for creatinine clearance levels of <20 ml/min.

Use of LIPANTIL Micro 67 is also to be preferred in elderly patients with renal impairment where dosage reduction may be required.

Serum transaminases: Moderately elevated levels of serum transaminases may be found in some patients but rarely interfere with treatment. However, it is recommended that serum transaminases should be monitored every three months during the first twelve months of treatment. Treatment should be interrupted in the event of SGPT elevation of more than one hundred international units.

Interactions:

Oral anti-coagulants: In patients receiving oral anti-coagulant therapy, the dose of anti-coagulant should be reduced by about one-third at the commencement of treatment and then gradually adjusted if necessary.

Other: No proven clinical interactions of fenofibrate with other drugs have been reported, although in vitro interaction studies suggest displacement of phenylbutazone from plasma protein binding sites. In common with other fibrates, fenofibrate induces microsomal mixed-function oxidases involved in fatty acid metabolism in rodents and may interact with drugs metabolised by these enzymes. Possible interactions with oral hypoglycaemic agents should also be considered.

Pregnancy and lactation: Fenofibrate has not been shown to be teratogenic in animals. However, signs of embryotoxicity have been seen in rats and it is therefore recommended that LIPANTIL Micro 200 should not be administered to women who are pregnant or are breast-feeding.

Effects on ability to drive and use machines: No effect noted to date.

Undesirable effects: Adverse reactions observed during LIPANTIL Micro 200 treatment are not very frequent (2–4% of cases); they are generally minor, transient and do not interfere with treatment. Most commonly reported are mild gastro-intestinal disturbances, skin reactions, headache, fatigue and vertigo.

Sexual asthenia and muscle toxicity (as seen with other systemic lipid modifying drugs) are reported less frequently. Examples of the latter include myositis, myopathy and marked elevations of creatine phosphokinase (CPK). Rhabdomyolysis during treatment with fenofibrate has also been reported rarely. Patients who are at risk of developing, or who show signs of muscle toxicity should be monitored closely and CPK levels checked. Treatment with fenofibrate should be stopped if myopathy is suspected or if CPK rises to ≥10 times the upper limit of normal. The risk of serious muscle toxicity is increased if fenofibrate is used concomitantly with HMG-CoA reductase inhibitors or other fibrates. Combination therapy should be used with caution, and patients monitored closely for signs of muscle toxicity.

Gallstones have occasionally been reported during fenofibrate treatment but any causal relationship remains inconclusive.

Moderately elevated levels of serum transaminases may be found in some patients but rarely interfere with treatment (see also section 4.4). Episodes of hepatitis have been reported rarely.

Photosensitivity reactions have been reported rarely.

Overdose: No reports of ill effects from overdosage have been reported. There are no specific antidotes and treatment of acute overdosage should be symptomatic. Gastric lavage and appropriate supportive care may be instituted if necessary.

Pharmacological properties

Pharmacodynamic properties: LIPANTIL Micro 200 is a formulation containing 200 mg of micronised fenofibrate; the administration of this product results in effective plasma concentrations identical to those obtained with 3 capsules of LIPANTIL Micro 67 containing 67 mg of micronised fenofibrate.

The lipid-lowering properties of fenofibrate seen in clinical practice have been explained *in vivo* in transgenic mice and in human hepatocyte cultures by activation of Peroxisome Proliferator Activated Receptor type α (PPARα). Through this mechanism, fenofibrate increases lipolysis and elimination of triglyceride rich particles from plasma by activating lipoprotein lipase and reducing production of Apoprotein C-III. Activation of PPARα also induces an increase in the synthesis of Apoproteins A-I, A-II and of HDL cholesterol.

Epidemiological studies have demonstrated a positive correlation between abnormally increased serum lipid levels and an increased risk of coronary heart disease. The control of such dyslipidaemia forms the rationale for treatment with LIPANTIL Micro 200. However the possible beneficial and adverse long term consequences of drugs used in the management of dyslipidaemia are still the subject of scientific discussion. Therefore the presumptive beneficial effect of LIPANTIL Micro 200 on cardiovascular morbidity and mortality is as yet unproven.

Studies with fenofibrate on lipoprotein fractions show decreases in levels of LDL and VLDL cholesterol. HDL cholesterol levels are frequently increased. LDL and VLDL triglycerides are reduced. The overall effect is a decrease in the ratio of low and very low density lipoproteins to high density lipoproteins, which epidemiological studies have correlated with a decrease in atherogenic risk. Apolipoprotein-A and apolipoprotein-B levels are altered in parallel with HDL and LDL and VLDL levels respectively.

Regression of xanthomata has been observed during fenofibrate therapy.

Plasma uric acid levels are increased in approximately 20% of hyperlipidaemic patients, particularly in those with type IV disease. LIPANTIL Micro 200 has a uricosuric effect and is therefore of additional benefit in such patients.

Patients with raised levels of fibrinogen and Lp(a) have shown significant reductions in these measurements during clinical trials with fenofibrate.

Pharmacokinetic properties: Absorption: The unchanged compound is not recovered in the plasma. Fenofibric acid is the major plasma metabolite. Peak plasma concentration occurs after a mean period of 5 hours following dosing.

Mean plasma concentration is 15 μg/ml for a daily dose of 200 mg of micronised fenofibrate, equivalent to 3 capsules of LIPANTIL Micro 67.

Steady state levels are observed throughout continuous treatments.

Fenofibric acid is highly bound to plasma albumin; it can displace antivitamin K compounds from protein binding sites and may potentiate their anti-coagulant effect.

The plasma half-life of elimination of fenofibric acid is approximately 20 hours.

Metabolism and excretion: the product is mainly excreted in the urine; 70% in 24 hours and 88% in 6 days, at which time the total excretion in urine and faeces reaches 93%. Fenofibrate is mainly excreted as fenofibric acid and its derived glucuroconjugate.

Kinetic studies after administration of repeated doses show absences of accumulation of the product.

Fenofibric acid is not eliminated during haemodialysis.

Preclinical safety data: —

Pharmaceutical particulars

List of excipients: Lactose, pregelatinised starch, sodium lauryl sulphate, crospovidone and magnesium stearate.

Composition of the capsule shell: gelatin, titanium dioxide (E171), ferrous oxide (E172) and erythrosine (E127).

Incompatibilities: No effect noted to date.

Shelf life: 3 years.

Special precautions for storage: Store below 25°C in a dry place. Protect from light.

Nature and contents of container: LIPANTIL Micro 200 is available in a pack containing 3 strips of 10 capsules per blister.

Instructions for use/handling: —

Marketing authorisation number PL 12509/0001.

Date of first authorisation/renewal of authorisation November 1993/November 1998.

Date of (partial) revision of text September 1998.

Legal category POM.

**Trade Mark*

Fujisawa Limited
CP House, 8th Floor
97–107 Uxbridge Road
London W5 5TL

☎ 0181 840 9520 🗋 0181 840 9521

Fujisawa Limited

PROGRAF*

Qualitative and quantitative composition
Capsules containing 1 mg and 5 mg tacrolimus (INN), respectively

Concentrate for intravenous infusion containing tacrolimus 5 mg per 1 ml

For excipients see *Pharmaceutical particulars.*

Pharmaceutical form Hard gelatin capsules. Concentrate for intravenous infusion.

Clinical particulars
Therapeutic indication: Primary immunosuppression in liver and kidney allograft recipients and liver and kidney allograft rejection resistant to conventional immunosuppressive regimens.

Posology and method of administration:
General considerations: The dosage recommendations given below for oral and intravenous administration are intended to act as a guideline. Prograf doses should be adjusted according to individual patient requirements. Only initial dosing is recommended and therefore therapy should be based on clinical judgement aided by measurement of tacrolimus concentrations in blood.

Route of administration: Dosing should commence orally, if necessary via an intranasal gastric tube. If the clinical condition of the patient does not allow oral therapy, initial intravenous dosing may be necessary.

Mode of intake:
Prograf Capsules 1 mg/Prograf Capsules 5 mg – Oral Dosing: It is recommended that the oral daily dose should be taken in two divided doses. The capsules should be swallowed with fluid, preferably water.

Based on pharmacokinetic considerations, the capsules should be taken on an empty stomach or at least 1 hour before or 2–3 hours after a meal to achieve maximal absorption (see *Interactions* and *Pharmacokinetic properties*).

The capsules should be taken out of the blister only immediately before intake. After opening of the aluminium wrapper, the capsules from the blisters must be used within 12 months.

Patients should be cautioned not to swallow desiccant contained within the aluminium wrapper.

Prograf Concentrate for Infusion 5 mg/ml – Intravenous Dosing: NB: Prograf Concentrate for Infusion 5 mg/ml must not be injected undiluted. The concentrate for infusion should be diluted in 5% dextrose solution or in physiological saline solution in polyethylene or glass bottles. The concentration of a solution for final infusion produced in this way should be in the range of 0.004 to 0.1 mg/ml. The total volume of infusion during 24 hours should be in the range of 20 to 250 ml. The solution should not be given as a bolus. The content of the concentrate for infusion is not compatible with PVC. The solution for final use should be used up within 24 hours.

Maximum whole blood concentration levels: Clinical study analysis suggests that the majority of patients can be successfully managed if the blood concentrations of tacrolimus are maintained below 20 ng/ml.

It is necessary to consider the clinical condition of the patient when interpreting whole blood level concentrations. If the blood levels are below the limit of quantification of the assay and the patient's clinical condition is satisfactory, then the dose should not be adjusted.

In clinical practice, 12 h trough whole blood levels are generally 5–20 ng/ml early post-transplant.

Duration of dosing: For oral dosing the capsules normally have to be taken continually to suppress graft rejection and no limit for therapy duration can be given.

Patients should be converted from intravenous to oral medication as soon as individual circumstances permit. Intravenous therapy should not be continued for more than 7 days.

Administration with other therapies: Prograf is normally administered together with other immunosuppressive agents. Prograf should not be given together with cyclosporin.

If allograft rejection or adverse events occur, alteration to the immunosuppressive regimen should be considered.

Dosage level recommendations: Initial dose level recommendation.

Primary immunosuppression dose levels – adults:
Liver and kidney transplantation: Oral tacrolimus therapy should commence at 0.10–0.20 mg/kg/day for liver transplantation and at 0.15–0.30 mg/kg/day for kidney transplantation administered as two divided doses. Administration should start approximately 6 hours after the completion of liver transplant surgery and within 24 hours of kidney transplant surgery.

If the clinical condition of the patient does not allow for oral dosing then intravenous tacrolimus therapy should be initiated as a continuous 24 hour infusion, at 0.01 to 0.05 mg/kg for liver transplants and 0.05 to 0.10 mg/kg for kidney transplants.

Primary immunosuppression dose levels – paediatric patients: Paediatric patients generally require doses 1½–2 times higher than the recommended adult doses to achieve the same blood levels. Experience with initial oral administration in paediatric patients is limited.

Liver and kidney transplantation: An initial dose of 0.3 mg/kg/day for liver and kidney transplantation should be administered in two divided doses. If the dose cannot be given orally, an initial intravenous dose of 0.05 mg/kg/day for liver transplantation or 0.1 mg/kg/day for kidney transplantation should be administered as a continuous 24-hour infusion.

Maintenance therapy dose levels: It is necessary to continue immunosuppression with oral Prograf to maintain graft survival. Dose can frequently be reduced during maintenance therapy. Dosing should be primarily based on clinical assessments of rejection and tolerability in each patient individually. During the course of the post-transplant improvement of the patient, it is likely that the pharmacokinetics of Prograf may be altered, requiring adjustment of the Prograf dose.

If progression of disease occurs (e.g. signs of acute rejection), alteration of the immunosuppressive regimen should be considered. Increase in the amount of corticosteroids, introduction of short courses of mono/polyclonal antibodies and increase in the dose of Prograf have all been used to manage rejection episodes. If signs of toxicity (e.g. pronounced adverse event, see *Undesirable effects*) are noted, the dose of Prograf should be reduced. Patients should be instructed not to decrease the dose without the consent of the treating physician.

When Prograf is administered in combination with a corticosteroid, these may often be reduced and in rare cases the treatment has continued as monotherapy.

Therapy dose levels for liver and kidney allograft rejection resistant to conventional immunosuppressive regimens: In patients experiencing rejection episodes which are unresponsive to conventional immunosuppressive therapy, Prograf treatment should begin with the initial dose recommended for primary immunosuppression in that particular allograft.

Co-administration of cyclosporin and Prograf may increase the half-life of cyclosporin and exacerbate any toxic effects. Prograf therapy should be initiated after considering cyclosporin blood concentrations and the clinical condition of the patient. In practice, Prograf therapy has been initiated 12–24 hours after discontinuation of cyclosporin. Monitoring of cyclosporin blood levels should be continued following conversion as the clearance of cyclosporin may be affected.

Compromised patients
Patients with liver impairment: A dose reduction may be necessary in patients with pre- and/or post-operative impairment, e.g. initial graft dysfunction.

Patients with renal impairment: The renal clearance of tacrolimus is low, hence no adjustment in dose is regarded as necessary on pharmacokinetic principles. However, owing to the nephrotoxic potential, careful monitoring of renal function, including serial creatinine estimations, calculations of creatinine clearance and monitoring of urine output, is recommended. The blood concentration of Prograf is not reduced by dialysis.

Elderly patients: Limited experience suggests that doses should be the same as for other adults.

Monitoring of whole blood concentrations: Various assays have been used to measure blood or plasma levels. Comparison of the levels in published literature with those found in clinical practice should be made with knowledge of the assay methods employed. In current clinical practice, blood levels are monitored using immunoassay methods.

Drug level monitoring is recommended during the early post-transplantation period, following dose adjustment of Prograf therapy after switching from another immunosuppressive regimen or following co-administration of drugs which are likely to lead to a drug to drug interaction. Trough blood levels of Prograf should also be monitored periodically during maintenance therary. The frequency of blood level monitoring should be based on clinical need. As tacrolimus has a long half-life, it can take several days for adjustments in Prograf dosing to be reflected in changes in blood levels.

Contra-indications:
Pregnancy
Known hypersensitivity to tacrolimus or other macrolides.
Prograf Capsules 1 mg and Prograf Capsules 5 mg in addition:
Known hypersensitivity to other ingredients of the capsules.
Prograf Concentrate for Infusion 5 mg/ml in addition:
Known hypersensitivity to polyoxyethylated castor oil (HC0–60) or structurally related compounds.

Special warnings and special precautions for use: Prograf therapy requires careful monitoring in units equipped and staffed with adequate laboratory and supportive medical resources. The drug should only be prescribed, and changes in immunosuppressive therapy should only be initiated, by physicians experienced in immunosuppressive therapy and the management of transplant patients. The physician responsible for maintenance therapy should have complete information requisite for the follow-up of the patient.

Dose and/or blood level adjustment should only be undertaken by the transplant centre responsible for the transplant patient.

Patients should be thoroughly controlled. In particular during the first months post-transplant, close monitoring of the patient is required.

Regular monitoring of the following parameters should be undertaken on a routine basis: blood pressure, ECG, visual status, blood glucose levels, blood levels of potassium and other electrolytes, creatinine, BUN, haematology parameters, coagulation values and liver function tests. If clinically relevant alterations of these parameters are seen, the dose of tacrolimus should be reviewed.

Renal function tests should be performed at frequent intervals. In particular during the first days post-transplant, monitoring of urinary output should be performed. If necessary the dose should be adjusted.

Several types of neurological and CNS disorders have been reported in association with Prograf therapy. For this reason, patients exhibiting such adverse events should be controlled very carefully. Occurrence of severe CNS symptoms should prompt immediate dose review. It has been reported that in some cases severe tremor and/or motoric (expressive) aphasia may be indicators for severe CNS disorders.

Ventricular hypertrophy or hypertrophy of the septum and rare cases of cardiomyopathy have been reported in association with administration of Prograf. Most of these have been reversible following dose reduction or drug discontinuation, occurring primarily in children having tacrolimus blood trough levels much higher than the recommended maximum levels. Factors which may increase the risk of this condition are pre-existing cardiac disease, corticosteroid usage, hypertension, renal or hepatic dysfunction, infections and fluid overload and oedema. Monitoring of cardiovascular function with echocardiography with or without ECG pre- and post-transplant (e.g. within the first 3 months and then at 9 months to 1 year) is advised for high risk patients. If abnormalities develop, dose reduction of Prograf therapy or discontinuation and change to alternative immunosuppressive therapy should be considered.

As with other potent immunosuppressive compounds, patients treated with Prograf have been reported to develop EBV-associated lymphoproliferative disorders. In patients switched to Prograf, this may be attributable to over-immunosuppression before commencing therapy with this agent. Patients switched to Prograf rescue therapy should not receive concomitantly anti-lymphocyte treatment. Very young (<2 years), EBV-sero-negative children have been reported to have an increased risk of developing a lymphoproliferative disorder. Therefore, in this patient group, EBV serology should be ascertained before starting treatment with Prograf. During treatment, careful monitoring is recommended.

In view of the potential risk of malignancies, patients who spend extended periods in the sun, or are otherwise exposed to UV light, should apply a high protection sun-cream.

If accidentally administered arterially or perivasally, Prograf Concentrate for Infusion 5 mg/ml may cause irritation.

Prograf should not be administered together with cyclosporin.

Prograf Concentrate for Infusion contains polyoxyethylated castor oil which has been reported to cause anaphylactoid reactions. These reactions consist of flushing of the face and upper thorax, acute respiratory distress with dyspnoea and wheezing, blood pressure changes and tachycardia. Caution is therefore necessary in patients who have previously received, by intravenous injection or infusion, preparations containing polyoxyethylated castor oil (such as HCO 60) and patients with an allergenic predisposition. Animal studies have shown that the risk of anaphylaxis may be reduced by slow infusion of polyoxyethylated castor oil containing drugs or by the prior administration of an antihistamine.

Interactions with other medicaments and other forms of interaction

Clinically observed drug interactions: Imidazole antimycotics (such as clotrimazole [from troches], fluconazole and ketoconazole), macrolide antibiotics (such as clarithromycin and erythromycin, for which up to 10-fold increase in blood trough levels has been observed), danazol and omeprazole have been reported to increase tacrolimus whole blood/plasma levels. Rifampicin has been shown to decrease tacrolimus whole blood and plasma levels.

Concomitant administration of methylprednisolone has been reported to increase and to decrease plasma levels of tacrolimus.

After combination of either amphotericin B or ibuprofen with Prograf enhanced nephrotoxicity has been observed.

Combination with cyclosporin: The half-life of cyclosporin has been shown to increase when Prograf is given simultaneously. In addition, synergistic/additive nephrotoxic effects can occur. For these reasons, the combined administration of cyclosporin and Prograf is not recommended and care should be taken when administering tacrolimus to patients who have previously received cyclosporin.

Drug interactions observed in animals: In rats, Prograf decreased the clearance and increased the half-life of pentobarbital and antipyrine.

Potential drug interactions based on the metabolic system for Prograf: Tacrolimus is cleared by hepatic metabolism. The cytochrome P450 3A4 family of enzymes is responsible for its metabolism. Concomitant use of drugs known to affect the cytochrome P450 3A system requires monitoring of tacrolimus blood levels and possible dose adjustment.

Drugs inhibiting the cytochrome P450 3A system: Substances known to inhibit cytochrome P450 3A may decrease the metabolism of Prograf with a resultant increase in tacrolimus blood levels.

Based on *in vitro* studies, the following drugs may be regarded as potential inhibitors of metabolism: bromocriptine, cortisone, dapsone, ergotamine, ethinyloestradiol, gestodene, itraconazole, josamycin, lidocaine, mephenytoin, miconazole, midazolam, nicardipine, nifedipine, nilvadipine, norethindrone, quinidine, tamoxifen, (triacetyl)oleandomycin, verapamil.

Naringenine (flavenoid in grapefruit juice) is known to inhibit the cytochrome P450 3A4 system.

Drugs inducing the cytochrome P450 3A system: Drugs known to induce cytochrome P450 3A might theoretically increase the metabolism of Prograf and hence decrease blood levels of tacrolimus. These include barbiturates (e.g. phenobarbitone), phenytoin, rifampicin, carbamazepine, metamizole and isoniazide.

Prograf inhibition of the cytochrome P450 3A system – mediated metabolism of other drugs: In vitro, Prograf showed a broad and powerful inhibitory effect on cytochrome P450 3A dependent metabolism. Prograf also demonstrated inhibition of cortisone and testosterone metabolism *in vitro.*

As Prograf might interfere with the metabolism of steroidal sexual hormones the efficacy of oral contraception may be decreased.

Potential drug interactions based on plasma protein binding: Prograf is extensively bound to plasma proteins. For this reason, possible interactions with other drugs known to have high affinity for plasma proteins (e.g. oral anticoagulants, oral antidiabetics) should be considered.

Other forms of interaction

Vaccines: During treatment with Prograf, vaccinations may be less effective and the use of live attenuated vaccines should be avoided.

Compounds with nephrotoxic/neurotoxic effects: Using Prograf with compounds known to have nephrotoxic or neurotoxic effects, (e.g. aminoglycosides, amphotericin B, gyrase inhibitors, vancomycin, cotrimoxazole and NSAIDs, ganciclovir or aciclovir) may increase toxic effects.

Potassium: As Prograf therapy may be associated with hyperkalaemia, or may increase pre-existing hyperkalaemia, high potassium intake or potassium-saving diuretics (e.g. amiloride, triamterene and spironolactone) should be avoided.

Food: Administration of Prograf with a meal of moderate fat content has been shown to reduce significantly the oral bioavailability or absorption of the drug. Therefore, it may be preferable to administer Prograf on an empty stomach or at least 1 hour before or 2–3 hours after a meal to achieve maximal absorption.

Pregnancy and lactation: Prograf is contra-indicated in pregnancy. In animal studies (rats and rabbits) Prograf has been shown to be teratogenic at doses which also demonstrated maternal toxicity.

Preclinical and human data show that the drug is able to cross the placenta. The possibility of pregnancy should therefore be excluded before initiating Prograf therapy.

As Prograf may alter the metabolism of oral contraceptives, other forms of contraception should be used.

Preclinical data in rats suggest that Prograf is excreted into breast milk. Human data on effects of the drug during the lactation period is limited. As detrimental effects on the newborn cannot be excluded, women should not breast-feed whilst receiving tacrolimus.

Effects on ability to drive and use machines: Prograf is associated with visual and neurological disturbances. Patients treated with Prograf who are affected by such disorders should not drive a car or operate dangerous machines. This effect may be enhanced when Prograf is given together with alcohol.

Undesirable effects: The adverse drug reactions (ADRs) profile associated with the use of immunosuppressive drugs is often difficult to establish owing to the presence of the mostly severe underlying disease and the concurrent use of many other medications.

There is evidence that many of the ADRs stated below are reversible and respond to dose reduction. Oral administration appears to be associated with a lower incidence of adverse events compared with intravenous use. The ADRs stated below have been arranged according to body system and within these according to frequency.

Cardiovascular system:

frequent:	hypertension
occasional:	angina pectoris, tachycardia, effusion (e.g. pericard, pleural)
rare:	hypotension including shock, abnormal ECG, cardiac arrhythmias, including atrial/ventricular fibrillations and cardiac arrest, thrombophlebitis, haemorrhage (e.g. gastrointestinal, cerebral), heart failure, cardiomegaly, bradycardia, ventricular and/or septal hypertrophy (including cardiomyopathy)
isolated:	thrombosis, embolus (e.g. pulmonary), ischaemia (e.g. cerebral), infarct (e.g. myocard; kidney; cerebrum), syncope, pericarditis and vascular disease

Nervous system/sensory system:

frequent:	tremor, headache, insomnia, perception disorder, visual disorders (e.g. cataract, amblyopia)
occasional:	depression, neuropathy, nervousness, anxiety, hypertonia, incoordination, emotional lability, amnesia, encephalopathy
rare:	migraine, confusion, dizziness, decreased reflexes, somnolence, hallucinations, dream and thinking abnormalities, agitation, psychosis, glaucoma, otological disturbances (e.g. tinnitus, deafness), photophobia
isolated:	paralysis (e.g. tetraplegia), coma, convulsion, stupor, speech disorders (e.g. aphasia, dysarthria), refraction disorder, hostility, retinopathy, cortical blindness, taste loss

Kidney

frequent:	abnormal kidney function (e.g. increase in creatinine, BUN and decrease/increase in urine output)
occasional:	lesion of kidney tissue (e.g. tubular necrosis)
rare:	dialysis-dependent renal failure, proteinuria, haematuria, hydronephrosis
isolated:	HUS, glomerulopathy (glomerulitis, nephritis)

Digestive system/liver:

frequent:	constipation, diarrhoea, nausea
occasional:	cholangitis, vomiting, abnormal liver function test, jaundice, weight and appetite changes, inflammatory disorders (e.g. ulcer), dysfunction of GI-tract (e.g. dyspepsia)
rare:	lesion of liver tissue (cirrhosis, necrosis), haematemesis, ileus, ascites, dysphagia
isolated:	pancreatitis, hepatomegaly, liver failure, bile duct abnormality

Metabolism and electrolytes:

frequent:	hypercalaemia, hyperglycaemia, hypophosphataemia
occasional:	diabetes mellitus, disorders of acid/base balance, hypervolaemia, hypokalaemia, hyperuricaemia (including gout), increased amylase
rare:	decrease in blood concentration of magnesium, calcium, protein, sodium; increase in blood concentration of calcium, phosphate; dehydration, hyperlipidaemia, hypoglycaemia
isolated:	hypermagnesaemia, increase of creatine phosphokinase

Musculoskeletal:

occasional:	cramps
rare:	osteoporosis
isolated:	myasthenia, avascular bone necrosis, arthritis, myopathy

Respiratory system:

occasional:	impairment of lung function (e.g. dyspnoea), atelectasis
rare:	asthma
isolated:	respiratory failure, pulmonary fibrosis

Skin:

occasional:	alopecia, pruritus, sweating, rash, photosensitivity
rare:	gynaecomastia, hirsutism, urticaria
isolated:	erythema (e.g. erythema nodosum)

Haematological and lymphatic system:

frequent:	leucocytosis
occasional:	leucopenia, anaemia (e.g. aplastic, haemolytic)
rare:	thrombocytopaenia, splenomegaly, eosinophilia, thrombocythaemia
isolated:	coagulation disorders, bone marrow depression (incl. pancytopenia), thrombotic thrombocytopenic purpura

Miscellaneous:

occasional:	oedema in various organ-systems (e.g. CNS, respiratory, cardiovascular), localised pain (e.g. arthralgia, neuralgia, abdominal pain, chest pain), asthenia, fever
isolated:	incontinence, prostatic disorder, thyroid and parathyroid disorder

Malignancies: Malignancies are known to occur with immunosuppressive therapy. Benign and malignant neoplasms (e.g. of the lymphatic and myeloid system epithelial and mesenchymal tissue) have been reported in isolated cases in association with tacrolimus treatment.

Autoimmune diseases: In isolated cases autoimmune processes (e.g. vasculitis, Lyell syndrome, Stevens-Johnson syndrome) were observed in patients receiving tacrolimus.

Allergic reactions: Allergic and anaphylactoid reactions were noted in patients being treated with tacrolimus, such as flush, pruritus and anaphylactic shock, in isolated cases.

Infections: As with other potent immunosuppressive drugs, the susceptibility to viral, bacterial, fungal and/or protozoal infection is increased in patients receiving tacrolimus. Overall, infections are reported frequently in patients being treated with tacrolimus. The course of pre-existing infectious diseases may also be aggravated. Both generalised (sepsis) and localised infections (abscess, pneumonia) can occur. The risk of over-immunosuppression may be increased if tacrolimus is administered along with other immunosuppressive medication.

Overdose: Experience of overdosage is limited.

Early clinical experience (when initial induction doses were 2 or 3 times greater than those currently recommended) suggested that symptoms of overdosage may include, renal, neurological and cardiac disturbances, effects on glucose intolerance, hypertension and electrolyte disorders (e.g. hyperkalaemia). Over-immunosuppression may increase the risk of severe infections.

Isolated reports on overdose of tacrolimus indicate that nausea, vomiting, tremor, increased liver enzyme values, headache, lethargy, urticaria, nephrotoxicity and infections may occur.

Liver function clearly influences all pre- and post-operative pharmacokinetic variables. Patients with failing liver grafts or those switched from other immunosuppressive therapy to Prograf should be monitored carefully to avoid overdosage.

No specific antidote to Prograf therapy is available. If overdosage occurs, general supportive measures and symptomatic treatment should be conducted.

Based on the poor aqueous solubility and extensive erythrocyte and plasma protein binding, it is anticipated that Prograf will not be dialysable. In isolated patients with very high plasma concentrations of tacrolimus, haemofiltration and haemodiafiltration have been reported to considerably decrease the tacrolimus levels. In cases of oral intoxication, gastric lavage and/or the use of absorbents (such as activated charcoal) may be helpful.

Pharmacological properties

Pharmacodynamic properties

Pharmacotherapeutic group: Immunosuppressive macrolide lactone.

Mechanism of action: On the molecular level, the effects of tacrolimus appear to be mediated by binding to a cytosolic protein (FKBP12) which is also responsible for the intracellular accumulation of the compound. The FKBP12-tacrolimus complex specifically and competitively binds to and inhibits calcinurin, which leads to a calcium-dependent inhibition of signal transduction pathways in T-cells, thereby preventing transcription of a discrete set of lymphokine genes.

Pharmacodynamic effects: Prograf is a highly immunosuppressive agent and has proven activity in both *in vitro* and *in vivo* experiments.

In particular, Prograf inhibits the formation of cytotoxic lymphocytes which are mainly responsible for graft rejection. The drug suppresses T-cell activation and T-helper-cell dependent B-cell proliferation, as well as the formation of lymphokines such as interleukins-2, -3 and γ-interfon and the expression of the interleukin-2 receptor. At the molecular level, the effects of Prograf appear to be mediated by binding to a cytosolic protein (FKBP) which is also responsible for the intracellular accumulation of the compound.

In *in vivo* studies, Prograf has been shown to be efficacious in transplantation of the liver and kidney.

Pharmacokinetic properties

General characteristics

Absorption: Studies in the rat have shown that tacrolimus is absorbed throughout the gastrointestinal tract. The major site of absorption was identified as the upper GI. In man, absorption of tacrolimus from the gastrointestinal tract after oral administration is variable. Peak concentrations (C_{max}) of tacrolimus in blood are achieved in approximately 1 to 3 hours. In some patients the drug appears to be continuously absorbed over a prolonged time period yielding more or less a flat absorption profile. Mean (±sd) absorption parameters of tacrolimus are listed in the table below.

After oral administration (0.15 mg/kg/bid) in liver transplant patients, steady state concentrations of tacrolimus were achieved within 3 days in most patients. The oral bioavailability of tacrolimus was reduced when it was administered after food containing a moderate fat content. There was a decrease in AUC (27%), C_{max} (50%) and an increase in t_{max} (173%) in whole blood. Both rate and extent of absorption were reduced when tacrolimus was given with food. Bile does not influence the absorption of tacrolimus and therefore commencement of tacrolimus therapy with an oral dose or early conversion of liver transplant patients from intravenous to oral therapy is possible. There is strong correlation between the area under the curve and the trough whole blood levels at steady state. Thus monitoring of trough whole blood levels provides a good estimate of systemic exposure.

Distribution and elimination: In man, the disposition of tacrolimus after intravenous infusion may be described as biphasic. In systemic circulation, tacrolimus binds strongly to erythrocytes resulting in the distribution of whole blood/plasma concentrations of tacrolimus of approximately 20:1. In plasma the drug is highly bound (>98.8%) to plasma proteins, mainly to serum albumin and α-1-acid glycoprotein.

Tacrolimus is extensively distributed in the body. The steady state volume of distribution based on plasma concentrations is approximately 1300 L (healthy subjects). Corresponding data based on whole blood data averaged 47.6 L. The total body clearance (TBC) of tacrolimus from blood is low. In healthy subjects the average TBC was estimated from whole blood concentrations to be 2.43 L/h. In adult liver transplant patients, TBC was 4.1 L/h. In paediatric liver patients, the TBC is approximately double the TBC in adult liver transplant patients. In kidney transplant patients, TBC was 6.7 L/h.

There is evidence that the pharmacokinetics of tacrolimus change with improving clinical condition of the patients. In liver transplant patients, the mean oral dose was decreased by 28% from day 7 to month 6 after transplantation, to maintain similar mean trough levels of tacrolimus. Changes in clearance and/or bioavailability were suggested as probable causes for this effect.

The half-life of tacrolimus is long and variable. In healthy volunteers the main half-life in whole blood is approximately 43 hours. In paediatric and adult liver transplant patients, it averaged 12.4 and 11.7 hours respectively. In adult kidney transplant patients, it averaged 15.6 hours.

Metabolism and biotransformation: Tacrolimus is cleared by hepatic metabolism. The cytochrome P450 3A4 is primarily responsible for its metabolism. There is also evidence of gastrointestinal metabolism.

Eight metabolites have so far been characterised. Of these, only one metabolite showed significant immunosuppressive activity, in comparison to tacrolimus.

Excretion: Following intravenous and oral administration of ^{14}C-labelled tacrolimus, most of the radioactivity was eliminated in the faeces. Approximately 2% of the radioactivity was eliminated in the urine. Less than 1% of unchanged tacrolimus was detected in the urine and the faeces. This indicates that tacrolimus is almost completely metabolised prior to elimination from the body and that bile is the principal route of elimination.

Characteristics in patients

Relationship between plasma/blood concentrations and therapeutic activity: As stated in *Posology and method of administration* section, individual dose adjustment controlled by monitoring of Prograf levels in whole blood may be helpful to achieve optimal therapy. Several immunoassays are available for determining Prograf concentrations in whole blood, including a fully automatic microparticle enzyme immunoassay (MEIA). Details are available on request.

Variations with respect to confounding factors – age, polymorphism, metabolism and concomitant pathological situations (renal failure, hepatic insufficiency): Based on limited experience, the kinetic properties of Prograf are not altered in elderly patients.

Children require a higher dose of Prograf, approximately 1½ to 2 times higher than that recommended for adults, possibly owing to a higher metabolic turnover.

Patients with liver dysfunction: Patients with liver dysfunction tended to have higher Prograf concentrations (and correspondingly longer half-lives and smaller clearance values) compared with patients with a normal liver function.

As the drug is extensively metabolised by the liver, patients with impaired liver function should be carefully monitored, and dose adjustment may be necessary.

Patients with kidney dysfunction: Since the drug is nearly completely metabolised, highly lipid-soluble, and has a molecular weight of 822, it is not expected to be dialysable. Also, less than 1% of an administered intravenous dose is excreted in the urine. Therefore, changes to the dosing regimen from the pharmacokinetic point of view are not necessary in patients with renal failure or in patients undergoing dialysis. However, dosage adjustment may be necessary in patients with evidence of drug-induced impairment of kidney function.

Preclinical safety data

Mutagenicity: Relevant *in vitro* and *in vivo* tests showed no signs of a mutagenic potential of Prograf.

Carcinogenicity: In chronic, 1-year toxicity studies (rats and baboons) and in long-term carcinogenicity studies (mouse 18 months and rat 24 months at maximum tolerable dose of 2.5–5 mg/kg/day) no signs of a direct tumorigenic potential of Prograf were seen.

However, as known from other immunosuppressive drugs, malignancies such as lymphomas and skin cancers can be expected but were seen rarely in patients.

Reproduction toxicity: In rats, fertility, embryonic and foetal development and the birth as well as the peri- and post-natal development were only impaired when receiving clearly toxic dosages (3.2 mg/kg/day). The only exception was a reversible reduction of the foetal birth weights at a dose of 0.1 mg/kg/day. Furthermore in rabbits, toxic effects on the embryos and on the foetus were observed. Again, these were limited to doses of 1.0 mg/kg/day which showed significant toxicity in maternal animals. Based on these observations, Prograf should not be administered to pregnant women.

Pharmaceutical particulars

List of excipients

Prograf Capsules 1 mg/Prograf Capsules 5 mg: Hydroxypropylmethylcellulose, croscarmellose sodium, lactose, magnesium stearate and titanium dioxide (E 171). Prograf Capsules 5 mg also contain red iron oxide (E 172).

Prograf Concentrate for Infusion 5 mg/ml: Polyoxyethylene hydrogenated castor oil, dehydrated alcohol.

Incompatibilities: Prograf is not compatible with PVC plastics. Mixed infusions between a solution prepared with Prograf Concentrate for Infusion 5 mg/ml and other drugs should be avoided. In particular mixed infusions with drugs exhibiting a marked alkaline reaction in solution (e.g. aciclovir, ganciclovir) must not be administered as tacrolimus can disintegrate in this condition.

Shelf life

Prograf Capsules 1 mg/Prograf Capsules 5 mg: Aluminium-wrapped blisters: 36 months. After opening of the aluminium wrapper the capsules are stable for 12 months.

Prograf Concentrate for Infusion 5 mg/ml: 24 months when protected from light and stored at temperatures up to 25°C. To be used within 24 hours when reconstituted with 5% dextrose solution or physiological saline in polyethylene or glass containers.

Special precautions for storage

Prograf Capsules 1 mg/ Prograf Capsules 5 mg: Once the aluminium wrapper is opened the capsules in the blister strips are stable for 12 months. The individual blister strips should be kept in a dry place. The patients should be instructed accordingly.

Prograf Concentrate for Infusion 5 mg/ml: Store below 25°C. Protect from light.

Nature and contents of container

Prograf Capsules 1 mg/Prograf Capsules 5 mg: Ten capsules per blister sheet. For Prograf Capsules 1 mg three, five or ten blisters and for Prograf Capsules 5 mg three or five blisters are packaged with one dessicant sachet in an aluminium wrapper.

The following pack sizes are currently available on the market:

Prograf Capsules 1 mg: cartons of 50 and 100 capsules

Prograf Capsules 5 mg: cartons of 50 capsules

Prograf Concentrate for Infusion 5 mg/ml: Concentrate for Infusion (solution) in transparent glass ampoules.

Instructions for use/handling: Tubing, syringes and any other equipment used to administer Prograf should not contain PVC.

Prograf Capsules 1 mg/Prograf Capsules 5 mg: To be used as directed. Patients should take the capsules immediately once they are taken out of the blister.

Prograf Concentrate for Infusion 5 mg/ml: Prograf Concentrate for Infusion should be prepared for infusion with 5% dextrose solution or physiological

Population	*Dose*	C^{max} *(ng/ml)*	T^{max} *(hours)*	*Bioavailability (%)*
Healthy subjects (Single dose)	1×5 mg 5×1 mg	28.6 (8.6) 36.2 (13.8)	1.4 (0.6) 1.3 (0.4)	14.4 (6.0) 17.4 (7.0)
Adult liver transplant (Steady state)	0.15 mg/kg/12 h	74.1	3.0	21.8 (6.3)
Paediatric liver transplant (Steady state)	0.15 mg/kg/12 h	37.0 (26.5)	2.1 (1.3)	25 (20)
Adult kidney transplant (Steady state)	0.15 mg/kg/12 h	44.3 (21.9)	1.5	20.1 (11.0)

saline in polyethylene or glass containers. After constitution, infusion solutions should be used within 24 hours. Opened ampoules should be disposed of immediately, if not used, to avoid contamination.

Marketing authorisation numbers

Prograf Capsules 1 mg	13424/0001
Prograf Capsules 5 mg	13424/0002
Prograf Concentrate for Infusion 5 mg/ml	13424/0003

Date of approval/revision of SPC 9 September 1997.

Legal category POM.

**Trade Mark*

Futuna Limited

57 Masonfield
Bamber Bridge
Preston PR5 8HP

☎ 0870 6012037 🗋 0870 6012036

SURMONTIL*

Qualitative and quantitative composition
Surmontil tablets 10 mg contain Trimipramine Maleate EP 14 mg equivalent to 10 mg trimipramine per tablet.

Surmontil tablets 25 mg contain Trimipramine Maleate EP 35.0 mg equivalent to 25 mg trimipramine per tablet.

Surmontil capsules 50 mg contain Trimipramine Maleate EP 69.75 mg per capsule.

Pharmaceutical form
Surmontil tablets are compression coated, white. The face is indented with the name and strength; the reverse is plain.

Surmontil capsules are white opaque with a green cap, printed 'SU50'.

Clinical particulars
Therapeutic indications: Surmontil has a potent antidepressant action similar to that of other tricyclic antidepressants. It also possesses pronounced sedative action. It is, therefore, indicated in the treatment of depressive illness, especially where sleep disturbance, anxiety or agitation are presenting symptoms. Sleep disturbance is controlled within 24 hours and true antidepressant action follows within 7 to 10 days.

Posology and method of administration: For oral use.

Adults: For depression 50–75 mg/day initially increasing to 150–300 mg/day in divided doses or one dose at night. The maintenance dose is 75–150 mg/day.

Elderly: 10–25 mg three times a day initially. The initial dose should be increased with caution under close supervision. Half the normal maintenance dose may be sufficient to produce a satisfactory clinical response.

Children: Not recommended.

Contra-indications: Recent myocardial infarction. Any degree of heart block or other cardiac arrhythmias. Mania. Severe liver disease. During breast feeding.

Special warnings and precautions for use: The elderly are particularly liable to experience adverse reactions, especially agitation, confusion and postural hypotension. Avoid if possible in patients with narrow angle glaucoma, symptons suggestive of prostatic hypertrophy and a history of epilepsy.

Patients posing a high suicidal risk require close initial supervision. Tricyclic antidepressants potentiate the central nervous depressant action of alcohol.

Anaesthetics given during tri/tetracyclic antidepressant therapy may increase the risk of arrhythmias and hypotension. If surgery is necessary, the anaesthetist should be informed that a patient is being so treated.

It may be advisable to monitor liver function in patients on long term treatment with Surmontil.

Interactions with other medicaments and other forms of interaction: Trimipramine should not be given concurrently with, or within 2 weeks of cessation of, therapy with monoamine oxidase inhibitors. Trimipramine may decrease the antihypertensive effect of guanethidine, debrisoquine, bethanidine and possibly clonidine. It would be advisable to review all antihypertensive therapy during treatment with tricyclic antidepressants.

Trimipramine should not be given with sympathomimetic agents such as adrenaline, ephedrine, isoprenaline, noradrenaline, phenylephrine and phenylpropanolamine.

Barbiturates may increase the rate of metabolism.

Surmontil should be administered with care in patients receiving therapy for hyperthyroidism.

Pregnancy and lactation: Do not use in pregnancy especially during the first and last trimesters unless there are compelling reasons. There is no evidence from animal work that it is free from hazard. Trimipramine is contra-indicated during lactation.

Effects on ability to drive and use machines: Trimipramine may initially impair alertness. Patients should be warned of the possible hazard when driving or operating machinery.

Undesirable effects: Cardiac arrhythmias and severe hypotension are likely to occur with high dosage or in deliberate overdosage. They may also occur in patients with pre-existing heart disease taking normal dosage.

The following adverse effects, although not necessarily all reported with trimipramine, have occurred with other tricyclic antidepressants. Atropine-like side effects including dry mouth, disturbance of accommodation, tachycardia, constipation and hesitancy of micturition are common early in treatment but usually lessen. Other common adverse effects include drowsiness, sweating, postural hypotension, tremor and skin rashes. Interference with sexual function may occur. Serious adverse effects are rare; the following have been reported: depression of bone marrow, including agranulocytosis, cholestatic jaundice, hypomania, convulsions and peripheral neuropathy. Psychotic manifestations including mania and paranoid delusions, may be exacerbated during treatment with tricyclic antidepressants. Withdrawal symptoms may occur on abrupt cessation of therapy and include insomnia, irritability and excessive perspiration. Adverse effects such as withdrawal symptoms, respiratory depression and agitation have been reported in neonates whose mothers had taken trimipramine during the last trimester of pregnancy.

Overdose: Acute overdosage may be accompanied by hypotensive collapse, convulsions and coma. Provided coma is not present, gastric lavage should be carried out without delay even though some time may have passed since the drug was ingested. Patients in coma should have an endotracheal tube passed before gastric lavage is started. Absorption of trimipramine is slow but, as cardiac effects may appear soon after the drug is absorbed, a saline purge should be given. Electrocardiography monitoring is essential.

It is important to treat acidosis as soon as it appears with, for example, 20 ml per kg of M/6 sodium lactate injection by slow intravenous injection. Intubation is necessary and the patient should be ventilated before convulsions develop. Convulsions should be treated with diazepam administered intravenously.

Ventricular tachycardia or fibrillation should be treated by electrical defibrillation. If supraventicular tachycardia develops, pyridostigmine bromide 1 mg (adults) intravenously or propranolol 1 mg (adults) should be administered at intervals as required.

Treatment should be continued for at least three days even if the patient appears to have recovered.

Pharmacological properties
Pharmacodynamic properties: Trimipramine is a tricyclic antidepressant. It has marked sedative properties.

Pharmacokinetic properties: Trimipramine undergoes high first-pass hepatic clearance, with a mean value for bioavailability of about 41% after oral administration.

The absolute volume of distribution is 31 litres/kg and total metabolic clearance is 16 ml/min/kg.

Plasma protein binding of trimipramine is about 95%. The plasma elimination half-life is around 23 hours. Trimipramine is largely metabolised by demethylation prior to conjugation yielding a glucuronide.

Pharmaceutical particulars
List of excipients: The tablets contain: Maize starch, Kaolin heavy, Dextrin white technical, Williams Ariavit Indigo Carmine C1 73015, Calcium Hydrogen Phosphate, Starch potato, Sodium Lauryl Sulphate, Magnesium Stearate.

The capsules contain Maize starch, Microcrystalline cellulose (E460), Magnesium stearate, Colloidal silicon dioxide. The shell contains Titanium dioxide, Indigo carmine, Iron oxide Yellow, Gelatine, Iron oxide black ink (E172).

Incompatibilities: None known.

Shelf life:
Tablets 60 months.
Capsules 36 months.

Special precautions for storage:
Tablets: Protect from light.
Capsules: Store in a dry place below 25°C and protect from light.

Nature and contents of container:
Surmontil tablets 10 mg: blister packs of 28 tablets.
Surmontil tablets 10 mg: blister packs of 84 tablets.
Surmontil tablets 25 mg: blister packs of 28 tablets.
Surmontil tablets 25 mg: blister packs of 84 tablets.
Surmontil capsules 50 mg: blister packs of 28 tablets.

Instructions for use/handling: None stated.

Marketing authorisation numbers

Surmontil Tablets 10 mg	PL 16457/0001
Surmontil Tablets 25 mg	PL 16457/0002
Surmontil Capsules 50 mg	PL 16457/0003

Date of approval/revision of SPC December 1997

Legal category POM

***Trade Mark*

Galderma (U.K.) Ltd

Leywood House
Woodside Road
Amersham
Bucks HP6 6AA

☎ 01494 432606 📠 01494 432607

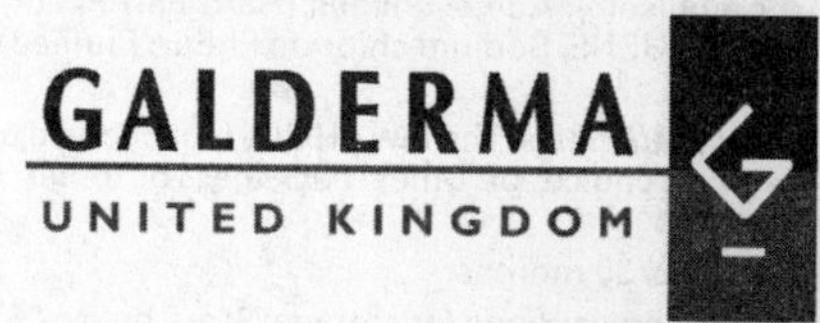

ACNECIDE* 5% GEL
ACNECIDE* 10% GEL

Qualitative and quantitative composition
Benzoyl Peroxide PhEur 5% w/w.
Benzoyl Peroxide PhEur 10% w/w.

Pharmaceutical Form Topical gel.

Clinical particulars
Therapeutic indications: Topical therapy for the treatment of acne vulgaris.

Posology and Method of Administration: For external use only.

Adults and children: After washing with a mild cleanser, apply once or twice daily or as directed to the affected areas. Initially Acnecide 5% should be used; treatment may be continued with Acnecide 10% provided Acnecide 5% has been well tolerated. The extent of any drying or peeling may be adjusted by modifying the dosage schedule.

Contra-indications: Persons having known sensitivity to benzoyl peroxide.

Special warnings and precautions for use: Avoid contact with the eyes, eyelids, and other mucous surfaces.

Interaction with other medicaments and other forms of interaction: None known.

Pregnancy and lactation: No known effects. Use at the discretion of the physician.

Effects on ability to drive and use machines: Not applicable.

Undesirable effects: None known.

Overdose: Not applicable.

Pharmacological particulars
Pharmacodynamic properties: Benzoyl peroxide is an established and effective keratolytic agent with antibacterial properties. It has been shown to be effective in reducing the local population of Propionibacterium acnes leading to a reduction in the production of irritant fatty acids in the sebaceous glands.

Pharmacokinetic properties: Not applicable. Acnecide is a topical preparation.

Preclinical safety data: In animal studies by the cutaneous route, benzoyl peroxide is associated with a minimal to moderate skin irritation potential including erythema and oedema. Phototoxic and photoallergic reactions have been reported for benzoyl peroxide therapy.

Pharmaceutical particulars
List of excipients: Docusate sodium; disodium edetate; poloxamer 182; carbomer 940; propylene glycol; acrylates copolymer or glycerol microsponge; glycerol; silicon dioxide; purified water; and sodium hydroxide to adjust the pH.

Incompatibilities: None known.

Shelf life: 36 months.

Special precautions for storage: Store below 25°C.

Nature and contents of container: White low density polyethylene tubes containing 60 g gel.

Instruction for use/handling: No special instructions.

Marketing authorisation number

Acnecide 5% Gel:	PL10590/0006
Acnecide 10% Gel:	PL10590/0007

Date of first authorisation/renewal of authorisation
13 July 1992/12 January 1998

Date of (partial) revision of the text April 1998 (UK Version 2)

Legal category: P

ALCODERM* CREAM
ALCODERM* LOTION

Qualitative and quantitative composition None.

Pharmaceutical form
Alcoderm Cream: Cream.
Alcoderm Lotion: Lotion.

Clinical particulars
Therapeutic indications: Dry, chafed or irritated skin– Alcoderm is indicated in any condition where the moisture content of the horny layer has decreased below the normal level and the skin is no longer soft and pliable.

Also recommended:

a) in acute inflammatory conditions where the skin is intact, such as sunburn and windburn.

b) as a soothing, hydrating agent in certain inflammatory skin conditions where there is dryness and scaling, such as ichthyosis, atopic eczema, winter itch, etc.

Posology and method of administration:
Dosage:
Adults, children and the elderly: Apply topically to the skin as required to alleviate the symptoms of dry, chafed or irritated skin conditions or as directed by a doctor.

Route of Administration: Apply topically to the skin.

Contra-indications: Hypersensitivity to the constituents of the preparation.

Special warnings and special precautions for use: Avoid contact with eyes.

If symptoms persist consult your physician.

In the rare event of a skin reaction, treatment should be discontinued.

Interaction with other medicaments and other forms of interaction: None.

Pregnancy and lactation: May be used during this period.

Effects on ability to drive and use machines: Not applicable.

Undesirable effects: Very rarely, a mild skin irritation can occur.

Overdose: Accidental ingestion is not anticipated to cause any harm to the patient.

Pharmacological properties
Pharmacodynamic properties: Not applicable.

Pharmacokinetic properties: Not applicable.

Preclinical safety data: Not relevant as the product has been in use for many years without apparent ill consequence.

Pharmaceutical particulars
List of excipients:

Alcoderm Cream:
Mineral Oil (Liquid Paraffin)
Isopropyl Palmitate Ph. Eur.
Sodium Lauryl Sulphate Ph. Eur.
Methylparaben Ph. Eur.
Propylparaben Ph. Eur.
Sorbitol solution (70%) Ph. Eur.
Cetyl Alcohol Ph. Eur.
Stearyl Alcohol Ph. Eur.
Sorbitan Monostearate Ph. Eur.
Spermaceti (Cetyl Esters Wax) USP/NF
Silicone Fluid (Dimeticone) Ph. Eur.
Perfume (Chemoderm 6435)
Citric Acid Anhydrous Ph. Eur., or Sodium Hydroxide Ph. Eur.
Purified Water Ph. Eur.

Alcoderm Lotion:
Mineral Oil (Liquid Paraffin)
Sodium Lauryl Sulphate Ph. Eur.
Methylparaben Ph. Eur.
Propylparaben Ph. Eur.
Cetyl Alcohol Ph. Eur.
Stearyl Alcohol Ph. Eur.
Sorbitan Monostearate Ph. Eur.
Triethanolamine
Carbomer 940
Perfume (Chemoderm 6435)
Purified Water Ph. Eur.

Incompatibilities: None.

Shelf life: 4 years.

Special precautions for storage: Store at room temperature.

Nature and contents of container: Alcoderm Cream: Polyethylene plastic tube with a white polypropylene screw cap as the closure.

Pack size: 60 g.

Alcoderm Lotion: Polyethylene plastic cylindrical container with a polypropylene screw cap as the closure.

Pack size: 200 ml.

Instructions for use/handling: Not relevant.

Marketing authorisation number

Alcoderm Cream:	PL 10590/0004
Alcoderm Lotion:	PL 10590/0005

Date of first authorisation/renewal of authorisation
21 January 1993/10 June 1998

Date of (partial) revision of text October 1997

Legal category P

CALMURID* CREAM

Qualitative and quantitative composition A white cream containing Urea PhEur 10.0 % w/w and Lactic Acid PhEur 5.0% w/w in a stabilising emulsified base.

Pharmaceutical form Cream for topical (cutaneous) use.

Clinical particulars
Therapeutic indications: To be applied topically for the correction of hyperkeratosis and dryness in ichthyosis and allied conditions characterised by dry, rough, scaly skin.

Posology and method of administration: For external use only.

Dosage and administration:
Adults, elderly and children: A thick layer of Calmurid is applied twice daily after washing the affected area. The cream is left on the skin for 3-5 minutes and then rubbed lightly in. Excess cream should be wiped off the skin with a tissue, not washed off. Frequency of application can be reduced as the patient progresses. In hyperkeratosis of the feet apply Calmurid as above after soaking the feet in warm water for 15 minutes and drying with a rough towel.

Contra-indications: Hypersensitivity to any constituent of the product.

Special warnings and special precautions for use: Calmurid is acidic and hypertonic and can cause smarting if applied to raw areas, fissures or mucous membranes. Where this is a barrier to therapy the use of Calmurid diluted 50% with aqueous cream B.P. for one week should result in freedom from smarting upon use of Calmurid.

Interaction with other medicaments and other forms of interaction: Low pH of cream might affect stability of other drugs.

Pregnancy and lactation: There is no specific data available regarding the use in pregnant women and during lactation.

Effects on ability to drive and use machines: None known.

Undesirable effects: Calmurid is acidic and hypertonic and can cause smarting if applied to raw areas, fissures or mucous membranes.

Overdose: Unlikely. In the case of smarting, wash the cream off.

Pharmacological properties
Pharmacodynamic properties: Urea at a concentration of 10% has keratolytic, anti microbial, anti pruritic and hydrating effects on the skin. Lactic acid has keratolytic, hydrating and anti microbial properties also. Treatment of ichthyotic patients shows a parallel between clinical improvement and increase in the otherwise depressed binding capacity of the horny layer.

Pharmacokinetic properties: Not applicable.

Preclinical safety data: Urea and lactic acid are long established materials, whose pre-clinical profile is known.

Pharmaceutical particulars
List of excipients: Glyceryl monostearate PhEur, Betaine monohydrate, Diethanolamine cetylphosphate ("Amphisol"), Adeps solidus (Hard Fat) PhEur, Cholesterol USNF, Sodium chloride PhEur, Purified water PhEur.
Incompatibilities: The low pH due to lactic acid means care in choice of other packages or other drugs admixed.
Shelf life: 30 months.
Special precautions for storage: Store below 25°C. Do not freeze. Do not put in alloy containers.
Nature and contents of container: Polythene tubes with polypropylene caps.
Package sizes: 100 g.
Plastic pump dispenser.
Package sizes: 500 g.
Instructions for use/handling: Not relevant.

Marketing authorisation number PL 10590/0009

Date of first authorisation/renewal of authorisation 9 February 1993/24 March 1998

Date of (partial) revision of text November 1997 (UK Version 4)

Legal category P

CALMURID HC* CREAM

Presentation A smooth, homogenous white oil in water cream containing: Urea PhEur 10% w/w, Lactic Acid PhEur 5% w/w and Hydrocortisone PhEur 1% w/w.

Uses To be used topically for the management of atopic eczema, Besniers prurigo, acute and chronic allergic eczema, neurodermatitis and other hyperkeratotic skin conditions with accompanying inflammation.

Dosage and administration For external use only.
Adults, elderly and children: Apply twice daily to the affected area after bathing or washing. Moist lesions should be treated as to dry them before using Calmurid HC.

Contra-indications, warnings, etc
Contra-indications: Skin tuberculosis, viral infections accompanied by dermal manifestations e.g. herpes simplex, vaccinia, chicken pox and measles. Syphilitic skin lesions. In concurrent mycotic infections, the cream should be complemented with antimycotic treatment.
Interactions: None known.
Side effects: If applied to open wounds or mucous membranes the hypertonic and acidic nature of the preparation may produce smarting. Where smarting is a barrier to therapy, dilute with an equal quantity of aqueous cream: after a week of treatment with this material, the normal strength should be tolerated.
Pregnancy and lactation
Pregnancy: Evidence from animal studies suggests that prolonged intensive therapy with steroids during pregnancy should be avoided.
Lactation: Given the slow uptake of hydrocortisone from the skin and the rapid destruction of hydrocortisone by the body, there would seem to be little risk of significant transfer at lactation.
Precautions and warnings: In infants, high surface area in relation to mass raises the likelihood of uptake of excessive amounts of steroid from the cream, even without occlusion, thus adrenal suppression is more likely. In infants, long term continuous topical therapy should be avoided.
Overdose: The barrier function in the skin to steroid uptake, the low toxicity of hydrocortisone and the natural mechanism for its rapid inactivation make overdose unlikely.

Pharmaceutical precautions Store below 25°C. Do not mix with other preparations, as the effect on the stability of each is unknown. Do not pack in alloy containers as they may react with the lactic acid.

Legal category POM.

Package quantities Collapsible polypropylene tubes of 30 g and 100 g.

Further information Urea at a concentration of 10% has keratolytic, anti-microbial, anti-pruritic and hydrating effects on the skin, properties also attributable to lactic acid.

Hydrocortisone 1% is the normal concentration of the drug used as a dermatological anti-inflammatory agent. In some patients with eczema, Calmurid HC cream may be as effective as fluorinated steroid creams.

The constituents of the base are: glycerol monostearate, betaine monohydrate, diethanolamine cetyl phosphate ('Amphisol'), adeps solidus (hard fat), cholesterol, sodium chloride and purified water.

Product licence number 10590/0010.

DIFFERIN* CREAM ▼

Qualitative and quantitative composition Adapalene (INN, BAN, USAN) 0.1% w/w.

Pharmaceutical form Cream for topical application.

Clinical particulars
Therapeutic indications: Differin Cream is proposed for the cutaneous treatment of mild to moderate acne vulgaris where comedones, papules and pustules predominate. Differin cream is best suited for use on dry and fair skin. Acne of the face, chest or back is appropriate for treatment.
Posology and method of administration: Differin cream should be applied to the acne affected areas once a day before retiring and after washing. A thin film of cream should be applied, with the fingertips, avoiding the eyes and lips (see *Special warnings and special precautions for use*, below). Ensure that the affected areas are dry before application.

Since it is customary to alternate therapies in the treatment of acne, it is recommended that the physician assess the continued improvement of the patient after three months of treatment with Differin Cream.

With patients for whom it is necessary to reduce the frequency of application or to temporarily discontinue treatment, frequency of application may be restored or therapy resumed once it is judged that the patient can again tolerate the treatment.

If patients use cosmetics, these should be non-comedogenic and non-astringent.

The safety and effectiveness of Differin Cream have not been studied in neonates and young children.
Contra-indications: Hypersensitivity to any ingredient of the product.
Special warnings and special precautions for use: If a reaction suggesting sensitivity or severe irritation occurs, use of the medication should be discontinued. If the degree of local irritation warrants, patients should be directed to use the medication less frequently, to discontinue use temporarily, or to discontinue use altogether. Differin Cream should not come into contact with the eyes, mouth, angles of the nose or mucous membranes.

If product enters the eye, wash immediately with warm water. The product should not be applied to either broken (cuts and abrasions) or eczematous skin, nor should it be used in patients with severe acne, or acne involving large areas of the body, especially in women of child bearing age who are not on effective contraception.
Interaction with other medicaments and other forms of interaction: There are no known interactions with other medications which might be used cutaneously and concurrently with Differin Cream; however, other retinoids or drugs with a similar mode of action should not be used concurrently with adapalene.
Adapalene is essentially stable to oxygen and light and is chemically non-reactive. Whilst extensive studies in animals and man have shown neither phototoxic nor photoallergic potential for adapalene, the safety of using adapalene during repeated exposure to sunlight or UV irradiation has not been established in either animals or man. Exposure to excessive sunlight or UV irradiation should be avoided.
Absorption of adapalene through human skin is low (see *Pharmacokinetic properties*) and therefore interaction with systemic medications is unlikely. There is no evidence that the efficacy of oral drugs such as contraceptives and antibiotics is influenced by the cutaneous use of Differin Cream.
Differin Cream has a potential for mild local irritation, and therefore it is possible that concomitant use of peeling agents, astringents or irritant products may produce additive irritant effects. However, cutaneous antiacne treatment e.g. erythromycin (up to 4%) or clindamycin phosphate (1% as the base) solutions or benzoyl peroxide water based gels up to 10% may be used in the morning when Differin Cream is used at night as there is no mutual degradation or cumulative irritation.
Pregnancy and lactation: No information on the effects of Adapalene in pregnant women is available and therefore this product should not be used during pregnancy, unless considered essential by the physician. Because of the risk of teratogenicity shown in animal studies and since there is no information on the use of adapalene in pregnant women, it should not be used in women of child bearing age unless they are using an effective means of contraception.

Adapalene produces teratogenic effects by the oral route in rats and rabbits. At cutaneous doses up to 200-fold the therapeutic dose, producing circulating plasma levels of adapalene at least 35 to 120 times higher than plasma levels demonstrated in therapeutic use, adapalene increased the incidence of additional ribs in rats and rabbits, without increasing the incidence of major malformations.

It is not known whether adapalene is secreted in animal or human milk. In animal studies, infant rats suckled by mother with circulating levels of adapalene at least 300 times those demonstrated in clinical use developed normally.

Its use in women breast feeding infants should be avoided but when it is used in breast feeding women, to avoid contact exposure of the infant, application of adapalene to the chest should be avoided.
Effects on ability to drive and use machines: Based upon the pharmacodynamic profile and clinical experience, performance related to driving and using machines should not be affected.
Undesirable effects: Side effects include skin irritation (erythema, dryness, scaling) and stinging at the site of application which is reversible when treatment is reduced in frequency or discontinued.
Overdosage: Differin Cream is not to be taken orally and is for cutaneous use only. If the medication is applied excessively, no more rapid or better results will be obtained and marked redness, peeling or discomfort may occur.

The acute oral dose of Differin Cream required to produce toxic effects in mice is greater than 10 g/kg. Nevertheless, unless the amount accidentally ingested is small, an appropriate method of gastric emptying should be considered.

Pharmacological properties
Pharmacodynamic properties: Adapalene is a retinoid-like compound which in, in vivo and in vitro models of inflammation, has been demonstrated to possess anti-inflammatory properties. Adapalene is essentially stable to oxygen and light and is chemically non-reactive. Mechanically, adapalene binds like tretinoin to specific retinoic acid nuclear receptors but, unlike tretinoin not to cytosolic receptor binding proteins.

Adapalene applied cutaneously is comedolytic in the rhino mouse model and also has effects on the abnormal processes of epidermal keratinisation and differentiation, both of which are present in the pathogenesis of acne vulgaris. The mode of action of adapalene is suggested to be a normalisation of differentiation of follicular epithelial cells resulting in decreased microcomedone formation.

Adapalene is superior to reference retinoids in standard anti-inflammatory assays, both in vivo and in vitro. Mechanistically, it inhibits chemotactic and chemokinetic responses of human polymorphonuclear leucocytes and also the metabolism by lipoxidation of arachidonic acid to pro-inflammatory mediators. This profile suggests that the cell mediated inflammatory component of acne may be modified by adapalene. Studies in human patients provide clinical evidence that cutaneous adapalene is effective in reducing the inflammatory components of acne (papules and pustules).
Pharmacokinetic properties: Absorption of adapalene through human skin is low, in clinical trials measurable plasma adapalene levels were not found following chronic cutaneous application to large areas of acneic skin with an analytical sensitivity of 0.15 ng/ml.
After administration of [^{14}C]-adapalene in rats (IV, IP, oral and cutaneous), rabbits (IV, oral and cutaneous) and dogs (IV and oral), radioactivity was distributed in several tissues, the highest levels being found in liver, spleen, adrenals and ovaries. Metabolism in animals has been tentatively identified as being mainly by O-demethylation, hydroxylation and conjugation, and excretion is primarily by the biliary route.
Preclinical safety data: In animal studies, adapalene was well tolerated on cutaneous application for periods of up to six months in rabbits and for up to two years in mice. The major symptoms of toxicity found in all animal species by the oral route were related to an hypervitaminosis A syndrome, and included bone dissolution, elevated alkaline phosphatase and a slight anaemia. Large oral doses of adapalene produced no adverse neurological, cardiovascular or respiratory effects in animals. Adapalene is not mutagenic. Lifetime studies with adapalene have been completed in mice at cutaneous doses of 0.6, 2 and 6 mg/kg/day and in rats at oral doses of 0.15, 0.5 and 1.5 mg/kg/day. The only significant finding was a statistically significant increase of benign phaeochromocytomas of the adrenal medulla among male rats receiving adapalene at 1.5 mg/kg/day. These changes are unlikely to be of relevance to the cutaneous use of adapalene.

Pharmaceutical particulars
List of excipients: Carbomer 934P, PEG-20 methyl glucose sesquistearate, Glycerol, Natural squalane, Methyl parahydroxybenzoate, Propyl parahydroxybenzoate, Disodium edetate, Methyl glucose sesquis-

tearate, Phenoxyethanol, Cyclomethicone, Sodium hydroxide, Purified water.

Incompatibilities: None known.

Shelf life: The shelf life expiry date for this product shall not exceed two years from the date of its manufacture.

Special precautions for storage: Warning: do not allow to freeze.
Store at a temperature not exceeding 25°C.
Keep out of reach of children.

Nature and contents of container: Collapsible Aluminium tube coated internally with an epoxy-phenolic resin and fitted with a white Polypropylene screw cap. Pack size 30 g.

Instructions for use/handling: A thin film of the cream should be applied, avoiding eyes, lips and mucous membranes.

Marketing authorisation number PL 10590/0029

Date of first authorisation/renewal of authorisation
9 January 1998

Date of (partial) revision of text October 1997

Legal category POM

DIFFERIN* GEL ▼

Qualitative and quantitative composition Adapalene (INN, BAN, USAN) 0.1% w/w.

Pharmaceutical form Topical gel.

Clinical particulars

Therapeutic indications: Differin Gel is proposed for the cutaneous treatment of mild to moderate acne where comedones, papules and pustules predominate. Acne of the face, chest or back is appropriate for treatment.

Posology and method of administration: Differin Gel should be applied to the acne affected areas once a day before retiring and after washing. A thin film of gel should be applied, with the fingertips, avoiding the eyes and lips (see *Special warnings and special precautions for use*, below). Ensure that the affected areas are dry before application.

Since it is customary to alternate therapies in the treatment of acne, it is recommended that the physician assess the continued improvement of the patient after three months of treatment with Differin Gel.

With patients for whom it is necessary to reduce the frequency of application or to temporarily discontinue treatment, frequency of application may be restored or therapy resumed once it is judged that the patient can again tolerate the treatment. If patients use cosmetics, these should be non-comedogenic and non-astringent. The safety and effectiveness of Differin Gel have not been studied in neonates and young children. Differin Gel should not be used in patients with severe acne.

Contra-indications: Hypersensitivity to any ingredient of the product.

Special warnings and special precautions for use: If a reaction suggesting sensitivity or severe irritation occurs, use of the medication should be discontinued. If the degree of local irritation warrants, patients should be directed to use the medication less frequently, to discontinue use temporarily, or to discontinue use altogether. Differin Gel should not come into contact with the eyes, mouth, angles of the nose or mucous membranes.

If product enters the eye, wash immediately with warm water. The product should not be applied to either broken (cuts and abrasions) or eczematous skin, nor should it be used in patients with severe acne involving large areas of the body, especially in women of child bearing age who are not on effective contraception.

Interaction with other medicaments and other forms of interaction: There are no known interactions with other medications which might be used cutaneously and concurrently with Differin Gel; however, other retinoids or drugs with a similar mode of action should not be used concurrently with adapalene.

Adapalene is essentially stable to oxygen and light and is chemically non-reactive. Whilst extensive studies in animals and man have shown neither phototoxic nor photoallergic potential for adapalene, the safety of using adapalene during repeated exposure to sunlight or UV irradiation has not been established in either animals or man. Exposure to excessive sunlight or UV irradiation should be avoided.

Absorption of adapalene through human skin is low (see *Pharmacokinetic properties*) and therefore interaction with systemic medications is unlikely. There is no evidence that the efficacy of oral drugs such as contraceptives and antibiotics is influenced by the cutaneous use of Differin Gel.

Differin Gel has a potential for mild local irritation, and therefore it is possible that concomitant use of peeling agents, abrasive cleansers, strong drying agents, astringents or irritant products (aromatic and alcoholic agents) may produce additive irritant effects. However, cutaneous antiacne treatment e.g. erythromycin (up to 4%) or clindamycin phosphate (1% as the base) solutions or benzoyl peroxide water based gels up to 10% may be used in the morning when Differin Gel is used at night as there is no mutual degradation or cumulative irritation.

Pregnancy and lactation: No information on the effects of Adapalene in pregnant women is available and therefore this product should not be used during pregnancy, unless considered essential by the physician. Because of the risk of teratogenicity shown in animal studies and since there is no information on the use of adapalene in pregnant women, it should not be used in women of child bearing age unless they are using an effective means of contraception.

Adapalene produces teratogenic effects by the oral route in rats and rabbits. At cutaneous doses up to 200-fold the therapeutic dose, producing circulating plasma levels of adapalene at least 35 to 120 times higher than plasma levels demonstrated in therapeutic use, adapalene increased the incidence of additional ribs in rats and rabbits, without increasing the incidence of major malformations.

It is not known whether adapalene is secreted in animal or human milk. In animal studies, infant rats suckled by mother with circulating levels of adapalene at least 300 times those demonstrated in clinical use developed normally.

Its use in women breast feeding infants should be avoided but when it is used in breast feeding women, to avoid contact exposure of the infant, application of adapalene to the chest should be avoided.

Effects on ability to drive and use machines: Based upon the pharmacodynamic profile and clinical experience, performance related to driving and using machines should not be affected.

Undesirable effects: Side effects include skin irritation, stinging and a feeling of warmth at the site of application.

The major undesirable effect which may occur is irritation of the skin which is reversible when treatment is reduced in frequency or discontinued.

Overdose: Differin Gel is not to be taken orally and is for cutaneous use only. If the medication is applied excessively, no more rapid or better results will be obtained and marked redness, peeling or discomfort may occur.

The acute oral dose of Differin Gel required to produce toxic effects in mice and rats is greater than 10 ml/kg. Nevertheless, unless the amount accidentally ingested is small, an appropriate method of gastric emptying should be considered.

Pharmacological properties

Pharmacodynamic properties: Adapalene is a retinoid-like compound which in, in-vivo and in-vitro models of inflammation, has been demonstrated to possess anti-inflammatory properties. Adapalene is essentially stable to oxygen and light and is chemically non-reactive.

Mechanically, adapalene binds like tretinoin to specific retinoic acid nuclear receptors, but unlike tretinoin, not to cytosolic receptor binding proteins.

Adapalene applied cutaneously is comedolytic in the rhino mouse model and also has effects on the abnormal processes of epidermal keratinisation and differentiation, both of which are present in the pathogenesis of acne vulgaris. The mode of action of adapalene is suggested to be a normalisation of differentiation of follicular epithelial cells resulting in decreased microcomedone formation.

Adapalene is superior to reference retinoids in standard anti-inflammatory assays, both in-vivo and in-vitro. Mechanistically, it inhibits chemotactic and chemokinetic responses of human polymorphonuclear leucocytes and also the metabolism by lipoxidation of arachidonic acid to pro-inflammatory mediators. This profile suggests that the cell mediated inflammatory component of acne may be modified by adapalene.

Pharmacokinetic properties: Absorption of adapalene through human skin is low. In clinical trial, measurable plasma adapalene levels were not found following chronic cutaneous application to large areas of acneic skin with an analytical sensitivity of 0.15 ng/ml.

After administration of [^{14}C]-adapalene in rats (IV, IP, oral and cutaneous), rabbits (IV, oral and cutaneous) and dogs (IV and oral), radioactivity was distributed in several tissues, the highest levels being found in liver, spleen, adrenals and ovaries. Metabolism in animals has been tentatively identified as being mainly by O-demethylation, hydroxylation and conjugation, and excretion is primarily by the biliary route.

Preclinical safety data: In animal studies, adapalene was well tolerated on cutaneous application for periods of up to six months in rabbits and for up to two years in mice. The major symptoms of toxicity found in all animal species by the oral route were related to an hypervitaminosis A syndrome, and included bone dissolution, elevated alkaline phosphatase and a slight anaemia. Large oral doses of adapalene produced no adverse neurological, cardiovascular or respiratory effects in animals. Adapalene is not mutagenic. Lifetime studies with adapalene have been completed in mice at cutaneous doses of 0.6, 2 and 6 mg/kg/day and in rats at oral doses of 0.15, 0.5 and 1.5 mg/kg/day. The only significant finding was a statistically significant increase of benign phaeochromocytomas of the adrenal medulla among male rats receiving adapalene at 1.5 mg/kg/day. These changes are unlikely to be of relevance to the cutaneous use of adapalene.

Pharmaceutical particulars

List of excipients: Carbomer 940, Methyl Parahydroxybenzoate PhEur, Propylene glycol PhEur, Phenoxyethanol PhEur, Poloxamer 182 PhEur, Sodium Hydroxide PhEur, Disodium Edetate PhEur and Purified Water PhEur.

Incompatibilities: None known.

Shelf life: The shelf life expiry date shall not exceed two years from the date of its manufacture.

Special precautions for storage: Store at room temperature not exceeding 25°C. Warning: do not allow to freeze. Keep out of reach of children.

Nature and contents of container: White low density polypropylene tube with a white polypropylene screw cap. Pack size 30 g.

Instructions for use/handling: A thin film of the gel should be applied, avoiding eyes, lips and mucous membranes.

Marketing authorisation number 10590/0015.

Date of approval/revision of SPC August 1996.

Legal category POM.

ERYACNE* 2
ERYACNE* 4

Qualitative and quantitative composition
Eryacne 2: Erythromycin (PhEur) 2% w/w
Eryacne 4: Erythromycin (PhEur) 4% w/w
expressed as erythromycin base with a potency of 1,000 IU/mg.

Pharmaceutical form Alcohol-based gel for topical (cutaneous) use.

Clinical particulars

Therapeutic indications: Eryacne is intended for the cutaneous treatment of acne vulgaris.

Posology and method of administration: Eryacne 4 (containing 4% w/w erythromycin) is recommended for the first four weeks of treatment. If the condition has improved after four weeks, Eryacne 2 (containing 2% w/w erythromycin) may be substituted.

A thin film of Eryacne should be applied to the affected areas twice daily, morning and evening. These areas should be washed and dried before the product is used.

As a rule, treatment is continued for eight weeks, although this period may be extended to obtain a satisfactory response.

Contra-indications: Eryacne is contra-indicated in persons known to be sensitive to any of the ingredients.

Special warnings and precautions for use: Eryacne is for external use only and should be kept away from the eyes, nose, mouth and other mucous membranes. If accidental contact does occur, the area should be washed with lukewarm water.

If a reaction suggesting sensitivity or a severe reaction occurs, use of the product should be discontinued. Depending upon the degree of irritation, the patient should be advised to use the product less frequently, to discontinue its use temporarily or to discontinue its use altogether.

Cross-resistance could occur with other antibiotics of the macrolide group.

Interactions with other medicaments and other forms of interaction: Concurrent topical acne therapy should be used with caution because a cumulative irritant effect could occur.

Concurrent use of exfoliants or medicated soaps or cosmetics containing alcohol could also cause a cumulative irritant or drying effect in patients using Eryacne.

Erythromycin and clindamycin topical preparations should not be used concurrently.

Pregnancy and Lactation: There is no evidence of risk from using erythromycin in human pregnancy. It has been in wide use for many years without apparent ill consequence. Animal reproduction studies have shown no risk.

If Eryacne is used during lactation, it should not be

applied on the chest to avoid accidental ingestion by the infant.

Effects on ability to drive and use machines: Performance related to driving and using machines should not be affected by use of Eryacne.

Undesirable effects: Adverse reactions reported to date with topical erythromycin therapy include dryness, irritation, pruritis, erythema, desquamation, oiliness and a burning sensation.

Most of these reactions appear to be caused by alcohol or other excipients rather than by erythromycin and are reversible when the frequency of application is reduced or treatment is discontinued.

Overdose: Eryacne is for cutaneous use only. If the product is applied excessively, no more rapid or better results will be obtained, and marked redness, peeling or discomfort could occur. If these effects should occur, the frequency of application could be reduced or treatment discontinued and appropriate symptomatic therapy instituted.

The acute oral toxicity in mice and rats is greater than 10 mL.kg^{-1}. Unless the amount accidentally ingested is small, an appropriate method of gastric emptying should be considered provided that this is carried out soon after ingestion. One unopened 30 g tube of Eryacne contains about 30 mL of alcohol.

Pharmacological properties

Pharmacodynamic properties: Erythromycin is a macrolide antibiotic active in vivo and in vitro against most aerobic and anaerobic gram-positive bacteria as well as some gram-negative bacilli.

Erythromycin is usually bacteriostatic in action, but may be bacteriocidal in high concentrations or against highly susceptible organisms.

Erythromycin appears to inhibit protein synthesis in susceptible organisms by reversible binding to 50S ribosomal subunits. Following application to the skin, the drug inhibits the growth of susceptible organisms (principally Propionibacterium acnes) on the surface of the skin and reduces the concentration of free fatty acids in the sebum.

The reduction of free fatty acids in sebum may be an indirect result of the inhibition of lipase-producing organisms that convert triglycerides into free fatty acids. It may also be a direct result of interference with lipase production in these organisms.

Free fatty acids are comedogenic and are believed to be a possible cause of the inflammatory lesions of acne, e.g. papules, pustules, nodules and cysts. However, other mechanisms may be involved in the clinical improvement of acne as a direct result of the anti-inflammatory action of erythromycin applied topically to the skin.

Pharmacokinetic properties: Erythromycin does not appear to be absorbed systemically following application of Eryacne to the skin, although it is not known whether it is absorbed from denuded or broken skin, wounds or mucous membranes.

Preclinical safety data: There is no evidence from toxicological studies that cutaneous application of the proposed clinical dose of erythromycin would be associated with the risk of significant adverse reactions in humans. Published data and information on the toxicity of erythromycin applied to the skin support this conclusion.

Pharmaceutical particulars

List of excipients: Butylhydroxytoluene, hydroxypropylcellulose and alcohol.

Incompatibilities: None known.

Shelf life: Twenty-four (24) months.

Special precautions for storage: Store below 25°C, and out of the sight and the reach of children.

Nature and contents of container: Eryacne is presented in collapsible aluminium tubes. Each tube has an internal coating of an epoxy-phenolic resin. It is closed with a polypropylene screw cap. This cap is used to pierce the tube before its first use. Each tube of Eryacne contains 30 g of product.

Instruction for use/handling: On first use, the screw cap is removed and is used to pierce the neck of the tube. Unscrew the cap, remove the plastic collar and screw the cap back onto the tube.

Marketing authorisation number
Eryacne 2: PL 10590/0021
Eryacne 4: PL 10590/0022

Date of first authorisation/renewal of authorisation 29 November 1996

Date of (partial) revision of the text 31 July 1995

Legal category POM

IONAX* SCRUB

Qualitative and quantitative composition
Polyoxyethylene (4) Lauryl Ether 4.18% w/w
Polyoxyethylene (23) Lauryl Ether 15.42% w/w
Benzalkonium Chloride Solution PhEur 0.53% w/w
Ethyl Alcohol (Denatured) 11.77% w/w
Polyethylene Granules 21.87% w/w

Pharmaceutical form Cream.

Clinical particulars

Therapeutic indications: An abradant cleanser for the control and hygiene of acne.

To cleanse the skin prior to acne or oily skin treatment.

For topical application to the skin.

Posology and method of administration:

Dosage: Adults and children: Use once or twice daily, or as directed by a physician.

Apply to wet face. Massage on the skin for one or two minutes, then rinse thoroughly.

Contra-indications: Hypersensitivity to any of the constituents of the product.

Special warnings and special precautions for use: Avoid contact with the eyes.

Upon accidental contact, flush with water and avoid rubbing.

If the skin becomes too dry or too reddened, discontinue use temporarily.

For external use only.

Interaction with other medicaments and other forms of interaction: None known.

Pregnancy and lactation: Not applicable.

Effects on ability to drive and use machines: Not applicable.

Undesirable effects: None known.

Overdose: None known.

Pharmacological properties

Pharmacodynamic properties: Not applicable.

Pharmacokinetic properties: Not applicable.

Preclinical safety data: Not relevant as the product has been in use for many years without apparent ill consequence.

Pharmaceutical particulars

List of excipients: Propylene glycol PhEur, Potassium sorbate PhEur, Silica 200 PhEur, Lauramine oxide, Colouring–D & C Yellow 10, Perfume–Givandan–W 33261, Purified water PhEur.

Incompatibilities: None

Shelf life: 36 months.

Special precautions for storage: None.

Nature and contents of container: Plastic tube fitted with a screw cap and packed into a cardboard carton. Package sizes: 60 g

Instructions for use/handling: Not relevant.

Marketing authorisation number PL 10590/0008

Date of first authorisation/renewal of authorisation 24 February 1993/24 March 1998

Date of (partial) revision of text October 1997 (UK Version 2)

Legal category P

IONIL T* SHAMPOO

Qualitative and quantitative composition Coal tar solution 4.25% w/w, salicylic acid 2.0% w/w, benzalkonium chloride 0.2% w/w, polyoxyethylene (4) lauryl ether 7.2% w/w and polyoxyethylene (23) lauryl ether 14.4% w/w.

Pharmaceutical form Hydro-alcoholic solution for topical (cutaneous) application as a shampoo.

Clinical particulars

Therapeutic indications: Psoriasis and seborrhoeic dermatitis of the scalp.

Posology and method of administration:

Adults, elderly and children: Massage Ionil T Shampoo into wet hair and rinse out (not too much lather will be produced on first application). Apply again, working into a lather, and allow to remain on the hair for five minutes before rinsing.

Repeat the treatment once or twice a week, or as directed by the doctor or pharmacist.

Contra-indications: None.

Special warnings and special precautions for use: Avoid contact with the eyes. Upon accidental contact, flush with clean, warm water.

Interaction with other medicaments and other forms of interaction: None known.

Pregnancy and lactation: No special precautions required.

Effects on ability to drive and use machines: None.

Undesirable effects: None known.

Overdose: Not applicable.

Pharmacological properties

Pharmacodynamic properties: The active constituents of Ionil T Shampoo provide the product with keratolytic, antiseptic and anti-pruritic properties to effect symptomatic relief of psoriasis and seborrhoeic dermatitis of the scalp.

In animal models, coal tar has been demonstrated to suppress epidermal cell DNA synthesis.

Pharmacokinetic properties: Not applicable.

Preclinical safety data: No specific information is presented given the widespread use of coal tar preparations on humans over many years.

Pharmaceutical particulars

List of excipients: Ethyl alcohol, tetrasodium edetate, citric acid and purified water.

Incompatibilities: None known.

Shelf life: Thirty six (36) months.

Special precautions for storage: Ionil T Shampoo should be stored below 25°C and away from direct heat. The product should be stored away from internal preparations and food.

As with all medicines, Ionil T Shampoo should be kept out of the sight and reach of children.

Nature and contents of container: White polypropylene flat bottle with a white polypropylene snap or screw cap as the closure; pack sizes 50 ml (physicians sample), 200 ml.

Instruction for use/handling: No special instructions.

Marketing authorisation number 10590/0003.

Date of approval/revision of SPC 7 March 1997.

Legal category P.

METROGEL*

Qualitative and quantitative composition Metronidazole BP 0.75%.

Pharmaceutical form Aqueous gel for cutaneous use.

Clinical particulars

Therapeutic indications: For the treatment of acute inflammatory exacerbation of rosacea.

For the deodorisation of the smell associated with malodorous fungating tumours.

Posology and method of administration:

For the treatment of rosacea:

Adults and elderly: Apply to the affected skin of the face in a thin film twice daily for a period of eight to nine weeks. Thereafter, further applications may be necessary depending upon the severity of the condition.

Children: Not recommended.

For the deodorisation of malodorous fungating tumours:

Adults and Elderly: Clean the wound thoroughly. Apply the gel over the complete area and cover with a non-adherent dressing. Use once or twice daily as necessary.

Children: Not recommended.

Contra-indications: In patients known to be hypersensitive to metronidazole or bronopol.

Special warnings and precautions for use: Avoid contact with the eyes. If contact occurs, the gel should be washed out carefully with water.

Interactions with other medicaments and other forms of interaction: The following statement takes into account the possibility that metronidazole may be absorbed after topical application. However, there is evidence to suggest that the systemic absorption of metronidazole following topical administration of Metrogel is slight. A disulfiram-like reaction has been reported in a small number of patients taking oral metronidazole and alcohol concomitantly.

Pregnancy and lactation: The safety of metronidazole in pregnancy and lactation had not been adequately established. The gel should therefore not be used in these circumstances unless the physician considers it essential. Medication should be stopped if pregnancy occurs.

Effects on ability to drive and use machines: None.

Undesirable effects: Dryness of the skin may be experienced after application.

Overdose: Overdose is extremely unlikely. If necessary, medication should be removed by washing with warm water.

Pharmacological properties

Pharmacodynamic properties: The etiology of rosacea is unknown although a variety of hypotheses have been reported.

Pharmacokinetic properties: The systemic concentration of Metronidazole following the topical administration of 1 g of a 0.75% Metronidazole gel to 10 patients with rosacea ranged from 25 ng/ml (limit of detection), to 66 mg/ml with a mean Cmax of 40.6 ng/ml.

The corresponding mean Cmax following the oral

administration of a solution containing 30 mg of metronidazole was 850 ng/ml (equivalent to 212 ng/ml if dose corrected. The mean Tmax for the topical formulation was 6.0 hours compared to 0.97 hours for the oral solution.

Preclinical safety data: Metronidazole is a well established pharmaceutical active ingredient and to the subject of pharmacopoeial monograph in both the BP and PhEur.

Pharmaceutical particulars
List of excipients: Bronopol BP, Hydroxybenzoic acid esters HSE, Hydroxyethylcellulose HSE, Propylene glycol PhEur, Phosphoric acid PhEur, Purified water PhEur.

Incompatibilities: None known.

Shelf life: 2 years.

Special precautions for storage: Store between 15°C and 25°C in a dry place.

Nature and contents of container:
Tube: Internally lacquered, membrane sealed aluminium.
Cap: low density polyethylene
Pack sizes available: 25 g and 40 g.

Instruction for use/handling: There are no special instructions for use/handling.

Marketing authorisation number PL 10590/0035

Date of first authorisation/renewal of authorisation 27 February 1998

Date of (partial) revision of the text March 1997

Legal category POM

MISTAMINE* ▼

Qualitative and quantitative composition Mizolastine (INN) 10 mg per tablet.

Pharmaceutical form Oblong, white film-coated modified release tablets with MZI10 engraved on one side.

Clinical particulars
Therapeutic indications: Mizolastine is a long-acting H1-antihistamine indicated for the symptomatic relief of seasonal allergic rhinoconjunctivitis (hay fever), perennial allergic rhinoconjunctivitis and urticaria.

Posology and method of administration:
Adults, including the elderly, and children 12 years of age and over: The recommended daily dose is one 10 mg tablet.

Contra-Indications: Hypersensitivity to mizolastine.

Concomitant administration of mizolastine with macrolide antibiotics or systemic imidazole antifungals.

Significantly impaired hepatic function.

Clinically significant cardiac disease or a history of symptomatic arrhythmias.

Patients with known or suspected QT prolongation or with electrolyte imbalance, in particular hypokalaemia.

Clinically significant bradycardia.

Drugs known to prolong the QT interval, such as Class I and III anti-arrhythmics.

Special warnings and precautions for use: Mizolastine has a weak potential to prolong the QT interval in a few individuals. The degree of prolongation is modest and has not been associated with cardiac arrhythmias.

The elderly may be particularly susceptible to the sedative effects of mizolastine and the potential effects of the drug on cardiac repolarisation.

Interactions with other medicaments and other forms of interaction: Although the bioavailability of mizolastine is high and the drug is principally metabolised by glucuronidation, systemically administered ketoconazole and erythromycin moderately increase the plasma concentration of mizolastine and their concurrent use is contraindicated. Concurrent use of other potent inhibitors or substrates of hepatic oxidation (cytochrome P450 3A4) with mizolastine should be approached with caution. These would include cimetidine, cyclosporin, and nifedipine.

Alcohol: In studies with mizolastine, no potentiation of the sedation and the alteration in performance caused by alcohol has been observed.

Pregnancy and lactation: The safety of mizolastine for use in human pregnancy has not been established. The evaluation of experimental animal studies does not indicate direct or indirect harmful effects with respect to the development of the embryo or foetus, the course of gestation and peri- and post-natal development. However, as with all drugs, mizolastine should be avoided in pregnancy, particularly during the first trimester.

In the absence of information on the levels of mizolastine which may appear in human breast milk after administration, mizolastine is not recommended during lactation.

Effects on ability to drive and use machines: Most patients taking mizolastine may drive or perform tasks requiring concentration. However, in order to identify sensitive people who have unusual reactions to drugs, it is advisable to check the individual response before driving or performing complicated tasks.

Undesirable effects: The following adverse reactions were reported in decreasing order of frequency in mizolastine-treated patients: drowsiness and asthenia, often transient in nature, and increased appetite associated with weight gain in some individuals. Dry mouth, diarrhoea, dyspepsia or headache may occur. Isolated cases of hypotension, anxiety and depression, low neutrophil count and raised liver enzymes have been reported rarely. There were reports of bronchospasm and aggravation of asthma but in view of the high frequency of asthma in the patient population being treated, a causal relationship remains uncertain.

Treatment with certain antihistamines has been associated with QT interval prolongation increasing the risk of serious cardiac arrhythmias in susceptible subjects.

Minor changes in blood sugar and electrolytes have been observed rarely. The clinical significance of these changes in otherwise healthy individuals remains unclear. Patients at risk (diabetics, those susceptible to electrolyte imbalance and cardiac arrhythmias) should be monitored periodically.

Overdose: In cases of overdosage, general symptomatic surveillance with cardiac monitoring including QT interval and cardiac rhythm for at least 24 hours is recommended, along with standard measures to remove any unabsorbed drug.

Studies in patients with renal insufficiency suggest that haemodialysis does not increase clearance of the drug.

Pharmacological properties
Pharmacodynamic properties: ATC Code: R06AX.

Mizolastine possesses antihistamine and antiallergic properties due to a specific and selective antagonism of peripheral histamine H1 receptors. It has also been shown to inhibit histamine release from mast cells (at 0.3 mg/kg orally) and the migration of neutrophils (at 3 mg/kg orally) in animal models of allergic reactions.

In man, histamine-induced wheal and flare studies have shown that mizolastine 10 mg is a rapid, potent (80 % inhibition after 4 hrs) and sustained (24hr) antihistamine. No tachyphylaxis occurred after long-term administration.

In both preclinical and clinical studies, no anticholinergic effect has been demonstrated.

Pharmacokinetic properties: Following oral administration mizolastine is rapidly absorbed. Peak plasma concentration is reached at a median time of 1.5 hours.

Bioavailability is 65% and linear kinetics have been demonstrated.
The mean elimination half-life is 13.0 hours with plasma protein binding of 98.4%.

In hepatic insufficiency the absorption of mizolastine is slower and the distribution phase longer, with a resulting moderate increase in AUC of 50%.

The principal metabolic pathway is glucuronidation of the parent compound. The cytochrome P450 3A4 enzyme system is involved in one of the additional metabolic pathways with formation of the hydroxylated metabolites of mizolastine. None of the identified metabolites contribute to the pharmacological activity of mizolastine.

An increase in mizolastine plasma levels, observed with systemic ketoconazole and erythromycin, led to concentrations equivalent to those obtained after a 15 to 20 mg dose of mizolastine alone.

In studies carried out in healthy volunteers, no clinically significant interaction has been recorded with food, warfarin, digoxin, theophylline, lorazepam, or diltiazem.

Preclinical safety data: Pharmacological studies in several species have shown an effect on cardiac repolarisation at doses in excess of 10-20 times the therapeutic dose. In conscious dogs, mizolastine has shown pharmacological interactions with ketoconazole at the electrocardiographic level at 70 times the therapeutic dose.

Pharmaceutical particulars
List of excipients:
Core: Hydrogenated castor oil, lactose monohydrate, microcrystalline cellulose, tartaric acid, povidone, anhydrous colloidal silica, magnesium stearate.
Film-coating: Hypromellose, titanium dioxide, propylene glycol.

Incompatibilities: None stated

Shelf life: 2 years in blisters.
3 years in polypropylene securitainers.

Special precautions for storage: Store in a dry place below 25°C.

Tablets should not be taken if they become discoloured.

Nature and contents of container: Aluminium/PVC blisters
Polypropylene tubes with polyethylene caps (securitainers)
Packs of 30 tablets

Instruction for use/handling: None stated.

Marketing authorisation number PL 10590/0031

Date of first authorisation/renewal of authorisation 2nd September 1997

Date of (partial) revision of the text 12th February 1998

Legal category POM

NUTRAPLUS* CREAM

Qualitative and quantitative composition Urea PhEur 10% w/w.

Pharmaceutical form Smooth white, almost odourless cream (water in oil emulsion).

Clinical particulars
Therapeutic indications: An emollient, moisturising and protective cream for the treatment of dry or damaged skin.

Posology and method of administration:
Adults, elderly and children: Apply evenly to the dry skin areas two to three times daily, or as directed by the physician or pharmacist.

Contra-indications: None.

Special warnings and special precautions for use: Avoid contact with the eyes. If irritation occurs, discontinue use temporarily.

Interaction with other medicaments and other forms of interaction: None known.

Pregnancy and lactation: No known effects. Use at the discretion of the physician or pharmacist.

Effects on ability to drive and use machines: Not applicable.

Undesirable effects: None known.

Overdose: Not applicable.

Pharmacological properties
Pharmacodynamic properties: Urea is a recognised hydrating agent that has been widely used topically to treat dry or damaged skin.

Pharmacokinetic properties: Not applicable. Nutraplus is a topical (cutaneous) preparation.

Preclinical safety data: No specific information is presented given the widespread use of topically applied urea on humans over many years.

Pharmaceutical particulars
List of excipients: Glycerol monostearate, octyl palmitate, myristyl lactate, mineral oil, promulgen D, propylene glycol, propyl parahydroxybenzoate, methyl parahydroxybenzoate, purified water.

Incompatibilities: None known.

Shelf life: Thirty six months.

Special precautions for storage: Nutraplus Cream should be stored below 25°C and away from direct heat. As with all medicines, Nutraplus Cream should be stored out of the sight and reach of children.

Nature and contents of container: White, polyethylene tube with a white polypropylene screw cap as the closure. Pack size 100 g.

Instruction for use/handling: No special instructions.

Marketing authorisation number 10590/0002.

Date of approval/revision of SPC 1 March 1996.

Legal category P.

PSORIGEL*

Qualitative and quantitative composition Psorigel contains Coal Tar Solution HSE 7.5% as the active ingredient.

Pharmaceutical form Hydro-alcoholic gel for topical (cutaneous) application.

Clinical particulars
Therapeutic indications: For the relief and treatment of inflammatory manifestations of tar responsive dermatoses. Among these are eczema, psoriasis, inflammation, erythema, scaling, pruritis and induration that accompany various forms of dermatitis.

Psorigel also helps relieve the itching that accompanies psoriasis and eczema, and helps control flaking and scaling.

For topical use on the affected areas of the skin and scalp.

Posology and method of administration: Adults, elderly and children: Rub Psorigel onto the affected areas once or twice daily. The gel may be applied more frequently if necessary. Rub the gel in well, allow it to dry and remove any excess by patting with a paper tissue.

Contra-indications: There are no contra-indications to the topical (cutaneous) use of Psorigel.

Special warnings and special precautions for use: Avoid contact with the eyes. Upon accidental contact, flush with water.

After using Psorigel, avoid exposure to direct sunlight unless specifically directed by the physician.

The product contains 33% alcohol. Do not use Psorigel on highly inflamed or on broken skin. If undue irritation occurs in use reduce the frequency of use, or discontinue use until the irritation subsides.

The staining potential of the product is minimal but if it does occur, standard laundry procedures will remove most stains.

Interaction with other medicaments and other forms of interaction: None known.

Pregnancy and lactation: No known effects. Coal tar preparations have been in wide use for many years without apparent deleterious effects. Use at the discretion of the physician or pharmacist.

Effects on ability to drive and to use machines: None known.

Undesirable effects: None known.

Overdose: Not pertinent to this topically applied product.

Pharmacological properties

Pharmacodynamic properties: The active ingredient of Psorigel is coal tar, which possesses both antipruritic and keratolytic properties. In animal models, coal tar has been demonstrated to suppress epidermal cell DNA synthesis.

Pharmacokinetic particulars: Not applicable. Psorigel is a topical (cutaneous) preparation.

Preclinical safety data: No specific information is presented given the widespread use of coal tar preparations on humans for many years.

Pharmaceutical particulars

List of excipients: Carbomer 940, propylene glycol, ethyl alcohol (95.6%), laureth 4, perfume M72-512, diisopropanolamine, purified water.

Incompatibilities: None known.

Shelf life: 36 months.

Special precautions for storage: Psorigel should be stored below 25°C and away from direct heat. As with all medicines, Psorigel should be kept out of the sight and reach of children.

Nature and contents of container: Brown HDPE tube with a polypropylene cap. Tubes of 100 g are available.

Instructions for use/handling: No special instructions.

Marketing authorisation number 10590/0001

Date of approval/revision of SPC 10 July 1997

Legal category P.

ROZEX* CREAM

Qualitative and quantitative composition Metronidazole PhEur 0.75% w/w.

Pharmaceutical form Cream.

Clinical particulars

Therapeutic indications: Indicated in the treatment of inflammatory papules, pustules and erythema of rosacea.

Posology and method of administration: For topical administration only.

The average period of treatment is three to four months. If a clear benefit has been demonstrated, continued therapy for a further three to four months period may be considered by the prescribing physician depending upon the severity of the condition. In clinical studies topical metronidazole therapy has been continued for up to 2 years. In the absence of a clear clinical improvement, therapy should be stopped.

Adults: A pea-sized amount of cream is applied to the affected areas of skin, twice daily, morning and evening. Areas to be treated should be washed with a mild cleanser before application.

Patients may use non-comedogenic and non-astringent cosmetics after application of Rozex cream.

Elderly: The dosage recommended in the elderly is the same as that recommended in adults.

Children: Not recommended. Safety and efficacy have not been established.

Contra-indications: Contraindicated in individuals with a history of hypersensitivity to Metronidazole, or other ingredients of the formulation.

Special warnings and precautions for use: Contact with eyes and mucous membranes should be avoided.

If a reaction suggesting local irritation occurs patients should be directed to use the medication less frequently, discontinue use temporarily and to seek medical advice if necessary.

Metronidazole is a nitroimidazole and should be used with caution in patients with evidence of, or history of, blood dyscrasia.

Unnecessary and prolonged use of this medication should be avoided.

Exposure of treated sites to ultraviolet or strong sunlight should be avoided during use of metronidazole.

Interactions with other medicaments and other forms of interaction: Interaction with systemic medication is unlikely because absorption of metronidazole following cutaneous application of Rozex cream is low.

Ingestion of alcohol during oral treatment with metronidazole may cause potentiation of the effects of the latter on the central nervous system and may induce a disulfiram-like reaction.

Drug interactions are less likely with topical administration but should be kept in mind when Rozex cream is prescribed for patients receiving anticoagulant treatment. Oral Metronidazole has been reported to potentiate the anti-coagulant effect of dicoumarin and warfarin, resulting in a prolongation of prothrombin time.

Pregnancy and lactation: There is no experience to date with the use of Rozex cream in pregnancy. Metronidazole crosses the placental barrier and rapidly enters the foetal circulation. There is inadequate evidence of the safety of Metronidazole in human pregnancy. In animals, Metronidazole was not teratogenic or embryotoxic unless administered at extremely high doses. Rozex cream should only be used in pregnancy when there is no safer alternative.

After oral administration, Metronidazole is excreted in breast milk in concentrations similar to those found in the plasma. Even though Metronidazole blood levels from topical administration are significantly lower than those achieved after oral administration, in nursing mothers, a decision should be made to discontinue nursing or to discontinue the drug, taking into account the importance of the drug to the mother.

Effects on ability to drive and use machines: Not applicable.

Undesirable effects: Because of the minimal absorption of metronidazole and consequently its insignificant plasma concentration after topical administration, the adverse experiences reported with the oral form of the drug have not been reported with Rozex cream. Adverse reactions reported with Rozex cream have been only local and mild, and include skin discomfort (burning and stinging), erythema, pruritis, and skin irritation. Rarely, worsening of rosacea has occurred. All individual events occurred in less than 3% of patients.

Overdose: There is no human experience with overdosage of Rozex cream. The acute oral toxicity of a gel formulation was determined to be greater than 5 g/kg (the highest dose given) in albino rats. No toxic effects were observed at this dose. This dose is equivalent to the intake of 12 30 g tubes of Rozex cream for an adult weighing 72 kg, and 2 tubes for a child weighing 12 kg.

Pharmacological properties

Pharmacodynamic properties: Metronidazole is an antiprotozoal and antibacterial agent which is active against a wide range of pathogenic micro-organisms. The mechanisms of action of metronidazole in rosacea are unknown but available evidence suggests that the effects may be antibacterial and/or anti-inflammatory.

Pharmacokinetic properties: Metronidazole is rapidly and nearly totally absorbed after oral administration. The drug is not significantly bound to serum proteins and distributes well to all body compartments with the lowest concentration found in the fat. Metronidazole is excreted primarily in the urine as parent drug, oxidative metabolites and conjugates.

Bioavailability studies with a topical 1 g application of Rozex cream to the face of normal subjects resulted in mean maximum serum concentrations of 32.9 ng/ml (range 14.8 to 54.4 ng/ml) which is approximately 100 times less than those attained after a single oral dose of 250 mg (mean Cmax=7248 ng/ml; range 4270–13970 ng/ml). The peak concentration occurred between 0.25–4 hours after oral dosing, and 6 to 24 hours after cutaneous application of Rozex cream. Following topical application of Rozex cream, serum concentrations of the major metabolite (the hydroxy metabolite 2-hydroxymethylmetronidazole) were below the quantifiable limit of the assay (<9.6 ng/ml) at most of the time points, ranging to a maximum of 17.5 ng/ml peak concentration between 8 and 24 hours after application. In comparison, the peak concentration following a 250 mg oral dose ranged from 626 to 1788 ng/ml between 4 and 12 hours after dosing.

The extent of exposure (Area under the curve, AUC) from a 1 g application of metronidazole administered topically was 1.36% of the AUC of a single oral 250 mg metronidazole dose (mean+912.7 ng.hr/ml and approximately 67207 ng.hr/ml respectively).

Preclinical safety data: No evidence for a primary dermal irritation was observed in rabbits following a single 24-hour cutaneous application of Rozex cream to abraded and non-abraded skin, under occlusion.

Metronidazole has shown mutagenic activity in several *in vitro* bacterial assay systems. In addition, a dose-response increase in the frequency of micronuclei was observed in mice after intraperitoneal injection and an increase in chromosome aberrations have been reported in patients with Crohn's disease who were treated with 200 to 1200 mg/day of oral metronidazole for 1 to 24 months. However the preponderance of evidence from these studies suggests that although metronidazole has a potential for producing mutations, this should not occur in well oxygenated mammalian cells, i.e., under normal aerobic conditions.

The carcinogenicity of metronidazole by the oral route of administration has been evaluated in rats, mice and hamsters. These studies showed that oral metronidazole caused an increased incidence of pulmonary tumours in mice and possibly other tumours, including liver tumours, in the rat. Conversely, two lifetime studies in hamsters produced negative results. Moreover, one study showed a significant enhancement of UV-induced skin tumours in hairless mice treated with metronidazole intraperitoneally (15 μg per g body weight and per day for 28 weeks).

Although the significance of these results to the cutaneous use of metronidazole for the treatment of rosacea is unclear, patients should be advised to avoid or minimise exposure to metronidazole cream-treated sites to sun. After several decades of systemic use no evidence has been published to suggest that metronidazole is associated with a carcinogenic potential in humans.

Pharmaceutical particulars

List of excipients: Emulsifying wax, benzyl alcohol, isopropyl palmitate, glycerol, sorbitol 70% (non-crystallising), lactic acid and/or sodium hydroxide, purified water.

Incompatibilities: None known.

Shelf life: Rozex cream has a shelf life when unopened of 24 months.

Special precautions for storage: Store at a temperature not exceeding 25°C. Do not refrigerate.

Nature and content of container: Aluminium tubes with epoxy phenolic lining, fitted with white polypropylene screw caps; pack sizes: 30 g

Instruction for use/handling: Replace cap tightly after use.

Marketing authorisation number PL 10590/0028

Date of first authorisation/renewal of authorisation 18 June 1997

Date of (partial) revision of text February 1997

Legal category POM

ROZEX* GEL

Qualitative and quantitative composition Metronidazole PhEur 0.75% w/w.

Pharmaceutical form Gel.

Clinical particulars

Therapeutic indications: Indicated in the treatment of inflammatory papules, pustules and erythema of rosacea.

Posology and method of administration: For topical administration only.

Adults: Apply and rub in a film of Gel twice daily, morning and evening, to entire affected area after washing.

Elderly: The dosage recommended in the elderly is the same as that recommended in adults.

Children: Not recommended.

Contra-indications: Contra-indicated in individuals with a history of hypersensitivity to metronidazole, parabens or other ingredients of the formulation.

Special warnings and special precautions for use: Rozex Gel has been reported to cause lacrimation of the eyes, therefore, contact with the eyes should be avoided. If a reaction suggesting local irritation occurs patients should be directed to use the medication less frequently, discontinue use temporarily or discontinue use until further instructions. Metronidazole is a nitroimidazole and should be used with care in patients with evidence of, or history of, blood dyscrasia. Exposure of treated sites to ultraviolet or strong sunlight should be avoided during use of metronidazole.

Interaction with other medicaments and other forms of interaction: Drug interactions are less likely with topical administration but should be kept in mind when Rozex Gel is prescribed for patients receiving anticoagulant treatment. Oral Metronidazole has been reported to potentiate the anti-coagulant effect of dicoumarin and warfarin, resulting in a prolongation of prothrombin time.

Pregnancy and lactation: There is no experience to date with the use of Rozex Gel in pregnancy. Metronidazole crosses the placental barrier and rapidly enters the foetal circulation. There is inadequate evidence of the safety of Metronidazole in human pregnancy. In animals, Metronidazole was not teratogenic or embryotoxic unless administered at extremely high doses. Rozex Gel should only be used in pregnancy when there is no safer alternative.

After oral administration, Metronidazole is excreted in breast milk in concentrations similar to those found in the plasma, Metronidazole blood levels from topical administration are significantly lower than those achieved after oral administration. A decision should be made to discontinue nursing or to discontinue the drug, taking into account the importance of the drug to the mother.

Effects on ability to drive and use machines: Not applicable.

Undesirable effects: Because of the minimal absorption of metronidazole and consequently its insignificant plasma concentration after topical administration, the adverse experiences reported with the oral form of the drug have not been reported with Rozex Gel. Adverse reactions reported with Rozex Gel include watery (tearing) eyes if the gel is applied too closely to this area, transient redness and mild dryness, burning, and skin irritation.

Overdosage: There is no human experience with overdosage of Rozex Gel. The acute oral toxicity of Rozex Gel was determined to be greater than 5 g/kg (the highest dose given) in albino rats.

Pharmacological properties

Pharmacodynamic properties: Metronidazole is an antiprotozoal and antibacterial agent which is active against a wide range of pathogenic micro-organisms. The mechanisms of action of metronidazole in rosacea are unknown but available evidence suggests that the effects may be antibacterial and/or anti-inflammatory.

Pharmacokinetic properties: Metronidazole is rapidly and nearly totally absorbed after oral administration. The drug is not significantly bound to serum proteins and distributes well to all body compartments with the lowest concentration found in the fat. Metronidazole is excreted primarily in the urine as parent drug, oxidative metabolites and conjugates.

Bioavailability studies with Rozex Gel in rosacea patients treated with 7.5 mg metronidazole applied topically to the face resulted in maximum serum concentrations of 66 ng/ml which is approximately 100 times less than those attained after a single oral dose of 250 mg. In most patients at most time points after Rozex Gel application, serum concentrations of metronidazole were below the detectable limits of the assay (25 ng/ml).

Preclinical safety data: The toxicity studies conducted with the Metronidazole 0.75% Topical Gel formulation demonstrate that the product is non-toxic in rats after acute oral administration of 5 g/kg and produced no ocular irritation in rabbit eyes. The formulation produced no observable effects in rabbits after dermal application of 13 mg/kg for 90 days. No compound-related dermal or systemic effects were observed in a 13-week cutaneous route toxicity study, in which Rozex gel containing Metronidazole 0.75% w/w was applied daily to rabbits at doses ranging between 0.13 and 13 mg/kg. Metronidazole has shown evidence of carcinogenic activity in a number of studies involving chronic, oral administration in mice and rats but not in studies involving hamsters.

One study showed a significant enhancement of UV induced skin tumours in hairless mice treated with Metronidazole intraperitoneally (15 µg per g body weight and per day for 28 weeks). Although the significance of these studies to man is not clear, patients should be advised to avoid or minimise exposure of metronidazole treated sites to sun. Metronidazole has shown mutagenic activity in several in vitro bacterial assay systems. In addition, a dose-response increase in the frequency of micronuclei was observed in mice after intraperitoneal injection and an increase in chromosome aberrations have been reported in patients with Crohn's disease who were treated with 200 to 1200 mg/day of metronidazole for 1 to 24 months. However, no excess chromosomal aberrations in circulating human lymphocytes have been observed in patients treated for 8 months.

Pharmaceutical particulars

List of excipients: Carbomer (Carbopol 940) BP, Disodium Edetate PhEur, Methyl Hydroxybenzoate PhEur, Propyl Hydroxybenzoate PhEur, Propylene Glycol PhEur, Sodium Hydroxide PhEur, Purified Water PhEur.

Incompatibilities: None known.

Shelf life: Rozex Gel has a shelf life when unopened of 36 months.

Special precautions for storage: Store at a temperature not exceeding 25°C, away from direct heat. Do not freeze.

Nature and contents of container: Aluminium tubes with epoxy phenolic lining, and white polypropylene or polyethylene screw caps; pack size: 30 g.

Instructions for use/handling: Not applicable.

Marketing authorisation number 10590/0016

Date of approval/revision of SPC July 1996.

Legal category POM.

TETRALYSAL* 300

Qualitative and quantitative composition Lymecycline BP 408 mg equivalent to 300 mg tetracycline base.

Pharmaceutical form Hard gelatin capsule.

Clinical particulars

Therapeutic indications: Tetralysal 300 is for the treatment of acne.

As Tetralysal 300 contains a broad spectrum antibiotic, it is also recommended for the treatment of infections caused by tetracycline-sensitive organisms and may be utilised in all conditions where tetracycline is indicated, including use in penicillin-sensitive patients for the treatment of staphylococcal infections. Typical indications include: ear, nose and throat infections; acute and chronic bronchitis (including prophylaxis); infections of the gastro-intestinal and urinary tracts; non-gonococcal urethritis of chlamydial origin and other chlamydial infections such as trachoma; rickettsial fevers; soft tissue infections.

Posology and method of administration: Adults: The usual dosage for the chronic treatment of acne is 1 capsule daily: treatment should be continued for at least 8 weeks.

For other infections, the usual dosage is 1 capsule b.d. If higher doses are required, 3-4 capsules may be given over 24 hours. Lower doses may be given for prophylaxis.

In the management of sexually transmitted disease both partners should be treated.

Elderly: As for other tetracyclines, no specific dose adjustment is required.

Children: Not recommended for children under the age of 12 years. For children over the age of 12 years the adult dosage may be given.

Contra-indications: As lymecycline is mainly excreted by the kidneys, Tetralysal 300 should not be administered to patients with overt renal insufficiency.

Its use is also contra-indicated in patients hypersensitive to tetracyclines.

Children under 12 years.

Pregnancy and lactation (see *Pregnancy and lactation*).

Special warnings and precautions for use: Prolonged use of broad spectrum antibiotics may result in the appearance of resistant organisms and superinfection.

Bulging fontanelles in infants and benign intracranial hypertension in adults has been reported during treatment with tetracyclines. Therefore treatment should cease if evidence of raised intracranial pressure develops during treatment with Tetralysal 300.

Care should be exercised in administering tetracyclines to patients with hepatic impairment.

Tetracyclines may rarely cause photosensitivity.

Interaction with other medicaments and other forms of interaction: The absorption of tetracyclines may be affected by the simultaneous administration of antacids and/or iron preparations. These products should not be taken within two hours before or after taking Tetralysal 300.

Unlike earlier tetracyclines, absorption of Tetralysal 300 is not significantly impaired by moderate amounts of milk.

Although not reported for Tetralysal 300, a few cases of pregnancy or breakthrough bleeding have been attributed to the concurrent use of tetracycline or oxytetracycline with oral contraceptives.

The anticoagulant effect of warfarin and phenindione may be enhanced by tetracyclines.

Co-administration of zinc salts may reduce the absorption of both tetracyclines and zinc.

Pregnancy and lactation: Tetracyclines are selectively absorbed by developing bones and teeth and may cause dental staining and enamel hypoplasia. In addition these compounds readily cross the placental barrier and therefore Tetralysal 300 should not be given to pregnant or lactating women.

Effects on ability to drive and use machines: None known.

Undesirable effects: Nausea, vomiting, diarrhoea, erythema (discontinue treatment); headache and visual disturbances may indicate benign intracranial hypertension; hepatotoxicity, pancreatitis and antibiotic associated colitis have been reported with tetracyclines.

Overdosage: There is no specific treatment, but gastric lavage should be performed as soon as possible. Supportive measures should be instituted as required and a high fluid intake maintained.

Pharmacological properties

Pharmacodynamic properties: Lymecycline has antimicrobial activity and uses similar to those of tetracycline hydrochloride.

It acts by interfering with bacterial protein synthesis and is active against a large number of Gram-positive and Gram-negative pathogenic bacteria including some which are resistant to penicillin.

Pharmacokinetic properties: Lymecycline is more readily absorbed from the gastro-intestinal tract than tetracycline, with a peak serum concentration of approximately 2 mg/L after 3 hours following a 300 mg dose. In addition, similar blood concentrations are achieved with smaller doses. When the dose is doubled an almost correspondingly higher blood concentration has been reported to occur.

The serum half-life of lymecycline is approximately 10 hours.

Preclinical safety data: No specific information is presented given the vast experience gained with the use of tetracyclines in humans over the last forty years.

Pharmaceutical particulars

List of excipients: Silica gel, magnesium stearate, gelatin, glyceryl mono-oleate, purified water.

Incompatibilities: None known.

Shelf life: Thirty-six (36) months (unopened).

Special precautions for storage: The capsules should be stored in the original container in which they were dispensed. The carton should be stored in a dry place, below 25°C and protected from light.

As with all medicines, Tetralysal 300 should be kept out of the sight and reach of children.

Nature and contents of container: Aluminium-PVC/PVDC calendar blister strips of 14 capsules; two strips per carton, pack size = 28 capsules.

Instructions for use/handling: No special instructions.

Marketing authorisation number PL 10590/0019

Date of first authorisation/renewal of authorisation 29th September 1995

Date of (partial) revision of text March 1998

Legal category POM.

**Trade Mark*

Glaxo Wellcome
Stockley Park West
Middlesex UB11 1BT
☎ 0181 990 9000 0181 990 4321

GlaxoWellcome

ALKERAN* TABLETS AND INJECTION

Presentation *Alkeran Tablets:* White, round, biconvex, compression-coated tablets impressed WELLCOME and A2A, each containing 2 mg Melphalan BP.

White, round, biconvex, compression-coated tablets impressed WELLCOME and B2A, each containing 5 mg Melphalan BP.

Alkeran Injection: Alkeran Injection is supplied as a unit pack comprising a vial containing a freeze-dried powder and a vial of solvent-diluent. Each Alkeran vial contains the equivalent of 50 mg of melphalan, in the form of the hydrochloride, as a sterile, white to off-white, freeze-dried powder which includes 20 mg povidone K12. Each vial of solvent-diluent provides 10 ml of buffer solution containing 60% v/v propylene glycol with sodium citrate and ethanol.

Uses *Alkeran Tablets* are indicated in the treatment of multiple myeloma and advanced ovarian adenocarcinoma.

Alkeran Tablets may be used in the treatment of:
breast carcinoma: Alkeran either alone or in combination with other drugs has a significant therapeutic effect in a proportion of patients suffering from advanced breast carcinoma; Alkeran has also been used as an adjuvant to surgery in the management of breast carcinoma.

polycythaemia rubra vera: Alkeran is effective in the treatment of a proportion of patients suffering from polycythaemia vera.

Alkeran Injection, administered by regional arterial perfusion, is indicated in the treatment of localised malignant melanoma of the extremities and localised soft tissue sarcoma of the extremities.

Alkeran Injection, at conventional intravenous dosage, may be used in the treatment of:

multiple myeloma: Alkeran Injection, either alone or in combination with other cytotoxic drugs, is as effective as the oral formulation in the treatment of multiple myeloma;

ovarian cancer: Alkeran Injection produces an objective response in approximately fifty percent of the patients with advanced ovarian adenocarcinoma, when given alone, or in combination with other cytotoxic drugs.

Alkeran Injection, at high intravenous dosage, may be used in the treatment of:

multiple myeloma: complete remissions have been achieved in up to fifty percent of patients given high dose Alkeran Injection, with or without autologous bone marrow rescue, either as first line treatment or to consolidate a response to conventional cytoreductive chemotherapy;

neuroblastoma in childhood: high dose Alkeran Injection with autologous bone marrow rescue has been used either alone, or combined with radiotherapy and/or other cytotoxic drugs, to consolidate a response to conventional treatment. A significant increase in the duration of disease-free survival was demonstrated in a prospective randomised trial of high dose Alkeran Injection versus no further treatment.

Mode of action: Melphalan is a bifunctional alkylating agent. Formation of carbonium intermediates from each of the two bis-2-chloroethyl groups enables alkylation through covalent binding with the 7-nitrogen of guanine on DNA, cross-linking the two DNA strands and thereby preventing cell replication.

Pharmacokinetics: The absorption of melphalan was found to be highly variable in 13 patients given 0.6 mg/kg orally, with respect to both the time to first appearance of the drug in plasma (range 0 to 336 minutes) and peak plasma concentration (range 70 to 630 ng/ml). In 5 of the patients who were given an equivalent intravenous dose, the mean bioavailability of melphalan was found to be 56±27%. The terminal plasma half-life was 90±57 minutes with 11% of the drug being recovered in the urine over 24 hours.

The administration of Alkeran Tablets immediately after food delayed the time to achieving peak plasma concentrations and reduced the area under the plasma concentration-time curves by between 39 and 45%.

The pharmacokinetics of intravenous Alkeran given at both conventional and high doses are best described by a bi-exponential, 2-compartment model. In 8 patients given a single bolus dose of 0.5 to 0.6 mg/kg, the composite initial and terminal half-lives were reported to be 7.7±3.3 minutes and 108±20.8 minutes respectively. Following injection of melphalan, monohydroxymelphalan and dihydroxymelphalan were detected in the patients' plasma, reaching peak levels at approximately 60 minutes and 105 minutes respectively. A similar half-life of 126±6 minutes was seen when melphalan was added to the patients' serum *in vitro* (37°C), suggesting that spontaneous degradation rather than enzymic metabolism may be the major determinant of the drug's half-life in man.

Following administration of a 2 minute infusion of doses ranging from 5 to 23 mg/m² (approximately 0.1 to 0.6 mg/kg) to 10 patients with ovarian cancer or multiple myeloma, the pooled initial and terminal half lives were, respectively, 8.1±6.6 minutes and 76.9±40.7 minutes. In this study, the mean volumes of distribution at steady state and central compartment were 29.1±13.6 litres and 12.2±6.5 litres, respectively, and a mean clearance of 342.7±96.8 ml/minute was recorded.

In 15 children and 11 adults given high-dose intravenous Alkeran (140 mg/m²) with forced diuresis, the mean initial and terminal half-lives were found to be 6.5±3.6 minutes and 41.4±16.5 minutes respectively. Mean initial and terminal half-lives of 8.8±6.6 minutes and 73.1±45.9 minutes, respectively, were recorded in 28 patients with various malignancies who were given doses of between 70 and 200 mg/m² as a 2 to 20 minute infusion. The mean volumes of distribution at steady state and central compartment were, respectively, 40.2±18.3 litres and 18.2±11.7 litres, and the mean clearance was 564.6±159.1 ml/minute.

Following hyperthermic (39°C) perfusion of the lower limb with 1.75 mg/kg bodyweight, mean initial and terminal half-lives of 3.6±1.5 minutes and 46.5±17.2 minutes, respectively, were recorded in 11 patients with advanced malignant melanoma. Mean volumes of distribution at steady state and central compartment were, respectively, 2.87±0.8 litres and 1.01±0.28 litres, and a mean clearance of 55.0±9.4 ml/minute was recorded.

Dosage and administration Alkeran is a cytotoxic drug which falls into the general class of alkylating agents. It should be prescribed only by physicians experienced in the management of malignant disease with such agents.

Since Alkeran is myelosuppressive, frequent blood counts are essential during therapy and the dosage should be delayed or adjusted if necessary (see *Precautions*).

The absorption of Alkeran after oral administration is variable. Dosage may need to be cautiously increased until myelosuppression is seen, in order to ensure that potentially therapeutic levels have been reached.

Multiple myeloma: Oral administration: A typical oral dosage schedule is 0.15 mg/kg bodyweight/day in divided doses for 4 days, repeated at intervals of six weeks. Numerous regimens have, however, been used and the scientific literature should be consulted for details. The administration of oral Alkeran and prednisone maybe more effective than Alkeran alone. The combination is usually given on an intermittent basis. Prolonging treatment beyond one year in responders does not appear to improve results.

Intravenous administration: Alkeran Injection has been used on an intermittent basis alone, or in combination with other cytotoxic drugs, at doses varying between 8 mg/m² body surface area and 30 mg/m² body surface area, given at intervals of between 2 to 6 weeks. Additionally, administration of prednisone has been included in a number of regimens. The literature should be consulted for precise details on treatment protocols.

When used as a single agent, a typical intravenous dosage schedule is 0.4 mg/kg bodyweight (16 mg/m² body surface area) repeated at appropriate intervals (e.g. once every 4 weeks), provided there has been recovery of the peripheral blood count during this period.

High-dose regimens generally employ single intravenous doses of between 100 and 200 mg/m² body surface area (approximately 2.5 to 5.0 mg/kg bodyweight), but autologous bone marrow rescue becomes essential following doses in excess of 140 mg/m² body surface area. In cases of renal impairment, the dose should be reduced by 50% (see *Dosage in renal impairment*). In view of the severe myelosuppression induced by high dose Alkeran Injection, treatment should be confined to specialist centres, with the appropriate facilities, and only be administered by experienced clinicians (see *Precautions*).

Ovarian adenocarcinoma: Oral administration: A typical regimen is 0.2 mg/kg bodyweight/day orally for 5 days. This is repeated every 4 to 8 weeks, or as soon as the peripheral blood count has recovered.

Intravenous administration: When used intravenously as a single agent, a dose of 1 mg/kg bodyweight (approximately 40 mg/m² body surface area) given at intervals of 4 weeks has often been used.

When combined with other cytotoxic drugs, intravenous doses of between 0.3 and 0.4 mg/kg bodyweight (12 to 16 mg/m² body surface area) have been used at intervals of 4 to 6 weeks.

Carcinoma of the breast: Alkeran has been given orally at a dose of 0.15 mg/kg bodyweight or 6 mg/m² body surface area/day for 5 days and repeated every 6 weeks. The dose was decreased if bone marrow toxicity was observed.

Malignant melanoma: Hyperthermic regional perfusion with Alkeran has been used as an adjuvant to surgery for early malignant melanoma and as palliative treatment for advanced but localised disease. The scientific literature should be consulted for details of perfusion technique and dosage used. A typical dose range for upper extremity perfusions is 0.6 to 1.0 mg/kg bodyweight and for lower extremity perfusions is 0.8 to 1.5 mg/kg bodyweight.

Soft tissue sarcoma: Hyperthermic regional perfusion with Alkeran has been used in the management of all stages of localised soft tissue sarcoma, usually in combination with surgery. Alkeran has also been given with actinomycin D and the scientific literature should be consulted for details of dosage regimens. A typical dose range for upper extremity perfusions is 0.6 to 1.0 mg/kg bodyweight and for lower extremity perfusions is 1 to 1.4 mg/kg bodyweight.

Polycythaemia rubra vera: For remission, induction doses of 6 to 10 mg daily for 5 to 7 days have been used, after which 2 to 4 mg daily were given until satisfactory disease control was achieved.

A dose of 2 to 6 mg once per week has been used for maintenance therapy.

In view of the possibility of severe myelosuppression if Alkeran is given on a continuous basis, it is essential that frequent blood counts are taken throughout therapy, with dosage adjustment or breaks in treatment, as appropriate, to maintain careful haematological control.

Advanced neuroblastoma: Doses of between 100 and 240 mg/m² body surface area (sometimes divided equally over 3 consecutive days) together with autologous bone marrow rescue, have been used either alone or in combination with radiotherapy and/or other cytotoxic drugs.

Preparation of Alkeran Injection Solution: Alkeran Injection should be prepared, AT ROOM TEMPERATURE, by reconstituting the freeze-dried powder with the Solvent-Diluent provided. 10 ml of this vehicle should be added, as a single quantity, and the vial immediately shaken VIGOROUSLY until solution is complete. The resulting solution contains the equivalent of 5 mg per ml anhydrous melphalan and has a pH of approximately 6.5.

Alkeran Injection solution has limited stability and should be prepared immediately before use. Any unused solution should be discarded (see *Pharmaceutical precautions*).

The reconstituted solution should not be refrigerated as this will cause precipitation.

Parenteral administration: Except in cases where regional arterial perfusion is indicated, Alkeran Injection is for intravenous use only.

For intravenous administration it is recommended that Alkeran Injection solution is injected slowly into a fast-running infusion solution via a swabbed injection port.

If direct injection into a fast-running infusion is not appropriate, Alkeran Injection solution may be administered diluted in an infusion bag.

Alkeran is not compatible with infusion solutions containing dextrose, and it is recommended that ONLY Sodium Chloride Intravenous Infusion 0.9% w/v is used.

When further diluted in an infusion solution, Alkeran Injection has reduced stability and the rate of degradation increases rapidly with rise in temperature. If administration occurs at a room temperature of approximately 25°C, the total time from preparation of the Injection solution to the completion of infusion should not exceed 1.5 hours.

Should any visible turbidity or crystallisation appear in the reconstituted or diluted solutions the preparation must be discarded.

Care should be taken to avoid possible extravasation of Alkeran and in cases of poor peripheral venous access, consideration should be given to use of a central venous line.

If high dose Alkeran Injection is administered with or without autologous bone marrow transplantation, administration via a central venous line is recommended.

For regional arterial perfusion, the literature should be consulted for detailed methodology.

Use in children: Alkeran, at conventional dosage, is only rarely indicated in children and dosage guidelines cannot be stated.

High dose Alkeran Injection, in association with bone marrow rescue, has been used in childhood neuroblastoma and dosage guidelines based on body surface area, as for adults, may be used.

Use in the elderly: Although Alkeran is frequently used at conventional dosage in the elderly, there is no specific information available relating to its administration to this patient sub-group.

Experience in the use of high dose Alkeran in elderly patients is limited. Consideration should therefore be given to ensure adequate performance status and organ function before using high dose Alkeran Injection in elderly patients.

Dosage in renal impairment: Alkeran clearance, though variable, is decreased in renal impairment.

Currently available pharmacokinetic data do not justify an absolute recommendation on dosage reduction when administering Alkeran Tablets to patients with renal impairment, but it may be prudent to use a reduced dosage initially until tolerance is established.

When Alkeran Injection is used at conventional intravenous dosage (8 to 40 mg/m² body surface area), it is recommended that the initial dose should be reduced by 50% in patients with moderate to severe renal impairment and subsequent dosage determined according to the degree of haematological suppression.

For high intravenous doses of Alkeran (100 to 240 mg/m² body surface area), the need for dose reduction depends upon the degree of renal impairment, whether autologous bone marrow stem cells are reinfused, and therapeutic need. As a guide, for moderate to severe renal impairment (EDTA clearance 30 to 50 ml/min) a dose reduction of 50% is usual. Adequate hydration and forced diuresis are also necessary. High dose Alkeran is not recommended in patients with more severe renal impairment (EDTA clearance less then 30 ml/min).

Contra-indications, warnings, etc

Contra-indications: Alkeran should not be given to patients who have suffered a previous hypersensitivity reaction to melphalan.

Precautions: ALKERAN IS AN ACTIVE CYTOTOXIC AGENT FOR USE UNDER THE DIRECTION OF PHYSICIANS EXPERIENCED IN THE ADMINISTRATION OF SUCH AGENTS.

Alkeran Injection solution may cause local tissue damage should extravasation occur, and consequently it should not be administered by direct injection into a peripheral vein. It is recommended that Alkeran Injection solution is administered by injecting slowly into a fast-running intravenous infusion via a swabbed injection port, or via a central venous line.

In view of the hazards involved and the level of supportive care required, the administration of high dose Alkeran Injection should be confined to specialist centres, with the appropriate facilities, and only be conducted by experienced clinicians.

In patients receiving high dose Alkeran Injection, consideration should be given to the prophylactic administration of anti-infective agents, the administration of blood products as required, and the maintenance of a high renal output during the period immediately following the administration of Alkeran by the use of hydration and forced diuresis.

Consideration should be given to ensure adequate performance status and organ function before using high dose Alkeran Injection.

Safe handling of Alkeran: The handling of Alkeran formulations should follow guidelines for the handling of cytotoxic drugs according to the Royal Pharmaceutical Society of Great Britain Working Party on the Handling of Cytotoxic Drugs.

Provided the outer coating of the tablet is intact, there is no risk in handling Alkeran Tablets.

Alkeran Tablets should not be divided.

Monitoring: Since Alkeran is a potent myelosuppressive agent, it is essential that careful attention should be paid to the monitoring of blood counts to avoid the possibility of excessive myelosuppression and the risk of irreversible bone marrow aplasia. Blood counts may continue to fall after treatment is stopped, so at the first sign of an abnormally large fall in leukocyte or platelet counts treatment should be temporarily interrupted. Alkeran should be used with caution in patients who have undergone recent radiotherapy or chemotherapy in view of increased bone marrow toxicity.

Renal impairment: Alkeran clearance may be reduced in patients with renal impairment, who may also have uraemic bone marrow suppression. Dose reduction may therefore be necessary (see **Dosage and administration**), and these patients should be closely observed.

Temporary significant elevation of the blood urea has been seen in the early stages of melphalan therapy in myeloma patients with renal damage.

Mutagenicity: Melphalan is mutagenic in animals and chromosome aberrations have been observed in patients being treated with the drug.

Carcinogenicity: Melphalan, in common with other alkylating agents, may be leukaemogenic in man. There have been reports of acute leukaemia occurring after prolonged melphalan treatment for diseases such as amyloid, malignant melanoma, multiple myeloma, macroglobulinaemia, cold agglutinin syndrome and ovarian cancer.

A comparison of patients with ovarian cancer who received alkylating agents with those who did not showed that the use of alkylating agents, including melphalan, significantly increased the incidence of acute leukaemia.

The leukaemogenic risk must be balanced against the potential therapeutic benefit when considering the use of melphalan.

Effects on fertility: Alkeran causes suppression of ovarian function in pre-menopausal women resulting in amenorrhoea in a significant number of patients.

There is evidence from some animal studies that Alkeran can have an adverse effect on spermatogenesis. Therefore, it is possible that Alkeran may cause temporary or permanent sterility in male patients.

Use in pregnancy and lactation: The teratogenic potential of Alkeran has not been studied. In view of its mutagenic properties and structural similarity to known teratogenic compounds, it is possible that melphalan could cause congenital defects in the offspring of patients treated with the drug.

As with all cytotoxic chemotherapy, adequate contraceptive precautions should be practised when either partner is receiving Alkeran.

The use of melphalan should be avoided whenever possible during pregnancy, particularly during the first trimester. In any individual case the potential hazard to the fetus must be balanced against the expected benefit to the mother.

Mothers receiving Alkeran should not breast feed.

Side- and adverse effects: The most common side-effect is bone marrow depression, leading to leucopenia and thrombocytopenia.

Gastro-intestinal effects such as nausea and vomiting have been reported in up to 30% of patients receiving conventional oral doses of Alkeran.

Stomatitis occurs rarely following conventional doses of Alkeran.

The incidence of diarrhoea, vomiting and stomatitis becomes the dose limiting toxicity in patients given high intravenous doses of Alkeran in association with autologous bone marrow transplantation. Cyclophosphamide pre-treatment appears to reduce the severity of gastro-intestinal damage induced by high dose Alkeran and the literature should be consulted for details.

Allergic reactions to Alkeran such as urticaria, oedema, skin rashes and anaphylactic shock have been reported uncommonly following initial or subsequent dosing, particularly after intravenous administration. Cardiac arrest has also been reported rarely in association with such events.

Maculopapular rashes and pruritus have occasionally been noted.

There have also been case reports of fatal pulmonary fibrosis and haemolytic anaemia occurring after melphalan treatment.

Alopecia has been reported but is uncommon at conventional doses.

A subjective and transient sensation of warmth and/or tingling was described in approximately two thirds of patients with haematological malignancies who were given high dose Alkeran Injection via a central line.

Drug interactions: Nalidixic acid together with high-dose intravenous melphalan has caused deaths in children due to haemorrhagic enterocolitis.

Impaired renal function has been described in bone marrow transplant patients who were conditioned with high dose intravenous melphalan and who subsequently received cyclosporin to prevent graft-versus-host disease.

Toxicity and treatment of overdosage: Gastro-intestinal effects, including nausea, vomiting and diarrhoea are the most likely signs of acute oral overdosage. The immediate effects of acute intravenous overdosage are nausea and vomiting. Damage to the gastro-intestinal mucosa may also ensue, and diarrhoea, sometimes haemorrhagic, has been reported after overdosage. The principal toxic effect is bone marrow suppression, leading to leucopenia, thrombocytopenia and anaemia.

General supportive measures, together with appropriate blood and platelet transfusions, should be instituted if necessary and consideration given to hospitalisation, antibiotic cover, and the use of haematological growth factors.

There is no specific antidote. The blood picture should be closely monitored for at least four weeks following overdosage until there is evidence of recovery.

Pharmaceutical precautions

Alkeran Tablets:	Store at 2 to 8°C. Keep dry.
Injection unit pack:	Store below 30°C. Protect from light.

Alkeran Tablets and Injection surplus to requirements should be destroyed in a manner appropriate to the prevailing local regulatory requirements for the disposal of cytotoxic drugs.

Legal category POM

Package quantities

Alkeran Tablets 2 mg:	Bottle of 25
Alkeran Tablets 5 mg:	Bottle of 25
Alkeran Injection unit pack:	Vial of Alkeran freeze-dried powder and vial of solvent-diluent.

Further information Nil.

Product licence numbers

Alkeran Tablets 2 mg:	0003/5008R
Alkeran Tablets 5 mg:	0003/5009R
Alkeran Injection:	0003/0323
Alkeran Solvent-Diluent:	0003/0324

ANECTINE* INJECTION

Qualitative and quantitative composition Suxamethonium Chloride Injection BP 100 mg in 2 ml.

Pharmaceutical form Injection.

Clinical particulars

Therapeutic indications: Used in anaesthesia as a muscle relaxant to facilitate endotracheal intubation, mechanical ventilation and a wide range of surgical and obstetric procedures.

It is also used to reduce the intensity of muscular contractions associated with pharmacologically or electrically-induced convulsions.

Posology and method of administration: Usually by bolus intravenous injection.

Adults: The dose is dependent on body weight, the degree of muscular relaxation required, the route of administration, and the response of individual patients.

To achieve endotracheal intubation Anectine is usually administered intravenously in a dose of 1 mg/kg. This dose will usually produce muscular relaxation in about 30 to 60 seconds and has a duration of action of about 2 to 6 minutes. Larger doses will produce more prolonged muscular relaxation, but doubling the dose does not necessarily double the duration of relaxation. Supplementary doses of Anectine of 50% to 100% of the initial dose administered at 5 to 10 minute intervals will maintain muscle relaxation during short surgical procedures performed under general anaesthesia.

For prolonged surgical procedures Anectine may be given by intravenous infusion as a 0.1% to 0.2% solution, diluted in 5% glucose solution or sterile isotonic saline solution, at a rate of 2.5 to 4 mg per minute. The infusion rate should be adjusted according to the response of individual patients.

The total dose of Anectine given by repeated intravenous injection or continuous infusion should ***not*** exceed 500 mg per hour.

Children: Infants and young children are more resistant to Anectine compared with adults.

The recommended intravenous dose of Anectine for neonates and infants is 2 mg/kg. A dose of 1 mg/kg in older children is recommended.

When Anectine is given as intravenous infusion in children, the dosage is as for adults with a proportionately lower initial infusion rate based on bodyweight.

Anectine may be given intramuscularly to infants at doses up to 4 to 5 mg/kg and in older children up to 4 mg/kg. These doses produce muscular relaxation within about 3 minutes. A total dose of 150 mg should ***not*** be exceeded.

Use in the elderly: Dosage requirements of Anectine in the elderly are comparable to those for younger adults.

The elderly may be more susceptible to cardiac arrhythmias, especially if digitalis-like drugs are also being taken. See also *Special warnings and precautions for use.*

Contra-indications: Anectine has no effect on the level of consciousness and should not be administered to a patient who is not fully anaesthetised.

Hypersensitivity to suxamethonium may exist in rare instances, and Anectine should not be administered to patients known to be hypersensitive to the drug.

As suxamethonium can act as a trigger of sustained myofibrillar contraction in susceptible individuals, Anectine is contra-indicated in patients with a personal or family history of malignant hyperthermia. If this condition occurs unexpectedly, all anaesthetic agents known to be associated with its development (including Anectine) must be immediately discontinued, and full supportive measures must be immediately instituted. Intravenous dantrolene sodium is the primary specific therapeutic drug and is recommended as soon as possible after the diagnosis is made.

Anectine is contra-indicated in patients known to have an inherited atypical plasma cholinesterase activity.

An acute transient rise in serum potassium often occurs following the administration of Anectine in normal individuals; the magnitude of this rise is of the order of 0.5 mmol/litre. In certain pathological states or conditions this increase in serum potassium following Anectine administration may be excessive and cause serious cardiac arrhythmias and cardiac arrest. For this reason the use of Anectine is contra-indicated in:

- Patients recovering from major trauma or severe burns; the period of greatest risk of hyperkalaemia is from about 5 to 70 days after the injury and may be further prolonged if there is delayed healing due to persistent infection.
- Patients with neurological deficits involving acute major muscle wasting (upper and/or lower motor neurone lesions); the potential for potassium release occurs within the first 6 months after the acute onset of the neurological deficit and correlates with the degree and extent of muscle paralysis. Patients who have been immobilised for prolonged periods of time may be at similar risk.
- Patients with pre-existing hyperkalaemia. In the absence of hyperkalaemia and neuropathy, renal failure is not a contra-indication to the administration of a normal single dose of Anectine Injection, but multiple or large doses may cause clinically significant rises in serum potassium and should not be used.

Suxamethonium causes a significant transient rise in intra-ocular pressure, and should therefore not be used in the presence of open eye injuries or where an increase in intra-ocular pressure is undesirable unless the potential benefit of its use outweighs the potential risk to the eye.

Anectine should be avoided in patients with a personal or family history of congenital myotonic diseases such as myotonia congenita and dystrophia myotonica since its administration may on occasion be associated with severe myotonic spasms and rigidity.

Anectine should be avoided in patients with Duchenne muscular dystrophy since its administration may be associated with rigidity, hyperthermia, hyperkalaemia, myoglobinaemia, cardiac arrest, and post-operative respiratory depression.

Special warnings and precautions for use: Anectine should be administered only by or under close supervision of an anaesthetist familiar with its action, characteristics and hazards, who is skilled in the management of artificial respiration and only where there are adequate facilities for immediate endotracheal intubation with administration of oxygen by intermittent positive pressure ventilation.

Anectine should not be mixed in the same syringe with any other agent, especially thiopentone.

During prolonged administration of Anectine, it is recommended that the patient is fully monitored with a peripheral nerve stimulator in order to avoid overdosage.

Anectine is rapidly hydrolysed by plasma cholinesterase which thereby limits the intensity and duration of the neuromuscular blockade.

Prolonged and intensified neuromuscular blockade following Anectine Injection may occur secondary to reduced plasma cholinesterase activity in the following states or pathological conditions: physiological variation as in pregnancy and the puerperium; genetically determined abnormal plasma cholinesterase; severe generalised tetanus, tuberculosis, other severe or chronic infections; following severe burns; chronic debilitating disease, malignancy, chronic anaemia and malnutrition; end-stage hepatic failure, acute or chronic renal failure; auto-immune diseases: myxoedema, collagen diseases; iatrogenic: following plasma exchange, plasmapheresis, cardiopulmonary bypass, and as a result of concomitant drug therapy (see *Interactions*).

If Anectine is given over a prolonged period, the characteristic depolarising neuromuscular (or Phase I) block may change to one with characteristics of a non-depolarising (or Phase II) block. Although the characteristics of a developing Phase II block resemble those of a true non-depolarising block, the former cannot always be fully or permanently reversed by anticholinesterase agents. When a Phase II block is fully established, its effects will then usually be fully reversible with standard doses of neostigmine accompanied by an anticholinergic agent.

Tachyphylaxis occurs after repeated administration of Anectine.

Caution should be exercised when using suxamethonium in children, since paediatric patients are more likely to have an undiagnosed myopathy or an unknown predisposition to malignant hyperthermia, which places them at increased risk of serious adverse events following suxamethonium.

In patients with severe sepsis, the potential for hyperkalaemia seems to be related to the severity and duration of infection.

It is inadvisable to administer Anectine to patients with advanced myasthenia gravis. Although these patients are resistant to suxamethonium they develop a state of Phase II block which can result in delayed recovery. Patients with myasthenic Eaton-Lambert syndrome are more sensitive than normal to Anectine, necessitating dosage reduction.

In healthy adults, Anectine occasionally causes a mild transient slowing of the heart rate on initial administration. Bradycardias are more commonly observed in children and on repeated administration of suxamethonium in both children and adults. Pretreatment with intravenous atropine or glycopyrrolate significantly reduces the incidence and severity of suxamethonium-related bradycardia.

In the absence of pre-existing or evoked hyperkalaemia, ventricular arrhythmias are rarely seen following suxamethonium administration. Patients taking digitalis-like drugs are however more susceptible to such arrhythmias. The action of suxamethonium on the heart may cause changes in cardiac rhythm including cardiac arrest.

Interaction with other medicaments and other forms of interaction: Certain drugs or chemicals are known to reduce normal plasma cholinesterase activity and may therefore prolong the neuromuscular blocking effects of Anectine. These include: organophosphorous insecticides and metriphonate; ecothiopate eye drops; trimetaphan; specific anticholinesterase agents: neostigmine, pyridostigmine, physostigmine, edrophonium; tachrine hydrochloride; cytotoxic compounds; cyclophosphamide, mechlorethamine, triethylene-melamine, and thiotepa; psychiatric drugs: phenelzine, promazine and chlorpromazine; anaesthetic agents and drugs: ketamine, morphine and morphine antagonists, pethidine, pancuronium, propanidid.

Other drugs with potentially deleterious effects on plasma cholinesterase activity include aprotinin, diphenhydramine, promethazine, oestrogens, oxytocin, high-dose steroids, and oral contraceptives, terbutaline and metoclopramide.

Certain drugs or substances may enhance or prolong the neuromuscular effects of Anectine by mechanisms unrelated to plasma cholinesterase activity. These include: magnesium salts; lithium carbonate; azathioprine; quinine and chloroquinine; antibiotics such as the aminoglycosides, clindamycin and polymyxins; antiarrhythmic drugs: quinidine, procainamide, verapamil, beta-blockers, lignocaine and procaine; volatile inhalational anaesthetic agents: halothane, enflurane, desflurane, isoflurane, diethylether and methoxyflurane have little effect on the Phase I block of Anectine injection but will accelerate the onset and enhance the intensity of a Phase II suxamethonium-induced block.

Patients receiving digitalis-like drugs are more susceptible to the effects of suxamethonium-exacerbated hyperkalaemia.

Pregnancy and lactation: Suxamethonium has no direct action on the uterus or other smooth muscle structures. In normal therapeutic doses it does not cross the placental barrier in sufficient amounts to affect the respiration of the infant.

The benefits of the use of suxamethonium as part of a rapid sequence induction for general anaesthesia normally outweigh the possible risk to the foetus.

Plasma cholinesterase levels fall during the first trimester of pregnancy to about 70 to 80% of their pre-pregnancy values; a further fall to about 60 to 70% of the pre-pregnancy levels occurs within 2 to 4 days after delivery. Plasma cholinesterase levels then increase to reach normal over the next 6 weeks. Consequently, a high proportion of pregnant and puerperal patients may exhibit mildly prolonged neuromuscular blockade following Anectine injection.

It is not known whether suxamethonium or its metabolites are excreted in human milk.

Effect on ability to drive and use machines: Not applicable.

Undesirable effects: Muscle pains are frequently experienced after administration of suxamethonium and most commonly occur in ambulatory patients undergoing short surgical procedures under general anaesthesia. There appears to be no direct connection between the degree of visible muscle fasciculation after Anectine administration and the incidence or severity of pain. The use of small doses of non-depolarising muscle relaxants given minutes before suxamethonium administration has been advocated for the reduction of incidence and severity of suxamethonium-associated muscle pains. This technique may require the use of doses of suxamethonium in excess of 1 mg/kg to achieve satisfactory conditions for endotracheal intubation.

The following adverse reactions have been reported after administration of Anectine:

Cardiovascular: bradycardia, tachycardia, hypertension, hypotension, arrhythmias;

Respiratory: bronchospasm, prolonged respiratory depression and apnoea;

Musculoskeletal: muscle fasciculation, post-operative muscle pains, myoglobinaemia, myoglobinuria;

Other: anaphylactic reactions, hyperthermia, increased intra-ocular pressure, increased intragastric pressure, rash, skin flushing, excessive salivation.

There are case reports of hyperkalaemia-related cardiac arrests following the administration of suxamethonium to patients with congenital cerebral palsy, tetanus, Duchenne muscular dystrophy, and closed head injury.

Overdose: Apnoea and prolonged muscle paralysis are the main serious effects of overdosage. It is essential, therefore, to maintain the airway and adequate ventilation until spontaneous respiration occurs.

The decision to use neostigmine to reverse a Phase II suxamethonium-induced block depends on the judgement of the clinician in the individual case. Valuable information in regard to this decision will be gained by monitoring neuromuscular function. If neostigmine is used its administration should be accompanied by appropriate doses of an anticholinergic agent such as atropine.

Pharmacological properties

Pharmacodynamic properties: Short-acting depolarising neuromuscular blocking agent.

Pharmacokinetic properties: None stated.

Preclinical safety data: None relevant to the prescriber additional to that already included in other sections.

Pharmaceutical particulars

List of excipients: Water for Injections EP.

Incompatibilities: None known.

Shelf life: 18 months.

Special precautions for storage: Store below 4°C. Do not freeze. Protect from light.

Nature and contents of container: Neutral glass. 2 ml ampoules.

Instructions for use/handling: For intravenous injection under medical direction.

Marketing authorisation number 0003/5203R

Date of approval/revision of SPC May 1997

BETNOVATE*-C CREAM

Qualitative and quantitative composition

Betamethasone Valerate BP 0.122% w/w.
Clioquinol BP 3.00% w/w.

Pharmaceutical form Aqueous Cream.

Clinical particulars

Therapeutic indications: Betamethasone valerate is

an active topical corticosteroid which produces a rapid response in those inflammatory dermatoses that are normally responsive to topical corticosteroid therapy, and is often effective in the less responsive conditions such as psoriasis.

Clioquinol is an anti-infective agent which has both antibacterial and anticandidal activity.

Betnovate-C preparations are indicated for the treatment of the following conditions where secondary bacterial and/or fungal infection is present, suspected, or likely to occur: eczema in children and adults, including atopic and discoid eczemas, prurigo nodularis; psoriasis (excluding widespread plaque psoriasis); neurodermatoses; seborrhoeic dermatitis; contact sensitivity reactions and discoid lupus erythematosus.

Betnovate-C can also be used in the management of secondary infected insect bites and anal and genital intertrigo.

Betnovate-C cream is often appropriate for moist or weeping surfaces and Betnovate-C ointment for dry, lichenified or scaly lesions, but this is not invariably so.

Posology and method of administration: A small quantity should be applied gently to the affected area two or three times daily until improvement occurs. It may then be possible to maintain improvement by applying once a day, or even less often.

Children: Courses should be limited to five days if possible. Occlusion should not be used.

For topical application.

Contra-indications: Rosacea, acne vulgaris and perioral dermatitis. Primary cutaneous viral infections (e.g. herpes simplex, chickenpox). Hypersensitivity to any component of the preparation or to iodine.

Use of Betnovate-C skin preparations is not indicated in the treatment of primarily infected skin lesions caused by infection with fungi (e.g. candidiasis, tinea); or bacteria (e.g. impetigo); primary or secondary, infections due to yeast; perianal or genital pruritus; dermatoses in children under 1 year of age, including dermatitis and napkin eruptions.

Special warnings and precautions for use: Long-term continuous topical therapy should be avoided where possible, particularly in infants and children, as adrenal suppression can occur even without occlusion.

The face, more than other areas of the body, may exhibit atrophic changes after prolonged treatment with potent topical corticosteroids. This must be borne in mind when treating such conditions as psoriasis, discoid lupus erythematosus and severe eczema with Betnovate. If applied to the eyelids, care is needed to ensure that the preparation does not enter the eye, as glaucoma might result.

If used in childhood, or on the face, courses should be limited to five days and occlusion should not be used.

Topical corticosteroids may be hazardous in psoriasis for a number of reasons including rebound relapses, development of tolerance, risk of generalised pustular psoriasis and development of local or systemic toxicity due to impaired barrier function of the skin. If used in psoriasis careful patient supervision is important.

If infection persists, systemic chemotherapy is required. Any spread of infection requires withdrawal of topical corticosteroid therapy. Bacterial infection is encouraged by the warm, moist conditions induced by occlusive dressings, and the skin should be cleansed before a fresh dressing is applied.

Do not continue for more than 7 days in the absence of clinical improvement, since occult extension of infection may occur due to the masking effect of the steroid.

Betnovate-C may stain hair, skin or fabric, and the application should be covered with a dressing to protect clothing.

Products which contain antimicrobial agents should not be diluted.

The least potent corticosteroid which will control the disease should be selected. These preparations do not contain lanolin or parabens.

Interaction with other medicaments and other forms of interaction: None.

Pregnancy and lactation: There is inadequate evidence of safety in human pregnancy. Topical administration of corticosteroids to pregnant animals can cause abnormalities of foetal development including cleft palate and intrauterine growth retardation. There may therefore be a very small risk of such effects in the human foetus.

Effects on ability to drive and use machines: None.

Undesirable effects: Prolonged and intensive treatment with highly active corticosteroid preparations may cause local atrophic changes in the skin such as thinning, striae, and dilatation of the superficial blood vessels, particularly when occlusive dressings are used or when skin folds are involved.

As with other topical corticosteroids, prolonged use of large amounts or treatment of extensive areas can result in sufficient systemic absorption to produce the features of hypercorticism and suppression of the HPA axis. These effects are likely to occur in infants and children, and if occlusive dressings are used. In infants the napkin may act as an occlusive dressing.

In rare instances, treatment of psoriasis with corticosteroids (or its withdrawal) is thought to have provoked the pustular form of the disease (see *Precautions*).

There are reports of pigmentation changes and hypertrichosis with topical steroids.

The Betnovate preparations are usually well tolerated, but if signs of hypersensitivity appear, application should be stopped immediately.

Exacerbation of symptoms may occur.

Overdose: Acute overdosage is very unlikely to occur, however, in the case of chronic overdosage or misuse the features of hypercorticism may appear and in this situation topical steroids should be discontinued.

Pharmacological properties

Pharmacodynamic properties: Betamethasone valerate is an active corticosteroid with topical anti-inflammatory activity.

Clioquinol is an anti-infective agent which has both anti-bacterial and anti-candidal activity.

Pharmacokinetic properties: The extent of percutaneous absorption of topical corticosteroid is determined by many factors including the vehicle, the integrity of the epidermal barrier, and the use of occlusive dressings.

Topical corticosteroids can be absorbed from normal intact skin. Inflammation and/or other disease processes in the skin increase percutaneous absorption. Occlusive dressings substantially increase the percutaneous absorption of topical corticosteroids.

Once absorbed through the skin, topical corticosteroids are handled through pharmacokinetic pathways similar to systematically administered corticosteroids. Corticosteroids are bound to plasma proteins in varying degrees. Corticosteroids are metabolised primarily by the liver and are then excreted by the kidneys.

Preclinical safety data: There are no preclinical data of relevance to the prescriber which are additional to that in other sections of the SmPC.

Pharmaceutical particulars

List of excipients: Chlorocresol BP, Cetomacrogol 1000 BP, Cetostearyl Alcohol BP, White Soft Paraffin BP, Liquid Paraffin BP, Sodium Acid Phosphate BP, Phosphoric Acid BP, Sodium Hydroxide BP, Purified Water BP.

Incompatibilities: None known.

Shelf life: 36 months.

Special precautions for storage: Store below 30°C.

Nature and contents of container: 15 gm and 30 gm collapsible aluminium tubes coated with an epoxy resin based lacquer with an aluminium membrane seal and a polyethylene cap.

Instructions for use/handling: No special instructions.

Marketing authorisation number PL 10949/0016

Date of first authorisation/renewal of authorisation 3/9/97

Date of (partial) revision of text March 1997

BETNOVATE*-C OINTMENT

Qualitative and quantitative composition
Betamethasone Valerate BP 0.122% w/w.
Clioquinol BP 3.00% w/w.

Pharmaceutical form Ointment.

Clinical particulars

Therapeutic indications: Betamethasone valerate is an active topical corticosteroid which produces a rapid response in those inflammatory dermatoses that are normally responsive to topical corticosteroid therapy, and is often effective in the less responsive conditions such as psoriasis.

Clioquinol is an anti-infective agent which has both antibacterial and anticandidal activity.

Betnovate-C preparations are indicated for the treatment of the following conditions where secondary bacterial and/or fungal infection is present, suspected, or likely to occur: eczema in children and adults, including atopic and discoid eczemas, prurigo nodularis; psoriasis (excluding widespread plaque psoriasis); neurodermatoses; seborrhoeic dermatitis; contact sensitivity reactions and discoid lupus erythematosus.

Betnovate-C can also be used in the management of secondary infected insect bites and anal and genital intertrigo.

Betnovate-C ointment is often appropriate for dry, lichenified or scaly lesions, but this is not invariably so.

Posology and method of administration: A small quantity of Betnovate should be applied gently to the affected area two or three times daily until improvement occurs. It may then be possible to maintain improvement by applying once a day, or even less often.

Children: Courses should be limited to five days, if possible. Occlusion should not be used.

For topical application.

Contra-indications: Rosacea, acne vulgaris and perioral dermatitis. Primary cutaneous viral infections (e.g. herpes simplex, chickenpox). Hypersensitivity to any component of the preparation or to iodine.

Use of Betnovate-C skin preparations is not indicated in the treatment of primarily infected skin lesions caused by infection with fungi (e.g. candidiasis, tinea); or bacteria (e.g. impetigo); primary or secondary, infections due to yeast; perianal or genital pruritus; dermatoses in children under 1 year of age, including dermatitis and napkin eruptions.

Special warnings and special precautions for use: Long-term continuous topical therapy should be avoided where possible, particularly in infants and children, as adrenal suppression can occur even without occlusion.

The face, more than other areas of the body, may exhibit atrophic changes after prolonged treatment with potent topical corticosteroids. This must be borne in mind when treating such conditions as psoriasis, discoid lupus erythematosus and severe eczema with Betnovate. If applied to the eyelids, care is needed to ensure that the preparation does not enter the eye, as glaucoma might result.

If used in childhood, or on the face, courses should be limited to five days and occlusion should not be used.

Topical corticosteroids may be hazardous in psoriasis for a number of reasons including rebound relapses, development of tolerance, risk of generalised pustular psoriasis and development of local or systemic toxicity due to impaired barrier function of the skin. If used in psoriasis careful patient supervision is important.

If infection persists, systemic chemotherapy is required. Any spread of infection requires withdrawal of topical corticosteroid therapy. Bacterial infection is encouraged by the warm, moist conditions induced by occlusive dressings, and the skin should be cleansed before a fresh dressing is applied.

Do not continue for more than 7 days in the absence of clinical improvement, since occult extension of infection may occur due to the masking effect of the steroid.

Betnovate-C may stain hair, skin or fabric, and the application should be covered with a dressing to protect clothing.

Products which contain antimicrobial agents should not be diluted.

The least potent corticosteroid which will control the disease should be selected. These preparations do not contain lanolin or parabens.

Interaction with other medicaments and other forms of interaction: None.

Pregnancy and lactation: There is inadequate evidence of safety in human pregnancy. Topical administration of corticosteroids to pregnant animals can cause abnormalities of foetal development including cleft palate and intrauterine growth retardation. There may therefore be a very small risk of such effects in the human foetus.

Effects on ability to drive and use machines: None.

Undesirable effects: Prolonged and intensive treatment with highly active corticosteroid preparations may cause local atrophic changes in the skin such as thinning, striae, and dilatation of the superficial blood vessels, particularly when occlusive dressings are used or when skin folds are involved.

As with other topical corticosteroids, prolonged use of large amounts or treatment of extensive areas can result in sufficient systemic absorption to produce the features of hypercorticism and suppression of the HPA axis. These effects are likely to occur in infants and children, and if occlusive dressings are used. In infants the napkin may act as an occlusive dressing.

In rare instances, treatment of psoriasis with corticosteroids (or its withdrawal) is thought to have provoked the pustular form of the disease (see *Precautions*).

There are reports of pigmentation changes and hypertrichosis with topical steroids.

The Betnovate preparations are usually well tolerated, but if signs of hypersensitivity appear, application should be stopped immediately.

Exacerbation of symptoms may occur.

Overdose: Acute overdosage is very unlikely to occur, however, in the case of chronic overdosage or misuse the features of hypercorticism may appear and in this situation topical steroids should be discontinued.

Pharmacological properties
Pharmacodynamic properties: Betamethasone valerate is an active corticosteroid with topical anti-inflammatory activity.

Clioquinol is an anti-infective agent which has both anti-bacterial and anti-candidal activity.

Pharmacokinetic properties: The extent of percutaneous absorption of topical corticosteroid is determined by many factors including the vehicle, the integrity of the epidermal barrier, and the use of occlusive dressings.

Topical corticosteroids can be absorbed from normal intact skin. Inflammation and/or other disease processes in the skin increase percutaneous absorption. Occlusive dressings substantially increase the percutaneous absorption of topical corticosteroids.

Once absorbed through the skin, topical corticosteroids are handled through pharmacokinetic pathways similar to systematically administered corticosteroids. Corticosteroids are bound to plasma proteins in varying degrees. Corticosteroids are metabolised primarily by the liver and are then excreted by the kidneys.

Preclinical safety data: There are no preclinical data of relevance to the prescriber which are additional to that in other sections of the SmPC.

Pharmaceutical particulars
List of excipients: Liquid Paraffin BP, White Soft Paraffin BP.

Incompatibilities: None known.

Shelf life: 36 months.

Special precautions for storage: Store below 30°C.

Nature and contents of container: 15 gm and 30 gm collapsible aluminium tubes coated with an epoxy resin based lacquer with an aluminium membrane seal and a polyethylene cap.

Instructions for use/handling: No special instructions.

Marketing authorisation number PL 10949/0017

Date of first authorisation/renewal of authorisation 24/10/97

Date of (partial) revision of text October 1997

BETNOVATE* CREAM

Qualitative and quantitative composition Betamethasone Valerate BP 0.122% w/w.

Pharmaceutical form Aqueous Cream.

Clinical particulars
Therapeutic indications: Betamethasone valerate is an active topical corticosteroid which produces a rapid response in those inflammatory dermatoses that are normally responsive to topical corticosteroid therapy, and is often effective in the less responsive conditions such as psoriasis.

Betnovate preparations are indicated for the treatment of eczema in children and adults, including atopic and discoid eczemas, prurigo nodularis, psoriasis (excluding widespread plaque psoriasis); neurodermatoses, including lichen simplex, lichen planus; seborrhoeic dermatitis; contact sensitivity reactions; discoid lupus erythematosus and they may be used as an adjunct to systemic steroid therapy in generalised erythroderma.

Posology and method of administration: A small quantity of Betnovate should be applied gently to the affected area two or three times daily until improvement occurs. It may then be possible to maintain improvement by applying once a day, or even less often, or by using the appropriate ready-diluted (1 in 4) preparation Betnovate RD. If no improvement is seen within two to four weeks, reassessment of the diagnosis, or referral, may be necessary.

Betnovate and Betnovate RD creams are especially appropriate for dry, lichenified or scaly lesions, but this is not invariably so.

In the more recent resistant lesions, such as the thickened plaques of psoriasis on elbows and knees, the effect of Betnovate can be enhanced, if necessary, by occluding the treatment area with polythene film. Overnight occlusion only is usually adequate to bring about a satisfactory response in such lesions; thereafter improvement can usually be maintained by regular application without occlusion.

Children: Courses should be limited to five days. Occlusion should not be used.

For topical administration.

Contra-indications: Rosacea, acne and perioral dermatitis. Primary cutaneous viral infections (e.g. herpes simplex, chickenpox). Hypersensitivity to any component of the preparation.

The use of Betnovate skin preparations is not indicated in the treatment of primarily infected skin lesions caused by infections with fungi (e.g. candidiasis, tinea); or bacteria (e.g. impetigo); primary or secondary infections due to yeast; peri-anal and genital pruritus; dermatoses in children under 1 year of age, including dermatitis and napkin eruptions.

Special warnings and precautions for use: Long-term continuous topical therapy should be avoided where possible, particularly in infants and children, as adrenal suppression can occur even without occlusion.

The face, more than other areas of the body, may exhibit atrophic changes after prolonged treatment with potent topical corticosteroids. This must be borne in mind when treating such conditions as psoriasis, discoid lupus erythematosus and severe eczema. If applied to the eyelids, care is needed to ensure that the preparation does not enter the eye, as glaucoma might result.

If used in childhood, or on the face, courses should be limited to five days and occlusion should not be used.

Topical corticosteroids may be hazardous in psoriasis for a number of reasons including rebound relapses, development of tolerance, risk of generalised pustular psoriasis and development of local or systemic toxicity due to impaired barrier function of the skin. If used in psoriasis careful patient supervision is important.

Appropriate antimicrobial therapy should be used whenever treating inflammatory lesions which have become infected. Any spread of infection requires withdrawal of topical corticosteroid therapy and systemic administration of antimicrobial agents. Bacterial infection is encouraged by the warm, moist conditions induced by occlusive dressings, and so the skin should be cleansed before a fresh dressing is applied.

Further information: The least potent corticosteroid which will control the disease should be selected. None of these preparations contain lanolin. Betnovate Cream and Ointment and the corresponding RD preparations do not contain parabens. Betnovate Lotion contains parabens.

Interaction with other medicaments and other forms of interaction: None known.

Pregnancy and lactation: There is inadequate evidence of safety in human pregnancy. Topical administration of corticosteroids to pregnant animals can cause abnormalities of foetal development including cleft palate and intra-uterine growth retardation. There may therefore be a very small risk of such effects in the human foetus.

Effects on ability to drive and use machines: None known.

Undesirable effects: Prolonged and intensive treatment with highly active corticosteroid preparations may cause local atrophic changes in the skin such as thinning, striae, and dilatation of the superficial blood vessels, particularly when occlusive dressings are used or when skin folds are involved.

As with other topical corticosteroids, prolonged use of large amounts or treatment of extensive areas can result in sufficient systemic absorption to produce the features of hypercorticism and suppression of the HPA axis. These effects are likely to occur in infants and children, and if occlusive dressings are used. In infants the napkin may act as an occlusive dressing.

There are reports of pigmentation changes and hypertrichosis with topical steroids.

In rare instances, treatment of psoriasis with corticosteroids (or its withdrawal) is thought to have provoked the pustular form of the disease (see *Precautions*).

The Betnovate and Betnovate RD preparations are usually well tolerated, but if signs of hypersensitivity appear, application should be stopped immediately.

Exacerbation of symptoms may occur.

Overdose: Acute overdosage is very unlikely to occur, however, in the case of chronic overdosage or misuse the features of hypercorticism may appear and in this situation topical steroids should be discontinued.

Pharmacological properties
Pharmacodynamic properties: Betamethasone valerate is an active corticosteroid with topical anti-inflammatory activity.

Pharmacokinetic properties: The extent of percutaneous absorption of topical corticosteroid is determined by many factors including the vehicle, the integrity of the epidermal barrier, and the use of occlusive dressings.

Topical corticosteroids can be absorbed from normal intact skin. Inflammation and/or other disease processes in the skin increase percutaneous absorption. Occlusive dressings on the skin increase percutaneous absorption. Occlusive dressings substantially increase the percutaneous absorption of topical corticosteroids.

Once absorbed through the skin, topical corticosteroids are handled through pharmacokinetic pathways similar to systematically administered corticosteroids. Corticosteroids are bound to plasma proteins in varying degrees. Corticosteroids are metabolised primarily by the liver and are then excreted by the kidneys.

Preclinical safety data: There are no preclinical data of relevance to the prescriber which are additional to that in other sections of the SmPC.

Pharmaceutical particulars
List of excipients: Chlorocresol BP, Cetomacrogol 1000 BP, Cetostearyl Alcohol BP, White Soft Paraffin BP, Liquid Paraffin BP, Sodium Acid Phosphate BP, Phosphoric Acid BP, Sodium Hydroxide BP, Purified Water BP.

Incompatibilities: None known.

Shelf life: Tubes: 36 months. 500 gm pots: 18 months.

Special precautions for storage: Store below 25°C.

Nature and contents of container: 15 gm, 30 gm and 100 gm collapsible aluminium tubes internally coated with an epoxy resin based lacquer and closed with a cap.

500 mg opaque high density polythene pots with black urea formaldehyde screw caps having a steran faced wad.

Instructions for use/handling: No special instructions.

Marketing authorisation number PL 10949/0014

Date of first authorisation/renewal of authorisation
MAA: 01/02/93
Renewal: 24/10/97

Date of (partial) revision of text October 1997

BETNOVATE* CREAM PUMP

Qualitative and quantitative composition Betamethasone Valerate BP 0.122% w/w.

Pharmaceutical form Cream.

Clinical particulars
Therapeutic indications: Betamethasone valerate is an active topical corticosteroid which produces a rapid response in those inflammatory dermatoses that are normally responsive to topical corticosteroid therapy, and is often effective in the less responsive conditions such as psoriasis.

Betnovate preparations are indicated for the treatment of: eczema in children and adults; including atopic and discoid eczemas; prurigo nodularis; psoriasis (excluding widespread plaque psoriasis); neurodermatoses, including lichen simplex, lichen planus; seborrhoeic dermatitis; contact sensitivity reactions; discoid lupus erythematosus and they may be used as an adjunct to systemic steroid therapy in generalised erythroderma.

Posology and method of administration: A small quantity of Betnovate should be applied to the affected area two or three times daily until improvement occurs. It may then be possible to maintain improvement by applying once a day, or even less often, or by using the appropriate ready-diluted (1 in 4) preparation Betnovate RD. If no improvement is seen within two or four weeks, reassessment of the diagnosis, or referral, may be necessary.

Betnovate and Betnovate RD ointments are especially appropriate for dry, lichenified scaly lesions, but this is not invariably so.

In the more resistant lesions, such as the thickened plaques of psoriasis on elbows and knees, the effect of Betnovate can be enhanced, if necessary, by occluding the treatment area with polythene film. Overnight occlusion only is usually adequate to bring about a satisfactory response in such lesions; thereafter improvement can usually be maintained by regular application without occlusion.

Children: Courses should be limited to five days if possible. Occlusion should not be used.

Contra-indications: Rosacea, acne vulgaris and perioral dermatitis. Primary cutaneous viral infections (e.g. herpes simplex, chickenpox). Hypersensitivity to the preparation. The use of Betnovate skin preparations is not indicated in the treatment of primarily infected skin lesions caused by infection with fungi (e.g. candidiasis, tinea), or bacteria (e.g. impetigo); primary or secondary infections due to yeast; perianal and genital pruritus; dermatoses in children under 1 year of age, including dermatitis and napkin eruptions.

Special warnings and special precautions for use: Long-term continuous topical therapy should be avoided where possible, particularly in infants and children, as adrenal suppression can occur even without occlusion.

The face, more than other areas of the body, may exhibit atrophic changes after prolonged treatment with potent topical corticosteroids. This must be borne in mind when treating such conditions as psoriasis, discoid lupus erythematosus and severe eczema. If applied to the eyelids, care is needed to ensure that the preparation does not enter the eye, as glaucoma might result.

If used in childhood or on the face, courses should be limited if possible to five days and occlusion should not be used.

Topical corticosteroids may be hazardous in psoriasis for a number of reasons including rebound relapses, development of tolerance, risk of generalised pustular psoriasis and development of local or systemic toxicity due to impaired barrier function of the skin. If used in psoriasis careful patient supervision is important.

Appropriate antimicrobial therapy should be used whenever treating inflammatory lesions which have become infected. Any spread of infection requires withdrawal of topical corticosteroid therapy and systemic administration of antimicrobial agents. Bacterial infection is encouraged by the warm, moist conditions induced by occlusive dressings, and so the skin should be cleansed before a fresh dressing is applied.

In rare instances, treatment of psoriasis with corticosteroids (or its withdrawal) is thought to have provoked the pustular form of the disease. Betnovate RD is usually well tolerated but if signs of hypersentivity appear, application should stop immediately.

Interaction with other medicaments and other forms of interaction: None known.

Pregnancy and lactation: Avoid extensive use in pregnancy. There is inadequate evidence of safety. Topical administration of corticosteroids to pregnant animals can cause abnormalities of foetal development including cleft palate and intrauterine growth retardation. There may therefore be a very small risk of such effects in the human foetus.

Effects on ability to drive and use machines: None known.

Undesirable effects: Prolonged and intensive treatment with highly active corticosteroid preparations may cause local atrophic changes in the skin such as striae, thinning, and dilatation of the superficial blood vessels, particularly when occlusive dressings are used or when skin folds are involved.

As with other topical corticosteroids, prolonged use of large amounts or treatment of extensive areas can result in sufficient systemic absorption to produce the features of hypercorticism and suppression of the HPA axis. These effects are likely to occur in infants and children, and if occlusive dressings are used. In infants the napkin may act as an occlusive dressing.

There are reports of pigmentation changes and hypertrichosis with topical steroids. In rare instances, treatment of psoriasis with corticosteroids (or its withdrawal) is thought to have provoked the pustular form of the disease (see *Precautions*).

The Betnovate and Betnovate RD preparations are usually well tolerated, but if signs of hypersensitivity appear, application should stop immediately.

Exacerbation of symptoms may occur.

Overdose: Acute overdosage is very unlikely to occur, however, in the case of chronic overdosage or misuse the features of hypercorticism may appear and in this situation topical steroids should be discontinued.

Pharmacological properties
Pharmacodynamic properties: Betamethasone is a corticosteroid with topical anti-inflammatory activity.

Pharmacokinetic properties: The extent of percutaneous absorption of topical corticosteroid is determined by many factors including the vehicle, the integrity of the epidermal barrier, and the use of occlusive dressings.

Topical corticosteroids can be absorbed from normal intact skin. Inflammation and/or other disease processes in the skin increase percutaneous absorption of topical corticosteroids.

Once absorbed through the skin, topical corticosteroids are handled through pharmacokinetic pathways similar to systematically administered corticosteroids. Corticosteroids are metabolised primarily by the liver and are then excreted by the kidneys.

Preclinical safety data: No additional data of relevance.

Pharmaceutical particulars
List of excipients: Cetostearyl Alcohol BP, Cetomacrogol 1000 BP, White Soft Paraffin BP, Liquid Paraffin BP, Chlorocresol BP, Sodium Acid Phosphate BP, Phosphoric Acid BP, Sodium Hydroxide BP, Purified Water BP.

Incompatibilities: None known.

Shelf life: 18 months.

Special precautions for storage: Store below 25°C.

Nature and contents of container: 100 gm pump dispenser pack. Polypropylene/polyethylene pump dispenser with translucent polypropylene body. Nozzle is sealed with a polyethylene/acetal tab. Pump is closed with a white opaque polypropylene overcap and overwrapped with a white opaque shrink wrap.

Instructions for use/handling: No special instructions.

Marketing authorisation number PL 10949/0128

Date of first authorisation/renewal of authorisation 1st December 1993

Date of (partial) revision of text June 1996

BETNOVATE* LOTION

Qualitative and quantitative composition Betamethasone Valerate 0.122% w/w.

Pharmaceutical form Lotion.

Clinical particulars
Therapeutic indications: Betamethasone valerate is an active topical corticosteroid which produces a rapid response in those inflammatory dermatoses that are normally responsive to topical corticosteroid therapy, and is often effective in the less responsive conditions such as psoriasis.

Betnovate preparations are indicated for the treatment of: eczema in children and adults; including atopic and discoid eczemas, prurigo nodularis; psoriasis (excluding widespread plaque psoriasis); neurodermatoses, including lichen simplex, lichen planus, seborrhoeic dermatitis; contact sensitivity reactions; discoid lupus erythematosus and they may be used as an adjunct to systemic steroid therapy in generalised erythroderma.

Posology and method of administration: A small quantity of Betnovate should be applied to the affected area two or three times daily until improvement occurs. It may then be possible to maintain improvement by applying once a day, or even less often. If no improvement is seen within two to four weeks, reassessment of the diagnosis or referral, may be necessary.

Betnovate lotion is particularly suitable when a minimal application to a large area is required.

In the more resistant lesions, such as the thickened plaques of psoriasis on elbows and knees, the effect of Betnovate can be enhanced, if necessary, by occluding the treatment area with polythene film. Overnight occlusion only is usually adequate to bring about a satisfactory response in such lesions. Thereafter improvement can usually be maintained by regular application without occlusion.

Children: Courses should be limited to five days if possible. Occlusion should not be used.

Contra-indications: Rosacea, acne vulgaris and perioral dermatitis. Primary cutaneous viral infections (e.g. herpes simplex, chickenpox). Hypersensitivity to the preparation.

The use of Betnovate skin preparations is not indicated in the treatment of primarily infected skin lesions caused by infection with fungi (e.g. candidiasis, tinea); or bacteria (e.g. impetigo); primary or secondary infections due to yeast; perianal and genital pruritus; dermatoses in children under 1 year of age, including dermatitis and napkin eruptions.

Special warnings and precautions for use: Long-term continuous topical therapy should be avoided where possible, particularly in infants and children, as adrenal suppression can occur even without occlusion.

The face, more than other areas of the body, may exhibit atrophic changes after prolonged treatment with potent topical corticosteroids. This must be borne in mind when treating such conditions as psoriasis, discoid lupus erythematosus and severe eczema. If applied to the eyelids, care is needed to ensure that the preparation does not enter the eye, as glaucoma might result.

If used in childhood, or on the face, courses should be limited if possible to five days and occlusion should not be used.

Topical corticosteroids may be hazardous in psoriasis for a number of reasons including rebound relapses, development of tolerance, risk of generalised pustular psoriasis and development of local or systemic toxicity due to impaired barrier function of the skin. If used in psoriasis careful patient supervision is important.

Appropriate antimicrobial therapy should be used whenever treating inflammatory lesions which have become infected. Any spread of infection requires withdrawal of topical corticosteroid therapy and systemic administration of antimicrobial agents.

Bacterial infection is encouraged by the warm moist conditions induced by occlusive dressings and so the skin should be cleansed before a fresh dressing is applied.

Further information: The least potent corticosteroid which will control the disease should be selected. None of these preparations contain lanolin. Betnovate cream and ointment and the corresponding RD preparations do not contain parabens. Betnovate lotion contains parabens.

Interaction with other medicaments and other forms of interaction: None known.

Pregnancy and lactation: There is inadequate evidence of safety in human pregnancy. Topical administration of corticosteroids to pregnant animals can cause abnormalities of foetal development including cleft palate and intrauterine growth retardation. There may therefore be a very small risk of such effects in the human foetus.

Effect on ability to drive and use machines: None known.

Undesirable effects: Prolonged and intensive treatment with highly active corticosteroid preparations may cause local atrophic changes in the skin such as thinning, striae and dilatation of the superficial blood vessels, particularly when occlusive dressings are used or when skin folds are involved.

As with other topical corticosteroids, prolonged use of large amounts or treatment of extensive areas can result in sufficient systemic absorption to produce features of hypercorticism and suppression of the HPA Axis. These effects are likely to occur in infants and children, and if occlusive dressings are used. In infants the napkin may act as an occlusive dressing.

In rare instances, treatment of psoriasis with corticosteroids (or its withdrawal) is thought to have provoked the pustular form of the disease (see *Precautions*).

There are reports of pigmentation changes and hypertrichosis with topical steroids.

The Betnovate and Betnovate RD preparations are usually well tolerated, but if signs of hypersensitivity appear, application should stop immediately.

Exacerbation of symptoms may occur.

Overdose: Acute overdosage is very unlikely to occur, however, in the case of chronic overdosage or misuse the features of hypercorticism may appear and in this situation topical steroids should be discontinued.

Pharmacological properties
Pharmacodynamic properties: Betamethasone valerate is an active corticosteroid with topical anti-inflammatory activity.

Pharmacokinetic properties: The extent of percutaneous absorption of topical corticosteroid is determined by many factors including the vehicle, the integrity of the epidermal barrier, and the use of occlusive dressings.

Topical corticosteroids can be absorbed from normal intact skin. Inflammation and/or other disease processes in the skin increase percutaneous absorption. Occlusive dressings substantially increase the percutaneous absorption of topical corticosteroids.

Once absorbed through the skin, topical corticosteroids are handled through pharmacokinetic pathways similar to systemically administered corticosteroids. Corticosteroids are bound to plasma proteins in varying degrees. Corticosteroids are metabolised primarily by the liver and are then excreted by the kidneys.

Preclinical safety data: There are no preclinical data of relevance to the prescriber which are additional to that in other sections of the SmPC.

Pharmaceutical particulars
List of excipients: Methyl Hydroxybenzoate BP, Xanthan Gum USP, Cetostearyl Alcohol BP, Liquid Paraffin BP, Isopropyl Alcohol BP, Glycerol BP, Cetomacrogol 1000 BP, Sodium citrate BP, Citric Acid Monohydrate BP, Purified Water BP.

Incompatibilities: None known.

Shelf life: 36 months.

Special precautions for storage: Store below 25°C.

Nature and contents of container: Polythene squeeze bottle with a polythene nozzle and a polystyrene or polyethylene cap.

Pack size: 20 ml; 100 ml.

Instructions for use/handling: No special instructions.

Marketing authorisation number PL 10949/0044

Date of first authorisation/renewal of authorisation 10/9/97

Date of (partial) revision of text March 1997

BETNOVATE*-N CREAM

Qualitative and quantitative composition
Betamethasone Valerate BP 0.122% w/w.
Neomycin Sulphate BP 0.5% w/w.

Pharmaceutical form Aqueous Cream.

Clinical particulars
Therapeutic indications: Betamethasone valerate is an active topical corticosteroid which produces a rapid response in those inflammatory dermatoses that are normally responsive to topical corticosteroid therapy, and is often effective in the less responsive conditions such as psoriasis.

Neomycin Sulphate is a broad-spectrum, bacterial antibiotic effective against the majority of bacteria commonly associated with skin infections.

Betnovate-N preparations are indicated for the treatment of the following conditions where secondary bacterial infection is present, suspected, or likely to occur: eczema in children and adults, including atopic and discoid eczemas, prurigo nodularis; psoriasis (excluding widespread plaque psoriasis); neurodermatoses; seborrhoeic dermatitis; contact sensitivity reactions and they may be used as an adjunct to systemic steroid therapy in generalised erythroderma.

Betnovate-N preparations can also be used in the management of secondarily infected insect bites and anal and genital intertrigo.

Betnovate-N Cream is especially appropriate for moist or weeping surfaces, and Betnovate-N Ointment for dry lichenified or scaly lesions, but this is not invariably so.

Posology and method of administration: A small quantity should be applied gently to the affected area two or three times daily until improvement occurs. It may then be possible to maintain improvement by applying once a day or even less often.

Children: Betnovate-N is suitable for use in children at the same dose as adults, but the dose should be reduced for use in infants.

Betnovate-N is not recommended for use in neonates (see *Precautions*).

Courses should be limited to five days. Occlusion should not be used.

For topical administration.

Contra-indications: Rosacea, acne vulgaris and perioral dermatitis. Primary cutaneous viral infections (e.g. herpes simplex, chickenpox). Hypersensitivity to any component of the preparation.

Application to large areas especially during pregnancy, in the elderly and in patients with impaired renal function due to a risk of ototoxicity.

A possibility of increased absorption exists in very young children thus Betnovate-N is not recommended for use in neonates.

Use of Betnovate-N skin preparations is not indicated in the treatment of primarily infected skin lesions caused by infection with fungi (e.g. candidiasis, tinea), or bacteria (e.g. impetigo), primary or secondary infections due to yeast; secondary infections due to pseudomonas or proteus species; perianal and genital pruritus; dermatoses in children under 1 year of age, including dermatitis and napkin eruptions.

Preparations containing neomycin should not be used for the treatment of otitis externa when the ear drum is perforated, because of the risk of ototoxicity.

Special warnings and precautions for use: Long-term continuous topical therapy should be avoided where possible, particularly in infants and children, as adrenal suppression can occur even without occlusion.

The face, more than other areas of the body, may exhibit atrophic changes after prolonged treatment with potent topical corticosteroids. This must be borne in mind when treating such conditions as psoriasis, discoid lupus erythematosus and severe eczema with Betnovate. If applied to the eyelids, care is needed to ensure that the preparation does not enter the eye, as glaucoma might result.

If used in childhood, or on the face, courses should be limited to five days and occlusion should not be used.

Topical corticosteroids may be hazardous in psoriasis for a number of reasons including rebound relapses, development of tolerance, risk of generalised pustular psoriasis and development of local or systemic toxicity due to impaired barrier function of the skin. If used in psoriasis careful patient supervision is important.

Do not continue for more than 7 days in the absence of clinical improvement, since occult extension of infection may occur due to the masking effect of the steroid. If bacterial infection persists, systemic chemotherapy is required. Any spread of infection requires withdrawal of topical corticosteroid therapy. Bacterial infection is encouraged by the warm, moist conditions induced by occlusive dressings, and the skin should be cleansed before a fresh dressing is applied.

In neonates and infants, absorption by immature skins may be enhanced and renal function may be immature (see *Contra-indications*).

Extended or recurrent application may increase the risk of contact sensitisation.

Products which contain antimicrobial agents should not be diluted.

Interaction with other medicaments and other forms of interaction: None known.

Pregnancy and lactation: There is little information to demonstrate the possible effect of topically applied neomycin in pregnancy and lactation. However, neomycin present in maternal blood can cross the placenta and may give rise to a theoretical risk of foetal toxicity, thus use of Betnovate-N is not recommended in pregnancy or lactation.

Effects on ability to drive and use machines: None known.

Undesirable effects: Prolonged and intensive treatment with highly active corticosteroid preparations may cause local atrophic changes in the skin such as thinning, striae, and dilatation of the superficial blood vessels, particularly when occlusive dressings are used or when skin folds are involved.

As with other topical corticosteroids, prolonged use of large amounts or treatment of extensive areas can result in sufficient systemic absorption to produce the features of hypercorticism and suppression of the HPA axis. These effects are likely to occur in infants and children, and if occlusive dressings are used. In infants the napkin may act as an occlusive dressing.

In rare instances, treatment of psoriasis with corticosteroids (or its withdrawal) is thought to have provoked the pustular form of the disease (see *Precautions*).

There are reports of pigmentation changes and hypertrichosis with topical steroids.

The Betnovate preparations are usually well tolerated, but if signs of hypersensitivity appear, application should be stopped immediately.

Exacerbation of symptoms may occur.

Overdose: Acute overdosage is very unlikely to occur, however, in the case of chronic overdosage or misuse the features of hypercorticism may appear and in this situation topical steroids should be discontinued.

Pharmacological properties

Pharmacodynamic properties: Betamethasone valerate is an active corticosteroid which produces a rapid response in those inflammatory dermatoses that are normally responsive to topical corticosteroid therapy, and is often effective in the less responsive conditions such as psoriasis.

Neomycin sulphate is a broad spectrum, bactericidal antibiotic effective against the majority of bacteria commonly associated with skin infections.

Pharmacokinetic properties: The extent of percutaneous absorption of topical corticosteroid is determined by many factors including the vehicle, the integrity of the epidermal barrier, and the use of occlusive dressings.

Topical corticosteroids can be absorbed from normal intact skin. Inflammation and/or other disease processes in the skin increase percutaneous absorption. Occlusive dressings substantially increase the percutaneous absorption of topical corticosteroids.

Once absorbed through the skin, topical corticosteroids are handled through pharmacokinetic pathways similar to systematically administered corticosteroids. Corticosteroids are bound to plasma proteins in varying degrees. Corticosteroids are metabolised primarily by the liver and are then excreted by the kidneys.

Preclinical safety data: There are no preclinical data of relevance to the prescriber which are additional to that in other sections of the SmPC.

Pharmaceutical particulars

List of excipients: Chlorocresol BP, Cetomacrogol 1000 BP, Cetostearyl Alcohol BP, White Soft Paraffin BP, Liquid Paraffin BP, Sodium Acid Phosphate BP, Phosphoric Acid BP, Sodium Hydroxide BP, Purified Water BP.

Incompatibilities: None known.

Shelf life: 36 months.

Special precautions for storage: Store below 25°C.

Nature and contents of container: 15 gm, 30 gm and 100 gm collapsible aluminium tubes internally coated with an epoxy resin based lacquer and closed with a wadless polypropylene cap.

Instructions for use/handling: No special instructions.

Marketing authorisation number PL 10949/0018

Date of first authorisation/renewal of authorisation 1 March 1993

Date of (partial) revision of text October 1997

BETNOVATE*-N OINTMENT

Qualitative and quantitative composition
Betamethasone Valerate BP 0.122% w/w.
Neomycin Sulphate BP 0.5% w/w.

Pharmaceutical form Ointment.

Clinical particulars

Therapeutic indications: Betamethasone valerate is an active topical corticosteroid which produces a rapid response in those inflammatory dermatoses that are normally responsive to topical corticosteroid therapy, and is often effective in the less responsive conditions such as psoriasis.

Neomycin Sulphate is a broad-spectrum, bactericidal antibiotic effective against the majority of bacteria commonly associated with skin infections.

Betnovate preparations are indicated for the treatment of the following conditions where secondary bacterial infection is present, suspected or likely to occur: eczema in children and adults, including atopic and discoid eczema, prurigo nodularis; psoriasis (excluding widespread plaque psoriasis); neurodermatoses; seborrhoeic dermatitis; contact sensitivity reactions and they may be used as an adjunct to systemic steroid therapy in generalised erythroderma.

Betnovate-N preparations can also be used in the management of secondarily infected insect bites and anal and genital intertrigo.

Betnovate-N ointment is especially appropriate for dry, lichenified or scaly lesions, but this is not invariably so.

Posology and method of administration: A small quantity should be applied gently to the affected area two or three times daily until improvement occurs. It may then be possible to maintain improvement by applying once a day, or even less often.

Betnovate-N is suitable for use in children at the same dose as adults, but the dose should be reduced for use in infants. Betnovate-N is not recommended for use in neonates (see *Precautions*).

Children: Courses should be limited to five days, if possible. Occlusion should not be used.

For topical application.

Contra-indications: Rosacea, acne vulgaris and perioral dermatitis. Primary cutaneous viral infections (e.g. herpes simplex, chickenpox). Hypersensitivity to any component of the preparation.

Application to large areas especially during pregnancy, in the elderly and in patients with impaired renal function due to a risk of ototoxicity.

A possibility of increased absorption exists in very young children thus Betnovate-N is not recommended for use in neonates.

Use of Betnovate-N skin preparations is not indicated in the treatment of primarily infected skin lesions caused by infection with fungi (e.g. candidiasis, tinea); or bacteria (e.g. impetigo); primary or secondary, infections due to yeast; secondary infections due to pseudomonas or proteus species; perianal and genital pruritus; dermatoses in children under 1 year of age, including dermatitis and napkin eruptions.

Preparations containing neomycin should not be used for the treatment of otitis externa when the ear drum is perforated, because of the risk of ototoxicity.

Special warnings and precautions for use: Long-term continuous topical therapy should be avoided where possible, particularly in infants and children, as adrenal suppression can occur even without occlusion.

The face, more than other areas of the body, may exhibit atrophic changes after prolonged treatment with potent topical corticosteroids. This must be borne in mind when treating such conditions as psoriasis, discoid lupus erythematosus and severe eczema. If applied to the eyelids, care is needed to ensure that the preparation does not enter the eye, as glaucoma might result.

If used in childhood, or on the face, courses should be limited to five days and occlusion should not be used.

Topical corticosteroids may be hazardous in psoriasis for a number of reasons including rebound relapses, development of tolerance, risk of generalised pustular psoriasis and development of local or systemic toxicity due to impaired barrier function of the skin. If used in psoriasis careful patient supervision is important.

Do not continue for more than 7 days in the absence of clinical improvement, since occult extension of infection may occur due to the masking effect of the steroid. If bacterial infection persists, systemic chemotherapy is required. Any spread of infection requires withdrawal of topical corticosteroid therapy. Bacterial infection is encouraged by the warm, moist conditions induced by occlusive dressings, and the skin should be cleansed before a fresh dressing is applied.

In neonates and infants absorption by immature skins may be enhanced and renal function may be immature (see *Contra-indications*).

Extended or recurrent application may increase the risk of contact sensitisation.

Products which contain antimicrobial agents should not be diluted.

Interaction with other medicaments and other forms of interaction: None known.

Pregnancy and lactation: There is little information to demonstrate the possible effect of topically applied neomycin in pregnancy and lactation. However, neomycin present in maternal blood can cross the placenta and may give rise to a theoretical risk of foetal toxicity, thus use of Betnovate-N is not recommended in pregnancy or lactation.

Effects on ability to drive and use machines: None known.

Undesirable effects: Prolonged and intensive treatment with highly active corticosteroid preparations may cause local atrophic changes in the skin such as thinning, striae, and dilatation of the superficial blood vessels, particularly when occlusive dressings are used or when skin folds are involved.

As with other topical corticosteroids, prolonged use of large amounts or treatment of extensive areas can result in sufficient systemic absorption to produce the features of hypercorticism and suppression of the HPA axis. These effects are likely to occur in infants and children, and if occlusive dressings are used. In infants the napkin may act as an occlusive dressing.

In rare instances, treatment of psoriasis with corticosteroids (or its withdrawal) is thought to have provoked the pustular form of the disease (see *Precautions*). There are reports of pigmentation changes and hypertrichosis with topical steroids.

The Betnovate preparations are usually well tolerated, but if signs of hypersensitivity appear, application should be stopped immediately.

Exacerbation of symptoms may occur.

Overdose: Acute overdosage is very unlikely to occur, however, in the case of chronic overdosage or misuse the features of hypercorticism may appear and in this situation topical steroids should be discontinued.

Pharmacological properties

Pharmacodynamic properties: Betamethasone valerate is a corticosteroid with topical anti-inflammatory activity.

Pharmacokinetic properties: The extent of percutaneous absorption of topical corticosteroids is determined by many factors including the vehicle, the integrity of the epidermal barrier, and the use of occlusive dressings.

Topical corticosteroids can be absorbed from normal intact skin. Inflammation and/or other disease processes in the skin increase percutaneous absorption. Occlusive dressings substantially increase the percutaneous absorption of topical corticosteroids.

Once absorbed through the skin, topical corticosteroids are handled through pharmacokinetic pathways similar to systematically administered corticosteroids. Corticosteroids are bound to plasma proteins in varying degrees. Corticosteroids are metabolised primarily by the liver and are then excreted by the kidneys.

Preclinical safety data: There are no preclinical data of relevance to the prescriber which are additional to that in other sections of the SmPC.

Pharmaceutical particulars

List of excipients: Liquid Paraffin BP, White Soft Paraffin BP.

Incompatibilities: None known.

Shelf life: 36 months.

Special precautions for storage: Store at temperatures not exceeding 30°C.

Nature and contents of container: 15 gm, 30 gm and 100 gm collapsible aluminium tubes internally coated with an epoxy resin based lacquer and closed with a wadless polypropylene cap.

Instructions for use/handling: No special instructions.

Marketing authorisation number PL 10949/0019

Date of first authorisation/renewal of authorisation 3/12/97

Date of (partial) revision of text December 1997

BETNOVATE* OINTMENT

Qualitative and quantitative composition Betamethasone Valerate BP 0.122% w/w.

Pharmaceutical form Ointment.

Clinical particulars

Therapeutic indications: Betamethasone valerate is an active topical corticosteroid which provides a rapid response in those inflammatory dermatoses that are often effective in the less responsive conditions such as psoriasis.

Betnovate preparations are indicated for the treatment of: eczema in children and adults; including atopic and discoid eczemas, prurigo nodularis; psoriasis (excluding widespread plaque psoriasis); neurodermatoses, including lichen simplex, lichen planus; seborrhoeic dermatitis; contact sensitivity reactions; discoid lupus erythematosus and they may be used as an adjunct to systemic steroid therapy in generalised erythroderma.

Posology and method of administration: A small quantity of Betnovate should be applied to the affected area two or three times daily until improvement occurs. It may then be possible to maintain improvement by applying once a day, or even less often, or by using the appropriate ready diluted (1 in 4) preparation, Betnovate RD. If no improvement is seen within two to four weeks, reassessment of the diagnosis, or referral, may be necessary.

Betnovate and Betnovate RD ointments are especially appropriate for dry, lichenified or scaly lesions, but this is not invariably so.

In the more resistant lesions, such as the thickened plaques of psoriasis on elbows and knees, the effect of Betnovate can be enhanced, if necessary, by occluding the treatment area with polythene film. Overnight occlusion only is usually adequate to bring about a satisfactory response in such lesions; thereafter improvement can usually be maintained by regular application without occlusion.

Children: Courses should be limited to five days if possible. Occlusion should not be used.

For topical application.

Contra-indications: Rosacea, acne vulgaris, perioral dermatitis, primary cutaneous viral infections (e.g. herpes simplex, chickenpox). Hypersensitivity to the preparation.

The use of Betnovate skin preparations is not indicated in the treatment of primarily infected skin lesions caused by infections with fungi (e.g. candidiasis, tinea); or bacteria (e.g. impetigo); primary or secondary infections due to yeast; peri-anal and genital pruritus; dermatoses in children under 1 year of age, including dermatitis and napkin eruptions.

Special warnings and special precautions for use: Long-term continuous topical therapy should be avoided where possible, particularly in infants and children, as adrenal suppression can occur even without occlusion.

The face, more than other areas of the body, may exhibit atrophic changes after prolonged treatment with potent topical corticosteroids. This must be borne in mind when treating such conditions as psoriasis, discoid lupus erythematosus and severe eczema. If applied to the eyelids, care is needed to ensure that the preparation does not enter the eye, as glaucoma might result.

If used in childhood, or on the face, courses should be limited if possible to five days and occlusion should not be used.

Topical corticosteroids may be hazardous in psoriasis for a number of reasons including rebound relapses, development of tolerance, risk of generalised postural psoriasis and development of local or systemic toxicity due to impaired barrier function of the skin. If used in psoriasis careful patient supervision is important.

Appropriate antimicrobial therapy should be used whenever treating inflammatory lesions which have become infected. Any spread of infection requires withdrawal of topical corticosteroid therapy and systemic administration of antimicrobial agents. Bacterial infection is encouraged by the warm, moist conditions induced by occlusive dressings, and so the skin should be cleansed before a fresh dressing is applied.

Interaction with other medicaments and other forms of interaction: None known.

Pregnancy and lactation: There is inadequate evidence of safety in human pregnancy. Topical administration of corticosteroids to pregnant animals can cause abnormalities of foetal development including cleft palate and intrauterine growth retardation. There may therefore be a very small risk of such effects in the human foetus.

Effects on ability to drive and use machines: None known.

Undesirable effects: Prolonged and intensive treatment with highly active corticosteroid preparations may cause local atrophic changes in the skin such as thinning, striae, and dilatation of the superficial blood vessels, particularly when occlusive dressings are used or when skin folds are involved.

As with other topical corticosteroids, prolonged use of large amounts or treatment of extensive areas can result in sufficient systemic absorption to produce the features of hypercorticism and suppression of the HPA axis. These effects are likely to occur in infants and children and if occlusive dressings are used. In infants the napkin may act as an occlusive dressing.

In rare instances, treatment of psoriasis with corticosteroids (or its withdrawal) is thought to have provoked the pustular form of the disease (see *Precautions*).

There are reports of pigmentation changes and hypertrichosis with topical steroids. The Betnovate and Betnovate RD preparations are usually well tolerated, but if signs of hypersensitivity appear, application should stop immediately.

Exacerbation of symptoms may occur.

Overdose: Acute overdosage is very unlikely to occur, however, in the case of chronic overdosage or misuse the features of hypercorticism may appear and in this situation topical steroids should be discontinued.

Pharmacological properties

Pharmacodynamic properties: Betamethasone valerate is an active corticosteroid with topical anti-inflammatory activity.

Pharmacokinetic properties: The extent of percutaneous absorption of topical corticosteroid is determined by many factors including the vehicle, the integrity of the epidermal barrier, and the use of occlusive dressings.

Topical corticosteroids can be absorbed from normal intact skin. Inflammation and/or other disease processes in the skin increase percutaneous absorption. Occlusive dressings substantially increase the percutaneous absorption of topical corticosteroids.

Once absorbed through the skin, topical corticosteroids are handled through pharmacokinetic pathways similar to systematically administered corticosteroids. Corticosteroids are bound to plasma proteins in varying degrees. Corticosteroids are metabolised primarily by the liver and are then excreted by the kidneys.

Preclinical safety data: There are no preclinical data of relevance to the prescriber which are additional to that in other sections of the SmPC.

Pharmaceutical particulars

List of excipients: Liquid Paraffin BP, White Soft Paraffin BP.

Incompatibilities: None known.

Shelf life: Tubes: 36 months. Pump Dispenser: 24 months.

Special precautions for storage: Tubes: Store below 30°C. Pumps: Store below 25°C.

Nature and contents of container: 30 gm and 100 gm collapsible aluminium tubes internally coated with an epoxy resin based lacquer and closed with a polypropylene cap.

100 gm polypropylene/polyethylene pump dispenser with natural (translucent) polypropylene body. The nozzle is sealed with a polyethylene acetyl tab. The pump is closed with an opaque polypropylene overcap and overwrapped with an opaque shrink-wrap.

Instructions for use/handling: No special instructions.

Marketing authorisation number PL 10949/0020

Date of first authorisation/renewal of authorisation 3/9/97

Date of (partial) revision of text March 1997

BETNOVATE* RD CREAM

Qualitative and quantitative composition Betamethasone Valerate BP. Equivalent to Betamethasone 0.025%.

Pharmaceutical form Cream.

Clinical particulars

Therapeutic indications: Betamethasone valerate is an active topical corticosteroid which produces a rapid response in those inflammatory dermatoses that are normally responsive to topical corticosteroid therapy, and is often effective in the less responsive conditions such as psoriasis.

Betnovate preparations are indicated for the treatment of: eczema in children and adults; including atopic and discoid eczemas; prurigo nodularis; psoriasis (excluding widespread plaque psoriasis); neurodermatoses, including lichen simplex, lichen planus; seborrhoeic dermatitis; contact sensitivity reactions; discoid lupus erythematosus and they may be used as an adjunct to systemic steroid therapy in generalised erythroderma.

Betnovate RD preparations are indicated for maintenance treatment when control has been achieved with Betnovate.

Posology and method of administration: A small quantity of Betnovate should be applied to the affected area two or three times daily until improvement occurs. It may then be possible to maintain improvement by applying once a day, or even less often, or by using the appropriate ready-diluted (1 in 4) preparation Betnovate RD. If no improvement is seen within two or four weeks, reassessment of the diagnosis, or referral, may be necessary.

Betnovate and Betnovate RD Creams are especially appropriate for moist or weeping surfaces but this is not invariably so.

In the more resistant lesions, such as the thickened plaques of psoriasis on elbows and knees, the effect of Betnovate can be enhanced, if necessary, by occluding the treatment area with polythene film. Overnight occlusion only is usually adequate to bring about a satisfactory response in such lesions; thereafter improvement can usually be maintained by regular application without occlusion.

Children: Courses should be limited to five days if possible. Occlusion should not be used.

Contra-indications: Rosacea, acne vulgaris and perioral dermatitis. Primary cutaneous viral infections (e.g. herpes simplex, chickenpox). Hypersensitivity to the preparation.

The use of Betnovate skin preparations is not indicated in the treatment of primarily infected skin lesions caused by infection with fungi (e.g. candidiasis, tinea), or bacteria (e.g. impetigo); primary or secondary infections due to yeast; peri-anal and genital pruritus; dermatoses in children under 1 year of age, including dermatitis and napkin eruptions.

Special warnings and special precautions for use: Long-term continuous topical therapy should be avoided where possible, particularly in infants and children, as adrenal suppression can occur even without occlusion.

The face, more than other areas of the body, may exhibit atrophic changes after prolonged treatment with potent topical corticosteroids. This must be borne in mind when treating such conditions as psoriasis, discoid lupus erythematosus and severe eczema. If applied to the eyelids, care is needed to ensure that the preparation does not enter the eye, as glaucoma might result.

If used in childhood or on the face, courses should be limited if possible to five days and occlusion should not be used.

Topical corticosteroids may be hazardous in psoriasis for a number of reasons including rebound relapses, development of tolerance, risk of generalised pustular psoriasis and development of local or systemic toxicity due to impaired barrier function of the skin. If used in psoriasis careful patient supervision is important.

Appropriate antimicrobial therapy should be used whenever treating inflammatory lesions which have become infected. Any spread of infection requires withdrawal of topical corticosteroid therapy and systemic administration of antimicrobial agents. Bacterial infection is encouraged by the warm, moist conditions induced by occlusive dressings, and so the skin should be cleansed before a fresh dressing is applied.

In rare instances, treatment of psoriasis with corticosteroids (or its withdrawal) is thought to have provoked the pustular form of the disease. Betnovate RD is usually well tolerated but if signs of hypersensitivity appear, application should stop immediately.

Interaction with other medicaments and other forms of interaction: None known.

Pregnancy and lactation: Avoid extensive use in pregnancy. There is inadequate evidence of safety. Topical administration of corticosteroids to pregnant animals can cause abnormalities of foetal development including cleft palate and intrauterine growth retardation. There may therefore be a very small risk of such effects in the human foetus.

Effects on ability to drive and use machines: None known.

Undesirable effects: Prolonged and intensive treatment with highly active corticosteroid preparations may cause local atrophic changes in the skin such as striae, thinning, and dilatation of the superficial blood vessels, particularly when occlusive dressings are used or when skin folds are involved.

As with other topical corticosteroids, prolonged use of large amounts or treatment of extensive areas can result in sufficient systemic absorption to produce the features of hypercorticism and suppression of the HPA axis. These effects are likely to occur in infants and children, and if occlusive dressings are used. In infants the napkin may act as an occlusive dressing.

There are reports of pigmentation changes and hypertrichosis with topical steroids. In rare instances, treatment of psoriasis with corticosteroids (or its withdrawal) is thought to have provoked the pustular form of the disease (see *Precautions*).

The Betnovate and Betnovate RD preparations are usually well tolerated, but if signs of hypersensitivity appear, application should stop immediately.

Exacerbation of symptoms may occur.

Overdose: Acute overdosage is very unlikely to occur, however, in the case of chronic overdosage or misuse the features of hypercorticism may appear and in this situation topical steroids should be discontinued.

Pharmacological properties
Pharmacodynamic properties: Betamethasone is a corticosteroid with topical anti-inflammatory activity.

Pharmacokinetic properties: The extent of percutaneous absorption of topical corticosteroid is determined by many factors including the vehicle, the integrity of the epidermal barrier, and the use of occlusive dressings.

Topical corticosteroids can be absorbed from normal intact skin. Inflammation and/or other disease processes in the skin increase percutaneous absorption of topical corticosteroids.

Once absorbed through the skin, topical corticosteroids are handled through pharmacokinetic pathways similar to systematically administered corticosteroids. Corticosteroids are metabolised primarily by the liver and are then excreted by the kidneys.

Preclinical safety data: No additional data of relevance.

Pharmaceutical particulars
List of excipients: Cetostearyl Alcohol BP, Cetomacrogol 1000 BP, White Soft Paraffin BP, Liquid Paraffin BP, Chlorocresol BP, Disodium Hydrogen Phosphate, Anhydrous, Citric Acid Monohydrate BP, Purified Water BP.

Incompatibilities: None known.

Shelf life: 36 months.

Special precautions for storage: Store below 25°C.

Nature and contents of container: 100 gm lacquered aluminium tubes with polypropylene screw caps.

Instructions for use/handling: No special instructions.

Marketing authorisation number PL 10949/0021

Date of first authorisation/renewal of authorisation 24th March 1993

Date of (partial) revision of text 18/6/96

BETNOVATE* RD OINTMENT

Qualitative and quantitative composition Betamethasone Valerate BP 0.0305%. Equivalent to Betamethasone 0.025%.

Pharmaceutical form Ointment.

Clinical particulars
Therapeutic indications: Betamethasone valerate is an active topical corticosteroid which produces a rapid response in those inflammatory dermatoses that are normally responsive to topical corticosteroid therapy, and is often effective in the less responsive conditions such as psoriasis.

Betnovate preparations are indicated for the treatment of: eczema in children and adults; including atopic and discoid eczemas; prurigo nodularis; psoriasis (excluding widespread plaque psoriasis); neurodermatoses, including lichen simplex, lichen planus; seborrhoeic dermatitis; contact sensitivity reactions; discoid lupus erythematosus and they may be used as an adjunct to systemic steroid therapy in generalised erythroderma.

Betnovate RD preparations are indicated for maintenance treatment when control has been achieved with Betnovate.

Posology and method of administration: A small quantity of Betnovate should be applied to the affected area two or three times daily until improvement occurs. It may then be possible to maintain improvement by applying once a day, or even less often, or by using the appropriate ready-diluted (1 in 4) preparation Betnovate RD. If no improvement is seen within two or four weeks, reassessment of the diagnosis, or referral, may be necessary.

Betnovate and Betnovate RD ointments are especially appropriate for dry, lichenified or scaly lesions, but this is not invariably so.

In the more resistant lesions, such as the thickened plaques of psoriasis on elbows and knees, the effect of Betnovate can be enhanced, if necessary, by occluding the treatment area with polythene film. Overnight occlusion only is usually adequate to bring about a satisfactory response in such lesions; thereafter improvement can usually be maintained by regular application without occlusion.

Children: Courses should be limited to five days if possible. Occlusion should not be used.

Contra-indications: Rosacea, acne vulgaris and perioral dermatitis. Primary cutaneous viral infections (e.g. herpes simplex, chickenpox). Hypersensitivity to the preparation.

The use of Betnovate skin preparations is not indicated in the treatment of primarily infected skin lesions caused by infection with fungi (e.g. candidiasis, tinea), or bacteria (e.g. impetigo); primary or secondary infections due to yeast; peri-anal and genital pruritus; dermatoses in children under 1 year of age, including dermatitis and napkin eruptions.

Special warnings and precautions for use: Long-term continuous topical therapy should be avoided where possible, particularly in infants and children, as adrenal suppression can occur even without occlusion.

The face, more than other areas of the body, may exhibit atrophic changes after prolonged treatment with potent topical corticosteroids. This must be borne in mind when treating such conditions as psoriasis, discoid lupus erythematosus and severe eczema. If applied to the eyelids, care is needed to ensure that the preparation does not enter the eye, as glaucoma might result.

If used in childhood or on the face, courses should be limited if possible to five days and occlusion should not be used.

Topical corticosteroids may be hazardous in psoriasis for a number of reasons including rebound relapses, development of tolerance, risk of generalised pustular psoriasis and development of local or systemic toxicity due to impaired barrier function of the skin. If used in psoriasis careful patient supervision is important.

Appropriate antimicrobial therapy should be used whenever treating inflammatory lesions which have become infected. Any spread of infection requires withdrawal of topical corticosteroid therapy and systemic administration of antimicrobial agents. Bacterial infection is encouraged by the warm, moist conditions induced by occlusive dressings and so the skin should be cleansed before a fresh dressing is applied.

In rare instances, treatment of psoriasis with corticosteroids (or its withdrawal) is thought to have provoked the pustular form of the disease. Betnovate RD is usually well tolerated but if signs of hypersensitivity appear, application should stop immediately.

Interaction with other medicaments and other forms of interaction: None known.

Pregnancy and lactation: Avoid extensive use in pregnancy. There is inadequate evidence of safety. Topical administration of corticosteroids to pregnant animals can cause abnormalities of foetal development including cleft palate and intrauterine growth retardation. There may therefore be a very small risk of such effects in the human foetus.

Effects on ability to drive and use machines: None known.

Undesirable effects: Prolonged and intensive treatment with highly active corticosteroid preparations may cause local atrophic changes in the skin such as striae, thinning, and dilatation of the superficial blood vessels, particularly when occlusive dressings are used or when skin folds are involved.

As with other topical corticosteroids, prolonged use of large amounts or treatment of extensive areas can result in sufficient systemic absorption to produce the features of hypercorticism and suppression of the HPA axis. These effects are likely to occur in infants and children, and if occlusive dressings are used. In infants the napkin may act as an occlusive dressing.

There are reports of pigmentation changes and hypertrichosis with topical steroids. In rare instances, treatment of psoriasis with corticosteroids (or its withdrawal) is thought to have provoked the pustular form of the disease (see *Precautions*).

The Betnovate and Betnovate RD preparations are usually well tolerated, but if signs of hypersensitivity appear, application should stop immediately.

Exacerbation of symptoms may occur.

Overdose: Acute overdosage is very unlikely to occur, however, in the case of chronic overdosage or misuse the features of hypercorticism may appear and in this situation topical steroids should be discontinued.

Pharmacological properties
Pharmacodynamic properties: Betamethasone is a corticosteroid with topical anti-inflammatory activity.

Pharmacokinetic properties: The extent of percutaneous absorption of topical corticosteroid is determined by many factors including the vehicle, the integrity of the epidermal barrier, and the use of occlusive dressings.

Topical corticosteroids can be absorbed from normal intact skin. Inflammation and/or other disease processes in the skin increase percutaneous absorption of topical corticosteroids.

Once absorbed through the skin, topical corticosteroids are handled through pharmacokinetic pathways similar to systematically administered corticosteroids. Corticosteroids are metabolised primarily by the liver and are then excreted by the kidneys.

Preclinical safety data: No additional data of relevance.

Pharmaceutical particulars
List of excipients: White Soft Paraffin BP, Liquid Paraffin BP.

Incompatibilities: None known.

Shelf life: 36 months.

Special precautions for storage: Store below 30°C.

Nature and contents of container: 100 gm lacquered aluminium tubes with polypropylene screw caps.

Instructions for use/handling: No special instructions.

Marketing authorisation number PL 10949/0022

Date of first authorisation/renewal of authorisation 17/01/97

Date of (partial) revision of text August 1996

BETNOVATE* RECTAL OINTMENT

Qualitative and quantitative composition

Betamethasone Valerate BP	0.05% w/w
Phenylephrine Hydrochloride BP	0.10% w/w
Lignocaine Hydrochloride BP	2.50% w/w

Pharmaceutical form Ointment.

Clinical particulars
Therapeutic indications: The clinical effectiveness of Betnovate Rectal Ointment is attributable to the marked local anti-inflammatory property of the corticosteroid betamethasone valerate, the analgesic effect of lignocaine, and the vasoconstrictor effect of phenylephrine.

Betnovate Rectal Ointment is indicated for: relief of the symptoms of itching, irritation, discomfort or pain associated with local non-infective anal or peri-anal conditions such as external haemorrhoids.

Posology and method of administration: Apply a small amount of ointment two or three times a day initially using the applicator if internal administration is required. When inflammation is subsiding, once daily application is sufficient in most cases.

A course of treatment should be limited to seven days.

For topical and rectal administration.

Contra-indications: Primary cutaneous viral infections (e.g. herpes simplex, chickenpox). Hypersensitivity to any component of the preparation.

The use of Betnovate Rectal Ointment is not indicated in the treatment of primarily infected skin lesions caused by infection with fungi (e.g.candidiasis, tinea); or bacteria (e.g. impetigo); dermatoses in children under 1 year of age, including dermatitis and napkin eruptions.

Special warnings and precautions for use: None.

Interaction with other medicaments and other forms of interaction: None.

Pregnancy and lactation: There is inadequate evidence of safety in human pregnancy. Topical administration of corticosteroids to pregnant animals can cause abnormalities of foetal development including cleft palate and intra-uterine growth retardation. There may therefore be a very small risk of such effects in the human foetus.

Effects on ability to drive and use machines: None.

Undesirable effects: As with all topical corticosteroids, if the Betnovate preparations are used for prolonged periods, the consequences of systemic absorption e.g. suppression of the HPA axis, should be considered, especially in children.

Prolonged and intensive treatment with active corticosteroid preparations may cause local atrophic changes in the skin. There are reports of pigmentation changes and hypertrichosis with topical steroids.

Overdose: Acute overdosage is very unlikely to occur, however, in the case of chronic overdosage or misuse the features of hypercorticism may appear and in this situation topical steroids should be discontinued.

Pharmacological properties

Pharmacodynamic properties: Betamethasone valerate is an active corticosteroid with topical anti-inflammatory activity.

Lignocaine has an analgesic effect and phenylephrine acts as a vasoconstrictor.

Pharmacokinetic properties: The extent of percutaneous absorption of topical corticosteroids is determined by many factors including the vehicle, the integrity of the epidermal barrier, and the use of occlusive dressings.

Topical corticosteroids can be absorbed from normal intact skin. Inflammation and/or other disease processes in the skin increase percutaneous absorption. Occlusive dressings substantially increase the percutaneous absorption of topical corticosteroids.

Once absorbed through the skin, topical corticosteroids are handled through pharmacokinetic pathways similar to systemically administered corticosteroids. Corticosteroids are bound to plasma proteins in varying degrees. Corticosteroids are metabolised primarily by the liver and are then excreted by the kidneys.

Lignocaine is readily absorbed from mucous membranes and damaged skin. Absorption of lignocaine through intact skin is poor. The pharmacokinetics of lignocaine may be altered by disease states and other factors. Lignocaine undergoes first-pass metabolism in the liver and metabolites are then excreted by the kidneys. Phenylephrine is subject to first-pass metabolism by mono-amine oxidase in the gut and liver.

Preclinical safety data: There are no preclinical data of relevance to the prescriber which are additional to that in other sections of the SmPC.

Pharmaceutical particulars

List of excipients: Microcrystalline Wax USNF, Liquid Paraffin BP.

Incompatibilities: None known.

Shelf life: 36 months.

Special precautions for storage: Store below 30°C.

Nature and contents of container: 25 gm and 30 gm collapsible aluminium tubes internally coated with an epoxy resin based lacquer and closed with a wadless polypropylene cap.

Instructions for use/handling: No special instructions.

Marketing authorisation number PL 10949/0024

Date of first authorisation/renewal of authorisation MAA: 1/2/93, Renewal: 24/10/97

Date of (partial) revision of text October 1997

BETNOVATE* SCALP APPLICATION

Qualitative and quantitative composition Betamethasone Valerate BP 0.122% w/w.

Pharmaceutical form Aqueous Suspension.

Clinical particulars

Therapeutic indications: Steroid responsive dermatoses of the scalp, such as psoriasis and seborrhoeic dermatitis.

Posology and method of administration: A small quantity of Betnovate Scalp Application should be applied to the scalp night and morning until improvement is noticeable. It may then be possible to sustain improvement by applying once a day, or less frequently.

For topical application.

Contra-indications: Infections of the scalp. Hypersensitivity to the preparation. Dermatoses in children under one year of age, including dermatitis.

Special warnings and precautions for use: Care must be taken to keep the preparation away from the eyes. Do not use near a naked flame.

Long-term continuous topical therapy should be avoided where possible, particularly in infants and children, as adrenal suppression can occur even with occlusion.

Topical corticosteroids may be hazardous in psoriasis for a number of reasons including rebound relapses, development of tolerance, risk of generalised pustular psoriasis and development of local or systemic toxicity due to impaired barrier function of the skin. If used in psoriasis careful patient supervision is important.

Development of secondary infection requires withdrawal of topical corticosteroid therapy and commencement of appropriate systemic antimicrobial therapy.

The least potent corticosteroid which will control the disease should be selected. The viscosity of the scalp application has been adjusted so that the preparation spreads easily without being too fluid. The specially-designed bottle and nozzle allow easy application direct to the scalp through the hair.

Interaction with other medicaments and other forms of interaction: None known.

Pregnancy and lactation: There is inadequate evidence of safety in human pregnancy. Topical administration of corticosteroids to pregnant animals can cause abnormalities of foetal development including cleft palate and intrauterine growth retardation. There may therefore be a very small risk of such effects in the human foetus.

Effects on ability to drive and use machines: None known.

Undesirable effects: Betnovate preparations are usually well tolerated, but if signs of hypersensitivity appear, application should be stopped immediately.

As with other topical corticosteroids, prolonged use of large amounts or treatment of extensive areas can result in sufficient systemic absorption to produce the features of hypercorticism and suppression of the HPA axis. These effects are likely to occur in infants and children, and if occlusive dressings are used. In infants the napkin may act as an occlusive dressing.

There are rare reports of pigmentation changes and hypertrichosis with topical steroids.

In rare instances, treatment of psoriasis with corticosteroids (or its withdrawal) is thought to have provoked the pustular form of the disease (see *Precautions*).

Overdose: Acute overdosage is very unlikely to occur, however, in the case of chronic overdosage or misuse the features of hypercorticism may appear and in this situation topical steroids should be discontinued.

Pharmacological properties

Pharmacodynamic properties: Betamethasone valerate is an active corticosteroid with topical anti-inflammatory activity.

Pharmacokinetic properties: The extent of percutaneous absorption of topical corticosteroids is determined by many factors including the vehicle, the integrity of the epidermal barrier, and the use of occlusive dressings.

Topical corticosteroids can be absorbed from normal intact skin. Inflammation and/or other disease processes in the skin increase percutaneous absorption. Occlusive dressings substantially increase the percutaneous absorption of topical corticosteroids.

Once absorbed through the skin, topical corticosteroids are handled through pharmacokinetic pathways similar to systemically administered corticosteroids. Corticosteroids are bound to plasma proteins in varying degrees. Corticosteroids are metabolised primarily by the liver and are then excreted by the kidneys.

Preclinical safety data: There are no preclinical data of relevance to the prescriber which are additional to that in other sections of the SPC.

Pharmaceutical particulars

List of excipients: Carbomer BP, Isopropyl Alcohol BP, Sodium Hydroxide BP, Purified Water BP.

Incompatibilities: None known.

Shelf life: 24 months.

Special precautions for storage: Store below 25°C.

Nature and contents of container: 30 ml and 100 ml polythene squeeze bottles with a polythene nozzle and a polystyrene or polyethylene cap.

Instructions for use/handling: No special instructions.

Marketing authorisation number PL 10949/0045.

Date of first authorisation/renewal of authorisation MAA: 1/4/93, Renewal: 9/12/97

Date of (partial) revision of the text June 1997

CEPOREX* CAPSULES 250 mg

Qualitative and quantitative composition Cephalexin BP 250 mg per capsule.

Pharmaceutical form Capsule.

Clinical particulars

Therapeutic indications: Ceporex is a bactericidal antibiotic of the cephalosporin group which is active against a wide range of Gram-positive and Gram-negative organisms. It is indicated for treatment of the following conditions, when caused by susceptible bacteria.

Respiratory tract infections: Acute and chronic bronchitis and infected bronchiectasis.

Ear, nose and throat infections: Otitis media, mastoiditis, sinusitis, follicular tonsillitis and pharyngitis.

Urinary tract infections: Acute and chronic pyelonephritis, cystitis and prostatitis. Prophylaxis of recurrent urinary tract infection.

Gynaecological and obstetric infections.

Skin, soft-tissue and bone infections.

Gonorrhoea (when Penicillin is unsuitable).

Dental procedures: Treatment of dental infections.

As prophylaxis treatment for patients with heart disease undergoing dental treatment as an alternative to penicillin.

Posology and method of administration:
Route of administration: Oral.

Many infections in adults will respond to oral dosage of 1 gram to 2 grams per day in divided doses; however, for most infections, the following simple dosage scheme will be found satisfactory:

Adults and children over 12 years: 1 g b.d.

The following additional information should also be considered:

Adults: For severe or deep-seated infections, especially when less sensitive organisms are involved, the dosage should be increased to 1 g t.d.s. or 3 g b.d. For prophylaxis of recurrent urinary tract infections in adults, a dose of 125 mg each night is recommended and may be continued for several months (the 125 mg/ 5 ml Suspension is suitable for this purpose).

Children: Ideally, dosage should be calculated on a body-weight basis, particularly in infants. The following dosage recommendations for children are derived from a normal dosage of 25 to 60 mg/kg/day. For chronic, severe or deep-seated infections, this should be increased to 100 mg/kg/day (maximum 4 g/day).

Children under 1 year	(25 to 60 mg/kg/day)
	62.5 to 125 mg b.d.
Children 1–6 years	250 mg–500 mg b.d.
Children 7–12 years	500 mg–1 g b.d.

Notes: For most acute infections, treatment should continue for at least two days after signs have returned to normal and symptoms have subsided, but in chronic, recurrent or complicated urinary tract infections, treatment for two weeks (giving 1 g b.d.) is recommended. For gonorrhoea, a single dose of 3 g with 1 g probenecid for males or 2 g with 0.5 g probenecid for females is usually effective. Concurrent administration of probenecid delays excretion of cephalexin and raises the serum levels by 50 to 100%.

Ceporex has not been shown to have a toxic effect on the kidney, but as with other antibiotics which are excreted mainly by the kidneys, unnecessary accumulation may occur in the body when renal function is below about half of normal. Therefore, the maximum recommended dosages (i.e. Adults 6 g/day, children 4 g/day) should be reduced proportionately in these patients.

In elderly patients, the possibility of renal impairment should be considered. Adult patients receiving intermittent dialysis should be given an additional 500 mg Ceporex after each dialysis, i.e., a total dosage of up to 1 g on that day. Children should receive an additional 8 mg per kg.

Contra-indications: Hypersensitivity to any ingredient of the preparation.

Special warnings and precautions for use: Ceporex is usually well-tolerated by patients allergic to penicillin, but cross-reaction has been encountered rarely.

As with other broad-spectrum antibiotics, prolonged use may result in the overgrowth of non-susceptible organisms (e.g. Candida, Enterococci, *Clostridium difficile*), which may require interruption of treatment. Pseudomembranous colitis has been reported with the use of broad-spectrum antibiotics, therefore, it is important to consider its diagnosis in patients who develop severe diarrhoea during or after antibiotic use.

As with other antibiotics that are excreted mainly by the kidneys, when renal function is poor, dosage of Ceporex should be suitably reduced (see *Posology and method of administration*).

Interaction with other medicaments and other forms of interaction: Concurrent treatment with high doses of cephalosporins and nephrotoxic drugs such as aminoglycosides or potent diuretics (e.g. Frusemide, ethacrynic acid and piretamide) may adversely affect renal function. Clinical experience has shown that it is not likely to be a problem with Ceporex at the recommended dosage levels.

In patients receiving Ceporex, a false-positive reaction for glucose in the urine may be given, with Benedict's or Fehling's solution, or with 'Clinitest' tablets, but not with enzyme-based tests. There are reports of positive Coombs' test.

Ceporex can interfere with the alkaline picrate assay for creatinine, giving a falsely high reading, but the degree of elevation is unlikely to be of clinical importance.

Pregnancy and lactation: Laboratory experiments and clinical experience show no evidence of teratogenicity, but it would be wise to proceed with caution during the early months of pregnancy, as with all drugs.

Effect on ability to drive and use machines: No effect.

Undesirable effects: A small proportion of patients receiving Ceporex experience gastro-intestinal disturbances such as nausea, vomiting and diarrhoea.

As with other broad-spectrum antibiotics, there have been rare reports of pseudomembranous colitis.

As with other antibiotics, prolonged use may result in the overgrowth of non-susceptible organisms, e.g., Candida. This may present as vulvo-vaginitis. Reversible neutropenia has occurred in a few patients, but is very rare. Drug rashes both urticarial and maculopapular.

Ceporex should be used with care in patients with a history of hypersensitivity to drugs.

Severe skin reactions including very rarely toxic epidermal necrolysis (exanthematic necrolysis), Stevens-Johnson Syndrome and hypersensitivity reactions including angioedema and anaphylaxis.

As with other cephalosporins there have been rare reports of reversible interstitial nephritis.

Overdose: Serum levels of cephalexin can be reduced greatly by peritoneal dialysis or haemodialysis.

Pharmacological properties

Pharmacodynamic properties: Ceporex is resistant to the action of staphylococcal penicillinase, and is therefore active against strains of *Staph. aureus* that are insensitive to penicillin (or ampicillin) through production of that enzyme. Ceporex is also active against the majority of ampicillin-resistant *E. coli*.

Pharmacokinetic properties: Absorption of Ceporex is almost complete, even in the presence of food, and is not adversely affected by coeliac disease, partial gastrectomy, achlorhydria, jaundice or diverticulosis (duodenal or jejunal). Ceporex is excreted in the urine in high concentration.

The serum half-life is normally about one hour, but is longer in the newborn (see *Posology and method of administration*). Ceporex has a wide margin of safety.

Preclinical safety data: None reported.

Pharmaceutical particulars

List of excipients: Magnesium stearate.

Capsule shells: Hard gelatin capsules size 2.

Colours: Caramel/grey.

Caramel body: 36: 11 Caramel opaque C11.

Grey cap: 10: 13 Standard grey opaque C13.

Incompatibilities: No incompatibilities have been reported.

Shelf life: 36 months.

Special precautions for storage: The product is stored at a temperature not exceeding 30°C, protected from light.

Nature and contents of container:

1. Tubular glass vial with polyethylene snap-plug closure.

2. Tamper evident polypropylene container with low density polyethylene lid. One or more cartridges of activated charcoal according to pack size are included.

3. Capsules are sealed into individual pockets in an aluminium/polyethylene/foil laminate (30 and 38 micrometres respectively).

4. Capsules are sealed into individual pockets in an aluminium foil blister with an aluminium lid (43 and 20 micrometres respectively).

All container presentations contain 20, 28, 100 or 500 tablets.

Instructions for use/handling: None stated.

Marketing authorisation number PL 10949/0129

Date of first authorisation/renewal of authorisation MAA: 30.09.93.

Date of (partial) revision of text June 1998. This is the first SmPC.

CEPOREX* CAPSULES 500 mg

Qualitative and quantitative composition Cephalexin BP 500 mg per capsule.

Pharmaceutical form Capsule.

Clinical particulars

Therapeutic indications: Ceporex is a bactericidal antibiotic of the cephalosporin group which is active against a wide range of Gram-positive and Gram-negative organisms. It is indicated for treatment of the following conditions, when caused by susceptible bacteria.

Respiratory tract infections: Acute and chronic bronchitis and infected bronchiectasis.

Ear, nose and throat infections: Otitis media, mastoiditis, sinusitis, follicular tonsillitis and pharyngitis.

Urinary tract infections: Acute and chronic pyelonephritis, cystitis and prostatitis. Prophylaxis of recurrent urinary tract infection.

Gynaecological and obstetric infections.

Skin, soft-tissue and bone infections.

Gonorrhoea (when Penicillin is unsuitable).

Dental procedures: Treatment of dental infections.

As prophylaxis treatment for patients with heart disease undergoing dental treatment as an alternative to penicillin.

Posology and method of administration:

Route of administration: Oral.

Many infections in adults will respond to oral dosage of 1 gram to 2 grams per day in divided doses; however, for most infections, the following simple dosage scheme will be found satisfactory:

Adults and children over 12 years: 1 g b.d.

The following additional information should also be considered:

Adults: For severe or deep-seated infections, especially when less sensitive organisms are involved, the dosage should be increased to 1 g t.d.s. or 3 g b.d. For prophylaxis of recurrent urinary tract infections in adults, a dose of 125 mg each night is recommended and may be continued for several months (the 125 mg/5 ml Suspension is suitable for this purpose).

Children: Ideally, dosage should be calculated on a body-weight basis, particularly in infants. The following dosage recommendations for children are derived from a normal dosage of 25 to 60 mg/kg/day. For chronic, severe or deep-seated infections, this should be increased to 100 mg/kg/day (maximum 4 g/day).

Children under 1 year	(25 to 60 mg/kg/day) 62.5 to 125 mg b.d.
Children 1–6 years	250 mg–500 mg b.d.
Children 7–12 years	500 mg–1 g b.d.

Notes: For most acute infections, treatment should continue for at least two days after signs have returned to normal and symptoms have subsided, but in chronic, recurrent or complicated urinary tract infections, treatment for two weeks (giving 1 g b.d.) is recommended. For gonorrhoea, a single dose of 3 g with 1 g probenecid for males or 2 g with 0.5 g probenecid for females is usually effective. Concurrent administration of probenecid delays excretion of cephalexin and raises the serum levels by 50 to 100%.

Ceporex has not been shown to have a toxic effect on the kidney, but as with other antibiotics which are excreted mainly by the kidneys, unnecessary accumulation may occur in the body when renal function is below about half of normal. Therefore, the maximum recommended dosages (i.e. Adults 6 g/day, children 4 g/day) should be reduced proportionately in these patients.

In elderly patients, the possibility of renal impairment should be considered. Adult patients receiving intermittent dialysis should be given an additional 500 mg Ceporex after each dialysis, i.e., a total dosage of up to 1 g on that day. Children should receive an additional 8 mg per kg.

Contra-indications: Hypersensitivity to any ingredient of the preparation.

Special warnings and precautions for use: Ceporex is usually well-tolerated by patients allergic to penicillin, but cross-reaction has been encountered rarely.

As with other broad-spectrum antibiotics, prolonged use may result in the overgrowth of non-susceptible organisms (e.g. Candida, Enterococci, *Clostridium difficile*), which may require interruption of treatment. Pseudomembranous colitis has been reported with the use of broad-spectrum antibiotics, therefore, it is important to consider its diagnosis in patients who develop severe diarrhoea during or after antibiotic use.

As with other antibiotics that are excreted mainly by the kidneys, when renal function is poor, dosage of Ceporex should be suitably reduced (see *Posology and method of administration*).

Interaction with other medicaments and other forms of interaction: Concurrent treatment with high doses of cephalosporins and nephrotoxic drugs such as aminoglycosides or potent diuretics (e.g. Frusemide, ethacrynic acid and piretamide) may adversely affect renal function. Clinical experience has shown that it is not likely to be a problem with Ceporex at the recommended dosage levels.

In patients receiving Ceporex, a false-positive reaction for glucose in the urine may be given, with Benedict's or Fehling's solution, or with 'Clinitest' tablets, but not with enzyme-based tests. There are reports of positive Coombs' test.

Ceporex can interfere with the alkaline picrate assay for creatinine, giving a falsely high reading, but the degree of elevation is unlikely to be of clinical importance.

Pregnancy and lactation: Laboratory experiments and clinical experience show no evidence of teratogenicity, but it would be wise to proceed with caution during the early months of pregnancy, as with all drugs.

Effect on ability to drive and use machines: No effect.

Undesirable effects: A small proportion of patients receiving Ceporex experience gastro-intestinal disturbances such as nausea, vomiting and diarrhoea.

As with other broad-spectrum antibiotics, there have been rare reports of pseudomembranous colitis.

As with other antibiotics, prolonged use may result in the overgrowth of non-susceptible organisms, e.g., Candida. This may present as vulvo-vaginitis. Reversible neutropenia has occurred in a few patients, but is very rare. Drug rashes both urticarial and maculopapular.

Ceporex should be used with care in patients with a history of hypersensitivity to drugs.

Severe skin reactions including very rarely toxic epidermal necrolysis (exanthematic necrolysis), Stevens-Johnson Syndrome and hypersensitivity reactions including angioedema and anaphylaxis.

As with other cephalosporins there have been rare reports of reversible interstitial nephritis.

Overdose: Serum levels of cephalexin can be reduced greatly by peritoneal dialysis or haemodialysis.

Pharmacological properties

Pharmacodynamic properties: Ceporex is resistant to the action of staphylococcal penicillinase, and is therefore active against strains of *Staph. aureus* that are insensitive to penicillin (or ampicillin) through production of that enzyme. Ceporex is also active against the majority of ampicillin-resistant *E. coli*.

Pharmacokinetic properties: Absorption of Ceporex is almost complete, even in the presence of food, and is not adversely affected by coeliac disease, partial gastrectomy, achlorhydria, jaundice or diverticulosis (duodenal or jejunal). Ceporex is excreted in the urine in high concentration.

The serum half-life is normally about one hour, but is longer in the newborn (see *Posology and method of administration*). Ceporex has a wide margin of safety.

Preclinical safety data: None reported.

Pharmaceutical particulars

List of excipients: Magnesium stearate.

Capsule shells: Hard gelatin capsules size 0.

Colours: Caramel/grey.

Caramel body: 36: 11 Caramel opaque C11.

Grey cap: 10: 13 Standard grey opaque C13.

Incompatibilities: No incompatibilities have been reported.

Shelf life: 36 months.

Special precautions for storage: The product is stored at a temperature not exceeding 30°C, protected from light.

Nature and contents of container:

1. Tubular glass vial with polyethylene snap-plug closure.

2. Tamper evident polypropylene container with low density polyethylene lid. One or more cartridges of activated charcoal according to pack size are included.

3. Capsules are sealed into individual pockets in an aluminium/polyethylene/foil laminate (30 and 38 micrometres respectively).

4. Capsules are sealed into individual pockets in an aluminium foil blister with an aluminium lid (43 and 20 micrometres respectively).

All container presentations contain 20, 28, 100 or 500 tablets.

Instructions for use/handling: None stated.

Marketing authorisation number PL 10949/0130

Date of first authorisation/renewal of authorisation MAA: 30.09.93.

Date of (partial) revision of text June 1998. This is the first SmPC.

CEPOREX* TABLETS 250 mg

Qualitative and quantitative composition Cephalexin PhEur 250 mg per tablet.

Pharmaceutical form Tablet.

Clinical particulars

Therapeutic indications: Ceporex is a bactericidal antibiotic of the cephalosporin group which is active against a wide range of Gram-positive and Gram-negative organisms. It is indicated for treatment of the following conditions, when caused by susceptible bacteria.

Respiratory tract infections: Acute and chronic bronchitis and infected bronchiectasis.

Ear, nose and throat infections: Otitis media, mastoiditis, sinusitis, follicular tonsillitis and pharyngitis.

Urinary tract infections: Acute and chronic pyelonephritis, cystitis and prostatitis. Prophylaxis of recurrent urinary tract infection.

Gynaecological and obstetric infections.
Skin, soft-tissue and bone infections.
Gonorrhoea (when Penicillin is unsuitable).
Dental procedures: Treatment of dental infections.

As prophylaxis treatment for patients with heart disease undergoing dental treatment as an alternative to penicillin.

Posology and method of administration:
Route of administration: Oral.

Many infections in adults will respond to oral dosage of 1 gram to 2 grams per day in divided doses; however, for most infections, the following simple dosage scheme will be found satisfactory:

Adults and children over 12 years: 1 g b.d.

The following additional information should also be considered:

Adults: For severe or deep-seated infections, especially when less sensitive organisms are involved, the dosage should be increased to 1 g t.d.s. or 3 g b.d. For prophylaxis of recurrent urinary tract infections in adults, a dose of 125 mg each night is recommended and may be continued for several months (the 125 mg/5 ml Suspension is suitable for this purpose).

Children: Ideally, dosage should be calculated on a body-weight basis, particularly in infants. The following dosage recommendations for children are derived from a normal dosage of 25 to 60 mg/kg/day. For chronic, severe or deep-seated infections, this should be increased to 100 mg/kg/day (maximum 4 g/day).

Children under 1 year	(25 to 60 mg/kg/day) 62.5 to 125 mg b.d.
Children 1–6 years	250 mg–500 mg b.d.
Children 7–12 years	500 mg–1 g b.d.

Notes: For most acute infections, treatment should continue for at least two days after signs have returned to normal and symptoms have subsided, but in chronic, recurrent or complicated urinary tract infections, treatment for two weeks (giving 1 g b.d.) is recommended. For gonorrhoea, a single dose of 3 g with 1 g probenecid for males or 2 g with 0.5 g probenecid for females is usually effective. Concurrent administration of probenecid delays excretion of cephalexin and raises the serum levels by 50 to 100%.

Ceporex has not been shown to have a toxic effect on the kidney, but as with other antibiotics which are excreted mainly by the kidneys, unnecessary accumulation may occur in the body when renal function is below about half of normal. Therefore, the maximum recommended dosages (i.e. Adults 6 g/day, children 4 g/day) should be reduced proportionately in these patients.

In elderly patients, the possibility of renal impairment should be considered. Adult patients receiving intermittent dialysis should be given an additional 500 mg Ceporex after each dialysis, i.e., a total dosage of up to 1 g on that day. Children should receive an additional 8 mg per kg.

Contra-indications: Hypersensitivity to any ingredient of the preparation.

Special warnings and precautions for use: Ceporex is usually well-tolerated by patients allergic to penicillin, but cross-reaction has been encountered rarely.

As with other broad-spectrum antibiotics, prolonged use may result in the overgrowth of non-susceptible organisms (e.g. Candida, Enterococci, *Clostridium difficile*), which may require interruption of treatment. Pseudomembranous colitis has been reported with the use of broad-spectrum antibiotics, therefore, it is important to consider its diagnosis in patients who develop severe diarrhoea during or after antibiotic use.

As with other antibiotics that are excreted mainly by the kidneys, when renal function is poor, dosage of Ceporex should be suitably reduced (see *Posology and method of administration*).

Interaction with other medicaments and other forms of interaction: Concurrent treatment with high doses of cephalosporins and nephrotoxic drugs such as aminoglycosides or potent diuretics (e.g. Frusemide, ethacrynic acid and piretamide) may adversely affect renal function. Clinical experience has shown that it is not likely to be a problem with Ceporex at the recommended dosage levels.

In patients receiving Ceporex, a false-positive reaction for glucose in the urine may be given, with Benedict's or Fehling's solution, or with 'Clinitest' tablets, but not with enzyme-based tests. There are reports of positive Coombs' test.

Ceporex can interfere with the alkaline picrate assay for creatinine, giving a falsely high reading, but the degree of elevation is unlikely to be of clinical importance.

Pregnancy and lactation: Laboratory experiments and clinical experience show no evidence of teratogenicity, but it would be wise to proceed with caution during the early months of pregnancy, as with all drugs.

Effect on ability to drive and use machines: No effect.

Undesirable effects: A small proportion of patients receiving Ceporex experience gastro-intestinal disturbances such as nausea, vomiting and diarrhoea.

As with other broad-spectrum antibiotics, there have been rare reports of pseudomembranous colitis.

As with other antibiotics, prolonged use may result in the overgrowth of non-susceptible organisms, e.g., Candida. This may present as vulvo-vaginitis. Reversible neutropenia has occurred in a few patients, but is very rare. Drug rashes both urticarial and maculopapular.

Ceporex should be used with care in patients with a history of hypersensitivity to drugs.

Severe skin reactions including very rarely toxic epidermal necrolysis (exanthematic necrolysis), Stevens-Johnson Syndrome and hypersensitivity reactions including angioedema and anaphylaxis.

As with other cephalosporins there have been rare reports of reversible interstitial nephritis.

Overdose: Serum levels of cephalexin can be reduced greatly by peritoneal dialysis or haemodialysis.

Pharmacological properties

Pharmacodynamic properties: Ceporex is resistant to the action of staphylococcal penicillinase, and is therefore active against strains of *Staph. aureus* that are insensitive to penicillin (or ampicillin) through production of that enzyme. Ceporex is also active against the majority of ampicillin-resistant *E. coli.*

Pharmacokinetic properties: Absorption of Ceporex is almost complete, even in the presence of food, and is not adversely affected by coeliac disease, partial gastrectomy, achlorhydria, jaundice or diverticulosis (duodenal or jejunal). Ceporex is excreted in the urine in high concentration.

The serum half-life is normally about one hour, but is longer in the newborn (see *Posology and method of administration*). Ceporex has a wide margin of safety.

Preclinical safety data: None reported.

Pharmaceutical particulars

List of excipients: Microcrystalline cellulose EP, Magnesium stearate EP.

Film coating: Hydroxypropyl methylcellulose EP, Macrogol 400 EP, Opadry OY-S-6927 In-house, Purified water BP.

Incompatibilities: No incompatibilities have been reported.

Shelf life: 36 months.

Special precautions for storage: The product is stored at a temperature not exceeding 30°C, protected from light.

Nature and contents of container:

1. Tubular glass vial with polyethylene snap-plug closure.
2. Tamper evident polypropylene container with low density polyethylene lid. One or more cartridges of activated charcoal according to pack size are included.
3. Tablets are sealed into individual pockets in an aluminium polyethylene/foil laminate (30 and 38 micrometres respectively).
4. Tablets are sealed into individual pockets in an aluminium foil blister with an aluminium lid (43 and 20 micrometres respectively).

All container presentations contain 20, 28, 100 or 500 tablets.

Instructions for use/handling: None stated.

Marketing authorisation number PL 10949/0134

Date of first authorisation/renewal of authorisation MAA: 31.08.93.

Date of (partial) revision of text September 1998

CEPOREX* TABLETS 500 mg

Qualitative and quantitative composition Cephalexin PhEur 500 mg per tablet.

Pharmaceutical form Tablet.

Clinical particulars

Therapeutic indications: Ceporex is a bactericidal antibiotic of the cephalosporin group which is active against a wide range of Gram-positive and Gram-negative organisms. It is indicated for treatment of the following conditions, when caused by susceptible bacteria.

Respiratory tract infections: Acute and chronic bronchitis and infected bronchiectasis.

Ear, nose and throat infections: Otitis media, mastoiditis, sinusitis, follicular tonsillitis and pharyngitis.

Urinary tract infections: Acute and chronic pyelonephritis, cystitis and prostatitis. Prophylaxis of recurrent urinary tract infection.

Gynaecological and obstetric infections.
Skin, soft-tissue and bone infections.
Gonorrhoea (when Penicillin is unsuitable).
Dental procedures: Treatment of dental infections.

As prophylaxis treatment for patients with heart disease undergoing dental treatment as an alternative to penicillin.

Posology and method of administration:
Route of administration: Oral.

Many infections in adults will respond to oral dosage of 1 gram to 2 grams per day in divided doses; however, for most infections, the following simple dosage scheme will be found satisfactory:

Adults and children over 12 years: 1 g b.d.

The following additional information should also be considered:

Adults: For severe or deep-seated infections, especially when less sensitive organisms are involved, the dosage should be increased to 1 g t.d.s. or 3 g b.d. For prophylaxis of recurrent urinary tract infections in adults, a dose of 125 mg each night is recommended and may be continued for several months (the 125 mg/5 ml Suspension is suitable for this purpose).

Children: Ideally, dosage should be calculated on a body-weight basis, particularly in infants. The following dosage recommendations for children are derived from a normal dosage of 25 to 60 mg/kg/day. For chronic, severe or deep-seated infections, this should be increased to 100 mg/kg/day (maximum 4 g/day).

Children under 1 year	(25 to 60 mg/kg/day) 62.5 to 125 mg b.d.
Children 1–6 years	250 mg–500 mg b.d.
Children 7–12 years	500 mg–1 g b.d.

Notes: For most acute infections, treatment should continue for at least two days after signs have returned to normal and symptoms have subsided, but in chronic, recurrent or complicated urinary tract infections, treatment for two weeks (giving 1 g b.d.) is recommended. For gonorrhoea, a single dose of 3 g with 1 g probenecid for males or 2 g with 0.5 g probenecid for females is usually effective. Concurrent administration of probenecid delays excretion of cephalexin and raises the serum levels by 50 to 100%.

Ceporex has not been shown to have a toxic effect on the kidney, but as with other antibiotics which are excreted mainly by the kidneys, unnecessary accumulation may occur in the body when renal function is below about half of normal. Therefore, the maximum recommended dosages (i.e. Adults 6 g/day, children 4 g/day) should be reduced proportionately in these patients.

In elderly patients, the possibility of renal impairment should be considered. Adult patients receiving intermittent dialysis should be given an additional 500 mg Ceporex after each dialysis, i.e., a total dosage of up to 1 g on that day. Children should receive an additional 8 mg per kg.

Contra-indications: Hypersensitivity to any ingredient of the preparation.

Special warnings and precautions for use: Ceporex is usually well-tolerated by patients allergic to penicillin, but cross-reaction has been encountered rarely.

As with other broad-spectrum antibiotics, prolonged use may result in the overgrowth of non-susceptible organisms (e.g. Candida, Enterococci, *Clostridium difficile*), which may require interruption of treatment. Pseudomembranous colitis has been reported with the use of broad-spectrum antibiotics, therefore, it is important to consider its diagnosis in patients who develop severe diarrhoea during or after antibiotic use.

As with other antibiotics that are excreted mainly by the kidneys, when renal function is poor, dosage of Ceporex should be suitably reduced (see *Posology and method of administration*).

Interaction with other medicaments and other forms of interaction: Concurrent treatment with high doses of cephalosporins and nephrotoxic drugs such as aminoglycosides or potent diuretics (e.g. Frusemide, ethacrynic acid and piretamide) may adversely affect renal function. Clinical experience has shown that it is not likely to be a problem with Ceporex at the recommended dosage levels.

In patients receiving Ceporex, a false-positive reaction for glucose in the urine may be given, with Benedict's or Fehling's solution, or with 'Clinitest' tablets, but not with enzyme-based tests. There are reports of positive Coombs' test.

Ceporex can interfere with the alkaline picrate assay for creatinine, giving a falsely high reading, but the degree of elevation is unlikely to be of clinical importance.

Pregnancy and lactation: Laboratory experiments and clinical experience show no evidence of teratogenicity, but it would be wise to proceed with caution during the early months of pregnancy, as with all drugs.

Effect on ability to drive and use machines: No effect.

Undesirable effects: A small proportion of patients receiving Ceporex experience gastro-intestinal disturbances such as nausea, vomiting and diarrhoea.

As with other broad-spectrum antibiotics, there have been rare reports of pseudomembranous colitis.

As with other antibiotics, prolonged use may result in the overgrowth of non-susceptible organisms, e.g., Candida. This may present as vulvo-vaginitis. Reversible neutropenia has occurred in a few patients, but is very rare. Drug rashes both urticarial and maculopapular.

Ceporex should be used with care in patients with a history of hypersensitivity to drugs.

Severe skin reactions including very rarely toxic epidermal necrolysis (exanthematic necrolysis), Stevens-Johnson Syndrome and hypersensitivity reactions including angioedema and anaphylaxis.

As with other cephalosporins there have been rare reports of reversible interstitial nephritis.

Overdose: Serum levels of cephalexin can be reduced greatly by peritoneal dialysis or haemodialysis.

Pharmacological properties

Pharmacodynamic properties: Ceporex is resistant to the action of staphylococcal penicillinase, and is therefore active against strains of *Staph. aureus* that are insensitive to penicillin (or ampicillin) through production of that enzyme. Ceporex is also active against the majority of ampicillin-resistant *E. coli*.

Pharmacokinetic properties: Absorption of Ceporex is almost complete, even in the presence of food, and is not adversely affected by coeliac disease, partial gastrectomy, achlorhydria, jaundice or diverticulosis (duodenal or jejunal). Ceporex is excreted in the urine in high concentration.

The serum half-life is normally about one hour, but is longer in the newborn (see *Posology and method of administration*). Ceporex has a wide margin of safety.

Preclinical safety data: None reported.

Pharmaceutical particulars

List of excipients: Microcrystalline cellulose EP, Magnesium stearate EP.

Film coating: Hydroxypropyl methylcellulose EP, Macrogol 400 EP, Opadry OY-S-6927 In-house, Purified water BP.

Incompatibilities: No incompatibilities have been reported.

Shelf life: 36 months.

Special precautions for storage: The product is stored at a temperature not exceeding 30°C, protected from light.

Nature and contents of container:

1. Tubular glass vial with polyethylene snap-plug closure.
2. Tamper evident polypropylene container with low density polyethylene lid. One or more cartridges of activated charcoal according to pack size are included.
3. Tablets are sealed into individual pockets in an aluminium polyethylene/foil laminate (30 and 38 micrometres respectively).
4. Tablets are sealed into individual pockets in an aluminium foil blister with an aluminium lid (43 and 20 micrometres respectively).

All container presentations contain 20, 28, 100 or 500 tablets.

Instructions for use/handling: None stated.

Marketing authorisation number PL 10949/0135

Date of first authorisation/renewal of authorisation MAA: 31.08.93.

Date of (partial) revision of text September 1998

CEPOREX* TABLETS 1 g

Qualitative and quantitative composition Cephalexin PhEur 1000 mg per tablet.

Pharmaceutical form Tablet.

Clinical particulars

Therapeutic indications: Ceporex is a bactericidal antibiotic of the cephalosporin group which is active against a wide range of Gram-positive and Gram-negative organisms. It is indicated for treatment of the following conditions, when caused by susceptible bacteria.

Respiratory tract infections: Acute and chronic bronchitis and infected bronchiectasis.

Ear, nose and throat infections: Otitis media, mastoiditis, sinusitis, follicular tonsillitis and pharyngitis.

Urinary tract infections: Acute and chronic pyelonephritis, cystitis and prostatitis. Prophylaxis of recurrent urinary tract infection.

Gynaecological and obstetric infections.

Skin, soft-tissue and bone infections.

Gonorrhoea (when Penicillin is unsuitable).

Dental procedures: Treatment of dental infections.

As prophylaxis treatment for patients with heart disease undergoing dental treatment as an alternative to penicillin.

Posology and method of administration:
Route of administration: Oral.

Many infections in adults will respond to oral dosage of 1 gram to 2 grams per day in divided doses; however, for most infections, the following simple dosage scheme will be found satisfactory:

Adults and children over 12 years: 1 g b.d.

The following additional information should also be considered:

Adults: For severe or deep-seated infections, especially when less sensitive organisms are involved, the dosage should be increased to 1 g t.d.s. or 3 g b.d. For prophylaxis of recurrent urinary tract infections in adults, a dose of 125 mg each night is recommended and may be continued for several months (the 125 mg/5 ml Suspension is suitable for this purpose).

Children: Ideally, dosage should be calculated on a body-weight basis, particularly in infants. The following dosage recommendations for children are derived from a normal dosage of 25 to 60 mg/kg/day. For chronic, severe or deep-seated infections, this should be increased to 100 mg/kg/day (maximum 4 g/day).

Children under 1 year	(25 to 60 mg/kg/day)
	62.5 to 125 mg b.d.
Children 1–6 years	250 mg–500 mg b.d.
Children 7–12 years	500 mg–1 g b.d.

Notes: For most acute infections, treatment should continue for at least two days after signs have returned to normal and symptoms have subsided, but in chronic, recurrent or complicated urinary tract infections, treatment for two weeks (giving 1 g b.d.) is recommended. For gonorrhoea, a single dose of 3 g with 1 g probenecid for males or 2 g with 0.5 g probenecid for females is usually effective. Concurrent administration of probenecid delays excretion of cephalexin and raises the serum levels by 50 to 100%.

Ceporex has not been shown to have a toxic effect on the kidney, but as with other antibiotics which are excreted mainly by the kidneys, unnecessary accumulation may occur in the body when renal function is below about half of normal. Therefore, the maximum recommended dosages (i.e. Adults 6 g/day, children 4 g/day) should be reduced proportionately in these patients.

In elderly patients, the possibility of renal impairment should be considered. Adult patients receiving intermittent dialysis should be given an additional 500 mg Ceporex after each dialysis, i.e., a total dosage of up to 1 g on that day. Children should receive an additional 8 mg per kg.

Contra-indications: Hypersensitivity to any ingredient of the preparation.

Special warnings and precautions for use: Ceporex is usually well-tolerated by patients allergic to penicillin, but cross-reaction has been encountered rarely.

As with other broad-spectrum antibiotics, prolonged use may result in the overgrowth of non-susceptible organisms (e.g. Candida, Enterococci, *Clostridium difficile*), which may require interruption of treatment. Pseudomembranous colitis has been reported with the use of broad-spectrum antibiotics, therefore, it is important to consider its diagnosis in patients who develop severe diarrhoea during or after antibiotic use.

As with other antibiotics that are excreted mainly by the kidneys, when renal function is poor, dosage of Ceporex should be suitably reduced (see *Posology and method of administration*).

Interaction with other medicaments and other forms of interaction: Concurrent treatment with high doses of cephalosporins and nephrotoxic drugs such as aminoglycosides or potent diuretics (e.g. Frusemide, ethacrynic acid and piretamide) may adversely affect renal function. Clinical experience has shown that it is not likely to be a problem with Ceporex at the recommended dosage levels.

In patients receiving Ceporex, a false-positive reaction for glucose in the urine may be given, with Benedict's or Fehling's solution, or with 'Clinitest' tablets, but not with enzyme-based tests. There are reports of positive Coombs' test.

Ceporex can interfere with the alkaline picrate assay for creatinine, giving a falsely high reading, but the degree of elevation is unlikely to be of clinical importance.

Pregnancy and lactation: Laboratory experiments and clinical experience show no evidence of teratogenicity, but it would be wise to proceed with caution during the early months of pregnancy, as with all drugs.

Effect on ability to drive and use machines: No effect.

Undesirable effects: A small proportion of patients receiving Ceporex experience gastro-intestinal disturbances such as nausea, vomiting and diarrhoea.

As with other broad-spectrum antibiotics, there have been rare reports of pseudomembranous colitis.

As with other antibiotics, prolonged use may result in the overgrowth of non-susceptible organisms, e.g., Candida. This may present as vulvo-vaginitis. Reversible neutropenia has occurred in a few patients, but is very rare. Drug rashes both urticarial and maculopapular.

Ceporex should be used with care in patients with a history of hypersensitivity to drugs.

Severe skin reactions including very rarely toxic epidermal necrolysis (exanthematic necrolysis), Stevens-Johnson Syndrome and hypersensitivity reactions including angioedema and anaphylaxis.

As with other cephalosporins there have been rare reports of reversible interstitial nephritis.

Overdose: Serum levels of cephalexin can be reduced greatly by peritoneal dialysis or haemodialysis.

Pharmacological properties

Pharmacodynamic properties: Ceporex is resistant to the action of staphylococcal penicillinase, and is therefore active against strains of *Staph. aureus* that are insensitive to penicillin (or ampicillin) through production of that enzyme. Ceporex is also active against the majority of ampicillin-resistant *E. coli*.

Pharmacokinetic properties: Absorption of Ceporex is almost complete, even in the presence of food, and is not adversely affected by coeliac disease, partial gastrectomy, achlorhydria, jaundice or diverticulosis (duodenal or jejunal). Ceporex is excreted in the urine in high concentration.

The serum half-life is normally about one hour, but is longer in the newborn (see *Posology and method of administration*). Ceporex has a wide margin of safety.

Preclinical safety data: None reported.

Pharmaceutical particulars

List of excipients: Microcrystalline cellulose EP, Magnesium stearate EP.

Film coating: Hydroxypropyl methylcellulose EP, Macrogol 400 EP, Opadry OY-S-6927 In-house, Purified water BP.

Incompatibilities: No incompatibilities have been reported.

Shelf life: 36 months.

Special precautions for storage: The product is stored at a temperature not exceeding 30°C, protected from light.

Nature and contents of container:

1. Tubular glass vial with polyethylene snap-plug closure.
2. Tamper evident polypropylene container with low density polyethylene lid. One or more cartridges of activated charcoal according to pack size are included.
3. Tablets are sealed into individual pockets in an aluminium polyethylene/foil laminate (30 and 38 micrometres respectively).
4. Tablets are sealed into individual pockets in an aluminium foil blister with an aluminium lid (43 and 20 micrometres respectively).

All container presentations contain 14 or 4 tablets.

Instructions for use/handling: None stated.

Marketing authorisation number PL 10949/0136

Date of first authorisation/renewal of authorisation MAA: 31 December 1993. Renewal: 21 August 1998.

Date of (partial) revision of text August 1998

CEPOREX* SYRUP 125 mg

Qualitative and quantitative composition Cephalexin BP 125 mg per 5 ml (Cephalexin BP (in granules) 3.90% w/w, Cephalexin BP (in dispensed syrup) 2.50% w/v).

Pharmaceutical form Pale orange granules.

Clinical particulars
Therapeutic indications: Ceporex is a bactericidal antibiotic of the cephalosporin group which is active against a wide range of Gram-positive and Gram-negative organisms. It is indicated for treatment of the following conditions, when caused by susceptible bacteria.

Respiratory tract infections: Acute and chronic bronchitis and infected bronchiectasis.

Ear, nose and throat infections: Otitis media, mastoiditis, sinusitis, follicular tonsillitis and pharyngitis.

Urinary tract infections: Acute and chronic pyelonephritis, cystitis and prostatitis. Prophylaxis of recurrent urinary tract infection.

Gynaecological and obstetric infections.

Skin, soft-tissue and bone infections.

Gonorrhoea (when Penicillin is unsuitable).

Dental procedures: Treatment of dental infections.

As prophylaxis treatment for patients with heart disease undergoing dental treatment as an alternative to penicillin.

Posology and method of administration:
Route of administration: Oral.

Many infections in adults will respond to oral dosage of 1 gram to 2 grams per day in divided doses; however, for most infections, the following simple dosage scheme will be found satisfactory:

Adults and children over 12 years: 1 g b.d.

The following additional information should also be considered:

Adults: For severe or deep-seated infections, especially when less sensitive organisms are involved, the dosage should be increased to 1 g t.d.s. or 3 g b.d. For prophylaxis of recurrent urinary tract infections in adults, a dose of 125 mg each night is recommended and may be continued for several months (the 125 mg/5 ml Suspension is suitable for this purpose).

Children: Ideally, dosage should be calculated on a body-weight basis, particularly in infants. The following dosage recommendations for children are derived from a normal dosage of 25 to 60 mg/kg/day. For chronic, severe or deep-seated infections, this should be increased to 100 mg/kg/day (maximum 4 g/day).

Children under 1 year	(25 to 60 mg/kg/day) 62.5 to 125 mg b.d.
Children 1–6 years	250 mg–500 mg b.d.
Children 7–12 years	500 mg–1 g b.d.

Notes: For most acute infections, treatment should continue for at least two days after signs have returned to normal and symptoms have subsided, but in chronic, recurrent or complicated urinary tract infections, treatment for two weeks (giving 1 g b.d.) is recommended. For gonorrhoea, a single dose of 3 g with 1 g probenecid for males or 2 g with 0.5 g probenecid for females is usually effective. Concurrent administration of probenecid delays excretion of cephalexin and raises the serum levels by 50 to 100%.

Ceporex has not been shown to have a toxic effect on the kidney, but as with other antibiotics which are excreted mainly by the kidneys, unnecessary accumulation may occur in the body when renal function is below about half of normal. Therefore, the maximum recommended dosages (i.e. Adults 6 g/day, children 4 g/day) should be reduced proportionately in these patients.

In elderly patients, the possibility of renal impairment should be considered. Adult patients receiving intermittent dialysis should be given an additional 500 mg Ceporex after each dialysis, i.e., a total dosage of up to 1 g on that day. Children should receive an additional 8 mg per kg.

Contra-indications: Hypersensitivity to any ingredient of the preparation.

Special warnings and precautions for use: Ceporex is usually well-tolerated by patients allergic to penicillin, but cross-reaction has been encountered rarely.

As with other broad-spectrum antibiotics, prolonged use may result in the overgrowth of non-susceptible organisms (e.g. Candida, Enterococci, *Clostridium difficile*), which may require interruption of treatment. Pseudomembranous colitis has been reported with the use of broad-spectrum antibiotics, therefore, it is important to consider its diagnosis in patients who develop severe diarrhoea during or after antibiotic use.

As with other antibiotics that are excreted mainly by the kidneys, when renal function is poor, dosage of Ceporex should be suitably reduced (see *Posology and method of administration*).

Interaction with other medicaments and other forms of interaction: Concurrent treatment with high doses of cephalosporins and nephrotoxic drugs such as aminoglycosides or potent diuretics (e.g. Frusemide, ethacrynic acid and piretamide) may adversely affect renal function. Clinical experience has shown that it is not likely to be a problem with Ceporex at the recommended dosage levels.

In patients receiving Ceporex, a false-positive reaction for glucose in the urine may be given, with Benedict's or Fehling's solution, or with 'Clinitest' tablets, but not with enzyme-based tests. There are reports of positive Coombs' test.

Ceporex can interfere with the alkaline picrate assay for creatinine, giving a falsely high reading, but the degree of elevation is unlikely to be of clinical importance.

Pregnancy and lactation: Laboratory experiments and clinical experience show no evidence of teratogenicity, but it would be wise to proceed with caution during the early months of pregnancy, as with all drugs.

Effect on ability to drive and use machines: No effect.

Undesirable effects: A small proportion of patients receiving Ceporex experience gastro-intestinal disturbances such as nausea, vomiting and diarrhoea.

As with other broad-spectrum antibiotics, there have been rare reports of pseudomembranous colitis.

As with other antibiotics, prolonged use may result in the overgrowth of non-susceptible organisms, e.g., Candida. This may present as vulvo-vaginitis. Reversible neutropenia has occurred in a few patients, but is very rare. Drug rashes both urticarial and maculopapular.

Ceporex should be used with care in patients with a history of hypersensitivity to drugs.

Severe skin reactions including very rarely toxic epidermal necrolysis (exanthematic necrolysis), Stevens-Johnson Syndrome and hypersensitivity reactions including angioedema and anaphylaxis.

As with other cephalosporins there have been rare reports of reversible interstitial nephritis.

Overdose: Serum levels of cephalexin can be reduced greatly by peritoneal dialysis or haemodialysis.

Pharmacological properties
Pharmacodynamic properties: Ceporex is resistant to the action of staphylococcal penicillinase, and is therefore active against strains of *Staph. aureus* that are insensitive to penicillin (or ampicillin) through production of that enzyme. Ceporex is also active against the majority of ampicillin-resistant *E. coli.*

Pharmacokinetic properties: Absorption of Ceporex is almost complete, even in the presence of food, and is not adversely affected by coeliac disease, partial gastrectomy, achlorhydria, jaundice or diverticulosis (duodenal or jejunal). Ceporex is excreted in the urine in high concentration.

The serum half-life is normally about one hour, but is longer in the newborn (see *Posology and method of administration*). Ceporex has a wide margin of safety.

Preclinical safety data: None reported.

Pharmaceutical particulars
List of excipients:
In granules and dispensed syrup: Sodium calcium edetate, Acacia powdered, Citric acid, Sodium citrate, Sunset yellow ariavit (311831) E110, Polvaromas orange-bramble flavour, Sucrose, Purified water.

Incompatibilities: No incompatibilities have been reported.

Shelf life:
Dispensed syrup: 24 months (unopened).

10 days when the bottle container is opened for the first time.

Sachets: 24 months.

Special precautions for storage: 24 months at a temperature not exceeding 25°C.

Nature and contents of container:
Bottles: 150 ml amber glass bottles with PVC lined aluminium roll on caps or polypropylene caps having Melinex/Aluminium pulpboard liners. Pack size: 100 ml.

Sachets: (single dose) The 125 mg sachets are made from a paper/aluminium foil/polyethylene laminate.

Instructions for use/handling: None stated.

Marketing authorisation number PL 10949/0131

Date of first authorisation/renewal of authorisation MAA: 26.09.93. Renewal: 16.10.98.

Date of (partial) revision of text June 1998. This is the first SmPC.

CEPOREX* SYRUP 250 mg

Qualitative and quantitative composition Cephalexin BP 250 mg per 5 ml (Cephalexin BP (in granules) 7.80% w/w, Cephalexin BP (in dispensed syrup) 5.00% w/v).

Pharmaceutical form Pale orange granules.

Clinical particulars
Therapeutic indications: Ceporex is a bactericidal antibiotic of the cephalosporin group which is active against a wide range of Gram-positive and Gram-negative organisms. It is indicated for treatment of the following conditions, when caused by susceptible bacteria.

Respiratory tract infections: Acute and chronic bronchitis and infected bronchiectasis.

Ear, nose and throat infections: Otitis media, mastoiditis, sinusitis, follicular tonsillitis and pharyngitis.

Urinary tract infections: Acute and chronic pyelonephritis, cystitis and prostatitis. Prophylaxis of recurrent urinary tract infection.

Gynaecological and obstetric infections.

Skin, soft-tissue and bone infections.

Gonorrhoea (when Penicillin is unsuitable).

Dental procedures: Treatment of dental infections.

As prophylaxis treatment for patients with heart disease undergoing dental treatment as an alternative to penicillin.

Posology and method of administration:
Route of administration: Oral.

Many infections in adults will respond to oral dosage of 1 gram to 2 grams per day in divided doses; however, for most infections, the following simple dosage scheme will be found satisfactory:

Adults and children over 12 years: 1 g b.d.

The following additional information should also be considered:

Adults: For severe or deep-seated infections, especially when less sensitive organisms are involved, the dosage should be increased to 1 g t.d.s. or 3 g b.d. For prophylaxis of recurrent urinary tract infections in adults, a dose of 125 mg each night is recommended and may be continued for several months (the 125 mg/5 ml Suspension is suitable for this purpose).

Children: Ideally, dosage should be calculated on a body-weight basis, particularly in infants. The following dosage recommendations for children are derived from a normal dosage of 25 to 60 mg/kg/day. For chronic, severe or deep-seated infections, this should be increased to 100 mg/kg/day (maximum 4 g/day).

Children under 1 year	(25 to 60 mg/kg/day) 62.5 to 125 mg b.d.
Children 1–6 years	250 mg–500 mg b.d.
Children 7–12 years	500 mg–1 g b.d.

Notes: For most acute infections, treatment should continue for at least two days after signs have returned to normal and symptoms have subsided, but in chronic, recurrent or complicated urinary tract infections, treatment for two weeks (giving 1 g b.d.) is recommended. For gonorrhoea, a single dose of 3 g with 1 g probenecid for males or 2 g with 0.5 g probenecid for females is usually effective. Concurrent administration of probenecid delays excretion of cephalexin and raises the serum levels by 50 to 100%.

Ceporex has not been shown to have a toxic effect on the kidney, but as with other antibiotics which are excreted mainly by the kidneys, unnecessary accumulation may occur in the body when renal function is below about half of normal. Therefore, the maximum recommended dosages (i.e. Adults 6 g/day, children 4 g/day) should be reduced proportionately in these patients.

In elderly patients, the possibility of renal impairment should be considered. Adult patients receiving intermittent dialysis should be given an additional 500 mg Ceporex after each dialysis, i.e., a total dosage of up to 1 g on that day. Children should receive an additional 8 mg per kg.

Contra-indications: Hypersensitivity to any ingredient of the preparation.

Special warnings and precautions for use: Ceporex is usually well-tolerated by patients allergic to penicillin, but cross-reaction has been encountered rarely.

As with other broad-spectrum antibiotics, prolonged use may result in the overgrowth of non-susceptible organisms (e.g. Candida, Enterococci, *Clostridium difficile*), which may require interruption of treatment. Pseudomembranous colitis has been reported with the use of broad-spectrum antibiotics, therefore, it is important to consider its diagnosis in patients who develop severe diarrhoea during or after antibiotic use.

As with other antibiotics that are excreted mainly by the kidneys, when renal function is poor, dosage of Ceporex should be suitably reduced (see *Posology and method of administration*).

Interaction with other medicaments and other forms of interaction: Concurrent treatment with high doses of cephalosporins and nephrotoxic drugs such as aminoglycosides or potent diuretics (e.g. Frusemide, ethacrynic acid and piretamide) may adversely affect renal function. Clinical experience has shown that it is not likely to be a problem with Ceporex at the recommended dosage levels.

In patients receiving Ceporex, a false-positive reaction for glucose in the urine may be given, with Benedict's or Fehling's solution, or with 'Clinitest' tablets, but not with enzyme-based tests. There are reports of positive Coombs' test.

Ceporex can interfere with the alkaline picrate assay for creatinine, giving a falsely high reading, but the degree of elevation is unlikely to be of clinical importance.

Pregnancy and lactation: Laboratory experiments and clinical experience show no evidence of teratogenicity, but it would be wise to proceed with caution during the early months of pregnancy, as with all drugs.

Effect on ability to drive and use machines: No effect.

Undesirable effects: A small proportion of patients receiving Ceporex experience gastro-intestinal disturbances such as nausea, vomiting and diarrhoea.

As with other broad-spectrum antibiotics, there have been rare reports of pseudomembranous colitis.

As with other antibiotics, prolonged use may result in the overgrowth of non-susceptible organisms, e.g., Candida. This may present as vulvo-vaginitis. Reversible neutropenia has occurred in a few patients, but is very rare. Drug rashes both urticarial and maculopapular.

Ceporex should be used with care in patients with a history of hypersensitivity to drugs.

Severe skin reactions including very rarely toxic epidermal necrolysis (exanthematic necrolysis), Stevens-Johnson Syndrome and hypersensitivity reactions including angioedema and anaphylaxis.

As with other cephalosporins there have been rare reports of reversible interstitial nephritis.

Overdose: Serum levels of cephalexin can be reduced greatly by peritoneal dialysis or haemodialysis.

Pharmacological properties

Pharmacodynamic properties: Ceporex is resistant to the action of staphylococcal penicillinase, and is therefore active against strains of *Staph. aureus* that are insensitive to penicillin (or ampicillin) through production of that enzyme. Ceporex is also active against the majority of ampicillin-resistant *E. coli.*

Pharmacokinetic properties: Absorption of Ceporex is almost complete, even in the presence of food, and is not adversely affected by coeliac disease, partial gastrectomy, achlorhydria, jaundice or diverticulosis (duodenal or jejunal). Ceporex is excreted in the urine in high concentration.

The serum half-life is normally about one hour, but is longer in the newborn (see *Posology and method of administration*). Ceporex has a wide margin of safety.

Preclinical safety data: None reported.

Pharmaceutical particulars

List of excipients:

In granules and dispensed syrup: Sodium calcium edetate, Acacia powdered, Citric acid, Sodium citrate, Sunset yellow ariavit (311831) E110, Polvaromas orange-bramble flavour, Sucrose, Purified water.

Incompatibilities: No incompatibilities have been reported.

Shelf life:

Dispensed syrup: 24 months (unopened).

10 days when the bottle container is opened for the first time.

Sachets: 24 months.

Special precautions for storage: 24 months at a temperature not exceeding 25°C.

Nature and contents of container:

Bottles: 150 ml amber glass bottles with PVC lined aluminium roll on caps or polypropylene caps having Melinex/Aluminium pulpboard liners. Pack size: 100 ml.

Sachets: (single dose) The 250 mg sachets are made from a paper/aluminium foil/polyethylene laminate.

Instructions for use/handling: None stated.

Marketing authorisation number PL 10949/0132

Date of first authorisation/renewal of authorisation
MAA: 26.09.93. Renewal: 16.10.98.

Date of (partial) revision of text
June 1998. This is the first SmPC.

CEPOREX* PAEDIATRIC DROPS
CEPOREX* SYRUP 500 mg/5 ml

Qualitative and quantitative composition Cephalexin BP 500 mg per 5 ml (Cephalexin BP (in granules) 15.61% w/w, Cephalexin BP (in dispensed syrup) 10.00% w/v).

Pharmaceutical form Pale orange granules.

Clinical particulars

Therapeutic indications: Ceporex is a bactericidal antibiotic of the cephalosporin group which is active against a wide range of Gram-positive and Gram-negative organisms. It is indicated for treatment of the following conditions, when caused by susceptible bacteria.

Respiratory tract infections: Acute and chronic bronchitis and infected bronchiectasis.

Ear, nose and throat infections: Otitis media, mastoiditis, sinusitis, follicular tonsillitis and pharyngitis.

Urinary tract infections: Acute and chronic pyelonephritis, cystitis and prostatitis. Prophylaxis of recurrent urinary tract infection.

Gynaecological and obstetric infections.

Skin, soft-tissue and bone infections.

Gonorrhoea (when Penicillin is unsuitable).

Dental procedures: Treatment of dental infections.

As prophylaxis treatment for patients with heart disease undergoing dental treatment as an alternative to penicillin.

Posology and method of administration:

Route of administration: Oral.

Many infections in adults will respond to oral dosage of 1 gram to 2 grams per day in divided doses; however, for most infections, the following simple dosage scheme will be found satisfactory:

Adults and children over 12 years: 1 g b.d.

The following additional information should also be considered:

Adults: For severe or deep-seated infections, especially when less sensitive organisms are involved, the dosage should be increased to 1 g t.d.s. or 3 g b.d. For prophylaxis of recurrent urinary tract infections in adults, a dose of 125 mg each night is recommended and may be continued for several months (the 125 mg/5 ml Suspension is suitable for this purpose).

Children: Ideally, dosage should be calculated on a body-weight basis, particularly in infants. The following dosage recommendations for children are derived from a normal dosage of 25 to 60 mg/kg/day. For chronic, severe or deep-seated infections, this should be increased to 100 mg/kg/day (maximum 4 g/day).

Children under 1 year	(25 to 60 mg/kg/day) 62.5 to 125 mg b.d.
Children 1–6 years	250 mg–500 mg b.d.
Children 7–12 years	500 mg–1 g b.d.

Notes: For most acute infections, treatment should continue for at least two days after signs have returned to normal and symptoms have subsided, but in chronic, recurrent or complicated urinary tract infections, treatment for two weeks (giving 1 g b.d.) is recommended. For gonorrhoea, a single dose of 3 g with 1 g probenecid for males or 2 g with 0.5 g probenecid for females is usually effective. Concurrent administration of probenecid delays excretion of cephalexin and raises the serum levels by 50 to 100%.

Ceporex has not been shown to have a toxic effect on the kidney, but as with other antibiotics which are excreted mainly by the kidneys, unnecessary accumulation may occur in the body when renal function is below about half of normal. Therefore, the maximum recommended dosages (i.e. Adults 6 g/day, children 4 g/day) should be reduced proportionately in these patients.

In elderly patients, the possibility of renal impairment should be considered. Adult patients receiving intermittent dialysis should be given an additional 500 mg Ceporex after each dialysis, i.e., a total dosage of up to 1 g on that day. Children should receive an additional 8 mg per kg.

Contra-indications: Hypersensitivity to any ingredient of the preparation.

Special warnings and precautions for use: Ceporex is usually well-tolerated by patients allergic to penicillin, but cross-reaction has been encountered rarely.

As with other broad-spectrum antibiotics, prolonged use may result in the overgrowth of non-susceptible organisms (e.g. Candida, Enterococci, *Clostridium difficile*), which may require interruption of treatment. Pseudomembranous colitis has been reported with the use of broad-spectrum antibiotics, therefore, it is important to consider its diagnosis in patients who develop severe diarrhoea during or after antibiotic use.

As with other antibiotics that are excreted mainly by the kidneys, when renal function is poor, dosage of Ceporex should be suitably reduced (see *Posology and method of administration*).

Interaction with other medicaments and other forms of interaction: Concurrent treatment with high doses of cephalosporins and nephrotoxic drugs such as aminoglycosides or potent diuretics (e.g. Frusemide, ethacrynic acid and piretamide) may adversely affect renal function. Clinical experience has shown that it is not likely to be a problem with Ceporex at the recommended dosage levels.

In patients receiving Ceporex, a false-positive reaction for glucose in the urine may be given, with Benedict's or Fehling's solution, or with 'Clinitest' tablets, but not with enzyme-based tests. There are reports of positive Coombs' test.

Ceporex can interfere with the alkaline picrate assay for creatinine, giving a falsely high reading, but the degree of elevation is unlikely to be of clinical importance.

Pregnancy and lactation: Laboratory experiments and clinical experience show no evidence of teratogenicity, but it would be wise to proceed with caution during the early months of pregnancy, as with all drugs.

Effect on ability to drive and use machines: No effect.

Undesirable effects: A small proportion of patients receiving Ceporex experience gastro-intestinal disturbances such as nausea, vomiting and diarrhoea.

As with other broad-spectrum antibiotics, there have been rare reports of pseudomembranous colitis.

As with other antibiotics, prolonged use may result in the overgrowth of non-susceptible organisms, e.g., Candida. This may present as vulvo-vaginitis. Reversible neutropenia has occurred in a few patients, but is very rare. Drug rashes both urticarial and maculopapular.

Ceporex should be used with care in patients with a history of hypersensitivity to drugs.

Severe skin reactions including very rarely toxic epidermal necrolysis (exanthematic necrolysis), Stevens-Johnson Syndrome and hypersensitivity reactions including angioedema and anaphylaxis.

As with other cephalosporins there have been rare reports of reversible interstitial nephritis.

Overdose: Serum levels of cephalexin can be reduced greatly by peritoneal dialysis or haemodialysis.

Pharmacological properties

Pharmacodynamic properties: Ceporex is resistant to the action of staphylococcal penicillinase, and is therefore active against strains of *Staph. aureus* that are insensitive to penicillin (or ampicillin) through production of that enzyme. Ceporex is also active against the majority of ampicillin-resistant *E. coli.*

Pharmacokinetic properties: Absorption of Ceporex is almost complete, even in the presence of food, and is not adversely affected by coeliac disease, partial gastrectomy, achlorhydria, jaundice or diverticulosis (duodenal or jejunal). Ceporex is excreted in the urine in high concentration.

The serum half-life is normally about one hour, but is longer in the newborn (see *Posology and method of administration*). Ceporex has a wide margin of safety.

Preclinical safety data: None reported.

Pharmaceutical particulars

List of excipients:

In granules and dispensed syrup: Sodium calcium edetate, Acacia powdered, Citric acid, Sodium citrate, Sunset yellow ariavit (311831) E110, Polvaromas orange-bramble flavour, Sucrose, Purified water.

Incompatibilities: No incompatibilities have been reported.

Shelf life: 24 months.

Special precautions for storage: Store at a temperature not exceeding 25°C.

Nature and contents of container:

1. 150 ml amber glass bottles with PVC lined aluminium roll on caps or polypropylene caps having Melinex/Aluminium pulpboard liners. Pack size: 100 ml.

2. 15 ml amber glass bottles with a white screw cap and polycone liner, together with a plastic dropper assembly, rubber teat and polypropylene screw cap. Pack size: 10 ml.

Instructions for use/handling: None stated.

Marketing authorisation number PL 10949/0133

Date of first authorisation/renewal of authorisation
MAA: 26.09.93. Renewal: 16.10.98.

Date of (partial) revision of text
June 1998. This is the first SmPC.

COMBIVIR FILM COATED TABLETS

Qualitative and quantitative composition Combivir contains 150 mg lamivudine and 300 mg zidovudine.

Pharmaceutical form Film coated tablets.

White to off-white, capsule-shaped tablets, engraved with GXFC3 on one side.

Clinical particulars

Therapeutic indications: Combivir is indicated in antiretroviral combination therapy for the treatment of HIV infected adults and adolescents >12 years of age.

Posology and method of administration:

Adults and adolescents over the age of 12 years: The recommended dose of Combivir is one tablet twice daily. Combivir may be administered with or without food.

Therapy should be initiated by a physician experienced in the management of HIV infection.

For situations where discontinuation of therapy with one of the active constituents of Combivir, or dose reduction is necessary separate preparations of lamivudine and zidovudine are available in tablets/capsules and oral solution.

Renal impairment: Lamivudine and zidovudine concentrations are increased in patients with renal impairment due to decreased clearance. Therefore as dosage adjustment of these may be necessary it is recommended that separate preparations of lamivudine and zidovudine be administered to patients with reduced renal function (creatinine clearance ≤50 ml/min).

Hepatic impairment: The influence of hepatic impairment on lamivudine levels is under investigation. Lamivudine clearance is largely renal. Based on preliminary safety data no dosage adjustment is necessary. However limited data in patients with cirrhosis suggest that accumulation of zidovudine may occur in patients with hepatic impairment because of decreased glucuronidation. Therefore as dosage adjustments for zidovudine may be necessary, it is recommended that separate preparations of lamivudine and zidovudine be administered to patients with severe hepatic impairment.

Dosage adjustments in patients with haematological adverse reactions: Dosage adjustment of zidovudine may be necessary if the haemoglobin level falls below 9 g/dl or 5.59 mmol/l or the neutrophil count falls below 1.0×10^9/l (see *Contra-indications*). This is more likely in patients with poor bone marrow reserve prior to treatment, particularly in patients with advanced HIV disease. As dosage adjustment of Combivir is not possible, separate preparations of zidovudine and lamivudine should be used. Physicians should refer to the individual prescribing information for these drugs.

Dosage in the elderly: No specific data are available, however special care is advised in this age group due to age associated changes such as the decrease in renal function and alteration of haematological parameters.

Contra-indications: The use of Combivir is contra-indicated in patients with known hypersensitivity to lamivudine, zidovudine or to any ingredient of the preparation.

Zidovudine is contra-indicated in patients with abnormally low neutrophil counts ($<0.75 \times 10^9$/l), or abnormally low haemoglobin levels (<7.5 g/dL or 4.65 mmol/l). Combivir is therefore contra-indicated in these patients (see *Special warnings and special precautions for use*).

Special warnings and special precautions for use: The special warnings and precautions relevant to both lamivudine and zidovudine are included in this section. There are no additional precautions and warnings relevant to the combination Combivir.

Special warnings: Patients receiving Combivir or any other antiretroviral therapy may continue to develop opportunistic infections and other complications of HIV infection. Therefore patients should remain under close clinical observation by physicians experienced in the treatment of HIV infection.

Patients should be advised that current antiretroviral therapy, including Combivir, has not been proven to prevent the risk of transmission of HIV to others through sexual contact or blood contamination. Appropriate precautions should continue to be employed.

Haematological: Anaemia, neutropenia and leucopenia (usually secondary to neutropenia) can be expected to occur in patients with advanced symptomatic HIV disease receiving zidovudine, therefore haematological parameters should be carefully monitored (see *Contra-indications*) in patients receiving Combivir. These haematological effects are not usually observed before four to six weeks therapy. For patients with advanced symptomatic HIV disease, it is generally recommended that blood tests are performed at least every two weeks for the first three months of therapy and at least monthly thereafter.

In patients with early HIV disease haematological adverse reactions are infrequent. Depending on the overall condition of the patient, blood tests may be performed less often, for example every one to three months. Decreases in the haemoglobin level of more than 25% from baseline and falls in the neutrophil count of more than 50% from baseline may require more frequent monitoring.

Additionally dosage adjustment of zidovudine may be required if severe anaemia or myelosuppression occurs during treatment with Combivir, or in patients with pre-existing bone marrow compromise e.g. haemoglobin <9 g/dL (5.59 mmol/l) or neutrophil count $<1.0 \times 10^9$/l (see *Posology and method of administration*). As dosage adjustment of Combivir is not possible separate preparations of zidovudine and lamivudine should be used. Physicians should refer to the individual prescribing information for these drugs.

Children: Combivir is not indicated for children <12 years old. Physicians should refer to the individual prescribing information for lamivudine and zidovudine.

Use in pregnancy: As the active substances of Combivir may inhibit cellular DNA replication, any use, especially during the first trimester of pregnancy, presents a potential risk to the foetus (see *Use during pregnancy and lactation*).

Pancreatitis: Cases of pancreatitis have occurred rarely in patients treated with lamivudine and zidovudine. However it is not clear whether these cases were due to drug treatment or to the underlying HIV disease. Treatment with Combivir should be stopped immediately if clinical signs, symptoms or laboratory abnormalities suggestive of pancreatitis occur.

Lactic acidosis and hepatomegaly with steatosis: Occurrences of lactic acidosis (in the absence of hypoxemia), usually associated with severe hepatomegaly and hepatic steatosis have been reported with the use of nucleoside analogues. Treatment should be discontinued in the setting of rapidly elevating aminotransferase levels, progressive hepatomegaly or metabolic/lactic acidosis of unknown etiology. Caution should be exercised when administering nucleoside analogues to any patient (particularly obese women) with hepatomegaly, hepatitis or other known risk factors for liver disease. These patients should be followed closely.

Special precautions for use: It is recommended that separate preparations of lamivudine and zidovudine should be administered in cases where dosage adjustment is necessary (see *Posology and administration*). In these cases the physician should refer to the individual prescribing information for these drugs.

Patients should be cautioned about the concomitant use of self-administered medications (see *Interactions with other medicinal products and other forms of interaction*).

Combivir should be used with caution in patients with advanced cirrhotic liver disease due to chronic Hepatitis B infection, as there is a small risk of rebound hepatitis if lamivudine is discontinued.

Interaction with other medicinal products and other forms of interaction: As Combivir contains lamivudine and zidovudine, any interactions that have been identified with these agents individually may occur with Combivir. The likelihood of metabolic interactions with lamivudine is low due to limited metabolism and plasma protein binding, and almost complete renal clearance. Similarly zidovudine has limited protein binding but is eliminated primarily by hepatic conjugation to an active glucuronidated metabolite.

The interactions listed below should not be considered exhaustive but are representative of the classes of drug where caution should be exercised.

Interactions relevant to lamivudine: The possibility of interactions with other drugs administered concurrently with Combivir should be considered, particularly when the main route of elimination is active renal secretion especially via the cationic transport system e.g. trimethoprim. Nucleoside analogues (e.g. zidovudine, didanosine and zalcitabine) and other drugs (e.g. ranitidine, cimetidine) are eliminated only in part by this mechanism and were shown not to interact with lamivudine.

Administration of prophylactic doses of co-trimoxazole results in a 40% increase in lamivudine exposure, because of the trimethoprim component; the sulfamethoxazole component does not interact. However, unless the patient has renal impairment, no dosage adjustment of lamivudine is necessary (see *Posology and method of administration*).

When concomitant administration with co-trimoxazole is warranted, patients should be monitored clinically. Co-administration of Combivir with high doses of co-trimoxazole for the treatment of *Pneumocystis carinii* pneumonia (PCP) and toxoplasmosis should be avoided. Lamivudine has no effect on the pharmacokinetics of co-trimoxazole at the doses studied.

Co-administration of lamivudine with intravenous ganciclovir or foscarnet is not recommended until further information is available.

Lamivudine metabolism does not involve CYP3A, making interactions with drugs metabolised by this system (e.g. protease inhibitors) unlikely.

Interactions relevant to zidovudine: A modest increase in C_{max} (28%) was observed for zidovudine when administered with lamivudine, however overall exposure (AUC) was not significantly altered. Zidovudine has no effect on the pharmacokinetics of lamivudine.

Phenytoin blood levels have been reported to be low in some patients receiving zidovudine, while in one patient a high level was noted. These observations suggest that phenytoin concentrations should be carefully monitored in patients receiving Combivir and phenytoin.

Paracetamol use during treatment with zidovudine in a placebo-controlled trial was associated with an increased incidence of neutropenia especially following chronic therapy. However, the available pharmacokinetic data indicate that paracetamol at the doses studied does not increase plasma levels of zidovudine or of its glucuronide metabolite.

Other drugs, including but not limited to, aspirin, codeine, morphine, indometacin, ketoprofen, naproxen, oxazepam, lorazepam, cimetidine, clofibrate, dapsone and isoprinosine, may alter the metabolism of zidovudine by competitively inhibiting glucuronidation or directly inhibiting hepatic microsomal metabolism. Careful thought should be given to the possibilities of drug interaction before using such drugs particularly for chronic therapy, in combination with Combivir.

Concomitant treatment, especially acute therapy, with potentially nephrotoxic or myelosuppressive drugs (e.g. systemic pentamidine, dapsone, pyrimethamine, co-trimoxazole, amphotericin, flucytosine, ganciclovir, interferon, vincristine, vinblastine and doxorubicin) may also increase the risk of adverse reactions to zidovudine. If concomitant therapy with Combivir and any of these drugs is necessary then extra care should be taken in monitoring renal function and haematological parameters and, if required, the dosage of one or more agents should be reduced.

The nucleoside analogue ribavirin antagonises the *in vitro* antiviral activity of zidovudine and therefore concomitant use of Combivir with this drug should be avoided.

Since some patients receiving Combivir may continue to experience opportunistic infections, concomitant use of prophylactic antimicrobial therapy may have to be considered. Such prophylaxis has included co-trimoxazole, aerosolised pentamidine, pyrimethamine and acyclovir. Limited data from clinical trials do not indicate a significantly increased risk of adverse reactions to zidovudine with these drugs.

Limited data suggest that probenecid increases the mean half-life and area under the plasma concentration curve of zidovudine by decreasing glucuronidation. Renal excretion of the glucuronide (and possibly zidovudine itself) is reduced in the presence of probenecid.

Pregnancy and lactation:

Pregnancy: In reproductive toxicity studies in animals both lamivudine and zidovudine were shown to cross the placenta. Lamivudine has demonstrated evidence of causing an increase in early embryonic deaths in the rabbit at relatively low systemic exposures, but not in the rat even at very high systemic exposure. Zidovudine had a similar effect in both species, but only at very high systemic exposures. Lamivudine was not teratogenic in animal studies. At maternally toxic doses, zidovudine given to rats during organogenesis resulted in an increased incidence of malformations, but no evidence of foetal abnormalities was observed at lower doses.

The safety of lamivudine in human pregnancy has not been established. The use in pregnant women of zidovudine alone, with subsequent treatment of the newborn infants, has been shown to reduce the rate of maternal-foetal transmission of HIV. However, no such data are available for lamivudine. Likewise, no data are available for the treatment with a combination of lamivudine and zidovudine in humans or animals. As the active substances of Combivir may inhibit cellular DNA replication, any use, especially during the first trimester of pregnancy, presents a potential risk to the foetus (see *Special warnings and special precautions for use*). Consequently the administration of Combivir during pregnancy should only be considered if expected benefits outweigh any possible risks.

Based on the animal carcinogenicity and mutagenicity findings a carcinogenic risk to humans cannot be excluded. The relevance of these animal data to both infected and uninfected infants exposed to zidovudine is unknown. However, pregnant women considering using Combivir during pregnancy should be made aware of these findings (see *Pre-clinical safety data*).

Neither zidovudine nor lamivudine have shown evidence of impairment of fertility in studies in male and female rats. There are no data on their effect on human female fertility. In men zidovudine has not been shown to affect sperm count, morphology or motility.

Lactation: It is not known if lamivudine or zidovudine are excreted in human milk. Since animal data suggest that the two substances may pass into breast milk, it is recommended that mothers taking Combivir do not breast feed their infants. Some health experts recommend that HIV infected women do not breast feed their infants under any circumstances in order to avoid transmission of HIV.

Effects on ability to drive and use machines: There have been no studies to investigate the effect of lamivudine or zidovudine on driving performance or the ability to operate machinery. Further, a detrimental effect on such activities cannot be predicted from the pharmacology of the drugs. Nevertheless, the clinical status of the patient and the adverse event profile of lamivudine and zidovudine should be borne in mind when considering the patient's ability to drive or operate machinery.

Undesirable effects: Adverse events have been reported during therapy for HIV disease with lamivudine and zidovudine separately or in combination. For many of these events it is unclear whether they are related to lamivudine, zidovudine, or to the wide range of drugs used in the management of HIV disease or as a result of the underlying disease process.

As Combivir contains lamivudine and zidovudine, the type and severity of adverse reactions associated with each of the compounds may be expected. There is no evidence of added toxicity following concurrent administration of the two compounds.

Cases of lactic acidosis, usually associated with severe hepatomegaly and hepatic steatosis, have been reported with the use of nucleoside analogues.

Lamivudine: The adverse events which have been commonly reported are headache, malaise, fatigue, nausea, diarrhoea, vomiting, abdominal pain or cramps, insomnia, cough, nasal symptoms and musculoskeletal pain.

Cases of pancreatitis and peripheral neuropathy (or paraesthesia) have been reported, although no relationship to the dose of lamivudine has been noted.

Neutropenia and anaemia (both occasionally severe) have occurred in combination with zidovudine. Thrombocytopenia, transient rises in liver enzymes (AST, ALT) and rises in serum amylase have been reported.

Zidovudine: The most serious adverse reactions include anaemia (which may require transfusions), neutropenia and leucopenia. These occur more frequently at higher doses (1200–1500 mg/day) and in patients with advanced HIV disease (especially when there is poor bone marrow reserve prior to treatment), and particularly in patients with CD_4 cell counts $<100/mm^3$. Dosage reduction or cessation of therapy may become necessary (see *Posology and method of administration*).

The incidence of neutropenia was also increased in those patients whose neutrophil counts, haemoglobin levels and serum vitamin B_{12} levels were low at the start of zidovudine therapy, and in those patients taking paracetamol concurrently (see *Interaction with other medicinal products and other forms of interaction*).

Other frequent adverse events reported in large placebo-controlled clinical trials included nausea, vomiting, anorexia, abdominal pain, headache, rash, fever, myalgia, paraesthesia, insomnia, malaise, asthenia and dyspepsia. Apart from nausea, which was significantly more common in all studies in patients receiving zidovudine, the other adverse events were not consistently reported to be more common than in the placebo recipients. Severe headache, myalgia and insomnia were more common in zidovudine-treated patients with advanced HIV disease, whilst vomiting, anorexia, malaise and asthenia were more common in zidovudine-treated patients with early HIV disease.

Other adverse events reported included somnolence, diarrhoea, dizziness, sweating, dyspnoea, flatulence, taste perversion, chest pains, loss of mental acuity, anxiety, urinary frequency, depression, generalised pain, chills, cough, urticaria, pruritus and an influenza-like syndrome. The incidence of these and other less frequent adverse events was similar in both zidovudine and placebo-treated patients. The available data from both placebo-controlled and open-labelled studies indicate that the incidence of nausea and other frequently reported clinical adverse events consistently decreases over time during the first few weeks of therapy with zidovudine.

The following events have also been reported in patients treated with zidovudine. The relationship between these events and the use of zidovudine is difficult to evaluate, particularly in the medically complicated situations which characterise advanced HIV disease:

Myopathy, pancytopenia with marrow hypoplasia and isolated thrombocytopenia, lactic acidosis in the absence of hypoxaemia, liver disorders such as severe hepatomegaly with steatosis, raised blood levels of liver enzymes and bilirubin, pancreatitis, nail, skin and oral mucosa pigmentation (see *Special warnings and special precautions for use*).

Convulsions and other cerebral events have also been reported in patients receiving open-label therapy with zidovudine. The weight of evidence however indicates an overall beneficial effect of zidovudine on HIV-associated neurological disorders.

If the severity of the symptoms warrants it, a reduction or suspension of zidovudine therapy may assist in the assessment and management of these conditions. In this situation Combivir should be discontinued and separate preparations of zidovudine and lamivudine should be administered (see *Special warnings and special precautions for use*).

Overdose: There is no experience of overdosage with Combivir. However, there are limited data available on the consequences of ingestion of acute overdoses of lamivudine and zidovudine in humans. No fatalities occurred, and all patients recovered. No specific signs or symptoms have been identified following such overdosage.

If overdosage occurs the patient should be monitored for evidence of toxicity (see *Undesirable effects*), and standard supportive treatment applied as necessary. Since lamivudine is dialysable, continuous haemodialysis could be used in the treatment of overdosage, although this has not been studied. Haemodialysis and peritoneal dialysis appear to have a limited effect on elimination of zidovudine, but enhance the elimination of the glucuronide metabolite. For more details physicians should refer to the individual prescribing information for lamivudine and zidovudine.

Pharmacological properties

Pharmacodynamic properties: Pharmacotherapeutic group – nucleoside analogue, ATC Code: JO5A B20.

Lamivudine and zidovudine are potent, selective inhibitors of HIV-1 and HIV-2. Lamivudine has been shown to be highly synergistic with zidovudine, inhibiting the replication of HIV in cell culture. Both drugs are metabolised sequentially by intracellular kinases to the 5′-triphosphate (TP). Lamivudine-TP and zidovudine-TP are substrates for and competitive inhibitors of HIV reverse transcriptase. However, their main antiviral activity is through incorporation of the monophosphate form into the viral DNA chain, resulting in chain termination. Lamivudine and zidovudine triphosphates show significantly less affinity for host cell DNA polymerases.

The relationship between *in vitro* susceptibility of HIV to lamivudine and/or zidovudine and the clinical response to therapy remain under investigation. *In vitro* sensitivity testing has not been standardised and results may vary according to methodological factors.

In clinical trials lamivudine in combination with zidovudine has been shown to reduce HIV-1 viral load and to increase CD_4 cell count. Clinical end-point data indicate that lamivudine in combination with zidovudine alone or in combination with zidovudine containing treatment regimens results in a significant reduction in the risk of disease progression and mortality.

Individually, lamivudine and zidovudine therapy has resulted in HIV clinical isolates which show reduced sensitivity *in vitro* to the nucleoside analogue to which they have been exposed. However *in vitro* studies also indicate that zidovudine-resistant virus isolates can become zidovudine sensitive when they simultaneously acquire resistance to lamivudine. Furthermore *in vivo* there is clinical evidence that lamivudine plus zidovudine delays the emergence of zidovudine resistance in anti-retroviral naive patients.

Pharmacokinetic properties:

Absorption: Lamivudine and zidovudine are well absorbed from the gastrointestinal tract. The bioavailability of oral lamivudine in adults is normally between 80–85% and for zidovudine 60–70%.

A bioequivalence study compared Combivir with lamivudine 150 mg and zidovudine 300 mg tablets taken together. The effect of food on the rate and extent of absorption was also studied. Combivir was shown to be bioequivalent to lamivudine 150 mg and zidovudine 300 mg given as separate tablets, when administered to fasting subjects.

Following Combivir administration, lamivudine and zidovudine C_{max} (95% confidence interval) values were 1.5 (1.3–1.8) µg/ml and 1.8 (1.5–2.2) µg/ml respectively. The median (range) lamivudine and zidovudine t_{max} values were 0.75 (0.50–2.00) hours and 0.50 (0.25–2.00) hours respectively. The extent of lamivudine and zidovudine absorption (AUC∞) and estimates of half-life following administration of Combivir with food were similar when compared to fasting subjects, although the rates of absorption (C_{max}, t_{max}) were slowed. Based on these data Combivir may be administered with or without food.

Distribution: Intravenous studies with lamivudine and zidovudine showed that the mean apparent volume of distribution is 1.3 and 1.6 l/kg respectively. Lamivudine exhibits linear pharmacokinetics over the therapeutic dose range and displays limited binding to the major plasma protein albumin (<36% serum albumin *in vitro*). Zidovudine plasma protein binding is 34% to 38%. Drug interactions involving binding site displacement are not anticipated with Combivir.

Data show that lamivudine and zidovudine penetrate the central nervous system (CNS) and reach the cerebrospinal fluid (CSF). The mean ratios of CSF/serum lamivudine and zidovudine concentrations 2–4 hours after oral administration were approximately 0.12 and 0.5 respectively. The true extent of CNS penetration of lamivudine and its relationship with any clinical efficacy is unknown.

Metabolism: Metabolism of lamivudine is a minor route of elimination. Lamivudine is predominately cleared by renal excretion of unchanged drug. The likelihood of metabolic drug interactions with lamivudine is low due to the small extent of hepatic metabolism (5–10%) and low plasma binding.

The 5′-glucuronide of zidovudine is the major metabolite in both plasma and urine, accounting for approximately 50–80% of the administered dose eliminated by renal excretion. 3′-amino-3′-deoxythymidine (AMT) has been identified as a metabolite of zidovudine following intravenous dosing.

Elimination: The observed lamivudine half-life of elimination is 5 to 7 hours. The mean systemic clearance of lamivudine is approximately 0.32 l/h/kg, with predominantly renal clearance (>70%) via the organic cationic transport system. Studies in patients with renal impairment show lamivudine elimination is affected by renal dysfunction. Dose reduction is required for patients with creatinine clearance ≤50 ml/min (see *Posology and method of administration*).

From studies with intravenous zidovudine, the mean terminal plasma half-life was 1.1 hours and the mean systemic clearance was 1.6 l/h/kg. Renal clearance of zidovudine is estimated to be 0.34 l/h/kg, indicating glomerular filtration and active tubular secretion by the kidneys. Zidovudine concentrations are increased in patients with advanced renal failure.

Preclinical safety data: No synergy of toxicity has been observed in studies with lamivudine in combination with zidovudine. The clinically relevant effects of the two drugs in combination are anaemia, neutropenia and leucopenia.

Neither lamivudine nor zidovudine are mutagenic in bacterial tests, but like many nucleoside analogues they show activity in *in vitro* mammalian tests such as the mouse lymphoma assay. Lamivudine has not shown any genotoxic activity in *in vivo* studies at doses that gave plasma concentrations up to 40–50 times higher than clinical plasma levels. Zidovudine showed clastogenic effects in an oral repeated dose micronucleus test in mice. Peripheral blood lymphocytes from AIDS patients receiving zidovudine treatment have also been observed to contain higher numbers of chromosome breakages. The clinical implications of these findings are unclear. The genotoxic potential of a combination of lamivudine and zidovudine has not been tested.

In long-term oral carcinogenicity studies in rats and mice, lamivudine did not show any carcinogenic potential. In zidovudine treated animals treatment-related effects were limited to late-appearing vaginal neoplasms. The carcinogenic potential of a combination of lamivudine and zidovudine has not been tested. The relevance for humans of the tumours induced by zidovudine in rodents is uncertain. However, metabolic, biological and physiological differences between rodents and humans suggest that a similar carcinogenic risk in humans is unlikely. Any theoretical risk of carcinogenicity should be balanced against the proven therapeutic benefit.

Pharmaceutical particulars

List of excipients:

Tablet core: Microcrystalline cellulose, Sodium starch glycollate, Colloidal silicon dioxide, Magnesium stearate.

Tablet film coat: Methylhydroxypropyl cellulose, Titanium Dioxide (E171), Macrogol 400, Polysorbate 80.

Incompatibilities: None reported.

Shelf life: 2 years.

Special precautions for storage: Store below 30°C.

Nature and contents of container: Tamper-evident cartons containing opaque polyvinyl chloride/foil blister packs or white high density polyethylene (HDPE) bottle with a child-resistant closure. Each pack type contains 60 coated tablets.

Instructions for use and handling: None required.

Marketing authorisation holder: Glaxo Group Ltd, Greenford Road, Greenford, Middlesex UB6 0NN, United Kingdom.

Marketing authorisation numbers

EU/1/98/058/001 (blisters)
EU/1/98/058/002 (bottle)

Date of first authorisation/renewal of the authorisation 18th March 1998

Date of revision of the text March 1998

CUTIVATE* CREAM 0.05%

Qualitative and quantitative composition Fluticasone Propionate (micronised) HSE 0.05% w/w.

Pharmaceutical form Cream.

Clinical particulars

Therapeutic indications: For the relief of the inflammatory and pruritic manifestations of corticosteroid-responsive dermatoses such as: eczema including atopic, infantile, and discoid eczemas; prurigo nodularis; psoriasis (excluding widespread plaque psoriasis); neurodermatoses including lichen simplex; lichen planus; seborrhoeic dermatitis; contact sensitivity reactions; discoid lupus erythematosus; an adjunct to systemic steroid therapy in generalised erythroderma; insect bite reactions; prickly heat.

Posology and method of administration:

Eczema/dermatitis: Apply a thin film of the cream to the affected skin areas once daily.

Other indications: Apply a thin film of the cream to the affected skin areas twice daily.

For topical administration.

Contra-indications: Rosacea, acne vulgaris, perioral dermatitis, primary cutaneous viral infections (e.g. herpes simplex, chickenpox). Hypersensitivity to any of the ingredients. Perianal and genital pruritus. The use of fluticasone propionate skin preparations is not indicated in the treatment of primarily infected skin lesions caused by infection with fungi or bacteria and dermatoses in children under one year of age, including dermatitis and napkin eruptions.

Special warnings and precautions for use: Fluticasone propionate has a very low propensity for systemic absorption, nevertheless, prolonged application of high doses to large areas of body surface, especially in infants and small children, might lead to adrenal suppression. Children may absorb proportionally larger amounts of topical corticosteroids and thus be more susceptible to systemic toxicity.

The face, more than other areas of the body may exhibit atrophic changes after prolonged treatment with potent topical corticosteroids. This must be borne in mind when treating such conditions as psoriasis, discoid lupus erythematosus and severe eczema.

If applied to the eyelids, care is needed to ensure that the preparation does not enter the eye so as to avoid the risk of local irritation or glaucoma.

Topical steroids may be hazardous in psoriasis for a number of reasons, including rebound relapses, development of tolerance, risk of generalised pustular psoriasis and development of local or systemic toxicity due to impaired barrier function of the skin. If used in psoriasis careful patient supervision is important.

Appropriate antimicrobial therapy should be used whenever treating inflammatory lesions which have become infected. Any infection requires withdrawal of topical corticosteroid therapy and systemic administration of antimicrobial agents. Bacterial infection is encouraged by the warm, moist conditions induced by occlusive dressing, and so the skin should be cleansed before a fresh dressing is applied.

Interaction with other medicaments and other forms of interaction: None known.

Pregnancy and lactation:

Pregnancy: Topical administration of corticosteroids to pregnant animals can cause abnormalities of foetal development. The relevance of this finding to human beings has not been established; however, administration of fluticasone propionate during pregnancy should only be considered if the expected benefit to the mother is greater than any possible risk to the foetus.

Lactation: The excretion of fluticasone propionate into human breast milk has not been investigated. When measurable, plasma levels were obtained in lactating laboratory rats following subcutaneous administration, there was evidence of fluticasone propionate in the breast milk. However, plasma levels in patients following dermal application of fluticasone propionate at recommended doses are likely to be low.

When fluticasone propionate is used in breast feeding mothers, the therapeutic benefits must be weighed against the potential hazards to mother and baby.

Effect on ability to drive and use machines: None known.

Undesirable effects: The fluticasone propionate preparation is usually well tolerated; local burning and pruritus have been reported. If signs of hypersensitivity appear, application should stop immediately.

Prolonged and intensive treatment with potent corticosteroid preparations may cause local atrophic changes in the skin such as thinning, striae, dilation of the superficial blood vessels, hypertrichosis and hypopigmentation.

Secondary infection, particularly when occlusive dressings are used or when skin folds are involved and allergic contact dermatitis have also been reported with corticosteroid use.

Exacerbation of the signs and symptoms of the dermatoses have been reported with corticosteroid use.

Prolonged use of large amounts of corticosteroids, or treatment of extensive areas, can result in sufficient systemic absorption to produce the features of hypercorticism. This effect is more likely to occur in infants and children, and if occlusive dressings are used. In infants, the napkin may act as an occlusive dressing.

In rare instances, treatment of psoriasis with a corticosteroid (or its withdrawal) is thought to have provoked the pustular form of the disease.

Overdose: Acute overdosage is very unlikely to occur, however, in the case of chronic overdosage or misuse, the features of hypercorticism may appear and in this situation, as with any corticosteroid, application should be discontinued. Overdose by ingestion of fluticasone propionate cream is extremely unlikely to occur due to the very low oral bioavailability of fluticasone propionate.

Pharmacological properties

Pharmacodynamic properties: Fluticasone propionate is a glucocorticoid with high topical anti-inflammatory potency but low HPA-axis suppressive activity after dermal administration. It therefore has a therapeutic index which is greater than most of the commonly available steroids.

It shows high systemic glucocorticoid potency after subcutaneous administration but very weak oral activity, probably due to metabolic inactivation. *In vitro* studies show a strong affinity for, and agonist activity at, human glucocorticoid receptors.

Fluticasone propionate has no unexpected hormonal effects, and no overt, marked effects upon the central and peripheral nervous systems, the gastrointestinal system, or the cardiovascular or respiratory systems.

Pharmacokinetic properties: Pharmacokinetic data for the rat and dog indicate rapid elimination and extensive metabolic clearance. Bioavailability is very low after topical or oral administration, due to limited absorption through the skin or from the gastrointestinal tract, and because of extensive first-pass metabolism. Distribution studies have shown that only minute traces of orally administered compound reach the systemic circulation, and that any systemically-available radiolabel is rapidly eliminated in the bile and excreted in the faeces.

Fluticasone propionate does not persist in any tissue, and does not bind to melanin. The major route of metabolism is hydrolysis of the S-fluoromethyl carbothioate group, to yield a carboxylic acid (GR36264), which has very weak glucocorticoid or anti-inflammatory activity. In all test animal species, the route of excretion of radioactivity is independent of the route of administration of radiolabelled fluticasone propionate. Excretion is predominantly faecal and is essentially complete within 48 hours.

In man too, metabolic clearance is extensive, and elimination is consequently rapid. Thus drug entering the systemic circulation via the skin, will be rapidly inactivated. Oral bioavailability approaches zero, due to poor absorption and extensive first-pass metabolism. Therefore systemic exposure to any ingestion of the topical formulation will be low.

Preclinical safety data: There are no preclinical data of relevance to the prescriber which are additional to that in other sections of the SmPC.

Pharmaceutical particulars

List of excipients: Liquid Paraffin PhEur, Cetostearyl Alcohol BP, Isopropyl Myristate BP, Cetomacrogol 1000 BP, Propylene Glycol PhEur, Imidurea USNF, Sodium Phosphate PhEur, Citric Acid Monohydrate PhEur, Purified Water PhEur.

Incompatibilities: None reported.

Shelf life: 24 months.

Special precautions for storage: Store below 30°C.

Nature and contents of container: 15 g, 30 g, 50 g and 100 g collapsible internally-laquered, blind-end aluminium tubes, with latex bands and closed with polypropylene caps.

Instructions for use/handling: No special instructions.

Marketing authorisation number PL 10949/0013.

Date of first authorisation/renewal of authorisation 17 February 1993.

Date of (partial) revision of text November 1997. This is the first SmPC.

Legal category POM.

CUTIVATE* OINTMENT 0.005%

Qualitative and quantitative composition Fluticasone Propionate (micronised) HSE 0.005% w/w.

Pharmaceutical form Ointment.

Clinical particulars

Therapeutic indications: For the relief of the inflammatory and pruritic manifestations of corticosteroid-responsive dermatoses such as: eczema including atopic, infantile, and discoid eczemas; prurigo nodularis; psoriasis (excluding widespread plaque psoriasis); neurodermatoses including lichen simplex; lichen planus; seborrhoeic dermatitis; contact sensitivity reactions; discoid lupus erythematosus; an adjunct to systemic steroid therapy in generalised erythroderma; insect bite reactions; prickly heat.

Posology and method of administration: Apply a thin film of fluticasone propionate ointment to the affected skin areas twice daily.

For topical administration.

Contra-indications: Rosacea, acne vulgaris, perioral dermatitis, primary cutaneous viral infections (e.g. herpes simplex, chickenpox). Hypersensitivity to any of the ingredients. Perianal and genital pruritus. The use of fluticasone propionate skin preparations is not indicated in the treatment of primarily infected skin lesions caused by infection with fungi or bacteria and dermatoses in children under one year of age, including dermatitis and napkin eruptions.

Special warnings and precautions for use: Prolonged applications of high doses to large areas of body surface, especially in infants and small children, might lead to adrenal suppression. Children may absorb proportionally larger amounts of topical corticosteroids and thus be more susceptible to systemic toxicity.

The face, more than other areas of the body may exhibit atrophic changes after prolonged treatment with potent topical corticosteroids. This must be borne in mind when treating such conditions as psoriasis, discoid lupus erythematosus and severe eczema.

If applied to the eyelids, care is needed to ensure that the preparation does not enter the eye so as to avoid the risk of local irritation or glaucoma.

Topical steroids may be hazardous in psoriasis for a number of reasons, including rebound relapses, development of tolerance, risk of generalised pustular psoriasis and development of local or systemic toxicity due to impaired barrier function of the skin. If used in psoriasis careful patient supervision is important.

Appropriate antimicrobial therapy should be used whenever treating inflammatory lesions which have become infected. Any infection requires withdrawal of topical corticosteroid therapy and systemic administration of antimicrobial agents. Bacterial infection is encouraged by the warm, moist conditions induced by occlusive dressing, and so the skin should be cleansed before a fresh dressing is applied.

Interaction with other medicaments and other forms of interaction: None known.

Pregnancy and lactation:

Pregnancy: Topical administration of corticosteroids to pregnant animals can cause abnormalities of foetal development. The relevance of this finding to human beings has not been established; however, administration of fluticasone propionate during pregnancy should only be considered if the expected benefit to the mother is greater than any possible risk to the foetus.

Lactation: The excretion of fluticasone propionate into human breast milk has not been investigated. When measurable, plasma levels were obtained in lactating laboratory rats following subcutaneous administration, there was evidence of fluticasone propionate in the breast milk. However, plasma levels in patients following dermal application of fluticasone propionate at recommended doses are likely to be low.

When fluticasone propionate is used in breast feeding mothers, the therapeutic benefits must be weighed against the potential hazards to mother and baby.

Effects on ability to drive and use machines: None known.

Undesirable effects: The fluticasone propionate preparation is usually well tolerated; local burning and pruritus have been reported. If signs of hypersensitivity appear, application should stop immediately.

Prolonged and intensive treatment with potent corticosteroid preparations may cause local atrophic changes in the skin such as thinning, striae, dilation of the superficial blood vessels, hypertrichosis and hypopigmentation.

Secondary infection, particularly when occlusive dressings are used or when skin folds are involved and allergic contact dermatitis have also been reported with corticosteroid use.

Exacerbation of the signs and symptoms of the dermatoses have been reported with corticosteroid use.

Prolonged use of large amounts of corticosteroids, or treatment of extensive areas, can result in sufficient systemic absorption to produce the features of hypercorticism. This effect is more likely to occur in infants and children, and if occlusive dressings are used. In infants, the napkin may act as an occlusive dressing.

In rare instances, treatment of psoriasis with a corticosteroid (or its withdrawal) is thought to have provoked the pustular form of the disease.

Overdose: Acute overdosage is very unlikely to occur, however, in the case of chronic overdosage or misuse, the features of hypercorticism may appear and in this situation, as with any corticosteroid, application should be discontinued.

Pharmacological properties

Pharmacodynamic properties: Fluticasone propionate is a glucocorticoid with high topical anti-inflammatory potency but low HPA-axis suppressive activity after dermal administration. It therefore has a therapeutic index which is greater than most of the commonly available steroids.

It shows high systemic glucocorticoid potency after subcutaneous administration but very weak oral activity, probably due to metabolic inactivation. *In vitro* studies show a strong affinity for, and agonist activity at, human glucocorticoid receptors.

Fluticasone propionate has no unexpected hormonal effects, and no overt, marked effects upon the central and peripheral nervous systems, the gastrointestinal system, or the cardiovascular or respiratory systems.

Pharmacokinetic properties: Pharmacokinetic data for the rat and dog indicate rapid elimination and extensive metabolic clearance. Bioavailability is very low after topical or oral administration, due to limited absorption through the skin or from the gastrointestinal tract, and because of extensive first-pass metabolism. Distribution studies have shown that only minute traces of orally administered compound reach the systemic circulation, and that any systemically-available radiolabel is rapidly eliminated in the bile and excreted in the faeces.

Fluticasone propionate does not persist in any tissue, and does not bind to melanin. The major route of metabolism is hydrolysis of the S-fluoromethyl carbothioate group, to yield a carboxylic acid (GR36264), which has very weak glucocorticoid or anti-inflammatory activity. In all test animal species, the route of excretion of radioactivity is independent of the route of administration of radiolabelled fluticasone propionate. Excretion is predominantly faecal and is essentially complete within 48 hours.

In man too, metabolic clearance is extensive, and elimination is consequently rapid. Thus drug entering the systemic circulation via the skin, will be rapidly inactivated. Oral bioavailability approaches zero, due to poor absorption and extensive first-pass metabolism. Therefore systemic exposure to any ingestion of the topical formulation will be low.

Preclinical safety data: There are no preclinical data of relevance to the prescriber which are additional to that in other sections of the SmPC.

Pharmaceutical particulars

List of excipients: Propylene Glycol PhEur, Sorbitan Sesquioleate HSE, Microcrystalline Wax USNF, Liquid Paraffin PhEur.

Incompatibilities: None reported.

Shelf life: 24 months.

Special precautions for storage: Store below 30°C.

Nature and contents of container: 15 g, 30 g, 50 g and 100 g collapsible blind-end aluminium tubes, with latex bands and closed with polypropylene caps.

Instructions for use/handling: None.

Marketing authorisation number PL 10949/0012

Date of first authorisation/renewal of authorisation 17 February 1993.

Date of (partial) revision of text November 1997. This is the first SmPC.

Legal category POM

CYCLIMORPH* 10 INJECTION
CYCLIMORPH* 15 INJECTION

Qualitative and quantitative composition

Ingredients per 1 ml of product:

	10	*15*
Morphine Tartrate	10 mg	15 mg
Cyclizine	39.01 mg	39.01 mg

Pharmaceutical form Injection.

Clinical particulars

Therapeutic indications: Cyclimorph Injection is indicated for the relief of moderate to severe pain in all suitable medical and surgical conditions (see *Contra-indications* and *Special warnings and special precautions*) in which reduction of the nausea and vomiting associated with the administration of morphine is required.

Posology and method of administration:

Use by injection in adults: The usual dose is 10–20 mg morphine tartrate, given subcutaneously, intramuscularly or intravenously.

Additional doses may not be given more frequently than 4-hourly.

Not more than 3 doses (representing 150 mg cyclizine: i.e. 3 ml of Cyclimorph 10 or Cyclimorph 15 Injection) should be given in any 24-hour period.

Use in the elderly: Morphine doses should be reduced in elderly patients and titrated to provide optimal pain relief with minimal side effects since:

- Increased duration of pain relief from a standard dose of morphine has been reported in elderly patients.
- A review of pharmacokinetic studies has suggested that morphine clearance decreases and half-life increases in older patients.
- The elderly may be particularly sensitive to the adverse effects of morphine.

Children: Cyclimorph Injection should not be used in children under 12 years of age.

Contra-indications: Cyclimorph Injection is contra-indicated in individuals with known hypersensitivity to morphine, cyclizine or any of the other constituents.

Cyclimorph Injection, like other opioid-containing preparations, is contra-indicated in patients with respiratory depression. Patients with excessive bronchial secretions should not be given Cyclimorph Injection as morphine diminishes the cough response.

Cyclimorph Injection should not be given during an attack of bronchial asthma or in heart failure secondary to chronic lung disease.

Cyclimorph Injection is contra-indicated in patients with head injury or raised intra-cranial pressure.

Renal impairment: Severe and prolonged respiratory depression may occur in patients with renal impairment given morphine; this is attributed to the accumulation of the active metabolite morphine-6-glucuronide. Therefore, Cyclimorph Injection should not be administerd to patients with moderate or severe renal impairment (glomerular filtration rate <20 ml/min).

Hepatic impairment: As with other opioid analgesic containing preparations Cyclimorph Injection should not be administered to patients with severe hepatic impairment as it may precipitate coma.

Cyclimorph Injection is contra-indicated in the presence of acute alcohol intoxication. The antiemetic properties of cyclizine may increase the toxicity of alcohol.

Cyclimorph Injection is contra-indicated in individuals receiving monoamine oxidase inhibitors or within 14 days of stopping such treatment.

Cyclimorph Injection, as with other opioid containing preparations, is contra-indicated in patients with ulcerative colitis, since such preparations may precipitate toxic dilation or spasm of the colon.

Cyclimorph Injection is contra-indicated in biliary and renal tract spasm.

Special warnings and special precautions for use: In common with the other opioid containing preparations, Cyclimorph Injection has the potential to produce tolerance and physical and psychological dependence in susceptible individuals. Abrupt cessation of therapy after prolonged use may result in withdrawal symptoms.

Cyclimorph Injection should be used with caution in the debilitated since they may be more sensitive to the respiratory depressant effects.

Cyclimorph Injection should be used with caution (including consideration of dose administered) in the presence of the following:

hypothyroidism
adrenocortical insufficiency
hypopituitarism
prostatic hypertrophy
shock
diabetes mellitus

Extreme caution should be exercised when administering Cyclimorph Injection to patients with phaeochromocytoma, since aggravated hypertension has been reported in association with diamorphine.

Cyclizine may cause a fall in cardiac output associated with increases in heart rate, mean arterial pressure and pulmonary wedge pressure. Cyclimorph Injection should therefore be used with caution in patients with severe heart failure.

Because cyclizine has anticholinergic activity it may precipitate incipient glaucoma. It should be used with caution and appropriate monitoring in patients with glaucoma and also in obstructive disease of the gastrointestinal tract.

Interaction with other medicaments and other forms of interaction: The central nervous system depressant effects of Cyclimorph Injection may be enhanced by other centrally-acting agents such as phenothiazines, hypnotics, neuroleptics, alcohol and muscle relaxants.

Monoamine oxidase inhibitors (MAOIs) may prolong and enhance the respiratory depressant effects of morphine. Opioids and MAOIs used together may cause fatal hypotension and coma (see *Contra-indications*).

Because of its anticholinergic activity cyclizine may enhance the side effects of other anticholinergic drugs.

The analgesic effect of opioids tends to be enhanced by co-administration of dexamphetamine, hydroxyzine, and some phenothiazines although respiratory depression may also be enhanced by the latter combination.

Morphine may reduce the efficacy of diuretics by inducing the release of antidiuretic hormone.

Propranolol has been reported to enhance the lethality of toxic doses of opioids in animals. Although the significance of this finding is not known for man, caution should be exercised when these drugs are administered concurrently.

Interference with laboratory tests: Morphine can react with Folin-Ciocalteau reagent in the Lowry method of protein estimation.

Morphine can also interfere with the determination of urinary 17-ketosteroids due to chemical structure effects in the Zimmerman procedure.

Use in pregnancy and lactation:

Pregnancy: There is no evidence on the safety of the combination in human pregnancy, nor is there evidence from animal work that the constituents are free from hazard. However, limited data from epidemiological studies of cyclizine and morphine in human pregnancies have found no evidence of teratogenicity. In the absence of definitive human data with the combination the use of Cyclimorph Injection in pregnancy is not advised.

Administration of morphine during labour may cause respiratory depression in the newborn infant.

Lactation: Cyclizine is excreted in human milk, however, the amount has not been quantified.

Morphine can significantly suppress lactation. Morphine is excreted in human milk, but the amount is generally considered to be less than 1% of any dose.

Effects on ability to drive and use machines: In common with other opioids, morphine may produce orthostatic hypotension and drowsiness in ambulatory patients. Sedation of short duration has been reported in patients receiving intravenous cyclizine. The CNS depressant effects of Cyclimorph Injection may be enhanced by combination with other centrally acting agents (see *Interactions*). Patients should therefore be cautioned against activities requiring vigilance including driving vehicles and operating machinery.

Undesirable effects: As Cyclimorph Injection contains morphine and cyclizine, the type and frequency of adverse effects associated with such compounds may be expected.

Adverse reactions attributable to morphine include respiratory depression, raised intra-cranial pressure, orthostatic hypotension, drowsiness, confusion, dysphoria, restlessness, miosis, constipation, nausea, vomiting, skin reactions (e.g. urticaria) biliary tract and renal spasm, vertigo and difficulty with micturition.

Adverse reactions attributable to cyclizine include urticaria, drug rash, drowsiness/sedation, dryness of the mouth, nose and throat, blurred vision, tachycardia, urinary retention, constipation, restlessness, nervousness, insomnia, auditory and visual hallucination and cholestatic jaundice.

A single case of anaphylaxis has been reported following intravenous administration of cyclizine co-administered in the same syringe as propanidid.

Anaphylactic shock is a rare adverse reaction to morphine.

An increase in excitatory phenomena (tremor and muscle movements) has been reported when cyclizine has been given before propanidid and methohexitone anaesthesia. A case of hyperactivity following intravenous administration of morphine during induction of anaesthesia has been reported.

A case of morphine-induced thrombocytopenia has been reported.

Morphine has a depressant effect on gonadal hormone secretion which can result in a reduction of testosterone leading to regression of secondary sexual characteristics in men on long-term therapy.

Overdose: Signs: The signs of overdosage with Cyclimorph Injection are those pathognomonic of opioid poisoning i.e. respiratory depression, pin point pupils, hypotension, circulatory failure and deepening coma. Mydriasis may replace miosis as asphyxia intervenes.

Drowsiness, floppiness, miosis and apnoea are signs of opioid overdosage in children as are convulsions.

Treatment: It is imperative to maintain and support respiration and circulation.

The specific opioid antagonist naloxone is the treatment of choice for the reversal of coma and restoration of spontaneous respiration, the literature should be consulted for details of appropriate dosage.

The use of a specific opioid antagonist in patients tolerant to morphine may produce withdrawal symptoms.

Patients should be monitored closely for at least 48 hours in case of relapse.

Pharmacological properties
Pharmacodynamic properties: Cyclizine is a histamine H_1 receptor antagonist of the piperazine class. It possesses anticholinergic and antiemetic properties. The exact mechanism by which cyclizine can prevent or suppress both nausea and vomiting from various causes is unknown. Cyclizine increases lower oesophageal sphincter tone and reduces the sensitivity of the labyrinthine apparatus.

Morphine is a competitive agonist at the μ-opioid receptor and is a potent analgesic. It is thought that activity at the μ-receptor subtype may mediate the analgesic and euphoric actions of morphine whilst activity at the μ2-receptor subtype may mediate respiratory depression and inhibition of gut motility. An action at the k-opioid receptor may mediate spinal analgesia.

Pharmacokinetic properties: In a healthy adult volunteer the administration of a single oral dose of 50 mg cyclizine resulted in a peak plasma concentration of approximately 70 ng/ml, occurring at about 2 hours after administration. Urine collected over 24 hours contained less than 1% of the total dose administered. In a separate study in one healthy adult volunteer the plasma elimination half-life of cyclizine was approximately 20 hours.

Cyclizine is metabolised to its N-dimethylated derivative norcyclizine, which has little antihistaminic (H_1) activity compared to cyclizine.

The mean elimination half-life for morphine in blood and plasma is 2.7 h (range 1.2–4.9 h) and 2.95 (range 0.8–5 h) respectively.

Morphine is extensively metabolised by hepatic biotransformation. In addition, the kidney has been shown to have the capacity to form morphine glucuronides. The major metabolite is morphine-3-glucuronide (approximately 45% of a dose). Morphine-6-glucuronide is a minor metabolite (approx. 5% of the dose) but is highly active. Although renal excretion is a minor route of elimination for unchanged morphine, it constitutes the major mechanism of elimination of conjugated morphine metabolites including the active morphine-6-glucuronide.

Morphine is bound to plasma proteins only to the extent of 25–35% and therefore functions that change the extent of protein binding will have only a minor impact on its pharmacodynamic effects.

Preclinical safety data:
A. Mutagenicity: Cyclizine was not mutagenic in an Ames test (at a dose level of 100 μg/plate), with or without metabolic activation.

No bacterial mutagenicity studies with morphine have been reported. A review of the literature has indicated that morphine was negative in gene mutation assays in *Drosphilia melanogaster*, but was positive in a mammalian spermatocyte test. The results of another study by the same authors has indicated that morphine causes chromosomal aberrations, in germ cells of male mice when given at dose levels of 10, 20, 40 or 60 mg/kg bodyweight for three consecutive days.

B. Carcinogenicity: No long term studies have been conducted in animals to determine whether cyclizine or morphine are potentially carcinogenic.

C. Teratogenicity: Some animal studies indicate that cyclizine may be teratogenic at dose levels up to 25 times the clinical dose level. In another study, cyclizine was negative at oral dose levels up to 65 mg/kg in rats and 75 mg/kg in rabbits.

Morphine was not teratogenic in rats when dosed for up to 15 days at 70 mg/kg/day. Morphine given subcutaneously to mice at very high doses (200, 300 or 400 mg/kg/day) on days eight or nine of gestation, resulted in a few cases of exencephaly and axial skeletal fusions. The hypoxic effects of such high doses could account for the defects seen.

Lower doses of morphine (40, 4.0 or 0.4 mg/ml) given to mice as a continuous i.v. infusion (at a dose volume of 0.3 ml/kg) between days seven and ten of gestation, caused soft tissue and skeletal malformations as shown in previous studies.

D. Fertility: In a study involving prolonged administration of cyclizine to male and female rats, there was no evidence of impaired fertility after continuous treatment for 90–100 days at dose levels of approximately 15 and 25 mg/kg/day.

Effects of morphine exposure on sexual maturation of male rats, their reproductive capacity and the development of their progeny have been examined. Results indicated that exposure during adolescence led to pronounced inhibition of several indices of sexual maturation (e.g. hormone levels, reduced gonad weights), smaller litters and selective gender specific effects on endocrine function in the offspring.

A disruption in ovulation and amenorrhoea can occur in women given morphine.

Pharmaceutical particulars
List of excipients: Tartaric acid; sodium metabisulphite; Water for Injections.

Incompatibilities: See *Interaction with other medicaments and other forms of interaction* and *Contra-indications.*

Shelf life: 3 years.

Special precautions for storage: Store below 30°C. Protect from light. Do not freeze.

Nature and contents of container: Ampoules which comply with the requirements of the European Pharmacopoeia for type 1 neutral glass.

Instructions for use/handling: No special instructions.

Pack sizes: Cyclimorph 10 injection: 1 ml ampoules: Box of 5. Cyclimorph 15 injection: 1 ml ampoules: Box of 5.

Marketing authorisation numbers
Cyclimorph 10 Injection 0003/5022
Cyclimorph 15 Injection 0003/5023

Date of approval/revision of SPC 28 June 1995

DARAPRIM* TABLETS

Qualitative and quantitative composition Pyrimethamine EP 25.0 mg.

Pharmaceutical form Tablet.

Clinical particulars
Therapeutic indications: Daraprim is indicated for chemoprophylaxis of malaria due to susceptible strains of Plasmodia. However, since resistance to pyrimethamine is increasing worldwide, Daraprim can only be considered suitable for use in individuals who are resident in areas where pyrimethamine is acknowledged to be effective. It is not suitable as a prophylactic for travellers.

Posology and method of administration
Adults: 1 tablet regularly each week.

Children: Over 10 years: 1 tablet regularly each week.

5 to 10 years: ½ tablet regularly each week.

Under 5 years: Formulation not applicable.

Daraprim is rapidly absorbed and therefore prophylactic cover can be expected shortly after the first dose. Prophylaxis should commence before arrival in an endemic area and be continued once weekly. On returning to a non-malarious area, dosage should be maintained for a further four weeks.

Route of administration: Oral.

Contra-indications: Daraprim should not be given to patients with a history of pyrimethamine sensitivity.

Special warnings and precautions for use: The recommended dosage should not be exceeded.

Daraprim should be used with caution in patients with hepatic or renal disorders.

During pregnancy and in other conditions predisposing to folate deficiency, a folate supplement should be given.

Daraprim, by its mode of action, may further depress folate metabolism in patients receiving treatment with other folate inhibitors. Occasional reports suggest that individuals taking pyrimethamine as malarial prophylaxis at doses in excess of 25 mg weekly may develop megaloblastic anaemia if co-trimoxazole is prescribed concurrently.

Daraprim may exacerbate folate deficiency due to innate disease or malnutrition.

Interaction with other medicaments and other forms of interaction: The concurrent administration of lorazepam and Daraprim may induce hepatotoxicity.

Pregnancy and lactation: While there is a theoretical risk of foetal abnormality with all folate inhibitors given during pregnancy, no such adverse effects have been reported with Daraprim. A folate supplement should be given to pregnant women receiving Daraprim. The amount of pyrimethamine excreted in breast milk is insufficient to contra-indicate its use in lactating mothers, but breast-fed infants should not receive other anti-folate agents.

Effect on ability to drive and use machines: None known.

Undesirable effects: At the recommended dose, side-effects are rare. Occasionally, rashes have been observed. Excessive doses may produce a macrocytic anaemia resembling that of folic acid deficiency.

Overdose: Symptoms reported have included vomiting, cyanosis, respiratory distress, convulsions and tachycardia. In less severe cases, gastric lavage, adequate fluids and general supportive measures are recommended. In severe cases, maintenance of a clear airway and control of convulsions are required. In addition, fresh blood transfusion to counteract blood dyscrasias should be available.

To counteract possible folate deficiency, calcium folinate 9–15 mg daily should be given until the signs of toxicity have subsided.

Pharmacological properties
Pharmacodynamic properties: Not available.

Pharmacokinetic properties: Not available.

Preclinical safety data:
A) *Mutagenicity*
There is insufficient information available to determine whether the active ingredients have mutagenic potential.
B) *Carcinogenicity*
There is insufficient information available to determine whether the active ingredients have carcinogenic potential.
C) *Teratogenicity*
There is insufficient information available to determine whether the active ingredients have teratogenic potential.
D) *Fertility*
There is insufficient information available to determine whether the active ingredients can affect fertility.

Pharmaceutical particulars
List of excipients: Lactose EP, Starches EP, Hydrolysed starch HSE, Docusate sodium USP, Magnesium stearate EP, Industrial methylated spirit or Ethanol (96%) BP, Purified water EP.

Incompatibilities: None known.

Shelf life: 5 years.

Special precautions for storage: Store below 35°C. Protect from light.

Nature and contents of container: Vinyl-lacquered aluminium foil strip-packs.

Pack size: 30 tablets.

Instructions for use/handling: No special instructions.

Marketing authorisation holder: The Wellcome Foundation Ltd, Glaxo Wellcome House, Berkeley Avenue, Greenford, Middlesex UB6 0NN.

Marketing authorisation number PL 0003/5026R

Date of first authorisation/renewal of authorisation
Product licence of right: 31.01.73.
Reviewed licence: 25.09.86.
Renewed licence: 13.09.91., 26.11.98.

Date of (partial) revision of text
This is the first SmPC (28 June 1996).

DERMOVATE* CREAM

Qualitative and quantitative composition Clobetasol propionate 0.0525% w/w.

Pharmaceutical form Cream.

Clinical particulars
Therapeutic indications: Clobetasol Propionate is a very active topical corticosteroid which is of particular value when used in short courses for the treatment of more resistant dermatoses such as psoriasis (excluding widespread plaque psoriasis) recalcitrant eczemas, lichen planus, discoid lupus erythematosus, and other conditions which do not respond satisfactorily to less active steroids.

Posology and method of administration: Apply sparingly to the affected area once or twice daily until improvement occurs. As with other highly active topical steroid preparations, therapy should be discontinued when control is achieved. In the more responsive conditions this may be within a few days.

If no improvement is seen within two to four weeks, reassessment of the diagnosis, or referral, may be necessary.

Repeated short courses of Dermovate may be used to control exacerbations. If continuous steroid treatment is necessary, a less potent preparation should be used.

In very resistant lesions, especially where there is hyperkeratosis, the anti-inflammatory effect of Dermovate can be enhanced, if necessary, by occluding the treatment area with polythene film. Overnight occlusion only is usually adequate to bring about a satisfactory response. Thereafter improvement can usually be maintained by application without occlusion.

For topical administration.

Contra-indications: Rosacea, acne vulgaris and perioral dermatitis. Primary cutaneous viral infections (e.g. herpes simplex, chickenpox). Hypersensitivity to the preparation.

The use of Dermovate skin preparations is not indicated in the treatment of primarily infected skin lesions caused by infection with fungi (e.g. candidiasis, tinea), or bacteria (e.g. impetigo), perianal and genital pruritus.

Dermatoses in children under one year of age, including dermatitis and napkin eruptions.

Special warnings and precautions for use: Long term continuous topical therapy should be avoided where possible, particularly in infants and children, as adrenal suppression can occur readily even without occlusion.

If used in childhood or on the face, courses should be limited if possible to five days and occlusion should not be used.

The face, more than other areas of the body, may exhibit atrophic changes after prolonged treatment with potent topical corticosteroids. This must be borne in mind when treating such conditions as psoriasis, discoid lupus erythematosus and severe eczema.

If applied to the eyelids, care is needed to ensure that the preparation does not enter the eye, as glaucoma might result.

Topical corticosteroids may be hazardous in psoriasis for a number of reasons including rebound relapses, development of tolerance, risk of generalised pustular psoriasis and development of local or systemic toxicity due to impaired barrier function of the skin. If used in psoriasis careful patient supervision is important.

Appropriate antimicrobial therapy should be used whenever treating inflammatory lesions which have become infected. Any spread of infection requires withdrawal of topical corticosteroid therapy and systemic administration of antimicrobial agents. Bacterial infection is encouraged by the warm, moist conditions induced by occlusive dressings, and so the skin should be cleansed before a fresh dressing is applied.

Interaction with other medicaments and other forms of interaction: None known.

Pregnancy and lactation: There is inadequate evidence of safety in human pregnancy. Topical administration of corticosteroids to pregnant animals can cause abnormalities of foetal development including cleft palate and intrauterine growth retardation. There may therefore be a very small risk of such effects in the human foetus.

Effect on ability to drive and use machines: None known.

Undesirable effects: As with other topical corticosteroids, prolonged use of large amounts, or treatment of extensive areas can result in sufficient systemic absorption to produce the features of hypercorticism.

Provided the weekly dosage is less than 50 g in adults, any suppression of the HPA axis is likely to be transient with a rapid return to normal values once the short course of steroid therapy has ceased. The same applies to children given proportionate dosage. Use of occlusive dressing increases the absorption of topical corticosteroids. In infants, the napkin may act as an occlusive dressing.

Prolonged and intensive treatment with a highly active corticosteroid preparation may cause local atrophic changes in the skin such as thinning, striae, and dilatation of the superficial blood vessels, particularly when occlusive dressings are used or when skin folds are involved.

In rare instances, treatment of psoriasis with corticosteroids (or its withdrawal) is thought to have provoked the pustular form of the disease (see *Precautions*).

There are reports of pigmentation changes and hypertrichosis with topical steroids.

Dermovate is usually well tolerated, but if signs of hypersensitivity appear, application should be stopped immediately. Exacerbation of symptoms may occur.

Overdose: Acute overdosage is very unlikely to occur, however, in the case of chronic overdosage or misuse, the features of hypercorticism may appear and in this situation topical steroids should be discontinued.

Pharmacological properties
Pharmacodynamic properties: Clobetasol Propionate is a highly active corticosteroid with topical anti-inflammatory activity.

Pharmacokinetic properties: The extent of percutaneous absorption of topical corticosteroid is determined by many factors including the vehicle, the integrity of the epidermal barrier, and the use of occlusive dressings.

Topical corticosteroids can be absorbed from normal intact skin. Inflammation and/or other disease processes in the skin increase percutaneous absorption. Occlusive dressings substantially increase the percutaneous absorption of topical corticosteroids.

Once absorbed through the skin, topical corticosteroids are handled through pharmacokinetic pathways similar to systemically administered corticosteroids. Corticosteroids are bound to plasma proteins in varying degrees. Corticosteroids are metabolised primarily by the liver and are then excreted by the kidneys.

Preclinical safety data: There are no preclinical data of relevance to the prescriber which are additional to that in other sections of the SmPC.

Pharmaceutical particulars
List of excipients: Cetostearyl alcohol BP; Glyceryl monostearate; Arlacel 165; Beeswax substitute BP; Propylene glycol BP; Chlorocresol BP; Sodium citrate BP; Citric acid monohydrate BP; Purified water BP.

Incompatibilities: None known.

Shelf life: 24 months.

Special precautions for storage: Store below 25°C.

Nature and contents of container: Collapsible latex banded aluminium tube internally coated with epoxy resin based lacquer, with polypropylene cap.

Pack size: 25 g, 30 g, 100 g.

Instructions for use/handling: No special instructions.

Marketing authorisation number PL 10949/0025

Date of first authorisation/renewal of authorisation
1 March 1993

Date of (partial) revision of text November 1997.

DERMOVATE* OINTMENT

Qualitative and quantitative composition Clobetasol 17-Propionate 0.05% w/w.

Pharmaceutical form Ointment.

Clinical particulars
Therapeutic indications: Clobetasol Propionate is a very active topical corticosteroid which is of particular value when used in short courses for the treatment of more resistant dermatoses such as psoriasis (excluding widespread plaque psoriasis) recalcitrant eczemas, lichen planus, discoid lupus erythematosus, and other conditions which do not respond satisfactorily to less active steroids.

Posology and method of administration: Apply sparingly to the affected area once or twice daily until improvement occurs. As with other highly active topical steroid preparations, therapy should be discontinued when control is achieved. In the more responsive conditions this may be within a few days.

If no improvement is seen within two to four weeks, reassessment of the diagnosis, or referral, may be necessary.

Repeated short courses of Dermovate may be used to control exacerbations. If continuous steroid treatment is necessary, a less potent preparation should be used.

In very resistant lesions, especially where there is hyperkeratosis, the anti-inflammatory effect of Dermovate can be enhanced, if necessary, by occluding the treatment area with polythene film. Overnight occlusion only is usually adequate to bring about a satisfactory response. Thereafter improvement can usually be maintained by application without occlusion.

For topical administration.

Contra-indications: Rosacea, acne vulgaris and perioral dermatitis. Primary cutaneous viral infections (e.g. herpes simplex, chickenpox). Hypersensitivity to the preparation.

The use of Dermovate skin preparations is not indicated in the treatment of primarily infected skin lesions caused by infection with fungi (e.g. candidiasis, tinea), or bacteria (e.g. impetigo), perianal and genital pruritus.

Dermatoses in children under one year of age, including dermatitis and napkin eruptions.

Special warnings and precautions for use: Long term continuous topical therapy should be avoided where possible, particularly in infants and children, as adrenal suppression can occur readily even without occlusion.

If used in childhood or on the face, courses should be limited if possible to five days and occlusion should not be used.

The face, more than other areas of the body, may exhibit atrophic changes after prolonged treatment with potent topical corticosteroids. This must be borne in mind when treating such conditions as psoriasis, discoid lupus erythematosus and severe eczema.

If applied to the eyelids, care is needed to ensure that the preparation does not enter the eye, as glaucoma might result.

Topical corticosteroids may be hazardous in psoriasis for a number of reasons including rebound relapses, development of tolerance, risk of generalised pustular psoriasis and development of local or systemic toxicity due to impaired barrier function of the skin. If used in psoriasis careful patient supervision is important.

Appropriate antimicrobial therapy should be used whenever treating inflammatory lesions which have become infected. Any spread of infection requires withdrawal of topical corticosteroid therapy and systemic administration of antimicrobial agents. Bacterial infection is encouraged by the warm, moist conditions induced by occlusive dressings, and so the skin should be cleansed before a fresh dressing is applied.

Interaction with other medicaments and other forms of interaction: None known.

Pregnancy and lactation: There is inadequate evidence of safety in human pregnancy. Topical administration of corticosteroids to pregnant animals can cause abnormalities of foetal development including cleft palate and intrauterine growth retardation. There may therefore be a very small risk of such effects in the human foetus.

Effect on ability to drive and use machines: None known.

Undesirable effects: As with other topical corticosteroids, prolonged use of large amounts, or treatment of extensive areas can result in sufficient systemic absorption to produce the features of hypercorticism.

Provided the weekly dosage is less than 50 g in adults, any suppression of the HPA axis is likely to be transient with a rapid return to normal values once the short course of steroid therapy has ceased. The same applies to children given proportionate dosage. Use of occlusive dressing increases the absorption of topical corticosteroids. In infants, the napkin may act as an occlusive dressing.

Prolonged and intensive treatment with a highly active corticosteroid preparation may cause local atrophic changes in the skin such as thinning, striae, and dilatation of the superficial blood vessels, particularly when occlusive dressings are used or when skin folds are involved.

In rare instances, treatment of psoriasis with corticosteroids (or its withdrawal) is thought to have provoked the pustular form of the disease (see *Precautions*).

There are reports of pigmentation changes and hypertrichosis with topical steroids.

Dermovate is usually well tolerated, but if signs of hypersensitivity appear, application should be stopped immediately. Exacerbation of symptoms may occur.

Overdose: Acute overdosage is very unlikely to occur, however, in the case of chronic overdosage or misuse, the features of hypercorticism may appear and in this situation topical steroids should be discontinued.

Pharmacological properties
Pharmacodynamic properties: Clobetasol Propionate is a highly active corticosteroid with topical anti-inflammatory activity.

Pharmacokinetic properties: The extent of percutaneous absorption of topical corticosteroid is determined by many factors including the vehicle, the integrity of the epidermal barrier, and the use of occlusive dressings.

Topical corticosteroids can be absorbed from normal intact skin. Inflammation and/or other disease processes in the skin increase percutaneous absorption. Occlusive dressings substantially increase the percutaneous absorption of topical corticosteroids.

Once absorbed through the skin, topical corticosteroids are handled through pharmacokinetic pathways similar to systemically administered corticosteroids. Corticosteroids are bound to plasma proteins in varying degrees. Corticosteroids are metabolised primarily by the liver and are then excreted by the kidneys.

Preclinical safety data: There are no preclinical data of relevance to the prescriber which are additional to that in other sections of the SmPC.

Pharmaceutical particulars
List of excipients: Propylene glycol BP; Sorbitan sesquioleate HSE; White soft paraffin BP.

Incompatibilities: None known.

Shelf life: 24 months.

Special precautions for storage: Store below 30°C.

Nature and contents of container: 25 g, 30 g and 100 g collapsible tubes either internally coated with epoxy resin based lacquer or uncoated with wadless polypropylene caps.

Instructions for use/handling: No special instructions.

Marketing authorisation number PL 10949/0028

Date of first authorisation/renewal of authorisation
1 May 1993

Date of (partial) revision of text November 1997.

DERMOVATE* SCALP APPLICATION

Presentation Dermovate Scalp Application is a transparent, slightly gelled solution containing 0.05% w/w clobetasol propionate. The vehicle contains 50% isopropyl alcohol, which has antibacterial activity.

Uses Psoriasis and recalcitrant eczemas of the scalp. Clobetasol propionate is a highly-active topical corticosteroid which is indicated for use in short courses for conditions which do not respond satisfactorily to less active steroids.

Dosage and administration Apply sparingly to the scalp night and morning until improvement occurs. As with other highly-active topical steroid preparations, therapy should be discontinued when control is achieved. Repeated short courses of Dermovate Scalp Application may be used to control exacerbations. If continuous steroid treatment is necessary, a less potent preparation should be used.

Contra-indications, warnings, etc
Contra-indications: Infections of the scalp. Hypersensitivity to the preparation. Dermatoses in children under one year of age, including dermatitis.

Precautions: Care must be taken to keep the preparation away from the eyes. Do not use near a naked flame.

Long-term continuous topical therapy should be avoided, particularly in infants and children, as adrenal suppression can occur readily even without occlusion.

Development of secondary infection requires withdrawal of topical corticosteroid therapy and commencement of appropriate systemic antimicrobial therapy.

Topical corticosteroids may be hazardous in psoriasis for a number of reasons including rebound relapses, development of tolerance, risk of generalised pustular psoriasis and development of local or systemic toxicity due to impaired barrier function of the skin. If used in psoriasis careful patient supervision is important.

Pregnancy: There is inadequate evidence of safety in human pregnancy. Topical administration of corticosteroids to pregnant animals can cause abnormalities of foetal development including cleft palate and intrauterine growth retardation. There may therefore be a very small risk of such effects in the human foetus.

Side-effects: Dermovate preparations are usually well tolerated, but if signs of hypersensitivity appear, application should be stopped immediately.

As with other topical corticosteroids, prolonged use of large amounts or treatment of extensive areas can result in sufficient systemic absorption to produce the features of hypercorticism and suppression of the HPA axis. These effects are more likely to occur in infants and children, and if occlusive dressings are used. Local atrophy may occur after prolonged treatment.

In rare instances, treatment of psoriasis with corticosteroids (or its withdrawal) is thought to have provoked the pustular form of the disease (see *Precautions*).

Overdosage: Acute overdosage is very unlikely to occur, however, in the case of chronic overdosage or misuse the features of hypercorticism may appear and in this situation topical steroids should be discontinued.

Pharmaceutical precautions None.

Legal category POM.

Package quantities Plastic squeeze bottle with elongated nozzle containing 30 or 100 ml.

Further information The least potent corticosteroid which will control the disease should be selected. The viscosity of the scalp application has been adjusted so that the preparation spreads easily without being too fluid. The specially-designed bottle and nozzle allow easy application direct to the scalp through the hair.

Product licence number 10949/0046

DERMOVATE*-NN CREAM

Qualitative and quantitative composition Dermovate-NN skin preparations contain clobetasol propionate 0.05% w/w, neomycin sulphate 0.5% and nystatin 100,000 units per gram.

Pharmaceutical form Cream for topical administration.

Clinical particulars
Therapeutic indications: Clobetasol propionate is a highly active topical corticosteroid which is of particular value when used in short courses for the treatment of recalcitrant eczemas, neurodermatoses, and other conditions which do not respond satisfactorily to less active steroids.

Dermovate-NN is indicated in more resistant dermatoses such as recalcitrant eczemas and psoriasis (excluding widespread plaque psoriasis) where secondary bacterial or candidal infection is present, suspected or likely to occur, as when using occlusive dressings.

Posology and method of administration: Apply sparingly to the affected area once or twice daily until improvement occurs. As with other highly-active topical steroid preparations, therapy should be discontinued when control is achieved. In the more responsive conditions this may be within a few days.

If a longer course is necessary, it is recommended that treatment should not be continued for more than four weeks without the patient's condition being reviewed.

Repeated short courses of Dermovate-NN may be used to control exacerbations. If continuous steroid treatment is necessary, a less potent preparation should be used.

In very resistant lesions, especially where there is hyperkeratosis, the anti-inflammatory effect of Dermovate-NN can be enhanced, if necessary, by occluding the treatment area with polythene. Overnight occlusion only is usually adequate to bring about a satisfactory response, thereafter improvement can usually be maintained by application without occlusion.

Dermovate-NN is suitable for use in children at the same dose as adults, but the dose should be reduced for use in infants. Dermovate-NN is not recommended for use in neonates.

Contra-indications: Rosacea, acne vulgaris and perioral dermatitis.

Primary cutaneous viral infections (e.g. herpes simplex, chickenpox).

Hypersensitivity to the preparations.

Use of Dermovate-NN skin preparations is not indicated in the treatment of primarily infected skin lesions caused by infection with fungi (e.g. candidiasis, tinea), bacteria (e.g. impetigo), or yeast; secondary infections due to Pseudomonas or Proteus species; perianal and genital pruritus, dermatoses in children under one year of age, including dermatitis and napkin eruptions.

Preparations containing neomycin should not be used for the treatment of otitis externa when the ear drum is perforated, because of the risk of toxicity.

Applications to large areas especially during pregnancy, in the elderly and in patients with impaired renal function due to a risk of ototoxicity.

A possibility of increased absorption exists in very young children, thus Dermovate-NN is not recommended for use in neonates.

Special warnings and precautions for use: Long-term continuous topical therapy should be avoided where possible, particularly in infants and children, as adrenal suppression can occur readily even without occlusion.

If used in childhood, or on the face, courses should be limited to five days and occlusion should not be used.

The face, more than other areas of the body, may exhibit atrophic changes after prolonged treatment with potent topical corticosteroids. This must be borne in mind when treating such conditions as psoriasis and severe eczema with Dermovate-NN. If applied to the eyelids, care is needed to ensure that the preparation does not enter the eye, as glaucoma might result.

Topical corticosteroids may be hazardous in psoriasis for a number of reasons, including rebound relapses, development of tolerance, risk of generalised pustular psoriasis and development of local or systemic toxicity due to impaired barrier function of the skin. If used in psoriasis careful patient supervision is important.

Do not continue for more than 7 days in the absence of clinical improvement, since occult extension of infection may occur due to the masking effect of the steroid.

If infection persists, systemic chemotherapy is required. Any spread of infection requires withdrawal of topical corticosteroid therapy. Bacterial infection is encouraged by the warm, moist conditions induced by occlusive dressings, and the skin should be cleansed before a fresh dressing is applied.

In neonates and infants, absorption by immature skins may be enhanced and renal function may be immature (see *Contra-indications*).

Extended or recurrent application may increase the risk of contact sensitisation.

Products which contain antimicrobial agents should not be diluted.

Interaction with other medicaments and other forms of interaction: None known.

Pregnancy and lactation: There is little information to demonstrate the possible effect of topically applied neomycin in pregnancy and lactation. However, neomycin present in maternal blood can cross the placenta and may give rise to a theoretical risk of foetal toxicity, thus use of Dermovate-NN is not recommended in pregnancy and lactation.

Effects on ability to drive and use machines: None known.

Undesirable effects: As with other topical corticosteroids prolonged use of large amounts or treatment of extensive areas can result in sufficient systemic absorption to produce the features of hypercorticism. Provided the weekly dosage is less than 50 g in adults, any suppression of the HPA axis is likely to be transient with a rapid return to normal values once the short course of steroid therapy has ceased. The same applies to children given proportionate dosage. Use of occlusive dressings increases the absorption of topical corticosteroids. In infants, the napkin may act as an occlusive dressing.

Prolonged and intensive treatment with highly active corticosteroid preparations may cause local atrophic changes in the skin such as thinning, striae, and dilatation of the superficial blood vessels, particularly when occlusive dressings are used, or when skin folds are involved.

In rare instances, treatment of psoriasis with corticosteroids (or its withdrawal) is thought to have provoked the pustular form of the disease (see *Precautions*).

There are reports of pigmentation changes and hypertrichosis with topical steroids.

Dermovate-NN is usually well tolerated, but if signs of hypersensitivity appear, application should be stopped immediately.

Exacerbation of symptoms may occur.

Overdose: Acute overdosage is very unlikely to occur, however, in the case of overdosage or misuse the features of hypercorticism may appear and in this situation topical steroids should be discontinued.

Pharmacological properties
Pharmacodynamic properties: Clobetasol propionate is a highly active corticosteroid with topical anti-inflammatory activity.

The use of nystatin in the local treatment of candidal infections of the skin and of neomycin as a broad spectrum antibiotic is well known.

The principal action of the preparation is based on the anti-inflammatory activity of the corticosteroid. The broad spectrum antibacterial and anti-candidal activity provided by the combination of neomycin and nystatin allow this effect to be utilised in the treatment of conditions which are or are likely to become infected.

Pharmacokinetic properties: Dermovate-NN has been shown to have a satisfactory pharmacokinetic profile by many years of successful clinical experience.

The extent of percutaneous absorption of topical corticosteroids is determined by many factors including the vehicle and the integrity of the epidermal barrier.

Topical corticosteroids can be absorbed from normal intact skin. Inflammation and/or other disease processes in the skin increase percutaneous absorption.

Once absorbed through the skin, topical corticosteroids are handled through pharmacokinetic pathways similar to systematically administered corticosteroids. Corticosteroids are bound to plasma proteins in varying degrees. Corticosteroids are metabolised primarily by the liver and are then excreted by the kidneys.

Preclinical safety data: No additional data of relevance.

Pharmaceutical particulars
List of excipients: Microcrystalline wax, Arachis oil, Polyoxyethylene cetyl ether, Beeswax/Beeswax substitute, Titanium dioxide, Propyl gallate, Liquid paraffin.

Incompatibilities: None known.

Shelf life: Cream: 18 months.

Special precautions for storage: Store below 25°C.

Nature and contents of container: Collapsible aluminium 25 or 30 gm tubes with polypropylene cap.

Instructions for use/handling: For detailed instructions for use refer to the Patient Information Leaflet in every pack.

Marketing authorisation number PL 10949/0026

Date of first authorisation/renewal of authorisation 11.12.95

Date of (partial) revision of the text June 1997

DERMOVATE*-NN OINTMENT

Qualitative and quantitative composition Dermovate-NN skin preparations contain clobetasol propionate 0.05% w/w, neomycin sulphate 0.5% and nystatin 100,000 units per gram.

Pharmaceutical form Ointment for topical administration.

Clinical particulars
Therapeutic indications: Clobetasol propionate is a highly active topical corticosteroid which is of particular value when used in short courses for the treatment of recalcitrant eczemas, neurodermatoses, and other conditions which do not respond satisfactorily to less active steroids.

Dermovate-NN is indicated in more resistant dermatoses such as recalcitrant eczemas and psoriasis (excluding widespread plaque psoriasis) where secondary bacterial or candidal infection is present, suspected or likely to occur, as when using occlusive dressings.

Posology and method of administration: Apply sparingly to the affected area once or twice daily until improvement occurs. As with other highly-active topical steroid preparations, therapy should be discontinued when control is achieved. In the more responsive conditions this may be within a few days.

If a longer course is necessary, it is recommended that treatment should not be continued for more than four weeks without the patient's condition being reviewed.

Repeated short courses of Dermovate-NN may be used to control exacerbations. If continuous steroid treatment is necessary, a less potent preparation should be used.

In very resistant lesions, especially where there is hyperkeratosis, the anti-inflammatory effect of Dermovate-NN can be enhanced, if necessary, by occluding the treatment area with polythene. Overnight occlusion only is usually adequate to bring about a satisfactory response, thereafter improvement can usually be maintained by application without occlusion.

Dermovate-NN is suitable for use in children at the same dose as adults, but the dose should be reduced for use in infants. Dermovate-NN is not recommended for use in neonates.

Contra-indications: Rosacea, acne vulgaris and perioral dermatitis.

Primary cutaneous viral infections (e.g. herpes simplex, chickenpox).

Hypersensitivity to the preparations.

Use of Dermovate-NN skin preparations is not indicated in the treatment of primarily infected skin lesions caused by infection with fungi (e.g. candidiasis, tinea), bacteria (e.g. impetigo), or yeast; secondary infections due to Pseudomonas or Proteus species; perianal and genital pruritus, dermatoses in children under one year of age, including dermatitis and napkin eruptions.

Preparations containing neomycin should not be used for the treatment of otitis externa when the ear drum is perforated, because of the risk of toxicity.

Applications to large areas especially during pregnancy, in the elderly and in patients with impaired renal function due to a risk of ototoxicity.

A possibility of increased absorption exists in very young children, thus Dermovate-NN is not recommended for use in neonates.

Special warnings and precautions for use: Long-term continuous topical therapy should be avoided where possible, particularly in infants and children, as adrenal suppression can occur readily even without occlusion.

If used in childhood, or on the face, courses should be limited to five days and occlusion should not be used.

The face, more than other areas of the body, may exhibit atrophic changes after prolonged treatment with potent topical corticosteroids. This must be borne in mind when treating such conditions as psoriasis and severe eczema with Dermovate-NN. If applied to the eyelids, care is needed to ensure that the preparation does not enter the eye, as glaucoma might result.

Topical corticosteroids may be hazardous in psoriasis for a number of reasons, including rebound relapses, development of tolerance, risk of generalised pustular psoriasis and development of local or systemic toxicity due to impaired barrier function of the skin. If used in psoriasis careful patient supervision is important.

Do not continue for more than 7 days in the absence of clinical improvement, since occult extension of infection may occur due to the masking effect of the steroid.

If infection persists, systemic chemotherapy is required. Any spread of infection requires withdrawal of topical corticosteroid therapy. Bacterial infection is encouraged by the warm, moist conditions induced by occlusive dressings, and the skin should be cleansed before a fresh dressing is applied.

In neonates and infants, absorption by immature skins may be enhanced and renal function may be immature (see *Contra-indications*).

Extended or recurrent application may increase the risk of contact sensitisation.

Products which contain antimicrobial agents should not be diluted.

Interaction with other medicaments and other forms of interaction: None known.

Pregnancy and lactation: There is little information to demonstrate the possible effect of topically applied neomycin in pregnancy and lactation. However, neomycin present in maternal blood can cross the placenta and may give rise to a theoretical risk of foetal toxicity, thus use of Dermovate-NN is not recommended in pregnancy and lactation.

Effects on ability to drive and use machines: None known.

Undesirable effects: As with other topical corticosteroids prolonged use of large amounts or treatment of extensive areas can result in sufficient systemic absorption to produce the features of hypercorticism. Provided the weekly dosage is less than 50 g in adults, any suppression of the HPA axis is likely to be transient with a rapid return to normal values once the short course of steroid therapy has ceased. The same applies to children given proportionate dosage. Use of occlusive dressings increases the absorption of topical corticosteroids. In infants, the napkin may act as an occlusive dressing.

Overdose: Acute overdosage is very unlikely to occur, however, in the case of overdosage or misuse the features of hypercorticism may appear and in this situation topical steroids should be discontinued.

Pharmacological properties

Pharmacodynamic properties: Clobetasol propionate is a highly active corticosteroid with topical anti-inflammatory activity.

The use of nystatin in the local treatment of candidal infections of the skin and of neomycin as a broad spectrum antibiotic is well known.

The principal action of the preparation is based on the anti-inflammatory activity of the corticosteroid. The broad spectrum antibacterial and anti-candidal activity provided by the combination of neomycin and nystatin allow this effect to be utilised in the treatment of conditions which are or are likely to become infected.

Pharmacokinetic properties: Dermovate-NN has been shown to have a satisfactory pharmacokinetic profile by many years of successful clinical experience.

The extent of percutaneous absorption of topical corticosteroids is determined by many factors including the vehicle and the integrity of the epidermal barrier.

Topical corticosteroids can be absorbed from normal intact skin. Inflammation and/or other disease processes in the skin increase percutaneous absorption.

Once absorbed through the skin, topical corticosteroids are handled through pharmacokinetic pathways similar to systematically administered corticosteroids. Corticosteroids are bound to plasma proteins in varying degrees. Corticosteroids are metabolised primarily by the liver and are then excreted by the kidneys.

Preclinical safety data: No additional data of relevance.

Pharmaceutical particulars

List of excipients: Titanium dioxide, Liquid paraffin, Soft white paraffin.

Incompatibilities: None known.

Shelf life: 36 months.

Special precautions for storage: Store below 25°C.

Nature and contents of container: Collapsible aluminium 25 or 30 gm tubes with polypropylene cap.

Instructions for use/handling: For detailed instructions for use refer to the Patient Information Leaflet in every pack.

Marketing authorisation number PL 10949/0027

Date of first authorisation/renewal of authorisation 31.08.94

Date of (partial) revision of the text June 1997.

DICONAL* TABLETS

Qualitative and quantitative composition Each tablet contains 10 mg of Dipipanone Hydrochloride BP and 30 mg of Cyclizine Hydrochloride BP, coloured deep pink, scored and coded 'WELLCOME F3A'.

Pharmaceutical form Tablet.

Clinical particulars

Therapeutic indications: Diconal Tablets are indicated for the management of moderate to severe pain in medical and surgical conditions in which morphine may be indicated.

Cyclizine is effective in preventing nausea and vomiting associated with the administration of narcotic analgesics.

Posology and method of administration:

Adults: The initial dose in all conditions is one tablet every 6 hours. It is unwise to exceed this dose in view of the difficulty in accurately predicting the initial central effects of dipipanone.

Should this dose fail to prove adequate analgesia, as in severe intractable pain or when other potent opioids have been used, it may be increased by half a tablet every six hours.

It is seldom necessary to exceed a dose of 30 mg dipipanone given 6-hourly (i.e. 12 tablets in 24 hours).

Children: There is no specific information on the use of Diconal in children. Diconal is very rarely indicated in childen and dosage guidelines cannot be stated.

Use in the elderly: There is no specific information on the use of Diconal in elderly patients. In common with opioid drugs, Diconal may be expected to cause confusion in this age group, and careful monitoring is advised (see *Special warnings and precautions*).

Contra-indications: Diconal is contra-indicated in individuals who are hypersensitive to dipipanone or cyclizine.

Diconal is generally contra-indicated in patients with respiratory depression, especially in the presence of cyanosis and excessive bronchial secretions.

Diconal should not be given during an attack of bronchial asthma.

Diconal is generally contra-indicated in the presence of acute alcoholism, head injury and raised intracranial pressure.

Diconal is contra-indicated in individuals receiving monoamine oxidase inhibitors, or within 14 days of stopping such treatment.

Diconal is contra-indicated in patients with ulcerative colitis since in common with other narcotic analgesics it may precipitate toxic dilatation or spasm of the colon.

As with all narcotic analgesics Diconal should not be administered to patients with severe hepatic impairment as it may precipitate hepatic encephalopathy.

In severe renal impairment Diconal, in common with all narcotic analgesics, may precipitate coma and should not be administered.

Diconal, in common with morphine and most other narcotics, may cause spasm of the biliary and renal tracts; it is contra-indicated in these conditions.

Special warnings and precautions for use: The repeated use of Diconal may lead to tolerance and physical dependence as well as to psychological dependence on the product.

Misuse of Diconal has been reported, particularly by young addicts who have previously been dependent on, or have misused other agents both opiate and non-opiate. Extreme caution is warranted when prescribing Diconal to this group of patients.

Diconal should be used with extreme caution in the presence of the following: hypothyroidism; adrenocortical insufficiency; prostatic hypertrophy; hypotension secondary to hypovolaemic shock; diabetes mellitus.

Diconal is metabolised in the liver and excreted along with its metabolites in the urine. Where not contra-indicated in patients with impaired hepatic and/or renal function, Diconal should be given at less than the usual recommended dose, and the patient's response used as a guide to further dosage requirements.

Extreme caution should be exercised when administering Diconal to patients with phaeochromocytoma, since hypertension has been reported in association with other potent opioids.

No data are available as to whether or not dipipanone has carcinogenic, mutagenic or teratogenic potential. It is not known whether cyclizine has carcinogenic or mutagenic potential. Some animal studies are interpreted as indicating that cyclizine may be teratogenic, but relevance to the human situation is not known.

In a study involving prolonged administration of cyclizine to male and female rats, there was no evidence of impaired fertility after continuous treatment for 90–100 days. There are no similar data for dipipanone. There is no information on the effect of Diconal on human fertility.

Interaction with other medicaments and other forms of interaction: The central nervous system depressant effects of Diconal may be increased by phenothiazine drugs, alcohol, sedatives and tricyclic antidepressants. Concurrent administration of some phenothiazines increases the respiratory depressant effects of narcotic analgesics and also produces hypotension.

Because of its anticholinergic activity, cyclizine may enhance the side effects of other anticholinergic agents.

Analgesic effects of opioid drugs tend to be enhanced by co-administration of dexamphetamine, however their use in combination is not recommended.

Pregnancy and lactation: The use of Diconal during pregnancy is not recommended. No data are available on the therapeutic use of Diconal in human pregnancy. It may be anticipated that if given in the last trimester, Diconal would cause withdrawal symptoms in the neonate.

Diconal is not recommended for use in labour because of its potential to cause respiratory depression in the neonate.

No data are available on the excretion of dipipanone, cyclizine or their metabolites in human milk.

Effect on ability to drive and use machines: Ambulatory patients receiving Diconal should be cautioned against driving cars or operating machinery in view of its tendency to cause drowsiness.

Undesirable effects: The adverse effects of dipipanone

are common to all opioid agents, and may include: respiratory depression; mental clouding, drowsiness and sedation, confusion, mood changes, euphoria, dysphoria, psychosis, restlessness, miosis and raised intracranial pressure; constipation, nausea and vomiting; sweating, facial flushing and hypotension; urticaria and rashes; difficulty with micturition; biliary and renal tract spasm; vertigo.

In addition, cyclizine may cause drowsiness which is potentiated by other sedative drugs including alcohol. Furthermore dryness of the mouth, nose and throat, blurred vision, tachycardia, urinary retention, restlessness, nervousness, insomnia and auditory and visual hallucinations have been reported, particularly when dosage recommendations have been exceeded. Cholestatic jaundice has occurred in association with cyclizine.

Following cyclizine administration, single case reports have been documented of: fixed drug eruption; generalised chorea; hypersensitivity hepatitis; agranulocytosis.

Overdose: The signs of overdosage with Diconal are typically those of opioid poisoning, i.e. respiratory depression, pin-point pupils, hypotension, circulatory failure and deepening coma. Mydriasis may replace miosis as asphyxia intervenes. Drowsiness, floppiness, miosis and apnoea have been reported in children, as have convulsions.

General supportive measures should be employed as required. Gastric lavage should be performed if indicated. The specific opioid antagonist naloxone is the treatment of choice for the reversal of coma and the restoration of spontaneous respiration; the literature should be consulted for details of appropriate dosage. Patients should be monitored closely for at least 48 hours after recovery in case of relapse, since the duration of action of the antagonist may be substantially shorter than that of dipipanone.

Pharmacological properties

Pharmacodynamic properties: The onset of analgesic action of dipipanone is approximately one hour and lasts for 4 to 6 hours. Cyclizine produces its anti-emetic effect within 2 hours and lasts for approximately 4 hours.

Pharmacokinetic properties: Dipipanone is absorbed from the gastro-intestinal tract. It is metabolised in the liver and excreted in the urine and faeces, although data on the proportions of parent compound and metabolites so excreted are lacking.

In healthy adult volunteers, the administration of a single oral dose of 50 mg cyclizine resulted in a peak plasma concentration of approximately 70 nanogram/ml occurring approximately 2 hours after drug administration. The plasma elimination half-life was approximately 20 hours.

The N-demethylated derivative, norcyclizine, has been identified as a metabolite of cyclizine. Norcyclizine has little antihistaminic (H_1) activity compared with cyclizine and has a plasma elimination half life of approximately 20 hours. After a single oral dose of 50 mg cyclizine given to a single adult male volunteer, urine collected over the following 24 hours contained less than 1% of the total dose administered.

Preclinical safety data: No additional data of relevance.

Pharmaceutical particulars

List of excipients: Lactose, starches, dye (FD and C Red No 3), gelatin, magnesium stearate. Methylated spirit, ethanol and purified water are all used in the manufacturing process but are not detected in the final formulation.

Incompatibilities: None stated.

Shelf life: 60 months.

Special precautions for storage: Store below 25°C. Protect from light. Keep dry.

Nature and contents of container: PVC/aluminium foil blister packs containing 50 tablets.

Instructions for use/handling: None stated.

Marketing authorisation number PL 0003/5027R

Date of approval/revision of SPC August 1996

EFCORTELAN* CREAM 0.5%

Qualitative and quantitative composition Hydrocortisone BP 0.5% w/w.

Pharmaceutical form Aqueous cream.

Clinical particulars

Therapeutic indications: Hydrocortisone has topical anti-inflammatory activities of value in the treatment of a wide variety of dermatological conditions, including the following: eczema, including atopic, infantile, discoid and stasis eczemas; prurigo nodularis, neurodermatoses, seborrhoeic dermatitis, intertrigo and contact sensitivity reactions.

Efcortelan preparations can also be used in the management of insect bites and otitis externa.

Efcortelan 0.5% preparations can be used as continuation therapy in mild cases of seborrhoeic or atopic eczema once the acute inflammatory phase has passed.

Posology and method of administration:

Adults, children and elderly: A small quantity should be applied to the affected area two or three times daily.

Efcortelan Cream is often appropriate for moist or weeping surfaces, and Efcortelan Ointment for dry, lichenified or scaly lesions, but this is not invariably so.

For topical application.

Contra-indications: Skin lesions caused by infection with viruses (e.g. herpes simplex, chickenpox), fungi (e.g. candidiasis, tinea) or bacteria (e.g. impetigo).

Hypersensitivity to the preparation.

Special warnings and precautions for use: In infants and children, long-term continuous topical therapy should be avoided where possible, as adrenal suppression can occur even without occlusion. In infants, the napkin may act as an occlusive dressing, and increase absorption. Treatment should therefore be limited, if possible, to a maximum of seven days.

Appropriate antimicrobial therapy should be used whenever treating inflammatory lesions which have become infected. Any spread of infection requires withdrawal of topical corticosteroid therapy, and systemic administration of antimicrobial agents.

As with all corticosteroids, prolonged application to the face is undesirable.

Interaction with other medicaments and other forms of interaction: None.

Pregnancy and lactation: There is inadequate evidence of safety in human pregnancy. Topical application of corticosteroids to pregnant animals can cause abnormalities of foetal development including cleft palate and intrauterine growth retardation. There may therefore be a very small risk of such effects in the human foetus.

Effects on ability to drive and use machines: None.

Undesirable effects: Efcortelan preparations are usually well tolerated, but if signs of hypersensitivity appear, application should be stopped immediately.

Local atrophic changes may occur where skin folds are involved, or in areas such as the nappy area in small children, where constant moist conditions favour the absorption of hydrocortisone. Sufficient systemic absorption may also occur in such sites to produce the features of hypercorticism and suppression of the HPA axis after prolonged treatment.

The effect is more likely to occur in infants and children, and if occlusive dressings are used.

There are reports of pigmentation changes and hypertrichosis with topical steroids.

Exacerbation of symptoms may occur.

Overdose: Acute overdosage is very unlikely to occur, however, in the case of chronic overdosage or misuse the features of hypercorticism may appear and in this situation topical steroids should be discontinued.

Pharmacological properties

Pharmacodynamic properties: Hydrocortisone is the main glucocorticoid secreted by the adrenal cortex. It is used topically for its anti-inflammatory effects which suppress the clinical manifestations of the disease in a wide range of disorders where inflammation is a prominent feature.

Pharmacokinetic properties: Hydrocortisone is absorbed through the skin particularly in denuded areas. Hydrocortisone is metabolised in the liver and most body tissues to hydrogenated and degraded forms such as tetrahydrocortisone and tetrahydrocortisol. These are excreted in the urine, mainly conjugated as glucuronides, together with a very small proportion of unchanged hydrocortisone.

Preclinical safety data: There are no preclinical data of relevance to the prescriber which are additional to that in other sections of the SmPC.

Pharmaceutical particulars

List of excipients: Chlorocresol BP, Cetomacrogol 1000 BP, Cetostearyl alcohol BP, White soft paraffin BP, Liquid paraffin BP, Sodium acid phosphate BP, Phosphoric acid BP, Sodium hydroxide BP, Purified water BP.

Incompatibilities: None known.

Shelf life: 24 months.

Special precautions for storage: Store below 25°C.

Nature and contents of container: 15 gm and 30 gm collapsible aluminium tubes internally coated with an epoxy resin based lacquer and closed with a wadless polypropylene cap.

Instructions for use/handling: No special instructions.

Marketing authorisation number PL 10949/0029

Date of first authorisation/renewal of authorisation 9/12/97

Date of (partial) revision of the text May 1997

EFCORTELAN* CREAM 1%

Qualitative and quantitative composition Hydrocortisone BP 1% w/w.

Pharmaceutical form Aqueous cream.

Clinical particulars

Therapeutic indications: Hydrocortisone has topical anti-inflammatory activities of value in the treatment of a wide variety of dermatological conditions, including the following: eczema, including atopic, infantile, discoid and stasis eczemas; prurigo nodularis, neurodermatoses, seborrhoeic dermatitis, intertrigo and contact sensitivity reactions.

Efcortelan preparations can also be used in the management of insect bites and otitis externa.

Efcortelan 0.5% preparations can be used as continuation therapy in mild cases of seborrhoeic or atopic eczema once the acute inflammatory phase has passed.

Posology and method of administration:

Adults, children and elderly: A small quantity should be applied to the affected area two or three times daily.

Efcortelan Cream is often appropriate for moist or weeping surfaces, and Efcortelan Ointment for dry, lichenified or scaly lesions, but this is not invariably so.

For topical application.

Contra-indications: Skin lesions caused by infection with viruses (e.g. herpes simplex, chickenpox), fungi (e.g. candidiasis, tinea) or bacteria (e.g. impetigo).

Hypersensitivity to the preparation.

Special warnings and precautions for use: In infants and children, long-term continuous topical therapy should be avoided where possible, as adrenal suppression can occur even without occlusion. In infants, the napkin may act as an occlusive dressing, and increase absorption. Treatment should therefore be limited, if possible, to a maximum of 7 days.

Appropriate antimicrobial therapy should be used whenever treating inflammatory lesions which have become infected. Any spread of infection requires withdrawal of topical corticosteroid therapy, and systemic administration of antimicrobial agents.

As with all corticosteroids, prolonged application to the face is undesirable.

Interaction with other medicaments and other forms of interaction: None.

Pregnancy and lactation: There is inadequate evidence of safety in human pregnancy. Topical application of corticosteroids to pregnant animals can cause abnormalities of foetal development including cleft palate and intrauterine growth retardation. There may therefore be a very small risk of such effects in the human foetus.

Effects on ability to drive and use machines: None.

Undesirable effects: Efcortelan preparations are usually well tolerated, but if signs of hypersensitivity appear, application should be stopped immediately.

Local atrophic changes may occur where skin folds are involved, or in areas such as the nappy area in small children, where constant moist conditions favour the absorption of hydrocortisone. Sufficient systemic absorption may also occur in such sites to produce the features of hypercorticism and suppression of the HPA axis after prolonged treatment.

The effect is more likely to occur in infants and children, and if occlusive dressings are used.

There are reports of pigmentation changes and hypertrichosis with topical steroids.

Exacerbation of symptoms may occur.

Overdose: Acute overdosage is very unlikely to occur, however, in the case of chronic overdosage or misuse the features of hypercorticism may appear and in this situation topical steroids should be discontinued.

Pharmacological properties

Pharmacodynamic properties: Hydrocortisone is the main glucocorticoid secreted by the adrenal cortex. It is used topically for its anti-inflammatory effects which suppress the clinical manifestations of the disease in a wide range of disorders where inflammation is a prominent feature.

Pharmacokinetic properties: Hydrocortisone is absorbed through the skin particularly in denuded areas. Hydrocortisone is metabolised in the liver and most body tissues to hydrogenated and degraded forms such as tetrahydrocortisone and tetrahydrocortisol. These are excreted in the urine, mainly conjugated as glucuronides, together with a very small proportion of unchanged hydrocortisone.

Preclinical safety data: There are no preclinical data of

relevance to the prescriber which are additional to that in other sections of the SmPC.

Pharmaceutical particulars
List of excipients: Chlorocresol BP, Cetomacrogol 1000 BP, Cetostearyl alcohol BP, White soft paraffin BP, Liquid paraffin BP, Sodium acid phosphate BP, Phosphoric acid BP, Sodium hydroxide BP, Purified water BP.

Incompatibilities: None known.

Shelf life: 24 months.

Special precautions for storage: Store below 25°C.

Nature and contents of container: 15 gm, 30 gm and 50 gm collapsible aluminium tubes internally coated with an epoxy resin based lacquer and closed with a wadless polypropylene cap.

Instructions for use/handling: No special instructions.

Marketing authorisation number PL 10949/0030

Date of first authorisation/renewal of authorisation 18 December 1997

Date of (partial) revision of the text This is the first SmPC (May 1997).

EFCORTELAN* CREAM 2.5%

Qualitative and quantitative composition Hydrocortisone BP 2.5% w/w.

Pharmaceutical form Aqueous cream.

Clinical particulars
Therapeutic indications: Hydrocortisone has topical anti-inflammatory activities of value in the treatment of a wide variety of dermatological conditions, including the following: eczema, including atopic, infantile, discoid and stasis eczemas; prurigo nodularis, neurodermatoses, seborrhoeic dermatitis, intertrigo and contact sensitivity reactions.

Efcortelan preparations can also be used in the management of insect bites and otitis externa.

Efcortelan 0.5% preparations can be used as continuation therapy in mild cases of seborrhoeic or atopic eczema once the acute inflammatory phase has passed.

Posology and method of administration:
Adults, children and elderly: A small quantity should be applied to the affected area two or three times daily.

Efcortelan Cream is often appropriate for moist or weeping surfaces, and Efcortelan Ointment for dry, lichenified or scaly lesions, but this is not invariably so.

For topical application.

Contra-indications: Skin lesions caused by infection with viruses (e.g. herpes simplex, chickenpox), fungi (e.g. candidiasis, tinea) or bacteria (e.g. impetigo).

Hypersensitivity to the preparation.

Special warnings and precautions for use: In infants and children, long-term continuous topical therapy should be avoided where possible, as adrenal suppression can occur even without occlusion. In infants, the napkin may act as an occlusive dressing, and increase absorption. Treatment should therefore be limited, if possible, to a maximum of 7 days.

Appropriate antimicrobial therapy should be used whenever treating inflammatory lesions which have become infected. Any spread of infection requires withdrawal of topical corticosteroid therapy, and systemic administration of antimicrobial agents.

As with all corticosteroids, prolonged application to the face is undesirable.

Interaction with other medicaments and other forms of interaction: None.

Pregnancy and lactation: There is inadequate evidence of safety in human pregnancy. Topical application of corticosteroids to pregnant animals can cause abnormalities of foetal development including cleft palate and intrauterine growth retardation. There may therefore be a very small risk of such effects in the human foetus.

Effects on ability to drive and use machines: None.

Undesirable effects: Efcortelan preparations are usually well tolerated, but if signs of hypersensitivity appear, application should be stopped immediately.

Local atrophic changes may occur where skin folds are involved, or in areas such as the nappy area in small children, where constant moist conditions favour the absorption of hydrocortisone. Sufficient systemic absorption may also occur in such sites to produce the features of hypercorticism and suppression of the HPA axis after prolonged treatment.

The effect is more likely to occur in infants and children, and if occlusive dressings are used.

There are reports of pigmentation changes and hypertrichosis with topical steroids.

Exacerbation of symptoms may occur.

Overdose: Acute overdosage is very unlikely to occur, however, in the case of chronic overdosage or misuse the features of hypercorticism may appear and in this situation topical steroids should be discontinued.

Pharmacological properties
Pharmacodynamic properties: Hydrocortisone is the main glucocorticoid secreted by the adrenal cortex. It is used topically for its anti-inflammatory effects which suppress the clinical manifestations of the disease in a wide range of disorders where inflammation is a prominent feature.

Pharmacokinetic properties: Hydrocortisone is absorbed through the skin particularly in denuded areas. Hydrocortisone is metabolised in the liver and most body tissues to hydrogenated and degraded forms such as tetrahydrocortisone and tetrahydrocortisol. These are excreted in the urine, mainly conjugated as glucuronides, together with a very small proportion of unchanged hydrocortisone.

Preclinical safety data: There are no preclinical data of relevance to the prescriber which are additional to that in other sections of the SmPC.

Pharmaceutical particulars
List of excipients: Chlorocresol BP, Cetomacrogol 1000 BP, Cetostearyl alcohol BP, White soft paraffin BP, Liquid paraffin BP, Sodium acid phosphate BP, Phosphoric acid BP, Sodium hydroxide BP, Purified water BP.

Incompatibilities: None known.

Shelf life: 24 months.

Special precautions for storage: Store below 25°C.

Nature and contents of container: 15 gm and 30 gm collapsible aluminium tubes internally coated with an epoxy resin based lacquer and closed with a wadless polypropylene cap.

Instructions for use/handling: No special instructions.

Marketing authorisation number PL 10949/0031

Date of first authorisation/renewal of authorisation 18 December 1997

Date of (partial) revision of the text This is the first SmPC (May 1997).

EFCORTELAN* OINTMENT 0.5%

Qualitative and quantitative composition Hydrocortisone BP 0.5% w/w.

Pharmaceutical form Ointment.

Clinical particulars
Therapeutic indications: Hydrocortisone has topical anti-inflammatory activities of value in the treatment of a wide variety of dermatological conditions, including the following: eczema, including atopic, infantile, discoid and stasis eczemas: prurigo nodularis, neurodermatoses, seborrhoeic dermatitis, intertrigo and contact sensitivity reactions.

Efcortelan preparations can also be used in the management of insect bites and otitis externa.

Efcortelan 0.5% preparations can be used as continuation therapy in mild cases of seborrhoeic or atopic eczema once the acute inflammatory phase has passed.

Posology and method of administration:
Adults, children and elderly: A small quantity should be applied to the affected area two or three times daily.

Efcortelan cream is often appropriate for moist or weeping surfaces, and Efcortelan Ointment for dry, lichenified or scaly lesions, but this is not invariably so. Efcortelan lotion is particularly suitable when a minimal application to a large area is required.

Route of administration: For topical application.

Contra-indications: Skin lesions, caused by infection with viruses (e.g. herpes simplex, chickenpox), fungi (e.g. candidiasis, tinea) or bacteria (e.g. impetigo). Hypersensitivity to the preparations.

Special warnings and precautions for use: In infants and children, long-term continuous topical therapy should be avoided where possible, as adrenal suppression can occur even without occlusion. In infants, the napkin may act as an occlusive dressing, and increase absorption. Treatment should therefore be limited if possible, to a maximum of seven days.

Appropriate antimicrobial therapy should be used whenever treating inflammatory lesions which have become infected. Any spread of infection requires withdrawal of topical corticosteroid therapy, and systemic administration of antimicrobial agents.

As with all corticosteroids, prolonged application to the face is undesirable.

Interaction with other medicaments and other forms of interaction: None known.

Pregnancy and lactation: There is inadequate evidence of safety in human pregnancy. Topical application of corticosteroids to pregnant animals can cause abnormalities of foetal development including cleft palate and intra-uterine growth retardation. There may, therefore, be a very small risk of such effects in the human foetus.

Effect on ability to drive and use machines: None known.

Undesirable effects: Efcortelan preparations are usually well tolerated, but if signs of hypersensitivity appear, application should stop immediately.

Exacerbation of symptoms may occur.

Local atrophic changes may occur where skin folds are involved, or in areas such as the nappy area in small children, where constant moist conditions favour the absorption of hydrocortisone. Sufficient systemic absorption may also occur in such sites to produce the features of hypercorticism and suppression of the HPA axis after prolonged treatment. This effect is more likely to occur in infants and children, and if occlusive dressings are used.

There are reports of pigmentation changes and hypertrichosis with topical steroids.

Overdose: Acute overdosage is very unlikely to occur, however, in the case of chronic overdosage or misuse the features of hypercorticism may appear and in this situation topical steroids should be discontinued.

Pharmacological properties
Pharmacodynamic properties: Hydrocortisone is the main glucocorticoid secreted by the adrenal cortex. It is used topically for its anti-inflammatory effects which suppress the clinical manifestations of the disease in a wide range of disorders where inflammation is a prominent feature.

Pharmacokinetic properties: Hydrocortisone is absorbed through the skin particularly in denuded areas. Hydrocortisone is metabolised in the liver and most body tissues to hydrogenated and degraded forms such as tetrahydrocortisone and tetrahydrocortisol. These are excreted in the urine, mainly conjugated as glucuronides, together with a very small proportion of unchanged hydrocortisone.

Preclinical safety data: There are no preclinical data of relevance to the prescriber which are additional to that in other sections of the SPC.

Pharmaceutical particulars
List of excipients: White soft paraffin BP, Liquid paraffin BP.

Incompatibilities: None known.

Shelf life: 36 months.

Special precautions for storage: Store below 25°C.

Nature and contents of container: 15 gm and 30 gm collapsible aluminium tubes internally uncoated or coated with an epoxy resin based lacquer and closed with a wadless polypropylene cap.

Instructions for use/handling: No special instructions.

Marketing authorisation number PL 10949/0032

Date of first authorisation/renewal of authorisation 1 March 1993

Date of (partial) revision of text This is the first SPC. July 1997.

EFCORTELAN* OINTMENT 1.0%

Qualitative and quantitative composition Hydrocortisone BP 1.0% w/w.

Pharmaceutical form Ointment.

Clinical particulars
Therapeutic indications: Hydrocortisone has topical anti-inflammatory activities of value in the treatment of a wide variety of dermatological conditions, including the following: eczema, including atopic, infantile, discoid and stasis eczemas: prurigo nodularis, neurodermatoses, seborrhoeic dermatitis, intertrigo and contact sensitivity reactions.

Efcortelan preparations can also be used in the management of insect bites and otitis externa.

Efcortelan 0.5% preparations can be used as continuation therapy in mild cases of seborrhoeic or atopic eczema once the acute inflammatory phase has passed.

Posology and method of administration:
Adults, children and elderly: A small quantity should be applied to the affected area two or three times daily.

Efcortelan cream is often appropriate for moist or weeping surfaces, and Efcortelan Ointment for dry, lichenified or scaly lesions, but this is not invariably so. Efcortelan lotion is particularly suitable when a minimal application to a large area is required.

Route of administration: For topical application.

Contra-indications: Skin lesions, caused by infection with viruses (e.g. herpes simplex, chickenpox), fungi (e.g. candidiasis, tinea) or bacteria (e.g. impetigo). Hypersensitivity to the preparations.

Special warnings and precautions for use: In infants

and children, long-term continuous topical therapy should be avoided where possible, as adrenal suppression can occur even without occlusion. In infants, the napkin may act as an occlusive dressing, and increase absorption. Treatment should therefore be limited if possible, to a maximum of seven days.

Appropriate antimicrobial therapy should be used whenever treating inflammatory lesions which have become infected. Any spread of infection requires withdrawal of topical corticosteroid therapy, and systemic administration of antimicrobial agents.

As with all corticosteroids, prolonged application to the face is undesirable.

Interaction with other medicaments and other forms of interaction: None known.

Pregnancy and lactation: There is inadequate evidence of safety in human pregnancy. Topical application of corticosteroids to pregnant animals can cause abnormalities of foetal development including cleft palate and intra-uterine growth retardation. There may, therefore, be a very small risk of such effects in the human foetus.

Effect on ability to drive and use machines: None known.

Undesirable effects: Efcortelan preparations are usually well tolerated, but if signs of hypersensitivity appear, application should stop immediately.

Exacerbation of symptoms may occur.

Local atrophic changes may occur where skin folds are involved, or in areas such as the nappy area in small children, where constant moist conditions favour the absorption of hydrocortisone. Sufficient systemic absorption may also occur in such sites to produce the features of hypercorticism and suppression of the HPA axis after prolonged treatment. This effect is more likely to occur in infants and children, and if occlusive dressings are used.

There are reports of pigmentation changes and hypertrichosis with topical steroids.

Overdose: Acute overdosage is very unlikely to occur, however, in the case of chronic overdosage or misuse the features of hypercorticism may appear and in this situation topical steroids should be discontinued.

Pharmacological properties

Pharmacodynamic properties: Hydrocortisone is the main glucocorticoid secreted by the adrenal cortex. It is used topically for its anti-inflammatory effects which suppress the clinical manifestations of the disease in a wide range of disorders where inflammation is a prominent feature.

Pharmacokinetic properties: Hydrocortisone is absorbed through the skin particularly in denuded areas. Hydrocortisone is metabolised in the liver and most body tissues to hydrogenated and degraded forms such as tetrahydrocortisone and tetrahydrocortisol. These are excreted in the urine, mainly conjugated as glucuronides, together with a very small proportion of unchanged hydrocortisone.

Preclinical safety data: There are no preclinical data of relevance to the prescriber which are additional to that in other sections of the SPC.

Pharmaceutical particulars

List of excipients: White soft paraffin BP, Liquid paraffin BP.

Incompatibilities: None known.

Shelf life: 36 months.

Special precautions for storage: Store below 25°C.

Nature and contents of container: 15 gm, 30 gm and 50 gm collapsible aluminium tubes internally uncoated or coated with an epoxy resin based lacquer and closed with a wadless polypropylene cap.

Instructions for use/handling: No special instructions.

Marketing authorisation number PL 10949/0033

Date of first authorisation/renewal of authorisation 1 March 1993

Date of (partial) revision of text This is the first SPC. July 1997.

EFCORTELAN* OINTMENT 2.5%

Qualitative and quantitative composition Hydrocortisone BP 2.5% w/w.

Pharmaceutical form Ointment.

Clinical particulars

Therapeutic indications: Hydrocortisone has topical anti-inflammatory activities of value in the treatment of a wide variety of dermatological conditions, including the following: eczema, including atopic, infantile, discoid and stasis eczemas: prurigo nodularis, neurodermatoses, seborrhoeic dermatitis, intertrigo and contact sensitivity reactions.

Efcortelan preparations can also be used in the management of insect bites and otitis externa.

Efcortelan 0.5% preparations can be used as continuation therapy in mild cases of seborrhoeic or atopic eczema once the acute inflammatory phase has passed.

Posology and method of administration:

Adults, children and elderly: A small quantity should be applied to the affected area two or three times daily.

Efcortelan cream is often appropriate for moist or weeping surfaces, and Efcortelan Ointment for dry, lichenified or scaly lesions, but this is not invariably so. Efcortelan lotion is particularly suitable when a minimal application to a large area is required.

Route of administration: For topical application.

Contra-indications: Skin lesions, caused by infection with viruses (e.g. herpes simplex, chickenpox), fungi (e.g. candidiasis, tinea) or bacteria (e.g. impetigo). Hypersensitivity to the preparations.

Special warnings and precautions for use: In infants and children, long-term continuous topical therapy should be avoided where possible, as adrenal suppression can occur even without occlusion. In infants, the napkin may act as an occlusive dressing, and increase absorption. Treatment should therefore be limited if possible, to a maximum of seven days.

Appropriate antimicrobial therapy should be used whenever treating inflammatory lesions which have become infected. Any spread of infection requires withdrawal of topical corticosteroid therapy, and systemic administration of antimicrobial agents.

As with all corticosteroids, prolonged application to the face is undesirable.

Interaction with other medicaments and other forms of interaction: None known.

Pregnancy and lactation: There is inadequate evidence of safety in human pregnancy. Topical application of corticosteroids to pregnant animals can cause abnormalities of foetal development including cleft palate and intra-uterine growth retardation. There may, therefore, be a very small risk of such effects in the human foetus.

Effects on ability to drive and use machines: None known.

Undesirable effects: Efcortelan preparations are usually well tolerated, but if signs of hypersensitivity appear, application should stop immediately.

Exacerbation of symptoms may occur.

Local atrophic changes may occur where skin folds are involved, or in areas such as the nappy area in small children, where constant moist conditions favour the absorption of hydrocortisone. Sufficient systemic absorption may also occur in such sites to produce the features of hypercorticism and suppression of the HPA axis after prolonged treatment. This effect is more likely to occur in infants and children, and if occlusive dressings are used.

There are reports of pigmentation changes and hypertrichosis with topical steroids.

Overdose: Acute overdosage is very unlikely to occur, however, in the case of chronic overdosage or misuse the features of hypercorticism may appear and in this situation topical steroids should be discontinued.

Pharmacological properties

Pharmacodynamic properties: Hydrocortisone is the main glucocorticoid secreted by the adrenal cortex. It is used topically for its anti-inflammatory effects which suppress the clinical manifestations of the disease in a wide range of disorders where inflammation is a prominent feature.

Pharmacokinetic properties: Hydrocortisone is absorbed through the skin particularly in denuded areas. Hydrocortisone is metabolised in the liver and most body tissues to hydrogenated and degraded forms such as tetrahydrocortisone and tetrahydrocortisol. These are excreted in the urine, mainly conjugated as glucuronides, together with a very small proportion of unchanged hydrocortisone.

Preclinical safety data: There are no preclinical data of relevance to the prescriber which are additional to that in other sections of the SPC.

Pharmaceutical particulars

List of excipients: White soft paraffin BP, Liquid paraffin BP.

Incompatibilities: None known.

Shelf life: 36 months.

Special precautions for storage: Store below 25°C.

Nature and contents of container: 15 gm and 30 gm collapsible aluminium tubes internally uncoated or coated with an epoxy resin based lacquer and closed with a wadless polypropylene cap.

Instructions for use/handling: No special instructions.

Marketing authorisation number PL 10949/0034

Date of first authorisation/renewal of authorisation 1 March 1993

Date of (partial) revision of text This is the first SPC. July 1997.

EFCORTESOL* INJECTION

Qualitative and quantitative composition Hydrocortisone Sodium Phosphate BP 13.39% w/v.

Pharmaceutical form Sterile aqueous solution.

Clinical particulars

Therapeutic indications: This presentation permits rapid use in emergency situations involving the following conditions.

Status asthmaticus and acute allergic reactions, including anaphylactic reaction to drugs. Efcortesol supplements the action of adrenaline.

Severe shock arising from surgical or accidental trauma or overwhelming infection.

Acute adrenal insufficiency caused by abnormal stress in Addison's disease, hypopituitarism, following adrenalectomy, and when adrenocortical function has been suppressed by prolonged corticosteroid therapy.

Soft-tissue lesions such as tennis elbow, tenosynovitis, or bursitis.

Note: Efcortesol does not replace other forms of therapy for the treatment of shock and status asthmaticus.

Posology and method of administration: Undesirable effects may be minimised by using the lowest effective dose for the minimum period. Frequent patient review is required to appropriately titrate the dose against disease activity (see *Precautions*).

Systemic therapy in adults: 100 to 500 mg hydrocortisone (1 to 5 ml) administered by slow intravenous injection, taking at least half to one minute. This dose can be repeated three or four times in 24 hours, depending upon the condition being treated and the patient's response. Alternatively, Efcortesol Injection may be given as an intravenous infusion. A clinical effect is seen in two to four hours, and it persists for up to eight hours after intravenous injection. The same dose can be given by intramuscular injection, but the response is likely to be less rapid, especially in shock.

Systemic therapy in children: As a guide, infants up to 1 year may be given 25 mg hydrocortisone intravenously; children 1 to 5 years, 50 mg; 6 to 12 years, 100 mg (1 ml). This dose can be repeated three or four times in 24 hours depending upon the condition being treated and the patient's response.

Other uses: Local treatment of soft-tissue lesions – 100 to 200 mg. This daily dose may be repeated on two or three occasions depending upon the patient's response.

Efcortesol Injection is not recommended for intrathecal use.

Route(s) of administration: Intravenous or intramuscular injection, or injection into soft tissues.

Contra-indications: Systemic infections, unless specific anti-infective therapy is employed. Live virus immunisation. Hypersensitivity to any component.

Efcortesol Injection should not be injected directly into tendons.

Special warnings and precautions for use: In patients who have received more than physiological doses of systemic corticosteroids (approximately 30 mg hydrocortisone) for greater than 3 weeks, withdrawal should not be abrupt. How dose reduction should be carried out depends largely on whether the disease is likely to relapse as the dose of systemic corticosteroids is reduced. Clinical assessment of disease activity may be needed during withdrawal. If the disease is unlikely to relapse on withdrawal of systemic corticosteroids but there is uncertainty about HPA suppression, the dose of systemic corticosteroid may be reduced rapidly to physiological doses. Once a daily dose of 30 mg hydrocortisone is reached, dose reduction should be slower to allow the HPA-axis to recover.

Abrupt withdrawal of systemic corticosteroid treatment, which has continued up to 3 weeks is appropriate if it is considered that the disease is unlikely to relapse. Abrupt withdrawal of doses of up to 160 mg hydrocortisone for 3 weeks is unlikely to lead to clinically relevant HPA-axis suppression, in the majority of patients. In the following patient groups, gradual withdrawal of systemic corticosteroid therapy should be *considered* even after courses lasting 3 weeks or less:

- Patients who have had repeated courses of systemic corticosteroids, particularly if taken for greater than 3 weeks,
- When a short course has been prescribed within one year of cessation of long-term therapy (months or years),
- Patients who may have reasons for adrenocortical insufficiency other than exogenous corticosteroid therapy,
- Patients receiving doses of systemic corticosteroid greater than 160 mg hydrocortisone,
- Patients repeatedly taking doses in the evening.

Suppression of the HPA axis and other undesirable effects may be minimised by using the lowest effective dose for the minimum period (see *Posology and method of administration*). The pronounced hormonal effects associated with prolonged corticosteroid therapy will probably not be seen when this injection is used for short term adjunctive therapy in shock. Frequent patient review is required to appropriately titrate the dose against disease activity.

Patients should carry 'steroid treatment' cards which give clear guidance on the precautions to be taken to minimise risk and which provide details of prescriber, drug, dosage and the duration of treatment.

Suppression of the inflammatory response and immune function increases the susceptibility to infections and their severity. The clinical presentation may often be atypical and serious infections such as septicaemia and tuberculosis may be masked and may reach an advanced stage before being recognised.

Chickenpox is of particular concern since this normally minor illness may be fatal in immunosuppressed patients. Patients without a definite history of chickenpox should be advised to avoid close personal contact with chickenpox or herpes zoster and if exposed they should seek urgent medical attention. If the patient is a child, parents must be given the above advice. Passive immunisation with varicella zoster immunoglobulin (VZIG) is needed by exposed non-immune patients who are receiving systemic corticosteroids or who have used them within the previous 3 months; this should be given within 10 days of exposure to chickenpox. If a diagnosis of chickenpox is confirmed, the illness warrants specialist care and urgent treatment. Corticosteroids should not be stopped and the dose may need to be increased.

Live vaccines should not be given to individuals with impaired immune responsiveness. The antibody response to other vaccines may be diminished.

Adrenal cortical atrophy develops during prolonged therapy and may persist for years after stopping treatment. Withdrawal of corticosteroids after prolonged therapy must therefore always be gradual to avoid acute adrenal insufficiency, being tapered off over weeks or months according to the dose and duration of treatment. During prolonged therapy any intercurrent illness, trauma or surgical procedure will require a temporary increase in dosage; if corticosteroids have been stopped following prolonged therapy they may need to be temporarily reintroduced.

Because of the possibility of fluid retention, care must be taken when corticosteroids are administered to patients with renal insufficiency or congestive heart failure.

Corticosteroids may worsen diabetes mellitus, osteoporosis, hypertension, glaucoma and epilepsy and therefore patients with these conditions or a family history should be monitored frequently.

Care is required and frequent patient monitoring necessary where there is a history of severe affective disorders (especially a previous history of steroid psychosis), previous steroid myopathy, peptic ulceration or patients with a history of tuberculosis.

In patients with liver failure, blood levels of corticosteroid may be increased, as with other drugs which are metabolised in the liver and therefore patients should be monitored frequently. Care and monitoring is also required in patients with renal insufficiency.

When treatment is to be discontinued, the dose should be reduced gradually over a period of several weeks or months depending on the dosage and duration of the therapy.

Interaction with other medicaments and other forms of interaction

Drug interactions: Rifampicin, rifabutin, carbamazepine, phenobarbitone, phenytoin, primidone, ephedrine and aminoglutethimide enhance the metabolism of corticosteroids and its therapeutic effects may be reduced.

The desired effects of hypoglycaemic agents (including insulin), anti-hypertensives and diuretics are antagonised by corticosteroids, and the hypokalaemic effects of acetazolamide, loop diuretics, thiazide diuretics and carbenoxolone are enhanced. The efficacy of coumarin anticoagulants may be enhanced by concurrent corticosteroid therapy and close monitoring of the INR or prothrombin time is required to avoid spontaneous bleeding.

The renal clearance of salicylates is increased by corticosteroids and steroid withdrawal may result in salicylate intoxication.

Steroids may reduce the effects of anticholinesterases in myasthenia gravis and cholecystographic X-ray media.

Pregnancy and lactation:

Pregnancy: The ability of corticosteroids to cross placenta varies between individual drugs, however, hydrocortisone readily crosses the placenta. Administration of corticosteroids to pregnant animals can cause abnormalities of foetal development including cleft palate, intra-uterine growth retardation and effects on brain growth and development. There is no evidence that corticosteroids result in an increased incidence of congenital abnormalities, such as cleft palate/lip in man. However, when administered for prolonged periods or repeatedly during pregnancy, corticosteroids may increase the risk of intra-uterine growth retardation. Hypoadrenalism may, in theory, occur in the neonate following prenatal exposure to corticosteroids but usually resolves spontaneously following birth and is rarely clinically important. As with all drugs, corticosteroids should only be prescribed when the benefits to the mother and child outweigh the risks. When corticosteroids are essential however, patients with normal pregnancies may be treated as though they were in the non-gravid state.

Patients with pre-eclampsia or fluid retention require close monitoring.

Depression of hormone levels has been described in pregnancy but the significance of this finding is not clear.

Lactation: Corticosteroids are excreted in breast milk, although no data are available for hydrocortisone. Doses of up to 160 mg daily of hydrocortisone are unlikely to cause systemic effects in the infant. Infants of mothers taking higher doses than this may have a degree of adrenal suppression but the benefits of breast feeding are likely to outweigh any theoretical risk.

Effect on ability to drive and use machines: None stated.

Undesirable effects:

Side-effects: Paraesthesia may occur following intravenous administration and is probably related to the rate of injection. It is often localised to the genital area but in some cases may radiate over the entire body. The unpleasant and sometimes painful sensation usually passes off within a few minutes and no sequelae have been reported. The effect seems to be related to the sodium phosphate salt of hydrocortisone.

The incidence of predictable undesirable effects, including hypothalamic-pituitary-adrenal suppression correlates with the relative potency of the drug, dosage, timing of administration and the duration of treatment (see *Special warnings and precautions for use*).

Endocrine/metabolic: Suppression of the hypothalamic-pituitary-adrenal axis, growth suppression in infancy, childhood and adolescence, menstrual irregularity and amenorrhoea, cushingoid faces, hirsutism, weight gain, impaired carbohydrate tolerance with increased requirement for anti-diabetic therapy. Negative protein and calcium balance. Increased appetite.

Anti-inflammatory and immunosuppressive effects: Increased susceptibility and severity of infections with suppression of clinical symptoms and signs, opportunistic infections, recurrence of dormant tuberculosis (see *Special warnings and precautions for use*).

Musculoskeletal: Osteoporosis, vertebral and long bone fractures, avascular osteonecrosis, tendon rupture. Proximal myopathy.

Fluid and electrolyte disturbance: Sodium and water retention, hypertension, potassium loss, hypokalaemic alkalosis.

Neuropsychiatric: Euphoria, psychological dependence, depression, insomnia and aggravation of schizophrenia, increased intra-cranial pressure with papilloedema in children (pseudotumour cerebri), usually after treatment withdrawal. Aggravation of epilepsy.

Ophthalmic: Increased intra-ocular pressure, glaucoma, papilloedema, posterior subcapsular cataracts, corneal or scleral thinning, exacerbation of ophthalmic viral or fungal diseases.

Gastrointestinal: Dyspepsia, peptic ulceration with perforation and haemorrhage, acute pancreatitis, candidiasis.

Dermatological: Impaired healing, skin atrophy, bruising, telangiectasia, striae, acne.

General: Hypersensitivity including anaphylaxis, has been reported. Leucocytosis. Thromboembolism.

Withdrawal symptoms and signs: Too rapid a reduction of corticosteroid dosage following prolonged treatment can lead to acute adrenal insufficiency, hypotension and death (see *Special warnings and precautions for use*).

A 'withdrawal syndrome' may also occur including, fever, myalgia, arthralgia, rhinitis, conjunctivitis, painful itchy skin nodules and loss of weight.

Use in children: Corticosteroids cause dose-related growth retardation in infancy, childhood and adolescence, which may be irreversible.

Use in the elderly: The common adverse effects of systemic corticosteroids may be associated with more serious consequences in old age, especially osteoporosis, hypertension, hypokalaemia, diabetes, susceptibility to infections and thinning of the skin. Close clinical supervision is required to avoid life-threatening reactions.

Overdose: None stated.

Pharmacological properties

Pharmacodynamic properties: Hydrocortisone is a glucocorticoid with anti-inflammatory properties.

Pharmacokinetic properties: Hydrocortisone is readily absorbed from the gastrointestinal tract and peak blood concentrations are attained in about an hour. It is more than 90% bound to plasma proteins.

Hydrocortisone is metabolised in the liver and most body tissues to hydrogenated and degraded forms such as tetrahydrocortisone and tetrahydrocortisol.

These are then excreted in the urine, mainly conjugated as glucuronides, together with a very small proportion of unchanged hydrocortisone.

Preclinical safety data: There are no preclinical data of relevance to the prescriber which are additional to that in other sections of the SPC.

Pharmaceutical particulars

List of excipients: Disodium edetate BP, Disodium hydrogen phosphate, anhydrous HSE, Sodium acid phosphate BP, Sodium formaldehyde bisulphite monohydrate HSE, Phosphoric acid (10% solution) BP, Water for injection BP.

Incompatibilities: None known.

Shelf life: 24 months.

Special precautions for storage: Store below 25°C. Protect from light.

Nature and contents of container: 1 ml and 5 ml neutral glass ampoules.

Instructions for use/handling: No special instructions.

Marketing authorisation number PL 10949/0098

Date of first authorisation/renewal of authorisation 11/12/97

Date of (partial) revision of text May 1998

EPIVIR* ORAL SOLUTION 

Qualitative and quantitative composition Epivir contains 10 mg/ml lamivudine in a solution containing 20% (w/v) sucrose, and preservatives (methyl parahydroxybenzoate and propyl parahydroxybenzoate).

Pharmaceutical form Oral solution. It is a clear, colourless to pale yellow solution.

Clinical particulars

Therapeutic indications: Epivir is indicated as part of antiretroviral combination therapy for the treatment of HIV infected adults and children.

Posology and method of administration:

Adults and adolescents over the age of 12 years: The recommended dose of Epivir is 150 mg (15 ml) twice daily.

Children:

Less than three months of age: The limited data available are insufficient to propose specific dosage recommendations (see *Pharmacokinetic properties*).

Three months to 12 years of age: The recommended dose is 4 mg/kg twice daily up to a maximum of 300 mg daily.

Epivir is also available as a tablet formulation.

Epivir may be administered with or without food.

The therapy should be initiated by a physician experienced in the management of HIV infection.

Renal impairment: Lamivudine levels are increased in patients with moderate–severe renal impairment due to decreased clearance. The dose should therefore be adjusted (see tables).

Dosing Recommendations – Adults and adolescents over 12 years:

Renal function (Clcr, ml/min)	*First dose*	*Maintenance dose*
Clcr≥50	150 mg (15 ml)	150 mg (15 ml) Twice daily
50>Clcr≥30	150 mg (15 ml)	150 mg (15 ml) Once daily
30>Clcr≥15	150 mg (15 ml)	100 mg (10 ml) Once daily
15>Clcr≥5	150 mg (15 ml)	50 mg (5 ml) Once daily
5>Clcr	50 mg (5 ml)	25 mg (2.5 ml) Once daily

There are no data available on the use of lamivudine in children with renal impairment. Based on the assumption that creatinine clearance and lamivudine clearance are correlated similarly in children as in adults it is recommended that the dosage in children with renal impairment may be reduced according to their creatinine clearance by the same proportion as in adults.

Dosing Recommendations – Children from 3 months to 12 years:

Renal function (Clcr, ml/min)	*First dose*	*Maintenance dose*
Clcr≥50	4 mg/kg	4 mg/kg twice daily
50>Clcr≥30	4 mg/kg	4 mg/kg once daily
30>Clcr≥15	4 mg/kg	2.6 mg/kg once daily
15>Clcr≥5	4 mg/kg	1.3 mg/kg once daily
5>Clcr	1.3 mg/kg	0.7 mg/kg once daily

Hepatic impairment: Data obtained in patients with moderate to severe hepatic impairment shows that lamivudine pharmacokinetics are not significantly affected by hepatic dysfunction. Based on these data, no dose adjustment is necessary in patients with moderate or severe hepatic impairment unless accompanied by renal impairment.

Contra-indications: The use of Epivir is contra-indicated in patients with known hypersensitivity to lamivudine or to any ingredient of the preparation.

Special warnings and special precautions for use:
Special warnings: Epivir is not recommended for use as monotherapy.

Cases of pancreatitis have occurred rarely. However it is not clear whether these cases were due to drug treatment or to the underlying HIV disease. Treatment with Epivir should be stopped immediately if clinical signs, symptoms or laboratory abnormalities suggestive of pancreatitis occur.

Occurrences of lactic acidosis (in the absence of hypoxemia), usually associated with severe hepatomegaly and hepatic steatosis have been reported with the use of nucleoside analogues. Treatment should be discontinued in the setting of rapidly elevating aminotransferase levels, progressive hepatomegaly or metabolic/lactic acidosis of unknown etiology. Caution should be exercised when administering nucleoside analogues to any patient (particularly obese women) with hepatomegaly, hepatitis or other known risk factors for liver disease. These patients should be followed closely.

Administration of Epivir is not recommended during the first 3 months of pregnancy (see *Pregnancy and lactation*).

Patients receiving Epivir or any other antiretroviral therapy may continue to develop opportunistic infections and other complications of HIV infection, and therefore should remain under close clinical observation by physicians experienced in the treatment of patients with associated HIV diseases.

Patients should be advised that current antiretroviral therapy, including Epivir, has not been proven to prevent the risk of transmission of HIV to others through sexual contact or blood contamination. Appropriate precautions should continue to be employed.

Special precautions for use: In patients with moderate–severe renal impairment, the terminal plasma half-life of lamivudine is increased due to decreased clearance, therefore the dose should be adjusted (see dosage in renal impairment, *Posology and method of administration*).

Patients co-infected with Hepatitis B virus: Clinical trial and marketed use of lamivudine, have shown that some patients with chronic hepatitis B virus (HBV) disease may experience clinical or laboratory evidence of recurrent hepatitis upon discontinuation of lamivudine, which may have more severe consequences in patients with decompensated liver disease. If Epivir is discontinued in patients co-infected with Hepatitis B virus, periodic monitoring of both liver function tests and markers of HBV replication should be considered.

Diabetic patients should be advised that each dose (150 mg = 15 ml) contains 3 g of sucrose.

Interaction with other medicaments and other forms of interaction: The likelihood of metabolic interactions is low due to limited metabolism and plasma protein binding and almost complete renal clearance.

A modest increase in C_{max} (28%) was observed for zidovudine when administered with lamivudine, however overall exposure (AUC) is not significantly altered. Zidovudine has no effect on the pharmacokinetics of lamivudine (see *Pharmacokinetic properties*).

The possibility of interactions with other drugs administered concurrently should be considered, particularly when the main route of elimination is active renal secretion via the organic cationic transport system e.g. trimethoprim. Other drugs (e.g. ranitidine, cimetidine) are eliminated only in part by this mechanism and were shown not to interact with lamivudine. The nucleoside analogues (e.g. didanosine and zalcitabine) like zidovudine, are not eliminated by this mechanism and are unlikely to interact with lamivudine.

Administration of trimethoprim as trimethoprim/sulphamethoxazole 160 mg/800 mg results in a 40% increase in lamivudine exposure, because of the trimethoprim component; the sulphamethoxazole component did not interact. However, unless the patient has renal impairment, no dosage adjustment of lamivudine is necessary (see *Posology and method of administration*). Lamivudine has no effect on the pharmacokinetics of trimethoprim or sulphamethoxazole. When concomitant administration is warranted, patients should be monitored clinically.

Co-administration of Epivir with high doses of co-trimoxazole for the treatment of *Pneumocystis carinii* pneumonia (PCP) and toxoplasmosis should be avoided.

Lamivudine metabolism does not involve CYP3A, making interactions with drugs metabolised by this system (e.g. protease inhibitors) unlikely.

Co-administration of Epivir with intravenous ganciclovir or foscarnet is not recommended until further information is available.

Use during pregnancy and lactation:
Pregnancy: The safety of lamivudine in human pregnancy has not been established. Reproductive studies in animals have not shown evidence of teratogenicity, and showed no effect on male or female fertility. Lamivudine induces early embryolethality when administered to pregnant rabbits at exposure levels comparable to those achieved in man. Consistent with passive transmission of the drug across the placenta, lamivudine concentrations in infant serum at birth were similar to those in maternal and cord serum at delivery.

Although animal reproductive studies are not always predictive of the human response, administration during the first three months of pregnancy is not recommended (see *Special warnings and special precautions for use*).

Lactation: Following oral administration lamivudine was excreted in breast milk at similar concentrations to those found in serum. Since lamivudine and the virus pass into breast milk, it is recommended that mothers taking Epivir do not breast feed their infants. Some health experts recommend that HIV infected women do not breast feed their infants under any circumstances in order to avoid transmission of HIV.

Effects on ability to drive and use machines: There have been no studies to investigate the effect of lamivudine on driving performance or the ability to operate machinery. Further, a detrimental effect on such activities cannot be predicted from the pharmacology of the drug. Nevertheless, the clinical status of the patient and the adverse event profile of Epivir should be borne in mind when considering the patient's ability to drive or operate machinery.

Undesirable effects: Adverse events have been reported during therapy for HIV disease with Epivir alone and in combination with zidovudine. With many it is unclear whether they are drug related or are as a result of the underlying disease process.

Adverse events which have been commonly reported are headache, fever, rash, malaise, fatigue, alopecia, nausea, diarrhoea, vomiting, abdominal pain or cramps, insomnia, cough, nasal symptoms and musculoskeletal pain.

Cases of pancreatitis and peripheral neuropathy (or paraesthesia) have been recorded, although no relationship to the dose of Epivir has been noted.

Neutropenia and anaemia (both occasionally severe) have occurred in combination with zidovudine. Thrombocytopenia, transient rises in liver enzymes (AST, ALT) and rises in serum amylase have been reported.

Cases of lactic acidosis, usually associated with severe hepatomegaly and hepatic steatosis, have been reported with the use of nucleoside analogues.

Overdose: Administration of lamivudine at very high dose levels in acute animal studies did not result in any organ toxicity. Limited data are available on the consequences of ingestion of acute overdoses in humans. No fatalities occurred, and the patients recovered. No specific signs or symptoms have been identified following such overdose.

If overdosage occurs the patient should be monitored, and standard supportive treatment applied as required. Since lamivudine is dialysable, continuous haemodialysis could be used in the treatment of overdosage, although this has not been studied.

Pharmacological properties
Pharmacodynamic properties: Pharmacotherapeutic group—nucleoside analogue, ATC Code: J05A B10.

Lamivudine is a nucleoside analogue. Lamivudine is metabolised intracellularly to lamivudine 5'-triphosphate, its main mode of action is as a chain terminator of HIV reverse transcription. The triphosphate has selective inhibitory activity against HIV-1 and HIV-2 replication *in vitro*, it is also active against zidovudine-resistant clinical isolates of HIV.

The relationships between *in vitro* susceptibility of HIV to lamivudine and the clinical response to therapy remain under investigation. *In vitro* sensitivity testing has not been standardised and results may vary according to methodological factors. In clinical trials, lamivudine in combination with zidovudine has been shown to reduce HIV-1 viral load and increases CD4 cell count. Clinical end-point data indicate that lamivudine in combination with zidovudine alone or in combination with zidovudine containing treatment regimens results in a significant reduction in the risk of disease progression and mortality.

Reduced *in vitro* sensitivity to lamivudine has been reported for HIV isolates from patients who have received Epivir therapy.

Lamivudine has been shown to be highly synergistic with zidovudine, inhibiting the replication of HIV in cell culture.

In vitro studies indicate that zidovudine-resistant virus isolates can become zidovudine sensitive when they simultaneously acquire resistance to lamivudine. Furthermore, *in vivo*, there is evidence showing that lamivudine plus zidovudine delays the emergence of zidovudine-resistant isolates in individuals with no prior antiretroviral therapy.

In vitro, lamivudine demonstrates low cytotoxicity to peripheral blood lymphocytes, to established lymphocyte and monocyte-macrophage cell lines and to a variety of bone marrow progenitor cells *in vitro*. Lamivudine therefore has, *in vitro*, a high therapeutic index.

Pharmacokinetic properties:
Absorption: Lamivudine is well absorbed from the gastrointestinal tract, and the bioavailability of oral lamivudine in adults is normally between 80 and 85%. Following oral administration, the mean time (t_{max}) to maximal serum concentrations (C_{max}) is about an hour. At therapeutic dose levels i.e. 4 mg/kg/day (as two 12-hourly doses), C_{max} is in the order of 1.5–1.9 mcg/ml.

Co-administration of lamivudine with food results in a delay of t_{max} and a lower C_{max} (decreased by 47%). However, the extent (based on the AUC) of lamivudine absorbed is not influenced.

Co-administration of zidovudine results in a 13% increase in zidovudine exposure and a 28% increase in peak plasma levels. This is not considered to be of significance to patient safety and therefore no dosage adjustments are necessary.

Distribution: From intravenous studies, the mean volume of distribution is 1.3 L/kg. The observed half-life of elimination is 5 to 7 hours. The mean systemic clearance of lamivudine is approximately 0.32 L/h/kg, with predominantly renal clearance (>70%) via the organic cationic transport system.

Lamivudine exhibits linear pharmacokinetics over the therapeutic dose range and displays limited binding to the major plasma protein albumin (<16%–36% to serum albumin in *in vitro* studies).

Limited data shows lamivudine penetrates the central nervous system and reaches the cerebrospinal fluid (CSF). The mean ratio CSF/serum lamivudine concentration 2–4 hours after oral administration was approximately 0.12. The true extent of penetration or relationship with any clinical efficacy is unknown.

Metabolism: Lamivudine is predominantly cleared by renal excretion of unchanged drug. The likelihood of metabolic drug interactions with lamivudine is low due to the small extent of hepatic metabolism (5–10%) and low plasma protein binding.

Elimination: Studies in patients with renal impairment show lamivudine elimination is affected by renal dysfunction. A recommended dosage regimen for patients with creatinine clearance below 50 ml/min is shown in the dosage section (see *Posology and method of administration*).

An interaction with trimethoprim, a constituent of co-trimoxazole, causes a 40% increase in lamivudine exposure at therapeutic doses. This does not require dose adjustment unless the patient also has renal impairment (see *Interaction with other medicaments and other forms of interaction*, and dosage adjustments in renal impairment in *Posology and method of administration*). Administration of co-trimoxazole with Epivir in patients with renal impairment should be carefully assessed.

Pharmacokinetics in children: In general, lamivudine pharmacokinetics in paediatric patients is similar to adults. However, absolute bioavailability (approximately 55–65%) was reduced in paediatric patients below 12 years of age. In addition, systemic clearance values were greater in younger paediatric patients and decreased with age approaching adult values around 12 years of age. Due to these differences, the recommended dose for children from three months to 12 years is 8 mg/kg/day, which will achieve similar adult and paediatric exposure (average AUC approximately 5000 ng.h/ml).

There are limited pharmacokinetic data for patients less than three months of age. In neonates one week of age, lamivudine oral clearance was reduced when compared to paediatric patients and is likely to be due to immature renal function and variable absorption. Therefore to achieve similar adult and paediatric exposure, the recommended dose for neonates is 4 mg/kg/day.

Pharmacokinetics in pregnancy: Following oral administration, lamivudine pharmacokinetics in late-pregnancy were similar to non-pregnant animals.

Preclinical safety data: Administration of lamivudine in animal toxicity studies at high doses was not associated with any major organ toxicity. At the highest dosage levels, minor effects on indicators of liver and kidney function were seen together with occasional reductions in liver weight. The clinically relevant effects noted were a reduction in red blood cell count and neutropenia.

Lamivudine was not mutagenic in bacterial tests but, like many nucleoside analogues, showed activity in an *in vitro* cytogenetic assay and the mouse lymphoma assay. Lamivudine was not genotoxic *in vivo* at doses that gave plasma concentrations around 40–50 times higher than the anticipated clinical plasma levels. As the *in vitro* mutagenic activity of lamivudine could not be confirmed in *in vivo* tests, it is concluded that lamivudine should not represent a genotoxic hazard to patients undergoing treatment.

The results of long-term carcinogenicity studies in rats and mice, lamivudine did not show any carcinogenic potential relevant for humans.

Pharmaceutical particulars

List of excipients: Sucrose PhEur (20% w/v); Methyl Parahydroxybenzoate PhEur (E218); Propyl Parahydroxybenzoate PhEur (E216); Citric Acid Anhydrous PhEur; Propylene Glycol PhEur; Sodium Citrate PhEur; Artificial Strawberry Flavour; Artificial Banana Flavour; Water Purified PhEur.

Incompatibilities: None reported.

Shelf life: 24 months.

Special precautions for storage: Store below 25°C.

Nature and contents of container: Cartons containing 240 ml lamivudine 10 mg/ml in a white high density polyethylene (HDPE) bottle, with a child resistant closure. A 10 ml polypropylene oral dosing syringe and a polyethylene adaptor are also included in the pack.

Instructions for use/handling: The oral dosing syringe is provided for accurate measurement of the prescribed dose of Oral Solution. Instructions for use are included in the pack.

Discard Oral Solution one month after first opening.

Marketing authorisation number EU/1/96/015/002

Date of approval/revision of SPC July 1998

Legal category POM.

EPIVIR TABLETS ▼

Qualitative and quantitative composition Epivir contains 150 mg lamivudine.

Pharmaceutical form Coated tablets. The tablets are white film coated, diamond shaped tablets engraved 'GX CJ7' on one face.

Clinical particulars

Therapeutic indications: Epivir is indicated as part of antiretroviral combination therapy for the treatment of HIV infected adults and children.

Posology and method of administration:

Adults and adolescents over the age of 12 years: The recommended dose of Epivir is 150 mg (one tablet) twice daily.

Children:

Less than three months of age: The limited data available are insufficient to propose specific dosage recommendations (see *Pharmacokinetic properties*).

Three months to 12 years of age: The recommended dose is 4 mg/kg twice daily up to a maximum of 300 mg daily.

Epivir is also available as an oral solution formulation.

Epivir may be administered with or without food.

The therapy should be initiated by a physician experienced in the management of HIV infection.

Renal impairment: Lamivudine concentrations are increased in patients with moderate–severe renal impairment due to decreased clearance. The dose should therefore be adjusted, using the oral solution presentation of Epivir for patients whose creatinine clearance falls below 30 ml/min (see tables).

Dosing Recommendations – Adults and adolescents over 12 years:

Renal function (Clcr, ml/min)	*First dose*	*Maintenance dose*
Clcr≥50	150 mg	150 mg Twice daily
50>Clcr≥30	150 mg	150 mg Once daily
Clcr<30	As doses below 150 mg are needed the use of the oral solution is recommended	

There are no data available on the use of lamivudine in children with renal impairment. Based on the assumption that creatinine clearance and lamivudine clearance are correlated similarly in children as in adults it is recommended that the dosage in children with renal impairment may be reduced according to their creatinine clearance by the same proportion as in adults.

Dosing Recommendations – Children from 3 months to 12 years:

Renal function (Clcr, ml/min)	*First dose*	*Maintenance dose*
Clcr≥50	4 mg/kg	4 mg/kg twice daily
50>Clcr≥30	4 mg/kg	4 mg/kg once daily
30>Clcr≥15	4 mg/kg	2.6 mg/kg once daily
15>Clcr≥5	4 mg/kg	1.3 mg/kg once daily
5>Clcr	1.3 mg/kg	0.7 mg/kg once daily

Hepatic impairment: Data obtained in patients with moderate to severe hepatic impairment shows that lamivudine pharmacokinetics are not significantly affected by hepatic dysfunction. Based on these data, no dose adjustment is necessary in patients with moderate or severe hepatic impairment unless accompanied by renal impairment.

Contra-indications: The use of Epivir is contra-indicated in patients with known hypersensitivity to lamivudine or to any ingredient of the preparation.

Special warnings and special precautions for use:

Special warnings: Epivir is not recommended for use as monotherapy.

Cases of pancreatitis have occurred rarely. However it is not clear whether these cases were due to drug treatment or to the underlying HIV disease. Treatment with Epivir should be stopped immediately if clinical signs, symptoms or laboratory abnormalities suggestive of pancreatitis occur.

Occurrences of lactic acidosis (in the absence of hypoxemia), usually associated with severe hepatomegaly and hepatic steatosis have been reported with the use of nucleoside analogues. Treatment should be discontinued in the setting of rapidly elevating aminotransferase levels, progressive hepatomegaly or metabolic/lactic acidosis of unknown etiology. Caution should be exercised when administering nucleoside analogues to any patient (particularly obese women) with hepatomegaly, hepatitis or other known risk factors for liver disease. These patients should be followed closely.

Administration of Epivir is not recommended during the first 3 months of pregnancy (see *Pregnancy and lactation*).

Patients receiving Epivir or any other antiretroviral therapy may continue to develop opportunistic infections and other complications of HIV infection, and therefore should remain under close clinical observation by physicians experienced in the treatment of patients with associated HIV diseases.

Patients should be advised that current antiretroviral therapy, including Epivir, has not been proven to prevent the risk of transmission of HIV to others through sexual conduct or blood contamination. Appropriate precautions should continue to be employed.

Special precautions for use: In patients with moderate–severe renal impairment, the terminal plasma half-life of lamivudine is increased due to decreased clearance, therefore the dose should be adjusted. (See dosage in renal impairment, in *Posology and method of administration* section).

Patients co-infected with Hepatitis B virus: Clinical trial and marketed use of lamivudine, have shown that some patients with chronic hepatitis B virus (HBV) disease may experience clinical or laboratory evidence of recurrent hepatitis upon discontinuation of lamivudine, which may have more severe consequences in patients with decompensated liver disease. If Epivir is discontinued in patients co-infected with Hepatitis B virus, periodic monitoring of both liver function tests and markers of HBV replication should be considered.

Interaction with other medicaments and other forms of interaction: The likelihood of metabolic interactions is low due to limited metabolism and plasma protein binding and almost complete renal clearance.

A modest increase in C_{max} (28%) was observed for zidovudine when administered with lamivudine, however overall exposure (AUC) is not significantly altered. Zidovudine has no effect on the pharmacokinetics of lamivudine (see *Pharmacokinetic properties* section).

The possibility of interactions with other drugs administered concurrently should be considered, particularly when the main route of elimination is active renal secretion via the organic cationic transport system e.g. trimethoprim. Other drugs (e.g. ranitidine, cimetidine) are eliminated only in part by this mechanism and were shown not to interact with lamivudine. The nucleoside analogues (e.g. didanosine and zalcitabine) like zidovudine, are not eliminated by this mechanism and are unlikely to interact with lamivudine.

Administration of trimethoprim/sulphamethoxazole 160 mg/800 mg results in a 40% increase in lamivudine exposure, because of the trimethoprim component; the sulphamethoxazole component did not interact. However, unless the patient has renal impairment, no dosage adjustment of lamivudine is necessary (see *Posology and method of administration*). Lamivudine has no effect on the pharmacokinetics of trimethoprim or sulphamethoxazole. When concomitant administration is warranted, patients should be monitored clinically. Co-administration of Epivir with high doses of co-trimoxazole for the treatment of *Pneumocystis carinii* pneumonia (PCP) and toxoplasmosis should be avoided.

Lamivudine metabolism does not involve CYP3A, making interactions with drugs metabolised by this system (e.g. protease inhibitors) unlikely.

Co-administration of Epivir with intravenous ganciclovir or foscarnet is not recommended until further information is available.

Use during pregnancy and lactation:

Pregnancy: The safety of lamivudine in human pregnancy has not been established. Reproductive studies in animals have not shown evidence of teratogenicity, and showed no effect on male or female fertility. Lamivudine induces early embryolethality when administered to pregnant rabbits at exposure levels comparable to those achieved in man. Consistent with passive transmission of the drug across the placenta, lamivudine concentrations in infant serum at birth were similar to those in maternal and cord serum at delivery.

Although animal reproductive studies are not always predictive of the human response, administration during the first three months of pregnancy is not recommended (see *Special warnings and special precautions for use*).

Lactation: Following oral administration lamivudine was excreted in breast milk at similar concentrations to those found in serum. Since lamivudine and the virus pass into breast milk, it is recommended that mothers taking Epivir do not breast feed their infants. Some health experts recommend that HIV infected women do not breast feed their infants under any circumstances in order to avoid transmission of HIV.

Effects on ability to drive and use machines: There have been no studies to investigate the effect of lamivudine on driving performance or the ability to operate machinery. Further, a detrimental effect on such activities cannot be predicted from the pharmacology of the drug. Nevertheless, the clinical status of the patient and the adverse event profile of Epivir should be borne in mind when considering the patient's ability to drive or operate machinery.

Undesirable effects: Adverse events have been reported during therapy for HIV disease with Epivir alone and in combination with zidovudine. With many it is unclear whether they are drug related or are as a result of the underlying disease process.

Adverse events which have been commonly reported are headache, fever, rash, malaise, fatigue, alopecia, nausea, diarrhoea, vomiting, abdominal pain or cramps, insomnia, cough, nasal symptoms and musculoskeletal pain.

Cases of pancreatitis and peripheral neuropathy (or paraesthesia) have been recorded, although no relationship to the dose of Epivir has been noted.

Neutropenia and anaemia (both occasionally severe) have occurred in combination with zidovudine. Thrombocytopenia, transient rises in liver enzymes (AST, ALT) and rises in serum amylase have been reported. Cases of lactic acidosis, usually associated with severe hepatomegaly and hepatic steatosis, have been reported with the use of nucleoside analogues.

Overdose: Administration of lamivudine at very high dose levels in acute animal studies did not result in any organ toxicity. Limited data are available on the consequences of ingestion of acute overdoses in humans. No fatalities occurred, and the patients recovered. No specific signs or symptoms have been identified following such overdose.

If overdosage occurs the patient should be monitored, and standard supportive treatment applied as required. Since lamivudine is dialysable, continuous haemodialysis could be used in the treatment of overdosage, although this has not been studied.

Pharmacological properties

Pharmacodynamic properties: Pharmacotherapeutic group—nucleoside analogue, ATC Code: J05A B10.

Lamivudine is a nucleoside analogue. Lamivudine is metabolised intracellularly to lamivudine 5'-triphosphate, its main mode of action is as a chain terminator of HIV reverse transcription. The triphosphate has selective inhibitory activity against HIV-1 and HIV-2 replication *in vitro*, it is also active against zidovudine-resistant clinical isolates of HIV.

The relationships between *in vitro* susceptibility of HIV to lamivudine and the clinical response to therapy remain under investigation. *In vitro* sensitivity testing has not been standardised and results may vary according to methodological factors. In clinical trials, lamivudine in combination with zidovudine has been shown to reduce the HIV-1 viral load and increases CD4 cell count. Clinical end-point data indicate that lamivudine in combination with zidovudine, alone or in combination with zidovudine treatment regimens results in a significant reduction in the risk of disease progression and mortality.

Reduced *in vitro* sensitivity to lamivudine has been reported for HIV isolates from patients who have received Epivir therapy.

Lamivudine has been shown to be highly synergistic with zidovudine, inhibiting the replication of HIV in cell culture.

In vitro studies indicate that zidovudine-resistant virus isolates can become zidovudine sensitive when they simultaneously acquire resistance to lamivudine. Furthermore, *in vivo*, there is evidence showing that lamivudine plus zidovudine delays the emergence of zidovudine-resistant isolates in individuals with no prior antiretroviral therapy.

In vitro, lamivudine demonstrates low cytotoxicity to peripheral blood lymphocytes, to established lymphocyte and monocyte-macrophage cell lines and to a variety of bone marrow progenitor cells *in vitro*. Lamivudine therefore has, *in vitro*, a high therapeutic index.

Pharmacokinetic properties:

Absorption: Lamivudine is well absorbed from the gastrointestinal tract, and the bioavailability of oral lamivudine in adults is normally between 80 and 85%. Following oral administration, the mean time (t_{max}) to maximal serum concentrations (C_{max}) is about an hour. At therapeutic dose levels i.e. 4 mg/kg/day (as two 12-hourly doses), C_{max} is in the order of 1.5–1.9 mcg/ml.

Co-administration of lamivudine with food results in a delay of t_{max} and a lower C_{max} (decreased by 47%). However, the extent (based on AUC) of lamivudine absorbed is not influenced.

Co-administration of zidovudine results in a 13% increase in zidovudine exposure and a 28% increase in peak plasma levels. This is not considered to be of significance to patient safety and therefore no dosage adjustments are necessary.

Distribution: From intravenous studies, the mean volume of distribution is 1.3 L/kg. The observed half-life of elimination is 5 to 7 hours. The mean systemic clearance of lamivudine is approximately 0.32 L/h/kg, with predominantly renal clearance (>70%) via the organic cationic transport system.

Lamivudine exhibits linear pharmacokinetics over the therapeutic dose range and displays limited binding to the major plasma protein albumin (<16%–36% to serum albumin in *in vitro* studies).

Limited data shows lamivudine penetrates the central nervous system and reaches the cerebro-spinal fluid (CSF). The mean ratio CSF/serum lamivudine concentration 2–4 hours after oral administration was approximately 0.12. The true extent of penetration or relationship with any clinical efficacy is unknown.

Metabolism: Lamivudine is predominantly cleared by renal excretion of unchanged drug. The likelihood of metabolic drug interactions with lamivudine is low due to the small extent of hepatic metabolism (5–10%) and low plasma protein binding.

Elimination: Studies in patients with renal impairment show lamivudine elimination is affected by renal dysfunction. A recommended dosage regimen for patients with creatinine clearance below 50 ml/min is shown in the dosage section (see *Posology and method of administration*).

An interaction with trimethoprim, a constituent of co-trimoxazole, causes a 40% increase in lamivudine exposure at therapeutic doses. This does not require dose adjustment unless the patient also has renal impairment (see *Interaction with other medicaments and other forms of interaction*, and dosage adjustments in renal impairment in *Posology and method of administration* section). Administration of co-trimoxazole with Epivir in patients with renal impairment should be carefully assessed.

Pharmacokinetics in children: In general, lamivudine pharmacokinetics in paediatric patients is similar to adults. However, absolute bioavailability (approximately 55–65%) was reduced in paediatric patients below 12 years of age. In addition, systemic clearance values were greater in younger paediatric patients and decreased with age approaching adult values around 12 years of age. Due to these differences, the recommended dose for children from three months to 12 years is 8 mg/kg/day, which will achieve similar adult and paediatric exposure (average AUC approximately 5000 ng.h/ml).

There are limited pharmacokinetic data for patients less than three months of age. In neonates one week of age, lamivudine oral clearance was reduced when compared to paediatric patients and is likely to be due to immature renal function and variable absorption. Therefore to achieve similar adult and paediatric exposure, the recommended dose for neonates is 4 mg/kg/day.

Pharmacokinetics in pregnancy: Following oral administration, lamivudine pharmacokinetics in late-pregnancy were similar to non-pregnant adults.

Preclinical safety data: Administration of lamivudine in animal toxicity studies at high doses was not associated with any major organ toxicity. At the highest dosage levels, minor effects on indicators of liver and kidney function were seen together with occasional reductions in liver weight. The clinically relevant effects noted were a reduction in red blood cell count and neutropenia.

Lamivudine was not mutagenic in bacterial tests but, like many nucleoside analogues, showed activity in an *in vitro* cytogenetic assay and the mouse lymphoma assay. Lamivudine was not genotoxic *in vivo* at doses that gave plasma concentrations around 40–50 times higher than the anticipated clinical plasma levels. As the *in vitro* mutagenic activity of lamivudine could not be confirmed in *in vivo* tests, it is concluded that lamivudine should not represent a genotoxic hazard to patients undergoing treatment.

The results of long-term carcinogenicity studies in rats and mice, lamivudine did not show any carcinogenic potential relevant for humans.

Pharmaceutical particulars

List of excipients: Tablet core: Cellulose, Microcrystalline PhEur (E460); Sodium Starch Glycollate BP; Magnesium Stearate PhEur (E572).

Tablet Film Coat: Methylhydroxypropyl Cellulose PhEur (E464); Titanium Dioxide PhEur (E171); Macrogol PhEur; Polysorbate 80 PhEur (E433); Purified Water PhEur.

Incompatibilities: None reported.

Shelf life: 24 months.

Special precautions for storage: Store between 2 and 30°C.

Nature and contents of container: Cartons containing 60 coated tablets in a white high density polyethylene (HDPE) bottle, with a child-resistant closure.

Instructions for use/handling: None required.

Marketing authorisation number EU/1/96/015/001

Date of approval/revision of SPC May 1997

Legal category POM.

EUMOVATE* CREAM AND EUMOVATE* OINTMENT

Qualitative and quantitative composition 0.05% clobetasone butyrate.

Pharmaceutical form Water miscible cream and paraffin based ointment.

Clinical particulars

Therapeutic indications: Eumovate is suitable for the treatment of eczema and dermatitis of all types including atopic eczema, photodermatitis, otitis externa, primary irritant and allergic dermatitis (including napkin rash), intertrigo, prurigo nodularis, seborrhoeic dermatitis and insect bite reactions. Eumovate may be used as maintenance therapy between courses of one of the more active topical steroids.

Posology and method of administration: Clobetasone butyrate is a topically active corticosteroid which provides an exceptional combination of activity and safety. When formulated as Eumovate, it is more effective in the treatment of eczemas than 1% hydrocortisone, or the less-active synthetic steroid preparations that are in common use, yet has little effect on hypothalamic-pituitary-adrenal function. This has been so even when Eumovate was applied to adults in large amounts under whole-body occlusion. All topical corticosteroids can cause cutaneous atrophy if grossly misused. However, studies in animal and human models indicate that Eumovate and hydrocortisone cause less thinning of the epidermis than the other topical steroids tested.

Eumovate should be applied to the affected area up to four times a day until improvement occurs, when the frequency of application may be reduced.

Contra-indications: Skin lesions caused by infection with viruses (e.g. herpes simplex, chickenpox), fungi (e.g. candidiasis, tinea) or bacteria (e.g. impetigo).

Special warnings and precautions for use: Hypersensitivity to the preparations.

Precautions: Although generally regarded as safe, even for long-term administration in adults, there is a potential for overdosage, and in infants and children this may result in adrenal suppression. Extreme caution is required in dermatoses in such patients and treatment should not normally exceed seven days. In infants, the napkin may act as an occlusive dressing, and increase absorption.

Appropriate antimicrobial therapy should be used whenever treating inflammatory lesions which have become infected. Any spread of infection requires withdrawal of topical corticosteroid therapy, and systemic administration of antimicrobial agents.

As with all corticosteroids, prolonged application to the face is undesirable.

Topical corticosteroids may be hazardous in psoriasis for a number of reasons including rebound relapses, development of tolerance, risk of generalised pustular psoriasis and development of local or systemic toxicity due to impaired barrier function of the skin. If used in psoriasis, careful patient supervision is important.

If applied to the eyelids, care is needed to ensure that the preparation does not enter the eye as glaucoma might result.

Interaction with other medicaments and other forms of interaction: None stated.

Pregnancy and lactation: There is inadequate evidence of safety in human pregnancy. Topical administration of corticosteroids to pregnant animals can cause abnormalities of foetal development including cleft palate and intra-uterine growth retardation. There may therefore be a very small risk of such effects in the human foetus.

Effects on ability to drive and use machines: None stated.

Undesirable effects:

Side-effects: In the unlikely event of signs of hypersensitivity appearing, application should stop immediately. When large areas of the body are being treated with Eumovate, it is possible that some patients will absorb sufficient steroid to cause transient adrenal suppression despite the low degree of systemic activity associated with clobetasone butyrate.

Local atrophic changes could possibly occur in situations where moisture increases absorption of clobetasone butyrate, but only after prolonged use.

There are reports of pigmentation changes and hypertrichosis with topical steroids.

Exacerbation of symptoms may occur.

Overdose: Acute overdosage is very unlikely to occur, however, in the case of chronic overdosage or misuse the features of hypercorticism may appear and in this situation topical steroids should be discontinued.

Pharmacological properties

Pharmacodynamic properties: Clobetasone butyrate is a topically active corticosteroid.

Clobetasone butyrate has little effect on hypothalamo-pituitary-adrenal function. This was so even when Eumovate was applied to adults in large amounts under whole body occlusion.

Clobetasone butyrate is less potent than other available corticosteroid preparations and has been shown not to suppress the hypothalamo-pituitary-adrenal axis in patients treated for psoriasis or eczema.

Pharmacological studies in man and animals have shown that clobetasone butyrate has a relatively high level of topical activity accompanied by a low level of systemic activity.

Pharmacokinetic properties: A single application of 30 g clobetasone butyrate 0.05% ointment to eight patients resulted in a measurable rise in plasma clobetasone butyrate levels during the first three hours but then the levels gradually decreased. The maximum plasma level reached in the first three hours was 0.6 ng/ml. This rise in levels was followed by a more gradual decline with plasma levels of clobetasone butyrate falling below 0.1 ng/ml (the lower limit of the assay) after 72 hours. The normal diurnal variation in plasma cortisol levels was not affected by the application of clobetasone butyrate ointment.

Preclinical safety data: No additional data included.

Pharmaceutical particulars

List of excipients:

Cream: Glycerol, Glycerol monostearate, Cetostearyl alcohol, Beeswax substitute 6621, Arlacel 165,

Dimethicone 20, Chlorocresol, Sodium citrate, Citric acid monohydrate and purified water.

Ointment: White soft paraffin and liquid paraffin.

Incompatibilities: None stated.

Shelf life:
Cream: 36 months stored below 25°C.
Ointment: 36 months stored below 25°C.

Special precautions for storage: Store below 25°C.

Nature and contents of container:
Cream: Internally lacquered aluminium tubes with latex band and wadless polypropylene cap.

Ointment: Collapsible aluminium tube with wadless polypropylene cap.

30 and 100 gm tubes are available (25 gm pack is also registered).

Instructions for use/handling: None.

Marketing authorisation numbers
PL 10949/0035 (Cream)
PL 10949/0037 (Ointment)

Date of first authorisation/renewal of authorisation 01.01.93

Date of (partial) revision of text March 1996

FORTUM* FOR INJECTION

Qualitative and quantitative composition Fortum for Injection: Vials contain either 250 mg, 500 mg, 1 g, 2 g or 3 g ceftazidime (as pentahydrate) with sodium carbonate (118 mg per gram of ceftazidime).

Fortum Monovial in a vial containing 2 g ceftazidime pentahydrate.

Pharmaceutical form Sterile powder for constitution for injection.

Clinical particulars

Therapeutic indications:
Single infections
Mixed infections caused by two or more susceptible organisms
Severe infections in general
Respiratory tract infections
Ear, nose and throat infections
Urinary tract infections
Skin and soft tissue infections
Gastrointestinal, biliary and abdominal infections
Bone and joint infections
Dialysis: infections associated with haemo– and peritoneal dialysis and with continuous peritoneal dialysis (CAPD)

In meningitis it is recommended that the results of a sensitivity test are known before treatment with ceftazidime as a single agent. It may be used for infections caused by organisms resistant to other antibiotics including aminoglycosides and many cephalosporins. When appropriate, however, it may be used in combination with an aminoglycoside or other β-lactam antibiotic for example, in the presence of severe neutropenia, or with an antibiotic active against anaerobes when the presence of *Bacteroides fragilis* is suspected. In addition, ceftazidime is indicated in the perioperative prophylaxis of transurethral prostatectomy.

Bacteriology: Ceftazidime is bactericidal in action, exerting its effect on target cell wall proteins and causing inhibition of cell wall synthesis. A wide range of pathogenic strains and isolates associated with hospital-acquired infections are susceptible to ceftazidime *in vitro,* including strains resistant to gentamicin and other aminoglycosides. It is highly stable to most clinically important β-lactamases produced by both gram-positive and gram-negative organisms and consequently is active against many ampicillin- and cephalothin-resistant strains. Ceftazidime has high intrinsic activity *in vitro* and acts within a narrow mic range for most genera with minimal changes in mic at varied inoculum levels. Ceftazidime has been shown to have *in vitro* activity against the following organisms:

Gram-negative: *Pseudomonas aeruginosa,* Pseudomonas spp (other), *Klebsiella pneumoniae,* Klebsiella spp (other), *Proteus mirabilis, Proteus vulgaris, Morganella morganii* (formerly *Proteus morganii*), *Proteus rettgeri,* Providencia spp, *Escherichia coli,* Enterobacter spp, Citrobacter spp, Serratia spp, Salmonella spp, Shigella spp, *Yersinia enterocolitica, Pasteurella multocida,* Acinetobacter spp, *Neisseria gonorrhoeae, Neisseria meningitidis, Haemophilus influenzae* (including ampicillin-resistant strains), *Haemophilus parainfluenzae* (including ampicillin-resistant strains).

Gram-positive: *Staphylococcus aureus* (methicillin-sensitive strains), *Staphylococcus epidermidis* (methicillin-sensitive strains), Micrococcus spp, *Streptococcus pyogenes,* Streptococcus group b, *Streptococcus pneumoniae, Streptococcus mitis,* Streptococcus spp (excluding *Enterococcus (Streptococcus) faecalis*).

Anaerobic strains: Peptococcus spp, Peptostreptococcus spp, Streptococcus spp, Propionibacterium spp, *Clostridium perfringens,* Fusobacterium spp, Bacteroides spp (many strains of *Bact. fragilis* are resistant).

Ceftazidime is not active *in vitro* against methicillin-resistant staphylococci, *Enterococcus (Streptococcus) faecalis* and many other enterococci, *Listeria monocytogenes,* Campylobacter spp or *Clostridium difficile.*

In vitro the activities of ceftazidime and aminoglycoside antibiotics in combination have been shown to be at least additive; there is evidence of synergy in some strains tested. This property may be important in the treatment of febrile neutropenic patients.

Posology and method of administration: Ceftazidime is to be used by the parenteral route, the dosage depending upon the severity, sensitivity and type of infection and the age, weight and renal function of the patient.

Adults: The adult dosage range for ceftazidime is 1 to 6 g per day 8 or 12 hourly (i.m. or i.v.). In the majority of infections, 1 g 8-hourly or 2 g 12-hourly should be given. In urinary tract infections and in many less serious infections, 500 mg or 1 g 12-hourly is usually adequate. In very severe infections, especially immunocompromised patients, including those with neutropenia, 2 g 8 or 12-hourly or 3 g 12-hourly should be administered.

When used as a prophylactic agent in prostatic surgery 1 g (from the 1 g vial) should be given at the induction of anaesthesia. A second dose should be considered at the time of catheter removal.

Elderly: In view of the reduced clearance of ceftazidime in acutely ill elderly patients, the daily dosage should not normally exceed 3 g, especially in those over 80 years of age.

Cystic fibrosis: In fibrocystic adults with normal renal function who have pseudomonal lung infections, high doses of 100 to 150 mg/kg/day as three divided doses should be used. In adults with normal renal function 9 g/day has been used.

Infants and children: The usual dosage range for children aged over two months is 30 to 100 mg/kg/day, given as two or three divided doses.

Doses up to 150 mg/kg/day (maximum 6 g daily) in three divided doses may be given to infected immunocompromised or fibrocystic children or children with meningitis.

Neonates and children up to 2 months of age: Whilst clinical experience is limited, a dose of 25 to 60 mg/kg/day given as two divided doses has proved to be effective. In the neonate the serum half-life of ceftazidime can be three to four times that in adults.

Dosage in impaired renal function: Ceftazidime is excreted by the kidneys almost exclusively by glomerular filtration. Therefore, in patients with impaired renal function it is recommended that the dosage of ceftazidime should be reduced to compensate for its slower excretion, except in mild impairment, i.e. glomerular filtration rate (GFR) greater than 50 ml/min. In patients with suspected renal insufficiency, an initial loading dose of 1 g of ceftazidime may be given. An estimate of GFR should be made to determine the appropriate maintenance dose.

Renal impairment: For patients in renal failure on continuous arteriovenous haemodialysis or high-flux haemofiltration in intensive therapy units, it is recommended that the dosage should be 1 g daily in divided doses. For low-flux haemofiltration it is recommended that the dosage should be that suggested under impaired renal function.

Recommended maintenance doses are shown below:

Recommended maintenance doses of ceftazidime in renal insufficiency:

Creatinine clearance ml/min	*Approx. serum creatinine* μmol/l (mg/dl)*	*Recommended unit dose of ceftazidime (g)*	*Frequency of dosing (hourly)*
50-31	150-200 (1.7-2.3)	1	12
30-16	200-350 (2.3-4.0)	1	24
15-6	350-500 (4.0-5.6)	0.5	24
<5	>500 (>5.6)	0.5	48

* These values are guidelines and may not accurately predict renal function in all patients especially in the elderly in whom the serum creatinine concentration may overestimate renal function.

In patients with severe infections, especially in neutropenics, who would normally receive 6 g of ceftazidime daily were it not for renal insufficiency, the unit dose given in the table above may be increased by 50% or the dosing frequency increased appropriately. In such patients it is recommended that ceftazidime serum levels should be monitored and trough levels should not exceed 40 mg/litre.

When only serum creatinine is available, the following formula (Cockcroft's equation) may be used to estimate creatinine clearance. The serum creatinine should represent a steady state of renal function:

Males:

$$\text{Creatinine clearance (ml/min)} = \frac{\text{Weight (kg)} \times (140 - \text{age in years})}{72 \times \text{serum creatinine (mg/dl)}}$$

Females:
0.85 x above value.

To convert serum creatinine in μmol/litre into mg/dl divide by 88.4.

In children the creatinine clearance should be adjusted for body surface area or lean body mass and the dosing frequency reduced in cases of renal insufficiency as for adults.

The serum half-life of ceftazidime during haemodialysis ranges from 3 to 5 hours. The appropriate maintenance dose of ceftazidime should be repeated following each haemodialysis period.

Dosage in peritoneal dialysis: Ceftazidime may also be used in peritoneal dialysis and continuous ambulatory peritoneal dialysis (CAPD). As well as using ceftazidime intravenously, it can be incorporated into the dialysis fluid (usually 125 to 250 mg for 2L of dialysis fluid).

Administration: Ceftazidime may be given intravenously or by deep intramuscular injection into a large muscle mass such as the upper outer quadrant of the gluteus maximus or lateral part of the thigh.

Contra-indications: Ceftazidime is contra-indicated in patients with known hypersensitivity to cephalosporin antibiotics.

Special warnings and special precautions for use:
Hypersensitivity reactions: As with other β-lactam antibiotics, before therapy with ceftazidime is instituted, careful inquiry should be made for a history of hypersensitivity reactions to ceftazidime, cephalosporins, penicillins or other drugs. Ceftazidime should be given only with special caution to patients with type I or immediate hypersensitivity reactions to penicillin. If an allergic reaction to ceftazidime occurs, discontinue the drug. Serious hypersensitivity reactions may require epinephrine (adrenaline), hydrocortisone, antihistamine or other emergency measures.

Renal function: Cephalosporin antibiotics at high dosage should be given with caution to patients receiving concurrent treatment with nephrotoxic drugs, e.g. aminoglycoside antibiotics, or potent diuretics such as frusemide, as these combinations are suspected of affecting renal function adversely. Clinical experience with ceftazidime has shown that this is not likely to be a problem at the recommended dose levels. There is no evidence that ceftazidime adversely affects renal function at normal therapeutic doses: however, as for all antibiotics eliminated via the kidneys, it is necessary to reduce the dosage according to the degree of reduction in renal function to avoid the clinical consequences of elevated antibiotic levels, e.g. neurological sequelae, which have occasionally been reported when the dose has not been reduced appropriately (see *Dosage in Impaired Renal Function*).

Overgrowth of non-susceptible organisms: As with other broad spectrum antibiotics, prolonged use of ceftazidime may result in the overgrowth of non-susceptible organisms (e.g. Candida, Enterococci) which may require interruption of treatment or adoption of appropriate measures. Repeated evaluation of the patient's condition is essential.

Interaction with other medicaments and other forms of interaction: Ceftazidime does not interfere with enzyme-based tests for glycosuria. Slight interference with copper reduction methods (Benedict's, Fehling's, Clinitest) may be observed. Ceftazidime does not interfere in the alkaline picrate assay for creatinine. The development of a positive Coombs' test associated with the use of ceftazidime in about 5% of patients may interfere with the cross-matching of blood.

Chloramphenicol is antagonistic *in vitro* with ceftazidime and other cephalosporins. The clinical relevance of this finding is unknown, but if concurrent administration of ceftazidime with chloramphenicol is proposed, the possibility of antagonism should be considered.

Pregnancy and lactation: There is no experimental evidence of embryopathic or teratogenic effects attributable to ceftazidime but, as with all drugs, it should be administered with caution during the early months of pregnancy and in early infancy. Use in pregnancy requires that the anticipated benefit be weighed against the possible risks.

Ceftazidime is excreted in human milk in low

concentrations and consequently caution should be exercised when ceftazidime is administered to a nursing mother.

Effects on ability to drive and use machines: None reported.

Undesirable effects: Clinical trial experience has shown that ceftazidime is generally well tolerated.

Adverse reactions are infrequent and include:

Local: phlebitis or thrombophlebitis with i.v. administration, pain and/or inflammation after i.m. injection.

Hypersensitivity: maculopapular or urticarial rash, fever, pruritus, and very rarely angioedema and anaphylaxis (including bronchospasm and/or hypotension).

As with other cephalosporins, there have been rare reports of toxic epidermal necrolysis.

Gastrointestinal: diarrhoea, nausea, vomiting, abdominal pain, and very rarely oral thrush or colitis. As with other cephalosporins, colitis may be associated with *Clostridium difficile* and may present as pseudomembranous colitis.

Other adverse events which may be related to ceftazidime therapy or of uncertain aetiology include:

Genito-urinary: Candidiasis, vaginitis.

Central nervous system: Headache, dizziness, paraesthesiae and bad taste. There have been reports of neurological sequelae including tremor, myoclonia, convulsions, and encephalopathy in patients with renal impairment in whom the dose of ceftazidime has not been appropriately reduced.

Laboratory test changes noted transiently during ceftazidime therapy include: eosinophilia, positive Coombs' test, very rarely haemolytic anaemia, thrombocytosis and elevations in one or more of the hepatic enzymes, ALT (SGPT), AST (SGOT), LDH, GGT and alkaline phosphatase.

As with some other cephalosporins, transient elevation of blood urea, blood urea nitrogen and/or serum creatinine have been observed occasionally. Very rarely, leucopenia, neutropenia, agranulocytosis, thrombocytopenia and lymphocytosis have been seen.

Overdose: Overdosage can lead to neurological sequelae including encephalopathy, convulsions and coma.

Serum levels of ceftazidime can be reduced by dialysis.

Pharmacological properties

Pharmacodynamic properties: Ceftazidime is a bactericidal cephalosporin antibiotic which is resistant to most β-lactamases and is active against a wide range of gram-positive and gram-negative bacteria.

Pharmacokinetic properties: Ceftazidime administered by the parenteral route reaches high and prolonged serum levels in man. After intramuscular administration of 500 mg and 1 g, serum mean peak levels of 18 and 37 mg/litre respectively are rapidly achieved. Five minutes after an intravenous bolus injection of 500 mg, 1 g or 2 g, serum mean levels are respectively 46, 87 and 170 mg/litre.

Therapeutically effective concentrations are still found in the serum 8 to 12 hours after both intravenous and intramuscular administration. The serum half-life is about 1.8 hours in normal volunteers and about 2.2 hours in patients with apparently normal renal function. The serum protein binding of ceftazidime is low at about 10%.

Ceftazidime is not metabolised in the body and is excreted unchanged in the active form into the urine by glomerular filtration. Approximately 80 to 90% of the dose is recovered in the urine within 24 hours. Less than 1% is excreted via the bile, significantly limiting the amount entering the bowel.

Concentrations of ceftazidime in excess of the minimum inhibitory levels for common pathogens can be achieved in tissues such as bone, heart, bile, sputum, aqueous humour, synovial and pleural and peritoneal fluids. Transplacental transfer of the antibiotic readily occurs. Ceftazidime penetrates the intact blood brain barrier poorly and low levels are achieved in the csf in the absence of inflammation. Therapeutic levels of 4 to 20 mg/litre or more are achieved in the csf when the meninges are inflamed.

Preclinical safety data: No additional data of relevance.

Pharmaceutical particulars

List of excipients: Sodium carbonate (anhydrous sterile).

Incompatibilities: Ceftazidime is less stable in Sodium Bicarbonate Injection than other intravenous fluids. It is not recommended as a diluent.

Ceftazidime and aminoglycosides should not be mixed in the same giving set or syringe.

Precipitation has been reported when vancomycin has been added to ceftazidime in solution. It is recommended that giving sets and intravenous lines are flushed between administration of these two agents.

Shelf life: Three years when stored below 25°C and protected from light. Two years for Fortum Monovials when stored below 30°C and protected from light.

Special precautions for storage: Fortum for Injection should be stored below 25°C and Fortum Monovial should be stored below 30°C. Protect from light.

Nature and contents of container: Individually cartoned vials containing 250 mg, 500 mg or 1 g ceftazidime (as pentahydrate) for intramuscular or intravenous use in packs of 5.

Individually cartoned vials containing 2 g ceftazidime (as pentahydrate) for intravenous use in packs of 5.

Individually cartoned vials containing 2 g ceftazidime (as pentahydrate) for intravenous infusion in packs of 5.

Individually cartoned Monovials containing 2 g ceftazidime (as pentahydrate) for intravenous infusion.

Individually cartoned vials containing 3 g ceftazidime (as pentahydrate) for intravenous and intravenous infusion use.

Individually packaged Fortum Saline Infusion Kit containing 2 g ceftazidime (as pentahydrate) with sodium carbonate (118 mg per gram ceftazidime), a 50 ml infusion bag of Sodium Chloride Intravenous Infusion, a transfer needle, a pre-injection swab, a sealing cap and a label for the infusion bag.

Instructions for use/handling: Instructions for constitution: See table for addition volumes and solution concentrations, which may be useful when fractional doses are required.

Preparation of solution

	Vial size	Amount of Diluent to be added (ml)	Approximate Concentration (mg/ml)
250 mg	Intramuscular	1.0	210
250 mg	Intravenous	2.5	90
500 mg	Intramuscular	1.5	260
500 mg	Intravenous	5.0	90
1 g	Intramuscular	3.0	260
1 g	Intravenous	10.0	90
2 g	Intravenous bolus	10.0	170
2 g	Intravenous Infusion	50.0*	40†
3 g	Intravenous bolus	15.0	170
3 g	Intravenous Infusion	75.0*	40†

*Note: Addition should be in two stages unless using the infusion kit (see text).

†Note: Use Sodium Chloride Injection 0.9%, Dextrose Injection 5% or other approved diluent (see *Pharmaceutical particulars*) as Water for Injections produces hypotonic solutions at this concentration.

All sizes of vials as supplied are under reduced pressure. As the product dissolves, carbon dioxide is released and a positive pressure develops. For ease of use, it is recommended that the following techniques of reconstitution are adopted.

250 mg i.m./i.v., 500 mg i.m./i.v., 1 g i.m./i.v., and 2 g and 3 g i.v. bolus vials:

1. Insert the syringe needle through the vial closure and inject the recommended volume of diluent. The vacuum may assist entry of the diluent. Remove the syringe needle.
2. Shake to dissolve: carbon dioxide is released and a clear solution will be obtained in about 1 to 2 minutes.
3. Invert the vial. With the syringe plunger fully depressed, insert the needle through the vial closure and withdraw the total volume of solution into the syringe (the pressure in the vial may aid withdrawal). Ensure that the needle remains within the solution and does not enter the head space. The withdrawn solution may contain small bubbles of carbon dioxide; they may be disregarded.

2 g and 3 g i.v. infusion vials:

This vial may be constituted for short intravenous infusion (e.g. up to 30 minutes) as follows:

1. Insert the syringe needle through the vial closure and inject 10 ml of diluent for 2 g vial and 15 ml for 3 g vial. The vacuum may assist entry of the diluent. Remove the syringe needle.
2. Shake to dissolve: carbon dioxide is released and a clear solution obtained in about 1 to 2 minutes.
3. Insert a gas relief needle through the vial closure to relieve the internal pressure and, with the gas relief in position, add a further 40 ml of diluent for 2 g vial and 60 ml for 3 g vial. Remove the gas relief needle and syringe needle; shake the vial and set up for infusion use in the normal way.

NOTE: To preserve product sterility, it is important that a gas relief needle is not inserted through the vial closure before the product has dissolved.

2 g i.v. infusion kit:

Throughout the reconstitution procedure, aseptic technique should be used.

1) Remove the overwrap from the infusion bag. Remove the plastic dust cover from the vial and disinfect the rubber closure by using the Glaxo pre-injection swab.

Break tip off red plastic protector of infusion bag additive port.

2) Grasp transfer needle by central collar and remove either cap from the transfer needle.

3) Keeping the bag uppermost, hold the bag by the additive port and insert the exposed end of the transfer needle into the drug additive port. Please ensure that the bag is not squeezed as this may allow non-sterile air to enter the bag or solution to be expelled.

4) Keeping the bag uppermost, hold the collar of the transfer needle and remove the cover from the other needle of the transfer device. Insert the exposed end of the transfer needle into the vial closure.

5) Hold the bag uppermost and approximately one-third fill the vial by repeatedly squeezing and releasing the bag.

The vial is supplied under reduced pressure.

6) Hold vial/bag assembly centrally and shake, or repeatedly invert to dissolve the powder in the vial. As the antibiotic dissolves, carbon dioxide is released causing frothing which clears quickly. The carbon dioxide will pressurise the bag and vial.

7) Invert the assembly so that the vial is held above the bag and return the solution to the bag by repeatedly squeezing and releasing the bag. Repeat steps 5, 6 and 7 to rinse the inside of the vial.

8) Remove the transfer needle and vial from the bag as a single unit, replace the needle guards and dispose of safely. Squeeze the bag to inspect for minute leaks and examine the solution for visible particles. If in doubt, consult hospital pharmacy.

9) Place clear plastic guard over additive port and push firmly to close. The additive port is now sealed.

10) Complete the patient and drug information label and apply to the unprinted side of the reconstituted infusion bag.

11) Twist off the plastic strip which covers the solution administration set port of the bag and insert a solution administration set connector into the port. Prepare solution administration set according to manufacturers' instructions. The bag will contain a larger gas space than is usually present in an infusion bag. This gas can be carefully vented in a laminar flow cabinet before the solution administration set is attached. If the infusion is given without venting the bag, care should be taken to ensure the infusion is stopped before the gas enters the i.v. line.

Fortum Monovial:

The contents of the Monovial are added to small volume infusion bags containing 0.9% Sodium Chloride Injection or 5% Dextrose Injection, or another compatible fluid.

The 2 g presentation must be constituted in not less than 100 ml infusion bag.

1) Peel off the removable top part of the label and remove the cap.

2) Insert the needle of the Monovial into the additive port of the infusion bag.

3) To activate, push the plastic needle holder of the Monovial down onto the vial shoulder until a 'click' is heard.

4) Holding it upright, fill the vial to approximately two-thirds capacity by squeezing the bag several times.

5) Shake the vial to reconstitute the Fortum.

6) On constitution, the Fortum will effervesce slightly.

7) With the vial uppermost, transfer the reconstituted Fortum into the infusion bag by squeezing and releasing the bag.

8) Repeat the steps 4 to 7 to rinse the inside of the vial. Dispose of the empty Monovial safely. Check that the powder is completely dissolved and that the bag has no leaks.

Fortum Monovial is for i.v. infusion only.

These solutions may be given directly into the vein or introduced into the tubing of a giving set if the patient is receiving parenteral fluids. Ceftazidime is compatible with the most commonly used intravenous fluids.

Vials of Fortum for Injection and Fortum Monovials as supplied are under reduced pressure; a positive pressure is produced on constitution due to the release of carbon dioxide.

Vials of Fortum for Injection should be stored at a temperature below 25°C.

Vials of Fortum for Injection do not contain any preservatives and should be used as single-dose preparations.

The combination pack is intended solely for the preparation of a saline infusion of ceftazidime.

In keeping with good pharmaceutical practice, it is preferable to use freshly constituted solutions of

Fortum for Injection. If this is not practicable, satisfactory potency is retained for 24 hours in the refrigerator (2–8°C) when prepared in Water for Injections BP or any of the injections listed below.

At ceftazidime concentrations between 1 mg/ml and 40 mg/ml in:

0.9% Sodium Chloride Injection BP

M/6 Sodium Lactate Injection BP

Compound Sodium Lactate Injection BP (Hartmann's Solution)

5% Dextrose Injection BP

0.225% Sodium Chloride and 5% Dextrose Injection BP

0.45% Sodium Chloride and 5% Dextrose Injection BP

0.9% Sodium Chloride and 5% Dextrose Injection BP

0.18% Sodium Chloride and 4% Dextrose Injection BP

10% Dextrose Injection BP

Dextran 40 Injection BP 10% in 0.9% Sodium Chloride Injection BP

Dextran 40 Injection BP 10% in 5% Dextrose Injection BP

Dextran 70 Injection BP 6% in 0.9% Sodium Chloride Injection BP

Dextran 70 Injection BP 6% in 5% Dextrose Injection BP

(Ceftazidime is less stable in Sodium Bicarbonate Injection than in other intravenous fluids. It is not recommended as a diluent.)

At concentrations of between 0.05 mg/ml and 0.25 mg/ml in Intraperitoneal Dialysis Fluid (Lactate) BPC 1973.

When reconstituted for intramuscular use with: 0.5% or 1% Lignocaine Hydrochloride Injection BP.

When admixed at 4 mg/ml with (both components retain satisfactory potency):

Hydrocortisone (hydrocortisone sodium phosphate) 1 mg/ml in 0.9% Sodium Chloride Injection BP or 5% Dextrose Injection BP

Cefuroxime (cefuroxime sodium) 3 mg/ml in 0.9% Sodium Chloride Injection BP

Cloxacillin (cloxacillin sodium) 4 mg/ml in 0.9% Sodium Chloride Injection BP

Heparin 10u/ml or 50u/ml in 0.9% Sodium Chloride Injection BP

Potassium Chloride 10 mEq/L or 40 mEq/L in 0.9% Sodium Chloride Injection BP

The contents of a 500 mg vial of Fortum for Injection, constituted with 1.5 ml water for injections, may be added to metronidazole injection (500 mg in 100 ml) and both retain their activity.

Solutions range from light yellow to amber depending on concentration, diluent and storage conditions used. Within the stated recommendations, product potency is not adversely affected by such colour variations.

Marketing authorisation numbers

250 mg vials	0004/0304
500 mg vials	0004/0292
1 gram vials	0004/0293
2 and 3 gram vials	0004/0294
Sodium Chloride Intravenous Infusion	3460/0015

Date of first authorisation/renewal of authorisation

	MAA	Renewal
PL 0004/0304	01.11.93	
PL 0004/0292	16.11.89	22.02.96
PL 0004/0293	16.11.89	22.02.96
PL 0004/0294	16.11.89	22.02.96
PL 3460/0015	01.09.92	

GRISOVIN* TABLETS 125 mg

Qualitative and quantitative composition Griseofulvin BP 125.0 mg.

Pharmaceutical form Tablets.

Clinical particulars

Therapeutic indications: The treatment of fungal infections of the skin, scalp, hair or nails where topical therapy is considered inappropriate or has failed.

When griseofulvin is given orally for systemic treatment of fungal infections, it enables newly-formed keratin of the skin, hair and nails to resist attack by the fungi. As the new keratin extends, the old infected keratin is shed. Grisovin is effective against the dermatophytes causing ringworm (tinea), including: *Microsporum canis* and *T. verrucosum.*

Grisovin is not effective in infections caused by *Candida albicans* (monilia), *Aspergilli, Malassezia furfur (Pityriasis versicolor)* and *Nocardia* species.

Posology and method of administration:

Route of administration: Oral.

Dosage and administration: Doses should be taken after meals, otherwise absorption is likely to be inadequate.

Adults: Normally 500 to 1,000 mg daily, but not less than 10 mg/kg bodyweight daily. A single dose daily is often satisfactory, but divided doses may be more effective in patients who respond poorly.

Children: Usually 10 mg/kg (5 mg/lb) bodyweight daily in divided doses.

Duration of treatment: This depends upon the thickness of keratin at the site of infection. For hair or skin at least four weeks' treatment is required, whereas toe or finger nails may need six to twelve months' treatment. Therapy should be continued for at least two weeks after all signs of infection have disappeared.

Contra-indications: Porphyria or severe liver disease. Griseofulvin may cause liver disease to deteriorate, and liver function should be monitored in such conditions.

Systemic lupus erythematosus: Griseofulvin has been reported to exacerbate the condition.

Hypersensitivity to any ingredient of the preparation.

There is no evidence of the safety of Grisovin in human pregnancy. Griseofulvin is teratogenic in animals and some case reports of human foetal abnormalities have been observed. Therefore, Grisovin should not be used in pregnancy, or in women intending to become pregnant within one month following cessation of treatment.

Males should not father children within six months of treatment with Grisovin.

Long term administration of high doses of griseofulvin with food has been reported to induce hepatomas in mice and thyroid tumours in rats but not hamsters.

The clinical significance of these findings in man is not known. In view of these data, Grisovin Tablets should not be used prophylactically.

Special warnings and precautions for use: None.

Interaction with other medicaments and other forms of interaction: Griseofulvin may decrease the effect of the coumarin anti-coagulants.

Absorption of griseofulvin is inhibited when phenobarbitone is taken concurrently. The blood level, and hence efficacy, of griseofulvin may also be impaired as the result of concurrent administration of substances such as phenylbutazone and sedative and hypnotic drugs which induce metabolising enzymes.

Patients should be warned that an enhancement of the effects of alcohol by griseofulvin has been reported.

Pregnancy and lactation: Concurrent treatment with griseofulvin may reduce the effectiveness of oral contraceptives, so additional contraceptive precautions should be taken during griseofulvin treatment and for a month after stopping griseofulvin. There is no evidence of its safety in human pregnancy (see *Contra-indications*). Griseofulvin has been shown to be teratogenic in mice and rats following administration to pregnant animals. Some case-reports suggest that it produces human foetal abnormalities.

As Grisovin is capable of inducing aneuploidy (abnormal segregation of chromosomes following cell division) in mammalian cells exposed to the compound *in vitro* and *in vivo*, women should be warned that they should not take the drug during pregnancy or become pregnant within one month following cessation of treatment.

Additionally, males should not father children within six months of treatment.

It is not known if griseofulvin is excreted in human milk. Safety in children of mothers who are breast-feeding has not been established.

Effect on ability to drive and use machines: In those rare cases where individuals are affected by drowsiness while taking griseofulvin, they should not drive vehicles or operate machinery.

Undesirable effects: Headache and gastric discomfort sometimes occur, but usually disappear as treatment continues. On rare occasions urticarial reactions, skin rashes and precipitation of Systemic Lupus Erythematosus have been reported.

Toxic epidermal necrolysis and erythema multiforme have been reported.

There have been reports of central nervous system effects e.g. confusion, dizziness, impaired co-ordination and peripheral neuropathy.

Leucopenia with neutropenia has been reported.

Photosensitivity reactions can occur on exposure to intense natural or artificial sunlight.

Overdose: Treatment is unlikely to be required in cases of acute overdosage.

Pharmacological properties

Pharmacodynamic properties:

Mode of action: Griseofulvin is an antifungal antibiotic which is active *in vitro* against common dermatophytes. It exerts its antifungal effect by disrupting the cell division spindle apparatus of fungal cells, thereby arresting cell division.

A prominent morphological manifestation of the action of griseofulvin is the production of multinucleate cells as the drug inhibits fungal mitosis. Griseofulvin causes disruption of the mitotic spindle by interacting with polymerised microtubules while the effects of the drug are thus similar to those of colchicine and vinca alkaloids, its binding sites on the microtubular protein are distinct.

Pharmacokinetic properties: The absorption of griseofulvin from the gastrointestinal tract is variable and incomplete. On average, less than 50% of the oral dose is absorbed, but fatty foods and a reduction in particle size will increase the rate and extent of the absorption.

After oral dosing there is a phase of rapid absorption followed by slower prolonged absorption. Peak plasma levels (0.5–1.5 micrograms after a 500 mg oral dose) are achieved by 4 hours and are maintained for 10–20 hours. The terminal plasma half-life ranges from 9.5–21 hours, there being considerable intersubject variability. In plasma griseofulvin is approximately 84% bound to plasma proteins, predominantly albumin.

The absorbed griseofulvin is excreted in the urine mainly as 6-desmethylgriseofulvin or its glucuronide conjugate.

There is selective deposition of griseofulvin in newly formed keratin of hair, nails and skin, which gradually moves to the surface of these appendages.

Preclinical safety data: Griseofulvin can induce aneuploidy and meiotic delay in mouse oocytes following oral administration of high doses, i.e. 250 mg/kg or greater. In addition, griseofulvin caused increases in numerical and structural chromosome aberrations in mouse spermatocytes at doses of 500 mg/kg and above. Aneuploidy was observed at doses of 1500 mg/kg. Griseofulvin administered to rats and mice during pregnancy has been associated with foetotoxicity and foetal malformations. Long-term administration of high doses of griseofulvin with food has been reported to induce hepatomas in mice and thyroid tumours in rats but not hamsters (see *Contra-indications*). The effects in mice may be due to a species specific effect on porphyrin metabolism.

Pharmaceutical particulars

List of excipients: Sodium lauryl sulphate BP, Povidone BP, Maize starch BP, Potato starch BP, Microcrystalline cellulose HSE, Magnesium stearate BP, Purified water BP.

Film coating: Hydroxypropylmethylcellulose HSE, Ethylcellulose HSE, Acetylated monoglyceride HSE, Polysorbate 80 BP, Propylene glycol BP, Methylene chloride HSE, Isopropyl alcohol HSE.

Incompatibilities: None.

Shelf life: 36 months.

Special precautions for storage: None.

Nature and contents of container: 100 tablets in a tubular glass vial with a polythene snap plug closure or, tamper evident polypropylene container with a low density polyethylene lid.

Instructions for use/handling: None.

Marketing authorisation number PL 10949/0100

Date of first authorisation/renewal of authorisation 01/10/93 06/03/98

Date of (partial) revision of text 28 October 1998

GRISOVIN* TABLETS 500 mg

Qualitative and quantitative composition Griseofulvin BP 500.0 mg.

Pharmaceutical form Tablets.

Clinical particulars

Therapeutic indications: The treatment of fungal infections of the skin, scalp, hair or nails where topical therapy is considered inappropriate or has failed.

When griseofulvin is given orally for systemic treatment of fungal infections, it enables newly-formed keratin of the skin, hair and nails to resist attack by the fungi. As the new keratin extends, the old infected keratin is shed. Grisovin is effective against the dermatophytes causing ringworm (tinea), including: *Microsporum canis* and *T. verrucosum.*

Grisovin is not effective in infections caused by *Candida albicans* (monilia), *Aspergilli, Malassezia furfur (Pityriasis versicolor)* and *Nocardia* species.

Posology and method of administration:

Route of administration: Oral.

Dosage and administration: Doses should be taken after meals, otherwise absorption is likely to be inadequate.

Adults: Normally 500 to 1,000 mg daily, but not less than 10 mg/kg bodyweight daily. A single dose daily is often satisfactory, but divided doses may be more effective in patients who respond poorly.

Children: Usually 10 mg/kg (5 mg/lb) bodyweight daily in divided doses.

Duration of treatment: This depends upon the thickness of keratin at the site of infection. For hair or skin at least four weeks' treatment is required, whereas toe or finger nails may need six to twelve months' treatment. Therapy should be continued for at least two weeks after all signs of infection have disappeared.

Contra-indications: Porphyria or severe liver disease. Griseofulvin may cause liver disease to deteriorate, and liver function should be monitored in such conditions.

Systemic lupus erythematosus: Griseofulvin has been reported to exacerbate the condition.

Hypersensitivity to any ingredient of the preparation.

There is no evidence of the safety of Grisovin in human pregnancy. Griseofulvin is teratogenic in animals and some case reports of human foetal abnormalities have been observed. Therefore, Grisovin should not be used in pregnancy, or in women intending to become pregnant within one month following cessation of treatment.

Males should not father children within six months of treatment with Grisovin.

Long term administration of high doses of griseofulvin with food has been reported to induce hepatomas in mice and thyroid tumours in rats but not hamsters.

The clinical significance of these findings in man is not known. In view of these data, Grisovin Tablets should not be used prophylactically.

Special warnings and precautions for use: None.

Interaction with other medicaments and other forms of interaction: Griseofulvin may decrease the effect of the coumarin anti-coagulants.

Absorption of griseofulvin is inhibited when phenobarbitone is taken concurrently. The blood level, and hence efficacy, of griseofulvin may also be impaired as the result of concurrent administration of substances such as phenylbutazone and sedative and hypnotic drugs which induce metabolising enzymes.

Patients should be warned that an enhancement of the effects of alcohol by griseofulvin has been reported.

Pregnancy and lactation: Concurrent treatment with griseofulvin may reduce the effectiveness of oral contraceptives, so additional contraceptive precautions should be taken during griseofulvin treatment and for a month after stopping griseofulvin. There is no evidence of its safety in human pregnancy (see *Contra-indications*). Griseofulvin has been shown to be teratogenic in mice and rats following administration to pregnant animals. Some case-reports suggest that it produces human foetal abnormalities.

As Grisovin is capable of inducing aneuploidy (abnormal segregation of chromosomes following cell division) in mammalian cells exposed to the compound *in vitro* and *in vivo*, women should be warned that they should not take the drug during pregnancy or become pregnant within one month following cessation of treatment.

Additionally, males should not father children within six months of treatment.

It is not known if griseofulvin is excreted in human milk. Safety in children of mothers who are breast-feeding has not been established.

Effect on ability to drive and use machines: In those rare cases where individuals are affected by drowsiness while taking griseofulvin, they should not drive vehicles or operate machinery.

Undesirable effects: Headache and gastric discomfort sometimes occur, but usually disappear as treatment continues. On rare occasions urticarial reactions, skin rashes and precipitation of Systemic Lupus Erythematosus have been reported.

Toxic epidermal necrolysis and erythema multiforme have been reported.

There have been reports of central nervous system effects e.g. confusion, dizziness, impaired co-ordination and peripheral neuropathy.

Leucopenia with neutropenia has been reported.

Photosensitivity reactions can occur on exposure to intense natural or artificial sunlight.

Overdose: Treatment is unlikely to be required in cases of acute overdosage.

Pharmacological properties

Pharmacodynamic properties:

Mode of action: Griseofulvin is an antifungal antibiotic which is active *in vitro* against common dermatophytes. It exerts its antifungal effect by disrupting the cell division spindle apparatus of fungal cells, thereby arresting cell division.

A prominent morphological manifestation of the action of griseofulvin is the production of multinucleate cells as the drug inhibits fungal mitosis. Griseofulvin causes disruption of the mitotic spindle by interacting with polymerised microtubules while the effects of the drug are thus similar to those of colchicine and vinca alkaloids, its binding sites on the microtubular protein are distinct.

Pharmacokinetic properties: The absorption of griseofulvin from the gastrointestinal tract is variable and incomplete. On average, less than 50% of the oral dose is absorbed, but fatty foods and a reduction in particle size will increase the rate and extent of the absorption.

After oral dosing there is a phase of rapid absorption followed by slower prolonged absorption. Peak plasma levels (0.5–1.5 micrograms after a 500 mg oral dose) are achieved by 4 hours and are maintained for 10–20 hours. The terminal plasma half-life ranges from 9.5–21 hours, there being considerable intersubject variability. In plasma griseofulvin is approximately 84% bound to plasma proteins, predominantly albumin.

The absorbed griseofulvin is excreted in the urine mainly as 6-desmethylgriseofulvin or its glucuronide conjugate.

There is selective deposition of griseofulvin in newly formed keratin of hair, nails and skin, which gradually moves to the surface of these appendages.

Preclinical safety data: Griseofulvin can induce aneuploidy and meiotic delay in mouse oocytes following oral administration of high doses, i.e. 250 mg/kg or greater. In addition, griseofulvin caused increases in numerical and structural chromosome aberrations in mouse spermatocytes at doses of 500 mg/kg and above. Aneuploidy was observed at doses of 1500 mg/kg. Griseofulvin administered to rats and mice during pregnancy has been associated with foetotoxicity and foetal malformations. Long-term administration of high doses of griseofulvin with food has been reported to induce hepatomas in mice and thyroid tumours in rats but not hamsters (see *Contra-indications*). The effects in mice may be due to a species specific effect on porphyrin metabolism.

Pharmaceutical particulars

List of excipients: Sodium lauryl sulphate BP, Povidone BP, Maize starch BP, Potato starch BP, Microcrystalline cellulose HSE, Magnesium stearate BP, Purified water BP.

Film coating: Hydroxypropylmethylcellulose HSE, Ethylcellulose HSE, Acetylated monoglyceride HSE, Polysorbate 80 BP, Propylene glycol BP, Methylene chloride HSE, Isopropyl alcohol HSE.

Incompatibilities: None.

Shelf life: 36 months.

Special precautions for storage: None.

Nature and contents of container: 100 tablets in a tubular glass vial with a polythene snap plug closure or, tamper evident polypropylene container with a low density polyethylene lid.

Instructions for use/handling: None.

Marketing authorisation number PL 10949/0101

Date of first authorisation/renewal of authorisation 01/10/93 17/03/98

Date of (partial) revision of text 28 October 1998

IMIGRAN* INJECTION
IMIGRAN* SUBJECT

Qualitative and quantitative composition Each pre-filled syringe contains 6 mg of sumatriptan base, as the succinate salt, in an isotonic solution of 0.5 ml.

Pharmaceutical form Pre-filled syringes for use in conjunction with an auto injector for subcutaneous injection.

Clinical particulars

Therapeutic indications: Subcutaneous Injection is indicated for the acute relief of migraine attacks, with or without aura, and for the acute treatment of cluster headache. Imigran should only be used where there is a clear diagnosis of migraine or cluster headache.

Posology and method of administration: Imigran should not be used prophylactically.

It is recommended to start the treatment at the first sign of a migraine headache or associated symptoms such as nausea, vomiting or photophobia. It is equally effective at whatever stage of the attack it is administered. Imigran Injection should be injected subcutaneously using an auto-injector. Patients should be advised to observe strictly the instruction leaflet for the Imigran auto-injector especially regarding the safe disposal of syringes and needles.

Migraine:

Adults: The recommended adult dose of Imigran is a single 6 mg subcutaneous injection. Patients who do not respond to this dose should not take a second dose of Imigran for the same attack. Imigran may be taken for subsequent attacks. Patients who respond initially but whose migraine returns may take a further dose at any time in the next 24 hours provided that one hour has elapsed since the first dose.

The maximum dose in 24 hours is two 6 mg injections (12 mg).

Imigran is recommended as monotherapy for the acute treatment of migraine and should not be given concomitantly with other acute migraine therapies. If a patient fails to respond to a single dose of Imigran there are no reasons, either on theoretical grounds or from limited clinical experience, to withhold products containing aspirin or non-steroidal anti-inflammatory drugs or paracetamol for further treatment of the attack.

Cluster headache:

Adults: The recommended adult dose is a single 6 mg subcutaneous injection for each cluster attack. The maximum dose in 24 hours is two 6 mg injections (12 mg) with a minimum interval of one hour between the two doses.

Children: The safety and effectiveness of Imigran in children has not yet been established.

Elderly (over 65): Experience of the use of Imigran in patients aged over 65 years is limited. The pharmacokinetics do not differ significantly from a younger population but, until further clinical data are available, the use of Sumatriptan in patients aged over 65 years is not recommended.

Contra-indications: Hypersensitivity to any component of the preparation.

Sumatriptan should not be given to patients who have had myocardial infarction or have ischaemic heart disease, coronary vasospasm (Prinzmetal's angina), peripheral vascular disease or patients who have symptoms or signs consistent with ischaemic heart disease.

Sumatriptan should not be administered to patients with a history of cerebrovascular accident (CVA) or transient ischaemic attack (TIA).

Sumatriptan should not be administered to patients with severe hepatic impairment.

The use of sumatriptan in patients with uncontrolled hypertension is contra-indicated.

The concomitant administration of ergotamine or derivatives of ergotamine (including methysergide) is contra-indicated (see *Interaction with other medicaments and other forms of interaction*).

Concurrent administration of monoamine oxidase inhibitors and sumatriptan is contra-indicated.

Imigran Injection must not be used within two weeks of discontinuation of therapy with monoamine oxidase inhibitors.

Special warnings and precautions for use:

Warnings: Imigran should only be used where there is a clear diagnosis of migraine or cluster headache.

Sumatriptan is not indicated for use in the management of hemiplegic, basilar or ophthalmoplegic migraine.

The recommended doses of Sumatriptan should not be exceeded.

Imigran Injection should not be given intravenously because of its potential to cause vasospasm. The vasospasm may result in arrhythmias, ischaemic ECG changes or myocardial infarction.

Before treating headaches in patients not previously diagnosed as migraineurs, and in migraineurs who present with atypical symptoms, care should be taken to exclude other potentially serious neurological conditions. It should be noted that migraineurs may be at risk of certain cerebrovascular events (e.g. cerebrovascular accident, transient ischaemic attack).

Following administration, Sumatriptan can be associated with transient symptoms including chest pain and tightness which may be intense and involve the throat. Where such symptoms are thought to indicate ischaemic heart disease appropriate evaluation should be carried out.

If the patient experiences symptoms which are severe or persistent or are consistent with angina, further doses should not be taken until appropriate investigations have been carried out to check for the possibility of ischaemic changes.

Sumatriptan should therefore not be given to patients in whom unrecognised cardiac disease is likely without a prior evaluation for underlying cardiovascular disease. Such patients include post menopausal women, males over 40 and patients with risk factors for coronary artery disease.

Precautions: Sumatriptan should be administered with caution to patients with controlled hypertension as transient increases in blood pressure and peripheral vascular resistance have been observed in a small proportion of patients.

There have been rare post-marketing reports describing patients with weakness, hyper-reflexia, and incoordination following the use of a selective serotonin reuptake inhibitor (SSRI) and sumatriptan. If concomitant treatment with sumatriptan and an SSRI is clinically warranted, appropriate observation of the patient is advised.

Sumatriptan should be administered with caution to patients with conditions which may affect significantly the absorption, metabolism or excretion of the drug e.g. impaired hepatic or renal function.

Patients with known hypersensitivity to sulphonamides may exhibit an allergic reaction following administration of Sumatriptan. Reactions may range from cutaneous hypersensitivity to anaphylaxis.

Evidence of cross-sensitivity is limited, however,

caution should be exercised before using sumatriptan in these patients.

Interaction with other medicaments and other forms of interaction: Studies in healthy subjects show that Imigran does not interact with propranolol, flunarizine, pizotifen or alcohol. Sumatriptan has the potential to interact with MAOIs, ergotamine and derivatives of ergotamine (see also *Contra-indications*).

Rarely an interaction may occur between sumatriptan and SSRIs (see *Special warnings and precautions for use*).

Prolonged vasospastic reactions have been reported with ergotamine. As these effects may be additive, 24 hours should elapse before sumatriptan can be taken following any ergotamine-containing preparation. Conversely, ergotamine-containing preparations should not be taken until 6 hours have elapsed following sumatriptan administration.

Pregnancy and lactation: The safety of this medicinal product for use in human pregnancy has not been established. Evaluation of experimental animal studies does not indicate direct teratogenic effects or harmful effects on peri- and postnatal development.

When administered to pregnant rabbits throughout the period of organogenesis sumatriptan has occasionally caused embryolethality at doses which were sufficiently high to produce maternal toxicity.

In a rat fertility study oral doses of sumatriptan resulting in plasma levels approximately 150 times those seen in man after a 6 mg subcutaneous dose were associated with a reduction in the success of insemination. This effect did not occur during a subcutaneous study where maximum plasma levels achieved approximately 100 times those in man by the subcutaneous route.

As yet, experience of the use of sumatriptan during human pregnancy is limited. Although animal reproduction studies are not always predictive of human response, administration of this drug is not recommended during pregnancy unless the expected benefit to the mother is greater than any possible risk to the foetus.

It has been demonstrated that following subcutaneous administration sumatriptan is excreted into breast milk. Infant exposure can be minimised by avoiding breast feeding for 24 hours after treatment.

Effect on ability to drive and use machines: Drowsiness may occur as a result of migraine or its treatment with Sumatriptan. Caution is recommended in patients performing skilled tasks, e.g., driving or operating machinery.

Undesirable effects:

General: The most common side effect associated with treatment with Imigran administered subcutaneously is transient pain at the site of injection. Stinging/burning, erythema, bruising and bleeding at the injection site have also been reported.

These symptoms are usually transient and may be intense and can affect any part of the body including the chest and throat: pain, sensations of tingling, heat, heaviness, pressure or tightness.

The following symptoms are mild to moderate in intensity and transient: flushing, dizziness and feelings of weakness.

Fatigue and drowsiness have been reported.

Cardiovascular: Hypertension, bradycardia, tachycardia, palpitations. Transient increases in blood pressure arising soon after treatment have been recorded. In extremely rare cases, serious coronary events have been reported which have included cardiac arrhythmias, ischaemic ECG changes or myocardial infarction.

Gastrointestinal: Nausea and vomiting occurred in some patients but the relationship to Imigran is not clear.

CNS: There have been rare reports of seizures following use of sumatriptan. Although some have occurred in patients with either a history of seizures or concurrent conditions predisposing to seizures there are also reports in patients where no such predisposing factors are apparent.

Eye disorders: Patients treated with Imigran rarely exhibit visual disorders like flickering and diplopia. Additionally, cases of nystagmus, scotoma and reduced vision have been observed. Very rarely a transient loss of vision has been reported. However, visual disorders may also occur during a migraine attack itself.

Hypersensitivity/skin: Hypersensitivity reactions ranging from cutaneous hypersensitivity to, in rare cases, anaphylaxis.

Laboratory values: Minor disturbances in liver function tests have occasionally been observed.

Overdose: There have been some reports of overdosage with Imigran Injection. Patients have received single injections of up to 12 mg subcutaneously without significant adverse effects. Doses in excess of 16 mg subcutaneously were not associated with side effects other than those mentioned.

If overdosage with Imigran occurs, the patient should be monitored for at least ten hours and standard supportive treatment applied as required.

It is unknown what effect haemodialysis or peritoneal dialysis has on the plasma concentrations of Imigran.

Pharmacological properties

Pharmacodynamic properties:

Pharmacotherapeutic group: Analgesics: Selective 5-HT_1 receptor agonists. ATC Code: N02CC01.

Sumatriptan has been demonstrated to be a specific and selective 5-hydroxytryptamine (5-HT_{1D}) receptor agonist with no effect on other 5-HT receptor (5-HT_2-5-HT_7) subtypes. The vascular 5-HT_{1D} receptor is found predominantly in cranial blood vessels and mediates vasoconstriction. In animals, sumatriptan selectively constricts the carotid arterial circulation but does not alter cerebral blood flow. The carotid arterial circulation supplies blood to the extracranial and intracranial tissues, such as the meninges and dilatation and/or oedema formation in these vessels is thought to be the underlying mechanism of migraine in man. In addition, experimental evidence from animal studies suggests that sumatriptan inhibits trigeminal nerve activity. Both these actions (cranial vasoconstriction and inhibition of trigeminal nerve activity) may contribute to the anti-migraine action of sumatriptan in humans.

Clinical response begins 10 to 15 minutes following a 6 mg subcutaneous injection.

Because of its route of administration Imigran Injection may be particularly suitable for patients who suffer with nausea and vomiting during an attack.

Pharmacokinetic properties: Following subcutaneous injection, sumatriptan has a high mean bioavailability (96%) with peak serum concentrations occurring in 25 minutes. Average peak serum concentration after a 6 mg subcutaneous dose is 72 ng/ml. The elimination phase half life is approximately two hours.

Plasma protein binding is low (14 to 21%), mean volume of distribution is 170 litres. Mean total plasma clearance is approximately 1, 160 ml/min and the mean renal plasma clearance is approximately 260 ml/min. Non-renal clearance accounts for about 80% of the total clearance. Sumatriptan is eliminated primarily by oxidative metabolism mediated by monoamine oxidase A.

The major metabolite, the indole acetic acid analogue of sumatriptan, is mainly excreted in the urine where it is present as a free acid and the glucuronide conjugate. It has no known 5-HT_1 or 5-HT_2 activity. Minor metabolites have not been identified.

In a pilot study no significant differences were found in the pharmacokinetic parameters between the elderly and young healthy volunteers.

Preclinical safety data: Sumatriptan was devoid of genotoxic and carcinogenic activity in *in vitro* systems and animal studies.

Pharmaceutical particulars

List of excipients: Sodium chloride, Water for injection.

Incompatibilities: None reported.

Shelf life: Two years when stored below 30°C and protected from light.

Special precautions for storage: Imigran Injection should be stored below 30°C and protected from light.

Nature and contents of container:

Treatment pack: 2 pre-filled syringes (in cases) plus an auto-injector, in a plastic tray within a carton.

Refill pack: 2 pre-filled syringes (in cases) in a carton.

Instructions for use/handling: None stated.

Marketing authorisation number PL 10949/0113

Date of first authorisation/renewal of authorisation 11/07/1997

Date of (partial) revision of text June 1998

Legal category POM

IMIGRAN* 20 NASAL SPRAY ▼

Qualitative and quantitative composition Imigran 20 Nasal Spray: Unit dose spray device for intranasal administration. The device delivers 20 mg of sumatriptan in 0.1 ml of an aqueous buffered solution.

Pharmaceutical form Nasal spray.

Clinical particulars

Therapeutic indications: Imigran Nasal Spray is indicated for the acute treatment of migraine attacks with or without aura.

Posology and method of administration: Imigran Nasal Spray should not be used prophylactically.

Imigran is recommended as monotherapy for the acute treatment of a migraine attack and should not be given concomitantly with ergotamine or derivatives of ergotamine (including methysergide) (see *Contra-indications*).

It is advisable that Imigran be given as early as possible after the onset of a migraine headache. It is equally effective at whatever stage of the attack it is administered.

Adults: The optimal dose of Imigran Nasal Spray is 20 mg for administration into one nostril. Although, due to inter/intra patient variability of both the migraine attacks and the absorption of sumatriptan, 10 mg may be effective in some patients.

If a patient does not respond to the first dose of Imigran, a second dose should not be taken for the same attack. However, the attack can be treated with paracetamol, aspirin or non-steroidal anti-inflammatory drugs. Imigran may be taken for subsequent attacks.

If the patient has responded to the first dose, but the symptoms recur, a second dose may be given in the next 24 hours, provided that there is a minimum interval of two hours between the two doses.

No more than two Imigran 20 mg Nasal Sprays to be used in any 24 hour period.

Children (under 18 years of age): The safety and effectiveness of Imigran Nasal Spray in children has not yet been established.

Elderly (over 65): There is no experience of the use of Imigran Nasal Spray in patients over 65. The kinetics in elderly patients have not been sufficiently studied. Therefore, the use of sumatriptan is not recommended until further data is available.

Contra-indications: Hypersensitivity to any component of the preparation.

Sumatriptan should not be given to patients who have had myocardial infarction or have ischaemic heart disease, coronary vasospasm (Prinzmetal's angina), peripheral vascular disease or patients who have symptoms or signs consistent with ischaemic heart disease.

Sumatriptan should not be administered to patients with a history of cerebrovascular accident (CVA) or transient ischaemic attack (TIA).

Sumatriptan should not be administered to patients with severe hepatic impairment.

The use of sumatriptan in patients with uncontrolled hypertension is contra-indicated.

The concomitant administration of ergotamine, or derivatives of ergotamine (including methysergide) is contra-indicated (see *Interactions*).

Concurrent administration of monoamine oxidase inhibitors and sumatriptan is contra-indicated.

Imigran must not be used within two weeks of discontinuation of therapy with monoamine oxidase inhibitors.

Special warnings and special precautions for use: Imigran Nasal Spray should only be used where there is a clear diagnosis of migraine. Sumatriptan is not indicated for use in the management of hemiplegic, basilar or ophthalmoplegic migraine.

As with other acute migraine therapies, before treating headaches in patients not previously diagnosed as migraineurs, and in migraineurs who present with atypical symptoms, care should be taken to exclude other potentially serious neurological conditions.

It should be noted that migraineurs may be at increased risk of certain cerebrovascular events (e.g. CVA, TIA).

Following administration, sumatriptan can be associated with transient symptoms including chest pain and tightness which may be intense and involve the throat (see *Side effects*). Where such symptoms are thought to indicate ischaemic heart disease, appropriate evaluation should be carried out.

Sumatriptan should not be given to patients in whom unrecognised cardiac disease is likely without a prior evaluation for underlying cardiovascular disease. Such patients include post-menopausal women, males over 40 and patients with risk factors for coronary artery disease.

Sumatriptan should be administered with caution to patients with controlled hypertension as transient increases in blood pressure and peripheral vascular resistance have been observed in a small proportion of patients.

There have been rare postmarketing reports describing patients with weakness, hyper-reflexia, and inco-ordination following the use of a selective serotonin reuptake inhibitor (SSRI) and sumatriptan. If concomitant treatment with sumatriptan and an SSRI is clinically warranted, appropriate observation of the patient is advised.

Sumatriptan should be administered with caution to patients with conditions which may affect significantly the absorption, metabolism or excretion of the drug, e.g. impaired hepatic or renal function.

Patients with known hypersensitivity to sulphonamides may exhibit an allergic reaction following administration of sumatriptan. Reactions may range from cutaneous hypersensitivity to anaphylaxis.

The recommended dose of Imigran should not be exceeded.

Interaction with other medicaments and other forms of interaction: There is no evidence of interactions with propranolol, flunarizine, pizotifen or alcohol.

There are limited data on an interaction with ergotamine containing preparations. The increased risk of coronary vasospasm is a theoretical possibility and concomitant administration is contra-indicated.

The period of time that should elapse between the use of sumatriptan and ergotamine containing preparations is not known. This will also depend on the doses and type of ergotamine containing products used. The effects may be additive. It is advised to wait at least 24 hours following the use of ergotamine containing preparations before administering sumatriptan. Conversely, it is advised to wait at least six hours following use of sumatriptan before administering an ergotamine containing product (see *Contra-indications*).

An interaction may occur between sumatriptan and MAOIs and concomitant administration is contra-indicated (see *Contra-indications*). Rarely an interaction may occur between sumatriptan and SSRIs.

Pregnancy and lactation: The safety of this medicinal product for use in human pregnancy has not been established. Evaluation of experimental animal studies does not indicate direct teratogenic effects or harmful effects on peri- and postnatal development.

However, embryofoetal viability might be affected in the rabbit. Because animal reproduction studies are not always predictive of human response, administration of this drug should only be considered if the expected benefit to the mother is greater than any possible risk to the foetus.

It has been demonstrated that following subcutaneous administration sumatriptan is secreted into breast milk. Infant exposure can be minimised by avoiding breast feeding for 24 hours after treatment.

Effects on ability to drive and use machines: No data are available. Drowsiness may occur as a result of migraine or its treatment with sumatriptan. This may influence the ability to drive and to operate machinery.

Undesirable effects:

General: The most frequently reported side effect following the use of Imigran Nasal Spray is its taste.

Following administration of Imigran Nasal Spray mild, transient irritation or a burning sensation in the nose or throat or epistaxis have been reported.

The following symptoms are usually transient and may be intense and can affect any part of the body including the chest and throat: pain, sensations of tingling, heat, heaviness, pressure or tightness.

The following symptoms are mostly mild to moderate in intensity and transient: flushing, dizziness, and feelings of weakness.

Fatigue and drowsiness have been reported.

Cardiovascular: Hypotension, bradycardia, tachycardia, palpitations.

Transient increases in blood pressure arising soon after treatment have been recorded.

In extremely rare cases serious coronary events have been reported which have included cardiac arrhythmias, transient ischaemic ECG changes or myocardial infarction.

Gastrointestinal: Nausea and vomiting occurred in some patients but the relationship to sumatriptan is not clear.

CNS: There have been rare reports of seizures, following use of sumatriptan. Although some have occurred in patients with either a history of seizures or concurrent conditions predisposing to seizures, there are also reports in patients where no such predisposing factors are apparent.

Eye disorders: Patients treated with Imigran rarely exhibit visual disorders like flickering and diplopia. Additionally cases of nystagmus, scotoma and reduced vision have been observed. Very rarely a transient loss of vision has been reported. However, visual disorders may also occur during a migraine attack itself.

Hypersensitivity/Skin: Hypersensitivity reactions ranging from cutaneous hypersensitivity to rare cases of anaphylaxis.

Laboratory values: Minor disturbances in liver function tests have occasionally been observed.

Overdose: Single doses, of sumatriptan, up to 40 mg intranasally and in excess of 16 mg subcutaneously and 400 mg orally have not been associated with side effects other than those mentioned.

In clinical studies volunteers have received 20 mg of sumatriptan by the intranasal route three times a day for a period of 4 days without significant adverse effects.

If overdosage occurs, the patient should be monitored for at least ten hours and standard supportive treatment applied as required. It is unknown what effect haemodialysis or peritoneal dialysis has on the plasma concentrations of sumatriptan.

Pharmacological properties

Pharmacodynamic properties: Pharmacotherapeutic group: Selective $5HT_1$ receptor agonists. ATC code: N02CC01.

Sumatriptan has been demonstrated to be a selective vascular 5-hydroxytryptamine-1-($5HT_{1d}$) receptor agonist with no effect at other 5HT receptor ($5HT_2$-$5HT_7$) subtypes. The vascular $5HT_{1d}$ receptor is found predominantly in cranial blood vessels and mediates vasoconstriction. In animals sumatriptan selectively constricts the carotid arterial circulation. The carotid arterial circulation supplies blood to the extracranial and intracranial tissues such as the meninges and dilatation and/or oedema formation in these vessels is thought to be the underlying mechanism of migraine in man. In addition, evidence from animal studies suggests that sumatriptan inhibits trigeminal nerve activity. Both these actions (cranial vasoconstriction and inhibition of trigeminal nerve activity) may contribute to the anti-migraine action of sumatriptan in humans.

Clinical response begins 15 minutes following a 20 mg dose given by intra-nasal administration.

Because of its route of administration Imigran Nasal Spray may be particularly suitable for patients who suffer with nausea and vomiting during an attack.

Pharmacokinetic properties: After intranasal administration, sumatriptan is rapidly absorbed, maximum plasma concentration occurring in 1–1.5 hours. After a 20 mg dose, the mean maximum concentration is 13 ng/ml. Mean intranasal bioavailability, relative to subcutaneous administration is about 16%, partly due to pre-systemic metabolism.

Following oral administration, pre-systemic clearance is reduced in patients with hepatic impairment resulting in increased plasma levels of sumatriptan, a similar increase would be expected following intranasal administration.

Plasma protein binding is low (14–21%), the mean total volume of distribution is 170 litres. The elimination half-life is approximately 2 hours. The mean plasma clearance is approximately 1160 ml/min and the mean renal plasma clearance is approximately 260 ml/min. Non-renal clearance accounts for about 80% of the total clearance. Sumatriptan is eliminated primarily by oxidative metabolism mediated by monoamine oxidase A. The major metabolite, the indole acetic acid analogue of sumatriptan is mainly excreted in urine, where it is present as a free acid and the glucuronide conjugate. It has no known $5HT_1$ or $5HT_2$ activity. Minor metabolites have not been identified. The pharmacokinetics of intra-nasal sumatriptan do not appear to be significantly affected by migraine attacks.

The kinetics in the elderly have been insufficiently studied to justify a statement on possible differences in kinetics between elderly and young volunteers.

Preclinical safety data: In studies carried out to test for local and ocular irritancy, following administration of sumatriptan nasal spray, there was no nasal irritancy seen in laboratory animals and no ocular irritancy observed when the spray was applied directly to the eyes of rabbits.

In a rat fertility study a reduction in success of insemination was seen at exposures sufficiently in excess of the maximum human exposure. In rabbits embryolethality, without marked teratogenic defects, was seen. The relevance for humans of these findings is unknown.

Sumatriptan was devoid of genotoxic and carcinogenic activity in *in vitro* systems and animal studies.

Pharmaceutical particulars

List of excipients: Potassium Dihydrogen Phosphate PhEur, Dibasic Sodium Phosphate Anhydrous USP, Sulphuric Acid BP, Sodium Hydroxide PhEur, Purified Water PhEur.

Incompatibilities: None reported.

Shelf life: 2 years.

Special precautions for storage: Imigran Nasal Spray should be stored between 2–30°C. It should be kept in the sealed blister, preferably in the box, to protect from light.

Nature and contents of container: The container consists of a vial with rubber stopper and applicator. Imigran Nasal 20 mg: unit dose spray device containing 0.1 ml solution. Pack with 2 and 6 sprays.

Instructions for use/handling: See patient information leaflet.

Marketing authorisation number 10949/0261

Date of approval/revision of SPC December 1996

IMIGRAN* TABLETS

Presentation Imigran Tablets 100 mg: white, capsule-shaped, biconvex film-coated tablets engraved 'Imigran' on one face and 'Glaxo' on the other. Each tablet contains 100 mg sumatriptan base (as the succinate salt).

Imigran Tablets 50 mg: pink, capsule-shaped, biconvex film-coated tablets engraved 'Imigran' on one face and '50' on the other. Each tablet contains 50 mg sumatriptan base (as the succinate salt). The 50 mg tablets may also be marked with '50' on one side and blank on the other.

Uses

Indications: Imigran Tablets are indicated for the acute relief of migraine attacks, with or without aura. Imigran should only be used where there is a clear diagnosis of migraine.

Mode of action/pharmacology: Sumatriptan has been demonstrated to be a selective 5-hydroxytryptamine-1D ($5\text{-}HT_{1D}$) receptor agonist with no effect on other 5-HT receptor ($5\text{-}HT_2$-$5\text{-}HT_7$) subtypes. The vascular 5-HT_{1D} receptor is found predominantly in cranial blood vessels and mediates vasoconstriction. In animals, sumatriptan selectively constricts the carotid arterial circulation but does not alter cerebral blood flow. The carotid arterial circulation supplies blood to the extracranial and intracranial tissues such as the meninges and dilatation of and/or oedema formation in these vessels is thought to be the underlying mechanism of migraine in man.

In addition, evidence from animal studies suggests that sumatriptan inhibits trigeminal nerve activity. Both these actions (cranial vasoconstriction and inhibition of trigeminal nerve activity) may contribute to the anti-migraine action of Sumatriptan in humans.

Clinical response begins around 30 minutes following a 100 mg oral dose.

Although the recommended dose of oral Sumatriptan is 50 mg, migraine attacks vary in severity both within and between patients. Doses of 25–100 mg have shown greater efficacy than placebo in clinical trials, but 25 mg is statistically significantly less effective than 50 and 100 mg.

Dosage and administration Imigran should not be used prophylactically.

Imigran should be given as early as possible after the onset of an attack of migraine but it is equally effective at whatever stage of the attack it is administered.

The recommended dose of oral Imigran is a single 50 mg tablet. Some patients may require 100 mg. If the patient has responded to the first dose but the symptoms recur a second dose may be given in the next 24 hours provided that there is a minimum interval of two hours between the two doses and not more than 300 mg is taken in any 24 hour period.

Patients who do not respond to the prescribed dose of Imigran should not take a second dose for the same attack. Imigran may be taken for subsequent attacks.

Imigran is recommended as monotherapy for the acute treatment of migraine and should not be given concomitantly with other acute migraine therapies. If a patient fails to respond to a single dose of Imigran there are no reasons, either on theoretical grounds or from limited clinical experience, to withhold products containing aspirin or non-steroidal anti-inflammatory drugs or paracetamol for further treatment of the attack.

The tablets should be swallowed whole with water.

Children: The safety and effectiveness of Imigran in children has not yet been established.

Elderly (Over 65): Experience of the use of Imigran in patients aged over 65 years is limited. The pharmacokinetics do not differ significantly from a younger population but until further clinical data are available, the use of Imigran in patients aged over 65 years is not recommended.

Contra-indications, warnings, etc

Contra-indications: Hypersensitivity to any component of the preparation.

Sumatriptan should not be given to patients who have had myocardial infarction or have ischaemic heart disease, coronary vasospasm (Prinzmetal's angina), peripheral vascular disease or patients who have symptoms or signs consistent with ischaemic heart disease.

Sumatriptan should not be administered to patients with a history of cerebrovascular accident (CVA) or transient ischaemic attack (TIA).

Sumatriptan should not be administered to patients with severe hepatic impairment.

The use of sumatriptan in patients with uncontrolled hypertension is contra-indicated.

The concomitant administration of ergotamine or derivatives of ergotamine (including methysergide) is contra-indicated (see *Interactions*).

Concurrent administration of monoamine oxidase inhibitors and sumatriptan is contra-indicated.

Imigran Injection must not be used within two weeks of discontinuation of therapy with monoamine oxidase inhibitors.

Warnings: Imigran should only be used where there is a clear diagnosis of migraine.

Sumatriptan is not indicated for use in the management of hemiplegic, basilar or ophthalmoplegic migraine.

The recommended doses of Sumatriptan should not be exceeded.

As with other migraine therapies, before treating headaches in patients not previously diagnosed as migraineurs, and in migraineurs who present with atypical symptoms, care should be taken to exclude other potentially serious neurological conditions.

It should be noted that migraineurs may be at risk of certain cerebrovascular events (e.g. cerebrovascular accident, transient ischaemic attack).

Following administration, sumatriptan can be associated with transient symptoms including chest pain and tightness which may be intense and involve the throat. Where such symptoms are thought to indicate ischaemic heart disease, appropriate evaluation should be carried out.

Sumatriptan should therefore not be given to patients in whom unrecognised cardiac disease is likely without a prior evaluation for underlying cardiovascular disease. Such patients include post menopausal women, males over 40 and patients with risk factors for coronary artery disease.

Drowsiness may occur as a result of migraine or its treatment with Sumatriptan. Caution is recommended in patients performing skilled tasks, e.g. driving or operating machinery.

Precautions: Sumatriptan should be administered with caution to patients with controlled hypertension as transient increases in blood pressure and peripheral vascular resistance have been observed in a small proportion of patients.

There have been rare post-marketing reports describing patients with weakness, hyperreflexia, and incoordination following the use of a selective serotonin reuptake inhibitor (SSRI) and sumatriptan. If concomitant treatment with sumatriptan and an SSRI is clinically warranted, appropriate observation of the patient is advised.

Sumatriptan should be administered with caution to patients with conditions which may affect significantly the absorption, metabolism or excretion of the drug e.g. impaired hepatic or renal function. A 50 mg dose should be considered in patients with hepatic impairment.

Patients with known hypersensitivity to sulphonamides may exhibit an allergic reaction following administration of sumatriptan. Reactions may range from cutaneous hypersensitivity to anaphylaxis. Evidence of cross-sensitivity is limited, however, caution should be exercised before using sumatriptan in these patients.

Pregnancy: The safety of this medicinal product for use in human pregnancy has not been established. Evaluation of experimental animal studies does not indicate direct teratogenic effects or harmful effects on peri- and postnatal development.

When administered to pregnant rabbits throughout the period of organogenesis sumatriptan has occasionally caused embryolethality at doses which were sufficiently high to produce maternal toxicity.

In a rat fertility study oral doses of sumatriptan resulting in plasma levels approximately 200 times those seen in man after a 100 mg oral dose were associated with a reduction in the success of insemination. This effect did not occur during a subcutaneous study where maximum plasma levels achieved approximately 150 times those in man by the oral route.

As yet, experience of the use of sumatriptan during human pregnancy is limited. Although animal reproduction studies are not always predictive of human response, administration of this drug is not recommended during pregnancy unless the expected benefit to the mother is greater than any possible risk to the foetus.

It has been demonstrated that following subcutaneous administration, sumatriptan is excreted into breast milk. Infant exposure can be minimised by avoiding breast feeding for 24 hours after treatment.

Side effects: Side effects which have been reported include the following:

General: Pain, sensations of tingling, heat, heaviness, pressure or tightness. These symptoms are usually transient and may be intense and can affect any part of the body including the chest and throat. Flushing, dizziness, paraesthesia, and feelings of weakness. These are mostly mild to moderate in intensity and transient. Fatigue and drowsiness have been reported.

Cardiovascular: Hypotension, bradycardia, tachycardia, palpitations.

Transient increases in blood pressure arising soon after treatment have been recorded.

In extremely rare cases, serious coronary events have been reported which have included cardiac arrhythmias, ischaemic ECG changes or myocardial infarction.

Gastrointestinal: Nausea and vomiting occurred in some patients but the relationship to Sumatriptan is not clear.

CNS: There have been rare reports of seizures following use of sumatriptan. Although some have occurred in patients with either a history of seizures or concurrent conditions predisposing to seizures there are also reports in patients where no such predisposing factors are apparent.

Eye disorders: Patients treated with Imigran rarely exhibit visual disorders like flickering and diplopia. Additionally, cases of nystagmus, scotoma and reduced vision have been observed. Very rarely, a transient loss of vision has been reported. However, visual disorders may occur during a migraine attack itself.

Hypersensitivity: Hypersensitivity reactions ranging from cutaneous hypersensitivity to, in rare cases, anaphylaxis.

Laboratory values: Minor disturbances in liver function tests have occasionally been observed.

Interactions: Studies in healthy subjects show that Sumatriptan does not interact with propranolol, flunarizine, pizotifen or alcohol. Sumatriptan has the potential to interact with MAOIs, ergotamine and derivatives of ergotamine. The increased risk of coronary vasospasm is a theoretical possibility and concomitant administration is contra-indicated (see also *Contra-indications*).

Prolonged vasospastic reactions have been reported with ergotamine. As these effects may be additive, 24 hours should elapse before sumatriptan can be taken following any ergotamine-containing preparation. Conversely, ergotamine-containing preparations should not be taken until 6 hours have elapsed following sumatriptan administration.

Rarely, an interaction may occur between sumatriptan and SSRIs (see *Contra-indications, warnings, etc*).

Overdosage: There have been some reports of overdosage with Imigran Tablets. Doses in excess of 400 mg orally were not associated with side effects other than those mentioned.

If overdosage with Imigran occurs, the patient should be monitored for at least ten hours and standard supportive treatment applied as required.

It is unknown what effect haemodialysis or peritoneal dialysis has on the plasma concentrations of Imigran.

Pharmaceutical precautions Imigran Tablets should be stored below 30°C.

Legal category POM.

Package quantities Imigran Tablets: A double foil blister pack of 2, 3, 6, or 12 tablets in a wallet with an outer carton.

Further information
Pharmacokinetics: Following oral administration, Imigran is rapidly absorbed, 70% of maximum concentration occurring at 45 minutes. After 100 mg dose the mean maximum plasma concentration is 54 ng/ml. Mean absolute oral bioavailability is 14% partly due to pre-systemic metabolism and partly due to incomplete absorption. The elimination phase half-life is approximately 2 hours, although there is an indication of a longer terminal phase. Plasma protein binding is low (14–21%), mean volume of distribution is 170 litres. Mean total plasma clearance is approximately 1160 ml/min and the mean renal plasma clearance is approximately 260 ml/min. Non-renal clearance accounts for about 80% of the total clearance. Sumatriptan is eliminated primarily by oxidative metabolism mediated by monoamine oxidase A. The major metabolite, the indole acetic acid analogue of sumatriptan is mainly excreted in the urine, where it is present as a free acid and the glucuronide conjugate. It has no known $5HT_1$ or $5HT_2$ activity. Minor metabolites have not been identified. The pharmacokinetics of oral sumatriptan do not appear to be significantly affected by migraine attacks.

In a pilot study no significant differences were found in the pharmacokinetic parameters between the elderly and young healthy volunteers.

Product licence numbers
Imigran Tablets 100 mg 10949/0231
Imigran Tablets 50 mg 10949/0222

IMURAN* INJECTION

Qualitative and quantitative composition Azathioprine EP 50 mg/ml.

Pharmaceutical form Injection.

Clinical particulars
Therapeutic indications: Imuran is used as an immunosuppressant antimetabolite either alone or, more commonly, in combination with other agents (usually corticosteroids) and procedures which influence the immune response. Therapeutic effect may be evident only after weeks or months and can include a steroid-sparing effect, thereby reducing the toxicity associated with high dosage and prolonged usage of corticosteroids.

Imuran, in combination with corticosteroids and/or other immunosuppressive agents and procedures, is indicated to enhance the survival of organ transplants, such as renal transplants, cardiac transplants, and hepatic transplants, and to reduce the corticosteroid requirements of renal transplant recipients.

Imuran, either alone or more usually in combination with corticosteroids and/or other drugs and procedures, has been used with clinical benefit (which may include reduction of dosage or discontinuation of corticosteroids) in a proportion of patients suffering from the following:

severe rheumatoid arthritis;
systemic lupus erythematosus;
dermatomyositis and polymyositis;
auto-immune chronic active hepatitis;
pemphigus vulgaris;
polyarteritis nodosa;
auto-immune haemolytic anaemia;
chronic refractory idiopathic thrombocytopenic purpura.

Posology and method of administration: Imuran Injection should be used ONLY when the oral route is impractical, and should be discontinued as soon as oral therapy is tolerated. It must be administered only by the intravenous route.

Specialist medical literature should be consulted for guidance as to clinical experience in particular conditions.

Dosage in transplantation – adults and children: Depending on the immunosuppressive regimen employed, a dosage of up to 5 mg/kg bodyweight/day may be given on the first day of therapy, either orally or intravenously.

Maintenance dosage should range from 1 to 4 mg/kg bodyweight/day and must be adjusted according to clinical requirements and haematological tolerance.

Evidence indicates that Imuran therapy should be maintained indefinitely, even if only low doses are necessary, because of the risk of graft rejection.

Dosage in other conditions – adults and children: In general, starting dosage is from 1 to 3 mg/kg bodyweight/day, and should be adjusted, within these limits, depending on the clinical response (which may not be evident for weeks or months) and haematological tolerance.

When therapeutic response is evident, consideration should be given to reducing the maintenance dosage to the lowest level compatible with the maintenance of that response. If no improvement occurs in the patient's condition within 3 months, consideration should be given to withdrawing Imuran.

The maintenance dosage required may range from less than 1 mg/kg bodyweight/day to 3 mg/kg bodyweight/day, depending on the clinical condition being treated and the individual patient response, including haematological tolerance.

In patients with renal and/or hepatic insufficiency, dosages should be given at the lower end of the normal range (see *Precautions* for further details).

Use in the elderly: (see *Renal and/or hepatic insufficiency*): There is a limited experience of the administration of Imuran to elderly patients. Although the available data do not provide evidence that the incidence of side effects among elderly patients is higher than that among other patients treated with Imuran, it is recommended that the dosages used should be at the lower end of the range.

Particular care should be taken to monitor haematological response and to reduce the maintenance dosage to the minimum required for clinical response.

Reconstitution and dilution of Imuran Injection: Precautions should always be taken when handling Imuran Injection (see *Instructions for use/handling*).

No antimicrobial preservative is included. Therefore, reconstitution and dilution must be carried out under full aseptic conditions, preferably immediately before use. Any unused solution should be discarded.

The contents of each vial should be reconstituted by the addition of 5 ml to 15 ml of Water for Injections BP. The reconstituted solution is stable for up to 5 days when stored between 5°C and 25°C.

When diluted on the basis of 5 ml of reconstituted solution to a volume of between 20 ml and 200 ml of one of the following infusion solutions, Imuran is stable for up to 24 hours at room temperature (15°C to 25°C):

Sodium Chloride Intravenous Infusion BP (0.45% w/v and 0.9% w/v).
Sodium Chloride (0.18% w/v) and Glucose (4.0% w/v) Intravenous Infusion BP.

Should any visible turbidity or crystallisation appear in the reconstituted or diluted solution the preparation must be discarded.

Imuran Injection should ONLY be reconstituted with the recommended volume of Water for Injections BP and should be diluted as specified above. Imuran Injection should not be mixed with other drugs or fluids, except those specified above, before administration.

Administration of Imuran Injection: Imuran Injection, when reconstituted as directed, is a very irritant solution with a pH of 10–12.

When the reconstituted solution is diluted as directed above, the pH of the resulting solution may be expected to be within the range pH 8.0 to 9.5 (the greater the dilution, the lower the pH).

Where dilution is not practicable, the reconstituted solution should be injected slowly over a period of not less than one minute and followed immediately by not less than 50 ml of one of the recommended infusion solutions.

Care must be taken to avoid perivenous injection which may produce tissue damage.

Contra-indications: Imuran is contra-indicated in patients known to be hypersensitive to azathioprine. Hypersensitivity to 6-mercaptopurine (6-MP) should alert the prescriber to probable hypersensitivity to Imuran.

Imuran therapy should not be initiated in patients who may be pregnant, or who are likely to become pregnant in the near future (see *Precautions*).

Special warnings and precautions for use: There are potential hazards in the use of Imuran. It should be prescribed only if the patient can be adequately monitored for toxic effects throughout the duration of therapy.

It is suggested that during the first 8 weeks of therapy, complete blood counts, including platelets, should be performed weekly or more frequently if high dosage is used or if severe renal and/or hepatic disorder is present. The blood count frequency may be reduced later in therapy, but it is suggested that complete blood counts are repeated monthly, or at least at intervals of not longer than 3 months.

Patients receiving Imuran should be instructed to report immediately any evidence of infection, unexpected bruising or bleeding or other manifestations of bone marrow depression.

There are rare individuals with an inherited deficiency of the enzyme thiopurine methyltransferase (TPMT) who may be unusually sensitive to the myelosuppressive effect of azathioprine and prone to developing rapid bone marrow depression following the initiation of treatment with Imuran.

Renal and/or hepatic insufficiency: It has been suggested that the toxicity of Imuran may be enhanced in the presence of renal insufficiency, but controlled studies have not supported this suggestion. Nevertheless, it is recommended that the dosages used should be at the lower end of the normal range and that haematological response should be carefully monitored. Dosage should be further reduced if haematological toxicity occurs.

Caution is necessary during the administration of Imuran to patients with hepatic dysfunction, and regular complete blood counts and liver function tests should be undertaken. In such patients the metabolism of Imuran may be impaired, and the dosage of Imuran should therefore be reduced to the lower end of the recommended range. Dosage should be further reduced if hepatic or haematological toxicity occurs.

Limited evidence suggests that Imuran is not beneficial to patients with hypoxanthine-guanine-phosphoribosyltransferase deficiency (Lesch-Nyhan syndrome). Therefore, given the abnormal metabolism in these patients, it is not prudent to recommend that these patients should receive Imuran.

Mutagenicity: Chromosomal abnormalities have been demonstrated in both male and female patients treated with Imuran. It is difficult to assess the role of Imuran in the development of these abnormalities.

Chromosomal abnormalities, which disappear with time, have been demonstrated in lymphocytes from the offspring of patients treated with Imuran. Except in extremely rare cases, no overt physical evidence of abnormality has been observed in the offspring of patients treated with Imuran. Azathioprine and long–wave ultraviolet light have been shown to have a synergistic clastogenic effect in patients treated with azathioprine for a range of disorders.

Teratogenicity: Studies in pregnant rats, mice and rabbits using azathioprine in dosages from 5 to 15 mg/kg bodyweight/day over the period of organogenesis have shown varying degrees of foetal abnormalities. Teratogenicity was evident in rabbits at 10 mg/kg bodyweight/day.

Evidence of the teratogenicity of Imuran in man is equivocal. As with all cytotoxic chemotherapy, adequate contraceptive precautions should be advised when either partner is receiving Imuran.

Carcinogenicity: There is no clear evidence that, in therapeutic doses, Imuran *per se* is oncogenic in man, but the issue remains unresolved.

The risk of developing post-transplant lymphomas is increased in patients who receive aggressive treatment with immunosuppressive drugs, and such therapy should be maintained at the lowest effective levels. The increased risk of developing lymphomas in immunosuppressed rheumatoid arthritis patients compared with the general population appears to be related at least in part to the disease itself. There have been reports of increased incidences of skin cancers in renal transplant recipients compared with the general population, which may be in part associated with immunosuppressive therapy.

Effects on fertility: Relief of chronic renal insufficiency by renal transplantation involving the administration of Imuran has been accompanied by increased fertility in both male and female transplant recipients.

Interaction with other medicaments and other forms of interaction:

Allopurinol/oxipurinol/thiopurinol: Xanthine oxidase activity is inhibited by allopurinol, oxipurinol and thiopurinol which results in reduced conversion of biologically active 6-thioinosinic acid to biologically inactive 6-thioric acid. When allopurinol, oxipurinol and/or thiopurinol are given concomitantly with 6-mercaptopurine or azathioprine, the dose of 6-mercaptopurine and azathioprine should be reduced to one-quarter of the original dose.

Neuromuscular blocking agents: Imuran can potentiate the neuromuscular blockade produced by depolarising agents such as succinylcholine and can reduce the blockade produced by non-depolarising agents such as tubocurarine. There is considerable variation in the potency of this interaction.

Warfarin: Inhibition of the anticoagulant effect of warfarin, when administered with azathioprine, has been reported.

Cytostatic/myelosuppressive agents: Where possible, concomitant administration of cytostatic drugs, or drugs which may have a myelosuppressive effect, such as penicillamine, should be avoided. There are conflicting clinical reports of interactions, resulting in serious haematological abnormalities, between Imuran and co-trimoxazole.

There has been a case report suggesting that haematological abnormalities may develop due to the concomitant administration of Imuran and captopril.

It has been suggested that cimetidine and indomethacin may have myelosuppressive effects which may be enhanced by concomitant administration of Imuran.

Other interactions: Frusemide has been shown to impair the metabolism of azathioprine by human hepatic tissue *in vitro*. The clinical significance is unknown.

Vaccines: The immunosuppressive activity of Imuran could result in an atypical and potentially deleterious response to live vaccines and so the administration of live vaccines to patients receiving Imuran therapy is contra-indicated on theoretical grounds.

A diminished response to killed vaccines is likely and such a response to hepatitis B vaccine has been observed among patients treated with a combination of azathioprine and corticosteroids.

A small clinical study has indicated that standard therapeutic doses of Imuran do not deleteriously affect the response to polyvalent pneumococcal vaccine, as assessed on the basis of mean anti-capsular specific antibody concentration.

Pregnancy and lactation: Imuran should not be given during pregnancy without careful assessment of risk versus benefit.

Azathioprine and/or its metabolites have been found in low concentrations in foetal blood and amniotic fluid after maternal administration of azathioprine.

Leucopenia and/or thrombocytopenia have been reported in a proportion of neonates whose mothers took azathioprine throughout their pregnancies. Extra care in haematological monitoring is advised during pregnancy.

6-mercaptopurine has been identified in the colostrum and breast-milk of women receiving azathioprine treatment.

Effects on ability to drive and use machines: None known.

Undesirable effects:

Hypersensitivity reactions: Several different clinical syndromes, which appear to be idiosyncratic manifestations of hypersensitivity, have been described occasionally following administration of Imuran. Clinical features include general malaise, dizziness, nausea, vomiting, diarrhoea, fever, rigors, exanthema, rash, myalgia, arthralgia, renal dysfunction and hypotension. In many cases, rechallenge has confirmed an association with Imuran.

Immediate withdrawal of azathioprine and institution of circulatory support where appropriate have led to recovery in the majority of cases. Other marked underlying pathology has contributed to the very rare deaths reported.

Following a hypersensitivity reaction to Imuran, the necessity for continued administration of Imuran should be carefully considered on an individual basis.

Haematopoiesis: Therapeutic use of Imuran may be associated with a dose-related, generally reversible, depression of bone marrow function, most frequently expressed as leucopenia, but also sometimes as anaemia and thrombocytopenia.

Reversible, dose-related increases in mean corpuscular volume and red cell haemoglobin content have occurred in association with Imuran therapy. Megaloblastic bone marrow changes have also been observed but severe megaloblastic anaemia and erythroid hypoplasia are rare.

Failure to reduce the dosage of Imuran in the presence of allopurinol can result in severe bone marrow suppression and pancytopenia.

Susceptibility to infection: Transplant recipients receiving Imuran and corticosteroids have shown increased susceptibility to viral, fungal and bacterial infections evident both in skin and other body systems. The use of Imuran in other conditions does not appear to give rise to a marked increase in susceptibility to such infections.

Gastro-intestinal reactions: A minority of patients experience nausea when first given Imuran. This appears to be relieved by administering the tablets after meals.

Serious complications, including colitis, diverticulitis and bowel perforation, have been described in transplant recipients receiving immunosuppressive therapy. However, the aetiology is not clearly established and high-dose corticosteroids may be implicated. Severe diarrhoea, recurring on rechallenge, has been reported in patients treated with Imuran for inflammatory bowel disease. The possibility that exacerbation of symptoms might be drug-related should be borne in mind when treating such patients.

Pancreatitis has been reported in a small percentage of patients on Imuran therapy, particularly in renal transplant patients and those diagnosed as having inflammatory bowel disease. There are difficulties in relating the pancreatitis to the administration of one particular drug, although rechallenge has confirmed an association with Imuran on occasions.

Cholestasis and deterioration of liver function have occasionally been reported in association with Imuran therapy and are usually reversible on withdrawal of therapy.

A rare, but life-threatening hepatic veno-occlusive disease associated with chronic administration of azathioprine has been described, primarily in transplant patients. In some cases withdrawal of azathioprine has resulted in either a temporary or permanent improvement in liver histology and symptoms.

Pulmonary reactions: Reversible pneumonitis has been described very rarely.

Alopecia: Hair loss has been described on a number of occasions in patients receiving azathioprine and other immunosuppressive agents. In many instances the condition resolved spontaneously despite continuing therapy. The relationship between alopecia and azathioprine treatment is uncertain.

Overdose:

Symptoms and signs: Unexplained infection, ulceration of the throat, bruising and bleeding are the main signs of overdosage with Imuran and result from bone marrow depression which may be maximal after 9 to 14 days. These signs are more likely to be manifest following chronic overdosage, rather than after a single acute overdose. There has been a report of a patient who ingested a single overdose of 7.5 g of azathioprine. The immediate toxic effects of this overdose were nausea, vomiting and diarrhoea, followed by mild leucopenia and mild abnormalities in liver function. Recovery was uneventful.

Treatment: There is no specific antidote. Gastric lavage has been used. Subsequent monitoring, including haematological monitoring, is necessary to allow prompt treatment of any adverse effects which may develop. The value of dialysis in patients who have taken an overdose of Imuran is not known, though azathioprine is partially dialysable.

Pharmacological properties

Pharmacodynamic properties: Azathioprine is an imidazole derivative of 6-mercaptopurine (6-MP). It is rapidly broken down *in vivo* into 6-MP and a methylnitroimidazole moiety. The 6-MP readily crosses cell membranes and is converted intracellularly into a number of purine thioanalogues, which include the main active nucleotide, thioinosinic acid. The rate of conversion varies from one person to another. Nucleotides do not traverse cell membranes and therefore do not circulate in body fluids. Irrespective of whether it is given directly or is derived *in vivo* from azathioprine, 6-MP is eliminated mainly as the inactive oxidised metabolite thiouric acid. This oxidation is brought about by xanthine oxidase, an enzyme which is inhibited by allopurinol. The activity of the methylnitroimidazole moiety has not been defined clearly. However, in several systems it appears to modify the activity of azathioprine as compared with that of 6-MP. Determinations of plasma concentrations of azathioprine or 6-MP have no prognostic value as regards effectiveness or toxicity of these compounds.

Mode of action: While the precise modes of action remain to be elucidated, some suggested mechanisms include:

1. The release of 6-MP which acts as a purine antimetabolite.
2. The possible blockade of -SH groups by alkylation.
3. The inhibition of many pathways in nucleic acid biosynthesis, hence preventing proliferation of cells involved in determination and amplification of the immune response.
4. Damage to deoxyribonucleic acid (DNA) through incorporation of purine thio-analogues.

Because of these mechanisms, the therapeutic effect of Imuran may be evident only after several weeks or months of treatment.

Imuran appears to be well absorbed from the upper gastro-intestinal tract.

Studies in mice with ^{35}S-azathioprine showed no unusually large concentration in any particular tissue, but there was very little ^{35}S found in brain.

Plasma levels of azathioprine and 6-mercaptopurine do not correlate well with the therapeutic efficacy or toxicity of Imuran.

Pharmacokinetic properties: Azathioprine is well absorbed following oral administration. After oral administration of ^{35}S-azathioprine, the maximum plasma radioactivity occurs at 1–2 hours and decays with half-life of 4–6 hours. This is not an estimate of the half-life of azathioprine itself, but reflects the elimination from plasma of azathioprine and the ^{35}S-containing metabolites of the drug. As a consequence of the rapid and extensive metabolism of azathioprine, only a fraction of the radioactivity measured in plasma is comprised of unmetabolised drug. Studies in which the plasma concentrations of azathioprine and 6-mercaptopurine have been determined following intravenous administration of azathioprine have estimated the mean plasma $T_{\frac{1}{2}}$ for azathioprine to be in the range of 6–28 minutes and the mean plasma $T_{\frac{1}{2}}$ for 6-MP to be in the range 38–114 minutes after iv administration of the drug.

Azathioprine is principally excreted as 6-thioric uric acid in the urine. 1-methyl-4-nitro-5-thioimidazole has also been detected in urine as a minor excretory product. This would indicate that, rather than azathioprine being exclusively cleaved by nucleophilic attack at the 5-position of the nitroimidazole ring to generate 6-mercaptopurine and 1-methyl-4-nitro-5-(s-glutathionyl)imidazole, a small proportion of the drug may be cleaved between the s-atom and the purine ring. Only a small amount of the dose of azathioprine administered is excreted unmetablished in the urine.

Preclinical safety data: None.

Pharmaceutical particulars

List of excipients: Sodium hydroxide pellets* BP 7.2 mg; Sodium hydroxide pellets* to adjust pH; Water for injections EP.

* In the form of a IM solution in water for injections.

Incompatibilities: Imuran Injection should ONLY be reconstituted with the recommended volume of Water for Injections BP and should be diluted as specified above. Imuran Injection should not be mixed with other drugs or fluids, except those specified above, before administration.

Shelf life: 3 years unopened.

5 days when reconstituted with 5 ml to 15 ml water for injections and stored at 5 to 25°C.

1 day for 5 ml of the reconstituted injection further diluted with between 20 ml and 200 ml of an appropriate infusion solution and stored at 15°C to 25°C.

Special precautions for storage: Store below 25°C. Keep dry. Protect from light.

Nature and contents of container: Neutral glass vials with synthetic butyl rubber closures and aluminium collars. Each vial contains the equivalent of 50 mg azathioprine.

Instructions for use/handling:

Safe handling of Imuran Injection: Health professionals who handle Imuran Injection should follow guidelines for the handling of cytotoxic drugs according to prevailing local recommendations and/or regulations (for example, the Royal Pharmaceutical Society of Great Britain Working Party Report on the Handling of Cytotoxic Drugs, 1983).

Marketing authorisation number PL 0003/5043R

Date of first authorisation/renewal of authorisation
MAA: 13.03.85 (reviewed licence)
Renewal: 28.03.91

Date of (partial) revision of text February 1997

IMURAN* TABLETS 25 mg
IMURAN* TABLETS 50 mg

Qualitative and quantitative composition Orange, round, biconvex, film-coated tablets, impressed 'L3C' and containing 25 mg Azathioprine BP in each tablet.

Yellow, round, biconvex, scored, film-coated tablets, impressed 'WELLCOME K7A' and containing 50 mg Azathioprine BP in each tablet.

Pharmaceutical form Tablet.

Clinical particulars

Therapeutic indications: Imuran tablets are used as an immunosuppressant antimetabolite either alone or, more commonly, in combination with other agents (usually corticosteroids) and procedures which influence the immune response. Therapeutic effect may be evident only after weeks or months and can include a steroid-sparing effect, thereby reducing the toxicity associated with high dosage and prolonged usage of corticosteroids.

Imuran, in combination with corticosteroids and/or other immunosuppressive agents and procedures, is indicated to enhance the survival of organ transplants, such as renal transplants, cardiac transplants, and hepatic transplants; and to reduce the corticosteroid requirements of renal transplant recipients.

Imuran, either alone or more usually in combination with corticosteroids and/or other drugs and procedures, has been used with clinical benefit (which may include reduction of dosage or discontinuation of corticosteroids) in a proportion of patients suffering from the following:

severe rheumatoid arthritis;
systemic lupus erythematosus;
dermatomyositis and polymyositis;
auto-immune chronic active hepatitis;
pemphigus vulgaris;
polyarteritis nodosa;
auto-immune haemolytic anaemia;
chronic refractory idiopathic thrombocytopenic purpura.

Route of administration: Oral.

Posology and method of administration:

Transplantation – adults and children: Depending on the immunosuppressive regimen employed, a dosage of up to 5 mg/kg bodyweight/day may be given on the first day of therapy, either orally or intravenously.

Maintenance dosage should range from 1 to 4 mg/kg bodyweight/day and must be adjusted according to clinical requirements and haematological tolerance.

Evidence indicates that Imuran therapy should be maintained indefinitely, even if only low doses are necessary, because of the risk of graft rejection.

Dosage in other conditions – adults and children: In general, starting dosage is from 1 to 3 mg/kg bodyweight/day, and should be adjusted, within these limits, depending on the clinical response (which may not be evident for weeks or months) and haematological tolerance.

When therapeutic response is evident, consideration should be given to reducing the maintenance dosage to the lowest level compatible with the maintenance of that response. If no improvement occurs in the patient's condition within 3 months, consideration should be given to withdrawing Imuran.

The maintenance dosage required may range from less than 1 mg/kg bodyweight/day to 3 mg/kg bodyweight/day, depending on the clinical condition being treated and the individual patient response, including haematological tolerance.

In patients with renal and/or hepatic insufficiency, dosages should be given at the lower end of the normal range (see *Special warnings and precautions for use* for further details).

Use in the elderly: (see *Renal and/or hepatic insufficiency*): There is a limited experience of the administration of Imuran to elderly patients. Although the available data do not provide evidence that the incidence of side effects among elderly patients is higher than that among other patients treated with Imuran, it is recommended that the dosages used should be at the lower end of the range.

Particular care should be taken to monitor haematological response and to reduce the maintenance dosage to the minimum required for clinical response.

Contra-indications: Imuran is contra-indicated in patients known to be hypersensitive to azathioprine. Hypersensitivity to 6-mercaptopurine (6-MP) should alert the prescriber to probable hypersensitivity to Imuran.

Imuran therapy should not be initiated in patients who may be pregnant, or who are likely to become pregnant in the near future (see *Special warnings and precautions for use*).

Special warnings and precautions for use:

Monitoring: There are potential hazards in the use of Imuran. It should be prescribed only if the patient can be adequately monitored for toxic effects throughout the duration of therapy.

It is suggested that during the first 8 weeks of therapy, complete blood counts, including platelets, should be performed weekly or more frequently if high dosage is used or if severe renal and/or hepatic disorder is present. The blood count frequency may be reduced later in therapy, but it is suggested that complete blood counts are repeated monthly, or at least at intervals of not longer than 3 months.

Patients receiving Imuran should be instructed to report immediately any evidence of infection, unexpected bruising or bleeding or other manifestations of bone marrow depression.

There are rare individuals with an inherited deficiency of the enzyme thiopurine methyltransferase (TPMT) who may be unusually sensitive to the myelosuppressive effect of azathioprine and prone to developing rapid bone marrow depression following the initiation of treatment with Imuran.

Renal and/or hepatic insufficiency: It has been suggested that the toxicity of Imuran may be enhanced in the presence of renal insufficiency, but controlled studies have not supported this suggestion. Nevertheless, it is recommended that the dosages used should be at the lower end of the normal range and that haematological response should be carefully monitored. Dosage should be further reduced if haematological toxicity occurs.

Caution is necessary during the administration of Imuran to patients with hepatic dysfunction, and regular complete blood counts and liver function tests should be undertaken. In such patients the metabolism of Imuran may be impaired, and the dosage of Imuran should therefore be reduced if hepatic or haematological toxicity occurs.

Limited evidence suggests that Imuran is not beneficial to patients with hypoxanthine-guanine-phosphoribosyltransferase deficiency (Lesch-Nyhan syndrome). Therefore, given the abnormal metabolism in these patients, it is not prudent to recommend that these patients should receive Imuran.

Effects on fertility: Relief of chronic renal insufficiency by renal transplantation involving the administration of Imuran has been accompanied by increased fertility in both male and female transplant recipients.

Interaction with other medicaments and other forms of interaction:

Allopurinol/oxipurinol/thiopurinol: Xanthine oxidase activity is inhibited by allopurinol, oxipurinol and thiopurinol which results in reduced conversion of biologically active 6-thioinosinic acid to biologically inactive 6-thiouric acid. When allopurinol, oxipurinol and/or thiopurinol are given concomitantly with 6-mercaptopurine or azathioprine, the dose of 6-mercaptopurine and azathioprine should be reduced to one-quarter of the original dose.

Neuromuscular blocking agents: Imuran can potentiate the neuromuscular blockade produced by depolarising agents such as succinylcholine and can reduce the blockade produced by non-depolarising agents such as tubocurarine. There is considerable variation in the potency of this interaction.

Warfarin: Inhibition of the anticoagulant effect of warfarin, when administered with azathioprine, has been reported.

Cytostatic/myelosuppressive agents: Where possible, concomitant administration of cytostatic drugs, or drugs which may have a myelosuppressive effect, such as penicillamine, should be avoided. There are conflicting clinical reports of interactions, resulting in serious haematological abnormalities, between Imuran and co-trimoxazole.

There has been a case report suggesting that haematological abnormalities may develop due to the concomitant administration of Imuran and captopril.

It has been suggested that cimetidine and indomethacin may have myelosuppressive effects which may be enhanced by concomitant administration of Imuran.

Other interactions: Frusemide has been shown to impair the metabolism of azathioprine by human hepatic tissue *in vitro*. The clinical significance is unknown.

Vaccines: The immunosuppressive activity of Imuran could result in an atypical and potentially deleterious response to live vaccines and so the administration of live vaccines to patients receiving Imuran therapy is contra-indicated on theoretical grounds.

A diminished response to killed vaccines is likely and such a response to hepatitis B vaccine has been observed among patients treated with a combination of azathioprine and corticosteroids.

A small clinical study has indicated that standard therapeutic doses of Imuran do not deleteriously affect the response to polyvalent pneumococcal vaccine, as assessed on the basis of mean anti-capsular specific antibody concentration.

Pregnancy and lactation: Imuran should not be given during pregnancy without careful assessment of risk versus benefit.

Azathioprine and/or its metabolites have been found in low concentrations in foetal blood and amniotic fluid after maternal administration of azathioprine.

Leucopenia and/or thrombocytopenia have been reported in a proportion of neonates whose mothers took azathioprine throughout their pregnancies. Extra care in haematological monitoring is advised during pregnancy.

6-mercaptopurine has been identified in the colostrum and breast-milk of women receiving azathioprine treatment.

Effects on ability to drive and use machines: None known.

Undesirable effects: Several different clinical syndromes, which appear to be idiosyncratic manifestations of hypersensitivity, have been described occasionally following administration of Imuran. Clinical features include general malaise, dizziness, nausea, vomiting, diarrhoea, fever, rigors, exanthema, rash, myalgia, arthralgia, renal dysfunction and hypotension. In many cases, rechallenge has confirmed an association with Imuran.

Immediate withdrawal of azathioprine and institution of circulatory support where appropriate have led to recovery in the majority of cases. Other marked underlying pathology has contributed to the very rare deaths reported.

Following a hypersensitivity reaction to Imuran, the necessity for continued administration of Imuran should be carefully considered on an individual basis.

Haematopoiesis: Therapeutic use of Imuran may be associated with a dose-related, generally reversible, depression of bone marrow function, most frequently expressed as leucopenia, but also sometimes as anaemia and thrombocytopenia.

Reversible, dose-related increases in mean corpuscular volume and red cell haemoglobin content have occurred in association with Imuran therapy. Megaloblastic bone marrow changes have also been observed but severe megaloblastic anaemia and erythroid hypoplasia are rare.

Failure to reduce the dosage of Imuran in the presence of allopurinol can result in severe bone marrow suppression and pancytopenia.

Susceptibility to infection: Transplant recipients receiving Imuran and corticosteroids have shown increased susceptibility to viral, fungal and bacterial infections evident both in skin and other body systems. The use of Imuran in other conditions does not appear to give rise to a marked increase in susceptibility to such infections.

Gastro-intestinal reactions: A minority of patients experience nausea when first given Imuran. This appears to be relieved by administering the tablets after meals.

Serious complications, including colitis, diverticulitis and bowel perforation, have been described in transplant recipients receiving immunosuppressive therapy. However, the aetiology is not clearly established and high-dose corticosteroids may be implicated. Severe diarrhoea, recurring on rechallenge, has been reported in patients treated with Imuran for inflammatory bowel disease. The possibility that exacerbation of symptoms might be drug-related should be borne in mind when treating such patients.

Pancreatitis has been reported in a small percentage of patients on Imuran therapy, particularly in renal transplant patients and those diagnosed as having inflammatory bowel disease. There are difficulties in relating the pancreatitis to the administration of one particular drug, although rechallenge has confirmed an association with Imuran on occasions.

Cholestasis and deterioration of liver function have occasionally been reported in association with Imuran therapy and are usually reversible on withdrawal of therapy.

A rare, but life-threatening hepatic veno-occlusive disease associated with chronic administration of azathioprine has been described, primarily in transplant patients. In some cases withdrawal of azathioprine has resulted in either a temporary or permanent improvement in liver histology and symptoms.

Pulmonary reactions: Reversible pneumonitis has been described very rarely.

Alopecia: Hair loss has been described on a number of occasions in patients receiving azathioprine and other immunosuppressive agents. In many instances the condition resolved spontaneously despite continuing therapy. The relationship between alopecia and azathioprine treatment is uncertain.

Overdose:

Symptoms and signs: Unexplained infection, ulceration of the throat, bruising and bleeding are the main signs of overdosage with Imuran and result from bone marrow depression which may be maximal after 9 to 14 days. These signs are more likely to be manifest following chronic overdosage, rather than after a single acute overdose. There has been a report of a patient who ingested a single overdose of 7.5 g of azathioprine. The immediate toxic effects of this overdose were nausea, vomiting and diarrhoea, followed by mild leucopenia and mild abnormalities in liver function. Recovery was uneventful.

Treatment: There is no specific antidote. Gastric lavage has been used. Subsequent monitoring, including haematological monitoring, is necessary to allow prompt treatment of any adverse effects which may develop. The value of dialysis in patients who have taken an overdose of Imuran is not known, though azathioprine is partially dialysable.

Pharmacological properties

Pharmacodynamic properties: Azathioprine is an imidazole derivative of 6-mercaptopurine (6-MP). It is rapidly broken down *in vivo* into 6-MP and a methylnitroimidazole moiety. The 6-MP readily crosses cell membranes and is converted intracellularly into a number of purine thioanalogues, which include the main active nucleotide, thioinosinic acid. The rate of conversion varies from one person to another. Nucleotides do not traverse cell membranes and therefore do not circulate in body fluids. Irrespective of whether it is given directly or is derived *in vivo* from azathioprine, 6-MP is eliminated mainly as the inactive oxidised metabolite thiouric acid. This oxidation is brought about by xanthine oxidase, an enzyme which is inhibited by allopurinol. The activity of the methylnitroimidazole moiety has not been defined clearly. However, in several systems it appears to modify the activity of azathioprine as compared with that of 6-MP. Determinations of plasma concentrations of azathioprine or 6-MP have no prognostic value as regards effectiveness or toxicity of these compounds.

While the precise modes of action remain to be elucidated, some suggested mechanisms include:

1. The release of 6-MP which acts as a purine antimetabolite.
2. The possible blockade of -SH groups by alkylation.
3. The inhibition of many pathways in nucleic acid biosynthesis, hence preventing proliferation of cells involved in determination and amplification of the immune response.
4. Damage to deoxyribonucleic acid (DNA) through incorporation of purine thio-analogues.

Because of these mechanisms, the therapeutic effect of Imuran may be evident only after several weeks or months of treatment.

Imuran appears to be well absorbed from the upper gastro-intestinal tract.

Studies in mice with ^{35}S-azathioprine showed no unusually large concentration in any particular tissue, but there was very little ^{35}S found in brain.

Plasma levels of azathioprine and 6-mercaptopurine do not correlate well with the therapeutic efficacy or toxicity of Imuran.

Pharmacokinetic properties: Azathioprine is well absorbed following oral administration. After oral administration of ^{35}S-azathioprine, the maximum plasma radioactivity occurs at 1–2 hours and decays with a half-life of 4–6 hours. This is not an estimate of the half-life of azathioprine itself, but reflects the elimination from plasma of azathioprine and the ^{35}S-containing metabolites of the drug. As a consequence of the rapid and extensive metabolism of azathioprine, only a fraction of the radioactivity measured in plasma is comprised of unmetabolised drug. Studies in which the plasma concentration of azathioprine and 6-mercaptopurine have been determined following intravenous administration of azathioprine have estimated the mean plasma $T_{\frac{1}{2}}$ for azathioprine to be in the range of 6–28 minutes and the mean plasma $T_{\frac{1}{2}}$ for 6-MP to be in the range 38–114 minutes after IV administration of the drug.

Azathioprine is principally excreted as 6-thiouric uric acid in the urine. 1-methyl-4-nitro-5-thioimidazole has also been detected in urine as a minor excretory product. This would indicate that, rather than azathioprine being exclusively cleaved by nucleophilic attack at the 5-position of the nitroimidazole ring to generate 6-mercaptopurine and 1-methyl-4-nitro-5-(S-glutathionyl)imidazole. A small proportion of the drug may be cleaved between the S atom and the purine ring. Only a small amount of the dose of azathioprine administered is excreted unmetabolised in the urine.

Preclinical safety data:

Mutagenicity: Chromosomal abnormalities have been demonstrated in both male and female patients treated with Imuran. It is difficult to assess the role of Imuran in the development of these abnormalities.

Chromosomal abnormalities, which disappear with time, have been demonstrated in lymphocytes from the offspring of patients treated with Imuran. Except in extremely rare cases, no overt physical evidence of abnormality has been observed in the offspring of patients treated with Imuran. Azathioprine and long-wave ultraviolet light have been shown to have a synergistic clastogenic effect in patients treated with azathioprine for a range of disorders.

Teratogenicity: Studies in pregnant rats, mice and rabbits using azathioprine in dosages from 5 to 15 mg/kg bodyweight/day over the period of organogenesis have shown varying degrees of foetal abnormalities. Teratogenicity was evident in rabbits at 10 mg/kg bodyweight/day.

Evidence of the teratogenicity of Imuran in man is equivocal. As with all cytotoxic chemotherapy, adequate contraceptive precautions should be advised when either partner is receiving Imuran.

Carcinogenicity: There is no clear evidence that, in therapeutic doses, Imuran *per se* is oncogenic in man, but the issue remains unresolved.

The risk of developing post-transplant lymphomas is increased in patients who receive aggressive treatment with immunosuppressive drugs, and such therapy should be maintained at the lowest effective levels. The increased risk of developing lymphomas in immunosuppressed rheumatoid arthritis patients compared with the general population appears to be related at least in part to the disease itself. There have been reports of increased incidences of skin cancers in renal transplant recipients compared with the general population, which may be in part associated with immunosuppressive therapy.

Pharmaceutical particulars

List of excipients:

Imuran 25 mg Tablets: Lactose, starches, hydrolysed starch, stearic acid, magnesium stearate, methylhydroxylpropyl cellulose, polyethylene glycol 400, titanium dioxide (E171), iron oxide, yellow (E172), iron oxide, red (E172), industrial methylated spirit, purified water.

Imuran 50 mg Tablets: Lactose, starches, hydrolysed starch, stearic acid, magnesium stearate, purified water, methylhydroxylpropyl cellulose, polyethylene glycol 400.

Incompatibilities: None known.

Shelf life: 5 years.

Special precautions for storage: Store below 25°C. Protect from light.

Nature and contents of container: Blister strips in a pack.

Imuran 25 mg Tablets pack size: 28, 30, 56, 60 and 100 tablets.

Imuran 50 mg Tablets pack size: 28, 30, 56, 60, 100 and 1000 tablets.

Instructions for use/handling: Health professionals who handle Imuran Injection should follow guidelines for the handling of cytotoxic drugs (for example, the Royal Pharmaceutical Society of Great Britain Working Party Report on the Handling of Cytotoxic Drugs, 1983).

Provided that the film-coating is intact, there is no risk in handling film-coated Imuran Tablets. Imuran Tablets should not be divided and, provided the coating is intact, no additional precautions are required when handling them.

Marketing authorisation numbers

Imuran Tablets 25 mg PL 0003/0225
Imuran Tablets 50 mg PL 0003/0226

Date of first authorisation/renewal of authorisation 20th March 1992.

Date of (partial) revision of text September 1997

Legal status POM.

LANVIS* TABLETS

Qualitative and quantitative composition 40 mg Thioguanine BP per tablet.

Pharmaceutical form Tablet.

Clinical particulars

Therapeutic indications: Lanvis is indicated primarily for the treatment of acute leukaemias especially acute myelogenous leukaemia and acute lymphoblastic leukaemia.

Lanvis is also used in the treatment of chronic granulocytic leukaemia.

Posology and method of administration:

Route of administration: Oral.

The exact dose and duration of administration will depend on the nature and dosage of other cytotoxic drugs given in conjunction with Lanvis.

Lanvis is variably absorbed following oral administration and plasma levels may be reduced following emesis or intake of food.

Induction therapy:

Adults: The usual dosage of Lanvis is between 100 and 200 mg/m² body surface area, per day on a single or twice-daily dosing regimen over a period of 5 to 20 days.

Children: Similar dosages to those used in adults, with appropriate correction for body surface area, have been used, although lower dosages of 60 to 75 mg/m² body surface area have been employed in some regimens.

Maintenance: For both adults and children, intermittent or continuous daily maintenance doses of between 60 and 200 mg/m² body surface area have been used.

Use in the elderly: There are no specific dosage recommendations in elderly patients (see *Dosage in renal or hepatic impairment*).

Lanvis has been used in various combination chemotherapy schedules in elderly patients with acute leukaemia at equivalent doses to those used in younger patients.

Dosage in renal or hepatic impairment: Consideration should be given to reducing the dosage in patients with impaired hepatic or renal function.

Contra-indications: In view of the seriousness of the indications there are no absolute contra-indications.

Special warnings and precautions for use: Lanvis is an active cytotoxic agent for use only under the direction of physicians experienced in the administration of such agents.

During remission induction, full blood counts must be carried out frequently.

The main side-effect of treatment with Lanvis is bone marrow suppression leading to leucopenia and thrombocytopenia. Patients must be carefully monitored during therapy. The leucocyte and platelet counts continue to fall after treatment is stopped, so at the first sign of an abnormally large fall in these counts, treatment should be temporarily discontinued. Bone marrow suppression is readily reversible if Lanvis is withdrawn early enough. During remission induction in acute myelogenous leukaemia the patient may frequently have to survive a period of relative bone marrow aplasia and it is important that adequate supportive facilities are available. There are individuals with an inherited deficiency of the enzyme thiopurine methyltransferase (TPMT) who may be unusually sensitive to the myelosuppressive effect of thioguanine and prone to developing rapid bone marrow depression following the initiation of treatment with Lanvis. This problem could be exacerbated by coadministration with drugs that inhibit TPMT, such as olsalazine, mesalazine or sulphasalazine.

Patients on myelosuppressive chemotherapy are particularly susceptible to a variety of infections.

During remission induction particularly, when rapid cell lysis is occurring, adequate precautions should be taken to avoid hyperuricaemia and/or hyperuricosuria and the risk of uric acid nephropathy.

In view of its action on cellular DNA, thioguanine is potentially mutagenic and carcinogenic.

It is recommended that the handling of Lanvis Tablets follows the 'Guidelines for the handling of cytotoxic drugs' issued by the Royal Pharmaceutical Society of Great Britain Working Party on the handling of cytotoxic drugs.

If halving of a tablet is required, care should be taken not to contaminate the hands or inhale the drug.

Since the enzyme hypoxanthine guanine phosphoribosyl transferase is responsible for the conversion of Lanvis to its active metabolite, it is possible that patients deficient in this enzyme, such as those suffering from Lesch-Nyhan Syndrome, may be resistant to the drug. Resistance to azathioprine (Imuran*), which has one of the same active metabolites as Lanvis, has been demonstrated in two children with Lesch-Nyhan Syndrome.

Interaction with other medicaments and other forms of interaction: The combination of busulphan and Lanvis has resulted in the development of nodular regenerative hyperplasia, portal hypertension and oesophageal varices. As there is *in vitro* evidence that aminosalicylate derivatives (e.g. olsalazine, mesalazine or sulphasalazine) inhibit the TPMT enzyme, they should be administered with caution to patients receiving concurrent Lanvis therapy (see *Special warnings and precautions for use*).

Pregnancy and lactation: Lanvis, like other cytotoxic agents, is potentially teratogenic. There have been isolated cases where men, who have received combinations of cytotoxic agents including Lanvis, have fathered children with congenital abnormalities. Its use should be avoided whenever possible during pregnancy, particularly during the first trimester. In any individual case the potential hazard to the foetus must be balanced against the expected benefit to the mother.

As with all cytotoxic chemotherapy, adequate contraceptive precautions should be advised when either partner is receiving Lanvis.

There are no reports documenting the presence of Lanvis or its metabolites in maternal milk. It is suggested that mothers receiving Lanvis should not breast feed.

Effects on ability to drive and use machines: None known.

Undesirable effects: Lanvis is usually one component of combination chemotherapy and, consequently, it is not possible to ascribe the side effects unequivocally to this drug alone.

The following side effects have been reported during treatment with thioguanine-containing regimens: gastro-intestinal intolerance; intestinal necrosis and perforation; liver function abnormalities and jaundice, which may be reversible if therapy is withdrawn; veno-occlusive disease (VOD) of the liver which, in most cases, was reversible on withdrawal of chemotherapy; one case of centrilobular hepatic necrosis in a patient who has been treated for acute myelogenous leukaemia with high cumulative doses of Lanvis and cytosine arabinoside. This patient was also taking oral contraceptives.

Overdose: The principal toxic effect is on the bone marrow, and haematological toxicity is likely to be more profound with chronic overdosage than with a single ingestion of Lanvis. As there is no known antidote the blood picture should be closely monitored and general supportive measures, together with appropriate blood transfusion instituted if necessary.

Pharmacological properties

Pharmacodynamic properties: Thioguanine is a sulphydryl analogue of guanine and behaves as a purine antimetabolite. It is activated to its nucleotide, thioguanylic acid. Thioguanine metabolites inhibit *de novo* purine synthesis and purine nucleotide interconversions. Thioguanine is also incorporated into nucleic acids and DNA (deoxyribonucleic acid) incorporation is claimed to contribute to the agent's cytotoxicity. Cross resistance usually exists between thioguanine and mercaptopurine, and it is not to be expected that patients resistant to one will respond to the other.

Pharmacokinetic properties: Thioguanine is extensively metabolised *in vivo*. There are two principal catabolic routes: methylation to 2-amino-6-methylthiopurine and deamination to 2-hydroxy-6-mercaptopurine, followed by oxidation to 6-thiouric acid.

Studies with radioactive thioguanine show that peak blood levels of total radioactivity are achieved about 8–10 hours after oral administration and decline slowly thereafter. Later studies using HPLC have shown 6-thioguanine to be the major thiopurine present for at least the first 8 hours after intravenous administration. Peak plasma concentrations of 61–118 nanomol (nmol)/ml are obtainable following intravenous administration of 1 to 1.2 g of 6-thioguanine/m^2 body surface area.

Plasma levels decay biexponentially with initial and terminal half lives of 3 and 5.9 hours respectively. Following oral administration of 100 mg/m^2, peak levels as measured by HPLC occur at 2–4 hours and lie in the range of 0.03–0.94 micromolar (0.03–0.94 nmol/ml). Levels are reduced by concurrent food intake (as well as vomiting).

Preclinical safety data: There are no preclinical data of relevance to the prescriber which are additional to that already included in other sections of the SPC.

Pharmaceutical particulars

List of excipients: Lactose NF; Starch, potato HSE; Acacia NF; Stearic acid NF; Magnesium stearate NF; Purified water USP.

Incompatibilities: None known.

Shelf life: 60 months (unopened).

Special precautions for storage: Store below 25°C. Keep dry. Protect from light.

Nature and contents of container: Amber glass bottles with child-resistant polyethylene/polypropylene closures. Pack size 25.

Instructions for use/handling: None.

Marketing authorisation number PL 0003/0083

Date of first authorisation/renewal of authorisation Renewal: 29 October 1997

Date of (partial) revision of text November 1998

LEUKERAN* TABLETS 2 mg
LEUKERAN* TABLETS 5 mg

Qualitative and quantitative composition Chlorambucil EP 2.0 mg or 5.0 mg.

Pharmaceutical form Tablet.

Clinical particulars

Therapeutic indications: Leukeran is indicated in the treatment of Hodgkin's disease, certain forms of non-Hodgkin's lymphoma, chronic lymphocytic leukaemia, Waldenstrom's macroglobulinaemia and advanced ovarian adenocarcinoma. Leukeran has a significant therapeutic effect in a proportion of patients with breast cancer.

Posology and method of administration:

Adults: Hodgkin's disease: Used as a single agent a typical dosage is 0.2 mg/kg/day for 4–8 weeks. Leukeran is usually included in combination therapy and a number of regimes have been used. Leukeran has been used as an alternative to nitrogen mustard with a reduction in toxicity but similar therapeutic results.

Non-Hodgkin's lymphoma: Used as a single agent the usual dosage is 0.1–0.2 mg/kg/day for 4–8 weeks initially, maintenance therapy is then given either by a reduced daily dosage or intermittent courses of treatment. Leukeran is useful in the management of patients with advanced diffuse lymphocytic lymphoma and those who have relapsed after radiotherapy. There is no significant difference in the overall response rate obtained with chlorambucil as lymphocytic lymphoma.

Chronic lymphocytic leukaemia: Treatment with Leukeran is usually started after the patient has developed symptoms or when there is evidence of impaired bone marrow function (but not bone marrow failure) as indicated by the peripheral blood count. Initially Leukeran is given at a dosage of 0.15 mg/kg/day until the total leucocyte count has fallen to 10,000 per μL. Treatment may be resumed 4 weeks after the end of the first course and continued at a dosage of 0.1 mg/kg/day.

In a proportion of patients, usually after about 2 years of treatment, the blood leucocyte count is reduced to the normal range, enlarged spleen and lymph nodes become impalpable and the proportion of lymphocytes in the bone marrow is reduced to less than 20 per cent. Patients with evidence of bone marrow failure should first be treated with prednisolone and evidence of marrow regeneration should be obtained before commencing treatment with Leukeran. Intermittent high dose therapy has been compared with daily Leukeran but no significant difference in therapeutic response or frequency of side effects was observed between the two treatment groups.

Waldenstrom's macroglobulinaemia: Leukeran is the treatment of choice in this indication. Starting doses of 6–12 mg daily until leucopenia occurs are recommended followed by 2–8 mg daily indefinitely.

Ovarian carcinoma: Used as a single agent a typical dosage is 0.2 mg/kg/day for 4–6 weeks. A dosage of 0.3 mg/kg/day has been given until leucopenia had been induced. Maintenance dosage of 0.2 mg/kg/day has been given aiming to keep the total leucocyte count below 4,000/mm^3. In practice, maintenance courses tend to last 2–4 weeks with intervals of 2–6 weeks between each course.

Advanced breast cancer: Used as a single agent a typical dosage is 0.2 mg/kg bodyweight per day for 6 weeks. Leukeran may be given in combination with prednisolone at a range of 14–20 mg daily, regardless of bodyweight, over 4–6 weeks provided there is no serious haemopoietic depression. Leukeran may be given in combination with methotrexate, 5-fluorouracil, and prednisolone at a dosage of 5 to 7.5 mg/m^2/day.

Children: Leukeran may be used in the management of Hodgkin's disease and non-Hodgkin's lymphomas in children. The dosage regimes are similar to those used in adults.

Use in the elderly: No specific studies have been carried out in the elderly, however, it may be advisable to monitor renal or hepatic function and if there is serious impairment then caution should be exercised.

Contra-indications: In view of the seriousness of the indications there are no absolute contra-indications.

Special warnings and special precautions for use: Leukeran is an active cytotoxic agent for use only under the direction of physicians experienced in the administration of such agents.

Safe handling of Leukeran Tablets: The handling of Leukeran Tablets should follow guidelines for the handling of cytotoxic drugs according to prevailing local recommendations and/or regulations (for example, Royal Pharmaceutical Society of Great Britain Working Party on the Handling of Cytotoxic Drugs).

Provided that the outer coating of the tablet is intact, there is no risk in handling Leukeran Tablets. Leukeran Tablets should not be divided.

Since Leukeran is capable of producing irreversible bone marrow suppression, blood counts should be closely monitored in patients under treatment.

At therapeutic dosage Leukeran depresses lymphocytes and has less effect on neutrophil and platelet counts and on haemoglobin levels. Discontinuation of Leukeran is not necessary at the first sign of a fall in neutrophils but it must be remembered that the fall may continue for 10 days or more after the last dose.

Leukeran should not be given to patients who have recently undergone radiotherapy or received other cytotoxic agents.

When lymphocytic infiltration of the bone marrow is present or the bone marrow is hypoplastic, the daily dose should not exceed 0.1 mg/kg bodyweight.

Patients with evidence of impaired renal function should be carefully monitored as they are prone to additional myelosuppression associated with azotaemia.

The metabolism of Leukeran is still under investigation and consideration should be given to dose reduction in patients with gross hepatic dysfunction.

Interaction with other medicaments and other forms of interaction: Patients receiving phenylbutazone may require a reduced dose of Leukeran.

Pregnancy and lactation: As with other cytotoxic agents Leukeran is potentially teratogenic. The use of Leukeran should be avoided whenever possible during pregnancy, particularly during the first trimester.

In any individual case, the potential hazard to the foetus must be balanced against the expected benefit to the mother.

As with all cytotoxic chemotherapy, adequate contraceptive precautions should be advised when either partner is receiving Leukeran.

Mothers receiving Leukeran should not breast feed.

Effects on ability to drive and use machines: None known.

Undesirable effects: The most common side-effect is bone marrow suppression. Although this frequently occurs, it is usually reversible if Leukeran is withdrawn early enough. However, irreversible bone marrow failure has been reported.

Gastro-intestinal disturbances such as nausea and vomiting, diarrhoea and oral ulceration occur infrequently. Other side-effects may be encountered but usually only when the therapeutic dosage has been exceeded.

Severe interstitial pulmonary fibrosis has occasionally been reported in patients with chronic lymphocytic leukaemia on long-term Leukeran therapy. However, this may be reversible on withdrawal of Leukeran.

Hepatotoxicity and jaundice have been reported after Leukeran treatment.

Skin rashes are uncommon but have on very rare occasions been reported to progress to serious conditions including Stevens-Johnson Syndrome and toxic epidermal necrolysis.

Other reported adverse reactions include fever, peripheral neuropathy, interstitial pneumonia and sterile cystitis.

Seizures have occurred in children with nephrotic syndrome treated with Leukeran and dose-related focal fits in adults have been reported.

Overdose: Reversible pancytopenia was the main finding of inadvertent overdoses of Leukeran. Neurological toxicity ranging from agitated behaviour and ataxia to multiple grand mal seizures has also occurred. As there is no known antidote the blood picture should be closely monitored and general supportive measures should be instituted, together with appropriate blood transfusion if necessary.

Pharmacological properties

Pharmacodynamic properties: Chlorambucil is an aromatic nitrogen mustard derivative which acts as a bifunctional alkylating agent. Alkylation takes place through the formation of a highly reactive ethylenimonium radical. A probable mode of action involves cross-linkage of the ethylenimonium derivative between 2 strands of helical DNA and subsequent interference with replication.

Pharmacokinetic properties: After oral administration of 14C chlorambucil, maximum plasma radioactivity occurs between 40 and 70 minutes later. Studies have shown that chlorambucil disappears from the plasma with a mean terminal phase life of 1.5 hours and that its urinary excretion is low. A high level of urinary radioactivity after oral or intravenous administration of 14C labelled chlorambucil indicates that the drug is well absorbed after oral dosage.

The metabolism of chlorambucil in man appears to be similar to that in laboratory animals and involves B-oxidation of the butyric acid side chain. BIS-2-chlorethyl-2(4-aminophenyl) acetic acid (or phenylacetic mustard) is a major metabolite of chlorambucil; its peak plasma concentration occurs within 2–4 hours after administration of the parent drug, it has a longer terminal phase half-life than chlorambucil and it contributes significantly to the alkylating activity of the drug.

Preclinical safety data:

A. Mutagenicity and Carcinogenicity: Leukeran has been shown to cause chromatid or chromosome damage in man. Development of acute leukaemia after Leukeran therapy for chronic lymphocytic leukaemia has been reported. However, it was not clear whether the acute leukaemia was part of the natural history of the disease or if the chemotherapy was the cause.

A comparison of patients with ovarian cancer who received alkylating agents with those who did not, showed that the use of alkylating agents, including Leukeran, significantly increased the incidence of acute leukaemia.

Acute myelogenous leukaemia has been reported in a small proportion of patients receiving Leukeran as long-term adjuvant therapy for breast cancer.

The leukaemogenic risk must be balanced against the potential therapeutic benefit when considering the use of Leukeran.

B. Teratogenicity: See information under *Pregnancy and lactation* section.

C. Fertility: Leukeran may cause suppression of ovarian function and amenorrhoea has been reported following Leukeran therapy.

Azoospermia has been observed as a result of therapy with Leukeran although it is estimated that a total dose of at least 400 mg is necessary.

Varying degrees of recovery of spermatogenesis have been reported in patients with lymphoma following treatment with Leukeran in total doses of 400–2600 mg.

Pharmaceutical particulars

List of excipients: Lactose EP; Sucrose EP; Magnesium stearate EP; Pregelatinised maize starch BP; Purified water EP; Maize starch EP; Quinoline yellow HSE.

Incompatibilities: None known.

Shelf life: 3 years.

Special precautions for storage: Store at temperatures between 2°C and 8°C. Keep dry.

Nature and contents of container: Amber glass bottle with low-density polyethylene snap-fit closures.

Instructions for use/handling: Leukeran is an active cytotoxic agent for use only under the direction of physicians experienced in the administration of such agents.

Safe handling of Leukeran Tablets: The handling of Leukeran Tablets should follow guidelines for the handling of cytotoxic drugs according to prevailing local recommendations and/or regulations (for example, Royal Pharmaceutical Society of Great Britain Working Party on the Handling of Cytotoxic Drugs).

Provided that the outer coating of the tablet is intact, there is no risk in handling Leukeran Tablets. Leukeran Tablets should not be divided.

Marketing authorisation numbers
2 mg: PL 0003/5264R
5 mg: PL 0003/5265R

Date of first authorisation/renewal of the authorisation
2 mg and 5 mg Reviewed licence: 12th September 1984
2 mg: Renewal: 13th February 1990
5 mg: Renewal: 12th February 1990

Date of (partial) revision of the text This is the first SmPC.

MALARONE* ▼

Qualitative and quantitative composition Each tablet contains: Atovaquone 250 mg and proguanil hydrochloride 100 mg.

Pharmaceutical form Round, biconvex, pink film coated tablets containing 250 mg atovaquone and 100 mg proguanil hydrochloride.

Clinical particulars

Therapeutic indications: Malarone is a fixed dose combination of atovaquone and proguanil hydrochloride which acts as a blood schizonticide. It is indicated for: Treatment of acute, uncomplicated *Plasmodium falciparum* malaria.

Because Malarone is effective against drug sensitive and drug resistant *P. falciparum* it is especially recommended for acute, uncomplicated *P. falciparum* malaria acquired in areas where the pathogen may be resistant to other antimalarials, such as chloroquine, halofantrine, mefloquine, amodiaquine and chloroquine plus pyrimethimene/sulphadoxine.

Posology and method of administration: The daily dose should be taken with food or a milky drink at the same time each day.

In the event of vomiting within 1 hour of dosing a repeat dose should be taken.

Dosage in adults: Four tablets as a single dose for three consecutive days.

Dosage in children:
11–20 kg bodyweight: One tablet daily for three consecutive days.
21–30 kg bodyweight: Two tablets as a single dose for three consecutive days.
31–40 kg bodyweight: Three tablets as a single dose for three consecutive days.
>40 kg bodyweight: Dose as for adults.

Dosage in the elderly: Although no studies have been carried out in the elderly, no special precautions or dosage adjustment are anticipated in this age group.

Dosage in hepatic impairment: Although no studies have been carried out, no special precautions or dosage adjustment are anticipated.

Dosage in renal impairment: Proguanil, and hence Malarone, should be administered with caution to patients with acute renal failure (see *Special warnings and precautions for use*).

Contra-indications: Malarone is contra-indicated in individuals with known hypersensitivity to atovaquone or proguanil hydrochloride or any component of the formulation.

Special warnings and precautions for use: Malarone has not been evaluated for the treatment of cerebral malaria or other severe manifestations of complicated malaria including hyperparasitaemia, pulmonary oedema or renal failure.

Parasite relapse occurred commonly when *P. vivax* malaria was treated with Malarone alone.

In the event of recrudescent infections due to *P. falciparum*, patients should be treated with a different blood schizonticide.

Because absorption of atovaquone may be reduced in patients with diarrhoea and vomiting, alternative therapy should be considered in such patients. If Malarone is used in these patients parasitaemia should be closely monitored.

Parasitaemia should be closely monitored in patients receiving concurrent metoclopramide or tetracycline (see *Interactions*).

The concomitant administration of Malarone and rifampicin is not recommended (see *Interactions*).

Proguanil, and hence Malarone, should be administered with caution to patients with acute renal failure (see *Posology and method of administration*).

Interaction with other medicaments and other forms of interaction: Concomitant treatment with metoclopramide and tetracycline have been associated with significant decreases in plasma concentrations of atovaquone (see *Special warnings and precautions for use*).

Concomitant administration of rifampicin is known to reduce atovaquone levels by approximately 50% (see *Special warnings and precautions for use*).

Atovaquone is highly protein bound (>99%) but does not displace other highly protein bound drugs *in vitro*, indicating significant drug interactions arising from displacement are unlikely.

Pregnancy and lactation: The safety of atovaquone and proguanil hydrochloride when administered concurrently for use in human pregnancy has not been established.

There is no evidence of teratogenicity in reproductive studies in rats with atovaquone alone. Segment II studies in rats with proguanil and atovaquone in combination up to a dose of atovaquone: proguanil (50:20) mg/kg/day show no indication of teratogenic effects.

However, as animal studies are not always predictive of human response the use of Malarone in pregnancy should only be considered if the expected benefit to the mother outweighs the risk to the foetus.

Lactation: The atovaquone concentrations in milk, in a rat study, were 30% of the concurrent atovaquone concentrations in maternal plasma. It is not known whether atovaquone is excreted in human milk.

Proguanil is excreted in human milk in small quantities.

It is not recommended that mothers receiving Malarone breast feed their babies.

Effects on ability to drive and use machines: There have been no studies to investigate the effect of Malarone on driving performance or the ability to operate machinery but a detrimental effect on such activities is not predicted from the pharmacology of the component drugs.

Undesirable effects: As Malarone contains atovaquone and proguanil hydrochloride, the type and severity of adverse reactions associated with each of the compounds may be expected. However, at the doses employed for the treatment of malaria, they are generally mild and of limited duration.

In a database comprising approximately 500 patients abdominal pain, headache, anorexia, nausea, vomiting, diarrhoea and coughing were the most commonly reported adverse experiences.

The only abnormalities noted in laboratory tests were occasional reversible abnormalities in liver function tests which were not associated with untoward clinical events.

Overdose: There have been no reports of overdosage with Malarone. In cases of suspected overdosage symptomatic and supportive therapy should be given as appropriate.

Pharmacological properties

Pharmacodynamic properties: Pharmacotherapeutic group – Antimalarials: biguanides–proguanil combinations. ATC Code: P01B B51.

Mode of action: The constituents of Malarone, atovaquone and proguanil hydrochloride, interfere with two different pathways involved in the biosynthesis of pyrimidines required for nucleic acid replication. Atovaquone is a selective and potent inhibitor of parasite mitochondrial electron transport. Proguanil hydrochloride primarily exerts its effect by means of the metabolite cycloguanil, a dihydrofolate reductase inhibitor. Inhibition of dihydrofolate reductase in the malaria parasite disrupts deoxythymidylate synthesis. These two mechanisms are believed to be the prime explanation of the synergy seen when used in combination.

Microbiology: Atovaquone has potent activity against

Plasmodium spp *in vitro* IC_{50} against *P. falciparum* 0.23–1.43 ng/ml.

The animalarial activity of proguanil is exerted via the primary metabolite cycloguanil (*in vitro* IC_{50} against various *P. falciparum* strains of 4–20 ng/ml; some activity of proguanil and another metabolite, 4-chlorophenylbiguanide, is seen *in vitro* at 600–3000 ng/ml).

In *in vitro* studies of *P. falciparum* the combination of atovaquone and proguanil was shown to be synergistic. This enhanced efficacy was also demonstrated in clinical studies in both immune and non-immune patients.

Pharmacokinetic properties: There are no pharmacokinetic interactions between atovaquone and proguanil at the recommended dose.

Absorption: Atovaquone is a highly lipophilic compound with low aqueous solubility. The bioavailability of atovaquone shows considerable inter-individual variability. Dietary fat taken with atovaquone increases the rate and extent of absorption, increasing AUC 2–3 times and C_{max} 5 times over fasting. Patients are recommended to take Malarone tablets with food (see *Posology and method of administration*).

Proguanil hydrochloride is rapidly and extensively absorbed regardless of food intake.

Distribution: Atovaquone is highly protein bound (>99%) but does not displace other highly protein bound drugs *in vitro*, indicating significant drug interactions arising from displacement are unlikely.

The volume of distribution of atovaquone is 0.62±0.19 l/kg.

Proguanil is 75% protein bound.

In human plasma the binding of atovaquone and proguanil were unaffected by the presence of the other.

Metabolism: There is no evidence that atovaquone is metabolised and there is negligible excretion of atovaquone in urine with the parent drug being predominantly (>90%) eliminated unchanged in faeces.

Proguanil hydrochloride is partially metabolised with less than 40% being excreted unchanged in the urine. Its metabolites cycloguanil and 4-chlorophenylbiguanide are also excreted in the urine.

During treatment of malaria with Malarone at recommended doses proguanil metabolism status appears to have no implications for treatment.

Elimination: The elimination half-life of atovaquone is about 2–3 days in adults and 1–2 days in children.

The clearance of atovaquone is 0.15±0.09 ml/min/kg.

The elimination half lives of proguanil and cycloguanil are about 12–15 hours in both adults and children.

Preclinical safety data:

Repeat dose toxicity: Results of repeat dose studies in rats and dogs at dosages of atovaquone: proguanil hydrochloride up to 100:40 mg/kg/day for 30 days either singly or in combination revealed reversible toxicity attributable to proguanil alone. There was no additional animal toxicity attributable to atovaquone alone or to the combination. Dosages of atovaquone: proguanil hydrochloride of 50:20 mg/kg/day was the no-effect dose.

Reproductive toxicity studies: Reproduction toxicity studies in animals did not indicate any teratogenic potential at dosages of atovaquone: proguanil hydrochloride of up to 50:20 mg/kg/day (see *Pregnancy and lactation*). In rabbits given atovaquone alone at dosages up to 1200 mg/kg/day, an increased incidence of resorptions and decreased length and weight of foetuses was noted. These effects were likely to be secondary to toxicity of atovaquone in maternal animals.

Mutagenicity: A wide range of mutagenicity tests have shown no evidence that atovaquone or proguanil have mutagenic activity as single agents.

Mutagenicity studies have not been performed with atovaquone in combination with proguanil.

Carcinogenicity: Oncogenicity studies of atovaquone alone in mice showed an increased incidence of hepatocellular adenomas and carcinomas. No such findings were observed in rats and mutagenicity tests were negative. These findings appear to be due to the inherent susceptibility of mice to atovaquone and are considered of no relevance in the clinical situation.

Oncogenicity studies on proguanil alone or in combination with atovaquone have not been undertaken.

Pharmaceutical particulars

List of excipients: Core: Poloxamer 188 BP; Microcrystalline Cellulose PhEur; Low-substituted Hydroxypropyl Cellulose USNF; Povidone K30 PhEur; Sodium Starch Glycollate PhEur; Magnesium Stearate PhEur.

Coating: Methylhydroxypropyl Cellulose PhEur; Titanium Dioxide PhEur; Iron Oxide Red E172; Macrogol 400 PhEur; Polyethylene Glycol 8000 USNF.

Incompatibilities: None known.

Shelf life: 3 years.

Special precautions for storage: None.

Nature and contents of container: PVC aluminium foil blister packs containing 12 tablets.

Instructions for use/handling: None.

Marketing authorisation number 10949/0258

Date of approval/revision of SPC 18 April 1997

MIVACRON* INJECTION

Presentation Mivacron Injection is a clear, pale yellow, sterile aqueous solution, in glass ampoules, containing 2 mg/ml mivacurium as mivacurium chloride. Each 5 ml ampoule contains 10 mg mivacurium and each 10 ml ampoule contains 20 mg mivacurium.

Uses Mivacron is a highly selective, short-acting, non-depolarising, neuromuscular blocking agent with a fast recovery profile. Mivacron is used as an adjunct to general anaesthesia to relax skeletal muscles and to facilitate tracheal intubation and mechanical ventilation.

This formulation contains no antimicrobial preservative and is intended for single patient use.

Pharmacokinetics: Mivacurium chloride is a mixture of three stereoisomers. The trans-trans and cis-trans stereoisomers comprise 92% to 96% of mivacurium chloride and when studied in cats their neuromuscular blocking potencies are not significantly different from each other or from mivacurium chloride. The cis-cis isomer has been estimated from studies in cats to have one-tenth of the neuromuscular blocking potency of the other two stereoisomers. Enzymatic hydrolysis by plasma cholinesterase is the primary mechanism for inactivation of mivacurium and yields a quaternary alcohol and a quaternary monoester metabolite. Pharmacological studies in cats and dogs have shown that the metabolites possess insignificant neuromuscular, autonomic or cardiovascular activity at concentrations higher than seen in man.

Dosage and administration

Use by injection in adults: Mivacron is administered by intravenous injection. The mean dose required to produce 95% suppression of the adductor pollicis single twitch response to ulnar nerve stimulation (ED_{95}) is 0.07 mg/kg (range 0.06 to 0.09) in adults receiving narcotic anaesthesia.

The recommended bolus dose range for healthy adults is 0.07 to 0.25 mg/kg. The duration of neuromuscular blockade is related to the dose. Doses of 0.07, 0.15, 0.20 and 0.25 mg/kg produce clinically effective block for approximately 13, 16, 20 and 23 minutes respectively.

Doses of up to 0.15 mg/kg may be administered over 5 to 15 seconds. Higher doses should be administered over 30 seconds in order to minimise the possibility of occurrence of cardiovascular effects.

The following dosage regimens are recommended for tracheal intubation:

i) A dose of 0.2 mg/kg, administered over 30 seconds, produces good to excellent conditions for tracheal intubation within 2 to 2.5 minutes.

ii) A dose of 0.25 mg/kg administered as a divided dose (0.15 mg/kg followed 30 seconds later by 0.1 mg/kg), produces good to excellent conditions for tracheal intubation within 1.5 to 2.0 minutes of completion of administration of the first dose portion.

With Mivacron, significant train-of-four fade is not seen during onset. It is often possible to intubate the trachea before complete abolition of the train-of-four response of the adductor pollicis muscle has occurred.

Full block can be prolonged with maintenance doses of Mivacron. Doses of 0.1 mg/kg administered during narcotic anaesthesia each provide approximately 15 minutes of additional clinically effective block. Successive supplementary doses do not give rise to accumulation of neuromuscular blocking effect.

The neuromuscular blocking action of Mivacron is potentiated by isoflurane or enflurane anaesthesia. If steady-state anaesthesia with isoflurane or enflurane has been established, the recommended initial Mivacron dose should be reduced by up to 25%. Halothane appears to have only a minimal potentiating effect on Mivacron and dose reduction is probably not necessary.

Once spontaneous recovery is underway it is complete in approximately 15 minutes and is independent of the size of the Mivacron dose administered.

The neuromuscular block produced by Mivacron can be reversed with standard doses of anticholinesterase agents. However, because spontaneous recovery after mivacurium is rapid, reversal may not be routinely required since it shortens recovery time by only 5 to 6 minutes.

Use as an infusion in adults: Continuous infusion of Mivacron may be used to maintain neuromuscular block. Upon early evidence of spontaneous recovery from an initial Mivacron dose, an infusion rate of 8 to 10 microgram/kg/min (0.5 to 0.6 mg/kg/hr) is recommended. The initial infusion rate should be adjusted according to the patient's response to peripheral nerve stimulation and clinical criteria. Adjustments of the infusion rate should be made in increments of approximately 1 microgram/kg/min (0.06 mg/kg/hr). In general, a given rate should be maintained for at least 3 minutes before a rate change is made. On average, an infusion rate of 6 to 7 microgram/kg/min will maintain neuromuscular block within the range of 89% to 99% for extended periods in adults receiving narcotic anaesthesia. During steady-state isoflurane or enflurane anaesthesia, reduction in the infusion rate by up to 40% should be considered. With halothane, smaller reductions in infusion rate may be required.

Spontaneous recovery after Mivacron infusion is independent of the duration of infusion and comparable to recovery reported for single doses.

Continuous infusion of Mivacron has not been associated with the development of tachyphylaxis or cumulative neuromuscular blockade.

Mivacron (2 mg/ml) may be used undiluted for infusion.

Mivacron is compatible with the following infusion fluids:

Sodium Chloride Intravenous Infusion (0.9% w/v)

Glucose Intravenous Infusion (5% w/v)

Sodium Chloride (0.18% w/v) and Glucose (4% w/v) Intravenous Infusion

Lactated Ringer's Injection, USP

When diluted with the listed infusion solutions in the proportion of 1 plus 3 (i.e. to give 0.5 mg/ml) Mivacron Injection has been shown to be chemically and physically stable for at least 48 hours at 30°C. However, since the product contains no antimicrobial preservative, dilution should be carried out immediately prior to use, administration should commence as soon as possible thereafter, and any remaining solution should be discarded.

Dose in children aged 2 months to 12 years: Mivacron has a faster onset, shorter clinically effective duration of action and more rapid spontaneous recovery in infants and children than in adults.

The ED_{95} in infants aged 2 to 6 months is approximately 0.07 mg/kg; and in infants and children aged 7 months to 12 years is approximately 0.1 mg/kg.

Pharmacodynamic data for recommended initial doses in infants and children are summarised in the following table:

Age	*Dose for Tracheal Intubation*	*Time to Maximum Neuromuscular Block (Min)*	*Duration of Clinically Effective Block (Min)*
2 to 6 Months[A]	0.15 mg/kg	1.4	9
7 Months to12 Years[B]	0.2 mg/kg	1.7	9

[A] Data obtained during halothane anaesthesia.
[B] Data obtained during halothane or narcotic anaesthesia.

Since maximum block is usually achieved within 2 minutes following administration of these doses, tracheal intubation should be possible within this time.

Infants and children generally require more frequent maintenance doses and higher infusion rates than adults. Pharmacodynamic data for maintenance doses are summarised in the table below together with recommended infusion rates:

Age	*Maintenance Dose*	*Duration of Clinically Effective Block (Min)*	*Average Infusion Rate Required to Maintain 89–99% Neuromuscular Block*
2 Months–12 Years[A]	0.1 mg/kg	6–9	11–14 micrograms/kg/min (0.7–0.9 mg/kg/hr)

[A] Data obtained during halothane or narcotic anaesthesia.

Once spontaneous recovery is underway, it is complete in approximately 10 minutes.

Dose in neonates and infants under 2 months of age: No dose recommendations for neonates and infants under 2 months of age can be made until further information becomes available.

Dose in the elderly: In elderly patients receiving single bolus doses of Mivacron, the onset time, duration of action and recovery rate may be extended relative to younger patients by 20 to 30%. Elderly patients may also require decreased infusion rates or smaller or less frequent maintenance bolus doses.

Dose in patients with cardiovascular disease: In patients with clinically significant cardiovascular disease, the initial dose of Mivacron should be administered over 60 seconds. Mivacron has been administered in this way with minimal haemodynamic effects to patients undergoing cardiac surgery.

Dose in patients with reduced renal function: In patients with end-stage renal failure, the clinically effective duration of block produced by 0.15 mg/kg is approximately 1.5 times longer than in patients with normal renal function. Subsequently, dosage should be adjusted according to individual clinical response.

Dose in patients with reduced hepatic function: In patients with end-stage liver failure the clinically effective duration of block produced by 0.15 mg/kg is approximately 3 times longer than in patients with normal hepatic function. This prolongation is related to the markedly reduced plasma cholinesterase activity seen in these patients. Subsequently, dosage should be adjusted according to individual clinical response.

Dose in patients with reduced plasma cholinesterase activity: Mivacurium is metabolised by plasma cholinesterase. Plasma cholinesterase activity may be diminished in the presence of genetic abnormalities of plasma cholinesterase (e.g. patients heterozygous or homozygous for the atypical plasma cholinesterase gene), in various pathological conditions and by the administration of certain drugs (see *Drug interactions*).

The possibility of prolonged neuromuscular block following administration of Mivacron must be considered in patients with reduced plasma cholinesterase activity. Mild reductions (i.e. within 20% of the lower limit of the normal range) are not associated with clinically significant effects on duration. In patients heterozygous for the atypical plasma cholinesterase gene, the clinically effective duration of block of 0.15 mg/kg Mivacron is approximately 10 minutes longer than in control patients.

Dose in obese patients: In obese patients (those weighing 30% or more above their ideal bodyweight for height), the initial dose of Mivacron should be based upon ideal bodyweight and not actual bodyweight.

Monitoring: In common with all neuromuscular blocking agents, monitoring of neuromuscular function is recommended during the use of Mivacron in order to individualise dosage requirements.

Contra-indications, warnings, etc

Contra-indications: Mivacron should not be administered to patients known to have an allergic hypersensitivity to the drug.

Mivacron is contra-indicated in pregnancy since there is no information on the use of Mivacron in pregnant women.

Mivacron is contra-indicated in patients known or suspected of being homozygous for the atypical plasma cholinesterase gene (see *Precautions*).

Precautions: In common with all the other neuromuscular blocking agents, Mivacron paralyses the respiratory muscles as well as other skeletal muscles but has no effect on consciousness. Mivacron should be administered only by or under close supervision of an experienced anaesthetist with adequate facilities for endotracheal intubation and artificial ventilation.

In common with suxamethonium/succinylcholine, adult and paediatric patients homozygous for the atypical plasma cholinesterase gene (1 in 2,500 patients) are extremely sensitive to the neuromuscular blocking effect of Mivacron. In three such adult patients, a small dose of 0.03 mg/kg (approximately the ED_{10-20} in genotypically normal patients) produced complete neuromuscular block for 26 to 128 minutes. Once spontaneous recovery had begun, neuromuscular block in these patients was antagonised with conventional doses of neostigmine (see *Dosage and administration* and *Use in patients with reduced plasma cholinesterase activity*).

In adults, doses of Mivacron of ≥0.2 mg/kg (≥3 x ED_{95}) have been associated with histamine release when administered by rapid bolus injection. However, the slower administration of the 0.2 mg/kg Mivacron dose and the divided administration of the 0.25 mg/kg Mivacron dose (see *Dosage and administration*) minimise the cardiovascular effects of these doses. Cardiovascular safety did not appear to be compromised in children given a rapid bolus dose of 0.2 mg/kg in clinical studies.

Caution should be exercised in administering Mivacron to patients with a history suggestive of an increased sensitivity to the effects of histamine, e.g. asthma. If Mivacron is used in this group of patients it should be administered over 60 seconds.

Mivacron should be administered over a period of 60 seconds to patients who may be unusually sensitive to falls in arterial blood pressure, for example those who are hypovolaemic.

Mivacron does not have significant vagal or ganglion blocking properties in the recommended dosage range. Recommended doses of Mivacron consequently have no clinically significant effects on heart rate and will not counteract the bradycardia produced by many anaesthetic agents or by vagal stimulation during surgery.

In common with other non-depolarising neuromuscular blocking agents, increased sensitivity to Mivacron can be expected in patients with myasthenia gravis, other forms of neuromuscular disease and cachectic patients. Severe acid-base or electrolyte abnormalities may increase or reduce sensitivity to Mivacron.

Mivacron solution is acidic (approximately pH 4.5) and should not be mixed in the same syringe or administered simultaneously through the same needle with highly alkaline solutions (e.g. barbiturate solutions). It has been shown to be compatible with some commonly used peri-operative drugs supplied as acidic solutions, e.g. fentanyl, alfentanil, sufentanil, droperidol and midazolam. Where other anaesthetic agents are administered through the same indwelling needle or cannula as used for Mivacron, and compatibility has not been demonstrated, it is recommended that each drug is flushed through with physiological saline.

Studies in malignant hyperthermia-susceptible pigs, indicated that Mivacron does not trigger this syndrome. Mivacron has not been studied in malignant hyperthermia-susceptible patients.

Patients with burns may develop resistance to non-depolarising neuromuscular blocking agents and require increased doses. However, such patients may also have reduced plasma cholinesterase activity, requiring dose reduction. Consequently, burn patients should be given a test dose of 0.015 to 0.020 mg/kg Mivacron followed by appropriate dosing guided by monitoring of block with a nerve stimulator.

No data are available on the long-term use of Mivacron in patients undergoing mechanical ventilation in the intensive care unit.

Mivacron has been evaluated in four short-term mutagenicity tests. Mivacron was non-mutagenic in the Ames Salmonella assay, the mouse lymphoma assay, the human lymphocyte assay and the *in vivo* rat bone marrow cytogenetic assay.

There is no information available on whether mivacurium has carcinogenic potential.

Fertility studies have not been performed.

Reversal of neuromuscular block: As with other neuromuscular blocking agents, evidence of spontaneous recovery should be observed prior to administration of reversal agent (e.g. neostigmine). The use of peripheral nerve stimulator to evaluate recovery prior to and following reversal of neuromuscular block is strongly recommended.

Side- and adverse effects: Associated with the use of Mivacron there have been reports of skin flushing, erythema, urticaria, mild transient hypotension, transient tachycardia or bronchospasm which have been attributed to histamine release. These effects are dose–related and more common following initial doses of ≥ 0.2 mg/kg or more when given rapidly and are reduced if Mivacron is injected over 30 to 60 seconds or in divided doses over 30 seconds.

Very rarely, severe anaphylactic or anaphylactoid reactions have been reported in patients receiving Mivacron in conjunction with one or more anaesthetic agents.

Use in pregnancy and lactation: Animal studies have indicated that mivacurium has no adverse effect on foetal development.

There is no information on the use of Mivacron in pregnant women (see *Contra-indications*).

There has been no experience with the use of Mivacron during Caesarean section.

It is not known whether Mivacron is excreted in human milk.

Drug interactions: The neuromuscular block produced by mivacurium may be increased by the concomitant use of inhalational anaesthetics such as enflurane, isoflurane and halothane.

Mivacron has been safely administered following suxamethonium-facilitated tracheal intubation. Evidence of spontaneous recovery from suxamethonium should be observed prior to administration of Mivacron.

In common with all non-depolarising neuromuscular blocking agents, the magnitude and/or duration of non-depolarising neuromuscular block may be increased and infusion requirements may be reduced as a result of interaction with: antibiotics, including the aminoglycosides, polymyxins, spectinomycin, tetracyclines, lincomycin and clindamycin; anti arrhythmic drugs: propranolol, calcium channel blockers, lignocaine, procainamide and quinidine; diuretics: frusemide and possibly thiazides, mannitol and acetazolamide; magnesium salts; ketamine; lithium salts; ganglion blocking drugs: trimetaphan, hexamethonium.

Drugs that may reduce plasma cholinesterase activity may also prolong the neuromuscular blocking action of Mivacron. These include anti-mitotic drugs, monoamine oxidase inhibitors, ecothiopate iodide, pancuronium, organophosphates, anticholinesterases, certain hormones, bambuterol.

Rarely, certain drugs may aggravate or unmask latent myasthenia gravis or actually induce a myasthenic syndrome; increased sensitivity to Mivacron would be consequent on such a development. Such drugs include various antibiotics, β-blockers, (propranolol, oxprenolol), anti-arrhythmic drugs (procainamide, quinidine), anti-rheumatic drugs (chloroquine, D-penicillamine), trimetaphan, chlorpromazine, steroids, phenytoin and lithium.

The administration of combinations of non-depolarising neuromuscular blocking agents in conjunction with Mivacron may produce a degree of neuromuscular blockade in excess of that which might be expected from an equipotent total dose of Mivacron. Any synergistic effect may vary between different drug combinations.

A depolarising muscle relaxant such as suxamethonium chloride should not be administered to prolong the neuromuscular blocking effects of non-depolarising agents, as this may result in a prolonged and complex block which can be difficult to reverse with anticholinesterase drugs.

Toxicity and treatment of overdosage: Prolonged muscle paralysis and its consequences are the main signs of overdosage with neuromuscular blocking agents. However, the risk of haemodynamic side-effects especially decreases in blood pressure, may be increased.

It is essential to maintain a patent airway together with assisted positive pressure ventilation until spontaneous respiration is adequate. Full sedation will be required since consciousness is not impaired. Recovery may be hastened by the administration of anticholinesterase agents accompanied by atropine or glycopyrrolate, once evidence of spontaneous recovery is present. Cardiovascular support may be provided by proper positioning of the patient and administration of fluids or vasopressor agents as required.

Pharmaceutical precautions Store below 25°C. Do not freeze. Protect from light.

Since no antimicrobial preservative is included, Mivacron must be used under full aseptic conditions and any dilution carried out immediately before use. Any unused solution in open ampoules should be discarded.

Mivacron Injection is acidic (approximately pH 4.5) and should not be mixed with highly alkaline solutions (e.g. barbiturates). Mivacron Injection has been shown to be compatible with some commonly used peri-operative drugs supplied as acidic solutions. Where such agents are administered through the same indwelling needle or cannula as used for Mivacron Injection, and compatibility has not been demonstrated, it is recommended that each drug is flushed through with physiological saline.

Legal category POM

Package quantities Ampoules of 5 ml and 10 ml in packs of 5.

Further information The termination of the neuromuscular blocking action of Mivacron is mainly dependent on hydrolysis by plasma pseudocholinesterase, which is present at high levels in human plasma.

Multiple degradation/elimination pathways appear to exist for Mivacron (e.g. hydrolysis by liver esterases, elimination in bile and renal excretion).

Product licence number 0003/0325.

MYLERAN* TABLETS 0.5 mg and 2 mg

Qualitative and quantitative composition Busulphan 0.5 mg or 2 mg per tablet.

Pharmaceutical form Tablet.

Clinical particulars

Therapeutic indications: Myleran is indicated for the palliative treatment of the chronic phase of chronic granulocytic leukaemia. Although not curative, Myleran is very effective in reducing the total granulocyte mass, relieving the symptoms of disease and improving the clinical state of the patient.

Myleran has been shown to be superior to splenic irradiation when judged by survival times and maintenance of haemoglobin levels and is as effective in controlling spleen size.

Myleran is ineffective once blast transformation has occurred.

Myleran is effective in producing prolonged remission in polycythaemia vera, particularly in cases with marked thrombocytosis.

Myleran may be useful in selected cases of essential thrombocythaemia and myelofibrosis.

Oral administration.

Posology and method of administration:
Induction in adults: Treatment is usually initiated as soon as the condition is diagnosed. The dose is 0.06 mg/kg/day, with an initial daily maximum of 4 mg, which may be given as a single dose.

There is individual variation in the response to Myleran and in a small proportion of patients the bone marrow may be extremely sensitive (see *Special warnings and precautions for use*).

The blood count must be monitored at least weekly during the induction phase and it may be helpful to plot counts on semilog graph paper.

The dose should be increased only if the response is inadequate after three weeks.

Treatment should be continued until the total leucocyte count has fallen to between 15 and 25×10^9 per litre (typically 12 to 20 weeks). Treatment may then be interrupted, following which a further fall in the leucocyte count may occur over the next two weeks. Continued treatment at the induction dose after this point, or following depression of the platelet count to below 100×10^9 per litre is associated with a significant risk of prolonged and possibly irreversible bone marrow aplasia.

Maintenance in adults: Control of the leukaemia may be achieved for long periods without further Myleran treatment; further courses are usually given when the leucocyte count rises to 50×10^9 per litre, or symptoms return.

Some clinicians prefer to give continuous maintenance therapy. Continuous treatment is more practical when the duration of unmaintained remissions is short. The usual maintenance dosage is 0.5 to 2 mg/day, but individual requirements may be much less. The aim is to maintain a leucocyte count of 10 to 15×10^9 per litre and blood counts must be performed at least every 4 weeks. The maintenance dose may also be adjusted by reducing the number of treatment days per week.

Lower doses of Myleran should be used if it is administered in conjunction with other cytotoxic agents (see also *Undesirable effects* and *Drug interactions*).

Children: Chronic granulocytic leukaemia is rare in the paediatric age group. Myleran may be used to treat Philadelphia chromosome positive (Ph' positive) disease, but the Ph' negative juvenile variant responds poorly.

Polycythaemia vera: The usual dose is 4 to 6 mg daily, continued for 4 to 6 weeks, with careful monitoring of the blood count, particularly the platelet count.

Further courses are given when relapse occurs; alternatively, maintenance therapy may be given using approximately half the induction dose.

If the polycythaemia is controlled primarily by venesection, short courses of Myleran may be given solely to control the platelet count.

Myelofibrosis: The usual initial dose is 2 to 4 mg daily.

Very careful haematological control is required because of the extreme sensitivity of the bone marrow in this condition.

Essential thrombocythaemia: The usual dose is 2 to 4 mg per day.

Treatment should be interrupted if the total leucocyte count falls below 5×10^9 per litre or the platelet count below 500×10^9 per litre.

Use in the elderly: No special comment.

Contra-indications: Myleran should not be used in patients whose disease has demonstrated resistance to busulphan.

Myleran should not be given to patients who have previously suffered a hypersensitivity reaction to the drug.

Special warnings and precautions for use: Myleran is an active cytotoxic agent for use **only** under the direction of physicians experienced in the administration of such agents.

Myleran should be discontinued if lung toxicity develops (see *Side-effects*).

Myleran should not generally be given in conjunction with or soon after radiotherapy.

If anaesthesia is required in patients with possible pulmonary toxicity, the concentration of inspired oxygen should be kept as low as safely as possible and careful attention given to post-operative respiratory care.

Hyperuricaemia and/or hyperuricosuria are not uncommon in patients with chronic granulocytic leukaemia and should be corrected before starting treatment with Myleran. During treatment, hyperuricaemia and the risk of uric nephropathy should be prevented by adequate prophylaxis, including adequate hydration and the use of allopurinol.

Very careful consideration should be given to the use of Myleran for the treatment of polycythaemia vera and essential thrombocythaemia in view of the drug's carcinogenic potential. The use of Myleran for these indications should be avoided in younger or asymptomatic patients. If the drug is considered necessary, treatment courses should be kept as short as possible.

Careful attention must be paid to monitoring the blood counts throughout treatment to avoid the possibility of excessive myelosuppression and the risk of irreversible bone marrow aplasia.

If high-dose Myleran is prescribed (see *Overdose*), patients should be given prophylactic anticonvulsant therapy, preferably with a benzodiazepine rather than phenytoin.

It is recommended that the handling of Myleran Tablets follows the 'Guidelines for the Handling of Cytotoxic Drugs' issued by the Royal Pharmaceutical Society of Great Britain Working Party on the Handling of Cytotoxic Drugs.

If halving of a tablet is required, care should be taken not to contaminate the hands or inhale the drug.

Busulphan has been shown to be mutagenic in various experimental systems, including bacteria, fungi, *Drosophila* and cultured mouse lymphoma cells.

In vivo cytogenetic studies in rodents have shown an increased incidence of chromosome aberrations in both germ cells and somatic cells after busulphan treatment.

Various chromosome aberrations have been noted in cells from patients receiving Myleran.

On the basis of short-term tests, Myleran has been classified as potentially carcinogenic by the IARC. The World Health Association has concluded that there is a causal relationship between busulphan exposure and cancer.

Widespread epithelial dysplasia has been observed in patients treated with long-term Myleran, with some of the changes resembling precancerous lesions.

A number of malignant tumours have been reported in patients who have received Myleran treatment.

The evidence is growing that Myleran, in common with other alkylating agents, is leukaemogenic. In a controlled prospective study in which 2 years' Myleran treatment was given as an adjuvant to surgery for lung cancer, long-term follow-up showed an increased incidence of acute leukaemia compared with the placebo-treated group. The incidence of solid tumours was not increased.

Although acute leukaemia is probably part of the natural history of polycythaemia vera, prolonged alkylating agent therapy may increase the incidence.

Ovarian suppression and amenorrhoea with menopausal symptoms commonly occur in premenopausal patients. In one case, recovery of ovarian function has been reported with continuing treatment.

Myleran treatment in a pre-adolescent girl prevented the onset of puberty due to ovarian failure.

Bulsulphan interferes with spermatogenesis in experimental animals, and there have been clinical reports of sterility, azoospermia and testicular atrophy in male patients.

Interaction with other medicaments and other forms of interaction: The combination of Myleran and thioguanine has resulted in the development of nodular regenerative hyperplasia, portal hypertension and oesophageal varices.

The effects of other cytotoxics producing pulmonary toxicity may be additive.

The administration of phenytoin to patients receiving high-dose Myleran (see *Overdose*) may result in a decrease in the myeloblative effect.

Pregnancy and lactation: As with all cytotoxic chemotherapy, adequate contraceptive precautions should be advised when either partner is receiving Myleran.

Busulphan is teratogenic in animal studies and potentially teratogenic in humans. A few cases of congenital abnormalities, not necessarily attributable to busulphan, have been reported and third trimester exposure may be associated with impaired intrauterine growth. However, there have also been many reported cases of apparently normal children born after exposure to Myleran *in utero*, even during the first trimester.

The use of Myleran should be avoided whenever possible during pregnancy, particularly during the first trimester. In every individual case the expected benefit of treatment to the mother must be weighed against the possible risks to the foetus.

It is not known whether Myleran or its metabolites are excreted in human breast milk. Mothers receiving Myleran should not breast feed their infants.

Effect on ability to drive and use machines: None known.

Undesirable effects: The main adverse reaction of Myleran treatment is bone marrow depression, particularly thrombocytopenia.

Gastro-intestinal effects such as nausea, vomiting and diarrhoea have been reported rarely at normal therapeutic doses and may possibly be ameliorated by using divided doses.

Diffuse interstitial pulmonary fibrosis, with progressive dyspnoea and a persistent, non-productive cough has occurred rarely, usually after prolonged treatment over a number of years.

Histological features include atypical changes of the alveolar and bronchiolar epithelium and the presence of giant cells with large hyperchromatic nuclei. Once pulmonary toxicity is established the prognosis is poor despite Myleran withdrawal and there is little evidence that corticosteroids are helpful. The onset is usually insidious but may also be acute. The lung pathology may be complicated by superimposed infections. Pulmonary ossification and dystrophic calcification have also been reported. It is possible that subsequent radiotherapy can augment subclinical lung injury caused by Myleran. Other cytotoxic agents may cause additive lung toxicity.

Hyperpigmentation is the most common skin reaction and occurs in 5 to 10% of patients, particularly those with a dark complexion. It is often most marked on the neck, upper trunk, nipples, abdomen and palmar creases. In a few cases following prolonged Myleran therapy, hyperpigmentation occurs as a part of a clinical syndrome resembling adrenal insufficiency (Addison's disease). It is characterised by weakness, severe fatigue, anorexia, weight loss, nausea and vomiting and hyperpigmentation of the skin, but without biochemical evidence of adrenal impairment or mucous membrane hyperpigmentation or hair loss. The syndrome has sometimes resolved when Myleran has been withdrawn.

Other rare skin reactions include urticaria, erythema multiforme, erythema nodosum, alopecia, porphyria cutanea tarda, an 'allopurinol-type' rash and excessive dryness and fragility of the skin with complete anhydrosis, dryness of the oral mucous membranes and cheilosis. Sjogren's syndrome has also been reported.

An increased cutaneous radiation effect has been observed in patients receiving radiotherapy soon after high-dose Myleran (see *Overdose*).

There have been occasional reports of cholestatic jaundice and liver function abnormalities, but Myleran is not generally considered to be significantly hepatotoxic at normal therapeutic doses. However, retrospective review of post-mortem reports of patients who had been treated with low-dose Myleran for at least two years for chronic granulocytic leukaemia showed evidence of centrilobular sinusoidal fibrosis. The combination of Myleran and thioguanine is associated with significant hepatotoxicity.

Hyperbilirubinaemia, jaundice, hepatic veno-occlusive disease and centrilobular sinusoidal fibrosis with hepatoceullular atrophy and necrosis have been observed after high-dose Myleran treatment (see *Overdose*).

Lens changes and cataracts, which may be bilateral, have been reported during Myleran therapy. Corneal thinning has been reported after bone marrow transplantation preceded by high-dose Myleran treatment (see *Overdose*).

Convulsions have been observed in adults who have received high-dose Myleran (see *Overdose, Interactions, Warnings and precautions*).

Cardiac tamponade has been reported in a small number of patients with thalassaemia who received high-dose Myleran (see *Overdose*).

Gynaecomastia has been reported as a side effect of Myleran, as have myasthenia gravis and haemorrhagic cystitis.

Many histological and cytological changes have been observed in patients treated with Myleran, including widespread dysplasia affecting uterine cervical, bronchial and other epithelia. Most reports relate to long-term treatment but transient epithelial abnormalities have been observed following short-term high-dose treatment.

Overdose: The acute dose-limiting toxicity of Myleran in man is myelosuppression. If high-dose Myleran is used in association with bone marrow transplantation (The usual total dose of Myleran, given in combination with other agents is 14 to 16 mg/kg given orally over 4 consecutive days (3.5 to 4 mg/kg/day in divided doses)), gastrointestinal toxicity becomes dose-limiting, with mucositis, nausea, vomiting, diarrhoea and anorexia. The main effect of chronic overdosage is bone marrow depression and pancytopenia.

There is no known antidote to Myleran. There are no data about the possible value of dialysis. Appropriate supportive treatment should be given during the period of haematological toxicity.

Pharmacological properties
Pharmacodynamic properties: Busulphan (1,4-Butanediol Dimethanesulfonate) is a bifunctional alkylating agent. Binding to DNA is believed to play a role in its mode of action and di-guanyl derivatives have been isolated but interstrand crosslinking has not been conclusively demonstrated.

The basis for the uniquely selective effect of busulphan on granulocytopoiesis is not fully understood.

Pharmacokinetic properties: Early studies were carried out with radioactive labelled busulphan. More recently, gas liquid chromatography with selected ion monitoring has been used to quantitate busulphan in biological fluids. Busulphan doses of 2 to 6 mg were well absorbed and the kinetic data could be fitted to a zero-order absorption, one-compartment open model. The mean half-life for drug elimination was 2.57 hours.

The pharmacokinetics of busulphan have also been studied in patients following high-dose administration (1 mg/kg every 6 hours for 4 days). Drug was assayed either using gas liquid chromatography with electron capture detection or by high-performance liquid chromatography (HPLC). Using the former technique, the mean elimination half-life was found to be 2.3 hours after the final busulphan dose, but 3.4 hours after the first dose.

This suggests that busulphan may increase its own metabolic rate on repeated treatment.

The mean steady-state plasma concentration was 1.1 microgram/ml after dosing. Due to the variable absorption kinetics observed, it was not possible to evaluate the order of kinetics.

Using HPLC, steady-state plasma levels of busulphan were found to range from 2 to 8 microM (approximately 0.5 to 2 microgram/ml respectively). Peak plasma levels ranged from 3.1 to 5.9 microgram/ml in a patient treated with total dose of 16 mg/kg, or from 3.8 to 9.7 microgram/ml in two patients treated with a total of 20 mg/kg.

The urinary metabolites of busulphan have been identified as 3-hydroxysulpholane, tetrahydrothiophene 1-oxide and sulpholane, in patients treated with high-dose busulphan. Very little busulphan is excreted unchanged in the urine. After low- and high-dose administration, values of 1 and 2% respectively of unchanged drug has been observed.

Busulphan given in high doses has recently been shown to enter the cerebrospinal fluid (CSF) in concentrations comparable to those found in plasma, with a mean CSF: plasma ratio of 1.3:1. The saliva: plasma distribution of busulphan was found to be 1.1:1.

The level of busulphan bound reversibly to plasma proteins has been variably reported to be insignificant or approximately 55%. Irreversible binding of drug to blood cells and plasma proteins has been reported to be 47% and 32% respectively.

Preclinical safety data: There are no preclinical data of relevance to the prescriber which are additional to that in other sections of this SmPC.

Pharmaceutical particulars
List of excipients: Lactose PhEur; Maize Starch PhEur; Povidone BP; Magnesium Stearate PhEur; Erythrosine, E127 – Aluminium Lake HSE; Industrial Methylated Spirit BP or Ethanol BP; Gelatine PhEur; Purified Water PhEur.

Incompatibilities: None known.

Shelf life: 3 years.

Special precautions for storage: Store between 2–8°C (0.5 mg). Keep dry. Store below 25°C (2 mg tablets).

Nature and contents of container: Amber glass bottles with low-density polyethylene snap-fit closures. Pack size of 25 tablets per bottle.

Instructions for use/handling: No special instructions.

Marketing authorisation numbers
Myleran Tablets 0.5 mg PL 0003/5113R
Myleran Tablets 2 mg PL 0003/5112R

Date of approval/revision of SPC September 1998

NARAMIG* TABLETS 2.5 mg ▼

Qualitative and quantitative composition Tablets containing 2.5 mg of naratriptan as naratriptan hydrochloride.

Pharmaceutical form Tablets

Clinical particulars
Therapeutic indications: Naramig Tablets are indicated for the acute treatment of migraine attacks with or without aura.

Posology and method of administration: Naramig Tablets are recommended as monotherapy for the acute treatment of a migraine attack.

Naramig Tablets should not be used prophylactically.

Naramig Tablets should be swallowed whole with water.

Adults (18–65 years of age): The recommended dose of Naramig Tablets is a single 2.5 mg tablet.

The total dose should not exceed two 2.5 mg tablets in any 24-hour period.

If symptoms of migraine should recur, following an initial response, a second dose may be taken provided that there is a minimum interval of four hours between the two doses.

If a patient does not respond to a first dose of Naramig Tablets a second dose should not be taken for the same attack, as it is unlikely to be of benefit. However, Naramig Tablets may be used for subsequent migraine attacks.

Adolescents (12–17 years of age): Efficacy of Naramig Tablets at single doses of 0.25, 1.0 and 2.5 mg was not demonstrated to be greater than placebo in a placebo-controlled study in adolescents (12 to 17 years). Therefore, the use of Naramig Tablets in patients under 18 years of age is not recommended.

Children (under 12 years of age): There are no data available on the use of naratriptan in children under 12 years of age, therefore its use in this age group is not recommended.

Elderly (over 65 years of age): The safety and effectiveness of naratriptan in individuals over age 65 have not been evaluated and, therefore, its use in this age group cannot be recommended. There is a moderate decrease in clearance with age (see *Pharmacokinetics*).

Renal impairment: Naramig should be used with caution in patients with renal impairment. The maximum dose in any 24-hour treatment period is a single 2.5 mg tablet. The use of Naramig is contra-indicated in patients with severe renal impairment (creatinine clearance <15 ml/min) (see *Contra-indications* and *Pharmacokinetics*).

Hepatic impairment: Naramig should be used with caution in patients with hepatic impairment. The maximum dose in any 24-hour treatment period is a single 2.5 mg tablet. The use of Naramig is contra-indicated in patients with severe hepatic impairment (Child-Pugh grade C) (see *Contra-indications* and *Pharmacokinetics*).

Contra-indications: Hypersensitivity to any component of the preparation.

As with other 5-hydroxytryptamine$_1$ (5-HT$_1$) receptor agonists naratriptan should not be used in patients who have had a myocardial infarction or have ischaemic heart disease, or Prinzmetal's angina/coronary vasospasm, peripheral vascular disease or patients who have symptoms or signs consistent with ischaemic heart disease.

Naratriptan should not be administered to patients with a history of cerebrovascular accident (CVA) or transient ischaemic attack (TIA).

The use of naratriptan in patients with uncontrolled hypertension is contra-indicated.

As with other 5-HT$_1$ receptor agonists the concomitant use of naratriptan and other 5HT$_1$ agonists is contra-indicated.

Naratriptan is contra-indicated in patients with severely impaired renal or hepatic function.

Special warnings and precautions for use: Naratriptan should only be used where there is a clear diagnosis of migraine.

Naratriptan is not indicated for use in the management of hemiplegic, basilar or ophthalmoplegic migraine.

As with other acute migraine therapies, before treating headaches in patients not previously diagnosed as migraineurs, and in migraineurs who present with atypical symptoms, care should be taken to exclude other potentially serious neurological conditions. It should be noted that migraineurs may be at risk of certain cerebrovascular events (e.g. CVA or TIA).

As with other 5-HT$_1$ receptor agonists, naratriptan should not be given to patients in whom unrecognised cardiac disease is likely without a prior evaluation for underlying cardiovascular disease. Such patients include postmenopausal women, males over 40 and patients with risk factors for coronary artery disease.

If symptoms consistent with ischaemic heart disease occur appropriate evaluation should be carried out.

The concomitant administration of ergotamine and derivatives of ergotamine (including methysergide) with naratriptan is not recommended.

Naratriptan contains a sulphonamide component. Therefore, there is a theoretical risk of a hypersensitivity reaction in patients with known hypersensitivity to sulphonamides.

The recommended dose of naratriptan should not be exceeded.

Interactions with other medicaments and other forms of interaction: There is no evidence of interactions with β-blockers, tricyclic antidepressants, selective serotonin reuptake inhibitors, alcohol or food.

Co-administration of naratriptan with ergotamine, dihydroergotamine, or sumatriptan did not result in clinically significant effects on blood pressure, heart rate or ECG or affect naratriptan exposure.

Naratriptan does not inhibit monoamine oxidase enzymes; therefore interactions with monoamine oxidase inhibitors are not anticipated. In addition, the limited metabolism of naratriptan and the wide range of cytochrome P450 isoenzymes involved suggest that significant drug interactions with naratriptan are unlikely (see *Pharmacokinetics*).

Pregnancy and lactation: The safe use of naratriptan in pregnant women has not been established. Evaluation of experimental animal studies does not indicate any direct teratogenic effects or harmful effects on peri- and postnatal development.

Because animal reproduction studies are not always predictive of human response administration of naratriptan should only be considered if the expected benefit to the mother is greater than any possible risk to the foetus.

Naratriptan and/or drug related metabolites are secreted into the milk of lactating rats. Caution should be exercised when considering administration of naratriptan to nursing women.

Effects on ability to drive and use machines: Caution is recommended in patients performing skilled tasks (e.g. driving or operating machinery) as drowsiness may occur as a result of migraine. Drowsiness was no more apparent with naratriptan than with placebo in clinical trials.

Undesirable effects: Naramig is well tolerated.

At therapeutic doses of naratriptan the incidence of side effects reported in clinical trials was similar to placebo.

Some of the symptoms may be part of the migraine attack.

Frequent (>1/100)

General: The following symptoms are usually transient, may be intense and can affect any part of the body including the chest and throat: sensations of tingling or heat. Malaise/fatigue, dizziness, drowsiness.

Gastrointestinal: Nausea, vomiting.

Less frequent (<1/100)

General: The following symptoms are usually transient, may be intense and can affect any part of the body including the chest and throat: pain, sensations of heaviness, pressure or tightness.

Cardiovascular: Bradycardia, tachycardia, palpitations.

Eye: Visual disturbance.

Overdosage: There is no experience of accidental overdosage. However, administration of a high dose of 25 mg naratriptan in one healthy male subject increased blood pressure by up to 71 mmHg and resulted in adverse events including light-headedness, tension in the neck, tiredness and a loss of coordination. Blood pressure returned to baseline by 8 hours after dosing without other pharmacological intervention.

It is unknown what effect haemodialysis or peritoneal dialysis has on the plasma concentrations of naratriptan.

Treatment: If overdosage with naratriptan occurs, the patient should be monitored for at least 24 hours and standard supportive treatment applied as required.

Pharmacological properties
Pharmacodynamic properties: Naratriptan has been shown to be a selective agonist for 5 hydroxytryptamine$_1$ (5-HT$_1$) receptors mediating vascular contraction. This receptor is found predominantly in intracranial (cerebral and dural) blood vessels. Naratriptan has high affinity for human cloned 5-HT$_{1B}$ and 5-HT$_{1D}$ receptors, the human 5-HT$_{1B}$ receptor is thought to correspond to the vascular 5-HT$_1$ receptor mediating contraction of intracranial blood vessels. Naratriptan has little or no effect at other 5-HT receptor (5-HT$_2$, 5-HT$_3$, 5-HT$_4$ and 5-HT$_7$) subtypes.

In animals, naratriptan selectively constricts the carotid arterial circulation. This circulation supplies blood to the extracranial and intracranial tissues such as the meninges, and dilatation and/or oedema formation in these vessels is thought to be the underlying mechanism of migraine in man. In addition, experimental evidence suggests that naratriptan inhibits trigeminal nerve activity. Both these actions may contribute to the anti-migraine action of naratriptan in humans.

In man, a meta-analysis of BP recordings in 15 studies showed that the population average maximum increases in systolic and diastolic blood pressure after a 2.5 mg dose of naratriptan tablets would be less than 5 mmHg and 3 mmHg respectively. The blood pressure response was unaffected by age, weight, hepatic or renal impairment.

Pharmacokinetic properties:
Absorption, distribution, metabolism and elimination: Following oral administration, naratriptan is rapidly absorbed with maximum plasma concentrations observed at 2–3 hours. After administration of a 2.5 mg naratriptan tablet C_{max} is approximately 8.3 ng/ml (95% CI:6.5 to 10.5 ng/ml) in women and 5.4 ng/ml (95% CI: 4.7 to 6.1 ng/ml) in men.

The oral bioavailability is 74% in women and 63% in men with no differences in efficacy and tolerability in clinical use. Therefore, a gender-related dose adjustment is not required.

Naratriptan is distributed in a volume of 170 l. Plasma protein binding is low (29%).

The mean elimination half-life ($t_{1/2}$) is 6 hours.

Mean clearance after intravenous administration was 470 ml/min in men and 380 ml/min in women. Renal clearance is similar in men and women at 220 ml/min and is higher than the glomerular filtration rate suggesting that naratriptan is actively secreted in the renal tubules. Naratriptan is predominantly excreted in the urine with 50% of the dose recovered as unchanged naratriptan and 30% recovered as inactive metabolites. *In vitro*, naratriptan was metabolised by a wide range of cytochrome P450 isoenzymes. Consequently, significant metabolic drug interactions with naratriptan are not anticipated (see *Interactions*).

Special patient populations:

Elderly: In healthy elderly subjects (n=12), clearance was decreased by 26% when compared to healthy young subjects (n=12) in the same study (see *Posology and method of administration*).

Gender: The naratriptan AUC and C_{max} were approximately 35% lower in males compared to females however, with no differences in efficacy and tolerability in clinical use. Therefore, a gender-related dose adjustment is not required (see *Posology and method of administration*).

Renal impairment: Renal excretion is the major route for the elimination of naratriptan. Accordingly exposure to naratriptan may be increased in patients with renal disease.

In a study in male and female renally-impaired patients (creatinine clearance 18 to 115 ml/min; n=15) matched for sex, age and weight with healthy subjects (n=8); renally-impaired patients had an approximately 80% increase in $t_{1/2}$ and an approximately 50% reduction in clearance (see *Posology and method of administration*).

Hepatic impairment: The liver plays a lesser role in the clearance of orally administered naratriptan. In a study in male and female hepatically-impaired patients (Child-Pugh grade A or B n=8) matched for sex, age and weight with healthy subjects who received oral naratriptan; hepatically-impaired patients had an approximately 40% increase in $t_{1/2}$ and an approximately 30% reduction in clearance (see *Posology and method of administration*).

Preclinical safety data: No clinically relevant findings were observed in preclinical studies.

Pharmaceutical particulars
List of excipients:
Tablet core: Microcrystalline cellulose; Anhydrous lactose; Croscarmellose sodium; Magnesium stearate.

Film coat: Methylhydroxypropylcellulose; Titanium dioxide (E171); Triacetin; Iron oxide yellow (E172); Indigo carmine aluminium lake (E132).

Incompatibilities: None reported.

Shelf life: 24 months.

Special precautions for storage: Store below 30°C.

Nature and contents of container: 2, 4, 6 or 12 tablets in a double-foil blister pack.

Instructions for use/handling: None.

Marketing authorisation number PL 10949/0273

Date of approval/revision of SPC April 1997/March 1998

Legal category POM

NIMBEX INJECTION 2 mg/ml
NIMBEX [FORTE] INJECTION 5 mg/ml

Qualitative and quantitative composition A sterile solution containing 2 mg cisatracurium (bis-cation) per ml as cisatracurium besilate (BAN, pINN). The product contains no antimicrobial preservative and is supplied in an ampoule.

A sterile solution containing 5 mg cisatracurium (bis-cation) per ml as cisatracurium besilate (BAN, pINN). The product contains no antimicrobial preservative and is supplied in a vial.

Chemical description: Nimbex (cisatracurium besilate), (1R, 1'R, 2R, 2'R,)-2,2'-(3, 11-Dioxo-4,10-dioxatridecamethylene) bis (1,2,3,4-tetrahydro-6,7-dimethoxy-2-methyl-1-veratryisoquinolinium) dibenzenesulfonate.

Cisatracurium besilate is one of the ten isomeric components of atracurium besilate comprising about 15% of the mixture.

Pharmaceutical form Solution for injection.

Clinical particulars Nimbex is an intermediate-duration, non-depolarising neuromuscular blocking agent for intravenous administration.

Therapeutic indications: Nimbex is indicated for use during surgical and other procedures and in intensive care. Nimbex can be used as an adjunct to general anaesthesia, or sedation in the Intensive Care Unit (ICU) to relax skeletal muscles, and to facilitate tracheal intubation and mechanical ventilation.

Posology and method of administration: Please note that Nimbex should not be mixed in the same syringe or administered simultaneously through the same needle as propofol injectable emulsion or with alkaline solutions such as sodium thiopentone (please refer to *Incompatibilities* section).

Nimbex contains no antimicrobial preservative and is intended for single patient use.

Monitoring advice: As with other neuromuscular blocking agents, monitoring of neuromuscular function is recommended during the use of Nimbex in order to individualise dosage requirements.

Use by intravenous bolus injection.

Dosage in adults: Tracheal Intubation. The recommended intubation dose of Nimbex for adults is 0.15 mg/kg (body weight). This dose produced good to excellent conditions for tracheal intubation 120 seconds after administration of Nimbex, following induction of anaesthesia with propofol.

Higher doses will shorten the time to onset of neuromuscular block.

Table 1 summarises mean pharmacodynamic data when Nimbex was administered at doses of 0.1 to 0.4 mg/kg/(body weight) to healthy adult patients during opioid (thiopentone/fentanyl/midazolam) or propofol anaesthesia.

Enflurane or isoflurane anaesthesia may extend the clinically effective duration of an initial dose of Nimbex by as much as 15%.

Maintenance: Neuromuscular block can be extended with maintenance doses of Nimbex. A dose of 0.03 mg/kg (body weight) provides approximately 20 minutes of additional clinically effective neuromuscular block during opioid or propofol anaesthesia.

Consecutive maintenance doses do not result in progressive prolongation of effect.

Spontaneous recovery: Once spontaneous recovery from neuromuscular block is underway, the rate is independent of the Nimbex dose administered. During opioid or propofol anaesthesia, the median times from 25 to 75% and from 5 to 95% recovery are approximately 13 and 30 minutes, respectively.

Reversal: Neuromuscular block following Nimbex administration is readily reversible with standard doses of anticholinesterase agents. The mean times from 25 to 75% recovery and to full clinical recovery (T_4:T_1 ratio ≥0.7) are approximately 4 and 9 minutes respectively, following administration of the reversal agent at an average of 10% T_1 recovery.

Dosage in children aged 2 to 12 years: The recommended initial dose of Nimbex in children aged 2 to 12 years, during opioid anaesthesia, is 0.1 mg/kg (bodyweight) administered over 5 to 10 seconds. Table 2 summarises mean pharmacodynamic data obtained during opioid or halothane anaesthesia. A dose of 0.1 mg/kg (bodyweight) has a faster onset time, a shorter clinically effective duration and a faster spontaneous recovery profile than those observed in adults under similar anaesthetic conditions.

Based on the tabulated data, halothane may be expected to potentiate the neuromuscular blocking effect of Nimbex by approximately 20%. No information is available on the use of Nimbex in children during isoflurane or enflurane anaesthesia but these agents may also be expected to extend the clinically effective duration of a dose of Nimbex by approximately 15–20%.

Tracheal intubation: Although intubation has not been specifically studied in this age group, onset is faster than in adults and therefore intubation should also be possible within 2 minutes of administration. No dosage recommendation for intubation in children can be made until further information becomes available.

Maintenance: Neuromuscular block can be extended with maintenance doses of Nimbex. A dose of 0.02 mg/kg (body weight) provides approximately 9 minutes of additional clinically effective neuromuscular block during halothane anaesthesia. Consecutive maintenance doses do not result in progressive prolongation of effect.

Spontaneous Recovery: During opioid anaesthesia, the median times from 25 to 75% and from 5 to 95% recovery are approximately 10 and 25 minutes, respectively.

Reversal: Neuromuscular block following Nimbex administration is readily reversible with standard doses of anti-cholinesterase agents. The mean times from 25 to 75% recovery and to full clinical recovery (T_4:T_1 ratio ≥0.7) are approximately 2 and 5 minutes respectively, following administration of the reversal agent at an average of 13% T_1 recovery.

Table 1

Initial Nimbex dose mg/kg (bodyweight)	*Anaesthetic background*	*Time to 90% T_1† suppression min*	*Time to maximum T_1† suppression min*	*Time to 25% spontaneous T_1† recovery min*
0.1	Opioid	3.4	4.8	45
0.15	Propofol	2.6	3.5	55
0.2	Opioid	2.4	2.9	65
0.4	Opioid	1.5	1.9	91

†T_1 Single twitch response as well as the first component of the Train-of-four response of the adductor pollicis muscle following supramaximal electrical stimulation of the ulnar nerve.

Table 2

Initial Nimbex dose mg/kg (bodyweight)	*Anaesthetic background*	*Time to 90% T_1† suppression min*	*Time to maximum T_1† suppression min*	*Time to 25% spontaneous T_1† recovery min*
0.1	Opioid	1.7	2.8	28
0.08	Halothane	1.7	2.5	31

†T_1 Single twitch response as well as the first component of the Train-of-four response of the adductor pollicis muscle following supramaximal electrical stimulation of the ulnar nerve.

Table 3
Infusion delivery rate of Nimbex injection 2 mg/ml

Patient (bodyweight) (kg)	*Dose (μg/kg/min)*				*Infusion rate*
	1.0	*1.5*	*2.0*	*3.0*	
20	0.6	0.9	1.2	1.8	ml/hr
70	2.1	3.2	4.2	6.3	ml/hr
100	3.0	4.5	6.0	9.0	ml/hr

Table 4
Infusion delivery rate of Nimbex FORTE injection 5 mg/ml

Patient (bodyweight) (kg)	*Dose (μg/kg/min)*				*Infusion rate*
	1.0	*1.5*	*2.0*	*3.0*	
70	0.8	1.2	1.7	2.5	ml/hr
100	1.2	1.8	2.4	3.6	ml/hr

Use by intravenous infusion:

Dosage in adults and children aged 2 to 12 years: Maintenance of neuromuscular block may be achieved by infusion of Nimbex. An initial infusion rate of 3 µg/kg (bodyweight)/min (0.18 mg/kg/hr) is recommended to restore 89 to 99% T_1 suppression following evidence of spontaneous recovery. After an initial period of stabilisation of neuromuscular block, a rate of 1 to 2 µg/kg (body weight)/min (0.06 to 0.12 mg/kg/hr) should be adequate to maintain block in this range in most patients.

Reduction of the infusion rate by up to 40% may be required when Nimbex is administered during isoflurane or enflurane anaesthesia (see *Interactions* section).

The infusion rate will depend upon the concentration of cisatracurium in the infusion solution, the desired degree of neuromuscular block, and the patient's weight. Tables 3 and 4 provide guidelines for delivery of undiluted Nimbex.

Steady rate continuous infusion of Nimbex is not associated with a progressive increase or decrease in neuromuscular blocking effect.

Following discontinuation of infusion of Nimbex, spontaneous recovery from neuromuscular block proceeds at a rate comparable to that following administration of a single bolus.

Dosage in children aged less than 2 years: No dosage recommendation for paediatric patients under 2 years of age can be made until further information becomes available.

Dosage in elderly patients: No dosing alterations are required in elderly patients. In these patients Nimbex has a similar pharmacodynamic profile to that observed in young adult patients but, as with other neuromuscular blocking agents, it may have a slightly slower onset.

Dosage in patients with renal impairment: No dosing alterations are required in patients with renal failure.

In these patients Nimbex has a similar pharmacodynamic profile to that observed in patients with normal renal function but it may have a slightly slower onset.

Dosage in patients with hepatic impairment: No dosing alterations are required in patients with end-stage liver disease. In these patients Nimbex has a similar pharmacodynamic profile to that observed in patients with normal hepatic function but it may have a slightly faster onset.

Dosage in patients with cardiovascular disease: When administered by rapid bolus injection (over 5 to 10 seconds) to adult patients with serious cardiovascular disease (New York Heart Association Class I-III) undergoing coronary artery bypass graft (CABG) surgery, Nimbex has not been associated with clinically significant cardiovascular effects at any dose studied (up to and including 0.4 mg/kg (8×ED_{95}). However, there are limited data for doses above 0.3 mg/kg in this patient population).

Dosage in intensive care unit (ICU) patients: Nimbex may be administered by bolus dose and/or infusion to adult patients in the ICU. An initial infusion rate of Nimbex of 3 µg/kg (body weight)/min (0.18 mg/kg/hr) is recommended for adult ICU patients. There may be wide interpatient variation in dosage requirements and these may increase or decrease with time. In clinical studies the average infusion rate was 3 µg/kg/min [range 0.5 to 10.2 µg/kg (body weight)/min (0.03 to 0.6 mg/kg/hr)].

The median time to full spontaneous recovery following long-term (up to 6 days) infusion of Nimbex in ICU patients was approximately 50 minutes.

The recovery profile after infusions of Nimbex to ICU patients is independent of duration of infusion.

Contra-indications: Nimbex is contra-indicated in patients known to be hypersensitive to cisatracurium, atracurium, or benzenesulfonic acid.

Nimbex is contra-indicated in pregnancy since there is no information on the use of Nimbex in pregnant women.

Nimbex is contra-indicated in children under 2 years of age since it has not been studied in this patient population.

Special warnings and special precautions for use: Cisatracurium paralyses the respiratory muscles as well as other skeletal muscles but has no known effect on consciousness or pain threshold. Nimbex should be only administered by or under the supervision of anaesthetists or other clinicians who are familiar with the use and action of neuromuscular blocking agents. Facilities for tracheal intubation, and maintenance of pulmonary ventilation and adequate arterial oxygenation have to be available.

Great caution should be exercised when administering Nimbex to patients who have shown allergic hypersensitivity to other neuromuscular blocking agents since cross-reactivity between neuromuscular blocking agents has been reported.

Cisatracurium does not have significant vagolytic or ganglion-blocking properties.

Consequently, Nimbex has no clinically significant effect on heart rate and will not counteract the bradycardia produced by many anaesthetic agents or by vagal stimulation during surgery.

Patients with myasthenia gravis and other forms of neuromuscular disease have shown greatly increased sensitivity to non-depolarising blocking agents. An initial dose of not more than 0.02 mg/kg Nimbex is recommended in these patients.

Severe acid-base and/or serum electrolyte abnormalities may increase or decrease the sensitivity of patients to neuromuscular blocking agents.

Cisatracurium has not been studied in patients with a history of malignant hyperthermia. Studies in malignant hyperthermia-susceptible pigs indicated that cisatracurium does not trigger this syndrome.

There have been no studies of cisatracurium in patients undergoing surgery with induced hypothermia (25 to 28°C). As with other neuromuscular blocking agents the rate of infusion required to maintain adequate surgical relaxation under these conditions may be expected to be significantly reduced.

Cisatracurium has not been studied in patients with burns; however, as with other non-depolarising neuromuscular blocking agents, the possibility of increased dosing requirements and shortened duration of action must be considered if Nimbex injection is administered to these patients.

Nimbex is hypotonic and must not be applied into the infusion line of a blood transfusion.

Intensive Care Unit (ICU) patients: When administered to laboratory animals in high doses, laudanosine, a metabolite of cisatracurium and atracurium, has been associated with transient hypotension and in some species, cerebral excitatory effects. In the most sensitive animal species, these effects occurred at laudanosine plasma concentrations similar to those that have been observed in some ICU patients following prolonged infusion of atracurium.

Consistent with the decreased infusion rate requirements of cisatracurium, plasma laudanosine concentrations are approximately one third those following atracurium infusion. There have been rare reports of seizures in ICU patients who have received atracurium and other agents. These patients usually had one or more medical conditions predisposing to seizures (e.g. cranial trauma, hypoxic encephalopathy, cerebral oedema, viral encephalitis, uraemia). A causal relationship to laudanosine has not been established.

Interaction with other medicaments and other forms of interaction: Many drugs have been shown to influence the magnitude and/or duration of action of non-depolarising neuromuscular blocking agents, including the following:

Increased effect: By anaesthetic agents such as enflurane, isoflurane, halothane (see *Posology and method of administration*) and ketamine, by other non-depolarising neuromuscular blocking agents or by other drugs such as antibiotics (including the aminoglycosides, polymyxins, spectinomycin, tetracyclines, lincomycin and clindamycin); anti-arrhythmic drugs (including propranolol, calcium channel blockers, lignocaine, procainamide and quinidine); diuretics (including frusemide and possibly thiazides, mannitol and acetazolamide); magnesium and lithium salts and ganglion blocking drugs (trimetaphan, hexamethonium).

A decreased effect is seen after prior chronic administration of phenytoin or carbamazepine.

Prior administration of suxamethonium has no effect on the duration of neuromuscular block following bolus doses of Nimbex or on infusion rate requirements.

Administration of suxamethonium to prolong the effects of non-depolarising neuromuscular blocking agents may result in a prolonged and complex block which can be difficult to reverse with anticholinesterases.

Rarely, certain drugs may aggravate or unmask latent myasthenia gravis or actually induce a myasthenic syndrome; increased sensitivity to non-depolarising neuromuscular blocking agents might result. Such drugs include various antibiotics, β-blockers (propranolol, oxprenolol), anti-arrhythmic drugs (procainamide, quinidine), anti-rheumatic drugs (chloroquine, D-penicillamine), trimetaphan, chlorpromazine, steroids, phenytoin and lithium.

Pregnancy and lactation: Nimbex is contra-indicated in pregnancy since there is no information on the use of Nimbex in pregnant women. Fertility studies have not been performed. Reproduction studies in rats have not revealed any adverse effects on foetal development of cisatracurium. The relevance of these studies is limited due to species differences in metabolism and low systemic exposure levels.

It is not known whether cisatracurium or its metabolites are excreted in human milk.

Effects on ability to drive and use machines: This precaution is not relevant to the use of Nimbex. However the usual precautions relating to performance of tasks following general anaesthesia still apply.

Undesirable effects: Adverse effects recorded following administration of Nimbex were cutaneous flushing or rash, bradycardia, hypotension and bronchospasm (see *Dosage in intensive care unit (ICU) patients* and *Pharmacodynamic properties*).

Anaphylactic reactions of varying degrees of severity have been observed after the administration of neuromuscular blocking agents. Very rarely, severe anaphylactic reactions have been reported in patients receiving Nimbex in conjunction with one or more anaesthetic agents.

There have been some reports of muscle weakness and/or myopathy following prolonged use of muscle relaxants in severely ill patients in the ICU. Most patients were receiving concomitant corticosteroids. These events have been reported infrequently in association with Nimbex and a causal relationship has not been established.

Overdosage: Symptoms and signs: Prolonged muscle paralysis and its consequences are expected to be the main signs of overdosage with Nimbex.

Management: It is essential to maintain pulmonary ventilation and arterial oxygenation until adequate spontaneous respiration returns. Full sedation will be required since consciousness is not impaired by Nimbex. Recovery may be accelerated by the administration of anti-cholinesterase agents once evidence of spontaneous recovery is present.

Pharmacological properties

Pharmacodynamic properties: Cisatracurium is an intermediate-duration, non-depolarising benzylisoquinolinium skeletal muscle relaxant.

Clinical studies in man indicated that Nimbex is not associated with dose-dependent histamine release even at doses up to and including 8×ED_{95}.

Mode of action: Cisatracurium binds to cholinergic receptors on the motor end-plate to antagonise the action of acetylcholine, resulting in a competitive block of neuromuscular transmission. This action is readily reversed by anti-cholinesterase agents such as neostigmine or edrophonium.

The ED_{95} (dose required to produce 95% depression of the twitch response of the adductor pollicis muscle to stimulation of the ulnar nerve) of cisatracurium is estimated to be 0.05 mg/kg bodyweight during opioid anaesthesia (thiopentone/fentanyl/midazolam).

The ED_{95} of cisatracurium in children during halothane anaesthesia is 0.04 mg/kg.

Pharmacokinetic properties: Cisatracurium undergoes degradation in the body at physiological pH and temperature by Hofmann elimination (a chemical process) to form laudanosine and the monoquaternary acrylate metabolite. The monoquaternary acrylate undergoes hydrolysis by non-specific plasma esterases to form the monoquaternary alcohol metabolite. Elimination of cisatracurium is largely organ independent but the liver and kidneys are primary pathways for the clearance of its metabolites.

These metabolites do not possess neuromuscular blocking activity.

Pharmacokinetics in adult patients: Non-compartmental pharmacokinetics of cisatracurium are independent of dose in the range studied (0.1 to 0.2 mg/kg, i.e. 2 to 4×ED_{95}).

Population pharmacokinetic modelling confirms and extends these findings up to 0.4 mg/kg (8×ED_{95}). Pharmacokinetic parameters after doses of 0.1 and 0.2 mg/kg Nimbex administered to healthy adult surgical patients are summarised in the table below:

Parameter	*Range of mean values*
Clearance	4.7 to 5.7 ml/min/kg
Volume of distribution at steady state	121 to 161 ml/kg
Elimination half-life	22 to 29 min

Pharmacokinetics in elderly patients: There are no clinically important differences in the pharmacokinetics of cisatracurium in elderly and young adult patients. The recovery profile is also unchanged.

Pharmacokinetics in patients with renal/hepatic impairment: There are no clinically important differences in the pharmacokinetics of cisatracurium in patients with end-stage renal failure or end stage liver disease and in healthy adult patients. Their recovery profiles are also unchanged.

Pharmacokinetics during infusions: The pharmacokinetics of cisatracurium after infusions of Nimbex are similar to those after single bolus injection. The recovery profile after infusion of Nimbex is independent of duration of infusion and is similar to that after single bolus injection.

Pharmacokinetics in intensive care unit (ICU) patients: The pharmacokinetics of cisatracurium in ICU patients receiving prolonged infusions are similar to those in healthy surgical adults receiving infusions or single bolus injections. The recovery profile after infusions of Nimbex in ICU patients is independent of duration of infusion.

Concentrations of metabolites are higher in ICU patients with abnormal renal and/or hepatic function (see *Special warnings and special precautions for use*). These metabolites do not contribute to neuromuscular block.

Preclinical safety data: Acute toxicity: Meaningful acute studies with cisatracurium could not be performed. For symptoms of toxicity see *Overdosage*.

Subacute toxicity: Studies with repeated administration for three weeks in dogs and monkeys showed no compound specific toxic signs.

Mutagenicity: Cisatracurium was not mutagenic in an *in vitro* microbial mutagenicity test at concentrations up to 5000 mcg/plate.

In an *in vivo* cytogenetic study in rats, no significant chromosomal abnormalities were seen at s.c doses up to 4 mg/kg.

Cisatracurium was mutagenic in an *in vitro* mouse lymphoma cell mutagenicity assay, at concentrations of 40 mcg/ml and higher.

A single positive mutagenic response for a drug used infrequently and/or briefly is of questionable clinical relevance.

Carcinogenicity: Carcinogenicity studies have not been performed.

Local tolerance: The result of an intra-arterial study in rabbits showed that Nimbex injection is well tolerated and no drug related changes were seen.

Pharmaceutical particulars

List of excipients: Benzenesulfonic Acid solution 32% w/v (Wellcome specification); Water for Injections (PhEur).

Incompatibilities: Degradation of cisatracurium besilate has been demonstrated to occur more rapidly in lactated Ringer's Injection and 5% Dextrose and lactated Ringer's Injection than in the infusion fluids listed in *Instructions for use/handling* section.

Therefore it is recommended that lactated Ringer's Injection and 5% Dextrose and lactated Ringer's Injection are not used as the diluent in preparing solutions of Nimbex for infusion.

Since Nimbex is stable only in acidic solutions it should not be mixed in the same syringe or administered simultaneously through the same needle with alkaline solutions, e.g., sodium thiopentone. It is not compatible with ketorolac trometamol or propofol injectable emulsion.

Shelf life: Shelf-life of the medicinal product as packaged for sale: 24 months at 2–8°C.

Shelf-life after dilution according to directions: The product contains no antimicrobial preservative and therefore should be used immediately on dilution, or failing this the aseptically prepared dilution should be stored at 2–8°C for no more than 24 hrs, after which time unused solution should be discarded.

Shelf-life after the first time the pack is opened: The pack is designed for use on a single occasion, injected or diluted immediately after opening, any remaining solution should be discarded.

Special precautions for storage: Do not freeze. Protect from light.

Nature and contents of container: Nimbex injection 2 mg/ml comes in boxes of 5×2.5 ml, 5 ml or 10 ml ampoules, 2×25 ml ampoules and Nimbex [Forte] injection 5 mg/ml as 1×30 ml vial.

Type I, clear, neutral glass ampoules.

Type I, clear, neutral glass vial with a polymeric coated synthetic bromobutyl rubber stopper and aluminium collar with plastic flip-top cover.

Instructions for use/handling: Use only clear and almost colourless up to slightly yellow/greenish yellow coloured solutions.

Diluted Nimbex is physically and chemically stable for at least 24 hours at 5°C and 25°C at concentrations between 0.1 and 2 mg/ml in the following infusion fluids, in either polyvinyl chloride or polypropylene containers:

Sodium Chloride (0.9% w/v) Intravenous Infusion.
Glucose (5% w/v) Intravenous Infusion.
Sodium Chloride (0.18% w/v) and Glucose (4% w/v) Intravenous Infusion.
Sodium Chloride (0.45% w/v) and Glucose (2.5% w/v) Intravenous Infusion.

However, since the product contains no antimicrobial preservative, dilution should be carried out immediately prior to use, or failing this be stored as directed under *Special precautions for storage.*

Nimbex has been shown to be compatible with the following commonly used peri-operative drugs, when mixed in conditions simulating administration into a running intravenous infusion via a Y-site injection port: alfentanil hydrochloride, droperidol, fentanyl citrate, midazolam hydrochloride and sufentanil citrate. Where other drugs are administered through the same indwelling needle or cannula as Nimbex, it is recommended that each drug be flushed through with an adequate volume of a suitable intravenous fluid, e.g. Sodium Chloride Intravenous Infusion (0.9% w/v).

As with other drugs administered intravenously, when a small vein is selected as the injection site, Nimbex should be flushed through the vein with a suitable intravenous fluid, e.g. sodium chloride intravenous infusion (0.9% w/v).

Marketing authorisation numbers
Nimbex Injection 2 mg/ml PL 0003/0364
Nimbex (Forte) Injection 5 mg/ml PL 0003/0365

Date of approval/revision of SPC July 1998

Legal category POM.

PREDNESOL* TABLETS

Qualitative and quantitative composition Small, pink, soluble tablets engraved 'Prednesol Glaxo' on one side and scored on the reverse. Each tablet contains 5 mg prednisolone as the sodium phosphate ester.

Pharmaceutical form Tablet.

Clinical particulars

Therapeutic indications: A wide variety of diseases may sometimes require corticosteroid therapy. Some of the principal indications are: bronchial asthma, severe hypersensitivity reactions, anaphylaxis; rheumatoid arthritis, systemic lupus erythematosus, dermatomyositis, mixed connective tissue disease (excluding systemic sclerosis), polyarteritis nodosa; inflammatory skin disorders, including pemphigus vulgaris, bullous pemphigoid and pyoderma gangrenosum; minimal change nephrotic syndrome, acute interstitial nephritis; ulcerative colitis, Crohn's disease; sarcoidosis; rheumatic carditis; haemolytic anaemia (autoimmune), acute and lymphatic leukaemia, malignant lymphoma, multiple myeloma, idiopathic thrombocytopenic purpura; immunosuppression in transplantation.

Posology and method of administration: Prednesol Tablets are best taken dissolved in water, but they can be swallowed whole without difficulty.

The lowest dosage that will produce an acceptable result should be used (see *Special warnings and precautions for use*); when it is possible to reduce the dosage, this must be accomplished by stages. During prolonged therapy any intercurrent illness, trauma or surgical procedure will require a temporary increase in dosage; if corticosteroids have been stopped following prolonged therapy they may need to be temporarily re-introduced.

Adults: The dose used will depend upon the disease, its severity, and the clinical response obtained. The following regimens are for guidance only. Divided dosage is usually employed.

Short-term treatment: 20 to 30 mg daily for the first few days, subsequently reducing the daily dosage by 2.5 or 5 mg every two to five days, depending upon the response.

Rheumatoid arthritis: 7.5 to 10 mg daily. For maintenance therapy the lowest effective dosage is used.

Most other conditions: 10 to 100 mg daily for one to three weeks, then reducing to the minimum effective dosage.

Children: Fractions of the adult dosage may be used (e.g. 75% at 12 years, 50% at 7 years and 25% at 1 year) but clinical factors must be given due weight.

Contra-indications: Systemic infections, unless specific anti-infective therapy is employed. Live virus immunisation. Hypersensitivity to any component of the tablets.

Special warnings and precautions for use: In patients who have received more than physiological doses of systemic corticosteroids (approximately 7.5 mg prednisolone or equivalent) for greater than 3 weeks, withdrawal should not be abrupt. How dose reduction should be carried out depends largely on whether the disease is likely to relapse as the dose of systemic corticosteroids is reduced. Clinical assessment of disease activity may be needed during withdrawal. If the disease is unlikely to relapse on withdrawal of systemic corticosteroids but there is uncertainty about HPA suppression, the dose of systemic corticosteroid may be reduced rapidly to physiological doses. Once a daily dose equivalent to 7.5 mg prednisolone is reached, dose reduction should be slower to allow the HPA-axis to recover.

Abrupt withdrawal of systemic corticosteroid treatment, which has continued up to 3 weeks is appropriate if it is considered that the disease is unlikely to relapse. Abrupt withdrawal of doses of up to 40 mg daily of prednisolone, or equivalent for 3 weeks is unlikely to lead to clinically relevant HPA-axis suppression, in the majority of patients. In the following patient groups, gradual withdrawal of systemic corticosteroid therapy should be *considered* even after courses lasting 3 weeks or less:

- Patients who have had repeated courses of systemic corticosteroids, particularly if taken for greater than 3 weeks.
- When a short course has been prescribed within one year of cessation of long-term therapy (months or years).
- Patients who may have reasons for adrenocortical insufficiency other than exogenous corticosteroid therapy.
- Patients receiving doses of systemic corticosteroid greater than 40 mg daily of prednisolone (or equivalent).
- Patients repeatedly taking doses in the evening.

Patients should carry 'Steroid treatment' cards which give clear guidance on the precautions to be taken to minimise risk and which provide details of prescriber, drug, dosage and the duration of treatment.

Adrenal cortical atrophy develops during prolonged therapy and may persist for years after stopping treatment. Withdrawal of corticosteroids after prolonged therapy must therefore always be gradual to avoid acute adrenal insufficiency, being tapered off over weeks or months according to the dose and duration of treatment. During prolonged therapy any intercurrent illness, trauma or surgical procedure will require a temporary increase in dosage; if corticosteroids have been stopped following prolonged therapy they may need to be temporarily re-introduced.

Suppression of the HPA axis and other undesirable effects may be minimised by using the lowest effective dose for the minimum period, and by administering the daily requirement as a single morning dose or, whenever possible, as a single morning dose on alternate days. Frequent patient review is required to appropriately titrate the dose against disease activity (see *Posology and method of administration*).

Suppression of the inflammatory response and immune function increases the susceptibility to infections and their severity. The clinical presentation may often be atypical and serious infections such as septicaemia and tuberculosis may be masked and may reach an advanced stage before being recognised.

Chickenpox is of particular concern since this normally minor illness may be fatal in immunosuppressed patients. Patients without a definite history of chickenpox should be advised to avoid close personal contact with chickenpox or herpes zoster and if exposed they should seek urgent medical attention. If the patient is a child parents must be given the above advice. Passive immunisation with varicella zoster immunoglobulin (VZIG) is needed by exposed non-immune patients who are receiving systemic corticosteroids or who have used them within the previous 3 months; this should be given within 10 days of exposure to chickenpox. If a diagnosis of chickenpox is confirmed, the illness warrants specialist care and urgent treatment. Corticosteroids should not be stopped and the dose may need to be increased.

Live vaccines should not be given to individuals with impaired immune responsiveness. The antibody response to other vaccines may be diminished.

Because of the possibility of fluid retention, care must be taken when corticosteroids are administered to patients with renal insufficiency or hypertension or congestive heart failure.

Corticosteroids may worsen diabetes mellitus, osteoporosis, hypertension, glaucoma and epilepsy and therefore patients with these conditions or a family history of them should be monitored frequently.

Care is required and frequent patient monitoring necessary where there is a history of severe affective disorders (especially a previous history of steroid psychosis), previous steroid myopathy, peptic ulceration or patients with a history of tuberculosis.

In patients with liver failure, blood levels of corticosteroid may be increased, as with other drugs which are metabolised in the liver. Frequent patient monitoring is therefore necessary.

Use in children: Corticosteroids cause dose-related growth retardation in infancy, childhood and adolescence, which may be irreversible.

Use in the elderly: The common adverse effects of systemic corticosteroids may be associated with more serious consequences in old age, especially osteoporosis, hypertension, hypokalaemia, diabetes, susceptibility to infection and thinning of the skin. Close clinical supervision is required to avoid life-threatening reactions.

Interaction with other medicaments and other forms of interaction: Rifampicin, rifabutin, carbamazepine, phenobarbitone, phenytoin, primidone, ephedrine and aminoglutethimide enhance the metabolism of corticosteroids and its therapeutic effects may be reduced.

The desired effects of hypoglycaemic agents (including insulin), anti-hypertensives and diuretics are antagonised by corticosteroids, and the hypokalaemic effects of acetazolamide, loop diuretics, thiazide diuretics and carbenoxolone are enhanced.

The efficacy of coumarin anticoagulants may be enhanced by concurrent corticosteroid therapy and close monitoring of the INR or prothrombin time is required to avoid spontaneous bleeding.

The renal clearance of salicylates is increased by corticosteroids and steroid withdrawal may result in salicylate intoxication.

Steroids may reduce the effects of anticholinesterases in myasthenia gravis and cholecystographic X-ray media.

Pregnancy and lactation: The ability of corticosteroids to cross placenta varies between individual drugs, however, 88% of prednisolone is inactivated as it crosses the placenta.

Administration of corticosteroids to pregnant animals can cause abnormalities of foetal development including cleft palate, intra-uterine growth retardation and effects on brain growth and development. There is no evidence that corticosteroids result in an increased incidence of congenital abnormalities, such as cleft palate/lip in man. However, when administered for prolonged periods or repeatedly during pregnancy, corticosteroids may increase the risk of intra-uterine growth retardation. Hypoadrenalism may, in theory, occur in the neonate following prenatal exposure to corticosteroids but usually resolves spontaneously following birth and is rarely clinically important. As with all drugs, corticosteroids should only be prescribed when the benefits to the mother and child outweigh the risks. When corticosteroids are essential however, patients with normal pregnancies may be treated as though they were in the non-gravid state.

Patients with pre-eclampsia or fluid retention require close monitoring.

Depression of hormone levels has been described in pregnancy but the significance of this finding is not clear.

Lactation: Corticosteroids are excreted in small amounts in breast milk. However doses of up to 40 mg daily of prednisolone are unlikely to cause systemic effects in the infant. Infants of mothers taking higher doses than this may have a degree of adrenal suppression but the benefits of breast feeding are likely to outweigh any theoretical risk.

Effects on ability to drive and use machines: None known.

Undesirable effects: The incidence of predictable undesirable effects, including hypothalamic-pituitary-adrenal suppression correlates with the relative potency of the drug, dosage, timing of administration and the duration of treatment (see *Special warnings and precautions for use*).

Endocrine/metabolic: Suppression of the hypothalamic-pituitary-adrenal axis, growth suppression in infancy, childhood and adolescence, menstrual irregularity and amenorrhoea. Cushingoid faces, hirsutism, weight gain, impaired carbohydrate tolerance with increased requirement for anti-diabetic therapy. Negative protein and calcium balance. Increased appetite.

Anti-inflammatory and immunosuppressive effects: Increased susceptibility and severity of infections with suppression of clinical symptoms and signs, opportunistic infections, recurrence of dormant tuberculosis (see *Special warnings and precautions for use*).

Musculoskeletal: Osteoporosis, vertebral and long bone fractures, avascular osteonecrosis particularly of the femoral head may occur after prolonged corticosteroid therapy or after repeat short courses involving high doses, tendon rupture. Proximal myopathy.

Fluid and electrolyte disturbance: Sodium and water retention, hypertension, potassium loss, hypokalaemic alkalosis.

Neuropsychiatric: Euphoria, psychological dependence, depression, insomnia and aggravation of schizophrenia. Increased intra-cranial pressure with papilloedema in children (pseudotumour cerebri), usually after treatment withdrawal. Aggravation of epilepsy.

Ophthalmic: Increased intra-ocular pressure, glaucoma, papilloedema, posterior subcapsular cataracts, corneal or scleral thinning, exacerbation of ophthalmic viral or fungal diseases.

Gastrointestinal: Dyspepsia, peptic ulceration with perforation and haemorrhage, acute pancreatitis, candidiasis.

Dermatological: Impaired healing, skin atrophy, bruising, telangiectasia, striae, acne.

General: Hypersensitivity including anaphylaxis, has been reported. Leucocytosis. Thrombo-embolism.

Withdrawal symptoms and signs: Too rapid a reduction of corticosteroid dosage following prolonged treatment can lead to acute adrenal insufficiency, hypotension and death (see *Special warnings and precautions for use*).

A 'withdrawal syndrome' may also occur including, fever, myalgia, arthralgia, rhinitis, conjunctivitis, painful itchy skin nodules and loss of weight.

Overdose: Treatment is unlikely to be needed in cases of acute overdosage.

Pharmacological properties

Pharmacodynamic properties: Prednesol tablets contain the equivalent of 5 mg of prednisolone in the form of the 21-disodium phosphate ester. Prednisolone sodium phosphate is a synthetic glucocorticoid with the same general properties as prednisolone itself and other compounds classified as corticosteroids. Prednisolone is four times as active as hydrocortisone on a weight-for-weight basis.

Prednisolone sodium phosphate is very soluble in water, and is therefore less likely to cause local gastric irritation than prednisolone alcohol, which is only slightly soluble. This is important when high dosages are required, as in immuno-suppressive therapy.

Pharmacokinetic properties: Prednisolone sodium phosphate has been shown to have a satisfactory pharmacokinetic profile by many years of successful clinical experience.

Preclinical safety data: No additional data of relevance.

Pharmaceutical particulars

List of excipients: Sodium acid citrate BP; Sodium bicarbonate PhEur; Saccharin sodium BP; Povidone BP; Erythorine E127 HSE; Sodium benzoate PhEur.

Incompatibilities: None known.

Shelf life: 2 years.

Special precautions for storage: Store below 25°C. Protect from light.

Nature and contents of container: The tablets are foil strip packed and supplied in cartons of 30 or 100 tablets.

Instructions for use/handling: For detailed instructions for use refer to the Patient Information Leaflet in every pack.

Marketing authorisation number PL 10949/0107

Date of first authorisation/renewal of authorisation 01.11.93

Date of (partial) revision of text June 1997

PROPADERM* SKIN PREPARATIONS

Presentation Propaderm Cream and Ointment are topical preparations of Beclomethasone Dipropionate BP. Beclomethasone Dipropionate BP is a potent anti-inflammatory steroid when applied topically to the skin.

Propaderm Cream: Beclomethasone Dipropionate BP 0.025% in a cream base.

Propaderm Ointment: Beclomethasone Dipropionate BP 0.025% in an ointment base.

Propaderm Cream is white in colour; Propaderm Ointment is yellowish.

Uses Propaderm Cream and Ointment are indicated for the treatment of the various forms of eczema in children and adults including atopic and discoid eczemas; primary irritant and allergic dermatitis; psoriasis (excluding widespread plaque psoriasis); neurodermatoses including lichen simplex; intertrigo; discoid lupus erythematosus.

Propaderm Cream is often appropriate for moist or weeping surfaces and Propaderm Ointment for dry, lichenified or scaly lesions but this is not invariably so.

Dosage and administration Propaderm preparations should be applied thinly over the whole of the affected area and gently rubbed in. Initially, application should be made twice daily, but when improvement is seen, the intervals between applications may be extended and treatment eventually stopped. If no improvement is seen within two to four weeks, reassessment of the diagnosis, or referral may be necessary. After cessation of treatment, should the condition recur, twice daily treatment should be re-instituted. However, when improvement is seen again, the intervals between application may be gradually extended until maintenance dosing of application every third or fourth day is achieved. This is likely to avoid subsequent reappearance of the condition. The beneficial effects may be enhanced by preliminary use of hot soaks, or by intermittent applications or occlusive dressings.

Contra-indications, warnings, etc.

Contra-indications: Propaderm should not be applied to the eyes. Rosacea, acne vulgaris; peri-oral dermatitis. Primary cutaneous viral infections (e.g. herpes simplex, chickenpox). Hypersensitivity to the preparation. Varicose ulcers or any other statis ulcers.

Use of Propaderm preparations is not indicated in the treatment of primarily infected skin lesions caused by infection with fungi (e.g. candidiasis, tinea) or bacteria (e.g. impetigo); primary or secondary infections due to yeasts; perianal and genital pruritus; dermatoses in children under 1 year of age, including dermatitis and napkin eruptions.

Precautions: Long-term continuous therapy should be avoided where possible, particularly in infants and children, as adrenal suppression can occur even without occlusion.

The face, more than the other areas of the body, may exhibit atrophic changes after prolonged treatment with potent topical corticosteroids. This must be borne in mind when treating such conditions as psoriasis, discoid lupus erythematosus and severe eczema. If applied to the eyelids, care is needed to ensure that the preparation does not enter the eye, as glaucoma might result.

If used in childhood, or on the face, courses should be limited if possible to five days and occlusion should not be used.

Topical corticosteroids may be hazardous in psoriasis for a number of reasons including rebound relapses, development of tolerance, risk of generalised pustular psoriasis and development of local or systemic toxicity due to impaired barrier function of the skin. If used in psoriasis careful patient supervision is important.

Appropriate antimicrobial therapy should be used whenever treating inflammatory lesions which have become infected. Any spread of infection requires withdrawal of topical corticosteroid therapy and systemic administration of antimicrobial agents.

Bacterial infection is encouraged by the warm, moist conditions induced by occlusive dressings, and so the skin should be cleansed before a fresh dressing is applied.

Pregnancy: There is inadequate evidence of safety in human pregnancy. Topical administration of corticosteroids to pregnant animals can cause abnormalities of foetal development including cleft palate and intrauterine growth retardation. There may therefore be a very small risk of such effects in the human foetus.

Side-effects: Prolonged and intensive treatment with highly active corticosteroid preparations may cause local atrophic changes in the skin such as thinning, striae, and dilatation of the superficial blood vessels, particularly when occlusive dressings are used or when skin folds are involved.

As with other topical corticosteroids, prolonged use of large amounts, or treatment of extensive areas, can result in sufficient systemic absorption to produce the features of hypercorticism. The effect is more likely to occur in infants and children, and if occlusive dressings are used. In infants, the napkin may act as an occlusive dressing.

Should systemic corticosteroid effects arise from application of Propaderm preparations topical treatment should be discontinued. If adrenal function is impaired the patient will need to be protected from any harmful effects of stress with oral corticosteroid preparations until normal adrenal function is established.

There are reports of pigmentation changes and hypertrichosis with topical steroids.

In rare instances, treatment of psoriasis with corticosteroids (or its withdrawal) is thought to have provoked the pustular form of the disease (see *Precautions*).

Propaderm Cream and Ointment are usually well tolerated, but if signs of hypersensitivity appear, application should stop immediately.

Exacerbation of symptoms may occur.

Overdosage: Acute overdosage is very unlikely to occur. However, in the case of chronic overdosage or misuse the features of hypercorticism may appear and in this situation topical steroids should be discontinued.

Pharmaceutical precautions

Storage: All Propaderm preparations should be stored at a temperature below 25°C and protected from light.

Dilution: Propaderm Cream may be diluted, if necessary, with Cetomacrogol Cream Formula A BPC. For Propaderm Ointment, dilution can be effected with White Soft Paraffin BP.

Legal category POM.

Package quantities Propaderm Cream is available in tubes of 30 g; Propaderm Ointment in tubes of 30 g.

Further information No Propaderm preparation contains lanolin or parabens.

Product licence numbers

Propaderm Cream 10949/0038
Propaderm Ointment 10949/0039

PURI-NETHOL* TABLETS

Qualitative and quantitative composition Mercaptopurine BP 50.0 mg/tablet.

Pharmaceutical form Tablet.

Clinical particulars

Therapeutic indications: Cytotoxic agent.

Puri-Nethol is indicated for the treatment of acute leukaemia. It is of value in remission induction and is particularly indicated for maintenance therapy in acute lymphoblastic leukaemia and acute myelogenous leukaemia. Puri-Nethol is used in the treatment of chronic granulocytic leukaemia.

Posology and method of administration: For oral administration.

For adults and children the usual dose is 2.5 mg/kg bodyweight per day, but the dose and duration of administration depend on the nature and dosage of other cytotoxic agents given in conjunction with Puri-Nethol. The dosage should be carefully adjusted to suit the individual patient. Puri-Nethol has been used in various combination therapy schedules for acute leukaemia and the literature should be consulted for details. Consideration should be given to reducing the dosage in patients with impaired hepatic or renal function. When Zyloric (allopurinol) and mercaptopurine are administered concomitantly it is essential that only a quarter of the usual dose of mercaptopurine is given since Zyloric (allopurinol) decreases the rate of catabolism of mercaptopurine.

Use in the elderly: No specific studies have been carried out in the elderly, however, it is advisable to monitor renal and hepatic function in these patients, and if there is any impairment, consideration should be given to reducing Puri-Nethol dosage.

Contra-indications: In view of the seriousness of the indications there are no absolute contra-indications.

Special warnings and special precautions for use: Puri-Nethol is an active cytotoxic agent for use only under the direction of physicians experienced in the administration of such agents.

Since Puri-Nethol is strongly myelosuppressive full blood counts must be taken daily during remission induction. Patients must be carefully monitored during therapy.

Treatment with Puri-Nethol causes bone marrow suppression leading to leucopenia and thrombocytopenia.

The leucocyte and platelet counts continue to fall after treatment is stopped, so at the first sign of an abnormally large fall in the counts, treatment should be interrupted immediately.

Bone marrow suppression is reversible if Puri-Nethol is withdrawn early enough.

During remission induction in acute myelogenous leukaemia the patient may frequently have to survive a period of relative bone marrow aplasia and it is important that adequate supportive facilities are available.

There are individuals with an inherited deficiency of the enzyme thiopurine methyltransferase (TPMT) who may be unusually sensitive to the myelosuppresive effect of 6-mercaptopurine and prone to developing rapid bone marrow depression following the initiation of treatment with Puri-Nethol. This problem could be exacerbated by coadministration with drugs that inhibit TPMT, such as olsalazine, mesalazine or sulphasalazine.

Puri-Nethol is hepatotoxic and liver function tests should be monitored weekly during treatment. More frequent monitoring may be advisable in those with pre-existing liver disease or receiving other potentially hepatotoxic therapy. The patient should be instructed to discontinue Puri-Nethol immediately if jaundice becomes apparent.

During remission induction when rapid cell lysis is occurring, uric acid levels in blood and urine should be monitored as hyperuricaemia and/or hyperuricosuria may develop, with the risk of uric acid nephropathy.

Puri-Nethol in common with other antimetabolites is potentially mutagenic and chromosome damage has been reported in rats and man. Increases in chromosomal aberrations were observed in the peripheral lymphocytes of leukaemia patients and in a hypernephroma patient who received an unstated dose of 6-mercaptopurine.

In view of its action on cellular deoxyribonucleic acid (DNA) 6-mercaptopurine is potentially carcinogenic and consideration should be given to the theoretical risk of carcinogenesis with this treatment. Three cases have been documented of the occurrence of acute nonlymphatic leukaemia in patients who received 6-mercaptopurine for non-neoplastic disorders.

A patient with Hodgkin's disease treated with 6-mercaptopurine and multiple additional cytotoxic agents developed acute myelogenous leukaemia. Twelve and a half years after 6-mercaptopurine treatment for myasthenia gravis a female patient developed chronic myeloid leukaemia.

Interaction with other medicaments and other forms of interaction: When Zyloric (allopurinol) and Puri-Nethol are administered concomitantly it is essential that only a quarter of the usual dose of Puri-Nethol is given since Zyloric decreases the rate of catabolism of Puri-Nethol.

Inhibition of the anticoagulant effect of warfarin, when given with Puri-Nethol, has been reported.

As there is *in vitro* evidence that aminosalicylate derivatives (e.g. olsalazine, mesalazine or sulphasalazine) inhibit the TPMT enzyme, they should be administered with caution to patients receiving concurrent Puri-Nethol therapy (see *Special warnings and precautions for use*).

Pregnancy and lactation: Puri-Nethol is embryotoxic in rats. This effect is dose dependent.

Normal offspring have been born after Puri-Nethol therapy during human pregnancy, but abortion, prematurity and malformation have been reported. A leukaemia patient treated with 6-mercaptopurine 100 mg/day (plus splenic irradiation) throughout pregnancy gave birth to a normal, premature baby. A second baby, born to the same mother, who was treated as before together with busulphan 4 mg/day, had multiple severe abnormalities, including corneal opacities, microphthalmia, cleft palate and hypoplasia of the thyroid and ovaries.

The small numbers involved do not allow an evaluation of the degree of risk of Puri-Nethol therapy during pregnancy and the possible hazard to the foetus must be balanced against the expected benefit in any individual case.

Transient profound oligospermia was observed in a young man who received 6-mercaptopurine 150 mg/day plus prednisone 80 mg/day for acute leukaemia. Two years after cessation of the chemotherapy he had a normal sperm count and fathered a normal child.

Mothers receiving Puri-Nethol should not breast feed.

Effects on ability to drive and use machines: Not applicable.

Undesirable effects: The main side-effect of treatment with Puri-Nethol is bone marrow suppression leading to leucopenia and thrombocytopenia. Puri-Nethol is hepatotoxic in animals and man. The histological findings in man have shown hepatic necrosis and biliary stasis. The incidence of hepatotoxicity varies considerably and can occur with any dose but more frequently when the recommended dose of 2.5 mg/kg bodyweight daily is exceeded. Monitoring of liver function tests may allow early detection of liver toxicity. This is usually reversible if Puri-Nethol therapy is stopped soon enough, but fatal liver damage has occurred.

Anorexia, nausea and vomiting have occasionally been noted.

Oral ulceration has been reported during Puri-Nethol therapy and rarely intestinal ulceration has occurred.

Rare complications are drug fever and skin rash.

Pancreatitis has been reported in association with the unlicensed use of 6-mercaptopurine in the treatment of inflammatory bowel disease.

Overdose: The principal toxic effects on the bone marrow and haematological toxicity is likely to be more profound with chronic overdosage than with a single ingestion of Puri-Nethol. The risk of overdosage is also increased when Zyloric is being given concomitantly with Puri-Nethol. As there is no known antidote the blood picture should be closely monitored and general supportive measures, together with appropriate blood transfusion, instituted if necessary.

Pharmacological properties

Pharmacodynamic properties: 6-mercaptopurine is an analogue of adenine, one of the bases required for nucleic acid biosynthesis, and of the purine base hypoxanthine. Hence Puri-Nethol acts as an antimetabolite and interferes with the synthesis of nucleic acids in proliferating cells. Its metabolites are also pharmacologically active.

Pharmacokinetic properties: Absorption of an oral dose of Puri-Nethol is incomplete and variable averaging about 50% of the administered dose. The half-life of 6-mercaptopurine in the circulation is of the order of 90 minutes. It is extensively metabolised and excreted via the kidneys and the active metabolites have a longer half-life than the parent drug. 6-mercaptopurine has pKa's of 7.7 and 11.0.

Preclinical safety data: There are no preclinical data of relevance to the prescriber which are additional to that in other sections of the SmPC.

Pharmaceutical particulars

List of excipients: Lactose PhEur, Maize Starch PhEur, Hydrolysed Starch HSE, Stearic Acid BPC, Magnesium Stearate PhEur, Purified Water PhEur.

Incompatibilities: None known.

Shelf life: 60 months.

Special precautions for storage: Store below 25°C. Keep dry. Protect from light.

Nature and contents of container: Amber glass bottles with low-density polythene snap-fit closures.

Pack size: 25 tablets.

Instructions for use/handling: It is advisable that care be taken when handling or halving these tablets not to contaminate hands or inspire drug.

Marketing authorisation number PL 0003/5227R

Date of first authorisation/renewal of authorisation Renewal: 27 April 1998.

Date of (partial) revison of text November 1998.

PYLORID* TABLETS ▼

Qualitative and quantitative composition Each tablet contains 400 mg of ranitidine bismuth citrate (INN).

Pharmaceutical form Light blue, film-coated, octagonal capsule-shaped tablets.

Clinical particulars

Therapeutic indications: Treatment of duodenal ulcer and benign gastric ulcer.

Eradication of *Helicobacter pylori* and prevention of relapse of peptic ulcer disease when administered in co-prescription with appropriate antibiotic(s). Treatment of duodenal ulcer and benign gastric ulcer.

Posology and method of administration: Pylorid should be taken twice daily, in the morning and evening, preferably with food.

Eradication of Helicobacter pylori and prevention of relapse of peptic ulcer disease: The following dosage regimens have been shown to be clinically effective. Selection of the appropriate regimen should be based on patient tolerability and local prescribing habits/availability of the antibiotic(s).

7 day triple therapy regimens: The recommended dose of Pylorid is 400 mg twice daily taken orally with antibiotics as detailed below:–

clarithromycin 500 mg twice daily with either metronidazole 400 mg or 500 mg twice daily or amoxycillin 1 g twice daily.

clarithromycin 250 mg twice daily with metronidazole 400 mg or 500 mg twice daily.

Alternatively, 14 day dual therapy regimens may be given as follows:

Pylorid 400 mg twice daily with either clarithromycin 500 mg two or three times daily or in cases where clarithromycin cannot be given, amoxycillin 500 mg four times daily, although the latter resulted in lower eradication rates.

If symptoms recur and the patient is *H. pylori* positive, a further course of Pylorid together with an alternative antibiotic regimen may be considered.

To facilitate ulcer healing, therapy with Pylorid 400 mg twice daily may be continued to 28 days.

Treatment of peptic ulcer disease:

Duodenal ulcer: Pylorid 400 mg b.d. for 4 weeks. Treatment may be extended for a further 4 weeks.

Benign gastric ulcer: Pylorid 400 mg b.d. for 8 weeks.

Pylorid is not indicated for long-term (maintenance) therapy; more than two 8-week courses in any one year should be avoided because of the possibility of accumulation of bismuth. If 4-week courses of therapy are given, up to a maximum of 16 weeks of treatment may be given in any one year.

Elderly patients: Ranitidine and bismuth exposure is increased in elderly patients as a result of decreased renal clearance (see *Renal impairment* and *Contra-indications*).

Children: There are no data available on the use of Pylorid Tablets in children. Therefore, they are not recommended for use in children.

Renal impairment: Ranitidine and bismuth exposure is increased in patients with renal impairment as a result of decreased clearance. As with other bismuth-containing drugs, Pylorid should not be used in patients with moderate to severe renal impairment i.e., creatinine clearance typically <25 ml/min (see *Contra-indications*).

Hepatic impairment: There is no information regarding the use of Pylorid Tablets in patients with hepatic impairment. However, as ranitidine and bismuth in the systemic circulation are eliminated mainly by renal clearance, no dosage adjustment is necessary in hepatically-impaired patients.

Contra-indications: Pylorid Tablets are contra-indicated in patients known to have hypersensitivity to any of the ingredients.

Pylorid is contra-indicated for long-term (maintenance) therapy.

As with other bismuth-containing drugs, Pylorid should not be used in patients with moderate to severe renal impairment i.e., creatinine clearance typically <25 ml/min.

Special warnings and precautions for use: The possibility of malignancy should be excluded before commencement of therapy in patients with gastric ulcer, as treatment with Pylorid Tablets may mask symptoms of gastric carcinoma.

Pylorid Tablets should be avoided in patients with a history of acute porphyria.

When co-prescription with antibiotic(s) is clinically indicated, the relevant prescribing information should be consulted prior to initiation of therapy.

Interaction with other medicaments and other forms of interaction: An increase in median trough plasma bismuth concentrations has been observed when Pylorid is co-administered with clarithromycin. However, this has not been associated with any adverse clinical sequelae in clinical trials. This increase was not observed in clinical studies in patients receiving 7 day triple therapy with Pylorid, clarithromycin and either metronidazole or amoxycillin. Clarithromycin levels are unaffected by the administration of ranitidine bismuth citrate, although systemic exposure to the active metabolite of clarithromycin is increased. The ranitidine absorption from Pylorid Tablets is increased when co-administered with clarithromycin. This enhanced ranitidine exposure is of no clinical concern due to the wide therapeutic index of ranitidine.

Food causes a decrease in bismuth absorption which is not of any clinical relevance. Limited data suggest increased ulcer healing when Pylorid Tablets are administered with food (see *Posology and method of administration*).

The co-administration of antacids with Pylorid Tablets does not result in any clinically relevant effect.

Pregnancy and lactation: The safety of ranitidine bismuth citrate in human pregnancy has not been established. As animal reproductive studies are not always predictive of human response, Pylorid Tablets should not be used in pregnancy.

It has been demonstrated in animal reproductive studies that during repeat dosing, low levels of ranitidine and bismuth cross the placenta. There was no evidence that ranitidine bismuth citrate induced any major malformations in either foetal rats or rabbits after maternal administration at high dose levels. Embryo/foetal lethality in rabbits, as a consequence of the maternal susceptibility to antimicrobial agents, together with minor effects of skeletal development in both rats and rabbits, were a result of dose levels considerably in excess of clinical exposure and were related to maternal toxicity.

It has been demonstrated that during repeat dosing of ranitidine bismuth citrate in the lactating rat, low levels of ranitidine and bismuth are secreted in the milk with consequent exposure of the pups. The passage of ranitidine bismuth citrate into human breast milk has not been evaluated.

Consequently, Pylorid Tablets should not be used by women who are breast feeding.

Effects on ability to drive and use machines: None reported.

Undesirable effects: Blackening of the stools is frequently reported with bismuth-containing drugs.

As with other medicines containing bismuth, ranitidine bismuth citrate may cause blackening of the tongue.

There have been rare reports of hypersensitivity reactions including pruritus, skin rash and anaphylaxis.

Gastro-intestinal disturbances, including diarrhoea, abdominal discomfort, and gastric pain may occur.

Headache.

Treatment with Pylorid Tablets may cause transient changes in the liver enzymes SGPT (ALT) and SGOT (AST).

Mild anaemia has been reported.

The following have been reported as adverse events in patients treated with ranitidine. Because ranitidine is used for longer treatment periods, their relevance to the clinical use of Pylorid Tablets is unknown.

There have been occasional reports of hepatitis (hepatocellular, hepatocanalicular or mixed) with or without jaundice. These were usually reversible. Acute pancreatitis has been rarely reported. Blood count changes (leucopenia, thrombocytopenia) have occurred in a few patients.

These are usually reversible. Rare cases of agranulocytosis or pancytopenia, sometimes with marrow hypoplasia or aplasia have been reported. As with other H_2-receptor antagonists, there have been rare reports of bradycardia and A-V Block. Dizziness has been reported in a very small proportion of patients. Rare cases of reversible mental confusion, depression and hallucinations have been reported, predominantly in severely ill and elderly patients. Rare cases of erythema multiforme have been reported. Musculoskeletal symptoms such as arthralgia and myalgia have been reported rarely. There have been a few reports of breast symptoms in men taking ranitidine.

Overdose: Administration of ranitidine bismuth citrate in acute animal studies at very high dosages has been associated with nephrotoxicity. In cases of overdose, gastric lavage and appropriate supportive therapy would be indicated. The ranitidine and bismuth components may be removed from the plasma by haemodialysis.

Pharmacological properties

Pharmacodynamic properties: Pharmaco-therapeutic group: Pylorid Tablets are histamine H_2-receptor antagonists, with anti-*H. pylori*, and mucosal protective activity.

Mechanism of action: Ranitidine bismuth citrate inhibits basal and stimulated secretion of gastric acid, reducing both the volume and the acid and pepsin content of the secretion, is bactericidal to *Helicobacter pylori in vitro*, and has gastric mucosal-protective actions.

These pharmacodynamic properties depend on the dissociation of ranitidine bismuth citrate into ranitidine and bismuth components. The biological and anti-*H. pylori* activity of the latter is related to the solubility of dissociated bismuth from ranitidine bismuth citrate. As the absorption of bismuth from ranitidine bismuth citrate is minimal (see *Pharmacokinetic properties*) the *H. pylori* activity is a local effect. Even in acidic conditions, which lead to precipitation of bismuth, sufficient bismuth from ranitidine bismuth citrate remains soluble to inhibit the growth of *H. pylori.*

Pharmacokinetic properties: Bismuth absorption from Pylorid Tablets is less than 1% of the bismuth dose administered, and is similar in healthy volunteers, male and female subjects, patients with peptic ulcer disease and gastritis patients. The rate of absorption of ranitidine and bismuth is rapid, the time to peak plasma levels typically being 1–3 h and 15–60 min, respectively. The absorption of bismuth from Pylorid Tablets is dependent on intragastric pH and increases if the intragastric pH is raised to ≥6 prior to dosing.

However, the co-administration of antacids has no clinically relevant effect (see *Interactions*).

Ranitidine is cleared primarily by renal clearance (approximately 500 ml/min). This accounts for approximately 70% of the total clearance, which is approximately 700 ml/min. Ranitidine is rapidly eliminated from the body, with a half-life of about 3 hours after oral dosing; and does not accumulate in the plasma with twice daily dosing.

Bismuth in the systemic circulation is cleared from the body mainly by renal clearance (approximately 50 ml/min). Multiple half-lives describe the distribution and elimination of bismuth. The mean terminal plasma half-life of bismuth is 20.7 days and the mean terminal half-life of bismuth urinary excretion is 45.1 days. Bismuth accumulates in plasma upon twice daily dosing with Pylorid Tablets. Within 3 months of completing a 4- or 8-week course of treatment with Pylorid, plasma concentrations and urinary excretion of bismuth have returned to pre-treatment levels in most patients.

Ranitidine and bismuth exposure is increased in patients with renal impairment and the elderly as a result of decreased renal clearance.

Patients with moderate to severe renal impairment (creatinine clearance typically <25 ml/min) should not be given Pylorid Tablets (see *Posology and method of administration* and *Contra-indications*).

Preclinical safety data: In acute animal studies at high dosages, nephrotoxicity was observed in all species studied.

In local tolerance studies ranitidine bismuth citrate was slightly irritating to abraded guinea pig skin. It was also a weak skin contact sensitiser in the guinea pig "split adjuvant" test.

No mutagenic activity was seen in standard genotoxicity tests with ranitidine bismuth citrate. A weak clastogenic effect was seen *in vitro*. This can be accounted for as an effect of a bismuth containing compound as it also occurred with bismuth citrate, at bismuth equivalent concentrations of 33 mcg/ml for ranitidine bismuth citrate compared to 26 mcg/ml for bismuth citrate. As no genotoxic activity was demonstrated *in vivo* these findings are not considered to be of any clinical significance.

Evidence of bismuth accumulation in tissues to steady state was observed following long-term repeat dosing in animal studies. To avoid the possibility of bismuth accumulation, ranitidine bismuth citrate is not indicated for maintenance therapy in man.

Pharmaceutical particulars

List of excipients: Tablet core: Sodium carbonate (anhydrous) USNF; Microcrystalline cellulose PhEur; Polyvidone K30 PhEur; Magnesium stearate PhEur.

Tablet film coat: Hydroxypropylmethyl cellulose PhEur (E464); Titanium dioxide PhEur (E171); Triacetin USP; Indigo carmine aluminium lake (E132).

Incompatibilities: None reported.

Shelf life: 3 years.

Special precautions for storage: Store Pylorid Tablets below 30°C.

Nature and contents of container: Cartons containing 14, 28 or 56 tablets in a double-foil blister pack.

The tablets are light blue, film-coated, octagonal capsule-shaped tablets identified by a logo on one face, containing 400 mg of ranitidine bismuth citrate.

Instructions for use/handling: None.

Marketing authorisation number 14213/0001

Date of approval/revision of SPC 17 April 1998

RAXAR* TABLETS 400 mg

Qualitative and quantitative composition Tablets containing 400 mg grepafloxacin base, present as the sesquihydrate of the hydrochloride salt.

Pharmaceutical form White, oval, biconvex, bevel edged film-coated tablets engraved with GX CK5.

Clinical particulars

Therapeutic indications: Raxar is indicated for the treatment of infections caused by strains of bacteria susceptible to grepafloxacin in the following diseases:

- Community-acquired pneumonia, except severe pneumonia requiring parenteral therapy
- Acute bacterial exacerbations of chronic bronchitis
- Uncomplicated gonorrhoea (urethritis and cervicitis)
- Urethritis and cervicitis caused by *Chlamydia trachomatis*

Consideration should be given to national and/or local guidance regarding the appropriate use of antibacterial agents.

Posology and method of administration: In adults: The recommended dose of Raxar for acute bacterial exacerbations of chronic bronchitis is 400 mg once daily. This may be increased to 600 mg once daily for patients with more severe infections. The recommended dose of Raxar for community acquired pneumonia is 600 mg once daily. The treatment duration is up to a maximum of 10 days depending on the patient's medical history and clinical characteristics. Treatment should normally continue for two or three days after symptoms have subsided.

For urethritis and cervicitis caused by *Chlamydia* the recommended dose is 400 mg once daily for 7 days. Uncomplicated gonorrhoea should be treated with a single 400 mg dose.

Renal impairment: Dosage reduction is not required as renal excretion of grepafloxacin is a minor pathway of elimination. There is no experience in patients undergoing haemodialysis.

Hepatic impairment: Grepafloxacin is cleared primarily in the liver. Patients with mild hepatic impairment should receive a maximum dose of 400 mg once a day (see *Pharmacokinetic properties*). Raxar is contraindicated in patients with moderate or severe hepatic impairment.

Raxar tablets can be taken with or without food and should be swallowed whole with an adequate amount of liquid.

Contra-indications: Raxar is contra-indicated for use in patients with the following conditions:

- known hypersensitivity to grepafloxacin, any of the excipients of Raxar or to other quinolone antibiotics;
- history of tendon disease with a fluoroquinolone;
- moderate or severe hepatic impairment.

Raxar is also contra-indicated in children or growing adolescents, and in pregnant or nursing mothers (see *Use during pregnancy and lactation*).

In selected patients Raxar may cause QT interval prolongation which may lead to torsade de pointes. Therefore Raxar is also contra-indicated in patients with any of the following conditions; congenital or documented acquired QT interval prolongation, disturbances in the electrolyte balance, especially hypokalemia, clinically relevant bradycardia, clinically relevant congestive heart failure with reduced left ventricular ejection fraction and patients with a history of symptomatic cardiac arrhythmias (see *Special warnings and special precautions for use*).

The concomitant use of drugs which prolong the QT interval e.g. class Ia and class III antiarrhythmics should be avoided.

Special warnings and special precautions for use: Grepafloxacin has been shown to inhibit the receptor binding of GABA, and therefore has the potential to induce convulsions. However, in pre-clinical studies grepafloxacin did not cause convulsions when co-administered with non-steroidal anti-inflammatory drugs. Raxar should be used with caution in patients with known or suspected CNS disorders which predispose to seizures (see *Interaction with other medicinal products and other forms of interaction*).

Quinolones have been associated with CNS stimulation therefore caution is recommended if Raxar is to be used in psychotic patients, or in patients with a history of psychiatric disease.

Tendon inflammation and rupture may occur with quinolone antibiotics. Such reactions have been observed particularly in older patients and those treated concurrently with corticosteroids. At first sign of pain or inflammation, patients should discontinue Raxar and rest the affected limbs.

Pseudomembranous colitis has been reported with the use of broad-spectrum antibiotics; therefore it is important to consider this diagnosis in patients who develop serious diarrhoea during or after antibiotic use. Products inhibiting peristalsis are contra-indicated in this clinical situation.

Quinolones have been shown to cause dose-dependent photosensitivity reactions. Grepafloxacin is a weak photosensitiser, nevertheless during treatment with Raxar patients should not expose themselves to sunlight and should avoid UV rays (solaria, sun lamps). Therapy should be discontinued if photosensitivity occurs.

Patients should be advised that if coadministration with antacids, sucralfate or iron containing preparations is necessary, then these preparations should not be taken within four hours before or four hours after taking Raxar.

Patients with a family history of, or actual defects in glucose-6-phosphate dehydrogenase activity are prone to haemolytic reactions when treated with quinolones. Therefore Raxar should be used with caution in these patients.

Patients taking theophylline during treatment with Raxar should have their maintenance dose halved, and their theophylline levels monitored as a guide to further dosage reduction.

Prolongation of the QTc-interval: In healthy volunteers who received grepafloxacin for study purposes a prolongation of the QTc-interval was observed. To date no cardiac arrhythmias could be attributed to treatment with grepafloxacin. Based on these findings there exists the possibility that in rare cases in particularly predisposed patients, that grepafloxacin can induce cardiac arrhythmias (e.g. torsade de pointes). If cardiac arrhythmias occur during treatment, Raxar should be stopped and an ECG should be performed.

Interaction with other medicaments and other forms of interaction:

Magnesium, calcium, aluminium, iron and zinc ions and sucralfate: Quinolones form chelates with alkaline earth and transition metal ions. Administration of quinolones with preparations that contain these e.g. antacids, multivitamins may substantially interfere with absorption of quinolones. These agents should not be taken within four hours before or four hours after taking Raxar. Where appropriate, patients should be advised not to self-medicate with these preparations during therapy with Raxar.

Drugs metabolised by cytochrome P450 enzymes: Grepafloxacin is metabolised primarily by the Cytochrome P450 enzymes, particularly the isoenzyme CYP1A2. Like most quinolone drugs, grepafloxacin may competitively inhibit their activity. This may result in impaired metabolism of other drugs that are also metabolised by this system, as demonstrated with theophylline.

Theophylline: In common with other quinolones, grepafloxacin is a competitive inhibitor of the metabolism of theophylline by the isoenzyme CYP1A2. Serum theophylline concentrations were increased by approximately 50% when grepafloxacin was given concurrently. This also resulted in an increase in theophylline-related adverse events.

In patients receiving theophylline concurrently with a multi-day course of Raxar, the theophylline maintenance dose should be halved for the period of concurrent use. Monitoring of theophylline serum levels should be initiated as a guide to further dosage adjustments.

Caffeine: Caffeine is also metabolised by the CYP1A2 isoenzyme. In some patients concurrent administration of Raxar may lead to a reduced clearance, prolongation of its half life, and enhanced effects of caffeine.

Warfarin and probenecid: Grepafloxacin did not alter the pharmacokinetics or pharmacodynamic effects of warfarin. Co-administration of probenecid had no effect on the pharmacokinetics of grepafloxacin.

Non-steroidal anti-inflammatory drugs (NSAIDs): Drug interactions resulting in seizures have been reported between some quinolones and NSAIDs. In pre-clinical studies, grepafloxacin did not induce seizures when administered with a variety of NSAIDs.

Pregnancy and lactation: The safe use of Raxar in pregnant women has not been established. However as with other quinolones, grepafloxacin has been shown to cause lesions in the cartilage of the weight bearing joints of immature animals. Limited evidence indicates that grepafloxacin is secreted in human milk (see *Contra-indications*).

Effects on ability to drive and use machines: Dizziness has been reported in up to 6% of patients receiving Raxar in clinical trials. If affected, patients should avoid driving or operating machinery.

Undesirable effects: The adverse reactions identified with recommended doses of Raxar are as follows:

Central nervous system/psychiatric:
Common (↓1% and <10%): Headache, dizziness, insomnia, nervousness, tiredness.

Gastrointestinal system:
Very common (↓10%): Nausea, unpleasant taste.
Common (↓1% and <10%): Abdominal pain, constipation, diarrhoea, dyspepsia, dry mouth, vomiting.

General:
Common (↓1% and <10%): Asthenia, anorexia, pruritus, rash, photosensitivity.
Uncommon (↓0.1% and <1%): Allergic reactions of varying severity up to anaphylactic shock, tendonitis.

Laboratory findings: Transient rises in creatinine, liver enzymes, BUN. Uricaemia, hyperlipidemia, thrombocytopenia, hyperglycaemia.

Most of the adverse events reported were transient in nature and mild to moderate in severity. The following adverse reactions have been reported rarely (<0.1%) during treatment with Raxar: Fever, arthralgia, myalgia, and less often vaginitis, exfoliative dermatitis, depression, hallucinations, confusions, disturbances in vision, hearing, taste and smell.

Side effects of fluoroquinolones which so far have not been observed following treatment with Raxar: The clinical experience to date with Raxar does not allow for a final assessment to be made of the side effects. It is presumed that the side effect spectrum will be similar to other fluoroquinolones. There have been isolated cases of the following side effects reported following treatment with other fluoroquinolones and these may also be seen with Raxar:

Cholestatic icterus, drug induced hepatitis, transient sight loss, disturbance in the sense of balance with the clinical symptoms of vertigo and ataxia, disturbance in taste lasting several months, hypoglycaemia, hypernatriemia, hypercalcaemia.

Haematological changes: These may include in connection with quinolone therapy leucocytosis, leucopenia, neutropenia, increased rate of blood sedimentation, anaemia and haemolysis.

Overdose: Information on overdosage is limited. In the event of overdosage it is recommended that appropriate supportive care should be instituted as dictated by the patient's clinical status. Adequate hydration should be maintained.

Pharmacological properties

Pharmacodynamic properties:

General properties: Grepafloxacin is a broad-spectrum fluoroquinolone antibiotic. It has bactericidal activity against a wide range of Gram-negative, Gram-positive and atypical bacteria. The bactericidal activity is due to inhibition of the bacterial enzymes DNA gyrase (topoisomerase II) and topoisomerase IV, which are essential enzymes for duplication, transcription, and repair of bacterial DNA.

This mode of action of quinolones differs from other classes of antibiotics, therefore bacteria resistant to other classes would generally retain their susceptibility to grepafloxacin. Beta-lactamases and alterations to penicillin binding proteins have no effect on grepafloxacin activity.

Breakpoints: The following MIC breakpoints for grepafloxacin, separating susceptible (S) from intermediately susceptible organisms, and intermediately susceptible from resistant (R) organisms have been set by the National Committee for Clinical Laboratory Standards in the USA (NCCLS):

Streptococcus pneumoniae: S≤0.5 μg/ml, R≥2 μg/ml;
Haemophilus influenzae: S≤0.5 μg/ml;
Neisseria gonorrhoeae: S≤0.06 μg/ml, R≥1 μg/ml;
Non-fastidious pathogens: S≤1 μg/ml, R≥4 μg/ml.

Susceptibility: The prevalence of resistance may vary geographically and with time for selected species. Local information on resistance is desirable, particularly when treating severe infections. This information gives only an approximate guidance on the probabilities whether microorganisms will be susceptible to grepafloxacin or not. The following table lists the susceptibilities of bacteria relevant to the therapeutic indications approved for Raxar:

Susceptible
Aerobic Gram-positive micro-organisms
Staphylococcus aureus – methicillin susceptible strains*
Streptococcus agalactiae
*Streptococcus pneumoniae**
Streptococcus pneumoniae (penicillin-intermediate and resistant)

Aerobic Gram-negative micro-organisms
Escherichia coli
Haemophilus influenzae – including beta-lactamase producing strains*
*Haemophilus parainfluenzae**
Klebsiella oxytoca
Klebsiella pneumoniae
Moraxella catarrhalis – including beta-lactamase producing strains*
Neisseria gonorrhoeae – including tetracycline and penicillin resistant strains*
Proteus mirabilis
Proteus vulgaris

Resistant
Aerobic Gram-positive organisms
Staphylococcus aureus (methicillin resistant)

Other organisms
Susceptible
Chlamydia pneumoniae
*Chlamydia trachomatis**
*Legionella pneumophila**
Mycoplasma hominis
*Mycoplasma pneumoniae**

Intermediate
Ureaplasma urealyticum

* Clinical efficacy has been demonstrated for susceptible organisms in approved indications.

Resistance: Resistance to grepafloxacin through spontaneous mutation *in vitro* occurs at a very low frequency. In clinical trials, grepafloxacin-resistant mutants were rarely encountered during the treatment of infection caused by susceptible isolates.

Anaerobes are generally resistant to grepafloxacin; in particular *Bacteroides fragilis* group and *Clostridium difficile.*

Other information: Certain organisms exhibit cross-resistance to grepafloxacin and some other fluoroquinolones. However, some organisms that are resistant to other quinolones may be susceptible to grepafloxacin. Cross-resistance to grepafloxacin and other classes of antimicrobial agents, including β-lactam antibiotics, macrolides and aminoglycosides has not generally been observed. Therefore, organisms resistant to the latter classes of drugs are expected to be susceptible to grepafloxacin.

Pharmacokinetic properties:

Absorption: Grepafloxacin is rapidly and extensively absorbed following oral administration. The absolute bioavailability of grepafloxacin has been estimated to be about 72%. The presence of food or increased gastric pH does not affect the rate or extent of grepafloxacin absorption.

After oral administration, peak plasma levels (C_{max}) were reached within two hours of dosing. Following multiple oral doses, steady-state was reached within 5 days of treatment and a 1.5–2 fold accumulation was observed. The C_{max} values at steady state after administration of 400 mg and 600 mg were 1.35 μg/ml, and 2.30 μg/ml respectively. The plasma levels for females were greater than for males. This variation was considered to be related mainly to differences in body weight (and in particular lean body mass), with grepafloxacin clearance unaffected. Although some mild side effects like nausea, vomiting and unpleasant taste were seen more often in women than in men, this difference in the pharmacokinetics is not considered clinically relevant.

Distribution: Binding of grepafloxacin to human plasma proteins is approximately 50%, and is not affected by advancing age or renal or hepatic impairment. The apparent volume of distribution after oral administration of 400 mg of grepafloxacin was 5 l/kg, suggesting that grepafloxacin is extensively distributed into the various tissues in the body.

Relative to plasma concentrations, grepafloxacin penetrates and concentrates in alveolar fluid, alveolar macrophages, bronchial mucosa, male and female genital tissues, bile, biliary, skin and tonsilar tissues.

Metabolism: After oral administration, grepafloxacin and five metabolites were identified in plasma, urine, and an additional sixth metabolite was identified in the faeces. Grepafloxacin appears to be eliminated by multiple pathways and therefore changes in its pharmacokinetics due to interaction with other drugs is less likely. In plasma, about 50% was unchanged grepafloxacin and 7.8% was present as the 4′-glucoronide; other metabolites ranged from 0.7–5.2%.

Studies in human hepatocytes *in vitro* showed that the CYP1A2 isoenzyme is involved in the oxidative metabolism of grepafloxacin, while CYP3A4 is marginally involved. The major oxidative metabolites showed weak antimicrobial activity compared to the parent compound, and no significant toxicity.

Excretion: The typical plasma elimination half-life of grepafloxacin is 12 hours. Average elimination half life values ranged between 10 and 13 hours after single doses and 10 to 16 hours after multiple doses of grepafloxacin. Grepafloxacin is eliminated principally through hepatic metabolism and biliary excretion, with only 5–14% renally excreted. Faecal excretion accounts for 27% of the oral dose.

Pharmacokinetics in demographic subpopulations:

Elderly: The pharmacokinetic profile of grepafloxacin was generally similar with increasing age.

Renal impairment: Renal insufficiency, including

that considered severe (Clcr<30 ml/min), did not substantially influence the pharmacokinetics of grepafloxacin. This finding is consistent with the elimination route. No dose adjustment of Raxar in patients with renal impairment is necessary.

Hepatic impairment: Higher grepafloxacin plasma concentrations were observed among subjects with hepatic disease when compared to subjects with normal liver function. The area under the curve (AUC) was increased by 56% and 137% for subjects with mild and moderate hepatic impairment, respectively. These findings are consistent with the elimination route of grepafloxacin, which is mainly by hepatic metabolism. Treatment with Raxar is contra-indicated in patients with moderate or severe hepatic impairment.

Preclinical safety data: Haemopoetic (decrease in the number of erythrocytes and leucocytes, especially neutrophils, which was reversible when the drug was discontinued) and lymphoid tissue changes (atrophic changes of lymph nodes, spleen, thymus) following treatment with quinolones are seen in rats and monkeys, but are rare in man. As with other quinolones hepatotoxicity and nephrotoxicity was seen (monkey, dog). The liver toxicity showed as raised liver enzymes and vacuolar degeneration. The nephrotoxicity seen were degenerative changes in the renal proximal tubules of monkeys. These changes were commonly seen only after prolonged treatment or treatment with high doses of grepafloxacin.

Although conventional long-term studies to determine the carcinogenic potential of grepafloxacin have not been performed, the drug has been subjected to a range of *in vitro* and *in vivo* genotoxicity tests. Negative results were obtained in Ames and V79 hprt mutation assays. The *in vitro* test in the Chinese hamster fibroblasts showed chromosomal abnormalities and polyploidy at low concentrations, under continuous and extended treatment conditions. However, *in vivo* genotoxicity tests at plasma concentrations higher than those at which induction of chromosome damage was observed *in vitro*, were negative. It is concluded that the negative *in vivo* results adequately reflect the *in vivo* situation in terms of genotoxicity.

Some quinolones have been shown to enhance the action of UVA-induced photocarcinogenicity when administered concurrently to mice exposed to ultraviolet light. Grepafloxacin induces chromosomal damage *in vitro* in the presence and in the absence of UV radiation. *In vivo* genotoxicity tests yielded negative results. Grepafloxacin did not enhance UV-induced tumourigenesis in hairless mice, but shortened slightly the latent period of development of skin tumours.

Phototoxicity has been reported for many quinolones. In animal models grepafloxacin seems to show less potency than many other quinolones, although it has a relatively long half life (505 h) in the skin of the pigmented rat (see *Special warnings and special precautions for use*).

Grepafloxacin binds to melanin with a relatively long half life (705 h). Toxicity tests in rats, dogs, and monkeys (repeated dosing up to six months) revealed no indication regarding an oculotoxic risk. A specific 52 weeks trial in monkeys showed no result. A further specific trial in pigmented rats showed no indication of a cataractogenic or co-cataractogenic effect.

Grepafloxacin caused in isolated cases ventricular arrhythmias in the rabbit after intravenous doses of ↓30 mg/kg. In the dog doses of ↓30 mg/kg orally caused prolongation of the QT-interval. In the monkey after intravenous doses of ↓75 mg/kg ventricular arrhythmias were observed.

Quinolones are known to cause lesions in the cartilage of the major diarthrodial joints in immature animals. In animal models grepafloxacin appears to have a relatively low potential for causing joint toxicity (see *Use in pregnancy and lactation*). The lowest dose of grepafloxacin causing joint toxicity in young dogs was seven times maximum recommended therapeutic dose (600 mg/50 kg person) on a mg/kg basis, with plasma concentrations in the same range as the therapeutic doses.

Reproductive studies performed in rats and rabbits indicate that placental transfer of grepafloxacin occurs. Studies in these species did not show any evidence of teratogenicity or impairment of fertility following administration of grepafloxacin. In rat, changes in the behaviour (increased spontaneous activity) of some female offspring were seen.

Pharmaceutical particulars

List of excipients:

Tablet core: Microcrystalline cellulose, Low substituted hydroxypropyl cellulose, Hydroxypropyl cellulose, Magnesium stearate.

Film-coat: Hypromellose, Titanium dioxide, Talc.

Incompatibilities: No incompatibilities are known to date.

Shelf life: 3 years.

Special precautions for storage: Store below 30°C.

Nature and contents of container: Cartons containing white opaque PVC/aluminium foil blister packs. The tablets are available in 400 mg and 600 mg strengths in packs of one, two, five, seven or ten tablets.

Instructions for use/handling: None.

Marketing authorisation number PL 10949/0299

Date of first authorisation/renewal of authorisation 9 December 1997

Date of revision of the text 9 December 1997.

RAXAR* TABLETS 600 mg

Qualitative and quantitative composition Tablets containing 600 mg grepafloxacin base, present as the sesquihydrate of the hydrochloride salt.

Pharmaceutical form White, oval, biconvex, bevel edged film-coated tablets engraved with GX CK7.

Clinical particulars

Therapeutic indications: Raxar is indicated for the treatment of infections caused by strains of bacteria susceptible to grepafloxacin in the following diseases:

- Community-acquired pneumonia, except severe pneumonia requiring parenteral therapy
- Acute bacterial exacerbations of chronic bronchitis
- Uncomplicated gonorrhoea (urethritis and cervicitis)
- Urethritis and cervicitis caused by *Chlamydia trachomatis*

Consideration should be given to national and/or local guidance regarding the appropriate use of antibacterial agents.

Posology and method of administration: In adults: The recommended dose of Raxar for acute bacterial exacerbations of chronic bronchitis is 400 mg once daily. This may be increased to 600 mg once daily for patients with more severe infections. The recommended dose of Raxar for community acquired pneumonia is 600 mg once daily. The treatment duration is up to a maximum of 10 days depending on the patient's medical history and clinical characteristics. Treatment should normally continue for two or three days after symptoms have subsided.

For urethritis and cervicitis caused by *Chlamydia* the recommended dose is 400 mg once daily for 7 days. Uncomplicated gonorrhoea should be treated with a single 400 mg dose.

Renal impairment: Dosage reduction is not required as renal excretion of grepafloxacin is a minor pathway of elimination. There is no experience in patients undergoing haemodialysis.

Hepatic impairment: Grepafloxacin is cleared primarily in the liver. Patients with mild hepatic impairment should receive a maximum dose of 400 mg once a day (see *Pharmacokinetic properties*). Raxar is contra-indicated in patients with moderate or severe hepatic impairment.

Raxar tablets can be taken with or without food and should be swallowed whole with an adequate amount of liquid.

Contra-indications: Raxar is contra-indicated for use in patients with the following conditions:

- known hypersensitivity to grepafloxacin, any of the excipients of Raxar or to other quinolone antibiotics;
- history of tendon disease with a fluoroquinolone;
- moderate or severe hepatic impairment.

Raxar is also contra-indicated in children or growing adolescents, and in pregnant or nursing mothers (see *Pregnancy and lactation*).

In selected patients Raxar may cause QT interval prolongation which may lead to torsade de pointes. Therefore Raxar is also contra-indicated in patients with any of the following conditions; congenital or documented acquired QT interval prolongation, disturbances in the electrolyte balance, especially hypokalemia, clinically relevant bradycardia, clinically relevant congestive heart failure with reduced left ventricular ejection fraction and patients with a history of symptomatic cardiac arrhythmias (see *Special warnings and special precautions for use*).

The concomitant use of drugs which prolong the QT interval e.g. class Ia and class III antiarrhythmics should be avoided.

Special warnings and special precautions for use: Grepafloxacin has been shown to inhibit the receptor binding of GABA, and therefore has the potential to induce convulsions. However, in pre-clinical studies grepafloxacin did not cause convulsions when co-administered with non-steroidal anti-inflammatory drugs. Raxar should be used with caution in patients with known or suspected CNS disorders which predispose to seizures (see *Interaction with other medicinal products and other forms of interaction*).

Quinolones have been associated with CNS stimulation therefore caution is recommended if Raxar is to be used in psychotic patients, or in patients with a history of psychiatric disease.

Tendon inflammation and rupture may occur with quinolone antibiotics. Such reactions have been observed particularly in older patients and those treated concurrently with corticosteroids. At first sign of pain or inflammation, patients should discontinue Raxar and rest the affected limbs.

Pseudomembranous colitis has been reported with the use of broad-spectrum antibiotics; therefore it is important to consider this diagnosis in patients who develop serious diarrhoea during or after antibiotic use. Products inhibiting peristalsis are contra-indicated in this clinical situation.

Quinolones have been shown to cause dose-dependent photosensitivity reactions. Grepafloxacin is a weak photosensitiser, nevertheless during treatment with Raxar patients should not expose themselves to sunlight and should avoid UV rays (solaria, sun lamps). Therapy should be discontinued if photosensitivity occurs.

Patients should be advised that if coadministration with antacids, sucralfate or iron containing preparations is necessary, then these preparations should not be taken within four hours before or four hours after taking Raxar.

Patients with a family history of, or actual defects in glucose-6-phosphate dehydrogenase activity are prone to haemolytic reactions when treated with quinolones. Therefore Raxar should be used with caution in these patients.

Patients taking theophylline during treatment with Raxar should have their maintenance dose halved, and their theophylline levels monitored as a guide to further dosage reduction.

Prolongation of the QTc-interval: In healthy volunteers who received grepafloxacin for study purposes a prolongation of the QTc-interval was observed. To date no cardiac arrhythmias could be attributed to treatment with grepafloxacin. Based on these findings there exists the possibility that in rare cases in particularly predisposed patients, that grepafloxacin can induce cardiac arrhythmias (e.g. torsade de pointes). If cardiac arrhythmias occur during treatment, Raxar should be stopped and an ECG should be performed.

Interaction with other medicaments and other forms of interaction:

Magnesium, calcium, aluminium, iron and zinc ions and sucralfate: Quinolones form chelates with alkaline earth and transition metal ions. Administration of quinolones with preparations that contain these e.g. antacids, multivitamins may substantially interfere with absorption of quinolones. These agents should not be taken within four hours before or four hours after taking Raxar. Where appropriate, patients should be advised not to self-medicate with these preparations during therapy with Raxar.

Drugs metabolised by cytochrome P450 enzymes: Grepafloxacin is metabolised primarily by the Cytochrome P450 enzymes, particularly the isoenzyme CYP1A2. Like most quinolone drugs, grepafloxacin may competitively inhibit their activity. This may result in impaired metabolism of other drugs that are also metabolised by this system, as demonstrated with theophylline.

Theophylline: In common with other quinolones, grepafloxacin is a competitive inhibitor of the metabolism of theophylline by the isoenzyme CYP1A2. Serum theophylline concentrations were increased by approximately 50% when grepafloxacin was given concurrently. This also resulted in an increase in theophylline-related adverse events.

In patients receiving theophylline concurrently with a multi-day course of Raxar, the theophylline maintenance dose should be halved for the period of concurrent use. Monitoring of theophylline serum levels should be initiated as a guide to further dosage adjustments.

Caffeine: Caffeine is also metabolised by the CYP1A2 isoenzyme. In some patients concurrent administration of Raxar may lead to a reduced clearance, prolongation of its half life, and enhanced effects of caffeine.

Warfarin and probenecid: Grepafloxacin did not alter the pharmacokinetics or pharmacodynamic effects of warfarin. Co-administration of probenecid had no effect on the pharmacokinetics of grepafloxacin.

Non-steroidal anti-inflammatory drugs (NSAIDs): Drug interactions resulting in seizures have been reported between some quinolones and NSAIDs. In pre-clinical studies, grepafloxacin did not induce seizures when administered with a variety of NSAIDs.

Pregnancy and lactation: The safe use of Raxar in pregnant women has not been established. However as with other quinolones, grepafloxacin has been shown to cause lesions in the cartilage of the weight bearing joints of immature animals. Limited evidence indicates that grepafloxacin is secreted in human milk (see *Contra-indications*).

Effects on ability to drive and use machines: Dizziness has been reported in up to 6% of patients receiving

Raxar in clinical trials. If affected, patients should avoid driving or operating machinery.

Undesirable effects: The adverse reactions identified with recommended doses of Raxar are as follows:

Central nervous system/psychiatric:
Common (↓1% and <10%): Headache, dizziness, insomnia, nervousness, tiredness.

Gastrointestinal system:
Very common: (↓10%): Nausea, unpleasant taste.
Common (↓1% and <10%): Abdominal pain, constipation, diarrhoea, dyspepsia, dry mouth, vomiting.

General:
Common (↓1% and <10%): Asthenia, anorexia, pruritus, rash, photosensitivity.
Uncommon (↓0.1% and <1%): Allergic reactions of varying severity up to anaphylactic shock, tendonitis.
Laboratory findings: Transient rises in creatinine, liver enzymes, BUN. Uricaemia, hyperlipidemia, thrombocytopenia, hyperglycaemia.

Most of the adverse events reported were transient in nature and mild to moderate in severity. The following adverse reactions have been reported rarely (<0.1%) during treatment with Raxar: Fever, arthralgia, myalgia, and less often vaginitis, exfoliative dermatitis, depression, hallucinations, confusions, disturbances in vision, hearing, taste and smell.

Side effects of fluoroquinolones which so far have not been observed following treatment with Raxar: The clinical experience to date with Raxar does not allow for a final assessment to be made of the side effects. It is presumed that the side effect spectrum will be similar to other fluoroquinolones. There have been isolated cases of the following side effects reported following treatment with other fluoroquinolones and these may also be seen with Raxar:

Cholestatic icterus, drug induced hepatitis, transient sight loss, disturbance in the sense of balance with the clinical symptoms of vertigo and ataxia, disturbance in taste lasting several months, hypoglycaemia, hypernatriemia, hypercalcaemia.

Haematological changes: These may include in connection with quinolone therapy leucocytosis, leucopenia, neutropenia, increased rate of blood sedimentation, anaemia and haemolysis.

Overdose: Information on overdosage is limited. In the event of overdosage it is recommended that appropriate supportive care should be instituted as dictated by the patient's clinical status. Adequate hydration should be maintained.

Pharmacological properties

Pharmacodynamic properties:

General properties: Grepafloxacin is a broad-spectrum fluoroquinolone antibiotic. It has bactericidal activity against a wide range of Gram-negative, Gram-positive and atypical bacteria. The bactericidal activity is due to inhibition of the bacterial enzymes DNA gyrase (topoisomerase II) and topoisomerase IV, which are essential enzymes for duplication, transcription, and repair of bacterial DNA.

This mode of action of quinolones differs from other classes of antibiotics, therefore bacteria resistant to other classes would generally retain their susceptibility to grepafloxacin. Beta-lactamases and alterations to penicillin binding proteins have no effect on grepafloxacin activity.

Breakpoints: The following MIC breakpoints for grepafloxacin, separating susceptible (S) from intermediately susceptible organisms, and intermediately susceptible from resistant (R) organisms have been set by the National Committee for Clinical Laboratory Standards in the USA (NCCLS):

Streptococcus pneumoniae: S≤0.5 μg/ml, R≥2 μg/ml;
Haemophilus influenzae: S≤0.5 μg/ml;
Neisseria gonorrhoeae: S≤0.06 μg/ml, R≥1 μg/ml;
Non-fastidious pathogens: S≤1 μg/ml, R≥4 μg/ml.

Susceptibility: The prevalence of resistance may vary geographically and with time for selected species. Local information on resistance is desirable, particularly when treating severe infections. This information gives only an approximate guidance on the probabilities whether microorganisms will be susceptible to grepafloxacin or not. The following table lists the susceptibilities of bacteria relevant to the therapeutic indications approved for Raxar:

Susceptible
Aerobic Gram-positive micro-organisms
Staphylococcus aureus – methicillin susceptible strains*
Streptococcus agalactiae
*Streptococcus pneumoniae**
Streptococcus pneumoniae (penicillin-intermediate and resistant)

Aerobic Gram-negative micro-organisms
Escherichia coli
Haemophilus influenzae – including beta-lactamase producing strains*
*Haemophilus parainfluenzae**
Klebsiella oxytoca
Klebsiella pneumoniae
Moraxella catarrhalis – including beta-lactamase producing strains*
Neisseria gonorrhoeae – including tetracycline and penicillin resistant strains*
Proteus mirabilis
Proteus vulgaris

Resistant
Aerobic Gram-positive organisms
Staphylococcus aureus (methicillin resistant)

Other organisms
Susceptible
Chlamydia pneumoniae
*Chlamydia trachomatis**
*Legionella pneumophila**
Mycoplasma hominis
*Mycoplasma pneumoniae**

Intermediate
Ureaplasma urealyticum

* Clinical efficacy has been demonstrated for susceptible organisms in approved indications.

Resistance: Resistance to grepafloxacin through spontaneous mutation *in vitro* occurs at a very low frequency. In clinical trials, grepafloxacin-resistant mutants were rarely encountered during the treatment of infection caused by susceptible isolates.

Anaerobes are generally resistant to grepafloxacin; in particular *Bacteroides fragilis* group and *Clostridium difficile.*

Other information: Certain organisms exhibit cross-resistance to grepafloxacin and some other fluoroquinolones. However, some organisms that are resistant to other quinolones may be susceptible to grepafloxacin. Cross-resistance to grepafloxacin and other classes of antimicrobial agents, including β-lactam antibiotics, macrolides and aminoglycosides has not generally been observed. Therefore, organisms resistant to the latter classes of drugs are expected to be susceptible to grepafloxacin.

Pharmacokinetic properties:

Absorption: Grepafloxacin is rapidly and extensively absorbed following oral administration. The absolute bioavailability of grepafloxacin has been estimated to be about 72%. The presence of food or increased gastric pH does not affect the rate or extent of grepafloxacin absorption.

After oral administration, peak plasma levels (C_{max}) were reached within two hours of dosing. Following multiple oral doses, steady-state was reached within 5 days of treatment and a 1.5–2 fold accumulation was observed. The C_{max} values at steady state after administration of 400 mg and 600 mg were 1.35 μg/ml, and 2.30 μg/ml respectively. The plasma levels for females were greater than for males. This variation was considered to be related mainly to differences in body weight (and in particular lean body mass), with grepafloxacin clearance unaffected. Although some mild side effects like nausea, vomiting and unpleasant taste were seen more often in women than in men, this difference in the pharmacokinetics is not considered clinically relevant.

Distribution: Binding of grepafloxacin to human plasma proteins is approximately 50%, and is not affected by advancing age or renal or hepatic impairment. The apparent volume of distribution after oral administration of 400 mg of grepafloxacin was 5 l/kg, suggesting that grepafloxacin is extensively distributed into the various tissues in the body.

Relative to plasma concentrations, grepafloxacin penetrates and concentrates in alveolar fluid, alveolar macrophages, bronchial mucosa, male and female genital tissues, bile, biliary, skin and tonsilar tissues.

Metabolism: After oral administration, grepafloxacin and five metabolites were identified in plasma, urine, and an additional sixth metabolite was identified in the faeces. Grepafloxacin appears to be eliminated by multiple pathways and therefore changes in its pharmacokinetics due to interaction with other drugs is less likely. In plasma, about 50% was unchanged grepafloxacin and 7.8% was present as the 4'-glucoronide; other metabolites ranged from 0.7–5.2%.

Studies in human hepatocytes *in vitro* showed that the CYP1A2 isoenzyme is involved in the oxidative metabolism of grepafloxacin, while CYP3A4 is marginally involved. The major oxidative metabolites showed weak antimicrobial activity compared to the parent compound, and no significant toxicity.

Excretion: The typical plasma elimination half-life of grepafloxacin is 12 hours. Average elimination half life values ranged between 10 and 13 hours after single doses and 10 to 16 hours after multiple doses of grepafloxacin. Grepafloxacin is eliminated principally through hepatic metabolism and biliary excretion, with only 5–14% renally excreted. Faecal excretion accounts for 27% of the oral dose.

Pharmacokinetics in demographic subpopulations:
Elderly: The pharmacokinetic profile of grepafloxacin was generally similar with increasing age.

Renal impairment: Renal insufficiency, including that considered severe (Clcr<30 ml/min), did not substantially influence the pharmacokinetics of grepafloxacin. This finding is consistent with the elimination route. No dose adjustment of Raxar in patients with renal impairment is necessary.

Hepatic impairment: Higher grepafloxacin plasma concentrations were observed among subjects with hepatic disease when compared to subjects with normal liver function. The area under the curve (AUC) was increased by 56% and 137% for subjects with mild and moderate hepatic impairment, respectively. These findings are consistent with the elimination route of grepafloxacin, which is mainly by hepatic metabolism. Treatment with Raxar is contra-indicated in patients with moderate or severe hepatic impairment.

Preclinical safety data: Haemopoetic (decrease in the number of erythrocytes and leucocytes, especially neutrophils, which was reversible when the drug was discontinued) and lymphoid tissue changes (atrophic changes of lymph nodes, spleen, thymus) following treatment with quinolones are seen in rats and monkeys, but are rare in man. As with other quinolones hepatotoxicity and nephrotoxicity was seen (monkey, dog). The liver toxicity showed as raised liver enzymes and vacuolar degeneration. The nephrotoxicity seen were degenerative changes in the renal proximal tubules of monkeys. These changes were commonly seen only after prolonged treatment or treatment with high doses of grepafloxacin.

Although conventional long-term studies to determine the carcinogenic potential of grepafloxacin have not been performed, the drug has been subjected to a range of *in vitro* and *in vivo* genotoxicity tests. Negative results were obtained in Ames and V79 hprt mutation assays. The *in vitro* test in the Chinese hamster fibroblasts showed chromosomal abnormalities and polyploidy at low concentrations, under continuous and extended treatment conditions. However, *in vivo* genotoxicity tests at plasma concentrations higher than those at which induction of chromosome damage was observed *in vitro,* were negative. It is concluded that the negative *in vivo* results adequately reflect the *in vivo* situation in terms of genotoxicity.

Some quinolones have been shown to enhance the action of UVA-induced photocarcinogenicity when administered concurrently to mice exposed to ultraviolet light. Grepafloxacin induces chromosomal damage *in vitro* in the presence and in the absence of UV radiation. *In vivo* genotoxicity tests yielded negative results. Grepafloxacin did not enhance UV-induced tumourigenesis in hairless mice, but shortened slightly the latent period of development of skin tumours.

Phototoxicity has been reported for many quinolones. In animal models grepafloxacin seems to show less potency than many other quinolones, although it has a relatively long half life (505 h) in the skin of the pigmented rat (see *Special warnings and special precautions for use*).

Grepafloxacin binds to melanin with a relatively long half life (705 h). Toxicity tests in rats, dogs, and monkeys (repeated dosing up to six months) revealed no indication regarding an oculotoxic risk. A specific 52 weeks trial in monkeys showed no result. A further specific trial in pigmented rats showed no indication of a cataractogenic or co-cataractogenic effect.

Grepafloxacin caused in isolated cases ventricular arrhythmias in the rabbit after intravenous doses of ↓30 mg/kg. In the dog doses of ↓30 mg/kg orally caused prolongation of the QT-interval. In the monkey after intravenous doses of ↓75 mg/kg ventricular arrhythmias were observed.

Quinolones are known to cause lesions in the cartilage of the major diarthrodial joints in immature animals. In animal models grepafloxacin appears to have a relatively low potential for causing joint toxicity (see *Use in pregnancy and lactation*). The lowest dose of grepafloxacin causing joint toxicity in young dogs was seven times maximum recommended therapeutic dose (600 mg/50 kg person) on a mg/kg basis, with plasma concentrations in the same range as the therapeutic doses.

Reproductive studies performed in rats and rabbits indicate that placental transfer of grepafloxacin occurs. Studies in these species did not show any evidence of teratogenicity or impairment of fertility following administration of grepafloxacin. In rat, changes in the behaviour (increased spontaneous activity) of some female offspring were seen.

Pharmaceutical particulars

List of excipients:
Tablet core: Microcrystalline cellulose, Low substituted hydroxypropyl cellulose, Hydroxypropyl cellulose, Magnesium stearate.
Film-coat: Hypromellose, Titanium dioxide, Talc.

Incompatibilities: No incompatibilities are known to date.

Shelf life: 3 years.

Special precautions for storage: Store below 30°C.

Nature and contents of container: Cartons containing white opaque PVC/aluminium foil blister packs. The tablets are available in 400 mg and 600 mg strengths in packs of one, two, five, seven or ten tablets.

Instructions for use/handling: None.

Marketing authorisation number PL 10949/0300

Date of first authorisation/renewal of authorisation 9 December 1997

Date of revision of the text 9 December 1997.

RETROVIR* IV FOR INFUSION

Qualitative and quantitative composition Zidovudine 200 mg.

Pharmaceutical form Retrovir IV for Infusion is a clear, nearly colourless, sterile aqueous solution in an amber glass vial containing 10 mg zidovudine per ml, with a pH of approximately 5.5. Each 20 ml vial contains 200 mg zidovudine.

Clinical particulars

Therapeutic indications: Retrovir IV for Infusion is indicated for the short-term management of serious manifestations of Human Immunodeficiency Virus (HIV) infection in patients with the Acquired Immune Deficiency syndrome (AIDS) or AIDS-related complex (ARC) who are unable to take Retrovir Oral Formulations. Evidence of efficacy has been demonstrated in AIDS patients who have recovered from their first episode of *Pneumocystis carinii* pneumonia within 4 months and ARC patients with multiple signs of HIV infection, including mucocutaneous candidiasis, weight loss (more than 10% or 14 pounds), lymphadenopathy and unexplained fever.

Retrovir should be considered for use in HIV-positive pregnant women (over 14 weeks of gestation) and their newborn infants as it has been shown to reduce the rate of maternal-foetal transmission of HIV (23% infection rate for placebo versus 8% for zidovudine).

Posology and method of administration: The required dose of Retrovir IV for Infusion must be administered by slow intravenous infusion of the diluted product.

Retrovir IV for Infusion must *NOT* be given intramuscularly.

Dilution: Retrovir IV for Infusion must be diluted prior to administration.

The required dose (see *Dosage*) should be added to and mixed with Glucose Intravenous Infusion (5% w/v) to give a final zidovudine concentration of either 2 mg/ml or 4 mg/ml. These dilutions are chemically and physically stable for up to 48 hours at both 5°C and 25°C.

Since no antimicrobial preservative is included, dilution must be carried out under full aseptic conditions, preferably immediately prior to administration, and any unused portion of the vial should be discarded. Should any visible turbidity appear in the product either before or after dilution or during infusion, the preparation should be discarded.

Dosage in adults: A dose for Retrovir IV for Infusion of 1 or 2 mg zidovudine/kg bodyweight every 4 hours approximately corresponds to an oral dose of 1.5 or 3.0 mg zidovudine/kg every 4 hours (600 or 1200 mg/day for a 70 kg patient).

The effectiveness of lower dosage in the treatment or prevention of HIV-associated neurological dysfunction and malignancies is unknown. Patients should receive Retrovir IV for Infusion only until oral therapy can be administered (see *Undesirable effects*).

Dosage adjustments in patients with haematological adverse reactions: Dosage adjustments may be necessary in patients with haematological adverse reactions. This is more likely in patients with poor bone marrow reserve prior to treatment. If the haemoglobin level falls to between 7.5 g/decilitre (4.65 mmol/litre) and 9 g/decilitre (5.59 mmol/litre) or the neutrophil count falls to between 0.75×10^9/litre and 1.0×10^9/litre, the daily dosage may be reduced until there is evidence of marrow recovery; alternatively, recovery may be enhanced by brief (2 to 4 weeks) interruption of Retrovir therapy. If dosage reduction is considered, the daily dosage may, for example, be halved and subsequently increased, depending on patient tolerance, up to the original dosage.

Therapy with Retrovir IV for Infusion should be discontinued if the haemoglobin level falls below 7.5 g/decilitre (4.65 mmol/litre) or if the neutrophil count falls to less than 0.75×10^9/litre. Marrow recovery is usually observed within 2 weeks after which time Retrovir therapy at a reduced dosage may be reinstituted. After a further 2 to 4 weeks the dosage of zidovudine may be gradually increased, depending on patient tolerance until the original dosage is reached, although data on the use of intravenous Retrovir for periods in excess of 2 weeks are limited.

Dosage in children: Limited data are available on the use of Retrovir IV for Infusion in children. A range of dosages between 80–160 mg/m² every 6 hours (320–640 mg/m²/day) has been used. Exposure following the 120 mg/m² dose every 6 hours approximately corresponds to the recommended oral dose of 180 mg/m² every 6 hours.

Dosage in the prevention of maternal-foetal transmission: Although the optimal dosage schedule has not been identified the following dosage regimen has been shown to be effective. Pregnant women (over 14 weeks of gestation) should be given 500 mg/day orally (100 mg five times a day) until the beginning of labour. During labour and delivery Retrovir should be administered intravenously at 2 mg/kg bodyweight given over 1 hour followed by a continuous intravenous infusion at 1 mg/kg/h until the umbilical cord is clamped. The newborn infants should be given 2 mg/kg bodyweight orally every 6 hours starting within 12 hours after birth and continuing until 6 weeks-old. Infants unable to receive oral dosing should be given Retrovir intravenously at 1.5 mg/kg bodyweight infused over 30 minutes every 6 hours.

IN CASE OF PLANNED CAESAREAN, THE INFUSION SHOULD BE STARTED 4 HOURS BEFORE THE OPERATION.

In the event of a false labour, the Retrovir infusion should be stopped and oral dosing restarted.

Dosage in the elderly: No data are available, however special care is advised in this age group due to age-associated changes such as the decrease in renal functions and alterations in haematological parameters.

Dosage in renal impairment: Compared to healthy subjects, patients with advanced renal failure have a 50% higher maximum plasma concentration after oral administration. Systemic exposure (measured as area under the zidovudine concentration time curve) is increased 100%; the half-life is not significantly altered. In renal failure there is substantial accumulation of the major glucuronide metabolite but this does not appear to cause toxicity. Patients with advanced renal failure should receive Retrovir at the lower end of the dosage range. Haematological parameters and clinical response, may influence the need for subsequent dosage adjustment. Haemodialysis and peritoneal dialysis have no significant effect on zidovudine elimination whereas elimination of the glucuronide metabolite is increased.

Dosage in hepatic impairment: Limited data in patients with cirrhosis given oral Retrovir suggest that accumulation of zidovudine may occur in patients with hepatic impairment because of decreased glucuronidation. Dosage adjustments may be necessary but precise recommendations cannot be made at present. If monitoring of plasma zidovudine levels is not feasible, physicians will need to pay particular attention to signs of intolerance and increase the interval between doses as appropriate.

Contra-indications: Retrovir IV for Infusion is contra-indicated in patients known to be hypersensitive to zidovudine, or to any of the components of the formulation.

Retrovir IV for infusion should not be given to patients with abnormally low neutrophil counts (less than 0.75×10^9/litre) or abnormally low haemoglobin levels (less than 7.5 g/decilitre or 4.65 mmol/litre).

Retrovir is contra-indicated in newborn infants with hyperbilirubinaemia requiring treatment other than phototherapy, or with increased transaminase levels of over five times the upper limit of normal.

Special warnings and precautions for use: Retrovir is not a cure for HIV infection and patients remain at risk of developing illnesses which are associated with immune suppression, including opportunistic infections and neoplasm. Whilst it has been shown to reduce the risk of opportunistic infections, data on the development of neoplasms, including lymphomas, are limited. The available data on patients treated for advanced HIV disease indicate that the risk of lymphoma development is consistent with that observed in untreated patients. In patients with early HIV disease on long term treatment the risk of lymphoma development is unknown. Retrovir should be administered under the supervision of a doctor with experience of treating patients with HIV infection or AIDS/ARC. An appropriate treatment procedure requires access to suitable facilities e.g. for performing haematological monitoring investigations, including determination of CD4+ lymphocytes and for provision of blood transfusions if necessary.

Haematological adverse reactions: Anaemia (usually occurring after 6 weeks of Retrovir therapy but occasionally earlier), neutropenia (usually occurring at any time after 4 weeks' therapy but sometimes earlier) and leucopenia (usually secondary to neutropenia) can be expected to occur frequently in patients receiving Retrovir IV for Infusion; therefore, haematological parameters should be carefully monitored. It is recommended that blood tests are performed at least weekly in patients receiving Retrovir IV for Infusion. Particular care should be taken in patients with pre-existing bone marrow compromise (e.g. haemoglobin less than 9 g/decilitre (5.59 mmol/litre) or neutrophil count less than 1.0×10^9/litre). Lower daily dosages from the start of treatment may be appropriate for some such patients.

If severe anaemia or myelosuppression occurs dosage adjustments are suggested (see *Posology and method of administration*). Such abnormalities are usually rapidly reversible on stopping therapy. In patients with significant anaemia, dosage adjustments do not necessarily eliminate the need for transfusions.

Lactic acidosis and severe hepatomegaly with steatosis: Rare occurrences of lactic acidosis, in the absence of hypoxaemia, and severe hepatomegaly with steatosis have been reported and are potentially fatal; it is not known whether these events are causally related to Retrovir, but they have been reported in HIV-positive patients without AIDS. Treatment with Retrovir should be suspended in the setting of rapidly elevating aminotransferase levels, progressive hepatomegaly, or metabolic/lactic acidosis of unknown aetiology (see *Undesirable effects*).

Caution should be exercised when administering Retrovir to any patient, particularly obese women, with hepatomegaly, hepatitis or other known risk factor for liver disease. These patients should be followed closely while on therapy with Retrovir.

Patients should be cautioned about the concomitant use of self-administered medications (see *Interaction with other medicaments*).

Patients should be advised that zidovudine therapy has not been shown to reduce the risk of transmission of HIV to others through sexual contact or blood contamination.

Interaction with other medicaments and other forms of interaction: As experience of drug with interactions with Retrovir is still limited, care should be taken when combining with other drug regimens. The interactions listed below should not be considered exhaustive but are representative of the classes of drug where caution should be exercised.

Limited data suggest that probenecid increases the mean half-life and area under the plasma concentration curve of zidovudine by decreasing glucuronidation. Renal excretion of the glucuronide (and possibly zidovudine itself) is reduced in the presence of probenecid.

Phenytoin blood levels have been reported to be low in some patients receiving Retrovir, while in one patient a high level was noted. These observations suggest that phenytoin levels should be carefully monitored in patients receiving both drugs.

Paracetamol use during treatment with Retrovir in a placebo-controlled trial was associated with an increased incidence of neutropenia especially following chronic therapy. However, the available pharmacokinetic data indicate that paracetamol does not increase plasma levels of zidovudine nor of its glucuronide metabolite.

Other drugs including but not limited to aspirin, codeine, morphine, indomethacin, ketoprofen, naproxen, oxazepam, lorazepam, cimetidine, clofibrate, dapsone and isoprinosine may alter the metabolism of zidovudine by competitively inhibiting glucuronidation or directly inhibiting hepatic microsomal metabolism. Careful thought should be given to the possibilities of drug interactions before using such drugs, particularly for chronic therapy, in combination with Retrovir IV for Infusion.

Concomitant therapy especially acute therapy with potentially nephrotoxic or myelosuppressive drugs (e.g. systemic pentamidine, dapsone, pyrimethamine, co-trimoxazole, amphotericin, flucytosine, ganciclovir, interferon, vincristine, vinblastine and doxorubicin) may also increase the risk of adverse reactions with Retrovir IV for Infusion. If concomitant therapy with any of these drugs is necessary then extra care should be taken in monitoring renal function and haematological parameters and if required, the dosage of one or more agents should be reduced.

The nucleoside analogue ribavirin antagonises the *in vitro* antiviral activity of zidovudine and so concomitant use of such drugs should be avoided.

Since some patients receiving Retrovir may continue to experience opportunistic infections, concomitant use of prophylactic antimicrobial therapy may have to be considered. Such therapy has included co-trimoxazole, aerosolised pentamidine, pyrimethamine and acyclovir. Limited data from controlled clinical trials do not indicate a significantly increased risk of adverse reactions to Retrovir with these drugs.

Use during pregnancy and lactation:

Pregnancy: The use of Retrovir in pregnant women over 14 weeks of gestation, with subsequent treatment of their newborn infants, has been shown to significantly reduce the rate of maternal-foetal transmission of HIV based on viral cultures in infants.

Interim analysis of the pivotal US placebo-controlled study indicated that Retrovir reduced maternal-foetal transmission by approximately 70%. In this study, pregnant women had CD4+ cell counts of 200 to 1818/mm^3 (median in treated group 560/mm^3) and began treatment therapy between weeks 14 and 34 of gestation and had no clinical indications for Retrovir therapy; their newborn infants received Retrovir until 6-weeks old. A decision to reduce the risk of maternal transmission of HIV should be based on the balance of potential benefits and potential risk. Pregnant women considering the use of Retrovir during pregnancy for prevention of HIV transmission to their infants should be advised that transmission may still occur in some cases despite therapy.

The efficacy of zidovudine to reduce the maternal-foetal transmission in women with previously prolonged treatment with zidovudine or other antiretroviral agents or women infected with HIV strains with reduced sensitivity to zidovudine is unknown.

It is unknown whether there are any long-term consequences of *in utero* and infant exposure to Retrovir. Based on the animal carcinogenicity/mutagenicity findings a carcinogenic risk to humans cannot be excluded (see *Preclinical safety data*). Zidovudine has been shown to be mutagenic in some, but not all, standard *in vitro* and *in vivo* assays. Although the predictive value of rodent carcinogenicity studies for humans is uncertain, late-occurring vaginal tumours (appearing after 19 months of continuous daily oral dosing) have been seen in rodents following lifetime dosing with zidovudine. The relevance of these findings to both infected and uninfected infants exposed to Retrovir is unknown. However, pregnant women considering using Retrovir during pregnancy should be made aware of these findings.

Given the limited data on the general use of Retrovir in pregnancy, Retrovir should only be used prior to the 14th week of gestation when the potential benefit to the mother outweighs the risk to the foetus. Studies in pregnant rats and rabbits given zidovudine orally at dosage levels up to 450 and 500 mg/kg/day respectively during the major period of organogenesis have revealed no evidence of teratogenicity. There was, however, a statistically significant increase in foetal-resorptions in rats given 150 to 450 mg/kg/day and in rabbits given 500 mg/kg/day. A separate study, reported subsequently, found that rats given a dosage of 3000 mg/kg/day, which is very near the oral median lethal dose (3683 mg/kg), caused marked maternal toxicity and an increase in the incidence of foetal malformations. No evidence of teratogenicity was observed in this study at the lower dosages tested (600 mg/kg/day or less).

Lactation: Limited data indicate that zidovudine is excreted in animal milk. It is not known if zidovudine is excreted in human milk.

Since the drug may pass into breast milk it is recommended that mothers taking Retrovir do not breast feed their infants.

Fertility: It is not known whether zidovudine can affect human fertility. There are no data on the effect of Retrovir on human female fertility. In men, Retrovir has not been shown to affect sperm count, morphology or motility.

Effects on ability to drive and use machines: Retrovir IV for Infusion is generally used in an in-patient hospital population and information on ability to drive and use machinery is not usually relevant. There have been no studies to investigate the effect of Retrovir on driving performance or the ability to operate machinery. Further, a detrimental effect on such activities cannot be predicted from the pharmacology of the drug. Nevertheless, the clinical status of the patient and the adverse events profile of Retrovir should be borne in mind when considering the patient's ability to drive or operate machinery.

Undesirable effects: The most serious adverse reactions include anaemia (which may require transfusions), neutropenia and leucopenia. These occur more frequently at higher doses (1200–1500 mg/day) and in AIDS than in ARC patients (especially when there is poor bone marrow reserve prior to treatment), and particularly in patients with CD4+ cell counts less than 100/mm^3. Dosage reduction or cessation of therapy may become more necessary (see *Posology and method of administration*). The incidence of neutropenia was also increased in those patients whose neutrophil counts, haemoglobin levels and vitamin B12 levels were low at the start of Retrovir therapy, and in those patients taking paracetamol concurrently (see *Interaction with other medicaments*).

Other frequent adverse events reported in a large placebo-controlled clinical trial of Retrovir included nausea, vomiting, anorexia, abdominal pain, headache, rash, fever, myalgia, paraesthesiae, insomnia, malaise, asthenia and dyspepsia. Apart from nausea, severe headaches, myalgia and insomnia, which were significantly more common in patients receiving Retrovir, the incidence of the other adverse events was only slightly higher than in the placebo recipients.

Other reported adverse events included, somnolence, diarrhoea, dizziness, sweating, dyspnoea, flatulence, taste perversion, chest pain, loss of mental acuity, anxiety, urinary frequency, depression, generalised pain, chills, cough, urticaria, pruritus and influenza-like syndrome. The incidence of these and other less frequent adverse events was generally similar in Retrovir and placebo-treated patients. The available data from studies of Retrovir Oral Formulations indicate that the incidence of nausea and other frequently reported clinical adverse events consistently decreases over time during the first few weeks of therapy with Retrovir.

The following events have been reported in patients treated with Retrovir. They may also occur as part of the underlying disease process or as a result of the wide range of drugs used in the management of HIV disease. The relationship between these events and use of Retrovir may therefore be difficult to evaluate, particularly in the medically complicated situations which characterise advanced HIV disease. If the severity of the symptoms warrants it, a reduction or suspension of Retrovir therapy may assist in the assessment and management of these conditions:

- myopathy;
- pancytopenia with marrow hypoplasia and isolated thrombocytopenia;
- lactic acidosis in the absence of hypoxaemia, liver disorders such as severe hepatomegaly with steatosis, raised blood levels of liver enzymes and bilirubin;
- pancreatitis;
- nail, skin and oral mucosa pigmentation.

Convulsions and other cerebral events have also been reported in patients receiving open-label therapy with Retrovir. However, the relationship between these events and the use of Retrovir is difficult to evaluate. Furthermore, the weight of evidence indicates an overall beneficial effect of Retrovir on HIV-associated neurological disorders.

Experience with Retrovir IV for Infusion treatment for periods in excess of 2 weeks is limited, although some patients have received treatment for up to 12 weeks. The most frequent adverse events were anaemia, neutropenia and leucopenia. Local reactions were infrequent.

Children: Limited data from open labelled studies in children, involving intravenous administration of a limited duration, do not contradict the adverse event profile of zidovudine in adults.

In a placebo-controlled trial, overall clinical adverse events and laboratory test abnormalities were similar for women in the Retrovir and placebo groups. However, there was a trend for mild and moderate anaemia to be seen more commonly prior to delivery in the zidovudine treated women.

In the same trial, haemoglobin concentrations in infants exposed to Retrovir for this indication were marginally lower than in infants in the placebo group, but transfusion was not required. Anaemia resolved within 6 weeks after completion of Retrovir therapy. Other clinical adverse events and laboratory test abnormalities were similar in the Retrovir and placebo groups. The long term consequences of *in utero* and infant exposure to Retrovir are unknown.

Overdosage: symptoms and signs: Dosages as high as 7.5 mg/kg by infusion every 4 hours for 2 weeks have been administered to 5 patients. One patient experienced an anxiety reaction while the other 4 had no untoward effects.

Limited data are available on the consequences of ingestion of acute oral overdoses in both adults and children. No fatalities occurred and all patients recovered. The highest recorded blood level of zidovudine was 185 μM (49.4 mcg/ml). No specific symptoms or signs have been identified following such overdosage.

Treatment: Patients should be observed closely for evidence of toxicity (see *Undesirable effects*) and given the necessary supportive therapy.

Haemodialysis and peritoneal dialysis appear to have a limited effect on elimination of zidovudine but enhances the elimination of the glucuronide metabolite.

Pharmacological properties

Pharmacodynamic properties:

(a) Mode of action: Zidovudine is an antiviral agent which is highly active *in vitro* against retroviruses including the Human Immunodeficiency Virus (HIV).

Zidovudine is phosphorylated in both infected and uninfected cells to the monophosphate (MP) derivative by cellular thymidine kinase. Subsequent phosphorylation of zidovudine-MP to the diphosphate (DP), and then the triphosphate (TP) derivative is catalysed by cellular thymidylate kinase and non-specific kinases respectively. Zidovudine-TP acts as an inhibitor of and substrate for the viral reverse transcriptase. The formation of further proviral DNA is blocked by incorporation of zidovudine-TP into the chain and subsequent chain termination.

Competition by zidovudine-TP for HIV reverse transcriptase is approximately 100-fold greater than for cellular DNA polymerase alpha.

(b) Microbiology: The relationships between *in vitro* susceptibility of HIV to zidovudine and clinical response to therapy remain under investigation. *In vitro* sensitivity testing has not been standardised and results may therefore vary according to methodological factors.

Reduced *in vitro* sensitivity to zidovudine has been reported for HIV isolates from patients who have received prolonged courses of Retrovir therapy. The available information indicates that the early HIV disease, the frequency and the degree of reduction of *in vitro* sensitivity is notably less than for advanced disease.

Pharmacokinetic properties:

(a) Pharmacokinetics in adults: Dose-independent kinetics were observed in patients receiving one-hour infusions of 1 to 5 mg/kg 3 to 6 times daily. Mean steady state peak (C^{ss}max) and trough (C^{ss}min) plasma concentrations in adults following a one-hour infusion of 2.5 mg/kg every 4 hours were 4.0 and 0.4 μM, respectively (or 1.1 and 0.1 mcg/ml).

The mean terminal plasma half life was 1.1 hours, the mean total body clearance was 27.1 ml/min/kg and the apparent volume of distribution was 1.6 litres/kg. Renal clearance of zidovudine greatly exceeds creatinine clearance, indicating significant tubular secretion takes place.

The 5'-glucuronide of zidovudine is the major metabolite in both plasma and urine accounting for approximately 50–80% of the administered dose eliminated by renal excretion. 3'-amino-3'-deoxythymidine (AMT) has been identified as a metabolite of zidovudine following intravenous dosing.

There are limited data concerning the pharmacokinetics of zidovudine in patients with renal or hepatic impairment (see *Posology and method of administration*). There are also limited data on the pharmacokinetics of zidovudine in pregnant women. No specific data are available on the pharmacokinetics of zidovudine in the elderly.

(b) Pharmacokinetics in children: In children over the age of 5–6 months, the pharmacokinetic profile of zidovudine is similar to that in adults. C^{ss}max levels were 1.46 mcg/ml following an intravenous dose of 80 mg zidovudine/m^2 body surface area, 2.26 mcg/ml following 120 mg/m^2 and 2.96 mcg/ml following 160 mg/m^2.

With intravenous dosing, the mean terminal plasma half-life and total body clearance were 1.5 hours and 30.9 ml/min/kg respectively. The major metabolite is the 5'-glucuronide. After intravenous dosing, 29% of the dose was recovered unchanged in the urine and 45% excreted as the glucuronide. Renal clearance of zidovudine greatly exceeds creatinine clearance indicating that significant tubular secretion takes place.

The limited data available on the pharmacokinetics in neonates and young infants indicate that glucuronidation of zidovudine is reduced with a consequent increase in bioavailability, reduction in clearance and longer half-life in infants less than 14 days-old but thereafter the pharmacokinetics appear similar to those reported in adults.

(c) Distribution: In adults the average cerebrospinal fluid/plasma zidovudine concentration ratio 2 to 4 hours after chronic intermittent oral dosing was found to be approximately 0.5. Limited data indicate that zidovudine crosses the placenta and is found in amniotic fluid and foetal blood. Zidovudine has also been detected in semen.

In children the mean cerebrospinal fluid/plasma zidovudine concentration ratio ranged from 0.52–0.85 as determined during oral therapy 0.5 to 4 hours after dosing and was 0.87 as determined during intravenous therapy 1–5 hours after a 1 hour infusion. During continuous intravenous infusion the mean steady-state cerebrospinal fluid/plasma concentration ratio was 0.24.

Plasma protein binding is relatively low (34 to 38%) and drug interactions involving binding site displacement are not anticipated.

Preclinical safety data:

(a) Mutagenicity: No evidence of mutagenicity was observed in the Ames test. However, zidovudine was weakly mutagenic in a mouse lymphoma assay. Clastogenic effects (chromosome damage) were observed in an *in vitro* study in human lymphocytes and in *in vivo* oral repeat dose micronucleus studies in rats and mice. An *in vivo* cytogenetic study in rats did not show chromosomal damage. A study of peripheral blood lymphocytes of eleven AIDS patients showed a higher chromosome breakage frequency in those who

had received Retrovir than in those who had not. The clinical significance of these findings is unclear.

(b) Carcinogenicity: Zidovudine was administered orally at three dosage levels to separate groups of mice and rats (60 females and 60 males in each group). Initial single daily doses were 30, 60 and 120 mg/kg/day and 80, 220 and 600 mg/kg/day in mice and rats, respectively. The doses in mice were reduced to 20, 30 and 40 mg/kg/day after Day 90 because of treatment-related anaemia, whereas in rats only the high dose was reduced (to 450 and then 300 mg/kg/day on Days 91 and 279, respectively).

In mice, seven late-appearing (after 19 months) vaginal neoplasms (5 squamous cell carcinomas, one squamous cell papilloma and one squamous polyp) occurred at the highest dose. One late-appearing squamous cell papilloma occurred in the vagina of a middle-dose animal. No vaginal tumours were found at the lowest dose.

In rats, two late-appearing (after 20 months) vaginal squamous cell carcinomas occurred in animals given the highest dose. No vaginal tumours occurred at the middle or low doses in rats.

There were no other drug-related tumours observed in either sex of either species.

The predictive value of rodent carcinogenicity studies for humans is uncertain and thus the clinical significance of these findings is unclear.

(c) Teratogenicity: See *Use during pregnancy and lactation.*

(d) Fertility: Zidovudine did not impair male or female fertility in rats given oral dosages up to 450 mg/kg/day.

Pharmaceutical particulars

List of excipients: Hydrochloric acid; sodium hydroxide; water for injections.

Incompatibilities: None.

Shelf life: 3 years.

Special precautions for storage: Store below 30°C. Protect from light.

Nature and contents of container: Glass vial containing 20 ml.

Instructions for use/handling: No special instructions are required.

Marketing authorisation number PL 0003/0332

Date of approval/revision of SPC October 1994

Legal category POM.

RETROVIR* ORAL FORMULATIONS

Qualitative and quantitative composition Capsules containing either 100 mg or 250 mg zidovudine. Tablets containing 300 mg zidovudine. Syrup containing 50 mg zidovudine per 5 ml.

Pharmaceutical form

Retrovir 100 mg Capsules: Hard gelatin capsules with opaque white cap and body and a central dark-blue band, printed 'Wellcome', '100' and coded 'Y9C' and each containing 100 mg zidovudine.

Retrovir 250 mg Capsules: Hard gelatin capsules with opaque blue cap, opaque white body and a central dark-blue band, printed 'Wellcome', '250' and coded H2F and each containing 250 mg zidovudine.

Retrovir Syrup: A clear, pale yellow, strawberry-flavoured, sugar-free oral solution containing 50 mg zidovudine in each 5 ml.

The pack contains a 10 ml oral-dosing syringe which should be fitted to the bottle before use and closed with the cap provided.

Retrovir 300 mg Tablets: White, round, biconvex, film-coated tablets, with a white to beige core scored and branded 'WELLCOME X4F' and each containing 300 mg zidovudine.

Clinical particulars

Therapeutic indications: Retrovir Oral Formulations are indicated for use in combination with other anti-retroviral agents (except when used in pregnant women) for the treatment of Human Immunodeficiency Virus (HIV) infection in adults and children.

Retrovir monotherapy is indicated for use in HIV-positive pregnant women (over 14 weeks of gestation) and their newborn infants for primary prophylaxis of maternal-foetal HIV-1 transmission.

Posology and method of administration:

Dosage in adults: The usual recommended dose of Retrovir in combination with other anti-retroviral agents is 500 or 600 mg/day in two or three divided doses. For treatment or prevention of HIV-associated neurological dysfunction the efficacy of doses of Retrovir below 1000 mg/day has not been proven.

Dosage in children:

3 months–12 years: The recommended dose of Retrovir is 360 to 480 mg/m² per day, in 3 or 4 divided doses in combination with other antiretroviral agents. For the treatment or prevention of HIV-associated neurological dysfunction, the effectiveness of dosages less than 720 mg/m² per day (180 mg/m² every six hours) is unknown. The maximum dosage should not exceed 200 mg every 6 hours.

<3 months: The limited data available are insufficient to propose specific dosage recommendations (see *Maternal-foetal transmission and Pharmacokinetic properties*).

Dosage in the prevention of maternal-foetal transmission: Although the optimal dosage schedule has not been identified the following dosage regimen has been shown to be effective. Pregnant women (over 14 weeks of gestation) should be given 500 mg/day orally (100 mg five times per day) until the beginning of labour. During labour and delivery Retrovir should be administered intravenously at 2 mg/kg bodyweight given over 1 hour followed by a continuous intravenous infusion at 1 mg/kg/h until the umbilical cord is clamped. The newborn infants should be given 2 mg/kg bodyweight orally every 6 hours starting within 12 hours after birth and continuing until 6-weeks-old. Infants unable to receive oral dosing should be given Retrovir intravenously at 1.5 mg/kg bodyweight infused over 30 minutes every 6 hours.

IN CASE OF PLANNED CAESAREAN, THE INFUSION SHOULD BE STARTED 4 HOURS BEFORE THE OPERATION.

In the event of a false labour, the Retrovir infusion should be stopped and oral dosing restarted.

Dosage adjustments in patients with haematological adverse reactions: Dosage reduction or interruption of Retrovir therapy may be necessary in patients whose haemoglobin level falls to between 7.5 g/decilitre (4.65 mmol/litre) and 9 g/dl (5.59 mmol/l) or whose neutrophil count falls to between 0.75×10⁹/litre and 1.0×10⁹/litre (see *Contra-indications and Special warnings and special precautions for use*).

Dosage in the elderly: Zidovudine pharmacokinetics have not been studied in patients over 65 years of age and no specific data are available.

However, since special care is advised in this age group due to age-associated changes such as the decrease in renal function and alterations in haematological parameters, appropriate monitoring of patients before and during use of Retrovir is advised.

Dosage in renal impairment: In patients with severe renal impairment, apparent zidovudine clearance after oral zidovudine administration was approximately 50% of that reported in healthy subjects with normal renal function. Therefore a dosage reduction to 300–400 mg daily is recommended for patients with severe renal impairment with creatinine clearance ≤10 ml/min.

Haemodialysis and peritoneal dialysis have no significant effect on zidovudine elimination whereas elimination of the glucuronide metabolite is increased.

Dosage in hepatic impairment: Data in patients with cirrhosis suggest that accumulation of zidovudine may occur in patients with hepatic impairment because of decreased glucuronidation. Dosage adjustments may be necessary but, as there is only limited data available, precise recommendations cannot be made. If monitoring of plasma zidovudine levels is not feasible, physicians will need to monitor for signs of intolerance and adjust the dose and/or increase the interval between doses as appropriate.

Contra-indications: Retrovir Oral Formulations are contra-indicated in patients known to be hypersensitive to zidovudine, or to any of the components of the formulations. Retrovir Oral Formulations should not be given to patients with abnormally low neutrophil counts (less than 0.75×10⁹/litre) or abnormally low haemoglobin levels (less than 7.5 g/decilitre or 4.65 mmol/litre).

Retrovir is contra-indicated in new born infants with hyperbilirubinaemia requiring treatment other than phototherapy, or with increased transaminase levels of over five times the upper limit of normal.

Special warnings and special precautions for use: Retrovir is not a cure for HIV infection and patients remain at risk of developing illnesses which are associated with immune suppression, including opportunistic infections and neoplasms. Whilst it has been shown to reduce the risks of opportunistic infections, data on the development of neoplasms, including lymphomas, are limited. The available data on patients treated for advanced HIV disease indicate that the risk of lymphoma development is consistent with that observed in untreated patients. In patients with early HIV disease on long-term treatment the risk of lymphoma development is unknown.

Retrovir should be administered under the supervision of a doctor with experience of treating patients with HIV infection or AIDS. An appropriate treatment procedure requires access to suitable facilities e.g. for performing haematological monitoring investigations, including determination of viral load CD4+ lymphocytes and for provision of blood transfusions if necessary.

Haematological adverse reactions: Anaemia (usually not observed before six weeks of Retrovir therapy but occasionally occurring earlier), neutropenia (usually not observed before four weeks' therapy but sometimes occurring earlier) and leucopenia (usually secondary to neutropenia) can be expected to occur in patients receiving Retrovir. These occurred more frequently at higher dosages (1200–1500 mg/day) and in patients with poor bone marrow reserve prior to treatment, particularly with advanced HIV disease.

Haematological parameters should be carefully monitored. For patients with advanced symptomatic HIV disease it is generally recommended that blood tests are performed at least every two weeks for the first three months of therapy and at least monthly thereafter. In patients with early HIV disease (where bone marrow reserve is generally good), haematological adverse reactions are infrequent. Depending on the overall condition of the patient, blood tests may be performed less often, for example every 1 to 3 months.

If the haemoglobin level falls to between 7.5 g/dl (4.65 mmol/l) and 9 g/dl (5.59 mmol/l) or the neutrophil count falls to between 0.75×10⁹/l and 1.0×10⁹/l, the daily dosage may be reduced until there is evidence of marrow recovery; alternatively, recovery may be enhanced by brief (2–4 weeks) interruption of Retrovir therapy. Marrow recovery is usually observed within 2 weeks after which time Retrovir therapy at a reduced dosage may be reinstituted. In patients with significant anaemia, dosage adjustments do not necessarily eliminate the need for transfusions (see *Contra-indications*).

Lactic acidosis and severe hepatomegaly with steatosis: Rare occurrences of lactic acidosis, in the absence of hypoxaemia, and severe hepatomegaly with steatosis have been reported and are potentially fatal; it is not known whether these events are causally related to Retrovir, but they have been reported in HIV-positive patients without AIDS. Treatment with Retrovir should be suspended in the setting of rapidly elevating aminotransferase levels, progressive hepatomegaly, or metabolic/lactic acidosis of unknown aetiology (see *Undesirable effects*).

Caution should be exercised when administering Retrovir to any patient, particularly obese women, with hepatomegaly, hepatitis, or other known risk factor for liver disease. These patients should be followed closely while on therapy with Retrovir.

Patients should be cautioned about the concomitant use of self-administered medications (see *Interactions with other medicaments and other forms of interaction*).

Patients should be advised that Retrovir therapy has not been proven to prevent the transmission of HIV to others through sexual contact or blood contamination.

Use in elderly and in patients with renal or hepatic impairment: See *Posology and method of administration.*

Interaction with other medicaments and other forms of interaction: Zidovudine is primarily eliminated by hepatic conjugation to an inactive glucuronidated metabolite. Drugs which are primarily eliminated by hepatic metabolism especially via glucuronidation may have the potential to inhibit metabolism of zidovudine. The interactions listed below should not be considered exhaustive but are representative of the classes of drug where caution should be exercised.

Limited data suggests that co-administration of zidovudine and rifampicin decreases the AUC of zidovudine by 48%±34%. However the clinical significance of this is unknown.

Limited data suggest that probenecid increases the mean half-life and area under the plasma concentration curve of zidovudine by decreasing glucuronidation. Renal excretion of the glucuronide (and possibly zidovudine itself) is reduced in the presence of probenecid.

A modest increase in C_{max} (28%) was observed for zidovudine when administered with lamivudine, however overall exposure (AUC) was not significantly altered. Zidovudine has no effect on the pharmacokinetics of lamivudine.

Phenytoin blood levels have been reported to be low in some patients receiving Retrovir, while in one patient a high level was noted. These observations suggest that phenytoin levels should be carefully monitored in patients receiving both drugs.

In a pharmacokinetic study co-administration of zidovudine and atovaquone showed a decrease in zidovudine oral clearance leading to a 35%±23% increase in plasma zidovudine AUC. Given the limited data available the clinical significance of this is unknown.

Valproic acid or methadone when co-administered with zidovudine have been shown to increase the

AUC and a corresponding decrease in its clearance. As only limited data is available the clinical significance is not known.

Other drugs, including but not limited to, aspirin, codeine, morphine, indomethacin, ketoprofen, naproxen, oxazepam, lorazepam, cimetidine, clofibrate, dapsone and isoprinosine, may alter the metabolism of zidovudine by competitively inhibiting glucuronidation or directly inhibiting hepatic microsomal metabolism. Careful thought should be given to the possibilities of drug interaction before using such drugs, particularly for chronic therapy, in combination with Retrovir.

Retrovir in combination with either ribavarin or stavudine are antagonistic *in vitro*. The concomitant use of either ribavarin or stavudine with Retrovir should be avoided.

Concomitant treatment, especially acute therapy, with potentially nephrotoxic or myelosuppressive drugs (e.g. systemic pentamidine, dapsone, pyrimethamine, co-trimoxazole, amphotericin, flucytosine, ganciclovir, interferon, vincristine, vinblastine and doxorubicin) may also increase the risk of adverse reactions to Retrovir. If concomitant therapy with any of these drugs is necessary then extra care should be taken in monitoring renal function and haematological parameters and, if required, the dosage of one or more agents should be reduced.

Since some patients receiving Retrovir may continue to experience opportunistic infections, concomitant use of prophylactic antimicrobial therapy may have to be considered. Such prophylaxis has included co-trimoxazole, aerosolised pentamidine, pyrimethamine and aciclovir. Limited data from clinical trials do not indicate a signficantly increased risk of adverse reactions to Retrovir with these drugs.

Use during pregnancy and lactation:
Pregnancy: The use of Retrovir in pregnant women over 14 weeks of gestation, with subsequent treatment of their newborn infants, has been shown to significantly reduce the rate of maternal-foetal transmission of HIV based on viral cultures in infants.

The results from the pivotal U.S. placebo-controlled study indicated that Retrovir reduced maternal-foetal transmission by approximately 70%. In this study, pregnant women had CD4+cell counts of 200 to 1818/mm^3 (median in treated group 560/mm^3) and began treatment therapy between weeks 14 and 34 of gestation and had no clinical indications for Retrovir therapy; their newborn infants received Retrovir until 6-weeks old.

A decision to reduce the risk of maternal transmission of HIV should be based on the balance of potential benefits and potential risk. Pregnant women considering the use of Retrovir during pregnancy for prevention of HIV transmission to their infants should be advised that transmission may still occur in some cases despite therapy.

The efficacy of zidovudine to reduce the maternal-foetal transmission in women with previously prolonged treatment with zidovudine or other antiretroviral agents or women infected with HIV strains with reduced sensitivity to zidovudine is unknown.

It is unknown whether there are any long-term consequences of *in utero* and infant exposure to Retrovir. Based on the animal carcinogenicity/mutagenicity findings a carcinogenic risk to humans cannot be excluded (see *Preclinical safety data*). The relevance of these findings to both infected and uninfected infants exposed to Retrovir is unknown. However, pregnant women considering using Retrovir during pregnancy should be made aware of these findings. Given the limited data on the general use of Retrovir in pregnancy, Retrovir should only be used prior to the 14th week of gestation when the potential benefit to the mother outweighs the risk to the foetus. Studies in pregnant rats and rabbits given zidovudine orally at dosage levels up to 450 and 500 mg/kg/day respectively during the major period of organogenesis have revealed no evidence of teratogenicity. There was, however, a statistically significant increase in foetal resorptions in rats given 150 to 450 mg/kg/day and in rabbits given 500 mg/kg/day. A separate study, reported subsequently, found that rats given a dosage of 3000 mg/kg/day, which is very near the oral median lethal dose (3683 mg/kg), caused marked maternal toxicity and an increase in the incidence of foetal malformations. No evidence of teratogenicity was observed in this study at the lower dosages tested (600 mg/kg/day or less).

Fertility: Zidovudine did not impair male or female fertility in rats given oral doses of up to 450 mg/kg/day.

There are no data on the effect of Retrovir on human female fertility. In men, Retrovir has not been shown to affect sperm count, morphology or motility.

Lactation: Some health experts recommend that women infected with HIV do not breast feed their infants in order to avoid the transmission of HIV. After administration of a single dose of 200 mg zidovudine to HIV-infected women, the mean concentration of zidovudine was similar in human milk and serum. Therefore, since the drug and the virus may pass into breast milk, it is recommended that mothers taking Retrovir do not breast feed their infants.

Effects on ability to drive and use machines: There have been no studies to investigate the effect of Retrovir on driving performance or the ability to operate machinery. Furthermore, a detrimental effect on such activities cannot be predicted from the pharmacology of the drug. Nevertheless, the clinical status of the patient and the adverse event profile of Retrovir should be borne in mind when considering the patient's ability to drive or operate machinery.

Undesirable effects: The adverse event profile appears similar for adults and children. The most serious adverse reactions include anaemia (which may require transfusions), neutropenia and leucopenia. These occurred more frequently at higher dosages (1200–1500 mg/day) and in patients with advanced HIV disease (especially when there is poor bone marrow reserve prior to treatment), and particularly in patients with CD4+ cell counts less than 100/mm^3. Dosage reduction or cessation of therapy may become necessary (see *Special warnings and special precautions for use*).

The incidence of neutropenia was also increased in those patients whose neutrophil counts, haemoglobin levels and serum vitamin B_{12} levels were low at the start of Retrovir therapy.

The following events have been reported in patients treated with Retrovir. They may also occur as part of the underlying disease process or in association with other drugs used in the management of HIV disease. The relationship between these events and use of Retrovir is therefore difficult to evaluate, particularly in the medically complicated situations which characterise advanced HIV disease. A reduction in dose or suspension of Retrovir therapy may be warranted in the management of these conditions:

Gastrointestinal tract: Nausea, vomiting, oral mucosa pigmentation, abdominal pain, dyspepsia, anorexia, diarrhoea, flatulence.

Haematological: Anaemia, neutropenia, leucopenia, thrombocytopenia, pancytopenia with marrow hypoplasia.

Liver/pancreas: Liver disorders such as severe hepatomegaly with steatosis, raised blood levels of liver enzymes and bilirubin, pancreatitis.

Metabolic/endocrine: Lactic acidosis in the absence of hypoxaemia.

Musculoskeletal: Myalgia, myopathy.

Neurological/psychiatry: Headache, dizziness, insomnia, paraesthesiae, somnolence, loss of mental acuity, convulsions, anxiety, depression.

Respiratory tract: Dyspnoea, cough.

Skin: Nail and skin pigmentation, rash, urticaria, pruritus, sweating.

Miscellaneous: Urinary frequency, taste perversion, fever, malaise, generalised pain, chills, chest pain, influenza-like syndrome, gynaecomastia, asthenia.

The available data from both placebo-controlled and open-label studies indicate that the incidence of nausea and other frequently reported clinical adverse events consistently decreases over time during the first few weeks of therapy with Retrovir.

Adverse reactions with Retrovir for the prevention of maternal-foetal transmission: In a placebo-controlled trial, overall clinical adverse events and laboratory test abnormalities were similar for women in the Retrovir and placebo groups. However, there was a trend for mild and moderate anaemia to be seen more commonly prior to delivery in the zidovudine treated women.

In the same trial, haemoglobin concentrations in infants exposed to Retrovir for this indication were marginally lower than in infants in the placebo group, but transfusion was not required. Anaemia resolved within 6 weeks after completion of Retrovir therapy. Other clinical adverse events and laboratory test abnormalities were similar in the Retrovir and placebo groups. The long term consequences of *in utero* and infant exposure to Retrovir are unknown.

Overdosage: Symptoms and signs: No specific symptoms or signs have been identified following acute overdose with zidovudine apart from those listed as undesirable effects such as fatigue, headache, vomiting, and occasional reports of haematological disturbances. Following a report where a patient took an unspecified quantity of zidovudine with blood levels consistent with an overdose of greater than 17 g there were no short term clinical, biochemical or haematological sequelae identified.

Treatment: Patients should be observed closely for evidence of toxicity (see *Undesirable effects*) and given the necessary supportive therapy.

Haemodialysis and peritoneal dialysis appear to have a limited effect on elimination of zidovudine but enhance the elimination of the glucuronide metabolite.

Pharmacological properties
Pharmacodynamic properties:
Mode of action: Zidovudine is an antiviral agent which is highly active *in vitro* against retroviruses including the Human Immunodeficiency Virus (HIV).

Zidovudine is phosphorylated in both infected and uninfected cells to the monophosphate (MP) derivative by cellular thymidine kinase. Subsequent phosphorylation of zidovudine-MP to the diphosphate (DP), and then the triphosphate (TP) derivative is catalysed by cellular thymidylate kinase and non-specific kinases respectively. Zidovudine-TP acts as an inhibitor of and substrate for the viral reverse transcriptase. The formation of further proviral DNA is blocked by incorporation of zidovudine-MP into the chain and subsequent chain termination.

Competition by zidovudine-TP for HIV reverse transcriptase is approximately 100-fold greater than for cellular DNA polymerase alpha.

Clinical virology: The relationships between *in vitro* susceptibility of HIV to zidovudine and clinical response to therapy remain under investigation. *In vitro* sensitivity testing has not been standardised and results may therefore vary according to methodological factors.

Reduced *in vitro* sensitivity to zidovudine has been reported for HIV isolates from patients who have received prolonged courses of Retrovir therapy. The available information indicates that for early HIV disease, the frequency and degree of reduction of *in vitro* sensitivity is notably less than for advanced disease.

The reduction of sensitivity with the emergence of zidovudine resistant strains limits the usefulness of zidovudine monotherapy clinically. In clinical studies, clinical end-point data indicate that zidovudine, particularly in combination with lamivudine, and also with didanosine or zalcitabine results in a significant reduction in the risk of disease progression and mortality. The addition of a protease inhibitor to a combination of zidovudine and lamivudine, has been shown to confer additional benefit in delaying disease progression, and improving survival compared to the double combination on its own.

The anti-viral effectiveness *in vitro* of combination of anti-retroviral agents are being investigated. Clinical and *in vitro* studies of zidovudine in combination with lamivudine indicate that zidovudine-resistant virus isolates can become zidovudine sensitive when they simultaneously acquire resistance to lamivudine. Furthermore there is clinical evidence that zidovudine plus lamivudine delays the emergence of zidovudine resistance in anti-retroviral naive patients.

In some *in vitro* studies zidovudine has been shown to act additively or synergistically with a number of anti-HIV agents, such as lamivudine, didanosine, and interferon-alpha, inhibiting the replication of HIV in cell culture. However, studies *in vitro* indicate that triple combinations of nucleoside analogues or two nucleoside analogues and a protease inhibitor are more effective in inhibiting HIV-1 induced cytopathic effects than one or two drug combinations.

Retrovir has been shown to be effective in reducing the rate of maternal-foetal transmission of HIV-1 (23% infection rate for placebo versus 8% for zidovudine) when administered to HIV-positive pregnant women (over 14 weeks of gestation) and their new-born infants.

Pharmacokinetic properties:
A. Pharmacokinetics in adults: Zidovudine is well absorbed from the gut and, at all dose levels studied, the bioavailability was 60–70%. From a Phase I study, mean steady state peak (C^{ss}max) and trough (C^{ss}min) plasma concentrations following oral administration of Retrovir (in solution) at doses of 5 mg/kg every four hours were 7.1 and 0.4 microMolar (μM) (or 1.9 and 0.1 microgram (mcg/ml) respectively. From a bioequivalence study, mean C^{ss}max and C^{ss}min levels following oral administration of Retrovir Capsules every 4 hours and dose normalised to 200 mg were 4.5 μM (or 1.2 mcg/ml) and 0.4 μM (or 0.1 mcg/ml) respectively.

From studies with intravenous Retrovir, the mean terminal plasma half-life was 1.1 hours, the mean total body clearance was 27.1 ml/min/kg and the apparent volume of distribution was 1.6 Litres/kg. Renal clearance of zidovudine greatly exceeds creatinine clearance, indicating that significant tubular secretion takes place.

The 5′-glucuronide of zidovudine is the major metabolite in both plasma and urine, accounting for approximately 50–80% of the administered dose eliminated by renal excretion. 3′-amino-3′-deoxythymidine (AMT) has been identified as a metabolite of zidovudine following intravenous dosing. There are limited data on the pharmacokinetics of zidovudine in patients with renal or hepatic impairment (see *Posology and method of administration*).

No specific data are available on the pharmacokinetics of zidovudine in the elderly.

B. Pharmacokinetics in children: In children over the age of 5–6 months, the pharmacokinetic profile of zidovudine is similar to that in adults.

Zidovudine is well absorbed from the gut and, at all dose levels studied, its bioavailability was 60–74% with a mean of 65%. $C^{ss}max$ levels were 4.45 μM (1.19 mcg/ml) following a dose of 120 mg Retrovir (in solution)/m² body surface area and 7.7 μM (2.06 mcg/ml) at 180 mg/m² body surface area. Dosages of 180 mg/m² four times daily in children produced similar systemic exposure (24 hour AUC 40.0 hr μM or 10.7 hr mcg/ml) as doses of 200 mg six times daily in adults (40.7 hr μM or 10.9 hr mcg/ml).

With intravenous dosing, the mean terminal plasma half-life and total body clearance were 1.5 hours and 30.9 ml/min/kg respectively. The major metabolite is 5'-glucuronide. After intravenous dosing, 29% of the dose was recovered unchanged in the urine and 45% excreted as the glucuronide. Renal clearance of zidovudine greatly exceeds creatinine clearance indicating that significant tubular secretion takes place.

The data available on the pharmacokinetics in neonates and young infants indicate that glucuronidation of zidovudine is reduced with a consequent increase in bioavailability, reduction in clearance and longer half life in infants less than 14 days old but thereafter the pharmacokinetics appear similar to those reported in adults.

Pharmacokinetics in pregnancy: The pharmacokinetics of zidovudine have been investigated in a study of eight women during the third trimester of pregnancy. As pregnancy progressed, there was no evidence of drug accumulation. The pharmacokinetics of zidovudine was similar to that of non-pregnant adults. Consistent with passive transmission of the drug across the placenta, zidovudine concentrations in infant plasma at birth were essentially equal to those in maternal plasma at delivery.

C. Distribution: In adults, the average cerebrospinal fluid/plasma zidovudine concentration ratio 2 to 4 hours after dosing was found to be approximately 0.5. Data indicate that zidovudine crosses the placenta and is found in amniotic fluid and foetal blood. Zidovudine has also been detected in semen and milk. In children the mean cerebrospinal fluid/plasma zidovudine concentration ratio ranged from 0.52–0.85, as determined during oral therapy 0.5 to 4 hours after dosing and was 0.87 as determined during intravenous therapy 1–5 hours after a 1 hour infusion. During continuous intravenous infusion, the mean steady-state cerebrospinal fluid/plasma concentration ratio was 0.24.

Plasma protein binding is relatively low (34 to 38%) and drug interactions involving binding site displacement are not anticipated.

Preclinical safety data:
Mutagenicity: No evidence of mutagenicity was observed in the Ames test. However, zidovudine was weakly mutagenic in a mouse lymphoma cell assay and was positive in an *in vitro* cell transformation assay. Clastogenic effects were observed in an *in vitro* study in human lymphocytes and in *in vivo* oral repeat dose micronucleus studies in rats and mice. An *in vivo* cytogenetic study in rats did not show chromosomal damage. A study of the peripheral blood lymphocytes of eleven AIDS patients showed a higher chromosome breakage frequency in those who had received Retrovir than in those who had not. The clinical significance of these findings is unclear.

Carcinogenicity: In oral carcinogenicity studies with zidovudine in mice and rats, late appearing vaginal epithelial tumours were observed. A subsequent intravaginal carcinogenicity study confirmed the hypothesis that the vaginal tumours were the result of long term local exposure of the rodent vaginal epithelium to high concentrations of unmetabolised zidovudine in urine. There were no other drug-related tumours observed in either sex of either species.

In addition, two transplacental carcinogenicity studies have been conducted in mice. One study, by the US National Cancer Institute, administered zidovudine at maximum tolerated doses to pregnant mice from day 12 to 18 of gestation. One year post-natally, there was an increase in the incidence of tumours in the lung, liver and female reproductive tract of offspring exposed to the highest dose level (420 mg/kg term body weight).

In a second study, mice were administered zidovudine at doses up to 40 mg/kg for 24 months, with exposure beginning prenatally on gestation day 10. Treatment related findings were limited to late-occurring vaginal epithelial tumours, which were seen with a similar incidence and time of onset as in the standard oral carcinogenicity study. The second study thus provided no evidence that zidovudine acts as a transplacental carcinogen.

It is concluded that the transplacental carcinogenicity data from the first study represents a hypothetical risk, whereas the reduction in risk of maternal transfection of HIV to the uninfected child by the use of zidovudine in pregnancy has been well proven.

Pharmaceutical particulars
List of excipients:
Retrovir Capsules: Starches; microcrystalline cellulose; sodium starch glycollate; magnesium stearate.

Retrovir Tablets
Tablet core: Microcrystalline cellulose; Sodium starch glycollate; Povidone K30; Magnesium stearate.
Tablet coating: Hypromellose, Titanium dioxide, Polyethylene glycol 400, Polyethylene glycol 8000.

Retrovir Syrup: Hydrogenated glucose syrup; glycerol; citric acid; sodium benzoate; saccharin sodium; flavour strawberry, flavour white sugar; purified water.

Incompatibilities: None.

Shelf life:

Retrovir Capsules 100 mg and 250 mg:	5 years
Retrovir Tablets 300 mg:	3 years
Retrovir Syrup:	2 years

Special precautions for storage:
Retrovir Capsules 100 mg and 250 mg: Store below 30°C. Keep dry. Protect from light.

Retrovir Tablets 300 mg:
Store below 30°C. Protect from light.

Retrovir Syrup: Store below 30°C.

Nature and contents of container:
Retrovir Capsules 100 mg: Amber glass bottle containing 100 capsules.

Retrovir Capsules 250 mg: PVC/aluminium foil blister pack containing 40 capsules.

Retrovir Tablets 300 mg: PVC/aluminium foil blister packs of 28 and 60 tablets. Amber glass bottle containing 28 tablets.

Retrovir Syrup: 200 ml amber glass bottle with metal roll-on closure and polyethylene wad and with a 10 ml oral-dosing syringe in the pack which should be fitted to the bottle before use and closed with the cap provided.

Instructions for use/handling: No special instructions are required.

Marketing authorisation numbers

Retrovir Capsules 100 mg	PL 0003/0239
Retrovir Capsules 250 mg	PL 0003/0240
Retrovir Tablets 300 mg	PL 0003/0357
Retrovir Syrup	PL 0003/0288

Date of approval/revision of SPC July 1998.

Legal category POM.

SEPTRIN* FOR INFUSION
Strong Sterile Co-trimoxazole Solution To make Co-trimoxazole Intravenous Infusion BP

Qualitative and quantitative composition Sulphamethoxazole EP 400 mg; Trimethoprim EP 80 mg per 5 ml.

Pharmaceutical form Solution for Infusion.

Clinical particulars
Therapeutic indications: Septrin is an antibacterial agent. Septrin is effective *in vitro* against a wide range of Gram-positive and Gram-negative organisms. It is not active against *Mycobacterium tuberculosis, Mycoplasma,* or *Treponema pallidum. Pseudomonas aeruginosa* is usually insensitive.

In general, the indications for the use of Septrin for Infusion are the same as those for oral presentations.

It is intended that Septrin for Infusion should be used only during such a period as the patient is unable to accept oral therapy, where initiation of treatment is particularly urgent or for convenience if the patient is already receiving intravenous fluids. Although intravenous co-trimoxazole is useful in critically ill patients, there may be no therapeutic advantage over the oral preparation.

Septrin for Infusion has been investigated clinically in the following indications amongst others:
Respiratory tract infections: Pneumonia and *Pneumocystis carinii* pneumonitis.
Genito-urinary infections
Gastro-intestinal tract infections: Shigellosis and typhoid fever.
Other bacterial infections caused by sensitive organisms: Brucellosis, septicaemia, intra-abdominal sepsis, meningitis, osteoarticular infections, paediatric soft tissue and skeletal infections.

Posology and method of administration: Septrin for Infusion is for administration only by the intravenous route and must be diluted before administration.

Dilution should be carried out immediately before use. After adding Septrin for Infusion to the infusion solution shake thoroughly to ensure complete mixing. If visible turbidity or crystallisation appears at any time before or during an infusion, the mixture should be discarded.

It is recommended that Septrin for Infusion is diluted according to the following schedules:
One ampoule (5 ml) to 125 ml infusion solution.
Two ampoules (10 ml) to 250 ml infusion solution.
Three ampoules (15 ml) to 500 ml infusion solution.

Septrin for Infusion is known to be compatible, when diluted as recommended above, with the following fluids:

Glucose Intravenous Infusion BP (5% w/v and 10% w/v).
Sodium Chloride Intravenous Infusion BP (0.9% w/v).
Sodium Chloride (0.18% w/v) and Glucose (4% w/v) Intravenous Infusion BP.
Dextran 70 Injection BP (6% w/v) in glucose (5% w/v) or normal saline.
Dextran 40 Injection BP (10% w/v) in glucose (5% w/v) or normal saline.
Ringer's Solution for Injection BPC 1959.

No other substance should be mixed with the infusion.

The duration of the infusion should be approximately one to one and a half hours, but this should be balanced against the fluid requirements of the patient.

When fluid restriction is necessary, Septrin for Infusion may be administered at a higher concentration, 5 ml diluted with 75 ml of glucose 5% w/v in water. The resultant solution, whilst being clear to the naked eye, may on occasion exceed the BP limits set for particulate matter in large volume parenterals. The solution should be infused over a period not exceeding one hour. Discard any unused solution.

Acute infections: Adults and children over 12 years: Standard dosage: 2 ampoules (10 ml) every 12 hours.

Children aged 12 years and under: The recommended dosage is approximately 6 mg trimethoprim and 30 mg sulphamethoxazole per kg bodyweight per 24 hours, given in two equally divided doses. As a guide the following schedules may be used diluted as described above.
6 weeks to 5 months: 1.25 ml every 12 hours.
6 months to 5 years: 2.5 ml every 12 hours.
6 to 12 years: 5.0 ml every 12 hours.

For severe infections in all age groups dosage may be increased by 50%.

Treatment should be continued until the patient has been symptom free for two days; the majority will require treatment for at least 5 days.

Special dosage recommendations:
Impaired renal function: Adults and children over 12 years (no information is available for children under 12 years of age):

Creatinine clearance (ml/min)	*Serum creatinine (μmol/l)*	*Recommended dosage*
Above 25	men <265 women <175	Standard dosage.
15 to 25	men 265 to 620 women 175 to 400	Standard dosage for maximum of 3 days followed by half the standard daily dosage.
Below 15	men >620 women >400	Not recommended unless haemodialysis facilities are available when half the standard daily dosage may be given.

Measurements of plasma concentrations of sulphamethoxazole at intervals of 2 to 3 days are recommended in samples obtained 12 hours after administration of Septrin for Infusion. If the concentration of total sulphamethoxazole exceeds 150 micrograms/ml then treatment should be interrupted until the value falls below 120 micrograms/ml.

Pneumocystis carinii pneumonitis: Treatment: 20 mg trimethoprim and 100 mg sulphamethoxazole per kg bodyweight per day in two or more divided doses. Therapy should be changed to the oral route as soon as possible and continued for a total treatment period of two weeks. The aim is to obtain peak plasma or serum levels of trimethoprim of ≥5 microgram/ml (see *Undesirable effects*).

Prevention: Standard dosage (i.v. or oral as appropriate) for the duration of the period at risk.

Acute brucellosis: It may be advisable to use a higher than standard dosage initially when the intravenous route may be preferred. Treatment should continue for a period of at least four weeks and repeated courses may be beneficial.

Use in the elderly: No specific studies have been

carried out in the elderly, although Septrin has been widely used in older people. See *Precautions* for further information.

Contra-indications: Septrin for Infusion should not be given to patients with a history of hypersensitivity to sulphonamides, trimethoprim or co-trimoxazole.

Septrin for Infusion is contra-indicated in patients showing marked liver parenchymal damage.

Except under careful supervision Septrin for Infusion should not be given to patients with serious haematological disorders. Co-trimoxazole has been given to patients receiving cytotoxic therapy with little or no additional effect on the bone marrow or peripheral blood.

Septrin for Infusion is contra-indicated in severe renal insufficiency where repeated measurements of the plasma concentration cannot be performed.

Septrin for Infusion should not be given to premature babies nor to full-term infants during the first six weeks of life.

Special warnings and precautions for use: Septrin for Infusion should be discontinued if a skin rash appears.

Septrin for Infusion contains sulphite. This may cause allergic-type reactions including anaphylactic symptoms and life-threatening or less severe asthmatic episodes in susceptible individuals.

Fluid overload is possible, especially when very high doses are being administered to patients with underlying cardiopulmonary disease.

An adequate urinary output should be maintained at all times. Evidence of crystalluria *in vivo* is rare, although sulphonamide crystals have been noted in cooled urine from treated patients. In patients suffering from malnutrition the risk may be increased.

For patients with known renal impairment special measures should be adopted (see *Dosage recommendations*).

Regular monthly blood counts are advisable when Septrin is given for long periods since there exists a possibility of asymptomatic changes in haematological laboratory indices due to lack of available folate. These changes may be reversed by administration of folinic acid (5 to 10 mg/day) without interfering with the antibacterial activity.

Particular care is always advisable when treating elderly patients because, as a group, they are more susceptible to adverse reactions and more likely to suffer serious side effects as a result.

Special care should be exercised in treating elderly or suspected folate-deficient patients; folate supplementation should be considered.

A folate supplement should also be considered with prolonged high dosage of Septrin.

In treatment of tonsillo-pharyngitis due to Group A beta-haemolytic streptococci, eradication of these organisms from the oropharynx is less effective than with penicillin.

Trimethoprim has been noted to impair phenylalanine metabolism but this is of no significance in phenylketonuric patients on appropriate dietary restriction.

The administration of Septrin to patients known or suspected to be at risk of acute porphyria should be avoided. Both trimethoprim and sulphonamides (although not specifically sulphamethoxazole) have been associated with clinical exacerbation of porphyria.

Interaction with other medicaments and other forms of interaction: In elderly patients concurrently receiving diuretics, mainly thiazides, there appears to be an increased risk of thrombocytopenia with or without purpura.

Occasional reports suggest that patients receiving pyrimethamine as malarial prophylaxis at doses in excess of 25 mg weekly may develop megaloblastic anaemia should co-trimoxazole be prescribed concurrently.

Co-trimoxazole has been shown to potentiate the anticoagulant activity of warfarin via stereo-selective inhibition of its metabolism. Sulphamethoxazole may displace warfarin from plasma-albumin protein-binding sites *in vitro*. Careful control of the anticoagulant therapy during treatment with Septrin is advisable.

Co-trimoxazole prolongs the half-life of phenytoin and if co-administered the prescriber should be alert for excessive phenytoin effect. Close monitoring of the patient's condition and serum phenytoin levels is advisable.

Interaction with sulphonylurea hypoglycaemic agents is uncommon but potentiation has been reported.

Concurrent use of rifampicin and Septrin results in a shortening of the plasma half life of trimethoprim after a period of about one week. This is not thought to be of clinical significance.

Reversible deterioration in renal function has been observed in patients treated with co-trimoxazole and cyclosporin following renal transplantation.

When trimethoprim is administered simultaneously with drugs that form cations at physiological pH, and are also partly excreted by active renal secretion (e.g. procainamide, amantadine), there is the possibility of competitive inhibition of this process which may lead to an increase in plasma concentration of one or both of the drugs.

Concomitant use of trimethoprim with digoxin has been shown to increase plasma digoxin levels in a proportion of elderly patients.

If Septrin is considered appropriate therapy in patients receiving other anti-folate drugs such as methotrexate, a folate supplement should be considered.

Pregnancy and lactation: The safety of Septrin in human pregnancy has not been established. The drug should not be given during pregnancy. Animal studies have shown teratogenic effects typical of a folate antagonist in rats but not rabbits at high doses; these were prevented by administration of dietary folates. Sulphonamide-containing products should not be administered in late pregnancy because of the risk of kernicterus.

The usual caution in prescribing any drug for women of child-bearing age should be exercised with Septrin.

Despite the excretion of sulphamethoxazole into breast milk, the administration of Septrin to lactating women represents a negligible risk to the suckling infant.

Effects on ability to drive and use machines: None known.

Undesirable effects: As Septrin contains trimethoprim and a sulphonamide, the type and frequency of adverse reactions associated with such compounds may be expected. At the recommended dosages Septrin is usually well tolerated.

Of the reported adverse reactions most are mild and comprise nausea, with or without vomiting, and skin rashes.

More severe skin sensitivity reactions such as erythema multiforme bullosa (Stevens-Johnson syndrome) and toxic epidermal necrolysis (Lyell syndrome) have occurred rarely; the latter condition carries a high mortality.

Haematological changes have been reported, the majority being mild and reversible when treatment was stopped. The changes are mainly leucopenia, neutropenia, thrombocytopenia and, less commonly, agranulocytosis, megaloblastic anaemia and purpura. Although most of the changes cause no clinical symptoms they may become severe in isolated cases, especially in the elderly, in those with hepatic or renal dysfunction or in those with poor folate status; such patients should be observed carefully. Septrin may induce haemolysis in certain susceptible G-6-PD deficient patients but this does not appear to be dose-related.

Hepatic changes including cholestatic jaundice and hepatic necrosis have been reported rarely and may be fatal.

Aseptic meningitis has been reported in association with the administration of co-trimoxazole. The condition was rapidly reversible on withdrawal of the drug, but recurred in a number of cases on re-exposure to either co-trimoxazole or to trimethoprim alone.

At the high dosages used for the therapy of *Pneumocystis carinii* pneumonitis in patients with Acquired Immune Deficiency Syndrome, rash, fever, neutropenia, thrombocytopenia and raised liver enzymes have been reported, necessitating cessation of therapy. Concomitant administration of intravenous diphenhydramine may permit continued infusion.

Impaired renal function has been reported rarely following the administration of co-trimoxazole, but its relationship to therapy remains unproven.

Allergic reactions including serum sickness and mild anaphylaxis have been reported rarely.

Local thrombophlebitis may occasionally be a problem at the site of injection.

Diarrhoea, glossitis and stomatitis are uncommon.

Pseudomembranous colitis has been reported rarely.

Monilial overgrowth is also very rare.

There have been a few reports of subjective experiences such as headache, depression, dizziness and hallucinations but their relationship to therapy remains unproven.

Overdose: The maximum tolerated dose in humans is unknown.

Nausea, vomiting, dizziness and confusion are likely symptoms of overdosage.

In cases of known, suspected or accidental overdosage, stop therapy.

Acidification of the urine will increase the elimination of trimethoprim. Inducing diuresis plus alkalinisation of urine will enhance the elimination of sulphamethoxazole. Alkalinisation will reduce the rate of elimination of trimethoprim. Calcium folinate (5 to 10 mg/day) will reverse any folate deficiency effect of trimethoprim on the bone marrow should this occur. General supportive measures are recommended.

Both trimethoprim and active sulphamethoxazole are dialysable by renal dialysis.

Pharmacological properties

Pharmacodynamic properties: Septrin is an antibacterial agent effective *in vitro* against a wide range of gram-positive and gram-negative organisms. Trimethoprim and sulphamethoxazole have separate, sequential inhibitory effects on dihydrofolate reduction and on folate synthesis in bacteria thereby producing synergistic inhibition of bacterial growth. The combination provides an extension of chemotherapeutic effectiveness to include organisms such as *Proteus bordatella, Haemophilus* and *Neisseris* species which show border line sensitivities to the individual drugs.

Trimethoprim and sulphamethoxazole separately and combined have little pharmacodynamic activity except at high dosage.

Pharmacokinetic properties: Peak plasma levels of trimethoprim and sulphamethoxazole are higher and achieved more rapidly after one hour of intravenous infusion of Septrin for Infusion than after oral administration of an equivalent dose of a Septrin oral presentation. Plasma concentrations, elimination half life and urinary excretion rates show no significant differences following either the oral or intravenous route of administration.

Trimethoprim is a weak base with a pKa of 7.3. It is lipophilic. Tissue levels of trimethoprim are generally higher than corresponding plasma levels, the lungs and kidneys showing especially high concentrations. Trimethoprim concentrations exceed those in plasma in the case of bile, prostatic fluid and tissue, sputum, and vaginal secretions. Levels in the aqueous humour, breast milk, cerebrospinal fluid, middle ear fluid, synovial fluid and tissue (interstitial) fluid are adequate for antibacterial activity. Trimethoprim passes into amniotic fluid and foetal tissues reaching concentrations approximating those at maternal serum.

Approximately 50% of trimethoprim in the plasma is protein bound. The half life in man is in the range 8.6 to 17 hours in the presence of normal renal function. It is increased by a factor of 1.5 to 3.0 when the creatinine clearance is less than 10 ml/minute. There appears to be no significant difference in the elderly compared with young patients.

The principal route of excretion of trimethoprim is renal and approximately 50% of the dose is excreted in the urine within 24 hours as unchanged drug. Several metabolites have been identified in the urine. Urinary concentrations of trimethoprim vary widely.

Sulphamethoxazole is a weak acid with a pKa of 6.0. The concentration of active sulphamethoxazole in amniotic fluid, aqueous humour, bile, cerebrospinal fluid, middle ear fluid, sputum, synovial fluid and tissue (interstitial) fluid is of the order of 20 to 50% of the plasma concentration. Approximately 66% of sulphamethoxazole in the plasma is protein bound. The half life in man is approximately 9 to 11 hours in the presence of normal renal function. There is no change in the half life of active sulphamethoxazole with a reduction in renal function but there is prolongation of the half life of the major, acetylated metabolite when the creatinine clearance is below 25 ml/minute.

The principal route of excretion of sulphamethoxazole is renal; between 15% and 30% of the dose recovered in the urine is in the active form. In elderly patients there is reduced renal clearance of sulphamethoxazole.

Preclinical safety data: No clinically relevant findings were observed in preclinical studies.

Pharmaceutical particulars

List of excipients: Propylene Glycol PhEur; Trometamine USP; Sodium Hydroxide BP; Sodium Metabisulphite BP; Ethanol BP; Water for Injections PhEur.

Incompatibilities: None known.

Shelf life: 36 months.

Special precautions for storage: Store below 30°C. Protect from light.

Nature and contents of container: Neutral glass ampoules (5 ml nominal fill volume). Pack size: 10×5 ml ampoules.

Instructions for use/handling: None.

Marketing authorisation number PL 0003/0095R

Date of first authorisation/renewal of authorisation 11/02/93

Date of (partial) revision of text November 1997

SEPTRIN* ADULT SUSPENSION

Presentation

Septrin Adult Suspension (Co-trimoxazole Mixture BP) contains 80 mg Trimethoprim BP and 400 mg

Sulphamethoxazole BP in each 5 ml. Off-white in colour.

Uses Septrin should only be used where, in the judgement of the physician, the benefits of treatment outweigh any possible risks; consideration should be given to the use of a single effective antibacterial agent.

The *in vitro* susceptibility of bacteria to antibiotics varies geographically and with time; the local situation should always be considered when selecting antibiotic therapy.

Treatment and prevention of *Pneumocystis carinii* pneumonitis (see *Dosage and administration* and *Side- and adverse effects*).

Treatment and prophylaxis of toxoplasmosis, treatment of nocardiosis.

Urinary tract infections: Acute uncomplicated urinary tract infections: Treatment of urinary tract infections where there is bacterial evidence of sensitivity to co-trimoxazole and good reason to prefer this combination to a single antibiotic.

Respiratory tract infections: Otitis media: Acute treatment of otitis media, where there is good reason to prefer co-trimoxazole to a single antibiotic.

Treatment of acute exacerbations of chronic bronchitis, where there is bacterial evidence of sensitivity to co-trimoxazole and good reason to prefer this combination to a single antibiotic.

Dosage and administration It may be preferable to take Septrin with some food or drink to minimise the possibility of gastrointestinal disturbances.

Acute infections: Adults and children over 12 years: Standard dosage Adult Suspension
10 ml every 12 hours.

Treatment should be continued until the patient has been symptom free for two days; the majority will require treatment for at least 5 days. If clinical improvement is not evident after 7 days' therapy, the patient should be reassessed.

As an alternative to *standard dosage* for acute uncomplicated lower urinary tract infections, short-term therapy of 1 to 3 days' duration has been shown to be effective.

Use in the elderly: Particular care is *always* advisable when treating elderly patients because, as a group, they are more susceptible to adverse reactions and more likely to suffer serious effects as a result particularly when complicating conditions exist, e.g. impaired kidney and/or liver function and/or concomitant use of other drugs.

Special dosage recommendations: Unless otherwise specified *standard dosage* applies.

Where dosage is expressed as 'tablets' this refers to the adult tablet, i.e. 80 mg Trimethoprim BP and 400 mg Sulphamethoxazole BP. If other formulations are to be used appropriate adjustment should be made.

Impaired renal function: Adults and children over 12 years: (no information is available for children under 12 years of age).

Creatinine clearance (ml/min)	*Recommended Dosage*
>30	standard dosage
15 to 30	Half the standard dosage
<15	Not recommended

Measurements of plasma concentration of sulphamethoxazole at intervals of 2 to 3 days are recommended in samples obtained 12 hours after administration of Septrin. If the concentration of total sulphamethoxazole exceeds 150 microgram/ml then treatment should be interrupted until the value falls below 120 microgram/ml.

Pneumocystis carinii pneumonitis: Treatment: 20 mg trimethoprim and 100 mg sulphamethoxazole per kg bodyweight per day in two or more divided doses for two weeks. The aim is to obtain peak plasma or serum levels of trimethoprim of ≥5 microgram/ml (verified in patients receiving 1-hour infusions of intravenous Septrin) (see *Side- and adverse effects*).

Prevention: Adults: The following dose schedules may be used:

160 mg trimethoprim/800 mg sulphamethoxazole daily 7 days per week.

160 mg trimethoprim/800 mg sulphamethoxazole three times per week on alternate days.

320 mg trimethoprim/1,600 mg sulphamethoxazole per day in two divided doses three times per week on alternate days.

Children: Standard dosage for the duration of the period at risk – either given 7 days per week or three days per week (on consecutive days).

This dosage approximates to 150 mg trimethoprim/m^2/day and 750 mg sulphamethoxazole/m^2/day to be given in equally divided doses twice a day. The total daily dose should not exceed 320 mg trimethoprim and 1,600 mg sulphamethoxazole.

Nocardiosis: There is no consensus on the most appropriate dosage. Adult doses of 6 to 8 tablets daily for up to 3 months have been used.

Toxoplasmosis: There is no consensus on the most appropriate dosage for the treatment or prophylaxis of this condition. The decision should be based on clinical experience. For prophylaxis, however, the dosages suggested for prevention of PCP may be appropriate.

Contra-indications, warnings, etc

Contra-indications: Septrin should not be given to patients with a history of hypersensitivity to sulphonamides, trimethoprim or co-trimoxazole.

Contra-indicated in patients showing marked liver parenchymal damage.

Contra-indicated in severe renal insufficiency where repeated measurements of the plasma concentration cannot be performed.

Except under careful supervision Septrin should not be given to patients with serious haematological disorders (see *Side- and adverse effects*). Co-trimoxazole has been given to patients receiving cytotoxic therapy with little or no additional effect on the bone marrow or peripheral blood.

Septrin should not be given to premature babies nor to full-term infants during the first 6 weeks of life except for the treatment/prophylaxis of PCP in infants 4 weeks of age or greater.

Precautions: Fatalities, although rare, have occurred due to severe reactions including Stevens-Johnson syndrome, Lyell syndrome (toxic epidermal necrolysis), fulminant hepatic necrosis, agranulocytosis, aplastic anaemia, other blood dyscrasias and hypersensitivity of the respiratory tract.

Septrin should be discontinued at the first appearance of skin rash (see *Side- and adverse effects*).

Particular care is *always* advisable when treating elderly patients because, as a group, they are more susceptible to adverse reactions and more likely to suffer serious effects as a result particularly when complicating conditions exist, e.g. impaired kidney and/or liver function and/or concomitant use of other drugs.

Special care should be exercised in treating elderly or suspected folate-deficient patients; folate supplementation should be considered.

An adequate urinary output should be maintained at all times. Evidence of crystalluria *in vivo* is rare, although sulphonamide crystals have been noted in cooled urine from treated patients. In patients suffering from malnutrition the risk may be increased.

Regular monthly blood counts are advisable when Septrin is given for long periods since there exists a possibility of asymptomatic changes in haematological laboratory indices due to lack of available folate. These changes may be reversed by administration of folinic acid (5 to 10 mg/day) without interfering with the antibacterial activity.

A folate supplement should also be considered with prolonged high dosage of Septrin (see *Drug interactions*).

In glucose-6-phosphate dehydrogenase (G-6-PD) deficient patients haemolysis may occur.

Septrin should be given with caution to patients with severe allergy or bronchial asthma.

Septrin should not be used in the treatment of streptococcal pharyngitis due to Group A beta-haemolytic streptococci; eradication of these organisms from the oropharynx is less effective than with penicillin.

Trimethoprim has been noted to impair phenylalanine metabolism but this is of no significance in phenylketonuric patients on appropriate dietary restriction.

The administration of Septrin to patients known or suspected to be at risk of acute porphyria should be avoided. Both trimethoprim and sulphonamides (although not specifically sulphamethoxazole) have been associated with clinical exacerbation of porphyria.

Use in pregnancy and lactation: The safety of Septrin in human pregnancy has not been established and as trimethoprim and sulphamethoxazole may interfere with folic acid metabolism, co-trimoxazole should not be used during pregnancy unless in the judgement of the clinician the potential benefit to the mother justifies the potential risk to the foetus.

At doses greatly in excess of the recommended human therapeutic dose, trimethoprim has been reported to be teratogenic in rats with effects typical of a folate antagonist and preventable by administration of dietary folate. No significant drug-related malformations have been demonstrated in rabbits but at doses approximately ten times in excess of the human therapeutic dose an increase in foetal deaths was noted.

Trimethoprim and sulphamethoxazole are excreted into breast milk, however, the administration of Septrin to lactating women represents a negligible risk to the suckling infant.

Side- and adverse effects: As Septrin contains trimethoprim and a sulphonamide the type and frequency of adverse reactions associated with such compounds may be expected. At the recommended dosages Septrin is usually well tolerated.

Of the reported adverse reactions most are mild and comprise nausea, with or without vomiting, and skin rashes.

Skin effects: Skin rashes with photosensitivity also reported. More severe skin sensitivity reactions such as exfoliative dermatitis, erythema multiforme, Stevens-Johnson syndrome and Lyell syndrome (toxic epidermal necrolysis) have occurred rarely; the last condition carries a high mortality.

Allergic effects: Other allergic reactions including serum sickness, anaphylaxis, allergic myocarditis, angioedema and drug fever have been reported rarely. Periarteritis nodosa and systemic lupus erythematosus have also been documented.

Effects associated with PCP management: At the high dosages used for the therapy of *Pneumocystis carinii* pneumonitis in patients with acquired immune deficiency syndrome (AIDS), rash, fever, neutropenia, thrombocytopenia, raised liver enzymes, hyperkalaemia and hyponatremia have been reported, necessitating cessation of therapy. If signs of bone marrow depression occur, the patient should be given calcium folinate supplementation (5 to 10 mg/day). Severe hypersensitivity reactions have also been reported in HIV-infected patients on re-exposure to co-trimoxazole, sometimes after a dosage interval of a few days.

Haematological effects: Haematological changes have been reported, the majority being mild and reversible when treatment was stopped. The changes are mainly leucopenia, neutropenia, thrombocytopenia and, less commonly, agranulocytosis, megaloblastic anaemia, aplastic anaemia, haemolytic anaemia and methaemoglobinaemia. Although most of the changes cause no clinical symptoms they may become severe in isolated cases especially in the elderly, in those with hepatic or renal dysfunction or in those with poor folate status. Fatalities have been recorded in at-risk patients and such patients should be observed carefully (see *Contra-indications*). Septrin may induce haemolysis in certain susceptible G-6-PD deficient patients.

Gastro-intestinal effects: Hepatic changes including elevation of serum transaminases and bilirubin levels. Cholestatic jaundice and hepatic necrosis have been reported rarely and may be fatal.

Diarrhoea, glossitis and stomatitis are uncommon. Anorexia has been reported. Pseudomembranous colitis and pancreatitis have been reported rarely.

Neurological effects: Aseptic meningitis has been reported in association with the administration of co-trimoxazole. The condition was rapidly reversible on withdrawal of the drug, but recurred in a number of cases on re-exposure to either co-trimoxazole or to trimethoprim alone.

Convulsions, peripheral neuritis, ataxia, vertigo, and tinnitus have also been reported. There have also been a few reports of subjective experiences such as headache, depression, dizziness and hallucinations.

Genito-urinary effects: Impaired renal function, including cases of interstitial nephritis, has been reported rarely following the administration of co-trimoxazole.

Respiratory effects: Cough, shortness of breath and pulmonary infiltrates have been reported. These may be early indicators of respiratory hypersensitivity which, while rare, has been fatal.

Metabolic effects: Hyperkalaemia and hyponatraemia have been reported occasionally in association with elderly patients or in patients taking high doses.

Musculoskeletal effects: Arthralgia and myalgia have been reported.

Miscellaneous: Monilial overgrowth is very rare.

Drug interactions: In elderly patients concurrently receiving diuretics, mainly thiazides, there appears to be an increased risk of thrombocytopenia.

Occasional reports suggest that patients receiving pyrimethamine at doses in excess of 25 mg weekly may develop megaloblastic anaemia should co-trimoxazole be prescribed concurrently.

Reversible deterioration in renal function has been observed in patients treated with co-trimoxazole and cyclosporin following renal transplantation.

Co-trimoxazole has been shown to potentiate the anticoagulant activity of warfarin via stereo-selective inhibition of its metabolism. Sulphamethoxazole may displace warfarin from plasma-albumin protein-binding sites *in vitro*. Careful control of the anticoagulant therapy during treatment with Septrin is advisable.

Co-trimoxazole prolongs the half-life of phenytoin and if co-administered could result in excessive phenytoin effect. Close monitoring of the patient's condition and serum phenytoin levels are advisable.

Interaction with sulphonylurea hypoglycaemic agents is uncommon but potentiation has been reported.

Concurrent use of rifampicin and Septrin results in a shortening of the plasma half-life of trimethoprim after a period of about one week. This is not thought to be of clinical significance.

When trimethoprim is administered simultaneously with drugs that form cations at physiological pH, and are also partly excreted by active renal secretion (e.g. procainamide, amantadine), there is the possibility of competitive inhibition of this process which may lead to an increase in plasma concentration of one or both of the drugs.

Concomitant use of trimethoprim with digoxin has been shown to increase plasma digoxin levels in a proportion of elderly patients.

If Septrin is considered appropriate therapy in patients receiving other anti-folate drugs such as methotrexate, a folate supplement should be considered (see *Precautions*).

Toxicity and treatment of overdosage: Nausea, vomiting, dizziness and confusion are likely signs/symptoms of overdosage. Bone marrow depression has been reported in acute trimethoprim overdosage.

If vomiting has not occurred, induction of vomiting may be desirable. Gastric lavage may be useful, though absorption from the gastrointestinal tract is normally very rapid and complete within approximately two hours. This may not be the case in gross overdosage. Dependent on the status of renal function administration of fluids is recommended if urine output is low.

Both trimethoprim and active sulphamethoxazole are moderately dialysable by haemodialysis. Peritoneal dialysis is not effective.

Further information *In vitro activity:* Sulphamethoxazole competitively inhibits the utilisation of para-aminobenzoic acid in the synthesis of dihydrofolate by the bacterial cell resulting in bacteriostasis. Trimethoprim reversibly inhibits bacterial dihydrofolate reductase (DHFR), an enzyme active in the folate metabolic pathway converting dihydrofolate to tetrahydrofolate. Depending on the conditions the effect may be bactericidal. Thus, trimethoprim and sulphamethoxazole block two consecutive steps in the biosynthesis of purines and therefore nucleic acids essential to many bacteria. This action produces marked potentiation of activity *in vitro* between the two agents.

Trimethoprim binds to plasmodial DHFR but less tightly than to the bacterial enzyme. Its affinity for mammalian DHFR is some 50,000 times less than for the corresponding bacterial enzyme.

Many of common pathogenic bacteria are sensitive *in vitro* to trimethoprim and sulphamethoxazole at concentrations well below those reached in blood, tissue fluids and urine after the administration of recommended doses. In common with other antibiotics, however, *in vitro* activity does not necessarily imply that clinical efficacy has been demonstrated and it must be noted that satisfactory sensitivity testing is achieved only with recommended media, free from inhibitory substances especially thymidine and thymine.

Pharmacokinetics: After oral administration, trimethoprim and sulphamethoxazole are rapidly and nearly completely absorbed. The presence of food does not appear to delay absorption. Peak levels in the blood occur between one and four hours after ingestion and the level attained is dose related. Effective levels persist in the blood for up to 24 hours after a therapeutic dose.

Trimethoprim is a weak base with a pKa of 7.4. It is lipophilic. Tissue levels of trimethoprim are generally higher than corresponding plasma levels, the lungs and kidneys showing especially high concentrations.

Approximately 50% of trimethoprim in the plasma is protein bound and the principal route of excretion of trimethoprim is renal. The half life in man is in the range 8.6 to 17 hours in the presence of normal renal function. It is increased by a factor of 1.5 to 3.0 when the creatinine clearance is less than 10 ml/minute. There appears to be no significant difference in the elderly compared with young patients.

Sulphamethoxazole is a weak acid with a pKa of 6.0. The concentration of active sulphamethoxazole in a variety of body fluids is of the order of 20 to 50% of the plasma concentration.

Approximately 66% of sulphamethoxazole in the plasma is protein bound and the principal route of excretion of sulphamethoxazole is renal. The half-life in man is approximately 9 to 11 hours in the presence of normal renal function. There is no change in the half-life of active sulphamethoxazole with a reduction in renal function but there is prolongation of the half life of the major, acetylated metabolite when the creatinine clearance is below 25 ml/minute.

In elderly patients there is a reduced renal clearance of sulphamethoxazole.

Pharmaceutical precautions
Store below 25°C. Protect from light.

Legal category POM.

Package quantities
Septrin Adult Suspension: Bottle of 100 ml.

Further information Trimethoprim interferes with assays for serum methotrexate when dihydrofolate reductase from *Lactobacillus casei* is used in the assay. No interference occurs if methotrexate is measured by radioimmune assay.

Trimethoprim may interfere with the estimation of serum/plasma creatinine when the alkaline picrate reaction is used. This may result in overestimation of serum/plasma creatinine of the order of 10%. Functional inhibition of the renal tubular secretion of creatinine may produce a spurious fall in the estimated rate of creatinine clearance.

Product licence number
Adult Suspension: 0003/5223R

SEPTRIN* FORTE TABLETS
SEPTRIN* TABLETS
SEPTRIN* PAEDIATRIC SUSPENSION

Qualitative and quantitative composition
Septrin Forte Tablets: Sulphamethoxazole 800 mg PhEur. Trimethoprim 160 mg PhEur.

Septrin Tablets: Sulphamethoxazole 400 mg PhEur. Trimethoprim 80 mg PhEur.

Septrin Paediatric Suspension: Sulphamethoxazole 200 mg PhEur. Trimethoprim 40 mg PhEur.

Pharmaceutical form Tablet/Suspension.

Clinical particulars
Therapeutic indications: Septrin should only be used where, in the judgement of the physician, the benefits of treatment outweigh any possible risks; consideration should be given to the use of a single effective antibacterial agent.

The *in vitro* susceptibility of bacteria to antibiotics varies geographically and with time; the local situation should always be considered when selecting antibiotic therapy.

Treatment and prevention of *Pneumocystis carinii* pneumonitis (see *Dosage and administration* and *Side- and adverse effects*).

Treatment and prophylaxis of toxoplasmosis, treatment of nocardiosis.

Urinary tract infections: Acute uncomplicated urinary tract infections: Treatment of urinary tract infections where there is bacterial evidence of sensitivity to co-trimoxazole and good reason to prefer this combination to a single antibiotic.

Respiratory tract infections: Otitis media: Acute treatment of otitis media, where there is good reason to prefer co-trimoxazole to a single antibiotic.

Treatment of acute exacerbations of chronic bronchitis, where there is bacterial evidence of sensitivity to co-trimoxazole and good reason to prefer this combination to a single antibiotic.

Posology and method of administration: Method of administration: Oral.

It may be preferable to take Septrin with some food or drink to minimise the possibility of gastrointestinal disturbances.

Acute infections: Adults and children over 12 years:
STANDARD DOSAGE
Forte Tablets: 1 every 12 hours.
Tablets: 2 every 12 hours.

Children aged 12 years and under:
STANDARD DOSAGE (Paediatric Suspension).

Age	
6–12 years	10 ml every 12 hours
6 months to 5 years	5 ml every 12 hours
6 weeks to 5 months	2.5 ml every 12 hours

This dosage approximates to 6 mg trimethoprim and 30 mg sulphamethoxazole per kilogram body weight per 24 hours.

Treatment should be continued until the patient has been symptom free for two days; the majority will require treatment for at least 5 days. If clinical improvement is not evident after 7 days' therapy, the patient should be reassessed.

As an alternative to STANDARD DOSAGE for acute uncomplicated lower urinary tract infections, short-term therapy of 1 to 3 days' duration has been shown to be effective.

Use in the elderly: Particular care is *always* advisable when treating elderly patients because, as a group, they are more susceptible to adverse reactions and more likely to suffer serious effects as a result particularly when complicating conditions exist, e.g. impaired kidney and/or liver function and/or concomitant use of other drugs.

Special dosage recommendations: Unless otherwise specified *standard dosage* applies.

Where dosage is expressed as 'tablets' this refers to the adult tablet, i.e. 80 mg Trimethoprim BP and 400 mg Sulphamethoxazole BP. If other formulations are to be used appropriate adjustment should be made.

Impaired renal function: Adults and children over 12 years: (no information is available for children under 12 years of age).

Creatinine clearance (ml/min)	*Recommended Dosage*
>30	STANDARD DOSAGE
15 to 30	Half the STANDARD DOSAGE
<15	Not recommended

Measurements of plasma concentration of sulphamethoxazole at intervals of 2 to 3 days are recommended in samples obtained 12 hours after administration of Septrin. If the concentration of total sulphamethoxazole exceeds 150 microgram/ml then treatment should be interrupted until the value falls below 120 microgram/ml.

Pneumocystis carinii pneumonitis: Treatment: 20 mg trimethoprim and 100 mg sulphamethoxazole per kg bodyweight per day in two or more divided doses for two weeks. The aim is to obtain peak plasma or serum levels of trimethoprim of ≥5 microgram/ml (verified in patients receiving 1-hour infusions of intravenous Septrin) (see *Side- and adverse effects*).

Prevention: Adults: The following dose schedules may be used:

160 mg trimethoprim/800 mg sulphamethoxazole daily 7 days per week.

160 mg trimethoprim/800 mg sulphamethoxazole three times per week on alternative days.

320 mg trimethoprim/1600 mg sulphamethoxazole per day in two divided doses three times per week on alternative days.

Children: Standard dosage for the duration of the period at risk – either given 7 days per week or three days per week (on consecutive days).

This dosage approximates to 150 mg trimethoprim/m²/day and 750 mg sulphamethoxazole/m²/day to be given in equally divided doses twice a day. The total daily dose should not exceed 320 mg trimethoprim and 1600 mg sulphamethoxazole.

Nocardiosis: There is no consensus on the most appropriate dosage. Adult doses of 6 to 8 tablets daily for up to 3 months have been used.

Toxoplasmosis: There is no consensus on the most appropriate dosage for the treatment or prophylaxis of this condition. The decision should be based on clinical experience. For prophylaxis, however, the dosages suggested for prevention of PCP may be appropriate.

Contra-indications: Septrin should not be given to patients with a history of hypersensitivity to sulphonamides, trimethoprim or co-trimoxazole.

Contra-indicated in patients showing marked liver parenchymal damage.

Contra-indicated in severe renal insufficiency where repeated measurements of the plasma concentration cannot be performed.

Except under careful supervision Septrin should not be given to patients with serious haematological disorders (see *Side- and adverse effects*). Co-trimoxazole has been given to patients receiving cytotoxic therapy with little or no additional effect on the bone marrow or peripheral blood.

Septrin should not be given to premature babies nor to full-term infants during the first 6 weeks of life except for the treatment/prophylaxis of PCP in infants 4 weeks of age or greater.

Special warnings and precautions for use:
Precautions: Fatalities, although rare, have occurred due to severe reactions including Stevens-Johnson Syndrome, Lyell Syndrome (toxic epidermal necrolysis), fulminant hepatic necrosis, agranulocytosis, aplastic anaemia, other blood dyscrasias and hypersensitivity of the respiratory tract.

Septrin should be discontinued at the first appearance of skin rash (see *Side- and adverse effects*).

Particular care is *always* advisable when treating elderly patients because, as a group, they are more susceptible to adverse reactions and more likely to suffer serious effects as a result particularly when complicating conditions exist, e.g. impaired kidney and/or liver function and/or concomitant use of other drugs.

Special care should be exercised in treating elderly or suspected folate-deficient patients; folate supplementation should be considered.

An adequate urinary output should be maintained at all times. Evidence of crystalluria *in vivo* is rare, although sulphonamide crystals have been noted in cooled urine from treated patients. In patients suffering from malnutrition the risk may be increased.

Regular monthly blood counts are advisable when Septrin is given for long periods since there exists a possibility of asymptomatic changes in haematological laboratory indices due to lack of available folate. These changes may be reversed by administration of folinic acid (5 to 10 mg/day) without interfering with the antibacterial activity.

A folate supplement should also be considered with prolonged high dosage of Septrin (see *Drug interactions*).

In glucose-6-phosphate dehydrogenase (G-6-PD) deficient patients haemolysis may occur.

Septrin should be given with caution to patients with severe allergy or bronchial asthma.

Septrin should not be used in the treatment of streptococcal pharyngitis due to Group A beta-haemolytic streptococci; eradication of these organisms from the oropharynx is less effective than with penicillin.

Trimethoprim has been noted to impair phenylalanine metabolism but this is of no significance in phenylketonuric patients on appropriate dietary restriction.

The administration of Septrin to patients known or suspected to be at risk of acute porphyria should be avoided. Both trimethoprim and sulphonamides (although not specifically sulphamethoxazole) have been associated with clinical exacerbation of porphyria.

Interaction with other medicaments and other forms of interaction:

Drug interactions: In elderly patients concurrently receiving diuretics, mainly thiazides, there appears to be an increased risk of thrombocytopenia with or without purpura.

Occasional reports suggest that patients receiving pyrimethamine at doses in excess of 25 mg weekly may develop megaloblastic anaemia should co-trimoxazole be prescribed concurrently.

Reversible deterioration in renal function has been observed in patients treated with co-trimoxazole and cyclosporin following renal transplantation.

Co-trimoxazole has been shown to potentiate the anticoagulant activity of warfarin via stereo-selective inhibition of its metabolism. Sulphamethoxazole may displace warfarin from plasma-albumin protein-binding sites *in vitro*. Careful control of the anticoagulant therapy during treatment with Septrin is advisable.

Co-trimoxazole prolongs the half life of phenytoin and if co-administered could result in excessive phenytoin effect. Close monitoring of the patient's condition and serum phenytoin levels are advisable.

Interaction with sulphonylurea hypoglycaemic agents is uncommon but potentiation has been reported.

Concurrent use of rifampicin and Septrin results in a shortening of the plasma half life of trimethoprim after a period of about one week. This is not thought to be of clinical significance.

When trimethoprim is administered simultaneously with drugs that form cations at physiological pH, and are also partly excreted by active renal secretion (e.g. procainamide, amantadine), there is the possibility of competitive inhibition of this process which may lead to an increase in plasma concentration of one or both of the drugs.

Concomitant use of trimethoprim with digoxin has been shown to increase plasma digoxin levels in a proportion of elderly patients.

If Septrin is considered appropriate therapy in patients receiving other anti-folate drugs such as methotrexate, a folate supplement should be considered (see *Precautions*).

Pregnancy and lactation:

Use in pregnancy and lactation: The safety of Septrin in human pregnancy has not been established and as trimethoprim and sulphamethoxazole may interfere with folic acid metabolism, co-trimoxazole should not be used during pregnancy unless in the judgement of the clinician the potential benefit to the mother justifies the potential risk to the foetus.

At doses greatly in excess of the recommended human therapeutic dose, trimethoprim has been reported to be teratogenic in rats with effects typical of a folate antagonist and preventable by administration of dietary folate. No significant drug-related malformations have been demonstrated in rabbits but at doses approximately ten times in excess of the human therapeutic dose an increase in foetal deaths was noted.

Trimethoprim and sulphamethoxazole are excreted into breast milk, however, the administration of Septrin to lactating women represents a negligible risk to the suckling infant.

Effects on ability to drive and use machines: There have been no studies to investigate the effect of Septrin on driving performance or the ability to operate machinery. Further a detrimental effect on such activities cannot be predicted from the pharmacology of the drug. Nevertheless the clinical status of the patient and the adverse events profile of Septrin should be borne in mind when considering the patient's ability to operate machinery.

Undesirable effects:

Side- and adverse effects: As Septrin contains trimethoprim and a sulphonamide the type and frequency of adverse reactions associated with such compounds may be expected. At the recommended dosages Septrin is usually well tolerated.

Of the reported adverse reactions most are mild and comprise nausea, with or without vomiting, and skin rashes.

Skin effects: Skin rashes with photosensitivity also reported. More severe skin sensitivity reactions such as exfoliative dermatitis, erythema multiforme, Stevens-Johnson syndrome and Lyell syndrome (toxic epidermal necrolysis) have occurred rarely; the last condition carries a high mortality.

Allergic effects: Other allergic reactions including serum sickness, anaphylaxis, allergic myocarditis, angioedema and drug fever have been reported rarely. Periarteritis nodosa and systemic lupus erythematosus have also been documented.

Effects associated with PCP management: At the high dosages used for the therapy of *Pneumocystis carinii* pneumonitis in patients with acquired immune deficiency syndrome (AIDS), rash, fever, neutropenia, thrombocytopenia, raised liver enzymes, hyperkalaemia and hyponatremia have been reported, necessitating cessation of therapy. If signs of bone marrow depression occur, the patient should be given calcium folinate supplementation (5 to 10 mg/day). Severe hypersensitivity reactions have also been reported in HIV-infected patients on re-exposure to co-trimoxazole, sometimes after a dosage interval of a few days.

Haematological effects: Haematological changes have been reported, the majority being mild and reversible when treatment was stopped. The changes are mainly leucopenia, neutropenia, thrombocytopenia and, less commonly, agranulocytosis, megaloblastic anaemia, aplastic anaemia, haemolytic anaemia and methaemoglobinaemia. Although most of the changes cause no clinical symptoms they may become severe in isolated cases especially in the elderly, in those with hepatic or renal dysfunction or in those with poor folate status. Fatalities have been recorded in at-risk patients and such patients should be observed carefully (see *Contra-indications*). Septrin may induce haemolysis in certain susceptible G-6-PD deficient patients.

Gastro-intestinal effects: Hepatic changes including elevation of serum transaminases and bilirubin levels. Cholestatic jaundice and hepatic necrosis have been reported rarely and may be fatal.

Diarrhoea, glossitis and stomatitis are uncommon. Anorexia has been reported. Pseudomembranous colitis and pancreatitis have been reported rarely.

Neurological effects: Aseptic meningitis has been reported in association with the administration of co-trimoxazole. The condition was rapidly reversible on withdrawal of the drug, but recurred in a number of cases on re-exposure to either co-trimoxazole or to trimethoprim alone.

Convulsions, peripheral neuritis, ataxia, vertigo and tinnitus have also been reported. There have also been a few reports of subjective experiences such as headache, depression, dizziness and hallucinations.

Genito-urinary effects: Impaired renal function, including cases of interstitial nephritis, has been reported rarely following the administration of co-trimoxazole.

Respiratory effects: Cough, shortness of breath and pulmonary infiltrates have been reported. These may be early indicators of respiratory hypersensitivity which, while rare, has been fatal.

Metabolic effects: Hyperkalaemia and hyponatraemia have been reported occasionally in association with elderly patients or in patients taking high doses.

Musculoskeletal effects: Arthralgia and myalgia have been reported.

Miscellaneous: Monilial overgrowth is very rare.

Overdose:

Toxicity and treatment of overdosage: Nausea, vomiting, dizziness and confusion are likely signs/symptoms of overdosage. Bone marrow depression has been reported in acute trimethoprim overdosage.

If vomiting has not occurred, induction of vomiting may be desirable. Gastric lavage may be useful, though absorption from the gastrointestinal tract is normally very rapid and complete within approximately two hours. This may not be the case in gross overdosage. Dependent on the status of renal function administration of fluids is recommended if urine output is low.

Both trimethoprim and active sulphamethoxazole are moderately dialysable by haemodialysis. Peritoneal dialysis is not effective.

Pharmacological properties

Pharmacodynamic properties: In vitro activity: Sulphamethoxazole competitively inhibits the utilisation of para-aminobenzoic acid in the synthesis of dihydrofolate by the bacterial cell resulting in bacteriostasis. Trimethoprim reversibly inhibits bacterial dihydrofolate reductase (DHFR), an enzyme active in the folate metabolic pathway converting dihydrofolate to tetrahydrofolate. Depending on the conditions the effect may be bactericidal. Thus, trimethoprim and sulphamethoxazole block two consecutive steps in the biosynthesis of purines and therefore nucleic acids essential to many bacteria. This action produces marked potentiation of activity *in vitro* between the two agents.

Trimethoprim binds to plasmodial DHFR but less tightly than to the bacterial enzyme. Its affinity for mammalian DHFR is some 50,000 times less than for the corresponding bacterial enzyme.

Many of common pathogenic bacteria are sensitive *in vitro* to trimethoprim and sulphamethoxazole at concentrations well below those reached in blood, tissue fluids and urine after the administration of recommended doses. In common with other antibiotics, however, *in vitro* activity does not necessarily imply that clinical efficacy has been demonstrated and it must be noted that satisfactory sensitivity testing is achieved only with recommended media, free from inhibitory substances especially thymidine and thymine.

Pharmacokinetic properties: Pharmacokinetics: After oral administration, trimethoprim and sulphamethoxazole are rapidly and nearly completely absorbed. The presence of food does not appear to delay absorption. Peak levels in the blood occur between one and four hours after ingestion and the level attained is dose related. Effective levels persist in the blood for up to 24 hours after a therapeutic dose.

Trimethoprim is a weak base with a pKa of 7.4. It is lipophilic. Tissue levels of trimethoprim are generally higher than corresponding plasma levels, the lungs and kidneys showing especially high concentrations.

Approximately 50% of trimethoprim in the plasma is protein bound and the principal route of excretion of trimethoprim is renal. The half life in man is in the range 8.6 to 17 hours in the presence of normal renal function. It is increased by a factor of 1.5 to 3.0 when the creatinine clearance is less than 10 ml/minute. There appears to be no significant difference in the elderly compared with young patients.

Sulphamethoxazole is a weak acid with a pKa of 6.0. The concentration of active sulphamethoxazole in a variety of body fluids is of the order of 20 to 50% of the plasma concentration.

Approximately 66% of sulphamethoxazole in the plasma is protein bound and the principal route of excretion of sulphamethoxazole is renal. The half life in man is approximately 9 to 11 hours in the presence of normal renal function. There is no change in the half life of active sulphamethoxazole with a reduction in renal function but there is prolongation of the half life of the major, acetylated metabolite when the creatinine clearance is below 25 ml/minute.

In elderly patients there is a reduced renal clearance of sulphamethoxazole.

Preclinical safety data: There are no preclinical data of relevance to the prescriber which are additional to that in other sections of the SPC.

Pharmaceutical particulars

List of excipients:

Forte Tablets: Povidone PhEur; Sodium Starch Glycollate BP; Magnesium Stearate PhEur; Docusate Sodium BP.

Tablets: Sodium starch glycollate; Povidone; *Dioctyl sodium sulphosuccinate; *Docusate sodium; Magnesium stearate.

* alternative ingredients.

Paediatric Suspension: Sorbitol solution 70% (non-crystallising) PhEur, Glycerol PhEur, Dispensible cellulose BP, Sodium carmellose BP, Polysorbate 80 PhEur, Methyl hydroxybenzoate PhEur, Sodium benzoate PhEur, Saccharin sodium BP, Ethanol (96%) BP, Flavour, Banana 81.605P HSE, Flavour, Vanilla 407 HSE, Purified Water to 5 ml PhEur.

Incompatibilities: None known.

Shelf life: 60 months (Tablets). 36 months (Paediatric Suspension).

Special precautions for storage: Store below 25°C. Protect from light.

Nature and contents of container:

Forte Tablets: Polypropylene container with polyethylene snap-fit closure. Pack size: 100.

Tablets: Amber glass bottles with low density polyethylene snap-fit closures. Pack size: 100.

Paediatric Suspension: Amber glass bottles with metal roll-on closures. Pack size: 100 ml.

Instructions for use/handling: Trimethoprim interferes with assays for serum methotrexate when dihydrofolate reductase from *Lactobacillus casei* is used in the assay. No interference occurs if methotrexate is measured by radioimmune assay.

Trimethoprim may interfere with the estimation of serum/plasma creatinine when the alkaline picrate reaction is used. This may result in overestimation of serum/plasma creatinine of the order of 10%. Functional inhibition of the renal tubular secretion of creatinine may produce a spurious fall in the estimated rate of creatinine clearance.

Marketing authorisation number

Forte Tablets:	0003/0121R
Tablets:	0003/0109R
Paediatric Suspension:	0003/5222R

Date of first authorisation/renewal of authorisation
Forte Tablets:
Date of first authorisation: 14th April 1997
Renewed: 16th July 1998

Tablets:
Date of first authorisation: 30th October 1986
Date of last renewal: 27th January 1997

Paediatric Suspension:
Date of first authorisation: 1st January 1972
Renewed: 30th March 1998

Date of (partial) revision of text July 1998

TRACRIUM* INJECTION

Presentation Tracrium Injection is a clear, faintly yellow, sterile aqueous solution in a glass ampoule containing 10 mg atracurium besylate per ml. Each 2.5 ml ampoule contains 25 mg atracurium besylate, each 5 ml ampoule contains 50 mg atracurium besylate and each 25 ml ampoule contains 250 mg atracurium besylate.

Uses Tracrium is a highly selective, competitive or non-depolarising neuromuscular blocking agent. It is used as an adjunct to general anaesthesia or sedation in the intensive care unit (ICU), to relax skeletal muscles, and to facilitate tracheal intubation and mechanical ventilation.

Dosage and administration
Use by injection in adults: Tracrium is administered by intravenous injection.

The dosage range recommended for adults is 0.3 to 0.6 mg/kg (depending on the duration of full block required) and will provide adequate relaxation for about 15 to 35 minutes.

Endotracheal intubation can usually be accomplished within 90 seconds from the intravenous injection of 0.5 to 0.6 mg/kg.

Full block can be prolonged with supplementary doses of 0.1 to 0.2 mg/kg as required. Successive supplementary dosing does not give rise to accumulation of neuromuscular blocking effect.

Spontaneous recovery from the end of full block occurs in about 35 minutes as measured by the restoration of the tetanic response to 95% of normal neuromuscular function.

The neuromuscular block produced by Tracrium can be rapidly reversed by standard doses of anticholinesterase agents, such as neostigmine and edrophonium, accompanied or preceded by atropine, with no evidence of recurarisation.

Use as an infusion in adults: After an initial bolus dose of 0.2 to 0.6 mg/kg, Tracrium can be used to maintain neuromuscular block during long surgical procedures by administration as a continuous infusion at rates of 0.3 to 0.6 mg/kg/hour.

Tracrium can be administered by infusion during cardiopulmonary bypass surgery at the recommended infusion rates. Induced hypothermia to a body temperature of 25° to 26°C reduces the rate of inactivation of atracurium, therefore full neuromuscular block may be maintained by approximately half the original infusion rate at these low temperatures.

Tracrium is compatible with the following infusion solutions for the times stated below:

Infusion solution	*Period of stability*
Sodium Chloride Intravenous Infusion BP (0.9% w/v)	24 hours
Glucose Intravenous Infusion BP (5% w/v)	8 hours
Ringer's Injection USP	8 hours
Sodium Chloride (0.18% w/v) and Glucose (4% w/v) Intravenous Infusion BP	8 hours
Compound Sodium Lactate Intravenous Infusion BP (Hartmann's Solution for Injection)	4 hours.

When diluted in these solutions to give atracurium besylate concentrations of 0.5 mg/ml and above, the resultant solutions will be stable in daylight for the stated periods at temperatures of up to 30°C.

Use in children: The dosage in children over the age of one month is similar to that in adults on a bodyweight basis.

Use in neonates: There are insufficient data to recommend a dose for use in neonates. However, this patient group is known to have increased sensitivity to non-depolarising muscle relaxants.

Use in the elderly: Tracrium may be used at standard dosage in elderly patients. It is recommended, however, that the initial dose be at the lower end of the range and that it be administered slowly.

Use in patients with reduced renal and/or hepatic function: Tracrium may be used at standard dosage at all levels of renal or hepatic function, including end stage failure.

Use in patients with cardiovascular disease: In patients with clinically significant cardiovascular disease, the initial dose of Tracrium should be administered over a period of 60 seconds.

Use in intensive care unit (ICU) patients: After an optional initial bolus dose of Tracrium of 0.3 to 0.6 mg/kg, Tracrium can be used to maintain neuromuscular block by administering a continous infusion at rates of between 11 and 13 microgram/kg/min (0.65 to 0.78 mg/kg/hr). There may be wide inter-patient variability in dosage requirements and these may increase or decrease with time. Infusion rates as low as 4.5 microgram/kg/min (0.27 mg/kg/hr) or as high as 29.5 microgram/kg/min (1.77 mg/kg/hr) are required in some patients.

The rate of spontaneous recovery from neuromuscular block after infusion of Tracrium in ICU patients is independent of the duration of administration. Spontaneous recovery to a train-of-four ratio >0.75 (the ratio of the height of the fourth to the first twitch in a train-of-four) can be expected to occur in approximately 60 minutes. A range of 32 to 108 minutes has been observed in clinical trials.

Monitoring: In common with all neuromuscular blocking agents, monitoring of neuromuscular function is recommended during the use of Tracrium in order to individualise dosage requirements.

Contra-indications, warnings, etc
Contra-indications: Tracrium should not be administered to patients known to have an allergic hypersensitivity to the drug.

Precautions: In common with all the other neuromuscular blocking agents, Tracrium paralyses the respiratory muscles as well as other skeletal muscles but has no effect on consciousness. Tracrium should be administered only with adequate general anaesthesia and only by or under the close supervision of an experienced anaesthetist with adequate facilities for endotracheal intubation and artificial ventilation.

In common with other neuromuscular blocking agents, the potential for histamine release exists in susceptible patients during Tracrium administration. Caution should be exercised in administering Tracrium to patients with a history suggestive of an increased sensitivity to the effects of histamine.

Monitoring of serial creatinine phosphate (cpk) values should be considered in asthmatic patients receiving high dose corticosteroids and neuromuscular blocking agents in ICU.

Tracrium does not have significant vagal or ganglionic blocking properties in the recommended dosage range. Consequently, Tracrium has no clinically significant effects on heart rate in the recommended dosage range and it will not counteract the bradycardia produced by many anaesthetic agents or by vagal stimulation during surgery.

In common with other non-depolarising neuromuscular blocking agents, increased sensitivity to atracurium may be expected in patients with myasthenia gravis and other forms of neuromuscular disease.

As with other neuromuscular blocking agents severe acid-base and/or serum electrolyte abnormalities may increase or decrease the sensitivity of patients to atracurium.

As with other non-depolarising neuromuscular blockers hypophosphataemia may prolong recovery. Recovery may be hastened by correcting this condition.

Tracrium should be administered over a period of 60 seconds to patients who may be unusually sensitive to falls in arterial blood pressure, for example those who are hypovolaemic.

Tracrium is inactivated by high pH and so must not be mixed in the same syringe with thiopentone or any alkaline agent.

When a small vein is selected as the injection site, Tracrium should be flushed through the vein with physiological saline after injection. When other anaesthetic drugs are administered through the same indwelling needle or cannula as Tracrium it is important that each drug is flushed through with an adequate volume of physiological saline. Atracurium besylate is hypotonic and must not be administered into the infusion line of a blood transfusion.

Studies in malignant hyperthermia in susceptible animals (swine), and clinical studies in patients susceptible to malignant hyperthermia indicate that Tracrium does not trigger this syndrome.

In common with other non-depolarising neuromuscular blocking agents, resistance may develop in patients suffering from burns. Such patients may require increased doses, dependent on the time elapsed since the burn injury and the extent of the burn.

Intensive Care Unit (ICU) patients: When administered to laboratory animals in high doses, laudanosine, a metabolite of atracurium has been associated with transient hypotension and, in some species, cerebral excitatory effects. Although seizures have been seen in ICU patients receiving atracurium, a causal relationship to laudanosine has not been established (see *Side- and adverse effects*).

Carcinogenicity: Carcinogenicity studies have not been performed.

Teratogenicity: Animal studies have indicated that Tracrium has no significant effects on foetal development.

Fertility: Fertility studies have not been performed.

Drug interactions: The neuromuscular block produced by Tracrium may be increased by the concomitant use of inhalational anaesthetics such as halothane, isoflurane and enflurane.

In common with all non-depolarising neuromuscular blocking agents the magnitude and/or duration of a non-depolarising neuromuscular block may be increased as a result of interaction with: antibiotics, including the aminoglycosides, polymyxins, spectinomycin, tetracyclines, lincomycin and clindamycin; antiarrhythmic drugs, propranolol, calcium channel blockers, lignocaine, procainamide and quinidine; diuretics: frusemide and possibly mannitol, thiazide diuretics and acetazolamide; magnesium sulphate, ketamine, lithium salts, ganglion blocking agents, trimetaphan, hexamethonium.

Rarely, certain drugs may aggravate or unmask latent myasthenia gravis or actually induce a myasthenic syndrome; increased sensitivity to Tracrium would be consequent on such a development. Such drugs include various antibiotics, β-blockers (propranolol, oxprenolol), antiarrhythmic drugs (procainamide, quinidine), anti-rheumatic drugs (chloroquine, D-penicillamine), trimetaphan, chlorpromazine, steroids, phenytoin and lithium.

The onset of non-depolarising neuromuscular block is likely to be lengthened and the duration of block shortened in patients receiving chronic anticonvulsant therapy.

The administration of combinations of non-depolarising neuromuscular blocking agents in conjunction with Tracrium may produce a degree of neuromuscular blockage in excess of that which might be expected were an equipotent total dose of Tracrium administered. Any synergistic effect may vary between different drug combinations.

A depolarising muscle relaxant such as suxamethonium chloride should not be administered to prolong the neuromuscular blocking effects of non-depolarising blocking agents such as atracurium, as this may result in a prolonged and complex block which can be difficult to reverse with anticholinesterase drugs.

Side- and adverse effects: Associated with the use of Tracrium there have been reports of skin flushing, and mild transient hypotension or bronchospasm, which have been attributed to histamine release. Very rarely, severe anaphylactoid reactions have been reported in patients receiving Tracrium in conjunction with one or more anaesthetic agents.

There have been rare reports of seizures in ICU patients who have been receiving atracurium concurrently with several other agents. These patients usually had one or more medical conditions predisposing to seizures (e.g. cranial trauma, cerebral oedema, viral encephalitis, hypoxic encephalopathy, uraemia). A causal relationship to laudanosine has not been established. In clinical trials, there appears to be no correlation between plasma laudanosine concentration and the occurrence of seizures.

There have been some reports of muscle weakness and/or myopathy following prolonged use of muscle relaxants in severely ill patients in the ICU. Most patients were receiving concomitant corticosteroids. These events have been seen infrequently in association with Tracrium. A causal relationship has not been established.

Use in pregnancy and lactation: In common with all neuromuscular blocking agents, Tracrium should be used during pregnancy only if the potential benefit to the mother outweighs any potential risk to the foetus.

Tracrium is suitable for maintenance of muscle relaxation during Caesarean section as it does not cross the placenta in clinically significant amounts following recommended doses.

It is not known whether Tracrium is excreted in human milk.

Toxicity and treatment of overdosage: Signs: Prolonged muscle paralysis and its consequences are the main signs of overdosage.

Treatment: It is essential to maintain a patent airway together with assisted positive pressure ventilation until spontaneous respiration is adequate. Full sedation will be required since consciousness is not impaired. Recovery may be hastened by the administration of anticholinesterase agents accompanied by atropine or glycopyrrolate, once evidence of spontaneous recovery is present.

Pharmaceutical precautions Store at 2°to 8°C. Protect from light. Do not freeze. Any unused Tracrium from opened ampoules should be discarded.

Short periods at temperatures up to 30°C are permissible but ONLY to allow transportation or temporary storage outside of a cold store. It is estimated that an 8% loss of potency would occur if Tracrium Injection was stored at 30°C for one month.

Legal category POM.

Package quantities Box of 5×2.5 ampoules (each ampoule containing 25 mg atracurium besylate).

Box of 5×5 ml ampoules (each ampoule containing 50 mg atracurium besylate).

Box of 2×25 ml ampoules (each ampoule containing 250 mg atracurium besylate).

Further information Tracrium is inactivated by Hofmann elimination, a non-enzymatic process which occurs at physiological pH and temperature, and by ester hydrolysis catalysed by non-specific esterases.

The termination of the neuromuscular blocking action of Tracrium is not dependent on its hepatic or renal metabolism or excretion. Its duration of action, therefore, is unlikely to be affected by impaired renal, hepatic or circulatory function.

Tests with plasma from patients with low levels of pseudochlolinesterase show that the inactivation of Tracrium proceeds unaffected.

Tracrium has no direct effect on intra-ocular pressure, and is therefore suitable for use in ophthalmic surgery.

Variations in the blood pH and body temperature of the patient within the physiological range will not significantly alter the duration of action of Tracrium.

Haemofiltration and haemodiafiltration have a minimal effect on plasma levels of atracurium and its metabolites, including laudanosine. The effects of haemodialysis and haemoperfusion on plasma levels of atracurium and its metabolites are unknown.

Product licence number 0003/0166.

TRIMOVATE* CREAM

Qualitative and quantitative composition Trimovate Cream is a yellow water-miscible cream containing clobetasone butyrate 0.05% w/w, oxytetracycline 3.0% w/w as calcium oxytetracycline and nystatin 100,000 units per gram.

Pharmaceutical form Cream for topical administration.

Clinical particulars

Therapeutic indications: Clobetasone butyrate is a topically active corticosteroid which provides an exceptional combination of activity and safety. Topical formulations have been shown to be more effective in the treatment of eczemas than 1% hydrocortisone, yet to have little effect on hypothalamic-pituitary-adrenal function.

The combination of the topically active antibiotics, nystatin and oxytetracycline, provides a broad spectrum of antibacterial and anticandidal activity against many of the organisms associated with infected dermatoses. Trimovate is indicated for the treatment and management of steroid responsive dermatoses where candidal or bacterial infection is present, suspected or likely to occur and the use of a more potent topical corticosteroid is not required. These include infected eczemas, intertrigo, napkin rash, anogenital pruritus and seborrhoeic dermatitis.

Posology and method of administration: Apply to the affected area up to four times a day.

Suitable for treating infants, children and adults.

Contra-indications: Primary cutaneous infections caused by viruses (e.g. herpes simplex, chickenpox) fungi and bacteria. Secondary infections due to dermatophytes, Pseudomonas or Proteus species.

Hypersensitivity to the preparation.

Special warnings and special precautions for use: Although generally regarded as safe, even for long term administration in adults, there is a potential for overdosage, and in children this may result in adrenal suppression. Extreme caution is required in dermatoses in such patients and treatment should not normally exceed seven days. In infants, the napkin may act as an occlusive dressing, and increase absorption.

If infection persists, systemic chemotherapy is likely to be required. Any spread of infection requires withdrawal of topical corticosteroid therapy. Bacterial infection is encouraged by the warm, moist conditions induced by occlusive dressings, and the skin should be cleansed before a fresh dressing is applied. Do not continue for more than seven days in the absence of clinical improvement, since occult extension of infection may occur due to the masking effect of the steroid.

As with all corticosteroids, prolonged application to the face is undesirable. If applied to the eyelids, care is needed to ensure that the preparation does not enter the eye, as glaucoma might result.

Trimovate may cause slight staining of hair, skin or fabric, but this can be removed by washing. The application may be covered with a non-occlusive dressing to protect clothing.

Extended or recurrent application may increase the risk of contact sensitisation.

Products which contain antimicrobial agents should not be diluted.

Interaction with other medicaments and other forms of interaction: None reported.

Pregnancy and lactation: There is inadequate evidence of safety in human pregnancy. Topical administration of corticosteroids to pregnant animals can cause abnormalities of foetal development including cleft palate and intra-uterine growth retardation. There may therefore be a very small risk of such effects in the human foetus.

Effects on ability to drive and use machines: None stated.

Undesirable effects: In the unlikely event of signs of hypersensitivity appearing, application should be stopped immediately.

If large areas of the body were to be treated with Trimovate, it is possible that some patients would absorb sufficient steroid to cause transient adrenal suppression despite the low degree of systemic activity associated with clobetasone butyrate.

Local atrophic changes could possibly occur in situations where moisture increases absorption of clobetasone butyrate, but only after prolonged use.

There are reports of pigmentation changes and hypertrichosis with topical steroids. Exacerbation of symptoms may occur with extensive use.

Overdose: Acute overdosage is very unlikely to occur, however, in the case of chronic overdosage or misuse the features of hypercorticism may appear and in this situation topical steroids should be discontinued.

Pharmacological properties

Pharmacodynamic properties: Clobetasone butyrate is a topically active corticosteroid.

Clobetasone butyrate is less potent than other available corticosteroid preparations and has been shown not to suppress the hypothalamic-pituitary-adrenal axis in patients treated for psoriasis or eczema. Pharmacological studies in man and animals have shown that clobetasone butyrate has a relatively high level of topical activity accompanied by a low level of systemic activity.

The use of nystatin in the local treatment of candidal infections of the skin and of the tetracyclines in localised bacterial infections is well known. Nystatin is included in Trimovate at the standard concentration recommended by the British Pharmaceutical codex for the topical preparation nystatin ointment (100,000 units/g), and oxytetracycline calcium is included at a concentration to give approximately the same level of activity as recommended for Oxytetracycline Ointment BPC (3.0% w/w).

The principal action of the preparation is based on the anti-inflammatory activity of the corticosteroid. The broad spectrum antibacterial and anti-candidal activity provided by the combination of oxytetracycline and nystatin allow this effect to be utilised in the treatment of conditions which are or are likely to become infected.

Pharmacokinetic properties: Trimovate has been shown to have a satisfactory pharmacokinetic profile by many years of successful clinical experience.

Preclinical safety data: No additional data of relevance.

Pharmaceutical particulars

List of excipients: Titanium dioxide, glyceryl monostearate, cetostearyl alcohol, white soft paraffin, polyoxyl 40 stearate, dimethicone 20, glycerol, chlorocresol, sodium metabisulphite, sodium acid phosphate, disodium hydrogen phosphate anhydrous, purified water.

Incompatibilities: None reported.

Shelf-life: 18 months.

Special precautions for storage: Store below 25°C.

Nature and contents of container: Collapsible latex-banded aluminium tube, internally coated with epoxy resin-based lacquer with polypropylene cap.

Instructions for use/handling: None stated.

Marketing authorisation number PL 10949/0040

Date of approval/revision of SPC March 1996

Legal category POM.

ULTIVA* FOR INJECTION ▼

Qualitative and quantitative composition Ultiva is a sterile, endotoxin-free, preservative-free, white to off white, lyophilised powder, to be reconstituted before use.

When reconstituted as directed, solutions of Ultiva are clear and colourless and contain 1 mg/ml of remifentanil base as remifentanil hydrochloride.

Ultiva for injection is available as glass vials containing 1 mg, 2 mg or 5 mg of remifentanil base.

Pharmaceutical form Lyophilised powder for reconstitution for intravenous administration.

Clinical particulars

Therapeutic indications: Ultiva is indicated as an analgesic agent for use during induction and/or maintenance of general anaesthesia under close supervision.

Posology and method of administration: Ultiva should be administered only in a setting fully equipped for the monitoring and support of respiratory and cardiovascular function, and by persons specifically trained in the use of anaesthetic drugs and the recognition and management of the expected adverse effects of potent opioids, including respiratory and cardiac resuscitation. Such training must include the establishment and maintenance of a patent airway and assisted ventilation.

Ultiva is for intravenous use only and must not be administered by epidural or intrathecal injection (see *Contra-indications*).

Ultiva is stable for 24 hours at room temperature after reconstitution and further dilution to concentrations of 20 to 250 mcg/ml with one of the following i.v. fluids listed below: 50 mcg/ml is the recommended dilution for general anaesthesia.

Sterilised Water for Injections
5% Dextrose Injection
5% Dextrose and 0.9% Sodium Chloride Injection
0.9% Sodium Chloride Injection
0.45% Sodium Chloride Injection

(See *Instructions for use/handling* for additional information, including tables to help titrate Ultiva to the patient's anaesthetic needs.)

The administration of Ultiva must be individualised based on the patient's response.

The table below summarises the starting infusion rates and dose range.

At the doses recommended below, remifentanil significantly reduces the amount of hypnotic agent required to maintain anaesthesia. Therefore, isoflurane and propofol should be administered as recommended above to avoid excessive depth of anaesthesia (see *Concomitant medication*).

Induction of anaesthesia: Ultiva should be administered with a hypnotic agent, such as propofol, thiopental, or isoflurane, for the induction of anaesthesia. Administering Ultiva after a hypnotic agent will reduce the incidence of muscle rigidity. Ultiva can be administered at an infusion rate of 0.5 to 1 mcg/kg/min, with or without an initial bolus infusion of 1 mcg/kg given over not less than 30 seconds. If endotracheal intubation is to occur more than 8 to 10 minutes after the start of the infusion of Ultiva, then a bolus infusion is not necessary.

Maintenance of anaesthesia: After endotracheal intubation, the infusion rate of Ultiva should be decreased, according to anaesthetic technique, as indicated in the table below. Due to the fast onset and short duration of action of Ultiva, the rate of administration during anaesthesia can be titrated upward in 25% to 100% increments or downward in 25% to 50% decrements, every 2 to 5 minutes to attain the desired level of μ-opioid response. In response to light anaesthesia, supplemental bolus infusions may be administered every 2 to 5 minutes.

Guidelines for discontinuation: Due to the very rapid offset of action of Ultiva no residual opioid activity will be present within 5 to 10 minutes after discontinuation. For those patients undergoing surgical procedures where post-operative pain is anticipated, analgesics should be administered prior to discontinuation of Ultiva. Sufficient time must be allowed to reach the maximum effect of the longer acting analgesic. The choice of analgesic should be appropriate for the patient's surgical procedure and the level of post-operative care.

Care should be taken to avoid inadvertent administration of Ultiva remaining in i.v. lines and cannulae (see *Special warnings and precautions for use*).

Concomitant medication: Ultiva decreases the amounts or doses of inhaled anaesthetics, hypnotics and benzodiazepines required for anaesthesia (see *Special warnings and precautions for use* and *Interaction with other medicaments and other forms of interaction*).

Doses of the following agents used in anaesthesia: isoflurane, thiopentone, propofol and temazepam have been reduced by up to 75% when used concurrently with remifentanil.

Dosing guidelines for Ultiva-based anaesthesia

Indication	*Bolus infusion (mcg/kg)*	*Continuous infusion (mcg/kg/min)*	
		Starting rate	*Range*
Induction of anaesthesia	1 (give over not less than 30 seconds)†	0.5 to 1	—
Maintenance of anaesthesia in ventilated patients			
• Nitrous oxide (66%)	0.5 to 1	0.4	0.1 to 2
• Isoflurane (starting dose 0.5 MAC)	0.5 to 1	0.25	0.05 to 2
• Propofol (starting dose 100 mcg/kg/min)	0.5 to 1	0.25	0.05 to 2

† When given by bolus infusion at induction Ultiva should be administered over not less than 30 seconds.

Spontaneous ventilation anaesthesia: In spontaneous ventilation anaesthesia respiratory depression is likely to occur. Special care is needed to adjust the dose to the patient and ventilatory support may be required. The recommended starting dose is 0.04 mcg/kg/min with titration to effect. A range of infusion rates from 0.025 to 0.1 mcg/kg/min has been studied. Bolus doses are not recommended.

Children (2–12 years of age): There are no data available on use in children under 2 years of age.

The pharmacokinetics of remifentanil in children 2 to 12 years of age are similar to those seen in adults after correction for body weight differences.

Clinical experience in a limited number of children 2 to 12 years of age has shown that doses required are similar to those recommended for adults on a weight-related basis. In the studies performed, remifentanil was only given after the children had been induced with an inhalation agent, intubated and had received an anti-cholinergic drug.

Elderly (over 65 years of age): Caution should be exercised in the administration of Ultiva in this population. The initial starting dose of Ultiva administered to patients over 65 should be half the recommended adult dose and then titrated to individual patient need as an increased sensitivity to the pharmacodynamic effects of remifentanil has been seen in this patient population.

ASA III/IV patients: As the haemodynamic effects of potent opioids can be expected to be more pronounced in ASA III/IV patients, caution should be exercised in the administration of Ultiva in this population. Initial dosage reduction and subsequent titration to effect is therefore recommended.

Obese patients: It is recommended that for obese patients the dosage of Ultiva should be reduced and based upon ideal bodyweight as the clearance and volume of distribution of remifentanil are better correlated with ideal bodyweight than actual bodyweight.

Renal impairment: No dosage adjustment, relative to that used in healthy adults, is necessary as the pharmacokinetic profile of remifentanil is unchanged in this patient population.

Hepatic impairment: No adjustment of the initial dose, relative to that used in healthy adults, is necessary as the pharmacokinetic profile of remifentanil is unchanged in this patient population. However, patients with severe hepatic impairment may be slightly more sensitive to the respiratory depressant effects of remifentanil. These patients should be closely monitored and the dose of Ultiva titrated to individual patient need.

Long-term use in the Intensive Care Unit (ICU): No data are available on the long-term (longer than 24 hours) use of Ultiva in ICU patients.

Contra-indications: As glycine is present in the formulation Ultiva is contra-indicated for epidural and intrathecal use.

Ultiva is contra-indicated in patients with known hypersensitivity to any component of the preparation and other fentanyl analogues.

Ultiva is contra-indicated for use as the sole agent for induction of anaesthesia.

Special warnings and precautions for use: Ultiva should be administered only in a setting fully equipped for the monitoring and support of respiratory and cardiovascular function, and by persons specifically trained in the use of anaesthetic drugs and the recognition and management of the expected adverse effects of potent opioids, including respiratory and cardiac resuscitation. Such training must include the establishment and maintenance of a patent airway and assisted ventilation.

Inadvertent administration: A sufficient amount of Ultiva may be present in the dead space of the i.v. line and/or cannula to cause respiratory depression, apnoea and/or muscle rigidity if the line is flushed with i.v. fluids or other drugs. This may be avoided by administering Ultiva into a fast flowing i.v. line or via a dedicated i.v. line which is removed when Ultiva is discontinued.

Muscle rigidity – prevention and management: At the doses recommended muscle rigidity may occur. As with other opioids, the incidence of muscle rigidity is related to the dose and rate of administration. Therefore, bolus infusions should be administered over not less than 30 seconds.

Muscle rigidity induced by remifentanil must be treated in the context of the patient's clinical condition with appropriate supporting measures including ventilatory support. Excessive muscle rigidity occurring during the induction of anaesthesia should be treated by the administration of a neuromuscular blocking agent and/or additional hypnotic agents. Muscle rigidity seen during the use of remifentanil as an analgesic may be treated by stopping or decreasing the rate of administration of remifentanil. Resolution of muscle rigidity after discontinuing the infusion of remifentanil occurs within minutes.

Respiratory depression – management: As with all potent opioids, profound analgesia is accompanied by marked respiratory depression. Therefore, remifentanil should only be used in areas where facilities for monitoring and dealing with respiratory depression are available. The appearance of respiratory depression should be managed appropriately, including decreasing the rate of infusion by 50%, or a temporary discontinuation of the infusion. Unlike other fentanyl analogues, remifentanil has not been shown to cause recurrent respiratory depression even after prolonged administration. However, as many factors may affect post-operative recovery it is important to ensure that full consciousness and adequate spontaneous ventilation are achieved before the patient is discharged from the recovery area.

Cardiovascular effects: Hypotension and bradycardia may be managed by reducing the rate of infusion of Ultiva or the dose of concurrent anaesthetics or by using i.v. fluids, vasopressor or anticholinergic agents as appropriate.

Debilitated, hypovolaemic, and elderly patients may be more sensitive to the cardiovascular effects of remifentanil.

Rapid offset of action: Due to the very rapid offset of action of Ultiva, no residual opioid activity will be present within 5–10 minutes after the discontinuation of Ultiva. For those patients undergoing surgical procedures where post-operative pain is anticipated, analgesics should be administered prior to discontinuation of Ultiva. Sufficient time must be allowed to reach the maximum effect of the longer acting analgesic. The choice of analgesic should be appropriate for the patient's surgical procedure and the level of post-operative care.

Drug abuse: As with other opioids remifentanil may produce dependency.

Interaction with other medicaments and other forms of interaction: Remifentanil is not metabolised by plasmacholinesterase, therefore, interactions with drugs metabolised by this enzyme are not anticipated.

As with other opioids remifentanil decreases the amounts or doses of inhaled and i.v. anaesthetics, and benzodiazepines required for anaesthesia (see *Posology and method of administration*).

Pregnancy and lactation: There are no adequate and well-controlled studies in pregnant women. Ultiva should be used during pregnancy only if the potential benefit justifies the potential risk to the foetus.

It is not known whether remifentanil is excreted in human milk. However, because fentanyl analogues are excreted in human milk and remifentanil-related material was found in rat milk after dosing with remifentanil, caution should be exercised when remifentanil is administered to a nursing mother.

For a summary of the reproductive toxicity study findings please refer to Preclinical safety data.

Labour and delivery: The safety profile of remifentanil during labour or delivery has not been demonstrated.

Effects on the ability to drive and use machines: If an early discharge is envisaged, following treatment using anaesthetic agents, patients should be advised not to drive or operate machinery.

Undesirable effects: The most common adverse events associated with remifentanil are direct extensions of µ-opioid agonist pharmacology. These are acute respiratory depression, bradycardia, hypotension and/or skeletal muscle rigidity. These adverse events resolve within minutes of discontinuing or decreasing the rate of remifentanil administration.

Post-operative shivering, nausea and vomiting have also been reported.

Overdose: As with all potent opioid analgesics, overdose would be manifested by an extension of the pharmacologically predictable actions of remifentanil. Due to the very short duration of action of Ultiva, the potential for deleterious effects due to overdose are limited to the immediate time period following drug administration. Response to discontinuation of the drug is rapid, with return to baseline within ten minutes.

In the event of overdose, or suspected overdose, take the following actions: discontinue administration of Ultiva; maintain a patent airway; initiate assisted or controlled ventilation with oxygen; maintain adequate cardiovascular function. If depressed respiration is associated with muscle rigidity, a neuromuscular blocking agent may be required to facilitate assisted or controlled respiration. Intravenous fluids and vasopressor for the treatment of hypotension and other supportive measures may be employed.

Intravenous administration of an opioid antagonist such as naloxone may be given as a specific antidote in addition to ventilatory support to manage severe respiratory depression. The duration of respiratory depression following overdose with Ultiva is unlikely to exceed the duration of action of the opioid antagonist.

Pharmacological properties

Pharmacodynamic properties: Remifentanil is a selective µ-opioid agonist with a rapid onset and very short duration of action. The µ-opioid activity, of remifentanil, is antagonised by narcotic antagonists, such as naloxone.

Assays of histamine in patients and normal volunteers have shown no elevation in histamine levels after administration of remifentanil in bolus doses up to 30 mcg/kg.

Pharmacokinetic properties: Following administration of the recommended doses of remifentanil, the effective biological half-life is 3–10 minutes. The average clearance of remifentanil in young healthy adults is 40 ml/min/kg, the central volume of distribution is 100 ml/kg and the steady-state volume of distribution is 350 ml/kg. Blood concentrations of remifentanil are proportional to the dose administered throughout the recommended dose range. For every 0.1 mcg/kg/min increase in infusion rate, the blood concentration of remifentanil will rise 2.5 ng/ml. Remifentanil is approximately 70% bound to plasma proteins.

Metabolism: Remifentanil is an esterase metabolised opioid that is susceptible to metabolism by non-specific blood and tissue esterases. The metabolism of remifentanil results in the formation of an essentially inactive carboxylic acid metabolite (1/4600th as potent as remifentanil). The half-life of the metabolite in healthy adults is 2 hours. Approximately 95% of remifentanil is recovered in the urine as the carboxylic acid metabolite. Remifentanil is not a substrate for plasma cholinesterase.

Renal impairment: The pharmacokinetics of remifentanil are not changed in patients with severe renal impairment (creatinine clearance<10 ml/minute). In anephric patients, the half-life of the carboxylic acid metabolite increases to approximately 30 hours. However, in light of the estimated potency ratio of the metabolite compared with the parent molecule (1:4,600), pharmacokinetic simulations indicate that the carboxylic acid metabolite will not accumulate to clinically active concentrations after remifentanil infusions of up to 2 mcg/kg/min for up to 12 hours.

Hepatic impairment: The pharmacokinetics of remifentanil are not changed in patients with severe hepatic impairment awaiting liver transplant, or during the anhepatic phase of liver transplant surgery. Patients with severe hepatic impairment may be slightly more sensitive to the respiratory depressant effects of remifentanil. These patients should be closely monitored and the dose of remifentanil should be titrated to the individual patient need.

Children: The pharmacokinetics of remifentanil in children 2–12 years of age are similar to those seen in adults after correcting for differences in body weight.

Elderly: The clearance of remifentanil is slightly reduced (approximately 25%) in elderly patients (>65 years) compared to young patients. The pharmacodynamic activity of remifentanil increases with increasing age. Elderly patients have a remifentanil EC50 for formation of delta waves on the electroencephalogram (EEG) that is 50% lower than young patients; therefore, the initial dose of remifentanil should be reduced by 50% in elderly patients and then carefully titrated to meet the individual patient need.

Table 1: Ultiva for Injection Infusion Rates (ml/kg/h)

Drug Delivery Rate (mcg/kg/min)	Infusion Delivery Rate (ml/kg/h) for Solution Concentrations of		
	25 mcg/ml 1 mg/40 ml	50 mcg/ml 1 mg/20 ml	250 mcg/ml 10 mg/40 ml
0.0125	0.03	0.015	not recommended
0.025	0.06	0.03	not recommended
0.05	0.12	0.06	0.012
0.075	0.18	0.09	0.018
0.1	0.24	0.12	0.024
0.15	0.36	0.18	0.036
0.2	0.48	0.24	0.048
0.25	0.6	0.3	0.06
0.5	1.2	0.6	0.12
0.75	1.8	0.9	0.18
1.0	2.4	1.2	0.24
1.25	3.0	1.5	0.3
1.5	3.6	1.8	0.36
1.75	4.2	2.1	0.42
2.0	4.8	2.4	0.48

Table 2: Ultiva for Injection Infusion Rates (ml/h) for a 25 mcg/ml Solution

Infusion Rate (mcg/kg/min)	Patient Weight (kg)							
	30	40	50	60	70	80	90	100
0.0125	0.9	1.2	1.5	1.8	2.1	2.4	2.7	3.0
0.025	1.8	2.4	3.0	3.6	4.2	4.8	5.4	6.0
0.05	3.6	4.8	6.0	7.2	8.4	9.6	10.8	12.0
0.075	5.4	7.2	9.0	10.8	12.6	14.4	16.2	18.0
0.1	7.2	9.6	12.0	14.4	16.8	19.2	21.6	24.0
0.15	10.8	14.4	18.0	21.6	25.2	28.8	32.4	36.0
0.2	14.4	19.2	24.0	28.8	33.6	38.4	43.2	48.0

Table 3: Ultiva for Injection Infusion Rates (ml/h) for a 50 mcg/ml Solution

Infusion Rate (mcg/kg/min)	Patient Weight (kg)							
	30	40	50	60	70	80	90	100
0.025	0.9	1.2	1.5	1.8	2.1	2.4	2.7	3.0
0.05	1.8	2.4	3.0	3.6	4.2	4.8	5.4	6.0
0.075	2.7	3.6	4.5	5.4	6.3	7.2	8.1	9.0
0.1	3.6	4.8	6.0	7.2	8.4	9.6	10.8	12.0
0.15	5.4	7.2	9.0	10.8	12.6	14.4	16.2	18.0
0.2	7.2	9.6	12.0	14.4	16.8	19.2	21.6	24.0
0.25	9.0	12.0	15.0	18.0	21.0	24.0	27.0	30.0
0.5	18.0	24.0	30.0	36.0	42.0	48.0	54.0	60.0
0.75	27.0	36.0	45.0	54.0	63.0	72.0	81.0	90.0
1.0	36.0	48.0	60.0	72.0	84.0	96.0	108.0	120.0
1.25	45.0	60.0	75.0	90.0	105.0	120.0	135.0	150.0
1.5	54.0	72.0	90.0	108.0	126.0	144.0	162.0	180.0
1.75	63.0	84.0	105.0	126.0	147.0	168.0	189.0	210.0
2.0	72.0	96.0	120.0	144.0	168.0	192.0	216.0	240.0

Table 4: Ultiva for Injection Infusion Rates (ml/h) for a 250 mcg/ml Solution

Infusion Rate (mcg/kg/min)	Patient Weight (kg)							
	30	40	50	60	70	80	90	100
0.1	0.72	0.96	1.20	1.44	1.68	1.92	2.16	2.40
0.15	1.08	1.44	1.80	2.16	2.52	2.88	3.24	3.60
0.2	1.44	1.92	2.40	2.88	3.36	3.84	4.32	4.80
0.25	1.80	2.40	3.00	3.60	4.20	4.80	5.40	6.00
0.5	3.60	4.80	6.00	7.20	8.40	9.60	10.80	12.00
0.75	5.40	7.20	9.00	10.80	12.60	14.40	16.20	18.00
1.0	7.20	9.60	12.00	14.40	16.80	19.20	21.60	24.00
1.25	9.00	12.00	15.00	18.00	21.00	24.00	27.00	30.00
1.5	10.80	14.40	18.00	21.60	25.20	28.80	32.40	36.00
1.75	12.60	16.80	21.00	25.20	29.40	33.60	37.80	42.00
2.0	14.40	19.20	24.00	28.80	33.60	38.40	43.20	48.00

Preclinical safety data: Intrathecal administration of the glycine formulation without remifentanil to dogs caused agitation, pain and hind limb dysfunction and inco-ordination. These effects are believed to be secondary to the glycine excipient. Glycine is a commonly used excipient in intravenous products and this finding has no relevance for intravenous administration of Ultiva.

Reproductive toxicity studies: Remifentanil has been shown to reduce fertility in male rats when administered daily by intravenous injection for at least 70 days at a dose of 0.5 mg/kg, or approximately 250 times the maximum recommended human bolus dose of 2 mcg/kg. The fertility of female rats was not affected at doses up to 1 mg/kg when administered for at least 15 days prior to mating. No teratogenic effects have been observed with remifentanil at doses up to 5 mg/kg in rats and 0.8 mg/kg in rabbits. Administration of remifentanil to rats throughout late gestation and lactation at doses up to 5 mg/kg i.v. had no significant effect on the survival, development, or reproductive performance of the F_1 generation.

Genotoxicity: Remifentanil was devoid of genotoxic activity in bacteria and in rat liver or mouse bone marrow cells *in vivo*. However, a positive response was seen *in vitro* in different mammalian cell systems in the presence of a metabolic activation system. This activity was seen only at concentrations more than three orders of magnitude higher than therapeutic blood levels.

Pharmaceutical particulars

List of excipients: Glycine PhEur; Hydrochloric acid PhEur.

Incompatibilities: Ultiva should only be admixed with those infusion solutions recommended (see *Instructions for use/handling*).

It should not be admixed with Lactated Ringer's Injection or Lactated Ringer's and 5% Dextrose Injection.

Ultiva should not be mixed with propofol in the same intravenous admixture solution.

Administration of Ultiva into the same intravenous line with blood/serum/plasma is not recommended. Non-specific esterase in blood products may lead to the hydrolysis of remifentanil to its inactive metabolite.

Ultiva should not be mixed with other therapeutic agents prior to administration.

Shelf life: 2 years for 1 mg/vial.
3 years for 2 mg/vial, 5 mg/vial.

Special precautions for storage: Store at or below 25°C.

The reconstituted solution of Ultiva is chemically and physically stable for 24 hours at room temperature. However, Ultiva does not contain an antimicrobial preservative and thus care must be taken to assure the sterility of prepared solutions. Reconstituted product should be used promptly, and any unused material discarded.

Nature and contents of container: Ultiva Injection for intravenous use is available as:

1 mg Remifentanil lyophilised powder in 3 ml vials in cartons of 5.

2 mg Remifentanil lyophilised powder in 5 ml vials in cartons of 5.

5 mg Remifentanil lyophilised powder in 10 ml vials in cartons of 5.

Instructions for use/handling: Ultiva is stable for 24 hours at room temperature after reconstitution and further dilution to concentrations of 20 to 250 mcg/ml with one of the following i.v. fluids listed below: 50 mcg/ml is the recommended dilution for general anaesthesia.

Sterilised Water for Injections
5% Dextrose Injection
5% Dextrose and 0.9% Sodium Chloride Injection
0.9% Sodium Chloride Injection
0.45% Sodium Chloride Injection

Ultiva has been shown to be compatible with the following intravenous fluids when administered into a running i.v. catheter:

Lactated Ringer's Injection
Lactated Ringer's and 5% Dextrose Injection

Ultiva has been shown to be compatible with propofol when administered into a running i.v. catheter.

The tables on this page give guidelines for infusion rates of Ultiva.

Marketing authorisation numbers
Ultiva for Injection 1 mg 14213/0002
Ultiva for Injection 2 mg 14213/0003
Ultiva for Injection 5 mg 14213/0004

Date of approval/revision of SPC August 1997

Legal category POM

VASOXINE* INJECTION

Qualitative and quantitative composition Methoxamine Hydrochloride BP 2% w/v.

Pharmaceutical form Injection.

Clinical particulars

Therapeutic indications: Methoxamine hydrochloride is a direct stimulant of α-adrenergic receptors and is indicated for counteraction of systemic hypotension. The most common clinical application for methoxamine is the prevention or correction of hypotension associated with the use of spinal anaesthetics or antihypertensive drugs.

Methoxamine hydrochloride can be used to increase blood pressure during cyclopropane anaesthesia for it does not increase the irritability of the cyclopropane-sensitised heart.

Posology and method of administration:

Adults: The usual intravenous dose for emergencies is 3–5 mg (0.15–0.25 ml) Vasoxine intravenously injected slowly (e.g. at a rate of 1 mg methoxamine hydrochloride/min). Intravenous doses may be supplemented by intramuscular injection of 10–15 mg (0.5–0.75 ml Vasoxine Injection), to provide a more prolonged effect.

For use shortly before or during administration of spinal anaesthesia, a dose of methoxamine hydrochloride of 10–20 mg (0.5–1.0 ml Vasoxine Injection) intramuscularly may be given to prevent or correct systemic hypotension. For a low spinal block, a 10 mg dose of methoxamine hydrochloride may be adequate. For a high spinal block with extensive sympathetic blockade, the tendency for blood pressure to fall is greater and so a dose of 15–20 mg methoxamine hydrochloride may be required. Repeated doses may be necessary, but about 15 minutes should be allowed for the previous intramuscular dose to act.

For cases of only moderate hypotension, 5–10 mg methoxamine hydrochloride (0.25–0.5 ml Vasoxine Injection) intramuscularly may be adequate.

Children up to 12 years of age: The efficacy of methoxamine in children has not been established.

However, if required, a dose of 40–70 mcg Vasoxine Injection/kg bodyweight administered intravenously or 70–280 mcg Vasoxine Injection/kg bodyweight by intramuscular injection would be considered appropriate.

Use in the elderly: No specific information is available on the use of methoxamine in the elderly. However, see *Special warnings and precautions for use* and *Undesirable effects.*

Route of administration: Intravenous or intramuscular.

Contra-indications: Known hypersensitivity to methoxamine. Vasoxine is contra-indicated in cases of pre-existent severe hypertension.

Special warnings and precautions for use: Methoxamine should not be administered unless facilities are available to make frequent measurements of systemic blood pressure.

The effect of increased arterial pressure on a patient with pre-existing vascular disease or impairment of myocardial function should be considered before administering Vasoxine.

Vasoxine Injection should be used with care in hyperthyroidism for there may be a marked pressor response.

When administered intravenously, large veins are preferred to prevent extravasation of Vasoxine Injection. Extravasation may cause necrosis and sloughing of surrounding tissue. The infusion site should be monitored closely for free flow.

Vasoxine should not be used in combination with local anaesthetics to prolong their action at local sites.

Use Vasoxine Injection with care in patients with poor left ventricular function as the increase in peripheral resistance which is brought about by methoxamine may cause or exacerbate cardiac failure.

The use of Vasoxine Injection is not a substitute for replacement of lost intravascular fluid and care should be taken to ensure adequate provision of intravenous fluid, plasma or blood before or during recourse to Vasoxine Injection.

There are no data available on whether or not methoxamine has a carcinogenic or mutagenic potential, or whether it may affect fertility.

Interaction with other medicaments and other forms of interaction: Concomitant use of Vasoxine with sympathomimetic agents, such as decongestants, some appetite suppressants and amphetamine-like psychostimulants may cause an exaggerated response to methoxamine.

The systemic pressor effect of methoxamine can be markedly potentiated in patients who are taking or who have taken monoamine oxidase inhibitors in the preceding two weeks. This effect may also occur in patients who are taking tricyclic antidepressants, ergot alkaloids, some oxytoxic drugs, β-adrenergic blocking agents, guanethidine or reserpine.

Pregnancy and lactation: It is reported that vasopressors with strong α-adrenergic activity diminish uterine blood flow and may adversely affect the foetus. Use of Vasoxine Injection to prevent and treat hypotension during spinal anaesthesia in obstetric patients cannot be recommended.

In the absence of adequate experience of administration to pregnant women, Vasoxine Injection should not be used during pregnancy unless the potential benefit to the mother outweighs any possible risk to the foetus.

It is not known if methoxamine is excreted in human milk.

Effects on ability to drive and use machines: None known.

Undesirable effects: Subjective effects reported by patients receiving methoxamine include dull headaches, feelings of cold and other skin sensations resulting from piloerection, sensation of fullness in neck and chest and desire to micturate.

Reflex bradycardia may occur with methoxamine which can be countered with standard doses of atropine given intravenously.

Vomiting and headache have been reported without severe hypertension.

Overdose: The hypertension caused by an overdose of Vasoxine Injection should be managed with an α-adrenergic blocking agent such as phentolamine, administered intravenously and repeated as necessary. Clinically significant bradycardia should be treated with intravenous atropine.

Pharmacological properties

Pharmacodynamic properties: Methoxamine is a vasopressor agent which produces a prompt and prolonged rise in blood pressure after parenteral administration. It acts by exclusively stimulating α-adrenergic receptors and hence causing vasoconstriction.

Pharmacokinetic properties: The usual time of onset of activity is one minute after intravenous injections and twenty minutes after the intramuscular injections. The usual duration of activity is about one hour after intravenous and somewhat longer after intramuscular administration. Actual plasma concentrations attained have never been measured, so the disposition and elimination rate have to be inferred from observation of biological activity. Methoxamine is not active after oral administration.

Preclinical safety data: There are no preclinical data of relevance to the prescriber which are additional to that in other sections of the SPC.

Pharmaceutical particulars

List of excipients: Sodium Chloride HSE*; Sodium Chloride PhEur*; Water for Injections PhEur.

* These ingredients are alternatives.

Incompatibilities: None known.

Shelf life: 60 months.

Special precautions for storage: Store at 25°C. Do not freeze.

Nature and contents of container: Neutral glass ampoules. 1 ml nominal fill volume. Pack size: 1.

Instructions for use/handling: Not applicable.

Marketing authorisation number PL 0003/5066R

Date of approval/revision of SPC September 1996.

WELLFERON* INJECTION

Qualitative and quantitative composition

Active ingredient: Human lymphoblastoid interferon, 3 Mega Units, 5 Mega Units or 10 Mega Units in 1 ml in each vial, (1 Mega Unit (MU) = 1×10^6 International Units of lymphoblastoid interferon by reference to the WHO International Reference Preparation of lymphoblastoid interferon Ga 23–901–532).

Pharmaceutical form A clear colourless solution which is administered by intramuscular or subcutaneous injection.

Clinical particulars

Therapeutic indication: Wellferon is indicated for the treatment of patients with hairy cell leukaemia.

Wellferon is indicated for the treatment of patients with chronic myeloid leukaemia in the chronic phase. Treatment has been shown to result in an improvement in overall survival when compared with conventinal cytotoxic chemotherapy. (Median survival 59 versus 38 months; overall survival p = 0.001.)

Wellferon is indicated for the treatment of adult patients with chronic active hepatitis B, who have markers for viral replication, e.g. those who are positive for HBV-DNA, DNA polymerase or HBeAg.

Wellferon is indicated for the treatment of patients with chronic hepatitis C (non A non B) infection. Efficacy has been established on the basis of normalisation of serum aminotransferases, clearance of serum HCV-RNA and improvements in liver histology.

Posology and method of administration for adults and children: The site of injection should be changed in succeeding injections.

Some patients appear to be less troubled by interferon-related side effects if the dose is administered in the evening.

The subcutaneous route is more acceptable and convenient for patient self-administration than the intramuscular route.

Dosage in adults

Hairy cell leukaemia: For remission induction, the dose recommended is 3 MU given daily by subcutaneous or intramuscular injection.

After initial improvement in peripheral haematological indices (commonly 12 to 16 weeks), the dose may be administered thrice weekly during which time further improvement in the bone marrow is to be anticipated.

Haematological recovery is to be expected in patients who have failed splenectomy as well as in those with palpable splenomegaly in whom a reduction in spleen size is to be anticipated.

Alternative dosage regimens have also been used with effect. A randomised study comparing dosing at 2.0 MU/m² body surface area daily for one month and then thrice weekly, and 0.2 MU/m² body surface area according to the same schedule, has shown a greater anti-leukaemic effect at one year using the higher dosage regimen, although side effects were less using the lower dose. See also Special Warnings.

Prolonged treatment for 6 months or more may be required to clear hairy cells from the bone marrow. Studies have suggested a broad correlation between the degree of reponse achieved and cumulative dose administered.

Chronic myeloid leukaemia: Wellferon treatment should be started once initial control of the white cell count has been achieved to a level of 4 to 20×10^9/l for a period of a least 4 weeks using cytotoxic chemotherapy e.g. conventional doses of busulphan or hydroxyurea. If busulphan is used for this purpose, there should be an interval of at least 4 weeks between stopping busulphan and starting Wellferon therapy. If either the leucocyte or platelet count is still falling after this interval the start of Wellferon treatment should be further delayed until the count is stable.

For the first 3 weeks of therapy, the dose recommended is 3 MU given daily by subcutaneous injection.

After 3 weeks, the dose is adjusted to achieve a leucocyte count between 2 and 5×10^9/l. Dose adjustment may be made by altering the daily dose and also by varying the number of days each week on which the dose is administered.

The median average weekly dose in long term clinical studies was approximately 21 MU per week.

In the event of intolerance or severe cytopenia the total weekly dose should be reduced.

If the leucocyte count falls below 2×10^9/l, the total dose per week should be reduced. Wellferon should be stopped if the leucocyte count falls below 1×10^9/l and restarted when the count exceeds 2×10^9/l.

If the platelet count falls below 50×10^9/l, the total dose per week should be reduced. Wellferon should be stopped if the platelet count falls below 25×10^9/l and restarted when the count exceeds 50×10^9/l.

If the leucocyte count rises above 30×10^9/l, chemotherapy with either hydroxyurea or busulphan at conventional dosage should be given in addition to Wellferon until the leucocyte count has re-established between 4 and 20×10^9/l for a period of 4 weeks. Chemotherapy is then discontinued, but administration is repeated in the same manner whenever the leucocyte count exceeds 30×10^9/l. Weekly blood counts are recommended when initiating combination treatment with Wellferon and cytotoxic drugs and if significant chemotherapy-related myelosuppression occurs, chemotherapy should be discontinued and withheld until haematological recovery in accordance with normal clinical practice. (See prescribing information for busulphan and hydroxyurea.)

Wellferon is continued indefinitely until the leucocyte count is no longer controlled (even despite additional chemotherapy), or evidence of acceleration or blast transformation is apparent.

Although there is limited clinical experience, doses of 3 MU or 6 MU (occasionally 9 MU) daily have been successfully used to achieve initial control of the white cell count. In the event of intolerance, dose reduction along the lines of those discussed above should be considered.

Prolonged treatment of at least 6 months and frequently longer, may be required to achieve a cytogenetic response in terms of suppression of the philadephia chromosome (PH) positive cells in the bone marrow.

Chronic hepatitis B infection: A twelve week course of thrice weekly subcutaneous or intramuscular injections of 10 to 15 MU (up to 7.5 MU/m² body surface area) is generally recommended.

Longer periods of treatment for up to six months at lower doses (5 to 10 MU or up to 5 MU/m² of body surface area thrice weekly) have been employed and may be preferred for patients who do not tolerate higher doses.

An initial period, employing escalating daily doses, usually over five days (but up to 28 days with the longer treatment), may be a convenient way of introducing treatment.

Chronic hepatitis C infection (non A non B): The optimal treatment schedule with Interferons for chronic hepatitis C (non A non B) has not yet been established.

A 48 week course of thrice weekly subcutaneous (or intramuscular) injection of 5 MU is recommended. A good response may still be achieved in some patients with an alternative dose such as 3 MU thrice weekly for 48 weeks. The 3 MU thrice weekly regimen may also be more appropriate in patients where tolerance of the higher dose is in doubt.

Clinical experience indicates that Wellferon therapy can result in an ALT response at the end of treatment in up to 50% of patients. Approximately half of these patients will maintain a sustained ALT response, post-treatment.

Almost 50% of HCV infected patients treated with Wellferon show sustained improvement in liver inflammation on histological examination.

Dosage in children:

Hairy cell leukaemia: Not known to occur in children.

Chronic Myeloid leukaemia: Wellferon has been used in the management of PH positive chronic myeloid leukaemia in children, using the adult dosing regimen, although data are limited.

Chronic hepatitis B infection: Up to 10 MU/m² body surface area has been administered to children with chronic hepatitis B. However, efficacy of therapy has not yet been demonstrated.

Chronic hepatitis C infection (non A non B): Chronic hepatitis C (non A non B) is rare in children. No information on treatment is available.

Dosage in the elderly: Elderly patients may be less tolerant of the side effects of interferon, particularly those effects which are cumulative. These patients should be seen frequently whilst receiving treatment; Wellferon dosage should be reduced or even stopped if patients are unduly sensitive to side effects.

Whilst vigilance is necessary in treating elderly Chronic Myeloid Leukaemia (CML) patients (≥65 years) clinical experience indicates that they gain simiilar survival benefit with comparable treatment tolerance to that of younger patients.

Contra-indications: Hairy cell leukaemia and phase chronic myeloid leukaemia: Wellferon should not be given to patients known to be hypersensitive to the preparation or any of its components. Other than known hypersensitivity there are no contra-indications to the use of Wellferon in hairy cell leukaemia or chronic myeloid leukaemia.

Chronic hepatitis B infection and chronic hepatitis C: A history of hypersensitivity to interferon alpha-nl (Ins), or any component of the preparation.

Severe pre-existing cardiac disease.

Severe renal or hepatic dysfunction.

Epilepsy and/or compromised central nervous system function.

Chronic hepatitis with advanced decompensated cirrhosis of the liver.

Chronic hepatitis in patients who are being or have recently been treated with immunosuppressive agents excluding short term 'steroid withdrawal'.

Special precautions for use: None.

Special warnings: Extreme caution is advised when using alpha interferons in the treatment of patients with concurrent renal, cardiovascular or severe hepatic disease, central nervous system disease, or patients with a history of pre-existing mental disturbance. In view of rare cases of cardiac arrhythmia or infarction occurring in patients receiving Wellferon it is prudent to perform an ECG before starting and during treatment in patients with pre-existing heart disease. Consideration should be given to dose reduction or temporary cessation of dosing if problems are encountered when treating patients suffering from concurrent diseases such as these.

It is important to monitor the blood count closely in patients during the first 6 weeks of treatment for hairy cell leukaemia, following which the suppressive effects of alpha interferons on the bone marrow will be overtaken by the improving leukaemic state, leading towards a normalisation of haematological parameters. In patients with profound or potentially life-threatening neutropenia or thrombocytopenia at the outset it may be preferable to initiate treatment with a lower dose of Wellferon, particularly for out-patients who are remote from immediate medical care.

During Wellferon treatment of chronic myeloid leukaemia the blood count should be monitored weekly in the first 3 weeks and thereafter at least once a month or more frequently if cytopenias occur. In the event of dose escalation above 3 MU daily the patient should be seen weekly until tolerance has been assessed.

Severe cytopenias, with or without bone marrow aplasia, have been observed very occasionally in patients with chronic myeloid leukaemia treated with Wellferon directly after busulphan therapy. Careful monitoring of the blood count in patients in whom busulphan induction is used is important to ensure that the leucocyte and platelet counts have stabilised before starting treatment with Wellferon.

Caution is advised if either busulphan or hydroxyurea is reintroduced in combination with Wellferon and weekly blood counts are recommended.

During Wellferon treatment of chronic hepatitis B infection and chronic hepatitis C infection it is similarly important to monitor blood count and liver function throughout treatment.

Care should be exercised in treating patients with certain pre-existing autoimmune diseases e.g. thyroid disorders, as rare occurrences of exacerbation of disease have been reported.

Efficacy against hepatitis B virus and hepatitis C (non A non B) virus infections has not yet been demonstrated in patients whose immune systems are compromised (e.g. by current or recent therapy with immunosuppressive drugs (excluding short term steroid pre treatment) or due to human immunodeficiency virus (HIV) infection).

As with other alpha interferon preparations, care should be exercised when using Wellferon in combination with vinblastine. With relatively high doses of vinblastine and Wellferon, life-threatening (rarely fatal) myelosuppression has been reported.

Care should be exercised in treating patients with asthma, as exacerbation of the disease has been reported on isolated occasions following alpha interferon administration.

It is prudent to ensure maintenance of adequate hydration.

Interaction with other medicaments and other forms of interaction: Alpha-interferons may alter the activity of certain enzymes. In particular, they reduce the activity of P-450 cytochromes. The metabolism of drugs such as cimetidine, phenytoin, warfarin, theophylline, diazepam and propranolol by these enzyme systems may therefore be impaired in patients receiving alpha interferon. Several cytotoxic drugs e.g. cyclophosphamide, are also metabolised by these enzymes.

Concurrent administration of a combination of relatively high doses of vinblastine with Wellferon has been shown to produce severe myelosuppression.

In the treatment of chronic myeloid leukaemia, the use of Wellferon immediately following busulphan has occasionally resulted in bone marrow aplasia and the combination should therefore be regarded as potentially severely myelotoxic. If chemotherapy is administered concurrently with Wellferon to maintain control of the leucocyte count the blood count should be checked frequently to ensure that severe myelosuppression does not occur.

In the treatment of chronic hepatitis B infection, the occurrence of an acute, hepatitis-like illness presents the theoretical risk of additive interaction with hepatotoxic drugs and of further impairment of hepatic drug metabolism.

Progressive renal failure has been reported in patients receiving concurrent high dose acyclovir. Concurrent administration of interferon with drugs which act on the central nervous system has occasionally resulted in unexpectedly severe changes in mental state.

Concurrent administration of immunosuppressive drugs (including corticosteroids), which may enhance viral replication, should be avoided during treatment of chronic hepatitis B infection with Wellferon.

Pregnancy and lactation: Offspring from pregnant rhesus monkeys given daily Wellferon dosages of up to 2.5 MU/kg bodyweight (from Day 21 through to Day 50 in one group and from Day 51 through to Day 130 in the second group) did not reveal teratogenic or other adverse effects, although there was an increased incidence of abortion and stillbirth in those animals who received the highest dose (2.5 MU/kg bodyweight daily).

No studies have been performed in animals to determine whether Wellferon may affect fertility.

No information is available on the use of Wellferon in human pregnancy. In view of the profound effects of the drug on human metabolism and physiology however, Wellferon should be considered as a drug which might result in damage to the foetus and patients should therefore be advised accordingly. The expected clinical benefit of treatment to the patient must be balanced against any possible hazard to the developing foetus. Adequate contraceptive precautions should be advised if either partner is receiving Wellferon. In view of the long clinical course of chronic hepatitis B infection and the availability of hepatitis B immunisation for the neonate, use of Wellferon to treat chronic hepatitis B infection during human pregnancy is not recommended.

There is no information on the excretion of interferon in human breast milk, following Wellferon therapy. In consequence lactating women should be advised accordingly and the possible risks balanced against the advantages of treatment.

Effects on ability to drive and use machines: As alpha interferons may affect central nervous system functions, patients should be warned not to drive a vehicle or operate machinery until their tolerance of treatment has been assessed.

Undesirable effects: Wellferon in common with other alpha-interferons is a highly active mediator of biological events and its use may be associated with severe side effects, particularly when large doses are administered.

The most frequently reported side effects of Wellferon and other alpha interferon preparations consist of fever, chills, occasionally rigors, headache, malaise and myalgia, all reminiscent of an attack of influenza. These acute side effects can usually be reduced or eliminated by concurrent administration of paracetamol and tend to diminish with continuing therapy. In contrast however, continuing therapy can lead to lethargy, weakness, arthralgia, and fatigue accompanied by anorexia and weight loss.

Alpha-interferons have a suppressive effect on the bone marrow leading to a fall in the white blood count, particularly the granulocytes, the platelet count and, less commonly, the haemoglobin concentration. Additionally, abnormalities in the blood-clotting mechanism have occurred. These effects can lead to an increased risk of infection and haemorrhage.

Marked effects on the central nervous system may occur; these include abnormal electroencephalograms with excess slow wave activity, severe depression, confusion, apathy and coma. Occasionally seizures occur which may be precipitated by fever in children. A few reports of movement disorders (including extrapyramidal and cerebellar dysfunction) have been reported in cancer patients receiving Wellferon.

The administration of alpha-interferons may give rise to hypotension, hypertension or arrhythmias in certain individuals. Severe cardiovascular events reported in patients receiving alpha interferons include myocardial infarction, cerebrovascular accident and peripheral ischaemia.

Nausea, vomiting and diarrhoea have occurred during therapy with alpha-interferons.

Alpha interferons can lead to an elevation in liver-related enzymes; this is usually transient but occasionally is marked and persistent. Hepatic necrosis has been reported on very rare occasions.

On rare occasions elevations of serum creatinine levels have been seen in Wellferon treated patients.

In patients with myelomatosis, there have been rare reports of renal failure/and or nephrotic syndrome in patients treated with Wellferon, all had varying degrees of prior renal dysfunction.

After repeated very high doses (100–200 MU) intravenously by infusion, hypocalcaemia and hyperkalaemia have occurred.

Reactions at injection sites have been reported in some patients.

Alopecia occurs occasionally as a late side effect.

Other uncommon events which have been reported in patients receiving alpha-interferons include Raynaud's phenomenon, dyspnoea, urticaria, erythema nodosum, skin rashes, pruritus, psoriasis, mucositis, isolated peripheral nerve defects, and disturbances of antidiuretic hormone levels.

Isolated cases of various autoimmune phenomena e.g. immune thrombocytopenia, haemolytic anaemia, hypothyroidism have occurred following alpha-interferon administration. In some patients with pre-existing autoimmune phenomena, isolated cases of exacerbation have been seen.

Overdose: There have been no reports of overdosage but repeated large doses of alpha interferons are associated with profound lethargy, fatigue, prostration and coma. Such patients should be hospitalised for observation, and appropriate supportive treatment given.

Pharmacological properties

Pharmacodynamic properties: The mode of action of alpha-interferon in hairy cell leukaemia is not understood. The rapid rate of clearance of hairy cells from the blood on commencing treatment suggests a direct effect of interferon following cellular binding, particularly since malignant hairy cells are known to bear prolific interferon receptors on their surface membranes. The resulting anti-leukaemic effect may be brought about by a reduction in the sensitivity of hairy cells to stimulation by growth factors produced by the same cells (autocrine loop) or different cells (paracrine loop) a change towards a more differentiated state and a decrease in cell proliferation.

The mechanism of action of alpha-interferon in chronic myeloid leukaemia is not fully understood. Possibilities include inhibition of the late progenitor cell stage of chronic myeloid leukaemia, either directly or by interruption of an autocrine feedback loop, enhancement of T-cells to inhibit the proliferation of chronic myeloid leukaemia cells and modulation of interactions between chronic myeloid leukaemia progenitor cells and bone marrow stromal cells, leading to growth arrest and repopulation of the marrow with normal progenitors.

The mode of action of alpha-interferon in the treatment of chronic hepatitis B is poorly understood but seems to consist of both a direct antiviral effect and immuno-modulatory actions.

The mode of action of alpha-interferon in the treatment of chronic hepatitis C (non A non B) has not yet been determined; however, it is currently thought to consist mainly of an antiviral effect supported by immunomodulatory effects.

Antibodies to Wellferon: Neutralising antibodies occur infrequently in patients receiving Wellferon which therefore appears to have low immunogenicity. An overall anti-interferon antibody incidence of 2.0% was found in follow-up sera from more than 1500 patients who had received Wellferon for benign and malignant diseases.

Pharmacokinetic properties: There is considerable inter-patient variability in the handling of alpha-interferons; furthermore, absolute serum levels may be less meaningful as a measure of alpha-interferon biological activity than the induction of certain cellular enzymes such as 2', 5'-oligoadenylate synthetase (2-

5A synthetase) or human Mx protein. Following intramuscular or subcutaneous administration, maximum serum levels are usually reached within 4 to 8 hours, but may merge into a plateau phase as a result of rate-limited absorption from the site of administration.

The measured serum half-life also varies considerably as a result of this, being in the approximate range of 4 to 12 hours although the true elimination half life can be estimated to be about 3 to 4 hours. Similar serum alpha-interferon levels and pharmacokinetics are found after intramuscular and subcutaneous administration of Wellferon. When Wellferon is administered at the recommended daily dose for the treatment of hairy cell leukaemia, steady state accumulation results in maximum serum values lying in the approximate range of 30 to 90 IU per ml. The range of doses suggested for the treatment of chronic hepatitis B infection can be expected to result in maximum serum concentrations of 200 to 300 IU per ml. Alpha-interferon is not detectable in the urine except rarely in cases of severe renal disease. In a study of 20 patients aged 29–81 years, with estimated creatinine clearances of 15 to >100 ml/min, there were no apparent effects of renal function or age on Wellferon pharmacokinetic parameters in the range 3 MU to 10 MU. Total body clearance estimates, uncorrected for bioavailability (CL/b), have been calculated for Wellferon; from two different studies mean values were found to be 57 ml/min/m², and approximately 2 ml/min/kg respectively.

Preclinical safety data: The alpha interferons are unusually restricted in their species specificity. Additionally administration of a heterologous protein to primates and rodents results in the production of circulating antibodies. These factors greatly limit the predictive value of pre-clinical information. The studies conducted in animals have not demonstrated any particular toxic or pharmacologic effects.

Carcinogenicity: No studies have been conducted in animals to determine whether Wellferon has carcinogenic potential.

Mutagenicity: Wellferon was not mutagenic in the Ames test.

Pharmaceutical particulars

List of excipients: Sodium Chloride PhEur; Tris (Tromethamine) USP; Glycine BP; Human Albumin Solution (equivalent to total protein) PhEur; Water for Injection PhEur.

Incompatibilities: Not applicable.

Shelf life: 3 years at 2–8°C. Wellferon contains no preservative, therefore any partly used vials should be discarded immediately after withdrawal of the required dose.

Special precautions for storage: Store between 2 and 8°C. Protect from light.

Nature and contents of container: Wellferon is filled in nominal 1 ml volumes into PhEur Type 1 glass (white neutral) vials, plugged with red butyl/natural rubber closures with an aluminium collar and polypropylene flip-off cap.

Instructions for use/handling: Not applicable.

Marketing authorisation number

3 MU	PL 0003/0221
5 MU	PL 0003/0281
10 MU	PL 0003/0220

Date of approval/revision of SPC November 1996.

Legal category POM.

WELLVONE* SUSPENSION ▼

Qualitative and quantitative composition Atovaquone 150 mg/ml. A unit dose of 5 ml contains 750 mg atovaquone.

Pharmaceutical form A bright yellow oral suspension containing 150 mg atovaquone/ml.

Clinical particulars

Therapeutic indications: Wellvone suspension is indicated for: Acute treatment of mild to moderate *Pneumocystis carinii* pneumonia (PCP) (alveolar-arterial oxygen tension difference $[(A\text{-}a)DO_2] \leq 45$ mmHg (6 kPa) and oxygen tension in arterial blood $(PaO_2) \geq 60$ mmHg (8 kPa) breathing room air) in patients who are intolerant of co-trimoxazole therapy (see *Special warnings and precautions for use*).

Posology and method of administration: The importance of taking the full prescribed dose of Wellvone **with food** should be stressed to patients. The presence of food, particularly high fat food, increases bioavailability by two to three fold.

Dosage in adults: Pneumocystis carinii pneumonia: The recommended oral dose is 750 mg twice a day (1×5 ml morning and evening) administered with food each day for 21 days.

Higher doses may be more effective and will be investigated (see *Pharmacokinetic properties*).

Dosage in children: Clinical efficacy has not been studied.

Dosage in the elderly: There have been no studies of Wellvone in the elderly (see *Special warnings and precautions for use*).

Renal or hepatic impairment: Wellvone has not been specifically studied in patients with significant hepatic or renal impairment (see *Pharmacokinetics in adults*). If it is necessary to treat such patients with Wellvone, caution is advised and administration should be closely monitored.

Contra-indications: Wellvone suspension is contra-indicated in individuals with known hypersensitivity to atovaquone or to any components of the formulation.

Special warnings and precautions for use: Diarrhoea at the start of treatment has been shown to be associated with significantly lower atovaquone plasma levels. These in turn correlated with a higher incidence of therapy failures and a lower survival rate. Therefore, alternative therapies should be considered for such patients and for patients who have difficulty taking Wellvone with food.

The concomitant administration of atovaquone and rifampicin is not recommended (see *Interaction with other medicaments*).

The efficacy of Wellvone has not been systematically evaluated (i) in patients failing other PCP therapy, including co-trimoxazole, (ii) for treatment of severe episodes of PCP $[(A\text{-}a)\ DO_2 > 45$ mmHg 6kPa] or (iii) as a prophylactic agent for PCP or (iv) versus intravenous pentamidine for treatment of PCP.

No data are available in non-HIV immunocompromised patients suffering with PCP.

As HIV infection is rarely observed in elderly patients, no clinical experience of atovaquone treatment has been gained. Therefore use in the elderly should be closely monitored.

Patients with pulmonary disease should be carefully evaluated for causes of disease other than PCP and treated with additional agents as appropriate. Wellvone is not expected to be effective therapy for other fungal, bacterial, mycobacterial or viral diseases.

Interaction with other medicaments and other forms of interaction: As experience is limited, care should be taken when combining other drugs with Wellvone.

Concomitant administration of rifampicin is known to reduce atovaquone levels by approximately 50% and could result in subtherapeutic plasma concentrations in some patients (see *Special warnings and precautions for use*).

Concomitant treatment with metoclopramide has been associated with significant decreases in plasma concentrations of atovaquone. Caution should be exercised in prescribing this drug with Wellvone until the potential interaction has been further studied.

In clinical trials of Wellvone small decreases in plasma concentrations of atovaquone (mean <3 mcg/ml) were associated with concomitant administration of paracetamol, benzodiazepines, acyclovir, opiates, cephalosporins, anti-diarrhoeals and laxatives. The causal relationship between the change in plasma concentrations of atovaquone and the administration of the drugs mentioned above is unknown.

Clinical trials have evaluated the interaction of Wellvone Tablets with:

Zidovudine – Zidovudine does not appear to affect the pharmacokinetics of atovaquone. However, pharmacokinetic data have shown that atovaquone appears to decrease the rate of metabolism of zidovudine to its glucuronide metabolite (steady state AUC of zidovudine was increased by 33% and peak plasma concentration of the glucuronide was decreased by 19%). At zidovudine dosages of 500 or 600 mg/day it would seem unlikely that a three week, concomitant course of Wellvone for the treatment of acute PCP would result in an increased incidence of adverse reactions attributable to higher plasma concentrations of zidovudine.

Didanosine (ddI) – ddI does not affect the pharmacokinetics of atovaquone as determined in a prospective multidose interaction study of atovaquone and ddI. However, there was a 24% decrease in the AUC for ddI when co-administered with atovaquone which is unlikely to be of clinical significance.

Nevertheless, the modes of interaction being unknown, the effects of atovaquone administration on zidovudine and ddI may be greater with atovaquone suspension. The higher concentrations of atovaquone possible with the suspension might induce greater changes in the AUC values for zidovudine or ddI than those observed. Patients receiving atovaquone and zidovudine should be regularly monitored for zidovudine associated adverse effects.

There are no data available for interaction of atovaquone with other anti-retroviral drugs.

In clinical trials of Wellvone the following medications were not associated with a change in steady state plasma concentrations of atovaquone: fluconazole, clotrimazole, ketoconazole, antacids, systemic corticosteroids, non-steroidal anti-inflammatory drugs, anti-emetics (excluding metoclopramide) and H_2-antagonists.

Atovaquone is highly bound to plasma proteins and caution should be used when administering Wellvone concurrently with other highly plasma protein bound drugs with narrow therapeutic indices. Atovaquone does not affect the pharmacokinetics, metabolism or extent of protein binding of phenytoin *in vivo. In vitro* there is no plasma protein binding interaction between atovaquone and quinine, phenytoin, warfarin, sulphamethoxazole, indomethacin or diazepam.

Pregnancy and lactation: There is no information on the effects of atovaquone administration during human pregnancy. Atovaquone should not be used during pregnancy unless the benefit of treatment to the mother outweighs any possible risk to the developing foetus.

Insufficient data are available from animal experiments to assess the possible risk to reproductive potential or performance.

It is not known whether atovaquone is excreted in human milk, and therefore breast feeding is not recommended.

Effects on ability to drive and use machines: There have been no studies to investigate the effect of Wellvone on driving performance or the ability to operate machinery but a detrimental effect on such activities is not predicted from the pharmacology of the drug.

Undesirable effects: Patients participating in clinical trials with Wellvone have often had complications of advanced Human Immunodeficiency Virus (HIV) disease and therefore the causal relationship between the adverse experiences and atovaquone is difficult to evaluate.

The most common adverse experiences reported while receiving treatment with Wellvone, regardless of attributability, are: rash, nausea, diarrhoea, headache, vomiting, fever and insomnia.

The most common abnormalities in laboratory parameters reported in patients receiving Wellvone, regardless of attributability, are: elevated liver enzyme levels, elevated amylase levels, hyponatraemia, neutropenia and anaemia.

Overdose: There have been no reports of overdosage from the administration of Wellvone in humans.

In the case of overdosage, treatment should be symptomatic.

Pharmacological properties

Pharmacodynamic properties:

(a) Mode of action: Atovaquone belongs to a new therapeutic class with a novel mechanism of action. It is a selective and potent inhibitor of the eukaryotic mitochondrial electron transport chain in a number of parasitic protozoa. The site of action appears to be the cytochrome bcl complex (complex III). The ultimate metabolic effect of such blockade is likely to be inhibition of nucleic acid and ATP synthesis.

(b) Microbiology: Atovaquone has potent antiprotozoal activity, both *in vitro* and in animal models, particularly against the parasitic protozoan-life fungus *Pneumocystis carinii* (IC_{50} 0.1–1.0 mcg/ml).

Pharmacokinetic properties: Atovaquone is a highly lipophilic compound with a low aqueous solubility. It is 99.9% bound to plasma proteins. The bioavailability of the drug demonstrates a relative decrease with single doses above 750 mg, and it shows considerable inter-individual variability. Average absolute bioavailability of a 750 mg single dose of atovaquone suspension administered with food to adult HIV positive males is 47% (compared to 23% for Wellvone tablets). Following the intravenous administration, the volume of distribution and clearance were calculated to be 0.62±0.19 l/kg and 0.15±0.09 ml/min/kg, respectively.

The bioavailability of atovaquone is greater when administered with food than in the fasting state. In healthy volunteers, a standardised breakfast (23 g fat; 610 kCal) increased bioavailability two to three-fold following a single 750 mg dose. The mean area under the atovaquone plasma concentration-time curve (AUC) was increased 2.5 fold and the mean C_{max} was increased 3.4 fold. The mean (±SD) AUC values for suspension were 324.3 (±115.0) mcg/ml.h fasted and 800.6 (±319.8) mcg/ml.h with food.

In a safety and pharmacokinetic study in patients with PCP, the following results were obtained.

Dose regimen	750 mg twice daily	1000 mg twice daily
Number of patients	18	9
C avg. ss (range)	22 mcg/ml (6–41)	25.7 mcg/ml (15–36)
% of patients with C Avg. ss>15 mcg/ml	67%	100%

Average steady state concentrations above 15 mcg/ml are predictive of a high (>90%) success rate.

In healthy volunteers and patients with AIDS atovaquone has a half-life of 2 to 3 days.

In healthy volunteers there is no evidence that the drug is metabolised and there is negligible excretion of atovaquone in the urine, with parent drug being predominantly (>90%) excreted unchanged in faeces.

Preclinical safety data:
(a) Carcinogenicity: Oncogenicity studies in mice showed an increased incidence of hepatocellular adenomas and carcinomas without determination of the no observed adverse effect level. No such findings were observed in rats and mutagenicity tests were negative. These findings appear to be due to the inherent susceptibility of mice to atovaquone and are not predictive of a risk in the clinical situation.

(b) Reproductive toxicity: In the dosage range of 600 to 1200 mg/kg studies in rabbits gave indications of maternal and embryotoxic effects.

Pharmaceutical particulars
List of excipients: Benzyl alcohol; xanthan gum; poloxamer 188; saccharin sodium; tutti frutti flavour (Firmenich 51.880/A); purified water.

Incompatibilities: None.

Shelf life: 2 years (after first opening, the suspension may be stored for up to 21 days).

Special precautions for storage: Store below 25°C. Do not freeze.

Nature and contents of container: A 240 ml high density polyethylene bottle with child resistant closure, containing 226 ml of atovaquone suspension.

A 5 ml measuring spoon (polypropylene) is included.

Instructions for use/handling: Do not dilute.

Marketing authorisation number PL 10949/0271

Date of approval/revision of SPC March 1997.

Legal category POM.

ZANTAC* INJECTION 50 mg/2 ml

Qualitative and quantitative composition Ranitidine Hydrochloride HSE 56.0 mg/2 ml equivalent to Ranitidine 50.0 mg/2 ml.

Pharmaceutical form Injection (Aqueous solution).

Clinical particulars
Therapeutic indications: Zantac Injection is indicated for the treatment of duodenal ulcer, benign gastric ulcer, post-operative ulcer, reflux oesophagitis, Zollinger-Ellison Syndrome and the following conditions where reduction of gastric secretion and acid output is desirable:

The prophylaxis of gastrointestinal haemorrhage from stress ulceration in seriously ill patients, the prophylaxis of recurrent haemorrhage in patients with bleeding peptic ulcers and before general anaesthesia in patients considered to be at risk of acid aspiration (Mendelson's Syndrome), particularly obstetric patients during labour. For appropriate cases, Zantac tablets are also available.

Posology and method of administration:
Adults (including elderly): Zantac Injection may be given either as a slow (over a period of at least two minutes) intravenous injection of 50 mg, after dilution to a volume of 20 ml per 50 mg dose, which may be repeated every six to eight hours; or as an intermittent intravenous infusion at a rate of 25 mg per hour for two hours; the infusion may be repeated at six to eight hour intervals, or as an intramuscular injection of 50 mg (2 ml) every six to eight hours.

In the prophylaxis of haemorrhage from stress ulceration in seriously ill patients or the prophylaxis of recurrent haemorrhage in patients bleeding from peptic ulceration, parenteral administration may be continued until oral feeding commences. Patients considered to be still at risk may then be treated with Zantac tablets 150 mg twice daily.

In the prophylaxis of upper gastro-intestinal haemorrhage from stress ulceration in seriously ill patients a priming dose of 50 mg as a slow intravenous injection followed by a continuous intravenous infusion of 0.125-0.250 mg/kg/hr may be preferred.

In patients considered to be at risk of developing acid aspiration syndrome, Zantac Injection 50 mg may be given intramuscularly or by slow intravenous injection 45 to 60 minutes before induction of general anaesthesia.

Children: The use of Zantac Injection in children has not been evaluated.

Route of administration: Intravenous or intramuscular injection.

Contra-indications: Ranitidine is contra-indicated for patients known to have hypersensitivity to any component of the preparation.

Special warnings and special precautions for use: Treatment with a histamine H_2-antagonist may mask the symptoms associated with carcinoma of the stomach and may therefore delay diagnosis of the condition. Accordingly, where gastric ulcer is suspected, the possibility of malignancy should be excluded before therapy with Zantac is instituted.

Ranitidine is excreted via the kidney and so plasma levels of the drug are increased in patients with renal impairment. Accordingly, it is recommended in such patients that Zantac be administered in doses of 25 mg.

Bradycardia in association with rapid administration of Zantac Injection has been reported rarely, usually in patients with factors predisposing to cardiac rhythm disturbances. Recommended rates of administration should not be exceeded.

It has been reported that the use of higher than recommended doses of intravenous H_2-antagonists has been associated with rises in liver enzymes when treatment has been extended beyond five days.

Although clinical reports of acute intermittent porphyria associated with ranitidine administration have been rare and inconclusive, ranitidine should be avoided in patients with a history of this condition.

Interaction with other medicaments and other forms of interaction: Ranitidine does not inhibit the hepatic cytochrome P450-linked mixed function oxygenase system. Accordingly, ranitidine does not potentiate the actions of drugs which are inactivated by this enzyme; these include diazepam, lignocaine, phenytoin, propranolol, theophylline and warfarin.

Pregnancy and lactation: Zantac crosses the placenta but therapeutic doses administered to obstetric patients in labour or undergoing caesarean section have been without any adverse effect on labour, delivery or subsequent neonatal progress. Zantac is also excreted in human breast milk. Like other drugs, Zantac should only be used during pregnancy and nursing if considered essential.

Effects on ability to drive and use machines: None known.

Undesirable effects: The following have been reported as events in clinical trials or in the routine management of patients treated with ranitidine. The relationship to ranitidine therapy has not been established in many cases.

Transient and reversible changes in liver function tests can occur. There have been occasional reports of hepatitis (hepatocellular, hepatocanalicular or mixed) with or without jaundice. These were usually reversible. Acute pancreatitis has been reported rarely.

Leucopenia and thrombocytopenia have occurred rarely in patients. These are usually reversible. Rare cases of agranulocytosis or of pancytopenia, sometimes with marrow hypoplasia, or aplasia have been reported.

Hypersensitivity reactions (urticaria, angioneurotic oedema, fever, bronchospasm, hypotension, anaphylactic shock) have been seen rarely following the parenteral and oral administration of ranitidine. These reactions have occasionally occurred after a single dose.

As with other H_2-receptor antagonists there have been rare reports of bradycardia, A-V block and asystole.

Headache, sometimes severe, and dizziness have been reported in a very small proportion of patients. Rare cases of reversible mental confusion, depression and hallucinations have been reported, predominantly in severely ill and elderly patients.

Skin rash has been reported, including rare cases of erythema multiforme. Musculoskeletal symptoms such as arthralgia and myalgia have been reported rarely.

No clinically significant interference with endocrine or gonadal function has been reported. There have been a few reports of breast symptoms (swelling and/or discomfort) in men taking ranitidine; some cases have resolved on continued ranitidine treatment. Discontinuation of therapy may be necessary in order to establish the underlying cause.

Overdose: Zantac is very specific in action and accordingly, no particular problems are expected following overdosage with the drug. Symptomatic and supportive therapy should be given as appropriate. If need be, the drug may be removed from the plasma by haemodialysis.

Pharmacological properties
Pharmacodynamic properties: Ranitidine is a specific, rapidly acting histamine H_2-antagonist. It inhibits basal and stimulated secretion of gastric acid, reducing both the volume and the acid and pepsin content of the secretion.

Pharmacokinetic properties: Absorption of ranitidine after intramuscular injection is rapid and peak plasma concentrations are usually achieved within 15 minutes of administration. Ranitidine is not extensively metabolised. Elimination of the drug is primarily by tubular secretion. The elimination half-life of ranitidine is 2–3 hours. In balance, studies with 150 mg 3H-ranitidine, 93% of an intravenous dose was excreted in urine and 5% in faeces. Analysis of urine excreted in the first 24 hours after dosing showed that 70% of the intravenous dose was eliminated unchanged. About 6% of the dose is excreted in the urine as the N-oxide, 2% as desmethyl ranitidine and 1–2% as the furoic acid analogue.

Preclinical safety data: There are no pre-clinical data of relevance to the prescriber which are additional to that already included in other sections of the SmPC.

Pharmaceutical particulars
List of excipients: Sodium chloride BP; Potassium Dihydrogen Orthophosphate HSE; Disodium Hydrogen Orthophosphate HSE; Water for Injection BP.

Incompatibilities: None.

Shelf life: 36 months unopened.

All unused admixtures of Zantac Injection with infusion fluids should be discarded 24 hours after preparation.

Special precautions for storage: Store below 25°C, protect from light.

Zantac Injection should not be autoclaved.

Nature and contents of container: 2 ml colourless Type I glass ampoules. Pack size: 5 ampoules.

Instructions for use/handling: None.

Marketing authorisation number PL 10949/0109

Date of first authorisation/renewal of authorisation 2 August 1993.

Date of (partial) revision of text December 1997. This is the first SmPC.

Legal classification POM.

ZANTAC* SYRUP

Qualitative and quantitative composition Ranitidine Hydrochloride 168.0 mg (equivalent to Ranitidine 150.0 mg).

Pharmaceutical form Syrup.

Clinical particulars
Therapeutic indications: Zantac syrup is indicated for the treatment of duodenal ulcer and benign gastric ulcer, including that associated with non-steroidal anti-inflammatory agents. In addition, Zantac syrup is indicated for the prevention of NSAID associated duodenal ulcers. Zantac syrup is also indicated for the treatment of post-operative ulcer, Zollinger-Ellison Syndrome and oesophageal reflux disease including long term management of healed oesophagitis. Other patients with chronic episodic dyspepsia, characterised by pain (epigastric or retrosternal) which is related to meals or disturbs sleep but is not associated with the preceding conditions may benefit from ranitidine treatment. Zantac syrup is indicated for the following conditions where reduction of gastric secretion and acid output is desirable; the prophylaxis of gastro-intestinal haemorrhage from stress ulceration in seriously ill patients, the prophylaxis of recurrent haemorrhage in patients with bleeding peptic ulcers and before general anaesthesia in patients considered to be at risk of acid aspiration (Mendelson's Syndrome), particularly obstetric patients during labour. For appropriate cases Zantac injection is also available (see separate SPC).

Posology and method of administration:
Route of administration: Oral.

Adults (including the elderly): The usual dosage is 150 mg twice daily, taken in the morning and evening. Alternatively, patients with duodenal ulceration, gastric ulceration or oesophageal reflux disease may be treated with a single bedtime dose of 300 mg. It is not necessary to time the dose in relation to meals. In most cases of duodenal ulcer, benign gastric ulcer and post operative ulcer, healing occurs in four weeks.

Healing usually occurs after a further 4 weeks of treatment in those patients whose ulcers have not fully healed after the initial course of therapy.

In ulcers following non-steroidal anti-inflammatory drug therapy or associated with continued non-steroidal anti-inflammatory drugs, 8 weeks treatment may be necessary.

For the prevention of non-steroidal anti-inflammatory drug associated duodenal ulcers ranitidine 150 mg twice daily may be given concomitantly with non-steroidal anti-inflammatory drug therapy.

In duodenal ulcer 300 mg twice daily for 4 weeks results in healing rates which are higher than those at 4 weeks with ranitidine 150 mg twice daily or 300 mg nocte. The increased dose has not been associated with an increased incidence of unwanted effects.

Maintenance treatment at a reduced dosage of 150 mg at bedtime is recommended for patients who have responded to short term therapy, particularly those with a history of recurrent ulcer.

In the management of oesophageal reflux disease, the recommended course of treatment is either 150 mg twice daily or 300 mg at bedtime for up to 8 weeks or if necessary 12 weeks.

In patients with moderate to severe oesophagitis, the dosage of ranitidine may be increased to 150 mg four times daily for up to twelve weeks. The increased dose has not been associated with an incidence of unwanted effects.

For the long-term management of oesophagitis the recommended adult oral dose is 150 mg twice daily. Long-term treatment is not indicated in the management of patients with unhealed oesophagitis with or without barrett's epithelium.

In patients with Zollinger-Ellison Syndrome, the starting dose is 150 mg three times daily and this may be increased as necessary. Patients with this syndrome have been given increasing doses up to 6 g per day and these doses have been well tolerated.

For patients with chronic episodic dyspepsia the recommended course of treatment is 150 mg twice daily for up to six weeks. Anyone not responding or relapsing shortly afterwards should be investigated.

In the prophylaxis of haemorrhage from stress ulceration in seriously ill patients or in the prophylaxis or recurrent haemorrhage in patients bleeding from peptic ulceration, treatment with Zantac tablets 150 mg twice daily may be substituted for Zantac injection once oral feeding commences in patients considered to be still at risk from these conditions.

In patients thought to be at risk of acid aspiration syndrome an oral dose of 150 mg can be given 2 hours before induction of general anaesthesia, and preferably also 150 mg the previous evening.

In obstetric patients at commencement of labour, an oral dose of 150 mg may be given followed by 150 mg at six hourly intervals. It is recommended that since gastric emptying and drug absorption are delayed during labour, any patient requiring emergency general anaesthesia should be given, in addition, a non-particulate antacid (e.g. sodium citrate) prior to induction of anaesthesia. The usual precautions to avoid acid aspiration should also be taken.

Children: The recommended oral dose for the treatment of peptic ulcer in children is 2 mg/kg to 4 mg/kg twice daily to a maximum of 300 mg ranitidine per day.

Contra-indications: Ranitidine is contra-indicated for patients known to have hypersensitivity to any component of the preparation.

Special warnings and precautions for use: Treatment with a histamine H_2-antagonist may mask symptoms associated with carcinoma of the stomach and may therefore delay diagnosis of the condition. Accordingly, where gastric ulcer has been diagnosed or in patients of middle age and over with new or recently changed dyspeptic symptoms the possibility of malignancy should be excluded before therapy with Zantac is instituted.

Ranitidine is excreted via the kidney and so plasma levels of the drug are increased in patients with severe renal impairment. Accordingly, it is recommended that the therapeutic regimen for Zantac in such patients be 150 mg at night for 4 to 8 weeks. The same dose should be used for maintenance treatment should this be deemed necessary. If an ulcer has not healed after treatment, the standard dosage regimen of 150 mg twice daily should be instituted, followed, if need be, by maintenance treatment of 150 mg at night.

Regular supervision of patients who are taking non-steroidal anti-inflammatory drugs concomitantly with ranitidine is recommended, especially in the elderly. Current evidence shows that ranitidine protects against NSAID associated ulceration in the duodenum and not in the stomach.

Although clinical reports of acute intermittent porphyria associated with ranitidine administration have been rare and inconclusive, ranitidine should be avoided in patients with a history of this condition.

Rates of healing of ulcers in clinical trial patients aged 65 and over have not been found to differ from those in younger patients. Additionally, there was no difference in the incidence of adverse effects.

Interaction with other medicaments and other forms of interaction: Ranitidine does not inhibit the hepatic cytochrome p450-linked mixed function oxygenase system. Accordingly, ranitidine does not potentiate the actions of drugs which are inactivated by this enzyme; these include Diazepam, Lignocaine, Phenytoin, Propranolol, Theophylline and Warfarin.

Pregnancy and lactation: Zantac crosses the placenta but therapeutic doses administered to obstetric patients in labour or undergoing caesarean section have been without any adverse effect on labour, delivery or subsequent neonatal progress. Zantac is also excreted in human breast milk. Like other drugs, Zantac should only be used during pregnancy and nursing if considered essential.

Effects on ability to drive and use machines: Not applicable.

Undesirable effects: The following have been reported as events in clinical trials or in the routine management of patients treated with ranitidine. The relationship to ranitidine therapy has not been established in many cases.

Transient and reversible changes in liver function tests can occur. There have been occasional reports of hepatitis (hepatocellular, hepatocanalicular or mixed) with or without jaundice. These were usually reversible. Acute pancreatitis has been reported rarely.

Leucopenia and thrombocytopenia have occurred rarely in patients. These are usually reversible. Rare cases of agranulocytosis or of pancytopenia, sometimes with marrow hypoplasia, or aplasia have been reported.

Hypersensitivity reactions (urticaria, angioneurotic oedema, fever, bronchospasm, hypotension, anaphylactic shock) have been seen rarely following the parenteral and oral administration of ranitidine. These reactions have occasionally occurred after a single dose.

As with other H_2 receptor antagonists there have been rare reports of bradycardia and a-v block.

Headache, sometimes severe, and dizziness have been reported in a very small proportion of patients. Rare cases of reversible mental confusion, depression and hallucinations have been reported, predominantly in severely ill and elderly patients.

Skin rash has been reported, including rare cases of erythema multiforme. Musculoskeletal symptoms such as arthralgia and myalgia have been reported rarely.

No clinically significant interference with endocrine or gonadal function has been reported. There have been a few reports of breast symptoms (swelling and/or discomfort) in men taking ranitidine; some cases have resolved on continued ranitidine treatment.

Discontinuation of therapy may be necessary in order to establish the underlying cause.

Overdose: Zantac is very specific in action and accordingly no particular problems are expected following overdosage with the drug. Symptomatic and supportive therapy should be given as appropriate. If need be, the drug may be removed from the plasma by haemodialysis.

Pharmacological properties

Pharmacodynamic properties: Zantac is a specific, rapidly acting H_2-antagonist. It inhibits basal and stimulated secretion of gastric acid, reducing both the volume of the acid and pepsin content of the secretion. Zantac has a relatively long duration of action and a single 150 mg dose effectively suppresses gastric acid secretion for twelve hours.

Pharmacokinetic properties: The bioavailability of ranitidine is consistently about 50%. Absorption of ranitidine after oral administration is rapid and peak plasma concentrations are usually achieved 2–3 hours after administration. Absorption is not significantly impaired by foods or antacids. Ranitidine is not extensively metabolised. Elimination of the drug is primarily by tubular secretion. The elimination half-life of ranitidine is 2–3 hours. In balance studies with 150 mg 3H-ranitidine 60–70% of an oral dose was excreted in urine and 26% in faeces. Analysis of urine excreted in the first 24 hours after dosing showed that 35% of the oral dose was eliminated unchanged. About 6% of the dose is excreted as the N-oxide, 2% as the S-oxide, 2% as desmethyl ranitidine and 1–2% as the furoic acid analogue.

Preclinical safety data: No clinically relevant findings were observed in preclinical studies.

Pharmaceutical particulars

List of excipients: Hydroxypropyl methylcellulose 2906 or 2910 USP; Ethanol (96%) BP; Propyl hydroxybenzoate BP; Butyl hydroxybenzoate BP; Potassium dihydrogen; Orthophosphate AR; Disodium hydrogen orthophosphate; Anhydrous AR; Sodium chloride BP; Saccharin sodium BP; Sorbitol solution 1973 BPC; Mint flavour IFF 17: 42: 3632; Purified water BP.

Incompatibilities: Not applicable.

Shelf life: 24 months.

Special precautions for storage: Zantac syrup should be stored at a temperature not exceeding 25°C.

Nature and contents of container: Amber glass bottles with polypropylene screw caps, or plastic child resistant closures, or plastic child resistant tamper evident closures with either pet faced/al foil/epe wads, or pet faced/al foil/folding box board.

Pack sizes: 300 ml, 2×150 ml.

Instructions for use/handling: None.

Marketing authorisation number PL 10949/108

Date of first authorisation/renewal of authorisation 14 December 1992

Date of (partial) revision of text August 1997

ZANTAC* TABLETS

Presentation Zantac Tablets 150 mg: 5-sided, white, film-coated, biconvex circular tablet, engraved on one face with ZANTAC 150 and on the other with GLAXO plus two linear lines. Each tablet contains ranitidine 150 mg (as hydrochloride).

Zantac Tablets 300 mg: White, capsule-shaped, film-coated tablet, engraved ZANTAC 300 on one face and GLAXO on the other. Each tablet contains ranitidine 300 mg (as hydrochloride).

Zantac Effervescent Tablets 150 mg: White to pale yellow, round, flat, bevel-edged tablets which effervesce on dissolution in water to give a clear, grapefruit/orange flavoured solution. Each tablet contains ranitidine 150 mg (as hydrochloride) and 14.3 mEq (328 mg) of sodium.

Zantac Effervescent Tablets 300 mg: White to pale yellow, round, flat, bevel-edged tablets which effervesce on dissolution in water to give a clear, grapefruit/orange flavoured solution. Each tablet contains ranitidine 300 mg (as hydrochloride) and 20.8 mEq (479 mg) of sodium.

Uses

Indications: Zantac Tablets are indicated for the treatment of duodenal ulcer and benign gastric ulcer, including that associated with non-steroidal anti-inflammatory agents. In addition, Zantac Tablets are indicated for the prevention of NSAID associated duodenal ulcers. Zantac Tablets are indicated for the treatment of duodenal ulcers associated with *Helicobacter pylori* infection.

Zantac Tablets are also indicated for the treatment of post-operative ulcer, Zollinger-Ellison syndrome, and oesophageal reflux disease including the long term management of healed oesophagitis as well as the symptomatic relief of gastro-oesophageal reflux disease. Other patients with chronic episodic dyspepsia, characterised by pain (epigastric or retrosternal) which is related to meals or disturbs sleep but is not associated with the preceding conditions may benefit from ranitidine treatment. Zantac Tablets are indicated for the following conditions where reduction of gastric secretion and acid output is desirable: the prophylaxis of gastrointestinal haemorrhage from stress ulceration in seriously ill patients; the prophylaxis of recurrent haemorrhage in patients with bleeding peptic ulcers and before general anaesthesia in patients considered to be at risk of acid aspiration (Mendelson's syndrome), particularly obstetric patients during labour. For appropriate cases Zantac Injection is also available (see separate SPC).

Mode of action: Zantac is a specific, rapidly acting histamine H_2-antagonist. It inhibits basal and stimulated secretion of gastric acid, reducing both the volume and the acid and pepsin content of the secretion. Zantac has a relatively long duration of action and so a single 150 mg dose effectively suppresses gastric acid secretion for twelve hours.

Dosage and administration Zantac Effervescent Tablets should be placed in half a glass of water (minimum 75 ml) and allowed to dissolve completely before swallowing. The effervescent tablets contain aspartame.

Adults: The usual dosage is 150 mg twice daily, taken in the morning and evening. Alternatively, patients with duodenal ulceration, gastric ulceration or oesophageal reflux disease may be treated with a single bedtime dose of 300 mg. It is not necessary to time the dose in relation to meals. In most cases of duodenal ulcer, benign gastric ulcer and post operative ulcer, healing occurs in four weeks. Healing usually occurs after a further four weeks of treatment in those patients whose ulcers have not fully healed after the initial course of therapy.

In ulcers following non-steroidal anti-inflammatory drug therapy or associated with continued non-steroidal anti-inflammatory drugs, eight week's treatment may be necessary.

For the prevention of non-steroidal anti-inflammatory drug-associated duodenal ulcers ranitidine 150 mg twice daily may be given concomitantly with non-steroidal anti-inflammatory drug therapy. In duodenal ulcer 300 mg twice daily for 4 weeks results in healing rates which are higher than those at 4 weeks with ranitidine 150 mg twice daily or 300 mg nocte. The increased dose has not been associated with an increased incidence of unwanted effects.

For duodenal ulcers associated with *Helicobacter pylori* infection Zantac 300 mg at bedtime or 150 mg twice daily may be given with oral amoxycillin 750 mg three times daily and metronidazole 500 mg three times daily for two weeks. Therapy with Zantac should continue for a further 2 weeks. This dose regimen significantly reduces the frequency of duodenal ulcer recurrence.

Maintenance treatment at a reduced dosage of 150 mg at bedtime is recommended for patients who have responded to short-term therapy, particularly those with a history of recurrent ulcer.

In patients with gastro-oesophageal reflux disease, a dose regimen of 150 mg twice daily for 2 weeks is recommended and this can be repeated in patients in whom the initial symptomatic response is inadequate.

In the management of oesophageal reflux disease, the recommended course of treatment is either 150 mg twice daily or 300 mg at bedtime for up to 8 weeks or if necessary 12 weeks.

In patients with moderate to severe oesophagitis, the dosage of ranitidine may be increased to 150 mg four times daily for up to twelve weeks.

The increased dose has not been associated with an increased incidence of unwanted effects. For the long-term treatment of healed oesophagitis, the recommended adult oral dose is 150 mg twice daily. Long-term treatment is not indicated in the management of patients with unhealed oesophagitis, with or without barrett's epithelium.

In patients with Zollinger-Ellison syndrome, the starting dose is 150 mg three times daily and this may be increased as necessary. Patients with this syndrome have been given increasing doses up to 6 g per day and these doses have been well tolerated.

For patients with chronic episodic dyspepsia the recommended course of treatment is 150 mg twice daily for up to six weeks. Anyone not responding or relapsing shortly afterwards should be investigated.

In the prophylaxis of haemorrhage from stress ulceration in seriously ill patients or the prophylaxis of recurrent haemorrhage in patients bleeding from peptic ulceration, treatment with Zantac Tablets 150 mg twice daily may be substituted for Zantac Injection (see separate SPC) once oral feeding commences in patients considered to be still at risk from these conditions.

In patients thought to be at risk of acid aspiration syndrome an oral dose of 150 mg can be given 2 hours before induction of general anaesthesia, and preferably also 150 mg the previous evening. Alternatively, Zantac Injection for intravenous and intramuscular use is also available (see separate SPC).

In obstetric patients at commencement of labour, an oral dose of 150 mg may be given followed by 150 mg at six-hourly intervals. It is recommended that since gastric emptying and drug absorption are delayed during labour, any patient requiring emergency general anaesthesia should be given, in addition, a non-particulate antacid (e.g. sodium citrate) prior to induction of anaesthesia. The usual precautions to avoid acid aspiration should also be taken.

Children: The recommended oral dose for treatment of peptic ulcer in children is 2 mg/kg to 4 mg/kg twice daily to a maximum of 300 mg ranitidine per day.

Contra-indications, warnings, etc

Contra-indications: Ranitidine is contra-indicated for patients known to have hypersensitivity to any component of the preparation.

Precautions: Treatment with a histamine H_2-antagonist may mask symptoms associated with carcinoma of the stomach and may therefore delay diagnosis of the condition. Accordingly, where gastric ulcer has been diagnosed or in patients of middle age and over with new or recently changed dyspeptic symptoms the possibility of malignancy should be excluded before therapy with Zantac Tablets is instituted.

Ranitidine is excreted via the kidney and so plasma levels of the drug are increased in patients with severe renal impairment. Accordingly, it is recommended that the therapeutic regimen for Zantac in such patients be 150 mg at night for 4 to 8 weeks. The same dose should be used for maintenance treatment should this be deemed necessary. If an ulcer has not healed after treatment the standard dosage regimen of 150 mg twice daily should be instituted, followed, if need be, by maintenance treatment of 150 mg at night.

Regular supervision of patients who are taking non-steroidal anti-inflammatory drugs concomitantly with ranitidine is recommended, especially in the elderly. Current evidence shows that ranitidine protects against NSAID associated ulceration in the duodenum and not in the stomach.

Although clinical reports of acute intermittent porphyria associated with ranitidine administration have been rare and inconclusive, ranitidine should be avoided in patients with a history of this condition.

Zantac Effervescent Tablets contain sodium (see Presentation section). Care should therefore be taken in treating patients in whom sodium restriction is indicated. As Zantac Effervescent Tablets contain aspartame they should be used with caution in patients with phenylketonuria.

Pregnancy and lactation: Zantac crosses the placenta but therapeutic doses administered to obstetric patients in labour or undergoing caesarean section have been without any adverse effect on labour, delivery or subsequent neonatal progress. Zantac is also excreted in human breast milk.

Like other drugs, Zantac should only be used during pregnancy and nursing if considered essential.

Side-effects: The following have been reported as events in clinical trials or in the routine management of patients treated with ranitidine. The relationship to ranitidine therapy has not been established in many cases.

Transient and reversible changes in liver function tests can occur. There have been occasional reports of hepatitis (hepatocellular, hepatocanalicular or mixed) with or without jaundice. These were usually reversible. Acute pancreatitis has been reported rarely.

Leucopenia and thrombocytopenia have occurred rarely in patients. These are usually reversible. Rare cases of agranulocytosis or of pancytopenia, sometimes with marrow hypoplasia, or aplasia have been reported.

Hypersensitivity reactions (urticaria, angioneurotic oedema, fever, bronchospasm, hypotension, anaphylactic shock) have been seen rarely following the parenteral and oral administration of ranitidine. These reactions have occasionally occurred after a single dose.

As with other H_2-receptor antagonists, there have been rare reports of bradycardia and A-V block.

Headache, sometimes severe, and dizziness have been reported in a very small proportion of patients. Rare cases of reversible mental confusion, depression and hallucinations have been reported, predominantly in severely ill and elderly patients.

Skin rash has been reported, including rare cases of erythema multiforme. Musculoskeletal symptoms such as arthralgia and myalgia have been reported rarely.

No clinically significant interference with endocrine or gonadal function has been reported. There have been a few reports of breast symptoms (swelling and/or discomfort) in men taking ranitidine; some cases have resolved on continued ranitidine treatment. Discontinuation of therapy may be necessary in order to establish the underlying cause.

Antibiotic associated diarrhoea may occur when amoxycillin and metronidazole are taken with ranitidine.

Use in elderly patients: Rates of healing of ulcers in clinical trial patients aged 65 and over have not been found to differ from those in younger patients. Additionally, there was no difference in the incidence of adverse effects.

Overdosage: Zantac is very specific in action and accordingly no particular problems are expected following overdosage. In the case of the effervescent formulations, clinicians should be aware of the sodium content (see Presentation section). Symptomatic and supportive therapy should be given as appropriate. If need be, the drug may be removed from the plasma by haemodialysis.

Pharmaceutical precautions Effervescent products should be stored below 30°C in a dry place.

Legal category POM.

Package quantities

Zantac Tablets 150 mg: Carton of 60 tablets, foil-wrapped (OP).

Zantac Tablets 300 mg: Carton of 30 tablets, foil-wrapped (OP).

Zantac Effervescent Tablets 150 mg: Carton of 4 polypropylene tubes, each containing 15 tablets (OP).

Zantac Effervescent Tablets 300 mg: Carton of 2 polypropylene tubes, each containing 15 tablets (OP).

Further information

Drug interactions: Ranitidine does not inhibit the hepatic cytochrome P450-linked mixed function oxygenase system. Accordingly, ranitidine does not potentiate the actions of drugs which are inactivated by this enzyme; these include amoxycillin, diazepam, lignocaine, phenytoin, metronidazole, propranolol, theophylline and warfarin. There is no evidence of an interaction between ranitidine and amoxycillin or metronidazole.

Pharmacokinetics: The bioavailability of ranitidine is consistently about 50%. Absorption of ranitidine after oral administration is rapid and peak plasma concentrations are usually achieved 2-3 hours after administration. Absorption is not significantly impaired by food or antacids. Ranitidine is not extensively metabolised. Elimination of the drug is primarily by tubular secretion. The elimination half-life of ranitidine is 2-3 hours. In balance studies with 150 mg 3H-ranitidine 60-70% of an oral dose was excreted in urine and 26% in faeces. Analysis of urine excreted in the first 24 hours after dosing showed that 35% of the oral dose was eliminated unchanged. About 6% of the dose is excreted as the N-oxide, 2% as the S-oxide, 2% as desmethyl ranitidine and 1-2% as the furoic acid analogue.

Use in renal transplants: Zantac has been used in patients with renal transplants.

Duodenal ulcers associated with Helicobacter pylori: Helicobacter pylori infects about 95% of patients with duodenal ulcer and 80% of patients with gastric ulcer.

Clinical evidence has shown that ranitidine combined with amoxycillin and metronidazole eradicates *Helicobacter pylori* in approximately 90% of patients. This combination therapy has been shown to significantly reduce duodenal ulcer recurrence.

Product licence numbers

Zantac Tablets 150 mg	10949/0042
Zantac Tablets 300 mg	10949/0043
Zantac Effervescent 150 mg Tablets	10949/0137
Zantac Effervescent 300 mg Tablets	10949/0138

Date of revision 6 January 1999.

ZINACEF*

Qualitative and quantitative composition Vials contain either 250 mg, 750 mg or 1.5 g cefuroxime (as sodium).

Pharmaceutical form Cefuroxime is a white to cream powder to which appropriate amounts of water are added to prepare an off-white suspension for intramuscular use or a yellowish solution for intravenous administration.

Clinical particulars

Therapeutic indications: Zinacef is a bactericidal cephalosporin antibiotic which is resistant to most β-lactamases and is active against a wide range of Gram-positive and Gram-negative organisms. It is indicated for the treatment of infections before the infecting organism has been identified or when caused by sensitive bacteria. In addition, it is an effective prophylactic against post-operative infection in a variety of operations. Usually Zinacef will be effective alone, but when appropriate it may be used in combination with an aminoglycoside antibiotic, or in conjunction with metronidazole, orally or by suppository or injection.

In situations where mixed aerobic and anaerobic infections are encountered or suspected (e.g. peritonitis, aspiration pneumonia, abscesses in the lung, pelvis and brain), or are likely to occur (e.g. in association with colorectal or gynaecological surgery) it is appropriate to administer Zinacef in combination with metronidazole.

Most of these infections will respond to an i.v. regimen of Zinacef (750 mg) plus metronidazole injection (500 mg/100 ml) administered eight-hourly for which the Zinacef/Metronidazole Infusion Kit may be appropriate. In more severe or well established mixed infections, an i.v. regimen of Zinacef (1.5 g) plus metronidazole injection (500 mg/100 ml) eight-hourly may be indicated. For the prophylaxis of infection in surgery (e.g. colorectal and gynaecological) a single dose of 1.5 g Zinacef plus metronidazole injection (500 mg/100 ml) is appropriate. Alternatively, this may be followed by two 750 mg doses of Zinacef plus metronidazole.

Indications include:

Respiratory tract infections for example, acute and chronic bronchitis, infected bronchiectasis, bacterial pneumonia, lung abscess and post operative chest infections.

Ear, nose and throat infections for example, sinusitis, tonsillitis and pharyngitis.

Urinary tract infections for example, acute and chronic pyelonephritis, cystitis and asymptomatic bacteriuria.

Soft-tissue infections for example, cellulitis, erysipelas, peritonitis and wound infections.

Bone and joint infections for example, osteomyelitis and septic arthritis.

Obstetric and gynaecological infections pelvic inflammatory diseases.

Gonorrhoea particularly when penicillin is unsuitable.

Other infections including septicaemia and meningitis.

Prophylaxis against infection in abdominal, pelvic, orthopaedic, cardiac, pulmonary, oesophageal and vascular surgery where there is increased risk from infection.

Posology and method of administration:

Intramuscular: Add 1 ml water for injections to 250 mg Zinacef or 3 ml water for injections to 750 mg Zinacef. Shake gently to produce an opaque suspension.

Intravenous: Dissolve Zinacef in water for injections using at least 2 ml for 250 mg, at least 6 ml for 750 mg or 15 ml for 1.5 g. For short intravenous infusion (e.g. up to 30 minutes), 1.5 g may be dissolved in 50 ml water for injections. These solutions may be given directly into the vein or introduced into the tubing of the giving set if the patient is receiving parenteral fluids.

Adults: Many infections will respond to 750 mg t.i.d. by i.m. or i.v. injection. For more severe infections, this dose should be increased to 1.5 g t.i.d. i.v. The frequency of i.m. or i.v. injection can be increased to six-hourly if necessary, giving total doses of 3 g to 6 g daily.

Infants and children: Doses of 30 to 100 mg/kg/day given as three or four divided doses. A dose of 60 mg/kg/day will be appropriate for most infections.

Neonates: Doses of 30 to 100 mg/kg/day given as two or three divided doses. In the first weeks of life the serum half-life of cefuroxime can be three to five times that in adults.

Elderly: See dosage in adults.

Other recommendations:
Gonorrhoea: 1.5 g should be given as a single dose. This may be given as 2×750 mg injections into different sites, e.g. each buttock.

Meningitis: Zinacef is suitable for sole therapy of bacterial meningitis due to sensitive strains. The following dosages are recommended:

Infants and children: 200 to 240 mg/kg/day i.v. in three or four divided doses. This dosage may be reduced to 100 mg/kg/day i.v. after three days or when clinical improvement occurs.

Neonates: The initial dose should be 100 mg/kg/day i.v. A reduction to 50 mg/kg/day i.v. may be made when clinically indicated.

Adults: 3 g i.v. every eight hours. Data are not yet sufficient to recommend a dose for intrathecal administration.

Prophylaxis: The usual dose is 1.5 g i.v. with induction of anaesthesia for abdominal, pelvic and orthopaedic operations, but may be supplemented with two 750 mg i.m. doses eight and sixteen hours later. In cardiac, pulmonary, oesophageal and vascular operations, the usual dose is 1.5 g i.v. with induction of anaesthesia continuing with 750 mg i.m. t.d.s. for a further 24 to 48 hours.

In total joint replacement, 1.5 g cefuroxime powder may be mixed dry with each pack of methyl methacrylate cement polymer before adding the liquid monomer.

Dosage in impaired renal function: Cefuroxime is excreted by the kidneys. Therefore, as with all such antibiotics, in patients with markedly impaired renal function it is recommended that the dosage of Zinacef should be reduced to compensate for its slower excretion. However, it is not necessary to reduce the dose until the creatinine clearance falls below 20 ml/min. In adults with marked impairment (creatinine clearance 10-20 ml/min) 750 mg b.d. is recommended and with severe impairment (creatinine clearance <10 ml/min) 750 mg once daily is adequate. For patients on haemodialysis a further 750 mg dose should be given at the end of each dialysis. When continuous peritoneal dialysis is being used, a suitable dosage is usually 750 mg twice daily.

For patients in renal failure on continuous arterio-venous haemodialysis or high-flux haemofiltration in intensive therapy units a suitable dosage is 750 mg twice daily. For low-flux haemofiltration follow the dosage recommended under impaired renal function.

Contra-indications: Hypersensitivity to cephalosporin antibiotics.

Special warnings and special precautions for use: Cephalosporin antibiotics may in general be given safely to patients who are hypersensitive to penicillins, although cross-reactions have been reported. Especial care is indicated in patients who have experienced an anaphylactic reaction to penicillin.

There may be some variation on the results of biochemical tests of renal function, but these do not appear to be of clinical importance. As a precaution, renal function should be monitored if this is already impaired.

Interaction with other medicaments and other forms of interaction: Cephalosporin antibiotics at high dosage should be given with caution to patients receiving concurrent treatment with potent diuretics such as frusemide and aminoglycosides, as these combinations are suspected of adversely affecting renal function. Clinical experience with Zinacef has shown that this is not likely to be a problem at the recommended dose levels.

Zinacef does not interfere in enzyme-based tests for glycosuria. Slight interference with copper reduction methods (Benedict's, Fehling's, Clinitest) may be observed. However, this should not lead to false-positive results, as may be experienced with some other cephalosporins.

It is recommended that either the glucose oxidase or hexokinase methods are used to determine blood/plasma glucose levels in patients receiving Zinacef. This antibiotic does not interfere in the alkaline picrate assay for creatinine.

Pregnancy and lactation: There is no experimental evidence of embryopathic or tetratogenic effects attributable to Zinacef but, as with all drugs, it should be administered with caution during the early months of pregnancy.

Cefuroxime is excreted in human milk, and consequently caution should be exercised when Zinacef is administered to a nursing mother.

Effect on ability to drive and use machines: None reported.

Undesirable effects: Adverse reactions to Zinacef have occurred relatively infrequently and have been generally mild and transient in nature.

Hypersensitivity reactions have been reported; these include skin rashes (maculopapular and urticarial), drug fever and very rarely anaphylaxis.

As with other antibiotics, prolonged use may result in the overgrowth of non-susceptible organisms, e.g. candida. Gastrointestinal disturbance, including, very rarely, symptoms of pseudomembranous colitis may occur during or after treatment. The principal changes in haematological parameters seen in some patients have been of decreased haemoglobin concentration and of eosinophilia, leukopenia and neutropenia. Cephalosporins as a class tend to be absorbed onto the surface of red cell membranes and react with antibodies directed against the drug to produce a positive Coombs test (which can interfere with cross-matching of blood) and very rarely haemolytic anaemia.

Although there are sometimes transient rises in serum liver enzymes or serum bilirubin, particularly in patients with pre-existing liver disease, there is no evidence of hepatic involvement.

Transient pain may be experienced at the site of intramuscular injection. This is more likely to occur with higher doses. However, it is unlikely to be a cause for discontinuation of treatment. Occasionally, thrombophlebitis may follow intravenous injection.

As with other cephalosporins, there have been very rare reports of thrombocytopenia.

Overdose: Overdosage of cephalosporins can cause cerebral irritation leading to convulsions. Serum levels of cefuroxime can be reduced by haemodialysis or peritoneal dialysis.

Pharmacological properties
Pharmacodynamic properties: Cefuroxime is a bactericidal cephalosporin antibiotic which is resistant to most β-lactamases and is active against a wide range of Gram-positive and Gram-negative organisms.

It is highly active against *Staphylococcus aureus*, including strains which are resistant to penicillin (but not the rare methicillin-resistant strains), *Staph. epidermidis, Haemophilus influenzae,* Klebsiella spp, Enterobacter spp, *Streptococcus pyogenes, Escherichia coli, Str. mitis (viridans group),* Clostridium spp, *Proteus mirabilis, Pr. rettgeri, Salmonella typhi, S. typhimurium* and other Salmonella spp, Shigella spp, Neisseria spp (including β-lactamase producing strains of *N. gonorrhoea*) and *Bordetella pertussis.* It is also moderately active against strains of *Pr. vulgaris, Morganella morganii* (formerly *Proteus morganii*) and *Bacteroides fragilis.*

The following organisms are not susceptible to cefuroxime: *Clostridium difficile,* Pseudomonas spp, Campylobacter spp, *Acinetobacter calcoaceticus,* Legionella spp and methicillin-resistant strains of *Staph. aureus* and *Staph. epidermidis.* Some strains of the following genera have also been found not to be susceptible to Zinacef: *Strep. faecalis, Morganella morganii, Proteus vulgaris,* Enterobacter spp, Citrobacter spp, Serratia spp and *Bacteroides fragilis.*

In vitro the activities of Zinacef and aminoglycoside antibiotics in combination have been shown to be at least additive with occasional evidence of synergy.

Metronidazole is active against a wide range of pathogenic micro-organisms notably species of Bacteroides, Fusobacteria, Clostridia, Eubacteria and anaerobic cocci. It is also active against *Gardnerella vaginalis, Trichomonas, Entamoeba histolytica, Giardia lamblia* and *Balantidium coli.*

Pharmacokinetic properties: Peak levels of cefuroxime are achieved within 30 to 45 minutes after intramuscular administration. The serum half-life after either intramuscular or intravenous injection is approximately 70 minutes. Concurrent administration of probenecid prolongs the excretion of the antibiotic and produces an elevated peak serum level. There is almost complete recovery of unchanged cefuroxime in the urine within 24 hours of administration, the major part being eliminated in the first six hours. Approximately 50% is excreted through the renal tubules and approximately 50% by glomerular filtration. Concentrations of cefuroxime in excess of the minimum inhibitory levels for common pathogens can be achieved in bone, synovial fluid and aqueous humor. Cefuroxime passes the blood-brain barrier when the meninges are inflamed.

Pharmaceutical particulars
List of excipients: None.

Incompatibilities: Cefuroxime is compatible with most commonly used intravenous fluids and electrolyte solutions.

The pH of 2.74% w/v Sodium Bicarbonate Injection BP considerably affects the colour of solutions and therefore this solution is not recommended for the dilution of Zinacef. However, if required, for patients receiving sodium bicarbonate injection by infusion, the Zinacef may be introduced into the tube of the giving set.

Zinacef should not be mixed in the syringe with aminoglycoside antibiotics.

Shelf life: Two years when stored below 25°C and protected from light.

Special precautions for storage: Store below 25°C and protect from light.

After constitution, Zinacef should be stored at 2 to 8°C for no longer than 24 hours.

Nature and contents of container:

(1) Moulded glass (type I or III) vials with bromobutyl or fluoro-resin laminated butyl rubber plug, overseal and flip-off cap containing either 250 mg, 750 mg or 1.5 g Zinacef.

(2) A kit containing 1 vial of Zinacef 750 mg and 1×50 ml infusion of normal saline (PL3460/0015), a transfer needle for the preparation of an intravenous infusion and a swab (Zinacef/saline infusion kit).

(3) A kit containing 1 vial of Zinacef 750 mg and 1×500 mg/100 ml infusion of metronidazole (PL5271/0047) a transfer needle, a port stopper and a swab; for the preparation of an intravenous infusion (Zinacef/metronidazole infusion kit).

(4) A bulk pack of 100 vials.

(5) Monovial containing either 750 mg or 1.5 g Zinacef with transfer needle.

Marketing authorisation number PL 0004/0263

Date of first authorisation/renewal of authorisation
MAA: 07.04.83
Renewal: 28.04.97

Date of (partial) revision of the text 26 November 1997

Legal category POM

ZINNAT* TABLETS AND SUSPENSION

Presentation Zinnat Tablets 125 mg: white, film-coated, capsule-shaped tablets engraved with 'Glaxo' on one side and '125' on the other. Each tablet contains cefuroxime 125 mg (as cefuroxime axetil).

Zinnat Tablets 250 mg: white, film-coated, capsule-shaped tablets engraved with 'Glaxo' on one side and '250' on the other. Each tablet contains cefuroxime 250 mg (as cefuroxime axetil).

Zinnat Suspension 125 mg: granules for oral suspension in multidose bottles and sachets. Constitution of the multidose bottles as directed yields a suspension containing 125 mg of cefuroxime (as cefuroxime axetil) in each 5 ml. Constitution of the contents of the sachets gives a suspension containing 125 mg of cefuroxime (as cefuroxime axetil).

Uses Cefuroxime axetil is an oral prodrug of the bactericidal cephalosporin antibiotic cefuroxime, which is resistant to most β-lactamases and is active against a wide range of Gram-positive and Gram-negative organisms. It is indicated for the treatment of infections caused by sensitive bacteria.

Indications include:
Lower respiratory tract infections: for example, acute bronchitis, acute exacerbations of chronic bronchitis and pneumonia.

Upper respiratory tract infections: for example, ear, nose, throat infections, such as otitis media, sinusitis, tonsillitis and pharyngitis.

Genito-urinary tract infections: for example, pyelonephritis, cystitis and urethritis.

Skin and soft-tissue infections: for example, furunculosis, pyoderma and impetigo.

Gonorrhoea: acute uncomplicated gonococcal urethritis, and cervicitis.

Treatment of early Lyme disease and subsequent prevention of late Lyme disease: in adults and children over 12 years old.

Microbiology: Cefuroxime axetil owes its *in vivo* bactericidal activity to the parent compound, cefuroxime. Cefuroxime is a well-characterised and effective antibacterial agent which has broad-spectrum bactericidal activity against a wide range of common pathogens, including β-lactamase-producing strains. Cefuroxime has good stability to bacterial β-lactamase and consequently, is active against many ampicillin-resistant and amoxycillin-resistant strains. The bactericidal action of cefuroxime results from inhibition of cell-wall synthesis by binding to essential target proteins.

Cefuroxime is usually active against the following organisms *in vitro*:

Aerobes, Gram-negative: *Haemophilus influenzae* (including ampicillin-resistant strains); *Haemophilus parainfluenzae; Moraxella catarrhalis; Escherichia coli;* Klebsiella spp; *Proteus mirabilis; Proteus inconstans;* Providencia spp; *Proteus rettgeri* and *Neisseria gonorrhoeae* (including penicillinase and non-penicillinase-producing strains).

Some strains of *Morganella morganii,* Enterobacter spp and Citrobacter spp have been shown by *in vitro* tests to be resistant to cefuroxime and other β-lactam antibiotics.

Aerobes, Gram-positive: *Staphylococcus aureus* (including penicillinase-producing strains but excluding methicillin-resistant strains); *Staphylococcus epidermidis* (including penicillinase producing strains but excluding methicillin-resistant strains); *Streptococcus pyogenes (*and β-haemolytic streptococci), *Streptococcus pneumoniae;* Streptococcus Group B (*Streptococcus agalactiae)* and Propionibacterium spp. Certain strains of enterococci, e.g. *Streptococcus faecalis,* are resistant.

Anaerobes, Gram-positive and Gram-negative cocci (including Peptococcus and Peptostreptococcus spp); Gram-positive bacilli (including Clostridium spp) and Gram-negative bacilli (including Bacteroides and Fusobacterium spp). Most strains of *Bacteroides fragilis* are resistant.

Other organisms, *Borrelia burgdorferi.*

Pseudomonas spp, Campylobacter spp, *Acinetobacter calcoaceticus, Listeria monocytogenes,* Legionella spp and most strains of Serratia and *Proteus vulgaris* and *Clostridium difficile* are resistant to many cephalosporins including cefuroxime.

Dosage and administration
Adults: Most infections will respond to 250 mg b.d. In mild to moderate lower respiratory tract infections e.g. bronchitis 250 mg b.d. should be given. For more severe lower respiratory tract infections, or if pneumonia is suspected then 500 mg b.d. should be given. For urinary tract infections a dose of 125 mg b.d. is usually adequate; in pyelonephritis the recommended dose is 250 mg b.d. A single dose of one gram is recommended for the treatment of uncomplicated gonorrhoea. Lyme disease in adults and children over the age of 12 years: the recommended dose is 500 mg b.d. for 20 days.

Children: The usual dose is 125 mg b.d. (1 x 125 mg tablet or 5 ml of suspension or 1 x 125 mg sachet), or 10 mg/kg b.d. to a maximum of 250 mg daily. For otitis media, in children less than 2 years of age the usual dosage is 125 mg b.d. (1 x 125 mg tablet or 5 ml of suspension or 1 x 125 mg sachet), or 10 mg/kg b.d. to a maximum of 250 mg daily and in children over 2 years of age, 250 mg b.d. (1 x 250 mg tablet or 10 ml of suspension or 2 x 125 mg sachets), or 15 mg/kg b.d. to a maximum of 500 mg daily. There is no experience in children under 3 months of age.

Zinnat Tablets should not be crushed. Therefore, in younger children the suspension is more appropriate.

No special precautions are necessary in patients with renal impairment or on renal dialysis or in the elderly at dosages up to the normal maximum of 1 g per day.

The usual course of therapy is seven days.

Zinnat should be taken after food for optimum absorption.

Contra-indications, warnings, etc
Contra-indications: Hypersensitivity to cephalosporin antibiotics.

Precautions: Cephalosporin antibiotics may in general be given safely to patients who are hypersensitive to penicillins, although cross-reactions have been reported. Special care is indicated in patients who have experienced an anaphylactic reaction to penicillins.

As with other antibiotics, prolonged use of cefuroxime axetil may result in the overgrowth of non-susceptible organisms (e.g. Candida, Enterococci, *Clostridium difficile*), which may require interruption of treatment. Pseudomembranous colitis has been reported with the use of broad-spectrum antibiotics, therefore, it is important to consider its diagnosis in patients who develop serious diarrhoea during or after antibiotic use.

There is no experimental evidence of embryopathic or teratogenic effects attributable to cefuroxime axetil but, as with all drugs, it should be administered with caution during early months of pregnancy. Cefuroxime is excreted in human milk, and consequently caution should be exercised when cefuroxime axetil is administered to a nursing mother.

It is recommended that either the glucose oxidase or hexokinase methods are used to determine blood/plasma glucose levels in patients receiving cefuroxime axetil. This antibiotic does not interfere in the alkaline picrate assay for creatinine.

The Jarisch-Herxheimer reaction has been seen following Zinnat treatment of Lyme disease. It results from the bactericidal activity of Zinnat on the causative organism of Lyme disease, the spirochaete *Borrelia burgdorferi.* Patients should be reassured that this is a common and usually self-limited consequence of antibiotic treatment of Lyme disease.

Side-effects: Adverse reactions to cefuroxime axetil have been generally mild and transient in nature.

As with other cephalosporins, there have been rare reports of interstitial nephritis erythema multiforme, Stevens-Johnson syndrome, toxic epidermal necrolysis (exanthematic necrolysis) and hypersensitivity reactions including skin rashes, urticaria, pruritus, drug fever, serum sickness, and very rarely anaphylaxis.

Gastrointestinal disturbances including diarrhoea and nausea and vomiting have been reported. Diarrhoea, although uncommon, is more likely to be associated with higher doses.

As with other broad-spectrum antibiotics, there have been occasional reports of pseudomembranous colitis.

Headache has also been reported.

There have been rare reports of thrombocytopenia and leucopenia (sometimes profound).

Eosinophilia and transient increases of hepatic enzyme levels [ALT (SGPT), AST (SGOT) and LDH] have been noted during Zinnat therapy. As with other cephalosporins, jaundice has been reported very rarely. Cephalosporins as a class tend to be absorbed onto the surface of red cell membranes and react with antibodies directed against the drug to produce a positive Coombs test (which can interfere with cross-matching of blood) and very rarely haemolytic anaemia.

Overdosage: Overdosage of cephalosporins can cause cerebral irritancy leading to convulsions.

Serum levels of cefuroxime can be reduced by haemodialysis or peritoneal dialysis.

Pharmaceutical precautions Zinnat Tablets should be stored below 30°C.

Zinnat Suspension granules should be stored below 30°C.

Directions for constituting suspension in bottles: Shake the bottle to loosen dry granules, add water as directed on the label and replace cap. INVERT bottle and shake granules down into water using a rocking action. Continue to shake the bottle until the suspension is well dispersed. If using a dosing syringe, allow the constituted suspension to stand for at least one hour before taking the first dose.

If desired the dose of the constituted suspension may be added to children's cold drinks such as fruit drinks or cold milk immediately prior to administration.

Directions for constituting suspension from sachets: Empty granules from sachet into a glass, add 10 ml water, or 10 ml children's cold drinks such as fruit drinks or milk, stir well and drink straight away.

The constituted suspension (in multidose bottles) should be stored below 25°C and preferably in a refrigerator. The constituted suspension (from sachets) and the further diluted suspension from multidose bottles in children's cold drinks should be taken immediately.

The constituted suspension (in multidose bottles) retains potency for up to 10 days when stored below 25°C.

Zinnat granules should not be constituted in hot drinks. The constituted suspension should not be mixed with hot drinks.

Legal category POM.

Package quantities Zinnat Tablets, both 125 mg and 250 mg strengths, are supplied in foil strips of 14 and 50.

Zinnat Suspension, 125 mg/5 ml, granules for oral suspension are supplied in multidose bottles of 70 ml and in 125 mg sachets packed in cartons of 14.

Further information After oral administration, cefuroxime axetil is absorbed from the gastrointestinal tract and rapidly hydrolysed in the intestinal mucosa and blood to release cefuroxime into the circulation. Optimum absorption occurs when it is administered after a meal. Peak serum cefuroxime levels occur approximately two to three hours after oral dosing. The serum half life is about 1.2 hours. Approximately 50% of serum cefuroxime is protein bound. Cefuroxime is not metabolised and is excreted by glomerular filtration and tubular secretion. Concurrent administration of probenecid increases the area under the mean serum concentration time curve by 50%. Serum levels of cefuroxime are reduced by dialysis.

Cefuroxime is also available as the sodium salt (Zinacef) for parenteral administration. This permits parenteral therapy with cefuroxime to be followed by oral therapy in situations where a change from parenteral to oral treatment is clinically indicated.

Product licence numbers
Zinnat Tablets 125 mg 10949/0095
Zinnat Tablets 250 mg 10949/0096
Zinnat Suspension 125 mg 10949/0094

ZOFRAN* INJECTION
ZOFRAN* FLEXI-AMP INJECTION

Qualitative and quantitative composition Zofran Injection 2 mg/ml: 2 ml glass ampoules each containing 4 mg ondansetron (as hydrochloride dihydrate) in aqueous solution for intramuscular or intravenous administration. 4 ml glass ampoules each containing 8 mg ondansetron (as hydrochloride dihydrate) in aqueous solution for intravenous or intramuscular administration.

Zofran Flexi-amp injection 2 mg/ml: 2 ml plastic ampoules each containing 4 mg ondansetron (as hydrochloride dihydrate) in aqueous solution for intramuscular or intravenous administration. 4 ml plastic ampoules each containing 8 mg ondansetron (as hydrochloride dihydrate) in aqueous solution for intravenous or intramuscular administration.

Pharmaceutical form Injection (aqueous solution).

Clinical particulars
Therapeutic indications: Zofran is indicated for the management of nausea and vomiting induced by cytotoxic chemotherapy and radiotherapy, and for the prevention and treatment of post-operative nausea and vomiting (PONV).

Posology and method of administration:
Chemotherapy and radiotherapy
Adults: The emetogenic potential of cancer treatment varies according to the doses and combinations of chemotherapy and radiotherapy regimens used. The route of administration and dose of Zofran should be flexible in the range of 8 to 32 mg a day and selected as shown below.

Emetogenic chemotherapy and radiotherapy. Zofran can be given either by rectal, oral (tablets or syrup), intravenous or intramuscular administration.

For most patients receiving emetogenic chemotherapy or radiotherapy, Zofran 8 mg should be administered as a slow intravenous or intramuscular injection immediately before treatment, followed by 8 mg orally twelve hourly.

To protect against delayed or prolonged emesis after the first 24 hours, oral or rectal treatment with Zofran should be continued for up to 5 days after a course of treatment.

Highly emetogenic chemotherapy: For patients receiving highly emetogenic chemotherapy, e.g. high-dose cisplatin, Zofran can be given either by rectal, intravenous or intramuscular administration. Zofran has been shown to be equally effective in the following dose schedules over the first 24 hours of chemotherapy.

A single dose of 8 mg by slow intravenous or intramuscular administration immediately before chemotherapy.

A dose of 8 mg by slow intravenous or intramuscular injection immediately before chemotherapy, followed by two further intravenous or intramuscular doses of 8 mg two to four hours apart, or by a constant infusion of 1 mg/hour for up to 24 hours.

A single dose of 32 mg diluted in 50 to 100 ml of saline or other compatible infusion fluid (see *Instructions for use/handling*) and infused over not less than 15 minutes immediately before chemotherapy.

The selection of dose regimen should be determined by the severity of the emetogenic challenge.

The efficacy of Zofran in highly emetogenic chemotherapy may be enhanced by the addition of a single intravenous dose of dexamethasone sodium phosphate, 20 mg administered prior to chemotherapy.

To protect against delayed or prolonged emesis after the first 24 hours, oral or rectal treatment with Zofran should be continued for up to 5 days after a course of treatment.

Children: Zofran may be administered as a single intravenous dose of 5 mg/m² immediately before chemotherapy, followed by 4 mg orally twelve hours later. 4 mg orally twice daily should be continued for up to 5 days after a course of treatment.

Elderly: Zofran is well tolerated by patients over 65 years and no alteration of dosage, dosing frequency or route of administration are required.

Patients with renal impairment: No alteration of daily dosage or frequency of dosing, or route of administration are required.

Patients with hepatic impairment: Clearance of Zofran is significantly reduced and serum half-life significantly prolonged in subjects with moderate or severe impairment of hepatic function. In such patients a total daily dose of 8 mg should not be exceeded.

Post-operative nausea and vomiting (PONV): Adults: For the prevention of PONV Zofran can be administered orally or by intravenous or intramuscular injection. Zofran may be administered as a single dose of 4 mg given by intramuscular or slow intravenous injection at induction of anaesthesia.

For treatment of established PONV a single dose of 4 mg given by intramuscular or slow intravenous injection is recommended.

Children (aged 2 years and over): For prevention of PONV in paediatric patients having surgery performed under general anaesthesia, ondansetron may be administered by slow intravenous injection at a dose of 0.1 mg/kg up to a maximum of 4 mg either prior to, at or after induction of anaesthesia.

For treatment of established PONV in paediatric patients, ondansetron may be administered by slow intravenous injection at a dose of 0.1 mg/kg up to a maximum of 4 mg.

There is limited data on the use of Zofran in the prevention and treatment of PONV in children under 2 years of age.

Elderly: There is limited experience in the use of Zofran in the prevention and treatment of PONV in the elderly, however, Zofran is well tolerated in patients over 65 years receiving chemotherapy.

Patients with renal impairment: No alteration of daily dosage or frequency of dosing, or route of administration are required.

Patients with hepatic impairment: Clearance of Zofran is significantly reduced and serum half life significantly prolonged in subjects with moderate or severe impairment of hepatic function. In such patients a total daily dose of 8 mg should not be exceeded.

Patients with poor sparteine/debrisoquine metabolism: The elimination half-life of ondansetron is not altered in subjects classified as poor metabolisers of sparteine and debrisoquine. Consequently in such patients repeat dosing will give drug exposure levels no different from those of the general population. No alteration of daily dosage or frequency of dosing are required.

Contra-indications: Hypersensitivity to any component of the preparation.

Special warnings and precautions for use: Hypersensitivity reactions have been reported in patients who have exhibited hypersensitivity to other selective $5HT_3$ receptor antagonists. As ondansetron is known to increase large bowel transit time, patients with signs of subacute intestinal obstruction should be monitored following administration.

Interaction with other medicaments and other forms of interaction: There is no evidence that ondansetron either induces or inhibits the metabolism of other drugs commonly co-administered with it. Specific studies have shown that ondansetron does not interact with alcohol, temazepam, frusemide, tramadol and propofol.

Pregnancy and lactation: The safety of ondansetron for use in human pregnancy has not been established. Evaluation of experimental animal studies does not indicate direct or indirect harmful effects with respect to the development of the embryo, or foetus, the course of gestation and peri- and post-natal development. However, as animal studies are not always predictive of human response the use of ondansetron in pregnancy is not recommended. Tests have shown that ondansetron passes into the milk of lactating animals. It is therefore recommended that mothers receiving Zofran should not breast-feed their baby.

Effects on ability to drive and use machines: In psychomotor testing ondansetron does not impair performance nor cause sedation.

Undesirable effects: Ondansetron is known to increase large bowel transit time and may cause constipation in some patients. The following side effects can occur: headache, a sensation of flushing or warmth, hiccups and occasional transient, asymptomatic increases in aminotransferases. There have been rare reports of immediate hypersensitivity reactions, sometimes severe, including anaphylaxis. Rare cases of transient visual disturbances (e.g. blurred vision) and dizziness have been reported during rapid intravenous administration of ondansetron. There have been rare reports suggestive of involuntary movement disorders without definitive evidence of persistent clinical sequelae and seizures have been rarely observed although no known pharmacological mechanism can account for ondansetron causing these effects. Chest pain, cardiac arrhythmias, hypotension and bradycardia have been rarely reported.

Occasionally, hypersensitivity reactions around the injection site (e.g. rash, urticaria, itching) may occur, sometimes extending along the drug administration vein.

Overdose: Little is known at present about overdosage with ondansetron, however, a limited number of patients received overdoses. Manifestations that have been reported include visual disturbances, severe constipation, hypotension and a vasovagal episode with transient second degree AV block. In all instances, the events resolved completely. There is no specific antidote for ondansetron, therefore in all cases of suspected overdose, symptomatic and supportive therapy should be given as appropriate.

Pharmacological properties

Pharmacodynamic properties: Ondansetron is a potent, highly selective $5HT_3$ receptor-antagonist. Its precise mode of action in the control of nausea and vomiting is not known. Chemotherapeutic agents and radiotherapy may cause release of 5HT in the small intestine initiating a vomiting reflex by activating vagal afferents via $5HT_3$ receptors. Ondansetron blocks the initiation of this reflex. Activation of vagal afferents may also cause a release of 5HT in the area postrema, located on the floor of the fourth ventricle, and this may also promote emesis through a central mechanism. Thus, the effect of ondansetron in the management of the nausea and vomiting induced by cytotoxic chemotherapy and radiotherapy is probably due to antagonism of $5HT_3$ receptors on neurons located both in the peripheral and central nervous system. The mechanisms of action in post-operative nausea and vomiting are not known but there may be common pathways with cytotoxic-induced nausea and vomiting.

Ondansetron does not alter plasma prolactin concentrations.

The role of ondansetron in opiate-induced emesis is not yet established,

Pharmacokinetic properties: Following oral administration, ondansetron is passively and completely absorbed from the gastrointestinal tract and undergoes first pass metabolism. Peak plasma concentrations of about 30 ng/ml are attained approximately 1.5 hours after an 8 mg dose. For doses above 8 mg the increase in ondansetron systemic exposure with dose is greater than proportional; this may reflect some reduction in first pass metabolism at higher oral doses. Bioavailability, following oral administration, is slightly enhanced by the presence of food but unaffected by antacids. Studies in healthy elderly volunteers have shown slight, but clinically insignificant, age-related increases in both oral bioavailability (65%) and half-life (5 hours) of ondansetron. Gender differences were shown in the disposition of ondansetron, with females having a greater rate and extent of absorption following an oral dose and reduced systemic clearance and volume of distribution (adjusted for weight).

The disposition of ondansetron following oral, intramuscular (IM) and intravenous (IV) dosing is similar with a terminal half-life of about 3 hours and steady state volume of distribution of about 140 L. Equivalent systemic exposure is achieved after IM and IV administration of ondansetron.

A 4 mg intravenous infusion of ondansetron given over 5 minutes results in peak plasma concentrations of about 65 ng/ml. Following intramuscular administration of ondansetron, peak plasma concentrations of about 25 ng/ml are attained within 10 minutes of injection.

Following administration of ondansetron suppository, plasma ondansetron concentrations become detectable between 15 and 60 minutes after dosing. Concentrations rise in an essentially linear fashion, until peak concentrations of 20–30 ng/ml are attained, typically 6 hours after dosing. Plasma concentrations then fall, but at a slower rate than observed following oral dosing due to continued absorption of ondansetron. The absolute bioavailability of ondansetron from the suppository is approximately 60% and is not affected by gender. The half life of the elimination phase following suppository administration is determined by the rate of ondansetron absorption, not systemic clearance and is approximately 6 hours. Females show a small, clinically insignificant, increase in half-life in comparison with males.

Ondansetron is not highly protein bound (70–76%). Ondansetron is cleared from the systemic circulation predominantly by hepatic metabolism through multiple enzymatic pathways. Less than 5% of the absorbed dose is excreted unchanged in the urine. The absence of the enzyme CYP2D6 (the debrisoquine polymorphism) has no effect on ondansetron's pharmacokinetics. The pharmacokinetic properties of ondansetron are unchanged on repeat dosing.

In a study of 21 paediatric patients aged between 3 and 12 years undergoing elective surgery with general anaesthesia, the absolute values for both the clearance and volume of distribution of ondansetron following a single intravenous dose of 2 mg (3–7 years old) or 4 mg (8–12 years old) were reduced. The magnitude of the change was age-related, with clearance falling from about 300 ml/min at 12 years of age to 100 ml/min at 3 years. Volume of distribution fell from about 75 L at 12 years to 17 L at 3 years. Use of weight-based dosing (0.1 mg/kg up to 4 mg maximum) compensates for these changes and is effective in normalising systemic exposure in paediatric patients.

In patients with renal impairment (creatinine clearance 15–60 ml/min), both systemic clearance and volume of distribution are reduced following IV administration of ondansetron, resulting in a slight, but clinically insignificant, increase in elimination half-life (5.4 h). A study in patients with severe renal impairment who required regular haemodialysis (studied between dialyses) showed ondansetron's pharmacokinetics to be essentially unchanged following IV administration.

Specific studies in the elderly or patients with renal impairment have been limited to IV and oral administration. However, it is anticipated that the half-life of ondansetron after rectal administration in these populations will be similar to that seen in healthy volunteers, since the rate of elimination of ondansetron following rectal administration is not determined by systemic clearance.

Following oral, intravenous or intramuscular dosing in patients with severe hepatic impairment, ondansetron's systemic clearance is markedly reduced with prolonged elimination half-lives (15–32 h) and an oral bioavailability approaching 100% due to reduced presystemic metabolism. The pharmacokinetics of ondansetron following administration as a suppository have not been evaluated in patients with hepatic impairment.

Preclinical safety data: No additional data of relevance.

Pharmaceutical particulars

List of excipients: Citric acid monohydrate, sodium citrate, sodium chloride, Water for Injections.

Incompatibilities: Zofran injection should not be administered in the same syringe or infusion as any other medication.

Shelf life: 36 months (unopened). 24 hours (dilutions stored 2–8°C).

Special precautions for storage: Protect from light. Store below 30°C.

Dilutions of Zofran Injection in compatible intravenous infusion fluids are stable under normal room lighting conditions or daylight for at least 24 hours, thus no protection from light is necessary while infusion takes place.

Nature and contents of container: Zofran Injection: Type I clear glass snap-ring ampoules.

Zofran Flexi-amp Injection: Polypropylene blow-fill-sealed ampoules with a twist-off top and overwrapped in a double foil blister.

Five ampoules are packed in a carton.

Instructions for use/handling: Zofran Injection and Zofran Flexi-amp Injection should not be autoclaved.

Compatibility with intravenous fluids: Zofran Injection should only be admixed with those infusion solutions which are recommended:
Sodium Chloride Intravenous Infusion BP 0.9% w/v
Glucose Intravenous Infusion BP 5% w/v
Mannitol Intravenous Infusion BP 10% w/v
Ringers Intravenous Infusion
Potassium Chloride 0.3% w/v and Sodium Chloride 0.9% w/v Intravenous Infusion BP
Potassium Chloride 0.3% w/v and Glucose 5% w/v Intravenous Infusion BP

In keeping with good pharmaceutical practice dilutions of Zofran injection in intravenous fluids should be prepared at the time of infusion or stored at 2–8°C for no more than 24 hours before the start of administration.

Compatibility studies have been undertaken in polyvinyl chloride infusion bags and polyvinyl chloride administration sets. It is considered that adequate stability would also be conferred by the use of polyethylene infusion bags or Type 1 glass bottles. Dilutions of Zofran in sodium chloride 0.9% w/v or in glucose 5% w/v have been demonstrated to be stable in polypropylene syringes. It is considered that Zofran Injection diluted with other compatible infusion fluids would be stable in polypropylene syringes.

Compatibility with other drugs: Zofran may be administered by intravenous infusion at 1 mg/hour, e.g. from an infusion bag or syringe pump. The following drugs may be administered via the Y-site of the Zofran giving set for ondansetron concentrations of 16 to 160 micrograms/ml (e.g. 8 mg/500 ml and 8 mg/50 ml respectively):

Cisplatin: Concentrations up to 0.48 mg/ml (e.g. 240 mg in 500 ml) administered over one to eight hours.

5-Fluorouracil: Concentrations up to 0.8 mg/ml (e.g. 2.4 g in 3 litres or 400 mg in 500 ml) administered at a rate of at least 20 ml per hour (500 ml per 24 hours). Higher concentrations of 5-fluorouracil may cause precipitation of ondansetron. The 5-fluorouracil infusion may contain up to 0.045% w/v magnesium chloride in addition to other excipients shown to be compatible.

Carboplatin: Concentrations in the range 0.18 mg/ml to 9.9 mg/ml (e.g. 90 mg in 500 ml to 990 mg in 100 ml), administered over ten minutes to one hour.

Etoposide: Concentrations in the range 0.14 mg/ml

to 0.25 mg/ml (e.g. 72 mg in 500 ml to 250 mg in 1 litre), administered over thirty minutes to one hour.

Ceftazidime: Doses in the range 250 mg to 2,000 mg reconstituted with Water for Injections BP as recommended by the manufacturer (e.g. 2.5 ml for 250 mg and 10 ml for 2 g ceftazidime) and given as an intravenous bolus injection over approximately five minutes.

Cyclophosphamide: Doses in the range 100 mg to 1 g, reconstituted with Water for Injections BP, 5 ml per 100 mg cyclophosphamide, as recommended by the manufacturer and given as an intravenous bolus injection over approximately five minutes.

Doxorubicin: doses in the range 10–100 mg reconstituted with Water for Injections BP, 5 ml per 10 mg doxorubicin, as recommended by the manufacturer and given as an intravenous bolus injection over approximately 5 minutes.

Dexamethasone: Dexamethasone sodium phosphate 20 mg may be administered as a slow intravenous injection over 2–5 minutes via the Y-site of an infusion set delivering 8 or 32 mg of ondansetron diluted in 50–100 ml of a compatible infusion fluid over approximately 15 minutes. Compatibility between dexamethasone sodium phosphate and ondansetron has been demonstrated supporting administration of these drugs through the same giving set resulting in concentrations in line of 32 microgram – 2.5 mg/ml for dexamethasone sodium phosphate and 8 microgram – 1 mg/ml for ondansetron.

Marketing authorisation number PL 0004/0375.

Date of approval/revision of SPC December 1997.

Legal category POM.

ZOFRAN* MELT 8 mg ▼
ZOFRAN* MELT 4 mg ▼

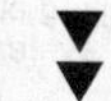

Qualitative and quantitative composition White, round, plano-convex, freeze dried, fast dispersing oral dosage form. Each Melt contains ondansetron 4 mg or 8 mg.

Pharmaceutical form Oral lyophilisate.

Clinical particulars

Therapeutic indications: The management of nausea and vomiting induced by cytotoxic chemotherapy and radiotherapy, and for the prevention of post-operative nausea and vomiting in adults.

Posology and method of administration: Place the Melt on top of the tongue, where it will disperse within seconds, then swallow.

Chemotherapy and radiotherapy induced nausea and vomiting

Adults: The emetogenic potential of cancer treatment varies according to the doses and combinations of chemotherapy and radiotherapy regimens used. The route of administration and dose of Zofran should be flexible and selected as shown below.

Emetogenic chemotherapy and radiotherapy: Zofran can be given either by rectal, oral (as Melt, tablets or syrup) intravenous or intramuscular administration.

For oral administration: 8 mg 1–2 hours before treatment, followed by 8 mg 12 hours later.

To protect against delayed or prolonged emesis after the first 24 hours, oral or rectal treatment with Zofran should be continued for up to 5 days after a course of treatment. The recommended dose for oral administration is 8 mg twice daily.

Highly emetogenic chemotherapy (e.g. high dose cisplatin): Zofran can be given either by rectal, intravenous or intramuscular administration.

To protect against delayed or prolonged emesis after the first 24 hours, oral or rectal treatment with Zofran should be continued for up to 5 days after a course of treatment. The recommended dose for oral administration is 8 mg twice daily.

Children: Zofran may be administered as a single intravenous dose of 5 mg/m² immediately before chemotherapy, followed by 4 mg orally twelve hours later. 4 mg orally twice daily should be continued for up to 5 days after a course of treatment.

Elderly: Zofran is well tolerated by patients over 65 years and no alteration of dosage, dosing frequency or route of administration are required.

Post operative nausea and vomiting (PONV):

Adults:

For the prevention of PONV: Zofran may be administered either orally (as Melt, tablets or syrup) or by intravenous or intramuscular injection.

For oral administration: 16 mg one hour prior to anaesthesia. Alternatively, 8 mg one hour prior to anaesthesia followed by two further doses of 8 mg at eight hourly intervals.

For the treatment of established PONV: Intravenous or intramuscular administration is recommended.

Children (aged 2 years and over):

For the prevention and treatment of PONV: Slow intravenous injection is recommended.

Elderly: There is limited experience in the use of Zofran in the prevention and treatment of PONV in the elderly, however Zofran is well tolerated in patients over 65 years receiving chemotherapy.

For both indications:

Patients with renal impairment: No special requirements.

Patients with hepatic impairment: Clearance of Zofran is significantly reduced and serum half life significantly prolonged in subjects with moderate or severe impairment of hepatic function. In such patients a total daily dose of 8 mg should not be exceeded.

Patients with poor sparteine/debrisoquine metabolism: The elimination half-life of ondansetron is not altered in subjects classified as poor metabolisers of sparteine and debrisoquine. Consequently in such patients repeat dosing will give drug exposure levels no different from those of the general population. No alteration of daily dosage or frequency of dosing are required.

Contra-indications: Hypersensitivity to any component of the preparation.

Special warnings and precautions for use: Hypersensitivity reactions have been reported in patients who have exhibited hypersensitivity to other selective $5HT_3$ receptor antagonists.

Patients with signs of subacute intestinal obstruction should be monitored following administration.

Caution in patients with phenylketonuria.

Interaction with other medicaments and other forms of interaction: There is no evidence that ondansetron either induces or inhibits the metabolism of other drugs commonly co-administered with it. Specific studies have shown that ondansetron does not interact with alcohol, tamazepam, frusemide, tramadol and propofol.

Pregnancy and lactation: The safety of ondansetron for use in human pregnancy has not been established. Evaluation of experimental animal studies does not indicate direct or indirect harmful effects with respect to the development of the embryo, or the foetus, the course of gestation and peri- and post-natal development. However, as animal studies are not always predictive of human response the use of ondansetron in pregnancy is not recommended.

Tests have shown that ondansetron passes into the milk of lactating animals. It is therefore recommended that mothers receiving Zofran should not breast-feed their babies.

Effects on ability to drive and use machines: None reported.

Undesirable effects: There have been rare reports of immediate hypersensitivity reactions, sometimes severe, including anaphylaxis.

Chest pain, cardiac arrhythmias, hypotension and bradycardia have been rarely reported.

There have been rare reports suggestive of involuntary movement disorders without definitive evidence of persistent clinical sequelae, and seizures have been rarely observed, although no known pharmacological mechanism can account for ondansetron causing these effects.

Ondansetron is known to increase large bowel transit time and may cause constipation in some patients.

The following side effects can occur: headache, a sensation of flushing or warmth, hiccups and occasional transient, asymptomatic increases in aminotransferases.

Overdose: Little is known at present about overdosage with ondansetron. However two patients who received doses of 84 and 145 mg intravenously reported only mild side-effects and required no active therapy. In cases of suspected overdose, symptomatic and supportive therapy should be given as appropriate.

The use of Ipecacuanha to treat overdose with ondansetron is not recommended as patients are unlikely to respond due to the anti-emetic action of Zofran itself.

Pharmacological properties

Pharmacodynamic properties: Ondansetron is a potent, highly selective $5HT_3$ receptor-antagonist. Its precise mode of action in the control of nausea and vomiting is not known. Chemotherapeutic agents and radiotherapy may cause release of 5HT in the small intestine initiating a vomiting reflex by activating vagal afferents via $5HT_3$ receptors. Ondansetron blocks the initiation of this reflex. Activation of vagal afferents may also cause a release of 5HT in the area postrema, located on the floor of the fourth ventricle, and this may also promote emesis through a central mechanism. Thus, the effect of ondansetron in the management of the nausea and vomiting induced by cytotoxic chemotherapy and radiotherapy is probably due to antagonism of $5HT_3$ receptors on neurons located both in the peripheral and central nervous system. The mechanisms of action in post-operative nausea and vomiting are not known but there may be common pathways with cytotoxic induced nausea and vomiting.

Ondansetron does not alter plasma prolactin concentrations.

The role of ondansetron in opiate-induced emesis is not yet established.

Pharmacokinetic properties: Following oral administration of ondansetron, absorption is rapid with maximum peak plasma concentrations of about 30 ng/ml being attained and achieved in approximately 1.5 hours after an 8 mg dose. The syrup and tablet formulations are bioequivalent and have an absolute oral bioavailability of 60%. The disposition of ondansetron following oral, intravenous and intramuscular dosing is similar with a terminal elimination half-life of approximately 3 hours and a steady-state volume of distribution of about 140 L. Ondansetron is not highly protein bound (70–76%) and is cleared from the systemic circulation predominantly by hepatic metabolism through multiple enzymatic pathways. Less than 5% of the absorbed dose is excreted unchanged in the urine. The absence of the enzyme CYP2D6 (the debrisoquine polymorphism) has no effect on the pharmacokinetics of ondansetron. The pharmacokinetic properties of ondansetron are unchanged on repeat dosing.

Studies in healthy elderly volunteers have shown slight but clinically insignificant, age-related increases in both oral bioavailability (65%) and half-life (5 h) of ondansetron. Gender differences were shown in the disposition of ondansetron, with females having a greater rate and extent of absorption following an oral dose and reduced systemic clearance and volume of distribution (adjusted for weight).

In a study of 21 paediatric patients aged between 3 and 12 years undergoing elective surgery with general anaesthesia, the absolute values for both the clearance and volume of distribution of ondansetron following a single intravenous dose of 2 mg (3–7 years old) or 4 mg (8–12 years old) were reduced. The magnitude of the change was age-related, with clearance falling from about 300 ml/min at 12 years of age to 100 ml/min at 3 years. Volume of distribution fell from about 75 L at 12 years to 17 L at 3 years. Use of weight-based dosing (0.1 mg/kg up to 4 mg maximum) compensates for these changes and is effective in normalising systemic exposure in paediatric patients.

In patients with renal impairment (creatinine clearance >15 ml/min), systemic clearance and volume of distribution are reduced, resulting in a slight, but clinically insignificant increase in elimination half-life (5.4 h). A study in patients with severe renal impairment who required regular haemodialysis (studied between dialyses) showed ondansetron's pharmacokinetics to be essentially unchanged.

In patients with severe hepatic impairment, systemic clearance is markedly reduced with prolonged elimination half-lives (15–32 h) and an oral bioavailability approaching 100% because of reduced pre-systemic metabolism.

Preclinical safety data: No additional data of relevance.

Pharmaceutical particulars

List of excipients: Gelatin, Mannitol, Aspartame, Sodium methyl hydroxybenzoate, Sodium propyl hydroxybenzoate, Strawberry flavour.

Incompatibilities: None reported.

Shelf life: 3 years.

Special precautions for storage: Store below 30°C.

Nature and contents of container: Double aluminium foil blister strip containing 10 tablets.

Instructions for use/handling: Do not attempt to push Zofran Melt through the lidding foil. Peel back the lidding foil of one blister and gently remove the Zofran Melt. Place the Melt on top of the tongue, where it will disperse within seconds then swallow.

Marketing authorisation numbers
PL 10949/0264 – Zofran Melt 8 mg
PL 10949/0263 – Zofran Melt 4 mg

Date of first authorisation/renewal of authorisation
3 April 1998

Date of (partial) revision of text June 1998

ZOFRAN* SUPPOSITORIES 16 mg ▼

Qualitative and quantitative composition White, torpedo-shaped suppositories containing 16 mg of ondansetron.

Pharmaceutical form Suppositories.

Clinical particulars

Therapeutic indications: The management of nausea and vomiting induced by cytotoxic chemotherapy and radiotherapy.

Posology and method of administration:

Adults (including the elderly): The emetogenic potential of cancer treatment varies according to the doses and combinations of chemotherapy and radiotherapy regimens used. The route of administation and dose of Zofran should be flexible and selected as shown below.

Emetogenic chemotherapy and radiotherapy: Zofran can be given either by rectal, oral (tablets or syrup) or intravenous or intramuscular administration.

For rectal administation: One suppository (16 mg ondansetron) 1–2 hours before treatment.

To protect against delayed or prolonged emesis after the first 24 hours, oral or rectal treatment with Zofran should be continued for up to 5 days after a course of treatment.

The recommended dose for rectal administration is one suppository daily.

Highly emetogenic chemotherapy (e.g. high-dose cisplatin): Zofran can be given either by rectal or intravenous or intramuscular administration.

For rectal administration: One suppository (16 mg ondansetron) 1–2 hours before treatment.

The efficacy of Zofran in highly emetogenic chemotherapy may be enhanced by the addition of a single intravenous dose of dexamethasone sodium phosphate 20 mg, administered prior to chemotherapy.

To protect against delayed or prolonged emesis after the first 24 hours, oral or rectal treatment with Zofran should be continued for up to 5 days after a course of treatment.

The recommended dose for rectal administration is one suppository daily.

Children: The use of Zofran Suppositories in children is not recommended.

Zofran may be administered as a single intravenous dose of 5 mg/m² immediately before chemotherapy, followed by 4 mg orally twelve hours later. 4 mg orally twice daily should be continued for up to 5 days after a course of treatment.

Patients with renal impairment: No special requirements.

Patients with hepatic impairment: Clearance of Zofran is significantly reduced and serum half-life significantly prolonged in subjects with moderate or severe impairment of hepatic function. In such patients a total daily dose of 8 mg should not be exceeded and therefore intravenous or oral administration is recommended.

Patients with poor sparteine/debrisoquine metabolism: The elimination half-life of ondansetron is not altered in subjects classified as poor metabolisers of sparteine and debrisoquine. Consequently, in such patients repeat dosing will give drug exposure levels no different from those of the general population. No alteration of daily dosage or frequency of dosing are required.

Contra-indications: Hypersensitivity to any ingredient.

Special warnings and precautions for use: Hypersensitivity reactions have been reported in patients who have exhibited hypersensitivity to other selective $5HT_3$ receptor antagonists. As ondansetron is known to increase large bowel transit time, patients with signs of subacute intestinal obstruction should be monitored following administration.

Interaction with other medicaments and other forms of interaction: There is no evidence that ondansetron either induces or inhibits the metabolism of other drugs commonly co-administered with it. Specific studies have shown that ondansetron does not interact with alcohol, temazepam, frusemide, tramadol and propofol.

Pregnancy and lactation: The safety of ondansetron for use in human pregnancy has not been established. Evaluation of experimental animal studies does not indicate direct or indirect harmful effects with respect to the development of the embryo, or foetus, the course of gestation and peri- and post-natal development. However, as animal studies are not always predictive of human response the use of ondansetron in pregnancy is not recommended. Tests have shown that ondansetron passes into the milk of lactating animals. It is therefore recommended that mothers receiving Zofran should not breast-feed their baby.

Effect on ability to drive and use machines: None reported.

Undesirable effects: There have been rare reports of immediate hypersensitivity reactions, sometimes severe, including anaphylaxis.

Chest pain, cardiac arrhythmias, hypotension and bradycardia have been rarely reported.

There have been rare reports suggestive of involuntary movement disorders without definitive evidence of persistent clinical sequelae, and seizures have been rarely observed, although no known pharmacological mechanism can account for ondansetron causing these effects.

Ondansetron is known to increase large bowel transit time and may cause constipation in some patients.

The following side effects can occur: headache, a sensation of flushing or warmth, hiccups and occasional transient, asymptomatic increases in aminotransferases.

There have been rare reports of a local anal/rectal burning sensation following insertion of a suppository.

Overdose: Little is known at present about overdosage with ondansetron, however, a limited number of patients received overdoses. Manifestations that have been reported include visual disturbances, severe constipation, hypotension and a vasovagal episode with transient second degree AV block. In all instances, the events resolved completely. There is no specific antidote for ondansetron, therefore in all cases of suspected overdose, symptomatic and supportive therapy should be given as appropriate.

Pharmacological properties

Pharmacodynamic properties: Ondansetron is a potent, highly selective $5HT_3$ receptor-antagonist. The precise mode of action in the control of nausea and vomiting is not known. Chemotherapeutic agents and radiotherapy may cause release of 5HT in the small intestine initiating a vomiting reflex by activating vagal afferents via $5HT_3$ receptors. Ondansetron blocks the initiation of this reflex. Activation of vagal afferents may also cause a release of 5HT in the area postrema, located on the floor of the fourth ventricle, and this may also promote emesis through a central mechanism. Thus, the effect of ondansetron in the management of the nausea and vomiting induced by cytotoxic chemotherapy and radiotherapy is probably due to antagonism of $5HT_3$ receptors on neurons located both in the peripheral and central nervous system. The mechanisms of action in post-operative nausea and vomiting are not known but there may be common pathways with cytotoxic-induced nausea and vomiting.

Ondansetron does not alter plasma prolactin concentrations.

The role of ondansetron in opiate-induced emesis is not yet established.

Pharmacokinetic properties: Following oral administration, ondansetron is passively and completely absorbed from the gastrointestinal tract and undergoes first pass metabolism. Peak plasma concentrations of about 30 ng/ml are attained approximately 1.5 hours after an 8 mg dose. For doses above 8 mg the increase in ondansetron systemic exposure with dose is greater than proportional; this may reflect some reduction in first pass metabolism at higher oral doses. Bioavailability, following oral administration, is slightly enhanced by the presence of food but unaffected by antacids. Studies in healthy elderly volunteers have shown slight, but clinically insignificant, age-related increases in both oral bioavailability (65%) and half-life (5 hours) of ondansetron. Gender differences were shown in the disposition of ondansetron, with females having a greater rate and extent of absorption following an oral dose and reduced systemic clearance and volume of distribution (adjusted for weight).

The disposition of ondansetron following oral, intramuscular (IM) and intravenous (IV) dosing is similar with a terminal half-life of about 3 hours and steady state volume of distribution of about 140 L. Equivalent systemic exposure is achieved after IM and IV administration of ondansetron.

A 4 mg intravenous infusion of ondansetron given over 5 minutes results in peak plasma concentrations of about 65 ng/ml. Following intramuscular administration of ondansetron, peak plasma concentrations of about 25 ng/ml are attained within 10 minutes of injection.

Following administration of ondansetron suppository, plasma ondansetron concentrations become detectable between 15 and 60 minutes after dosing. Concentrations rise in an essentially linear fashion, until peak concentrations of 20–30 ng/ml are attained, typically 6 hours after dosing. Plasma concentrations then fall, but at a slower rate than observed following oral dosing due to continued absorption of ondansetron. The absolute bioavailability of ondansetron from the suppository is approximately 60% and is not affected by gender. The half life of the elimination phase following suppository administration is determined by the rate of ondansetron absorption, not systemic clearance and is approximately 6 hours. Females show a small, clinically insignificant, increase in half-life in comparison with males.

Ondansetron is not highly protein bound (70–76%). Ondansetron is cleared from the systemic circulation predominantly by hepatic metabolism through multiple enzymatic pathways. Less than 5% of the absorbed dose is excreted unchanged in the urine. The absence of the enzyme CYP2D6 (the debrisoquine polymorphism) has no effect on ondansetron's pharmacokinetics. The pharmacokinetic properties of ondansetron are unchanged on repeat dosing.

In a study of 21 paediatric patients aged between 3 and 12 years undergoing elective surgery with general anaesthesia, the absolute values for both the clearance and volume of distribution of ondansetron following a single intravenous dose of 2 mg (3–7 years old) or 4 mg (8–12 years old) were reduced. The magnitude of the change was age-related, with clearance falling from about 300 ml/min at 12 years of age to 100 ml/min at 3 years. Volume of distribution fell from about 75 L at 12 years to 17 L at 3 years. Use of weight-based dosing (0.1 mg/kg up to 4 mg maximum) compensates for these changes and is effective in normalising systemic exposure in paediatric patients.

In patients with renal impairment (creatinine clearance 15–60 ml/min), both systemic clearance and volume of distribution are reduced following IV administration of ondansetron, resulting in a slight, but clinically insignificant, increase in elimination half-life (5.4 h). A study in patients with severe renal impairment who required regular haemodialysis (studied between dialyses) showed ondansetron's pharmacokinetics to be essentially unchanged following IV administration.

Specific studies in the elderly or patients with renal impairment have been limited to IV and oral administration. However, it is anticipated that the half-life of ondansetron after rectal administration in these populations will be similar to that seen in healthy volunteers, since the rate of elimination of ondansetron following rectal administration is not determined by systemic clearance.

Following oral, intravenous or intramuscular dosing in patients with severe hepatic impairment, ondansetron's systemic clearance is markedly reduced with prolonged elimination half-lives (15–32 h) and an oral bioavailability approaching 100% due to reduced presystemic metabolism. The pharmacokinetics of ondansetron following administration as a suppository have not been evaluated in patients with hepatic impairment.

Preclinical safety data: No additional data of relevance.

Pharmaceutical particulars

List of excipients: Witepsol S58.

Incompatibilities: None reported.

Shelf life: 3 years.

Special precautions for storage: Store below 30°C.

Nature and contents of container: Each suppository is in an individually sealed cavity enclosed in a perforated cardboard mount and packed into a carton.

Instructions for use/handling: Insert into the rectum.

For detailed instructions see the patient information leaflet included in every pack.

Marketing authorisation number PL 10949/0247.

Date of approval/revision of SPC December 1997.

Legal category POM.

ZOFRAN* SYRUP ▼

Qualitative and quantitative composition Sugar-free strawberry flavoured liquid.

Each 5 ml contains 4 mg of ondansetron as the hydrochloride dihydrate.

Pharmaceutical form Oral solution.

Clinical particulars

Therapeutic indications: The management of nausea and vomiting induced by cytotoxic chemotherapy and radiotherapy, and for the prevention of post-operative nausea and vomiting in adults.

Posology and method of administration:

Chemotherapy and radiotherapy-induced nausea and vomiting – Adults (including the elderly): The emetogenic potential of cancer treatment varies according to the doses and combinations of chemotherapy and radiotherapy regimens used. The route of administration and dose of Zofran should be flexible and selected as shown below.

Emetogenic chemotherapy and radiotherapy: Zofran can be given either by rectal, oral (tablets or syrup) or intravenous or intramuscular administration.

For oral administation: 8 mg 1–2 hours before treatment, followed by 8 mg 12 hours later.

To protect against delayed or prolonged emesis after the first 24 hours, oral or rectal treatment with Zofran should be continued for up to 5 days after a course of treatment.

The recommended dose for oral administration is 8 mg twice daily.

Highly emetogenic chemotherapy (e.g. high dose cisplatin): Zofran can be given either by rectal, intravenous or intramuscular administration.

To protect against delayed or prolonged emesis after the first 24 hours, oral or rectal treatment with Zofran should be continued for up to 5 days after a course of treatment.

The recommended dose for oral administration is 8 mg twice daily.

Children: Zofran may be administered as a single intravenous dose of 5 mg/m^2 immediately before chemotherapy, followed by 4 mg orally twelve hours later. 4 mg orally twice daily should be continued for up to 5 days after a course of treatment.

Post operative nausea and vomiting (PONV):
Adults: For the prevention of PONV: Zofran can be administered orally or by intravenous or intramuscular injection.

For oral administration: 16 mg one hour prior to anaesthesia. Alternatively, 8 mg one hour prior to anaesthesia followed by two further doses of 8 mg at eight-hourly intervals.

For the treatment of established PONV: Intravenous or intramuscular administration is recommended.

Children (aged 2 years and over): For the prevention and treatment of PONV: Slow intravenous injection is recommended.

Elderly: There is limited experience in the use of Zofran in the prevention and treatment of PONV in the elderly. However, Zofran is well tolerated in patients over 65 years receiving chemotherapy.

For both indications

Patients with renal impairment: No special requirements.

Patients with hepatic impairment: Clearance of Zofran is significantly reduced and serum half-life significantly prolonged in subjects with moderate or severe impairment of hepatic function. In such patients a total daily dose of 8 mg should not be exceeded.

Patients with poor sparteine/debrisoquine metabolism: The elimination half-life of ondansetron is not altered in subjects classified as poor metabolisers of sparteine and debrisoquine. Consequently, in such patients repeat dosing will give drug exposure levels no different from those of the general population. No alteration of daily dosage or frequency of dosing are required.

Contra-indications: Hypersensitivity to any ingredient.

Special warnings and precautions for use: Hypersensitivity reactions have been reported in patients who have exhibited hypersensitivity to other selective 5HT$_3$ receptor antagonists. As ondansetron is known to increase large bowel transit time, patients with signs of subacute intestinal obstruction should be monitored following administration.

Interaction with other medicaments and other forms of interaction: There is no evidence that ondansetron either induces or inhibits the metabolism of other drugs commonly co-administered with it. Specific studies have shown that ondansetron does not interact with alcohol, temazepam, frusemide, tramadol and propofol.

Pregnancy and lactation: The safety of ondansetron for use in human pregnancy has not been established. Evaluation of experimental animal studies does not indicate direct or indirect harmful effects with respect to the development of the embryo, or foetus, the course of gestation and peri- and post-natal development. However, as animal studies are not always predictive of human response the use of ondansetron in pregnancy is not recommended. Tests have shown that ondansetron passes into the milk of lactating animals. It is therefore recommended that mothers receiving Zofran should not breast-feed their baby.

Effect on ability to drive and use machines: None reported.

Undesirable effects: There have been rare reports of immediate hypersensitivity reactions, sometimes severe, including anaphylaxis.

Chest pain, cardiac arrhythmias, hypotension and bradycardia have been rarely reported.

There have been rare reports suggestive of involuntary movement disorders without definitive evidence of persistent clinical sequelae, and seizures have been rarely observed, although no known pharmacological mechanism can account for ondansetron causing these effects.

Ondansetron is known to increase large bowel transit time and may cause constipation in some patients.

The following side effects can occur: headache, a sensation of flushing or warmth, hiccups and occasional transient, asymptomatic increases in aminotransferases.

Overdose: Little is known at present about overdosage with ondansetron, however, a limited number of patients received overdoses. Manifestations that have been reported include visual disturbances, severe constipation, hypotension and a vasovagal episode with transient second degree AV block. In all instances, the events resolved completely. There is no specific antidote for ondansetron, therefore in all cases of suspected overdose, symptomatic and supportive therapy should be given as appropriate.

Pharmacological properties

Pharmacodynamic properties: Ondansetron is a potent, highly selective 5HT$_3$ receptor-antagonist. Its precise mode of action in the control of nausea and vomiting is not known. Chemotherapeutic agents and radiotherapy may cause release of 5HT in the small intestine initiating a vomiting reflex by activating vagal afferents via 5HT$_3$ receptors. Ondansetron blocks the initiation of this reflex. Activation of vagal afferents may also cause a release of 5HT in the area postrema, located on the floor of the fourth ventricle, and this may also promote emesis through a central mechanism. Thus, the effect of ondansetron in the management of the nausea and vomiting induced by cytotoxic chemotherapy and radiotherapy is probably due to antagonism of 5HT$_3$ receptors on neurons located both in the peripheral and central nervous system. The mechanisms of action in post-operative nausea and vomiting are not known but there may be common pathways with cytotoxic-induced nausea and vomiting.

Ondansetron does not alter plasma prolactin concentrations.

The role of ondansetron in opiate-induced emesis is not yet established.

Pharmacokinetic properties: Following oral administration, ondansetron is passively and completely absorbed from the gastrointestinal tract and undergoes first pass metabolism. Peak plasma concentrations of about 30 ng/ml are attained approximately 1.5 hours after an 8 mg dose. For doses above 8 mg the increase in ondansetron systemic exposure with dose is greater than proportional; this may reflect some reduction in first pass metabolism at higher oral doses. Bioavailability, following oral administration, is slightly enhanced by the presence of food but unaffected by antacids. Studies in healthy elderly volunteers have shown slight, but clinically insignificant, age-related increases in both oral bioavailability (65%) and half-life (5 hours) of ondansetron. Gender differences were shown in the disposition of ondansetron, with females having a greater rate and extent of absorption following an oral dose and reduced systemic clearance and volume of distribution (adjusted for weight).

The disposition of ondansetron following oral, intramuscular (IM) and intravenous (IV) dosing is similar with a terminal half-life of about 3 hours and steady state volume of distribution of about 140 L. Equivalent systemic exposure is achieved after IM and IV administration of ondansetron.

A 4 mg intravenous infusion of ondansetron given over 5 minutes results in peak plasma concentrations of about 65 ng/ml. Following intramuscular administration of ondansetron, peak plasma concentrations of about 25 ng/ml are attained within 10 minutes of injection.

Following administration of ondansetron suppository, plasma ondansetron concentrations become detectable between 15 and 60 minutes after dosing. Concentrations rise in an essentially linear fashion, until peak concentrations of 20–30 ng/ml are attained, typically 6 hours after dosing. Plasma concentrations then fall, but at a slower rate than observed following oral dosing due to continued absorption of ondansetron. The absolute bioavailability of ondansetron from the suppository is approximately 60% and is not affected by gender. The half life of the elimination phase following suppository administration is determined by the rate of ondansetron absorption, not systemic clearance and is approximately 6 hours. Females show a small, clinically insignificant, increase in half-life in comparison with males.

Ondansetron is not highly protein bound (70–76%). Ondansetron is cleared from the systemic circulation predominantly by hepatic metabolism through multiple enzymatic pathways. Less than 5% of the absorbed dose is excreted unchanged in the urine. The absence of the enzyme CYP2D6 (the debrisoquine polymorphism) has no effect on ondansetron's pharmacokinetics. The pharmacokinetic properties of ondansetron are unchanged on repeat dosing.

In a study of 21 paediatric patients aged between 3 and 12 years undergoing elective surgery with general anaesthesia, the absolute values for both the clearance and volume of distribution of ondansetron following a single intravenous dose of 2 mg (3–7 years old) or 4 mg (8–12 years old) were reduced. The magnitude of the change was age-related, with clearance falling from about 300 ml/min at 12 years of age to 100 ml/min at 3 years. Volume of distribution fell from about 75 L at 12 years to 17 L at 3 years. Use of weight-based dosing (0.1 mg/kg up to 4 mg maximum) compensates for these changes and is effective in normalising systemic exposure in paediatric patients.

In patients with renal impairment (creatinine clearance 15–60 ml/min), both systemic clearance and volume of distribution are reduced following IV administration of ondansetron, resulting in a slight, but clinically insignificant, increase in elimination half-life (5.4 h). A study in patients with severe renal impairment who required regular haemodialysis (studied between dialyses) showed ondansetron's pharmacokinetics to be essentially unchanged following IV administration.

Specific studies in the elderly or patients with renal impairment have been limited to IV and oral administration. However, it is anticipated that the half-life of ondansetron after rectal administration in these populations will be similar to that seen in healthy volunteers, since the rate of elimination of ondansetron following rectal administration is not determined by systemic clearance.

Following oral, intravenous or intramuscular dosing in patients with severe hepatic impairment, ondansetron's systemic clearance is markedly reduced with prolonged elimination half-lives (15–32 h) and an oral bioavailability approaching 100% due to reduced presystemic metabolism. The pharmacokinetics of ondansetron following administration as a suppository have not been evaluated in patients with hepatic impairment.

Preclinical safety data: No additional data of relevance.

Pharmaceutical particulars

List of excipients: Citric acid; sodium citrate dihydrate; sodium benzoate; sorbitol solution; strawberry flavour; purified water.

Incompatibilities: None reported.

Shelf life: 2 years.

Special precautions for storage: Store upright below 30°C. Do not refrigerate.

Nature and contents of container: 60 ml amber glass bottle with a child-resistant cap containing 50 ml of Zofran Syrup.

Instructions for use/handling: For oral administration. For detailed information see the patient information leaflet included in every pack.

Marketing authorisation number PL 10949/0246.

Date of approval/revision of SPC December 1997.

Legal category POM.

ZOFRAN* TABLETS 4 mg 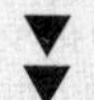
ZOFRAN* TABLETS 8 mg ▼

Qualitative and quantitative composition Each Zofran Tablet 4 mg is a yellow, oval, film-coated tablet engraved 'GLAXO' on one face and '4' on the other. Each tablet contains ondansetron 4 mg (as hydrochloride dihydrate).

Each Zofran Tablet 8 mg is a yellow, oval, film-coated tablet engraved 'GLAXO' on one face and '8' on the other. Each tablet contains ondansetron 8 mg (as hydrochloride dihydrate).

Pharmaceutical form Film-coated tablet.

Clinical particulars

Therapeutic indications: Zofran is indicated for the management of nausea and vomiting induced by cytotoxic chemotherapy and radiotherapy, and for the prevention and treatment of post-operative nausea and vomiting.

Posology and method of administration:
Chemotherapy and radiotherapy-induced nausea and vomiting: Adults: The emetogenic potential of cancer treatment varies according to the doses and combinations of chemotherapy and radiotherapy regimens used. The route of administration and dose of Zofran should be flexible in the range of 8–32 mg a day and selected as shown below.

Emetogenic chemotherapy and radiotherapy: Zofran can be given either by rectal, oral (tablets or syrup), intravenous or intramuscular administration.

To protect against delayed or prolonged emesis after the first 24 hours, oral or rectal treatment with Zofran should be continued for up to 5 days after a course of treatment.

The recommended dose for oral administration is 8 mg twice daily.

Highly emetogenic chemotherapy: For patients receiving highly emetogenic chemotherapy, e.g. high-dose cisplatin, Zofran can be given either by rectal, intravenous or intramuscular administration.

To protect against delayed or prolonged emesis after the first 24 hours, oral or rectal treatment with Zofran should be continued for up to 5 days after a course of treatment.

The recommended dose for oral administration is 8 mg twice daily.

Children: Zofran may be administered as a single intravenous dose of 5 mg/m^2 immediately before chemotherapy, followed by 4 mg orally twelve hours later. 4 mg orally twice daily should be continued for up to 5 days after a course of treatment.

Elderly: Zofran is well tolerated by patients over 65 years and no alteration of dosage, dosing frequency or route of administration are required.

Patients with renal impairment: No alteration of daily dosage or frequency of dosing, or route of administration are required.

Patients with hepatic impairment: Clearance of Zofran is significantly reduced and serum half-life significantly prolonged in subjects with moderate or severe impairment of hepatic function. In such patients a total daily dose of 8 mg should not be exceeded.

Post operative nausea and vomiting (PONV):
Adults: For the prevention of PONV: Zofran can be administered orally or by intravenous or intramuscular injection.

For oral administration: 16 mg one hour prior to anaesthesia. Alternatively, 8 mg one hour prior to anaesthesia followed by two further doses of 8 mg at eight hourly intervals.

For the treatment of established PONV: Intravenous or intramuscular administration is recommended.

Children (aged 2 years and over): For the prevention and treatment of PONV, slow intravenous injection is recommended.

Elderly: There is limited experience in the use of Zofran in the prevention and treatment of PONV in the elderly. However, Zofran is well tolerated in patients over 65 years receiving chemotherapy.

Patients with renal impairment: No alteration of daily dosage or frequency of dosing, or route of administration are required.

Patients with hepatic impairment: Clearance of Zofran is significantly reduced and serum half-life significantly prolonged in subjects with moderate or severe impairment of hepatic function. In such patients a total daily dose of 8 mg should not be exceeded.

Patients with poor sparteine/debrisoquine metabolism: The elimination half-life of ondansetron is not altered in subjects classified as poor metabolisers of sparteine and debrisoquine. Consequently, in such patients repeat dosing will give drug exposure levels no different from those of the general population. No alteration of daily dosage or frequency of dosing are required.

Contra-indications: Hypersensitivity to any component of the preparation.

Special warnings and precautions for use: Hypersensitivity reactions have been reported in patients who have exhibited hypersensitivity to other selective $5HT_3$ receptor antagonists. As ondansetron is known to increase large bowel transit time, patients with signs of subacute intestinal obstruction should be monitored following administration.

Interaction with other medicaments and other forms of interaction: There is no evidence that ondansetron either induces or inhibits the metabolism of other drugs commonly coadministered with it. Specific studies have shown that ondansetron does not interact with alcohol, temazepam, frusemide, tramadol and propofol.

Pregnancy and lactation: The safety of ondansetron for use in human pregnancy has not been established. Evaluation of experimental animal studies does not indicate direct or indirect harmful effects with respect to the development of the embryo, or foetus, the course of gestation and peri- and post-natal development. However, as animal studies are not always predictive of human response the use of ondansetron in pregnancy is not recommended. Tests have shown that ondansetron passes into the milk of lactating animals. It is therefore recommended that mothers receiving Zofran should not breast-feed their baby.

Effect on ability to drive and use machines: In psychomotor testing ondansetron does not impair performance nor cause sedation.

Undesirable effects: Ondansetron is known to increase large bowel transit time and may cause constipation in some patients. The following side effects can occur: headache, a sensation of flushing or warmth, hiccups and occasional transient, asymptomatic increases in aminotransferases. There have been rare reports of immediate hypersensitivity reactions sometimes severe including anaphylaxis. Rare cases of transient visual disturbances (e.g. blurred vision) and dizziness have been reported during rapid intravenous administration of ondansetron. There have been rare reports suggestive of involuntary movement disorders without definitive evidence of persistent clinical sequelae and seizures have been rarely observed although no known pharmacological mechanism can account for ondansetron causing these effects. Chest pain, cardiac arrhythmias, hypotension and bradycardia have been rarely reported.

Overdose: Little is known at present about overdosage with ondansetron, however, a limited number of patients received overdoses. Manifestations that have been reported include visual disturbances, severe constipation, hypotension and a vasovagal episode with transient second degree AV block. In all instances, the events resolved completely. There is no specific antidote for ondansetron, therefore in all cases of suspected overdose, symptomatic and supportive therapy should be given as appropriate.

Pharmacological properties

Pharmacodynamic properties: Ondansetron is a potent, highly selective $5HT_3$ receptor-antagonist. Its precise mode of action in the control of nausea and vomiting is not known. Chemotherapeutic agents and radiotherapy may cause release of 5HT in the small intestine initiating a vomiting reflex by activating vagal afferents via $5HT_3$ receptors. Ondansetron blocks the initiation of this reflex. Activation of vagal afferents may also cause a release of 5HT in the area postrema, located on the floor of the fourth ventricle, and this may also promote emesis through a central mechanism. Thus, the effect of ondansetron in the management of the nausea and vomiting induced by cytotoxic chemotherapy and radiotherapy is probably due to antagonism of $5HT_3$ receptors on neurons located both in the peripheral and central nervous system. The mechanisms of action in post-operative nausea and vomiting are not known but there may be common pathways with cytotoxic-induced nausea and vomiting.

Ondansetron does not alter plasma prolactin concentrations.

Pharmacokinetic properties: Following oral administration, ondansetron is passively and completely absorbed from the gastrointestinal tract and undergoes first pass metabolism. Peak plasma concentrations of about 30 ng/ml are attained approximately 1.5 hours after an 8 mg dose. For doses above 8 mg the increase in ondansetron systemic exposure with dose is greater than proportional; this may reflect some reduction in first pass metabolism at higher oral doses. Bioavailability, following oral administration, is slightly enhanced by the presence of food but unaffected by antacids. Studies in healthy elderly volunteers have shown slight, but clinically insignificant, age-related increases in both oral bioavailability (65%) and half-life (5 hours) of ondansetron. Gender differences were shown in the disposition of ondansetron, with females having a greater rate and extent of absorption following an oral dose and reduced systemic clearance and volume of distribution (adjusted for weight).

The disposition of ondansetron following oral, intramuscular (IM) and intravenous (IV) dosing is similar with a terminal half-life of about 3 hours and steady state volume of distribution of about 140 L. Equivalent systemic exposure is achieved after IM and IV administration of ondansetron.

A 4 mg intravenous infusion of ondansetron given over 5 minutes results in peak plasma concentrations of about 65 ng/ml. Following intramuscular administration of ondansetron, peak plasma concentrations of about 25 ng/ml are attained within 10 minutes of injection.

Following administration of ondansetron suppository, plasma ondansetron concentrations become detectable between 15 and 60 minutes after dosing. Concentrations rise in an essentially linear fashion, until peak concentrations of 20–30 ng/ml are attained, typically 6 hours after dosing. Plasma concentrations then fall, but at a slower rate than observed following oral dosing due to continued absorption of ondansetron. The absolute bioavailability of ondansetron from the suppository is approximately 60% and is not affected by gender. The half life of the elimination phase following suppository administration is determined by the rate of ondansetron absorption, not systemic clearance and is approximately 6 hours. Females show a small, clinically insignificant, increase in half-life in comparison with males.

Ondansetron is not highly protein bound (70–76%). Ondansetron is cleared from the systemic circulation predominantly by hepatic metabolism through multiple enzymatic pathways. Less than 5% of the absorbed dose is excreted unchanged in the urine. The absence of the enzyme CYP2D6 (the debrisoquine polymorphism) has no effect on ondansetron's pharmacokinetics. The pharmacokinetic properties of ondansetron are unchanged on repeat dosing.

In a study of 21 paediatric patients aged between 3 and 12 years undergoing elective surgery with general anaesthesia, the absolute values for both the clearance and volume of distribution of ondansetron following a single intravenous dose of 2 mg (3–7 years old) or 4 mg (8–12 years old) were reduced. The magnitude of the change was age-related, with clearance falling from about 300 ml/min at 12 years of age to 100 ml/min at 3 years. Volume of distribution fell from about 75 L at 12 years to 17 L at 3 years. Use of weight-based dosing (0.1 mg/kg up to 4 mg maximum) compensates for these changes and is effective in normalising systemic exposure in paediatric patients.

In patients with renal impairment (creatinine clearance 15–60 ml/min), both systemic clearance and volume of distribution are reduced following IV administration of ondansetron, resulting in a slight, but clinically insignificant, increase in elimination half-life (5.4 h). A study in patients with severe renal impairment who required regular haemodialysis (studied between dialyses) showed ondansetron's pharmacokinetics to be essentially unchanged following IV administration.

Specific studies in the elderly or patients with renal impairment have been limited to IV and oral administration. However, it is anticipated that the half-life of ondansetron after rectal administration in these populations will be similar to that seen in healthy volunteers, since the rate of elimination of ondansetron following rectal administration is not determined by systemic clearance.

Following oral, intravenous or intramuscular dosing in patients with severe hepatic impairment, ondansetron's systemic clearance is markedly reduced with prolonged elimination half-lives (15–32 h) and an oral bioavailability approaching 100% due to reduced presystemic metabolism. The pharmacokinetics of ondansetron following administration as a suppository have not been evaluated in patients with hepatic impairment.

Preclinical safety data: No additional data of relevance.

Pharmaceutical particulars

List of excipients: Lactose, microcrystalline cellulose, pre-gelatinised maize starch, magnesium stearate, methylhydroxypropylcellulose, titanium dioxide (E171), iron oxide (E172).

Incompatibilities: None reported.

Shelf life: 36 months.

Special precautions for storage: Store below 30°C.

Nature and contents of container:

Zofran 4 mg Tablets: Blister packs of 30 tablets comprising PVC film and aluminium foil lidding.

Zofran 8 mg Tablets: Blister packs of 10 tablets comprising PVC film and aluminium foil lidding.

Instructions for use/handling: None stated.

Marketing authorisation numbers
Zofran 4 mg Tablets PL 10949/0110
Zofran 8 mg Tablets PL 10949/0111

Date of approval/revision of SPC December 1997.

Legal category POM.

**Trade Mark*

Glenwood Laboratories Ltd
Jenkins Dale
Chatham
Kent ME4 5RD
☎ 01634 830535 🗋 01634 831345

MYOTONINE*

Qualitative and quantitative composition 10 mg tablet weighs 400 mg; active ingredient 10 mg Bethanechol Chloride USPXXII.

25 mg tablet weighs 450 mg; active ingredient 25 mg Bethanechol Chloride USPXXII.

Other ingredients: see *List of excipients.*

Pharmaceutical form

Tablet: 10 mg white, flat bevelled edge and single scored.

Tablet: 25 mg white, flat bevelled edge and cross scored.

Clinical particulars

Therapeutic indications: Urinary retention: acute post-operative, postpartum and neurogenic. Reflux oesophagitis.

Posology and method of administration: Administration orally by tablets.

Adults: 10 mg–25 mg 3–4 times daily. Taken ½ hr before food. Occasionally it may be felt necessary to initiate therapy with a 50 mg dose.

Children: The experience with children is limited; therefore no recommended dose is given.

Elderly: Adult dosage administered with caution.

Contra-indications: Intestinal or urinary obstruction, recent myocardial infarction, recent intestinal anastomosis.

Special warnings and special precautions for use: A severe cholinergic reaction is likely to occur if Bethanechol Chloride is administered IV or IM. This reaction has also rarely occurred in cases of hypersensitivity or overdose.

Interaction with other medicaments and other forms of interaction: Pharmacological interactions may occur with the following when bethanechol is administered.

Quinidine and procainamide which may antagonise cholinergic effects, cholinergic drugs which may have an additive effect, particularly cholinesterase inhibitors.

When administered to patients receiving ganglionic compounds, a critical fall in blood pressure may occur preceded by severe abdominal symptoms.

Pregnancy and lactation: Should not be used during pregnancy or lactation.

Effects on ability to drive and use machines: In some cases the ability to drive and operate machinery may be impaired.

Undesirable effects: Nausea, vomiting, sweating and intestinal colic.

Overdose:

Symptoms: Include nausea, salivation, lachrymation, eructation, involuntary defecation and urination, transient dyspnoea, palpitation, bradycardia and peripheral vasodilation leading to hypertension, transient heart block and a feeling of constriction under the sternum.

Procedure: The stomach should be emptied by aspiration and lavage. Give atropine sulphate 1–2 mg intravenously, intramuscularly or subcutaneously to control muscarinic effects. This dose may be repeated every 2–4 hours as necessary. Supportive treatment includes intravenous administration of diazepam 5–10 mg; muscle twitching may be controlled by small doses of tubocurarine (together with assisted respiration); oxygen may be required.

Pharmacological properties

Pharmacodynamic properties: Bethanechol is a synthetic choline ester of carbamic acid which possesses a significant acetylcholine-like activity. It is active after oral administration. As a consequence of the very slow hydrolysation by acetylcholinesterase, bethanechol has a prolonged action as has been demonstrated on the urinary tract.[1] The onset of action after oral administration of bethanechol chloride occurs within an hour.[2,3]

The major pharmacological effects of bethanechol result from interaction of the drug with muscarinic receptor sites of smooth muscles, especially those of the urinary bladder and gastrointestinal tract.[1,4,5] In addition, minor but important nicotine effects have been noted.

In usual therapeutic doses, bethanechol does not cross the blood brain barrier.[6] Studies addressing pharmacokinetic-pharmacodynamic association are not available.

References

1. Draper J.W., Zorgniotta A.W. The effects of banthine and similar agents on the urinary tract. N.Y. State *J. Med.* 1954; 54; 77.
2. Boas E., Comarr A.E. *Neurological Urology.* Baltimore, University Park Press 1971; 215.
3. Lapides J., Friend C.R., Ajemian E.P., Sonda L.P. Comparison of action of oral and parenteral bethanechol chloride upon the urinary bladder. *Invest. Urol.* 1963; 1:94.
4. Paul D.A., Icardi J.A., Parkman H.P., Ryan J.P. Development changes in gastric fundus smooth muscle contractility and involvement of extracellular calcium in foetal and adult guinea pigs. *Paediatr. Res.* 1994; 36:642–646.
5. Ursillo R.C. Rationale for drug therapy in bladder dysfunction. In. Boyarsk s. *The Neurogenic Bladder.* Baltimore, The Williams and Wilkins CO. 1967; 187.
6. Goodman Gilman. *The Pharmacological Basis of Therapeutics.* Editors: Goodman, Gilman A; Rale T.W., Nies A.S., Taylor P., New York. Pergamon Press. 8th Edition 1991.

Preclinical safety data Not applicable.

Pharmaceutical particulars

List of excipients: Calcium Sulphate Hemihydrate BP; Maize Starch BP; Talc BP (iron free); Magnesium Stearate BP.

Incompatibilities: Major – none known.

Shelf life: The shelf life of Myotonine tablets is currenctly two years from date of manufacture.

Storage: Store below 20°C. Keep out of reach of children and away from direct heat or light sources. Store in areas free from the risk of dampness.

Nature and contents of container: The container is of polypropylene with a tamper-evident polyethylene cap and closure. A filla may be inserted to reduce the risk of tablet breakage due to ullage.

Each container is filled with 100 tablets.

Marketing authorisation number

Myotonine 10 mg 00245/5009R
Myotonine 25 mg 00245/5010R.

Date of approval/revision of SPC April 1996.

Legal category POM.

POTABA* (Potassium para-aminobenzoate)

Composition Capsules: white/white gelatin capsule shell containing the active ingredient 500 mg of potassium para-aminobenzoate powder.

Pharmaceutical form

Capsules: White/white size zero gelatin capsules containing 500 mg potassium para-aminobenzoate).

Clincal particulars

Therapeutic indications: Peyronie's Disease. Scleroderma.

Posology and method of administration: Potaba capsules should be taken orally; six capsules four times daily with food.

Children: Not recommended.

Contra-indications: Potaba should not be given to patients taking sulphonamides as it will inactivate this medication.

Special warnings and precautions: Treatment with Potaba should be interrupted during periods of low food intake (e.g. during fasting, anorexia, nausea). This is to avoid the possible development of hypoglycaemia.

Potaba treatment should be given cautiously to patients with renal impairment and treatment discontinued if a hypersensitivity reaction occurs.

Potaba should not be taken by patients on sulphonamides; Potaba may cause inactivation of this medication.

Interactions: With the exception of sulphonamides, no interactions with other medicaments have been established.

Pregnancy and breast feeding: No information is available on this, therefore, it is not recommended.

Effects on ability to drive and use machines: There is no evidence that Potaba has any effect on ability to drive or use machines.

Undesirable effects: Treatment with Potaba should be interrupted during periods of low food intake, (e.g. during fasting, anorexia, nausea). This is to avoid the possible development of hypoglycaemia. No serious adverse effects have been reported in patients treated with Potaba.

Overdose: No particular problems are expected following overdosage with Potaba. Symptomatic and supportive therapy should be given as appropriate.

Pharmacological properties

Pharmacodynamic properties: P. Aminobenzoate is considered a member of the Vitamin B complex. Small amounts are found in cereal, eggs, milk and meats. Detectable amounts are normally present in human blood, spinal fluid, urine and sweat. The pharmacological action of this chemical has not been clearly established, but it has been suggested that the antifibrosis activity of Potaba is brought about by the drug increasing oxygen uptake at the tissue level. Fibrosis is believed to occur from either too much serotonin or too little monoamine oxidase activity over a period of time. The activity of monoamine oxidase is dependant on an adequate oxygen supply. By increasing oxygen supply at tissue level Potaba enhances monoamine oxidase activity thereby preventing or bringing about regression of fibrosis.

Pharmacokinetics: Potaba is rapidly absorbed and metabolised as food. Excretion is through renal function.

Preclinical safety data: N/A.

Pharmaceutical particulars

Excipients: None.

Incompatibilities: Sulphonamides.

Shelf life: Capsules: three years from date of manufacture.

Storage: Store below 25°C.

Nature and contents of containers: White polypropylene tube with tamper-evident polyethylene cap. A filla may be inserted to reduce ullage.

Containers of 240 × 500 mg capsules.

Marketing authorisation number 0245/5001R

Date of revision of text November 1998, December 1997, November 1996, June 1996 (revised from December 1995).

POTABA* (Potassium para-aminobenzoate)

Composition Envules: foil laminate sachets containing 3 g of potassium para-aminobenzoate.

Pharmaceutical form

Envule: contains 3 g potassium para-aminobenzxoae; white/off-white powder.

Clincal particulars

Therapeutic indications: Peyronie's Disease. Scleroderma.

Posology and method of administration: Potaba envules should be taken orally; four times daily with food; dissolve the powder in fruit juice.

Children: Not recommended.

Contra-indications: Potaba should not be given to patients taking sulphonamides as it will inactivate this medication.

Special warnings and precautions: Treatment with Potaba should be interrupted during periods of low food intake (e.g. during fasting, anorexia, nausea). This is to avoid the possible development of hypoglycaemia.

Potaba treatment should be given cautiously to patients with renal impairment and treatment discontinued if a hypersensitivity reaction occurs.

Potaba should not be taken by patients on sulphonamides; Potaba may cause inactivation of this medication.

Interactions: With the exception of sulphonamides,

no interactions with other medicaments have been established.

Pregnancy and breast feeding: No information is available on this, therefore, it is not recommended.

Effects on ability to drive and use machines: There is no evidence that Potaba has any effect on ability to drive or use machines.

Undesirable effects: Treatment with Potaba should be interrupted during periods of low food intake, (e.g. during fasting, anorexia, nausea). This is to avoid the possible development of hypoglycaemia. No serious adverse effects have been reported in patients treated with Potaba.

Overdose: No particular problems are expected following overdosage with Potaba. Symptomatic and supportive therapy should be given as appropriate.

Pharmacological properties

Pharmacodynamic properties: P. Aminobenzoate is considered a member of the Vitamin B complex. Small amounts are found in cereal, eggs, milk and meats. Detectable amounts are normally present in human blood, spinal fluid, urine and sweat. The pharmacological action of this chemical has not been clearly established, but it has been suggested that the antifibrosis activity of Potaba is brought about by the drug increasing oxygen uptake at the tissue level. Fibrosis is believed to occur from either too much serotonin or too little monoamine oxidase activity over a period of time. The activity of monoamine oxidase is dependant on an adequate oxygen supply. By increasing oxygen supply at tissue level Potaba enhances monoamine oxidase activity thereby preventing or bringing about regression of fibrosis.

Pharmacokinetics: Potaba is rapidly absorbed and metabolised as food. Excretion is through renal function.

Preclinical safety data: N/A.

Pharmaceutical particulars

Excipients: None in this presentation.

Incompatibilities: Sulphonamides.

Shelf life: Envules: five years from date of manufacture.

Storage: Store below 25°C.

Nature and contents of containers: Cardboard outer containing 40 × 3 g foil laminate sachets.

Marketing authorisation number 0245/5000R

Date of revision of text November 1998, December 1997, June 1996 (revised from December 1995).

POTABA*
(Potassium para-aminobenzoate)

Presentation Tablets: white/off-white tablet containing 500 mg of potassium para-aminobenzoate and excipients as under *Excipients.*

Pharmaceutical form Tablet: contains 500 mg of potassium para-aminobenzoate; white/off-white plain deep concave 11.00 mm in diameter.

Clinical particulars

Therapeutic indications: Peyronie's Disease, Scleroderma.

Posology and method of administration: Potaba tablets should be taken orally; six tablets, crushed in juice, four times daily with food.

Children: not recommended.

Contra-indications: Potaba should not be given to patient taking sulphonamides as it will inactivate this medication.

Special warnings and precautions: Treatment with Potaba should be interrupted during periods of low food intake (e.g., during fasting, anorexia, nausea). This is to avoid the possible development of hypoglycaemia.

Potaba treatment should be given cautiously to patients with renal impairment and treatment discontinued if a hypersensitivity reaction occurs.

Potaba should not be taken by patients on sulphonamides; Potaba may cause inactivation of this medication.

Interactions: With the exception of sulphonamides, no interactions with other medicaments have been established.

Pregnancy and breast feeding: No information is available on this therefore it is not recommended.

Effects on ability to drive and use machines: There is no evidence that Potaba has any effect on ability to drive or use machines.

Undesirable effects: Treatment with Potaba should be interrupted during periods of low food intake, (e.g. during fasting, anorexia, nausea). This is to avoid the possible development of hypoglycaemia. No serious adverse effects have been reported in patients treated with Potaba.

Overdose: No particular problems are expected following overdosage with Potaba. Symptomatic and supportive therapy should be given as appropriate.

Pharmacological properties

P. Aminobenzoate is considered a member of the Vitamin B complex. Small amounts are found in cereal, eggs, milk and meats. Detectable amounts are normally present in human blood, spinal fluid, urine and sweat. The pharmacological action of this chemical has not been clearly established, but it has been suggested that the antifibrosis activity of Potaba is brought about by the drug increasing oxygen uptake at the tissue level. Fibrosis is believed to occur from either too much serotonin or too little monoamine oxidase activity over a period of time. The activity of monoamine oxidase is dependant on an adequate oxygen supply. By increasing oxygen supply at tissue level Potaba enhances monoamine oxidase activity thereby preventing or bringing about regression of fibrosis.

Pharmacokinetics: Potaba is rapidly absorbed and metabolised as food. Excretion is through renal function.

Preclinical safety data: N/A.

Pharmaceutical particulars

Excipients: Sucrose BP; Acacia BP; Ethocol 200; Industrial Methylated Spirit (11 litres/100,000 tablets); Magnesium stearate BP; Stearic acid BPC; Maize starch BP.

Incompatibilities: Sulphonamides.

Shelf life: Tablets: three years from date of manufacture.

Storage: Store below 25°C.

Nature and contents of containers: White polypropylene tube with tamper-evident polyethylene cap. A filla may be inserted to reduce ullage.

Containers of 120×500 mg tablets and also 1,000×500 mg tablets.

Marketing authorisation number 0245/5002R.

Date of revision of text November 1998; December 1997, November 1996, June 1996 (revised from December 1995).

**Trade Mark*

Goldshield Pharmaceuticals Ltd
NLA Tower
12–16 Addiscombe Road
Croydon
CR0 0XT

☎ 0181 649 8500   🖷 0181 686 0807

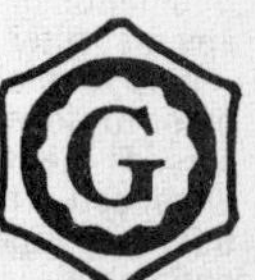

DINDEVAN* TABLETS

Presentation
Dindevan Tablets 10 mg: White tablets engraved D10, each tablet containing Phenindione BP 10 mg.

Dindevan Tablets 25 mg: Green tablets engraved D25, each tablet containing Phenindione BP 25 mg.

Dindevan Tablets 50 mg: White tablets engraved D50, each tablet containing Phenindione BP 50 mg.

Uses Dindevan (Phenindione BP) is a synthetic anticoagulant which acts by interfering with the formation of clotting factors II, VII, IX and X. It produces its effect in 36 to 48 hours after the initial dose: the effect wanes over a period of 48 to 72 hours after Dindevan is stopped.

Anticoagulant therapy can be initiated with heparin and Dindevan together.

Indications: Prophylaxis of systemic embolisation in patients with rheumatic heart disease and atrial fibrillation.

Prophylaxis after insertion of prosthetic heart valves. Prophylaxis and treatment of venous thrombosis and pulmonary embolism.

Dosage and administration *Initial loading dose:* Usually 200 mg, followed on the second day with a dose of 100 mg.

Maintenance therapy: Dosage must be adjusted, from the third day, in accordance with the results of appropriate coagulation tests. Concomitant heparin therapy affects the results of control tests and should be discontinued at least six hours before the first test is carried out.

Control tests must be made at regular intervals and the dosage further adjusted according to the results obtained. As a general guide, a maintenance dosage of between 50 and 150 mg per day will prove satisfactory in most cases. Occasionally, a resistant patient may need 200 mg or more per day; on the other hand a sensitive patient may need less than 50 mg per day.

Contra-indications, warnings, etc
Contra-indications: Pregnancy. Infants should not be fed with breast milk from mothers being treated with Dindevan. Known hypersensitivity to phenindione. Dindevan should not be given in the presence of severe hepatic or renal disease, bacterial endocarditis, actual or potential haemorrhagic conditions, or to patients with uncontrolled hypertension. Its use within 24 hours following surgery or labour should be undertaken with caution, if at all.

Precautions: (See Drug interactions) The following factors may exaggerate the effects of Dindevan and necessitate a reduction in dosage: loss in weight; elderly subject; acute illness, impaired renal function; decreased dietary intake of vitamin K and administration of certain drugs (see 'Drug interactions').

Factors which may call for an increase in maintenance dosage include weight gain, diarrhoea and vomiting, increased intake of vitamin K, fats and oils and administration of certain drugs (see 'Drug interactions').

Administration of vitamin K can lead to resistance to the action of Dindevan for some days. For this reason, fresh-frozen plasma should be administered to patients with prosthetic heart valves where haemorrhage has occurred.

Pregnancy: Oral anticoagulants should not be used in pregnancy particularly because of possible teratogenicity and the risk of foetal haemorrhage near term. It is therefore suggested that heparin (which does not cross the placenta) be used during the first trimester and after 37 weeks gestation. However, the use of heparin in pregnancy is not absolutely safe and specialist guidance is advisable for those who are pregnant and who need anti-coagulant therapy. Women of child-bearing age who are receiving treatment with Dindevan should be cautioned about the possible complications of pregnancy. Infants should not be fed with breast milk from mothers being treated with Dindevan.

Side-effects: The following effects have been reported: hypersensitivity including skin rashes, alopecia, exanthema, skin necrosis, exfoliative dermatitis, fever, leucopenia and agranulocytosis, diarrhoea, vomiting, hepatitis and renal damage with tubular necrosis. Micro-adenopathy, jaundice, albuminuria, eosinophilia, a leukaemoid blood picture or cytopenia or haemothorax may also be observed. If any of these are observed administration of Dindevan should stop immediately and full investigations of blood and of liver and kidney function should be carried out. Possible sensitivity to other drugs should be considered. Other anticoagulants, such as warfarin, are usually tolerated by patients sensitive to Dindevan. If therapy is controlled as recommended then bleeding due to overdosage of anticoagulant is rare. An episode of bleeding occurring during anticoagulant therapy must therefore be investigated fully and not regarded automatically as a manifestation of overdosage.

NB. The metabolites of Dindevan often colour the urine pink or orange. This may be distinguished from discolouration caused by haemoglobin by the addition of a few drops of dilute acetic acid to the urine. If the colour is due to Dindevan it will disappear immediately.

Drug interactions: Care is required in the concomitant use of all drugs in patients receiving oral anticoagulant therapy. Known interactions include the following, but prescribers of other or newly available medicines should refer to the manufacturers prescribing information or the appropriate monograph. The following may exaggerate the effects of Dindevan: ACTH, allopurinol, amiodarone, amitriptyline/nortriptyline, anabolic steroids, azapropazone, aztreonam, broad spectrum antibiotics, ciprofloxacin, cimetidine, clofibrate, corticosteroids, co-trimoxazole, dextropropoxyphene, diflunisal, dipyridamole, disulfiram, feprazone, flurbiprofen, gemfibrozil, glucagon, hepato-toxic drugs, indomethacin, metronidazole, NSAIDS, oxyphenbutazone, phenformin, phenylbutazone, quinidine, salicylates, sulindac, sulphinpyrazone, thyroid compounds, tolbutamide. Monitoring and reduction of the dose of Dindevan may be necessary.

The following may reduce the effects of Dindevan: alcohol in large amounts, carbamazepine, cholestyramine, dichloralphenazone, glutethimide, griseofulvin, phenobarbitone, phenytoin, rifampicin. Monitoring and increase of the dose of Dindevan may be necessary.

Overdosage: If haemorrhage occurs or a potential bleeding state arises, excessive depression of the coagulation activity can be corrected by temporary withdrawal of Dindevan accompanied, if necessary, by infusion of fresh-frozen plasma or whole blood. Vitamin K, 5 to 10 mg intravenously, may be required to supplement specific treatment with factor concentrates.

Pharmaceutical precautions No special requirements or precautions.

Legal category POM.

Package quantities Dindevan Tablets 10 mg, 25 mg and 50 mg are each available in containers of 100 tablets (OP).

Further information Also contains Lactose BP.

Product licence numbers

Dindevan Tablets 10 mg	10972/0037
Dindevan Tablets 25 mg	10972/0038
Dindevan Tablets 50 mg	10972/0039

ELTROXIN* TABLETS

Presentation Small white tablets engraved 'Eltroxin 50' or 'Eltroxin 100' containing 50 micrograms (0.05 mg) or 100 micrograms (0.1 mg) anhydrous thyroxine sodium respectively. The lower-strength tablets are scored. Eltroxin Tablets comply with the specification for Thyroxine Tablets BP.

Uses Hypothyroidism.

Dosage and administration *Adults:* Initially 50 to 100 micrograms daily, preferably taken before breakfast, and adjusted at three to four weeks intervals by 50 micrograms until normal metabolism is steadily maintained; this may require doses of 100 to 200 micrograms daily. With patients aged over 50 years, it is not advisable to exceed 50 micrograms a day initially, and where there is cardiac disease, 25 micrograms daily, or 50 micrograms on alternate days, is more suitable. In this condition the daily dosage may be increased by 25 micrograms at intervals of perhaps four weeks.

In younger patients, and in the absence of heart disease, a serum thyroxine (T4) level of about 70 to 160 nanomols per litre, or a serum thyrotrophin level of less than 5 milli-units per litre, should be aimed at. In those aged over 50, and/or in the presence of heart disease, clinical response is probably a more acceptable criterion of dosage than serum levels.

A pre-therapy ECG is valuable, as changes induced by hypothyroidism may be confused with ECG evidence of ischaemia. If too rapid an increase of metabolism is produced (causing diarrhoea, nervousness, rapid pulse, insomnia, tremors and sometimes anginal pain where there is latent myocardial ischaemia), dosage must be reduced or withheld for a day or two, then begun again at a lower level.

Congenital hypothyroidism and juvenile myxoedema: The largest dose consistent with freedom from toxic effects should be given. The dosage is guided by clinical response, growth assessment and appropriate thyroid function tests – clinically normal pulse rate and absence of diarrhoea or constipation are the most useful indicators.

Thyrotrophin levels may remain elevated during the first year of life in children with neonatal hypothyroidism due to re-setting of the hypothalamic-pituitary axis. For infants with congenital hypothyroidism, a suitable starting dose is 25 micrograms Eltroxin daily, with increments of 25 micrograms every two to four weeks until mild toxic symptoms appear. Dosage is then slightly reduced. The same applies to juvenile myxoedema, except that the starting dose for children older than one year may be 2.5 to 5 micrograms/kg/day.

Contra-indications, warnings, etc
Contra-indications: Thyrotoxicosis. Hypersensitivity to any component of the preparation.

Precautions: Patients with panhypopituitarism or other causes predisposing to adrenal insufficiency may react unfavourably to thyroxine treatment, and it is advisable to initiate corticosteroid therapy before giving thyroxine in these cases.

Special care is needed in the elderly and in patients with symptoms of myocardial insufficiency or ECG evidence of myocardial infarction.

Thyroid replacement therapy may result in an increase in dosage requirement of insulin or other antidiabetic therapy. Care is needed in patients with diabetes mellitus or diabetes insipidus.

Use in pregnancy and lactation: The safety of thyroxine during pregnancy is unknown but any possible risk of congenital abnormalities should be weighed up against the risk to the foetus of untreated hypothyroidism.

Thyroxine is excreted into breast milk in low concentrations and it is contentious whether this may interfere with neonatal screening programs.

Side-effects: The following effects are indicative of excessive dosage and usually disappear on reduction of dosage or withdrawal of treatment for a few days. Anginal pain, cardiac arrhythmias, palpitation, and cramps in skeletal muscle; also tachycardia, diarrhoea, vomiting, tremors, restlessness, excitability, insomnia, headache, flushing, sweating, excessive loss of weight and muscular weakness.

Drug interactions: Thyroxine increases the effect of anticoagulants and it may be necessary to reduce the dose of anticoagulant if excessive hypoprothrombinaemia and bleeding are to be avoided. Phenytoin levels may be increased by thyroxine. Anticonvulsants such as carbamazepine and phenytoin enhance the metabolism of thyroid hormones and may displace them from plasma proteins.

Initiation or discontinuation of anticonvulsant therapy may alter thyroxine dose requirements.

If co-administered with cardiac glycosides, adjustment of dosage of cardiac glycoside may be necessary. The effect of sympathomimetic agents is also enhanced. Thyroxine raises blood sugar levels and this may upset the stability of patients receiving antidiabetic agents. Thyroxine increases receptor sensitivity to catecholamines thus accelerating the response to tricyclic antidepressants. Cholestyramine given concurrently reduces the gastrointestinal absorption of thyroxine.

Co-administration of oral contraceptives may result in an increased dosage requirement of thyroid therapy.

A number of drugs may affect thyroid function tests and this should be borne in mind when monitoring a patient on thyroxine therapy.

Overdosage: Gastric lavage or emesis is required if the patient is seen within several hours of taking the dose. In addition to exaggeration of side effects the following symptoms may be seen: agitation, confusion, irritability, hyperactivity, sweating, mydriasis, tachycardia, arrhythmias, tachypnoea, pyrexia, increased bowel movements and convulsions. The appearance of clinical hyperthyroidism may be delayed for up to five days.

Treatment is symptomatic, and tachycardia has been controlled in an adult by 40 mg doses of propranolol given every six hours and other symptoms by diazepam and/or chlorpromazine as appropriate.

Pharmaceutical precautions Protect from light.

Legal category POM.

Package quantities Bottles of 100 and 1,000 tablets.

Further information 100 micrograms thyroxine is equivalent in activity to 20 to 30 micrograms liothyronine or 60 mg Thyroid BP. Also contains Lactose BP.

Product licence numbers

Tablets 50 micrograms	10972/0031
Tablets 100 micrograms	10972/0032

MAREVAN* TABLETS

Presentation Marevan Tablets are Warfarin Tablets BP.

Marevan Tablets 1 mg: Brown tablets engraved M1, each tablet containing Warfarin Sodium BP 1 mg.

Marevan Tablets 3 mg: Blue tablets engraved M3, each tablet containing Warfarin Sodium BP 3 mg.

Marevan Tablets 5 mg: Pink tablets engraved M5, each tablet containing Warfarin Sodium BP 5 mg.

Uses Marevan is a synthetic anti-coagulant of the coumarin series and acts by inhibiting the formation of active clotting factors II, VII, IX and X. An effect on prothrombin time is produced in 24 to 36 hours after the initial dose. This reaches a maximum in 36 to 48 hours and is maintained for 48 hours or more after administration is stopped.

Indications: Prophylaxis of systemic embolisation in patients with rheumatic heart disease and atrial fibrillation.

Prophylaxis after insertion of prosthetic heart valves. Prophylaxis and treatment of venous thrombosis and pulmonary embolism.

Transient cerebral ischaemic attacks.

Dosage and administration *Adults and the elderly:* The typical induction dose of Marevan is 10 mg daily for 2 days, but this should be tailored to individual requirement.

The daily maintenance dose of Marevan is usually 3 to 9 mg taken at the same time each day. The exact maintenance dose for an individual is dependent on the prothrombin time or other appropriate coagulation tests.

The maintenance dose is omitted if the prothrombin time is excessively prolonged. Once the maintenance dose is stabilised in the therapeutic range, it is rarely necessary to alter it.

In emergencies, anticoagulant therapy should be initiated with heparin and Marevan together. Where there is less urgency, as in patients disposed to or at special risk of thromboembolism, anticoagulant therapy may be initiated with Marevan alone.

Concomitant heparin therapy affects the results of control tests and should be discontinued at least six hours before the first test is carried out.

Control tests must be made at regular intervals and Marevan maintenance dosage further adjusted according to the results obtained.

Children: The dosage of Marevan which may be used in children has not yet been established.

Contra-indications, warnings, etc

Contra-indications: Pregnancy (see below). Known hypersensitivity to warfarin. Marevan should not be given in the presence of severe hepatic or renal disease, bacterial endocarditis, actual or potential haemorrhagic conditions, eg. peptic ulcer, or to patients with uncontrolled hypertension. Its use within 24 hours following surgery or labour should be undertaken with caution, if at all.

Precautions: The following factors may exaggerate the effects of Marevan and necessitate a reduction in dosage; loss of weight, elderly subject, acute illness, deficient renal function, decreased dietary intake of vitamin K, administration of certain drugs (see 'Drug interactions').

Factors which may call for an increase in maintenance dosage include weight gain, diarrhoea and vomiting, increased intake of vitamin K, fats and oils, and the administration of certain drugs (see 'Drug interactions').

Careful additional laboratory control is necessary if the patient is to be changed from one formulation to another.

Reversal of warfarin anticoagulation by vitamin K takes several days. In emergency situations fresh-frozen plasma should be given.

Pregnancy: Oral anticoagulants should not be used in pregnancy particularly because of possible teratogenicity and the risk of foetal haemorrhage near term. It is therefore suggested that heparin (which does not cross the placenta) be used during the first trimester and after 37 weeks gestation. However, the use of heparin in pregnancy is not absolutely safe and specialist guidance is advisable for those who are pregnant and who need anticoagulant therapy. Women of child bearing age who are receiving treatment with Marevan should be cautioned about the possible complications of pregnancy.

Side-effects: The following effects have been reported: hypersensitivity, skin rashes, alopecia, diarrhoea, an unexplained drop in haematocrit, a 'purple toes' syndrome, jaundice and hepatic dysfunction.

Skin necrosis within a few days of starting treatment has been infrequently reported. Most subjects are obese, elderly women. The first sign is an erythematous swollen patch. Administration of vitamin K at this stage may prevent the development of ecchymosis and infarction.

Purpura, fever, nausea, vomiting, pancreatitis, haemothorax and epistaxis may also be observed. If any of these are observed administration of Marevan should stop immediately. Possible sensitivity to other drugs should be considered. Other anticoagulants are often tolerated by patients sensitive to Marevan. If therapy is controlled as recommended then bleeding due to overdosage of anticoagulant is rare. An episode of bleeding occurring during anticoagulant therapy must therefore be investigated fully and not regarded automatically as a manifestation of overdosage.

Drug interactions: Care is required in the concomitant use of all drugs in patients receiving oral anticoagulant therapy. Known interactions include the following, but prescribers of other or newly available medicines should refer to the manufacturer's information or appropriate monograph.

The activity of warfarin may be potentiated by amiodarone, amitriptyline/nortriptyline, anabolic steroids, azapropazone, bezafibrate, cephamandole, chloral hydrate, chloramphenicol, cimetidine, clofibrate, co-trimoxazole, danazol, dextropropoxyphene, dextrothyroxine, dipyridamole, erythromycin, feprazone, glucagon, latamoxef, metronidazole, miconazole, neomycin, oxyphenbutazone, phenformin, phenylbutazone, phenyramidol, quinidine, salicylates, sulphonamides (eg. sulphaphenazole, sulphinpyrazone), tamoxifen, tolbutamide and tricolofos.

Potentiation may also occur with the following drugs, aztreonam, ciprofloxacin, diflunisel, fluconazole, flurbiprofen, fluroxamine, gemfibrocil, indomethacin, mefenamic acid, piroxicam, sulindac and possibly other anti-inflammatory analgesics, ketoconazole, nalidixic acid, norfloxacin, omeprazole, propafenone, tetracyclines and other broad spectrum antibiotics.

Anticoagulant activity may be possibly increased by allopurinol, disulfiram, methylphenidate, paracetamol, thyroid drugs, and any potentially hepatoxic drug.

Both potentiation and inhibition of anticoagulant effect have been reported with phenytoin, ACTH and corticosteroids.

Anticoagulant activity may also be increased with large amounts of chronic ingestion of alcohol, particularly in patients with impaired liver function.

Warfarin absorption is impaired and activity decreased by cholestyramine and sulcralfate. Cholestyramine, however, may also decrease absorption of vitamin K and thus increase coumarin anticoagulant activity. Anticoagulant effect may be decreased by administration of vitamin K (eg. as a constituent of some enteral feeds).

The anticoagulant activity of warfarin may be inhibited by drugs which induce liver enzymes such as aminoglutethimide, barbiturates, carbamazepine, ethchlorvynol, glutethimide, primidone, griseofulvin, dichloralphenazone, rifampicin and oral contraceptives.

Overdosage: If haemorrhage occurs or a potential bleeding state arises, excessive depression of the coagulation activity can be corrected by temporary withdrawal of Marevan accompanied, if necessary, by infusion of fresh-frozen plasma or whole blood. Vitamin K, 5 to 10 mg orally or intravenously, may be required to supplement specific treatment with factor concentrates.

Pharmaceutical precautions Replace cap securely and protect from light.

Legal category POM.

Package quantities Marevan Tablets 1 mg are available in containers of 100 (OP) and 500.

Marevan Tablets 3 mg are available in containers of 100 (OP) and 500.

Marevan Tablets 5 mg are available in containers of 100 (OP) and 500.

Further information Also contains Lactose BP.

Product licence numbers

Marevan Tablets 1 mg	10972/0034
Marevan Tablets 3 mg	10972/0035
Marevan Tablets 5 mg	10972/0036

**Trade Mark*

Grifols UK Ltd
Howlett Way
Thetford
Norfolk
IP24 1HZ

☎ 01842 761942/764260 🖷 01842 766661

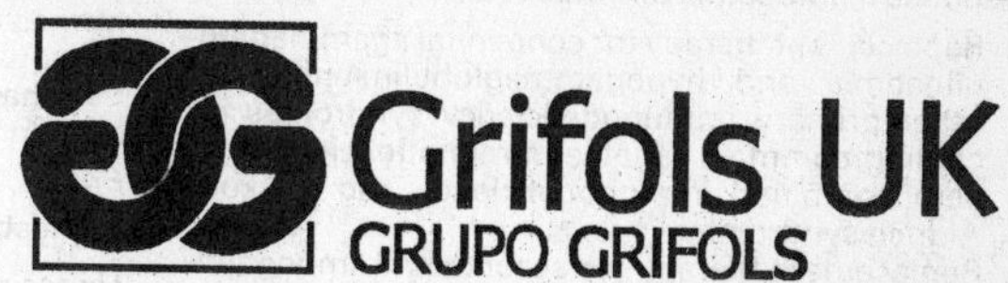

ALBUTEIN* 5%

Presentation Albutein 5% is Albumin Solution BP 5% and each 100 ml of solution contains 5 g of human serum albumin. It is a clear, almost colourless to amber sterile aqueous solution for single dose intravenous administration.

Uses Albumin is a highly soluble globular protein (MW 66,500) which is important in regulating the osmotic pressure of plasma. Albutein 5% solution supplies the oncotic equivalent of approximately its own volume of normal human plasma and will increase the circulating plasma volume by an amount equal to the volume infused. The degree and duration of volume expansion depend upon the initial blood volume. The effect of infused albumin persists longer in patients with diminished blood volume than in individuals with normal blood volume. Albumin is also a transport protein and binds naturally occurring, therapeutic and toxic materials in the circulation. The binding properties of albumin may in special circumstances provide an indication for its clinical use. For such purposes, however, Albutein 20% or Albutein 25% should be used.

Albutein 5% is indicated:

1. For the treatment of hypovolaemic shock.
2. In conditions in which there is severe hypoalbuminaemia. However unless the pathologic condition responsible for the hypoalbuminaemia can be corrected, administration of albumin can afford only symptomatic or supportive relief.
3. For the treatment of burns.
4. As an adjunct in cardiopulmonary bypass procedures.

In those conditions in which the colloid requirement is high and there is less need for fluid, albumin should be administered as the 20% or 25% solutions.

Dosage and administration Albutein 5% is intended for intravenous administration. The total dosage will vary with the individual.

Adults: An initial infusion of 500 ml is suggested. This may be repeated in 15–30 minutes if the initial dose is inadequate. Additional amounts should be administered as clinically indicated.

The rate of administration should be 1–2 ml per minute in patients with slightly low or normal blood volume. In patients with shock and/or greatly reduced blood volume, Albutein 5% may be administered as rapidly as necessary.

Children: Dosage will vary with clinical state and body weight. A dose of one-quarter to one-half of the adult dose may be administered or dosage may be calculated on the basis of 3–5 ml per kilogram body weight.

The rate of administration should be calculated on one-quarter of the adult rate.

Contra-indications, warnings, etc Albutein 5% is contra-indicated in patients with severe anaemia or cardiac failure in the presence of normal or increased intravascular volume and in patients with a history of allergic reactions to albumin products.

Albutein 5% should be administered with caution to patients with low cardiac reserve. Additional fluids may be required for patients with marked dehydration. Rapid infusion may cause vascular overload with resultant pulmonary oedema. Patients should be closely monitored for signs of increased venous pressure. A rapid rise in blood pressure following infusion necessitates careful observation of injured or postoperative patients to detect and treat severed blood vessels that may not have bled at a lower pressure.

Do not use for control of haemorrhage due to deficiencies or defects in the clotting mechanism.

Albumin naturally binds a variety of therapeutic and toxic materials and thus administration of Albutein 5% may modify the pre-existing distribution of certain substances.

Adverse reactions are rare. However allergic or pyrogenic reactions, characterised primarily by fever and chills, nausea, vomiting, tachycardia and hypotension have been reported.

If such reactions occur the infusion should be discontinued and appropriate therapy (eg. antihistamine) or specific support treatment should be given.

Reproduction studies have not been conducted with albumin. Human albumin should be given to a pregnant woman only if clearly needed.

Administration of large quantities of albumin may require supplementation with red cell concentrates to help overcome any resulting relative anaemia.

Pharmaceutical precautions Do not use if the solution appears turbid or contains a deposit. Since the solution does not contain a preservative it should be used within 3 hours of penetration of the container. Discard any unused portion.

Do not administer protein hydrolysates or alcohol via the same administration set used for Albutein 5%.

Albutein 5% should be stored between 2°C and 25°C protected from light.

Legal category POM.

Package quantities Albutein 5% is supplied in:
250 ml glass vials containing 12.5 g of albumin.
500 ml glass vials containing 25.0 g of albumin.

Further information Albutein 5% is prepared from plasma obtained from carefully selected and rigorously screened donors. The final product is heated at 60°C for 10 hours. However as with all blood products the risk of viral transmission with this product cannot be absolutely excluded. Nevertheless there are no known cases of viral transmission resulting from the administration of Albutein 5%.

Product licence number 4447/0007.

ALBUTEIN* 20%

Presentation Albutein 20% is Albumin Solution BP 20% and each 100 ml of solution contains 20 g of human serum albumin. It is a clear, almost colourless to amber sterile aqueous solution for single dose intravenous administration.

Uses Albumin is a highly soluble globular protein (MW 66,500) which is important in regulating the osmotic pressure of plasma. Albutein 20% solution supplies the oncotic equivalent of approximately 4 times its own volume of normal human plasma. It will increase the circulating plasma volume by an amount approximately 2.5 times the volume infused within 15 minutes, if the recipient is adequately hydrated. The degree and duration of volume expansion depend upon the initial blood volume. The effect of infused albumin persists longer in patients with diminished blood volume than in individuals with normal blood volume. Albumin is also a transport protein and binds naturally occurring, therapeutic and toxic materials in the circulation. The binding properties of albumin may in special circumstances provide an indication for its clinical use.

Albutein 20% is indicated:

1. For the treatment of hypovolaemic shock.
2. In conditions in which there is severe hypoalbuminaemia. However unless the pathologic condition responsible for the hypoalbuminaemia can be corrected, administration of albumin can afford only symptomatic or supportive relief.
3. For the treatment of burns.
4. As an adjunct in cardiopulmonary bypass procedures.
5. In conjunction with exchange transfusion in the treatment of neonatal hyperbilirubinaemia.

Dosage and administration Albutein 20% is intended for intravenous administration. The total dosage will vary with the individual.

Adults: An initial infusion of 100 ml is suggested. This may be repeated in 15–30 minutes if the initial dose is inadequate. Additional amounts should be administered as clinically indicated.

The rate of administration should be 1 ml per minute in patients with slightly low or normal blood volume. In patients with shock and/or greatly reduced blood volume, Albutein 20% may be administered as rapidly as necessary.

Children: Dosage will vary with clinical state and body weight. Dosage may be calculated on the basis of 1 ml per kilogram body weight for Albutein 20%.

The rate of administration should be calculated on one-quarter to one-half of the adult rate.

Contra-indications, warnings, etc Albutein 20% is contra-indicated in patients with severe anaemia or cardiac failure in the presence of normal or increased intravascular volume and in patients with a history of allergic reactions to albumin products.

Albutein 20% should be administered with caution to patients with low cardiac reserve. Additional fluids may be required for patients with marked dehydration. Rapid infusion may cause vascular overload with resultant pulmonary oedema. Patients should be closely monitored for signs of increased venous pressure. A rapid rise in blood pressure following infusion necessitates careful observation of injured or postoperative patients to detect and treat severed blood vessels that may not have bled at a lower pressure.

Do not use for control of haemorrhage due to deficiencies or defects in the clotting mechanism.

Albumin naturally binds a variety of therapeutic and toxic materials and thus administration of Albutein 20% may modify the pre-existing distribution of certain substances.

Adverse reactions are rare. However allergic or pyrogenic reactions, characterised primarily by fever and chills, nausea, vomiting, tachycardia and hypotension have been reported.

If such reactions occur the infusion should be discontinued and appropriate therapy (eg. antihistamine) or specific support treatment should be given.

Reproduction studies have not been conducted with albumin. Human albumin should be given to a pregnant woman only if clearly needed.

Administration of large quantities of albumin may require supplementation with red cell concentrates to help overcome any resulting relative anaemia.

Pharmaceutical precautions Do not use if the solution appears turbid or contains a deposit. Since the solution does not contain a preservative it should be used within 3 hours of penetration of the container. Discard any unused portion.

Do not administer protein hydrolysates or alcohol via the same administration set used for Albutein 20%.

Albutein 20% should be stored between 2°C and 25°C protected from light.

Legal category POM.

Package quantities Albutein 20% is supplied in:
50 ml glass vials containing 10 g of albumin.
100 ml glass vials containing 20 g of albumin.

Further Information Albutein 20% is prepared from plasma obtained from carefully selected and rigorously screened donors. The final product is heated at 60°C for 10 hours. However as with all blood products the risk of viral transmission with this product cannot be absolutely excluded. Nevertheless there are no known cases of viral transmission resulting from the administration of Albutein 20%.

Product licence number 4447/0008.

ALPHAGLOBIN*

Qualitative and quantitative composition Alphaglobin is available in 4 sizes containing 0.5 g, 2.5 g, 5.0 g, or 10.0 g immunoglobulin per vial.

Pharmaceutical form Alphaglobin is a sterile, pasteurised, 50 g/litre solution of highly purified intact human normal immunoglobulin for intravenous infusion. The solution contains an immunoglobulin G subclass distribution that approximates to the distribution found in normal plasma and contains not more than 0.05 mg/ml IgA. The product is stabilised by 5% D-sorbitol.

Clinical particulars

Therapeutic indications: Alphaglobin has been used as substitution/replacement therapy in primary and secondary antibody deficiency disorders and for the prevention and treatment of infections associated with these conditions. Alphaglobin has also been used to modify or control the individual's immune response in idiopathic thrombocytopenic purpura.

1. Replacement therapy for congenital agammaglobulinaemia and hypogammaglobulinaemia and other primary immunodeficiency syndromes including common variable immunodeficiency, severe combined immunodeficiency and Wiskott-Aldrich syndrome.
2. Replacement therapy for secondary immunodeficiency disorders.
3. Treatment of idiopathic thrombocytopenic purpura (ITP).
4. Prophylactic use in children with symptomatic HIV infection who have recurrent bacterial infections.

Posology and method of administration:
Posology: Immunodeficiency Syndromes: The usual dosage of Alphaglobin in immunodeficiency syndromes is 200 mg/kg bodyweight usually administered once a month by intravenous infusion. If the clinical response is inadequate or the level of serum IgG achieved is felt to be insufficient the dose may be increased to 300–400 mg/kg bodyweight or the infusion may be repeated more frequently than once a month.

Idiopathic Thrombocytopenic Purpura: The usual treatment regimen is 400 mg/kg bodyweight daily for 5 days. Maintenance doses of 400 mg/kg bodyweight may be given every few weeks as required to maintain the platelet count.

Elderly: There is no evidence to suggest that the dosage regimens used for adults are inappropriate for the elderly.

Administration: Alphaglobin should be infused at a rate of 0.01–0.02 ml/kg bodyweight per minute for the first thirty minutes. If the patient does not experience any discomfort the rate may be increased up to 0.07 ml/kg per minute and if tolerated subsequent infusions to the same patient may be at the higher rate. If adverse effects occur the rate should be reduced or the infusion interrupted until the symptoms subside. The infusion may then be resumed at a rate which is tolerated by the patient.

Contra-indications: Alphaglobin is contra-indicated in individuals with a history of anaphylactic or severe systematic response to intramuscular or intravenous immune globulin preparations.

Although only containing trace quantities of IgA, Alphaglobin, as with all blood products containing IgA, is contra-indicated in patients with selective IgA deficiency who possess antibody to IgA.

Special warnings and special precautions for use: Patients with agamma- or extreme hypogammaglobulinaemia who have never before received immunoglobulin therapy or whose time from last treatment is greater than 8 weeks may be at risk of developing inflammatory reactions on infusion of Alphaglobin. Such reactions appear to be related to the rate of infusion. They are manifested by a rise in temperature, chills, nausea and vomiting. Vital signs should be monitored continuously and the patient should be carefully observed throughout the infusion.

The rate of administration specified in Section relating to *Posology and method of administration* should be closely followed, at least until the physician has had sufficient experience with a given patient. Adrenaline should be available for treatment of any acute anaphylactoid reaction.

This product is prepared from pooled units of human plasma which have been individually tested and found non-reactive for hepatitis B surface antigen, antibodies to hepatitis C and antibodies to human immunodeficiency viruses HIV-1 and -2. The plasma used in the preparation of this product has also been screened for alanine aminotransferase (ALT) and each unit used in manufacture has been found to have an ALT level of less than twice the upper limit of normal for the test. Other screening procedures are used to eliminate high risk plasma donors.

The manufacturing process of Alphaglobin includes a 60°C 10 hour pasteurisation process specifically designed to inactivate any contaminating viruses. The results from *in vitro* studies on various stages of the manufacturing process including the cold ethanol fractionation, pasteurisation, polyethylene glycol precipitation and DEAE Sephadex filtration steps, indicate that considerable quantities of HIV-1 and model viruses of other blood borne infections are both inactivated and partitioned during the process.

However, despite all precautions taken by the manufacturer the risk of transmission of infection, of blood borne viruses, by intravenous immunoglobulin preparations cannot be entirely excluded.

Interaction with other medicaments: Alphaglobin is supplied as a sterile 5% solution. It should not be mixed with any other drugs or intravenous fluids. It should be administered by a separate intravenous line.

Pregnancy and lactation: Animal reproduction studies using Alphaglobin indicate that there appear to be no harmful effects to either the mother or the offspring. However, the safety of this product in pregnant women has not been established in controlled clinical trials.

Alphaglobin should, therefore, be given to pregnant women only if clearly indicated.

Effect on ability to drive and use machines: Not applicable.

Undesirable effects: Clinical investigations have confirmed that Alphaglobin is well tolerated and not likely to produce side effects when infused at the recommended rates. However, the first infusion of immunoglobulin particularly in previously untreated agamma- and hypogammaglobulinaemic patients or patients who have previously received another immunoglobulin preparation may lead to systemic side effects. Some of the effects may occur as a result of a reaction between the antibodies administered and free antigens in the blood and tissues of the patient.

Adverse reactions such as headache, chills, fever, nausea, vomiting, allergic reactions, rash, arthralgia and mild back pain may occur occasionally. As with other intravenous immune globulin preparations, Alphaglobin has been associated at high doses with rare occurrences of aseptic meningitis and haemolytic anaemia.

Rarely immunoglobulins may cause a fall in blood pressure and, in isolated cases, anaphylactic shock, even when the patient has shown no sensitivity to previous administration.

Overdose: Overdosage with Alphaglobin has not been reported but is unlikely to have any harmful effects.

Pharmacological properties
Pharmacodynamic properties: Alphaglobin is a high purity human immunoglobulin class G (IgG) preparation which contains antibodies against the wide spectrum of antigens to which the plasma donor population has been exposed.

Alphaglobin retains the biological functions of endogenous gammaglobulin and has very low anticomplementary activity.

Pharmacokinetic properties: As Alphaglobin is administered intravenously, the dose is immediately bioavailable in the circulation.

Alphaglobin has a half-life of about 46 days (range 33–65 days). This half-life may vary from patient to patient.

Preclinical safety data: Not applicable.

Pharmaceutical particulars
List of excipients: 5% D-sorbitol, Water for Injections.

Incompatibilities: Alphaglobin should not be mixed with any other drugs or intravenous fluids. It should be administered by a separate intravenous line.

Shelf life: The shelf life of Alphaglobin is 2 years if stored below 25°C and protected from light.

Special precautions for storage: Alphaglobin should be stored below 25°C and protected from light. The contents must **not** be frozen.

Nature and contents of container: Alphaglobin is supplied in Type II clear glass vials, 10 ml, 50 ml, 100 ml and 200 ml.

Instructions for use/handling: Ensure aseptic technique is used during attachment of infusion lines.

Pharmaceutical precautions: If large volumes are to be administered it is advisable to ensure the solution is near to body temperature prior to infusion.

Do not use after expiry date.

Marketing authorisation number 4447/0031

Date of approval/revision of SPC 1 February 1997

Legal category POM

ALPHANATE*

Qualitative and quantitative composition Alphanate is a high purity, solvent detergent and heat treated, freeze dried human coagulation Factor VIII, PhEur.

Active ingredient (Nominal)	*Specification*	*Quantity*
Human coagulation Factor VIII	PhEur	250 IU/vial
Human coagulation Factor VIII	PhEur	500 IU/vial
Human coagulation Factor VIII	PhEur	1000 IU/vial
Human coagulation Factor VIII	PhEur	1500 IU/vial

Each container is labelled with the number of International Units of Factor VIII activity.

Pharmaceutical form Sterile, non-pyrogenic, white/slightly yellow lyophilisate that is reconstituted with the Water for Injections BP/PhEur diluent (PL 4447/0016) supplied with the product. For intravenous administration.

Clinical particulars
Therapeutic indications: Alphanate is indicated for the treatment and prophylaxis of bleeding in patients with moderate or severe Factor VIII deficiency due to congenital haemophilia A or acquired Factor VIII deficiency.

Posology and method of administration: The dose and dosing schedule for Alphanate must be adjusted according to the needs of the individual patient, taking into account the severity of the haemostatic disorder, the location and extent of the bleeding and the clinical condition.

Posology : Factor VIII replacement therapy: The required dosage may be estimated using the following formula as a guide:

Body weight (kg) × Desired increase in Factor VIII (%) × 0.5 = Number of Factor VIII units required (IU)

Example:
50 kg×30%×0.5=750 IU Alphanate

This calculation is based on the empirical finding that 1 IU of Factor VIII per kg body weight raises the plasma Factor VIII activity by approximately 2% (i.e. 0.5 IU/kg required for a 1% increase in plasma Factor VIII level).

The patient's plasma Factor VIII levels should be determined and monitored during treatment with Alphanate. This is particularly important in the case of surgical procedures.

Treatment schedules:
Haemorrhagic Events: If not prescribed otherwise by the attending physician, the following dosage schedule is recommended. For each of the following haemorrhagic events, the Factor VIII activity should not fall below the given plasma activity level (in % of normal) over the corresponding period.

Haemorrhagic event	*Therapeutically effective plasma level of Factor VIII activity*	*Period that therapeutic plasma level of Factor VIII activity should be maintained*
Minor haemorrhage: (Including haemorrhage into joints)	30%	At least 1 day, depending on the severity of the haemorrhage.
Major haemorrhage: (Including haemorrhage into muscles; tooth extraction; mild trauma capitis; minor operations; haemorrhages in the oral cavity)	40 – 50%	3–4 days or until adequate wound healing has been achieved.
Life-threatening haemorrhage: (Including major operations; gastro-intestinal bleeding; intracranial, intra-abdominal or intra-thoracic haemorrhages; fractures)	60 – 100%	For 7 days. Factor VIII therapy should continue for at least another 7 days until adequate healing has been achieved.

Under certain circumstances larger amounts than those calculated will be required, especially for the initial dose.

Prophylaxis: For long-term prophylaxis against bleeding in patients with severe haemophilia A, Alphanate should be administered at doses of 10 to 50 IU/kg at intervals of 2 to 3 days. In some cases, especially in younger patients, shorter dosage intervals or higher doses may be necessary.

Elderly patients: The dosage regimens recommended for adults are appropriate for the elderly.

Administration: Alphanate is intended for intravenous administration only. Once reconstituted with the diluent supplied, Alphanate may be administered at a rate of no more than 10 ml/minute by injection or infusion. (For full details of reconstitution and use refer to the *Instructions for use/handling* section).

Contra-indications: None known.

Special warnings and special precautions for use: If allergic or anaphylactic reactions occur, administration should be stopped immediately. Subsequent treatment, where necessary, should follow the current specific guidelines for shock therapy.

After repeated treatment with Factor VIII concentrate, the level of inhibitor in the plasma should be determined.

Patients receiving Factor VIII concentrates should be vaccinated against hepatitis A and B.

Interaction with other medicaments and other forms of interaction: As Factor VIII is a constituent of normal plasma, no such interactions are anticipated.

Pregnancy and lactation: The safety of human coagulation Factor VIII for use in human pregnancy has not been established in controlled clinical trials. Experimental animal studies are insufficient to assess safety with respect to reproduction, development of the embryo or foetus, the course of gestation and peri- and postnatal development. Therefore, Factor VIII concentrates should only be used if clearly needed during pregnancy and lactation.

Effects on ability to drive and use machines: As Factor VIII is a constituent of normal plasma no effects on ability to drive or use machines are anticipated.

Undesirable effects:

1. Occasionally, mild reactions occur following the administration of Factor VIII concentrates. These may include allergic reactions, urticaria, fever, chills, nausea, vomiting, headache, somnolence or lethargy.
2. Very rarely, anaphylactic reactions occur following the administration of Factor VIII concentrates.
3. Patients receiving Factor VIII concentrates may develop antibodies (inhibitors) to the Factor VIII protein. In these patients, the response to Alphanate may be much less than would otherwise be expected, and larger doses are often required. The management of patients with inhibitors requires careful monitoring, especially if surgical procedures are indicated.
4. With products derived from human plasma, the transmission of infectious diseases due to the transmission of pathogens cannot be totally excluded.

This product is prepared from pooled units of human plasma derived from fully screened donors. Each unit has been individually tested and found nonreactive for hepatitis B surface antigen, antibodies to human immunodeficiency viruses (HIV-1 and -2) and antibodies to hepatitis C virus (HCV). Each unit has also been tested and found to have alanine aminotransferase (ALT) levels less than twice the upper limit of normal for the test.

The manufacturing process for Alphanate includes an organic solvent, tri-(n-butyl)-phosphate, and detergent, polysorbate-80, virus inactivation step designed to reduce the risk of transmitting infective agents. This process has been shown to be effective against a wide range of lipid-enveloped viruses. The manufacturing process also includes a heat-treatment step in which lyophilised Alphanate is heated at 80°C for 72 hours. This second inactivation step is designed to further reduce the risk of transmitting infective agents, in particular non-lipid-enveloped viruses.

As with all drugs, the risks associated with use must be weighed against the benefits of therapy.

Overdose: Massive doses of Factor VIII have, rarely, resulted in acute haemolytic anaemia, increased bleeding tendency or hyperfibrinogenaemia. In the case of overdose the patient should be carefully monitored and supportive treatment given.

Pharmacological properties

Pharmacodynamic properties: Factor VIII is a constituent of normal plasma as the Factor VIII/von Willebrand Factor complex and forms part of the clotting process. As a cofactor for Factor IX, it accelerates the conversion of Factor X to activated Factor X. Activated Factor X converts prothrombin into thrombin. Thrombin then converts fibrinogen into fibrin and a clot can be formed. The Factor VIII activity is greatly reduced in patients with haemophilia A or acquired Factor VIII deficiency. The administration of Factor VIII concentrates such as Alphanate to these patients therefore temporarily corrects their blood clotting mechanism and minimises the hazards of haemorrhage.

Pharmacokinetic properties: After injection of the product, approximately two thirds to three quarters of the Factor VIII remains in the circulation. The achieved Factor VIII activity in the plasma should be between 80–120 percent of the predicted value.

Plasma Factor VIII activity probably decreases by a two-phase exponential decay. In the initial phase, distribution between the intravascular and other compartments (body fluids) occurs with a half-life of elimination from the plasma of 3–6 hours. In the subsequent slower phase (which probably reflects the consumption of Factor VIII) the half-life varies between 8–20 hours, with an average of 12 hours. This appears to correspond to the true biological half-life.

In clinical studies, the Factor VIII half life of Alphanate was estimated at approximately 12 hours. Mean recovery was approximately 87%.

Preclinical safety data: As Alphanate is purified from pooled human plasma it is considered to act in the same manner as endogenous Factor VIII. Toxicity testing is therefore of no relevance.

Immunoelectrophoretic and immunoprecipitation studies on rabbit antisera raised against Alphanate indicate that no detectable new antigenic determinants were generated by heat-treatment.

Pharmaceutical particulars

List of excipients:

Material	*Specification*
Albumin	PhEur
Histidine	USP
Arginine	USP
Water for Injections (Diluent)	BP/PhEur

Incompatibilities: Alphanate should not be mixed with other drugs before administration.

Use only approved injection/infusion sets because treatment may fail as a consequence of adsorption to the internal surface of some infusion equipment.

Shelf life: Lyophilised Alphanate has a shelf life of 24 months at 2–8°C. Storage at no more than 30°C for 6 months within this period is acceptable.

Reconstituted Alphanate has a shelf life of 3 hours at 25°C.

Special precautions for storage: Lyophilised Alphanate should be stored under refrigeration (2–8°C), protected from light. Do not freeze.

Reconstituted Alphanate should not be stored prior to administration.

Nature and contents of containers: Alphanate is supplied as lyophilisate in clear Type I/II glass, single dose vials with rubber stoppers and aluminium caps (bearing the lot number) with plastic flip-off top. Water for Injections diluent (5 ml for 250/500 IU/vial; 10 ml for 1000/1500 IU/vial) is provided in a separate vial.

Instructions for use/handling: Alphanate is for intravenous administration after reconstitution with the Water for Injections diluent provided.

Use aseptic technique during reconstitution and administration.

Usually the reconstituted solution is clear or slightly opalescent–do not use solutions which are cloudy or have deposits.

Alphanate should be used immediately after reconstitution.

Any unused solution must be discarded appropriately.

All reconstitution and administration equipment must be discarded appropriately.

Reconstitution: Use only the diluent and devices provided.

1. Warm diluent and concentrate vials to at least room temperature (but not above 37°C).

2. Remove plastic flip-off tops from the diluent and concentrate vials.

3. Swab the exposed rubber surfaces with alcohol. Do not leave excess cleaning agent in indentation on the stopper.

3. Remove covering from the vented filter spike. Remove plastic sheath from pointed end of vented filter spike and insert point through rubber stopper of concentrate vial. Air will be drawn through the sterile filter into the vial, thus releasing the vacuum. Leave the device inserted in the stopper.

4. Using the needle provided draw up the required volume of Water for Injections into the syringe.

5. Remove the plastic cap from the top of the vented filter spike. Insert the filled syringe into the exposed Luer end of the device. Depress the syringe plunger to transfer all the diluent into the concentrate vial. DO NOT REMOVE THE SYRINGE FROM THE VENTED FILTER SPIKE, DO NOT REMOVE THE DEVICE FROM THE STOPPER. Maintain the concentrate vial and spike/syringe assembly in the vertical position.

6. Holding the entire assembly securely, GENTLY SWIRL the diluent until all concentrate is dissolved. When the reconstitution procedure is strictly followed a few small particles may occasionally remain. The microaggregate filter built into the filter spike will retain any remaining particles, without reducing the label potency.

Administration: By syringe:

1. Invert the vial and withdraw the reconstituted product into the syringe via the vented filter spike with inbuilt microaggregate filter.

2. Detach the syringe from the filter spike and discard the empty concentrate vial with the filter spike attached.

3. Attach the syringe to the infusion set, expel air from the syringe and infusion set. Perform venepuncture and administer slowly.

4. If the patient is to receive more than one vial of concentrate, the infusion set will allow this to be performed with a single venepuncture.

By administration set:

1. Close clamp on the administration set. Remove the filter spike from the vial.

2. With vial upright, insert the piercing pin of the administration set straight through the stopper centre. Do not twist or angle.

3. Immediately invert vial to automatically establish a proper fluid level in drip chamber (half full).

4. Attach infusion set, open the clamp and allow the solution to expel air from the tubing and needle, then close the clamp.

5. Perform venepuncture, release the clamp and administer slowly.

Marketing authorisation number 4447/0005

Date of approval/revision of SPC 20 September 1996

Legal category POM

ALPHANINE*

Qualitative and quantitative composition: High purity, solvent detergent and nanofiltered human coagulation Factor IX, freeze dried in vials containing 500 IU, 1000 IU or 1500 IU (nominal sizes). Each container is labelled with the number of International Units of Factor IX activity.

Pharmaceutical form: Sterile, non-pyrogenic, white/ slightly yellow friable powder that is reconstituted with the Water for Injections BP/PhEur diluent (PL 4447/0016) supplied with the product. For intravenous administration only.

Clinical particulars

Therapeutic indications: For the prevention and control of bleeding in patients with Factor IX deficiency due to haemophilia B.

Posology and method of administration: The dose of AlphaNine for a particular patient depends upon the level of plasma Factor IX which is to be achieved. The desired plasma level of Factor IX will vary according to the patient's age and clinical condition, and as such should be decided upon by the physician, based on clinical experience. The patient's plasma Factor IX level should be determined and monitored during treatment.

The following formula provides a guide for dosage calculations:

Body weight (kg) × 1.0 × Desired increase in Factor IX (%) = Number of Factor IX units required

Infusions are generally required daily.

Contra-indications: There are no known contra-indications to the use of AlphaNine.

Special warnings and special precautions for use: This product is prepared from pooled units of human plasma derived from screened donors. Each unit has been individually tested and found non-reactive for hepatitis B surface antigen, antibodies to HIV-1, HIV-2 and hepatitis C virus, and also to have an alanine amino-transferase level of less than twice the upper limit of normal for the test. Incubation in an organic solvent / detergent mixture during manufacture is designed to reduce the risk of transmitting infection with lipid-enveloped viruses. The specific viral filtration step in AlphaNine manufacture has been demonstrated to remove substantial amounts of non-lipid enveloped viruses.

However, testing methods are not yet sufficiently sensitive to detect all units of potentially infectious plasma, and no treatment during manufacture has been shown to eliminate totally the risk of viral infectivity. Therefore, despite the rigorous precautions taken by the manufacturer, it cannot be assumed that this product is totally free of viral contamination.

As with all drugs the risks associated with use must be weighed against the benefits of therapy.

Patients receiving Factor IX concentrates should be vaccinated against hepatitis A and B.

Occasionally haemophilia B sufferers develop inhibitors to Factor IX. In these patients the response to AlphaNine may be much less than would otherwise be expected and larger doses would be required. The management of patients with inhibitors requires careful monitoring, especially if surgical procedures are indicated.

AlphaNine is not suitable for the reversal of anticoagulant over-dosage.

Interaction with other medicaments and other forms of interaction: As Factor IX is a constituent of normal plasma, no interactions are anticipated.

Pregnancy and lactation: Animal reproduction studies have not been conducted with AlphaNine. AlphaNine should be given to a pregnant or lactating woman only if clearly indicated.

Effects on ability to drive and use machines: As Factor IX is a constituent of normal plasma, no effects on ability to drive or use machines are anticipated.

Undesirable effects: Occasionally, mild reactions occur following the administration of Factor IX concentrates. These may include allergic reactions, mild chills, nausea or stinging at the infusion site. Slowing the infusion rate will usually relieve the symptoms. For highly reactive individuals who require additional AlphaNine, product from a different lot should be administered.

Thrombosis or disseminated intravascular coagulation have been reported following the administration of Prothrombin Complex Concentrates (PCCs) especially to patients with liver disease or undergoing surgery. The thrombogenic potential of AlphaNine has been shown in clinical trials to be very considerably reduced from that of PCCs (data available for single doses only). However patients in high risk groups receiving AlphaNine should be closely observed for signs of intravascular coagulation.

Overdose: In the event of an overdose the patient should be carefully monitored and supportive treatment given.

Pharmacological properties

Pharmacodynamic properties: AlphaNine is human coagulation Factor IX derived from human plasma. Its actions are understood to mimic exactly those of endogenous circulating Factor IX. The administration of AlphaNine increases the plasma levels of Factor IX, which in haemophilia B sufferers temporarily corrects their blood clotting disorder and minimises the hazards of haemorrhage.

Pharmacokinetic properties: Following administration by intravenous infusion, distribution of Factor IX between the intra- and extra-vascular compartments occurs resulting in equilibration. The elimination of Factor IX, which reflects its actual biological usage, then takes place. The median half life of Factor IX from AlphaNine has been estimated to be approximately 21 hours.

Preclinical safety data: The thrombogenic potential of purified Factor IX preparations such as AlphaNine has been examined in various animal models including the Wessler stasis rabbit model, porcine, canine and rodent models. The results have been compared with PCC preparations, which carry a known clinical risk of thromboembolic episodes. Purified Factor IX preparations have been shown to be associated with a very substantial reduction in thrombogenic activity compared with PCCs, even at doses many times higher than those which are employed in the clinical setting.

Pharmaceutical particulars

List of excipients: AlphaNine is Coagulation Factor IX purified from human plasma.

The other components may be listed as follows:

Dextrose	PhEur
Heparin	PhEur
Sodium hydroxide	PhEur
Hydrochloric acid	PhEur

Incompatibilities: AlphaNine is supplied in glass vials, each with a vial of diluent (Water for Injections). No data on incompatibilities with other containers or solutions are available. It is therefore recommended that AlphaNine be reconstituted only with the diluent provided.

Shelf life: Lyophilised AlphaNine has a shelf life of 24 months at 2–8°C. Storage at no more than 30°C for 1 month within this period is acceptable.

Reconstituted AlphaNine has a shelf life of 3 hours at 25°C.

Special precautions for storage: Lyophilised AlphaNine should be stored under refrigeration (2–8°C), protected from light. Do not freeze.

Nature and contents of container: AlphaNine is a white/slightly yellow friable powder containing 500 IU, 1000 IU or 1500 IU of Factor IX (nominal sizes). The actual assay value is printed on the vial label. The container is Type I glass and is closed with a grey butyl rubber stopper, aluminium crimp seal (bearing the lot number) and plastic "Flip-Off" dust cover.

Each vial of AlphaNine is supplied with a separate diluent vial containing 10 ml Water for Injections (PL 4447/0016).

Instructions for use/handling: AlphaNine must be reconstituted with the diluent provided, before administration. AlphaNine is intended for intravenous use only and should be used within three hours of reconstitution. It is recommended that the solution be administered at less than 10 ml/minute. Aseptic technique must be employed.

Check assay value on label carefully before use.

Reconstitution:

1. Warm the diluent and concentrate vials to at least room temperature (but not above 37°C). This may take up to 45 minutes following removal from refrigerator, depending on the temperature of the room.
2. Remove the plastic flip-off caps from the diluent and concentrate vials.
3. Swab the exposed rubber surfaces with alcohol. Do not leave excess cleaning agent in the indentation on the stoppers.
4. Remove the covering from one end of a double-ended needle to expose the short needle. Insert this exposed short needle through the depression in the centre of the stopper in the vial of diluent.
5. Remove the plastic cap from the upper end of the double-ended needle now seated in the stopper of the diluent vial. Holding the concentrate vial in one hand, invert the vial of diluent in the other hand and push the exposed end of the needle through the depression in the centre of the stopper, making certain that the diluent is always above the vial of concentrate. There should be enough vacuum in the vial to draw in all of the diluent.
6. Disconnect the two vials by removing the needle from the concentrate vial stopper. Swirl the concentrate vial until all concentrate is dissolved: do not shake. Reconstitution normally requires less than five minutes. When the reconstitution procedure is strictly followed a few small particles may occasionally remain. The microaggregate filter will retain particles and the labelled potency will not be reduced.

Administration:

1. Peel the cover from the microaggregate filter package and securely install the syringe into the exposed luer inlet of the filter using a slight clockwise twisting motion.
2. Remove the filter from the packaging. Remove the protective sleeve from the spike end of the filter using a clockwise twisting motion.
3. Pull back the plunger to aspirate sufficient air into the syringe to allow the reconstituted product to be withdrawn as described in the next step.
4. Insert the spike end of the filter into the reconstituted concentrate vial. Inject air and aspirate the reconstituted product from the vial into the syringe.
5. Remove and discard the filter from the syringe. Attach the syringe to an infusion set. Expel the air from the syringe and the infusion set. Perform venepuncture and administer slowly.
6. If the patient is to receive more than one vial of concentrate, the infusion set will allow this to be performed with a single venepuncture.
7. Discard all administration equipment after use.

By administration set:

1. Close the clamp on the administration set.
2. With the vial upright, insert the piercing pin straight through the stopper centre. Do not twist or angle.
3. Immediately invert the vial to automatically establish a proper fluid level in the drip chamber (half full).
4. Attach an infusion set, open the clamp and allow the solution to expel air from the tubing and needle, then close the clamp.
5. Perform venepuncture and adjust the flow, not to exceed 10 ml/minute.
6. Discard all administration equipment after use.

Marketing authorisation numbers

500 IU/Vial	4447/0030
1000 IU/Vial	4447/0035
1500 IU/Vial	4447/0036

Date of approval/revision of SPC February 1997

Legal category POM

ALPHAPARIN*

Qualitative and quantitative composition

Pre-filled syringes: Certoparin sodium 3000 IU (as anti-Xa) in 0.3 ml Water for Injections.

Ampoules: Certoparin sodium 3000 IU (as anti-Xa) and sodium chloride 1.69 mg in 0.5 ml Water for Injections.

Pharmaceutical form Pre-filled syringes and ampoules for subcutaneous injection.

Clinical particulars

Therapeutic indications: The prophylaxis of peri- and post-operative venous thromboembolism.

Posology and method of administration:

Adults: 3000 IU per day. The first injection should be given 1 to 2 hours before surgery. Injections should then be given once daily for 7 to 10 days or until the patient is mobile. At each injection, the entire contents of the pre-filled syringe or ampoule should be administered.

Elderly: There is no reason, based on clinical trials, why elderly patients should require dosages other than those stated above.

Children: No studies have been carried out in children.

Contra-indications: Major bleeding disorders, bleeding ulcers of the stomach or intestine, severe hypertension (>200/120 mm Hg), hypersensitivity to heparin, subacute bacterial endocarditis, severe renal and/or hepatic dysfunction.

Special warnings and precautions for use: Alphaparin must not be administered by the intramuscular route.

Like heparin, this product may cause the following misleading results: simulation of low cholesterol values in the serum; high T3 and T4 values in non-fasting patients; high blood sugar values; false positive bromsulphthalein test. It is recommended that the platelet count should be monitored before surgery, during therapy and at the end of treatment.

As the different low molecular weight heparins have differing characteristics, it is not recommended that similar preparations are given during treatment.

Interactions with other medicaments and other forms of interaction: As with the use of unfragmented heparin, the following interactions should be considered:

- Potentiation of effect by non-steroidal anti-inflammatory drugs as well as dicoumarols, dipyridamole, dextrans, ethacrynic acid and cytostatic agents.
- Reduction of effect by antihistamines, digitalis preparations, tetracyclines and ascorbic acid.

Pregnancy and lactation: A study in 60 pregnant women showed no passage of certoparin across the placenta. It is also known from unfractionated heparin and other low molecular weight heparins that they do not pass across the placenta, nor are they excreted in breast milk. Alphaparin should only be used in such patients if the theoretical advantages are considered to outweigh the potential risks.

Effects on ability to drive and use machines: Not applicable.

Undesirable effects: Minor bleeding at the injection site may be seen. In isolated cases there have been reports of hypersensitivity reactions (e.g. allergic skin reactions with swelling, pruritis or rash) at the site of injection or over the entire body. Other side effects which are associated with treatment with unfragmented heparin may also occur and include thrombocytopenia, raised liver enzymes and osteoporosis.

Overdose: Due to the mode of administration, overdosage is not likely to occur. Acute haemorrhage and cutaneous and mucosal bleeding would be expected. The effect of overdosage can be neutralised by slow iv injection of protamine sulphate, 1500 IU for each dose of Alphaparin. The effect on aPTT and prothrombin time is rapidly reversed, whilst the anti-Xa activity returns to normal more slowly.

Pharmacological properties

Pharmacodynamic properties: Certoparin is a low molecular weight heparin with anti-thrombotic activity similar to unfractionated heparin. It has a powerful inhibitory effect on factor Xa but only a slight effect on aPTT. At the recommended doses, it does not significantly influence platelet aggregation.

Pharmacokinetic properties: Measured by the inhibition of factor Xa, which reaches its maximum after approximately 2 to 4 hours, subcutaneously administered certoparin is quickly absorbed. The mean half life of factor Xa inhibition is calculated to be 4.3 hours, compared with a mean half life of 2.2 hours for unfractionated heparin.

Toxicological results: The results of acute single dose and repeat dose toxicological studies showed that the tolerance of Alphaparin at high doses is limited only by its anticoagulant effect. The LD_{50} was found to be at least 30 times higher than the recommended human dose. Chronic toxicity studies revealed no toxic effect on any organ. No measurable transplacental passage was detected.

Pharmaceutical properties

List of excipients:

Pre-filled syringes: Water for Injections.

Ampoules: Sodium chloride, Water for Injections.

Incompatibilities: Do not mix Alphaparin with other injections or infusions.

Shelf life: 24 months.

Storage conditions: Store at room temperature below 25°C.

Nature and contents of container:

Pre-filled syringes: PhEur type I glass syringe of 0.5 ml volume with chlorinated butyl rubber stopper and natural rubber cap.

Ampoules: PhEur type I glass ampoules of 1 ml volume.

Instructions for use/handling: Subcutaneous injection, usually into the peritoneal fold. With the patient supine, a fold of skin between the navel and the iliac crest should be lifted (not squeezed), the full length of the needle inserted and held vertically throughout the injection.

The injection can be administered at other sites if deemed necessary.

Marketing authorisation numbers

Pre-filled syringes	4447/0033
Ampoules	4447/0034

Date of approval/revision of SPC November 1995.

Legal category POM

**Trade Mark*

Hawgreen Ltd
4 Priory Hall
Stillorgan Road
Stillorgan
C. Dublin
☎ 353 1 283 6602 353 1 283 6658

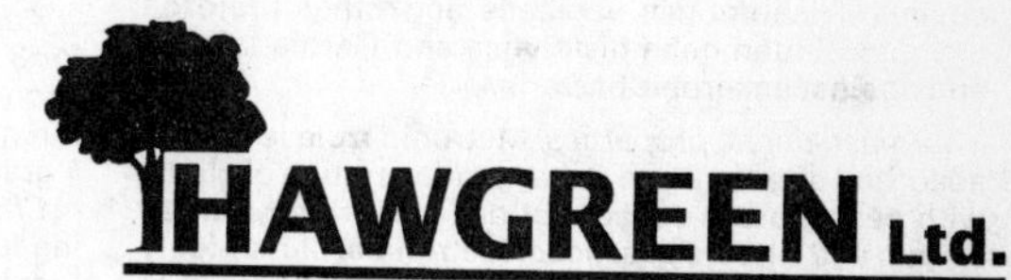

FLAGYL* & FLAGYL-S* SUSPENSION

Qualitative and quantitative composition Flagyl Tablets 200 mg Contain metronidazole BP 200 mg.

Flagyl Tablets 400 mg Contain metronidazole BP 400 mg.

Flagyl S Suspension Contains 320 mg/5 ml metronidazole benzoate equivalent to 200 mg/5 ml metronidazole

Pharmaceutical form

Flagyl tablets: White to off-white, circular biconvex, film coated tablets. The 200 mg tablets are impressed 'FLAGYL 200' on one face, plain reverse, and the 400 mg tablets are impressed 'FLAGYL 400' on one face, plain reverse.

Flagyl S Suspension: White to cream suspension with a slight yellow tinge and an odour of orange and lemon.

Clinical particulars

Therapeutic indications: Flagyl is indicated in the prophylaxis and treatment of infections in which anaerobic bacteria have been identified or are suspected to be the cause.

Flagyl is active against a wide range of pathogenic micro-organisms notably species of Bacteroides, Fusobacteria, Clostridia, Eubacteria, anaerobic cocci and Gardnerella vaginalis. It is also active against Trichomonas, Entamoeba histolytica, Giardia lamblia and Balantidium.

Used by the oral route Flagyl is indicated in: 1. the prevention of postoperative infections due to anaerobic bacteria, particularly species of bacteroides and anaerobic streptococci. 2. treatment of established anaerobic infections (septicaemia, bacteraemia, peritonitis, brain abscess, necrotising pneumonia, osteomyelitis, puerperal sepsis, pelvic abscess, pelvic cellulitis, and post-operative wound infections from which pathogenic anaerobes have been isolated). 3. treatment of urogenital trichomoniasis in the female (trichomonal vaginitis) and in the male. 4. treatment of bacterial vaginosis (also known as non-specific vaginitis, anaerobic vaginosis or Gardnerella vaginitis). 5. treatment of all forms of amoebiasis (intestinal and extra-intestinal disease and that of symptomless cyst passers). 6. treatment of giardiasis. 7. treatment of acute ulcerative gingivitis. 8. treatment of anaerobically-infected leg ulcers and pressure sores. 9. treatment of acute dental infections (e.g. acute pericoronitis and acute apical infections).

Posology and method of administration: For oral administration. All dosages are given in terms of metronidazole or metronidazole equivalent. Flagyl tablets should be swallowed with water (not chewed). It is recommended that the tablets be taken during or after a meal and that Flagyl S suspension be taken at least one hour before a meal. For dosages see table.

Oral Dosages of Flagyl:

1. Prevention of post-operative infections due to anaerobic bacteria:

Adults: 400 mg 8 hourly during 24 hours immediately preceding operation then intravenous or rectal administration until patient is able to take oral form.

Children and infants: 7.5 mg/kg 8 hourly

2. Treatment of established anaerobic infection:*

Adults: 800 mg followed by 400 mg 8 hourly

Children and infants: 7.5 mg/kg 8 hourly

*For the prevention and treatment of anaerobic infections the duration of dosing is about 7 days but, depending on the seriousness of the patient's condition assessed clinically and bacteriologically, this may be prolonged.

3. Treatment of urogenital trichomoniasis (where reinfection of adults is likely the partner should be treated concurrently)

Adults: Either: 300 mg three times daily for 7 days Or: 400 mg twice daily for 7 days

Or: 800 mg morning and 1200 mg evening for 2 days Or: 2 g as a single dose

Children 7–10 years: 100 mg three times daily

Children 3–7 years: 100 mg twice daily

Children 1–3 years: 50 mg three times daily

4. Treatment of bacterial vaginosis:

Adults Either: 400 mg twice daily for 7 days Or: 2.0 g as a single dose

5. Treatment of amoebiasis:

Invasive intestinal disease in susceptible patients

Adults: 800 mg three times daily for 5 days

Children 7–10 years: 400 mg three times daily for 5 days

Children 3–7 years: 200 mg four times daily for 5 days

Children 1–3 years: 200 mg three times daily for 5 days

Intestinal disease in less susceptible patients and chronic amoebic hepatitis

Adults: 400 mg three times daily for 5–10 days

Children 7–10 years: 200 mg three times daily for 5–10 days

Children 3–7 years: 100 mg four times daily for 5–10 days

Children 1–3 years: 100 mg three times daily for 5–10 days

Extra-intestinal amoebiasis

Adults: 400 mg three times daily for 5 days

Children 7–10 years: 200 mg three times daily for 5 days

Children 3–7 years: 100 mg four times daily for 5 days

Children 1–3 years: 100 mg three times daily for 5 days

Symptomless cyst passers

Adults: 400–800 mg three times daily for 5–10 days

Children 7–10 years: 200–400 mg three times daily for 5–10 days

Children 3–7 years: 100–200 mg four times daily for 5–10 days

Children 1–3 years: 100–200 mg three times daily for 5–10 days

6. Treatment of gardiasis

Adults: 2.0 g once daily for 3 days

Children 7–10 years: 1.0 g once daily for 3 days

Children 3–7 years: 600–800 mg once daily for 3 days

Children 1–3 years: 500 mg once daily for 3 days

7. Treatment of acute ulcerative gingivitis

Adults: 200 mg three times daily for 3 days

Children 7–10 years: 100 mg three times daily for 3 days

Children 3–7 years: 100 mg twice daily for 3 days

Children 1–3 years: 50 mg three times daily for 3 days

8. Treatment of anaerobically infected leg ulcers and pressure sores

Adults: 400 mg three times daily for 7 days

9. Treatment of acute dental infections

Adults: 200 mg three times daily for 3 to 7 days

Infants and children: weighing less than 10 kg should receive proportionally smaller dosages.

Elderly: Flagyl is well tolerated by the elderly but a pharmacokinetic study suggests cautious use of high dosage regimens in this age group.

Contra-indications: Known hypersensitivity to metronidazole.

Special warnings and special precautions for use: Metronidazole has no direct activity against anaerobic or facultative anaerobic bacteria. Regular clinical and laboratory monitoring are advised if administration of Flagyl for more than 10 days is considered to be necessary.

There is a possibility that after Trichomonas vaginalis has been eliminated a gonococcal infection might persist. The elimination half-life of metronidazole remains unchanged in the presence of renal failure. The dosage of metronidazole therefore needs no reduction. Such patients however retain the metabolites of metronidazole. The clinical significance of this is not known at present. In patients undergoing haemodialysis metronidazole and metabolites are efficiently removed during an eight hour period of dialysis. Metronidazole should therefore be re-administered immediately after haemodialysis. No routine adjustment in the dosage of Flagyl need be made in patients with renal failure undergoing intermittent peritoneal dialysis (IDP) or continuous ambulatory peritoneal dialysis (CAPD). Metronidazole is mainly metabolised by hepatic oxidation. Substantial impairment of metronidazole clearance may occur in the presence of advanced hepatic insufficiency. Significant cumulation may occur in patients with hepatic encephalopathy and the resulting high plasma concentrations of metronidazole may contribute to the symptoms of the encephalopathy. Flagyl should therefore, be administered with caution to patients with hepatic encephalopathy. The daily dosage should be reduced to one third and may be administered once daily. Aspartate amino transferase assays may give spuriously low values in patients being treated with metronidazole depending on the method used. Flagyl should be used with caution in patients with active disease of the CNS.

Interaction with other medicaments and other forms of interaction: Patients should be advised not to take alcohol during metronidazole therapy and for at least 48 hours afterwards because of the possibility of a disulfiram-like (antabuse effect) reaction. Some potentiation of anticoagulant therapy has been reported when metronidazole has been used with the warfarin type oral anticoagulants. Dosage of the latter may require reducing. Prothrombin times should be monitored. There is no interaction with heparin. Lithium retention accompanied by evidence of possible renal damage has been reported in patients treated simultaneously with lithium and metronidazole. Lithium treatment should be tapered or withdrawn before administering metronidazole. Plasma concentrations of lithium, creatinine and electrolytes should be monitored in patients under treatment with lithium while they receive metronidazole. Patients receiving phenobarbitone metabolise metronidazole at a much greater rate than normally, reducing the half-life to approximately 3 hours.

Pregnancy and lactation: There is inadequate evidence of the safety of metronidazole in pregnancy but it has been in wide use for many years without apparent ill consequence.

Nevertheless Flagyl, like other medicines, should not be given during pregnancy or during lactation unless the physician considers it essential; in these circumstances the short, high-dosage regimens are not recommended.

Effects on ability to drive and use machines: Therapy with Flagyl does not affect a patient's ability to drive or operate machines.

Undesirable effects: During intensive and/or prolonged metronidazole therapy, a few instances of peripheral neuropathy or transient epileptiform seizures have been reported.

In most cases neuropathy disappeared after treatment was stopped or when dosage was reduced. A moderate leucopenia has been reported in some patients but the white cell count has always returned to normal before or after treatment has been completed. Clinicians who contemplate continuous therapy for the relief of chronic conditions for periods longer than those recommended are advised to consider the possible therapeutic benefit against the risk of peripheral neuropathy. Serious adverse reactions occur rarely with standard recommended regimens. Unpleasant taste in the mouth, furred tongue, nausea, vomiting, gastro-intestinal disturbances, urticaria and angioedema occur occasionally. Anaphylaxis may occur rarely. Erythema multiforme may occur, which may be reversed on drug withdrawal. Abnormal liver function tests, cholestatic hepatitis and jaundice, reversible on drug withdrawal, have been reported very rarely. Agranulocytosis, neutropenia, thrombocytopenia and pancytopenia, often reversible on drug withdrawal, have very rarely been reported, although fatalities have occurred. Drowsiness, dizziness, headaches, ataxia, skin rashes, pruritus, inco-ordination of movement, darkening of urine (due to metronidazole metabolite) myalgia and arthralgia have been reported but very rarely.

Overdose: There is no specific treatment for gross overdosage of Flagyl

Pharmacological properties
Pharmacodynamic properties: Metronidazole has antiprotozoal and antibacterial actions and is effective against Trichomonas vaginalis and other protozoa including Entamoeba histolytica and Gardia lambila and against anaerobic bacteria.

Pharmacokinetic properties: Metronidazole is rapidly absorbed after oral and rectal administration of Flagyl with peak plasma concentrations occurring between 20 min and 3 hours post dose. Metronidazole is widely distributed in body tissues. The plasma half life is of the order of 8.5 hours with at least half the dose being excreted in the urine as metronidazole and its metabolites. Metronidazole can be used in chronic renal failure; it is rapidly removed from the plasma by dialysis. Metronidazole diffuses across the placenta and is excreted in breast milk with levels equivalent to those seen in serum.

Preclinical safety data: There are no pre-clinical data of relevance to the prescriber which are additional to that already included in other sections of the SPC.

Pharmaceutical particulars
List of excipients: Flagyl tablets (200 mg and 400 mg): Calcium hydrogen phosphate (E341), starch maize, Povidone K30 (E1201), magnesium stearate (E572), hydroxypropylmethylcellulose (E464), polyethylene glycol 400, and demineralised water.

Flagyl S Suspension: Liquid sugar granular liquors, sodium dihydrogen phosphate or sodium acid phosphate crystalline, Veegum HV, methyl hydroxybenzoate (E218), propyl hydroxybenzoate (E216), ethanol, lemon flavour, oil orange terpenless, demineralised water.

Incompatibilities: None known.

Shelf life: Flagyl tablets (200 mg and 400 mg): 60 months.

Flagyl S Suspension: 36 months. After dilution with Syrup BP the diluted suspension may be stored for 14 days.

Special precautions for storage: Flagyl tablets (200 mg and 400 mg): Protect from light.

Flagyl S Suspension: Store below 25°C, protect from light

Nature and contents of container: Flagyl tablets 200 mg are available in blisters packs of 21 tablets

Flagyl tablets 400 mg are available in blisters packs of 14 tablets

Flagyl S Suspension is available in glass bottles containing 100 ml

Instructions for use/handling: None.

Marketing authorisation numbers

Flagyl tablets 200 mg	PL 17077/0002
Flagyl tablets 400 mg	PL 17077/0003
Flagyl S Suspension	PL 17077/0001

Date of approval/revision of SPC September 1998.

Legal category POM.

FLAGYL* SUPPOSITORIES

Qualitative and quantitative composition Flagyl Suppository 500 mg Contain metronidazole BP 500 mg.

Flagyl Suppositories 1 g Contain metronidazole BP 1 g.

Pharmaceutical form A cream coloured, smooth, torpedo-shaped suppositories.

Clinical particulars
Therapeutic indications: Flagyl is indicated in the prophylaxis and treatment of infections in which anaerobic bacteria have been identified or are suspected to be the cause.

Flagyl is active against a wide range of pathogenic micro-organisms notably species of Bacteroides, Fusobacteria, Clostridia, Eubacteria, anaerobic cocci and Gardnerella vaginalis. It is also active against Trichomonas, Entamoeba histolytica, Giardia lamblia and Balantidium coli. Used by the rectal route Flagyl is indicated in the: 1. prevention of postoperative infections due to anaerobic bacteria, particularly species of Bacteroides and anaerobic streptococci. 2. treatment of established anaerobic infections (septicaemia, bacteraemia, peritonitis, brain abscess, necrotising pneumonia, osteomyelitis, puerperal sepsis, pelvic abscess, pelvic cellulitis, and post-operative wound infections from which pathogenic anaerobes have been isolated).

Posology and method of administration: For rectal administration. All dosages are given in terms of metronidazole. For dosages see table.

Dosages of Flagyl Suppositories
1. Prevention of post-operative infections due to anaerobic bacteria:

Adults and children over 10 years: 1 gram suppository inserted 2 hours before surgeryrepeated 8 hourly until patient is able to take oral form.

Children (5–10 years): 500 mg 8 hourly until oral medication becomes possible

2. Treatment of established anaerobic infection:

Adults and children over 10 years: 1 gram 8 hourly for 3 days. Oral medication should be substituted as soon as possible. If rectal administration continued for more than 3 days dose should be reduced to 1 gram 12 hourly.

Children (5–10 years): 500 mg suppository according to adult schedule. Oral medication should be substituted as soon as feasible

Children 1–5 years: 250 mg (one half 500 mg suppository) according to adult schedule. Oral medication should be substituted as soon as feasible.

Infants under 1 years: 125 mg (one quarter of 500 mg suppository) according to adult schedule. Oral medication should be substituted as soon as feasible.

Contra-indications: Known hypersensitivity to metronidazole.

Special warnings and special precautions for use: Metronidazole has no direct activity against anaerobic or facultative anaerobic bacteria. Regular clinical and laboratory monitoring are advised if administration of Flagyl for more than 10 days is considered to be necessary.

There is a possibility that after Trichomonas vaginalis has been eliminated a gonococcal infection might persist. The elimination half-life of metronidazole remains unchanged in the presence of renal failure. The dosage of metronidazole therefore needs no reduction. Such patients however retain the metabolites of metronidazole. The clinical significance of this is not known at present. In patients undergoing haemodialysis metronidazole and metabolites are efficiently removed during an eight hour period of dialysis. Metronidazole should therefore be re-administered immediately after haemodialysis. No routine adjustment in the dosage of Flagyl need be made in patients with renal failure undergoing intermittent peritoneal dialysis (IDP) or continuous ambulatory peritoneal dialysis (CAPD). Metronidazole is mainly metabolised by hepatic oxidation. Substantial impairment of metronidazole clearance may occur in the presence of advanced hepatic insufficiency. Significant cumulation may occur in patients with hepatic encephalopathy and the resulting high plasma concentrations of metronidazole may contribute to the symptoms of the encephalopathy. Flagyl should therefore, be administered with caution to patients with hepatic encephalopathy. The daily dosage should be reduced to one third and may be administered once daily. Aspartate amino transferase assays may give spuriously low values in patients being treated with metronidazole depending on the method used. Flagyl should be used with caution in patients with active disease of the CNS.

Interaction with other medicaments and other forms of interaction: Patients should be advised not to take alcohol during metronidazole therapy and for at least 48 hours afterwards because of the possibility of a disulfiram-like (antabuse effect) reaction. Some potentiation of anticoagulant therapy has been reported when metronidazole has been used with the warfarin type oral anticoagulants. Dosage of the latter may require reducing. Prothrombin times should be monitored. There is no interaction with heparin. Lithium retention accompanied by evidence of possible renal damage has been reported in patients treated simultaneously with lithium and metronidazole. Lithium treatment should be tapered or withdrawn before administering metronidazole. Plasma concentrations of lithium, creatinine and electrolytes should be monitored in patients under treatment with lithium while they receive metronidazole. Patients receiving phenobarbitone metabolise metronidazole at a much greater rate than normally, reducing the half-life to approximately 3 hours.

Pregnancy and lactation: There is inadequate evidence of the safety of metronidazole in pregnancy but it has been in wide use for many years without apparent ill consequence. Nevertheless Flagyl, like other medicines, should not be given during pregnancy or during lactation unless the physician considers it essential; in these circumstances the short, high-dosage regimens are not recommended.

Effects on ability to drive and use machines: Therapy with Flagyl does not affect a patient's ability to drive or operate machines.

Undesirable effects: During intensive and/or prolonged metronidazole therapy, a few instances of peripheral neuropathy or transient epileptiform seizures have been reported.

In most cases neuropathy disappeared after treatment was stopped or when dosage was reduced. A moderate leucopenia has been reported in some patients but the white cell count has always returned to normal before or after treatment has been completed. Clinicians who contemplate continuous therapy for the relief of chronic conditions for periods longer than those recommended are advised to consider the possible therapeutic benefit against the risk of peripheral neuropathy. Serious adverse reactions occur rarely with standard recommended regimens. Unpleasant taste in the mouth, furred tongue, nausea, vomiting, gastro-intestinal disturbances, urticaria and angioedema occur occasionally. Anaphylaxis may occur rarely. Erythema multiforme may occur, which may be reversed on drug withdrawal. Abnormal liver function tests, cholestatic hepatitis and jaundice, reversible on drug withdrawal, have been reported very rarely. Agranulocytosis, neutropenia, thrombocytopenia and pancytopenia, often reversible on drug withdrawal, have very rarely been reported, although fatalities have occurred. Drowsiness, dizziness, headaches, ataxia, skin rashes, pruritus, inco-ordination of movement, darkening of urine (due to metronidazole metabolite) myalgia and arthralgia have been reported but very rarely.

Overdose: There is no specific treatment for gross overdosage of Flagyl

Pharmacological properties
Pharmacodynamic properties: Metronidazole has antiprotozoal and antibacterial actions and is effective against Trichomonas vaginalis and other protozoa including Entamoeba histolytica and Gardia lambila and against anaerobic bacteria.

Pharmacokinetic properties: Metronidazole is rapidly absorbed after oral and rectal administration of Flagyl with peak plasma concentrations occurring between 20 min and 3 hours post dose. Metronidazole is widely distributed in body tissues. The plasma half life is of the order of 8.5 hours with at least half the dose being excreted in the urine as metronidazole and its metabolites. Metronidazole can be used in chronic renal failure; it is rapidly removed from the plasma by dialysis. Metronidazole diffuses across the placenta and is excreted in breast milk with levels equivalent to those seen in serum.

Preclinical safety data: There are no pre-clinical data of relevance to the prescriber which are additional to that already included in other sections of the SPC.

Pharmaceutical particulars
List of excipients: Suppository base E75 and suppository base W35

Incompatibilities: None known.

Shelf life: 36 months.

Special precautions for storage: Store below 20°C, protect from light.

Nature and contents of container: Flagyl suppositories are available PVC/polyethylene bandoliers containing 10 suppositories.

Instructions for use/handling: None.

Marketing authorisation numbers

Flagyl Suppositories 500 mg	PL 17077/0004
Flagyl Suppositories 1.0 g	PL 17077/0005

Date of approval/revision of SPC September 1998.

Legal category POM.

FLAGYL* COMPAK

Qualitative and quantitative composition The active component of the tablets is metronidazole 400 mg, the active component of the vaginal inserts is nystatin BP 42 mg.

Pharmaceutical form Flagyl tablets 400 mg: White to off-white, biconvex, circular, film coated tablets impressed 'FLAGYL 400' on one face, plain reverse.

Nystatin vaginal inserts 100,00 units: Yellowish-cream, almond shaped, marked M&B on one face, other plain. Both surfaces are slightly convex.

Clinical particulars
Therapeutic indications: Flagyl is a potent trichomonacide. It is also active against other protozoa and anaerobic bacteria. Nystatin is a fungistatic and fungicidal antibiotic which is actively topically against Candida albicans. Flagyl Compak is indicated in the treatment of vaginitis where a mixed trichomonal/candidal infection is diagnosed or suspected. Presenting symptoms may include vaginal discharge, pruritus vulvae and dyspareunia

Posology and method of administration: Flagyl tablets: For oral administration.

Nyastatin inserts: For vaginal administration.

Adults including the elderly: One Flagyl 400 tablet to be swallowed whole, with half a glass of water during or after meals, twice daily for seven days. Concurrently, one nystatin vaginal insert to be moistened and introduced high into the vagina, night and morning for seven days. Some physicians may prefer to instruct patients to use one insert nightly, before retiring for fourteen nights. Full patient instructions for use of the applicator are included in each Compak.

This product is not recommended for girls under 10 years of age. Where cross infection with Trichomonas vaginalis is confirmed or suspected the male consort should be treated concurrently with one Flagyl 400 tablet by mouth twice daily for seven days.

Contra-indications: Known hypersensitivity to metronidazole.

Special warnings and special precautions for use: Regular clinical and laboratory monitoring are advised if administration of Flagyl for more than 10 days is considered to be necessary. There is a possibility that after Trichomonas vaginalis has been eliminated a gonococcal infection might persist. The elimination half-life of metronidazole remains unchanged in the presence of renal failure. The dosage of metronidazole therefore needs no reduction. Such patients however retain the metabolites of metronidazole. The clinical significance of this is not known at present.

Metronidazole is mainly metabolised by hepatic oxidation. Substantial impairment of metronidazole clearance may occur in the presence of advanced hepatic insufficiency. Significant cumulation may occur in patients with hepatic encephalopathy and the resulting high plasma concentrations of metronidazole may contribute to the symptoms of the encephalopathy. Flagyl should therefore, be administered with caution to patients with hepatic encephalopathy. The daily dosage should be reduced to one third and may be administered once daily.

Interaction with other medicaments and other forms of interaction: Patients should be advised not to take alcohol during metronidazole therapy and for at least 48 hours afterwards because of the possibility of a disulfiram-like (antabuse effect) reaction. Some potentiation of anticoagulant therapy has been reported when metronidazole has been used with the warfarin type oral anticoagulants. Dosage of the latter may require reducing. Prothrombin times should be monitored. There is no interaction with heparin. Lithium retention accompanied by evidence of possible renal damage has been reported in patients treated simultaneously with lithium and metronidazole. Lithium treatment should be tapered or withdrawn before administering metronidazole. Plasma concentrations of lithium, creatinine and electrolytes should be monitored in patients under treatment with lithium while they receive metronidazole. Patients receiving phenobarbitone metabolise metronidazole at a much greater rate than normally, reducing the half-life to approximately 3 hours.

Pregnancy and lactation: There is inadequate evidence of the safety of metronidazole in pregnancy but it has been in wide use for many years without apparent ill consequence. Nevertheless Flagyl, like other medicines, should not be given during pregnancy or during lactation unless the physician considers it essential; in these circumstances the short, high-dosage regimens are not recommended.

Effects on ability to drive and use machines: None stated.

Undesirable effects: During intensive and/or prolonged metronidazole therapy, a few instances of peripheral neuropathy or transient epileptiform seizures have been reported. In most cases neuropathy disappeared after treatment was stopped or when dosage was reduced. A moderate leucopenia has been reported in some patients but the white cell count has always returned to normal before or after treatment has been completed. Serious adverse reactions occur rarely with standard recommended regimens. Unpleasant taste in the mouth, furred tongue, nausea, vomiting, gastro-intestinal disturbances, urticaria and angioedema occur occasionally. Anaphylaxis may occur rarely. Drowsiness, dizziness, headaches, ataxia, skin rashes, pruritus, inco-ordination of movement, darkening of urine (due to metronidazole metabolite), myalgia and arthralgia have been reported but very rarely.

Overdose: There is no specific treatment for gross overdosage of Flagyl.

Pharmacological properties

Pharmacodynamic properties: Flagyl is a potent trichomonacide. It is also active against other protozoa and anaerobic bacteria. Nystatin is a fungistatic and fungicidal antibiotic which is active topically against Candida albicans.

Pharmacokinetic properties: Metronidazole is rapidly and almost completely absorbed from the tablets leading to peak plasma concentrations after 20 minutes to 3 hours. Metronidazole is excreted in milk but the intake of a suckling infant of a mother receiving normal dosage would be considerably less than the therapeutic dosage for infants. Nystatin is not absorbed through the skin or mucous membranes when applied topically

Preclinical safety data: There are no pre-clinical data of relevance to the prescriber which are additional to that already included in other sections of the SPC.

Pharmaceutical particulars

List of excipients: Flagyl tablets: calcium hydrogen phosphate (E341), starch maize, povidone K30 (E1201), magnesium stearate (E572), hydroxypropylmethylcellulose (E464), polyethylene glycol 400, and french chalk powdered (E553(b)).

Nystatin vaginal inserts: lactose anhydrous, sodium starch glycollate and magnesium stearate.

Incompatibilities: None known.

Shelf life: 36 months.

Special precautions for storage: Store below 20°C, protect from light.

Nature and contents of container: Blister containing 14 Flagyl 400 tablets and 14 nystatin vaginal inserts.

Instructions for use/handling: None.

Marketing authorisation number PL 17077/0006

Date of approval/revision of SPC September 1998.

Legal category POM.

LARGACTIL* INJECTION

Qualitative and quantitative composition Largactil injection contains 2.5% w/v chlorpromazine hydrochloride BP.

Pharmaceutical form Largactil injection is a sterile solution for injection.

Clinical particulars

Therapeutic indications: Largactil is a phenothiazine neuroleptic. It is indicated in the following conditions: Schizophrenia and other psychoses (especially paranoid) mania and hypomania.

Anxiety, psychomotor agitation, excitement, violent or dangerously impulsive behaviour. Largactil is used as an adjunct in the short-term treatment of these conditions.

Intractable hiccup. Nausea and vomiting of terminal illness (where other drugs have failed or are not available). Induction of hypothermia is facilitated by largactil which prevents shivering and causes vasodilation. Childhood schizophrenia and autism.

Posology and method of administration: Deep intramuscular injection.

Oral route of administration should be used wherever possible. Parenteral formulations may be used in emergencies. They may only be administered by deep intramuscular injection. Largactil is too irritant to give subcutaneously. Repeated injections should be avoided if possible.

Adults: A single deep intramuscular injection of 25–50 mg followed by oral therapy will suffice in many cases, but the intramuscular dose may be repeated if required at 6 to 8 hour intervals. As soon as possible oral administration should be substituted.

Elderly: Should be started on half or even quarter of the adult dosage.

Dosage of chlorpromazine in schizophenia, other psychoses, anxiety and agitation, childhood schizophrenia and autism

Route: Intramuscular

Adult: For acute relief of symptoms 25–50 mg every 6–8 hours.

Children under 1 year: Do not use unless need is life saving.

Children 1–5 years: 0.5 mg/kg bodyweight every 6–8 hours. Dosage is not advised to exceed 40 mg daily.

Children 6–12 years: 0.5 mg/kg bodyweight every 6–8 hours. Dosage is not advised to exceed 75 mg daily.

Elderly or debilitated patients: Doses in the lower range for adults should be sufficient to control symptoms. i.e. 25 mg 8 hourly.

Hiccup, induction of hypothermia to prevent shivering.

Indication: Hiccups

Adults: 25–50 mg and if this fails 25–50 mg in 500–1000 ml sodium chloride injection by slow intravenous infusion.

Children under 1 year: No information available.

Children 1–5 years: No information available.

Children 6–12 years: No information available.

Elderly or debilitated patients: No information available.

Induction of hypothermia to prevent shivering

Adults: 25–50 mg every 6–8 hours.

Children under 1 year: Do not use.

Children 1–5 years: Initial dose 0.5 to 1 mg/kg. Maintenance 0.5 mg/kg every 4–6 hours.

Children 6–12 years: Initial dose 0.5 to 1 mg/kg. Maintenance 0.5 mg/kg every 4–6 hours.

Elderly or debilitated patient: No data available.

Nausea and vomiting of terminal illness

Adults: 25 mg initially then 25–50 mg every 3-4 hours until vomiting stops then drug to be taken orally.

Children under 1 year: Do not use unless need is life saving.

Children 1–5 years: 0.5 mg/kg 6–8 hourly. It is advised that maximum daily dosage should not exceed 40 mg.

Children 6–12 years: 0.5 mg/kg every 6–8 hours. It is advised that maximum daily dosage should not exceed 75 mg.

Elderly or debilitated patient: Not recommended.

Contra-indications: None stated.

Special warnings and special precautions for use: Largactil should be avoided in patients with liver or renal dysfunction, epilepsy, Parkinson's disease, hypothyroidism, cardiac failure, phaechromcytoma, myasthenia gravis and prostate hypertrophy. It should be avoided in patients known to be hypersensitive to phenothiazines or with a history of narrow angle glaucoma. It should be used with caution in the elderly, particularly during very hot or cold weather (risk of hyper-, hypothermia). Postural hypotension with tachycardia as well as local pain or nodule formation may occur after intramuscular administration. The patient should be kept supine and blood pressure monitored when receiving parenteral chlorpromazine. The elderly are particularly susceptible to postural hypotension.

Interaction with other medicaments and other forms of interaction: The CNS depressant actions of Largactil and other neuroleptic agents may be intensified (additively) by alcohol, barbiturates and other sedatives. Respiratory depression may occur. The hypotensive effect of most antihypertensive drugs especially alpha adrenceptor blocking agents may be exaggerated by Largactil. The mild anticholinergic effect of Largactil may be enhanced by other anticholinergic drugs possibly leading to constipation, heat stroke, etc. The action of some drugs may be opposed by Largactil; these include amphetamine, levodopa, clonidine, guanethidine, adrenaline. Anticholinergic agents may reduce the antipsychotic effect of Largactil. Some drugs interfere with absorption of neuroleptic agents: antacids, anti-Parkinson, lithium. Increases or decreases in the plasma concentrations of a number of drugs, e.g. propranalol, phenobarbitone have been observed but were not of clinical significance. High doses of Largactil reduce the response to hypoglycaemic agents the dosage of which might have to be raised. Documented adverse clinically significant interactions occur with alcohol. Guanethidine and hypoglycaemic agents. Adrenaline must not be used in patients overdosed with Largactil. Other interactions are of a theoretical nature and not serious. Simultaneous administration of desferroxamine and prochlorperazine has been observed to induce a transient metabolic encephalopathy characterised by loss of consciousness for 48–72 hours. It is possible this may occur with Largactil since it shares many of the pharmacological properties of prochlorperazine.

Pregnancy and lactation: There is inadequate evidence of the safety of Largactil in human pregnancy but it has been widely used for many years without apparent ill consequence. There is evidence of harmful effects in animals. Like other drugs it should be avoided in pregnancy unless the physician considers it essential. It may occasionally prolong labour and at such time should be withheld until the cervix is dilated 3–4 cm. Possible adverse effect on the foetus include lethargy or paradoxical hyperexcitability, tremor and low Apgar score. Largactil being excreted in milk, breast-feeding should be suspended during treatment.

Effects on ability to drive and use machines: Patients should be warned about drowsiness during the early days of treatment and advised not to drive or operate machinery.

Undesirable effects: Minor side effects are nasal stuffiness, dry mouth, insomnia, agitation.

Liver effects: Jaundice, usually transient, occurs in a very small percentage of patients taking chlorpromazine. A premonitory sign may be a sudden onset of fever after one to three weeks of treatment followed by the development of jaundice. Chlorpromazine jaundice has the biochemical and other characteristics of obstructive jaundice and is associated with obstructions of the canaliculi by bile thrombi; the frequent presence of an accompanying eosinophilia indicates the allergic nature of this phenomenon. Treatment should be withheld on the development of jaundice.

Skin and eyes: Contact skin sensitisation is a serious but rare complication in those frequently handling preparations of chlorpromazine: the greatest care must be taken to avoid contact of the drug with the skin. Skin rashes of various kinds may also be seen in patients treated with the drug. Patients on high dosage may develop photosensitivity in sunny weather and should avoid exposure to direct sunlight. Ocular changes and the development of a metallic greyish-mauve coloration of exposed skin have been noted in some individuals, mainly females, who have received chlorpromazine continuously for long periods (four to eight years).

Cardiorespiratory: Hypotension, usually postural,

commonly occurs. Elderly or volume depleted subjects are particularly susceptible: it is more likely to occur after intramuscular administration. Cardiac arrhythmia's including atrial arrhythmia, A-V block, ventricular tachycardia and fibrillation have been reported during neuroleptic therapy, possibly related to dosage. Pre-existing cardiac disease, old age, hypokalaemia and concurrent tricyclic antidepressant may predispose.

ECG changes, usually benign, including widened QT interval, ST depression, U-waves and T-wave changes. Respiratory depression is possible in susceptible patients.

Blood picture: A mild leucopenia occurs in up to 30% of patients on prolonged high dosage.

Agranulocytosis may occur rarely; it is not dose related. The occurrence of unexplained infections or fever requires immediate haematological investigation.

Extrapyramidal: Acute dystonias or dyskinesias, usually transitory are more common in children and young adults and usually occur within the first 4 days of treatment or after dosage increases. Akathisia characteristically occurs after large initial doses. Parkinsonism is more common in adults and the elderly. It usually develops after weeks or months of treatment. One or more of the following may be seen: tremor, rigidity, akinesia or other features of Parkinsonism. Commonly just tremor.

Tardive dyskinesia: If this occurs it is usually, but not necessarily, after prolonged high dosage.

It can even occur after treatment has been stopped. Dosage should therefore be kept low whenever possible.

Endocrine: Hyperprolactinaemia which may result in galactorrhoea, gynaecomastia, amenorrhoea and impotence. Neuroleptic malignant syndrome (hyperthermia, rigidity, autonomic dysfunction and altered consciousness) may occur with any neuroleptic. Allergic phenomena such as angiodema, bronchospasm, and urticaria have occurred with phenothiazines but anaphylactic reactions have been exceedingly rare.

Overdose: Symptoms of chlorpromazine overdosage include drowsiness or loss of consciousness, hypotension, tachycardia, ECG changes, ventricular arrhythmia's and hypothermia. Severe extra-pyramidal dyskinesias may occur. If the patient is seen sufficiently soon (up to 6 hours) after ingestion of a toxic dose, gastric lavage may be attempted. Pharmacological induction of emesis is unlikely to be of any use. Activated charcoal should be given. There is no specific antidote. Treatment is supportive. Generalised vasodilation may result in circulatory collapse; raising the patient's legs may suffice. In severe cases, volume expansion by intravenous fluids may be needed; infusion fluids should be warmed before administration in order not to aggravate hypothermia. Positive inotropic agents such as dopamine may be tried if fluid replacement is insufficient to correct the circulatory collapse. Peripheral vasoconstriction agents are not generally recommended; avoid the use of adrenaline. Ventricular or supraventricular tachyarrhythmias usually respond to restoration of normal body temperature and correction of circulatory or metabolic disturbances. If persistent or life threatening, appropriate anti-arrhythmic therapy may be considered. Avoid lignocaine and, as far as possible, long acting anti-arrhythmic drugs. Pronounced central nervous system depression requires airway maintenance or, in extreme circumstances, assisted respiration. Severe dystonic reactions usually respond to procyclidine (5-10 mg) or orphenadrine (20-40 mg) administered intramuscularly or intravenously. Convulsions should be treated with intravenous diazepam. Neuroleptic malignant syndrome should be treated with cooling. Dantrolene sodium may be tried.

Pharmacological properties

Pharmacodynamic properties: Largactil is a phenothiazine neuroleptic.

Pharmacokinetic properties: Chlorpromazine is rapidly absorbed and widely distributed in the body. It is metabolised in the liver and excreted in the urine and bile. Whilst plasma concentration of chlorpromazine itself rapidly declines excretion of chlorpromazine metabolites is very slow. The drug is highly bound to plasma protein. It readily diffuses across the placenta. Small quantities have been detected in milk from treated women. Children require smaller dosages per kg than adults.

Preclinical safety data: There are no preclinical data of relevance to the prescriber which are additional to that already included in other sections of the SPC.

Pharmaceutical particulars

List of excipients: Sodium sulphite anhydrous BP (E221), Sodium citrate BP, Sodium metabisulphite powder BP (E223), Water for Injections, Sodium chloride Ph Eur.

Incompatibilities: Largactil injection solutions have a pH of 5.0-6.5; they are incompatible with benzylpenicillin potassium, phenobarbitone sodium and phenobarbitone sodium.

Shelf life: 60 months.

Special precautions for storage: Largactil Injection should be stored protected from light. Discoloured solution should not be used.

Nature and contents of container: Largactil Injection 2.5% w/v is supplied in boxes containing 10×2 ml in glass ampoules.

Instructions for use/handling: None.

Marketing authorisation number PL 17077/0011.

Date of approval/revision of SPC September 1998.

Legal category POM.

LARGACTIL* TABLETS, SYRUP AND FORTE SUSPENSION

Qualitative and quantitative composition *Largactil tablets 10 mg* contain 10 mg chlorpromazine hydrochloride. *Largactil tablets 25 mg* contain 25 mg chlorpromazine hydrochloride. *Largactil tablets 50 mg* contain 50 mg chlorpromazine hydrochloride. *Largactil tablets 100 mg* contain 100 mg chlorpromazine hydrochloride. *Largactil syrup* contains 0.5% w/v Chlorpromazine Hydrochloride BP (25 mg chlorpromazine hydrochloride in 5 ml).

Largactil forte suspension contains 2.9% w/v chlorpromazine embonate, equivalent to 100 mg/5 ml of chlorpromazine hydrochloride.

Pharmaceutical form Largactil tablets are white to off-white circular, biconvex, film coated tablets: one face impressed [LG] and the strength, and the reverse face plain. Largactil syrup is a clear, bright golden-brown syrup, Largactil Forte suspension is an orange coloured suspension.

Clinical particulars

Therapeutic indications: Largactil is a phenothiazine neuroleptic. It is indicated in the following conditions:

Schizophrenia and other psychoses (especially paranoid) mania and hypomania.

Anxiety, psychomotor agitation, excitement, violent or dangerously impulsive behaviour. Largactil is used as an adjunct in the short-term treatment of these conditions.

Intractable hiccup.

Nausea and vomiting of terminal illness (where other drugs have failed or are not available).

Childhood schizophrenia and autism.

Posology and method of administration: Route of administration: Oral. Oral administration should be used whenever possible. Route of administration: oral. Patients unwilling to swallow tablets may be treated with suspension or syrup. Dosages should be low to begin with and gradually increased under close supervision until the optimum dosage within the recommended range, for the individual is reached. Individuals vary considerably and the optimum dose may be affected by the formulation used.

Contra-indications: None stated.

Special warnings and special precautions for use: Largactil should be avoided in patients with liver or renal dysfunction, epilepsy, Parkinson's disease, hypothyroidism, cardiac failure, phaechromcytoma, myasthenia gravis and prostate hypertrophy. It should be avoided in patients known to be hypersensitive to phenothiazines or with a history of narrow angle glaucoma. It should be used with caution in the elderly, particularly during very hot or cold weather (risk of hyper-, hypothermia). The elderly are particularly susceptible to postural hypotension.

Interaction with other medicaments and other forms of interaction: The CNS depressant actions of Largactil and other neuroleptic agents may be intensified (additively) by alcohol, barbiturates and other sedatives. Respiratory depression may occur. The hypotensive effect of most antihypertensive drugs especially alpha adrenceptor blocking agents may be exaggerated by Largactil. The mild anticholinergic effect of Largactil may be enhanced by other anticholinergic drugs possibly leading to constipation, heat stroke, etc. The action of some drugs may be opposed by Largactil; these include amphetamine, levodopa, clonidine, guanethidine, adrenaline. Anticholinergic agents may reduce the antipsychotic effect of Largactil. Some drugs interfere with absorption of neuroleptic agents: antacids, anti-Parkinson, lithium. Increases or decreases in the plasma concentrations of a number of drugs, e.g. propranalol, phenobarbitone have been observed but were not of clinical significance. High doses of Largactil reduce the response to hypoglycaemic agents the dosage of which might have to be raised. Documented adverse clinically significant interactions occur with alcohol. Guanethidine and hypoglycaemic agents. Adrenaline must not be used in patients overdosed with Largactil. Other interactions are of a theoretical nature and not serious. Simultaneous administration of desferroxamine and prochlorperazine has been observed to induce a transient metabolic encephalopathy characterised by loss of consciousness for 48–72 hours. It is possible this may occur with Largactil since it shares many of the pharmacological properties of prochlorperazine.

Pregnancy and lactation: There is inadequate evidence of the safety of Largactil in human pregnancy but it has been widely used for many years without apparent ill consequence. There is evidence of harmful effects in animals. Like other drugs it should be avoided in pregnancy unless the physician considers it essential. It may occasionally prolong labour and at such time should be withheld until the cervix is dilated 3–4 cm. Possible adverse effect on the foetus include lethargy or paradoxical hyperexcitability, tremor and low Apgar score. Largactil being excreted in milk, breast-feeding should be suspended during treatment.

Effects on ability to drive and use machines: Patients should be warned about drowsiness during the early days of treatment and advised not to drive or operate machinery.

Undesirable effects: Minor side effects are nasal stuffiness, dry mouth, insomnia, agitation.

Liver effects: Jaundice, usually transient, occurs in a very small percentage of patients taking chlorpromazine. A premonitory sign may be a sudden onset of fever after one to three weeks of treatment followed by the development of jaundice. Chlorpromazine jaundice has the biochemical and other characteristics of obstructive jaundice and is associated with obstructions of the canaliculi by bile thrombi; the frequent presence of an accompanying eosinophilia indicates the allergic nature of this phenomenon. Treatment should be withheld on the development of jaundice.

Skin and eyes: Contact skin sensitisation is a serious but rare complication in those frequently handling preparations of chlorpromazine: the greatest care must be taken to avoid contact of the drug with the skin. Skin rashes of various kinds may also be seen in patients treated with the drug. Patients on high dosage may develop photosensitivity in sunny weather and should avoid exposure to direct sunlight. Ocular changes and the development of a metallic greyish-mauve coloration of exposed skin have been noted in some individuals, mainly females, who have received chlorpromazine continuously for long periods (four to eight years).

Cardiorespiratory: Hypotension, usually postural, commonly occurs. Elderly or volume depleted subjects are particularly susceptible: it is more likely to occur after intramuscular administration.. Cardiac arrhythmia's including atrial arrhythmia, A-V block, ventricular tachycardia and fibrillation have been reported during neuroleptic therapy, possibly related to dosage. Pre-existing cardiac disease, old age, hypokalaemia and concurrent tricyclic antidepressant may predispose. ECG changes, usually benign, including widened QT interval, ST depression, U-waves and T-wave changes. Respiratory depression is possible in susceptible patients.

Blood picture: A mild leucopenia occurs in up to 30% of patients on prolonged high dosage. Agranulocytosis may occur rarely; it is not dose related. The occurrence of unexplained infections or fever requires immediate haematological investigation.

Extrapyramidal: Acute dystonias or dyskenias, usually transitory are more common in children and young adults and usually occur within the first 4 days of treatment or after dosage increases. Akathisia characteristically occurs after large initial doses. Parkinsonism is more common in adults and the elderly. It usually develops after weeks or months of treatment. One or more of the following may be seen: tremor, rigidity, akinesia or other features of Parkinsonism. Commonly just tremor.

Tardive dyskinesia: If this occurs it is usually, but not necessarily, after prolonged high dosage. It can even occur after treatment has been stopped. Dosage should therefore be kept low whenever possible.

Endocrine: Hyperprolactinaemia which may result in galactorrhoea, gynaecomastia, amenorrhoea and impotence.

Neuroleptic malignant syndrome: (hyperthermia, rigidity, autonomic dysfunction and altered consciousness) may occur with any neuroleptic.

Overdose: Symptoms of chlorpromazine overdosage include drowsiness or loss of consciousness, hypotension, tachycardia, ECG changes, ventricular arrhythmia's and hypothermia. Severe extra-pyramidal dyskinesias may occur. If the patient is seen sufficiently soon (up to 6 hours) after ingestion of a toxic dose, gastric lavage may be attempted. Pharmacological induction of emesis is unlikely to be of any use. Activated charcoal should be given. There is no specific antidote. Treatment is supportive. Generalised vasodilation may result in circulatory collapse; raising the patient's legs may suffice. In severe cases,

Dosage of chlorpromazine in:
Schizophrenia, other psychoses, anxiety, childhood schizophrenia and autism.

Adult	*Children under 1 year*	*Children 1–5 years*	*Children 6–12 years*	*Elderly or debilitated patients*
Initially 25 mg t.d.s. or 75 mg at bedtime increasing by daily amounts of 25 mg to an effective maintenance dose. This is usually in the range 75 to 300 mg daily, but some patients may require up to 1 g daily.	Do not use unless need is life saving.	0.5 mg/kg bodyweight every 4–6 hours to a maximum recommended dose of 40 mg daily.	1/3 to 1/2 the adult dose to a maximum recommended dose of 75 mg daily.	Start with 1/3 to 1/2 the usual adult dose with a more gradual increase in dosage.

Hiccup:

Adult	*Children under 1 year*	*Children 1–5 years*	*Children 6–12 years*	*Elderly or debilitated patients*
25–50 mg t.d.s or q.d.s	No information available			

Nausea and vomiting of terminal illness

Adults	*Children under 1 year*	*Children 1–5 years*	*Children 6–12 years*	*Elderly or debilitated patients*
10–25 mg every 4–6 hours	Do not use unless need is life saving	0.5 mg/kg 4–6 hours. Maximum daily dosage should not exceed 40 mg	0.5 mg/Kg 4–6 hours. maximum daily dosage should not exceed 75 mg	Initially 1/3 to 1/2 the adult dose. The physician should then use his clinical judgement to obtain control.

volume expansion by intravenous fluids may be needed; infusion fluids should be warmed before administration in order not to aggravate hypothermia. Positive inotropic agents such as dopamine may be tried if fluid replacement is insufficient to correct the circulatory collapse. Peripheral vasoconstriction agents are not generally recommended; avoid the use of adrenaline. Ventricular or supraventricular tachyarrhythmias usually respond to restoration of normal body temperature and correction of circulatory or metabolic disturbances. If persistent or life threatening, appropriate anti-arrhythmic therapy may be considered. Avoid lignocaine and, as far as possible, long acting anti-arrhythmic drugs. Pronounced central nervous system depression requires airway maintenance or, in extreme circumstances, assisted respiration. Severe dystonic reactions usually respond to procyclidine (5–10 mg) or orphenadrine (20–40 mg) administered intramuscularly or intravenously. Convulsions should be treated with intravenous diazepam. Neuroleptic malignant syndrome should be treated with cooling. Dantrolene sodium may be tried.

Pharmacological properties
Pharmacodynamic properties: Largactil is a phenothiazine neuroleptic.

Pharmacokinetic properties: Chlorpromazine is rapidly absorbed and widely distributed in the body. It is metabolised in the liver and excreted in the urine and bile. Whilst plasma concentration of chlorpromazine itself rapidly declines excretion of chlorpromazine metabolites is very slow. The drug is highly bound to plasma protein. It readily diffuses across the placenta. Small quantities have been detected in milk from treated women. Children require smaller dosages per kg than adults.

Preclinical safety data: There are no preclinical data of relevance to the prescriber which are additional to that already included in other sections of the SPC.

Pharmaceutical particulars
List of excipients:
Largactil tablets: Lactose, maize starch, Aerosil 200 (E464), magnesium sterate; Tablet coating: Hydroxypropylmethylcellulose, polyethylene glycol 200, Opaspray M-1-7111B (contains E171 and E646).
Largactil syrup: Liquid sugar gran. liquors, Oil peppermint Chinese, Fruit flavouring, Sodium citrate gran. (E331), Sodium sulphite anhydrous (E221), Caramel flavour, Demineralised water, Tween 20, Oil spearmint, Citric acid anhydrous (E330), Ascorbic acid (E300), Sodium metabisulphite powder (E223), Sodium benzoate (E211).
Largactil forte suspension: Sorbitol solution or sorbitol powder (E420), Sodium benzoate (E211), Sodium citrate gran, Standacol sunset yellow dye (E110), Propylene glycol, Povidone K30 (E1201), Veegum RG, Citric acid anhydrous (E330), Saccharin sodium, Oil Orange terpenless, Sodium alginate (E401), Demineralised water.
Incompatibilities: None stated.

Shelf life: 36 months. Largactil Forte Suspension: After opening for the first time the shelf life is 6 months. After dilution with Simple Syrup BP the shelf life is 7 days. Largactil Syrup: After opening for the first time the shelf life is 1 month. After dilution the shelf life is 14 days.

Special precaution for storage: Protect from light. Store below 30°C.

Nature and contents of container:
Largactil tablets 10 mg 25 mg 50 mg and 100 mg are available in blisters of 56 tablets.
Largactil syrup is available in glass bottles containing 100, ml.
Largactil forte suspension is available in glass bottles containing 100 ml.

Instructions for use/handling: None.

Marketing authorisation numbers

Largactil tablets 10 mg	PL 17077/0007
Largactil tablets 25 mg	PL 17077/0008
Largactil tablets 50 mg	PL 17077/0009
Largactil tablets 100 mg	PL 17077/0010
Largactil syrup	PL 17077/0012
Largactil forte suspension	PL 17077/0013

Date of approval/revision of SPC September 1998.

Legal category POM.

ORUDIS*

Presentation Capsules each containing 50 mg ketoprofen, bicoloured (opaque green/opaque purple) with each half printed 'Orudis 50' in white. Capsules each containing 100 mg ketoprofen (flesh opaque) printed 'Orudis 100' in black. The capsules also contain lactose.

Cream coloured suppositories each containing 100 mg ketoprofen.

Uses Orudis is recommended in the management of rheumatoid arthritis, osteoarthritis, ankylosing spondylitis, acute articular and periarticular disorders (bursitis, capsulitis, synovitis, tendonitis), fibrositis, cervical spondylitis, low back pain (strain, lumbago, sciatica, fibrositis), painful musculo-skeletal conditions, dysmenorrhoea, acute gout and control of pain and inflammation following orthopaedic surgery. Orudis suppositories are *not* recommended for treatment of dysmenorrhoea.

Orudis is a potent non-steroidal anti-inflammatory analgesic agent and a strong inhibitor of prostaglandin synthetase.

Orudis reduces joint pain and inflammation, and facilitates increase in mobility and functional independence. As with other non-steroidal anti-inflammatory agents, it does not cure the underlying disease.

Kinetics: Ketoprofen is completely absorbed from Orudis capsules and maximum plasma concentration occurs after ½–1 hour. It declines thereafter with an elimination half-life of about 2–3 hours. There is no accumulation on continued daily dosing. Ketoprofen is rapidly absorbed from the suppository dosage form with maximum plasma concentrations at 1–2 hours with an elimination half-life of 2–3 hours. Plasma levels obtained are comparable to those obtained from equal oral doses. Ketoprofen is very highly bound to plasma protein.

Dosage and administration Orudis is administered orally and/or rectally; to limit occurrence of gastrointestinal disturbance, capsules should always be taken with food (milk, meals).

Oral dosage is 50–100 mg twice daily, depending on patient weight and on severity of symptoms; medication should be taken early in the morning and late at night.

Rectal dosage is one suppository (100 mg) late at night supplemented as required with Orudis capsules during the daytime.

Orudis suppositories are especially appropriate for controlling overnight symptoms (severity of night and morning pain; duration and severity of morning stiffness). Suppositories administered late at night provide more consistent effective control of overnight symptoms than oral medication.

Best results are obtained by titrating dosage to suit each patient; start with a low dosage in mild chronic disease and a high dosage in acute or severe disease. Some patients derive greater benefit by treatment with capsules only; some with a combined capsule/suppository regimen; and others with a higher dosage at night-time than at early morning. Where patients require a maximum oral dosage initially, an attempt should be made to reduce this dosage for maintenance, since lower dosage might be better tolerated for purposes of long-term treatment.

Elderly: As with other medications, it is generally advisable to begin ketoprofen therapy at the lower end of the dose range and to maintain such patients on the lowest effective dosage.

Paediatric: Dosage is not established.

Contra-indications, warnings, etc Active peptic ulceration; a history of recurrent peptic ulceration or chronic dyspepsia; severe renal dysfunction; disease in children (safety/dosage during long-term treatment has not been established).

Suppositories should not be used following recent proctitis or in association with haemorrhoids.

Ketoprofen should not be given to patients with a known hypersensitivity to ketoprofen or to aspirin or other non-steroidal anti-inflammatory agents. Severe bronchospasm might be precipitated in these subjects, and in patients suffering from, or with a history of, bronchial asthma or allergic disease.

Precautions
Use in pregnancy: No embryopathic effects have been demonstrated in animals and there is epidemiological evidence of the safety of ketoprofen in human pregnancy. Nevertheless, it is recommended to avoid ketoprofen unless considered essential in which case it should be discontinued within one week of expected confinement when NSAIDs might cause premature closure of the ductus arteriosus or persistent pulmonary hypertension in the neonate. They also may delay labour. Trace amounts of ketoprofen are also excreted in breast milk; avoid use of ketoprofen unless considered essential.

Warnings: Inhibition of renal prostaglandin synthesis by non-steroidal anti-inflammatory agents may interfere with renal function especially in the presence of existing renal disease. Ketoprofen should therefore be used with caution in patients with renal impairment.

Orudis capsules should always be prescribed 'To be taken with food' to minimise gastric intolerance.

Interactions: Ketoprofen is highly protein-bound. Concomitant use of other protein-binding drugs, e.g. anticoagulants, sulphonamides, hydantoins, might necessitate modification of dosage in order to avoid increased levels of such drugs resulting from competition for plasma protein-binding sites. Similar acting drugs such as aspirin or other non-steroidal anti-inflammatory agents should not be administered concomitantly with ketoprofen as the potential for adverse reactions is increased.

Serious interactions have been recorded after the use of high dose methotrexate with non-steroidal anti-inflammatory agents including ketoprofen.

Adverse effects: Minor adverse effects, frequently transient, consist for the most part of gastrointestinal effects such as indigestion, dyspepsia, nausea, constipation, diarrhoea, heartburn and various types of abdominal discomfort. Other minor effects such as headache, dizziness, mild confusion, vertigo, drowsiness, oedema, mood change and insomnia may occur less commonly.

Major gastrointestinal adverse effects such as peptic ulceration, haemorrhage or perforation may rarely occur.

Major adverse effects involving other organ systems such as haematological reactions including thrombocytopenia, hepatic or renal damage, dermatological and photosensitivity reactions, bronchospasm and anaphylaxis are exceedingly rare.

In all cases of major adverse effects Orudis should be withdrawn at once.

Use of suppositories is sometimes associated with change in stool consistency mostly of mild softening. In a study of 64 patients treated for up to six months with one suppository each night (supplemented during daytime with Orudis capsules), local intolerance to suppositories sufficiently severe to discontinue treatment occurred in only four subjects.

Overdosage: Like other propionic acid derivatives, ketoprofen is of low toxicity in overdosage; symptoms after acute ketoprofen intoxication are largely limited to drowsiness, abdominal pain and vomiting, but adverse effects seen after overdosage with propionic acid derivatives such as hypotension, bronchospasm and gastrointestinal haemorrhage should be anticipated. Treatment is otherwise supportive and symptomatic.

Pharmaceutical precautions Store in a dry place, below 25°C.

Legal category POM.

Package quantities Orudis 50: Containers of 112×50 mg.

Orudis 100: Containers of 56×100 mg capsules.

Blister pack of 7×100 mg suppositories.

Further information Nil.

Marketing Authorisation numbers

50 mg capsules	PL 17077/0015
100 mg capsules	PL 17077/0016
100 mg suppositories	PL 17077/0017

ORUVAIL*

Qualitative and quantitative composition Oruvail 100 contain in terms of the active ingredient Ketoprofen BP 100 mg.

Oruvail 150 contain in terms of the active ingredient Ketoprogen BP 150 mg.

Oruvail 200 contain in terms of the active ingredient Ketoprofen BP 200 mg.

Pharmaceutical form Controlled release capsules.

Clinical particulars

Therapeutic indications: Oruvail is recommended in the management of rheumatoid arthritis, osteoarthritis, ankylosing spondylitis, acute articular and periarticular disorders, (bursitis, capsulitis, synovitis, tendinitis), cervical spondylitis, low back pain (strain, lumbago, sciatica, fibrositis), painful musculoskeletal conditions, acute gout, dysmenorrhoea and control of pain and inflammation following orthopaedic surgery.

Oruvail reduces joint pain and inflammation and facilitates increase in mobility and functional independence. As with other non-steroidal anti-inflammatory agents, it does not cure the underlying disease.

Posology and method of administration:

Adults: 100–200 mg once daily, depending on patient weight and on severity of symptoms.

Elderly: There is no evidence of an excess of adverse reactions in the elderly. However, as with other medication, it is generally advisable in the elderly to begin ketoprofen therapy at the lower end of the dose range and to maintain such patients on the lowest effective dosage.

Paediatric dosage: Not established.

Oruvail capsules are for oral administration.

The capsules should always be prescribed, 'to be taken with food' to minimise gastric intolerance.

Contra-indications: Active peptic ulceration, a history of recurrent peptic ulceration or chronic dyspepsia, severe renal dysfunction. Ketoprofen should not be given to patients sensitive to aspirin or other non-steroidal anti-inflammatory agents. Severe bronchospasm might be precipitated in these subjects and in patients suffering from or with a history of, bronchial asthma or allergic disease.

Special warnings and special precautions for use: Inhibition of renal prostaglandin synthesis by non-steroidal anti-inflammatory agents may interfere with renal function especially in the presence of existing renal disease. Ketoprofen should therefore be used with caution in patients with renal impairment.

Interaction with other medicaments and other forms of interaction: Ketoprofen is highly protein bound. Concomitant use of other protein-binding drugs e.g. anticoagulants, sulphonamides, hydantoins, might necessitate modification of dosage in order to avoid increased levels of such drugs resulting from competition for plasma protein-binding sites.

Similar acting drugs such as aspirin or other NSAIDS should not be administered concomitantly with ketoprofen as the potential for adverse reactions is increased.

Serious interactions have been recorded after the use of high dose methotrexate with non-steroidal anti-inflammatory agents, including ketoprofen.

Pregnancy and lactation: No embryopathic effects have been demonstrated in animals and there is epidemiological evidence of the safety of ketoprofen in human pregnancy. Nevertheless, it is recommended to avoid ketoprofen unless considered essential in which case it should be discontinued within one week of expected confinement when NSAIDS might cause premature closure of the ductus arteriosus or persistent pulmonary hypertension in the neonate. They may also delay labour.

Trace amounts of ketoprofen are excreted in breast milk. Avoid use of ketoprofen unless it is considered essential.

Effects on ability to drive and use machines: CNS side effects have been observed in some patients (see *Undesirable effects*) If affected patients should not drive or operate machinery.

Undesirable effects: Adverse effects: Minor adverse effects, frequently transient, consist for the most part of gastrointestinal effects such as indigestion, dyspepsia, nausea, constipation, diarrhoea, heartburn and various types of abdominal discomfort. Other minor effects, such as headache, dizziness, mild confusion, vertigo, drowsiness, oedema, mood change and insomnia may occur less commonly.

Major gastrointestinal adverse effects such as peptic ulceration, haemorrhage, or perforation may rarely occur.

Major adverse effects involving other organ systems such as haematological reactions including thrombocytopenia, hepatic or renal damage, dermatological and photosensitivity reactions, bronchospasm and anaphylaxis are exceedingly rare.

In all cases of major effects Oruvail should be withdrawn at once.

Overdose: Like other propionic acid derivatives, ketoprofen is of low toxicity in overdosage; symptoms after acute ketoprofen intoxication are largely limited to drowsiness, abdominal pain and vomiting, but adverse effects seen after overdosage with propionic acid derivatives such as hypotension, bronchospasm and gastro-intestinal haemorrhage should be anticipated. Owing to the slow release characteristics of Oruvail, it should be expected that ketoprofen will continue to be absorbed for up to 16 hours after ingestion. Gastric lavage, aimed at recovering pellets that may still be in the stomach should be performed if the patient is seen soon after ingestion. It should be possible to identify the pellets in the gastric contents. Treatment is otherwise supportive and symptomatic. Administration of activated charcoal in an attempt to reduce absorption of slowly-released ketoprofen should be considered.

Pharmacological properties

Pharmacodynamic properties: Ketoprofen overall has the properties of a potent non-steroidal anti-inflammatory agent. It has the following pharmacological effects:

Anti-inflammatory: It inhibits the development of carageenan-induced abscesses in rats at 1 mg/kg and UV-radiation induced erythema in guinea pigs at 6 mg/kg. It is also a potent inhibitor of PGE_2 and $PGF_2\alpha$ synthesis in guinea pig and human chopped lung preparations.

Analgesic: Ketoprofen effectively reduced visceral pain in mice caused by phenyl benzoquinone or by bradykinin following p.o. administration at about 6 mg/kg.

Antipyretic: Ketoprofen (2 and 6 mg/kg) inhibited hyperthermia caused by s.c injection of brewer's yeast in rats and, at 1 mg/kg hyperthermia caused by i.v. administration of anticoagulant vaccine to rabbits.

Ketoprofen at 10 mg/kg i.v. did not affect the cardiovascular, respiratory, central nervous system or autonomic nervous systems.

Pharmacokinetic properties: Ketoprofen is slowly but completely absorbed from Oruvail capsules. Maximum plasma concentration occurs after 6–8 hours. It declines thereafter with a half-life of about 8 hours. There is no accumulation on continued daily dosing. Ketoprofen is very highly bound to plasma protein

Preclinical safety data: No additional pre-clinical data of relevance to the prescriber.

Pharmaceutical particulars

List of excipients: Pellets: Sugar Spheres NF, Colloidal Silicon Dioxide EP, Shellac NF, Ethyl Cellulose NF, Talc EP, *Capsule Shell - body* Erythrocine (EEC 127), Gelatin, *Capsule Shell - Cap* Erythrocine (EEC 127), Patent Blue V (EEC 131), Titanium Dioxide (EEC 171), Gelatin.

Incompatibilities: None known.

Shelf life: 36 months.

Special precautions for storage: Store below 25°C in a dry place. Protect from light.

Nature and contents of container: Cardboard cartons containing blister packs of 56 capsules (100 mg) and 28 capsules (150 mg and 200 mg).

Instructions for use/handling: None.

Marketing authorisation numbers

Oruvail capsules 100 mg	PL 17077/0020
Oruvail capsules 150 mg	PL 17077/0018
Oruvail capsules 200 mg	PL 17077/0019

Date of approval/revision of SPC September 1998.

Legal category POM.

ORUVAIL* I.M. INJECTION

Qualitative and quantitative composition Ketoprofen BP 100mg in 2 ml.

Pharmaceutical form Solution for IM injection.

Clinical particulars

Therapeutic indications: Oruvail injection is recommended in the management of acute exacerbations of : Rheumatoid arthritis, osteoarthritis, ankylosing spondylitis.

Periarticular conditions such as fibrositis, bursitis, capsulitis, tendinitis and tenosynovitis.

Low back pain of musculoskeletal origin and sciatica. Other painful musculoskeletal conditions. Acute gout. Control of pain and inflammation following orthopaedic surgery.

Posology and method of administration:

Adults: 50 to 100 mg every four hours, repeated up to a maximum of 200 mg in twenty-four hours. Following a satisfactory response, oral therapy should be instituted with Oruvail capsules. It is recommended that the injection should not normally be continued for longer than three days.

Elderly: As with other medications it is generally advisable in the elderly to begin ketoprofen therapy at the lower end of the dose range and to maintain such patients on the lowest effective dosage.

Paediatric dosage: Not established.

Oruvail IM Injection is for intramuscular injection. It must not be given intravenously.

Contra-indications: Active peptic ulceration, a history of recurrent peptic ulceration or chronic dyspepsia, severe renal dysfunction, sensitivity to aspirin or other non-steroidal anti-inflammatory agents.

Special warnings and special precautions for use: Inhibition of renal prostaglandin synthesis by non-steroidal anti-inflammatory agents may interfere with renal function especially in the presence of existing renal disease. Ketoprofen should therefore be used with caution in patients with renal impairment. Severe bronchospasm might be precipitated in patients with a history of bronchial asthma or allergic disease.

Oruvail injection must not be given intravenously.

Interaction with other medicaments and other forms of interaction: Ketoprofen is highly protein bound. Concomitant use of other protein-binding drugs e.g. anticoagulants, sulphonamides, hydantoins, might necessitate modification of dosage in order to avoid increased levels of such drugs resulting from competition for plasma protein-binding sites.

Similar acting drugs such as aspirin or other NSAIDs should not be administered concomitantly with ketoprofen as the potential for adverse reactions is increased.

Serious interactions have been recorded after the use of high dose methotrexate with non-steroidal anti-inflammatory agents, including ketoprofen.

Pregnancy and lactation: No embryopathic effects have been demonstrated in animals and there is epidemiological evidence of the safety of ketoprofen in human pregnancy. Nevertheless, it is recommended to avoid ketoprofen unless considered essential in which case it should be discontinued within one week of expected confinement when NSAIDs might cause premature closure of the ductus arteriosus or persistent pulmonary hypertension in the neonate. They may also delay labour.

Effects on ability to drive and use machines: CNS side effects have been observed in some patients (see *Undesirable effects*). If affected patients should not drive or operate machinery.

Undesirable effects: Adverse effects: Minor adverse effects, frequently transient, consist for the most part of gastrointestinal effects such as indigestion, dyspepsia, nausea, constipation, diarrhoea, heartburn and various types of abdominal discomfort. Other minor effects, such as headache, dizziness, mild confusion, vertigo, drowsiness, oedema, mood change and insomnia may occur less commonly.

Major gastrointestinal adverse effects such as peptic ulceration, haemorrhage, or perforation may rarely occur. Major adverse effects involving other organ systems such as haematological reactions including thrombocytopenia, hepatic or renal damage, dermatological and photosensitivity reactions, bronchospasm and anaphylaxis are exceedingly rare. Local reactions can occur and may include pain or a burning sensation. In all cases of major adverse effects Oruvail should be withdrawn at once.

Overdose: Like other propionic acid derivatives, ketoprofen is of low toxicity in overdosage. Symptoms after acute ketoprofen intoxication are largely limited to drowsiness, abdominal pain and vomiting, but adverse effects seen after overdosage with propionic acid derivatives such as hypotension, bronchospasm and gastro-intestinal haemorrhage should be anticipated. Treatment is otherwise supportive and symptomatic.

Pharmacological properties

Pharmacodynamic properties: Ketoprofen is a pharmacopoeial non-steroidal anti-inflammatory drug (NSAID). It is a strong inhibitor of prostaglandin synthetase and potent analgesic agent. Studies in vitro and in vivo show that ketoprofen possesses powerful anti-inflammatory, antipyretic, antibradykinin and lysosomal membrane stabilising properties.

Pharmacokinetic properties: Peak concentrations of approximately 10 mg/L are reached at about 0.5-0.75 H after a 100 mg dose. The elimination half life is approximately 1.88 H. Apart from earlier Tmax values, there are no significant differences between the pharmacokinetics of Oruvail IM injection and conventional release capsules (Orudis).

Preclinical safety data: No additional pre-clinical data of relevance to the prescriber.

Pharmaceutical particulars

List of excipients: Arginine BP, Benzyl Alcohol BP, Citric Acid anhydrous (E330) BP, Water For Injections BP.

Incompatibilities: None known.

Shelf life: 36 months.

Special precautions for storage: Store below 30°C. Protect from light.

Nature and contents of container: Carton containing 10×2 ml ampoules.

Instructions for use/handling: None.

Marketing authorisation number PL 17077/0021.

Date of approval/revision of SPC September 1998.

Legal category POM.

**Trade Mark*

Helios Healthcare Ltd
11A Ferraidy Street
Peyki
Attikis
Greece

☎ 301 524 6955 🗋 301 524 5249

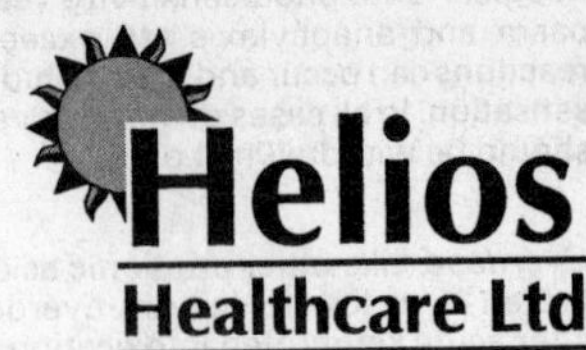

FRUMIL*, FRUMIL LS*

Presentation
Frumil: Orange tablets with a breakline, marked Frumil each containing 40 mg Frusemide BP and Amiloride Hydrochloride BP equivalent to amiloride hydrochloride anhydrous 5 mg. Other ingredients include lactose, sunset yellow (E110).

Frumil LS (low strength): Orange tablets marked 'LS' containing 20 mg Frusemide BP and Amiloride Hydrochloride BP equivalent to amiloride hydrochloride anhydrous 2.5 mg.

Uses Frumil is indicated where a prompt diuresis is required. It is of particular value in conditions where potassium conservation is important: congestive cardiac failure, nephrosis, corticosteroid therapy, oestrogen therapy. Ascites associated with cirrhosis.

Dosage and administration The tablets should be taken in the morning.

Frumil: The normal adult dose is one tablet although this may be increased to two tablets.

Frumil LS: When weaker diuresis is required one Frumil LS tablet (equivalent to half a Frumil tablet) should be taken.

Elderly: The dosage should be adjusted according to diuretic response: serum electrolytes and urea should be carefully monitored.

Contra-indications, warnings, etc
Contra-indications: Hyperkalaemia (serum potassium >5.3 mmol/litre), Addison's disease, acute renal failure, anuria, severe progressive renal disease, electrolyte imbalance, precomatose states associated with cirrhosis, concomitant potassium supplements or potassium-sparing diuretics, known sensitivity to frusemide or amiloride.

Frumil is contra-indicated in children as safety in this age group has not been established.

Warnings: Hyperkalaemia has been observed in patients receiving amiloride hydrochloride. As ACE inhibitors may elevate serum potassium levels, especially in the presence of renal impairment, combination with Frumil is best avoided in elderly patients or in any others in whom renal function may be compromised. If use of the combination is deemed essential, clinical condition and serum electrolytes must be carefully and continuously monitored.

Frusemide may cause latent diabetes to become manifest. It may be necessary to increase the dose of hypoglycaemic agents in diabetic patients.

Patients with prostatic hypertrophy or impairment of micturition have an increased risk of developing acute urinary retention during diuretic therapy.

Serum uric acid levels may rise during treatment with Frumil and acute attacks of gout may be precipitated.

Cephaloridine nephrotoxicity may be increased by concomitant administration of potent diuretics such as Frumil.

Precautions: Patients who are being treated with this preparation require regular supervision, with monitoring of fluid and electrolyte states to avoid excessive loss of fluid.

Frumil should be used with particular caution in elderly patients or those with potential obstruction of the urinary tract or disorders rendering electrolyte balance precarious.

Hyponatraemia, hypochloraemia and raised blood urea nitrogen may occur during vigorous diuresis, especially in seriously ill patients. Careful monitoring of serum electrolytes and urea should therefore be undertaken in these patients.

The dosage of concurrently administered cardiac glycosides, lithium, non-depolarising muscle relaxants or antihypertensive agents may require adjustment.

Frumil should be discontinued before a glucose tolerance test.

Pregnancy and lactation: The safety of Frumil use during pregnancy and lactation has not been established.

Side effects: Malaise, gastric upset, nausea, vomiting, diarrhoea, and constipation may occur.

If skin rashes or pruritus occur, treatment should be withdrawn.

Rare complications may include minor psychiatric disturbances, disturbances in liver function tests and ototoxicity.

Bone marrow depression occasionally complicates treatment, necessitating withdrawal of the product. The haematopoietic state should be regularly monitored during treatment.

Treatment of overdosage: Treatment of overdosage should be aimed at reversing dehydration and correcting electrolyte imbalance, particularly hyperkalaemia. Emesis should be induced or gastric lavage performed. Treatment is symptomatic and supportive. If hyperkalaemia is seen, appropriate measures to reduce serum potassium must be instituted.

Pharmaceutical precautions Store below 25°C in a dry place, protect from light.

Package quantities Frumil: Cartons of 28 tablets consisting of 2 calendar foils of 14 tablets (OP).

Cartons of 56 tablets consisting of 4 calendar foils of 14 tablets (OP).

Frumil LS: Cartons of 28 tablets consisting of 2 calendar foils of 14 tablets (OP).

Cartons of 56 tablets consisting of 4 calendar foils of 14 tablets (OP).

Further information Frumil is particularly suitable for patients at risk from hypokalaemia and causes significantly less potassium excretion than frusemide during the 12 hours after administration. The daily loss of potassium with Frumil is equivalent to normal potassium excretion.

Marketing authorisation numbers

Frumil	PL 17076/0001
Frumil LS	PL 17076/0002

Legal category POM.

FRUMIL FORTE*

Qualitative and quantitative composition The active ingredient is Frusemide BP (Furosemide INN) 80.0 mg and Amiloride.

Hydrochloride equivalent to 10.0 mg anhydrous Amiloride Hydrochloride BP.

Pharmaceutical form Tablets for oral administration.

Clinical particulars
Therapeutic indications: Frumil Forte is a potassium sparing diuretic which is indicated where a prompt diuresis is required. It is of particular value in conditions where potassium conservation is important: congestive cardiac failure, nephrosis, corticosteroid therapy, oestrogen therapy and for ascites associated with cirrhosis.

Posology and method of administration: Adults: One tablet to be taken in the morning.

Children: Not recommended.

Elderly: The dosage should be adjusted according to the diuretic response; serum electrolytes and urea should be carefully monitored.

Contra-indications: Hyperkalaemia (serum potassium >5.3 mmol/litre), Addison's disease, renal failure, anuria, severe progressive renal disease, electrolyte imbalance, precomatose states associated with cirrhosis, concomitant potassium supplements or potassium sparing diuretics, known sensitivity to frusemide or amiloride.

Frumil Forte is contraindicated in children as safety in this age group has not been established.

Special warnings and special precautions for use: Frumil Forte should be discontinued before a glucose tolerance test. Patients who are being treated with this preparation require supervision, with monitoring of fluid electrolyte states to avoid excessive loss of fluid. Frumil Forte should be used with particular caution in elderly patients or those with potential obstruction of the urinary tract or disorders rendering electrolyte balance precarious.

Interaction with other medicaments and other forms of interaction: Cephaloridine nephrotoxicity may be increased by concomitant administration of potent diuretics such as Frumil Forte. The dosage of concurrently administered cardiac glycosides, lithium, non-depolarising muscle relaxants or antihypertensive agents may require adjustment.

Pregnancy and lactation: The safety of Frumil Forte during pregnancy and lactation has not been established.

Effects on ability to drive and use machines: None stated.

Undesirable effects: Serum uric acid levels may rise during treatment with Frumil Forte and acute attacks of gout may be precipitated.

Malaise, gastric upset, nausea, vomiting, diarrhoea and constipation may occur.

If skin rashes or pruritis occur treatment should be withdrawn.

Rare complications may include minor psychiatric disturbances, disturbances in liver function tests and ototoxicity. Bone marrow depression occasionally complicates treatment, necessitating withdrawal of the product. The haematopoetic state should be regularly monitored during treatment. Hyponatraemia, hypochloraemia and raised blood urea nitrogen may occur during vigorous diuresis, especially in seriously ill patients. Careful monitoring of serum electrolytes and urea should therefore be undertaken in these patients. Hyperkalaemia has been observed in patients receiving amiloride hydrochloride.

As ACE inhibitors may elevate serum potassium levels, especially in the presence of renal impairment, combination with Frumil Forte is best avoided in elderly patients or in any others in whom renal function may be compromised. If use of the combination is deemed essential clinical condition and serum electrolytes must be continuously monitored.

Frusemide may cause latent diabetes to become manifest. It may be necessary to increase the dose of hypoglycaemic agents in diabetic patients. Patients with prostatic hypertrophy or impairment of microturition have an increased risk of developing acute urinary retention during diuretic therapy.

Overdose: Treatment of overdosage should be aimed at reversing dehydration and correcting electrolyte imbalance, particularly hyperkalaemia. Emesis should be induced or gastric lavage performed. Treatment should be symptomatic and supportive. If hyperkalaemia is seen, appropriate measures to reduce serum potassium must be instituted.

Pharmacological properties
Pharmacodynamic properties: Frusemide: Frusemide is a loop diuretic which acts primarily to inhibit electrolyte reabsorption in the thick ascending Loop of Henle.

Excretion of sodium, potassium and chloride ions is increased and water excretion enhanced.

Amiloride: Amiloride is a mild diuretic which moderately increases the excretion of sodium and chloride and reduces potassium excretion, and appears to act mainly on the distal renal tubules. It does not appear to act by inhibition of aldosterone and does not inhibit carbonic anhydrase. Amiloride adds to the natiuretic but diminishes the kaliuretic effect of other diuretics.

A combination of Frusemide and Amiloride is a diuretic which reduces the potassium loss of frusemide alone while avoiding the possible gastro-intestinal disturbances of potassium supplements.

Pharmacokinetic properties: Frusemide: Approximately 65% of the dose is absorbed after oral administration. The plasma half-life is biphasic with a terminal elimination phase of about $1\frac{1}{2}$ hours. Frusemide is up to 99% bound to plasma proteins and is mainly excreted in the urine, largely unchanged, but also excreted in the bile, non-renal elimination being considerably increased in renal failure. Frusemide crosses the placental barrier and is excreted in the milk.

Amiloride: Approximately 50% of the dose is absorbed after oral administration and peak serum concentrations are achieved by about 3–4 hours. The serum half-life is estimated to be about 6 hours. Amiloride is not bound to plasma proteins. Amiloride is not metabolised and is excreted unchanged in the urine.

Preclinical safety data: No further information available.

Pharmaceutical particulars

List of excipients: Frumil Forte tablets contain the following excipients: Lactose BP, starch maize BP microcrystalline cellulose BP, sodium starch glycollate BP, Sunset yellow dye (E110), French chalk powdered BP, colloidal anhydrous silica BP, magnesium stearate BP.

Incompatibilities: None known.

Shelf life: 36 months.

Special precautions for storage: Store below 25°C in a dry place. Protect from light.

Nature and contents of container: Frumil Forte–blister packs of 28 and 56 tablets.

Instructions for use/handling: None.

Marketing authorisation number PL 17076/0003

Date of approval/revision of SPC September 1998

Legal category POM.

**Trade Mark*

HK Pharma Limited
PO Box 105
HITCHIN
Herts SG5 2GG

☎ 07071 880292 07070 604101

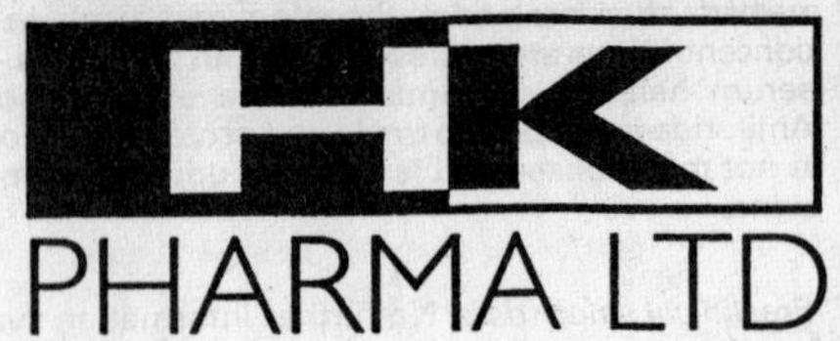

PHOSPHATE SANDOZ*
Effervescent Tablets

Qualitative and quantitative composition Phosphate Sandoz Effervescent Tablets containing 1.936 g of sodium acid phosphate, anhydrous, 0.35 g sodium bicarbonate Ph.Eur, 0.315 g potassium bicarbonate USP.

Pharmaceutical form Effervescent Tablets

Clinical particulars
Therapeutic indications: Hypercalcaemia associated with such conditions as hyperparathyroidism, multiple myelomatosis and malignancy.

Hypophosphataemia associated with vitamin D resistant rickets and vitamin D resistant hypophosphataemic osteomalacia.

Posology and method of administration: Phosphate Sandoz Effervescent should be dissolved in $\frac{1}{3}$ to $\frac{1}{2}$ a tumblerful of water and taken orally.

Dosage should be adjusted to suit the requirements of individual patients. Excessive dosage has been reported to produce hypocalcaemia in isolated cases. Particular care should therefore be taken to ensure appropriate dosage in the elderly.

Adults: Hypercalcaemia: up to 6 tablets daily (adjustment being made according to requirements).

Vitamin D resistant hypophosphateaemic osteomalacia: 4-6 tablets daily.

Children under 5 years: Hypercalcaemia: up to 3 tablets daily (adjustment being made according to requirements).

Vitamin D resistant rickets: 2-3 tablets daily.

Contra-indications: None.

Special warnings and special precautions for use: In cases of impaired renal function associated with hypercalcaemia and in cases where restricted sodium intake is required, eg. congestive cardiac failure, hypertension or pre-eclamptic toxaemia, the sodium (20.4 mmol per tablet) and potassium (3.1 mmol per tablet) content of Phosphate Sandoz should be taken into consideration. In cases of hypercalcaemia associated with impaired renal function and hyperphosphataemia, the main effect of oral phosphate is to bind calcium in the gut and thus reduce calcium absorption.

The effect of oral phosphate on serum phosphate is likely to be minimal, but close monitoring of serum levels is recommended.

Soft tissue calcification and nephrocalcinosis have been reported in isolated cases following intravenous therapy with phosphate.

This is thought to be a function of dosage and rapidity of phosphate administration. While such effects appear less likely to occur with oral phosphates, careful surveillance of patients is recommended, especially if on long term therapy.

Interactions with other medicaments and other forms of interaction: Concurrent administrations of antacids, containing agents such as aluminium hydroxide, may result in displacement of calcium from binding to oral phosphate, thus reducing efficacy.

Use during pregnancy and lactation: The safety of Phosphate Sandoz in human pregnancy has not been formally studied, but the drug has been widely used for many years without ill-consequence.

Effects on ability to drive and use machines: None

Undesirable effects: Apart from gastro-intestinal upsets, nausea and diarrhoea, very few side effects have been reported.

Overdose: Excessive dosage has been reported to produce hypocalcaemia in isolated cases. This has proved reversible when dosage has been adjusted.

Pharmacological properties
Pharmacodynamic properties: Oral administration of inorganic phosphates produces a fall in serum calcium in patients with hypercalcaemia. Phosphate Sandoz Effervescent Tablets also contain sodium ions which aid the correction of the dehydration and sodium depletion seen in hypercalcaemia.

Pharmacokinetic properties: Approximately two thirds of ingested phosphate is absorbed from the gastro-intestinal tract; most of the absorbed phosphate is then filtered by the glomeruli and subsequently undergoes reabsorption. Parathyroid hormone and vitamin D stimulate absorption of phosphate from the small intestine and its reabsorption from the proximal tubule. Virtually all absorbed phosphate is eventually excreted in the urine, the remainder being excreted in the faeces.

Preclinical safety data: Phosphate Sandoz Effervescent Tablets contain sodium acid phosphate, anhydrous, sodium bicarbonate and potassium bicarbonate (all of which are subject to pharmacopoeial monographs). The physiological, pharmacological and clinical toxicity of potassium salts are well documented and limited animal data are therefore available.

Pharmaceutical particulars
List of excipients: Sodium saccharin, orange flavour 52.570 TP, polyehtylene glycol 4000, sugar, icing CP, citric acid anhydrous, water.

Incompatibilities: None.

Shelf life: 60 months.

Special precautions for storage: This container must be kept tightly close and protected from heat and moisture.

Nature and contents of container: Polypropylene tubes of 20 effervescent tablets in boxes of 5 tubes (100 tablets).

Marketing authorisation number PL 16784/0001

Date of approval/revision of SPC April 1998

Legal category GSL.

SANDO-K*

Qualitative and quantitative composition Effervescent Tablets containing 0.6 g potassium chloride Ph.Eur., 0.4 g potassium bicarbonate USP

Pharmaceutical form Flat, round, white effervescent tablet with a slightly rough surface, weighing 2.4 g and of 22 mm diameter and 4.25 mm thick

Clinical particulars
Therapeutic indications: Prevention and treatment of hypokalaemic states such as those associated with:

i) Use of drugs which can induce potassium depletion eg. frusemide, thiazide diuretics, corticosteroids, carbenoxolone and cardiac glycosides, especially in combination with diuretics;

ii) Potassium loss resulting from severe diarrhoea, vomiting or fistulas;

iii) Acid-base disturbances e.g. alkalosis, renal tubular acidosis, states in which there is aldosterone excess, Cushing syndrome;

iv) Decreased intake of potassium e.g. malnutrition, alcoholism, some elderly patients with deficient diets;

v) Since SANDO-K Effervescent Tablets contain Cl^- they may be used in the treatment of hypokalaemia associated with hypochloraemic alkalosis.

Posology and method of administration: Oral administration, after dissolution of the tablet in water. May be taken with food if preferred.

Adults and children: Dosage is dependent upon the clinical conditions and diet of the patient, however the administration of 2 to 4 tablets daily (24 to 48 mmol K^+) is likely to provide an adequate prophylactic or therapeutic dose in most patients. Large doses may be indicated in more severe hypokalaemic conditions when the dose should be regulated by the patient's response as determined by serum electrolyte levels and acid-base studies.

Dosage guidelines: A drop in serum potassium level of 1 mmol/l represents a loss of about 100-200 mmol of potassium from body stores. While serum potassium levels below 2 mmol/l may warrant intravenous replacement therapy, following are approximate guidelines in less severe potassium depletion:

For serum levels between 2-3 mmol/l, a maximum daily dose of 100-200 mmol K^+ (8-16 tablets) and for serum levels between 3-4 mmol/l, a maximum daily dose of 50-100 mmol K^+ (4-8 tablets) should be considered.

Elderly: No evidence exists that elderly patients require different dosages or show different side-effects than younger patients. However, such patients should be carefully supervised as factors sometimes associated with ageing, such as poor diet or impaired renal function, may indirectly affect the dosage or tolerability.

Contra-indications: Severe renal impairment with oliguria, inadequately treated Addison's disease, hyperkalaemia from any cause, crush injuries and acute dehydration.

Special warnings and special precautions for use: Periodic evaluation of the patient's clinical status, serum electrolytes and the ECG should be carried out when replacement therapy is undertaken. This is particularly important in patients with cardiac disease and in those receiving digitalis. Care should be taken to avoid dosage in excess of requirements for patients with impaired renal function. Caution is also necessary in patients receiving potassium-sparing diuretics and ACE-inhibitors, and in patients with myotonia congenita or severe haemolysis. In patients with acidosis, the acid-base balance should be monitored. In patients with hypertension, it should be remembered that correction of hypokalaemia may lower blood pressure.

Interactions with other medicaments and other forms of interaction: If co-administered with potassium-sparing diuretics and ACE-inhibitors, the risk of hyperkalaemia must be considered.

Use during pregnancy and lactation: No clinical problems have been encountered during pregnancy and lactation. Nevertheless, the benefit of treatment should be considered in relation to the risks before SANDO-K is given to pregnant or nursing women.

Effects on ability to drive and use machines: No effects known.

Undesirable effects: Abdominal discomfort, diarrhoea, nausea and vomiting may occur. If there are any signs of gastric irritancy, SANDO-K, in common with all other potassium salts, should be given with or after food. Gastric irritancy has occurred but this is rare since the tablets dissolve in water and are taken in solution, thus preventing high local concentrations. A moderate hyperkalaemia may be asymptomatic; if suspected reference to the section on overdosage is recommended.

Overdose: Hyperkalaemia. Poisoning is usually minimal below 6.5 mmol per litre but may be severe above 8 mmol per litre. However, comparatively low doses may cause adverse effects when excretion is delayed as in renal insufficiency. The absolute toxicity is dependent on other electrolytes and acid-base levels.

Hyperkalaemic symptoms include paraesthesia of the extremities, listlessness, mental confusion, weakness, paralysis, hypotension, cardiac arrhythmias, heart block and cardiac arrest.

Hyperkalaemia is often asymptomatic. However, increasing serum potassium levels can be detected by changes in the ECG; initially the appearance of tall, peaked T waves, followed by a widening of the QRS complex bending into the abnormal T waves. P-wave voltage decreases and the PR interval is prolonged.

Severe cardiac toxicity may be treated with calcium gluconate (10-20 ml of a 10% injection given over 1-5 minutes with ECG monitoring). The effect may be transient and the injection may need to be repeated.

Raised serum potassium levels respond to administration of dextrose (300-500 ml/hr of 10 or 25% solution), dextrose and insulin (as for dextrose with 10 units of insulin per 20 g dextrose), or sodium bicarbonate solution.

Cation exchange resins may be used, or in severe cases peritoneal dialysis or haemodialysis may be necessary.

Caution should be exercised in patients who are digitalised and who may experience acute digitalis intoxication in the course of potassium removal.

Pharmacological properties
Pharmacodynamic properties: The potassium ion is essential to the maintenance of body function, being involved in the synthesis of protein, metabolism of carbohydrate and storage of energy reserves. It

interacts with sodium in the operation of the trans-membrane pump and at the site of exchange in the kidney, exchanges with sodium ion to maintain body homeostasis. A close relationship between potassium ion and magnesium ion has also been noted; a deficit in one ion has been associated with low levels of the other.

The diet of a healthy adult will provide an adequate intake of potassium (considered to be 20.5 to 33.3 mmol potassium daily) from a total intake of 60-100 mmol potassium. Total body potassium in an adult is about 3,500 mmol depending on the non-fat body tissues. A deficient intake or failure to conserve potassium leads to symptoms of hypokalaemia.

Pharmacokinetic properties: Unless a deficiency is present, requiring a supplement, sufficient potassium is taken into the body through the daily diet. The chloride salt of potassium is readily absorbed from the gastro-intestinal tract. Potassium enters the intra-cellular fluid to maintain a concentration of about 150 mEq/l and the normal range of concentration of potassium in the plasma is considered to be 3.5–5 mEq/l.

Excretion of potassium is mainly by the distal tubules of the kidney, by the faeces (5 to 10 mmol/day) and a smaller amount in perspiration.

Metabolic, drug induced, or dietary deficiencies in potassium intake may require administration of a supplement.

Preclinical safety data: SANDO-K Effervescent Tablets contain potassium chloride and postassium bicarbonate (both of which are the subject of pharmacopoeial monographs). The physiological, pharmacological and clinical toxicity of potassium salts are well documented and limited animal data are therefore available.

Pharmaceutical particulars

List of excipients: Dioctyle sodium sulphosuccinate BPC, Colloidal anhydrous silica EP,

Talc (acid washed) EP, Sodium saccharin BP, Icing sugar, CP HSE, Pulverised sugar, EP,

Citric acid anhydrous 30/60 EP, Polyethylene glycol 4000 EP, Purified water EP

Incompatibilities: Not applicable.

Shelf life: 48 months.

Special precautions for storage: Store in a cool dry place.

Nature and contents of container: High density polypropylene tube with polyethylene bellowed stopper containing integral silica gel dessicant capsule

Marketing authorisation number PL 16784/0002

Date of approval/revision of SPC April 1998

Legal category P.

SLOW SODIUM*

Qualitative and quantitative composition The active ingredient is Sodium Chloride PhEur Sodium Chloride contains not less than 99.0 per cent and not more than 100.5 per cent of NaCl.

One coated tablet contains 600 mg sodium chloride.

Pharmaceutical form Coated tablets.

Clinical particulars

Therapeutic indications: For the treatment and prophylaxis of sodium chloride deficiency.

Posology and method of administration: It is important that the tablets should be swallowed whole with water (approx. 70 ml per tablet where kidney function is normal to avoid hypernatraemia), and not chewed.

Adults: For prophylaxis 4-8 tablets per day. For treatment dosage to be adjusted to individual needs up to a maximum of 20 tablets per day in cases of severe salt depletion.

For control of muscle cramps during routine maintenance haemodialysis usually 10-16 tablets per dialysis. In cases of chronic renal salt-wasting up to 20 tablets per day may be required with appropriate fluid intake.

Children: Dosage should be adjusted to individual needs.

Elderly: No special dosage adjustment.

Contra-indications: Slow Sodium is contra-indicated in any situation where salt retention is undesirable, such as oedema, heart disease, cardiac decompensation and primary or secondary aldosteronism; or where therapy is being given to produce salt and water loss.

Special warnings and special precautions for use: Use of Slow Sodium without adequate water supplementation can produce hypernatraemia. The matrix (ghost) is often eliminated intact and owing to the risk of obstruction Slow Sodium should not be given to patients suffering from Crohn's disease or any other intestinal condition where strictures or diverticula may form.

Interactions with other medicaments and other forms of interaction: In hypertensive patients with chronic renal failure Slow Sodium may tend to impair the efficacy of antihypertensive drugs.

Use during pregnancy and lactation: No additional precautions required.

Effects on ability to drive and use machines: No effects known.

Undesirable effects: No side effects have been reported with Slow Sodium at the recommended dosage.

Overdose: Excessive intake of sodium chloride can result in hypernatraemia. Symptoms of hypernatraemia include restlessness, weakness, thirst, reduced salivation and lachrymation, swollen tongue, flushing of the skin, pyrexia, dizziness, headache, oliguria, hypertension, tachycardia, delirium, hyperpnoea and respiratory arrest.

Treatment requires the use of sodium-free liquids and the cessation of excessive sodium intake. In the event of a significant overdose serum sodium levels should be evaluated as soon as possible and appropriate steps taken to correct any abnormalities. The use of a loop diuretic e.g. frusemide (with potassium supplementation as required) may be appropriate in severe cases of hypernatraemia. Levels should be monitored until they return to normal.

Pharmacological properties

Pharmacodynamic properties:

Mode of action: Sodium chloride is the principle salt involved in maintaining the osmotic tension of blood and tissues, changes in osmotic tension influence the movement of fluids and diffusion of salts in cellular tissue.

Slow Sodium provides a source of sodium (in the form of sodium chloride) where a deficiency exists.

Pharmacokinetic properties: Sodium chloride is readily absorbed from the gastro-intestinal tract. It is present in all body fluids but especially in the extracellular fluid. The amount of sodium lost (as sweat) is normally small. Osmotic balance is maintained by excretion of surplus amounts in the urine.

Preclinical safety data: No information available.

Pharmaceutical particulars

List of excipients: The coated tablets contain cetostearyl alcohol, gelatin, magnesium stearate, acacia, talc, titanium dioxide and polyethylene glycol.

Incompatibilities: None known.

Shelf life: Five years.

Special precautions for storage: Protect from moisture and store below 30°C.

The tablets should be dispensed in moisture proof containers.

Medicines should be kept out of reach of children.

Nature and contents of container: The tablets are white, biconvex, polished, coated tablets about 11.4 mm in diameter, printed 'CIBA' on one side and available in containers of 100 tablets.

Marketing authorisation number PL 16784/0003

Date of approval/revision of SPC April 1998

Legal category P.

*Trade Mark

Hoechst Marion Roussel Ltd
Broadwater Park
Denham
Uxbridge
Middlesex UB9 5HP
☎ 01895 834343 🖷 01895 834479

Hoechst Marion Roussel

Hoechst

Hoechst Marion Roussel
The Pharmaceutical Company of Hoechst

AMARYL* ▼

Qualitative and quantitative composition Amaryl contains as active ingredient the sulfonylurea glimepiride (INN). Tablets of 1 mg, 2 mg, 3 mg and 4 mg glimepiride are available.

Pharmaceutical form Tablet

Clinical particulars

Therapeutic indications: Amaryl is indicated for type II diabetes mellitus, when diet, physical exercise and weight reduction alone are not adequate.

Posology and method of administration: The basis for successful treatment of diabetes is a good diet, regular physical activity, as well as routine checks of blood and urine. Tablets or insulin can not compensate if the patient does not keep to the recommended diet.

Dosage is determined by the results of blood and urinary glucose determinations.

The starting dose is 1 mg glimepiride per day. If good control is achieved this dosage should be used for maintenance therapy.

If control is unsatisfactory the dosage should be increased, based on the glycaemic control, in a stepwise manner with an interval of about 1-2 weeks between each step, to 2, 3 or 4 mg glimepiride per day.

A dosage of more than 4 mg glimepiride per day gives better results only in exceptional cases.

The maximum recommended dose is 6 mg glimepiride per day.

Normally a single daily dose of glimepiride is sufficient. It is recommended that this dose be taken shortly before or during a substantial breakfast or–if none is taken–shortly before or during the first main meal.

If a dose is forgotten, this should not be corrected by increasing the next dose.

Tablets should be swallowed whole with some liquid.

If a patient has a hypoglycaemic reaction on 1 mg glimepiride daily, this indicates that they can be controlled by diet alone.

In the course of treatment, as an improvement in control of diabetes is associated with higher insulin sensitivity, glimepiride requirements may fall. To avoid hypoglycaemia timely dose reduction or cessation of therapy must therefore be considered. Change in dosage may also be necessary, if there are changes in weight or life style of the patient, or other factors that increase the risk of hypo-or hyperglycaemia.

Switch over from other oral hypoglycaemic agents to Amaryl:

A switch over from other oral hypoglycaemic agents to Amaryl can generally be done. For the switch over to Amaryl the strength and the half life of the previous medication has to be taken into account. In some cases, especially in antidiabetics with a long half life (e.g. chlorpropamide), a wash out period of a few days is advisable in order to minimise the risk of hypoglycaemic reactions due to the additive effect. The recommended starting dose is 1 mg glimepiride per day.

Based on the response the glimepiride dosage may be increased stepwise, as indicated earlier.

Switch over from Insulin to Amaryl:

In exceptional cases, where type II diabetic patients are regulated on insulin, a changeover to Amaryl may be indicated.

The changeover should generally be undertaken in a hospital.

Contra-indications: Amaryl should not be used in the following cases: insulin dependent diabetes, diabetic coma, ketoacidosis, severe renal or hepatic function disorders, hypersensitivity to glimepiride, other sulfonylureas or sulphonamides or excipients in the tablet.

In case of severe renal or hepatic function disorders, a change over to insulin is required.

Amaryl is contra-indicated in pregnancy and lactation.

Special warnings and special precautions for use: Amaryl must be taken shortly before or during a meal.

When meals are taken at irregular hours or skipped altogether, treatment with Amaryl may lead to hypoglycaemia. Possible symptoms of hypoglycaemia include: headache, ravenous hunger, nausea, vomiting, lassitude, sleepiness, disordered sleep, restlessness, aggressiveness, impaired concentration, alertness and reaction time, depression, confusion, speech and visual disorders, aphasia, tremor, paresis, sensory disturbances, dizziness, helplessness, loss of self-control, delirium, cerebral convulsions, somnolence and loss of consciousness up to and including coma, shallow respiration and bradycardia.

In addition, signs of adrenergic counter-regulation may be present such as sweating, clammy skin, anxiety, tachycardia, hypertension, palpitations, angina pectoris and cardiac arrhythmias.

The clinical picture of a severe hypoglycaemic attack may resemble that of a stroke.

Symptoms can almost always be promptly controlled by immediate intake of carbohydrates (sugar). Artificial sweeteners have no effect.

It is known from other sulfonylureas that, despite initially successful countermeasures, hypoglycaemia may recur.

Severe hypoglycaemia or prolonged hypoglycaemia, only temporarily controlled by the usual amounts of sugar, require immediate medical treatment and occasionally hospitalisation.

Factors favouring hypoglycaemia include:

- unwillingness or (more commonly in older patients) incapacity of the patient to co-operate
- undernutrition, irregular mealtimes or missed meals or periods of fasting
- alterations in diet
- imbalance between physical exertion and carbohydrate intake
- consumption of alcohol, especially in combination with skipped meals
- impaired renal function
- serious liver dysfunction
- overdosage with Amaryl
- certain uncompensated disorders of the endocrine system affecting carbohydrate metabolism or counterregulation of hypoglycaemia (as for example in certain disorders of thyroid function and in anterior pituitary or adrenocortical insufficiency)
- concurrent administration of certain other medicines (see Interactions)

Treatment with Amaryl requires regular monitoring of glucose levels in blood and urine. In addition determination of the proportion of haemoglobin A1 and possibly of fructosamine is recommended.

Regular hepatic and haematological monitoring (especially leucocytes and thrombocytes) are required during treatment with Amaryl.

In stress-situations (e.g. accidents, acute operations, infections with fever, etc.) a temporary switch to insulin may be indicated.

No experience has been gained concerning the use of Amaryl in patients with severe impairment of liver function or dialysis patients. In patients with severe impairment of renal or liver function change over to insulin is indicated.

Interaction with other medicaments and other forms of interaction: If Amaryl is taken simultaneously with certain other medicines, both undesired increases and decreases in the hypoglycaemic action of glimepiride can occur. For this reason, other medicines should only be taken with the knowledge (or at the prescription) of the doctor.

Based on the experience with Amaryl and with other sulphonylurea the following interactions have to be mentioned.

Potentiation of the blood-glucose-lowering effect and, thus, in some instances hypoglycaemia may occur when one of the following drugs is taken, for example:

phenylbutazone, azapropazon and oxyfenbutazone
insulin and oral antidiabetic products
metformin
salicylates and p-amino-salicylic acid
anabolic steroids and male sex hormones
chloramphenicol
coumarin anticoagulants
fenfluramine
fibrates
ACE inhibitors
fluoxetine
allopurinol
sympatholytics
cyclo-, tro- and iphosphamides
sulphinpyrazone
certain long acting sulphonamides
tetracyclines
MAO-inhibitors
quinolone antibiotics
probenecid
miconazol
pentoxyfylline (high dose parenteral)
tritoqualine

Weakening of the blood-glucose-lowering effect and, thus raised blood glucose levels may occur when one of the following drugs is taken, for example:

- oestrogens and progestagens,
- saluretics, thiazide diuretics,
- thyroid stimulating agents, glucocorticoids,
- fenothiazine derivates, chlorpromazine,
- adrenaline and sympathicomimetics,
- nicotinic acid (high dosages) and nicotinic acid derivatives,
- laxatives (long term use),
- phenytoin, diazoxide,
- glucagon, barbiturates and rifampicin,
- acetozolamide

H_2 antagonists, betablockers, clonidine and reserpine may lead to either potentiation or weakening of the blood glucose lowering effect.

Under the influence of sympatholytic drugs such as betablockers, clonidine, guanethidine and reserpine, the signs of adrenergic counter regulation to hypoglycaemia may be reduced or absent.

Alcohol intake may potentiate or weaken the hypoglycaemic action of glimepiride in an unpredictable fashion.

Glimepiride may either potentiate or weaken the effects of coumarin derivatives.

Pregnancy and lactation: Amaryl is contra-indicated during pregnancy. The use of insulin is required under such circumstances. Patients who consider pregnancy should inform their physician.

In reproduction toxicity studies embryotoxicity, teratogenicity and development toxicity occurred. All reproduction toxicity effects are probably due to pharmacodynamic effects of extremely high doses and these are not substance-specific.

Because sulfonylurea-derivatives like glimepiride pass into the breast milk, Amaryl must not be taken by breast-feeding women.

Effects on ability to drive and use machines: Alertness and reaction time may be impaired due to hypo- or hyperglycaemia, especially when beginning or after altering treatment or when Amaryl is not taken regularly. This may, for example, affect the ability to drive or to operate machinery.

Undesirable effects: Based on experience with Amaryl and with other sulphonylureas the following side effects have to be mentioned.

Hypoglycaemia: In rare cases hypoglycaemic reactions have been observed after administration of Amaryl. These reactions mostly occur immediately, may be severe and are not always easy to correct. The occurrence of such reactions depends, as with other hypoglycaemic therapies, on individual factors such as dietary habits and the dosage (see further under *Special warnings and special precautions for use*).

Eyes: Transient visual disturbances may occur especially on initiation of treatment, due to changes in blood glucose levels.

Gastro-intestinal: Complaints like nausea, vomiting and diarrhoea, pressure or a feeling of fullness in the stomach and abdominal pain are very rare and seldom lead to discontinuation of therapy.

In isolated cases increase in liver enzyme values have been reported during treatment with sulphonylureas and also worsening of liver function with cholestasis, icterus and hepatitis. The symptoms generally disappear upon discontinuation of therapy, but severe hepatitis may progress to liver insufficiency.

Allergy: Hypersensitivity reactions of the skin may occur as itching, rash and urticaria. In isolated cases mild reactions may develop into serious reactions with dyspnoea, fall in blood pressure and sometimes shock. In isolated cases hypersensitivity to light may occur. Allergic vasculitis is possible in isolated cases.

Crossallergenicity with sulphonylureas, sulphonamides or related substances is possible.

Haematology: Changes in haematology are rare during Amaryl treatment. Moderate to severe thrombocytopenia, leucopenia, erythrocytopenia, agranulocytopenia, agranulocytosis, haemolytic anaemia and pancytopenia may occur.

These are in general reversible upon discontinuation of medication.

Various: A decrease in the sodium serum concentrations may occur.

In placebo-controlled studies upper respiratory tract infections were more frequent with glimepiride (14.2%) than with placebo (7.8%). This was in no case considered treatment related by the investigator. Incidence of upper respiratory tract infections was similar between glimepiride (4.6%) and glibenclamide (4.2%).

Overdose: After ingestion of an overdosage hypoglycaemia may occur, lasting from 12 to 72 hours, and may recur after an initial recovery. Symptoms may not be present for up to 24 hours after ingestion. In general observation in hospital is recommended. Nausea, vomiting and epigastric pain may occur. The hypoglycaemia may in general be accompanied by neurological symptoms like restlessness, tremor, visual disturbances, co-ordination problems, sleepiness, coma and convulsions.

Treatment primarily consists of preventing absorption by inducing vomiting and then drinking water or lemonade with activated charcoal (adsorbant) and sodium-sulphate (laxative). If large quantities have been ingested, gastric lavage is indicated, followed by activated charcoal and sodium-sulphate. In case of (severe) overdosage hospitalisation in an intensive care department is indicated. Start the administration of glucose as soon as possible, if necessary by a bolus intravenous injection of 50 ml of a 50% solution, followed by an infusion of a 10% solution with strict monitoring of blood glucose. Further treatment should be symptomatic.

In particular when treating hypoglycaemia due to accidental intake of Amaryl in infants and young children, the dose of glucose given must be carefully controlled to avoid the possibility of producing dangerous hyperglycaemia. Blood glucose should be closely monitored.

Pharmacological properties

Pharmacodynamic properties: Glimepiride is an orally active hypoglycaemic substance belonging to the sulphonylurea group. It may be used in non-insulin dependent diabetes mellitus.

Glimepiride acts mainly by stimulating insulin release from pancreatic beta cells.

As with other sulfonylureas this effect is based on an increase of responsiveness of the pancreatic beta cells to the physiological glucose stimulus. In addition, glimepiride seems to have pronounced extrapancreatic effects also postulated for other sulfonylureas.

Insulin release: Sulfonylureas regulate insulin secretion by closing the ATP-sensitive potassium channel in the beta cell membrane. Closing the potassium channel induces depolarisation of the beta cell and results–by opening of calcium channels–in an increased influx of calcium into the cell.

This leads to insulin release through exocytosis.

Glimepiride binds with a high exchange rate to a beta cell membrane protein which is associated with the ATP-sensitive potassium channel but which is different from the usual sulfonylurea binding site.

Extrapancreatic activity: The extrapancreatic effects are for example an improvement of the sensitivity of the peripheral tissue for insulin and a decrease of the insulin uptake by the liver.

The uptake of glucose from blood into peripheral muscle and fat tissues occurs via special transport proteins, located in the cells membrane. The transport of glucose in these tissues is the rate limiting step in the use of glucose. Glimepiride increases very rapidly the number of active glucose transport molecules in the plasma membranes of muscle and fat cells, resulting in stimulated glucose uptake.

Glimepiride increases the activity of the glycosyl-phosphatidylinositol-specific phospholipase C which may be correlated with the drug-induced lipogenesis and glycogenesis in isolated fat and muscle cells.

Glimepiride inhibits the glucose production in the liver by increasing the intracellular concentration of fructose-2,6-bisphosphate, which in its turn inhibits the gluconeogenesis.

General: In healthy persons, the minimum effective oral dose is approximately 0.6 mg. The effect of glimepiride is dose-dependent and reproducible. The physiological response to acute physical exercise, reduction of insulin secretion, is still present under glimepiride.

There was no significant difference in effect regardless of whether the drug was given 30 minutes or immediately before a meal. In diabetic patients, good metabolic control over 24 hours can be achieved with a single daily dose.

Although the hydroxy metabolite of glimepiride caused a small but significant decrease in serum glucose in healthy persons, it accounts for only a minor part of the total drug effect.

Pharmacokinetic properties: The bioavailability of glimepiride after oral administration is complete. Food intake has no relevant influence on absorption, only absorption rate is slightly diminished. Maximum serum concentrations (C_{max}) are reached approx. 2.5 hours after oral intake (mean 0.3 mg/ml during multiple dosing of 4 mg daily) and there is a linear relationship between dose and both C_{max} and AUC (area under the time/concentration curve). Glimepiride has a very low distribution volume (approx. 8.8 litres) which is roughly equal to the albumin distribution space, high protein binding (> 99%), and a low clearance (approx. 48 ml/min). Mean dominant serum half-life, which is of relevance for the serum concentrations under multiple-dose conditions, is about 5 to 8 hours. After high doses, slightly longer half-lives were noted.

After a single dose of radio labelled glimepiride, 58% of the radioactivity was recovered in the urine, and 35% in the faeces. No unchanged substance was detected in the urine. Two metabolites–most probably resulting from hepatic metabolism–were identified both in urine and faeces: the hydroxy derivative and the carboxy derivative. After oral administration of glimepiride, the terminal half-lives of these metabolites were 3 to 6 and 5 to 6 hours respectively.

Comparison of single and multiple once-daily dosing revealed no significant differences in pharmacokinetics, and the intraindividual variability was very low. There was no relevant cumulation.

Pharmacokinetics were similar in males and females, as well as in young and elderly (above 65 years) patients. In patients with low creatinine clearance, there was a tendency for glimepiride clearance to increase and for average serum concentrations to decrease, most probably resulting from a more rapid elimination because of lower protein binding. Renal elimination of the two metabolites was impaired. Overall no additional risk of cumulation is to be assumed in such patients.

Pharmacokinetics in five non-diabetic patients after bile duct surgery were similar to those in healthy persons.

In animals, glimepiride is excreted in milk.

Glimepiride is transferred to the placenta. Passage of the blood brain barrier is low.

Preclinical safety data: In subchronic and chronic toxicity studies in rats, mice and dogs, a decline in serum glucose as well as a degranulation of the beta cells of the pancreas were noted; these were shown to be, in principle, reversible and are regarded as signs of the pharmacodynamic effect.

In a chronic toxicity study in dogs, two of the animals receiving the highest dose (320 mg/kg body weight) developed cataract. In vitro studies in the bovine lens and investigations in rats demonstrated no cataractogenic or co-cataractogenic potential.

Glimepiride did not show any mutagenic or genotoxic effects.

Glimepiride caused a slight increased incidence of uterine adenocarcinomas in rats receiving the highest dose (345 mg/kg body weight). The safety factors based on a comparison of systemic exposure (AUC values) of female rats and humans are high enough (about 20 x) to exclude a risk to patients at the proposed clinical doses.

In mice, there was an increased incidence of islet cell hyperplasia and of islet cell adenomas; these are regarded as resulting from the chronic stimulation of the beta cells.

Administration to rats revealed no effects on fertility, course of pregnancy or delivery. Malformations (e.g. eye malformations, fissures and bone anomalies) occurred in rats and rabbits, and–in rabbits only–the numbers of abortions and intrauterine deaths were increased.

Pharmaceutical particulars

List of excipients: Lactose, sodium-starch-glycolate, magnesium stearate, cellulose and polyvidon 25000.

Further as colouring agents in Amaryl 1 mg red iron oxide (E172), in Amaryl 2 mg yellow iron oxide (E172) and indigo-carmine aluminium lake (E132), in Amaryl 3 mg yellow iron oxide (E172) and in Amaryl 4 mg indigo-carmine aluminium lake (E132).

Incompatibilities: Not applicable

Shelf life: 3 years.

Special precautions for storage: Store below 25°C and keep out of reach of children.

Nature and contents of container: Blister packs of 30 tablets (3 foils of 10). The tablets are oblong and scored on both sides. The Amaryl 1.0 tablets are 8x4 mm. The other Amaryl tablets are 10x5 mm.

Amaryl 1 mg is pink, Amaryl 2 mg is green, Amaryl 3 mg is pale yellow, Amaryl 4 mg is light blue.

Instructions for use/handling: No special information

Marketing authorisation numbers

AMARYL Tablets, 1.0 mg:	PL 13402/0006
AMARYL Tablets, 2.0 mg:	PL 13402/0007
AMARYL Tablets, 3.0 mg:	PL 13402/0008
AMARYL Tablets, 4.0 mg:	PL 13402/0009

Date of approval/revision of SPC 8 November 1996

Legal category POM

CEFROM* 1g IV INJECTION
CEFROM* 2g IV INJECTION

Qualitative and quantitative composition

	Cefpirome sulphate	*Corresponding amount of cefpirome base*
	(mg)	*(mg)*
Cefrom 1.0 g	*1191*	*1000*
Cefrom 2.0 g	*2382*	*2000*

Pharmaceutical form Cefpirome is supplied as a powder for reconstitution in vials for intravenous injection.

Clinical particulars

Therapeutic indications: Cefrom is indicated for the treatment of infections, either before the infecting organism has been identified or when caused by bacteria of established sensitivity, as follows:

Lower respiratory tract infections (bronchopneumonia and lobar pneumonia).

Complicated upper (pyelonephritis) and lower urinary tract infections.

Skin and soft tissue infections (cellulitis, skin abscess and wound infections).

Infections in neutropenic patients.

Bacteraemia/septicaemia.

Severe infections, as listed above.

Posology and method of administration: Cefrom is to be used by the parenteral route, the dosage, mode of administration and duration of treatment depending upon the severity of the infection, sensitivity of the pathogens, condition of the patient and renal function. The following dosages are recommended for moderate to severe infections in patients with normal renal function:

Indication	*Unit dose (g)*	*Dosage interval (hours)*	*Total daily dose (g)*
Complicated upper and lower urinary tract infections	1.0	12	2.0
Skin and soft tissue infections	1.0	12	2.0
Lower respiratory tract infections	1.0 or 2.0	12	2.0 or 4.0
Bacteraemia/Septicaemia and severe infections	2.0	12	4.0
Infections in neutropenic patients	2.0	12	4.0

For urinary tract and skin and soft tissue infections, the unit dose may be increased to 2 g in very severe cases.

Elderly: No adjustment is required unless renal impairment is present.

Children: There is insufficient evidence on which to base an appropriate dosage regimen in children under 12 years of age. Therefore, Cefrom is not recommended for this age group.

Dosage in patients with impaired renal function: Cepirome is excreted principally by the kidney. The dose must therefore be reduced in patients with impaired renal function to compensate for the slower excretion. The following doses are recommended:

Creatinine clearance	*Dose in normal renal function*	
>50 ml/min	1.0 g b.i.d.	2.0 g b.i.d.
	Dose Adjustment	
	1.0 g loading dose then	2.0 g loading dose then
50–20 ml/min	0.5 g b.i.d.	1.0 g b.i.d.
20–5 ml/min	0.5 g once daily	1.0 g once daily
<5 ml/min (haemodialysis patients)	0.5 g daily+0.25 g immediately after dialysis	1.0 g daily+0.5 g immediately after dialysis

Method of administration: Intravenous injection: The contents of one vial of 1.0 or 2.0 g cefpirome are dissolved in 10 or 20 ml sterile water for injections respectively, and then injected over 3–5 minutes either directly into a vein or into the distal section of a clamped-off infusion tube. For patients with renal impairment, 0.25 or 0.5 g Cefrom are dissolved in 2 or 5 ml water for injections respectively.

Short intravenous infusion: The contents of one 1.0 g or 2.0 g vial of cefpirome are dissolved in 100 ml of sterile water for injections and then infused over 20-30 minutes.

The following infusion solutions may also be used: 0.9% sodium chloride solution, Ringers solution, standard electrolyte infusions, 5 and 10% glucose solution, 5% fructose solution, 6% glucose + 0.9% sodium chloride solution.

Contra-indications: Hypersensitivity to cephalosporins.

Special warnings and precautions for use: Renal function: Caution should be exercised if cefpirome is administered together with aminoglycosides or loop diuretics. Renal function must be monitored in all such cases.

Renal insufficiency: The dosage of Cefrom should be adapted according to creatinine clearance.

Pseudomembranous colitis: Severe and persistent diarrhoea has been observed during and after treatment with antibiotics of several different classes. This may be symptomatic of pseudomembranous colitis (in most cases due to *Clostridium difficile*) which may be fatal. This is a rare complication with cephalosporins. Once pseudomembranous colitis is suspected as the diagnosis, confirmed by sigmoidoscopy, cefpirome treatment must be stopped immediately and specific antibiotic therapy must be started (e.g. vancomycin or metronidazole). Products which may cause faecal stasis are contra-indicated.

Preliminary enquiry to previous hypersensitivity to beta-lactam antibiotics is required.

The use of cefpirome is strictly contraindicated in subjects with a previous history of immediate hypersensitivity to cephalosporins. In any doubt, it is essential that a physician is present at the first administration in order to treat any possible anaphylactic reaction.

Cross sensitivity: As there is a cross allergy between penicillin and cephalosporins in 5 to 10% of cases, use of cefpirome should be undertaken with extreme care in penicillin sensitive patients. Careful surveillance is necessary from the first administration.

Hypersensitivity reactions (anaphylaxis) occurring with these two classes of antibiotics may be serious or even fatal.

Occurrence of a hypersensitivity reaction requires treatment to be stopped.

Blood constituents: For courses of treatment lasting longer than 10 days, blood count should be monitored and in the event of neutropenia developing treatment should be discontinued.

Cefrom should not be used in children until adequate clinical experience has been gained.

Interactions with other medicaments and other forms of interaction: Drug interactions: Drug interactions have not been observed with Cefrom. Although there is no evidence that cefpirome adversely affects renal function at normal therapeutic doses, cephalosporin antibiotics may potentiate the nephrotoxic effects of certain drugs (e.g. aminoglycosides) if administered concomitantly.

Probenecid interferes with renal tubular transfer of cefpirome, delaying its excretion and increasing the plasma concentration.

Other interactions: A false-positive Coombs test may be obtained in rare cases during treatment with cefpirome. Glycosuria should be determined by enzymatic methods during treatment as non-enzymatic methods may give a false-positive result.

Cefrom gives a strong, creatinine-like reaction in creatinine assays based on the picrate method. The use of an enzyme method is recommended to avoid falsely high levels of creatinine. If an enzyme method is not available, blood sampling should be done immediately before the next administration of cefpirome because if the recommended dosage and dosage intervals are followed, the serum level of cefpirome at that time is expected to be below the interference limit.

Pregnancy and lactation: In vitro studies have shown that cefpirome crosses the human placenta. Cefrom should therefore not be used during pregnancy. An evaluation of experimental animal studies has not indicated direct or indirect harmful effects with respect to reproduction, development of the embryo or foetus, the course of gestation and perinatal and postnatal development.

As cefpirome is excreted in human breast milk, either cefpirome treatment should be discontinued or breast feeding ceased.

Effects on ability to drive and use machines: There is no evidence that Cefrom impairs the ability to drive or operate machines.

Undesirable effects: The following may be observed during treatment with cephalosporins:

Hypersensitivity reactions: Allergic skin reactions; rash, urticaria, pruritus, drug fever; severe acute allergic reactions (anaphylaxis): angioedema, bronchospasm may occur and require emergency treatment. As with other cephalosporins, isolated cases of bullous reactions such as erythema multiforme, Stevens-Johnson syndrome, toxic epidermal necrolysis have been reported.

Effects on the gastrointestinal tract: Nausea and vomiting; diarrhoea; in very rare cases, pseudomembranous colitis (see Special warnings and precautions for use).

Effects on liver function: Increase in liver enzymes in the serum (e.g. ASAT [GOT], ALAT [GPT], alkaline phosphatase), Gamma GT, LDH and/or bilirubin. These laboratory abnormalities, which may also be explained by the infection, may rarely exceed twice the upper limit of the normal range and elicit a pattern of liver injury, usually cholestasis and most often asymptomatic.

Effects on renal function: Slight increases in serum creatinine and urea may be observed, but were only rarely a reason for discontinuing treatment. Interstitial nephritis has been observed in rare instances during treatment with other cephalosporins. Very rarely acute renal failure may occur.

Changes in blood constituents: Thrombocytopenia; eosinophilia; very rarely, haemolytic anaemia. As with other β-lactam antibiotics, granulocytopenia and, more rarely, agranulocytosis may develop during treatment with cefpirome, particularly if given over long periods. For courses of treatment lasting longer than 10 days, the blood count should be monitored (see Special warnings and precautions for use).

Local reactions: Inflammatory irritation of the venous wall and pain at the site of injection.

Neurological effects: A very few cases of convulsions have been reported. As with other cephalosporins, reversible encephalopathy may occur with high dose treatment, especially in patients with renal insufficiency.

Superinfection: As with other cephalosporins, Cefrom, especially with prolonged use may result in the overgrowth of non-susceptible organisms including moniliasis (candidiasis). Repeated evaluation of the condition of the patient is essential. If secondary infection occurs, appropriate measures should be taken.

Others: Taste and/or smell disturbances shortly after injection, headache, fever.

Overdose: In cases of overdosage, particularly in patients with renal insufficiency, encephalopathy may occur. The encephalopathy is usually reversible once plasma drug levels have fallen. Serum levels of cefpirome can be reduced by peritoneal dialysis and haemodialysis. Approximately 50% of the cefpirome present in the body is elimated in a four hour haemodialysis session.

Pharmacological properties

Pharmacodynamic properties: Cefrom is a bactericidal β-lactamase-stable cephalosporin antibiotic. As a β-lactam, it acts by disturbing the synthesis of the main bacterial cell-wall polymer, peptidoglycan. It is bactericidal at low concentrations against an extremely broad spectrum of Gram-negative and Gram-positive pathogens because it penetrates the cell wall of bacteria extremely rapidly and binds to the target enzymes (penicillin-binding proteins) with high affinity.

This has been demonstrated in numerous *in vitro* studies with hospital and community acquired pathogens throughout the world and recent studies show no change in the pattern of sensitivity. Many strains resistant to other injectable cephalosporins or aminoglycosides are sensitive to Cefrom.

Antibacterial activity: The following organisms show *in vitro* sensitivity to cefpirome:

Gram-positive: *Staphylococcus aureus* (including penicillin-resistant strains), coagulase-negative *Staphylococcus* spp. (including penicillin-resistant but not methicillin-resistant strains), *Streptococcus* Groups A (*Streptococcus pyogenes*), B (*Streptococcus agalactiae*), C, F and G, *Streptococcus mitis, Streptococcus sanguis, Streptococcus viridans, Streptococcus pneumoniae, Propionibacterium acnes, Peptostreptococcus anaerobius, Corynebacterium diphtheriae, Corynebacterium pyogenes.*

Gram-negative: *Citrobacter* spp., *Escherichia coli, Salmonella* spp., *Shigella* spp., *Klebsiella* spp. (indole-positive and indole-negative), *Enterobacter* spp., *Hafnia alvei, Serratia* spp., *Proteus mirabilis, Proteus vulgaris, Proteus rettgeri, Morganella morganii, Providencia* spp., *Yersinia enterocolitica, Pasteurella multocida, Haemophilus influenzae, Haemophilus ducreyi, Moraxella catarrhalis, Neisseria meningitidis, Neisseria gonorrhoeae, Aeromonas hydrophila.*

Most strains of the following species show sensitivity to cefpirome *in vitro*:

Gram positive: *Clostridium* spp.

Gram negative: *Pseudomonas aeruginosa; Pseudomonas* spp (non-aeruginosa), *Bacteroides fragilis* (non-β-lactamase-producing strains).

Most strains of the following species are resistant to cefpirome in vitro:

Gram-Positive: *Enterococcus faecium, Listeria monocytogenes, Clostridium difficile.*

Gram-Negative: *Xanthomonas maltophilia, Fusobacterium varium, Bacteroides fragilis* (β-lactamase-producing strains).

Cefpirome shows synergistic activity with aminoglycosides against many bacteria.

Infections caused by the following pathogens have been successfully treated in clinical trials:

Gram-positive: *Staphylococcus aureus* and coagulase-negative *Staphylococcus* spp. (*Staphylococcus epidermidis, Staphylococcus saprophyticus, Staphylococcus hominis, Staphylococcus warneri*), haemolytic and non-haemolytic streptococci, *Streptococcus pyogenes* (Group A), streptococci of serogroups B and F, *Streptococcus pneumoniae, Streptococcus agalactiae*, streptococci of the viridans group, *Corynebacterium* spp.

Gram-negative: *Escherichia coli, Enterobacter* spp., indole-positive and indole-negative *Klebsiella* spp. and *Proteus* spp., *Morganella morganii, Providencia* spp., *Citrobacter* spp., *Salmonella* spp., *Hafnia alvei, Serratia marcescens, Pasturella multocida, Haemophilus influenzae* and other *Haemophilus* species, *Moraxella catarrhalis, Neisseria* spp., *Alcaligenes* spp., *Pseudomonas aeruginosa* and other *Pseudomonas* species, *Bacteroides* spp.

Pharmacokinetic properties:

Bioavailability and absorption: Bioavailability after i.m. administration was greater than 90%.

Distribution: The average peak ($C_{5\ min}$) serum level after single i.v. doses of 1 g was 80–90 mg/l. Pharmacokinetics were dose linear. The volume of distribution is 14–19 L. No accumulation was seen after multiple dosing. The elimination half-life in serum is 1.8–2.2 hours. Serum protein binding was less than 10% and is dose independent. Rapid penetration into the following body tissues and fluids was observed. (See table overleaf).

Biotransformation and excretion: Cefpirome was principally eliminated by the kidney; 80–90% of the administered drug was recovered in the urine. Radioactive counts recovered in the urine consist of 98–99% unchanged Cefpirome. Approximately 30% of a 1.0 g dose was eliminated by haemodialysis.

Special groups: Elderly (>65 years): The $C_{5\ min}$ serum level after a single i.v. dose of 2.0 g to healthy elderly subjects was 174 mg/l. The elimination half-life in serum was 3.4 hours and urinary excretion of the unchanged product was 71% after 24 hours. In patients older than 65 years $C_{5\ min}$ after i.v. doses of 1 and 2 g amounts to 127.1 and 231.1 mg/l respectively. The elimination half-lives after the same doses amounted to 4.4±1.4 and 4.5±1.6 hours respectively.

Renally impaired patients: The average elimination half-lives after single doses of 2.0 g i.v. to patients with different degrees of renal impairment were as follows:

Cefpirome elimination in renally impaired patients

	Creatinine clearance (ml/min)			
	>50	*20–50*	*10–20*	*<10*
Elimination half-life (h)	2.6	9.2	9.8	14.5

Dose adjustments are required in renally impaired patients only at creatinine clearance levels below 50 ml/min.

Preclinical safety data: Not applicable.

Pharmaceutical particulars

List of excipients: Anhydrous sodium carbonate.

Incompatibilities: Cefrom should not be administered in sodium bicarbonate solution.

Cefpirome should not be mixed with other antibiotics in the same syringe, this applies particularly in the case of aminoglycosides.

Shelf life: Finished product (sterile powder): 3 years.

Reconstituted solution: Up to 24 hours refrigerated. See 'Special precautions for storage' below for further details.

Special precautions for storage: Finished product: Store finished product (sterile powder) below 25°C. Protect from light. Some intensification of colour may occur on storage. However, provided the recommended storage conditions are observed, this does not indicate any change in potency or safety.

Reconstituted solution: In keeping with good pharmaceutical practice, it is preferable to use freshly constituted solutions of Cefrom. Cefrom can be stored for up to 24 hours refrigerated (2—8°C) when prepared in Water for Injections BP.

Cefrom tissue distribution

Tissue/fluid	Dose (g)	Mean concentration			Tissue: Serum or fluid: serum ratio		
		2 h	<8 h	12 h	2 h	<8 h	12 h
Tissue (mg/kg)							
Prostate	1.0	12.9	6.1	1.7	0.3	0.4	0.6
Bronchial mucosa	1.0	33.0	15.7	—	0.6	0.6	—
Fluid (mg/l)							
Interstitial	1.0	32.9	13.3	2.9	1.9	2.3	3.0
Peritoneal	1.0	46.3	10.6	—	1.1	1.0	—
Meninges							
Inflamed	2.0	2.7	3.6	2.3	0.05	0.9	0.7
Non-inflamed	2.0	0.5	0.8	—	0.01	0.13	—

Peak plasma levels were above the MICs for commonly encountered pathogens.

Cefrom is compatible with several other commonly used intravenous infusion fluids and will retain satisfactory potency for up to 24 hrs when refrigerated (2–8°C) in the following fluids:

Water for Injections BP, 0.9% Sodium chloride Injection, 5% glucose solution, 10% glucose solution, 5% fructose solution, Ringers Solution BPC.

Some intensification of colour may occur on storage of the reconstituted solution. However, provided the recommended storage conditions are observed, this does not indicate a change in potency or safety.

No data is yet available to support the mixing of reconstituted Cefrom with any other drugs or infusion solutions other than those specified.

Nature and contents of container: Cefrom powder for reconstitution is presented in glass, type III vials with coated rubber stoppers sealed with aluminium caps.

Vials are individually packed.

Instructions for use/handling: The vials are manufactured under slight negative pressure. The negative pressure facilitates the addition of the solvent. Carbon dioxide is released when the solvent and the powder for reconstitution are mixed and an increase in pressure occurs. The solution may still contain bubbles of carbon dioxide, but these have no adverse effects on efficacy. The vials containing the solvent and powder for reconstitution should be held horizontal when preparing the infusion solution and the cannula should be inserted rapidly.

Effervesence occurs on dissolution of cefpirome and the vial has to be tipped gently from side to side for approximately 1 minute before cefpirome is completely dissolved.

Marketing authorisation numbers
Cefrom 1 g IV injection PL 13402/0063
Cefrom 2 g IV injection PL 13402/0064

Date of approval/revision of SPC 13 February 1998

Legal category POM

CIDOMYCIN* ADULT INJECTABLE 80 mg/2 ml

Qualitative and quantitative composition Each ampoule or vial (2 ml) contains 82.80 mg Gentamicin Sulphate BP equivalent to 80 mg Gentamicin base.

Pharmaceutical form Injection

Clinical particulars
Therapeutic indications: Gentamicin is an aminoglycoside antibiotic with broad-spectrum bactericidal activity. It is usually active against most strains of the following organisms: *Escherichia coli*, *Klebsiella* spp., *Proteus* spp. (indole positive and indole negative), *Pseudomonas aeruginosa*, Staphylococci, *Enterobacter* spp., *Citrobacter* spp and *Providencia* spp.

Gentamicin injection and gentamicin paediatric injection are indicated in urinary-tract infections, chest infections, bacteraemia, septicaemia, severe neonatal infections and other systemic infections due to sensitive organisms.

Posology and method of administration:
Adults: Serious infections: If renal function is not impaired, 5 mg/kg/daily in divided doses at six or eight hourly intervals. The total daily dose may be subsequently increased or decreased as clinically indicated.

Systemic infections: If renal function is not impaired, 3-5 mg/kg/day in divided doses according to severity of infection, adjusting according to clinical response and body weight.

Urinary tract infections: As "Systemic infections". Or, if renal function is not impaired, 160 mg once daily may be used.

Children: Premature infants or full term neonates up to 2 weeks or age: 3 mg/kg 12 hourly. 2 weeks to 12 years: 2 mg/kg 8 hourly.

The elderly: There is some evidence that elderly patients may be more susceptible to aminoglycoside toxicity whether secondary to previous eighth nerve impairment or borderline renal dysfunction. Accordingly, therapy should be closely monitored by frequent determination of gentamicin serum levels, assessment of renal function and signs of ototoxicity.

Renal impairment: Gentamicin is excreted by simple glomerular filtration and therefore reduced dosage is necessary where renal function is impaired. Nomograms are available for the calculation of dose, which depends on the patient's age, weight and renal function. The following table may be useful when treating adults.

Blood urea (mg/100 ml)	(mmol/l)	Creatinine clearance (GFR) (ml/min)	Dose and frequency of administration
<40	6–7	>70	80 mg* 8-hourly
40–100	6–17	30–70	80 mg* 12-hourly
100–200	17–34	10–30	80 mg* daily
>200	>34	5–10	80 mg* every 48 hours
Twice-weekly intermittent haemodialysis		<5	80 mg* after dialysis

*60 mg if body weight <60 kg. Frequency of dosage in hours may also be approximated as serum creatinine (mg%)x eight or in SI units, as serum creatinine (micromol/l) divided by 11. If these dosage guides are used peak serum levels must be measured. Peak levels of gentamicin occur approximately one hour after intramuscular injection and intravenous injection. Trough levels are measured just prior to the next injection. Assay of peak serum levels gives confirmation of adequacy of dosage and also serves to detect levels above 10 mg/l, at which the possibility of ototoxicity should be considered. One hour concentrations of gentamicin should not exceed 10 mg/l (but should reach 4 mg/l), while the pre dose trough concentration should be less than 2 mg/l.

The recommended dose and precautions for intramuscular and intravenous administration are identical. Gentamicin when given intravenously should be injected directly into a vein or into the drip set tubing over no less than three minutes. If administered by infusion, this should be over no longer than 20 minutes and in no greater volume of fluid than 100 ml.

Contra-indications: Hypersensitivity; Myasthenia Gravis.

Special warnings and special precautions for use: Ototoxicity has been recorded following the use of gentamicin. Groups at special risk include patients with impaired renal function and possibly the elderly. Consequently, renal, auditory and vestibular functions should be monitored in these patients and serum levels determined so as to avoid peak concentrations above 10 mg/l and troughs above 2 mg/l. As there is some evidence that risk of both ototoxicity and nephrotoxicity is related to the level of total exposure, duration of therapy should be the shortest possible compatible with clinical recovery. In some patients with impaired renal function there has been a transient rise in blood-urea-nitrogen which has usually reverted to normal during or following cessation of therapy. It is important to adjust the frequency of dosage according to the degree of renal function.

Interactions with other medicaments and other forms of interaction: Concurrent administration of gentamicin and other potentially ototoxic or nephrotoxic drugs should be avoided. Potent diuretics such as ethacrynic acid and frusemide are believed to enhance the risk of ototoxicity whilst amphotericin B, cisplatin and cyclosporin are potential enhancers of nephrotoxicity.

Any potential nephrotoxicity of cephalosporins, and in particular cephaloridine, may also be increased in the presence of gentamicin. Consequently, if this combination is used monitoring of kidney function is advised.

Neuromuscular blockade and respiratory paralysis have been reported from administration of aminoglycosides to patients who have received curare-type muscle relaxants during anaesthesia.

Pregnancy and lactation: There are no proven cases of intrauterine damage caused by gentamicin. However, in common with most drugs known to cross the placenta, usage in pregnancy should only be considered in life threatening situations where expected benefits outweigh possible risks. In the absence of gastro-intestinal inflammation, the amount of gentamicin ingested from the milk is unlikely to result in significant blood levels in breast-fed infants.

Effects on ability to drive and use machines: Not known

Undesirable effects: See *Special warnings and special precautions for use.*

Overdose: Haemodialysis and peritoneal dialysis will aid the removal from blood but the former is probably more efficient. Calcium salts given intravenously have been used to counter the neuromuscular blockade caused by gentamicin.

Pharmacological properties
Pharmacodynamic properties: Gentamicin is a mixture of antibiotic substances produced by the growth of *Micromonospora purpurea*. It is bactericidal with greater antibacterial activity than streptomycin, neomycin or kanamycin.

Gentamicin exerts a number of effects on cells of susceptible bacteria. It affects the integrity of the plasma membrane and the metabolism of RNA, but its most important effect is inhibition of protein synthesis at the level of the 30s ribosomal subunit.

Pharmacokinetic properties: Gentamicin is not readily absorbed from the gastro-intestinal tract. Gentamicin is 70-85% bound to plasma albumin following administration and is excreted 90% unchanged in urine. The half-life for its elimination in normal patients is 2 to 3 hours.

Effective plasma concentration is 4-8 μg/ml.
The volume of distribution (vd) is 0.3 l/kg.
The elimination rate constant is:
0.02/hr for anuric patients*
0.30/hr normal

* Therefore in those with anuria care must be exercised following the usual initial dose, any subsequent administration being reduced in-line with plasma concentrations of gentamicin.

Preclinical safety data: Not applicable

Pharmaceutical Particulars
List of excipients: Methylhydroxybenzoate BP, Propylhydroxybenzoate BP, Disodium edetate BP, Water for Injections BP

Incompatibilities: In general, gentamicin injection should not be mixed. In particular the following are incompatible in mixed solution with gentamicin injection: penicillins, cephalosporins, erythromycin, heparins, sodium bicarbonate.* Dilution in the body will obviate the danger of physical and chemical incompatibility and enable gentamicin to be given concurrently with the drugs listed above either as a bolus injection into the drip tubing, with adequate flushing, or at separate sites. In the case of carbenicillin, administration should only be at a separate site.

* Carbon dioxide may be liberated on addition of the two solutions. Normally this will dissolve in the solution but under some circumstances small bubbles may form.

Shelf life: 36 months

Special precautions for storage: Store below 25°C. Do not refrigerate.

Nature and contents of container: Cidomycin Adult Injectable is supplied in ampoules and vials.
Instruction for use/handling: Not applicable.

Marketing authorisation holder: Roussel Laboratories Ltd., Broadwater Park, Denham, Uxbridge, Middlesex, UB9 5HP

Marketing authorisation number PL 0109/5065R

Date of approval/revision of SPC October 1997

Legal category POM

CIDOMYCIN* EYE/EAR DROPS

Qualitative and quantitative composition Gentamicin Sulphate BP (equivalent to gentamicin base) 0.3% w/v

Pharmaceutical form Sterile Aqueous Solution (Eye/Ear Drops)

Clinical particulars
Therapeutic indications: Gentamicin is an aminoglycoside antibiotic with broad-spectrum bactericidal activity against most gram positive and gram negative bacteria.

In the eye: Cidomycin drops are effective in the treatment of external bacterial infections of the eye, including conjunctivitis, blepharitis, styes, corneal ulcers, and for prophylaxis in trauma.

In the ear: Cidomycin drops are also effective in the treatment of external ear infections due to sensitive organisms.

Posology and method of administration: For adults and children:
In the eye: One to three drops should be instilled into the affected eye three or four times daily, or as required.

In the ear: Following cleansing of the affected ear, two to four drops should be instilled three to four times daily and at night.

No specific recommendations for the elderly.

Contra-indications: The product is contra-indicated where there is known hypersensitivity to any of the ingredients. Use in the ear is contraindicated if the drum is perforated.

Special warnings and precautions for use: If irritation, sensitization, or super-infection develop, treatment with Cidomycin should be discontinued and appropriate therapy instituted.

Interactions with other medicaments and other forms of interaction: Gentamicin is pharmaceutically incompatible with amphotericin, cephalosporins, erythromycin, heparin, penicillins, sodium bicarbonate and sulphadiazine sodium.

Use in pregnancy and lactation: There are no proven cases of intrauterine damage caused by gentamicin. However, as with most drugs known to cross the placenta, usage in pregnancy should be considered where benefits outweigh possible risks. In the absence of gastro-intestinal inflammation, the amount of gentamicin ingested from breast milk is unlikely to result in significant blood levels in infants.

Effects on ability to drive and to use machines: Topical eye preparations may cause transient blurring of vision on instillation. Patients should be warned not to drive or operate hazardous machinery unless vision is clear.

Undesirable effects: Gentamicin drops may cause transient eye irritation. Severe dose related ototoxicity can occur with gentamicin in susceptible patients, particularly those with renal impairment. Vestibular damage is more common than hearing loss. Reversible nephrotoxicity may occur and acute nerve failure has been reported, often in association with concurrent administration of cephalosporins.

Overdose: Haemodialysis or peritoneal dialysis will aid the removal of gentamicin from the blood.

Pharmacological properties
Pharmacodynamic properties: Gentamicin is a mixture of antibiotic substances produced by the growth of *Micromonospora purpurea*. It is bactericidal with greater antibacterial activity than streptomycin, neomycin or kanamycin.

Gentamicin exerts a number of effects on cells of susceptible bacteria. It affects the integrity of the plasma membrane and the metabolism of RNA. Its most important effects is inhibition of protein synthesis at the level of the 30s ribosomal subunit.

Pharmacokinetic properties: Gentamicin is not readily absorbed from the gastro-intestinal tract. It is 70-85% bound to plasma albumin following administration and is excreted 90% unchanged in urine. The half-life for its elimination in normal patients is 2 to 3 hours.

Effective plasma concentration is 4-8 μg/ml.
The volume of distribution (Vd) is 0.3 l/kg.
The elimination rate constant is:
0.02/hr for anuric patients
0.30/hr for normal

Preclinical safety data: Not applicable.

Pharmaceutical particulars
List of excipients: Disodium edetate, sodium metabisulphite, benzalkonium chloride solution, sodium phosphate, sodium acid phosphate and purified water.

Incompatibilities: Potent diuretics such as ethacrynic acid and frusemide are believed to enhance any risk of ototoxicity. Amphotericin B, cisplatin and cyclosporin are potential enhancers of nephrotoxicity.

Neuromuscular blockade and respiratory paralysis have been reported from the administration of aminoglycosides to patients who have received curare-type muscle relaxants during anaesthesia.

Shelf-life: 60 months. Discard contents 28 days after opening.

Special precautions for storage: Store below 25°C.

Nature and contents of container: EP Type I neutral amber glass vial. Bromobutyl rubber teat held to vial by a low density polyethylene collar (lower cap). Lower density polyethylene upper cap (with a pilferproof tear strip). Pack size of 8 ml.

Instructions for use/handling: Not applicable.

Marketing authorisation holder: Roussel Laboratories Ltd., Broadwater Park, Denham, Uxbridge, Middlesex UB9 5HP

Marketing authorisation number PL 0109/0114

Date of approval/revision of SPC February 1998

Legal category POM

CIDOMYCIN* INJECTIONS

Presentation Cidomycin for parenteral use is available as:

Cidomycin Paediatric Injectable in 2 ml vials each containing the equivalent of 20 mg gentamicin base as Gentamicin Sulphate BP.

Cidomycin Intrathecal Injection in 1 ml ampoules each containing 5 mg gentamicin base as Gentamicin Sulphate BP.

Uses Gentamicin is an aminoglycoside antibiotic with broad-spectrum bactericidal activity. It is usually active against most strains of the following organisms: *Escherichia coli, Klebsiella* spp., *Proteus* spp. (indole positive and indole negative), *Pseudomonas aeruginosa,* staphylococci, *Enterobacter* spp., *Citrobacter* spp and *Providencia* spp.

Gentamicin paediatric injection is indicated in urinary-tract infections, chest infections, bacteraemia, septicaemia, severe neonatal infections, and other systemic infections due to sensitive organisms.

Gentamicin intrathecal injection is indicated as a supplement to systemic therapy in bacterial meningitis, ventriculitis and other bacterial infections of the central nervous system.

Dosage and administration
Gentamicin intramuscular/intravenous injection:
Adults: Serious infections: If renal function is not impaired, 5 mg/kg daily in divided doses at six or eight hourly intervals. The total daily dose may be subsequently increased or decreased as clinically indicated.

Systemic infections: If renal function is not impaired, 3-5 mg/kg/day in divided doses according to severity of infection, adjusting according to clinical response and body weight.

Urinary-tract infections: As 'Systemic infections'. Or, if renal function is not impaired, 160 mg once daily may be used.

Children: Premature infants or full term neonates up to 2 weeks of age: 3 mg/kg 12-hourly. 2 weeks to 12 years: 2 mg/kg 8-hourly.

The elderly: There is some evidence that elderly patients may be more susceptible to aminoglycoside toxicity whether secondary to previous eighth nerve impairment or borderline renal dysfunction. Accordingly, therapy should be closely monitored by frequent determination of gentamicin serum levels, assessment of renal function and signs of ototoxicity.

Gentamicin intrathecal injection: Bacterial meningitis and ventriculitis: the starting dose of gentamicin intrathecal injection for both children and adults is 1 mg daily, intrathecally or intraventricularly, together with 1 mg/kg every eight hours intramuscularly. The MIC of the infecting organism in the CSF should be assessed and, if necessary, the intrathecal/intraventricular dose increased to 5 mg daily, whilst keeping the intramuscular dose at 1 mg/kg eight-hourly. Treatment should be continued for at least seven days but longer if necessary. Periodic serum and CSF gentamicin assays should be carried out to ensure that adequate antibiotic levels are maintained and that serum and CSF levels do not exceed 10 mg/l.

Renal impairment: Gentamicin is excreted by simple glomerular filtration and therefore is given in reduced doses in cases of renal impairment. Nomograms are available for the calculation of dose, which depends on the patient's age, weight and renal function. The following table may be useful when treating adults.

Blood urea		*Creatinine clearance (GFR)*	*Dose and frequency of administration*
(mg/100 ml)	*(mmol/l)*	*(ml/min)*	
<40	6–7	>70	80 mg* 8-hourly
40–100	6–17	30–70	80 mg* 12-hourly
100–200	17–34	10–30	80 mg* daily
>200	>34	5–10	80 mg* every 48 hours
Twice-weekly intermittent haemodialysis		<5	80 mg* after dialysis

*60 mg if body weight <60 kg. Frequency of dosage in hours may also be approximated as serum creatinine (mg%)× eight or in SI units, as serum creatinine (micromol/l) divided by 11. If these dosage guides are used peak serum levels must be measured. Peak levels of gentamicin occur approximately one hour after intramuscular injection and intravenous injection. Trough levels are measured just prior to the next injection. Assay of peak serum levels gives confirmation of adequacy of dosage and also serves to detect levels above 10 mg/l, at which the possibility of ototoxicity should be considered. One-hour concentrations of gentamicin should not exceed 10 mg/l (but should reach 4 mg/l), while the pre-dose trough concentration should be less than 2 mg/l.

The recommended dose and precautions for intramuscular and intravenous administration are identical. Gentamicin when given intravenously should be injected directly into a vein or into the drip set tubing over no less than three minutes. If administered by infusion, this should be over no longer than 20 minutes and in no greater volume of fluid than 100 ml.

Contra-indications, warnings, etc.
Contra-indications: Hypersensitivity; myasthenia gravis.

Warnings: Ototoxicity has been recorded following the use of gentamicin. Groups at special risk include patients with impaired renal function and possibly the elderly. Consequently, renal, auditory and vestibular functions should be monitored in these patients and serum levels determined so as to avoid peak concentrations above 10 mg/l and troughs above 2 mg/l. As there is some evidence that risk of both ototoxicity and nephrotoxicity is related to the level of total exposure, duration of therapy should be the shortest possible compatible with clinical recovery. In some patients with impaired renal function there has been a transient rise in blood-urea-nitrogen which has usually reverted to normal during or following cessation of therapy. It is important to adjust the frequency of dosage according to the degree of renal function (see table).

Pregnancy and lactation: There are no proven cases of intrauterine damage caused by gentamicin. However, in common with most drugs known to cross the placenta, usage in pregnancy should only be considered in life-threatening situations where the expected benefits outweigh possible risks. In the absence of gastro-intestinal inflammation, the amount of gentamicin ingested from the milk is unlikely to result in significant blood levels in breast-fed infants.

Interaction with other substances: Concurrent administration of gentamicin and other potentially ototoxic or nephrotoxic drugs should be avoided. Potent diuretics such as ethacrynic acid and frusemide are believed to enhance the risk of ototoxicity whilst amphotericin B, cisplatin and cyclosporin are potential enhancers of nephrotoxicity. Any potential nephrotoxicity of cephalosporins, and in particular cephaloridine, may also be increased in the presence of gentamicin. Consequently, if this combination is used monitoring of kidney function is advised.

Neuromuscular blockade and respiratory paralysis have been reported from administration of aminoglycosides to patients who have received curare-type muscle relaxants during anaesthesia.

Overdosage: Haemodialysis and peritoneal dialysis will aid removal from blood but the former is probably more efficient. Calcium salts given intravenously have been used to counter the neuromuscular blockade caused by gentamicin.

Pharmaceutical precautions Cidomycin Paediatric Injectable: Store below 25°C. Do not refrigerate. Cidomycin Intrathecal injection: Store below 25°C. Gentamicin is a remarkably stable antibiotic and does not require refrigeration. Avoid freezing.

In general gentamicin injection should not be mixed. In particular the following are incompatible in mixed solution with gentamicin injection: penicillins, cephalosporins, erythromycin, heparins, sodium bicarbonate (Carbon dioxide may be liberated on addition of the two solutions. Normally this will dissolve in the solution but under some circumstances small bubbles may form). Dilution in the body will obviate the danger of physical and chemical incompatibility and enable gentamicin to be given concurrently with the drugs listed above either as a bolus injection into the drip tubing, with adequate flushing, or at separate sites. In the case of carbenicillin, administration should only be at a separate site.

Legal category POM.

Package quantities
Cidomycin Paediatric Injectable: Packs of 5×2 ml vials.

Cidomycin Intrathecal Injection: Packs of 5×1 ml ampoules.

Further information Cidomycin Paediatric Injectable contains methylhydroxybenzoate, propylhydroxybenzoate and disodium edetate. Cidomycin Intrathecal Injection contains sodium chloride.

Marketing authorisation numbers
Cidomycin Paediatric Injectable PL 0109/5066R
Cidomycin Intrathecal Injection PL 0109/0057R

Marketing authorisation holder: Roussel Laboratories Limited, Broadwater Park, Denham, Uxbridge, Middlesex UB9 5HP.

CLAFORAN*

Qualitative and quantitative composition
250 mg vial: Contains cefotaxime sodium PhEur equivalent to 250 mg cefotaxime base.

500 mg vial: Contains cefotaxime sodium PhEur equivalent to 500 mg cefotaxime base.
1 g vial: Contains cefotaxime sodium PhEur equivalent to 1 g cefotaxime base.
2 g vial: Contains cefotaxime sodium PhEur equivalent to 2 g cefotaxime base.
Each gram of Claforan contains approximately 48 mg (2.09 mmol) of sodium.

Pharmaceutical form Vials containing powder for injection or infusion. Claforan is supplied as a white to slightly creamy powder, which when dissolved in Water for Injections PhEur forms a straw-coloured solution suitable for IV or IM injection. Variations in the intensity of colour of the freshly prepared solution do not indicate a change in potency or safety.

Clinical particulars
Therapeutic indications: Properties: Claforan is a broad-spectrum bactericidal cephalosporin antibiotic. Claforan is exceptionally active in vitro against Gram-negative organisms sensitive or resistant to first or second generation cephalosporins. It is similar to other cephalosporins in activity against Gram-positive organisms.

Claforan is indicated in the treatment of the following infections either before the infecting organism has been identified or when caused by bacteria of established sensitivity.

Septicaemias

Respiratory tract infections such as acute and chronic bronchitis, bacterial pneumonia, infected bronchiectasis, lung abscess and post-operative chest infections.

Urinary tract infections such as acute and chronic pyelonephritis, cystitis and asymptomatic bacteriuria.

Soft-tissue infections: such as cellulitis, peritonitis and wound infections.

Bone and joint infections such as osteomyelitis, septic arthritis.

Obstetric and gynaecological infections such as pelvic inflammatory disease.

Gonorrhoea: particularly when penicillin has failed or is unsuitable.

Other bacterial infections: meningitis and other sensitive infections suitable for parenteral antibiotic therapy.

Prophylaxis: The administration of Claforan prophylactically may reduce the incidence of certain post-operative infections in patients undergoing surgical procedures that are classified as contaminated or potentially contaminated or in clean operations where infection would have serious effects.

Protection is best ensured by achieving adequate local tissue concentrations at the time contamination is likely to occur. Claforan should therefore be administered immediately prior to surgery and if necessary continued in the immediate post-operative period.

Administration should usually be stopped within 24 hours since continuing use of any antibiotic in the majority of surgical procedures does not reduce the incidence of subsequent infection.

Bacteriology: The following organisms have shown in vitro sensitivity to Claforan.

Gram positive: Staphylococci, including coagulase-positive, coagulase-negative and penicillinase-producing strains. β-haemolytic and other streptococci such as *Streptococcus mitis* (*viridans*) (many strains of enterococci, e.g. *Streptococcus faecalis*, are relatively resistant). *Streptococcus* (Diplococcus) *pneumoniae. Clostridium* spp.

Gram negative: *Escherichia coli, Haemophilus influenzae* including ampicillin resistant strains, *Klebsiella* spp, *Proteus* spp (both indole positive and indole negative), *Enterobacter* spp, *Neisseria* spp. (including β-lactamase producing strains of *N. gonorrhoeae), Salmonella* spp. (including *Sal. typhi*), *Shigella* spp, *Providencia* spp, *Serratia* spp, *Citrobacter* spp. Claforan has frequently exhibited useful in vitro activity against *Pseudomonas* and *Bacteroides* species although some strains of *Bacteroides fragilis* are resistant.

There is in vitro evidence of synergy between Claforan and aminoglycoside antibiotics such as gentamicin against some species of Gram-negative bacteria including some strains of *Pseudomonas*. No in vitro antagonism has been noted. In severe infections caused by *Pseudomonas* spp. the addition of an aminoglycoside antibiotic may be indicated.

Posology and method of administration: Dosage: Claforan may be administered intravenously, by bolus injection or infusion or intramuscularly. The dosage, route and frequency of administration should be determined by the severity of infection, the sensitivity of causative organisms and condition of the patient. Therapy may be initiated before the results of sensitivity tests are known.

Adults: The recommended dosage for mild to moderate infections is 1 g 12 hourly. However, dosage may be varied according to the severity of the infection, sensitivity of causative organisms and condition of the patient. Therapy may be initiated before the results of sensitivity tests are known.

In severe infections dosage may be increased up to 12 g daily given in 3 or 4 divided doses. For infections caused by sensitive *Pseudomonas* spp. daily doses of greater than 6 g will usually be required.

Children: The usual dosage range is 100-150 mg/kg/day in 2 to 4 divided doses. However, in very severe infections doses of up to 200 mg/kg/day may be required.

Neonates: The recommended dosage is 50 mg/kg/day in 2 to 4 divided doses. In severe infections 150-200 mg/kg/day, in divided doses, have been given.

Dosage in gonorrhoea: A single injection of 1 g may be administered intramuscularly or intravenously.

Dosage in renal impairment: Because of extra-renal elimination, it is only necessary to reduce the dosage of Claforan in severe renal failure (GFR < 5 ml/min = serum creatinine approximately 751 micromol/litre). After an initial loading dose of 1 g, daily dose should be halved without change in the frequency of dosing, i.e. 1 g 12 hourly becomes 0.5 g 12 hourly, 1 g 8 hourly becomes 0.5 g 8 hourly, 2 g 8 hourly becomes 1 g 8 hourly etc. As in all other patients, dosage may require further adjustment according to the course of the infection and the general condition of the patient.

Administration:

Intravenous and intramuscular administration: Reconstitute Claforan with Water for Injection PhEur as given in the Dilution Table. Shake well until dissolved and then withdraw the entire contents of the vial into the syringe and use immediately.

Dilution table:

Vial size	*Diluent to be added*
250 mg	2 ml
500 mg	2 ml
1 g	4 ml
2 g	10 ml

Intravenous infusion: Claforan may be administered by intravenous infusion. 1-2 g are dissolved in 40-100 ml of Water for Injection PhEur or in the infusion fluids listed under 'Pharmaceutical particulars'. The prepared infusion may be administered over 20-60 minutes. To produce an infusion using vials with an infusion connector, remove the safety cap and directly connect the infusion bag. The needle in the closure will automatically pierce the vial stopper. Pressing the infusion bag will transfer solvent in to the vial. Reconstitute by shaking the vial and finally, transfer the reconstituted solution back to the infusion bag ready for use.

Contra-indications: Known or suspected hypersensitivity to cephalosporins.

Special warnings and precautions for use: Preliminary enquiry about hypersensitivity to penicillin and other β-lactam antibiotics is necessary before prescribing cephalosporins since cross allergy occurs in 5-10% of cases.

Hypersensitivity reactions (anaphylaxis) occuring with the two types of antibiotics can be serious and occasionally fatal. Hypersensitivity requires that treatment be stopped.

Patients with severe renal dysfunction should be placed on the dosage schedule recommended under 'Posology and Method of Administration'.

As with other antibiotics, the use of Claforan, especially if prolonged, may result in overgrowth of non susceptible organisms, such as *Enterococcus* spp. Repeated evaluation of the condition of the patient is essential. If superinfection occurs during treatment with Claforan, specific antimicrobial therapy should be instituted if considered clinically necessary. Claforan constituted with lignocaine must never be used:

- By the intravenous route
- In infants under 30 months
- In subjects with a previous history of hypersensitivity to this product
- In patients who have an unpaced heart block
- In patients with severe heart failure

The sodium content of Claforan (2.09 mmol/gram) should be taken into account when prescribing to patients requiring sodium restriction.

Claforan may predispose patients to pseudomembranous colitis. Although any antibiotic may predispose to pseudomembranous colitis, the risk is higher with broad spectrum drugs, such as cephalosporins. This side effect, which may occur more frequently in patients receiving higher doses for prolonged periods, should be considered as potentially serious. The presence of *C. difficile* toxin should be investigated, and treatment with Claforan stopped in cases of suspected colitis. Diagnosis can be confirmed by toxin detection and specific antibiotic therapy (e.g. oral vancomycin or metronidazole) should be initiated if considered clinically necessary. The administration of products which cause faecal stasis should be avoided.

Interactions with other medicaments and other forms of interaction: Cephalosporin antibiotics at high dosage should be given with caution to patients receiving aminoglycoside antibiotics or potent diuretics such as frusemide as these combinations are suspected to adversely affect renal function. However, at the recommended doses, enhancement of nephrotoxicity is unlikely to be a problem with Claforan.

Probenecid interferes with renal tubular transfer of Claforan delaying its excretion and increasing the plasma concentration.

Interference with Laboratory Tests: A positive Coombs test may be seen during treatment with cephalosporins. This phenomenon may occur during treatment with cefotaxime.

A false positive reaction to glucose may occur with reducing substances but not with the use of specific glucose oxidase methods.

Pregnancy and lactation: Pregnancy: It is known that Claforan crosses the placental barrier. Although studies in animals have not shown an adverse effect on the developing foetus, the safety of Claforan in human pregnancy has not been established. Consequently, Claforan should not be administered during pregnancy especially during the first trimester, without carefully weighing the expected benefit against possible risks.

Lactation: Claforan is excreted in the milk.

Effects on ability to drive and use machines: There is no evidence that cefotaxime directly impairs the ability to drive or to operate machines.

Undesirable effects: Adverse reactions to Claforan have occurred relatively infrequently and have generally been mild and transient. Effects reported include candidiasis, nausea, vomiting, abdominal pain, diarrhoea (diarrhoea may sometimes be a symptom of pseudomembranous colitis (see warnings)), transient rises in liver transaminase, alkaline phosphatase and/or bilirubin.

As with other cephalosporins, changes in renal function have been rarely observed with high doses of Claforan, particularly when co-prescribed with aminoglycosides. Rare cases of interstitial nephritis have been reported in patients treated with Claforan. Administration of high doses of cephalosporins, particularly in patients with renal insufficiency may result in encephalopathy (e.g. impairment of consciousness, abnormal movements and convulsions).

Hypersensitivity reactions have been reported. These include skin rashes, pruritis and less frequently urticaria, drug fever and very rarely anaphylaxis (e.g. angioedema, bronchospasm possibly culminating in shock).

As with other cephalosporins, occasional cases of bullous reactions such as Stevens Johnson syndrome, toxic epidermal necrolysis and erythema multiforme have also been reported.

As with other β-lactam antibiotics, granulocytopenia and more rarely agranulocytosis may develop during treatment with Claforan, particularly if given over long periods. A few cases of eosinophilia and neutropenia have been observed, reversible when treatment is ceased. Some cases of rapidly reversible eosinophilia and thrombocytopenia on stopping treatment have been reported. Rare cases of haemolytic anaemia have been reported. For cases of treatment lasting longer than 10 days, blood count should, therefore, be monitored.

Transient pain may be experienced at the site of injection. This is more likely to occur with higher doses. Occasionally, phlebitis has been reported in patients receiving intravenous Claforan. However, this has rarely been a cause for discontinuation of treatment.

A very small number of cases of arrythmias have occurred following rapid bolus infusion through a central venous catheter.

The following symptoms have occurred after several weeks of treatment for Borreliosis (Lyme's Disease): skin rash, itching, fever, leucopenia, increases in liver enzymes, difficulty of breathing, joint discomfort. To some extent these manifestations are consistent with the symptoms of the underlying disease, for which the patient is being treated.

Overdose: Serum levels of Claforan may be reduced by peritoneal dialysis or haemodialysis. In the case of overdosage, particularly in renal insufficiency there is a risk of reversible encephalopathy.

Pharmacological properties
Pharmacodynamic properties: Claforan is a broad spectrum bactericidal cephalosporin antibiotic. Claforan is exceptionally active in vitro against Gram-negative organisms sensitive or resistant to first or second generation cephalosporins. It is similar to other cephalosporins in activity against Gram-positive bacteria.

Pharmacokinetic properties: After a 1000 mg intravenous bolus, mean peak plasma concentrations of cefotaxime usually range between 81 and 102 microgram/ml. Doses of 500 mg and 2000 mg produce plasma concentrations of 38 and 200 microgram/ml, respectively. There is no accumulation following administration of 1000 mg intravenously or 500 mg intramuscularly for 10 or 14 days.

The apparent volume of distribution at steady-state of cefotaxime is 21.6 litres/1.73 m² after 1 g intravenous 30 minute infusion.

Concentrations of cefotaxime (usually determined by non-selective assay) have been studied in a wide range of human body tissues and fluids. Cerebrospinal fluid concentrations are low when the meninges are not inflamed, but are between 3 and 30 microgram/ml in children with meningitis. Cefotaxime usually passes the blood-brain barrier in levels above the MIC of common sensitive pathogens when the meninges are inflamed. Concentrations (0.2-5.4 microgram/ml), inhibitory for most Gram-negative bacteria, are attained in purulent sputum, bronchial secretions and pleural fluid after doses of 1 or 2 g. Concentrations likely to be effective against most sensitive organisms are similarly attained in female reproductive organs, otitis media effusions, prostatic tissue, interstitial fluid, renal tissue, peritoneal fluid and gall bladder wall, after usual therapeutic doses. High concentrations of cefotaxime and desacetyl-cefotaxime are attained in bile.

Cefotaxime is partially metabolised prior to excretion. The principal metabolite is the microbiologically active product, desacetyl-cefotaxime. Most of a dose of cefotaxime is excreted in the urine about 60% as unchanged drug and a further 24% as desacetyl-cefotaxime. Plasma clearance is reported to be between 260 and 390 ml/minute and renal clearance 145 to 217 ml/minute.

After intravenous administration of cefotaxime to healthy adults, the elimination half-life of the parent compound is 0.9 to 1.14 hours and that of the desacetyl metabolite, about 1.3 hours.

In neonates the pharmacokinetics are influenced by gestational and chronological age, the half-life being prolonged in premature and low birth weight neonates of the same age.

In severe renal dysfunction the elimination half-life of cefotaxime itself is increased minimally to about 2.5 hours, whereas that of desacetyl-cefotaxime is increased to about 10 hours. Total urinary recovery of cefotaxime and its principal metabolite decreases with reduction in renal function.

Preclinical safety data: Not applicable.

Pharmaceutical particulars
List of excipients: None.

Incompatibilities: None stated.

Shelf life: Finished Product: 24 months. Reconstituted Solution: 24 hours.

Special precautions for storage: Finished Product: Store below 25°C. Protect from light.

Reconstituted Solution: Whilst it is preferable to use only freshly prepared solutions for both intravenous and intramuscular injection, Claforan is compatible with several commonly used intravenous infusion fluids and will retain satisfactory potency for up to 24 hours refrigerated in the following:
Water for Injections PhEur
Sodium Chloride Injection BP
5% Dextrose Injection BP
Dextrose and Sodium Chloride Injection BP
Compound Sodium Lactate Injection BP (Ringer-lactate Injection).

After 24 hours any unused solution should be discarded.

Claforan is also compatible with 1% lignocaine, however freshly prepared solutions should be used.

Claforan is also compatible with metronidazole infusion (500 mg/100 ml) and both will maintain potency when refrigerated (2–8°C) for up to 24 hours. Some increase in colour of prepared solutions may occur on storage. However, provided the recommended storage conditions are observed, this does not indicate change in potency or safety.

Nature and contents of container: Claforan is supplied in tubular or moulded glass vials PhEur, closed with a grey elastomer stopper and sealed with either an aluminium cap fitted with a detachable flip top, or an infusion connector closure.

The bottles are boxed individually and in packs of 10, 25 or 50.

Instruction for use/handling: Not applicable.

Marketing authorisation holder: Roussel Laboratories Ltd, Broadwater Park, Denham, Uxbridge, Middlesex UB9 5HP UK

Marketing authorisation number PL 0109/0074

Date of approval/revision of SPC February 1998

Legal category POM

CLOMID*

Qualitative and quantitative composition Clomiphene Citrate BP 50 mg

Pharmaceutical form Tablet.

Clinical particulars
Therapeutic indications: Indications: Clomid (Clomiphene Citrate BP) is indicated for the treatment of ovulatory failure in women desiring pregnancy. Clomid is indicated only for patients in whom ovulatory dysfunction is demonstrated. Other causes of infertility must be excluded or adequately treated before giving Clomid. Good levels of endogenous oestrogen (as estimated from vaginal smears, endometrial biopsy, assay of urinary oestrogen, or endometrial bleeding in response to progesterone) provide a favourable prognosis for ovulatory response induced by Clomid. A low level of oestrogen, although clinically less favourable, does not preclude successful outcome of therapy. Clomid therapy is ineffective in patients with primary pituitary or primary ovarian failure. Clomid therapy cannot be expected to substitute for specific treatment of other causes of ovulatory failure, such as thyroid or adrenal disorders. For hyperprolactinaemia there is other preferred specific treatment. Clomid is not first line treatment for low weight related amenorrhoea, with infertility, and has no value if a high FSH blood level is observed following an early menopause.

Route of administration: oral

Posology and method of administration:
Adults only: The recommended dose for the first course of Clomid (Clomiphene Citrate BP) is 50 mg (1 tablet) daily for 5 days. Therapy may be started at any time in the patient who has had no recent uterine bleeding. If progestin-induced bleeding is planned, or if spontaneous uterine bleeding occurs before therapy, the regimen of 50 mg daily for 5 days should be started on or about the fifth day of the cycle. When ovulation occurs at this dosage, there is no advantage to increasing the dose in subsequent cycles of treatment.

If ovulation appears not to have occurred after the first course of therapy, a second course of 100 mg daily (two 50 mg tablets given as a single daily dose) for 5 days should be given. This course may be started as early as 30 days after the previous one. *Increase of the dosage or duration of therapy beyond 100 mg/day for 5 days should not be undertaken.*

The majority of patients who are going to respond will respond to the first course of therapy, and 3 courses should constitute an adequate therapeutic trial. If ovulatory menses have not yet occurred, the diagnosis should be re-evaluated. Treatment beyond this is not recommended in the patient who does not exhibit evidence of ovulation.

Long-term cyclic therapy: Not recommended. The relative safety of long-term cyclic therapy has not been conclusively demonstrated and, since the majority of patients will ovulate following 3 courses, long-term cyclic therapy is not recommended, i.e. beyond a total of about 6 cycles (including 3 ovulatory cycles).

Contra-indications:
Pregnancy: See *Pregnancy and lactation.*

Liver disease: Clomid (Clomiphene Citrate BP) therapy is contra-indicated in patients with liver disease or a history of liver dysfunction.

Abnormal uterine bleeding: Clomid is contra-indicated in patients with hormone-dependent tumours or in patients with abnormal uterine bleeding of undetermined origin.

Ovarian cyst: Clomid should not be given in the presence of an ovarian cyst, except polycystic ovary, since further enlargement of the cyst may occur. Patients should be evaluated for the presence of ovarian cyst prior to each course of treatment.

Special warnings and special precautions for use:
Warnings:

Ovarian hyperstimulation syndrome: Ovarian hyperstimulation syndrome (OHSS) has been reported in patients receiving Clomid therapy for ovulation induction. In some cases, OHSS occurred following the cyclic use of Clomid therapy or when Clomid was used in combination with gonadotropins. The following symptoms have been reported in association with this syndrome during Clomid therapy: pericardial effusion, anasarca, hydrothorax, acute abdomen, renal failure, pulmonary oedema, ovarian haemorrhage, deep venous thrombosis, torsion of the ovary and acute respiratory distress. If conception results, rapid progression to the severe form of the syndrome may occur.

To minimise the hazard of the abnormal ovarian enlargement associated with Clomid therapy, the lowest dose consistent with expectation of good results should be used. The patient should be instructed to inform the physician of any abdominal or pelvic pain, weight gain, discomfort or distension after taking Clomid. Maximal enlargement of the ovary may not occur until several days after discontinuation of the course of Clomid. Some patients with polycystic ovary syndrome who are unusually sensitive to gonadotropin may have an exaggerated response to usual doses of Clomid.

The patient who complains of abdominal or pelvic pain, discomfort, or distension after taking Clomid should be examined because of the possible presence of an ovarian cyst or other cause. Due to fragility of enlarged ovaries in severe cases, abdominal and pelvic examination should be performed very cautiously. If abnormal enlargement occurs Clomid should not be given until the ovaries have returned to pre-treatment size. Ovarian enlargement and cyst formation associated with Clomid therapy usually regress spontaneously within a few days or weeks after discontinuing treatment. Most of these patients should be managed conservatively. The dosage and/or duration of the next course of treatment should be reduced.

Visual symptoms: Patients should be advised that blurring or other visual symptoms may occasionally occur during or shortly after therapy with Clomid. Patients should be warned that visual symptoms may render such activities as driving a car or operating machinery more hazardous than usual, particularly under conditions of variable lighting. The significance of these visual symptoms is not understood. If the patient has any visual symptoms, treatment should be discontinued and ophthalmologic evaluation performed.

Precautions:

Multiple pregnancy: There is an increased chance of multiple pregnancy when conception occurs in relationship to Clomid therapy. During the clinical investigation studies, the incidence of multiple pregnancy was 7.9% (186 of 2369 Clomid associated pregnancies on which outcome was reported). Among these 2369 pregnancies, 165 (6.9%) twin, 11 (0.5%) triplet, 7 (0.3%) quadruplet and 3 (0.13%) quintuplet. Of the 165 twin pregnancies for which sufficient information was available, the ratio of monozygotic twins was 1:5.

Ectopic pregnancy: There is an increased chance of ectopic pregnancy (including tubal and ovarian sites) in women who conceive following Clomid therapy. Ectopic pregnancy associated with Clomid involves a multiple pregnancy with coexisting extrauterine and intrauterine gestations.

Uterine fibroids: Caution should be exercised when using Clomid in patients with uterine fibroids due to potential for further enlargement of the fibroids.

Pregnancy wastage and birth anomalies: The overall incidence of reported birth anomalies from pregnancies associated with maternal Clomid ingestion (before or after conception) during the investigational studies was within the range of that reported in the published references for the general population. Among the birth anomalies spontaneously reported in the published literature as individual cases, the proportion of neural tube defects has been high among pregnancies associated with ovulation induced by Clomid, but this has not been supported by data from population based studies.

The physician should explain so that the patient understands the assumed risk of any pregnancy whether the ovulation was induced with the aid of Clomid or occurred naturally.

The patient should be informed of the greater pregnancy risks associated with certain characteristics or conditions of any pregnant woman: e.g. age of female and male partner, history of spontaneous abortions, Rh genotype, abnormal menstrual history, infertility history (regardless of cause), organic heart disease, diabetes, exposure to infectious agents such as rubella, familial history of birth anomaly, and other risk factors that may be pertinent to the patient for whom Clomid is being considered. Based upon the evaluation of the patient, genetic counselling may be indicated.

Population based reports have been published on possible elevation of risk of Down's Syndrome in ovulation induction cases and of increase in trisomy defects among spontaneously aborted foetuses from subfertile women receiving ovulation inducing drugs (no women with Clomid alone and without additional inducing drug). However, as yet, the reported observations are too few to confirm or not confirm the presence of an increased risk that would justify amniocentesis other than for the usual indications because of age and family history.

The experience from patients of all diagnoses during clinical investigation of Clomid shows a pregnancy (single and multiple) wastage or foetal loss rate of 21.4% (abortion rate of 19.0%), ectopic pregnancies, 1.18%, hydatiform mole, 0.17%, foetus papyraceous, 0.04% and of pregnancies with one or more stillbirths, 1.01%.

Clomid therapy after conception was reported for 158 of the 2369 delivered and reported pregnancies in the clinical investigations. Of these 158 pregnancies 8 infants (born of 7 pregnancies) were reported to have birth defects.

There was no difference in reported incidence of birth defects whether Clomid was given before the 19th day after conception or between the 20th and 35th day after conception. This incidence is within the anticipated range of general population.

Ovarian cancer: There have been rare reports of ovarian cancer with fertility drugs; infertility itself is a primary risk factor. Epidemiological data suggest that prolonged use of Clomid may increase this risk. Therefore the recommended duration of treatment should not be exceeded (see *Posology and method of administration*).

Interactions with other medicaments and other forms of interaction: None stated.

Pregnancy and lactation: Clomid is not indicated during pregnancy. Although there is no evidence that Clomid has a harmful effect on the human foetus, there is evidence that Clomid has a deleterious effect on rat and rabbit foetuses when given in high doses to the pregnant animal. To avoid inadvertent Clomid administration during early pregnancy, appropriate tests should be utilised during each treatment cycle to determine whether ovulation occurs. The patient should have a pregnancy test before the next course of Clomid therapy.

It is not known whether clomiphene citrate is excreted in human milk. Clomiphene may reduce lactation.

Effects on ability to drive and use machines: Patients should be warned that visual symptoms may render such activities as driving a car or operating machinery more hazardous than usual, particularly under conditions of variable lighting. (See *Special warnings and special precautions for use*).

Undesirable effects:
Symptoms/signs/conditions: Adverse effects appeared to be dose-related, occurring more frequently at the higher dose and with the longer courses of treatment used in investigational studies. At recommended dosage, adverse effects are not prominent and infrequently interfere with treatment.

During the investigational studies, the more common reported adverse effects included ovarian enlargement (13.6%), vasomotor flushes (10.4%), abdominal-pelvic discomfort (distension, bloating) (5.5%), nausea and vomiting (2.2%), breast discomfort (2.1%), visual symptoms (1.5%), headache (1.3%) and intermenstrual spotting or menorrhagia (1.3%).

Ovarian enlargement: At recommended dosage, abnormal ovarian enlargement is infrequent although the usual cyclic variation in ovarian size may be exaggerated. Similarly, cyclic ovarian pain (mittelschmerz) may be accentuated. With higher or prolonged dosage, more frequent ovarian enlargement and cyst formation may occur, and the luteal phase of the cycle may be prolonged.

Rare instances of massive ovarian enlargement are recorded. Such an instance has been described in a patient with polycystic ovary syndrome whose Clomid therapy consisted of 100 mg daily for 14 days. Abnormal ovarian enlargement usually regresses spontaneously; most of the patients with this condition should be treated conservatively.

Eye/visual symptoms: Symptoms described usually as "blurring" or spots or flashes (scintillating scotomata) increase in incidence with increasing total dose and usually disappear within periods ranging from a few days to a few weeks after Clomid is discontinued.

These symptoms appear to be due to intensification and prolongation of after-images. After-images as such have also been reported. Symptoms often first appear or are accentuated with exposure to a bright-light environment.

Ophthalmologically definable scotomata, phosphenes and reduced visual acuity have been reported. There are rare reports of cataracts and optic neuritis.

Genitourinary: There are reports of new cases of endometriosis and exacerbation of pre-existing endometriosis during Clomid therapy.

Multiple pregnancies, including simultaneous intrauterine and extrauterine pregnancies, have been reported.

Tumours/neoplasms: Isolated reports have been received on the occurrence of endocrine-related or dependent neoplasms or their aggravation. Ovarian cancer: See *Special warnings and special precautions for use.*

Central nervous system: Convulsions have been reported; patients with a history of seizures may be predisposed. In investigational patients, CNS symptoms/signs, conditions of dizziness, light-headedness/vertigo (0.9%), nervous tension/insomnia (0.8%) and fatigue/depression (0.7%) were reported. After prescription availability, there were isolated additional reports of these conditions and also reports of other conditions such as syncope/fainting, cerebrovascular accident, cerebral thrombosis, psychotic reactions including paranoid psychosis, neurologic impairment, disorientation and speech disturbance.

Dermatoses: Dermatitis and rash were reported by investigational patients. Conditions such as rash and urticaria were the most common ones reported after prescription availability but also reported were conditions such as allergic reaction, erythema multiforme, ecchymosis and angioneurotic oedema. Hair thinning has been reported very rarely.

Liver function: Bromsulphalein (BSP) retention of greater than 5% was reported in 32 of 141 patients in whom it was measured, including 5 of 43 patients who took approximately the dose of Clomid now recommended. Retention was usually minimal unless associated with prolonged continuous Clomid administration or with apparently unrelated liver disease. Other liver function tests were usually normal. In a later study in which patients were given 6 consecutive monthly courses of Clomid (50 or 100 mg daily for 3 days) or matching placebo, BSP tests were done on 94 patients. Values in excess of 5% retention were recorded in 11 patients, 6 of whom had taken drug and 5 placebo.

In a separate report, one patient taking 50 mg of Clomid daily developed jaundice on the 19th day of treatment; liver biopsy revealed bile stasis without evidence of hepatitis.

Overdose: Toxic effects of acute overdosage of Clomid have not been reported but the number of overdose cases recorded is small. In the event of overdose, appropriate supportive measures should be employed.

Pharmacological properties
Pharmacodynamic properties: Clomid is a triarylethylene compound (related to chlorotrianisene and triparanol). It is a non-steroidal agent which stimulates ovulation in a high percentage of appropriately selected anovulatory women.

Pharmacokinetic properties: Orally administered ^{14}C labelled clomiphene citrate was readily absorbed when administered to humans. Cumulative excretion of the ^{14}C label by way of urine and faeces averaged about 50% of the oral dose after 5 days in 6 subjects, with mean urinary excretion of 7.8% and mean faecal excretion of 42.4%. A mean rate of excretion of 0.73% per day of the ^{14}C dose after 31 days to 35 days and 0.45% per day of the ^{14}C dose after 42 days to 45 days was seen in faecal and urine samples collected from 6 subjects for 14 to 53 days after clomiphene citrate ^{14}C administration. The remaining drug/metabolites may be slowly excreted from a sequestered enterohepatic recirculation pool.

Animal safety studies: None stated.

Pharmaceutical particulars
List of excipients: Sucrose PhEur, Lactose PhEur, Soluble starch HSE, Maize starch PhEur, Magnesium stearate PhEur, Iron oxide yellow E172 HSE, Purified Water BP

Incompatibilities: Not applicable.

Shelf-life: 5 years.

Special precautions for storage: Protect from light, moisture and excessive heat.

Nature and contents of container: Blister pack: Base: 250 micron PVC; Foil: 20 micron hard-tempered aluminium (in cardboard cartons). Pack sizes: 30 and 100 tablets.

Instructions for use/handling: None.

Marketing authorisation holder: Marion Merrell Ltd, Broadwater Park, Denham, Uxbridge, Middlesex, UB9 5HP

Marketing authorisation number PL 04425/5900

Date of approval/revision of SPC September 1997

Legal category POM

DAONIL* TABLETS
SEMI-DAONIL* TABLETS

Presentation Daonil Tablets each contain 5 mg Glibenclamide BP. Daonil is presented as white oblong tablets, scored in the middle, one half bearing the Hoechst insignia, the other bearing the letters LDI. The tablet is 10 mm in length and 5 mm wide.

Semi-Daonil Tablets each contain 2.5 mg Glibenclamide BP. Semi-Daonil is presented as white circular biplanar tablets, 6 mm in diameter, one side bearing the Hoechst insignia, the other scored and bearing the letters LBG on either side of the score mark.

Excipients include lactose.

Uses Daonil is a hypoglycaemic agent, indicated for the oral treatment of patients with non-insulin dependent diabetes who respond inadequately to dietary measures alone.

Dosage and administration
1. *Treatment of previously untreated diabetics:* Stabilisation can be started with one 5 mg tablet of Daonil daily. The dose should be taken by mouth, with or immediately after breakfast or the first main meal. Where control is satisfactory, 1 tablet is continued as the maintenance dose. If control is unsatisfactory, the dose can be adjusted by increments of 2.5 or 5 mg at weekly intervals. The total daily dosage rarely exceeds 15 mg and increasing the daily dosage above this does not generally produce any additional effect. The total daily requirement should normally be administered as a single dose at breakfast, or with the first main meal; due consideration should be given to the patient's dietary habits and daily activity in apportioning the dosage.

Elderly: In debilitated or aged patients, who may be more liable to hypoglycaemia, treatment should be initiated with one Semi-Daonil tablet daily.

2. *Change-over from other oral anti-diabetics:* The change over to Daonil from other drugs with a similar mode of action can be carried out without any break in therapy. Daonil treatment should be started with one 5 mg tablet daily and adjusted by increments of 2.5-5 mg to achieve control. For patients not adequately controlled on other oral agents, treatment is commenced with the equivalent dose of Daonil, without exceeding an initial dose of 10 mg. If response is inadequate, the dose can be raised in a stepwise fashion to 15 mg daily. One 5 mg tablet of Daonil is approximately equivalent to 1 g tolbutamide or glymidine, 250 mg chlorpropamide or tolazamide, 500 mg acetohexamide, 25 mg glibornuride or 5 mg glipizide.

3. *Change-over from biguanides:* Daonil treatment should be started with 1 tablet of Semi-Daonil (2.5 mg) and the biguanide withdrawn. The dosage should then be adjusted by increments of 2.5 mg to achieve control.

Combination with biguanides: If adequate control is not possible with diet and 15 mg of Daonil, control can often be re-established by combined administration of Daonil and a biguanide derivative.

4. *Change-over from insulin:* While it is appreciated that most patients who are on insulin therapy will continue to need it, there may be a few patients, particularly those on low daily doses, who will remain stabilised if transferred from insulin to Daonil.

The tablets should always be taken with, or immediately after, the first main meal.

Children: As non-insulin dependent diabetes is not usually a disease of childhood, Daonil is not recommended for use in children.

Contra-indications, warnings, etc
Contra-indications: Daonil should not be used in patients who have or have ever had diabetic ketoacidosis or diabetic/coma pre-coma or in patients who have insulin-dependant diabetes mellitus, serious impairment of renal, hepatic or adrenocortical function, in patients who are hypersensitive to glibenclamide, or in circumstances of unusual stress, e.g. surgical operations or during pregnancy, when dietary measures and insulin are essential.

Warnings: The hypoglycaemic effect of glibenclamide may be enhanced by ACE inhibitors, anabolic steroids, beta-adrenergic blocking agents, benzafibrate, chloramphenicol, clofibrate, coumarin derivatives, cyclophosphamide, disopyramide, fenfluramine, fluoxetine, guanethidine, MAO inhibitors, miconazole, phenylbutazone, probenecid, quinolone antibacterials, salicylates, sulphinpyrazone, sulphonamides and tetracycline compounds or diminished by clonidine, corticosteroids, diazoxide, diuretics, glucagon, laxative abuse, nicotinic acid (high dose), oral contraceptives, phenothiazine derivatives, phenytoin, sympathomimetic agents and thyroid hormones.

Both a potentiation and a reduction in the blood sugar-lowering effect have been reported in patients treated concomitantly with clonidine or H2 receptor antagonists.

The warning symptoms of a hypoglycaemic attack may be masked during concomitant treatment with beta-adrenergic blocking agents, clonidine or guanethidine.

There is no information on the use of Daonil in human pregnancy but it has been in wide, general use for many years without apparent ill consequence. Animal studies have shown no hazard.

Nursing mothers: It has not yet been established whether glibenclamide is transferred to human milk. However, other sulphonylureas have been found in milk and there is no evidence to suggest that glibenclamide differs from the group in this respect.

Overdosage: Hypoglycaemia may be treated in the conscious patient by the administration of glucose, or three to four lumps of table sugar with water. This may be repeated as necessary.

If the patient is comatose, glucose should be administered as an intravenous infusion and the patient monitored. Bolus glucose injections are not recommended because of the possibility of rebound hypoglycaemia which may be delayed. Alternatively, glucagon may be administered in a dose of 1 mg subcutaneously or intramuscularly to restore consciousness.

Side-effects: Adverse reactions serious enough to warrant discontinuation of treatment are uncommon, but mild gastro-intestinal or allergic skin reactions have occurred. Cross sensitivity to sulphonamides or their derivatives may occur. Transient visual disturbances may occur at the start of treatment. Reversible leucopenia and thrombocytopenia have been reported but are rare. Agranulocytosis, pancytopenia and haemolytic anaemia have been reported very rarely. Treatment with sulphonylureas has been associated with occasional disturbances of liver function and cholestatic jaundice. If hepatitis or cholestatic jaundice occurs, glibenclamide should be discontinued. Hypoglycaemic symptoms have occasionally been reported when the dose has been administered without due regard to the patient's dietary habits.

Pharmaceutical precautions Daonil Tablets should be stored below 25°C in a dry place protected from light and in containers similar to those of the manufacturer.

Legal category POM.

Package quantities Daonil and Semi-Daonil Tablets are available in blister (calendar) packs of 28 (OP).

Further information Orally administered Daonil is rapidly absorbed. It is substantially metabolised prior to its excretion in urine and bile. Some of the metabolites have hypoglycaemic activity, markedly reduced in comparison with the parent compound and usually without clinical significance.

Maketing authorisation numbers
Daonil Tablets 5 mg PL 13402/0027
Semi-Daonil Tablets 2.5 mg PL 13402/0028.

Date of approval/revision of SPC September 1997

EUGLUCON*

Qualitative and quantitative composition Each Euglucon tablet contains: either 2.5 mg or 5 mg of Glibenclamide.

Pharmaceutical form Tablets for oral use.

Clinical particulars

Therapeutic indications: Euglucon is indicated for the treatment of maturity-onset diabetes which is not adequately controlled by dietary measures alone.

Posology and method of administration:

Adults and the elderly: Euglucon should be taken with or immediately after food. The total daily dosage is preferably given as a single dose at breakfast or with the first main meal, but due consideration should be given to the patient's meal habits and daily activity when apportioning dosage.

New diabetics: In maturity-onset diabetes of mild to moderate severity, treatment should be started with 5 mg daily or 2.5 mg in debilitated or elderly patients. If this dosage is not sufficient for proper control it should be increased by 2.5 mg at intervals of one week or as directed by the clinician. The total daily dose of Euglucon rarely exceeds 15 mg. Increasing dosage beyond this point is unlikely to produce further response.

Transfer from other sulphonylureas: Transfer to Euglucon can usually be carried out without any break in therapy. Euglucon treatment should be started with 5 mg daily and, if necessary, adjusted in steps of 2.5 mg or 5 mg. For patients not adequately controlled on other oral agents, treatment is commenced with the equivalent dose of Euglucon. Without exceeding an initial dose of 10 mg the dose can be raised in a stepwise fashion to 15 mg daily. A dose of 5 mg Euglucon is approximately equivalent to 1000 mg tolbutamide or glymidine, 250 mg chlorpropamide or tolazamide, 500 mg acetohexamide, 25 mg glibornuride or 5 mg glipizide.

Change-over from biguanides: Euglucon treatment should be started with 2.5 mg of Euglucon and the biguanide withdrawn. The dosage should then be adjusted by increments of 2.5 mg to achieve control.

Combination with biguanides: If adequate control is not possible with diet and 15 mg of Euglucon, control can often be re-established by combination of Euglucon and a biguanide derivative.

Euglucon and insulin: While it is appreciated that most patients who are on insulin therapy will continue to need it, there may be a few patients, particularly those on low daily dosages, who will remain stabilised if transferred to Euglucon.

As non insulin dependant diabetes is not usually a disease of childhood, Euglucon is not recommended for use in children.

Contra-indications: Euglucon is contra-indicated in:

1. The treatment of insulin dependent diabetes mellitus.
2. Patients who have had serious metabolic decompensation with ketosis and, in particular, in diabetic pre-coma and coma.
3. Serious impairment of renal, hepatic, thyroid or adrenocortical function.
4. Unusual stress e.g. surgical operations or during pregnancy when dietary measures and insulin are essential. After pregnancy Euglucon therapy can be started or resumed.
5. Hypersensitivity to Glibenclamide.

Special warnings and precautions for use: Both a potentiation and a reduction in the blood sugar-lowering effect have been reported in patients treated concomitantly with clonidine or H2-receptor antagonists.

The warning symptoms of a hypoglycaemic attack may be masked during concomitant treatment with beta adrenergic blocking agents, clonidine or guanethidine.

Interactions with other medicaments and other forms of interaction: The hypoglycaemic action of oral antidiabetic agents including Euglucon may be enhanced by ACE-Inhibitors, anabolic steroids, beta-blocking agents, benzafibrate, chloramphenicol, clofibrate, coumarin derivatives, cyclophosphamide, disopyramide, fenfluramine, fluoxetine, guanethidine, mono-amine oxidase inhibitors, miconazole, phenylbutazone, probenicid, quinolone antibiotics, salicylates, sulphinpyrazone, sulphonamides, tetracyclines. Conversely, clonidine, corticosteroids, diazoxide, ethacrynic acid, frusemide, glucagon, laxative abuse, nicotinic acid (high dosage), oral contraceptives containing oestrogens/gestagens, phenothiazine derivatives, phenytoin, sympathomimetics, thiazide diuretics, thyroid hormones may diminish hypoglycaemic activity. Hypoglycaemic activity may also be affected by tuberculostatics.

In patients suffering from intercurrent infections or trauma, the dosage of Euglucon may need to be increased. If such complications are severe, diabetic control may be lost necessitating withdrawal of Euglucon and maintenance of diabetic control with insulin. Euglucon should be re-introduced when the patient has recovered from the infection or trauma.

Pregnancy and lactation: Pregnancy: There is no information on the use of Euglucon in human pregnancy but it has been in wide, general use for many years without apparent ill consequence. Animal studies have shown no hazard.

Nursing mothers: It has not been established whether glibenclamide is excreted in human milk. Other sulphonylureas have been found in milk. There is no evidence that glibenclamide differs from the group in this respect.

Effects on ability to drive and to use machines: Patients should be warned about the possible adverse effects of hypoglycaemia. Alertness and reactions may be impaired by hypoglycaemic or hyperglycaemic episodes, especially when beginning or after treatment or when Euglucon is not taken regularly. This may affect the ability to drive or operate machinery.

Undesirable effects (frequency and seriousness): Euglucon is well tolerated and side effects serious enough to necessitate withdrawal are uncommon. Gastro-intestinal symptoms (nausea, anorexia and diarrhoea) are uncommon and allergic skin reactions are seldom encountered. Cross sensitivity to sulphonamides and their derivatives may occur. Transient visual disturbances may occur at the start of treatment.

Reversible leucopenia and thrombocytopenia have been reported but are rare. Agranulocytosis, pancytopenia and haemolytic anaemia have been reported very rarely. Treatment with sulphonylureas has been associated with occasional disturbances of liver function and cholestatic jaundice. If hepatitis or cholestatic jaundice occurs, glibenclamide should be discontinued. As with other agents, hypoglycaemia can occur with Euglucon, but is not usually prolonged and responds to appropriate therapeutic measures.

Overdose: If a hypoglycaemic reaction should occur, the conscious patient may be treated with dextrose or 3–4 lumps of table sugar with water. This may be repeated, if necessary, in 15 minutes.

If the patient is comatose, glucose should be administered as an intravenous infusion and the patient monitored. Alternatively, sucrose or dextrose may be given by a stomach tube or dextrose given intravenously. Bolus glucose injections are not recommended because of the possibility of rebound hypoglycaemia which may be delayed. Glucagon may be administered in a dose of 1 mg subcutaneously or intramuscularly to regain consciousness.

Pharmacological properties

Pharmacodynamic properties: Euglucon is an oral hypoglycaemic agent of the sulphonylurea type.

Pharmacokinetic properties: Absorption studies in healthy human volunteers using labelled glibenclamide formulated as Euglucon tablets showed a mean absorption of 84 plus or minus 9%.

The half-life is about 10 hours

Excretion was approximately 50% in the urine and 50% in the faeces. Absorbed glibenclamide was completely metabolised and the three isolated metabolites in the concentrations found had no significant hypoglycaemic activity.

Pharmaceutical particulars

List of excipients: The product contains: Lactose, Maize Starch, Aerosil, (Colloidal Silicon Dioxide), Talc, Magnesium Stearate, Purified Water

Incompatibilities: None

Shelf-life: 60 Months

Special precautions for storage: Store below 25°C.

Nature and contents of container: Euglucon 2.5 mg and 5 mg tablets are supplied in blister packs of 28 and 100.

Instructions for use/handling: None.

Marketing authorisation numbers
Euglucon 2.5 mg PL 13402/0058
Euglucon 5 mg PL 13402/0059

Date of approval/revision of SPC January 1998

Legal category POM

FERTIRAL*

Presentation Fertiral contains Gonadorelin BP (luteinising hormone releasing hormone) 500 micrograms in 1 ml aqueous solution presented as a 2 ml ampoule containing 1000 micrograms. The solution also contains sodium chloride, sodium dihydrogen phosphate and benzyl alcohol as excipients.

Uses Amenorrhoea and infertility associated with:

1. Hypogonadotrophic hypogonadism.
2. Multifollicular ovaries: where this finding implies that pulse frequency and amplitude of endogenous LHRH are abnormal, e.g. in patients in whom weight related amenorrhoea has been corrected.

Dosage and administration Gonadorelin is given by means of an intermittent pulsatile pump, a pulse being delivered every 90 minutes over the entire 24 hour period. Treatment should be initiated by subcutaneous infusion but in some patients intravenous therapy may be required. Dosage should be determined individually but a starting dose of 10–20 micrograms given over 1 minute every 90 minutes is recommended. Treatment should be continued until conception occurs, or for a maximum of 6 months. Ultrasound of ovary or oestradiol or urinary oestrogen levels or basal body temperature measurements may be used to monitor treatment. (*See also Pharmaceutical Precautions*).

Contra-indications, warnings, etc Gonadorelin should not be used in patients with endometriotic cysts or polycystic disease of the ovaries. Treatment with gonadorelin should not be started in women with weight related amenorrhoea until the weight has been corrected and the ponderal index is above 19.5. Gonadorelin may be discontinued once evidence of conception has been obtained. Pituitary adenoma is a relative contra-indication because in isolated cases haemorrhagic infarction with symptoms of neurologic deficiency has been observed.

Side-effects: Side-effects are very rare. Skin rashes have been reported at the infusion site. The following reactions have been reported after treatment with the high dose diagnostic preparation of gonadorelin: Abdominal pain, nausea, headache and increased menstrual bleeding.

Overdosage: Treatment of overdose should be symptomatic.

Pharmaceutical precautions Gonadorelin should be infused using a pulsatile pump e.g. Graseby MS 27 with an infusion set of minimum volume e.g. Butterfly 25 or Butterfly 19 cannulae (Abbott). For intravenous administration heparin is added to the gonadorelin solution at a concentration of 150 IU/ml.

Store below 25°C. Use normal saline to dilute if necessary; use immediately after dilution. The solution is stable in the pump, at about body temperature, for 4 days.

Fertiral contains benzyl alcohol 1% as a preservative.

Legal category POM.

Package quantities Fertiral is available in packs of 5×2 ml ampoules.

Further information Results from clinical studies show a rate of multiple pregnancy very similar to that of the normal population.

Product licence number 13402/0029

FRISIUM*

Qualitative and quantitative composition Clobazam 10 mg

Pharmaceutical form Tablet

Clinical particulars
Therapeutic indications: Frisium is a 1,5–benzodiazepine indicated for the short-term relief (2–4 weeks) only of anxiety that is severe, disabling or subjecting the individual to unacceptable distress, occurring alone or in association with insomnia or short-term psychosomatic, organic or psychotic illness. The use of Frisium to treat short-term "mild" anxiety is inappropriate and unsuitable. Frisium may be used as adjunctive therapy in epilepsy.

Posology and method of administration: The usual anxiolytic dose for adults is 20–30 mg daily in divided doses or as a single dose given at night. Doses of up to 60 mg daily have been used in the treatment of adult in-patients with severe anxiety.

The lowest dose that can control symptoms should be used. It should not be used for longer than 4 weeks. Long term chronic use as an anxiolytic is not recommended. Treatment should always be withdrawn gradually. Patients who have taken Frisium for a long time may require a longer period during which doses are reduced.

Epilepsy: In epilepsy a starting dose of 20–30 mg/day is recommended, increasing as necessary up to a maximum of 60 mg daily. A break in therapy may be beneficial if drug exhaustion develops, recommencing therapy at a low dose.

Elderly: Doses of 10–20 mg daily in anxiety may be used in the elderly, who are more sensitive to the effects of psychoactive agents.

Children: When prescribed for children over three years of age, dosage should not exceed half the recommended adult dose. There is insufficient experience of the use of Frisium in children under three years of age to enable any dosage recommendation to be made.

Benzodiazepines should be used in reduced doses in patients with impaired renal or hepatic function.

Contra-indications: Frisium should not be used in patients known to be hypersensitive to benzodiazepines, or any of the excipients or in patients with a history of drug dependence.

Frisium should not be used in phobic and obsessional states or for the treatment of chronic psychosis. It should not be used alone to treat depression or anxiety associated with depression as suicide may be precipitated in such patients.

Special warnings and special precautions for use: Amnesia may occur with benzodiazepines. In cases of loss or bereavement psychological adjustment may be inhibited by benzodiazepines.

Special caution is necessary if Frisium is used in patients with myasthenia gravis, spinal or cerebellar ataxia or sleep apnoea.

Disinhibiting effects may be manifested in various ways. Suicide may be precipitated in patients who are depressed and aggressive behaviour towards self and others may be precipitated. Extreme caution should therefore be used in prescribing benzodiazepines in patients with personality disorders.

Withdrawal from benzodiazepines may be associated with physiological and psychological symptoms. Withdrawal symptoms occur with benzodiazepines following normal therapeutic doses given for short periods of time.

Respiratory function should be monitored in patients with acute severe respiratory insufficiency.

Interactions with other medicaments and other forms of interaction: Frisium is a benzodiazepine derivative and, in common with other members of this group, may potentiate the effects of central nervous system depressant drugs, such as alcohol, analgesics, hypnotics and neuroleptics.

Addition of Frisium to established anticonvulsant medication may cause a change in plasma levels of these drugs. If used as an adjuvant in epilepsy the dosage of Frisium should be determined by monitoring the EEG and the plasma levels of the drugs checked.

The effects of muscle relaxants, analgesics and nitrous oxide may be enhanced.

Concurrent treatment with drugs that inhibit the mono-oxygenase system (e.g. cimetidine) may enhance the effect of clobazam.

Pregnancy and lactation: If the product is prescribed to a woman of childbearing potential, she should be warned to contact her physician regarding discontinuation of the product if she intends to become pregnant or suspects that she is pregnant.

If, for compelling medical reasons, the product is administered during the late phase of pregnancy, or during labour at high doses, effects on the neonate such as hypothermia, hypotonia and moderate respiratory depression, can be expected due to the pharmacological action of the compound.

Moreover, infants born to mothers who took benzodiazepines during the latter stage of pregnancy may have developed physical dependence and may be at some risk for developing withdrawal symptoms in the postnatal period.

Since benzodiazepines are found in the breast milk, benzodiazepines should not be given to breast feeding mothers.

Effects on ability to drive and use machines: The ability to drive or operate machinery may be impaired in individuals who are particularly sensitive to the effects of Frisium or in patients taking high doses.

Undesirable effects: Side-effects such as drowsiness, dizziness or dryness of the mouth, constipation, loss of appetite, nausea, or a fine tremor of the fingers have been reported. These are more likely to occur at the beginning of treatment and often disappear with continued treatment or a reduction in dose. Paradoxical reactions, such as restlessness, irritability or difficulty in sleeping, may occur. Isolated cases of skin reactions, such as rashes or urticaria, have been observed.

Slowing of reaction time, ataxia, confusion and headaches may occasionally occur.

After prolonged use of benzodiazepines, impairment of consciousness, sometimes combined with respiratory disorders, has been reported in very rare cases, particularly in elderly patients: it sometimes persists for some length of time. These disorders have not been seen so far under clobazam treatment.

When used as an adjuvant in the treatment of epilepsy, this preparation may in rare cases cause restlessness and muscle weakness.

As with other benzodiazepines, the therapeutic benefit must be balanced against the risk of habituation and dependence during prolonged use.

Overdose: Muscle weakness, ataxia, drowsiness and sedation may occur and, after very high doses, the patient may lose consciousness. The treatment of overdosage is symptomatic. The stomach should be emptied as soon as possible by gastric lavage and general supportive measures should be undertaken as necessary. Consideration should be given to the use of flumazenil as a benzodiazepine antagonist. Forced diuresis or haemodialysis are ineffective.

Pharmacological properties
Pharmacodynamic properties: Clobazam is a 1,5-benzodiazepine. In single doses up to 20 mg or in divided doses up to 30 mg, clobazam does not affect psychomotor function, skilled performance, memory or higher mental functions.

Pharmacokinetic properties: Absorption of clobazam is virtually complete after oral administration. Approximately 85% is protein bound in man. It is metabolised by demethylation and hydroxylation. It is excreted unchanged and as metabolites in the urine (87%) and faeces.

Preclinical safety data: None applicable

Pharmaceutical particulars
List of excipients: Lactose monohydrate, maize starch, colloidal silicon dioxide, talc, magnesium stearate.

Incompatibilities: None

Shelf life: Five years

Special precautions for storage: Store below 25°C

Nature and contents of container: Blister pack (Alufoil/PVC) containing 30 tablets

Instruction for use/handling: None

Marketing authorisation number PL 13402/0030

Date of approval/revison of SPC August 1998

Legal Category POM

HAEMACCEL* INFUSION SOLUTION

Qualitative and quantitative composition Haemaccel contains 35 g Polygeline as active ingredient in 1000 ml.

Pharmaceutical form Solution for infusion

Clinical particulars
Therapeutic indications:

1. As a plasma volume substitute in the initial treatment of hypovolaemic shock due to:
   (a) Haemorrhage (visible or concealed)
   (b) Burns, peritonitis, pancreatitis, crush injuries
2. Fluid replacement in plasma exchange
3. Extra-corporeal circulation
4. Isolated organ perfusion
5. As a carrier solution for insulin.

Posology and method of administration: Route of Administration: Intravenous infusion.

Haemaccel should be administered intravenously in a volume approximately equal to the estimated blood loss.

See 'Instructions for Use/Handling' section under 'Pharmaceutical particulars'.

Infusion rate: The rate of infusion is determined by the condition of the patient. Normally, 500 ml will be infused in not less than 60 minutes but, in emergencies, Haemaccel can be rapidly infused. Losses of up to 25% of the blood volume can be replaced by Haemaccel alone.

Hypovolaemic shock: 500-1,000 ml Haemaccel should be infused intravenously initially. Up to 1,500 ml blood loss can be replaced entirely by Haemaccel. For between 1,500 ml and 4,000 ml blood loss, fluid replacement should be with equal volumes of Haemaccel and blood, given separately (see Pharmaceutical precautions). For losses over 4,000 ml, the separate infusion should be in the ratio of two parts blood to one part Haemaccel. The Haematocrit should not be allowed to fall below 25%.

Burns: It is suggested that at least 1 ml Haemaccel be infused per kg of body weight. Multiplied by the % of body surface burned for each 24 hours for two days, e.g. if a 70 kg person has burns covering 10% of body surface, then the dosage of Haemaccel should be at least 1 (ml) x 70 (kg) x 10 (%) = 700 ml/24 hours. Additional crystalloid solutions should be given to cover the normal fluid loss, i.e. about 2,000 ml per 24 hours. In severe burns, additional protein and vitamin therapy may be required. The volume of colloid and crystalloid given should be varied according to the clinical response of the patient, the urine volume, its specific gravity and osmolality etc.

Plasma exchange: Haemaccel should be given either alone or in combination with other replacement fluids in a volume adequate to replace the plasma removed. Up to 2 litres have been given as sole replacement fluid.

Contra-indications: Haemaccel is contra-indicated in patients with a known hypersensitivity to constituents of the preparation and/or patients with existing anaphylactoid reactions.

Special warnings and precautions for use: In the following cases, Haemaccel is indicated to a restricted extent only; if the physician considers the infusion necessary, it should be given taking special precautions.

All conditions in which an increase in intravascular volume and its consequences (e.g. increased stroke volume, elevated blood pressure), or an increase in interstitial fluid volume, or haemodilution could represent a special risk for the patient. Examples of such conditions are: congestive heart failure, hypertension, oesophageal varices, pulmonary oedema, haemorrhagic diathesis, renal and post-renal anuria.

In all patients at an increased risk of histamine release (e.g. allergic persons and patients with a history of histamine response; also patients who in the previous 7 days have received a drug which releases histamine). In the latter cases, Haemaccel may be given only after taking appropriate prophylactic steps. Reactions caused by histamine release can be avoided by the prophylactic use of H_1 and H_2 receptor antagonists.

Inappropriate rapid administration of Haemaccel, especially to normovolaemic patients may cause the release of vasoactive substances. The exact mechanism of this histamine release has not been clearly defined.

Interactions with other medicaments and other forms of interaction: Haemaccel contains calcium ions and caution should be observed in patients being treated with cardiac glycosides.

Haemaccel may be mixed with other infusion solutions (e.g. saline, dextrose, Ringer's solution etc.) or with heparinised blood. Sterility must be maintained. Compatible water-soluble drugs may be infused in Haemaccel, e.g. insulin, streptokinase etc. Any additive should be injected into the bottle through a small hole located next to the pull-ring.

Pregnancy and lactation: Haemorrhage around the time of childbirth or blood loss during other obstetric or gynaecological procedures may necessitate plasma volume replacement. Haemaccel has been used for many years for the initial treatment in such cases without apparent ill consequence. If plasma volume replacement is needed during pregnancy, Haemaccel may be used if blood is not available.

Effects on ability to drive and use machines: Not applicable.

Undesirable effects: During or after the infusion of volume-expanding solutions, transient urticarial skin reactions (wheals), hypotension, tachycardia, bradycardia, nausea/vomiting, dyspnoea, increases in temperature and/or shivering may occasionally occur.

Rare cases of severe hypersensitivity reactions including shock have been observed. Treatment will depend on the nature and severity of the reaction.

Mild reactions: administer corticosteroids and antihistamines.

In the event of anaphylactic shock, the infusion should be discontinued and adrenalin (5-10 ml of 1:10,000 by slow i.v. injection or 0.5-1.0 ml of 1:1,000 by i.m./s.c. injection) should immediately be given. Administration of adrenalin should be repeated every 15 minutes until improvement occurs. Circulatory collapse requires volume replacement, preferably monitored by a central venous pressure line. Large volumes of electrolyte solution may be necessary because, in severe anaphylactic shock, plasma loss may constitute up to 40% of the plasma volume. A slow i.v. injection of an H_1 antagonist such as 10-20 mg chlorpheniramine may be given.

Histamine release has been shown to be a cause of anaphylactic side-effects associated with infusions of Haemaccel.

These reactions may occur as a result of the cumulative effect of several histamine-releasing drugs (e.g. anaesthetics, muscle relaxants, analgesics, ganglia blockers and anticholinergic drugs).

Due to the calcium content of Haemaccel, the serum calcium concentrations may be found to be slightly elevated for a temporary period – especially when large amounts of Haemaccel are administered by rapid infusion. So far, no reports have been received of cases involving clinical signs of hypercalcaemia resulting from an infusion of Haemaccel.

The infusion of Haemaccel may result in a temporary increase in the erythrocyte sedimentation rate.

Overdose: Not applicable

Pharmacological properties

Pharmacodynamic properties: Haemaccel is a gelatin derivative with a mean molecular weight of 30,000. It is iso-oncotic with plasma and has a viscosity and pH similar to plasma. It has very little pharmacological action and does not interfere with cross matching or blood typing tests.

Pharmacokinetic properties: Haemaccel has a mean half-life of about 5 hours. About 74% is excreted via the kidneys four days after administration. It is metabolised into smaller peptides and amino acids by proteolytic enzymes.

Preclinical safety data: None

Pharmaceutical particulars

List of excipients: Sodium Chloride, Ph.Eur. 8.5 g; Potassium Chloride, Ph.Eur. 0.38 g; Callcium Chloride, Ph.Eur. 0.7 g; Water for Injections, Ph.Eur. to 1.0 Litre

Incompatibilities: Citrated blood should NOT be mixed with Haemaccel since clotting of the blood may occur due to the presence of calcium ions in Haemaccel. However, citrated blood may be infused before or after Haemaccel provided that there is adequate flushing of the infusion set.

Shelf-life: 5 years

Special precautions for storage: None.

Nature and contents of container: 500 ml plastic bottles.

Instructions for use/handling: In common with all intravenous infusion, Haemaccel should, if possible, be warmed to body temperature before use. However, in emergencies, it may be infused at ambient temperature. For technical reasons, there is a residual air volume in the container. Thus, pressure infusions with the plastic infusion bottle must be carried out under controlled conditions only, as the risk of an air embolism cannot be excluded.

Marketing authorisation number PL 13402/0031

Date of approval/revision of SPC October 1998

Legal category POM

LOPRAZOLAM TABLETS 1 mg

Presentation Loprazolam tablets 1 mg. Pale yellow, biconvex tablets, 7 mm in diameter, marked Dormonoct* 1 on one face with breakline on reverse. Each tablet contains loprazolam mesylate equivalent to 1 mg loprazolam.

Uses Loprazolam is indicated for the short-term treatment of insomnia including difficulty in falling asleep and/or frequent nocturnal awakenings. Benzodiazepines should be used to treat insomnia only when it is severe, disabling or subjecting the individual to extreme distress. An underlying cause for insomnia should be sought before deciding upon the use of benzodiazepines for symptomatic relief.

Dosage and administration

Adults: The recommended dose is 1 mg at bedtime. This may be increased to 1.5 mg or 2 mg if necessary.

Elderly: Dosage in the elderly should be limited to 1 mg at bedtime.

Frail, debilitated or aged patients: A starting dose of a half tablet may be appropriate. Dosage should not exceed 1 mg.

Treatment should if possible be intermittent.

The lowest dose to control symptoms should be used. Treatment should not normally be continued beyond 4 weeks.

Long-term chronic use is not recommended.

Treatment should always be tapered off gradually.

Patients who have taken benzodiazepines for a long time may require a longer period during which doses are reduced.

Children: There is insufficient evidence to recommend the use of Loprazolam in children.

Contra-indications, warnings, etc

Contra-indications: Sensitivity to benzodiazepines, acute pulmonary insufficiency, severe respiratory insufficiency, myasthenia gravis, phobic or obsessional states and sleep apnoea syndrome. Monotherapy in depression or anxiety associated with depression and chronic psychosis and alcohol intake.

Pregnancy and lactation: If the product is prescribed to a woman of child bearing potential, she should be warned to contact her physician regarding discontinuance of the product if she intends to become or suspects she is pregnant.

If, for compelling medical reasons, the product is administered during the late phase of pregnancy, or during labour at high doses, effects on the neonate, such as hypothermia, hypotonia and moderate respiratory depression can be expected due to the pharmacological action of the compound.

Moreover, infants born to mothers who took benzodiazepines chronically during the latter stages of pregnancy may have developed physical dependancy and may be at some risk for developing withdrawal symptoms in the post natal period.

Since benzodiazepines are found in the breast milk, they should not be given to breast feeding mothers.

Precautions: Attention should be drawn to the risk of drowsiness, sedation, impaired concentration and muscular weakness., especially in drivers of vehicles and operators of machines when taking the product.

Loprazolam may be potentiated by alcohol, or other drugs acting on the CNS or with cisapride. Additive synergy has been observed with neuromuscular depressants (curare-like drugs and muscle relaxants). Combination with CNS depressants e.g. antipsychotics, hypnotics, anxiolytics/sedatives, anitidepressant agents, narcotic analgesics, anti-epileptic drugs, anaesthetics and sedative antihistamines, causes enhancement of the central depressive effects of loprazolam.

The risk of a withdrawal syndrome occurring is increased when loprazolam is combined with other benzodiazepines prescribed as anxiolytics or hypnotics.

Disinhibiting effects may be manifested in various ways. Suicide may be precipitated in patients who are depressed and who exhibit aggressive behaviour towards self and others. Extreme caution should therefore be used in prescribing benzodiazepines in patients with personality disorders.

In general, the dependence potential of benzodiazepines is low but this increases when high doses are attained, especially when given over long periods, and particularly in patients with a history of alcoholism or drug abuse. However, withdrawal symptoms occur even with normal therapeutic doses given for short periods of time. Withdrawal from benzodiazepines may be associated with physiological and psychological symptoms of withdrawal including depression, anxiety, tension, restlessness, confusion, unreliability and headaches. Patients receiving benzodiazepines should be regularly monitored.

Rebound insomnia may also occur. It may be accompanied by other reactions such as changes of mood, anxiety, sleep disturbances and restlessness.

Loprazolam should be used with caution in chronic pulmonary insufficiency, cerebrovascular disease and chronic renal or hepatic impairment.

Side-effects: In general, loprazolam is very well tolerated. However, the common side effects of benzodiazepines, including headaches, nausea, drowsiness, hypotonia, blurring of vision, dizziness and ataxia may occur on the following day, particularly in unusually sensitive patients or when dosage has been excessive.

Rare behavioural adverse effects of benzodiazepines include paradoxical aggressive outbursts, excitement, confusion, and the uncovering of depression with suicidal tendencies. If these reactions should occur, use of the drug should be discontinued. Even more rare side effects reported with some benzodiazepines have been hypotension, gastrointestinal and visual disturbances, skin rashes, urinary retention, changes in libido, blood dyscrasias and jaundice.

Benzodiazepines may induce anterograde amnesia. In cases of loss or bereavement psychological adjustment may be inhibited by benzodiazepines.

Overdosage: As with other benzodiazepines, overdosage does not usually present a threat to life. Treatment is symptomatic and gastric lavage may be of use if performed shortly after ingestion. Use of a specific antidote such as flumazenil in association with symptomatic treatment in hospital should be considered.

Pharmaceutical precautions Store below 25°C in a dry place. Protect from light.

Legal category CD(Sch 4) POM.

Package quantities Loprazolam Tablets 1 mg are blister packed and presented in OP cartons of 28.

Further information Loprazolam is an intermediate acting benzodiazepine. There are no long-lived sedative metabolites. Therefore there is a reduced likelihood of the occurrence of daytime drowsiness or impairment in the performance of skilled tasks, associated with the long acting products. Equally, there is less likelihood of rebound insomnia, which may occur with the ultra-short acting benzodiazepines.

Loprazolam was previously known as Dormonoct*.

Loprazolam tablets contain lactose.

Product licence number PL 13402/0060.

MOLIPAXIN*

Molipaxin Capsules, 50 mg Size No. 3, opaque violet/green capsules printed R365B and [logo]. Each capsule contains 50 mg trazodone hydrochloride. Molipaxin Capsules, 100 mg Size No. 2, opaque violet/fawn capsules printed R365C and [logo]. Each capsule contains 100 mg trazodone hydrochloride.

Uses

Properties: Molipaxin is a potent antidepressant. It also has anxiety reducing activity. Molipaxin is a triazolopyridine derivative chemically unrelated to known tricyclic, tetracyclic and other antidepressant agents. The available data show that at low, subtherapeutic, doses trazodone acts as a 5-HT reuptake antagonist and at higher, therapeutic, doses inhibits 5-HT reuptake. These effects and the effects of trazodone on noradrenergic transmission probably underlie the antidepressant actions of Molipaxin. The importance of the effects on each transmitter is unknown.

Indications: Relief of symptoms in anxiety and all types of depressive illness including depressive illness accompanied by anxiety. Symptoms of depressive illness likely to respond in the first week of treatment include depressed mood, insomnia, anxiety, somatic symptoms and hypochondriasis.

Dosage and administration

Anxiety: 75 mg/day increasing to 300 mg/day as necessary.

Adults: The starting dose of Molipaxin is 150 mg/day after food or as a single dose on retiring.

This may be increased to 300 mg/day, the major portion of which is preferably taken on retiring. In hospitalised patients, dosage may be further increased to 600 mg/day in divided doses.

Elderly: Dosage in the elderly or frail should be started at 100 mg/day in divided doses or as a single night time dose.

Dosage may be increased, under supervision, according to efficacy and tolerance. Doses above 300 mg/day are unlikely to be required.

Tolerability may be improved by taking Molipaxin after food.

In conformity with current psychiatric opinion, it is suggested that Molipaxin be continued for several months after remission. Cessation of Molipaxin treatment should be gradual.

Children: There are insufficient data to recommend the use of Molipaxin in children.

Contra-indications, warnings, etc

Contra-indications: Known hypersensitivity to trazodone.

Precautions: As with all other drugs acting on the central nervous system, patients should be warned against the risk of handling machinery and driving.

Although no untoward effects have been reported, Molipaxin may enhance the effects of muscle relaxants and volatile anaesthetics. Similar considerations apply to combined administration with sedative and antidepressant drugs, including L-tryptophan and alcohol. Molipaxin has been well tolerated in depressed schizophrenic patients receiving standard phenothiazine therapy and also in depressed parkinsonian patients receiving therapy with levodopa.

Possible interactions with monoamine oxidase inhibitors have occasionally been reported, therefore, concurrent administration with MAOIs is not recommended. Giving Molipaxin within two weeks of stopping MAOIs or giving MAOIs within one week of stopping Molipaxin are not recommended.

Since Molipaxin is only a very weak inhibitor of noradrenaline re-uptake and does not modify the blood pressure response to tyramine, interference with the hypotensive action of guanethidine-like compounds is unlikely. However, studies in laboratory animals suggest that Molipaxin may inhibit most of the acute actions of clonidine. In the case of other types of antihypertensive drug, although no clinical interactions have been reported, the possibility of potentiation should be considered.

Concurrent use with trazodone may result in elevated serum levels of digoxin or phenytoin. Monitoring of serum levels should be considered in these patients.

Current clinical experience suggest that Molipaxin does not cause seizures. Nevertheless, care should be exercised when administering Molipaxin to patients suffering epilepsy, avoiding in particular, abrupt increases or decreases in dosage.

Molipaxin should be administered with care in patients with severe hepatic, renal or cardiac disease.

Pregnancy and lactation: Although studies in animals have not shown any direct teratogenic effect, the safety of Molipaxin in human pregnancy has not been established. On basic principles, therefore, its use during the first trimester should be avoided. The possibility of Molipaxin being excreted in the milk should also be considered in nursing mothers.

Side-effects: Molipaxin is a sedative antidepressant, but the drowsiness sometimes experienced during the first days of treatment usually disappears on continued therapy.

Anticholinergic-like symptoms do occur but the incidence is similar to placebo.

The following symptoms, most of which are commonly reported in cases of untreated depression, have also been recorded in small numbers of patients receiving Molipaxin therapy: dizziness, headache, nausea and vomiting, weakness, decreased altertness, weight loss, tremor, dry mouth, bradycardia, tachycardia, postural hypotension, oedema, constipation, diarrhoea, blurred vision, restlessness, confusional states, insomnia and skin rash.

Blood dyscrasias, including agranulocytosis, thrombocytopenia and anaemia, have been reported on rare occasions. Adverse effects on hepatic function, including jaundice and hepatocellular damage, sometimes severe, have been rarely reported. Should such effects occur, Molipaxin should be discontinued immediately.

As with other drugs with alpha-adrenolytic activity, Molipaxin has very rarely been associated with priapism. This may be treated with an intracavernosum injection of an alpha-adrenergic agent such as adrenaline or metaraminol. However there are reports of trazodone-induced priapism which have required surgical intervention or led to permanent sexual dysfunction. Patients developing this suspected adverse reaction should cease Molipaxin therapy immediately.

Clinical studies in patients with pre-existing cardiac disease indicate that trazodone may be arrhythmogenic in some patients in that population. Arrhythmias identified include isolated premature ventricular contractions, ventricular couplets, and short episodes (3-4 beats) of ventricular tachycardia.

Overdosage: The most frequently reported reactions to overdose have included drowsiness, dizziness and vomiting. There is no specific antidote to Molipaxin. The stomach should be emptied as quickly as possible followed by the oral administration of activated charcoal. Treatment should be symptomatic and supportive in the case of hypotension and excessive sedation.

Pharmaceutical precautions Store below 30°C in a dry place.

Legal category POM.

Package quantities Molipaxin 50 mg and 100 mg are presented in blister strips of 14 in pack sizes of 84 and 56 respectively.

Further information In contrast to the tricyclic antidepressants, Molipaxin is devoid of anticholinergic activity. Consequently, troublesome side effects such as dry mouth, blurred vision and urinary hesitancy have occurred no more frequently than in patients receiving placebo therapy. This may be of importance when treating depressed patients who are at risk from conditions such as glaucoma, urinary retention and prostatic hypertrophy.

Studies in animals have shown that Molipaxin is less cardiotoxic than the tricyclic antidepressants and clinical studies suggest that the drug may be less likely to cause cardiac arrhythmias in man.

Molipaxin has had no effect on arterial blood pCO2 or pO2 levels in patients with severe respiratory insufficiency due to chronic bronchial or pulmonary disease.

Product licence numbers Molipaxin 50 mg Capsules: 0109/0045. Molipaxin 100 mg Capsules: 0109/0046

Product authorisation holder: Roussel Laboratories Ltd., Broadwater Park, Denham, Uxbridge UB9 5HP

MOLIPAXIN CR 150 mg Tablets*

Qualitative and quantitative composition Tablet containing 150 mg of trazodone hydrochloride.

Pharmaceutical form Controlled release tablets.

Clinical particulars

Therapeutic indications: Relief of symptoms in all types of depression including depression accompanied by anxiety.

Posology and method of administration: Route of Administration: Oral

Adults: Starting dose 150 mg/day. This may be increased to 300 mg/day in hospitalised patients, dosage may be more easily achieved with Molipaxin CR 150 mg tablet.

Elderly or frail: Starting dose 100 mg/day i.e. Molipaxin CR 100 mg tablet, single dose. This may be increased under supervision, according to efficacy and tolerance. Doses above 300 mg/day are unlikely to be required.

Children: There are insufficient data to recommend the use of Molipaxin in children.

Molipaxin controlled release tablets should be swallowed whole and not chewed. Tolerability may be improved by taking Molipaxin after food.

Contra-indications: Known hypersensitivity to trazodone.

Special warnings and precautions for use: Care should be exercised when administering Molipaxin to patients suffering epilepsy, avoiding in particular, abrupt increases or decreases in dosage.

Molipaxin should be administered with care in patients with severe hepatic, renal or cardiac disease.

Interactions with other medicaments and other forms of interaction: Although no untoward effects have been reported, Molipaxin may enhance the effects of muscle relaxants and volatile anaesthetics. Similar considerations apply to combined administration with sedative and anti-depressant drugs, including alcohol. Molipaxin has been well tolerated in depressed schizophrenic patients receiving standard phenothiazine therapy and also in depressed Parkinsonian patients receiving therapy with levodopa.

Possible interactions with monoamine oxidase inhibitors have occasionally been reported. Although some clinicians do give both concurrently, we do not recommend concurrent administration with MAOIs, or within two weeks of stopping treatment with these compounds. Nor do we recommend giving MAOIs within one week of stopping Molipaxin.

Since Molipaxin is only a very weak inhibitor of noradrenaline re-uptake and does not modify the blood pressure response to tyramine, interference with the hypotensive action of guanethidine-like compounds in unlikely. However, studies in laboratory animals suggest that Molipaxin may inhibit most of the acute actions of clonidine. In the case of other types of antihypertensive drug, although no clinical interactions have been reported, the possibility of potentiation should be considered.

Concurrent use with trazodone may result in elevated serum levels of digoxin or phenytoin. Monitoring of serum levels should be considered in these patients.

Pregnancy and lactation: Although studies in animals have not shown any direct teratogenic effect, the safety of Molipaxin in human pregnancy has not been established. On basic principles, therefore, its use during the first trimester should be avoided. The possibility of Molipaxin being excreted in the milk should also be considered in nursing mothers.

Effects on ability to drive and to use machines: As with all other drugs acting on the central nervous system, patients should be warned against the risk of handling machinery and driving.

Undesirable effects: Molipaxin is a sedative antidepressant and drowsiness sometimes experienced during the first days of treatment, usually disappears on continued therapy.

Anticholinergic-like symptoms do occur but the incidence is similar to placebo.

The following symptoms, most of which are commonly reported in cases of untreated depression, have also been recorded in small numbers of patients receiving Molipaxin therapy: dizziness, headache, nausea and vomiting, weakness, decreased alertness, weight loss, tremor, dry mouth, bradycardia, tachycardia, postural–hypotension, oedema, constipation, diarrhoea, blurred vision, restlessness, confusional states, insomnia and skin rash.

Blood dyscrasias, including agranulocytosis, thrombocytopenia and anaemia, have been reported on rare occasions. Adverse effects on hepatic function, including jaundice and hepatocellular damage, sometimes severe, have been rarely reported. Should such effects occur, Molipaxin should be discontinued immediately.

As with other drugs with alpha-adrenolytic activity, Molipaxin has very rarely been associated with priapism. This may be treated with an intracavernosum injection of an alpha-adrenergic agent such as adrenaline or metaraminol. However there are reports of trazodone-induced priapism which have required surgical intervention or led to permanent sexual dysfunction. Patients developing this suspected adverse reaction should cease Molipaxin immediately.

In contrast to the tricyclic antidepressants, Molipaxin is devoid of anticholinergic activity. Consequently, troublesome side effects such as dry mouth, blurred vision and urinary hesitancy have occurred no more frequently than in patients receiving placebo therapy. This may be of importance when treating depressed patients who are at risk from conditions such as glaucoma, urinary retention and prostatic hypertrophy.

Studies in animals have shown that Molipaxin is less cardiotoxic than the tricyclic antidepressants and clinical studies suggest that the drug may be less likely to cause cardiac arrhythmias in man. Clinical studies in patients with pre-existing cardiac disease indicate that trazodone may be arrhythmogenic in some patients in that population. Arrhythmias identified include isolated premature ventricular contractions, ventricular couplets, and short episodes (3-4 beats) of ventricular tachycardia.

Molipaxin has had no effect on arterial blood pCO_2 or O_2 levels in patients with severe respiratory insufficiency due to chronic bronchial or pulmonary disease.

Overdose: The most frequently reported reactions to overdose have included drowsiness, dizziness and vomiting. There is no specific antidote to Molipaxin. The stomach should be emptied as quickly as possible followed by the oral administration of activated charcoal. Treatment should be symptomatic and supportive in the case of hypotension and excessive sedation.

Pharmacological properties

Pharmacodynamic properties: Molipaxin is a potent antidepressant. It also has anxiety reducing activity. Molipaxin is a triazolopyridine derivative chemically unrelated to known tricyclic, tetracyclic and other antidepressant agents. The available data show that at sub-therapeutic dose, trazodone acts as a 5-HT re-uptake antagonist and at higher, therapeutic doses inhibits 5-HT re-uptake. These effects and the effects of trazodone on noradrenergic transmission probably underlie the antidepressant actions of Molipaxin. The importance of the effects on each transmitter is not known.

Pharmacokinetic properties:

Cmax	Single dose	0.9	1.87 μg/ml
Tmax	Single dose	4.0	5.6 hours
AUC_{24}	Single dose	10.3	19.8 μg hours/ml
$t_{\frac{1}{2}}$	Single dose	7.5	10.3 hours

Preclinical safety data: None applicable.

Pharmaceutical particulars

List of excipients: The tablets also contain caster sugar, carnauba wax, povidone, magnesium stearate, hydroxypropyl methyl cellulose, propylene glycol, sorbitan monolaurate, indigo carmine lake (E132) and titanium dioxide (E171).

Incompatibilities: None stated.

Shelf-life: Amber glass bottles: 60 months. Blister packs: 36 months

See below for details of containers.

Special precautions for storage: Store below 25 °C in a dry place. Protect from light. N.B. 'in a dry place' applies to blister pack only.

Nature and contents of container: i) Amber glass bottles with Jay-caps, pack sizes: 28, 56 or 84 tablets. ii) Blister packs (250 μm PVdC coated blisters backed by 20 μm foil): pack sizes 28, 56 or 84 tablets.

Instructions for use/handling: None.

Marketing authorisation holder: Roussel Laboratories Ltd., Broadwater Park, Denham, Uxbridge, Middlesex UB9 5HP

Marketing authorisation number PL 0109/0214

Date of approval/revision of SPC October 1997

Legal category POM

MOLIPAXIN TABLETS 150 mg*

Qualitative and quantitative composition Tablet containing 150 mg of trazodone hydrochloride.

Pharmaceutical form Tablets.

Clinical particulars

Therapeutic indications: Relief of symptoms in all types of depression including depression accompanied by anxiety.

Posology and method of administration: Route of administration: oral

Depression: Adults: Initially 150 mg/day in divided dose after food or as a single dose on retiring.

This may be increased up to 300 mg/day in a single or divided dose: the major portion of a divided dose to be taken on retiring. The dose may be further increased to 600 mg/day in divided dose in hospitalised patients.

Elderly: For very elderly or frail patients initially 100 mg/day in divided doses or a single night-time dose. This may be increased, under supervision, according to efficacy and tolerance. It is unlikely that 300 mg/day will be exceeded.

Depression accompanied by anxiety: As for Depression.

Anxiety: 75 mg/day increasing to 300 mg/day as necessary.

Tolerability may be improved by taking Molipaxin after food.

Contra-indications: Known sensitivity to Trazodone.

Special warnings and precautions for use: Care should be exercised when administering Molipaxin to patients suffering epilepsy, avoiding in particular, abrupt increases or decreases in dosage.

Molipaxin should be administered with care in patients with severe hepatic, renal or cardiac disease.

Interactions with other medicaments and other forms of interaction: Although no untoward effects have been reported, Molipaxin may enhance the effects of muscle relaxants and volatile anaesthetics. Similar considerations apply to combined administration with sedative and anti-depressant drugs, including alcohol. Molipaxin has been well tolerated in depressed schizophrenic patients receiving standard phenothiazine therapy and also in depressed Parkinsonian patients receiving therapy with levodopa.

Possible interactions with monoamine oxidase inhibitors have occasionally been reported. Although some clinicians do give both concurrently, we do not recommend concurrent administration with MAOIs, or within two weeks of stopping treatment with these compounds. Nor do we recommend giving MAOIs within one week of stopping Molipaxin.

Since Molipaxin is only a very weak inhibitor of noradrenaline re-uptake and does not modify the blood pressure response to tyramine, interference with the hypotensive action of guanethidine-like compounds in unlikely. However, studies in laboratory animals suggest that Molipaxin may inhibit most of the acute actions of clonidine. In the case of other types of antihypertensive drug, although no clinical interactions have been reported, the possibility of potentiation should be considered.

Concurrent use with trazodone may result in elevated serum levels of digoxin or phenytoin. Monitoring of serum levels should be considered in these patients.

Pregnancy and lactation: Although studies in animals have not shown any direct teratogenic effect, the safety of Molipaxin in human pregnancy has not been established. On basic principles, therefore, its use during the first trimester should be avoided. The possibility of Molipaxin being excreted in the milk should also be considered in nursing mothers.

Effects on ability to drive and to use machines: As with all other drugs acting on the central nervous system, patients should be warned against the risk of handling machinery and driving.

Undesirable effects: Molipaxin is a sedative antidepressant and drowsiness sometimes experienced during the first days of treatment, usually disappears on continued therapy.

Anticholinergic-like symptoms do occur but the incidence is similar to placebo.

The following symptoms, most of which are commonly reported in cases of untreated depression, have also been recorded in small numbers of patients receiving Molipaxin therapy: dizziness, headache, nausea and vomiting, weakness, decreased alertness, weight loss, tremor, dry mouth, bradycardia, tachycardia, postural–hypotension, oedema, constipation, diarrhoea, blurred vision, restlessness, confusional states, insomnia and skin rash.

Blood dyscrasias, including agranulocytosis, thrombocytopenia and anaemia, have been reported on rare occasions. Adverse effects on hepatic function, including jaundice and hepatocellular damage, sometimes severe, have been rarely reported. Should such effects occur, Molipaxin should be discontinued immediately.

As with other drugs with alpha-adrenolytic activity, Molipaxin has very rarely been associated with priapism. This may be treated with an intracavernosum injection of an alpha-adrenergic agent such as adrenaline or metaraminol. However there are reports of trazodone-induced priapism which have required surgical intervention or led to permanent sexual dysfunction. Patients developing this suspected adverse reaction should cease Molipaxin immediately.

In contrast to the tricyclic antidepressants, Molipaxin is devoid of anticholinergic activity. Consequently, troublesome side effects such as dry mouth, blurred vision and urinary hesitancy have occurred no more frequently than in patients receiving placebo therapy. This may be of importance when treating depressed patients who are at risk from conditions such as glaucoma, urinary retention and prostatic hypertrophy.

Studies in animals have shown that Molipaxin is less cardiotoxic than the tricyclic antidepressants and clinical studies suggest that the drug may be less likely to cause cardiac arrhythmias in man. Clinical studies in patients with pre-existing cardiac disease indicate that trazodone may be arrhythmogenic in some patients in that population. Arrhythmias identified include isolated premature ventricular contractions, ventricular couplets, and short episodes (3-4 beats) of ventricular tachycardia.

Molipaxin has had no effect on arterial blood pCO_2 or O_2 levels in patients with severe respiratory insufficiency due to chronic bronchial or pulmonary disease.

Overdose: The most frequently reported reactions to overdose have included drowsiness, dizziness and vomiting. There is no specific antidote to Molipaxin. The stomach should be emptied as quickly as possible followed by the oral administration of activated charcoal. Treatment should be symptomatic and supportive in the case of hypotension and excessive sedation.

Pharmacological properties

Pharmacodynamic properties: Molipaxin is a potent antidepressant. It also has anxiety reducing activity. Molipaxin is a triazolopyridine derivative chemically unrelated to known tricyclic, tetracyclic and other antidepressant agents. It has negligible effect on noradrenaline re-uptake mechanisms. Whilst the mode of action of Molipaxin is not known precisely, its antidepressant activity may concern noradrenergic potentiation by mechanisms other than uptake blockade. A central antiserotonin effect may account for the drug's anxiety reducing properties.

Pharmacokinetic particulars: Trazodone is rapidly absorbed from the gastro-intestinal tract and extensively metabolised. Paths of metabolism of trazodone include n-oxidation and hydroxylation. The metabolic m-chlorophenylpiperazine is action. Trazodone is excreted in the urine almost entirely in the form of its metabolites, either in free or in conjugated form. The elimination of trazodone is biphasic, with a terminal elimination half-life of 5 to 13 hours. Trazodone is excreted in breast milk.

There was an approximate two-fold increase in terminal phase half-life and significantly higher plasma concentrations of trazodone in 10 subjects aged 65 to 74 years compared with 12 subjects aged 23 to 30 years following a 100 mg dose of trazodone. It was suggested that there is an age-related reduction in the hepatic metabolism of trazodone.

Preclinical safety data: None stated

List of excipients: The tablets also contain lactose, calcium hydrogen phosphate, microcrystalline cellulose, maize starch, sodium starch glycollate, povidone and magnesium stearate. The film coating contains hydroxypropyl methyl cellulose, propylene glycol, red iron oxide E172 and titanium dioxide.

Incompatibilities: None stated.

Shelf-life: 60 Months

Special precautions for storage: Glass bottles: store below 30°C. Blister packs: store in a dry place below 30°C.

Nature and contents of container: i) Amber glass bottles with Jay-caps, pack sizes: 28, 30 or 100 tablets. ii) Blister packs: pack sizes 28 or 100 tablets.

Instructions for use/handling: None.

Marketing authorisation holder: Roussel Laboratories Ltd., Broadwater Park, Denham, Uxbridge, Middlesex UB9 5HP

Marketing authorisation numbers PL 0109/0133

Date of approval/revision of SPC June 1997

Legal category POM

MOLIPAXIN* LIQUID (50 mg/5 ml)

Qualitative and quantitative composition Each 5 ml contaims 50 mg of trazodone hydrochloride.

Pharmaceutical form Clear, colourless solution with an orange odour and taste.

Clinical particulars

Therapeutic indications: Relief of symptoms in all types of depression including depression accompanied by anxiety.

Symptoms of depression likely to respond in the first week of treatment include depressed mood, insomnia, anxiety, somatic symptoms and hypchondriasis.

Posology and method of administration: Route of Administration: Oral

Adults: Starting dose is 150 mg/day in divided doses after food or as a single dose before retiring. This may be increased to 300 mg/day, the major portion of which is preferably taken on retiring. In hospitalised patients dosage may be increased further to 600 mg/day.

Children: There is insufficient data to recommend the use of Molipaxin in children.

Elderly or frail: For elderly or very frail patients initial starting dose 100 mg/day in divided doses or as a single night-time dose. This may be increased, under supervision, according to efficacy and tolerance. Doses above 300 mg/day are unlikely to be required.

Tolerability may be improved by taking Molipaxin after food.

In conformity with current psychiatric opinion, it is suggested that Molipaxin be continued for several months after remission. Cessation of Molipaxin treatment should be gradual.

Contra-indications: Known sensitivity to trazodone.

Special warnings and precautions for use: Molipaxin should be administered with care in patients with severe hepatic, renal or cardiac disease.

Care should be exercised when administering Molipaxin to patients suffering epilepsy, avoiding in particular, abrupt increases or decreases in dosage.

Blood dyscrasias, including agranulocytosis, thrombocytopenia and anaemia, have been reported on rare occasions. Adverse effects on hepatic function, including jaundice and hepatocellular damage, sometimes severe, have been rarely reported. Should such effects occur, Molipaxin should be discontinued immediately.

Interactions with other medicaments and other forms of interaction: Although no untoward effects have been reported, Molipaxin may enhance the effects of muscle relaxants and volatile anaesthetics. Similar considerations apply to combined administration with sedative and anti-depressant drugs, including alcohol.

Molipaxin has been well tolerated in depressed schizophrenic patients receiving standard phenothiazine therapy and also in depressed parkinsonian patients receiving therapy with levodopa.

Possible interactions with monoamine oxidase inhibitors have occasionally been reported. Although some clinicians do give both concurrently, we do not recommend concurrent administration with MAOIs, or within two weeks of stopping treatment with these compounds. Nor do we recommend giving MAOIs within one week of stopping Molipaxin.

Since Molipaxin is only a very weak inhibitor of noradrenaline re-uptake and does not modify the blood pressure response to tyramine, interference with the hypotensive action of guanethidine-like compounds in unlikely. However, studies in laboratory animals suggest that Molipaxin may inhibit most of the acute actions of clonidine. In the case of other types of antihypertensive drug, although no clinical, interactions have been reported, the possibility of potentiation should be considered.

Concurrent use with trazodone may result in elevated serum levels of digoxin or phenytoin. Monitoring of serum levels should be considered in these patients.

Molipaxin has had no effect on arterial blood pCO_2 or pO_2 levels in patients with severe respiratory insufficiency due to chronic bronchial or pulmonary disease.

Pregnancy and lactation: Although studies in animals have not shown any direct teratogenic effect, the safety of Molipaxin in human pregnancy has not been established. On basic principles, therefore, its use during the first trimester should be avoided. The possibility of Molipaxin being excreted in the milk should also be considered in nursing mothers.

Trazodone should only be administered during pregnancy and lactation if considered essential by the physician.

Effects on ability to drive and use machines: As with all other drugs acting on the central nervous system, patients should be warned against the risk of handling machinery and driving.

Undesirable effects: Molipaxin is a sedative antidepressant and drowsiness sometimes experienced during the first days of treatment, usually disappears on continued therapy.

Anticholinergic-like symptoms do occur but the incidence is similar to placebo.

The following symptoms, most of which are commonly reported in cases of untreated depression, have also been recorded in small numbers of patients receiving Molipaxin therapy: Dizziness, headache, nausea and vomiting, weakness, decreased alertness, weight loss, tremor, dry mouth, bradycardia, tachycardia, postural hypotension, oedema, constipation, diarrhoea, blurred vision, restlessness, confusional states, insomnia and skin rash.

As with other drugs with alpha-adrenolytic activity, Molipaxin has very rarely been associated with priapism. This may be treated with an intracavernosum injection of an alpha-adrenergic agent such as adrenaline or metaraminol. However there are reports of trazodone-induced priapism which have required surgical intervention or led to permanent sexual dysfunction. Patients developing this suspected adverse reaction should cease Molipaxin immediately.

In contrast to the tricyclic antidepressants, Molipaxin is devoid of anticholinergic activity. Consequently, troublesome side effects such as dry mouth, blurred vision and urinary hesitancy have occurred no more frequently than in patients receiving placebo therapy. This may be of importance when treating depressed patients who are at risk from conditions such as glaucoma, urinary retention and prostatic hypertrophy.

Studies in animals have shown that Molipaxin is less cardiotoxic than the tricyclic antidepressants and clinical studies suggest that the drug may be less likely to cause cardiac arrhythmias in man. Clinical studies in patients with pre-existing cardiac disease indicate that trazodone may be arrhythmogenic in some patients in that population. Arrhythmias identified include isolated premature ventricular contractions, ventricular couplets, and short episodes (3-4 beats) of ventricular tachycardia.

Overdose: The most frequently reported reactions to overdose have included drowsiness, dizziness and vomiting. There is no specific antidote to Molipaxin. The stomach should be emptied as quickly as possible followed by the oral administration of activated charcoal. Treatment should be symptomatic and supportive in the case of hypotension and excessive sedation.

Pharmacological properties

Pharmacodynamic properties: Trazodone is a triazolopyridine derivative which differs chemically from other currently available antidepressants. Although trazodone bears some resemblance to the benzodiazepines, phenothiazines and tricyclic antidepressants, its pharmacological profile differs from each of these classes of drugs. The basic idea for the development of trazodone was the hypothesis that depression involves an imbalance of the mechanism responsible for the emotional integration of unpleasant experiences. Consequently, new animal models of depression consisting of responses to unpleasant or noxious stimuli, instead of the current tests related to the aminergic theory of depression, were used in studying the drug. Trazodone inhibits serotonin uptake into rat brain synaptosomes and by rat platelets at relatively high concentrations and inhibits brain uptake of noradrenaline in vitro only at very high concentrations. It possesses antiserotonin-adrenergic blocking and analgesic effects. The anticholinergic activity of trazodone is less than that of the tricyclic antidepressants in animal studies and this has been confirmed in therapeutic trials in depressant patients.

The electroencephalographic profile of trazodone in humans is distinct from that of the tricyclic antidepressants or the benzodiazepines, although bearing some resemblance to these agents in its effect in certain wavebands. Studies of the cardiovascular effects of trazodone in humans. His bundle and surface electrocardiograms in dogs and experience with overdosage in man indicate that trazodone is less liable than imipramine to cause important adverse effects on the heart. However, studies in depressed patients with significant cardiac impairment suggest that trazodone may aggravate existing ventricular arrhythmias in a small undefined subgroup of such patients.

Trazodone is less liable than imipramine to cause important adverse effects on the heart. However, studies in depressed patients with significant cardiac impairment suggest that trazodone may aggravate existing ventricular arrhythmias in a small undefined subgroup of such patients.

Pharmacokinetic properties: Peak plasma concentrations are attained about 1.5 hours after oral administration of trazodone. Absorption is delayed and somewhat enhanced by food. The area under the plasma concentration-time curve is directly proportional to dosage after oral administration of 25 to 100 mg. Trazodone is extensively metabolised, less than 1% of an oral dose being excreted unchanged in the urine. The main route of elimination is via the kidneys with 70 to 75% of an oral dose being recovered in the urine within the first 72 hours of ingestion. The elimination half-life for unchanged drug has been reported to be about 7 hours.

Preclinical safety data: None stated

Pharmaceutical particulars

List of excipients: Glycerol, sorbitol, benzoic acid, saccharin sodium, orange flavour FC 901775, sodium hydroxide solution 1N and purified water.

Incompatibilities: None stated.

Shelf-life: 60 Months

Special precautions for storage: Store below 25°C and protect from light.

Nature and contents of container: Type III PhEur amber glass sealed with a polypropylene screw cap, containing 150 ml of solution.

Instructions for use/handling: None.

Marketing authorisation holder: Roussel Laboratories Ltd., Broadwater Park, Denham, Uxbridge, Middlesex UB9 5HP, UK

Marketing authorisation number PL 0109/0117

Date of approval/revision of SPC September 1998

Legal category POM

NORPLANT*

Qualitative and quantitative composition Norplant consists of six flexible closed capsules for subdermal implantation designed to release the progestin levonorgestrel over a period of five years. The capsules are made of a medicinal grade elastomer (polydimethylsiloxane), measure about 34 mm in length and 2.44 mm in diameter and each contains 38 mg Levonorgestrel B.P.

Pharmaceutical form Subdermal implant.

Clinical particulars

Therapeutic indications: Contraception. Norplant is a long term (up to five years) reversible contraceptive system. The efficacy of Norplant in preventing pregnancy is comparable to or greater than that of other hormonally based and non–hormonally based reversible methods of contraception. The efficacy of Norplant does not depend on patient compliance but may be slightly reduced in heavier women.

Posology and method of administration: Norplant is recommended for insertion into women aged from 18 to 40 years.

Norplant should be inserted or removed only by a Health Care Professional who has completed, (or is participating under supervision in), a training programme such as that leading to a Letter of Competence in Subdermal Contraceptive Implants offered by the Faculty of Family Planning and Reproductive Healthcare of the Royal College of Obstetricians and Gynaecologists.

One Norplant set consists of six capsules in a sterile pouch. Insertion is performed using a trocar to place the capsules under the skin. Strict asepsis must be observed. The capsules should be inserted in the inner aspect of the upper non–dominant arm approximately 6–8cm above the fold in the elbow. Prior to insertion the skin should be cleaned; the insertion area should be anaesthetised with local anaesthetic; a 2 mm transverse incision should be made in the skin using a scalpel. Using the trocar provided the capsules should be inserted subdermally, caudally and in a fan shape. The skin incision should be cleaned and dressed. Care should be taken that capsules are not nicked, cut or broken during insertion or removal.

Starting Norplant: Norplant should be inserted ideally on day 1 of a menstrual cycle, but may be inserted from days 2 to 5 of the menstrual cycle, and, additional non–hormonal contraceptive precautions must be used for 7 days afterwards.

If Norplant is inserted at any other time, pregnancy must be excluded prior to insertion and additional non–hormonal contraceptive cover used for 7 days afterwards.

After abortion: Norplant should be inserted immediately post–abortion and not more than 5 days later. If inserted after this time additional non–hormonal contraceptive precautions must be used for 7 days afterwards.

After childbirth: In line with the recommendations for other progestogen only contraceptive methods, Norplant may be inserted from day 21 after birth. If inserted after this time, additional non–hormonal contraceptive precautions must be used for 7 days afterwards.

Removal: Norplant should be removed within 5 years of insertion. Removal may be done at any time in the menstrual cycle. Loss of contraceptive effect should be viewed in practice as immediate and a new method commenced as appropriate. After the skin has been cleaned local anaesthetic should be infiltrated. A 4 mm skin incision should be made with a scalpel over the apex of the fan according to the requirements of the specific technique that you have been trained to use. The capsules should be removed using small forceps (e.g. mosquito's). Removal usually takes 20–30 minutes. On rare occasions one or more of the capsules may prove difficult to remove. If it is not possible to remove all 6 capsules at once, further visits may be required when the area has healed (4–6 weeks later). In overseas experience removal difficulties have been observed in approximately 5% of cases. If the patient wishes to continue using the method, a new set of Norplant capsules can be inserted through the same incision, but in the opposite direction.

Contra-indications: Known or suspected pregnancy; sensitivity to levonorgestrel; undiagnosed vaginal bleeding; known or suspected sex hormone dependent neoplasia; acute liver disease; benign or malignant liver tumours; existence or past history of thromboembolic disease; past history or evidence of severe arterial disease; risk of ischaemic heart disease, (family history and plasma cholesterol above 6.5 mmol/L); recent trophoblastic disease before levels of human chorionic gonadotrophin have returned to normal.

Special warnings and special precautions for use: Warnings: In patients with a history of thromboembolic disease Norplant should only be used if other methods are unsuitable and after a careful assessment of the risk benefit ratio. Patients who develop arterial thrombotic or embolic disease should have Norplant capsules removed.

The effects of Norplant on clotting factors and plasma lipids have been inconsistent.

Caution should be observed when using Norplant in patients with recognised risk factors for arterial disease or any form of migraine. If focal or crescendo type migraine develop or become worse during use, the removal of Norplant capsules should be considered.

Women who become significantly depressed or have a history of depression, should be carefully observed and removal of Norplant considered.

Benign intracranial hypertension has been reported on rare occasions in Norplant users. Although a causal relationship to the use of Norplant has not been established, this diagnosis should be considered if significant episodes of headache or visual disturbance occur. If the diagnosis is confirmed, Norplant should be removed.

Variation in menstrual bleeding patterns may occur. Irregular menstrual bleeding, intermenstrual bleeding, prolonged episodes of bleeding and spotting and amenorrhoea occur in some women. Overall these irregularities diminish with continuing use. Although, when severe and/or poorly tolerated, they may lead to request for removal of Norplant before the end of five years of use. Significant blood loss is rare and haemoglobin concentrations normally rise slightly in Norplant users.

Since some users of Norplant experience periods of amenorrhoea, missed menstrual periods should not be relied on as the sole means of diagnosing pregnancy. Pregnancy tests should be performed whenever a pregnancy is suspected. Six or more weeks of amenorrhoea after a period of regular menses may indicate pregnancy. The capsules must be removed if pregnancy occurs.

Ectopic pregnancies have been reported amongst Norplant users. The incidence of ectopic pregnancies in Norplant users was however below that estimated to occur in the UK in non–contraceptive users. The risk of ectopic pregnancy may be increased in years 4 and 5 after Norplant insertion and possibly in heavier women. Any patient who presents with lower abdominal pain or pregnancy should be evaluated to exclude ectopic pregnancy.

When follicular development occurs with Norplant, atresia of the follicle is sometimes delayed and the follicle may continue to grow beyond the normal size. In the majority of women enlarged follicles will disappear spontaneously. Rarely they may cause abdominal pain by, for example, twisting or rupturing. Even in the presence of symptoms conservative management is indicated but ectopic pregnancy must be excluded. Only in unusual circumstances is surgical intervention warranted.

Precautions: Any hormonally based method of contraception should only be used under regular medical supervision. Examination of the pelvic organs and breasts and blood pressure measurements should be made at suitable intervals.

Major or Minor Surgery: As with other methods of contraception which have no oestrogen component, Norplant may be continued during surgical procedures but in cases of high risk of thrombosis consideration should be given to standard prophylactic measures.

Interactions with other medicaments and other forms of interaction: As is the case with combined and progestogen–only contraceptive pills the efficacy of Norplant may be reduced by carbamazepine, barbiturates, phenytoin, primidone, phenylbutazone, rifampicin and griseofulvin. Though not established for non–orally systemically administered contraceptive steroids, these and other hepatic enzyme inducers must be presumed to increase the risk of method failure. This will normally mean that the method is inappropriate in long term users of such drugs. A supplementary contraceptive method should be used during short term treatment with such drugs and for seven days thereafter rising to 28 days if the drug was used more than four weeks or at all in the case of rifampicin.

Antibiotics, except rifampicin and griseofulvin, are thought not to reduce the effectiveness of Norplant.

Pregnancy and lactation: There have been reports of foetal congenital malformations when progestogens have been used in pregnant women. If pregnancy occurs Norplant capsules should be removed. Levonorgestrel is excreted in breast milk in small quantities. The long term effects on the nursing infant are unknown.

Effects on ability to drive and use machines: There are no known effects on the ability to drive or use machines.

Undesirable effects: Frequent, irregular or prolonged menstrual bleeding; spotting; amenorrhoea. Pain or itching near implant site; infection at implant site; difficulty in removal. Controlled clinical trials suggest the following adverse effects are associated with the use of Norplant: headache, nervousness, nausea, dizziness, adnexal enlargement, dermatitis, acne, change of appetite, mastalgia, weight changes, hirsutism, hypertrichosis and scalp hair loss. Other events possibly associated with the use of Norplant include breast discharge, cervicitis, mood changes, depression, musculoskeletal pain, abdominal discomfort, vaginitis and vaginal discharge.

Hypertension has occurred in a small percentage of women taking oral hormonal contraceptives. This is usually reversible on discontinuing treatment.

Although there is evidence that combined oral contraceptives may increase the risk of arterial thrombosis, such as myocardial or cerebral infarction, the association of progestogen only methods, like Norplant to this risk is not known.

Overdose: There is no experience of overdose with Norplant.

Pharmacological properties

Pharmacodynamic properties: The active principle, levonorgestrel, is a progestogen. Levonorgestrel released from Norplant has been shown to have effects on ovarian function ranging from absent follicular and luteal activity through cyclical follicular but no luteal activity, normal follicular activity but deficient luteal activity, to normal ovulatory patterns. It suppresses the endometrium possibly preventing implantation of the blastocyst and causes thickening of the cervical mucus preventing passage of spermatozoa into the uterus.

Pharmacokinetic properties: Norplant is a progestogen–only contraceptive system which is implanted subdermally and has been shown to provide contraceptive cover for periods in excess of five years. During the intended five year lifetime of the product, the daily release rate of levonorgestrel ranges from a peak in the first few days of at most 160 mcg/day reducing to 85 mcg/day for the first month and subsequently to 30 mcg/day. It is known that the bio–availability of oral levonorgestrel products approaches 100%. Norplant has, therefore, been designed to provide a systemically available dosage of levonorgestrel in the same range as is provided by the oral products.

Preclinical safety data: None stated.

Pharmaceutical particulars

Excipients: None

Capsule components: Polydimethylsiloxane tubing, Medical Adhesive Type A

Incompatibilities: None known

Shelf-life: 60 months

Special precautions for storage: Store at a temperature not exceeding 25°C. Protect from sunlight and excess moisture.

Nature and contents of container: Six implants contained in a tyvek pouch, enclosed in a carton.

Instructions for use/handling: Information on implantation is provided in *Posology and method of administration.* Further information on implantation is contained in the package insert for doctors and is also available from the product licence holder.

Marketing authorisation number PL 13402/0088

Date of approval/revision of SPC December 1997

Legal category POM

ODRIK*

Qualitative and quantitative composition

0.5 mg capsule contains 0.5 mg of Trandolapril.
1.0 mg capsule contains 1.0 mg of Trandolapril.
2.0 mg capsule contains 2.0 mg of Trandolapril.

Pharmaceutical form

0.5 mg opaque red/yellow capsules.
1.0 mg opaque red/orange capsules.
2.0 mg opaque red/red capsules.

Clinical particulars

Therapeutic indications: Mild or moderate hypertension. Left ventricular dysfunction after myocardial infarction.

It has been demonstrated that Odrik improves survival following myocardial infarction in patients with left ventricular dysfunction (ejection fraction ≤35 percent), with or without symptoms of heart failure, and/or, with or without residual ischaemia. Long-term treatment with Odrik significantly reduces overall cardiovascular mortality. It significantly decreases the risk of sudden death and the occurrence of severe or resistant heart failure.

Posology and method of administration:

Adults: *Mild or moderate hypertension:* For adults not taking diuretics, without congestive heart failure and without renal or hepatic insufficiency; the recommended initial dosage is 0.5 mg as a single daily dose. A 0.5 mg dose will only achieve a therapeutic response in a minority of patients. Dosage should be doubled incrementally at intervals of 2 to 4 weeks, based on patient response, up to a maximum of 4 mg as a single daily dose. The usual maintenance dose range is 1 to 2 mg as a single daily dose. If the patient response is still unsatisfactory at a dose of 4 mg Odrik, combination therapy should be considered.

Left ventricular dysfunction after myocardial infarction: Following a myocardial infarction, therapy may be initiated as early as on the third day. Treatment should be initiated at a daily dose of 0.5 mg. The dose should be progressively increased to a maximum of 4 mg as a single daily dose. Depending upon the tolerability such as symptomatic hypotension, this forced titration can be temporarily suspended.

In the event of hypotension, all concomitant hypotensive therapies such as vasodilators including nitrates, diuretics, must be carefully checked and if possible their dose reduced.

The dose of Odrik should be lowered only if the previous measures are not effective or not feasible.

Elderly: The dose in elderly patients is the same as in adults. There is no need to reduce the dose in elderly patients with normal renal and hepatic function. Caution in elderly patients with concomitant use of diuretics, congestive heart failure or renal or hepatic insufficiency. The dose should be titrated according to the need for the control of blood pressure.

Prior diuretic treatment: In patients who are at risk from a stimulated renin-angiotensin system (e.g. patients with water and sodium depletion) the diuretic should be discontinued 2-3 days before beginning therapy with 0.5 mg trandolapril to reduce the likelihood of symptomatic hypotension. The diuretic may be resumed later if required.

Cardiac failure: In hypertensive patients who also have congestive heart failure, with or without associated renal insufficiency, symptomatic hypotension has been observed after treatment with ACE inhibitors. In these patients therapy should be started at a dose of 0.5 mg Odrik once daily under close medical supervision in hospital.

Dosage adjustment in renal impairment: For patients with mild or moderate renal impairment (creatinine clearance of 10-70 ml/min) the usual adult and elderly doses are recommended.

For patients with severe renal impairment (creatinine clearance of <10 ml/min) the usual adult and elderly starting doses are also recommended but the maximum daily dose should not exceed 2 mg. In these patients therapy should be under close medical supervision.

Dialysis: It is not known for certain if trandolapril or trandolaprilat are removed by dialysis. However, it would be expected that dialysis could remove the active moiety, trandolaprilat, from the circulation, resulting in a possible loss of control of blood pressure. Therefore careful monitoring of the patient's blood pressure during dialysis is required, and the dosage of trandolapril adjusted if needed.

Dosage adjustment in hepatic impairment: In patients with severely impaired liver function a decrease in the metabolic clearance of the parent compound trandolapril and the active metabolite trandolaprilat results in a large increase in plasma trandolapril levels and to a lesser extent an increase in trandolaprilat levels. Treatment with Odrik should therefore be initiated at a dose of 0.5 mg once daily under close medical supervision.

Children: Odrik has not been studied in children and therefore use in this age group is not recommended.

Contra-indications: Known hypersensitivity to trandolapril. History of angioneurotic oedema associated with administration of an ACE inhibitor. Hereditary/idiopathic angioneurotic oedema. Pregnancy or lactation. Use in children.

Special warnings and precautions for use: Odrik should not be used in patients with aortic stenosis or outflow obstruction.

Assessment of renal function: Evaluation of the patient should include assessment of renal function prior to initiation of therapy and during treatment. Proteinuria may occur if renal impairment is present prior to therapy or relatively high doses are used.

Impaired renal function: Patients with severe renal insufficiency may require reduced doses of Odrik; their renal function should be closely monitored. In the majority, renal function will not alter. In patients with renal insufficiency, congestive heart failure or unilateral or bilateral renal artery stenosis, in the single kidney as well as after renal transplantation, there is a risk of impairment of renal function. If recognised early, such impairment of renal function is reversible upon discontinuation of therapy.

Some hypertensive patients with no apparent pre-existing renal disease may develop minor and usually transient increases in blood urea nitrogen and serum creatinine when Odrik is given concomitantly with a diuretic. Dosage reduction of Odrik and/or discontinuation of the diuretic may be required. Additionally, in patients with renal insufficiency the risk of hyperkalaemia should be considered and the patient's electrolyte status checked regularly.

Impaired liver function: As trandolapril is a prodrug metabolised to its active moiety in the liver, particular caution and close monitoring should be applied to patients with impaired liver function.

Symptomatic hypotension: In patients with uncomplicated hypertension, symptomatic hypotension has been observed rarely after the initial dose of Odrik as well as after increasing the dose of Odrik. It is more likely to occur in patients who have been volume- and salt-depleted by prolonged diuretic therapy, dietary salt restriction, dialysis, diarrhoea or vomiting. Therefore, in these patients, diuretic therapy should be discontinued and volume and/or salt depletion should be corrected before initiating therapy with Odrik.

If symptomatic hypotension occurs, the patient should be placed in a supine position and, if necessary, receive an intravenous infusion of physiological saline. Intravenous atropine may be necessary if there is associated bradycardia. Treatment with Odrik may usually be continued following restoration of effective blood volume and blood pressure.

Surgery/anaesthesia: In patients undergoing surgery or during anaesthesia with agents producing hypotension, Odrik may block angiotensin II formation secondary to compensatory renin release. If hypotension occurs and is considered to be due to this mechanism, it can be corrected by appropriate treatment.

Agranulocytosis and bone marrow depression: In patients on angiotensin converting enzyme inhibitors, agranulocytosis and bone marrow depression have been seen rarely. They are more frequent in patients with renal impairment, especially if they have a collagen vascular disease. However, regular monitoring of white blood cell counts and protein levels in urine should be considered in patients with collagen vascular disease (e.g. lupus erythematosus and scleroderma), especially associated with impaired renal function and concomitant therapy particularly with corticosteroids and antimetabolites.

Hyperkalaemia: Elevated serum potassium has been observed very rarely in hypertensive patients. Risk factors for the development of hyperkalaemia include renal insufficiency, potassium sparing diuretics, the concomitant use of agents to treat hypokalaemia, diabetes mellitus and/or left ventricular dysfunction after myocardial infarction.

Angioneurotic oedema: Rarely, ACE inhibitors (such as trandolapril) may cause angioneurotic oedema that includes swelling of the face, extremities, tongue, glottis and/or larynx. Patients experiencing angioneurotic oedema must immediately discontinue Odrik therapy and be monitored until oedema resolution.

Angioneurotic oedema to the face will usually resolve spontaneously. Oedema involving not only the face but also the glottis may be life-threatening because of the risk of airway obstruction.

Angioneurotic oedema involving the tongue, glottis or larynx requires immediate sub-cutaneous administration of 0.3-0.5 ml of adrenaline solution (1:1000) along with other therapeutic measures as appropriate.

Caution must be exercised in patients with a history of idiopathic angioneurotic oedema and Odrik is contraindicated if angioneurotic oedema was an adverse reaction to an ACE inhibitor (see Contraindications section).

Cough: During treatment with an ACE inhibitor, a dry and non-productive cough may occur which disappears after discontinuation.

Interactions with other medicaments and other forms of interaction: Drug interactions: Combination with diuretics or other antihypertensive agents may potentiate the antihypertensive response to Odrik. Adrenergic-blocking drugs should only be combined with trandolapril under careful supervision.

Potassium sparing diuretics (spironolactone, amiloride, triamterene) or potassium supplements may increase the risk of hyperkalaemia particularly in renal failure. Odrik may attenuate the potassium loss caused by thiazide-type diuretics. If concomitant use of these agents is indicated, they should be given with caution and serum potassium should be monitored regularly.

Antidiabetic agents: As with all ACE-inhibitors, concomitant use of antidiabetic medicines (insulin or oral hypoglycaemic agents) may cause an increased blood glucose lowering effect with greater risk of hypoglycaemia. Therefore, blood glucose should be closely monitored in diabetics treated with a hypoglycaemic agent and trandolapril, particularly when starting or increasing the dose of ACE-inhibitor, or in patients with impaired renal function.

Combinations necessitating a warning: In some patients already receiving diuretic treatment, particularly if this treatment has been recently instituted, the fall in blood pressure on initiation of treatment with Odrik may be excessive. The risk of symptomatic hypotension may be reduced by stopping the diuretic a few days before starting treatment with Odrik. If it is necessary to continue the diuretic treatment, the patient should be monitored, at least after the initial administration of Odrik. As with all antihypertensives, combination with a neuroleptic or tricyclic antidepressant increases the risk of orthostatic hypotension. Odrik may reduce the elimination of lithium and serum levels of lithium should be monitored.

Anaphylactoid reactions to high-flux polyacrylonitrile membranes used in haemodialysis have been reported in patients treated with ACE inhibitors. As with other antihypertensives of this chemical class this combination should be avoided when prescribing ACE inhibitors to renal dialysis patients.

The effects of certain anaesthetics may be enhanced by ACE inhibitors.

Allopurinol, cytostatic or immunosuppresive agents, systemic corticosteroids or procainamide may increase the risk of leucopenia, if used concomitantly with ACE inhibitors.

The antihypertensive effect of ACE inhibitors may be reduced by the administration of NSAIDs. an additive effect on serum potassium increase has been described when NSAIDs and ACE inhibitors have been used concomitantly, while renal function may be reduced.

Antacids cause reduced bioavailability of ACE inhibitors.

The antihypertensive effects of ACE inhibitors may be reduced by sympathomimetics, patients should be carefully monitored.

No clinical interaction has been observed in patients with left ventricular dysfunction after myocardial infarction when Odrik has been concomitantly administered with thrombolytics, aspirin, beta blockers, calcium channel blockers, nitrates, anticoagulants, diuretics or digoxin.

Use in pregnancy and lactation: The use of Odrik is contra-indicated in pregnancy and lactation. Pregnancy should be excluded before start of treatment and avoided during treatment. Exposure of the mother to ACE inhibitors in mid or late pregnancy has been associated with oligohydramnios and neonatal hypotension with anuria or renal failure.

In the rat and particularly in the rabbit, trandolapril caused maternal toxicity together with fetotoxicity at high doses. Neither embryotoxicity nor teratogenicity was observed in the rat, rabbit or monkey.

Effects on ability to drive and to use machines: Given the pharmacological properties of Odrik, no particular effect is expected. However, in some individuals, ACE inhibitors may affect the ability to drive or operate machinery particularly at the start of treatment, when changing over from other medication or during concomitant use of alcohol. Therefore, after the first dose, or subsequent increases in dose it is not advisable to drive or operate machinery for several hours.

Undesirable effects (frequency and seriousness): The following adverse events have been reported with ACE inhibitors as a class. Not all will have been reported in association with Odrik.

In long term studies the most frequently reported adverse events were cough, headaches, asthenia and dizziness.

Respiratory: Dyspnoea, sinusitis, rhinitis, glossitis, bronchitis and bronchospasm have been reported, but rarely in association with treatment with ACE inhibitors.

Cardiovascular: Tachycardia, palpitations, arrhythmias, angina pectoris, myocardial infarction, transient ischaemic attacks and cerebral haemorrhage have been reported in association with hypotension during treatment with ACE inhibitors.

Gastrointestinal: Nausea, vomiting, abdominal pain, indigestion, diarrhoea, constipation and dry mouth have occurred occasionally during treatment with ACE inhibitors.

There have been reports of individual incidents of cholestatic jaundice, hepatitis, pancreatitis and ileus connected with the use of ACE inhibitors.

Hypersensitivity: Allergic hypersensitivity reactions such as pruritis and rash have been reported. Urticaria, erythema multiform, Stevens-Johnson Syndrome, toxic epidermal necrolysis, psoriasis-like efflorescences and alopecia, which may be accompanied by fever, myalgia, arthralgia, eosinophilia and/or increased ANA (anti-nuclear antibody)-titres have been occasionally reported with ACE inhibitor treatment.

Angioneurotic oedema: In very rare cases angioneurotic oedema has occurred. If laryngeal stridor or angioedema of the face, tongue or glottis occurs treatment with Odrik must be discontinued and appropriate therapy instituted immediately.

Renal: Deterioration of renal function and acute renal failure have been reported with the use of ACE inhibitors.

Drug/laboratory parameters: Reversible (on stopping treatment) increases in blood urea and plasma creatinine may result, particularly if renal insufficiency, severe heart failure or renovascular hypertension are present.

Decreased haemoglobin, haematocrit, platelets and white cell count, and individual cases of agranulocytosis or pancytopenia, have been reported with ACE inhibitor treatment : also evaluate liver enzymes and serum bilirubin. Haemolytic anaemia has been reported in some patients with a congenital deficiency concerning g-6 PDH (glucose-6-phosphate dehydrogenase) during treatment with ACE inhibitors.

Overdose: Symptoms expected with ACE inhibitors are severe hypotension, shock, stupor, bradycardia, electrolyte disturbance and renal failure. In the event of overdosage following recent ingestion, consideration should be given to emptying the stomach contents. Blood pressure should be monitored and if hypotension develops, volume expansion should be considered.

Pharmacological properties

Pharmacodynamic properties: Odrik capsules contain the prodrug trandolapril, a non-peptide angiotensin converting enzyme (ACE) inhibitor with a carboxyl group but without a sulphydryl group. Trandolapril is rapidly absorbed and then non-specifically hydrolysed to its potent, long-acting active metabolite, trandolaprilat.

Trandolaprilat binds tightly and in a saturable manner to ACE.

The administration of trandolapril causes decreases in the concentrations of angiotensin II, aldosterone and atrial natriuretic factor and increases in plasma renin activity and concentrations of angiotensin I. Odrik thus modulates the renin-angiotensin-aldosterone system which plays a major part in regulating blood volume and blood pressure and consequently has a beneficial antihypertensive effect.

The administration of usual therapeutic doses of Odrik to hypertensive patients produces a marked reduction of both supine and erect blood pressure. The antihypertensive effect is evident after 1 hour, with a peak effect between 8 and 12 hours, persisting for at least 24 hours.

The properties of trandolapril might explain the results obtained in the regression of cardiac hypertrophy with improvement of diastolic function, and improvement of arterial compliance in humans. In addition a decrease in vascular hypertrophy has been shown in animals.

Pharmacokinetic properties: Trandolapril is very rapidly absorbed after oral administration. The amount absorbed is equivalent to 40 to 60% of the administered dose and is not affected by food consumption.

The peak plasma concentration of trandolapril is observed 30 minutes after administration. Trandolapril disappears rapidly from the plasma with a half-life of less than one hour.

Trandolapril is hydrolysed to trandolaprilat, a specific angiotensin converting enzyme inhibitor. The amount of trandolaprilat formed is not modified by food consumption. The peak plasma concentration of trandolaprilat is reached after 4 to 6 hours.

In the plasma trandolaprilat is more than 80% protein-bound. It binds saturably, with a high affinity, to angiotensin converting enzyme. The major proportion of circulating trandolaprilat is also non-saturably bound to albumin.

After repeated administration of Odrik in a single daily dose, steady state is reached on average in four days, both in healthy volunteers and in young or elderly hypertensives. The effective half-life of trandolaprilat is between 16 and 24 hours. The terminal half life of elimination is between 47 and 98 hours, depending on dose. This terminal phase probably represents binding/dissociation kinetics of the trandolaprilat/ACE complex.

Trandolaprilat eliminated in the urine in the unchanged form accounts for 10 to 15% of the dose of trandolapril administered. After oral administration of the labelled product in man, 33% of the radioactivity is found in the urine and 66% in the faeces.

The renal clearance of trandolaprilat is proportional to the creatinine clearance. The plasma concentrations of trandolaprilat are significantly higher in patients with a creatinine clearance less than or equal to 30 ml/min. However, after repeated dosing in patients with chronic renal failure steady state is also reached on average in four days, whatever the degree of renal failure.

Preclinical safety data: Acute oral toxicity studies of trandolapril and its active metabolite, trandolaprilat, in rats and mice showed both compounds to be non-toxic with respective LD_{50} values of > 4000 mg/kg and >5000 mg/kg.

Repeat dose oral toxicity was evaluated in the rat and dog with studies of up to 18 and 12 months duration respectively. The principal observations in these studies were of anaemia (doses of 20 mg/kg/day and above in the rat 30 day study and 25 mg/kg/day and above in the dog 6 month study), gastric irritation and ulceration (doses of 20 mg/kg/day and above in the rat 30 day study and 125 mg/kg/day in the dog 6 month study) and renal lesions (20 mg/kg/day and above in the rat 30 day study and 10 mg/kg/day in the dog 30 day study): renal lesions were also seen in the 6 month studies in the rat and dog (from doses of 0.25 and 25 mg/kg/day respectively)–these were reversible on cessation of treatment.

Reproduction toxicity studies showed effects on renal development in offspring with increased incidence of renal pelvic dilation; this was seen at doses of 10 mg/kg/day and above in the rat but these changes did not affect the normal development of the offspring.

Trandolapril was not mutagenic or carcinogenic.

Pharmaceutical particulars

List of excipients: Corn starch, lactose, povidone, sodium stearyl fumarate and printing ink (Shellac, industrial methylated spirit, purified water, soya lecithin, 2-ethoxyethanol, dimethyl polysiloxane and black iron oxide).

Incompatibilities: None.

Shelf-life:

Odrik 0.5 mg:

PVC/Al blister pack	24 months
Aluminium blister pack	24 months
Colourless glass bottle	24 months

Odrik 1 mg & 2 mg:

PVCA/Al blister pack	36 months
Aluminium blister pack	36 months
Colourless glass bottle	36 months

Special precautions for storage: For PVCA/Aluminium blisters: Store in a dry place

Nature and contents of container: PVCA/Al Blister packs containing 28 or 56 capsules or Aluminium blister packs containing 28 or 56 capsules or colourless glass bottles containing 250 capsules.

Instructions for use/handling: None.

Marketing authorisation holder: Roussel Laboratories Ltd., Broadwater Park, Denham, Uxbridge, Middlesex UB9 5HP

Marketing authorisation numbers

Odrik 0.5 mg capsule	PL 0109/0237
Odrik 1 mg capsule	PL 0109/0238
Odrik 2 mg capsule	PL 0109/0239

Date of approval/revision of SPC March 1998

Legal category POM

OESTROGEL* PUMP PACK

Qualitative and quantitative composition Oestrogel contains oestradiol as active ingredient, 0.06% w/w.

Pharmaceutical form Hydro-alcoholic gel.

Clinical particulars

Therapeutic indications: As oestrogen replacement therapy for the relief of symptoms due to natural or surgically induced menopause, such as vasomotor symptoms (hot flushes and sweating), atrophic vaginitis and atrophic urethritis.

Prevention of postmenopausal osteoporosis in women considered at risk of developing fractures. Where several risk factors are present hormone replacement therapy should be considered. Epidemiological studies have suggested that a number of risk factors may contribute to postmenopausal osteoporosis, and these include early menopause (either naturally or surgically induced); family history of osteoporosis; recent prolonged corticosteroid therapy; a small, thin frame; excessive cigarette consumption.

Bone mineral density meausrements may help to confirm the presence of low bone mass. For a maximum prophylactic benefit, treatment should commence as soon as possible after menopause.

Posology and method of administration:

Adults and the elderly: Menopausal symptoms: Each measure from the dispenser is 1.25 g of Oestrogel. Two measures (2.5 g) of Oestrogel once daily (1.5 mg 17β-oestradiol) is the usual starting dose, which in the majority of women will provide effective relief of symptoms. If after one month's treatment effective relief is not obtained, the dosage may be increased accordingly to a maximum of four measures (5 g) of Oestrogel daily (3.0 mg 17β-oestradiol).

Prevention of osteoporosis: The minimum effective dose is 2.5 g of Oestrogel once daily for most patients.

The lowest effective dose should be used for maintenance therapy. In women with an intact uterus the recommended dose of a progestogen should be administered for 12 days of each month, in accordance with the manufacturers recommendations. Oestrogel should be administered daily on a continuous basis.

The correct dose of gel should be dispensed and applied to clean, dry, intact areas of skin e.g. on the arms and shoulders, or inner thighs. The area of application should be at least 750 cm², twice the area of the template provided. One measure from the dispenser, or half the prescribed dose, should be applied to each arm/shoulder (or thigh). Oestrogel should NOT be applied on or near the breasts or on the vulval region.

Oestrogel should be allowed to dry for 5 minutes before covering the skin with clothing.

Children: Not recommended for children.

Contra-indications: Pregnancy and lactation. Known or suspected cancer of the breast, genital tract or other oestrogen dependent neoplasia. Severe hepatic, renal or cardiac disease. Porphyria. Active deep vein thrombosis, thromboembolic disorders, or a confirmed history of these conditions. Endometrial hyperplasia, undiagnosed vaginal bleeding.

Special warnings and precautions for use: Before commencing any oestrogen therapy, the patient should have a complete physical and gynaecological examination, including blood pressure, breasts, abdomen and pelvic organs, and endometrial assessment where necessary. This should be repeated at regular intervals.

Prolonged use of unopposed oestrogens may increase the risk of endometrial carcinoma. In women with an intact uterus the addition of a progestogen is therefore considered essential. Caution should be exercised in prescribing oestrogens for patients with mastopathy or a strong family history of breast cancer.

In patients with hypertension, or a history of it, blood pressure should be monitored at regular intervals. If hypertension develops in patients receiving oestrogens, treatment should be discontinued.

Epidemiological studies have suggested that hormone replacement therapy (HRT) is associated with an increased relative risk of developing venous thromboembolism (VTE) i.e. deep vein thrombosis or pulmonary embolism. The studies find a 2-3 fold increase for users compared with non-users which for healthy women amounts to a low risk of one extra case of VTE each year for every 5000 patients taking HRT.

Generally recognised risk factors for VTE include a personal or family history and severe obesity (Body Mass Index >30 kg/m²). In women with these factors the benefits of treatment with HRT need to be carefully weighed against risks.

The risk of VTE may be temporarily increased with prolonged immobilisation, major trauma or major surgery. In women on HRT scrupulous attention should be given to prophylactic measures to prevent VTE following surgery. Where prolonged immobilisation is liable to follow elective surgery, particularly abdominal or orthopaedic surgery to the lower limbs, consideration should be given to temporarily stopping HRT 4 weeks earlier.

If venous thromboembolism develops after initiating therapy the drug should be discontinued.

Care should be taken with patients with cholelithiasis, a history of endometriosis, diabetes mellitus, migraine, otosclerosis or any other condition which is known to deteriorate during pregnancy.

The gel should be applied by the patient herself, not by anyone else, and skin contact, particularly with a male partner, should be avoided for one hour after application. Washing the skin or contact with other skin products should be avoided until at least one hour after application of Oestrogel.

Interactions with other medicaments and other forms of interaction: Treatment with surface active agents, (e.g. sodium lauryl sulphate) or other drugs which alter barrier structure or function, could remove drug bound to the skin, altering transdermal flux. Therefore patients should avoid the use of strong skin cleansers and detergents (e.g. benzalkonium or benzothonium chloride products), skin care products of high alcoholic content (astringents, sunscreens) and keratolytics (e.g. salicylic acid, lactic acid).

The use of any concomitant skin medication which alters skin production (e.g. cytotoxic drugs) should be avoided.

Pregnancy and lactation: Use is contraindicated in pregnancy and during lactation.

Effects on ability to drive and use machines: None known.

Undesirable effects: Irritation, reddening of the skin or mild and transient erythema at the site of application have been occasionally reported. In this instance a different site of application should be used, but if the topical side-effects continue, consideration should be given to discontinuation of treatment.

Systemic side-effects with Oestrogel are rare but the following have been reported with oral oestrogen therapy:

Genito-urinary tract: increase in the size of uterine fibromyomata, excessive production of cervical mucus.

Breast: pain, enlargement and secretion.

Gastrointestinal tract: nausea

CNS: headache, migraine and mood changes.

Overdose: Pain in the breasts or excessive production of cervical mucus may be indicative of too high a dosage, but acute overdosage has not been reported and is unlikely to be a problem. Overdosages of oestrogen may cause nausea, and withdrawal bleeding may occur. There are no specific antidotes and treatment should be symptomatic.

Pharmacological properties

Pharmacodynamic properties: As the major oestrogen secreted by the human ovary, oestradiol is crucial to the development and maintenance of the female reproductive system and secondary sex characteristics, it promotes growth and development of the vagina, uterus and fallopian tubes, and enlargement of the breasts. Indirectly it contributes to the shaping of the skeleton, maintenance of tone and elasticity of urogenital structures, changes in the epiphyses of the long bones that allow for pubertal growth spurt and its termination, growth of axillary and pubic hair and pigmentation of the nipples and genitals.

The onset of menopause results from a decline in the secretion of oestradiol and other oestrogens by the ovary resulting initially in the cessation of menstruation, followed by menopausal symptoms such as vasomotor symptoms (hot flushes and sweating), muscle cramps, myalgias, arthralgias, anxiety, atrophic vaginitis and kraurosis vulvae. Oestrogens are also an important factor in preventing bone loss and after the menopause women lose bone mineral content at an average rate of 15-20% in a ten year period.

Pharmacokinetic properties: Pharmacokinetic studies indicate that, when applied topically to a large area of skin in a volatile solvent, approximately 10% of the oestradiol is percutaneously absorbed into the vascular system, regardless of the age of the patient. Daily application of 2.5 g or 5 g Oestrogel over a surface area of 400-750cm² results in a gradual increase in oestrogen blood levels to steady state after approximately 3-5 days and provides circulating levels of both oestradiol and oestrone equivalent in absolute concentrations and in their respective ratio to those obtained during the early-mid follicular phase of the menstrual cycle.

Avoidance of first pass metabolism by the percutaneous route not only results in a physiologic ratio of oestradiol and oestrone, but also reduces the impact on hepatic biosynthesis of protein that has been demonstrated with orally administered oestrogens.

Preclinical safety data: No relevant information additional to that already contained in the SPC.

Pharmaceutical particulars

List of excipients: Ethanol, carbomer, triethanolamine and purified water.

Incompatibilities: None known.

Shelf life: 18 months

Special precautions for storage: Store below 25°C.

Nature and contents of container: Rigid plastic container enclosing a LDPE bag fitted with a metering valve and closed with a polypropylene cap, containing 80 g.

Instruction for use/handling: Not applicable.

Marketing authorisation number PL 13402/0020

Date of approval/revision of SPC November 1998

Legal category POM

ORELOX* TABLETS

Qualitative and quantitative composition Each Orelox tablet contains 130.45 mg of cefpodoxime proxetil (equivalent to 100 mg cefpodoxime).

Pharmaceutical form Tablets for oral use.

Clinical particulars

Therapeutic indications: Orelox is a bactericidal cephalosporin antibiotic active against a wide variety of Gram-negative and Gram-positive organisms. It is indicated for the treatment of the following infections either before the infecting organism has been identified or when caused by bacteria of established sensitivity.

Upper respiratory tract infections caused by organisms sensitive to cefpodoxime including sinusitis. In tonsillitis and pharyngitis, Orelox should be reserved for recurrent or chronic infections, or for infections where the causative organism is known or suspected to be resistant to commonly used antibiotics.

Lower respiratory tract infections caused by organisms sensitive to cefpodoxime, including acute bronchitis, relapses or exacerbations of chronic bronchitis, and bacterial pneumonia

Upper and lower urinary tract infections including cystitis and acute pyelonephritis.

Skin and soft tissue infections caused by organisms sensitive to cefpodoxime such as abscesses, cellulitis, infected wounds, furuncles, folliculitis, paronychia, carbuncles and ulcers.

Gonorrhoea – uncomplicated gonococcal urethritis.

Posology and method of administration: Route of administration: oral.

Adults: Adults with normal renal function:

Upper respiratory tract infections: For upper respiratory tract infections, caused by organisms sensitive to cefpodoxime including sinusitis. In tonsillitis and pharyngitis, Orelox should be reserved for recurrent or chronic infections, or for infections where the causative organism is known or suspected to be resistant to commonly used antibiotics. Sinusitis: 200 mg twice daily. Other upper respiratory tract infections: 100 mg twice daily.

Lower respiratory tract infections: For lower respiratory tract infections caused by organisms sensitive to cefpodoxime, including acute bronchitis, relapses or exacerbations of chronic bronchitis and bacterial pneumonia; 100-200 mg twice daily, dependent on the severity of the infection.

Urinary tract infections: Uncomplicated lower urinary tract infections: 100 mg should be taken twice daily.

Uncomplicated upper urinary tract infections: 200 mg should be taken twice daily.

Uncomplicated gonococcal urethritis*:* 200 mg should be taken as a single dose.

Skin and soft tissue infections: 200 mg should be taken twice daily.

Tablets should be taken during meals for optimum absorption.

Elderly: It is not necessary to modify the dose in elderly patients with normal renal function.

Children: Orelox Paediatric is available to treat infants (over 15 days old) and children. Please refer to the separate Summary of Product Characteristics for details.

Hepatic impairment: The dosage does not require modification in cases of hepatic impairment.

Renal impairment: The dosage of Orelox does not require modification if creatinine clearance exceeds 40 ml/min. Below this value, pharmacokinetic studies indicate an increase in plasma elimination half life and maximum plasma concentrations, and hence the dosage should be adjusted appropriately.

Creatinine clearance (ml/min)	
39–10	Unit dose[1] administered as a single dose every 24 hours (i.e. half of the usual adult dose).
<10	Unit dose[1] administered as a single dose every 48 hours (i.e. quarter of the usual adult dose).
Haemodialysis patients	Unit dose[1] administered after each dialysis session.

Note: [1] The unit dose is either 100 mg or 200 mg, depending on the type of infection.

Contra-indications: Hypersensitivity to cephalosporin antibiotics.

Special warnings and precautions for use: Preliminary enquiry about allergy to penicillin is necessary before prescribing cephalosporins since cross allergy to penicillins occurs in 5-10% of cases.

Particular care will be needed in patients sensitive to penicillin: strict medical surveillance is necessary from the very first administration. Where there is doubt, medical assistance, should be available at the initial administration, in order to treat any anaphylactic episode.

In patients who are allergic to other cephalosporins, the possibility of cross-allergy to Orelox should be borne in mind. Orelox should not be given to those patients with a previous history of immediate type hypersensitivity to cephalosporins.

Hypersensitivity reactions (anaphylaxis) occuring with beta-lactam antibiotics can be serious and occasionally fatal.

The onset of any manifestation of hypersensitivity indicates that treatment should be stopped.

Orelox is not the preferred antibiotic for the treatment of staphylococcal pneumonia and should not be used in the treatment of atypical pneumonia caused by organisms such as *Legionella, Mycoplasma* and *Chlamydia*.

In cases of severe renal insufficiency it may be necessary to reduce the dosage regimen dependent on the creatinine clearance.

Possible side effects include gastrointestinal disorders such as nausea, vomiting and abdominal pain. Antibiotics should always be prescribed with caution in patients with a history of gastrointestinal disease, particularly colitis. Orelox may induce diarrhoea, antibiotic-associated colitis and pseudomembranous colitis. These side-effects, which may occur more frequently in patients receiving higher doses for prolonged periods, should be considered as potentially serious. The presence of *C. difficile* should be investigated. In all potential cases of colitis the treatment should be stopped immediately. The diagnosis should be confirmed by sigmoidoscopy and specific antibiotic therapy (vancomycin) substituted if considered clinically necessary. The administration of products which cause faecal stasis must be avoided. Although any antibiotic may cause pseudomembranous colitis, the risk may be higher with broad-spectrum drugs, such as the cephalosporins.

As with all beta-lactam antibiotics, neutropenia and more rarely, agranulocytosis may develop particularly during extended treatment. For cases of treatment lasting longer than 10 days, blood count should therefore be monitored and treatment discontinued if neutropenia is found.

Cephalosporins may be absorbed onto the surface of red cell membranes and react with antibodies directed against the drug. This can produce a positive Coomb's test and very rarely, haemolytic anaemia. Cross-reactivity may occur with penicillin for this reaction.

Changes in renal function have been observed with antibiotics of the same class, particularly when given concurrently with potentially nephrotoxic drugs such as aminoglycosides and/or potential diuretics. In such cases, renal function should be monitored.

As with other antibiotics, the prolonged use of cefpodoxime proxetil may result in the overgrowth of non-susceptible organisms. With oral antibiotics the normal colonic flora may be altered, allowing overgrowth by Clostridia with consequent pseudomembranous colitis. Repeated evaluation of the patient is essential, and if superinfection occurs during therapy, appropriate measures should be taken.

Interactions with other medicaments and other forms of interaction: No clinically significant drug interactions have been reported during the course of clinical studies.

As with other cephalosporins, isolated cases showing development of a positive Coomb's test have been reported (see precautions).

Studies have shown that bioavailability is decreased by approximately 30% when Orelox is administered with drugs which neutralise gastric pH or inhibit acid secretions. Therefore, such drugs as antacids of the mineral type and H_2 blockers such as ranitidine, which can cause an increase in gastric pH, should be taken 2 to 3 hours after Orelox administration.

The bioavailability increases if the product is administered during meals.

A false positive reaction for glucose in urine may occur with Benedicts or Fehlings solution or with copper sulphate test tablets, but not with tests based on ezymatic glucose oxidase reactions.

Pregnancy and lactation: Studies carried out in several animal species have not shown any teratogenic or fetotoxic effects. However, the safety of cefpodoxime proxetil in pregnancy has not been established, and, as with all drugs, it should be administered with caution during the early months of pregnancy.

Cefpodoxime is excreted in human milk. Either breastfeeding or treatment of the mother should be stopped.

Effects on ability to drive and use machines: Attention should be drawn to the risk of dizzy sensations.

Undesirable effects: Possible side-effects include gastrointestinal disorders such as diarrhoea, nausea, vomiting and abdominal pain. Occasional cases have been reported of headaches, dizziness, tinnitus, parasthesia, asthema and malaise. Rare cases of allergic reactions including hypersensitivity, mucocutaneous reactions, skin rashes and pruritus. Occasional cases of bullous reactions such as Stevens Johnson Syndrome, toxic epidermal necrolysis and erythema multiforme have also been received. Transient moderate elevations of ASAT, ALAT and alkaline phosphatases and/or bilirubin have been reported. These laboratory abnormalities which may be explained by the infection, may rarely exceed twice the upper limit of the named range and elicit a pattern of liver injury, usually chlolestatic and most often asymptomatic. Slight increases in blood urea and creatinine have been reported. Exceptionally rare are the occurrence of liver damage and of haematological disorders such as reduction in haemoglobin, thrombocytosis, thrombocytopenia, leucopenia and eosinophilia. Haemolytic anaemia has been reported.

As with other cephalosporins, there have been rare reports of anaphylactic reactions, bronchospasm, purpura and angioedema.

Overdose: In the event of overdosage with Orelox, supportive and symptomatic therapy is indicated.

In cases of overdosage, particularly in patients with renal insufficiency, encephalopathy may occur. The encephalopathy is usually reversible once cefpodoxime plasma levels have fallen.

Pharmacological properties

Pharmacodynamic properties: Cefpodoxime proxetil is a beta-lactam antibiotic, a 3rd generation oral cephalosporin. It is the prodrug of cefpodoxime.

Following oral administration, Orelox is taken up by the gastro-intestinal wall where it is rapidly hydrolysed to cefpodoxime, a bactericidal antibiotic, which is then absorbed systemically.

Bacteriology: The mechanism of action of cefpodoxime is based on inhibition of bacterial cell wall synthesis. It is stable to numerous beta-lactamases.

Antibacterial acitivity: Cefpodoxime has been shown to possess in vitro bactericidal activity against numerous Gram-positive and Gram-negative bacteria.

It is highly active against the Gram-positive organisms: *Streptococcus pneumoniae*, streptococci of groups A *(S. pyogenes)*, B *(S. agalactiae)*, C, F and G, other streptococci *(S. mitis, S. sanguis and S. salivarius), Corynebacterium diphtheriae*.

It is highly active against the Gram-negative organisms: *Haemophilus influenzae* (beta-lactamase and non beta-lactamase producing strains), *Haemophilus para-influenzae* (beta-lactamase and non beta-lactamase producing strains), *Branhamella catarrhalis* (beta-lactamase and non beta-lactamase producing strains), *Neisseria meningitidis, Neisseria gonorrhoeae, Escherichia coli, Klebsiella* spp, *(K. pneumoniae, K. oxytoca), Proteus mirabilis*.

It is moderately active against: Methicillin-sensitive staphylococci, penicillinase and non-penicillinase producing strains *(S. aureus and S. epidermidis)*.

In addition, as with many cephalosporins, the following are resistant to cefpodoxime: enterococci, methicillin-resistant staphylococci *(S. aureus and S. epidermidis), Staphylococcus saprophyticus, Pseudomonas aeruginosa* and *Pseudomonas* spp., *Clostridium difficile, Bacteroides fragilis* and related species.

As with all antibiotics, whenever possible, sensitivity should be confirmed by *in-vitro* testing.

Pharmacokinetic properties: Orelox is taken up in the intestine and is hydrolysed to the active metabolite cefpodoxime. When cefpodoxime proxetil is administered orally to fasting subjects as a tablet corresponding to 100 mg of cefpodoxime, 51.5% is absorbed and absorption is increased by food intake. The volume of distribution is 32.3 litres and peak plasma levels of cefpodoxime occur 2 to 3 hours after dosing. The maximum plasma concentration is 1.2 mg/litre and 2.5 mg/litre after doses of 100 mg and 200 mg respectively. Following administration of 100 mg and 200 mg twice daily over 14.5 days, the plasma pharmacokinetic parameters of cefpodoxime remain unchanged.

Serum protein binding of cefpodoxime is 40%, principally to albumin. This binding is non saturable in type.

Concentrations of cefpodoxime in excess of the minimum inhibitory levels (MIC) for common pathogens can be achieved in lung parenchyma, bronchial mucosa, pleural fluid, tonsils, interstitial fluid and prostate tissue.

As the majority of cefpodoxime is eliminated in the urine, the concentration is high. (Concentrations in 0-4, 4-8, 8-12 hour fractions after a single dose exceed MIC_{90} of common urinary pathogens). Good diffusion of cefpodoxime is also seen into renal tissue, with concentrations above MIC_{90} of the common urinary pathogens, 3-12 hours after an administration of a single 200 mg dose (1.6-3.1 microgram/g). Concentrations of cefpodoxime in the medullary and cortical tissues is similar.

Studies in healthy volunteers show median concentrations of cefpodoxime in the total ejaculate 6-12 hours following administration of a single 200 mg daily dose to be above the MIC_{90} of *N gonorrhoeae*.

The main route of excretion is renal, 80% is excreted unchanged in the urine, with an elimination half life of approx 2.4 hours.

Preclinical safety data: Not applicable.

Pharmaceutical particulars

List of excipients: The product contains magnesium stearate, carboxymethylcellulose-calcium hydoypropylcellulose, sodium lauryl sulphate, lactose, ethyl alcohol and purified water. The coating contains titanium dioxide, talc and hydroxypropylmethyl-cellulose 6CP

Incompatibilities: None reported during clinical studies.

Shelf life: 36 months.

Special precautions for storage: Store below 25°C

Nature and contents of container: Orelox tablets are supplied in blister packs of 2,10 and 20 tablets.

Instruction for use/handling: None.

Marketing authorisation number PL 13402/0067

Date of approval/revision of SPC April 1998

Legal category POM

ORELOX* PAEDIATRIC GRANULES FOR ORAL SUSPENSION

Qualitative and quantitative composition When reconstituted, each 5 ml volume contains 52 mg of cefpodoxime proxetil (equivalent to 40 mg cefpodoxime).

Pharmaceutical form Granules for the preparation of an oral suspension.

Clinical particulars

Therapeutic indications: Orelox is a bactericidal cephalosporin antibiotic active against a wide range of Gram-negative and Gram-positive organisms. It is indicated for the treatment of the following infections either before the infecting organism has been identified or when caused by bacteria of established sensitivity.

Indications include:

Upper respiratory tract infections caused by organisms sensitive to cefpodoxime including acute otitis media, sinusitis, tonsillitis and pharyngitis.

Orelox should be reserved for recurrent or chronic infections, or for infections where the causative organism is known or suspected to be resistant to commonly used antibiotics.

Lower respiratory tract infections caused by organisms sensitive to cefpodoxime. Including pneumonia, acute bronchitis and when bacterial super-infection complicates bronchiolitis.

Upper and lower urinary tract infections caused by organisms sensitive to cefpodoxime including cystitis and acute pyelonephritis.

Skin and soft tissue infections caused by organisms sensitive to cefpodoxime such as abscesses, cellulitis, infected wounds, furuncles, folliculitis, paronychia, carbuncles and ulcers.

Posology and method of administration: Route of administration: oral.

Adult and elderly: not applicable for this product.

Children: The recommended mean dosage for children is 8 mg/kg/day administered in two divided doses at 12 hour intervals.

The following dosage regimen is proposed as a guide to prescribing:

Below 6 months:	8 mg/kg/day in 2 divided doses
6 months–2years:	5.0 ml twice daily
3—8 years:	10.0 ml twice daily
Above 9 years:	12.5 ml twice daily or 100 mg tablet twice daily

Orelox should not be used in infants less than 15 days old, as no experience yet exists in this age group.

A measuring spoon (5 ml) is provided with the bottle to aid correct dosing. One measuring spoon (5 ml) contains the equivalent of 40 mg cefpodoxime.

This product should be taken during meals for optimal absorption.

Renal impairment: The dosage of Orelox does not require modification if creatinine clearance exceeds 40 ml/min/1.73 m².

Below this value, pharmacokinetic studies indicate an increase in plasma elimination half life and maximum plasma concentrations, and hence the dosage should be adjusted appropriately.

Creatinine clearance (ml/min)	
39–10	Unit dose[1] administered as a single dose every 24 hours (i.e. half of the usual adult dose).
<10	Unit dose[1] administered as a single dose every 48 hours (i.e. quarter of the usual adult dose).
Haemodialysis patients	Unit dose[1] administered after each dialysis session.

Note: [1] The unit dose is either 100 mg or 200 mg, depending on the type of infection.

Hepatic impairment: The dosage does not require modification in cases of hepatic impairment.

Instructions for reconstitution: Before preparing the suspension the silica gel dessicant contained in a capsule inside the cap must be removed and disposed of. The suspension is prepared by adding water to the bottle up to the calibrated mark and shaking thoroughly to obtain an evenly dispersed suspension.

Contra-indications: Patients with hypersensitivity to cephalosporin antibiotics.

Patients with phenylketonuria since the product contains aspartame.

Special warnings and precautions for use: Preliminary enquiry about allergy to penicillin is necessary before prescribing cephalosporins since cross allergy to penicillins occurs in 5-10% of cases.

Particular care will be needed in patients sensitive to penicillin: strict medical surveillance is necessary from the very first administration. Where there is doubt, medical assistance, should be available at the initial administration, in order to treat any anaphylactic episode.

In patients who are allergic to other cephalosporins, the possibility of cross-allergy to Orelox should be borne in mind. Orelox should not be given to those patients with a previous history of immediate type hypersensitivity to cephalosporins.

Hypersensitivity reactions (anaphylaxis) observed with beta-lactam antibiotics can be serious and occasionally fatal.

The onset of any manifestation of hypersensitivity indicates that treatment should be stopped.

Orelox is not the preferred antibiotic for the treatment of staphylococcal pneumonia and should not be used in the treatment of atypical pneumonia caused by organisms such as *Legionella, Mycoplasma* and *Chlamydia.*

In cases of severe renal insufficiency it may be necessary to reduce the dosage regimen dependent on the creatinine clearance.

Antibiotics should always be prescribed with caution in patients with a history of gastrointestinal disease, particularly colitis. Orelox may induce diarrhoea, antibiotic-associated colitis and pseudomembranous colitis. These side-effects, which may occur more frequently in patients receiving higher doses for prolonged periods, should be considered as potentially serious. The presence of *C. difficile* should be investigated. In all potential cases of colitis the treatment should be stopped immediately. The diagnosis should be confirmed by sigmoidoscopy and specific antibiotic therapy (vancomycin) substituted if considered clinically necessary. The administration of products which cause faecal stasis must be avoided. Although any antibiotic may cause pseudomembranous colitis, the risk may be higher with broad-spectrum drugs, such as the cephalosporins.

As with all beta-lactam antibiotics, neutropenia and more rarely, agranulocytosis may develop particularly during extended treatment. For cases of treatment lasting longer than 10 days, blood count should therefore be monitored and treatment discontinued if neutropenia is found.

Cephalosporins may be absorbed onto the surface of red cell membranes and react with antibodies directed against the drug. This can produce a positive Coomb's test and, very rarely, haemolytic anaemia. Cross-reactivity may occur with penicillin for this reaction.

The product should not be used in infants less than 15 days old, as no clinical trial data in this age group yet exists.

Changes in renal function have been observed with antibiotics of the same class, particularly when given concurrently with potentially nephrotoxic drugs such as aminoglycosides and/or potent diuretics. In such cases, renal function should be monitored.

As with other antibiotics, the prolonged use of cefpodoxime proxetil may result in the overgrowth of non-susceptible organisms. With oral antibiotics the normal colonic flora may be altered, allowing overgrowth by clostridia with consequent pseudomembranous colitis. Repeated evaluation of the patient is essential and if superinfection occurs during therapy, appropriate measures should be taken.

Interactions with other medicaments and other forms of interaction: No clinically significant drug interactions have been reported during the course of clinical studies.

As with other cephalosporins, isolated cases showing development of a positive Coomb's test have been reported. (See *Precautions*).

Studies have shown that bioavailability is decreased by approximately 30% when Orelox is administered with drugs which neutralise gastric pH or inhibit acid secretions. Therefore, such drugs as antacids of the mineral type and H_2 blockers such as ranitidine, which cause an increase in gastric pH, should be taken 2 or 3 hours after Orelox administration.

In contrast, drugs which decrease gastric pH such as pentagastrine will increase bioavailability. The clinical consequences remain to be established.

The bioavailability increases if the product is administered during meals.

A false positive reaction for glucose in urine may occur with Benedicts or Fehlings solution or with copper sulphate test tablets, but not with tests based on ezymatic glucose oxidase reactions.

Pregnancy and lactation: Not applicable.

Effects on ability to drive and use machines: Not applicable.

Undesirable effects: Possible side effects include gastrotrointestinal disorders such as diarrhoea, nausea, vomiting and abdominal pain and rash, urticaria and itching.

Occasional cases have been reported of headaches, dizziness, tinnitus, parethesia, asthenia and malaise. Rare cases of allergic reactions including hypersensitivity, mucocutaneous reactions, skin rashes and pruritus. Occasional cases of bullous reactions including Stevens Johnson Syndrome, toxic epidermal necrolysis and erythema multiforme have also been received. Transient moderate elevations of ASAT, ALAT and alkaline phosphatases and/or bilirubin have been reported. These laboratory abnormalities which may also be explained by the infection, may rarely exceed twice the upper limit of the named range and elicit a pattern of liver injury, usually cholestatic and often symptomatic. Slight increases in blood urea and creatinine have also been reported. Exceptionally rare are the occurrence of liver damage and of haematological disorders such as reduction in haemoglobin, thrombocytosis, thrombocytopenia and eosinophilia. Haemolytic anaemia has extremely rarely been reported.

As with other cephalosporins, there have been rare reports of anaphylactic reactions, bronchospasm, purpura and angioedema.

Overdosage: In the event of overdosage with Orelox, supportive and symptomatic therapy is indicated.

In cases of overdosage, particularly in patients with renal insufficiency, encephalopathy may occur. The encephalopathy is usually reversible once cefpodoxime plasma levels have fallen.

Pharmacological properties

Pharmacodynamic properties: Orelox (cefpodoxime proxetil) is a beta-lactam antibiotic, a 3rd generation oral cephalosporin. It is the prodrug of cefpodoxime.

Following oral administration, Orelox is taken up by the gastro-intestinal wall where it is rapidly hydrolysed to cefpodoxime, a bactericidal antibiotic, which is then absorbed systemically.

Bacteriology: The mechanism of action of cefpodoxime is based on inhibition of bacterial cell wall synthesis. It is stable to numerous beta-lactamases.

Cefpodoxime has been shown to possess in vitro bactericidal activity against numerous Gram-positive and Gram-negative bacteria.

Antibacterial activity: It is highly active against the Gram-positive organisms: *Streptococcus pneumoniae,* streptococci of groups A *(S. pyogenes),* B *(S. agalactiae),* C, F and G, other streptococci *(S. mitis, S. sanguis and S. salivarius), Propionibacterium acnes, Corynebacterium diphtheriae.*

It is highly active against the Gram-negative organisms: *Haemophilus influenzae* (beta-lactamase and non beta-lactamase producing strains), *Haemophilus para-influenzae* (beta-lactamase and non beta-lactamase producing strains), *Moraxella catarrhalis* (beta-lactamase and non beta-lactamase producing strains), *Escherichia coli, Klebsiella* spp, *(K. pneumoniae), Proteus mirabilis.*

It is moderately active against: Methicillin-sensitive staphylococci, penicillinase and non-penicillinase producing strains (*S. aureus and S. epidermidis*).

In addition, as with many cephalosporins, the following are resistant to cefpodoxime: enterococci, methicillin-resistant staphylococci (*S. aureus* and *S. coagulase* (negative)), *Staphylococcus saprophyticus, Pseudomonas aeruginosa* and *Pseudomonas* spp., *Clostridium difficile, Bacteroides fragilis* and related species.

As with all antibiotics, whenever possible, sensitivity should be confirmed by in-vitro testing.

Pharmacokinetic properties: Orelox is taken up in the intestine and is hydrolysed to the active metabolite cefpodoxime. When cefpodoxime proxetil is administered orally to fasting subjects as a tablet corresponding to 100 mg of cefpodoxime, 51.5% is absorbed and absorption is increased by food intake. The volume of distribution is 32.3 litres and peak plasma levels of cefpodoxime occur 2 to 3 hours after dosing. The maximum plasma concentration is 1.2 mg/litre and 2.5 mg/litre after doses of 100 mg and 200 mg respectively. Following administration of 100 mg and 200 mg twice daily over 14.5 days, the plasma pharmacokinetic parameters of cefpodoxime remain unchanged.

Serum protein binding of cefpodoxime, 40% principally to albumin. This binding is non saturable in type.

Concentrations of cefpodoxime in excess of the minimum inhibitory levels (MIC) for common pathogens can be achieved in lung parenchyma, bronchial mucosa, pleural fluid, tonsils, interstitial fluid and prostate tissue.

As the majority of cefpodoxime is eliminated in the urine, the concentration is high. (Concentrations in 0-4, 4-8, 8-12 hour fractions after a single dose exceed MIC_{90} of common urinary pathogens). Good diffusion of cefpodoxime is also seen into renal tissue, with concentrations above MIC_{90} of the common urinary pathogens, 3-12 hours after an administration of a single 200 mg dose (1.6–3.1 microgram/g). Concentrations of cefpodoxime in the medullary and cortical tissues is similar.

Studies in healthy volunteers show median concentrations of cefpodoxime in the total ejaculate 6-12 hours following administration of a single 200 mg dose to be above the MIC_{90} of *N gonorrhoeae.*

The main route of excretion is renal, 80% is excreted unchanged in the urine, with an elimination half life of approx 2.4 hours.

Children: In children, studies have shown the maximum plasma concentration occurs approximately 2—4 hours after dosing. A single 5 mg/kg dose in 4-12 year olds produced a maximum concentration similar to that in adults given a 200 mg dose.

In patients below 2 years receiving repeated doses of 5 mg/kg 12 hourly, the average plasma concentrations, 2 hours post dose, are between 2.7 mg/litre (1-6 months) and 2.0 mg/litre (7 months-2 years).

In patients between 1 month and 12 years receiving repeated doses of 5 mg/kg 12 hourly, the residual plasma concentrations at steady state are between 0.2—0.3 mg/l (1 month—2 years) and 0.1 mg/l (2—12 years).

Preclinical safety data: Not applicable.

Pharmaceutical particulars

List of excipients: The product contains anhydrous colloidal silica, aspartame, banana flavour, carboxymetyhylcellulose-calcium, carboxymethylcellulose-sodium, citric acid monohydrate, hydroxypropylcellulose, yellow iron oxide, lactose monohydrate, monosodium glutamate, potassium sorbate, sodium chloride, sorbitan trioleate, sucrose and talc.

Incompatibilities: None reported during clinical studies.

Shelf life: 24 months. Reconstituted suspension: can be stored for up to 10 days refrigerated (2–8°C).

Special precautions for storage: Bottles: unreconstituted product should be stored below 30°C.

Nature and contents of container: Amber glass bottles with a calibration marking. This is fitted with a polyethylene dehydrating capsule containing silica gel, closed by a cardboard disc make up part of the closure. There is a polyethene pilfer and childproof screw cap fitted with a triseal joint.

Pack sizes of 50 ml, 75 ml, 100 ml or 125 ml of suspension.

A 5 ml plastic spoon is supplied with the pack.

Instruction for use/handling: Before preparing the suspension, the silica gel dessicant contained in the capsule inside the cap must be removed and disposed of. The suspension is prepared by adding water to the bottle up to the calibrated mark and shaking thoroughly to obtain an evenly dispersed suspension.

Marketing authorisation number PL 13402/0068

Date of approval/revision of SPC September 1998

Legal category POM

PERFAN* INJECTION

Qualitative and quantitative composition 5 mg/ml solution of enoximone presented in ampoules containing 20 ml.

Pharmaceutical form Solution for injection

Clinical particulars

Therapeutic indications: Perfan Injection is indicated for the treatment of congestive heart failure, typically where cardiac output is reduced and filling pressures increased, in patients who require intravenous therapy and who can be closely monitored. The duration of therapy should depend on the patient's continued positive and beneficial response. Sustained haemodynamic and clinical effects have been observed in patients treated for up to 48 hours.

Posology and method of administration: Perfan Injection is for intravenous administration (slow injection or continuous infusion) and must be diluted before use. Dilutions should be used immediately and any unused portion discarded.

Dilution: The pH of Perfan Injection is approximately 12.0. Perfan Injection must be diluted with an equal volume of 0.9% Sodium Chloride Injection or Water for Injections before administration.

Do not use more dilute solutions or other diluents, particularly dextrose injection, as crystal formation may occur.

Since crystal formation has been observed within approximately 1 hour after mixing Perfan Injection in glass containers or syringes, only plastic containers or syringes should be used for dilutions.

Administration: The following procedure is recommended for the administration of the diluted Perfan Injection.

Initial Therapy: Therapy should be initiated with a dose of 0.5–1.0 mg/kg given as a slow injection (not faster than 12.5 mg/min); further doses of 0.5 mg/kg may be given similarly every 30 minutes until a satisfactory response is achieved or a total initial dose of 3.0 mg/kg is reached. Alternatively treatment may be initiated as an infusion at a rate of 90 micrograms/kg/minute administered over 10 to 30 minutes until the required haemodynamic response is achieved.

Maintenance Therapy: To maintain the effects of Perfan Injection the initial dose (not more than 3.0 mg/kg) may be repeated as required every 3–6 hours and adjusted according to the response of the patient. Alternatively, a continuous or intermittent infusion at a rate of 5 to 20 micrograms/kg/minute may be instituted. Total dose over 24 hours should not normally exceed 24.0 mg/kg. In patients with renal impairment the dosage or dosage frequency may need to be reduced.

Precautions should be taken to avoid venous extravasation during administration.

This dosing regimen will produce, in the majority of patients, a 30% or greater increase in cardiac output and/or decreases in pulmonary capillary wedge pressure of about 30% and right atrial pressure of about 40%. It should be noted that the initial haemodynamic response determines the subsequent rate of administration as well as the duration of treatment.

Use in children: Safety and effectiveness in children have not been established.

Contra-indications: Perfan Injection is contra-indicated in patients with a known hypersensitivity to Perfan or its components.

Special warnings and precautions for use: Perfan Injection should be used cautiously when heart failure is associated with hypertrophic cardiomyopathy, stenotic or obstructive valvular disease or other outlet obstruction. Blood pressure and heart rate should be closely monitored during intravenous administration of Perfan Injection. In patients who show symptomatic decreases in blood pressure, Perfan Injection should be administered at a reduced rate or, if necessary, should be terminated.

Patients with severe congestive heart failure have a high incidence of arrhythmias and are particularly vulnerable to the development of arrhythmias. It is recommended that patients to be observed closely while receiving Perfan Injection.

Electrolyte and Fluid Balance: Fluid and electrolyte status and renal function should be assessed during therapy with Perfan Injection. Improvement in cardiac output with associated diuresis may require a reduction in the dose of diuretic drugs. Abnormal serum potassium levels (which may be due to excessive diuresis) may predispose patients to arrhythmias, especially those on digitalis. Therefore, serum potassium levels should be monitored carefully and corrective measures should be instituted before or during therapy with Perfan Injection. Hypovolaemia with inadequate cardiac filling pressure (which may be due to diuretic therapy) may prevent patients from responding adequately to Perfan Injection. Fluid and electrolyte status should be continuously monitored and corrective measures should be instituted before or during therapy with Perfan Injection.

Management of Adverse Reactions: Arrhythmias: The occurrence of severe supraventricular and ventricular arrhythmias may require immediate discontinuation of Perfan Injection and institution of appropriate antiarrhythmic therapy.

Platelet Count Reduction: Platelet counts before and during therapy are recommended.

Gastrointestinal Side Effects: Severe gastrointestinal side effects may be managed by reducing dosage, or if necessary, administration of Perfan Injection may be temporarily interrupted.

Increases in Hepatic Enzyme Levels: It is recommended to monitor patients for changes in hepatic enzyme levels. If clinically significant increases in hepatic enzymes occur following the intravenous administration of Perfan Injection, therapy should be discontinued.

Interactions with other medicaments and other forms of interaction: No clinical manifestations of untoward drug interaction were observed in patients receiving Perfan Injection most of whom concomitantly received one or more of the following: diuretics (amiloride, triamterene, frusemide and spironolactone), digitalis glycosides (digoxin), potassium supplements, antiarrhythmics (diltiazem, propranolol, lignocaine, nifedipine, procainamide and quinidine), vasodilators (captopril, hydralazine, nitroprusside and nitrates), anticoagulants (warfarin and heparin), analgesics (acetylsalicylic acid, paracetamol and codeine), sedatives (chloral hydrate, diazepam and lorazepam) and positive inotropic agents (dobutamine and dopamine).

In general, administration of Perfan Injection has not been associated with clinically significant alterations in laboratory tests. However, some changes have been noted in platelet counts (reduction in a small percentage of patients) and hepatic enzyme levels (a few patients with minor abnormalities). Monitoring of these parameters is recommended.

Pregnancy and lactation: There is no evidence of animal teratogenicity with oral therapy. Reproduction studies performed in rats at doses up to 300 mg/kg/day and 100 mg/kg/day have revealed reductions in maternal food consumption, maternal body weight gain and in pup weight at weaning and sexual maturity when enoximone was administered throughout pregnancy and lactation. Sexual behaviour and reproductive capability were unaltered by enoximone treatment. There are no adequate and well-controlled studies in pregnant women. Perfan Injection should be used during pregnancy only if the potential benefit justifies the potential risk.

It is not known whether this drug is excreted in human milk. Because many drugs are excreted in human milk, caution should be exercised when Perfan Injection is administered to a nursing mother.

Effects on ability to drive and use machines: Not applicable as the product is used in hospitalised patients.

Undesirable effects: Whilst Perfan Injection has not been shown to be arrhythmogenic in electrophysiological studies, ectopic beats have been observed in some patients during or after Perfan Injection administration. Ventricular tachycardias or supraventricular arrhythmias have been reported less frequently and are more likely to occur in patients with pre-existing arrhythmias. Perfan Injection may induce hypotension as a consequence of its vasodilator activity. Temporary discontinuation of treatment or a reduction in dosage will usually reverse these conditions.

Other side-effects reported include headache, insomnia, nausea and/or vomiting and diarrhoea.

Isolated cases of chills, oliguria, fever, urinary retention and upper and lower extremity pain have also been reported.

Overdose: Intravenous administration of Perfan Injection has been shown to produce reductions in blood pressure with occasional instances of hypotensive symptoms. If symptomatic hypotension is observed, administration of Perfan Injection should be reduced or discontinued. No specific antidote is known, but general measures for circulatory support should be taken.

Perfan Injection has been shown to have a low degree of acute toxicity in rats and mice. The oral LD_{50} of enoximone suspension exceeded 5000 mg/kg in both male and female rats and mice, while the intraperitoneal LD_{50} exceeded 2500 mg/kg in male and female rats and male mice; in female mice it was between 1600 and 2500 mg/kg. The true acute intravenous LD_{50} could not be determined because of the toxicity of the vehicle (approximately 12 ml/kg).

Pharmacological properties

Pharmacodynamic properties: Enoximone is an inodilator, possessing both positive inotropic and vasodilator properties. It differs in structure and mode of action from digitalis glycosides and catecholamines.

The exact mechanism of the inotropic and vasodilator effects of enoximone is not completely understood; however, animal studies have shown that the positive inotropic activity is direct and apparently results, at least in part, from a selective inhibition of cardiac phosphodiesterase III with a subsequent increase in cellular levels of cAMP. Enoximone has no significant direct effect on adenylate cyclase activity, Na^+, K^+-ATPase activity, CA^{++}-uptake by sarcoplasmic reticulum. The vasodilation activity is also direct and does not involve either blockade or stimulation of adrenergic receptors.

Pharmacokinetic properties: The median elimination half-life of enoximone was 4.2 hours in normal subjects and 6.2 hours in congestive heart failure patients. In the latter group who received single i.v. doses of 0.5 to 3.0 mg/kg, apparent total body clearance ranged from 3.7 to 13.0 ml/min/kg, and volume of distribution at steady state ranged from 1.1 to 3.6 l/kg. With continuous infusion at higher doses, the median clearance and median elimination half-life were 6.3 ml/min/kg and about eight hours, respectively. In patients with congestive heart failure a loading dose of 90 micrograms/kg/min over 20-60 minutes followed by an average maintenance infusion of 1.0 mg/min (range 0.5-1.25) over 48 hours maintained mean plasma levels at about 3.6 micrograms/ml and 9.7 micrograms/ml for the parent compound and active sulphoxide metabolite, respectively.

The primary route of elimination in man is via the kidney (or urine) following biotransformation to the sulphoxide, the principal urinary excretion product. On average, 78% of an oral dose is recoverable as the cardioactive sulphoxide metabolite in an eight-hour urine collection.

Enoximone is approximately 85% plasma protein bound and it is unlikely therefore that clinically significant drug interactions will occur as a result of displacement from protein binding.

Preclinical safety data: Not applicable

Pharmaceutical particulars

List of excipients: Alcohol (95%), sodium hydroxide, propylene glycol and Water for Injections.

Incompatibilities: Perfan Injection must only be diluted with 0.9% sodium chloride injection or water for injections. Do not use other diluents, particularly dextrose injection, as crystal formation has been observed after mixing.

Perfan injection must not be mixed in glass containers or syringes as crystal formation has been observed within approximately 1 hour after mixing. Only plastic containers or syringes should be used for dilutions.

Other drugs or fluids must not be mixed in the same container or administered concomitantly in the same infusion line as Perfan Injection.

Shelf life: 36 months unopened. 24 hours once diluted.

Special precautions for storage: Store at or below 20°C.

After dilution, the product must be stored at room temperature. Dilutions must not be refrigerated as crystal formation may occur.

Nature and contents of container: Glass ampoules (Type I Ph. Eur.) of 10 ml (50 mg enoximone/ampoule), 20 ml (100 mg enoximone/ampoule) or 25 ml (125 mg enoximone/ampoule) in cartons containing 10 ampoules.

Instructions for use/handling: No special information.

Marketing authorisation holder: Marion Merrell Ltd., Broadwater Park, Denham, Uxbridge, Middlesex UB9 5HP

Marketing authorisation number PL 4425/0086

Date of approval/revision of SPC August 1998

Legal category POM

PROCTOSEDYL*

Presentation Proctosedyl is available as smooth, off-white suppositories and as an odourless, yellowish-white, translucent, greasy ointment. Each suppository or gram of ointment contains the following active ingredients:

Cinchocaine Hydrochloride (micro) BP	5 mg
Hydrocortisone (micro) PhEur	5 mg

Uses The local anaesthetic cinchocaine relieves pain and relaxes sphincteric spasm. Pruritus and inflammation are relieved by hydrocortisone, which also decreases serous discharge.

Proctosedyl is therefore useful for the short term relief (not more than 7 days) of pain, irritation and pruritus associated with haemorrhoids and pruritus ani.

Dosage and administration A suppository is inserted morning and evening, and after each stool.

Apply the ointment in small quantities with the finger, on the painful or pruritic area, morning and evening and after each stool. For deep application attach cannula to tube, insert to full extent and squeeze tube gently from lower end whilst withdrawing.

The ointment may be used separately or concurrently with the suppositories.

Contra-indications, warnings, etc.

Contra-indications: Known hypersensitivity to any of the ingredients. Not for use in the presence of infection.

Pregnancy: In pregnant animals, administration of corticosteroids can cause abnormalities of foetal development. The relevance of this finding to human beings has not been established. However, topical steroids should not be used extensively in pregnancy, i.e. in large amounts or for long periods.

Precautions: Apply only to the region of the rectum and anus and surrounding skin. Hydrocortisone can cause thinning and damage of the skin especially of the face. As with all preparations containing topical steroids, the possibility of systemic absorption should be considered. In particular, long-term continuous therapy should be avoided in infants. Adrenal suppression can occur even without occlusion.

Side-effects: In persons sensitive to any of the

ingredients, skin rash may occur. Although less likely to cause adrenal suppression when applied topically, Hydrocortisone, applied to a large enough area, especially of damaged skin for long enough, or if under occlusive dressing, may have this adverse effect.

Pharmaceutical precautions Ointment: Store below 25°C. Suppositories: Store below 25°C.

Legal category POM.

Package quantities Proctosedyl Suppositories: Packs of 12. Proctosedyl Ointment: Tubes of 30 g (with cannula).

Further information Proctosedyl ointment contains white soft paraffin, liquid paraffin and wool fat. Proctosedyl suppositories contain Suppocire AM.

Product licence numbers
Proctosedyl Ointment PL 13402/0093
Proctosedyl Suppositories PL 13402/0109

REFLUDAN* ▼

Qualitative and quantitative composition
Lepirudin (INN) 50 mg
(Lepirudin is a recombinant DNA product derived from yeast cells)

Pharmaceutical form Powder for solution for injection or infusion

Clinical particulars
Therapeutic indications: Anticoagulation in adult patients with heparin-associated thrombocytopenia (HAT) type II and thromboembolic disease mandating parenteral antithrombotic therapy.

The diagnosis should be confirmed by the HIPAA (*h*eparin *i*nduced *p*latelet *a*ctivation *a*ssay) or an equivalent test.

Posology and method of administration: Treatment with Refludan should be initiated under the guidance of a physician with experience in coagulation disorders.

Please note: Recommendations for the initial dosage of Refludan are given in subsection 'Initial doage'. Dose modifications are to be derived from monitoring of aPTT (see *'Monitoring and modification of the Refludan dosage regime'*).

Initial dosage: Anticoagulation in adult patients with HAT type II and thromboembolic disease:

- 0.4 mg / kg bw intravenously as a bolus dose
- followed by 0.15 mg / kg bw / hour as a continuous intravenous infusion for 2 - 10 days or longer if clinically needed.

Normally, the dosage depends on the patient's body weight (bw). This is valid up to a bw of 110 kg. In patients with a bw exceeding 110 kg the dosage should not be increased beyond the 110 kg bw dose (see also 'see *'Monitoring and modification of the Refludan dosage regime'* and *'Method of administration'* and tables 2 and 3, below).

Monitoring and modification of the Refludan dosage regimen:

1. Standard recommendations
Monitoring:

- In general, the **dosage** (infusion rate) **should be adjusted to the** activated partial thromboplastin time, **aPTT.**
- The **first aPTT determination** should be done **4 hours after start** of Refludan therapy.
- The **aPTT** should be **monitored at least once daily.**
- **Target range** (therapeutic window) for the **aPTT:**
- Using 'Actin FS' or 'Neothromtin' on automated coagulometers the target range for the aPTT is 1.5 fold to 3 fold prolongation of the normal control value.
- With other reagents, the upper limit of the therapeutic aPTT window should be reduced to 2.5 fold prolongation of the normal control value.
- To obtain specific and exact aPTT limits, the laboratory equipment / test reagent used may be calibrated by spiking standardized human plasma with 0.15 μg/ml lepirudin (lower limit) and 1.5 μg/ml lepirudin (upper limit).

Dose modifications:

- **Any aPTT value out of the target range is to be confirmed at once** before drawing conclusions with respect to dose modifications, unless there is a clinical need to react immediately.
- If the **confirmed aPTT value** is **above** the target range, the infusion should be stopped for two hours. At restart, the infusion speed should be decreased by 50 % (no additional i.v. bolus should be administered). The aPTT should be determined again 4 hours later.
- If the **confirmed aPTT value** is **below** the target range, the infusion speed should be increased by 20 %. The aPTT should be determined again 4 hours later.

2. Recommendations for use in patients scheduled for a switch to oral anticoagulation
If a patient is scheduled to receive coumarin derivatives (vitamin K antagonists) for oral anticoagulation after Refludan therapy, the dose of Refludan should first be gradually reduced in order to reach an aPTT ratio just above 1.5 before initiating oral anticoagulation. As soon as an INR value of 2.0 is reached, Refludan therapy should be stopped.

3. Recommendations for use in patients with renal impairment
As lepirudin is almost exclusively excreted and metabolised renally (see also *Pharmacokinetic properties* section), the individual renal function should be considered prior to administration. In case of renal impairment relative overdose might occur even under standard dosage regimen. Therefore, the infusion rate must be reduced in case of known or suspected renal insufficiency (creatinine clearance below 60 ml/min or creatinine value above 1.5 mg/dl [133 μmol/l]).

Refludan has not been therapeutically administered to HAT type II patients with significant renal impairment. The following dosage recommendations are based on single-dose studies in a small number of patients with renal impairment. Therefore, these recommendations are only tentative.

Whenever available, dose adjustments should preferably be based on creatinine clearance values as obtained from a reliable method (24 h urine sampling). In all other cases the dose adjustment is based on the creatinine value.

In any case, the bolus dose must be reduced to 0.2 mg / kg bw.

The infusion rate given under *Initial dosage* section (and *Method of administration*, table 3) must be reduced according to table 1. Additional aPTT monitoring is mandatory.

Table 1: Reduction of infusion rate in patients with renal impairment

Creatinine clearance [ml/min]	*Creatinine value [mg/dl (μmol/l)]*	*Adjusted infusion rate [% of original dose]*
45–60	1.6–2.0 (141–177)	50 %
30–44	2.1–3.0 (178–265)	30 %
15–29	3.1–6.0 (266–530)	15 %
Below 15*	above 6.0 (530)*	avoid or STOP infusion*

*In haemodialysis patients or in case of acute renal failure (creatinine clearance below 15 ml/min or creatinine value above 6.0 mg/dl [530 μmol/l]), infusion of Refludan is to be avoided or stopped.

Only if aPTT values have fallen below the lower therapeutic limit (see *Monitoring and modification of the Refludan dosage regimen:* Monitoring: target range), further i.v. bolus doses of 0.1 mg / kg bw may be considered every other day.

Method of administration
Reconstitute the lyophilisate as described under *Instructions for use and handling.*

1. Initial i.v. bolus:

For i.v. bolus injection, a solution with a *concentration of 5 mg/ml* is needed. Intravenous **injection** is to be carried out **slowly.**

Table 2: Examples for standard injection volume according to body weight.

Body weight [kg]	*Injection volume [ml]* Dosage 0.4 mg/kg bw	Dosage 0.2 mg/kg bw
50	4.0	2.0
60	4.8	2.4
70	5.6	2.8
80	6.4	3.2
90	7.2	3.6
100	8.0	4.0
≥110	8.8	4.4

2. Intravenous infusion:

For continuous i.v. infusion, a solution with a *concentration of 2 mg/ml* is needed.

The **speed of the perfusor automate** [ml per hour] is to be set in a **body weight dependent** fashion.

Table 3: Examples for standard infusion speed according to body weight.

Body weight [kg]	*Infusion speed [ml/h]* Dosage 0.15 mg/kg bw/h	Dosage 0.1 mg/kg bw/h
50	3.8	2.5
60	4.5	3.0
70	5.3	3.5
80	6.0	4.0
90	6.8	4.5
100	7.5	5.0
≥110	8.3	5.5

Contra-indications: Refludan should not be used in the following situations:

- Known hypersensitivity to hirudins or other constituents of Refludan
- Pregnancy and lactation (see *'Use during pregnancy and lactation'*)

In the case of bleeding tendency it is generally not advisable to administer Refludan. In the individual case careful assessment weighing the risk of Refludan administration versus its anticipated benefit must be made by the treating physician.

This particularly includes the following:

- Recent puncture of large vessels or organ biopsy
- Anomaly of vessels or organs
- Recent cerebrovascular accident, stroke, or intracerebral surgery
- Severe uncontrolled hypertension
- Bacterial endocarditis
- Advanced renal impairment (see also *Recommendation for use in patients with renal impairment* under the *Monitoring and modification of the Refludan dosage regimen* in the *Posology and administration* section.)
- Haemorrhagic diathesis
- Recent major surgery
- Recent bleeding (e.g. intracranial, gastrointestinal, intraocular, pulmonary)
- Overt signs of bleeding.

Special warnings and special precautions for use:

- In case of renal impairment relative overdose might occur even under standard dosage regimen. Therefore, the rate of infusion must be reduced in case of known or suspected renal insufficiency (see *'Monitoring and modification of the Refludan dosage regimen'*: 3., and *'Pharmacokinetic properties'*). There is no experience with Refludan in patients with significant liver impairment. Liver cirrhosis may also affect the renal excretion of lepirudin.
- Formation of anti-hirudin antibodies was observed in about 40 % of HAT type II patients. This may result in a possibly enhanced anticoagulant effect of lepirudin. Therefore, strict monitoring of aPTT is necessary also during prolonged therapy. No evidence of a neutralisation of lepirudin or of an allergic reaction associated with the positive antibody test results was found.
- Re-exposure: So far, clinical trials have provided limited information to address recommendations for re-exposure. No adverse experience has been observed in relation to re-exposure of patients to Refludan. Nevertheless, special attention should be paid to patients receiving a second course of Refludan.
- Experience of combined therapy with thrombolytic agents in patients with HAT type II is very limited. Since the risk of serious bleeding is considerable in this situation, the dosage of Refludan should be substantially reduced. The optimal dose regimen of Refludan in these circumstances is not known.

Interactions with other medicinal products and other forms of interaction: No formal interaction studies have been performed.

Concomitant treatment with thrombolytics (e.g. rt-PA or streptokinase) may

- increase the risk of bleeding complications
- considerably enhance the effect of Refludan on aPTT prolongation.

Concomitant treatment with coumarin derivatives (vitamin K antagonists) may also increase the risk of bleeding.

Pregnancy and lactation: The safety of Refludan for use in human pregnancy or lactation has not been established.

In a standard embryo-foetal toxicity trial, decreased pup and maternal survival was observed.

There is currently no information available on the use of Refludan during lactation.

Refludan should therefore not be administered to pregnant women or nursing mothers (see also *'Contraindications'*).

Effects on ability to drive and use machines: Not applicable.

Undesirable effects:

1. The following safety information is based on 198 HAT type II patients treated with Refludan:

a) Bleeding:

- Bleeding from puncture sites and wound bleeding were observed in 6 % and 9 % of patients, respectively.
- Epistaxis or gastrointestinal bleeding occurred in 4 % and 1 % of patients, respectively.
- Haematuria and rectal bleeding were reported for 7 % and 3 % of patients, respectively.

- Haematoma were observed in 7 % of patients treated with Refludan.
- Postoperative haemothorax was observed in 3 % of patients.
- Lung bleeding and vaginal bleeding were reported for 1 % and 2 % of patients, respectively.
- Anemia or drop in haemoglobin value without obvious source of bleeding occurred in 12 % of patients.

All other bleeding events (esophageal bleeding, haematemesis, haemoperitoneum, haemoptysis, haemorrhagic gastritis, liver haemorrhage, mouth bleeding, petechiae, retroperitoneal bleeding) occurred in a single patient each.

In patients with HAT type II and thromboembolic disease treated with Refludan (n = 125), the overall bleeding rate was 39 % and major bleeds were recorded in 11 % of the patients.

b) Allergic reactions:

Allergic reactions, including skin reactions (eczema, maculopapular rash or rash) were reported in 4 % of patients.

c) Other reactions:

- Fever was observed in 7 % of patients.
- Injection site reactions occurred in 0.5 % of patients.
- Kidney failure was reported in 2 % of patients without evidence of a causal relationship.

2. Further undesirable effects[1] have been observed in studies with more than 900 patients treated with Refludan in other indications:

a) Bleeding:

Intracranial bleeding following lysis therapy with rt-PA or streptokinase is infrequent but may be life-threatening.

b) Allergic reactions:

Reports of allergic reactions including the terms:

- anaphylactoid reaction, anaphylactic reaction
- pruritus, urticaria, maculopapular rash, rash, hot flushes, isolated chills
- isolated cough, bronchospasm, stridor, isolated dyspnoea
- face edema, tongue edema, larynx edema, angioedema

have been documented frequently.

[1] The CIOMS III standard categories for verbal classification of frequencies are used:

Very common:	10 % or more	Uncommon (infrequent):	0.1 - 1 %
Common (frequent):	1 - 10 %	Rare:	0.01 - 0.1 %
		Very rare:	0.01% or less

Overdose: In case of overdose the risk of bleeding may be increased.

Currently, no specific antidote against lepirudin is available. If life-threatening bleeding occurs and excessive plasma levels of lepirudin are suspected, the following recommendations should be followed:

- Immediately STOP Refludan administration
- Determine aPTT and other coagulation parameters as appropriate
- Determine haemoglobin and prepare for blood transfusion
- Follow the current guidelines of shock-therapy.

Additionally, individual case reports and *in-vitro* data suggest that either haemofiltration or haemodialysis (using high flux dialysis membranes with a cut-off point of 50,000 Dalton, e.g. 'Polysulfon F60S', 'Polyamid/Polyflux-11', or 'AN/69 HF') may be useful in this situation.

Results from studies in pigs showed that the application of von Willebrand Factor (vWF, 66 I.U./kg bw) markedly reduced the bleeding time.

Pharmacological properties

Pharmacodynamic properties: Pharmacotherapeutic group: Antithrombotic drug (ATC Code: B01AX [Other Anticoagulants])

Lepirudin ([Leu1, Thr2]-63-desulfohirudin) is a recombinant hirudin derived from yeast cells. The polypeptide composed of 65 amino acids has a molecular weight of 6979.5 Dalton. Natural hirudin is produced in trace amounts as a family of highly homologous iso-polypeptides by the leech *Hirudo medicinalis.*

Lepirudin is a highly specific direct inhibitor of thrombin. Its activity is measured in a chromogenic assay. One anti-thrombin unit (ATU) is the amount of hirudin that neutralises one unit of WHO preparation 89/588 of thrombin. The specific activity of lepirudin is approximately 16,000 ATU/mg.

Its mode of action is independent of antithrombin III. Platelet factor 4 does not inhibit lepirudin. One molecule of hirudin binds to one molecule of thrombin and thereby blocks the thrombogenic activity of thrombin.

As a result all thrombin dependent coagulation assays are affected, e.g. the aPTT values increase in a dose-dependent fashion.

The clinical information on HAT type II in this SPC is based upon the data of two prospective trials comprising a total of 198 HAT type II patients treated with Refludan. In the indication HAT type II with thromboembolic disease (125 patients) the overall mortality during the study period was approximately 9 % while amputations and new thromboembolic complications were recorded in 6 % and 10 %, respectively.

Pharmacokinetic properties: The pharmacokinetic properties of lepirudin following i.v. administration are well described by a two-compartment model. Distribution is essentially confined to extra-cellular fluids and is characterized by an initial half-life of approximately 10 minutes. Elimination follows a first order process and is characterized by a terminal half-life of about 1.3 hours in young healthy volunteers.

Both, excretion and metabolism take place in the kidney, and about 45 % of the dose administered is detectable in the urine. About 35 % of the dose is excreted as unchanged compound.

The systemic clearance of lepirudin decreases in proportion to the existing glomerular filtration rate. In female patients the systemic clearance is about 25 % lower as compared to male patients.

In elderly patients the systemic clearance of lepirudin is about 25 % lower as compared to younger patients. Age alone causes a 7 % reduction in clearance from the age of 30 to 70 years. The majority of the difference in clearance between young and elderly patients is due to the differences in renal function. In patients with terminal renal insufficiency prolonged elimination half-lives of about 2 days were observed.

Preclinical safety data:

General toxicity: Single and repeat-dose toxicity studies in mice, rats and monkeys showed the adverse responses that could be expected from an exaggerated pharmacodynamic impact of lepirudin. In monkeys retinal haemorrhages occurred. Moreover, in rats slight to moderate sinushistiocytosis of the regional lymph nodes and decreased haemosiderin deposits in the spleen were observed. Antibodies against hirudin which appeared in several of the treated monkeys resulted in prolongation of the terminal half-life and an increase in systemic exposure to lepirudin.

Mutagenicity: Lepirudin was not mutagenic or clastogenic in standard assays for such effects.

Pharmaceutical particulars

List of excipients: 1 vial Refludan contains 90 mg freeze dried material

- 40 mg Mannitol
- Sodium hydroxide for adjustment to pH 7

Incompatibilities: Refludan should not be mixed with other drugs except for water for injections, isotonic-saline or glucose 5 %.

Shelf life: The shelf-life is 24 months.

Special precautions for storage: Refludan should be stored below +25 °C. Refludan should not be frozen.

Once reconstituted (as described under '*Instructions for use/handling*') Refludan is to be used immediately.

Keep out of the reach of children.

Nature and contents of container:

Injection vial: Colourless tubular glass vial (glass type I according to Ph.Eur.) sealed with rubber infusion stopper, plastic flip-off cap and aluminium cap.

Presentations:

- Pack with 1 vial Refludan containing 50 mg lepirudin
- Pack with 10 vials Refludan, each containing 50 mg lepirudin.

Instruction for use/handling and disposal (if appropriate): Refludan must not be used after the expiry date given on the pack and container.

General recommendations:

- Reconstitution and further dilution must be carried out under sterile conditions.
- For reconstitution water for injections or isotonic-saline are to be used.
- For further dilution isotonic saline or glucose 5 % are suitable.
- For rapid, complete reconstitution, inject 1 ml of diluent into the vacuum vial and shake it gently. On reconstitution a clear, colourless solution is usually obtained within less than 3 minutes.
- Do not use solutions which are cloudy or contain particles.
- The reconstituted solution is to be used immediately.
- The preparation should be warmed to room temperature before administration.
- Any unused solution must be discarded appropriately.
- For injection only polypropylene syringes may be used.

Preparation of a Refludan solution with a concentration of 5mg/ml: For i.v. bolus injection a solution with a concentration of 5 mg/ml is needed:

- Reconstitute one vial (50 mg of lepirudin) with 1 ml of either water for injections or isotonic saline.
- The final concentration of 5 mg/ml is obtained by transfer into a sterile, single-use syringe (of at least 10 ml capacity) and further dilution to a total volume of 10 ml using isotonic saline or glucose 5 %.
- The final solution is to be administered in a body weight-dependent fashion (see '*Posology and method of administration*').

Preparation of a Refludan solution with a concentration of 2mg/ml: For continuous i.v. infusion, a solution with a concentration of 2 mg/ml is needed:

- Reconstitute two vials (each containing 50 mg of lepirudin) with 1 ml each using either water for injections or isotonic saline.
- The final concentration of 2 mg/ml is obtained by transfer of both solutions into one sterile, single-use perfusor syringe (50 ml capacity) and further dilution to a total volume of 50 ml using isotonic-saline or glucose 5 %.

  The infusion speed of the perfusor automate is to be set in a body weight-dependent fashion (see '*Posology and method of administration*').
- The perfusor syringe must be changed at least every 12 hours after the start of the infusion.

Marketing authorisation holder: Hoechst Marion Roussel Ltd., Hoechst Marion Roussel Deutschland GmbH, D-65926 Frankfurt am Main.

Marketing authorisation number EU/1/97/035/001&2

Date of approval/revision of SPC 13 March 1997

Legal category POM

RELEFACT* LH-RH

Qualitative and quantitative composition Gonadorelin 100 microgram

Pharmaceutical form Solution for Injection

Clinical Particulars

Therapeutic indications: Intravenous injection of Relefact LH-RH causes release of LH (luteinizing hormone) and FSH (follicle-stimulating hormone) from the pituitary gland. It provides a means of assessing the reserve of LH and FSH in the pituitary glands of patients with suspected pituitary impairment. In addition, Relefact LH-RH may be of value in the differential diagnosis of delayed puberty and hypogonadism.

Posology and method of administration: Relefact LH-RH should be administered intravenously to adults or children as a single dose of 100 microgram. The test is based upon the pituitary response to this dose measured as serum LH and FSH levels. Qualitative data may be obtained from a single test but each laboratory must establish its own normal range for values of serum LH and FSH to obtain quantitative assessment of pituitary reserve.

Contra-indications: Relefact LH-RH should not be administered in pregnancy. There is a theoretical possibility of induction of ovulation following the administration of LH-RH. Pituitary adenoma is a relative contra-indication.

Special warnings and special precautions for use: None known

Interactions with other medicaments and other forms of interaction: None known

Pregnancy and lactation: Relefact LH-RH should not be administered in pregnancy

Effects on ability to drive and use machines: None known

Undesirable effects: Side-effects of any description are rare, but the following reactions have been reported in isolated cases in healthy women: abdominal pain, nausea, headache and increased menstrual bleeding.

Overdose: Overdosage with Relefact LH-RH has never been reported and is unlikely to be a problem.

Pharmacological properties

Pharmacodynamic properties: LH-RH, a decapeptide, is a hypothalamic releasing hormone which stimulates the synthesis of follicle-stimulating hormone and luteinising hormone in the anterior lobe of the pituitary as well as their release. LH-RH secretion is controlled by several factors including circulating sex hormones.

Hence, it is used in the assessment of the reserve of LH and FSH in the pituitary glands of patients with suspected pituitary impairment. In addition, it may be of value in the differential diagnosis of delayed puberty and hypogonadism.

Pharmacokinetic properties: LH-RH is rapidly hydrolysed in plasma ($t_{\frac{1}{2}}$ = 4 minutes) and about half of the dose has been detected in the urine as metabolites within the hour.

Preclinical safety data: Not applicable

Pharmaceutical particulars

List of excipients: Mannitol, sodium dihydrogen phosphate, sodium chloride and water for injections

Incompatibilities: Do not dilute or mix with any additive

Shelf life: Three years

Special precautions for storage: Store below 25°C

Nature and contents of container: 1 ml glass ampoule containing 100 microgram gonadorelin in 1 ml aqueous solution

Available in packs of 10 ampoules

Instruction for use/handling: Test procedure:

1. Obtain venous blood sample for control value of LH and, if facilities are available for its measurement, FSH.
2. Rapid intravenous injection of 100 microgram Relefact LH-RH.
3. Obtain venous blood sample 20 minutes after injection for measurement of LH/FSH response.

Interpretation of results:

1. *Normal response:* Following the administration of Relefact LH-RH there is a rise in serum LH within two minutes of injection; the response is dose-dependent. Peak levels are achieved 20–30 minutes after injection and baseline levels are approached six hours after a dose of 100 microgram. The FSH response is similar but of lesser magnitude (except a. prior to puberty when, in both sexes, the FSH response is higher than the LH response and b. in some patients with hypothalamic-pituitary dysfunction, e.g. anorexia nervosa). The normal female response to Relefact LH-RH shows cyclical variation, the response in the luteal phase being about twice that seen in the early follicular phase.
   It is important for each laboratory to establish its own normal ranges of LH and FSH according to the time of the menstrual cycle before attempting to obtain quantitative results.
2. *Assessment of pituitary function:* Relefact LH-RH is a very sensitive index of pituitary function. Consequently, many patients with pituitary tumours, who do not respond to other dynamic tests of pituitary function (such as the growth hormone response to hypoglycaemia), will show a normal response to Relefact LH-RH; others will show an impaired or absent response. A normal response to the Relefact LH-RH test in clinically hypogonadal patients with pituitary abnormalities indicates that their pituitary glands are capable of producing LH and FSH in response to therapy. Similar responses may be seen in patients with hypothalamic tumours such as craniopharyngiomas.
3. *Assessment of primary and secondary hypogonadism:* Patients with primary hypogonadism resulting from gonadal failure or gonadal dysgenesis will have an exaggerated response to Relefact LH-RH. The majority of these patients will also have elevated basal values. The test is of particular value in those cases where basal levels are normal.
   The majority of patients with congenital hypogonadotrophic hypogonadism with or without hyposmia (Kallman's syndrome) show a normal or impaired response to single doses of Relefact LH-RH.
   These results indicate that, in most cases of isolated pituitary gonadotrophin deficiency, there is a reduced output of hypothalamic hormone releasing factor. An absent response to a single injection, however, is not necessarily indicative of pituitary failure, as more than one injection may be required in order to produce a response.
4. *Assessment of delayed puberty:* In simple delayed puberty the LH and FSH responses are within the normal range, whereas patients with hypogonadotrophic hypogonadism or hypopituitarism have an absent or impaired response. Patients with primary gonadal failure will have an exaggerated response

Marketing authorisation number PL 13402/0043

Date of approval/revision of SPC December 1997

Legal category POM

RIFADIN* CAPSULES 150 mg
RIFADIN* CAPSULES 300 mg
RIFADIN* SYRUP 100 mg/5 ml

Qualitative and quantitative composition

Rifadin Capsules 150 mg:	Rifampicin Ph Eur 150 mg
Rifadin Capsules 300 mg:	Rifampicin Ph Eur 300 mg
Rifadin Syrup 100 mg/5 ml:	Rifampicin Ph Eur 100 mg

Pharmaceutical form

Rifadin Capsules 150 mg:	Blue and red hard gelatin capsules.
Rifadin Capsules 300 mg:	Red hard gelatin capsules.
Rifadin Syrup 100 mg/ 5 ml:	Raspberry coloured and flavoured suspension.

Clinical particulars

Therapeutic indications: Indications for use

Tuberculosis: In combination with other active anti-tuberculosis drugs in the treatment of all forms of tuberculosis, including fresh, advanced, chronic and drug-resistant cases. Rifadin is also effective against most atypical strains of *Mycobateria*.

Leprosy: In combination with at least one other active anti-leprosy drug in the management of multi-bacillary and paucibacillary leprosy to effect conversion of the infectious state to a non-infectious state.

Other Infections: In the treatment of Brucellosis, Legionnaires Disease, and serious staphylococcal infections. To prevent emergence of resistant strains of the infecting organisms, Rifadin should be used in combination with another antibiotic appropriate for the infection.

Prophylaxis of meningococcal meningitis: For the treatment of asymptomatic carriers of *N. meningitidis* to eliminate meningococci from the nasopharynx.

Haemophilus influenzae: For the treatment of asymptomatic carriers of *H.influenzae* and as chemoprophylaxis of exposed children, 4 years of age or younger.

Posology and method of administration: Recommended Dosage

For oral administration

The daily dose of Rifadin, calculated from the patient's body weight, should preferably be taken at least 30 minutes before a meal or 2 hours after a meal to ensure rapid and complete absorption.

Tuberculosis: Rifadin should be given with other effective anti-tuberculosis drugs to prevent the possible emergence of rifampicin-resistant strains of Mycobacteria.

Adults: The recommended single daily dose in tuberculosis is 8-12 mg/kg.

Usual daily dose: Patients weighing less than 50 kg–450 mg. Patients weighing 50 kg or more–600 mg.

Children: In children, oral doses of 10-20 mg/kg body weight daily are recommended, although a total daily dose should not usually exceed 600 mg.

Leprosy: 600 mg doses of rifampicin should be given once per month. Alternatively, a daily regimen may be used. The recommended single daily dose is 10 mg/kg.

Usual daily dose: Patients weighing less than 50 kg–450 mg. Patients weighing 50 kg or more–600 mg.

In the treatment of leprosy, rifampicin should always be used in conjunction with at least one other antileprosy drug.

Brucellosis, Legionnaires Disease or serious staphylococcal infections: Adults: The recommended daily dose is 600-1200 mg given in 2 to 4 divided doses, together with another appropriate antibiotic to prevent the emergence of resistant strains of the infecting organisms.

Prophylaxis of meningococcal meningitis: Adults: 600 mg twice daily for 2 days.

Children (1–12 years): 10 mg/kg twice daily for 2 days.

Children (3 months–1 year): 5 mg/kg twice daily for 2 days.

Prophylaxis of Haemophilus influenzae: Adults and children: For members of households exposed to *H. influenzae* B disease when the household contains a child 4 years of age or younger, it is recommended that all members (including the child) receive rifampicin 20 mg/kg once daily (maximum daily dose 600 mg) for 4 days.

Index cases should be treated prior to discharge from hospital.

Neonates (1 month): 10 mg/kg daily for 4 days.

Impaired liver function: A daily dose of 8 mg/kg should not be exceeded in patients with impaired liver function.

Use in the elderly: In elderly patients, the renal excretion of rifampicin is decreased proportionally with physiological decrease of renal function; due to compensatory increase of liver excretion, the terminal half-life in serum is similar to that of younger patients. However, as increased blood levels have been noted in one study of rifampicin in elderly patients, caution should be exercised in using rifampicin in such patients, especially if there is evidence of impaired liver function.

Contra-indications: Rifadin is contra-indicated in the presence of jaundice, and in patients who are hypersensitive to the rifamycins.

Special warnings and special precautions for use: Rifampicin should be given under the supervision of a respiratory or other suitably qualified physician.

Patients with impaired liver function should only be given rifampicin in cases of necessity, and then with caution and under close medical supervision. In these patients, lower doses of rifampicin are recommended and careful monitoring of liver function, especially serum glutamic pyruvic transaminase (SGPT) and serum glutamic oxaloacetic transaminase (SGOT) should initially be carried out prior to therapy, weekly for two weeks, then every two weeks for the next six weeks. If signs of hepatocellular damage occur, rifampicin should be withdrawn.

Rifampicin should also be withdrawn if clinically significant changes in hepatic function occur. The need for other forms of antituberculosis therapy and a different regimen should be considered. Urgent advice should be obtained from a specialist in the management of tuberculosis. If rifampicin is re-introduced after liver function has returned to normal, liver function should be monitored daily.

In patients with impaired liver function, elderly patients, malnourished patients, and possibly, children under two years of age, caution is particularly recommended when instituting therapeutic regimens in which isoniazid is to be used concurrently with Rifadin. If the patient has no evidence of pre-existing liver disease and normal pre-treatment liver function, liver function tests need only be repeated if fever, vomiting, jaundice or other deterioration in the patient's condition occur.

In some patients hyperbilirubinsemia can occur in the early days of treatment. This results from competition between rifampicin and bilirubin for hepatic excretion.

An isolated report showing a moderate rise in bilirubin and/or transaminase level is not in itself an indication for interrupting treatment; rather the decision should be made after repeating the tests, noting trends in the levels and considering them in conjunction with the patient's clinical condition.

All tuberculosis patients should have pre-treatment measurements of liver function.

Because of the possibility of immunological reaction (see side effects) occurring with intermittent therapy (less than 2 to 3 times per week) patients should be closely monitored. Patients should be cautioned against interrupting treatment.

Rifampicin has enzyme-inducing properties including induction of delta amino levulinic acid synthetase. Isolated reports have associated porphyria exacerbation with rifampicin administration.

Interactions with other medicaments and other forms of interaction: Rifampicin has been shown in animals and man to have liver enzyme inducing properties and may reduce the activity of anticoagulants, corticosteroids, cyclosporin, digitalis preparations, oral contraceptives, oral hypoglycaemic agents, dapsone, phenytoin, quinidine, narcotics and analgesics. It may be necessary to adjust the dosage of these drugs if they are given concurrently with Rifadin, particularly when it is initiated or withdrawn.

Patients on oral contraceptives should be advised to use alternative, non-hormonal methods of birth control during Rifadin therapy. Also diabetes may become more difficult to control.

If *p*-aminosalicylic acid and rifampicin are both included in the treatment regimen, they should be given not less than eight hours apart to ensure satisfactory blood levels.

Therapeutic levels of rifampicin have been shown to inhibit standard microbiological assays for serum folate and Vitamin B12. Thus alternative assay methods should be considered. Transient elevation of BSP and serum bilirubin have been reported. Therefore, these tests should be performed before the morning dose of rifampicin.

Pregnancy and lactation: At very high doses in animals rifampicin has been shown to have teratogenic effects. There are no well controlled studies with rifampicin in pregnant women. Therefore, Rifadin should be used in pregnant women or in women of child bearing potential only if the potential benefit justifies the potential risk to the foetus. When Rifadin is administered during the last few weeks of pregnancy it may cause post-natal haemorrhages in the mother and infant for which treatment with Vitamin K1 may be indicated.

Rifampicin is excreted in breast milk, patients receiving rifampicin should not breast feed unless in the physician's judgement the potential benefit to the patient outweighs the potential risk to the infant.

Effects on ability to drive and use machines: None stated.

Undesirable effects: Reactions occurring with either daily or intermittent dosage regimens include:

Cutaneous reactions which are mild and self-limiting and do not appear to be hypersensitivity reactions. Typically they consist of flushing and itching with or without a rash.

Gastrointestinal reactions consist of anorexia, nausea, vomiting, abdominal discomfort, and diarrhoea. Pseudomembranous colitis has been reported with rifampicin therapy.

Hepatitis can be caused by rifampicin and liver function tests should be monitored (see Precautions).

Thrombocytopenia with or without purpura may occur, usually associated with intermittent therapy, but is reversible if drug is discontinued as soon as purpura occurs. Cerebral haemorrhage and fatalities have been reported when rifampicin administration has been continued or resumed after the appearance of purpura.

Eosinophilia, leucopenia, oedema, muscle weakness and myopathy have been reported to occur in a small percentage of patients treated with rifampicin.

Reactions usually occurring with intermittent dosage regimens and probably of immunological origin include:

- 'Flu Syndrome' consisting of episodes of fever, chills, headache, dizziness, and bone pain appearing most commonly during the 3rd to the 6th monthly of therapy. The frequency of the syndrome varies but may occur in up to 50 % of patients given once-weekly regimens with a dose of rifampicin of 25 mg/kg or more.
- Shortness of breath and wheezing.
- Decrease in blood pressure and shock.
- Acute haemolytic anaemia.
- Acute renal failure usually due to acute tubular necrosis or acute interstitial nephritis.

If serious complications arise, e.g. renal failure, thrombocytopenia or haemolytic anaemia, rifampicin should be stopped and never restarted.

Occasional disturbances of the menstrual cycle have been reported in women receiving long-term anti-tuberculosis therapy with regimens containing rifampicin.

Rifampicin may produce a reddish discolouration of the urine, sputum and tears. The patient should be forewarned of this. Soft contact lenses may be permanently stained.

Overdose: In cases of overdose with Rifadin, gastric lavage should be performed as soon as possible. Intensive supportive measures should be instituted and individual symptoms treated as they arise.

Pharmacological properties

Pharmacodynamic properties: Rifampicin is an active bactericidial antituberculosis drug which is particularly active against the rapidly growing extracellular organisms and also has bactericidial activity intracellularly. Rifampicin has activity against slow and intermittently-growing *M. Tuberculosis*.

Rifampicin inhibits DNA-dependent RNA polymerase activity in susceptible cells. Specifically, it interacts with bacterial RNA polymerase but does not inhibit the mammalian enzyme. Cross-resistance to rifampicin has only been shown with other rifamycins.

Pharmacokinetic properties: In normal subjects the biological half-life of rifampicin in serum averages about 3 hours after a 600 mg dose and increases to 5.1 hours after a 900 mg dose. With repeated administration, the half-life decreases and reaches average values of approximately 2-3 hours. If does not differ in patients with renal failure and consequently, no dosage adjustment is required.

Rifampicin is rapidly eliminated in the bile and an enterophepatic circulation ensues. During this process, rifampicin undergoes progressive deacetylation, so that nearly all the drug in the bile is in this form in about 6 hours. This metabolite retains essentially complete antibacterial activity. Intestinal absorption is reduced by deacetylation and elimination is facilitated. Up to 30% of a dose is excreted in the urine, with about half of this being unchanged drug.

Rifampicin is widely distributed throughout the body. It is present in effective concentrations in many organs and body fluids, including cerebrospinal fluid. Rifampicin is about 80 % protein bound. Most of the unbound fraction is not ionized and therefore is diffused freely in tissues.

Preclinical safety data: Not applicable

Pharmaceutical particulars

List of excipients:

Rifadin Capsules 150 mg and 300 mg:

Corn starch PhEur
Magnesium stearate PhEur

Rifadin Syrup 100 mg/5 ml:

Agar PhEur
Sucrose PhEur
Methyl-p-hydroxybenzoate PhEur
Propyl-p-hydroxybenzoate PhEur
Potassium sorbate PhEur
Sodium metabisulphite PhEur
Tween 80 PhEur
Raspberry essence HSE
Saccharin USNF
Diethanolamine USNF
Purified water PhEur

Incompatibilities: None stated

Shelf life:

Rifadin capsules 150 mg and 300 mg: 4 years from date of manufacture

Rifadin syrup 100 mg/5 ml: 3 years from date of manufacture

Special precautions for storage:

Rifadin capsules 150 mg and 300 mg: Store below 25°C. Protect from light and moisture.

Rifadin syrup 100 mg/5 ml: Store below 30°C. Do not dilute. Dispense in clear or amber glass bottles.

Nature and contents of container:

Rifadin capsules 150 mg and 300 mg: Amber glass bottles of 100 tablets.Blister packs of 100 tablets in cardboard cartons. Blister material is aluminium foil / PVDC (Aluminium 0.025 mm; PVDC 20 gsm) and PVC / PVDC foil (PVC 0.25 mm; PVDC 60 gsm).

Rifadin syrup 100 mg/5 ml: 120 ml in amber glass bottles

Instruction for use/handling: Not applicable

Marketing authorisation holder: Marion Merrell Ltd., Broadwater Park, Denham, Uxbridge, Middlesex UB9 5HP

Marketing authorisation numbers

Rifadin capsules 150 mg	PL 4425/5915R
Rifadin capsules 300 mg	PL 4425/5916R
Rifadin syrup 100 mg/5 ml	PL 4425/5917R

Date of approval/revision of SPC May 1997

Legal category POM

RIFADIN* FOR INFUSION

Presentation 20 ml vial containing 600 mg Rifampicin BP (red lyophilised powder) and 10 ml ampoule of clear colourless solvent solution (pyrogen free water plus polysorbate 81).

Uses

Mode of action: Rifadin is a semi-synthetic antibiotic with bactericidal activity against most Mycobacteria and Gram-positive organisms. Rifadin is also active against Gram-negative organisms at higher concentrations.

Indications: Rifadin for Infusion is indicated for acutely ill patients who are unable to tolerate oral therapy e.g. post operative or comatose patients or patients in whom gastrointestinal absorption is impaired.

Oral therapy should be used where possible. As soon as patients are able to accept oral medication, they should be transferred to Rifadin Capsules or Syrup.

Tuberculosis: Rifadin, used in combination with other active anti-tuberculosis drugs, is indicated in the treatment of all forms of tuberculosis, including fresh, advanced, chronic and drug-resistant cases. Rifadin is also effective against most atypical strains of Mycobacteria.

Leprosy: Rifadin, used in combination with at least one other active anti-leprosy drug, is indicated in the management of multibacillary and paucibacillary leprosy to effect conversion of the infectious state to a non-infectious state.

Other infections: Rifadin is indicated in the treatment of Brucellosis, Legionnaires Disease, and serious staphylococcal infections. To prevent emergence of resistant strains of the infecting organisms, Rifadin should be used in combination with another antibiotic appropriate for the infection.

Preparation of infusion: Rifadin for Infusion is prepared by aseptically adding the solvent to the vial of rifampicin powder and shaking vigorously and continuously for about 30 seconds. When the powder has completely dissolved, the solution should be immediately diluted in 500 ml 5% glucose solution, or other suitable infusion fluid (see 'Pharmaceutical precautions'). It is suggested that the infusion is administered over a period of 2–3 hours. Rifadin solution should be used within 6 hours of preparation.

Dosage and administration Treatment with Rifadin for Infusion should include concomitant use of other appropriate antibacterials to prevent the emergence of resistant strains of the causative organism.

Tuberculosis:

Adults: A single daily administration of 600 mg given by intravenous infusion over 2 to 3 hours has been found to be effective and well tolerated for adult patients. Serum concentrations following this dosage regimen are similar to those obtained after 600 mg by mouth.

Children: The usual paediatric regimen is a single daily dose of up to 20 mg/kg bodyweight; the total daily dose should not normally exceed 600 mg.

Leprosy: The recommended daily dose is 10 mg/kg.

Usual daily dose: Patients weighing less than 50 kg – 450 mg. Patients weighing 50 kg or more – 600 mg. Alternatively, 600 mg doses of rifampicin may be given once per month.

In the treatment of leprosy, rifampicin should always be used in conjunction with at least one other antileprosy drug.

Brucellosis, Legionnaires Disease or serious staphylococcal infections:

Adults: The recommended daily dose is 600 – 1200 mg given in 2 to 4 divided doses, together with another antibacterial agent with similar properties to prevent the emergence of resistant strains.

Impaired liver function: A daily dose of 8 mg/kg should not be exceeded in patients with impaired liver function.

Use in the elderly: In elderly patients, the renal excretion of rifampicin is decreased proportionally with physiological decrease of renal function; due to compensatory increase of liver excretion, the serum terminal half-life is similar to that of younger patients. However, as increased blood levels have been noted in one study of rifampicin in elderly patients, caution should be exercised in using rifampicin in such patients, especially if there is evidence of liver function impairment.

When patients are able to accept oral medication, they should be transferred to Rifadin capsules or syrup.

Contra-indications, warnings, etc

Contra-indications: Rifadin for Infusion is contra-indicated in patients who are hypersensitive to rifamycins.

Although not recommended for use in patients with jaundice, the therapeutic benefit of Rifadin for Infusion should be weighed against the possible risks.

Use in pregnancy and lactation: At very high doses in animals rifampicin has been shown to have teratogenic effects. There are no well controlled studies with rifampicin in pregnant women. Therefore, Rifadin for Infusion should be used in pregnant women or in women of child bearing potential only if the potential benefit justifies the potential risk to the foetus. When rifampicin is administered during the last few weeks of pregnancy it may cause post-natal haemorrhages in the mother and infant for which treatment with Vitamin K1 may be indicated.

Rifampicin is excreted in breast milk and infants should not be breast fed by a patient receiving rifampicin unless in the physician's judgement the potential benefit to the patient outweighs the potential risk to the infant.

Precautions: Patients with impaired liver function should only be given rifampicin in cases of necessity, and then with caution and under close medical supervision. In these patients, lower doses of rifampicin are recommended and careful monitoring of liver function, especially serum glutamic pyruvic transaminase (SGPT) and serum glutamic oxaloacetic transaminase (SGOT) should be carried out. If signs of hepatocellular damage occur, rifampicin should be withdrawn. In patients with impaired liver function, elderly patients, malnourished patients, and possibly, children under two years of age, caution is particularly recommended when instituting therapeutic regimens in which isoniazid is to be used concurrently with rifampicin.

It is rarely necessary, in the absence of clinical findings, to increase the frequency of performing routine liver function tests in patients with normal pretreatment liver function. In the presence of complete renal failure, rifampicin is excreted entirely in the bile: provided hepatic function is not impaired the dosage of rifampicin need not be adjusted.

In some patients hyperbilirubinaemia resulting from competition between rifampicin and bilirubin for excretory pathways of the liver at the cell level can occur in the early days of treatment. An isolated report showing a moderate rise in bilirubin and/or transaminase level is not in itself an indication for interrupting treatment; rather the decision should be made after repeating the tests, noting trends in the levels and considering them in conjunction with the patient's clinical condition.

Rifampicin has enzyme-inducing properties including induction of delta amino levulinic acid synthetase. Isolated reports have associated porphyria exacerbation with rifampicin administration.

Drug/laboratory interactions: Rifampicin has been shown in animals and man to have liver enzyme inducing properties and may reduce the activity of anticoagulants, corticosteroids, cyclosporin, digitalis preparations, oral contraceptives, oral hypoglycaemic agents, dapsone, phenytoin, quinidine, narcotics and analgesics. It may be necessary to adjust the dosage of these drugs if they are given concurrently with Rifadin, particularly when it is initiated or withdrawn.

Therapeutic levels of rifampicin have been shown

to inhibit standard microbiological assays for serum folate and Vitamin B12. Thus alternative assay methods should be considered. Transient elevation of BSP and serum bilirubin have been reported. Therefore, these tests should be performed before the daily administration of Rifadin for Infusion.

Side-effects: Rifadin for Infusion is generally well tolerated and accepted by patients, although hypersensitivity reactions have been described and occasionally patients have experienced fever, skin rashes and nausea/vomiting.

Occasional instances of phlebitis and pain at the infusion site have been reported.

Reactions occurring with either daily or intermittent dosage regimens include:

Cutaneous reactions which are mild and self-limiting may occur and do not appear to be hypersensitivity reactions. Typically they consist of flushing and itching with or without a rash.

Gastro-intestinal reactions consist of anorexia, nausea, vomiting, abdominal discomfort, and diarrhoea. Pseudomembranous colitis has been reported with rifampicin therapy.

Hepatitis can be caused by rifampicin and liver function tests should be monitored (see Precautions).

Thrombocytopenia with or without purpura may occur, usually associated with intermittent therapy, but is reversible if the drug is discontinued as soon as purpura occurs. Cerebral haemorrhage and fatalities have been reported when rifampicin administration has been continued or resumed after the appearance of purpura.

Eosinophilia, leucopenia, oedema, muscle weakness and myopathy have been reported to occur in a small percentage of patients treated with rifampicin.

Reactions usually occurring with intermittent dosage regimens and probably of immunological origin include:

- 'Flu Syndrome' consisting of episodes of fever, chills, headache, dizziness, and bone pain appearing most commonly during the 3rd to the 6th month of therapy. The frequency of the syndrome varies but may occur in up to 50% of patients given once-weekly regimens with a dose of rifampicin of 25 mg/kg or more.
- Shortness of breath and wheezing.
- Decrease in blood pressure and shock.
- Acute haemolytic anaemia.
- Acute renal failure usually due to acute tubular necrosis or acute interstitial nephritis.

If serious complications arise, (renal failure, thrombocytopenia or haemolytic anaemia), rifampicin should be stopped and never restarted.

Occasional disturbances of the menstrual cycle have been reported in women receiving long term anti-tuberculosis therapy with regimens containing rifampicin.

Rifampicin may produce a reddish discolouration of the urine, sputum and tears. The patient should be forewarned of this. Soft contact lenses may be permanently stained.

Overdose: In cases of overdosage with rifampicin, intensive supportive measures should be instituted and individual symptoms treated as they arise.

Pharmaceutical precautions Rifadin for Infusion should be freshly prepared. Store below 25°C.

Compatibilities: Rifadin for Infusion is compatible with the following infusion solutions for up to 6 hours: Mannitol 10% and 20%, Macrodex with Saline Solution, Macrodex with Glucose Solution, Rheomacrodex, Sodium Bicarbonate 1.4%, Laevulose 5% and 10%, Ringer Lactate, Ringer Acetate, Dextrose 5% and 10%, Saline Solution.

Incompatibilities: Rifadin for Infusion is incompatible with the following: Perfudex, Sodium Bicarbonate 5%, Sodium Lactate 0.167M, Ringer Acetate with Dextrose.

Legal category POM

Package quantities Combined pack of one vial containing 600 mg Rifampicin BP, and one ampoule containing 10 ml solvent.

Further information Nil.

Product licence number PL 4425/0051

Product licence holder: Marion Merrell Ltd., Broadwater Park, Denham, Uxbridge, Middlesex UB9 5HP

RIFATER*

Presentation Smooth, round, shiny, light pink, sugar coated tablets containing Isoniazid PhEur 50 mg, Pyrazinamide PhEur 300 mg and Rifampicin PhEur 120 mg.

Uses Rifater is indicated in the treatment of pulmonary tuberculosis.

Dosage and administration Rifater is recommended in the initial intensive phase of the short-course treatment of pulmonary tuberculosis. During this phase, which lasts for 2 months, Rifater should be administered on a daily continuous basis. The concomitant administration of ethambutol or intramuscular streptomycin over the same period of time is advised.

Each Rifater tablet contains isoniazid (INH), pyrazinamide (Z) and rifampicin (RAMP) in such a ratio that the administration of 9–12 mg/kg RAMP, 4–5 mg/kg INH and 23–30 mg/kg Z can be achieved by giving 3 tablets daily to patients weighing less than 40 kg, 4 tablets to patients weighing 40–49 kg, 5 tablets to patients weighing 50–64 kg and 6 tablets to patients weighing 65 kg or more.

Rifater should be given as a single dose and preferably on an empty stomach at least 30 minutes before a meal or 2 hours after a meal to ensure rapid and complete absorption.

Once the initial intensive phase of treatment has been completed treatment can be continued with the combination rifampicin-isoniazid (Rifinah*) always on a daily basis.

This regimen, if correctly applied, is 100% effective with very few, if any, relapses. The clinical evidence indicates that these occur generally in the first 6 months after stopping treatment with bacilli fully sensitive to the drugs employed, so that changes in the drugs to be utilised for further treatment are not required. The regimen has been found to be fully effective also in the presence of a bacillary population resistant to isoniazid, to streptomycin or to both drugs.

Children: The ratio of the three drugs in Rifater may not be appropriate in children (e.g. higher mg/kg doses of INH are usually given in children than in adults). Rifater can be used only in special cases, after careful consideration of the mg/kg dose of each component.

Use in the elderly: Caution should be exercised in such patients, in view of the possible decrease of the excretory function of the kidney and of the liver.

Contra-indications, warnings, etc

Contra-indications: Rifater is contra-indicated in patients who are hypersensitive to any one of the components of the combination. Rifater is contra-indicated in the presence of jaundice.

Use in pregnancy and lactation: At very high doses in animals rifampicin has been shown to have teratogenic effects. There are no well controlled studies with Rifater in pregnant women. Therefore, Rifater should be used in pregnant women or in women of child-bearing potential only if the potential benefit justifies the potential risk to the foetus. When administered during the last few weeks of pregnancy, Rifater may cause post-natal haemorrhages in the mother and infant, for which treatment with Vitamin K1 may be indicated.

Rifampicin and isoniazid are excreted in breast milk and infants should not be breast fed by a patient receiving Rifater unless in the physician's judgement the potential benefit to the patient outweighs the potential risk to the infant.

Precautions: The precautions for the use of Rifater are the same as those considered when a triple individual administration of rifampicin, isoniazid and pyrazinamide is required. Each of these drugs has been associated with liver dysfunction. Patients with impaired liver function should only be given Rifater in cases of necessity and then with caution and under strict medical supervision. In these patients, careful monitoring of liver function, especially serum glutamic pyruvic transaminase (SGPT) and serum glutamic oxaloacetic transaminase (SGOT) should be carried out prior to therapy and then every two to four weeks during therapy. If signs of hepatocellular damage occur, Rifater should be withdrawn. Care should be exercised in the treatment of elderly or malnourished patients who may also require Vitamin B6 supplementation with the isoniazid therapy.

In some cases hyperbilirubinaemia resulting from competition between rifampicin and bilirubin for excretory pathways of the liver at the cell level can occur in the early days of treatment. An isolated report showing a moderate rise in bilirubin and/or transaminase level is not in itself an indication for interrupting treatment; rather, the decision should be made after repeating the tests, noting trends in the levels and considering them in conjunction with the patient's clinical condition.

Rifater should be used with caution in patients with a history of gout. If hyperuricaemia accompanied by an acute gouty arthritis occurs, the patient should be transferred to a regimen not containing pyrazinamide (e.g. Rifinah 150 or 300).

The possibility of pyrazinamide having an adverse effect on blood clotting time or vascular integrity should be borne in mind in patients with haemoptysis.

Because of the possibility of immunological reaction (see 'Side-effects') occurring with intermittent rifampicin therapy (less than 2 to 3 per week) patients should be closely monitored. Patients should be cautioned against interruption of dosage regimens since these reactions may occur.

Drug/laboratory interactions: Rifampicin has liver enzyme-inducing properties and may reduce the activity of a number of drugs including anticoagulants, corticosteroids, cyclosporin, digitalis preparations, quinidine, oral contraceptives, oral hypoglycaemic agents, dapsone, narcotics and analgesics. It may be necessary to adjust the dosage of these drugs if they are given concurrently with Rifater.

Patients using oral contraceptives should be advised to change to non-hormonal methods of birth control during Rifater therapy. Also diabetes may become more difficult to control.

If p-aminosalicylic acid and rifampicin are both included in the treatment regimen, they should be given not less than eight hours apart to ensure satisfactory blood levels.

Therapeutic levels of rifampicin have been shown to inhibit standard microbiological assays for serum folate and Vitamin B12. Thus alternative assay methods should be considered. Transient elevation of BSP and serum bilirubin have been reported. Therefore, these tests should be performed before the morning dose of rifampicin. Isoniazid may decrease the excretion of phenytoin or may enhance its effects. Appropriate adjustment of the anti-convulsant dose should be made.

Side-effects: Rifampicin: Reactions occurring with either daily or intermittent dosage regimens include: *Cutaneous reactions* which are mild and self-limiting and do not appear to be hypersensitivity reactions. Typically they consist of flushing and itching with or without a rash.

Gastro-intestinal reactions consist of anorexia, nausea, vomiting, abdominal discomfort, and diarrhoea. Pseudomembranous colitis has been reported with rifampicin therapy.

Hepatitis can be caused by rifampicin and liver function tests should be monitored. (See 'Precautions').

Thrombocytopenia with or without purpura may occur, usually associated with intermittent therapy, but is reversible if drug is discontinued as soon as purpura occurs. Cerebral haemorrhage and fatalities have been reported when rifampicin administration has been continued or resumed after the appearance of purpura.

Eosinophilia, leucopenia, oedema, muscle weakness and myopathy have been reported to occur in a small percentage of patients treated with rifampicin.

Reactions usually occurring with intermittent dosage regimens and probably of immunological origin include:

- 'Flu Syndrome' consisting of episodes of fever, chills, headache, dizziness, and bone pain appearing most commonly during the 3rd to the 6th month of therapy. The frequency of the syndrome varies but may occur in up to 50% of patients given once-weekly regimens with a dose of rifampicin of 25 mg/kg or more.
- Shortness of breath and wheezing.
- Decrease in blood pressure and shock.
- Acute haemolytic anaemia.
- Acute renal failure usually due to acute tubular necrosis or to acute interstitial nephritis.

If serious complications arise, (renal failure, thrombocytopenia or haemolytic anaemia), Rifater should be stopped and never restarted.

Occasional disturbances of the menstrual cycle have been reported in women receiving long term anti-tuberculosis therapy with regimens containing rifampicin.

Rifampicin may produce a reddish discolouration of the urine, sputum and tears. The patient should be forewarned of this. Soft contact lenses may be permanently stained.

Isoniazid: Severe and sometimes fatal hepatitis may occur with isoniazid therapy. Polyneuritis associated with isoniazid, presenting as paraesthesia, muscle weakness, loss of tendon reflexes etc., is unlikely to occur with the recommended daily dose of Rifater. Various haematological disturbances have been identified during treatment with isoniazid, including eosinophilia, agranulocytosis, and anaemia. High doses of isoniazid can cause convulsions. The possibility that the frequency of seizures may be increased in patients with epilepsy should be borne in mind.

Pyrazinamide: Adverse reactions, other than hepatic reactions, which have been attributed to pyrazinamide are active gout (pyrazinamide has been reported to reduce urate excretion), sideroblastic anaemia, arthralgia, anorexia, nausea and vomiting, dysuria, malaise, fever, urticaria and aggravation of peptic ulcer. The hepatic reaction is the most common adverse reaction and varies from a symptomless abnormality of hepatic cell function detected only through laboratory liver function tests, through a mild syndrome of fever, malaise and liver tenderness, to more serious reactions such as clinical jaundice and rare cases of acute yellow atrophy and death.

Overdosage: In cases of overdosage with Rifater, gastric lavage should be instituted and individual symptoms treated as they arise. Parenteral pyridoxine (Vitamin B6) should be given. Symptoms are more likely to be related to isoniazid, including coma, respiratory distress, hyperglycaemia and metabolic ketoacidosis.

Pharmaceutical precautions None.

Legal category POM.

Package quantities Blister strips of 20's in packs of 100's.

Further information Nil.

Product licence number PL 4425/0060.

Product licence holder: Marion Merrell Ltd., Broadwater Park, Denham, Uxbridge, Middlesex UB9 5HP

RIFINAH*

Presentation

Rifinah 300: orange, smooth, shiny, capsule-shaped sugar coated tablets containing 300 mg Rifampicin PhEur and 150 mg Isoniazid PhEur.

Rifinah 150: cyclamen, smooth, shiny, round, curved sugar coated tablets containing 150 mg Rifampicin PhEur and 100 mg Isoniazid PhEur.

Uses Rifinah 300 and Rifinah 150 are indicated in the treatment of all forms of tuberculosis, including fresh, advanced and chronic cases.

Dosage and administration Another anti-tuberculosis drug may be given concurrently with Rifinah until the susceptibility of the infecting organism to rifampicin and isoniazid has been confirmed.

Adults: Patients should be given the following single daily dose preferably on an empty stomach at least 30 minutes before a meal or 2 hours after a meal:
Rifinah 150: Patients weighing less than 50 kg – 3 tablets.

Rifinah 300: Patients weighing 50 kg or more – 2 tablets.

Use in the elderly: Caution should be exercised in such patients especially if there is evidence of liver impairment.

Contra-indications, warnings, etc

Contra-indications: Rifinah 300 and Rifinah 150 are contra-indicated in the presence of jaundice. Rifinah 300 and Rifinah 150 are contra-indicated in patients who are hypersensitive to rifamycins or isoniazid.

Use in pregnancy and lactation: Rifampicin has been shown to be teratogenic in rodents when given in large doses. There are no well controlled studies with Rifinah in pregnant women. Therefore, Rifinah should be used in pregnant women or in women of child bearing potential only if the potential benefit justifies the potential risk to the foetus.

When administered during the last few weeks of pregnancy, rifampicin can cause post-natal haemorrhages in the mother and infant, for which treatment with Vitamin K1 may be indicated.

Rifampicin and isoniazid are excreted in breast milk and infants should not be breast fed by a patient receiving Rifinah, unless in the physician's judgement the potential benefit to the patient outweighs the potential risk to the infant.

Precautions: Rifinah is a combination of 2 drugs, each of which has been associated with liver dysfunction.

Patients with impaired liver function should only be given Rifinah in cases of necessity, and then with caution and under close medical supervision. In these patients, careful monitoring of liver function, especially serum glutamic pyruvic transaminase (SGPT) and serum glutamic oxaloacetic transaminase (SGOT) should be carried out prior to therapy and then every two to four weeks during therapy. Similar care should be exercised in elderly patients, malnourished patients and children under two years of age. If signs of hepatocellular damage occur, Rifinah should be withdrawn. Care should be exercised in the treatment of elderly or malnourished patients who may also require Vitamin B6 supplementation with the isoniazid therapy.

In some cases hyperbilirubinaemia resulting from competition between rifampicin and bilirubin for excretory pathways of the liver at the cell level can occur in the early days of treatment. An isolated report showing a moderate rise in bilirubin and/or transaminase level is not in itself an indication for interrupting treatment; rather the decision should be made after repeating the tests, noting trends in the levels and considering them in conjunction with the patient's clinical condition.

Because of the possibility of immunological reaction (see *Side-effects*) occurring with intermittent rifampicin therapy (less than 2 to 3 times per week) patients should be closely monitored. Patients should be cautioned against interruption of dosage regimens since these reactions may occur.

Drug/laboratory interactions: Rifampicin has liver enzyme inducing properties and may reduce the activity of a number of drugs including anticoagulants, corticosteroids, cyclosporin, digitalis preparations, quinidine, oral contraceptives, oral hypoglycaemic agents, dapsone, narcotics and analgesics. It may be necessary to adjust the dosage of these drugs if they are given concurrently with Rifinah. Patients using oral contraceptives should be advised to change to non-hormonal methods of birth control during Rifinah therapy. Also, diabetes may become more difficult to control. When rifampicin is taken with para-aminosalicylic acid (P.A.S.), rifampicin levels in the serum may decrease. Therefore the drugs should be taken at least eight hours apart. Therapeutic levels of rifampicin have been shown to inhibit standard microbiological assays for serum folate and Vitamin B12. Thus, alternative assay methods should be considered. Transient elevation of BSP and serum bilirubin have been reported. Therefore, these tests should be performed before the morning dose of rifampicin. Isoniazid may decrease the excretion of phenytoin or may enhance its effects. Appropriate adjustments of the anticonvulsant dose should be made.

Side-effects:

Rifampicin: Reactions to rifampicin occurring with either daily or intermittent dosage regimens include:
Cutaneous reactions which are mild and self-limiting may occur and do not appear to be hypersensitivity reactions. Typically they consist of flushing and itching with or without a rash. More serious hypersensitivity cutaneous reactions occur but are uncommon.

Gastro-intestinal reactions consist of anorexia, nausea, vomiting, abdominal discomfort, and diarrhoea. Pseudomembranous colitis has been reported with rifampicin therapy.

Hepatitis can be caused by rifampicin and liver function tests should be monitored. (See 'Precautions').

Thrombocytopenia with or without purpura may occur, usually associated with intermittent therapy, but is reversible if drug is discontinued as soon as purpura occurs. Cerebral haemorrhage and fatalities have been reported when rifampicin administration has been continued or resumed after the appearance of purpura.

Eosinophilia, leucopenia, oedema, muscle weakness and myopathy have been reported to occur in a small percentage of patients treated with rifampicin.

Reactions usually occurring with intermittent dosage regimens and probably of immunological origin include:

- 'Flu Syndrome' consisting of episodes of fever, chills, headache, dizziness, and bone pain appearing most commonly during the 3rd to the 6th month of therapy. The frequency of the syndrome varies but may occur in up to 50% of patients given once-weekly regimens with a dose of rifampicin of 25 mg/kg or more.
- Shortness of breath and wheezing.
- Decrease in blood pressure and shock.
- Acute haemolytic anaemia.
- Acute renal failure usually due to acute tubular necrosis or to acute interstitial nephritis.

If serious complications arise (renal failure, thrombocytopenia or haemolytic anaemia) rifampicin should be stopped and never restarted.

Occasional disturbances of the menstrual cycle have been reported in women receiving long term antituberculosis therapy with regimens containing rifampicin.

Rifampicin may produce a reddish discolouration of the urine, sputum and tears. The patient should be forewarned of this. Soft contact lenses may be permanently stained.

Isoniazid: Severe and sometimes fatal hepatitis may occur with isoniazid therapy. Polyneuritis associated with isoniazid, presenting as paraesthesia, muscle weakness, loss of tendon reflexes etc., is unlikely to occur with the recommended daily dose of Rifinah. Various haematological disturbances have been identified during treatment with isoniazid, including eosinophilia, agranulocytosis, and anaemia. High doses of isoniazid can cause convulsions. The possibility that the frequency of seizures may be increased in patients with epilepsy should be borne in mind.

Overdosage: In cases of overdosage with Rifinah 300 or Rifinah 150, gastric lavage should be performed as soon as possible. Intensive supportive measures should be instituted and individual symptoms treated as they arise. Parenteral pyridoxine (Vitamin B6) should be given. Symptoms are more likely to be related to isoniazid, including coma, respiratory distress, hyperglycaemia and metabolic ketoacidosis.

Pharmaceutical precautions Store below 25°C.

If it proves necessary to open a blister pack, Rifinah 300 and Rifinah 150 should be dispensed in amber glass or plastic containers. Protect from moisture.

Legal category POM.

Package quantities Rifinah 300: Original packs of 56 tablets (4 weeks calendar packs); Blister packs of 100 tablets.

Rifinah 150: Original packs of 84 tablets (4 weeks calendar packs); Blister packs of 100 tablets.

Further information The recommended daily dose of Rifinah 300 or Rifinah 150 produces therapeutically effective blood levels of rifampicin and isoniazid, two of the most powerful antituberculosis drugs. Serum concentrations and the biological half-life of the two component drugs do not differ significantly from values obtained when the drugs are given alone.

Product licence numbers
Rifinah 150 PL 4425/0041
Rifinah 300 PL 4425/0042

Product licence holder: Marion Merrell Ltd., Broadwater Park, Denham, Uxbridge, Middlesex UB9 5HP

SABRIL* SACHETS

Qualitative and quantitative composition Each sachet contains vigabatrin 0.5 g

Pharmaceutical form Powder

Clinical particulars

Therapeutic indications: Recommended for the treatment of epilepsy which is not satisfactorily controlled by another antiepileptic drug.

Recommended as monotherapy for management of infantile spasms (West's syndrome).

Posology and method of administration: Sabril is for oral administration once or twice daily and may be taken before or after meals.

Sabril should be added to the patient's current therapeutic regimen.

Adults: Maximal efficacy is usually seen in the 2–4 g/day range. A starting dose of 1 g daily should be added to the patient's current anti-epileptic drug regimen. The daily dose should then be titrated in 0.5 g increments at weekly intervals depending on clinical response and tolerability. Although a slight increase in efficacy has been observed in some patients treated with up to a maximum of 6 g/day, this dose has been associated with an increased incidence of adverse effects. Doses above 4 g/day should only be used in exceptional circumstances with close monitoring for adverse effects.

There is no direct correlation between plasma concentration and efficacy. The duration of the effects of the drug are dependent on the rate of enzyme resynthesis rather than the concentration of the drug in the plasma.

Children: The recommended starting dose in children is 40 mg/kg/day increasing to 80–100 mg/kg/day depending on response. Convenient recommendations in relation to body weight are:

Bodyweight:	
10–15 kg	½–1 g/day
15–30 kg	1–1½ g/day
30–50 kg	1½–3 g/day
>50 kg	2–4 g/day

Infants: Monotherapy for infantile spasms (West's Syndrome): The recommended dose is between 60–100 mg/kg/day depending on the severity of the spasms. This may be titrated over a period of one week if necessary. Doses of up to 150 mg/kg/day have been used with good tolerability.

Elderly and patients with renal impairment: Since vigabatrin is eliminated via the kidney, caution should be exercised when administering the drug to the elderly and more particularly in patients with creatinine clearance less than 60 ml/min. Adjustment of dose or frequency of administration should be considered. Such patients may respond to a lower maintenance dose.

Contra-indications: Pregnant women (see 'Pregnancy and lactation') and patients who have a history of hypersensitivity to vigabatrin or its product components.

Special warnings and special precautions for use: In view of the results of animal safety studies, it is recommended that patients treated with Sabril are closely observed for adverse effects on neurological function. Intensive monitoring of neurological function in patients treated with Sabril, including 300 patients followed for 12 months or longer, has not given any indication of the development of neurotoxicity.

As with other antiepileptic drugs abrupt withdrawal may lead to rebound seizures. If a patient is to be withdrawn from Sabril treatment, it is recommended that this is done by gradually reducing the dose.

Sabril should be used with caution in patients with a history of psychosis or behavioural problems.

Visual field defects have been reported in patients receiving vigabatrin. The onset of symptoms has varied between 1 month and several years after the start of treatment. In most cases, visual field defects persisted even after discontinuation of treatment.

Visual field testing should be performed at baseline and during routine follow up of patients on vigabatrin. Patients should be instructed to report any new vision problems. If visual symptoms develop, then the patient should be referred to an opthalmologist for further evaluation and consideration given to discontinuation of the drug.

Interaction with other medicaments and other forms of interaction: As Sabril is neither metabolised, nor protein bound and is not an inducer of hepatic cytochrome P450 drug-metabolising enzymes, interactions with other drugs are unlikely. However, during controlled clinical studies a gradual reduction of about 20% in the plasma concentrations of phenytoin has been observed. The exact nature of this interaction is presently not understood, however, in the majority of cases it is unlikely to be of therapeutic significance.

The plasma concentrations of carbamazepine, phenobarbitone and sodium valproate have also been monitored during controlled clinical trials and no clinically significant interactions have been detected.

Pregnancy and lactation: As little data are available on the use of Sabril during pregnancy, it is currently contra-indicated in pregnant women.

Studies in animals have shown that vigabatrin does not adversely affect fertility, foetal development or pup development, nor is it teratogenic in the rat at doses up to 150 mg/kg or the rabbit at doses up to 100 mg/kg. However, in the rabbit at doses of 150 and 200 mg/kg, a slight increase in the incidence of cleft palate was observed.

There are no adequate and well-controlled studies in pregnant women. Congenital anomalies have been reported in the off-spring of mothers using vigabatrin during pregnancy. No trends in the type of abnormal pregnancy outcome are evident from the available data.

In the absence of data on the excretion of vigabatrin in human milk, breast feeding during Sabril treatment is not recommended.

Effects on ability to drive and use machines: As a general rule, uncontrolled epileptic patients are not allowed to drive or handle potentially dangerous machinery. In view of the fact that drowsiness has been observed in clinical trials with Sabril, patients should be warned of this possibility at the start of treatment.

Undesirable effects: Adverse reactions are mainly CNS related and probably a secondary consequences of the increase in GABA caused by Sabril. The most commonly reported adverse reactions are drowsiness and fatigue except in children where excitation/agitation are more frequent. Other CNS-related reactions that have been reported include dizziness, nervousness, irritability, headache, nystagmus, ataxia, tremor, paraesthesia, impaired or decreased concentration or alertness and less commonly confusion, memory disturbance and vision complaints such as diplopia. Rare cases of visual field defect, and retinal disorders (such as peripheral retinal atrophy) and very rare cases of optic neuritis or atrophy have been reported.

Psychiatric reactions (agitation, aggression, depression, abnormal thinking, paranoid reactions) have been reported during vigabatrin therapy. These reactions occurred in patients with and without a psychiatric history and were usually reversible when vigabatrin doses were reduced or gradually discontinued (see 'Special warnings and special precautions for use'). Depression was a common psychiatric reaction but seldom required discontinuation of vigabatrin. Less common reactions included psychotic symptoms. Hypomania and mania have been reported rarely.

The sedative effect of vigabatrin usually decreases with continuing treatment. However, rare instances of patients developing marked sedation/stupor/confusion in association with non-specific slow wave activity on electroencephalogram have been described soon after the introduction of vigabatrin. Such reactions have been fully reversible following dose reduction or discontinuation of vigabatrin.

Other adverse reactions reported include weight gain, oedema, minor gastro-intestinal side-effects and alopecia. Allergic reactions such as rash and urticaria have been reported rarely.

As with other antiepileptic drugs, some patients may experience an increase in seizure frequency with vigabatrin. Patients with myoclonic seizures may be particularly liable to this effect.

Laboratory data indicate that Sabril treatment does not lead to renal or hepatic toxicity. Decreases in SGOT or SGPT, which are considered to be a result of inhibition of these transaminases by Sabril, have been observed. Chronic treatment with Sabril may be associated with a slight decrease in haemoglobin which rarely attains clinical significance.

Overdose: There is no specific antidote and the usual supportive measures should be employed. Vigabatrin overdose has been reported. When provided, doses were most commonly between 7.5 g to 30 g; however ingestions up to 65 g have been reported. Nearly half of the cases involved multiple drug ingestions. None of the overdoses resulted in death.

Activated charcoal has been shown not to significantly absorb vigabatrin in an *in-vitro* study. The effectiveness of haemodialysis in the treatment of vigabatrin overdose is unknown.

Pharmacological properties

Pharmacodynamic properties: Sabril is an antiepileptic drug with a clearly defined mechanism of action. Treatment with Sabril leads to an increase in the concentration of GABA (gamma amino butyric acid), the major inhibitory neurotransmitter in the brain. This is because vigabatrin, the active ingredient in Sabril, was designed rationally as a selective reversible inhibitor of GABA-transaminase, the enzyme responsible for the breakdown of GABA.

Controlled and long-term clinical trials have shown that Sabril is an effective anticonvulsant agent when given as add-on therapy in patients with epilepsy not controlled satisfactorily by conventional therapy. This efficacy is particularly marked in patients with seizures of partial origin.

Pharmacokinetic properties: Vigabatrin is a water soluble compound. The absorption of Sabril is rapid and complete, with the presence of food having no effect. The drug is widely distributed with an apparent volume of distribution slightly greater than total body water. Plasma and CSF concentrations are linearly related to dose over the recommended dose range.

There is no direct correlation between plasma concentration and efficacy. This is a consequence of the mechanism of action of vigabatrin, the duration of the effects of the drug being dependent on the rate of enzyme resynthesis rather than on the concentration of drug in the plasma.

Sabril is eliminated from the plasma with a terminal half-life of 5–8 hours with approximately 70% of a single oral dose being recovered as unchanged drug in the urine in the first 24 hours post-dose. No metabolites have been identified.

Sabril does not induce the hepatic cytochrome P450 enzymes nor is it metabolised or protein bound. Therefore drug interactions are unlikely.

Preclinical safety data: Animal safety studies carried out in the rat, mouse, dog and monkey have indicated that vigabatrin has no significant adverse effects on the liver, kidney, lung, heart or gastrointestinal tract. In the brain, microvacuolation has been observed in white matter tracts of rat, mouse and dog at doses of 30–50 mg/kg/day.

In the monkey these lesions are minimal or equivocal. This effect is caused by a separation of the outer lamellar sheath of myelinated fibres, a change characteristic of intramyelinic oedema. In both rat and dog the intramyelinic oedema was reversible on stopping vigabatrin treatment and even with continued treatment histologic regression was observed. However, in rodents, minor residual changes consisting of swollen axons (eosinophilic spheroids) and mineralised microbodies have been observed. In the dog, the results of an electrophysiological study indicate that intramyelinic oedema is associated with an increase in the latency of the somatosensory evoked potential which is reversible when the drug is withdrawn.

In humans, there is no evidence of intramyelinic oedema. Tests done to confirm lack of significant adverse effect on neurological function include evoked potentials, CAT scans, magnetic resonance imaging, CSF analyses and in a small number of cases, neuropathological examinations of brain specimens.

Pharmaceutical particulars

List of excipients: Polyvinylpyrrolidone PhEur

Incompatibilities: Not applicable

Shelf life: 3 years

Special precautions for storage: None stated

Nature and contents of the container:
Containers(s): Sachets (paper, polythene/aluminium foil/laminated) packed in cardboard cartons.
Pack size: 50 sachets.

Instructions for use/handling: Not applicable

Marketing authorisation holder: Marion Merrell Ltd., Broadwater Park, Denham, Uxbridge, Middlesex UB9 5HP

Marketing authorisation number PL4425/0119

Date of first approval/revision of SPC January 1998

Legal category POM

SABRIL* TABLETS

Presentation
White, oval, biconvex, film-coated tablets with a breakline on one side and SABRIL on the other. Each tablet contains 500 mg vigabatrin.

Uses
Mode of action: Vigabatrin is a selective, irreversible inhibitor of GABA-transaminase. Treatment with Sabril leads to an increase in brain levels of GABA (gamma aminobutyric acid), the major inhibitory neurotransmitter in the brain.

Indications: Sabril is indicated for the treatment of epilepsy which is not satisfactorily controlled by another antiepileptic drug.

Sabril is recommended as monotherapy for the management of infantile spasms (West's Syndrome).

Dosage and administration Sabril is for oral administration once or twice daily and may be taken before or after meals. Sabril should be added to the patient's current therapeutic regimen.

Adults: Maximal efficacy is usually seen in the 2–4 g/day range. A starting dose of 1 g daily should be added to the patient's current antiepileptic drug regimen. The daily dose should then be titrated in 0.5 g increments at weekly intervals depending on clinical response and tolerability. Although a slight increase in efficacy has been observed in some patients treated with up to a maximum of 6 g/day, this dose has been associated with an increased incidence of adverse effects. Doses above 4 g/day should only be used in exceptional circumstances with close monitoring for adverse effects.

There is no direct correlation between plasma concentration and efficacy. The duration of the effects of the drug are dependent on the rate of enzyme resynthesis rather than the concentration of drug in the plasma.

Children: The recommended starting dose in children is 40 mg/kg/day increasing to 80–100 mg/kg/day depending on response. Convenient recommendations in relation to body weight are:

Bodyweight:	10–15 kg	1–2 tablets/day
	15–30 kg	2–3 tablets/day
	30–50 kg	3–6 tablets/day
	>50 kg	4–8 tablets/day

Infants: Monotherapy for infantile spasms (West's Syndrome): The recommended dose is between 60–100 mg/kg/day depending on the severity of the spasms. This may be titrated over a period of one week if necessary. Doses of up to 150 mg/kg/day have been used with good tolerability.

Elderly and patients with renal impairment: Since vigabatrin is eliminated via the kidney, caution should be exercised when administering the drug to the elderly and more particularly in patients with creatinine clearance less than 60 ml/min. Adjustment of dose or frequency of administration should be considered. Such patients may respond to a lower maintenance dose.

Contra-indications, warnings, etc
Contra-indications: Pregnant women (see *Use in pregnancy and lactation*); patients who have a history of hypersensitivity to vigabatrin or its product components.

Use in pregnancy and lactation: As little data are available on the use of Sabril during pregnancy, it is currently contra-indicated in pregnant women.

Studies in animals have shown that vigabatrin does not adversely affect fertility, foetal development or pup development, nor is it teratogenic in the rat at doses up to 150 mg/kg or the rabbit at doses up to 100 mg/kg. However, in the rabbit at doses of 150 and 200 mg/kg, a slight increase in the incidence of cleft palate was observed.

There are no adequate and well controlled studies in pregnant women. Congenital anomalies have been reported in the off-spring of some mothers using vigabatrin during pregnancy. No trends in the type of abnormal pregnancy outcome are evident from available data.

In the absence of data on the excretion of vigabatrin in human milk, breast-feeding during Sabril treatment is not recommended.

Precautions: As with other antiepileptic drugs abrupt withdrawal may lead to rebound seizures. If treatment is to be discontinued it is recommended that this is done by gradually reducing the dose.

Sabril should be used with caution in patients with a history of psychosis or behavioural problems.

Visual field defects have been reported in patients receiving vigabatrin. The onset of symptoms has varied between 1 month and several years after the start of treatment. In most cases, visual field defects persisted even after discontinuation of treatment.

Visual field testing should be performed at baseline and during routine follow up of patients on vigabatrin.

Patients should be instructed to report any new vision problems. If visual symptoms develop, then the patient should be referred to an opthalmologist for further evaluation and consideration given to discontinuation of the drug.

Warning: In view of the results of animal safety studies, it is recommended that patients treated with Sabril are closely observed for adverse effects on neurological function. Intensive monitoring of neurological function in patients treated with Sabril, including 300 patients followed for 12 months or longer, has not given any indication of the development of neurotoxicity.

Effects on driving ability: As a general rule, uncontrolled epileptic patients are not allowed to drive or handle potentially dangerous machinery. In view of the fact that drowsiness has been observed in clinical trials with Sabril, patients should be warned of this possibility at the start of treatment.

Side-effects: Adverse reactions are mainly CNS related and probably a secondary consequence of the increase in GABA caused by Sabril. The most commonly reported adverse reactions are drowsiness and fatigue except in children where excitation/agitation are more frequent. Other CNS-related reactions that have been reported include dizziness, nervousness, irritability, headache, nystagmus, ataxia, tremor, paraesthesia, impaired or decreased concentration or alertness and less commonly confusion, memory disturbance and vision complaints such as diplopia. Rare cases of visual field defect and retinal disorders (such as peripheral retinal atrophy) and very rare cases of optic neuritis or atrophy have been reported.

Psychiatric reactions (agitation, aggression, depression, abnormal thinking, paranoid reactions) have been reported during vigabatrin therapy. These reactions occurred in patients with and without a psychiatric history and were usually reversible when vigabatrin doses were reduced or gradually discontinued (See *Precautions*). Depression was a common psychiatric reaction but seldom required discontinuation of vigabatrin. Less common reactions included psychotic symptoms. Hypomania and mania have been reported rarely.

The sedative effect of vigabatrin usually decreases with continuing treatment. However, rare instances of marked sedation/stupor/confusion in association with non-specific slow wave activity on electroencephalogram have been described soon after the introduction of vigabatrin. Such reactions have been fully reversible following dose reduction or discontinuation of vigabatrin.

Other adverse reactions reported include weight gain, oedema, minor gastrointestinal side-effects and alopecia. Allergic reactions such as rash and urticaria have been reported rarely.

As with other antiepileptic drugs, some patients may experience an increase in seizure frequency with vigabatrin. Patients with myoclonic seizures may be particularly liable to this effect.

Laboratory data indicate that Sabril treatment does not lead to renal or hepatic toxicity. Decreases in SGOT and SGPT have been observed and may be a result of inhibition of these transaminases by Sabril. Chronic treatment with Sabril may be associated with a slight decrease in haemoglobin which rarely attains clinical significance.

Drug interactions: As Sabril is neither metabolised, nor protein bound and is not an inducer of hepatic cytochrome P450 drug-metabolising enzymes, interactions with other drugs are unlikely. However, during controlled clinical studies a gradual reduction of about 20% in the plasma concentrations of phenytoin has been observed. The exact nature of this interaction is presently not understood, however, in the majority of cases, it is unlikely to be of therapeutic significance.

The plasma concentrations of carbamazepine, phenobarbitone and sodium valproate have also been monitored during controlled clinical trials and no clinically significant interactions have been detected.

Overdose: There is no specific antidote and the usual supportive measures should be employed. Vigabatrin overdose has been reported. When provided, doses were most commonly between 7.5 g to 30 g; however, ingestions up to 65 g have been reported. Nearly half of the cases involved multiple drug ingestions. None of the overdoses resulted in death.

Activated charcoal has been shown not to significantly absorb vigabatrin in an *in-vitro* study. The effectiveness of haemodialysis in the treatment of vigabatrin overdose is unknown.

Pharmaceutical precautions None.

Legal category POM.

Package quantities Sabril Tablets: Blister strips of 10 in cartons of 100.

Further information Animal safety studies carried out in rat, mouse, dog and monkey have indicated that vigabatrin has no significant adverse effects on the liver, kidney, lung, heart or gastrointestinal tract. In the brain, microvacuolation has been observed in white matter tracts of rat, mouse and dog at doses of 30–50 mg/kg/day. In the monkey these lesions are minimal or equivocal. This effect is caused by a separation of the outer lamellar sheath of myelinated fibres, a change characteristic of intramyelinic oedema. In both rat and dog the intramyelinic oedema was reversible on stopping vigabatrin treatment and even with continued treatment histologic regression was observed. However, in rodents, minor residual changes consisting of swollen axons (eosinophilic spheroids) and mineralised microbodies have been observed. In the dog, the results of an electrophysiological study indicate that intramyelinic oedema is associated with an increase in the latency of the somatosensory evoked potential which is reversible when the drug is withdrawn.

In humans, there is no evidence of intramyelinic oedema. Tests done to confirm lack of significant adverse effect on neurological function include evoked potentials, CAT scans, magnetic resonance imaging, CSF analysis and in a small number of cases, neuropathological examinations of brain specimens.

Product licence numbers
Sabril Tablets 4425/0098

Product licence holder: Marion Merrell Ltd., Broadwater Park, Denham, Uxbridge, Middlesex UB9 5HP

SOFRA-TULLE*

Qualitative and quantitative composition Each unit is impregnated with Framycetin Sulphate BP 1% (Soframycin).

Pharmaceutical form A sterile, lightweight, lanoparaffin gauze dressing 10x10cm or gauze strip 30x10cm impregnated with Framycetin Sulphate BP 1% (Soframycin).

Clinical particulars
Therapeutic indications: Sofra-tulle has a wide range of antibacterial activity and is an ideal dressing for immediate use in a variety of infected lesions.

Thermal: Burns, scalds.

Traumatic: Lacerations, abrasions, bites, puncture, wounds, crush injuries.

Ulcerative: Varicose, diabetic, decubitus and tropical ulcers.

Elective: Skin grafts (donor and receptors sites) avulsion of finger and/or toe nails, circumcision, suture lines.

Miscellaneous: Secondary infected skin conditions (e.g. eczema, dermatitis, herpes zoster), colostomies, ileostomies, tracheostomies, incised abscesses, incised perionychia.

Posology and method of administration:

Adults, children and the elderly: If necessary, the lesion should first be cleansed, then a single layer of Sofra-tulle applied and covered with a suitable dressing.

When dressing ulcers, the tulle should be shaped to fit the ulcer crater.

If the lesion exudes profusely it is advisable to change the dressings at least once a day.

Contra-indications: Sofra-tulle is contra-indicated where there is known allergy to lanolin or to Soframycin, or where organisms are known to be resistant to the latter.

Special warnings and special precautions for use: In most cases, absorption of the antibiotic is negligible. However, where large body areas are involved e.g. 30% or more body burns, the possibility of ototoxicity being produced by prolonged applications should be borne in mind.

Interactions with other medicaments and other forms of interaction: None.

Use in pregnancy and lactation: There is inadequate evidence of safety in human pregnancy.

Effects on ability to drive and to use machines: None.

Undesirable effects (frequency and seriousness): Cross-sensitisation to Soframycin may occur in patients known to be allergic to streptomyces-derived antibiotics (neomycin, paramomycin, kanamycin).

Overdose: Unlikely to occur (refer to *Special warnings and special precautions for use*).

Pharmacological properties
Pharmacodynamic properties: Framycetin Sulphate has broad spectrum bactericidal activity against most Gram-positive and Gram-negative rods and many Gram-positive and Gram-negative cocci including some but not all streptococci.

Like other aminoglycoside antibiotics framycetin sulphate interferes with protein synthesis by specifically and irreversibly binding to the 30S subunit of sensitive 70S ribosomes resulting in misreading of m RNA. The precise mechanisms are unknown.

Pharmacokinetic properties: Absorption is negligible through the skin except for large burn areas. If there is absorption of framycetin sulphate, it is excreted unchanged in the urine by glomerular filtration.

Preclinical safety data: Not applicable.

Pharmaceutical particulars
List of excipients: The product contains Lanolin BP and White Soft Paraffin BP.

Incompatibilities: Not applicable.

Shelf-life: 36 Months.

Special precautions for storage: Store flat below 25°C.

Nature and contents of container: Each unit pack contains one sterile antibiotic gauze dressing 10cm x 10cm packed in cartons of 10 and 50 units.

Also available as: each unit pack contains one sterile antibiotic gauze strip 30cmx10cm packed in cartons of 10 units.

Instructions for use/handling: None.

Marketing authorisation holder: Roussel Laboratories Ltd., Broadwater Park, Denham, Uxbridge, Middlesex UB9 5HP

Marketing authorisation number 0109/5047R

Date of approval/revision of SPC January 1995

Legal category POM

STREPTASE* INJECTION 250000 IU
STREPTASE* INJECTION 750000 IU

Qualitative and quantitative composition Streptase Injection contains purified streptokinase as active ingredient. Each vial contains 250,000 or 750,000 International Units.

Pharmaceutical form Freeze dried powder for reconstitution into solution for infusion.

Clinical particulars
Therapeutic indications: Intravascular dissolution of thrombi and emboli in: extensive deep vein thrombosis; pulmonary embolism; acute or sub-acute occlusion of peripheral arteries; central retinal venous or arterial thrombosis.

Posology and method of administration: Streptase should be given by intravenous infusion in physiological saline, Haemaccel, 5% glucose, 5% fructose or ringer-lactate solution.

Loading dose: Since human exposure to streptococci is common, antibodies to streptokinase (streptokinase resistance) are found normally. Thus, a loading dose of Streptase sufficient to neutralise the resistance is required. A dose of 250,000 units of Streptase infused into a peripheral vein over 30 minutes has been found appropriate in over 90% of patients.

Maintenance dose: A maintenance dose infusion of 100,000 units/hour is given following the loading dose. Administer the maintenance dose of 100,000 units per hour for 72 hours for the treatment of deep vein thrombosis, for 24 hours for the treatment of pulmonary embolism (up to 72 hours if concurrent deep vein thrombosis is suspected), for 24–72 hours for the treatment of arterial thrombosis and for up to 12 hours for central retinal thrombosis.

Control of therapy: If the thrombin time of any other parameter of lysis after 4 hours of therapy is less than approximately 1.5 times the normal control value, discontinue Streptase as excessive resistance to streptokinase is present.

Children: In children, in whom it is always advisable to estimate the initial dose by means of the streptokinase resistance test, the recommended maintenance dose per hour is 20 units/ml blood volume.

Patient monitoring: Before commencing thrombolytic therapy, it is desirable to obtain a thrombin time (TT), activated partial thromboplastin time (aPTT), haematocrit and platelet count to obtain the haemostatic status of the patient. If heparin has been given, it should be discontinued and the TT or aPTT should be less than twice the normal control value before thrombolytic therapy is started.

In patients previously treated with coumarin derivatives, the INR (International Normalised Ratio) should be below 1.7 before starting therapy with streptokinase.

During the infusion, decreases in the plasminogen and fibrinogen level and an increase in the level of fibrin degradation products (FDP) (the latter two serving to prolong the clotting times of coagulation tests) will generally confirm the existence of a lytic state. Therefore therapy can be monitored by performing the TT or aPTT approximately 4 hours after initiation of therapy.

Anticoagulation after terminating intravenous streptokinase therapy: At the end of Streptase therapy, treatment with heparin by continuous intravenous infusion is recommended to prevent recurrent thrombosis. Heparin treatment (without a loading dose)

should not begin until the thrombin time has decreased to less than twice the normal control value (approximately 3 to 4 hours). (See manufacturer's prescribing information for proper use of heparin). This should be followed by oral anticoagulation in the conventional manner.

Contra-indications: Contra-indications to Streptase treatment include all conditions that are likely to be associated with existing or very recent haemorrhage, for example:

- active internal bleeding
- recent cerebrovascular accident
- intracranial or intraspinal surgery
- known intracranial neoplasm
- recent trauma to the head
- severe uncontrollable hypertension
- uncontrollable clotting disorders
- previous severe allergic reactions, including vasculitic purpura, to streptokinase or streptokinase-containing products.

Other contra-indications include:

Existing or very recent haemorrhage associated with:

- all forms of reduced blood coagulability, in particular spontaneous fibrinolysis
- local lesions with risk of bleeding (e.g. gastrointestinal conditions with existing haemorrhage, previous translumbar aortography, puncture of large arteries, intramuscular injection, indwelling catheters or endotracheal tubes)
- recent operations (up to the 6th post-operative day, depending on the extent of the procedure) and recent severe trauma
- recent abortion or delivery
- diseases of the urogenital tract with existing or potential sources of bleeding.

Recent streptococcal infections which have produced high anti-streptokinase titres (e.g. acute rheumatic fever, acute glomerulonephritis), or recent streptokinase therapy more than 5 days and less than 12 months previously.

Subacute bacterial endocarditis.

Pericarditis. In isolated cases pericarditis has been misdiagnosed as an acute nyocardial infarction and treated with Streptase leading to pericardial effusions and cardiac tamponade.

Severe hypertension with systolic values over 200 mmHg or diastolic values over 100 mmHg or hypertensive retinal changes Grades III/IV.

Severe liver or kidney damage.

Disorders of cerebral blood flow or recent cerebral haemorrhage.

Pulmonary disease with cavitation (e.g. open tuberculosis) or severe bronchitis.

Acute pancreatitis.

Advanced age with suspicion of arteriosclerotic degeneration.

Septic thrombotic disease.

Pregnancy (see *Precautions*).

Special warnings and precautions for use: Caution is necessary in patients with mitral valve defects or atrial fibrillation because of the danger of cerebral embolisation from the left side of the heart.

The risks of therapy must be weighed against the dangers of the disease.

Caution is necessary in patients with diabetic retinopathy as there may be an increased risk of local bleeding.

Streptokinase is unlikely to be effective in the following conditions:

- deep vein thrombosis more than 14 days old
- occlusion of central retinal artery more than 6–8 hours old and thrombosis of retinal vein more than 10 days old

Interactions with other medicaments and other forms of interaction: There is an increased risk of haemorrhage in patients who are receiving or have recently been treated with anticoagulants or any drugs which affect platelet formation or function. Simultaneous treatment with dextrans also increases the danger of haemorrhage. The effects of drugs which act upon platelet formation or function should be allowed to subside before starting long-term lysis with Streptase (see *Patient monitoring*).

If the patient has been given heparin, its effects can be neutralised by giving protamine sulphate.

In patients previously treated with coumarin derivatives, the INR should be below 1.7 before starting treatment with streptokinase.

Pregnancy and lactation: Streptase is contra-indicated in pregnancy.

There is no evidence from the drug's safety in pregnancy nor is there any evidence from animal work that it is free from hazard. Bleeding and anaphylactic reactions might cause abortion and fetal death, especially when Streptase is given within the first 18 weeks of pregnancy. Use only when there is no safer alternative and when the disease (as, for example, in individual cases of massive pulmonary embolism) carries a high risk for the mother.

Effects on ability to drive and use machines: Not applicable.

Undesirable effects:

1. Early reactions: Fever and chills, asthenia, malaise, headache, gastrointestinal symptoms or musculoskeletal pain may occur but usually respond well to symptomatic therapy.

If hypotension occurs, it can usually be controlled by temporarily slowing the infusion rate. Tachycardia or bradycardia have been observed occasionally.

Patients may develop allergic reactions (e.g. rash, flushing, dyspnoea, bronchospasm). Allergic reactions can be largely avoided by giving the initial intravenous dose slowly. Corticosteroids can also be given prophylactically (e.g. 100–250 mg methylprednisolone ten minutes before starting streptokinase therapy). If an allergic reaction occurs the infusion should be discontinued and the patient given intravenous corticosteroids together with adrenaline and an antihistamine. Once the symptoms have subsided treatment can be continued.

Streptokinase administration has been associated with low back pain. This may indicate an allergic response, and it may be appropriate to discontinue the infusion. In some cases, without other features of allergy, infusion has been continued with analgesic cover, without adverse consequence.

Anaphylactic reactions have been observed rarely. If an anaphylactic reaction occurs discontinue the infusion immediately and give adrenaline immediately by slow intravenous injection. In addition high doses of corticosteroids by slow intravenous injection may be given.

2. Haemorrhage: Minor bleeding may occur at infusion sites. Discontinuation of treatment is not necessary.

In serious haemorrhagic complications, streptokinase therapy should be discontinued and a proteinase inhibitor, e.g. aprotinin should be given in the following dosages:

Initially inject 500,000 KIU to one million KIU by slow intravenous injection or infusion (maximum rate 5 ml/min). If necessary, this should be followed by 200,000 KIU four-hourly until the bleeding stops.

In addition, combination with synthetic antifibrinolytics is recommended. If necessary, clotting factors can be substituted.

Severe haemorrhages including gastrointestinal and liver haemorrhages, splenic rupture, urogenital haemorrhages, rare cases of intracranial haemorrhages with their complications (also with fatal outcome) or retroperitoneal haemorrhages have been observed.

During thrombolytic treatment of acute myocardial infarction, haemorrhages into the pericardium including myocardial rupture can occur in individual cases.

Haemorrhage can occur in any tissue and organ in the body, and can present with symptoms affecting any body system, including the abdomen and cardiovascular, joints and CNS. Haemorrhage should be considered as a potential cause of unusual symptoms occurring after administration.

3. Other reactions: In a few sporadic cases, neuroallergic symptoms (Guillane-Barre syndrome, polyneuropathy) have been reported in temporal coincidence with Streptase administration.

Uveitis has been reported in temporal association with streptokinase administration.

Serum sickness has been reported but is rare. Arthritis, vasculitis and nephritis have been reported in temporal association with streptokinase administration.

Persistent angina pectoris and cardiac failure, possibly leading to cardiac and respiratory arrest, may occur during thrombolytic therapy of acute myocardial infarction.

The risk of pulmonary embolis in patients with deep vein thrombosis is not greater during treatment with streptokinase than during treatment with heparin alone. If acute or recurrent pulmonary embolism occurs during the treatment, the course of streptokinase should be continued as originally planned so as to lyse the emboli.

Non-cardiogenic pulmonary oedema has been observed in a few cases, mainly after intracoronary thrombolytic therapy in patients with extensive myocardial infarction.

Transient increases in liver function tests or bilirubin have been reported. Jaundice may occur as a consequence of bilirubin increase. A few cases of cholesterol embolism have been described in temporal coincidence with thrombolytic therapy, particularly in patients undergoing angiography.

Individual cases of cerebral convulsions have been reported under thrombolytic therapy, and in temporal coincidence with cardiovascular hypoxia and cerebral haemorrhage.

Overdose: Long term overdose of streptokinase may induce the risk of rethrombosis by prolonged decrease of plasminogen. (See also *Side-effects, Haemorrhages*).

Pharmacological properties

Pharmacodynamic properties: Streptokinase is an enzyme obtained from β haemolytic streptococci of the lancefield group C. It is a potent activator of the fibrinolytic enzyme system in man and it acts directly by complexing with plasminogen to form an activator complex which then reacts with plasminogen to form plasmin.

Pharmacokinetic properties: Streptokinase has a very short half-life, the first rapid clearance from the plasma is due to the formation of the complex between streptokinase and streptokinase antibody. The complex is biochemically inert and is cleared rapidly from the circulation. Once the antibody has been neutralised , the streptokinase activates plasminogen and the resulting complex acts on non complexed plasminogen to form plasmin. During these events the streptokinase is proteolytically modified into several lower molecular weight fragments.

Peak fibrinolytic activity is found in the blood about 20 minutes after dosing activity is detected in the urine 2 hours after dosing.

Preclinical safety data: Extensive studies in different species of laboratory animals have shown that multiple human doses do not have an acute toxic dose.

Pharmaceutical particulars

List of excipients: Human albumin, sodium-L-hydrogen glutamate monohydrate and polygeline.

Incompatibilities: Other drugs should not be added to the infusion solution.

Shelf-life: Three years.

Special precautions for storage: Streptase should be stored below +25°C. Once dissolved in physiological saline Streptase can be stored for 24 hours at +2 to +8°C without loss of activity.

Nature and contents of container: 5 ml multidose glass vials, containing 250,000 or 750,000 International Units of streptokinase.

Instructions for use/handling: To ensure that the contents of the vial are rapidly and completely dissolved, 5 ml physiological saline should be injected into the vial and the residual vacuum removed by briefly loosening the needle from the syringe.

Marketing authorisation numbers

Streptase 250,000 IU	PL 13402/0045
Streptase 750,000 IU	PL 13402/0046

Date of approval/revision of SPC December 1997

Legal category POM

STREPTASE* INJECTION 1.5 Million IU

Qualitative and quantitative composition Streptase contains purified streptokinase as active ingredient. Each vial contains 1.5 million International Units.

Pharmaceutical form Freeze dried powder for reconstitution into solution for infusion.

Clinical particulars

Therapeutic indication: Treatment of acute myocardial infarction

Posology and method of administration:

Adults: Streptase should be given by intravenous infusion in 50-200 ml physiological saline

or 5% glucose, 5% fructose, Ringer-lactate solution or Haemaccel as soon as possible after the onset of symptoms. The efficacy of Streptase therapy is diminished if treatment is delayed. The benefit/risk profile of treatment initiated more than 12 hours after the onset of a myocardial infarction is uncertain. A single dose of 1.5 million IU streptokinase should be infused over one hour. No laboratory controls are necessary.

Children: There are no recommendations for the use of Streptase in acute myocardial infarction in children.

Adjuvant therapy: Treatment with aspirin (150 mg daily) for at least 4 weeks is recommended for prophylaxis after streptokinase therapy for acute myocardial infarction.

The first dose should be given as soon as possible after the myocardial infarction.

Contra-indications: Contra-indications to Streptase treatment include all conditions that are likely to be associated with existing or very recent haemorrhage. Absolute contra-indications include:

- Active internal bleeding
- Recent cerebrovascular accident
- Intracranial or intra-spinal surgery
- Recent trauma to the head
- Known intracranial neoplasm
- Severe uncontrollable hypertension
- Uncontrollable clotting disorders (with the exception of consumption coagulopathy)

– Previous severe allergic reactions, including vasculitic purpura, to streptokinase or streptokinase-containing products.

The following conditions would normally be considered to be contraindications to Streptase therapy. However, in certain situations the benefits of treatment may be considered to outweigh the potential risks. 'Relative' contra-indications of this nature include:

Existing or very recent haemorrhage:

- All forms of reduced blood coagulability, in particular spontaneous fibrinolysis.
- Local lesions with risk of bleeding (e.g. gastrointestinal conditions with existing haemorrhage, previous translumbar aortography, puncture of large arteries, intramuscular injections, indwelling catheters or endotracheal tubes).
- Recent operations (up to the 6th post-operative day, depending on the extent of the procedure) and recent severe trauma.
- Recent abortion or delivery.
- Diseases of the urogenital tract with existing or potential sources of bleeding.

Recent streptococcal infections which have produced high anti-streptokinase titres (e.g. acute rheumatic fever, acute glomerulonephritis), or recent streptokinase therapy more than 5 days and less than 12 months previously.

Subacute bacterial endocarditis.

Pericarditis. In isolated cases pericarditis has been misdiagnosed as an acute myocardial infarction and treated with Streptase, leading to pericardial effusions and cardiac tamponade.

Severe hypertension with systolic values over 200 mm/Hg or diastolic values over 100 mg/Hg or hypertensive retinal changes grades III/IV.

Severe liver or kidney damage.

Disorders of cerebral blood flow or recent cerebral haemorrhage.

Pulmonary diseases with cavitation (e.g. open tuberculosis) or severe bronchitis.

Acute pancreatitis.

Advanced age with suspicion of arteriosclerotic degeneration.

Septic thrombotic disease.

Pregnancy (see *Precautions*).

Special warnings and special precautions for use: Caution is necessary in patients with mitral valve defects or atrial fibrillation, because of the danger of cerebral embolisation from the left side of the heart.

The risk of therapy must be weighed against the dangers of the disease.

Caution is necessary in patients with diabetic retinopathy as there may be an increased risk of local bleeding.

Interaction with other medicaments and other forms of interaction: There is an increased risk of haemorrhage in patients who are receiving or who have recently been treated with anticoagulants or any drugs which affect platelet formation or function. Simultaneous treatment with dextrans also increased the danger of haemorrhage.

If the patient has previously been receiving heparin, its effects can be neutralised by giving protamine sulphate.

In patients previously treated with coumarin derivatives, the INR should be below 1.7 before starting treatment with streptokinase.

Pregnancy and lactation: Streptase is contra-indicated in pregnancy.

There is no evidence of the drug's safety in pregnancy, nor is there evidence from animal work that it is free from hazard. Bleeding and anaphylactic reactions might cause abortion and fetal death, especially when Streptase is given within the first 18 weeks of pregnancy. Use only when there is no safer alternative.

Effects on ability to drive and use machines: Not applicable.

Undesirable effects:

Haemorrhages: Minor bleeding may occur at infusion sites. Discontinuation of treatment is not necessary.

In serious haemorrhagic complications, streptokinase therapy should be discontinued and a proteinase inhibitor, e.g. aprotinin should be given in the following dosages:

Initially inject 500,000 KIU to one million KIU by slow intravenous injection of infusion

(maximum rates 5 ml/min). If necessary, this should be followed by 200,000 KIU four-hourly until the bleeding stops.

In addition, combination with synthetic antifibrinolytics is recommended. If necessary, clotting factors can be substituted.

Severe haemorrhages including gastrointestinal and liver haemorrhages, splenic rupture, urogenital haemorrhages, rare cases of intracranial haemorrhages with their complications (also with fatal outcome) or retroperitoneal haemorrhages have been observed.

During thrombolytic treatment of acute myocardial infarction, haemorrhages into the pericardium including myocardial rupture can occur in individual cases.

Haemorrhage can occur in any tissue and organ in the body and can present with symptoms affecting any body system, including the abdomen and cardiovascular system, joints and CNS.

Haemorrhage should be considered as a potential cause of unusual symptoms occurring after administration.

Early reactions: Early reactions such as fever and chills, asthenia, malaise, headache, gastrointestinal symptoms or musculoskeletal pain are less likely to occur after a single infusion of Streptase than during prolonged therapy. Such reactions usually respond well to symptomatic therapy.

Patients may develop allergic reactions (e.g. rash, flushing, dyspnoea, bronchospasm). Allergic reactions can be largely avoided by giving the initial intravenous dose slowly. Corticosteroids can also be given prophylactically (e.g. 100–250 mg methylprednisolone 10 minutes before starting streptokinase treatment). If an allergic reaction occurs the infusion should be discontinued and the patient given intravenous corticosteroids together with adrenaline and an antihistamine. Once the symptoms have subsided, treatment can be continued.

Streptokinase administration has been associated with low back pain. This may indicate an allergic response, and it may be appropriate to discontinue the infusion. In some cases, without other features of allergy, infusion has been continued with analgesic cover, without adverse consequence.

Anaphylactic reactions have been observed rarely. If an anaphylactic reaction occurs discontinue the infusion immediately and give adrenaline immediately by slow intravenous

injection. In addition, high doses of corticosteroids by slow intravenous injection may be given.

Other reactions: In a few sporadic cases, neuroallergic symptoms (Guillane-Barre Syndrome, polyneuropathy) have been reported in temporal coincidence with Streptase administration.

Uveitis has been reported in temporal association with streptokinase administration.

Serum sickness has been reported but is rare. Arthritis, vasculitis and nephritis have been reported in temporal association with streptokinase administration.

Arrhythmias and transient hypotension have been noted, particularly after high dose, short-term therapy. Tachycardia and bradycardia have been observed occasionally.

Persistent angina pectoris and cardiac failure, possibly leading to cardiac and respiratory arrest, may occur during thrombolytic therapy of acute myocardial infarction.

Non-cardiogenic pulmonary oedema has been observed in a few cases, mainly after intracoronary thrombolytic therapy in patients with extensive myocardial infarction.

Transient increases in liver function tests or bilirubin have been reported. Jaundice may occur as a consequence of bilirubin increase. A few cases of cholesterol embolism have been described in temporal coincidence with thrombolytic therapy, particularly in patients undergoing angiography.

Individual cases of cerebral convulsion were reported under thrombolytic therapy, and in temporal coincidence with cardiovascular hypoxia and cerebral haemorrhage.

Overdose: Long-term overdosage of streptokinase may induce the risk of rethrombosis by prolonged decrease of plasminogen. See also *Side-effects, Haermorrhages.*

Pharmacological properties

Pharmacodynamic properties: Strepokinase is an enzyme obtained from β haemolytic streptococci of Lancefield group C. It is a potent activator of the fibrinolytic enzyme system in man and it acts indirectly by complexing with plasminogen to form an activator complex which then reacts with more plasminogen to form plasmin.

Pharmacokinetic properties: Streptokinase has a very short half-life, the first rapid clearance from the plasma is due to the formation of the complex between stretokinase and stretokinase antibody. This complex is biochemically inert and is cleared rapidly from the circulation. Once the antibody has been neutralised, the streptokinase activates plasminogen and the resulting complex acts on non complexed plasminogen to form plasmin. During these events the streptokinase is proteolytically modified into several lower molecular weight fragments.

Peak fibrinolytic activity is found in the blood about 20 minutes after dosing activity is detected in the urine 2 hours after dosing.

Preclinical safety data: Extensive studies in different species of laboratory animals have shown that the multiple human doses have no acute toxic effect.

Pharmaceutical particulars

List of excipients: Human albumin, sodium-L-hydrogen glutamate monohydrate, polygeline

Incompatibilities: Other drugs should not be added to the infusion solution.

Shelf-life: Three years.

Special precautions for storage: Streptase is to be stored below 25°C. Once dissolved in sterile physiological saline Streptase can be stored for 24 hours at +2 to +8°C without loss of activity.

Nature and contents of container: Multidose glass vial sealed with rubber infusion stopper, plastic disc and aluminium cap, containing 1.5 million International Units of streptokinase.

Instructions for use/handling: For rapid, complete reconstitution, inject 5 ml of physiological saline into the vacuum vial and remove the residual vacuum by briefly loosening the needle from the syringe.

Marketing authorisation number PL 13402/0044

Date of approval/revision of SPC 31st December 1997

Legal category POM

TARGOCID*

Presentation For intravenous or intramuscular injection or intravenous infusion.

Targocid 200 mg: Each vial provides 200 mg teicoplanin presented as a lyophilisate for reconstitution. Each pack contains an ampoule of diluent (Water for Injections PhEur).

Targocid 400 mg: Each vial provides 400 mg teicoplanin presented as a lyophilisate for reconstitution. Each pack contains an ampoule of diluent (Water for Injections PhEur).

The vials do not contain any preservative.

Uses

Properties: Teicoplanin is a bactericidal, glycopeptide antibiotic, produced by fermentation of *Actinoplanes teichomyceticus.* It is active against both aerobic and anaerobic Gram-positive bacteria.

Species usually sensitive (MIC less than or equal to 16 mg/l): *Staphylococcus aureus* and coagulase negative staphylococci (sensitive or resistant to methicillin), streptococci, enterococci, *Listeria monocytogenes,* micrococci, *Eikenella corrodens,* group *JK* corynebacteria and Gram-positive anaerobes including *Clostridium difficile,* and peptococci.

Species usually resistant (MIC superior to 16 mg/l): *Nocardia asteroides, Lactobacillus* spp, *Leuconostoc* and all Gram-negative bacteria. Bactericidal synergy has been demonstrated *in vitro* with aminoglycosides against group D streptococci and staphylococci. *In vitro* combinations of teicoplanin with rifampicin or fluorinated quinolones show primarily additive effects and sometimes synergy.

One-step resistance to teicoplanin could not be obtained *in vitro* and multi-step resistance was only reached *in vitro* after 11–14 passages.

Teicoplanin does not show cross-resistance with other classes of antibiotics.

Susceptibility testing: Sensidiscs are charged with 30 micrograms of teicoplanin. Strains showing an inhibition zone diameter of 14 mm or more are susceptible, and those of 10 mm or less are resistant.

Indications: Targocid is indicated in potentially serious Gram-positive infections including those which cannot be treated with other antimicrobial drugs, e.g. penicillins and cephalosporins.

Targocid is useful in the therapy of serious staphylococcal infections in patients who cannot receive or who have failed to respond to the penicillins and cephalosporins, or who have infections with staphylococci resistant to other antibiotics.

The effectiveness of teicoplanin has been documented in the following infections: Skin and soft tissue infections, urinary tract infections, lower respiratory tract infections, joint and bone infections, septicaemia, endocarditis and peritonitis related to continuous ambulatory peritoneal dialysis.

Targocid may be used for antimicrobial prophylaxis in orthopaedic surgery at risk of Gram-positive infection.

Dosage and administration

Preparation of injection: The entire contents of the water ampoule should be slowly added to the vial of Targocid and the vial rolled gently until the powder is completely dissolved, taking care to avoid formation of foam. If the solution does become foamy then allow to stand for about 15 minutes for the foam to subside.

A calculated excess is included in each vial of Targocid so that, when prepared as described above, a full dose of 200 mg or 400 mg (depending on the strength of the vial) will be obtained if all the reconstituted solution is withdrawn from the vial by a syringe. The concentration of teicoplanin in these injections will be 100 mg in 1.5 ml (from the 200 mg vial) and 400 mg in 3 ml (from the 400 mg vial).

Administration: The reconstituted Targocid injection may be administered directly either intravenously or intramuscularly. The intravenous injection may be administered either as a bolus or as a 30 minute infusion. Dosage is usually once daily but, in cases of severe infection, a second injection should be administered on the first day in order to reach more rapidly the required serum concentrations. The majority of patients with infections caused by organisms sensitive to the antibiotic show a therapeutic response within 48–72 hours. The total duration of therapy is determined by the type and severity of the infection and the clinical response of the patient. In endocarditis and osteomyelitis, treatment for three weeks or longer is recommended.

Determination of teicoplanin serum concentrations may optimise therapy. In severe infections, trough serum concentrations should not be less than 10 mg/l (see *Further information*). Peak concentrations measured one hour after a 400 mg intravenous dose are usually in the range of 20–50 mg/l; peak serum concentrations of up to 250 mg/l have been reported after intravenous doses of 25 mg/kg. A relationship between serum concentration and toxicity has not been established.

Therapeutic dosage:
Adult or elderly patients with normal renal function:

Prophylaxis: 400 mg intravenously as a single dose at induction of anaesthesia.

Moderate infections: skin and soft tissue infection, urinary tract infection, lower respiratory tract infection.

Loading dose: one single i.v. or i.m. injection of 400 mg on the first day.

Maintenance dose: a single i.v. or i.m. injection of 200 mg daily.

Severe infections: joint and bone infection, septicaemia, endocarditis.

Loading dose: Three 400 mg i.v. injections administered 12 hours apart.

Maintenance dose: a single i.v. or i.m. injection of 400 mg daily.

In some clinical situations, such as infected, severely burned patients or *Staphylococcus aureus* endocarditis, unit maintenance doses of up to 12 mg/kg have been administered (intravenously).

NB: Standard doses of 200 and 400 mg equate respectively to mean doses of 3 and 6 mg/kg. In patients weighing more than 85 kg it is recommended to adapt the dosage to the weight following the same therapeutic schedule: moderate infection 3 mg/kg, severe infection 6 mg/kg.

Children: Teicoplanin can be used to treat Gram positive infections in children from the age of 2 months. For severe infections and neutropenic patients the recommended dose is 10 mg/kg every 12 hours for the first three doses; thereafter a dose of 10 mg/kg should be administered by either intravenous or intramuscular injection as a single dose each day. For moderate infections the recommended dose is 10 mg/kg every twelve hours for the first three doses: thereafter a dose of 6 mg/kg should be administered by either intravenous or intramuscular injection as a single dose each day.

Neonates: The recommended dosage for neonates is a single loading dose of 16 mg/kg on the first day of treatment followed on subsequent days by a maintenance dose of 8 mg/kg once daily. The doses should be given as intravenous infusion over thirty minutes.

Adults and elderly patients with renal insufficiency: For patients with impaired renal function, reduction of dosage is not required until the fourth day of Targocid treatment. Measurement of the serum concentration of teicoplanin may optimise therapy (see *Administration*).

From the fourth day of treatment:
In mild renal insufficiency: Creatinine clearance between 40 and 60 ml/min, Targocid dose should be halved, either by administering the initial unit dose every two days, or by administering half of this dose once a day.

In severe renal insufficiency: Creatinine clearance less than 40 ml/min, and in haemodialysed patients, Targocid dose should be one third of the normal either by administering the initial unit dose every third day, or by administering one third of this dose once a day. Teicoplanin is not removed by dialysis.

In continuous ambulatory peritoneal dialysis: After a single loading iv dose of 400 mg if the patient is febrile, the recommended dosage is 20 mg/l per bag in the first week, 20 mg/l in alternate bags in the second week, and 20 mg/l in the overnight dwell bag only during the third week.

Contra-indications, warnings, etc
Contra-indications: Teicoplanin is contra-indicated in patients who have exhibited previous hypersensitivity to the drug.

Warnings: Targocid should be administered with caution in patients known to be hypersensitive to vancomycin since cross hypersensitivity may occur. However, a history of the 'Red Man Syndrome' that can occur with vancomycin is not a contra-indication to Targocid.

Thrombocytopenia has been reported with teicoplanin, especially at higher doses than those usually recommended. It is advisable for periodic haematological studies to be performed during treatment. Liver and renal function tests are advised during treatment.

Serial renal and auditory function tests should be undertaken in the following circumstances:

- prolonged treatment in patients with renal insufficiency.
- concurrent and sequential use of other drugs which may have neurotoxic and/or nephrotoxic properties. These include aminoglycosides, colistin, amphotericin B, cyclosporin, cisplatin, frusemide and ethacrynic acid.

However, there is no evidence of synergistic toxicity with combinations with Targocid.

Dosage must be adapted in patients with renal impairment (see *Dosage*).

Precautions: Superinfection: as with other antibiotics, the use of teicoplanin, especially if prolonged, may result in overgrowth of non-susceptible organisms. Repeated evaluation of the patient's condition is essential. If superinfection occurs during therapy, appropriate measures should be taken.

Use in pregnancy: Animal reproduction studies have not shown evidence of impairment of fertility or teratogenic effects. At high doses in rats there was an increased incidence of stillbirths and neonatal mortality. It is recommended that Targocid should not be used during confirmed or presumed pregnancy or during lactation unless a physician considers that the potential benefits outweigh any possible risk. There is no information about the excretion of teicoplanin in milk or placental transfer of the drug.

Interactions: Targocid should be used with care in conjunction with or sequentially with other drugs with known nephrotoxic or ototoxic potential. Of particular concern are streptomycin, neomycin, kanamycin, gentamicin, amikacin, tobramycin, cephaloridine, colistin. In clinical trials teicoplanin has been administered to many patients already receiving various medications including other antibiotics, antihypertensives, anaesthetic agents, cardiac drugs, and antidiabetic agents without evidence of adverse interaction. Animal studies have shown lack of interaction with diazepam, thiopentone, morphine, neuromuscular blocking agents or halothane.

Side-effects: Targocid is generally well tolerated. Side-effects rarely require cessation of therapy and are generally mild and transient; serious side-effects are rare. The following adverse events have been reported:
Local reactions: erythema, local pain, thrombophlebitis, injection site abscess

Hypersensitivity: rash, pruritus, fever, bronchospasm, anaphylactic reactions, anaphylactic shock, rigors, urticaria, angioedema, rare reports of exfoliative dermatitis, toxic epidermal necrolysis, rare cases of erythema multiforme including Stevens-Johnson Syndrome. In addition, infusion-related events such as erythema or flushing of the upper body, have been rarely reported in which the events occurred without a history of previous teicoplanin exposure and did not recur on re-exposure when the infusion rate was slowed and/or concentration rate decreased. These events were not specific to any concentration or rate of infusion.

Gastro-intestinal: nausea, vomiting, diarrhoea.

Blood: eosinophilia, leucopenia, thrombocytopenia, thrombocytosis, neutropenia, rare cases of reversible agranulocytosis.

Liver function: increases in serum transaminases and/or serum alkaline phosphatase.

Renal function: transient elevations of serum creatinine, renal failure.

Central nervous system: dizziness and headache.

Auditory/vestibular: Mild hearing loss, tinnitus and vestibular disorder.

Other: Superinfection (overgrowth of non-susceptible organisms).

Overdosage: Targocid is not removed by haemodialysis. Treatment of overdosage should be symptomatic. Several overdoses of 100 mg/kg day have been administered in error to two neutropenic paediatric patients, aged 4 and 8 years. Despite high plasma concentrations of teicoplanin up to 300 mg/l, there were no symptoms or laboratory abnormalities.

Pharmaceutical precautions In keeping with good clinical and pharmaceutical practice reconstituted vials of Targocid should be used immediately and any unused portion discarded. On the few occasions when changing circumstances make this impracticable reconstituted solutions should be kept at 4°C and discarded within 24 hours.

The reconstituted solution may be injected directly, or alternatively diluted with: 0.9% Sodium Chloride Injection; Compound Sodium Lactate Injection (Ringer-Lactate Solution, Hartmanns Solution); 5% Dextrose Injection; 0.18% Sodium Chloride and 4% Dextrose Injection; Peritoneal dialysis solution containing 1.36% or 3.86% Dextrose.

Solutions of teicoplanin and aminoglycosides are incompatible when mixed directly and should not be mixed before injection.

Vials of dry Targocid should be stored below 25°C.

Legal category POM.

Package quantities
Targocid 200 mg: Combined pack of one vial providing 200 mg teicoplanin and one ampoule containing Water for Injections, PhEur.

Targocid 400 mg: Combined pack of one vial providing 400 mg teicoplanin and one ampoule containing Water for Injections, PhEur.

Further information
Pharmacokinetics: Following injection teicoplanin rapidly penetrates into tissues, including skin, fat and bone, and reaches the highest concentrations in the kidney, trachea, lungs and adrenals. Teicoplanin does not readily penetrate into the cerebrospinal fluid (CSF).

In man the plasma level profile after intravenous administration indicates a biphasic distribution (with a rapid distribution phase having a half life of about 0.3 hour, followed by a more prolonged distribution phase having a half life of about 3 hours), followed by slow elimination (with a terminal elimination half life of about 150 hours). At 6 mg/kg administered intravenously at 0, 12, 24 hours and every 24 hours thereafter as a 30 minute infusion, a predicted trough serum concentration of 10 mg/l would be reached by Day 4. The steady state volume of distribution after 3 to 6 mg/kg intravenously ranges from 0.94 l/kg to 1.4 l/kg. The volume of distribution in children is not substantially different from that in adults.

Approximately 90–95% teicoplanin is bound with weak affinity to plasma proteins. Teicoplanin penetrates readily into blister exudates and into joint fluid; it penetrates neutrophils and enhances their bactericidal activity; it does not penetrate red blood cells.

No metabolites of teicoplanin have been identified; more than 97% of the administered teicoplanin is excreted unchanged.

The elimination of teicoplanin from the plasma is prolonged with a terminal half life of elimination in man of about 150 hours. Teicoplanin is excreted mainly in the urine.

Marketing authorisation numbers

Targocid	200 mg vial	PL 4425/0088
	400 mg vial	PL 4425/0089
Water for Injections PhEur		PL 4425/0090

Marketing authorisation holder: Marion Merrell Ltd., Broadwater Park, Denham, Uxbridge, Middlesex UB9 5HP

TARIVID* I.V. INFUSION SOLUTION

Qualitative and quantitative composition Ofloxacin, 2 mg/ml.

Pharmaceutical form Solution for Infusion.

Clinical particulars
Therapeutic indications: Ofloxacin is a synthetic 4-fluoroquinolone antibacterial agent with bactericidal activity against a wide range of Gram-negative and Gram-positive organisms. It is indicated for the treatment of the following infections when caused by sensitive organisms:

Lower Respiratory Tract: Acute and chronic infections.

Upper and Lower Urinary Tract: Acute and chronic lower urinary tract infections; acute and chronic upper urinary tract infections (pyelonephritis).

Septicaemia.

Skin and soft tissue infections.

Microbiological results indicate that the following pathogens may be regarded as sensitive: *Staphylococcus aureus* (including methicillin resistant staphylococci), *Staphylococcus epidermidis, Neisseria* species, *Escherichia coli, Citrobacter, Klebsiella, Enterobacter, Hafnia, Proteus* (indole-negative and indole-positive strains), *Salmonella, Shigella, Acinetobacter, Yersinia enterocolitica, Campylobacter jejuni, Aeromonas, Plesiomonas, Vibrio cholerae,*

Vibrio parahaemolyticus, Haemophilus influenzae, Chlamydiae, *Legionella, Gardenerella.*

Variable sensitivity is shown by Streptococci, *Serratia marcescens, Pseudomonas aeruginosa, Clostridium* species and Mycoplasmas.

Anaerobic bacteria (e.g. *Fusobacterium* species, *Bacteroides* species, *Eubacterium* species, Peptococci, Peptostreptococci) are normally resistant.

Tarivid is not active against *Treponema pallidum.*

Posology and method of administration: General dosage recommendations: The dose of ofloxacin is determined by the type and severity of the infection.

Adults: The usual intravenous dosages in adults are:

Complicated urinary tract infection: 200 mg daily.
Lower respiratory tract infection: 200 mg twice daily
Septicaemia: 200 mg twice daily.
Skin and soft tissue infections: 400 mg twice daily.

The infusion time for Tarivid I.V. should not be less than 30 minutes for 200 mg. Generally, individual doses are to be given at approximately equal intervals.

The dose may be increased to 400 mg twice daily in severe or complicated infections.

Impaired renal function: Following a normal initial dose, dosage should be reduced in patients with impairment of renal function. When creatinine clearance is 20–50 ml/minute (serum creatinine 1.5–5.0 mg/dl) the dosage should be reduced by half (100–200 mg daily). If creatinine clearance is less than 20 ml/minute (serum creatinine greater than 5 mg/dl) 100 mg should be given every 24 hours. In patients undergoing haemodialysis or peritoneal dialysis, 100 mg should be given every 24 hours.

Impaired liver function: The excretion of ofloxacin may be reduced in patients with severe hepatic dysfunction.

Children: Ofloxacin is not indicated for use in children or growing adolescents.

Elderly: No adjustment of dosage is required in the elderly, other than that imposed by consideration of renal or hepatic function.

Duration of treatment: The duration of treatment is determined according to the response of the causative organisms and the clinical picture. As with all antibacterial agents, treatment with Tarivid should be continued for at least 3 days after the body temperature has returned to normal and the symptoms have subsided.

In most cases of acute infection, a course of treatment lasting 7 to 10 days is sufficient. Once the patient's condition has improved, the mode of administration should be changed from parenteral to oral, normally at the same total daily dose.

Treatment should not exceed 2 months duration.

Contra-indications: Ofloxacin should not be used in patients with known hypersensitivity to 4-quinolone antibacterials, or any of the excipients.

Ofloxacin should not be used in patients with a past history of tendinitis.

Ofloxacin, like other 4-quinolones, is contra-indicated in patients with a history of epilepsy or with a lowered seizure threshold. Ofloxacin is contra-indicated in children or growing adolescents, and in pregnant or breast-feeding women, since animal experiments do not entirely exclude the risk of damage to the cartilage of joints in the growing subject.

Patients with latent or actual defects in glucose-6-phosphate dehydrogenase activity may be prone to haemolytic reactions when treated with quinolone antibacterial agents.

Special warnings and precautions for use: Patients being treated with ofloxacin should not expose themselves unnecessarily to strong sunlight and should avoid UV rays (sunlamps, solaria). Caution is recommended if the drug is to be used in psychotic patients or in patients with a history of psychiatric disease.

Sudden reductions in blood pressure may occur when Tarivid I.V. is administered with hypotensive agents. In such cases, or if the drug is given concomitantly with barbiturate anaesthetics, cardiovascular function should be monitored.

Administration of antibiotics, especially if prolonged, may lead to proliferation of resistant microorganisms. The patient's condition must therefore be checked at regular intervals. If a secondary infection occurs, appropriate measures must be taken.

Interactions with other medicaments and other forms of interaction: Prolongation of bleeding time has been reported during concomitant administration of Tarivid and anticoagulants.

There may be a further lowering of the cerebral seizure threshold when quinolones are given concurrently with other drugs which lower the seizure threshold e.g. theophylline. However, ofloxacin is not thought to cause a pharmacokinetic interaction with theophylline, unlike some other fluoroquinolones.

Further lowering of the cerebral seizure threshold may also occur with certain nonsteroidal anti-inflammatory drugs.

Ofloxacin may cause a slight increase in serum concentrations of glibenclamide administered concurrently; patients treated with this combination should be closely monitored.

With high doses of quinolones, impairment of excretion and an increase in serum levels may occur when co-administered with other drugs that undergo renal tubular secretion (e.g. probenecid, cimetidine, frusemide and methotrexate).

Interactions with laboratory tests: Determination of opiates or porphyrins in urine may give false-positive results during treatment with ofloxacin.

Pregnancy and lactation: The safety of this medicinal product for use in human pregnancy has not been established. Reproduction studies performed in rats and rabbits did not reveal any evidence of teratogenicity, impairment of fertility or impairment of peri- and post-natal development. However, as with other quinolones, ofloxacin has been shown to cause arthropathy in immature animals and therefore its use during pregnancy is not recommended. Studies in rats have indicated that ofloxacin is secreted in milk. It should therefore not be used during lactation.

Effects on ability to drive and use machines: Since there have been occasional reports of somnolence, impairment of skills, dizziness and visual disturbances, patients should know how they react to Tarivid before they drive or operate machinery. These effects may be enhanced by alcohol.

Undesirable effects: In rare cases after i.v. infusion, a reduction in blood pressure may occur. If this effect is marked, the infusion should be stopped. Pain, reddening of the infusion site and thrombophlebitis have been reported in rare cases.

The overall frequency of adverse reactions from the clinical trial data base is about 7%. The commonest events involved the gastrointestinal system (about 5.0%) and the nervous system (about 2.0%).

The following provides a tabulation based on post marketing experience where occasional represents a frequency of 0.1-1.0%, rare <0.1%, very rare <0.01% and isolated cases <<0.01%.

Digestive and Liver side effects:

Occasional: Nausea and vomiting, diarrhoea, abdominal pain, gastric symptoms. (Diarrhoea may sometimes be a symptom of enterocolitis which may, in some cases, be haemorrhagic).

Rare: Loss of appetite, increase in liver enzymes and/or bilirubin.

Very rare: cholestatic jaundice, hepatitis or severe liver damage may develop. A particular form of enterocolitis that can occur with antibiotics is pseudomembranous colitis (in most cases due to Clostridium difficile). Even if Clostridium difficile is only suspected, administration of ofloxacin should be discontinued immediately, and appropriate treatment given. Drugs that inhibit peristalsis should not be administered in such cases.

Central nervous system:

Occasional: Headache, dizziness, sleep disorders, restlessness.

Rare: Confusion, nightmares, anxiety, depression, hallucinations and psychotic reactions, drowsiness, unsteady gait and tremor (due to disorders of muscular co-ordination), neuropathy, numbness and paraesthesia or hypaesthesiae, visual disturbances, disturbances of taste and smell (including, in exceptional cases, loss of function), extrapyramidal symptoms

Very rare: Convulsions, hearing disorders (including, in exceptional cases, loss of hearing).

These reactions have occurred in some patients after the first dose of ofloxacin. In such cases, discontinue treatment immediately.

Cardiovascular system:

Tachycardia and a temporary decrease in blood pressure have been reported.

Rare: circulatory collapse (due to pronounced drop in blood pressure).

Haematological side effects:

Very rare: anaemia, leucopenia (including agranulocytosis), thrombocytopenia, pancytopenia. Only in some cases are these due to bone marrow depression. In very rare cases, haemolytic anaemia may develop.

Renal side effects: Rare: Disturbances of kidney function.

Isolated cases: Acute interstitial nephritis, or an increase in serum creatinine, which may progress to acute renal failure.

Allergic and skin side effects: Occasional: Skin rash, itching.

Very rare: Rash on exposure to strong sunlight, other severe skin reactions. Hypersensitivity reactions, immediate or delayed, usually involving the skin (e.g. erythema multiforme, Stevens-Johnson syndrome, Lyell's syndrome and vasculitis) may occur. In exceptional circumstances, vasculitis can lead to skin lesions including necrosis and may also involve internal organs. There are rarely other signs of anaphylaxis such as tachycardia, fever, dyspnoea, shock, angioneurotic oedema, vasculitic reactions, eosinophilia. In these cases treatment should be discontinued immediately and where appropriate, supportive treatment given.

Isolated cases: Pneumonitis.

Other side effects: Rare: Malaise.

Very rare: Excessive rise or fall in blood-sugar levels. Weakness, joint and muscle pains (in isolated cases these may be symptoms of rhabdomyolysis).

Isolated cases: Tendon discomfort, including inflammation and rupture of tendons (e.g. the Achilles tendon) particularly in patients treated concurrently with corticosteroids. In the event of signs of inflammation of a tendon, treatment with Tarivid must be halted immediately and appropriate treatment must be initiated for the affected tendon.

The possibility cannot be ruled out that ofloxacin may trigger an attack of porphyria in predisposed patients.

Except in very rare instances (e.g. isolated cases of smell, taste and hearing disorders) the adverse effects observed subsided after discontinuation of ofloxacin.

Overdose: The most important signs to be expected following acute overdosage are CNS symptoms such as confusion, dizziness, impairment of consciousness and convulsive seizures, as well as gastrointestinal reactions such as nausea and mucosal erosions.

Elimination of ofloxacin may be increased by forced diuresis.

Pharmacological properties

Pharmacodynamic properties: Ofloxacin is a quinolone-carboxylic acid derivative with a wide range of antibacterial activity against both gram negative and gram positive organisms. It inhibits bacterial DNA replication by blocking DNA topo-isomerases, in particular DNA gyrase.

Therapeutic doses of ofloxacin are devoid of pharmacological effects on the voluntary or autonomic nervous systems.

Pharmacokinetic properties: Maximum plasma concentrations occur within five minutes of the end of the infusion. The plasma half life is about five hours. Ofloxacin is primarily excreted unchanged in the urine.

Urinary clearance is reduced in renal insufficiency.

Preclinical safety data: None stated.

Pharmaceutical particulars

List of excipients: Sodium chloride, hydrochloric acid and water for injections.

Incompatibilities: Tarivid IV should be administered alone unless compatibility with other infusion fluids has been demonstrated. Compatible infusion solutions include isotonic sodium chloride, Ringer's solution and 5 % glucose solution. Heparin and ofloxacin are incompatible.

Shelf-life: 3 years.

Special precautions for storage: Tarivid IV presented in glass infusion bottles should be protected from light.

Nature and contents of container: Clear, colourless Type I glass vials with grey chlorobutyl rubber closures and aluminium caps containing either 50 ml, 100 ml or 200 ml infusion solution.

Instructions for use/handling: None.

Marketing authorisation number PL 13402/0052

Date of approval/revision of SPC October 1998

Legal category POM

TARIVID* TABLETS 200 mg
TARIVID* TABLETS 400 mg

Qualitative and quantitative composition Tarivid Tablets 200 mg contain 200 mg of ofloxacin.

Tarivid Tablets 400 mg contain 400 mg of ofloxacin.

Pharmaceutical form Film coated tablets.

Clinical particulars

Therapeutic indications: Ofloxacin is a synthetic 4-fluoroquinolone antibacterial agent with bactericidal activity against a wide range of Gram-negative and Gram-positive organisms. It is indicated for the treatment of the following infections when caused by sensitive organisms: Upper and lower urinary tract infections; lower respiratory tract infections; uncomplicated urethral and cervical gonorrhoea; non-gonococcal urethritis and cervicitis, skin and soft tissue infections.

Posology and method of administration: General dosage recommendations: The dose of ofloxacin is determined by the type and severity of the infection. The dosage range for adults is 200 mg to 800 mg daily. Up to 400 mg may be given as a single dose, preferably in the morning, larger doses should be given as two divided doses. Generally, individual doses are to be given at approximately equal intervals. Tarivid tablets should be swallowed with liquid; they should not be taken within two hours of magnesium/

aluminium containing antacids, sucralfate or iron preparations since reduction of absorption of ofloxacin can occur.

Lower urinary tract infection: 200–400 mg daily.

Upper urinary tract infection: 200–400 mg daily increasing, if necessary, to 400 mg twice a day.

Lower respiratory tract infection: 400 mg daily increasing, if necessary, to 400 mg twice daily.

Uncomplicated urethral and cervical gonorrhoea: A single dose of 400 mg.

Non-gonococcal urethritis and cervicitis: 400 mg daily in single or divided doses.

Skin and soft tissue infections: 400 mg twice daily.

Impaired renal function: Following a normal initial dose, dosage should be reduced in patients with impairment of renal function. When creatinine clearance is 20–50 ml/minute (serum creatinine 1.5–5.0 mg/dl) the dosage should be reduced by half (100–200 mg daily). If creatinine clearance is less than 20 ml/minute (serum creatinine greater than 5 mg/dl) 100 mg should be given every 24 hours. In patients undergoing haemodialysis or peritoneal dialysis, 100 mg should be given every 24 hours.

Impaired liver function: The excretion of ofloxacin may be reduced in patients with severe hepatic dysfunction.

Elderly: No adjustment of dosage is required in the elderly, other than that imposed by consideration of renal or hepatic function.

Children: Ofloxacin is not indicated for use in children or growing adolescents.

Duration of treatment: Duration of treatment is dependent on the severity of the infection and the response to treatment. The usual treatment period is 5–10 days except in uncomplicated gonorrhoea, where a single dose is recommended.

Treatment should not exceed 2 months duration.

Contra-indications: Ofloxacin should not be used in patients with known hypersensitivity to 4-quinolone antibacterials or any of the tablet excipients.

Ofloxacin should not be used in patients with a past history of tendinitis.

Ofloxacin, like other 4-quinolones, is contra-indicated in patients with a history of epilepsy or with a lowered seizure threshold. Ofloxacin is contra-indicated in children or growing adolescents, and in pregnant or breast-feeding women, since animal experiments do not entirely exclude the risk of damage to the cartilage of joints in the growing subject.

Patients with latent or actual defects in glucose-6-phosphate dehydrogenese activity may be prone to haemolytic reactions when treated with quinolone antibacterial agents.

Special warnings and special precautions for use: Patients being treated with ofloxacin should not expose themselves unnecessarily to strong sunlight and should avoid UV rays (sun lamps, solaria). Caution is recommended if the drug is to be used in psychotic patients or in patients with a history of psychiatric disease.

Administration of antibiotics, especially of prolonged, may lead to proliferation of resistant micro-organisms. The patient's condition must therefore be checked at regular intervals. If a secondary infection occurs, appropriate measures must be taken.

Interactions with other medicaments and other forms of interaction: Co-administered magnesium/aluminium antacids, sucralfate or iron preparations can reduce absorption. Therefore, ofloxacin should be taken 2 hours before such preparations. Prolongation of bleeding time has been reported during concomitant administration of Tarivid and anticoagulants.

There may be a further lowering of the cerebral seizure threshold when quinolones are given concurrently with other drugs which lower the seizure threshold, e.g. theophylline. However ofloxacin is not thought to cause a pharmacokinetic interaction with theophylline, unlike some other fluoroquinolones.

Further lowering of the cerebral seizure threshold may also occur with certain nonsteroidal anti-inflammatory drugs.

Ofloxacin may cause a slight increase in serum concentrations of glibenclamide administered concurrently; patients treated with this combination should be closely monitored.

With high doses of quinolones, impairment of excretion and an increase in serum levels may occur when co-administered with other drugs that undergo renal tubular secretion (e.g. probenecid, cimetidine, frusemide and methotrexate).

Interaction with laboratory tests: Determination of opiates or porphyrins in urine may give false-positive results during treatment with ofloxacin.

Pregnancy and lactation: The safety of this medicinal product for use in human pregnancy has not been established. Reproduction studies performed in rats and rabbits did not reveal any evidence of teratogenicity, impairment of fertility or impairment of peri- and post-natal development. However, as with other quinolones, ofloxacin has been shown to cause arthropathy in immature animals and therefore its use during pregnancy is not recommended. Studies in rats have indicated that ofloxacin is secreted in milk. It should therefore not be used during lactation.

Effects on ability to drive and use machines: Since there have been occasional reports of somnolence, impairment of skills, dizziness and visual disturbances, patients should know how they react to Tarivid before they drive or operate machinery. These effects may be enhanced by alcohol.

Undesirable effects: The overall frequency of adverse reactions from the clinical trial database is about 7%. The commonest events involved the gastrointestinal system (about 5.0%) and the nervous system (about 2.0%).

The following provides a tabulation based on post marketing experience where occasional represents a frequency of 0.1–1.0%, rare <0.1%, very rare <0.01% and isolated cases <<0.01%:

Digestive and Liver side effects: Occasional: Nausea and vomiting, diarrhoea, abdominal pain, gastric symptoms. (Diarrhoea may sometimes be a symptom of enterocolitis which may, in some cases, be haemorrhagic).

Rare: Loss of appetite, increase in liver enzymes and/or bilirubin.

Very rare: cholestatic jaundice; hepatitis or severe liver damage may develop. A particular form of enterocolitis that can occur with antibiotics is pseudomembranous colitis (in most cases due to *Clostridium difficile*). Even if *Clostridium difficile* is only suspected, administration of ofloxacin should be discontinued immediately and appropriate treatment given. Drugs that inhibit peristalsis should not be administered in such cases.

Central nervous system: Occasional: Headache, dizziness, sleep disorders, restlessness.

Rare: Confusion, nightmares, anxiety, depression, hallucinations and psychotic reactions, drowsiness, unsteady gait and tremor (due to disorders of muscular co-ordination), neuropathy, numbness and paraesthesia or hypaesthesiae, visual disturbances, disturbances of taste and smell (including, in exceptional cases, loss of function), extrapyramidal symptoms.

Very rare: Convulsions, hearing disorders (including, in exceptional cases, loss of hearing). These reactions have occurred in some patients after the first dose of ofloxacin. In such cases, discontinue treatment immediately.

Cardiovascular system: Tachycardia and a temporary decrease in blood pressure have been reported.

Rare: circulatory collapse (due to pronounced drop in blood pressure).

Haematological side effects: Very rare: anaemia, leucopenia (including agranulocytosis), thrombocytopenia, pancytopenia. Only in some cases are these due to bone marrow depression. In very rare cases, haemolytic anaemia may develop.

Renal side effects: Rare: Disturbances of kidney function.

Isolated cases: Acute interstitial nephritis, or an increase in serum creatinine, which may progress to acute renal failure.

Allergic and skin side effects: Occasional: Skin rash, itching.

Very rare: Rash on exposure to strong sunlight, other severe skin reactions. Hypersensitivity reactions, immediate or delayed, usually involving the skin (e.g. erythema multiforme, Stevens-Johnson syndrome, Lyell's syndrome, and vasculitis) may occur. In exceptional circumstances, vasculitis can lead to skin lesions including necrosis and may also involve internal organs. There are rarely other signs of anaphylaxis such as tachycardia, fever, dyspnoea, shock, angioneurotic oedema, vasculitic reactions, eosinophilia. In these cases treatment should be discontinued immediately and where appropriate, supportive treatment given.

Isolated cases: Pneumonitis.

Other side effects: Rare: Malaise.

Very rare: Excessive rise or fall in blood-sugar levels. Weakness, joint and muscle pains (in isolated cases these may be symptoms of rhabdomyolysis).

Isolated cases: Tendon discomfort including inflammation and rupture of tendons (e.g. the Achilles tendon) particularly in patients treated concurrently with corticosteroids. In the event of signs of inflammation of a tendon, treatment with Tarivid must be halted immediately and appropriate treatment must be initiated for the affected tendon.

The possibility cannot be ruled out that ofloxacin may trigger an attack of porphyria in predisposed patients.

Except in very rare instances (e.g. isolated cases of smell, taste and hearing disorders) the adverse effects observed subsided after discontinuation of ofloxacin.

Overdose: The most important signs to be expected following acute overdosage are CNS symptoms such as confusion, dizziness, impairment of consciousness and convulsive seizures as well as gastrointestinal reactions such as nausea and mucosal erosions.

In the case of overdose steps to remove any unabsorbed ofloxacin eg gastric lavage, administration of adsorbants and sodium sulphate, if possible during the first 30 minutes, are recommended; antacids are recommended for protection of the gastric mucosa.

Elimination of ofloxacin may be increased by forced diuresis.

Pharmacological properties

Pharmacodynamic properties: Ofloxacin is a quinolone-carboxylic acid derivative with a wide range of antibacterial activity against both gram negative and gram positive organisms. It is active after oral administration. It inhibits bacterial DNA replication by blocking DNA topo-isomerases, in particular DNA gyrase.

Therapeutic doses of ofloxacin are devoid of pharmacological effects on the voluntary or autonomic nervous systems.

Microbiological results indicate that the following pathogens may be regarded as sensitive: *Staphylococcus aureus* (including methicillin resistant staphylococci), *Staphylococcus epidermidis, Neisseria* species, *Escherichia coli, Citrobacter, Klebsiella, Enterobacter, Hafnia, Proteus* (indole-negative and indole-positive strains), *Haemophilus influenzae*, Chlamydiae, *Legionella, Gardnerella.*

Variable sensitivity is shown by Streptococci, *Serratia marcescens, Pseudomonas aeruginosa* and Mycoplasmas.

Anaerobic bacteria (e.g. Fusobacterium species, Bacteroides species, *Eubacterium* species, Peptococci, Peptostreptococci) are normally resistant.

Tarivid is not active against *Treponema pallidum.*

Pharmacokinetic properties: Ofloxacin is almost completely absorbed after oral administration. Maximal blood levels occur 1–3 hours after dosing and the elimination half-life is 4–6 hours. Ofloxacin is primarily excreted unchanged in the urine.

In renal insufficiency the dose should be reduced.

No clinically relevant interactions were seen with food and no interaction was found between ofloxacin and theophylline.

Preclinical safety data: Not applicable

Pharmaceutical particulars

List of excipients:

Tarivid 200 mg Tablets: Maize starch, lactose, hyprolose, carmellose NS300, magnesium stearate, hypromellose (2910), titanium dioxide (E171) talc, macrogol 8000.

Tarivid 400 mg Tablets: Lactose, maize starch, sodium starch glycolate, hyprolose, magnesium stearate, hypromellose, macrogol 8000, talc, titanium dioxide (E171), yellow ferric oxide (E172), purified water.

Incompatibilities: None known.

Shelf life:

Tarivid 200 mg Tablets 5 years
Tarivid 400 mg Tablets 3 years

Special precautions for storage: Store in a dry place.

Nature and contents of container:

Tarivid 200 mg Tablets: Blister packs of 10, 20 and 100 tablets

Tarivid 400 mg Tablets: Aluminium/PVC blister pack with aluminium foil 20 microgram and PVC (bluish clear) 250 microgram.

Pack sizes: 1 tablet (starter pack), 5, 10 and 50 tablets.

Instructions for use/handling: None.

Marketing authorisation numbers

Tarivid 200 mg tablets PL 13402/0053
Tarivid 400 mg tablets PL 13402/0054

Date of approval/revision of SPC October 1998

Legal category POM

TAVANIC* i.v. ▼

Qualitative and quantitative composition Each 50 ml bottle of Tavanic solution for infusion contains 250 mg (5 mg/ml) of levofloxacin as active ingredient.

Each 100 ml bottle of Tavanic solution for infusion contains 500 mg (5 mg/ml) of levofloxacin as active ingredient.

Pharmaceutical form Solution for infusion.

Clinical particulars

Therapeutic indications: In adults for whom intravenous therapy is considered to be appropriate, Tavanic solution for infusion is indicated for the treatment of the following infections when due to levofloxacin-susceptible micro-organisms:

Community-acquired pneumonia

Complicated urinary tract infections including pyelonephritis

Skin and soft tissue infections

Consideration should be given to national and/or local guidance on the appropriate use of antibacterial agents.

Posology and method of administration: Tavanic solution is administered by **slow** intravenous infusion once or twice daily. The dosage depends on the type and severity of the infection and the sensitivity of the presumed causative pathogen. It is usually possible to switch from initial intravenous treatment to the oral route after a few days (Tavanic 250 or 500 mg tablets), according to the condition of the patient. Given the bioequivalence of the parenteral and oral forms, the same dosage can be used.

Duration of treatment: The duration of therapy varies according to the course of the disease. As with antibiotic therapy in general, administration of Tavanic (solution for infusion or tablets) should be continued for a minimum of 48 to 72 hours after the patient has become afebrile or evidence of bacterial eradication has been obtained.

Method of administration: Tavanic solution for infusion is only intended for **slow** intravenous infusion; it is administered once or twice daily with a maximum treatment duration of 14 days. The infusion time must be **at least 30 minutes for 250 mg or 60 minutes for 500 mg Tavanic solution for infusion** (see 'Special warnings and precautions for use'). It is possible to switch from an initial intravenous application to the oral route at the same dosage after a few days, according to the condition of the patient. For incompatibilities please see 'Incompatibilities' and compatibility with other infusion solutions see 'Instructions for use/handling'.

The following dose recommendations can be given for Tavanic:

Dosage in patients with normal renal function (creatinine clearance >50 ml/min).

Indication	*Daily dose regimen (according to severity)*
Community–acquired pneumonia	500 mg once or twice daily
Complicated urinary tract infections including pyelonephritis	250 mg[1] once daily
Skin and soft tissue infections	500 mg twice daily

[1] consideration should be given to increasing the dose in severe infection

Dosage in patients with impaired liver function: No adjustment of dosage is required since levofloxacin is not metabolised to any relevant extent by the liver and is mainly excreted by the kidneys.

Dosage in patients with impaired renal function (creatinine clearance ≤50 ml/min)

	Dose regimen		
	250 mg/24 h	500 mg/24 h	500 mg/12 h
Creatinine clearance	first dose 250 mg	first dose 500 mg	first dose 500 mg
50–20 ml/min	then: 125 mg/24 h	then: 250 mg/24 h	then: 250 mg/12 h
19–10 ml/min	then: 125 mg/48 h	then: 125 mg/24 h	then: 125 mg/12 h
<10 ml/min (including haemodialysis and CAPD)[1]	then: 125 mg/48 h	then: 125 mg/24 h	then: 125 mg/24 h

[1] No additional doses are required after haemodialysis or continuous ambulatory peritoneal dialysis (CAPD).

Dosage in elderly: No adjustment of dosage is required in the elderly, other than that imposed by consideration of renal function.

Contra-indications: Tavanic solution for infusion must not be used :
in patients hypersensitive to levofloxacin, or any other quinolone, or any of the excipients,
in patients with epilepsy,
in patients with history of tendon disorders related to fluoroquinolone administration,
in children or growing adolescents,
during pregnancy,
in breast-feeding women.

Special warnings and special precautions for use: In the most severe cases of pneumococcal pneumonia Tavanic may not be the optimal therapy.

Nosocomial infections due to *P. aeruginosa* may require combination therapy.

Infusion time: The recommended infusion time of at least 30 minutes for 250 mg or 60 minutes for 500 mg Tavanic solution for infusion should be observed. It is known for ofloxacin that during infusion, tachycardia and a temporary decrease in blood pressure may develop. In rare cases, as a consequence of a profound drop in blood pressure, circulatory collapse may occur. Should a conspicuous drop in blood pressure occur during infusion of levofloxacin, (*l*-isomer of ofloxacin) the infusion must be halted immediately.

Clostridium difficile-associated disease: Diarrhoea, particularly if severe, persistent and/or bloody, during or after treatment with Tavanic solution for infusion, may be symptomatic of Clostridium difficile-associated disease, the most severe form of which is pseudomembranous colitis. If pseudomembranous colitis is suspected, Tavanic solution for infusion must be stopped immediately and patients should be treated with supportive measures ± specific therapy without delay (e.g. oral vancomycin). Products inhibiting the peristalsis are contraindicated in this clinical situation.

Tendinitis: Tendinitis, rarely observed with quinolones, may occasionally lead to rupture, involving Achilles tendon in particular. Elderly patients are more prone to tendinitis. The risk of tendon rupture may be increased by coadministration of corticosteroids. If tendinitis is suspected, treatment with Tavanic solution for infusion must be halted immediately, and appropriate treatment (e.g. immobilisation) must be initiated for the affected tendon.

Patients predisposed to seizures: Tavanic solution for infusion is contra-indicated in patients with a history of epilepsy and, as other quinolones, should be used with extreme caution in patients predisposed to seizures, such as patients with pre-existing central nervous system lesions, concomitant treatment with fenbufen and similar non-steroidal anti-inflammatory drugs or with drugs which lower the cerebral seizure threshold, such as theophylline (see 'Interactions with other medicaments and other forms of interaction').

Patients with G-6- phosphate dehydrogenase deficiency: Patients with latent or actual defects in glucose-6-phosphate dehydrogenase activity may be prone to hemolytic reactions when treated with quinolone antibacterial agents, and so levofloxacin should be used with caution.

Patients with renal impairment: Since levofloxacin is excreted mainly by the kidneys, the dose of Tavanic should be adjusted in patients with renal impairment.

Prevention of photosensitisation: Although photosensitisation is very rare with levofloxacin, it is recommended that patients should not expose themselves unnecessarily to strong sunlight or to artificial UV rays (e.g. sunray lamp, solarium), in order to prevent photosensitisation.

Interactions with other medicaments and other forms of interaction:

Theophylline, fenbufen or similar non-steroidal anti-inflammatory drugs: No pharmacokinetic interactions of levofloxacin were found with theophylline in a clinical study. However, a pronounced lowering of the cerebral seizure threshold may occur when quinolones are given concurrently with theophylline, non-steroidal anti-inflammatory drugs, or other agents which lower the seizure threshold.

Levofloxacin concentrations were about 13% higher in the presence of fenbufen than when administered alone.

Probenecid and cimetidine: Probenecid and cimetidine had a statistically significant effect on the elimination of levofloxacin. The renal clearance of levofloxacin was reduced by cimetidine (24%) and probenecid (34%). This is because both drugs are capable of blocking the renal tubular secretion of levofloxacin. However, at the tested doses in the study, the statistically significant kinetic differences are unlikely to be of clinical relevance.

Caution should be exercised when levofloxacin is coadministered with drugs that effect the tubular renal secretion such as probenecid and cimetidine, especially in renally impaired patients.

Cyclosporin: The half life of cyclosporin was increased by 33% when coadministered with levofloxacin.

Other relevant information: Clinical pharmacology studies were carried out to investigate possible pharmacokinetic interactions between levofloxacin and commonly prescribed drugs. The pharmacokinetics of levofloxacin were not affected to any clinically relevant extent when levofloxacin was administered together with the following drugs: calcium carbonate, digoxin, glibenclamide, ranitidine, warfarin.

Pregnancy and lactation:

Pregnancy: Reproductive studies in animals did not raise specific concern. However in the absence of human data and due to the experimental risk of damage by fluoroquinolones to the weight-bearing cartilage of the growing organism, Tavanic must not be used in pregnant women.

Lactation: In the absence of human data and due to the experimental risk of damage by fluoroquinolones to the weight-bearing cartilage of the growing organism, Tavanic solution for infusion must not be used in breast-feeding women.

Effects on ability to drive and use machines: Some undesirable effects (e.g., dizziness/vertigo, drowsiness, visual disturbances) may impair the patient's ability to concentrate and react, and therefore may constitute a risk in situations where these abilities are of special importance (e.g. driving a car or operating machinery).

Undesirable effects: The information given below is based on data from clinical studies in more than 5000 patients and on extensive post marketing experience. The following frequency rating has been used: (See table overleaf).

Overdose: According to toxicity studies in animals, the most important signs to be expected following acute overdosage of Tavanic solution for infusion are central nervous system symptoms such as confusion, dizziness, impairment of consciousness, and convulsive seizures.

In the event of relevant overdose, symptomatic treatment should be implemented. Haemodialysis, including peritoneal dialysis and CAPD, are not effective in removing levofloxacin from the body. No specific antidote exists.

Pharmacological properties

Pharmacodynamic properties: Levofloxacin is a synthetic antibacterial agent of the fluoroquinolone class (ATC code J01MA) and is the S (-) enantiomer of the racemic drug substance ofloxacin.

Mode of action: As a fluoroquinolone antibacterial agent, levofloxacin acts on the DNA–DNA-gyrase complex and topoisomerase IV.

Breakpoints: The preliminary NCCLS (US National Committee on Clinical Laboratory Standards) recommended MIC breakpoints for levofloxacin, separating susceptible from intermediately susceptible organisms and intermediately susceptible from resistant organisms are:

susceptible ≤2 mg/L, resistant ≥8 mg/L

Antibacterial spectrum: The prevalence of resistance may vary geographically and with time for selected species and local information on resistance is desirable, particularly when treating severe infections. Therefore, the information presented provides only an approximate guidance on probabilities as to whether microorganisms will be susceptible to levofloxacin or not. Only microorganisms relevant to the given clinical indications are presented here.

Susceptible micro-organisms:

Aerobic Gram-positive:
*Enterococcus faecalis**
*Staphylococcus aureus** methi-S
Staphylococcus haemolyticus methi-S
Staphylococcus saprophyticus
Streptococci, group C and G
Streptococcus agalactiae
Streptococcus pneumoniae pen-I/S/R*
*Streptococcus pyogenes**

Aerobic Gram-negative:
*Acinetobacter baumannii**
*Citrobacter freundii**
Eikenella corrodens
Enterobacter aerogenes
Enterobacter agglomerans
*Enterobacter cloacae**
*Escherichia coli**
Haemophilus influenzae ampi-S/R*
*Haemophilus para-influenzae**
Klebsiella oxytoca
*Klebsiella pneumoniae**
Moraxella catarrhalis β+/β-*
*Morganella morganii**
Pasteurella multocida
*Proteus mirabilis**
Proteus vulgaris
Providencia rettgeri
Providencia stuartii
*Pseudomonas aeruginosa**
*Serratia marcescens**

Anaerobic:
Bacteroides fragilis
Clostridium perfringens
Peptostreptococcus

"Other":
*Chlamydia pneumoniae**
Chlamydia psittaci
*Legionella pneumophila**
*Mycoplasma pneumoniae**

Intermediately susceptible microorgansisms:

Aerobic Gram-positive:
Staphylococcus haemolyticus methi-R

Aerobic Gram-negative:
Burkholderia cepacia

Anaerobic:
Bacteroides ovatus
Bacteroides thetaiotamicron
Bacteroides vulgatus
Clostridium difficile

Resistant microorganisms:

Aerobic Gram-positive:
Staphylococcus aureus methi-R

*clinical efficacy has been proven in clinical studies

Other information: The main mechanism of resistance

Very common	more than		10 %
common	1 %	to	10 %
uncommon	0.1%	to	1%
rare	0.01%	to	0.1%
very rare	less than		0.01%
isolated cases			

Allergic reactions

Uncommon: Pruritus, rash
Rare: Urticaria, bronchospasm/dyspnoea
Very rare: Angio-oedema, hypotension, anaphylactic-like shock; photosensitisation
Isolated cases: Severe bullous eruptions such as Stevens Johnson syndrome, toxic shock, epidermal necrolysis (Lyell's syndrome) and erythema exsudativum multiforme

Muco-cutaneous, anaphylactic/-oid reactions may sometimes occur even after the first dose.

Gastro-intestinal, metabolism

Common: Nausea, diarrhoea
Uncommon: Anorexia, vomiting, abdominal pain, dyspepsia
Rare: Bloody diarrhoea which in very rare cases may be indicative of enterocolitis, including pseudomembranous colitis
Very rare: Hypoglycaemia, particularly in diabetic patients

Neurological

Uncommon: Headache, dizziness/vertigo, drowsiness, insomnia
Rare: Paraesthesia, tremor, anxiety, agitation, confusion, convulsion,
Very rare: Hypoaesthesia, visual and auditory disturbances, disturbances of taste and smell, hallucinations

Cardiovascular

Rare: Tachycardia, hypotension
Very rare: Shock (anaphylactic-like)

Musculo-skeletal

Rare: Arthralgia, myalgia, tendon disorders, incl. tendinitis, (e.g. Achille's tendon)
Very rare: Tendon rupture (e.g. Achille's tendon), as with other fluoroquinolones this undesirable effect may occur within 48 hours of starting treatment and may be bilateral. Muscular weakness, which may be of special importance in patients with myasthenia gravis
Isolated cases: Rhabdomyolysis

Liver, kidney

Common: Increases in liver enzymes (e.g. ALT/AST)
Uncommon: Increase in bilirubin, increase in serum creatinine
Very rare: Liver reactions, such as hepatitis; acute kidney failure (e.g. due to interstitial nephritis)

Blood

Uncommon: Eosinophilia,leukopenia
Rare: Neutropenia, thrombocytopenia,
Very rare: Agranulocytosis
Isolated cases: Haemolytic anaemia, pancytopenia

Others:

Common: Pain, reddening of the infusion site and phlebitis
Uncommon: Asthenia, fungal overgrowth and proliferation of other resistant micro-organisms
Very rare: Allergic pneumonitis, fever

Other undesirable effects which have been associated with fluoroquinolone administration include:

* psychotic reactions such as acute confusional states and depressive mood changes (these reactions may occur even after the first dose)
* extrapyramidal symptoms and other disorders of muscular coordination
* hypersensitivity vasculitis
* attacks of porphyria in patients with porphyria.

is due to a *gyr-A* mutation. In vitro there is a cross-resistance between levofloxacin and other fluoroquinolones.

Acquired resistance with levofloxacin has recently been documented in 1997:

- *S. pneumoniae* France ≤ 1%
- *H. influenzae: rare.*

Due to the mechanism of action, there is generally no cross-resistance between levofloxacin and other classes of antibacterial agents.

Nosocomial infections due to *P. aeruginosa* may require combination therapy.

Pharmacokinetic properties:

Absorption: Orally administered levofloxacin is rapidly and almost completely absorbed with peak plasma concentrations being obtained within 1 hour. The absolute bioavailability is approximately 100 %. Levofloxacin obeys linear pharmacokinetics over a range of 50 to 600 mg.

Food has little effect on the absorption of levofloxacin.

Distribution: Approximately 30–40% of levofloxacin is bound to serum protein. 500 mg once daily multiple dosing with levofloxacin showed negligible accumulation. There is modest but predictable accumulation of levofloxacin after doses of 500 mg twice daily. Steady-state is achieved within 3 days.

Penetration into tissues and body fluids:

Penetration into Bronchial Mucosa, Epithelial Lining Fluid (ELF): Maximum levofloxacin concentrations in bronchial mucosa and epithelial lining fluid after 500 mg po were 8.3µg/g and 10.8µg/ml respectively. These were reached approximately one hour after administration.

Penetration into lung tissue: Maximum levofloxacin concentrations in lung tissue after 500 mg po were approximately 11.3µg/g and were reached between 4 and 6 hours after administration. The concentrations in the lungs consistently exceeded those in plasma.

Penetration into blister fluid: Maximum levofloxacin concentrations of about 4.0 and 6.7µg/ml in the blister fluid were reached 2–4 hours after administration following 3 days treatment at 500 mg once or twice daily, respectively.

Penetration into Cerebro-Spinal Fluid: Levofloxacin has poor penetration into cerebro-spinal fluid.

Concentration in urine: The mean urine concentrations 8 -12 hours after a single oral dose of 150 mg, 300 mg or 500 mg levofloxacin were 44 mg/L, 91 mg/L and 200 mg/L, respectively.

Metabolism: Levofloxacin is metabolised to a very small extent, the metabolites being desmethyl-levofloxacin and levofloxacin N-oxide. These metabolites account for < 5 % of the dose excreted in urine. Levofloxacin is stereochemically stable and does not undergo chiral inversion.

Elimination: Following oral and intravenous administration of levofloxacin, it is eliminated relatively slowly from the plasma ($t_{½}$: 6–8 hours). Excretion is primarily by the renal route (> 85 % of the administered dose).

There are no major differences in the pharmacokinetics of levofloxacin following intravenous and oral administration, suggesting that the oral and intravenous routes are interchangeable.

Subjects with renal insufficiency: The pharmacokinetics of levofloxacin are affected by renal impairment. With decreasing renal function renal elimination and clearance are decreased, and elimination half-lives increased as shown in the table below:

Cl_{cr} [ml/min]	< 20	20–40	50–80
Cl_R [ml/min]	13	26	57
$t_{1/2}$ [h]	35	27	9

Elderly subjects: There are no significant differences in levofloxacin kinetics between young and elderly subjects, except those associated with differences in creatinine clearance.

Gender differences: Separate analysis for male and female subjects showed small to marginal gender differences in levofloxacin pharmacokinetics. There is no evidence that these gender differences are of clinical relevance.

Preclinical safety data:

Acute toxicity: The median lethal dose (LD_{50}) values obtained in mice and rats after intravenous administration of levofloxacin were in the range 250–400 mg/kg, in dogs the LD_{50} value was approximately 200 mg/kg with one of two animals which received this dose dying.

Repeated dose toxicity: Studies of one months duration with intravenous administration have been carried out in the rat (20, 60, 180 mg/kg/day) and monkey (10, 25, 63 mg/kg/day) and a three month study has also been carried out in the rat (10, 30, 90 mg/kg/day).

The "No Observed Adverse Effects Levels" (NOEL) in the rat studies were concluded to be 20 and 30 mg/kg/day in the one-month and three-month studies respectively. Crystal deposits in urine were seen in both studies at doses of 20 mg/kg/day and above. High doses (180 mg/kg/day for 1 month or 30 mg/kg/day and above for 3 months) slightly decreased food consumption and body weight gain. Haematological examination showed reduced erythrocytes and increased leucocytes and reticulocytes at the end of the 1 month, but not the 3 months study.

The NOEL in the monkey study was concluded to be 63 mg/kg/day with only minor reduction in food and water consumption at this dose.

Reproductive toxicity: Levofloxacin caused no impairment of fertility or reproductive performance in rats at oral doses as high as 360 mg/kg/day or intravenous doses up to 100 mg/kg/day. Levofloxacin was not teratogenic in rats at oral doses as high as 810 mg/kg/day, or at intravenous doses as high as 160 mg/kg/day. No teratogenicity was observed when rabbits were dosed orally with up to 50 mg/kg/day or intravenously with up to 25 mg/kg/day.

Levofloxacin had no effect on fertility and its only effect on fetuses was delayed maturation as a result of maternal toxicity.

Genotoxicity: Levofloxacin did not induce gene mutations in bacterial or mammalian cells but did induce chromosome aberrations in Chinese hamster lung (CHL) cells in vitro at or above 100µg/ml, in the absence of metabolic activation. In vivo tests (micronucleus, sister chromatid exchange, unscheduled DNA synthesis, dominant lethal tests) did not show any genotoxic potential.

Phototoxic potential: Studies in the mouse after both oral and intravenous dosing showed levofloxacin to have phototoxic activity only at very high doses. Levofloxacin did not show any genotoxic potential in a photomutagenicity assay, and it reduced tumour development in a photocarcinogenicity assay.

Carcinogenic potential: No indication of carcinogenic potential was seen in a two year study in the rat with dietary administration (0, 10, 30 and 100 mg/kg/day).

Toxicity to joints: In common with other fluoroquinolones, levofloxacin showed effects on cartilage (blistering and cavities) in rats and dogs. These findings were more marked in young animals.

Pharmaceutical particulars

List of excipients: Tavanic solution for infusion contains the following excipients: Sodium chloride; sodium hydroxide; hydrochloric acid; *(qs: pH 4.8)* and water for injection. (Na^+ concentration: 154 mmol/litre).

Incompatibilities: Tavanic solution for infusion should not be mixed with heparin or alkaline solutions (e.g. sodium hydrogen carbonate).

Shelf life: Shelf-life as packaged for sale: 36 months.

Shelf-life after removal of the outer packaging: 3 days (under indoor light conditions)

Shelf-life after perforation of the rubber stopper: (see *Instructions for use/handling*)

Special precautions for storage: Protection from light is required and guaranteed by storage in the outer packaging.

Nature and contents of container: Type I glass vial (50 or 100 ml) with a chlorbutyl rubber stopper containing a clear, greenish yellow solution.

Pack sizes for 50 ml bottles: 1, 5 as commercially available.

Pack sizes for 100 ml bottles: 1, 5, 20 as commercially available.

Instruction for use/handling: Tavanic solution for infusion should be used immediately (within 3 hours) after perforation of the rubber stopper in order to prevent any bacterial contamination. No protection from light is necessary during infusion.

Mixture with other solutions for infusion: Tavanic solution for infusion is compatible with the following solutions for infusion:

0.9% sodium chloride USP
5% dextrose injection, USP
2.5% dextrose in Ringer solution
combination solutions for parenteral nutrition (amino acids, carbohydrates, electrolytes).

See *Incompatibilities* for incompatibilities.

Marketing authorisation number PL 13402/0013

Date of approval/revision of SPC September 1998

Legal category POM

TAVANIC* 250 mg TABLETS ▼
TAVANIC* 500 mg TABLETS ▼

Qualitative and quantitative composition 250 mg tablet: Each film-coated tablet of Tavanic contains 250 mg of levofloxacin as active ingredient corresponding to 256.23 mg of levofloxacin hemihydrate. 500 mg tablet: Each film-coated tablet of TAVANIC contains 500 mg of levofloxacin as active ingredient corresponding to 512.46 mg of levofloxacin hemihydrate.

Pharmaceutical form Film coated tablet.

Clinical particulars

Therapeutic indications: In adults with infections of mild to moderate severity Tavanic tablets are indicated for the treatment of the following infections when due to levofloxacin-susceptible micro-organisms:

Acute sinusitis

Acute exacerbation of chronic bronchitis

Community-acquired pneumonia

Complicated urinary tract infections including pyelonephritis

Skin and soft tissue infections

Consideration should be given to national and/or local guidance on the appropriate use of antibacterial agents.

Posology and method of administration: Tavanic tablets are administered once or twice daily. The dosage depends on the type and severity of the infection and the sensitivity of the presumed causative pathogen.

Duration of treatment: The duration of therapy varies according to the course of the disease with a maximum duration of treatment of 14 days. As with antibiotic therapy in general, administration of Tavanic tablets should be continued for a minimum of 48 to 72 hours after the patient has become afebrile or evidence of bacterial eradication has been obtained.

Method of administration: Tavanic tablets should be swallowed without crushing and with sufficient amount of liquid. They may be divided at the score line to adapt the dosage. The tablets may be taken during meals or between meals. Tavanic tablets should be taken at least two hours before or after iron salts, antacids and sucralfate administration since reduction of absorption can occur (see *Interactions with other medicaments and other forms of interaction*).

The following dose recommendations can be given for Tavanic:

Dosage in patients with normal renal function (creatinine clearance >50 ml/min)

Indication	*Daily dose regimen (according to severity)*	*Duration of treatment*
Acute sinusitis	500 mg once daily	10–14 days
Acute exacerbation of chronic bronchitis	250 to 500 mg once daily	7–10 days
Community–acquired pneumonia	500 mg once or twice daily	7–14 days
Complicated urinary tract infections including pyelonephritis	250 mg once daily	7–10 days
Skin and soft tissue infections	250 mg once daily or 500 mg once or twice daily	7–14 days

Dosage in patients with impaired renal function (creatinine clearance <50 ml/min)

	Dose regimen		
	250 mg/24 h	**500 mg/24 h**	**500 mg/12 h**
Creatinine clearance	first dose 250 mg	first dose 500 mg	first dose 500 mg
50–20 ml/min	then: 125 mg/24 h	then: 250 mg/24 h	then: 250 mg/12 h
19–10 ml/min	then: 125 mg/48 h	then: 125 mg/24 h	then: 125 mg/12 h
<10 ml/min (including hemodialysis and CAPD)[1]	then: 125 mg/48 h	then: 125 mg/24 h	then: 125 mg/24 h

[1] No additional doses are required after hemodialysis or continuous ambulatory peritoneal dialysis (CAPD).

Dosage in patients with impaired liver function: No adjustment of dosage is required since levofloxacin is not metabolised to any relevant extent by the liver and is mainly excreted by the kidneys.

Dosage in elderly: No adjustment of dosage is required in the elderly, other than that imposed by consideration of renal function.

Contra-indications: Tavanic tablets must not be used: in patients hypersensitive to levofloxacin, other quinolones, or any of the excipients; in patients with epilepsy; in patients with history of tendon disorders related to fluoroquinolone administration; in children or growing adolescents; during pregnancy; in breast-feeding women.

Special warnings and special precautions for use: In the most severe cases of pneumococcal pneumonia Tavanic may not be the optimal therapy. Nosocomial infections due to *P. aeruginosa* may require combination therapy.

Clostridium difficile-associated disease: Diarrhoea, particularly if severe, persistent and/or bloody, during or after treatment with Tavanic tablets, may be symptomatic of Clostridium difficile-associated disease, the most severe form of which is pseudomembranous colitis. If pseudomembranous colitis is suspected, Tavanic tablets must be stopped immediately and patients should be treated with supportive measures ± specific therapy without delay (e.g. oral vancomycin). Products inhibiting the peristalsis are contraindicated in this clinical situation.

Tendinitis: Tendinitis, rarely observed with quinolones, may occasionally lead to rupture, involving Achilles tendon in particular. Elderly patients are more prone to tendinitis. The risk of tendon rupture may be increased by coadministration of corticosteroids. If tendinitis is suspected, treatment with Tavanic tablets must be halted immediately, and appropriate treatment (e.g. immobilisation) must be initiated for the affected tendon.

Patients predisposed to seizures: Tavanic tablets are contra-indicated in patients with a history of epilepsy and, as other quinolones, should be used with extreme caution in patients predisposed to seizures, such as patients with pre-existing central nervous system lesions, concomitant treatment with fenbufen and similar non-steroidal anti-inflammatory drugs or with drugs which lower the cerebral seizure threshold, such as theophylline (see 'Interactions with other medicaments and other forms of interaction').

Patients with G-6- phosphate dehydrogenase deficiency: Patients with latent or actual defects in glucose-6-phosphate dehydrogenase activity may be prone to haemolytic reactions when treated with quinolone antibacterial agents, and so levofloxacin should be used with caution.

Patients with renal impairment: Since levofloxacin is excreted mainly by the kidneys, the dose of Tavanic should be adjusted in patients with renal impairment.

Prevention of photosensitisation: Although photosensitisation is very rare with levofloxacin, it is recommended that patients should not expose themselves unnecessarily to strong sunlight or to artificial UV rays (e.g. sunray lamp, solarium), in order to prevent photosensitisation.

Interactions with other medicaments and other forms of interaction:

Iron salts, magnesium- or aluminium-containing antacids: Levofloxacin absorption is significantly reduced when iron salts, or magnesium- or aluminium-containing antacids are administered concomitantly with Tavanic tablets. It is recommended that preparations containing divalent or trivalent cations such as iron salts, or magnesium- or aluminium-containing antacids should not be taken 2 hours before or after Tavanic tablet administration. No interaction was found with calcium carbonate.

Sucralfate: The bioavailability of Tavanic tablets is significantly reduced when administered together with sucralfate. If the patient is to receive both sucralfate and Tavanic, it is best to administer sucralfate 2 hours after the Tavanic tablet administration.

Theophylline, fenbufen or similar non-steroidal anti-inflammatory drugs: No pharmacokinetic interactions of levofloxacin were found with theophylline in a clinical study. However, a pronounced lowering of the cerebral seizure threshold may occur when quinolones are given concurrently with theophylline, non-steroidal anti-inflammatory drugs, or other agents which lower the seizure threshold.

Levofloxacin concentrations were about 13% higher in the presence of fenbufen than when administered alone.

Probenicid and cimetidine: Probenicid and cimetidine had a statistically significant effect on the elimination of levofloxacin. The renal clearance of levofloxacin was reduced by cimetidine (24%) and probenicid (34%). This is because both drugs are capable of blocking the renal tubular secretion of levofloxacin. However, at the tested doses in the study, the statistically significant kinetic differences are unlikely to be of clinical relevance.

Caution should be exercised when levofloxacin is coadministered with drugs that effect the tubular renal secretion such as probenicid and cimetidine, especially in renally impaired patients.

Cyclosporin: The half life of cyclosporin was increased by 33% when coadministered with levofloxacin.

Meals: There is no clinically relevant interaction with food. Tavanic tablets may therefore be administered regardless of food intake.

Other relevant information: Clinical pharmacology studies were carried out to investigate possible pharmacokinetic interactions between levofloxacin and commonly prescribed drugs. The pharmacokinetics of levofloxacin were not affected to any clinically relevant extent when levofloxacin was administered together with the following drugs: calcium carbonate, digoxin, glibenclamide, ranitidine, warfarin.

Pregnancy and lactation:

Pregnancy: Reproductive studies in animals did not raise specific concern. However in the absence of human data and due to the experimental risk of damage by fluoroquinolones to the weight-bearing cartilage of the growing organism, Tavanic tablets must not be used in pregnant women.

Lactation: In the absence of human data and due to the experimental risk of damage by fluoroquinolones to the weight-bearing cartilage of the growing organism, Tavanic tablets must not be used in breast-feeding women.

Effects on ability to drive and use machines: Some undesirable effects (e.g., dizziness/vertigo, drowsiness, visual disturbances) may impair the patient's ability to concentrate and react, and therefore may constitute a risk in situations where these abilities are of special importance (e.g. driving a car or operating machinery).

Undesirable effects: The information given below is based on data from clinical studies in more than 5000 patients and on extensive post marketing experience. The following frequency rating has been used: (see table overleaf).

Overdose: According to toxicity studies in animals, the most important signs to be expected following acute overdosage of Tavanic tablets are central nervous system symptoms such as confusion, dizziness, impairment of consciousness, and convulsive seizures, as well as gastro-intestinal reactions such as nausea and mucosal erosions.

In the event of relevant overdose, gastric lavage should be considered and symptomatic treatment should be implemented. Antacids may be used for protection of gastric mucosa. Haemodialysis, including peritoneal dialysis and CAPD, are not effective in removing levofloxacin from the body. No specific antidote exists.

Pharmacological properties

Pharmacodynamic properties: Levofloxacin is a synthetic antibacterial agent of the fluoroquinolone class (ATC code J01MA) and is the S (-) enantiomer of the racemic drug substance ofloxacin.

Mode of action: As a fluoroquinolone antibacterial agent, levofloxacin acts on the DNA–DNA-gyrase complex and topoisomerase IV.

Break points: The preliminary NCCLS (US National Committee on Clinical Laboratory Standards) recommended MIC breakpoints for levofloxacin, separating susceptible from intermediately susceptible organisms and intermediately susceptible from resistant organisms are:

susceptible ≤ 2 mg/L, resistant ≥ 8 mg/L

Antibacterial spectrum: The prevalence of resistance may vary geographically and with time for selected species and local information on resistance is desirable, particularly when treating severe infections. Therefore, the information presented provides only an approximate guidance on probabilities as to whether microorganisms will be susceptible to levofloxacin or not. Only microorganisms relevant to the given clinical indications are presented here.

Susceptible micro-organisms:

Aerobic Gram-positive:

*Enterococcus faecalis**

*Staphylococcus aureus** methi-S

Staphylococcus haemolyticus methi-S

Staphylococcus saprophyticus

Streptococci, group C and G

Streptococcus agalactiae

*Streptococcus pneumoniae** peni-I/S/R

Streptococcus pyogenes

Aerobic Gram-negative:

*Acinetobacter baumannii**

*Citrobacter freundii**

Eikenella corrodens

Enterobacter aerogenes

Enterobacter agglomerans

*Enterobacter cloacae**

*Escherichia coli**

Haemophilus influenzae ampi-S/R*

*Haemophilus para-influenzae**

Klebsiella oxytoca

*Klebsiella pneumoniae**

Moraxella catarrhalis β+/β-*

*Morganella morganii**

Pasteurella multocida

*Proteus mirabilis**
Proteus vulgaris
Providencia rettgeri
Providencia stuartii
*Pseudomonas aeruginosa**
*Serratia marcescens**
Anaerobic:
Bacteroides fragilis
Clostridium perfringens
Peptostreptococcus
"Other":
*Chlamydia pneumoniae**
Chlamydia psittaci
*Legionella pneumophila**
*Mycoplasma pneumoniae**

Intermediately susceptible microorgansisms:
Aerobic Gram-positive:
Staphylococcus haemolyticus methi-R
Aerobic Gram-negative:
Burkholderia cepacia
Anaerobic:
Bacteroides ovatus
Bacteroides thetaiotamicron
Bacteroides vulgatus
Clostridium difficile

Resistant microorganisms:
Aerobic Gram-positive:
Staphylococcus aureus methi-R

*clinical efficacy has been proven in clinical studies

Other information: The main mechanism of resistance is due to a *gyr-A* mutation. In vitro there is a cross-resistance between levofloxacin and other fluoroquinolones.

Acquired resistance with levofloxacin has recently been documented in 1997:
- *S. pneumoniae* France ≤ 1%
- *H. influenzae: rare.*

Due to the mechanism of action, there is generally no cross-resistance between levofloxacin and other classes of antibacterial agents.

Nosocomial infections due to *P. aeruginosa* may require combination therapy.

Pharmacokinetic properties:
Absorption: Orally administered levofloxacin is rapidly and almost completely absorbed with peak plasma concentrations being obtained within 1 h. The absolute bioavailability is approximately 100%. Levofloxacin obeys linear pharmacokinetics over a range of 50 to 600 mg.

Food has little effect on the absorption of levofloxacin.

Distribution: Approximately 30–40% of levofloxacin is bound to serum protein. 500 mg once daily multiple dosing with levofloxacin showed negligible accumulation. There is modest but predictable accumulation of levofloxacin after doses of 500 mg twice daily. Steady-state is achieved within 3 days.

Penetration into tissues and body fluids:
Penetration into Bronchial Mucosa, Epithelial Lining Fluid (ELF): Maximum levofloxacin concentrations in bronchial mucosa and epithelial lining fluid after 500 mg po were 8.3µg/g and 10.8µg/ml respectively. These were reached approximately one hour after administration.

Penetration into lung tissue: Maximum levofloxacin concentrations in lung tissue after 500 mg po were approximately 11.3µg/g and were reached between 4 and 6 hours after administration. The concentrations in the lungs consistently exceeded those in plasma.

Penetration into blister fluid: Maximum levofloxacin concentrations of about 4.0 and 6.7µg/ml in the blister fluid were reached 2–4 hours after administration following 3 days treatment at 500 mg once or twice daily, respectively.

Penetration into Cerebro-Spinal Fluid: Levofloxacin has poor penetration into cerebro-spinal fluid.

Concentration in urine: The mean urine concentrations 8 -12 hours after a single oral dose of 150 mg, 300 mg or 500 mg levofloxacin were 44 mg/L, 91 mg/L and 200 mg/L, respectively.

Metabolism: Levofloxacin is metabolised to a very small extent, the metabolites being desmethyl-levofloxacin and levofloxacin N-oxide. These metabolites account for < 5 % of the dose excreted in urine. Levofloxacin is stereochemically stable and does not undergo chiral inversion.

Elimination: Following oral and intravenous administration, levofloxacin is eliminated relatively slowly from the plasma ($t_{\frac{1}{2}}$: 6–8 hours). Excretion is primarily by the renal route (>85 % of the administered dose).

There are no major differences in the pharmacokinetics of levofloxacin following intravenous and oral administration, suggesting that the oral and intravenous routes are interchangeable.

Subjects with renal insufficiency: The pharmacokinetics of levofloxacin are affected by renal impairment. With decreasing renal function renal elimination and clearance are decreased, and elimination half-lives increased as shown in the table below:

Very common	more than		10 %
common	1 %	to	10 %
uncommon	0.1%	to	1%
rare	0.01%	to	0.1%
very rare	less than		0.01%
isolated cases			

Allergic reactions
Uncommon: Pruritus, rash
Rare: Urticaria, bronchospasm/dyspnoea
Very rare: Angio-oedema, hypotension, anaphylactic-like shock; photosensitisation
Isolated cases: Severe bullous eruptions such as Stevens Johnson syndrome, toxic shock, epidermal necrolysis (Lyell's syndrome) and erythema exsudativum multiforme

Muco-cutaneous, anaphylactic/ -oid reactions may sometimes occur even after the first dose.

Gastro-intestinal, metabolism
Common: Nausea, diarrhoea
Uncommon: Anorexia, vomiting, abdominal pain, dyspepsia
Rare: Bloody diarrhoea which in very rare cases may be indicative of enterocolitis, including pseudomembranous colitis
Very rare: Hypoglycaemia, particularly in diabetic patients

Neurological
Uncommon: Headache, dizziness/vertigo, drowsiness, insomnia
Rare: Paraesthesia, tremor, anxiety, agitation, confusion, convulsion,
Very rare: Hypoaesthesia, visual and auditory disturbances, disturbances of taste and smell, hallucinations

Cardiovascular
Rare: Tachycardia, hypotension
Very rare: Shock (anaphylactic-like)

Musculo-skeletal
Rare: Arthralgia, myalgia, tendon disorders, incl. tendinitis, (e.g. Achille's tendon)
Very rare: Tendon rupture (e.g. Achille's tendon), as with other fluoroquinolones this undesirable effect may occur within 48 hours of starting treatment and may be bilateral. Muscular weakness, which may be of special importance in patients with myasthenia gravis
Isolated cases: Rhabdomyolysis

Liver, kidney
Common: Increases in liver enzymes (e.g. ALT/AST)
Uncommon: Increase in bilirubin, increase in serum creatinine
Very rare: Liver reactions, such as hepatitis; acute kidney failure (e.g. due to interstitial nephritis)

Blood
Uncommon: Eosinophilia, leukopenia
Rare: Neutropenia, thrombocytopenia,
Very rare: Agranulocytosis
Isolated cases: Haemolytic anaemia, pancytopenia

Others
Uncommon: Asthenia, fungal overgrowth and proliferation of other resistant micro-organisms
Very rare: Allergic pneumonitis, fever

Other undesirable effects which have been associated with fluoroquinolone administration include:
* psychotic reactions such as acute confusional states and depressive mood changes (these reactions may occur even after the first dose)
* extrapyramidal symptoms and other disorders of muscular coordination
* hypersensitivity vasculitis
* attacks of porphyria in patients with porphyria.

Cl_{cr} [ml/min]	< 20	20–40	50–80
Cl_R [ml/min]	13	26	57
$t_{1/2}$ [h]	35	27	9

Elderly subjects: There are no significant differences in levofloxacin kinetics between young and elderly subjects, except those associated with differences in creatinine clearance.

Gender differences: Separate analysis for male and female subjects showed small to marginal gender differences in levofloxacin pharmacokinetics. There is no evidence that these gender differences are of clinical relevance.

Preclinical safety data:
Acute toxicity: The median lethal dose (LD_{50}) values obtained in mice and rats after oral administration of levofloxacin were in the range 1500-2000 mg/kg.

Administration of 500 mg/kg p.o. to monkeys induced little effect apart from vomiting.

Repeated dose toxicity: Studies of one and six months duration by gavage have been carried out in the rat and monkey. Doses were 50, 200, 800 mg/kg/day and 20, 80, 320 mg/kg/day for 1 and 6 months in the rat and 10, 30, 100 mg/kg/day and 10, 25, 62.5 mg/kg/day for 1 and 6 months in the monkey.

Signs of reaction to treatment were minor in the rat with slight effects principally at 200 mg/kg/day and above in reducing food consumption and slightly altering haematological and biochemical parameters. The No Observed Adverse Effect Level (NOEL) in these studies were concluded to be 200 and 20 mg/kg/day after 1 and 6 months respectively.

Toxicity after oral dosing in the monkey was minimal with reduced body weight at 100 mg/kg/day together with salivation, diarrhoea and decreased urinary pH in some animals at this dose. No toxicity was seen in the 6 month study. The NOELs were concluded to be 30 and 62.5 mg/kg/day after 1 and 6 months respectively.

The " No Observed Adverse Effect Levels " (NOEL) in the six-month studies were concluded to be 20 and 62.5 mg/kg/day in the rat and monkey respectively.

Reproductive toxicity: Levofloxacin caused no impairment of fertility or reproductive performance in rats at oral doses as high as 360 mg/kg/day or intravenous doses up to 100 mg/kg/day. Levofloxacin was not teratogenic in rats at oral doses as high as 810 mg/kg/day, or at intravenous doses as high as 160 mg/kg/day. No teratogenicity was observed when rabbits were dosed orally with up to 50 mg/kg/day or intravenously with up to 25 mg/kg/day.

Levofloxacin had no effect on fertility and its only effect on foetuses was delayed maturation as a result of maternal toxicity.

Genotoxicity: Levofloxacin did not induce gene mutations in bacterial or mammalian cells but did induce chromosome aberrations in Chinese hamster lung cells in vitro at or above 100 µg/ml, in the absence of metabolic activation. In vivo tests (micronucleus, sister chromatid exchange, unscheduled DNA synthesis, dominant lethal tests) did not show any genotoxic potential.

Phototoxic potential: Studies in the mouse after both oral and intravenous dosing showed levofloxacin to have phototoxic activity only at very high doses. Levofloxacin did not show any genotoxic potential in a photomutagenicity assay, and it reduced tumour development in a photocarcinogenicity assay.

Carcinogenic potential: No indication of carcinogenic potential was seen in a two year study in the rat with dietary administration (0, 10, 30 and 100 mg/kg/day).

Toxicity to joints: In common with other fluoroquinolones, levofloxacin showed effects on cartilage (blistering and cavities) in rats and dogs. These findings were more marked in young animals.

Pharmaceutical particulars
List of excipients: Tavanic 250 mg and 500 mg film-coated tablet contain the following excipients for a weight of 315 mg and 630 mg respectively:
Tablet core: Crospovidone; methylhydroxypropylcellulose; microcrystalline cellulose and sodium stearyl fumarate.

Tablet coating: Methylhydroxypropylcellulose; titanium dioxide (E 171); talc; polyethylene glycol; yellow ferric oxide (E 172) and red ferric oxide (E 172).

Incompatibilities: Not applicable.

Shelf life: Film-coated tablet 250 mg and 500 mg: 36 months.

Special precautions for storage: No special conditions for storage.

Nature and contents of container: PVC aluminium blisters containing film coated tablets.

Pack sizes for 250 mg tablets: 1, 5, 7, 10, 50 and 200 as commercially available.

Pack sizes for 500 mg tablets: 1, 5, 7, 10, 50, 200 and 500 as commercially available.

Instruction for use/handling: A score line allows adaptation of the dose in patients with impaired renal function.

Marketing authorisation numbers

PL 13402/0011 250 mg Tablet
PL 13402/0012 500 mg Tablet

Date of approval/revision of SPC September 1998

Legal category POM

TELFAST* 120 & 180 ▼

Qualitative and quantitative composition

Telfast 120: Active ingredient: fexofenadine base 112 mg (as fexofenadine hydrochloride 120 mg).
Telfast 180: Active ingredient: fexofenadine base 168 mg (as fexofenadine hydrochloride 180 mg).

Pharmaceutical form

Telfast 120: Film-coated tablets.
Telfast 180: Film-coated tablets.

Clinical particulars

Therapeutic indications:
Telfast 120: Relief of symptoms associated with seasonal allergic rhinitis.
Telfast 180: Relief of symptoms associated with chronic idiopathic urticaria.

Posology and method of administration:
Adults and children aged 12 years and over:
Telfast 120: The recommended dose of fexofenadine hydrochloride for adults and children aged 12 years and over is 120 mg once daily.
Telfast 180: The recommended dose of fexofenadine hydrochloride for adults and children aged 12 years and over is 180 mg once daily.

Fexofenadine is a pharmacologically active metabolite of terfenadine.

Children under 12 years of age: The efficacy and safety of fexofenadine hydrochloride has not been studied in children under 12.

Special risk groups: Studies in special risk groups (elderly, renally or hepatically impaired patients) indicate that it is not necessary to adjust the dose of fexofenadine hydrochloride in these patients.

Contra-indications: The product is contraindicated in patients with known hypersensitivity to any of its ingredients.

Special warnings and precautions for use: As with most new drugs there is only limited data in the elderly and renally or hepatically impaired patients. Fexofenadine hydrochloride should be administered with care in these special groups.

Interaction with other medicaments and other forms of interaction: Fexofenadine does not undergo hepatic biotransformation and therefore will not interact with other drugs through hepatic mechanisms. Coadministration of fexofenadine hydrochloride with erythromycin or ketoconazole has been found to result in a 2-3 times increase in the level of fexofenadine in plasma. The changes were not accompanied by any effects on the QT interval and were not associated with any increase in adverse events compared to the drugs given singly.

Animal studies have shown that the increase in plasma levels of fexofenadine observed after coadministration of erythromycin or ketoconazole, appears to be due to an increase in gastrointestinal absorption and either a decrease in biliary excretion or gastrointestinal secretion, respectively.

No interaction between fexofenadine and omeprazole was observed. However, the administration of an antacid containing aluminium and magnesium hydroxide gels 15 minutes prior to fexofenadine hydrochloride caused a reduction in bioavailability, most likely due to binding in the gastrointestinal tract. It is advisable to leave 2 hours between administration of fexofenadine hydrochloride and aluminium and magnesium hydroxide containing antacids.

Pregnancy and lactation: No animal reproduction studies have been performed with fexofenadine hydrochloride. Supportive pharmacokinetic studies with terfenadine have been performed and show exposure to fexofenadine at the high dose level in animal reproduction studies performed with terfenadine to be higher than is achieved at the recommended clinical fexofenadine dose. In these studies no evidence of teratogenicity or effects on male fertility were observed. Effects on female fertility and on peri and post natal development were seen only at maternally toxic doses.

There is no experience with fexofenadine hydrochloride in pregnant women. As with other medications fexofenadine hydrochloride should not be used during pregnancy unless the expected benefit to the patient outweighs any possible risk to the foetus.

There are no data on the content of human milk after administering fexofenadine hydrochloride. However, when terfenadine was administered to nursing mothers fexofenadine was found to cross into human breast milk. Therefore fexofenadine hydrochloride is not recommended for mothers breast feeding their babies.

Effects on ability to drive and use machines: On the basis of the pharmacodynamic profile and reported adverse events it is unlikely that fexofenadine hydrochloride tablets will produce an effect on the ability to drive or use machines. In objective tests, Telfast has been shown to have no significant effects on central nervous system function. This means that patients may drive or perform tasks that require concentration. However, in order to identify sensitive people who have an unusual reaction to drugs, it is advisable to check the individual response before driving or performing complicated tasks.

Undesirable effects: In controlled clinical trials the most commonly reported adverse events were headache (7.3%), drowsiness (2.3%), nausea (1.5%), dizziness (1.5%) and fatigue (0.9%). The incidence of these events observed with fexofenadine was similar to that observed with placebo.

Overdose: There has been no reported case of an acute overdose of fexofenadine hydrochloride. Standard measures should be considered to remove any unabsorbed drug. Haemodialysis does not effectively remove fexofenadine hydrochloride from blood.

Pharmacological properties

Pharmacodynamic properties: Fexofenadine hydrochloride is a non-sedating H_1 antihistamine. Fexofenadine is a pharmacologically active metabolite of terfenadine.

Human histamine wheal and flare studies following single and twice daily doses of fexofenadine hydrochloride demonstrate that the drug exhibits an antihistaminic effect beginning within one hour, achieving maximum at 6 hours and lasting 24 hours. There was no evidence of tolerance to these effects after 28 days of dosing. A positive dose-response relationship between doses of 10 mg to 130 mg taken orally was found to exist. In this model of antihistaminic activity, it was found that doses of at least 130 mg were required to achieve a consistent effect that was maintained over a 24 hour period. Maximum inhibition in skin wheal and flare areas were greater than 80%. Clinical studies conducted in seasonal allergic rhinitis have shown that a dose of 120 mg is sufficient for 24 hour efficacy.

No significant differences in QT_c intervals were observed in seasonal allergic rhinitis patients given fexofenadine hydrochloride up to 240 mg twice daily for 2 weeks when compared to placebo. Also, no significant change in QT_c intervals was observed in healthy subjects given fexofenadine hydrochloride up to 60 mg twice daily for 6 months, 400 mg twice daily for 6.5 days and 240 mg once daily for 1 year, when compared to placebo. Fexofenadine at concentrations 32 times greater than the therapeutic concentration in man had no effect on the delayed rectifier K^+ channel cloned from human heart.

Fexofenadine hydrochloride (5-10 mg/kg p.o.) inhibited antigen induced bronchospasm in sensitised guinea pigs and inhibited histamine release at supratherapeutic concentrations (10-100 microMolar) from peritoneal mast cells.

Pharmacokinetic properties: Fexofenadine hydrochloride is rapidly absorbed into the body following oral administration, with T_{max} occurring at approximately 1-3 hours post dose. The mean C_{max} value was approximately 427 ng/ml following the administration of a 120 mg dose once daily and approximately 494 ng/ml following the administration of a 180 mg dose once daily.

Fexofenadine is 60-70% plasma protein bound. Fexofenadine undergoes negligible metabolism (hepatic or non-hepatic), as it was the only major compound identified in urine and faeces of animals and man. The plasma concentration profiles of fexofenadine follow a bi-exponential decline with a terminal elimination half-life ranging from 11 to 15 hours after multiple dosing. The single and multiple dose pharmacokinetics of fexofenadine are linear for oral doses up to 120 mg b.i.d. A dose of 240 mg b.i.d. produced slightly greater than proportional increase (8.8%) in steady state area under the curve, indicating that fexofenadine pharmacokinetics are practically linear at these doses between 40 and 240 mg taken daily. The major route of elimination is believed to be via biliary excretion while up to 10% of ingested dose is excreted unchanged through the urine.

Preclinical safety data: Dogs tolerated 450 mg/kg administered twice daily for 6 months and showed no toxicity other than occasional emesis. Also, in single dose dog and rodent studies, no treatment-related gross findings were observed following necropsy.

Radiolabelled fexofenadine hydrochloride in tissue distribution studies of the rat indicated that fexofenadine did not cross the blood brain barrier.

Fexofenadine hydrochloride was found to be non-mutagenic in various *in vitro* and *in vivo* mutagenicity tests.

The carcinogenic potential of fexofenadine hydrochloride was assessed using terfenadine studies with supporting pharmacokinetic studies showing fexofenadine hydrochloride exposure (via plasma AUC values). No evidence of carcinogenicity was observed in rats and mice given terfenadine (up to 150 mg/kg/day).

Pharmaceutical particulars

List of excipients: Tablet core: Microcrystalline Cellulose, Pregelatinised Maize Starch, Croscarmellose Sodium, Magnesium Stearate

Film coat: Hypromellose, Povidone, Titanium Dioxide (E171), Colloidal Anhydrous Silica, Macrogol 400, Iron oxide (E172).

Incompatibilities: None.

Shelf life: 24 months.

Special precautions for storage: None.

Nature and contents of container: White opaque polyvinylchloride blisters (pharmaceutical grade) 200 micrometers thick with a polyvinylidine chloride coating of 90 g/m² on the internal surface of the blister. The PVC/PE/PVDC is sealed to hard tempered aluminium foil 20 micrometer thick with a vinyl heat seal coating. The blisters are packaged into cardboard boxes.

Telfast 120: The number of peach modified capsule-shaped tablets, per package are 2 (sample only), 7, 10, 15, 20, 30, 50, 100 and 200 (as 10×20), as available.

Telfast 180: The number of peach, capsule-shaped tablets, per package are 2 (sample only), 10, 15, 20, 30, 50, 100 and 200 (as 10×20), as available.

Instructions for use/handling: No special instructions.

Marketing authorisation holder: Marion Merrell Ltd., Broadwater Park, Denham, Uxbridge, Middlesex, UB9 5HP

Marketing authorisation numbers

Telfast 120: 4425/0157
Telfast 180: 4425/0158

Date of approval/revision of SPC January 1998

Legal category POM.

TRITACE*

Qualitative and quantitative composition

1.25 mg ramipril
2.5 mg ramipril
5.0 mg ramipril
10.0 mg ramipril

Pharmaceutical form

1.25 mg:Yellow opaque/white opaque hard gelatin capsules.
2.5 mg: Orange opaque / white opaque hard gelatin capsules.
5.0 mg: Scarlet opaque / white opaque hard gelatin capsules.
10.0 mg: Blue opaque/ white opaque hard gelatin capsules.

Capsules are marked with the strength and the Hoechst logo.

Clinical particulars

Therapeutic indications: Tritace is indicated in the treatment of mild to moderate hypertension.

Congestive heart failure as adjunctive therapy to diuretics with or without cardiac glycosides.

Tritace has been shown to reduce mortality when given to patients surviving acute myocardial infarction with clinical evidence of heart failure.

Oral administration.

Posology and method of administration:
Dosage and administration:

Hypertension: The recommended initial dosage in patients not on diuretics and without congestive heart failure is 1.25 mg Tritace once a day. Dosage should be increased incrementally at intervals of 1–2 weeks, based on patient response, up to a maximum of 10 mg once a day.

A 1.25 mg dose will only achieve a therapeutic response in a minority of patients. The usual maintenance dose is 2.5–5 mg as a single daily dose. If the patient response is still unsatisfactory at a dose of 10 mg Tritace, combination treatment is recommended.

In diuretic-treated patients, the diuretic should be discontinued 2–3 days before beginning therapy with Tritace to reduce the likelihood of symptomatic hypotension. It may be resumed later if required.

In hypertensive patients who also have congestive heart failure, with or without associated renal insufficiency, symptomatic hypotension has been observed after treatment with ACE inhibitors. In these patients therapy should be started at a dose of 1.25 mg under close medical supervision in hospital.

Congestive heart failure: Recommended initial dose: In patients stabilised on diuretic therapy the initial dose is 1.25 mg once daily. Depending on the patient's response, the dose may be increased. It is recommended that the dose, if increased, be doubled at intervals of 1 to 2 weeks. If a daily dose of 2.5 mg or more is required, this may be taken as a single dose or as two divided doses. Maximum permitted daily dose: 10 mg.

In order to minimise the possibility of symptomatic hypotension, patients on previous high dose diuretics should have the diuretic dose reduced before starting Tritace.

Post myocardial infarction: Initiation of therapy: Treatment must be started in hospital between day 3 and day 10 following AMI. The starting dose is 2.5 mg twice a day which is increased to 5 mg twice a day after 2 days. If the initial 2.5 mg dose is not tolerated a dose of 1.25 mg twice a day should be given for two days before increasing to 2.5 mg and 5.0 mg twice a day. If the dose cannot be increased to 2.5 mg twice a day treatment should be withdrawn.

Maintenance dose: 2.5 to 5.0 mg twice a day.

Dosage adjustment in renal impairment: The usual dose of Tritace is recommended for patients with a creatinine clearance >30 ml/min (serum creatinine <165 micromol/litre). For patients with a creatinine clearance <30 ml/min (serum creatinine >165 micromol/litre) the initial dose is 1.25 mg Tritace once daily and the maximum dose 5 mg Tritace once daily.

In patients with severe renal impairment (creatinine clearance <10 ml/min and serum creatinine of 400-650 micromol/litre), the recommended initial dose is also 1.25 mg Tritace once a day, but the maintenance dose should not exceed 2.5 mg Tritace once a day.

Dosage in hepatic impairment: In patients with impaired liver function the metabolism of the parent compound ramipril, and therefore the formation of the bioactive metabolite ramiprilat, is delayed due to diminished activity of esterases in the liver, resulting in elevated plasma ramipril levels. Treatment with Tritace should therefore be initiated at a dose of 1.25 mg under close medical supervision in patients with impaired liver function.

Elderly: Caution in elderly patients with concomitant use of diuretics, congestive heart failure or renal or hepatic insufficiency. The dose should be titrated according to need for the control of blood pressure.

Children: Tritace has not been studied in children, and therefore use in this age group is not recommended.

Tritace should be taken with a glass of water. The absorption of ramipril is not affected by food.

Contra-indications: Hypersensitivity to ramipril or any of the excipients. History of angioneurotic oedema, haemodynamically relevant renal artery stenosis, hypotensive or haemodynamically unstable patients. Pregnancy. Lactation.

Special warnings and special precautions for use:
Warnings: Tritace should not be used in patients with aortic or mitral valve stenosis or outflow obstruction.

Precautions: Assessment of renal function: Evaluation of the patient should include assessment of renal function prior to initiation of therapy and during treatment.

Impaired renal function: Patients with renal insufficiency may require reduced or less frequent doses of Tritace; their renal function should be closely monitored. In the majority, renal function will not alter. There is a risk of impairment of renal function, particularly in patients with renal insufficiency, congestive heart failure, bilateral renal artery stenosis and unilateral renal artery stenosis in the single kidney as well as after renal transplantation. If recognised early, such impairment of renal function is reversible upon discontinuation of therapy.

Patients haemodialysed using high flux polyacrylonitrile ('AN69') membranes are highly likely to experience anaphylactoid reactions if they are treated with ACE inhibitors. This combination should therefore be avoided, either by use of alternative antihypertensive drugs or alternative membranes for dialysis.

Similar reactions have been observed during low-density lipoprotein apheresis with dextran sulphate. This method should, therefore, not be used in patients treated with ACE inhibitors.

Some hypertensive patients with no apparent pre-existing renal disease, may develop minor and usually transient increases in blood urea nitrogen and serum creatinine when Tritace is given, in particular concomitantly with a diuretic. Dosage reduction of Tritace and/or discontinuation of the diuretic may be required. Additionally, in patients with renal insufficiency, there is a risk of hyperkalaemia.

Impaired liver function: As ramipril is a prodrug metabolised to its active moiety in the liver, particular caution and close monitoring should be applied to patients with impaired liver function. The metabolism of the parent compound, and therefore the formation of the bioactive metabolite ramiprilat, may be diminished resulting in markedly elevated plasma levels of the parent compound (due to the reduced activity of esterases in the liver).

Symptomatic hypotension: In patients with uncomplicated hypertension, symptomatic hypotension has been observed rarely after the initial dose of Tritace as well as after increasing the dose of Tritace. It is more likely to occur in patients who have been volume-and salt-depleted by prolonged diuretic therapy, dietary salt restriction, dialysis, diarrhoea, vomiting or in patients with severe heart failure. Therefore, in these patients, diuretic therapy should be discontinued and volume and/or salt depletion should be corrected before initiating therapy with Tritace.

If symptomatic hypotension occurs, the patient should be placed in a supine position and, if necessary, receive an intravenous infusion of physiological saline. Intravenous atropine may be necessary if there is associated bradycardia. Treatment with Tritace may usually be continued following restoration of effective blood volume and blood pressure.

Surgery/anaesthesia: In patients undergoing surgery or during anaesthesia with agents producing hypotension, Tritace may block angiotensin II formation secondary to compensatory renin release. If hypotension occurs and is considered to be due to this mechanism, it can be corrected by appropriate treatment.

Agranulocytosis and bone marrow depression: In patients on angiotensin converting enzyme inhibitors agranulocytosis and bone marrow depression have been seen rarely, as well as a reduction in red cell count, haemoglobin content and platelet count. These are more frequent in patients with renal impairment, especially if they have a collagen vascular disease. Regular monitoring of white blood cell counts and protein levels in urine should be considered in patients with collagen vascular disease (e.g. lupus erythematosus and scleroderma), especially associated with impaired renal function and concomitant therapy particularly with corticosteroids and antimetabolites. Patients on allopurinol, immunosuppressants and other substances that may change the blood picture also have increased likelihood of other blood picture changes.

Hyperkalaemia: Elevated serum potassium has been observed very rarely in hypertensive patients. Risk factors for the development of hyperkalaemia include renal insufficiency, potassium sparing diuretics and the concomitant use of agents to treat hypokalaemia.

Interactions with other medicaments and other forms of interaction: Combination with diuretics or other antihypertensive agents may potentiate the antihypertensive response to Tritace. Adrenergic-blocking drugs should only be combined with ramipril under careful supervision.

Potassium sparing diuretics (spironolactone, amiloride, triamterene) or potassium supplements may increase the risk of hyperkalaemia. Tritace may attenuate the potassium loss caused by thiazide-type diuretics. If concomitant use of these agents is indicated, they should be given with caution and serum potassium should be monitored regularly.

When antidiabetic agents (insulin and sulphonylurea derivatives) are used concurrently, the possibility of increased blood-sugar reduction must be considered.

If Tritace is given with lithium, an increase in serum lithium concentration may occur.

When ACE inhibitors are administered simultaneously with non-steroidal anti-inflammatory drugs (e.g. acetylsalicylic acid and indomethacin), attenuation of the antihypertensive effect may occur.

The protein binding of ramipril is about 73% and of ramiprilat about 56%.

Pregnancy and lactation: Pregnancy should be excluded before start of treatment with Tritace and avoided during treatment; exposure of the mother to ACE inhibitors in mid or late pregnancy has been associated with oligohydramnios and neonatal hypotension with anuria or renal failure.

From animal experiments it is known that use of ramipril may cause a decreased utero-placental perfusion. There is also a potential risk of fetal or post-natal effect as ACE inhibitors also influence the local renin-angiotensin system. In peri-post natal studies increased renal pelvic dilatation was observed in the first generation offspring. However, ramipril was not fetotoxic in our studies although ACE inhibitors have shown fetotoxicity in some species.

Tritace should not be used during lactation.

Effects on ability to drive and use machines: In individual cases, as a result of a reduction in blood pressure, treatment with Tritace may affect the ability to drive and operate machinery. This occurs especially at the start of treatment, when changing over from other preparations and during concomitant use of alcohol. After the first dose or subsequent increases in dose it is not advisable to drive or operate machinery for several hours.

Undesirable effects: Generally, adverse reactions have been mild and transient, and do not required discontinuation of therapy. The most frequently reported adverse reactions are nausea, dizziness and headache.

Cardiovascular: Symptomatic hypotension accompanied by dizziness, weakness and nausea may occur after the initial dose of Tritace and after an increase in the dose of Tritace. It has been rarely observed, but may occur in severely salt/volume-depleted patients such as those treated with diuretics, patients on dialysis and in patients with severe congestive heart failure. Syncope has also been observed rarely.

Myocardial infarction or cerebrovascular accident possibly secondary to severe hypotension in high risk patients, chest pain, palpitations, rhythm disturbances, angina pectoris may occur.

Renal: Treatment with Tritace may impair renal function.

Gastrointestinal: Treatment with Tritace may be associated with symptoms in the digestive tract, e.g. dryness of the mouth, irritation or inflammation of the oral mucosa, digestive disturbances, constipation, diarrhoea, nausea, and vomiting, (gastritis-like) stomach pain, upper abdominal discomfort (sometimes with increased levels of pancreatic enzymes), increases in hepatic enzymes and/or serum bilirubin, jaundice due to impaired excretion of bile pigment (cholestatic jaundice), other forms of impaired liver function, and hepatitis.

Pancreatitis has been reported rarely in patients treated with ACE inhibitors; in some cases this has proved fatal.

Allergic: Hypersensitivity reactions accompanied by pruritus, rash, shortness of breath and sometimes fever may occur, but usually resolve spontaneously after withdrawal of Tritace.

In addition, the following cutaneous and mucosal reaction may occur: reddening of skin areas with accompanying heat sensation, conjunctivitis, itching, urticaria, other skin or mucosal eruptions (maculopapular and lichenoid exanthema and enanthema, erythema multiforme), sometimes pronounced hair loss, and precipitation or intensification of Raynaud's phenomenon. With other ACE inhibitors psoriasiform and pemphigoid exanthema and enanthema, hypersensitivity of the skin to light, and onycholysis have been observed.

Vasculitis, muscle and joint pains, fever, or eosinophilia may occur. Raised titres of antinuclear antibodies have been seen with other ACE inhibitors.

Angioneurotic oedema: In very rare cases angioneurotic oedema has occurred during therapy with ACE inhibitors including Tritace. If laryngeal stridor or angioedema of the face, tongue or glottis occurs, treatment with Tritace must be discontinued and appropriate therapy instituted immediately.

Respiratory tract: A dry tickling cough may occur. This is possibly due to the desired ACE inhibition as are the following adverse effects: rhinitis, sinusitis, bronchitis and, especially in patients with tickling cough, bronchospasm.

Other adverse reactions: Disturbances of balance, headache, nervousness, restlessness, tremor, sleep disorders, confusion, loss of appetite, depressed mood, feeling of anxiety, paraesthesiae, taste change, taste reduction and sometimes loss of taste, muscle cramps, erectile impotence and reduced sexual desire may occur.

Laboratory test findings: Increases in blood urea nitrogen and serum creatinine may occur, in particular with renal insufficiency or in patients pretreated with a diuretic. Pre-existing proteinuria may deteriorate.

Serum sodium levels may decrease. Elevation of serum potassium may occur, since Tritace leads to a decrease in aldosterone secretion; potassium-sparing diuretics (spironolactone, amiloride, triamterene) or potassium supplements should therefore be avoided.

Overdose: In case of overdosage prolonged hypotension is to be expected. Treatment with an intravenous infusion of physiological saline and/or angiotensin II may be required.

Pharmacological properties
Pharmacodynamic properties: Ramipril is a prodrug which, after absorption from the gastrointestinal tract, is hydrolysed in the liver to form the active angiotensin converting enzyme (ACE) inhibitor, ramiprilat which is a potent and long acting ACE inhibitor. Administration of ramipril causes an increase in plasma renin activity and a decrease in plasma concentrations of angiotensin II and aldosterone. The beneficial haemodynamic effects resulting from ACE inhibition are

a consequence of the reduction in angiotensin II causing dilatation of peripheral vessels and reduction in vascular resistance. There is evidence suggesting that tissue ACE particularly in the vasculature, rather than circulating ACE, is the primary factor determining the haemodynamic effects.

Angiotensin converting enzyme is identical with kininase II, one of the enzymes responsible for the degradation of bradykinin. There is evidence that ACE inhibition by ramiprilat appears to have some effects on the kallikrein-kinin-prostaglandin systems. It is assumed that effects on these systems contribute to the hypotensive and metabolic activity of ramipril.

Administration of Tritace to hypertensive patients results in reduction of both supine and standing blood pressure. The antihypertensive effect is evident within one to two hours after the drug intake; peak effect occurs 3-6 hours after drug intake and has been shown to be maintained for at least 24 hours after usual therapeutic doses.

Pharmacokinetic properties: Following oral administration ramipril is rapidly absorbed from the gastrointestinal tract, peak plasma concentrations of ramipril are reached within one hour. Peak plasma concentrations of the active metabolite, ramiprilat, are reached within 2–4 hours.

Plasma concentrations of ramiprilat decline in a polyphasic manner. The effective half-life of ramiprilat after multiple once daily administration of ramipril is 13–17 hours for 5–10 mg ramipril and markedly longer for lower doses, 1.25–2.5 mg ramipril. This difference is related to the long terminal phase of the ramiprilat concentration time curve observed at very low plasma concentrations. This terminal phase is independent of the dose, indicating a saturable capacity of the enzyme to bind ramiprilat. Steady-state plasma concentrations of ramiprilat after once daily dosing with the usual doses of ramipril are reached by about the fourth day of treatment.

Ramipril is almost completely metabolised and the metabolites are excreted mainly via the kidneys. In addition to the bioactive metabolite, ramiprilat, other, inactive metabolites have been identified, including diketopiperazine ester, diketopiperazine acid and conjugates.

Preclinical safety data: Reproduction toxicology studies in the rat, rabbit and monkey did not disclose any teratogenic properties. Fertility was not impaired either in male or in female rats. The administration of ramipril to female rats during the fetal period and lactation produced irreversible renal damage (dilatation of the renal pelvis) in the offspring at daily doses of 50 mg/kg body weight and higher.

Pharmaceutical particulars

List of excipients: Pregelatinised starch, Gelatin, Colours include: E171, E172 (1.25 mg), E127, E171, E172 (2.5 mg); E127, E131, E171 (5 mg); E127, E132, E171, E172 (10 mg) in the capsule shell.

Incompatibilities: None known.

Shelf life: 2 years.

Special precautions for storage: Tritace capsules should be stored below 25°C. They should be kept away from children.

Nature and contents of container: Blister (calendar) pack of 28 or 30 capsules. Glass bottles with screw cap with 50 or 100 capsules

Instruction for use/handling: None.

Marketing authorisation numbers

1.25 mg capsules	PL 13402/0021
2.5 mg capsules	PL 13402/0022
5.0 mg capsules	PL 13402/0023
10.0 mg capsules	PL 13402/0024

Date of approval/revision of SPC November 1997

Legal Category POM

**Trade Mark*

Hyland Immuno
Baxter Healthcare Ltd
Wallingford Road
Compton
nr Newbury
Berkshire
RG20 7QW

☎ 01635 206265 01635 206126

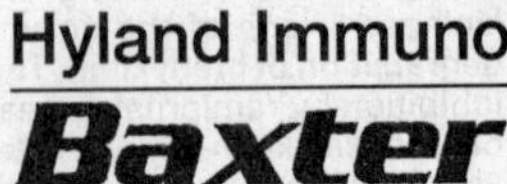

FEIBA* IMMUNO (Factor VIII Inhibitor Bypassing Fraction Human) Vapour Heated

Presentation FEIBA in its lyophilised form is an amorphous powder. After reconstitution with Water for Injections BP it is a clear yellowish solution.

It is produced from pooled human venous plasma. Only plasma units which are non reactive in tests for HBsAg and antibody to HIV1, HIV2 and HCV are used in the manufacture of FEIBA. All plasma units are further tested for ALT.

The product is subjected to in-process virus inactivation where vapour is first applied for 10 hours at 60°C ± 0.5°C and an excess pressure of 190 ± 20 mbar followed by one hour at 80°C ± 0.5°C and an excess pressure of 370 ± 30 mbar.

FEIBA contains an anti-inhibitor coagulant complex with standardised FEIB-activity (Factor Eight Inhibitor Bypassing Activity):

1 mg of protein contains 0.7 to 2.5 units FEIBA.

FEIBA also contains factors II, IX and X mainly in non-activated form as well as activated factor VII: factor VIII coagulant antigen (FVIII C:Ag) is present in a concentration of up to 0.1 U/1 U FEIBA. The factors of the kallikrein-kinin system are present in trace amounts or absent.

1 unit of FEIBA is defined as that amount of factor VIII inhibitor bypassing activity which shortens the activated partial thromboplastin time (APTT) of a high titre factor VIII inhibitor plasma to 50% of the buffer value (blank).

The state of the art suggests that it cannot be precluded with certainty that both known or unknown viruses, which may occur in plasma, are transmitted through factor concentrates.

Uses FEIBA is indicated for the control of bleeding episodes in haemophilia A patients with Factor VIII Inhibitors and also in patients with acquired Factor VIII Inhibitors.

Dosage and administration FEIBA should only be administered intravenously. Do not exceed an injection/infusion rate of 2 units of FEIBA per kg bodyweight per minute.

As a general guide a dose of 50 to 100 units of FEIBA per kg bodyweight is recommended, however, not exceeding a daily dose of 200 U/ kg bodyweight.

Dosage is independent of the patient's inhibitor titre. Since the response to treatment may differ from patient to patient the dosage recommendations are only guidelines.

Coagulation tests such as the whole blood clotting time (WBCT), the thromboelastogram (TEG, r-value), and the APTT usually show only a minor shortening and need not correlate with clinical improvement. For this reason these tests have only very limited value for monitoring FEIBA therapy.

1. SPONTANEOUS BLEEDING

Joint muscle and soft tissue haemorrhage: For minor to moderate bleeds a dose of 50–75 U/ kg bodyweight is recommended at 12-hour intervals. Treatment should be continued until clear signs of clinical improvement appear, such as relief of pain, reduction of swelling or mobilisation of the joint.

For major muscle and soft tissue haemorrhage, such as retroperitoneal bleeding, doses of 100 U/ kg bodyweight at 12 hour intervals are recommended.

Mucous membrane bleeding: A dose of 50 U/ kg bodyweight is recommended to be given every 6 hours with careful monitoring of the patient (visible bleeding site, repeated measurements of haematocrit). Again if haemorrhage does not stop, the dose may be increased to 100 U/ kg bodyweight taking care not to exceed the maximum daily dose of 200 U/ kg bodyweight.

Other severe haemorrhage: Severe haemorrhage, such as CNS bleeding has been effectively treated with doses of 100 U/ kg bodyweight at 12 hour intervals. In individual cases FEIBA may be given at intervals of 6 hours until clear clinical improvement is achieved. (Do not exceed the maximum daily dose).

2. SURGERY

Taking care not to exceed the maximum daily dose, 50–100 U/ kg bodyweight should be given at intervals of up to 6 hours.

The above dosage schedule applies equally to children and the elderly.

Use in the elderly:

No specific precautions have to be taken into account when using FEIBA in the elderly. Attention is, however, drawn to the fact that in patients with a tentative or definitive diagnosis of coronary heart disease the use of FEIBA is only indicated in life-threatening bleeding events.

Use in pregnancy:

Animal reproduction studies have not been conducted with FEIBA. It is also not known whether the product can cause fetal harm when administered to a pregnant woman or can affect reproduction capacity.

Contra-indications, warnings, etc

Contra-indications:

Disseminated intravascular coagulation (DIC): Laboratory and/or clinical symptoms which are clearly indicative of DIC.

Laboratory, histological and/or clinical signs of liver damage: due to the delayed clearance of activated coagulation factors such patients are at an increased risk of developing DIC.

Myocardial infarction, acute thrombosis and/or embolism: Except in cases of life threatening bleeding where no other form of therapy is likely to bring about satisfactory results.

Precautions and warnings: In rare cases allergic reactions such as fever, urticarial rashes, nausea and retching as well as other anaphylactoid reactions of varying severity have been observed after administration of FEIBA. Severe allergic and anaphylactoid reactions may necessitate the interruption of substitution treatment. Mild reactions can be managed with antihistamines: severe reactions require immediate intervention. In patients with a history of hypersensitivity reactions to plasma derivatives the prophylactic administration of antihistamines may be indicated.

In individual instances myocardial infarction was found to occur after high doses and/or prolonged administration and/or in the presence of risk factors predisposing to cardiovascular disease.

Single doses of 100 units FEIBA per kg bodyweight and daily doses of 200 units FEIBA per kg bodyweight should not be exceeded. Patients given single doses of 100 units FEIBA per kg bodyweight should be monitored for the development of DIC or symptoms of acute coronary ischaemia.

High doses of FEIBA should be given only as long as absolutely necessary to stop bleeding.

Disseminated intravascular coagulation (DIC): After administration of high doses (single doses of more than 100 units FEIBA per kg bodyweight, and daily doses of more than 200 units per kg bodyweight) laboratory signs such as the presence of fibrinopeptide A, Fibrin/Fibrinogen degradation products, or prolonged activated partial thromboplastin time (APTT), thrombin time and prothrombin time indicative of DIC were observed in a few cases.

If clinical signs of intravascular coagulation occur, which include changes in blood pressure, pulse rate, respiratory distress, chest pain and cough, the infusion should be stopped immediately and the patient monitored for DIC by appropriate laboratory tests.

Laboratory tests and clinical efficacy: In vitro tests to control efficacy such as APTT, whole blood clotting time and thromboelastogram (TEG) need not correlate with clinical improvement. For this reason, attempts at normalising these values by increasing the dose of FEIBA may not be successful and are strongly discouraged because of the potential hazard of producing DIC by overdosage.

Significance of platelet count: In case of inadequate or reduced response to FEIBA treatment it is recommended that a platelet count be performed, since a sufficient number of functionally intact platelets is considered to be necessary for the efficacy of FEIBA.

Antifibrinolytics: If treatment with both antifibrinolytics such as epsilon-aminocaproic acid and FEIBA is to be carried out, the interval between the administration of either product should be a least 6 hours.

Treatment of overdosage: Occasionally biological and/or clinical signs of DIC have been observed following the administration of high doses of FEIBA.

In such cases administration of the product should be stopped promptly.

If the coagulation parameters indicative of DIC do not quickly return to normal once administration of FEIBA is halted, it should be attempted to control the consumption reaction with Heparin or with antifibrinolytics in the case of secondary hyperfibrinolysis.

Pharmaceutical precautions FEIBA must be stored between +2°C and +8°C when it will have a shelf life of 2 years. The product may be stored at room temperature (maximum 25°C) for six months within the two year shelf life period.

Legal category POM

Package quantities FEIBA is supplied in packs containing 500 and 1000 FEIBA units together with a separate vial containing 20 ml Water for Injections BP as solvent. All packs contain sufficient equipment for reconstitution and administration.

Further information

1. Effect on laboratory tests: Inherent in its mechanism of action FEIBA causes a shortening of the following clotting times: activated partial thromboplastin time (APTT), whole blood clotting time (WBCT), activated clotting time (ACT), thromboelastogram (TEG).

Coagulation tests measuring the extrinsic coagulation system such as the prothrombin time, which is usually normal in haemophiliacs remained unchanged after treatment with FEIBA. Overdosage of the product may result in laboratory signs of DIC such as the presence of fibrinopeptide A, fibrin/fibrinogen degradation products, a fall in fibrinogen, a prolonged APTT, thrombin time and prothrombin time.

2. *Interactions:* It is not recommended to use antifibrinolytics such as epsilon-aminocaproic acid in combination with FEIBA treatment (see *Precautions and warnings*).

3. FEIBA is only available to Haemophilia Treatment Centres.

Product licence numbers 0215/0021-22

GAMMABULIN* Normal Immunoglobulin Injection BP

Presentation Gammabulin is a concentrate of antibodies present in the IgG fraction of human plasma. It is produced from pooled human plasma of venous origin. Only plasma units which are non-reactive in tests for HBsAg and antibodies to HIV1, HIV2 and HCV are used in the manufacture of Gammabulin. All plasma units are further tested for ALT.

Gammabulin is a clear pale yellow to light brown solution.

Gammabulin has a protein content of 16% of which 90% is gamma globulin. Glycine is added as a stabiliser at a concentration of 2.25%. There is no preservative added to the product.

Uses Gammabulin is used in the treatment of:

Antibody deficiency syndrome and recurring bacterial infections in dys-, hypo- and agammaglobulinaemia.

Hepatitis A prophylaxis.
Prevention or modification of measles infection.
Treatment of susceptible pregnant women exposed to Rubella infection in whom continuing pregnancy places the fetus at risk.

Dosage and administration Gammabulin must be administered by the intramuscular route.

All recommendations and doses given below refer to the 16% solution and are expressed in ml.

Antibody deficiency syndrome in dys-, hypo- and agammaglobulinaemia: By intramuscular administration of Gammabulin antibody concentrate the frequency and severity of recurring bacterial infections can be reduced. For treatment of immunoglobulin deficiency, it is necessary to achieve and maintain an immunoglobulin level of approximately 200 mg per 100 ml serum.
Initial dosage: 1.8 ml per kg bodyweight, e.g. in three single administrations of 0.6 ml/ kg bodyweight each at intervals of 24 hours.
Maintenance dose: 0.6 ml per kg bodyweight monthly.

Hepatitis A: Gammabulin is an efficient agent for the prevention or modification of Hepatitis A. It must be pointed out that after immunoglobulin administration an anicteric course of Hepatitis has been observed. Because of this, regular monitoring of transaminase levels may be warranted.
Dosage for children: 0.02-0.04 ml per kg bodyweight. If exposure continues, repeat the dose after 4-6 months.
Dosage for adults: (a) for a short period of exposure of less than 2 months: 0.02 to 0.04 ml per kg bodyweight. (b) for longer periods of exposure: 0.08 to 0.12 ml per kg bodyweight. If exposure continues, repeat the dose after 4 to 6 months.
Note: No benefit may be expected if administered after the onset of clinical symptoms.

Measles: Gammabulin should be given as soon as possible at a dose of 0.25 ml/ kg bodyweight to prevent or modify measles in a susceptible person exposed less than six days previously. Gammabulin may be especially indicated for susceptible household contacts of measles patients, particularly with children under one year of age or children who are immunosuppressed or have an immune deficiency disease and should not receive measles vaccine or any other live viral vaccine.
Prophylaxis: 0.2 ml per kg bodyweight. With continued or repeated exposure repeat after 3 weeks.
Mitigation without influence on the immunising effect: 0.04 ml per kg bodyweight.

Rubella (German Measles): The routine use of Gammabulin prophylaxis of Rubella in early pregnancy is of dubious value and cannot be justified. Some studies suggest that the use of Gammabulin in exposed, susceptible women can lessen the likelihood of infection and fetal damage, therefore 20 ml of Gammabulin may benefit those women in whom continuing pregnancy places the fetus at risk.

Use in the elderly: No special precautions need to be observed in the elderly.

Use in pregnancy: See *Interactions* with live vacines e.g. Rubella. According to present knowledge, no influence of immunoglobulin administrations in temporal connection with Rho prophylaxis with anti-D immunoglobulin can be proved. The diaplacental passage of administered immunoglobulin G into the fetus may be assumed.

Contra-Indications, warnings, etc Gammabulin is generally well tolerated without reactions. On very rare occasions (e.g. in special forms of a- or hypogammaglobulinaemia) anaphylactoid reactions may occur in patients who have antibodies against Immunoglobulin A (IgA) or who have shown atypical reaction after blood transfusion or following administration of blood derivatives.

Gammabulin must be not administered intravenously.

Treatment of overdosage: Gammabulin is a homologous protein, the antibody spectrum and protein structure of which corresponds qualitatively to that of an average donor population. Overdosage need not be expected to lead to more frequent or more severe adverse reactions than the recommended dose.

Pharmaceutical precautions Gammabulin should be stored between +2°C and +8°C when it will have a shelf life of 3 years. Gammabulin should be protected from the light.

Legal category POM

Package quantitites Rubber capped vials containing 2 ml, 5 ml or 10 ml.

Further information Gammabulin should be used immediately after drawing up the vial contents. Gammabulin vials are intended for single dose use only.

Effect on laboratory tests: Laboratory tests, as far as antibody determinations are concerned, are influenced inasmuch as the application of Gammabulin may lead to an increased or new appearance of types of antibodies (e.g. antibacterial, antiviral or antitoxic antibodies). In cases of very high doses, determinations of serum complement may give reduced values (consumption). Phagocytosis (phagocytosis index) may be increased.

Interactions: Active immunization with live virus vaccines (e.g. measles, mumps or rubella) should be postponed until 3 months after the last administration of Gammabulin, as the efficacy of the live virus vaccines may be impaired.

Administration of Gammabulin should be postponed until 2-4 weeks after the first complete cycle of immunization with live virus vaccines and 2 weeks after booster injection.

Product licence number 0215/0018

HUMAN ALBUMIN SOLUTION 4.5% BP IMMUNO*

Presentation Human Albumin Solution 4.5% BP Immuno is a sterile solution of protein for intravenous administration prepared from human plasma of venous origin. Only plasma units which are non reactive in tests for HBsAg and antibodies to HIV1, HIV2 and HCV are used in the manufacture of Human Albumin Solution 4.5% BP Immuno. All plasma units are further tested for ALT. It is heat treated for 10 hours at 60°C in the final container in accordance with international guidelines. The product contains a minimum of 96% albumin and is stabilised with 3.6 mmol/l sodium caprylate and sodium acetyltryptophanate.

Uses Human Albumin Solution 4.5% BP Immuno is indicated for volume replacement in hypovolaemic shock, as a replacement fluid during therapeutic plasmapheresis and in hypoalbuminaemia associated with an oncotic deficit.

Dosage and administration

Hypovolaemic shock: The dosage is largely determined by the duration and severity of hypovolaemia.
Adults: 500 ml/hr (125 drops/ min) in severe shock up to 1000 ml/hour (rapid infusion).
Children: For shock due to hypovolaemia and/or dehydration 20-30 ml/ kg bodyweight infused at a rate of 5-10 ml/ min.

If the haematocrit drops below 25%, packed red cells or whole blood should be given in conjunction with Human Albumin Solution 4.5% B.P. Immuno to maintain the oxygen transport capacity of the blood.

Hypoalbuminaemia with oncotic deficit:
Adults: 3.5–7.0 ml/ kg bodyweight daily infused at a rate of 250-500 ml/hr.
Children: 5–10 ml/ kg bodyweight per day given slowly.

Use in the elderly: In elderly patients careful haemodynamic and respiratory monitoring is essential throughout the administration of Human Albumin Solution 4.5% B.P. Immuno as a circulatory overload may lead to decompensation of the haemodynamic system.

In dehydrated patients only low concentrated protein solutions (up to 5% protein content) should be administered.

Use in pregnancy: As some patients show renal insufficiency during pregnancy, concentrated human albumin should be administered only when absolutely indicated and with utmost caution. Based on a persisting hypertension careful haemodynamic monitoring is essential to avoid an overloading syndrome which may lead to cardiac decompensation.

Contra-indications, warnings, etc Do not use if the solution is cloudy or contains a deposit.

Once the container has been penetrated the contents should be used within three hours and any unused preparation discarded.

Adequate precautions should be taken against circulatory overload. If symptoms of hypervolaemia develop the rate of infusion should be slowed or even halted.

Though side effects are extremely rare, such reactions as flushing, chills, fever, tachycardia, hypotension, urticarial skin rash and nausea may occur.

In these cases, the infusion of Human Albumin Solution 4.5% BP Immuno should be interrupted (or replaced by Ringer's solution) and antihistamines and/or corticosteroids should be administered intravenously (e.g. 50-200 mg prednisolone).

Human Albumin has been reported to contain trace amounts of Aluminium. In accordance with the limits laid down by the British Pharmacopoeia Human Albumin Solution 4.5% BP Immuno contains less than 200 micrograms per litre. It is therefore suitable for use in patients undergoing dialysis and premature infants.

Nevertheless, accumulation of aluminium in patients with chronic renal insufficiency has led to toxic effects such as hypercalcaemia, Vitamin D refractory osteodystrophy, anaemia and severe progressive encephalopathy.

When large volumes of Human Albumin solutions are contemplated for administration to such patients the potential risks as compared to the expected benefits should be carefully evaluated.

Treatment of overdosage: Interrupt infusion immediately and carefully watch the patient's haemodynamic parameters.

The half life of human albumin in the tissue is approximately 16-18 days. The disappearance rate of intravascular albumin depends on the permeability of the vascular system and on the catabolic rate.

Pharmaceutical precautions Human Albumin Solution 4.5% BP Immuno should be stored between +2°C and +25°C. It must be protected from light. The shelf life is 3 years.

Legal category POM

Package quantities Human Albumin Solution 4.5% BP Immuno is supplied in 50 ml, 100 ml, and 400 ml infusion bottles.

Further information Human Albumin Solution 4.5% BP Immuno is compatible with whole blood or packed red cells as well as the usual electrolyte and carbohydrate solutions intended for intravenous use. However, it should not be mixed with protein hydrolysates, amino acid mixtures or solutions containing alcohol. Human Albumin Solution 4.5% BP Immuno must not be given through infusion sets which have been used, or are intended, for simultaneous infusion of protein hydrolysates, amino acid mixtures, or solutions containing alcohol. Only clear solutions of slightly yellowish colour should be administered.

Effect on Laboratory Tests: As a consequence of haemodilution patients' blood samples taken during or shortly after infusion show lower laboratory test results (e.g. haematocrit) corresponding to the amount of Human Albumin Solution 4.5% BP Immuno administered to the patient (calculation based on isotonic solutions). Human Albumin Solution 4.5% BP Immuno does not interfere with the determination of patients' Rh-factors nor is there any adverse effect on thrombocyte function or blood coagulation.

Product licence number 0215/0002

HUMAN ALBUMIN SOLUTION 20% BP IMMUNO*

Presentation Human Albumin Solution 20% BP Immuno is a solution in water of human albumin containing a low proportion of salt and is described as Salt Poor Albumin. It is a clear liquid varying in colour from amber to orange-brown and is presented as a solution for intravenous injection or infusion. It is prepared from pooled human plasma of venous origin. Only plasma units which are non reactive in tests for HBsAg and antibodies to HIV1, HIV2 and HCV are used in the manufacture of Human Albumin Solution 20% BP Immuno. All plasma units are further tested for ALT. The product contains 20% protein of which at least 96% is albumin, the rest being thermostable alpha and beta globulins.

It is stabilised with 16 mmol/l sodium caprylate and 16 mmol/l sodium acetyltryptophanate and heat treated for 10 hours at 60°C in the final container in accordance with international guidelines. There is no preservative added to the solution.

Uses Human Albumin Solution 20% BP Immuno is administered as an injection or an infusion in the treatment of acute oedema: hypoalbuminaemia. For the treatment of the acute phase of burns or haemorrhagic shock, Human Albumin Solution 20% BP Immuno is diluted 1:4 with dextrose 5% or isotonic electrolyte solutions and the resulting 5% solution administered by infusion.

Dosage and administration
Acute oedema: There is an increased tendency for oedema to occur in patients with hypoalbuminaemia. Attempts should be made to bring about diuresis using the appropriate dose of Human Albumin Solution 20% BP Immuno. A reduction in oedema may then result.

Recommended dosage: Adults 100 ml Human Albumin Solution 20% BP Immuno (20 g). *Children* 2 ml Human Albumin Solution 20% BP Immuno (0.4 g) per kg bodyweight.

Pre- and post-operative hypoproteinaemia: In debilitated patients stabilisation of the protein balance with Human Albumin Solution 20% B.P. Immuno may considerably improve the pre-operative condition of the patient. The catabolism of albumin can be severely disturbed after operations on the gastro-intestinal tract and hypoproteinaemia may result. The normal average albumin breakdown of 70 g per week may be enhanced under pathological conditions. Additional loss of protein and diminished albumin synthesis might lead to severe albumin deficiency.

Repeated post-operative infusions of Human Albumin Solution 20% B.P. Immuno can be most valuable in such cases.

Recommended dosage for pre- and post-operative hypoproteinaemia: Adults 100 to 200 ml Human Albumin Solution 20% BP Immuno (20 to 40 g) daily in concentrated or diluted form depending on the plasma volume and serum albumin level of the patient. The dosage and duration of this substitution therapy depends on the amount of protein lost and should be continued until the serum concentration returns to normal. *Children* 1.5 to 3 ml Human Albumin Solution 20% BP Immuno (0.3 to 0.6 g) per kg bodyweight daily in concentrated form or diluted to a 5% solution. In hypoproteinaemia multiple administration of albumin might be necessary until the plasma protein level has returned to normal.

Attention must be paid to the oncotic activity of albumin which may lead to an increased blood volume.

See *Precautions*.

Other hypoalbuminaemia

(a) Hepatic cirrhosis with diffuse loss of parenchyma leads to diminished production of albumin and a resulting hypoalbuminaemia which, as a consequence, enhances the formation of ascites and oedema. Treatment with albumin results in the disappearance of oedema and a reduction of ascites.

Recommended dosage: Adults 100 to 200 ml Human Albumin Solution 20% BP Immuno (20 to 40 g) daily. *Children and Infants* 1.5 to 3 ml Human Albumin Solution 20% BP Immuno (0.3 to 0.6 g) per kg bodyweight.

(b) Nephrotic Syndrome. In cases of nephrotic syndrome particularly with patients who do not respond at all, or only slightly, to diuretics, the administration of Human Albumin Solution 20% BP Immuno will induce diuresis and therefore bring about a reduction of the oedema.

Recommend dosage: Adults 200 to 400 ml Human Albumin Solution 20% BP Immuno (40 to 80 g) daily. *Children and Infants* 3 to 6 ml Human Albumin Solution 20% BP Immuno (0.6 to 1.2 g) per kg bodyweight in concentrated form.

The dose should be infused over a period of 60 to 90 minutes.

Shock: Shock due to blood loss should be treated with whole blood, red cell concentrates, fresh frozen plasma, or with albumin diluted with isotonic electrolyte and/or dextrose solution 5%. *Adults* 50 to 200 ml Human Albumin Solution 20% BP Immuno (10 to 40 g) diluted 1:4 with isotonic electrolyte and/or dextrose solution 5%. *Children* 1 to 2 ml Human Albumin Solution 20% BP Immuno (0.2 g to 0.4 g) per kg bodyweight diluted 1:4 with isotonic electrolyte and/ or dextrose solution 5%.

Burns: Return of fluid from the extravascular compartment to the circulation must be ensured in cases of burns with associated hypoalbuminaemia.

In these cases hyperoncotic Human Albumin Solution 20% BP Immuno can be used with careful control of the oncotic pressure and the haemodynamic parameters.

Recommended dosage: Adults 50 to 200 ml Human Albumin Solution 20% BP Immuno (10 to 40 g). *Children* 1 to 2 ml Human Albumin Solution 20% BP Immuno (0.2 to 0.4 g) per kg bodyweight.

The initial dose should be infused over a period of 5 to 15 minutes.

In cases of extensive and severe burns with an increased haematocrit value, normalisation of the circulatory conditions can be achieved very effectively with Human Albumin Solution 20% BP Immuno diluted with dextrose 5% and/or isotonic electrolyte solutions.

Recommended initial dosage: Adults 200 to 400 ml Human Albumin Solution 20% BP Immuno (40 to 80 g) diluted 1:4 corresponding to 800 to 1600 ml of a 5% albumin solution. *Children* 4 ml Human Albumin Solution 20% BP Immuno per kg bodyweight diluted 1:4 corresponding to 16 ml of a 5% albumin solution.

The total dosage over the first 24 hours can be determined in accordance with the formula: 2 ml x bodyweight (kg) × % of surface burned + 1500 ml.

After the acute stage has been brought under control, considerable protein deficiency, largely of albumin, may occur. This hypoalbuminaemia can be corrected by administration of the following doses: *Adults* 50 ml Human Albumin Solution 20% BP Immuno (10 g) twice a day. *Children* 1 ml Human Albumin Solution 20% BP Immuno (0.2 g) per kg bodyweight twice a day.

Use in the elderly: In elderly patients careful haemodynamic and respiratory monitoring is essential throughout the administration of Human Albumin Solution 20% BP Immuno as a circulatory overload may lead to decompensation of the haemodynamic system.

In dehydrated patients only low concentrated protein solutions (up to 5% protein content) should be administered.

Use in pregnancy: As some patients show renal insufficiency during pregnancy, concentrated human albumin should be administered only when absolutely indicated and with utmost caution. Based on a persisting hypertension, monitoring is essential to avoid an overloading syndrome which may lead to cardiac decompensation.

Contra-indications, warnings, etc

1. Human Albumin Solution 20% BP Immuno must not be used if the solution is cloudy or contains a deposit.

Once the container has been penetrated, the contents must be used within 3 hours and any unused preparation discarded.

2. With patients suffering from hypertension or in cases of latent or manifest cardiac insufficiency, caution is indicated in the administration of Human Albumin Solution 20% BP Immuno. The single doses should be reduced to relatively small amounts and the infusion given slowly. A careful watch must be kept for the possible development of pulmonary oedema. If pulmonary oedema occurs, the infusion must be stopped immediately.

3. In all cases of considerable blood loss, whole blood or packed red cells must be given in addition to Human Albumin Solution 20% BP Immuno.

4. Intolerance reactions are extremely rare with Human Albumin Solution 20% BP Immuno.

5. Human Albumin has been reported to contain trace amounts of aluminium. In accordance with the limits laid down by the British Pharmacopoeia Human Albumin Solution 20% BP Immuno contains less than 200 micrograms per litre. It is therefore suitable for use in patients undergoing dialysis and premature infants.

Nevertheless, accumulation of Aluminium in patients with chronic renal insufficiency has led to toxic effects such as hypercalcaemia, Vitamin D refractory osteodystrophy, anaemia and severe progressive encephalopathy.

When large volumes of Human Albumin solutions are contemplated for administration to such patients the potential risks as compared to the expected benefits should be carefully evaluated.

Treatment of overdosage: Interrupt infusion immediately and carefully watch the patient's haemodynamic parameters.

The half life of human albumin in the tissue is approximately 16–18 days. The disappearance rate of intravascular albumin depends on the permeability of the vascular system and on the catabolic rate.

Pharmaceutical precautions Human Albumin Solution 20% BP Immuno should be stored between + 2°C and + 8°C. It must be protected from light. The shelf life is 3 years.

Legal category: POM

Package quantities Human Albumin Solution 20% BP Immuno is supplied in rubber capped vials of 10 ml, 50 ml and 100 ml.

Further information Human Albumin Solution 20% BP Immuno is compatible with whole blood or packed red cells as well as the usual electrolyte and carbohydrate solutions intended for intravenous use. However, it should not be mixed with protein hydrolysates, amino acid mixtures or solutions containing alcohol. Human Albumin Solution 20% BP Immuno must not be given through infusion sets which have been used, or are intended, for simultaneous infusion of protein hydrolysates, amino acid mixtures, or solutions containing alcohol. Only clear solutions of slightly yellowish colour should be administered.

Effect on laboratory tests: As a consequence of haemodilution patients' blood samples taken during or shortly after infusion show lower laboratory test results (e.g. haematocrit) corresponding to the amount of Human Albumin Solution 20% BP Immuno administered to the patient (calculation based on isotonic solutions). Human Albumin Solution 20% BP Immuno does not interfere with the determination of patients' Rh-factors nor is there any adverse effect on thrombocyte function or blood coagulation.

Product licence number 0215/0009

ANTI-D(RHO) IMMUNOGLOBULIN B.P. IMMUNO
ANTI-D(RHO) IMMUNOGLOBULIN INJECTION BP

Presentation Anti-D(Rho) Immunoglobulin B.P. Immuno is a clear liquid varying in colour from pale yellow to light brown. Each pre-loaded syringe contains 1,250 iu (250 micrograms) Anti-D in 1 ml of solution. It is prepared from pooled human venous plasma with a high content of Anti-D antibodies. Only plasma units which are non reactive in tests for HBsAg and antibodies to HIV1, HIV2 and HCV are used in the manufacture of Anti-D(Rho) Immunoglobulin B.P. Immuno. All plasma units are further tested for ALT. Glycine and Sodium Chloride are added as stabilisers. There is no preservative added to the product.

Uses Anti-D(Rho) Immunoglobulin B.P. Immuno is used for the prevention of D(Rh_o) sensitisation.

Dosage and administration Anti-D(Rho) Immunoglobulin B.P. Immuno must be administered by the intramuscular route. Anti-D(Rho) Immunoglobulin B.P. Immuno is indicated to prevent D(Rh_o) sensitisation in the situations described below when the blood groups of mother/recipient and fetus/child/transfused blood are as follows or when the rhesus factor of the fetus/child is unknown or cannot be determined:

Mother/recipient	*Fetus/child/transfused blood*
D(Rh_o)-negative	*D(Rh_o)-positive*
D(Rh_o)-negative	*D^u-positive*
D^u-positive	*D(Rh_o)-positive*

(a) Abortion and miscarriage: Following every abortion or miscarriage where D(Rh_o) sensitisation may be expected, 1,250 iu should be administered immediately or at the latest within 72 hours.

(b) Antenatal prophylaxis: As sensitisation can also occur during preganacy, 1,250 iu may be administered during weeks 28 and 34 of pregnancy in D(Rh_o) negative or D^u positive mothers.

In addition, after any potentially sensitising episode such as amniocentesis, external cephalic version, abdominal trauma, antepartum haemorrhage, ectopic pregnancy or chorionic villus sampling, 1,250 iu should be administered immediately or at the latest within 72 hours.

Note: Where antenatal prophylaxis has been given, a further dose should routinely be administered to the mother within 72 hours of birth.

(c) Parturition: In first deliveries and all subsequent deliveries where D(Rh_o) sensitisation may be expected 1,250 iu should be administered immediately or at the latest within 72 hours.

(d) Macrotransfusion: In all deliveries where a transplacental haemorrhage of more than 25 ml fetal blood (1% of fetal erythrocytes according to the elution method of Kleihauer and Betke) into the maternal blood occurs and a D(Rh_o) incompatibility exists, a dose of 5,000 iu (i.e. 4 preloaded syringes of Anti-D(Rho) Immunoglobulin B.P. Immuno) or 50 iu per ml of fetal blood is recommended.

Such macroinfiltrations occur in less than 1% of cases.

(e) D(Rh_o) incompatible blood transfusion: Following the transfusion of D(Rh_o) incompatible blood an i.m. injection of 50 to 100 iu Anti-D(Rh_o) Immunoglobulin per ml of transfused blood is recommended. Recent findings underline the necessity of starting the treatment as soon as possible. Some authors are using considerably higher doses and monitoring the disappearance of D(Rh_o) positive cells and also determining the antibody excess.

Use in the elderly: Use in the elderly is normally limited to the prevention of sensitisation following incompatible transfusion. Under these circumstances no special precautions or dosage amendments need to be observed in the elderly.

Use in pregnancy: The use of Anti-D(Rho) Immunoglobulin B.P. Immuno during pregnancy as described under Indications and Dosage does not usually produce antibody titres in the maternal circulation that might threaten the fetus. Exceptions are possible, for example, if anti-D immunoglobulin is given repeatedly at short intervals. In general, the antibody titre in the maternal blood should not exceed 1:2 (Coombs Test).

Contra-indications, warnings, etc Anti-D(Rho) Immunoglobulin B.P. Immuno must not be administered intravenously. Anti-D(Rho) Immunoglobulin B.P. Immuno must not be administered to D(Rh_o) positive individuals or D(Rh_o) positive newborns.

Anti-D(Rho) Immunoglobulin B.P. Immuno is generally well tolerated without reactions. On very rare occasions (e.g. in special forms of a- or Hypogammaglobulinaemia), anaphylactoid reactions may occur in people who have antibodies against immune globulin A (IgA) or have shown atypical reaction after blood transfusion or following administration of blood derivatives.

Interactions: Active Immunisation with live virus vaccines (e.g. Measles, Mumps or Rubella) should be postponed until 3 months after the last administration of Anti-D(Rho) Immunoglobulin B.P. Immuno, as the efficacy of the live virus vaccine may be impaired.

If Anti-D(Rho) Immunoglobulin B.P. Immuno needs to be administered within 2-4 weeks of a live virus vaccination, then the efficacy of such a vaccination may be impaired.

Treatment of overdosage: In rhesus negative individuals overdosage need not be expected to lead to more frequent or more severe adverse reactions than the normal dose. It has been observed that even an accidental injection of the preparation into the newborn does not necessarily lead to adverse reaction.

Pharmaceutical precautions Anti-D(Rho) Immunoglobulin B.P. Immuno should be stored between +2°C and +8°C when it will have a shelf life of three years.

Legal category POM

Package quantities Pre-loaded syringes containing 1,250 iu (250 micrograms) Anti-D in 1 ml.

Further information Anti-D(Rho) Immunoglobulin B.P. Immuno should be administered immediately following removal of the protective needle cover. Anti-D(Rho) Immunoglobulin B.P. Immuno syringes are intended for single dose use only.

Effect on laboratory tests: Passively introduced D(Rh_o) antibodies may be detected in the blood of the mother several weeks and even months after an injection of Anti-D(Rho) Immunoglobulin B.P. Immuno. Therefore, any previous administration of Anti-D(Rho) Immunoglobulin B.P. Immuno must be taken into account when examining maternal blood for its content of D(Rh_o) antibody and when evaluating these tests.

The presence of additional antibodies (e.g. Rubella) in Anti-D(Rho) Immunoglobulin B.P. Immuno may lead to false positive reactions in tests for such antibodies.

Product licence number 0215/0026

TETABULIN*
Tetanus Immunoglobulin BP Immuno

Qualitative and quantitative composition
Active ingredient: Tetanus antitoxin
Quantitative composition: 1 ml of solution contains Tetanus antitoxin 250iu

Pharmaceutical form Solution for intramuscular administration.

Clinical particulars
Therapeutic indications: Prophylaxis in persons with recent injuries who have no immunity, incomplete or unknown immunity against tetanus.
Therapy of clinically manifest tetanus.

Posology and method of administration:
Posology: Passive immunisation against tetanus is recommended in all cases of injury where a risk of tetanus infection is involved and where active protection against tetanus is insufficient, i.e. when immunisation is incomplete, when the immune response is reduced or following severe loss of blood or plasma. Tetanus Immunoglobulin BP Immuno is also indicated when the status of immunisation is unknown or when active immunisation is contraindicated.

Besides thorough debridement and cleansing of the wound along with the injection of Tetanus Immunoglobulin BP Immuno, active immunisation with tetanus vaccine should be started simultaneously at a separate injection site unless active immunisation is contraindicated.

It is recommended that the physician determines if a minor wound is 'tetanus-prone', based on the likelihood that *Clostridium tetani* was present on the object which caused the wound.

The same dose applies to both children and adults.

a. *Prophylaxis of tetanus:* 250 iu by intramuscular injection

This dose should be doubled in cases where the wound is heavily contaminated or older than 12 hours and in patients weighing more than 90 kg. Patients with antibody deficiency syndrome such as dys-, hypo- or agammaglobulinaemia or with a reduced capacity of antibody formation (after radiotherapy or steroid treatment, burns, etc.) should receive another dose of Tetanus Immunoglobulin BP Immuno 3 to 4 weeks after the first dose as a prophylaxis against the delayed onset of tetanus.

A further dose should also be given after 3 to 4 weeks where simultaneous vaccination is contraindicated.

b. *Therapy of tetanus:* Several studies suggest the value of HTIG in the treatment of active tetanus using doses of between 30 and 300iu per kg bodyweight i.m. in combination with other appropriate clinical procedures.

The absence of thiomersal as a preservative theoretically allows intrathecal administration although efficacy and safety in children and adults have not yet been definitely assessed.

Method of administration: Slow injection by the i.m. route only.

If large doses (>5 ml) are required, it is advisable to administer them in divided doses at different sites.

Contra-indications: The lethal risk associated with tetanus rules out any potential contraindication (see *Warnings* below).

Special warnings and special precautions for use: The warnings and precautions described for human normal immunoglobulin (i.m.) may be applied for Tetanus Immunoglobulin BP Immuno and are described below.

Do not give this product intravascularly (possibility of shock). Therefore, it is necessary to verify that the needle has not penetrated a blood vessel.

Give with caution in highly allergic individuals due to the potential risk of hypersensitivity reactions such as anaphylactoid shock.

Measures against allergic and anaphylactoid reactions require immediate discontinuation of the injection. If allergic reactions persist after discontinuation of the injection, then appropriate treatment with, for example, antihistamines and/or corticosteroids is recommended.

In anaphylactoid shock, treatment should follow the guidelines of shock therapy.

Interaction with other medicaments and other forms of interaction:
Live attenuated virus vaccines: If the patient has received live attenuated virus vaccines (measles, rubella, mumps, varicella) within the two previous weeks, an assay of protective post-vaccinal antibodies may be of value before giving a possible booster.

After injection of immunoglobulin, wait at least 6 weeks (and preferably 3 months) prior to administering any live attenuated virus vaccines (measles, rubella, mumps, varicella).

The efficacy of the virus vaccines may be impaired by the antibodies contained in the immunoglobulin preparation.

Interpretation of blood typing and antibody testing: After injection of immunoglobulin, take into account the possible and transitory cross-reactions of the antibodies administered which may lead to false-positive results in serological testing.

Pregnancy and lactation: The safety of this medicinal product for use in pregnancy has not been established in controlled clinical trials. Long lasting clinical experience with immunoglobulin, in particular the routine administration of anti-D immunoglobulin, does indicate that no harmful effects on the course of pregnancy, on the fetus and the neonate are to be expected (category A).

Experimental animal studies are inappropriate with respect to the product which is heterologous for animals (immunological incompatibility).

Immunoglobulins are excreted into the milk and may contribute to the transfer of protective antibodies to the neonate.

Effects on ability to drive and use machines: There are no known restrictions.

Undesirable effects: The undesirable effects described for human normal immunoglobulin (i.m.) may be applied for Tetanus Immunoglobulin BP Immuno and are described below.

Pain and discomfort may be observed at the site of administration; this local pain can be prevented by giving smaller volumes more frequently.

Occasionally, fever, cutaneous reactions, chills may occur. In rare instances nausea, vomiting, hypotension, tachycardia, allergic reactions have been reported.

Serious effects such as anaphylactoid shock have been observed in isolated cases.

Overdose: Overdosage with Tetanus Immunoglobulin BP Immuno is not known.

Pharmacological properties

Pharmacodynamic properties: Tetanus Immunoglobulin BP Immuno is a sterile preparation that contains antibodies to tetanus toxin.

Tetanus Immunoglobulin BP Immuno is prepared from pooled plasma containing specific antibodies against the toxin of *Clostridium tetani.*

Pharmacokinetic properties: Measurable levels of antibodies are obtained approximately 20 minutes after i.m. injection. Peak serum levels are usually achieved 2 to 3 days later.

The half-life is 3 to 4 weeks.

Preclinical safety data:
Viral safety: The respective national guidelines on the collection of human plasma in their effective versions are observed. In addition, several steps of the manufacturing process contribute to the viral safety of human immunoglobulins. They result in extensive partitioning and/or inactivation of potentially contaminating viruses.

Toxicological properties: Immunoglobulins are normal constituents of the human body. Repeated dose toxicity testing in animals is impracticable due to interference with developing antibodies.

Tetanus Immunoglobulin BP Immuno has not been reported to be associated with embryo-fetal toxicity, oncogenic or mutagenic potential.

Pharmaceutical particulars

List of excipients: 1 ml of solution contains:

Protein (>90% gamma globulin)	100–170 mg
Glycine	22.5 mg
Sodium Chloride	3.0 mg

Incompatibilities: Tetanus Immunoglobulin BP Immuno must not be mixed with other pharmaceutical products.

Shelf life: 3 years when stored between +2°C and +8°C.

Once a container has been opened, its contents should be used immediately.

Special precautions for storage: Store at a temperature of between +2°C and +8°C. Protect from light. Do not freeze. Do not use after the expiry date indicated on the label.

Nature and contents of container: Preloaded syringe of neutral glass, hydrolytic type 1, each containing 1 ml of solution.

Instructions for use/handling: Tetanus Immunoglobulin BP Immuno should be administered immediately following removal of the protective needle cover from the preloaded syringe. Tetanus Immunoglobulin BP Immuno syringes are intended for single dose use only. Do not use solutions which are cloudy or have deposits.

Marketing authorisation number 0215/0030

Date of approval/revision August 1993

Legal category POM

**Trade Mark*

ICN Pharmaceuticals Ltd

1 Elmwood
Chineham Business Park
Crockford Lane
Basingstoke
Hants RG24 8WG

☎ 01256 707744 🗋 01256 707334

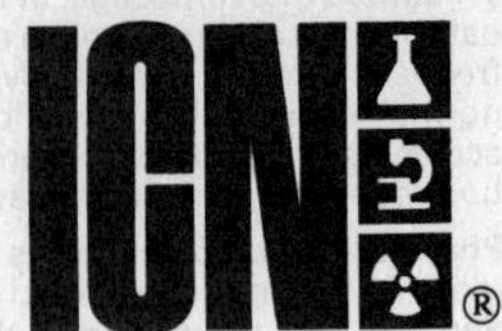

ALCOBON

Presentation Infusion bottles containing 2.5g flucytosine Ph. Eur. in 250ml isotonic sodium chloride solution. Other excipients are tromethamine and hydrochloric acid 25%. The solution is colourless to slightly yellow.

Uses
Pharmacological properties: Alcobon is a fluorinated pyrimidine effective in the treatment of certain systemic fungal infections. In fungi sensitive to the preparation, it acts as a competitive inhibitor of uracil metabolism.

Pharmacokinetics: Alcobon is widely distributed in body tissues and fluids (including cerebrospinal fluid). Binding to plasma proteins is minimal. Half-life of elimination is 3-6 hours in patients with normal renal function but this value increases in renal failure. About 90% of the dose administered is excreted unchanged in the urine. Flucytosine is metabolised to 5-fluorouracil. The area under the curves (AUC) ratio of 5-fluorouracil to flucytosine is 4%. Flucytosine can be removed by haemodialysis.

Indications: Alcobon is indicated for the treatment of systemic yeast and fungal infections due to sensitive organisms: such infections include cryptococcosis, candidiasis, chromomycosis and infections due to *Torulopsis glabrata* and *Hansenula*.

In the treatment of cryptococcal meningitis and severe systemic candidiasis it is recommended that Alcobon should be given in combination with amphotericin-B. Amphotericin-B may also be given in combination with Alcobon in severe or long-standing infections due to other organisms. In cases of cryptococcal meningitis, where toxicity of amphotericin-B, or a combination of flucytosine with amphotericin-B is dose limiting, a combination of flucytosine with fluconazole has demonstrated successful cure, but at a lower rate than in combination with amphotericin-B.

Dosage and administration
Adults and children: Alcobon for Infusion should be administered using a giving set. It may be administered directly into a vein, through a central venous catheter, or by intra-peritoneal infusion. The recommended daily dosage in adults and children is 200mg/kg body-weight divided into four doses over the 24 hours. In patients harbouring extremely sensitive organisms a total daily dose of 100 to 150mg/kg body-weight may be sufficient. Adequate effects can, however, often be obtained with a lower dose. It is suggested that the duration of the infusion should be of the order of 20 to 40 minutes provided this is balanced with the fluid requirements of the patient. As a rule, treatment with Alcobon for Infusion should rarely be required for periods of more than one week. Since Alcobon is excreted primarily by the kidneys, patients with renal impairment should be given smaller doses. The following is suggested as a guide for dosage in patients with severe infection associated with renal impairment:
In patients with:

creatinine clearance < 40 to > 20ml/min: 50mg/kg every 12 hours.

creatinine clearance < 20 to > 10ml/min: 50mg/kg every 24 hours.

creatinine clearance < 10ml/min: an initial single dose of 50mg/kg; subsequent doses should be calculated according to the results of regular monitoring of the serum concentration of the drug, which should not be allowed to exceed 80 micrograms/ml. Blood levels of 25 to 50 micrograms/ml are normally effective.

The duration of treatment should be determined on an individual basis.

The outcome of therapy will be affected by variations in the sensitivity of the infecting organism, its accessibility and its susceptibility to Alcobon, as well as by differences in the response of individual patients. In cases of cryptococcal meningitis, treatment should last for at least four months.

Neonates: The dose in neonates should be calculated in the same way as for adults and children, but the high possibility of renal impairment should be considered in this group either as intrinsic to their age or as a result of other nephrotoxic therapies. It is advised to closely monitor the serum levels of flucytosine in this group and adjust the dose according to levels. In cases where renal impairment is present the dose interval should be extended (as with adults and children). Where renal impairment is not a feature but serum levels are above those recommended, the dose should be reduced but the dosing interval should remain the same.

Use in the elderly: Although no specific studies have been performed to establish the use of Alcobon in the elderly, documented use indicates that the dosage requirements and side-effects profile are similar to those of younger patients. Particular attention should be paid to renal function in this group.
Alcobon for Infusion is for intravenous or intraperitoneal administration.
Alcobon for Infusion may be given concurrently with other infusions of normal saline, glucose or glucose/saline. No other agent should be added to or mixed with Alcobon for Infusion.

Contra-indications, warnings etc
Contra-indications: Alcobon is contra-indicated in patients who have shown hypersensitivity to flucytosine or any of the excipients.

Use in pregnancy and lactation: Teratogenic effects have been seen in rats, in which species flucytosine is metabolised to fluorouracil. The metabolism may differ in man: nevertheless, the use of Alcobon in pregnancy and in women of childbearing age requires that the potential benefits of therapy be weighed against its possible hazards. The drug should not be given to women breast feeding infants.

Precautions: The product should be used with great caution in patients with depression of bone marrow function or blood dyscrasias. Blood counts and tests of renal and hepatic function should be performed before and during treatment. This should occur at least weekly in patients with renal insufficiency or blood dyscrasias.

Alcobon should not be used in patients with impaired renal function in the absence of facilities for monitoring blood levels of the drug.

When measuring drug serum levels, it should be noted that levels of the drug in blood samples, taken during or immediately after administration of Alcobon for Infusion, are not a reliable guide to subsequent levels; it is advisable to remove blood for monitoring of blood levels of Alcobon shortly before starting the next infusion.

In calculating the fluid and electrolyte intake of patients with impaired renal function, cardiac failure or electrolyte imbalance, due allowance should be made for the volume and sodium content (138 millimole/litre) of Alcobon for Infusion.

Side-effects and adverse reactions: Nausea, vomiting, diarrhoea and skin rashes may occur but are usually of a transient nature.

Less frequently observed side-effects include allergic reactions, Lyell's Syndrome, myocardial toxicity and ventricular dysfunction, confusion, hallucinations, convulsions, headache, sedation and vertigo. Alterations in tests of liver function are generally dose related and reversible but hepatitis and hepatic necrosis have been reported. Acute liver injury with possible fatal outcome in debilitated patients may occur in isolated cases.

Haematological changes, mainly leucopenia, thrombocytopenia, agranulocytosis or aplastic anaemia have been reported. These are more common when serum levels of flucytosine are high in patients with renal impairment and when amphotericin-B has been co-prescribed. In isolated cases, bone marrow toxicity has been reported. This toxicity may be irreversible and could lead to death in patients with pre-existing immunosuppression.

Local irritation or phlebitis does not appear to be a problem with Alcobon for Infusion.

Drug interactions: There is contradictory evidence concerning a drug interaction between Alcobon and cytarabine. Strict monitoring of blood levels is required if the two medicines are given concurrently.

Treatment of overdosage: Haemodialysis produces a rapid fall in the serum concentration of Alcobon.

Pharmaceutical precautions
Storage: Alcobon for Infusion should be stored between 18°C and 25°C. If stored below 18°C, precipitation of Alcobon substance may occur, which should be redissolved by heating to 80°C for not more than 30 minutes.

Prolonged storage above 25°C could lead to the decomposition of Alcobon resulting in the formation of 5-fluorouracil.

Additives: Alcobon for Infusion may be given concurrently with other infusions of Sodium Chloride Intravenous infusion (0.9% w/v) BP, Glucose Intravenous Infusion (5% w/v) BP, or Sodium Chloride (0.18% w/v) and Glucose (4% w/v) Intravenous infusion BP. No other agent should be added to or mixed with Alcobon for Infusion.

Legal category POM.

Package quantities Alcobon for Infusion 2.5g in 250ml in packs of 5.

Further information
Availability: Alcobon for Infusion is available to hospitals only.

Sensitivity testing: It is recommended that cultures for sensitivity testing be taken before treatment and repeated at regular intervals during therapy. However, it is not necessary to delay treatment until results of these tests are known.

To determine sensitivities, the methods of Shadomy (Appl. Microbiol., 1969, 17, 871) and Scholer (Mykosen, 1970, 13, 179) are recommended.
For sensitivity testing it is essential that culture media are free of antagonists to flucytosine.

Creatinine measurement: Flucytosine may interfere with the dual-slide enzymatic measurement of creatinine used with the manual, desk-top Vitros DT60 analyser, giving the false impression of azotemia. Other suitable methods should be used for creatinine assessment. The current creatinine method used with automated Vitros analysers is not affected by flucytosine.

Product licence number PL 15142/0002

EFUDIX

Presentation Efudix cream contains the substance with the approved name fluorouracil. It is chemically described as 5-fluorouracil.

Presentation White, opaque cream containing 5% w/w fluorouracil.

Uses
Properties: Efudix is a topical cytostatic preparation which exerts a beneficial therapeutic effect on neoplastic and pre-neoplastic skin lesions without damaging normal skin. The pattern of response follows this sequence: erythema, vesiculation, erosion, ulceration, necrosis and epithelisation.

Pharmacokinetics: Animal studies have shown that after topical application of fluorouracil, less than 10% is systemically absorbed. This may be metabolised by catabolic or anabolic routes which are similar to that of endogenous uracil.

Indications: Efudix is used for the topical treatment of superficial pre-malignant and malignant skin lesions; keratoses including senile, actinic and arsenical forms; keratoacanthoma; Bowen's disease; superficial basal-cell carcinoma. Deep, penetrating or nodular basal cell and squamous cell carcinomas do not usually respond to Efudix therapy. It should be used only as a palliative therapy in such cases where no other form of treatment is possible.

Dosage and administration
Pre-malignant conditions: The cream should be applied thinly to the affected area once or twice daily; an occlusive dressing is not essential.

Malignant conditions: The cream should be applied once or twice daily under an occlusive dressing where this is practicable.
The cream should not harm healthy skin. Treatment should be continued until there is marked inflammatory response from the treated area, preferably with some erosion in the case of pre-malignant conditions. Severe discomfort may be alleviated by the use of topical steroid cream. The usual duration of treatment for an initial course of therapy is three to four weeks, but this may be prolonged. Lesions on the face usually respond more quickly than those on the trunk or lower limbs whilst lesions on the hands and forearms respond more slowly. Healing may not be complete until one or two months after therapy is stopped.

Elderly: Many of the conditions for which Efudix is indicated are common in the elderly. No special precautions are necessary.

Children: In view of the lack of clinical data available, Efudix is not recommended for use in children.

Efudix cream is for topical application.

Contra-indications and warnings
Contra-indications: Efudix is contra-indicated in patients with known hypersensitivity to Efudix or parabens.

Use in pregnancy and lactation: There is evidence from animal work that fluorouracil is teratogenic and there is no evidence as to drug safety in human pregnancy. Therefore the use of Efudix is contra-indicated during pregnancy. It should also be regarded as contra-indicated in mothers who are breast-feeding.

Precautions: Efudix is for topical use only and care should be taken to avoid contact with mucous membranes or the eyes. The hands should be washed carefully after applying the cream.
The total area of skin being treated with Efudix at any one time should not exceed 500cm^2 (approx. 23 x 23cm). Larger areas should be treated a section at a time.

Drug interactions: No significant drug interactions with Efudix have been reported.

Side-effects and adverse reactions: Efudix is well tolerated. Transient erythema may occur in healthy skin surrounding the area being treated. Pre-existing subclinical lesions may become apparent. Exposure to sunlight may increase the intensity of the reaction. Dermatitis, allergic skin reactions and, rarely, erythema multiforme have been reported.

Percutaneous absorption of fluorouracil should not lead to clinically significant systemic toxicity when Efudix is administered as directed. However, this possibility should be borne in mind if the product is used excessively, especially on ulcerated or broken skin.

Treatment of overdosage: If Efudix is accidentally ingested, signs of fluorouracil overdosage may include nausea, vomiting and diarrhoea. Stomatitis and blood dyscrasias may occur in severe cases. Appropriate measures should be taken for the prevention of systemic infection and daily white cell counts should be performed.

Pharmaceutical precautions
Storage: The recommended maximum storage temperature for Efudix cream is 30°C.
Dilution: Efudix cream should not be diluted.

Legal category POM

Package quantities Efudix cream in tubes of 20g.

Further information
Availability
Efudix cream is available through hospital pharmacies for use in hospitals and hospital clinics and can be supplied to retail pharmacies for dispensing prescriptions for patients whose treatment has been initiated by a specialist in oncology or dermatology, in the NHS or otherwise, whose bona fide can be identified by the dispensing pharmacist.

Efudix should be used only under specialist medical supervision.

Product licence number PL 15142/0003

LIBRIUM

Qualitative and quantitative composition Each 5mg capsule contains 5mg of the active ingredient chlordiazepoxide hydrochloride BP. Each 10mg capsule contains 10mg of the active ingredient chlordiazepoxide hydrochloride BP.

Pharmaceutical form Librium Capsules 5mg and Librium Capsules 10mg.

Clinical particulars
Therapeutic indications: Short-term (2-4 weeks) symptomatic treatment of anxiety that is severe, disabling or subjecting the individual to unacceptable distress, occurring alone or in association with insomnia or short-term psychosomatic, organic or psychotic illness.
Muscle spasm of varied aetiology.
Symptomatic relief of acute alcohol withdrawal.

Posology and method of administration
Adults: Anxiety states
Usual dose: Up to 30mg daily in divided doses.
Maximum dose: Up to 100mg daily in divided doses. Adjusted on an individual basis.
Insomnia associated with anxiety 10 to 30mg before retiring.
Symptomatic relief of acute alcohol withdrawal 25 to 100mg repeated if necessary in 2 to 4 hours.
Muscle spasm of varied aetiology 10 to 30mg daily in divided doses.

Elderly: Elderly or debilitated patients: doses should not exceed half those normally recommended.

Children: Librium is not for paediatric use.

The lowest dose which can control symptoms should be used. Treatment should not be continued at the full dose beyond four weeks.
Long-term chronic use is not recommended.
Treatment should always be tapered off gradually. Patients who have taken benzodiazepines for a prolonged time may require a longer period during which doses are reduced. Specialist help may be appropriate.
Librium capsules are for oral administration.
Treatment should be kept to a minimum and given only under close medical supervision. Little is known regarding the efficacy or safety of benzodiazepines in long-term use.

Contra-indications: Patients with known sensitivity to benzodiazepines; acute pulmonary insufficiency; respiratory depression; phobic or obsessional states; chronic psychosis.

Special warnings and special precautions for use: In patients with chronic pulmonary insufficiency, and in patients with chronic renal or hepatic disease, dosage may need to be reduced.
Librium should not be used alone to treat depression or anxiety associated with depression, since suicide may be precipitated in such patients.
Amnesia may occur.
In cases of loss or bereavement, psychological adjustment may be inhibited by benzodiazepines.
The dependence potential of the benzodiazepines is low, particularly when limited to short-term use, but this increases when high doses are used, especially when given over long periods. This is particularly so in patients with a history of alcoholism or drug abuse or in patients with marked personality disorders. Regular monitoring in such patients is essential, routine repeat prescriptions should be avoided and treatment should be withdrawn gradually. Symptoms such as depression, nervousness, rebound insomnia, irritability, sweating, and diarrhoea have been reported following abrupt cessation of treatment in patients receiving even normal therapeutic doses for short periods of time.
In rare instances, withdrawal following excessive dosages may produce confusional states, psychotic manifestations and convulsions.
Abnormal psychological reactions to benzodiazepines have been reported. Rare behavioural effects include paradoxical aggressive outbursts, excitement, confusion, and the uncovering of depression with suicidal tendencies. Extreme caution should therefore be used in prescribing benzodiazepines to patients with personality disorders.

Interaction with other medicaments and other forms of interaction: If Librium is combined with centrally-acting drugs such as neuroleptics, tranquillisers, antidepressants, hypnotics, analgesics and anaesthetics, the sedative effects are likely to be intensified. The elderly require special supervision.
When Librium is used in conjunction with anti-epileptic drugs, side-effects and toxicity may be more evident, particularly with hydantoins or barbiturates or combinations including them. This requires extra care in adjusting dosage in the initial stages of treatment.
Known inhibitors of hepatic enzymes, e.g. cimetidine, have been shown to reduce the clearance of benzodiazepines and may potentiate their action and known inducers of hepatic enzymes, e.g. rifampicin, may increase the clearance of benzodiazepines.

Pregnancy and lactation: There is no evidence as to drug safety in human pregnancy, nor is there evidence from animal work that it is free from hazard. Do not use during pregnancy, especially during the first and last trimesters, unless there are compelling reasons.
If the product is prescribed to a woman of child-bearing potential, she should be warned to contact her physician regarding discontinuance of the product if she intends to become or suspects that she is pregnant.
The administration of high doses or prolonged administration of low doses of benzodiazepines in the last trimester of pregnancy has been reported to produce irregularities in the foetal heart rate, and hypotonia, poor sucking and hypothermia in the neonate.
Moreover, infants born to mothers who took benzodiazepines chronically during the latter stages of pregnancy may have developed physical dependence and may be at some risk for developing withdrawal symptoms in the postnatal period. Chlordiazepoxide may appear in breast milk. If possible, the use of Librium should be avoided during lactation.

Effects on ability to drive and use machines: Patients should be advised that, like all medicaments of this type, Librium may modify patients' performance at skilled tasks (driving, operating machinery, etc.) to a varying degree depending upon dosage, administration and individual susceptibility. Patients should further be advised that alcohol may intensify any impairment and should therefore be avoided during treatment.

Undesirable effects: Common adverse effects include drowsiness, sedation, unsteadiness and ataxia; these are dose-related and may persist into the following day even after a single dose. The elderly are particularly sensitive to the effects of centrally-depressant drugs and may experience confusion, especially if organic brain changes are present; the dosage of Librium should not exceed one-half that recommended for other adults.
Other adverse effects are rare and include headache, vertigo, hypotension, gastro-intestinal upsets, skin rashes, visual disturbances, changes in libido, and urinary retention. Isolated cases of blood dyscrasias and jaundice have also been reported.

Overdose: When taken alone in overdosage Librium presents few problems in management. Signs may include drowsiness, ataxia and dysarthria, with coma in severe cases. Treatment is symptomatic. Gastric lavage is useful only if performed soon after ingestion.
The value of dialysis has not been determined. Anexate is a specific IV antidote for use in emergency situations. Patients requiring such intervention should be monitored closely in hospital (see separate prescribing information).
If excitation occurs, barbiturates should not be used.
When taken with centrally-acting drugs, especially alcohol, the effects of overdosage are likely to be more severe and, in the absence of supportive measures, may prove fatal.

Pharmacological properties
Pharmacodynamic properties: Librium has anxiolytic and central muscle relaxant properties. It has little autonomic activity.

Pharmacokinetic properties: Librium is well absorbed, with peak blood levels being achieved one or two hours after administration. The drug has a half-life of 6-30 hours. Steady-state levels are usually reached within three days.
Chlordiazepoxide is metabolised to desmethylchlordiazepoxide. Demoxepam and desmethyldiazepam are also found in the plasma of patients on continuous treatment. The active metabolite desmethylchlordiazepoxide has an accumulation half-life of 10-18 hours; that of demoxepam has been recorded as 21-78 hours.
Steady-state levels of these active metabolites are reached after 10-15 days, with metabolite concentrations which are similar to those of the parent drug.
No clear correlation has been demonstrated between the blood levels of Librium and its clinical effects.

Preclinical safety data: None stated

Pharmaceutical particulars
List of excipients: 5mg capsules contain the following excipients: gelatin, starch maize white, talc purified, lactose, yellow iron oxide E172, indigo carmine E132, titanium dioxide E171, quinoline yellow E104 and erythrosine E127.
10mg capsules contain the following excipients: gelatin, starch maize white, talc purified, lactose, black iron oxide E172, titanium dioxide E171, yellow iron oxide E172 and indigo carmine E 132.

Incompatibilities: None.

Shelf life: For both Librium Capsules 5mg and 10mg:
PVDC blister pack - 36 months.
HDPE bottle - 60 months.
Plastic bottle - 60 months.
Amber glass bottle - 60 months.

Special precautions for storage: Librium capsules should not be stored above 30°C.

Nature and contents of container: For both Librium Capsules 5mg and 10mg:
- PVDC blister pack containing 10 capsules.

- HDPE bottle with jay-cap (snap-fit) closure containing 100 capsules.
- Plastic bottle with screw cap containing 100 capsules.
- Amber glass bottle with screw cap containing 100 capsules.

Instructions for use/handling: None.

Marketing authorisation number
Librium Capsules 5mg PL 15142/0004
Librium Capsules 10mg PL 15142/0005

Legal category POM.

MESTINON

Qualitative and quantitative composition Each tablet contains 62.5mg pyridostigmine bromide (equivalent to 60.0mg of the base).

Pharmaceutical form Tablets for oral administration.

Clinical particulars
Therapeutic indications: Myasthenia gravis, paralytic ileus and post-operative urinary retention.

Posology and method of administration
Myasthenia gravis: Adults: Doses of 30 to 120mg are given at intervals throughout the day when maximum strength is needed (for example, on rising and before mealtimes). The usual duration of action of a dose is 3 to 4 hours in the daytime but a longer effect (6 hours) is often obtained with a dose taken on retiring for bed.

The total daily dose is usually in the range of 5-20 tablets but doses higher than these may be needed by some patients.

Children: Children under 6 years old should receive an initial dose of half a tablet (30mg) of Mestinon; children 6-12 years old should receive one tablet (60mg). Dosage should be increased gradually, in increments of 15-30mg daily, until maximum improvement is obtained. Total daily requirements are usually in the range of 30-360mg.

The requirement for Mestinon is usually markedly decreased after thymectomy or when additional therapy (steroids, immunosuppressant drugs) is given.

When relatively large doses of Mestinon are taken by myasthenic patients it may be necessary to give atropine or other anticholinergic drugs to counteract the muscarinic effects. It should be noted that the slower gastro-intestinal motility caused by these drugs may affect the absorption of Mestinon.

In all patients the possibility of "cholinergic crisis", due to overdosage of Mestinon, and its differentiation from "myasthenic crisis" due to increased severity of the disease, must be borne in mind. Both types of crisis are manifested by increased muscle weakness, but whereas myasthenic crisis may require more intensive anticholinesterase treatment, cholinergic crisis calls for immediate discontinuation of this treatment and institution of appropriate supportive measures, including respiratory assistance.

Other indications
Adults: The usual dose is 1 to 4 tablets (60-240mg).

Children: 15-60mg.

The frequency of these doses may be varied according to the needs of the patient.

Elderly: There are no specific dosage recommendations for Mestinon in elderly patients.

Contra-indications: Mestinon should not be given to patients with mechanical gastro-intestinal or urinary obstruction.
Mestinon is contra-indicated in patients with known hypersensitivity to the drug and to bromides.

Special warnings and special precautions for use: Extreme caution is required when administering Mestinon to patients with bronchial asthma.

Care should also be taken in patients with bradycardia, recent coronary occlusion, hypotension, vagotonia, peptic ulcer, epilepsy or Parkinsonism.

There is no evidence to suggest that Mestinon has any special effects on the elderly. However, elderly patients may be more susceptible to dysrhythmias than the young adult.

Mestinon is mainly excreted unchanged by the kidney, therefore lower doses may be required in patients with renal disease and treatment should be based on titration of drug dosage to effect.

Interaction with other medicaments and other forms of interaction: None known.

Pregnancy and lactation: The safety of Mestinon during pregnancy or lactation has not been established. Although the possible hazards to mother and child must be weighed against the potential benefits in every case, experience with Mestinon in pregnant patients with myasthenia gravis has revealed no untoward effect of the drug on the course of pregnancy.

As the severity of myasthenia gravis often fluctuates considerably, particular care is required to avoid cholinergic crisis, due to overdosage of the drug, but otherwise management is no different from that in non-pregnant patients.

Observations indicate that only negligible amounts of Mestinon are excreted in breast milk; nevertheless, due regard should be paid to possible effects on the breast-feeding infant.

Effects on ability to drive and use machines: None known.

Undesirable effects: These may include nausea and vomiting, increased salivation, diarrhoea and abdominal cramps.

Overdose: Signs of overdosage due to muscarinic effects may include abdominal cramps, increased peristalsis, diarrhoea, nausea and vomiting, increased bronchial secretions, salivation, diaphoresis and miosis. Nicotinic effects consist of muscular cramps, fasciculations and general weakness. Bradycardia and hypotension may also occur.

Artificial ventilation should be instituted if respiration is severely depressed. Atropine sulphate 1 to 2mg intravenously is an antidote to the muscarinic effects.

Pharmacological properties
Pharmacodynamic properties: Mestinon is an antagonist to cholinesterase, the enzyme which normally destroys acetylcholine. The action of Mestinon can briefly be described, therefore, as the potentiation of naturally occurring acetylcholine. Mestinon has a more prolonged action than Prostigmin (neostigmine) although it is somewhat slower to take effect (generally taking 30 – 60 minutes). Because it has a weaker "muscarinic" action than Prostigmin, it is usually much better tolerated by myasthenic patients in whom the longer action is also an advantage.

Pharmacokinetic properties: Oral pyridostigmine is poorly absorbed. Maximum plasma concentrations occur at 1 to 2 hours and it is eliminated by the kidney largely unchanged with a half-life of 3 to 4 hours.

Preclinical safety data: Not applicable.

Pharmaceutical particulars
List of excipients
Each tablet contains: Lactose BP, Starch BP, Precipitated Silica Talc BP, Magnesium Stearate BP, Purified Water BP

Incompatibilities: None known.

Shelf life: 3 years.

Special precautions for storage: Recommended maximum storage temperature 25°C. Protect from light and moisture.

Nature and contents of container: Amber glass bottles with aluminium screw caps and desiccant, containing 200 tablets.

Instructions for use/handling: No special requirements.

Marketing authorisation number PL 15142/0006

Legal category POM

VIRAZOLE (Ribavirin) Aerosol (previously called Virazid)

Qualitative and quantitative composition Ribavirin 6g
International non-proprietary name (INN): Ribavirin
Chemical name: 1-Beta-D-Ribofuranosyl-1H, 2, 4-triazole-3-carboxamide

Pharmaceutical form Powder for inhalation solution.

Clinical particulars
Therapeutic indications: Virazole is indicated in the treatment of infants and children with severe respiratory syncytial virus (RSV) bronchiolitis.

Important: Ribavirin aerosol is more effective when instituted within the first 3 days of the treatment of bronchiolitis. Treatment early in the course of the disease may be necessary to achieve efficacy.

Treatment with Virazole must be accompanied by, and does not replace, standard supportive respiratory and fluid management for infants and children with severe respiratory tract infection.

Nebulised bronchodilators, when clinically indicated, should be administered with the SPAG generator turned off.

Posology and method of administration: Ribavirin aerosol is only recommended for use in infants and children.

Aerosol administration or nebulisation should be carried out in a small particle aerosol generator (SPAG). Before use read the SPAG Operator's Manual for instructions.

Treatment is carried out for 12-18 hours per day for at least 3 and no more than 7 days and is part of a total treatment programme.

The daily dose is prepared by dissolving 6g of Ribavirin in a minimum of 75ml Water for Injection BP. Shake well. Transfer dissolved drug and dilute to a total volume of 300ml of distilled water in the reservoir of the aerosol generator.

The concentration of ribavirin in the reservoir is 20mg/ml in the SPAG unit and the average concentration for a 7 hours period is 190 µg/l of air.

Method of administration: Please see *Instructions for use/handling* for instructions on preparation of the aerosol solution.

The aerosol is delivered to an infant oxygen hood from the SPAG aerosol generator. Administration by face mask or oxygen tent may be necessary if a hood cannot be employed (see SPAG Operator's Manual). However, the volume of distribution and condensation area are larger in a tent and the efficacy of this method of administration has been evaluated only in a small number of patients.

Contra-indications: Ribavirin is contra-indicated in females who are or may become pregnant and it should be noted that ribavirin can be detected in human blood even four weeks after oral administration has ceased.

Special warnings and special precautions for use: Precipitation of the drug in respiratory equipment and consequent accumulation of fluid in the tubing has caused difficulties for patients requiring assisted ventilation.

In infants requiring assisted ventilation, Virazole should only be used when there is a constant monitoring of both patients and equipment.

Directions for use during assisted ventilation are given in the SPAG manual which should be read carefully before such administration.

The teratogenic risk of Virazole to humans is unknown. As a precaution, women who are pregnant or trying to become pregnant should avoid exposure to the Virazole aerosol. Health care workers directly providing care to patients receiving aerosolised Virazole should be aware that ribavirin has been shown to be teratogenic in rabbits and rodents but not in baboons. However, no reports of teratogenicity in the offspring of mothers who were exposed to Virazole aerosol during pregnancy have been confirmed.

Nebulised Virazole may potentially escape into the hospital environment during therapy. However, ribavirin was not detected in the erythocytes, plasma or urine of subjects exposed for a mean of 25 hours during 5 consecutive days.

It is good practice to avoid unnecessary occupational exposure to chemicals whenever possible. Several methods have been employed to lower environmental exposure during Virazole use. The most practical of these is to turn the SPAG device off for 5 to 10 minutes prior to prolonged contact.

Interaction with other medicaments and other forms of interaction: None known.

Pregnancy and lactation: Ribavirin is contra-indicated in females who are or may become pregnant, and in nursing mothers. Ribavirin can be detected in human blood four weeks after administration has ceased. Although there are no pertinent human data, oral ribavirin has been found to be teratogenic in tested rodent species. Pregnant baboons given up to 120mg/kg/day orally over a 4 week period and within 20 days of gestation failed to exhibit any teratogenic effects.

Effects on ability to drive and use machines: None known.

Undesirable effects (frequency and seriousness)
Side-effects: Several serious adverse events occurred in severely ill infants with life-threatening underlying disease, many of whom required assisted ventilation. These events included worsening of respiratory status, bacterial pneumonia and pneumothorax. The role of ribavirin aerosol in these events has not been determined.

Anaemia (often of a haemolytic variety) and reticulocytosis have been reported with oral and intravenous administration. Rarely, cases of non-specific anaemia and haemolysis have been reported spontaneously in association with the aerosol administration of Virazole.

Overdose: No overdoses have been reported.

Pharmacological properties
Pharmacodynamic properties: Ribavirin has anti-viral inhibitory activity *in vitro* against respiratory syncytial virus, influenzae virus and herpes simplex virus. Ribavirin is also active against respiratory syncytial virus in experimentally infected cotton rats.

The inhibitory activity of ribavirin on RSV in cell cultures is selective. The mechanism of action is unknown, but there is evidence that ribavirin interferes with protein translation by mRNA of several other RNA viruses, possibly the result of interference with formation of the 5′ cap structure of mRNA.

Pharmacokinetic properties: Assay for ribavirin in human materials is by a radioimmunoassay which detects ribavirin and at least one metabolite.

Ribavirin administered by aerosol is absorbed systemically. Four paediatric patients inhaling ribavirin aerosol administered by face mask for 2.5 hours each day had plasma concentrations ranging from 0.44 to 1.44μM, with a mean concentration of 0.76μM. The plasma half-life was reported to be 9.5 hours. Three paediatric patients inhaling ribavirin aerosol administered by face mask or mist tent for 20 hours each day for 5 days had plasma concentrations ranging from 1.5 to 14.3μM, with a mean concentration of 6.8μM.

It is likely that the concentration of ribavirin in respiratory tract secretions is much higher than plasma concentrations in view of the route of administration.

The bioavailability of ribavirin is unknown and may depend on the mode of aerosol delivery. After aerosol treatment, peak plasma concentrations are less than the concentration that reduced RSV plaque formation in tissue cultures by 85 to 98%. After aerosol treatment, respiratory tract secretions are likely to contain ribavirin in concentrations many fold higher than those required to reduce plaque formation. However, RSV is an intracellular virus and serum concentrations may better reflect intracellular concentrations in the respiratory tract than respiratory secretion concentrations.

Preclinical safety data: Pertinent information is included in the Pregnancy and Lactation section.

Pharmaceutical particulars

List of excipients: Not applicable.

Incompatibilities: None known.

Shelf-life: 5 years. After reconstitution in Water for Injections, Virazole should be used within 24 hours.

Special precautions for storage: Store in a dry place at 15-20°C.

Nature and contents of containers: 100ml Type 1 glass serum bottle with butyl rubber closure and aluminium seal with tear-off septum. Each bottle contains 6g ribavirin as a lyophilised white cake. Virazole is packaged in cartons of three bottles.

Instructions for use/handling: By aseptic technique dissolve the powder in a minimum of 75ml Water for Injections BP in the 100ml vial. The solution should be adequately mixed to ensure complete dissolution. Shake well. It is not recommended that this solution is heated during dissolution. Transfer to the clean, sterilised 500ml flask and dilute to a final volume of 300ml with Water for Injections BP. The final concentration should be 20mg/ml.

The Water for Injections BP used to make up the Virazole solution should not have any antimicrobial agent or any other substance added and all solutions should be inspected for particulate matter and discolouration prior to administration.

See guidelines for avoiding unwanted exposure to Virazole aerosol under *Special warnings and special precautions for use.*

Marketing authorisation number PL 15142/0001

Legal category POM.

International Medication Systems (UK) Ltd

Medeva House
Regent Park
Kingston Road
Leatherhead
Surrey KT22 7PQ

☎ 01372 364000 🖷 01372 364190

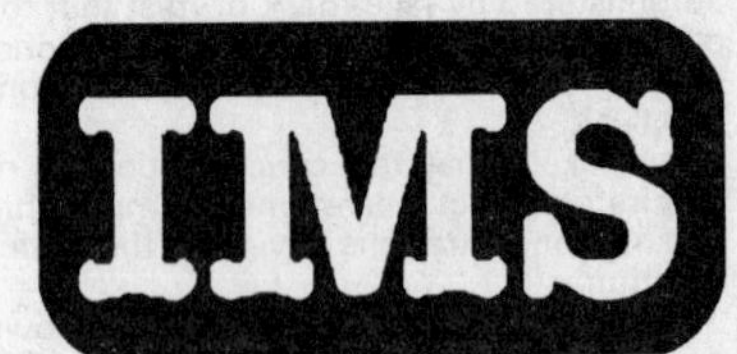

EPINEPHRINE (ADRENALINE) INJECTION 1:1000 MINIJET*

Qualitative and quantitative composition Epinephrine USP 1 mg per ml.

Pharmaceutical form Sterile aqueous solution for intramuscular or subcutaneous administration.

Clinical particulars

Therapeutic indications: Emergency treatment of anaphylaxis or acute angioneurotic oedema with airways obstruction, or acute allergic reactions.

Posology and method of administration: For the relief of life-threatening angioneurotic oedema and anaphylactic shock, epinephrine should be administered by intramuscular injection.

For acute allergic reactions due to insect stings etc: Intramuscular or subcutaneous injection.

Adults: 0.5 to 1.0 ml (0.5-1.0 mg), administered slowly. The dose may be repeated every 5 to 15 minutes as needed.

Elderly: As for adults, use with caution.

Children (up to age of 12): 0.01 ml/kg bodyweight (0.01 mg/kg), up to a maximum of 0.5 ml. This can be repeated twice at 15 minute intervals, then every 4 hours as needed. The actual amount varies according to whether the child is small, medium or large for his/her age:

Volume of epinephrine 1:1,000 for intramuscular injection in anaphylactic shock:

Age	Volume of epinephrine (ml)
Under 1 year	0.05
1 year	0.1
2 years	0.2
3-4 years	0.3
5 years	0.4
6-12 years	0.5

These doses are for robust children. If underweight use half these doses.

Care should be taken when administering small volumes of the product.

Contra-indications: Contra-indications are relative as this product is intended for use in life-threatening emergencies.

Other than in the emergency situation, the following contra-indications should be considered: hyperthyroidism, hypertension, ischaemic heart disease, diabetes mellitus and closed angle glaucoma.

Special warnings and precautions for use: These special warnings and precautions are relative as this product is intended for use in life-threatening situations.

Administer slowly with caution to elderly patients and to patients with ischaemic heart disease, hypertension, diabetes mellitus, hyperthyroidism or psychoneurosis. Anginal pain may be induced when coronary insufficiency is present. Use with caution in patients with closed angle glaucoma.

Interaction with other medicaments and other forms of interaction: The effects of epinephrine may be potentiated by tricyclic antidepressants. Halothane and other anaesthetics such as cyclopropane and trichloroethylene, increase the risk of epinephrine-induced ventricular arrhythmias and acute pulmonary oedema, if hypoxia is present. Severe hypertension and bradycardia may occur with non-selective beta-blocking drugs, such as propranolol. Propranolol also inhibits the bronchodilator effect of epinephrine. The risk of cardiac arrhythmias is higher when epinephrine is given to patients receiving digoxin or quinidine. Epinephrine-induced hypoglycaemia may lead to loss of blood-sugar control in diabetic patients treated with hypoglycaemic agents.

Pregnancy and lactation : Epinephrine crosses the placenta. There is some evidence of a slightly increased incidence of congenital abnormalities. Injection of epinephrine may cause foetal tachycardia, cardiac irregularities, extrasystoles and louder heart sounds. In labour, epinephrine may delay the second stage. Epinephrine should only be used in pregnancy if the potential benefits outweigh the risks to the foetus.

Epinephrine is excreted in breast milk but, as pharmacologically active plasma concentrations are not achieved by the oral route, the use of epinephrine in breast-feeding mothers is presumed to be safe.

Effect on ability to drive and use machinery: Not applicable; this preparation is intended for use only in emergencies.

Undesirable effects: The potentially severe adverse effects of epinephrine arise from its effect upon blood pressure and cardiac rhythm. Ventricular fibrillation may occur and severe hypertension may lead to cerebral haemorrhage and pulmonary oedema. Symptomatic adverse effects are anxiety, dyspnoea, restlessness, palpitations, tachycardia, tremor, weakness, dizziness, headache and cold extremities. Biochemical effects include inhibition of insulin secretion and hypoglycaemia (even with low doses), gluconeogenesis, glycolysis, lipolysis and ketogenesis.

Overdose:

Symptoms: cardiac arrhythmias leading to ventricular fibrillation and death, severe hypertension leading to pulmonary oedema and cerebral haemorrhage.

Treatment: combined alpha- and beta-adrenergic blocking agents such as labetalol may counteract the effects of epinephrine, or a beta-blocking agent may be used to treat any supraventricular arrhythmias and phentolamine to control the alpha-mediated effects on the peripheral circulation. Rapidly acting vasodilators such as nitrates and sodium nitroprusside may also be helpful.

Immediate resuscitation support must be available.

Pharmacological properties

Pharmacodynamic properties: Epinephrine is a direct-acting sympathomimetic agent exerting its effect on alpha- and beta-adrenoceptors. Major effects are increased systolic blood pressure, reduced diastolic pressure, tachycardia, hyperglycaemia and hypokalaemia. It is a powerful cardiac stimulant. It has vasopressor properties and is a bronchodilator.

Pharmacokinetic properties: Epinephrine is rapid in onset and of short duration and is rapidly distributed to the heart, spleen, several glandular tissues and adrenergic nerves. It crosses the placenta and is excreted in breast milk. It is approximately 50% bound to plasma proteins. The onset of action is rapid and after intravenous infusion, the half-life is approximately 5-10 minutes.

Epinephrine is rapidly metabolised in the liver and tissues by oxidative deamination and O-methylation followed by reduction or by conjugation with glucuronic acid or sulphate. Up to 90% of the intravenous dose is excreted in the urine as metabolites.

Preclinical safety data: Not applicable since Epinephrine (Adrenaline) Injection has been used in clinical practice for many years and its effects in man are well known.

Pharmaceutical particulars

List of excipients: Citrate Acid Monohydrate USP, Sodium Citrate Dihydrate USP, Sodium Chloride USP, Sodium Bisulphite USP, Hydrochloric Acid 10% w/v USP, Water for Injection USP.

Incompatibilities: Epinephrine should not be mixed with sodium bicarbonate; the solution is oxidised to adrenochrome and then forms polymers.

Shelf life: 9 months.

Special precautions for storage: Store below 25°C. Protect from light.

Nature and contents of container: The solution is contained in a USP type I glass vial with an elastomeric closure which meets all the relevant USP specifications. The product is available either as 0.5 ml or 1 ml.

Instructions for use/handling: The container is specially designed for use with the IMS Minijet injector.

Marketing authorisation number 3265/0030

Date of approval/revision of SPC May 1997

Legal category POM

**Trade Mark*

Ipsen Ltd
1 Bath Road
Maidenhead
Berkshire SL6 4UH
☎ 01628 771447 🗋 01628 770199

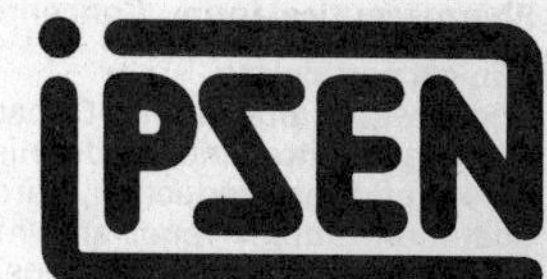

DE-CAPEPTYL SR* ▼

Qualitative and quantitative composition Triptorelin 4.2 mg.

Pharmaceutical form A 5 ml slightly tinted transparent Type I glass vial fitted with a crimped elastomer stopper containing a sterile, practically white crumbly cake which when reconstituted as directed with the clear, colourless, sterile liquid in the accompanying 2 ml clear Type I glass ampoule yields a sterile suspension for intramuscular injection.

Clinical particulars
Therapeutic indications:
Treatment of advanced prostate cancer.
Treatment of endometriosis.
Treatment of uterine fibroids prior to surgery or when surgery is not appropriate.

Posology and method of administration:
Advanced prostate cancer: One intramuscular injection should be administered every 4 weeks (28 days). No dosage adjustment is necessary in the elderly.

Endometriosis and uterine fibroids: One intramuscular injection every 28 days. For the treatment of endometriosis and uterine fibroids the treatment must be initiated in the first five days of the cycle. The maximum duration of treatment should be 6 months. For patients with uterine fibroids De-capeptyl SR should be administered for a minimum of 3 months.

A second course of treatment by De-capeptyl SR or by other GnRH analogues should not be undertaken due to concerns about bone density losses.

Contra-indications: In prostate cancer, De-capeptyl SR should not be prescribed in patients presenting with spinal cord compression or evidence of spinal metastases.

In endometriosis and uterine fibroid treatment, confirm that the patient is not pregnant before beginning treatment.

Special warnings and special precautions for use:
Advanced prostate cancer: Initially, De-capeptyl SR causes a transient increase in serum testosterone and consequent worsening of symptoms including increase in bone pain (and acid phosphatase levels). Consideration should be given to the use of an anti-androgen for three days prior to De-capeptyl SR treatment, to counteract this initial rise in serum testosterone levels. During the first month of treatment, patients presenting with, or at particular risk of developing, ureteric obstruction should be carefully monitored, as should those at risk of developing spinal cord compression. Continued treatment with De-capeptyl SR leads to suppression of testosterone (and dihydrotestosterone) and consequent improvement in the disease.

Endometriosis and uterine fibroids: Regular administration, every 28 days of one vial of De-capeptyl SR causes a persistent hypogonadotrophic amenorrhoea. During the first month of treatment, a non-hormonal contraception should be given. A supervening metrorrhagia in the course of treatment, other than in the first month, should lead to measurement of plasma oestradiol levels. Should this level be less than 50 pg/ml, possible associated organic lesions should be sought. After withdrawal of treatment, ovarian function resumes and ovulation occurs on average 58 days after the last injection, with first menses occurring on average 70 days after the last injection. Contraception may therefore be required. Due to concerns about bone density losses, De-capeptyl SR should be used with caution in women with known metabolic bone disease.

Interactions with other medicaments and other forms of interaction: Drugs which raise prolactin levels should not be prescribed concomitantly as they reduce the level of LHRH receptors in the pituitary.

Pregnancy and lactation: Reproductive studies in primates have shown no maternal toxicity or embryotoxicity, and there was no effect on parturition. Inadvertent administration of triptorelin during human pregnancy has not demonstrated a teratogenic or other foetal risk. However it is recommended that De-capeptyl SR should not be used during pregnancy or lactation.

Effect on ability to drive and use machines: There is no evidence that De-capeptyl SR has any effect on the ability to drive or operate machinery.

Undesirable effects:
Prostate cancer: In prostate cancer patients, the most frequent side-effects of hot flushes, decreased libido, and impotence are a result of the decrease in testosterone levels. Bone pain, as a result of 'disease flare', occurs occasionally. Pain and erythema at injection site, phlebitis and moderate and transient hypertension have been reported. On rare occasions the following have been reported: gynaecomastia, gastralgia, dry mouth, headaches, recurrence of asthma, increased dysuria, fever, pruritus, sweating, paresthesias, dizziness, insomnia, excessive salivation, gastric disturbance, nausea, vertigo, slight hair loss, induration at injection site.

Endometriosis and uterine fibroid patients: In endometriosis and uterine fibroid patients, adverse effects such as hot flushes, menorrhagia and vaginal dryness, reflect the efficacy of pituitary-ovarian blockade. Cutaneous rash, hair loss, asthenia, headache, weight gain, oedema, arthralgia, myalgia, transient sight disturbances and temporary hypertension may occur. As with any GnRH analogue, a small loss in bone density, specifically trabecular bone density, occurs during six months of De-capeptyl SR treatment. Clinical data suggests that this loss is reversible.

In the studies of uterine fibroids surgical intervention, as a result of an increase in vaginal haemorrhage was a rare complication of GnRH therapy.

With uterine fibroid patients it is important to monitor the early response to GnRH analogues and if there is no change or even an increase in uterine volume then the possibility of uterine leiomyosarcoma should be considered.

Overdose: There is no human experience of overdosage. Animal data do not predict any effects other than those on sex hormone concentration and consequent effect on the reproductive tract. If overdosage occurs, symptomatic management is indicated.

Pharmacological properties
Pharmacodynamic properties: Triptorelin is a decapeptide analogue of LHRH which initially stimulates release of pituitary gonadotrophins.

Prostate cancer patients: This results in an increase in peripheral circulating levels of testosterone and dihydrotestosterone. Continued administration (over 7 days) however, leads to suppression of gonadotrophins and a consequent fall in plasma testosterone. In prostate cancer patients, plasma testosterone levels fall to castrate levels after 2–3 weeks of treatment, frequently resulting in an improvement of function and objective symptoms.

Endometriosis and uterine fibroid patients: Continued administration of De-capeptyl SR induces suppression of oestrogen secretion and thus enables resting of ectopic endometrial tissue. In pre-operative therapy for uterine fibroids there appears to be a beneficial effect on the blood loss at surgery. Studies have demonstrated a consistent and marked reduction in uterine and/or fibroid volume becoming maximal in a three to six month treatment period. Clinical studies have shown that 90–100% of fibroid patients become amenorrhoeic within two months of treatment and triptorelin provides relief from the symptoms of abdominal pain, dysmenorrhoea and menorrhagia associated with uterine fibroids.

Pharmacokinetic properties:
Subcutaneous form: In healthy volunteers:
Subcutaneously administered triptorelin (100 μg) is rapidly absorbed (Tmax = 0.63±0.26 hr for peak plasma concentration = 1.85±0.23 ng/ml). Elimination is effected with a biological half-life of 7.6±1.6 hr, after a 3 to 4 hr distribution phase. Total plasma clearance is: 161±28 ml/min. Distribution volume is 104.1±11.7 litres.

In prostate cancer patients: With subcutaneous administration (100 μg), triptorelin blood levels oscillate between maximum values of 1.28±0.24 ng/ml (Cmax) obtained in general one hour after injection (Tmax) and minimum values of 0.28±0.15 ng/ml (Cmin) obtained 24 hrs after injection.

The biological half-life is on average 11.7±3.4 hr but varies according to patients. Plasma clearance (118±32 ml/min) reflects slower elimination in patients, whilst distribution volumes are close to those of healthy volunteers (113.4±21.6 litres).

Sustained release form:
Prostate cancer patients: Following intramuscular injection of the sustained release form, an initial phase of release of the active principle present on the surface of the microspheres is observed, followed by further fairly regular release (Cmax = 0.32±0.12 ng/ml), with a mean rate of release of triptorelin of 46.6±7.1 μg/day. The bioavailability of the microparticles is approximately 53% at one month.

Endometriosis and uterine fibroid patients: After intramuscular injection of De-capeptyl SR in endometriosis and uterine fibroid patients the maximum blood level of triptorelin is obtained between 2 to 6 hours after injection, the peak value reached is 11 ng/ml. There was no evidence of accumulation of the product following monthly injections over six months. The minimum blood level oscillates between 0.1 and 0.2 ng/ml. The bioavailability of the sustained release product is approximately 50%.

Preclinical safety data: Preclinical findings were only those related to the expected pharmacological activity of triptorelin, namely down-regulation of the hypothalamic-pituitary-gonadal axis. These included atrophy of the testes and genital tract, with resultant suppression of spermatogenesis, together with decreased weight of the prostate gland. These findings were largely reversible within the recovery period. In a small number of rats, in a 24 months oncogenicity study, a low incidence of benign histological changes were seen in the non-glandular part of the fore stomach. Erosions, ulcers, necrosis and inflammation were seen at varying degrees of severity. The clinical relevance of these findings is unknown. The increased incidence of adenomatous tumours in the rat pituitary observed with De-capeptyl following long-term repeated dosing is thought to be a class specific action of GnRH analogues due to an hormonally-mediated mechanism and has not been found in the mouse nor has it been described in man.

Standard mutagenicity testing revealed no mutagenic activity of triptorelin.

Pharmaceutical particulars
List of excipients:
a) *Powder:* D,L-lactide/glycolide copolymer, mannitol, sodium carboxymethylcellulose, polysorbate 80.
b) *Suspension vehicle:* mannitol, water for injections.

Incompatibilities: None.
Shelf life: The shelf-life of the powder for injection shall not exceed 18 months.

The shelf-life of the injection vehicle shall not exceed 3 years.

The product should be used immediately after reconstitution.

Special precautions for storage: The product should be stored below 25°C, away from direct heat.

Nature and contents of container: A 5 ml slightly tinted, transparent, Type I glass vial with a crimped, elastomer stopper containing a sterile, practically white, crumbly cake and a 2 ml, type I glass ampoule containing a clear, colourless, sterile liquid.

Instructions for use/handling: The vehicle should be drawn into the syringe provided and transferred to the vial containing the powder for injection. The vial should be gently shaken and the mixture then drawn back into the syringe without inverting the vial. The needle should then be changed and the injection administered immediately.

Marketing authorisation numbers:

De-capeptyl SR	10829/0002
Mannitol solution	10829/0003

Date of approval/revision of SPC April 1998.

Legal category POM.

DOPACARD*

Qualitative and quantitative composition Dopexamine hydrochloride as a 1% solution (w/v). Each 5 ml ampoule contains 50 mg of dopexamine hydrochloride.

Pharmaceutical form Concentrate for infusion.

Clinical particulars

Therapeutic indications: Dopacard is indicated for short-term intravenous administration to patients in whom afterload reduction, (through peripheral vasodilatation, and/or renal and mesenteric vasodilatation), combined with a mild positive inotropic effect is required for the treatment of exacerbations of chronic heart failure, or heart failure associated with cardiac surgery.

Posology and method of administration: Dopacard must be diluted before use.

Dosage

Adults and the elderly: Infusion should begin at a dose of 0.5 microgram/kg/min and may be increased to 1 microgram/kg/min and then in increments (0.5–1 microgram/kg/min) up to 6 micrograms/kg/min at not less than 15 minute intervals according to the patient's haemodynamic and clinical response. Smaller increments (0.5 microgram/kg/min) may be justified in certain patients according to haemodynamic and clinical response.

Children: The safety and efficacy of Dopacard for use in children have not been established.

Administration Dopacard should only be administered intravenously by infusion through a cannula or catheter in a central or large peripheral vein. Contact with metal parts in infusion apparatus should be minimised. A device which provides accurate control of the rate of flow is essential.

Central administration: Dopacard can be administered via a cannula or catheter sited in a central vein. The concentration of the infusion solution for administration via this route must not exceed 4 mg/ml.

Peripheral administration: Dopacard can be administered via a cannula in a large peripheral vein. The concentration of the infusion solution for administration via this route must not exceed 1 mg/ml. Thrombophlebitis has been reported with peripheral administration using concentrations of Dopacard exceeding 1 mg/ml.

During the administration of Dopacard, as with any parenteral catecholamine, the rate of administration and duration of therapy should be adjusted according to the patient's response as determined by heart rate and rhythm (ECG), blood pressure, urine flow and, whenever possible, measurement of cardiac output.

It is recommended that the infusion of Dopacard is reduced gradually rather than withdrawn abruptly.

The duration of therapy is dependent upon the patient's overall response to treatment. Extended therapy beyond 48 hours has not been fully evaluated.

Contra-indications: Known hypersensitivity to dopexamine hydrochloride or excipients (disodium edetate). Patients who are receiving monoamine oxidase inhibitors (MAOIs). Phaeochromocytoma. Thrombocytopenia. Patients with left ventricular outlet obstruction such as hypertrophic obstructive cardiomyopathy or aortic stenosis. In such patients, positive inotropic activity may increase left ventricular outflow obstruction and sudden vasodilatation may cause hypotension.

Special warnings and precautions for use: Correction of hypovolaemia must be achieved prior to administration of Dopacard.

Care should be exercised so as to restrict the sodium and fluid load during administration of Dopacard.

Dopacard should not be administered to patients with severe hypotension or a markedley reduced systemic vascular resistance until specific resuscitative measures have been taken to restore blood pressure to a clinically acceptable level.

In patients with a marked reduction in systemic vascular resistance, Dopacard should not be used as a direct substitute for pressor agents or other inotropes.

As with other catecholamines, Dopacard should be administered with caution to patients with a clinical history of ischaemic heart disease especially following acute myocardial infarction or recent episodes of angina pectoris as a tachycardia may increase myocardial oxygen demand and further exacerbate myocardial ischaemia.

As has been observed with other β_2-adrenergic agonists, a small reversible fall in circulating platelet numbers has been observed in some patients. No adverse effects attributable to alterations in platelet count have been seen in clinical studies.

Care must be exercised when administering Dopacard in the presence of hypokalaemia or hyperglycaemia. In common with other β_2-agonists, Dopacard depresses plasma potassium and raises plasma glucose. These effects are minor and reversible. Monitoring of potassium and glucose is advisable in patients likely to be at risk from such changes, e.g. diabetics, patients with myocardial infarction or patients being treated with diuretics or cardiac glycosides.

Benign arrhythmias such as ventricular premature beats and, more rarely, serious arrhythmias have been reported in some patients. If excessive tachycardia occurs during Dopacard administration, then a reduction or temporary discontinuation of the infusion should be considered.

As with other parenteral catecholamines, there have been occasional reports of partial tolerance, with some attenuation of the haemodynamic response developing during long-term infusions of Dopacard.

The risk of thrombophlebitis and local necrosis may be increased if the concentration of Dopacard administered via a peripheral vein exceeds 1 mg/ml. Thrombophlebitis is rare when the concentration of drug used for peripheral administration is less than 1 mg/ml.

Interaction with other medicaments and other forms of interaction: As Dopacard inhibits the Uptake-1 mechanism, it may potentiate the effects of exogenous catecholamines such as noradrenaline. Caution is recommended when these agents are administered concomitantly with Dopacard or soon after its discontinuation.

There is no evidence of an interaction with dopamine, other than possible attenuation of the indirect sympathomimetic inotropic effects of higher doses of dopamine due to Uptake-1 blockade by Dopacard.

Concomitant use with β_2-adrenergic and dopamine receptor antagonists requires caution since possible attenuation of the pharmacological effects of Dopacard may occur.

Pregnancy and lactation: There is no experience of the use of Dopacard in pregnant or lactating women and therefore its safety in these situations has not been established. There is insufficient evidence from animal studies to indicate it is free from hazard. Dopacard is not therefore currently recommended for use in pregnant or lactating women.

Effects on ability to drive and use machines: Not applicable.

Undesirable effects: The most common undesirable effect reported with Dopacard administration in studies of use in heart failure is tachycardia (11.8% in studies of exacerbations of chronic heart failure; 19.4% in studies of use in cardiac surgery). The increases in heart rate are dose-related and, in most cases, not clinically significant.

Hypertension and transient hypotension have been reported after cardiac surgery (at an incidence of 8.8% and 7.0% respectively). These events, however, are not uncommon as compensatory mechanisms following cardiac surgery. Transient hypotension was reported in studies of exacerbations of chronic heart failure at an incidence of 6.3%.

Other undesirable effects reported in clinical trials in both exacerbations of chronic heart failure and cardiac surgery at an incidence of 1% or more include:

Cardiovascular: A number of tachyarrhythmias such as premature ventricular contractions (PVCs) and atrial fibrillation, bradycardia, both sinus and nodal, worsening heart failure leading to asystole and cardiac arrest, angina, myocardial infarction, cardiac enzyme changes and non-specific ECG changes have occurred.

Non-cardiovascular: Nausea and vomiting, tremor, headache, diaphoresis and dyspnoea.

Careful titration of the dose may minimise the incidence of adverse events.

More rarely a number of serious adverse events have been reported in patients undergoing cardiac surgery: renal failure, respiratory failure, acute respiratory distress syndrome (ARDS), pulmonary oedema, pulmonary hypertension, bleeding and septicaemia. However, such events may also be due to the condition of the patients in such populations.

Overdose: The half-life of Dopacard in blood is short. Consequently, the effects of overdosage are likely to be short-lived provided that administration is discontinued. However, in some cases, it may be necessary to initiate prompt supportive measures.

Effects of overdosage are likely to be related to the pharmacological actions and include tachycardia, tremulousness and tremor, nausea and vomiting, and anginal pain. Treatment should be supportive and directed to these symptoms.

Pharmacological properties

Pharmacodynamic properties: The primary actions of Dopacard (dopexamine hydrochloride) are the stimulation of adrenergic β_2-receptors and peripheral dopamine receptors of DA_1 and DA_2 subtypes. In addition, Dopacard is an inhibitor of neuronal reuptake of noradrenaline (Uptake-1). These pharmacological actions result in an increase in cardiac output mediated by afterload reduction (β_2, DA_1) and mild positive inotropism (β_2, Uptake-1 inhibition) together with an increase in blood flow to vascular beds (DA1) such as the renal and mesenteric beds. Dopacard therefore provides an increase in systemic and regional oxygen delivery. Dopacard is not an α-adrenergic agonist and does not cause vasoconstriction and is not a pressor agent.

Pharmacokinetic properties: Dopacard is rapidly eliminated from blood with a half-life of approximately 6-7 minutes in healthy volunteers and around 11 minutes in patients with cardiac failure. Subsequent elimination of the metabolites is by urinary and biliary excretion. The response to Dopacard is rapid in onset and effects subside rapidly on discontinuation of the infusion.

Pre-clinical safety data: There is no information relevant to the prescriber, which has not been included in other sections of this Summary of Product Characteristics.

Pharmaceutical particulars

List of excipients: Disodium edetate, Hydrochloric acid, Water for Injections.

Incompatibilities: Dopacard should only be diluted with 0.9% Sodium Chloride Injection, 5% Dextrose Injection, Hartmann's Solution (Compound Sodium Lactate Intravenous Infusion) or Dextrose 4%/Saline 0.18% Injection, and should not be added to sodium bicarbonate or any other strongly alkaline solutions as inactivation will occur

Dopacard should not be mixed with any other drugs before administration.

Contact with metal parts, in infusion apparatus for example, should be minimised.

Shelf life: The shelf life of unopened ampoules is 3 years.

Prepared intravenous solutions in 0.9% Sodium Chloride Injection or 5% Dextrose Injection are stable for 24 hours at room temperature.

Special precautions for storage: Store below 25°C, protect from light.

Nature and contents of container: Box of 10 clear glass ampoules each containing 5 ml of 1% (w/v) solution of dopexamine hydrochloride (50 mg per ampoule).

Instructions for use/handling: The contents of four ampoules (20 ml) should be injected aseptically into one of the following:

0.9% Sodium Chloride Injection	500 or 250 ml
5% Dextrose Injection	500 or 250 ml

These dilutions give a concentration for administration as follows:-

4 ampoules of Dopacard diluted to 500 ml = 400 micrograms/ml

4 ampoules of Dopacard diluted to 250 ml = 800 micrograms/ml

Dopacard, in common with other catecholamines, may turn slightly pink in prepared solutions. There is no significant loss of potency associated with this change.

Marketing authorisation number 6958/0008

Date of approval/revision of SPC April 1998.

Legal category POM.

DYSPORT*

Qualitative and quantitative composition

Active constituent	*per vial*
Clostridium botulinum type A toxin-haemagglutinin complex	500U‡
Other constituents	
Albumin solution 20%	125 micrograms
Lactose	2.5 mg

‡ One unit (U) is defined as the median lethal peritoneal dose in mice.

Pharmaceutical form Injection.

Clinical particulars

Therapeutic indications: For the treatment of blepharospasm, hemifacial spasm and spasmodic torticollis.

Posology and method of administration when treating blepharospasm and hemifacial spasm

Adults and elderly: In the treatment of bilateral blepharospasm the recommended initial dose is 120 units per eye.

Injection of 0.1 ml (20 units) should be made medially and of 0.2 ml (40 units) should be made laterally into the junction between the preseptal and orbital parts of both the upper and lower orbicularis oculi muscles of each eye.

For injections into the upper lid the needle should be directed away from its centre to avoid the levator muscle. A diagram to aid placement of these injections is provided below. The relief of symptoms may be expected to begin within two to four days with maximal effect within two weeks.

Injections should be repeated approximately every eight weeks or as required to prevent recurrence of symptoms. On such subsequent administrations the dose may need to be reduced to 80 units per eye, viz. 0.1 ml (20 units) medially and 0.1 ml (20 units) laterally above and below each eye in the manner previously described. The dose may be further reduced to 60 units per eye by omitting the medial lower lid injection.

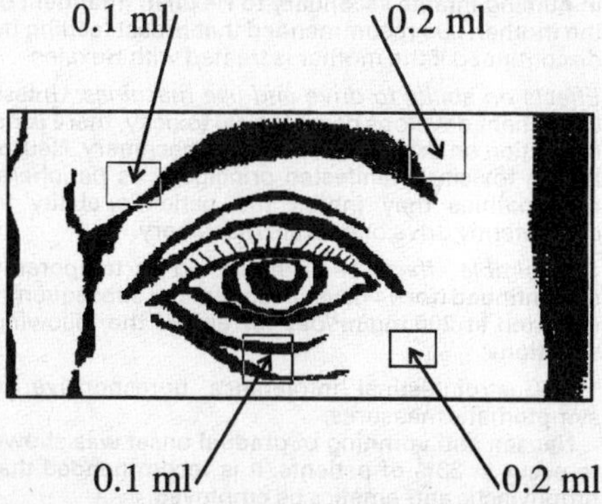

In cases of unilateral blepharospasm the injections should be confined to the affected eye. Patients with hemifacial spasm should be treated as for unilateral blepharospasm. The doses recommended are applicable to adults of all ages including the elderly.

Posology and method of administration when treating spasmodic torticollis: The doses recommended for torticollis are applicable to adults of all ages providing the adults are of normal weight with no evidence of low neck muscle mass. A reduced dose may be appropriate if the patient is markedly underweight or in the elderly where reduced muscle mass may exist.

The initial recommended dose for the treatment of spasmodic torticollis is 500 units (1 ml) per patient given as a divided dose and administered to the two or three most active neck muscles.

For rotational torticollis distribute the 500 units by administering 350 units into the splenius capitis muscle, ipsilateral to the direction of the chin/head rotation and 150 units into the sternomastoid muscle, contralateral to the rotation.

For laterocollis, distribute the 500 units by administering 350 units into the ipsilateral splenius capitis muscle and 150 units into the ipsilateral sternomastoid muscle. In cases associated with shoulder elevation the ipsilateral trapezoid or levator scapulae muscles may also require treatment, according to visible hypertrophy of the muscle or electromyographic (EMG) findings. Where injections of three muscles are required, distribute the 500 units as follows, 300 units splenius capitis, 100 units sternomastoid and 100 units to the third muscle.

For retrocollis distribute the 500 units by administering 250 units into each of the splenius capitis muscles. This may be followed by bilateral trapezius injections (up to 250 units per muscle) after 6 weeks, if there is insufficient response. Bilateral splenii injections may increase the risk of neck muscle weakness.

All other forms of torticollis are highly dependent on specialist knowledge and EMG to identify and treat the most active muscles. EMG should be used diagnostically for all complex forms of torticollis, for reassessment after unsuccessful injections in non complex cases, and for guiding injections into deep muscles or in overweight patients with poorly palpable neck muscles.

On subsequent administration, the doses may be adjusted according to the clinical response and side effects observed. Doses within the range of 250–1000 units are recommended, although the higher doses may be accompanied by increase in side effects, particularly dysphagia. Doses above 1000 units are not recommended.

The relief of symptoms of torticollis may be expected within a week after the injection. Injections should be repeated approximately every eight to twelve weeks or as required to prevent recurrence of symptoms.

Children: The safety and effectiveness of Dysport in children has not been demonstrated.

Method of administration: The exposed central portion of the rubber stopper should be cleaned with alcohol immediately prior to piercing the septum. A sterile 23 or 25 gauge needle should be used.

When treating blepharospasm and hemifacial spasm Dysport is reconstituted with 2.5 ml of sodium chloride injection BP (0.9%) to yield a solution containing 200 units per ml of Dysport.

Dysport is administered by subcutaneous injection medially and laterally into the junction between the preseptal and orbital parts of both the upper and lower orbicularis oculi muscles of the eyes.

When treating spasmodic torticollis Dysport is reconstituted with 1 ml of sodium chloride injection BP (0.9%) to yield a solution containing 500 units per ml of Dysport. Dysport is administered by intramuscular injection as above when treating spasmodic torticollis.

The units of Dysport are specific to the preparation and are not interchangeable with other preparations of botulinum toxin.

Contra-indications, warnings, etc
Contra-indications: Dysport is contra-indicated in pregnancy.

Special warnings and special precautions: For the treatment of spasmodic torticollis, Dysport should only be injected by specialists experienced in the diagnosis and management of this condition and who have received training on the administration of Dysport.

Careful consideration should be given before the re-injection of patients who have experienced a previous allergic reaction. The risk of a further allergic reaction must be considered in relation to the benefit of treatment.

Dysport should only be used with caution under close supervision in patients with subclinical or clinical evidence of marked defective neuromuscular transmission. Such patients may have an increased sensitivity to agents such as Dysport which may result in excessive muscle weakness.

Training: Ipsen will facilitate training in administration of Dysport injections.

There are no reports of any immune response after the local administration of *Clostridium botulinum* Type A toxin-haemagglutinin complex in accordance with the doses recommended when treating blepharospasm and hemifacial spasm. Antibody formation to botulinum toxin has been noted in a small number of patients receiving therapy with Dysport for torticollis. Clinically, this has been detected by substantial deterioration in response to therapy or a need for consistently increasing high doses.

This product contains a small amount of human albumin. The risk of transmission of viral infection cannot be excluded with absolute certainty following the use of human blood or blood products.

Interaction with other medicaments and other forms of interaction: No interactions of clinical significance have been reported.

Pregnancy and lactation: Teratological and other reproductive studies have not been performed with Dysport. The safety of its use in pregnant or lactating women has not been demonstrated.

Effects on ability to drive and use machines: None known.

Undesirable effects when treating blepharospasm and hemifacial spasm: Side-effects may occur from deep or misplaced injections of Dysport, temporarily paralysing other nearby muscle groups. They may also occur from exacerbation of pre-existing eyelid abnormalities or from an initial over-correction. Ptosis is the most common unwanted effect. A few patients may also experience diplopia or symptoms from spread of paralytic effect to mid-facial muscles. These side effects may be expected to resolve within two to four weeks. Keratitis and dry eyes due to reduced blinking have also been reported for which the use of artificial tears could be considered. Minor bruising and lid swelling may occur but are short lived. Reversible external ophthalmoplegia has been reported after excessive dosing.

The injections have been associated with a burning sensation which lasts for 1–2 minutes after injection.

Allergic reactions such as skin rashes and influenza-like symptoms have occasionally been noted.

Undesirable effects when treating spasmodic torticollis: Side-effects may occur mainly from deep or misplaced injections temporarily paralysing other nearby muscle groups. The injections have been associated with a burning sensation which lasts for 1–2 minutes after injection.

In patients treated for torticollis dysphagia is the most frequently reported adverse event. In a double-blind placebo controlled trial the incidence of dysphagia was 29% following treatment with 500 units of Dysport and 10% in the placebo group. This appears to be dose related and occurs most frequently following injection into the sternomastoid muscle. A soft diet may be required until symptoms resolve. In those patients severely affected, laryngoscopy has identified pooling of saliva. Aspiration may occur rarely and be of potential concern in those patients with pre-existing respiratory problems. Less frequently reported events include weakness of the neck muscles, dryness of mouth and voice changes. A more generalised weakness and visual disturbances (including diplopia and blurred vision) have occasionally been reported. Respiratory difficulties have been noted on rare occasions in association with high doses.

These side-effects may be expected to resolve within two to four weeks.

Allergic reactions such as skin rashes and influenza-like symptoms have occasionally been noted.

Overdose: Excessive doses may produce distant and profound neuromuscular paralysis. Respiratory support may be required where excessive doses cause paralysis of respiratory muscles. There is no specific antidote; antitoxin should not be expected to be beneficial and general supportive care is advised.

Pharmacological properties
Pharmacodynamic properties: Clostridium botulinum type A toxin-haemagglutinin complex blocks peripheral cholinergic transmission at the neuromuscular junction by a presynaptic action at a site proximal to the release of acetylcholine. The toxin acts within the nerve ending to antagonise those events that are triggered by Ca^{2+} which culminate in transmitter release. It does not affect postganglionic cholinergic transmission or postganglionic sympathetic transmission.

The action of toxin involves an initial binding step whereby the toxin attaches rapidly and avidly to the presynaptic nerve membrane. Secondly there is an internalisation step in which toxin crosses the presynaptic membrane, without causing onset of paralysis. Finally the toxin inhibits the release of acetylcholine by disrupting the Ca^{2+} mediated acetylcholine release mechanism, thereby diminishing the endplate potential and causing paralysis.

Recovery of impulse transmission occurs gradually as new nerve terminals sprout and contact is made with the post synaptic motor endplate, a process which takes 6–8 weeks in the experimental animal.

Pharmacokinetic properties: Pharmacokinetic studies with botulinum toxin pose problems in animals because of the high potency, the minute doses involved, the large molecular weight of the compound and the difficulty of labelling toxin to produce sufficiently high specific activity. Studies using I^{125} labelled toxin have shown that the receptor binding is specific and saturable, and the high density of toxin receptors is a contributory factor to the high potency. Dose and time responses in monkeys showed that at low doses there was a delay of 2–3 days with peak effect seen 5–6 days after injection. The duration of action, measured by changes of ocular alignment and muscle paralysis varied between 2 weeks and 8 months. This pattern is also seen in man, and is attributed to the process of binding, internalisation and changes at the neuromuscular junction.

Pharmaceutical particulars
List of excipients: Albumin and lactose.

Incompatibilities: None known.

Shelf life: The shelf life of the packaged product is 12 months.

The reconstituted product should be used within one hour of reconstitution.

Special precautions for storage: Unopened vials must be maintained at temperatures between 2°C and 8°C. Dysport must be stored in a refrigerator at the hospital where the injections are to be carried out and should not be given to the patient to store.

Dysport should not be frozen.

Nature and contents of container
Nature of container/closure: Type 1 glass vials 3 ml capacity. 13 mm chlorbutyl freeze-drying closures oversealed by 13 mm aluminium overseals with centre hole, crimped over.

Contents of container: A white lypophilised powder for reconstitution.

Instructions for use/handling: Immediately after treatment of the patient, any residual Dysport which may be present in either vial or syringe should be inactivated with dilute hypochlorite solution (1% available chlorine). Thereafter, all items should be disposed of in accordance with standard hospital practice.

Spillage of Dysport should be wiped up with an absorbent cloth soaked in dilute hypochlorite solution.

Marketing authorisation number 6958/0005.

Date of approval/revision of SPC March 1998.

Legal category POM.

ERWINASE*

Qualitative and quantitative composition Crisantaspase (Asparaginase from *Erwinia chrysanthemi*; Erwinia L-asparaginase), 10,000 Units/vial.

Pharmaceutical form Freeze-dried powder for reconstitution.

Clinical particulars
Therapeutic indications: Erwinase is used in combination with other anti-neoplastic agents to treat acute lymphoblastic leukaemia. It may also be used in other neoplastic conditions where depletion of asparagine might be expected to have a useful effect. Patients receiving treatment with L-asparaginase from *Escherichia coli*, and who develop hypersensitivity to that enzyme may be able to continue treatment with

Erwinase as the enzymes are immunologically distinct.

Dosage and method of administration: Erwinase solution can be given by intravenous injection or infusion or by intramuscular or subcutaneous injection.

For all patients the usual dose is 6,000 Units/m² body surface area (200 Units/kg of body weight), three times a week for three weeks.

Therapy may be further intensified according to protocol.

Reference to current Medical Research Council protocols on leukaemia therapy should be made for information on dose, route and frequency of treatment.

Contra-indications, warnings, etc
Contra-indications: Previous allergic reaction to Erwinia asparaginase.

Special warnings and special precautions for use
Warnings: Asparaginase is a bacterial protein and repeated use can, therefore, lead to sensitisation reactions.

Special precautions for use: Erwinase should preferably be given without interruption. If, however, an interruption cannot be avoided, treatment should be resumed with a low dose, 10 Units/kg/day, and increased to the full dose over five days if tolerated. Anaphylaxis is rare but facilities should be made available for its management during administration.

Interaction with other medicaments and other forms of interaction: Asparaginase must not be mixed with any other drugs prior to administration.

Pregnancy and lactation: Asparaginase should not be given to women who are, or likely to become, pregnant.

Effects on ability to drive and use machinery: None known.

Undesirable effects: Neurotoxicity, life-threatening sepsis and severe hypersensitivity have been described in patients treated with L-asparaginases. Other effects reported with both enzymes include fever; nausea; vomiting; CNS depression; hypersensitivity and various plasma biochemical changes including increased BSP retention and elevation of bilirubin, SGOT, alkaline phosphatase and cholesterol levels; decreases in fibrinogen and some clotting factors. For these reasons, careful monitoring is therefore necessary and urine should be tested for glucose to exclude hyperglycaemia.

Undesirable effects are generally reversible and are less common with Erwinia L-asparaginase than with *E. coli.* asparaginase.

Overdose: No specific measures are recommended.

Pharmacological properties
Pharmacodynamic properties: Neoplastic cells associated with Acute Lymphoblastic Leukaemia (ALL), Acute Myeloid Leukaemia (AML) and Lymphoblastic Lymphosarcoma (LSA) are asparagine-dependent. Reduction of plasma asparagine levels achieved by administration of L-asparaginase produces an anti-neoplastic effect.

The animal studies carried out with Erwinase provide only an approximate indication of the human dose required when comparisons are made on a mg/kg basis. However, clinical studies have used doses in the range 500 to 60,000 Units/m²/day. The upper dose level is made possible by the intrinsically low toxicity of the Erwinia enzyme.

Pharmacokinetic properties: Peak levels of Erwinase are achieved in blood in 1 to 2 hours. The fall in enzyme levels follows first order kinetics with a half-life of 7 to 13 hours.

Pre-clinical safety data: No further relevant data.

Pharamceutical particulars
List of excipients: Sodium chloride BP; dextrose monohydrate BP.

Incompatibilities: See '*Interaction with other medicaments and other forms of interaction*'.

Shelf-life
Shelf-life of product as packed for sale: 3 years.
Shelf-life following reconstitution according to directions: 15 minutes in the original container, 8 hours in a glass or polypropylene syringe (See section *Instructions for use/handling*).

Special precautions for storage: Store between 2°C and 8°C.

Nature and contents of container: Type I clear neutral glass vials of 3 ml nominal capacity, closed with 13 mm halobutyl freeze-drying stoppers and aluminium overseals, containing a white lyophilised solid.

Instructions for use/handling: The contents of each vial should be reconstituted in 1 ml to 2 ml of Sodium Chloride for Injection BP and dissolved by gentle mixing.

The solution should be administered within 15 minutes of reconstitution. If a delay of more than 15 minutes between reconstitution and administration is unavoidable, the solution should be withdrawn into a glass or polypropylene syringe for the period of the delay. The solution should be used within 8 hours.

Erwinase is not a cytotoxic drug (such as vincristine or methotrexate) and does not require the special precautions needed for manipulating such agents. It should be handled in the same way as other therapeutic enzymes such as hyaluronidase.

Name and address of the marketing authorisation holder: Microbiological Research Authority, Centre for Applied Microbiology and Research, Porton Down, Salisbury, Wiltshire SP4 0JG.

Marketing authorisation number 13663/0001

Date of approval/revision of SPC January 1998.

Legal category POM.

HEXALEN* CAPSULES ▼

Qualitative and quantitative composition

	Unit and/or percentage formula	
Active ingredient	*% w/w*	*mg/capsule*
Altretamine	19.6	50.0

Pharmaceutical form Clear transparent capsules containing 50 mg altretamine for oral administration.

Clinical particulars
Therapeutic indications: Hexalen is indicated for the treatment of advanced ovarian cancer as second line therapy in patients who have failed other treatments.

Posology and method of administration: Hexalen is administered orally. Doses are calculated on the basis of body surface area.

Hexalen should be administered only as a single agent for 14 consecutive days in a 28 day cycle at a dose of 260 mg/m²/day. The total daily dose should be rounded to the nearest 50 mg and may be given as 4 divided oral doses, given after meals and at bedtime. Hexalen should be administered for 12 cycles or until disease progression or unacceptable toxicity develops.

For dosage modifications please see *Undesirable effects* section.

Impaired renal function: No studies have been conducted in patients with impaired renal function.

Impaired hepatic function: There have been no studies of Hexalen metabolism or pharmacokinetics in patients with evidence of liver disease.

Elderly: Dose modifications should be based on adult toxicity guidelines described in *Undesirable effects* section, rather than age.

Contra-indications, warnings, etc
Contra-indications: Hexalen is contra-indicated in patients who have shown hypersensitivity to it. Hexalen should not be used in patients with pre-existing severe bone marrow depression or severe neurological toxicity.

Due to Hexalen's embryotoxic and teratogenic potential it is contra-indicated during pregnancy (see '*Use during pregnancy and lactation*').

Special warnings and precautions: Hexalen should only be given under the supervision of a physician experienced in the use of anti-neoplastic agents.

Peripheral blood counts should be monitored at least monthly, prior to the initiation of each course of Hexalen, and as clinically indicated.

Because of the possibility of Hexalen-related neurotoxicity, neurological examination should be performed regularly during Hexalen administration.

Concurrent administration of Hexalen and antidepressants of the monoamine oxidase inhibitor (MAOI) and tricyclic classes may cause severe orthostatic hypotension.

The carcinogenic potential of Hexalen has not been studied in animals, but drugs with similar mechanisms of action have been reported to be carcinogenic. Hexalen was weakly mutagenic when tested in strain TA100 of *Salmonella typhimurium*. With continuous, high dose administration, Hexalen adversely affected fertility in male rats.

Interactions: Concurrent administration of Hexalen and antidepressants of the MAO inhibitor or tricyclic classes may cause severe orthostatic hypotension. Cimetidine, an inhibitor of microsomal drug metabolism, increased altretamine's half-life and toxicity in a rat model.

Data from a randomised trial of Hexalen and cisplatin plus or minus pyridoxine in ovarian cancer indicated that pyridoxine significantly reduced neurotoxicity, however, it adversely affected response duration suggesting that pyridoxine should not be administered with Hexalen.

Use during pregnancy and lactation: No data are available on the use of Hexalen in human pregnancy. Hexalen has been shown to be embryotoxic and teratogenic in rats and rabbits. Due to Hexalen's embryotoxic and teratogenic potential, it is contraindicated during pregnancy. Women of childbearing potential should be advised to avoid becoming pregnant.

It is not known whether altretamine is excreted in human milk. Because there is a possibility of toxicity in nursing infants secondary to Hexalen treatment of the mother, it is recommended that breast feeding be discontinued if the mother is treated with Hexalen.

Effects on ability to drive and use machines: Unless the patient develops neurological toxicity, there is no restriction on driving or operating machinery. Neurological toxicity, manifested principally as peripheral neuropathies may inhibit the patient's ability to competently drive or operate machinery.

Undesirable effects: Hexalen should be temporarily discontinued (for 14 days or longer) and subsequently restarted at 200 mg/m²/day for any of the following situations:

1. Gastrointestinal intolerance unresponsive to symptomatic measures.

Nausea and vomiting of gradual onset was shown to occur in 33% of patients. It is recommended that prophylactic anti-emetics be employed.

Approximately 15% of patients may require dose interruptions or reductions and 5–10% of patients may require discontinuation of Hexalen therapy due to nausea and vomiting.

2. Myelosuppression defined as neutrophils $<2\times10^9$/l or platelets $<100\times10^9$/l.

Myelosuppression is dose related to Hexalen. At this dose and schedule Hexalen should not cause significant myelosuppression.

Hexalen should be withheld until neutrophils are $\geq2\times10^9$/l and platelets $\geq100\times10^9$/l before restarting at the reduced dose. If at the reduced dose neutrophils are $<1\times10^9$/l or platelets $<50\times10^9$/l Hexalen should be discontinued indefinitely.

Approximately 5% of patients may require dose interruptions or reductions due to neuropenia defined as $<2\times10^9$/l. Less than 1% of patients had neutropenia below $<1\times10^9$/l, following dose reduction. These patients were discontinued from Hexalen therapy.

Approximately 9% of patients may require dose interruptions or dose reductions due to thrombocytopenia defined as platelets $<100\times10^9$/l. Less than 3% of patients had thrombocytopenia below 50×10^9/l following dose reduction. These patients were discontinued from Hexalen therapy.

3. Progressive neurotoxicity during therapy.

Approximately 10% of patients may require dose interruptions or reductions. Neurotoxicity is dose and time dependent. If neurological symptoms fail to stabilise on the reduced dose schedule, Hexalen should be discontinued indefinitely.

Peripheral neuropathy and central nervous system symptoms (mood disorders, disorders of consciousness, ataxia, dizziness, vertigo) have been reported. Neurological toxicity may be reversible when therapy is discontinued.

Less than 5% of patients required discontinuation of Hexalen therapy.

4. Renal toxicity, defined as serum creatinine levels ≥1.6 mg/dL.

Dose interruptions or reductions were required in 7% of patients with increased serum creatinine levels (1.6–3.75 mg/dL).

Hexalen should be discontinued indefinitely if renal toxicity (serum creatinine levels ≥1.6 mg/dL) recurs on the reduced dose schedule and known nephrotoxic agents e.g. nephrotoxic anti-biotics have been discontinued.

Following dose interruptions or dose reductions less than 1% of patients required discontinuation of Hexalen therapy due to renal toxicity.

Other toxicities: Rare events included hepatic toxicity, skin rash, pruritus and alopecia; each were reported in <1% of patients treated. Less than 1% of patients had mild to moderate anaemia (haemoglobin 8–10 gm/dl) and less than 1% had severe anaemia (haemoglobin 6.5–7.9 gm/dl).

Overdose: No reports of overdosage are available. The most likely reaction would be severe nausea and vomiting and myelosuppression.

In the event of an overdose patients should be observed carefully and should signs of fever and infection arise, be treated along conventional lines.

Pharmacological properties
Pharmacodynamic properties: The precise mechanism by which Hexalen exerts its cytotoxic effect is unknown, although a number of theoretical possibilities have been studied. Structurally, Hexalen resembles the alkylating agent triethylenemelamine, yet in vitro tests for alkylating activity of Hexalen and its metabolites have been negative. Metabolism of altretamine is a requirement for cytotoxicity. Synthetic monohydroxymethylmelamines and products of altretamine metabolism, in vitro and in vivo, can form covalent adducts with tissue macromolecules includ-

ing DNA, but the relevance of these reactions to antitumour activity is unknown.

Pharmacokinetic properties: Urinary recovery and bioavailability data demonstrate that Hexalen is well absorbed following oral administration in humans, but undergoes rapid and extensive demethylation in the liver, producing variation in Hexalen plasma levels.

After oral administration in doses of 120–300 mg/m^2, peak plasma levels (as measured by gas-chromatographic assay) varying from 0.2 to 20.8 μg/ml were reached between 0.5 and 3 hours. Half-life of the β-phase of elimination ranged from 4.7 to 10.2 hours. There was no plasma accumulation of ^{14}C-radiolabelled hexamethylmelamine after daily treatment for 14 to 21 days.

Preclinical safety data: After intraperitoneal administration of ^{14}C-ring-labelled altretamine to mice, tissue distribution was rapid in all organs, reaching a maximum at 30 minutes. The excretory organs (liver and kidney) and the small intestine showed high concentrations of radioactivity, whereas relatively low concentrations were found in other organs, including the brain.

The carcinogenic potential of Hexalen has not been studied in animals, but drugs with similar mechanisms of action have been shown to be carcinogenic. Hexalen was weakly mutagenic when tested in strain TA100 of *Salmonella typhimurium*. Hexalen administered to female rats 14 days prior to breeding through the gestation period had no adverse effect on fertility, but decreased post-natal survival at 120 mg/m^2/day and was embryocidal at 240 mg/m^2/day. Administration of 120 mg/m^2/day Hexalen to male rats for 60 days prior to mating resulted in testicular atrophy, reduced fertility and a possible dominant lethal mutagenic effect. Male rats treated with Hexalen at 450 mg/m^2/day for 10 days had decreased spermatogenesis, atrophy of testes, seminal vesicles and ventral prostate.

Treatment of male rats with doses ≥60 mg/m^2/day for 60 days produced a marked increase in plasma glucose levels accompanied by morphological changes in pancreatic beta cells (vacuolisation).

Pharmaceutical particulars

List of excipients: Anhydrous lactose and calcium stearate.

Incompatibilities: No major incompatibilities are known.

Shelf life: 48 months.

Special precautions for storage: Hexalen capsules should be stored at a temperature not exceeding 25°C.

Procedures for the proper handling and disposal of anticancer drugs should be considered.

Packaging quantities: Hexalen 50 mg capsules are available in blister packs of 60 capsules. Each pack consists of six blister cards of ten capsules (6 × 10). The blister cards are packaged in a cardboard carton.

Name and address of holder of the marketing authorisation: US Bioscience Inc, Suites 9, 10 and 11, Awberry Court, Croxley Business Park, Watford, Hertfordshire WD1 8YJ.

Marketing authorisation number 11284/0001.

Date of approval/revision of SPC March 1998.

Legal category POM.

HYATE*:C

Presentation Hyate:C is a highly purified freeze-dried concentrate of porcine antihaemophilic factor (Porcine Factor VIII:C) for intravenous administration. Hyate:C is in the form of a white lyophilised powder for reconstitution with 20 ml Water for Injections PhEur per vial. Each vial contains between 400 and 700 units of Factor VIII:C. The assayed amount of activity is stated on the label.

Uses Hyate:C is intended for the treatment or prevention of bleeding in patients with inhibitory antibodies to human Factor VIII:C. These inhibitors may have developed as a complication of hereditary haemophilia or may have arisen spontaneously in previously non-haemophilic patients (Acquired haemophilia).

Hyate:C has not been known to transmit hepatitis or human immunodeficiency virus (1). It may therefore be justified to consider Hyate:C as a primary treatment option, particularly in patients with spontaneously acquired antibodies to human Factor VIII:C and no previous exposure to human blood products.

Dosage and administration The clinical efficiency of Hyate:C has been reported to be as good as that achieved with the administration of human Factor VIII:C in non-antibody patients for similar Factor VIII:C levels and similar bleeding episodes (2, 3). Therefore, the general objectives for treatment with Hyate:C for the prevention or control of bleeding, joint mobilisation, wound healing and surgical cover are essentially the same as those employed with the use of human Factor VIII:C concentrates.

The dosage of Hyate:C varies for individual patients, but is dependent upon the patient's weight, the level of circulating antibody, the type and severity of haemorrhage and the desired plasma Factor VIII:C level.

The required dose is determined by administering an initial dose of Hyate:C and assaying the post-infusion level of Factor VIII:C in the patient's plasma. According to the response, the dosage can then be either increased or decreased for subsequent infusions.

Initial Dose: An estimate of the dose of Hyate:C required for the initial infusion can be made in the following ways:

1. It is recommended that the patient's antibody titre against Porcine Factor VIII:C is determined using the Bethesda assay (4).

If the anti-Porcine Factor VIII:C level is less than 20 Bethesda units per ml an initial dose of 25 - 50 units/kg body weight is recommended for a mild to moderate joint or muscle bleed and 50 - 100 units/kg body weight for a severe bleed.

If the anti-Porcine Factor VIII:C inhibitor level is greater than 20 Bethesda units per ml a minimum initial dose of 100 units/kg body weight is suggested for all indications.

2. If the patient's antibody titre against Hyate:C is known, a prediction of the dose of Hyate:C required to neutralise the circulating antibody completely can be made using the formula:

Neutralising dose
= Plasma volume (ml) x antibody titre (Bethesda units/ml)

An incremental dose must then be added to this neutralising dose to increase plasma Factor VIII:C level by the desired amount. This increment can be calculated by assuming that 1 unit of Hyate:C per kg body weight will give rise to a 1.5 units/decilitre increase in plasma Factor VIII:C activity (2).

3. If the patient's antibody titre against Porcine Factor VIII:C is not known but the anti-human Factor VIII:C is less than 50 Bethesda units per ml, an initial dose of 25 - 50 units/kg body weight is recommended for a moderately severe joint or muscle bleed, or 50 - 100 units/kg body weight for a major bleed.

If the patient's antibody titre to human Factor VIII:C is greater than 50 Bethesda units per ml, an initial dose of at least 100 units/kg body weight is suggested (5).

4. If the patient has previously been treated with Hyate:C this may provide a guide to the likely response and therefore assist in estimation of the initial dose.

Subsequent Dose Administration: Subsequent doses should be based on the post-infusion levels of Factor VIII:C achieved. It has been reported that recovery of Factor VIII:C can increase during the course of treatment probably as a result of saturation of circulating antibody (2, 5). Monitoring of pre- and post-infusion levels of Factor VIII:C for each dose is therefore recommended.

If measurable post-infusion Factor VIII:C levels are not achieved Hyate:C therapy should still be continued as long as clinical efficacy is judged to be sufficient (6).

Frequency of Administration: Based upon the reported half-disappearance time for Hyate:C of 10 - 11 hours (5), it is recommended that the product is administered by intermittent intravenous infusion every 6 - 8 hours.

Determination of the Activity of Inhibitor Against Hyate:C: A modification of the Bethesda assay (4) is recommended. Hyate:C should be diluted to 1 unit per ml in Factor VIII depleted plasma and used as a substrate in the Bethesda assay.

Reconstitution and Administration: 1. Warm the unopened vials of Hyate:C to between 20°C and 37°C.

2. Clean the exposed central portion of the rubber stopper with antiseptic immediately prior to piercing.

3. Using a sterile needle and syringe slowly inject 20 ml of Water for Injections PhEur into the vial.

4. Withdraw the needle and shake the vial gently, avoiding frothing, until the powder is completely dissolved. This usually takes less than 1 minute.

5. The concentration of Hyate:C in units/ml should be calculated from the units/vial printed on the vial label.

6. Withdraw the solution into a syringe using a filter needle.

7. Replace the filter needle with a sterile injection needle and administer intravenously at a rate of not more than 2 - 5 ml per minute.

Contra-indications, warnings, etc

Contra-indications: Previous occurrence of an acute infusion reaction.

Acute Infusion Reactions: On rare occasions Hyate:C may give rise to acute infusion reactions, such as anaphylactic shock.

Adrenaline, hydrocortisone and facilities for resuscitation should be available in case these reactions occur.

Mild Infusion Reactions: Hyate:C may occasionally give rise to reactions such as fever, chills, headache, nausea, vomiting and skin rashes. These reactions are more common after the first infusion of a course of treatment, and tend to lessen in frequency and severity as further infusions are given. Hydrocortisone and/or antihistamine may alleviate these effects and may be prescribed as a precautionary measure.

Immune Response to Hyate:C: Infusion of Hyate:C may be followed by a rise in plasma levels of inhibitor to both human and Porcine Factor VIII:C. Inhibitor levels to both human and Porcine Factor VIII:C should be monitored during and after treatment.

Effect on the platelet count: A significant fall in the patient's platelet count occurs on rare occasions after infusion of Hyate:C. However, monitoring of platelet count during the treatment period is recommended.

Pharmaceutical precautions Hyate:C should be stored between a temperature of minus 15°C to minus 20°C and should be used before the expiry date on the package. Reconstituted Hyate:C must not be stored and should be used within 3 hours.

Legal category POM.

Package quantities Vials contain between 400 and 700 units of Porcine Factor VIII:C. The number of units in each vial is printed on the vial label.

Further information The ease of reconstitution of Hyate:C in 20 ml Water for Injections PhEur makes it suitable for syringe administration facilitating high dose therapy.

References:[1] Lusher J.M Annals N.Y Acad Sci 509:89-102, 1987

[2] Gatti L and Mannucci P.M Thromb and Haemostas 51:379-384, 1984

[3] Ciavarella N et al B.J Haematol 58:641-648, 1984

[4] Kasper C.K et al Thrombos Diathes Haemorrh 34:869-872, 1975

[5] Kernoff P.B.A et al Blood 63:31-41, 1984

[6] Brettler D.B et al Arch Intern Med 149:1381-1385, 1989

Product licence number 3070/0007

NEUTREXIN* ▼

Qualitative and quantitative composition

Active ingredient	*mg/vial*
Trimetrexate	25.0

Pharmaceutical form Concentrate for infusion.

Clinical particulars

Therapeutic indication: Neutrexin (trimetrexate glucuronate for injection) with concurrent leucovorin administration (leucovorin protection) is indicated as an alternative therapy for the treatment of moderate to severe *Pneumocystis carinii* pneumonia in patients with Acquired Immunodeficiency Syndrome (AIDS), who are intolerant of or refractory to standard therapy or for whom standard therapy is contra-indicated.

In comparative studies as first-line treatment of pneumocystis carinii pneumonia in AIDS patients. Neutrexin with concurrent leucovorin was less effective than trimethoprim/sulphamethoxazole. Comparative studies versus IV pentamidine have not yet been performed.

Caution: Leucovorin must be administered daily during treatment with Neutrexin and for 72 hours past the last dose of Neutrexin in order to avoid potentially serious or life threatening toxicities.

Posology and method of administration: Neutrexin is administered at a dose of 45 mg/m^2 once daily by intravenous infusion over 60–90 minutes. Leucovorin must be administered daily during treatment with Neutrexin and for 72 hours past the last dose of Neutrexin . Leucovorin may be administered intravenously at a dose of 20 mg/m^2 over 5 to 10 minutes every 6 hours for a total daily dose of 80 mg/m^2, or orally as 4 doses of 20 mg/m^2 spaced equally throughout the day. The recommended course of therapy is 21 days of Neutrexin and 24 days of leucovorin. Leucovorin protection may be administered prior to or following Neutrexin. The daily dosage of leucovorin has to be modified according to haematologic toxicities (see '*Dosage modifications*').

Efforts should be made by the physician to continue patients on Neutrexin plus concurrent leucovorin therapy for a minimum of 14 days before discontinuation for lack of response to allow sufficient time for patients to respond. Patients should continue to receive corticosteroid therapy, supplemental oxygen, intubation and mechanical ventilation or other supportive care as necessary throughout Neutrexin therapy. To allow for full therapeutic doses of Neutrexin to be administered, treatment with azidothymidine

Neutrexin/Leucovorin dose modifications for haematological toxicity

Toxicity grade	Neutrophils (Polys and Bands)	Platelets	Recommended dosage of Neutrexin	Recommended dosage of Leucovorin
1	>1000/mm^3	>75,000/mm^3	45 mg/m^2 once daily	20 mg/m^2 every 6 hours
2	750–1000/mm^3	50,000–75,000.mm^3	45 mg/m^2 once daily	40 mg/m^2 every 6 hours
3	500–749/mm^3	25,000–49,999/mm^3	22 mg/m^2 once daily	40 mg/m^2 every 6 hours
4	<500/mm^3	<25,000/mm^3	Day 1–9 Discontinue Day 10–21 Interrupt up to 96 hours[a]	40 mg/m^2 every 6 hours

[a] If Grade 4 haematologic toxicity occurs prior to Day 10, Neutrexin should be discontinued. Leucovorin (40 mg/m^2, q6h) should be administered for an additional 72 hours. If Grade 4 haematologic toxicity occurs at Day 10 or later, Neutrexin may be held up to 96 hours to allow counts to recover. If counts recover to Grade 3 within 96 hours, Neutrexin should be administered at a dose of 22 mg/m^2 and leucovorin maintained at 40 mg/m^2, q6h. When counts recover to Grade 2 toxicity, Neutrexin dose may be increased to 45 mg/m^2, but the leucovorin dose should be maintained at 40 mg/m^2 for the duration of treatment. If counts do not improve to ≤Grade 3 toxicity within 96 hours, Neutrexin should be discontinued. Leucovorin at a dose of 40 mg/m^2, q6h should be administered for 72 hours following the last dose of Neutrexin.

(AZT) and other myelosuppressive agents should be discontinued during Neutrexin therapy.

Hepatic or renal insufficiency: Patients should be treated with trimetrexate under careful monitoring conditions. Dose modifications should be based on toxicity guidelines described hereafter.

Dosage modification

Haematologic toxicity: Neutrexin and leucovorin doses should be modified for haematologic toxicities according to the table below. These guidelines were based upon empirical data from clinical trials utilizing initial doses of Neutrexin, 45 mg/m^2 per day and leucovorin, 20 mg/m^2, 4 times a day. Therapy should then continue with the adjusted dosage for the remainder of the patient's treatment.

Hepatic toxicity: Transient elevations of transaminases and alkaline phosphatase have been observed in patients treated with Neutrexin. Interruption of treatment is advisable if transaminase levels or alkaline phosphatase levels increase to >5 times the upper limit of normal range.

Renal toxicity: Interruption of treatment is advisable if serum creatinine levels increase to >2.5 mg/dL.

Other toxicities: Interruption of treatment is advisable in patients who experience severe mucosal toxicity which interferes with oral intake. Treatment should be discontinued for fever (oral temperature ≥105°F/ 40.5°C) that cannot be controlled with antipyretics.

Elderly: Dose modifications should be based on toxicity guidelines described above, rather than age.

Children: The safety and effectiveness of Neutrexin in children has not been established.

Contra-indications, warnings, etc

Contra-indications: Neutrexin is contra-indicated in patients with known sensitivity to trimetrexate or to other quinazoline-containing compounds. Neutrexin must not be used without concurrent leucovorin, therefore Neutrexin is contra-indicated in patients with known sensitivity to leucovorin. Due to Neutrexin's fetotoxic and teratogenic potential (see *'Use during pregnancy and lactation'*), it is contra-indicated during pregnancy.

Special warnings and precautions

Warnings: **Neutrexin must be used with concurrent leucovorin (leucovorin protection) to avoid potentially serious or life threatening complications including bone marrow suppression, oral and gastrointestinal mucosal ulceration, and renal and hepatic dysfunction. Leucovorin therapy must extend for 72 hours past the last dose of Neutrexin.** Patients should be informed that failure to take the recommended dose and duration of leucovorin can lead to fatal toxicity. Patients should be closely monitored for the development of serious haematologic adverse reactions (see *'Precautions'* and *'Posology and method of administration'*).

Neutrexin should only be prescribed by clinicians experienced in treating patients with AIDS or with immunocompromised states due to other underlying condition.

Both females of childbearing age and males should take contraceptive measures during and at least 6 months after cessation of therapy.

Anaphylaxis In cancer clinical trials, anaphylactoid reactions have been observed very rarely in patients receiving trimetrexate as an intravenous bolus injection. At present, it is not known whether any specific clinical condition or co-indications contributed to the occurrence of these reactions. Therefore, it is recommended that trimetrexate be administered as an intravenous infusion over 60–90 minutes.

Precautions: Patients receiving Neutrexin may experience severe haematologic, hepatic, renal and gastrointestinal toxicities; hence these parameters should be closely monitored in all patients. Special caution should be used in treating patients with impaired haematologic, hepatic or renal function. These patients and patients who require concomitant therapy with myelosuppressive, hepatotoxic or nephrotoxic drugs should be treated with Neutrexin under careful monitoring conditions.

Laboratory tests: Patients receiving Neutrexin with leucovorin protection should be closely monitored throughout therapy. Blood tests to monitor the following parameters should be performed at least twice a week during therapy: haematology (absolute neutrophil counts [ANC], platelets, haemoglobin), renal function (serum creatinine, BUN), hepatic function (SGOT, SGPT, alkaline phosphatase). In addition, haemoglobin levels should be monitored before, during and after therapy as anaemia may develop in some patients.

Drug interactions: The metabolism of trimetrexate both with and without the administration of folinic acid is poorly understood. There is therefore a significant potential for serious drug-drug interactions over a wide range of potential therapeutic agents. This is particularly the case for agents which may utilise, inhibit or induce hepatic cytochrome P450 mechanisms. Such agents may also affect the ratio of trimetrexate to folinic acid in individual tissue subsets. Thus, when ANY comedication is considered mandatory, additional care in monitoring of adverse events, hemopoietic and hepatic toxicities is advised. Agents which may enhance the liver clearance of trimetrexate may also result in diminished efficacy of the trimetrexate-folonic acid combination.

Trimetrexate and its metabolites are partially cleared renally, therefore nephrotoxic agents may also interact with trimetrexate when co-administered. Drugs which may affect protein binding may also affect the pharmacodynamics of trimetrexate and vice versa (see 'Preclinical safety data').

Experience with concomitant corticosteroids and trimetrexate-folinic acid administration has been obtained only in open clinical studies. In these there was no obvious interference with the efficacy of the combination regimen and little or no detectable potentiation of the described toxicities. It is therefore considered that steroids may be co-prescribed in accordance with clinical practice.

Use during pregnancy and lactation: The safe use of Neutrexin during pregnancy has not been established. Neutrexin has been shown to be fetotoxic and teratogenic in animals (see 'Preclinical safety data' section); it is therefore contra-indicated during pregnancy.

When Neutrexin is considered to be therapeutically necessary in women of child bearing potential, appropriate procedures should be followed to establish whether pregnancy might have occurred. The patient should be appraised of the risks of becoming pregnant during treatment and take adequate contraceptive measures (see 'Special warnings and precautions' section). Men who are treated with Neutrexin should also take contraceptive measures during treatment and for a period of six months after completing therapy.

It is not known if trimetrexate is secreted in human breast milk. Because there is a possibility of toxicity to nursing infants secondary to Neutrexin treatment of the mother, it is recommended that breast feeding should be terminated and artificial feeding substituted if the mother is treated with Neutrexin.

Effects on ability to drive and use machines: Unless the patient develops severe toxicity (see *'Undesirable effects'*), Neutrexin itself, should not impair the patient's ability to drive or operate machinery; this is more likely to be influenced by the patient's overall state of well being.

Undesirable effects: As many patients who receive Neutrexin already have complications of advanced HIV disease, it is difficult to distinguish adverse events caused by Neutrexin from those resulting from underlying medical conditions. The toxicities reported hereafter refer to patients with morphologically confirmed PCP who received Neutrexin, 45 mg/m^2 per day for 21 days and leucovorin, 80 mg/m^2 per day for 24 days (n=182). These clinical trials included dose modifications to the Neutrexin-Leucovorin combination for toxicity as described under *'Posology and method of administration'*. These toxicities were similar in frequency and severity to the combined analysis of all patients treated in clinical studies.

Haematological: The most frequently reported abnormal haematological parameters have been low granulocytes, haemoglobin and platelets. In clinical trials, these effects were classed as severe in approximately 15%, 9% and 3% of patients respectively. However following dose modifications outlined under 'Posology and method of administration', less than 4% of patients had to discontinue Neutrexin therapy due to haematologic toxicity.

Gastrointestinal: Emesis and diarrhoea have been reported in 3.8% and 1.6% of patients, occasionally resulting in withdrawal of therapy.

Cutaneous: The most common cutaneous reaction reported is rash which occurs in approximately 8% of patients; itching and injection site reaction have been reported rarely.

Fever: In clinical trials, this was reported in approximately 11% of patients, but in only 1% of patients was it of sufficient severity to warrant withdrawal of therapy.

Neurologic: Confusion was reported in 3% of patients. Seizure has rarely been reported; a causal relationship between seizure and trimetrexate has not been established.

Hepatic toxicity: Transiently raised transaminases (SGOT and SGPT) and alkaline phosphatase have been reported; in 14%, 13% and 5% of patients respectively.

Laboratory abnormalities: These have rarely been reported, and have included increased and decreased calcium and potassium, magnesium and GGT levels. No clinical signs of hypocalcaemia have been reported.

Anaphylaxis: Anaphylactoid reactions have been observed very rarely (see under *Warnings*).

Overdose: Neutrexin administered without concurrent leucovorin can cause lethal complications. There has been little experience in humans receiving single intravenous doses of trimetrexate greater than 90 mg/m^2/day without concurrent leucovorin. The toxicities seen at this dose were primarily haematologic. In the event of overdose, Neutrexin should be stopped and leucovorin should be administered at a dose of 40 mg/m^2 every 6 hours for 3 days.

Pharmacological properties

Pharmacodynamic properties: In vitro studies have shown that trimetrexate is a potent, competitive inhibitor of dihydrofolate reductase (DHFR) from bacterial, protozoan and mammalian sources, including *Pneumocystis carinii.* DHFR catalyzes the reduction of intracellular dihydrofolate to the active cofactor tetrahydrofolate. Inhibition of DHFR results in the depletion of this cofactor, leading directly to interference with thymidylate biosynthesis, as well as interference with folate-dependent formyltransferase, with consequent reduction in purine biosynthesis. The end result is disruption of DNA, RNA and protein synthesis, with consequent cell death.

Leucovorin (folinic acid) is readily transported into mammalian cells by a carrier-mediated active transport process and can be assimilated into cellular folate pools following its metabolism. In vitro studies have shown that leucovorin provides a source of reduced folates necessary for normal cellular biosynthetic processes. Because the *Pneumocystis carinii* organism lacks the reduced folate carrier-mediated transport system, leucovorin is prevented from entering the organism. Therefore, the concurrent administration of leucovorin with trimetrexate protects normal host cells from the cytotoxic effect of trimetrexate without impairing the antifolate's inhibition of *Pneumocystis carinii.* The active transport of leucovorin into mammalian cells but not into the *Pneumocystis carinii* organism allows the concurrent use of leucovorin to protect normal host cells from the cytotoxicity of trimetrexate without inhibiting the antifolate's inhibition of *Pneumocystis carinii.*

Pharmacokinetic properties

Absorption: No detailed kinetic studies have been performed in patients with AIDS utilising the advised regimen administered by infusion. However, steady-state peak and trough levels were measured in patients administered 30 mg/m^2/day by i.v. bolus with leucovorin 80 mg/m^2/day (given in 4 equally divided doses). In these subjects the mean 'peak' 1 hour post-dosing level of trimetrexate, using an in-vitro DHFR inhibition assay, was 11.8±6.0 μM. Similarly, the mean 23 hour trough level was 1.9±1.4 μM. In 6 of these patients a terminal half-life in the order of 11 h was observed. More extensive data are available on cancer patients receiving 10–20 hours. Furthermore despite a marked inter-individual variation in pharmacokinetic characteristics a linear relationship between dose and trimetrexate steady state plasma level/AUC was suggested.

Distribution: Binding of trimetrexate to plasma proteins is extensive (>97%). The concentration of trimetrexate in the cerebrospinal fluid accounted for less than 2% of the plasma level.

Metabolism: The metabolism of trimetrexate in man with or without the coadministration of leucovorin has not yet been completely elucidated. Preclinical data suggest that oxidative O-demethylation, followed by conjugation to either the glucuronide or the sulphate is involved. It appears that N-demethylation and oxidation is a related minor pathway. The exact P450 enzyme catalysing O-demethylation is unknown. Some of the metabolites formed are active in the in vitro cell-free DHFR inhibition assay. Whether these metabolites are also active against *Pneumocystis carinii* infection was not examined. The active metabolites may however contribute to trimetrexate's cytotoxic effects towards host cells.

Elimination: Urinary recovery of trimetrexate using an HPLC assay averaged about 10–20% of the dose, over a 24–48 hour period. Part of the trimetrexate metabolites formed, including part of the metabolites that are active in the DHFR-inhibition assay, are renally excreted. Faecal excretion of trimetrexate and its active metabolites appears to be low. To date, the fate of 50% of a trimetrexate dose administered to man remains unknown. Although the low urinary recovery of trimetrexate suggests that clearance is predominantly non-renal, significant retention of trimetrexate may occur in patients with impaired renal function.

No formal studies have evaluated the kinetic behaviour of trimetrexate in patients with renal or hepatic impairment. These patients should be closely monitored.

Preclinical safety data

Drug interactions: Animal studies suggest that there is a potential for serious drug interactions in man when trimetrexate-folinic acid are prescribed with drugs of the imidazol class (clotrimazole, ketoconazole, micronazole). See *Pharmacodynamic properties* for further details.

Carcinogenesis and mutagenicity: Negative results have been observed for trimetrexate in gene mutation systems with bacterial and mammalian cells. Other systems, however, have shown that trimetrexate induces very efficient chromosomal damage, a type of genetic damage which could be expected from the mechanism of action of trimetrexate. Although trimetrexate showed no genotoxic or carcinogenic effects in the limited test procedures utilised in vivo, the compound should be considered as possibly mutagenic and carcinogenic in vivo.

Impairment of fertility: No studies have been conducted to evaluate the potential of trimetrexate to impair fertility. However, during standard toxicity studies conducted in mice and rats, degeneration of the testes and spermatocytes including the arrest of spermatogenesis was observed. Therefore, the potential for distribution in male fertility cannot be excluded. As the ova are formed long before ovulation, it is possible that the level of fertility in females will not be affected, but other early stages after fertilisation will be at risk because of the inhibition of DHFR.

Teratogenic effects: Maternal and foetal toxicity were observed in both rats and rabbits. Rats administered 1.5 and 2.5 mg/kg/day intravenously on gestational days 6–15 showed substantial post-implantation loss and severe inhibition of maternal weight gain. Trimetrexate administered intravenously to rats at 0.5 and 1.0 mg/kg/day on gestational days 6–15 retarded normal fetal development and was teratogenic. Rabbits administered trimetrexate intravenously at daily doses of 2.5 and 5.0 mg/kg/day on gestational days 6–15 resulted in significant maternal and fetotoxicity. In rabbits, trimetrexate at 0.1 mg/kg/day was teratogenic in the absence of significant maternal toxicity. These effects were observed using doses $\frac{1}{20}$ to $\frac{1}{2}$ the equivalent human therapeutic dose based on a mg/m² basis. Teratogenic effects included skeletal, visceral, ocular and cardiovascular abnormalities.

Drug interactions: Based on an in vitro rat liver model, nitrogen substituted imidazole drugs (clotrimazole, ketoconazole, miconazole) were potent, non-competitive inhibitors of trimetrexate metabolism. A number of agents might be co-administered with trimetrexate in AIDS patients for other indications that could elicit this activity including erythromycin, rifampicin, ketoconazole, fluconazole and others.

Pharmaceutical particulars

List of excipients: D-glucuronic acid 15.35 mg per vial.

Incompatibilities: **Caution: Since Neutrexin forms a precipitate instantly upon contact with chloride or Leucovorin, it should not be added to solutions containing sodium chloride or other anions. Neutrexin and Leucovorin solutions must be administered separately. Intravenous lines should be flushed with at least 10 mL of 5% Glucose Injection BP, between Neutrexin and Leucovorin infusions.**

Compatibility with other anions: In a study to determine the potential for precipitation of Neutrexin upon contact with other anions, Neutrexin 2 mg/ml solution in sterile water at ambient temperature for 24 hours precipitated a 1% solution of bicarbonate but did NOT form a precipitate with acetate, lactose or phosphate. However, Neutrexin at a higher concentration of 6.25 mg/ml caused precipitation with all four anions studied.

Shelf-life: 24 months for the product as packaged for sale.

After reconstitution, the solution should be used immediately; however, the solution is stable under refrigeration (2–8°C) for 24 hours or at room temperature (15°C–25°C) for up to six hours. [NOTE: This is justified based on acceptable challenge test after incubation with various test organisms.] It must be assumed that like any parenteral product, Neutrexin will be reconstituted aseptically.

Special precautions for storage: Neutrexin should be stored at room temperature (15–25°C).

Nature and contents of container: Neutrexin is contained in a 5 cc Type I flint glass tubing vial, fitted with a grey rubber stopper and sealed with an aluminium seal, covered with a white polypropylene flip off cap. Each vial of lyophilized powder contains trimetrexate glucuronate equivalent to 25 mg of trimetrexate.

Vials will be supplied in nested white chipboard cartons, shrink wrapped and placed in brown corrugated cartons, in quantities of 10, 25, 50 and 100.

N.B. Only the 25 vial pack presentation will be available in the UK.

Instructions for use/handling: Neutrexin should be reconstituted with 2 ml of 5% Glucose Injection BP or Sterile Water for Injection PhEur to yield a concentration of 12.5 mg of trimetrexate per ml (reconstitution time up to two minutes). The reconstituted product must be inspected visually for particulate matter prior to dilution. Do not use if cloudiness or precipitate is observed.

Reconstituted solution should be further diluted with 5% Glucose Injection BP to yield a final concentration of 0.25 to 2 mg of trimetrexate per ml.

Do not freeze reconstituted solution. Discard the unused portion after 24 hours.

If Neutrexin contacts the skin or mucosa, immediately wash thoroughly with soap and water. Procedures for the proper handling and disposal of cytotoxic drugs should be considered.

Name and address of holder of marketing authorisation: US Bioscience Inc, Suites 9, 10 and 11, Awberry Court, Croxley Business Park, Watford, Hertfordshire WD1 8YJ.

Marketing authorisation number 11284/0006.

Date of approval/revision of SPC March 1998.

Legal category POM.

PHOTOFRIN* 15 ▼

Qualitative and quantitative composition Each vial of Photofrin 15 contains 15 mg of porfimer sodium.

Pharmaceutical form Powder for solution for injection.

Clinical particulars

Therapeutic indications: Photodynamic therapy (PDT) with Photofrin is indicated for:

- palliative treatment of obstructing endobronchial nonsmall cell lung cancer;
- palliative treatment of obstructing oesophageal cancer.

Posology and method of administration: Photodynamic therapy (PDT) with Photofrin is a two-stage process requiring administration of both drug and light. Physicians should be trained in the use of photodynamic therapy. The first stage of PDT is the intravenous injection of Photofrin at a dose of 2 mg/kg. The second stage of therapy is illumination with laser light 40–50 hours following injection with Photofrin. Patients may receive a second laser light application 96–120 hours after drug administration. Therefore, one course of PDT consists of one injection plus one or two light applications. Up to 2 more courses of drug and light may be given, with each injection separated by a minimum of 30 days.

Photofrin administration: Photofrin should be reconstituted according to the directions given in instructions for use/handling, and administered as a single slow intravenous injection over 3 to 5 minutes at 2 mg/kg body weight. As with all intravenous injections, care should be taken to prevent extravasation at the injection site. If extravasation does occur, the area should be protected from light for a minimum of 30 days. There is no known benefit from injecting the extravasation site with another substance.

Photoactivation of Photofrin: Photofrin is activated by light in the spectral region of 630 nm. Approximately 40–50 hours after Photofrin administration, laser light should be delivered to the tumour by a cylindrical fibre optic diffuser or a microlens fibre optic passed through the operating channel of an endoscope/bronchoscope.

Light doses: Photoactivation of Photofrin is controlled by the total light energy (light dose) delivered to the tumour site and depends on the indication and the means of light delivery, as follows:

- For endobronchial tumours, the cylindrical diffuser will be suitable for most tumours. The light dose for endobronchial tumours using the cylindrical diffuser is 200 joules/cm of tumour length. Alternatively, the microlens fibre optic may be appropriate for small, flat, non-circumferential tumours. The light dose using the microlens fibre optic is 100 joules/cm².
- For oesophageal tumours, a light dose of 300 joules/cm of tumour length should be delivered using a cylindrical diffuser.

Cylindrical Diffuser (Endobronchial or Oesophageal Lesions): The cylindrical diffuser uniformly distributes laser light radially in a cylindrical pattern over the entire length of the fibre optic tip. The following light dosimetry equation applies.

$$\text{Light dose (J/cm)} = \frac{\text{Total power output from diffuser (W)} \times \text{Treatment time (seconds)}}{\text{Diffuser length (cm)}}$$

For example, the total power output from the diffuser, as measured by a suitable integrating sphere power meter, could be set to [400 mW/cm x length of diffuser in cm] which will deliver the appropriate dose using exposure times of either 8 minutes, 20 seconds (endobronchial tumours, 200 J/cm) or 12 minutes, 30 seconds (oesophageal tumours, 300 J/cm).

Cylindrical diffusers are available in several lengths and the diffuser tip length should be chosen to match the length of the tumour. Tumours with lengths that differ from available diffuser lengths may require multiple use of a single diffuser or the use of two or more diffusers of differing lengths. Diffuser length should be sized to avoid exposure of non-malignant tissue to light and to prevent overlapping of previously treated malignant tissue. Diffusers or combinations of diffusers should be selected to minimise patient treatment time.

The cylindrical diffusers may be used either interstitially or intraluminally. For non-circumferential endobronchial tumours that are soft enough to penetrate, interstitial fibre placement is preferred to intraluminal activation, since this method produces better efficacy and results in less exposure of normal bronchial mucosa to the light. When the interstitial technique is used, up to 90% of the length of the diffuser should be inserted into the tumour mass.

Microlens (Endobronchial lesions only): The microlens fibre optic delivers a diverging, forward-directed beam of light similar to that produced by a torch. It is used to treat small lesions by positioning the microlens tip so that the lesion is uniformly illuminated by a circular spot. The diameter of the spot can be increased or decreased by moving the microlens tip further from or nearer to the lesion. The following light dosimetry equation applies:

$$\text{Light dose (J/cm2)} = \frac{\text{Total power output at fibre tip (W)} \times \text{Treatment time (seconds)}}{\text{Treatment area (cm2)}}$$

For example, the power output at the microlens fibre tip, as measured by a power meter, could be set to [200 mW/cm² x tumour area in cm²]. This will deliver the dose of 100 J/cm² of tumour using an exposure time of 8 minutes, 20 seconds per area treated.

Debridement and retreatment: In patients with endobronchial tumours, debridement is mandatory to remove necrotic tumour debris and clear secretions or mucous plugs, thereby preventing possible dyspnoea, obstruction, atelectasis and infection. For oesophageal cancer, debridement is optional since the residua will be removed naturally by peristaltic action. Debridement of residua should be performed 2 days after light treatment. Patients with residual tumour may be retreated with laser light at the time of debridement at the same dose as used for the initial treatment. The second light dose should be administered 96 to 120 hours after the Photofrin injection.

Patients may receive a second course of PDT a minimum of 30 days after the initial therapy; up to three courses of PDT (each injection separated by a minimum of 30 days) can be given. Before each course of treatment, patients should be evaluated for the presence of a tracheo-oesophageal or broncho-oesophageal fistula or for the possibility that the tumour may be eroding into a major blood vessel (see Contraindications).

Use in children: Safety and effectiveness in children

have not been established. Photofrin should not be used in children until further data are available.

Use in elderly patients: Approximately 70% of the patients treated with PDT using Photofrin in clinical trials were over 60 years of age. There was no apparent difference in effectiveness or safety in these patients compared to younger people. Dose modification based upon age is not required.

Use in patients with impaired hepatic or renal function: The influence of impaired hepatic function on Photofrin disposition has not been evaluated. No special precautions are necessary in patients with renal impairment because excretion is primarily via the faecal route.

Contra-indications: PDT with Photofrin is contraindicated in patients with porphyria or in patients with known hypersensitivity to porphyrins.

PDT with Photofrin is contraindicated in patients with severe hepatic impairment.

PDT is contraindicated in patients with tracheo-oesophageal or broncho-oesophageal fistula.

PDT is contraindicated in patients with suspected erosion of major blood vessels due to risk of massive, potentially fatal haemorrhage.

PDT is not suitable for emergency treatment of patients with severe acute respiratory distress caused by an obstructing endobronchial lesion because 40 to 50 hours are required between injection with Photofrin and laser light treatment.

Special warnings and precautions for use: Photodynamic therapy with Photofrin should be used only in clinics or centres with experience of endoscopic laser procedures.

All patients who receive Photofrin will be photosensitive and must observe precautions to avoid exposure of skin and eyes to direct sunlight or bright indoor light (from examination lamps, including dental lamps, operating room lamps, unshaded light bulbs at close proximity, etc.) for 30 days. The photosensitivity is due to residual drug which will be present in all parts of the skin. Exposure of the skin to ambient indoor light is, however, beneficial because the remaining drug will be inactivated gradually and safely through a photobleaching reaction. Therefore, patients should not stay in a darkened room during this period and should be encouraged to expose their skin to ambient indoor light. The level of photosensitivity will vary for different areas of the body, depending on the extent of previous exposure to light. Before exposing any area of skin to direct sunlight or bright indoor light, the patient should test it for residual photosensitivity. A small area of skin should be exposed to sunlight for 10 minutes. If no photosensitivity reaction (erythema, oedema, blistering) occurs within 24 hours, the patient can gradually resume normal outdoor activities, initially continuing to exercise caution and gradually allowing increased exposure. If some photosensitivity reaction occurs with the limited skin test, the patient should continue precautions for another 2 weeks before retesting. The tissue around the eyes may be more sensitive, and therefore, it is not recommended that the face be used for testing. If patients travel to a different geographical area with greater sunshine, they should retest their level of photosensitivity. **UV (ultraviolet) sunscreens are of no value in protecting against photosensitivity reactions because photoactivation is caused by visible light.**

As the result of PDT treatment, patients may complain of substernal chest pain because of inflammatory responses within the area of treatment. Such pain may be of sufficient intensity to warrant the short-term prescription of opiate analgesics.

If PDT is to be used before or after radiotherapy, sufficient time should be allowed between the therapies to ensure that the inflammatory reaction produced by the first treatment has subsided prior to commencement of the second treatment.

As Photofrin is a biological material, possibility of acute hypersensitivity reaction including anaphylaxis cannot be ruled out (see undersirable effects). In case of allergic reaction, treatment should be stopped immediately and appropriate emergency measures initiated.

Oesophageal cancer: If the oesophageal tumour is eroding into the trachea or bronchial tree, the likelihood of tracheo-oesophageal or broncho-oesophageal fistula resulting from treatment is sufficiently high that PDT is not recommended.

Patients with oesophageal varices should be treated with extreme caution. Light should not be given directly to the variceal area because of the high risk of bleeding.

Lung cancer: If the endobronchial tumour invades deeply into the bronchial wall, the possibility exists for fistula formation upon resolution of tumour.

PDT should be used with extreme caution for endobronchial tumours in locations where treatment-induced inflammation could obstruct the main airway, e.g., long or circumferential tumours of the trachea, tumours of the main carina that involve both mainstem bronchi circumferentially, or circumferential tumours in the remaining mainstem bronchus of patients with prior pneumonectomy.

Patients with endobronchial lesions must be closely monitored between the laser light therapy and the mandatory debridement bronchoscopy for any evidence of respiratory distress (see posology and method of administration). Inflammation and mucositis may result from exposure of normal tissue to too much light. Necrotic debris may also obstruct the airway. If respiratory distress occurs, the physician should be prepared to carry out immediate bronchoscopy to remove secretions and debris to open the airway.

Interaction with other medicaments and other forms of interaction: There have been no formal interaction studies of Photofrin and any other drugs. However, it is possible that concomitant use of other photosensitising agents (e.g., tetracyclines, sulphonamides, phenothiazines, sulphonylurea hypoglycaemic agents, thiazide diuretics, and griseofulvin) could increase the photosensitivity reaction.

Photofrin PDT causes direct intracellular damage by initiating radical chain reactions that damage intracellular membranes and mitochondria. Tissue damage also results from ischaemia secondary to vasoconstriction, platelet activation and aggregation and clotting. Research in animals and in cell culture has suggested that many drugs could influence the effects of PDT, possible examples of which are described below. There are no human data that support or rebut these possibilities.

Compounds that quench active oxygen species or scavenge radicals, such as dimethyl sulphoxide, b-carotene, ethanol, formate and mannitol would be expected to decrease PDT activity. Preclinical data also suggest that tissue ischaemia, allopurinol, calcium channel blockers and some prostaglandin synthesis inhibitors could interfere with Photofrin PDT. Drugs that decrease clotting, vasoconstriction or platelet aggregation, e.g., thromboxane A_2 inhibitors, could decrease the efficacy of PDT. Glucocorticoid hormones given before or concomitant with PDT may decrease the efficacy of the treatment.

Pregnancy and lactation: Photofrin was not teratogenic in rats or rabbits at doses comparable to those used in clinical situations. Foetotoxicity was observed only at maternally toxic doses. There are no adequate and well-controlled studies in pregnant women. Women of childbearing potential should practice an effective method of contraception during therapy. Photofrin may be used during pregnancy only if the potential benefit outweighs the potential risk to the foetus.

It is not known whether this drug is excreted in human milk. Therefore, women receiving Photofrin must not breast feed.

Effects on ability to drive and use machines: Photofrin causes no adverse effects that could impair the patient's ability to drive or use machines

Undesirable effects: Systemically induced effects associated with PDT with Photofrin consist of photosensitivity and mild constipation. All patients who receive Photofrin will be photosensitive and must observe precautions to avoid sunlight and bright indoor light (see special warnings and special precautions for use). Photosensitivity reactions consist mainly of mild erythema on the face and hands.

Most toxicities associated with this therapy are local effects seen in the region of illumination and occasionally in surrounding tissues. The local adverse reactions are characteristic of an inflammatory response induced by the photodynamic effect.

No cases of anaphylaxis have been reported although occasionally rashes have been observed.

Endobronchial cancer: Adverse events reported in 5% or more of patients (n=99) with obstructing endobronchial nonsmall cell lung cancer were most commonly associated with the respiratory system; their relationship to therapy is unclear: dyspnoea (32%), nonfatal haemoptysis (12%), coughing (17%), pneumonia (13%), bronchitis (11%), fatal massive haemoptysis (10%), increased sputum (9%) and respiratory insufficiency (7%). Other frequent events were photosensitivity reaction (20%), fever (15%), chest pain (9%), insomnia (7%), anxiety (5%) and constipation (5%). Inflammatory reactions manifested as fever, bronchitis and chest pain. Coughing, dyspnoea, haemoptysis and increased sputum, while reported as adverse events, are also symptoms of the disease. Fatal massive haemoptysis, with or without prior radiotherapy, has been observed with greater frequency in the PDT-treated group. In half of the patients with fatal haemoptysis, the event occurred more than 30 days after the last treatment procedure and was judged by the investigator to be unrelated to PDT. Fatal massive haemoptysis may be due to disease progression or due to resolution of tumour eroding into a major blood vessel (see contraindications).

Serious and other notable adverse events observed in less than 5% of PDT-treated patients with endobronchial cancer included pleural effusion, pulmonary thrombosis, pulmonary embolism and lung abscess. Their relationship to therapy is uncertain.

Oesophageal cancer: The following adverse events were reported in at least 5% of patients (n=127) with partially or completely obstructing oesophageal cancer; the relationship of many of these events to PDT is uncertain.

Gastrointestinal: constipation (23%), nausea (21%), abdominal pain (18%), vomiting (16%), dysphagia (9%), haematemesis (9%), diarrhoea (7%), oesophageal oedema (6%), oesophageal stricture (6%), oesophageal tumour bleeding (6%), dyspepsia (6%).

Respiratory: pleural effusion (28%), pneumonia (17%), dyspnoea (17%), respiratory insufficiency (11%), pharyngitis (10%), tracheo-oesophageal fistula (9%).

Cardiovascular: atrial fibrillation (8%), tachycardia (6%), cardiac failure (6%).

Other: fever (32%), anaemia (25%), chest pain (24%), pain (23%), photosensitivity reaction (19%), insomnia (14%), urinary tract infection (8%), moniliasis (8%), back pain (8%) dehydration (6%), generalised oedema (6%), peripheral oedema (6%), hypotension (6%), hypertension (6%), sepsis (6%), anorexia (6%), weight decrease (6%), confusion (6%), asthenia (5%).

These effects were generally mild or moderate in severity and easily managed. Anaemia was not due to myelosuppression, but rather it was due to tumour bleeding and was more common in patients with large tumours (>10 cm) and with tumours in the lower third of the oesophagus. Tumour bleeding may be exacerbated by vigorous debridement. Debridement is optional in patients with oesophageal cancer (see posology and method of administration). The syndrome of respiratory insufficiency included one patient who experienced upper airway oedema (1%) and one who experienced bronchospasm during debridement (1%); the remaining events (8%) did not appear to be related to PDT. Fever and pleural effusion, as well as pain, oesophageal oedema and atrial fibrillation are thought to be manifestations of a local/regional inflammatory reaction. Oesophageal oedema occurred more frequently when the tumour was located in the upper third of the oesophagus; atrial fibrillation was more likely to occur when the tumour was in the middle third of the oesophagus.

Serious and other notable adverse events observed in less than 5% of patients include the following; their relationship to therapy is uncertain. In the gastrointestinal system, oesophagitis, oesophageal perforation, gastric ulcer, ileus, jaundice, and peritonitis have occurred. Cardiovascular events have included angina pectoris, bradycardia, myocardial infarction, sick sinus syndrome, and supraventricular tachycardia. Respiratory events of bronchitis, pneumonitis, pulmonary haemorrhage, pulmonary oedema, respiratory failure, and stridor have occurred. Vision-related events of abnormal vision, diplopia, eye pain and photophobia have been reported.

Overdose:

Overdose of Photofrin: There is no information on overdosage situations involving Photofrin. Higher than recommended drug doses of two 2 mg/kg doses given two days apart (10 patients) and three 2 mg/kg doses given within two weeks (1 patient) were tolerated without notable adverse reactions. Effects of overdosage on the duration of photosensitivity are unknown. Laser treatment should not be given if an overdose of Photofrin is administered. In the event of an overdose, patients should protect their eyes and skin from direct sunlight or bright indoor lights for 30 days. At this time, patients should test for residual photosensitivity (see special warnings and special precautions for use). Photofrin is not dialysable.

Overdose of laser light following Photofrin: Light doses of two to three times the recommended dose have been administered to a few patients with superficial endobronchial tumours. One patient experienced life-threatening dyspnoea and the others had no notable complications. Increased symptoms and damage to normal tissue might be expected following an overdose of light.

Pharmacological properties

Pharmacodynamic properties: The cytotoxic and antitumour actions of Photofrin (ATC code L01X X15) are light and oxygen-dependent. Photodynamic therapy (PDT) with Photofrin is a 2-stage process. The first stage is the intravenous injection of Photofrin. Clearance from a variety of tissues occurs over 40-72 hours, but tumours, skin, and organs of the reticuloendothelial system (including liver and spleen) retain Photofrin for a longer period. Illumination with 630 nm wavelength laser light constitutes the second stage of therapy. Tumour selectivity in treatment occurs through a combination of selective retention of Photofrin and selective delivery of light. Cellular damage caused by Photofrin PDT is a consequence of the propagation of free radical reactions. Radical initiation may occur after Photofrin absorbs light to form a porphyrin excited state. Spin transfer from Photofrin to molecular oxygen may then generate singlet oxygen. Subsequent free radical reactions can form superoxide and hydroxyl radicals. Tumour death also occurs through ischaemic necrosis secondary to vascular occlusion that appears to be partly mediated by thromboxane A_2 release. The laser treatment induces a photochemical, not a thermal, effect. The necrotic reaction and associated inflammatory response evolve over several days.

Pharmacokinetic properties:

General characteristics: A pharmacokinetic study was conducted in 12 endobronchial cancer patients given 2 mg/kg of Photofrin intravenously. Samples of plasma were obtained out to 56 days (1,344 hours) post injection and total porphyrin units determined. The mean peak plasma concentration (C_{max}) immediately following injection was 79.6 µg/ml (C.V. 61%, range 39-222); the mean $T_{1/2}$ was 515 hours, i.e. 21.5 days (C.V. 26%, range 264-672). Thus, porfimer sodium is cleared slowly from the body, with a mean CL_T of 0.859 mL/h/kg (C.V. 53%).

In vitro binding of Photofrin to human serum protein is around 90% and independent of concentration between 20 and 100 µg/mL. Preclinical studies indicate that the excretion of Photofrin components occurs primarily via the faecal route.

Characteristics in patients: No special precautions in renally impaired patients are necessary because excretion is primarily via the faecal route.

The influence of impaired hepatic function on Photofrin disposition has not been evaluated.

Preclinical safety data: In vitro, Photofrin PDT did not cause mutations in the Ames test, nor did it cause chromosome aberrations or mutations (HGPRT locus) in Chinese hamster ovary (CHO) cells. Photofrin caused <2-fold, but significant, increases in sister chromatid exchange in CHO cells irradiated with visible light and a 3-fold increase in Chinese hamster lung fibroblasts irradiated with near UV light. Photofrin PDT caused an increase in thymidine kinase mutants and DNA-protein cross-links in mouse L5178Y cells, but not mouse LYR83 cells. Photofrin PDT caused a light-dose dependent increase in DNA-strand breaks in malignant human cervical carcinoma cells, but not in normal cells. *In vivo,* Photofrin did not cause chromosomal aberrations in the mouse micronucleus test. Therefore, the overall mutagenic potential of Photofrin is considered minimal.

Pharmaceutical particulars

List of excipients: Hydrochloric acid and/or sodium hydroxide may be added during manufacture to adjust pH. The product contains no other excipients or antimicrobial preservatives.

Incompatibilities: Reconstitute Photofrin with 5% glucose intravenous as described under instructions for use/handling. Do not use other diluents. Do not mix Photofrin with other drugs in the same solution.

Shelf life: 36 months.

Special precautions for storage: Do not store above 25°C. Keep container in the outer carton.

After reconstitution, use immediately (within 3 hours). Protect from light following reconstitution.

Nature and contents of container: Vial: Flint, type I glass, treated, 7 mL capacity.

Closure: Grey butyl stopper.

Vial contents: A dark red to reddish brown lyophilised powder (or cake) for reconstitution.

Pack size: 1 vial.

Instructions for use/handling: Photofrin 15 should be reconstituted with 6.6 mL of 5% glucose intravenous infusion, resulting in a final concentration of 2.5 mg/mL. Do not use other diluents. Do not mix Photofrin with other drugs in the same solution. Sufficient vials of Photofrin should be reconstituted to provide the patient with a dose of 2 mg/kg using the calculation below. For most patients (up to 75 kg) two vials of Photofrin 75 (M.A. No.: PL 05980/0018) will suffice. Each Photofrin 15 vial will treat an additional 7.5 kg of body weight.

$$\text{Photofrin (mL)} = \frac{\text{Patient's weight (kg)} \times 2\text{ mg/kg}}{2.5\text{ mg/mL}} = 0.8 \times \text{Patient's weight}$$

Marketing authorisation number 05980/0017

Date of approval/revision of SPC December 1998.

Legal category POM.

PHOTOFRIN* 75 ▼

Qualitative and quantitative composition Each vial of Photofrin 75 contains 75 mg of porfimer sodium.

Pharmaceutical form Powder for Solution for Injection.

Clinical particulars

Therapeutic indications: Photodynamic therapy (PDT) with Photofrin is indicated for:

- palliative treatment of obstructing endobronchial nonsmall cell lung cancer;
- palliative treatment of obstructing oesophageal cancer.

Posology and method of administration: Photodynamic therapy (PDT) with Photofrin is a two-stage process requiring administration of both drug and light. Physicians should be trained in the use of photodynamic therapy. The first stage of PDT is the intravenous injection of Photofrin at a dose of 2 mg/kg. The second stage of therapy is illumination with laser light 40–50 hours following injection with Photofrin. Patients may receive a second laser light application 96–120 hours after drug administration. Therefore, one course of PDT consists of one injection plus one or two light applications. Up to 2 more courses of drug and light may be given, with each injection separated by a minimum of 30 days.

Photofrin administration: Photofrin should be reconstituted according to the directions given in instructions for use/handling, and administered as a single slow intravenous injection over 3 to 5 minutes at 2 mg/kg body weight. As with all intravenous injections, care should be taken to prevent extravasation at the injection site. If extravasation does occur, the area should be protected from light for a minimum of 30 days. There is no known benefit from injecting the extravasation site with another substance.

Photoactivation of Photofrin: Photofrin is activated by light in the spectral region of 630 nm. Approximately 40–50 hours after Photofrin administration, laser light should be delivered to the tumour by a cylindrical fibre optic diffuser or a microlens fibre optic passed through the operating channel of an endoscope/bronchoscope.

Light Doses: Photoactivation of Photofrin is controlled by the total light energy (light dose) delivered to the tumour site and depends on the indication and the means of light delivery, as follows:

- For endobronchial tumours, the cylindrical diffuser will be suitable for most tumours. The light dose for endobronchial tumours using the cylindrical diffuser is 200 joules/cm of tumour length. Alternatively, the microlens fibre optic may be appropriate for small, flat, non-circumferential tumours. The light dose using the microlens fibre optic is 100 joules/cm².
- For oesophageal tumours, a light dose of 300 joules/cm of tumour length should be delivered using a cylindrical diffuser.

Cylindrical Diffuser (Endobronchial or Oesophageal Lesions): The cylindrical diffuser uniformly distributes laser light radially in a cylindrical pattern over the entire length of the fibre optic tip. The following light dosimetry equation applies.

$$\text{Light dose (J/cm)} = \frac{\text{Total power output from diffuser (W)} \times \text{Treatment time (seconds)}}{\text{Diffuser length (cm)}}$$

For example, the total power output from the diffuser, as measured by a suitable integrating sphere power meter, could be set to [400 mW/cm × length of diffuser in cm] which will deliver the appropriate dose using exposure times of either 8 minutes, 20 seconds (endobronchial tumours, 200 J/cm) or 12 minutes, 30 seconds (oesophageal tumours, 300 J/cm).

Cylindrical diffusers are available in several lengths and the diffuser tip length should be chosen to match the length of the tumour. Tumours with lengths that differ from available diffuser lengths may require multiple use of a single diffuser or the use of two or more diffusers of differing lengths. Diffuser length should be sized to avoid exposure of non-malignant tissue to light and to prevent overlapping of previously treated malignant tissue. Diffusers or combinations of diffusers should be selected to minimise patient treatment time.

The cylindrical diffusers may be used either interstitially or intraluminally. For non-circumferential endobronchial tumours that are soft enough to penetrate, interstitial fibre placement is preferred to intraluminal activation, since this method produces better efficacy and results in less exposure of normal bronchial mucosa to the light. When the interstitial technique is used, up to 90% of the length of the diffuser should be inserted into the tumour mass.

Microlens (Endobronchial lesions only): The microlens fibre optic delivers a diverging, forward-directed beam of light similar to that produced by a torch. It is used to treat small lesions by positioning the microlens tip so that the lesion is uniformly illuminated by a circular spot. The diameter of the spot can be increased or decreased by moving the microlens tip further from or nearer to the lesion. The following light dosimetry equation applies:

$$\text{Light dose (J/cm}^2) = \frac{\text{Total power output at fibre tip (W)} \times \text{Treatment time (seconds)}}{\text{Treatment area (cm}^2)}$$

For example, the power output at the microlens fibre tip, as measured by a power meter, could be set to [200 mW/cm² x tumour area in cm²]. This will deliver the dose of 100 J/cm² of tumour using an exposure time of 8 minutes, 20 seconds per area treated.

Debridement and retreatment: In patients with endobronchial tumours, debridement is mandatory to remove necrotic tumour debris and clear secretions or mucous plugs, thereby preventing possible dyspnoea, obstruction, atelectasis and infection. For oesophageal cancer, debridement is optional since the residua will be removed naturally by peristaltic action. Debridement of residua should be performed 2 days after light treatment. Patients with residual tumour may be retreated with laser light at the time of debridement at the same dose as used for the initial treatment. The second light dose should be administered 96 to 120 hours after the Photofrin injection.

Patients may receive a second course of PDT a minimum of 30 days after the initial therapy; up to three courses of PDT (each injection separated by a minimum of 30 days) can be given. Before each course of treatment, patients should be evaluated for the presence of a tracheo-oesophageal or broncho-oesophageal fistula or for the possibility that the tumour may be eroding into a major blood vessel (see contraindications).

Use in children: Safety and effectiveness in children have not been established. Photofrin should not be used in children until further data are available.

Use in elderly patients: Approximately 70% of the patients treated with PDT using Photofrin in clinical trials were over 60 years of age. There was no apparent difference in effectiveness or safety in these patients compared to younger people. Dose modification based upon age is not required.

Use in patients with impaired hepatic or renal function: The influence of impaired hepatic function on Photofrin disposition has not been evaluated. No special precautions are necessary in patients with renal impairment because excretion is primarily via the faecal route.

Contra-indications: PDT with Photofrin is contraindicated in patients with porphyria or in patients with known hypersensitivity to porphyrins.

PDT with Photofrin is contraindicated in patients with severe hepatic impairment.

PDT is contraindicated in patients with tracheo-oesophageal or broncho-oesophageal fistula.

PDT is contraindicated in patients with suspected erosion of major blood vessels due to risk of massive, potentially fatal haemorrhage.

PDT is not suitable for emergency treatment of patients with severe acute respiratory distress caused by an obstructing endobronchial lesion because 40 to 50 hours are required between injection with Photofrin and laser light treatment.

Special warnings and precautions for use: Photodynamic therapy with Photofrin should be used only in clinics or centres with experience of endoscopic laser procedures.

All patients who receive Photofrin will be photosensitive and must observe precautions to avoid exposure of skin and eyes to direct sunlight or bright indoor light (from examination lamps, including dental lamps, operating room lamps, unshaded light bulbs at close proximity, etc.) for 30 days. The photosensitivity is due to residual drug which will be present in all parts of the skin. Exposure of the skin to ambient indoor light is, however, beneficial because the remaining drug will be inactivated gradually and safely through a photobleaching reaction. Therefore, patients should not stay in a darkened room during this period and should be encouraged to expose their skin to ambient indoor light. The level of photosensitivity will vary for different areas of the body, depending on the extent of previous exposure to light. Before exposing any area of skin to direct sunlight or bright indoor light, the patient should test it for residual photosensitivity. A small area of skin should be exposed to sunlight for 10 minutes. If no photosensitivity reaction (erythema, oedema, blistering) occurs within 24 hours, the patient can gradually resume normal outdoor activities, initially continuing to exercise caution and gradually allowing increased exposure. If some photosensitivity reaction occurs with the limited skin test, the patient should continue precautions for another 2 weeks before retesting. The tissue around the eyes may be more sensitive, and therefore, it is not recommended that the face be used for testing. If patients travel to a different geographical area with greater sunshine, they should retest their level of photosensitivity. **UV (ultraviolet) sunscreens are of no value in protecting against photosensitivity reactions because photoactivation is caused by visible light.**

As the result of PDT treatment, patients may complain of substernal chest pain because of inflammatory responses within the area of treatment. Such pain may be of sufficient intensity to warrant the short-term prescription of opiate analgesics.

If PDT is to be used before or after radiotherapy, sufficient time should be allowed between the therapies to ensure that the inflammatory reaction produced by the first treatment has subsided prior to commencement of the second treatment.

As Photofrin is a biological material, possibility of acute hypersensitivity reaction including anaphylaxis cannot be ruled out (see undesirable effects). In case of allergic reaction, treatment should be stopped immediately and appropriate emergency measures initiated.

Oesophageal cancer: If the oesophageal tumour is eroding into the trachea or bronchial tree, the likelihood of tracheo-oesophageal or broncho-oesophageal fistula resulting from treatment is sufficiently high that PDT is not recommended.

Patients with oesophageal varices should be treated with extreme caution. Light should not be given directly to the variceal area because of the high risk of bleeding.

Lung cancer: If the endobronchial tumour invades deeply into the bronchial wall, the possibility exists for fistula formation upon resolution of tumour.

PDT should be used with extreme caution for endobronchial tumours in locations where treatment-induced inflammation could obstruct the main airway, e.g., long or circumferential tumours of the trachea, tumours of the main carina that involve both mainstem bronchi circumferentially, or circumferential tumours in the remaining mainstem bronchus of patients with prior pneumonectomy.

Patients with endobronchial lesions must be closely monitored between the laser light therapy and the mandatory debridement bronchoscopy for any evidence of respiratory distress (see posology and method of administration). Inflammation and mucositis may result from exposure of normal tissue to too much light. Necrotic debris may also obstruct the airway. If respiratory distress occurs, the physician should be prepared to carry out immediate bronchoscopy to remove secretions and debris to open the airway.

Interaction with other medicaments and other forms of interaction: There have been no formal interaction studies of Photofrin and any other drugs. However, it is possible that concomitant use of other photosensitising agents (e.g., tetracyclines, sulphonamides, phenothiazines, sulphonylurea hypoglycaemic agents, thiazide diuretics, and griseofulvin) could increase the photosensitivity reaction.

Photofrin PDT causes direct intracellular damage by initiating radical chain reactions that damage intracellular membranes and mitochondria. Tissue damage also results from ischaemia secondary to vasoconstriction, platelet activation and aggregation and clotting. Research in animals and in cell culture has suggested that many drugs could influence the effects of PDT, possible examples of which are described below. There are no human data that support or rebut these possibilities.

Compounds that quench active oxygen species or scavenge radicals, such as dimethyl sulphoxide, b-carotene, ethanol, formate and mannitol would be expected to decrease PDT activity. Preclinical data also suggest that tissue ischaemia, allopurinol, calcium channel blockers and some prostaglandin synthesis inhibitors could interfere with Photofrin PDT. Drugs that decrease clotting, vasoconstriction or platelet aggregation, e.g., thromboxane A_2 inhibitors, could decrease the efficacy of PDT. Glucocorticoid hormones given before or concomitant with PDT may decrease the efficacy of the treatment.

Pregnancy and lactation: Photofrin was not teratogenic in rats or rabbits at doses comparable to those used in clinical situations. Foetotoxicity was observed only at maternally toxic doses. There are no adequate and well-controlled studies in pregnant women. Women of childbearing potential should practice an effective method of contraception during therapy. Photofrin may be used during pregnancy only if the potential benefit outweighs the potential risk to the foetus.

It is not known whether this drug is excreted in human milk. Therefore, women receiving Photofrin must not breast feed.

Effects on ability to drive and use machines: Photofrin causes no adverse effects that could Impair the patient's ability to drive or use machines.

Undesirable effects: Systemically induced effects associated with PDT with Photofrin consist of photosensitivity and mild constipation. All patients who receive Photofrin will be photosensitive and must observe precautions to avoid sunlight and bright indoor light (see special warnings and special precautions for use). Photosensitivity reactions consist mainly of mild erythema on the face and hands.

Most toxicities associated with this therapy are local effects seen in the region of illumination and occasionally in surrounding tissues. The local adverse reactions are characteristic of an inflammatory response induced by the photodynamic effect.

No cases of anaphylaxis have been reported although occasionally rashes have been observed.

Endobronchial cancer: Adverse events reported in 5% or more of patients (n=99) with obstructing endobronchial nonsmall cell lung cancer were most commonly associated with the respiratory system; their relationship to therapy is unclear: dyspnoea (32%), nonfatal haemoptysis (12%), coughing (17%), pneumonia (13%), bronchitis (11%), fatal massive haemoptysis (10%), increased sputum (9%) and respiratory insufficiency (7%). Other frequent events were photosensitivity reaction (20%), fever (15%), chest pain (9%), insomnia (7%), anxiety (5%) and constipation (5%). Inflammatory reactions manifested as fever, bronchitis and chest pain. Coughing, dyspnoea, haemoptysis and increased sputum, while reported as adverse events, are also symptoms of the disease. Fatal massive haemoptysis, with or without prior radiotherapy, has been observed with greater frequency in the PDT-treated group. In half of the patients with fatal haemoptysis, the event occurred more than 30 days after the last treatment procedure and was judged by the investigator to be unrelated to PDT. Fatal massive haemoptysis may be due to disease progression or due to resolution of tumour eroding into a major blood vessel (see contraindications).

Serious and other notable adverse events observed in less than 5% of PDT-treated patients with endobronchial cancer included pleural effusion, pulmonary thrombosis, pulmonary embolism and lung abscess. Their relationship to therapy is uncertain.

Oesophageal cancer: The following adverse events were reported in at least 5% of patients (n=127) with partially or completely obstructing oesophageal cancer; the relationship of many of these events to PDT is uncertain.

Gastrointestinal: constipation (23%), nausea (21%), abdominal pain (18%), vomiting (16%), dysphagia (9%), haematemesis (9%), diarrhoea (7%), oesophageal oedema (6%), oesophageal stricture (6%), oesophageal tumour bleeding (6%), dyspepsia (6%).

Respiratory: pleural effusion (28%), pneumonia (17%), dyspnoea (17%), respiratory insufficiency (11%), pharyngitis (10%), tracheo-oesophageal fistula (9%).

Cardiovascular: atrial fibrillation (8%), tachycardia (6%), cardiac failure (6%).

Other: fever (32%), anaemia (25%), chest pain (24%), pain (23%), photosensitivity reaction (19%), insomnia (14%), urinary tract infection (8%), moniliasis (8%), back pain (8%) dehydration (6%), generalised oedema (6%), peripheral oedema (6%), hypotension (6%), hypertension (6%), sepsis (6%), anorexia (6%), weight decrease (6%), confusion (6%), asthenia (5%).

These effects were generally mild or moderate in severity and easily managed. Anaemia was not due to myelosuppression, but rather it was due to tumour bleeding and was more common in patients with large tumours (>10 cm) and with tumours in the lower third of the oesophagus. Tumour bleeding may be exacerbated by vigorous debridement. Debridement is optional in patients with oesophageal cancer (see posology and method of administration). The syndrome of respiratory insufficiency included one patient who experienced upper airway oedema (1%) and one who experienced bronchospasm during debridement (1%); the remaining events (8%) did not appear to be related to PDT. Fever and pleural effusion, as well as pain, oesophageal oedema and atrial fibrillation are thought to be manifestations of a local/regional inflammatory reaction. Oesophageal oedema occurred more frequently when the tumour was located in the upper third of the oesophagus; atrial fibrillation was more likely to occur when the tumour was in the middle third of the oesophagus.

Serious and other notable adverse events observed in less than 5% of patients include the following; their relationship to therapy is uncertain. In the gastrointestinal system, oesophagitis, oesophageal perforation, gastric ulcer, ileus, jaundice, and peritonitis have occurred. Cardiovascular events have included angina pectoris, bradycardia, myocardial infarction, sick sinus syndrome, and supraventricular tachycardia. Respiratory events of bronchitis, pneumonitis, pulmonary haemorrhage, pulmonary oedema, respiratory failure, and stridor have occurred. Vision-related events of abnormal vision, diplopia, eye pain and photophobia have been reported.

Overdose:

Overdose of Photofrin: There is no information on overdosage situations involving Photofrin. Higher than recommended drug doses of two 2 mg/kg doses given two days apart (10 patients) and three 2 mg/kg doses given within two weeks (1 patient) were tolerated without notable adverse reactions. Effects of overdosage on the duration of photosensitivity are unknown. Laser treatment should not be given if an overdose of Photofrin is administered. In the event of an overdose, patients should protect their eyes and skin from direct sunlight or bright indoor lights for 30 days. At this time, patients should test for residual photosensitivity (see *Special warnings and special precautions for use*). Photofrin is not dialysable.

Overdose of laser light following Photofrin: Light doses of two to three times the recommended dose have been administered to a few patients with superficial endobronchial tumours. One patient experienced life-threatening dyspnoea and the others had no notable complications. Increased symptoms and damage to normal tissue might be expected following an overdose of light.

Pharmacological properties

Pharmacodynamic properties: The cytotoxic and antitumour actions of Photofrin (ATC code L01X X15) are light and oxygen-dependent. Photodynamic therapy (PDT) with Photofrin is a 2-stage process. The first stage is the intravenous injection of Photofrin. Clearance from a variety of tissues occurs over 40–72 hours, but tumours, skin, and organs of the reticuloendothelial system (including liver and spleen) retain Photofrin for a longer period. Illumination with 630 nm wavelength laser light constitutes the second stage of therapy. Tumour selectivity in treatment occurs through a combination of selective retention of Photofrin and selective delivery of light. Cellular damage caused by Photofrin PDT is a consequence of the propagation of free radical reactions. Radical initiation may occur after Photofrin absorbs light to form a porphyrin excited state. Spin transfer from Photofrin to molecular oxygen may then generate singlet oxygen. Subsequent free radical reactions can form superoxide and hydroxyl radicals. Tumour death also occurs through ischaemic necrosis secondary to vascular occlusion that appears to be partly mediated by thromboxane A_2 release. The laser treatment induces a photochemical, not a thermal, effect. The necrotic reaction and associated inflammatory response evolve over several days.

Pharmacokinetic properties:

General characteristics: A pharmacokinetic study was conducted in 12 endobronchial cancer patients given 2 mg/kg of Photofrin intravenously. Samples of plasma were obtained out to 56 days (1,344 hours) post injection and total porphyrin units determined. The mean peak plasma concentration (C_{max}) immediately following injection was 79.6 µg/ml (C.V. 61%, range 39-222); the mean $T_{1/2}$ was 515 hours, i.e. 21.5 days (C.V. 26%, range 264-672). Thus, porfimer sodium is cleared slowly from the body, with a mean CL_T of 0.859 mL/h/kg (C.V. 53%).

In vitro binding of Photofrin to human serum protein is around 90% and independent of concentration between 20 and 100 µg/mL. Preclinical studies indicate that the excretion of Photofrin components occurs primarily via the faecal route.

Characteristics in patients: No special precautions in renally impaired patients are necessary because excretion is primarily via the faecal route.

The influence of impaired hepatic function on Photofrin disposition has not been evaluated.

Preclinical safety data: In vitro, Photofrin PDT did not cause mutations in the Ames test, nor did it cause chromosome aberrations or mutations (HGPRT locus) in Chinese hamster ovary (CHO) cells. Photofrin caused <2-fold, but significant, increases in sister chromatid exchange in CHO cells irradiated with visible light and a 3-fold increase in Chinese hamster lung fibroblasts irradiated with near UV light. Photofrin PDT caused an increase in thymidine kinase mutants and DNA-protein cross-links in mouse L5178Y cells, but not mouse LYR83 cells. Photofrin PDT caused a light-dose dependent increase in DNA-strand breaks in malignant human cervical carcinoma cells, but not in normal cells. *In vivo,* Photofrin did not cause chromosomal aberrations in the mouse micronucleus test. Therefore, the overall mutagenic potential of Photofrin is considered minimal.

Pharmaceutical particulars

List of excipients: Hydrochloric acid and/or sodium hydroxide may be added during manufacture to adjust pH. The product contains no other excipients or antimicrobial preservatives.

Incompatibilities: Reconstitute Photofrin with 5% glucose intravenous as described under *instructions for use/handling.* Do not use other diluents. Do not mix Photofrin with other drugs in the same solution.

Shelf life: Photofrin is stable for 36 months.

Special precautions for storage: Do not store above 25°C. Keep container in the outer carton.

After reconstitution, use immediately (within 3 hours). Protect from light following reconstitution.

Nature and contents of container: Vial: Flint, type I glass, treated, 40 mL capacity.

Closure: Grey butyl stopper.

Vial contents: A dark red to reddish brown lyophilised powder (or cake) for reconstitution.

Pack size: 1 vial.

Instructions for use/handling: Photofrin 75 should be reconstituted with 31.8 mL of 5% glucose intravenous infusion, resulting in a final concentration of 2.5 mg/mL. Do not use other diluents. Do not mix Photofrin with other drugs in the same solution. Sufficient vials of Photofrin should be reconstituted to provide the patient with a dose of 2 mg/kg using the calculation below. For most patients (up to 75 kg) two vials of Photofrin 75 will suffice. Each Photofrin 15 (M.A. No.: PL 05980/0017) vial will treat an additional 7.5 kg of body weight.

Photofrin (mL)

$$= \frac{\text{Patient's weight (kg)} \times 2\ \text{mg/kg}}{2.5\ \text{mg/mL}}$$

$$= 0.8 \times \text{Patient's weight}$$

Marketing authorisation number 05980/0018

Date of approval/revision of SPC December 1998.

Legal category POM.

SOMATULINE* LA ▼

Qualitative and quantitative composition Lanreotide (I.N.N., B.A.N.) 0.030 g*.

* Each vial is filled with a quantity of microparticles of lanreotide acetate and co-polymers corresponding to 40 mg of lanreotide base, which ensures the actual injection of 30 mg of lanreotide.

Pharmaceutical form Powder for suspension for injection.

Clinical particulars

Therapeutic indications: Somatuline LA is indicated for the treatment of acromegaly when the circulating levels of growth hormone remain abnormal after surgery and/or radiotherapy. Somatuline LA is also indicated for the relief of symptoms associated with neuroendocrine (particularly carcinoid) tumours.

Posology and method of administration: Initially, one intramuscular injection should be given every 14 days. The frequency of subsequent injections may be varied in accordance with the individual patient's response (as judged by a reduction in symptoms and/or a reduction in GH and/or IGF-1 levels,) such that injections can be given every 7 to 10 days as necessary. No dose modification is required in elderly patients. As there is no experience of the use of the product in children, the use of Somatuline LA in children cannot be advised.

Contra-indications: Somatuline LA should not be prescribed during pregnancy and lactation, nor in patients presenting with hypersensitivity to the peptide or related peptides.

Special warnings and special precautions for use: Pharmacological studies in animals and humans show that lanreotide, like somatostatin and its analogues, inhibit secretion of insulin and glucagon. Hence, diabetic patients treated by Somatuline LA may experience a slight transient decrease of blood glucose levels. Blood sugar levels should be checked in order to adjust the anti-diabetic treatment if necessary.

Lanreotide may reduce gall bladder motility and therefore, gall bladder echography is advised at the start of treatment and every six months thereafter. If gallstones do occur, they are generally asymptomatic. Symptomatic stones should be treated as medically indicated.

In patients with hepatic/renal dysfunction, kidney and liver function should be regularly monitored and the dose interval adjusted if necessary.

Interaction with other medicaments and other forms of interaction: The gastrointestinal effects of Somatuline LA may reduce the intestinal absorption of co-administered drugs. As with other somatostatin analogues, Somatuline LA may reduce the intestinal absorption of cyclosporin A. Interactions with highly plasma bound drugs are unlikely in view of the moderate binding of lanreotide to serum proteins (78 % mean serum binding).

Pregnancy and lactation: Studies in animals showed transitory growth retardation of offspring prior to weaning. Although no teratogenic effects have been observed in animals, in the absence of clinical experience, lanreotide must not be administered to pregnant or lactating women.

Effects on ability to drive and use machine: Therapy with Somatuline LA is unlikely to impair a patient's ability to drive or use machinery.

Undesirable effects

Clinical tolerance: the side effects of Somatuline LA reported in the clinical trials are mainly local and gastrointestinal.

Local tolerance: moderate, transitory pain at the injection site is sometimes associated with local redness.

General tolerance: gastrointestinal side effects are the most common and include: diarrhoea or soft stools, abdominal pain, flatulence, anorexia, nausea and vomiting. In general, all these side effects are mild to moderate in intensity; in most cases the frequency and the intensity of such effects appear to diminish or to resolve with continued therapy.

Cases of asymptomatic and symptomatic gallbladder lithiasis have been reported in patients during prolonged treatment. A precautionary statement is included under special warnings and special precautions for use.

Biological tolerance: Altered glucose regulation was reported in healthy volunteers, however, this finding was not reflected in the patient studies.

Overdose: There is no human experience of overdosage. Animal data do not predict any effects other than those on insulin and glucagon secretion and the gastrointestinal system. If overdosage occurs, symptomatic management is indicated.

Pharmacological properties

Pharmacodynamic properties: Like natural somatostatin, lanreotide is a peptide inhibitor of a number of endocrine, neuroendocrine, exocrine and paracrine functions. It shows good affinity for peripheral somatostatin receptors (anterior pituitary and pancreatic). In contrast, its affinity for central receptors is much lower. This profile confers a good specificity of action at the level of growth hormone and digestive hormone secretion.

Lanreotide shows a much longer duration of action than natural somatostatin. In addition, its marked selectivity for the secretion of growth hormone, compared to that of insulin, makes it a suitable candidate for the treatment of acromegaly. Furthermore, the inhibitory action of lanreotide on intestinal exocrine secretion, digestive hormones and cellular proliferation mechanisms is suited to the symptomatic treatment of endocrine digestive tumours, especially carcinoids.

Pharmacokinetic properties: The plasma profile of lanreotide administered intramuscularly in healthy volunteers, is characterised by an initial rapid release phase (phase 1) followed by a prolonged slow release phase (phase 2). The first plasma peak (C_{max1}: 6.8±3.8 µg/l) occurs at 1.4±0.8 hours and the second (C_{max2} : 2.5±0.9 µg/l) at 1.9±1.8 days. The absolute bioavailability is 46.1±16.7%. The mean residence time of 8.0±1.0 days and the apparent half-life of 5.2±2.5 days, confirm the prolonged release of the product.

After a single administration in acromegaly patients, a comparable pharmacokinetic profile is observed and the levels of growth hormone and IGF-1 are significantly reduced for a period of about 14 days. With repeated administration over several months, there is no evidence of accumulation of lanreotide.

Preclinical safety data: In vitro and animal toxicology studies have not shown any specific toxic potential for lanreotide. The observed effects are related to the pharmacological properties of lanreotide on the endocrine system. The resorption of Somatuline LA is complete in 45–60 days.

Pharmaceutical particulars

List of excipients: Lactide-glycolide copolymer, Lactic-glycolic copolymer, Mannitol, Carmellose (Na), Polysorbate 80

Incompatibilities: Somatuline LA must be made up immediately prior to use, using only the solution supplied in the package.

Shelf life: 2 years

Special precautions for storage: Store at a temperature between +2°C and 8°C (in the refrigerator), do not freeze.

Nature and contents of container: Type I, clear, slightly tinted, glass vial containing sterile Somatuline LA. Box of 1 vial, 1 ampoule (vehicle), 2 needles and 1 syringe. Box of 2 vials, 2 ampoules (vehicle), 4 needles and 2 syringes. Box of 6 vials, 6 ampoules (vehicle), 12 needles and 6 syringes.

Instructions for use/handling: Somatuline LA must be made up in the supplied solution immediately before injection, by shaking the vial, gently, 20 to 30 times, in order to obtain a homogenous suspension with a milky appearance. This must not be mixed **with other medications.**

NB: It is important that injection of this product is performed according to the instructions in the leaflet.

Marketing authorisation numbers

Somatuline LA	10829/0006
Mannitol solution	10829/0003

Date of approval/revision of SPC January 1998.

Legal category POM.

**Trade Mark*

Janssen-Cilag Ltd
Saunderton
High Wycombe
Bucks HP14 4HJ

☎ 01494 567567 🖷 01494 567568

ANQUIL*

Presentation White, uncoated tablets marked 'JANSSEN' on one side and 'A/0.25' on the reverse. Each tablet contains 0.25 mg benperidol. The tablets also contain lactose.

Uses Anquil is a neuroleptic of the butyrophenone series for the control of deviant anti-social sexual behaviour.

Dosage and administration Anquil is intended for oral administration to adults only. The recommended daily dose is 0.25-1.5 mg in divided doses. Dosage is best initiated and adjusted under close clinical supervision, as individual response to neuroleptic drugs is variable.

In determining dosage, consideration should be given to the patient's age, severity of symptoms and previous response to other neuroleptic drugs.

In adolescents a lower dose may be advisable.

Use in children: Not recommended.

Use in the elderly: Patients who are elderly or debilitated, or those with previously reported adverse reactions to neuroleptic drugs, may require less Anquil, and half the normal starting dose may be sufficient for therapeutic response.

Contra-indications, warnings, etc
Contra-indications: Comatose states, patients with extrapyramidal symptoms, CNS depression, hypersensitivity to any of the ingredients of Anquil or other butyrophenones, depressive disorders or Parkinson's disease.

Precautions: Rare cases of sudden and unexplained death have been reported in psychiatric patients receiving antipsychotic drugs. However, Anquil has not been clearly implicated in any case.

Acute withdrawal symptoms, including nausea, vomiting and insomnia, have very rarely been described after abrupt cessation of high doses of anti-psychotic drugs. Relapse may also occur and gradual withdrawal is advisable.

Where prolonged treatment with Anquil is envisaged, it would be a reasonable precaution to carry out regular blood counts and tests of liver function.

Caution is advised in patients with liver disease, renal failure, cardiovascular disease, epilepsy, and conditions predisposing to epilepsy or convulsions.

Use during pregnancy and lactation: The safety of Anquil in pregnancy has not been established, although studies in animals have not demonstrated teratogenic effects. As with other drugs, it is not advisable to administer Anquil in pregnancy.

Butyrophenones are excreted in breast milk and are not recommended during lactation. If the use of Anquil is considered essential, breast feeding should be discontinued.

Effects on driving ability and operation of machinery: Anquil may interfere with activities requiring mental alertness. Therefore, patients should be advised not to drive or operate machinery until their individual susceptibility is known.

Interactions: In common with all neuroleptics, Anquil can increase the central nervous system depression produced by other CNS-depressant drugs, including alcohol, hypnotics, sedatives, strong analgesics or sedating antihistamines and may antagonise the action of adrenaline and other sympathomimetic agents.

Certain agents (eg phenobarbitone, carbamazepine, phenytoin), as well as smoking and alcohol consumption, which stimulate metabolising enzymes in the liver, may theoretically enhance the metabolic breakdown of neuroleptics, necessitating an increased dose.

Anquil may impair the anti-Parkinson effects of levodopa and other dopamine agonists. The dosage of anti-convulsants may need to be increased to take account of the lowered seizure threshold.

The risk of hypotension with antihypertensive drugs may be increased when Anquil is given concomitantly.

Enhanced CNS effects when combined with methyldopa have been reported for some butyrophenones.

Adverse effects:
Central nervous system: In common with all neuroleptics, extrapyramidal symptoms may occur. Acute dystonias may occur early in treatment. Parkinsonian rigidity, tremor and akathisia tend to appear less rapidly. Oculogyric crises and laryngeal dystonias have been reported.

Anti-Parkinson agents should only be given as required; they should not be prescribed routinely because of the possible risk of impairing the therapeutic efficacy of Anquil.

Tardive dyskinesia may occur during administration or after withdrawal of neuroleptic drugs, including Anquil. The syndrome is common among patients treated with moderate to high doses of anti-psychotic drugs for prolonged periods of time and may prove irreversible, particularly in patients over the age of 50.

It is unlikely to occur in the short-term when low or moderate doses of Anquil are used as recommended, but the risk increases with age and increasing dosage. Anquil should be given in the minimal effective dose for the minimum possible time.

The potential seriousness and unpredictability of tardive dyskinesia and the fact that it has occasionally been reported to occur when neuroleptic anti-psychotic drugs have been prescribed for relatively short periods in low dosage means that the prescribing of such agents requires especially careful assessment of risks versus benefit. Tardive dyskinesia can be precipitated or aggravated by anti-Parkinson drugs. Tardive dyskinesias may occur after abrupt drug withdrawal.

It has been reported that fine vermicular movements of the tongue may be an early sign of tardive dyskinesia and that the full syndrome may not develop if the medication is stopped at that time. If signs and symptoms of tardive dyskinesia appear, the discontinuation of all neuroleptic drugs should be considered.

As with other neuroleptics, rare cases of Neuroleptic Malignant Syndrome, an idiosyncratic response characterised by hyperthermia, muscle rigidity, autonomic instability, altered consciousness, coma and elevated CPK levels, have been reported. Signs of autonomic dysfunction such as tachycardia, labile arterial pressure and sweating may precede the onset of hyperthermia, acting as early warning signs. Antipsychotic treatment should be withdrawn immediately and appropriate supportive therapy and careful monitoring instituted.

Anquil, even in low dosage in susceptible (especially non-psychotic) individuals, may cause unpleasant subjective feelings of being mentally dulled or slowed down, dizziness, headache, or paradoxical effects of excitement, agitation or insomnia.

Depression and seizures have been reported rarely. A causal relationship with Anquil has not been unequivocally established.

Confusional or agitated states have been reported rarely.

Gastrointestinal system: Nausea, vomiting, loss of appetite, constipation and dyspepsia have been reported.

Endocrinological system: Hormonal effects of anti-psychotic neuroleptic drugs include hyper-prolactinaemia, which may cause galactorrhoea, gynaecomastia and oligo- or amenorrhoea.

Cardiovascular system: Dose-related hypotension is uncommon but can occur, particularly in the elderly who are more susceptible to the sedative and hypotensive effects. Benign tachycardia has occasionally been reported.

Other adverse reactions: Jaundice or transient abnormalities of liver function in the absence of jaundice have been reported. The following effects have been reported rarely: oedema, skin rashes or hypersensitivity reactions such as exanthema and pruritus. Blood dyscrasias, including granulocytopenia, have been reported occasionally. Weight changes may occur. Isolated cases of excessive salivation have been reported.

Overdosage:
Symptoms: In general, the manifestations of Anquil overdosage are an extension of its pharmacological action. In patients who have received daily doses of 160 mg, the most prominent side-effects were extrapyramidal symptoms such as oculogyric crisis, excessive salivation, muscle rigidity, akinesia and akathisia. Drowsiness or paradoxical excitement may occur.

Treatment: There is no specific antidote to Anquil. Treatment consists of supportive and symptomatic measures combined with standard measures to remove any unabsorbed drug. Extrapyramidal symptoms should be treated with anti-Parkinson drugs as required.

Pharmaceutical precautions Protect from light.

Legal category POM.

Package quantities Anquil tablets, each containing 0.25 mg benperidol, are supplied in packs of 100.

Further information Nil.

Product licence number 0242/0014R.

BINOVUM*

Qualitative and quantitative composition BiNovum are tablets for oral administration.

Each white tablet contains norethisterone PhEur 0.5 mg and ethinyloestradiol PhEur 0.035 mg.

Each peach coloured tablet contains norethisterone PhEur 1.0 mg and ethinyloestradiol PhEur 0.035 mg.

Pharmaceutical form Tablets.

The white tablets are small, round and engraved C 535 on both faces.

The peach-coloured tablets are small, round and engraved C 135 on both faces.

Clinical particulars
Therapeutic indications: Contraception and the recognised indications for such oestrogen/progestogen combinations.

Posology and method of administration:
Adults: It is preferable that tablet intake from the first pack is started on the first day of menstruation in which case no extra contraceptive precautions are necessary.

If menstruation has already begun (that is 2, 3 or 4 days previously), tablet taking should commence on day 5 of the menstrual period. In this case additional contraceptive precautions must be taken for the first 7 days of tablet taking.

If menstruation began more than 5 days previously then the patient should be advised to wait until her next menstrual period before starting to take BiNovum.

How to take BiNovum: One tablet is taken daily at the same time (preferably in the evening) without interruption for 21 days, followed by a break of 7 tablet-free days. (A white tablet is taken every day for 7 days, then a peach coloured tablet is taken every day for 14 days, then 7 tablet-free days). Each subsequent pack is started after the 7 tablet-free days have elapsed. Additional contraceptive precautions are not then required.

Elderly: Not applicable.

Children: Not recommended.

Contra-indications:
Absolute contra-indications:
- pregnancy or suspected pregnancy (that cannot yet be excluded).
- circulatory disorders (cardiovascular or cerebrovascular) such as thrombophlebitis and thromboembolic processes (or a history of these conditions), moderate to severe hypertension, hyperlipoproteinaemia. In addition the presence of more than one of the risk factors for arterial disease.
- severe liver disease, cholestatic jaundice or hepatitis (viral or non-viral) or a history of these conditions if the results of liver function tests have failed to return to normal, and for 3 months after liver function tests have been found to be normal; a history of jaundice of pregnancy or jaundice due to the use of steroids, Rotor syndrome and Dubin-Johnson syndrome, hepatic cell tumours and porphyria.
- cholelithiasis.
- known or suspected oestrogen-dependent tum-

ours; endometrial hyperplasia; undiagnosed vaginal bleeding.
- systemic lupus erythematosus or a history of this condition.
- a history during pregnancy or previous use of steroids of:
- severe pruritus
- herpes gestationis
- a manifestation or deterioration of otosclerosis

Relative contra-indications: If any relative contraindications listed below are present, the benefits of oestrogen/progestogen containing preparations must be weighed against the possible risk for each individual case and the patient kept under close supervision. In case of aggravation or appearance of any of these conditions whilst the patient is taking the pill, its use should be discontinued.

- conditions implicating an increasing risk of developing venous thrombo-embolic complications, e.g. severe varicose veins or prolonged immobilisation or major surgery. Disorders of coagulation.
- presence of any risk factor for arterial disease e.g. smoking, hyperlipidaemia or hypertension.
- other conditions associated with an increased risk of circulatory disease such as latent or overt cardiac failure, renal dysfunction, or a history of these conditions.
- epilepsy or a history of this condition.
- migraine or a history of this condition.
- a history of cholelithiasis.
- presence of any risk factor for oestrogen-dependent tumours; oestrogen-sensitive gynaecological disorders such as uterine fibromyomata and endometriosis.
- diabetes mellitus.
- severe depression or a history of this condition. If this is accompanied by a disturbance in tryptophan metabolism, administration of vitamin B6 might be of therapeutic value.
- sickle cell haemoglobinopathy, since under certain circumstances, e.g. during infections or anoxia, oestrogen containing preparations may induce thromboembolic process in patients with this condition.
- if the results of liver function tests become abnormal, use should be discontinued.

Special warnings and special precautions for use:
Post partum administration: Following a vaginal delivery, oral contraceptive administration to non-breast-feeding mothers can be started 21 days post-partum provided the patient is fully ambulant and there are no puerperal complications. No additional contraceptive precautions are required. If post partum administration begins more than 21 days after delivery, additional contraceptive precautions are required for the first 7 days of pill-taking.

If intercourse has taken place post-partum, oral contraceptive use should be delayed until the first day of the first menstrual period.

After miscarriage or abortion administration should start immediately in which case no additional contraceptive precautions are required.

Changing from a 21 day pill or another 22 day pill to BiNovum: All tablets in the old pack should be finished. The first BiNovum tablet is taken the next day i.e. no gap is left between taking tablets nor does the patient need to wait for her period to begin. Tablets should be taken as instructed in 'How to take BiNovum'. Additional contraceptive precautions are not required. The patient will not have a period until the end of the first BiNovum pack, but this is not harmful, nor does it matter if she experiences some bleeding on tablet-taking days.

Changing from a combined every day pill (28 day tablet) to BiNovum: BiNovum should be started after taking the last active tablet from the 'Every day Pill' pack (i.e. after taking 21 or 22 tablets). The first BiNovum tablet is taken the next day i.e. no gap is left between taking tablets nor does the patient need to wait for her period to begin. Tablets should be taken as instructed in 'How to take BiNovum'. Additional contraceptive precautions are not required. Remaining tablets from the every day (ED) pack should be discarded.

The patient will not have a period until the end of the first BiNovum pack, but this is not harmful, nor does it matter if she experiences some bleeding on tablet-taking days.

Changing from a progestogen-only pill (POP or mini pill) to BiNovum: The first BiNovum tablet should be taken on the first day of the period, even if the patient has already taken a mini pill on that day. Tablets should be taken as instructed in 'How to take BiNovum'. Additional contraceptive precautions are not required. All the remaining progestogen-only pills in the mini pill pack should be discarded.

If the patient is taking a mini pill, then she may not always have a period, especially when she is breast-feeding. The first BiNovum tablet should be taken on the day after stopping the mini pill. All remaining pills in the mini pill packet must be discarded. Additional contraceptive precautions must be taken for the first 7 days.

To skip a period: To skip a period, a new pack of BiNovum should be started on the day after finishing the current pack (the patient skips the tablet-free days). Tablet-taking should be continued in the usual way.

During the use of the second pack she may experience slight spotting or break-through bleeding but contraceptive protection will not be diminished provided there are no tablet omissions.

The next pack of BiNovum is started after the usual 7 tablet-free days, regardless of whether the period has completely finished or not.

Reduced reliability: When BiNovum is taken according to the directions for use the occurrence of pregnancy is highly unlikely. However the reliability of oral contraceptives may be reduced under the following circumstances:

Forgotten tablets: If the patient forgets to take a tablet, she should take it as soon as she remembers and take the next one at the normal time. This may mean that two tablets are taken in one day. Provided she is less than 12 hours late in taking her tablet, BiNovum will still give contraceptive protection during this cycle and the rest of the pack should be taken as usual.

If she is more than 12 hours late in taking one or more tablets then she should take the last missed pill as soon as she remembers but leave the other missed pills in the pack. She should continue to take the rest of the pack as usual but must use extra precautions (e.g. sheath, diaphragm, plus spermicide) and follow the '7-day rule' (see Further Information for the 7 day rule).

If there are 7 or more pills left in the pack after the missed and delayed pills then the usual 7-day break can be left before starting the next pack. If there are less than 7 pills left in the pack after the missed and delayed pills then when the pack is finished the next pack should be started the next day. If withdrawal bleeding does not occur at the end of the second pack then a pregnancy test should be performed.

Vomiting or diarrhoea: If after tablet intake vomiting or diarrhoea occurs, a tablet may not be absorbed properly by the body. If the symptoms disappear within 12 hours of tablet-taking, the patient should take an extra tablet from a spare pack and continue with the rest of the pack as usual.

However, if the symptoms continue beyond those 12 hours, additional contraceptive precautions are necessary for any sexual intercourse during the stomach or bowel upset and for the following 7 days (the patient must be advised to follow the '7-day rule').

Change in bleeding pattern: If after taking BiNovum for several months there is a sudden occurrence of spotting or breakthrough bleeding (not observed in previous cycles) or the absence of withdrawal bleeding, contraceptive effectiveness may be reduced. If withdrawal bleeding fails to occur and none of the above mentioned events have taken place, pregnancy is highly unlikely and oral contraceptive use can be continued until the end of the next pack.

(If withdrawal bleeding fails to occur at the end of the second cycle, tablet intake should be discontinued and pregnancy excluded before oral contraceptive use can be resumed). However, if withdrawal bleeding is absent and any of the above mentioned events has occurred, tablet intake should be discontinued and pregnancy excluded before oral contraceptive use can be resumed.

Medical examination/consultation: A complete medical history and physical examination should be taken prior to the initiation or reinstitution of oral contraceptives and should be repeated periodically.

These physical examinations should include special reference to blood pressure, breasts, abdomen and pelvic organs, including cervical cytology and, where indicated by the medical or family history, relevant laboratory tests. Caution should be observed when prescribing oral contraceptives to young women whose cycles are not yet stabilised.

Surgery, varicose veins or immobilisation: In patients using oestrogen-containing preparations the risk of deep vein thrombosis may be temporarily increased when undergoing a major operation (e.g. abdominal, orthopaedic), and surgery to the legs, medical treatment for varicose veins or prolonged immobilisation. Therefore, it is advisable to discontinue oral contraceptive use at least 4 to 6 weeks prior to these procedures if performed electively and to (re)start not less than 2 weeks after full ambulation. The latter is also valid with regard to immobilisation after an accident or emergency surgery. In case of emergency surgery, thrombotic prophylaxis is usually indicated e.g. with subcutaneous heparin.

Chloasma: Chloasma may occasionally occur, especially in women with a history of chloasma gravidarum. Women with a tendency to chloasma should avoid exposure to the sun or ultraviolet radiation whilst taking this preparation. Chloasma is often not fully reversible.

Laboratory tests: The use of steroids may influence the results of certain laboratory tests. In the literature, at least a hundred different parameters have been reported to possibly be influenced by oral contraceptive use, predominantly by the oestrogenic component. Among these are: biochemical parameters of the liver, thyroid, adrenal and renal function, plasma levels of (carrier) proteins and lipid/lipoprotein fractions and parameters of coagulation and fibrinolysis.

Further information:
Additional contraceptive precautions: When additional contraceptive precautions are required the patient should be advised either not to have sex, or to use a cap plus spermicide or for her partner to use a condom. Rhythm methods should not be advised as the pill disrupts the usual cyclical changes associated with the natural menstrual cycle e.g. changes in temperature and cervical mucus.

The 7-day rule: If any one tablet is forgotten for more than 12 hours.

If the patient has vomiting or diarrhoea for more than 12 hours.

If the patient is taking any of the drugs listed under 'Interactions':

The patient should continue to take her tablets as usual and:

– Additional contraceptive precautions must be taken for the next 7 days.

But–if these 7 days run beyond the end of the current pack: the next pack must be started as soon as the current one is finished, i.e. no gap should be left between packs. (This prevents an extended break in tablet taking which may increase the risk of the ovaries releasing an egg and thus reducing contraceptive protection). The patient will not have a period until the end of 2 packs but this is not harmful nor does it matter if she experiences some bleeding on tablet taking days.

Interactions: Irregular cycles and reduced reliability of oral contraceptives may occur when these preparations are used concomitantly with drugs such as anticonvulsants, barbiturates, antibiotics, (e.g. tetracyclines, ampicillin, rifampicin, etc), griseofulvin, activated charcoal and certain laxatives. Special consideration should be given to patients being treated with antibiotics for acne. They should be advised to use a non-hormonal method of contraception, or to use an oral contraceptive containing a progestogen showing minimal androgenicity, which have been reported as helping to improve acne without using an antibiotic. Oral contraceptives may diminish glucose tolerance and increase the need for insulin or other antidiabetic drugs in diabetics.

Pregnancy and lactation: BiNovum is contra-indicated for use during pregnancy or suspected pregnancy, since it has been suggested that combined oral contraceptives, in common with many other substances, might be capable of affecting the normal development of the child in the early stages of pregnancy. It can be concluded, however, that, if a risk of abnormality exists at all, it must be very small.

Mothers who are breast-feeding should be advised not to use the combined pill since this may reduce the amount of breast-milk, but may be advised instead to use a progestogen-only pill (POP).

Effects on ability to drive and use machines: Not applicable.

Undesirable effects: Various adverse reactions have been associated with oral contraceptive use. The first appearance of symptoms indicative of any one of these reactions necessitates immediate cessation of oral contraceptive use while appropriate diagnostic and therapeutic measures are undertaken.

Serious adverse reactions:

- There is a general opinion, based on statistical evidence that users of combined oral contraceptives experience more often than non-users various disorders of the coagulation. How often these disorders occur in users of modern low-oestrogen oral contraceptives is unknown, but there are reasons for suggesting that they may occur less often than with the older types of pill which contain more oestrogen.
- Various reports have associated oral contraceptive use with the occurrence of deep venous thrombosis, pulmonary embolism and other embolisms. Other investigations of these oral contraceptives have suggested an increased risk of oestrogen and/or progestogen dose-dependent coronary and cerebrovascular accidents, predominantly in heavy smokers. Thrombosis has very rarely been reported to occur in other veins or arteries, e.g. hepatic, mesenteric, renal or retinal.

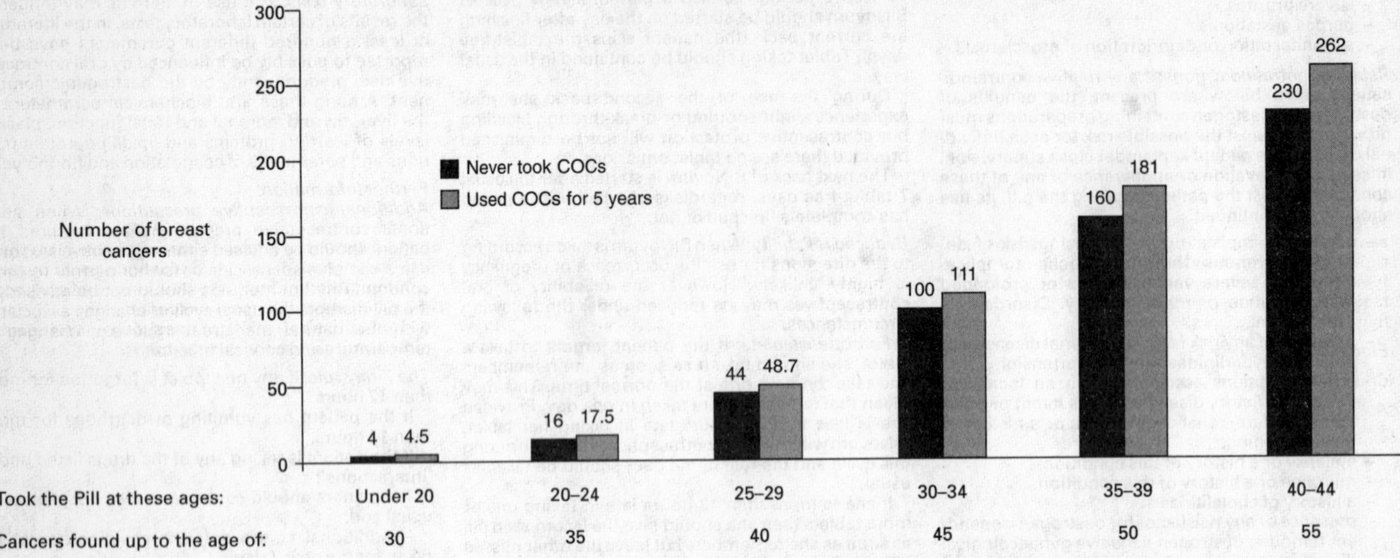

- It should be noted that there is no consensus about often contradictory findings obtained in early studies. The physician should bear in mind the possibility of vascular accidents occurring and that there may not be full recovery from such disorders and they may be fatal. The physician should take into account the presence of risk factors for arterial disease and deep venous thrombosis when prescribing oral contraceptives. Risk factors for arterial disease include smoking, the presence of hyperlipidaemia, hypertension or diabetes.
- Signs and symptoms of a thrombotic event may include: sudden severe pain in the chest, whether or not reaching to the left arm; sudden breathlessness; and unusual severe, prolonged headache, especially if it occurs for the first time or gets progressively worse, or is associated with any of the following symptoms: sudden partial or complete loss of vision or diplopia, aphasia, vertigo, a bad fainting attack or collapse with or without focal epilepsy, weakness or very marked numbness suddenly affecting one side or one part of the body, motor disturbances; severe pain in the calf of one leg; acute abdomen.
- Cigarette smoking increases the risk of serious cardiovascular adverse reactions to oral contraceptive use. The risk increases with age and with heavy smoking and is more marked in women over 35 years of age. Women who use oral contraceptives should be strongly advised not to smoke.
- The use of oestrogen-containing oral contraceptives may promote growth of existing sex steroid dependent tumours. For this reason, the use of these oral contraceptives in patients with such tumours is contraindicated. Numerous epidemiological studies have been reported on the risk of ovarian, endometrial, cervical and breast cancer in women using combined oral contraceptives.
- The evidence is clear that combined oral contraceptives offer substantial protection against both ovarian and endometrial cancer. An increased risk of cervical cancer in long term users of combined oral contraceptives has been reported in some studies, but there continues to be controversy about the extent to which this is attributable to the confounding effects of sexual behaviour and other factors.
- A meta-analysis from 54 epidemiological studies reported that there is a slightly increased relative risk (RR = 1.24) of having breast cancer diagnosed in women who are currently using combined oral contraceptives (COCs). The observed pattern of increased risk may be due to an earlier diagnosis of breast cancer in COC users, the biological effects of COCs or a combination of both. The additional breast cancers diagnosed in current users of COCs or in women who have used COCs in the last 10 years are more likely to be localised to the breast than those in women who never used COCs.
- Breast cancer is rare among women under 40 years of age whether or not they take COCs. Whilst this background risk increases with age, the excess number of breast cancer diagnoses in current and recent COC users is small in relation to the overall risk of breast cancer (see bar chart).
- The most important risk factor for breast cancer in COC users is the age women discontinue the COC; the older the age at stopping, the more breast cancers are diagnosed. Duration of use is less important and the excess risk gradually disappears during the course of the 10 years after stopping COC use such that by 10 years there appears to be no excess.
- The possible increase in risk of breast cancer should be discussed with the user and weighed against the benefits of COCs taking into account the evidence that they offer substantial protection against the risk of developing certain other cancers (e.g. ovarian and endometrial cancer).
- Malignant hepatic tumours have been reported on rare occasions in long-term users of oral contraceptives. Benign hepatic tumours have also been associated with oral contraceptive usage. A hepatic tumour should be considered in the differential diagnosis when upper abdominal pain, enlarged liver or signs of intra-abdominal haemorrhage occur.
- The use of oral contraceptives may sometimes lead to the development of cholestatic jaundice or cholelithiasis.
- On rare occasions the use of oral contraceptives may trigger or reactivate systemic lupus erythematosus.
- A further rare complication of oral contraceptive use is the occurrence of chorea which can be reversed by discontinuing the pill. The majority of cases of oral contraceptive-induced chorea show a pre-existing predisposition which often relates to acute rheumatism.

Other adverse reactions:

Cardiovascular system: Rise of blood pressure. If hypertension develops, treatment should be discontinued.

Genital tract: Intermenstrual bleeding, post-medication amenorrhoea, changes in cervical secretion, increase in size of uterine fibromyomata, aggravation of endometriosis, certain vaginal infections, e.g. candidiasis.

Breast: Tenderness, pain, enlargement, secretion.

Gastro-intestinal tract: Nausea, vomiting, cholelithiasis, cholestatic jaundice.

Skin: Erythema nodosum, rash, chloasma, erythema multiforme, hirsutism, loss of scalp hair.

Eyes: Discomfort of the cornea if contact lenses are used.

CNS: Headache, migraine, mood changes, depression.

Metabolic: Fluid retention, change in body weight, reduced glucose tolerance.

Other: Changes in libido, leg cramp, premenstrual-like syndrome.

Overdose: There have been no reports of serious ill-health from overdosage even when a considerable number of tablets have been taken by a small child. In general, it is therefore unnecessary to treat overdosage. However, if overdosage is discovered within two or three hours and is large, then gastric lavage can be safely used. There are no antidotes and further treatment should be symptomatic.

Pharmacological properties

Pharmacodynamic properties: BiNovum Oral Contraceptive Tablets act through the mechanism of gonadotrophin suppression by the oestrogenic and progestational actions of the ethinyloestradiol and norethisterone. The primary mechanism of action is inhibition of ovulation, but alterations to the cervical mucus and to the endometrium may also contribute to the efficacy of the product.

Pharmacokinetic properties: Norethisterone and ethinyloestradiol are absorbed from the gastro-intestinal tract and metabolised in the liver. To obtain maximal contraceptive effectiveness the tablet should be taken as directed and at approximately the same time each day.

Because the active ingredients are metabolised in the liver, reduced contraceptive efficacy has been associated with concomitant use of oral contraceptives and rifampicin. A similar association has been suggested with oral contraceptives and barbiturates, phenytoin sodium, phenylbutazone, griseofulvin and ampicillin.

Preclinical safety data: The toxicology of norethisterone and ethinyloestradiol has been extensively investigated in animal studies and through long term clinical experience with widespread use in contraceptives.

Pharmaceutical particulars

List of excipients:
Lactose
Magnesium stearate
Pregelatinised starch
Methanol (does not appear in final product)
Purified water (peach coloured tablets only; does not appear in final product)
FD & C yellow No 6 (peach coloured tablets only)

Incompatibilities (major): Not applicable.

Shelf-life: Three years.

Special precautions for storage: Store at room temperature (below 25°C). Protect from light.

Nature and contents of container: Carton containing 3 PVC/foil blister strips of 21 tablets each.

Marketing authorisation number 0242/0208

Date of approval/revision of SPC 18 March 1996/ January 1998.

Legal category POM.

CILEST* 250/35 ORAL CONTRACEPTIVE TABLETS

Qualitative and quantitative composition Cilest are tablets for oral administration.

Each tablet contains norgestimate 0.25 mg and ethinyloestradiol PhEur 0.035 mg.

Pharmaceutical form Tablets (small, round, dark blue, engraved 'C 250' on both faces).

Clinical particulars

Therapeutic indications: Contraception and the recognised indications for such oestrogen/progestogen combinations.

Posology and method of administration: For oral administration.

Adults: It is preferable that tablet intake from the first pack is started on the first day of menstruation in which case no extra contraceptive precautions are necessary.

If menstruation has already begun (that is 2, 3 or 4 days previously), tablet taking should commence on day 5 of the menstrual period. In this case additional contraceptive precautions must be taken for the first 7 days of tablet taking.

If menstruation began more than 5 days previously then the patient should be advised to wait until her next menstrual period before starting to take Cilest.

How to take Cilest: One tablet is taken daily at the same time (preferably in the evening) without interruption for 21 days, followed by a break of 7 tablet-free days. Each subsequent pack is started after the 7 tablet-free days have elapsed. Additional contraceptive precautions are not then required.

Elderly: Not applicable.

Children: Not recommended

Absolute contra-indications:

- pregnancy or suspected pregnancy (that cannot yet be excluded).
- circulatory disorders (cardiovascular or cerebrovascular) such as thrombophlebitis and thromboembolic processes (or a history of these conditions), moderate to severe hypertension, hyperlipoproteinaemia. In addition the presence of more than one of the risk factors for arterial disease.
- severe liver disease, cholestatic jaundice or hepatitis (viral or non-viral) or a history of these conditions if the results of liver function tests have failed to return to normal, and for 3 months after liver function tests have been found to be normal; a history of jaundice of pregnancy or jaundice due to the use of steroids, Rotor syndrome and Dubin-Johnson syndrome, hepatic cell tumours and porphyria.
- cholelithiasis.
- known or suspected oestrogen-dependent tumours; endometrial hyperplasia; undiagnosed vaginal bleeding.
- systemic lupus erythematosus or a history of this condition.
- a history during pregnancy or previous use of steroids of:
- severe pruritus.
- herpes gestationis.
- a manifestation or deterioration of otosclerosis.

Relative contra-indications: If any relative contraindications listed below is present, the benefits of oestrogen/progestogen-containing preparations must be weighed against the possible risk for each individual case and the patient kept under close supervision. In case of aggravation or appearance of any of these conditions whilst the patient is taking the pill, its use should be discontinued.

- conditions implicating an increasing risk of developing venous thrombo-embolic complications, e.g. severe varicose veins or prolonged immobilisation or major surgery.
- disorders of coagulation.
- presence of any risk factor for arterial disease e.g. smoking, hyperlipidaemia or hypertension.
- other conditions associated with an increased risk of circulatory disease such as latent or overt cardiac failure, renal dysfunction, or a history of these conditions.
- epilepsy or a history of this condition.
- migraine or a history of this condition.
- a history of cholelithiasis.
- presence of any risk factor for oestrogen-dependent tumours; oestrogen-sensitive gynaecological disorders such as uterine fibromyomata and endometriosis.
- diabetes mellitus.
- severe depression or a history of this condition. If this is accompanied by a disturbance in tryptophan metabolism, administration of vitamin B6 might be of therapeutic value.
- sickle cell haemoglobinopathy, since under certain circumstances, e.g. during infections or anoxia, oestrogen-containing preparations may induce thromboembolic process in patients with this condition.
- if the results of liver function tests become abnormal, use should be discontinued.

Special warnings and special precautions for use:
Post partum administration: Following a vaginal delivery, oral contraceptive administration to non-breast-feeding mothers can be started 21 days post-partum provided the patient is fully ambulant and there are no puerperal complications. No additional contraceptive precautions are required. If post-partum administration begins more than 21 days after delivery, additional contraceptive precautions are required for the first 7 days of pill-taking.

If intercourse has taken place post-partum, oral contraceptive use should be delayed until the first day of the first menstrual period.

After miscarriage or abortion administration should start immediately in which case no additional contraceptive precautions are required.

Changing from a 21 day pill or another 22 day pill to Cilest: All tablets in the old pack should be finished. The first Cilest tablet is taken the next day i.e. no gap is left between taking tablets nor does the patient need to wait for her period to begin. Tablets should be taken as instructed in 'How to take Cilest'. Additional contraceptive precautions are not required. The patient will not have a period until the end of the first Cilest pack, but this is not harmful, nor does it matter if she experiences some bleeding on tablet-taking days.

Changing from a combined every day pill (28 day tablets) to Cilest: Cilest should be started after taking the last active tablet from the 'Every day Pill' pack (i.e. after taking 21 or 22 tablets). The first Cilest tablet is taken the next day i.e. no gap is left between taking tablets nor does the patient need to wait for her period to begin. Tablets should be taken as instructed in 'How to take Cilest'. Additional contraceptive precautions are not required. Remaining tablets from the every day (ED) pack should be discarded.

The patient will not have a period until the end of the first Cilest pack, but this is not harmful, nor does it matter if she experiences some bleeding on tablet-taking days.

Changing from a progestogen-only pill (POP or mini pill) to Cilest: The first Cilest tablet should be taken on the first day of the period, even if the patient has already taken a mini pill on that day. Tablets should be taken as instructed in 'How to take Cilest'. Additional contraceptive precautions are not required. All the remaining progestogen-only pills in the mini pill pack should be discarded.

If the patient is taking a mini pill, then she may not always have a period, especially when she is breast-feeding. The first Cilest tablet should be taken on the day after stopping the mini pill. All remaining pills in the mini pill packet must be discarded. Additional contraceptive precautions must be taken for the first 7 days.

To skip a period: To skip a period, a new pack of Cilest should be started on the day after finishing the current pack (the patient skips the tablet-free days). Tablet-taking should be continued in the usual way.

During the use of the second pack she may experience slight spotting or break-through bleeding but contraceptive protection will not be diminished provided there are no tablet omissions.

The next pack of Cilest is started after the usual 7 tablet-free days, regardless of whether the period has completely finished or not.

Reduced reliability: When Cilest is taken according to the directions for use the occurrence of pregnancy is highly unlikely. However, the reliability of oral contraceptives may be reduced under the following circumstances:

Forgotten tablets: If the patient forgets to take a tablet, she should take it as soon as she remembers and take the next one at the normal time. This may mean that two tablets are taken in one day. Provided she is less than 12 hours late in taking her tablet, Cilest will still give contraceptive protection during this cycle and the rest of the pack should be taken as usual.

If she is more than 12 hours late in taking one or more tablets then she should take the last missed pill as soon as she remembers but leave the other missed pills in the pack. She should continue to take the rest of the pack as usual but must use extra precautions (e.g. sheath, diaphragm, plus spermicide) and follow the '7-day rule' (see Further Information for the 7 day rule).

If there are 7 or more pills left in the pack after the missed and delayed pills then the usual 7-day break can be left before starting the next pack. If there are less than 7 pills left in the pack after the missed and delayed pills then when the pack is finished the next pack should be started the next day. If withdrawal bleeding does not occur at the end of the second pack then a pregnancy test should be performed.

Vomiting or diarrhoea: If after tablet intake vomiting or diarrhoea occurs, a tablet may not be absorbed properly by the body. If the symptoms disappear within 12 hours of tablet-taking, the patient should take an extra tablet from a spare pack and continue with the rest of the pack as usual.

However, if the symptoms continue beyond those 12 hours, additional contraceptive precautions are necessary for any sexual intercourse during the stomach or bowel upset and for the following 7 days (the patient must be advised to follow the '7-day rule').

Change in bleeding pattern: If after taking Cilest for several months there is a sudden occurrence of spotting or breakthrough bleeding (not observed in previous cycles) or the absence of withdrawal bleeding, contraceptive effectiveness may be reduced. If withdrawal bleeding fails to occur and none of the above mentioned events has taken place, pregnancy is highly unlikely and oral contraceptive use can be continued until the end of the next pack.

(If withdrawal bleeding fails to occur at the end of the second cycle, tablet intake should be discontinued and pregnancy excluded before oral contraceptive use can be resumed). However, if withdrawal bleeding is absent and any of the above mentioned events has occurred, tablet intake should be discontinued and pregnancy excluded before oral contraceptive use can be resumed.

Medical examination/consultation: A complete medical history and physical examination should be taken prior to the initiation or reinstitution of oral contraceptives and should be repeated periodically.

These physical examinations should include special reference to blood pressure, breasts, abdomen and pelvic organs, including cervical cytology and, where indicated by the medical or family history, relevant laboratory tests. Caution should be observed when prescribing oral contraceptives to young women whose cycles are not yet stabilised.

Surgery, varicose veins or immobilisation: In patients using oestrogen-containing preparations the risk of deep vein thrombosis may be temporarily increased when undergoing a major operation (e.g. abdominal, orthopaedic), and surgery to the legs, medical treatment for varicose veins or prolonged immobilisation. Therefore, it is advisable to discontinue oral contraceptive use at least 4 to 6 weeks prior to these procedures if performed electively and to (re)start not less than 2 weeks after full ambulation. The latter is also valid with regard to immobilisation after an accident or emergency surgery. In case of emergency surgery, thrombotic prophylaxis is usually indicated e.g. with subcutaneous heparin.

Chloasma: Chloasma may occasionally occur, especially in women with a history of chloasma gravidarum. Women with a tendency to chloasma should avoid exposure to the sun or ultraviolet radiation whilst taking this preparation. Chloasma is often not fully reversible.

Laboratory tests: The use of steroids may influence the results of certain laboratory tests. In the literature, at least a hundred different parameters have been reported to possibly be influenced by oral contraceptive use, predominantly by the oestrogenic component. Among these are: biochemical parameters of the liver, thyroid, adrenal and renal function, plasma levels of (carrier) proteins and lipid/lipoprotein fractions and parameters of coagulation and fibrinolysis.

Further information:
Additional contraceptive precautions: When additional contraceptive precautions are required the patient should be advised either not to have sex, or to use a cap plus spermicide or for her partner to use a condom. Rhythm methods should not be advised as the pill disrupts the usual cyclical changes associated with the natural menstrual cycle e.g. changes in temperature and cervical mucus.

The 7-day rule: If any one tablet is forgotten for more than 12 hours.

If the patient has vomiting or diarrhoea for more than 12 hours.

If the patient is taking any of the drugs listed under 'Interactions':

The patient should continue to take her tablets as usual and:

– Additional contraceptive precautions must be taken for the next 7 days.

But–if these 7 days run beyond the end of the current pack: the next pack must be started as soon as the current one is finished, i.e. no gap should be left between packs. (This prevents an extended break in tablet taking which may increase the risk of the ovaries releasing an egg and thus reducing contraceptive protection). The patient will not have a period until the end of 2 packs but this is not harmful nor does it matter if she experiences some bleeding on tablet taking days.

Interaction with other medicaments and other forms of interaction: Irregular cycles and reduced reliability of oral contraceptives may occur when these preparations are used concomitantly with drugs such as anticonvulsants, barbiturates, antibiotics, (e.g. tetracyclines, ampicillin, rifampicin, etc), griseofulvin, activated charcoal and certain laxatives. Special consideration should be given to patients being treated with antibiotics for acne. They should be advised to use a non-hormonal method of contracep-

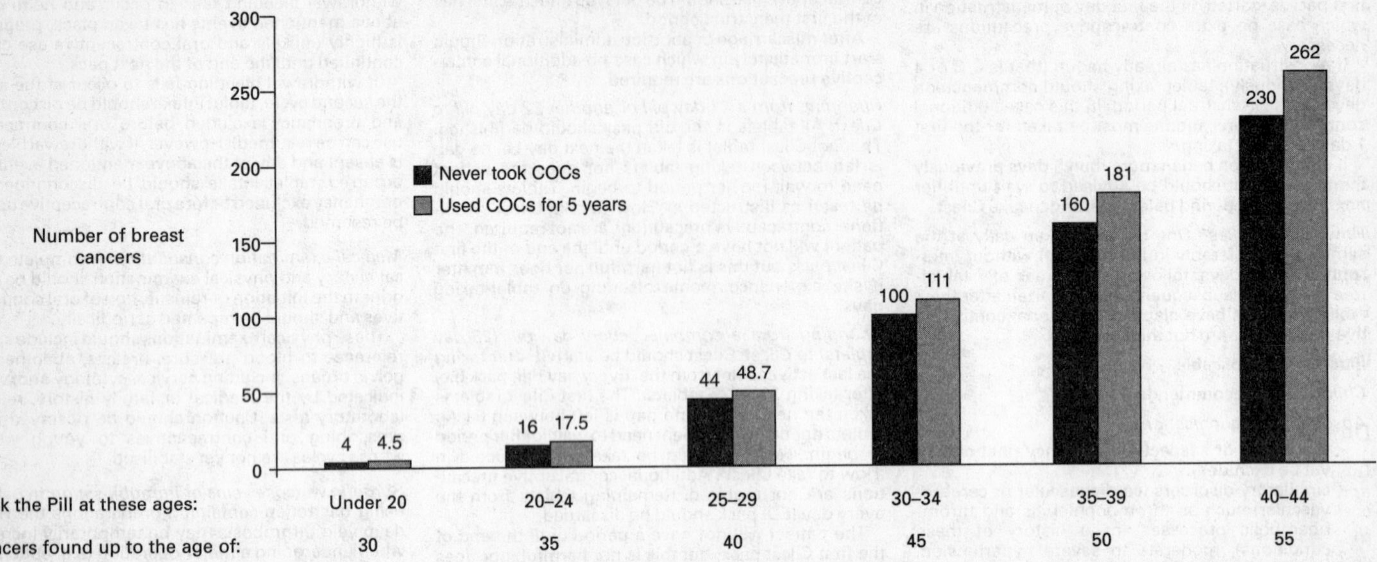

tion, or to use an oral contraceptive containing a progestogen showing minimal androgenicity, which have been reported as helping to improve acne without using an antibiotic. Oral contraceptives may diminish glucose tolerance and increase the need for insulin or other antidiabetic drugs in diabetics.

Pregnancy and lactation: Cilest is contra-indicated for use during pregnancy or suspected pregnancy, since it has been suggested that combined oral contraceptives, in common with many other substances, might be capable of affecting the normal development of the child in the early stages of pregnancy. It can be definitely concluded, however, that, if a risk of abnormality exists at all, it must be very small.

Mothers who are breast-feeding should be advised not to use the combined pill since this may reduce the amount of breast-milk, but may be advised instead to use a progestogen-only pill (POP).

Effects on ability to drive and use machines: Not applicable.

Undesirable effects: Various adverse reactions have been associated with oral contraceptive use. The first appearance of symptoms indicative of any one of these reactions necessitates immediate cessation of oral contraceptive use while appropriate diagnostic and therapeutic measures are undertaken.

Serious adverse reactions:

- There is a general opinion, based on statistical evidence, that users of combined oral contraceptives experience more often than non-users various disorders of the coagulation. How often these disorders occur in users of modern low-oestrogen oral contraceptives is unknown, but there are reasons for suggesting that they may occur less often than with the older types of pill which contain more oestrogen.
- Various reports have associated oral contraceptive use with the occurrence of deep venous thrombosis, pulmonary embolism and other embolisms. Other investigations of these oral contraceptives have suggested an increased risk of oestrogen and/or progestogen dose-dependent coronary and cerebrovascular accidents, predominantly in heavy smokers. Thrombosis has very rarely been reported to occur in other veins or arteries, e.g. hepatic, mesenteric, renal or retinal.
- It should be noted that there is no consensus about often contradictory findings obtained in early studies. The physician should bear in mind the possibility of vascular accidents occurring and that there may not be full recovery from such disorders and they may be fatal. The physician should take into account the presence of risk factors for arterial disease and deep venous thrombosis when prescribing oral contraceptives. Risk factors for arterial disease include smoking, the presence of hyperlipidaemia, hypertension or diabetes.
- Signs and symptoms of a thrombotic event may include: sudden severe pain in the chest, whether or not reaching to the left arm; sudden breathlessness; and unusual severe, prolonged headache, especially if it occurs for the first time or gets progressively worse, or is associated with any of the following symptoms: sudden partial or complete loss of vision or diplopia, aphasia, vertigo, a bad fainting attack or collapse with or without focal epilepsy, weakness or very marked numbness suddenly affecting one side or one part of the body, motor disturbances; severe pain in the calf of one leg; acute abdomen.

  Cigarette smoking increases the risk of serious cardiovascular adverse reactions to oral contraceptive use. The risk increases with age and with heavy smoking and is more marked in women over 35 years of age. Women who use oral contraceptives should be strongly advised not to smoke.
- The use of oestrogen-containing oral contraceptives may promote growth of existing sex steroid dependent tumours. For this reason, the use of these oral contraceptives in patients with such tumours is contraindicated. Numerous epidemiological studies have been reported on the risk of ovarian, endometrial, cervical and breast cancer in women using combined oral contraceptives. The evidence is clear that combined oral contraceptives offer substantial protection against both ovarian and endometrial cancer. An increased risk of cervical cancer in long term users of combined oral contraceptives has been reported in some studies, but there continues to be controversy about the extent to which this is attributable to the confounding effects of sexual behaviour and other factors.
- A meta-analysis from 54 epidemiological studies reported that there is a slightly increased relative risk (RR = 1.24) of having breast cancer diagnosed in women who are currently using combined oral contraceptives (COCs). The observed pattern of increased risk may be due to an earlier diagnosis of breast cancer in COC users, the biological effects of COCs or a combination of both. The additional breast cancers diagnosed in current users of COCs or in women who have used COCs in the last 10 years are more likely to be localised to the breast than those in women who never used COCs.
- Breast cancer is rare among women under 40 years of age whether or not they take COCs. Whilst this background risk increases with age, the excess number of breast cancer diagnoses in current and recent COC users is small in relation to the overall risk of breast cancer (see bar chart).
- The most important risk factor for breast cancer in COC users is the age women discontinue the COC; the older the age at stopping, the more breast cancers are diagnosed. Duration of use is less important and the excess risk gradually disappears during the course of the 10 years after stopping COC use such that by 10 years there appears to be no excess.
- The possible increase in risk of breast cancer should be discussed with the user and weighed against the benefits of COCs taking into account the evidence that they offer substantial protection against the risk of developing certain other cancers (e.g. ovarian and endometrial cancer).
- Malignant hepatic tumours have been reported on rare occasions in long-term users of oral contraceptives. Benign hepatic tumours have also been associated with oral contraceptive usage. A hepatic tumour should be considered in the differential diagnosis when upper abdominal pain, enlarged liver or signs of intra-abdominal haemorrhage occur.
- The use of oral contraceptives may sometimes lead to the development of cholestatic jaundice or cholelithiasis.
- On rare occasions the use of oral contraceptives may trigger or reactivate systemic lupus erythematosus.
- A further rare complication of oral contraceptive use is the occurrence of chorea which can be reversed by discontinuing the pill. The majority of cases of oral contraceptive-induced chorea show a pre-existing predisposition which often relates to acute rheumatism.

Other adverse reactions:

Cardiovascular system: Rise of blood pressure. If hypertension develops, treatment should be discontinued.

Genital tract: Intermenstrual bleeding, post-medication amenorrhoea, changes in cervical secretion, increase in size of uterine fibromyomata, aggravation of endometriosis, certain vaginal infections, e.g. candidiasis.

Breast: Tenderness, pain, enlargement, secretion.

Gastro-intestinal tract: Nausea, vomiting, cholelithiasis, cholestatic jaundice.

Skin: Erythema nodosum, rash, chloasma, erythema multiforme.

Eyes: Discomfort of the cornea if contact lenses are used.

CNS: Headache, migraine, mood changes, depression.

Metabolic: Fluid retention, change in body weight, reduced glucose tolerance.

Other: Changes in libido.

Overdose: There have been no reports of serious ill-health from overdosage even when a considerable number of tablets have been taken by a small child. In general, it is therefore unnecessary to treat overdosage. However, if overdosage is discovered within two or three hours and is large, then gastric lavage can be safely used. There are no antidotes and further treatment should be symptomatic.

Pharmacological properties

Pharmacodynamic properties: Cilest acts through the mechanism of gonadotrophin suppression by the oestrogenic and progestational actions of ethinyloestradiol and norgestimate. The primary mechanism of action is inhibition of ovulation, but alterations to the cervical mucus and to the endometrium may also contribute to the efficacy of the product.

Pharmacokinetic properties: Norgestimate and ethinyloestradiol are absorbed from the gastro-intestinal tract and metabolised in the liver. To obtain maximal contraceptive effectiveness the tablets should be taken as directed and at approximately the same time each day.

Because the active ingredients are metabolised in the liver, reduced contraceptive efficacy has been associated with concomitant use of oral contraceptives and rifampicin. A similar association has been suggested with oral contraceptives and barbiturates, phenytoin sodium, phenylbutazone, griseofulvin and ampicillin.

Preclinical safety data: The toxicology of norgestimate and ethinyloestradiol has been extensively investigated in animal studies and through long term clinical experience with widespread use in contraceptives.

Pharmaceutical particulars
List of excipients: Lactose (anhydrous); magnesium stearate; pregelatinised starch; F.D. & C. Blue No. 2 Lake; methanol (does not appear in final product).

Incompatibilities (major): Not applicable.

Shelf-life: Three years.

Special precautions for storage: Store at room temperature (below 25°C). Protect from light.

Nature and contents of container: Carton containing 3 PVC/foil blister strips of 21 tablets each.

Marketing authorisation number 0242/0209

Date of approval/revision of the text 18 November 1995/January 1998.

Legal category POM.

DAKTACORT*

Qualitative and quantitative composition *Cream and ointment:* miconazole nitrate 2% w/w and hydrocortisone 1% w/w.

Pharmaceutical form *Cream:* White, homogenous cream. *Ointment:* White, odourless, fatty ointment.

Clinical particulars
Therapeutic indications: For the topical treatment of inflamed dermatoses where infection by susceptible organisms and inflammation co-exist, eg intertrigo and infected eczema.

Moist or dry eczema or dermatitis including atopic eczema, primary irritant or contact allergic eczema or seborrhoeic eczema including that associated with acne.

Intertriginous eczema including inframammary intertrigo, perianal and genital dermatitis.

Organisms which are susceptible to miconazole are dermatophytes and pathogenic yeasts (eg *Candida* spp.). Also many Gram-positive bacteria including most strains of *Streptococcus* and *Staphylococcus*.

The properties of Daktacort indicate it particularly for the initial stages of treatment. Once the inflammatory symptoms have disappeared (after about 7 days), treatment can be continued where necessary with Daktarin Cream or Daktarin Powder.

Posology and method of administration: For topical administration.

Cream: Apply the cream two or three times a day to the affected area, rubbing in gently until the cream has been absorbed by the skin.

Ointment: Daktacort ointment should be applied topically two or three times daily.

The same dosage applies to both adults and children.

Use in elderly: Natural thinning of the skin occurs in the elderly, hence corticosteroids should be used sparingly and for short periods of time.

In infants, long term continuous topical corticosteroid therapy should be avoided.

If after about 7 days' application, no improvement has occurred, cultural isolation of the offending organism should be followed by appropriate local or systemic antimicrobial therapy.

Contra-indications: True hypersensitivity to any of the ingredients. Tubercular or viral infections of the skin or those caused by Gram-negative bacteria.

Special warnings and precautions for use: As with any topical corticosteroid, care is advised with infants and children when Daktacort is to be applied to extensive surface areas or under occlusive dressings including baby napkins; similarly, application to the face should be avoided.

In infants, long term continuous topical corticosteroid therapy should be avoided. Adrenal suppression can occur even without occlusion.

Interaction with other medicaments and other forms of interaction: None known.

Pregnancy and lactation: In animals, miconazole nitrate has shown no teratogenic effects but is foetotoxic at high oral doses and administration of corticosteroids to pregnant animals can cause abnormalities of foetal development. The relevance of these findings to humans has not been established. However, combinations of topical steroids with imidazoles should be used in pregnant women only if the practitioner considers it to be necessary.

Effects on ability to drive and use machines: None known.

Undesirable effects: Rarely, local sensitivity may occur requiring discontinuation of treatment.

Overdose: Topically applied corticosteroids can be absorbed in sufficient amounts to produce systemic effects. If accidental ingestion of large quantities of the product occurs, an appropriate method of gastric emptying may be used if considered necessary.

Pharmacological properties
Pharmacodynamic properties: Miconazole nitrate is active against dermatophytes and pathogenic yeasts, and many gram-positive bacteria. Hydrocortisone has anti-inflammatory activity.

Pharmacokinetic properties: Not applicable.

Preclinical safety data: Not applicable.

Pharmaceutical particulars
List of excipients:

Cream: PEG-6, PEG-32 and glycol stearate; polyoxyethylene glycol glycerides; mineral oil; benzoic acid; disodium edetate; butylated hydroxyanisole; purified water.

Ointment: Polyethylene 5.5% liquid paraffin.

Incompatibilities: None known.

Shelf life: 36 months.

Special precautions for storage: Cream: Store in a refrigerator (2-8°C).

Ointment: Store at or below 25°C.

Nature and contents of container: Aluminium tube with polypropylene cap.

Cream: Each tube contains 30 g cream.

Ointment: Each tube contains 30 g ointment.

Instructions for use/handling: None.

Marketing authorisation numbers
Daktacort Cream 0242/0042
Daktacort Ointment 0242/0130

Date of approval/revision of SPC
Cream: April 1997
Ointment: April 1998

Legal category POM.

DAKTARIN* CREAM

Presentation White, non-staining, water miscible cream containing miconazole nitrate PhEur 2% w/w. The cream also contains macrogol stearate, glycol stearate, unsaturated polyglycolysed glycerides, liquid paraffin, benzoic acid (E210), butylated hydroxyanisole (E320) and purified water.

Uses Miconazole nitrate is a synthetic imidazole antifungal agent with a broad spectrum of activity against pathogenic fungi (including yeasts and dermatophytes) and Gram-positive bacteria (*Staphylococcus* and *Streptococcus* spp.). Daktarin cream is used for the topical treatment of fungal infections of the skin and super infections due to Gram-positive bacteria.

These include athlete's foot, ringworm (tinea infections), intertrigo, candida nappy rash, paronychia, erythrasma, fungal infection of the outer ear and pityriasis versicolor. Daktarin cream may also be used for nail infections.

Dosage and administration The dosage is the same for all ages.

In skin infections, apply to the affected area twice daily. In nail infections, apply to the infected nail(s) once or twice daily.

To prevent relapse, treatment should be continued for ten days after all the lesions have disappeared.

Use in elderly: As above.

Contra-indications, warnings, etc
Contra-indications: None stated.

Use in pregnancy: In animals, miconazole nitrate has shown no teratogenic effects but is foetotoxic at high oral doses. Only small amounts of miconazole nitrate are absorbed following topical administration. However, as with other imidazoles, miconazole nitrate should be used with caution during pregnancy.

Side effects: Occasionally irritation has been reported. Rarely local sensitisation or hypersensitivity may occur in which case administration of the product should be discontinued.

Overdosage: Daktarin cream is intended for topical use. If accidental ingestion of large quantities of the product occurs, an appropriate method of gastric emptying may be used if considered desirable.

Pharmaceutical precautions Store at 25°C or below.

Legal category P.

Package quantities 30 g tube.

Further information A leaflet outlining to the patient the hygiene routines to be observed and the correct method of application of Daktarin is included in each pack of cream.

Product licence number 0242/0016

DAKTARIN* ORAL GEL

Qualitative and quantitative composition Each gram of Daktarin Oral Gel contains 20 mg of miconazole.

Pharmaceutical form White gel with orange taste.

Clinical particulars
Therapeutic indications: Oral treatment and prevention of fungal infections of the oropharynx and gastrointestinal tract, and of superinfections due to gram-positive bacteria.

Posology and method of administration: For oral administration.

Dosage is based on 15 mg/kg/day (0.625 ml/kg/day).
Adults: 1–2 spoonfuls of gel four times per day.
Elderly: As for adults.
Children aged 6 years and over: One spoonful of gel four times per day.
Children aged 2-6 years: One spoonful of gel twice per day.
Infants under 2 years: Half a spoonful of gel twice per day.

Alternatively, in localised lesions of the mouth, a small amount of gel may be applied directly to the affected area with a clean finger.

For topical treatment of the oropharynx, the gel should be kept in the mouth for as long as possible.

Treatment should be continued for up to 2 days after the symptoms have cleared.

For oral candidosis, dental prostheses should be removed at night and brushed with the gel.

Contra-indications: Known hypersensitivity to miconazole or to any of the excipients. Liver dysfunction. The drugs terfenadine, astemizole and cisapride should not be given concurrently with Daktarin Oral Gel. (See also interactions.)

Special warnings and precautions for use: If the concomitant use of Daktarin and anticoagulants is envisaged, the anti-coagulant effect should be carefully monitored and titrated. It is advisable to monitor miconazole and phenytoin levels, if they are used concomitantly.

Interaction with other medicaments and other forms of interaction: Miconazole can inhibit the metabolism of drugs metabolised by the cytochrome P450-3A and -2C9 families. This can result in an increase and/or prolongation of their effects, including side effects. Examples are:

- terfenadine, astemizole and cisapride. The metabolism of these drugs was inhibited by miconazole in *in vitro* studies. Therefore, they should not be used in patients treated with Daktarin Oral Gel.

- oral anticoagulants, cyclosporin, phenytoin, oral hypoglycaemics and possibly tacrolimus. It is advisable to reduce the dosage of such drugs, if necessary.

Pregnancy and lactation: In animals, miconazole has shown no teratogenic effects but is foetotoxic at high oral doses. The significance of this to man is unknown. However, as with other imidazoles, Daktarin Oral Gel should be avoided in pregnant women if possible. The potential hazards should be balanced against the possible benefits.

It is not known whether miconazole is excreted in human milk. Caution should be exercised when prescribing Daktarin Oral Gel to nursing mothers.

Effects on ability to drive and use machines: Daktarin should not affect alertness or driving ability.

Undesirable effects: Occasionally, nausea and vomiting have been reported, and with long term treatment, diarrhoea. In rare instances, allergic reactions have been reported. There are isolated reports of hepatitis, for which the causal relationship with Daktarin has not been established.

Overdose: Symptoms: In general, miconazole is not highly toxic. In the event of accidental overdosage, vomiting and diarrhoea may occur.

Treatment: Treatment is symptomatic and supportive. A specific antidote is not available.

Pharmacological properties
Pharmacodynamic properties: The active ingredient, miconazole, is a synthetic imidazole anti-fungal agent with a broad spectrum of activity against pathogenic fungi (including yeast and dermatophytes) and gram-positive bacteria (*Staphylococcus* and *Streptococcus* spp). It may act by interfering with the permeability of the fungal cell membranes.

Pharmacokinetic properties: When administered orally, miconazole is incompletely absorbed from the gastrointestinal tract, peak plasma levels of about 1 µg per ml have been achieved after a dose of 1 g per day.

Miconazole is inactivated in the body and 10–20%

of an oral dose is excreted in the urine, mainly as metabolites, within 6 days. About 50% of an oral dose may be excreted unchanged in the faeces.

Preclinical safety data: Not applicable.

Pharmaceutical particulars
List of excipients: Purified water PhEur; Pregelatinised starch PhEur; Alcohol BP; Polysorbate 20 PhEur; Sodium saccharin BP; Arome cacao blanc 43B/IFF; Arome orange 67601/GIV; Glycerin PhEur.

Incompatibilities: None known.

Shelf life: 5 years.

Special precautions for storage: Store at or below 30°C.

Nature and contents of container: Aluminium tubes containing 15 g or 80 g gel.

A 5 ml plastic spoon, marked with a 2.5 ml graduation is provided.

Instructions for use/handling: Not applicable.

Marketing authorisation number 0242/0048

Date of approval/revision of SPC April 1998

Legal category POM/P.
External use: Pharmacy Medicine Only.
Other: Prescription Only Medicine.

DAKTARIN* ORAL TABLETS

Qualitative and quantitative composition Each tablet contains miconazole 250 mg.

Pharmaceutical form Tablet.

Clinical particulars
Therapeutic indications: Oral treatment and prevention of fungal infections of the oropharynx and gastrointestinal tract and of superinfections due to gram-positive bacteria.

Posology and method of administration: For oral administration.

Dosage is based on 15 mg/kg/day.

Daktarin Oral Tablets should be taken after meals.

Adults: One 250 mg tablet four times per day for 10 days, or for up to 2 days after the symptoms have cleared.

Elderly: As for adults.

Children: Use Daktarin Oral Gel.

Topical treatment of the oropharynx may be achieved by sucking the tablet, allowing it to dissolve slowly in the mouth.

Treatment should be continued for up to 2 days after the symptoms have cleared.

Contra-indications: Known hypersensitivity to miconazole or to any of the excipients. Liver dysfunction. The drugs terfenadine, astemizole and cisapride should not be given concurrently with Daktarin Oral Tablets. (See also interactions.)

Special warnings and precautions for use: If the concomitant use of Daktarin and anticoagulants is envisaged, the anti-coagulant effect should be carefully monitored and titrated. It is advisable to monitor miconazole and phenytoin levels, if they are used concomitantly.

Interaction with other medicaments and other forms of interaction: Miconazole can inhibit the metabolism of drugs metabolised by the cytochrome P450-3A and -2C9 families. This can result in an increase and/or prolongation of their effects, including side effects. Examples are:

- terfenadine, astemizole and cisapride. The metabolism of these drugs was inhibited by miconazole in *in vitro* studies. Therefore, they should not be used in patients treated with Daktarin Oral Tablets.
- oral anticoagulants, cyclosporin, phenytoin, oral hypoglycaemics and possibly tacrolimus. It is advisable to reduce the dosage of such drugs, if necessary.

Pregnancy and lactation: In animals, miconazole has shown no teratogenic effects but is foetotoxic at high oral doses. The significance of this to man is unknown. However, as with other imidazoles, Daktarin Oral Tablets should be avoided in pregnant women if possible. The potential hazards should be balanced against the possible benefits.

It is not known whether miconazole is excreted in human milk. Caution should be exercised when prescribing Daktarin Oral Tablets to nursing mothers.

Effects on ability to drive and use machines: Daktarin should not affect alertness or driving ability.

Undesirable effects: Occasionally, nausea and vomiting have been reported, and with long term treatment, diarrhoea. In rare instances, allergic reactions have been reported. There are isolated reports of hepatitis, for which the causal relationship with Daktarin has not been established.

Overdose: Symptoms: In general, miconazole is not highly toxic. In the event of accidental overdosage, vomiting and diarrhoea may occur.

Treatment: Treatment is symptomatic and supportive. A specific antidote is not available.

Pharmacological properties
Pharmacodynamic properties: The active ingredient, miconazole, is a synthetic imidazole anti-fungal agent with a broad spectrum of activity against pathogenic fungi (including yeast and dermatophytes) and gram-positive bacteria (*Staphylococcus* and *Streptococcus* spp). It may act by interfering with the permeability of the fungal cell membranes.

Pharmacokinetic properties: When administered orally, miconazole is incompletely absorbed from the gastrointestinal tract. Peak plasma levels of about 1 μg per ml have been achieved after a dose of 1 g per day.

Miconazole is inactivated in the body and 10-20% of an oral dose is excreted in the urine, mainly as metabolites, within 6 days. About 50% of an oral dose may be excreted unchanged in the faeces.

Preclinical safety data: Not applicable.

Pharmaceutical particulars
List of excipients: Lactose; sucrose; microcrystalline cellulose; maize starch; rice starch; sodium saccharin; polyvidone K90; magnesium stearate; colloidal anhydrous silica; sodium lauryl sulphate; purified water (not present in final product).

Incompatibilities: None known.

Shelf life: 5 years.

Special precautions for storage: None stated.

Nature and contents of container: Blister packs of 20 tablets, comprising aluminium foil; PVC genotherm glass.

Instructions for use/handling: Not applicable.

Marketing authorisation number 0242/0047

Date of approval/revision of SPC September 1997

Legal category POM.

DAKTARIN* POWDER

Qualitative and quantitative composition Daktarin powder contains miconazole nitrate PhEur 2.0% w/w.

Pharmaceutical form Topical powder.

Clinical particulars
Therapeutic indications: For the treatment of mycotic infections of the skin and superinfections due to gram-positive bacteria.

Posology and method of administration: Daktarin powder is for topical administration.

Adults: Twice daily application of powder to the lesions, treatment being prolonged for some 10 days after all lesions have disappeared to prevent relapse.

Elderly and children: As for adults.

Contra-indications: The powder should not be recommended for the treatment of infections of the hair and nails.

Special warnings and precautions for use: None.

Interaction with other medicaments and other forms of interaction: None known.

Pregnancy and lactation: In animals, miconazole nitrate has shown no teratogenic effects but is foetotoxic at high oral doses. Only small amounts of miconazole nitrate are absorbed following topical administration. However, as with other imidazoles, miconazole nitrate should be used with caution during pregnancy.

Effects on ability to drive and use machines: None known.

Undesirable effects: Hypersensitivity has rarely been recorded, if it should occur the treatment should be discontinued.

Overdose: Daktarin powder is intended for topical use. If accidental ingestion of large quantities of product occurs, an appropriate method of gastric emptying may be used if considered desirable.

Pharmacological properties
Pharmacodynamic properties: Miconazole is an imidazole antifungal agent and may act by interfering with the permeability of the fungal cell membrane. It possesses a wide antifungal spectrum and has some antibacterial activity.

Pharmacokinetic properties: There is little absorption through skin or mucous membranes when miconazole nitrate is applied topically.

When administered orally miconazole is incompletely absorbed from the gastro-intestinal tract. Peak plasma concentrations occur at about 4 hours after administration. Miconazole disappears from the plasma in a triphasic manner with a biological half life of about 24 hours. Over 90% is reported to be bound to plasma proteins.

Preclinical safety data: Not applicable.

Pharmaceutical particulars
List of excipients: Talc; zinc oxide; colloidal silicon dioxide.

Incompatibilities: Not applicable.

Shelf life: 5 years.

Special precautions for storage: Store at room temperature.

Nature and contents of container: High density polyethylene bottle with a polypropylene dredger-cap and screw-cap containing 20 gram of powder.

Instructions for use/handling: Not applicable.

Marketing authorisation number 0242/0017

Date of approval/revision of SPC 21 May 1996

Legal category P.

DELFEN* CONTRACEPTIVE FOAM

Qualitative and quantitative composition Contains 12.5% w/w of nonoxynol-9.

Pharmaceutical form Foam.

Clinical particulars
Therapeutic indications: For use as a spermicidal contraceptive in conjunction with barrier methods of contraception.

Posology and method of administration: For topical intravaginal administration.

For use by adult females only.

Insert one applicatorful intravaginally prior to coitus. A fresh application of foam must be made if intercourse is repeated or delayed for more than one hour. The diaphragm must be allowed to remain *in situ* for at least six to eight hours after coitus.

Douching is not recommended, but if desired it should be deferred for at least six hours after intercourse.

Contra-indications: Hypersensitivity to nonoxynol-9 or to any component of the preparation.

Patients with absent vaginal sensation, eg paraplegics and quadriplegics.

Special warnings and special precautions for use: Spermicidal intravaginal preparations are intended for use in conjunction with barrier methods of contraception such as condoms, diaphragms and caps.

Where avoidance of pregnancy is important the choice of contraceptive method should be made in consultation with a doctor or a family planning clinic.

If vaginal or penile irritation occurs discontinue use. If symptoms worsen or continue for more than 48 hours medical advice should be sought.

Interaction with other medicaments and other forms of interaction: None known.

Pregnancy and lactation: There is no evidence from animal and human studies that nonoxynol-9 is teratogenic. Human epidemiological studies have not shown any firm evidence of adverse effects on the foetus, however some studies have shown that nonoxynol-9 may be embryotoxic in animals. This product should not be used if pregnancy is suspected or confirmed. Animal studies have detected nonoxynol-9 in milk after intravaginal administration. Use by lactating women has not been studied.

Effects on ability to drive and use machines: None known.

Undesirable effects: May cause irritation of the vagina or penis.

Overdose: If taken orally the surfactant properties of this preparation may cause gastric irritation. General supportive therapy should be carried out. Hepatic and renal function should be monitored if medically indicated.

Pharmacological properties
Pharmacodynamic properties: The standard *in vitro* test (Sander-Cramer) evaluating the effect of nonoxynol-9 on animal sperm motility has shown the compound to be a potent spermicide.

The site of action of nonoxynol-9 has been determined as the sperm cell membrane. The lipoprotein membrane is disrupted, increasing permeability, with subsequent loss of cell components and decreased motility. A similar effect on vaginal epithelial and bacterial cells is also found.

Pharmacokinetic properties: The intravaginal absorption and excretion of radiolabelled (^{14}C) nonoxynol-9 has been studied in non-pregnant rats and rabbits and in pregnant rats. No appreciable difference was found in the extent or rate of absorption in pregnant and non-pregnant animals. Plasma levels peaked at about one hour and recovery from urine as unchanged nonoxynol-9 accounted for approximately 15-25% and faeces approximately 70% of the administered dose as unchanged nonoxynol-9. Less than 0.3% was found in the milk of lactating rats. No metabolites were detected in any of the samples analysed.

Preclinical safety data: Not applicable.

Pharmaceutical particulars
List of excipients: Acetic acid glacial; benzoic acid (E 210); cetyl alcohol; methyl parahydroxybenzoate (E 218); phosphoric acid; polyvinyl alcohol; propylene glycol; sodium carboxymethylcellulose; stearic acid; diethylaminoethyl stearamide; Van Dyke Perfume No. 6301; purified water; isobutane (propellant).

Incompatibilities: Not applicable.

Shelf life: 3 years.

Special precautions for storage: Store at room temperature (at or below 25°C). Caution: contents under pressure, with flammable propellant. Do not burn or puncture.

Nature and contents of container: Aluminium aerosol can containing a minimum of 20 doses of Delfen foam. An applicator is also provided in the pack.

Instructions for use/handling: Not applicable.

Marketing authorisation number 0242/0211

Date of approval/revision of SPC October 1996.

Legal category GSL.

DROLEPTAN*

Qualitative and quantitative composition *Droleptan Injection:* droperidol 5 mg per ml; *Droleptan Tablets:* each tablet contains droperidol 10 mg per tablet; *Droleptan liquid:* droperidol 1 mg per ml.

Pharmaceutical form *Droleptan Injection:* ampoules; *Droleptan Tablets:* tablet; *Droleptan Liquid:* liquid.

Clinical particulars
Therapeutic indications: Droleptan is a major tranquilliser of the butyrophenone series for use in psychiatry to rapidly calm the manic, agitated patient.

Injection only: In anaesthesia

(a) in conjunction with a narcotic analgesic in the technique of neuroleptanalgesia,

(b) either alone or in combination with a narcotic analgesic for premedication,

(c) for post-operative nausea and vomiting.

For treatment of chemotherapy-induced nausea and vomiting.

Posology and method of administration:
Method of administration: Droleptan Injection: Intravenous (bolus or infusion) or intramuscular injection. *Droleptan Tablets and Liquid:* Oral use.

In psychiatry:

Tablets and Liquid: Adults: 5-20 mg. The dosage may be repeated at intervals of 4-8 hours.

Children: 0.5-1.0 mg/day. Adjust according to response.

Injection: Adults: 5-15 mg iv; up to 10 mg im. The dosage may be repeated at intervals of 4-6 hours (im or iv).

Children: 0.5-1.0 mg/day im adjusted according to response.

In psychiatry, dosage should be determined on an individual basis and is best initiated and titrated under close medical supervision. To determine the initial dose, the patient's age, symptom severity, and previous response to other neuroleptic drugs should be taken into account.

Elderly or debilitated patients or individuals with a history of adverse reactions to neuroleptic drugs may require less Droleptan and half the normal starting dose in psychiatry may be sufficient for therapeutic response. The optimal response in such patients is usually obtained with more gradual titration and at lower dose levels. In adolescents a lower starting dose may be recommended.

Injection only:

Neuroleptanalgesia: Adults: 5-15 mg iv at induction of anaesthesia with a narcotic analgesic.

Premedication in anaesthesia: Adults: up to 10 mg im 30-60 minutes before an operation or diagnostic procedure.

The dosage should be adapted to each individual case. The factors to be considered here include age, bodyweight, the use of other drugs, the type of anaesthesia to be used and the surgical procedure involved.

Vital signs should be monitored routinely.

Elderly or debilitated patients or individuals with previously reported adverse reactions to neuroleptic drugs may require less Droleptan, and half the normal dose may be sufficient for a therapeutic response.

Anti-emetic:

Post-operative: Adults: 5 mg iv or im.

Children: Doses used have ranged between 0.02-0.075 mg/kg im or iv dependent on emetic stimulus.

In cancer chemotherapy: Adults: Out-patients or those on mildly emetic therapy should receive the lowest recommended dose. Patients on more aggressive chemotherapy may require doses in the upper range of those recommended. Dosage must always be determined individually.

A loading dose of 1-10 mg im or iv should be given 30 minutes before commencement of therapy, followed either by a continuous infusion of 1-3 mg/hour or 1-5 mg im or iv every 1-6 hours as required.

Children: Doses used have ranged between 0.02-0.075 mg/kg im or iv depending on emetic stimulus. Dosage must be determined individually using minimum effective dose.

Contra-indications: Droleptan is contra-indicated in patients with known hypersensitivity to the product, in patients with severe depression, in comatose individuals or in patients with Parkinson's disease.

Special warnings and special precautions for use: Caution is advised in patients with liver disease, renal failure, epilepsy, and conditions predisposing to epilepsy or convulsions.

Any patient subjected to anaesthesia and receiving potent CNS depressant drugs or showing CNS depression should be monitored closely.

In anaesthesia intravenous induction agents will generally be required in lower dosage where Droleptan is used as part of the anaesthetic technique, and the effects of heavy sedative premedication may be potentiated. When using Droleptan at induction of anaesthesia provision should be made for rapid infusion of intravenous fluid to correct any large fall in blood pressure, which, if it occurs, is due to relative hypovolaemia and is more common in the elderly or untreated hypertensives.

Mild to moderate hypotension and occasionally (reflex) tachycardia have been observed following administration of Droleptan. This reaction usually subsides spontaneously. However, should hypotension persist, the possibility of hypovolaemia should be considered and appropriate fluid replacement administered.

Since there is a risk of QT prolongation, Droleptan should only be used with caution in patients with hypokalaemia or in patients with pre-existing prolonged QT-interval.

Acute withdrawal symptoms, including nausea, vomiting and insomnia, have very rarely been described after abrupt cessation of high doses of antipsychotic drugs. Relapse may also occur and gradual withdrawal is advisable.

In patients with diagnosed/suspected phaeochromocytoma, severe hypertension and tachycardia have been observed after the administration of Droleptan. Therefore the use of Droleptan should be avoided in such patients.

Interaction with other medicaments and other forms of interaction: In common with all neuroleptics Droleptan can increase the central nervous system depression produced by other CNS-depressant drugs, including alcohol, hypnotics, sedatives or strong analgesics; and may antagonise the action of adrenaline and other sympathomimetic agents.

Like other sedative drugs, Droleptan may potentiate respiratory depression caused by opioids.

Droleptan may potentiate the action of antihypertensive agents, so that orthostatic hypotension may ensue.

Since droperidol blocks dopamine receptors, it may inhibit the action of dopamine agonists, such as bromocriptine, lisuride and levodopa.

The dosage of anti-convulsants may need to be increased to take account of the lowered seizure threshold.

Enhanced CNS effects, when combined with methyldopa, have been reported for some butyrophenones.

Theoretically, certain agents (eg phenobarbitone, carbamazepine, phenytoin), as well as smoking and alcohol consumption, which stimulate metabolising enzymes in the liver, may enhance the metabolic breakdown of neuroleptics, possibly necessitating adjustment of the dose.

Pregnancy and lactation: The safety of Droleptan in pregnancy has not been established, although studies in animals have not demonstrated teratogenic effects. As with other drugs, it is not advisable to administer Droleptan in pregnancy.

Butyrophenones are excreted in breast milk and are not recommended during lactation. If the use of Droleptan is essential, breast feeding should be discontinued.

Effects on ability to drive and use machines: Some degree of sedation or impairment of alertness may occur, particularly with higher doses and at the start of treatment and may be potentiated by alcohol. Patients should be advised not to drive or operate machinery during treatment until their susceptibility is known, or on the day following administration if early discharge is envisaged.

Undesirable effects: In common with all neuroleptics, extrapyramidal symptoms may occur. Acute dystonias may occur early in treatment. Parkinsonian rigidity, tremor and akathisia tend to appear less rapidly. Oculogyric crises and laryngeal dystonias have been reported. Extrapyramidal symptoms are less common at the low single doses used in anaesthesia, or as an anti-emetic.

These symptoms are usually reversible by treatment with an anticholinergic antiparkinsonian drug.

Anti-Parkinson agents should, however, only be given as required; they should not be prescribed routinely because of the possible risk of impairing the therapeutic efficacy of Droleptan.

Tardive dyskinesia may occur during administration or after withdrawal of neuroleptic drugs, including Droleptan, and can be precipitated or aggravated by anti-Parkinson drugs. Tardive dyskinesia has not been reported following anti-emetic or anaesthetic uses of Droleptan.

The syndrome is unlikely to occur in the short-term when low or moderate doses of Droleptan are used as recommended, but since its occurrence may be related to duration of treatment, as well as daily dose, Droleptan should be given in the minimum effective dose for the minimum possible time.

The potential seriousness and unpredictability of tardive dyskinesia, and the fact that it has occasionally been reported to occur when neuroleptic antipsychotic drugs have been prescribed for relatively short periods in low doses, means that the prescribing of such agents requires especially careful assessment of risks versus benefits.

The syndrome is mainly characterised by involuntary rhythmical movements of the tongue, face, mouth or jaw. The symptoms may persist in some patients. The syndrome may be masked when treatment is reinstituted, when the dosage is increased or when a switch is made to a different antipsychotic drug. Treatment should be discontinued as soon as possible.

Gastrointestinal symptoms, nausea, loss of appetite and dyspepsia, have been reported.

Hormonal effects of antipsychotic neuroleptic drugs include hyperprolactinaemia, which may cause galactorrhoea, gynaecomastia and oligo-or amenorrhoea.

Very rare cases of syndrome of inappropriate ADH secretion have been reported.

Dose-related mild to moderate hypotension and occasionally (reflex) tachycardia have been observed following administration of droperidol, particularly in the elderly who are more susceptible to the sedative and hypotensive effects. As with other neuroleptics, ventricular arrhythmias and sudden death have been reported very rarely. They may occur more frequently with high doses and in predisposed patients.

Droleptan, even in low dosage in susceptible (especially non-psychotic) individuals, may cause unpleasant subjective feelings of being mentally dulled or slowed down, dizziness, headache, or paradoxical effects of excitement, agitation, insomnia or hallucination.

In common with other antipsychotics, Droleptan may be associated with rare cases of neuroleptic malignant syndrome, an idiosyncratic response characterised by hyperthermia, generalised muscle rigidity, autonomic instability, altered consciousness, coma and elevated creatine phosphokinase levels. Hyperthermia together with other evidence of autonomic dysfunction may occur as early warning signs of this syndrome. In such cases, Droleptan treatment should be discontinued immediately and appropriate supportive therapy initiated. Recovery usually occurs within five to seven days of antipsychotic withdrawal. Affected patients should be carefully monitored and treated as appropriate.

The following effects have been reported rarely: angio-oedema, various skin rashes and reactions, hypersensitivity, body temperature dysregulation, jaundice or transient abnormalities of liver function in the absence of jaundice; anxiety or confusional states or epileptic fits, vision disturbances, sweating.

Blood dyscrasias have been reported very rarely.

Overdose: Symptoms: In general, the manifestations of Droleptan overdosage are an extension of its pharmacological actions, the most prominent of which would be severe extrapyramidal symptoms, hypotension and psychic indifference with a transition to sleep. The risk of cardiac arrhythmias should be considered. The patient may appear comatose with respiratory depression and hypotension which could be severe enough to produce a shock-like state. Convulsions may also occur.

Treatment: There is no specific antidote to droperidol. However, when an extra-pyramidal reaction occurs, an anticholinergic should be administered. A patent airway should be established and maintained with mechanically assisted ventilation if necessary. In view of isolated observations of arrhythmia following high doses of droperidol, ECG monitoring is mandatory. Hypotension and circulatory collapse should be treated by plasma volume expansion and other appropriate measures. Adrenaline should not be used. The patient should be monitored carefully for 24 hours or longer, body warmth and adequate fluid intake should be maintained.

Pharmacological properties
Pharmacodynamic properties: Droleptan is a butyrophenone neuroleptic. Its pharmacological profile is characterised mainly by dopamine-blocking and α_1-adrenolytic effects. Droleptan is devoid of anticholinergic and antihistaminic activity.

Pharmacokinetic properties: The relative bioavailability of the oral form is 75% compared with iv administration, the peak concentration being reached after 1-2 hours.

The action of a single intramuscular and intravenous dose commences 3-10 minutes after administration, although the peak effect may not be apparent for up to 30 minutes. The tranquillising and sedative effects tend to persist for 2 to 4 hours, although alertness may be affected for up to 12 hours.

Preclinical safety data: There are no pre-clinical data of relevance to the prescriber which are additional to that already included in other sections of the SPC.

Pharmaceutical particulars
List of excipients: Injection: Lactic acid; mannitol; water for injections; *Tablets:* Lactose hydrous; corn starch; magnesium stearate, quinoline yellow (E104); *Liquid:* Lactic acid; methyl parahydroxybenzoate; propyl parahydroxybenzoate; water.

Incompatibilities: Injection: Droleptan injection is chemically incompatible with the induction agent thiopentone and methohexitone because of the wide difference in pH. *Tablets and Liquid:* Not applicable.

Shelf life: 5 years (all products).

Special precautions for storage: Protect from light.

Nature and contents of container: Injection: One-point-cut ampoules containing 2 ml clear, colourless to slightly yellow solution. The ampoules are packed in cardboard cartons, in packs of 10 ampoules. *Tablets:* Blister packs consisting of aluminium foil, hermetalu and polyvinyl chloride glass clear. The blister strips are packed in cardboard cartons to contain 50 tablets. *Liquid:* Amber glass bottles containing 100 ml or 500 ml.

Instructions for use/handling: Not applicable

Marketing authorisation numbers
Droleptan Injection 0242/5003R
Droleptan Tablets 0242/5004R
Droleptan Liquid 0242/0080

Date of approval/revision of SPC June 1998

Legal category POM.

DUROGESIC*

Presentation Durogesic is a transdermal drug delivery system comprising a transparent, self-adhesive patch containing a drug reservoir of fentanyl. Each system is designed to release fentanyl into the systemic circulation over a period of 72 hours. There are four different strengths:

Durogesic 25, with a delivery rate of approximately 25 micrograms/hour fentanyl (active surface area 10 cm², fentanyl content 2.5 mg, and printed 'Durogesic 25 µg fentanyl/h' in pink)

Durogesic 50, with a delivery rate of approximately 50 micrograms/hour fentanyl (active surface area 20 cm², fentanyl content 5 mg, and printed 'Durogesic 50 µg fentanyl/h' in green)

Durogesic 75, with a delivery rate of approximately 75 micrograms/hour fentanyl (active surface area 30 cm², fentanyl content 7.5 mg, and printed 'Durogesic 75 µg fentanyl/h' in blue)

Durogesic 100, with a delivery rate of approximately 100 micrograms/hour fentanyl (active surface area 40 cm², fentanyl content 10 mg, and printed 'Durogesic 100 µg fentanyl/h' in grey)

The drug reservoir also contains ethanol BP, hydroxyethylcellulose PhEur and purified water PhEur. The contact adhesive is silicone medical adhesive.

Uses
Indications: Durogesic is indicated in the management of chronic intractable pain due to cancer.

Properties: Fentanyl is an opioid analgesic with a high affinity for the µ-opioid receptor.

Durogesic provides continuous systemic delivery of fentanyl over the 72 hour administration period. After the first Durogesic application, serum fentanyl concentrations increase gradually, generally levelling off between 12 and 24 hours and remaining relatively constant for the remainder of the 72-hour application period. The serum fentanyl concentrations attained are proportional to the Durogesic patch size. For all practical purposes by the second 72-hour application, a steady state serum concentration is reached and is maintained during subsequent applications of a patch of the same size.

After Durogesic is removed, serum fentanyl concentrations decline gradually, falling approximately 50% in 17 (range 13-22) hours. Continued absorption of fentanyl from the skin accounts for a slower disappearance of the drug from the serum than is seen after an iv infusion. Fentanyl is metabolised primarily in the liver. Around 75% of fentanyl is excreted into the urine, mostly as metabolites, with less than 10% as unchanged drug. About 9% of the dose is recovered in the faeces, primarily as metabolites. The major metabolite, norfentanyl, is inactive. Mean values for unbound fractions of fentanyl in plasma are estimated to be between 13 and 21%.

Dosage and administration Durogesic should be applied to non-irritated and non-irradiated skin on a flat surface of the torso or upper arm. A non-hairy area should be selected. If the site of Durogesic application requires to be cleansed prior to application of the system, this should be done with water. Soaps, oils, lotions or any other agent that might irritate the skin or alter its characteristics should not be used. The skin should be completely dry before the system is applied.

Durogesic should be applied immediately after removal from the sealed pouch. Following removal of the protective layer, the transdermal system should be pressed firmly in place with the palm of the hand for approximately 30 seconds, making sure the contact is complete, especially around the edges.

Durogesic should be worn continuously for 72 hours. A new system should then be applied to a different skin site after removal of the previous transdermal system. Several days should elapse before a new patch is applied to the same area of skin.

Adults:
Initial dose selection: The initial Durogesic dose should be based on the patient's opioid history, including the degree of opioid tolerance, if any, as well as on the current general condition and medical status of the patient.

In strong opioid-naive patients: The lowest Durogesic dose, 25 micrograms/h, should be used as the initial dose.

In opioid-tolerant patients: The initial dose of Durogesic should be based on the previous 24 hour opioid analgesic requirement. A recommended conversion scheme from oral morphine to Durogesic is given below:

Oral 24-hour morphine (mg/day)	*Durogesic (micrograms/h)*
<135	25
135-224	50
225-314	75
315-404	100
405-494	125
495-584	150
585-674	175
675-764	200
765-854	225
855-944	250
945-1034	275
1035-1124	300

For both strong opioid-naive and opioid-tolerant patients, the initial evaluation of the analgesic effect of Durogesic should not be made before the system has been worn for 24 hours due to the gradual increase in serum fentanyl concentrations up to this time. Previous analgesic therapy should therefore be phased out gradually from the time of the first patch application until analgesic efficacy with Durogesic is attained.

Dose titration and maintenance therapy: The Durogesic patch should be replaced every 72 hours. The dose should be titrated individually until analgesic efficacy is attained. If analgesia is insufficient at the end of the initial application period the dose may be increased. Dose adjustment, when necessary, should normally be performed in 25 micrograms/h increments, although the supplementary analgesic requirements (oral morphine 90 mg/day ≈ Durogesic 25 micrograms/h) and pain status of the patient should be taken into account. More than one Durogesic system may be used for doses greater than 100 micrograms/h. Patients may require periodic supplemental doses of a short-acting analgesic for 'breakthrough' pain. Additional or alternative methods of analgesia should be considered when the Durogesic dose exceeds 300 micrograms/h.

Discontinuation of Durogesic: If discontinuation of Durogesic is necessary, any replacement with other opioids should be gradual, starting at a low dose and increasing slowly. This is because fentanyl levels fall gradually after Durogesic is removed; it may take 17 hours or more for the fentanyl serum concentration to decrease by 50%. As a general rule, the discontinuation of opioid analgesia should be gradual.

Use in elderly patients: Data from intravenous studies with fentanyl suggest that elderly patients may have reduced clearance, a prolonged half-life and they may be more sensitive to the drug than younger patients. Studies of Durogesic in elderly patients demonstrated fentanyl pharmacokinetics which did not differ significantly from young patients although serum concentrations tended to be higher. Elderly, cachectic, or debilitated patients should be observed carefully for signs of fentanyl toxicity and the dose reduced if necessary.

Use in children: The safety and efficacy of Durogesic in children has not been established and is therefore not recommended.

Contra-indications, warnings, etc
Contra-indications: Durogesic is contra-indicated in patients with known hypersensitivity to fentanyl or to the adhesive in the system.

Durogesic is a sustained-release preparation indicated for the treatment of chronic intractable cancer pain and is contraindicated in acute pain because of the lack of opportunity for dosage titration in the short term and the resultant possibility of significant respiratory depression.

Warnings and precautions: Patients who have experienced serious adverse events should be monitored for up to 24 hours after Durogesic removal since serum fentanyl concentrations decline gradually and are reduced by about 50% in approximately 17 (range 13-22) hours.

Durogesic should be kept out of the reach of children at all times before and after use.

Respiratory depression: As with all potent opioids, some patients may experience significant respiratory depression with Durogesic; patients must be observed for these effects. Respiratory depression may persist beyond the removal of the Durogesic system. The incidence of respiratory depression increases as the Durogesic dose is increased. See also 'Overdosage' concerning respiratory depression. CNS active drugs may increase the respiratory depression (see 'Interactions').

Chronic pulmonary disease: Fentanyl, like other opioids, may have more severe adverse effects in patients with chronic obstructive or other pulmonary disease. In such patients, they may decrease respiratory drive and increase airway resistance.

Drug dependence: Tolerance and physical and psychological dependence may develop upon repeated administration of opioids such as fentanyl. Iatrogenic addiction following opioid administration is rare.

Increased intracranial pressure: Durogesic should be used with caution in patients who may be particularly susceptible to the intracranial effects of CO_2 retention such as those with evidence of increased intracranial pressure, impaired consciousness or coma. Durogesic should be used with caution in patients with brain tumours.

Cardiac disease: Fentanyl may produce bradycardia and Durogesic should therefore be administered with caution to patients with bradyarrhythmias.

Hepatic disease: Because fentanyl is metabolised to inactive metabolites in the liver, hepatic disease might delay its elimination. In patients with hepatic cirrhosis, the pharmacokinetics of a single application of Durogesic were not altered although serum concentrations tended to be higher in these patients. Patients with hepatic impairment should be observed carefully for signs of fentanyl toxicity and the dose of Durogesic reduced if necessary.

Renal disease: Less than 10% of fentanyl is excreted unchanged by the kidney and, unlike morphine, there are no known active metabolites eliminated by the kidney. Data obtained with intravenous fentanyl in patients with renal failure suggest that the volume of distribution of fentanyl may be changed by dialysis. This may affect serum concentrations. If patients with renal impairment receive Durogesic, they should be observed carefully for signs of fentanyl toxicity and the dose reduced if necessary.

Patients with fever/external heat: Patients who develop fever should be monitored for opioid side effects since significant increases in body temperature can potentially increase fentanyl delivery rate.

Patients should also be advised to avoid exposing the Durogesic application site to direct external heat sources such as heating pads, hot water bottles, electric blankets, heat lamps, saunas or hot whirlpool spa baths while wearing the system, since there is potential for temperature dependent increases in release of fentanyl from the system.

Pregnancy and lactation: The safety of fentanyl in pregnancy has not been established. Durogesic should not be used in women of child-bearing potential without adequate contraception unless in the judgement of the doctor the potential benefits outweigh the possible hazards.

Fentanyl is excreted into breast milk hence Durogesic should not be used by women who are breast-feeding.

Effects on driving and operating machinery: Durogesic may impair the mental or physical ability required to perform potentially hazardous tasks such as driving or operating machinery.

Drug interactions: The concomitant use of other CNS depressants, including opioids, anxiolytics, hypnotics, general anaesthetics, antipsychotics, skeletal muscle relaxants, sedating antihistamines and alcoholic beverages may produce additive depressant effects; hypoventilation, hypotension and profound sedation or coma may occur. Therefore, the use of any of these drugs concomitantly with Durogesic requires special care and observation.

Fentanyl is metabolised mainly via the human cytochrome P450 3A4 enzyme. However, no *in vivo* inhibition by itraconazole (a known cytochrome P450 3A4 enzyme inhibitor) has been observed, most probably because of the high hepatic extraction ratio of fentanyl.

Patch disposal: Used patches may contain significant residues of active substance. After removal, therefore, used patches should be folded firmly in half, adhesive side inwards, so that the release membrane is not exposed, and then discarded safely and out of the reach of children according to the instructions in the pack.

Side effects: The most serious adverse reaction, as with all potent opioids, is hypoventilation. Other opioid-related adverse reactions include: nausea; vomiting; constipation; hypotension; somnolence; confusion; hallucinations; euphoria; pruritus and urinary retention.

Skin reactions such as rash, erythema and itching have occasionally been reported. These reactions usually resolve within 24 hours of removal of the patch.

Overdosage: Symptoms: The symptoms of fentanyl overdosage are an extension of its pharmacological actions, the most serious effect being respiratory depression.

Treatment: For management of respiratory depression, immediate countermeasures include removing Durogesic and physically or verbally stimulating the patient. These actions can be followed by administration of a specific opioid antagonist such as naloxone. The interval between iv opioid antagonist doses should be carefully chosen and repeated administration or a continuous infusion of naloxone may be necessary because of continued absorption of fentanyl from the skin after patch removal, which may result in prolonged respiratory depression. Reversal of the narcotic effect may result in acute onset of pain and release of catecholamines.

A patent airway should be established and maintained. An oropharyngeal airway or endotracheal tube and oxygen should be administered and respiration assisted or controlled, as appropriate. Adequate body temperature and fluid intake should be maintained.

If severe or persistent hypotension occurs, hypovolaemia should be considered, and the condition should be managed with appropriate parenteral fluid therapy.

Pharmaceutical precautions Store below 25°C.

Legal category CD (Schedule 2) POM

Package quantities Durogesic 25, 50, 75, 100: Cartons of 5 patches individually packaged in pouches.

Further information None.

Product licence numbers

Durogesic 25	0242/0192
Durogesic 50	0242/0193
Durogesic 75	0242/0194
Durogesic 100	0242/0195

EPREX*

Presentation Eprex is a sterile, buffered protein solution for intravenous or subcutaneous injection, containing varying quantities of epoetin alfa between 1,000 and 10,000 IU.

Eprex is also available as a sterile, phosphate buffered protein solution, formulated with 0.03% polysorbate 80 and 0.5% glycine, in vials containing 1,000 IU/0.5 ml, 2,000 IU/1.0 ml, 4,000 IU/1.0 ml and 10,000 IU/1.0 ml.

Eprex is further available as a sterile, phosphate buffered protein solution, formulated with 0.03% polysorbate 80 and 0.5% glycine, in graduated, pre-filled syringes containing 1,000 IU/0.5 ml, 2,000 IU/0.5 ml, 3,000 IU/0.3 ml, 4,000 IU/0.4 ml and 10,000 IU/1.0 ml.

Uses Eprex is indicated for the treatment of anaemia associated with chronic renal failure in children and adults on haemodialysis and adults on peritoneal dialysis.

Eprex is also indicated for the treatment of severe anaemia of renal origin accompanied by clinical symptoms in adults with renal insufficiency not yet undergoing dialysis, ie non-dialysis patients.

Eprex is indicated for the treatment of anaemia in adult cancer patients receiving platinum-containing chemotherapy regimens.

Eprex can be used to increase the yield of autologous blood from patients in a predonation programme initiated to avoid the use of homologous blood. Treatment is indicated in patients with moderate anaemia (PCV approximately 33 to 39%, no iron deficiency) if blood conserving procedures are not available or insufficient either:

a) When the scheduled major elective surgery requires a large volume of blood (4 or more units of blood for females or 5 or more units for males).

or

b) When the period necessary to obtain the required volume of autologous blood is too short.

Dosage and administration In patients with chronic renal failure and clinically evident ischaemic heart disease or congestive heart failure, maintenance haemoglobin concentration should not exceed the upper limit of the target haemoglobin concentration.

Adult dialysis patients:

Haemodialysis: Recommended starting dose 50 IU/kg, three times weekly (total 150 IU/kg per week).

Administer by intravenous injection or subcutaneous injection.

Dosage may be increased in 25 IU/kg increments three times weekly at 4 week intervals, until desired response achieved, ie Haemoglobin (Hb) 10-12 g/dl or Haematocrit (HCT) 30-35%.

Maintenance dose (100-300 IU/kg per week) should be divided into two or three injections.

Maximum dosage should not exceed 200 IU/kg three times weekly (total 600 IU/kg per week).

Peritoneal dialysis: Recommended starting dose 50 IU/kg twice weekly.

Administer by subcutaneous injection.

Dosage may be increased in 25 IU/kg increments twice weekly in 4 week intervals until desired response achieved, ie Hb 10-12 g/dl or HCT 30-35%.

Maintenance dose, 50-100 IU/kg per week, divided into two equal injections.

Paediatric patients:

Haemodialysis: Recommended starting dose is 50 IU/kg, three times weekly.

Administer by intravenous injection.

Dosage may be increased in 25 IU/kg increments three times weekly in 4 week intervals until desired response achieved; Hb 9.5-11 g/dl.

Maintenance dose recommended as follows (based on available clinical data).

Dose (IU/kg given 3 x/week)

Weight (kg)	Median	Usual maintenance dose
<10	100	75-150
10-30	75	60-150
>30	33	30-100

Generally, children under 30 kg require higher maintenance doses.

Clinical data also suggests higher maintenance doses required by those patients with an initial Hb <6.8 g/dl than those with Hb>6.8 g/dl.

Adult non-dialysis patients: Recommended starting dose 50 IU/kg, three times weekly (total 150 IU/kg per week).

Subcutaneous administration is preferred to intravenous administration.

Dosage may be increased in 25 IU/kg increments, three times weekly at 4 week intervals, until desired response achieved, ie Hb 10-12 g/dl or HCT 30-35%.

Maintenance dose 50-100 IU/kg per week divided into three doses.

Maximum dosage should not exceed 200 IU/kg three times a week (total 600 IU/kg per week).

Based on information available to date, correction of anaemia with Eprex in pre-dialysis patients does not accelerate the rate of progression of renal insufficiency.

Adult cancer patients: The subcutaneous route of administration should be used.

Epoetin alfa therapy should be administered to patients with anaemia (eg Hb < 10.5 g/dl [6.5 mmol/l]). The Hb concentration aimed for is approximately 12 g/dl (7.5 mmol/l).

The initial dose is 150 IU/kg given subcutaneously 3 times per week.

If the Hb has increased by at least 1 g/dl (0.62 mmol/l) or the reticulocyte count has increased ≥40,000 cells/µl (40 x 10^9 cells/litre) above baseline after 4 weeks of treatment, the dose should remain at 150 IU/kg.

If the Hb increase is <1 g/dl (<0.62 mmol/l) and the reticulocyte count has increased by <40,000 cells/µl (40 x 10^9 cells/litre) above baseline, after 4 weeks of treatment, increase the dose to 300 IU/kg. After an additional 4 weeks of therapy at 300 IU/kg, if the Hb has increased ≥1 g/dl (≥0.62 mmol/l) or the reticulocyte count has increased by ≥40,000 cells/µl (40 x 10^9 cells/litre) the dose should remain at 300 IU/kg. However, if the Hb has increased <1 g/dl (<0.62 mmol/l) and the reticulocyte count has increased by <40,000 cells/µl (40 x 10^9 cells/litre) above baseline, response is unlikely and treatment should be discontinued.

Dose adjustment: A rate of rise in Hb of greater than 2 g/dl (1.25 mmol/l) per month or Hb levels of >14 g/dl (>8.7 mmol/l) should be avoided.

If the Hb is rising by more than 2 g/dl (1.25 mmol/l) per month, reduce the dose of Eprex by about 25-50% depending upon the rate of rise of Hb.

If the Hb exceeds 14 g/dl (8.7 mmol/l) discontinue therapy until it falls below 12 g/dl (7.5 mmol/l) and then reinstitute epoetin alfa at a dose 25% below the previous dose.

Therapy with Eprex should continue until one month after the end of chemotherapy.

Adult patients in an autologous predonation programme: The intravenous route of administration should be used.

Mildly anaemic patients (HCT of 33-39%) requiring predeposit of 4 units of blood should be treated with Eprex at 600 IU/kg 2 times weekly for 3 weeks prior to surgery.

N.B. Using this regimen, it was possible to withdraw 4 units of blood from 81% of patients treated with Eprex compared to 37% of placebo-treated patients. Therapy with Eprex reduced the risk of exposure to homologous blood by 50% compared to patients not receiving Eprex.

Iron supplementation: All patients being treated with Eprex should receive adequate iron supplementation (eg 200 mg oral elemental iron daily) throughout the course of Eprex treatment.

Iron supplementation should be started as soon as possible, even several weeks prior to initiating the autologous predeposit, in order to achieve high iron stores prior to starting therapy with Eprex.

General administration advice: Parenteral drug products should be visually inspected for particulate matter and discolouration prior to administration.

Eprex pre-filled syringes are ready for use.

Prepare Eprex vials for injection by drawing solution into syringe from a single use vial. Attach needle for injection.

Intravenous injections should be administered over 1-2 minutes; slow injection over 5 minutes may be beneficial to patients who experience flu-like symptoms.

Do not administer Eprex by intravenous infusion or in conjunction with other drug solutions.

For the subcutaneous route, a maximum volume of 1 ml at one injection site should generally not be exceeded. In the case of larger volumes more than one site should be chosen for the injection.

A gradual increase in Hb of less than 2 g/dl per month is recommended. All patients receiving Eprex should have the level of their Hb measured frequently (weekly) until it is stable. Thereafter the level should be measured periodically. When Eprex is discontinued, the Hb concentration decreases by approximately 0.5 g/dl weekly.

Administration advice–dialysis patients: Eprex injection should follow the dialysis procedure for dialysis patients.

If Hb rise exceeds 2 g/dl per month at 50 IU/kg three times weekly, doses should be adjusted downward by omitting one of the weekly doses.

Non-response to therapy with Eprex should prompt a search for causative factors which include: iron, folate or Vitamin B_{12} deficiency, aluminium intoxication, intercurrent infections, inflammatory or traumatic episodes, occult blood loss, haemolysis, bone marrow fibrosis.

Increase in urea and creatinine prior to dialysis may occur in individual patients as a result of increased protein intake, in which case dialysis regimen modification may be necessary.

Changing between subcutaneous and intravenous administration: The subcutaneous (maintenance) dose is generally approximately 20-30% lower than the intravenous. When changing route of administration the same dose should be used and the Hb followed carefully (eg weekly) so that appropriate Eprex dose alterations can be made to keep Hb within desired range.

Available data indicate higher maintenance dose levels may be required by adult patients with pre-treatment Hb levels of less than 6 g/dl compared to adult patients with pre-treatment Hb levels of more than 8 g/dl.

Contra-indications: Eprex is contra-indicated in uncontrolled hypertension.

All contra-indications associated with autologous blood predonation programmes should be respected in patients being supplemented with Eprex.

Warnings and precautions: All special warnings and special precautions associated with autologous predonation programmes should be respected in patients being supplemented with Eprex. In patients with chronic renal failure and clinically evident ischaemic heart disease or congestive heart failure, maintenance haemoglobin concentration should not exceed the upper limit of the target haemoglobin concentration as recommended under Dosage and Administration. Iron status should be evaluated for all patients prior to and during treatment and iron supplementation administered if necessary. In most cases, serum ferritin values fall simultaneously with the rise in packed cell volume. Therefore, oral iron substitution for 200-300 mg/day (100-200 mg/day for paediatric patients) is recommended for all patients whose serum ferritin levels are below 100 ng/ml.

Other causes of anaemia, such as vitamin B_{12} or folate deficiency should be excluded before instituting therapy with Eprex.

Eprex should be used with caution in the presence of untreated, inadequately treated or poorly controllable hypertension (close monitoring is required to detect any changes in blood pressure and serum electrolytes). It may be necessary to add or increase anti-hypertensive treatment. If blood pressure cannot be controlled, treatment with Eprex treatment should be discontinued.

Eprex should also be used with caution in those patients with ischaemic vascular disease, or history of seizures, and in the presence of epilepsy, thrombocytosis, chronic liver failure and known hypersensitivity to the medication.

Hyperkalaemia has been observed in dialysis patients in isolated cases.

Growth factor potential: Epoetin alfa is a growth factor that primarily stimulates red blood cell production. However, the possibility that epoetin alfa can act as a growth factor for any tumour type, particularly myeloid malignancies, cannot be excluded.

Pregnancy and lactation: Eprex has been shown to decrease foetal body weight, delay ossification and increase mortality in animals when given in weekly doses of approximately 20 times the recommended human weekly dose. These changes are believed to be secondary to decreased maternal body weight gain.

There are no adequate and well controlled studies in pregnant women. In chronic renal failure patients, Eprex should be used in pregnancy and lactation only if the potential benefit justifies the potential risk to the foetus. In pregnancy or lactating surgical patients participating in an autologous blood predonation programme, the use of Eprex is not recommended.

Side effects: The following adverse events have been reported:

'Flu-like' symptoms such as headaches, joint pains, feelings of weakness, dizziness, tiredness and chills may occur, especially at the start of treatment.

The most frequent adverse reaction during treatment is a dose-dependent increase in blood pressure or aggravation of existing hypertension. These increases in blood pressure can be treated with drugs. Moreover, monitoring of blood pressure is recommended, particularly at the start of therapy.

The following reactions may also occur in isolated patients with normal or low blood pressure: hypertensive crisis with encephalopathy-like symptoms (eg headaches, confused state) and generalised tonic-clonic seizures, requiring the immediate attention of a physician and intensive medical care. Particular attention should be paid to sudden stabbing migraine-like headaches as a possible warning signal.

The following adverse effects have also been occasionally observed: seizures, skin reactions, palpebral oedema, possibly allergic in nature.

There may be a moderate dose-dependent rise in the platelet count within the normal range during treatment with Eprex. This regresses during the course of continued therapy. Development of thrombocytosis is very rare. It is recommended that the platelet count is regularly monitored during the first eight weeks of therapy.

Chronic renal failure patients: Serum potassium levels should be regularly monitored during therapy with Eprex. Potassium elevation has been exhibited in a few predialysis patients receiving Eprex though causality has not been established. If an elevated (or rising) serum potassium level is observed then consideration should be given to ceasing Eprex administration until hyperkalaemia has been corrected.

Shunt thromboses may occur, particularly in patients with a tendency to hypotension or whose arteriovenous fistulae exhibits complications (eg stenosis, aneurysms, etc). Early shunt revision and thrombosis prophylaxis by administration of aspirin for example is recommended in these patients.

An increase in heparin dose during dialysis is frequently required during the course of therapy with Eprex as a result of the increased packed cell volume. Occlusion of the dialysis system is possible if heparinisation is not optimum.

Anaemic adult cancer patients receiving platinum-based chemotherapy: As hypertension may occur in some patients treated with Eprex, Hb and blood pressure should be closely monitored.

Surgery patients in autologous predonation programmes: Independent of treatment with Eprex, routine volume replacement should be performed in surgical patients with underlying cardiovascular disease following repeated phlebotomy as thrombotic and vascular events may occur.

Interactions: Eprex should not be administered by intravenous infusion or in conjunction with other drug solutions.

No evidence exists indicating that treatment with Eprex alters the metabolism of other drugs. However, since cyclosporin is bound by red blood cells there is potential for drug interaction. If Eprex is given concomitantly with cyclosporin, blood levels of cyclosporin should be monitored, and the dose of cyclosporin adjusted as the HCT rises.

The efficacy of Eprex should be potentiated by the simultaneous administration of a haematinic agent where a deficiency state existed.

No evidence exists that indicates an interaction between Eprex and G-CSF or GM-CSF with regard to haematological differentiation or proliferation of tumour biopsy specimens *in vitro.*

Overdosage: The therapeutic margin of Eprex is very wide. Even at very high serum levels, no symptoms of poisoning have been observed. Response to Eprex is dose related and individualised.

Incompatibilities: Do not administer by intravenous infusion or in conjunction with other drug solutions. See 'Interactions' above.

Further information Erythropoietin is an endogenous glycoprotein hormone that regulates red blood cell production. Its production primarily occurs in, and is regulated by, the kidney in response to changes in tissue oxygenation.

Measurement of epoetin alfa following multiple dose intravenous administration revealed a half life of approximately four hours in normal patients and five hours in renal failure patients. A half-life of approximately six hours has been reported in children.

Following subcutaneous injection, serum levels are much lower than those achieved by intravenous injection. The levels increase slowly, reaching a peak between twelve and eighteen hours post dosing. The peak is always well below the peak achieved using the intravenous route. There is no accumulation, levels remaining the same whether determined twenty four hours after the first or last injection.

The half life is difficult to evaluate for the subcutaneous route and is estimated at about twenty four hours. The bioavailability of subcutaneously injected erythropoietin is approximately 20% that of the drug when administered intravenously.

Pharmaceutical precautions Store at 2°C to 8°C. Do not freeze or shake. Protect from light. Eprex is a sterile but unpreserved product. Under no circumstances should more than one dose be administered per vial or syringe.

Legal category POM.

Package quantities Packages of 6 vials containing: 1,000 IU/0.5 ml, 2,000 IU/ ml, 4,000 IU/ml or 10,000 IU/ml of epoetin alfa.

Packages of 6 pre-filled syringes containing: 1,000 IU/0.5 ml, 2,000 IU/0.5 ml, 3,000 IU/0.3 ml, 4,000 IU/0.4 ml or 10,000 IU/ml of epoetin alfa.

Product licence numbers

Eprex 1,000 IU/0.5 ml	0242/0218
Eprex 2,000 IU/ml	0242/0218
Eprex 4,000 IU/ml	0242/0221
Eprex 10,000 IU/ml	0242/0215
Eprex pre-filled syringes 1,000 IU/0.5 ml	0242/0297
Eprex pre-filled syringes 2,000 IU/0.5 ml	0242/0298
Eprex pre-filled syringes 3,000 IU/0.3 ml	0242/0299
Eprex pre-filled syringes 4,000 IU/0.4 ml	0242/0299
Eprex pre-filled syringes 10,000 IU/ml	0242/0299

EVOREL* CONTI AND SEQUI

Qualitative and quantitative composition Evorel Conti and Sequi are both Transdermal Delivery Systems (TDS).

Evorel Conti contains:
3.2 mg of estradiol hemihydrate
11.2 mg of norethisterone acetate

Evorel Sequi consists of:
a) 4 Evorel 50 TDSs, each containing:
3.2 mg of estradiol hemihydrate
b) 4 Evorel Conti TDSs, each containing:
3.2 mg of estradiol hemihydrate
11.2 mg of norethisterone acetate

Pharmaceutical form Evorel 50, Evorel Conti And Evorel Sequi are Transdermal Delivery Systems (TDS), or transdermal patches, composed of a flat two-layer laminate which is 0.1 mm in thickness. The first layer is a flexible, translucent, and nearly colourless backing film. The second layer is a monolayer adhesive film (matrix) composed of acrylic adhesive and guar gum and contains the hormones. This system is protected by a polyester foil release liner, which is affixed to the adhesive matrix and is removed prior to application of the patch to the skin. The polyester foil used is coated with silicone on both sides. The release liner has a S-shaped opening to facilitate its removal prior to use. Each TDS is enclosed in a protective, hermetically-sealed sachet.

Evorel Conti has a surface area of 16 sq cm and contains 3.2 mg of estradiol corresponding to a nominal release of 50 micrograms of estradiol per 24 hours and 11.2 mg of norethisterone acetate corresponding to a nominal release of 170 micrograms of norethisterone acetate per 24 hours. Each TDS is marked in the centre of the lower margin on the outside of the backing film: CEN1.

Evorel 50 has a surface area of 16 sq cm and contains 3.2 mg of estradiol corresponding to a nominal release of 50 micrograms of estradiol per 24 hours. The release liner of Evorel 50 is aluminised on one side. Each TDS is marked in the centre of the lower margin of the outside of the backing film: CE50.

Clinical particulars

Therapeutic indications: Hormone replacement therapy for the relief of menopausal symptoms.

Prevention and management of post-menopausal osteoporosis in women considered at risk of developing fractures. Epidemiological studies have suggested that there are a number of risk factors associated with post-menopausal osteoporosis such as early menopause, a family history of osteoporosis, prolonged exposure to corticosteroid therapy, small and thin skeletal frame and excessive cigarette smoking.

Posology and method of administration:
Adults
Menopausal symptoms:
Evorel Conti

Evorel Conti TDS should be applied individually without interruption.

Each Evorel Conti TDS should be applied twice weekly, every three to four days, to the trunk below the waist.

Insufficient data are available to guide dose adjustments for patients with severe liver or kidney function impairment.

Evorel Sequi

Evorel Sequi comprises four Evorel 50 TDSs and four Evorel Conti TDSs.

Evorel 50 and Evorel Conti should be applied individually in the following sequence: four Evorel 50 TDSs followed by four Evorel Conti TDSs. This cycle should be repeated without interruption. TDSs should be applied twice weekly, every three to four days, to the trunk below the waist.

Insufficient data are available to guide dose adjustments for patients with severe liver or kidney function impairment.

It is important that the TDS be used in the correct sequence to ensure regular cyclic bleeding. Most patients will experience vaginal bleeding after the start of the progestogen therapy.

Post-menopausal osteoporosis: Evorel Conti and Sequi are recommended as an effective bone-sparing dose, with lower doses of estradiol slowing but not halting bone loss.

Children: Evorel Conti and Evorel Sequi (Evorel 50 and Evorel Conti) are not indicated in children.

Elderly: Data are insufficient in regard to the use of Evorel Conti and Evorel Sequi in the elderly (>65 years old).

Administration: The sachet containing one TDS should be opened and one part of the protective foil removed at the S-shaped incision. The TDS should be applied to clean, dry, healthy, intact skin as soon as it is removed from the sachet. The patient should avoid contact between fingers and the adhesive part of the

TDS during application. Each application should be made to a different area of the skin, on the trunk below the waist. **Evorel Conti and SEQUI should not be applied on or near the breasts.**

Should a TDS fall off, it should be replaced immediately with a new equivalent Evorel 50 or Evorel Conti TDS. However, the usual day of changing TDSs should be maintained.

Contra-indications:

- Hypersensitivity to any component of this product.
- Malignant tumours of the breast.
- Genital tract or other oestrogen-dependent neoplasia.
- Undiagnosed vaginal bleeding.
- Pregnancy or lactation.
- Severe hepatic or renal disease.
- Active thrombophlebitis.
- Active deep venous thrombosis, thromboembolic disorders, or a history of confirmed venous thromboembolism.
- Endometriosis.

Special warnings and special precautions for use: Prior to commencing, and periodically during oestrogen replacement therapy, it is recommended that the patient be given a thorough physical and gynaecological examination. A complete medical and family history should be taken. Repeated breakthrough bleeding, unexplained vaginal bleeding and changes noticed during breast examination require further evaluation.

At the present time, the results of epidemiological studies suggest an increase in the relative risk of breast cancer in postmenopausal women receiving long-term hormone replacement therapy. Concurrent progestogen does not appear to protect for this risk. Therefore, a careful appraisal of the risk/benefit ratio should be undertaken before the initiation of long-term treatment.

Epidemiological studies have suggested that hormone replacement therapy (HRT) is associated with an increased relative risk of developing venous thromboembolism (VTE), i.e. deep vein thrombosis or pulmonary embolism. The studies find a 2–3 fold increase for users compared with non-users which for healthy women amounts to a low risk of one extra case of VTE each year for every 5,000 patients taking HRT.

Generally recognised risk factors for VTE include a personal or family history and severe obesity (body mass index >30 kg/m²). In women with these factors the benefits of treatment with HRT need to be carefully weighed against risks.

The risk of VTE may be temporarily increased with prolonged immobilisation, major trauma or major surgery. In women on HRT scrupulous attention should be given to prophylactic measures to prevent VTE following surgery. Where prolonged immobilisation is liable to follow elective surgery, particularly abdominal or orthopaedic surgery to the lower limbs, consideration should be given to temporarily stopping HRT 4 weeks earlier, if this is possible.

If venous thromboembolism develops after initiating therapy the drug should be discontinued.

Appropriate monitoring is recommended in patients with cardiac impairment, epilepsy, diabetes mellitus, hypertension, disturbances or impairment of liver or kidney function, mastopathy, a family history of breast cancer, or a history of cholestatic jaundice.

Administration of unopposed oestrogen in patients with an intact uterus has been reported to increase the risk of endometrial hyperplasia and of endometrial carcinoma. Therefore oestrogen in combination with continuous administration of a progestogen as in Evorel Conti, or with sequential administration of a progestogen as in Evorel Sequi, is recommended in women with an intact uterus in order to reduce the risk of hyperplasia or endometrial carcinoma.

Evorel Conti and Evorel Sequi are not to be used as contraception.

The TDSs should be kept away from children and pets.

Interaction with other medicaments and other forms of interaction: Drugs which induce microsomal liver enzyme activity may alter oestrogen and progestogen metabolism. Examples of such drugs are barbiturates, hydantoins, carbamazepine, meprobamate, phenylbutazone, and rifampicin. On a theoretical basis, the effects of liver enzyme induction on the metabolism of transdermally administered estradiol and norethisterone acetate should be minimised by the avoidance of the first pass liver metabolism.

Pregnancy and lactation: The use of Evorel Conti and Evorel Sequi is contra-indicated in pregnancy and lactation.

Effects on ability to drive and use machines: There are no known data on the effects of Evorel Conti and Evorel Sequi on the ability to drive or use machinery.

Undesirable effects: The most commonly reported adverse events reported in clinical trials with Evorel Conti and Evorel Sequi include vaginal bleeding, spotting, breast tenderness, headache, and abdominal cramps/bloating. These adverse events reflect the known profile of oestrogen or oestrogen/progestogen therapy.

Skin reactions reported include transient erythema and irritation with or without pruritus at the site of TDS application. Very rarely, contact dermatitis, reversible post-inflammatory pigmentation, generalised pruritus, and exanthema occurred in studies with Evorel 50.

Rare adverse events reported in association with **oral** progestogen or oestrogen replacement therapy include: thromboembolic events, cholestasis, benign or malignant breast disease, uterine carcinoma, aggravation of epilepsy, liver adenoma and galactorrhoea. If such events occur, Evorel Conti and Evorel Sequi should be discontinued immediately.

Overdose: Symptoms of overdose of oestrogen and progestogen therapy may include nausea, break-through bleeding, breast tenderness, abdominal cramps and/or bloating. These symptoms can be reversed by removing the TDS.

Pharmacological properties

Pharmacodynamic properties: Evorel Conti and Evorel Sequi belong to pharmacotherapeutic class G 03 F B 05, according to the ATC classification.

The active hormone of Evorel Conti and Evorel Sequi is 17β-estradiol, the biologically most potent oestrogen produced by the ovary. Its synthesis in the ovarian follicles is regulated by pituitary hormones. Like all steroid hormones, estradiol diffuses freely into target cells, where it binds to specific macromolecules (receptors). The estradiol-receptor complex then interacts with genomic DNA to alter transcriptional activity. This results in increases or decreases in protein synthesis and in changes of cellular functions.

Estradiol is secreted at different rates during the menstrual cycle. The endometrium is highly sensitive to estradiol, which regulates endometrial proliferation during the follicular phase of the cycle and together with progesterone, induces secretory changes during the luteal phase. Around the menopause estradiol secretion becomes irregular and eventually ceases altogether. The absence of estradiol is associated with menopausal symptoms such as vasomotor instability, sleep disturbances, depressive mood, signs of vulvovaginal and urogenital atrophy and with increased bone loss. In addition, there is growing evidence for an increased incidence in cardiovascular disease in the absence of oestrogen.

Oestrogen replacement therapy has been found effective in most postmenopausal women to compensate for the endogenous oestrogen depletion. It has been demonstrated that transdermal estradiol administration of 50 micrograms/day, is effective in the treatment of menopausal symptoms and of postmenopausal bone loss.

In postmenopausal women, Evorel Conti and Evorel Sequi increases estradiol to early follicular levels, with a consequent significant decrease in hot flushes, improvement in Kupperman Index and beneficial changes in vaginal cytology.

However, there is substantial evidence that oestrogen replacement therapy is associated with an increase in endometrial cancer. There is also compelling evidence that adjunctive progestogen treatment protects against oestrogen-induced endometrial cancer. Therefore, women with a uterus should receive combination oestrogen-progestogen hormone replacement therapy.

Norethisterone acetate, used in Evorel Conti and Evorel Sequi is rapidly hydrolysed to norethisterone, a synthetic 19-nortestosterone derivative of the 13-methyl gonane group, with potent progestational activity. Transdermal norethisterone acetate administration prevents oestrogen-related endometrial proliferation. Combined 17β-estradiol-norethisterone acetate therapy is effective in treating the deficits associated with menopause.

Pharmacokinetic properties: Estradiol is readily absorbed from the gastrointestinal tract but is extensively metabolised by the intestinal mucosa and the liver during the first hepatic passage. Transdermal delivery of estradiol is sufficient to cause a systemic effect.

Estradiol distributes widely in body tissues and is bound to albumin (~60-65%) and sex-hormone-binding globulin (~35-45%) in serum. Serum protein-binding fractions remain unaltered following transdermal delivery of estradiol. Estradiol is promptly eliminated from the systemic circulation. The elimination half-life is ~1 hour following intravenous administration. Estradiol is metabolised principally into the less pharmacologically active estrone and its conjugates. Estradiol, estrone and estrone sulphate are interconverted to each other and are excreted in urine as glucuronides and sulphates. The skin metabolises estradiol only to a small extent.

In a single and multiple application study in postmenopausal women, serum estradiol concentrations increased rapidly from pretreatment levels (~ 5 pg/ml) after application of a Evorel Conti TDS. At four hours after application, the mean serum estradiol concentration was ~19 pg/ml. A mean peak serum estradiol concentration of ~41 pg/ml above the pretreatment level was observed at about 23 hours following application. Serum estradiol concentrations remained elevated for the 3.5-day application period. Concentrations returned rapidly to pretreatment levels within 24 hours following removal of the TDS. A serum half-life of ~6.6 hours was determined following removal of the TDS, indicative of the skin depot effect. Multiple application of the Evorel Conti TDS resulted in little or no accumulation of estradiol in the systemic circulation. Higher circulating levels of estradiol were attained from Evorel 50. Both formulations were shown to be effective in achieving serum estradiol concentration typically seen in premenopausal women.

Prior to treatment, the mean serum estradiol to estrone concentration ratio (E_2/E_1) was less than 0.3 in the postmenopausal women studied. During use of Evorel Conti TDS the E_2/E_1 ratios increased rapidly and were maintained at the physiological levels that approximated 1. The E_2/E_1 ratios returned to pretreatment levels within 24 hours after removal of the TDS. An average E_2/E_1 ratio that approximated 1 was also maintained over an entire 3.5-day application period following Evorel 50 application.

Norethisterone acetate is rapidly hydrolysed to the active progestogen, norethisterone. After oral administration, norethisterone is subject to pronounced first-pass metabolism which reduces the bioavailability. Transdermal delivery of norethisterone acetate produces a sustained and effective level of norethisterone in the systemic circulation.

Norethisterone distributes widely in body tissues and is bound to albumin (~61%) and sex-hormone-binding globulin (~36%) in serum. The elimination half-life is ~6 to 12 hours following oral administration which is not altered following long-term therapy. Norethisterone is primarily metabolised in the liver by reduction of the α,β-unsaturated ketone structure in ring A of the molecule. Among the four possible stereoisomeric tetrahydrosteroids, the 5β-, 3α-hydroxy-derivative appears to be the predominant metabolite. These compounds are primarily excreted in urine and faeces as sulphate and glucuronide conjugates.

In a single and multiple application study in postmenopausal women, serum norethisterone concentrations rose within 1 day after application of a Evorel Conti TDS to a mean steady-state level of ~199 pg/ml. Mean steady-state serum norethisterone concentrations ranging between ~141 to 224 pg/ml were maintained for the entire 3.5-day application period following multiple application. Mean concentrations declined rapidly to the lower limit of assay quantitation at 24 hours after removal of the TDS. A serum half-life of ~15 hours was determined following removal of the TDS, indicative of the skin depot effect. As expected from transdermal delivery of most drugs, only a transient and limited increase in serum norethisterone concentrations was observed following multiple application of the TDS.

Preclinical safety data: Estradiol is a naturally occurring hormone and norethisterone acetate is a synthetic derivative of 19-nortestosterone. The pharmacology and toxicology of estradiol and norethisterone acetate are well documented.

Additional toxicity studies which include local tolerance studies in rabbits and dermal sensitisation studies in guinea pigs have been conducted to support registration of Evorel Conti and Evorel Sequi. These studies indicate that the Evorel Conti TDS caused mild local skin irritation. It is recognised that test studies on rabbits over-predict skin irritation which occurs in humans. Evorel Conti appeared to be a weak sensitiser to the guinea pig model. Clinical trial experience with a duration of TDS use over more than one year revealed no evidence of a clinically relevant sensitisation potential in humans.

Pharmaceutical particulars

List of excipients:

Adhesive: acrylate-vinylacetate copolymer (Duro-Tak 387-2287); Guar gum. Backing film: polyethylene terephthalate foil (Hostaphan MN19); Release liner: siliconised polyethylene terephthalate foil, is removed before application.

Incompatibilities: No creams, lotions, or powders should be applied to the skin area where the TDS is to be applied to prevent interference with the adhesive properties of Evorel 50 TDS and Evorel Conti TDS.

Shelf life: Evorel Conti and Evorel Sequi have a shelf-life of 24 months when stored at or below 25 degrees Celsius. The product can be used until the expiration date mentioned on the container.

Special precautions for storage: Store at room temperature, at or below 25°C, within the original sachet and box.

Keep out of reach of children. This also applies to used and disposed TDSs.

Nature and contents of container:
Evorel Conti:

Each carton box has 8 TDSs in individual foil-lined sachets. The sachet comprises a 4 layer laminate including:

surlyn-ionomer film on the inside,
- then aluminium foil,
- then polyethylene film,
- with a layer of bleached reinforced paper on the outside.

Evorel Sequi:

Each carton box has 8 TDSs in individual foil-lined sachets. The sachet comprises a 4 layer laminate including:

- surlyn-ionomer film on the inside,
- then aluminium foil,
- then polyethylene film,
- with a layer of bleached reinforced paper on the outside.

One Evorel Sequi box contains 4 Evorel 50 TDSs and 4 Evorel Conti TDSs.

Instructions for use/handling: The TDSs should be placed on a clean, dry area of skin on the trunk of the body below the waist. Creams, lotions, or powders may interfere with the adhesive properties of the Evorel Conti and Evorel Sequi TDS. The TDS should not be applied on or near to the breasts. The area of application should be changed, with an interval of at least one week allowed between applications to a particular site. The skin area selected should not be damaged or irritated. The waistline should not be used because excessive rubbing of the TDS may occur.

The TDS should be used immediately after opening the sachet. Remove one part of the protecting foil. Apply the exposed part of adhesive to the application site from the edge to the middle; avoid wrinkling of the TDS. The second part of the protective foil should now be removed and the freshly exposed adhesive applied. Wrinkling should again be avoided and the palm of the hand used to press the TDS onto the skin and to bring the TDS to skin temperature at which the adhesive effect is optimised. Do not touch the adhesive part of the TDS.

When using Evorel Sequi for the first two weeks, one of the Evorel 50 TDSs should be applied and changed twice weekly. During the following two weeks of Evorel Sequi, one of the Evorel Conti TDSs should be applied, also to be changed twice weekly. The patient then starts again with a new box of Evorel Sequi.

To remove the EVOREL TDS, peel away an edge of the patch and pull smoothly away from the skin.

Any gum that remains on the skin after removal of EVOREL TDS may be removed by rubbing it off with the fingers or washing with soap and water.

The EVOREL TDS should be disposed of in household waste (do not flush down the toilet).

Marketing authorisation numbers
Evorel Conti 0242/0319
Evorel Sequi 0242/0320

Date of approval/revision of SPC June 1998.

Legal category POM.

EVOREL* PAK

Presentation Evorel Pak is a calendar pack comprising:

8 'Evorel 50' patches–each patch is a square shaped, transparent, self-adhesive transdermal delivery system of surface area 16 sq cm and 0.2 mm thickness, for application to the skin surface. Each consists of a monolayered adhesive matrix throughout which 17β-oestradiol is uniformly distributed and each contains 3.2 mg of oestradiol corresponding to a release rate of 50 micrograms of oestradiol in 24 hours. Patches are marked 'CE 50'.

12 white tablets each containing 1 mg norethisterone. The tablets are round with C over 1 engraved on both faces.

Uses Hormone replacement therapy for the symptomatic relief of menopausal symptoms.

Prevention and management of post-menopausal osteoporosis in women considered at risk of developing fractures. Epidemiological studies have suggested that there are a number of risk factors associated with post-menopausal osteoporosis such as early menopause, a family history of osteoporosis, prolonged exposure to corticosteroid therapy, small and thin skeletal frame and excessive cigarette smoking.

Mode of action: Oestrogen substitution effectively prevents the characteristic symptomatic, metabolic and atrophic changes associated with loss of ovarian function due to natural or surgical menopause.

Evorel releases oestradiol transdermally into the circulation. In post-menopausal women Evorel increases oestradiol levels to early and mid-follicular phase levels.

Norethisterone tablets, an oral progestogen, is used to oppose the oestrogenic effects on the endometrium by converting the oestrogen primed proliferative endometrium into secretory endometrium which, on withdrawal of norethisterone at the end of each cycle, causes a withdrawal bleed in most patients thus eliminating the possibility of endometrial hyperplasia.

Pharmacokinetics: With Evorel therapeutic serum oestradiol levels are achieved approximately four hours after application to the skin. From 10 hours onwards, the serum levels remain stable and at early to mid-follicular levels throughout the duration of the application (3 to 4 days).

Twenty four hours following removal of Evorel oestradiol levels return to baseline.

Norethisterone is rapidly and completely absorbed from the gastrointestinal tract; mean peak plasma levels are observed at 1–2 hours post-dose and the elimination half-life is 7-9 hours.

Dosage and administration
Adults:

Menopausal symptoms:

Therapy should be started with one Evorel 50 patch (delivering 50 micrograms of estradiol/24 hours) and the dose adjusted after the first month if necessary depending on efficacy and signs of over-oestrogenisation (e.g. breast tenderness). For maintenance therapy the lowest effective dose should be used; a maximum dose of 100 micrograms of estradiol/24 hours should not be exceeded.

Post-menopausal osteoporosis:

Evorel 50 is recommended as an effective bone-sparing dose, with lower doses of estradiol slowing but not halting bone loss.

Evorel should be applied twice weekly on a continuous basis, each patch being renewed after 3 to 4 days and a fresh patch applied. Evorel should be applied to the skin as soon as it is removed from the wrapper. Recommended application sites are on clean, dry, healthy, intact skin and each application should be made to a slightly different area of skin on the trunk below waistline. Evorel should not be applied on or near the breasts. Evorel should remain in place during bathing and showering. Should it fall off during bathing or showering the patient should wait until cutaneous vasodilation ceases before applying a replacement patch to avoid potential excessive absorption. Should a patch fall off at other times it should be replaced immediately.

Patients can be advised to use baby oil to help remove any gum/glue which may remain on their skin after patch removal.

Children: Evorel Pak is not indicated in children.

Use in pregnancy and lactation: Evorel Pak is contra-indicated in pregnancy or lactation.

Contra-indications, warnings, etc
Contra-indications: Known or suspected malignant tumours of the breast, genital tract or other oestrogen dependent neoplasia. Undiagnosed vaginal bleeding, known or suspected pregnancy and lactation, severe hepatic, renal or cardiac disease, Rotor syndrome or Dubin-Johnson syndrome, active thrombophlebitis or thromboembolic disorders, endometriosis, hypersensitivity to any of the excipients. History during pregnancy of idiopathic jaundice, severe pruritus or pemphigoid gestationis.

Precautions and warnings: At the present time there is suggestive evidence of an overall change in the relative risk of breast cancer in post menopausal women receiving hormone replacement therapy. Some studies have reported an increased risk of breast cancer in long-term users, others, however, have shown no such increase. It is not known whether concurrent progestogen use influences the risk of breast cancer. A careful appraisal of the risk/benefit ratio should be undertaken before treating for longer than 5 years.

Administration of unopposed oestrogen therapy in patients with an intact uterus has been reported to increase the risk of endometrial hyperplasia. Consequently, prior to commencing and periodically during oestrogen replacement therapy, it is recommended that the patient should be given a thorough physical and gynaecological examination and a complete medical and family history taken. Repeated breakthrough bleeding should be investigated, including endometrial biopsy.

Epidemiological studies have suggested that hormone replacement therapy (HRT) is associated with an increased relative risk of developing venous thromboembolism (VTE), i.e. deep vein thrombosis or pulmonary embolism. The studies find a 2–3 fold increase for users compared with non-users which for healthy women amounts to a low risk of one extra case of VTE each year for every 5,000 patients taking HRT.

Generally recognised risk factors for VTE include a personal or family history and severe obesity (body mass index >30 kg/m²). In women with these factors the benefits of treatment with HRT need to be carefully weighed against risks.

The risk of VTE may be temporarily increased with prolonged immobilisation, major trauma or major surgery. In women on HRT scrupulous attention should be given to prophylactic measures to prevent VTE following surgery. Where prolonged immobilisation is liable to follow elective surgery, particularly abdominal or orthopaedic surgery to the lower limbs, consideration should be given to temporarily stopping HRT 4 weeks earlier, if this is possible.

If venous thromboembolism develops after initiating therapy the drug should be discontinued.

Close monitoring is recommended in patients with epilepsy, diabetes or hypertension (as oestrogens may cause fluid retention), disturbances or impairment of liver function, mastopathy or a strong family history of breast cancer, fibrocystic disease, uterine fibromyomata, cholelithiasis, otosclerosis, multiple sclerosis, systemic lupus erythematosus, porphyria, melanoma, migraine, asthma, as these conditions may be worsened by oestrogen therapy.

Consideration should be given to discontinuing treatment at least four weeks prior to surgery or during periods of prolonged immobilisation. Also, if hypertension develops after initiating therapy, consider discontinuing Evorel Pak while the cause is investigated.

Drug interactions: Barbiturates, hydantoins, carbamazepine, meprobamate, phenylbutazone, antibiotics (including rifampicin) and activated charcoal, may impair the activity of oestrogen and progestogens (irregular bleeding and recurrence of symptoms may occur). In transdermal administration of oestradiol, a first pass effect via the liver is avoided.

Evorel Pak is not to be used for contraception.

Side effects: Minor effects of oestrogen and combined oestrogen/progestogen hormone replacement therapy which do not usually preclude continuation of therapy include headaches, nausea and breast-tenderness. The following side effects have been reported with oestrogen/progestogen therapy:

Genito-urinary system: Pre-menstrual-like syndrome, increase in size of uterine fibromyomata, vaginal candidiasis, change in cervical erosion and degree of cervical secretion, cystitis-like syndrome.

Breasts: Tenderness, enlargement, secretion.

Gastrointestinal: Nausea, vomiting, abdominal cramps, bloating, cholestatic jaundice.

Skin: Chloasma which may persist when drug is discontinued, erythema multiforme, erythema nodosum, haemorrhagic eruption, loss of scalp hair, hirsutism.

Eyes: Steepening of corneal curvature, intolerance to contact lenses.

CNS: Headaches, migraine, dizziness, mental depression, chorea.

Miscellaneous: Increase or decrease in weight, reduced carbohydrate tolerance, aggravation of porphyria, oedema, changes in libido, leg cramps.

In clinical studies with 'Evorel 50' patches, the following side effects were seen: breast tenderness (less than 2%), bleeding (less than 2%) and intermittent bleeding/spotting (less than 5%). None were serious and they reflect the known profile of oestrogen or oestrogen/progestogen therapy. Skin reactions were reported by less than 6% of patients over six treatment cycles.

Overdosage: There have been no reports of serious ill-effects from overdosage with Evorel or norethisterone and treatment is usually unnecessary. Nausea and vomiting may occur in the event of a norethisterone overdosage. There is no special antidote and treatment should be symptomatic. The most commonly observed symptoms of overdose with oestrogen therapy are breast tenderness, nausea and breakthrough bleeding. Effects of Evorel overdosage can be reversed by removal of the patch.

Pharmaceutical precautions Protect from light. Store below 25°C.

Legal category POM.

Package quantities Evorel Pak contains: 8 'Evorel 50' patches, each presented in a sealed protective pouch; 12 norethisterone 1 mg tablets; Patient Information Booklet.

Product licence numbers 0242/0223 and 0232/0241

EVOREL* 25, EVOREL 50, EVOREL 75 AND EVOREL 100 PATCH

Qualitative and quantitative composition Each Evorel 25 patch contains 1.6 mg estradiol, each 50 patch contains 3.2 mg estradiol, each Evorel 75 patch contains 4.8 mg estradiol and each Evorel 100 patch contains 6.4 mg estradiol.

Pharmaceutical form Evorel is a square shaped, transparent, self-adhesive transdermal delivery system (patch) of 0.2 mm thickness for application to the skin surface. It consists of a monolayered adhesive matrix throughout which 17β oestradiol is uniformly distributed. The adhesive matrix is protected on the outside surface (from clothes etc) by a polyethylene terephthalate backing foil, while the adhesive surface of the patch is covered by a polyester sheet (the release liner) which is removed before placing the patch on the body surface. This release liner has an S-shaped incision which facilitates easy removal from the patch.

Evorel is available in four sizes corresponding to four different concentrations:

Evorel 25 is marked 'CE25', has a surface area of 8 sq cm and contains 1.6 mg oestradiol corresponding to a release rate of 25 micrograms of oestradiol in 24 hours.

Evorel 50 is marked 'CE50', has a surface area of 16 sq cm and contains 3.2 mg oestradiol corresponding to a release rate of 50 micrograms of oestradiol in 24 hours.

Evorel 75 is marked 'CE75', has a surface area of 24 sq cm and contains 4.8 mg oestradiol corresponding to a release rate of 75 micrograms of oestradiol in 24 hours.

Evorel 100 is marked 'CE100', has a surface area of 32 sq cm and contains 6.4 mg oestradiol corresponding to a release rate of 100 micrograms of oestradiol in 24 hours.

Clinical particulars

Therapeutic indications: Oestrogen replacement for the symptomatic relief of menopausal symptoms.

Evorel 50, 75 and 100 only: Prevention and management of post-menopausal osteoporosis in women considered at risk of developing fractures. Epidemiological studies have suggested that there are a number of risk factors associated with post-menopausal osteoporosis such as early menopause, a family history of osteoporosis, prolonged exposure to corticosteroid therapy, small and thin skeletal frame and excessive cigarette smoking.

Posology and method of administration:
Menopausal symptoms:

Therapy should be started with one Evorel 50 patch (delivering 50 micrograms of estradiol/24 hours) and the dose adjusted after the first month if necessary depending on efficacy and signs of over-oestrogenisation (e.g. breast tenderness). For maintenance therapy the lowest effective dose should be used; a maximum dose of 100 micrograms of estradiol/24 hours should not be exceeded.

Evorel 50, 75 and 100 only:
Post-menopausal osteoporosis:

Evorel 50, 75 and 100 are recommended as an effective bone-sparing dose, with lower doses of estradiol slowing but not halting bone loss.

Evorel should be applied twice weekly on a continuous basis, each patch being renewed after 3 to 4 days and a fresh patch applied. Evorel should be applied to the skin as soon as it is removed from the wrapper.

Recommended application sites are on clean, dry, healthy, intact skin and each application should be made to a slightly different area of skin on the trunk below waistline. **Evorel should not be applied on or near the breasts.** Evorel should remain in place during bathing and showering. Should it fall off during bathing or showering the patient should wait until cutaneous vasodilation ceases before applying a replacement patch to avoid potential excessive absorption. Should a patch fall off at other times it should be replaced immediately.

Patients can be advised to use baby oil to help remove any gum/glue which may remain on their skin after patch removal.

Unopposed oestrogen therapy is not recommended unless the patient has had hysterectomy. Where a progestogen is considered necessary, the appropriate dose should be administered for not less than 12 days each month.

Children: Evorel is not indicated in children.

Contra-indications: Known or suspected malignant tumours of the breast, genital tract or other oestrogen dependent neoplasia. Undiagnosed vaginal bleeding, known or suspected pregnancy and lactation, severe hepatic, renal or cardiac disease, Rotor syndrome or Dubin-Johnson syndrome, active thrombophlebitis, active deep venous thrombosis, thromboembolic disorders, or a history of confirmed venous thromboembolism, endometriosis, hypersensitivity to any of the excipients.

Special warnings and special precautions for use: At the present time there is suggestive evidence of an overall change in the relative risk of breast cancer in the post menopausal women receiving hormone replacement therapy. A careful appraisal of the risk/benefit ratio should be undertaken before treating for longer than 5 years.

Administration of unopposed oestrogen therapy in patients with an intact uterus has been reported to increase the risk of endometrial hyperplasia. Consequently, prior to commencing and periodically during oestrogen replacement therapy, it is recommended that the patient should be given a thorough physical and gynaecological examination and a complete medical and family history taken. Repeated breakthrough bleeding should be investigated, including endometrial biopsy.

Close monitoring is recommended in patients with: epilepsy, diabetes or hypertension (as oestrogens may cause fluid retention), disturbances or impairment of liver function, mastopathy or a strong family history of breast cancer, fibrocystic disease, uterine fibromyomata, cholelithiasis, otosclerosis, multiple sclerosis, systemic lupus erythematosus, porphyria, melanoma, migraine, and asthma, as these conditions may be worsened by oestrogen therapy.

Consideration should be given to discontinuing treatment at least four weeks prior to surgery or during periods of prolonged immobilisation. Also, if hypertension develops after initiating therapy, consider discontinuing Evorel while the cause is investigated.

Epidemiological studies have suggested that hormone replacement therapy (HRT) is associated with an increased relative risk of developing venous thromboembolism (VTE), i.e. deep vein thrombosis or pulmonary embolism. The studies find a 2–3 fold increase for users compared with non-users which for healthy women amounts to a low risk of one extra case of VTE each year for every 5,000 patients taking HRT.

Generally recognised risk factors for VTE include a personal or family history and severe obesity (body mass index >30 kg/m^2). In women with these factors the benefits of treatment with HRT need to be carefully weighed against risks.

The risk of VTE may be temporarily increased with prolonged immobilisation, major trauma or major surgery. In women on HRT scrupulous attention should be given to prophylactic measures to prevent VTE following surgery. Where prolonged immobilisation is liable to follow elective surgery, particularly abdominal or orthopaedic surgery to the lower limbs, consideration should be given to temporarily stopping HRT 4 weeks earlier, if this is possible.

If venous thromboembolism develops after initiating therapy the drug should be discontinued.

Evorel is not to be used for contraception.

Interaction with other medicaments and other forms of interaction: Drugs which cause liver enzyme induction may alter oestrogen action. Examples of such drugs include barbiturates, hydantoins, carbamazepine, meprobamate, phenylbutazole and rifampicin. In transdermal administration of estradiol, a first pass effect via the liver is avoided.

There have been no reports of interaction with Evorel although the clinical exposure has been very limited.

Pregnancy and lactation: Evorel is contra-indicated in pregnancy and lactation.

Effects on ability to drive and use machines: In normal use, Evorel would not be expected to have any effect on the ability to drive or use machinery.

Undesirable effects: Although side effects are rare, minor effects which do not usually preclude continuation of therapy include headaches, nausea, breast tenderness, and intermittent bleeding.

In clinical studies with Evorel (50 µg/24 hours) the following side effects were seen: breast tenderness (less than 2%), bleeding (less than 21%), and intermittent bleeding/spotting (less than 5%). None were serious, reflecting the known profile of oestrogen or oestrogen/progestogen therapy. Skin reactions were reported by less than 6% of patients over six treatment cycles. Rarely, dizziness, bloating, oedema, weight gain and leg cramps may occur.

Overdose: By virtue of the mode of administration of Evorel, overdosage is unlikely, but effects can if necessary be reversed by removal of the patch. The most commonly observed symptoms of overdose with oestrogen therapy are breast tenderness, nausea and breakthrough bleeding.

Pharmacological properties

Pharmacodynamic properties: Estradiol is a naturally occurring oestrogenic hormone. It is formed in the ovarian follicles under the influence of the pituitary gland. In the female it stimulates the accessory reproductive organs and causes development of the secondary sexual changes in the endometrium during the first half of the menstrual cycle.

Estradiol is readily and completely absorbed from the gastro-intestinal tract through the skin and mucous membranes. Metabolism is primarily in the liver. Excretion of the less active metabolites, primarily oestrone and oestriol is via the urine.

Evorel releases estradiol transdermally into the circulation in pre-menopausal physiological amounts.

In post-menopausal women Evorel increased estradiol levels to early and mid-follicular phase levels. The transcutaneous route avoids the first pass hepatic effect seen with orally administered oestrogens.

In contrast with oral oestrogens, stimulation of hepatic protein synthesis is largely avoided with consequent lack of effect on circulating levels of renin substrate, thyroid binding globulin, sex hormone binding globulin and cortisol binding globulin. Similarly coagulation factors also appear to be unaffected (eg fibrinopeptide A etc). Transdermal estradiol does not affect circulating levels of renin.

Studies with Evorel have shown a significant decrease in hot flushes, improvement in Kupperman Index and vaginal cytology.

Local tolerance with Evorel has been very good. The adhesive matrix used has a low irritation index.

Pharmacokinetic properties:

General characteristics: Oestrogens are in general readily absorbed from the gastro-intestinal tract, through the skin and mucous membranes. Absorption from the gastro-intestinal tract is prompt and complete. Transdermal absorption of oestrogens is sufficient to cause a systemic effect. Inactivation of oestrogens is related to first pass hepatic metabolism and not to poor absorption. A certain proportion of oestrogen is excreted into the bile and then reabsorbed from the intestine. During the enterohepatic circulation, estradiol is readily oxidised to the less pharmacologically active oestrone which may in turn then be hydrated to form oestriol (also pharmacologically less than estradiol). Estradiol circulates in the blood in association with sex hormone-binding globulin and albumin.

Characteristics in patients: With Evorel therapeutic serum estradiol levels are achieved approximately four hours after application to the skin. From 10 hours onwards, the serum levels remain stable and at early to mid-follicular levels throughout the duration of the application (3 to 4 days).

Twenty four hours following removal of the transdermal therapeutic system estradiol levels return to baseline.

Preclinical safety data: Not applicable.

Pharmaceutical particulars

List of excipients: Adhesive acrylic polymer (Duro-Tak 387-2287); Guar gum (meyprogat 90); Hostaphan MN19 (polyester film–removed before application).

Incompatibilities: None known.

Shelf life: Evorel 25 patch, 70 patch and 100 patch: 18 months for the product as packed for sale.

Evorel 50 patch: 24 months for the product as packed for sale.

Special precautions for storage: Store below 25°C.

Nature and contents of container: Each Evorel patch size is presented in a sealed protective pouch. The pouches are packed in a cardboard carton.

Instructions for use/handling: None.

Marketing authorisation numbers

Evorel 25	0242/0293
Evorel 50	0242/0223
Evorel 75	0242/0294
Evorel 100	0242/0295

Date of approval/revision of SPC June 1998

Legal category POM.

GYNE-T* 380 INTRAUTERINE COPPER CONTRACEPTIVE DEVICE

Presentation Each device consists of a polyethylene 'T' shaped support with 180 mg pure copper wire (providing a surface area of 320 mm^2) wound around the vertical section of the 'T' and one collar with 70 mg pure copper providing an exposed surface area of 30 mm^2 on the distal portion of each transverse arm. The support is impregnated with a radiopaque substance and has a polyethylene suture attached to the base of the 'T'.

Uses Contraception.

Dosage and administration One device is inserted by its introducer into the uterus preferably at the end of the menstrual period. The device should be removed after ten years of use. If continued contraception is required a new device may be inserted.

Contra-indications, warnings, etc.

Contra-indications:

Pregnancy or suspected pregnancy.

Malignancy of the genital tract.

Undiagnosed vaginal bleeding.
Unresolved abnormal cervical smear.
Active pelvic inflammatory disease or a history of repeated pelvic inflammatory disease.
Copper allergy or Wilson's disease.
Postpartum endometriosis or septic abortion in the past 3 months.
Distortion of uterine cavity.
Untreated acute cervicitis or vaginitis.
Leukaemia.

Warnings and precautions:
Prior to insertion: A thorough history and physical examination, including a pelvic examination and cervical cytology (if a smear has not recently been taken) should be performed, to exclude pregnancy, infection, other abnormalities of the uterus and to determine the size and position of the uterus.

Vaginal or cervical infection should be appropriately treated before insertion is considered.

IUCDs should also be used with caution in patients with hypermenorrhoea, or receiving coagulopathy.

It has been reported that IUCDs may be less effective in insulin-dependent diabetics.

Insertion: Insertion should be as early as possible in the menstrual cycle unless alternative methods of effective contraception have been used throughout the cycle.

If the device is being inserted into a patient with known or suspected cardiac abnormalities then antibiotic cover is required both at insertion and removal.

The possibility of a seizure being precipitated in an epileptic, at or shortly after insertion should be borne in mind.

Insertion of an IUCD into a uterine cavity measuring less than 6.5 cm by sounding may increase the incidence of expulsion, bleeding pain and perforation. Expulsion rate can also be increased when insertions are made before normal uterine involution occurs following delivery.

Precautions in use: The patient should be re-examined 3 months after insertion, and thereafter at yearly intervals to ensure the device is still in place. If a partial expulsion occurs, removal is indicated and a new IUCD may be inserted.

The patient should be advised to contact her doctor immediately if she misses a menstrual period, has any other reason to think she may be pregnant, or if any other unwanted symptoms develop.

If pregnancy should occur with an IUCD *in situ* and the threads are visible, in the absence of reasons to the contrary, it is recommended that the device be removed as soon as possible even though removal may increase the chances of miscarriage. If the patient elects to maintain the pregnancy, she should be warned that there may be an increased risk of abortion or premature labor and delivery and/or sepsis.

The risk of ectopic pregnancy may be greater in women who conceive with an IUCD *in situ*. Therefore women who become pregnant while using an IUCD should be carefully evaluated for the possibility of an ectopic pregnancy.

Abnormal bleeding in an established IUCD user is not necessarily due to the device and should always be fully investigated to exclude other pathology.

Medical diathermy or ultrasonic therapy must not be applied to the user's abdomen or sacral region, since heating of the copper may cause injury.

Removal of Ortho Gyne-T 380
The device should be removed for the following reasons:
Uterine or cervical perforation.
Partial downward displacement of the device within the cervical canal.
Endometrial or cervical malignancy.
Uncontrolled pelvic infection.
Menorrhagia and/or metrorrhagia producing significant anaemia.
Intractable pain often aggravated by intercourse.
Dyspareunia.
Pregnancy (if thread is visible).
Genital actinomycosis.

Lost threads: The patient should check periodically, particularly after menstruation to ensure that the threads still protrude from the cervix. She should return to her doctor if she becomes aware that the device has been expelled.

In the absence of a detectable thread, a uterine sound should be introduced into the endometrial cavity following the same technique as for insertion. In most cases the IUCD can be detected by the sound. If the threads have retracted into the uterine cavity, they may be brought back down through the cervix and into the vagina. In such cases there is usually no need to replace the device providing there is no evidence of infection.

If the device cannot be detected by the sound, ultrasound or X-ray techniques may be required.

Pregnancy and lactation: Use is contra-indicated in pregnancy.

Insertions within 48 hours postpartum are associated with an increased risk of expulsion. Insertions from 48 hours to 4 weeks are associated with an increased risk of perforation.

An IUCD can be inserted from 4 weeks to 8 weeks postpartum without an apparent increase in pregnancy rate, expulsion, uterine perforation or removals for bleeding and/or pain.

Side effects: The following adverse effects have been reported with the use of IUCDs:
Uterine or cervical perforation.
Pregnancy with an IUCD *in situ* or when an IUCD has been partially or completely expelled.
On insertion some cramping usually for no more than a few minutes duration; however some women may experience residual cramping for several hours or even days).
Intermenstrual spotting or bleeding or prolonged or increased menstrual flow.
Pelvic inflammatory disease including salpingitis with tubal damage or occlusion.
Urticarial allergic skin reactions.
Other adverse effects reported include: Amenorrhoea or delayed menses, backaches, cervical erosion, cystic masses in the pelvis, vaginitis, dyspareunia, endometritis, spontaneous abortion, septic abortion, septicaemia, leukorrhea, infection of reproductive organs, ectopic pregnancy, difficult removal, uterine embedment, anaemia, abdominal or pelvic pain, neurovascular episodes including bradycardia and syncope associated with insertion or removal, dysmenorrhoea, infection with actinomyces, fragmentation of the copper wire on the IUCD and breakage of the IUCD and/or the string.

Overdosage: Not applicable.

Pharmaceutical precautions If the seal of the sterile pack is broken the device inside should not be used.

Package quantities Each sterile Gyne-T 380 Intrauterine Copper Contraceptive Device unit is supplied in a sealed transparent pouch. Full fitting instructions and advice for the patient are supplied with each device.

Further information Nil.

GYNO-DAKTARIN* 1

Qualitative and quantitative composition Miconazole nitrate 1200 mg.

Pharmaceutical form White, egg-shaped soft gelatin Scherer capsule.

Clinical particulars
Therapeutic indications: For the local treatment of vulvovaginal candidosis and superinfections due to gram-positive bacteria.

Posology and method of administration: Gyno-Daktarin 1 is for intravaginal administration.

Adults and elderly: One ovule to be inserted high in the vagina at night, as a single dose.

Children: Not recommended.

Contra-indications: None known.

Special warnings and special precautions for use: None known.

Interaction with other medicaments and other forms of interaction: Contact should be avoided between contraceptive diaphragms or sheaths and Gyno-Daktarin 1 since the rubber may be damaged by the emollient base.

Pregnancy and lactation: In animals, miconazole nitrate has shown no teratogenic effects but is foetotoxic at high oral doses. The significance of this to man is unknown as there is no evidence of increased risk when taken in human pregnancy. However, as with other imidazoles, Gyno-Daktarin 1 should be used in pregnant women only if the practitioner considers it to be necessary.

Effects on ability to drive and use machines: None.

Undesirable effects: Occasionally, irritation has been reported. Rarely, local sensitisation may occur requiring discontinuation of treatment.

Overdose: Gyno-Daktarin 1 is for intravaginal use only. If accidental ingestion of large quantities occurs, an appropriate method of gastric emptying may be used if considered desirable.

Pharmacological properties
Pharmacodynamic properties: Miconazole is a synthetic imidazole antifungal agent with a broad spectrum of activity against pathogenic fungi (including yeasts and dermatophytes) and gram-positive bacteria (*Staphylococcus* and *Streptococcus* spp).

Pharmacokinetic properties: There is little absorption through mucous membranes when miconazole nitrate is applied topically.

Preclinical safety data: Not applicable.

Pharmaceutical particulars
List of excipients: Liquid paraffin; white petrolatum; lecithin. The capsule itself contains: Gelatin; glycerol; titanium dioxide; sodium ethylparahydroxybenzoate; sodium propyl parahydroxybenzoate and medium chain triglycerides.

Incompatibilities: None known.

Shelf life: 60 months.

Special precautions for storage: Store at room temperature.

Nature and contents of container: Blister packs.

Instructions for use/handling: None.

Marketing authorisation number 0242/0121

Date of approval/revision of SPC July 1998

Legal category POM.

GYNO-DAKTARIN*

Presentation *Cream:* White, non-staining, water miscible cream containing miconazole nitrate PhEur 2% w/w. Cream also contains benzoic acid (E210), butylated hydroxyanisole (E320), liquid paraffin, macrogol 6-32 stearate, glycol stearate, unsaturated polyglycolysed glycerides and purified water.

Pessary: White, non-staining pessaries each containing 100 mg miconazole nitrate PhEur.

Combi-pack: White, non-staining pessaries each containing 100 mg miconazole nitrate PhEur plus white, non-staining, water miscible cream containing miconazole nitrate PhEur 2% w/w.

Uses Miconazole is a synthetic imidazole antifungal agent with a broad spectrum of activity against pathogenic fungi (including yeasts and dermatophytes) and gram-positive bacteria (*Staphylococcus* and *Streptococcus* spp).

Gyno-Daktarin is for the local treatment of vulvovaginal candidosis and superinfection due to susceptible Gram-positive bacteria.

Dosage and administration Gyno-Daktarin cream may be used in both adults and children. Gyno-Daktarin pessaries are for use in adults only.

Cream: 5 g once daily into vagina for 10–14 days or twice daily for 7 days. For vulvitis the cream should be applied topically twice daily.

Continue treatment for a few days after symptomatic relief has been achieved.

Pessary: One pessary to be inserted high into the vagina as a single dose at night for 14 days, or twice daily for 7 days. The cream should also be applied to the vulva twice daily.

Contra-indications, warnings, etc
Contra-indications: None known.

Interactions: Contact between contraceptive diaphragms or condoms and the cream or pessaries must be avoided since the rubber may be damaged by this preparation.

Use in pregnancy: In animals miconazole nitrate has shown no teratogenic effects but is foetotoxic at high oral doses. The significance of this to man is unknown as there is no evidence of an increased risk when taken in human pregnancy. However as with other imidazoles, Gyno-Daktarin should be used in pregnant women only if the practitioner considers it to be necessary.

Side effects: Occasionally, irritation has been reported. Rarely, local sensitisation may occur requiring discontinuation of treatment.

Precautions: Contact should be avoided between contraceptive diaphragms or sheaths and Gyno-Daktarin pessaries since the rubber may be damaged by the emollient base.

Overdosage: Gyno-Daktarin preparations are for intravaginal or topical use only. If accidental ingestion of large quantities occurs, an appropriate method of gastric emptying may be used if considered desirable.

Pharmaceutical precautions *Cream and pessaries:* Store at or below 25°C.

Legal category POM.

Package quantities *Cream:* Gyno-Daktarin cream is supplied in 78 g tubes with disposable applicators – seven days' treatment. *Combi-pack:* Gyno-Daktarin combi-pack consists of 14 pessaries plus 15 g topical cream.

Further information Gyno-Daktarin may be used in 'problem vaginitis' as seen in diabetic patients and in women using oral contraceptives.

A leaflet instructing the patient on the correct use is included in each package of Gyno-Daktarin.

Product licence numbers

Gyno-Daktarin Cream	0242/0015
Gyno-Daktarin Combi-Pack	0242/0015
	0242/0037

GYNO-DAKTARIN* PESSARIES

Qualitative and quantitative composition Miconazole nitrate 100 mg.

Pharmaceutical form Vaginal pessary.

Clinical particulars
Therapeutic indications: For the local treatment of vulvovaginal candidosis and superinfections due to gram-positive bacteria.

Posology and method of administration:
Adults and elderly: One pessary to be inserted in the vagina once daily for 14 days or 1 pessary twice daily for 7 days.

Children: Not recommended.

Method of administration: Vaginal administration.

Contra-indications: None known.

Special warnings and special precautions for use: None.

Interaction with other medicaments and other forms of interaction: Contact should be avoided between contraceptive diaphragms or sheaths and Gyno-Daktarin pessaries since the rubber may be damaged by the emollient base.

Pregnancy and lactation: In animals, miconazole nitrate has shown no teratogenic effects but is foetotoxic at high oral doses. The significance of this to man is unknown as there is no evidence of increased risk when taken in human pregnancy. However, as with other imidazoles, Gyno-Daktarin should be used in pregnant women only if the practitioner considers it to be necessary.

Effects on ability to drive and use machines: None.

Undesirable effects: Occasionally, irritation has been reported. Rarely, local sensitisation may occur requiring discontinuation of treatment.

Overdose: Gyno-Daktarin pessaries are for intravaginal use only. In the unlikely event of oral ingestion, an appropriate method of gastric emptying may be used if considered desirable.

Pharmacological properties
Pharmacodynamic properties: Miconazole is a synthetic imidazole antifungal agent with a broad spectrum of activity against pathogenic fungi (including yeasts and dermatophytes) and gram-positive bacteria (*Staphylococcus* and *Streptococcus* spp).

Pharmacokinetic properties: There is little absorption through mucous membranes when miconazole nitrate is applied topically.

Preclinical safety data: Not applicable.

Pharmaceutical particulars
List of excipients: Hard fat.

Incompatibilities: Not applicable.

Shelf life: 60 months.

Special precautions for storage: Store at or below 25°C.

Nature and contents of container: Cardboard cartons containing 14 pessaries packed in PVC-polyethylene strips.

Combination pack: 1 x pessary pack as above and Gyno-Daktarin Cream pack(s) as for PL 0242/0015.

Instructions for use/handling: The following information will appear in the Patient Information Leaflet:

1. Each of the Gyno-Daktarin pessaries is individually wrapped to protect it and keep it clean. To remove a pessary, tear down the groove separating two pessaries and peel back the plastic wrapping, starting at the smooth end.
2. Lie on your back with your knees up and your legs apart. Holding the pessary between your thumb and first finger, insert the pessary as high into the vagina as possible with your finger.
3. Always wash your hands with soap and warm water after inserting the pessary.

Marketing authorisation number 0242/0037

Date of approval/revision of SPC April 1997.

Legal category POM.

GYNO-PEVARYL* CREAM

Presentation A white non-perfumed cream containing 1% w/w econazole nitrate.

Uses For the treatment of mycotic vulvovaginitis and mycotic balanitis.

Dosage and administration
Females: One applicatorful (approximately 5 g) intravaginally once daily at night for not less than 14 days. The cream should also be applied to the vulva. The full 14 days treatment should be carried out even if the symptoms of vaginal itching or discharge have disappeared. The sexual partner should also be treated.

Contra-indications, warnings, etc Hypersensitivity to any imidazole preparation (or other vaginal antifungal products).

Side effects: Rarely, transient local mild irritation may occur immediately after application.

Precautions: Hypersensitivity has rarely been recorded, if it should occur, administration should be discontinued.

Gyno-Pevaryl Cream should be used only by those women who have symptoms of candidosis, and think that they might have candidosis.

If they believe or suspect that they might have some other sexually transmitted disease, either as well as, or instead of, candidosis, they should consult a Genitourinary Medicine Clinic or their own doctor.

The preparation should not be used if they are pregnant, or think that they might be pregnant, without first consulting a doctor.

It should not be used by those under 16 years of age or over 60 years without first consulting a doctor.

The woman should see her doctor if, after treatment:
- There is not complete relief of symptoms within 7 days.
- There is recurrence of symptoms within 4 weeks of treatment.
- She has more than two episodes of infection within a 6 month period, even if it completely resolves with treatment.
- Adverse effects such as redness, irritation or swelling, associated with the treatment occur.

Self medication should not be undertaken if the woman has:
- Any abnormal or irregular vaginal bleeding.
- Any blood staining of a vaginal discharge.
- Any vulval or vaginal sores, ulcers or blisters.
- Any associated lower abdominal pain or dysuria.

In all of these cases she should consult her doctor.

Contact between contraceptive diaphragms and this product must be avoided since the rubber may be damaged by this preparation.

In animals, econazole nitrate has shown no teratogenic effects, but is foetotoxic at high doses. The significance of this to man is unknown as there is no evidence of increased risk when taken in human pregnancy. However, as with other imidazoles, econazole should only be used in pregnancy if the practitioner considers it to be necessary.

Overdosage: Gyno-Pevaryl Cream is intended for intravaginal/penile use. If accidental ingestion of large quantities of the product occurs, an appropriate method of gastric emptying may be used if considered desirable.

Pharmaceutical precautions Store at room temperature, not exceeding 25°C.

Legal category P.

Package quantities Tubes of 15 g and 30 g. An applicator is not included in the pack. It can be purchased separately.

Further information Anogenital hygiene is important to help prevent reinfection.

Product licence number 0242/0229.

GYNO-PEVARYL* 1 VAGINAL PESSARY
GYNO-PEVARYL* 1 VAGINAL PESSARY AND CREAM C.P. PACK

Presentation *Pessary:* Light beige bullet shaped pessary containing 150 mg econazole nitrate PhEur.

C.P. Pack: A combination pack comprising a Gyno-Pevaryl 1 Vaginal Pessary (containing 150 mg econazole nitrate) and a 15 g tube of Gyno-Pevaryl Cream (containing 1% w/w econazole nitrate).

Uses
Pessary: Vaginitis due to *Candida albicans* and other yeasts.

C.P. Pack: Pessary as above; cream to treat mycotic vulvovaginitis and mycotic balanitis.

Dosage and administration
Pessary: The pessary should be inserted as high as possible into the vagina in the evening prior to retiring.

C.P. Pack: Pessary as above. One applicatorful (approximately 5 g) intravaginally once daily at night for not less than 14 days. The cream should also be applied to the vulva. The full 14 days treatment should be carried out even if the symptoms of vaginal itching or discharge have disappeared. The sexual partner should also be treated.

Contra-indications, warnings, etc
Contra-indications: Hypersensitivity to any imidazole preparation (or other vaginal antifungal products).

Side effects: Rarely, transient local mild irritation may occur immediately after application.

Precautions: Hypersensitivity has rarely been recorded, if it should occur, administration of the product should be discontinued.

Gyno-Pevaryl Cream should be used only by those women who have symptoms of candidosis, and think that they might have candidosis.

If they believe or suspect that they might have some other sexually transmitted disease, either as well as, or instead of, candidosis, they should consult a Genitourinary Medicine Clinic or their own doctor.

The preparation should not be used if they are pregnant, or think that they might be pregnant, without first consulting a doctor.

It should not be used by those under 16 years of age or over 60 years without first consulting a doctor.

The woman should see her doctor if, after treatment:
- There is not complete relief of symptoms within 7 days.
- There is recurrence of symptoms within 4 weeks of treatment.
- She has more than two episodes of infection within a 6 month period, even if it completely resolves with treatment.
- Adverse effects such as redness, irritation or swelling, associated with the treatment occur.

Self medication should not be undertaken if the woman has:
- Any abnormal or irregular vaginal bleeding.
- Any blood staining of a vaginal discharge.
- Any vulval or vaginal sores, ulcers or blisters.
- Any associated lower abdominal pain or dysuria.

In all of these cases she should consult her doctor.

Contact between contraceptive diaphragms and this product must be avoided since the rubber may be damaged by this preparation.

In animals econazole nitrate has shown no teratogenic effects, but is foetotoxic at high doses. The significance of this in man is unknown as there is no evidence of an increased risk when taken in human pregnancy. However, as with other imidazoles, econazole should be used in pregnancy only if the practitioner considers it to be necessary.

Overdosage: Gyno-Pevaryl 1 Vaginal Pessary and Cream are intended for intravaginal use. Cream is also for penile use. If accidental ingestion of large quantities of the product occurs, an appropriate method of gastric emptying may be used if considered desirable.

Pharmaceutical precautions Store at room temperature, not exceeding 25°C.

Legal category P.

Package quantities *Pessaries:* Each pack contains one pessary with a plastic vaginal applicator and a patient instruction leaflet. The pessary is individually sealed in a white plastic strip marked Gyno-Pevaryl 1.

C.P. Pack: Each pack contains one pessary, a 15 g tube of cream and a patient instruction leaflet.

Further information Anogenital hygiene is important to help prevent re-infection.

Due to the differing nature of the pessary base of Gyno-Pevaryl 1, substitution of a single Gyno-Pevaryl 150 pessary from the three pessary treatment must not be made.

Product licence numbers

Gyno-Pevaryl	0242/0226
Combipack	0242/0226 and 0242/0229

GYNO-PEVARYL*150 VAGINAL PESSARIES

Qualitative and quantitative composition Vaginal pessaries each containing 150 mg econazole nitrate.

Pharmaceutical form Pessaries (creamy, white to yellowish, bullet-shaped).

Clinical particulars
Therapeutic indications: Vaginitis due to Candida albicans and other yeasts

Posology and method of administration: Gyno-Pevaryl 150 mg Vaginal Pessaries are for vaginal administration.

One pessary should be inserted high into the vagina each evening for three consecutive days.

This product should not be used by those under 16 years of age or over 60 years of age without first consulting a doctor.

Contra-indications: Hypersensitivity to any imidazole preparation or other vaginal antifungal products.

Special warnings and precautions for use: Hypersensitivity has rarely been recorded; if it should occur administration should be discontinued.

Gyno-Pevaryl 150 mg Vaginal Pessaries should be used only by those women who have symptoms of candidosis, and think that they might have candidosis.

If a woman believes or suspects that she might have some other sexually transmitted disease, either as well as, or instead of, candidosis, she should consult a genitourinary medicine clinic or her own doctor.

Gyno-Pevaryl should not be used by those under 16 years of age or over 60 years of age without first consulting a doctor.

The woman should see her doctor if, after treatment:

- There is not complete relief of symptoms within 7 days
- There is the recurrence of symptoms within 4 weeks of treatment
- She has more than two episodes of infection within a 6 month period, even if they completely resolve with treatment.
- Adverse effects such as redness, irritation or swelling, associated with the treatment occur.

Self medication should not be undertaken if the woman has:

- Any abnormal or irregular vaginal bleeding
- Any blood staining of a vaginal discharge
- Any vulval or vaginal sores, ulcers or blisters
- Any associated lower abdominal pain or dysuria.

In all of these cases the woman should consult her doctor.

Interaction with other medicaments and other forms of interaction: Contact between contraceptive diaphragms and this product must be avoided since the rubber may be damaged by this preparation.

Pregnancy and lactation: In animals, econazole nitrate has shown no teratogenic effects but is foetotoxic at high dose. The significance of this to man is unknown as there is no evidence of an increased risk when taken in human pregnancy. However, as with other imidazoles, econazole should be used in pregnancy only if the practitioner considers it to be necessary.

Effects on ability to drive and use machines: None known.

Undesirable effects: Rarely, transient local mild irritation may occur immediately after application.

Overdose: Gyno-Pevaryl 150 mg Vaginal Pessaries are intended for intra-vaginal use and by that route overdose is extremely unlikely. If accidental ingestion of large quantities of the product occurs an appropriate method of gastric emptying may be used if considered desirable.

Pharmacological properties
Pharmacodynamic properties: Econazole nitrate has no anti-inflammatory action, no effects on the circulation, no central or autonomic nervous effects, no effects on respiration, no effect on α or β adrenergic receptors, no anticholinergic or antiserotonic reactions.

A broad spectrum of antimycotic activity has been demonstrated against dermatophytes, yeasts and moulds. A clinically relevant action against Gram positive bacteria has also been found.

Econazole acts by damaging cell membranes. The permeability of the fungal cell is increased. Subcellular membranes in the cytoplasm are damaged. The site of action is most probably the unsaturated fatty acid acyl moiety of membrane phospholipids.

Pharmacokinetic properties: Econazole nitrate is poorly absorbed from the vagina and skin. No active drug has been detected in the serum, but radio labelling has shown that absorption is less than 0.1%. When administered orally, peak serum levels occur two hours after dosing. About 90% of the absorbed dose is bound to plasma proteins. Metabolism is limited, but primarily occurs in the liver. Metabolites are excreted in the urine. Five major and two minor metabolites have been identified.

Preclinical safety data: Not applicable.

Pharmaceutical particulars
List of excipients: Wecobee M; Wecobee FS

Incompatibilities: None known.

Shelf life: Five years.

Special precautions for storage: Store at room temperature (not exceeding 25°C).

Nature and contents of container: Available in PVC/PE strips containing three pessaries.

Instructions for use/handling: Not applicable.

Marketing authorisation number 0242/0227

Date of approval/revision of SPC May 1997

Legal category P

GYNO-PEVARYL*150 VAGINAL PESSARIES AND CREAM COMBIPACK

Presentation A combination pack comprising 3 Gyno-Pevaryl vaginal pessaries (each containing 150 mg econazole nitrate) plus a 15 g tube of Gyno-Pevaryl cream (containing 1% w/w econazole nitrate).

Uses Pessaries: Vaginitis due to *Candida albicans* and other yeasts; cream to treat mycotic vulvovaginitis and mycotic balanitis.

Dosage and administration Pessaries: One pessary should be inserted high into the vagina each evening for three consecutive days. The cream should also be applied to the area around the vaginal opening and the vulva. The full 14 days treatment should be carried out even if the symptoms of vaginal itching or discharge have disappeared. The sexual partner should also be treated with the cream.

Contra-indications, warnings, etc
Contra-indications: Hypersensitivity to any imidazole preparation (or other vaginal antifungal products).

Side effects: Rarely, transient local mild irritation may occur immediately after application.

Precautions: Hypersensitivity has rarely been recorded, if it should occur, administration should be discontinued.

Gyno-Pevaryl Cream should be used only by those women who have symptoms of candidosis, and think that they might have candidosis.

If they believe or suspect that they might have some other sexually transmitted disease, either as well as, or instead of, candidosis, they should consult a Genitourinary Medicine Clinic or their own doctor.

The preparation should not be used if they are pregnant, or think that they might be pregnant, without first consulting a doctor.

It should not be used by those under 16 years of age or over 60 years without first consulting a doctor.

The woman should see her doctor if, after treatment:

- There is not complete relief of symptoms within 7 days.
- There is recurrence of symptoms within 4 weeks of treatment.
- She has more than two episodes of infection within a 6 month period, even if it completely resolves with treatment.
- Adverse effects such as redness, irritation or swelling, associated with the treatment occur.

Self medication should not be undertaken if the woman has:

- Any abnormal or irregular vaginal bleeding.
- Any blood staining of a vaginal discharge.
- Any vulval or vaginal sores, ulcers or blisters.
- Any associated lower abdominal pain or dysuria.

In all of these cases she should consult her doctor.

Contact between contraceptive diaphragms and this product must be avoided since the rubber may be damaged by this preparation.

In animals econazole nitrate has shown no teratogenic effects, but is foetotoxic at high doses. The significance of this in man is unknown as there is no evidence of an increased risk when taken in human pregnancy. However, as with other imidazoles, econazole should be used in pregnancy only if the practitioner considers it to be necessary.

Overdosage: Gyno-Pevaryl Vaginal Pessaries and Cream are intended for intravaginal use. If accidental ingestion of large quantities of the product occurs, an appropriate method of gastric emptying may be used if considered desirable.

Pharmaceutical precautions Store at room temperature, not exceeding 25°C.

Legal category P.

Package quantities Each pack contains 3 pessaries, a 15 g tube of cream and a patient instruction leaflet.

Further information Anogenital hygiene is important to help prevent re-infection.

Product licence numbers 0242/0227 and 0242/0229

GYNOL* II CONTRACEPTIVE JELLY

Qualitative and quantitative composition The gel contains 2.0% w/w of nonoxynol-9.

Pharmaceutical form Vaginal jelly.

Clinical particulars
Therapeutic indications: For use as a spermicidal contraceptive in conjunction with barrier methods of contraception.

Posology and method of administration: For topical intravaginal administration.

For use by adult females only.

The gel should be spread over the surface of the diaphragm which will be in contact with the cervix, and on the rim. The diaphragm and spermicide must be allowed to remain undisturbed for at least six to eight hours after coitus. A fresh application of gel or other spermicides eg Orthoforms Contraceptive pessaries must be made prior to any subsequent acts of coitus within this period of time, without removing the diaphragm. (A vaginal applicator should be used for inserting more jelly).

Douching is not recommended, but if desired it should be deferred for at least six hours after intercourse.

Contra-indications: Hypersensitivity to nonoxynol-9 or to any component of the preparation. Patients with absent vaginal sensation eg paraplegics and quadriplegics.

Special warnings and special precautions for use: Spermicidal intravaginal preparations are intended for use in conjunction with barrier methods of contraception such as condoms, diaphragms and caps.

Where avoidance of pregnancy is important the choice of contraceptive method should be made in consultation with a doctor or a family planning clinic.

If vaginal or penile irritation occurs discontinue use. If symptoms worsen or continue for more than 48 hours medical advice should be sought.

Interaction with other medicaments and other forms of interaction: None known.

Pregnancy and lactation: There is no evidence from animal and human studies that nonoxynol-9 is teratogenic. Human epidemiological studies have not shown any firm evidence of adverse effects on the foetus, however some studies have shown that nonoxynol-9 may be embryotoxic in animals. This product should not be used if pregnancy is suspected or confirmed. Animal studies have detected nonoxynol-9 in milk after intravaginal administration. Use by lactating women has not been studied.

Effects on ability to drive and use machines: None known.

Undesirable effects: May cause irritation of the vagina or penis.

Overdose: If taken orally the surfactant properties of this preparation may cause gastric irritation. General supportive therapy should be carried out. Hepatic and renal function should be monitored if medically indicated.

Pharmacological properties
Pharmacodynamic properties: The standard *in vitro* test (Sander-Cramer) evaluating the effect of nonoxynol-9 on animal sperm motility has shown the compound to be a potent spermicide.

The site of action of nonoxynol-9 has been determined as the sperm cell membrane. The lipoprotein membrane is disrupted, increasing permeability, with subsequent loss of cell components and decreased motility. A similar effect on vaginal epithelial and bacterial cells is also found.

Pharmacokinetic properties: The intravaginal absorption and excretion of radiolabelled (^{14}C) nonoxynol-9 has been studied in non-pregnant rats and rabbits and in pregnant rats. No appreciable difference was found in the extent or rate of absorption in pregnant and non-pregnant animals. Plasma levels peaked at about one hour and recovery from urine as unchanged nonoxynol-9 accounted for approximately 15-25% and faeces approximately 70% of the administered dose as unchanged nonoxynol-9. Less than 0.3% was found in the milk of lactating rats. No metabolites were detected in any of the samples analysed.

Preclinical safety data: Not applicable.

Pharmaceutical particulars
List of excipients: Methyl parahydroxybenzoate (E 218); sorbitol solution (E 420); lactic acid; povidone K30; propylene glycol; sodium carboxymethylcellulose; sorbic acid (E 200); purified water

Incompatibilities: Not applicable.

Shelf life: 2 years.

Special precautions for storage: Store at room temperature (at or below 25°C).

Nature and contents of container: Epoxy resin lined aluminium tubes with polyethylene caps. Available in 81 gram packs; an applicator is available separately if required.

Instructions for use/handling: Not applicable.

Marketing authorisation number 0242/0225

Date of approval/revision of SPC July 1996

Legal category GSL.

HALDOL*

Presentation Clear, colourless, odourless liquid containing 2 mg haloperidol BP per ml for oral administration. The liquid also contains methyl paraben as an inactive ingredient.

Amber glass ampoules containing 5 mg haloperidol BP in 1 ml aqueous solution for injection also containing lactic acid and water for injection as inactive ingredients.

Uses Haldol is a neuroleptic butyrophenone drug with a wide range of actions, indicated in the following conditions:

Adults:

- Schizophrenia: treatment of symptoms and prevention of relapse (oral and im).
- Other psychoses, especially paranoid (oral and im).
- Mania and hypomania (oral and im).
- Mental or behavioural problems such as aggression, hyperactivity and self-mutilation in the mentally retarded and in patients with organic brain damage (oral and im).
- As an adjunct to short-term management of moderate to severe psychomotor agitation, excitement, violent or dangerously impulsive behaviour (oral and im).
- Intractable hiccup (oral).
- Restlessness and agitation in the elderly (oral).
- Gilles de la Tourette syndrome and severe tics (oral).
- Nausea and vomiting (im).

Children (oral administration only):

- Childhood behavioural disorders especially when associated with hyperactivity and aggression.
- Gilles de la Tourette syndrome.
- Childhood schizophrenia.

Dosage and administration Dosage for all indications should be individually determined and is best initiated and titrated under close clinical supervision. To determine the initial dose, consideration should be given to the patient's age, severity of symptoms and previous response to other neuroleptics.

Patients who are elderly or debilitated or those with previously reported adverse reactions to neuroleptic drugs may require less haloperidol. The normal starting dose should be halved, followed by a gradual titration to achieve optimal response.

Oral administration:

Adults:

Schizophrenia, Psychoses, Mania and Hypomania, Mental or Behavioural Problems, Psychomotor Agitation, Excitement, Violent or Dangerously Impulsive Behaviour, Organic Brain Damage.

Initial dosage: Moderate symptomatology 1.5-3.0 mg bd or tds.

Severe symptomatology/resistant patients 3.0-5.0 mg bd or tds.

The same starting doses may be employed in adolescents or resistant schizophrenics, who, in certain cases, may require up to 30 mg/day.

Maintenance dosage: Once satisfactory control of symptoms has been achieved dosage, should be gradually reduced to the lowest effective maintenance dose, often as low as 5 or 10 mg/day. Too rapid a dosage reduction should be avoided.

Restlessness or Agitation in the Elderly: Initial dose 1.5-3.0 mg bd or tds titrated as required, to attain an effective maintenance dose (1.5-50 mg daily).

Gilles de la Tourette Syndrome, Severe Tics, Intractable Hiccup: Starting dose 1.5 mg tds. adjusted according to response. A daily maintenance dose of 10 mg may be required in Gilles de la Tourette syndrome.

Children

Childhood Behavioural Disorders/Schizophrenia: Total daily maintenance dose of 0.025-0.05 mg/kg/day. Half the total dose should be given in the morning and the other half in the evening, up to a maximum of 10 mg daily.

Gilles de la Tourette Syndrome: Oral maintenance doses of up to 10 mg/day in most patients.

Parenteral Administration

Adults

Schizophrenia, Psychoses, Mania and Hypomania, Mental or Behavioural Problems, Psychomotor Agitation, Excitement, Violent or Dangerously Impulsive Behaviour, Organic Brain Damage: For control of acutely agitated patients with moderate symptoms: 2-10 mg im.

Depending on the response of the patient, subsequent doses may be given every 4-8 hours, until sufficient symptom control is achieved or up to a maximum of 18 mg/day.

Infrequently, severely disturbed patients may require an initial dose of up to 18 mg.

Oral treatment should succeed intramuscular administration as soon as practicable. Bioavailability from the oral route is about 60% of that from the im route, and readjustment of dose may be required.

Haldol can also be administered by the iv route.

Nausea and vomiting: 1-2 mg im.

Children: Not recommended for parenteral use in children.

Contra-indications, warnings etc

Contra-indications: Comatose states; CNS depression; Parkinson's disease; known hypersensitivity to haloperidol; lesions of the basal ganglia.

Use in pregnancy and lactation: The safety of haloperidol in pregnancy has not been established. There is some evidence of harmful effects in some but not all animal studies. There have been a number of reports of birth defects following foetal exposure to haloperidol for which a causal role for haloperidol cannot be excluded. Haldol should be used during pregnancy only if the anticipated benefit outweighs the risk and the administered dose and duration of treatment should be as low and as short as possible.

Haloperidol is excreted in breast milk. There have been isolated cases of extrapyramidal symptoms in breast-fed children. If the use of Haldol is essential, the benefits of breast feeding should be balanced against its potential risks.

Effects on ability to drive and use machines: Some degree of sedation or impairment of alertness may occur, particularly with higher doses and at the start of treatment, and may be potentiated by alcohol or other CNS depressants. Patients should be advised not to undertake activities requiring alertness such as driving or operating machinery during treatment, until their susceptibility is known.

Precautions and warnings: Please also refer to Drug Interactions section.

Caution is advised in patients with liver disease, renal failure, phaeochromocytoma, epilepsy, and conditions predisposing to epilepsy (eg alcohol withdrawal and brain damage) or convulsions. Haloperidol should only be used with great caution in patients with disturbed thyroid function. Antipsychotic therapy in those patients must always be accompanied by adequate management of the underlying thyroid dysfunction.

Cases of sudden death have been reported in psychiatric patients receiving antipsychotic drugs, including haloperidol. The risk-benefit of haloperidol treatment should be fully assessed before treatment is commenced and patients with risk factors for ventricular arrhythmias such as cardiac disease, subarachnoid haemorrhage, metabolic abnormalities such as hypokalaemia, hypocalcaemia or hypomagnesemia, starvation, alcohol abuse or those receiving concomitant therapy with other drugs known to prolong the QT interval, should be monitored carefully (ECGs and potassium levels), particularly during the initial phase of treatment, to obtain steady plasma levels.

Acute withdrawal symptoms including nausea, vomiting and insomnia have very rarely been described after abrupt cessation of high doses of antipsychotic drugs. Relapse may also occur and gradual withdrawal is advisable.

In schizophrenia, the response to antipsychotic drug treatment may be delayed. If drugs are withdrawn, recurrence of symptoms may not become apparent for several weeks or months.

As with all antipsychotic agents, haloperidol should not be used alone where Depression is predominant. It may be combined with antidepressants to treat those conditions in which Depression and psychosis coexist. Haloperidol may impair the metabolism of tricyclic antidepressants (clinical significance unknown).

If concomitant antiparkinson medication is required, it may have to be continued after haloperidol is discontinued to take account of any differences in excretion rates. The physician should keep in mind the possible anticholinergic effects associated with antiparkinson agents.

Drug interactions: In common with all neuroleptics, haloperidol can increase the central nervous system depression produced by other CNS-depressant drugs, including alcohol, hypnotics, sedatives or strong analgesics. An enhanced CNS effect, when combined with methyldopa, has been reported.

Haloperidol may antagonise the action of adrenaline and other sympathomimetic agents and reverses the blood pressure lowering effects of adrenergic-blocking agents such as guanethidine.

The dosage of anticonvulsants may need to be increased to take account of the lowered seizure threshold. Coadministration of enzyme-inducing drugs such as carbamazepine, phenobarbitone and rifampicin with haloperidol may result in a significant reduction of haloperidol plasma levels. The haloperidol dose may therefore need to be increased, according to the patient's response. After stopping such drugs, it may be necessary to readjust the dosage of haloperidol.

Haloperidol may impair the metabolism of tricyclic antidepressants (clinical significance unknown) and the antiparkinson effects of levodopa.

In pharmacokinetic studies, increased haloperidol levels have been reported when haloperidol was given concomitantly with the following drugs: quinidine, buspirone and fluoxetine. Haloperidol plasma levels should therefore be monitored and reduced if necessary.

Antagonism of the effect of phenindione has been reported.

In rare cases, an encephalopathy-like syndrome has been reported in combination with lithium and haloperidol. It remains controversial whether these cases represent a distinct clinical entity or whether they are in fact cases of NMS and/or lithium toxicity. Signs of encephalopathy-like syndrome include confusion, disorientation, headache, disturbances of balance and drowsiness. One report showing symptomless EEG abnormalities on the combination has suggested that EEG monitoring might be advisable. When lithium and haloperidol therapy are used concomitantly, haloperidol should be given in the lowest effective dosage and lithium levels should be monitored and kept below 1 mmol/l. If symptoms of encephalopathy-like syndrome occur, therapy should be stopped immediately.

Adverse effects: Central nervous system: In common with all neuroleptics, extrapyramidal symptoms may occur, eg tremor, rigidity, hypersalivation, bradykinesia, akathisia, acute dystonia, oculogyric crisis and laryngeal dystonia. Anti-Parkinson agents should not be prescribed routinely.

As with all antipsychotic agents, tardive dyskinesia may appear in some patients on long-term therapy or after drug discontinuation.

The syndrome is mainly characterised by rhythmical involuntary movements of the tongue, face, mouth or jaw. The manifestations may be permanent in some patients. The syndrome may be masked when treatment is reinstituted, when the dosage is increased or when a switch is made to a different antipsychotic drug. Treatment should be discontinued as soon as possible.

However since its occurrence may be related to duration of treatment, as well as daily dose, Haldol should be given in the minimum effective dose for the minimum possible time, unless it is established that long term administration for the treatment of schizophrenia is required.

It has been reported that fine vermicular movements of the tongue may be an early sign of tardive dyskinesia and that the full syndrome may not develop if the medication is stopped at that time.

The following effects have been reported rarely: confusional states or epileptic fits, depression, sedation, agitation, drowsiness, insomnia, headache, vertigo and apparent exacerbation of psychotic symptoms.

In common with other antipsychotic drugs, haloperidol has been associated with rare cases of neuroleptic malignant syndrome (CMS), an idiosyncratic response characterised by hyperthermia, generalised muscle rigidity, autonomic instability, altered consciousness, coma and elevated CPK. Signs of autonomic dysfunction such as tachycardia, labile arterial pressure and sweating may precede the onset of hyperthermia, acting as early warning signs. Antipsychotic treatment should be withdrawn immediately and appropriate supportive therapy and careful monitoring instituted.

Haloperidol, even in low dosage in susceptible (especially non-psychotic) individuals, may cause unpleasant subjective feelings of being mentally dulled or slowed down, dizziness, headache or paradoxical effects of excitement, agitation or insomnia.

Gastrointestinal system: Gastrointestinal symptoms, nausea, loss of appetite, constipation and dyspepsia have been reported.

Endocrinological system: Hormonal effects of antipsychotic neuroleptic drugs include hyperprolactinaemia, which may cause galactorrhoea, gynaecomastia and oligo- or amenorrhoea. Hypoglycaemia and the syndrome of inappropriate antidiuretic hormone secretion have been reported rarely. Impairment of sexual function including erection and ejaculation has also been occasionally reported.

Cardiovascular system: Tachycardia and dose related hypotension are uncommon, but can occur, particularly in the elderly, who are more susceptible to the sedative and hypotensive effects. Less commonly hypertension has also been reported. Cardiac effects such as QT-interval prolongation, Torsade de Pointes and/or ventricular arrhythmias have been reported rarely. They may occur more frequently with high doses, intravenous administration and in predisposed patients (see Precautions and Warnings).

Autonomic nervous system: Dry mouth as well as excessive salivation, blurred vision, urinary retention and hyperhidrosis have been reported.

Dermatological system: The following effects have been reported rarely: oedema, various skin rashes and reactions including urticaria, exfoliative dermatitis and erythema multiforme. Photosensitive skin reactions have been reported very rarely.

Other adverse reactions: The following effects have been reported rarely: jaundice, cholestatic hepatitis or transient abnormalities of liver function in the absence of jaundice; priapism and weight changes may occur. Temperature disorders may also occur, characteristically hyperthermia associated with NMS, although hypothermia has also been reported.

The following have been reported very rarely: blood dyscrasias, including agranulocytosis, thrombocytopenia and transient leucopenia; hypersensitivity reactions including anaphylaxis.

Overdose

Symptoms: In general, the manifestations of haloperidol overdosage are an extension of its pharmacological actions, the most prominent of which would be severe extrapyramidal symptoms, hypotension and psychic indifference with a transition to sleep. The risk of ventricular arrhythmias possibly associated with QT-prolongation should be considered. The patient may appear comatose with respiratory depression and hypotension which could be severe enough to produce a shock-like state. Paradoxically hypertension rather than hypotension may occur. Convulsions may also occur.

Treatment: There is no specific antidote to haloperidol. A patent airway should be established and maintained with mechanically assisted ventilation if necessary. In view of isolated reports of arrhythmia ECG monitoring is strongly advised. Hypotension and circulatory collapse should be treated by plasma volume expansion and other appropriate measures. Adrenaline should not be used. The patient should be monitored carefully for 24 hours or longer, body temperature and adequate fluid intake should be maintained.

In cases of severe extrapyramidal symptoms, appropriate antiparkinson medication should be administered.

Pharmaceutical precautions Store tablets in a cool dry place. Haldol oral liquid should be stored at room temperature. Ampoules should be protected from light.

Legal category POM.

Further information Haldol is rapidly absorbed after oral administration with a mean bioavailability of 44-74% (approximately 60%). Variable bioavailability is likely due to inter-individual differences in GI absorption and extent of first-pass hepatic metabolism.

Distribution is rapid to extravascular tissues, especially liver and adipose tissue. It is approximately 92% bound to plasma proteins. Haloperidol crosses the blood-brain barrier and is excreted in human breast milk.

Haloperidol is extensively metabolised by oxidative dealkylation, and ultimately conjugated with glycine. Half life is approximately 20 hours.

A 10 mg iv dose of haloperidol given over 2 minutes produced a peak serum concentration of 34 µg/ml at the end of infusion, declining to 1 µg/ml by 40 hours. Following im administration of 2 mg, peak plasma concentrations were similar to after oral, ie 10 µg/ml, but are reached within 20 minutes.

Package quantities

5 mg/ml injectable solution	5 × 1 ml ampoules
2 mg/ml oral solution	100 ml amber glass bottles with calibrated pipette

Product licence numbers

5 mg/ml injectable solution	0242/0036R
2 mg/ml oral liquid	0242/0035R

HALDOL* TABLETS 5 mg and 10 mg

Qualitative and quantitative composition Haloperidol 5 mg; haloperidol 10 mg.

Pharmaceutical form Tablets.

Clinical particulars

Therapeutic indications:

Adults:

Schizophrenia: treatment of symptoms and prevention of relapse.

Other psychoses: especially paranoid.

Mania and hypomania.

Mental or behavioural problems such as aggression, hyperactivity and self mutilation in the mentally retarded and in patients with organic brain damage.

As an adjunct to short term management of moderate to severe psychomotor agitation, excitement, violent or dangerously impulsive behaviour.

Intractable hiccup.

Restlessness and agitation in the elderly.

Gilles de la Tourette Syndrome and severe tics.

Children (oral administration only)

Childhood behavioural disorders, especially when associated with hyperactivity and aggression.

Gilles de la Tourette Syndrome.

Childhood schizophrenia.

Posology and method of administration: Dosage for all indications should be individually determined and is best initiated and titrated under close clinical supervision. To determine initial dose, consideration should be given to the patient's age, severity of symptoms and previous response to neuroleptic drugs.

Patients who are elderly or debilitated or those with previously reported adverse reactions to neuroleptic drugs may require less Haldol. The normal starting dose should be halved, followed by a gradual titration to achieve optimal response.

Oral administration

Adults

Schizophrenia, Psychoses, Mania and Hypomania, Mental or Behavioural Problems, Psychomotor Agitation, Excitement, Violent or Dangerously Impulsive Behaviour, Organic Brain Damage.

Initial dose:

Moderate symptomatology–1.5–3.0 mg bd or tds.

Severe symptomatology/resistant patients–3.0–5.0 mg bd or tds.

The same starting dose may be employed in adolescents, who in certain cases, may require up to 30 mg.

Maintenance dosage:

Once satisfactory control of symptoms has been achieved dosage should be gradually reduced to the lowest effective maintenance dose, often as low as 5 or 10 mg/day. Too rapid a dosage reduction should be avoided.

Restlessness or agitation in the elderly:

Initial dose: 1.5–3.0 mg bd or tds titrated as required, to attain an effective maintenance dose (1.5-30 mg daily).

Gilles de la Tourette Syndrome, Severe Tics, Intractable Hiccup

Starting dose 1.5 mg tds adjusted according to response. A daily maintenance dose of 10 mg may be required in Gilles de la Tourette Syndrome.

Children

Childhood Behavioural Disorders and Schizophrenia

Total daily maintenance dose of 0.025-0.05 mg/kg/day. Half the total dose should be given in the morning and the other half in the evening, up to a maximum of 10 mg daily.

Gilles de la Tourette Syndrome

Oral maintenance doses up to 10 mg/day in most patients.

Contra-indications: Comatose states, CNS depression, Parkinson's disease, known hypersensitivity to haloperidol, lesions of basal ganglia.

Special warnings and special precautions for use: Caution is advised in patients with liver disease, renal failure, phaeochromocytoma, epilepsy, and conditions predisposing to epilepsy (eg alcohol withdrawal and brain damage) or convulsions. Haloperidol should only be used with great caution in patients with disturbed thyroid function. Antipsychotic therapy in those patients must always be accompanied by adequate management of the underlying thyroid dysfunction.

Cases of sudden death have been reported in psychiatric patients receiving antipsychotic drugs, including haloperidol. The risk-benefit of haloperidol treatment should be fully assessed before treatment is commenced and patients with risk factors for ventricular arrhythmias such as cardiac disease, subarachnoid haemorrhage, metabolic abnormalities such as hypokalaemia, hypocalcaemia or hypomagnesemia, starvation, alcohol abuse or those receiving concomitant therapy with other drugs known to prolong the QT interval, should be monitored carefully (ECGs and potassium levels), particularly during the initial phase of treatment, to obtain steady plasma levels.

Acute withdrawal symptoms including nausea, vomiting and insomnia have very rarely been described after abrupt cessation of high doses of antipsychotic drugs. Relapse may also occur and gradual withdrawal is advisable.

In schizophrenia, the response to antipsychotic drug treatment may be delayed. If drugs are withdrawn, recurrence of symptoms may not become apparent for several weeks or months.

As with all antipsychotic agents, haloperidol should not be used alone where depression is predominant. It may be combined with antidepressants to treat those conditions in which depression and psychosis coexist. Haloperidol may impair the metabolism of tricyclic antidepressants (clinical significance unknown).

If concomitant antiparkinson medication is required, it may have to be continued after haloperidol is discontinued to take account of any differences in excretion rates. The physician should keep in mind the possible anticholinergic effects associated with antiparkinson agents.

Interaction with other medicaments and other forms of interaction: In common with all neuroleptics, haloperidol can increase the central nervous system depression produced by other CNS-depressant drugs, including alcohol, hypnotics, sedatives or strong analgesics.

Haloperidol may antagonise the action of adrenaline and other sympathomimetic agents and reverses the blood pressure lowering effects of adrenergic-blocking agents such as guanethidine.

Haloperidol may impair the antiparkinson effects of levodopa. In pharmacokinetic studies, increased haloperidol levels have been reported when haloperidol was given concomitantly with the following drugs: quinidine, buspirone and fluoxetine. Haloperidol plasma levels should therefore be monitored and reduced if necessary. The dosage of anticonvulsants may need to be increased to take account of the lowered seizure threshold.

Coadministration of enzyme-inducing drugs such as carbamazepine, phenobarbitone and rifampicin with haloperidol may result in a significant reduction of haloperidol plasma levels. The haloperidol dose may therefore need to be increased, according to the patient's response. After stopping such drugs, it may be necessary to readjust the dosage of haloperidol.

An enhanced CNS effect, when combined with methyldopa, has been reported.

In rare cases, an encephalopathy-like syndrome has been reported in combination with lithium and haloperidol. It remains controversial whether these cases represent a distinct clinical entity or whether they are in fact cases of NMS and/or lithium toxicity. Signs of encephalopathy-like syndrome include confusion, disorientation, headache, disturbances of balance and drowsiness. One report showing symptomless EEG abnormalities on the combination has suggested that EEG monitoring might be advisable. When lithium and haloperidol therapy are used concomitantly, haloperidol should be given in the lowest effective dosage and lithium levels should be monitored and kept below 1 mmol/l. If symptoms of encephalopathy-like syndrome occur, therapy should be stopped immediately.

Haloperidol may impair the metabolism of tricyclic antidepressants (clinical significance unknown). Antagonism of the effect of phenindione has been reported.

Pregnancy and lactation: The safety of haloperidol in pregnancy has not been established. There is some evidence of harmful effects in some, but not all animal studies. There have been a number of reports of birth defects following foetal exposure to haloperidol for which a causal role for haloperidol cannot be excluded. Haldol should be used during pregnancy only if the anticipated benefit outweighs the risk and the administered dose and duration of treatment should be as low and as short as possible.

There have been isolated cases of extrapyramidal symptoms in breast-fed children. If the use of Haldol is essential, the benefits of breast feeding should be balanced against its potential risks.

Effects on ability to drive and use machines: Some degree of sedation or impairment of alertness may occur, particularly with higher doses and at the start of treatment, and may be potentiated by alcohol or other CNS depressants. Patients should be advised not to undertake activities requiring alertness such as driving or operating machinery during treatment, until their susceptibility is known.

Undesirable effects:

Central nervous system: In common with all neuroleptics, extrapyramidal symptoms may occur, eg tremor, rigidity, hypersalivation, bradykinesia, akathisia, acute dystonia, oculogyric crisis and laryngeal dystonia.

Anti-Parkinson agents should not be prescribed routinely.

As with all antipsychotic agents, tardive dyskinesia may appear in some patients on long-term therapy or after drug discontinuation.

The syndrome is mainly characterised by rhythmical involuntary movements of the tongue, face, mouth or jaw. The manifestations may be permanent in some patients. The syndrome may be masked when treatment is reinstituted, when the dosage is increased or when a switch is made to a different antipsychotic drug. Treatment should be discontinued as soon as possible.

However, since its occurrence may be related to duration of treatment, as well as daily dose, haloperidol should be given in the minimum effective dose for the minimum possible time, unless it is established that long term administration for the treatment of schizophrenia is required.

It has been reported that fine vermicular movements of the tongue may be an early sign of tardive dyskinesia and that the full syndrome may not develop if the medication is stopped at that time.

The following effects have been reported rarely: confusional states or epileptic fits, depression, sedation, agitation, drowsiness, insomnia, headache, vertigo and apparent exacerbation of psychotic symptoms.

In common with other antipsychotic drugs, haloperidol has been associated with rare cases of neuroleptic malignant syndrome (NMS), an idiosyncratic response characterised by hyperthermia, generalised muscle rigidity, autonomic instability, altered consciousness, coma and elevated CPK. Signs of autonomic dysfunction such as tachycardia, labile arterial pressure and sweating may precede the onset of hyperthermia, acting as early warning signs. Antipsychotic treatment should be withdrawn immediately and appropriate supportive therapy and careful monitoring instituted.

Haloperidol, even in low dosage in susceptible (especially non-psychotic) individuals, may cause unpleasant subjective feelings of being mentally dulled or slowed down, dizziness, headache or paradoxical effects of excitement, agitation or insomnia.

Gastrointestinal system: Gastrointestinal symptoms, nausea, loss of appetite, constipation and dyspepsia have been reported.

Endocrinological system: Hormonal effects of antipsychotic neuroleptic drugs include hyper-prolactinaemia, which may cause galactorrhoea, gynaecomastia and oligo- or amenorrhoea. Hypoglycaemia and the syndrome of inappropriate antidiuretic hormone secretion have been reported rarely. Impairment of sexual function including erection and ejaculation has also been occasionally reported.

Cardiovascular system: Tachycardia and dose related hypotension is uncommon, but can occur, particularly in the elderly, who are more susceptible to the sedative and hypotensive effects. Less commonly hypertension has also been reported. Cardiac effects such as QT-interval prolongation, Torsade de Pointes and/or ventricular arrhythmias have been reported rarely. They may occur more frequently with high doses, intravenous administration and in predisposed patients (see Precautions and Warnings).

Autonomic nervous system: Dry mouth as well as excessive salivation, blurred vision, urinary retention and hyperhidrosis have been reported.

Dermatological system: The following effects have been reported rarely: oedema, various skin rashes and reactions including urticaria, exfoliative dermatitis and erythema multiforme. Photosensitive skin reactions have been reported very rarely.

Other adverse reactions: The following effects have been reported rarely: jaundice, cholestatic hepatitis or transient abnormalities of liver function in the absence of jaundice; priapism and weight changes. Temperature disorders may also occur, characteristically hyperthermia associated with NMS, although hypothermia has also been reported.

The following have been reported very rarely: blood dyscrasias, including agranulocytosis, thrombocytopenia and transient leucopenia; hypersensitivity reactions including anaphylaxis.

Overdose:
Symptoms: In general, the manifestations of haloperidol overdosage are an extension of its pharmacological actions, the most prominent of which would be severe extrapyramidal symptoms, hypotension and psychic indifference with a transition to sleep. The risk of ventricular arrhythmias possibly associated with QT-prolongation should be considered. The patient may appear comatose with respiratory depression and hypotension which could be severe enough to produce a shock-like state. Paradoxically hypertension rather than hypotension may occur. Convulsions may also occur.

Treatment: There is no specific antidote to haloperidol. A patent airway should be established and maintained with mechanically assisted ventilation if necessary. In view of isolated reports of arrhythmia ECG monitoring is strongly advised. Hypotension and circulatory collapse should be treated by plasma volume expansion and other appropriate measures. Adrenaline should not be used. The patient should be monitored carefully for 24 hours or longer, body temperature and adequate fluid intake should be maintained.

In cases of severe extrapyramidal symptoms, appropriate antiparkinsonian medication should be administered.

Pharmacological properties
Pharmacodynamic properties: Haloperidol acts as a central and peripheral dopamine receptor antagonist it also has some anticholinergic activity and binds to opiate receptors.

Pharmacokinetic properties: Haloperidol is rapidly absorbed after oral administration with a bioavailability of 44-74% (mean 60%) after tablets. Variable bioavailability is likely due to inter-individual differences in GI absorption and extent of first-pass hepatic metabolism.

Distribution is rapid to extravascular tissue, haloperidol crosses the blood-brain barrier and is excreted in human breast milk.

Metabolism is by oxidative dealkylation. The elimination half-life is approximately 20 hours, with considerable diurnal variation.

Preclinical safety data: Not applicable.

Pharmaceutical particulars
List of excipients:
10 mg tablet: Calcium phosphate dihydrate; corn starch; calcium stearate; quinoline yellow (E104); purified water (not present in final product).

5 mg tablet: Lactose; maize starch; talc; hydrogenated vegetable oil; indigo carmine (E132); purified water (not present in final product).

Incompatibilities: Not applicable.

Shelf life: 60 months.

Special precautions for storage: Store in a cool, dry place.

Nature and contents of container: Blister packs of aluminium foil and polyvinylchloride genotherm glass clear.

The strips are packed in cardboard cartons containing 100 tablets per pack.

Instructions for use/handling: None specific.

Marketing authorisation numbers
5 mg Tablets 0242/0031R
10 mg Tablets 0242/0039R

Date of approval/revision of SPC 5 mg Tablets: March 1998; 10 mg Tablets: May 1997

Legal category POM.

HALDOL* DECANOATE

Qualitative and quantitative composition Haldol decanoate 50 mg/ml: haloperidol decanoate 70.52 mg, equivalent to 50 mg haloperidol base, per millilitre. Haldol decanoate 100 mg/ml: haloperidol decanoate 141.04 mg, equivalent to 100 mg haloperidol base, per millilitre.

Pharmaceutical form Straw-coloured viscous solution for intramuscular injection.

Clinical particulars
Therapeutic indications: Haldol decanoate is indicated for long term maintenance treatment where a neuroleptic is required; for example in schizophrenia, other psychoses (especially paranoid), and other mental or behavioural problems where maintenance treatment is clearly indicated.

Posology and method of administration: By intramuscular administration.

Haldol decanoate is for use in adults only and has been formulated to provide one month's therapy for most patients following a single deep intramuscular injection in the gluteal region. Haldol decanoate should not be administered intravenously.

Since individual response to neuroleptic drugs is variable, dosage should be individually determined and is best initiated and titrated under close clinical supervision.

The size of the initial dose will depend on both the severity of the symptomatology and the amount of oral medication required to maintain the patient before starting depot treatment.

An initial dose of 50 mg every four weeks is recommended, increasing if necessary by 50 mg increments to 300 mg every four weeks. If, for clinical reasons, two-weekly administration is preferred, these doses should be halved.

In patients with severe symptomatology, or in those who require large oral doses as maintenance therapy, higher doses of Haldol decanoate will be required. However, clinical experience with Haldol decanoate at doses greater than 300 mg per month is limited.

Routine administration of volumes greater than 3 mls at any one injection site is not recommended as larger volumes of injection are uncomfortable for the patient.

Haldol decanoate should be administered by deep intramuscular injection using an appropriate needle, preferably 2-2.5 inches long, of at least 21 gauge. Local reactions and medication oozing from the injection site may be reduced by the use of a good injection technique, eg the 'Z-track' method. As with all oily injections, it is important to ensure, by aspiration before injection, that intravenous entry has not occurred.

For patients previously maintained on oral neuroleptics, an approximate guide to the starting dose of Haldol decanoate is as follows: 500 mg of chlorpromazine a day is equivalent to 100 mg of Haldol decanoate monthly.

The approximate equivalence for transferring patients previously maintained on fluphenazine decanoate or flupenthixol decanoate is as follows: 25 mg of fluphenazine decanoate 2-weekly or 40 mg of flupenthixol decanoate 2-weekly is equivalent to 100 mg of Haldol decanoate monthly. This dose should be adjusted to suit the individual patient's response.

Use in elderly: It is recommended to start with low doses, for example 12.5 mg - 25 mg every four weeks, only increasing the dose according to the individual patient's response.

Contra-indications: Comatose states, CNS depression, Parkinson's disease, known hypersensitivity to haloperidol, lesions of basal ganglia.

Special warnings and special precautions for use: Caution is advised in patients with liver disease, renal failure, phaeochromocytoma, epilepsy, and conditions predisposing to epilepsy (eg alcohol withdrawal and brain damage) or convulsions. Haloperidol should only be used with great caution in patients with disturbed thyroid function. Antipsychotic therapy in those patients must always be accompanied by adequate management of the underlying thyroid dysfunction.

Cases of sudden death have been reported in psychiatric patients receiving antipsychotic drugs, including haloperidol.

The risk-benefit of Haldol decanoate treatment should be fully assessed before treatment is commenced and patients with risk factors for ventricular arrhythmias such as cardiac disease, subarachnoid haemorrhage, metabolic abnormalities such as hypokalaemia, hypocalcaemia or hypomagnesemia, starvation, alcohol abuse or those receiving concomitant therapy with other drugs known to prolong the QT interval, should be monitored carefully (ECGs and potassium levels), particularly during the initial phase of treatment, to obtain steady plasma levels.

In schizophrenia, the response to antipsychotic drug treatment may be delayed. If drugs are withdrawn, recurrence of symptoms may not become apparent for several weeks or months.

As with all antipsychotic agents, haloperidol should not be used alone where depression is predominant. It may be combined with antidepressants to treat those conditions in which depression and psychosis coexist. Haloperidol may impair the metabolism of tricyclic antidepressants (clinical significance unknown).

If concomitant antiparkinson medication is required, it may have to be continued after haloperidol is discontinued to take account of any differences in excretion rates. The physician should keep in mind the possible anticholinergic effects associated with antiparkinson agents.

Interaction with other medicaments and other forms of interaction: In common with all neuroleptics, haloperidol can increase the central nervous system depression produced by other CNS-depressant drugs, including alcohol, hypnotics, sedatives or strong analgesics. An enhanced CNS effect, when combined with methyldopa, has been reported.

Haloperidol may antagonise the action of adrenaline and other sympathomimetic agents and reverses the blood pressure lowering effects of adrenergic-blocking agents such as guanethidine.

Haloperidol may impair the metabolism of tricyclic antidepressants (clinical significance unknown) and the antiparkinson effects of levodopa. In pharmacokinetic studies, increased haloperidol levels have been reported when haloperidol was given concomitantly with the following drugs: quinidine, buspirone and fluoxetine. Haloperidol plasma levels should therefore be monitored and reduced if necessary. The dosage of anticonvulsants may need to be increased to take account of the lowered seizure threshold.

Coadministration of enzyme-inducing drugs such as carbamazepine, phenobarbitone and rifampicin with haloperidol may result in a significant reduction of haloperidol plasma levels. The haloperidol dose may therefore need to be increased or the dosage interval reduced, according to the patient's response. After stopping such drugs, it may be necessary to readjust the dosage of haloperidol.

Antagonism of the effect of phenindione has been reported.

In rare cases, an encephalopathy-like syndrome has been reported in combination with lithium and Haldol decanoate. It remains controversial whether these cases represent a distinct clinical entity or whether they are in fact cases of NMS and/or lithium toxicity. Signs of encephalopathy-like syndrome include confusion, disorientation, headache, disturbances of balance and drowsiness. One report showing symptomless EEG abnormalities on the combination has suggested that EEG monitoring might be advisable. When lithium and haloperidol therapy are used concomitantly, haloperidol should be given in the lowest effective dosage and lithium levels should be monitored and kept below 1 mmol/l. If symptoms of encephalopathy-like syndrome occur, therapy should be stopped immediately.

Pregnancy and lactation: The safety of haloperidol in pregnancy has not been established. There is some evidence of harmful effects in some, but not all, animal studies. There have been a number of reports of birth defects following foetal exposure to haloperidol for which a causal role for haloperidol cannot be excluded. Haldol decanoate should be used during pregnancy only if the anticipated benefit outweighs the risk and the administered dose and duration of treatment should be as low and as short as possible.

Haloperidol is excreted in breast milk. There have been isolated cases of extrapyramidal symptoms in breast-fed children. If the use of Haldol decanoate is essential, the benefits of breast feeding should be balanced against its potential risks.

Effects on ability to drive and use machines: Some degree of sedation or impairment of alertness may occur, particularly with higher doses and at the start of treatment, and may be potentiated by alcohol or other CNS depressants. Patients should be advised not to undertake activities requiring alertness such as driving or operating machinery during treatment, until their susceptibility is known.

Undesirable effects:
Central nervous system: In common with all neuroleptics, extrapyramidal symptoms may occur, eg tremor, rigidity, hypersalivation, bradykinesia, akathisia, acute dystonia, oculogyric crisis and laryngeal dystonia. Antiparkinson agents should not be prescribed routinely. Preliminary results suggest that withdrawal of antiparkinson medication may be attempted following transfer from oral medication to monthly depot injections of Haldol decanoate.

As with all antipsychotic agents, tardive dyskinesia may appear in some patients on long-term therapy or after drug discontinuation.

The syndrome is mainly characterised by rhythmical involuntary movements of the tongue, face, mouth or jaw. The manifestations may be permanent in some patients. The syndrome may be masked when treatment is reinstituted, when the dosage is increased or when a switch is made to a different antipsychotic drug. Treatment should be discontinued as soon as possible.

However, since its occurrence may be related to duration of treatment, as well as dose, haloperidol should be given in the minimum effective dose for the minimum possible time, unless it is established that long term administration for the treatment of schizophrenia is required.

It has been reported that fine vermicular movements of the tongue may be an early sign of tardive dyskinesia and that the full syndrome may not develop if the medication is stopped at that time.

The following effects have been reported rarely with haloperidol: confusional states or epileptic fits, depression, sedation, agitation, drowsiness, insomnia, headache, vertigo and apparent exacerbation of psychotic symptoms.

In common with other antipsychotic drugs, haloperidol has been associated with rare cases of neuroleptic malignant syndrome (NMS), an idiosyncratic response characterised by hyperthermia, generalised muscle rigidity, autonomic instability, altered consciousness, coma and elevated CPK. Signs of autonomic dysfunction such as tachycardia, labile arterial pressure and sweating may precede the onset of hyperthermia, acting as early warning signs. Antipsychotic treatment should be withdrawn immediately and appropriate supportive therapy and careful monitoring instituted.

Haloperidol, even in low dosage in susceptible (especially non-psychotic) individuals, may cause unpleasant subjective feelings of being mentally dulled or slowed down, dizziness, headache or paradoxical effects of excitement, agitation or insomnia.

Gastrointestinal system: Gastrointestinal symptoms, nausea, loss of appetite, constipation and dyspepsia have been reported with haloperidol.

Endocrinological system: Hormonal effects of antipsychotic neuroleptic drugs include hyperprolactinaemia, which may cause galactorrhoea, gynaecomastia and oligo- or amenorrhoea. Hypoglycaemia and the Syndrome of Inappropriate Antidiuretic Hormone Secretion have been reported rarely. Impairment of sexual function including erection and ejaculation has also been occasionally reported.

Cardiovascular system: Tachycardia and dose related hypotension is uncommon, but can occur with haloperidol, particularly in the elderly, who are more susceptible to the sedative and hypotensive effects. Less commonly hypertension has also been reported. Cardiac effects such as QT-interval prolongation, torsade de pointes and/or ventricular arrhythmias have been reported rarely. They may occur more frequently with high doses, intravenous administration and in predisposed patients (see Precautions and Warnings).

Autonomic nervous system: Dry mouth as well as excessive salivation, blurred vision, urinary retention and hyperhidrosis have been reported with haloperidol.

Dermatological system: The following effects have been reported rarely with haloperidol: oedema, various skin rashes and reactions, including urticaria, exfoliative dermatitis and erythema multiforme. Photosensitive skin reactions have been reported very rarely.

Other adverse reactions: The following effects have been reported rarely with haloperidol: jaundice, cholestatic hepatitis or transient abnormalities of liver function in the absence of jaundice; priapism and weight changes may occur. Temperature disorders may also occur, characteristically hyperthermia associated with NMS, although hypothermia has also been reported.

The following have been reported very rarely with haloperidol: blood dyscrasias, including agranulocytosis, thrombocytopenia and transient leucopenia; hypersensitivity reactions including anaphylaxis. Occasional local reactions such as erythema, swelling or tender lumps have been reported.

Overdose: Symptoms: In general, the manifestations of haloperidol overdosage are an extension of its pharmacological actions, the most prominent of which would be severe extrapyramidal symptoms, hypotension and psychic indifference with a transition to sleep. The risk of ventricular arrhythmias possibly associated with QT-prolongation should be considered. The patient may appear comatose with respiratory depression and hypotension which could be severe enough to produce a shock-like state. Paradoxically, hypertension rather than hypotension may occur. Convulsions may also occur.

Treatment: There is no specific antidote to haloperidol. A patent airway should be established and maintained with mechanically assisted ventilation if necessary. In view of isolated reports of arrhythmia, ECG monitoring is strongly advised. Hypotension and circulatory collapse should be treated by plasma volume expansion and other appropriate measures. Adrenaline should not be used. The patient should be monitored, body temperature and adequate fluid intake should be maintained.

In cases of severe extrapyramidal symptoms, appropriate antiparkinson medication should be administered.

Pharmacological properties
Pharmacodynamic properties: The antipsychotic activity of haloperidol is principally due to its central dopamine blocking activity.

It has some activity against noradrenaline and less against serotonin. There is only very minimal activity against histamine and acetylcholine receptors.

Pharmacokinetic properties: Haloperidol decanoate in solution is slowly released from the injection site and enters the systemic circulation, where it is hydrolysed by esterases to haloperidol. After an initial dose of 30-300 mg of haloperidol decanoate, plasma concentrations ranged from 0.8-3.2 ng/ml. After the second dose they were raised to 2.8 ng/ml which was steady state. A monthly dose of approximately 20 times the previous oral maintenance dose has been shown to be approximately clinically equivalent. Blood levels will vary considerably between patients.

Preclinical safety data: No relevant information additional to that contained elsewhere in the Summary of Product Characteristics.

Pharmaceutical particulars
List of excipients: Benzyl alcohol; sesame oil.

Incompatibilities: None known.

Shelf life: 5 years.

Special precautions for storage: Haldol decanoate should be protected from light and stored at room temperature. In common with other depot neuroleptics, if stored for long periods in the cold, precipitation may occur which may clear on storage at room temperature. If precipitate does not clear, the contents of the ampoule should be discarded. Do not store below room temperature.

Nature and contents of container: 1 ml amber glass ampoules, in packs containing 5 ampoules.

Instructions for use/handling: Not applicable.

Marketing authorisation numbers
Haldol decanoate 50 mg/ml 0242/0094
Haldol decanoate 100 mg/ml 0242/0095

Date of approval/revision of SPC January 1998

Legal category POM.

HISMANAL* TABLETS

Presentation White, biconvex, half-scored, uncoated tablets. Each tablet is marked 'Janssen' on one side and 'Ast/10' on the reverse, and contains astemizole 10 mg. Hismanal tablets also contain lactose.

Uses Hismanal is a long acting antihistamine (H_1-antagonist) characterised by a lack of sedative potential.

Hismanal is indicated for allergic rhinitis and conjunctivitis and other conditions normally responsive to antihistamines, including allergic skin reactions (urticaria).

Dosage and administration
Adults and children over 12 years: The daily dose is 10 mg (one tablet or 10 ml) as a single intake, which should not be exceeded.

Children 6–12 years: The daily dose is 5 mg (half a tablet or 5 ml), which should not be exceeded.

Children under 6 years: There have been no specific studies in children under 6 years, therefore the drug is not indicated in this age group.

Use in elderly: There have been no specific studies in the elderly.

Contra-indications, warnings, etc
Contra-indications:
- Pregnancy.
- Known hypersensitivity to astemizole or any of the inactive ingredients.
- Since Hismanal is Hismanal is extensively metabolised by the liver, the use of Hismanal in patients with hepatic dysfunction is contra-indicated.
- Concomitant administration of any of the following:
  - an oral or parenteral formulation of azole antifungals;
  - macrolide antibiotics except azithromycin;
  - selective serotonin reuptake inhibitors (SSRIs);
  - HIV protease inhibitors;
  - mibefradil;
  - therapeutic doses of quinine.
- Pre-existing prolongation of the QT-interval.
- Hypokalaemia.
- Concurrent use of other medications which may predispose to arrhythmias (such as anti-arrhythmic agents, neuroleptics, tricyclic antidepressants, terfenadine).

(see *Interactions*)

Precautions: Because of the risk of developing serious ventricular arrhythmias at high doses, the recommended dose of Hismanal should not be exceeded.

Because of the potential of some diuretics to produce hypokalaemia, care should be taken if it is proposed to administer diuretics concurrently with Hismanal.

Adequate contraceptive precautions should be taken by women of childbearing potential during therapy, and, in view of the prolonged half-life, for several weeks after stopping treatment.

Interactions: The main metabolic pathway of astemizole is through CYP3A4, and to a lesser extent other P-450 isoforms, i.e. CYP2D6 and CYP2A6. The concomitant use of drugs that significantly inhibit these enzymes may theoretically result in increased plasma levels of astemizole, which could increase the risk of QT-interval prolongation. Therefore, the use of such drugs is contra-indicated. Examples include the following:
- an oral or parenteral formulation of azole antifungals;
- macrolide antibiotics except azithromycin (see below);
- selective serotonin reuptake inhibitors.

  An *in vitro* study with nefazodone suggests a clinically significant interaction.
- HIV protease inhibitors, such as ritonavir and indinavir – *in vitro* studies suggest that saquinavir is a weak inhibitor;
- mibefradil.

An interaction with therapeutic doses of quinine has also been established.

Macrolides: Arrythmias have been reported rarely in association with the combination of erythromycin and astemizole.

A human volunteer study suggests a potentially clinically relevant drug interaction with the macrolide clarithromycin, although another *in vivo* study has shown that azithromycin has a negligible effect on the bioavailability of astemizole.

The combination of astemizole and macrolide antibiotics (with the exception of azithromycin) should be avoided. (See *Contra-indications.*)

Astemizole may also interact with other drugs with arrhythmogenic potential (see *Contra-indications*).

There is no evidence to suggest the need for any modification of oral contraceptive dosage in users of Hismanal.

Use in pregnancy: Like many other antihistamines, Hismanal has been associated with adverse effects on the maintenance of pregnancy in rats. No teratogenic effects were observed in animal studies with Hismanal. The safety of Hismanal in human pregnancy has not been established. Therefore it is contra-indicated during pregnancy.

Since astemizole is excreted in breast milk, it should not be used by nursing mothers.

Adverse reactions: Ventricular arrhythmias have occurred at high doses including QT-prolongation and torsades de pointes. In some cases, severe arrhythmias have been preceded by or associated with one or more episodes of syncope. Therefore, syncope in patients receiving astemizole should lead to immediate discontinuation of treatment and appropriate clinical evaluation, including electrocardiography.

As might be expected with Hismanal's lack of sedative potential, sedation has been reported extremely rarely. It should be recognised that, in controlled clinical trials, the incidence of sedation with Hismanal has been no greater than that with placebo. Weight gain has occasionally been reported.

Rare cases, spontaneously reported from post-marketing experience with Hismanal include hypersensitivity reactions such as angio-oedema, bronchospasm, photosensitivity, pruritus, rash and anaphylactoid reactions. There have also been isolated cases of convulsions, benign paraesthesias, myalgia/arthralgia, oedema, mood disturbances, insomnia, nightmares, transaminase elevation and hepatitis. In most cases, a causal relationship with Hismanal is unclear.

Overdosage: Symptoms: In patients exceeding the recommended dose, cases of serious, life-threatening cardiovascular adverse events including QT-prolongation, torsades de pointes, and other ventricular arrhythmias have been observed. While the majority of such events have occurred following substantial overdoses of astemizole, arrhythmias, including torsades de pointes, have very rarely occurred at reported doses as low as 20-30 mg daily (2-3 times the recommended daily dose).

Treatment: Supportive measures including gastric lavage and emesis should be employed, followed by the administration of activated charcoal. In these patients the ECG should be carefully monitored. If the QT-interval is prolonged the monitoring should continue as long as it remains prolonged. The terminal half-life is 1-2 days for astemizole and 9-13 days for desmethylastemizole (the active metabolite). Studies in patients with renal insufficiency suggest that haemodialysis does not increase the clearance of the drug.

Pharmaceutical precautions Store at or below 25°C.

Legal category POM.

Package quantities Supplied in packs of 30 tablets.

Further information Although clinical trials have shown no interaction between Hismanal and diazepam or alcohol, care should be taken to caution the patient against excessive alcohol intake while on medication. Controlled clinical trials with placebo and reference antihistamines have demonstrated that Hismanal is non-sedative, and should not therefore interfere with activities requiring mental alertness, for example, driving or operating machinery. Nevertheless as with other medications, patients should exert caution when undertaking such activities following the first dose of Hismanal.

Pharmacokinetic studies in man demonstrate that astemizole is rapidly absorbed, peak plasma concentrations are attained within 1-2 hours. There is extensive first-pass metabolism and significant tissue distribution. At steady state, the average peak plasma concentration of astemizole plus its metabolite desmethylastemizole (considered together to represent the pharmacologically active fraction in plasma) is 3-5 ng/ml. The terminal half-life is 1-2 days for astemizole and 9-13 days for desmethylastemizole.

Astemizole is excreted as metabolites mainly within the bile.

Receptor binding studies have shown that astemizole, at pharmacological doses, provides complete occupancy of peripheral, H_1-receptors and does not reach the H_1-receptors in the brain, because the drug does not readily cross the blood-brain barrier.

In spite of the long half-life of astemizole and its metabolites, the pharmacokinetics are linear after single and chronic dosing.

Astemizole does not induce human liver enzymes.

Product licence number 0242/0086

HISMANAL* SUSPENSION

Qualitative and quantitative composition Astemizole 5 mg/5 ml.

Pharmaceutical form Suspension.

Clinical particulars

Therapeutic indications: Non-sedative anti-histamine indicated in adults and children over 5 for allergic rhinitis and conjunctivitis and other conditions normally responsive to antihistamines, including allergic skin reactions (urticaria).

Posology and method of administration: Adults and children over 12 years: The daily dose is 10 mg (10 ml) as a single intake, which should not be exceeded.

Children 6-12 years: The daily dose is 5 mg (5 ml) as a single intake, which should not be exceeded.

Children under 6 years: There have been no specific studies of astemizole in children under 6 years, therefore, the drug is not indicated in this age group.

Use in elderly: There have been no specific studies of astemizole in the elderly.

Method of administration: Suspension for oral administration.

Contra-indications:

- Pregnancy.
- Known hypersensitivity to astemizole or any of the inactive ingredients.
- Since Hismanal is extensively metabolised by the liver, the use of Hismanal in patients with hepatic dysfunction is contra-indicated.
- Concomitant administration of any of the following:
- an oral or parenteral formulation of azole antifungals;
- macrolide antibiotics except azithromycin;
- selective serotonin reuptake inhibitors (SSRIs);
- HIV protease inhibitors;
- mibefradil;
- therapeutic doses of quinine.
- Pre-existing prolongation of the QT-interval;
- Hypokalaemia;
- Concurrent use of other medications which may predispose to arrhythmias (such as anti-arrhythmic agents, neuroleptics, tricyclic antidepressants, terfenadine).

(see *Interactions*)

Special warnings and special precautions for use: The following sentence will be included in the patient information leaflet "In some circumstances it is very important not to take Hismanal and these are listed below. If you ignore these instructions, this medicine could affect your heart rhythm".

Because of the risk of developing serious ventricular arrhythmias at high doses, the recommended dose of astemizole should not be exceeded.

Adequate contraceptive precautions should be taken by women of child bearing potential during therapy, and, in view of the prolonged half-life, for several weeks after stopping treatment.

The pack labelling and leaflet for all packs will state (in a box): "IMPORTANT WARNING: Please follow these instructions carefully. If you do not, this medicine could affect your heart rhythm.

If you have heart or liver problems or are taking any other medicines, you should talk to your doctor or pharmacist before taking Hismanal. As with all drugs, Hismanal should only be taken at the recommended dose. Overdosing is dangerous. If an overdose is suspected, see a doctor at once."

Because of the potential of some diuretics to produce hypokalaemia, care should be taken if it is proposed to administer diuretics concurrently with Hismanal.

Hismanal is extensively metabolised by the liver to the active metabolite desmethylastemizole and to other inactive metabolites. The terminal half-life is 1-2 days for astemizole and 9-13 days for desmethylastemizole.

Interaction with other medicaments and other forms of interaction: The main metabolic pathway of astemizole is through CYP3A4, and to a lesser extent other P-450 isoforms, ie CYP2D6 and CYP2A6. The concomitant use of drugs that significantly inhibit these enzymes may theoretically result in increased plasma levels of astemizole, which could increase the risk of QT-interval prolongation. Therefore, the use of such drugs is contra-indicated. Examples include the following:

- an oral or parenteral formulation of azole antifungals;
- macrolide antibiotics except azithromycin (see below);
- selective serotonin reuptake inhibitors;

  An *in vitro* study with nefazodone suggests clinically significant interaction.
- HIV protease inhibitors, such as ritonavir and indinavir – *in vitro* studies suggest that saquinavir is a weak inhibitor;
- mibefradil.

An interaction with therapeutic doses of quinine has also been established.

Macrolides: Arrhythmias have been reported rarely in association with the combination of erythromycin and astemizole.

A human volunteer study suggests a potentially clinically relevant drug interaction with the macrolide clarithromycin, although an *in vivo* study has shown that azithromycin has a negligible effect on the bioavailability of astemizole.

The combination of astemizole and macrolide antibiotics (with the exception of azithromycin) should be avoided. (See contra-indications.)

Astemizole may also interact with other drugs with arrhythmogenic potential (see contra-indications).

There is no evidence to suggest the need for any modification of oral contraceptive dosage in users of Hismanal.

Although clinical trials have shown no interaction between astemizole and diazepam or alcohol, care should be taken to caution the patient against excessive alcohol intake whilst on medication.

Pregnancy and lactation: Like many other antihistamines, astemizole has been associated with adverse effects on the maintenance of pregnancy in rats. No teratogenic effects were observed in animal studies with astemizole. The safety in human pregnancy has not been established and, therefore, astemizole is contra-indicated in women who are pregnant.

Since astemizole is excreted in breast milk, it should not be used by nursing mothers.

Effects on ability to drive and use machines: Controlled clinical trials with placebo and reference antihistamines have demonstrated that astemizole is non-sedative and should not, therefore, interfere with activities requiring mental alertness, for example driving or operating machinery. Nevertheless, as with other medications, patients should exert caution when undertaking such activities following the first dose of astemizole.

Undesirable effects: Ventricular arrhythmias have occurred at high doses including QT-interval prolongation and torsades de pointes. In some cases, severe arrhythmias have been preceded by or associated with one or more episodes of syncope. Therefore syncope in patients receiving astemizole should lead to immediate discontinuation of treatment and appropriate clinical evaluation, including electrocardiography.

As might be expected with astemizole's lack of sedative potential, sedation has been reported extremely rarely. It should be recognised that, in controlled clinical trials, the incidence of sedation with astemizole has been no greater than that with placebo. Weight gain has occasionally been reported.

Rare cases, spontaneously reported from post-marketing experience with Hismanal include hypersensitivity reactions such as angio-oedema, bronchospasm, photosensitivity, pruritus, rash and anaphylactoid reactions. There have also been isolated cases of convulsions, benign paraesthesias, myalgia/arthralgia, oedema, mood disturbances, insomnia, nightmares, transaminase elevation and hepatitis. In most cases a causal relationship with Hismanal is unclear.

Overdose: Symptoms: In patients exceeding the recommended dose, cases of serious, life-threatening cardiovascular adverse events including QT-interval prolongation, torsades de pointes and other ventricular arrhythmias have been observed. While the majority of such events have occurred following substantial overdoses of astemizole, arrhythmias including torsades de pointes, have very rarely occurred at reported doses as low as 20-30 mg (2-3 times the recommended daily dose).

Treatment: Supportive measures including gastric lavage and emesis should be employed, followed by the administration of activated charcoal. In these patients the ECG should be carefully monitored. If the QT-interval is prolonged the monitoring should continue as long as it remains prolonged. The terminal half-life is 1-2 days for astemizole and 9-13 days for desmethylastemizole (the active metabolite). Studies in patients with renal insufficiency suggest that haemodialysis does not increase the clearance of the drug.

Pharmacological properties

Pharmacodynamic properties: Astemizole is an orally active antiallergic agent which acts by specifically blocking peripheral H_1 receptors. Astemizole is a long-acting antihistamine characterised by a lack of sedative potential.

Pharmacokinetic properties: Astemizole is rapidly and completely absorbed in man. Plasma levels of unchanged astemizole are low after single and chronic dosing due to extensive first pass metabolism and considerable distribution to the tissues.

In spite of the long half-life of astemizole and its metabolites, the pharmacokinetics are linear after single and chronic dosing.

Astemizole does not induce human liver enzymes.

Preclinical safety data: Not applicable.

Pharmaceutical particulars

List of excipients: Sorbitol solution; alcohol; propylene glycol; microcrystalline cellulose and sodium carmellose; disodium hydrogen phosphate anhydrous; polysorbate 20, raspberry flavour; sodium saccharin;

sodium dihydrogen phosphate monohydrate; sodium hydroxide; redcurrant flavour; purified water.

Incompatibilities: Not applicable.

Shelf life: 60 months.

Special precautions for storage: Store at room temperature.

Nature and contents of container: Amber glass bottle with a pilfer-proof screw cap, or child-resistant polypropylene screw cap lined inside with a LDPE insert, and separate measuring cup or spoon.

Spoon–standard plastic 5 ml spoon.

Hismanal Suspension may be presented in a bottle size of 200 ml.

Instructions for use/handling: Not applicable.

Marketing authorisation number 0242/0111

Date of approval/revision of SPC June 1998

Legal category POM.

HYPNOMIDATE*

Presentation Clear colourless solution containing 2 mg/ml etomidate. The aqueous vehicle contains 35% propylene glycol and water for injection.

Uses

Indications: Intravenous induction of anaesthesia.

Properties: Hypnomidate is a short-acting hypnotic agent. It is an imidazole-derivative, chemically unrelated to other intravenous hypnotics.

Dosage and administration *Adults:* A dose of 0.3 mg/kg given intravenously at induction of anaesthesia gives sleep lasting from 6 to 10 minutes.

Elderly: A dose of 0.15-0.2 mg/kg bodyweight should be given and the dose should be further adjusted according to effects.

Children up to 15 years old: The dosage may be increased by up to 30% of the adult dose because it is sometimes necessary in order to obtain the same depth and duration of sleep.

Since Hypnomidate has no analgesic action, appropriate analgesics should be used in procedures involving painful stimuli.

Do not exceed a total dose of 30 ml (3 ampoules).

Hypnomidate should only be given by slow intravenous injection.

Hypnomidate may be diluted with sodium chloride infusion BP or dextrose infusion BP but it is not compatible with compound sodium lactate infusion BP (Hartmann's solution). Combinations with pancuronium bromide may show a very slight opalescence; for this reason the two should not be mixed together.

Contra-indications, warnings, etc

Contra-indications: Hypnomidate is contra-indicated in patients with known hypersensitivity to etomidate.

Warnings: Hypnomidate should not be administered to patients with evidence, or suggestion of, reduced adrenal cortical function.

Reduced serum cortisol levels, unresponsive to ACTH injections, have been reported in some patients during induction of anaesthesia but particularly during maintenance of anaesthesia with etomidate; for this reason etomidate should not be used for maintenance. However when etomidate is used for induction, the post-operative rise in serum cortisol which has been observed after thiopentone induction is delayed for approximately 3-6 hours.

In cases of adrenocortical gland dysfunction and during very long surgical procedures, a prophylactic cortisol supplement may be required (for example 50 to 100 mg hydrocortisone).

Convulsions may occur in unpremedicated patients.

In patients with liver cirrhosis, or in those who have already received neuroleptic, opiate or sedative agents, the dose of etomidate should be reduced.

When Hypnomidate is used, resuscitation equipment should be readily available to manage apnoea.

Precautions: Hypnomidate should only be given by slow intravenous injection.

Side effects: The use of narcotic analgesics or diazepam as premedication and during surgery will reduce the uncontrolled spontaneous muscle movements shown by some patients after Hypnomidate administration.

Pain can occur after injection into the small veins of the dorsum of the hand. Use of larger veins or an intravenous application of a small dose of fentanyl 1 to 2 minutes before induction reduces pain on injection.

Nausea and/or vomiting may occur although these are mainly as a result of concurrent use of opiates. Coughing, hiccup and/or shivering may also be experienced. Allergic reactions, including rare cases of bronchospasm and anaphylactoid reactions, have been reported. Rare cases of laryngospasm, cardiac arrhythmias and convulsions have also been reported.

A slight and transient drop in blood pressure may occur due to a reduction of the peripheral vascular resistance. In vulnerable patients, special care should be exercised to minimise this effect.

Respiratory depression and apnoea may occur.

Precautions: Hypnomidate should only be given by slow intravenous injection.

Interactions: Sedative drugs potentiate the hypnotic effect of Hypnomidate.

Hypnomidate is pharmacologically compatible with the muscle relaxants, premedicant drugs and inhalation anaesthetics in current clinical use.

Use in pregnancy: Hypnomidate has no primary effect on fertility, nor primary embryotoxic or teratogenic effects. At maternally toxic doses in rats, decreased survival was noted. Safety in human pregnancy has not been established. As with other drugs, the possible risks should be weighed against the potential benefits before the drug is administered during pregnancy. Hypnomidate may cross the placental barrier during obstetric anaesthesia.

Lactation: It is not known whether Hypnomidate is excreted in human milk. However, caution should be exercised when Hypnomidate is administered to a nursing mother.

Effects on ability to drive and use machinery: Not applicable but no effects likely. After very short surgical procedures (up to 15 minutes) the patient regains normal alertness 30 to 60 minutes after waking. After long operations, normal alertness is regained after 4 to 24 hours, depending on the duration of the operation.

Overdosage: Overdosing is likely to result in prolonged anaesthesia with the possibility of respiratory depression and even arrest. Hypotension has also been observed. General supportive measures and close observation are recommended. In addition, administration of 50-100 mg hydrocortisone (not ACTH) may be required for depression of cortisol secretion.

Pharmaceutical precautions Store at room temperature.

Legal category POM.

Package quantities Hypnomidate is supplied as 10 ml ampoules in packs of 10.

Further information Hypnomidate is rapidly metabolised and eliminated and recovery of consciousness from a single dose is rapid and complete.

Product licence number 0242/0019.

IMODIUM* CAPSULES AND SYRUP

Qualitative and quantitative composition *Capsules:* Loperamide hydrochloride 2 mg.

Syrup: Loperamide hydrochloride 0.2 mg/ml.

Pharmaceutical form Capsules and syrup for oral administration.

Clinical particulars

Therapeutic indications:

Capsules:

P Classification: For the symptomatic treatment of acute episodes of diarrhoea associated with Irritable Bowel Syndrome in adults following initial diagnosis by a doctor.

P and GSL Classification: For the symptomatic treatment of acute diarrhoea in adults and children aged 12 years and over.

POM Classification: For the symptomatic treatment of acute diarrhoea of any aetiology including acute exacerbations of chronic diarrhoea for periods of up to 5 days in adults and children over 8 years. For the symptomatic treatment of chronic diarrhoea in adults.

Syrup:

P Classification: For the symptomatic treatment of acute diarrhoea in adults and children aged 12 years and over.

POM Classification: For the symptomatic treatment of acute diarrhoea of any aetiology including acute exacerbations of chronic diarrhoea for periods of up to 5 days in adults and children over 4 years. For the symptomatic treatment of chronic diarrhoea in adults.

Posology and method of administration:

Acute diarrhoea:

GSL: Adults and children over 12: Two capsules initially followed by one capsule after every loose stool. The maximum daily dose should not exceed six capsules.

P and POM: Adults and children over 12: Two capsules or four 5 ml spoonfuls initially, followed by one capsule or two 5 ml spoonfuls after each loose stool. The usual dose is 3-4 capsules a day. The total daily dose should not exceed eight capsules or sixteen spoonfuls.

Children: The following doses should not be exceeded.

Children 9 to 12 years: One capsule or two 5 ml spoonfuls four times daily until diarrhoea is controlled (up to 5 days).

POM: Children 4–8 years: Use syrup: One 5 ml spoonful three or four times daily with the duration limited to 3 days.

Not recommended for children under 4 years of age.

Further investigation into the cause of the diarrhoea should be considered if there is no improvement within two days of starting treatment with Imodium.

Chronic diarrhoea POM:

Adults: Patients may need widely differing amounts of Imodium. The starting dose should be between two and four capsules, or four and eight 5 ml spoonfuls per day in divided doses, depending on severity. If required this dose can be adjusted up to a maximum of eight capsules or sixteen 5 ml spoonfuls daily.

Having established the patient's daily maintenance dose, Imodium may be administered on a twice daily regimen. Tolerance has not been observed and therefore subsequent dosage adjustment should be unnecessary.

Symptomatic treatment of acute episodes of diarrhoea associated with Irritable Bowel Syndrome in adults (P): Two capsules to be taken initially. The usual dose is between two and four capsules per day in divided doses, depending on severity. If required, this dose can be adjusted according to result, up to a maximum of 8 capsules daily.

Use in elderly: As for adults.

Method of administration: Oral Use.

Contra-indications: Imodium should not be used in children less than 4 years of age. Imodium must not be used when inhibition of peristalsis is to be avoided, in particular when ileus or constipation are present or when abdominal distension develops particularly in severely dehydrated children or in patients with acute ulcerative colitis or pseudomembranous colitis associated with broad spectrum antibiotics. Imodium should not be used **alone** in acute dysentery, which is characterised by blood in stools and elevated body temperatures.

Imodium should not be used in patients with a known hypersensitivity to loperamide or any of the constituents.

GSL – not for use when inflammatory bowel disease is present.

Special warnings and special precautions for use: In patients with diarrhoea, especially young children, fluid and electrolyte depletion may occur. Use of Imodium does not preclude the administration of appropriate fluid and electrolyte replacement therapy.

Since persistent diarrhoea can be an indicator of potentially more serious conditions, Imodium should not be used for prolonged periods until the underlying cause of the diarrhoea has been investigated.

Imodium must be used with caution when the hepatic function necessary for the drug's metabolism is defective (eg in cases of severe hepatic disturbance), as this might result in a relative overdose.

Also for P use only: If symptoms persist for more than 24 hours, consult your doctor.

If you are taking Imodium to control episodes of diarrhoea associated with Irritable Bowel Syndrome diagnosed by your doctor, you should return to him/her if the pattern of your symptoms changes. You should also return to your doctor if your episodes of acute symptoms continue for more than two weeks or there is a need for continuous treatment of more than two weeks.

Also for GSL use only: The first line of treatment in acute diarrhoea is the prevention or treatment of fluid and electrolyte depletion. This is of particular importance in frail and elderly patients with acute diarrhoea.

If symptoms persist for more than 24 hours, consult your doctor.

Interaction with other medicaments and other forms of interaction: None stated.

Pregnancy and lactation: Safety in human pregnancy has not been established although studies in animals have not demonstrated any teratogenic effects. As with other drugs, it is not advisable to administer Imodium in pregnancy. Although the fraction of Imodium secreted in human breast milk is extremely low, caution is advised if Imodium is to be administered to a nursing mother.

Effects on ability to drive and use machines: None stated.

Undesirable effects: Abdominal cramps, nausea, vomiting, tiredness, drowsiness, dizziness, dry mouth and skin reactions, including urticaria have been reported.

On occasions paralytic ileus, bloating and constipation have been reported.

Overdose: In case of overdosage the following effects may be observed: constipation, ileus and neurological symptoms (myosis, muscular hypertonia, somnolence and bradypnoea). If intoxication is suspected, naloxone may be given as an antidote. Since the duration of action of Imodium is longer than that of naloxone, the patient should be kept under constant observation for at least 48 hours in order to detect any possible depression of the central nervous system. Children, and patients with hepatic dysfunction, may be more sensitive to CNS effects. Gastric lavage, or induced emesis and /or enema or laxatives may be recommended.

Pharmacological properties

Pharmacodynamic properties: Loperamide binds to the opiate receptor in the gut wall, reducing propulsive peristalsis and increasing intestinal transit time. Loperamide increases the tone of the anal sphincter.

Pharmacokinetic properties: The half-life of loperamide in man is 10.8 hours with a range of 9–14 hours. Studies on distribution in rats show high affinity for the gut wall with preference for binding to the receptors in the longitudinal muscle layer. Loperamide is well absorbed from the gut, but is almost completely extracted and metabolised by the liver where it is conjugated and excreted via the bile. Due to its high affinity for the gut wall and its high first pass metabolism, very little loperamide reaches the systemic circulation.

Preclinical safety data: Not applicable.

Pharmaceutical particulars

List of excipients:

Capsules: Lactose; maize starch; talc; magnesium stearate.

Capsule cap: Titanium dioxide; yellow ferric oxide; indigotindisulphonate sodium; gelatin.

Capsule body: Titanium dioxide; black ferrous oxide; indigotindisulphonate sodium; erythrosin; gelatin.

Syrup: Glycerol; sodium saccharin; methyl parahydroxybenzoate; propyl parahydroxybenzoate; cochineal red A; raspberry flavour; redcurrant flavour; alcohol; citric acid monohydrate; purified water.

Incompatibilities: Not applicable.

Shelf life: 60 months (both products).

Special precautions for storage: None.

Nature and contents of container: Capsules: Blister packs consisting of aluminium foil, hermetalu and polyvinyl chloride genotherm glass clear.

The blister strips are packed in cardboard cartons to contain 2, 8, 12, 18 or 30 capsules.

OR

Tubs of capsules containing 250 capsules.

Syrup: Amber glass bottle with either a pilfer-proof aluminium screw cap coated on the inside with PVC or a child resistant polypropylene screw cap lined inside with an LDPE insert and a 5 ml or 10 ml polypropylene measuring cup.

Instructions for use/handling: Not applicable.

Marketing authorisation numbers

Imodium Capsules 0242/0028
Imodium Syrup 0242/0040

Date of approval/revision of SPC *Capsules:* October 1997.

Syrup: December 1995.

Legal category *Capsules:* POM/P/GSL; *Syrup:* POM/P.

LEUSTAT* INJECTION

Qualitative and quantitative composition Leustat (cladribine) Injection is a synthetic antineoplastic agent for continuous intravenous infusion. It is a clear, colourless, sterile, preservative-free, isotonic solution. Leustat Injection is available in single-use vials containing 10 mg (1 mg/ml) of 2-chloro-2′-deoxy-β-D-adenosine, or cladribine, a chlorinated purine nucleoside analogue. Each millilitre of Leustat Injection contains 1 mg of the active ingredient, cladribine, and 9 mg (0.15 mEq) of sodium chloride as an inactive ingredient. The solution has pH range of 5.5 to 8.0. Phosphoric acid and/or dibasic sodium phosphate may have been added to adjust the pH.

The chemical name of cladribine is 2-chloro-6-amino-9 (2-deoxy-β-D-erythropento-furanosyl) purine.

Pharmaceutical form A sterile, buffered solution in vials containing 10 mg (1 mg/ml) of 2-chloro-2′-deoxy-β-D-adenosine (cladribine) for dilution and subsequent continuous intravenous infusion.

Clinical particulars

Therapeutic indications: Leustat Injection is indicated for the primary or secondary treatment of patients with Hairy Cell Leukaemia (HCL).

Leustat is also indicated for the treatment of patients with B-cell chronic lymphocytic leukaemia (CLL) who have not responded to, or whose disease has progressed during or after, treatment with at least one standard alkylating-agent-containing regimen.

Posology and method of administration:

HCL: The recommended treatment for Hairy Cell Leukaemia is a single course of Leustat given by continuous intravenous infusion for 7 consecutive days at a dose of 0.09 mg/kg/day (3.6 mg/m²/day). Deviations from this dosage regimen are not advised. Physicians should consider delaying or discontinuing the drug if neurotoxicity or renal toxicity occurs.

CLL: In patients with CLL, the recommended treatment consists of a continuous intravenous infusion of Leustat for 2 hours on days 1 to 5 of a 28 day cycle at a dose of 0.12 mg/kg/day (4.8 mg/m²/day). The patient's response to therapy should be determined every two cycles of treatment. It is recommended that Leustat Injection be administered in responding patients for 2 cycles after maximum response has occurred, up to a maximum of 6 cycles. Therapy should be discontinued after 2 cycles in non-responding patients. Response for this treatment decision is defined as a lymphocyte reduction of 50% or more, ie if lymphocyte count decreases by 50% or more, administer 2 more cycles and re-evaluate response for decision whether to continue with 2 more cycles up to a maximum of 6 cycles.

Children: Safety and efficacy in children have not been established.

Specific risk factors predisposing to increased toxicity from Leustat have not been defined. In view of the known toxicities of agents of this class, it would be prudent to proceed carefully in patients with known or suspected renal insufficiency or severe bone marrow impairment of any aetiology. Patients should be monitored closely for haematological and renal and hepatic toxicity.

Preparation and administration of intravenous solutions: Leustat Injection must be diluted with the designated diluent prior to administration. Since the drug product does not contain any anti-microbial preservative or bacteriostatic agent, aseptic technique and proper environmental precautions must be observed in preparation of a solution of Leustat. For full details concerning preparation of an infusion solution, see Instructions for Use/Handling.

Contra-indications: Leustat Injection is contra-indicated in those patients who are hypersensitive to this drug or any of its components. Leustat is contra-indicated in pregnant women and nursing mothers.

Special warnings and special precautions for use: Leustat Injection is a potent antineoplastic agent with potentially significant toxic side effects. It should be administered under the supervision of a qualified physician experienced in the use of antineoplastic therapy.

CLL: Patients should be monitored closely for infections. Patients with active infection should be treated for the underlying condition prior to receiving therapy with Leustat Injection. Patients who are or who become Coombs' positive should be monitored carefully for occurrence of haemolysis.

Patients with high tumour burden or who are considered at risk for the development of hyperuricaemia as a result of tumour breakdown should receive appropriate prophylactic treatment.

Bone marrow suppression: Suppression of bone marrow function should be anticipated. This is usually reversible and appears to be dose dependent. Severe bone marrow suppression, including neutropenia, anaemia and thrombocytopenia, has been commonly observed in patients treated with Leustat, especially at high doses. At initiation of treatment, most patients in the clinical studies had haematological impairment as a manifestation of active Hairy Cell Leukaemia or Chronic Lymphocytic Leukaemia. Following treatment with Leustat, further haematological impairment occurred before recovery of peripheral blood counts began. Proceed carefully in patients with severe bone marrow impairment of any aetiology since further suppression of bone marrow function should be anticipated.

HCL: During the first two weeks after treatment initiation, mean platelet count, absolute neutrophil count (ANC), and haemoglobin concentration declined and then subsequently increased with normalisation of mean counts by day 15, week 5 and week 8, respectively. The myelosuppressive effects of Leustat were most notable during the first month following treatment. Forty three percent (43%) of patients received transfusions with RBCs and 13% received transfusions with platelets during month 1. Careful haematological monitoring, especially during the first 4 to 8 weeks after treatment with Leustat is recommended. (See Undesirable Effects).

CLL: During the first 2 cycles of therapy with Leustat Injection, haemoglobin concentration, platelet count and absolute neutrophil count declined to a nadir usually observed in Cycle 2. There appeared to be no cumulative toxicity upon administration of further cycles of therapy. Careful haematological monitoring is recommended throughout administration of Leustat Injection.

Neurotoxicity: Serious neurological toxicity (including irreversible paraparesis and quadraparesis) has been reported in patients who received Leustat Injection by continuous infusion at high doses (4 to 9 times the recommended dose for hairy cell leukaemia). Neurological toxicity appears to demonstrate a dose relationship; however, severe neurological toxicities have been reported rarely with the recommended dose. Physicians should consider delaying or discontinuing therapy if neurotoxicity occurs.

Fever/Infection: HCL: Fever (temperature greater than or equal to 37.8°C) was associated with the use of Leustat in approximately 72% (89/124) of patients. Most febrile episodes occurred during the first month. Although seventy percent (70%) of patients were treated empirically with parenteral antibiotics, less than a third of febrile events were associated with documented infection.

CLL: Pyrexia was reported in 22-24% of CLL patients during Cycle 1 of therapy with Leustat Injection, and in less than 3% of patients during subsequent cycles. Forty of 123 patients (32.5%) reported at least one infection during Cycle 1. Infections that occurred in 5% or more were: respiratory infection/inflammation (8.9%), pneumonia (7.3%), bacterial infection (5.7%), and viral skin infections (5.7%). Approximately 70% of patients had at least one infection during the overall study period of 6 years, including treatment and follow-up.

Since the majority of fevers occurred in neutropenic patients, patients should be closely monitored during the first month of treatment and empirical antibiotics should be initiated as clinically indicated. Given the known myelosuppressive effects of Leustat, practitioners should carefully evaluate the risks and benefits of administering this drug to patients with active infections. Since fever may be accompanied by increased fluid loss, patients should be kept well hydrated (See Undesirable effects).

Rare cases of tumour lysis syndrome have been reported in patients with haematological malignancies having a high tumour burden.

Effect on renal and hepatic function: Acute renal insufficiency has developed in some patients receiving high doses of Leustat. In addition, there are inadequate data on dosing of patients with renal or hepatic insufficiency. Until more information is available, caution is advised when administering the drug to patients with known or suspected renal or hepatic insufficiency. All patients should have their renal and hepatic function monitored regularly. (See Effects of high doses).

Leustat Injection must be diluted in a designated intravenous solution prior to administration (See Instructions for use/handling for full details concerning preparation of an infusion solution).

Laboratory tests: During and following treatment, the patient's haematological profile should be monitored regularly to determine the degree of haematopoietic suppression. In HCL patients, bone marrow aspiration and biopsy should be performed to confirm response to treatment with Leustat after peripheral counts have normalised. Febrile events should be investigated with appropriate laboratory and radiological studies. As with other potent chemotherapeutic agents, monitoring of renal and hepatic function should be performed as clinically indicated, especially in patients with underlying kidney or liver dysfunction.

Carcinogenesis/mutagenesis: No animal carcinogenicity studies have been conducted with Leustat. Cladribine is mutagenic in mammalian cells in culture. Cladribine was not mutagenic to bacteria and did not induce unscheduled DNA synthesis in primary rat hepatocyte cultures.

Impairment of fertility: When administered intravenously to Cynomolgus monkeys, Leustat (cladribine) has been shown to cause suppression of rapidly generating cells, including testicular cells. The effect on human fertility is unknown.

Extravasation: Should the drug accidentally be given extravenously, local tissue damage is unlikely. If extravasation occurs, the administration should be stopped immediately and restarted in another vein. Other recommended local measures include elevating the arm and applying an ice pack to reduce swelling.

Interaction with other medicaments and other forms of interaction: Caution should be exercised if Leustat Injection is administered following or in conjunction with other drugs known to cause myelosuppression. Following administration of Leustat Injection, caution should be exercised before administering other immunosuppressive or myelosuppressive therapy. (See Bone marrow suppression)

Pregnancy and lactation: Leustat Injection is teratogenic in mice and rabbits and consequently has the potential to cause foetal harm when administered to a pregnant woman. There are no human data, but Leustat Injection is contra-indicated in pregnancy.

A significant increase in foetal variations was

observed in mice receiving 1.5 mg/kg/day (4.5 mg/m²) and increased resorptions, reduced litter size and increased foetal malformations were observed when mice received 3.0 mg/kg/day (9 mg/m²). Foetal death and malformations were observed in rabbits that received 3.0 mg/kg/day (33.0 mg/m²). No foetal effects were seen in mice at 0.5 mg/kg/day (1.5 mg/m²) or in rabbits at 1.0 mg/kg/day (11.0 mg/m²).

Although there is no evidence of teratogenicity in humans due to Leustat, other drugs which inhibit DNA synthesis (eg methotrexate and aminopterin) have been reported to be teratogenic in humans. Leustat has been shown to be embryotoxic in mice when given at doses equivalent to the recommended dose.

It is not known whether this drug is excreted in human milk. Because it may be excreted in human milk and because there is potential for serious adverse reactions in nursing infants, Leustat should not be given to a nursing mother.

Effects on ability to drive and use machines: Given the patients underlying medical condition and the safety profile of Leustat Injection, caution should be exercised when a patient is performing activities requiring substantial physical well-being (See Undesirable effects).

Undesirable effects:

Overview: HCL: The following safety data are based on 124 patients with HCL enrolled in the pivotal studies. Severe neutropenia was noted in 70% of patients in month 1; fever in 72% at anytime; and infection was documented in 31% of patients in month 1. Other adverse experiences reported frequently during the first 14 days after initiating treatment included: fatigue (49%), nausea (29%), rash (31%), headache (23%) and decreased appetite (23%). Most non-haematological adverse experiences were mild to moderate in severity.

During the first 14 days, events reported by greater than 5% but less than 20% of patients included:

Body as a whole	Chills (13%), asthenia (11%), diaphoresis (11%), malaise (8%), trunk pain (7%).
Gastro-intestinal	Vomiting (14%), constipation (14%), diarrhoea (12%), abdominal pain (8%), flatulence (7%).
Haemic/lymphatic	Purpura (12%), petechia (9%).
Nervous system	Dizziness (13%), insomnia (8%), anxiety (7%).
Cardiovascular system	Oedema (8%), tachycardia (8%), heart murmur (7%).
Respiratory system	Abnormal breath sounds (14%), cough (12%), abnormal chest sounds (12%), shortness of breath (7%).
Skin/subcutaneous tissue	Injection site reaction (15%), pruritus (9%), pain (9%), erythema (8%).
Musculoskeletal system	Myalgia (8%).

Injection site reactions (ie redness, swelling, pain), thrombosis and phlebitis appear usually to be related to the infusion procedure and/or indwelling catheter, rather than to the medication or the vehicle.

From day 15 to the last day of follow-up, the following effects were reported in greater than 5% of patients: fatigue (14%), rash (10%), headache (7%), oedema (7%), arthralgia (7%), malaise (6%), diaphoresis (6%).

CLL: The following safety data are based on 124 patients with CLL enrolled in an open-label safety study. Haematological parameters declined during Cycle 1 and Cycle 2, reaching nadir values in Cycle 2; the percentage of patients having a haemoglobin level below 8.5 g/dL in Cycle 2 was 46.1%. The percentage of patients with platelet counts below 20 x 10(9)/L was 22.5% during Cycle 2. Absolute neutrophil count was below 500 x 10(6)/L in 61.8% of patients in Cycle 2. Adverse experiences reported frequently during the first 14 days after initiating treatment included: skin reaction at the injection site (22.8%), pyrexia (17.9%), fatigue (16.3%), oedema (13.8%), headache (13.0%), cough (11.4%), purpura (10.6%), diaphoresis (8.9%), diarrhoea (7.3%), nausea (6.5%), coagulation defect (6.5%), abnormal breath sounds (5.7%), pneumonia (5.7%), and abnormal chest sounds (5.7%). Adverse experiences that occurred in 5% or more of patients during the remainder of follow-up for Cycle 1 were: pyrexia (6.7%), and preterminal events (6.7%). Drug-related adverse experiences reported during cycles of therapy subsequent to Cycle 1 were limited to the following: skin reaction at medication site (22.8%), phlebitis (5.0%), bacterial skin infection (2.0%), cellulitis (1.0%), nausea (1.0%), skin pain (1.0%), and bacterial infection (1.0%). Skin reactions at the injection site were felt to be more likely related to the indwelling IV catheter and not study drug related. Leustat Injection was not associated with renal or hepatic toxicities.

Bone marrow suppression: HCL: Myelosuppression was frequently observed during the first month after starting treatment with Leustat Injection. Neutropenia (ANC less than 500 x 10⁶/L) was noted in 69% of patients, compared with 25% in whom it was present initially. Severe anaemia (haemoglobin less than 8.5 g/dL) occurred in 41.1% of patients, compared with 12% initially and thrombocytopenia (platelets less than 20x10⁹/L) occurred in 15% of patients, compared to 5% in whom it was noted initially.

Analysis of lymphocyte subsets indicates that treatment with cladribine is associated with prolonged depression of the CD4 counts. Prior to treatment, the mean CD4 count was 766/µl. The mean CD4 count nadir, which occurred 4 to 6 months following treatment, was 272/µl. Fifteen (15) months after treatment, mean CD4 counts remained below 500/µl. CD8 counts behaved similarly, though increasing counts were observed after 9 months. There were no serious opportunistic infections reported during this time. The clinical significance of the prolonged CD4 lymphopenia is unclear.

Prolonged bone marrow hypocellularity (< 35%) was observed. It is not known whether the hypocellularity is the result of disease related marrow fibrosis or Leustat Injection toxicity.

CLL: Patients with CLL treated with Leustat Injection were more severely myelosuppressed prior to therapy than HCL patients; increased myelo-suppression was observed during Cycle 1 and Cycle 2 of therapy, reaching a nadir during Cycle 2. The percentage of patients having a haemoglobin level below 8.5 g/dL was 16.9% at baseline, 37.9% in Cycle 1, and 46.1% in Cycle 2. The percentage of patients with platelet counts below 20 x 10(9)/L was 4.0% at baseline, 20.2% during Cycle 1, and 22.5% during Cycle 2. Absolute neutrophil count was below 500 x 10(6)/L in 19.0% of patients at baseline, 56.5% in Cycle 1, 61.8% in Cycle 2, 59.3% in Cycle 3 and 55.9% in Cycle 4. There appeared to be no cumulative toxicity upon administration of multiple cycles of therapy. Marked blood chemistry abnormalities noted during the study were pre-existing, or were isolated abnormalities which resolved, or were associated with death due to the underlying disease.

Fever/infection: HCL: As with other agents having known immunosuppressive effects, opportunistic infections have occurred in the acute phase of treatment due to the immunosuppression mediated by cladribine. Fever was a frequently observed side effect during the first month of study.

During the first month, 12% of patients experienced severe fever (i.e. greater than or equal to 40°C). Documented infections were noted in fewer than one-third of all febrile episodes. Of the 124 patients treated, 11 were noted to have a documented infection in the month prior to treatment. In the month following treatment, 31% of patients had a documented infection: 13.7% of patients had bacterial infection, 6.5% had viral and 6.5% had fungal infections. Seventy percent (70%) of these patients were treated empirically with antibiotics.

During the first month, serious infections (eg septicaemia, pneumonia), were reported in 7% of all patients; the remainder were mild or moderate. During the second month, the overall rate of documented infection was 8%; these infections were mild to moderate and no severe systemic infections were seen. After the third month, the monthly incidence of infection was either less than or equal to that of the months immediately preceding Leustat therapy.

CLL: During Cycle 1, 23.6% of patients experienced pyrexia, and 32.5% experienced at least one documented infection. Infections that occurred in 5% or more of the patients during Cycle 1 were: respiratory infection/inflammation (8.9%), pneumonia (7.3%), bacterial infection (5.6%), and viral skin infections (5.7%). In Cycles 2 through 9, 71.3% of the patients had at least one infection. Infections that occurred in 10% or more of patients were: pneumonia (28.7%), bacterial infection (21.8%), viral skin infection (20.8%), upper respiratory infection (12.9%), other intestinal infection/inflammation (12.9%), oral candidiasis (11.9%), urinary tract infection (11.9%), and other skin infections (11.9%). Overall, 72.4% of the patients had at least one infection during therapy with Leustat Injection. Of these, 32.6% had been administered concomitant immunosuppressive therapy (prednisone).

Effects of high doses: In a Phase 1 study with 31 patients in which Leustat Injection was administered at high doses (4 to 9 times that recommended for hairy cell leukaemia) for 7 to 14 days in conjunction with cyclophosphamide and total body irradiation as preparation for bone marrow transplantation, acute nephrotoxicity, delayed onset neurotoxicity, severe bone marrow suppression with neutropenia, anaemia, and thrombocytopenia and gastrointestinal symptoms were reported.

Nephrotoxicity: Six patients (19%) developed manifestations of acute renal dysfunction/insufficiency (eg acidosis, anuria, elevated serum creatinine, etc) within 7 to 13 days after starting treatment with Leustat, 5 of the affected patients required dialysis. Renal insufficiency was reversible in 2 of these patients. Evidence of tubular damage was noted at autopsy in 2 (of 4) patients whose renal function had not recovered at the time of death. Several of these patients had also been treated with other medications having known nephrotoxic potential.

Neurotoxicity: Eleven patients (35%) experienced delayed onset neurological toxicity. In the majority, this was characterised by progressive irreversible motor weakness, of the upper and/or lower extremities (paraparesis/quadraparesis), noted 35 to 84 days after starting high dose therapy.

Non-invasive neurological testing was consistent with demyelinating disease.

Post-marketing experience: The following additional adverse events have been reported since the drug became commercially available. These adverse events have been reported primarily in patients who received multiple courses of Leustat Injection:

Haematological: bone marrow suppression with prolonged pancytopenia, including some reports of aplastic anaemia; haemolytic anaemia, which was reported in patients with lymphoid malignancies, occurring within the first few weeks following treatment; hypereosinophilia.

Hepatic: reversible, generally mild, increases in bilirubin and transaminases.

Nervous system: confusion, neuropathy, ataxia, insomnia and somnolence.

Respiratory system: pulmonary interstitial infiltrates, in most cases an infectious aetiology was identified.

Skin/subcutaneous: urticaria.

Opportunistic infections have occurred in the acute phase of treatment due to the immunosuppression mediated by Leustat Injection.

Overdose: High doses of Leustat have been associated with serious neurological toxicity (including irreversible paraparesis/quadraparesis), acute nephrotoxicity, and severe bone marrow suppression resulting in neutropenia, anaemia and thrombocytopenia. (See Special warnings and special precautions for use). There is no known specific antidote to overdosage. It is not known whether the drug can be removed from the circulation by dialysis or haemofiltration. Treatment of overdosage consists of discontinuation of Leustat Injection, careful observation and appropriate supportive measures.

Pharmacological properties

Pharmacodynamic properties: Leustat Injection (also known as 2-chloro-2′-deoxy-β-D-adenosine or 2-CdA or cladribine) is a synthetic antineoplastic agent.

Cellular resistance and sensitivity: The selective toxicity of 2-chloro-2′-deoxy-β-D-adenosine towards certain normal and malignant lymphocyte and monocyte populations is based on the relative activities of deoxycytidine kinase, deoxynucleotidase and adenosine deaminase. It is postulated that cells with high deoxycytidine kinase and low deoxynucleotidase activities will be selectively killed by 2-chloro-2′-deoxy-β-D-adenosine as toxic deoxynucleotides accumulate intracellularly.

Cells containing high concentrations of deoxynucleotides are unable to properly repair single-strand DNA breaks. Leustat Injection can be distinguished from other chemotherapeutic agents affecting purine metabolism in that it is cytotoxic to both actively dividing and quiescent lymphocytes and monocytes, inhibiting both DNA synthesis and repair.

Pharmacokinetic properties: When Leustat Injection was given by continuous intravenous infusion over 7 days the mean steady-state serum concentration was estimated to be 6 ng/ml with an estimated systemic clearance of 640 ml/h/kg. Accumulation of Leustat over the seven day treatment period was not noted.

Plasma concentrations are reported to decline multi-exponentially after intravenous infusions with terminal half-lives ranging from approximately 3-22 hours. In general, the apparent volume of distribution of cladribine is very large (mean approximately 9l/kg), indicating an extensive distribution of cladribine in body tissues. The mean half-life of cladribine in leukaemic cells has been reported to be 23 hours.

There is little information available on the metabolism or route of excretion of cladribine in man. Based on animal data, it is expected that cladribine is cleared by the kidneys. However, information on the contribution of renal clearance to total body clearance is not available. The effect of renal and hepatic impairment on the elimination of cladribine has not been investigated in humans.

Cladribine penetrates into cerebrospinal fluid. One report indicates that concentrations are approximately 25% of those in plasma.

Cladribine is bound approximately 20% to plasma proteins.

Preclinical safety data: Preclinical safety data has been included in specific sections of SPC.

Pharmaceutical particulars

List of excipients: 9.0 mg (0.15 mEq) of sodium chloride as an inactive ingredient. Phosphoric acid and/or dibasic sodium phosphate to adjust the pH to a range of 5.5 to 8.0.

Incompatibilities: Since limited compatibility data are available, adherence to the recommended diluents and infusion systems is advised.

Solutions containing Leustat Injection should not be mixed with other intravenous drugs or additives or infused simultaneously via a common intravenous line, since compatibility testing has not been performed.

If the same intravenous line is used for sequential infusion of several different drugs, the line should be flushed with a compatible diluent before and after infusion of Leustat.

The use of 5% dextrose as a diluent is not recommended because of increased degradation of cladribine.

Shelf life: When stored in refrigerated conditions between 2° to 8°C (36° to 46°F) protected from light, unopened vials of Leustat Injection are stable until the expiration date indicated on the package. Freezing does not adversely affect the solution.

If freezing occurs, thaw naturally to room temperature. DO NOT heat or microwave. Once thawed, the vial of Leustat Injection is stable until expiry if refrigerated. *DO NOT REFREEZE.*

Once diluted, solutions containing Leustat Injection should be administered promptly or stored in the refrigerator (2° to 8°C) for no more than 8 hours prior to start of administration.

Special precautions for storage: Store refrigerated at 2° to 8°C (36° to 46°F). Protect from light during storage.

Nature and contents of container: Leustat Injection is supplied as a sterile, preservative-free, isotonic solution containing 10 mg (1 mg/ml) of cladribine (as 10 ml) in a single-use, flint glass 20 ml vial.

Instructions for use/handling: Preparation and administration of intravenous solutions: Leustat Injection must be diluted with the designated diluent prior to administration. Since the drug product does not contain any anti-microbial preservative or bacteriostatic agent, aseptic technique and proper environmental precautions must be observed in preparation of a solution of Leustat.

Parental drug products should be inspected visually for particulate matter and discoloration prior to administration, whenever solution and container permit. A precipitate may occur during the exposure of Leustat to low temperatures; it may be resolubilised by allowing the solution to warm naturally to room temperature and by shaking vigorously. *DO NOT HEAT OR MICROWAVE.*

Care must be taken to assure the sterility of prepared solutions. Once diluted, solutions of Leustat Injection should be administered promptly or stored in the refrigerator (2° to 8°C) for no more than 8 hours prior to start of administration. Vials of Leustat Injection are for single-use only. Any unused portion should be discarded in an appropriate manner.

The potential hazards associated with cytotoxic agents are well established and proper precautions should be taken when handling, preparing, and administering Leustat Injection. The use of disposable gloves and protective garments is recommended. If Leustat Injection contacts the skin or mucous membranes, wash the involved surface immediately with copious amounts of water.

Preparation of a single daily dose: HCL: Add the calculated dose for a 24 hours period (0.09 mg/kg or 0.09 ml/kg or 3.6 mg/m²) of Leustat Injection to an infusion bag containing 100 ml to 500 ml of 0.9% sodium chloride injection (PhEur). Infuse intravenously continuously over 24 hours. Repeat daily for a total of 7 consecutive days.

CLL: Add the calculated dose for a 2 hours' period (0.12 mg/kg or 4.8 mg/m²) of Leustat Injection to an infusion bag containing 100 ml to 500 ml of 0.9% sodium chloride injection (PhEur). Infuse intravenously continuously over 2 hours. Repeat daily for a total of 5 consecutive days.

The use of 5% dextrose as a diluent is not recommended because of increased degradation of cladribine. Admixtures of Leustat Injection are chemically and physically stable for at least 24 hours at room temperature under normal room fluorescent light in most commonly available PVC infusion containers.

	Dose of Leustat	*Recommended diluent*	*Quantity of diluent*
HCL: 24-hour infusion method	0.09 mg/kg/day	0.9% sodium chloride injection PhEur	100 ml to 500 ml
CLL: 2-hour infusion method	0.12 mg/kg/day	0.9% sodium chloride injection PhEur	100 ml to 500 ml

Marketing authorisation number 0242/0232

Date of approval/revision of SPC March 1998

Legal category POM.

MICRONOR* HRT

Presentation Micronor HRT tablets are round white tablets engraved C over 1 on both faces. Each tablet contains 1 mg of norethisterone.

Uses The progestogenic opposition of menopausal oestrogen replacement therapy.

Mode of Action: Micronor HRT tablets convert the oestrogen primed proliferative endometrium into secretory endometrium which, on withdrawal of norethisterone at the end of each cycle, causes a withdrawal bleed in most patients thus eliminating endometrial hyperplasia.

Dosage and administration
Adult females: One tablet should be taken by mouth each day on days 15-26 of each 28 day cycle of oestrogen replacement therapy.

Children: Micronor HRT tablets are not indicated for use in children.

Use in pregnancy and lactation: Micronor HRT is contraindicated.

Contra-indications, warnings, etc
Contra-indications: Micronor HRT tablets should not be used for contraception. Use is not recommended during pregnancy or lactation, severe disturbance of liver function, Dubin-Johnson and Rotor Syndromes, history during pregnancy of idiopathic jaundice, severe pruritus or pemphigoid gestationis.

Warnings and precautions: Prior to commencing and regularly during oestrogen replacement therapy, it is recommended that the patient should be given a thorough physical and gynaecological examination and a complete medical and family history should be taken. Close monitoring is recommended in patients with epilepsy, diabetes or hypertension, disturbances or impairment of liver function, mastopathy, or a strong family history of mammary cancer, uterine fibroids, cholelithiasis, multiple sclerosis, systemic lupus erythematosus, porphyria, melanoma and asthma. Repeated breakthrough bleeding should be investigated including endometrial biopsy.

At present there is suggestive evidence of an overall change in the relative risk of breast cancer in the post menopausal women receiving hormone replacement therapy. Some studies have reported an increased risk of breast cancer in long-term users, others, however, have shown no such increase. It is not known whether concurrent progestogen use influences the risk of breast cancer. A careful appraisal of the risk-benefit ratio should be undertaken before treatment for longer than 5 years. Administration of unopposed oestrogen therapy in patients with an intact uterus has been reported to increase the risk of endometrial hyperplasia.

There is no indication from published studies that the risk of thromboembolic disease, including myocardial infarction, stroke and thrombophlebitis is increased with hormone replacement therapy at the current recommended low dosage in apparently normal women. However, treatment should be discontinued immediately following the occurrence of an acute vascular thromboembolic event during therapy. There is no evidence that a past history of deep vein thrombosis, pulmonary embolism, stroke, or myocardial infarction should be a contra-indication to hormone replacement therapy when associated with recognised risk factors such as immobilisation (eg post-partum or post-trauma) or post-operative (e.g. in particular after pelvic surgery) but in the absence of specific data, hormone replacement therapy should be used with caution.

Drug interactions: Barbiturates, hydantoins, carbamazepine, meprobamate, phenylbutazone, antibiotics, (including rifampicin) and activated charcoal, may impair the activity of oestrogen and progestogens (irregular bleeding and recurrence of symptoms may occur).

Side effects: Minor effects of oestrogen and combined oestrogen/progestogen hormone replacement therapy which do not usually preclude continuation of therapy include headaches, nausea and breast-tenderness. The following side effects have been reported with oestrogen/progestogen therapy:

Genito-urinary system: Pre-menstrual-like syndrome, increase in size of uterine fibromyomata, vaginal candidiasis, change in cervical erosion and degree of cervical secretion, cystitis-like syndrome.

Breasts: Tenderness, enlargement, secretion.

Gastrointestinal: Nausea, vomiting, abdominal cramps, bloating, cholestatic jaundice.

Skin: Chloasma which may persist when drug is discontinued, erythema multiforme, erythema nodosum, haemorrhagic eruption, loss of scalp hair, hirsutism.

Eyes: Steepening of corneal curvature, intolerance to contact lenses.

CNS: Headaches, migraine, dizziness, mental depression, chorea.

Miscellaneous: Increase or decrease in weight, reduced carbohydrate tolerance, aggravation of porphyria, oedema, changes in libido, leg cramps.

Overdosage: There have been no reports of serious ill-effects from overdosage with norethisterone and treatment is usually unnecessary. Nausea and vomiting may occur.

There is no special antidote and treatment should be symptomatic.

Pharmaceutical precautions Protect from light. Store at room temperature (at or below 25°C).

Legal category POM.

Package quantities Carton containing 3 aluminium/PVC blister strips of 12 tablets each.

Further information Nil.

Product licence number 0242/0241.

MICRONOR* ORAL CONTRACEPTIVE TABLETS

Qualitative and quantitative composition Each tablet contains norethisterone 0.35 mg.

Pharmaceutical form Small, round, white tablet, engraved C035 on both faces.

Clinical particulars
Therapeutic indications: Oral contraceptive.

Posology and method of administration: For oral administration.

Adults: Tablet intake from the first pack is started on the first day of menstruation; no extra contraceptive precautions are necessary.

One tablet is taken at the same time each day, every day of the year, whether menstruation occurs or not.

Elderly: Not applicable.

Children: Not recommended.

Contra-indications:

- Existing thrombophlebitis
- Existing thrombo-embolic disorders
- Cerebrovascular disease or a past history of this condition
- Myocardial infarction or a past history of this condition
- Markedly impaired liver function
- Known or suspected hormone dependent neoplasia
- Known or suspected carcinoma of the breast
- Undiagnosed abnormal genital tract bleeding
- Known or suspected pregnancy
- Cholestatic jaundice of pregnancy or jaundice with prior pill use
- Hepatic adenomas or carcinomas

Special warnings and special precautions for use: There is a general opinion, based on statistic evidence, that users of **combined** oral contraceptives (ie oestrogen plus progestogen) experience more often than non-users various disorders of the circulation of blood, including strokes (blood clots in, and haemorrhages from, the blood vessels of the brain), heart attacks (coronary thromboses) and blood clots obstructing the arteries of the lungs (pulmonary emboli). There may not be a full recovery from such disorders and it should be realised that in a few cases they may be fatal.

To date no association between these disorders and progestogen only oral contraceptives (such as Micronor oral contraceptive tablets) has been shown. However there is a risk that the users of such progestogen only oral contraceptives will (like users of the combined oral contraceptive) be exposed to an increased risk of suffering from these disorders.

Reasons for stopping oral contraceptives immediately:

- Early manifestations of thrombotic or thrombo-embolic disorders, thrombophlebitis
- Cerebrovascular disorders (including haemorrhage)
- Myocardial infarction
- Pulmonary embolism
- Gradual or sudden, partial or complete loss of vision
- Proptosis or diplopia
- Onset or aggravation of migraine or development of headaches of a new pattern which are recurrent, persistent or severe
- Papilloedema or any evidence of retinal vascular lesions
- During periods of immobility (eg after accidents)
- Pregnancy
- Manifestations of liver tumours

Examination of the pelvic organs, breasts and blood

pressure should precede the prescribing of any oral contraceptive and should be repeated regularly.

Because of a possible increased risk of post surgery thrombo-embolic complications in oral contraceptive users, therapy should be discontinued six weeks prior to elective surgery.

When Micronor is administered during the post-partum period, the increased risk of thrombo-embolic disease associated with the post-partum period must be considered.

The following are some of the medical conditions reported to be influenced by the combined pill, and may be affected by Micronor. The physician will have to exercise medical judgement to commence, continue or discontinue therapy as appropriate. The worsening or first appearance of any of these conditions may indicate that Micronor should be discontinued.

1. Pre-existing uterine fibromyomata may increase in size.
2. A decrease in glucose tolerance in a significant number of women.
3. An increase in blood pressure in a small but significant number of women.
4. Cholestatic jaundice. Patients with a history of cholestatic jaundice of pregnancy are more likely to develop cholestatic jaundice during oral contraceptive therapy.
5. Amenorrhoea during and after oral contraceptive therapy. Temporary infertility after discontinuation of treatment.
6. Depression.
7. Fluid retention. Conditions which might be influenced by this factor including epilepsy, migraine, asthma, cardiac or renal dysfunction.
8. Varicose veins.
9. Multiple sclerosis.
10. Porphyria.
11. Tetany.
12. Intolerance to contact lenses.

Or any condition that is prone to worsening during pregnancy.

Ectopic pregnancy: Pregnancies in progestogen-only pill (POP) users are more likely to be ectopic than are pregnancies occurring in the general population since POPs offer less protection against ectopic pregnancy than against intra-uterine pregnancy.

Changing from another oral contraceptive: Start Micronor on the day following completion of the previous oral contraceptive pack without a break (or, in the case of the ED pill, omitting the inactive pills). No extra contraceptive precautions are required.

Post-partum administration: Micronor can be started on the 21st day after childbirth. This will ensure the patient is protected immediately. If there is any delay in taking the first dose, contraception may not be established until 7 days after the first tablet has been taken. In these circumstances patients should be advised that extra contraceptive precautions (non-hormonal methods) are necessary.

After miscarriage or abortion: Patients can take Micronor on the day after miscarriage or abortion, in which case no additional contraceptive precautions are required.

Missed tablets: If a tablet is missed within 3 hours of the correct dosage time, then the missed tablet should be taken as soon as possible; this will ensure that contraceptive protection is maintained. If one (for longer than 3 hours) or more tablets are missed, it is recommended that the patient takes the last missed tablet as soon as possible and continues to take the rest of the tablets as usual. Additional means of contraception (non-hormonal) should be used for the next seven days.

If the patient does not have a period within 45 days of her last period, Micronor should be discontinued and pregnancy should be excluded.

Vomiting and diarrhoea: Additional contraceptive measures (non-hormonal) should be employed during the period of gastro-intestinal upset and for the next seven days.

Laboratory tests: The following laboratory determinations may be altered in patients using oral contraceptives.

Hepatic: increased BSP retention and other tests.

Coagulation: increased prothrombin, factors VII, VIII, IX and X, decreased antithrombin III, increased platelet aggregability.

Endocrine: increased PBI and butanol extractable protein bound iodine and decreased T3 uptake, increased glucose blood levels.

Other: increased phospholipids and triglycerides, decreased serum folate values and disturbance in tryptophan metabolism, decreased pregnanediol excretion, reduced response to metapyrone test.

These tests usually return to pre-therapy values after discontinuing oral contraceptive use. However, the physician should be aware that these altered determinations may mask an underlying disease.

Interaction with other medicaments and other forms of interaction: Reduced efficacy and increased incidence of breakthrough bleeding have been associated with concomitant use of oral contraceptives and rifampicin. A similar association has been suggested with oral contraceptives and barbiturates, phenytoin sodium, ampicillin, tetracyclines and griseofulvin.

Pregnancy and lactation: Masculinisation of the female foetus has occurred when progesterones have been used in pregnant women, although this has been observed at doses much higher than that contained in Micronor. Pregnancy should be ruled out before continuing administration of Micronor to patients who have gone 45 days without a menstrual period.

A small fraction of the active ingredient in oral contraceptives has been identified in the milk of mothers receiving these drugs. The effects, if any, on the breast-fed child have not been determined. If possible the use of oral contraceptives should be deferred until the infant is weaned.

Effects on ability to drive and use machines: Not applicable.

Undesirable effects: Side effects are usually self-limiting and of relatively short duration. Amongst the symptoms reported are:

- Headaches/migraine
- Nausea
- Vomiting
- Breast changes
- Change in weight
- Changes in libido
- Chloasma
- Breakthrough bleeding and spotting
- Rash
- Depression
- Irregular cycle length (particularly in early cycles of therapy). It is important that patients should be advised that whilst on Micronor therapy they may experience that variation in cycle length and that they should continue taking a tablet every day whether they have a period or not. However, patients should be advised to discontinue Micronor and to consult their doctor if they have gone 45 days without having a period.

Malignant hepatic tumours have been reported on rare occasions in long-term users of oral contraceptives. Benign hepatic tumours have also been associated with oral contraceptive use. A hepatic tumour should be considered in the differential diagnosis when upper abdominal pain, enlarged liver or signs of intra-abdominal haemorrhage occur.

A meta-analysis from 54 epidemiological studies reported that there is a slightly increased relative risk of having breast cancer diagnosed in women who are currently using oral contraceptives (OC). The observed pattern of increased risk may be due to an earlier diagnosis of breast cancer in OC users, the biological effects of OCs or a combination of both. The additional breast cancers diagnosed in current users of OCs or in women who have used OCs in the last 10 years are more likely to be localised to the breast than those in women who have never used OCs.

Breast cancer is rare among women under 40 years of age whether or not they take OCs. Whilst the background risk increases with age, the excess number of breast cancer diagnoses in current and recent progesterone-only pill (POP) users is small in relation to the overall risk of breast cancer, possibly of similar magnitude to that associated with combined OCs. However, for POPs, the evidence is based on much smaller populations of users and so is less conclusive than that for combined OCs.

The most important risk factor for breast cancer in POP users is the age women discontinue the POP; the older the age at stopping, the more breast cancers are diagnosed. Duration of use is less important and the excess risk gradually disappears during the course of the 10 years after stopping POP use, such that by 10 years there appears to be no excess.

The evidence suggests that compared with never-users, among 10,000 women who use POPs for up to five years but stop by age 20, there would be much less than one extra case of breast cancer diagnosed up to 10 years afterwards. For those stopping by age 30 after 5 years use of the POP, there would be an estimated 2-3 extra cases (additional to the 44 cases of breast cancer per 10,000 women in this age group never exposed to oral contraceptives). For those stopping by age 40 after 5 years use, there would be an estimated 10 extra cases diagnosed up to 10 years afterwards (additional to the 160 cases of breast cancer per 10,000 never-exposed women in this age group).

It is important to inform patients that users of all contraceptive pills appear to have a small increase in the risk of being diagnosed with breast cancer, compared with non-users of oral contraceptives, but that this has to be weighed against the known benefits.

Overdose: Serious ill effects have not been reported following acute ingestion of large doses of oral contraceptives by young children. Overdosage may cause nausea and withdrawal bleeding may occur in females. An appropriate method of gastric emptying may be used if considered desirable.

Pharmacological properties

Pharmacodynamic properties: Micronor oral contraceptive tablets have a progestational effect on the endometrium and the cervical mucus.

Pharmacokinetic properties: Norethisterone is absorbed from the gastro-intestinal tract and metabolised in the liver. To obtain maximal contraceptive effectiveness, the tablets should be taken at the same time each day, every day.

Preclinical safety data: No relevant information additional to that contained elsewhere in the Summary of Product Characteristics.

Pharmaceutical particulars

List of excipients: Lactose; magnesium stearate; pregelatinised starch.

Incompatibilities: Not applicable.

Shelf life: 36 months.

Special precautions for storage: Store at room temperature (below 25°C).

Nature and contents of container: PVC/aluminium foil blister strips with or without a card wallet in cardboard carton, containing 3 x 28 tablets.

Instructions for use/handling: Not applicable.

Marketing authorisation number 0242/0234

Date of approval/revision of SPC March 1998

Legal category POM.

NIZORAL* TABLETS

Qualitative and quantitative composition Ketoconazole 200 mg.

Pharmaceutical form Tablet.

Clinical particulars

Therapeutic indications: Systemic mycoses, eg systemic candidosis, paracoccidioidomycosis, coccidioidomycosis, histoplasmosis.

Serious chronic mucocutaneous candidosis (including exceptionally disabling paronychia) not responsive to other therapy or when the organism is resistant to other therapy.

Serious mycoses of the gastrointestinal tract not responsive to other therapy or when organisms are resistant to other therapy.

Chronic vaginal candidosis not responsive to other therapy.

Prophylactic treatment to prevent mycotic infection in patients with reduced immune responses, eg in cancer, during treatment with immunosuppressive medication, or with burns.

Culturally determined dermatophyte infections of skin or finger nails which have failed to respond to adequate dose regimes of conventional anti-dermatophyte agents (excluding fungal infection of toe nails). Nizoral is not indicated for pityriasis versicolor, usually an asymptomatic skin rash.

Posology and method of administration: Nizoral tablets should be taken orally with meals to ensure maximum absorption.

Adults:

Mycoses and dermatophyte infections (except vaginal infections): One tablet once daily, usually for 14 days.

If an adequate response has not been achieved after 14 days, treatment can be continued until at least one week after symptoms have cleared and cultures have become negative. The dose may also be increased to 400 mg once daily if necessary.

As nail infections always require long term therapy, they should only be treated when a clinical rather than a purely cosmetic problem exists and only after alternative treatment has failed.

Prophylaxis and maintenance treatment: One tablet daily.

Chronic vaginal candidosis: Two tablets once daily for 5 days.

Children: Dosage should be reduced to 50 or 100 mg depending on body weight (ie approximately 3 mg/kg), for example:

Age 1–4 years: 50 mg

Age 5–12 years: 100 mg

Elderly: In the absence of specific data, chronic vaginal candidosis–as for adults; All other indications–200 mg daily.

Method of administration: oral.

Contra-indications: Nizoral should not be used in patients with a known hypersensitivity to ketoconazole or to any other imidazole antifungal.

Since it cannot be excluded that patients with pre-existing liver disease may be at greater risk of developing hepatic damage, oral ketoconazole treatment is contra-indicated in these patients. In patients suspected of having pre-existing liver disease, liver function tests should be performed prior to treatment and ketoconazole should not be used if significant abnormalities are observed. When administered in high doses (>80 mg/kg) to pregnant rats, ketoconazole has been shown to cause abnormalities of foetal development. The relevance of this finding to humans has not been established and consequently Nizoral is contraindicated in pregnancy.

Astemizole or terfenadine should not be given concurrently with oral ketoconazole.

Special warnings and special precautions for use: Hepatitis has been reported. The risk of hepatitis is greater in patients on long term treatment (>14 days). In patients receiving long term treatment, the benefits must be weighed against the possible risks.

In patients in whom long term treatment (ie >14 days) with ketoconazole is indicated, LFTs should be performed prior to starting treatment.

Asymptomatic elevations in serum transaminase can occur early during treatment with ketoconazole. These may either be insignificant and transient, or can represent early evidence of hepatotoxicity. Patients should therefore be monitored clinically and biochemically with serum transaminase determinations after the first 2 weeks of treatment, at 4 weeks and at monthly intervals thereafter. If significantly elevated levels are observed, liver function tests (LFTs) should be performed at weekly intervals until transaminase levels return to normal. If significant progressive elevation occurs or the patient develops symptoms of hepatitis (malaise, fever, dark urine, pale stools or jaundice), treatment with ketoconazole should be stopped immediately. The patient should then be monitored both clinically and biochemically for at least 2 months or until enzyme levels return to normal. Patients should also be told to consult their doctor if any of the above symptoms develop.

Hepatic damage has usually been reversible on discontinuation of treatment. Rarely, however, fatalities have been reported following ketoconazole treatment, usually where therapy has been continued despite development of symptoms of hepatitis.

The risk factors for the development of hepatitis includes age over 50 (especially women), known drug intolerance or prior administration of potentially hepatotoxic agents and history of liver disease.

Interaction with other medicaments and other forms of interaction: The concomitant administration of terfenadine or astemizole, with oral ketoconazole is contra-indicated. Ketoconazole is extensively bound to plasma proteins. Since ketoconazole inhibits certain hepatic oxidase enzymes, it may decrease the elimination of co-administered drugs whose metabolism depends on such enzymes. Increased levels of such drugs, when used together with ketoconazole, have been associated with an increase in side-effects. Known examples of serious interactions include those with cyclosporin, astemizole, terfenadine, anticoagulants, corticosteroids and, possibly, busulphan. The plasma levels or effects of cyclosporin, anticoagulants, corticosteroids and busulphan should be carefully monitored, if co-administered with oral ketoconazole, and the dosage reduced if necessary. Terfenadine or astemizole should not be taken concomitantly with oral ketoconazole (see contra-indications). Exceptional cases of a disulfiram-like reaction to alcohol, characterised by flushing, rash, peripheral oedema, nausea and headache, have been reported. All symptoms resolved completely within a few hours.

Concomitant use of rifampicin with ketoconazole may reduce the blood levels of both drugs. Similarly concomitant isoniazid treatment reduces the plasma levels of ketoconazole. If these combinations are to be used plasma levels should be carefully monitored.

Concomitant use of ketoconazole and phenytoin may alter the metabolism of one or both drugs.

Absorption of ketoconazole is maximal when taken during a meal, as it depends on stomach acidity. Concomitant treatment with agents that reduce gastric secretion (anti-cholinergic drugs, antacids, H_2 antagonists, proton pump inhibitors) should be avoided and, if indicated, such drugs should be taken not less than two hours after Nizoral.

Pregnancy and lactation: Nizoral is contra-indicated in pregnancy. Nizoral may be excreted in breast milk and therefore it is not advisable to breast feed whilst being treated with Nizoral.

Effects on ability to drive and use machines: None known.

Undesirable effects: Alterations in liver function tests have occurred in patients on ketoconazole; these changes may be transient, cases of hepatitis have been reported (see Warnings section). In rare cases, anaphylactoid reactions have been reported after the first dose. Hypersensitivity reactions including urticaria and angio-oedema have also been reported. The most commonly observed side effects are gastric upsets (nausea, vomiting, abdominal pain), rash, urticaria, pruritus and headache. Thrombocytopenia, paraesthesia, photophobia, exanthema, dizziness and alopecia have been reported rarely. Ketoconazole, 200 mg once daily, produces a transient decrease in plasma testosterone levels during the first 4–6 hours after intake of the drug. During long-term therapy at this dose, testosterone levels are usually not significantly different from controls. In rare instances, gynaecomastia and oligospermia have been reported. A few cases of menstrual irregularities have been reported when ketoconazole has been co-administered with the oral contraceptive. Although impaired response of plasma cortisol to ACTH has been described, clinically significant symptoms of adrenal insufficiency are unlikely to occur at recommended doses. However, patients with impaired adrenal function, or who may be under periods of stress (eg major surgery, intensive care, etc), should have their adrenal function monitored.

Overdose: Cases should be treated symptomatically with supportive measures or gastric lavage as necessary.

Pharmacological properties

Pharmacodynamic properties: Ketoconazole is an imidazole-dioxolane anti-mycotic which is effective after oral administration and has a broad spectrum of activity against dermatophytes, yeasts and other pathogenic fungi.

Pharmacokinetic properties: Ketoconazole is incompletely absorbed by the gastro-intestinal tract; absorption is reduced when gastric acidity is reduced. Peak plasma levels are obtained 2 hours after oral administration.

Ketoconazole is extensively bound to plasma proteins. Penetration into cerebrospinal fluid is poor. Ketoconazole is extensively metabolised in the body and is excreted in the urine as inactive metabolites and unchanged drug. It is also excreted in the faeces.

Preclinical safety data: Not applicable.

Pharmaceutical particulars

List of excipients: Maize starch; lactose; polyvidone; microcrystalline cellulose; colloidal anhydrous silica; magnesium stearate; purified water (not present in final product).

Incompatibilities: None.

Shelf life: Five years.

Special precautions for storage: Store in a dry place. Store between 15°C and 30°C.

Nature and contents of container: Blister packs containing 30 tablets.

Instructions for use/handling: Not applicable.

Marketing authorisation number 0242/0083

Date of approval/revision of SPC July 1997.

Legal category POM.

NIZORAL* SUSPENSION

Presentation Pink, cherry flavoured suspension in 100 ml amber glass bottles containing 20 mg ketoconazole per ml. The suspension also contains microcrystalline cellulose, carboxymethylcellulose sodium, sodium saccharin dihydrate and erythrosine sodium (E127).

Uses Nizoral is an imidazole-dioxolane antimycotic which is effective after oral administration and has a broad spectrum of activity against dermatophytes, yeasts and other pathogenic fungi.

The indications for Nizoral are:

In adults and children

1. Systemic mycoses, eg systemic candidosis, paracoccidioidomycosis, coccidioidomycosis, histoplasmosis.

2. Serious chronic mucocutaneous candidosis (including exceptionally disabling paronychia) not responsive to other therapy or when the organism is resistant to other therapy.

3. Serious mycoses of the gastrointestinal tract not responsive to other therapy or when organisms are resistant to other therapy.

4. Chronic vaginal candidosis not responsive to other therapy.

5. Prophylactic treatment to prevent mycotic infection in patients with reduced immune responses, e.g. in cancer, during treatment with immunosuppressive medication, or with burns.

6. Dermatophyte infections confirmed by culture of skin or finger nails which have failed to respond to adequate dose regimes of conventional anti-dermatophyte agents (excluding fungal infection of toe nails). Nizoral suspension, unlike the shampoo and cream formulations, is not indicated for pityriasis versicolor.

Dosage and administration Nizoral is for oral administration and should always be taken with meals.

The risk of hepatitis (see 'Warnings') may increase in relation to the duration of treatment, if therapy is continued for more than 14 days the benefits must be weighed against the possible risks.

In adults:

Mycoses and dermatophyte infections (except vaginal candidosis): Two 5 ml doses of suspension (200 mg) once daily, with food, usually for 14 days.

If an adequate response has not been achieved after 14 days, treatment may be continued until at least one week after symptoms have cleared and cultures have become negative. The dose may be increased to 400 mg once daily if necessary.

As nail infections always require long term therapy they should only be treated when a clinical rather than a purely cosmetic problem exists and only after alternative treatment has failed.

Prophylaxis and maintenance treatment: Two 5 ml doses of suspension (200 mg) once daily with food.

Chronic vaginal candidosis: Four 5 ml doses of suspension (400 mg) once daily with food for 5 days.

Use in children: Dosage should be reduced to 50 or 100 mg depending on bodyweight (ie approximately 3 mg/kg), for example:

Age 1–4 years—50 mg (2.5 ml) daily with food
Age 5–12 years—100 mg (5 ml) daily with food

Use in elderly: In the absence of specific data, chronic vaginal candidosis – as for adults; all other indications – 200 mg daily with food.

Contra-indications, warnings, etc

Contra-indications: Nizoral should not be used in patients with a known hypersensitivity to ketoconazole or to any other imidazole antifungal.

Since it cannot be excluded that patients with pre-existing liver disease may be at greater risk of developing hepatic damage, oral ketoconazole treatment is contra-indicated in these patients.

In patients suspected of having pre-existing liver disease, liver function tests should be performed prior to treatment and ketoconazole should not be used if significant abnormalities are observed.

Nizoral is contra-indicated in pregnancy (see 'Use in pregnancy' section).

Astemizole or terfenadine should not be given concurrently with oral ketoconazole.

Warnings and precautions: Hepatitis has been reported. The risk of developing hepatitis is greater in patients on long term treatment (>14 days). In patients receiving long term treatment, the benefits must be weighed against possible risks.

In patients in whom long term treatment (ie >14 days) with ketoconazole is indicated, LFTs should be performed prior to starting treatment.

Asymptomatic elevations in serum transaminase can occur early during treatment with ketoconazole. These may either be insignificant and transient, or can represent early evidence of hepatotoxicity. Patients should therefore be monitored clinically and biochemically with serum transaminase determinations after the first 2 weeks of treatment, at 4 weeks and at monthly intervals thereafter. If significantly elevated levels are observed, liver function tests (LFTs) should be performed at weekly intervals until transaminase levels return to normal. If significant progressive elevation occurs or the patient develops symptoms of hepatitis (malaise, fever, dark urine, pale stools or jaundice), treatment with ketoconazole should be stopped immediately. The patient should then be monitored both clinically and biochemically for at least 2 months or until enzyme levels return to normal. Patients should also be told to consult their doctor if any of the above symptoms develop.

The risk factors for the development of hepatitis include age over 50 (especially women), known drug intolerance or prior administration of potentially hepatotoxic agents and history of liver disease.

Hepatic damage has usually been reversible on discontinuation of treatment. Rarely, however, fatalities have been reported following ketoconazole treatment, usually where therapy has been continued despite development of symptoms of hepatitis.

Drug interactions: The concomitant administration of terfenadine or astemizole with oral ketoconazole is contraindicated.

Absorption of Nizoral is maximal when taken during a meal, as it depends on stomach acidity. Concomitant treatment with agents that reduce gastric secretion (anti-cholinergic drugs, antacids, H_2 antagonists, proton pump inhibitors) should be avoided and, if indicated, such drugs should be taken not less than two hours after Nizoral.

Ketoconazole is extensively bound to plasma proteins.

Since ketoconazole inhibits certain hepatic oxidase enzymes, it may decrease the elimination of co-administered drugs whose metabolism depends on such enzymes. Increased levels of such drugs, when used together with ketoconazole, have been associated with an increase in side-effects. Known examples of serious interactions include those with cyclosporin, astemizole, terfenadine, anticoagulants, corticosteroids and, possibly, busulphan. The plasma levels or effects of cyclosporin, anticoagulants, corticosteroids and busulphan should be carefully monitored, if co-administered with oral ketoconazole, and the dosage reduced if necessary. Terfenadine or astemizole should not be taken concomitantly with oral ketoconazole (see contra-indications). Exceptional cases of a disulfiram-like reaction to alcohol, characterised by flushing, rash, peripheral oedema, nausea and headache have been reported. All symptoms resolved completely within a few hours.

Concomitant use of rifampicin with ketoconazole may reduce the blood levels of both drugs. Similarly, concomitant isoniazid treatment reduces the plasma levels of ketoconazole. If these combinations are to be used, plasma levels should be carefully monitored.

Concomitant use of ketoconazole and phenytoin may alter the metabolism of one or both drugs.

Use in pregnancy and lactation: When administered in high doses (>80 mg/kg) to pregnant rats, Nizoral has been shown to cause abnormalities of foetal development. The relevance of this finding to humans has not been established, although Nizoral is contra-indicated in pregnancy.

Nizoral may be excreted in breast milk and therefore it is not advisable to breast feed whilst being treated with Nizoral.

Side effects: Alterations in liver function tests have occurred in patients on ketoconazole; these changes may be transient. Cases of hepatitis have been reported (see 'Warnings' section).

In rare cases, anaphylactoid reactions have been reported after the first dose. Hypersensitivity reactions including urticaria and angio-oedema have also been reported. The most commonly observed side-effects are gastric upsets (nausea, vomiting, abdominal pain), rash, urticaria, pruritus and headache. Thrombocytopenia, paraesthesia, photophobia, exanthema, dizziness and alopecia have been reported rarely.

Ketoconazole, 200 mg once daily, produces a transient decrease in plasma levels of testosterone during the first 4–6 hours after intake of the drug. During long term therapy at this dose, testosterone levels are usually not significantly different from controls. In rare instances, gynaecomastia and oligospermia have been reported. A few cases of menstrual irregularities have been reported when ketoconazole has been co-administered with the oral contraceptive. Although impaired response of plasma cortisol to ACTH has been described, clinically significant symptoms of adrenal insufficiency are unlikely to occur at recommended doses. However, patients with impaired adrenal function, or who may be under periods of stress (eg major surgery, intensive care, etc) should have their adrenal function monitored.

Overdosage: In the event of overdosage, cases should be treated symptomatically with supportive measures or gastric lavage as necessary.

Pharmaceutical precautions None.

Legal category POM.

Package quantities Nizoral suspension is supplied 100 ml bottles.

Further information Nil.

Product licence number 0242/0101

NIZORAL* CREAM

Presentation White, non-staining, water miscible cream containing ketoconazole 2% w/w. The cream also contains propylene glycol, cetyl alcohol and stearyl alcohol, sorbitan monostearate, polysorbate 60 and 80, sodium sulphite, isopropyl myristate and water.

Uses Nizoral has a potent antimycotic activity against dermatophytes and yeasts. Nizoral cream acts rapidly on pruritus which is commonly seen in dermatophyte and yeast infections. This symptomatic improvement often occurs before the first signs of healing are observed.

After topical application, Nizoral is not systemically absorbed and does not produce detectable plasma concentrations.

Nizoral cream is indicated for topical application in the treatment of dermatophyte infections of the skin such as tinea corporis, tinea cruris, tinea manus and tinea pedis infections due to *Trichophyton* spp., *Microsporum* spp. and *Epidermophyton* spp.

Nizoral cream is also indicated for the treatment of cutaneous candidosis (including external application in vulvitis), pityriasis versicolor, and seborrhoeic dermatitis caused by *Pityrosporum* spp.

Dosage and administration Nizoral cream should be applied to the infected areas once or twice daily, depending on the severity of the infection.

The treatment should be continued until a few days after the disappearance of all signs and symptoms. The usual duration of treatment is: pityriasis versicolor 2–3 weeks, tinea corporis 3–4 weeks, tinea pedis 4–6 weeks.

The diagnosis should be reconsidered if no clinical improvement is noted after 4 weeks. General measures in regard to hygiene should be observed to control sources of infection or reinfection.

Seborrhoeic dermatitis is a chronic condition and relapse is highly likely.

Contra-indications, warnings, etc
Contra-indications: Nizoral cream is contra-indicated in patients who have shown hypersensitivity to any of the ingredients or to ketoconazole itself.

Warnings: Not for ophthalmic use.

If a potent topical corticosteroid has been used previously in the treatment of seborrhoeic dermatitis, a recovery period of 2 weeks should be allowed before using Nizoral cream, as an increased incidence of steroid induced skin sensitisation has been reported when no recovery period is allowed.

Side effects: A few instances of irritation, dermatitis, and burning sensation have been observed during treatment with Nizoral cream.

Use in pregnancy: After topical application, Nizoral cream is not systemically absorbed and does not produce detectable plasma concentrations. However as with any medication, Nizoral cream should only be used in pregnant women if its use is considered essential.

Overdosage: If accidental ingestion of Nizoral cream occurs, an appropriate method of gastric emptying may be used if considered appropriate.

Pharmaceutical precautions Store at 25°C or below.

Legal category POM.

Package quantities 30 g tubes.

Further information Dermatophytes and yeast infections of the skin such as tinea corporis, tinea cruris, tinea manus, tinea pedis, pityriasis versicolor, seborrhoeic dermatitis and cutaneous candidosis, are common infections in patients with HIV infection and AIDS. These patients may also be treated with Nizoral cream.

Product licence number 0242/0107.

NIZORAL* SHAMPOO

Presentation 120 ml viscous pink liquid in plastic bottles containing ketoconazole 20 mg/ml. Nizoral shampoo also contains sodium lauryl ether sulphate, disodium monolauryl ether sulphosuccinate, coconut fatty acid diethanolamide, laurdimonium hydrolysed animal collagen, macrogol 120 methyl glucose dioleate, sodium chloride, sodium hydroxide, imidurea, hydrochloric acid, erythrosine (E127) and purified water.

Uses Ketoconazole has a potent antimycotic activity against pathogenic dermatophytes and yeasts including *Pityrosporum spp.* Nizoral shampoo rapidly relieves the scaling and pruritus usually associated with seborrhoeic dermatitis, pityriasis capitis (dandruff) and pityriasis versicolor.

Nizoral shampoo is not systemically absorbed after topical administration, as blood levels are not detectable after chronic use. Nizoral shampoo is indicated for the prevention and treatment of seborrhoeic dermatitis, dandruff and pityriasis versicolor.

Dosage and administration
Adults and children: Shake the bottle well. Wash the hair or affected areas of the skin with Nizoral shampoo. Leave in contact for 3-5 minutes before rinsing thoroughly.

Seborrhoeic dermatitis and dandruff: Treatment: Use Nizoral shampoo twice weekly for 2-4 weeks.

Prophylaxis: Use Nizoral shampoo once every 1-2 weeks.

Pityriasis versicolor: Treatment: Use Nizoral shampoo once daily for a maximum of 5 days.

Prophylaxis: As patches of pityriasis versicolor become more apparent on exposure to the sun, Nizoral shampoo may be used once daily for a maximum of 3 days in a single treatment course before exposure to sunshine.

Contra-indications, warnings, etc
Contra-indications: Hypersensitivity to any of the ingredients.

Interactions: To prevent a rebound effect after stopping prolonged treatment with topical corticosteroids, it is recommended to continue applying the topical corticosteroid together with Nizoral shampoo and to subsequently and gradually withdraw the steroid therapy over a period of 2-3 weeks.

Precautions: Seborrhoeic dermatitis and dandruff are often associated with increased hair shedding, and this has also been reported, although rarely, with the use of Nizoral shampoo.

Keep out of the eyes. If the shampoo should get into the eyes, they should be bathed with water.

Use in pregnancy: Since no ketoconazole is detected in plasma following topical administration, pregnancy and lactation are not a contra-indication for the use of Nizoral shampoo.

Side effects: As with other shampoos, a local burning sensation, itching, irritation and oily/dry hair may occur, but are rare, when using Nizoral shampoo. In rare instances, mainly in patients with chemically damaged hair or grey hair, a discolouration of the hair has been observed.

Accidental ingestion: In the event of accidental ingestion, only supportive measures should be carried out. In order to avoid aspiration, neither emesis nor gastric lavage should be instigated.

Pharmaceutical precautions Store at 25°C or below.

Legal category POM.

Package quantities 120 ml bottles.

Further information Seborrhoeic dermatitis, pityriasis capitis (dandruff) and pityriasis versicolor are common infections in patients with HIV infection and AIDS. These patients may also be treated with Nizoral shampoo.

Product licence number 0242/0139

ORAP*

Qualitative and quantitative composition *Orap 2 mg Tablets:* each tablet contains pimozide 2 mg; *Orap 4 mg Tablets:* each tablet contains pimozide 4 mg; *Orap 10 mg Tablets:* each tablet contains pimozide 10 mg.

Pharmaceutical form *Orap 2 mg Tablets:* White, circular, biconvex, normally arched tablets with one side 0/2 inscription and 'JANSSEN' inscription on the other side. *Orap 4 mg Tablets:* Green, circular, biconvex, normally arched tablets, cross-scored on one side and 'JANSSEN' on the other side. *Orap 10 mg Tablets:* White, circular, flat, bevel-edged tablets with 0/10 inscription on one side and 'JANSSEN' inscription on the other side.

Clinical particulars
Therapeutic indications: Orap is an antipsychotic of the diphenylbutyl-piperidine series and is indicated in:

Chronic schizophrenia, for the treatment of symptoms and prevention of relapse.

Other psychoses, especially paranoid and monosymptomatic hypochondriacal psychoses (eg delusional parasitosis).

Posology and method of administration: Orap is intended for once daily oral administration in adults and children over 12 years of age.

Since individual response to antipsychotic drugs is variable, dosage should be individually determined and is best initiated and titrated under close clinical supervision. In determining the initial dose, consideration should be given to the patient's age, severity of symptoms and previous response to other neuroleptic drugs. Dose increases should be made at weekly intervals or longer, and by increments of 2-4 mg in the daily dose.

The patient should be reviewed regularly to ensure the minimum effective dose is being used.

Chronic schizophrenia: The dose ranges between 2 and 20 mg daily, with 2 mg as a starting dose. This may be increased according to response and tolerance to achieve an optimum response.

Other psychoses, paranoid states and monosymptomatic hypochondriacal psychoses (MHP): An initial dose of 4 mg daily which may then be gradually increased, if necessary, according to response, to a maximum of 16 mg daily.

Use in elderly: Elderly patients require half the normal starting dose of pimozide.

Contra-indications: In common with several other neuroleptics, pimozide has been reported to prolong the QT-interval. It is, therefore, contra-indicated in patients with a pre-existing congenital prolongation of QT and in patients with a history of cardiac arrhythmias.

Orap is also contra-indicated in patients with severe central nervous system depression and in patients with a known hypersensitivity to pimozide or other diphenylbutyl-piperidine derivatives. It should not be used in patients with depression or Parkinson's syndrome.

The concomitant use of orally or parenterally administered cytochrome P450 CYP 3A4 inhibiting drugs such as azole antimycotics, antiviral protease inhibitors and macrolide antibiotics is contra-indicated. The concomitant use of CYP 2D6 inhibiting drugs such as quinidine is also contra-indicated. The inhibition of either or both cytochrome P450 systems, may result in the elevation of pimozide blood concentration and increase the possibility of QT-prolongation.

Special warnings and special precautions for use: A patient information leaflet is supplied with this product.

Please also refer to Drug Interactions section.

Caution is advised in patients with hepatic or renal dysfunction, phaeochromocytoma, thyrotoxicosis, epilepsy and conditions predisposing to epilepsy (eg alcohol withdrawal and brain damage).

It is recommended that a baseline ECG is undertaken in all patients prior to commencing treatment with pimozide in view of the cardiac contra-indications and in order to identify possible subsequent electrocardiographic changes.

It is further recommended that an ECG is repeated annually, or earlier if clinically indicated. Periodic assessment of cardiac function should be undertaken in those patients receiving pimozide in excess of 16 mg daily. If repolarisation changes (prolongation of QT-interval, T-wave or U-wave changes) appear or arrhythmias develop, treatment should be reviewed and either gradually withdrawn or the dose reduced under close supervision.

Drugs which may prolong the QT-interval (such as certain antimalarials, anti-arrhythmics and certain antihistamines), or cause electrolyte disturbance, are not recommended in patients receiving long-term pimozide (please also refer to the Drug Interactions section.)

Electrolyte disturbances, notably hypokalaemia, should also be considered a risk factor.

As with other neuroleptics, cases of sudden unexpected death have been rarely reported with pimozide (generally in doses in excess of the current recommended maximum of 20 mg per day). Whilst the cause of death in these cases is not known with certainty, it is postulated that the QT prolongation seen with pimozide in some patients may have made the patients susceptible to some form of fatal arrhythmia (eg torsades de pointes). Whilst some of these patients were taking pimozide as a sole therapy, the remainder were also taking other drugs, including neuroleptics, implicated in the aetiology of arrhythmias.

In schizophrenia, the response to antipsychotic drug treatment may be delayed. If drugs are withdrawn, recurrence of symptoms may not become apparent for several weeks or months.

Acute withdrawal symptoms, including nausea, vomiting and insomnia, have very rarely been described after abrupt cessation of high doses of antipsychotic drugs. Gradual withdrawal is advisable.

Interaction with other medicaments and other forms of interaction: Please also refer to the Precautions and Warnings section.

As with other neuroleptics, Orap may increase the central nervous system depression produced by other CNS depressant drugs, including alcohol, hypnotics, sedatives or strong analgesics.

Orap may impair the anti-Parkinson effect of levodopa. The dosage of anticonvulsants may need to be increased to take account of lowered seizure threshold.

Concurrent treatment with neuroleptics should be kept to a minimum as they may predispose to the cardiotoxic effects of pimozide. Particular care should be exercised in patients who are using depot neuroleptics. Low potency neuroleptics such as chlorpromazine and thioridazine should not be used concomitantly with pimozide.

Concurrent use of pimozide with drugs which also have arrhythmogenic potential (such as anti-arrhythmic agents and tricyclic antidepressants) is not recommended.

Pimozide is metabolised mainly via the cytochrome P450 subtype 3A4 (CYP 3A4) enzyme system and, to a lesser extent, via the CYP 2D6 subtype.

In vitro data indicate that highly potent inhibitors of CYP 3A4 enzyme system, such as azole antimycotics, antiviral protease inhibitors and macrolide antibiotics will inhibit the metabolism of pimozide, resulting in markedly elevated plasma levels of pimozide.

In vitro data also indicated that quinidine diminishes the CYP 2D6 dependent metabolism of pimozide.

Elevated pimozide levels may enhance the risk of QT-prolongation.

Drugs which may prolong the QT-interval, such as quinine and mefloquine, amiodarone, bretylium, disopyramide, procainamide, quinidine and sotalol, terfenadine and astemizole, are not recommended in patients receiving long-term pimozide treatment.

Concurrent use of drugs causing electrolyte imbalance is not recommended and hypokalaemia should be avoided. Diuretics should be avoided but, if necessary, potassium-sparing diuretics are preferred.

Pregnancy and lactation: The safety of Orap in human pregnancy has not been established. Studies in animals have not demonstrated teratogenic effects. As with other drugs, it is not advisable to administer Orap in pregnancy.

Orap may be excreted in breast milk. If the use of Orap is considered essential, breast feeding should be discontinued.

Effects on ability to drive and use machines: Orap may impair alertness, especially at the start of treatment. These effects may be potentiated by alcohol. Patients should be warned of the risks of sedation and advised not to drive or operate machinery during treatment until their susceptibility is known.

Undesirable effects: In common with all neuroleptics, extrapyramidal symptoms may occur. Anti-parkinson agents should not be prescribed routinely because of the possible risk of impairing pimozide's efficacy. They should only be given as required.

Tardive dyskinesia is common among patients treated with moderate to high doses of antipsychotic drugs for prolonged periods of time and may prove irreversible, particularly in patients over 50 years of age.

The potential seriousness and unpredictability of tardive dyskinesia, and the fact that it has occasionally been reported to occur when neuroleptic antipsychotic drugs have been prescribed for a relatively short period in low dosage, means that the prescribing of such agents requires especially careful assessment of risk versus benefit. Tardive dyskinesia can be precipitated or aggravated by anti-Parkinson drugs. Short-term dyskinesia may occur after abrupt drug withdrawal.

Epileptic fits have been reported even in low dosage. The elderly may be more liable to experience adverse effects.

Dose-related side effects, including drowsiness, insomnia, anxiety and gastro-intestinal symptoms, such as nausea, constipation or dyspepsia may occur. Dizziness, vertigo, weakness, excessive sweating, headache, dry mouth, loss of libido, impotence and hypotension have been reported, but autonomic symptoms are infrequent. QT-interval prolongation and/or ventricular arrhythmias have rarely been reported, and predominantly with high doses and in predisposed patients. Hypersensitivity reactions such as skin rash, itching, shortness of breath or swollen face have also rarely been reported.

Hormonal effects of antipsychotic neuroleptic drugs include hyperprolactinaemia, which may cause galactorrhoea, gynaecomastia and oligo- or amenorrhoea. Very rarely, cases have been reported of hyponatraemia, either due to polydipsia or to the syndrome of inappropriate secretion of anti-diuretic hormone. Neuroleptics may very rarely be associated with body temperature dysregulation.

Glycosuria has been reported.

In common with other antipsychotics, pimozide has been associated with rare cases of Neuroleptic Malignant Syndrome, an idiosyncratic response characterised by hyperthermia, muscle rigidity, autonomic instability, altered consciousness and coma. Signs of autonomic dysfunction such as tachycardia, labile arterial pressure and sweating may precede the onset of hyperthermia, acting as early warning signs. Recovery usually occurs within five to seven days of antipsychotic withdrawal. Affected patients should be carefully monitored. Dantrolene sodium, bromocriptine mesylate and ECT have all been reported as offering benefit in some patients with Neuroleptic Malignant Syndrome.

Overdose: In general, the signs and symptoms of overdose with Orap would be an exaggeration of known pharmacological effects, the most prominent of which would be severe extrapyramidal symptoms, hypotension or sedation. The risk of cardiac arrhythmias, possibly associated with QT-prolongation, should be considered. The patient may appear comatose with respiratory depression and hypotension which could be severe enough to produce a shock-like state.

Treatment: There is no specific antidote to pimozide. Gastric lavage, establishment of a patent airway and, if necessary, mechanically assisted respiration are advised. Electrocardiographic monitoring should commence immediately and continue until the ECG returns to normal. Hypotension and circulatory collapse may be counteracted by the use of intravenous fluids, plasma or concentrated albumin, and vasopressor agents such as noradrenaline.

Adrenaline should not be used.

In cases of severe extrapyramidal symptoms, anti-Parkinson medication should be administered.

Because of the long half-life of pimozide, patients who have taken an overdose should be observed for at least 4 days.

Pharmacological properties

Pharmacodynamic properties: Pimozide is an orally active neuroleptic drug which blocks central dopaminergic receptors. Pimozide antagonises many of the actions of amphetamine and apomorphine.

Pharmacokinetic properties: The mean serum elimination half-life in schizophrenic patients is approximately 55 hours. This is highly variable and may be as long as 150 hours in some individuals. There is a 13-fold interindividual difference in the area under the serum pimozide concentration-time curve and an equivalent degree of variation in peak serum levels among patients studied. The significance of this is unclear since there are few correlations between plasma levels and clinical findings.

Preclinical safety data: No relevant information additional to that contained elsewhere in the Summary of Product Characteristics.

Pharmaceutical particulars

List of excipients: Orap 2 mg Tablets: Lactose; maize starch; sucrose; magnesium stearate; polyvidone K30; purified water (not in final product). *Orap 4 mg Tablets:* Calcium hydrogen phosphate dihydrate; maize starch; microcrystalline cellulose; polyvidone K30; talc; hydrogenated vegetable oil Type I; ferric oxide (E172); indigotindisulphonate (E132) – aluminium lake; purified water (not in final product); *Orap 10 mg Tablets:* Lactose; maize starch; microcrystalline cellulose; pregelatinised potato starch; polyvidone K90; magnesium stearate; colloidal anhydrous silica; purified water (not in final product).

Incompatibilities: None known.

Shelf life: 5 years (all products).

Special precautions for storage: None stated.

Nature and contents of container: Orap 2 mg and 4 mg Tablets: PVC/aluminium foil blister packs, containing 100 tablets. *Orap 10 mg Tablets:* White, polypropylene bottle with white, low density polyethylene cap, containing 100 tablets.

Instructions for use/handling: Not applicable.

Marketing authorisation numbers

Orap 2 mg Tablets	0242/5010R
Orap 4 mg Tablets	0242/0038R
Orap 10 mg Tablets	0242/0069R

Date of approval/revision of SPC March 1998

Legal category POM.

ORTHO* DIENOESTROL CREAM

Presentation A white non-staining cream containing 0.01% w/w dienoestrol.

Uses For intravaginal use only. Indicated in the treatment of atrophic vaginitis and kraurosis vulvae in post menopausal women, and for the treatment of pruritus vulvae and dyspareunia when associated with the atrophic vaginal epithelium.

Dosage and administration Given for short term use only. The lowest dose that will control symptoms should be chosen and medication should be discontinued as promptly as possible.

Attempts to discontinue or taper medication should be made at three to six month intervals, following physical examination. The usual dosage range is one or two applicatorfuls per day for one or two weeks, then gradually reduced to one half initial dosage for a similar period. A maintenance dose of one applicatorful, one to three times a week, may be used after restoration of the vaginal mucosa has been achieved. If the treatment is continued, treated patients with an intact uterus should be monitored closely for signs of endometrial cancer and appropriate diagnostic measures should be taken to rule out malignancy in the event of persistent or recurring abnormal vaginal bleeding.

Studies of the addition of a progestin for seven or more days of a cycle of oestrogen administration have reported a lowered incidence of endometrial hyperplasia. Morphological and biochemical studies of endometrium suggest that 10 to 13 days of progestin are needed to provide maximal maturation of the endometrium and to eliminate any hyperplastic changes. In women with an intact uterus the addition of a progestogen is essential. There are possible additional risks which may be associated with the inclusion of progestin in oestrogen replacement regimens. The potential risks include adverse effects on carbohydrate and lipid metabolism.

As a general rule it is advisable that patients receiving any form of oestrogen replacement therapy should have a complete physical examination at least once a year.

Contra-indications, warnings, etc Pregnancy is an absolute contra-indication to the use of Dienoestrol cream since it may be harmful to the developing foetus.

Oestrogens should not be used in women with any of the other following conditions: known or suspected oestrogen-dependent neoplasia; endometrial hyperplasia; uterine fibromyomata; undiagnosed abnormal genital bleeding; cardiovascular disorders, eg thrombophlebitis; active deep venous thrombosis, thromboembolic disorders or a history of confirmed venous thromboembolism; severe liver disease; porphyria, hypersensitivity to peanuts or arachis oil.

Thromboembolic disorders: While an increased rate of thromboembolic and thrombotic disease in post-menopausal users of oestrogen has not been found this does not rule out the possibility that such an increase may be present or that subgroups of women who have underlying risk factors or who are receiving relatively large doses of oestrogen may have increased risk. Therefore oestrogens should not be used in persons with active thrombophlebitis or thromboembolic disorders, and they should not be used (except in treatment of malignancy) in persons with a history of such disorders.

Prolonged exposure to unopposed oestrogen may increase the risk of development of endometrial carcinoma, induction of other malignant neoplasms, and the risk of cancer of the breast: long term continuous administration of natural and synthetic oestrogens in certain animal species increases the frequency of carcinomas of the breast, cervix, vagina and liver. There is now evidence that oestrogens increase the risk of carcinoma of the endometrium in humans. At the present time there is no satisfactory evidence that oestrogens given to post-menopausal women increase the risk of cancer of the breast, although a recent long-term follow up of a single physician has raised this possibility. However, because of animal data there is a need for caution in prescribing oestrogens for women with a strong family history of breast cancer or who have breast nodules, fibrocystic disease, or abnormal mammograms.

Gall bladder disease: A recent study has reported a two to three-fold increase in the risk of surgically confirmed gall bladder disease in women receiving post-menopausal oestrogens, similar to the two-fold increase previously noted in users of oral contraceptives.

Hepatic adenoma: Benign hepatic adenomas appear to be associated with the use of oral contraceptives. Although benign, and rare, these may rupture and may cause death through intra-abdominal haemorrhage. Such lesions have not yet been reported in association with other oestrogen or progestogen preparations but should be considered in oestrogen users having abdominal pain and tenderness, abdominal mass, or hypovolemic shock.

Elevated blood pressure: It has been reported that this may occur with the use of oestrogens in the menopause and blood pressure should be monitored with oestrogen use, especially if high doses are used.

Epidemiological studies have suggested that hormone replacement therapy (HRT) is associated with an increased relative risk of developing venous thromboembolism (VTE), i.e. deep vein thrombosis or pulmonary embolism. The studies find a 2–3 fold increase for users compared with non-users which for healthy women amounts to a low risk of one extra case of VTE each year for every 5000 patients taking HRT.

Generally recognised risk factors for VTE include a personal or family history and severe obesity (body mass index > 30 kg/m^2). In women with these factors the benefits of treatment with HRT need to be carefully weighed against risks.

The risk of VTE may be temporarily increased with prolonged immobilisation, major trauma or major surgery. In women on HRT scrupulous attention should be given to prophylactic measures to prevent VTE following surgery. Where prolonged immobilisation is liable to follow elective surgery, particularly abdominal or orthopaedic surgery to the lower limbs, consideration should be given to temporarily stopping HRT four weeks earlier, if this is possible.

If venous thromboembolism develops after initiating therapy the drug should be discontinued.

Precautions: A complete medical and family history should be taken prior to the initiation of any oestrogen therapy. The pretreatment and periodic physical examinations should include special reference to blood pressure, breasts, abdomen, and pelvic organs, and should include a Papanicolaou smear.

A pathologist should be advised of oestrogen therapy when relevant specimens are submitted. Certain endocrine and liver function tests may be affected by oestrogen containing products. These are:

Increased BSP retention.

Increased prothrombin and factors VII, VIII, IX, and X; decreased antithrombin 3, increased norepinephrine-induced platelet aggregability.

Impaired glucose tolerance.

Increased thyroid binding globulin (TBG) leading to increased circulating total thyroid hormone, as measured by PBI, T4 by column or T4 by RIA. Free T3 resin uptake is decreased, reflecting the elevated TRG; free T4 is unaltered.

Decreased pregnanediol excretion.

Reduced response to metyrapone.

Reduced serum folate concentration.

Increased serum triglyceride and phospholipid concentration.

Certain patients may develop undesirable manifestations of excessive oestrogenic stimulations, such as abnormal or excessive uterine bleeding, mastodynia, etc. Pre-existing uterine fibroids may increase in size during oestrogen use.

Patients with a past history of jaundice during pregnancy have an increased risk of recurrence of jaundice while receiving oestrogen. The medication should be discontinued while the cause is investigated.

Oestrogens may cause fluid retention. Conditions possibly affected by this factor such as epilepsy, migraine and cardiac or renal dysfunction require careful monitoring.

Oestrogens should be used with caution in patients with:

Metabolic bone diseases that are associated with hypercalcaemia.

Impaired liver function.

A history of mental depression.

Diabetes.

Contact lenses.

Oestrogens should be used judiciously in patients in whom bone growth is not complete.

Ortho Dienoestrol is generally well tolerated. There have been occasional reports of burning, itching and irritation. The doctor should also be aware of those adverse reactions reported to occur with systemic administration of oestrogens.

Genito-urinary tract: intermenstrual bleeding, increase in the size of uterine fibromyomata, change in amount of cervical secretion.

Breast: tenderness, enlargement, secretion.

Gastrointestinal tract: nausea, vomiting, cholestatic jaundice.

Skin: erythema nodosum, rash, chloasma.

Eyes: corneal discomfort if contact lenses are used.

CNS: headache, migraine, mood changes.

Metabolic: reduced glucose tolerance and changes in body weight.

Other events normally associated with the use of oral contraceptives may result from prolonged use of unopposed oestrogens.

Overdosage: Ortho Dienoestrol Cream is intended for intravaginal use. If accidental ingestion of large quantities of the product occurs, an appropriate method of gastric emptying may be used if considered desirable. Overdosage may cause nausea, and in females withdrawal bleeding may occur.

Pharmaceutical precautions Store at room temperature, not exceeding 25°C.

Legal category POM.

Package quantities Tube containing 78 g with the Ortho Plastic Vaginal Applicator.

Further information Nil.

Product licence number 0242/0244.

ORTHO-GYNEST* CREAM

Presentation White to faint yellowish cream with fat like odour containing 0.01% w/w oestriol.

Uses Oestriol is a naturally occurring oestrogen which exerts specific actions on the vulva, vagina and cervix.

Ortho-Gynest Cream is indicated for the treatment of atrophic vaginitis and kraurosis vulvae in post menopausal women, and for the treatment of pruritus vulvae and dyspareunia when associated with atrophic vaginal epithelium.

For intravaginal use only.

Dosage and administration The lowest dose that will control symptoms should be chosen and medication should be discontinued as promptly as possible. Attempts to taper and discontinue medication should be made at three to six month intervals following initiation of therapy and in conjunction with physical examination.

The recommended initial daily dose is one applicatorful inserted high into the vagina, preferably in the evening.

A maintenance dose of one applicatorful twice a week may be used after restoration of the vaginal mucosa has been achieved.

Contra-indications, warnings, etc. Prolonged exposure to unopposed oestrogens may increase the risk of development of endometrial carcinoma. Although publications indicate that oestriol may occupy a somewhat different position with respect to mammary and endometrial carcinomas than other oestrogens, contra-indications for treatment with Ortho-Gynest Cream should be the same as for other oestrogen products.

Oestrogens should not be used in women with any of the following conditions: known or suspected cancer of the breast, known or suspected oestrogen-dependent neoplasia, undiagnosed abnormal genital bleeding, active thrombophlebitis or thromboembolic disorders, a past history of thrombophlebitis, active deep venous thrombosis, thromboembolic disorders, or a history of confirmed venous thromboembolism. Markedly impaired liver function. Congenital or existing disorders of lipid metabolism. History during pregnancy of idiopathic jaundice, severe pruritus, herpes gestationis or otosclerosis. Dubin-Johnson syndrome. Rotor syndrome. Ortho-Gynest Cream is contra-indicated in women with hypersensitivity to arachis oil or peanuts.

Ortho-Gynest Cream is contra-indicated in pregnancy; therapy should be discontinued immediately pregnancy is suspected.

An increased risk of gall-bladder disease has been reported in women receiving post-menopausal oestrogens, similar to the increase noted in users of oral contraceptives.

Benign hepatic adenomas appear to be associated with the use of oral contraceptives and although rare, these may rupture and cause death, through intra-abdominal haemorrhage. Such lesions have not yet been reported in association with other oestrogen or progestogen preparations but should be considered in oestrogen users having abdominal pain and tenderness, abdominal mass or hypovolemic shock.

It has been reported that elevated blood pressure may occur with the use of oestrogens in menopausal women and blood pressure should be monitored with oestrogen use.

Interactions: Contact between contraceptive diaphragms or condoms and the cream must be avoided since the rubber may be damaged by this preparation.

Precautions: A complete medical and family history should be taken prior to the initiation of any oestrogen therapy. The pre-treatment and periodic physical examinations should include special reference to blood pressure, breasts, abdomen, and pelvic organs and should include a Papanicolaou smear.

A pathologist should be advised of oestrogen therapy when relevant specimens are submitted.

Certain patients may develop undesirable manifestations of excessive oestrogenic stimulation such as abnormal or excessive uterine bleeding, mastodynia etc. Bleeding occurring during therapy should be investigated to exclude serious concomitant pathology. Pre-existing uterine fibroids may increase in size during oestrogen use.

Oestrogen may aggravate cases of porphyria.

Patients with a past history of jaundice during pregnancy have an increased risk of recurrence of jaundice while receiving oestrogen therapy. If jaundice develops in any patient receiving oestrogen, the medication should be discontinued while the cause is investigated.

Oestrogens should be used with caution in patients with endometriosis.

Epidemiological studies have suggested that hormone replacement therapy (HRT) is associated with an increased relative risk of developing venous thromboembolism (VTE), i.e. deep vein thrombosis or pulmonary embolism. The studies find a 2–3 fold increase for users compared with non-users which for healthy women amounts to a low risk of one extra case of VTE each year for every 5,000 patients taking HRT.

Generally recognised risk factors for VTE include a personal or family history and severe obesity (body mass index >30 kg/m^2). In women with these factors the benefits of treatment with HRT need to be carefully weighed against risks.

The risk of VTE may be temporarily increased with prolonged immobilisation, major trauma or major surgery. In women on HRT scrupulous attention should be given to prophylactic measures to prevent VTE following surgery. Where prolonged immobilisation is liable to follow elective surgery, particularly abdominal or orthopaedic surgery to the lower limbs, consideration should be given to temporarily stopping HRT 4 weeks earlier, if this is possible.

If venous thromboembolism develops after initiating therapy the drug should be discontinued.

Overdosage: Ortho-Gynest Cream is intended for intravaginal use. If accidental ingestion of large quantities of the product occurs, an appropriate method of gastric emptying may be used if considered desirable.

Pharmaceutical precautions Store at room temperature (not exceeding 25°C).

Legal category POM.

Package quantities Tube containing 80 g with the Ortho* Plastic Vaginal Applicator.

Further information Nil.

Product licence number 0242/0249

ORTHO-GYNEST* PESSARIES

Qualitative and quantitative composition Oestriol 0.5 mg.

Pharmaceutical form Pessary.

Clinical particulars

Therapeutic indications: Treatment of atrophic vaginitis and kraurosis vulvae in post-menopausal women.

Treatment of pruritus vulvae and dyspareunia associated with atrophic vaginal epithelium.

Posology and method of administration: For intravaginal administration.

The recommended initial dose is one pessary inserted high into the vagina, preferably in the evening. A maintenance dose of one pessary twice a week may be used after restoration of the vaginal mucosa has been achieved.

The lowest dose that will control symptoms should be chosen and medication should be discontinued as promptly as possible. Attempts to taper and discontinue medication should be made at three to six month intervals following physical examination.

Contra-indications: Although publications indicate that Oestriol may occupy a somewhat different position with respect to mammary and endometrial carcinomas than other estrogens, contra-indications for treatment with Ortho-Gynest should be the same as for other estrogen products.

Estrogens should not be used in women with any of the following conditions: Known or suspected cancer of the breast, known or suspected estrogen-dependent neoplasia, undiagnosed abnormal genital bleeding, active thrombophlebitis or thromboembolic disorders, a past history of thrombophlebitis, active deep venous thrombosis, thromboembolic disorders, or a history of confirmed venous thromboembolism. Markedly impaired liver function. Congenital or existing disorders of lipid metabolism. History during pregnancy of idiopathic jaundice, severe pruritus, herpes gestationis or otosclerosis. Dubin-Johnson Syndrome. Rotor Syndrome. Pregnancy.

Special warnings and special precautions for use: A complete medical and family history should be taken prior to the initiation of any estrogen therapy. The pre-treatment and periodic physical examination should include special reference to blood pressure, breasts, abdomen and pelvic organs, and should include a Papanicolaou smear.

A pathologist should be advised of estrogen therapy when relevant specimens are submitted.

If jaundice develops in any patient receiving estrogen, the medication should be discontinued while the cause is investigated.

Therapy should be discontinued immediately if pregnancy is suspected.

Epidemiological studies have suggested that hormone replacement therapy (HRT) is associated with an increased relative risk of developing venous thromboembolism (VTE), ie deep vein thrombosis or pulmonary embolism. The studies find a 2-3 fold increase for users compared with non-users which for healthy women amounts to a low risk of one extra case of VTE each year for every 5,000 patients taking HRT.

Generally recognised risk factors for VTE include a personal or family history and severe obesity (body mass index >30 kg/m^2). In women with these factors the benefits of treatment with HRT need to be carefully weighed against risks.

The risk of VTE may be temporarily increased with prolonged immobilisation, major trauma or major surgery. In women on HRT scrupulous attention should be given to prophylactic measures to prevent VTE following surgery. Where prolonged immobilisation is liable to follow elective surgery, particularly abdominal or orthopaedic surgery to the lower limbs, consideration should be given to temporarily stopping HRT 4 weeks earlier, if this is possible.

If venous thromboembolism develops after initiating therapy the drug should be discontinued.

Interaction with other medicaments and other forms of interaction: None known.

Pregnancy and lactation: Ortho-Gynest Pessaries are contra-indicated in pregnancy.

Effects on ability to drive and use machines: None known.

Undesirable effects: An increased risk of gall bladder disease has been reported in women receiving post-menopausal estrogens.

Prolonged exposure to unopposed estrogens may increase the risk of development of endometrial carcinoma.

Benign hepatic adenomas appear to be associated with the use of oral contraceptives and, although rare, these may rupture and cause death through intra-abdominal haemorrhage. Such lesions have not yet been reported in association with other estrogen or progestogen preparations, but should be considered in estrogen users having abdominal pain and tenderness, abdominal mass or hypovolaemic shock.

Elevated blood pressure may occur with the use of estrogens in menopausal women.

Estrogens may aggravate cases of porphyria.

Certain patients may develop undesirable manifestations of excessive estrogenic stimulation such as abnormal or excessive uterine bleeding, mastodynia, etc. Pre-existing uterine fibroids may increase in size during estrogen use.

Patients with a past history of jaundice during pregnancy have an increased risk of recurrence of jaundice while receiving estrogen therapy.

Overdose: If accidental ingestion of large quantities of the product occurs, an appropriate method of gastric emptying may be used if considered desirable.

Pharmacological properties

Pharmacodynamic properties: Oestriol is a naturally occurring estrogen which exerts specific actions on the vulva, vagina and cervix.

Pharmacokinetic properties: Oestriol is rapidly absorbed from the vaginal mucosa. Peak plasma oestriol levels are achieved within 2 hours of therapy and remain elevated for at least 6 hours in the recumbent patient.

Preclinical safety data: There are no pre-clinical data of relevance to the prescriber which are additional to that already included in other sections of the Summary of Product Characteristics.

Pharmaceutical particulars

List of excipients: Benzoic acid; butylated hydroxytoluene; polyethylene glycol 400; polyethylene glycol 1000, sorbitan monostearate, Witepsol S55.

Incompatibilities: None known.

Shelf life: Three years.

Special precautions for storage: Store at room temperature (maximum 25°C).

Nature and contents of container: PVC or PVC/PE moulds, containing 15 pessaries.

Instructions for use/handling: None.

Marketing authorisation number 0242/0250

Date of approval/revision of SPC December 1997

Legal category POM.

ORTHO-CREME* CONTRACEPTIVE CREAM

Qualitative and quantitative composition Contains 2.0% w/w of nonoxynol-9.

Pharmaceutical form Cream.

Clinical particulars

Therapeutic indications: For use as a spermicidal contraceptive in conjunction with barrier methods of contraception.

Posology and method of administration: For topical intravaginal administration.

For use by adult females only.

The cream should be spread over the surface of the diaphragm which will be in contact with the cervix and on the rim. The diaphragm must be allowed to remain *in situ* for at least six to eight hours after coitus. A fresh application of cream or other spermicides, eg Orthoforms Contraceptive Pessaries, must be made prior to any subsequent act of coitus within this period of time, without removing the diaphragm. (A vaginal applicator should be used for inserting more cream.)

Douching is not recommended, but if it is desired it should be deferred for at least six hours after intercourse.

Contra-indications: Hypersensitivity to nonoxynol-9 or to any component of the preparation.

Patients with absent vaginal sensation, eg paraplegics and quadriplegics.

Special warnings and special precautions for use: Spermicidal intravaginal preparations are intended for use in conjunction with barrier methods of contraception such as condoms, diaphragms and caps.

Where avoidance of pregnancy is important the choice of contraceptive method should be made in consultation with a doctor or a family planning clinic.

If vaginal or penile irritation occurs discontinue use. If symptoms worsen or continue for more than 48 hours medical advice should be sought.

Interaction with other medicaments and other forms of interaction: None known.

Pregnancy and lactation: There is no evidence from animal and human studies that nonoxynol-9 is teratogenic. Human epidemiological studies have not shown any firm evidence of adverse effects on the foetus. However some studies have shown that nonoxynol-9 may be embryotoxic in animals. This product should not be used if pregnancy is suspected or confirmed. Animal studies have detected nonoxynol-9 in milk after intravaginal administration. Use by lactating women has not been studied.

Effects on ability to drive and use machines: None known.

Undesirable effects: May cause irritation of the vagina or penis.

Overdose: If taken orally the surfactant properties of this preparation may cause gastric irritation. General supportive therapy should be carried out. Hepatic and renal function should be monitored if medically indicated.

Pharmacological properties

Pharmacodynamic properties: The standard *in vitro* test (Sander-Cramer) evaluating the effect of nonoxynol-9 on animal sperm motility has shown the compound to be a potent spermicide.

The site of action of nonoxynol-9 has been determined as the sperm cell membrane. The lipoprotein membrane is disrupted, increasing permeability, with subsequent loss of cell components and decreased motility. A similar effect on vaginal epithelial and bacterial cells is also found.

Pharmacokinetic properties: The intravaginal absorption and excretion of radiolabelled (^{14}C) nonoxynol-9 has been studied in non-pregnant rats and rabbits and in pregnant rats. No appreciable difference was found in the extent or rate of absorption in pregnant and non-pregnant animals. Plasma levels peaked at about one hour and recovery from urine as unchanged nonoxynol-9 accounted for approximately 15-25% and faeces approximately 70% of the administered dose as unchanged nonoxynol-9. Less than 0.3% was found in the milk of lactating rats. No metabolites were detected in any of the samples analysed.

Preclinical safety data: Not applicable.

Pharmaceutical particulars

List of excipients: Benzoic acid (E 210); cetyl alcohol; lavender compound 13091; methyl hydroxybenzoate (E218); propyl hydroxybenzoate (E216); propylene glycol; sodium carboxymethylcellulose; sodium lauryl sulphate; stearic acid; triethanolmine; acetic acid glacial; castor oil; potassium hydroxide; sorbic acid (E200); purified water.

Incompatibilities: Not applicable.

Shelf life: 3 years.

Special precautions for storage: Store at room temperature (at or below 25°C).

Nature and contents of container: Epoxy-resin lined aluminium tubes of 70 g with polyethylene cap.

Instructions for use/handling: Not applicable.

Marketing authorisation number 0242/0248

Date of approval/revision of SPC October 1996

Legal category GSL.

ORTHOFORMS* CONTRACEPTIVE PESSARIES

Qualitative and quantitative composition Nonoxynol-9, 5.0% w/w.

Pharmaceutical form Pessary.

Clinical particulars

Therapeutic indications: For use as a spermicide contraceptive in conjunction with barrier methods of contraception.

Posology and method of administration: For topical intravaginal administration.

For use by adult females only.

The Orthoforms Contraceptive Pessary should be inserted as high as possible into the vagina approximately 10 minutes before intercourse to permit the pessary to melt.

Any subsequent acts of intercourse should not be undertaken before the insertion of an additional pessary.

Contra-indications: Hypersensitivity to nonoxynol-9 or to any component of the preparation.

Patients with absent vaginal sensation e.g. paraplegics and quadriplegics.

Special warnings and special precautions for use: Spermicidal intravaginal preparations are intended for use in conjunction with barrier methods of contraception such as condoms, diaphragms and caps.

Where avoidance of pregnancy is important the choice of contraceptive method should be made in consultation with a doctor or family planning clinic.

If vaginal or penile irritation occurs, discontinue

use. If symptoms worsen or continue for more than 48 hours, medical advice should be sought.

Interaction with other medicaments and other forms of interaction: None known.

Pregnancy and lactation: There is no evidence from animal or human studies that nonoxynol-9 is teratogenic. Human epidemiological studies have not shown any firm evidence of adverse effects on the foetus. However, some studies have shown that nonoxynol-9 may be embryotoxic in animals. This product should not be used if pregnancy is suspected or confirmed.

Animal studies have detected nonoxynol-9 in milk after intravaginal administration. Use by lactating women has not been studied.

Effects on ability to drive and use machines: None known.

Undesirable effects: Orthoforms Contraceptive Pessaries may cause irritation of the vagina or penis.

Overdose: If taken orally, the surfactant properties of this preparation may cause gastric irritation. General supportive therapy should be carried out. Hepatic and renal function should be monitored if medically indicated.

Pharmacological properties

Pharmacodynamic properties: The standard *in vitro* test (Sander-Cramer) evaluating the effect of nonoxynol-9 on animal sperm motility has shown the compound to be a potent spermicide.

The site of action of nonoxynol-9 has been determined as the sperm cell membrane. The lipoprotein membrane is disrupted, increasing permeability, with subsequent loss of cell components and decreased motility. A similar effect on vaginal epithelial and bacterial cells is also found.

Pharmacokinetic properties: The intravaginal absorption and excretion of radiolabelled (^{14}C) nonoxynol-9 has been studied in non-pregnant rats and rabbits and in pregnant rats. No appreciable difference was found in the extent or rate of absorption in pregnant and non-pregnant animals. Plasma levels peaked at about one hour and recovery from urine as unchanged nonoxynol-9 accounted for approximately 15-25% and faeces approximately 70% of the administered dose as unchanged nonoxynol-9. Less than 0.3% was found in the milk of lactating rats. No metabolites were detected in any of the samples analysed.

Preclinical safety data: See 'Pregnancy and lactation'.

Pharmaceutical particulars

List of excipients: Cetomacrogol 1000 BP; citric acid monohydrate PhEur; polyethylene glycol 1500; polyethylene glycol 1000 BP; purified water PhEur.

Incompatibilities: None known.

Shelf life: 36 months.

Special precautions for storage: Store in a cool place (8-15°C).

Nature and contents of container: Immediate container: polyvinylchloride/polyethylene laminate moulds.

Three strips of 5 pessaries are packed in an outer cardboard carton.

Instructions for use/handling: None stated.

Marketing authorisation number 0242/0247

Date of approval/revision of SPC October 1996

Legal category GSL.

OVYSMEN* ORAL CONTRACEPTIVE TABLETS

Qualitative and quantitative composition Ovysmen are tablets for oral administration.

Each tablet contains norethisterone 0.5 mg and ethinyloestradiol 0.035 mg.

Pharmaceutical form Tablets.

Clinical particulars

Therapeutic indications: Contraception and the recognised indications for such oestrogen/progestogen combinations.

Posology and method of administration: For oral administration.

Adults: It is preferable that tablet intake from the first pack is started on the first day of menstruation in which case no extra contraceptive precautions are necessary.

If menstruation has already begun (that is 2, 3 or 4 days previously), tablet taking should commence on day 5 of the menstrual period. In this case additional contraceptive precautions must be taken for the first 7 days of tablet taking.

If menstruation began more than 5 days previously then the patient should be advised to wait until her next menstrual period before starting to take Ovysmen.

How to take Ovysmen: One tablet is taken daily at the same time (preferably in the evening) without interruption for 21 days, followed by a break of 7 tablet-free days. Each subsequent pack is started after the 7 tablet-free days have elapsed. Additional contraceptive precautions are not then required.

Elderly: Not applicable

Children: Not recommended

Contra-indications:
Absolute contra-indications:

- pregnancy or suspected pregnancy (that cannot yet be excluded)
- circulatory disorders (cardiovascular or cerebrovascular) such as thrombophlebitis and thromboembolic processes (or a history of these conditions), moderate to severe hypertension, hyperlipoproteinaemia.

In addition the presence of more than one of the risk factors for arterial disease.

- severe liver disease, cholestatic jaundice or hepatitis (viral or non-viral) or a history of these conditions if the results of liver function tests have failed to return to normal, and for 3 months after liver function tests have been found to be normal; a history of jaundice of pregnancy or jaundice due to the use of steroids, Rotor syndrome and Dubin-Johnson syndrome, hepatic cell tumours and porphyria.
- cholelithiasis
- known or suspected oestrogen-dependent tumours; endometrial hyperplasia; undiagnosed vaginal bleeding.
- systemic lupus erythematosus or a history of this condition.
- a history during pregnancy or previous use of steroids of:
  · severe pruritus
  · herpes gestationis
  · a manifestation or deterioration of otosclerosis

Relative contra-indications: If any relative contra-indications listed below is present, the benefits of oestrogen/progestogen-containing preparations must be weighed against the possible risk for each individual case and the patient kept under close supervision. In case of aggravation or appearance of any of these conditions whilst the patient is taking the pill, its use should be discontinued.

- conditions implicating an increasing risk of developing venous thrombo-embolic complications, eg severe varicose veins or prolonged immobilisation or major surgery. Disorders of coagulation.
- presence of any risk factor for arterial disease e.g. smoking, hyperlipidaemia or hypertension.
- other conditions associated with an increased risk of circulatory disease such as latent or overt cardiac failure, renal dysfunction, or a history of these conditions.
- epilepsy or a history of this condition.
- migraine or a history of this condition.
- a history of cholelithiasis.
- presence of any risk factor for oestrogen-dependent tumours; oestrogen-sensitive gynaecological disorders such as uterine fibromyomata and endometriosis.
- diabetes mellitus.
- severe depression or a history of this condition. If this is accompanied by a disturbance in tryptophan metabolism, administration of vitamin B6 might be of therapeutic value.
- sickle cell haemoglobinopathy, since under certain circumstances, eg during infections or anoxia, oestrogen-containing preparations may induce thromboembolic process in patients with this condition.
- if the results of liver function tests become abnormal, use should be discontinued.

Special warnings and special precautions for use:
Post partum administration: Following a vaginal delivery, oral contraceptive administration to non-breast-feeding mothers can be started 21 days post-partum provided the patient is fully ambulant and there are no puerperal complications. No additional contraceptive precautions are required. If post-partum administration begins more than 21 days after delivery, additional contraceptive precautions are required for the first 7 days of pill-taking.

If intercourse has taken place post-partum, oral contraceptive use should be delayed until the first day of the first menstrual period.

After miscarriage or abortion administration should start immediately in which case no additional contraceptive precautions are required.

Changing from a 21 day pill or another 22 day pill to Ovysmen: All tablets in the old pack should be finished. The first Ovysmen tablet is taken the next day, ie no gap is left between taking tablets nor does the patient need to wait for her period to begin. Tablets should be taken as instructed in 'How to take Ovysmen'. Additional contraceptive precautions are not required. The patient will not have a period until the end of the first Ovysmen pack, but this is not harmful, nor does it matter if she experiences some bleeding on tablet-taking days.

Changing from a combined every day pill (28 day tablets) to Ovysmen: Ovysmen should be started after taking the last active tablet from the 'Every day Pill' pack (i.e. after taking 21 or 22 tablets). The first Ovysmen tablet is taken the next day, ie no gap is left between taking tablets nor does the patient need to wait for her period to begin. Tablets should be taken as instructed in 'How to take Ovysmen' (see 4.2). Additional contraceptive precautions are not required. Remaining tablets from the every day (ED) pack should be discarded.

The patient will not have a period until the end of the first Ovysmen pack, but this is not harmful, nor does it matter if she experiences some bleeding on tablet-taking days.

Changing from a progestogen-only pill (POP or mini pill) to Ovysmen: The first Ovysmen tablet should be taken on the first day of the period, even if the patient has already taken a mini pill on that day. Tablets should be taken as instructed in 'How to take Ovysmen'. Additional contraceptive precautions are not required. All the remaining progestogen-only pills in the mini pill pack should be discarded.

If the patient is taking a mini pill, then she may not always have a period, especially when she is breast-feeding. The first Ovysmen tablet should be taken on the day after stopping the mini pill. All remaining pills in the mini pill packet must be discarded. Additional contraceptive precautions must be taken for the first 7 days.

To skip a period: To skip a period, a new pack of Ovysmen should be started on the day after finishing the current pack (the patient skips the tablet-free days). Tablet-taking should be continued in the usual way.

During the use of the second pack she may experience slight spotting or break- through bleeding but contraceptive protection will not be diminished provided there are no tablet omissions. The next pack of Ovysmen is started after the usual 7 tablet-free days, regardless of whether the period has completely finished or not.

Reduced reliability: When Ovysmen is taken according to the directions for use the occurrence of pregnancy is highly unlikely. However, the reliability of oral contraceptives may be reduced under the following circumstances:

(i) Forgotten tablets: If the patient forgets to take a tablet, she should take it as soon as she remembers and take the next one at the normal time. This may mean that two tablets are taken in one day. Provided she is less than 12 hours late in taking her tablet, Ovysmen will still give contraceptive protection during this cycle and the rest of the pack should be taken as usual.

If she is more than 12 hours late in taking one or more tablets then she should take the last missed pill as soon as she remembers but leave the other missed pills in the pack. She should continue to take the rest of the pack as usual but must use extra precautions (eg sheath, diaphragm, plus spermicide) and follow the '7-day rule' (see Further Information for the 7 day rule).

If there are 7 or more pills left in the pack after the missed and delayed pills then the usual 7-day break can be left before starting the next pack. If there are less than 7 pills left in the pack after the missed and delayed pills then when the pack is finished the next pack should be started the next day. If withdrawal bleeding does not occur at the end of the second pack then a pregnancy test should be performed.

(ii) Vomiting or diarrhoea: If after tablet intake vomiting or diarrhoea occurs, a tablet may not be absorbed properly by the body. If the symptoms disappear within 12 hours of tablet-taking, the patient should take an extra tablet from a spare pack and continue with the rest of the pack as usual.

However, if the symptoms continue beyond those 12 hours, additional contraceptive precautions are necessary for any sexual intercourse during the stomach or bowel upset and for the following 7 days (the patient must be advised to follow the '7-day rule').

(iii) Change in bleeding pattern: If after taking Ovysmen for several months there is a sudden occurrence of spotting or breakthrough bleeding (not observed in previous cycles) or the absence of withdrawal bleeding, contraceptive effectiveness may be reduced. If withdrawal bleeding fails to occur and none of the above mentioned events has taken place, pregnancy is highly unlikely and oral contraceptive use can be continued until the end of the next pack. (If withdrawal

Estimated cumulative numbers of breast cancers per 10,000 women diagnosed in 5 years of use and up to 10 years after stopping COCs, compared with numbers of breast cancers diagnosed in 10,000 women who had never used COCs

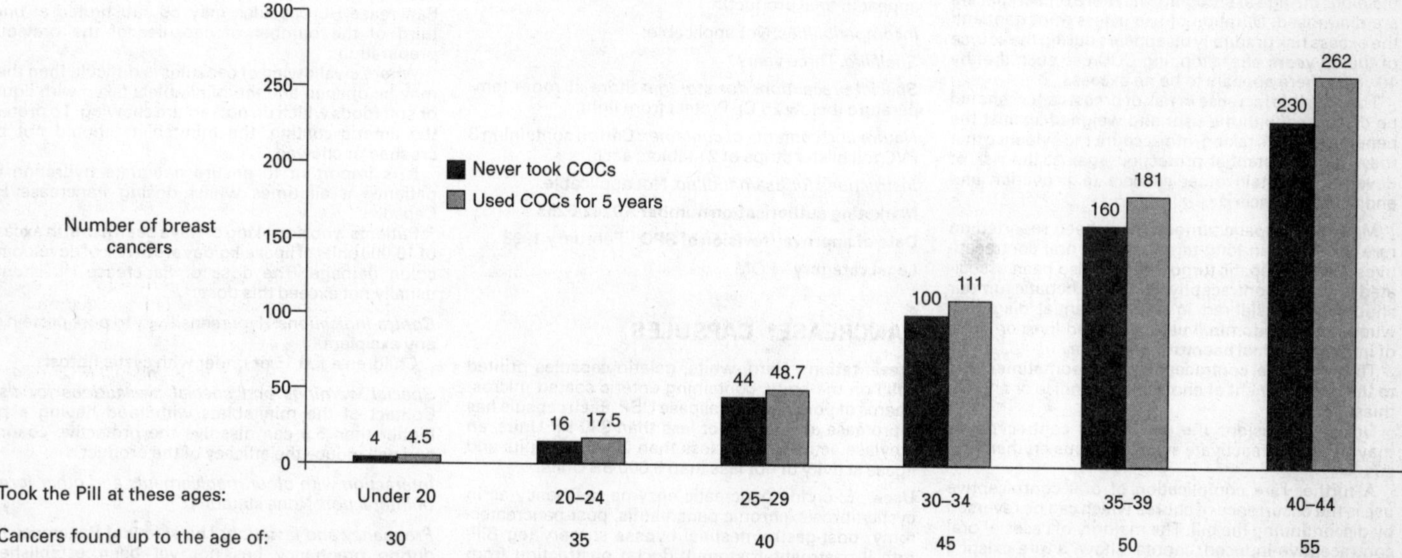

bleeding fails to occur at the end of the second cycle, tablet intake should be discontinued and pregnancy excluded before oral contraceptive use can be resumed). However, if withdrawal bleeding is absent and any of the above mentioned events has occurred, tablet intake should be discontinued and pregnancy excluded before oral contraceptive use can be resumed.

Medical examination/consultation: A complete medical history and physical examination should be taken prior to the initiation or reinstitution of oral contraceptives and should be repeated periodically.

These physical examinations should include special reference to blood pressure, breasts, abdomen and pelvic organs, including cervical cytology and, where indicated by the medical or family history, relevant laboratory tests. Caution should be observed when prescribing oral contraceptives to young women whose cycles are not yet stabilised.

Surgery, varicose veins or immobilisation: In patients using oestrogen-containing preparations the risk of deep vein thrombosis may be temporarily increased when undergoing a major operation (eg abdominal, orthopaedic), and surgery to the legs, medical treatment for varicose veins or prolonged immobilisation. Therefore, it is advisable to discontinue oral contraceptive use at least 4 to 6 weeks prior to these procedures if performed electively and to (re)start not less than 2 weeks after full ambulation. The latter is also valid with regard to immobilisation after an accident or emergency surgery. In case of emergency surgery, thrombotic prophylaxis is usually indicated eg with subcutaneous heparin.

Chloasma: Chloasma may occasionally occur, especially in women with a history of chloasma gravidarum. Women with a tendency to chloasma should avoid exposure to the sun or ultraviolet radiation whilst taking this preparation. Chloasma is often not fully reversible.

Laboratory tests: The use of steroids may influence the results of certain laboratory tests. In the literature, at least a hundred different parameters have been reported to possibly be influenced by oral contraceptive use, predominantly by the oestrogenic component. Among these are: biochemical parameters of the liver, thyroid, adrenal and renal function, plasma levels of (carrier) proteins and lipid/lipoprotein fractions and parameters of coagulation and fibrinolysis.

Further information:

Additional contraceptive precautions: When additional contraceptive precautions are required the patient should be advised either not to have sex, or to use a cap plus spermicide or for her partner to use a condom. Rhythm methods should not be advised as the pill disrupts the usual cyclical changes associated with the natural menstrual cycle, eg changes in temperature and cervical mucus.

The 7-day rule

If any one tablet is forgotten for more than 12 hours.

If the patient has vomiting or diarrhoea for more than 12 hours.

If the patient is taking any of the drugs listed under 'Interactions':-

The patient should continue to take her tablets as usual and:

- Additional contraceptive precautions must be taken for the next 7 days.

But - if these 7 days run beyond the end of the current pack, the next pack must be started as soon as the current one is finished, ie no gap should be left between packs. (This prevents an extended break in tablet taking which may increase the risk of the ovaries releasing an egg and thus reducing contraceptive protection.) The patient will not have a period until the end of 2 packs but this is not harmful nor does it matter if she experiences some bleeding on tablet taking days.

Interaction with other medicaments and other forms of interaction: Irregular cycles and reduced reliability of oral contraceptives may occur when these preparations are used concomitantly with drugs such as anticonvulsants, barbiturates, antibiotics (eg tetracyclines, ampicillin, rifampicin, etc), griseofulvin, activated charcoal and certain laxatives. Special consideration should be given to patients being treated with antibiotics for acne. They should be advised to use a non-hormonal method of contraception, or to use an oral contraceptive containing a progestogen showing minimal androgenicity, which have been reported as helping to improve acne without using an antibiotic. Oral contraceptives may diminish glucose tolerance and increase the need for insulin or other antidiabetic drugs in diabetics.

Pregnancy and lactation: Ovysmen is contraindicated for use during pregnancy or suspected pregnancy, since it has been suggested that combined oral contraceptives, in common with many other substances, might be capable of affecting the normal development of the child in the early stages of pregnancy. It can be definitely concluded, however, that, if a risk of abnormality exists at all, it must be very small.

Mothers who are breast-feeding should be advised not to use the combined pill since this may reduce the amount of breast-milk, but may be advised instead to use a progestogen-only pill (POP).

Effects on ability to drive and use machines: Not applicable.

Undesirable effects: Various adverse reactions have been associated with oral contraceptive use. The first appearance of symptoms indicative of any one of these reactions necessitates immediate cessation of oral contraceptive use while appropriate diagnostic and therapeutic measures are undertaken.

Serious adverse reactions: There is a general opinion, based on statistical evidence, that users of combined oral contraceptives experience more often than non-users various disorders of the coagulation. How often these disorders occur in users of modern low-oestrogen oral contraceptives is unknown, but there are reasons for suggesting that they may occur less often than with the older types of pill which contain more oestrogen.

Various reports have associated oral contraceptive use with the occurrence of deep venous thrombosis, pulmonary embolism and other embolisms. Other investigations of these oral contraceptives have suggested an increased risk of oestrogen and/or progestogen dose-dependent coronary and cerebrovascular accidents, predominantly in heavy smokers. Thrombosis has very rarely been reported to occur in other veins or arteries, eg hepatic, mesenteric, renal or retinal.

It should be noted that there is no consensus about often contradictory findings obtained in early studies. The physician should bear in mind the possibility of vascular accidents occurring and that there may not be full recovery from such disorders and they may be fatal. The physician should take into account the presence of risk factors for arterial disease and deep venous thrombosis when prescribing oral contraceptives. Risk factors for arterial disease include smoking, the presence of hyperlipidaemia, hypertension or diabetes.

Signs and symptoms of a thrombotic event may include: sudden severe pain in the chest, whether or not reaching to the left arm; sudden breathlessness; and unusual severe, prolonged headache, especially if it occurs for the first time or gets progressively worse, or is associated with any of the following symptoms: sudden partial or complete loss of vision or diplopia, aphasia, vertigo, a bad fainting attack or collapse with or without focal epilepsy, weakness of very marked numbness suddenly affecting one side or one part of the body, motor disturbances; severe pain in the calf of one leg; acute abdomen.

Cigarette smoking increases the risk of serious cardiovascular adverse reactions to oral contraceptive use. The risk increases with age and with heavy smoking and is more marked in women over 35 years of age. Women who use oral contraceptives should be strongly advised not to smoke.

The use of oestrogen-containing oral contraceptives may promote growth of existing sex steroid dependent tumours. For this reason, the use of these oral contraceptives in patients with such tumours is contraindicated. Numerous epidemiological studies have been reported on the risk of ovarian, endometrial, cervical and breast cancer in women using combined oral contraceptives. The evidence is clear that combined oral contraceptives offer substantial protection against both ovarian and endometrial cancer. An increased risk of cervical cancer in long term users of combined oral contraceptives has been reported in some studies, but there continues to be controversy about the extent to which this is attributable to the confounding effects of sexual behaviour and other factors.

A meta-analysis from 54 epidemiological studies reported that there is a slightly increased relative risk (RR = 1.24) of having breast cancer diagnosed in women who are currently using combined oral contraceptives (COCs). The observed pattern of increased risk may be due to an earlier diagnosis of breast cancer in COC users, the biological effects of COCs or a combination of both. The additional breast cancers diagnosed in current users of COCs or in women who have used COCs in the last 10 years are more likely to be localised to the breast than those in women who never used COCs.

Breast cancer is rare among women under 40 years of age whether or not they take COCs. Whilst this background risk increases with age, the excess number of breast cancer diagnoses in current and recent COC users is small in relation to the overall risk of breast cancer (see bar chart).

The most important risk factor for breast cancer in COC users is the age women discontinue the COC; the older the age at stopping, the more breast cancers are diagnosed. Duration of use is less important and the excess risk gradually disappears during the course of the 10 years after stopping COC use such that by 10 years there appears to be no excess.

The possible increase in risk of breast cancer should be discussed with the user and weighed against the benefits of COCs taking into account the evidence that they offer substantial protection against the risk of developing certain other cancers (e.g. ovarian and endometrial cancer).

Malignant hepatic tumours have been reported on rare occasions in long-term users of oral contraceptives. Benign hepatic tumours have also been associated with oral contraceptive usage. A hepatic tumour should be considered in the differential diagnosis when upper abdominal pain, enlarged liver or signs of intra-abdominal haemorrhage occur.

The use of oral contraceptives may sometimes lead to the development of cholestatic jaundice or cholelithiasis.

On rare occasions the use of oral contraceptives may trigger or reactivate systemic lupus erythematosus.

A further rare complication of oral contraceptive use is the occurrence of chorea which can be reversed by discontinuing the pill. The majority of cases of oral contraceptive-induced chorea show a pre-existing predisposition which often relates to acute rheumatism.

Other adverse reactions:
Cardiovascular system: Rise of blood pressure. If hypertension develops, treatment should be discontinued.

Genital tract: Intermenstrual bleeding, post-medication amenorrhoea, changes in cervical secretion, increase in size of uterine fibromyomata, aggravation of endometriosis, certain vaginal infections, eg candidiasis.

Breast: Tenderness, pain, enlargement, secretion.

Gastro-intestinal tract: Nausea, vomiting, cholelithiasis, cholestatic jaundice.

Skin: Erythema nodosum, rash, chloasma, erythema multiforme, hirsutism, loss of scalp hair.

Eyes: Discomfort of the cornea if contact lenses are used.

CNS: Headache, migraine, mood changes, depression.

Metabolic: Fluid retention, change in body weight, reduced glucose tolerance.

Other: Changes in libido, leg cramps.

Overdose: There have been no reports of serious ill-health from overdosage even when a considerable number of tablets have been taken by a small child. In general, it is therefore unnecessary to treat overdosage. However, if overdosage is discovered within two or three hours and is large, then gastric lavage can be safely used. There are no antidotes and further treatment should be symptomatic.

Pharmacological properties
Pharmacodynamic properties: Ovysmen acts through the mechanism of gonadotrophin suppression by the oestrogenic and progestational actions of ethinyloestradiol and norethisterone. The primary mechanism of action is inhibition of ovulation, but alterations to the cervical mucus and to the endometrium may also contribute to the efficacy of the product. If a patient misses more than one tablet she should begin taking tablets again as soon as remembered and an additional reliable method of contraception used until the next withdrawal bleed. The patient should be advised that during the first 14 days of the first course of tablets, she should use an additional reliable non-hormonal form of contraception.

Pharmacokinetic properties: Norethisterone and ethinyloestradiol are absorbed from the gastro-intestinal tract and metabolised in the liver. To obtain maximal contraceptive effectiveness the tablets should be taken as directed and at approximately the same time each day. If the patient has vomiting or diarrhoea absorption of the hormones will be impaired, making it advisable to use an additional reliable method of contraception until her next menstrual period.

Because the active ingredients are metabolised in the liver, reduced contraceptive efficacy has been associated with concomitant use of oral contraceptives and rifampicin. A similar association has been suggested with oral contraceptives and barbiturates, phenytoin sodium, phenylbutazone, griseofulvin and ampicillin.

Preclinical safety data: The toxicology of norethisterone and ethinyloestradiol has been extensively investigated in animal studies and through long term clinical experience with widespread use in contraceptives.

Pharmaceutical particulars
List of excipients: Lactose (anhydrous); magnesium stearate; pregelatinised starch; methanol (does not appear in final product).

Incompatibilities: Not applicable.

Shelf life: Three years.

Special precautions for storage: Store at room temperature (below 25°C). Protect from light.

Nature and contents of container: Carton containing 3 PVC/foil blister strips of 21 tablets each.

Instructions for use/handling: Not applicable.

Marketing authorisation number 0242/0253

Date of approval/revision of SPC February 1998

Legal category POM.

PANCREASE* CAPSULES

Presentation Hard, white, gelatin capsules printed 0095 on the body, containing enteric coated microspheres of porcine Pancrelipase USP. Each capsule has a protease activity of not less than 330 BP Units, an amylase activity of not less than 2,900 BP Units and lipase activity of not less than 5,000 BP Units.

Uses Exocrine pancreatic enzyme deficiency as in cystic fibrosis, chronic pancreatitis, post-pancreatectomy, post-gastrointestinal bypass surgery (eg Billroth II gastroenterostomy), ductal obstruction from neoplasm (eg of the pancreas or common bile duct).

The enzymes catalyse the hydrolysis of fats into glycerol and fatty acids, protein into proteoses and derived substances and starch into dextrins and sugars.

Dosage and administration For adults and children 1 or 2 capsules during each meal and one capsule with snacks. Occasionally a third capsule with meals may be required depending upon individual requirements. Where swallowing of capsules is difficult, they may be opened and the microspheres taken with liquids or soft foods which do not require chewing. To protect the enteric coating the microspheres should not be crushed or chewed.

Contra-indications, warnings, etc Hypersensitivity to pork protein. The safety of Pancrease during pregnancy has not yet been established. Such use is not recommended.

The most frequently reported adverse reactions to Pancrease Capsules are gastrointestinal in nature. Less frequently allergic-type reactions have also been observed.

Extremely high doses of exogenous pancreatic enzymes have been associated with hyperuricosuria and hyperuricaemia.

Contact of the microspheres with food having a pH higher than 5.5 can dissolve the protective enteric shell.

Pharmaceutical precautions Keep bottle tightly closed. Store at room temperature in a dry place. Do not refrigerate.

Legal category P.

Package quantities Containers of 100 capsules.

Further information The enteric coated Pancrease microspheres resist gastric inactivation and deliver predictable, high levels of biologically active enzymes into the duodenum.

Product licence number 0242/0254.

PANCREASE* HL CAPSULES

Qualitative and quantitative composition Each capsule contains pancreatin BP 387.45 mg, equivalent to not less than 25000 BP units of lipase, 22500 BP units of amylase and 1250 BP units of protease.

Pharmaceutical form Size 0, elongated hard gelatin capsule, with a white opaque body and a white opaque cap, each ringed with a red band and the letters HL in red, containing enterically coated minitablets.

Clinical particulars
Therapeutic indications: Exocrine pancreatic enzyme deficiency as in cystic fibrosis, chronic pancreatitis, post pancreatectomy, post gastrointestinal bypass surgery (eg Billroth II gastroenterostomy), and ductal obstruction from neoplasm (eg of the pancreas or common bile duct).

Posology and method of administration: For oral administration.

Adults and children: One or two capsules during each meal and one capsule with snacks. The interindividual response to pancreatin supplements is variable and the number of capsules may need to be titrated to the individual based upon parameters of steatorrhoea and symptomatology. Further dose increases, if required, should be added slowly, with careful monitoring of response and symptomatology.

Where patients are already in receipt of lower unit dose enteric coated pancreatin supplements, then Pancrease HL Capsules may be substituted at one-third of the number of capsules of the previous preparation.

Where swallowing of capsules is difficult, then they may be opened and the minitablets taken with liquid or soft foods which do not require chewing. To protect the enteric coating, the minitablets should not be crushed or chewed.

It is important to ensure adequate hydration of patients at all times whilst dosing Pancrease HL Capsules.

Patients who are taking or have been given in excess of 10,000 units of lipase/kg/day are at risk of developing colon damage. The dose of Pancrease HL should usually not exceed this dose.

Contra-indications: Hypersensitivity to pork protein or any excipient.

Children aged 15 or under with cystic fibrosis.

Special warnings and special precautions for use: Contact of the minitablets with food having a pH higher than 5.5 can dissolve the protective coating and will reduce the efficacy of the product.

Interaction with other medicaments and other forms of interaction: None stated/

Pregnancy and lactation: The safety of Pancrease HL during pregnancy has not yet been established. Consequently, use of the product in pregnancy is therefore not recommended.

Effects on ability to drive and use machines: None stated.

Undesirable effects: The most frequently reported adverse reactions are gastrointestinal in nature such as abdominal discomfort, nausea and vomiting. Less frequently, allergic-type reactions of the skin have also been observed. Very high doses of exogenous pancreatic enzymes have been associated with hyperuricosuria and hyperuricaemia.

Stricture of the ileo-caecum and large bowel and colitis have been reported in children with cystic fibrosis taking Pancrease HL.

Abdominal symptoms (not usually experienced by the patient) or changes in abdominal symptoms should be reviewed to exclude the possibility of colonic damage, especially if the patient is taking in excess of 10,000 units of lipase/kg/day.

Overdose: Overdosage is unlikely and has not been experienced to date with Pancrease HL. Inappropriately large doses could result in symptoms such as abdominal discomfort, nausea, vomiting, perianal irritation or inflammation.

Pharmacological properties
Pharmacodynamic properties: The enzymes catalyse the hydrolysis of fats into glycerol and fatty acids, protein into proteoses and derived substances, and starch into dextrins and sugars.

Pharmacokinetic properties: Pancreatin is not systemically absorbed from the gastrointestinal tract.

Preclinical safety data: No relevant information additional to that contained elsewhere in the Summary of Product Characteristics.

Pharmaceutical particulars
List of excipients: Caster oil, hydrogenated NF; silicon dioxide, colloidal PhEur; magnesium stearate PhEur; sodium carboxymethylcellulose PhEur; cellulose microcrystalline PhEur.

Coat composition: Simethicone emulsion USP; methacryllic acid copolymer type C NF; talc PhEur; triethyl citrate NF; purified water PhEur.

Capsule composition (body and cap): Titanium dioxide PhEur; gelatin PhEur.

Ink composition: Shellac; industrial methylated spirits; purified water PhEur; soya lecithin (food grade); 2-ethoxyethanol; dimethylpolysiloxane; red iron oxide (E172).

Incompatibilities: None stated.

Shelf life: 2 years.

Special precautions for storage: Keep bottle tightly closed. Store at room temperature (10°C-25°C) in a dry place. Do not refrigerate.

Nature and contents of container: High density polyethylene bottles with a low density polyethylene snap top lid, containing 100 or 500 capsules.

Instructions for use/handling: Not applicable.

Marketing authorisation number 0242/0255

Date of approval/revision of SPC September 1997

Legal category POM.

PEVARYL* TOPICAL CREAM
PEVARYL* TOPICAL LOTION

Presentation *Cream:* A soft, white, water-miscible cream containing 1% w/w econazole nitrate.

Lotion: A milky white homogeneous lotion containing 1% econazole nitrate.

Uses For the treatment of fungal infections of the skin.

Dosage and administration *Cream:* Apply to the affected area 2 times daily and rub in gently. Continue the application until all skin lesions are healed.

In nail infections, apply once daily and cover with an occlusive dressing.

Lotion: As for Pevaryl Cream.

In order to prevent relapse, treatment should be continued for 2 weeks after clinical cure.

Contra-indications, warnings, etc
Contra-indications: Lotion and Cream: Care should be taken in the presence of eczematous dermatitis.

Side effects: Rarely, transient local mild irritation may occur immediately after application.

Precautions: Cream and Lotion: Hypersensitivity has rarely been recorded, if it should occur, administration of the product should be discontinued.

Incompatibilities: None known.

Overdosage: Pevaryl Topical Cream and Lotion are intended for topical application only. If accidental ingestion of large quantities of the product occurs, an appropriate method of gastric emptying may be used if considered desirable.

Use in pregnancy: Only small amounts of the drug are absorbed through the skin and no teratogenic effects have been observed in animals. Hence, the product may be used with caution during pregnancy.

Pharmaceutical precautions *Cream and Lotion:* None.

Legal category P.

Package quantities *Cream:* Each tube contains 30 g. *Lotion:* Each bottle contains 30 ml.

Further information Nil.

Product licence numbers
Cream 0242/0259
Lotion 0242/0260

PEVARYL* TC CREAM

Presentation Pevaryl TC cream is a soft white water-miscible cream containing 1% w/w Econazole nitrate and 0.1% w/w triamcinolone acetonide.

Uses For the topical treatment of inflammatory dermatomycoses and inflammatory skin conditions complicated by or threatened by bacterial or fungal skin infection.

Econazole nitrate is a broad spectrum antifungal agent with activity against many gram positive bacteria.

Triamcinolone acetonide is a potent corticosteroid with anti-inflammatory, antipruritic and antiallergic activity.

Dosage and administration The cream should be applied by gently rubbing into the skin with the finger twice daily for 14 days OR apply twice daily to the affected area OR as directed by your doctor.

Contra-indications, warnings, etc
Contra-indications: Like all preparations containing corticosteroids, Pevaryl TC cream should not be used on tubercular or luetic skin infections or in viral diseases (eg herpes, vaccinia, varicella). Pevaryl TC cream should not be administered to patients who have previously exhibited hypersensitivity to imidazoles or corticosteroids.

Long-term continuous steroid therapy should be avoided since adrenal suppression can occur, particularly when infants or children are treated or when occlusive dressings are applied. In addition, long term therapy with corticosteroids can cause skin lesions such as atrophy, telangiectasia and striae.

Pregnancy: Topical administration of corticosteroids to pregnant animals can cause foetal abnormalities. The relevance of this finding to human beings has not been established. However, topical steroids should not be used extensively in pregnancy, ie in large amounts or for prolonged periods.

Side effects: Transient local mild irritation at the application site has been reported. Hypersensitivity has rarely been reported. Discontinuation of therapy usually results in cessation of the symptoms.

Pharmaceutical precautions Store at room temperature (at or below 25°C).

Legal category POM.

Package quantities 15 g tube.

Further information Nil.

Product licence number 0242/0263.

PREPULSID* TABLETS

Presentation White, biconvex, scored tablets, engraved CIS/10 on one side and JANSSEN on the reverse. Each tablet contains cisapride monohydrate equivalent to 10 mg of cisapride. The tablets contain lactose.

Uses
Properties: Prepulsid is a gastrointestinal prokinetic agent which stimulates lower oesophageal, gastric, small intestinal and colonic motility.

Prepulsid probably acts by enhancing the release of acetylcholine at the level of the myenteric plexus in the gut wall, and therefore its effects on motility can largely be abolished by atropine. *In vitro* studies have shown that cisapride is a serotonin (5-HT_4) receptor agonist. The mechanism by which acetylcholine release is enhanced is unclear. There is no direct evidence of direct cholinergic effects.

Prepulsid has no effect on gastric secretion.

In patients with gastro-oesophageal reflux, Prepulsid increases the resting tone of the lower oesophageal sphincter, and increases the amplitude of lower oesophageal contractions. Prepulsid has also been shown, by using pH monitoring, to reduce the duration of reflux episodes.

In patients with dyspepsia, impaired gastric emptying and GORD, Prepulsid improves gastric emptying of liquid and solid meals, and shortens mouth to caecum transit time.

Prepulsid also stimulates colonic propulsive peristalsis and accelerates colonic transit.

Indications: Treatment of symptoms (eg heartburn, regurgitation) and mucosal lesions associated with gastro-oesophageal reflux. Prepulsid may also be used for the maintenance treatment of reflux oesophagitis.

The management of symptoms of dyspepsia (eg epigastric pain or burning, early satiety, bloating), where peptic ulcer or other lesions have been excluded from the diagnosis.

Relief of symptoms (eg nausea, early satiety, anorexia, bloating, epigastric pain) of impaired gastric motility secondary to disturbed and delayed gastric emptying associated with diabetes, systemic sclerosis and autonomic neuropathy.

Dosage and administration Prepulsid should preferably be taken 15-30 minutes before a meal in order to ensure maximum plasma levels immediately after food intake.

Adults and children aged 12 years and over
Dyspepsia: 10 mg Prepulsid three times daily. The usual course of treatment is 4 weeks.

Gastro-oesophageal reflux: 10 mg Prepulsid three times daily. Night time symptoms can be treated with an extra 10 mg dose at bedtime. Alternatively, 20 mg Prepulsid twice daily (before breakfast and at bedtime). Healing of oesophageal lesions has been reported following treatment with 10 mg qds or 20 mg bd. A 12 week course of treatment is recommended to give maximum benefit.

For maintenance treatment, 20 mg Prepulsid once daily (at bedtime) or 10 mg Prepulsid twice daily (before breakfast and at bedtime) is recommended. It may be necessary to increase this dose to 20 mg Prepulsid twice daily in patients whose lesions were initially very severe.

Impaired gastric motility: 10 mg Prepulsid three or four times daily. An initial course of 6 weeks is recommended, but longer periods of treatment may be required.

Use in children: Clinical experience with Prepulsid in children younger than 12 years is limited. Hence the drug can only be recommended for use in children aged 12 years and older.

Use in elderly: Repeated dosing in elderly patients with Prepulsid produced steady state plasma levels which were generally higher than those reported in younger patients, due to a moderate prolongation of the elimination half life. Therapeutic doses, however, are similar to those used in younger patients. Therefore it is recommended that when Prepulsid is used in elderly patients, a starting dose similar to that used in other adults is prescribed initially. This can then be adapted depending on the therapeutic effects or possible side effects of the treatment.

Abnormal renal or liver function: Because of the importance of the hepatic metabolism and renal excretion of Prepulsid, the dosage should initially be halved in patients with hepatic or renal insufficiency. Subsequently the dose can be adapted depending on individual clinical response.

Contra-indications, warnings etc
Contra-indications: Prepulsid is contra-indicated in pregnancy (see Use in pregnancy section) and in patients in whom gastrointestinal stimulation might be dangerous, eg gastrointestinal haemorrhage, mechanical obstruction or perforation.

Prepulsid is also contra-indicated in patients known to be hypersensitive to the product.

The concomitant oral or parenteral use of potent CYP3A4 inhibiting drugs including:

- azole antifungals;
- macrolide antibiotics such as erythromycin, clarithromycin, troleandomycin;
- HIV protease inhibitors such as ritonavir and indinavir.
- nefazodone;

Cisapride in contra-indicated in patients with the following risk factors for cardiac arrhythmia: patients with a personal or family history of QT-interval prolongation (such as congenital long QT syndrome, idiopathic QT-interval prolongation, QT-interval prolongation associated with diabetes mellitus), with a previous history of ventricular arrhythmia or torsades de pointes, combination with medicines known to prolong the QT-interval such as certain anti-malarials, antiarrhythmics, certain antihistamines, tricyclic antidepressants and certain antipsychotic medicines (see interactions).

Prepulsid should not be used in prematurely born infants (born at gestational age of less than 36 weeks) for up to 3 months after birth, due to the risk of QT-interval prolongation in this age group.

Warnings: Abnormal renal or liver function (see dosage section).

The recommended dose of Prepulsid should not be exceeded.

It is advisable to avoid the use of cisapride in patients with other risk factors for arrhythmia such as those who have clinically significant heart disease (second or third degree atrioventricular block, congestive heart failure, ischaemic heart disease), uncorrected electrolyte (potassium/magnesium) disturbances (such as seen in patients taking potassium-wasting diuretics or in association with the administration of insulin in acute settings), renal failure (particularly when on chronic dialysis), significant chronic obstructive pulmonary disease or respiratory failure.

Patients with, or suspected of having, the above risk factors should be evaluated prior to administration of cisapride and benefits should be weighed against potential risks. An ECG should be part of this evaluation to exclude a prolonged QT-interval.

Drug interactions: Since Prepulsid accelerates gastric emptying, the absorption from the stomach of concomitantly administered drugs may be diminished, whereas absorption of drugs from the small intestine may be accelerated. For drugs that require careful individual titration, such as anticonvulsants, it may be useful to measure their plasma concentration.

Prepulsid does not affect psychomotor performance nor does it induce sedation or drowsiness. However, the sedative effects of benzodiazepines and alcohol may be accelerated when administered concomitantly with Prepulsid.

The beneficial effects of Prepulsid on gastrointestinal motility are largely antagonised by anticholinergic drugs.

In patients receiving anticoagulants, the prothrombin time may be increased. It is advisable to check the prothrombin time within the first few days of initiating or discontinuing Prepulsid treatment, and to adapt the dose of anticoagulant if necessary.

The drug exhibits extensive binding to plasma proteins, mainly to albumin.

The main metabolic pathway of cisapride is through CYP3A4. The concomitant oral or parenteral use of drugs that significantly inhibit these enzymes may result in increased plasma levels of cisapride, and could increase the risk of QT-interval prolongation.

Therefore, the use of such drugs is contra-indicated. Examples include the following:

- azole antifungals;
- macrolide antibiotics such as erythromycin, clarithromycin or troleandomycin;
- HIV protease inhibitors, such as ritonavir and indinavir;
- nefazodone;

Cisapride may increase the rate of absorption of ethanol.

Drugs which prolong the QT-interval such as quinine, halofantrine, amiodarone, bretylium, disopyramide, procainamide, quinidine, sotalol, terfenadine, astemizole, thioridazine, pimozide, chlorpromazine, haloperidol, lithium, sertindole, amitriptyline and pentamidine are contra-indicated in patients receiving cisapride (see Contra-indications).

Cimetidine co-administration leads to an increased peak plasma concentration and AUC of cisapride. There is no effect on cisapride absorption when it is co-administered with ranitidine. The gastrointestinal absorption of cimetidine and ranitidine is accelerated when they are co-administered with cisapride. The level of change is unlikely to be clinically significant.

In a study of 12 subjects, it was shown that grapefruit juice may increase the oral bioavailability of cisapride with wide interindividual variation, ie change in C_{max} and AUC. The values in C_{max} and AUC in the presence of grapefruit juice were within the range expected in its absence.

Use in pregnancy: In animals Prepulsid has shown no teratogenic or primary foetotoxic effects. In a study of 129 women exposed to Prepulsid there was no increase in foetal abnormalities compared to matched controls. Cisapride should only be used during pregnancy when there is a clear therapeutic benefit in the knowledge that the risks, especially during the first trimester, have not been fully evaluated.

Use in lactation: Although the excretion of Prepulsid in human breast milk is minimal (milk to serum ratio of 0.045), it is not advisable to breast feed while taking Prepulsid.

Side effects: The most frequent side effects reported with Prepulsid are gastrointestinal: abdominal cramps, borborygmi and diarrhoea. They are mainly transient and rarely require discontinuation of treatment. Should severe abdominal cramps occur with single administrations of 20 mg Prepulsid, it is recommended that the dose per administration is halved and the frequency of dosing doubled so that the total daily dose is unaltered.

Less frequent side effects include headaches and lightheadedness. Cases of hypersensitivity including rash, pruritus and urticaria, and bronchospasm have occasionally been reported. Reports of convulsions, extrapyramidal effects and dose related increase in urinary frequency have been received.

Rare cases of cardiac arrhythmia, including ventricular tachycardia, ventricular fibrillation, torsades de pointes, and QT-interval prolongation have been reported. Most of these patients had been receiving multiple other medications and had pre-existing cardiac disease or risk factors for arrhythmias.

Exceptional cases of reversible liver function abnormalities, with or without cholestasis, have been reported. Hyperprolactinaemia which may cause gynaecomastia and galactorrhoea has also been reported, however, in large scale surveillance studies the incidence (<0.1%) has not exceeded that commonly reported in the general population.

Overdosage: The symptoms that occur most frequently after overdosing are abdominal cramping and increased stool frequency. Rare cases of QT-interval prolongation and ventricular arrhythmia have been reported. In infants (<1 year of age), mild sedation, apathy and atony were also observed.

In case of overdosage, the administration of activated charcoal and close observation of the patient are recommended. It is also recommended that patients are evaluated for possible QT-interval prolongation and for factors such as electrolyte disturbances (especially hypokalaemia or hypomagnesaemia) and bradycardia that can predispose to the occurrence of torsades de pointes.

Pharmaceutical precautions Store at room temperature in a dry place and protect from light.

Legal category POM.

Package quantities 10 mg tablets: packs of 120 tablets.

Further information Prepulsid is rapidly absorbed, with peak plasma levels 1 to 2 hours after dosing, and an elimination half-life of approximately 10 hours.

It undergoes extensive first-pass metabolism in the liver and gut wall, with the main metabolic pathways being oxidative N-dealkylation and aromatic hydroxylation. Excretion is mainly as metabolites (90%) with approximately equal amounts in both urine and faeces.

Product licence number 0242/0136

PREPULSID* SUSPENSION

Qualitative and quantitative composition Cisapride monohydrate equivalent to cisapride 1 mg/ml.

Pharmaceutical form White, oral suspension.

Clinical particulars
Therapeutic indications: Treatment of symptoms and mucosal lesions associated with gastro-oesophageal reflux. Prepulsid may also be used for the maintenance treatment of reflux oesophagitis.

Relief of symptoms of impaired gastric motility secondary to disturbed and delayed gastric emptying associated with diabetes, systemic sclerosis and autonomic neuropathy.

The management of symptoms of dyspepsia where peptic ulcer or other lesions have been excluded from the diagnosis.

Posology and method of administration: For oral administration.

Prepulsid should preferably be taken 15-30 minutes before a meal in order to ensure maximum plasma levels immediately after food intake. When an additional dose is required to control night time symptoms, the suspension should be taken at bedtime.

Adults and children aged 12 years and over:
Gastro-oesophageal reflux: 10 mg Prepulsid three or four times daily, depending upon the symptoms being treated and the clinical response. Alternatively, 20 mg twice daily (before breakfast and at bedtime). Healing of oesophageal lesions has been reported following treatment with 10 mg qds or 20 mg bd for 12 weeks. A 12 week course of treatment is recommended to obtain maximum benefit.

For maintenance treatment, 10 mg Prepulsid twice daily (before breakfast and at bedtime) or 20 mg Prepulsid once daily (at bedtime) is recommended. It may be necessary to increase this dose to 20 mg Prepulsid twice daily in patients whose lesions were initially very severe.

Impaired gastric motility: 10 mg Prepulsid three or four times daily. An initial course of 6 weeks is recommended, but longer periods of treatment may be required.

Dyspepsia: 10 mg Prepulsid three times daily. The usual course of treatment is 4 weeks.

Use in children: Clinical experience with Prepulsid in children younger than 12 years is limited. Hence the drug can only be recommended for use in children aged 12 years and older.

Use in elderly: Repeated dosing in elderly patients with Prepulsid produced steady state plasma levels, which were generally higher than those reported in younger patients, due to a moderate prolongation of the elimination half life. Therapeutic doses, however, are similar to those used in younger patients. Therefore it is recommended that when Prepulsid is used in elderly patients, a starting dose similar to that used in other adults is prescribed initially. This can then be adapted depending on the therapeutic effects or possible side effects of the treatment.

Abnormal renal or liver function: Because of the importance of the hepatic metabolism and renal excretion of Prepulsid, the dosage should initially be halved in patients with hepatic or renal insufficiency. Subsequently the dose can be adapted depending on individual clinical response.

Contra-indications: Prepulsid is contra-indicated in patients in whom gastrointestinal stimulation might be dangerous, eg gastrointestinal haemorrhage, mechanical obstruction or perforation. Prepulsid is also contra-indicated in patients known to be hypersensitive to the product.

The concomitant oral or parenteral use of potent CYP3A4 inhibiting drugs including:

- azole antifungals;
- macrolide antibiotics such as erythromycin, clarithromycin, troleandomycin;
- HIV protease inhibitors such as ritonavir and indinavir;
- nefazodone;

Cisapride is contra-indicated in patients with the following risk factors for cardiac arrhythmia: patients with a personal or family history of QT-interval prolongation (such as congenital long QT syndrome, idiopathic QT-interval prolongation, QT-interval prolongation associated with diabetes mellitus), with a previous history of ventricular arrhythmia or torsades de pointes, combination with medicines known to prolong the QT-interval such as certain anti-malarials, antiarrhythmics, certain antihistamines, tricyclic antidepressants and certain antipsychotic medicines (see Interactions).

Prepulsid should not be used in prematurely born infants (born at a gestational age of less than 36 weeks) for up to 3 months after birth, due to the risk of QT-interval prolongation in this age group.

Special warnings and special precautions for use: For use in renal and liver disease, see under Dosage.

The recommended dose of Prepulsid should not be exceeded.

It is advisable to avoid the use of cisapride in patients with other risk factors for arrhythmia such as those who have clinically significant heart disease (second or third degree atrioventricular block, congestive cardiac failure, ischaemic heart disease), uncorrected electrolyte (potassium/magnesium) disturbances (such as seen in patients taking potassium-wasting diuretics or in association with the administration of insulin in acute settings), renal failure (particularly when on chronic dialysis), significant chronic obstructive pulmonary disease or respiratory failure.

Patients with, or suspected of having, the above risk factors should be carefully evaluated prior to administration of cisapride and benefits should be weighed against potential risks. An ECG should be part of this evaluation to exclude a prolonged QT-interval.

Interaction with other medicaments and other forms of interaction: Since Prepulsid accelerates gastric emptying, the absorption from the stomach of concomitantly administered drugs may be diminished, whereas absorption of drugs from the small intestine may be accelerated.

Prepulsid does not affect psychomotor performance nor does it induce sedation or drowsiness when administered alone. However, the sedative effects of benzodiazepines and alcohol may be enhanced when administered concomitantly with Prepulsid.

The beneficial effects of Prepulsid on gastrointestinal motility are largely antagonised by anticholinergic drugs.

In patients receiving anticoagulants, the prothrombin time may be increased. It is advisable to check the prothrombin time within the first few days of initiating or discontinuing Prepulsid treatment, and to adapt the dose of anticoagulant if necessary.

For drugs that require careful individual titration, such as anticonvulsants, it may be useful to monitor their plasma concentrations.

The main metabolic pathway of cisapride is through CYP3A4. The concomitant oral or parenteral use of drugs that significantly inhibit these enzymes may result in increased plasma levels of cisapride, and could increase the risk of QT-interval prolongation. Therefore, the use of such drugs is contra-indicated. Examples include the following:

- azole antifungals;
- macrolide antibiotics such as erythromycin, clarithromycin or troleandomycin;
- HIV protease inhibitors, such as ritonavir and indinavir;
- nefazodone;

Cisapride may increase the rate of absorption of ethanol.

Drugs which prolong the QT-interval such as quinine, halofantrine, amiodarone, bretylium, disopyramide, procainamide, quinidine, sotalol, terfenadine, astemizole, thioridazine, pimozide, chlorpromazine, haloperidol, lithium, sertindole, amitriptyline and pentamidine are contra-indicated in patients receiving cisapride (see Contra-indications).

Cimetidine co-administration leads to an increased peak plasma concentration and AUC of cisapride. There is no effect on cisapride absorption when it is co-administered with ranitidine. The gastrointestinal absorption of cimetidine and ranitidine is accelerated when they are co-administered with cisapride. The level of change is unlikely to be clinically significant.

In a study of 12 subjects, it was shown that grapefruit juice may increase the oral bioavailability of cisapride with wide interindividual variation ie change in C_{max} and AUC. The values in C_{max} and AUC in the presence of grapefruit juice were within the range expected in its absence.

Pregnancy and lactation: In animals, Prepulsid has shown no teratogenic or primary foetotoxic effects. In a study of 129 women exposed to Prepulsid there was no increase in foetal abnormalities compared to matched controls. Cisapride should only be used during pregnancy when there is a clear therapeutic benefit in the knowledge that the risks, especially during the first trimester, have not been fully evaluated.

Use in lactation: although the excretion of Prepulsid in human breast milk is minimal (milk to serum ratio of 0.045), it is not advisable to breast feed while taking Prepulsid

Effects on ability to drive and use machines: None stated.

Undesirable effects: The most frequent side effects reported with Prepulsid are gastrointestinal: abdominal cramps, borborygmi and diarrhoea. They are mainly transient and rarely require discontinuation of treatment. Should severe abdominal cramps occur with single administrations of 20 mg Prepulsid, it is recommended that the dose per administration is halved and the frequency of dosing doubled so that the total daily dose is unaltered.

Less frequent side effects include headaches and lightheadedness. Cases of hypersensitivity including rash, pruritus and urticaria, and bronchospasm have occasionally been reported. Reports of convulsions, extrapyramidal effects and dose related increase in urinary frequency have been received. Rare cases of cardiac arrhythmia, including ventricular tachycardia, ventricular fibrillation, torsades de pointes, and QT-interval prolongation have been reported. Most of these patients had been receiving multiple other medications and had pre-existing cardiac disease or risk factors for arrhythmias. Exceptional cases of reversible liver function abnormalities, with or without cholestasis have been reported. Hyperprolactinaemia which may cause gynaecomastia and galactorrhoea has also been reported, however, in large scale surveillance studies the incidence (<0.1%) has not exceeded that commonly reported in the general population.

Overdose: The symptoms that occur most frequently after overdosing are abdominal cramps and increased stool frequency. Rare cases of QT-interval prolongation and ventricular arrhythmia have been reported. In infants (<1 year of age), mild sedation, apathy and atony were also observed.

In case of overdosage, the administration of activated charcoal and close observation of the patient are recommended. It is also recommended that patients are evaluated for possible QT-interval prolongation and for factors such as electrolyte disturbances (especially hypokalaemia or hypomagnesaemia) and bradycardia that can predispose to the occurrence of torsades de pointes.

Pharmacological properties

Pharmacodynamic properties: Prepulsid, which stimulates lower oesophageal, gastric antral, small intestinal and colonic motility, is a gastrointestinal prokinetic agent.

Prepulsid probably acts by enhancing the release of acetylcholine at the level of the myenteric plexus in the gut wall, and therefore its effects on motility can largely be abolished by atropine. *In vitro* studies have shown that cisapride is a serotonin (5-HT_4) receptor agonist. It is devoid of direct cholinergic effects, and has no effect on gastric secretion. In patients with gastro-oesophageal reflux, Prepulsid increases the resting tone of the lower oesophageal sphincter and increases the amplitude of lower oesophageal contractions. Using pH monitoring, Prepulsid has also been shown to reduce the duration of reflux episodes.

Prepulsid increases antral and duodenal motility, accelerates gastric emptying of liquid and solid meals, and shortens mouth to caecum transit time. It stimulates colonic propulsive peristalsis and accelerates colonic transit.

Pharmacokinetic properties: Prepulsid is rapidly absorbed in man with peak plasma levels 1 to 2 hours after dosing, and an elimination half-life of approximately 10 hours. It undergoes extensive first pass metabolism in the liver and gut wall, with the main metabolic pathways being oxidative N-dealkylation and aromatic hydroxylation. Excretion is mainly as metabolites (90%) with approximately equal amounts in both urine and faeces. Prepulsid is highly plasma bound, mainly to albumin.

Preclinical safety data: Not applicable.

Pharmaceutical particulars

List of excipients: Sucrose; microcrystalline carboxymethyl cellulose and sodium carboxymethyl cellulose; hypromellose; polysorbate 20; sodium chloride; methyl parahydroxybenzoate; propyl parahydroxybenzoate; cherry cream flavour; purified water.

Incompatibilities: None stated.

Shelf life: 60 months.

Special precautions for storage: Store at room temperature (below 25°C).

Nature and contents of container: 500 ml amber glass bottle with

- white, polypropylene, child-resistant screw cap with LDPE insert, or
- black bakelite screw-cap with a glued cardboard layer coated with PVC.

The product is provided with a polypropylene measuring cup.

Instructions for use/handling: None stated.

Marketing authorisation number 0242/0157

Date of approval/revision of SPC September 1998

Legal category POM.

PREPULSID* QUICKLET TABLETS

Qualitative and quantitative composition Fast dissolving tablets. *Prepulsid Quicklet Tablets 10 mg:* Cisapride monohydrate equivalent to 10 mg cisapride per tablet. *Prepulsid Quicklet Tablets 20 mg:* Cisapride monohydrate equivalent to 20 mg cisapride per tablet.

Pharmaceutical form Oral lyophilisate.

Clinical particulars

Therapeutic indications: Treatment of symptoms (eg heartburn, regurgitation) and mucosal lesions associated with gastro-oesophageal reflux. Prepulsid may also be used for the maintenance treatment of reflux oesophagitis.

Relief of symptoms (eg nausea, early satiety, anorexia, bloating, epigastric pain) of impaired gastric motility secondary to disturbed and delayed gastric emptying associated with diabetes, systemic sclerosis and autonomic neuropathy.

The symptoms of dyspepsia where peptic ulcer or other lesions have been excluded from the diagnosis.

Posology and method of administration: Prepulsid Quicklet is put on the tongue. It disintegrates within seconds on the surface and can be swallowed with saliva. No fluid intake is needed.

Prepulsid should preferably be taken 15-30 minutes before a meal in order to ensure maximum plasma levels immediately after food intake. When an additional dose is required to control nighttime symptoms, the tablets should be taken at bedtime.

Adults and children aged 12 years and over:

Gastro-oesophageal reflux: 10 mg Prepulsid three or four times daily, depending upon the symptoms being treated and the clinical response. Alternatively, 20 mg twice daily (before breakfast and at bedtime). Healing of oesophageal lesions has been reported following treatment with 10 mg qds or 20 mg bd for 12 weeks. A 12 week course of treatment is recommended to obtain maximum benefit.

For maintenance treatment, 10 mg Prepulsid twice daily (before breakfast and at bedtime) or 20 mg Prepulsid once daily (at bedtime) is recommended. It may be necessary to increase this dose to 20 mg Prepulsid twice daily in patients whose lesions were initially very severe.

Impaired gastric motility: 10 mg Prepulsid three or four times daily. An initial course of 6 weeks is recommended, but longer periods of treatment may be required.

Dyspepsia: 10 mg Prepulsid three times daily. The usual course of treatment is 4 weeks.

Use in children: Clinical experience with Prepulsid in children younger than 12 years is limited. Hence the drug can only be recommended for use in children aged 12 years and older.

Use in elderly: Repeated dosing in elderly patients with Prepulsid produced steady state plasma levels, which were generally higher than those reported in younger patients, due to a moderate prolongation of the elimination half life. Therapeutic doses, however, are similar to those used in younger patients. Therefore it is recommended that when Prepulsid is used in elderly patients, a starting dose similar to that used in other adults is prescribed initially. This can then be adapted depending on the therapeutic effects or possible side effects of the treatment.

Abnormal renal or liver function: Because of the importance of the hepatic metabolism and renal excretion of Prepulsid, the dosage should initially be halved in patients with hepatic or renal insufficiency. Subsequently the dose can be adapted depending on individual clinical response.

Method of administration: Oral use.

Contra-indications: Prepulsid is contra-indicated in patients in whom gastrointestinal stimulation might be dangerous, eg gastrointestinal haemorrhage, mechanical obstruction or perforation. Prepulsid is also contra-indicated in patients known to be hypersensitive to the product.

The concomitant oral or parenteral use of potent CYP3A4 inhibiting drugs including:

- azole antifungals;
- macrolide antibiotics such as erythromycin, clarithromycin, troleandomycin;
- HIV protease inhibitors such as ritonavir and indinavir;
- nefazodone;

Cisapride is contra-indicated in patients with the following risk factors for cardiac arrhythmia: patients with a personal or family history of QT-interval prolongation (such as congenital long QT syndrome, idiopathic QT-interval prolongation, QT-interval prolongation associated with diabetes mellitus), with a previous history of ventricular arrhythmia or torsades de pointes, combination with medicines known to prolong the QT-interval such as certain anti-malarials, antiarrhythmics, certain antihistamines, tricyclic antidepressants and certain antipsychotic medicines (see Interactions).

Prepulsid should not be used in prematurely born infants (born at a gestational age of less than 36 weeks) for up to 3 months after birth, due to the risk of QT-interval prolongation in this age group.

Special warnings and special precautions for use: For use in renal and liver disease, see under Dosage.

The recommended dose of Prepulsid should not be exceeded.

It is advisable to avoid the use of cisapride in patients with other risk factors for arrhythmia such as those who have clinically significant heart disease (second or third degree atrioventricular block, congestive cardiac failure, ischaemic heart disease), uncorrected electrolyte (potassium/magnesium) disturbances (such as seen in patients taking potassium-wasting diuretics or in association with the administration of insulin in acute settings), renal failure (particularly when on chronic dialysis), significant chronic obstructive pulmonary disease or respiratory failure.

Patients with, or suspected of having, the above risk factors should be carefully evaluated prior to administration of cisapride and benefits should be weighed against potential risks. An ECG should be part of this evaluation to exclude a prolonged QT-interval.

Prepulsid Quicklet contains aspartame and therefore care should be taken in phenylketonuria.

Interaction with other medicaments and other forms of interaction: Since Prepulsid accelerates gastric emptying, the absorption from the stomach of concomitantly administered drugs may be diminished, whereas absorption of drugs from the small intestine may be accelerated.

Prepulsid does not affect psychomotor performance nor does it induce sedation or drowsiness when administered alone. However, the sedative effects of benzodiazepines and alcohol may be enhanced when administered concomitantly with Prepulsid.

The beneficial effects of Prepulsid on gastrointestinal motility are largely antagonised by anticholinergic drugs.

In patients receiving anticoagulants, the prothrombin time may be increased. It is advisable to check the prothrombin time within the first few days of initiating or discontinuing Prepulsid treatment, and to adapt the dose of anticoagulant if necessary.

For drugs that require careful individual titration, such as anticonvulsants, it may be useful to monitor their plasma concentrations.

The main metabolic pathway of cisapride is through CYP3A4. The concomitant oral or parenteral use of drugs that significantly inhibit these enzymes may result in increased plasma levels of cisapride, and could increase the risk of QT-interval prolongation. Therefore, the use of such drugs is contra-indicated. Examples include the following:

- azole antifungals;
- macrolide antibiotics such as erythromycin, clarithromycin or troleandomycin;
- HIV protease inhibitors, such as ritonavir and indinavir;
- nefazodone;

Cisapride may increase the rate of absorption of ethanol.

Drugs which prolong the QT-interval such as quinine, halofantrine, amiodarone, bretylium, disopyramide, procainamide, quinidine, sotalol, terfenadine, astemizole, thioridazine, pimozide, chlorpromazine, haloperidol, lithium, sertindole, amitriptyline and pentamidine are contra-indicated in patients receiving cisapride (see Contra-indications).

Cimetidine co-administration leads to an increased peak plasma concentration and AUC of cisapride. There is no effect on cisapride absorption when it is co-administered with ranitidine. The gastrointestinal absorption of cimetidine and ranitidine is accelerated when they are co-administered with cisapride. The level of change is unlikely to be clinically significant.

In a study of 12 subjects, it was shown that grapefruit juice may increase the oral bioavailability of cisapride with wide interindividual variation ie change in C_{max} and AUC. The values in C_{max} and AUC in the presence of grapefruit juice were within the range expected in its absence.

Pregnancy and lactation: In animals, Prepulsid has shown no teratogenic or primary foetotoxic effects. In a study of 129 women exposed to Prepulsid there was no increase in foetal abnormalities compared to matched controls. Cisapride should only be used during pregnancy when there is a clear therapeutic benefit in the knowledge that the risks, especially during the first trimester, have not been fully evaluated.

Use in lactation: although the excretion of Prepulsid in human breast milk is minimal (milk to serum ratio of 0.045), it is not advisable to breast feed while taking Prepulsid.

Effects on ability to drive and use machines: None stated.

Undesirable effects: The most frequent side effects reported with Prepulsid are gastrointestinal: abdominal cramps, borborygmi and diarrhoea. They are mainly transient and rarely require discontinuation of treatment. Should severe abdominal cramps occur with single administrations of 20 mg Prepulsid, it is recommended that the dose per administration is halved and the frequency of dosing doubled so that the total daily dose is unaltered.

Less frequent side effects include headaches and lightheadedness. Cases of hypersensitivity including rash, pruritus and urticaria, and bronchospasm have occasionally been reported. Reports of convulsions, extrapyramidal effects and dose related increase in urinary frequency have been received. Rare cases of cardiac arrhythmia, including ventricular tachycardia, ventricular fibrillation, torsades de pointes, and QT-interval prolongation have been reported. Most of these patients had been receiving multiple other medications and had pre-existing cardiac disease or risk factors for arrhythmias. Exceptional cases of reversible liver function abnormalities, with or without cholestasis have been reported. Hyperprolactinaemia which may cause gynaecomastia and galactorrhoea has also been reported, however, in large scale surveillance studies the incidence (<0.1%) has not exceeded that commonly reported in the general population.

Overdose: The symptoms that occur most frequently after overdosing are abdominal cramps and increased stool frequency. Rare cases of QT-interval prolongation and ventricular arrhythmia have been reported. In infants (<1 year of age), mild sedation, apathy and atony were also observed.

In case of overdosage, the administration of activated charcoal and close observation of the patient are recommended. It is also recommended that patients are evaluated for possible QT-interval prolongation and for factors such as electrolyte disturbances (especially hypokalaemia or hypomagnesaemia) and bradycardia that can predispose to the occurrence of torsades de pointes.

Pharmacological properties

Pharmacodynamic properties: Prepulsid, which stimulates lower oesophageal, gastric antral, small intestinal and colonic motility, is a gastrointestinal prokinetic agent.

Prepulsid probably acts by enhancing the release of acetylcholine at the level of the myenteric plexus in the gut wall, and therefore its effects on motility can largely be abolished by atropine. *In vitro* studies have shown that cisapride is a serotonin (5-HT_4) receptor agonist. It is devoid of direct cholinergic effects, and has no effect on gastric secretion. In patients with gastro-oesophageal reflux, Prepulsid increases the resting tone of the lower oesophageal sphincter and increases the amplitude of lower oesophageal contractions. Using pH monitoring, Prepulsid has also been shown to reduce the duration of reflux episodes.

Prepulsid increases antral and duodenal motility, accelerates gastric emptying of liquid and solid meals, and shortens mouth to caecum transit time. It stimulates colonic propulsive peristalsis and accelerates colonic transit.

Pharmacokinetic properties: Prepulsid is rapidly absorbed in man with peak plasma levels 1 to 2 hours after dosing, and an elimination half-life of approximately 10 hours. It undergoes extensive first pass metabolism in the liver and gut wall, with the main metabolic pathways being oxidative N-dealkylation and aromatic hydroxylation. Excretion is mainly as metabolites (90%) with approximately equal amounts in both urine and faeces. Prepulsid is highly plasma bound, mainly to albumin.

Preclinical safety data: Not applicable.

Pharmaceutical particulars

List of excipients: Carbomer 934P; sodium hydroxide; mannitol; aspartame; glycine; simethicone; sodium calcium EDTA; xanthan gum; gelatin; peppermint oil; spearmint flavour; indigotin disulphonate (E132)–aluminium lake.

Incompatibilities: None.

Shelf life: 24 months.

Special precautions for storage: Protect from light. Store at room temperature (below 25°C) in a dry place.

Nature and contents of container: Packs contain 56 tablets in Aclar/aluminium foil blisters.

Instructions for use/handling: Since the fast dissolving tablets are fragile, they are not to be pushed through the blister as this would damage them.

To take the tablets out of the blister:

Pull up the edge of the foil and peel foil completely off.

Push up tablet.

Remove tablet.

Marketing authorisation numbers

Prepulsid Quicklet Tablets 10 mg	0242/0330
Prepulsid Quicklet Tablets 20 mg	0242/0331

Date of approval/revision of SPC September 1998

Legal category POM.

RAPIFEN*

Presentation Clear, colourless, preservative-free, aqueous injection presented in 2 ml and 10 ml ampoules. Each millilitre contains 500 micrograms of alfentanil as the hydrochloride. Rapifen also contains sodium chloride and water for injection.

Uses Rapifen is a potent, opioid analgesic with a very rapid and short-lived action. This makes it especially suitable for use as an adjunct to anaesthesia in short operative procedures and out-patient surgery, requiring spontaneous respiration.

Rapifen may also be administered to ventilated patients undergoing longer operative procedures, either as a bolus followed by iv. increments or infusion, or as an iv. infusion throughout.

Dosage Rapifen by the intravenous route can be administered to both adults and children. The dosage of Rapifen should be individualised according to age, bodyweight, physical status, underlying pathological condition, use of other drugs and type of surgery and anaesthesia. The usual recommended dosage regimen is as follows:

	Initial	*Supplemental*
Adults		
Spontaneous respiration	up to 500 mcg	250 mcg
Assisted ventilation	30-50 mcg/kg	15 mcg/kg
Children		
Assisted ventilation	30-50 mcg/kg	15 mcg/kg

In spontaneously breathing patients, the initial bolus dose should be given slowly over about 30 seconds (dilution may be helpful).

Use in children: Children may require higher or more frequent dosing owing to a shorter half life of Rapifen in this age group.

Use in elderly: and debilitated patients: Lower or less frequent dosing may be required owing to a longer half life (dilution may be helpful).

After intravenous administration in unpremedicated adult patients, 1 ml Rapifen may be expected to have a peak effect in 90 seconds and to provide analgesia for 5-10 minutes. Periods of more painful stimuli may be overcome by the use of small increments of Rapifen. For procedures of longer duration additional increments will be required.

In ventilated patients undergoing longer procedures, Rapifen may be infused at a rate of 0.5-1 microgram/kg/minute. Adequate plasma concentrations of alfentanil will only be achieved rapidly if this infusion is preceded by a loading dose of 50-100 micrograms/kg given as a bolus or fast infusion over 10 minutes. Even lower doses may be adequate, for example, in geriatric patients or where anaesthesia is being supplemented by other agents. The infusion should be discontinued up to 30 minutes before the anticipated end of surgery. Increasing the infusion rate may prolong recovery. Therefore supplementation of the anaesthetic if required is best managed by extra bolus doses of Rapifen (1-2 ml) or low concentrations of a volatile agent for brief periods. In ventilated patients, the last bolus dose should not be given later than about 10 minutes before the end of surgery to avoid the continuation of respiratory depression after surgery is complete.

Also see precautions and drug interactions.

Contra-indications, warnings, etc

Contra-indications: Obstructive airways disease or respiratory depression if not ventilating.

Concurrent administration with monoamine oxidase inhibitors or within 2 weeks of their discontinuation.

Administration in labour or before clamping of the cord during Caesarean section due to the possibility of respiratory depression in the new-born infant.

Patients with a known intolerance to alfentanil or other morphinomimetics.

Warnings: Following administration of Rapifen, a transient fall in blood pressure may occur. The magnitude of this effect may be exaggerated in the hypovolaemic patient or in the presence of concomitant sedative medication. Appropriate measures to maintain a stable arterial pressure should be taken.

Significant respiratory depression will occur following administration of Rapifen in doses in excess of 1 mg. This and the other pharmacological effects of Rapifen are usually of short duration and can be reversed by specific opioid antagonists (eg naloxone). Additional doses of the antagonists may be necessary because the respiratory depression may last longer than the duration of action of the opioid antagonist.

Like other opioids, alfentanil may cause bradycardia, an effect that may be marked and rapid in onset but which can be antagonised by atropine. Particular care must be taken following treatment with drugs which may depress the heart or increase vagal tone, such as anaesthetic agents or beta-blockers since they may predispose to bradycardia or hypotension. Heart rate and blood pressure should therefore be monitored carefully. If hypotension or bradycardia occur, appropriate measures should be instituted.

Asystole following bradycardia has been reported on very rare occasions in non-atropinised patients. Therefore it is advisable to be prepared to administer an anticholinergic drug.

Precautions: It is wise to reduce the dosage in the elderly and debilitated patients. In hypothyroidism, pulmonary disease, decreased respiratory reserve, alcoholism and liver or renal impairment the dosage should be titrated with care and prolonged monitoring may be required.

Patients on chronic opioid therapy or with a history of opioid abuse may require higher doses.

Rapifen may induce muscle rigidity during induction. Rigidity, which may also involve the thoracic muscles, can be avoided by the following measures:

- slow iv. injection (usually sufficient for lower doses);
- premedication with a benzodiazepine;
- administration of a muscle relaxant just prior to administration of Rapifen;

As with all potent opioids, profound analgesia is accompanied by marked respiratory depression, which may persist into or recur in the early postoperative period. Care should be taken after infusions or large doses of alfentanil to ensure that adequate spontaneous breathing has been established and maintained in the absence of stimulation before discharging the patient from the recovery area. Resuscitation equipment and narcotic antagonists should be readily available. Hyperventilation during anaesthesia may alter the patient's response to CO_2, thus affecting respiration postoperatively.

The use of rapid bolus injections of opioids should be avoided in patients with compromised intracerebral compliance; in such patients a transient decrease in the mean arterial pressure has occasionally been accompanied by a transient reduction of the cerebral perfusion pressure.

Drug interactions: Alfentanil is metabolised mainly via the human cytochrome P450 3A4 enzyme. Available human pharmacokinetic data indicate that the metabolism of alfentanil may be inhibited by fluconazole, erythromycin, diltiazem and cimetidine (known cytochrome P450 3A4 enzyme inhibitors). *In vitro* data suggest that other potent cytochrome P450 3A4 enzyme inhibitors (e.g. ketoconazole, itraconazole, ritonavir) may also inhibit the metabolism of alfentanil. This could increase the risk of prolonged or delayed respiratory depression. The concomitant use of such drugs requires special patient care and observation; in particular, it may be necessary to lower the dose of Rapifen.

Treatment with drugs which may depress the heart or increase vagal tone, such as beta-blockers and anaesthetic agents, may predispose to bradycardia or hypotension. Bradycardia and possibly asystole can occur when Rapifen is combined with non-vagolytic muscle relaxants.

The use of opioid premedication, barbiturates, benzodiazepines, neuroleptics, halogenic gases and other non-selective CNS depressants may enhance or prolong the respiratory depressant effects of alfentanil.

If other narcotic or CNS depressant drugs are used concurrently with alfentanil, the effects of the drugs can be expected to be additive. When patients have received such drugs the dose of alfentanil required will be less than usual. Likewise, following the administration of alfentanil, the dose of other CNS-depressant drugs should be reduced.

Effects on driving ability and operation of machinery: Where early discharge is envisaged patients, should be advised not to drive or operate machinery for 24 hours following administration.

Side effects: The most common adverse reactions reported with alfentanil are respiratory depression, apnoea and bradycardia.

Nausea and vomiting and dizziness have been reported.

In patients receiving doses of Rapifen large enough to require assisted ventilation, myoclonic movements and muscle rigidity (possibly involving the thoracic muscles) have rarely been reported shortly after the administration of Rapifen.

Other reported adverse reactions are laryngospasm, slight transient hypotension, allergic reactions (such as anaphylaxis, bronchospasm and urticaria), asystole and arrhythmias.

Use in pregnancy and lactation: Safety in human pregnancy has not been established although studies in animals have not demonstrated teratogenic or acute embryotoxic effects. As with other drugs, risk should be weighed against potential benefit to the patient.

Limited data suggest that alfentanil may appear in breast milk. It is therefore recommended that breast feeding is not initiated within 24 hours of treatment.

Overdosage: The manifestations of alfentanil overdose are generally an extension of its pharmacological action, which include the following:-

Action:

Bradycardia: Anticholinergics such as atropine or glycopyrrolate;

Hypoventilation or apnoea: O_2 administration, assisted or controlled respiration and an opioid antagonist may be required;

Muscle rigidity: Intravenous neuromuscular blocking agent may be given.

A specific opioid antagonist (eg naloxone) should

be available to treat respiratory depression. If hypotension is severe or persists, the possibility of hypovolaemia should be considered and controlled with appropriate parenteral fluid administration.

The suggested treatments given above do not preclude the use of other clinically indicated countermeasures.

Body temperature and adequate fluid intake should be maintained and the patient observed for 24 hours.

Pharmaceutical precautions If desired, Rapifen can be mixed with Sodium Chloride Injection BP, Dextrose Injection BP or Compound Sodium Lactate Injection BP (Hartmann's Solution). Such dilutions are compatible with plastic bags and giving sets. These dilutions should be used within 24 hours of preparation.

Rapifen should be stored at or below 25°C.

Legal category CD (Sch 2), POM.

Package quantities Rapifen is supplied in 2 ml ampoules (0.5 mg/ml) in packs of 10 and in 10 ml ampoules (0.5 mg/ml) in packs of 10.

Further information The analgesic potency of Rapifen is one quarter that of fentanyl. The duration of action of Rapifen is one third that of an equianalgesic dose of fentanyl and is clearly dose-related. Its depressant effects on respiratory rate and alveolar ventilation are also of shorter duration than those of fentanyl.

The onset of action of Rapifen is four times more rapid than that of an equianalgesic dose of fentanyl. The peak analgesic and respiratory depressant effects occur within 90 seconds.

Product licence number 0242/0091.

RAPIFEN* INTENSIVE CARE

Presentation Clear, colourless, preservative-free, aqueous injection presented in 1 ml ampoules. Each millilitre contains 5 mg of alfentanil as the hydrochloride. Rapifen Intensive Care also contains sodium chloride and water for injection.

Uses Rapifen Intensive Care is a potent, opioid analgesic with a very rapid onset of action. It is indicated for analgesia and suppression of respiratory activity and to provide analgesic cover for painful manoeuvres in mechanically ventilated patients on intensive care. It will aid compliance with mechanical ventilation, and tolerance of the endotracheal tube. Intravenous bolus doses of Rapifen (0.5 mg/ml) may be used to provide additional pain relief during brief painful procedures in intensive care such as physiotherapy, endotracheal suction etc.

Patients may appear to be awake in the presence of adequate analgesia. At the proposed doses, Rapifen Intensive Care has no sedative activity. Therefore supplementation with an appropriate hypnotic or sedative agent is recommended. As alfentanil and the sedative drug need to be titrated separately admixture of the two drugs is not recommended.

Alfentanil given by infusion should only be used in areas where facilities are available to deal with respiratory depression and where continuous monitoring is performed. Alfentanil should only be prescribed by physicians familiar with the use of potent opioids when given by continuous iv infusion.

Dosage and administration Once the patient has been intubated, mechanical ventilation can be initiated using the following dosage regimes:

The recommended initial infusion rate for mechanically ventilated adult patients is 2 mg per hour (equivalent to 0.4 mls per hour of undiluted Rapifen Intensive Care). The product should be diluted using the standard infusion solutions. For a 70 kg patient, this corresponds to approximately 30 micrograms/kg/hour. More rapid control may initially be gained by using a loading dose. For example, a dose of 5 mg may be given in divided doses over a period of 10 minutes, during which time careful monitoring of blood pressure and heart rate should be performed. If hypotension or bradycardia occur, the rate of administration should be reduced accordingly and other appropriate measures instituted.

The dose to produce the desired effects should then be individually determined and reassessed regularly to ensure that the optimum dose is being used. In clinical trials, patient requirements have generally been met with doses of 0.5 to 10 mg alfentanil per hour.

Additional bolus doses of 0.5–1.0 mg alfentanil may be given to provide analgesia during short painful procedures.

Elderly and debilitated patients may require lower doses. In hypothyroidism, pulmonary disease, decreased respiratory reserve, alcoholism and liver impairment the dosage should be titrated with care and prolonged monitoring may be required.

Present data suggest that clearance of alfentanil is unaltered in renal failure. However there is an increased free fraction and hence dosage requirements may be less than in the patient with normal renal function.

Patients on chronic opioid therapy or with a history of opioid abuse may require higher doses. Obese patients may require a dose based on their lean body mass.

Adolescents and young adults will require higher than average doses. There is little experience of use of alfentanil to treat children in intensive care.

The maximum recommended duration of treatment with alfentanil infusions is 4 days.

See also precautions and drug interactions.

Contra-indications, warnings, etc
Contra-indications: Known intolerance to alfentanil or other morphinomimetics.

Warnings: Following administration of Rapifen Intensive Care, a transient fall in blood pressure may occur. The magnitude of this effect may be exaggerated in the hypovolaemic patient or in the presence of concomitant sedative medication. Appropriate measures to maintain a stable arterial pressure should be taken.

Like other opioids, alfentanil may cause bradycardia, an effect which may be marked and rapid in onset but which can be antagonised by atropine. Particular care must be exerted following treatment with drugs which may depress the heart or increase vagal tone, such as anaesthetic agents or beta blockers which may predispose to bradycardia or hypotension. Heart rate and blood pressure should therefore be monitored carefully. If hypotension or bradycardia occur, the rate of administration of alfentanil should be reduced and other appropriate measures instituted.

Asystole following bradycardia has been reported on very rare occasions in non-atropinised patients. Therefore it is advisable to be prepared to administer an anticholinergic drug.

Care must be taken if the patient has received monoamine oxidase inhibitors within the previous 2 weeks.

Significant respiratory depression will occur following administration of alfentanil in doses in excess of 1 mg. If necessary for assessment purposes, naloxone or other specific antagonists may be administered to reverse the opioid respiratory depression and other pharmacological effects of alfentanil. More than one dose of naloxone may be required in view of its short half life.

Muscle rigidity (morphine-like effect) may occur, in which case neuromuscular blocking drugs may be helpful.

Precautions: It is wise to reduce the dosage in the elderly and debilitated patient. In hypothyroidism, pulmonary disease, decreased respiratory reserve, alcoholism and liver or renal impairment the dosage should be titrated with care and prolonged monitoring may be required.

Patients on chronic opioid therapy or with a history of opioid abuse may require higher doses.

As with all potent opioids, profound analgesia is accompanied by marked respiratory depression, which may persist into or recur in the early post infusion period. Care should therefore be taken throughout the weaning period and adequate spontaneous respiration should be established and maintained in the absence of stimulation or ventilatory support. Following cessation of the infusion the patient should be closely observed for at least six hours. Prior use of opioid premedication may enhance or prolong the respiratory depressant effects of alfentanil.

The use of rapid bolus injections of opioids should be avoided in patients with compromised intracerebral compliance; in such patients a transient decrease in the mean arterial pressure has occasionally been accompanied by a transient reduction of the cerebral perfusion pressure.

Effects on driving ability and operation of machinery: Where early discharge is envisaged, patients should be advised not to drive or operate machinery for the 24 hours following administration.

Drug interactions: Alfentanil is metabolised mainly via the human cytochrome P450 3A4 enzyme. Available human pharmacokinetic data indicate that the metabolism of alfentanil may be inhibited by fluconazole, erythromycin, diltiazem and cimetidine (known cytochrome P450 3A4 enzyme inhibitors). *In vitro* data suggest that other potent cytochrome P450 3A4 enzyme inhibitors (e.g. ketoconazole, itraconazole, ritonavir) may also inhibit the metabolism of alfentanil. This could increase the risk of prolonged or delayed respiratory depression. The concomitant use of such drugs requires special patient care and observation; in particular, it may be necessary to lower the dose of Rapifen Intensive Care.

Treatment with drugs which may depress the heart or increase vagal tone, such as beta-blockers and anaesthetic agents, may predispose to bradycardia or hypotension. Bradycardia and possibly asystole can occur when Rapifen Intensive Care is combined with non-vagolytic muscle relaxants.

Prior use of opioid premedication, barbiturates, benzodiazepines, neuroleptics, halogenic gases and other non-selective CNS depressants may enhance or prolong the respiratory depressant effects of alfentanil.

If other narcotic or CNS depressant drugs are used concurrently with alfentanil, the effects of the drugs can be expected to be additive. When patients have received such drugs, the dose of alfentanil required will be less than usual. Likewise, following the administration of alfentanil, the dose of other CNS-depressant drugs should be reduced.

Side-effects: The most common adverse reactions reported with alfentanil are respiratory depression, apnoea and bradycardia.

Nausea and vomiting and dizziness have been reported.

In patients receiving doses of alfentanil large enough to require assisted ventilation, myoclonic movements and muscle rigidity (possibly involving the thoracic muscles) have rarely been reported shortly after the administration of alfentanil.

Other reported adverse reactions are laryngospasm, slight transient hypotension, allergic reactions (such as anaphylaxis, bronchospasm and urticaria), asystole and arrhythmias.

Use in pregnancy and lactation: Safety in human pregnancy has not been established although studies in animals have not demonstrated teratogenic or acute embryotoxic effects. As with other drugs possible risk should be weighed against potential benefit to the patient.

Limited data suggest that alfentanil may appear in breast milk. It is therefore recommended that breast feeding is not initiated within 24 hours of treatment.

Overdosage: The manifestations of alfentanil overdose are generally an extension of its pharmacological action, which include the following:-

Action:

Bradycardia: Anticholinergics such as atropine or glycopyrrolate;

Hypoventilation or apnoea: O_2 administration, assisted or controlled respiration and an opioid antagonist may be required;

Muscle rigidity: Intravenous neuromuscular blocking agent may be given.

A specific opioid antagonist (eg naloxone) should be available to treat respiratory depression. If hypotension is severe or persists, the possibility of hypovolaemia should be considered and controlled with appropriate parenteral fluid administration.

The suggested treatments given above do not preclude the use of other clinically indicated counter measures.

Body temperature and adequate fluid intake should be maintained and the patient observed for 24 hours.

Pharmaceutical precautions Rapifen Intensive Care should be diluted with Sodium Chloride Intravenous Infusion BP, Glucose Intravenous Infusion BP or Compound Sodium Lactate Intravenous Infusion BP (Hartmann's solution). Such dilutions are compatible with plastic bags and giving sets. These dilutions should be used within 24 hours of preparation.

Store at or below 25°C.

Legal category CD (Sch 2), POM.

Package quantities Rapifen Intensive Care 5 mg/ml is supplied in 1 ml ampoules in packs of 10 ampoules.

Further information Nil.

Product licence number 0242/0137.

RETIN-A* LOTION, GEL, CREAM

Qualitative and quantitative composition *Retin-A Cream:* Tretinoin 0.025% w/w. *Retin-A Lotion:* Tretinoin 0.025% w/w. *Retin-A Gel 0.01%:* Tretinoin 0.01% w/w. *Retin-A Gel 0.025%:* Tretinoin 0.025% w/w.

Pharmaceutical form *Retin-A Cream:* Cream. *Retin-A Lotion:* Cutaneous solution. *Retin-A Gel 0.01% and 0.025%:* Topical gel.

Clinical particulars
Therapeutic indications: Acne vulgaris and other keratotic conditions.

Posology and method of administration: For topical administration.

Retin-A should be applied once or twice daily to the area of skin where the acne lesions occur.

Only apply sufficient to cover the affected areas lightly, using a gauze swab, cotton wool or the tips of clean fingers. Avoid over-saturation to the extent that excess medication could run into the eyes, angles of the nose or other areas where treatment is not intended.

Initial application may cause transitory stinging and a feeling of warmth. The correct frequency of administration should produce a slight erythema similar to that of mild sunburn.

If Retin-A is applied excessively, no more rapid or better results will be obtained and marked redness, peeling or discomfort may occur. Should this occur accidentally or through over enthusiastic use, application should be discontinued for a few days.

Patience is needed in this treatment, since the therapeutic effects will not usually be observed until after 6-8 weeks of treatment. During the early weeks of treatment, an apparent exacerbation of inflammatory lesions may occur. This is due to the action of the medication on deep, previously unseen comedones and papules.

Once the acne lesions have responded satisfactorily, it should be possible to maintain the improvement with less frequent applications.

Moisturisers and cosmetics may be used during treatment with Retin-A but should not be applied to the skin at the same time. The skin should be thoroughly washed before application of Retin-A. Astringent toiletries should be avoided.

Contra-indications: History of sensitivity/hypersensitivity reactions to any of the components, pregnancy, personal or familial history of cutaneous epithelioma.

Special warnings and special precautions for use: *Local irritation:* The presence of cutaneous irritative signs (eg erythema, peeling, pruritus, sunburn, etc) should prohibit initiation or recommencement of treatment with Retin-A until the symptoms resolve.

In certain sensitive individuals, topical use may induce severe local erythema, swelling, pruritus, warmth, burning or stinging, blistering, crusting and/or peeling at the site of application. If the degree of local irritation warrants, the patient should be directed to apply the medication less frequently or discontinue its use temporarily. If a patient experiences severe or persistent irritation, the patient should be advised to discontinue application of Retin-A completely and, if necessary, consult a physician.

Weather extremes, such as wind or cold, also may be irritating to patients being treated with Retin-A.

Tretinoin has been reported to cause severe irritation on eczematous skin and should be used with utmost caution in patients with this condition.

Exposure to sunlight: Exposure to sunlight, including ultraviolet sunlamps, should be avoided or minimised during the use of tretinoin. Patients with sunburn should be advised not to use the product until fully recovered because of potential severe irritation to skin. A patient who experiences considerable sun exposure due to occupational duties and/or anyone inherently sensitive to the sun should exercise particular caution. When exposure to sunlight cannot be avoided, use of sunscreen products and protective clothing over treated areas is recommended.

General precautions for use: Before application of Retin-A, areas to be treated should be cleansed thoroughly.

Abstain from washing the treated area frequently: twice daily is sufficient. Use of mild soap is recommended. Dry skin without rubbing.

Avoid contact with eyes, eyelids, nostrils, mouth and mucous membranes. If contact in these areas occurs, careful washing with water is recommended.

Warning: The weight of evidence indicates that topical tretinoin is not carcinogenic. In a lifetime study of CD-1 mice, a low incidence of skin tumours was seen at 100 and 200 times the estimated clinical dose but, although no such tumours were seen in the study controls, the incidence in these treated animals was within the historic control range for CD-1 mice. Studies in hairless albino mice suggest that tretinoin may accelerate the tumorigenic potential of UVB light from a solar simulator. In other studies, when lightly pigmented hairless mice treated with tretinoin were exposed to carcinogenic doses of UVB light, photocarcinogenic effects of tretinoin were not observed. Due to significantly different experimental conditions, no strict comparison of these disparate data is possible. Although the significance of these studies in man is not clear, patients should avoid or minimise exposure to sunlight.

The weight of evidence indicates that topical tretinoin is not mutagenic. The mutagenic potential of tretinoin was evaluated in the Ames assay and the *in vivo* mouse micronucleus assay, both of which showed negative findings.

Interactions with other medicaments and other forms of interaction: Retin-A should be used with caution in the presence of:

- concomitant topical medications
- toiletry preparations having a strong drying, abrasive or desquamative effect.

Following prolonged use of a peeling agent it is advisable to "rest" a patient's skin until the effects of the peeling agent subside before use of Retin-A is begun. When Retin-A and peeling agents are alternated, contact dermatitis may result and the frequency of application may have to be reduced.

Pregnancy and lactation: The topical human dose used in a 50 kg adult applying a maximum volume of 500 mg of 0.05% Retin-A cream is 0.005 mg/kg. In animal reproductive studies, oral tretinoin is known to be teratogenic and has been shown to be foetotoxic in rats when given in doses 500 times the topical human dose. In reproduction studies in rats and rabbits, topical tretinoin, when used at doses 500 and 320 times the topical human dose, respectively, induced minor skeletal abnormalities, eg irregularly contoured or partially ossified skull bones. These changes may be considered variants of normal development and are usually corrected after weaning. Retin-A should not be used during pregnancy.

It is not known whether tretinoin is excreted in human milk, therefore caution should be exercised when Retin-A is administered to a nursing mother.

Effects on ability to drive and use machines: Retin-A is administered topically and is unlikely to have an effect on one's ability to drive or operate machinery.

Undesirable effects: Local reactions frequently reported during therapy included: dry or peeling skin, burning, stinging, warmth, erythema, pruritus, rash and temporary hypo- and hyper-pigmentation. These skin reactions were usually mild to moderate and were generally well-tolerated. They usually occurred early in therapy and, except for dry or peeling skin which persisted during therapy, generally decreased over the course of therapy. Rarely reported undesirable effects are blistering and crusting of the skin, eye irritation and oedema.

True contact allergy to topical tretinoin is rarely encountered. Heightened susceptibility to either sunlight or other sources of UVB light has been reported.

Overdose: Excessive application of Retin-A does not improve the results of treatment and may induce marked irritation, eg erythema, peeling, pruritus, etc. Oral ingestion of Retin-A may lead to the same effects associated with excessive oral intake of Vitamin A (eg pruritus, dry skin, arthralgias, anorexia, vomiting). In the event of accidental ingestion, if the ingestion is recent, an appropriate method of gastric emptying should be used as soon as possible.

Pharmacological properties

Pharmacodynamic properties: Tretinoin (β-*all trans* retinoic acid, Vitamin A acid) produces profound metabolic changes in keratinising epithelia. Tretinoin increases the proliferative activity of epidermal cells in *in vivo* and *in vitro* studies, and cellular differentiation (keratinisation and cornification) is also altered.

Pharmacokinetic properties: Topical administration of Retin-A products produces dose-dependent erythema, peeling and irritation, and excessive use of the products should be avoided. 0.1% w/w Retin-A did not produce an allergic response when tested in 160 subjects by the Draize test. The percutaneous absorption of 0.1% w/w ^{14}C labelled retinoic acid was studied in 6 adult male volunteers; between 0.3% and 2.18% of the retinoic acid was absorbed through the skin following a single topical application of the ^{14}C retinoic acid formulation. No systemic toxic effects have been reported following topical application of Retin-A formulations.

Preclinical safety data: No relevant information other than that contained elsewhere in the Summary of Product Characteristics.

Pharmaceutical particulars

List of excipients: Retin-A Cream: Butylated hydroxytoluene; isopropyl myristate; polyoxyl 40 stearate; sorbic acid; stearic acid; stearyl alcohol; xanthan gum; purified water. *Retin-A Lotion:* Butylated hydroxytoluene; ethanol pharma; undenatured polyethylene glycol 400. *Retin-A Gel 0.01% and 0.025%:* Butylated hydroxytoluene, hydroxypropyl cellulose; undenatured ethanol.

Incompatibilities: Avoid or minimise exposure of Retin-A treated areas to sunlight or sunlamps during the course of treatment.

Shelf life: Retin-A Cream: 36 months. *Retin-A Lotion:* 24 months. *Retin-A Gel 0.01%:* 36 months. *Retin-A Gel 0.025%:* 24 months.

Special precautions for storage: Store below 25°C. The lotion should also be protected from light.

Nature and contents of container: Retin-A Cream, Retin-A Gel 0.01% and 0.025%: Aluminium tube lined with epoxy resin or epoxy resin with wax. Tube cap of polyethylene or urea resin. Available in a tube size of 60 g. *Retin-A Lotion:* Amber glass bottle containing 100 ml.

Instructions for use/handling: None stated.

Marketing authorisation numbers

Cream	0242/0266
Lotion	0242/0269
Gel 0.01%	0242/0265
Gel 0.025%	0242/0268

Date of approval/revision of SPC October 1998

Legal category POM.

RISPERDAL*

Qualitative and quantitative composition *Tablets:* risperidone 1, 2, 3, 4 and 6 mg.

Liquid: risperidone 1 mg/ml.

Pharmaceutical form

1 mg: White, oblong tablets, marked Ris 1.

2 mg: Pale orange, oblong tablets, marked Ris 2.

3 mg: Yellow, oblong tablets, marked Ris 3.

4 mg: Green, oblong tablets, marked Ris 4.

6 mg: Yellow, circular tablets, marked Ris 6.

Oral liquid.

Clinical particulars

Therapeutic indications: Risperdal is indicated for the treatment of acute and chronic schizophrenic psychoses, and other psychotic conditions, in which positive symptoms (such as hallucinations, delusions, thought disturbances, hostility, suspiciousness), and/or negative symptoms (such as blunted affect, emotional and social withdrawal, poverty of speech) are prominent. Risperdal also alleviates affective symptoms (such as depression, guilt feelings, anxiety) associated with schizophrenia.

Posology and method of administration: 1 ml of Risperdal liquid contains 1 mg risperidone. If necessary Risperdal liquid may be diluted with mineral water, orange juice or black coffee. When diluted in this way, the product should be used immediately. The liquid should not be mixed with tea (See Pharmaceutical Particulars).

Switching from other antipsychotics: where medically appropriate, gradual discontinuation of the previous treatment while Risperdal therapy is initiated is recommended. Where medically appropriate when switching patients from depot antipsychotics, consider initiating Risperdal therapy in place of the next scheduled injection. The need for continuing existing antiparkinson medication should be re-evaluated periodically.

Adults: Risperdal may be given once or twice daily. Patients should be titrated to 6 mg/day gradually over three days. All patients, whether acute or chronic, should start with 2 mg/day Risperdal. The dosage should be increased to 4 mg/day on the second day and 6 mg/day on the third day. However, some patients such as first episode patients may benefit from a slower rate of titration. From then on the dosage can be maintained unchanged, or further individualised, if needed. The usual effective dosage is 4 to 8 mg/day although in some patients an optimal response may be obtained at lower doses.

Doses above 10 mg/day generally have not been shown to provide additional efficacy to lower doses and may increase the risk of extrapyramidal symptoms. Doses above 10 mg/day should only be used in individual patients if the benefit is considered to outweigh the risk. Doses above 16 mg/day have not been extensively evaluated for safety and therefore should not be used.

Elderly: A starting dose of 0.5 mg bd is recommended. This dosage can be individually adjusted with 0.5 mg bd increments to 1 to 2 mg bd

Risperdal is well tolerated by the elderly.

Children: Not recommended in children aged less than 15 years.

Renal and liver disease: A starting dose of 0.5 mg bd is recommended. This dosage can be individually adjusted with 0.5 mg bd increments to 1 to 2 mg bd

Risperdal should be used with caution in this group of patients until further experience is gained.

Method of administration Oral use.

Contra-indications: Risperdal is contra-indicated in patients with a known hypersensitivity to the product.

Special warnings and precautions for use: Due to the alpha-blocking activity of Risperdal, orthostatic hypotension can occur, especially during the initial dose-titration period. Risperdal should be used with caution in patients with known cardiovascular disease. A dose reduction should be considered if hypotension occurs.

If further sedation is required, an additional drug (such as a benzodiazepine) should be administered rather than increasing the dose of Risperdal.

Drugs with dopamine receptor antagonistic properties have been associated with the induction of tardive dyskinesia, characterised by rhythmical involuntary movements, predominantly of the tongue and/or face. It has been reported that the occurrence of extrapyramidal symptoms is a risk factor for the development of tardive dyskinesia. If signs and symptoms of tardive dyskinesia appear, the discontinuation of all antipsychotic drugs should be considered.

It is recommended to halve both the starting dose and the subsequent dose increments in geriatric patients and in patients with renal or liver insufficiency.

Caution should also be exercised when prescribing Risperdal to patients with Parkinson's disease since, theoretically, it may cause a deterioration of the disease.

Classical neuroleptics are known to lower the seizure threshold. Caution is recommended when treating patients with epilepsy.

As with other antipsychotics, patients should be advised of the potential for weight gain.

Interaction with other medicaments and other forms of interaction: Possible interactions of Risperdal with other drugs have not been systematically evaluated. Given the primary CNS effects of Risperdal it should be used with caution in combination with other centrally acting drugs.

Risperdal may antagonise the effect of levodopa and other dopamine-agonists.

Carbamazepine has been shown to decrease the plasma levels of the antipsychotic fraction of Risperdal. A similar effect might be anticipated with other drugs which stimulate metabolising enzymes in the liver. On initiation of carbamazepine or other hepatic enzyme-inducing drugs, the dosage of Risperdal should be re-evaluated and increased if necessary. Conversely, on discontinuation of such drugs, the dosage of Risperdal should be re-evaluated and decreased if necessary.

Phenothiazines, tricyclic antidepressants and some beta-blockers may increase the plasma concentrations of risperidone but not those of the antipsychotic fraction. Based on *in vitro* studies, the same interaction may occur with haloperidol and fluoxetine.

When Risperdal is taken together with other highly protein-bound drugs, there is no clinically relevant displacement of either drug from the plasma proteins.

Food does not affect the absorption of Risperdal.

Pregnancy and lactation: Although, in experimental animals, risperidone did not show direct reproductive toxicity, some indirect, prolactin- and CNS-mediated effects were observed, typically delayed oestrus and changes in mating and nursing behaviour in rats. No teratogenic effect of risperidone was noted in any study. The safety of Risperdal for use during human pregnancy has not been established. Therefore, Risperdal should only be used during pregnancy if the benefits outweigh the risks.

In animal studies, risperidone and 9-hydroxyrisperidone are excreted in the milk. It is not known whether Risperdal is excreted in human milk. Therefore, women receiving Risperdal should not breast feed.

Effects on ability to drive and use machines: Risperdal may interfere with activities requiring mental alertness. Therefore, patients should be advised not to drive or operate machinery until their individual susceptibility is known.

Undesirable effects: Risperdal is generally well tolerated and in many instances it has been difficult to differentiate adverse events from symptoms of the underlying disease. Adverse events observed in association with the use of Risperdal include:

Common: insomnia, agitation, anxiety, headache.

Less common: somnolence, fatigue, dizziness, impaired concentration, constipation, dyspepsia, nausea/vomiting, abdominal pain, blurred vision, priapism, erectile dysfunction, ejaculatory dysfunction, orgasmic dysfunction, urinary incontinence, rhinitis, rash and other allergic reactions.

The incidence and severity of extrapyramidal symptoms are significantly less than with haloperidol. However, in some cases the following extrapyramidal symptoms may occur: tremor, rigidity, hypersalivation, bradykinesia, akathisia, acute dystonia. If acute in nature, these symptoms are usually mild and are reversible upon dose reduction and/or administration of antiparkinson medication, if necessary.

As with other neuroleptics, rare cases of neuroleptic malignant syndrome, characterised by hyperthermia, muscle rigidity, autonomic instability, altered consciousness and elevated CPK levels, have been reported. In such an event, all antipsychotic drugs, including Risperdal, should be discontinued.

Occasionally, orthostatic dizziness, hypotension including orthostatic, tachycardia including reflex tachycardia and hypertension have been observed following administration of Risperdal.

Risperdal can induce a dose-dependent increase in plasma prolactin concentration. Possible associated manifestations are: galactorrhoea, gynaecomastia, disturbances of the menstrual cycle and amenorrhoea.

Weight gain, oedema and increased hepatic enzyme levels have been observed during treatment with Risperdal.

A mild fall in neutrophil and/or thrombocyte count has been reported.

As with classical neuroleptics, rare cases of the following have been reported in schizophrenic patients: water intoxication with hyponatraemia, either due to polydipsia or to the syndrome of inappropriate secretion of antidiuretic hormone; tardive dyskinesia, body temperature dysregulation and seizures.

Overdose: Overdosages of up to 360 mg have been reported. In general, reported signs and symptoms have been those resulting from an exaggeration of the drug's known pharmacological effects. These include drowsiness and sedation, tachycardia and hypotension, and extrapyramidal symptoms. A prolonged QT interval was reported in a patient with concomitant hypokalaemia who had ingested 360 mg. The patient made an uneventful recovery. In case of acute overdosage, the possibility of multiple drug involvement should be considered.

Establish and maintain a clear airway, and ensure adequate oxygenation and ventilation. Gastric lavage (after intubation, if the patient is unconscious) and administration of activated charcoal together with a laxative should be considered. Cardiovascular monitoring should commence immediately and should include continuous electrocardiographic monitoring to detect possible arrhythmias.

There is no specific antidote to Risperdal. Therefore appropriate supportive measures should be instituted. Hypotension and circulatory collapse should be treated with appropriate measures such as intravenous fluids and/or sympathomimetic agents. In case of severe extrapyramidal symptoms, anticholinergic medication should be administered. Close medical supervision and monitoring should continue until the patient recovers.

Pharmacological properties

Pharmacodynamic properties: Risperdal is a novel antipsychotic belonging to a new class of antipsychotic agents, the benzisoxazole-derivatives.

Risperdal is a selective monoaminergic antagonist with a high affinity for both serotonergic 5-HT_2 and dopaminergic D_2 receptors. Risperdal binds also to alpha$_1$-adrenergic receptors and, with lower affinity, to H_1-histaminergic and alpha$_2$-adrenergic receptors. Risperdal has no affinity for cholinergic receptors. Although Risperdal is a potent D_2 antagonist, an activity which is considered to improve the positive symptoms of schizophrenia, it causes less depression of motor activity and induction of catalepsy than classical neuroleptics. Balanced central serotonin and dopamine antagonism may reduce the tendency to cause extrapyramidal side effects, and extend the therapeutic activity to the negative and affective symptoms of schizophrenia.

Pharmacokinetic properties: Risperdal is completely absorbed after oral administration, reaching peak plasma concentrations within 1 to 2 hours. The absorption is not affected by food.

The most important route of metabolism of Risperdal is hydroxylation to 9-hydroxy-risperidone which has a similar pharmacological activity to risperidone. This hydroxylation is subject to debrisoquine-type genetic polymorphism but this does not affect the active antipsychotic fraction since this consists of risperidone and its active metabolite 9-hydroxyrisperidone. After oral administration, the elimination half-life of the active antipsychotic fraction is 24 hours.

A single-dose study showed higher active plasma concentrations and a slower elimination of Risperdal in the elderly and in patients with renal insufficiency. Risperdal plasma concentrations were normal in patients with liver insufficiency.

Preclinical safety data: Not applicable.

Pharmaceutical particulars

List of excipients: Tablets: All four tablet strengths contain the following excipients.

Lactose; maize starch; microcrystalline cellulose; hypromellose 2910 5 mPa.s; magnesium stearate; colloidal anhydrous silica; sodium lauryl sulphate; purified water*

* not present in the final product.

In addition, the tablets also contain the following excipients:

1 mg: Hypromellose 2910 15 mPa.s, propylene glycol.

2 mg: Hypromellose 2910 15 mPa.s, titanium dioxide, talc, propylene glycol, orange yellow S (E110) aluminium lake.

3 mg: Hypromellose 2910 15 mPa.s, titanium dioxide (E171), talc, propylene glycol, quinoline yellow (E104).

4 mg: Hypromellose 2910 15 mPa.s, titanium dioxide (E171), talc, propylene glycol, quinoline yellow (E104), indigotine disulphonate (E132), aluminium lake.

6 mg: Titanium dioxide (E171); talc; propylene glycol; quinoline yellow (E104); orange yellow S (E110).

Liquid: Tartaric acid, benzoic acid, sodium hydroxide, purified water.

Incompatibilities: Tablets: Not applicable.

Liquid: Risperdal Liquid should only be diluted with those beverages listed in Posology and method of administration.

Shelf life: 1, 2, 3 and 4 mg Tablets: 36 months. *6 mg Tablets:* 24 months.

Liquid: The unopened bottles have a shelf life of 36 months. Once opened, the contents of the bottle should be used within 3 months.

Special precautions for storage: Tablets: Store below 30°C.

Liquid: Store below 30°C; protect from freezing.

Nature and contents of container: Tablets: Blister strips consisting of polyvinylchloride (PVC)/low density polyethylene (LDPE)/polyvinylidene chloride (PVDC) and aluminium foil. The strips are packed in cardboard cartons to contain either 6 (1 mg tablets only), 20 (1 mg tablets only) 60 tablets (2, 3 and 4 mg tablets) per pack or 28 tablets (6 mg tablets) per pack.

Liquid: Amber glass bottle with a plastic child-resistant and tamper-evident cap. Each bottle contains 100 ml.

Instructions for use/handling: Tablets: Not applicable.

Liquid: A special dosing pipette is supplied with each pack of Risperdal Liquid.

Instructions for using the pipette with Risperdal liquid:

1. Remove the child-proof cap from the bottle by pushing down on the cap while turning it anti-clockwise (Fig. 1)

Fig. 1

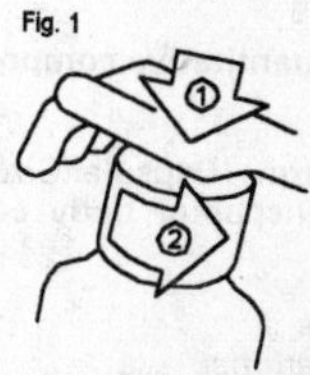

2. Place the bottle on a flat surface.
3. Pull the pipette out of its case (Fig. 2).

Fig. 2

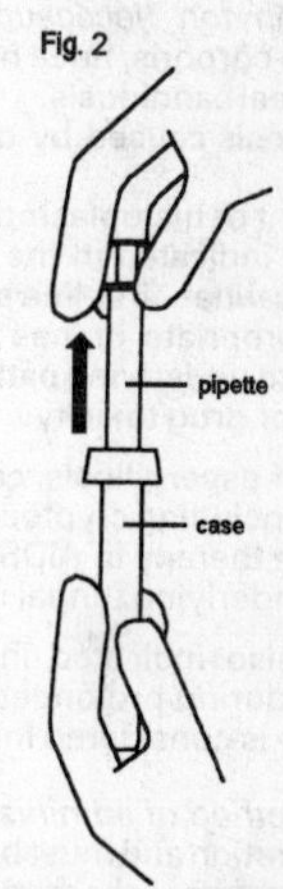

4. Insert the pipette into the liquid in the bottle.
5. While holding the lower ring, pull the top ring upwards until the mark that matches the number of mg or ml to be taken is just visible (Fig. 3).

Fig 3

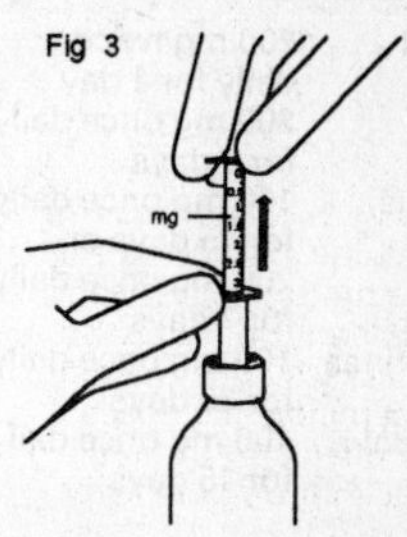

6. Holding the lower ring, remove the whole pipette from the bottle (Fig. 4).

Fig. 4

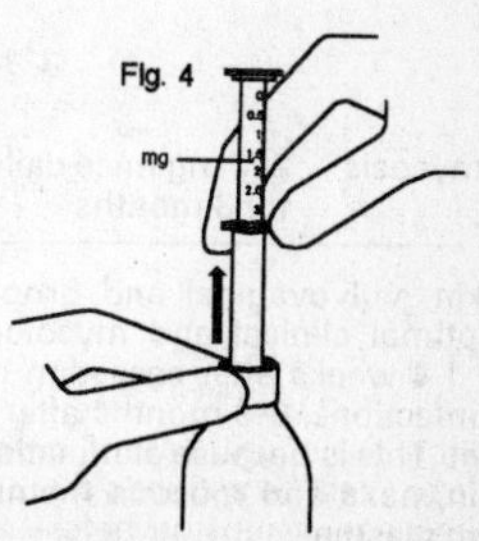

7. To empty the pipette, push down on the top ring while still holding the lower ring.

8. The contents of the pipette may be emptied directly into the mouth or into a drink of mineral water, orange juice or black coffee.

9. Put the empty pipette back in its case.

10. Replace the child-proof cap on the bottle by screwing it down clockwise.

Marketing authorisation numbers

1 mg tablets	0242/0186
2 mg tablets	0242/0187
3 mg tablets	0242/0188
4 mg tablets	0242/0189
6 mg tablets	0242/0317
1 mg/ml liquid	0242/0199

Date of approval/revision of SPC
Tablets: May 1997.
Liquid: May 1997.

Legal category POM.

SPORANOX*

Qualitative and quantitative composition Itraconazole 100 mg.

Pharmaceutical form Capsule (Size 0): opaque blue cap and pink transparent body containing coated beads.

Clinical particulars
Therapeutic indications:

1. Vulvovaginal candidosis.
2. Pityriasis versicolor.
3. Dermatophytoses caused by organisms susceptible to itraconazole *(Trichophyton spp., Microsporum spp., Epidermophyton floccosum)* eg tinea pedis, tinea cruris, tinea corporis, tinea manuum.
4. Oropharyngeal candidosis.
5. Onychomycosis caused by dermatophytes and/or yeasts.
6. The treatment of histoplasmosis.
7. Sporanox is indicated in the following systemic fungal conditions when first-line systemic anti-fungal therapy is inappropriate or has proved ineffective. This may be due to underlying pathology, insensitivity of the pathogen or drug toxicity.

- Treatment of aspergillosis, candidosis and cryptococcosis (including cryptococcal meningitis);
- Maintenance therapy in AIDS patients to prevent relapse of underlying fungal infection.

Sporanox is also indicated in the prevention of fungal infection during prolonged neutropenia when standard therapy is considered inappropriate.

Posology and method of administration: Sporanox is for oral administration and must be taken immediately after a meal for maximal absorption.

Treatment schedules in adults for each indication are as follows:

Indication	*Dose*	*Remarks*
Vulvovaginal candidosis	200 mg twice daily for 1 day	
Pityriasis versicolor	200 mg once daily for 7 days	
Tinea corporis, tinea cruris	100 mg once daily for 15 days or 200 mg once daily for 7 days	
Tinea pedis, tinea manuum	100 mg once daily for 30 days	
Oropharyngeal candidosis	100 mg once daily for 15 days	Increase dose to 200 mg once daily for 15 days in AIDS or neutropenic patients because of impaired absorption in these groups.
Onychomycosis	200 mg once daily for 3 months	

For skin, vulvovaginal and oropharyngeal infections, optimal clinical and mycological effects are reached 1-4 weeks after cessation of treatment and for nail infections, 6–9 months after the cessation of treatment. This is because elimination of itraconazole from skin, nails and mucous membranes is slower than from plasma.

The length of treatment for systemic fungal infections should be dictated by the mycological and clinical response to therapy:

Indication	*Dose*	*Remarks*
Aspergillosis	200 mg once daily	Increase dose to 200 mg twice daily in case of invasive or disseminated disease
Candidosis	100-200 mg once daily	Increase dose to 200 mg twice daily in case of invasive or disseminated disease
Non-meningeal cryptococcosis	200 mg once daily	
Cryptococcal meningitis	200 mg twice daily	
Histoplasmosis	200 mg once daily - 200 mg twice daily	
Maintenance in AIDS	200 mg once daily	See note on impaired absorption below
Prophylaxis in neutropenia	200 mg once daily	See note on impaired absorption below

Impaired absorption in AIDS and neutropenic patients may lead to low itraconazole blood levels and lack of efficacy. In such cases blood level monitoring and if necessary an increase in itraconazole dose to 200 mg twice daily is indicated.

In children (below 12 years): There are inadequate data on Sporanox in children for its use to be recommended, unless the potential benefits outweigh the risks.

In elderly: As for use in children.

Contra-indications: When administered at high doses to pregnant rats (40 mg/kg/day) and mice (80 mg/kg/day), itraconazole was shown to cause abnormalities of foetal development. No data are available in human pregnancy, and itraconazole is therefore contra-indicated in pregnancy. Adequate contraceptive precautions should be taken by women of childbearing potential during therapy and for one menstrual cycle after stopping therapy.

Itraconazole is also contraindicated in patients who have shown hypersensitivity to itraconazole, other azole antifungal agents or any of the excipients.

The drugs terfenadine, astemizole, cisapride, HMG-CoA reductase inhibitors such as simvastatin, oral midazolam or triazolam should not be given concurrently with itraconazole (see also interactions).

Special warnings and special precautions for use: Absorption is impaired when gastric acidity is decreased. In patients also receiving acid neutralising medicines (eg aluminium hydroxide) these should be administered at least 2 hours after the intake of Sporanox. In patients with achlorhydria such as certain AIDS patients and patients on secretion suppressors (eg H2-antagonists, proton-pump inhibitors), it is advisable to administer Sporanox with a cola beverage.

Rarely cases of hepatitis and cholestatic jaundice have been reported, mainly in patients treated for longer than one month. It is therefore advisable to monitor liver function in patients receiving continuous treatment of more than one month's duration. Additionally, if during treatment (other than single-day therapy for vulvovaginal candidosis) patients develop symptoms suggestive of hepatitis such as anorexia, nausea, vomiting, fatigue, abdominal pain or dark urine, liver enzymes should be monitored promptly. If these are abnormal, treatment should be stopped. In patients with raised liver enzymes, or with a known history of liver disease, or who have experienced liver toxicity with other drugs, treatment should not be started unless the expected benefit exceeds the risk of hepatic injury. In such instances liver enzyme monitoring is necessary.

Itraconazole is predominantly metabolised in the liver. A slight decrease in oral bioavailability in cirrhotic patients has been observed, although this was not of statistical significance. The terminal half-life was however significantly increased. It is advised to monitor the itraconazole plasma concentrations in such patients and to adapt the dose when necessary.

The oral bioavailability of itraconazole may be lower in some patients with renal insufficiency (eg those receiving continuous ambulatory peritoneal dialysis). Monitoring of the itraconazole plasma levels and dose adaptation are advisable.

Isolated cases of peripheral neuropathy have been reported, predominantly during long-term treatment and in severely compromised patients. The causal relationship to Sporanox was uncertain. If neuropathy occurs which may be attributable to Sporanox, treatment should be discontinued.

In systemic candidosis, if fluconazole-resistant strains of *Candida* species are suspected, it cannot be assumed that these are sensitive to itraconazole, hence their sensitivity should be tested before the start of Sporanox therapy.

Interaction with other medicaments and other forms of interaction:
Drug-interactions: Enzyme-inducing drugs such as rifampicin and phenytoin significantly reduce the oral bioavailability of itraconazole. Consequently, monitoring of the itraconazole plasma concentration is advised when enzyme-inducing agents are co-administered.

Itraconazole can inhibit the metabolism of drugs metabolised by the cytochrome 3A family. This can result in an increase and/or a prolongation of their effects, including side effects. Known examples are:

- Terfenadine, astemizole and cisapride, resulting in increased plasma levels of these drugs and predisposing to serious arrhythmias. Combination of itraconazole with terfenadine, astemizole or cisapride is contraindicated.
- Midazolam and triazolam, resulting in increased plasma levels of these drugs. Combination of itraconazole with oral midazolam or triazolam is contraindicated. If midazolam is administered intravenously (eg as premedication in surgical or investigative procedures) special care should be observed since the sedative effect may be prolonged.
- HMG-CoA reductase inhibitors such as simvastatin. These drugs should not be used during treatment with Sporanox.
- Oral anticoagulants, digoxin, cyclosporin A, systemic methylprednisolone, vinca-alkaloids and possibly tacrolimus. Co-administration of itraconazole and digoxin has led to increased levels of the latter drug. A rise in cyclosporin levels has also been reported in patients treated with high doses of itraconazole for several weeks. Plasma levels of digoxin and cyclosporin should therefore be monitored during concomitant administration of itraconazole and the doses adjusted accordingly. *In vitro* studies indicate that a similar interaction may occur with tacrolimus. With respect to oral anticoagulants, similar interactions have been reported and it is advisable to monitor prothrombin time and reduce the dosage of oral anticoagulants if necessary. Co-administration of itraconazole and vinca-alkaloids may potentiate the toxic effects of the latter drugs and should this occur, co-administration of these drugs should be reconsidered.
- Dihydropyridine calcium channel blockers and quinidine. Patients should be monitored for side effects, eg oedema and tinnitus/decreased hearing, respectively. If necessary, the dose of these drugs should be reduced.

Despite the fact that itraconazole is 99.8% bound to plasma proteins, there are no *in vitro* interactions on the plasma protein binding between itraconazole and imipramine, propanolol, diazepam, cimetidine, indomethacin, tolbutamide or sulphadimidine.

Itraconazole does not appear to affect the metabolism of ethinyloestradiol and norethisterone. Reports suggest that there is no interaction of itraconazole with the oral pharmacokinetics of AZT (zidovudine).

Pregnancy and lactation:
Pregnancy: Sporanox is contra-indicated in pregnancy (see Contra-indications section for further details).

Lactation: Only small amounts of itraconazole are excreted in human milk. The expected benefits of therapy should be weighed against the risks to the infant.

Effects on ability to drive and use machines: None known.

Undesirable effects: The most frequently reported adverse experiences in association with the use of Sporanox are of gastro-intestinal origin, such as dyspepsia, nausea, abdominal pain and constipation. Less frequently reported adverse experiences include headache, reversible increases in hepatic enzymes, menstrual disorder, dizziness and allergic reactions (such as pruritus, rash, urticaria and angio-oedema). Isolated cases of peripheral neuropathy and of Stevens-Johnson syndrome have also been reported; a causality for the latter was not established.

Mainly in patients receiving prolonged treatment (ie approximately one month), most of whom had major underlying pathology and multiple concomitant medications, cases of hypokalaemia, oedema and hair loss have been observed. Hepatitis and cholestatic jaundice have been reported rarely, mainly in patients treated for longer than one month.

Overdose: In the event of overdosage, patients should be treated symptomatically with supportive measures and gastric lavage as necessary. No specific antidote is available. Itraconazole cannot be removed by haemodialysis.

Pharmacological properties
Pharmacodynamic properties: Itraconazole is a substituted triazole antimycotic with a broad spectrum of activity against *Candida* spp and other yeasts, dermatophytes and pathogenic fungi. It acts by impairing the synthesis of ergosterol in fungal cell membranes.

Pharmacokinetic properties: Peak plasma concentrations of itraconazole in the region of 1 mcg equiv/ml are reached 1.5-3 hrs after administration. In man the elimination half life is about 20 hrs. Oral intake immediately after a meal doubled the peak level 3–4 hrs after intake.

Peak concentrations of itraconazole in keratinous tissues, especially skin, are up to 3 times higher than in plasma. Therapeutic levels in the skin persist for up to 2–4 weeks after stopping treatment as elimination is related to epidermal regeneration, rather than redistribution into the systemic circulation. Itraconazole is extensively metabolised by the liver to a large number of metabolites, which constitute 40% of the excreted dose. Faecal excretion of parent drug varies from 3-18% of the dose, and urinary excretion of unchanged drug is less than 0.03%.

Preclinical safety data: Not applicable.

Pharmaceutical particulars
List of excipients: Sugar spheres; hypromellose 2910 5 mPa.s; macrogol 20000. *Capsule shell:* Titanium dioxide; indigo carmine; gelatin; erythrosine.

Incompatibilities: None known.

Shelf life: 36 months.

Special precautions for storage: Protect from light. Store in a dry place. Store between 15°C and 30°C.

Nature and contents of container: Perlalux tristar blister–plastic foil consisting of 3 layers
Polyvinylchloride on the inner side;
Low density polyethylene in the middle;
Polyvinylidenechloride on the inside;
Aluminium foil (thickness 20 μm) coated on the inner side with colourless heat-seal Lacquer: pvc mixed polymers with acrylates, 6 g/m².
or
PVC blister consisting of -
Polyvinylchloride 'genotherm' glass clear, thickness 250 μm;
Aluminium foil (thickness 20 μm) coated on the inner side with a colourless heat-seal Lacquer: pvc mixed polymers with acrylates, 6 g/m².
Pack sizes: 4, 15, 60 capsules.

Instructions for use/handling: Not applicable.

Marketing authorisation number 0242/0142.

Date of approval/revision of SPC February 1997.

Legal category POM.

SPORANOX* LIQUID

Qualitative and quantitative composition Itraconazole 10 mg/ml.

Pharmaceutical form Oral solution containing 10 mg itraconazole/ml.

Clinical particulars
Therapeutic indications: Sporanox liquid is indicated:
For the treatment of oral and/or oesophageal candidosis in HIV-positive or other immunocompromised patients.

As prophylaxis of deep fungal infections anticipated to be susceptible to itraconazole, when standard therapy is considered inappropriate, in patients with haematological malignancy or undergoing bone marrow transplant, and who are expected to become neutropenic (ie < 500 cells/μl). At present there are insufficient clinical efficacy data in the prevention of aspergillosis.

Consideration should be given to national and/or local guidance regarding the appropriate use of antifungal agents.

Posology and method of administration: For optimal absorption, Sporanox liquid should be taken without food (patients are advised to refrain from eating for at least one hour after intake).

For the treatment of oral and/or oesophageal candidosis, the liquid should be swished around the oral cavity (approx. 20 seconds) and swallowed. There should be no rinsing after swallowing (patients are advised to refrain from eating for at least one hour after intake).

Treatment of oral and/or oesophageal candidosis: 200 mg (2 measuring cups) per day in one or two intakes for 1 week. If there is no response after 1 week, treatment should be continued for another week.

Treatment of fluconazole resistant oral and/or oesophageal candidosis: 100 to 200 mg (1–2 measuring cups) twice daily for 2 weeks. If there is no response after 2 weeks, treatment should be continued for another 2 weeks. The 400 mg daily dose should not be used for longer than 14 days if there are no signs of improvement.

Prophylaxis of fungal infections: 5 mg/kg per day administered in two intakes. In clinical trials, prophylaxis treatment was started immediately prior to the cytostatic treatment and generally one week before transplant procedure. Almost all proven deep fungal infections occurred in patients reaching neutrophil counts below 100 cells/μl. Treatment was continued until recovery of neutrophils (ie > 1000 cells/μl).

Pharmacokinetic parameters from clinical studies in neutropenic patients demonstrate considerable intersubject variation. Blood level monitoring should be considered particularly in the presence of gastrointestinal damage, diarrhoea and during prolonged courses of Sporanox liquid.

Use in children: See *Special warnings and precautions for use.*

Prophylaxis of fungal infections: there are no efficacy data available in neutropenic children. Limited safety experience is available with a dose of 5 mg/kg per day administered in two intakes. The incidence of adverse events such as diarrhoea, abdominal pain, vomiting, fever, rash and mucositis was higher than in adults.

Use in elderly and in patients with renal or hepatic impairment: See *Special warnings and precautions for use.*

Contra-indications: Sporanox liquid is contraindicated in patients who have shown hypersensitivity to the drug or its excipients.

Terfenadine, astemizole, cisapride, HMG-CoA reductase inhibitors such as simvastatin and lovastatin, oral midazolam and triazolam are contra-indicated with Sporanox liquid.

Sporanox liquid should only be given to pregnant women in life-threatening cases and when in these cases the potential benefit outweighs the potential harm to the foetus. Adequate contraceptive precautions should be taken by women of childbearing potential using Sporanox liquid until the next menstrual period following the end of Sporanox therapy.

Special warnings and special precautions for use: Sporanox has a potential for clinically important drug interactions in patients receiving immunosuppressive therapy (eg cyclosporin, rapamycin, tacrolimus) or antiretroviral therapy with protease inhibitors (eg indinavir, ritonavir, saquinavir). (See *Interaction with other medicaments and other forms of interaction).*

Paediatric use: Since clinical data on the use of Sporanox liquid in paediatric patients is limited, its use in children is not recommended.

Use in elderly: Since clinical data on the use of Sporanox liquid in elderly patients is limited, it is advised to use Sporanox liquid in these patients only if the potential benefit outweighs the potential risks.

It is advisable to monitor liver function in patients receiving continuous treatment of more than one month and promptly in patients developing symptoms suggestive of hepatitis such as anorexia, nausea, vomiting, fatigue, abdominal pain or dark urine. If abnormal, treatment should be stopped. In patients with raised liver enzymes or an active liver disease, or who have experienced liver toxicity with other drugs, treatment should not be started unless the expected benefit exceeds the risk of hepatic injury. In such cases, liver enzyme monitoring is necessary.

Hepatic impairment: Itraconazole is predominantly metabolised in the liver. The terminal half-life of itraconazole in cirrhotic patients is somewhat prolonged. A decrease in the oral bioavailability of itraconazole from Sporanox capsules was observed in cirrhotic patients. This can also be expected with Sporanox liquid. A dose adjustment may be considered.

Renal impairment: A decrease in the oral bioavailability of itraconazole from Sporanox capsules was observed in some patients with renal insufficiency. This can also be expected with Sporanox liquid. A dose adjustment may be considered.

Prophylaxis in neutropenic patients: in clinical trials diarrhoea was the most frequent adverse event. This disturbance of the gastrointestinal tract may result in impaired absorption and may alter the microbiological flora potentially favouring fungal colonisation. Consideration should be given to discontinuing Sporanox liquid in these circumstances.

If neuropathy occurs that may be attributable to Sporanox liquid, the treatment should be discontinued.

There is no information regarding cross hypersensitivity between itraconazole and other azole antifungal agents. Caution should be used in prescribing Sporanox liquid to patients with hypersensitivity to other azoles.

Interaction with other medicaments and other forms of interaction: Interaction studies have only been performed with the capsule formulation of Sporanox.

Enzyme-inducing drugs such as rifampicin, carbamazepine, isoniazid and phenytoin significantly reduce the oral bioavailability of itraconazole.

Itraconazole can inhibit the metabolism of drugs metabolised by the cytochrome 3A family. This can result in an increase and/or a prolongation of their effects, including side effects. Examples are:

Terfenadine, astemizole, cisapride, HMG-CoA reductase inhibitors such as simvastatin and lovastatin, oral midazolam and triazolam. These agents should not be used by patients during treatment with Sporanox liquid. If midazolam is administered iv, special care is required since the sedative effects may be prolonged.

Oral anticoagulants digoxin, Cyclosporin A, systemic methylprednisolone, vinca-alkaloids and possibly tacrolimus. The plasma levels or the effects of these drugs should be monitored. Their dosage, if co-administered with itraconazole, should be reduced if necessary.

Dihydropyridine calcium channel blockers and quinidine. Patients should be monitored for side effects, e.g. oedema and tinnitus/decreased hearing, respectively. If necessary, the dose of these drugs should be reduced.

No interaction studies have been performed with HIV protease inhibitors. A dose reduction could be necessary for HIV protease inhibitors when used in combination with itraconazole, or for itraconazole when used in combination with ritonavir.

In vitro studies have shown that there are no interactions on the plasma protein binding between itraconazole and imipramine, propranolol, diazepam, cimetidine, indomethacin, tolbutamide and sulfamethazine.

No interaction of itraconazole with AZT (zidovudine) has been observed.

No inducing effects of itraconazole on the metabolism of ethinyloestradiol and norethisterone were observed.

Pregnancy and lactation: When administered at high doses to pregnant rats (40 mg/kg/day or higher) and mice (80 mg/kg/day or higher), itraconazole was shown to increase the incidence of foetal abnormalities and did produce adverse effects on the embryo.

No studies are available on the use of Sporanox liquid in pregnant women. Therefore, Sporanox liquid should only be given in life-threatening cases and when in these cases the potential benefit outweighs the potential harm to the foetus.

Only a very small amount of itraconazole is excreted in human milk. The expected benefits of treatment with Sporanox liquid should therefore be weighed against the potential risk of breast-feeding. In case of doubt the patient should not breast feed.

Effects on ability to drive and use machines: No effects have been observed.

Undesirable effects: Adverse experiences reported in association with the use of Sporanox liquid:

The most frequently reported were of gastrointestinal origin, such as diarrhoea, nausea, abdominal pain and vomiting. Less frequently reported adverse experiences include headache, reversible increases in hepatic enzymes, dizziness and allergic reactions (such as pruritus, rash, urticaria and angiooedema).

Adverse experiences reported in association with the use of Sporanox 100 mg capsules. The most frequently reported were of a gastro-intestinal origin, such as dyspepsia, nausea, abdominal pain and constipation. Less frequently reported adverse experiences include headache, reversible increases in hepatic enzymes, menstrual disorder, dizziness and allergic reactions (such as pruritus, rash, urticaria and angio-oedema).

Isolated cases of peripheral neuropathy and of Stevens-Johnson syndrome have also been reported; a causality for the latter was not established.

Especially in patients receiving prolonged (= approximately 1 month) treatment, most of whom had major underlying pathology and multiple concomitant medications, cases of hypokalaemia, oedema, hepatitis and hair loss have been observed

Overdose: No data are available. In the event of accidental overdosage, supportive measures should be employed. Within the first hour after ingestion, gastric lavage may be performed. Activated charcoal may be given if considered appropriate. Itraconazole cannot be removed by haemodialysis. No specific antidote is available.

Pharmacological properties
Pharmacodynamic properties: Pharmacotherapeutic classification: J02A C02 (Antimycotics for systemic use, triazole derivatives).

In vitro studies demonstrate that itraconazole, a triazole derivative, inhibits the growth of a broad range of fungi pathogenic for humans at concentrations usually ranging from ≤ 0.025–0.8 μg/ml. These include: *Candida albicans*, many *Candida non-albicans* spp., *Aspergillus* spp., *Trichosporon* spp., *Geotrichum* spp., *Cryptococcus neoformans*, dermatophytes and many dematiaceous fungi such as *Fonsecaea* spp., *Histoplasma* spp., Pseudallescheria boydii and Penicullium marneffei.

Candida glabrata and *Candida tropicalis* are generally the least susceptible Candida species, with some isolates showing unequivocal resistance to itraconazole *in vitro*.

The principal fungus types that are not inhibited by itraconazole are *Zygomycetes* (eg *Rhizopus* spp., *Rhizomucor* spp., *Mucor* spp. and *Absidia* spp.), *Fusarium* spp., *Scedosporium* spp. and *Scopulariopsis* spp. *In vitro* studies have demonstrated that itraconazole impairs the synthesis of ergosterol in fungal cells. Ergosterol is a vital cell membrane component in fungi. Impairment of its synthesis ultimately results in an anti-fungal effect.

Pharmacokinetic properties: The oral bioavailability of Sporanox liquid is maximal when it is taken without food. During chronic administration, steady-state is reached after 1–2 weeks. Peak plasma levels are observed 2 hours (fasting for at least 2 hours) to 5 hours (with food) following the oral administration. After repeated once a day administration of itraconazole 200 mg in fasting condition, steady-state plasma concentrations of itraconazole fluctuated between 1 and 2 μg/ml (trough to peak). When the oral solution is taken with food, steady-state plasma concentrations of itraconazole are about 25% lower.

The plasma protein binding of itraconazole is 99.8%. Itraconazole is extensively distributed into tissues which are prone to fungal invasion. Concentrations in lung, kidney, liver, bone, stomach, spleen and muscle were found to be two to three times higher than the corresponding plasma concentration.

Itraconazole is extensively metabolised by the liver into a large number of metabolites. One of the metabolites is hydroxy-itraconazole, which has in vitro a comparable antifungal activity to itraconazole. Plasma levels of hydroxy-itraconazole are about twice as high as those of itraconazole.

After repeated oral administration, elimination of itraconazole from plasma is biphasic with a terminal half-life of 1.5 days. Faecal excretion of the parent drug varies between 3-18% of the dose. Renal excretion of the parent drug is less than 0.03% of the dose. About 35% of the dose is excreted as metabolites in the urine within 1 week.

Preclinical safety data: Hydroxypropyl-β-cyclodextrin (HP-β-CD)

Single and repeated dose toxicity studies in mice, rats and dogs indicate a wide safety margin after oral and intravenous administration of HP-β-CD. Most effects were adaptive in nature (histological changes in the urinary tract, softening of faeces related to the osmotic water retention in the large intestine, activation of the mononuclear phagocyte system) and showed good reversibility. Slight liver changes occurred at doses of about 30 times the proposed human dose of HP-β-CD.

HP-β-CD has no antifertile, no direct embryotoxic and no teratogenic effect, and is not mutagenic.

In the rat carcinogenicity study, an increased incidence of neoplasms in the large intestine (at 5000 mg/kg/day) and in the exocrine pancreas (from 500 mg/kg/day) were seen.

Development of the pancreatic tumours is related to the mitogenic action of cholecystokinin in rats. This finding was not observed in the mouse carcinogenicity study, nor in a 12-month toxicity study in dogs or in a 2-year toxicity study in female cynomolgus monkeys. There is no evidence that cholecystokinin has a mitogenic action in man. Based on body surface comparisons, the exposure to humans of HP-β-CD at the recommended clinical dose of Sporanox liquid, is approximately equivalent to 1.7 times the exposure at the lowest dose in the rat study.

Pharmaceutical particulars

List of excipients: Hydroxypropyl-β-cyclodextrin; sorbitol; propylene glycol; hydrochloric acid; cherry flavour 1; cherry flavour 2; caramel; sodium saccharin; sodium hydroxide; purified water.

Incompatibilities: None known.

Shelf life: 12 months as packaged for sale.
1 month after first opening the container.

Special precautions for storage: Store at 25°C or below.

Nature and contents of container: 150 ml amber glass bottle, with child resistant polypropylene screw cap and LDPE liner ring.

Instructions for use/handling: Sporanox liquid is supplied in bottles with a child-proof cap, and should be opened as follows: push the plastic screw cap down while turning it counter clockwise.

Marketing authorisation number 0242/0307

Date of approval/revision of SPC July 1998

Legal category POM.

SPORANOX*-PULSE

Qualitative and quantitative composition Itraconazole 100 mg.

Pharmaceutical form Capsule (Size 0): opaque blue cap and pink transparent body containing cream coloured coated beads.

Clinical particulars

Therapeutic indications: Onychomycosis caused by dermatophytes and/or yeasts.

Tinea pedis and/or tinea manuum.

Posology and method of administration: Sporanox-Pulse is for oral administration and must be taken immediately after a meal for maximal absorption.

Treatment schedules in adults are as follows:

Indication	*Dose*	*Remarks*
Tinea pedis and/ or tinea manuum	1 pulse treatment	A pulse treatment consists of 200 mg bd for 7 days.
Onychomycosis – fingernails	2 pulse treatments	Pulse treatments are separated by a 3-week drug-free interval
Onychomycosis – toenails	3 pulse treatments	

Impaired absorption in AIDS and neutropenic patients may lead to low itraconazole blood levels and lack of efficacy. In such cases blood level monitoring is indicated.

In children (below 12 years): There are inadequate data on Sporanox-Pulse in children for its use to be recommended, unless the potential benefits outweigh the risks.

In elderly: As for use in children.

Contra-indications: When administered at high doses to pregnant rats (40 mg/kg/day) and mice (80 mg/kg/day), itraconazole was shown to cause abnormalities of foetal development. No data are available in human pregnancy, and itraconazole is therefore contraindicated in pregnancy. Adequate contraceptive precautions should be taken by women of childbearing potential during therapy and for one menstrual cycle after stopping therapy.

Itraconazole is also contraindicated in patients who have shown hypersensitivity to itraconazole, other azole antifungal agents or any of the excipients.

The drugs terfenadine, astemizole, cisapride, HMG-CoA reductase inhibitors such as simvastatin, oral midazolam or triazolam should not be given concurrently with itraconazole (see also interactions).

Special warnings and special precautions for use: Absorption is impaired when the gastric acidity is decreased. In patients also receiving acid neutralising medicines (eg aluminium hydroxide) these should be administered at least 2 hours after the intake of Sporanox-Pulse. In patients with achlorhydria such as certain AIDS patients and patients on secretion suppressors (eg H_2-antagonists, proton-pump inhibitors) it is advisable to administer Sporanox-Pulse with a cola beverage.

Rarely cases of hepatitis and cholestatic jaundice have been reported, mainly in patients treated for longer than one month. It is therefore advisable to monitor liver function in patients receiving continuous treatment of more than one month's duration. If during treatment patients develop symptoms suggestive of hepatitis such as anorexia, nausea, vomiting, fatigue, abdominal pain or dark urine, liver enzymes should be monitored promptly. If these are abnormal, treatment should be stopped. In patients with raised liver enzymes, or with a known history of liver disease, or who have experienced liver toxicity with other drugs, treatment should not be started unless the expected benefit exceeds the risk of hepatic injury. In such instances liver enzyme monitoring is necessary.

Itraconazole is predominantly metabolised in the liver. A slight decrease in oral bioavailability in cirrhotic patients has been observed, although this was not of statistical significance. The terminal half-life was however significantly increased. It is advised to monitor the itraconazole plasma concentrations in such patients and to adapt the dose when necessary.

The oral bioavailability of itraconazole may be lower in some patients with renal insufficiency (eg those receiving continuous ambulatory peritoneal dialysis). Monitoring of the itraconazole plasma levels and dose adaptation are advisable.

Isolated cases of peripheral neuropathy have been reported, predominantly during long-term treatment and in severely compromised patients. The causal relationship to itraconazole was uncertain. If neuropathy occurs which may be attributable to Sporanox-Pulse, treatment should be discontinued.

Interaction with other medicaments and other forms of interaction: Drug-interactions: Enzyme-inducing drugs such as rifampicin and phenytoin significantly reduce the oral bioavailability of itraconazole. Consequently, monitoring of the itraconazole plasma concentration is advised when enzyme-inducing agents are co-administered.

Itraconazole can inhibit the metabolism of drugs metabolised by the cytochrome 3A family. This can result in an increase and/or a prolongation of their effects, including side effects. Known examples are:

-Terfenadine, astemizole and cisapride, resulting in increased plasma levels of these drugs and predisposing to serious arrhythmias. Combination of itraconazole with terfenadine, astemizole or cisapride is contraindicated.

-Midazolam and triazolam, resulting in increased plasma levels of these drugs. Combination of itraconazole with oral midazolam or triazolam is contraindicated. If midazolam is administered intravenously (eg as premedication in surgical or investigative procedures) special care should be observed since the sedative effect may be prolonged.

- HMG-CoA reductase inhibitors such as simvastatin. These drugs should not be used during treatment with Sporanox-Pulse.
- Oral anticoagulants, digoxin, Cyclosporin A, systemic methylprednisolone, vinca-alkaloids and possibly tacrolimus. Co-administration of itraconazole and digoxin has led to increased levels of the latter drug. A rise in cyclosporin levels has also been reported in patients treated with high doses of itraconazole for several weeks. Plasma levels of digoxin and cyclosporin should therefore be monitored during concomitant administration of itraconazole and the doses adjusted accordingly. *In vitro* studies indicate that a similar interaction may occur with tacrolimus. With respect to oral anticoagulants, similar interactions have been reported and it is advisable to monitor prothrombin time and reduce the dosage of oral anticoagulants if necessary. Co-administration of itraconazole and vinca-alkaloids may potentiate the toxic effects of the latter drugs and should this occur, co-administration of these drugs should be reconsidered.
- Dihydropyridine calcium channel blockers and quinidine. Patients should be monitored for side effects, eg oedema and tinnitus/decreased hearing, respectively. If necessary, the dose of these drugs should be reduced.

Despite the fact that itraconazole is 99.8% bound to plasma proteins, there are no *in vitro* interactions on the plasma protein binding between itraconazole and imipramine, propanolol, diazepam, cimetidine, indomethacin, tolbutamide or sulphadimidine.

Itraconazole does not appear to affect the metabolism of ethinyloestradiol and norethisterone. Reports suggest that there is no interaction of itraconazole with the oral pharmacokinetics of AZT (zidovudine).

Pregnancy and lactation:

Pregnancy: Sporanox-Pulse is contra-indicated in pregnancy (see Contraindications section for further details).

Lactation: Only small amounts of itraconazole are excreted in human milk. The expected benefits of therapy should be weighed against the risks to the infant.

Effects on ability to drive and use machines: None known.

Undesirable effects: The most frequently reported adverse experiences in association with the use of Sporanox-Pulse are of gastro-intestinal origin, such as dyspepsia, nausea, abdominal pain and constipation. Less frequently reported adverse experiences include headache, reversible increases in hepatic enzymes, menstrual disorder, dizziness and allergic reactions (such as pruritus, rash, urticaria and angio-oedema). Isolated cases of peripheral neuropathy and of Stevens-Johnson syndrome have also been reported; a causality for the latter was not established.

Mainly in patients receiving prolonged treatment (ie approximately one month), most of whom had major underlying pathology and multiple concomitant medications, cases of hypokalaemia, oedema and hair loss have been observed. Hepatitis and cholestatic jaundice have been reported rarely, mainly in patients treated for longer than one month.

Overdose: In the event of overdosage, patients should be treated symptomatically with supportive measures and gastric lavage as necessary. No specific antidote is available. Itraconazole cannot be removed by haemodialysis.

Pharmacological properties

Pharmacodynamic properties: Itraconazole is a substituted triazole antimycotic with a broad spectrum of activity against Candida spp and other yeasts, dermatophytes and pathogenic fungi. It acts by impairing the synthesis of ergosterol in fungal cell membranes.

Pharmacokinetic properties: Peak plasma concentrations of itraconazole in the region of 1 mcg equiv/ml are reached 1.5–3 hrs after administration. In man the elimination half life is about 20 hrs. Oral intake immediately after a meal doubled the peak level 3–4 hrs after intake.

Peak concentrations of itraconazole in keratinous tissues, especially skin, are up to 3 times higher than in plasma. Therapeutic levels in the skin persist for up to 2–4 weeks after stopping treatment as elimination is related to dermal regeneration, rather than redistribution into the systemic circulation.

Itraconazole is extensively metabolised by the liver to a large number of metabolites, which constitute 40% of the excreted dose. Faecal excretion of parent drug varies from 3–18% of the dose, and urinary excretion of unchanged drug is less than 0.03%.

Preclinical safety data: No relevant information additional to that contained elsewhere in the Summary of Product Characteristics.

Pharmaceutical particulars
List of excipients: Sugar spheres NF; hypromellose 2910 5 mPa.s PhEur; macrogol 20000 PhEur. *Capsule shell:* titanium dioxide E171; indigo carmine E132; gelatin PhEur; erythrosine E127.

Incompatibilities: None known.

Shelf life: 36 months.

Special precautions for storage: Protect from light. Store in a dry place. Store between 15°C and 30°C.

Nature and contents of container: Perlalux tristar blister–plastic foil consisting of 3 layers:

- Polyvinylchloride on the outside;
- Low density polyethylene in the middle;
- Polyvinylidenechloride on the inside;

Aluminium foil (thickness 20 µm) coated on the inner side with colourless heat-seal Lacquer: PVC mixed polymers with acrylates, 6 g/m².

or:

PVC blister consisting of:

Polyvinylchloride 'genotherm' glass clear, thickness 250 µm;

Aluminium foil (thickness 20 µm) coated on the inner side with a colourless heat-seal Lacquer: PVC mixed polymers with acrylates, 6 g/m².

Pack size: 28 capsules.

Instructions for use/handling: Not applicable.

Marketing authorisation number 0242/0334

Date of approval/revision of SPC July 1998

Legal category POM.

STUGERON*

Presentation White, uncoated, scored tablets marked 'JANSSEN' on one side and S above 15 on the reverse. Each tablet contains 15 mg cinnarizine. Stugeron tablets also contain lactose and sucrose but do not contain any colours.

Uses Stugeron is used for the control of vestibular disorders such as vertigo, tinnitus, nausea and vomiting as seen in Meniere's disease.

Dosage and administration Stugeron is for oral administration and may be sucked, chewed or swallowed whole by both adults and children according to the following dosage regimen :

Vestibular symptoms: Adults and children over 12: 2 tablets three times a day.

Children 5-12 years: one half the adult dose.

Use in elderly: As for adults.

Stugeron should preferably be taken after meals. These doses should not be exceeded.

Contra-indications, warnings, etc
Contra-indications: Stugeron should not be given to patients with known hypersensitivity to cinnarizine.

Warnings: As with other antihistamines, Stugeron may cause epigastric discomfort; taking it after meals may diminish gastric irritation. In patients with Parkinson's disease, Stugeron should only be given if the advantages outweigh the possible risk of aggravating this disease.

Stugeron may cause drowsiness especially at the start of treatment; patients affected in this way should not drive or operate machinery.

Drug interactions: Concurrent use of alcohol, CNS depressants or tricyclic antidepressants may potentiate the sedative effects of either these drugs or of Stugeron.

Because of its antihistamine effect, Stugeron may prevent an otherwise positive reaction to dermal reactivity indicators if used within 4 days prior to skin testing.

Use in pregnancy: The safety of Stugeron in human pregnancy has not been established although studies in animals have not demonstrated teratogenic effects. As with other drugs, it is not advisable to administer Stugeron in pregnancy.

Use in lactation: There are no data on the excretion of Stugeron in human breast milk: use of Stugeron is not recommended in nursing mothers.

Side effects: Drowsiness and gastro-intestinal disturbances may occur. These are usually transient.

In rare cases, headache, dry mouth, weight gain, perspiration or allergic reactions may occur. Very rare cases of lichen planus, lupus-like skin reactions and cholestatic jaundice have been reported.

Rare cases of aggravation or appearance of extrapyramidal symptoms (sometimes associated with depressive feelings) have been described, predominantly in elderly people during prolonged therapy. The treatment should be discontinued in such cases.

Overdosage: Vomiting, drowsiness, coma, tremor and hypotonia may occur.

There is no specific antidote to Stugeron but in the event of overdosage, gastric lavage and the administration of activated charcoal may help.

Pharmaceutical precautions Store at room temperature.

Legal category P.

Package quantities Stugeron tablets each containing 15 mg cinnarizine are supplied in packs of 100.

Further information Nil.

Product licence number 0242/5009R.

Legal category P.

STUGERON* FORTE 75 mg

Qualitative and quantitative composition Each capsule contains cinnarizine 75 mg.

Pharmaceutical form Orange and yellow capsule.

Clinical particulars
Therapeutic indications: Long term management of symptoms of peripheral arterial disease, including intermittent claudication, rest pain, muscular cramps and vasospastic disorders, eg Raynaud's disease.

Posology and method of administration: For oral administration.

Stugeron Forte should preferably be taken after meals.

Adults: Starting dose: One capsule three times daily.

Maintenance dose: Once capsule two or three times daily, according to response.

These doses should not be exceeded.

Peripheral arterial disease is slow to improve with any form of drug treatment. Maximum benefit with Stugeron Forte will not be felt until after several weeks of continuous treatment, although significant improvement in blood flow has frequently been demonstrated after one week.

Elderly: As for adults.

Children: Not recommended.

Contra-indications: Stugeron Forte should not be given to patients with known hypersensitivity to cinnarizine.

Special warnings and special precautions for use: Stugeron Forte has not been found to reduce blood pressure significantly. However, the drug should be used with reasonable caution in hypotensive patients.

As with other antihistamines, Stugeron Forte may cause epigastric discomfort; taking it after meals may diminish gastric irritation.

In patients with Parkinson's disease, Stugeron Forte should only be given if the advantages outweigh the possible risk of aggravating this disease.

Interaction with other medicaments and other forms of interaction: Concurrent use of alcohol, CNS depressants or tricyclic antidepressants may potentiate the sedative effects of either these drugs or of Stugeron Forte.

Because of its antihistamine effect, Stugeron Forte may prevent an otherwise positive reaction to dermal reactivity indicators if used within 4 days prior to testing.

Pregnancy and lactation: The safety of Stugeron Forte in human pregnancy has not been established although studies in animals have not demonstrated teratogenic effects. As with other drugs, it is not advisable to administer Stugeron Forte in pregnancy.

There are no data on the excretion of Stugeron Forte in human breast milk. Use of Stugeron Forte is not recommended in nursing mothers.

Effects on ability to drive and use machines: Stugeron Forte may cause drowsiness, especially at the start of treatment. Patients affected in this way should not drive or operate machinery.

Undesirable effects: Drowsiness and gastro-intestinal disturbances may occur. These are usually transient.

Rare cases of weight gain, headache, dry mouth, perspiration or allergic reactions may occur.

Very rare cases of lichen planus, lupus-like skin reactions and cholestatic jaundice have been reported.

Rare cases of aggravation or appearance of extrapyramidal symptoms (sometimes associated with depressive feelings) have been described, predominately in elderly people during prolonged treatment. The treatment should be discontinued in such cases.

Overdose: Vomiting, drowsiness, coma, tremor and hypotonia may occur.

There is no specific antidote to Stugeron Forte but in the event of overdosage, gastric lavage and the administration of activated charcoal may help.

Pharmacological properties
Pharmacodynamic properties: Cinnarizine's actions in the treatment of peripheral vascular disease are due to its anti-vasoconstrictor properties, its action on blood hyperviscosity and its anti-ischaemic effect. Anti-vasoconstriction is thought to be through a calcium blocker mechanism, and is evident selectively in vascular smooth muscle. Increased peripheral muscle blood flow may be mediated by prevention of calcium entry into ischaemic erythrocytes, thereby preserving flexibility.

Pharmacokinetic properties: After a single 75 mg dose of cinnarizine, peak plasma levels of 160 ± 130 ng/ml occurred after a mean time of 3.4 hours. Plasma concentrations declined with a half life of 3.04 hours. The mean area under the curve was 925 ± 603 µg/ml/hr. Absorption may be varied between subjects–the highest peak concentrations being 19 times the lowest value in one study. Less than 20% of isotopically labelled cinnarizine appears in the urine and about 40% in the faeces.

Preclinical safety data: No relevant information additional to that contained elsewhere in the Summary of Product Characteristics.

Pharmaceutical particulars
List of excipients: Lactose, hydrous PhEur; corn starch PhEur; talc PhEur; magnesium stearate PhEur. *Capsule cap:* titanium dioxide (E171) PhEur; orange yellow S (E110) PhEur; erythrosine (E127) FP; gelatin PhEur. *Capsule body:* titanium dioxide (E171) PhEur; yellow ferric oxide (E172) NF; gelatin PhEur.

Incompatibilities: None known.

Shelf life: 60 months.

Special precautions for storage: None.

Nature and contents of container: Blisters consisting of: Aluminium foil hermetalu, thickness 20 µm; Perlalux tristar, PVC 200 µm, LDPE 25 µm and PVDC 90 g/m², containing 100 capsules.

Instructions for use/handling: Not applicable.

Marketing authorisation number 0242/0008

Date of approval/revision of SPC August 1997

Legal category P.

SUBLIMAZE*

Qualitative and quantitative composition Fentanyl citrate 78.5 micrograms equivalent to 50 micrograms per ml fentanyl base.

Pharmaceutical form Injection.

Clinical particulars
Therapeutic indications: Sublimaze is a narcotic analgesic used:

a. In low doses to provide analgesia during short surgical procedures.

b. In high doses as an analgesic/respiratory depressant in patients requiring assisted ventilation.

c. In combination with a neuroleptic in the technique of neuroleptanalgesia.

d. In the treatment of severe pain, such as the pain of myocardial infarction.

Posology and method of administration:
Route of administration

Intravenous administration either as a bolus or by infusion.

Intramuscular administration.

Sublimaze, by the intravenous route, can be administered as a bolus or as an infusion to both adults and children. The dose of Sublimaze should be individualised according to age, body weight, physical status, underlying pathological condition, use of other drugs and type of surgery and anaesthesia. The usual dose is as follows:

	ADULTS		*CHILDREN*	
	Initial	*Supplemental*	*Initial*	*Supplemental*
Spontaneous respiration	50-200 mcg	50 mcg	3-5 mcg/kg	1 mcg/kg
Assisted ventilation	300-3500 mcg	100-200 mcg	15 mcg/kg	1-3 mcg/kg

Doses in excess of 200 mcg are for use in anaesthesia only. As a premedicant, 1-2 ml Sublimaze may be given intramuscularly 45 minutes before induction of anaesthesia.

After intravenous administration in unpremedicated adult patients 2 ml Sublimaze may be expected to provide sufficient analgesia for 10–20 minutes in surgical procedures involving low pain intensity. 10 ml Sublimaze injected as a bolus gives analgesia lasting about one hour. The analgesia produced is sufficient for surgery involving moderately painful procedures. Giving a dose of 50 mcg/kg Sublimaze will provide intense analgesia for some four to six hours, for intensely stimulating surgery.

Sublimaze may also be given as an infusion. In ventilated patients, a loading dose of Sublimaze may be given as a fast infusion of approximately 1 mcg/kg/min may be given for the first 10 minutes followed by an infusion of approximately 0.1 mcg/kg/min. Alternatively the loading dose of Sublimaze may be given as a bolus. Infusion rates should be titrated to individual patient response, lower infusion rates may be adequate. Unless it is planned to ventilate post-operatively, the infusion should be terminated at about 40 minutes before the end of surgery.

Lower infusion rates eg 0.05–0.08 mcg/kg/minute are necessary if spontaneous ventilation is to be maintained. Higher infusion rates (up to 3 mcg/kg/minute) have been used in cardiac surgery.

When judging the dose it is important to assess the likely degree of surgical stimulation, the effect of premedicant drugs, and the duration of the procedure.

Use in elderly and debilitated patients: It is wise to reduce the dosage in the elderly and debilitated patients. The effect of the initial dose should be taken into account in determining supplemental doses.

Contra-indications: Respiratory depression, obstructive airways disease. Concurrent administration with monoamine inhibitors, or within 2 weeks of their discontinuation. Known intolerance to fentanyl or other morphinomimetics.

Special warnings and special precautions for use: Tolerance and dependence may occur. Following intravenous administration of fentanyl, a transient fall in blood pressure may occur, especially in hypovolaemic patients. Appropriate measures to maintain a stable arterial pressure should be taken.

Significant respiratory depression will occur following the administration of fentanyl in doses in excess of 200 mcg. This, and the other pharmacological effects of fentanyl, can be reversed by specific narcotic analgesics (eg naloxone). Additional doses of the latter may be necessary because the respiratory depression may last longer than the duration of action of the opioid antagonist.

Bradycardia and possibly asystole can occur in non-atropinised patients, and can be antagonised by atropine.

Muscular rigidity (morphine-like effect) may occur.

Rigidity, which may also involve the thoracic muscles, can be avoided by the following measures:

- Slow iv injection (usually sufficient for lower doses).
- Premedication with benzodiazepines.
- Use of muscle relaxants.

As with all opioid analgesics, care should be observed when administering fentanyl to patients with Myasthenia Gravis.

It is wise to reduce dosage in the elderly and debilitated patients.

In hypothyroidism, pulmonary disease, decreased respiratory reserve, alcoholism and liver or renal impairment the dosage should be titrated with care and prolonged monitoring may be required.

Patients on chronic opioid therapy or with a history of opioid abuse may require higher doses.

Administration in labour may cause respiratory depression in the new born infant.

As with all potent opioids, profound analgesia is accompanied by marked respiratory depression, which may persist into or recur in the early post-operative period. Care should be taken after large doses or infusions of fentanyl to ensure that adequate spontaneous breathing has been established and maintained before discharging the patient from the recovery area.

Resuscitation equipment and opioid antagonists should be readily available Hyperventilation during anaesthesia may alter the patients response to CO_2, thus affecting respiration postoperatively.

The use of rapid bolus injections of opioids should be avoided in patients with compromised intracerebral compliance; in such patients the transient decrease in the mean arterial pressure has occasionally been accompanied by a transient reduction of the cerebral perfusion pressure.

Interaction with other medicaments and other forms of interaction: The use of opioid premedication, barbiturates, benzodiazepines, neuroleptics, halogenic gases and other non-selective CNS depressants (eg alcohol) may enhance or prolong the respiratory depression of fentanyl.

When patients have received CNS-depressants, the dose of fentanyl required will be less than usual. Likewise, following the administration of fentanyl the dose of other CNS-depressant drugs should be reduced.

Bradycardia and possibly asystole can occur when fentanyl is combined with non-vagolytic muscle relaxants.

The concomitant use of droperidol can result in a higher incidence of hypotension.

Pregnancy and lactation: Although no teratogenic or acute embryotoxic effects have been observed in animal experiments, insufficient data are available to evaluate any harmful effects in humans. As with other drugs, possible risks should be weighed against potential benefits to the patient.

Administration during childbirth (including caesarean section) is not recommended because fentanyl crosses the placenta and the foetal respiratory centre is particularly sensitive to opioids. If fentanyl is nevertheless administered, an antidote for the child should always be at hand.

Fentanyl may enter the maternal milk. It is therefore recommended that breast feeding is not initiated within 24 hours of treatment.

Effects on ability to drive and use machines: Where early discharge is envisaged, patients should be advised not to drive or operate machinery for 24 hours following administration.

Undesirable effects: The side effects are those associated with intravenous opioids eg. respiratory depression, apnoea, muscular rigidity (which may also involve thoracic muscles), myoclonic movements, bradycardia, transient hypotension, nausea, vomiting and dizziness.

Other less frequently reported adverse reactions are:

- laryngospasm;
- allergic reactions (eg anaphylaxis, bronchospasm, pruritus, urticaria) and asystole although it is uncertain whether there is a causal relationship as several drugs were co-administered;
- secondary rebound respiratory depression has rarely been reported.

When a neuroleptic such as droperidol is used with fentanyl, the following adverse reactions may be observed: chills and/or shivering, restlessness, post-operative hallucinatory episodes and extrapyramidal symptoms.

Overdose:

Symptoms: The manifestations of fentanyl overdosage are generally an extension of its pharmacological action. Depending on the individual sensitivity, the clinical picture is determined primarily by the degree of respiratory depression, which varies from bradypnoea to apnoea.

Treatment:

- hypoventilation or apnoea: O_2 administration, assisted or controlled respiration.
- respiratory depression: Specific narcotic antagonist (eg naloxone). This does not preclude the use of immediate countermeasures.
- muscular rigidity: Intravenous neuromuscular blocking agent.

The patient should be carefully observed; body warmth and adequate fluid intake should be maintained. If hypotension is severe or if it persists, the possibility of hypovolaemia should be considered, and if present, it should be controlled with appropriate parenteral fluid administration.

Pharmacological properties

Pharmacodynamic properties: Fentanyl is a synthetic opiate with a clinical potency of 50 to 100 times that of morphine. Its onset of action is rapid and its duration of action is short. In man, a single iv dose of 0.5-1 mg/70 kg body weight immediately produces a pronounced state of surgical analgesia, respiratory depression, bradycardia and other typical morphine-like effects. The duration of action of the peak effects is about 30 minutes. All potent morphine-like drugs produce relief from pain, ventilatory depression, emesis, constipation, physical dependence, certain vagal effects and varying degrees of sedation. Fentanyl, however, differs from morphine not only by its short duration of action but also by its lack of emetic effect and minimal hypotensive activity in animals.

Pharmacokinetic properties: Some pharmacokinetic parameters for fentanyl are as follows:

Urinary excretion = 8%
Bound in plasma = 80%
Clearance (ml . min^{-1} . Kg^{-1}) = 13±2
Volume of distribution (litres/kg) = 4.0±0.4
Half life (hours) = 3.7±0.4

Preclinical safety data: Not applicable.

Pharmaceutical particulars

List of excipients: Sodium chloride; water for injections; sodium hydroxide; hydrochloric acid.

Incompatibilities: The product is chemically incompatible with the induction agents thiopentone and methohexitone because of the wide differences in pH.

Shelf life: 36 months.

Special precautions for storage: Protect from light.

Nature and contents of container: Colourless glass ampoules (PhEur, USP Type 1).

Pack size: packs of 10 of 2 ml and 10 ml ampoules.

Instructions for use/handling: Not applicable (store as a CD).

Marketing authorisation number 0242/5001R

Date of approval/revision of SPC March 1997

Legal category POM.

SULTRIN* TRIPLE SULFA CREAM

Qualitative and quantitative composition Sulphabenzamide 3.7% w/w; sulphacetamide 2.86% w/w; sulphathiazole 3.42%w/w.

Pharmaceutical form White to off-white cream.

Clinical particulars

Therapeutic indications: Treatment of infections caused by *Haemophilus vaginalis.*

Posology and method of administration: For intravaginal administration.

One applicatorful intravaginally twice daily for ten days. The dosage may then be reduced to once a day, if necessary.

Contra-indications: Sulphonamide sensitivity. Kidney disease. Known hypersensitivity to peanuts. Throughout pregnancy and during the nursing period because sulphonamides cross the placenta, are excreted in breast milk and may cause kernicterus.

Special warnings and special precautions for use: The safety and effectiveness for use in children have not been established.

Caution should be used in prescribing the product to elderly patients who potentially may have impaired renal function.

Patients should be observed for skin rash or evidence of systemic toxicity and, if these develop, the medication should be discontinued.

Interaction with other medicaments and other forms of interaction: Contact should be avoided between contraceptive diaphragms or latex condoms and Sultrin Triple Sulfa Cream, since the rubber may be damaged.

Pregnancy and lactation: The safe use of sulphonamides in pregnancy has not been established. The teratogenic potential of most sulphonamides has not been thoroughly investigated in either animals or humans. However, a significant increase in the incidence of cleft palate and other bony abnormalities of offspring has been observed when certain sulphonamides of the short, intermediate and long-acting types were given to pregnant rats and mice at high oral doses (7 to 25 times the human therapeutic dose).

Because sulphonamides are excreted in breast milk and may cause serious adverse reactions in breast feeding infants, a decision should be made whether to discontinue breast feeding or to discontinue Sultrin, depending on the importance of the drug to the mother.

See *Contra-indications.*

Effects on ability to drive and use machines: None.

Undesirable effects: Local irritation and/or allergy have occasionally been reported. As sulphonamides may be absorbed from the vaginal mucosa, the following adverse effects associated with such compounds should be borne in mind:

Hypersensitivity reactions: Skin rashes; severe and potentially fatal skin reactions such as toxic epidermal necrolysis (Lyell's Syndrome) and erythema multiforme bullosa (Stevens-Johnson Syndrome).

Blood dyscrasias: Including agranulocytosis and aplastic anaemia.

Renal failure.

Overdose: If accidental ingestion of large quantities of the product occurs, an appropriate method of gastric emptying may be used if considered desirable. Elimination of sulphonamides in the urine may be assisted by giving alkalis, such as sodium bicarbonate, and increasing fluid intake.

Pharmacological properties

Pharmacodynamic properties: Sulphonamides are structural analogs and competitive antagonists of para-aminobenzoic acid (PABA) and prevent normal bacterial utilisation of PABA for the synthesis of folic acid. Sulphonamides are competitive inhibitors of the bacterial enzyme responsible for the incorporation of PABA into dihydropteroic acid, the immediate precursor of folic acid. The three sulphonamides exert optimal bacteriostatic action at different pH levels, as follows: Sulphathiazole pH 7.0; Sulphacetamide pH 5.2; Sulphabenzamide pH 4.6.

Pharmacokinetic properties: Studies with sulphacetamide and sulphathiazole have indicated that sulphonamides are absorbed in low and variable amounts from the vagina. Once absorbed, sulphonamides become distributed throughout the tissues and pass the placental barrier.

Elimination occurs partly as unchanged drug and partly as metabolites with the major route of elimination via the urine. Small amounts are excreted in the faeces, bile and milk.

Preclinical safety data: No relevant information additional to that contained elsewhere in the Summary of Product Characteristics.

Pharmaceutical particulars

List of excipients: Arachis oil; cetyl alcohol; cholesterol; Clearate™ paste (lecithin); Tegacid™; Regular (glyceryl monostearate) (E471); wool fat (anhydrous lanolin); methyl parahydroxybenzoate (E218); phosphoric acid (E338); propylene glycol; propyl parahydroxybenzoate (E216); stearic acid (E570); diethylaminoethyl stearamide; urea; purified water.

Incompatibilities: None known.

Shelf life: 36 months.

Special precautions for storage: Store at room temperature (not exceeding 25°C).

Nature and contents of container: Tube of epoxy resin lacquered aluminium, with polyethylene cap, containing 80 g cream.

Instructions for use/handling: Not applicable.

Marketing authorisation number 0242/0273

Date of approval/revision of SPC August 1998

Legal category POM.

TOPAMAX* 

Qualitative and quantitative composition Topamax (topiramate) is available in tablets for oral administration containing 25, 50, 100 and 200 mg of topiramate.

Pharmaceutical form Topamax is available as embossed, round, coated tablets in the following strengths and colours: 25 mg white, 50 mg light yellow, 100 mg yellow and 200 mg salmon. The tablets will be imprinted as follows:

25 mg "TOP" on one side; "25" on the other
50 mg "TOP" on one side; "50" on the other
100 mg "TOP" on one side; "100" on the other
200 mg "TOP" on one side; "200" on the other

Clinical particulars

Therapeutic indications: Topamax is indicated as adjunctive therapy for adults and children over 2 years of age who are inadequately controlled on conventional first line antiepileptic drugs for: partial seizures with or without secondarily generalised seizures; seizures associated with Lennox Gastaut Syndrome and primary generalised tonic-clonic seizures.

Posology and method of administration: The minimal effective dose is 200 mg per day. The usual total daily dose is 200 mg to 400 mg in two divided doses. Some patients may require doses up to 800 mg per day which is the maximum recommended dose. It is recommended that therapy be initiated at a low dose, followed by titration to an effective dose.

Titration should begin at 50 mg daily for one week. A lower dose may be used. The total daily dose should then be increased by 50 mg increments at weekly intervals and should be taken in two divided doses. If the patient is unable to tolerate the titration regimen then lower increments or longer intervals between increments may be used. Dose titration should be guided by clinical outcome.

Children aged 2–16 years: The recommended total daily dose of Topamax (topiramate) is approximately 5 to 9 mg/kg/day in two divided doses. Titration should begin at 25 mg nightly for the first week. The dosage should then be increased at 1- or 2-week intervals by increments of 1 to 3 mg/kg/day (administered in two divided doses), to achieve optimal clinical response. Dose titration should be guided by clinical outcome.

Daily doses up to 30 mg/kg/day have been studied and were generally well tolerated.

Tablets should not be broken. Topamax can be taken without regard to meals.

It is not necessary to monitor topiramate plasma concentrations to optimise Topamax therapy.

These dosing recommendations apply to children and to all adults, including the elderly, in the absence of underlying renal disease. (See SPECIAL WARNINGS AND SPECIAL PRECAUTIONS FOR USE).

Since Topamax is removed from plasma by haemodialysis, a supplemental dose of Topamax equal to approximately one-half the daily dose should be administered on haemodialysis days. The supplemental dose should be administered in divided doses at the beginning and completion of the haemodialysis procedure. The supplemental dose may differ based on the characteristics of the dialysis equipment being used.

Contra-indications: Hypersensitivity to any component of this product.

Special warnings and special precautions for use: Antiepileptic drugs, including Topamax, should be withdrawn gradually to minimise the potential of increased seizure frequency. In clinical trials, dosages were decreased by 100 mg/day at weekly intervals. In some patients, withdrawal was accelerated without complications.

The major route of elimination of unchanged topiramate and its metabolites is via the kidney. Renal elimination is dependent on renal function and is independent of age. Patients with moderate or severe renal impairment may take 10 to 15 days to reach steady-state plasma concentrations as compared to 4 to 8 days in patients with normal renal function.

As with all patients, the titration schedule should be guided by clinical outcome (ie seizure control, avoidance of side effects) with the knowledge that subjects with known renal impairment may require a longer time to reach steady state at each dose.

Some patients, especially those with a predisposition to nephrolithiasis, may be at increased risk for renal stone formation. Adequate hydration is recommended to reduce this risk.

Risk factors for nephrolithiasis include prior stone formation, a family history of nephrolithiasis and hypercalciuria. None of these risk factors can reliably predict stone formation during topiramate treatment. In addition, patients taking other medication associated with nephrolithiasis may be at increased risk.

In hepatically impaired patients, topiramate should be administered with caution as the clearance of topiramate may be decreased.

A dietary supplement or increased food intake may be considered if the patient is losing weight or has inadequate weight gain while on this medication.

Interaction with other medicaments and other forms of interaction:

Effects of Topamax on other antiepileptic drugs: The addition of Topamax to other antiepileptic drugs (phenytoin, carbamazepine, valproic acid, phenobarbital, primidone) has no clinically significant effect on their steady-state plasma concentrations, except in some patients where the addition of Topamax to phenytoin may result in an increase of plasma concentrations of phenytoin. Consequently, it is advised that any patient on phenytoin should have phenytoin levels monitored.

Effects of other antiepileptic drugs on Topamax: Phenytoin and carbamazepine decrease the plasma concentration of topiramate. The addition or withdrawal of phenytoin or carbamazepine to Topamax therapy may require an adjustment in dosage of the latter. This should be done by titrating to clinical effect.

The addition or withdrawal of valproic acid does not produce clinically significant changes in plasma concentrations of topiramate and, therefore, does not warrant dosage adjustment of Topamax.

The results of these interactions are summarised in the following table:

AED Coadministered	*AED Concentration*	*Topiramate Concentration*
Phenytoin	<->**	↓
Carbamazepine (CBZ)	<->	↓
Valproic Acid	<->	<->
Phenobarbital	<->	NS
Primidone	<->	NS

<-> = No effect on plasma concentration
** = Plasma concentrations increase in some patients
↓ = Plasma concentrations decrease
NS = Not studied
AED = antiepileptic drug

Other drug interactions

Digoxin: In a single-dose study, serum digoxin area under plasma concentration curve (AUC) decreased 12% due to concomitant administration of Topamax. The clinical relevance of this observation has not been established. When Topamax is added or withdrawn in patients on digoxin therapy, careful attention should be given to the routine monitoring of serum digoxin.

Oral contraceptives: In an interaction study with a combined oral contraceptive, Topamax increased plasma clearance of the oestrogenic component significantly. Consequently, and bearing in mind the potential risk of teratogenicity, patients should receive a preparation containing not less than 50 μg of oestrogen or use some alternative non-hormonal method of contraception. Patients taking oral contraceptives should be asked to report any change in their bleeding patterns.

Others: Topamax, when used concomitantly with other agents predisposing to nephrolithiasis, may increase the risk of nephrolithiasis. While using Topamax, agents like these should be avoided since they may create a physiological environment that increases the risk of renal stone formation. The interaction with benzodiazepines has not been studied.

Pregnancy and lactation: As with other antiepileptic drugs, topiramate was teratogenic in mice, rats and rabbits. In rats, topiramate crosses the placental barrier.

There are no studies using Topamax in pregnant women. However, Topamax should not be used during pregnancy unless, in the opinion of the physician, the potential benefit outweighs the potential risk to the foetus. It is recommended that women of child bearing potential use adequate contraception. Topamax should not be used during breast feeding.

Effects on ability to drive and use machines: As with all antiepileptic drugs, Topamax may produce central nervous system related adverse events. Drowsiness is likely and Topamax may be more sedating than other antiepileptic drugs. These adverse events could potentially be dangerous in patients driving a vehicle or operating machinery, particularly until such time as the individual patient's experience with the drug is established.

Undesirable effects: Adults: Since Topamax has most frequently been co-administered with other antiepileptic agents, it is not possible to determine which agents, if any, are associated with adverse effects. In double blind clinical trials, some of which included a rapid titration period, adverse events which occurred with a frequency greater than or equal to 5% and with a higher incidence in the topiramate-treated adult patients than in placebo included: abdominal pain, ataxia, anorexia, asthenia, confusion, difficulty with concentration/attention, difficulty with memory, diplopia, dizziness, fatigue, language problems, nausea, nystagmus, paraesthesia, psychomotor slowing, somnolence, speech disorders/related speech problems, abnormal vision and weight decrease. Topamax may cause agitation and emotional lability (which may manifest mood problems and nervousness) and depression. Other less common adverse effects include, gait abnormal, aggressive reaction, apathy, cognitive problems, co-ordination problems, leucopenia, psychotic symptoms (such as hallucinations) and taste perversion.

Isolated cases of venous thromboembolic events have been reported. A causal association with the drug has not been established.

Paediatrics: In double blind clinical trials, some of which included a rapid titration period, adverse events which occurred with a frequency greater than or equal to 5% and with a higher incidence in the topiramate-treated paediatric patients than in placebo included: somnolence, anorexia, fatigue, insomnia, nervousness, personality disorder (behaviour problems), difficulty with concentration/attention, aggressive reaction, weight decrease, gait abnormal, mood problems, ataxia, saliva increased, nausea, difficulty with memory, hyperkinesia, dizziness, speech disorders/related speech problems and paraesthesia.

Adverse events that occurred less frequently but were considered potentially medically relevant included: emotional lability, agitation, apathy, cognitive problems, psychomotor slowing, confusion, hallucination, depression and leucopenia.

Topamax increases the risk of nephrolithiasis especially in those with a predisposition (see Special Warnings and Special Precautions for Use). In the initial clinical trials none of the calculi required open surgery and three-quarters were passed spontaneously. Most of the patients opted to continue treatment despite nephrolithiasis.

Overdose: In acute overdose with Topamax, if the ingestion is recent, the stomach should be emptied immediately by lavage or by induction of emesis. *In vitro*, activated charcoal has not been shown to absorb topiramate, therefore, its use in overdosage is not recommended. Supportive treatment should be used as appropriate. Haemodialysis is an effective means of removing topiramate from the body. However, in cases of acute overdosage, including doses of over 20 g in one individual, haemodialysis has not been necessary.

Pharmacological properties

Pharmacodynamic properties: Topiramate is a novel antiepileptic agent classified as a sulphamate-substituted monosaccharide. Three pharmacological properties of topiramate have been identified that may contribute to its anticonvulsant activity:

Topiramate reduces the frequency at which action

potentials are generated when neurones are subjected to a sustained depolarisation indicative of a state-dependent blockade of voltage-sensitive sodium channels.

Topiramate markedly enhances the activity of GABA at some types of GABA receptors but has no apparent effect on the activity of N-methyl-D-aspartate (NMDA) at the NMDA receptor subtype.

Topiramate weakly antagonises the excitatory activity of kainate/AMPA subtype of glutamate receptor.

In addition, topiramate inhibits some isoenzymes of carbonic anhydrase. This pharmacologic effect is much weaker than that of acetazolamide, a known carbonic anhydrase inhibitor, and is not thought to be a major component of topiramate's antiepileptic activity.

Pharmacokinetic properties: Topiramate is rapidly and well absorbed. Based on recovery of radioactivity from the urine, the mean extent of absorption of a 100 mg dose of ^{14}C topiramate was at least 81%. There is no clinically significant effect of food on topiramate. Generally 13-17% of topiramate is bound to plasma proteins. The mean apparent volume of distribution has been measured as 0.55-0.8 L/kg for single doses up to 1200 mg. There is an effect of gender on the volume of distribution. Values for females are circa 50% of those for males.

Topiramate is not extensively metabolised (≈20%) in healthy volunteers. Topiramate is metabolised up to 50% in patients receiving concomitant antiepileptic therapy with known inducers of drug metabolising enzymes. Six metabolites have been isolated, characterised and identified from plasma, urine and faeces of humans. Two metabolites, which retained most of the structure of topiramate, were tested and found to have little or no anticonvulsant activity.

In humans, the major route of elimination of unchanged topiramate and its metabolites is via the kidney. Overall, plasma clearance is approximately 20 to 30 ml/min in humans following oral administration.

Topiramate exhibits low intersubject variability in plasma concentrations and, therefore, has predictable pharmacokinetics. The pharmacokinetics of topiramate are linear with plasma clearance remaining constant and area under the plasma concentration curve increasing in a dose-proportional manner over a 100 to 400 mg single oral dose range in healthy subjects. Patients with normal renal function may take 4 to 8 days to reach steady-state plasma concentrations. The mean Cmax following multiple, twice a day oral doses of 100 mg to healthy subjects was 6.76 µg/ml. Following administration of multiple doses of 50 mg and 100 mg of topiramate twice a day, the mean plasma elimination half-life was approximately 21 hours.

The plasma and renal clearance of topiramate are decreased in patients with impaired renal function (CL_{CR} ≤ 60 ml/min), and the plasma clearance is decreased in patients with end-stage renal disease.

Plasma clearance of topiramate is unchanged in elderly subjects in the absence of underlying renal disease.

Plasma clearance of topiramate is decreased in patients with moderate to severe hepatic impairment.

The pharmacokinetics of topiramate in children, as in adults receiving add-on therapy, are linear, with clearance independent of dose and steady-state plasma concentrations increasing in proportion to dose. Children, however, have a higher clearance and shorter elimination half-life. Consequently, the plasma concentrations of topiramate for the same mg/kg dose may be lower in children compared to adults. As in adults, hepatic enzyme inducing anti-epileptic drugs decrease the steady-state plasma concentrations.

Preclinical safety data: Acute and long-term exposure of mice, rats, dogs and rabbits to topiramate was well-tolerated.

As with other antiepileptic drugs, topiramate was teratogenic in mice, rats and rabbits. Overall numbers of fetal malformations in mice were increased for all drug-treated groups, but no significant differences or dosage-response relationships were observed for overall or specific malformations, suggesting that other factors such as maternal toxicity may be involved.

In a battery of *in vitro* and *in vivo* mutagenicity assays, topiramate did not show genotoxic potential.

Pharmaceutical particulars
List of excipients: Topamax contains the following inactive ingredients:
Lactose hydrous PhEur
Pregelatinized starch (modified) PhEur
Pregelatinized starch PhEur
Purified water
Carnauba wax PhEur
Microcrystalline cellulose PhEur
Sodium starch glycolate PhEur
Magnesium stearate PhEur
OPADRY White, Yellow, Pink, Red (depending on the colour, contains hydroxypropyl methylcellulose, titanium dioxide, polyethylene glycol, synthetic iron oxide and polysorbate 80).

Incompatibilities: None known.

Shelf life: 36 months.

Special precautions for storage: Store in a dry place at or below 25°C.

Nature and contents of container: Available in opaque containers with tamper-evident closures containing 60 tablets.

Instructions for use/handling: Not applicable

Marketing authorisation numbers
Topamax 25 mg 0242/0301
Topamax 50 mg 0242/0302
Topamax 100 mg 0242/0303
Topamax 200 mg 0242/0304

Date of approval/revision March 1998.

Legal category POM.

TRINOVUM* ORAL CONTRACEPTIVE TABLETS

Presentation Trinovum oral contraceptive tablets are 1/4 inch diameter, circular tablets with flat faces and bevelled edges. The 7 white tablets contain 500 µg norethisterone and 35 µg ethinyloestradiol and are engraved C over 535 on each face. The 7 light peach coloured tablets contain 750 µg norethisterone and 35 µg ethinyloestradiol and are engraved C over 735 on each face. The 7 peach coloured tablets contain 1.0 mg norethisterone PhEur and 35 µg ethinyloestradiol and are engraved C over 135 on each face.

Uses Contraception and the recognised indications for such oestrogen/progestogen combinations.

Action Through the mechanism of gonadotrophin suppression by the oestrogenic and progestational actions of the ingredients.

Although the primary mechanism of action is inhibition of ovulation, alterations to the cervical mucus and to the endometrium may also contribute to the efficacy of the product.

Dosage and administration It is preferable that tablet intake from the first pack is started on the first day of menstruation in which case no extra contraceptive precautions are necessary.

If menstruation has already begun (that is 2, 3 or 4 days previously), tablet taking should commence on day 5 of the menstrual period. In this case additional contraceptive precautions must be taken for the first 7 days of tablet taking. (See further information for additional contraceptive precautions).

If menstruation began more than 5 days previously then the patient should be advised to wait until her next menstrual period before starting to take Trinovum.

How to take Trinovum: One tablet is taken daily at the same time (preferably in the evening) without interruption for 21 days, followed by a break of 7 tablet-free days (a white tablet is taken every day for 7 days, then a pale peach coloured tablet every day for 7 days, then a peach coloured tablet every day for 7 days, then 7 tablet-free days). Each subsequent pack is started after the 7 tablet-free days have elapsed. Additional contraceptive precautions are not then required.

Use during pregnancy: Trinovum is contra-indicated for use during pregnancy or suspected pregnancy, since it has been suggested that combined oral contraceptives, in common with many other substances, might be capable of affecting the normal development of the child in the early stages of pregnancy. It can be definitely concluded, however, that, if a risk of abnormality exists at all, it must be very small.

Post-partum administration: Following a vaginal delivery, oral contraceptive administration to non-breast feeding mothers can be started 21 days post-partum, provided the patient is fully ambulant and there are no puerperal complications. No additional contraceptive precautions are required. If post-partum administration begins more than 21 days after delivery, additional contraceptive precautions are required for the first 7 days of pill-taking. If intercourse has taken place post-partum, oral contraceptive use should be delayed until the first day of the first menstrual period.

N.B. Mothers who are breast feeding should be advised not to use the combined pill since this may reduce the amount of breast-milk, but may be advised instead to use a progestogen-only pill (POP).

After miscarriage or abortion administration should start immediately in which case no additional contraceptive precautions are required.

Changing from a 21 day pill or another 22 day pill to Trinovum: All tablets in the old pack should be finished. The first Trinovum tablet is taken the next day i.e. no gap is left between taking tablets nor does the patient need to wait for her period to begin. Tablets should be taken as instructed in 'How to take Trinovum. Additional contraceptive precautions are not required. The patient will not have a period until the end of the first Trinovum pack, but this is not harmful, nor does it matter if she experiences some bleeding on tablet-taking days.

Changing from a combined Every Day Pill (28 day tablets) to Trinovum: Trinovum should be started after taking the last active tablet from the 'Every Day Pill' pack (ie after taking 21 or 22 tablets). The first Trinovum tablet is taken the next day ie no gap is left between taking tablets nor does the patient need to wait for her period to begin. Tablets should be taken as instructed in 'How to take Trinovum'. Additional contraceptive precautions are not required. Remaining tablets from the Every Day (ED) pack should be discarded. The patient will not have a period until the end of the first Trinovum pack, but this is not harmful, nor does it matter if she experiences some bleeding on tablet-taking days.

Changing from a Progestogen-only Pill (POP or Mini Pill) to Trinovum: The first Trinovum tablet should be taken on the first day of the period, even if the patient has already taken a mini pill on that day. Tablets should be taken as instructed in 'How to take Trinovum'. Additional contraceptive precautions are not required. All the remaining progestogen-only pills in the mini pill pack should be discarded.

If the patient is taking a (mini) pill, then she may not always have a period, especially when she is breast feeding. The first Trinovum tablet should be taken on the day after stopping the mini pill. All remaining pills in the mini pill packet must be discarded. Additional contraceptive precautions must be taken for the first 7 days.

To skip a period: To skip a period, a new pack of Trinovum should be started on the day after finishing the current pack (the patient skips the tablet-free days). Tablet-taking should be continued in the usual way. During the use of the second pack she may experience slight spotting or break-through bleeding but contraceptive protection will not be diminished provided there are no tablet omissions.

The next pack of Trinovum is started after the usual 7 tablet-free days, regardless of whether the period has completely finished or not.

Reduced reliability: The reliability of Trinovum may be reduced under the following circumstances.

Forgotten tablets: For further advice on the above please see precautions and warnings.

Vomiting or diarrhoea: For further advice on the above, please see precautions and warnings.

Interactions: For further advice on the above, please see precautions and warnings.

Contra-indications, warnings, etc
Absolute contra-indications: Pregnancy or suspected pregnancy (that cannot yet be excluded).

Circulatory disorders (cardiovascular or cerebrovascular) such as thrombophlebitis and thromboembolic processes (or a history of these conditions), moderate to severe hypertension, hyperlipoproteinaemia. In addition the presence of more than one of the risk factors for arterial disease which are discussed under 'Serious adverse reactions'.

Severe liver disease, cholestatic jaundice or hepatitis (viral or non-viral) or a history of these conditions if the results of liver function tests have failed to return to normal, and for 3 months after liver function tests have been found to be normal; a history of jaundice of pregnancy or jaundice due to the use of steroids, Rotor syndrome and Dubin-Johnson syndrome, hepatic cell tumours and porphyria.

Cholelithiasis.

Known or suspected oestrogen-dependent tumours, (see 'Serious Adverse Reactions'); endometrial hyperplasia; undiagnosed vaginal bleeding.

Systemic lupus erythematosus or a history of this condition.

A history during pregnancy or previous use of steroids of: severe pruritus; herpes gestationis; a manifestation or deterioration of otosclerosis.

Relative contra-indications: If any of the relative contra-indications listed below is present, the benefits of oestrogen/progestogen-containing preparations must be weighed against the possible risk for each individual case and the patient kept under close supervision. In case of aggravation or appearance of any of these conditions whilst the patient is taking the pill, its use should be discontinued.

- Conditions implicating an increasing risk of developing venous thromboembolic complications, eg severe varicose veins or prolonged immobilisation or major surgery (see Precautions and Warnings).
- Disorders of coagulation.
- Presence of any risk factor for arterial disease eg

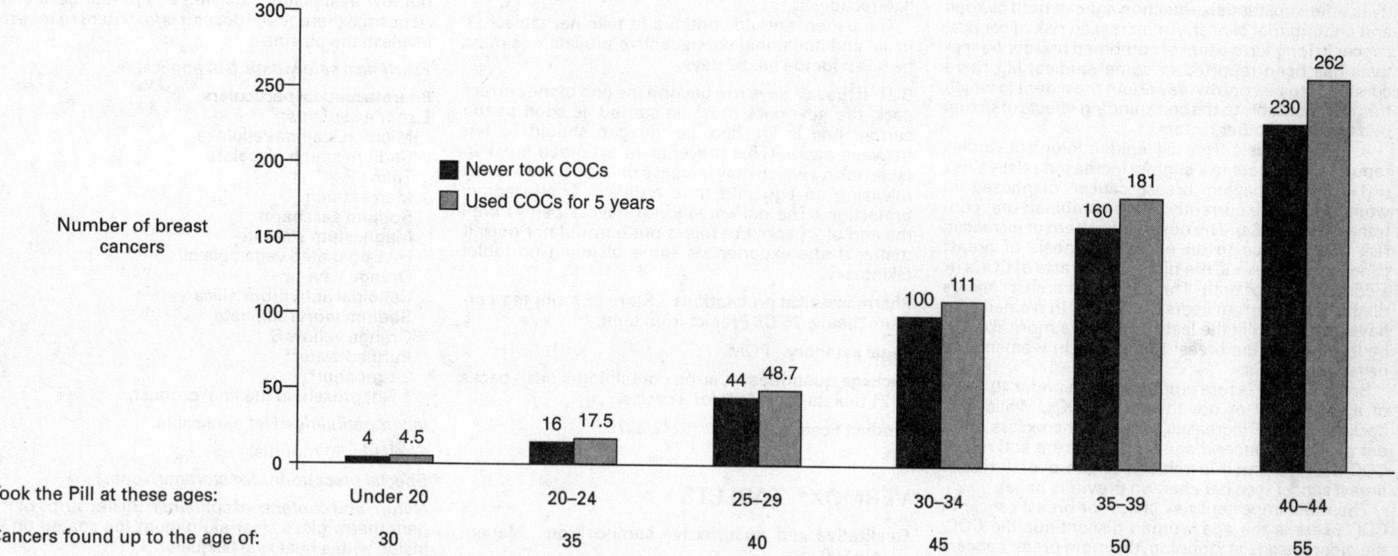

smoking, hyperlipidaemia or hypertension (see 'Serious Adverse Reactions').

- Other conditions associated with an increased risk of circulatory disease such as latent or overt cardiac failure, renal dysfunction, or a history of these conditions.
- Epilepsy or a history of this condition.
- Migraine or a history of this condition.
- A history of cholelithiasis.
- Presence of any risk factor for oestrogen-dependent tumours; oestrogen-sensitive gynaecological disorders such as uterine fibromyomata and endometriosis (see also under 'Serious Adverse Reactions').
- Diabetes mellitus.
- Severe depression or a history of this condition. If this is accompanied by a disturbance in tryptophan metabolism, administration of vitamin B6 might be of therapeutic value.
- Sickle cell haemoglobinopathy, since under certain circumstances, e.g. during infections or anoxia, oestrogen-containing preparations may induce thromboembolic process in patients with this condition.
- If the results of liver function tests become abnormal, use should be discontinued.

Precautions and warnings

Reduced reliability: When Trinovum is taken according to the directions for use the occurrence of pregnancy is highly unlikely. However, the reliability of oral contraceptives may be reduced under the following circumstances:

Forgotten tablets: If the patient forgets to take a tablet, she should take it as soon as she remembers and take the next one at the normal time. This may mean that two tablets are taken in one day. Provided she is less than 12 hours late in taking her tablet, Trinovum will still give contraceptive protection during this cycle and the rest of the pack should be taken as usual.

If she is more than 12 hours late in taking one or more tablets then she should take the last missed pill as soon as she remembers but leave the other missed pills in the pack. She should continue to take the rest of the pack as usual but must use extra precautions (e.g. sheath, diaphragm plus spermicide) and follow the '7-day rule' (see further information for 7-day rule). If there are 7 or more pills left in the pack after the missed and delayed pills then the usual 7-day break can be left before starting the next pack. If there are less than 7 pills left in the pack after the missed and delayed pills then when the pack is finished the next pack should be started the next day. If withdrawal bleeding does not occur at the end of the second pack then a pregnancy test should be performed.

Vomiting or diarrhoea: If after tablet intake vomiting or diarrhoea occurs, a tablet may not be absorbed properly by the body. If the symptoms disappear within 12 hours of tablet-taking, the patient should take an extra tablet from a spare pack and continue with the rest of the pack as usual.

However, if the symptoms continue beyond those 12 hours, additional contraceptive precautions are necessary for any sexual intercourse during the stomach or bowel upset and for the following 7 days (the patient must be advised to follow the '7-day rule').

Change in bleeding pattern: If after taking Trinovum for several months there is a sudden occurrence of spotting or break-through bleeding (not observed in previous cycles) or the absence of withdrawal bleeding, contraceptive effectiveness may be reduced. If withdrawal bleeding fails to occur and none of the above mentioned events has taken place, pregnancy is highly unlikely and oral contraceptive use can be continued until the end of the next pack.

(If withdrawal bleeding fails to occur at the end of the second cycle, tablet intake should be discontinued and pregnancy excluded before oral contraceptive use can be resumed). However, if withdrawal bleeding is absent and any of the above mentioned events has occurred, tablet intake should be discontinued and pregnancy excluded before oral contraceptive use can be resumed.

Interactions: Irregular cycles and reduced reliability of oral contraceptives may occur when these preparations are used concomitantly with drugs such as anticonvulsants, barbiturates, antibiotics, (eg tetracyclines, ampicillin, rifampicin, etc), griseofulvin, activated charcoal and certain laxatives. Special consideration should be given to patients being treated with antibiotics for acne. They should be advised to use a non-hormonal method of contraception, or to use an oral contraceptive containing a progestogen showing minimal androgenicity, which have been reported as helping to improve acne without using an antibiotic. Oral contraceptives may diminish glucose tolerance and increase the need for insulin or other antidiabetic drugs in diabetics.

Medical examination/consultation: A complete medical history and physical examination should be taken prior to the initiation or reinstitution of oral contraceptives and should be repeated periodically.

These physical examinations should include special reference to blood pressure, breasts, abdomen and pelvic organs, including cervical cytology and, where indicated by the medical or family history, relevant laboratory tests. Caution should be observed when prescribing oral contraceptives to young women whose cycles are not yet stabilised.

Surgery, varicose veins or immobilisation: In patients using oestrogen-containing preparations the risk of deep vein thrombosis may be temporarily increased when undergoing a major operation (e.g. abdominal, orthopaedic), any surgery to the legs, medical treatment for varicose veins or prolonged immobilisation. Therefore, it is advisable to discontinue oral contraceptive use at least 4 to 6 weeks prior to these procedures if performed electively and to (re)start not less than 2 weeks after full ambulation. The latter is also valid with regard to immobilisation after an accident or emergency surgery. In case of emergency surgery, thrombotic prophylaxis is usually indicated e.g. with subcutaneous heparin.

Chloasma: Chloasma may occasionally occur, especially in women with a history of chloasma gravidarum. Women with a tendency to chloasma should avoid exposure to the sun or ultraviolet radiation whilst taking this preparation. Chloasma is often not fully reversible.

Laboratory tests: The use of steroids may influence the results of certain laboratory tests. In the literature, at least a hundred different parameters have been reported to possibly be influenced by oral contraceptive use, predominantly by the oestrogenic component. Among these are: biochemical parameters of the liver, thyroid, adrenal and renal function, plasma levels of (carrier) proteins and lipid/lipoprotein fractions and parameters of coagulation and fibrinolysis.

Adverse reactions: Various adverse reactions have been associated with oral contraceptive use. The serious reactions are dealt with in more detail. The first appearance of symptoms indicative of any one of these reactions necessitates immediate cessation of oral contraceptive use while appropriate diagnostic and therapeutic measures are undertaken.

Serious adverse reactions: There is a general opinion, based on statistical evidence that users of combined oral contraceptives experience more often than non-users various disorders of the circulation. How often these disorders occur in users of modern low-oestrogen oral contraceptives is unknown, but there are reasons for suggesting that they may occur less often than with the older types of pill which contain more oestrogen.

Various reports have associated oral contraceptive use with the occurrence of deep venous thrombosis, pulmonary embolism and other embolisms. Other investigations of these oral contraceptives have suggested an increased risk or oestrogen and /or progestogen dose-dependent coronary and cerebrovascular accidents, predominantly in heavy smokers. Thrombosis has very rarely been reported to occur in other veins or arteries, e.g. hepatic, mesenteric, renal or retinal.

It should be noted that there is no consensus about the often contradictory findings obtained in early studies. The physician should bear in mind the possibility of vascular accidents occurring and that there may not be full recovery from such disorders and they may be fatal. The physician should take into account the presence of risk factors for arterial disease and deep venous thrombosis when prescribing oral contraceptives. Risk factors for arterial disease include smoking, the presence of hyperlipidaemia, hypertension or diabetes.

Signs and symptoms of a thrombotic event may include: sudden severe pain in the chest, whether or not reaching to the left arm; sudden breathlessness; any unusual severe, prolonged headache, especially if it occurs for the first time or gets progressively worse, or is associated with any of the following symptoms: sudden partial or complete loss of vision or diplopia, aphasia, vertigo, a bad fainting attack or collapse with or without focal epilepsy, weakness or very marked numbness suddenly affecting one side or one part of the body, motor disturbances; severe pain in the calf of one leg; acute abdomen.

Cigarette smoking increases the risk of serious cardiovascular adverse reactions to oral contraceptive use. The risk increases with age and with heavy smoking and is more marked in women over 35 years of age. Women who use oral contraceptives should be strongly advised not to smoke.

The use of oestrogen-containing oral contraceptives may promote growth of existing sex steroid dependent tumours. For this reason, the use of these oral contraceptives in patients with such tumours is contra-indicated. Numerous epidemiological studies have been reported of the risk or ovarian, endometrial, cervical and breast cancer in women using combined oral contraceptives.

The evidence is clear that combined oral contraceptives offer substantial protection against both ovarian and endometrial cancer. An increased risk of cervical cancer in long term users of combined oral contraceptives has been reported in some studies, but there continues to be controversy about the extent to which this is attributable to the confounding effects of sexual behaviour and other factors.

A meta-analysis from 54 epidemiological studies reported that there is a slightly increased relative risk (RR=1.24) of having breast cancer diagnosed in women who are currently using combined oral contraceptives (COCs). The observed pattern of increased risk may be due to an earlier diagnosis of breast cancer in COC users, the biological effects of COCs or a combination of both. The additional breast cancers diagnosed in current users of COCs or in women who have used COCs in the last 10 years are more likely to be localised to the breast than those in women who never used COCs.

Breast cancer is rare among women under 40 years of age whether or not they take COCs. Whilst this background risk increases with age, the excess number of breast cancer diagnoses in current and recent COC users is small in relation to the overall risk of breast cancer (see bar chart on previous page).

The most important risk factor for breast cancer in COC users is the age women discontinue the COC; the older the age at stopping, the more breast cancers are diagnosed. Duration of use is less important and the excess risk gradually disappears during the course of the 10 years after stopping COC use such that by 10 years there appears to be no excess.

The possible increase in risk of breast cancer should be discussed with the user and weighed against the benefits of COCs taking into account the evidence that they offer substantial protection against the risk of developing certain other cancers (e.g. ovarian and endometrial cancer).

Malignant hepatic tumours have been reported on rare occasions in long-term users of oral contraceptives. Benign hepatic tumours have also been associated with oral contraceptive usage. A hepatic tumour should be considered in the differential diagnosis when upper abdominal pain, enlarged liver or signs of intra-abdominal haemorrhage occur.

The use of oral contraceptives may sometimes lead to the development of cholestatic jaundice or cholelithiasis.

On rare occasions the use of oral contraceptives may trigger or reactivate systemic lupus erythematosus.

A further rare complication of oral contraceptive use is the occurrence of chorea which can be reversed by discontinuing the pill. The majority of cases of oral-contraceptive-induced chorea show a pre-existing predisposition which often relates to acute rheumatism.

Other adverse reactions:
Cardiovascular system: Rise of blood pressure. If hypertension develops, treatment should be discontinued

Genital tract: Intermenstrual bleeding, post-medication amenorrhoea, changes in cervical secretion, increase in size of uterine fibromyomata, aggravation of endometriosis, certain vaginal infections, e.g. candidiasis.

Breast: Tenderness, pain, enlargement, secretion.

Gastrointestinal tract: Nausea, vomiting, cholelithiasis, cholestatic jaundice.

Skin: Erythema nodosum, rash, chloasma, erythema multiforme, hirsutism, loss of scalp hair.

Eyes: Discomfort of the cornea if contact lenses are used.

CNS: Headache, migraines, mood changes, depression

Metabolic: Fluid retention, change in body weight, reduced glucose tolerance.

Other: Changes in libido, leg cramps, premenstrual -like syndrome.

Overdosage: There have been no reports of serious ill-health from overdosage even when a considerable number of tablets have been taken by a small child. In general, it is therefore unnecessary to treat overdosage. However, if overdosage is discovered within 2 or 3 hours and is large, then gastric lavage can be safely used. There are no antidotes and further treatment should be symptomatic.

Further information
Additional contraceptive precautions: When additional contraceptive precautions are required the patient should be advised either not to have sex, or to use a cap plus spermicide or for her partner to use a condom. Rhythm methods should not be advised as the pill disrupts the usual cyclical changes associated with the natural menstrual cycle e.g. changes in temperature and cervical mucus.

The 7-day rule: If any one tablet is forgotten for more than 12 hours:

If the patient has vomiting or diarrhoea for more than 12 hours:

If the patient is taking any of the drugs listed under 'Interactions':

The patient should continue to take her tablets as usual and additional contraceptive precautions must be taken for the next 7 days.

BUT–if these 7 days run beyond the end of the current pack, the next pack must be started as soon as the current one is finished, i.e. no gap should be left between packs. (This prevents an extended break in tablet taking which may increase the risk of the ovaries releasing an egg and thus reducing contraceptive protection.) The patient will not have a period until the end of 2 packs but this is not harmful nor does it matter if she experiences some bleeding on tablet taking days.

Pharmaceutical precautions Store at room temperature (below 25°C). Protect from light.

Legal category POM.

Package quantities Carton containing 3 push packs of 21 tablets–sufficient for 3 cycles.

Product licence number 0242/0279.

VERMOX* TABLETS

Qualitative and quantitative composition Mebendazole 100 mg.

Pharmaceutical form Tablet.

Clinical particulars
Therapeutic indications: For the treatment of *trichuris trichiura* (whipworm), *enterobius vermicularis* (pinworm), *ascaris lumbricoides* (roundworm), *ancylostoma duodenale* (common hookworm), *necator americanus* (American hookworm) in single or mixed infections.

Posology and method of administration:
Adults and children over 2 years: For the control of trichuriasis, ascaris and hookworm infections, one tablet bd for three consecutive days.

For the control of enterobiasis a single tablet is administered. It is highly recommended that a second tablet is taken after two weeks, if reinfection is suspected.

Method of administration: Oral.

Contra-indications: Vermox is contra-indicated in pregnancy and in patients who have shown hypersensitivity to the product or any components.

Special warnings and special precautions for use: Not recommended in the treatment of children under 2 years.

Interaction with other medicaments and other forms of interaction: Concomitant treatment with cimetidine may inhibit the metabolism of mebendazole in the liver, resulting in increased plasma concentrations of the drug especially during prolonged treatment.

Pregnancy and lactation:
Pregnancy: Since Vermox is contraindicated in pregnancy patients who think they are or may be pregnant should not take this preparation.

Lactation: As it is not known whether Vermox is excreted in human milk it is not advisable to breast feed following administration of Vermox

Effects on ability to drive and use machines: None stated.

Undesirable effects: Side effects reported for Vermox have been minor. Transient abdominal pain and diarrhoea have been reported, only rarely, in cases of massive infestation and expulsion of worms. Hypersensitivity reactions including exanthema, rash, urticaria and angio-oedema have rarely been observed.

Overdose: In the event of accidental overdosage, abdominal cramps, nausea, vomiting and diarrhoea may occur. Cases should be treated symptomatically with supportive measures and gastric lavage with activated charcoal as necessary. Although the maximum treatment duration of Vermox is limited to three days there have been rare reports of reversible liver function disturbances, hepatitis and neutropenia described in patients who were treated for hydatid disease with large doses for prolonged periods of time.

Pharmacological properties
Pharmacodynamic properties: In vitro and *in vivo* work suggests that mebendazole blocks the uptake of glucose by adult and larval forms of helminths, in a selective and irreversible manner. Inhibition of glucose uptake appears to lead to endogenous depletion of glycogen stores within the helminth. Lack of glycogen leads to decreased formation of ATP and ultrastructural changes in the cells.

Pharmacokinetic properties: Using a tracer dose of ^{3}H-mebendazole the pharmacokinetics and bioavailability of a solution and iv drug have been examined. After oral administration the half life was 0.93 hours. Absorption of this tracer dose was almost complete but low availability indicated a high first pass effect. At normal therapeutic doses it is very hard to measure levels in the plasma.

Preclinical safety data: Not applicable.

Pharmaceutical particulars
List of excipients:
Microcrystalline cellulose
Sodium starch glycolate
Talc
Maize starch
Sodium saccharin
Magnesium stearate
Hydrogenated vegetable oil
Orange flavour
Colloidal anhydrous silica
Sodium lauryl sulphate
Orange yellow S
Purified water*
2-propanol*
* Not present in the final product.

Incompatibilities: Not applicable.

Shelf life: 60 months.

Special precautions for storage: None.

Nature and contents of container: Blister strips of PVC genotherm glass clear aluminium foil coated on the inside with a heat seal lacquer.

Pack sizes: 1 and 6 tablet packs.

Instructions for use/handling: Not applicable.

Marketing authorisation number 0242/0011

Date of approval/revision of SPC June 1996

Legal category POM.

VERMOX* SUSPENSION

Qualitative and quantitative composition Each 5 ml of suspension contains mebendazole PhEur 100 mg.

Pharmaceutical form White homogeneous suspension.

Clinical particulars
Therapeutic indications: Broad spectrum anthelmintic indicated for the treatment of: *Enterobius vermicularis* (threadworm/pinworm); *Oxyuris vermicularis*; *Trichuris trichuria* (whipworm); *Ascaris lumbricoides* (large roundworm); *Ancylostoma duodenale* (common hookworm); *Necator americanus* (American hookworm).

Posology and method of administration: For oral administration.

Adults and children over 2 years:
Enterobiasis: 1 x 5 ml spoonful.

It is highly recommended that a second dose is taken after two weeks, if reinfection is suspected.

Ascariasis, trichuriasis, ancylostomiasis, necatoriasis and mixed infections: 1 x 5 ml spoonful bd for three days.

Contra-indications: Vermox is contra-indicated in pregnancy and in patients who have shown hypersensitivity to the product or any components.

Special warnings and special precautions for use: Not recommended in the treatment of children under 2 years.

Interaction with other medicaments and other forms of interaction: Concomitant treatment with cimetidine may inhibit the metabolism of mebendazole in the liver, resulting in increased plasma concentrations of the drug, especially during prolonged treatment.

Pregnancy and lactation: Since Vermox is contra-indicated in pregnancy, patients who think they are or may be pregnant should not take this preparation.

As it is not known whether Vermox is excreted in human milk, it is not advisable to breast feed following administration of Vermox.

Effects on ability to drive and use machines: None known.

Undesirable effects: Side effects reported for Vermox have been minor. Transient abdominal pain and diarrhoea have been reported, only rarely, in cases of massive infestation and expulsion of worms. Hypersensitivity reactions including exanthema, rash, urticaria and angio-oedema have rarely been observed.

Overdose: In the event of accidental overdosage, abdominal cramps, nausea, vomiting and diarrhoea may occur. Cases should be treated symptomatically with supportive measures and gastric lavage with activated charcoal as necessary. Although the maximum treatment duration of Vermox is limited to three days, there have been rare reports of reversible liver function disturbances, hepatitis and neutropenia described in patients who were treated for hydatid disease with large doses for prolonged periods of time.

Pharmacological properties

Pharmacodynamic properties: In vitro and *in vivo* work suggests that mebendazole blocks the uptake of glucose by adult and larval forms of helminths, in a selective and irreversible manner. Inhibition of glucose uptake appears to lead to endogenous depletion of glycogen stores within the helminth. Lack of glycogen leads to decreased formation of ATP and ultrastructural changes in the cells.

Pharmacokinetic properties: Using a tracer dose of ^{3}H-mebendazole, the pharmacokinetics and bioavailability of a solution and iv drug have been examined. After oral administration the half life was 0.93 hours. Absorption of this tracer dose was almost complete but low availability indicated a high first pass effect. At normal therapeutic doses, it is very hard to measure levels in the plasma.

Preclinical safety data: No relevant information additional to that contained elsewhere in the Summary of Product Characteristics.

Pharmaceutical particulars

List of excipients: Sucrose; microcrystalline cellulose and sodium carboxymethyl cellulose; methylcellulose 15 mPa.s; methylparaben; propylparaben; sodium lauryl sulphate; banana 51452T; citric acid, monohydrate; purified water.

Incompatibilities: None known.

Shelf life: 5 years.

Special precautions for storage: Shake well before use.

Nature and contents of container: Amber glass flask containing 30 ml suspension, with either:

Pilfer-proof screw cap. Cork insert in cap is coated on both sides with polyvinylchloride

or

Child-resistant polypropylene screw cap, lined inside with a LDPE insert.

Instructions for use/handling: Not applicable.

Marketing authorisation number 0242/0050

Date of approval/revision of SPC December 1997

Legal category POM.

**Trade Mark*

JHC Healthcare Ltd
5 Lower Merrion Street
Dublin 2
Eire

☎ 00 3531 283 66 46   🗋 00 3531 283 66 46

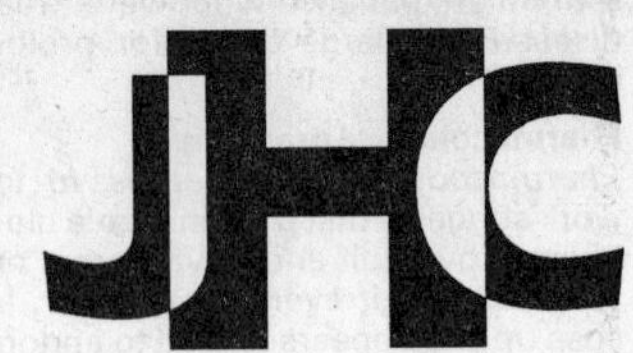

MYOCRISIN*

Qualitative and quantitative composition Sodium aurothiomalate BP 50 mg in 0.5 ml (10%), Sodium aurothiomalate BP 10 mg in 0.5 ml (2%) and Sodium aurothiomalate BP 20 mg in 0.5 ml (4%).

Pharmaceutical form Injection.

Clinical particulars
Therapeutic indications: Myocrisin is used in the management of active progressive rheumatoid arthritis and progressive juvenile chronic arthritis especially if polyarticular or seropositive.

Posology and method of administration: Do not use a darkened solution (more than pale yellow).

Myocrisin should be administered only by deep intramuscular injection followed by gentle massage of the area. The patient should remain under medical observation for a period of 30 minutes after drug administration.

Adults: An initial test dose of 10 mg should be given in the first week followed by weekly doses of 50 mg until signs of remission occur. At this point 50 mg doses should be given at two week intervals until full remission occurs. With full remission the interval between injections should be increased progressively to three, four and then, after 18 months to 2 years, to six weeks.

If after reaching a total dose of 1 g (excluding the test dose), no major improvement has occurred and the patient has not shown any signs of gold toxicity, six 100 mg injections may be administered at weekly intervals. If no sign of remission occurs after this time other forms of treatment are to be considered.

Elderly: There are no specific dosage recommendations. Elderly patients should be monitored with extra caution.

Children: Progressive juvenile chronic arthritis:

Weekly doses of 1 mg/kg should be given but not exceeding a maximum weekly dose of 50 mg. Depending on urgency, this dose may be preceded by a smaller test dose such as 1/10 or 1/5 of the full dose for 2-3 weeks. Continue weekly doses until signs of remission appear then increase the intervals between injections to two weeks. With full remission increase the interval to three then four weeks. In the absence of signs of remission after twenty weeks consider raising the dose slightly or changing to another therapy.

Treatment should be continued for six months. Response can be expected at the 300-500 mg level. If patients respond, maintenance therapy should be continued with the dosage administered over the previous 2-4 weeks, for 1-5 years.

Contra-indications: Pregnancy (see *Pregnancy and lactation*)

Myocrisin is contraindicated in patients with gross renal or hepatic disease, a history of blood dyscrasias, exfoliative dermatitis or systemic lupus erythematosus.

The absolute contraindications should be positively excluded before considering gold therapy.

Special warnings and special precautions for use: As with other gold preparations, reactions which resemble anaphylactoid effects have been reported. These effects may occur after any course of therapy within the first ten minutes following drug administration (see administration). If anaphylactoid effects are observed, treatment with Myocrisin should be discontinued.

Myocrisin should be administered with extra caution in the elderly and in patients with a history of urticaria, eczema or colitis. Extra caution should also be exercised if phenylbutazone or oxyphenbutazone are administered concurrently.

Before starting treatment and again before each injection, the urine should be tested for protein, the skin inspected for rash and a full blood count performed, including a numerical platelet count (not an estimate) and the readings plotted. Blood dyscrasias are most likely to occur when between 400 mg and 1 g of gold have been given, or between the 10th and 20th week of treatment, but can also occur with much lower doses or after only 2-4 weeks of therapy.

The presence of albuminura, pruritus or rash, or an eosinophilia, are indications of developing toxicity. The Myocrisin should be withheld for one or two weeks until all signs have disappeared when the course may be restarted on a test dose followed by a decreased frequency of gold injections.

A complaint of sore throat, glossitis, buccal ulceration and/or easy bruising or bleeding, demands an immediate blood count, followed if indicated, by appropriate treatment for agrananulocytosis, aplastic anaemia and/or thrombocytopenia. Every patient treated with Myocrisin should be warned to report immediately the appearance of pruritis, metallic taste, sore throat or tongue, buccal ulceration or easy bruising, purpura, epistaxis, bleeding gums, menorrhagia or diarrhoea.

Interaction with other medicaments and other forms of interaction: Concurrent gold administration may exacerbate aspirin-induced hepatic dysfunction. Caution should be exercised if phenylbutazone or oxyphenbutazone are administered concurrently.

Pregnancy and lactation: The safety of Myocrisin in the foetus and the new-born has not been established. Female patients receiving Myocrisin should be instructed to avoid pregnancy. Pregnant patients should not be treated with Myocrisin. Lactating mothers under treatment with Myocrisin excrete significant amounts of gold in their breast milk and should not breast feed their infants.

Effects on ability to drive and use machines: None

Undesirable effects: Hepatotoxicity with cholestatic jaundice is a rare complication which may occur early in the course of treatment. It subsides on withdrawing Myocrisin. A rare but severe form of enterocolitis has been described.

Diffuse unilateral or bilateral pulmonary fibrosis very rarely occurs. This progressive condition usually responds to drug withdrawal and steroid therapy. An annual x-ray is recommended and attention should be paid to unexplained breathlessness and dry cough.

Side effects may be largely avoided by the indicated careful titration of dosage. Minor reactions, usually manifest as skin rashes are the most frequent and commonly benign, but as such reactions may be the forerunners of severe gold toxicity they must never be treated lightly. Significant skin complications are almost exclusively pruritic. Irreversible skin pigmentation can occur in sun-exposed areas after prolonged treatment with Myocrisin. Rare reports of alopecia exist. Nephrotic syndrome has been rarely reported.

Overdose: Minor side effects resolve spontaneously on withdrawal of Myocrisin. Symptomatic treatment of pruritus with antihistamines may be helpful. Major skin lesions and serious blood dyscrasias demand hospital admission when dimercaprol or penacillamine may be used to enhance gold excretion. Fresh blood and/or platelet transfusions, corticosteroids and androgenic steroids may be required in the management of severe blood dyscrasias

Pharmacological properties
Pharmacological properties: The precise mode of action of sodium aurothiomalate is not yet known. Treatment with gold has been shown to be accompanied by a fall in ESR and C-reactive protein, an increase in serum histidine and sulphydryl levels and a reduction in serum immunoglobulins, rheumatoid factor titres and Clq-binding activity.

Numerous experimental observations have been recorded including physico-chemical changes in collagen and interference with complement activation, gammaglobulin aggregation, prostaglandin biosythesis, inhibition of cathepsin and production of superoxide radicals by activated polymophonuclear leukocytes.

Pharmacokinetics properties: Sodium aurothiomalate is absorbed readily after intramuscular injection and becomes bound to plasma proteins. With doses of 50 mg weekly the steady-state serum concentration of gold is about 3 to 5 microgram per ml. It is widely distributed and accumulates in the body. Concentrations in synovial fluid have been shown to be similar or slightly less than those in plasma. Sodium aurothiomalate is mainly excreted in the urine with smaller amounts in the faeces. The serum half-life of gold clearance is about 5 or 6 days but after a course of treatment, gold may be found in the urine for up to a year or more owing to its presence in deep body compartments.

Gold has been detected in the foetus following administration of sodium aurothiomalate to the mother. Gold has been detected in the breast fed child where the mother has received sodium aurothiomalate.

Preclinical safety data: No additional pre-clinical data of relevance to the prescriber.

Pharmaceutical particulars
List of excipients: Phenylmercuric nitrate BP, Water for Injections BP.

Incompatibilities: None Known

Shelf life: 36 months

Special precautions for storage: Store below 25°C. Protect from light

Nature and contents of container: Boxes of 10 x 10 mg, 20 mg and 50 mg ampoules

Instructions for use/handling: None stated

Marketing authorisation numbers
Injection 10 mg 16186/0007
Injection 20 mg 16186/0008
Injection 50 mg 16186/0009

Date of approval/revision of SPC March 1997

Legal category POM

NEULACTIL* TABLETS

Qualitative and quantitative composition
Pericyazine 10 mg
Pericyazine 2.5 mg

Pharmaceutical form
2.5 mg–Circular, very pale lime-yellow tablet, with one face impressed 'Neulactil' just inside the perimeter, breakline on reverse

10 mg–Circular, very pale lime-yellow tablet, with one face impressed 'Neulactil' just inside the perimeter around a central '10'. Breakline on reverse

Clinical particulars
Therapeutic indications: In adults with schizophrenia or other psychoses, for the treatment of symptoms or prevention of relapse.

In anxiety, psychomotor agitation, violent or dangerously impulsive behaviour. Neulactil is used as an adjunct to the short-term management of these conditions.

Posology and method of administration:

Route of administration: Oral.

Dosage requirement varies with the individual and the severity of the condition being treated. Initial dosage should be low with progressive increases until the desired response is obtained, after which dosage should be adjusted to maintain control of the symptoms.

Severe conditions: Schizophrenia and other psychoses. Adults: Initially 75 mg per day in divided doses. Dosage should be increased by 25 mg per day at weekly intervals until the optimum effect is achieved. Maintenance therapy would not normally be expected to exceed 300 mg per day. *Elderly:* Initially 15-30 mg per day in divided doses. If this is well tolerated the dosage may be increased if necessary for optimum control of behaviour.

Mild or moderate conditions: In anxiety: Adults: Initially 15-30 mg daily, divided into two portions with a larger dose being given in the evening. *Elderly:* 5–10 mg per day is suggested as a starting dose. It may be divided so that a larger portion is given in the evening. Half or quarter the normal adult dose may be sufficient for maintenance therapy.

Neulactil tablets are not recommended for children.

Contra-indications: See use in pregnancy below.

Special warnings and precautions for use: Neuroleptics should be avoided in patients with liver or renal dysfunction, epilepsy, Parkinson's disease, hypothyroidism, cardiac failure, phaeochromocytoma, myasthenia gravis, prostrate hypertrophy. It should be avoided in patients known to be hypersensitive to phenothiazines or with a history of narrow angle glaucoma. It should be used with caution in the elderly, particularly during very hot or very cold weather (risk of hyper-hypothermia).

Interactions with other medicaments and other forms of interaction: The following interactions are common to all phenothiazine neuroleptics. These interactions are a theoretical nature and are not serious.

The CNS depressant actions of neuroleptic agents may be intensified (additively) by alcohol, barbiturates and other sedatives. Respiratory depression may occur.

The hypotensive effect of most antihypertensive drugs, especially alpha adrenoceptor blocking agents may be exaggerated by neuroleptics.

The mild anticholinergic effect of neuroleptics may be exchanged by other anticholinergic drugs, possibly leading to constipation, heat stroke, etc.

The action of some drugs may be opposed by neuroleptics; these include amphetamine, levodopa, clonidine, guanethidine, adrenaline.

Anticholinergic agents may reduce the antipsychotic effect of neuroleptics.

Some drugs interfere with absorption of neuroleptic agents: antacids, anti-Parkinson drugs, lithium. Increases or decreases in the plasma concentrations of a number of drugs, eg: propranolol, phenobarbitone have been observed but were not of clinical significance.

High doses of neuroleptics may reduce the response to hypoglycaemic agents the dosage of which might have been raised.

Adrenaline must not be used in patients overdosed with neuroleptics. Most of the above interactions are of a theoretical nature and not serious.

Simultaneous administration of desferrioxamine and prochlorperazine has been observed to induce a transient metabolic encephalopathy characterised by loss of consciousness for 48-72 hours. It is possible this may occur with 'Neulactil' since it shares many of the pharmacological properties of prochlorperazine.

Pregnancy and lactation: There is inadequate evidence of the safety of Neulactil in human pregnancy but it has been widely used for many years without apparent ill consequence. There is evidence with some neuroleptics of harmful effects in animals. Like other drugs 'Neulactil' should be avoided in pregnancy unless the physician considers it essential. It may occasionally prolong labour and at such a time should be withheld until the cervix is dilated 3-4cm. Possible adverse effects on the foetus include lethargy or paradoxical hyperexcitability, tremor and low Apgar score.

Phenothiazines may be excreted in milk, therefore breastfeeding should be suspended during treatment.

Effects on ability to drive and use machines: Patients should be warned about drowsiness during early days of treatment, and advised not to drive or operate machinery. The elderly are particularly susceptible to postural hypotension

Undesirable effects: Liver function: jaundice, occurs in a very small percentage of patients taking neuroleptics. A premonitory sign may be a sudden onset of fever after one to three weeks of treatment followed by the development of jaundice. Neuroleptic jaundice has the biochemical and other characteristics of obstructive jaundice and is associated with obstruction of the canaliculi by bile thrombi; the frequent presence of an accompanying eosinophilia indicates the allergic nature of this phenomenon. Treatment should be withheld on the development of jaundice. Cardiorespiratory: hypotension, usually postural, commonly occurs. Elderly or volume depleted subjects are particularly susceptible. Cardiac arrhythmias, including atrial arrhythmia, A-V block, ventricular tachycardia and fibrillation have been reported during neuroleptic therapy, possibly related to dosage. Pre-existing cardiac disease, old age, hypokalaemia and concurrent tricyclic anti-depressants may predispose. ECG changes, usually benign, include widened QT interval, ST depression, U-waves and T-wave changes. Respiratory depression is possible in susceptible patients. *Blood picture:* A mild leukopenia occurs in up to 30% of patients on prolonged high dosage of neuroleptics: Agranulocytosis may occur rarely; it is not dose related. The occurrence of unexplained infections or fever requires immediate haematological investigation. Extraphyramidal: acute dystonias or dyskinesias, usually transitory are commoner in children and young adults, and usually occur within the first four days of treatment or after dosage increases. Akathisia characteristically occurs after large initial doses. Parkinsonism is commoner in adults and the elderly. It usually develops after weeks or months of treatment. One or more of the following may be seen: tremor, rigidity, akinesia, or other features of Parkinsonism. Commonly just tremor. Tardive dyskinesia: if this occurs it is usually, but not necessarily after prolonged or high dosage. It can even occur after treatment has been stopped. Dosage should therefore be kept low whenever possible. *Skin and eyes:* contact skin sensitation is a serious but rare complication in those frequently handling preparations of phenothiazines; The greatest care must be taken to avoid contact of the drug with the skin. Skin rashes of various kinds may also be seen in patients treated with the drug. Patients on high dosage should be warned that they may develop photosensitivity in sunny weather and should avoid exposure to direct sunlight. *Endocrine:* hyperprolactinaemia which may result in galactorrhoea, gynaecomastia, amenorrhoea; impotence. Neuroleptic malignant syndrome (hyperthermia, rigidity autonomic dysfunction and altered consciousness) may occur with any neuroleptic. Minor side effects are nasal stuffiness, dry mouth, insomnia, agitation

Overdose: Toxicity and treatment of overdosage: Symptoms of neuroleptic overdosage include drowsiness or loss of consciousness, hypotension, tachycardia, ECG changes, ventricular arrhythmias and hypothermia. Severe extra-pyramidal dyskinesias may occur. If the patient is seen sufficiently soon (up to 6 hours) after ingestion of a toxic dose, gastric lavage may be attempted. Pharmacological induction of emesis is unlikely to be of any use. Activated charcoal should be given. There is no specific antidote. Treatment is supportive. Generalised vasodilatation may result in circulatory collapse; raising the patient's legs may suffice, in severe cases, volume expansion by intravenous fluids may be needed; infusion fluids should be warmed before administration in order not to aggravate hypothermia. Positive inotropic agents such as dopamine may be tried if fluid replacement is insufficient to correct the circulatory collapse. Peripheral vasoconstrictor agents are not generally recommended; avoid the use of adrenaline. Ventricular or supraventricular tachy-arrhythmias usually respond to restoration of normal body temperature and correction of circulatory or metabolic disturbances. If persistent or life threatening, appropriate anti-arrhythmic therapy may be considered. Avoid lignocaine, and as far as possible long acting, anti-arrhythmic drugs. Pronounced central nervous system depression requires airway maintenance or, in extreme circumstances, assisted respiration. Severe dystonic reactions usually respond to procyclidine (5-10 mg) or orphenedrine (20-40 mg) administered intramuscularly or intravenously. Convulsions should be treated with intravenous diazepam. Neuroleptic malignant syndrome should be treated with cooling. Dantrolene sodium may be tried.

Pharmacological properties

Pharmacodynamic properties: Pericyazine is a neuroleptic with cardiovascular and antihistamine effects similar to those of chlorpromazine, but it has a stronger antiserotonin effect and a powerful central sedative effect.

Pharmacokinetic properties: Kinetics: there is little information about plasma concentrations, distribution and excretion in humans. The rate of metabolism and excretion of phenothiazines decreases in old age.

Preclinical safety data: There are no pre-clinical data of relevance to the prescriber which are additional to that already included in other sections of the SPC.

List of excipients: Lactose Anhydrous USP, Microcrystalline cellulose (E460), Sodium starch glycollate, Magnesium sterateBP, Colloidal silicon dioxide (E551), Methylhydroxybenzoate BP (E218)

Incompatibilities: None known.

Shelf-life: 60 months

Special precautions for storage: Protect from light.

Nature and contents of container: Containers of 84×2.5 mg (OP) and 10 mg tablets.

Instructions for use in handling: None stated

Marketing authorisation numbers

Tablets 2.5 mg 16186/0003
Tablets 10 mg 16186/0004

Date of approval/revision of SPC: February 1997

Legal category POM

NEULACTIL FORTE SYRUP

Qualitative and quantitative composition Pericyazine 10 mg/5 ml.

Pharmaceutical form Forte Syrup, clear orange brown syrupy liquid.

Clinical particulars

Therapeutic indications: In adults with schizophrenia or other psychoses, for the treatment of symptoms or prevention of relapse.

In anxiety, psychomotor agitation, violent or dangerously impulsive behaviour. Neulactil is used as an adjunct to the short-term management of these conditions.

In children with behaviour disorders or schizophrenia.

Posology and method of administration:

Route of administration: Oral. Dosage requirement varies with the individual and the severity of the condition being treated. Initial dosage should be low with progressive increases until the desired response is obtained, after which dosage should be adjusted to maintain control of the symptoms.

Schizophrenia and other psychoses: Adults: Initially 75 mg per day in divided doses. Dosage should be increased by 25 mg per day at weekly intervals until the optimum effect is achieved. Maintenance therapy would not normally be expected to exceed 300 mg per day. *Elderly:* Initially 15-30 mg per day in divided doses. If this is well tolerated the dosage may be increased if necessary for optimum control of behaviour. *Children* The initial daily dose should be calculated on bodyweight. A child weighing 10 kg should receive 0.5 milligram and this initial dose should be increased by 1 mg for each additional 5 kg of bodyweight up to a total daily dose of 10 mg daily. This dosage may be gradually increased until the desired effect is achieved, but the daily maintenance dose should not exceed twice the initial amount.

Neulactil is not recommended for use in children below 1 year of age.

Anxiety, psychomotor agitation, violent or dangerously impulsive behaviour.: Adults: Initially 15-30 mg daily, divided into two portions with a larger dose being given in the evening. *Elderly:* 5–10 mg per day is suggested as a starting dose. It may be divided so that a larger portion is given in the evening. Half or quarter the normal adult dose may be sufficient for maintenance therapy. *Children: Not recommended for children.*

Contra-indications: None stated

Special warnings and precautions for use: Neuroleptics should be avoided in patients with liver or renal dysfunction, epilepsy, Parkinson's disease, hypothyroidism, cardiac failure, phaeochromocytoma, myasthenia gravis, prostrate hypertrophy. It should be avoided in patients known to be hypersensitive to phenothiazines or with a history of narrow angle glaucoma. It should be used with caution in the elderly, particularly during very hot or very cold weather (risk of hyper-hypothermia).

Interactions with other medicaments and other forms of interaction: The following interactions are common to all phenothiazine neuroleptics. These interactions are mainly of a theoretical nature and not serious.

The CNS depressant actions of neuroleptic agents may be intensified (additively) by alcohol, barbiturates and other sedatives. Respiratory depression may occur.

The hypotensive effect of most antihypertensive drugs, especially alpha adrenoceptor blocking agents may be exaggerated by neuroleptics.

The mild anticholinergic effect of neuroleptics may be enhanced by other anticholinergic drugs, possibly leading to constipation, heat stroke, etc.

The action of some drugs may be opposed by neuroleptics; these include amphetamine, levodopa, clonidine, guanethidine, adrenaline.

Anticholinergic agents may reduce the antipsychotic effect of neuroleptics.

Some drugs interfere with absorption of neuroleptic agents: antacids, anti-Parkinson drugs, lithium. Increases or decreases in the plasma concentrations of a number of drugs, eg: propranolol, phenobarbitone have been observed but were not of clinical significance.

High doses of neuroleptics may reduce the response to hypoglycaemic agents the dosage of which might have been raised.

Adrenaline must not be used in patients overdosed with neuroleptics.

Simultaneous administration of desferrioxamine and prochlorperazine has been observed to induce a transient metabolic encephalopathy characterised by loss of consciousness for 48-72 hours. It is possible this may occur with Neulactil since it shares many of the pharmacological properties of prochlorperazine

Pregnancy and lactation: There is inadequate evidence of the safety of Neulactil in human pregnancy but it has been widely used for many years without apparent ill consequence. There is evidence with some neuroleptics of harmful effects in animals. Like other drugs Neulactil should be avoided in pregnancy unless the physician considers it essential. It may occasionally prolong labour and at such a time should be withheld until the cervix is dilated 3-4cm. Possible adverse effects on the foetus include lethargy or paradoxical hyperexcitability, tremor and low Apgar score.

Phenothiazines may be excreted in milk, therefore breastfeeding should be suspended during treatment.

Effects on ability to drive and use machines: Patients should be warned about drowsiness during early days of treatment, and advised not to drive or operate machinery. The elderly are particularly susceptible to postural hypotension

Undesirable effects: Liver function: jaundice occurs in a very small percentage of patients taking neuroleptics. A premonitory sign may be a sudden onset of fever after one to three weeks of treatment followed by the development of jaundice. Neuroleptic jaundice has the biochemical and other characteristics of obstructive jaundice and is associated with obstruction of the canaliculi by bile thrombi; the frequent presence of an accompanying eosinophilia indicates the allergic nature of this phenomenon. Treatment should be withheld on the development of jaundice. *Cardiorespiratory:* hypotension, usually postural, commonly occurs. Elderly or space depleted subjects are particularly susceptible. Cardiac arrhythmias, including atrial arrhythmia, A-V block, ventricular tachycardia and fibrillation have been reported during neuroleptic therapy, possibly related to dosage. Pre-existing cardiac disease, old age, hypokalaemia and concurrent tricyclic anti-depressants may predispose. ECG changes, usually benign, include widened QT interval, ST depression, U-waves and T-wave changes. Respiratory depression is possible in susceptible patients. *Blood picture:* A mild leukopenia occurs in up to 30% of patients on prolonged high dosage of neuroleptics: Agranulocytosis may occur rarely; it is not dose-related. The occurrence of unexplained infections or fever requires immediate haematological investigation. *Extrapyramidal:* acute dystonias or dyskinesias, usually transitory are commoner in children and young adults, and usually occur within the first four days of treatment or after dosage increases. Akathisia characteristically occurs after large initial doses. Parkinsonism is commoner in adults and the elderly. It usually develops after weeks or months of treatment. One or more of the following may be seen: tremor, rigidity, akinesia, or other features of Parkinsonism. Commonly just tremor. *Tardive dyskinesia:* if this occurs it is usually, but not necessarily after prolonged or high dosage. It can even occur after treatment has been stopped. Dosage should therefore be kept low whenever possible. *Skin and eyes:* Skin rashes of various kinds may also be seen in patients treated with the drug. Patients on high dosage should be warned that they may develop photosensitivity in sunny weather and should avoid exposure to direct sunlight. *Endocrine:* hyperprolactinaemia which may result in galactorrhoea, gynaecomastia, amenorrhoea; impotence. Neuroleptic malignant syndrome (hyperthermia, rigidity autonomic dysfunction and altered consciousness) may occur with any neuroleptic. Minor side effects are nasal stuffiness, dry mouth, insomnia, agitation.

Overdose: Symptoms of neuroleptic overdosage include drowsiness or loss of consciousness, hypotension, tachycardia, ECG changes, ventricular arrhythmias and hypothermia. Severe extra-pyramidal dyskinesias may occur.

If the patient is seen sufficiently soon (up to 6 hours) after ingestion of a toxic dose, gastric lavage may be attempted. Pharmacological induction of emesis is unlikely to be of any use. Activated charcoal should be given. There is no specific antidote. Treatment is supportive.

Generalised vasodilatation may result in circulatory collapse; raising the patient's legs may suffice, in severe cases, volume expansion by intravenous fluids may be needed; infusion fluids should be warmed before administration in order not to aggravate hypothermia.

Positive inotropic agents such as dopamine may be tried if fluid replacement is insufficient to correct the circulatory collapse. Peripheral vasoconstrictor agents are not generally recommended; avoid the use of adrenaline.

Ventricular or supraventricular tachy-arrhythmias usually respond to restoration of normal body temperature and correction of circulatory or metabolic disturbances. If persistent or life threatening, appropriate anti-arrhythmic therapy may be considered. Avoid lignocaine, and as far as possible long acting, anti-arrhythmic drugs.

Pronounced central nervous system depression requires airway maintenance or, in extreme circumstances, assisted respiration. Severe dystonic reactions usually respond to procyclidine (5-10 mg) or orphenedrine (20-40 mg) administered intramuscularly or intravenously. Convulsions should be treated with intravenous diazepam.

Neuroleptic malignant syndrome should be treated with cooling. Dantrolene sodium may be tried.

Pharmacological properties
Pharmacodynamic properties: Pericyazine is a neuroleptic with cardiovascular and antihistamine effects similar to those of chlorpromazine, but it has a stronger antiserotonin effect and a powerful central sedative effect.

Pharmacokinetic properties: Kinetics: there is little information about plasma concentrations, distribution and excretion in humans. The rate of metabolism and excretion of phenothiazines decreases in old age.

Preclinical safety data: There are no pre-clinical data of relevance to the prescriber which are additional to that already included in other sections of the SPC.

Pharmaceutical particulars
List of excipients: Sugar, Caramel Flavour, Spearmint Oil, Peppermint Oil, Fruit cup 868, 'Tween' 20 (Polysorbate 20), Citric acid anhydrous, Sodium citrate gran., Sodium sulphite anhydrous, Sodium metabisulphite powder, Ascorbic acid, Sodium benzoate, Demineralised water BP(E218)

Incompatibilities: None known

Shelf-life: 24 months unopened, 1 month after opening.

Special precautions for storage: Protect from light

Nature and contents of container: Amber glass bottle containing 100 ml. HDPE/polypropylene child resistant cap with tamper evident band or rolled on pilfer proof aluminium cap and a PVDC emulsion coated wad.

Instructions for use in handling: Care must be taken to avoid contact of the drug with skin. Contact sensitisation is a serious but rare complication in those frequently handling preparations of phenothiazines.

Marketing authorisation number 16186/0005

Date of approval/revision of SPC May 1997

Legal category POM

PENTACARINAT*

Qualitative and quantitative composition Pentacarinat 300 mg contain Pentamidine Isethionate BP 300 mg (Equivalent to 172.4 mg pentamidine base)

Pharmaceutical form Sterile powder for use after reconstitution

Clinical particulars
Therapeutic indications: Pentamidine is indicated in the treatment of: Pneumonia due to Pneumocystis carinii (PCP), Leishmaniasis including visceral and cutaneous, Early phase African sleeping sickness caused by Trypanosoma gambiense, All indications can be treated by deep intramuscular injection or intravenous injection.

Pneumocystis carinii pneumonia can also be treated by the inhalation route.

Pentacarinat is also indicated in the prevention of Pneumocystis carinii pneumonia in patients infected by the human immunodeficiency virus (HIV) who have experienced a previous episode of PCP. Administration is by the inhalation route.

Posology and method of administration: Pentamidine powder is reconstituted before use with Water for Injections BP. For intravenous use the required dose of pentamidine isethionate is diluted further in 50-250 ml of glucose intravenous infusion BP or 0.9% (normal) Sodium Chloride Injection BP.

The following dosage regimens are recommended for adults, children and infants.

Treatment: Pneumocystis carinii pneumonia: By slow iv infusion, 4 mg/kg bodyweight of pentamidine isethionate once daily for at least 14 days. If administered by inhalation, two 300 mg vials are dissolved in 6 ml of water for injection and the resultant solution administered by a suitable nebuliser once daily for three weeks.

Leishmaniasis: Visceral: 3-4 mg/kg bodyweight of pentamidine isethionate on alternate days to a maximum of 10 injections, preferably by im injection. A repeat course may be necessary. Cutaneous: 3-4 mg/kg bodyweight, once or twice weekly by im injection until the condition resolves.

Trypanosomiasis: 4 mg/kg bodyweight of pentamidine isethionate once daily or on alternate days to a total of 7-10 injections. The im or iv infusion route may be used.

There are no specific dosage recommendations for the elderly.

In renal failure the following recommendations are made for a creatinine clearance of less than 10 ml/min.:

P. carinii pneumonia: in life threatening cases, 4 mg/kg bodyweight once daily for 7 to 10 days, then 4 mg/kg bodyweight on alternate days, to complete the course of at least 14 doses. In less severe cases, 4 mg/kg bodyweight on alternate days, to complete the course of at least 14 doses.

No dosage reductions are necessary in renally impaired patients with leishmaniasis or trypanosomiasis.

Hepatic failure: no specific dosage recommendations.

Prevention: Dissolve the contents of one pentacarinat vial (300 mg pentamidine isethionate) in 4-6 ml water for injections BP. In the prophylaxis of P. carinii pneumonia, the adult dosage is 300 mg every 4 weeks or 150 mg every 2 weeks.

Contra-indications: The drug should not be administered to patients with a known hypersensitivity to pentamidine.

Special warnings and precautions for use: Pentamidine isethionate should be used with particular caution in patients with hepatic and/or renal dysfunction, hypertension or hypotension, hyperglycaemia or hypoglycaemia, leucopenia, thrombocytopenia or anaemia. Fatalities due to severe hypotension, hypoglycaemia, acute pancreatitis and cardiac arrhythmias have been reported in patients treated with pentamidine isethionate, by both the intramusclar and intravenous routes. Baseline blood pressure should be established and patients should receive the drug lying down. Blood pressure should be closely monitored during administration and at regular intervals until treatment is concluded. Therefore patients receiving pentamidine by inhalation should be closely monitored for the development of severe adverse reactions.

Laboratory monitoring: The following tests should be carried out before, during and after therapy by the parenteral route:

Blood urea, nitrogen and serum creatinine daily during therapy.

Complete blood and platelet counts daily during therapy.

Fasting blood glucose measurements daily during therapy, and at regular intervals after completion of therapy. Hyperglycaemia and diabetes mellitus, with or without preceding hypoglycaemia have occurred up to several months after cessation of therapy.

Liver function tests (LFTS) including bilirubin, alkaline phosphatase, aspartate aminotransferase (AST/GOT), and alkaline aminotransferase (ALT/GPT). If baseline measurements are normal and remain so during therapy, test weekly. When there is baseline elevation in LFTS and/or LFTS increase during therapy, continue monitoring weekly unless the patient is on other hepatotoxic agents, when monitoring every 3-5 days is appropriate.

Serum calcium, test weekly.

Electrocardiograms at regular intervals.

The benefit of aerosolised pentamidine therapy in patients at high risk of a pneumothorax should be weighed against the clinical consequences of such a manifestation.

Interactions with other medicaments and other forms of interaction: There are no documented interactions with other medicaments.

Pregnancy and lactation: There is no evidence of the safety of pentamidine isethionate in human pregnancy. A miscarriage within the first trimester of pregnancy has been reported following aerosolised prophylactic administration. Pentamidine isethionate should not be administered to pregnant patients unless considered essential. *Lactation:* The use of pentamidine isethionate is contra-indicated in breast feeding mothers unless considered essential by the physician.

Effects on ability to drive and use machines: Pentamidine has no known effect on the ability to drive and use machines.

Undesirable effects: Parenteral Route: Severe reactions which may be life threatening include hypotension, hypoglycaemia, pancreatitis, cardiac arrythmias, leucopenia, thrombocytopenia, acute renal failure, hypocalcaemia. A possible case of Stevens-Johnson syndrome has been reported.

Less severe reactions include azotemia, abnormal liver function tests, leucopenia, anaemia, thrombocytopenia, hyperkalaemia, nausea and vomiting, hypotension, dizziness, syncope, flushing, hypoglycaemia, hyperglycaemia, rash, taste disturbances.

Local reactions can occur ranging in severity from discomfort and pain to induration, abscess formation and muscle necrosis.

Reversible renal side effects occur with the highest frequency (over 20% of patients) with a slightly lower frequency of local reactions.

Side effects including metabolic disturbances, hepatic, haematological, or hypotensive episodes occur much less frequently (5-10% patients).

Inhalation route: Bronchospasm has been reported to occur following use of the nebuliser. This has been particularly noted in patients who have a history of smoking or asthma. This can usually be controlled by prior use of bronchodilators.

The occurrence of cases of pneumothorax has been reported in patients presenting a history of PCP. Although the aetiology of the pneumothorax was not linked primarily to the aerosolised administration of pentamidine in the majority of cases, a causal relationship to pentamidine cannot be ruled out.

Local reactions involving the upper respiratory tract can occur ranging in severity from cough, shortness of breath and wheezing to bronchospasms.

Other side effects reported were hypotention, hypoglycaemia, acute pancreatitis, renal insufficiency rash, fever, decrease in appetite, taste disturbances, fatigue, light-headedness and nausea.

Overdosage: Treatment is symptomatic. No cases of overdosage have been recorded with pentamidine isethionate.

Pharmacological properties
Pharmacodynamic properties: Pentamidine isethionate is an aromatic diamine. It is an antiprotozoal agent which acts by interfering with DNA and folate transformation, and by the inhibition of RNA and protein synthesis.

Pharmacokinetic properties: After intravenous infusion, plasma levels of pentamidine fall rapidly during the first two hours to one twentieth of peak levels, followed by a much slower decline thereafter. After intramuscular administration, the apparent volume of distribution of pentamidine is significantly greater (>3 times) than that observed following intravenous administration.

Elimination of half-lives after parenteral administration were estimated to be about 6 hours after intravenous infusion in patients with a normal renal function. The elimination of half-life following intramuscular injection was found to be about 9 hours.

Following parenteral administration, pentamidine appears to be widely distributed in the body and probably accumulates in tissue, particularly the liver and kidney. Only a small amount is excreted unchanged in the urine.

When administered by the use of a nebuliser, human kinetic studies revealed significant differences when compared to parenteral administration. Aerosol administration resulted in a 10-fold increase in bronchial alveolar lavage (BAL) supernatant fluid and an 80-fold increase in BAL sediment concentrations in comparison with those seen with equivalent intravenous doses.

Limited data suggests that the half-life of pentamidine in BAL fluid is greater than 10 to 14 days. Peak plasma concentrations after inhalation therapy were found to be approximately 10% of those observed with equivalent intramuscular doses and less than 5% of those observed following intravenous administration. This suggests that systemic effects by the inhalation route are less likely.

Long term pulmonary parenchymal effects of aerosolised pentamidine are not known. Lung volume and alveolar capillary diffusion, however, have not been shown to be affected by high doses of pentamidine administered by inhalation to AIDS patients.

Preclinical safety data: No additional data of relevance to the prescriber

Pharmaceutical particulars
List of excipients: Not applicable.

Incompatibilities: Pentamidine isethionate solution should not be mixed with any injection solutions other than Water for Injections BP, Glucose Intravenous Infusion BP and 0.9% (normal) Sodium Chloride Injection BP.

Shelf life: 60 months when unopened. After reconstitution 24 hours.

Special precautions for storage: Store the dry product below 30°C.

Store the reconstituted product (for intravenous infusion) at 2-8°C. Use within 24 hours.

Nature and contents of container: Cardboard carton containing 5 x 10 ml glass vials each with rubber bung and aluminium ring. Each vial contains 300 mg Pentamidine Isethionate BP.

Instructions for use/handling: This product should be reconstituted in a fume cupboard. Store the dry product below 30°C. Store dilute reconstituted drug solutions between 2-8°C, and discard all unused portions within 24 hours of preparation. Concentrated solutions for administration by the inhalation or intramuscular routes should be used immediately.

After reconstitution with Water for Injections BP, pentacarinat should not be mixed with any injection solutions other than Glucose Intravenous Infusion 5% BP and 0.9% (normal) Sodium Chloride Injection BP.

The optimal particle size for alveolar deposition is between 1 and 2 microns.

The freshly prepared solution should be administered by inhalation using a suitable nebuliser such as a Respirgard II (trade mark of Marquest Medical Products Inc.), Modified Acorn system 22 (trade mark of Medic-Aid) or an equivalent device with either a compressor or piped oxygen at a flow rate of 6 to 10 Litres/Minute.

The nebuliser should be used in a vacated , well ventilated room. Only staff wearing adequate protective clothing (mask, goggles, gloves) should be in the room when nebulisers are being used.

A suitable well fitted one-way system should be employed such that the nebuliser stores the aerosolised drug during exhalations and disperses exhaled pentamidine into a reservoir. A filter should be fitted to the exhaust line to reduce atmospheric pollution. It is advisable to use a suitable exhaust tube which vents directly through a window to the external atmosphere. Care should be taken to ensure that passers-by will not be exposed to the exhaust.

All bystanders including medical personnel, women of child bearing potential, pregnant women, children, and people with a history of asthma, should avoid exposure to atmospheric pentamidine resulting from nebuliser usage.

Dosage equivalence: 4 mG of pentamidine isethionate contains 2.3 mG pentamidine base; 1 mg of pentamidine base is equivalent to 1.74 mG pentamidine isethionate.

Displacement value: 300 mG of pentamidine isethionate displace approximately 0.15 ml of water.

Marketing authorisation number 16186/0001

Date of approval/revision of SPC February 1997

Legal category POM

PENTACARINAT READY-TO-USE SOLUTION

Qualitative and quantitative composition In terms of the active ingredient Pentamidine Isethionate BP 300 mg (Equivalent to 172.4 mg Pentamidine base)

Pharmaceutical form Nebuliser Solution

Clinical particulars
Therapeutic indications: Pentacarinat Ready-to-Use Solution is indicated in the treatment of Pneumocystis carinii pneumonia (PCP) in patients infected by the human immunodeficiency virus (HIV).

Pentacarinat Ready-to-Use Solution is also indicated for the prevention of Pneumocystis carinii pneumonia in patients infected by the human immunodeficiency virus who have experienced a previous episode of PCP.

Posology and method of administration:
Adults:
Treatment of Pneumocystis carinii pneumonia: 600 mg, (two bottles) given once daily for 3 weeks, administered by a suitable nebuliser.

Prevention of Pneumocystis carinii pneumonia: 300 mg given once a month or 150 mg given every two weeks, administered using a suitable nebuliser.

There are no specific dosage recommendations for the elderly.

Hepatic failure: No information is available.

Contra-indications: The drug should not be administered to patients with a known hypersensitivity to pentamidine.

Special warnings and special precautions for use: Fatalities due to severe hypotension, hypoglycaemia, acute pancreatitis and cardiac arrhythmias have been reported in patients treated with pentamidine isethionate, by both the intramuscular and intravenous routes. Therefore patients receiving pentamidine by inhalation should be closely monitored for the development of severe adverse reactions.

Pentamidine isethionate should be used with particular caution in patients with hepatic and/or renal dysfunction, hypertension, hyperglycaemia, hypoglycaemia, leucopenia, thrombocytopenia or anaemia. Bronchospasm has been reported to occur following the use of the nebuliser. This has been particularly noted in patients who have a history of smoking or asthma. This can be controlled by prior use of bronchodilators.

The benefit of aerosolised pentamidine therapy in patients at high risk of a pneumothorax should be weighed against the clinical consequences of such a manifestation.

Interactions with other medicaments and other forms of interaction: There are no documented interactions with other medicaments.

Use during pregnancy and lactation: There is no evidence on the safety of aerosolised pentamidine in human pregnancy. A miscarriage within the first trimester of pregnancy has been reported following aerosolised prophylactic administration. Pentamidine isethionate should not be administered to pregnant patients unless considered essential. The use of pentamidine isethionate is contraindicated in breast feeding mothers unless considered essential by the physician.

Effects on ability to drive and use machines: Pentamidine has no known effect on the ability to drive and use

Undesirable effects: Cases of pneumothorax have been reported in patients with a history of PCP. Although the aetiology of the pneumothorax was not linked primarily to the aerosolised administration of pentamidine in the majority of cases, a causal relationship cannot be ruled out. Local reactions involving the respiratory tract can occur, ranging in severity from cough, shortness of breath and wheezing to bronchospasms. Other adverse effects reported with the use of aerosolised pentamidine are rash, hypotension, hypoglycaemia, acute pancreatitis, renal insufficiency, fever, decrease in appetite, taste disturbances, fatigue, lightheadedness and nausea.

Overdose: No cases of overdosage have been recorded with pentamidine. Should overdosage occur, treatment is symptomatic.

Pharmacological properties
Pharmacodynamic properties: Pentamidine isethionate is an aromatic diamine. It is an antiprotozoal agent which acts by interfering with DNA and folate transformation, and by the inhibition of RNA and protein synthesis.

Pharmacokinetic properties: When administered by the use of a nebuliser, human kinetic studies revealed significant differences when compared to parenteral administration. Aerosol administration resulted in a 10-fold increase in bronchial alveolar lavage (BAL) supernatant fluid and an 80-fold increase in BAL sediment concentrations in comparison with those seen with equivalent parenteral doses.

Limited data suggests that the half life of pentamidine in BAL fluid is greater than 10-14 days.

Long term pulmonary parenchymal effects of aerosolised pentamidine are not known. Lung volume and alveolar capillary diffusion, however, have not been shown to be affected by high doses of pentamidine administered by inhalation to AIDS patients.

Preclinical safety data: No additional data of relevance to the prescriber

Pharmaceutical particulars
List of excipients: Glucose EP, Sodium acetate EP, Glacial acetic acid BP, Water for Injections EP.

Incompatibilities: Pentamidine nebuliser solution should not be mixed with any other solution.

Shelf life: 12 months

Special precautions for storage: Store below 25°C. Do not refrigerate. See Instructions for Use/Handling Section

Nature and contents of container: Low density polyethylene bottles and plug with yellow high density polyethylene tamper evident caps.

Instructions for Use/Handling: Any solid material evident in the polyethylene bottle should be redissolved by gentle warming in the hand before use. The solution placed in the nebuliser reservoir should be visually inspected prior to use. Any solution containing particulate matter should be discarded and the nebuliser reservoir rinsed with sterile water prior to re-use

The optimal particle size for alveolar deposition is between 1 and 2 microns.

The solution containing the required dosage should be administered by inhalation using a suitable nebuliser such as a Respirgard II (trade mark of Marquest Medical Products inc.), modified Acorn system 22 (trade mark of Medic-Aid) or an equivalent device with either a compressor or piped oxygen at a flow rate of 6 to 10 litres/minute.

The nebuliser should be used in a vacated well ventilated room. Only staff wearing adequate protective clothing (mask, goggles, gloves) should be in the room when nebulisers are being used.

A suitable well fitted one way system should be employed such that the nebuliser stores the aerosolised drug during exhalations and disperses exhaled pentamidine into a reservoir. A filter should be fitted to the exhaust line to reduce atmospheric pollution. It is advisable to use a suitable exhaust tube which vents directly through a window to the external atmosphere. Care should be taken to ensure that passers-by will not be exposed to the exhaust. All bystanders including medical personnel, women of child bearing potential, pregnant women, children and people with a history of asthma should avoid exposure to atmospheric pentamidine resulting from nebuliser usage.

Dosage equivalence: 4 mg pentamidine isethionate contain 2.3 mg pentamidine base. 1 mg pentamidine base is equivalent to 1.74 mg pentamidine isethionate.

Marketing authorisation number PL 16186/0002

Date of approval/revision of SPC October 1998

Legal category POM

PIPORTIL* DEPOT INJECTION

Qualitative and quantitative composition pipothiazine palmitate HSE 5.0% w/v

Pharmaceutical form Depot injection.

Clinical particulars
Therapeutic indications: For the maintenance treatment of schizophrenia and paranoid psychoses and

prevention of relapse, especially where compliance with oral medication is a problem

Posology and method of administration: Patients should be stabilised on Piportil Depot under psychiatric supervision. Administration should be by deep intramuscular injection into the gluteal region. Wide variation of response can be expected. The following dosage recommendations are suitable for either indication.

Adults: Initially 25 mg should be given to assess the response of the patient to the drug. Further doses should be administered at appropriate intervals, increasing by increments of 25 or 50 mg until a satisfactory response is obtained. In clinical practice, Piportil Depot has been shown to have a long duration of action, allowing intervals of 4 weeks between injections for maintenance therapy. Dosage should be adjusted under close supervision to suit each individual patient in order to obtain the best therapeutic response compatible with tolerance. The duration of action depends on the dose administered, allowing dosage intervals to be varied to suit individual circumstances. Most patients respond favourably to a dose of 50-100 mg every 4 weeks, the maximum recommended dose is 200 mg every four weeks.

Elderly: Neuroleptics should be used cautiously in the elderly: A reduced starting dose is recommended, ie 5-10 mg might be considered.

Children: Not recommended for use in children.

Contra-indications: Piportil Depot should not be administered to patients in a comatose state or with marked cerebral atherosclerosis, phaeochromocytoma, renal or liver failure, severe cardiac insufficiency or hypersensitivity to other phenothiazine derivatives.

Special warnings and special precautions for use: Piportil Depot should be used with caution in patients suffering from or who have a history of, the following conditions: severe respiratory disease, epilepsy, alcohol withdrawal symptoms, brain damage, Parkinson's disease or marked extrapyramidal symptoms with previously used neuroleptics, personal or family history of narrow angle glaucoma, hypothyroidism, myasthenia gravis, prostatic hypertrophy, thyrotoxicosis. Care is required in very hot or very cold weather particularly in elderly frail patients.

Interactions with other medicaments and other forms of interaction: The CNS depressant actions of neuroleptic agents may be intensified (additively) by alcohol, barbiturates and other sedatives. Respiratory depression may occur.

The hypotensive effect of most antihypertensive drugs especially alpha adrenoceptor blocking agents may be exaggerated by neuroleptics.

The mild anticholinergic effect of neuroleptics may be enhanced by other anticholinergic drugs possibly leading to constipation, heat stroke, etc.

The action of some drugs may be opposed by phenothiazine neuroleptics; these include amphetamine, levodopa, clonidine, guanethidine, adrenaline.

Anticholinergic agents may reduce the antipsychotic effect of neuroleptics.

Some drugs interfere with absorption of neuroleptic agents: antacids, anti-Parkinson drugs, lithium. Increases or decreases in the plasma concentrations of a number of drugs, e.g. propranolol, phenobarbitone have been observed but were not of clinical significance.

High doses of neuroleptics reduce the response to hypoglycaemic agents, the dosage of which might have to be raised.

Adrenaline must not be used in patients overdosed with phenothiazine neuroleptics. Most of the above interactions are of a theoretical nature and not dangerous.

Simultaneous administration of desferrioxamine and prochlorperazine has been observed to induce a transient metabolic encephalopathy characterised by loss of consciousness for 48–72 hours.

It is possible that this may occur with Piportil since it shares many of the pharmacological properties of prochlorperazine.

Pregnancy: There is inadequate evidence of safety of Piportil Depot in human pregnancy, although animal studies have shown no hazard. The drug should not be used during pregnancy or lactation unless the physician considers it essential.

Effect on ability to drive and use machines: None stated

Undesirable effects: Minor side effects of neuroleptics are nasal stuffiness, dry mouth, insomnia, agitation and weight gain. Other possible adverse effects are listed below.

Liver function: jaundice, usually transient, occurs in a very small percentage of patients taking neuroleptics. A premonitory sign may be a sudden onset of fever after one to three weeks of treatment followed by the development of jaundice. Neuroleptic jaundice has the biochemical and other characteristics of obstructive jaundice and is associated with obstructions of the canaliculi by bile thrombi; the frequent presence of an accompanying eosinophilia indicates the allergic nature of this phenomenon. Treatment should be withheld on the development of jaundice.

Cardiorespiratory: Hypotension, usually postural, commonly occurs. Elderly or volume depleted subjects are particularly susceptible; it is more likely to occur after intramuscular administration.

Cardiac arrhythmias, including atrial arrhythmia, A-V block, ventricular tachycardia and fibrillation have been reported during neuroleptic therapy, possibly related to dosage. Pre-existing cardiac disease, old age, hypokalaemia and concurrent tricyclic antidepressants may predispose. ECG changes, usually benign, include widened QT interval, ST depression, U-waves and T-wave changes.

Respiratory depression is possible in susceptible patients.

Blood picture: A mild leukopenia occurs in up to 30% of patients on prolonged high dosage of neuroleptics. Agranulocytosis may occur rarely; it is not dose-related. The occurrence of unexplained infections or fever requires immediate haematological investigation.

Extrapyramidal: Acute dystonias or dyskinesias, usually transitory, are commoner in children and young adults, and usually occur within the first 4 days of treatment or after dosage increases. Akathisia characteristically occurs after large initial doses. Parkinsonism is commoner in adults and the elderly. It usually develops after weeks or months of treatment. One or more of the following may be seen: tremor, rigidity, akinesia or other features of Parkinsonism. Commonly just tremor. Tardive dyskinesia: If this occurs it is usually, but not necessarily, after prolonged or high dosage. It can even occur after treatment has been stopped. Dosage should therefore be kept low whenever possible.

Skin and eyes: contact skin sensitisation is a serious but rare complication in those frequently handling preparations of phenothiazines; the greatest care must be taken to avoid contact of the drug with the skin. Skin rashes of various kinds may also be seen in patients treated with these drugs. Patients on high dosage should be warned that they may develop photosensitivity in sunny weather and should avoid exposure to direct sunlight.

Ocular changes and the development of a metallic greyish-mauve coloration of exposed skin have been noted in some individuals mainly females, who have received chlorpromazine continuously for long periods (four to eight years). Other neuroleptics have been implicated but less frequently.

Endocrine: hyperprolactinaemia which may result in galactorrhoea, gynaecomastia, amenorrhoea; impotence.

Neuroleptic malignant syndrome (hyperthermia, rigidity, autonomic dysfunction and altered consciousness) may occur with any neuroleptic.

Overdose: Symptoms of phenothiazine overdosage include drowsiness or loss of consciousness, hypotension, tachycardia, ECG changes, ventricular arrhythmias and hypothermia. Severe extrapyramidal dyskinesias may occur.

Generalised vasodilatation may result in circulatory collapse; raising the patient's legs may suffice, in severe cases, volume expansion by intravenous fluids may be needed; infusion fluids should be warmed before administration in order not to aggravate hypothermia.

Positive inotropic agents such as dopamine may be tried if fluid replacement is insufficient to correct the circulatory collapse. Peripheral vasoconstrictor agents are not generally recommended; avoid the use of adrenaline.

Ventricular or supraventricular tachy-arrhythmias usually respond to restoration of normal body temperature and correction of circulatory or metabolic disturbances. If they are persistent or life threatening, appropriate anti-arrhythmic therapy may be considered. Avoid lignocaine and, as far as possible, long acting anti-arrhythmic drugs.

Pronounced central nervous system depression requires airway maintenance or, in extreme circumstances, assisted respiration. Severe dystonic reactions usually respond to procyclidine (5–10 mg) or orphenadrine (20–40 mg) administered intramuscularly or intravenously. Convulsions should be treated with intravenous diazepam.

Neuroleptic malignant syndrome should be treated with cooling. Dantrolene sodium may be tried.

Pharmacological particulars

Pharmacodynamic properties: Slow release phenothiazine neuroleptic.

Pharmacokinetics properties: There is little information about blood levels, distribution and excretion in humans. The rate of metabolism and excretion of phenothiazines decreases in old age

Preclinical safety data: There are no pre-clinical data of relevance to the prescriber which are additional to that already included in other sections of the SPC.

Pharmaceutical particulars

List of excipients: Sesame oil (peroxide-free).

Incompatibilities: Piportil Depot injection should not be admixed with any other substance.

Shelf-life: 60 months.

Special precautions for storage: Protect from light.

Nature and contents of container: 1 and 2 ml clear glass ampoules- pack containing 10 ampoules.

Instructions for Use/handling: None stated.

Marketing authorisation number 16186/0006

Date of approval/revision of SPC February 1997

Legal category POM

**Trade Mark*

Knoll Limited
9 Castle Quay
Castle Boulevard
Nottingham, NG7 1FW

☎ 0115 912 5000 🗋 0115 912 5069

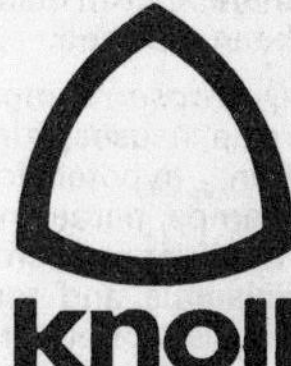

AKINETON*

Presentation White tablets each containing 2 mg biperiden hydrochloride, quartered by score lines on one side with the Knoll logo on the reverse side.

Akineton is also available in 1 ml ampoules containing 5 mg of Biperiden Lactate BP.

Uses Akineton is an anticholinergic drug used for the treatment of drug–induced extrapyramidal symptoms and all other types of parkinsonism.

Dosage and administration
Adults
Tablets: Initially half a tablet (1 mg) twice daily, increasing gradually to 1 tablet three times daily. After maintenance at this level for a few days, increase the dose gradually until no further symptomatic improvement is obtained. Decrease cautiously to lowest dose which adequately controls symptoms. The optimum maintenance dose varies from 3—12 mg daily. If a reduction in salivation occurs, the tablets are best taken after meals. Otherwise, tablets should be taken during meals.
Ampoules: 0.5—1 ampoule as a single dose to a maximum of 4 ampoules in one day, by intramuscular or slow intravenous injection.

Children: Not recommended.

Contra-indications, warnings, etc
Contra-indications: Akineton is absolutely contra-indicated in the presence of untreated narrow angle glaucoma, mechanical stenoses in the gastrointestinal tract and in megacolon. Prostatic adenoma and diseases that can lead to perilous tachycardia are relative contra-indications. The use of Akineton is also contra-indicated in patients hypersensitive to Akineton or any of the inactive ingredients.

Interactions with other medicaments and other forms of interaction: The administration of Akineton in combination with other anticholinergic psychotropic drugs, antihistamines, antiparkinsonian drugs and antispasmodics can potentiate the CNS and peripheral side effects. The concomitant intake of quinidine may potentiate the anticholinergic effect (especially AV conduction). The concurrent administration of levodopa and Akineton may potentiate dyskinesia. Tardive dyskinesia induced by neuroleptics may be intensified by Akineton. Parkinsonian symptoms in the presence of existing tardive dyskinesia are occasionally so serious as to mandate continued anticholinergic therapy.

As a centrally-acting drug, Akineton may potentiate the effect of alcohol.

The effect of metoclopramide and compounds with similar activity on the gastrointestinal tract is attenuated by anticholinergics such as Akineton.

Effects on ability to drive and to use machines: Occasionally, drowsiness may occur. These effects may possibly be enhanced by the additional administration of other antiparkinsonism drugs, antihistamines, tricyclic antidepressants, neuroleptics or quinidine. Patients who drive a car or operate potentially dangerous machinery which requires concentration should be warned that side-effects of this type are a possibility.

Other undesirable effects (frequency and seriousness): Central nervous system side-effects may take the form of fatigue, dizziness and drowsiness; at higher doses, restlessness and confusion, occasionally impairment of memory and in rare cases, hallucinations. Peripheral side-effects include dry mouth, disturbances of accommodation, hypohidrosis, constipation, gastric symptoms and an increase in heart rate; very rarely, a decrease in heart rate. Parenteral administration may be followed by a fall in blood pressure. Allergic skin rash and dyskinesia have also been observed occasionally following the administration of Akineton. In some cases, especially in patients with prostatic adenoma, Akineton may cause micturition difficulties (a dose reduction is recommended) and, more rarely, retention of urine (antidote: carbachol).

Use in pregnancy and lactation: There is no evidence to suggest that Akineton presents a particular teratogenic risk. In view of the lack of experience with the use of Akineton in pregnancy, the drug should only be used with great caution in such cases, especially during the first trimester.

Anticholinergics can inhibit lactation. No data on this subject are available for Akineton. Akineton transfers to human milk, and concentrations equal to those found in the maternal plasma may be reached. Since the type and extent of metabolism in neonates are not known and since pharmacological/toxicological effects cannot be excluded, breast-feeding is not generally recommended.

Other special warnings and precautions: Side-effects occur especially in the early stages of treatment and if the dose is increased too rapidly. Except in the case of vital complications, abrupt discontinuation of the drug is to be avoided due to the risk of excessive counter-regulation. Elderly patients, particularly those with cerebral lesions of a vascular or degenerative nature, may frequently exhibit increased sensitivity even to therapeutic doses of the substance. As the results of animal studies have demonstrated, centrally-acting anticholinergic drugs like Akineton may lead to an increased tendency to cerebral seizure. Physicians should therefore take account of this fact in the management of predisposed persons.

Akineton abuse has been observed.

Especially when Akineton is taken in combination with other centrally-acting drugs, anticholinergics or alcohol, central nervous and peripheral side-effects may impair the ability to drive and to operate machinery.

Combined treatment: In some cases, the response of tremor to Akineton alone may be inadequate. In such cases, combined therapy with an additional preparation effective against tremor should be considered.

Overdosage (symptoms, emergency procedures, antidotes): The symptoms of overdose are anticholinergic effects such as mydriasis, dryness of mucous membranes, flushing, rise in heart rate, reduction of bowel motility, reduction in ureter and bladder tone, increased temperature, excitation, confusion, clouding of consciousness and/or hallucinations. In severe overdose, cardiac and respiratory depression may occur.

Treatment: Gastric lavage or emesis should be considered. As an antidote, anticholinesterase inhibitors are recommended. Vital signs should be closely monitored and appropriate supportive measures taken. Artificial ventilation, reduction of fever, and the application of a bladder-emptying catheter may be necessary. In the event of cardiac depression, a cardiac stimulant drug such as dobutamine may be considered.

Incompatibilities: None.

Pharmaceutical precautions Store in a cool place, protected from light.

Legal category POM

Package quantities Akineton 2 mg tablets in blister packs of 100 tablets. Akineton 5 mg/ml ampoules in boxes of 5 x 1 ml ampoules.

Further information Metabolisable carbohydrate content: Approx. 0.16 g per tablet. Sodium content: 0.13 mmol per ampoule (0.13 mmol per ml).

Product licence numbers
Tablets 0169/0009
Ampoules 0169/0010

APRINOX

Qualitative and quantitative composition
Aprinox Tablets 2.5 mg: Bendrofluazide BP 2.5 mg.
Aprinox Tablets 5.0 mg: Bendrofluazide BP 5.0 mg.

Pharmaceutical form White tablets.

Clinical particulars
Therapeutic indications: For the treatment of oedema and hypertension. Aprinox may also be used to suppress lactation.

Posology and method of administration: For oral administration.

Diuretic: Initially 5 to 10 mg once daily or on alternate days. Maintenance: 5 to 10 mg once or twice weekly. The dose should be taken early in the morning so as to complete diuresis by bedtime.

Antihypertensive: 2.5 to 5 mg once daily. When Aprinox is used concurrently with other antihypertensive agents, the dose of the latter should be halved.

Suppression of lactation: 5 mg in the morning and 5 mg at midday for about five days.

Children: Dosage in children may be up to 400 microgram/kg bodyweight initially, reducing to 50–100 microgram/kg bodyweight daily for maintenance.

Elderly: The dosage of thiazide diuretics may need to be reduced in the elderly, particularly when renal function is impaired, because of the possibility of electrolyte imbalance.

Contra-indications: Aprinox is contra-indicated in severe renal failure and in patients with known hypersensitivity to thiazides.

Special warnings and special precautions for use: Bendrofluazide should be used with caution in patients with Addison's disease, hypercalcaemia and hepatic or renal impairment. Renal function should be continuously monitored during thiazide therapy. Thiazide diuretics may exacerbate or activate systemic lupus erythematosus in susceptible patients.

All thiazide diuretics can produce a degree of electrolyte imbalance, especially in patients with renal or hepatic impairment or when dosage is high or prolonged. Serum electrolytes should be checked for abnormalities, particularly hypokalaemia, and the latter corrected by the addition of a potassium supplement to the regimen.

Interaction with other medicaments and other forms of interaction: Sensitivity to digitalis glycosides may be increased by the hypokalaemic effect of concurrent bendrofluazide. Patients should be observed for signs of digitalis intoxication, in particular arrhythmias, and if these appear, the dosage of the digitalis glycoside should be temporarily reduced and a potassium supplement given to restore stability.

Serum lithium concentrations may be increased by concurrent use of thiazide diuretics.

Non-steroidal anti-inflammatory agents may blunt the diuretic and antihypertensive effects of thiazide diuretics.

ACTH, corticosteroids, acetazolamide and carbenoxolone may exacerbate the hypokalaemia associated with thiazide use. Thiazide diuretics may enhance the neuromuscular blocking effects of the non-depolarising muscle relaxants, e.g. tubocurarine.

Thiazides may enhance the effects of antihypertensive agents, while postural hypotension associated with therapy may be enhanced by concomitant ingestion of alcohol, barbiturates or opioids.

Bendrofluazide may interfere with a number of laboratory tests, including estimation of serum protein-bound iodine and tests of parathyroid function.

Pregnancy and lactation: Diuretics are best avoided for the management of oedema of pregnancy or hypertension in pregnancy as their use may be associated with hypokalaemia, increased blood viscosity and reduced placental perfusion.

There is inadequate evidence of safety in human pregnancy and foetal bone marrow depression and thrombocytopenia have been described. Foetal and neonatal jaundice have also been described.

As diuretics pass into breast milk and bendrofluazide can suppress lactation, its use should be avoided in mothers who wish to breast feed.

Effects on ability to drive and use machines: No adverse effects known.

Undesirable effects: All thiazide diuretics can produce a degree of electrolyte imbalance, e.g. hypokalaemia.

Thiazide diuretics may raise the serum uric acid levels with subsequent exacerbation of gout in susceptible subjects.

Thiazide diuretics sometimes lower carbohydrate tolerance and the insulin dosage of the diabetic patient may require adjustment. Care is necessary when bendrofluazide is administered to those with a known predisposition to diabetes.

Rarely, blood dyscrasias, including agranulocytosis, aplastic anaemia, thrombocytopenia and leucopenia, and pancreatitis have been reported with long-term therapy. Skin rashes and impotence have occasionally been reported.

Overdose: Symptoms of overdosage include anorexia, nausea, vomiting, diarrhoea, diuresis, dehydration, hypotension, dizziness, weakness, muscle cramps, paraesthesia, tetany, gastrointestinal bleeding, hyponatraemia, hypo- or hyperglycaemia, hypokalaemia and metabolic alkalosis. Initial treatment consists of either emesis or gastric lavage, if appropriate. Otherwise treatment should be symptomatic and supportive including the correction of fluid and electrolyte imbalance. Blood pressure should also be monitored. There is no specific antidote.

Pharmacological properties
Pharmacodynamic properties: Bendrofluazide is a thiazide diuretic which reduces the absorption of electrolytes from the renal tubules, thereby increasing the excretion of sodium and chloride ions, and consequently of water. The excretion of other electrolytes, notably potassium and magnesium, is also increased. The excretion of calcium is reduced. Thiazides also reduce carbonic anhydrase activity so that bicarbonate excretion is increased, but this effect is generally small and does not appreciably alter the acid-base balance or the pH of the urine. Thiazides also have a hypotensive effect, due to a reduction in peripheral resistance and enhance the effects of other antihypertensive agents.

Pharmacokinetic properties: Bendrofluazide is completely absorbed from the gastrointestinal tract and it is fairly extensively metabolised. About 30% is excreted unchanged in the urine. The onset of diuretic action of the thiazides following oral administration occurs within two hours and the peak effect between three and six hours after administration. The duration of the diuretic action of bendrofluazide is between 18 and 24 hours. The onset of the hypotensive action is generally three or four days.

Preclinical safety data: Not applicable.

Pharmaceutical particulars
List of excipients: Lactose, maize starch, stearic acid, French chalk for tablets.

Incompatibilities: Not applicable.

Shelf life: 36 months.

Special precautions for storage: None.

Nature and contents of container: Amber glass bottle having a tin-plate cap with a waxed aluminium-faced pulpboard liner. Pack sizes: 500 tablets.

Instructions for use/handling: None.

Marketing authorisation number
Aprinox Tablets 2.5 mg 00169/0045
Aprinox Tablets 5.0 mg 00169/0046

Date of approval/revision of SPC February 1996

Legal category POM

Further information can be obtained from Sovereign Healthcare.

ARYTHMOL*

Qualitative and quantitative composition Each film-coated tablet contains 150 mg propafenone hydrochloride or 300 mg propafenone hydrochloride.

Pharmaceutical form Film-coated tablets for oral use.

Clinical particulars
Therapeutic indications:

1. The prophylaxis and treatment of paroxysmal supraventricular tachyarrhythmias which include paroxysmal atrial flutter/fibrillation and paroxysmal re-entrant tachycardias involving the AV node or accessory bypass tracts when standard therapy has failed or is contra-indicated.

2. The prophylaxis and treatment of ventricular arrhythmias.

Posology and method of administration: It is recommended that Arythmol therapy should be initiated under hospital conditions, by a physician experienced in the treatment of arrhythmias. The individual maintenance dose should be determined under cardiological surveillance, including ECG monitoring and blood pressure control. If the QRS interval is prolonged by more than 20%, the dose should be reduced or discontinued until the ECG returns to normal limits.

Adults: Initially 150 mg three times daily, increasing at a minimum of three-day intervals to 300 mg twice daily and, if necessary, to a maximum of 300 mg three times daily.

The tablets should be swallowed whole and taken with a drink after food. A reduction in the total daily dose is recommended for patients below 70 kg bodyweight.

Elderly patients: Higher plasma concentrations of propafenone have been noted during treatment. Elderly patients may therefore respond to a lower dose.

Children: A suitable dosage form of Arythmol for children is not available.

Dosage in impaired liver function: Propafenone is extensively metabolised via a saturable hepatic oxidative pathway. In view of the increased bioavailability and elimination half-life of propafenone, a reduction in the recommended dose may be necessary.

Dosage in impaired renal function: Although the elimination of propafenone and its major metabolite is not affected by renal impairment, Arythmol should be administered cautiously.

Contra-indications: Uncontrolled congestive heart failure, cardiogenic shock (except arrhythmia-induced), severe bradycardia, uncontrolled electrolyte disturbances, severe obstructive pulmonary disease, marked hypotension.

Arythmol may worsen myasthenia gravis.

Unless patients are adequately paced (see Precautions), Arythmol should not be used in the presence of sinus node dysfunction, atrial conduction defects, second degree or greater AV block, bundle branch block or distal block. Minor prolongation of PR interval and intraventricular conduction defects (QRS duration of less than 20%) are to be expected during treatment with Arythmol and do not warrant dose reduction or drug withdrawal.

Special warnings and precautions for use: The weak negative inotropic effect of Arythmol may assume importance in patients predisposed to cardiac failure. In common with other anti-arrhythmic drugs, Arythmol has been shown to alter sensitivity and pacing threshold. In patients with pacemakers, appropriate adjustments may be required. Because of the beta-blocking effect, care should be exercised in the treatment of patients with obstructive airways disease or asthma. Patients with structural heart disease may be predisposed to serious adverse effects.

Interaction with other medicaments and other forms of interaction: The effects of propafenone may be potentiated if it is given in combination with other local anaesthetic agents or agents which depress myocardial activity.

Propafenone has been shown to increase the plasma levels of digoxin and caution should be exercised with regard to digitalis toxicity.

Propafenone has been shown to increase the plasma levels of warfarin with an accompanying increase in prothrombin time, which may require reduction of the dose of warfarin.

Plasma levels of propafenone may be increased by concomitant administration of cimetidine.

Increased propranolol and metoprolol plasma levels have been observed when these beta-blockers were used concurrently with propafenone. Thus, dose reduction of these beta-blockers may be required. Details of interactions with other beta-blockers are not known.

Concomitant administration of propafenone and quinidine may result in decreased oral clearance with an increase in the steady-state plasma concentration of propafenone. There has been a report of the lowering of propafenone levels by rifampicin, via the hepatic mixed oxidase system. This reduction may lead to breakthrough arrhythmias.

Cases of possible interactions with cyclosporin (levels increased with deterioration in renal function), theophylline (levels increased), desipramine (levels increased) have also been reported.

Due to the arrhythmogenic effects of tricyclic and related antidepressants, and/or neuroleptics, these drugs may interact adversely when used concomitantly with antiarrhythmic drugs including propafenone.

Pregnancy and lactation: Animal studies have not shown any teratogenic effects but, as there is no experience of the use of the drug in human pregnancy, Arythmol should not be used during pregnancy and lactation.

Effects on ability to drive and use machines: Blurred vision, dizziness, fatigue and postural hypotension may affect the patient's speed of reaction and impair the individual's ability to operate machinery or motor vehicles.

Undesirable effects: Arythmol may produce minor nervous system and cardiovascular side-effects but is generally well tolerated. Occasionally and particularly with higher doses, gastrointestinal disorders (i.e. anorexia, bloating, nausea and vomiting, constipation, diarrhoea, retching), dizziness, bitter taste, headache, blurred vision, dry mouth and vertigo have been reported. Very rarely, fatigue, restlessness, nightmares, sleep disorders, psychological disorders such as states of anxiety and confusion, and extrapyramidal symptoms may occur. Allergic skin reactions such as reddening, pruritus, exanthema or urticaria may occur infrequently. Postural hypotension is occasionally seen, particularly in the elderly. These effects disappear after reduction of the dose or discontinuation of the drug. Bradycardia, sinoatrial, atrioventricular or intraventricular block may occur (see Overdosage). In common with other anti-arrhythmic drugs, there is a small risk of proarrhythmic effects. Convulsions have been observed extremely rarely in cases of overdosage. Rare cases of individual hypersensitivity reactions (manifested by cholestasis, blood dyscrasias, lupus syndrome) and seizures have been reported. All were reversible on discontinuation of treatment. In some cases, a diminution of potency and a drop in sperm count have been observed after high doses of Arythmol. This phenomenon is reversible when treatment is discontinued. However, since treatment with Arythmol may be vital, the drug must not be discontinued due to this adverse reaction without consulting the attending physician. Very rarely, a fully reversible decrease of the white cell, granulocyte and platelet counts has been observed. Isolated cases of agranulocytosis have been reported.

Overdose: Experience with overdosage is limited. No specific antidote is known. Procedures to enhance drug elimination from the body by haemodialysis or haemoperfusion are unlikely to succeed because of the large volume of drug distribution. The usual emergency measures for acute cardiovascular collapse should be applied. In severe conduction disturbance associated with a compromised cardiac function, atropine, isoprenaline or pacemaker therapy may be required. If electrical stimulation is not possible, an attempt should be made to shorten the QRS duration and increase the heart rate with high doses of isoprenaline. Bundle branch block by itself is not an indication for isoprenaline. Hypotension may require inotropic support. Convulsions should be treated with I.V. diazepam.

Pharmacological properties
Pharmacodynamic properties: Propafenone is a class 1c anti-arrhythmic agent.

It has a stabilising action on myocardial membranes, reduces the fast inward current carried by sodium ions with a reduction of depolarisation rate, and prolongs the impulse conduction time in the atrium, AV node and, primarily, in the His-Purkinje system.

Impulse conduction through accessory pathways, as in WPW syndrome, is inhibited either by a prolongation of the refractory period or by a blockade of the conduction pathway, both in anterograde but mostly retrograde direction.

At the same time, spontaneous excitability is reduced by an increase of the myocardial stimulus threshold while electrical excitability of the myocardium is decreased by an increase of the ventricular fibrillation threshold.

Anti-arrhythmic effects: Slowing of upstroke velocity of the action potential, decrease of excitability, homogenisation of conduction rates, suppression of ectopic automaticity, lowered myocardial disposition to fibrillation.

Propafenone has moderate β_1 sympatholytic activity without clinical relevance. However, the possibility exists that high daily doses (900–1200 mg) may trigger a sympatholytic (anti-adrenergic) effect.

In the ECG, propafenone causes a slight prolongation of P, PR and QRS intervals while the QT_c interval remains unaffected as a rule.

In digitalised patients with an ejection fraction of 35–50%, contractility of the left ventricle is slightly decreased. In patients with acute transmural infarction and heart failure, the intravenous administration of propafenone may markedly reduce the left ventricular ejection fraction but to an essentially lesser extent in patients in the acute stages of infarction without heart failure. In both cases, pulmonary arterial pressure is minimally raised. Peripheral arterial pressure does not show any significant changes. This demonstrates that propafenone does not exert an unfavourable effect on left ventricular function which would be of clinical relevance. Clinically-relevant reduction of left ventricular function is to be expected only in patients with pre-existing poor ventricular function.

Untreated heart failure might then deteriorate, possibly resulting in decompensation.

Pharmacokinetic properties: Following oral administration, propafenone is nearly completely absorbed in the gastrointestinal tract in a dose-dependent manner and distributed rapidly in the body. After a single dose of one tablet, bioavailability is about 50%. With repeated doses, plasma concentration and bioavailability rise disproportionately due to saturation of the first-pass metabolism in the liver. Steady state is reached after 3 or 4 days when bioavailability is increased to about 100%.

Therapeutic plasma levels are in the range of 150 ng/ml to 1500 ng/ml. In the therapeutic concentration range, more than 95% of propafenone is bound to plasma proteins. Comparing cumulative urinary excretion over 24 hours demonstrated that 1.3% of intravenous (70 mg) and 0.65% of oral (600 mg) propafenone is excreted unchanged in the urine, i.e.

propafenone is almost exclusively metabolised in the liver. Even in the presence of impaired renal function, reduced elimination of propafenone is not likely, which is confirmed by case reports and single kinetic studies in patients undergoing chronic haemodialysis: clinical chemistry values did not differ from those of patients with uncompromised kidneys.

The terminal elimination half-life in patients is 5–7 hours, 12 hours in single cases, following repeated doses. A close positive correlation between plasma level and AV conduction time was seen in the majority of both healthy volunteers and patients.

At a concentration of 500 ng/ml, the PR interval is statistically significantly prolonged as compared to baseline values which allows for dose titration and monitoring of the patients with the help of ECG readings. The frequency of ventricular extrasystoles decreases as plasma concentrations increase. Adequate anti-arrhythmic activity has in single cases been observed at plasma levels as low as <500 ng/ml.

Preclinical safety data: Intravenous administration of propafenone at doses within the toxic range has caused reversible disorders of spermatogenesis at irregular intervals in monkeys, dogs and rabbits.

Pharmaceutical particulars
List of excipients: Microcrystalline cellulose, maize starch, hydroxypropylmethylcellulose, croscarmellose sodium, polyethylene glycol 6000, titanium dioxide, polyethylene glycol 400.

Incompatibilities: None.

Shelf-life: The recommended shelf-life is 5 years.

Special precautions for storage: Store at room temperature (i.e. below 25°C).

Nature and contents of container: PVC/aluminium blister strips. Arythmol 150 mg tablets: pack of 90. Arythmol 300 mg tablets: pack of 60.

Instructions for use/handling: Due to the bitter taste and local anaesthetic action of propafenone, the tablets should be taken whole together with some liquid after meals.

Marketing authorisation numbers
150 mg 0169/0015
300 mg 0169/0016

Date of approval/revision of SPC March 1996.

Legal category POM.

BRUFEN*

Presentation *Tablets:* Brufen is available as sugar-coated tablets containing either 200 mg or 400 mg (Brufen 400) Ibuprofen BP. It is also available as Brufen 600, film-coated tablets each containing 600 mg of Ibuprofen BP.

The tablets are light magenta in colour. The 200 mg tablets bear the overprint 'Brufen' in black; the 400 mg tablets are overprinted 'Brufen 400' and the 600 mg tablets 'Brufen 600', also in black.

Granules: Brufen Granules are packed in sachets, each one containing 600 mg of Ibuprofen BP. One sachet dispersed in water makes an effervescent, orange-flavoured drink.

Syrup: For children, and for adults who have difficulty in swallowing tablets, Brufen is presented as Brufen Syrup, an orange-flavoured liquid containing 100 mg of Ibuprofen BP in each 5 ml.

Inactive ingredients: Brufen (200 mg) – sodium benzoate; sucrose; erythrosine. Brufen 400 – sodium benzoate; sucrose; erythrosine. Brufen 600 – erythrosine. Brufen Granules – sucrose; microcrystalline cellulose; saccharin. Brufen Syrup – sucrose; sorbitol; methyl hydroxybenzoate; propyl hydroxybenzoate; sodium benzoate; sunset yellow.

Uses Brufen is indicated for its analgesic and anti-inflammatory effects in the treatment of rheumatoid arthritis (including juvenile rheumatoid arthritis or Still's disease), ankylosing spondylitis, osteoarthritis and other non-rheumatoid (seronegative) arthropathies.

In the treatment of non-articular rheumatic conditions, Brufen is indicated in periarticular conditions such as frozen shoulder (capsulitis), bursitis, tendinitis, tenosynovitis and low back pain; Brufen can also be used in soft-tissue injuries such as sprains and strains.

Brufen is indicated for its analgesic effect in the relief of mild to moderate pain such as dysmenorrhoea, dental and post-operative pain and for the symptomatic relief of headache including migraine headache.

Brufen Syprup is indicated in short-term use for the treatment of pyrexia in children over one year of age.

Dosage and administration
Adults: The recommended dosage of Brufen is 1200–1800 mg daily in divided doses. Some patients can be maintained on 600–1200 mg daily. In severe or acute conditions, it can be advantageous to increase the dosage until the acute phase is brought under control, provided that the total daily dosage does not exceed 2400 mg in divided doses.

Children: The daily dosage of Brufen is 20 mg/kg of bodyweight in divided doses. This can be achieved as follows using the syrup:
1–2 years: One 2.5 ml spoonful (50 mg) three to four times a day.
3–7 years: One 5 ml spoonful (100 mg) three to four times a day.
8–12 years: Two 5 ml spoonfuls (200 mg) three to four times a day.

In juvenile rheumatoid arthritis, up to 40 mg/kg of bodyweight daily in divided doses may be taken in severe cases. Not recommended for children weighing less than 7 kg.

Brufen Granules are not recommended for children under 12 years of age.

Elderly: No special dosage modifications are required for elderly patients, unless renal or hepatic function is impaired, in which case dosage should be assessed individually.

Contra-indications, warnings, etc
Contra-indications: Brufen should not be administered to patients with a history of, or active, peptic ulceration (see *Adverse events*).

Brufen is contra-indicated in patients who have previously shown hypersensitivity reactions (e.g. asthma, rhinitis or urticaria) in response to ibuprofen, aspirin or other non-steroidal anti-inflammatory drugs (NSAIDs; see *Adverse events*).

Precautions: Caution is required if Brufen is administered to patients suffering from, or with a previous history of, bronchial asthma since ibuprofen has been reported to cause bronchospasm in such patients (see *Adverse events*).

Brufen should only be given with care to patients with a history of gastrointestinal disease (see *Adverse events*).

Caution is required in patients with renal, hepatic or cardiac impairment since the use of NSAIDs may result in deterioration of renal function (see *Adverse events*). The dose should be kept as low as possible and renal function should be monitored in these patients.

Brufen should be given with care to patients with a history of heart failure or hypertension since oedema has been reported in association with ibuprofen administration (see *Adverse events*).

Each Brufen Granules sachet contains 197 mg (approximately 9 mEq) sodium. This should be considered in patients whose overall intake of sodium must be markedly restricted.

Adverse events:
Gastrointestinal: The most commonly-observed adverse events are gastrointestinal in nature. Nausea, vomiting, diarrhoea, dyspepsia, abdominal pain, melaena, haematemesis, ulcerative stomatitis and gastrointestinal haemorrhage have been reported following ibuprofen administration. Less frequently, gastritis, duodenal ulcer, gastric ulcer and gastrointestinal perforation have been observed. Epidemiological data indicate that of the seven most widely used oral, non-aspirin NSAIDs, ibuprofen presents the lowest risk of upper gastrointestinal toxicity.

Hypersensitivity: Hypersensitivity reactions have been reported following treatment with ibuprofen. These may consist of (a) non-specific allergic reaction and anaphylaxis, (b) respiratory tract reactivity comprising asthma, aggravated asthma, bronchospasm or dyspnoea, or (c) assorted skin disorders, including rashes of various types, pruritus, urticaria, purpura, angioedema and, less commonly, bullous dermatoses (including epidermal necrolysis and erythema multiforme).

Cardiovascular: Oedema has been reported in association with ibuprofen treatment.

Other adverse events reported less commonly and for which causality has not necessarily been established include:

Renal: Nephrotoxicity in various forms, including interstitial nephritis, nephrotic syndrome and renal failure.

Hepatic: Abnormal liver function, hepatitis and jaundice.

Neurological and special senses: Visual disturbances, optic neuritis, headaches, paraesthesia, depression, confusion, hallucinations, tinnitus, vertigo, dizziness, malaise, fatigue and drowsiness.

Haematological: Thrombocytopenia, neutropenia, agranulocytosis, aplastic anaemia and haemolytic anaemia.

Dermatological: Photosensitivity (see *Hypersensitivity* for other skin reactions).

Use in pregnancy and lactation: Whilst no teratogenic effects have been demonstrated in animal toxicology studies, the use of ibuprofen during pregnancy should, if possible, be avoided. Congenital abnormalities have been reported in association with ibuprofen administration in man; however, these are low in frequency and do not appear to follow any discernible pattern. In view of the known effects of NSAIDs on the foetal cardiovascular system (closure of ductus arteriosus), use in late pregnancy should be avoided.

In the limited studies so far available, ibuprofen appears in the breast milk in very low concentrations and is unlikely to adversely affect the breast-fed infant.

Drug interactions: Care should be taken in patients treated with any of the following drugs as interactions have been reported in some patients.

Antihypertensives: Reduced antihypertensive effect.

Diuretics: Reduced diuretic effect. Diuretics can increase the risk of nephrotoxicity of NSAIDs.

Cardiac glycosides: NSAIDs may exacerbate cardiac failure, reduce GFR and increase plasma cardiac glycoside levels.

Lithium: Decreased elimination of lithium.

Methotrexate: Decreased elimination of methotrexate.

Cyclosporin: Increased risk of nephrotoxicity with NSAIDs.

Mifepristone: NSAIDs should not be used for 8–12 days after mifepristone administration as NSAIDs can reduce the effects of mifepristone.

Other analgesics: Avoid concomitant use of two or more NSAIDs.

Corticosteroids: Increased risk of gastrointestinal bleeding.

Anticoagulants: Enhanced anticoagulant effect.

Quinolone antibiotics: Animal data indicate that NSAIDs can increase the risk of convulsions associated with quinolone antibiotics. Patients taking NSAIDs and quinolones may have an increased risk of developing convulsions.

Treatment of overdosage: Gastric lavage and, if necessary, correction of serum electrolytes and appropriate supportive measures. There is no specific antidote to ibuprofen.

Pharmaceutical precautions Brufen 600 (600 mg tablets), Brufen Granules and Brufen Syrup should be stored below 25°C. Brufen Syrup should be protected from light.

Legal category POM.

Package quantities
Brufen Tablets (200 mg): Pack of 100.
Brufen 400 (400 mg tablets): Pack of 100; pack of 250.
Brufen 600 (600 mg tablets): Pack of 100.
Brufen Granules (600 mg sachets): Box of 20 sachets.
Brufen Syrup: Bottle of 500 ml.

Further information Taken on an empty stomach, peak serum levels of ibuprofen occur 45 minutes after ingestion whereas, taken after a meal, the peak may occur up to 90 minutes post-ingestion. Since most people can take Brufen on an empty stomach without gastric discomfort, the initial dose of the day will be more rapidly effective if taken before food. This is particularly valuable in providing relief of the morning stiffness associated with arthritis.

Product licence numbers

Brufen Tablets 200 mg	0169/0049
Brufen Tablets 400 mg	0169/0050
Brufen Tablets 600 mg	0169/0051
Brufen Granules	0169/0047
Brufen Syrup	0169/0048

BRUFEN RETARD

Qualitative and quantitative composition Ibuprofen BP (800 mg)

Pharmaceutical form Sustained-release tablets.

Clinical particulars
Therapeutic indications: Brufen Retard is indicated for its analgesic and anti-inflammatory effects in the treatment of rheumatoid arthritis (including juvenile rheumatoid arthritis or Still's disease), ankylosing spondylitis, osteoarthritis and other non-rheumatoid (seronegative) arthropathies.

In the treatment of non-articular rheumatic conditions, Brufen Retard is indicated in periarticular conditions such as frozen shoulder (capsulitis), bursitis, tendinitis, tenosynovitis and low back pain; Brufen Retard can also be used in soft-tissue injuries such as sprains and strains.

Brufen Retard is also indicated for its analgesic effect in the relief of mild to moderate pain such as dysmenorrhoea, dental and post-operative pain and for symptomatic relief of headache including migraine headache.

Posology and method of administration: For oral administration.

Adults: Two tablets taken as a single daily dose, preferably in the early evening well before retiring to bed. The tablets should be swallowed whole with plenty of fluid. In severe or acute conditions, total daily dosage may be increased to three tablets in two divided doses.

Children: Not recommended for children under 12 years.

Elderly: No special dosage modifications are required unless renal or hepatic function is impaired, in which case dosage should be assessed individually.

Contra-indications: Patients with a history of, or active, peptic ulceration. Patients who have previously shown hypersensitivity reactions (e.g. asthma, rhinitis or urticaria) in response to ibuprofen, aspirin or other non-steroidal anti-inflammatory drugs (NSAIDs).

Special warnings and precautions for use: Caution is required if Brufen Retard is administered to patients suffering from, or with a previous history of, bronchial asthma since ibuprofen has been reported to cause bronchospasm in such patients. Brufen Retard should only be given with care to patients with a history of gastrointestinal disease.

Caution is required in patients with renal, hepatic or cardiac impairment since the use of NSAIDs may result in deterioration of renal function. The dose should be kept as low as possible and renal function should be monitored in these patients.

Brufen Retard should be given with care to patients with a history of heart failure or hypertension since oedema has been reported in association with ibuprofen administration.

Interactions with other medicaments and other forms of interaction: Care should be taken in patients treated with any of the following drugs as interactions have been reported in some patients.

Antihypertensives: Reduced antihypertensive effect.

Diuretics: Reduced diuretic effect. Diuretics can increase the risk of nephrotoxicity of NSAIDs.

Cardiac glycosides: NSAIDs may exacerbate cardiac failure, reduce GFR and increase plasma cardiac glycoside levels.

Lithium: Decreased elimination of lithium.

Methotrexate: Decreased elimination of methotrexate.

Cyclosporin: Increased risk of nephrotoxicity with NSAIDs.

Mifepristone: NSAIDs should not be used for 8–12 days after mifepristone administration as NSAIDs can reduce the effects of mifepristone.

Other analgesics: Avoid concomitant use of two or more NSAIDs.

Corticosteroids: Increased risk of gastrointestinal bleeding.

Anticoagulants: Enhanced anticoagulant effect.

Quinolone antibiotics: Animal data indicate that NSAIDs can increase the risk of convulsions associated with quinolone antibiotics. Patients taking NSAIDs and quinolones may have an increased risk of developing convulsions.

Pregnancy and lactation: Whilst no teratogenic effects have been demonstrated in animal toxicology studies, the use of ibuprofen during pregnancy should, if possible, be avoided. Congenital abnormalities have been reported in association with ibuprofen administration in man; however, these are low in frequency and do not appear to follow any discernible pattern. In view of the known effects of NSAIDs on the foetal cardiovascular system (closure of ductus arteriosus), use in late pregnancy should be avoided.

In the limited studies so far available, ibuprofen appears in the breast milk in very low concentrations and is unlikely to adversely affect the breast-fed infant.

Effects on ability to drive and use machines: No adverse effects known.

Undesirable effects:

Gastrointestinal: The most commonly-observed adverse events are gastrointestinal in nature. Nausea, vomiting, diarrhoea, dyspepsia, abdominal pain, melaena, haematemesis, ulcerative stomatitis and gastrointestinal haemorrhage have been reported following ibuprofen administration. Less frequently, gastritis, duodenal ulcer, gastric ulcer and gastrointestinal perforation have been observed. Epidemiological data indicate that of the seven most widely-used oral, non-aspirin NSAIDs, ibuprofen presents the lowest risk of upper gastrointestinal toxicity.

Hypersensitivity: Hypersensitivity reactions have been reported following treatment with ibuprofen. These may consist of (a) non-specific allergic reactions and anaphylaxis, (b) respiratory tract reactivity comprising asthma, aggravated asthma, bronchospasm or dyspnoea, or (c) assorted skin disorders, including rashes of various types, pruritus, urticaria, purpura, angioedema and, less commonly, bullous dermatoses (including epidermal necrolysis and erythema multiforme).

Cardiovascular: Oedema has been reported in association with ibuprofen treatment.

Other adverse events reported less commonly and for which causality has not necessarily been established include:

Renal: Nephrotoxicity in various forms, including interstitial nephritis, nephrotic syndrome and renal failure.

Hepatic: Abnormal liver function, hepatitis and jaundice.

Neurological & special senses: Visual disturbances, optic neuritis, headaches, paraesthesia, depression, confusion, hallucinations, tinnitus, vertigo, dizziness, malaise, fatigue and drowsiness.

Haematological: Thrombocytopenia, neutropenia, agranulocytosis, aplastic anaemia and haemolytic anaemia.

Dermatological: Photosensitivity (see 'Hypersensitivity' for other skin reactions).

Overdose: Symptoms include nausea, vomiting, dizziness and rarely, loss of consciousness. Large overdoses are generally well tolerated when no other drugs are involved.

Gastric lavage may be of value for a considerable time after ingestion. The tablets may not be totally retrieved. If necessary, correct serum electrolytes and implement appropriate supportive measures.

There is no specific antidote to ibuprofen.

Pharmacological Properties

Pharmacodynamic properties: Ibuprofen is a propionic acid derivative with analgesic, anti-inflammatory and antipyretic activity. The drug's therapeutic effect as an NSAID is thought to result from its inhibitory effect on the enzyme cyclo-oxygenase, which results in a marked reduction in prostaglandin synthesis.

Pharmacokinetic properties: The pharmacokinetic profile of Brufen Retard compared with that of conventional-release 400 mg tablets showed that the sustained-release formulation reduced the peaks and troughs characteristic of the conventional-release tablets and gave higher levels at 5, 10, 15 and 24 hours. Compared with conventional-release tablets, the area under the plasma concentration time curve for sustained-release tablets was almost identical.

Both mean plasma profiles and the pre-dose plasma levels showed no major differences between the young and elderly age groups. In several studies, Brufen Retard produced a double peak plasma profile when taken under fasting conditions. The elimination half-life of ibuprofen is approximately 2 hours. Ibuprofen is metabolised in the liver to two inactive metabolites and these, together with unchanged ibuprofen, are excreted by the kidney either as such or as conjugates. Excretion by the kidney is both rapid and complete. Ibuprofen is extensively bound to plasma proteins.

Preclinical safety data: None stated.

Pharmaceutical Particulars

List of excipients: Colloidal silicon dioxide, isopropyl alcohol, povidone, stearic acid, xanthan gum, French chalk for tablets (talc), hydroxypropylmethylcellulose, purified water, Opaspray White M-1-7111B (Solids), Opacode S-1-9460 HV Brown, industrial methylated spirit or industrial alcohol.

Incompatibilities: None.

Shelf life: 30 months.

Special precautions for storage: Store in a cool, dry place below 25°C.

Nature and contents of container: A blister consisting of 250 micrometre opaque PVC/40 gsm PVDC bonded to 20 micrometre aluminium foil. The blisters are packed in a cardboard carton. Pack size: 56.

Instruction for use/handling: None.

Marketing authorisation number 00169/0053

Date of approval/revision of SPC November 1995

Legal category POM

CHYMODIACTIN 4000 UNITS

Warning Chymodiactin should only be used in a hospital setting by clinicians experienced in the diagnosis and management of all spinal disorders and who have received specialised training in chemonucleolysis.

The proper selection of patients for the appropriate use of Chymodiactin in chemonucleolysis requires precise diagnosis in order to eliminate conditions other than herniated lumbar discs which may produce similar signs and symptoms of nerve root compression.

Chymodiactin should be used only in facilities where supporting personnel as well as clinicians are qualified and equipped to diagnose and manage all potential complications in the use of Chymodiactin, including anaphylaxis.

Presentation Chymodiactin is a sterile lyophilised powder of the proteolytic enzyme chymopapain. The product is available in 2 ml vials exhibiting 4000 picoKatals activity (=4,000 Smith BAPNA assay units) of chymopapain with 1·4 mg L-cysteine hydrochloride monohydrate as activator.

The proteolytic enzyme chymopapain is derived from the crude latex of Carica papaya and is purified by column chromatography.

Other ingredients: Sodium hydroxide and/or hydrochloric acid as pH adjusters.

Uses Chymodiactin Injection is indicated for the treatment of patients with clinically-confirmed herniated lumbar intervertebral discs whose symptoms and signs have not responded to an adequate period or periods of conservative therapy.

Dosage and administration

Adults: The lumbar intervertebral disc should be treated with a single injection of Chymodiactin on one occasion directly into the nucleus pulposus (see under 'Procedure').

Vials of Chymodiactin Injection 4000 picoKatals are reconstituted with 2 ml Water for Injections BP, the resulting solution containing 2000 picoKatals chymopapain per ml.

Recommended dosage is 2000–4000 picoKatals (1–2 ml) per disc, preferably 3000 picoKatals (1·5 ml) per disc. The maximum dose in a single patient with multiple disc herniation is 8000 picoKatals (4 ml).

Children: The safety and efficacy of Chymodiactin has not been studied in paediatric patients. Its use is therefore not recommended in this patient group.

Elderly: There is insufficient evidence to recommend use in patients over the age of 60 years.

Contra-indications, warnings, etc

Contra-indications: Chymodiactin is contra-indicated in patients with a known sensitivity to chymopapain, papaya or other papaya derivatives. It is also contra-indicated in severe spondylolisthesis, progressive paralysis or other increasing neurological dysfunction, and in patients with evidence of spinal cord tumour or a cauda equina lesion.

Chymopapain is a foreign protein and, as such, its injection has the potential to generate an immunological response. Therefore, patients who have previously received an injection of chymopapain must not be re-injected with Chymodiactin.

Patients with congestive cardiac failure, coronary artery disease or respiratory failure should be excluded from chymopapain therapy because of the cardiovascular risk in shock should an anaphylactic reaction occur. Additionally, patients on beta-blockers should be excluded due to the blocking effects on rescue adrenaline, should this be required, and because such agents significantly potentiate the liberation of chemical mediators of anaphylaxis.

Chymodiactin is contra-indicated in patients in whom a pre-operative sensitivity screening test is performed and found to be positive.

Warnings and precautions: 1. Anaphylactic reactions have been observed in a small proportion of patients after injection with Chymodiactin. In post-marketing surveillance conducted in the USA, such reactions occurred in 0.5% of cases overall, but a major European survey has revealed an incidence of 0.14% in contemporary clinical practice.

The reaction can be immediate or delayed for up to one hour after injection and may be life-threatening if not treated promptly. At least one open intravenous line must always be in place for such an occurrence. The reaction may commence with almost immediate hypotension and/or bronchospasm, the former being more common.

Subsequently, laryngeal oedema, cardiac arrhythmia/arrest, coma and death may ensue. Speed in diagnosis and treatment is critical since the clinical signs, severity of progression and duration of an anaphylactic reaction are highly unpredictable. Other signs of allergic response must be watched for, e.g. erythema, pilomotor erection, rash, pruritus, urticaria, conjunctivitis, vasomotor rhinitis, angioedema and various gastrointestinal disturbances, which may herald the imminent onset of a major reaction.

Post-marketing surveillance data from the United States indicates that females are more likely to develop anaphylactic reactions than males, the rates being 0.9% and 0.3%, respectively. There was a statistically significant difference in the frequency of anaphylaxis dependent on whether local or general anaesthesia was used for the procedure, rates of 0.4% and 0.6% being noted, respectively. However, such a difference was not confirmed in the European survey, as both forms of anaesthesia were associated with a recorded incidence of 0.14%.

2. Acute transverse myelitis/acute transverse myelopathy has been reported in association with the

injection of chymopapain at a rate of about 1 in 18,000 patients. Although a cause/effect relationship to the injection of chymopapain itself has not been established, the reported rate is significantly higher than the background incidence reported in the medical literature. These patients are characterised clinically by the delayed (2–3 weeks) onset of paraplegia or paraparesis without prior signs or symptoms. Patients receiving injections at more than one disc space appear to be at increased risk.

Paraplegia, cerebral haemorrhage and other serious neurological complications have been reported soon after chymopapain injection in a small number of patients. Causal relationships to the drug when properly injected have not been established. Needle trauma and/or introduction of chymopapain and contrast media into the spinal fluid may be causal in some of these cases. Less severe neurological reactions have included sacral burning, leg pain, hypalgesia, leg weakness, bilateral cramp, pain in the opposite leg and paraesthesia.

3. The drug is extremely toxic when injected intrathecally in animals. Therefore, great caution must be exercised in ensuring that Chymodiactin is not introduced into the dural canal either directly or by leakage.

4. Several deaths have been reported in association with Chymodiactin injection. These have been related to complications secondary to anaphylaxis, to staphylococcal meningitis with disc abscess or of unknown aetiology. The mortality rate associated with Chymodiactin is estimated at 1 in 4,500 patients (0·02%).

5. Discitis, both bacterial and aseptic, has been reported in several patients.

6. Less severe, but more frequent, adverse reactions include back pain/stiffness/soreness in approximately 50% of treated patients and/or back spasm in approximately 30%. Less frequent adverse reactions include rash, itching, urticaria, nausea, paralytic ileus, urinary retention, headache and dizziness.

7. Certain radio-opaque contrast media are neurotoxic. It has been suggested that the toxicity of these materials may be enhanced by the co-administration of Chymodiactin. Intrathecal administration of Chymodiactin results in capillary disruption and bleeding which may again potentiate the neurotoxicity of contrast agents.

Consequently, it is recommended that discography is not performed as part of the chemonucleolysis procedure unless the operating surgeon determines that the risks of discography are outweighed by the benefits in a particular clinical situation.

8. *Pregnancy and lactation:* As adequate studies have not been performed in either pregnant or lactating women, Chymodiactin is not recommended for use in these patient groups.

Procedure

1. Pre-Treatment: Because of the possibility of anaphylaxis during chemonucleolysis with Chymodiactin, a careful history should be conducted to determine if the patient has multiple allergies, especially a known allergy to papaya or papaya derivatives.

Pre-dose sensitivity testing to detect patients likely to be hypersensitive to Chymodiactin is recommended prior to Chymodiactin chemonucleolysis. Skin and serum testing methods are available.

The following pre-treatment may reduce the incidence, or decrease the severity, of any anaphylactic reaction.

(a) H_1 antagonist – e.g. chlorpheniramine – 4 mg orally, 6 hourly for 24 hours prior to chemonucleolysis to block H_1 effects.

(b) H_2 antagonist – e.g. cimetidine – 4–5 mg/kg bodyweight orally 2 hours prior to chemonucleolysis to block H_2 effects.

(c) Adequate hydration should be maintained throughout the procedure. A secure, wide-bore venous access must be established pre-operatively and maintained for at least one hour after injection of the enzyme, to facilitate emergency intervention if required.

(d) Corticosteroid – e.g. hydrocortisone – orally or intravenously immediately prior to injection may stabilise membranes, decrease permeability and mediator release. Doses from 500–1,000 mg have been recommended.

(a), (b) and (c) are recommended and (d) is optional.

2. Anaesthesia: The choice of anaesthesia for a specific patient should be made by the attending surgeon and anaesthetist. However, **it is recommended that supplemented local anaesthesia be used for chemonucleolysis whenever possible.**

Local anaesthesia: The use of supplemented local anaesthesia in preference to general anaesthesia provides an awake patient, more likely to be alert to pain, particularly if the needle impinges on nerve tissue. In addition, it is likely that a patient under local anaesthetic will not tolerate an excessive number of attempts to place the needle.

General anaesthesia: The advantages of general anaesthesia are thought to be: ease of airway management if anaphylaxis should develop; more precise patient positioning for injection; less patient discomfort.

If halothane anaesthesia is used, it should be noted that if adrenaline is required for treatment of an anaphylactic reaction, there is a potential for arrhythmogenic interaction of the two drugs.

3. Needle placement: Needle placement for the intradiscal administration of Chymodiactin should be made by clinicians experienced in needle placement. Needle placement should be via the lateral approach to avoid puncture of the dura mater. Serious neurological toxicity has been reported using a posterior transdural approach. Therefore, this latter method should not be used.

Great care must be taken to ensure that the dura is not penetrated and that chymopapain or contrast agents (if used) do not enter the subarachnoid space. If there is any question regarding needle tip location within the nucleus of the disc, or if the contrast agent extravasates into the subarachnoid space, the procedure should be abandoned and chymopapain should not be injected.

Prior to injection of Chymodiactin, visualisation of the needle tip position in the disc must be confirmed using an X-ray image intensifier for both the anteroposterior and lateral views.

As an additional aid to needle tip visualisation, surgeons performing chemonucleolysis may wish to consider the injection of saline or water into the nucleus pulposus (saline or water acceptance test). The use of this procedure does not supplant careful evaluation of high quality anteroposterior and lateral X-ray views of the disc.

Discography is not recommended at the time of the Chymodiactin injection unless the attending surgeon considers the risks to be outweighed by the benefits in the particular clinical situation. If, however, discography is considered to be essential, it should be performed using non-ionic water soluble contrast media. At least 15 minutes should elapse after the administration of the radio-opaque contrast medium to allow for diffusion and absorption of the medium before injection of Chymodiactin through the same needle after removal of the obturator.

A volume of less than 0·5 ml of the contrast medium is ordinarily sufficient in determining the location of the needle tip.

If high quality X-ray equipment including an image intensifier is not available to perform chemonucleolysis, the procedure should not be carried out. If there is any question about satisfactory needle placement or if needle placement is difficult, requiring repeated attempts, the procedure should be abandoned.

4. Injection: (a) For 3 minutes prior to Chymodiactin injection, 100% oxygen (O_2) may be administered to the patient by the anaesthetist to maximise oxygenation in case of anaphylaxis.

(b) Based on the increased frequency of neurological adverse reactions in patients with two or more disc level injections, **chemonucleolysis should be limited to the one disc producing the patient's symptoms unless definitive signs, symptoms and diagnostic procedure indicate that more than one disc is at fault.**

Treatment of anaphylaxis: Clinical judgement, speed of therapy and choice of agents all enter into the treatment of anaphylaxis. It must be emphasised that adrenaline is the definitive therapeutic agent in the immediate treatment of the condition. Beta-blocker therapy may antagonise the action of adrenaline, and if halothane is used for general anaesthesia, there is a potential for an arrhythmogenic interaction with adrenaline.

The recommended treatment for severe anaphylactic reaction includes the immediate administration of a vasopressor such as 0·5–1·0 ml of 1:1,000 adrenaline, generally by the intramuscular route. Aminophylline and corticosteroids may be administered intravenously to relieve bronchospasm.

The severe manifestations of anaphylaxis include a sudden fall in blood pressure due to generalised vasodilation and increased capillary permeability, angioedema (including laryngeal oedema), and bronchospasm. Milder signs and symptoms include rhinitis, pruritus, urticaria, vomiting, diarrhoea and abdominal pain. The fall in cardiac output which accompanies a reduced venous return may cause secondary myocardial and tissue hypoxia, with cardiac arrhythmias and a metabolic acidosis completing a vicious circle in severe cases.

Immediate therapy of acute reaction: (a) The keystone of effective treatment is adrenaline. As soon as the reaction is recognised 500–1000 micrograms (0·5 to 1·0 ml of 1:1,000 solution) should be injected intramuscularly (not subcutaneously).

(b) Intramuscular injections of adrenaline should be repeated every 15 minutes until improvement occurs.

(c) A slow intravenous injection of 20 mg of the H_1 antagonist, chlorpheniramine should be given immediately after intramuscular adrenaline and repeated over the subsequent 24 to 48 hours to prevent relapse.

Intravenous corticosteroids (e.g. hydrocortisone) have little place in the immediate management. Their beneficial effects are delayed for several hours. In severely ill patients, however, early administration may help prevent deterioration after the primary treatment has been given. Most patients respond to the combination of intramuscular adrenaline and an intravenous H_1-antagonist.

Continuation therapy: Continuing deterioration with circulatory collapse, bronchospasm or laryngeal oedema requires further treatment. Circulatory collapse requires volume replacement by intravenous fluids monitored, if possible, by a central venous pressure line. If electrolyte solutions are used, large volumes may be necessary because in severe anaphylactic shock the plasma loss may constitute 20–40% of the plasma volume. Colloid solutions such as plasma protein fraction or dextran are theoretically preferable but may themselves release histamine, though in severe anaphylaxis intracellular stores of histamine are likely to have been depleted. Bronchospasm refractory to intramuscular adrenaline requires treatment with intravenous aminophylline, a nebulised beta$_2$-agonist (such as salbutamol or terbutaline), oxygen, and (if necessary) assisted ventilation. Respiratory obstruction due to laryngeal oedema may require emergency tracheostomy.

Effective treatment of anaphylactic shock clearly depends on the severity of the clinical condition and the circumstances under which it occurs.

Pharmaceutical precautions Chymodiactin lyophilised powder should be stored under refrigeration (2–8°C), although it is stable at room temperature (25°C) for periods of time up to 18 months without loss of potency.

The drug should be used within 2 hours of its reconstitution. A vial should be used for only one patient and unused drug discarded and not stored for future use.

Since inactivation of the enzyme will occur with some bacteriostatic agents in common use, diluents containing such agents should not be used.

Legal category POM.

Package quantities Cartons containing 1 vial of Chymodiactin Injection 4000 picoKatals together with a leaflet for the information of the medical profession and a patient information leaflet.

Further information Chymodiactin has been shown to dissolve the nucleus pulposus of dogs and rabbits at doses as low as 50 units/disc and 100 units/disc, respectively. Doses of 3,000 units/disc cause thinning of the inner portion of the annulus in rabbits but do not penetrate the entire structure, while doses as high as 24,000 units/disc in dogs resulted in no apparent significant change in the peripheral portion of the annulus. In vitro studies demonstrated that chymopapain solubilised the glycosaminoglycan protein complex of human nucleus pulposus, but did not attack the collagen of this structure.

When chymopapain was injected into dogs and rabbits, doses up to 100 times greater than that required to remove the nucleus pulposus were well tolerated when injected intravenously, intradiscally and epidurally. The drug is extremely toxic when injected intrathecally; the approximate LD_{50} is 15 units/kg in rabbits, 150 units/kg in dogs and 200 units/kg in baboons. Therefore, great caution must be exercised to ensure that Chymodiactin is not injected intrathecally into the dural canal in the human.

In experiments in baboons, the serial injection of contrast agents (Renografin, Conray or Amipaque) into the spinal fluid, followed by Chymodiactin 15 minutes later produced serious neurotoxicity, including weakness, paralysis and death in doses that were harmless or only slightly toxic when administered as single agents. This information supports the clinical observation that the documented entry of contrast agent and presumed entry of chymopapain into the spinal fluid can produce serious neurotoxicity including paraplegia and cerebral haemorrhage.

Product licence number 0169/0055

DELTASTAB* INJECTION

Presentation Deltastab Injection is a sterile suspension of 25 mg/ml Prednisolone Acetate BP 1963.

Other ingredients: Water for injections; benzyl alcohol; sodium carboxymethylcellulose; polysorbate 80; sodium chloride; with sodium hydroxide and/or hydrochloric acid as pH adjusters.

Uses Prednisolone is a glucocorticoid which has anti-inflammatory activity. Deltastab Injection is intended for the local treatment by intra-articular or periarticular injection of the following conditions:

rheumatoid arthritis, osteoarthritis, synovitis not associated with infection, tennis elbow, golfer's elbow, bursitis.

Deltastab Injection is suitable for administration by the intramuscular route in conditions requiring systemic corticosteroids, e.g. suppression of inflammatory and allergic disorders such as bronchial asthma, anaphylaxis, ulcerative colitis and Crohn's disease.

Dosage and administration

Adults: For articular injection: 5–25 mg depending upon the size of the joint. The injections may be repeated when relapse occurs. Not more than three joints should be treated in any one day.

For intramuscular injection: Dosage will depend upon the clinical circumstances and the judgement of the physician. Suggested dose 25–100 mg once or twice weekly.

Children: Corticosteroids cause growth retardation in infancy, childhood and adolescence, which may be irreversible. Treatment should be limited to the minimum dosage for the shortest possible time.

Elderly: Steroids should be used cautiously in the elderly since adverse effects are enhanced by old age (see Warnings).

Note: When long-term treatment is to be discontinued, the dose administered should be gradually reduced over a period of weeks or months depending on dosage and duration of therapy (see Warnings).

Undesirable effects may be minimised by using the lowest effective dose for the minimum period, and by administering the daily requirement as a single morning dose or whenever possible as a single morning dose on alternate days. Frequent patient review is required to appropriately titrate the dose against disease activity.

Contra-indications, warnings, etc

Contra-indications: Deltastab Injection is contra-indicated in patients with known hypersensitivity to any of the ingredients, and in patients with systemic infections, unless specific anti-infective therapy is employed. It is also contra-indicated in patients vaccinated with live vaccines (see Warnings).

Intra-articular and periarticular injections of Deltastab Injection are contra-indicated when the joint or surrounding tissues are infected. The presence of infection also precludes injection into tendon sheaths and bursae. Deltastab Injection must not be injected directly into tendons, nor should it be injected into the spinal or other non-diarthrodial joints.

Precautions: A patient information leaflet should be supplied with this product.

Intra-articular corticosteroids are associated with a substantially increased risk of inflammatory response in the joint, particularly bacterial infection introduced with the injection. Great care is required that all intra-articular steroid injections should be undertaken under aseptic conditions.

Warnings:

Adrenal suppression: Adrenal cortical atrophy develops during prolonged therapy and may persist for years after stopping treatment. Withdrawal of corticosteroids after prolonged therapy must therefore always be gradual to avoid acute adrenal insufficiency, being tapered off over weeks or months according to the dose and duration of treatment. During prolonged therapy, any intercurrent illness, trauma or surgical procedure will require a temporary increase in dosage. If corticosteroids have been stopped following prolonged therapy they may need to be temporarily re-introduced.

Patients should carry 'Steroid Treatment' cards which give clear guidance on the precautions to be taken to minimise risk and which provide details of prescriber, drug, dosage and the duration of treatment.

Anti-inflammatory/immunosuppressive effects and infection: Suppression of inflammatory response and immune function increases the susceptibility to infections and their severity. The clinical presentation may often be atypical and serious infections such as septicaemia and tuberculosis may be masked and may reach an advanced stage before being recognised. New infections may appear during the use of corticosteroids.

Chickenpox is of particular concern since this normally minor illness may be fatal in immunosuppressed patients. Patients (or parents of children) without a definite history of chickenpox should be advised to avoid close personal contact with chickenpox or herpes zoster and if exposed they should seek urgent medical attention. Passive immunisation with varicella zoster immunoglobulin (VZIG) is needed by exposed non-immune patients who are receiving systemic corticosteroids or who have used them within the previous 3 months. This should be given within 10 days of exposure to chickenpox. If a diagnosis of chickenpox is confirmed, the illness warrants specialist care and urgent treatment. Corticosteroids should not be stopped and the dose may need to be increased.

Live vaccines should not be given to individuals with impaired immune responsiveness. Killed vaccines or toxoids may be given though their effects may be attenuated.

Particular care is required when prescribing systemic corticosteroids in patients with the following conditions and frequent patient monitoring is necessary:

(a) Osteoporosis (post-menopausal females are particularly at risk).
(b) Hypertension or congestive heart failure.
(c) Existing or previous history of severe affective disorders (especially previous history of steroid psychosis).
(d) Diabetes mellitus (or a family history of diabetes).
(e) Previous history of tuberculosis or characteristic appearance on chest X-ray. The emergence of active tuberculosis can, however, be prevented by the prophylactic use of antituberculous therapy.
(f) Glaucoma (or a family history of glaucoma).
(g) Previous corticosteroid-induced myopathy.
(h) Liver failure.
(i) Renal insufficiency.
(j) Epilepsy.
(k) Peptic ulceration.

During treatment, the patient should be observed for psychotic reactions, muscular weakness, electrocardiographic changes, hypertension and untoward hormonal effects.

Corticosteroids should be used with caution in patients with hypothyroidism.

Use in children: Corticosteroids cause growth retardation in infancy, childhood and adolescence, which may be irreversible. Treatment should be limited to the minimum dosage for the shortest possible time, in order to minimise suppression of the hypothalamo-pituitary-adrenal axis and growth retardation.

Use in the elderly: The common adverse effects of systemic corticosteroids may be associated with more serious consequences in old age, especially osteoporosis, hypertension, hypokalaemia, diabetes, susceptibility to infection and thinning of the skin. Close clinical supervision is required to avoid life-threatening reactions.

Withdrawal: In patients who have received more than physiological doses of systemic corticosteroids (approximately 7.5 mg prednisolone or equivalent) for greater than 3 weeks, withdrawal should not be abrupt. How dose reduction should be carried out depends largely on whether the disease is likely to relapse as the dose of systemic corticosteroids is reduced. Clinical assessment of disease activity may be needed during withdrawal. If the disease is unlikely to relapse on withdrawal of systemic corticosteroids but there is uncertainty about HPA suppression, the dose of systemic corticosteroid *may* be reduced rapidly to physiological doses. Once a daily dose equivalent to 7.5 mg of prednisolone is reached, dose reduction should be slower to allow the HPA-axis to recover.

Abrupt withdrawal of systemic corticosteroid treatment which has continued up to 3 weeks is appropriate if it is considered that the disease is unlikely to relapse. Abrupt withdrawal doses of up to 40 mg daily of prednisolone (or equivalent) for 3 weeks is unlikely to lead to clinically relevant HPA-axis suppression in the majority of patients. In the following patient groups, gradual withdrawal of systemic corticosteroid therapy should be *considered* even after courses lasting 3 weeks or less:

- Patients who have had repeated courses of systemic corticosteroids, particularly if taken for greater than 3 weeks,
- When a short course has been prescribed within one year of cessation of long-term therapy (months or years),
- Patients who may have reasons for adrenocortical insufficiency other than exogenous corticosteroid therapy,
- Patients receiving doses of systemic corticosteroid greater than 40 mg daily of prednisolone (or equivalent),
- Patients repeatedly taking doses in the evening.

Drug interactions: The effectiveness of anticoagulants may be increased or decreased with concurrent corticosteroid therapy, and close monitoring of the INR or prothrombin time is required to avoid spontaneous bleeding.

Serum levels of salicylates may increase considerably if corticosteroid therapy is withdrawn, possibly causing intoxication. Since both salicylates and corticosteroids are ulcerogenic, it is possible that there will be an increased rate of gastrointestinal ulceration.

The desired actions of hypoglycaemic drugs (including insulin), antihypertensives and diuretics will be antagonised by corticosteroids.

The potassium-depleting effects of amphotericin, carbenoxolone and diuretics (acetazolamide, loop diuretics and thiazides) are enhanced by corticosteroids and signs of hypokalaemia should be looked for during their concurrent use.

There is a small amount of evidence that use of corticosteroids and methotrexate simultaneously may cause increased methotrexate toxicity and possibly death, although this combination of drugs has been used very successfully.

The metabolism of corticosteroids may be enhanced and the therapeutic effects reduced by certain barbiturates (e.g. phenobarbitone) and by phenytoin, rifampicin, rifabutin, primidone, carbamazepine and aminoglutethimide.

Use in pregnancy and lactation:

Pregnancy: The ability of corticosteroids to cross the placenta varies between individual drugs. However, 88% of prednisolone is inactivated as it crosses the placenta.

Administration of corticosteroids to pregnant animals can cause abnormalities of foetal development including cleft palate, intra-uterine growth retardation and effects on brain growth and development. There is no evidence that corticosteroids result in an increased incidence of congenital abnormalities such as cleft palate/lip in man. However, when administered for prolonged periods or repeatedly during pregnancy, corticosteroids may increase the risk of intra-uterine growth retardation. Hypoadrenalism may, in theory, occur in the neonate following pre-natal exposure to corticosteroids but usually resolves spontaneously following birth and is rarely clinically important. As with all drugs, corticosteroids should only be prescribed when the benefits to the mother and child outweigh the risks. When corticosteroids are essential, however, patients with normal pregnancies may be treated as though they were in the non-gravid state.

Lactation: Corticosteroids are excreted in small amounts in breast milk. However, doses of up to 40 mg daily of prednisolone are unlikely to cause systemic effects in the infant. Infants of mothers taking higher doses than this may have a degree of adrenal suppression but the benefits of breast feeding are likely to outweigh any theoretical risk.

Undesirable effects: With intra-articular or other local injections, the principal side-effect encountered is a temporary local exacerbation with increased pain and swelling. Normally this subsides after a few hours.

The incidence of predictable undesirable effects, including hypothalamic-pituitary-adrenal suppression, correlates with the relative potency of the drug, dosage, timing of administration and the duration of treatment (see Warnings).

The following side-effects may be associated with the long-term systemic use of corticosteroids.

Anti-inflammatory and immunosuppressive effects: Increased susceptibility and severity of infections with suppression of clinical symptoms and signs, opportunistic infections, recurrence of dormant tuberculosis (see Warnings).

Gastrointestinal: Dyspepsia, peptic ulceration with perforation and haemorrhage, abdominal distension, oesophageal ulceration, candidiasis, acute pancreatitis.

Musculoskeletal: Proximal myopathy, osteoporosis, vertebral and long bone fractures, avascular osteonecrosis, tendon rupture.

Fluid and electrolyte disturbance: Sodium and water retention, hypertension, potassium loss, hypokalaemic alkalosis.

Dermatological: Impaired healing, skin atrophy, bruising, striae, acne, telangiectasia.

Endocrine/metabolic: Suppression of the hypothalamo-pituitary-adrenal axis, growth suppression in infancy, childhood and adolescence, menstrual irregularity and amenorrhoea. Cushingoid facies, hirsutism, weight gain, impaired carbohydrate tolerance with increased requirement for antidiabetic therapy. Negative protein and calcium balance. Increased appetite.

Neuropsychiatric: Euphoria, psychological dependence, depression, insomnia and aggravation of schizophrenia. Increased intracranial pressure with papilloedema in children (pseudotumour cerebri), usually after treatment withdrawal. Aggravation of epilepsy.

Ophthalmic: Increased intra-ocular pressure, glaucoma, papilloedema, posterior subcapsular cataracts, corneal or scleral thinning, exacerbation of ophthalmic viral or fungal diseases.

General: Hypersensitivity, including anaphylaxis has been reported. Nausea, malaise, leucocytosis, thromboembolism.

Withdrawal symptoms and signs: Too rapid a reduction of corticosteroid dosage following prolonged treatment can lead to acute adrenal insufficiency, hypotension and death (see Warnings).

A 'withdrawal syndrome' may also occur including fever, myalgia, arthralgia, rhinitis, conjunctivitis, painful itchy skin nodules and loss of weight.

Treatment of overdosage: Overdosage is unlikely with Deltastab Injection but there is no specific antidote available. Treatment should be symptomatic.

Pharmaceutical precautions Store between 15°C and 25°C. Protect from light. Shake well before use.

Legal category POM.

Package quantities 10 ampoules of 1 ml. Each pack contains a leaflet for the information of the medical profession and a patient information leaflet.

Further information Nil.

Product licence number 0169/0058.

Further information can be obtained from Sovereign Healthcare.

DIMERCAPROL INJECTION BP

Qualitative and quantitative composition Dimercaprol PhEur 5.0% w/v (50 mg/ml)

Pharmaceutical form Solution for injection.

Clinical particulars

Therapeutic indications: Dimercaprol Injection is indicated in the treatment of acute poisoning by certain heavy metals: arsenic, mercury, gold, bismuth, antimony and possibly thallium. Although dimercaprol has not been successful in the treatment of lead poisoning when used alone, there is evidence that used in conjunction with sodium calcium edetate, it can be used successfully in the treatment of lead poisoning, particularly in children.

Posology and method of administration: For intramuscular injection.

Adults: 400–800 mg, in divided doses, on the first day. 200–400 mg, in divided doses, on the second and third days. 100–200 mg, in divided doses, on subsequent days.

Within the above dose range, individual dosage should be calculated on a bodyweight basis and will depend upon the severity of symptoms and the causative agent. As a general guide, single doses should not exceed 3 mg/kg bodyweight. However, in severe acute poisoning, single doses up to 5 mg/kg bodyweight may be required initially.

Children: Dimercaprol Injection is well tolerated by children and the dosage should be calculated on the basis of bodyweight, using the same unit dose/kg of bodyweight as for an adult under similar clinical circumstances.

Elderly: There are no specific data on the use of dimercaprol in the elderly but since it is eliminated via the kidney, it should be used with caution in this age group.

Contra-indications: Dimercaprol Injection is contra-indicated in poisoning by iron, cadmium or selenium, in the presence of impaired hepatic function unless due to arsenic poisoning and in patients hypersensitive to dimercaprol.

Special warnings and special precautions for use: Dimercaprol Injection should be used with care in patients with hypertension or impaired renal function. It should be discontinued or continued with extreme caution if acute renal insufficiency develops during therapy. Dimercaprol Injection may not be effective in cases of concomitant renal failure, e.g. in arsine poisoning and some cases of arsenic poisoning. Any abnormal reaction (e.g. pyrexia) occurring after the initial injection of dimercaprol should be assessed before continuing treatment. The use of Dimercaprol Injection does not eliminate the need for the general treatment of poisoning due to the particular heavy metal.

Interaction with other medicaments and other forms of interaction: Iron supplements must not be taken during dimercaprol therapy as iron forms toxic complexes with it.

Pregnancy and lactation: Dimercaprol Injection has been used in Wilson's disease with successful full-term pregnancies, but since there is no other experience of its use in pregnancy or lactation, it should be prescribed with caution during these periods.

Effects on ability to drive and use machines: No adverse effects known.

Undesirable effects: Side effects are relatively frequent, but at the therapeutic dosage employed, are seldom severe enough to warrant cessation of treatment and are almost invariably reversible. There is some evidence to indicate that 30–60 mg of ephedrine sulphate by mouth, given half an hour before each injection of dimercaprol, will reduce these reactions. Also, a minimum interval of four hours between doses appears to reduce side effects. Dimercaprol may cause the following side effects, particularly at the higher dosage levels: elevation of blood pressure accompanied by tachycardia, nausea and possibly vomiting, burning sensation of the lips, mouth, throat and eyes, salivation and lacrimation, conjunctivitis, rhinorrhoea, muscle pain and spasm, abdominal pain, headache, tingling of the hands and other extremities, a feeling of constriction in the chest and throat, sweating of the forehead and hands. Local pain may occur at the site of injection and gluteal abscess has occasionally been encountered.

A side effect apparently peculiar to children is a fever which develops after the second or third injection, and persists until treatment with dimercaprol is terminated.

Overdose: Symptoms of overdosage include malaise, nausea, vomiting, lacrimation and salivation, burning sensation of lips, mouth, throat and eyes with headache. A sense of constriction of the throat and chest. Increased blood pressure maximal after 15–20 minutes. Transient effects lasting about four hours.

Treatment consists of the subcutaneous administration of diphenhydramine 50 mg or ephedrine 30 mg or ephedrine in a dosage of 30–60 mg orally if time permits.

Pharmacological properties

Pharmacodynamic properties: Dimercaprol is a chelating agent used in the treatment of acute poisoning by heavy metals. The sulphydryl groups of dimercaprol compete with endogenous sulphydryl groups on proteins such as enzymes to combine with these metals; chelation by dimercaprol therefore prevents or reverses any inhibition of the sulphydryl enzymes by the metal and the dimercaprol-metal complex formed is readily excreted by the kidney.

Pharmacokinetic properties: After intramuscular injection, maximum plasma concentrations of dimercaprol may be attained within one hour. Dimercaprol is rapidly metabolised and the metabolites and dimercaprol-metal chelates are excreted in the urine and bile. Elimination is essentially complete within four hours of a single dose.

Preclinical safety data: Not applicable.

Pharmaceutical particulars

List of excipients: Benzyl benzoate, arachis oil, 5N alcoholic ammonia, nitrogen.

Incompatibilities: None known.

Shelf life: 36 months.

Special precautions for storage: Store at 2°–25°C. Protect from light.

Nature and contents of container: A 2 ml clear neutral glass ampoule with ceramic breakring. Pack size: 10 ampoules packed in a polystyrene pack within a cardboard sleeve.

Instructions for use/handling: Special precautions for disposal: react with weak aqueous solution (up to 15% of calcium hypochlorite). Leave for 24 hours. Neutralise and discharge to drain with copious quantities of water.

Marketing authorisation number 00169/0061

Date of approval/revision of SPC October 1995

Legal category POM

FROBEN*

Presentation Yellow, sugar-coated tablets containing either 50 mg or 100 mg of Flurbiprofen BP. The 50 mg tablets are overprinted 'F50' in black; the 100 mg tablets are overprinted 'F100' in black.

White wax suppositories containing 100 mg of flurbiprofen.

Inactive ingredients: Tablets – lactose; sucrose; sunset yellow; quinoline yellow; sodium benzoate; glucose; titanium dioxide. *Suppository* – Witepsol.

Uses Froben is a non-steroidal anti-inflammatory drug (NSAID) which has significant anti-inflammatory, analgesic and antipyretic properties and is indicated in the treatment of rheumatoid disease, osteoarthritis, ankylosing spondylitis, musculoskeletal disorders and trauma such as periarthritis, frozen shoulder, bursitis, tendinitis, tenosynovitis, low back pain, sprains and strains. Froben is also indicated for its analgesic effect in the relief of mild to moderate pain, in conditions such as dental pain, post-operative pain, dysmenorrhoea and migraine.

Dosage and administration

Adults: The recommended daily dose is 150–200 mg in divided doses.

In patients with severe symptoms or disease of recent origin, or during acute exacerbations, the total daily dosage may be increased to 300 mg in divided doses.

Dysmenorrhoea: A dosage of 100 mg (in the form of tablets or suppositories) to be administered at the start of symptoms, followed by 50 or 100 mg (in the form of tablets) given at 4–6 hourly intervals. The maximum total daily dosage should not exceed 300 mg.

Children: Not recommended for use in children under 12 years.

Elderly: Although Froben is generally well tolerated in the elderly, some patients, especially those with impaired renal function, may eliminate NSAIDs more slowly than normal. In these cases, Froben should be used with caution and dosage should be assessed individually.

Contra-indications, warnings, etc Froben is contra-indicated in patients with peptic ulceration, gastrointestinal haemorrhage and ulcerative colitis.

Froben should not be given to patients with a history of asthma or to patients who have experienced bronchospasm, anaphylactic reactions, angioedema or other hypersensitivity-type reactions from use of aspirin or other NSAIDs.

Froben Suppositories are contra-indicated in patients with inflammatory diseases of the rectum and peri-anal area.

Caution is necessary if given to patients with a history of heart failure, hypertension or non-allergic asthma.

As it has been shown that Froben may prolong bleeding time, it should be used with caution in patients with a potential for abnormal bleeding.

NSAIDs have been reported to cause nephrotoxicity in various forms, including interstitial nephritis, nephrotic syndrome and renal failure. In patients with renal, cardiac or hepatic impairment, caution is required since the use of NSAIDs may result in deterioration of renal function. The dose should be kept as low as possible and renal function should be monitored in these patients.

Side-effects: Dyspepsia, nausea, vomiting, gastrointestinal haemorrhage, diarrhoea, mouth ulcers, fluid retention and oedema have been reported. Exacerbation of peptic ulceration and perforation have also been reported.

Urticaria, angioedema and rashes of varying description have been reported.

Very rarely, cholestatic jaundice and thrombocytopenia have been reported. These are usually reversible on withdrawal of the drug.

Very rarely, aplastic anaemia and agranulocytosis have been reported in association with the use of flurbiprofen but causality has not been established.

Occasional symptoms due to local irritation with the suppositories may occur, e.g. diarrhoea and pruritus.

Use in pregnancy and lactation: Preclinical studies have not revealed any teratogenic effects, although Froben should not be prescribed during pregnancy unless the benefits outweigh the possible risks. If Froben is used during early pregnancy, the lowest effective dosage should be employed. During the third trimester of pregnancy, regular use of NSAIDs has been associated with delayed and prolonged parturition and premature closure of the foetal ductus arteriosus in utero and possibly persistent pulmonary hypertension of the newborn.

The amounts of flurbiprofen secreted into the breast milk during lactation are considered to be too small to be harmful and therefore, breast feeding would not be contra-indicated.

Drug interactions: The diuretic response to frusemide can occasionally be reduced by flurbiprofen. Similarly, interference with the action of anticoagulants has occasionally been reported.

Other studies have failed to show any interaction between flurbiprofen and digoxin, tolbutamide or antacids.

Interference with laboratory tests: There is no evidence that flurbiprofen interferes with standard laboratory tests.

Treatment of overdosage: Gastric lavage and, if necessary, correction of serum electrolytes. There is no specific antidote to flurbiprofen.

Pharmaceutical precautions Suppositories: Store in a cool place.

Legal category POM.

Package quantities
50 mg Tablets: Packs of 100 (strips of 10).
100 mg Tablets: Packs of 100 (strips of 10).
100 mg Suppositories: Packs of 12 (strips of 6).

Further information Flurbiprofen is a potent inhibitor of prostaglandin synthetase which most probably explains its pharmacological effects.

Product licence numbers

Froben 50 mg Tablets	0169/0066
Froben 100 mg Tablets	0169/0067
Froben 100 mg Suppositories	0169/0064

FROBEN SR*

Presentation A hard gelatin capsule with a yellow opaque cap and a transparent yellow body containing white to off-white beads, printed 'FSR' in black. Each capsule contains 200 mg flurbiprofen in sustained-release form.

Inactive ingredients: Microcrystalline cellulose; quinoline yellow; titanium dioxide.

Uses Froben SR is a non-steroidal anti-inflammatory drug (NSAID) which has significant analgesic and anti-inflammatory properties and is indicated in the treatment of osteoarthritis, rheumatoid disease, ankylosing spondylitis, musculoskeletal disorders and trauma such as periarthritis, frozen shoulder, bursitis, tendinitis, tenosynovitis, low back pain, sprains and strains.

Dosage and administration
Adults: The recommended daily dose is one 200 mg capsule, taken preferably in the evening, after food.

Children: Froben SR is not recommended for children under 12 years.

Elderly: Although flurbiprofen is well tolerated in the elderly, some patients, especially those with impaired renal function, may eliminate NSAIDs more slowly than normal. In these cases, Froben SR should be used with caution and dosage should be assessed individually, using the standard formulation if necessary.

Contra-indications, warnings, etc Froben SR is contra-indicated in patients with peptic ulceration, gastrointestinal haemorrhage and ulcerative colitis.

Froben SR should not be given to patients with a history of asthma or to patients who have experienced bronchospasm, anaphylactic reactions, angioedema or other hypersensitivity-type reactions from use of aspirin or other NSAIDs.

Caution is necessary if given to patients with a history of heart failure, hypertension or non-allergic asthma.

As it has been shown that flurbiprofen may prolong bleeding time, it should be used with caution in patients with a potential for abnormal bleeding.

NSAIDs have been reported to cause nephrotoxicity in various forms, including interstitial nephritis, nephrotic syndrome and renal failure. In patients with renal, cardiac or hepatic impairment, caution is required since the use of NSAIDs may result in deterioration of renal function. The dose should be kept as low as possible and renal function should be monitored in these patients.

Side-effects: Dyspepsia, nausea, vomiting, gastrointestinal haemorrhage, diarrhoea, mouth ulcers, fluid retention and oedema have been recorded with flurbiprofen. Exacerbation of peptic ulceration and perforation have also been reported.

Urticaria, angioedema and rashes of varying description have been reported.

Very rarely, cholestatic jaundice and thrombocytopenia have been reported. These are usually reversible on withdrawal of the drug.

Very rarely, aplastic anaemia and agranulocytosis have been reported in association with the use of flurbiprofen but causality has not been established.

Use in pregnancy and lactation: Preclinical studies have not revealed any teratogenic effects, although Froben SR should not be prescribed during pregnancy unless the benefits outweigh the possible risks. During the third trimester of pregnancy, regular use of NSAIDs has been associated with delayed and prolonged parturition and premature closure of the foetal ductus arteriosus in utero and possibly persistent pulmonary hypertension of the newborn.

The amounts of flurbiprofen secreted into the breast milk during lactation are considered to be too small to be harmful and therefore, breast feeding would not be contra-indicated.

Drug interactions: The diuretic response to frusemide can occasionally be reduced by flurbiprofen. Similarly, interference with the action of anticoagulants has occasionally been reported.

Other studies have failed to show any interaction between flurbiprofen and digoxin, tolbutamide or antacids.

Interference with laboratory tests: There is no evidence that flurbiprofen interferes with standard laboratory tests.

Treatment of overdosage: Gastric lavage and, if necessary, correction of serum electrolytes. There is no specific antidote to flurbiprofen.

Pharmaceutical precautions No special storage conditions are necessary.

Legal category POM.

Package quantities HDPE bottle of 30 capsules.

Further information Flurbiprofen is a potent inhibitor of prostaglandin synthetase which most probably explains its pharmacological effects.

Taken once a day, preferably in the evening, Froben SR is particularly suitable for those patients where compliance may be a problem and for better control of morning stiffness.

Product licence number 0169/0068.

FURAMIDE

Qualitative and quantitative composition Diloxanide Furoate BP 500 mg

Pharmaceutical form A flat, white tablet, scored and with a characteristic engraving E/F on one face.

Clinical particulars
Therapeutic indications: For the treatment of acute and chronic intestinal amoebiasis.

Posology and method of administration: For oral administration.

Adults: One tablet three times daily for ten days.

Children: 20 mg/kg bodyweight daily in divided doses for ten days. Furamide is not suitable for use in children weighing less than 25 kg.

Elderly: There is no need for a dosage reduction in the elderly.

If required, a second course of treatment may be prescribed.

Contra-indications: Hypersensitivity to diloxanide furoate.

Special warnings and special precautions for use: None.

Interaction with other medicaments and other forms of interaction: No clinically-significant drug interactions known.

Pregnancy and lactation: The safety of Furamide during pregnancy and lactation has not been established and use during these periods should therefore be avoided.

Effects on ability to drive and use machines: No adverse effects known.

Undesirable effects: No serious side effects have been reported and the bacterial flora of the gut is not upset. Flatulence sometimes occurs but may usually be disregarded. Occasionally, vomiting, pruritus and urticaria may occur.

Overdose: Furamide tablets are unlikely to constitute a hazard in overdosage. In severe overdosage, early gastric lavage is recommended. There is no specific antidote. Treatment should be symptomatic and supportive.

Pharmacological properties
Pharmacodynamic properties: Diloxanide furoate is a luminal amoebicide acting principally in the bowel lumen, although its mode of action is not known.

Pharmacokinetic properties: In the gut, diloxanide furoate is largely, if not wholly, hydrolysed into diloxanide and furoic acid under the combined action of bacterial and gut esterases. After absorption, diloxanide is very rapidly conjugated to form a glucuronide. In circulating blood, it is present to about 99% as a glucuronide and 1% as free diloxanide. Diloxanide is predominantly excreted in the urine. It is believed that the unabsorbed diloxanide is the active anti-amoebic substance, up to 10% remaining in the gut which is subsequently excreted as diloxanide in the faeces.

Preclinical safety data: Not applicable.

Pharmaceutical particulars
List of excipients: Maize starch, pregelatinized maize starch, dried maize starch, magnesium stearate, purified water.

Incompatibilities: None known.

Shelf life: 36 months.

Special precautions for storage: None.

Nature and contents of container: A white aluminium tube with a polythene foam disc and a white aluminium screw cap with flowed-in PVC. Pack size: 15 tablets.

Instructions for use/handling: Not applicable.

Marketing authorisation number 00169/0070

Date of approval/revision of SPC October 1995

Legal category POM

GOPTEN

Qualitative and quantitative composition
Gopten Capsules 0.5 mg Trandolapril 0.5 mg
Gopten Capsules 1.0 mg Trandolapril 1.0 mg
Gopten Capsules 2.0 mg Trandolapril 2.0 mg

Pharmaceutical form
Gopten Capsules 0.5 mg Opaque red/yellow capsules
Gopten Capsules 1.0 mg Opaque red/orange capsules
Gopten Capsules 2.0 mg Opaque red/red capsules

Clinical particulars
Therapeutic indications: Mild or moderate hypertension.

Left ventricular dysfunction after myocardial infarction.

It has been demonstrated that Gopten improves survival following myocardial infarction in patients with left ventricular dysfunction (ejection fraction ≤35 percent), with or without symptoms of heart failure, and/or with or without residual ischaemia.

Long-term treatment with Gopten significantly reduces the overall cardiovascular mortality. It significantly decreases the risk of sudden death and the occurrence of severe or resistant heart failure.

Posology and method of administration: For oral administration.

Hypertension: For adults not taking diuretics, without congestive heart failure and without renal or hepatic insufficiency, the recommended initial dosage is 0.5 mg as a single daily dose. A 0.5 mg dose will only achieve a therapeutic response in a minority of patients. Dosage should be doubled incrementally at intervals of 2 to 4 weeks, based on patient response, up to a maximum of 4 mg as a single daily dose.

The usual maintenance dose range is 1 to 2 mg as a single daily dose. If the patient response is still unsatisfactory at a dose of 4 mg Gopten, combination therapy should be considered.

Left ventricular dysfunction after myocardial infarction: Following a myocardial infarction, therapy may be initiated as early as the third day. Treatment should be initiated at a daily dose of 0.5 mg. The dose should be progressively increased to a maximum of 4 mg as a single daily dose. Depending upon the tolerability such as symptomatic hypotension, this forced titration can be temporarily suspended.

In the event of hypotension, all concomitant hypotensive therapies such as vasodilators, including nitrates and diuretics must be carefully checked and if possible, their dose reduced.

The dose of Gopten should be lowered only if the previous measures are not effective or not feasible.

Elderly: The dose in elderly patients is the same as in adults. There is no need to reduce the dose in elderly patients with normal renal and hepatic function. Caution is required in elderly patients with concomitant use of diuretics, congestive heart failure or renal or hepatic insufficiency. The dose should be titrated according to the need to control blood pressure.

Prior diuretic treatment: In patients who are at risk from a stimulated renin-angiotensin system (e.g. patients with water and sodium depletion), the diuretic should be discontinued 2–3 days before beginning therapy with 0.5 mg trandolapril to reduce the likelihood of symptomatic hypotension. The diuretic may be resumed later if required.

Cardiac failure: In hypertensive patients who also have congestive heart failure, with or without associated renal insufficiency, symptomatic hypotension has been observed after treatment with ACE inhibitors. In these patients, therapy should be started at a dose of 0.5 mg Gopten once daily under close medical supervision in hospital.

Dosage adjustment in renal impairment: For patients with mild or moderate renal impairment (creatinine clearance of 10–70 ml/min), the usual adult and elderly doses are recommended. For patients with severe renal impairment (creatinine clearance of <10 ml/min), the usual adult and elderly starting doses are also recommended but the maximum daily dose should not exceed 2 mg. In these patients, therapy should be under close medical supervision.

Dialysis: It is not known for certain if trandolapril or trandolaprilat are removed by dialysis. However it would be expected that dialysis could remove the active moiety, trandolaprilat, from the circulation, resulting in a possible loss of control of blood pressure. Therefore careful monitoring of the patient's blood pressure during dialysis is required, and the dosage of trandolapril adjusted if needed.

Dosage adjustment in hepatic impairment: In patients with severely impaired liver function, a decrease in the metabolic clearance of the parent compound, trandolapril and the active metabolite, trandolaprilat results in a large increase in plasma trandolapril levels and to a lesser extent, an increase in trandolaprilat levels. Treatment with Gopten should therefore be initiated at a dose of 0.5 mg once daily under close medical supervision.

Children: Gopten has not been studied in children and therefore use in this age group is not recommended.

Contra-indications: Known hypersensitivity to trandolapril. History of angioneurotic oedema associated with administration of an ACE inhibitor. Hereditary/idiopathic angioneurotic oedema. Pregnancy or lactation. Use in children.

Special warnings and special precautions for use: Gopten should not be used in patients with aortic stenosis or outflow obstruction.

Assessment of renal function: Evaluation of the patient should include assessment of renal function prior to initiation of therapy and during treatment. Proteinuria may occur if renal impairment is present prior to therapy or relatively high doses are used.

Impaired renal function: Patients with severe renal insufficiency may require reduced doses of Gopten; their renal function should be closely monitored. In the majority, renal function will not alter. In patients with renal insufficiency, congestive heart failure or unilateral or bilateral renal artery stenosis, in the single kidney as well as after renal transplantation, there is a risk of impairment of renal function. If recognised early, such impairment of renal function is reversible upon discontinuation of therapy.

Some hypertensive patients with no apparent pre-existing renal disease may develop minor and usually transient increases in blood urea nitrogen and serum creatinine when Gopten is given concomitantly with a diuretic. Dosage reduction of Gopten and/or discontinuation of the diuretic may be required. Additionally, in patients with renal insufficiency, the risk of hyperkalaemia should be considered and the patient's electrolyte status checked regularly.

Impaired liver function: As trandolapril is a prodrug metabolised to its active moiety in the liver, particular caution and close monitoring should be applied to patients with impaired liver function.

Symptomatic hypotension: In patients with uncomplicated hypertension, symptomatic hypotension has been observed rarely after the initial dose of Gopten, as well as after increasing the dose of Gopten. It is more likely to occur in patients who have been volume- and salt-depleted by prolonged diuretic therapy, dietary salt restriction, dialysis, diarrhoea or vomiting. Therefore, in these patients, diuretic therapy should be discontinued and volume and/or salt depletion should be corrected before initiating therapy with Gopten.

If symptomatic hypotension occurs, the patient should be placed in a supine position and, if necessary, receive an intravenous infusion of physiological saline. Intravenous atropine may be necessary if there is associated bradycardia. Treatment with Gopten may usually be continued following restoration of effective blood volume and blood pressure.

Surgery/anaesthesia: In patients undergoing surgery or during anaesthesia with agents producing hypotension, Gopten may block angiotensin II formation secondary to compensatory renin release. If hypotension occurs and is considered to be due to this mechanism, it can be corrected by appropriate treatment.

Agranulocytosis and bone marrow depression: In patients on ACE inhibitors, agranulocytosis and bone marrow depression have been seen rarely. They are more frequent in patients with renal impairment, especially if they have a collagen vascular disease. However, regular monitoring of white blood cell counts and protein levels in urine should be considered in patients with collagen vascular disease (e.g. lupus erythematosus and scleroderma), especially associated with impaired renal function and concomitant therapy, particularly with corticosteroids and antimetabolites.

Hyperkalaemia: Elevated serum potassium has been observed very rarely in hypertensive patients. Risk factors for the development of hyperkalaemia include renal insufficiency, potassium-sparing diuretics, the concomitant use of agents to treat hypokalaemia, diabetes mellitus and/or left ventricular dysfunction after myocardial infarction.

Angioneurotic oedema: Rarely, ACE inhibitors (such as trandolapril) may cause angioneurotic oedema that includes swelling of the face, extremities, tongue, glottis, and/or larynx. Patients experiencing angioneurotic oedema must immediately discontinue Gopten therapy and be monitored until oedema resolution.

Angioneurotic oedema to the face will usually resolve spontaneously. Oedema involving not only the face but also the glottis may be life-threatening because of the risk of airway obstruction.

Angioneurotic oedema involving the tongue, glottis or larynx requires immediate subcutaneous administration of 0.3–0.5 ml of adrenaline solution (1:1000) along with other therapeutic measures as appropriate.

Caution must be exercised in patients with a history of idiopathic angioneurotic oedema, and Gopten is contra-indicated if angioneurotic oedema was an adverse reaction to an ACE inhibitor (see Contra-indications).

Cough: During treatment with an ACE inhibitor, a dry and non-productive cough may occur which disappears after discontinuation.

Interaction with other medicaments and other forms of interaction: Drug interactions: Combination with diuretics or other antihypertensive agents may potentiate the antihypertensive response to Gopten. Adrenergic-blocking drugs should only be combined with trandolapril under careful supervision.

Potassium-sparing diuretics (spironolactone, amiloride, triamterene) or potassium supplements may increase the risk of hyperkalaemia, particularly in renal failure. Gopten may attenuate the potassium loss caused by thiazide-type diuretics. If concomitant use of these agents is indicated, they should be given with caution and serum potassium should be monitored regularly.

Antidiabetic agents: As with all ACE inhibitors, concomitant use of antidiabetic medicines (insulin or oral hypoglycaemic agents) may cause an increased blood glucose lowering effect with greater risk of hypoglycaemia. Therefore, blood glucose should be closely monitored in diabetics treated with a hypoglycaemic agent and Gopten, particularly when starting or increasing the dose of ACE inhibitor, or in patients with impaired renal function.

Combinations necessitating a warning: In some patients already receiving diuretic treatment, particularly if this treatment has been recently instituted, the fall in blood pressure on initiation of treatment with Gopten may be excessive. The risk of symptomatic hypotension may be reduced by stopping the diuretic a few days before starting treatment with Gopten. If it is necessary to continue the diuretic treatment, the patient should be monitored, at least after the initial administration of Gopten. As with all antihypertensives, combination with a neuroleptic or tricyclic antidepressant increases the risk of orthostatic hypotension. Gopten may reduce the elimination of lithium and serum levels of lithium should be monitored.

Anaphylactoid reactions to high-flux polyacrylonitrile membranes used in haemodialysis have been reported in patients treated with ACE inhibitors. As with other antihypertensives of this chemical class, this combination should be avoided when prescribing ACE inhibitors to renal dialysis patients.

The effects of certain anaesthetics may be enhanced by ACE inhibitors .

Allopurinol, cytostatic or immunosuppressive agents, systemic corticosteroids or procainamide may increase the risk of leucopenia , if used concomitantly with ACE inhibitors.

The antihypertensive effect of ACE inhibitors may be reduced by the administration of NSAIDs. An additive effect on serum potassium increase has been described when NSAIDs and ACE inhibitors have been used concomitantly, while renal function may be reduced.

Antacids cause reduced bioavailability of ACE inhibitors.

The antihypertensive effects of ACE inhibitors may be reduced by sympathomimetics. Patients should be carefully monitored.

No clinical interaction has been observed in patients with left ventricular dysfunction after myocardial infarction when Gopten has been concomitantly administered with thrombolytics, aspirin, beta-blockers, calcium channel blockers, nitrates, anticoagulants, diuretics or digoxin.

Pregnancy and lactation: The use of Gopten is contra-indicated in pregnancy and lactation. Pregnancy should be excluded before start of treatment and avoided during treatment. Exposure of the mother to ACE inhibitors in mid or late pregnancy has been associated with oligohydramnios and neonatal hypotension with anuria or renal failure.

In the rat and particularly in the rabbit, trandolapril caused maternal toxicity together with foetotoxicity at high doses. Neither embryotoxicity nor teratogenicity was observed in the rat, rabbit or monkey.

Effects on ability to drive and use machines: Given the pharmacological properties of Gopten, no particular effect is expected. However, in some individuals, ACE inhibitors may affect the ability to drive or operate machinery, particularly at the start of treatment, when changing over from other medication or during concomitant use of alcohol. Therefore, after the first dose or subsequent increases in dose, it is not advisable to drive or operate machinery for several hours.

Undesirable effects: The following adverse events have been reported with ACE inhibitors as a class. Not all will have been reported in association with Gopten.

In long-term studies with Gopten, the most frequently reported adverse events were cough, headaches, asthenia and dizziness.

Respiratory: Dyspnoea, sinusitis, rhinitis, glossitis, bronchitis and bronchospasm have been reported, but rarely in association with treatment with ACE inhibitors.

Cardiovascular: Tachycardia, palpitations, arrhythmias, angina pectoris, myocardial infarction, transient ischaemic attacks and cerebral haemorrhage have been reported in association with hypotension during treatment with ACE inhibitors.

Gastrointestinal: Nausea, vomiting, abdominal pain, indigestion, diarrhoea, constipation and dry mouth have occurred occasionally during treatment with ACE inhibitors.

There have been reports of individual incidents of cholestatic jaundice, hepatitis, pancreatitis, and ileus connected with the use of ACE inhibitors.

Hypersensitivity: Allergic hypersensitivity reactions such as pruritus and rash have been reported. Urticaria, erythema multiforme, Stevens-Johnson syndrome, toxic epidermal necrolysis, psoriasis-like efflorescences and alopecia, which may be accompanied by fever, myalgia, arthralgia, eosinophilia and/or increased ANA (anti-nuclear antibody)-titres have been occasionally reported with ACE inhibitor treatment.

Angioneurotic oedema: In very rare cases, angioneurotic oedema has occurred. If laryngeal stridor or angioedema of the face, tongue or glottis occurs, treatment with Gopten must be discontinued and appropriate therapy instituted immediately.

Renal: Deterioration of renal function and acute renal failure have been reported with the use of ACE inhibitors.

Drug/Laboratory parameters: Reversible (on stopping treatment) increases in blood urea and plasma creatinine may result, particularly if renal insufficiency, severe heart failure, or renovascular hypertension are present.

Decreased haemoglobin, haematocrit, platelets and white cell count, and individual cases of agranulocytosis or pancytopenia, have been reported with ACE inhibitor treatment; also evaluate liver enzymes and serum bilirubin. Haemolytic anaemia has been reported in some patients with a congenital deficiency concerning G-6-PDH (glucose-6-phosphate dehydrogenase) during treatment with ACE inhibitors.

Overdose: Symptoms expected with ACE inhibitors are severe hypotension, shock, stupor, bradycardia, electrolyte disturbance and renal failure. In the event of overdosage following recent ingestion, consideration should be given to emptying the stomach contents. Blood pressure should be monitored and if hypotension develops, volume expansion should be considered.

Pharmacological properties

Pharmacodynamic properties: Gopten capsules contain the prodrug, trandolapril, a non-peptide ACE inhibitor with a carboxyl group but without a sulphydryl group. Trandolapril is rapidly absorbed and then non-specifically hydrolysed to its potent, long-acting active metabolite, trandolaprilat.

Trandolaprilat binds tightly and in a saturable manner to ACE. The administration of trandolapril causes decreases in the concentrations of angiotensin II, aldosterone and atrial natriuretic factor and increases in plasma renin activity and concentrations of angiotensin I. Gopten thus modulates the renin-angiotensin-aldosterone system which plays a major part in regulating blood volume and blood pressure and consequently has a beneficial antihypertensive effect.

The administration of usual therapeutic doses of Gopten to hypertensive patients produces a marked reduction in both supine and erect blood pressure. The antihypertensive effect is evident after 1 hour, with a peak effect between 8 and 12 hours, persisting for at least 24 hours.

The properties of trandolapril might explain the results obtained in the regression of cardiac hypertrophy with improvement of diastolic function, and improvement of arterial compliance in humans. In addition, a decrease in vascular hypertrophy has been shown in animals.

Pharmacokinetic properties: Trandolapril is very rapidly absorbed after oral administration. The amount absorbed is equivalent to 40 to 60% of the administered dose and is not affected by food consumption.

The peak plasma concentration of trandolapril is observed 30 minutes after administration. Trandolapril disappears rapidly from the plasma with a half-life of less than one hour.

Trandolapril is hydrolysed to trandolaprilat, a specific ACE inhibitor. The amount of trandolaprilat formed is not modified by food consumption. The peak plasma concentration of trandolaprilat is reached after 4 to 6 hours.

In the plasma, trandolaprilat is more than 80% protein-bound. It binds saturably, with a high affinity, to ACE. The major proportion of circulating trandolaprilat is also non-saturably bound to albumin.

After repeated administration of Gopten in a single daily dose, steady state is reached on average in four days, both in healthy volunteers and in young or elderly hypertensives. The effective half-life of trandolaprilat is between 16 and 24 hours. The terminal half-life of elimination is between 47 hours and 98 hours depending on dose. This terminal phase probably represents binding/dissociation kinetics of the trandolaprilat/ACE complex.

Trandolaprilat eliminated in the urine in the unchanged form accounts for 10 to 15% of the dose of trandolapril administered. After oral administration of the labelled product in man, 33% of the radioactivity is found in the urine and 66% in the faeces.

The renal clearance of trandolaprilat is proportional to the creatinine clearance. The plasma concentrations of trandolaprilat are significantly higher in patients with a creatinine clearance less than or equal to 30 ml/min. However, after repeated dosing in patients with chronic renal failure, steady state is also reached on average in four days, whatever the degree of renal failure.

Preclinical safety data: Acute oral toxicity studies of trandolapril and its active metabolite, trandolaprilat, in rats and mice showed both compounds to be non-toxic with respective LD50 values of > 4000 mg/kg and > 5000 mg/kg.

Repeat dose oral toxicity was evaluated in the rat and dog with studies of up to 18 and 12 months' duration, respectively. The principal observations in these studies were of anaemia (doses of 20 mg/kg/day and above in the rat 30-day study and 25 mg/kg/day and above in the dog 6-month study), gastric irritation and ulceration (doses of 20 mg/kg/day and above in the rat 30-day study and 125 mg/kg/day in the dog 6-month study) and renal lesions (20 mg/kg/day and above in the rat 30-day study and 10 mg/kg/day in the dog 30-day study). Renal lesions were also seen in the 6-month studies in the rat and dog (from doses of 0.25 and 25 mg/kg/day, respectively); these were reversible on cessation of treatment.

Reproduction toxicity studies showed effects on renal development in offspring with increased incidence of renal pelvic dilation; this was seen at doses of 10 mg/kg/day and above in the rat but these changes did not affect the normal development of the offspring.

Trandolapril was not mutagenic or carcinogenic.

Pharmaceutical particulars
List of excipients: Corn starch PhEur, lactose PhEur, povidone PhEur, sodium stearyl fumarate USNF, printing ink (shellac, industrial methylated spirit, purified water, soya lecithin, 2-ethoxyethanol, dimethylpolysiloxane, black iron oxide), E171 (titanium dioxide), E127 (erythrosine), E172 (yellow iron oxide), gelatin.

Incompatibilities: None.

Shelf life: Gopten 0.5 mg: 24 months. Gopten 1.0 mg, 2.0 mg: 36 months.

Special precautions for storage: Store in a dry place.

Nature and contents of container: Gopten 0.5 mg: PVC/Al calendar pack containing 14 capsules. Gopten 1.0 mg, 2.0 mg: PVC/Al calendar pack containing 28 capsules.

Instructions for use/handling: None.

Marketing authorisation number
Gopten Capsules 0.5 mg 00169/0031
Gopten Capsules 1.0 mg 00169/0030
Gopten Capsules 2.0 mg 00169/0029

Date of approval/revision of SPC January 1997

Legal category POM

HYDROCORTISTAB INJECTION

Qualitative and quantitative composition Hydrocortisone Acetate PhEur 2.5% w/v (25 mg/ml)

Pharmaceutical form Suspension for injection.

Clinical particulars
Therapeutic indications: Hydrocortistab Injection is indicated for the local treatment, by intra-articular or periarticular injection, of arthritic conditions such as rheumatoid arthritis and osteoarthritis when few joints are involved. It is also suitable for the symptomatic conditions such as inflamed tendon sheaths and bursae.

Hydrocortistab Injection is not suitable for the production of systemic effects.

Posology and method of administration: For intra-articular or periarticular injection.

Adults: 5–50 mg daily, depending on the size of the joint.

Children: 5–30 mg daily in divided doses.

Elderly: Steroids should be used cautiously in the elderly, since adverse effects are enhanced in old age.

No more than three joints should be treated in one day. The injection may be repeated at intervals of about three weeks.

Contra-indications: Hydrocortistab Injection is contra-indicated in patients with known hypersensitivity to any of the ingredients, and in patients with systemic infections, unless specific anti-infective therapy is employed.

Intra-articular and periarticular injections of Hydrocortistab Injection are contra-indicated when the joint or surrounding tissues are infected. The presence of infection also precludes injection into tendon sheaths and bursae. Hydrocortistab Injection must not be injected directly into tendons, nor should it be injected into spinal or any other true non-diarthrodial joints.

Special warnings and special precautions for use: Intra-articular corticosteroids are associated with a substantially increased risk of inflammatory response in the joint, particularly bacterial infection introduced with the injection. Great care is required that all intra-articular steroid injections should be undertaken under aseptic conditions.

Caution is necessary when prescribing corticosteroids in patients with the following conditions:

(a) Previous history of tuberculosis or characteristic appearance on chest X-ray. The emergence of active tuberculosis can, however, be prevented by the prophylactic use of antituberculous therapy.
(b) Diabetes mellitus (or a family history of diabetes).
(c) Osteoporosis (postmenopausal females are particularly at risk).
(d) Hypertension.
(e) History of severe affective disorders (especially previous history of steroid psychosis).
(f) Glaucoma (or a family history of glaucoma).
(g) Previous steroid myopathy.
(h) Peptic ulceration.
(i) Epilepsy.
(j) Vaccination with live vaccines.

Use in children: Corticosteroids cause growth retardation in infancy, childhood and adolescence. Treatment should be limited to the minimum dosage for the shortest possible time, in order to minimise suppression of the hypothalamo-pituitary-adrenal axis and growth retardation.

Use in the elderly: Treatment of elderly patients, particularly if long-term, should be planned bearing in mind the more serious consequences of the common side effects of corticosteroids in old age, especially osteoporosis, diabetes, hypertension, susceptibility to infection and thinning of the skin.

Interaction with other medicaments and other forms of interaction: The effectiveness of anticoagulants may be increased or decreased with concurrent corticosteroid therapy.

Serum levels of salicylates may increase considerably if corticosteroid therapy is withdrawn, possibly causing intoxication. Since both salicylates and corticosteroids are ulcerogenic, it is possible that there will be an increased rate of gastrointestinal ulceration.

The actions of hypoglycaemic drugs will be antagonised by the hyperglycaemic actions of corticosteroids.

Since amphotericin, diuretics (acetazolamide, loop diuretics and thiazides) and corticosteroids have potassium-depleting effects, signs of hypokalaemia should be looked for during their concurrent use.

There is a small amount of evidence that the simultaneous use of corticosteroids and methotrexate may cause increased methotrexate toxicity and possibly death, although this combination of drugs has been used very successfully.

The therapeutic effects of corticosteroids may be reduced by certain barbiturates (particularly when given at high doses), phenytoin and rifampicin.

The concurrent use of corticosteroids with antacids, cimetidine or theophylline appears to have no effect on the therapeutic use of either drug.

Pregnancy and lactation: There is evidence of harmful effects in pregnancy in animals.

There is inadequate evidence of safety in human pregnancy and there may be a very small risk of cleft palate and intra-uterine growth retardation in the foetus.

Trace amounts of hydrocortisone have been measured in breast milk but it is doubtful if these amounts are clinically significant. However, in lactation, continuous therapy with high doses could possibly affect the child's adrenal function. Monitor carefully.

The decision to use Hydrocortistab Injection during pregnancy and lactation must be made by weighing up the relative risks associated with the use of the drug against the potential benefits in maternal disease.

Effects on ability to drive and use machines: No adverse effects known.

Undesirable effects: With intra-articular or other local injections, the principal side effect encountered is a temporary local exacerbation with increased pain and swelling. This normally subsides after a few hours.

In certain circumstances, particularly after high or prolonged local dosage, corticosteroids can be absorbed in amounts sufficient to produce systemic effects.

The following side effects may be associated with the long-term systemic use of corticosteroids.

Gastrointestinal: Dyspepsia, peptic ulceration with perforation and haemorrhage, abdominal distension, oesophageal ulceration, oesophageal candidiasis, acute pancreatitis.

Musculoskeletal: Proximal myopathy, osteoporosis, vertebral and long bone fractures, avascular osteonecrosis, tendon rupture.

Fluid and electrolyte disturbance: Sodium and water retention, hypertension, hypokalaemic alkalosis.

Dermatological: Impaired healing, skin atrophy, bruising, striae, acne, telangiectasia.

Endocrine/metabolic: Suppression of the hypothalamo-pituitary-adrenal axis, growth suppression in childhood and adolescence, menstrual irregularity and amenorrhoea. Cushingoid facies, hirsutism, weight gain, impaired carbohydrate tolerance with increased requirement for antidiabetic therapy, negative nitrogen balance.

Neuropsychiatric: Euphoria, psychological dependence, depression, insomnia. Intracranial hypertension in children. Aggravation of schizophrenia.

Ophthalmic: Increased intra-ocular pressure, glaucoma, papilloedema, cataracts, corneal or scleral thinning, exacerbation of ophthalmic viral disease.

General: Opportunistic infection, recurrence of dormant tuberculosis, leucocytosis, hypersensitivity, thromboembolism, increased appetite, nausea, malaise.

Withdrawal symptoms and signs: Fever, myalgia, arthralgia, adrenal insufficiency.

Overdose: Overdosage is unlikely with Hydrocortistab Injection but there is no specific antidote available. Treatment should be symptomatic.

Pharmacological properties
Pharmacodynamic properties: Hydrocortisone has both glucocorticoid and mineralocorticoid activity.

Pharmacokinetic properties: Absorption following intra-articular or soft tissue injection is slow. Systemic absorption occurs slowly after local, intra-articular injection. Hydrocortisone is more than 90% bound to plasma proteins. Hydrocortisone is metabolised in the liver and most body tissues to hydrogenated and degraded forms, such as tetrahydrocortisone and tetrahydrocortisol. These are excreted in the urine, mainly conjugated as glucuronides, together with a very small proportion of unchanged hydrocortisone.

Preclinical safety data: Not applicable.

Pharmaceutical particulars
List of excipients: Water for injections, benzyl alcohol, sodium chloride for injections, sodium carboxymethylcellulose, polysorbate 80, with sodium hydroxide and/or hydrochloric acid as pH adjusters.

Incompatibilities: Not applicable.

Shelf life: 36 months.

Special precautions for storage: Store at 15–25°C and protect from light. Do not freeze.

Nature and contents of container: Glass ampoules. Pack size: 10×1 ml ampoules.

Instructions for use/handling: Shake the ampoule well before use. Do not freeze.

Marketing authorisation number 00169/0074

Date of approval/revision of SPC April 1996

Legal category POM

Further information can be obtained from Sovereign Healthcare.

KAODENE*

Presentation Kaodene is an aqueous suspension containing Codeine Phosphate PhEur 10 mg and Light Kaolin BP 3 g in each 10 ml. It is an off-white liquid with the odour and flavour of aniseed.

Other ingredients: Purified water; chloroform; xanthan gum; blanose sodium carboxymethylcellulose; vanilla essence; methyl hydroxybenzoate; anise oil; propyl hydroxybenzoate; sodium saccharin; peppermint oil.

Uses Kaodene is indicated for the symptomatic relief of simple diarrhoea.

Dosage and administration *Adults, elderly and children over 12 years:* 20 ml three or four times daily.

Children from 5 to 12 years: 10 ml three or four times daily.
Children under 5 years: Not recommended.

Contra-indications, warnings, etc Kaodene is contra-indicated in patients with pseudomembranous colitis, diverticular disease or respiratory depression.

It should be used with caution in patients with ulcerative colitis and hepatic or renal dysfunction.

The long-term administration of Kaodene, particularly in the elderly, is not recommended.

It cannot be used as a substitute for rehydration therapy.

Codeine phosphate is a narcotic analgesic and, given in large doses, may induce tolerance and psychological and physical dependence.

It may occasionally cause drowsiness, nausea, vomiting and constipation.

Large doses of codeine may cause drowsiness and CNS depression, but this should not be a problem with the recommended doses of Kaodene.

Effects on ability to drive and use machines: Kaodene may cause drowsiness and may therefore influence the ability to drive and use machines.

Use in pregnancy and lactation: The safety of Kaodene during pregnancy has not been established and therefore use of the product during this period should be avoided, unless under medical supervision. In limited studies, codeine appears in the breast milk in very low concentrations and is unlikely to affect the breast-fed infant adversely.

Drug interactions: Kaodene may interfere with the absorption of some drugs from the gastrointestinal tract, including certain antibiotics and digoxin. The depressant effects of codeine are enhanced by alcohol. May interact with monoamine oxidase inhibitors.

Interference with laboratory tests: Administration of Kaodene may interfere with laboratory estimations of serum amylase and certain liver function tests.

Overdosage: Symptoms of overdosage include the adverse effects given above. In addition, large overdoses may produce respiratory depression, hypotension, circulatory failure and deepening coma. Initial treatment includes emptying the stomach by aspiration and lavage. Intensive supportive therapy may be required to correct respiratory failure and shock. In addition the narcotic antagonist, naloxone hydrochloride, may be used to counteract very rapidly the severe respiratory depression and coma. A dose in adults of 0.4–2 mg is given intravenously or intramuscularly, repeated at intervals of 2–3 minutes if necessary up to 10 mg. In children, doses of naloxone of 5–10 micrograms/kg bodyweight may be given intravenously or intramuscularly.

Pharmaceutical precautions No special storage conditions are necessary.

Legal category CD (Sch 5), P.

Package quantities Bottle of 250 ml.

Further information Nil.

Product licence number 0169/0078.

Further information can be obtained from Sovereign Healthcare.

MUSTINE HYDROCHLORIDE FOR INJECTION BP

Qualitative and quantitative composition Mustine Hydrochloride BP 10 mg

Mustine hydrochloride is di (2-chloroethyl) methylamine hydrochloride. It is also known as Chlormethine Hydrochloride (INN), Nitrogen Mustard and Mustargen Hydrochloride.

Pharmaceutical form Mustine hydrochloride is a white or almost white powder.

Clinical Particulars

Therapeutic indications: Mustine is a powerful cytotoxic agent used in the treatment of several neoplastic conditions. It is an alkylating agent and also possesses immunosuppressant properties.

The principal use of mustine is as part of combination treatment for Hodgkin's disease. It is sometimes used for the treatment of non-Hodgkin's lymphomas and carcinoma of bronchus, ovary and breast.

It may be applied locally for the treatment of mycosis fungoides.

Posology and method of administration: For intravenous injection or topical application.

Under no circumstances should mustine be given intramuscularly.

Intravenous injection

Recommended dose and dosage schedule: A single dose of 0.4 mg/kg bodyweight, or a course of four daily doses of 0.1 mg/kg bodyweight. The term 'bodyweight' is defined, in this case, as the actual bodyweight at the time of treatment. A repeat course of mustine therapy should not be undertaken for at least six weeks or until the bone marrow has recovered its haemopoietic activity.

Dosage adjustment for oedema: The recommended dose corresponds to the actual bodyweight of the patient at the time of treatment. In cases where the bodyweight has been artificially increased by oedema, ascites or other fluid collections, the weight of the body before the increase should be used in calculating the dose.

Elderly: The dose for elderly patients is the same as for adults. Elderly patients with generalised vascular disease may be more prone to local vascular and extravascular toxicity.

Preparation of intravenous injection: A fresh solution is prepared by dissolving 10 mg of mustine hydrochloride in 10 ml of Sodium Chloride Injection BP 0.9% w/v, or Water for Injections BP.

The best method of administration is to set up an intravenous drip of Sodium Chloride Injection BP 0.9% w/v or Dextrose Injection BP 5% w/v; the required dose of mustine, prepared as above, should then be injected into the tubing. This avoids the hazards of extravasation during injection. The drip rate should be fast, at approximately 60 drops per minute, and the injection of mustine should be carried out over 2 minutes. The drip rate should then be reduced to 20 drops per minute.

Alternatively, the concentrated solution of mustine hydrochloride should be freshly prepared as above and transferred aseptically to 500 ml of Sodium Chloride Injection BP 0.9% w/v.

Topical use: Mycosis fungoides may be treated by topical application of a dilute solution of mustine hydrochloride. Various strengths of mustine hydrochloride have been used, but 20 mg in 100 ml of Sodium Chloride Injection BP 0.9% w/v or Water for Injections BP is frequently recommended. This solution should be applied to the affected cutaneous area using a gauze pad. The person applying the solution should wear polyvinylchloride gloves to give protection.

Contra-indications: The use of mustine is contra-indicated during pregnancy and lactation since the drug possesses foetotoxic and teratogenic potential. Mustine should not be used in patients with severe leucopenia, thombocytopenia or anaemia nor should it be used in patients with co-existent or suspected granuloma.

Special warnings and precautions for use: Extravasation during injection should be avoided as this may cause severe tissue necrosis. Infusion should be stopped immediately if local pain is experienced. Where doubt occurs as to whether significant leakage has occurred, the infusion should be discontinued and the cannula resited in another vein. If extravasation does occur during injection, the area involved should be infiltrated with isotonic sodium thiosulphate injection followed by the intermittent application of an ice compress for six to twelve hours. Management of extravasation must be carried out quickly because of mustine's rapid local toxic effects.

Interactions with other medicaments and other forms of interaction: No clinically-significant drug interactions are known.

Pregnancy and lactation: The use of mustine in pregnancy or lactation is contra-indicated. The drug possesses foetotoxic and teratogenic potential.

Effects on ability to drive and use machines: No adverse effects known.

Undesirable effects:

Intravenous use: The most common side-effects are nausea, emesis, fever and/or leucopenia.

Prolonged use of alkylating agents, particularly when combined with extensive radiation, is associated with a marked increase in the incidence of acute non-lymphocytic leukaemia.

Subsequent to mustine administration, extensive and rapid development of amyloidosis may occur in the presence of acute and chronic suppurative inflammation.

Gastrointestinal: Nausea and vomiting often occur during the eight hours following injection. Appropriate sedation and anti-emetics should be prescribed 10–30 minutes before mustine is injected. Transient anorexia has been reported, as well as diarrhoea and peptic ulcers.

Haematological: Severe bone marrow depression may occur following treatment with mustine, with lymphocytopenia, granulocytopenia and occasionally, agranulocytosis. These conditions are more likely to occur in patients who have been given a course of treatment which exceeds 0.4 mg/kg bodyweight and in those who have had previous treatment with other antineoplastic agents or recent radiotherapy. The bone marrow depression may lead to severe anaemia and thrombocytopenia. Peripheral blood counts should be checked prior to each treatment. Leucocyte and platelet counts start to fall approximately one week after treatment, with lowest levels occurring between 14 and 18 days. During the same period, there is a fall in haemoglobin levels. Both leucocyte and platelet counts return to normal before the end of the fourth week.

Skin and connective tissue: Skin reactions and alopecia have been reported. Herpes zoster may develop in patients with latent herpes infection.

Vein irritation leading to discolouration may occur, even in the absence of extravasation. Thrombophlebitis and venous thrombosis are potential complications of mustine therapy.

Neurological: Light-headedness, headache, drowsiness, tinnitus and deafness may occur.

Reproductive and urinary: In non-pregnant women, delayed menstruation or temporary amenorrhoea may follow treatment. In males, a reduction of active spermatogenesis has been reported.

Hyperuricaemia may develop in patients with large tumour masses.

Topical use: Patients may develop a contact dermatitis. Systemic side-effects have not been reported.

Overdose: If given immediately, sodium thiosulphate will neutralise an injection of mustine hydrochloride. Each 10 mg of mustine hydrochloride requires 640 mg of sodium thiosulphate, given as an isotonic solution. This is equivalent to approximately 1.5 ml of a 50% injection of sodium thiosulphate diluted with 20 ml of sodium chloride 0.9% solution or approximately 21 ml of a 3% sodium thiosulphate injection.

Pharmacological properties

Pharmacodynamic properties: Mustine is a cytotoxic drug with alkylating properties. It also possesses weak immunosuppressant properties.

Pharmacokinetic properties: Mustine is only partially absorbed from serous surfaces. Following intravenous injection, it is rapidly converted to a reactive ethyleneimmonium ion. It usually disappears from the blood within approximately 10 minutes. Less than 0.01% of the drug is excreted unchanged in the urine.

Preclinical safety data: None stated.

Pharmaceutical Particulars

List of excipients: None.

Incompatibilities: A 0.2% solution of mustine hydrochloride has a pH of 3 to 5. It is therefore recommended that mustine is administered in 0.9% sodium chloride or 5% dextrose as it becomes rapidly unstable in alkaline solutions.

Shelf life: 24 months.

Special precautions for storage: Store at 2°C to 15°C.

Nature and contents of container: Glass vials sealed with a rubber plug and oversealed with lacquered aluminium. Each vial contains 10 mg mustine hydrochloride.

Instructions for use/handling:

Handling:

(a) Only trained personnel should reconstitute this drug.

(b) Reconstitution should be carried out in a designated area, which has good general and local ventilation.

(c) The work surface should be covered with disposable, plastic backed absorbent paper.

(d) Polyvinylchloride gloves should be worn. Rubber and polyethylene gloves should not be used as these do not give sufficient protection.

(e) Mustine hydrochloride is a potent vesicant and local irritant to skin and mucous membranes. It can cause severe damage to the eyes and the vapour irritates the respiratory tract. Precautions should be taken to avoid accidental contact with the skin, eyes and clothing. Avoid inhalation or ingestion.

(f) Mustine hydrochloride should not be handled by pregnant staff.

(g) Adequate care and precautions should be taken in the disposal of items (syringes, needles etc.) used in the reconstitution and administration of mustine.

(h) Use Luèr-lock fittings on all syringes and sets. Large bore needles are recommended to minimise pressure and the possible formation of aerosols. The latter may also be reduced by the use of a venting needle.

(i) After treatment, all apparatus, including PVC gloves, should be washed. A 2.5% solution of sodium carbonate is particularly suitable or the use of the following solution:

Decontamination solution: Distilled water, 3 litres; caustic soda solution SG 1.50, 1 litre; Industrial Methylated Spirit (IMS) 66 OP, 4.5 litres. This solution should be prepared at least 24 hours before use and should be placed under the work bench, near the ventilation exhaust. All equipment should be dismantled as far as possible and immersed in the decontamination solution for at least 48 hours. The solution should then be decanted into the sluice and the equipment washed three times with clean water prior to disposal. Note: the equipment may be temporarily stored prior to decontamination on a suitable tray which is then placed inside a plastic bag and securely tied.

First Aid measures:

(i) Eyes–Irrigate immediately with large amounts of water or a 2% solution of sodium bicarbonate for at least 10 minutes and obtain urgent medical attention. The person affected should then be seen by an ophthalmologist.

(ii) Skin–Wash immediately with large amounts of water, a solution of sodium bicarbonate or an isotonic solution of sodium thiosulphate.

(iii) If accidentally ingested, wash out the mouth thoroughly with water and give water to drink.

(iv) If inhaled, remove to fresh air.

Urgent medical attention should be sought after any of these occurrences.

Marketing authorisation number 00169/0081

Date of approval/revision of SPC September 1998

Legal category POM

NIVEMYCIN

Qualitative and quantitative composition Each tablet contains an amount of Neomycin Sulphate PhEur equivalent to 550 mg of material having a potency of 700 units/mg.

Pharmaceutical form Tablets.

Clinical particulars

Therapeutic indications: Nivemycin (Neomycin Sulphate PhEur) is indicated for pre-operative sterilisation of the bowel and may be useful in the treatment of impending hepatic coma, including portal systemic encephalopathy.

Posology and method of administration: For oral administration.

Pre-operative sterilisation of the bowel:

Adults: Two tablets every hour for 4 hours, then 2 tablets every 4 hours for two or three days before the operation.

Children over 12 years: Two tablets every 4 hours for two or three days before the operation.

Children from 6 to 12 years: A half to one tablet every 4 hours for two or three days before the operation.

For practical reasons, use of the tablets in children under 6 years is not recommended.

In hepatic coma, the adult dose is 4–12 g/day in divided doses for a period of 5–7 days. For children, 50–100 mg/kg/day in divided doses appears appropriate. Chronic hepatic insufficiency may require up to 4 g/day over an indefinite period.

The elderly dose is the same as for adults.

Contra-indications: Nivemycin should not be given when intestinal obstruction is present. Hypersensitivity to aminoglycosides. Infants under 1 year.

Special warnings and special precautions for use: The absorption of neomycin is poor from the alimentary tract, with about 97% of an orally-administered dose being excreted unchanged in the faeces. However, impaired GI motility may increase absorption of the drug and it is therefore possible, as with other broad-spectrum antibiotics, that prolonged therapy could result in ototoxicity and nephrotoxicity, particularly in patients with a degree of renal failure.

When used as an adjunct in the management of hepatic coma, care should be taken that administration is of the minimal period necessary, since prolonged exposure to the drug may result in malabsorption. Neomycin should be used with caution in patients with neuromuscular disorders and parkinsonism. There is almost complete cross-resistance between neomycin, kanamycin, paromomycin and framycetin. Cross-resistance with gentamicin has also been reported.

Since prolonged therapy may result in the overgrowth of non-sensitive organisms, treatment should not be continued longer than necessary to prevent superinfection due to the overgrowth of non-sensitive organisms.

Interaction with other medicaments and other forms of interaction: Neomycin may impair absorption of other drugs including phenoxymethylpenicillin and digoxin. The efficacy of oral contraceptives may be reduced. Care should be taken when considering the use of neomycin concurrently with drugs with a potential to cause nephrotoxicity or ototoxicity and with drugs with neuromuscular-blocking activity.

Pregnancy and lactation: The use of neomycin in pregnancy is not recommended unless the benefits outweigh the potential risks.

There are no reports linking the use of neomycin to congenital defects. However, small amounts of the drug are absorbed when given orally and neomycin and other aminoglycosides may have harmful effects on the foetus following oral absorption during pregnancy.

In some circumstances, neomycin may enter the breast milk of lactating mothers. There is little risk of ototoxicity in the infant, but abnormal development of the gut flora may occur. The use of neomycin in lactating mothers is not recommended unless the benefits outweigh the potential risks.

Effects on ability to drive and use machines: Not applicable.

Undesirable effects: Nausea, vomiting, diarrhoea, increased salivation, stomatitis, nephrotoxicity, ototoxicity, rise in serum levels of hepatic enzymes and bilirubin, blood dyscrasias, haemolytic anaemia, confusion, paraesthesia, disorientation, nystagmus, hypersensitivity reactions including dermatitis, pruritus, drug fever and anaphylaxis.

Overdose: In overdose, exacerbation of the adverse events reported for neomycin (nausea, diarrhoea, nephrotoxicity, ototoxicity etc) is expected.

Monitor renal and auditory function. If these are impaired, haemodialysis is indicated. Prolonged assisted ventilation may also be required.

Pharmacological properties

Pharmacodynamic properties: Neomycin is an aminoglycoside antibiotic. Neomycin acts by binding to polysomes, inhibiting protein synthesis and generating errors in the transcription of the genetic code.

Pharmacokinetic properties: The absorption of neomycin from the alimentary tract is poor: only ~3% of an oral dose is absorbed. Neomycin is rapidly excreted by the kidneys in the unchanged form. The plasma half-life in healthy adults is approximately 2–3 hours. Oral doses of 3 g produce peak plasma concentrations of up to 4 microgram/ml.

Preclinical safety data: Not applicable.

Pharmaceutical particulars

List of excipients: Plasdone K29-32, isopropyl alcohol, calcium stearate.

Incompatibilities: Not applicable.

Shelf life: 3 years.

Special precautions for storage: Store below 30°C in a dry place. Protect from light.

Nature and contents of container: An amber glass bottle having a tin-plate screw cap with a waxed aluminium-faced pulpboard liner. The ullage is filled with cotton wool. Pack size: 100 tablets.

Instructions for use/handling: Not applicable.

Marketing authorisation number 00169/0083

Date of approval/revision of SPC January 1996

Legal category POM

Further information can be obtained from Sovereign Healthcare.

PHENYLEPHRINE INJECTION BP 10 mg/ml

Qualitative and quantitative composition Phenylephrine Hydrochloride Ph Eur 1.0% w/v

Pharmaceutical form Sterile solution.

Clinical particulars

Therapeutic indications: For the treatment of hypotensive states, e.g. circulatory failure, during spinal anaesthesia or drug-induced hypotension.

Posology and method of administration: For subcutaneous, intramuscular, slow intravenous injection or intravenous infusion.

Adults: Phenylephrine Injection may be administered subcutaneously or intramuscularly in a dosage of 2 to 5 mg with further doses of 1 to 10 mg if necessary according to response, or in a dose of 100 to 500 micrograms by slow intravenous injection as a 0.1% solution, repeated as necessary after at least 15 minutes.

Alternatively, 10 mg in 500 ml of glucose 5% injection or sodium chloride 0.9% injection may be infused intravenously, initially at a rate of up to 180 micrograms per minute, reduced according to response to 30–60 micrograms per minute.

Children: 100 microgram/kg bodyweight subcutaneously or intramuscularly.

Elderly: There is no need for dosage reduction in the elderly.

Contra-indications: Patients taking monoamine oxidase inhibitors, or within 14 days of ceasing such treatment. Severe hypertension and hyperthyroidism.

Special warnings and special precautions for use: Great care should be exercised in administering Phenylephrine Injection to patients with pre-existing cardiovascular disease such as ischaemic heart disease, arrhythmias, occlusive vascular disease including arteriosclerosis, hypertension or aneurysms. Anginal pain may be precipitated in patients with angina pectoris.

Care is also required when given to patients with diabetes mellitus or closed-angle glaucoma.

Interaction with other medicaments and other forms of interaction: Phenylephrine may interact with cyclopropane and halothane and other halogenated inhalational anaesthetics, to induce ventricular fibrillation. An increased risk of arrhythmias may also occur if Phenylephrine Injection is given to patients receiving cardiac glycosides, quinidine or tricyclic antidepressants.

Phenylephrine may increase blood pressure and consequently reverse the action of many antihypertensive agents. Interactions of phenylephrine with alpha- and beta-receptor blocking drugs may be complex.

Pregnancy and lactation: The safety of phenylephrine during pregnancy and lactation has not been established. Administration of phenylephrine in late pregnancy or labour may cause foetal hypoxia and bradycardia. Excretion of phenylephrine in breast milk appears to be minimal.

Effects on ability to drive and use machines: No adverse effects known.

Undesirable effects: Extravasation of Phenylephrine Injection may cause tissue necrosis. Phenylephrine will cause a rise in blood pressure with headache and vomiting and this may produce cerebral haemorrhage and pulmonary oedema. There may also be a reflex bradycardia or tachycardia, other cardiac arrhythmias, anginal pain, palpitations and cardiac arrest, hypotension with dizziness, and fainting and flushing. Phenylephrine may induce difficulty in micturition and urinary retention, dyspnoea, altered metabolism including disturbances of glucose metabolism, sweating, hypersalivation, transient tingling and coolness of the skin and temporary fullness of the head. Phenylephrine is without significant stimulating effects on the central nervous system at usual doses.

Overdose: Symptoms of overdosage include headache, vomiting, hypertension and reflex bradycardia and other cardiac arrhythmias.

Treatment should consist of symptomatic and supportive measures. The hypertensive effects may be treated with an alpha-adrenoceptor blocking drug, such as phentolamine, 5 to 60 mg i.v. over 10–30 minutes, repeated as necessary.

Pharmacological properties

Pharmacodynamic properties: Phenylephrine Injection is a sympathomimetic agent with mainly direct effects on adrenergic receptors. It has predominantly alpha-adrenergic activity and is without significant stimulating effects on the central nervous system at usual doses. After injection it produces peripheral vasoconstriction and increased arterial pressure. It also causes reflex bradycardia.

Pharmacokinetic properties: When injected subcutaneously or intramuscularly, phenylephrine takes 10 to 15 minutes to act. Subcutaneous and intramuscular injections are effective for up to about one hour and two hours, respectively. Intravenous injections are effective for up to about 20 minutes. Phenylephrine is metabolised in the liver by monoamine oxidase. The metabolites, their route and rate of excretion have not been identified.

Preclinical safety data: Not applicable.

Pharmaceutical particulars

List of excipients: N/1 sodium hydroxide for SP, N/1 hydrochloric acid for SP, Water for Injections Ph Eur, sterile N/1 sodium hydroxide for SP, sterile N/1 hydrochloric acid for SP.

Incompatibilities: Phenylephrine Injection has been stated to be incompatible with alkalis, ferric salts, phenytoin sodium and oxidising agents.

Shelf life: 24 months.

Special precautions for storage: Store at 2–25°C. Protect from light.

Nature and contents of container: 1 ml neutral glass ampoule with ceramic breakring. Pack size: 10 ampoules.

Instructions for use/handling: Not applicable.

Marketing authorisation number 00169/0084

Date of approval/revision of SPC August 1995

Legal category POM

PROTAMINE SULPHATE INJECTION BP 1%

Qualitative and quantitative composition Protamine Sulphate Injection BP 1% contains protamine sulphate 10 mg/ml in sodium chloride 0.9% w/v.

Pharmaceutical form Sterile solution for injection.

Clinical particulars

Therapeutic indications: Protamine sulphate neutralises the anticoagulant action of heparin. It is given by intravenous injection to restore the original coagulation time of the blood in patients receiving heparin, and in the treatment of haemorrhage due to heparin overdosage.

Posology and method of administration: For intravenous injection.

The dose is calculated from the results of determinations of the amount required to produce an acceptable blood clotting time in the patient.

Protamine sulphate is given by slow intravenous injection, being administered at the rate of 5 ml of the 1% solution over a period of ten minutes. 1 ml of Protamine Sulphate Injection BP 1% is required to neutralise the anticoagulant activity of approximately 850 Units of heparin (lung) or 1100 Units of heparin (mucous) that has been injected within the previous fifteen minutes.

As more time elapses after the heparin injection, so proportionately less protamine sulphate is required. Ideally, the dosage of protamine sulphate should be controlled by serial measurements of the patient's coagulation time. This helps to avoid an excess of protamine sulphate which, having some anticoagulant effect itself, can prolong coagulation time.

The anticoagulant effect of Heparin Retard injection can be counteracted by the intravenous injection of up to 5 ml of Protamine Sulphate Injection BP 1% over ten minutes. Because of the prolonged action of Heparin Retard, the dosage of protamine sulphate is best controlled by measurements of coagulation time.

Contra-indications: Protamine Sulphate Injection is contra-indicated in patients who are known to be hypersensitive to protamine.

Special warnings and special precautions for use: Protamine sulphate should be used with caution in patients with a known hypersensitivity to fish, in vasectomised or infertile males, and in patients who have received protamine-containing insulin or previous protamine sulphate therapy.

Not more than 50 mg of protamine sulphate, ie 5 ml of Protamine Sulphate Injection BP 1%, should usually be given at any one time. Protamine sulphate is a specific antidote to heparin and is not suitable for reversing the action of indirect anticoagulants such as coumarin and indanedione derivatives.

Interaction with other medicaments and other forms of interaction: Protamine sulphate may increase the magnitude and/or duration of action of non-depolarising neuromuscular blocking agents.

Pregnancy and lactation: The safety of protamine sulphate during pregnancy and lactation has not been established.

Neither animal nor human reproduction studies have been conducted, and therefore the drug should only be used during pregnancy when clearly needed. It is not known whether protamine sulphate is distributed into breast milk and the drug should be used with caution during lactation.

Effects on ability to drive and use machines: No adverse effects known.

Undesirable effects: Intravenous injections of protamine sulphate, particularly if given rapidly, may cause hypotension, bradycardia and dyspnoea. A sensation of warmth, transitory flushing, nausea, vomiting and lassitude may also occur. Occasionally, hypersensitivity reactions including urticaria, angioedema, pulmonary oedema, anaphylaxis and anaphylactoid reactions have been reported.

Overdose: Protamine sulphate is a weak anticoagulant and overdosage may theoretically result in bleeding. Usually, no specific therapy is required.

Pharmacological properties

Pharmacodynamic properties: Protamine sulphate is strongly basic and acts as a heparin antagonist by complexing with the strongly acidic heparin sodium or heparin calcium to form a stable complex.

Pharmacokinetic properties: Protamine sulphate has a rapid onset of action. Following intravenous administration, neutralisation of heparin occurs within 5 minutes. Although the metabolic fate of the protamine-heparin complex is not known, it appears that the complex is partially degraded, thus freeing heparin.

Preclinical safety data: Not applicable.

Pharmaceutical particulars

List of excipients: Water for injections, sodium chloride for injections, sodium hydroxide and/or hydrochloric acid as pH adjusters.

Incompatibilities: Protamine sulphate is incompatible with certain antibiotics, including several penicillins and cephalosporins.

Shelf life: 36 months.

Special precautions for storage: Store at 15 to 25°C. Do not refrigerate.

Nature and contents of container: One point cut ampoule. Pack size: 6×10 ml ampoules.

Instructions for use/handling: None.

Marketing authorisation number 00169/0085

Date of approval/revision of SPC April 1996

Legal category POM

PROTHIADEN

Qualitative and quantitative composition Each Prothiaden tablet contains 75 mg Dothiepin Hydrochloride BP. Each Prothiaden capsule contains 25 mg Dothiepin Hydrochloride BP.

Pharmaceutical form Red, sugar-coated tablets, bearing the overprint 'P75' in white; red/brown, hard gelatin capsules bearing the overprint 'P25' in white.

Clinical particulars

Therapeutic indications: Prothiaden is indicated in the treatment of symptoms of depressive illness, especially where an anti-anxiety effect is required.

Posology and method of administration: For oral administration.

Adults: Initially 75 mg/day in divided doses or as a single dose at night, increasing to 150 mg/day. In certain circumstances, *e.g.* in hospital use, dosages up to 225 mg daily have been used.

Suggested regimens: 25 or 50 mg three times daily or, alternatively, 75 or 150 mg as a single dose at night. Should the regimen of 150 mg as a single night-time dose be adopted, it is better to give a smaller dose for the first few days.

Elderly: 50 to 75 mg daily initially. As with any antidepressant, the initial dose should be increased with caution under close supervision. Half the normal adult dose may be sufficient to produce a satisfactory clinical response.

Children: Not recommended.

Contra-indications: Prothiaden is contra-indicated following recent myocardial infarction, and in patients with any degree of heart block or other cardiac arrhythmias. It is also contra-indicated in mania and severe liver disease.

Special warnings and special precautions for use: It may be two to four weeks from the start of treatment before there is an improvement in the patient's depression; the subject should be monitored closely during this period. The anxiolytic effect may be observed within a few days of commencing treatment.

The elderly are particularly liable to experience adverse effects with antidepressants, especially agitation, confusion and postural hypotension. Patients posing a high risk of suicide require close supervision.

Prothiaden should be avoided in patients with a history of epilepsy and in patients with narrow-angle glaucoma or symptoms suggestive of prostatic hypertrophy. Use with caution in patients with cardiovascular disorders.

Tricyclic antidepressants potentiate the central nervous depressant action of alcohol. Anaesthetics given during tri/tetracyclic antidepressant therapy may increase the risk of arrhythmias and hypotension. If surgery is necessary, the anaesthetist should be informed that a patient is being so treated.

On stopping treatment, it is recommended that antidepressants should be withdrawn gradually, wherever possible.

Interaction with other medicaments and other forms of interaction: Prothiaden should not be given concurrently with a monoamine oxidase inhibitor, nor within fourteen days of ceasing such treatment. The concomitant administration of Prothiaden and SSRIs should be avoided since increases in plasma tricyclic antidepressant levels have been reported following the co-administration of some SSRIs.

Prothiaden may alter the pharmacological effect of some concurrently administered drugs including CNS depressants such as alcohol and narcotic analgesics; the effect of these will be potentiated as will be the effects of adrenaline and noradrenaline (some local anaesthetics contain these sympathomimetics). Anaesthetics given during tri/tetracyclic antidepressant therapy may increase the risk of arrhythmias and hypotension.

Prothiaden has quinidine-like actions on the heart. For this reason, its concomitant use with other drugs which may affect cardiac conduction (*e.g.* sotalol, terfenadine, astemizole, halofantrine) should be avoided.

The hypotensive activity of certain antihypertensive agents (*e.g.* bethanidine, debrisoquine, guanethidine) may be reduced by Prothiaden. It is advisable to review all antihypertensive therapy during treatment with tricyclic antidepressants.

Barbiturates may decrease and methylphenidate may increase the serum concentration of dothiepin and thus affect its antidepressant action.

There is no evidence that dothiepin interferes with standard laboratory tests.

Pregnancy and lactation: Treatment with Prothiaden should be avoided during pregnancy, unless there are compelling reasons. There is inadequate evidence of safety of the drug during human pregnancy.

There is evidence that dothiepin is secreted in breast milk but this is at levels which are unlikely to cause problems.

Effects on ability to drive and use machines: Initially, Prothiaden may impair alertness; patients likely to drive vehicles or operate machinery should be warned of this possibility.

Undesirable effects: The following adverse effects, although not necessarily all reported with dothiepin, have occurred with other tricyclic antidepressants:

Atropine-like side effects including dry mouth, disturbances of accommodation, tachycardia, constipation and hesitancy of micturition are common early in treatment, but usually lessen.

Other adverse effects include drowsiness, sweating, postural hypotension, tremor and skin rashes. Interference with sexual function may occur.

Potentially serious adverse effects are rare. These include depression of the bone marrow, agranulocytosis, hepatitis (including altered liver function), cholestatic jaundice, convulsions and inappropriate ADH secretion.

Psychotic manifestations, including mania and paranoid delusions, may be exacerbated during treatment with tricyclic antidepressants.

Withdrawal symptoms may occur on abrupt cessation of tricyclic therapy and include insomnia, irritability and excessive perspiration. Similar symptoms in neonates whose mothers received tricyclic antidepressants during the third trimester have also been reported.

Cardiac arrhythmias and severe hypotension are likely to occur with high dosage or in deliberate overdosage. They may also occur in patients with pre-existing heart disease taking normal dosage.

Overdose: Symptoms of overdosage may include dryness of the mouth, excitement, ataxia, drowsiness, loss of consciousness, muscle twitching, convulsions, widely dilated pupils, hyperreflexia, sinus tachycardia, cardiac arrhythmias, hypotension, hypothermia, depression of respiration, visual hallucinations, delirium, urinary retention, paralytic ileus, and respiratory or metabolic alkalosis.

Treatment should consist of gastric lavage. When the patient is unconscious or the cough reflex depressed, the lungs should be protected by a cuffed endotracheal tube. Repeated gastric/intestinal aspiration or repeated administration of activated charcoal may remove drug and metabolites excreted into the gut via the bile. Continuous ECG monitoring is advisable. Abnormalities of cardiac rhythm and epileptic convulsions may occur and should be treated accordingly. Forced diuresis is not recommended. Bed rest is advisable, even after recovery.

Pharmacological properties

Pharmacodynamic properties: Dothiepin is a tricyclic antidepressant which acts by increasing transmitter levels at central synapses, so producing a clinical antidepressant effect.

Dothiepin, in common with other tricyclics, inhibits the reuptake of noradrenaline and 5-hydroxytryptamine, with a significantly greater action on the reuptake of noradrenaline. In addition, dothiepin inhibits the neuronal uptake of dopamine.

As a consequence of its effects on monoamine levels, dothiepin appears to produce adaptive changes in the brain by reducing or down-regulating both noradrenaline receptor numbers and noradrenaline-induced cyclic-AMP formation.

Pharmacokinetic properties: Dothiepin is readily absorbed from the gastrointestinal tract and extensively metabolised in the liver. Metabolites include northiaden, dothiepin-S-oxide and northiaden-S-oxide. Dothiepin is excreted in the urine, mainly in the form of metabolites; appreciable amounts are also excreted in the faeces. A half-life of about 50 hours has been reported for dothiepin and its metabolites.

Preclinical safety data: Not applicable.

Pharmaceutical particulars

List of excipients: Tablets: Refined sugar, tricalcium phosphate, maize starch, talc, povidone, liquid glucose, magnesium stearate, sandarac or sandarac tablet varnish, ponceau 4R, sunset yellow, titanium dioxide, shellac, white beeswax, sodium benzoate, polydimethylsiloxane, soya lecithin.

Capsules: Maize starch, magnesium stearate, gelatin, glycerin, ponceau 4R, yellow iron oxide, black iron oxide, red iron oxide, titanium dioxide, shellac, polydimethylsiloxane, soya lecithin.

Incompatibilities: Not applicable.

Shelf life: Tablets: 36 months. Capsules: 36 months.

Special precautions for storage: Tablets: None. Capsules: None.

Nature and contents of container: Tablets: Blister pack containing 28 tablets. Plastic bottle containing 500 tablets. Capsules: Amber glass bottle containing 100 or 600 tablets.

Instructions for use/handling: None.

Marketing authorisation number

Prothiaden Tablets 75 mg 00169/0087
Prothiaden Capsules 25 mg 00169/0086

Date of approval/revision of SPC February 1996

Legal category POM

PROTIUM ▼

Qualitative and quantitative composition Pantoprazole sodium sesquihydrate 45.1 mg (equivalent to pantoprazole 40 mg).

Pharmaceutical form Enteric-coated tablets for oral use.

Clinical particulars
Therapeutic indications: For symptomatic improvement and healing of gastrointestinal diseases which require a reduction in acid secretion:
- duodenal ulcer
- gastric ulcer
- moderate and severe reflux oesophagitis

Note: Prior to treatment of gastric ulcer, the possibility of malignancy should be excluded as treatment with Protium may alleviate the symptoms of malignant ulcers and can thus delay diagnosis.

Posology and method of administration: For oral administration.

The recommended oral dosage is one enteric-coated tablet per day. Protium should not be chewed or crushed, and should be swallowed whole with water either before or during breakfast.

The safety of longer-term use is generally well established. Long-term administration of pantoprazole has a safety profile similar to that observed with short-term treatment, and is well tolerated.

Extensive clinical experience has shown that a successful course of treatment rarely needs to exceed 8 weeks and, in most patients, freedom from symptoms is achieved rapidly. In a few instances, there may be benefit in extending treatment beyond 8 weeks to ensure healing.

Duodenal ulcer: Duodenal ulcers generally heal within 2 weeks. If a 2-week period of treatment is not sufficient, healing will be achieved in almost all cases within a further 2 weeks.

Gastric ulcer: A 4-week period is usually required for the treatment of gastric ulcers. If this is not sufficient, healing will usually be achieved within a further 4 weeks.

Gastro-oesophageal reflux: A 4-week period is usually required for the treatment of gastro-oesophageal reflux. If this is not sufficient, healing will usually be achieved within a further 4 weeks.

Elderly: No dose adjustment is necessary in the elderly.

Patients with impaired renal function: No dose adjustment is necessary in patients with renal impairment.

Patients with hepatic cirrhosis: Due to an increased AUC and a modified metabolism of pantoprazole in patients with hepatic cirrhosis, the dose regimen should be reduced to one tablet every other day.

Children: There is no information on the use of pantoprazole in children. Therefore Protium should not be used in children.

Contra-indications: Protium may not be used in cases of known hypersensitivity to any of its constituents.

Special warnings and special precautions for use: None.

Interaction with other medicaments and other forms of interaction: No drug interactions have been reported so far.

Pregnancy and lactation:

Use during pregnancy: There is no information about the safety of pantoprazole during pregnancy in humans. Animal experiments have revealed no signs of foetal damage, but reproduction studies have revealed reduced litter weight and delayed development of the skeleton at doses above 15 mg/kg.

During pregnancy, Protium should not be used unless the benefit exceeds the potential risk.

Use during lactation: There is no information about the safety of pantoprazole during breast-feeding in humans. In the rat, not more than 0.02% of the administered dose is excreted via the breast milk.

During breast-feeding, Protium should not be used unless the benefit exceeds the potential risk.

Effects on ability to drive and use machines: Pantoprazole does not affect the ability to drive and use machines.

Undesirable effects: Treatment with Protium can occasionally lead to headache (1.3%) or diarrhoea (1.5%).

Skin rashes (0.4%), pruritus (0.5%) and dizziness (0.7%) were observed rarely.

Overdose: There are no known symptoms of overdosage in man. However, pantoprazole is very specific in action and no particular problems are anticipated. Doses up to 240 mg i.v. were administered without obvious adverse effects.

As pantoprazole is extensively protein bound, it is not readily dialysable. Apart from symptomatic and supportive treatment, no specific therapeutic recommendations can be made.

Pharmacological properties
Pharmacodynamic properties: Pantoprazole is a proton pump inhibitor, i.e. it inhibits specifically and dose-proportionally the gastric H^+/K^+-ATPase enzyme which is responsible for acid secretion in the parietal cells of the stomach.

The substance is a substituted benzimidazole which accumulates in the acidic environment of the parietal cells after absorption. There it is converted into the active form, a cyclic sulphenamide, which binds to the H^+/K^+-ATPase, thus inhibiting the proton pump and causing potent and long-lasting suppression of basal and stimulated gastric acid secretion. As pantoprazole acts distally to the receptor level, it can inhibit gastric acid secretion irrespective of the nature of the stimulus (acetylcholine, histamine, gastrin).

Pantoprazole's selectivity is due to the fact that it can only exert its full effect in a strongly acidic environment (pH<3), remaining mostly inactive at higher pH values. As a result, its complete pharmacological and thus therapeutic effect can only be achieved in the acid-secretory parietal cells. By means of a feedback mechanism, this effect is diminished at the same rate as acid secretion is inhibited.

Pantoprazole has the same effect whether administered orally or intravenously.

Following intravenous or oral administration, pantoprazole inhibits the pentagastrin-stimulated gastric acid secretion. In volunteers, acid secretion was inhibited by 56% following the first i.v. administration of 30 mg and by 99% after 5 days. With an oral dose of 40 mg, inhibition was 51% on day 1 and 85% on day 7. Basal 24-hour acidity was reduced by 37% and 98%, respectively.

The fasting gastrin values increased under pantoprazole but in most cases they did not exceed the normal upper limit. Following completion of a course of oral treatment, the median gastrin levels clearly declined again.

Pharmacokinetic properties:

General pharmacokinetics: Pantoprazole is rapidly absorbed and the maximal plasma concentration is achieved even after one single 40 mg oral dose. On average, the maximum serum concentrations are approximately 2–3 microgram/ml about 2.5 hours post-administration and these values remain constant after multiple administration. Terminal half-life is about 1 hour. Volume of distribution is about 0.15 litre/kg and clearance is about 0.1 litre/h/kg. There were a few cases of subjects with delayed elimination. Because of the specific activation within the parietal cell, the elimination half-life does not correlate with the much longer duration of action (inhibition of acid secretion). Pharmacokinetics do not vary after single or repeated administration. The plasma kinetics of pantoprazole are linear after both oral and intravenous administration.

Studies with pantoprazole in humans reveal no interaction with the cytochrome P450-system of the liver. There was no induction of the P450-system seen as tested after chronic administration with antipyrine as a marker. Also, no inhibition of metabolism was observed after concomitant administration of pantoprazole with either antipyrine, diazepam, phenytoin, nifedipine, theophylline, digoxin, oral contraceptives, caffeine, diclofenac, carbamazepine, metoprolol, glibenclamide and ethanol. Concomitant administration of pantoprazole with warfarin has no influence on warfarin's effect on the coagulation factors.

The absolute bioavailability of the tablet is about 77%. Concomitant intake of food or antacids had no influence on AUC, maximum serum concentrations and thus bioavailability.

Pantoprazole's plasma protein binding is about 98%. The substance is almost exclusively metabolised in the liver. Renal elimination represents the major route of excretion (about 80%) for the metabolites of pantoprazole; the rest are excreted in the faeces. The main metabolite in both the plasma and urine is desmethylpantoprazole which is conjugated with sulphate. The half-life of the main metabolites (about 1.5 hours) is not much longer than that of pantoprazole.

Characteristics in patients/special groups of subjects: Although for patients with hepatic cirrhosis (classes A and B according to Child) the half-life values increased to between 7 and 9 hours and the AUC values increased by a factor of 5 to 7, the maximum plasma concentration only increased slightly by a factor of 1.5 compared with healthy subjects. Therefore the dose regimen in patients with hepatic cirrhosis should be reduced to one tablet every other day.

No dose reduction is required when pantoprazole is administered to patients with impaired kidney function (including dialysis patients). As with healthy subjects, pantoprazole's half-life is short. Only very small amounts of pantoprazole are dialysed. Although the main metabolite has a moderately delayed half-life (2–3 hours), excretion is still rapid and thus accumulation does not occur.

A slight increase in AUC and Cmax in elderly volunteers compared with younger counterparts is also not clinically relevant.

Preclinical safety data:

Acute toxicity: In acute toxicity studies in mice, the LD_{50} values were found to be 370 mg/kg bodyweight for i.v. administration and around 700 mg/kg bodyweight for oral administration.

In the rat, the corresponding values were around 240 mg/kg for i.v. administration and 900 mg/kg for oral administration.

Chronic toxicity: Hypergastrinaemia and morphologic changes of the mucosa were observed in studies investigating repeated administration for up to 12 months in the rat and dog. Most of the effects were reversible and attributable solely to the drug action, i.e. suppression of acid secretion.

In long-term studies in the rat and dog, there was an increase in stomach and liver weights, the increase being reversible after the substance was discontinued. The increase in liver weight following highly toxic doses was seen as a result of the induction of drug-metabolising enzymes.

Thyroid activation in two rat experiments is due to the rapid metabolism of thyroid hormones in the liver and has also been described in a similar form for other drugs. Changes in the thyroid and associated reduced degradation of cholesterol have been observed in one-year studies in the rat and dog. Hypertrophy of the thyroid and increases in cholesterol levels are reversible.

In studies in the dog, a species-specific pulmonary oedema was observed. The animal-specific metabolite which was responsible for the oedema could not be identified in man.

Carcinogenicity: In a 2-year carcinogenicity study in rats–which corresponds to lifetime treatment for rats–ECL cell carcinoids were found. The mechanism leading to the formation of gastric carcinoids by substituted benzimidazoles has been carefully investigated and allows the conclusion that it is a secondary reaction to the massively elevated serum gastrin levels occurring in the rat during treatment. In addition, rats have more ECL cells in the mucosa of the glandular stomach than man, so that a larger number of responder cells for the increased gastrin values can become active.

ECL cell neoplasms were not observed in either the study in mice (24 months) or in long-term studies in the dog. In clinical studies (40–80 mg for 1 year), ECL cell density slightly increased.

In the two-year studies, an increased number of neoplastic changes of the liver was observed in rats and female mice and was interpreted as being due to pantoprazole's high rate of metabolism in the liver.

A slight increase of neoplastic changes of the thyroid was observed in the group of rats receiving the highest dose. The occurrence of these neoplasms is associated with the pantoprazole-induced changes in the breakdown of thyroxine in the rat liver. In man, no changes in the thyroid hormones, T3, T4 and TSH were observed. This high dose phenomenon in the rat is therefore not relevant for man.

Mutagenicity: In mutagenicity studies, there were no indications of a mutagenic action *in vivo* or *in vitro*.

Reproduction toxicology: Investigations revealed no evidence of impaired fertility or teratogenic effects. Penetration of the placenta was investigated in the rat and was found to increase with advanced gestation. As a result, the concentration of pantoprazole in the foetus is increased shortly before birth, regardless of the route of administration.

In humans, there is no experience of the use of the drug during pregnancy.

Pharmaceutical particulars
List of excipients: Crospovidone, mannitol, hydroxypropyl methylcellulose, poly (ethylacrylate, methacrylic acid) 1:1, anhydrous sodium carbonate, propylene glycol, polyvidone K90, calcium stearate, triethyl citrate, polyvidone K25, titanium dioxide (E171), polysorbate 80, sodium lauryl sulphate, yellow iron oxide (E172).

Incompatibilities: None.

Shelf life: Pantoprazole tablets are stable over a period of 3 years.

Special precautions for storage: Store below 30°C.

Nature and contents of container: Protium is presented as a patient pack of 28 tablets, available in PE bottles packed in cardboard boxes.

Instructions for use/handling: None.

Marketing authorisation number 04889/0010

Date of approval/revision of SPC June 1998

Legal category POM

PROTIUM I.V. ▼

Qualitative and quantitative composition Pantoprazole sodium lyophile 42.3 mg (prepared from 45.1 mg pantoprazole sodium sesquihydrate, and corresponding to 40 mg pantoprazole)

Pharmaceutical form Lyophilised powder for injection.

Clinical particulars

Therapeutic indications: For symptomatic improvement and healing of gastrointestinal diseases which require a reduction in acid secretion:

– duodenal ulcer
– gastric ulcer
– moderate and severe reflux oesophagitis

Note: Prior to treatment of gastric ulcer, the possibility of malignancy should be excluded as treatment with Protium i.v. may alleviate the symptoms of malignant ulcers and can thus delay diagnosis.

Posology and method of administration: Protium i.v. is for intravenous administration ONLY and must NOT be given by any other route.

The recommended intravenous dosage is one vial (40 mg) of Protium i.v. per day.

A ready-to-use i.v. solution is prepared by injecting 10 ml of physiological sodium chloride solution into the vial containing the lyophilised powder. The reconstituted injection solution has a pH of 9–10.

The freshly prepared solution is designed for use as an i.v. injection or infusion, and the duration of administration should be 2 to 15 minutes.

After preparation, the reconstituted solution must be used immediately (within 3 hours) and the unused portion discarded.

In most patients, freedom from symptoms is achieved rapidly.

Data are available on i.v. use for up to 7 days. After this period, treatment should be continued with the same dose (40 mg) of the oral dosage form (Protium tablets), in compliance with the approved dosage regimen.

Duodenal ulcer: Duodenal ulcers generally heal within 2 weeks. If a 2-week period of treatment is not sufficient, healing will be achieved in almost all cases within a further 2 weeks.

Gastric ulcer: A 4-week period is usually required for the treatment of gastric ulcers. If this is not sufficient, healing will usually be achieved within a further 4 weeks.

Gastro-oesophageal reflux: A 4-week period is usually required for the treatment of gastro-oesophageal reflux. If this is not sufficient, healing will usually be achieved within a further 4 weeks.

Elderly: No dose adjustment is necessary in the elderly.

Patients with impaired renal function: No dose adjustment is necessary in patients with renal impairment.

Patients with hepatic cirrhosis: Due to an increased AUC and a modified metabolism of pantoprazole in patients with hepatic cirrhosis, the dose regimen should be reduced to one vial every other day.

Children: There is no information on the use of pantoprazole in children. Therefore Protium i.v. should not be used in children.

Contra-indications: Protium i.v. may not be used in cases of known hypersensitivity to any of its constituents.

Special warnings and special precautions for use: Protium i.v. is for intravenous administration ONLY and must NOT be given by any other route.

Interaction with other medicaments and other forms of interaction: No drug interactions have been reported so far.

Pregnancy and lactation:

Use during pregnancy: There is no information about the safety of pantoprazole during pregnancy in humans. Animal experiments have revealed no signs of foetal damage, but reproduction studies have revealed reduced litter weight and delayed development of the skeleton at doses above 15 mg/kg.

During pregnancy, Protium i.v. should not be used unless the benefit exceeds the potential risk.

Use during lactation: There is no information about the safety of pantoprazole during breast-feeding in humans. In the rat, not more than 0.02% of the administered dose is excreted via the breast milk.

During breast-feeding, Protium i.v. should not be used unless the benefit exceeds the potential risk.

Effects on ability to drive and use machines: Pantoprazole does not affect the ability to drive and use machines.

Undesirable effects: The most common undesirable effects seen with pantoprazole were headache and diarrhoea. Uncommon undesirable effects include skin rashes, pruritus and dizziness.

Overdose: There are no known symptoms of overdosage in man. However, pantoprazole is very specific in action and no particular problems are anticipated. Doses up to 240 mg i.v. were administered without obvious adverse effects.

As pantoprazole is extensively protein bound, it is not readily dialysable. Apart from symptomatic and supportive treatment, no specific therapeutic recommendations can be made.

Pharmacological properties

Pharmacodynamic properties: Pantoprazole is a proton pump inhibitor, i.e. it inhibits specifically and dose-proportionally the gastric H^+/K^+-ATPase enzyme which is responsible for acid secretion in the parietal cells of the stomach.

The substance is a substituted benzimidazole which accumulates in the acidic environment of the parietal cells after absorption. There it is converted into the active form, a cyclic sulphenamide, which binds to the H^+/K^+-ATPase, thus inhibiting the proton pump and causing potent and long-lasting suppression of basal and stimulated gastric acid secretion. As pantoprazole acts distally to the receptor level, it can inhibit gastric acid secretion irrespective of the nature of the stimulus (acetylcholine, histamine, gastrin).

Pantoprazole's selectivity is due to the fact that it can only exert its full effect in a strongly acidic environment (pH<3), remaining mostly inactive at higher pH values. As a result, its complete pharmacological and thus therapeutic effect can only be achieved in the acid-secretory parietal cells. By means of a feedback mechanism, this effect is diminished at the same rate as acid secretion is inhibited.

Pantoprazole has the same effect whether administered orally or intravenously.

Following intravenous or oral administration, pantoprazole inhibits the pentagastrin-stimulated gastric acid secretion. In volunteers, acid secretion was inhibited by 56% following the first i.v. administration of 30 mg and by 99% after 5 days. With an oral dose of 40 mg, inhibition was 51% on day 1 and 85% on day 7. Basal 24-hour acidity was reduced by 37% and 98%, respectively.

The fasting gastrin values increased under pantoprazole but in most cases they did not exceed the normal upper limit. Following completion of a course of oral treatment, the median gastrin levels clearly declined again.

Pharmacokinetic properties:

General pharmacokinetics: Terminal half-life is about 1 hour. Volume of distribution is about 0.15 litre/kg, clearance is about 0.1 litre/h/kg and Cmax is approximately 5.53 mg/litre.

Pharmacokinetics do not vary after single or repeated administration. The plasma kinetics of pantoprazole are linear after both oral and intravenous administration.

Studies with pantoprazole in humans reveal no interaction with the cytochrome P450-system of the liver. There was no induction of the P450-system seen as tested after chronic administration with antipyrine as a marker. Also, no inhibition of metabolism was observed after concomitant administration of pantoprazole with either antipyrine, diazepam, phenytoin, nifedipine, theophylline, digoxin or oral contraceptives. Concomitant administration of pantoprazole with warfarin has no influence on warfarin's effect on the coagulation factors.

Pantoprazole's plasma protein binding is about 98%. The substance is almost exclusively metabolised in the liver. Renal elimination represents the major route of excretion (about 80%) for the metabolites of pantoprazole; the rest are excreted in the faeces. The main metabolite in both the plasma and urine is desmethylpantoprazole which is conjugated with sulphate. The half-life of the main metabolites (about 1.5 hours) is not much longer than that of pantoprazole.

Characteristics in patients/special groups of subjects: Although for patients with hepatic cirrhosis (classes A and B according to Child) the half-life values increased to between 7 and 9 hours and the AUC values increased by a factor of 5 to 7, the maximum plasma concentration only increased slightly by a factor of 1.5 compared with healthy subjects. As pantoprazole has a good safety profile and is well tolerated it can be given to patients with mild to moderate liver impairment.

No dose reduction is required when pantoprazole is administered to patients with impaired kidney function (including dialysis patients). As with healthy subjects, pantoprazole's half-life is short. Only very small amounts of pantoprazole are dialysed. Although the main metabolite has a moderately delayed half-life (2–3 hours), excretion is still rapid and thus accumulation does not occur.

A slight increase in AUC and Cmax in elderly volunteers compared with younger counterparts is also not clinically relevant.

Preclinical safety data:

Acute toxicity: In acute toxicity studies in mice, the LD_{50} values were found to be 370 mg/kg bodyweight for i.v. administration and around 700 mg/kg bodyweight for oral administration.

In the rat, the corresponding values were around 240 mg/kg for i.v. administration and 900 mg/kg for oral administration.

Chronic toxicity: Hypergastrinaemia and morphologic changes of the mucosa were observed in studies investigating repeated administration for up to 12 months in the rat and dog. Most of the effects were reversible and attributable solely to the drug action, i.e. suppression of acid secretion.

In long-term studies in the rat and dog, there was an increase in stomach and liver weights, the increase being reversible after the substance was discontinued. The increase in liver weight following highly toxic doses was seen as a result of the induction of drug-metabolising enzymes.

Thyroid activation in two rat experiments is due to the rapid metabolism of thyroid hormones in the liver and has also been described in a similar form for other drugs. Changes in the thyroid and associated reduced degradation of cholesterol have been observed in one-year studies in the rat and dog. Hypertrophy of the thyroid and increases in cholesterol levels are reversible.

In studies in the dog, a species-specific pulmonary oedema was observed. The animal-specific metabolite which was responsible for the oedema could not be identified in man.

Carcinogenicity: In a 2-year carcinogenicity study in rats–which corresponds to lifetime treatment for rats–ECL cell carcinoids were found. The mechanism leading to the formation of gastric carcinoids by substituted benzimidazoles has been carefully investigated and allows the conclusion that it is a secondary reaction to the massively elevated serum gastrin levels occurring in the rat during treatment. In addition, rats have more ECL cells in the mucosa of the glandular stomach than man, so that a larger number of responder cells for the increased gastrin values can become active.

ECL cell neoplasms were not observed in either the study in mice (24 months) or in long-term studies in the dog. In clinical studies (40–80 mg for 1 year), ECL cell density slightly increased.

In the two-year studies, an increased number of neoplastic changes of the liver was observed in rats and female mice and was interpreted as being due to pantoprazole's high rate of metabolism in the liver.

A slight increase of neoplastic changes of the thyroid was observed in the group of rats receiving the highest dose. The occurrence of these neoplasms is associated with the pantoprazole-induced changes in the breakdown of thyroxine in the rat liver. In man, no changes in the thyroid hormones, T3, T4 and TSH were observed. This high dose phenomenon in the rat is therefore not relevant for man.

Mutagenicity: In mutagenicity studies, there were no indications of a mutagenic action *in vivo* or *in vitro*.

Reproduction toxicology: Investigations revealed no evidence of impaired fertility or teratogenic effects. Penetration of the placenta was investigated in the rat and was found to increase with advanced gestation. As a result, the concentration of pantoprazole in the foetus is increased shortly before birth, regardless of the route of administration.

In humans, there is no experience of the use of the drug during pregnancy.

Pharmaceutical particulars

List of excipients: None.

Incompatibilities: Protium i.v. is not compatible with acidic solutions.

Shelf life: Protium i.v. is stable over a period of 3 years.

The reconstituted solution must be used immediately (i.e within 3 hours). Any unused portion should be discarded.

Special precautions for storage: Store at room temperature, not exceeding 25°C.

Nature and contents of container: Protium i.v. is presented as a lyophilised powder in a 10 ml glass vial, with an aluminium cap and rubber stopper. It is distributed for sale packed in carton boxes.

Protium i.v. is available in single vials packed in outers of 5.

Instructions for use/handling: A ready-to-use injection solution is prepared by injecting 10 ml of Sodium Chloride Injection BP into the vial containing the lyophilised powder. The reconstituted injection solution has a pH of 9–10.

The reconstituted solution must be used immediately (i.e within 3 hours). The freshly prepared solution is designed for use as an i.v. injection or infusion, and the duration of administration should be 2 to 15 minutes. Any unused portion should be discarded.

Marketing authorisation number 04889/0011

Date of approval/revision of SPC February 1998

Legal category POM

SECURON*

Presentation Securon tablets containing 40 mg Verapamil Hydrochloride PhEur are white, film-coated tablets impressed with 40 on one side and the Knoll logo on the other.

Securon tablets containing 80 mg Verapamil Hydrochloride PhEur are white, film-coated tablets impressed with SECURON 80 on one side and KNOLL above the score-line on the other.

Securon tablets containing 120 mg Verapamil Hydrochloride PhEur are white, film-coated tablets impressed with Securon 120 on one side and KNOLL above the score-line on the other.

Inactive ingredients: Lactose.

Uses Securon is a calcium antagonist which blocks the inward movement of calcium ions in cardiac muscle cells, in smooth muscle cells of the coronary and systemic arteries and in the cells of the intracardiac conduction system. Securon lowers peripheral vascular resistance with no reflex tachycardia. Its efficacy in reducing both raised systolic and diastolic blood pressure is thought to be due to this mode of action. The decrease in systemic and coronary vascular resistance and the sparing effect on intracellular oxygen consumption appear to explain the antianginal properties of the drug. Because of its effect on the movement of calcium in the intracardiac conduction system, Securon reduces automaticity, decreases conduction velocity and increases the refractory period.

Securon is indicated for

(1) the treatment of mild to moderate hypertension;
(2) the treatment and prophylaxis of chronic stable angina, vasospastic angina and unstable angina;
(3) the treatment and prophylaxis of paroxysmal supraventricular tachycardia and the reduction of ventricular rate in atrial flutter/fibrillation. Verapamil should not be used when atrial flutter/fibrillation complicates Wolff-Parkinson-White syndrome (see Precautions).

Dosage and administration
Adults
Hypertension: Initially 120 mg b.d. increasing to 160 mg b.d. when necessary. In some cases, dosages of up to 480 mg daily, in divided doses, have been used. A further reduction in blood pressure may be obtained by combining Securon with other antihypertensive agents, in particular diuretics. For concomitant administration with beta-blockers see Precautions.

Angina: 120 mg t.d.s. is recommended. 80 mg t.d.s. can be completely satisfactory in some patients with angina of effort. Less than 120 mg t.d.s. is not likely to be effective in variant angina.

Supraventricular tachycardias: 40–120 mg t.d.s. according to the severity of the condition.

Children: Up to 2 years: 20 mg, 2–3 times a day.

2 years and above: 40–120 mg, 2-3 times a day, according to age and effectiveness.

Elderly patients: The adult dose is recommended unless liver or renal function is impaired (see Precautions).

Contra-indications, warnings etc
Contra-indications: Cardiogenic shock; acute myocardial infarction complicated by bradycardia, hypotension or left ventricular failure; second or third degree atrioventricular block; sino-atrial block; sick sinus syndrome; uncompensated heart failure; bradycardia of less than 50 beats/minute; hypotension of less than 90 mmHg systolic. Concomitant intake of grapefruit juice.

Interactions with other medicaments and other forms of interaction: Interactions between verapamil and the following medications have been reported:

Digoxin: Verapamil has been shown to increase the serum concentration of digoxin and caution should be exercised with regard to digitalis toxicity. The digitalis level should be determined and the glycoside dose reduced, if required.

Beta-blockers, anti-arrhythmic agents or inhaled anaesthetics: The combination with Securon may lead to additive cardiovascular effects (e.g. AV block, bradycardia, hypotension, heart failure). Intravenous beta-blockers should not be given to patients under treatment with Securon.

Carbamazepine, cyclosporin and theophylline: Use of verapamil has resulted in increased serum levels of these medications, which could lead to increased side-effects.

Rifampicin, phenytoin and phenobarbitone: Serum levels of verapamil reduced.

Lithium: Serum levels of lithium may be reduced (pharmacokinetic effect); there may be increased sensitivity to lithium causing enhanced neurotoxicity (pharmacodynamic effect).

Cimetidine: Increase in verapamil serum level is possible.

Neuromuscular blocking agents employed in anaesthesia: The effects may be potentiated.

The effects of Securon may be additive to other hypotensive agents.

Effects on the ability to drive and use machines: Depending on individual susceptibility, the patient's ability to drive a vehicle or operate machinery may be impaired. This is particularly true in the initial stages of treatment, or when changing over from another medication. Like many other common medicines, verapamil has been shown to increase the blood levels of alcohol and slow its elimination. Therefore, the effects of alcohol may be exaggerated.

Other undesirable effects (frequency and seriousness): Particularly when given in high doses or in the presence of previous myocardial damage, some cardiovascular effects of verapamil may occasionally be greater than therapeutically desired: bradycardic arrhythmias, such as sinus bradycardia, sinus arrest with asystole, second and third degree AV block, bradyarrhythmia in atrial fibrillation, hypotension, development or aggravation of heart failure.

Securon is generally well tolerated. Side-effects are usually mild and transient and discontinuation of therapy is rarely necessary. Constipation may occur. Flushing is observed occasionally and headaches, nausea, vomiting, dizziness, fatigue and ankle oedema have been reported rarely. Allergic reactions (e.g. erythema, pruritus, urticaria, Quincke's oedema, Stevens-Johnson syndrome) are very rarely seen. A reversible impairment of liver function, characterised by an increase in transaminase and/or alkaline phosphatase may occur on very rare occasions during verapamil treatment and is most probably a hypersensitivity reaction.

On very rare occasions, gynaecomastia has been observed in elderly male patients under long-term verapamil treatment, which was fully reversible in all cases when the drug was discontinued.

Gingival hyperplasia may very rarely occur when the drug is administered over prolonged periods, and is fully reversible when the drug is discontinued. Erythromelalgia and paraesthesia may occur. In very rare cases, there may be myalgia and arthralgia. Rises in prolactin levels have been reported.

Use in pregnancy and lactation: Although animal studies have not shown any teratogenic effects, verapamil should not be given during the first trimester of pregnancy unless, in the clinician's judgement, it is essential for the welfare of the patient.

Verapamil is excreted into the breast milk in small amounts and is unlikely to be harmful. However, rare hypersensitivity reactions have been reported with verapamil and, therefore, it should only be used during lactation if, in the clinician's judgement, it is essential for the welfare of the patient.

Other special warnings and precautions: Since verapamil is extensively metabolised in the liver, careful dose titration of verapamil is required in patients with liver disease. The disposition of verapamil in patients with renal impairment has not been fully established and therefore careful patient monitoring is recommended. Verapamil is not removed during dialysis.

Verapamil may affect impulse conduction and therefore Securon should be used with caution in patients with first degree AV block. Patients with atrial flutter/fibrillation in association with an accessory pathway (e.g. WPW syndrome) may develop increased conduction across the anomalous pathway and ventricular tachycardia may be precipitated. Securon may affect left ventricular contractility; this effect is small and normally not important but cardiac failure may be precipitated or aggravated. In patients with incipient cardiac failure, therefore, Securon should be given only after such cardiac failure has been controlled with appropriate therapy, e.g. digitalis. When treating hypertension with verapamil, monitoring of the patient's blood pressure at regular intervals is required.

Overdosage (symptoms, emergency procedures, antidotes): The course of symptoms in verapamil intoxication depends on the amount taken, the point in time at which detoxification measures are taken and myocardial contractility (age-related). The main symptoms are as follows: blood pressure fall (at times to values not detectable), shock symptoms, loss of consciousness, 1st and 2nd degree AV block (frequently as Wenckebach's phenomenon with or without escape rhythms), total AV block with total AV dissociation, escape rhythm, asystole, sinus bradycardia, sinus arrest. The therapeutic measures to be taken depend on the point in time at which verapamil was taken and the type and severity of intoxication symptoms. Gastric lavage, taking the usual precautionary measures may be appropriate. The usual intensive resuscitation measures, such as extrathoracic heart massage, respiration, defibrillation and/or pacemaker therapy. Specific measures to be taken: Elimination of cardiodepressive effects, hypotension or bradycardia. The specific antidote is calcium, e.g. 10–20 ml of a 10% calcium gluconate solution administered intravenously (2.25–4.5 mmol), repeated if necessary or given as a continuous drip infusion (e.g. 5 mmol/hour). The following measures may also be necessary: In case of 2nd or 3rd degree AV block, sinus bradycardia, asystole: atropine, isoprenaline, orciprenaline or pacemaker therapy. In case of hypotension after appropriate positioning of the patient: dopamine, dobutamine, noradrenaline. If there are signs of continuing myocardial failure: dopamine, dobutamine, cardiac glycosides or if necessary, repeated calcium gluconate injections.

Incompatibilities: None.

Pharmaceutical precautions Store in a dry place at room temperature (below 25°C).

Legal category POM

Package quantities Securon 120 mg tablets: blister pack of 60 tablets.

Securon 80 mg, 40 mg tablets: blister packs of 100 tablets.

Further information Nil.

Product licence numbers
Securon tablets 40 mg 0169/0003
Securon tablets 80 mg 0169/0004
Securon tablets 120 mg 0169/0005

SECURON* IV

Presentation Securon IV is an aqueous solution of Verapamil Hydrochloride BP in a concentration of 2.5 mg/ml. Each ampoule contains 5 mg of Verapamil Hydrochloride BP in 2 ml of intravenous injection solution.

Uses Securon is a calcium antagonist which blocks the inward movement of calcium ions in cardiac muscle cells, in smooth muscle cells of the coronary and systemic arteries and in the cells of the intracardiac conduction system. Because of its effect on the movement of calcium in the intracardiac conduction system, Securon reduces automaticity, decreases conduction velocity, and increases the refractory period.

Securon IV is indicated in the treatment of paroxysmal supraventricular tachycardia and the reduction of ventricular rate in atrial flutter/fibrillation. Verapamil should not be used when atrial flutter/fibrillation complicates Wolff-Parkinson-White syndrome (see 'Contra-indications').

Dosage and administration
Adults: 5–10 mg by slow intravenous injection over a period of 2 minutes. The patient should be observed continuously preferably under ECG and blood pressure control. If necessary, e.g. in paroxysmal tachycardia, a further 5 mg may be given after 5–10 minutes.

Children: Securon IV must always be administered under ECG monitoring in young patients.

0–1 year: 0.1–0.2 mg/kg bodyweight (usual single dose range 0.75–2 mg).

1–15 years: 0.1–0.3 mg/kg bodyweight (usual single dose range 2–5 mg).

The dose may be repeated after 30 minutes if necessary. Many cases are controlled by doses at the lower end of the range. The injection should be stopped at the onset of the desired effect.

Elderly: The dosage should be administered over 3 minutes to minimise the risk of adverse effects.

Dosage in impaired liver and renal function: Significant hepatic and renal impairment should not increase the effects of a single intravenous dose but may prolong its duration of action.

For use with beta-blocker therapy see *Contra-indications* and *Precautions*.

Contra-indications, warnings, etc
Contra-indications: Cardiogenic shock; acute myocardial infarction complicated by bradycardia, marked hypotension or left ventricular failure; second or third degree AV block; sino-atrial block; sick sinus syndrome; uncompensated heart failure; marked bradycardia of less than 50 beats/minute; marked hypotension of less than 90 mmHg systolic; patients with atrial flutter/fibrillation in the presence of an accessory pathway (e.g. WPW syndrome) may develop increased conduction across the anomalous pathway and ventricular tachycardia may be precipitated; simultaneous administration of intravenous beta-blockers.

Interactions with other medicaments and other forms of interaction: The effects of Securon IV, beta-blockers and anti-arrhythmic agents may be additive both with respect to conduction and contraction. Securon IV should not be given in combination with intravenous beta-blocker therapy and care must be exercised if Securon IV is combined with oral beta-blocker therapy or anti-arrhythmic agents by any route. Securon IV and inhaled anaesthetics may have additive cardiovascular effects. Securon IV may reduce blood pressure and an additive effect with antihypertensive drugs may be seen.

Verapamil hydrochloride has been shown to increase the serum concentration of digoxin and caution should be exercised with regard to digitalis toxicity.

Interactions with verapamil have been reported for carbamazepine (potentiated by verapamil), rifampicin (effects of verapamil attenuated), cyclosporin and theophylline (increase of plasma levels by verapamil). Neurotoxic interactions have been reported with lithium. The effect of muscle relaxants employed in anaesthesia may be potentiated.

Effects on the ability to drive and use machines: None stated.

Other undesirable effects (frequency and seriousness): Securon IV is generally well tolerated but due to the drug's mode of action, undesired cardiovascular effects may occur, particularly at high doses and in patients with AV block and/or impaired myocardial function. Decreased heart rate, hypotension and decreased myocardial contractility have been reported. On rare occasions, second or third degree AV block may occur and, in extreme cases, this may lead to asystole. The asystole is usually of short duration and cardiac action returns spontaneously after a few seconds, usually in the form of sinus rhythm. If necessary, the procedures for the treatment of overdosage should be followed as described below. A slight transient fall in blood pressure, due to a reduction in peripheral resistance, may be seen. In rare cases this may lead to severe hypotension. On rare occasions, dizziness, headache, nausea, vomiting, nervousness and flushing have been reported. Allergic reactions (erythema, pruritus, urticaria, bronchospasm) are extremely rare.

A reversible impairment of liver function, characterised by an increase of transaminase and/or alkaline phosphatase may occur on very rare occasions during verapamil treatment and is most probably a hypersensitivity reaction.

On very rare occasions, gynaecomastia has been observed in elderly male patients under long term verapamil treatment, which was fully reversible in all cases when the drug was discontinued.

Gingival hyperplasia may very rarely occur when the drug is administered over prolonged periods, and is fully reversible when the drug is discontinued.

Use in pregnancy and lactation: Although animal studies have not shown any teratogenic effects, verapamil should not be given during the first trimester of pregnancy unless, in the clinician's judgement, it is essential for the welfare of the patient.

Verapamil is excreted into the breast milk in small amounts and is unlikely to be harmful. However, rare hypersensitivity reactions have been reported with verapamil and, therefore, it should only be used during lactation if, in the clinician's judgement, it is essential for the welfare of the patient.

Other special warnings and precautions: Verapamil may affect impulse conduction and therefore Securon IV should be used with caution in patients with first degree AV block. Securon IV may affect left ventricular contractility; this effect is small and normally not important but cardiac failure may be precipitated or aggravated. In patients with poor ventricular function, therefore, Securon IV should only be given after cardiac failure has been controlled with appropriate therapy, e.g. digitalis and/or diuretics.

Overdose (symptoms, emergency procedures, antidotes): The symptoms of overdosage include hypotension, shock, loss of consciousness, first and second degree AV block (frequently as Wenckebach's phenomenon with or without escape rhythms), total AV block with total AV dissociation, escape rhythm, asystole, sinus bradycardia, sinus arrest.

Treatment of overdosage depends on the type and severity of symptoms. The specific antidote is calcium, e.g. 10–20 ml of 10% calcium gluconate solution i.v. (2.25–4.5 mmol) if necessary by repeated injection or continuous infusion (e.g. 5 mmol/hr). The usual emergency measures for acute cardiovascular collapse should be applied and followed by intensive care. Similarly in the case of second and third degree AV block, atropine, isoprenaline and, if required, pacemaker therapy should be considered. If there are signs of myocardial insufficiency, dopamine, dobutamine, cardiac glycosides or calcium gluconate (10–20 ml of a 10% solution) can be administered.

In the case of hypotension, after appropriately positioning the patient, dopamine, dobutamine or noradrenaline may be given.

Incompatibilities: None stated.

Pharmaceutical precautions Store at room temperature. Protect from light.

Legal category POM

Package quantities 5x2 ml ampoule.

Further information Each ampoule contains 17 mg sodium chloride (8.5 mg/ml).

Following intravenous infusion in man, verapamil is eliminated bi-exponentially with a rapid distribution phase (half-life about 4 mins) and a slower terminal elimination phase (half-life 2–5 hours).

Product licence number 0169/0017.

SECURON SR/HALF SECURON SR

Qualitative and quantitative composition Securon SR: Verapamil Hydrochloride PhEur 240 mg. Half Securon SR: Verapamil Hydrochloride PhEur 120 mg.

Pharmaceutical form Film-coated, sustained-release tablets.

Securon SR tablets are oblong, pale green, scored and embossed with two Knoll logos (triangles) on one side. Half Securon SR tablets are round, white, unscored and embossed with 'KNOLL' on one side and '120 SR' on the reverse.

Clinical particulars

Therapeutic indications: Securon SR and Half Securon SR are indicated for the treatment of mild to moderate hypertension and the treatment and prophylaxis of angina pectoris.

Secondary prevention of re-infarction after an acute myocardial infarction in patients without heart failure, and not receiving diuretics (apart from low-dose diuretics when used for indications other than heart failure), and where beta-blockers are not appropriate. Treatment is to be started at least one week after an acute myocardial infarction.

Posology and method of administration: For oral administration.

Securon SR and Half Securon SR tablets should not be chewed. Securon SR tablets are scored and may be halved without damaging the sustained-release formulation.

Adults: Hypertension: One tablet of Securon SR (240 mg) daily. For patients new to verapamil therapy, the physician should consider halving the initial dose to 120 mg (Half Securon SR). Most patients respond to 240 mg daily (one tablet Securon SR) given as a single dose. If control is not achieved after a period of at least one week, the dosage may be increased to a maximum of two Securon SR tablets daily (one in the morning and one in the evening at an interval of about twelve hours). A further reduction in blood pressure may be achieved by combining Securon SR tablets with other antihypertensive agents, in particular diuretics. Half Securon SR tablets may be used for dose titration purposes.

Angina pectoris: One tablet of Securon SR twice daily. A small number of patients respond to a lower dose and where indicated, adjustment down to one tablet of Securon SR daily could be made. Half Securon SR tablets may be used for dose titration purposes.

Secondary prevention of re-infarction after an acute myocardial infarction in patients without heart failure, and not receiving diuretics (apart from low-dose diuretics when used for indications other than heart failure), and where beta-blockers are not appropriate: Treatment is to be started at least one week after an acute myocardial infarction. 360 mg/day in divided doses, to be taken either as one Half Securon SR (120 mg) three times daily, or as one Securon SR (240 mg) to be taken in the morning and one Half Securon SR (120 mg) tablet in the evening, on a daily basis.

Elderly patients: The adult dose is recommended unless liver or renal function is impaired (see Precautions).

Children: Securon SR and Half Securon SR tablets are not recommended for children.

Contra-indications: Cardiogenic shock; acute myocardial infarction complicated by bradycardia, marked hypotension, left ventricular failure; second or third degree atrioventricular block; sino-atrial block; sick sinus syndrome; uncompensated heart failure; bradycardia of less than 50 beats/minute; hypotension of less than 90 mmHg systolic.

Concomitant ingestion of grapefruit juice.

Special warnings and special precautions for use: Since verapamil is extensively metabolised in the liver, careful dose titration of verapamil is required in patients with liver disease. The disposition of verapamil in patients with renal impairment has not been fully established and therefore careful patient monitoring is recommended. Verapamil is not removed during dialysis.

Verapamil may affect impulse conduction and should therefore be used with caution in patients with first degree atrioventricular block. Patients with atrial flutter/fibrillation in association with an accessory pathway (e.g. WPW-syndrome) may develop increased conduction across the anomalous pathway and ventricular tachycardia may be precipitated. Verapamil may affect left ventricular contractility. This effect is small and normally not important but cardiac failure may be precipitated or aggravated. In patients with incipient cardiac failure, therefore, verapamil should be given only after such cardiac failure has been controlled with appropriate therapy, e.g. digitalis.

When treating hypertension with verapamil, monitoring of the patient's blood pressure at regular intervals is required.

Interaction with other medicaments and other forms of interaction: Verapamil has been shown to increase the serum concentration of digoxin and caution should be exercised with regard to digitalis toxicity. The digitalis level should be determined and the glycoside dose reduced, if required. The combination of verapamil and beta-blockers, anti-arrhythmic agents or inhaled anaesthetics may lead to additive cardiovascular effects (e.g. AV block, bradycardia, hypotension, heart failure). Intravenous beta-blockers should not be given to patients under treatment with verapamil. The effects of verapamil may be additive to other hypotensive agents.

Interactions between verapamil and the following have been reported:

Carbamazepine, cyclosporin and theophylline: Use of verapamil has resulted in increased serum levels of these medications, which could lead to increased side effects.

Rifampicin, phenytoin and phenobarbitone: Serum levels of verapamil reduced.

Lithium: Serum levels of lithium may be reduced (pharmacokinetic effect); there may be increased sensitivity to lithium causing enhanced neurotoxicity (pharmacodynamic effect).

Cimetidine: Increase in verapamil serum level is possible.

Neuromuscular blocking agents employed in anaesthesia: The effects may be potentiated.

Grapefruit juice: Increase in verapamil serum level has been reported.

Alcohol: Increase in blood alcohol has been reported.

Pregnancy and lactation: Although animal studies have not shown any teratogenic effects, verapamil should not be given during the first trimester of pregnancy unless, in the clinician's judgement, it is essential for the welfare of the patient.

Verapamil is excreted into the breast milk in small amounts and is unlikely to be harmful. However, rare hypersensitivity reactions have been reported with verapamil and, therefore, it should only be used during lactation if, in the clinician's judgement, it is essential for the welfare of the patient.

Effects on ability to drive and use machines: Depending on individual susceptibility, the patient's ability to drive a vehicle or operate machinery may be impaired. This is particularly true in the initial stages of treatment, or when changing over from another drug. Like many other common medicines, verapamil has been shown to increase the blood levels of alcohol and slow its elimination. Therefore, the effects of alcohol may be exaggerated.

Undesirable effects: Particularly when given in high doses or in the presence of previous myocardial damage, some cardiovascular effects of verapamil may occasionally be greater than therapeutically desired: bradycardic arrhythmias, such as sinus bradycardia, sinus arrest with asystole, second and third degree AV block, bradyarrhythmia in atrial fibrillation, hypotension, development or aggravation of heart failure.

Securon SR and Half Securon SR tablets are generally well tolerated. Side-effects are usually mild and transient and discontinuation of therapy is rarely necessary. Constipation may occur. There have been rare reports of flushing, headache, nausea, vomiting, dizziness, fatigue and ankle oedema. Allergic reactions (e.g. erythema, pruritus, urticaria, Quincke's oedema, Stevens-Johnson syndrome) are very rarely seen. A reversible impairment of liver function, characterised by an increase of transaminases and/or alkaline phosphatase may occur on very rare occasions during verapamil treatment and is most probably a hypersensitivity reaction.

On very rare occasions, gynaecomastia has been observed in elderly male patients under long-term verapamil treatment, which was fully reversible in all cases when the drug was discontinued.

Gingival hyperplasia may very rarely occur when the drug is administered over prolonged periods, and is fully reversible when the drug is discontinued.

Erythromelalgia and paraesthesia may occur. In very rare cases, there may be myalgia and arthralgia. Rises in prolactin levels have been reported.

Overdose: The course of symptoms in verapamil intoxication depends on the amount taken, the point in time at which detoxication measures are taken and myocardial contractility (age-related). The main symptoms are as follows: blood pressure fall (at times to values not detectable), shock symptoms, loss of consciousness, 1st and 2nd degree AV block (frequently as Wenckebach's phenomenon with or without escape rhythms), total AV block with total AV dissociation, escape rhythm, asystole, sinus bradycardia, sinus arrest. The therapeutic measures to be taken depend on the point in time at which verapamil was taken and the type and severity of intoxication symptoms. In intoxications with large amounts of slow-release preparations (Securon SR and Half Securon SR), it should be noted that the release of the active drug and the absorption in the intestine may take more than 48 hours. Depending on the time of ingestion, it should be taken into account that there may be some lumps of incompletely-dissolved tablets along the entire length of the gastrointestinal tract, which function as active drug depots.

General measures to be taken: gastric lavage with the usual precautions, even later than 12 hours after ingestion, if no gastrointestinal motility (peristaltic sounds) is detectable. Where intoxication by Securon SR or Half Securon SR tablets is suspected, extensive elimination measures are indicated, such as induced vomiting, removal of the contents of the stomach and the small intestine under endoscopy, intestinal lavage, laxative, high enemas. The usual intensive resuscitation measures, such as extrathoracic heart massage, respiration, defibrillation and/or pacemaker therapy.

Specific measures to be taken: elimination of cardiodepressive effects, hypotension or bradycardia. The specific antidote is calcium, e.g. 10–20 ml of a 10% calcium gluconate solution administered intravenously (2.25–4.5 mmol), repeated if necessary or given as a continuous drip infusion (e.g. 5 mmol/hour).

The following measures may also be necessary: in case of 2nd or 3rd degree AV block, sinus bradycardia, asystole: atropine, isoprenaline, orciprenaline or pacemaker therapy. In case of hypotension: dopamine, dobutamine, noradrenaline. If there are signs of continuing myocardial failure: dopamine, dobutamine, if necessary repeated calcium injections.

Pharmacological properties
Pharmacodynamic properties: Verapamil, a phenylalkylamine calcium antagonist, has a balanced profile of cardiac and peripheral effects. It lowers heart rate, increases myocardial perfusion and reduces coronary spasm. In a clinical study in patients after myocardial infarction, verapamil reduced total mortality, sudden cardiac death and reinfarction rate.

Verapamil reduces total peripheral resistance and lowers high blood pressure by vasodilation without reflex tachycardia. Because of its use-dependent action on the voltage-operated calcium channel, the effects of verapamil are more pronounced on high than on normal blood pressure.

As early as day one of treatment, blood pressure falls; the effect is found to persist also in long-term therapy. Verapamil is suitable for the treatment of all types of hypertension: for monotherapy in mild to moderate hypertension; combined with other antihypertensives (in particular with diuretics and, according to more recent findings, with ACE inhibitors) in more severe types of hypertension. In hypertensive diabetic patients with nephropathy, verapamil in combination with ACE inhibitors led to a marked reduction of albuminuria and to an improvement of creatinine clearance.

Pharmacokinetic properties: Absorption: More than 90% of an orally-administered dose of verapamil is absorbed. Due to an intensive hepatic first-pass metabolism, the absolute bioavailability is about 22%, with a variability of about 10–35%. Under multiple dosing, bioavailability increases by about 30%. Bioavailability is not affected by food consumption.

Distribution/Biotransformation/Elimination: Plasma concentrations reach their peak 4–8 hours after drug intake. Plasma protein binding of verapamil is more than 90%. The elimination half-life is about 5–8 hours. The mean residence time of sustained-release verapamil is 13 hours. After repeated single daily doses, steady-state conditions are reached between 3–4 days.

Within 5 days, approximately 70% of an orally-administered dose is excreted in the urine and about 16% with the faeces. Only 3–4% is eliminated renally as unchanged drug. Norverapamil, one of the 12 metabolites identified in urine, which represents about 6% of the dose eliminated, has 10–20% of the activity of verapamil. Norverapamil can reach steady-state plasma concentrations approximately equal to those of verapamil itself.

At-risk Patients: In patients with liver cirrhosis, bioavailability is increased and elimination half-life is prolonged. In patients with compensated hepatic insufficiency, no influence on the kinetics of verapamil was observed. The disposition of verapamil in patients with renal impairment has not been fully established.

Preclinical safety data: Not applicable.

Pharmaceutical particulars
List of excipients: Securon SR: Sodium alginate, microcrystalline cellulose, povidone, purified water, talc, titanium dioxide (E171), hydroxypropyl methylcellulose, magnesium stearate, polyethylene glycol 400, polyethylene glycol 6000, montan glycol wax, L-green lake (E104, E132).

Half Securon SR: Sodium alginate, microcrystalline cellulose, povidone, purified water, talc, titanium dioxide (E171), hydroxypropyl methylcellulose, magnesium stearate, polyethylene glycol 400, polyethylene glycol 6000, montan glycol wax.

Incompatibilities: There are no major incompatibilities listed.

Shelf life: 60 months from date of manufacture.

Special precautions for storage: Store in a dry place, away from direct sunlight, below 25°C.

Nature and contents of container: PVC/PVDC blister packs, in a cardboard outer container, containing 28 tablets.

Instructions for use/handling: There are no special instructions for use/handling.

Marketing authorisation number

Securon SR	00169/0007
Half Securon SR	00169/0026

Date of approval/revision of SPC April 1997

Legal category POM

TARKA ▼

Qualitative and quantitative composition Each Tarka 180/2 capsule contains 180 mg of verapamil hydrochloride in a sustained-release form and 2 mg of trandolapril.

Pharmaceutical form Capsules. Pink in colour.

Clinical particulars
Therapeutic indications: Essential hypertension in patients whose blood pressure has been normalised with the individual components in the same proportion of doses.

Posology and method of administration: For oral administration.

The usual dosage is one Tarka capsule once daily, taken the morning, before, with or after breakfast.

Dosage in children: Tarka is contra-indicated in children (see *Contra-indications*).

Dosage in the elderly: See *Special warnings and special precautions for use.*

Contra-indications: Known hypersensitivity to trandolapril or any other ACE inhibitor and/or verapamil; history of angioneurotic oedema associated with previous ACE inhibitor therapy; hereditary/idiopathic angioneurotic oedema; cardiogenic shock; recent myocardial infarction with complications; second or third degree AV block without pacemaker; SA block; sick sinus syndrome; bradycardia of less than 50 beats/minute; congestive heart failure; severe renal impairment (creatinine clearance <10 ml/min); dialysis; liver cirrhosis with ascites; aortic or mitral stenosis; obstructive hypertrophic cardiomyopathy; pregnancy; lactation; children. Tarka should not be taken with grapefruit juice (see *Interaction with other medicaments and other forms of interaction*).

Special warnings and special precautions for use: Evaluation of the patients should include assessment of renal function prior to initiation of therapy and during treatment.

Blood pressure readings for evaluation of therapeutic response to Tarka should always be taken before the next dose.

Symptomatic hypotension: Under certain circumstances, Tarka may occasionally produce symptomatic hypotension. This risk is elevated in patients with a stimulated renin-angiotensin-aldosterone system (e.g. volume or salt depletion, due to the use of diuretics, a low-sodium diet, dialysis, diarrhoea or vomiting, decreased left ventricular function, renovascular hypertension).

Such patients should have their volume or salt depletion corrected beforehand and therapy should preferably be initiated in a hospital setting. Patients experiencing hypotension during titration should lie down and may require volume expansion by oral fluid supply or intravenous administration of normal saline. Tarka therapy can usually be continued once blood volume and pressure have been effectively corrected.

Renal impairment: See also *Contra-indications.*

Patients with moderate renal impairment should have their kidney function monitored.

Tarka may produce hyperkalaemia in patients with renal dysfunction.

Acute deterioration of kidney function (acute renal failure) may occur, especially in patients with preexisting renal impairment or congestive heart failure.

There is insufficient experience with Tarka in secondary hypertension and particularly in renovascular hypertension. Tarka should not be administered to these patients.

Patients with bilateral renal artery stenosis or unilateral renal artery stenosis in individuals with a single functioning kidney (e.g. renal transplant patients) are at risk of acute loss of renal function.

Proteinuria: Proteinuria may occur, particularly in patients with existing renal impairment or on relatively high doses of ACE inhibitors.

Severe hepatic impairment: See also *Contra-indications.*

Since there is insufficient therapeutic experience in these patients, the use of Tarka cannot be recommended.

Angioneurotic oedema: Rarely, ACE inhibitors (such as trandolapril) may cause angioneurotic oedema that includes swelling of the face, extremities, tongue, glottis, and/or larynx. Patients experiencing angioneurotic oedema must immediately discontinue Tarka therapy and be monitored until oedema resolution.

Angioneurotic ooedema to the face will usually resolve spontaneously. Oedema involving not only the face but also the glottis may be life-threatening because of the risk of airway obstruction.

Angioneurotic oedema involving the tongue, glottis or larynx requires immediate subcutaneous administration of 0.3–0.5 ml of adrenaline solution (1:1000) along with other therapeutic measures as appropriate.

Caution must be exercised in patients with a history of idiopathic angioneurotic oedema, and Tarka is contra-indicated if angioneurotic oedema was an adverse reaction to an ACE inhibitor (see *Contra-indications).*

Cough: During treatment with an ACE inhibitor, a dry and non-productive cough may occur which disappears after discontinuation.

Elderly: Tarka has been studied in a limited number of elderly hypertensive patients only. Pharmacokinetic data show that the systemic availability of Tarka is higher in elderly compared to younger hypertensives.

Some elderly patients might experience a more pronounced blood pressure lowering effect than others. Evaluation of renal function at the beginning of treatment is recommended.

Hyperkalaemia: Hyperkalaemia may occur during treatment with an ACE inhibitor, especially in the presence of renal insufficiency and/or heart failure. Potassium supplements or potassium-sparing diuretics are generally not recommended, since they may lead to significant increases in serum potassium. If concomitant use of the above mentioned agents is deemed appropriate, they should be used with frequent monitoring of serum potassium.

Surgical patients: In patients undergoing major surgery requiring general anaesthesia, ACE inhibitors may produce hypotension, which can be corrected by plasma volume expanders.

Neutropenia/agranulocytosis: The risk of neutropenia appears to be dose-and type-related and is dependent on the patient's clinical status. It is rarely seen in uncomplicated patients but may occur in patients with some degree of renal impairment, especially when it is associated with collagen vascular disease (e.g. systemic lupus erythematosus or scleroderma) and in patients receiving therapy with immunosuppressive agents. It is reversible after discontinuation of the ACE inhibitor.

Primary aldosteronism: Patients with primary aldosteronism should not be treated with Tarka as their renin-angiotensin system is affected by the primary disease.

Desensitisation: Anaphylactoid reactions (in some cases life threatening) may develop in patients receiving ACE inhibitor therapy and concomitant desensitisation against animal venoms.

LDL-apheresis: Life threatening anaphylactoid reactions have been noted when patients on LDL-apheresis take ACE inhibitors at the same time.

Conduction disturbances: Tarka should be used with caution in patients with first degree atrioventricular block and patients with atrial flutter/fibrillation in association with an accessory pathway (e.g. WPW-syndrome).

Haemodialysis patients: See also *Contra-indications.*

Patients on concurrent ACE inhibitor therapy and haemodialysis with polyacrylonitrile methallyl sulfonate high-flux membranes (e.g. 'AN 69') have experienced anaphylactoid reactions. Such membranes should therefore not be used in these patients.

Bradycardia: See also *Contra-indications.* Tarka should be used with caution in patients with bradycardia.

Interaction with other medicaments and other forms of interaction:

–Potassium-sparing diuretics or potassium supplements: ACE inhibitors attenuate diuretic induced potassium loss. Potassium-sparing diuretics (e.g. spironolactone, triamterene and amiloride), potassium supplements and potassium-containing salt substitutes may lead to significant increases in serum potassium, particularly in the presence of renal impairment. If concomitant use is indicated because of demonstrated hypokalaemia, they should be used with caution and with frequent monitoring of serum potassium.

–The simultaneous use of verapamil with dantrolene is not recommended.

–Antihypertensive agents: Increase in the hypotensive effect of Tarka.

–Diuretics: Patients on diuretics and especially those who are volume- and/or salt-depleted may experience an excessive reduction of blood pressure after initiation of therapy with an ACE inhibitor. The possibility of hypotensive effects can be reduced by discontinuation of the diuretic, by increasing volume or salt before starting therapy and by initiation of therapy with low doses. Further increases in dosage should be performed with caution.

–Lithium: There have been reports of both an increase and a reduction in the effects of lithium when used concurrently with verapamil. The concomitant administration of ACE inhibitors with lithium may reduce the excretion of lithium. Serum lithium levels should be monitored frequently.

–Anaesthetic drugs: Tarka may enhance the hypotensive effects of certain anaesthetic drugs.

–Narcotic drugs/antipsychotics: Postural hypotension may occur.

–Allopurinol, cytostatic or immunosuppressive agents, systemic corticosteroids or procainamide: Concomitant administration with ACE inhibitors may lead to an increased risk of leucopenia.

–Cardiodepressive drugs: The concurrent use of verapamil and cardiodepressive drugs, i.e. drugs that inhibit cardiac impulse generation and conduction (e.g. beta-adrenergic blocking agents, antiarrhythmic drugs, inhalation anaesthetics), may produce undesirable additive effects.

–Quinidine: The concomitant use of quinidine and oral verapamil in patients with hypertrophic (obstructive) cardiomyopathy has resulted in hypotension and pulmonary oedema in a small number of cases.

–Digoxin: Concurrent use of digoxin and verapamil has been reported to result in 50–75% higher digoxin plasma concentrations, requiring reduction of the digoxin dosage.

–Muscle relaxants: The effects of muscle relaxants may be enhanced.

–Tranquillisers/antidepressant agents: As with all antihypertensive drugs, there is an elevated risk of orthostatic hypotension when combining Tarka with major tranquillisers or tricyclic antidepressants.

–Non-steroidal anti-inflammatory drugs: The administration of a non-steroidal anti-inflammatory agent may reduce the antihypertensive effect of an ACE inhibitor. Furthermore, NSAIDs and ACE inhibitors may exert an additive effect on the increase in serum potassium, whereas renal function may decrease. These effects are in principle reversible, and occur especially in patients with compromised renal function.

–Antacids: Induce decreased bioavailability of ACE inhibitors.

–Sympathomimetics: May reduce the antihypertensive effects of ACE inhibitors; patients should be carefully monitored to confirm that the desired effect is being obtained.

–Tarka may increase the plasma concentrations of carbamazepine, cyclosporin, theophylline and alcohol.

–Rifampicin, phenytoin, and phenobarbital reduce the efficacy of verapamil, whereas cimetidine may increase the effect of Tarka.

–Antidiabetics: A dose adjustment of antidiabetics or of Tarka may be necessary in individual cases, especially at the start of therapy due to increased reduction of blood glucose.

–Grapefruit juice has been shown to increase the plasma levels of verapamil, which is a component of Tarka. Grapefruit juice should therefore not be ingested with Tarka.

Pregnancy and lactation: The safe use of Tarka in pregnant women is inadequately documented. However, there have been anecdotal reports of neonatal lung hypoplasia, intra-uterine growth retardation, persistent ductus arteriosus, and cranial hypoplasia following exposure of the foetus to ACE inhibitors. In addition, the pharmacologic activity of ACE inhibitors is compatible with the possibility of foetal hypotension, which may be associated with foetal/neonatal anuria and oligohydramnios (see *Preclinical safety data*).

Teratogenic effects are primarily expected when ACE inhibitors are used in the second and third trimesters of pregnancy, and it is not known whether exposure of the embryo/foetus to an ACE inhibitor only in the first trimester is teratogenic or embryotoxic/foetotoxic. Women who wish to get pregnant or are pregnant must consult their doctor without delay, so an alternative pharmacologic treatment can be prescribed.

Doctors should instruct women of child-bearing potential accordingly before prescribing an ACE inhibitor.

Nursing mothers on Tarka therapy should be discouraged from breast feeding.

Effects on ability to drive and use machines: Depending on individual susceptibility, the patient's ability to drive a vehicle or operate machinery may be impaired, especially in the initial stages of treatment.

Tarka may increase the blood levels of alcohol and slow its elimination. Therefore the effects of alcohol may be exaggerated.

Undesirable effects: New undesirable effects not yet described for either of the two component drugs of Tarka have not been reported.

The following side effects have been associated with ACE inhibitors therapy.

–Cardiovascular system: Severe hypotension has occurred after initiation of therapy. This occurs especially in certain risk groups (see *Special warnings and special precautions for use*). Symptoms like dizziness, feeling of weakness, impaired vision, rarely with disturbance of consciousness (syncope) can occur. Individual cases of tachycardia, palpitations, arrhythmias, angina pectoris, myocardial infarction, transient ischaemic attacks and cerebral haemorrhage have been reported for ACE inhibitors in association with hypotension.

–Renal system: Renal insufficiency may occur or be intensified. Acute renal failure has been reported (see *Special warnings and special precautions for use*).

–Respiratory system: ACE inhibitors have been documented to induce cough in a substantial number of patients. Rarely, dyspnoea, sinusitis, rhinitis, glossitis, bronchitis and bronchospasm have been reported. In individual cases, angioneurotic oedema involving the upper airway has caused fatal airway obstruction (see *Special warnings and special precautions for use*).

–Gastrointestinal tract: Occasionally nausea, abdominal pain, indigestion, vomiting, diarrhoea, constipation and dry mouth can occur.

Individual cases of cholestatic jaundice, hepatitis, pancreatitis and ileus have been described in relation to therapy with ACE inhibitors.

–Skin, vessels: Occasionally, allergic and hypersensitivity reactions can occur, e.g. rash, pruritus, urticaria, erythema multiforme, Stevens-Johnson syndrome, toxic epidermal necrolysis, psoriasis-like efflorescences, alopecia. This can be accompanied by fever, myalgia, arthralgia, eosinophilia and/or increased ANA-titers. ACE inhibitors have been associated with the onset of angioneurotic oedema in a small subset of patients involving the face and oropharyngeal tissues (see *Special warnings and special precautions for use*).

–Nervous system: Occasionally, headaches, dizziness, weariness, rarely depression, sleep disorders, paraesthesias, impotence, disorders of balance, confusion, tinnitus, blurred vision and taste disturbances.

–Drug/laboratory parameters: Increases in serum potassium levels, blood urea and plasma creatinine, reversible on discontinuation, may occur, especially in the presence of renal insufficiency, severe heart failure and renovascular hypertension. Decreases in haemoglobin, haematocrit, platelets and white cell count, and in individual cases, agranulocytosis or pancytopenia, as well as elevation of liver enzymes and serum bilirubin have been reported in a few patients. In patients with a congenital deficiency of G-6-PDH, individual cases of haemolytic anaemia have been reported.

The following side effects have been reported for verapamil:

–Cardiovascular system: Hypotension, bradycardia, heart failure. There have been rare reports of high-grade AV block, which, in extreme cases, may result in asystole. Excessive hypotension in patients with angina pectoris or cerebrovascular disease could result in myocardial infarction or cerebrovascular accident.

–Gastrointestinal tract: Mainly constipation, rarely nausea. Gingival hyperplasia following long-term treatment is extremely rare and reversible after discontinuation of therapy.

–Skin, vessels: Rarely, ankle oedema and flushing. There have been very rare reports of gynaecomastia in elderly patients, especially after long-term therapy. Hyperprolactinaemia and galactorrhoea, as well as Stevens-Johnson syndrome and erythromelalgia have been described. Allergic skin reactions (erythema, pruritus) have been reported in isolated instances.

–Nervous system: Rarely headache, nervousness, dizziness, fatigue, paraesthesia.

–Musculoskeletal system: There have been isolated reports of myalgia or arthralgia.

–Drugs/laboratory parameters: There have been isolated reports of transaminase and/or alkaline phosphatase elevation during verapamil therapy, probably as a consequence of allergic hepatitis.

Overdose: There have as yet been no reports of overdosage with the combination product.

The highest dose used in clinical trials was 16 mg of trandolapril. This dose produced no signs or symptoms of intolerance.

The most important symptom to be expected after a significant overdose of trandolapril is hypotension. Administration of normal saline solution is recommended in this case.

The most important signs and symptoms of a verapamil overdose are due to the pharmacological activity of the drug on the cardiovascular system and include hypotension arising from peripheral vasodilation and a negative inotropic effect, depression of impulse generation in the sinus node and cardiac impulse conduction disturbances that may result in sinus bradycardia, sinus arrest, AV block, and asystole.

Following oral verapamil overdosage, the patient must be monitored and treated in an intensive care setting. Overdose management must be aimed at preventing the further absorption of verapamil from the gastrointestinal tract, providing symptomatic treatment of the toxic effects (see above), and compensating for the calcium-antagonistic effects of this drug. Further absorption of verapamil from the gastrointestinal tract can be prevented by gastric lavage, administration of adsorbent material (activated charcoal) and a cathartic (sodium sulphate). Apart from general supportive measure in response to severe hypotension (to the point of shock), i.e., maintenance of an adequate circulating blood volume by administering plasma or a plasma expander, it may be necessary to stimulate the heart muscle with positive inotropic drugs such as dopamine, dobutamine or isoprenaline.

Atropine (or methylatropine) may be useful in the management of sinus bradycardia.

AV block should be treated with sympathomimetic drugs (isoprenaline or orciprenaline) or a pacemaker. Asystole should be handled by the usual measures including cardiopulmonary resuscitation, cardiac pacing, etc. The calcium-antagonistic effect can be offset by parenteral administration of calcium, for instance as calcium gluconate.

Pharmacological properties

Pharmacodynamic properties:

Verapamil: The pharmacological action of verapamil is due to inhibition of the influx of calcium ions through the slow channels of the cell membrane of vascular smooth muscle cells and of the conductile and contractile cells in the heart.

The mechanism of action of verapamil produces the following effects:

1. Arterial vasodilation. Verapamil reduces arterial pressure both at rest and at a given level of exercise by dilating peripheral arterioles.This reduction in total peripheral resistance (afterload) reduces myocardial oxygen requirements and energy consumption

2. Reduction of myocardial contractility. The negative inotropic activity of verapamil can be compensated by the reduction in total peripheral resistance. The cardiac index will not be decreased except in patients with pre-existing left ventricular dysfunction. Verapamil does not interfere with sympathetic regulation of the heart because it does not block the beta-adrenergic receptors. Asthma and similar conditions, therefore, are not contra-indications to verapamil.

Trandolapril: Trandolapril suppresses the plasma renin-angiotensin-aldosterone system. Renin is an endogenous enzyme synthesised by the kidneys and released into the circulation where it converts angiotensinogen to angiotensin I, a relatively inactive decapeptide.

Angiotensin I is then converted by angiotensin converting enzyme (ACE), a peptidyldipeptidase, to angiotensin II. Angiotensin II is a potent vasoconstrictor responsible for arterial vasoconstriction and increased blood pressure, as well as for stimulation of the adrenal gland to secrete aldosterone. Inhibition of ACE results in decreased plasma angiotensin II, which leads to decreased vasopressor activity and to reduced aldosterone secretion. Although the latter decrease is small, small increases in serum potassium concentrations may occur, along with sodium and fluid loss. The cessation of the negative feedback of angiotensin II on the renin secretion results in an increase of the plasma renin activity.

Another function of the converting enzyme is to degrade the potent vasodepressive kinin peptide, bradykinin, to inactive metabolites. Therefore inhibition of ACE results in an increased activity of circulating and local kallikrein-kinin system which contributes to peripheral vasodilation by activating the prostaglandin system. It is possible that this mechanism is involved in the hypotensive effects of ACE inhibitors and is responsible for certain side effects. In patients with hypertension, administration of ACE inhibitors results in a reduction of supine and standing blood pressure to about the same extent with no compensatory increase in heart rate. Peripheral arterial resistance is reduced with either no change or an increase in cardiac output.

There is an increase in renal blood flow and glomerular filtration rate is usually unchanged. Achievement of optimal blood pressure reduction may require several weeks of therapy in some patients. The antihypertensive effects are maintained during long-term therapy. Abrupt withdrawal of therapy has not been associated with a rapid increase in blood pressure.

The antihypertensive effect of trandolapril sets in one hour post-dose and lasts for at least 24 hours, but trandolapril does not interfere with the circadian blood pressure pattern.

Tarka: Neither animal studies nor healthy volunteer studies could demonstrate pharmacokinetic or renin-angiotensin system interactions between verapamil and trandolapril. The observed synergistic activity of these two drugs must therefore be due to their complementary pharmacodynamic actions.

In clinical trials, Tarka was more effective in reducing high blood pressure than either drug alone. In long-term trials, safety and tolerability of Tarka were adequate.

Pharmacokinetic properties:

Verapamil: Absorption: About 90% of orally-administered verapamil is absorbed. The mean bioavailability is as low as 22% because of extensive hepatic first-pass extraction, and shows great variation (10–35%). The mean bioavailability following repeated administration may increase to 30%.

The presence of food has no effect on the bioavailability of verapamil.

Distribution and biotransformation:

The mean time to peak plasma concentration is 4 hours. The peak plasma concentration of norverapamil is attained about 6 hours post-dose.

Steady state after multiple once-daily dosing is reached after 3–4 days.

Plasma protein binding of verapamil is about 90%.

Elimination:

The mean elimination half-life after repeated administration is 8 hours. 3–4% of a dose is excreted renally as unchanged drug. Metabolite excretion is in the urine (70%) and in the faeces (16%). Norverapamil is one of twelve metabolites identified in urine, has 10–20% of the pharmacologic activity of verapamil, and accounts for 6% of excreted drug. The steady-state plasma concentrations of norverapamil and verapamil are similar. Verapamil kinetics are not altered by renal impairment.

The bioavailability and elimination half-life of verapamil are increased in patients with liver cirrhosis. Verapamil kinetics are, however, unchanged in patients with compensated hepatic dysfunction. Kidney function has no effect on verapamil elimination.

Trandolapril: Absorption: Orally-administered trandolapril is absorbed rapidly. Bioavailability is 40–60% and independent of the presence of food.

The time to peak plasma concentration is about 30 minutes.

Distribution and biotransformation: Trandolapril disappears very rapidly from plasma, and its half-life is less than one hour.

Trandolapril is hydrolysed in plasma to form trandolaprilat, a specific ACE inhibitor. The amount of trandolaprilat formed is independent of food intake.

The time to peak plasma concentration of trandolaprilat is 4–6 hours.

Plasma protein binding of trandolaprilat is greater than 80%. Trandolaprilat binds with great affinity to ACE, and this is a saturable process. Most of circulating trandolaprilat binds to albumin in a nonsaturable process. Steady state after multiple once-daily dosing is reached after about 4 days in healthy volunteers as well as in younger and elderly hypertensive patients.

The effective half-life is between 16–24 hours. The terminal half-life of elimination is between 47 and 98 hours depending on dose. This terminal phase probably represents binding/dissociation kinetics of the trandolaprilat/ACE complex.

Elimination: 10–15% of an administered trandolapril dose is excreted as unchanged trandolaprilat in urine. Following oral administration of radioactive-labelled trandolapril, 33% of radioactivity is recovered in urine and 66% in faeces.

The renal clearance of trandolaprilat shows a linear correlation with creatinine clearance. The trandolaprilat plasma concentration is significantly higher in patients whose creatinine clearance is < 30 ml/min. Following repeated administration to patients with chronic renal dysfunction, steady state is, however, also reached after four days, independently of the extent of renal impairment.

The trandolapril plasma concentration may be 10 times higher in patients with liver cirrhosis than in healthy volunteers. The plasma concentration and renal extraction of trandolaprilat are also increased in cirrhotic patients, albeit to a lesser extent.

Trandolapril(at) kinetics are unchanged in patients with compensated hepatic dysfunction.

Tarka: As there are no known kinetic interactions between verapamil and trandolapril or trandolaprilat, the single-agent kinetic parameters of these two drugs apply to the combination product as well.

Preclinical safety data: General toxicity effects were observed in animals only at exposures that were sufficiently in excess of the maximum human exposure to make any concern for human safety negligible. Genotoxicity assays revealed no special hazard for humans.

Animal studies have shown that ACE inhibitors tend to have an adverse effect on late foetal development, resulting in foetal death and congenital abnormalities of the skull in particular. These cranial abnormalities are thought to be due to the pharmacological activity of these drugs and be related to ACE inhibitor-induced oligohydramnios.

Pharmaceutical particulars

List of excipients: Tarka also contains maize starch, povidone, sodium stearyl fumarate, lactose, microcrystalline cellulose, sodium alginate, magnesium stearate, methylhydroxypropylcellulose, polyethylene glycol 400 and 6000, docusate sodium, sodium lauryl sulphate, talc, colloidal anhydrous silica, titanium dioxide (E171), iron oxide (E172), and gelatin.

Incompatibilities: There are as yet no known incompatibilities with Tarka.

Shelf life: Tarka is stable for 3 years. The expiry date is shown on the package.

The strips show 'Exp.' followed by several numbers. 'Exp.' means 'Do not use after', and the numbers indicate the month and year.

Special precautions for storage: The capsules should be stored at 10–25°C (room temperature).

Nature and contents of container: Box of 28 capsules in blister strips.

The capsules are pink.

The blister strips consist of PVC/PVDC-aluminium.

Instructions for use/handling: The capsules are taken with some water before, during or after meals once daily and should be swallowed whole.

Marketing authorisation number 00169/0106

Date of approval/revision of SPC May 1997

Legal category POM

**Trade Mark*

Kyowa Hakko UK Ltd
258 Bath Road
Slough
Berkshire SL1 4DX

☎ 01753 566020 🗋 01753 566030

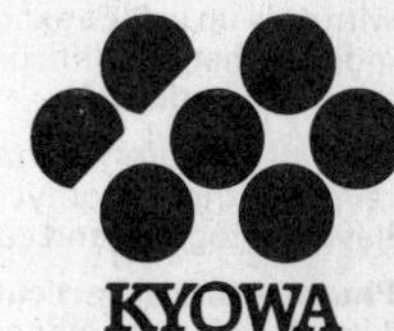

BLEO-KYOWA*

Qualitative and quantitative composition Bleomycin Sulphate equivalent to 15,000 IU (15×10³ IU).

Pharmaceutical form Freeze dried powder in a glass ampoule for reconstitution and administration by infusion, injection or instillation.

Clinical particulars
Therapeutical indications:

a. Squamous cell carcinoma affecting the mouth, nasopharynx and paranasal sinuses, larynx, oesophagus, external genitalia, cervix or skin. Well differentiated tumours usually respond better than anaplastic ones.
b. Hodgkin's disease and other malignant lymphomas, including mycosis fungoides.
c. Testicular teratoma.
d. Malignant effusions of serous cavities.
e. Secondary indications in which bleomycin has been shown to be of some value (alone or in combination with other drugs) include metastatic malignant melanoma, carcinoma of the thyroid, lung and bladder.

Posology and method of administration
Adults: Routes of administration: Bleomycin is usually administered intramuscularly but may be given intravenously (bolus or drip), intra-arterially, intrapleurally or intraperitoneally as a solution in physiological saline. Local injection directly into the tumour may occasionally be indicated.

Recommended dose and dosage schedules
1. *Squamous cell carcinoma and testicular teratoma:* Used alone the normal dosage is 15×10³ IU (1 ampoule) three times a week or 30×10³ IU (2 ampoules) twice a week, either intramuscularly or intravenously. Treatment may continue on consecutive weeks, or more usually at intervals of 3–4 weeks, up to a total cumulative dose of 500×10³ IU although young men with testicular tumours have frequently tolerated twice this amount. Continuous intravenous infusion at a rate of 15×10³ IU (1 ampoule) per 24 hours for up to 10 days, or 30×10³ IU (2 ampoules) per 24 hours for up to 5 days may produce a therapeutic effect more rapidly. The development of stomatitis is the most useful guide to the determination of individual tolerance of maximum therapeutic response. The dose may need to be adjusted when bleomycin is used in combination chemotherapy. Use in elderly or children – see below.

2. *Malignant lymphomas:* Used alone the recommended dosage regimen is 15×10³ IU (1 ampoule) once or twice a week, intramuscularly, to a total dose of 225×10³ IU (15 ampoules). Dosage should be reduced in the elderly. The dose may need to be adjusted when bleomycin is used in combination chemotherapy. Use in elderly or children – see below.

3. *Malignant effusions:* After drainage of the affected serous cavity 60×10³ IU (4 ampoules) bleomycin dissolved in 100 ml physiological saline is introduced via the drainage needle or cannula. After instillation, the drainage needle or cannula may be withdrawn. Administration may be repeated if necessary subject to a total cumulative dose of 500×10³ IU (about 33 ampoules). Use in the elderly or children – see below.

Combination therapy: Bleomycin is commonly used in conjunction with radiotherapy, particularly in treatment of cancer of the head and neck region. Such a combination may enhance mucosal reactions if full doses of both forms of treatment are used and bleomycin dosage may require reduction, e.g. to 5×10³ IU at the time of each radiotherapy fraction five days a week. Bleomycin is frequently used as one of the drugs multiple chemotherapy regimens (e.g. squamous cell carcinoma, testicular teratoma, lymphoma). The mucosal toxicity of bleomycin should be borne in mind in the selection and dosage of drugs with similar toxic potential use in such combinations.

Elderly patients: The total dose of bleomycin used in the treatment of squamous cell carcinoma, testicular teratoma or malignant effusions should be reduced as indicated.

Age in years	*Total dose (IU)*	*Dose per week (IU)*
80 and over	100×10³	16×10³
70–79	150–200×10³	30×10³
60–69	200–300×10³	30–60×10³
Under 60	500×10³	30–60×10³

Children: Until further data are available, administration of bleomycin to children should take place only under exceptional circumstances and in special centres. The dosage should be based on that recommended for adults and adjusted to body surface area or body weight.

Reduced kidney function: With serum creatinine values of 2–4 mg%†, it is recommended to half the above dosages. With serum creatinine above 4 mg%, a further reduction in dose is indicated.

† Under reduced kidney function on the SPC the serum creatinine values of 2–4 mg% converts to the more standard measurement of 177–354 mmol (micro mols per litre).

Preparation of solution: For intramuscular injections the required dose is dissolved in up to 5 ml of suitable solvents such as physiological saline. If pain occurs at the site of injection a 1% solution of lignocaine may be used as a solvent.

For intravenous injections the dose required is dissolved in 5–200 ml of physiological saline and injected slowly or added to the reservoir of a running intravenous infusion. For intra-arterial administration a slow infusion in physiological saline is used. For intra-cavity injection 60×10³ IU is dissolved in 100 ml of normal saline.

For local injections bleomycin is dissolved in physiological saline to make a 1–3×10³ IU/ml solution.

Contra-indications: Bleomycin is contra-indicated in patients with acute pulmonary infection or greatly reduced lung function.

Special warnings and precautions for use: Patients undergoing treatment with bleomycin should have chest X-rays weekly. These should continue to be taken for up to 4 weeks after completion of the course. If breathlessness or infiltrates appear, not obviously attributable to tumour or to co-existent lung disease administration of the drug must be stopped immediately and patients should be treated with a corticosteroid and a broad spectrum antibiotic.

Interactions with other medicaments and other forms of interaction: When bleomycin is used as one of the drugs in multiple chemotherapy regimens the toxicity of bleomycin should be borne in mind in the selection and dosage of drugs with similar toxic potential. The addition of other cytotoxic drugs can necessitate changes and dose alterations.

Previous or concurrent radiotherapy to the chest is an important factor in increasing the incidence and severity of lung toxicity.

Because of bleomycin's sensitisation of lung tissue, patients who have received bleomycin pre-operatively are at greater risk of developing pulmonary toxicity when oxygen is administered at surgery and a reduction in inspired oxygen concentration during operation and post-operatively is recommended.

In patients treated for testicular cancer with a combination of bleomycin and vinca alkaloids a syndrome had been reported correspondingly to morbus Raynaud, ischaemia which can lead to necrosis of peripheral parts of the body (fingers, toes, nose tip).

No specific clinical incompatibilities with other drugs or food have been encountered.

Pregnancy and lactation: Bleomycin should not normally be administered to patients who are pregnant or to mothers who are breast-feeding.

Animal experiences have revealed that bleomycin, like most cytotoxics, may have teratogenic and carcinogenic potential.

Effects on ability to drive and use machines: This depends on the patient's condition and should be considered in co-operation with the doctor.

Undesirable effects: Like most cytotoxic agents bleomycin can give rise both to immediate and to delayed toxic effects. The most immediate effect is fever on the day of injection. Anorexia, tiredness or nausea also may occur. Pain at the injection site, or in the region of the tumour, has occasionally been reported, and other rare adverse effects are hypotension and local thrombophlebitis after intravenous administration.

The majority of patients who receive a full course of bleomycin develop lesions of the skin or oral mucosa. Induration, hyperkeratotis, reddening, tenderness and swelling of the tips of the fingers, ridging of the nails, bulla formation over pressure points such as elbows, loss of hair and stomatitis are rarely serious and usually disappear soon after completion of the course.

The most serious delayed effect is interstitial pneumonia, which may develop during, or occasionally after, a course of treatment. This condition may sometimes develop into fatal pulmonary fibrosis, although such an occurrence is rare at recommended doses. Previous or concurrent radiotherapy to the chest is an important factor in increasing the incidence and severity of lung toxicity.

A few cases of acute fulminant reactions with hyperpyrexia and cardiorespiratory collapse have been observed after intravenous injections of doses higher than those recommended. Hypotension, hyperpyrexia and drug-related deaths have been reported rarely following intra-cavitary instillation of bleomycin.

Overdose: The acute reaction to an overdosage of bleomycin would probably include hypotension, fever, rapid pulse and general symptoms of shock. Treatment is purely symptomatic. In the event of respiratory complications the patient should be treated with a corticosteroid and a broad-spectrum antibiotic. There is no general antidote to bleomycin.

Pharmacological properties
Pharmacodynamic properties: Bleomycin is a basic soluble glycopeptide with cytotoxic activity. The mechanism of action of bleomycin is believed to involve single-strand scission of DNA, leading to inhibition of cell division, of growth and of DNA synthesis in tumour cells.

Apart from its antibacterial and antitumour properties, bleomycin is relatively free from biological activity. When injected intravenously it may have a histamine-like effect on blood pressure and may cause a rise in body temperature.

Pharmacokinetic properties: Bleomycin is administered parenterally. After intravenous (IV) administration of a bolus dose of 15×10³ IU/m² body surface, peak concentrations of 1 to 10 IU are achieved in plasma. Following the intramuscular (IM) injection of 15×10³ IU peak plasma concentrations of about 1 IU/ml have been reported. The peak plasma concentration is reached 30 minutes after an IM injection. Continuous infusion of bleomycin 30×10³ IU daily, for 4 to 5 days, resulted in an average steady state plasma concentration of 100–300 milli IU/ml. After IV injections of bleomycin in a dose of 15×10³ IU/m² body surface, the area under the serum concentration curve is, on an averafe, 300 milli IU×min×ml⁻¹.

Bleomycin is only bound to plasma proteins to a slight extent. Bleomycin is rapidly distributed in body tissues, with the highest concentrations in skin, lungs, peritoneum and lymph. Low concentrations are seen in the bone marrow. Bleomycin could not be detected in cerebrospinal fluid after intravenous injection. Bleomycin appears to cross the placental barrier.

The mechanism for bio-transformation is not yet fully known. Inactivation takes place during enzymatic breakdown by bleomycin hydrolase, primarily in plasma, liver and other organs and, to a much lesser degree, in skin and lungs. When bleomycin was administered as an IV bolus injection in a dose of 15×10³ IU/m² body surface, initial and terminal half-lives were 0.5 and 4 hours respectively. Given as a continuous intravenous infusion in a dose of 30×10³ IU daily for 4 to 5 days bleomycin disappears from plasma with initial and terminal half-lives of about 1.3 hours and 9 hours, respectively. About two thirds of the administered drug is excreted unchanged in the urine, probably by glomerular filtration. Approximately 50% is recovered in the urine in the 24 hours following an IV or IM injection. The rate of excretion, therefore, is highly influences by renal function;

concentration in plasma are greatly elevated if usual doses are given to patients with renal impairment with only up to 20% excreted in 24 hours. Observations indicate that it is difficult to eliminate bleomycin from the body by dialysis.

Preclinical safety data: Animal experiences have revealed that bleomycin, like most cytotoxics, may have teratogenic and carcinogenic potential.

Pharmaceutical particulars
List of excipients: None.

Incompatibilities: Bleomycin solution should not be mixed with solutions of essential amino acids, riboflavine, ascorbic acid, dexamethasone, aminophylline or frusemide.

Shelf life: Three years.

Special precautions for storage: Protect from light.

Nature and contents of container: 5 ml colourless glass ampoule of the snap-ring type containing freeze dried bleomycin sulphate equivalent to 15,000 IU. Ten ampoules per carton.

Instructions for use/handling: Bleomycin should be handled with care. Precautions should be taken to avoid bleomycin coming into contact with skin, mucous membranes or eyes, but in the event of contamination the affected part should be washed with water.

Marketing authorisation number PL 12196/0005

Date of first authorisation/renewal of authorisation 14 April 1998

Date of (partial) revision of the text October 1998

MITOMYCIN-C KYOWA*

Presentation Purple crystalline powder for intravenous injection containing Mitomycin-C Kyowa 2 mg potency with 48 mg sodium chloride, 10 mg potency with 240 mg sodium chloride, 20 mg potency with 480 mg sodium chloride for reconstitution with water for injections using the volume recommended for each strength.

Uses Mitomycin-C Kyowa is an antitumour antibiotic that is activated in the tissues to an alkylating agent which disrupts deoxyribonucleic acid (DNA) in cancer cells by forming a complex with DNA and also acts by inhibiting division of cancer cells by interfering with the biosynthesis of DNA. *In vivo,* Mitomycin-C Kyowa is rapidly cleared from the serum after intravenous administration. The time required to reduce the serum concentration by 50 per cent after a 30 mg bolus injection is 17 minutes. After injection of 30 mg, 20 mg, or 10 mg intravenously, the maximal serum concentrations were 2.4 micrograms/ml, 1.7 micrograms/ml and 0.52 micrograms/ml respectively. Clearance is effected primarily by metabolism in the liver but metabolism occurs in other tissues as well. The rate of clearance is inversely proportional to the maximal serum concentration because, it is thought, of saturation of the degradative pathways. Approximately 10 per cent of a dose of Mitomycin-C Kyowa is excreted unchanged in the urine. Since metabolic pathways are saturated at relatively low doses, the percentage dose excreted in the urine increases with increasing dose. In children, excretion of intravenously administered Mitomycin-C Kyowa is similar to that in adults.

Clinical indications: Antimitotic and Cytotoxic.

Mitomycin-C Kyowa is recommended for certain types of cancer in combination with other drugs or after primary therapy has failed. It has been successfully used to improve subjective and objective symptoms in a wide range of neoplastic conditions.

As a single agent in the treatment of superficial bladder cancer. In addition it has been shown that post-operative instillations of Mitomycin-C Kyowa can reduce recurrence rates in newly diagnosed patients with superficial bladder cancer.

As a single agent and in combination with other drugs in metastatic breast cancer.

In combination with other agents in advanced squamous cell carcinoma of the uterine cervix.

It shows a degree of activity as part of combination therapy in carcinoma of the stomach, pancreas and lung (particularly non-small cell).

It shows a degree of activity as a single agent and in combination in liver cancer when given by the intra-arterial route.

It has a possible role in combination with other cytotoxic drugs in colorectal cancer.

It shows a degree of activity as a single agent or part of combination therapy in cancer of the head and neck.

It shows a degree of activity as a single agent in cancer of the prostate.

It has a possible role in skin cancer.

It has a degree of activity in leukaemia and non-solid tumours.

It has a possible role in sarcomas.

It has been successfully used in combination with surgery, pre-operatively (oesophageal, squamous cell carcinoma) and post-operatively (gastric cancer).

It has been shown to be effective when used in combination with radiotherapy.

Dosage and administration Intravenously, the dose should be given with great care in order to avoid extravasation.

The usual dose is in the range of 4 to 10 mg potency (0.06 to 0.15 mg/kg) given at 1 to 6 weekly intervals depending on whether other drugs are given in combination and on bone marrow recovery.

In a number of combination schedules, the dose is 10 mg potency/m^2 of body surface area, the course being repeated at intervals for as long as required. A course ranging from 40 to 80 mg potency (0.58 to 1.2 mg/kg) is often required for a satisfactory response when used alone or in combination.

A higher dosage course may be given when used alone or as part of a particular combination schedule and total cumulative doses exceeding 2 mg/kg have been given.

For administration into specific tissues, Mitomycin-C Kyowa can be given by the intra-arterial route directly into the tumours.

Because of cumulative myelosuppression, patients should be fully re-evaluated after each course and the dose reduced if the patient has experienced any toxic effects. Individual doses greater than 0.06 mg/kg have not been shown to be more effective and are more toxic than lower doses.

Treatment of superficial urinary bladder tumours: In the treatment of superficial bladder tumours, the usual dose is 20 to 40 mg potency dissolved in 20 to 40 ml of Water for Injections, instilled into the bladder through a urethral catheter, weekly or three times a week for a total of 20 doses.

In the prevention of recurrent superficial bladder tumours, various doses have been used. These include 20 mg in 20 ml of Water for Injections every two weeks and 40 mg in 40 ml of Water for Injections monthly or three monthly. The dose is instilled into the bladder through a urethral catheter.

In both cases the dose should be adjusted in accordance with the age and condition of the patient.

Contra-indications, warnings, etc
Contra-indications: Mitomycin-C Kyowa is contraindicated in patients who have demonstrated a hypersensitive or idiosyncratic reaction to it in the past.

Precautions: Mitomycin-C Kyowa should be administered under the supervision of a physician experienced in cytotoxic cancer chemotherapy. Patients should be monitored closely during each course of treatment, paying particular attention to peripheral blood count including platelet count.

No repeat dosage should be given until leucocyte count has returned to 3.0×10^9 per litre and platelet count to 90.0×10^9 per litre. If disease progression continues after two courses of treatment, the drug should be stopped since the chances of response are then minimal.

The person administering the injection of Mitomycin-C Kyowa should not allow the solution to come into contact with his or her skin.

Side and adverse effects: The principal toxicity of Mitomycin-C Kyowa is bone marrow suppression, particularly thrombocytopenia and leucopenia. The nadir is usually around four weeks after treatment and toxicity is cumulative, with increasing risk after each course of treatment.

Severe renal toxicity has occasionally been reported after treatment and renal function should be monitored before starting treatment and again after each course. Nausea and vomiting are sometimes experienced immediately after treatment but these are usually mild and of short duration. Local ulceration and cellulitis may be caused by tissue extravasation during intravenous injection and utmost care should be taken in administration. In the event of extravasation following an intravenous injection of Mitomycin-C Kyowa it is recommended that 5 ml of sodium bicarbonate 8.4% solution is immediately infiltrated into the area where extravasation has occurred, followed by an injection of 4 mg dexamethasone. In addition a systemic injection of 200 mg vitamin B6 may be of some value in promoting the regrowth of tissues that have been damaged.

Use in pregnancy and lactation: Mitomycin-C Kyowa should not normally be administered to patients who are pregnant or to mothers who are breast feeding. Teratological changes have been noted in animal studies. The effect of Mitomycin-C Kyowa on fertility is unknown.

Treatment of skin or eye contact: Any Mitomycin-C Kyowa substance or solution in contact with the skin should be washed several times with 8.4% sodium bicarbonate solution, followed by washing with soap and water. Use of handcreams or other emollient preparations is inappropriate as this may assist the penetration of any traces of Mitomycin-C Kyowa into the epidermal tissue.

Contact with the eye. The eye should be rinsed several times with sodium bicarbonate eye lotion and the eye examined for several days after contact for evidence of corneal damage. If this occurs, appropriate treatment should be instituted.

Pharmaceutical precautions The contents of the vial should be reconstituted with water for injections or 20% dextrose solution, 5 ml for the 2 mg vial, at least 10 ml for the 10 ml vial and at least 20 ml for the 20 mg vial.

Unreconstituted Mitomycin-C Kyowa remains stable for four years after manufacture when stored at room temperature. Reconstitution, as directed, should be accomplished using aseptic technique and the resulting solutions are best used immediately. If reconstituted Mitomycin-C Kyowa must be stored prior to use, it should be protected from light and kept in a cool place – it should not be refrigerated. Solutions stored in this way should be discarded if unused after 24 hours.

When reconstituted solution is added to infusion fluids, especially where these contain dextrose, the resulting solution should be used immediately.

Legal category POM.

Package quantities 2 mg, 10 mg and 20 mg vials for intravenous injection, in packs of ten, one and one respectively.

Further information Mitomycin-C Kyowa vials are available through hospital pharmacies and can be supplied to retail pharmacists for dispensing against prescriptions for patients whose treatment has been initiated in hospital practice.

Product licence numbers

2 mg	12196/0001
10 mg	12196/0002
20 mg	12196/0003.

*Trade Mark

Laboratories for Applied Biology Limited

91 Amhurst Park
London N16 5DR

☎ 0181 800 2252 🗋 0181 809 6884

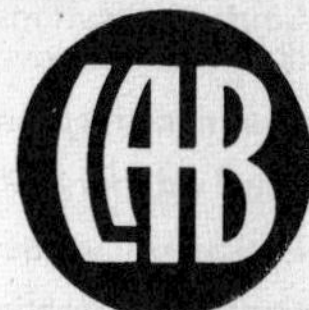

CERUMOL* EAR DROPS

Presentation A clear oily preparation containing:

Arachis (Peanut) oil BP	57.3% w/v
Chlorobutanol BP	5.0% w/v
p-Dichlorobenzene	2.0% w/v

Excipients: The product also contains o-Dichlorobenzene, Oil of Turpentine, and 3-Methoxybutyl acetate (Butoxyl).

Uses Occlusion or partial occlusion of external auditory meatus by either a collection of soft wax or a harder wax plug.

Dosage and administration *At home:* With the head inclined, 5 drops are put into the ear. This may cause a harmless tingling sensation. A plug of cotton wool moistened with Cerumol should then be applied to retain the liquid. One hour later, or the next morning, the plug is removed. The procedure is repeated twice a day for three days; the loosened wax may then come out on its own making syringing unnecessary. If any wax remains the doctor should be consulted so that syringing of the softened residue may be carried out.

At the surgery: If there has been no prior treatment with Cerumol, 5 drops are instilled as described above and left for at least 20 minutes. Then syringing or a probe tipped with cotton wool may be employed.

Contra-indications, warnings, etc Otitis externa, seborrhoeic dermatitis, eczema affecting the external ear and perforated ear drum. Arachis Oil BP is a refined oil free of protein and is extremely unlikely to cause a reaction in subjects with peanut allergy. Such individuals did not react to Arachis Oil BP given by mouth in a randomised double-blind trial. There have not been any reports of reactions to Cerumol by subjects with peanut allergy; individuals with this allergy might nevertheless not wish to use Cerumol.

Use in pregnancy: No side-effects have been reported.

Other special warnings: Not to be taken internally. Do not use for more than three days. If the condition persists consult your doctor.

Overdosage: As the product is applied topically, overdosage as such is not possible. In the case of accidental ingestion, the amounts of the majority of ingredients in the 11 ml bottle are too small to give rise to toxic effects. The 550 mg of chlorbutol in the whole bottle might cause excessive sedation in a child.

Pharmaceutical precautions No special storage precautions.

Legal category P

Package quantities 11 ml vial with separate dropper.

Further information Nil.

Product licence number 0118/0013.

EMESIDE* CAPSULES AND SYRUP

Presentation Soft orange gelatin capsules each containing 250 mg of Ethosuximide BP.

Blackcurrant-flavoured syrup containing 250 mg of Ethosuximide BP per 5 ml.

Uses Emeside gives selective control of absence seizures (petit-mal) even when complicated by grandmal. It is also indicated for myoclonic seizures. The reduction of seizure frequency is thought to be achieved by depression of the motor cortex and elevation of the threshold to convulsive stimuli as seen by the suppression of the characteristic spike and wave EEG pattern. Emeside may be prescribed together with other anticonvulsants such as phenobarbitone, phenytoin, primidone or sodium valproate where grandmal or other forms of epilepsy may require additional treatment.

Dosage and administration *Adults and children over 6 years:* Start with a small dose – 500 mg daily with increments of 250 mg every five to seven days until control is achieved usually with 1,000–1,500 mg (4–6 capsules) daily. Occasionally 2,000 mg daily in divided dose may be necessary.

The half life of ethosuximide in the plasma is about 60 hours in adults but the daily dose if large is more comfortably divided between morning and evening.

If Emeside is being substituted for another antiepileptic drug the latter must not be withdrawn abruptly but the replacement made gradually with overlap of the preparations otherwise petit mal may break through; the slow withdrawal applies to Emeside when another drug is to replace it.

Children and infants under six years: Begin with a daily dose of 250 mg (5 ml syrup) and increase the dose gradually by small increments every few days until control is achieved, the maximum dose should be 1,000 mg.

Peak concentrations occur in plasma 1–7 hours after ingestion and the plasma half life is about 30 hours in children and 60 hours in adults. Plasma levels of ethosuximide to be effective lie between 40 and 85 microgram per ml but the clinical response should be the criterion for regulation of dosage. Because young children metabolise ethosuximide more rapidly than adults higher and more frequent doses may be necessary.

Contra-indications, warnings, etc Plasma concentrations are not accurately predictable and since compliance is variable, monitoring of plasma concentrations can be of value in unresponsive cases. Known hypersensitivity to succinimides. Exercise caution with regular appropriate tests in patients with hepatic or renal disease and monitor drug plasma concentrations. Porphyrias. Ethosuximide may be excreted into breast milk. Mothers receiving the drug should not breastfeed. There is a recognised small increase in the incidence of congenital malformations in children born to mothers receiving anti-convulsants. For women planning pregnancy or who are already pregnant the risk should be weighed carefully against the benefit of treatment.

As with all syrups it is advisable to brush the teeth or rinse the mouth after taking Emeside syrup.

Side Effects: Nausea, vomiting, anorexia and epigastric pain are common at first and generally subside. High dosage may cause sedation or confusion. Unusual symptoms are headache, fatigue, drowsiness, dizziness, ataxia, dyskinesia, hiccough, photophobia, depression and skin rash. Isolated reports have been made of erythema nodosum, erythema multiforme, agranulocytosis, aplastic anaemia. In some instances, patients who become leucopenic on other anticonvulsant therapy have been treated satisfactorily with ethosuximide. Lupus-like reactions have been reported in children given ethosuximide. They vary in severity from systemic immunological disorders, which include the nephrotic syndrome, to the asymptomatic presence of antinuclear antibodies.

Drug Interaction: The plasma concentrations of ethosuximide are reduced by carbamazepine and increased by isoniazid, phenytoin and sodium valproate.

Overdosage: Where more than 2 g has been thought to be ingested gastric lavage may be employed, if the time lapse is less than four hours.

Routine observation of respiration and circulation will indicate the need for supportive measures.

Pharmaceutical precautions Store in a cool dry place. Recommended diluent – unpreserved Syrup BP; use within 14 days.

Legal category POM.

Package quantities *Capsules:* 112.
Syrup (blackcurrant flavour): Bottles of 200 ml.

Further information As with all syrups it is advisable to brush the teeth or rinse the mouth after taking Emeside syrup.

Product licence numbers

Emeside Capsules	0118/5002
Emeside Syrup blackcurrant	0118/5004.

HALYCITROL* VITAMIN EMULSION

Presentation Orange flavoured emulsion containing 27,600 microgram (92,000 iu)/100 ml Vitamin A and 190 microgram (7,600 iu) Vitamin D per 100 ml. This is equivalent to 1,380 microgram (4,600 iu) of Vitamin A and 9.5 microgram (380 iu) of Vitamin D in a 5 ml daily dose.

Uses For prevention of vitamin A and D deficiency.

Dosage and administration *Adults and children above 6 months:* 5 ml daily.

Infants up to six months: 2.5 ml daily.

Pregnancy: Vitamin A supplements should only be taken during pregnancy when deficiency is demonstrated or anticipated, e.g. due to malabsorption or restricted diets.

Contra-indications, warnings, etc Prolonged excessive ingestion of vitamins A and D can lead to hypervitaminosis states.

Hypervitaminosis A: Symptoms include dry rough skin, painful joint swellings, anorexia and vomiting.

Hypervitaminosis D: Infants already receiving vitamin D from such sources as vitaminised margarine and cereals can develop infantile hypercalcaemia from excessive vitamin D intake.

In children and adults the symptoms of hypercalcaemia are weakness, anorexia, abdominal pain, constipation, thirst and polyuria with the development of nephrocalcinosis, renal stones and renal failure. Individuals with renal disease and Sarcoidosis are particularly susceptible.

Pharmaceutical precautions Store in a cool place.

Legal category GSL.

Package quantities Bottles of 114 ml.

Further information This is a preparation of fish oil devoid of any fish odour or taste.

Product licence number 0118/0015.

LABITON* TONIC

Presentation A brown liquid containing vitamin B_1 0.75 mg, dried extract of kola nuts 6.05 mg, alcohol 2.8 ml, caffeine (total) 7 mg per 10 ml.

Uses The kola nut contains complex catechine-caffeinates which give central stimulation, increase muscular performance and reduce fatiguability. Vitamin B_1 is included to make up deficiency resulting from recent illness or anorexia. Labiton is indicated for use as a tonic for fatigue, anorexia and debility in convalescence after infections such as influenza and after operations.

Dosage and administration 10–20 ml twice daily, before or after meals, with or without water.

Not intended for administration to children.

Contra-indications, warnings, etc Undesirable in cases of hepatitis and patients taking sedatives. Car drivers should be made aware of the presence of alcohol and should be advised not to exceed the recommended dosage, especially if taking tranquillisers or remedies for allergies that have sedative side effects.

Drug interactions: Alcohol can cause flushing or a disulfiram-like reaction with metronidazole and chlorpropamide; this is dose-related in susceptible individuals. Interaction with Labiton has not been reported with any drug and is unlikely with correct dosage. With excessive dosage there could be potentiation of CNS depressants and potentiation of the hypoglycaemic effect of insulin.

Overdosage: Treatment is that for alcohol with correction of dehydration, attendance to the airway and other supportive measures for coma.

Pharmaceutical precautions Store in a cool place. Use within nine months of opening.

Legal category GSL.

Package quantities Supplied in bottles of 200 ml and 1 litre.

Further information Nil.

Product licence number 0118/5005.

LABOSEPT* PASTILLES

Presentation Hexagonal red pastilles each containing Dequalinium Chloride BP 0.25 mg in a slow dissolving gelatine base.

Uses For bacterial and fungal infections of the mouth and throat.

Dosage and administration *Adults and children:* To be sucked slowly every three or four hours. For maximum benefit pastilles should be lodged comfortably between gum and cheek rather than be chewed. The daily dose should not exceed eight pastilles.

Contra-indications, warnings, etc Side effects and ill-effects from overdosage have not been reported.

Pharmaceutical precautions No special precautions.

Legal category P.

Package quantities Carton containing 20 pastilles.

Further information Contains no sugar.

Product licence number 0118/0012.

MONPHYTOL*

Presentation A colourless, rapidly drying, non-greasy paint containing chlorbutol 3%, methyl undecylenate 5%, propyl undecylenate 0.7%, salicylic acid 3%, methyl salicylate 25%, and propyl salicylate 5%.

Uses Monphytol is indicated for tinea pedis, tinea unguium, tinea circinata, erosio interdigitalis, intertrigo.

Dosage and administration *Adults over 12:* Twice daily moisten brush with Monphytol and apply to the affected parts, reaching gently into the folds of the skin. Treatment should be repeated from time to time after the condition has subsided to prevent reinfection.

Children under 12, pregnant and lactating women: The safety of this product has not been demonstrated for these groups. Its use must be at the physician's discretion.

Contra-indications, warnings, etc Monphytol may sting sensitive weeping areas of acutely inflamed skin. Other treatment (to reduce inflammation and exudation) may first be necessary. Monphytol should not be used on bleeding areas.

Pharmaceutical precautions During use avoid contact of liquid with plastics. Store away from heat.

Legal category P.

Package quantities Bottles containing 18 ml.

Further information Nil.

Product licence number 0118/5010R.

**Trade Mark*

Lagap Pharmaceuticals Ltd
Woolmer Way
Bordon
Hants GU35 9QE

☎ 01420 478301 🗋 01420 474427

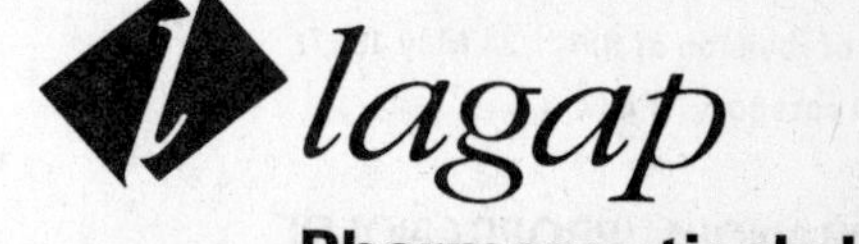

BACLOFEN TABLETS BP 10 mg

Qualitative and quantitative composition Each tablet contains Baclofen BP 10 mg.

Pharmaceutical form Tablets.

Clinical particulars

Therapeutic indications: Baclofen is indicated for the relief of spasticity of voluntary muscle resulting from such disorders as: multiple sclerosis, other spinal lesions e.g.: tumours of the spinal cord, syringomyelia, motor neurone disease, transverse myelitis, traumatic partial section of the cord.

Baclofen is also indicated in adults and children for the relief of spasticity of voluntary muscle arising from e.g.: cerebrovascular accidents, cerebral palsy, meningitis, traumatic head injury.

Patient selection is most important when initiating baclofen therapy; it is likely to be of most benefit in patients whose spasticity constitutes a handicap to activities and/or physiotherapy. Treatment should not be commenced until the spastic state has been stabilised.

Posology and method of administration: Oral administration.

The possible extent of clinical improvement to the patient should be assessed prior to the initiation of baclofen therapy. Titrated doses should be carefully administered in gradually increasing quantities until the patient's condition is stable (this is particularly important in elderly patients). If the dosage is too high or has been increased too quickly, side effects may ensue, especially in patients who are mobile to minimise muscle weakness in unaffected limbs or where some degree of spasticity is required.

Adults: The following slowly increasing dosage regimen is suggested, but may be adjusted to suit the patient.

5 mg 3 times a day for 3 days.
10 mg 3 times a day for 3 days.
15 mg 3 times a day for 3 days.
20 mg 3 times a day for 3 days.

Doses up to 60 mg a day usually provide satisfactory control of symptoms, though careful adjustment according to the requirements of each patient is frequently necessary. Small, more frequent doses of baclofen may prove better in some cases than larger, less frequent doses. If required, the dose may be increased slowly. A maximum daily dose of more than 100 mg is not recommended, unless the patient is hospitalised and under close supervision. Once this maximum recommended dose is reached, if the therapeutic effects are not evident in 6 weeks, it may not be of benefit for the patient to continue on baclofen therapy.

Some patients may benefit from the use of baclofen just at night to oppose painful flexor spasm. Also, a single dose about an hour before carrying out tasks like dressing, washing, shaving and physiotherapy will often augment a patient's motility.

Elderly: The elderly may be more susceptible to side effects, especially when first introducing baclofen. Initially, small doses are advised, with gradual adjustment under careful supervision. The eventual average maximum dose is as for adults, but caution should be exercised especially in patients with impaired renal function (see below).

Children: Dosages in the range of 0.75 to 2 mg/kg body weight should be used. In children over 10 years of age, a maximum daily dosage of 2.5 mg/kg body weight may be given. Treatment usually commences with 2.5 mg 4 times a day. Dosage should be cautiously raised at approximately 3 day intervals until the child's individual requirements are met.

Maintenance therapy:

Children aged 12 months to 2 years:	10 to 20 mg
Children aged 2 to 6 years:	20 to 30 mg
Children aged 6 to 10 years:	30 to 60 mg.

Patients with impaired renal function: A low dosage of baclofen should be given, i.e. approximately 5 mg a day, in patients with impaired renal function or who are undergoing chronic haemodialysis.

Patients with spastic states of cerebral origin: A very cautious dosage schedule should be adopted and patients should be carefully monitored as unwanted effects are more likely to occur in these patients.

Contra-indications: Peptic ulceration and hypersensitivity to baclofen.

Special warnings and special precautions for use: Psychotic disorders, confusional states or schizophrenia may be worsened by treatment with baclofen. Therefore, patients with these conditions should be kept under close observation and treatment should be administered cautiously.

Epileptic manifestations may be exacerbated with baclofen treatment, but may be used if appropriate supervision and anticonvulsive therapy are maintained.

Caution should be exercised with baclofen therapy in patients suffering from renal, hepatic or respiratory impairment or who have had a cerebrovascular accident.

Patients with neurogenic disturbances affecting emptying of the bladder may show improvement in their condition whilst taking baclofen. However, patients with pre-existing sphincter hypertonia may suffer with acute urine retention during treatment with baclofen; as a result it should be used cautiously in these patients.

Appropriate laboratory tests should be carried out on patients with hepatic dysfunction or diabetes mellitus to make sure that no drug-induced changes to the underlying diseases have resulted with concomitant baclofen therapy as, rarely, elevated SGOT, alkaline phosphatase and glucose levels in serum have been recorded.

Baclofen therapy should always be gradually discontinued, unless serious adverse effects have occurred, by reducing the dose over a period of 1–2 weeks. Anxiety, confusion, hallucinations, psychosis, mania, paranoia, convulsions, tachycardia, and, as a rebound phenomenon, temporary aggravation of spasticity, have all been reported on abrupt withdrawal.

Interactions with other medicaments and other forms of interaction: There have been reports of hallucinations, agitation and mental confusion with the use of baclofen with levodopa and carbidopa in Parkinson's disease.

Use of tricyclic antidepressants and baclofen may result in the potentiation of the effect of baclofen, resulting in pronounced muscular hypotonia.

Baclofen excretion may be reduced by drugs which produce renal insufficiency, e.g. ibuprofen, resulting in toxic effects.

Concomitant use of drugs acting on the CNS or alcohol with baclofen may lead to increased sedation.

Fentanyl induced analgesia may be extended by pretreatment with baclofen.

Hyperkinetic symptoms in patients receiving lithium may be exacerbated by baclofen.

Antihypertensive therapy may require adjustment as an increased fall in blood pressure may result with concomitant treatment with baclofen.

Pregnancy and lactation: Not recommended in pregnancy as fetal malformations have been reported as having occurred in rats but not mice or rabbits. Where treatment is necessary, the benefits for the mother should be carefully considered against the possible risks to the child, particularly in the first trimester when baclofen should only be used if essential. Baclofen is not recommended whilst breast-feeding as it is known to be present in the milk.

Effects on ability to drive and use machines: Patients taking baclofen should not take charge of vehicles, other means of transport, or machinery where loss of attention may lead to accidents.

Undesirable effects: Undesirable effects occur predominantly with initial treatment, with large doses, if the dose is increased too quickly or in the treatment of the elderly. These effects rarely necessitate withdrawal of the medication and are frequently of short duration. Modifying the dosage may lessen or eliminate the effects.

It may be difficult to distinguish between drug-induced undesirable effects and those caused by the diseases being treated.

Gastro-intestinal tract: Mild gastro-intestinal disturbances such as constipation or diarrhoea may occasionally occur. Dry mouth, nausea and vomiting have also been reported. Should nausea continue despite reduced dosage, baclofen should be taken with food or a milk drink.

Genito-urinary tract: Increased frequency of micturition, dysuria and enuresis have rarely been reported.

Cardio-respiratory system: Hypotension and cardiovascular or respiratory depression have been reported occasionally.

Central nervous system: Especially at the beginning of treatment, effects including drowsiness and daytime sedation may occur with occasional reports of lassitude, exhaustion, light-headedness, confusion, dizziness, headache and insomnia.

A lower convulsion threshold and seizures may occur, particularly in patients with epilepsy.

Other neurological effects which have been reported include paraesthesiase, muscle weakness, myalgia, ataxia, tremor, nystagmus and accommodation disorders. Reported psychiatric effects include euphoria, hallucinations, nightmares and depressive states.

Other unwanted effects: There have been very rare reports of skin rash, hyperhidrosis, visual disturbance, changes in taste sensation and a deterioration in liver function tests.

Increased spasticity as a contradictory response to the medication has been reported in some patients.

Some patients may experience greater difficulty in walking or coping for themselves as a result of excessive hypotonia. This may be alleviated by altering the dosage schedule.

Overdosage: Symptoms: Primarily, these are signs of central nervous depression: including drowsiness, consciousness impairment, respiratory depression, coma. Also likely are confusion, agitation, hallucinations, eye accommodation disorders, absent pupillary reflex, generalised muscular hypotonia, myoclonia, hyporeflexia or areflexia, convulsions, peripheral vasodilatation, hypotension, bradycardia, hypothermia, nausea, vomiting, diarrhoea, hypersalivation and elevated LDH, SGOT and AP values.

Deterioration in the condition may occur if various substances/drugs acting on the CNS, e.g. alcohol, tricyclic antidepressants or diazepam, have been taken at the same time.

Treatment: No specific antidote is known. Removal of the drug from the gastro-intestinal tract should be attempted by inducing vomiting or gastric lavage. Comatose patients need to be intubated prior to gastric lavage. Activated charcoal or, if necessary, a saline aperient may be given. In respiratory depression, artificial respiration and measures to support cardiovascular functions should be applied. Large quantities of fluid should be given, possibly with a diuretic, since baclofen is excreted mainly through the kidneys. If convulsions occur, intravenous diazepam should be administered.

Pharmacological properties

Pharmacodynamic properties: Baclofen is an analogue of aminobutyric acid. Its mode of action is not fully understood. It inhibits monosynaptic and polysynaptic transmission at the spinal level and also depresses the CNS.

Pharmacokinetic properties: The following mean values were obtained for Baclofen Tablets 10 mg in healthy volunteers.

$T_{\frac{1}{2}}$ (hours)	3.301
T_{max} (hours)	1.549
C_{max} (ng/ml)	102
AUC (ng/ml hours)	674

Pharmaceutical particulars

List of excipients: Lactose, potato starch, microcrystalline cellulose, sodium starch glycollate and magnesium stearate.

Incompatibilities: Not known.

Shelf life: 3 years.

Special precautions for storage: Store in a cool dry place and protect from light.

Nature and contents of container: Securitainer with polyethylene closure. Pack sizes: 28, 84 and 100.

Instructions for use/handling: Not applicable.

Marketing authorisation number 4416/0160.

Date of revision of SPC 21 May 1997.

Legal category POM.

BEDRANOL* (PROPRANOLOL HYDROCHLORIDE) SR CAPSULES 160 mg

Qualitative and quantative composition Each capsule contains propranolol hydrochloride BP 160 mg.

Pharmaceutical form Sustained release capsule.

Clinical particulars
Therapeutic indications: Bedranol SR is a competitive blocking agent of adrenergic β-receptor sites. It is used in the treatment of hypertension and angina.

Posology and method of administration:
Adults: Hypertension. The initial dose is one capsule daily taken orally in the morning or evening. An adequate response is seen by most patients at this dosage. If necessary, the dose can be increased to 2 capsules. A further reduction in blood pressure may be achieved by combining Bedranol SR with other anti-hypertensive agents.

Angina. Most patients will respond to one capsule daily taken orally in the morning or evening.

Elderly patients: The evidence concerning the relationship between blood level and age is conflicting. For patients already established on 160 mg propranolol daily, one capsule of Bedranol SR may be given. It is suggested that elderly patients being started off on propranolol treatment may need smaller initial doses and in these circumstances an alternative preparation should be used.

Children: Bedranol SR is not suitable for use in children.

Method of administration: Oral.

Contra-indications: Bedranol SR must not be used if any of the following conditions are present:
- hypersensitivity to propranolol or any of the other ingredients
- a history of bronchospasm or asthma
- bradycardia
- second or third degree heart block
- sick sinus syndrome
- cardiogenic shock
- uncontrolled heart failure
- hypotension
- severe peripheral circulatory disturbances
- Prinzmetal's angina
- untreated phaeochromocytoma
- prolonged fasting, or
- metabolic acidosis

Special warnings and special precautions for use: Patients with a history of wheezing or asthma should not take propranolol unless it is considered essential. The label will carry the following warning: 'Do not take this medicine if you have a history of wheezing or asthma'. The patient information leaflet will state 'Do not take this medicine if you have a history of wheezing or asthma. Consult your doctor or pharmacist first.'

Intolerance to propranolol, shown as bradycardia and hypotension may occur, in which case propranolol should be withdrawn. If necessary, treatment for overdose should be started.

Beta-blockers may increase both the sensitivity towards allergens and the seriousness of anaphylactic reactions.

Withdrawal of the drug for any reason should be gradual.

In patients with ischaemic heart disease treatment must not be discontinued abruptly. Either the equivalent dose of another beta-blocker may be substituted, or the withdrawal of Bedranol SR should be gradual. This can be carried out by substituting the equivalent dose in propranolol 40 mg tablets and then reducing the dose.

Bedranol SR should be used with caution in patients whose cardiac reserve is poor.

Bedranol SR may aggravate periperal arterial circulatory disturbances.

As propranolol has a negative effect on conduction time, care must be taken when giving it to patients with first degree heart block.

Care must be taken in patients with renal or hepatic dysfunction when beginning treatment and choosing the initial dose.

Bedranol SR should be used with care in patients with decompensated cirrhosis.

In patients with portal hypertension, liver function may deteriorate. There have been reports that treatment with propranolol may increase the risk of developing hepatic encephalopathy.

Interactions with other medicaments and other forms of interaction: Care should be taken when prescribing beta-adrenoceptor blocking drugs with Class 1 antidysrhythmic agents, e.g. disopyramide.

Beta-adrenoceptor blocking drugs should be used with caution in combination with calcium channel blockers such as verapamil or diltiazem in patients with impaired ventricular function. These should not be given to patients with conduction abnormalities. Beta-blockers or calcium channel blockers should not be given intravenously within 48 hours of discontinuing either one or the other.

Use with nifedipine or other dihydropyridines may cause an increased risk of hypotension, and heart failure may occur in patients with undiscovered cardiac insufficiency.

Propranolol modifies the tachycardia of hypoglycaemia and care should be taken when treating diabetic patients with Bedranol SR whether or not they are also taking hypoglycaemic agents. Propranolol may prolong the hypoglycaemic response to insulin.

Use of adrenaline or other sympathomimetics with propranolol may counteract the effects of propranolol. Care should be taken in giving parenteral administration of adrenaline to patients taking beta-blocking drugs as, rarely, vasoconstriction, hypertension and bradycardia may result.

Rebound hypertension which can follow after withdrawal of clonidine may be exacerbated by beta-blockers. Therefore, if the patient is transferring from clonidine to propranolol, the latter treatment should be started several days after clonidine has been stopped. If Bedranol SR and clonidine are given together, clonidine should be discontinued several days after stopping treatment with Bedranol SR.

Digitoxin or digoxin taken at the same time as beta-blockers can increase atrioventricular conduction time.

Ergotamine, dihydroergotamine or related compounds given with propranolol have resulted in reports of vasospastic reactions in some patients.

The hypotensive effects of propranolol may be decreased if the patient also takes prostaglandin synthetase inhibitors, e.g. ibuprofen or indomethacin.

If propranolol is taken with chlorpromazine, plasma levels of both agents may be increased, leading to enhanced antipsychotic and elevated antihypertensive effects.

Concomitant administration of rifampicin with propranolol may result in reduced plasma concentrations of propranolol. Thyroxine taken at the same time as propranolol also has this effect.

Cimetidine taken at the same time as propranolol will increase propranolol plasma levels. Fluvoxamine taken with propranolol also has this effect.

Alcohol will decrease the plasma levels of propranolol.

It may be necessary to withdraw Bedranol SR before surgery (24 hours should be allowed to elapse between the last dose and anaesthesia). If Bedranol SR is continued throughout surgery the anaesthetist should be told and care should be taken in selecting and using suitable anaesthetic agents. An anaesthetic agent with as little myocardial depression as possible should be used. Beta-blockers used with anaesthetic agents may result in attenuation of reflex tachycardia and the risk of hypotension may increase.

Propranolol may affect lignocaine infusion by increasing the plasma concentration of lignocaine by approximately a third and therefore this should be avoided.

Interference with laboratory tests: Propranolol has been reported to interfere with the estimation of serum bilirubin by the diazo method and with the determination of catecholamines by methods using fluorescence.

Pregnancy and lactation: Although there is no evidence that propranolol is teratogenic, Bedranol SR should not be used in pregnancy unless absolutely necessary. Beta-blockers reduce placental perfusion which may result in intra-uterine foetal death, immature or premature deliveries. Bradycardia may occur in the foetus and there may be an increased risk of cardiac and pulmonary problems in the post-natal period. Hypoglycaemia or bradycardia may occur in the neonate.

Breast-feeding is not recommended as beta-blockers taken by the mother will pass into the breast-milk.

Effects on ability to drive and use machines: Bedranol SR should not impair ability to drive and use machines. However, sometimes dizziness or tiredness may occur. If so, the patient should not drive or operate machines.

Undesirable effects: The following undesirable effects may occur.

Cardiovascular: deterioration of heart failure, bradycardia, postural hypotension with or without syncope may occur. Heart block, intermittent claudication or Raynaud's phenomenon may be precipitated or exacerbated. Cold extremities may occur.

Central nervous system: dizziness, confusion, mood changes, depression or psychosis and hallucinations, sleep disturbances or nightmares may occur.

Reports of visual disturbances or dry eyes have been made.

Peripheral nervous system: peripheral neuropathy or myopathies or paraesthesia may occur.

Gastrointestinal: GI disturbance including nausea, vomiting, diarrhoea, constipation or abdominal cramps have been reported.

Haematological: thrombocytopenia, purpura and rarely agranulocytosis. Eosinophilia may occur which passes quickly.

Hepatic: propranolol treatment may increase the risk of developing hepatic encephalopathy.

Respiratory: bronchospasm may occur in patients with bronchial asthma or a history of asthma. Fatalities have been reported.

Skin and hair: exacerbation of psoriasis, psoriasiform skin reactions, skin rashes, pruritus or alopecia may occur.

Miscellaneous: fatigue (commonly), lassitude (often passing quickly), and an increase in antinuclear antibodies have been observed. There have been isolated reports of a myasthenia gravis-like syndrome or aggravation of myasthenia gravis.

Intolerance to propranolol, shown as bradycardia and hypotension may occur, in which case propranolol should be withdrawn. If necessary, treatment for overdose should be started.

Propranolol should be discontinued gradually if the patient's well-being is adversely affected by any undesirable effects.

Overdosage: Symptoms of overdose: bradycardia, hypotension, bronchospasm and acute cardiac insufficiency.

General supportive measures should be employed such as gastric lavage, activated charcoal and a laxative to stop any remaining drug being absorbed. Shock treatment, if required should be given. Excessive bradycardia may be countered with 1–2 mg IV atropine, followed if necessary by glucagon 10 mg IV. This may be repeated, or followed by an intravenous infusion of glucagon 1–10 mg/hour according to response. Alternatively, a beta-receptor stimulant such as isoprenaline 25 mcg IV, orciprenaline 500 mcg (0.5 mg) IV or dobutamine 2.5–10 mcg/kg/minute IV may be given.

Pharmacological properties
Pharmacodynamic properties: Propranolol is a competitive blocker of beta-adrenergic receptor sites.

Pharmacokinetic properties: Following oral administration Bedranol SR peak plasma levels occur approximately 7 to 8.5 hours after an oral dose. Individual plasma concentrations vary. The plasma half-life of propranolol is about 3 to 6 hours. Propranolol binds well to plasma proteins. It has high lipid solubility, and crosses the blood-brain barrier, placenta and enters breast milk.

Propranolol is absorbed almost completely from the gastrointestinal tract, but binds to hepatic tissue where it is subject to first-pass metabolism.

Propranolol is metabolised in the liver, and excreted in the urine as metabolites and unchanged drug.

Preclinical safety data: There are no preclinical safety data of relevance to the prescriber.

Pharmaceutical particulars
List of excipients: Sucrose, corn starch, shellac, talc, gelatin, titanium dioxide (E171) and erythrosine (E127).

Incompatibilities: Not known.

Shelf life: 36 months.

Special precautions for storage: Store in a cool dry place and protect from light.

Nature and contents of container: Polypropylene securitainers with polyethylene closures. Pack sizes: 28, 56 and 100.

Instructions for use/handling: Not applicable.

Marketing authorisation number PL 4416/0068

Date of revision of the text August 1998

Legal category POM.

CAPTOPRIL TABLETS BP

Qualitative and quantitative composition Each Captopril Tablet contains Captopril BP 12.5 mg, 25 mg or 50 mg.

Pharmaceutical form Uncoated tablets.

Clinical particulars
Therapeutic indications:
Hypertension: For the treatment of mild to moderate hypertension. Captopril may be used in severe hypertension when standard therapy is inadequate or ineffective.

Congestive heart failure: In the treatment of congestive heart failure, Captopril should be used in association with diuretics and, if appropriate, digitalis.

Myocardial infarction: Following myocardial infarction in patients with left ventricular dysfunction, Captopril may be used to improve prognosis. Cardiac function should be assessed by echocardiography or radionuclide studies before starting treatment with Captopril.

Posology and method of administration: For oral administration only.

Hypertension: Captopril may be used alone or in combination with other therapies for the treatment of hypertension. Treatment should be started at a low dose and increased gradually at 2 to 4 week intervals until an adequate effect is achieved. The starting dose should be 12.5 mg twice daily and, in order to avoid a precipitous drop in blood pressure in some patients, the first dose should be given at bedtime. If possible, diuretics should be discontinued for a few days before commencing Captopril. In those patients who are still on diuretics, or who are elderly or have renal impairment, the starting dose should be 6.25 mg twice daily.

The maintenance dose is usually 25 mg to 50 mg twice daily but in more severe cases, up to 50 mg three times daily may be needed.

Congestive heart failure: In the treatment of heart failure, Captopril should be started under close medical supervision. A low initial dose of 6.25 mg or 12.5 mg twice daily will minimise hypotensive effects. The dose should be gradually increased at intervals of not less than 14 days until a satisfactory therapeutic response is attained. The maximum daily dose is usually 50 mg three times a day.

Myocardial infarction: A starting dose of 6.25 mg should be increased to a maximum of 150 mg daily over several weeks. The patient's tolerance will determine the dose used but symptomatic hypotension indicates the need to reduce the dose. Captopril may be used in conjunction with other post-infarction treatments including thrombolytics, aspirin and beta-blockers.

In renal impairment: As Captopril is largely excreted via the kidneys, the dosage and dose frequency should be reduced in patients with renal impairment (creatinine clearance of less than 30 ml/min or plasma creatinine above 150 μmol/l). As ACE inhibitors may reduce or abolish glomerular filtration in patients with renovascular disease they should not be used in such patients unless careful monitoring of renal function is available.

Captopril is removed by haemodialysis.

Elderly patients: The lowest dose of Captopril which achieves a satisfactory therapeutic effect should be used in elderly patients, particularly those with evidence of renal or other organ dysfunction.

Children: The use of Captopril is not recommended for the treatment of mild to moderate hypertension in children.

Experience in neonates, particularly premature infants, is limited. Because renal function in infants is not equivalent to that of older children and adults lower doses of Captopril should be used with the patients under close medical supervision. The starting dose may be 0.3 mg/kg bodyweight daily increasing to a maximum of 6 mg/kg in two or three divided doses.

Contra-indications: Hypersensitivity to Captopril, other ACE inhibitors or any of the tablet ingredients. Captopril is contra-indicated in pregnancy and lactation.

Special warnings and precautions for use: Captopril should not be used in patients with aortic stenosis or outflow tract obstruction. Renal function should be assessed before starting treatment with Captopril and at intervals during the course of therapy. Patients with bilateral renovascular disease should not be treated with ACE inhibitors except under very careful supervision. It is considered that patients with peripheral vascular disease or generalised atherosclerosis may be at higher risk of renovascular disease and care should be taken in those with systemic lupus erythematosus or scleroderma.

Hypotensive episodes may occur after the first one or two doses and this is usually relieved by lying the patient down or starting therapy at bedtime. Patients with severe hypertension or those with renin dependent hypertension may be more likely to develop hypotensive episodes and a lower starting dose may be appropriate. In patients on diuretics, reduction of the dose or withdrawal of the diuretic for a few days prior to starting treatment with Captopril may reduce the chance of hypotension occurring.

Potassium supplements or potassium sparing diuretics should not normally be used with ACE inhibitors because they decrease aldosterone production. A rise in serum potassium levels may occur in patients with renal impairment.

Anaphylactoid reactions have been reported in patients on ACE inhibitors undergoing renal dialysis using polyacrylonitrile membranes. The combined use of such membranes and ACE inhibitors should be avoided.

Interactions with other medicaments and other forms of interaction: Diuretics potentiate the anti-hypertensive action of Captopril. Potassium sparing diuretics or potassium supplements may cause an increase in serum potassium.

The response to other vasodilator drugs may be enhanced by Captopril and this should be borne in mind when adding Captopril to existing therapy.

Patients previously treated with clonidine may have a delayed response when they are changed to Captopril.

Indomethacin may reduce the anti-hypertensive effect of Captopril and this may occur with other non-steroidal anti-inflammatory drugs.

Probenecid reduces the renal clearance of Captopril.

Lithium serum levels may be increased when lithium is given with Captopril.

Allopurinol and procainamide have been reported to cause neutropenia and/or Stevens-Johnson syndrome when given concomitantly with Captopril. Care should be taken when using such combinations of drugs, particularly in patients with impaired renal function.

Azathioprine and cyclophosphamide given with Captopril have been associated with blood dyscrasias, especially in patients with renal failure.

A false-positive test for acetone in the urine may be caused by Captopril.

Polyacrylonitrile dialysis membranes have been associated with anaphylactoid reactions in patients taking ACE inhibitors.

Hypotension occurring during surgery or general anaesthesia as a result of angiotensin II blockade in patients treated with Captopril should be corrected by volume expansion.

Pregnancy and lactation: Captopril is contra-indicated in pregnancy. Captopril is known to be fetotoxic in some animal species and has been associated with oligohydramnios and hypotension and/or anuria in the neonate when given to pregnant women in the second or third trimesters. Women of child-bearing potential should take adequate contraceptive precautions if being treated with Captopril.

Captopril is excreted in breast milk and therefore should not be given to nursing mothers.

Effects on ability to drive and use machines: Patients should be warned to avoid driving or operating machinery if they experience any dizziness or fatigue when taking Captopril.

Undesirable effects: Adverse effects are usually dose related and more frequent in patients with impaired renal function. The more common side effects include skin rashes which occur with pruritus, hypotension; cough; taste disturbance and renal side effects. Reports in the literature indicate that the incidence of occurrence of these side effects varies up to 5%. The main exception to this is the incidence of rash occurring and up to 7% has been recorded for patients with impaired renal function.

Renal: proteinuria, hyperkalaemia. Some deterioration in renal function has been seen with raised blood urea and creatinine levels and reversible renal failure may occur in patients with existing renovascular disease.

Cardiovascular: tachycardia and hypotention may occur, particularly early in treatment, in patients with heart failure or volume or salt depleted such as those already on diuretics.

Gastro-intestinal: stomatitis, gastric irritation or abdominal pain, weight loss associated with taste disturbance. Transient increases in liver enzymes have been noted and, rarely, cholestatic jaundice or hepatocellular injury has occurred. Pancreatitis has been rarely reported in patients on ACE inhibitors.

Haematological: neutropenia, agranulocytosis, thrombocytopenia, anaemia and aplastic anaemia have been reported, more often in patients with renal impairment. Patients should be warned to report any unexpected bleeding, bruising or sore throats and appropriate haematological tests should be performed.

Dermatological: itchy skin rashes, urticaria, and vesicular or bullous rashes have been reported. Photosensitivity has occurred.

Other effects: headache, angioedema, paraesthesiae of extremities, serum sickness, lymphadenopathy, bronchospasm have been reported with Captopril.

Overdose: Blood pressure should be monitored and, if necessary, hypotension can be corrected by volume expansion. Captopril is readily eliminated by haemodialysis.

Pharmacological properties

Pharmacodynamic properties: Captopril is a highly specific competitive inhibitor of angiotensin I converting enzyme thus reducing angiotensin II levels. It reduces peripheral vascular resistance, lowering blood pressure, and by reducing both pre-load and after-load it is useful in the treatment of heart failure.

Pharmacokinetic properties: Captopril is fairly well absorbed and although blood levels are reduced when taken with food, its antihypertensive effect does not seem to be altered. There is some reversible binding to plasma proteins. About 50% is metabolised and the drug is mostly excreted via the kidneys either as metabolites or unchanged drug within about 6 hours. There is some accumulation with chronic dosing and renal impairment reduces clearance.

Preclinical safety data: It is reported that studies carried out in rabbits revealed that captopril had an embryocidal effect. However, no teratogenic or carcinogenic effects were observed. Captopril is reported to have a lethal effect in sheep foetuses. No toxic effects have been observed in hamster or rat foetuses.

It is reported that studies carried out in dogs revealed that bone marrow suppression occurred which was dose related. Anaemia is reported to have occurred at lower doses while leucopenia and thrombocytopenia were observed at higher doses only. Studies carried out in monkeys, rats and mice have shown anaemia to occur at very high doses which exceed the maximum dose in humans.

Pharmaceutical particulars

List of excipients: Lactose PhEur; Maize Starch PhEur; Microcrystalline Cellulose PhEur; Stearic Acid BP.

Incompatibilities: Not applicable.

Shelf life: 3 years.

Special precautions for storage: Store at a temperature not exceeding 25°C.

Nature and contents of container: Captopril tablets are available in blister strips composed of PVC/Aluminium.

Pack size: 56 tablets.

Instructions for use/handling: Not applicable.

Marketing authorisation numbers

Captopril Tablets BP 12.5 mg	4416/0271
Captopril Tablets BP 25 mg	4416/0272
Captopril Tablets BP 50 mg	4416/0273

Date of approval/revision of SPC July 1997.

Legal category POM.

CARBO-DOME* CREAM

Qualitative and quantitative composition Each 100 g of cream contain Coal Tar Solution BP 10 g.

Pharmaceutical form Cream.

Clinical particulars

Therapeutic indications: The coal tar solution in Carbo-Dome Cream has a keratoplastic and antipruritic effect in psoriasis.

Indications: Psoriasis.

Posology and method of administration: For topical application only. Apply to the affected areas two or three times daily. This dosage is recommended for both children and adults.

Contra-indications: Coal tar should not be used when a patient has known sensitivity to coal tar or any of the other ingredients. It should not be used on broken or highly inflamed skin.

Special warnings and precautions for use: For topical administration only.

Coal tar should be used with caution on the face (avoiding the eyes), skin flexures or genitalia. If it gets in the eyes, rinse them thoroughly with water.

Avoid exposure to direct sunlight and UV lamps after applying, unless its action is specifically required – see *Interactions* below.

Interactions with other medicaments and other forms of interaction: Ultraviolet-B (UVB) light increases the effect of coal tar in the treatment of psoriasis.

Pregnancy and lactation: Although there is no direct evidence of the safety of coal tar used topically in pregnancy and lactation, has been used over many years without known ill effects.

Effects on ability to drive and use machines: None known.

Undesirable effects: Coal tar may cause photosensitivity and patients should be warned to avoid exposure to sunlight or UV lamps after treatment (unless this is specifically intended).

Coal tar may cause irritation, acneiform eruptions or folliculitis, and may cause staining.

Overdosage: Not applicable.

Pharmacological properties

Pharmacodynamic properties: Coal tar as presented in this product is an antipruritic keratoplastic and weak antiseptic.

Pharmacokinetic properties: The product is designed

for external use only. Absorption of the coal tar is not reported in 'Martindale' and therefore the pharmacokinetics is not addressed.

Preclinical safety data: There are no pre-clinical data of relevance to the prescriber which are additional to that already included in other sections of the SPC.

Pharmaceutical particulars
List of excipients: Dehydag wax SX, beeswax, white soft paraffin, light liquid paraffin, glycerol, sodium lauryl sulphate, methyl-p-hydroxybenzoate and purified water.

Incompatibilities: None recorded.

Shelf life: 36 months.

Special precautions for storage: Store in cool place.

Nature and contents of container: Tubes (aluminium). Pack sizes: 30 g and 100 g.

Instructions for use/handling: Not applicable.

Marketing authorisation number 4416/0106.

Date of revision of SPC March 1996.

Legal category GSL.

CO-AMILOFRUSE TABLETS BP

Qualitative and quantitative composition Each tablet contains Frusemide BP 40 mg and Amiloride Hydrochloride BP equivalent to anhydrous amiloride hydrochloride 5 mg.

Pharmaceutical form Tablet.

Clinical particulars
Therapeutic indications: For the treatment of oedematous conditions where rapid diuresis with potassium conservation is required.

This includes congestive cardiac failure, oedema due to renal disease, corticosteroid therapy, and ascites associated with cirrhosis.

Posology and method of administration:
Adults: The normal dose is one tablet a day, to be taken in the morning. This can be increased to two tablets daily, if necessary.

Elderly: The dose may require adjustment according to the patient's diuretic response. If necessary, a lower dose (e.g. half a tablet) may be taken. Creatinine and serum electrolytes should be monitored carefully.

Children: Not recommended for use in children.

Oral administration.

Contra-indications: Known sensitivity to frusemide, amiloride hydrochloride or any of the other ingredients, acute renal failure or severe progressive renal disease. Addison's disease, hyperkalaemia (serum potassium >5.3 mmol/litre), anuria, electrolyte imbalance, precomatose states associated with cirrhosis, concomitant potassium supplements or potassium sparing diuretics. Co-amilofruse is also contra-indicated in children as safety has not been established.

Special warnings and precautions for use: Tests should be performed to monitor kidney function and serum electrolyte levels. This is particularly important in the treatment of the elderly, patients with impaired kidney function, potential obstruction of the urinary tract or fragile electrolyte balance, where a reduced dosage may be required.

Frusemide may cause latent diabetes to become manifest. It may be necessary to increase the dose of hypoglycaemic agents in diabetic patients. Patients suffering from diabetes mellitus are at an increased risk of developing hyperkalaemia. Treatment with co-amilofruse should be discontinued three days prior to glucose tolerance tests.

Co-amilofruse should be used with caution in patients with prostatic hypertrophy or impaired micturition as acute urinary retention may occur.

Interactions with other medicaments and other forms of interaction: Concurrent use of ACE inhibitors, non-steroidal anti-inflammatory drugs, cyclosporin, trilostane, potassium salts and hypoglycaemic agents may lead to an increased risk of hyperkalaemia.

The potential risk of nephrotoxicity may be increased when cephaloridine, NSAIDs, or aminoglycoside antibiotics are used concurrently. Ototoxicity may also occur with concurrent use of aminoglycoside antibiotics.

The dosage of cardiac glycosides, lithium, non-depolarising muscle relaxants, antihypertensive agents and hypoglycaemic agents may require adjustment.

Pregnancy and lactation: Use in pregnancy and lactation should be avoided as safety has not been established.

Effects on ability to drive and use machines: Reduced mental alertness and confusion may affect ability to drive. Other activities requiring full alertness should be avoided.

Undesirable effects: Side effects which may occur include nausea, vomiting, abdominal pain, diarrhoea or constipation, parasthesia, thirst, dizziness, skin rash (although rare may be severe), pruritus, weakness, muscle cramps, headache and minor psychiatric or visual changes.

Tinnitus and deafness and hypersensitivity reactions including interstitial nephritis occur rarely.

Hyperuricaemia may occur, precipitating attacks of gout in some patients. Pancreatitis has been reported with high doses and cholestatic jaundice has also been reported.

Bone marrow depression has occurred rarely: agranulocytosis, thrombocytopenia and leucopenia have been reported. The patients haematopoetic state should be regularly monitored throughout treatment.

Overdose: Symptoms of overdosage include dehydration, electrolyte imbalance (particularly hyperkalaemia). If possible, emesis should be induced or gastric lavage performed. In order to correct electrolyte changes and dehydration, sodium chloride and water should be administered. If there is evidence of hyperkalaemia, measures should be taken to reduce serum potassium levels.

Pharmacological properties
Pharmacodynamic properties: Frusemide is a high ceiling diuretic which acts on the ascending limb of the loop of Henle, inhibiting sodium and chloride re-absorption. It causes an increase in urinary excretion of sodium, chloride, water, potassium, calcium and magnesium. It also increases the excretion of bicarbonate, resulting in a rise in urinary pH.

Frusemide increases ammonia excretion via the kidney and decreases the secretion of uric acid, resulting in increased blood urate levels, which may precipitate gout.

Amiloride is a diuretic acting primarily in the distal tubule and promotes the excretion of sodium in the urine without decreasing the potassium levels in plasma. When excretion of potassium is increased by other diuretics, amiloride causes a noticeable decrease in potassium excretion. Amiloride also decreases urinary excretion of calcium and magnesium.

Pharmacokinetic properties: Frusemide is readily absorbed from the gastro-intestinal tract and is about 60% bioavailable. It is extensively bound to plasma proteins. The elimination half-life is approximately 1–2 hours and produces a duration of action of 3–6 hours. Approximately 50% of an oral dose of amiloride is absorbed which is not significantly bound to plasma protein. Absorption is reduced by food and the elimination half-life is 6–9 hours with peak serum levels at 3–4 hours.

Preclinical safety data: Not relevant.

Pharmaceutical particulars
List of excipients: Lactose, polyvinylpyrrolidone, orange E110 soluble, orange E110 insoluble, microcrystalline cellulose, sodium starch glycollate, magnesium stearate and purified water.

Incompatibilities: Not known.

Shelf life: 36 months.

Special precautions for storage: Store in dry place. Protect from light.

Nature and contents of container: Pack sizes: 28 and 56 tablets.

Blister strips composed of: 250 μm PVC/PVdC coated foil, 20 μm aluminium foil. Blister strips will be packed in cartons.

Instructions for use/handling: Not applicable.

Marketing authorisation number 04416/0267.

Date of approval/revision of SPC April 1996.

Legal category POM.

CO-CODAMOL EFFERVESCENT TABLETS

Qualitative and quantative composition Each effervescent tablet contains:

Paracetamol BP	500.0 mg
Codeine phosphate BP	8.0 mg

Pharmaceutical form Effervescent tablets.

Clinical Particulars
Therapeutic indications: For the relief of mild to moderate pain including headache, migraine, neuralgia, toothache, rheumatic, muscular and period pains.

The symptomatic relief of feverishness.

Posology and method of administration:
For oral administration:

Adults and children over 12 years: One or two tablets to be taken every four to six hours if necessary. Do not exceed 8 tablets in 24 hours.

Not to be given to children under 12 years.

Elderly patients: Normal adult dose unless there is impaired kidney or liver function.

Directions: The tablets must be dissolved in half a glass of water (l00 ml). The tablets dissolve more quickly in warm water or if stirred.

Contra-indications: Caution should be taken in patients with impaired kidney or liver function, or previous hypersensitivity to paracetamol, codeine or other ingredients.

Special warnings and special precautions for use:
Warnings: The patient must not exceed the stated dose.

This product contains paracetamol.

If symptoms persist for more than three days the patient should consult a doctor.

If the patient is pregnant she should consult her doctor before taking this preparation.

Care is advised in the administration of paracetamol-containing products to patients with severe renal or severe hepatic impairment and in those with non-cirrhotic alcoholic liver disease. The hazards of overdose are greater in those with alcoholic liver disease.

Patients should be advised not to take other paracetamol-containing products concurrently.

Keep out of the reach of children.

Each tablet contains 438.0 mg (19.1 millimoles) of sodium. This sodium should be taken into account when prescribing for patients on a sodium restricted diet.

Immediate medical advice should be sought in the event of an overdose, even if the patient feels well, because of the risk of delayed, serious liver damage.

Interactions with other medicaments and other forms of interaction:

i) Alcohol, barbiturates, anticonvulsants and tricyclic antidepressants may increase the hepatotoxicity of paracetamol, particularly after an overdose.
ii) chloramphenicol - paracetamol may increase the half-life of chloramphenicol.
iii) cholestyramine - may reduce absorption of paracetamol.
iv) metoclopramide - may potentiate the effect of paracetamol.
v) The anticoagulant effect of warfarin and other coumarins may be enhanced by prolonged regular use of paracetamol with increased risk of bleeding.

Pregnancy and lactation: There is inadequate evidence for the safety of codeine in pregnancy but there is epidemiological evidence for the safety of paracetamol. Both substances have been used for many years without apparent ill consequences and animal studies have not shown any hazard. Nonetheless, careful consideration should be given before giving co-codamol tablets to pregnant mothers particularly during the first trimester. Paracetamol has been detected in breast milk, although it is estimated that less than 0.1% of the maternal dose appears in l00 ml of breast milk. Codeine has also been shown to be excreted in breast milk, although the quantity was not determined.

Effects on ability to drive and use machines: Codeine can occasionally cause drowsiness, if affected the patient should not drive or operate machinery.

Undesirable effects: If given in therapeutic doses side effects are very rare. Haematological reaction, thrombocytopenia, agranulocytosis and acute pancreatitis have been reported. Skin rashes and other allergic reactions may occur occasionally. Most reports of adverse reactions to paracetamol relate to overdosage with the drug. Codeine can cause constipation, nausea, drowsiness and confusion.

Overdosage: In excess of 20 tablets.
Symptoms:

Due to Paracetamol Overdose: Symptoms of paracetamol overdosage in the first 24 hours are pallor, nausea, vomiting, anorexia and abdominal pain. Liver damage may become apparent 12 to 48 hours after ingestion. Abnormalities of glucose metabolism and metabolic acidosis may occur. In severe poisoning, hepatic failure may progress to encephalopathy, coma and death. Acute renal failure with acute tubular necrosis may develop even in the absence of severe liver damage. Cardiac arrhythmias have been reported.

Liver damage is likely in adults who have taken 10 g or more of paracetamol. It is considered that excess quantities of a toxic metabolite (usually adequately detoxified by glutathione when normal doses of paracetamol are ingested), become irreversibly bound to liver tissue.

Immediate treatment is essential in the management of paracetamol overdose. Despite a lack of significant early symptoms, patients should be referred to hospital urgently for immediate medical attention and any patient who had ingested around 7.5 g or more of paracetamol in the preceding 4 hours should undergo gastric lavage. Administration of oral methionine or intravenous n-acetylcysteine which may have a beneficial effect up to at least 48 hours after the overdose, may be required. General supportive measures must be available.

Due to Codeine: Respiratory depression and hypotension with circulatory failure and deepening coma. Convulsion may occur in infants and children.

Treatment: When over 4 hours have lapsed after overdosing, plasma paracetamol concentration should be measured. Specific treatment is required if the concentration falls above a line drawn between the point 200 mg per litre at 4 hours and 30 mg per litre at 15 hours after the overdose. Acetylcysteine should be given intravenously or alternatively, methionine may be given by mouth unless the patient is vomiting or is unconscious; both agents are of little value more than 15 hours after the overdose. Patients at risk of hepatic failure should receive a glucose infusion intravenously to prevent hypoglycaemia and established hepatic or renal failure should be managed conventionally. T J Metedith et al, Br Med J, 1986, 293, 345. Further reviews on paracetamol overdosage and its management: L F Prescott, Drugs, 1983, 25, 290: (official use only). R J Flanagan, Med Toxicol 1987, 2.

Naloxone hydrochloride – 400 µg is given iv repeated at intervals of 2 to 3 minutes if necessary. In children a dose of 5 to 10 µg per kg body weight may be given.

Pharmocological properties
Pharmacodynamic properties: Analgesic/antipyretic.

Pharmacokinetic properties:

Paracetamol: Paracetamol is rapidly absorbed from the upper gastrointestinal tract after oral administration.

Peak plasma levels of 15–20 micrograms per ml after 1 g oral dose occur within 30–90 minutes, depending on dosage form. It is rapidly distributed throughout the body and is primarily metabolised in the liver. About 85% is by conjugation with glucuronide and sulphate and about 10% by conjugation with glutathione.

Excretion of the biotransformation products is via the kidney. The elimination half-life is approximately 2–3 hours.

In overdose glucuronide pathways become saturated and excess paracetamol is metabolised via the glutathione pathway. Hepatic glutathione is rapidly depleted and an intermediate hydroxylamine metabolite accumulates and binds to liver protems causing irreversible damage.

Codeine: Codeine is rapidly absorbed from the gastro-intestinal tract following oral administration. Peak plasma levels are achieved in about 1 hour following oral ingestion and the half-life in plasma is about 24 hours.

Codeine is metabolised in the liver by O- and N-demethylation to morphine norcodeine, normorphine, hydrocodone and other metabolites. Approximately 10% of a dose of codeine is converted to morphine and accounts for most of the analgesic effect.

Urinary excretion is the main route of elimination of codeine and its metabolites which are mostly excreted as glucuronide conjugates.

Preclinical safety data: Paracetamol.

Acute Toxicity: Paracetamol hepatotoxicity is directly dependent on the plasma concentration related to time. Plasma concentrations above 1.2 mmo1/l at 4 hours, 0.6 mmol/l at 8 hours and 0.3 mmol/l at 12 hours are criteria for treatment with acetylcysteine to prevent irreversible liver damage.

Chronic Toxicity: In animal experiments the subchronic and chronic toxicity of paracetamol occurred in rats and mice as lesions in the gastro-intestinal tract, blood-count changes, degeneration and even necrosis of the hepatic and renal parenchyma. The metabolites that are assumed to have the toxic effects and the organic changes associated with them have been proven in humans as well.

Therefore, paracetamol should not be taken for a long period of time and in excessive doses. Oral daily doses with clearly hepatotoxic effects are around 5.8 g for non-alcoholics, symptoms of intoxication can occur as soon as 3 weeks after administration.

Mutagenic and tumorigenic potential: In mammalian cell cultures paracetamol induces chromosome mutations depending on its concentration. *In-vivo* tests show negative as well as slightly positive results. Due to the insufficient relevance of the most part of the *in-vivo* tests no final evaluation is possible at this time.

Long-term studies in rats and mice have yielded no indications of a carcinogenic effect.

Reproductive toxicology: Paracetamol passes the placental barrier. Animal studies and experience to date in humans reveal no evidence of embryotoxicity.

Codeine.
Acute animal toxicity: LD_{50} values for mice, rabbits and rats using different methods of administration are as follows:

	LD_{50} (mg kg^{-1})		
	Mice	Rabbits	Rats
Intravenous	ranges from 55-70		
Oral	400	120	500
Intraperitoneal		approximately 100	

Reproductive toxicology: There is no information on the carcinogenic or teratogenic potential of codeine in animal species. From studies, it has been reported that children born to mothers exposed to narcotic analgesics during months 1–4 of their pregnancy, may show a possible link between codeine exposure and respiratory malformations.

Codeine is excreted in the breast milk of nursing mothers. It has been reported that respiratory malformation in neonates may be associated with codeine exposure during pregnancy.

Clinical Toxicity: It is difficult to state an exact amount of an opioid product that would be toxic or fatal to man because chronic administration may lead to the development of tolerance. Serious toxicity has been reported in non-tolerant individuals following oral ingestion of 40–60 mg methadone. Older literature suggests that a normal healthy adult will not die after a l20 mg oral dose of morphine, or suffer from serious toxicity with less than a parenteral dose of 30 mg.

Caution should be employed in the treatment of patients with liver or kidney disease as under these conditions the pharmacokinetics of drug metabolism are significantly altered. This may lead to increased bioavailability and cumulative effects.

Morphine-like opioids should also be used with caution in patients with:
– reduced blood volume as these agents can aggravate hypovolaemic shock.
– reduced respiratory reserve as further depressant effects may occur.

As the dose is increased, the toxic effects, including respiratory depression become more pronounced. It has been reported that in acute overdosage producing respiratory depression, hypotension, circulatory failure and deepening coma, blood concentrations of codeine ranged from 1.4 to 5.6 mg/l.

Pharmaceutical particulars
List of excipients: Citric acid anhydrous, povidone, sodium saccharin, sodium bicarbonate, sodium carbonate anhydrous, simethicone, polysorbate 80 and aspartame.

Incompatibilities: None known.

Shelf life: 24 months.

Special precautions for storage: Store in a dry place, at or below 25°C.

Nature and contents of container: Strip pack using PPFM laminate constructed of: 40 gsm MGBK paper, l6 gsm LDPE, 9µ aluminium foil, 34.5 gsm LDPE. Strips are packed into an outer carton. Pack size: 100.

Instructions for use/handling: The following text appears on the outer packaging.

Indications: For the relief of mild to moderate pain including headache, migraine, neuralgia, toothache, rheumatic, muscular and period pains. The symptomatic relief of feverishness.

Dosage: Adults and children over 12 years: One or two tablets to be taken every four to six hours if necessary.

Do not exceed 8 tablets in 24 hours.

This dose may be given to the elderly unless there is impaired kidney or liver function.

Not to be given to children under 12 years.

Directions: Dissolve the tablets in half a glass of water (l00 ml). The tablet will dissolve more quickly in warm water or if stirred.

Warnings See *Special warnings and special precautions for use.*

Marketing authorisation number PL 4416/0253

Date of revision of the text September 1997

Legal category P.

DIAZEPAM SYRUP 2 mg/5 ml DIAZEPAM FORTE SYRUP 5 mg/5 ml

Presentation Bottles contain either diazepam BP 2 mg in 5 ml or diazepam BP 5 mg in 5 ml. The non-active ingredients include ethanol, sucrose, microcrystalline cellulose, ponceau 4R (E124), potassium sorbate, flavour, and methylhydroxybenzoate and propylhydroxybenzoate as preservatives.

Actions Diazepam has anticonvulsant, anxiolytic, sedative, muscle relaxant and amnesic properties. It is indicated:

Adults:

(i) for the short-term relief (2–4 weeks only) of anxiety that is severe, disabling or subjecting the individual to unacceptable distress, occurring alone or in association with insomnia or short-term psychosomatic, organic or psychotic illness;

(ii) as a sedative and premedicant;

(iii) as an anticonvulsant in the management of status epilepticus, febrile convulsions and poisoning;

(iv) in the control of muscle spasms as in tetanus;

(v) in the management of alcohol withdrawal symptoms;

(vi) in selected cases it may be useful in the management of cerebral spasticity.

Children:

(i) night terrors and somnambulism;

(ii) premedication;

(iii) in the control of muscle spasms as in tetanus;

(iv) in selected cases, it may be useful in controlling tension and irritabilty in cerebral spasticity.

The use of diazepam to treat short-term anxiety is inappropriate and unsuitable. Diazepam should be used to treat insomnia only when it is severe, disabling or subjecting the individual to extreme stress.

Dosage and administration For oral administration.

The lowest dose that can control the symptoms should be used and treatment should not be continued beyond 4 weeks.

Adults: Anxiety states: 2 mg three times daily up to 30 mg daily in divided doses.

Insomnia associated with anxiety: 5 mg to 15 mg before retiring.

Muscle spasms: 2 mg to 15 mg daily in divided doses up to 60 mg in severe spastic disorders such as cerebral spasticity, epilepsy and muscle spasms associated with upper-motor neurone disease.

In the control of muscle spasms as in tetanus: 3 mg to 10 mg/kg bodyweight daily.

Alcohol withdrawal symptoms: 5 mg to 20 mg repeated within 2 to 4 hours if necessary.

Premedication in dental patients: 5 mg the night before, 5 mg on waking and another 5 mg two hours before the appointment.

Children: Night terrors and somnabulism: 1 mg to 5 mg daily before retiring.

Premedication: 2 mg to 10 mg.

Management of cerebral spasticity: 2 mg to 40 mg daily in divided doses.

In the control of muscle spasms in tetanus: 3 mg to 10 mg/kg bodyweight daily.

Elderly or debilitated patients: The dosage should be half that recommended to adults.

Doses should be repeated only on medical advice. Long-term chronic use is not recommended and treatment should always be tapered off gradually. When a benzodiazepine is used as a hypnotic, treatment should, if possible, be intermittent.

Contra-indications, warnings, etc
Contra-indications: Patients with a known sensitivity to benzodiazepines; acute pulmonary insufficiency; respiratory depression.

Use in pregnancy and lactation: If the product is prescribed to a woman of childbearing potential, she should be warned to contact her physician regarding discontinuance of the product if she intends to become or suspects that she is pregnant. If, for compelling reasons, the product is administered during the late phase of pregnancy, or during labour at high doses, effects on the neonate, such as hypothermia, hypotonia and moderate respiratory depression, can be expected, due to the pharmacological action of the compound.

Moreover, infants born to mothers who took benzodiazepines chronically during the latter stages of pregnancy may have developed physical dependence and may be at some risk for developing withdrawal symptoms in the postnatal period.

Since benzodiazepines are found in the breast milk, benzodiazepines should not be given to breast feeding mothers.

Warnings: The lowest dose that can control the symptoms should be used and treatment should not be continued beyond 4 weeks. The risk of dependence increases when high dosages are attained, especially when given over long periods. This is particularly so in patients with a history of alcoholism, drug abuse or in patients with marked personality disorders.

Treatment should always be tapered off gradually. Sudden cessation of treatment can result in symptoms such as depression, nervousness, rebound insomnia, irritability, sweating and diarrhoea even in patients receiving normal therapeutic doses for short periods of time. Abrupt withdrawal following high dosage may produce confusion, toxic psychosis, convulsions or a condition resembling delirium tremens.

Diazepam should not be used to treat chronic psychoses or phobic or obsessional states. Because diazepam-induced disinhibition may precipitate suicidal or aggressive behaviour, it should not be used alone to treat depression or anxiety related depression. Caution must be exercised when treating patients with personality disorders.

Elderly or debilitated patients may be more prone

to adverse effects and care must be taken in patients with impaired liver or kidney function. Care is also required in patients with organic brain disease (particularly arteriosclerosis).

Diazepam should be avoided in cases of loss or bereavement as psychological adjustment may be inhibited by benzodiazepines.

Patients should be advised to avoid driving or operating machinery as diazepam, particularly when combined with alcohol, can reduce alertness and performance of skilled tasks.

Interactions: Sedation, or respiratory or cardiovascular depression may be enhanced if diazepam is combined with centrally acting drugs such as alcohol, anaesthetics, analgesics, antidepressants, hypnotics, neuroleptics and tranquillisers. Diazepam is primarily metabolised by hepatic microsomal oxidation and drugs which affect liver enzymes, such as cimetidine and phenobarbitone, may alter its pharmacokinetics. Diazepam has been reported to be displaced from protein-binding sites by sodium valproate.

Side-effects: Diazepam may cause drowsiness, sedation, blurring of vision, unsteadiness and ataxia. These may occur after a single as well as repeated doses and persist to the following day. Less common effects include vertigo, headache, confusion, slurred speech, visual disturbance, tremor, changes in libido, skin rashes and gastro-intestinal upset. Jaundice or blood dyscrasias have been reported rarely. High doses may be associated with respiratory depression or hypotension.

Abnormal psychological reactions to benzodiazepines have been reported. Rare behavioural adverse effects include paradoxical aggressive outbursts, excitement, confusion and the uncovering of depression with suicidal tendencies.

Overdosage: The symptoms of overdosage may include drowsiness, ataxia and dysarthria with coma or cardio-respiratory depression in very severe cases. Treatment should be symptomatic. Flumazenil is a specific antidote for use in emergency situations under close hospital supervision.

Pharmaceutical precautions Diazepam Syrup and Diazepam Forte Syrup should be stored below 25°C, protected from light.

Legal category CD (Sch 4), POM.

Package quantities Syrup 2 mg/5 ml: Bottles of 100 ml and 500 ml
Forte Syrup 5 mg/5 ml: Bottles of 100 ml

Further information Nil.

Product licence numbers

Syrup 2 mg/5 ml	4416/0026
Forte Syrup 5 mg/5 ml	4416/0067

DIAZEPAM RECTAL TUBES

Presentation Polyethylene tube containing 5 mg or 10 mg diazepam, in approximately 2.5 ml volume. The non-active ingredients include benzoic acid, sodium benzoate, ethanol, propylene glycol, benzyl alcohol and water.

Actions: Diazepam has a anticonvulsant, anxiolytic, sedative, muscle relaxant and amnesic properties.

It is indicated:

(i) for the short-term relief (2–4 weeks only) of anxiety that is severe, disabling or subjecting the individual to unacceptable distress, occurring alone or in association with insomnia or short-term psychosomatic, organic or psychotic illness;
(ii) as a sedative and premedicant;
(iii) as an anticonvulsant in the management of status epilepticus, febrile convulsions and poisoning;
(iv) in the control of muscle spasms as in tetanus;
(v) in the management of alcohol withdrawal symptoms.

The use of diazepam to treat short-term anxiety is inappropriate and unsuitable. Diazepam should be used to treat insomnia only when it is severe, disabling or subjecting the individual to extreme stress.

Dosage and administration For rectal administration only. Tubes are for single use only.

The lowest dose that can control the symptoms should be used and treatment should not be continued beyond 4 weeks.

Adults and children over 3 years: One 10 mg tube. If a child is particularly small, then consideration should be given to reducing the dose to one 5 mg tube and reducing the depth of insertion.

Children 1 to 3 years: One 5 mg tube. Insert the tube to about half-nozzle length (approx 2.5 cm).

Children under 1: Not recommended.

Elderly and debilitated patients: The dosage should be half that recommended for adults.

For acute muscle spasm, acute anxiety or agitation use 10 mg and repeat if necessary after 4 hours.

For sedative cover during dental or other surgical and medical procedures, give a dose dependent on patient's response using 0.2 mg/kg body weight as a guide.

Doses should be repeated only on medical advice. Long-term chronic use is not recommended and treatment should always be tapered off gradually. When a benzodiazepine is used as a hypnotic, treatment should, if possible, be intermittent.

Contra-indications, warnings, etc

Contra-indications: Patients with a known sensitivity to benzodiazepines; acute pulmonary insufficiency; respiratory depression.

Use in pregnancy and lactation: If the product is prescribed to a woman of childbearing potential, she should be warned to contact her physician regarding discontinuance of the product if she intends to become or suspects that she is pregnant. If, for compelling reasons, the product is administered during the late phase of pregnancy, or during labour at high doses, effects on the neonate, such as hypothermia, hypotonia and moderate respiratory depression, can be expected, due to the pharmacological action of the compound.

Moreover, infants born to mothers who took benzodiazepines chronically during the latter stages of pregnancy may have developed physical dependence and may be at some risk for developing withdrawal symptoms in the postnatal period.

Since benzodiazepines are found in the breast milk, benzodiazepines should not be given to breast feeding mothers.

Warnings: The lowest dose that can control the symptoms should be used and treatment should not be continued beyond 4 weeks. The risk of dependence increases when high dosages are attained, especially when given over long periods. This is particularly so in patients with a history of alcoholism, drug abuse or in patients with marked personality disorders.

Treatment should always be tapered off gradually. Sudden cessation of treatment can result in symptoms such as depression, nervousness, rebound insomnia, irritability, sweating and diarrhoea even in patients receiving normal therapeutic doses for short periods of time. Abrupt withdrawal following high dosage may produce confusion, toxic psychosis, convulsions or a condition resembling delirium tremens.

Diazepam should not be used to treat chronic psychoses or phobic or obsessional states. Because diazepam-induced disinhibition may precipitate suicidal or aggressive behaviour, it should not be used alone to treat depression or anxiety related depression. Caution must be exercised when treating patients with personality disorders.

Elderly or debilitated patients may be more prone to adverse effects an care must be taken in patients with impaired liver or kidney function. Care is also required in patients with organic brain disease (particularly arteriosclerosis).

Diazepam should be avoided in cases of loss or bereavement as psychological adjustment may be inhibited by benzodiazepines.

Patients should be advised to avoid driving or operating machinery as diazepam, particularly when combined with alcohol, can reduce alertness and performance of skilled tasks.

Interactions: Sedation, or respiratory or cardiovascular depression may be enhanced if diazepam is combined with centrally acting drugs such as alcohol, anaesthetics, analgesics, antidepressants, hypnotics, neuroleptics and tranquillisers. Diazepam is primarily metabolised by hepatic microsomal oxidation and drugs which affect liver enzymes, such as cimetidine and phenobarbitone, may alter its pharmacokinetics. Diazepam has been reported to be displaced from protein-binding sites by sodium valproate.

Side-effects: Diazepam may cause drowsiness, sedation, blurring of vision, unsteadiness and ataxia. These may occur after a single as well as repeated doses and persist to the following day. Less common effects include vertigo, headache, confusion, slurred speech, visual disturbance, tremor, changes in libido, skin rashes and gastro-intestinal upset. Jaundice or blood dyscrasias have been reported rarely. High doses may be associated with respiratory depression or hypotension.

Abnormal psychological reactions to benzodiazepines have been reported. Rare behavioural adverse effects include paradoxical aggressive outbursts, excitement, confusion and the uncovering of depression with suicidal tendencies.

Overdosage: The symptoms of overdosage may include drowsiness, ataxia and dysarthria with coma or cardio-respiratory depression in very severe cases. Treatment should be symptomatic. Flumazenil is a specific antidote for use in emergency situations under close hospital supervision.

Pharmaceutical precautions Store in cool dry place below 22°C.

Legal category CD (Sch 4), POM.

Package quantities Pack of 5 tubes.

Further information Nil.

Product licence numbers

5 mg rectal tube	4416/0027
10 mg rectal tube	4416/0028

DOXYLAR*/DOXYCYCLINE CAPSULES BP 50 mg

Qualitative and quantative composition Each capsule contains Doxycycline Hydrochloride BP equivalent to 50 mg Doxycycline.

Pharmaceutical form Capsule.

Clinical particulars

Therapeutic indications: Doxycycline is clinically useful in the treatment of a variety of infections caused by susceptible strains of gram-positive and gram-negative bacteria and certain other micro-organisms. These include:

Respiratory tract infections: Lower respiratory tract infections including pneumonia, due to susceptible strains of *Haemophilis influenzae*, *Klebsiella pneumoniae*, *Streptococcus pneumoniae* and other organisms. *Mycoplasma pneumoniae* pneumonia. The treatment of chronic bronchitis and sinusitis.

Dermatological infections: Doxycycline can be used in the treatment of acne vulgaris in cases where antibiotic therapy is considered necessary.

Urinary infections: Infections caused by susceptible strains of Klebsiella, Enterobacter, *Escherichia coli*, *Streptococcus faecalis* and other organisms.

Sexually transmitted diseases: Infections including uncomplicated urethral, endocervical or rectal infections due to *Chlamydia trachomatis*, non-gonoccal urethritis, caused by *Ureaplasma urealyticum* (t-mycoplasma). Doxycycline can also be used to treat chancroid and infections due to *Calymmatobacterium granulomatis* or as an alternative drug for the treatment of gonorrhoea and syphilis.

As a member of the tetracycline group of antibiotics, Doxycycline may be useful in the treatment of infections due to other tetracycline-sensitive micro-organisms such as:

Ophthalmic infections: Due to *Haemophilus influenzae* and susceptible strains of gonococci and staphylococci. Doxycycline is indicated in the treatment of trachoma. Inclusion conjunctivitis may be treated with oral doxycycline alone, or in combination with topical medication.

Rickettsial infections: Tick fevers, Q fever, rocky mountain spotted fever, coxiella endocarditis and typhus group.

Prophylaxis: Doxycycline is also indicated in the prophylactic treatment of leptospirosis, scrub typhus, travellers' diarrhoea (entero-toxigenic *Escherichia coli*).

Miscellaneous: Psittacosis, leptospirosis, cholera, meliodosis, other infections due to susceptible strains of yersinia species, brucella species (in combination with streptomycin), clostridium species, *Francisella tularensis* and chloroquine-resistant falciparum malaria.

Posology and method of administration:

Adults: 200 mg on the first day (administered as a single dose or divided into 2 equal doses with a 12 hour interval) followed by a maintenance dose of 100 mg/day. For more severe infections (particularly chronic infections of the urinary tract) 200 mg should be given throughout the treatment.

Children over 12 years of age: Normal adult dose should be given. Not recommended for use for children under 12 years of age (see *contra-indications*).

Elderly: Doxycyline may be prescribed in the usual dose with no special precautions. No dosage adjustment is necessary in the presence of renal impairment.

It is recommended that patients over 70 years of age are specifically instructed regarding the administration of doxycycline.

An adequate volume of fluid should be taken when administering Doxycycline capsules; this should preferably be taken in an upright position and not immediately before going to bed.

If gastric irritation occurs Doxycyline should be given with food or milk.

Treatment should be continued at least 24 to 48 hours after fever and symptoms have subsided. When used in Streptococcal infections, therapy should be continued for 10 days to prevent the development of rheumatic fever or glomerulo-nephritis.

Specific infections: Acne vulgaris: 50 mg daily with food or fluid for 6 to 12 weeks.

Sexually transmitted diseases: For the treatment of

uncomplicated gonococcal infections (except anorectal infections in males), uncomplicated urethral, endocervical or rectal infections caused by *Chlamydia trachomatis*, or non-gonococcal urethritis caused by *Ureaplasma urealyticum*, 100 mg should be taken twice daily for 7 days.

For the treatment of acute epididymo-orchitis caused by *Chlamydia trachomatis* or *Neisseria gonorrhoeae*; 100 mg twice daily for 10 days.

For the treatment of primary and secondary syphilis: 300 mg a day in divided doses for at least 10 days.

Louse and tick-borne relapsing fevers: A single dose of 100 mg or 200 mg according to severity.

Chloroquine-resistant falciparum malaria: 200 mg to be taken daily for at least 7 days. A quick-acting schizonticide such as quinine should be used in conjunction with Doxycycline because of the potential severity of the infection. Recommended dosages for quinine vary in different areas.

Prophylaxis: For the prevention of travellers' diarrhoea in adults: 200 mg on the first day of travel (administered as a single dose or as 100 mg every 12 hours), followed by 100 mg daily throughout the stay in the area.

For the prevention of scrub typhus: 200 mg to be taken as a single dose.

For the prevention of Leptospirosis: 200 mg to be taken once a week throughout the stay in the area and 200 mg at the end of the trip.

Contra-indications: Doxycycline should not be administered to patients who have shown hypersensitivity to tetracyclines.

Doxycycline is also contra-indicated in pregnancy, infancy and childhood up to 12 years of age. The use of tetracyclines during tooth development may cause permanent discolouration of the teeth (yellow-grey-brown). This reaction is more common during long term use of the drug but has been observed following repeated short term courses. Enamel hypoplasia has also been reported.

As for other tetracyclines, Doxycyline forms a stable calcium complex in any bone-forming tissue. A decrease in the fibula growth rate has been observed in prematures given oral tetracycline in doses of 25 mg/kg every 6 hours. This reaction was shown to be reversible when the drug was discontinued.

Special warnings and precautions for use: Doxycycline should be administered with caution to patients with hepatic impairment or those receiving potentially hepatotoxic drugs.

Care should be taken in the treatment of patients with myasthenia gravis who may be at risk of neuromuscular blockade.

Patients taking Doxycycline should be warned that exposure to strong sunlight or ultraviolet light may experience photosensitivity appearing as a severe sunburn reaction. Treatment should cease at the first sign of skin erythema.

In the treatment of venereal disease where co-existent syphilis is suspected, formal diagnostic procedures including dark-field examinations should be employed and monthly serological tests should be conducted for at least 4 months.

Infections due to group A beta haemolytic streptococci should be treated for at least 10 days.

Overgrowth of non-susceptible organisms may occur when using antibiotics. Continued observation of the patient is necessary and if a resistant organism appears, antibiotic therapy should be discontinued and appropriate measures instituted.

Interactions with other medicaments and other forms of interaction: Patients on anticoagulant therapy may require a reduction in anticoagulant dosage as tetracyclines have been shown to depress plasma prothrombin activity.

Since bacteriostatic drugs may interfere with the bactericidal action of penicillin, Doxycycline should not be administered in conjunction with penicillins.

Antacids containing aluminium, calcium, magnesium or zinc, bismuth chelates, sucralfate and iron-containing compounds impair absorption and should therefore not be given to patients taking Doxycycline.

The concurrent use of tetracyclines and methoxyflurane has been reported to result in fatal renal toxicity.

Barbiturates, carbamazepine, primidone and phenytoin have been reported to decrease the half-life of Doxycycline.

A few cases of pregnancy or breakthrough bleeding have been attributed to the concurrent use of tetracycline or oxytetracycline with oral contraceptives.

Doxycycline used concurrently with cyclosporins has been reported to increase the plasma concentration of cyclosporin.

Pregnancy and lactation: Use of Doxycycline is contra-indicated during pregnancy as it can have toxic effects on the developing foetus.

Tetracyclines are also found in the milk of lactating women receiving Doxycycline therapy and should therefore not be used in nursing mothers (see *Contra-indications* about tooth development).

Effects on ability to drive and use machines: Nausea has been reported.

Undesirable effects: Doxycycline is almost completely absorbed and therefore gastro-intestinal side-effects are infrequent. The following undesirable effects have been observed in patients receiving tetracyclines.

Gastro-intestinal: Nausea, vomiting, anorexia, dysphagia, glossitis, diarrhoea, enterocolitis and inflammatory lesions with monilial overgrowth in the ano-genital region. Oesophagitis and oesophageal ulceration have also been reported. A high proportion of these occurrences involved the hydrochloride salt in capsule form and taking medication immediately before going to bed.

Skin: Maculo papular and erythematous rashes. Skin photosensitivity is addressed under *Other special warnings and precautions*. Exfoliative dermatitis has been reported but is uncommon.

Renal: An apparently dose related rise in blood urea has been reported with tetracyclines.

Blood: Thrombocytopenia, neutropenia, haemolytic anaemia and eosinophilia have been reported with tetracyclines.

Hypersensitivity reactions: Exacerbation of systemic lupus erythematosus, anaphylaxis, anaphylactoid purpura, pericarditis, urticaria and angioneurotic oedema.

Other: Bulging fontanelles in infants and benign intracranial hypertension in adults has been reported with the use of tetracyclines. Treatment should cease if evidence of raised intracranial pressure develops. These conditions disappeared rapidly when the drug was discontinued.

Brown-black microscopic discolouration of thyroid tissue has been reported with long-term use of tetracyclines. Thyroid function is normal.

Overdose: Acute overdosage with antibiotics is rare. In the event of overdosage, gastric lavage and other supportive measures are indicated.

Pharmacological properties

Pharmacodynamic properties: Doxycycline is a broad-spectrum antibiotic.

Pharmacokinetic properties: Doxycycline hydrochloride is readily absorbed from the gastro-intestinal tract and absorption is not significantly affected by the presence of food. Following an oral dose of 200 mg, the plasma concentration of the drug reaches a level of 2.6 µg/ml after 2 hours, falling to 1.45 µg/ml at 24 hours. Up to 95% is bound to plasma protein and the half life ranges from 15–25 hours.

Excretion is largely in the faeces as an inactive conjugate or chelate, and approximately 40% may be excreted in the urine.

Preclinical safety data: Not required.

Pharmaceutical particulars

List of Excipients: Maize starch, magnesium stearate, talc, lactose.

Capsule Shell: Green cap: yellow iron oxide (E 172), indigotine (E132), titanium dioxide (E 171) gelatin. White body: titanium dioxide (E 171), gelatin.

Incompatibilities: Not known.

Shelf life: 3 years.

Special precautions for storage: Store in a dry place.

Nature and contents of container: Blister strips composes of 300 µm polypropylene 16 µm aluminium foil packed in outer cartons.

Pack size: 28.

Instruction for use/handling: Not applicable.

Marketing authorisation number: PL 04416/0264.

Date of (partial) revision of the text May 1995.

Legal category POM.

DOXYLAR*/DOXYCYCLINE CAPSULES BP 100 mg

Presentation Dark green capsules printed LAGAP DOX 100, containing Doxycycline Hydrochloride BP equivalent to 100 mg Doxycycline.

Uses

Indications: Doxycycline is clinically useful in the treatment of a variety of infections caused by susceptible strains of gram-positive and gram-negative bacteria and certain other micro-organisms. These include:

Respiratory tract infections: lower respiratory tract infections including pneumonia, due to susceptible strains of *Haemophilus influenzae, Klebsiella pneumoniae, Streptococcus pneumoniae* and other organisms. *Mycoplasma pneumoniae* pneumonia. The treatment of chronic bronchitis and sinusitis.

Urinary infections: Infections caused by susceptible strains of klebsiella, enterobactor, *Escherichia coli, Streptococcus faecaelis* and other organisms.

Sexually transmitted diseases: Infections including uncomplicated urethral, endocervical or rectal infections due to *Chlamydia trachomatis*, non-gonoccal urethritis, caused by *Ureaplasma urelyticulum* (T-mycoplasma). Doxycycline can also be used to treat chancroid and infections due to *Calymmatobacterium granulomatis* or as an alternative drug for the treatment of gonorrhoea and syphilis.

As a member of the tetracycline group of antibiotics, doxycycline may be useful in the treatment of infections due to other tetracycline-sensitive micro-organisms such as:

Ophthalmic infections: Due to *Haemophilus influenzae* and susceptible strains of gonococci and staphylococci. Doxycycline is indicated in the treatment of trachoma. Inclusion conjunctivitis may be treated with oral doxycycline alone, or in combination with topical medication.

Rickettsial infections: Tick Fevers, Q Fever, Rocky Mountain Spotted Fever, Coxiella endocarditis and typhus group.

Prophylaxis: Doxycycline is also indicated in the prophylactic treatment of leptospirosis, scrub typhus and travellers' diarrhoea (entero-toxigenic *Escherichia coli*).

Miscellaneous: Psittacosis, leptospirosis, cholera, meliodosis, other infections due to susceptible strains of yersinia species, brucella species (in combination with streptomycin), clostridum species, *Francisella tularensis* and chloroquine-resistant falciparum malaria.

Dosage and administration

Recommended doses:

Adults: 200 mg on the first day (administered as a single dose or divided into 2 equal doses with a 12 hour interval) followed by a maintenance dose of 100 mg/day. For more severe infections (particularly chronic infections of the urinary tract) 200 mg should be given throughout the treatment.

Children (over 12 years of age): Normal adult dose should be given. Not recommended for use for children under 12 years of age (see *Contra-indications*).

Elderly: Doxycyline may be prescribed in the usual dose with no special precautions. No dosage adjustment is necessary in the presence of renal impairment.

It is recommended that patients over 70 years of age are specifically instructed regarding the administration of doxycycline.

An adequate volume of fluid should be taken when administering doxycycline capsules; this should preferably be taken in an upright position and *not* immediately before going to bed.

If gastric irritation occurs doxycycline should be given with food or milk.

Treatment should be continued at least 24 to 48 hours after fever and symptoms have subsided. When used in streptococcal infections, therapy should be continued for 10 days to prevent the development of rheumatic fever or glomerulo-nephritis.

Specific infections: Sexually transmitted diseases: For the treatment of uncomplicated gonococcal infections (except anorectal infections in males), uncomplicated urethral, endocervical or rectal infections caused by *Chlamydia trachomatis*, or non-gonococcal urethritis caused by *Ureaplasma urealyticum*, 100 mg should be taken twice daily for 7 days.

For the treatment of acute epididymo-orchitis caused by *Chlamydia trachomatis* or *Neisseria gonorrhoeae*; 100 mg twice daily for 10 days.

For the treatment of primary and secondary syphilis: 300 mg a day in divided doses for at least 10 days.

Louse and tick-borne relapsing fevers: A single dose of 100 mg or 200 mg according to severity.

Chloroquine-resistant falciparum malaria: 200 mg to be taken daily for at least 7 days. A quick-acting schizonticide such as quinine should be used in conjunction with doxycycline because of the potential severity of the infection. Recommended dosages for quinine vary in different areas.

Prophylaxis: For the prevention of travellers' diarrhoea in adults: 200 mg on the first day of travel (administered as a single dose or as 100 mg every 12 hours), followed by 100 mg daily throughout the stay in the area.

For the prevention of scrub typhus: 200 mg to be taken as a single dose.

For the prevention of leptospirosis: 200 mg to be taken once a week throughout the stay in the area and 200 mg at the end of the trip.

Contra-indications, warnings, etc

Contra-indications: Doxycycline should not be administered to patients who have shown hypersensitivity to tetracyclines.

Doxycycline is also contra-indicated in pregnancy, lactation, infancy and childhood up to 12 years of age. The use of tetracyclines during tooth development may cause permanent discolouration of the teeth (yellow-grey-brown). This reaction is more common during long term use of the drug but has been observed following repeated short term courses. Enamel hypoplasia has also been reported.

As for other tetracyclines, doxycyline forms a stable calcium complex in any bone-forming tissue. A decrease in the fibula growth has been observed in prematures given oral tetracyclines in doses of 25 mg/kg every 6 hours. This reaction was shown to be reversible when the drug was discontinued.

Interactions with other medicaments and other forms of interaction: Patients on anticoagulant therapy may require a reduction in anticoagulant dosage as tetracyclines have been shown to depress plasma prothrombin activity.

Since bacteriostatic drugs may interfere with the bactericidal action of penicillin, doxycycline should not be administered in conjunction with penicillins.

Antacids containing aluminium, calcium, magnesium or zinc, bismuth chelates, sucralfate or iron-containing compounds impair absorption and should therefore not be given to patients taking doxycycline.

The concurrent use of tetracyclines and methoxyflurane has been reportd to result in fatal renal toxicity.

Barbiturates, carbamazepine, primidone and phenytoin have been reported to decrease the half-life of doxycycline.

A few cases of pregnancy or breakthrough bleeding have been attributed to the concurrent use of tetracycline or oxytetracycline with oral contraceptives.

Doxycycline used concurrently with cyclosporins has been reported to increase the plasma concentration of cyclosporin.

Effects on ability to drive and to use machines: Nausea has been reported.

Other undesirable effects: Doxycycline is almost completely absorbed and therefore gastro-intestinal side-effects are infrequent. The following undesirable effects have been observed in patients receiving tetracyclines.

Gastro-intestinal: Nausea, vomiting, anorexia, dysphagia, glossitis, diarrhoea, enterocolitis and inflammatory lesions with monilial overgrowth in the ano-genital region. Oesophagitis and oesophageal ulceration have also been reported. A high proportion of these occurrences involved the hydrochloride salt in capsule form and taking medication immediately before going to bed.

Skin: Maculo papular and erythematous rashes. Skin photosensitivity is addressed under *Other special warnings and precautions.* Exfoliative dermatitis has been reported but is uncommon.

Renal: An apparently dose related rise in blood urea has been reported with tetracyclines.

Blood: Thrombocytopenia, neutropenia, haemolytic anaemia and eosinophilia have been reported with tetracyclines.

Hypersensitivity reactions: Exacerbation of systemic lupus erythematosus, anaphylaxis, anaphylactoid purpura, pericarditis, urticaria and angioneurotic oedema.

Other: Bulging fontanelles in infants and benign intracranial hypertension in adults has been reported with the use of tetracyclines. Treatment should cease if evidence of raised intracranial pressure develops. These conditions disappeared rapidly when the drug was discontinued.

Brown-black microscopic discolouration of thyroid tissue has been reported with long-term use of tetracyclines. Thyroid function is normal.

Use in pregnancy and lactation: Use of doxycycline is contra-indicated during pregnancy as it can have toxic effects on the developing foetus.

Tetracyclines are also found in the milk of lactating women receiving doxycycline therapy and should therefore not be used in nursing mothers (see *Contra-indications* about tooth development).

Other special warnings and precautions: Doxycycline should be administered with caution to patients with hepatic impairment, acute porphyria or those receiving potentially hepatotoxic drugs.

Care should be taken in the treatment of patients with myasthenia gravis who may be at risk of neuromuscular blockade.

Patients taking doxycycline should be warned that exposure to strong sunlight or ultraviolet light may experience photosensitivity appearing as a severe sunburn reaction. Treatment should cease at the first sign of skin erythema.

In the treatment of venereal disease where co-existent syphilis is suspected, formal diagnostic procedures including dark-field examinations should be employed and monthly serological tests should be conducted for at least 4 months.

Infections due to a group A beta haemolytic streptococci should be treated for at least 10 days.

Overgrowth of non-susceptible organisms may occur when using antibiotics. Continued observation of the patient is necessary and if a resistant organism appears, antibiotic therapy should be discontinued and appropriate measures instituted.

Overdose: Acute overdosage with antibiotics is rare. In the event of overdosage, gastric lavage and other supportive measures are indicated.

Incompatibilities: Not known.

Pharmaceutical precautions Store in a cool dry place. Protect from light.

Legal category POM.

Package quantities Packs of 8 and 50 capsules.

Further information Nil.

Product licence number 4416/0007.

HYPOLAR* RETARD 20

Qualitative and quantitative composition Each tablet contains 20 mg nifedipine PhEur in a modified release formulation.

Pharmaceutical form Modified release tablets.

Clinical particulars

Therapeutic indications: Hypolar Retard 20 tablets are indicated for the treatment of hypertension and the prophylaxis of chronic stable angina pectoris.

Hypolar Retard 20 has no therapeutic antiarrhythmic effect.

Posology and route of administration: These tablets should be swallowed with a glass of water. They must be swallowed whole and not broken or chewed.

Adults: The recommended starting dose of nifedipine is 10 mg every 12 hours swallowed with water with subsequent titration of dosage according to response. The dose may be adjusted to 40 mg every 12 hours.

Elderly: The pharmacokinetics of nifedipine are altered in the elderly so that lower maintenance doses of nifedipine may be required compared to younger patients.

Nifedipine is metabolised primarily by the liver and therefore patients with liver dysfunction should be carefully monitored. Patients with renal impairment should not require adjustment of dosage.

Treatment with Hypolar Retard 20 may be continued long term.

Children: Nifedipine is not recommended for use in children.

Route of administration: Oral.

Contra-indications: Nifedipine has been shown to be teratogenic in animals and therefore Hypolar Retard 20 tablets should not be administered to women who are pregnant or may become pregnant and to nursing mothers.

Other contra-indications:

- Patients with cardiogenic shock.
- Hypersensitivity to nifedipine or other dihydropyridines because of the theoretical risk of cross reactivity.
- Nifedipine should not be used in clinically significant aortic stenosis, unstable angina, or during or within one month of a myocardial infarction.
- Nifedipine should not be used for the treatment of acute attacks of angina.
- The safety of nifedipine in malignant hypertension has not been established.
- Nifedipine should not be used for secondary prevention of myocardial infarction.
- Nifedipine should not be administered concomitantly with rifampicin since effective plasma levels of nifedipine may not be achieved owing to enzyme induction.

Special warnings and special precautions for use: Hypolar Retard 20 should be used with caution in patients with severe hypotension and in patients whose cardiac reserve is poor.

Cardiac ischaemic pain has been reported to have occurred in some patients within 1 to 4 hours of receiving nifedipine. In such cases treatment should be discontinued.

Caution should be exercised when Hypolar Retard 20 is given to diabetic patients as they may require adjustment of their diabetic therapy.

In patients with malignant hypertension and hypovolaemia who are on dialysis, a significant decrease in blood pressure can occur.

Interactions with other medicaments and other forms of interaction: Hypolar Retard 20 may be used in combined therapy with other antihypertensive agents including beta-blockers where an additive or synergistic hypotensive effect is to be expected. Withdrawal of any previous antihypertensive agents should be gradual as nifedipine will not compensate for any possible rebound effects.

As with other dihydropyridines, nifedipine should not be taken with grapefruit juice because bioavailability is increased.

Cimetidine may potentiate the antihypertensive effect of Hypolar Retard 20 if it is administered simultaneously.

Nifedipine should not be administered concomitantly with rifampicin since effective plasma levels of nifedipine, may not be achieved owing to enzyme induction (see *Contra-indications*).

It is reported that serum quinidine levels have been shown to be reduced when it is used in combination with nifedipine.

The simultaneous administration of nifedipine and digoxin may lead to reduced digoxin clearance and hence an increase in the plasma digoxin. Digoxin levels should be monitored and, if necessary, the digoxin dose reduced.

Other reactions reported include increased plasma levels of theophylline and phenytoin when used in combination with nifedipine and the enhanced effect of non-polarising muscle relaxants such as tubocurarine.

Pregnancy and lactation: As nifedipine has been shown to be teratogenic in animals, Hypolar Retard 20 should not be administered to women who are pregnant or may become pregnant and to nursing mothers.

Effects on ability to drive and use machines: Nausea, headaches, lethargy and dizziness have been reported to occur and therefore the patient should be warned of these possible effects.

Undesirable effects: Exacerbation of angina pectoris may occur rarely at the start of treatment with modified release formulations of nifedipine. The occurrence of myocardial infarction has been described although it is not possible to distinguish such an event from the natural course of ischaemic heart disease.

The most common side effects reported are dizziness, flushing, headaches, hypotension, tachycardia and palpitations and ankle swelling. Other less common side effects include gastrointestinal disturbances, increased micturition, rash, pruritus and urticaria, nausea, lethargy, paraesthesiae, myalgia, tremor and visual disturbances. Gingival hyperplasia has been reported to occur, and in older men gynaecomastia following long term therapy, however both these conditions are reversible on withdrawal of the drug.

There have been reports of rare cases of hypersensitivity-type jaundice. Liver function disturbances such as intra-hepatic cholestasis may also occur. Discontinuation of therapy will result in regression of these side effects.

Overdosage: This may be associated with severe hypotension, tachycardia or bradycardia and unconsciousness although there are few reports and the symptoms are not necessarily dose-related.

The metabolic disturbances which can occur include hyperglycaemia, metabolic acidosis and hypo- or hyperkalaemia. The cardiac effects which may occur include heart block, AV dissociation and asystole and cardiogenic shock with pulmonary oedema.

Other effects include drowsiness, dizziness, confusion, nausea, vomiting, lethargy, flushing and hypoxia.

In the treatment of overdosage it is important to restore stable cardiovascular conditions as soon as possible and achieve total elimination of nifedipine.

Gastric lavage and charcoal instillation may be of assistance if the patient is found early after the overdose. Gastric lavage may be necessary in combination with irrigation of the small intestine. Ipecacuanha should be given to children.

Activated charcoal should be given in 4 hourly doses of 25 g for adults and 10 g for children. The patient should be carefully monitored.

Hypotension should be treated by placing the patient in the supine position with the feet raised and the use of plasma expanders, as appropriate. If necessary, intravenous administration of 10% calcium gluconate 10–20 ml over a period of 5–10 minutes may be appropriate. Beta-sympathomimetics may be given e.g.: isoprenaline. If the blood pressure response is inadequate with calcium and isoprenaline, vasoconstricting sympathomimetics such as dopamine or noradrenaline should be administered. The patient's response should determine the dosage of these drugs.

If bradycardia persists the patient may be treated with atropine, beta-sympathomimetics or a temporary cardiac pacemaker.

It has also been reported that the use of metaraminol combined with calcium salts has been beneficial.

Care should be exercised with any additional fluids given to avoid cardiac overload.

Pharmacological properties

Pharmacodynamic properties: Nifedipine is a dihydropyridine and is a potent antagonist of calcium influx through the slow channel of the cell membrane of cardiac and smooth muscle cells. Nifedipine also binds to intracellular calcium binding proteins. Calcium is normally released from the sarcoplasmic reticulum intracellularly and this combined with the influx of extracellular calcium results in enhanced binding calcium to calmodulin. Calcium channel blockers such as nifedipine act as arteriolar dilators by inhibiting this calcium entry into the channel. The effects are more pronounced on vascular smooth muscle because depolarisation of cardiac muscle cells is dependent on both sodium ion influx and calcium ion influx and also nifedipine has little effect on the rate of recovery of the slow calcium channel.

Nifedipine is known to be an effective and relatively well tolerated treatment for angina and mild to severe hypertension.

The antihypertensive effects of nifedipine are achieved by causing peripheral vasodilatation resulting in a reduction in peripheral resistance. Nifedipine reduces blood pressure in hypertension but has little or no effect in normotensive individuals.

Nifedipine produces its effects in the treatment of angina by reducing peripheral and coronary vascular resistance, leading to an increase in coronary blood flow, cardiac output and stroke volume and causing a decrease in after-load.

Pharmacokinetic properties: Nifedipine is rapidly and almost completely absorbed from the gastro-instestinal tract after oral administration, however due to extensive hepatic first pass metabolism the resultant bioavailability lies between 45% and 75%.

Hypolar Retard 20 is a modified release preparation designed to release Nifedipine over a period of time. Following a pharmacokinetic study in volunteers it was found that the average time to reach maximum plasma concentration was 2.2 hours and the mean peak plasma concentration was found to be 58.5 ng/ml. The average elimination half-life was found to be 17.3 hours. Nifedipine is highly bound to plasma protein.

Preclinical safety data: Not required.

Pharmaceutical particulars

List of excipients: Microcrystalline cellulose, lactose, corn starch, talc, hydroxypropyl methyl cellulose, magnesium stearate, polysorbate 80, polyethylene glycol 4000, iron oxide (E172), and titanium dioxide (E171).

Incompatibilities: None reported.

Shelf life: 3 years.

Special precautions for storage: Store in dry place below 25°C. Protect from light.

Nature and contents of container: Blister strips composed of PVC foil 250 μm±5%, PVdC 25 μm±5%, aluminium foil 25 μm±8%, PVdC 20 μm±10%.

Pack size: 56.

Instructions for use/handling: Not applicable.

Marketing authorisation number 4416/0245.

Date of revision of SPC 5 December 1997.

Legal category POM.

INDOLAR* SR

Presentation Blue/colourless capsules containing white sustained release beads. Each capsule containing 75 mg Indomethacin BP.

Inactive ingredients: Sucrose; Lactose.

Uses Non-steroidal analgesic and anti-inflammatory agent indicated in active rheumatoid arthritis, osteoarthritis, ankylosing spondylitis, degenerative joint disease of the hip, acute musculo-skeletal disorders and low back pain. Also indicated in periarticular disorders such as bursitis, tendinitis, synovitis, tenosynovitis and capsulitis. Also indicated in inflammation, pain and oedema following orthopaedic procedures and the treatment of pain and associated symptoms of primary dysmenorrhoea.

Dosage and administration Indolar SR Capsules should always be given with food or milk to reduce the chance of gastro-intestinal disturbance.

To minimise the evolution of unwanted reactions it is helpful in chronic conditions to start the therapy with a low dosage, increasing as required.

Adults: One capsule once or twice daily, depending on patient needs and response.

Dosage in dysmenorrhoea: One capsule a day, starting with the onset of cramps or bleeding, and continuing for as long as symptoms usually last.

Children: Safety in children has not been established.

Elderly: Particular care should be taken with older patients who are more susceptible to side-effects from indomethacin.

Contra-indications, warnings, etc

Contra-indications: Patients with angioneurotic oedema or who have, with aspirin or other non-steroidal anti-inflammatory drugs experienced acute asthmatic attacks, urticaria or rhinitis.

Active peptic ulcer, a history of recurrent gastro-intestinal lesions, sensitivity to indomethacin or to aspirin.

Not to be used during pregnancy or during lactation as indomethacin is secreted in breast milk.

Safety in children has not been established.

Side-effects: The most common side-effects are headache, dizziness and dyspepsia; patients should be warned that they may experience dizziness and should therefore avoid driving or undertaking other activities which require full alertness. If headache persists even after dosage reduction indomethacin should be withdrawn.

Gastro-intestinal disorders which occur can be reduced by giving indomethacin with food, milk or antacids. Ulceration of the oesophagus, stomach or duodenum may also occur, accompanied by haemorrhage and perforation (a few fatalities have been reported).

Intestinal ulceration has rarely been associated with stenosis and obstruction. Also, bleeding without obvious ulceration and perforation of pre-existing sigmoid lesions (such as a diverticulum or carcinoma) have occurred; and increased abdominal pain in patients with ulcerative colitis (or the development of this condition) and regional ileitis have been rarely reported. If gastro-intestinal bleeding does occur treatment with indomethacin should be discontinued.

Blood dyscrasias, particularly thrombocytopenia have been reported.

Oedema and increased blood pressure also sometimes occur, as does haematuria.

Hypersensitivity reactions include pruritus, urticaria, angiitis, erythema nodosum. Skin rash and hair loss may also occur.

Acute respiratory distress, including sudden dyspnoea and asthma, have been reported on rare occasions. Bronchospasm may be precipitated in patients suffering from, or with a previous history of, bronchial asthma or allergic disease.

Indomethacin should be used with caution in patients with hepatic or renal dysfunction. Hepatitis and jaundice have been reported rarely.

Non-steroidal anti-inflammatory drugs may precipitate renal decompensation in those with renal or hepatic dysfunction, diabetes mellitus, advanced age, extracellular volume depletion, congestive cardiac failure, sepsis or concomitant use of other nephrotoxic drugs. Also, there have been reports of acute interstitial nephritis with haematuria, proteinuria and occasionally the nephrotic syndrome in long-term therapy with indomethacin.

In common with other anti-inflammatory analgesic antipyretic agents, indomethacin may mask the signs and symptoms of infectious disease and this should be borne in mind in order to avoid delay in starting treatment for infection.

Indomethacin should be used with caution in patients with an existing, albeit controlled infection.

Particular care should be taken with older patients who are more susceptible to side-effects from indomethacin.

Interactions: Co-administration of diflunisal with Indomethacin increases the plasma level of Indomethacin by about a third with a concomitant decrease in renal clearance. Fatal gastro-intestinal haemorrhage has occurred. The combination should not be used.

Use of indomethacin with aspirin or other salicylates is not recommended because there is no enhancement of therapeutic effect while the incidence of gastro-intestinal side-effects is increased. Moreover, co-administration of aspirin may decrease the blood concentration of indomethacin.

Indomethacin may decrease the tubular secretion of methotrexate thus potentiating toxicity; simultaneous use should be undertaken with caution.

Patients receiving anticoagulants should be observed carefully for alteration of prothrombin time even though clinical studies suggest no influence from indomethacin on hypoprothrombinaemia induced by anticoagulants.

Indomethacin can inhibit platelet aggregation – an effect which disappears within 24 hours of discontinuation; the bleeding time may be prolonged and this effect may be exaggerated in patients with an underlying haemostatic defect.

Indomethacin and triamterene should not be administered together since reversible renal failure may be induced.

Co-administration of probenecid may increase plasma levels of Indomethacin.

Because Indomethacin may reduce the antihypertensive effect of beta-blockers, patients receiving dual therapy should have the antihypertensive effect of their therapy reassessed.

If the patient is receiving corticosteroids concomitantly, a reduction in dosage of these may be possible, but should only be effected slowly under supervision.

Indomethacin is an inhibitor of prostaglandin synthesis and therefore the following drug interactions may occur; Indomethacin may raise plasma lithium levels and reduce renal lithium clearance in subjects with steady state plasma lithium concentrations. At the onset of such combined therapy, plasma lithium concentration should be monitored more frequently.

Indomethacin may reduce the diuretic and antihypertensive effect of thiazides and frusemide in some patients. Indomethacin may cause blocking of the frusemide-induced increase in plasma renin activity.

It is reported that a few patients receiving non-steroidal anti-inflammatory drugs manifest borderline elevations in liver function test results; if these persist or worsen or symptoms of liver disease, a rash or eosinophilia develop, treatment with indomethacin should be stopped. Periodic assessments to detect, at an early stage, unwanted effects on peripheral blood (anaemia) and liver function are advisable. The dexamethasone suppression test may give false negative results. An increase in plasma potassium concentration (including hyperkalaemia) has been reported even in the absence of renal impairment. Since indomethacin is eliminated primarily by the kidney, patients with impaired renal function should be monitored closely and a lower daily dosage may be needed to avoid accumulation.

Warnings and adverse reactions:

CNS: Headache, dizziness or lightheadedness, depression, vertigo and fatigue are not uncommon; infrequently there may be confusion, anxiety or other psychiatric disturbance, drowsiness, convulsions, neuropathy or paraesthesia, involuntary movements, insomnia, aggravation of epilepsy or Parkinsonism. All are often transient and likely to abate or disappear with reduced or ceased dosage.

Gastro-intestinal: Nausea, anorexia, vomiting, epigastric discomfort or abdominal pain, constipation or diarrhoea all have been reported; more rarely, stomatitis, flatulence, ulceration at any point in the gastro-intestinal tract (even with resultant stenosis and obstruction), bleeding (even without obvious ulceration or from a diverticulum) and perforation of pre-existing sigmoid lesions have all been reported.

Hepatic: Rarely hepatitis and jaundice (some fatalities have been reported).

Cardiovascular/renal: Oedema, increased blood pressure, hypotension, tachycardia, chest pain, arrhythmia, palpitations, congestive cardiac failure, elevation of blood urea and haematuria all have been reported infrequently.

In patients with renal, cardiac or hepatic impairment caution is required since the use of non-steroidal anti-inflammatory drugs may result in deterioration of renal function. The dose should be kept as low as possible and renal function should be monitored.

Non-steroidal anti-inflammatory drugs have been reported to cause nephrotoxicity in various forms and their use can lead to interstitial nephritis, nephrotic syndrome and renal failure.

Dermatological/hypersensitivity: Itching, urticaria, angioneurotic oedema, angiitis, erythema nodosum, rash and exfoliative dermatitis all have been reported infrequently – as have Stevens Johnson syndrome, erythema multiforme, toxic epidermal necrolysis, hair loss, acute anaphylaxis (including acute loss of blood pressure) and acute respiratory distress (including sudden dyspnoea, asthma and pulmonary oedema). There may be bronchospasm in patients with a history of bronchial asthma or other allergic disease.

Haematological: Blood dyscrasias (thrombocytopenia, leucopenia, petechiae, ecchymosis, purpura, aplastic or haemolytic anaemia, agranulocytosis and bone marrow depression, disseminated intravascular coagulation) may occur infrequently.

Ocular: Blurred vision and orbital and peri-orbital pain are seen infrequently. Corneal deposits and retinal disturbances have been reported in some patients with rheumatoid arthritis on prolonged therapy with indomethacin, and ophthalmic examinations are desirable in patients given prolonged treatment.

Aural: Tinnitus, or hearing disturbance (rarely deafness) have been reported.

Genito-urinary: Proteinuria, nephrotic syndrome, interstitial nephritis, renal insufficiency or failure all have been reported.

Other: Hyperglycaemia, glycosuria, hyperkalaemia, vaginal bleeding, epistaxis, breast changes (enlargement, tenderness, gynaecomastia), flushing, sweating and ulcerative stomatitis all have been reported rarely.

Overdosage: Many of the unwanted symptoms associated with indomethacin therapy may be seen. Treatment is symptomatic and supportive – emptying the stomach by induction of vomiting and/or lavage and use of activated charcoal. Antacid therapy may be useful. Close monitoring thereafter is required because intestinal ulceration may develop. It can be noted that indomethacin has a biphasic plasma elimination with the terminal phase showing a half-life ranging between 2 and 12 hours.

Pharmaceutical precautions Store in a cool, dry place and protect from light.

Legal category POM.

Package quantities 28, 56 and 100 capsules.

Further information Nil.

Product licence number 4416/0066.

KETOPROFEN CAPSULES BP 50 mg and 100 mg

Qualitative and quantitative composition Each capsule contains Ketoprofen BP 50 mg or 100 mg.

Pharmaceutical form Capsule.

Clinical particulars
Therapeutic indications: Ketoprofen capsules are recommended for the management of rheumatoid arthritis, osteoarthritis, ankylosing spondylitis, acute articular and periarticular disorders, fibrositis, cervical spondylitis, low back pain, painful musculoskeletal conditions and dysmenorrhoea. Ketoprofen reduces joint pain and inflammation, and facilitates increase in mobility and functional independence. As with other non-steroidal anti-inflammatory agents, it does not cure the underlying disease.

Posology and method of administration: Ketoprofen capsules should always be taken with food to reduce the occurrence of gastrointestinal disturbance.

Adults: 50–100 mg twice daily. The dosage can be altered depending on the patient weight and on the severity of symptoms.

Dysmenorhoea: 50 mg up to 3 times a day. Three to 4 days treatment is normally required from the outset of menstruation or symptoms of dysmenorrhoea.

Elderly: Caution should be used in treating the elderly. It is recommended that treatment be started at the lowest adult dose.

Children: Dosage has not been established.

Contra-indications: Ketoprofen should not be given to patients sensitive to aspirin or other non-steroidal anti-inflammatory agents. In such patients and in those suffering from, or with a history of, bronchial asthma or allergic disease, severe bronchospasm might be precipitated.

Ketoprofen is contra-indicated in patients with active peptic ulceration, a history of recurrent peptic ulceration or chronic dyspepsia, severe renal dysfunction.

Special warnings and special precautions for use: Ketoprofen capsules should always be given with food to limit gastrointestinal disturbance.

Ketoprofen should be used with caution in patients with cardiac, hepatic and renal impairment. Inhibition of renal prostaglandin synthesis by non-steroidal anti-inflammatory agents may interfere with renal function especially in the presence of existing renal disease.

Ketoprofen should also be used with caution in patients who have a history of bronchial asthma.

Interactions with other medicaments and other forms of interaction: Ketoprofen is highly protein-bound. If used concomitantly with other protein-binding drugs such as anticoagulants, sulphonamides or hydantoins an alteration in dosage level may be required to avoid increased levels of such drugs resulting from competition for plasma protein-binding sites. Similar acting drugs such as aspirin or other non-steroidal anti-inflammatory agents should not be administered concomitantly with ketoprofen as the potential for adverse reactions is increased.

Serious interactions have been recorded after the use of non-steroidal anti-inflammatory agents including ketoprofen with high dose methotrexate.

The use of more than one NSAID at the same time should be avoided due to an increased risk of adverse effects.

Concomitant admininstration of lithium or cardiac glycosides with NSAIDs such as ketoprofen may result in increased plasma concentrations of lithium, or cardiac glycosides.

If ketoprofen and corticosteroids are co-administered, there is an increased risk of gastro-intestinal bleeding and ulceration.

It is recommended that NSAIDs such as ketoprofen are avoided for 8–12 days after mifepristone administration.

Co-administration of NSAIDs such as ketoprofen and quinolone antibiotics are associated with an increased risk of convulsions.

If NSAIDs are taken with angiotensin-converting enzyme inhibitors, beta blockers, or diuretics, the antihypertensive effects of these drugs may be reduced.

The concurrent use of NSAIDs and cyclosporin, or diuretics may lead to an increased risk of nephrotoxicity.

Pregnancy and lactation: Studies in animals have not demonstrated any embryopathic effects. It is recommended to avoid ketoprofen unless considered absolutely essential, in which case it is advised to discontinue treatment within one week of expected confinement when non-steroidal anti-inflammatory drugs might cause premature closure of the ductus arteriosus or persistent pulmonary hypertension in the neonate. Labour could also be delayed. Trace amounts of ketoprofen are also excreted in breast milk.

The use of ketoprofen during pregnancy and lactation should be avoided unless considered essential.

Effects on ability to drive and use machines: Dizziness, mild confusion, vertigo and drowsiness have been reported, therefore patients who drive or operate machinery should be advised of this.

Undesirable effects: Adverse effects reported are frequently transient and are mainly gastrointestinal effects such as indigestion, dyspepsia, nausea, constipation, diarrhoea, heartburn and various types of abdominal discomfort. Other minor effects such as headache, dizziness, mild confusion, vertigo, drowsiness, oedema, mood change and insomnia have been reported to occur less commonly.

Major gastrointestinal adverse effects such as peptic ulceration, haemorrhage or perforation may rarely occur.

Major adverse effects involving other organ systems such as haematological reactions including thrombocytopenia, renal and hepatic damage, dermatological reactions, bronchospasm and anaphylaxis are rare.

It is advisable in all cases of major adverse effects for ketoprofen to be withdrawn at once.

Overdosage: Ketoprofen is of low toxicity in overdosage, symptoms after acute ketoprofen intoxication are largely limited to drowsiness, abdominal pain and vomiting, but adverse effects seen after overdosage with propionic acid derivatives such as hypotension, bronchospasm and gastrointestinal haemorrhage should be anticipated.

Treatment is otherwise supportive and symptomatic.

Pharmacological properties
Pharmacodynamic properties: Ketoprofen is a potent non-steroidal anti-inflammatory analgesic agent and is a strong inhibitor of prostaglandin synthetase.

Pharmacokinetic properties: In a bioequivalence study in healthy volunteers the following values were obtained for Ketoprofen Capsules 50 mg:
C_{max} 12.27±4.96 mg/l
T_{max} 1.17±0.48 hours.

Preclinical safety data: Not relevant.

Pharmaceutical particulars
List of excipients: Magnesium stearate and lactose. The 50 mg capsule shells contain gelatin, erythrosine (E127), indigotine (E132), titanium dioxide (E171) and quinoline yellow (E104). The 100 mg capsule shells contain gelatin, red iron oxide (E172) and titanium dioxide (E171).

Incompatibilities: Not recorded.

Shelf life: 50 mg: 60 months. 100 mg: 36 months.

Special precautions for storage: Store in a dry place not above 25°C.

Nature and contents of container: Amber glass bottles.
Ketoprofen 50 mg capsules – pack sizes: 28 and 100.
Ketoprofen 100 mg capsules – pack sizes: 56 and 100.

Instructions for use/handling: Not applicable.

Marketing authorisation numbers
Ketoprofen Capsules BP 50 mg 4416/0139
Ketoprofen Capsules BP 100 mg 4416/0140

Date of approval/revision of SPC March 1998.

Legal category POM.

LACTULOSE SOLUTION BP

Qualitative and quantitative composition Each 5 ml contains lactulose solution BP 100% w/v (equivalent to 62% to 74% w/v of lactulose).

Pharmaceutical form Liquid for oral use.

Clinical particulars
Therapeutic indications: Constipation; hepatic encephalopathy (portal systemic encephalopathy).

Posology and method of administration:
Constipation:
Adults: Initially 15 ml twice daily.
Children: 1 to 5 years - 5 ml twice daily.
5 to 10 years - 10 ml twice daily.

Dosage may vary depending on the condition. The above dosage serves as a guide. Eventually the dose should be adjusted, usually reduced to meet the needs of the individual.

Hepatic encephalopathy: Initially 30 ml to 50 ml, 3 times daily; adjust dose to produce 2 or 3 soft stools daily.

Method of administration: Oral.

Contra-indications: Contra-indicated where there is evidence of gastro-intestinal obstruction and in patients who require a galactose-free diet.

Special warnings and special precautions for use: The product should be administered with care to patients who are intolerant to lactose.

Due to the product's physiological mode of action it may take up to 48 hours before effects are obtained, however the product does exhibit a "carry-over" effect which may enable the patient to reduce the dose gradually over a period of time.

Interactions with other medicaments and other forms of interaction: Not applicable.

Pregnancy and lactation: The product should only be administered on the advice of a physician during pregnancy or lactation.

Effects on ability to drive and use machines: Not applicable.

Undesirable effects: In the event of diarrhoea, adequate fluid intake should be maintained during treatment and the dosage reduced to prevent loss of fluid and potassium and exacerbation of encephalopathy. The product may give rise temporarily to flatulence and abdominal cramping.

Overdosage: Patients should be given plenty of fluids. An anticholinergic preparation such as atropine methonitrate would help to offset the excessive intestinal motility.

Pharmacological properties
Pharmacodynamic properties: The action of lactulose in treating constipation depends on the inability of the enzymes in the small intestine to hydrolyse the synthetic disaccharide, lactulose, into its component molecules of fructose and galactose.

Therefore, as lactulose is virtually unabsorbed, it passes into the large bowel chemically unchanged and forms a substrate for commensal saccharolytic bacteria.

The resulting breakdown products, simple organic compounds like lactic and acetic acid, give rise to increased intra-colonic osmotic pressure, with consequent increased faecal bulk, and stimulate peristalsis. The growth of saccharolytic bacteria is favoured and the normal colonic flora restored.

A soft stool is formed and normal bowel action encouraged without irritation or direct interference with the gut mucosa.

In patients with hepatic encephalopathy larger doses of lactulose are used; a significant reduction in the pH of the colonic contents results, which reduces markedly the formation and absorption of ammonium ions and other nitrogenous toxins into the portal circulation. Rapid decrements in blood ammonia concentration have been reported following lactulose treatment.

Pharmacokinetic properties: No pharmacokinetic particulars are presented as lactulose is not absorbed by the body.

Preclinical safety data: Not required.

Pharmaceutical particulars
List of excipients: Lactose, D-galactose, fructose, D-tagatose and epilactose.

Incompatibilities: Not applicable.

Shelf life: 36 months, unopened and 36 months, after opening.

Special precautions for storage: This product should be stored at a temperature not exceeding 20°C. Do not freeze.

Nature and contents of container: Opaque, high density polythene bottles. Pack sizes: 300 ml 500 ml and 1,000 ml.

Instructions for use/handling: Not applicable.

Marketing authorisations number PL 4416/0218.

Date of revision of the text 6 June 1997.

Legal category P.

LARAFEN* CR CAPSULES

Presentation Gelatin capsule with opaque pink cap and transparent body printed LAGAP on one half with KET200CR on the other half in black ink. Each capsule contains 200 mg Ketoprofen BP in whitish pH-sensitive controlled-release pellets.

Uses Larafen CR is an analgesic, anti-inflammatory and antipyretic; and is recommended for the treatment of rheumatoid arthritis, osteoarthritis, ankylosing spondylitis and other musculoskeletal conditions including bursitis, capsulitis, synovitis and tendinitis, fibrositis and low back pain. It is also useful to relieve the pain of sciatica, acute gout and dysmenorrhoea.

Pharmacokinetics: Larafen CR Capsule is a controlled release formulation which is designed to release Ketoprofen over a period of time. Following a pharmacokinetic study in volunteers it was found that the average time to achieve maximum plasma concentration was 6.9 hours. The average half-life was found to be 7.4 hours, with a range of 5.5 to 8.0 hours. The average mean residence time was about 14 hours with an average clearance of 2.4 litres per hour. The study carried out over a five day period at the proposed dosage of once daily indicates that there is no accumulation on continued daily dosing. Ketoprofen is very highly bound to plasma protein.

Dosage and administration
Adults: One 200 mg Larafen CR capsule to be taken orally once daily with a little food.

Elderly: As for adult dosage as there is no evidence that that the pharmacokinetics of ketoprofen are altered in the elderly.

Children: There are no recommendations for the use of Larafen CR in children.

Contra-indications, warnings, etc
Contra-indications: Larafen CR should not be given to patients with active peptic ulceration or a history of recurrent peptic ulceration or chronic dyspepsia; known hypersensitivity to Ketoprofen, aspirin or other non-steroidal anti-inflammatory agents; severe renal dysfunction.

Warnings: Some patients with a history of bronchial asthma or allergic disease may suffer bronchospasm, particularly those with a history of allergy to Ketoprofen and related compounds. As non-steroidal anti-inflammatory agents can inhibit renal prostaglandin synthesis and interfere with renal function, care should be taken when using Larafen CR in patients with renal impairment. NSAIDs have been reported to cause nephrotoxicity in various forms; interstitial nephritis, nephrotic syndrome and renal failure. In patients with renal cardiac or hepatic impairment caution is required since the use of NSAIDs may result in deterioration of renal function: the dose should be kept as low as possible and renal function should be monitored. As with other drugs in the same therapeutic category, patients should be advised to take Larafen CR with food.

Interactions: The active ingredient of Larafen CR, ketoprofen, is highly protein bound, therefore alteration of the dosage of other protein bound drugs such as anticoagulants, sulphonamides and hydantoins such as phenytoin may be necessary when taken together. Serious interactions have been reported with methotrexate, digoxin, lithium and diuretics. To avoid the risk of increased side-effects, Larafen CR should not be given with other non-steroidal anti-inflammatory agents.

Pregnancy and lactation: There is no evidence of teratogenic effects of ketoprofen but as with all drugs, administration during pregnancy should be avoided unless essential. Because Ketoprofen interferes with prostaglandin synthesis, there may be premature closure of the ductus arteriosus or persistent pulmonary hypertension in the neonate, or delay in labour if Larafen CR is administered within a few days before the delivery. Small amounts of ketoprofen are excreted in breast milk so use in nursing mothers should be avoided.

Side-effects: The most common adverse effects relate to the gastrointestinal tract, mainly indigestion, dyspepsia, heartburn, various types of abdominal discomfort, nausea, constipation and diarrhoea. Other effects such as headache, dizziness, confusion, drowsiness, oedema, change of mood and insomnia occur less commonly. Peptic ulceration, perforation and gastrointestinal haemorrhage may rarely occur. Other rare adverse events reported include haematological reactions such as thrombocytopenia, hepatic or renal damage, dermatological reactions, bronchospasm and anaphylaxis. Should any severe adverse event occur, treatment with Larafen CR should be stopped immediately. Patients should be warned of the potential side effects.

Overdosage: As with other propionic acid derivatives, ketoprofen demonstrates less toxicity than aspirin or paracetamol. The most likely symptoms of overdosage are drowsiness, abdominal pain and vomiting but hypotension, bronchospasm and gastro-intestinal haemorrhage may occur. Because Larafen CR is a controlled release preparation, continued absorption from capsules in the gastro-intestinal tract, may be expected. Treatment should be symptomatic and may include gastric washout and the use of activated charcoal.

Pharmaceutical precautions Store in a dry place below 25°C. Protect from light.

Legal category POM.

Package quantities Blister packs of 28.

Further information Nil.

Product licence number 4416/0221

METROLYL* (METRONIDAZOLE) SUPPOSITORIES 500 mg AND 1 g

Qualitative and quantitative composition Each 500 mg suppository contains metronidazole BP 500 mg or 1 g.

Pharmaceutical form Suppository.

Clinical particulars
Therapeutic indications: Treatment of infections in which anaerobic bacteria have been identified or are suspected as pathogens, particularly *Bacteroides fragilis* and other species of bacteroides and including other species for which metronidazole is bactericidal e.g. Fusobacteria, Eubacteria, Clostridia and anaerobic cocci.

Metrolyl can be used in septicaemia, bacteraemia, brain abscess, necrotising pneumonia, osteomyelitis, puerperal sepsis, pelvic abscess, peritonitis and post-operative wound infection from which one or more of these anaerobes have been isolated.

Prevention of post operative infections due to anaerobic bacteria.

Use in treatment of acute ulcerative gingivitis and acute dental, pericoronitis and apical infections.

Trichomonas infections.

Amoebiasis.

Giardiasis.

Posology and method of administration: Seven day's treatment should be satisfactory for most patients. Prolonged treatment can be used if the physician considers it to be necessary.

Recommended doses are given as a guideline based on experience. If therapy is to continue for longer than 10 days, clinical and laboratory monitoring is advised.

Rectal medication using Metrolyl Suppositories can be used in patients for whom oral medication is not possible or is contraindicated. The suppositories may be administered alone or concurrently with other bacteriologically appropriate antibacterial agents.

Treatment of anaerobic infections:
Adults and children over 10 years: 2×500 mg suppositories or 1×1 g suppository inserted into the rectum 8-hourly for 3 days. If rectal medication must be continued for more than 3 days, the suppositories should be inserted at 12 hourly intervals.

Children aged 5 to 10 years: As for adults but with 500 mg suppositories, 3 times daily.

Infants and children under 5 years: As for children aged 5 to 10 years, but with appropriate reduction in dosage of suppositories (one-half of a 500 mg suppository for children aged 1 to 5 years and one-quarter of a 500 mg suppository for infants under 1 year).

Prevention of Anaerobic Infections:
Appendicectomy:
Adults and children over 10 years: 1 gram suppository inserted into the rectum 2 hours before surgery and repeated at 8 hourly intervals. If rectal medication is necessary after the third post-operative day, the frequency of administration should be reduced to 12 hourly.

Children aged 5 to 10 years: 500 mg suppositories, administered as for Adults.

Method of administration: For rectal use.

Contra-indications: Known sensitivity to metronidazole is an absolute contra-indication.

Special warnings and precautions for use: Clinicians considering continuous therapy for relief of chronic conditions are advised to consider the therapeutic benefit against risk of peripheral neuropathy.

Underlying gonococcal infection may persist after elimination of *Trichomonos vaginalis.*

No dose modification is needed in renal failure since the elimination half life of metronidazole is unchanged in this condition. The clinical significance of retained metabolites is not known; their efficient removal occurs during dialysis so that metronidazole should be re-administered after haemodialysis. No dosage adjustment is needed for patients undergoing intermittent or continuous ambulatory peritoneal dialysis.

Impairment of metronidazole clearace may occur in patients with advanced hepatic insufficiency since the drug is mainly metabolised by hepatic oxidation. High concentrations of metronidazole may contribute to the symptoms of hepatic encephalopathy - a condition in which significant cumulation my occur. Dose reduction to one-third once daily may be needed.

Metronidazole has no activity against aerobic or facultative anaerobic bacteria.

Interactions with other medicaments and other forms of interaction: The consumption of alcohol during metronidazole therapy should be avoided since there could be a disulfiram-like reaction.

Potentiation of warfarin-type (but not heparin) anticoagulant therapy has been reported so that dose adjustment of the anticoagulant may be needed.

The half-life of metronidazole is reduced from 7–8 hours to about 3 hours in patients receiving phenobarbitone.

In patients taking metronidazole, the assay of aspartate amino transferase may give spuriously low values; this depends on the method used.

Lithium retention with evidence of possible renal damage has been reported where this compound and metronidazole have been used concurrently. Preferably, apart from monitoring lithium, creatinine and electrolyte concentration, lithium therapy should be tapered and or withdrawn before use of metronidazole

Pregnancy and lactation: The safety of use of metronidazole in pregnancy has not been established and its use should be avoided; if essential, short high-dose regimes should *not* be used. Metronidazole is excreted in milk and no adverse effects in the new-born have been reported: the intake by the suckling infant of a mother receiving normal dosage is less than a therapeutic dose for infants.

Effects on ability to drive and use machines: Patients should be warned not to drive or operate machinery if they become dizzy or drowsy.

Undesirable effects: Serious reactions are rare.

An unpleasant taste in the mouth, furred tongue, nausea, vomiting or other gastro-intestinal disturbance have been reported. There is evidence that metronidazole has been associated with abnormal liver function tests, cholestatic hepatitis and jaundice which may be reversed upon drug withdrawal.

Urticaria, skin rash, pruritus, angioedema and rarely anaphylaxis have occurred. Erythema multiforme has been reported but this resolves on drug withdrawal.

Drowsiness, dizziness, headache, ataxia and darkening of the urine (due to metabolites) have been reported rarely.

Peripheral neuropathy and/or transient epileptiform seizures have occurred during prolonged or intensive treatment but in most cases neuropathy disappears on cessation of therapy.

There have been reports of bone marrow depression disorders such as agranulocytosis, leucopenia, neutropenia, thrombocytopenia and pancytopenia which may be reversed on drug withdrawal, although fatalities have been reported.

Overdosage: There is no specific treatment and uneventful recovery has followed ingestion of up to 12 g.

Pharmacological properties
Pharmocodynamic properties: Metronidazole has antiprotozoal and antibacterial actions and is effective against *Trichomonas vaginalis* and other protozoa including *Entamoeba histolytica* and *Giardia lamblia*; and against anaerobic bacteria.

Pharmacokinetic properties: In a controlled cross-over study healthy adult males were given a total of 3 doses of suppositories, viz; 500 mg, 1,000 mg and 2×1,000 mg.

The suppositories gave the following mean results:

	500 mg Suppository	1,000 mg Suppository	2×1,000 mg Suppositories
AUC 0-36μg/ml hours	88.1	165.9	292.5 (by chemical assay)
	80.1	163.6	255.4 (by microbiological assay)
Urinary excretion rate (% of dose)	8.7	8.5	7.2 (by chemical assay)
	10.5	11.0	8.4 (by microbiological assay)

Preclinical safety data: Not required.

Pharmaceutical particulars
List of excipients: Hard fat (Witepsol E75 and W35).

Incompatibilities: Not known.

Shelf life: 36 months.

Special precautions for storage: Store in a cool dry place and protect from light.

Nature and contents of container: Sealed PVC moulds containing the suppositories inside a cardboard carton.
Pack size: 10

Instructions for use/handling: Not applicable.

Marketing authorisation numbers
500 mg PL 4416/0053
1 g: PL 4416/0054

Date of (partial) revision of the text 30 April 1997.

Legal category POM.

MODISAL 60 XL*

Qualitative and quantitative composition Isosorbide-5-mononitrate 60 mg.

Pharmaceutical form Tablets (modified release).

Clinical particulars
Therapeutic indications: Prophylactic treatment of angina pectoris.

Posology and method of administration:
Adults: One tablet (60 mg) once daily given in the morning. The dose may be increased to two tablets (120 mg), the whole dose to be given together. The dose can be titrated to minimise the possibility of

headache by initiating treatment with half a tablet (30 mg) for the first two to four days. The tablets should not be chewed or crushed and should be swallowed with half a glass of fluid.

Children: The safety and efficacy of Modisal 60 XL modified release tablets has not been established.

Elderly: No need for routine dosage adjustment in the elderly has been found, but special care may be needed in those with increased susceptibility to hypotension or marked hepatic or renal insufficiency.

Contra-indications: Severe cerebrovascular insufficiency. Hypotension.

Special warnings and precautions for use: Modisal 60 XL modified release tablets are not indicated for relief of acute anginal attacks; in the event of an acute attack, sublingual or buccal glyceryl trinitrate tablets should be used.

Interactions with other medicaments and other forms of interaction: There is a possibility that ISMN may enhance the hypotensive effect of hydrazaline.

Pregnancy and lactation: The safety and efficacy of Modisal 60 XL modified release tablets during pregnancy or lactation has not been established.

Effects on ability to drive and use machines: The patient should be warned not to drive or operate machinery if hypotension or dizziness occurs.

Undesirable effects: Headache may occur when treatment is initiated, but usually disappears after 1–2 weeks of treatment. Hypotension with symptoms such as dizziness or nausea has occasionally been reported. These symptoms generally disappear during long-term treatment.

Overdose: Treatment should be symptomatic. The main symptom is likely to be hypotension.

Pharmacological properties
Pharmacodynamic properties: Organic nitrates (including GTN, ISDN and ISMN) are potent relaxers of smooth muscle. They have a powerful effect on vascular smooth muscle with less effect on bronchiolar, gastrointestinal, ureteral and uterine smooth muscle. Low concentrations dilate both arteries and veins.

Venous dilatation pools blood in the periphery leading to a decrease in venous return, central blood volume, and ventricular filling volumes and pressures. Cardiac output may remain unchanged or it may decline as a result of the decrease in venous return. Arterial blood pressure usually declines secondary to a decrease in cardiac output or arteriolar vasodilatation, or both. A modest reflex increase in heart rate results from the decrease in arterial blood pressure. Nitrates can dilate epicardial coronary arteries including atherosclerotic stenoses.

The cellular mechanism of nitrate-induced smooth muscle relaxation has become apparent in recent years. Nitrates enter the smooth muscle cell and are cleaved to inorganic nitrate and eventually to nitric oxide. This cleavage requires the presence of sulphydryl groups, which apparently come from the amino acid cysteine. Nitric oxide undergoes further reduction to nitrosothiol by further interaction with sulphydryl groups. Nitrosothiol activates guanylate cyclase in the vascular smooth muscle cells, thereby generating cyclic guanosine monophosphate (CGMP). It is this latter compound, CGMP, that produces smooth muscle relaxation by accelerating the release of calcium from these cells.

Pharmacokinetic properties:
Absorption: Isosorbide-5-mononitrate is readily absorbed from the gastro-intestinal tract.

Distribution: Following administration of conventional tablets, peak plasma levels are reached in about 1 hour. Unlike isosorbide dinitrate, ISMN does not undergo first-pass hepatic metabolism and bioavailability is 100%. ISMN has a volume of distribution of about 40 litres and is not significantly protein bound.

Elimination: ISMN is metabolised to inactive metabolites including isosorbide and isosorbide glucuronide. The pharmacokinetics are unaffected by the presence of heart failure, renal or hepatic insufficiency. Only 20% of ISMN is excreted unchanged in the urine. An elimination half life of about 4–5 hours has been reported.

Preclinical safety data: Not applicable.

Pharmaceutical particulars
List of excipients: Stearic acid, carnauba wax, hydroxypropylmethylcellulose, lactose, magnesium stearate, talc, purified siliceous earth, polyethylene glycol 4000, E171, E172.

Incompatibilities: None known.

Shelf life: 3 years.

Special precautions for storage: Store in a dry place at or below 25°C. Protect from light.

Nature and contents of container: The tablets are packed in aluminium foil/PVC blisters packed in boxes of 28 oval, cream-coloured tablets, half-scored on both sides and marked 60 on one side.

Instructions for use/handling: The tablets should be swallowed whole with half a glass of water. They must not be chewed or crushed.

Marketing authorisation holder: Valpharma s.a., Via Ranco 112, 47031 Serravalle, Republic of San Marino.

Marketing authorisation number 11102/0007.

Date of approval/revision of SPC October 1996.

Legal category P.

MONOVENT* SYRUP

Qualitative and quantitative composition Each 5 ml spoonful of syrup contains Terbutaline Sulphate BP 1.5 mg.

Pharmaceutical form Syrup.

Clinical particulars
Therapeutic indications: Terbutaline sulphate is a selective β_2-adrenergic agonist recommended for use in the following indications: prophylactic treatment and relief of an acute attack of allergic, intrinsic and exercise-induced asthma; chronic bronchitis; emphysema; other bronchopulmonary disorders in which bronchospasm is a complicating factor; for the management of uncomplicated premature labour.

Posology and method of administration:
Use in bronchospasm: Monovent Syrup has a duration of action of 7 to 8 hours. Therefore, the minimum recommended dosage interval is 7 hours.

Adults and elderly patients: The starting dose should be 2×5 ml spoonfuls, 3 times in 24 hours. This may be increased to 3×5 ml spoonfuls, 3 times in 24 hours, if necessary.

Children: A dosage of 0.075 mg (0.25 ml) per kilogram of the child's weight, 3 times in a 24 hour period, is recommended, e.g.

Body weight (kg)	*Dosage*
14	3.5 ml×3
16	4 ml×3
18	4.5 ml×3
20	5 ml×3
24	6 ml×3
28	7 ml×3
32	8 ml×3
36	9 ml×3
40	10 ml×3

Use in the management of labour:
Adults: Oral treatment should not be used initially in an attempt to arrest premature labour.

After contractions have been controlled by intravenous infusion or subcutaneous injections of terbutaline sulphate, maintenance therapy may be continued with Monovent Syrup at a dose of 5 mg, 3 times in a 24 hour period. Oral treatment may be continued for as long as the doctor considers it necessary to delay labour or delivery.

Route of administration: Oral.

Contra-indications: Monovent is contra-indicated in patients with a history of hypersensitivity to any of its constituents.

Although Monovent can be used in the management of uncomplicated premature labour, its use in the following conditions is contra-indicated: any condition of the mother or foetus in which prolongation of the pregnancy is hazardous, e.g. severe toxaemia, ante-partum haemorrhage, intra-uterine infection, ablatio placentae, threatened abortion during the first and second trimesters, or cord compression.

Special warnings and precautions for use: Care should be taken with patients suffering from myocardial insufficiency or thyrotoxicosis.

Due to the hyperglycaemic effects of β_2-stimulants, additional blood glucose controls are initially recommended when Monovent therapy is commenced in diabetic patients.

If treatment becomes less effective or shorter acting the patient's general condition should be reviewed.

Potentially serious hypokalaemia may result from β_2 agonist therapy. Particular caution is advised in severe asthma as this effect may be potentiated by concomitant treatment with xanthine derivatives, steroids, diuretics and by hypoxia. It is recommended that serum potassium levels are monitored in such situations.

Due to the positive inotropic effect of β_2-agonists, terbutaline sulphate should not be used in patients with hypertrophic cardiomyopathy.

During infusion treatment in pregnant women with β_2-stimulants, in combination with corticosteroids, a rare complication with a pathological picture resembling pulmonary oedema, has been reported.

An increased tendency to uterine bleeding in connection with Caesarean section has been reported. This can be stopped effectively by administering 1–2 mg of propranolol intravenous injection.

Interactions with other medicaments and other forms of interaction: Non-selective β-blocking agents such as propranolol may partially or totally inhibit the effect of β-stimulants. Therefore Monovent Syrup and non-selective β-blockers should not normally be administered concurrently. Monovent should be used with caution in patients receiving other sympathomimetics.

Pregnancy and lactation: Although no teratogenic effects have been reported in animals or in patients Monovent should only be administered with caution during the first trimester of pregnancy.

Terbutaline sulphate is secreted via breast milk but influence on the infant is unlikely at therapeutic doses.

Effects on ability to drive and use machines: In view of tht fact that tremor and palpitations have been reported it is felt that patients who drive or operate machinery should be advised of this.

Undesirable effects: The frequency of side-effects is low at the recommended doses. Side-effects which have been recorded such as tremor, headache, tonic cramp and palpitations are all characteristic of sympathomimetic amines. A few patients feel tense; this is also due to the effects on skeletal muscle and not to direct CNS stimulation. Whenever these side-effects have occurred the majority have usually been spontaneously reversible within the first week of treatment. Urticaria and exanthema may occur.

In children, sleep and behavioural disturbances have been seen.

Potentially serious hypokalaemia may result from β_2-agonist therapy.

Overdose: Possible symptoms and signs: headache, anxiety, tremor, tonic cramp, palpitations, arrhythmia. A fall in blood pressure sometimes occurs. Laboratory findings: hypokalaemia, hyperglycaemia and lacto-acidosis sometimes occur.

Treatment: (a) Mild and moderate cases: Reduce the dose. Then increase the dose more slowly if the bronchodilator effect is insufficient.

(b) Severe cases: Gastric lavage, activated charcoal. Determination of acid-base balance, blood sugar and electrolytes. Monitoring of heart rate and rhythm and blood pressure. Metabolic changes should be corrected. A cardioselective β-blocker (e.g. metoprolol) is recommended for the treatment of arrhythmias causing a haemodynamic deterioration. The β-blocker should be used with care because of the possibility of inducing bronchoconstriction. If the β_2-medicated reduction in peripheral vascular resistance significantly contributes to the fall in blood pressure, a volume expander should be given.

Pharmacological properties
Pharmacodynamic properties: Terbutaline sulphate is a selective β_2-adrenergic agonist.

Pharmacokinetic properties: Terbutaline sulphate is incompletely absorbed from the gastro-intestinal tract and is also subject to fairly extensive first-pass metabolism by sulphate (and some glucuronide) conjugation in the liver and possibly gut wall. It is excreted in the urine partly as the inactive conjugates and partly as unchanged terbutaline the ratio of this depends on the method of administration.

Preclinical safety data: Not relevant.

Pharmaceutical particulars
List of excipients: Citric acid, disodium edetate, ethanol, glycerol, sodium hydroxide, sorbitol, sodium benzoate, lemon limette flavouring, raspberry flavouring, purified water.

Incompatibilties: No other major incompatibilities are reported.

Shelf life: 36 months.

Special precautions for storage: Store below 25°C.

Nature and contents of container: Amber glass bottle with plastic cap or plastic bottle and cap. Pack size: 100 ml and 300 ml.

Instructions for use/handling: Not applicable.

Marketing authorisation number 4416/0100

Date of approval/revision of SPC 7 September 1998.

Legal category POM.

NAPROXEN TABLETS BP 250 mg AND 500 mg

Qualitative and quantitative composition Each tablet contains 250 mg or 500 mg naproxen BP.

Pharaceutical form Tablets.

Clinical particulars

Therapeutic indications: Naproxen is used in the treatment of rheumatoid arthritis and other rheumatic or musculoskeletal disorders, dysmenorrhoea and acute gout.

Posology and method of administration: In rheumatic disorders the usual initial dose of naproxen is 250 mg, twice daily, adjusted to 500 mg to 1 g daily in two divided doses.

A dose of 10 mg per kg body weight daily, in two divided doses has been used in children over 5 years of age with juvenile rheumatoid arthritis.

In acute gout, an initial dose of 750 mg followed by 250 mg every 8 hours has been suggested; while in dysmenorrhoea 500 mg may be given initially, followed by 250 mg every 6 to 8 hours.

Oral administration.

Contra-indications:

1. In patients with acute peptic ulceration.
2. In patients with known hypersensitivity to naproxen or naproxen sodium formulations.
3. Since the potential exists for cross-sensitivity reactions, naproxen should not be given to patients in whom aspirin or other non-steroidal anti-inflammatory/analgesic drugs induce asthma, rhinitis, or urticaria.

Special warnings and precautions for use: Naproxen has been found to be well tolerated by patients exhibiting dyspepsia with other similar agents. None the less, episodes of gastro-intestinal bleeding have been reported in patients with naproxen therapy. Naproxen should be given under close supervision to patients with a history of gastro-intestinal disease. Bronchospasm may be precipitated in patients suffering from or with a history of bronchial asthma or allergic disease. Naproxen decreases platelet aggregation and prolongs bleeding time.

Use in patients with impaired renal function: As naproxen is eliminated to a large extent (95%) by urinary excretion via glomerular filtration, it should be used with great caution in patients with significantly impaired renal function and the monitoring of serum creatinine and/or creatinine clearance is advised in these patients. Naproxen should not be used chronically in patients having baseline creatinine clearance less than 20 ml/minute. Certain patients, specifically those where renal blood flow is compromised, such as in extracellular volume depletion, cirrhosis of the liver, sodium restriction, congestive heart failure and pre-existing renal disease should have renal function assessed before and during naproxen therapy. Some elderly patients in whom impaired renal function may be expected, could also fall within this category. A reduction in the daily dosage should be considered to avoid the possibility of excessive accumulation of naproxen metabolites in the patients.

Use in patients with impaired liver function: Chronic alcoholic liver disease and probably other forms of cirrhosis reduce the total plasma concentration of naproxen but the plasma concentration of unbound naproxen is increased, so caution is advised when high doses are required.

Interactions with other medicaments and other forms of interaction:

1) Due to the plasma protein binding of naproxen, patients simultaneously receiving hydantoins, anticoagulants, or a highly protein bound sulphonamide should be observed for signs of overdosage of these drugs.
2) The natriuretic effect of frusemide and other thiazide-like diuretics have been reported to be inhibited by some drugs of this class.
3) Inhibition of renal lithium clearance leading to increase in plasma lithium concentration has also been reported.
4) Naproxen can reduce the anti-hypertensive effect of propranolol and other beta blocking agents.
5) Probenecid given concurrently increases naproxen plasma levels and extends its plasma half life considerably.
6) Caution is advised when methotrexate is administered concurrently because of possible enhancement of its toxicity since naproxen has been reported to reduce the tubular secretion of methotrexate in the animal model.

Pregnancy and lactation: Good medical practice indicates minimal drug usage in pregnancy and the use of this class of therapeutic agent requires cautious balancing of possible benefit against potential risk to mother and foetus, especially in the first and third trimesters. Naproxen has been found to affect the human foetal cardiovascular system (closure of the ductus arteriosus).

Naproxen delays the onset and increases the duration of labour.

The use of naproxen should be avoided in patients who are breast-feeding.

Effects on ability to drive and use machines: Patients are advised not to drive or operate machinery because naproxen may cause an inability to concentrate.

Undesirable effects: Occasional skin rashes and angio-oedema have been reported.

Side effects which occasionally occur are nausea, vomiting, abdominal discomfort, epigastric distress, headache, inability to concentrate, insomnia, tinnitus and vertigo. Rarely, thrombocytopenia, granulocytopenia, jaundice, aplastic anaemia, haemolytic anaemia, peptic ulceration, fatal hepatitis, hearing impairment, cognitive dysfunction, anaphylactic reactions to naproxen, and nephropathy. Mild peripheral oedema has been observed. Sodium retention may occur in patients with questionable or compromised cardiac function when taking naproxen.

Overdose: Significant overdosage of the drug may be characterised by drowsiness, heartburn, indigestion, nausea or vomiting. Should a patient ingest a large amount of naproxen the stomach may be emptied and usual supportive measures employed (it is not known what dose of drug would be life threatening).

Pharmacological properties

Pharmacodynamic properties: Naproxen has analgesic, anti-inflammatory and anti-pyretic actions.

Pharmacokinetic properties: Naproxen is readily absorbed from the gastro-intestinal tract. It is extensively bound to plasma proteins and has a half life of about 14 hours. About half of the dose is excreted in the urine in 24 hours and about 94% in 5 days largely as the glucuronide.

Preclinical safety data: Not applicable.

Pharmaceutical particulars

List of excipients: Lactose, starch (maize), polyvinyl pyrrolidone, sodium starch glycollate, magnesium stearate and quinoline yellow (E104).

Incompatibilities: Not known.

Shelf life: 36 months.

Special precautions for storage: Store in a dry place below 25°C. Protect from light. Keep container tightly closed.

Nature and contents of container: Tamper evident container comprised of polyethylene and polypropylene.

Pack sizes: 250 mg: 56 and 250 and 500 mg: 56 and 100.

Instruction for use/handling: Not applicable.

Marketing authorisation numbers

Naproxen Tablets BP 250 mg: PL 4416/0265
Naproxen Tablets BP 500 mg: PL 4416/0266

Date of (partial) revision of the text 23 October 1997.

Legal Category POM.

NYSTATIN ORAL SUSPENSION BP

Qualitative and quantitative composition Each ml contains 100,000 I.U. Nystatin BP.

Pharmaceutical form Oral suspension.

Clinical particulars

Therapeutic indications: Suspension for the prevention and treatment of candidal infections of the oral cavity, oesophagus and intestinal tract. It provides effective prophylaxis against oral candidosis in those born of mothers with vaginal candidosis.

Posology and method of administration:

Adults: For the treatment of denture sores, and oral infections in adults caused by *Candida albicans.* 1 ml of the suspension should be dropped into the mouth four times daily; it shoud be kept in contact with the affected areas as long as possible.

For the treatment of intestinal candidosis 5 ml of the suspension should be dropped into the mouth four times daily.

For prophylaxis a total daily dosage of 1 million units has been found to suppress the overgrowth of *Candida albicans* in patients receiving broad-spectrum antibiotic therapy.

Administration should be continued for 48 hours after clinical cure to prevent relapse.

Children: In intestinal and oral candidosis (thrush) in infants and children 1 ml should be dropped into the mouth four times a day. The longer the suspension is kept in contact with the affected area in the mouth before swallowing, the greater will be its effect.

Administration should be continued for 48 hours after clinical cure to prevent relapse.

For prophylaxis in the newborn the suggested dose is 1 ml once daily.

Elderly: No specific dosage recommendation or precautions.

Route of administration: Oral.

Contra-indications: Known sensitivity to any of the ingredients.

Special warnings and special precautions for use: Side effects: Nausea, vomiting and diarrhoea have occasionally been reported with doses of nystatin exceeding 4 to 5 million units daily. No systemic effects or allergic reactions have been assoiciated with its oral use.

The label states the following warnings:

Caution – do not use if seal is broken.
Shake well before use.
Store in a cool place. Avoid freezing.
Caution – contains sugar – should not be given to children with disaccharide intolerance.

The product should be protected from light.
The product should not be diluted.

Interactions with other medicaments and other forms of interaction: Not known.

Pregnancy and lactation: Absorption of Nystatin from the gastro-intestinal tract is negligible, therefore no special precautions apply in pregnancy.

Effects on ability to drive and use machines: No known effects.

Undesirable effects: Nystatin Oral Suspension BP contains sugar and should not be given to children with disaccharide intolerance.

Overdosage: Since the absorption of Nystatin from the gastro-intestinal tract is negligible, overdosage causes no systemic toxicity.

Pharmacological properties

Pharmacodynamic properties: Nystatin is a mixture of antifungal polyenes produced by the growth of certain strains of *Streptomyces noursei,* or by any other means. It consists largely of Nystatin A_1.

Pharmacokinetic properties: Nystatin is a tetraene macrolide. There is no data available on the pharmacokinetics as it is not absorbed from the gastro-intestinal tract, skin or vagina and most of the use is topical. Microbial growth-inhibiting concentrations have been shown to be in the range 3–6 mg/l.

Preclinical safety data: Not required.

Pharmaceutical particulars

List of excipients: Sodium carboxymethylcellulose, methyl p-hydroxybenzoate, propyl p-hydroxybenzoate, sodium metabisulphite, sucrose, saccharin sodium, sodium citrate, permaseal aniseed flavour, purified water.

Incompatibilities: Not known.

Shelf life: 36 months.

Special precautions for storage: Store in a cool place – avoid freezing.

Nature and contents of container: 30 g amber glass bottle fitted with a

(i) phenolic resin plastic cap and tin-foil covered melinex liner *or*
(ii) child-resistant cap.

Pack size: 30 ml.

Instructions for use/handling: Shake well before use.

Marketing authorisation number 4416/0161

Date of approval/revision of SPC September 1996.

Legal category POM.

RHUMALGAN* CR 75
RHUMALGAN* CR 100

Qualitative and quantative composition

Rhumalgan CR 75: Each tablet contains 75 mg diclofenac sodium BP.

Rhumalgan CR 100: Each tablet contains 100 mg diclofenac sodium BP.

Pharmaceutical form Controlled Release Tablets.

Clinical particulars

Therapeutic indications: Rheumatoid arthritis; osteo-arthritis; low back pain; acute gout; relief of pain in fractures; acute musculo-skeletal disorders and trauma including periarthritis (particularly frozen shoulder), bursitis, tendinitis, tenosynovitis, dislocations, sprains and strains; ankylosing spondylitis; and the control of pain and inflammation in orthopaedic, dental and other minor surgery.

Posology and method of administration:

For oral administration:

Adults: One 100 mg tablet a day or one 75 mg tablet once or twice a day. Tablets should be swallowed whole preferably with food.

Children: Not suitable for use in children.

Elderly: Care should be used when treating patients who are frail or have a low body weight as they will in general be more susceptible to adverse reactions. The lowest effective dose should be used in these patients.

The standard adult dose may be used for other elderly patients.

Contra-indications: Hypersensitivity to diclofenac sodium. Active or suspected peptic ulcer; gastro intestinal bleeding. Patients who when taking aspirin or other non-steroidal anti-inflammatory drugs suffer attacks of asthma, urticaria or acute rhinitis.

Special warnings and special precautions for use: Patients with a history of gastro-intestinal ulceration, haematemesis, or melaena, should be carefully observed, and care should be taken when treating patients with ulcerative colitis, Crohn's disease, haematological abnormalities, or bleeding diathesis. Elderly patients and those with renal, hepatic or cardiac impairment should also be carefully monitored as renal function may be reduced by NSAID therapy. Renal function should be monitored and the lowest effective dose used.

In patients with impairment of cardiac or renal function, those recovering from major surgery or those being treated with diuretics, prostaglandins are important for the maintenance of renal blood flow. The possibility of inhibition of prostaglandin synthetase should be considered when giving diclofenac to these patients. On stopping diclofenac, effects on renal function are usually reversible.

Diclofenac should be stopped if liver function tests show abnormalities which persist or worsen, or if liver disease develops or if other symptoms such as eosinophilia or rash occur.

Diclofenac sodium may trigger an attack in patients with hepatic porphyria.

Monitoring of renal function, hepatic function (elevation of liver enzymes may occur) and blood counts should be performed on long-term NSAID patients, as a precautionary measure.

Interactions with other medicaments and other forms of interaction: Diclofenac may increase plasma concentrations of lithium (by the impairment of its excretion from the kidneys) and digoxin.

Methotrexate and NSAIDs should only be administered within 24 hours of each other if given with extreme caution. NSAIDs are reported to increase the plasma levels of methotrexate resulting in increased toxicity.

If other NSADs are given concomitantly with diclofenac sodium the frequency of the side effects may be increased.

NSAIDs may increase cyclosporin nephrotoxicity as a result of their effect on renal prostaglandins.

There is an increased risk of convulsions if quinolone antibiotics are given while NSAIDs are being taken, and caution is advised when considering their use.

The activity of diuretics may be inhibited by some NSAIDs. Increased serum potassium levels may result when diclofenac is given concomitantly with potassium-sparing diuretics. Serum potassium levels should therefore be monitored.

Care is required when giving anticoagulants with NSAIDs as diclofenac may reversibly inhibit platelet aggregation. Monitoring is recommended to ensure the desired response to the anticoagulant is maintained as there are rare reports of increased risk of haemorrhage with combined diclofenac and anticoagulant therapy.

It has been reported that hypo- and hyperglycaemic effects have occurred rarely when diclofenac and oral antidiabetic agents have been given together and adjustment of the hypoglycaemic may be required.

Pregnancy and lactation: Diclofenac sodium should only be used during pregnancy and lactation if considered essential.

Diclofenac sodium is reported to cross the placenta in mice and rats but there have not been any studies reported for humans.

Effects on ability to drive and use machines: Patients should not drive or operate machinery if they experience dizziness or other central nervous system disturbances.

Undesirable effects: Common side effects include nausea, headache, diarrhoea, epigastric pain, anorexia, dyspepsia, flatulence, abdominal cramps, vertigo and dizziness. Serious effects such as peptic ulcer, gastro-intestinal bleeding and bloody diarrhoea have occasionally been reported, and there are reports of isolated cases of lower gut disorders (exacerbation of ulcerative colitis or Crohn's proctocolitis and non-specific haemorrhagic colitis), glossitis, constipation, pancreatitis, oesophageal lesions and aphthous stomatitis.

Skin rashes and eruptions have occasionally been reported and rarely urticaria. There are also rare reports of erythema multiforme, Stevens-Johnson syndrome, Lyell's syndrome, bullous reactions, eczema, erythroderma, hair loss, photosensitivity reactions and purpura.

Isolated effects on the central nervous system include drowsiness, tiredness, impaired hearing, insomnia, convulsions, irritability, anxiety, depression, psychotic reactions, tremors, memory disturbance, vertigo, disturbance of sensation, disorientation, disturbance of vision, tinnitus, nightmares and taste alterations.

Occasional effects on the kidney include acute renal insufficiency, urinary abnormalities (e.g. haematuria, proteinuria), nephrotic syndrome, papillary necrosis and interstitial nephritis.

Effects on the liver include occasional reports of elevation of serum aminotransferase enzymes (ALT, AST) and rarely, liver function disorders including hepatitis with or without jaundice.

Leucopenia, haemolytic anaemia, thrombocytopenia, aplastic anaemia and agranulocytosis have rarely been reported. Other rarely reported reactions include hypersensitivity reactions (anaphylactic/anaphylactoid systemic reactions, hypotension, bronchospasm), oedema, palpitation, impotence, chest pain and hypertension.

Overdosage: Gastric lavage and treatment with activated charcoal should be used as soon as possible after overdosage in order to prevent absorption of the drug.

Further treatment is supportive and symptomatic. Complications that might be encountered include renal failure, hypotension, convulsions, respiratory depression, and gastro-intestinal irritation.

Pharmacodynamic properties: Diclofenac sodium is a non-steroidal anti-inflammatory drug (NSAID) with analgesic and antipyretic properties. It is an inhibitor of prostaglandin synthetase.

Pharmacokinetic properties: Rhumalgan CR tablets are extended release preparations designed to release diclofenac over a period of time. Following a pharmacokinetic study with the 100 mg tablets in volunteers it was found that the average time to reach maximum plasma concentration was 6.05 hours. The average elimination half life was found to be 6.75 hours. The average maximum plasma concentration was found to be 262 ng/ml.

Pharmacokinetic properties

a) *General characteristics of the active substance:* Diclofenac sodium is almost totally absorbed after oral administration, and it is subject to significant first-pass metabolism with only approximately 60% of an oral dose reaching the systemic circulation.

Diclofenac sodium is highly protein bound (>99%). It is mainly excreted in the form of metabolites via the urine but also in the bile.

The main metabolite has minimal anti-inflammatory activity compared to the parent drug.

b) *Characteristics in patients:* Plasma concentrations of unchanged diclofenac are not reported to be significantly affected by age, renal or hepatic impairment. The metabolite concentrations may be increased by severe renal impairment.

Preclinical safety data: None stated.

Pharmaceutical particulars

List of excipients: Both strengths: Talc PhEur, ethylcellulose PhEur, magnesium stearate PhEur, povidone PhEur, stearic acid USP, hydroxypropyl methylcellulose PhEur, diethyl phthalate USP, titanium dioxide PhEur and polyethylene glycol BP.

Rhumagan CR 100 only: Iron oxide USP:

Incompatibilities: Not applicable.

Shelf life: 36 months.

Special precautions for storage: Store in a dry place below 25°C. Protect from light.

Nature and contents of container: PVdC/PVC/aluminium/PVdC blister strip

Number of tablets per carton: 100 mg: 28, 75 mg: 28 or 56.

Instructions for use/handling: Not applicable.

Marketing authorisation numbers

Rhumalgan CR 75: 4416/0242
Rhumalgan CR 100: 4416/0243

Date of revision of the text July 1998.

Legal category POM.

SALBUTAMOL SYRUP 2 MG/5 ML

Qualitative and quantitative composition Each 5 ml of syrup contains salbutamol sulphate equivalent to salbutamol BP 2 mg.

Pharmaceutical form Syrup.

Clinical particulars

Therapeutic indications: Salbutamol is a highly selective beta-agonist.

Salbutamol is indicated for the management of asthma, bronchospasm and/or reversible airways obstruction.

Posology and method of administration:

Adults: 4 mg (10 ml of syrup), 3 or 4 times per day is the usual effective dose. If adequate bronchodilatation is not obtained each single dose may be gradually increased to as much as 8 mg.

However, it has been established that some patients obtain adequate relief with 2 mg, 3 or 4 times daily. In elderly patients or in those known to be unusually sensitive to beta-adrenergic stimulant drugs, it is advisable to initiate treatment with 2 mg, 3 or 4 times per day.

Children: The following doses should be administered 3 or 4 times daily:

Age	*Dose*
2 to 6 years	1 mg to 2 mg, as 2.5 ml to 5 ml syrup.
6 to 12 years	2 mg, as 5 ml syrup.
Over 12 years	2 mg to 4 mg, as 5 ml to 10 ml syrup.

The drug is well tolerated by children, so that if necessary, these dosages may be cautiously increased.

Method of administration: Oral.

Contra-indications: Salbutamol Syrup is contra-indicated in patients with a history of hypersensitivity to any of its components. Salbutamol Syrup should not be used for threatened abortion during the first and second trimesters of pregnancy.

Special warnings and special precautions for use: Salbutamol should be administered cautiously to patients suffering from thyrotoxicosis.

Potentially serious hypokalaemia may result from beta$_2$-agonist therapy. Particular caution is advised in severe asthma as this effect may be potentiated by concomitant treatment with xanthine derivatives, steroids, diuretics and by hypoxia. It is recommended that serum potassium levels are monitored in such situations.

Patients should be instructed to seek medical advice should the prescribed dose become less effective. Dosage or frequency of administration should only be increased under medical supervision.

Interactions with other medicaments and other forms of interaction: Salbutamol oral preparations and non-selective beta-blocking drugs such as propranolol, should not usually be prescribed together. See also *Special warnings and special precautions for use.*

Pregnancy and lactation: Salbutamol Syrup should be avoided if possible.

Potentially serious hypokalaemia may result from beta$_2$-agonist therapy.

Effects on ability to drive and use machines: See *Undesirable effects.*

Undesirable effects: Salbutamol Syrup may cause fine tremor of the skeletal muscle which occurs in some patients, usually the hands are most obviously affected. This effect is dose related and is common to all beta-adrenergic stimulants. A few patients feel tense; this is also due to the effects on skeletal muscle and not to direct CNS stimulation. With doses of salbutamol higher than those recommended or in patients who are unusually sensitive to beta-adrenergic stimulants, peripheral vasodilation and a compensatory small increase in heart rate may occur. Occasionally headaches have been reported.

There have been very rare reports of transient muscle cramps. Hypersensitivity reactions including angioedema, urticaria, bronchospasm, hypotension and collapse have been reported very rarely.

Overdosage: The preferred antidote for overdosage with salbutamol is a cardio-selective beta-blocking agent, but beta-blocking drugs should be used with caution in patients with a history of bronchospasm.

Pharmacological properties

Pharmacodynamic properties: Salbutamol BP is a beta-adrenergic stimulant which has a highly selective action on the receptors in bronchial muscle and in therapeutic dosage, little or no action on the cardiac receptors.

Pharmacokinetic properties: Absorption of salbutamol takes place readily from the gastro-intestinal tract. It is subject to first-pass metabolism in the liver; about a half is excreted in the urine as an inactive sulphate conjugate following oral administration, the rest being unchanged as salbutamol.

It has been estimated that the plasma half-life of salbutamol ranges from about 2 to 7 hours. This covers all routes of administration, the intermediate values represent oral administration.

Preclinical safety data: There are no preclinical safety data of relevance to the prescriber.

Pharmaceutical particulars

List of excipients: Sodium benzoate, saccharin sodium, ethanol, citric acid monohydrate, xanthan gum, lime and apricot flavours and purified water.

Incompatibilities: Not known.

Shelf life: 36 months.

Special precautions for storage: Store below 25°C. Protect from light.

Nature and contents of container: A pharmaceutical grade amber glass bottle with polyethylene liner and tamper-evident aluminium cap.
Pack size: 150 ml.

Instructions for use/handling: Not applicable.

Marketing authorisation number PL 4416/0192.

Date of revision of the text 8 January 1998.

Legal category POM.

TEMAZEPAM TABLETS 10 mg and 20 mg

Qualitative and quantitative composition Each tablet contains: 10 mg or 20 mg Temazepam BP.

Pharmaceutical form Tablet.

Clinical particulars

Therapeutic indications: For the short-term treatment of insomnia in cases where it is severe, disabling or subjecting the individual to extreme distress. Temazepam is also indicated for pre-operative medication prior to minor surgery or other similar procedures.

Posology and method of administration: The recommended doses are as follows:

Insomnia:

Adults – 10–20 mg. In extreme cases this may be increased to 30–40 mg.

Elderly – 10 mg. In extreme cases this may be increased to 20 mg.

Tablets should be taken approximately 30 minutes before retiring to bed.

Premedication:

Adults – The normal dose is 20–40 mg, half an hour to an hour before the procedure.

Elderly – 10–20 mg.

Children: Temazepam tablets are not recommended for use in children.

The lowest possible dose should be used. Treatment should not be continued beyond four weeks and treatment should be tapered off gradually (see *Special warnings and precautions*).

Oral administration.

Contra-indications: Temazepam is contra-indicated in the treatment of patients suffering from severe respiratory or hepatic insufficiency, myasthenia gravis or sleep apnoea syndrome. It is also contra-indicated for use in those who have previously experienced hypersensitivity to this or other benzodiazepines.

Special warnings and precautions for use: The cause for insomnia should be determined prior to the use of temazepam, and it should not be used for first line treatment of psychotic illness. Temazepam should also not be used on its own to treat depression or anxiety accompanying depression.

The duration of treatment should be as short as possible (less than 4 weeks) including the tapering off process. More long-term treatment is not advised without re-assessment of the condition. Treatment should be discontinued gradually to minimise the risk of withdrawal or rebound phenomena where the symptoms requiring the treatment recur in an enhanced form.

Temazepam should also be used cautiously in patients with a history of alcohol or drug abuse, or severe hepatic or renal insufficiency.

When used to treat insomnia patients should ensure that they will be able to have 7–8 hours of uninterrupted sleep in order to reduce the risk of anterograde amnesia occurring. If insufficient sleep does occur, this could lead to impaired alertness. Sedation, amnesia, impaired concentration and impaired muscular function may adversely affect the ability to drive or to use machines.

When temazepam is used for pre-medication, patients should be accompanied home afterwards.

There is a risk of drug dependency developing with the use of temazepam. This risk increases in severity with increasing dose and duration of treatment. There is also a greater risk in patients with a history of alcohol or drug abuse, or personality disorder.

If dependence does develop, abrupt discontinuation of treatment will be accompanied by withdrawal symptoms. These may consist of headaches, muscle pain, extreme anxiety, tension, restlessness, confusion and irritability.

The use of benzodiazepines in patients also suffering from depression may unveil suicidal tendencies. Amnesia may occur and in cases of loss and bereavement, psychological adjustment may be inhibited by benzodiazepines.

Interactions with other medicaments and other forms of interaction: The concomitant use of temazepam and alcohol may enhance the sedative effect and is therefore not recommended.

Concurrent use of antipsychotics, antidepressants, narcotic analgesics, hypnotics, anxiolytics/sedatives, sedative antihistamines, anaesthetics and antiepileptic drugs may further enhance the central depressive effect.

Enhanced euphoria may also occur with combined use of temazepam and narcotic analgesics, therefore possibly increasing the risk of dependence.

Pregnancy and lactation: If the product is prescribed to a woman of childbearing potential, she should be warned to contact her physician regarding continuance of the product if she intends to become or suspects that she is pregnant.

If, for compelling medical reasons, the product is administered during the last phase of pregnancy, or during labour at high doses, effects on the neonate, such as hypothermia, hypotonia and moderate respiratory depression, can be expected, due to the pharmacological action of the compound.

Moreover, infants born to mothers who took benzodiazepines chronically during the latter stages of pregnancy may have developed physical dependence and may be at some risk for developing withdrawal symptoms in the postnatal period.

Since benzodiazepines are found in the breast milk, benzodiazepines should not be given to breast feeding mothers.

Effects on ability to drive and use machines: Temazepam may result in impaired alertness, if this occurs, patients should avoid driving or operating machinery.

Undesirable effects: At the start of treatment patients may suffer from drowsiness, reduced alertness, dizziness, confusion, fatigue, muscle weakness, numbed emotions, headache, ataxia or double vision. These will normally disappear with continued treatment.

More rarely, vivid dreams/nightmares, restless sleep, palpitations, change in libido, skin reactions, sedation, impaired muscular function, dry mouth and gastrointestinal disturbances may occur.

Pre-existing depression may be unmasked during treatment with temazepam.

Blood dyscrasias, urinary retention, increased liver enzymes, jaundice and visual disturbances have also been reported to occur occasionally. If any of these effects do occur, treatment should be discontinued.

Other effects, including delusions, psychoses, hallucinations, irritability and restlessness, aggressiveness and rages or other inappropriate behaviour have also been reported to occur, predominantly in elderly patients. If any of these effects occur, treatment should be discontinued.

Overdose: Overdose of temazepam usually results in some form of central nervous system depression ranging from drowsiness to coma.

Flumazenil may be used as antidote therapy.

Overdose with temazepam on its own should not present a threat to life. Temazepam overdose combined with the use of other CNS depressants or alcohol should be treated immediately.

Vomiting or gastric lavage should be induced within one hour. If emptying of the stomach is not advantageous then activated charcoal should be administered to reduce absorption of the drug.

In intensive care treatment, special attention should be given to respiratory and cardiovascular functions.

Pharmacological properties

Pharmacodynamic properties: Temazepam is known to have hypnotic/sedative and anxiolytic properties. It therefore results in anxiolysis, muscle relaxation and central nervous system sedation. It has been suggested that a close molecular association between the sites and action for gamma-aminobutyric acid (GABA) and benzodiazepines and potentiation of GABA may be responsible for these effects.

Other neurotransmitters may also be affected.

Pharmacokinetic properties: Temazepam is readily and almost completely absorbed from the gastrointestinal tract and has been reported to be relatively extensively bound to plasma proteins (75–95%). Peak plasma concentrations are reached approximately one hour after dosing. The majority of a dose of temazepam is metabolised to inactive glucuronides, which are then excreted in the urine.

Preclinical safety data: Not relevant.

Pharmaceutical particulars

List of excipients: Lactose monohydrate, maize starch, pregelled starch, sodium starch glycollate, microcrystalline cellulose and magnesium stearate.

Incompatibilities: Not known.

Shelf life: 24 months.

Special precautions for storage: Store at or below 25°C in a dry place. Protect from light.

Nature and contents of container: 10 mg strength: packs of 28 and 500 tablets. 20 mg strength: packs of 28 and 250. Polypropylene plastic tablet container, with tamper evident lid.

Instructions for use/handling: Not applicable.

Marketing authorisation numbers
Temazepam Tablets 10 mg 4416/0269
Temazepam Tablets 20 mg 4416/0270

Date of approval/revision of SPC 7 August 1997.

Legal category CD (Sch 3), POM.

**Trade Mark*

Lederle Laboratories

Cyanamid of Great Britain Limited
Fareham Road
Gosport, Hants PO13 OAS
☎ 01628 604377 📠 01628 666368

Please refer to Wyeth Laboratories.

Leo Laboratories Limited
Longwick Road
Princes Risborough
Bucks. HP27 9RR
☎ 01844 347333 🖷 01844 342278

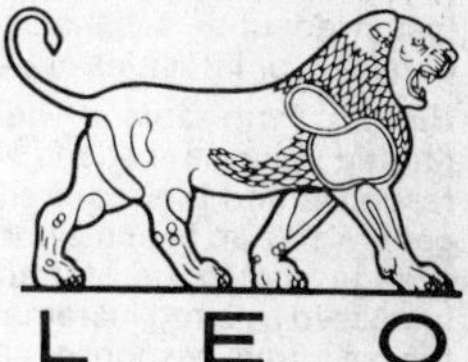

BETIM* TABLETS

Presentation White, flat circular tablets engraved with '102' on the scored face and with an Assyrian lion on the reverse. Each tablet contains Timolol Maleate PhEur 10 mg.

Uses

Mode of action: Betim is a beta-adrenergic receptor blocking agent. The competitive antagonism of adrenergic transmitters at beta receptors blocks beta-sympathomimetic activity particularly in the heart, the bronchi and blood vessels.

Betim has been shown to be a highly specific beta-adrenergic blocking drug and it does not block the chronotropic or inotropic effects of calcium, glucagon, theophylline or digitalis. It does not have significant local anaesthetic or direct myocardial depressant activity nor any significant intrinsic beta-adrenergic stimulant effect.

Betim reduces heart rate and force of myocardial contraction and therefore myocardial oxygen consumption. Modification of the cardiovascular responses to stress or exercise is therapeutically useful in the treatment of angina pectoris.

The beta blocking action of Betim is also of therapeutic value in hypertension although the exact mechanism of action is unclear.

Timolol maleate is rapidly and nearly completely absorbed following oral administration. Beta blocking activity is apparent within 30 minutes of administration and the duration of action, though dependent on dose, has been shown to last for up to 24 hours. Dose proportionality has been established. Plasma half life is approximately 2.7–5.0 hours with a peak plasma concentration occurring approximately 2 hours post dose. Timolol undergoes significant hepatic metabolism, but 'first pass metabolism' is low.

5% of timolol is excreted unchanged by the kidneys.

These pharmacokinetic parameters are unchanged in hypertensive patients and following multiple dosages.

The rate of timolol metabolism varies between individuals; poor metabolisers (approximately 10%) show higher plasma levels and slower elimination of timolol than extensive metabolisers. Within individuals, however, plasma concentrations and half-life are reproducible. As the therapeutic response and some adverse effects are related to plasma concentrations of timolol, poor metabolisers may require lower than normal doses.

Indications: Betim is indicated in angina pectoris due to ischaemic heart disease, for the treatment of hypertension and to reduce mortality and reinfarction in patients surviving acute myocardial infarction. Betim is also indicated in the prophylactic treatment of migraine in order to reduce the number of attacks.

Dosage and administration

For angina: The recommended dose range is 5–30 mg twice daily. The initial dose should be 5 mg twice daily, increasing the daily dose by 10 mg every 3–4 days to achieve optimum results.

Hypertension: The recommended dose range is 10–60 mg daily.

Most hypertensive patients will be controlled by 10–30 mg timolol which can be administered once daily or in two divided doses if preferred. Doses in excess of 30 mg daily should be given in two equally divided doses. The dose of Betim may need adjustment when used in conjunction with other antihypertensive drugs.

After myocardial infarction: Start with 5 mg (½ tablet) twice daily for two days. If there are no adverse effects, increase dosage to 10 mg twice daily and maintain at this dose.

For the prophylactic treatment of migraine: 10 to 20 mg once daily or in two divided doses.

Dosage in the elderly: Initiate treatment with lowest adult dose and thereafter adjust according to response.

Children: Safety and efficacy in children has not been established.

Contra-indications, warnings, etc

Contra-indications: Heart failure, unless adequately controlled. Sinus bradycardia or heart block. Cardiogenic shock. Bronchial asthma, chronic obstructive pulmonary disease. Patients receiving monoamine oxidase inhibitors. Pregnancy. Sick sinus syndrome, severe peripheral vascular disease or Raynaud's disease, hypersensitivity to timolol or any other ingredients.

Precautions: Although Betim has no direct myocardial depressant activity, the continued depression of sympathetic drive through beta blockade may lead to cardiac failure. All patients should be observed for evidence of cardiac failure; if it occurs, then treatment with beta blockers should be gradually withdrawn. If it is not possible to withdraw beta blocker treatment, then digitalisation and diuretic therapy should be considered.

Betim may be used safely in diabetes. It may however interfere with the cardiovascular and possibly the metabolic responses to hypoglycaemia and therefore should be used with caution in diabetic patients treated with insulin or oral hypoglycaemic agents as well as in patients subject to spontaneous hypoglycaemia.

Betim should be administered with caution to patients with impaired renal function or impaired hepatic function.

Drug interactions: Caution is recommended when Betim is administered to patients on catecholamine depleting drugs such as reserpine or guanethidine.

The bioavailability of Betim will be increased by co-administration with cimetidine and reduced with rifampicin.

Some non-steroidal anti-inflammatory agents have been shown to impair the anti-hypertensive effect of beta blocking drugs.

Betim may be prescribed with vasodilators, but increased gastro-intestinal blood flow may affect absorption and metabolism of timolol.

Betim should be used with caution in patients already receiving other hypotensive drugs, including clonidine.

The effect of sympathomimetic agents, eg isoprenaline, salbutamol, will be reduced by concomitant use of beta blockers.

The depressant effect of beta blocking drugs on myocardial contractility and on intracardiac conduction may be increased by concomitant use with other drugs having similar effects. Serious effects have been reported with verapamil, disopyramide, lignocaine and tocainide and may be anticipated with any of the Class 1 antiarrhythmic agents. Special care is necessary when any of these agents are given intravenously in patients who are beta blocked.

The adverse vasoconstrictor effects of ergot preparations may be potentiated during the treatment of migraine with beta blocking drugs.

Anaesthesia: The withdrawal of beta blocking drugs prior to surgery is not necessary in the majority of patients. However, anaesthetic agents such as ether, cyclopropane and trichloroethylene should not be used whereas halothane, isoflurane, nitrous oxide, intravenous induction agents, muscle relaxants, narcotic analgesics and local anaesthetic agents are all compatible with beta adrenergic blockade. Local anaesthetics with added vasoconstrictors, eg adrenaline, should be avoided.

Use in pregnancy: Betim is contraindicated in pregnancy. Timolol maleate appears in breast milk (milk: plasma ratio 0.8) and its use by nursing mothers requires caution. The neonate should be observed for any side-effects.

Side-effects: Betim is usually well tolerated in normal use. General symptoms resulting from beta blockade include fatigue and weakness.

Cardiovascular: bradycardia, heart failure, coldness of the limb extremities, hypotension, heart block.

Digestive: epigastric distress, nausea and vomiting.

CNS: dizziness, disorientation, vertigo, paraesthesiae, headache, hallucinations, nightmares, insomnia, somnolence, depression.

Respiratory: Dyspnoea, broncho-spasm.

Retroperitoneal fibrosis, allergic skin reactions, including erythematous or psoriaform rashes and arthralgia, have been rarely reported.

Warning: There have been reports of skin rashes and/or dry eyes associated with the use of beta-adrenergic blocking drugs. The reported incidence is rare and in most cases the symptoms have cleared when treatment was withdrawn.

Discontinuance of the drug should be considered if any such reaction is not otherwise explicable. Cessation of therapy with the beta-blocker should be gradual although withdrawal symptoms with timolol are infrequent.

Overdosage: Poisoning due to an overdose of Betim may lead to severe hypotension, sinus bradycardia, atrioventricular block, heart failure, cardiogenic shock, cardiac arrest, bronchospasm, impairment of consciousness, coma, occasionally, hyperkalaemia. The first manifestations usually appear 20 minutes to 2 hours after drug ingestion.

Treatment should include close monitoring of cardiovascular, respiratory and renal function, and blood glucose and electrolytes. Further absorption may be prevented by induction of vomiting, gastric lavage or administration of activated-charcoal if ingestion is recent. Cardiovascular complications should be treated symptomatically, which may require the use of sympathomimetic agents (eg noradrenaline, metariminol), atropine or inotropic agents, (eg dopamine, dobatamine). Temporary pacing may be required for AV block. Glucagon can reverse the effects of excessive beta-blockage, given in a dose of 1–10 mg intravenously. Intravenous B_2-stimulants, eg terbutaline may be required to relieve bronchospasm.

Timolol cannot be effectively removed by haemodialysis.

Pharmaceutical precautions Nil.

Legal category POM.

Package quantities Packs of 30 tablets.

Further information Nil.

Product licence number 0043/0035R.

BURINEX* TABLETS

Presentation *Tablets 1 mg:* Each tablet contains 1 mg bumetanide – a white, flat, circular, uncoated tablet marked with the number 133 on the scored face and with an Assyrian Lion on the reverse.

Tablets 5 mg: Each tablet contains 5 mg bumetanide – a white, flat, circular, uncoated, bevelled-edge tablet marked with a score line and '5 mg' on one face.

Uses

Mode of action: Burinex (bumetanide) is a potent, high ceiling loop diuretic with a rapid onset and a short duration of action. The primary site of action is the ascending limb of the Loop of Henlé where it exerts inhibiting effects on electrolyte reabsorption causing the diuretic and natriuretic action observed.

After oral administration of 1 mg Burinex, diuresis begins within 30 minutes with a peak effect between one and two hours. The diuretic effect is virtually complete in three hours after a 1 mg dose.

Pharmacokinetics: Burinex is well absorbed after oral administration with the bioavailability reaching between 80 and 95%. The elimination half life ranges from between 0.75 to 2.6 hours. No active metabolites are known. Renal excretion accounts for approximately half the clearance with hepatic excretion responsible for the other half. There is an increase in half-life and a reduced plasma clearance in the presence of renal or hepatic disease. In patients with chronic renal failure the liver takes more importance as an excretory pathway although the duration of action is not markedly prolonged.

Indications: Burinex is indicated whenever diuretic therapy is required in the treatment of oedema, e.g. that associated with congestive heart failure, cirrhosis of the liver and renal disease including the nephrotic syndrome.

In oedema of cardiac or renal origin where high doses of a potent short acting diuretic are required, Burinex 5 mg tablets may be used.

Dosage and administration

Burinex 1 mg tablets: Most patients require a daily dose of 1 mg which can be given as a single morning or early evening dose. Depending on the patient's response, a second dose can be given six to eight hours later. In refractory cases, the dose can be increased until a satisfactory diuretic response is obtained, or infusions of Burinex can be given.

Burinex 5 mg tablets: The dose should be carefully titrated in each patient according to the patient's response and the required therapeutic activity. As a general rule, in patients not controlled on lower doses, dosage should be started at 5 mg daily and then increased by 5 mg increments every 12–24 hours until the required response is obtained or side-effects appear.

Consideration should be given to a twice daily dosage rather than once daily. Direct substitution of Burinex for frusemide in a 1:40 ratio at high doses should be avoided. Treatment should be initiated at a lower equivalent dose and gradually increased in 5 mg increments.

Children: Not recommended for children under 12 years of age.

Dosage in the elderly: Adjust dosage according to response; a dose of 0.5 mg bumetanide per day may be sufficient in some elderly patients.

Contra-indications, warnings, etc
Contra-indications: Although Burinex can be used to induce diuresis in renal insufficiency, any marked increase in blood urea or the development of oliguria or anuria during treatment of severe progressing renal disease are indications for stopping treatment with Burinex.

Hypersensitivity to Burinex. Burinex is contra-indicated in hepatic coma and care should be taken in states of severe electrolyte depletion.

As with other diuretics, Burinex should not be administered concurrently with lithium salts. Diuretics can reduce lithium clearance resulting in high serum levels of lithium.

Precautions: Excessively rapid mobilisation of oedema particularly in elderly patients may give rise to sudden changes in cardiovascular pressure-flow relationships with circulatory collapse. This should be borne in mind when Burinex is given in high doses intravenously or orally. Electrolyte disturbances may occur particularly in those patients taking a low-salt diet. Regular checks of serum electrolytes, in particular sodium, potassium, chloride and bicarbonate should be performed and replacement therapy instituted where indicated.

Like other diuretics, Burinex shows a tendency to increase the excretion of potassium which can lead to an increase in the sensitivity of the myocardium to the toxic effects of digitalis. Thus the dose may need adjustment when given in conjunction with cardiac glycosides.

Burinex may potentiate the effects of antihypertensive drugs. Therefore, the dose of the latter may need adjustment when Burinex is used to treat oedema in hypertensive patients.

As with other diuretics, Burinex may cause an increase in blood uric acid. Periodic checks on urine and blood glucose should be made in diabetics and patients suspected of latent diabetes.

Patients with chronic renal failure on high doses of Burinex should remain under constant hospital supervision.

Certain non-steroidal anti-inflammatory drugs have been shown to antagonise the action of diuretics.

Warnings: Encephalopathy may be precipitated in patients with pre-existing hepatic impairment.

Burinex should be used with caution in patients already receiving nephrotoxic or ototoxic drugs.

Use in pregnancy and lactation: Although tests in four animal species have shown no teratogenic effects, the ordinary precaution of avoiding use of Burinex in the first trimester of pregnancy should at present be observed.

Since it is not known whether bumetanide is distributed into breast milk, a nursing mother should either stop breast feeding or observe the infant for any adverse effects if the drug is absolutely necessary for the mother.

Adverse effects: Reported reactions include abdominal pain, vomiting, dyspepsia, diarrhoea, stomach and muscle cramps, arthralgia, dizziness, fatigue, hypotension, headache, nausea, encephalopathy (in patients with pre-existing hepatic disease), fluid and electrolyte depletion, dehydration, hyperuricaemia, raised blood urea and serum creatinine, hyperglycaemia, abnormalities of serum levels of hepatic enzymes, skin rashes, pruritus, urticaria, thrombocytopenia, gynaecomastia and painful breasts. Bone marrow depression associated with the use of Burinex has been reported rarely but it has not been proven definitely to be attributed to the drug. Hearing disturbance after administration of Burinex is rare and reversible.

High dose therapy: In patients with severe chronic renal failure given high doses of Burinex, there have been reports of severe, generalised musculoskeletal pain sometimes associated with muscle spasm, occurring one to two hours after administration and lasting up to 12 hours. The lowest reported dose causing this type of adverse reaction was 5 mg by intravenous injection and the highest was 75 mg orally in a single dose. All patients recovered fully and there was no deterioration in their renal function. The cause of this pain is uncertain but it may be a result of varying electrolyte gradients at the cell membrane level.

Experience suggests that the incidence of such reactions is reduced by initiating treatment at 5–10 mg daily and titrating upwards using a twice daily dosage regimen at doses of 20 mg per day or more.

Overdosage: Symptoms would be those caused by excessive diuresis. Empty stomach by gastric lavage or emesis. General measures should be taken to restore blood volume, maintain blood pressure and correct electrolyte disturbance.

Pharmaceutical precautions Nil.

Legal category POM.

Package quantities
1 mg tablets – calendar pack of 28 (OP).
5 mg tablets – calendar pack of 28 (OP).

Further information Burinex is also available as Burinex K tablets, each containing 0.5 mg bumetanide and 573 mg potassium chloride in a slow release core.

Product licence numbers
Burinex 1 mg 0043/0021R
Burinex 5 mg 0043/0043R

BURINEX* INJECTION

Presentation A solution containing 0.5 mg bumetanide per ml in amber glass ampoules of 2 ml, 4 ml and 10 ml, each ampoule containing 1 mg, 2 mg and 5 mg bumetanide respectively. Other ingredients: xylitol, disodium hydrogen phosphate dihydrate, sodium dihydrogen phosphate dihydrate and water for injections.

Uses
Mode of action: Burinex (bumetanide) is a potent high ceiling diuretic with a rapid onset and a short duration of action.

After intravenous injection, diuresis usually starts within a few minutes and ceases in about two hours.

In most patients 1 mg of Burinex produces a similar diuretic effect to 40 mg of frusemide.

Burinex excretion in the urine shows a good correlation with the diuretic response. In patients with chronic renal failure the liver takes more importance as an excretory pathway, although the duration of action in such patients is not markedly prolonged.

Indications: Burinex is indicated whenever diuretic therapy is required in the treatment of oedema, e.g. that associated with congestive heart failure, cirrhosis of the liver and renal disease including the nephrotic syndrome.

For those oedematous conditions where a prompt diuresis is required, Burinex Injection may be used, e.g. acute pulmonary oedema, acute and chronic renal failure. Burinex Injection can be given intravenously or intramuscularly to those patients who are unable to take Burinex tablets or who fail to respond satisfactorily to oral therapy.

Dosage and administration
Pulmonary oedema: Initially 1–2 mg by intravenous injection. This can be repeated, if necessary, 20 minutes later.

In those conditions in which an infusion is appropriate, 2–5 mg may be given in 500 ml infusion fluid over 30–60 minutes. (See pharmaceutical precautions.)

When intramuscular administration is considered appropriate, a dose of 1 mg should be given initially and the dose then adjusted according to diuretic response.

Children: Not recommended for children under 12 years of age.

Dosage in the elderly: Adjust dosage according to response; a dose of 0.5 mg bumetanide per day may be sufficient in some elderly patients.

Contra-indications, warnings, etc
Contra-indications: Although Burinex can be used to induce diuresis in renal insufficiency, any marked increase in blood urea or the development of oliguria or anuria during treatment of severe progressing renal disease are indications for stopping treatment with Burinex.

Hypersensitivity to Burinex. Burinex is contra-indicated in hepatic coma and care should be taken in states of severe electrolyte depletion.

As with other diuretics, Burinex should not be administered concurrently with lithium salts. Diuretics can reduce lithium clearance resulting in high serum levels of lithium.

Precautions: Excessively rapid mobilisation of oedema particularly in elderly patients may give rise to sudden changes in cardiovascular pressure-flow relationships with circulatory collapse. This should be borne in mind when Burinex is given in high doses intravenously or orally. Electrolyte disturbances may occur, particularly in those patients taking a low-salt diet. Regular checks of serum electrolytes, in particular sodium, potassium, chloride and bicarbonate should be performed and replacement therapy instituted where indicated.

Like other diuretics, Burinex shows a tendency to increase the excretion of potassium which can lead to an increase in the sensitivity of the myocardium to the toxic effects of digitalis. Thus the dose may need adjustment when given in conjunction with cardiac glycosides.

Burinex may potentiate the effects of antihypertensive drugs. Therefore, the dose of the latter may need adjustment when Burinex is used to treat oedema in hypertensive patients.

As with other diuretics, Burinex may cause an increase in blood uric acid. Periodic checks on urine and blood glucose should be made in diabetics and patients suspected of latent diabetes.

Patients with chronic renal failure on high doses of Burinex should remain under constant hospital supervision.

Pregnancy: Although tests in four animal species have shown no teratogenic effects, the ordinary precaution of avoiding use of Burinex in the first trimester of pregnancy should at present be observed. Since it is not known whether bumetanide is distributed into breast milk, a nursing mother should either stop breast feeding or observe the infant for any adverse reactions if the drug is absolutely necessary for the mother.

Adverse Reactions: Reported reactions include skin rashes and muscular cramps in the legs, abdominal discomfort, thrombocytopenia and gynaecomastia. Bone marrow depression associated with the use of Burinex has been reported rarely, but it has not been proven definitely to be attributed to the drug. Hearing disturbance after administration of Burinex is rare and reversible. The possibility of hearing disturbance must be considered, particularly when Burinex is injected too quickly and in high doses.

High Dose Therapy: In patients with severe chronic renal failure given high doses of Burinex, there have been reports of severe, generalised, musculoskeletal pain sometimes associated with muscle spasm, occurring one to two hours after administration and lasting up to 12 hours. The lowest reported dose causing this type of adverse reaction was 5 mg by intravenous injection and the highest was 75 mg orally in a single dose. All patients recovered fully and there was no deterioration in their renal function.

The cause of this pain is uncertain but it may be a result of varying electrolyte gradients at the cell membrane level.

Experience suggests that the incidence of such reactions is reduced by initiating treatment at 5–10 mg daily and titrating upwards using a twice daily dosage regimen at doses of 20 mg per day or more.

Overdosage: Symptoms would be those caused by excessive diuresis. General measures should be taken to restore blood volume, maintain blood pressure and correct electrolyte disturbance.

Pharmaceutical precautions Burinex is presented in amber glass containers to protect against deterioration due to exposure to light.

When an intravenous infusion is required, Burinex Injection may be added to Dextrose Injection BP, Sodium Chloride Injection BP or Sodium Chloride and Dextrose Injection BP.

When 25 mg bumetanide (as Burinex Injection) was added to 1 litre of these infusion fluids, no evidence of precipitation was observed over a period of 72 hours. Higher concentrations of Burinex in these infusion fluids may cause precipitation. It is good practice to inspect all infusion fluids containing Burinex from time to time. Should cloudiness appear, the infusion should be discarded.

Legal category POM.

Package quantities Packs of 5×2 ml, 5×4 ml and 5×10 ml glass ampoules.

Further information Nil.

Product licence number 0043/0060

BURINEX* LIQUID

Presentation An opalescent, pale green, viscous, aqueous solution for oral administration containing 1 mg bumetanide in 5 ml (0.2 mg per ml).

Uses
Mode of action: Burinex (bumetanide) is a potent high ceiling diuretic with a rapid onset and a short duration of action. After oral administration of 1 mg Burinex, diuresis begins within 30 minutes with a peak effect between one and two hours. The diuretic effect is virtually complete in three hours after a 1 mg dose. In most patients 1 mg of Burinex produces a similar diuretic effect to 40 mg frusemide.

Burinex is well absorbed after oral administration. Burinex excretion in the urine shows good correlation with the diuretic response. In patients with chronic renal failure the liver takes more importance as an excretory pathway although the duration of action in such patients is not markedly prolonged.

Indications: Burinex is indicated whenever diuretic therapy is required in the treatment of oedema, e.g. that associated with congestive heart failure, cirrhosis of the liver and renal disease including the nephrotic syndrome.

Burinex Liquid may be more appropriate in patients who have difficulty swallowing tablets.

Dosage and administration Usually 1 mg (5 ml) as a single oral dose given morning or early evening. The dosage should be adjusted according to the patient's response.

Children: Not recommended for children under 12 years of age.

Dosage in the elderly: Adjust dosage according to response; a dose of 0.5 mg bumetanide per day may be sufficient in some elderly patients.

Contra-indications, warnings, etc
Contra-indications: Although Burinex can be used to induce diuresis in renal insufficiency, any marked increase in blood urea or the development of oliguria or anuria during treatment of severe progressing renal disease are indications for stopping treatment with Burinex.

Burinex is contra-indicated in hepatic coma and care should be taken in states of severe electrolyte depletion.

As with other diuretics, Burinex should not be administered concurrently with lithium salts. Diuretics can reduce lithium clearance resulting in high serum levels of lithium.

Precautions: Excessively rapid mobilisation of oedema particularly in elderly patients may give rise to sudden changes in cardiovascular pressure flow relationships with circulatory collapse. This should be borne in mind when Burinex is given in high doses intravenously or orally. Electrolyte disturbances may occur, particularly in those patients taking a low salt diet. Regular checks of serum electrolytes, in particular sodium, potassium, chloride and bicarbonate should be performed and replacement therapy instituted where indicated.

Like other diuretics, Burinex shows a tendency to increase the excretion of potassium which can lead to an increase in the sensitivity of the myocardium to the toxic effects of digitalis. Thus the dose may need adjustment when given in conjunction with cardiac glycosides.

Burinex may potentiate the effects of antihypertensive drugs. Therefore, the dose of the latter may need adjustment when Burinex is used to treat oedema in hypertensive patients.

As with other diuretics, Burinex may cause an increase in blood uric acid. Periodic checks on urine and blood glucose should be made in diabetics and patients suspected of latent diabetes.

Patients with chronic renal failure on high doses of Burinex should remain under constant hospital supervision.

Pregnancy: Although tests in four animal species have shown no teratogenic effects, the ordinary precaution of avoiding use of Burinex in the first trimester of pregnancy should at present be observed.

Adverse reactions: Reported reactions include skin rashes and muscular cramps in the legs, abdominal discomfort, thrombocytopenia, and gynaecomastia.

High dose therapy: In patients with severe chronic renal failure given high doses of Burinex, there have been reports of severe, generalised, musculoskeletal pain sometimes associated with muscle spasm, occurring one or two hours after administration and lasting up to 12 hours. The lowest reported dose causing this type of adverse reaction was 5 mg by intravenous injection and the highest was 75 mg orally in a single dose. All patients recovered fully and there was no deterioration in their renal function.

The cause of this pain is uncertain but it may be a result of varying electrolyte gradients at the cell membrane level.

Experience suggests that the incidence of such reactions is reduced by initiating treatment at 5–10 mg daily and titrating upwards using a twice daily dosage regimen at doses of 20 mg per day or more.

Overdosage: Symptoms would be those caused by excessive diuresis. Empty stomach by gastric lavage or emesis. General measures should be taken to restore blood volume, maintain blood pressure and correct electrolyte disturbance.

Pharmaceutical precautions Burinex is presented in amber glass containers to protect against deterioration due to exposure to light. Store below 25°C.

Legal category POM.

Package quantities Bottles of 150 ml (OP). A measure-spoon graduated at 2.5 ml and 5 ml is supplied.

Further information Nil.

Product licence number 0043/0075

BURINEX* A TABLETS

Qualitative and quantitative composition Each tablet contains Bumetanide BP 1 mg and Amiloride Hydrochloride BP 5 mg.

Pharmaceutical form Tablet.

Clinical particulars
Therapeutic indications: Burinex A is indicated where a prompt diuresis is required. It is particularly of value in conditions where potassium conservation is important.

Posology and method of administration
For oral administration:
Adults: The normal adult dose is 1 to 2 tablets daily. The dose may be adjusted according to response.
Elderly: The dose should be adjusted according to needs and serum electrolytes and urea should be monitored carefully.
Children: Not recommended for use in children.

Contra-indications: Hyperkalaemia (serum potassium >5.3 mmol/litre, severe electrolyte imbalance, acute renal insufficiency, severe progressive renal disease, anuria, severe liver disease, adrenocortical insufficiency (Addison's Disease), precomatose states associated with cirrhosis, known sensitivity to bumetanide or amiloride or to Burinex A. Burinex A should not be given concurrently with potassium supplements or potassium-sparing agents. Burinex A is contra-indicated in children as safety in this age group has not been established.

Burinex A is contra-indicated in hepatic coma and care should be taken in states of severe electrolyte depletion.

Special warnings and special precautions for use: Serum uric acid levels may be increased and acute attacks of gout may be precipitated. Patients with prostatic hypertrophy or impaired micturition may be at risk of developinig acute retention.

Burinex A should be discontinued before a glucose tolerance test. Burinex A may cause latent diabetes to become manifest. It may be necessary to increase the dose of hypoglycaemic agents in diabetic patients.

Burinex A should be used with caution in patients already receiving nephrotoxic or ototoxic drugs.

Patients who are being treated with this preparation require regular supervision with monitoring of fluid and electrolyte status to avoid excessive fluid loss.

In common with other potent diuretics, Burinex A should be used with caution in elderly patients or those with disorders rendering electrolyte balance precarious. Hyponatraemia, hypochloraemia and raised blood urea may occur during vigorous diuresis especially in seriously ill patients. Careful monitoring of serum electrolytes and urea should be undertaken in these patients.

Interactions with other medicaments and other forms of interaction: Hyperkalaemia has been observed in patients receiving amiloride and therefore concurrent use of Burinex A with potassium conserving diuretics is not recommended.

In common with other diuretics serum lithium levels may be increased when lithium is given concurrently with Burinex A necessitating adjustment of the lithium dosage.

As ACE inhibitors may elevate serum potassium levels, especially in the presence of renal impairment, combination with Burinex A is best avoided in elderly patients or in those in whom renal function may be compromised. If use of the combination is considered essential the clinical condition and serum electrolytes must be carefully and continuously monitored.

The dose of cardiac glycosides or hypotensive agents may require adjustment.

Certain non-steroidal anti-inflammatory drugs have been shown to antagonise the action of diuretics.

Pregnancy and lactation: The safety of the use of Burinex A during pregnancy has not been established. Since it is not known whether bumetanide or amiloride are distributed into breast milk, a nursing mother should either stop breast feeding or stop taking Burinex A. The decision depends on the importance of the drug to the mother.

Effects on ability to drive and use machines: None known.

Undesirable effects: Bumetanide and amiloride are generally well tolerated. Side effects which may occur include: abdominal pain, nausea and vomiting, dyspepsia, diarrhoea, stomach and muscle cramps, arthralgia, dizziness, fatigue, hypotension, headache, encephalopathy (in patients with pre-existing hepatic disease), fluid and electrolyte depletion, dehydration, hyperuricaemia, increased blood urea and serum creatinine, hyperglycaemia, abnormalities of serum levels of hepatic enzymes, skin rashes, pruritus, urticaria, thrombocytopenia, gynaecomastia and painful breasts. Bone marrow depression associated with the use of Burinex has been reported rarely but it has not been proven definitely to be attributed to the drug. Hearing disturbance after administration of Burinex is rare and reversible.

Overdosage: Symptoms would be those caused by excessive diuresis such as dehydration, electrolyte imbalance, particularly hyperkalaemia, and hypotension and treatment should be aimed at reversing these. No specific antidote is available. Treatment is symptomatic and supportive. If hyperkalaemia is present appropriate measures must be instituted to reduce serum potassium.

Pharmacological properties
Pharmacodynamic properties: Burinex A combines the potent loop diuretic bumetanide with the potassium sparing diuretic amiloride.

The action of bumetanide starts within 30 minutes and is virtually complete within 3 hours. The addition of amiloride will reduce any tendency towards hypokalaemia and its mild natriuretic effect will be additive to that of bumetanide.

Pharmacokinetic properties: The product contains a short acting diuretic and a potassium sparing diuretic with a more prolonged action.

After administration of one tablet containing bumetanide 1 mg and amiloride hydrochloride 5 mg to healthy volunteers, a C_{max} of 48.60±19.08 ng/ml was found for bumetanide at T_{max} 0.91±0.31 hours.

The corresponding data for amiloride hydrochloride was C_{max} 10.47±4.02 ng/ml at T_{max} 2.92±0.78 hours.

Preclinical safety data: There are no preclinical data of relevance to the prescriber which are additional to that already included in other sections of the SPC.

Pharmaceutical properties
List of excipients: Microcrystalline cellulose, lactose, magnesium stearate, maize starch.

Incompatibilities: None known.

Shelf life: 3 years.

Special precautions for storage: None.

Nature and contents of container: Blister packs of 28 tablets.

Instructions for use/handling: None.

Marketing authorisation number 0043/0161

Date of first authorisation/renewal of authorisation United Kingdom 25.9.90.

Date of revision of the text September 1998

Legal category POM

BURINEX* K TABLETS

Qualitative and quantitative composition Each tablet contains Bumetanide BP 0.5 mg and Potassium Chloride PhEur 573 mg.

Pharmaceutical form Tablet.

Clinical particulars
Therapeutic indications: For the treatment of oedema where potassium supplementation is necessary.

Posology and method of administration: For oral administration.

Adults: The recommended initial dose is 2 tablets to be taken once daily (morning or evening). This may be increased up to 4 tablets daily (given as a single dose or in divided doses if preferred), or reduced to 1 tablet daily according to clinical response. If more than 4 tablets are to be taken daily, it is preferred to administer the diuretic and potassium supplement as two separate preparations.

Elderly: Adjust dosage according to response. A dose of 1 tablet per day may be sufficient in some elderly patients.

Burinex K tablets must be swallowed whole and never chewed. The tablets should be swallowed whole with at least 100 ml of water.

Children: Not recommended in children under 12 years.

Contra-indications: The product should not be used with potassium-sparing diuretics (e.g. spironolactone, triamterene or amiloride) or in patients with renal insufficiency.

As with other diuretics, Burinex K should not be administered concurrently with lithium salts. Diuretics can reduce lithium clearance resulting in high serum levels of lithium.

All solid forms of potassium medication are contra-indicated in the presence of obstruction in the digestive tract (e.g. resulting from compression of the oesophagus due to dilation of the left atrium or from stenosis of the gut).

Anuria, Crohns Disease, hyperkalaemia, precomatose states associated with liver cirrhosis, Addison's Disease, known hypersensitivity to bumetanide or Burinex.

Special warnings and special precautions for use: The 15.4 mmol of potassium included in the usual dose of Burinex K (2 tablets daily) should help to prevent hypokalaemia in many patients. Certain patients, however, as for example those with hepatic ascites or those on a very low potassium diet, may require considerably more potassium than this. Periodic checks should, therefore, be made on the serum potassium level in patients on long-term therapy.

The diuretic in Burinex K may potentiate the effect of antihypertensive drugs, increase blood uric acid and (though rarely) affect carbohydrate metabolism. Certain non-steroidal anti-inflammatory drugs have been shown to antagonise the action of diuretics.

Non-specific small bowel lesions characterised by stenosis and possibly accompanied by ulceration have been associated with the oral administration of tablets and capsules containing potassium salts. Symptoms and signs which indicate ulceration or obstruction of the small bowel in patients taking tablets or capsules containing potassium salts are indications for stopping treatment with such preparations immediately.

Patients with prostatic hypertrophy or impairment of micturition have an increased risk of developing acute retention. Where indicated, steps should be taken to correct hypotension or hyperkalaemia before commencing therapy. ACE inhibitors should not be used with combination diuretic potassium products, such as Burinex K, as serum potassium levels may be increased. The toxic effects of nephrotoxic antibiotics may be increased by concomitant administration of potent diuretics such as bumetanide.

Interactions with other medicaments and other forms of interaction: See *Special warnings and special precautions for use* above.

Pregnancy and lactation: Although tests in four animal species have shown no teratogenic effects, the ordinary precaution of avoiding use of Burinex in the first trimester of pregnancy should at present be observed.

Since it is not known whether bumetanide is distributed into breast milk, a nursing mother should either stop breast feeding or observe the infant for any adverse effects if the drug is absolutely necessary for the mother.

Effects on ability to drive and use machines: None known.

Undesirable effects: Reported reactions include skin rashes and muscular cramps in the legs, abdominal discomfort, thrombocytopenia and gynaecomastia. As with other diuretics, fluid and electrolyte balance may be disturbed as a result of diuresis after prolonged therapy. This may cause symptoms such as headache, hypotension and myalgia.

Bone marrow depression associated with the use of Burinex has been reported rarely but it has not been proven definitely to be attributed to the drug. Hearing disturbance after administration of Burinex is rare and reversible.

Overdosage: General measures should be taken to restore blood volume and maintain blood pressure. Any electrolyte imbalance should be corrected.

Pharmacological properties

Pharmacodynamic properties: Burinex K combines the very potent high ceiling diuretic bumetanide with a slow-release potassium chloride supplement. Bumetanide has a rapid onset and a short duration of action. As with most diuretics, long-term therapy may be associated with potassium depletion.

Pharmacokinetic properties: The potassium supplement in Burinex K will help to maintain normal levels of potassium, especially in those patients whose dietary intake of potassium is inadequate.

The formulation of Burinex K presents the following advantages. The diuretic is coated around the tablet from which it is rapidly released. The diuretic and saluretic effects begin within 30 minutes after oral administration, peak at one to two hours, and are largely complete within three hours. In contrast, the potassium chloride, which is included in an inert wax core, is released only slowly over a period of six hours after oral ingestion. This slow release minimises the risk of gastro-intestinal intolerance as well as that of ulceration and stenosis resulting from localised high concentrations of potassium salts in the small bowel.

Preclinical safety data: There are no pre-clinical data of relevance to the prescriber which are additional to that already included in other sections of the SPC.

Pharmaceutical particulars

List of excipients: Ethyl cellulose, ferric oxide brown, glycerol, magnesium stearate, stearyl alcohol, hydroxypropylmethylcellulose, polyvidone K25, sucrose, talc, titanium dioxide.

Incompatibilities: None known.

Shelf life: 3 years.

Special precautions for storage: None.

Nature and contents of container: Blister packs of 28.

Instructions for use/handling: None.

Marketing authorisation number 0043/0027R.

Date of approval/revision of SPC December 1996.

Legal category POM.

DOVONEX* CREAM

Qualitative and quantitative composition
Calcipotriol 50 micrograms per g (as the hydrate).

Pharmaceutical form Cream.

Clinical particulars

Therapeutic indications: Dovonex Cream is indicated for the topical treatment of plaque psoriasis (psoriasis vulgaris) amenable to topical therapy.

Posology and method of administration:

Adults: Dovonex Cream should be applied to the affected area once or twice daily. For maximum benefit use the cream twice daily. Maximum weekly dose should not exceed 100 g.

Children over 12 years: Dovonex Cream should be applied to the affected area twice daily. Maximum weekly dose should not exceed 75 g.

Children aged 6 to 12 years: Dovonex Cream should be applied to the affected area twice daily. Maximum weekly dose should not exceed 50 g.

Children under 6 years: There is limited experience of the use of Dovonex in this age group. A maximum safe dose has not been established.

These dose recommendations are based on extensive experience in adults. In respect of children, clinical experience in children has shown Dovonex to be safe and effective over eight weeks at a mean dose of 15 g per week but with wide variability in dose among patients. Individual dose requirement depends on the extent of psoriasis but should not exceed the above recommendations.

Contra-indications: Dovonex Cream is contraindicated in patients with known disorders of calcium metabolism. As with other topical preparations, Dovonex Cream is contra-indicated in patients with hypersensitivity to any of the ingredients.

Special warnings and special precautions for use: Dovonex Cream should not be used on the face. Patients should be advised to wash their hands after applying the cream and to avoid inadvertent transfer to other body areas, especially the face. Care should be exercised in patients with other types of psoriasis, since hypercalcaemia, which rapidly reversed on cessation of treatment, has been reported in patients with generalised pustular or erythrodermic exfoliative psoriasis.

Interaction with other medicaments and other forms of interaction: There is no interaction between calcipotriol and sunlight or UV light. There is no experience of concomitant therapy with other antipsoriatic products applied to the same skin area at the same time.

Pregnancy and lactation: Safety for use during human pregnancy has not yet been established, although studies in experimental animals have not shown teratogenic effects. Avoid use in pregnancy unless there is no safer alternative. It is not known whether calcipotriol is excreted in breast milk.

Effects on ability to drive and use machines: Not applicable.

Undesirable effects: The most common side effect is transient local irritation which seldom requires discontinuation of treatment. Other local reactions may occur including dermatitis, pruritus, erythema, aggravation of psoriasis, photosensitivity. Facial or perioral dermatitis may occur rarely.

Overdose: Hypercalcaemia should not occur at the recommended dose of Dovonex Cream.

Excessive use may cause elevated serum calcium which rapidly subsides when the treatment is discontinued.

Pharmacological properties

Pharmacodynamic properties: Calcipotriol is a vitamin D derivative. *In vitro* data suggests that calcipotriol induces differentiation and suppresses proliferation of keratinocytes. This is the proposed basis for its effect in psoriasis.

Pharmacokinetic properties: Not applicable.

Preclinical safety data: The effect on calcium metabolism is approximately 100 times less than that of the hormonally active form of vitamin D_3.

Pharmaceutical particulars

List of excipients: Cetamacrogol 1000, cetostearyl alcohol, chloroallylhexaminium chloride, disodium edetate, disodium phospate dihydrate, glycerol 85%, liquid paraffin, purified water, white soft paraffin.

Incompatibilities: None known.

Shelf life: 2 years.

Special precautions for storage: Store below 25°C.

Nature and contents of container: Aluminium tubes of 30 g (OP), 60 g (OP) and 120 g (OP).

Instructions for use/handling: None.

Marketing authorisation number PL 0043/0188

Date of first authorisation/renewal of authorisation
10 August 1993

Date of (partial) revision of the text July 1998

Legal category POM

DOVONEX* OINTMENT

Qualitative and quantitative composition
Calcipotriol 50 micrograms/g.

Pharmaceutical form Ointment.

Clinical particulars

Therapeutic indications: Dovonex Ointment is indicated for the topical treatment of plaque psoriasis (psoriasis vulgaris) amenable to topical therapy.

Posology and method of administration:

Adults: Dovonex Ointment should be applied to the affected area once or twice daily. For maximum benefit use the ointment twice daily. Maximum weekly dose should not exceed 100 g.

Children over 12 years: Dovonex Ointment should be applied to the affected area twice daily. Maximum weekly dose should not exceed 75 g.

Children aged 6 to 12 years: Dovonex Ointment should be applied to the affected area twice daily. Maximum weekly dose should not exceed 50 g.

Children under 6 years: There is limited experience of the use of Dovonex Ointment in this age group. A maximum safe dose has not been established.

These dose recommendations are based on extensive experience in adults. In respect of children, clinical experience in children has shown Dovonex to be safe and effective over eight weeks at a mean dose of 15 g per week but with wide variability in dose among patients. Individual dose requirement depends on the extent of psoriasis but should not exceed the above recommendations.

Contra-indications: Dovonex Ointment is contra-indicated in patients with known disorders of calcium metabolism. As with other topical preparations, Dovonex Ointment is contra-indicated in patients with hypersensitivity to any of its constituents.

Special warnings and special precautions for use: Dovonex Ointment should not be used on the face. Patients should be advised to wash their hands after applying the ointment and to avoid inadvertent transfer to other body areas, especially the face. Patients should be advised to use no more than the recommended dose (see section on *Posology and method of administration*) since hypercalcaemia, which rapidly reverses on cessation of treatment, may occur.

Interaction with other medicaments and other forms of interaction: There is no interaction between calcipotriol and sunlight or UV light. There is no experience of concomitant therapy with other antipsoriatic products applied to the same skin area at the same time.

Pregnancy and lactation: Safety for use during human pregnancy has not yet been established, although studies in experimental animals have not shown teratogenic effects. Avoid use in pregnancy unless there is no safer alternative. It is not known whether calcipotriol is excreted in breast milk.

Effects on ability to drive and use machines: Not applicable.

Undesirable effects: The most common side-effect is transient local irritation which seldom requires discontinuation of treatment. Other local reactions may occur including dermatitis, pruritus, erythema, aggravation of psoriasis, photosensitivity. Facial or perioral dermatitis may occur rarely.

Overdose: Hypercalcaemia may occur in patients with plaque psoriasis who use more than the recommended dose of Dovonex Ointment weekly and has been reported at lower doses in patients with generalised pustular or erythrodermic exfoliative psoriasis.

Pharmacological properties

Pharmacodynamic properties: Calcipotriol is a vitamin D derivative. *In vitro* data suggest that calcipotriol induces differentiation and suppresses proliferation of keratinocytes. This is the proposed basis for its effect in psoriasis.

Pharmacokinetic properties: Data from a single study containing 5 evaluable patients with psoriasis treated with 0.3–1.7 g of a 50 micrograms/g tritium labelled calcipotriol ointment suggested that less than 1% of the dose was absorbed.

However, total recovery of the tritium label over a 96 hour period ranged from 6.7 to only 32.6%, figures maximised by uncorrected chemiluminescence. There were no data on ^{3}H tissue distribution or excretion from the lungs.

Preclinical safety data: The effect on calcium metabolism is approximately 100 times less than that of the hormonally active form of vitamin D_3.

Pharmaceutical particulars

List of excipients: Disodium edetate, disodium phosphate dihydrate, DL-α-tocopherol, liquid paraffin, polyoxyethylene-(2)-stearyl ether, propylene glycol, purified water and white soft paraffin.

Incompatibilities: Not applicable.

Shelf life: 2 years.

Special precautions for storage: Store below 25°C.

Nature and contents of container: Lacquered aluminium tube with polypropylene screw cap. Pack sizes: 30, 60, 120 g.

Instructions for use/handling: None.

Marketing authorisation number 0043/0177.

Date of approval/revision of SPC July 1998.

Legal category POM.

DOVONEX* SCALP SOLUTION

Qualitative and quantitative composition Calcipotriol 50 micrograms per ml (as the hydrate).

Pharmaceutical form Solution.

Clinical particulars

Therapeutic indications: Dovonex Scalp Solution is indicated for the topical treatment of scalp psoriasis.

Posology and method of administration:

Adults: Dovonex Scalp Solution should be applied twice daily (morning and evening) to the affected areas. Maximum weekly dose should not exceed 60 ml.

When used together with Dovonex Cream or Ointment, the total dose of calcipotriol should not exceed 5 mg in any week, e.g. 60 ml of Scalp Solution plus one 30 g tube of Cream or Ointment, or 30 ml of Scalp Solution plus 60 g (two 30 g tubes) of Cream or Ointment.

Children: Not recommended as there is no experience of the use of Dovonex Scalp Solution in children.

Contra-indications: Dovonex Scalp Solution is contra-indicated in patients with known disorders of calcium metabolism. As with other topical preparations, Dovonex Scalp Solution is contra-indicated in patients with hypersensitivity to any of its constituents.

Special warnings and special precautions for use: Application of Dovonex to the face may cause local irritation. Dovonex Scalp Solution should not therefore be applied directly to the face. Patients should be advised to wash their hands after applying the scalp solution and to avoid inadvertent transfer to the face. Patients should be advised to use no more than the maximum weekly dose since hypercalcaemia, which rapidly reverses on cessation of treatment, may occur.

Interaction with other medicaments and other forms of interaction: There is no interaction between calcipotriol and UV light. There is no experience of concomitant therapy with other antipsoriatic products applied to the same area.

Pregnancy and lactation: Safety for use during human pregnancy has not yet been established, although studies in experimental animals have not shown teratogenic effects. Avoid use in pregnancy unless there is no safer alternative. It is not known whether calcipotriol is excreted in breast milk.

Effects on ability to drive and use machines: Not applicable.

Undesirable effects: The most common side-effect is local irritation on the scalp or face. Facial or perioral dermatitis may occur. Other local reactions may occur. Reactions which have been reported with Dovonex Ointment include dermatitis, pruritus, erythema, aggravation of psoriasis, photosensitivity, and rarely hypercalcaemia or hypercalciuria.

Overdose: Hypercalcaemia may occur in patients with plaque psoriasis who use more than 100 g of Dovonex Ointment weekly and has been reported at lower doses in patients with generalised pustular or erythrodermic exfoliative psoriasis.

Pharmacological properties

Pharmacodynamic properties: Calcipotriol is a vitamin D derivative. *In vitro* data suggest that calcipotriol induces differentiation and suppresses proliferation of keratinocytes. This effect is the proposed basis for its effect in psoriasis.

Pharmacokinetic properties: Not applicable.

Preclinical safety data: The effect on the calcium metabolism is approximately 100 times less than that of the hormonally active form of vitamin D_3.

Pharmaceutical particulars

List of excipients: Hydroxypropyl cellulose, isopropanol, levomenthol, sodium citrate, propylene glycol, purified water.

Incompatibilities: None known.

Shelf life: 2 years.

Special precautions for storage: Store below 25°C. The alcohol base is flammable.

Nature and contents of container: 60 ml polyethylene bottle with nozzle.

Instructions for use/handling: None.

Marketing authorisation number 0043/0190.

Date of approval/revision of SPC February 1996.

Legal category POM.

FUCIDIN* TABLETS FUCIDIN* SUSPENSION

Presentation

Fucidin Tablets: White, oval film coated tablet with an Assyrian lion on one side and the number 121 on the other. Each tablet contains 250 mg Sodium Fusidate PhEur (equivalent to 240 mg fusidic acid). Sodium fusidate is the sodium salt of fusidic acid.

Fucidin Suspension: Each 5 ml of white to off-white, banana-flavoured aqueous suspension contains 250 mg Fusidic Acid PhEur.

Uses

Mode of action: Fusidic acid and its salts are potent anti-staphylococcal agents with unusual ability to penetrate tissue. Bactericidal levels have been assayed in bone and necrotic tissue. Blood levels are cumulative, reaching concentrations of 20–35 micrograms/ml after oral administration of 250 mg twice daily for seven days and 50–100 microgram/ml after oral administration of 1.5 g daily for three to four days. Concentrations of 0.03–0.12 micrograms/ml inhibit nearly all strains of *Staphylococcus aureus.* Fusidic acid is active against *Staphylococcus epidermidis* and methicillin resistant staphylococci.

Fucidin is excreted mainly in the bile, little or none being excreted in the urine.

In severe or deep-seated infections and when prolonged therapy may be required, systemic Fucidin should generally be given concurrently with other anti-staphylococcal antibiotic therapy.

Indications: Fucidin is indicated in the treatment of all staphylococcal infections due to susceptible organisms, such as: cutaneous infections; osteomyelitis; pneumonia; septicaemia; wound infections; endocarditis; superinfected cystic fibrosis.

Fucidin should be administered intravenously whenever oral therapy is inappropriate, which includes cases where absorption from the gastro-intestinal tract is unpredictable.

Dosage and administration

Fucidin Tablets: For staphylococcal cutaneous infections:

Adult: standard dose: 250 mg (one tablet) sodium fusidate (equivalent to 240 mg fusidic acid) twice daily for 5–10 days.

For staphylococcal infections such as osteomyelitis; pneumonia; septicaemia; wound infections; endocarditis; superinfected cystic fibrosis:

Adult: standard dose: 500 mg (two tablets) sodium fusidate (equivalent to 480 mg fusidic acid) three times daily.

In severe cases of fulminating infections, the dosage may be doubled or appropriate combined therapy may be used.

Fucidin Suspension: For all staphylococcal infections. Each 5 ml of Fucidin Suspension is therapeutically equivalent to 175 mg of sodium fusidate owing to its lower oral bioavailability. Therefore the following dosages are recommended:

Adult dose: 15 ml three times daily.

Children: 0–1 year: 1 ml/kg bodyweight daily, divided into 3 equal doses.
1–5 years: 5 ml three times daily.
5–12 years: 10 ml three times daily.

Since Fucidin is excreted in the bile, no dosage modifications are needed in renal impairment.

The dosage in patients undergoing haemodialysis needs no adjustment as Fucidin is not significantly dialysed.

Dosage in the elderly: No dosage alterations are necessary in the elderly.

Contra-indications, warnings, etc

Contra-indications: Contra-indicated in patients with known hypersensitivity to fusidic acid and its salts.

Precautions: Caution should be exercised with other antibiotics which have similar biliary excretion pathways, e.g. lincomycin and rifampicin. Periodic liver function tests should be carried out when high oral doses are used, when the drug is given for prolonged periods and in patients with liver dysfunction.

Fucidin displaces bilirubin from its albumin binding site *in vitro*. The clinical significance of this finding is uncertain and kernicterus has not been observed in neonates receiving Fucidin. However, this observation should be borne in mind when the drug is given to pre-term, jaundiced, acidotic or seriously ill neonates.

Pregnancy and lactation: There is inadequate evidence of safety in human pregnancy. Animal studies and many years of clinical experience suggest that fusidic acid is devoid of teratogenic effects. There is evidence to suggest that when given systemically fusidic acid can cross the placental barrier. If the administration of Fucidin to pregnant patients is considered essential, its use requires that the potential benefits be weighed against the possible hazards to the foetus.

Safety in nursing mothers has not been established. When fusidic acid (as the sodium salt) has been given systemically, levels have been detected in the breast milk. Caution is, therefore, required when Fucidin is used in mothers who wish to breast feed.

Adverse reactions: In some patients given Fucidin, particularly the young and elderly, a reversible jaundice has been reported. Jaundice has been seen most frequently in patients receiving intravenous Fucidin in high dosage, or where the drug has been infused too rapidly or at too high a concentration in the infusion fluid. In some instances instituting oral therapy may be beneficial.

If the jaundice persists Fucidin should be withdrawn, following which the serum bilirubin will invariably return to normal.

Reported reactions are gastro-intestinal upsets and, rarely, skin rashes and haematological disorders including bone marrow depression and neutropenia. Acute renal failure has been described in patients with jaundice, particularly in the presence of other factors predisposing to renal failure.

Overdosage: There has been no experience of overdosage with Fucidin. Treatment should be restricted to symptomatic and supportive measures. Dialysis is of no benefit, since the drug is not significantly dialysed.

Pharmaceutical precautions

Fucidin Tablets: Nil.

Fucidin Suspension: Protect from direct sunlight and heat. The Suspension should be shaken before use and dilution is not recommended.

Legal category POM.

Package quantities *Tablets:* Bottles of 100. *Suspension:* Bottles of 50 ml (OP).

Further information Both oral and intravenous Fucidin have been given concurrently with other antibiotics, e.g. cloxacillin, flucloxacillin, ampicillin, methicillin and erythromycin.

Fusidic acid and its salts exhibit no cross hypersensitivity or cross resistance with other antibiotics in clinical use.

Despite many years of clinical use, resistance to fusidic acid amongst *Staphylococcus aureus* remains low.

Product licence numbers

Tablets	0043/5000R
Suspension	0043/5014R

FUCIDIN* FOR INTRAVENOUS INFUSION

Presentation A pack of 2 vials. One vial contains Sodium Fusidate PhEur, 500 mg (equivalent to 480 mg fusidic acid) as a dry powder. The second vial of 10 ml sterile phosphate-citrate buffer solution (pH 7.4–7.6), contains disodium hydrogen phosphate, citric acid, disodium edetate and water for injections. When reconstituted contains 3.1 mMol sodium and 1.1 mMol phosphate.

Uses
Mode of action: Fusidic acid and its salts are potent anti-staphylococcal agents with unusual ability to penetrate tissue. Bactericidal levels have been assayed in bone and necrotic tissue. Concentrations of 0.03–1.12 micrograms/ml inhibit nearly all strains of *Staphylococcus aureus*. Fusidic acid is active against *Staphylococcus epidermidis* and methicillin-resistant staphylococci.

In severe or deep-seated infections and when prolonged therapy may be required, systemic Fucidin should generally be given concurrently with other anti-staphylococcal antibiotic therapy.

Pharmacokinetics: 500 mg of sodium fusidate given as a single infusion over 2 hours results in a Cmax of 52 micrograms/ml. Blood levels are cumulative, reaching concentrations of 60–120 micrograms/ml after repeated infusion of 500 mg sodium fusidate every 8 hours for 2–3 days.

The plasma half-life is approximately 10–15 hours.

Fucidin is excreted mainly in the bile, little or none being excreted in the urine.

Indications: Fucidin is indicated in the treatment of all staphylococcal infections due to susceptible organisms such as: osteomyelitis, pneumonia, septicaemia, wound infections, endocarditis, superinfected cystic fibrosis, cutaneous infections.

Fucidin should be administered intravenously whenever oral therapy is inappropriate, which includes cases where absorption from the gastro-intestinal tract is unpredictable.

Dosage and administration
Adults weighing more than 50 kg: 500 mg sodium fusidate three times daily.

Children and adults weighing less than 50 kg: 6–7 mg sodium fusidate per kg bodyweight three times daily.

Recommended procedure: To reconstitute, dissolve the contents of one vial containing 500 mg sodium fusidate powder (equivalent to 480 mg of fusidic acid) in the 10 ml buffer provided.

For adults weighing more than 50 kg: Add the 10 ml fusidate/buffer solution to 500 ml of infusion fluid.

For children and adults weighing less than 50 kg: Add the 10 ml fusidate/buffer solution to 500 ml of infusion fluid. Each dose corresponds to 6–7 ml of the resulting solution per kg bodyweight.

The diluted fluid should be infused via a central venous line over 2 hours. If a superficial vein is employed a more prolonged period of at least 6 hours is advisable.

Since Fucidin is excreted in the bile, no dosage modifications are needed in renal impairment.

The dosage in patients undergoing haemodialysis needs no adjustment as Fucidin is not significantly dialysed.

Dosage in the elderly: No dosage alterations are necessary in the elderly.

If additional antibacterial therapy is to be employed, it is recommended that for parenteral administration, separate infusion fluids be used.

Contra-indications, warnings, etc
Contra-indications: Contraindicated in patients with known hypersensitivity to fusidic acid and its salts. Intravenous Fucidin should not be infused with amino acid solutions or in whole blood. Due to local tissue injury, Fucidin should not be administered intramuscularly or subcutaneously.

Precautions: Caution should be exercised with other antibiotics which have similar biliary excretion pathways, e.g. lincomycin and rifampicin. Periodic liver function tests should be carried out when high oral doses are used, when the drug is given for prolonged periods and in patients with liver dysfunction.

Fucidin displaces bilirubin from its albumin binding site in vitro. The clinical significance of this finding is uncertain and kernicterus has not been observed in neonates receiving Fucidin. However, this observation should be borne in mind when the drug is given to pre-term, jaundiced, acidotic or seriously ill neonates.

Pregnancy and lactation: There is inadequate evidence of safety in human pregnancy. Animal studies and many years of clinical experience suggest that fusidic acid is devoid of teratogenic effects. There is evidence to suggest that when given systemically, fusidic acid can cross the placental barrier. If the administration of Fucidin to pregnant patients is considered essential, it requires that the potential benefits be weighed against the possible hazards to the foetus.

Safety in nursing mothers has not been established. When fusidic acid (as the sodium salt) has been given systemically, levels have been detected in the breast milk. Caution is, therefore, required when Fucidin is used in mothers who wish to breast feed.

Adverse reactions: In some patients given Fucidin, particularly the young and elderly, a reversible jaundice has been reported. Jaundice has been seen most frequently in patients receiving intravenous Fucidin in high dosage, or where the drug has been infused too rapidly or at too high a concentration in the infusion fluid. In some instances, instituting oral therapy may be beneficial. If the jaundice persists, Fucidin should be withdrawn, following which the serum bilirubin will invariably return to normal. Reported reactions are thrombophlebitis and, rarely, skin rashes and haematological disorders including bone marrow depression and neutropenia. Acute renal failure has been described in patients with jaundice, particularly in the presence of other factors predisposing to renal failure.

Overdosage: There has been no experience of overdosage with Fucidin. Treatment should be restricted to symptomatic and supportive measures. Dialysis is of no benefit since the drug is not significantly dialysed.

Pharmaceutical precautions Fucidin dry powder is stable for 3 years when stored at room temperature (below 25°C) and protected from light. When the buffer solution is transferred to the powder vial, this vial should be regarded as a unit dose. The required amount of Fucidin/buffer solution should be used once only and any unused portion discarded.

In vitro compatibility studies of Fucidin for Intravenous Infusion with commonly used infusion solutions have been carried out.

The results showed that sodium fusidate reconstituted at 50 mg/ml in buffer solution is physically and chemically compatible for at least 24 hours at room temperature with the following infusion solutions (the figure in parenthesis shows the concentration of sodium fusidate in the final admixture):

Sodium Chloride Intravenous Infusion BP 0.9% (1–2 mg/ml)

Dextrose Intravenous Infusion BP 5% (1–2 mg/ml)

Compound Sodium Lactate Intravenous Infusion ("Ringer-Lactate Solution") (1 mg/ml)

Sodium Lactate Intravenous Infusion BP (1 mg/ml)

Sodium Chloride (0.18%) and Dextrose (4%) Intravenous Infusion BP (1 mg/ml)

Potassium Chloride (0.3%) and Dextrose (5%) Intravenous Infusion BP (1 mg/ml)

Sodium Fusidate reconstituted at 50 mg/ml in buffer solution is physically incompatible with infusion fluids containing 20% or more of dextrose, lipid infusions and peritoneal dialysis fluids. Precipitation may occur in dilutions which result in a pH of less than 7.4.

Legal category POM.

Package quantities Pack containing a single pair of vials.

Further information Fucidin should be administered intravenously into a wide bore vein with a good blood flow. Excessive doses may cause venospasm and haemolysis of erthrocytes. Both oral and intravenous Fucidin have been given concurrently with other antibiotics, e.g. cloxacillin, flucloxacillin, ampicillin, methicillin and erythromycin.

Fusidic acid and its salts exhibit no cross hypersensitivity or cross resistance with other antibiotics in clinical use.

Despite many years of clinical use, resistance to fusidic acid amongst *Staphylococcus aureus* remains low.

Product licence number 0043/0184.

FUCIDIN* CREAM
FUCIDIN* OINTMENT
FUCIDIN* GEL
FUCIDIN* INTERTULLE

Presentation *Fucidin Cream* contains Fusidic Acid PhEur 2% in a cream base. Other ingredients: potassium sorbate 0.27% as preservative, butylated hydroxyanisole, cetyl alcohol, glycerol, liquid paraffin, polysorbate 60, purified water and white soft paraffin.

Fucidin Ointment contains Fusidic Acid, as the sodium salt, PhEur 2% in an ointment base (no preservative). Other ingredients: cetyl alcohol, lanolin, liquid paraffin and white soft paraffin.

Fucidin Gel contains Fusidic Acid PhEur 2% in a water-miscible base. Other ingredients: methyl paraben 0.27% and propyl paraben 0.03% as preservatives, carbomer, dimeticone, polysorbate 80, trolamine and water for injections.

Fucidin Intertulle: Sterile gauze squares each impregnated with Fusidic Acid, as the sodium salt, PhEur 2% (Fucidin Ointment) in an ointment base and enclosed between two leaves of sterile parchment in a sealed foil pack.

Uses *Mode of Action:* Fusidic acid is a potent topical antibacterial agent. Fusidic acid and its salts show fat and water solubility and strong surface activity and exhibit unusual ability to penetrate intact skin. Concentrations of 0.03–0.12 micrograms/ml inhibit nearly all strains of *Staphylococcus aureus*. Topical application of fusidic acid is also effective against Streptococci, Corynebacteria, Neisseria and certain Clostridia.

Indications: Indicated either alone or in combination with systemic therapy, in the treatment of primary and secondary skin infections caused by sensitive strains of *Staphylococcus aureus*, Streptococcus spp and *Corynebacterium minutissimum*. Primary skin infections that may be expected to respond to treatment with fusidic acid applied topically include: impetigo contagiosa, superficial folliculitis, sycosis barbae, paronychia and erythrasma; also such secondary skin infections as infected eczematoid dermatitis, infected contact dematitis and infected cuts/abrasions.

Dosage and administration *Fucidin Cream, Fucidin Gel and Fucidin Ointment: Adults and children:* Uncovered lesions – apply gently, three or four times daily. Covered lesions – less frequent applications may be adequate.

Fucidin Intertulle: Usually, once a day application but frequency of application will vary with clinical circumstances. The intertulle should be covered with a suitable dressing which should be renewed frequently.

Contra-indications, warnings, etc
Contra-indications: Infection caused by non-susceptible organisms, in particular, *Pseudomonas aeruginosa*.

Fucidin Cream, Ointment, Gel and Intertulle are contra-indicated in patients with hypersensitivity to fusidic acid and its salts.

Precautions: Bacterial resistance has been reported to occur with the use of fusidic acid applied topically. As with all topical antibiotics extended or recurrent application may increase the risk of contact sensitisation and the development of antibiotic resistance.

Fusidic acid does not appear to cause conjunctival irritation in experimental animals. Caution should, however, still be exercised when using Fucidin Cream or Gel near the eye. The sodium salt of fusidic acid has been shown to cause conjunctival irritation. The Ointment and Intertulle should not be used in or near the eye.

Pregnancy and lactation: There is inadequate evidence of safety in human pregnancy. Animal studies and many years of clinical experience have suggested that fusidic acid is devoid of teratogenic effects. There is evidence to suggest that when given systemically, fusidic acid can penetrate the placental barrier. The use of topical Fucidin in pregnancy requires that the potential benefits be weighed against the possible hazards to the foetus.

Safety in nursing mothers has not been established. When fusidic acid (as the sodium salt) has been given systemically, levels have been detected in breast milk but with topical use the possible amount of drug present is unlikely to affect the infant.

Adverse reactions: Hypersensitivity reactions to the active ingredient in the form of skin rashes and mild stinging and irritation on application, have been reported rarely.

Overdosage: Not applicable.

Pharmaceutical precautions *Fucidin Cream and Ointment:* Nil.

Fucidin Gel: Store below 25°C but do not freeze.

Fucidin Intertulle: Store below 25°C.

Legal category POM.

Package quantities *Fucidin Cream, Fucidin Ointment and Fucidin Gel:* Tubes of 15 g (OP) and 30 g (OP).
Fucidin Intertulle: Box of 10 foil packs, each containing one tulle piece (10 cm×10 cm) (OP).

Further information Fusidic acid and its salts exhibit no cross hypersensitivity with other antibiotics in clinical use.

Despite many years of clinical use, resistance to fusidic acid amongst *Staphylococcus aureus*, remains low.

The ointment base contains lanolin.

The gel base is non-staining and contains no lanolin or other fatty constituents.

The cream base is a vanishing base and contains no lanolin.

Product licence numbers

Fucidin Cream	0043/0065
Fucidin Ointment	0043/5005R
Fucidin Gel	0043/5018R
Fucidin Intertulle	0043/5007R

FUCIDIN* H CREAM
FUCIDIN* H OINTMENT
FUCIDIN* H GEL

Presentation Fucidin H cream contains Fusidic Acid PhEur 2% and Hydrocortisone Acetate PhEur 1% in a cream base. Other ingredients: potassium sorbate

0.27% as preservative, butylated hydroxyanisole, cetyl alcohol, glycerol, liquid paraffin, polysorbate 60, purified water and white soft paraffin.

Fucidin H Ointment contains Fusidic Acid, as the sodium salt PhEur 2% and Hydrocortisone Acetate PhEur 1% in an ointment base. Other ingredients: cetyl alcohol, lanolin, liquid paraffin and white soft paraffin.

Fucidin H Gel contains Fusidic Acid PhEur 2% and Hydrocortisone Acetate PhEur 1% in a water-miscible gel base. Other ingredients: methyl paraben 0.27% and propyl paraben 0.03% as preservatives, carbomer, dimeticone, polysorbate 80, trolamine and water for injections.

Uses *Mode of Action:* Fucidin H Cream, H Ointment and H Gel combine the potent topical antibacterial action of fusidic acid with the anti-inflammatory and antipruritic effects of hydrocortisone. Concentrations of 0.03–0.12 micrograms fusidic acid per ml inhibit nearly all strains of *Staphylococcus aureus.* Topical application of fusidic acid is also effective against Streptococci, Corynebacteria, Neisseria and certain Clostridia.

Indications: Fucidin H Cream, H Ointment and H Gel are indicated in eczema and dermatitis with secondary bacterial infections, including atopic eczema, primary irritant dermatitis and allergic and seborrhoeic dermatitis when the organisms responsible are known to be or believed to be sensitive to fusidic acid.

Dosage and administration *Adults and children:* Uncovered lesions – apply gently, three or four times daily. Covered lesions – less frequent applications may be adequate.

Contra-indications, warnings, etc

Contra-indications: As with other topical corticosteroid preparations, Fucidin H Cream, H Ointment and H Gel are contra-indicated in primary bacterial, viral and fungal skin infections.

Fucidin H Cream, H Ointment and H Gel are contra-indicated in patients with hypersensitivity to fusidic acid and its salts.

Precautions: Fucidin H Ointment should not be used in or near the eye, as sodium fusidate causes conjunctival irritation.

Fusidic acid does not appear to cause conjunctival irritation in experimental animals. Caution should still be exercised, however, when Fucidin H Cream or Fucidin H Gel is used near the eye.

Steroid-antibiotic combinations should not be continued for more than 7 days in the absence of any clinical improvement since in this situation occult extension of the infection may occur due to the masking of the steroid. Similarly, steroids may also mask hypersensitivity reactions.

Bacterial resistance has been reported to occur with the use of fusidic acid applied topically. As with all topical antibiotics, extended or recurrent application may increase the risk of contact sensitisation and the development of antibiotic resistance.

Pregnancy and lactation: There is inadequate evidence of safety in human pregnancy.

Topical administration of corticosteroids to pregnant animals can cause abnormalities of foetal development including cleft palate and intra-uterine growth retardation. There may, therefore, be a very small risk of such effects in the human foetus.

Animal studies and many years of clinical experience have suggested that fusidic acid is devoid of teratogenic effects. There is evidence to suggest that when given systemically, fusidic acid can penetrate the placental barrier. The use of topical Fucidin in pregnancy requires that the potential benefits be weighed against the possible hazards to the foetus.

Safety in nursing mothers has not been established.

When fusidic acid (as the sodium salt) has been given systemically, levels have been detected in breast milk, but with topical use the possible amount of drug present is unlikely to affect the infant.

In infants, long-term continuous topical therapy with corticosteroids should be avoided. Adrenal suppression can occur even without occlusion.

Adverse reactions: Hypersensitivity reactions to the active ingredient in the form of skin rashes and mild stinging and irritation on application, have been reported rarely.

Overdosage: Not applicable.

Pharmaceutical precautions *Fucidin H Cream and H Ointment:* Nil. *Fucidin H Gel:* Store below 25°C but do not freeze.

Legal category POM.

Package quantities Tubes of 15 g (OP) and 30 g (OP).

Further information Fusidic acid and its salts exhibit no cross hypersensitivity with other antibiotics in clinical use.

Despite many years of clinical use, resistance to fusidic acid amongst *Staphylococcus aureus,* remains low.

The ointment base contains lanolin.

The gel base is non-staining and contains no lanolin or other fatty constituents.

The cream base is a vanishing base and contains no lanolin.

Product licence numbers

Fucidin H Cream	0043/0093
Fucidin H Gel	0043/0024R
Fucidin H Ointment	0043/5012R

FuciBET* CREAM

Presentation FuciBET cream contains betamethasone 0.1% (as the valerate ester) and Fusidic Acid PhEur 2% in a smooth white to off-white water miscible base. Other ingredients: chlorocresol 0.1% as preservative, cetomacrogol 1000, cetostearyl alcohol, liquid paraffin, purified water, sodium dihydrogen phosphate and white soft paraffin.

Uses FuciBET combines the well-known anti-inflammatory and antipruritic effects of betamethasone with the potent topical antibacterial action of fusidic acid.

Betamethasone valerate is a topical steroid rapidly effective in those inflammatory dermatoses which normally respond to this form of therapy. More refractory conditions can often be treated successfully.

When applied topically, fusidic acid is effective against *Staphylococcus aureus,* Streptococci, Corynebacteria, Neisseria and certain Clostridia and Bacteroides. Concentrations of 0.03 to 0.12 microgram per ml inhibit nearly all strains of *S. aureus.* The antibacterial activity of fusidic acid is not diminished in the presence of betamethasone.

Indications: FuciBET is indicated for the treatment of eczematous dermatoses including atopic eczema, infantile eczema, discoid eczema, stasis eczema, contact eczema and seborrhoeic eczema when secondary bacterial infection is confirmed or suspected.

Dosage and administration A small quantity should be applied to the affected area two or three times daily until a satisfactory response is obtained. It may then be possible to maintain improvement by less frequent application or by the use of a less potent topical steroid/antibacterial preparation such as Fucidin H Ointment or Fucidin H Gel.

In the more resistant lesions the effect of FuciBET can be enhanced by occlusion with polythene film. Overnight occlusion is usually adequate.

Contra-indications, warnings, etc

Contra-indications: Acne rosacea and peri-oral dermatitis. Skin lesions of viral, fungal or bacterial origin. Hypersensitivity to the preparation.

Precautions: Long-term continuous topical therapy should be avoided, particularly in infants and children. Adrenal suppression can occur even without occlusion. Atrophic changes may occur on the face and to a lesser degree in other parts of the body, after prolonged treatment with potent topical steroids.

Caution should be exercised if FuciBET is used near the eye. Glaucoma might result if the preparation enters the eye. Systemic chemotherapy is required if bacterial infection persists.

Pregnancy: Topical administration of any corticosteroid to pregnant animals can cause abnormalities of foetal development. The relevance of this finding to human beings has not been established; however, topical steroids should not be used extensively in pregnancy, i.e. in large amounts or for prolonged periods.

Adverse reactions: Prolonged and intensive treatment with potent corticosteroids may cause local atrophic changes in the skin, including striae, thinning and dilation of superficial blood vessels, particularly when applied to the flexures or when occlusion is employed.

As with other topical corticosteroids sufficient systemic absorption to produce hypercorticism can occur with prolonged or extensive use. Infants and children are at particular risk, more so if occlusive dressings are used. A napkin may act as an occlusive dressing in infants.

Hypersensitivity reactions to fusidic acid are rare and FuciBET does not contain lanolin. However, if signs of hypersensitivity occur, treatment should be withdrawn.

Overdosage: Not applicable.

Pharmaceutical precautions Nil.

Legal category POM.

Package quantities Tubes of 15 g (OP), 30 g (OP) and 60 g (OP).

Further information The least potent corticosteroid, which controls the disease, should be used.

Product licence number 0043/0091.

FUCITHALMIC*

Qualitative and quantitative composition Each gram contains fusidic acid, hemihydrate PhEur 10 mg.

Pharmaceutical form Sterile viscous eye drops.

Clinical particulars

Therapeutic indications: Fucithalmic is indicated for the topical treatment of bacterial conjunctivitis where the organism is known to be sensitive to the antibiotic.

Posology and method of administration: For all ages: One Fucithalmic drop to be instilled into the eye twice daily. Treatment should be continued for at least 48 hours after the eye returns to normal.

Contra-indications: Hypersensitivity to any of its components.

Special warnings and precautions for use: Should not be used when contact lenses are being worn.

Interactions with other medicaments and other forms of interaction: Not applicable.

Pregnancy and lactation: Not applicable.

Effects on ability to drive and use machines: Not applicable.

Undesirable effects: Transient stinging after application has been encountered. Hypersensitivity may occur.

Overdosage: Not applicable.

Pharmacological properties

Pharmacodynamic properties: Fucithalmic is active against a wide range of gram-positive organisms, particularly *Staphylococcus aureus.* Other species against which Fucithalmic has been shown to have *in vitro* activity include *Streptococcus, Neisseria, Haemophilus, Moraxella* and *Corynebacteria.*

Pharmacokinetic properties: The sustained release formulation of Fucithalmic ensures a prolonged contact with the conjunctival sac. Twice daily application provides sufficient fusidic acid concentrations in all relevant tissues of the eye. Fusidic acid penetrates well into the aqueous humour.

Preclinical safety data: There are no pre-clinical data of relevance to the prescriber which are additional to that already included in other sections of the SPC.

Pharmaceutical particulars

List of excipients: Benzalkonium chloride, disodium edetate, mannitol, carbomer sodium hydroxide, water for injections.

Incompatibilities: None known.

Shelf life: 3 years.

Special precautions for storage: Store below 25°C. Keep the tube tightly closed. The tube should be discarded one month after opening.

Nature and contents of container: Available in 5 g tubes.

Instructions for use/handling: None.

Marketing authorisation number 0043/0137

Date of first authorisation/renewal of authorisation United Kingdom 10.8.1987

Date of (partial) revision of the text June 1997.

Legal category POM.

HEPARIN (MUCOUS) INJECTION BP

Presentation Heparin (Mucous) Injection BP 1,000 units per ml: each ml contains 1,000 units heparin sodium. (Presented in 5 ml vials with 1% benzyl alcohol, 0.1% methylparahydroxybenzoate and 0.02% propylparahydroxybenzoate as preservatives. Also contains sodium citrate, sodium chloride and water for injections.)

Heparin (Mucous) Injection BP 5,000 units per ml: each ml contains 5,000 units heparin sodium. (Presented in 5 ml vials with 1% benzyl alcohol, 0.1% methylparahydroxybenzoate and 0.02% propylparahydroxybenzoate as preservatives. Also contains sodium citrate, sodium chloride and water for injections.)

Heparin (Mucous) Injection BP 25,000 units per ml: each ml contains 25,000 units heparin sodium. (Presented in 5 ml vials with 1% benzyl alcohol, 0.1% methylparahydroxybenzoate and 0.02% propylparahydroxybenzoate as preservatives. Also contains sodium citrate and water for injections.)

Uses *Mode of action:* Heparin is a naturally occurring anticoagulant which prevents the coagulation of blood *in vivo* and *in vitro.* It potentiates the inhibition of several activated coagulation factors, including thrombin and factor X.

Indications: Treatment of thrombo-embolic disorders such as deep vein thrombosis, acute arterial embolism or thrombosis, thrombophlebitis, pulmonary embolism and fat embolism.

Prophylaxis against deep vein thrombosis and thromboembolic events in susceptible patients.

Dosage and administration

Treatment dosage

Intravenous administration: 5,000–10,000 units every 4 hours or 500 units/kg bodyweight daily as a continuous infusion in sodium chloride injection or dextrose injection. The dose should be individually adjusted according to coagulation tests.

Subcutaneous administration: The initial dose is 250 units/kg bodyweight. Further doses should be given every 12 hours and individually adjusted according to coagulation tests.

Dosage adjustment: It is recommended that dosages be adjusted to maintain a thrombin clotting time, whole blood clotting time or activated partial thromboplastin time 1.5–2 times that of control on blood withdrawn 4–6 hours after the first injection or commencement of infusion and at similar intervals until the patient is stabilised.

Prophylactic dosage

Administration is by subcutaneous injection.

Patients undergoing major elective surgery: 5,000 units should be given 2 hours pre-operatively and then every 8–12 hours post-operatively for 10–14 days or until the patient is ambulant whichever is the longer.

Following myocardial infarction: 5,000 units should be given twice daily for 10 days or until the patient is mobile.

Other patients: 5,000 units should be given every 8–12 hours.

These standard prophylactic regimens do not require routine control.

Dosage in children

Treatment dosage: Standard treatment dosages should be given initially. Subsequent dosages and/or dosage intervals should be individually adjusted according to changes in thrombin clotting time, whole blood clotting time and/or activated partial thromboplastin time.

Dosage in the elderly

Treatment dosage: Lower treatment dosages may be required, however, standard treatment dosages should be given initially and then subsequent dosages and/or dosage intervals should be individually adjusted according to changes in thrombin clotting time, whole blood clotting time and/or activated partial thromboplastin time.

Prophylactic dosage: Dosage alterations are unnecessary for prophylaxis in the elderly.

Pregnancy

Treatment dosage: Standard treatment dosages should be given initially by continuous intravenous infusion or every 12 hours by subcutaneous injection. Intermittent intravenous injections are not advised. Subsequent dosages and/or dosage intervals should be individually adjusted according to changes in thrombin clotting time, whole blood clotting time and/or activated partial thromboplastin time.

Prophylactic dosage: It is recommended that plasma heparin levels be maintained below 0.4 units/ml, as determined by specific anti-Xa assay. A suggested dosage is 5,000 units every 12 hours in early pregnancy, increasing to 10,000 units every 12 hours in the last trimester. The dosage should be reduced during labour and the standard prophylactic dosage is suitable in the puerperium.

Contra-indications, warnings, etc

Contra-indications: Haemorrhagic disorders and patients with an actual or potential bleeding site e.g. peptic ulcer. Patients with bacterial endocarditis and those with severe hypertension.

Precautions: Heparin therapy should be given with caution to patients with impaired renal or hepatic function.

Oral anticoagulants or drugs which interfere with platelet function, eg aspirin and dextran solutions should be administered with caution.

Pregnancy and lactation: Although animal studies have not been performed, epidemiological studies indicate that if drug therapy is needed in pregnancy, the use of heparin in the recommended dosage is acceptable. Heparin does not cross the placenta or appear in breast milk.

Adverse reactions: Hypersensitivity and acute reversible thrombocytopenia may occur rarely. Osteoporosis and alopecia have been reported after prolonged therapy.

Overdosage: The effect of heparin can be reversed immediately by intravenous administration of a 1% protamine sulphate solution. The dose of protamine sulphate required for neutralisation should be determined accurately by titrating the patient's plasma. It is important to avoid overdosage of protamine sulphate because protamine itself has anticoagulant properties. A single dose of protamine sulphate should never exceed 50 mg. Intravenous injection of protamine may cause a sudden fall in blood pressure, bradycardia, dyspnoea and transitory flushing, but these may be avoided or diminished by slow and careful administration.

Pharmaceutical precautions Store below 25°C. Heparin has been reported to be incompatible in aqueous solutions with certain substances, eg, some antibiotics, hydrocortisone, phenothiazines, narcotic analgesics and some antihistamines.

Legal category POM.

Package quantities *Heparin 1,000 units per ml:* 5 ml vials. Packs of 10.

Heparin 5,000 units per ml: 5 ml vials. Packs of 10.

Heparin 25,000 units per ml: 5 ml vials. Packs of 5.

Further information Nil.

Product licence numbers

1,000 units (with preservative)	0043/0041R
5,000 units (with preservative)	0043/0038R
25,000 units (with preservative)	0043/0039R

HEP-FLUSH*

Presentation Heparin flush solution, each ml containing 100 units sodium heparin in saline. Also contains 1% benzyl alcohol, 0.1% methylparahydroxybenzoate and 0.02% propylparahydroxybenzoate as preservatives, sodium citrate and water for injections. Available as ampoules of 200 units in 2 ml.

Uses

Mode of action: Heparin is a naturally occurring anticoagulant which prevents the coagulation of blood *in vivo* and *in vitro.* It potentiates the inhibition of several activated coagulation factors, including thrombin and factor X.

Indications: To maintain the patency of in-dwelling intravenous lines. It is not recommended for therapeutic use.

Dosage and administration For routine use, 2 ml containing 200 units of heparin should be administered into the catheter/cannula every 4 to 8 hours or as required.

Contra-indications, warnings, etc When used as recommended the low dose of heparin reaching the blood should have no systemic effects.

Pharmaceutical precautions Store below 25°C. Hep-Flush is compatible with normal saline. Heparin has been reported to be incompatible in aqueous solution with certain substances, e.g. some antibiotics, hydrocortisone, phenothiazines, narcotic analgesics and antihistamines.

Legal category POM.

Package quantities Packs of 10×2 ml ampoules.

Further information Nil.

Product licence number 0043/0057

HEPLOK*

Presentation Heparin flush solution; 5 ml ampoule, each ml containing 10 units heparin sodium in saline (no preservative), (i.e. 50 units per ampoule).

Uses

Mode of action: Heparin is a naturally occurring anticoagulant which prevents the coagulation of blood *in vivo* and *in vitro.* It potentiates the inhibition of several activated coagulation factors, including thrombin and factor X.

Indications: To maintain the patency of in-dwelling intravenous lines. It is not recommended for therapeutic use.

Dosage and administration For routine use 1–5 ml (10–50 units heparin) should be administered into the catheter/cannula every 4 to 8 hours or as required.

Contra-indications, warnings, etc When used as recommended the low dose of heparin reaching the blood should have no systemic effects.

Pharmaceutical precautions Store below 25°C. Heplok is compatible with normal saline. Heparin has been reported to be incompatible in aqueous solution with certain substances, e.g. some antibiotics, hydrocortisone, phenothiazines, narcotic analgesics and antihistamines.

Legal category POM.

Package quantities Packs of 10×5 ml ampoules.

Further information Nil.

Product licence number 0043/0092.

INNOHEP* 20,000 IU/ML ▼
INNOHEP* SYRINGE 20,000 IU/ML ▼

Qualitative and quantitative composition Tinzaparin sodium 20,000 anti-Factor Xa IU/ml.

Pharmaceutical form Solution for injection.

Clinical particulars

Therapeutic indications: Treatment of deep-vein thrombosis and of pulmonary embolus.

Posology and method of administration: Administration is by subcutaneous injection only.

Adults: 175 anti-Factor Xa IU/kg bodyweight once daily, for at least 6 days and until adequate oral anticoagulation is established.

There is no need to monitor the Innohep treatment.

Use in the elderly: No dose modifications are necessary.

Use in children: There is no experience of use in children.

Contra-indications: Known hypersensitivity to constituents. Generalised haemorrhagic tendency, uncontrolled severe hypertension, active peptic ulcer, septic endocarditis. Thrombocytopenia in patients with a positive *in vitro* aggregation test in the presence of tinzaparin.

Special warnings and precautions for use: Care should be taken when Innohep is administered to patients with severe liver or kidney insufficiency. In such cases a dose reduction should be considered.

Innohep should not be administered by intramuscular injection due to the risk of haematoma.

Innohep should be used with caution in patients with a history of asthma due to the presence of sodium bisulphite.

Care should be taken when Innohep is administered to patients who have recently suffered from cerebral haemorrhage, trauma and/or had recent surgery to the central nervous system.

Innohep should be used with caution in patients with hypersensitivity to heparin or to other low molecular weight heparins.

For some patients with pulmonary embolism (e.g. those with severe haemodynamic instability) alternative treatment, such as surgery or thrombolysis may be indicated.

Interaction with other medicaments and other forms of interaction: Any drug which affects platelet function or aggregation or blood coagulation, e.g. salicylates, non-steroidal anti-inflammatory drugs, vitamin K antagonists (such as warfarin) and dextran, should be used with caution in patients receiving Innohep.

Pregnancy and lactation: No transplacental passage of Innohep was found (assessed by anti-Factor Xa and anti-Factor IIa activity) in patients given a dose of 35–40 anti-Factor Xa IU/kg in the second trimester of pregnancy. In rabbits, no transplacental passage of anti-Factor Xa or anti-Factor IIa activity was observed after doses of 1750 anti-Factor Xa IU/kg. Toxicological studies in rats have shown no embryotoxic or teratogenic effects, although a lower birthweight was found.

Although these animal studies show no hazard, as a precaution Innohep should not be used in pregnancy unless no safer alternative is available.

It is not known whether Innohep is excreted in breast milk. However, patients are advised to stop breast-feeding while receiving Innohep.

Effects on ability to drive and use machines: No adverse effects to be expected.

Undesirable effects: Skin rashes and minor bruising at the site of injection have occurred occasionally. Systemic allergic reactions have been reported extremely rarely.

Innohep, like heparin, has been shown to increase the risk of haemorrhage. However, at the recommended dose this risk is low. As with heparin, thrombocytopenia may occur rarely.

As for heparin, a transient increase in aminotransferase levels is frequently seen. Cessation of treatment is not usually required.

Overdose: Overdose of Innohep may be complicated by haemorrhage. With recommended dosages there should be no need for an antidote but in the event of accidental administration of an overdose, the effect of Innohep can be reversed by intravenous administration of 1% protamine sulphate solution.

The dose of protamine sulphate required for neutralisation should be accurately determined by titrating with the patient's plasma. As a rule, 1 mg of protamine sulphate neutralises the effect of 100 anti-Factor Xa IU tinzaparin. The anti-Factor Xa activity of tinzaparin is only partially neutralised by protamine sulphate and the anti-Factor Xa and anti-factor IIa (APTT) activities are seen to return 3 hours after its reversal.

It is recommended that protamine sulphate (1 mg/100 anti-Factor Xa IU of tinzaparin) should be given as intermittent injections or continuous infusion.

Potential side-effects of protamine sulphate must be considered and patients carefully observed.

Transfusion of fresh plasma may be used, if necessary. Plasma anti-Factor Xa and anti-Factor IIa activity should be measured during the management of overdose situations.

Phamacological properties

Pharmacodynamic properties: Innohep is an antithrombotic agent. It potentiates the inhibition of several activated coagulation factors, especially Factor Xa, its activity being mediated via antithrombin III.

Pharmacokinetic properties: The pharmacokinetics/pharmacodynamic activity of Innohep is monitored by anti-Factor Xa activity. Following a subcutaneous injection of Innohep, anti-Factor Xa activity reaches a maximum at 4–6 hours (peak anti-Factor Xa activity, after administration of 175 anti-Factor Xa IU/kg bodyweight once daily, is approximately 0.5–1.0 IU/ml). Detectable anti-Factor Xa activity persists for 24 hours.

Preclinical safety data: There are no preclinical data of relevance to the prescriber which are additional to that already included in other sections of the SPC.

Pharmaceutical particulars

List of excipients:

Innohep 20,000 IU/ml – Sodium metabisulphite, benzyl alcohol, sodium hydroxide, water for injections.

Innohep Syringe 20,000 IU/ml – Sodium metabisulphite, sodium hydroxide, water for injections.

Incompatibilities: Innohep should be given by subcutaneous injection only. It should not be mixed with any other injection.

Shelf life: 2 years.

Special precautions for storage: To be stored at room temperature.

Nature and contents of container:

Innohep 20,000 IU/ml – A 2 ml vial containing 20,000 anti-Factor Xa IU/ml in packs of 1 vial.

Innohep Syringe 20,000 IU/ml – A prefilled variable dose graduated syringe containing: 0.5 ml (10,000 anti-Factor Xa IU), 0.7 ml (14,000 anti-Factor Xa IU), 0.9 ml (18,000 anti-Factor Xa IU) in packs of 2 and 6 syringes.

Instructions for use/handling:

Innohep 20,000 IU/ml – The vial should be discarded 14 days after first use.

Innohep Syringe 20,000 IU/ml – Contains no bactericide, any portion of the contents not used at once should be discarded together with the syringe.

Marketing authorisation numbers

Innohep 20,000 IU/ml – PL 0043/0192.

Innohep Syringe 20,000 IU/ml – PL 0043/0197.

Date of first authorisation/renewal of authorisation

Innohep 20,000 IU/ml – 18 October 1994.

Innohep Syringe 20,000 IU/ml – 3 October 1996.

Date of (partial) revision of the text August 1998.

Legal category POM.

INNOHEP* SYRINGE 10,000 IU/ml

Qualitative and quantitative composition Tinzaparin sodium 10,000 anti-Factor Xa IU/ml.

Pharmaceutical form Solution for injection.

Clinical particulars

Therapeutic indications: For the prevention of thromboembolic events, including deep vein thrombosis in patients undergoing general and orthopaedic surgery.

Posology and method of administration: Administration is by subcutaneous injection only.

Adults at low to moderate risk, e.g. patients undergoing general surgery: 3,500 anti-Factor Xa IU two hours before surgery and then once daily for 7 to 10 days post-operatively.

Adults at high risk, e.g. patients undergoing orthopaedic surgery: In this high risk group the recommended dose is either a fixed dose of 4,500 anti-Factor Xa IU given 12 hours before surgery followed by a once daily dose, or 50 anti-Factor Xa IU/kilogram body weight 2 hours before surgery followed by a once daily dose for 7 to 10 days post-operatively.

Use in the elderly: No dose modifications are necessary.

Use in children: There is no experience of use in children.

Contra-indications: Known hypersensitivity to constituents. Generalised haemorrhagic tendency, uncontrolled severe hypertension, active peptic ulcer, septic endocarditis. Thrombocytopenia in patients with a positive *in vitro* aggregation test in the presence of tinzaparin.

Special warnings and precautions for use: Care should be taken when Innohep is administered to patients with severe liver or kidney insufficiency.

Innohep should not be administered by intramuscular injection due to the risk of haematoma. Care should be taken when Innohep is administered to patients who have recently suffered from cerebral haemorrhage, trauma and/or had recent surgery to the central nervous system.

Innohep should be used with caution in patients with hypersensitivity to heparin or to other low molecular weight heparins.

Interaction with other medicaments and other forms of interaction: Any drug which affects platelet function or aggregation or blood coagulation, e.g. salicylates, non-steroidal anti-inflammatory drugs, vitamin K antagonists (such as warfarin) and dextran should be used with caution in patients receiving Innohep.

Pregnancy and lactation: No transplacental passage of Innohep was found (assessed by anti-Factor Xa and anti-Factor IIa activity) in patients given a dose of 35 to 40 anti-Factor Xa IU/kg in the second trimester of pregnancy. In rabbits, no transplacental passage of anti-Factor Xa or anti-Factor IIa activity was observed after doses of 1750 anti-Factor Xa IU/kg. Toxicological studies in rats have shown no embryotoxic or teratogenic effects, although a lower birthweight was found.

Although these animal studies show no hazard, as a precaution Innohep should not be used in pregnancy unless no safer alternative is available.

It is not known whether Innohep is excreted in breast milk. However, patients are advised to stop breast-feeding while receiving Innohep.

Effects on ability to drive and use machines: No adverse effects to be expected.

Undesirable effects: Skin rashes and minor bruising at the site of injection have occurred occasionally. Systemic allergic reactions have been reported extremely rarely.

Innohep, like heparin, has been shown to increase the risk of haemorrhage. However, at the recommended dose this risk is low. As with heparin, thrombocytopenia may occur rarely.

As for heparin, a transient increase in aminotransferase levels is frequently seen. Cessation of treatment is not usually required.

Overdose: Overdose of Innohep may be complicated by haemorrhage. With recommended dosages there should be no need for an antidote but in the event of accidental administration of an overdose, the effect of Innohep can be reversed by intravenous administration of 1% protamine sulphate solution.

The dose of protamine sulphate required for neutralisation should be accurately determined by titrating with the patient's plasma. As a rule, 1 mg of protamine sulphate neutralises the effect of 100 anti-Factor Xa IU tinzaparin. The anti-Factor Xa activity of tinzaparin is only partially neutralised by protamine sulphate and the anti-Factor Xa and anti-Factor IIa (APTT) activities are seen to return 3 hours after its reversal.

It is recommended that protamine sulphate (1 mg/100 anti-Factor Xa IU of tinzaparin) should be given as intermittent injections or continuous infusion. Potential side-effects of protamine sulphate must be considered and patients carefully observed.

Transfusion of fresh plasma may be used, if necessary. Plasma anti-Factor Xa and anti-Factor IIa activity should be measured during the management of overdose situations.

Pharmacological properties

Pharmacodynamic properties: Innohep is an antithrombotic agent. It potentiates the inhibition of several activated coagulation factors, especially Factor Xa, its activity being mediated via antithrombin III.

Pharmacokinetic properties: The pharmacokinetics/pharmacodynamic activity of Innohep is monitored by anti-Factor Xa activity. Innohep has a bioavailability of around 90% following a subcutaneous injection. The absorption half-life is 200 minutes, peak plasma activity being observed after 4 to 6 hours. The elimination half-life is about 90 minutes. There is a linear dose response relationship between plasma activity and the dose administered.

Preclinical safety data: There are no preclinical data of relevance to the prescriber which are additional to that already included in other sections of the SPC.

Pharmaceutical particulars

List of excipients: Sodium acetate, water for injections. As pH adjusters: sodium hydroxide or hydrochloric acid.

Incompatibilities: Innohep should be given by subcutaneous injection only. It should not be mixed with any other injection.

Shelf life: 2 years.

Special precautions for storage: To be stored below 25°C.

Nature and contents of container: A prefilled unit dose syringe containing: 3,500 anti-Factor Xa IU in 0.35 ml, 4,500 anti-Factor Xa IU in 0.45 ml, in packs of 10 syringes.

Instructions for use/handling: Contains no preservative, any portion of the contents not used at once should be discarded with the syringe.

Marketing authorisation number PL 0043/0204.

Date of first authorisation/renewal of authorisation 20 November 1997.

Date of (partial) revision of the text March 1998.

Legal category POM.

INNOHEP* 5,000 IU IN 0.5 ML

Qualitative and quantitative composition Tinzaparin sodium 5,000 anti-Factor Xa IU in 0.5 ml.

Pharmaceutical form Solution for injection.

Clinical particulars

Therapeutic indications: For the prevention of thromboembolic events including deep vein thrombosis in patients undergoing general and orthopaedic surgery.

Posology and method of administration: Administration is by subcutaneous injection.

Adults at low to moderate risk, e.g. patients undergoing general surgery: 3,500 anti-Factor Xa IU two hours before surgery and then once daily for 7 to 10 days, post-operatively.

Adults at high risk, e.g. patients undergoing orthopaedic surgery: In this high risk group the recommended dose is either a fixed dose of 4,500 anti-Factor Xa IU given 12 hours before surgery followed by a once daily dose, or 50 anti-Factor Xa IU/kilogram body weight two hours before surgery followed by a once daily dose for 7 to 10 days post-operatively.

Use in the elderly: No dose modifications are necessary.

Use in children: There is no experience of use in children.

Contra-indications: Known hypersensitivity to constituents. Generalised haemorrhagic tendency, uncontrolled severe hypertension, active peptic ulcer, septic endocarditis. Thrombocytopenia in patients with a positive *in vitro* aggregation test in the presence of tinzaparin.

Special warnings and precautions for use: Care should be taken when Innohep is administered to patients with severe liver or kidney insufficiency. In such cases a dose reduction should be considered.

Innohep should not be administered by intramuscular injection due to the risk of haematoma. Innohep should be used with caution in patients with a history of asthma due to the presence of sodium bisulphite.

Care should be taken when Innohep is administered to patients who have recently suffered from cerebral haemorrhage, trauma and/or had recent surgery to the central nervous system.

Innohep should be used with caution in patients with hypersensitivity to heparin or to other low molecular weight heparins.

Interaction with other medicaments and other forms of interaction: Any drug which affects platelet function or aggregation or blood coagulation, e.g. salicylates, non-steroidal anit-inflammatory drugs, vitamin K antagonists (such as warfarin) and dextran, should be used with caution in patients receiving Innohep.

Pregnancy and lactation: No transplacental passage of Innohep was found (assessed by anti-factor Xa and anti-Factor IIa activity) in patients given a dose of 35–40 anti-Factor Xa IU/kg in the second trimester of pregnancy. In rabbits, no transplacental passage of anti-Factor Xa or anti-Factor IIa activity was observed after doses of 1750 anti-Factor Xa IU/kg. Toxicological studies in rats have shown no embryotoxic or teratogenic effects, although a lower birthweight was found.

Although these animal studies show no hazard, as a precaution Innohep should not be used in pregnancy unless no safer alternative is available.

It is not known whether Innohep is excreted in breast milk. However, patients are advised to stop breast-feeding while receiving Innohep.

Effects on ability to drive and use machines: No adverse effects to be expected.

Undesirable effects: Skin rashes and minor bruising at the site of injection have occurred occasionally. Systemic allergic reactions been reported extremely rarely.

Innohep, like heparin, has been shown to increase the risk of haemorrhage. However, at the recommended dose this risk is low. As with heparin, thrombocytopenia may occur rarely.

As for heparin, a transient increase in aminotransferase levels is frequently seen. Cessation of treatment is not usually required.

Overdose: Overdose of Innohep may be complicated by haemorrhage. With recommended dosages there should be no need for an antidote but in the event of accidental administration of an overdose, the effect of

Innohep can be reversed by intravenous administration of 1% protamine sulphate solution.

The dose of protamine sulphate required for neutralisation should be accurately determined by titrating with the patient's plasma. As a rule, 1 mg of protamine sulphate neutralises the effect of 100 anti-Factor Xa IU tinzaparin. The anti-Factor Xa activity of tinzaparin is only partially neutralised by protamine sulphate and the anti-Factor Xa and anti-Factor IIa (APTT) activities are seen to return 3 hours after its reversal.

It is recommended that protamine sulphate (1 mg/100 anti-Factor Xa IU of tinzaparin) should be given as intermittent injections or continuous infusion. Potential side-effects of protamine sulphate must be considered and patients carefully observed.

Transfusion of fresh plasma may be used, if necessary. Plasma anti-Factor Xa and anti-Factor IIa activity should be measured during the management of overdose situations.

Pharmacological properties
Pharmacodynamic properties: Innohep is an anti-thrombotic agent. It potentiates the inhibition of several activated coagulation factors, especially Factor Xa, its activity being mediated via antithrombin III.

Pharmacokinetic properties: The pharmacokinetics/pharmacodynamic activity of Innohep is monitored by anti-Factor Xa activity. Innohep has a bioavailability of around 90% following a subcutaneous injection. The absorption half-life is 200 minutes, peak plasma activity being observed after 4 to 6 hours. The elimination half-life is about 90 minutes. There is a linear dose response relationship between plasma activity and the dose administered.

Preclinical safety data: There are no preclinical data of relevance to the prescriber which are additional to that already included in other sections of the SPC.

Pharmaceutical particulars
List of excipients: Sodium metabisulphite, sodium hydroxide and water for injections.

Incompatibilities: None known.

Shelf life: 2 years.

Special precautions for storage: To be stored at room temperature.

Nature and contents of container: A 1 ml ampoule containing 5,000 anti-Factor Xa IU in 0.5 ml in packs of 10 ampoules.

Instructions for use/handling: Contains no bactericide, any portion of the contents not used at once should be discarded with the ampoule.

Marketing authorisation number PL 0043/0166.

Date of first authorisation/renewal of authorisation 5 June 1992.

Date of (partial) revision of the text July 1998.

Legal category POM.

MINIHEP*

Presentation
Minihep: Heparin (Mucous) Injection BP. Single dose ampoules containing sodium heparin 5,000 iu in 0.2 ml (no preservative). Other ingredients: water for injections.

Uses
Mode of action: Heparin is a naturally occurring anticoagulant which prevents the coagulation of blood *in vivo* and *in vitro.* It potentiates the inhibition of several activated coagulation factors, including thrombin and factor X.

Indications: Prophylaxis against deep vein thrombosis and thromboembolic events in susceptible patients.

Dosage and administration Administration is by subcutaneous injection.

Patients undergoing major elective surgery: 5,000 iu in 0.2 ml should be given two hours pre-operatively and then every 8–12 hours post-operatively for 10–14 days, or until the patient is ambulant, whichever is the longer.

Following myocardial infarction: 5,000 iu in 0.2 ml should be given twice daily for 10 days, or until the patient is mobile.

Other patients: 5,000 iu in 0.2 ml should be given every 8–12 hours.

These standard dosage regimens do not require routine control.

Dosage in the elderly: Dosage alterations are unnecessary for prophylaxis in the elderly.

Pregnancy: It is recommended that plasma heparin levels be maintained below 0.4 iu/ml as determined by specific anti-Xa assay. A suggested dosage is 5,000 iu every 12 hours in early pregnancy increasing to 10,000 iu every 12 hours in the last trimester. The dosage should be reduced during labour and the standard prophylactic dosage is suitable in the puerperium.

Contra-indications, warnings, etc
Contra-indications: Haemorrhagic disorders and patients with an actual or potential bleeding site, e.g. peptic ulcer. Patients with bacterial endocarditis and those with severe hypertension.

Precautions: Heparin therapy should be given with caution to patients with impaired renal or hepatic function.

Oral anticoagulants or drugs which interfere with platelet function, e.g. aspirin and dextran solutions, should be administered with caution.

Pregnancy and lactation: Although animal studies have not been performed, epidemiological studies indicate that if drug therapy is needed in pregnancy, the use of heparin in the recommended dosage is acceptable. Heparin does not cross the placenta or appear in breast milk.

Adverse reactions: Hypersensitivity and acute reversible thrombocytopenia may occur rarely. Osteoporosis and alopecia have been reported after prolonged therapy.

Overdosage: The effect of heparin can be reversed immediately by intravenous administration of a 1% protamine sulphate solution. The dose of protamine sulphate required for neutralisation should be determined accurately by titrating with the patient's plasma.

It is important to avoid overdosage of protamine sulphate because protamine itself has anticoagulant properties. A single dose of protamine sulphate should never exceed 50 mg. Intravenous injection of protamine may cause a sudden fall in blood pressure, bradycardia, dyspnoea and transitory flushing, but these may be avoided or diminished by slow and careful administration.

Pharmaceutical precautions Store below 25°C.

Legal category POM.

Package quantities
Packs of 10×0.2 ml ampoules.

Further information Nil.

Product licence number 0043/0088.

MINIHEP* SYRINGE

Qualitative and quantitative composition Heparin sodium 25,000 IU/ml (5,000 iu in 0.2 ml).

Pharmaceutical form Solution for injection.

Clinical particulars
Therapeutic indications: Prophylaxis against deep vein thrombosis and thromboembolic events in susceptible patients.

Posology and method of administration: Administration is by subcutaneous injection.

Patients undergoing major elective surgery: 5,000 iu in 0.2 ml should be given 2 hours pre-operatively and then every 8–12 hours post-operatively for 10–14 days or until the patient is ambulant, whichever is the longer.

Following myocardial infarction: 5,000 iu in 0.2 ml should be given twice daily for 10 days or until the patient is mobile.

Other patients: 5,000 iu in 0.2 ml should be given every 8–12 hours.

These standard dosage regimens do not require routine control.

Dosage in the elderly: Dosage alterations are unnecessary for prophylaxis in the elderly.

Pregnancy: It is recommended that plasma heparin levels be maintained below 0.4 iu/ml as determined by specific anti-Xa assay. A suggested dosage regimen is 5,000 iu every 12 hours in early pregnancy, increasing to 10,000 iu every 12 hours in the last trimester.

The dosage should be reduced during labour and the standard prophylactic dosage is suitable in the puerperium.

Contra-indications: Haemorrhagic disorders and patients with an actual or potential bleeding site, e.g. peptic ulcer. Patients with bacterial endocarditis and those with severe hypertension.

Special warnings and special precautions for use: Heparin therapy should be given with caution to patients with impaired renal or hepatic function.

Interaction with other medicaments and other forms of interaction: Oral anticoagulants or drugs which interfere with platelet function, e.g. aspirin and dextran solutions, should be administered with caution.

Pregnancy and lactation: Although animal studies have not been performed, epidemiological studies indicate that if drug therapy is needed in pregnancy, the use of heparin in the recommended dosage is acceptable. Heparin does not cross the placenta or appear in breast milk.

Effects on ability to drive and use machines: None known.

Undesirable effects: Hypersensitivity and acute reversible thrombocytopenia may occur rarely. Osteoporosis and alopecia have been reported after prolonged therapy.

Overdose: The effect of heparin can be reversed immediately by intravenous administration of a 1% protamine sulphate solution. The dose of protamine sulphate required for neutralisation should be determined accurately by titrating the patient's plasma.

It is important to avoid overdosage of protamine sulphate because protamine itself has anticoagulant properties.

A single dose of protamine sulphate should never exceed 50 mg. Intravenous injection of protamine may cause a sudden fall in blood pressure, bradycardia, dyspnoea and transitory flushing, but these may be avoided or diminished by slow and careful administration.

Pharmacological properties
Pharmacodynamic properties: Heparin is a naturally occurring anticoagulant which prevents the coagulation of blood *in-vivo* and *in-vitro.* It potentiates the inhibition of several activated coagulation factors, including thrombin and factor X.

Pharmacokinetic properties: The increase in clotting time provided by heparin becomes apparent immediately after administration and lasts for about 8 hours after subcutaneous injection.

Preclinical safety data: There are no pre-clinical data of relevance to the prescriber which are additional to that already included in other sections of the SPC.

Pharmaceutical particulars
List of excipients: Water for injections.

Incompatibilities: Not applicable.

Shelf life: 2 years.

Special precautions for storage: Store below 25°C.

Nature and contents of containers: 10×unit dose syringe (containing 0.2 ml solution).

Instructions for use/handling: Contains no bactericide, any portion of the contents not used at once should be discarded together with the syringe.

Marketing authorisation number PL 0043/0164.

Date of first authorisation/renewal of authorisation 14 January 1992.

Date of revision of the text December 1997.

Legal category POM.

ONE-ALPHA* INJECTION

Presentation One-Alpha Injection is a clear, colourless solution containing 2 micrograms/ml of alfacalcidol. Available in amber glass ampoules containing 0.5 ml or 1.0 ml to provide dose units of 1 microgram and 2 micrograms, respectively. Other ingredients: citric acid, ethanol, sodium citrate, propylene glycol and water for injections.

Uses
Mode of action: Alfacalcidol (One-Alpha) is converted rapidly in the liver to 1,25 dihydroxyvitamin D. This is the metabolite of vitamin D which acts as a regulator of calcium and phosphate metabolism. Since this conversion is rapid, the clinical effects of One-Alpha and1,25 dihydroxyvitamin D are very similar.

Impaired 1α hydroxylation by the kidneys reduces endogenous 1,25 dihydroxyvitamin D production. This contributes to the disturbances in mineral metabolism found in several disorders, including renal bone disease, hypoparathyroidism, neonatal hypocalcaemia and vitamin D dependent rickets. These disorders, which require high doses of parent vitamin D for their correction, will respond to small doses of One-Alpha.

The delay in response and high dosage required in treating these disorders with parent vitamin D makes dosage adjustment difficult. This can result in unpredictable hypercalcaemia which may take weeks or months to reverse. The major advantage of One-Alpha is the more rapid onset of response, which allows a more accurate titration of dosage. Should inadvertent hypercalcaemia occur it can be reversed within days of stopping treatment.

Indications: One-Alpha is indicated in all conditions where there is a disturbance of calcium metabolism due to impaired 1α hydroxylation such as when there is reduced renal function.

The main indications are:

(a) Renal osteodystrophy
(b) Hyperparathyroidism (with bone disease)
(c) Hypoparathyroidism
(d) Neonatal hypocalcaemia

(e) Nutritional and malabsorptive rickets and osteomalacia
(f) Pseudo-deficiency (D dependent) rickets and osteomalacia
(g) Hypophosphataemic vitamin D resistant rickets and osteomalacia

Dosage and administration One-Alpha Injection should be administered intravenously as a bolus over approximately 30 seconds.

The dosage of One-Alpha Injection is the same as for One-Alpha in its oral presentations.

Initial dose

Adults	1 microgram/day
Dosage in the elderly	0.5 microgram/day
Neonates and premature infants	0.05–0.1 microgram/kg/day
Children under 20 kg bodyweight	0.05 microgram/kg/day
Children over 20 kg bodyweight	1 microgram/day

The dose of One-Alpha should be adjusted thereafter to avoid hypercalcaemia according to the biochemical response.

Indices of response include plasma levels of calcium (ideally corrected for protein binding), alkaline phosphatase, parathyroid hormone, as well as radiographic and histological investigations.

Maintenance doses are generally in the range of 0.25–1 microgram/day.

When administered as intravenous injection to patients undergoing haemodialysis the initial dosage for adults is 1 microgram per dialysis. The maximum dose recommended is 6 micrograms per dialysis and not more than 12 micrograms per week. The injection should be administered into the return line from the haemodialysis machine at the end of each dialysis.

(a) Renal bone disease: Patients with relatively high initial plasma calcium levels may have autonomous hyperparathyroidism, often unresponsive to One-Alpha. Other therapeutic measures may be indicated.

Before and during treatment with One-Alpha, phosphate binding agents should be considered to prevent hyperphosphataemia. It is particularly important to make frequent plasma calcium measurements in patients with chronic renal failure because prolonged hypercalcaemia may aggravate the decline of renal function.

(b) Hyperparathyroidism: In patients with primary or tertiary hyperparathyroidism about to undergo parathyroidectomy, pre-operative treatment with One-Alpha for 2–3 weeks alleviates bone pain and myopathy without aggravating pre-operative hypercalcaemia. In order to decrease post-operative hypocalcaemia, One-Alpha should be continued until plasma alkaline phosphatase levels fall to normal or hypercalcaemia occurs.

(c) Hypoparathyroidism: In contrast to the response to parent vitamin D, low plasma calcium levels are restored to normal relatively quickly with One-Alpha. Severe hypocalcaemia is corrected more rapidly with higher doses of One-Alpha (eg 3–5 micrograms) together with calcium supplements.

(d) Neonatal hypocalcaemia: Although the normal starting dose of One-Alpha is 0.05–0.1 microgram/kg/day (followed by careful titration) in severe cases doses of up to 2 microgram/kg/day may be required. Whilst ionised serum calcium levels may provide a guide to response, measurement of plasma alkaline phosphatase activity may be more useful. Levels of alkaline phosphatase approximately 7.5 times above the adult range indicates active disease.

(e) Nutritional and malabsorptive rickets and osteomalacia: Nutritional rickets and osteomalacia can be cured rapidly with One-Alpha. Malabsorptive osteomalacia (responding to large doses of IM or IV parent vitamin D) will respond to small doses of One-Alpha.

(f) Pseudo-deficiency (D-dependent) rickets and osteomalacia: Although large doses of parent vitamin D would be required, effective doses of One-Alpha are similar to those required to heal nutritional Vitamin D deficiency rickets and osteomalacia.

(g) Hypophosphataemic vitamin D-resistant rickets and osteomalacia: Neither large doses of parent vitamin D nor phosphate supplements are entirely satisfactory. Treatment with One-Alpha at normal dosage rapidly relieves myopathy when present and increases calcium and phosphate retention. Phosphate supplements may also be required in some patients.

Contra-indications, warnings, etc
Precautions: During treatment with One-Alpha Injection serum calcium should be monitored regularly.

One-Alpha Injection should be avoided in patients with known sensitivity to injections containing propylene glycol and it should be used with caution in small premature infants.

Drug interactions: Patients taking barbiturates or anticonvulsants may require larger doses of One-Alpha to produce the desired effect.

Pregnancy and lactation: There is inadequate evidence of safety of One-Alpha in human pregnancy but it has been in wide use for many years without apparent ill consequences. Animal studies have shown no hazard. If drug therapy is needed in pregnancy, One-Alpha can be used if there is no alternative.

Although it has not been established, it is likely that increased amounts of 1,25 dihydroxyvitamin D will be found in the milk of lactating mothers treated with One-Alpha. This may influence calcium metabolism in the infant.

Side-effects: Rarely hypercalcaemia occurs during treatment with One-Alpha Injection. This can be rapidly corrected by stopping treatment until plasma calcium levels return to normal (about 1 week). Treatment may then be restarted at a reduced dose.

Overdosage: Hypercalcaemia is treated by stopping One-Alpha. Severe hypercalcaemia may be additionally treated with a "loop" diuretic and intravenous fluids, or with corticosteroids.

Pharmaceutical precautions Store in a cool place (below 15°C).

Legal category POM.

Package quantities Amber glass ampoules containing 0.5 ml or 1 ml solution. Packs of 10 ampoules of 0.5 ml or 10 ampoules of 1 ml.

Further information Nil.

Product licence number 0043/0183.

ONE-ALPHA* CAPSULES
ONE-ALPHA* SOLUTION

Presentation *One-Alpha Capsules:* Capsules contain alfacalcidol (1α hydroxy-vitamin D) in two strengths: Brown capsule – contains 1 microgram alfacalcidol; white capsule – contains 0.25 microgram alfacalcidol. *One-Alpha Solution:* A clear or slightly opalescent solution, one ml contains 0.2 microgram alfacalcidol.

Uses
Mode of action: Alfacalcidol (One-Alpha) is converted rapidly in the liver to 1,25 dihydroxyvitamin D. This is the metabolite of vitamin D which acts as a regulator of calcium and phosphate metabolism. Since this conversion is rapid, the clinical effects of One-Alpha and 1,25 dihydroxyvitamin D are very similar.

Impaired 1α hydroxylation by the kidneys reduces endogenous 1,25 dihydroxyvitamin D production. This contributes to the disturbances in mineral metabolism found in several disorders, including renal bone disease, hypoparathyroidism, neonatal hypocalcaemia and vitamin D dependent rickets. These disorders, which require high doses of parent vitamin D for their correction, will respond to small doses of One-Alpha.

The delay in response and high dosage required in treating these disorders with parent vitamin D makes dosage adjustment difficult. This can result in unpredictable hypercalcaemia which may take weeks or months to reverse. The major advantage of One-Alpha is the more rapid onset of response, which allows a more accurate titration of dosage. Should inadvertent hypercalcaemia occur it can be reversed within days of stopping treatment.

Indications: One-Alpha is indicated in all conditions where there is a disturbance of calcium metabolism due to impaired 1α hydroxylation such as when there is reduced renal function.

The main indications are:

(a) Renal osteodystrophy
(b) Hyperparathyroidism (with bone disease)
(c) Hypoparathyroidism
(d) Neonatal hypocalcaemia
(e) Nutritional and malabsorptive rickets and osteomalacia
(f) Pseudo-deficiency (D dependent) rickets and osteomalacia
(g) Hypophosphataemic vitamin D resistant rickets and osteomalacia

Dosage and administration One-Alpha may be administered as capsules or solution. One-Alpha Solution should be administered using the enclosed oral dispenser. Initial dose for all indications:

Adults	1 microgram/day
Dosage in the elderly	0.5 microgram/day
Neonates and premature infants	0.05–0.1 microgram/kg/day
Children under 20 kg bodyweight	0.05 microgram/kg/day
Children over 20 kg bodyweight	1 microgram/day

The dose of One-Alpha should be adjusted thereafter to avoid hypercalcaemia according to the biochemical response.

Indices of response include plasma levels of calcium (ideally corrected for protein binding), alkaline phosphatase, parathyroid hormone, as well as radiographic and histological investigations.

Plasma levels should initially be measured at weekly intervals. The daily dose of One-Alpha may be increased by increments of 0.25–0.5 microgram. When the dose is stabilised, measurements may be taken every 2–4 weeks.

Most adult patients respond to doses between 1 and 3 micrograms per day. When there is biochemical or radiographic evidence of bone healing (and in hypoparathyroid patients when normal plasma calcium levels have been attained), the dose generally decreases. Maintenance doses are generally in the range of 0.25 to 1 microgram per day. If hypercalcaemia occurs, One-Alpha should be stopped until plasma calcium returns to normal (approximately 1 week) then restarted at half the previous dose.

(a) Renal bone disease: Patients with relatively high initial plasma calcium levels may have autonomous hyperparathyroidism, often unresponsive to One-Alpha. Other therapeutic measures may be indicated.

Before and during treatment with One-Alpha, phosphate binding agents should be considered to prevent hyperphosphataemia. It is particularly important to make frequent plasma calcium measurements in patients with chronic renal failure because prolonged hypercalcaemia may aggravate the decline of renal function.

(b) Hyperparathyroidism: In patients with primary or tertiary hyperparathyroidism about to undergo parathyroidectomy, pre-operative treatment with One-Alpha for 2–3 weeks alleviates bone pain and myopathy without aggravating pre-operative hypercalcaemia. In order to decrease post-operative hypocalcaemia, One-Alpha should be continued until plasma alkaline phosphatase levels fall to normal or hypercalcaemia occurs.

(c) Hypoparathyroidism: In contrast to the response to parent vitamin D, low plasma calcium levels are restored to normal relatively quickly with One-Alpha. Severe hypocalcaemia is corrected more rapidly with higher doses of One-Alpha (e.g. 3–5 micrograms) together with calcium supplements.

(d) Neonatal hypocalcaemia: Although the normal starting dose of One-Alpha is 0.05–0.1 microgram/kg/day (followed by careful titration) in severe cases doses of up to 2 microgram/kg/day may be required. Whilst ionised serum calcium levels may provide a guide to response, measurement of plasma alkaline phosphatase activity may be more useful. Levels of alkaline phosphatase approximately 7.5 times above the adult range indicates active disease.

A dose of 0.1 microgram/kg/day of One-Alpha has proven effective as prophylaxis against early neonatal hypocalcaemia in premature infants.

(e) Nutritional and malabsorptive rickets and osteomalacia: Nutritional rickets and osteomalacia can be cured rapidly with One-Alpha. Malabsorptive osteomalacia (responding to large doses of IM or IV parent vitamin D) will respond to small doses of One-Alpha.

(f) Pseudo-deficiency (D-dependent) rickets and osteomalacia: Although large doses of parent vitamin D would be required, effective doses of One-Alpha are similar to those required to heal nutritional Vitamin D deficiency rickets and osteomalacia.

(g) Hypophosphataemic vitamin D-resistant rickets and osteomalacia: Neither large doses of parent vitamin D nor phosphate supplements are entirely satisfactory. Treatment with One-Alpha at normal dosage rapidly relieves myopathy when present and increases calcium and phosphate retention. Phosphate supplements may also be required in some patients.

Contra-indications, warnings, etc
Precautions and side-effects: If hypercalcaemia occurs during treatment with One-Alpha this can be rapidly corrected by stopping treatment until plasma calcium levels return to normal (about 1 week). One-Alpha may then be restarted at half the previous dose.

Patients taking barbiturates or anticonvulsants may require larger doses of One-Alpha to produce the desired effect.

Pregnancy and lactation: There is inadequate evidence of safety of One-Alpha in human pregnancy but it has been in wide use for many years without apparent ill consequences. Animal studies have shown no hazard. If drug therapy is needed in pregnancy, One-Alpha can be used if there is no alternative.

Although it has not been established, it is likely that increased amounts of 1,25 dihydroxyvitamin D will be found in the milk of lactating mothers treated with One-Alpha. This may influence calcium metabolism in the infant.

Overdosage: Hypercalcaemia is treated by stopping One-Alpha. Severe hypercalcaemia may be additionally treated with a 'loop' diuretic and intravenous fluids, or with corticosteroids.

Pharmaceutical precautions One-Alpha capsules: Store at room temperature (below 25°C).

One-Alpha solution: Protect from direct sunlight and store in a cool place (below 15°C).

Legal category POM.

Package quantities Capsules: Blisters of 30 capsules. Solution: Amber glass bottle of 60 ml (OP); an oral dispenser is enclosed.

Further information One-Alpha Solution is sugar free and contains no colouring agents.

Product licence numbers

Capsules 1 microgram	0043/0050
Capsules 0.25 microgram	0043/0052
Solution	0043/0133

PRESTIM* TABLETS

Qualitative and quantitative composition Each tablet contains Timolol Maleate PhEur 10 mg and Bendroflumethiazide PhEur (Bendrofluazide) 2.5 mg.

Pharmaceutical form Tablet.

Clinical particulars

Therapeutic indications: Prestim tablets are indicated for the treatment of mild to moderate hypertension.

Posology and method of administration: Prestim tablets are for oral administration.

The recommended dosage range is 1 to 4 tablets daily. The dosage can be taken in the morning or in two divided doses, morning and evening.

If blood pressure control is not achieved on 4 tablets daily, consideration should be given to titrating timolol and bendrofluazide separately or adding another agent with hypotensive activity.

Dosage in the elderly: Initiate treatment with 1 tablet daily and thereafter adjust according to response.

Contra-indications: Anuria. Prestim should not be used in patients with renal failure.

Uncontrolled heart failure, bradycardia, cardiogenic shock, history of bronchospasm, bronchial asthma, chronic obstructive pulmonary disease, patients receiving adrenergic augmenting drugs (monoamine oxidase inhibitors and tricyclic antidepressants), sick sinus syndrome, Prinzmetals angina, untreated phaeochromocytoma, hypersensitivity to any of the constituents. Anaesthesia with agents that produce myocardial depression, such as chloroform and ether.

Pregnancy.

Special warnings and special precautions for use:

Precautions: The continued depression of sympathetic drive through beta-blockade may lead to cardiac failure. All patients should be observed for evidence of cardiac failure, and if it occurs, digitalisation should be considered.

Caution should be exercised in patients with diabetes mellitus, spontaneous hypoglycaemia, impaired renal or hepatic function and in patients receiving catecholamine depleting drugs, such as reserpine or guanethidine.

Warnings: There have been reports of skin rashes and/or dry eyes associated with the use of beta-adrenergic blocking drugs. The reported incidence is small and in most cases the symptoms have cleared when treatment was withdrawn. Discontinuance of the drug should be considered if any such reaction is not otherwise explicable, cessation of therapy with the beta-blocker should be gradual.

Interaction with other medicaments and other forms of interaction: As with other diuretics, Prestim should not be administered concurrently with lithium salts. Diuretics can reduce lithium clearance resulting in high serum levels of lithium.

Pregnancy and lactation: Prestim is contra-indicated in pregnancy. Both constituents cross the placenta and appear in breast milk.

Effects on ability to drive and use machines: None known.

Undesirable effects: Side-effects associated with beta blockade, e.g. gastro-intestinal symptoms, dizziness, insomnia, sedation, depression, weakness, dyspnoea, bradycardia, heart block, bronchospasm and heart failure. Thiazide diuretics may cause excessive depletion of fluid and electrolytes during prolonged or intense use. Symptoms are muscle pain or fatigue, thirst and oliguria. With thiazide diuretics hypokalaemia is more severe in patients already depleted of potassium, as in renal or hepatic insufficiency. Coma may be precipitated in hepatic cirrhosis. The thiazides may induce hyperglycaemia and glycosuria in diabetic and other susceptible patients. The thiazides increase blood urea, which is most pronounced in patients with renal disease and pre-existing retention of nitrogen. Hyperuricaemia sometimes can occur. Reports of other adverse reactions to the thiazides include skin rashes with associated photosensitivity, necrotising vasculitis, acute pancreatitis, blood dyscrasias and aggravation of pre-existing myopia.

Overdose: The most common signs of overdosage are bradycardia, hypotension, bronchospasm and acute cardiac failure. Suggested treatments are as follows:

Severe bradycardia: I.V. atropine sulphate 0.25–2 mg. If bradycardia persists, I.V. isoprenaline 25 micrograms may be given.

Severe hypotension: I.V. noradrenaline or adrenaline.

Bronchospasm: Isoprenaline hydrochloride, orciprenaline or salbutamol.

Acute cardiac failure: Digitalis, diuretics and oxygen. In refractory cases I.V. aminophylline and I.V. glucagon 0.5–1 mg have been reported useful.

General measures should be taken to restore blood volume, maintain blood pressure and correct electrolyte imbalance.

Pharmacological properties

Pharmacodynamic properties: Bendrofluazide, a thiazide diuretic, has a moderate, but established action in the treatment of hypertension.

Timolol maleate is a beta-adrenergic receptor blocking agent with marked hypotensive activity. It has been shown that the combination of a beta-blocking agent with a thiazide diuretic gives an enhanced antihypertensive effect. This means that a relatively lower dose of the beta-blocker is required.

Pharmacokinetic properties: Timolol and bendrofluazide are rapidly absorbed from the gut. The beta-blocking effect of timolol is apparent within 30 minutes of administration and has been shown to last for up to 24 hours. The diuretic effect of bendrofluazide is usually complete in 12–18 hours.

Preclinical safety data: There are no pre-clinical data of relevance to the prescriber which are additional to that already included in other sections of the SPC.

Pharmaceutical particulars

List of excipients: Microcrystalline cellulose, starch, magnesium stearate.

Incompatibilities: None known.

Shelf life: The shelf life of Prestim tablets is three years.

Special precautions for storage: Store below 25°C.

Nature and contents of container: Glass bottle of 30 tablets.

Instructions for use/handling: None.

Marketing authorisation number PL 0043/0047.

Date of first authorisation/renewal of authorisation 6 June 1979/29 August 1991

Date of (partial) revision of the text November 1997.

Legal category POM.

PUMP-HEP*
Heparin for Continuous Infusion

Presentation Heparin (Mucous) Injection BP 1000 units/ml. Single dose ampoules of 20 ml, 10 ml or 5 ml containing 1,000 units sodium heparin per ml without preservative (i.e. 20,000, 10,000 or 5,000 units per ampoule respectively). Other ingredients: sodium chloride, sodium citrate and water for injections.

Uses

Mode of action: Heparin is a naturally occurring anticoagulant which prevents the coagulation of blood *in vivo* and *in vitro*. It potentiates the inhibition of several activated coagulation factors, including thrombin and factor X.

Indications: Treatment of thrombo-embolic disorders such as: deep vein thrombosis, acute arterial embolism or thrombosis, thrombophlebitis, pulmonary embolism, fat embolism.

Dosage and administration Pump-Hep may be used when heparin is being administered intravenously as an alternative to diluting heparin taken from multidose vials.

500 units/kg bodyweight daily or 5,000–10,000 units every 4 hours as a continuous infusion in sodium chloride injection or dextrose injection. The dose should be individually adjusted according to coagulation tests.

Dosage adjustment: It is recommended that the dosages be adjusted to maintain a thrombin clotting time, whole blood clotting time or activated partial thromboplastin time 1.5 to 2 times that of control on blood withdrawn 4–6 hours after commencement of infusion and at similar intervals until the patient is stabilised.

Dosage in the elderly: Lower dosages may be required, however, standard dosages should be given initially and then subsequent dosages and/or dosage intervals should be individually adjusted according to changes in thrombin clotting time, whole blood clotting time and/or activated partial thromboplastin time.

Pregnancy: Standard dosages should be given initially. Intermittent intravenous injections are not advised. Subsequent dosages and/or dosage intervals should be individually adjusted according to changes in thrombin clotting time, whole blood clotting time and/or activated partial thromboplastin time.

Contra-indications, warnings, etc

Contra-indications: Haemorrhagic disorders and patients with an actual or potential bleeding site, eg, peptic ulcer. Patients with bacterial endocarditis and those with severe hypertension.

Precautions: Heparin therapy should be given with caution to patients with impaired renal or hepatic functions.

Oral anticoagulants or drugs which interfere with platelet function, eg aspirin and dextran solutions should be administered with caution.

Pregnancy and lactation: Although animal studies have not been performed, epidemiological studies indicate that if drug therapy is needed in pregnancy, the use of heparin in the recommended dosage is acceptable. Heparin does not cross the placenta or appear in breast milk.

Adverse reactions: Hypersensitivity and acute thrombocytopenia may occur rarely. Osteoporosis and alopecia have been reported after prolonged therapy.

Overdosage: The effect of heparin can be reversed immediately by intravenous administration of a 1% protamine sulphate solution. The dose of protamine sulphate required for neutralisation should be determined accurately by titrating the patient's plasma.

It is important to avoid overdosage of protamine sulphate because protamine itself has anticoagulant properties. A single dose of protamine sulphate should never exceed 50 mg. Intravenous injection of protamine may cause a sudden fall in blood pressure, bradycardia, dyspnoea and transitory flushing, but these may be avoided or diminished by slow and careful administration.

Pharmaceutical precautions Store below 25°C.

Heparin has been reported to be incompatible in aqueous solutions with certain substances, eg some antibiotics, hydrocortisone, phenothiazines, narcotic analgesics and some antihistamines.

Legal category POM.

Package quantities Packs of 10×20 ml ampoules; 10×10 ml ampoules; 10×5 ml ampoules.

Further information Nil.

Product licence number 0043/0149.

UNIHEP* LEO 1,000
UNIHEP* LEO 5,000
UNIHEP* LEO 10,000
UNIHEP* LEO 25,000

Presentation

Unihep Leo 1,000: Heparin (Mucous) Injection BP 1,000 units per ml. Single dose ampoules containing sodium heparin 1,000 units in 1 ml (no preservative). Other ingredients: sodium chloride, sodium citrate and water for injections.

Unihep Leo 5,000: Heparin (Mucous) Injection BP 5,000 units per ml. Single dose ampoules containing sodium heparin 5,000 units in 1 ml (no preservative). Other ingredients: water for injections.

Unihep Leo 10,000: Heparin (Mucous) Injection BP 10,000 units per ml. Single dose ampoules containing sodium heparin 10,000 units in 1 ml (no preservative). Other ingredients: water for injections.

Unihep Leo 25,000: Heparin (Mucous) Injection BP 25,000 units per ml. Single dose ampoules containing sodium heparin 25,000 units in 1 ml (no preservative). Other ingredients: water for injections.

Uses

Mode of action: Heparin is a naturally occurring anticoagulant which prevents the coagulation of blood *in vivo* and *in vitro*. It potentiates the inhibition of several activated coagulation factors, including thrombin and factor X.

Indications: Treatment of thromboembolic disorders such as: deep vein thrombosis, acute arterial embolism or thrombosis, thrombophlebitis, pulmonary embolism and fat embolism.

Prophylaxis against deep vein thrombosis and thromboembolic events in susceptible patients.

Dosage and administration

Treatment dosage

Intravenous administration: 5,000–10,000 units every 4 hours or 500 units/kg bodyweight daily as a continuous infusion in sodium chloride injection or dextrose injection. Doses should be individually adjusted according to coagulation tests.

Subcutaneous administration: The initial dose is

250 units/kg bodyweight. Further doses should be given every 12 hours and individually adjusted according to coagulation tests.

Dosage adjustment: It is recommended that dosages be adjusted to maintain a thrombin clotting time, whole blood clotting time or activated partial thromboplastin time 1.5 to 2 times that of control on blood withdrawn 4–6 hours after the first injection or commencement of infusion, and at similar intervals until the patient is stabilised.

Prophylactic dosage
Administration is by subcutaneous injection.

Patients undergoing major elective surgery: 5,000 units should be given 2 hours pre-operatively and then every 8–12 hours post-operatively for 10–14 days or until the patient is ambulant whichever is the longer.

Following myocardial infarction: 5,000 units should be given twice daily for 10 days or until the patient is mobile.

Other patients: 5,000 units should be given every 8–12 hours.

These standard prophylactic regimens do not require routine control.

Dosage in children
Treatment dosage: Standard treatment dosages should be given initially. Subsequent dosages and/or dosage intervals should be individually adjusted according to changes in thrombin clotting time, whole blood clotting time and/or activated partial thromboplastin time.

Dosage in the elderly
Treatment dosage: Lower treatment dosages may be required, however, standard treatment dosages should be given initially and then subsequent dosages and/or dosage intervals should be individually adjusted according to changes in thrombin clotting time, whole blood clotting time and/or activated partial thromboplastin time.

Prophylactic dosage: Dosage alterations are unnecessary for prophylaxis in the elderly.

Pregnancy
Treatment dosage: Standard treatment dosages should be given initially by continuous intravenous infusion or every 12 hours by subcutaneous injection. Intermittent intravenous injections are not advised. Subsequent dosages and/or dosage intervals should be individually adjusted according to changes in thrombin clotting time, whole blood clotting time and/or activated partial thromboplastin time.

Prophylactic dosage: It is recommended that plasma heparin levels be maintained below 0.4 units/ml, as determined by specific anti-Xa assay. A suggested dosage is 5,000 units every 12 hours in early pregnancy increasing to 10,000 units every 12 hours in the last trimester. The dosage should be reduced during labour and the standard prophylactic dosage is suitable in the puerperium.

Contra-indications, warnings, etc
Contra-indications: Haemorrhagic disorders and patients with an actual or potential bleeding site, e.g. peptic ulcer. Patients with bacterial endocarditis and those with severe hypertension.

Precautions: Heparin therapy should be given with caution to patients with impaired renal or hepatic function.

Oral anticoagulants or drugs which interfere with platelet function, e.g. aspirin and dextran solutions should be administered with caution.

Pregnancy and lactation: Although animal studies have not been performed, epidemiological studies indicate that if drug therapy is needed in pregnancy, the use of heparin in the recommended dosage is acceptable. Heparin does not cross the placenta or appear in breast milk.

Adverse reactions: Hypersensitivity and acute reversible thrombocytopenia may occur rarely. Osteoporosis and alopecia have been reported after prolonged therapy.

Overdosage: The effect of heparin can be reversed immediately by intravenous administration of a 1% protamine sulphate solution. The dose of protamine sulphate required for neutralisation should be determined accurately by titrating with the patient's plasma.

It is important to avoid overdosage of protamine sulphate because protamine itself has anticoagulant properties. A single dose of protamine sulphate should never exceed 50 mg. Intravenous injection of protamine may cause a sudden fall in blood pressure, bradycardia, dyspnoea and transitory flushing but these may be avoided or diminished by slow and careful administration.

Pharmaceutical precautions Store below 25°C. Heparin has been reported to be incompatible in aqueous solutions with certain substances, e.g. some antibiotics, hydrocortisone, phenothiazines, narcotic analgesics and some antihistamines.

Legal category POM.

Package quantities

Unihep Leo 1,000:	Packs of 5×10 ampoules
Unihep Leo 5,000:	Packs of 5×10 ampoules
Unihep Leo 10,000:	Packs of 10 ampoules
Unihep Leo 25,000:	Packs of 10 ampoules

Further information Nil.

Product licence numbers

Unihep Leo 1,000	0043/0085
Unihep Leo 5,000	0043/0086
Unihep Leo 10,000	0043/0064
Unihep Leo 25,000	0043/0087

UROKINASE 5,000 AND UROKINASE 25,000

Qualitative and quantitative composition Urokinase vials contain urokinase in a sterile, white, freeze-dried powder form. Each vial contains 5,000 IU or 25,000 IU of urokinase.

Pharmaceutical form Powder for injection after reconstitution with solvent.

Clinical particulars
Therapeutic indications: Urokinase is indicated for the lysis of clots in the following conditions:

(i) Thromboembolic occlusive vascular disease such as deep vein thrombosis (DVT), pulmonary embolism (PE) and peripheral vascular occlusion.

(ii) Hyphaema (haemorrhage into the anterior chamber of the eye).

(iii) Arterio-venous haemodialysis shunts and intravenous cannulae which are blocked by fibrin clots.

Posology and method of administration: Urokinase should be reconstituted with a small amount of sterile Water for Injections or saline and then further diluted with normal saline to the desired volume for administration.

Adults:
(i) Thromboembolic occlusive vascular disease
Deep vein thrombosis: A recommended dosage regimen consists of an initial loading dose of 4,400 IU/kg body weight in 15 ml solution, given over 10 minutes followed by an intravenous infusion of 4,400 IU/kg/hour for 12–24 hours.

Pulmonary embolism: A recommended dosage regimen consists of an initial loading dose of 4,400 IU/kg body weight in 15 ml solution, given over 10 minutes followed by an intravenous infusion of 4,400 IU/kg/hour for 12 hours.

Alternatively, a 50 ml bolus injection of urokinase into the pulmonary artery, repeated for up to 3 doses, at 24 hour intervals, has been employed. The initial dosage of 15,000 IU/kg body weight may be adjusted if necessary for subsequent injections, dependent upon the plasma fibrinogen concentration produced by the previous injection.

Peripheral vascular occlusion: A recommended dosage regimen involves the infusion of a 2,500 IU/ml solution of urokinase (500,000 IU in 200 ml) into the clot, using angiography to monitor the progress of treatment. Urokinase should be infused into the clot at a dose rate of 4,000 IU/minute (96 ml/hr) for 2 hours followed by repeat angiography. The catheter is then advanced into the remaining occluded segment and urokinase infused at 4,000 IU/min for a further 2 hours; this may be repeated up to 4 times if antegrade flow has not occurred. After lysing a channel through the occlusion the catheter is withdrawn until it is proximal to the remaining clot lining the vessel wall. Urokinase is given at a dose rate of 1,000 IU/min (0.4 ml) until the clot has completely lysed. A dose of 500,000 IU given over approximately 8 hours should be sufficient to achieve this.

If the clot is not reduced in length by more than 25% after the initial infusion of 500,000 IU and by an incremental 10% by subsequent infusions of 500,000 IU, consideration should be given to discontinuation of treatment.

After fibrinolytic therapy has been completed, treatment may be continued with suitable anticoagulant therapy.

(ii) Hyphaema: When saline irrigation is unsuccessful in removing the blood clot, urokinase may be considered for the management of hyphaema, particularly when the clot completely fills the anterior chamber and there is an accompanying rise in intraocular pressure. The following general technique is used: an incision of about 3 mm is made inside the temporal limbus of the cornea. 5,000 IU urokinase is dissolved in Sodium Chloride Injection BP (2 ml) and drawn up into a syringe fitted with a suitable irrigator. The tip of the irrigator is introduced through the incision so as to be over the iris rather than the pupillary space (thus avoiding risk of damage to the lens), with the aperture directed towards the corneal endothelium or parallel to the plane of the iris. The solution is injected and withdrawn repeatedly with minimal pressure. Clot disintegration commonly begins within five minutes, facilitating injection of the solution and aspiration of the clot. The chamber is then washed out with saline. If residual clot remains, a small quantity of the solution (e.g. 0.3 ml) may be left in the anterior chamber to facilitate further dissolution of the clot over the next 24–48 hours.

(iii) Clotted arterio-venous shunts: Generally, 5,000–25,000 IU urokinase in 2–3 ml Sodium Chloride Injection BP is instilled into the affected limb of the shunt which is then clamped off for 2–4 hours. The lysate is then aspirated. This may be repeated if necessary. For the venous side an infusion of 5,000 IU in 200 ml, run in over 30 minutes, has been used but this may be less satisfactory than the use of more concentrated solutions.

Dosage in the elderly: Initially no dosage alterations are recommended, however, thereafter, the dosage should be adjusted as necessary, according to response.

Dosage in children: Initially no dosage alterations are recommended, however, thereafter, the dosage should be adjusted as necessary, according to response.

Contra-indications: Urokinase is contra-indicated in any situation where bleeding has occurred, or is likely to occur.

Recent surgery (including biopsy): administration of urokinase for thromboembolic occlusive vascular disease is not recommended for 72 hours following surgery because of the risk of bleeding from the operation site.

Severe hypertension (with systolic bp > 200 mmHg and/or diastolic bp > 120 mmHg): in patients with severe hypertension, administration of urokinase carries the risk of cerebral haemorrhage.

Urokinase is contra-indicated in pregnancy and the immediate post-partum period.

Severe hepatic or renal insufficiency.

When used in 'local' situations, the above contra-indications may not be relevant.

Special warnings and special precautions for use: If bleeding occurs following systemic use, the infusion should be stopped immediately. However, this contra-indication is relative. The benefits of the continued use of urokinase must be weighed against the risks of stopping therapy, for example, in the situation where vascular occlusion can be life-threatening. For treatment of bleeding see 'Overdose'. When used in the eye, a normal gonioscopy result should be evident. Systemic urokinase should be used with caution in patients with gastrointestinal lesions such as peptic ulceration, which may be prone to haemorrhage, and in patients who have had multiple intracardiac and intravascular punctures as a consequence of cardio-pulmonary resuscitation.

Interactions with other medicaments and other forms of interaction: In glucose solution there is a measurable (< 10%) reduction in the activity of urokinase after 8 hours. Concomitant administration of dextran sulphate may prolong the activity of urokinase.

Pregnancy and lactation: Urokinase is contra-indicated in pregnancy and the immediate post-partum period.

Effects on ability to drive and use machines: None known.

Undesirable effects: The following side-effects have been associated with urokinase use in the listed indications:

Hyphaema – none reported.

Arteriovenous shunts – warmth, initial severe pain and dull ache in shunt limb have been reported occasionally.

Thromboembolic occlusive vascular disease – overt bleeding, haemorrhagic complications may occur. Temporary increase in temperature (when a high yield of lysis degradation products are produced) and haematuria have been reported occasionally.

Overdose: If severe haemorrhage occurs, treatment with urokinase must be stopped. Aprotinin and synthetic inhibitors such as epsilon-aminocaproic acid, tranexamic acid or p-aminomethylbenzoic acid can be used to inhibit the fibrinolytic action of urokinase. In serious cases, human fibrinogen, Factor XIII, Cohn-Fraction I, packed red cells or whole blood can be given, as appropriate.

Pharmacological properties
Pharmacodynamic properties: Urokinase is a preparation of urokinase, which is an enzyme extracted from human adult male urine. As urokinase is of human origin, it is not antigenic in man.

Urokinase brings about the dissolution of blood clots by promoting the activation of plasminogen; the latter is the inactive precursor of plasmin, the proteolytic enzyme responsible for the breakdown of fibrin into small soluble peptides which are dispersible through the blood stream.

Pharmacokinetic properties: Following intravenous administration, urokinase is rapidly cleared from the blood. The *in-vivo* half-life of urokinase activity in normal subject is about 10 to 15 minutes.

In cirrhotic patients, the elimination half-life is clearly increased up to about 30 minutes.

In subjects with kidney disease, elimination of endogenous urokinase is markedly decreased, even if the glomerular filtration rate is only moderately impaired.

The liver appears to perform an important function in the metabolism and elimination of urokinase.

The major part of urokinase activity has been found to be excreted in the bile, with peak activity achieved 35 to 60 minutes after injection and falling to unmeasurable levels after 140 to 190 minutes.

Preclinical safety data: Being extracted from human urine, urokinase is species-homologous and is free from inherent toxicity in man.

In animal toxicology studies, single i.v. doses up to 1 MIU/kg were not lethal and did not produce symptoms of intoxication or histological changes in any important organs. With repeated administration in increasing doses, no practical relevant toxic changes or lethal effects were observed.

Pharmaceutical particulars The activity of urokinase is expressed in International Units (IU), which are approximately equivalent to one Committee on Thrombolytic Agents (CTA) unit.

List of excipients:

Mannitol
Disodium edetate
Disodium hydrogen phosphate

Incompatibilities: None known.

Shelf life: 24 months.

Special precautions for storage: Urokinase, in the lyophilised form, should be stored below 25°C. When reconstituted, urokinase is stable for 24 hours when stored below 25°C.

Nature and content of container: 5 ml vials of colourless neutral glass type 1. The product is packed as single vials.

Instructions for use/handling: The lyophilised material should be reconstituted with a small amount of saline or Water for Injections, and then further diluted with saline.

Marketing authorisation holder: Serono Laboratories (UK) Limited, 99 Bridge Road East, Welwyn Garden City, Hertfordshire AL7 1BG.

Marketing authorisation number

Urokinase 5,000: PL 3400/0001R
Urokinase 25,000: PL 3400 0026R

Date of first authorisation/renewal of authorisation

Reviewed licences granted: 12-11-91

Date of (partial) revision of text April 1998.

Legal category POM.

**Trade Mark*

Eli Lilly and Company Limited

Kingsclere Road
Basingstoke
Hants. RG21 6XA

☎ 01256 315000 🗋 01256 315858

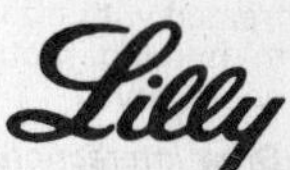

AXID*

Presentation Capsules (pale yellow and dark yellow, coded 3144) containing 150 mg nizatidine INN.

Capsules (pale yellow and brown, coded 3145) containing 300 mg nizatidine INN.

Uses For the treatment of the following diseases where reduction of gastric acid is indicated: Duodenal ulcer; benign gastric ulcer; prevention of duodenal or benign gastric ulcer recurrence; gastric oesophageal reflux disease (including erosions, ulcerations and associated heartburn); gastric and/or duodenal ulcer associated with concomitant use of non-steroidal anti-inflammatory drugs.

Dosage and administration Axid is administered orally.

Adults: For treatment of duodenal ulcer, the recommended daily dose is 300 mg in the evening. Treatment should continue for four weeks, although this period may be reduced if healing is confirmed earlier by endoscopy. Most ulcers will heal within four weeks, but if complete ulcer healing has not occurred after four weeks therapy, patients should continue therapy for a further four weeks.

For the treatment of benign gastric ulcer, the recommended daily dose is 300 mg in the evening for four or, if necessary, eight weeks. Prior to treatment with nizatidine, care should be taken to exclude the possibility of gastric cancer.

If preferred, the 300 mg daily dose for the treatment of duodenal or benign gastric ulcer may be given as two divided doses of 150 mg in the morning and evening.

For the prevention of duodenal or benign gastric ulcer recurrence (prophylactic maintenance therapy) the recommended daily dose is 150 mg in the evening.

For the treatment of gastric oesophageal reflux disease, the recommended dosage is from 150 mg twice daily, up to 300 mg twice daily. Therapy for up to 12 weeks is indicated for erosions and ulcerations, and associated heartburn.

For the treatment of gastric and/or duodenal ulcer associated with concomitant use of non-steroidal anti-inflammatory drugs, the recommended daily dose is 150 mg daily (either 300 mg at bedtime or 150 mg twice daily, in the morning and in the evening) for up to 8 weeks. In most patients, the ulcers will heal within 4 weeks. During treatment, the use of non-steroidal anti-inflammatory drugs may continue.

The elderly: Age does not significantly influence efficacy or safety. Normally dosage modification is not required except in patients who have moderate to severe renal impairment (creatinine clearance less than 50 ml/min).

Children: Not recommended, as safety and efficacy have not been established.

Patients with impaired renal function: Nizatidine is principally excreted via the kidneys.

For patients who have moderate renal impairment (creatinine clearance less than 50 ml/min) or patients who have severe renal impairment (creatinine clearance less than 20 ml/min), the dosage should be reduced as follows:

DOSAGE RECOMMENDED

No Renal Impairment	*Moderate Renal Impairment (Reduce Dose By 50%)*	*Severe Renal Impairment (Reduce Dose By 75%)*
600 mg	150 mg twice daily	150 mg daily
300 mg	150 mg in the evening	150 mg on alternate days
150 mg	150 mg on alternate days	150 mg every third day

Contra-indications, warnings, etc

Contra-indication: Known hypersensitivity to H_2-receptor antagonists.

Warnings

Usage in pregnancy: The safety of nizatidine for use during pregnancy has not been established. Animal studies have shown no evidence of impaired fertility or teratogenicity attributable to nizatidine. Nizatidine should only be used in pregnant women, or in those planning pregnancy, if considered absolutely necessary, and then with caution.

Usage in lactation: Studies conducted in lactating women have shown that 0.1% of the administered oral dose of nizatidine is secreted in human milk in proportion to plasma concentrations. Because of the growth depression in pups reared by lactating rats treated with nizatidine, Axid should be administered to nursing mothers only if considered absolutely necessary.

Drug interactions: There is evidence that nizatidine does not affect the serum levels of concomitantly administered aminophylline, theophylline, chlordiazepoxide, diazepam, lignocaine, phenytoin, ibuprofen, metoprolol, warfarin or lorazepam. Nizatidine does not inhibit the hepatic cytochrome P450-linked drug metabolising enzyme system, but may increase absorption of salicylates when they are used in very high dosage. Approximately 35 per cent of nizatidine is bound to plasma protein. Warfarin, diazepam, paracetamol, propantheline, phenobarbitone and propranolol did not affect plasma protein binding of nizatidine *in vitro*.

Absorption of nizatidine is not clinically significantly affected by food intake, anticholinergic agents or antacids.

Precautions: As nizatidine is partially metabolised by the liver and principally excreted by the kidneys, patients with impaired liver or kidney function should be treated with caution. (See *Dosage and administration* section.)

Symptomatic response to nizatidine therapy does not preclude the presence of gastric malignancy.

Side-effects: In large scale clinical trials, anaemia, sweating and urticaria were significantly more common in nizatidine treated patients when compared with placebo. In these trials, 1.9 per cent of treated patients experienced somnolence, compared to 1.6 per cent of placebo patients (non–significant).

In the same trials, patients treated with both nizatidine and placebo had mild, transient, asymptomatic elevations of transaminases or alkaline phosphatase; rare instances of marked elevations (>500 iu/l) occurred in nizatidine treated patients. The overall rate of occurrences of elevated liver enzymes and elevations to 3 times the upper limit of normal, however, did not differ significantly from placebo. All abnormalities were reversible after discontinuation of nizatidine. Since introduction hepatitis and jaundice have been reported. Rare cases of cholestatic or mixed hepatocellular and cholestatic injury with jaundice have been reported, with reversal of the abnormalities after discontinuation.

The following effects have also been rarely reported, although a causal relationship has not always been established: thrombocytopenic purpura, fatal thrombocytopenia, exfoliative dermatitis, vasculitis, arthralgia, myalgia, gynaecomastia, impotence, hyperuricaemia, fever, nausea and reversible mental confusion.

Rare episodes of hypersensitivity reactions (e.g. bronchospasm, laryngeal oedema, rash, pruritus and eosinophilia), serum sickness and anaphylaxis have been reported.

Overdosage: There is little experience of overdose in humans. Tested at very high doses in animals, nizatidine has been shown to be relatively non-toxic. Animal studies suggest that cholinergic-type effects, including lacrimation, salivation, emesis, miosis and diarrhoea, may occur following very large oral doses. *Treatment:* Symptomatic and supportive therapy is recommended. Activated charcoal, emesis or lavage may reduce nizatidine absorption. The ability of haemodialysis to remove nizatidine from the body has not been conclusively demonstrated. However, this method is not expected to be efficient, since nizatidine has a large volume of distribution.

Pharmaceutical precautions Store below 25°C.

Legal category POM.

Package quantities
Capsules 150 mg: Blister packs of 30
Capsules 150 mg: Blister packs of 28 (hospitals only)
Capsules 300 mg: Blister packs of 30
Capsules 300 mg: Blister packs of 28 (hospitals only)

Further information Nizatidine is a potent, selective, competitive and fully reversible histamine H_2-receptor antagonist with a rapid onset of action. It significantly decreases acid concentration together with the volume of basal and stimulated gastric secretion. In clinical trials, nizatidine usually abolished ulcer pain within the first week of therapy. Nizatidine 300 mg at bedtime significantly reduced overnight gastric secretion, but did not increase subsequent basal or meal stimulated gastrin production. Intrinsic factor is not decreased in subjects administered nizatidine.

Nizatidine has no significant effect on the serum concentrations of gonadotrophins, prolactin, growth hormone, antidiuretic hormone, cortisol, tri-iodothyronine, thyroxine, testosterone, 5a-dihydrotestosterone, androstenedione or oestradiol.

Experience in clinical trials indicates that nizatidine has no greater potential than placebo for antiandrogenic effects.

Product licence numbers
Capsules 150 mg: 0006/0230
Capsules 300 mg: 0006/0231

AXID* INJECTION

Presentation Ampoules containing 100 mg nizatidine in 4 ml.

Nizatidine solution is a clear and colourless to yellow liquid that tends to darken slightly. It has a pH of 6.5 to 7.5. Each 1 ml contains 25 mg nizatidine.

Uses Nizatidine injection is indicated in hospitalised patients as an alternative to the oral dosage form, for short-term use in peptic ulcer patients until oral medication is indicated.

For appropriate cases the oral dosage form, Axid capsules, is also available (see separate data sheet).

Dosage and administration

Continuous intravenous infusion: Dilute 300 mg (12 ml) in 150 ml of compatible i.v. solution and infuse the solution at a rate to achieve a dose of 10 mg/hr.

Intermittent intravenous infusion: Dilute 100 mg (4 ml) in 50 ml of compatible i.v. solution and infuse over a 15 minute period three times daily.

The total daily dose of nizatidine should not exceed 480 mg. To maintain gastric pH ≥4, a continuous infusion of 10 mg/hr is recommended. Nizatidine should not be given by rapid i.v. infusion.

Compatible solutions include 0.9% Sodium Chloride Intravenous Infusion BP, 5% Dextrose Intravenous Infusion BP, Compound Sodium Lactate Intravenous Infusion BP or 5% Sodium Bicarbonate Intravenous Infusion BP.

The elderly: Age does not significantly influence efficacy or safety. Normally dosage modification is not required except in patients who have moderate to severe renal impairment (creatinine clearance less than 50 ml/min).

Children: Not recommended, as safety and efficacy have not been established.

Patients with impaired renal function: Nizatidine is principally excreted via the kidneys. For patients with moderate renal impairment (creatinine clearance 20-50 ml/min), the dose should be reduced to 120–150 mg daily. For patients with severe renal impairment (creatinine clearance less than 20 ml/min), the dose should be reduced to 75 mg daily. The clinical effects of this dosage reduction, in patients with renal failure, have not been evaluated.

Contra-indications, warnings, etc

Contra-indication: Known hypersensitivity to H_2-receptor antagonists.

Warnings

Usage in pregnancy: The safety of nizatidine for use during pregnancy has not been established. Animal studies have shown no evidence of impaired fertility or teratogenicity attributable to nizatidine. Nizatidine should only be used in pregnant women, or in those planning pregnancy, if considered absolutely necessary, and then with caution.

Usage in lactation: Studies conducted in lactating

women have shown that 0.1% of the administered oral dose of nizatidine is secreted in human milk in proportion to plasma concentrations. Because of the growth depression in pups reared by lactating rats treated with nizatidine, Axid should be administered to nursing mothers only if considered absolutely necessary.

Drug interactions: There is evidence that oral nizatidine does not affect the serum levels of concomitantly administered aminophylline, theophylline, chlordiazepoxide, diazepam, lignocaine, phenytoin, metoprolol, warfarin or lorazepam. Nizatidine does not inhibit the hepatic cytochrome P450-linked drug metabolising enzyme system, but may increase absorption of salicylates when they are used in very high dosage. Approximately 35 per cent of nizatidine is bound to plasma protein. Warfarin, diazepam, paracetamol, propantheline, phenobarbitone and propranolol did not affect plasma protein binding of nizatidine *in vitro.*

Precautions: As nizatidine is partially metabolised by the liver and principally excreted by the kidneys, patients with impaired liver or kidney function should be treated with caution. (See *Dosage and administration* section.)

Symptomatic response to nizatidine therapy does not preclude the presence of gastric malignancy.

Side-effects: Pain and minor bruising at the injection site were reported in clinical trials.

In large scale clinical trials, anaemia, sweating and urticaria were significantly more common in patients treated with oral nizatidine when compared with placebo. In these trials, 1.9 per cent of treated patients experienced somnolence, compared to 1.6 per cent of placebo patients (non-significant).

In the same trials, patients treated with both nizatidine and placebo had mild, transient, asymptomatic elevations of transaminases or alkaline phosphatase; rare instances of marked elevations (>500iu/l) occurred in nizatidine treated patients. The overall rate of occurrences of elevated liver enzymes and elevations to 3 times the upper limit of normal, however, did not differ significantly from placebo. All abnormalities were reversible after discontinuation of nizatidine. Since introduction hepatitis and jaundice have been reported. Rare cases of cholestatic or mixed hepatocellular and cholestatic injury with jaundice have been reported, with reversal of the abnormalities after discontinuation.

Intravenous nizatidine was not associated with abnormalities in liver test results.

Rare occurrences of tachycardia, bradycardia, postural hypotension and syncope were reported with rapid i.v. injection.

The following effects have also been rarely reported, although a causal relationship has not always been established: thrombocytopenic purpura, fatal thrombocytopenia, exfoliative dermatitis, vasculitis, arthralgia, myalgia, gynaecomastia, impotence, hyperuricaemia, fever, nausea and reversible mental confusion.

Rare episodes of hypersensitivity reactions (e.g. bronchospasm, laryngeal oedema, rash, pruritus and eosinophilia), serum sickness and anaphylaxis have been reported.

Overdosage: There is little experience of overdose in humans. Tested at very high doses in animals, nizatidine has been shown to be relatively non-toxic. Animal studies suggest that cholinergic-type effects, including lacrimation, salivation, emesis, miosis and diarrhoea, may occur following very large oral doses. *Treatment:* Symptomatic and supportive therapy is recommended. The ability of haemodialysis to remove nizatidine from the body has not been conclusively demonstrated. However, this method is not expected to be efficient, since nizatidine has a large volume of distribution.

Pharmaceutical precautions
Unreconstituted ampoules: Store below 25°C. Protect from light.

Reconstituted ampoules: Nizatidine injection is stable for 24 hours at 2–8°C when added to, or diluted with, an appropriate solution (see *Dosage and administration*). In accordance with recognised practices, infusion fluids containing nizatidine should not be used after this period.

Parenteral drug products should be inspected visually for particulate matter and discolouration before administration, whenever solution and container permit. Nizatidine injection tends to darken but this does not adversely affect potency.

Legal category POM.

Package quantity 100 mg ampoules in packs of 5.

Further information Nizatidine is a potent, selective, competitive and fully reversible histamine H_2-receptor antagonist with a rapid onset of action. It significantly decreases acid concentration together with the volume of basal and stimulated gastric secretion. Intrinsic factor is not decreased in subjects administered nizatidine.

Nizatidine has no significant effect on the serum concentrations of gonadotrophins, prolactin, growth hormone, antidiuretic hormone, cortisol, tri-iodothyronine, thyroxine, testosterone, 5a–dihydrotestosterone, androstenedione or oestradiol.

Experience in clinical trials indicates that nizatidine has no greater potential than placebo for antiandrogenic effects.

Product licence number 0006/0256.

BRIETAL* Sodium

Presentation Brietal Sodium (methohexitone sodium for injection), in crystalline form, is supplied as follows: 500 mg (with anhydrous Sodium Carbonate BP 30 mg) in 50 ml rubber-stoppered vials.

Uses
Action: Methohexitone sodium is a rapid, ultrashort-acting barbiturate anaesthetic agent.

Indications: Brietal Sodium is an intravenous anaesthetic agent for the induction of anaesthesia. It is used alone for short surgical procedures, or in combination with other agents for more prolonged anaesthesia.

Dosage and administration Pre-anaesthetic medication is generally advisable. Brietal Sodium may be used with any recognised pre-anaesthetic medications, but the phenothiazines are less satisfactory than the combination of an opiate and a belladonna derivative.

This drug should be administered by persons qualified in the use of intravenous anaesthetics. Facilities for assisting respiration and administering oxygen are necessary adjuncts for intravenous anaesthesia. Since cardiorespiratory arrest may occur, patients should be observed carefully during and after use of Brietal Sodium. Resuscitative equipment (i.e. intubation and cardioversion equipment, oxygen, suction and a secure intravenous line) and personnel qualified in its use must be immediately available.

Brietal Sodium is administered by intravenous injection (not infusion), usually in a 1% solution (10 mg per ml). Higher concentrations markedly increase the incidence of muscular movements and irregularities in respiration and blood pressure. Higher concentrations should normally be avoided.

Adults: As an initial guide, an injection rate of 1 ml of a 1% solution (10 mg) in five seconds may be used – although a faster rate than this is preferred by some anaesthetists. The dose usually ranges between 5 and 12 ml (50–120 mg, with an average of about 70 mg), but it must be adjusted to the needs of the individual patient. The induction dose maintains unconsciousness for about five to seven minutes.

The elderly: Onset of anaesthesia may be slow due to sluggish circulation, therefore methohexitone should be injected slowly.

Children: The dose should be adjusted for age and/or weight. Doses of approximately 1 mg/kg are usually satisfactory.

Maintenance: Brietal Sodium is best used simply as an induction agent. If further injection for maintenance is needed the dose must be individualised; but, as a guide, 2–4 ml of a 1% solution (20 to 40 mg) every four to seven minutes may be used. Other parenteral agents, usually narcotic analgesics, are usually employed with methohexitone during longer procedures.

Preparation of solutions: The recommended diluent for Brietal Sodium is Water for Injections PhEur. Solutions may also be prepared in Sodium Chloride Intravenous Infusion BP or 5% Dextrose Intravenous Infusion BP. Brietal Sodium is not compatible with Compound Sodium Lactate Intravenous Infusion BP or diluents containing bacteriostats.

For a 1% solution (10 mg per ml) vial contents should be diluted as follows:
500 mg: Add 50 ml diluent.

Contra-indications, warnings, etc
Contra-indications: Hypersensitivity to barbiturates. When general anaesthesia is contra–indicated, Brietal Sodium should not be used. Patients with latent or manifest porphyria should not receive barbiturates in any form.

Warnings: Because the liver is involved in demethylation and oxidation of methohexitone and because barbiturates may enhance pre-existing circulatory depression, severe hepatic dysfunction, severe cardiovascular instability, or a shock-like condition, may be reason for selecting another induction agent.

Methohexitone is not recommended for use in patients in status asthmaticus or in individuals with a history of epilepsy. Psychomotor seizures may be elicited in susceptible individuals.

Danger of intra-arterial injection: Unintended intra-arterial injection of barbiturate solutions may be followed by the production of platelet aggregates and thrombosis, starting in arterioles distal to the site of injection. The resulting necrosis may lead to gangrene, which may require amputation. The first sign in conscious patients may be a complaint of fiery burning that roughly follows the injected artery. If noted, the injection should be stopped immediately. *Transient* bleaching *may* or may not be noted very early. Blotchy cyanosis and dark discolouration may then be the first sign in anaesthetised patients. There is no established treatment, other than prevention. Animal experiments and published individual cases concerned with a variety of arteriolar irritants, including barbiturates, suggest that one or more of the following *may* be of benefit in reducing the area of necrosis: (a) arterial injection of heparin at the site of injury, followed by systemic anticoagulation; (b) sympathetic blockade (or brachial plexus blockade in the arm); (c) intra-arterial glucocorticoid injection at the site of injury, followed by systemic steroids; (d) a case report of non-barbiturate injury suggested that intra-arterial urokinase may promote fibrinolysis, even if administered late in treatment.

If extravasation occurs, the injection should be discontinued. Local irritation may result; subcutaneous swelling may also serve as a sign of arterial or periarterial placement of the catheter.

Drug interactions: Barbiturates may influence the absorption and elimination of other concomitantly used drugs, such as diphenylhydantoin, halothane, anticoagulants, corticosteroids, ethanol and propylene glycol-containing solutions.

The central nervous system depressant effect of methohexitone may be additive with that of other CNS depressants, including alcohol and antihistamines.

Prolonged administration may result in cumulative effects, including extended somnolence, protracted unconsciousness and respiratory and cardiovascular depression. Respiratory depression in the presence of an impaired airway may lead to hypoxia, cardiac arrest and death.

Usage in pregnancy: The safety of methohexitone sodium for use during pregnancy has not been established. Brietal Sodium should not be used in the pregnant patient unless, in the opinion of the clinician, the expected benefit outweighs the possible risk. Animal studies have shown no evidence of teratogenicity or of impaired fertility.

Labour and delivery: Methohexitone sodium has been used in caesarean section delivery but, because of its solubility, it readily and rapidly traverses the placenta and may therefore cause respiratory depression in the newly delivered baby. The obstetrician and paediatrician should be aware of this fact.

Nursing mothers: Caution should be exercised when methohexitone is administered to a nursing woman.

Precautions: Brietal Sodium should be administered only by persons who are experienced in general anaesthesia and who have appropriate equipment on hand for the prevention and treatment of anaesthetic emergencies. Respiratory depression, laryngospasm, apnoea, hypotension or cardiorespiratory arrest may occur owing to individual variations in tolerance or to the physical status of the patient. Caution should be exercised in debilitated patients, in those with severe anaemia or extreme obesity, or in those with impaired function of respiratory, circulatory, renal, hepatic or endocrine systems. It is essential that a free airway be maintained at all times. As with any potent anaesthetic agent, pulmonary ventilation should be maintained if prolonged apnoea occurs. Too rapid induction, inadequate dosage, or insufficient or unsuitable pre-anaesthetic medication may result in skeletal muscle hyperactivity, laryngospasm, cough, sneezing or hiccups. Hiccups, coughing and/or muscle twitching may also impair pulmonary ventilation.

Following induction, temporary hypotension and tachycardia may occur.

The patient's stomach should be empty. The usual pre-anaesthetic medications may be administered for the production of sedation and inhibition of secretions. If increased muscular relaxation is required for the performance of certain surgical procedures, it may be accomplished by the concomitant use of Brietal Sodium and skeletal muscle relaxants.

Postanaesthetic shivering may occur.

When appropriate, patients should be instructed as to the hazards of drowsiness that may follow use of methohexitone sodium. Outpatients should be released in the company of another individual, and no skilled activities, such as operating machinery or driving a motor vehicle, should be engaged in for at least 24 hours.

Liver function studies may be influenced by administration of a single dose of barbiturates.

Excretion occurs via the kidneys through glomerular filtration.

Side-effects: Side-effects associated with methohexitone sodium are extensions of pharmacological effects and include:

Cardiovascular: Circulatory depression, thrombophlebitis, hypotension, peripheral vascular collapse and convulsions in association with cardiorespiratory arrest.

Respiratory: Respiratory depression (including apnoea), cardiorespiratory arrest, laryngospasm, bronchospasm, hiccups and dyspnoea.

Neurological: Skeletal-muscle hyperactivity (twitching), injury to nerves adjacent to injection site, and seizures.

Psychiatric: Emergence delirium, restlessness and anxiety may occur, especially in the presence of postoperative pain.

Gastro-intestinal: Nausea, emesis and abdominal pain.

Allergic: Erythema, pruritus, urticaria and cases of anaphylaxis have been reported rarely.

Other: Other adverse reactions include pain at injection site, salivation, headache and rhinitis.

Drug abuse and dependence: Methohexitone sodium may be habit forming.

Overdosage: The onset of toxicity following an overdose of intravenously administered methohexitone will be within seconds. If methohexitone is administered rectally or is ingested, the onset of toxicity may be delayed. The manifestations include central nervous system depression, respiratory depression, hypotension, loss of peripheral vascular resistance, and muscular hyperactivity ranging from twitching to convulsive-like movements or actual convulsions. Other findings may include allergic reactions. Following massive exposure to any barbiturate, pulmonary oedema, circulatory collapse with loss of peripheral vascular tone, and cardiac arrest may occur.

Management: No specific antidote is known. Treatment consists of the usual life supporting measures.

Pharmaceutical precautions The pH of a 1% solution of Brietal Sodium is between 10 and 11. Owing to differences in pH, solutions of Brietal Sodium should not be mixed with acid solutions such as atropine sulphate, tubocurarine and succinylcholine chloride.

Do not use solvents containing bacteriostats, as these may cause precipitation.

Vials of Brietal Sodium should be stored below 25°C.

After reconstitution: Solutions of methohexitone sodium should be freshly prepared and used promptly. Reconstituted solutions are chemically stable at room temperature (15°–25°C) for 24 hours.

Parenteral drug products should be inspected visually for particulate matter and discolouration prior to administration, whenever solution and container permit.

Legal category POM.

Package quantity
500 mg in 50 ml vial: Single vials.

Further information Nil.

Product licence number
500 mg: 0006/5051

CEFUROXIME

Qualitative and quantitative composition Each vial contains, as the active ingredient, Cefuroxime Sodium for Injection equivalent to 250 mg, 750 mg or 1.5 g of cefuroxime.

Pharmaceutical form Vials containing an off-white to slightly yellow sterile powder for reconstitution for injection or infusion.

Clinical particulars

Therapeutic indications: Cefuroxime is indicated for the treatment of infections caused by susceptible strains of the designated micro-organisms, or before the infecting organism has been identified, in the diseases listed below.

Respiratory tract infections, for example, acute and chronic bronchitis, infected bronchiectasis, bacterial pneumonia, lung abscess and post operative chest infections.

Ear, nose and throat infections, for example, sinusitis, tonsillitis and pharyngitis.

Urinary tract infections, for example, acute and chronic pyelonephritis, cystitis and asymptomatic bacteriuria.

Soft tissue infections, for example, cellulitis, erysipelas, peritonitis and wound infections.

Bone and joint infections, for example, osteomyelitis and septic arthritis.

Obstetric and gynaecological infections, pelvic inflammatory disease.

Gonorrhoea, particularly if penicillin is unsuitable.

Other infections, including septicaemia and meningitis.

Prophylaxis against infection in abdominal, pelvic, orthopaedic, cardiac, pulmonary, oesophageal and vascular surgery where there is increased risk from infection.

Posology and method of administration: Usually cefuroxime is effective when administered alone, but when appropriate it may be used in combination with metronidazole or an aminoglycoside.

General dosage:
Adults: Many infections will respond to 750 mg three times daily by intramuscular or intravenous injection. For more severe infections this dose should be increased to 1.5 g three times daily intravenously. The frequency of dosage may be increased to six-hourly injections, intramuscular or intravenous, giving total daily doses of 3 g to 6 g.

Infants and children: Doses of 30 to 100 mg/kg/day given in three or four divided doses. A dose of 60 mg/kg/day will be appropriate for most infections.

Neonates: Doses of 30 to 100 mg/kg/day given in two or three divided doses. In the first weeks of life the serum half-life of cefuroxime can be three to five times that in adults.

Gonorrhoea: 1.5 g should be given as a single dose or as two 750 mg injections into different sites, eg, each buttock.

Meningitis: Cefuroxime therapy is suitable for sole therapy of bacterial meningitis due to sensitive strains.
Infants and children: 200 to 240 mg/kg/day intravenously in three or four divided doses. This dosage may be reduced to 100 mg/kg/day after three days or when clinical improvement occurs.

Neonates: The initial dosage should be 100 mg/kg/day intravenously. This dosage may be reduced to 50 mg/kg/day after three days or when clinical improvement occurs.

Adults: 3 g intravenously every eight hours. No data is currently available to recommend a dose for intrathecal administration.

Prophylaxis: The usual dose is 1.5 g intravenously with induction of anaesthesia. For orthopaedic, pelvic and abdominal operations this may be followed with two 750 mg doses 8 and 16 hours later. For vascular, cardiac, oesophageal and pulmonary operations this may be supplemented with 750 mg intramuscularly three times a day for a further 24 to 48 hours.

In total joint replacement, 1.5 g cefuroxime powder may be mixed dry with each pack of methyl methacrylate cement polymer before adding the liquid monomer.

Dosage in impaired renal function: As cefuroxime is excreted by the kidneys, the dosage should be reduced to allow for slower excretion in patients with impaired renal function, once creatinine clearance falls below 20 ml/min, as follows.

Marked impairment (creatinine clearance 10 to 20 ml/min)	750 mg twice daily
Severe impairment (creatinine clearance of less than 10 ml/min)*	750 mg once daily
Continuous peritoneal dialysis	750 mg twice daily
Renal failure on continuous arteriovenous haemodialysis or high-flux haemofiltration in intensive therapy units	750 mg twice daily
Low-flux haemofiltration	As for impaired renal function

*For patients on haemodialysis, a further 750 mg should be given at the end of each dialysis session.

Contra-indications: Contra-indicated in patients hypersensitive to the cephalosporin group of antibiotics.

Special warnings and precautions for use: Cephalosporin antibiotics may, in general, be given safely to patients who are hypersensitive to penicillins, although cross-reactions have been reported. Special care is indicated in patients who have experienced an anaphylactic reaction to penicillin.

Cephalosporin antibiotics at high dosage should be given with caution to patients receiving potent diuretics or aminoglycosides, as these combinations are suspected of adversely affecting renal function. Clinical experience has shown that this is not likely to be a problem at the recommended dose levels.

Interactions with other medicaments and other forms of interaction: Concurrent administration of probenecid prolongs the excretion of cefuroxime and produces an elevated peak serum level.

Interference with laboratory tests: Slight interference may occur with the copper reduction methods (Fehling's, Benedict's) but this should not lead to false-positive results. Cefuroxime does not interfere with the enzyme based tests for glycosuria, or with the alkaline picrate method for creatinine. It is recommended that either the hexokinase or glucose oxidase methods are used for determination of blood/plasma glucose levels.

Pregnancy and lactation: Studies in animals revealed no evidence of embryopathic or teratogenic effects due to cefuroxime, but, as with all drugs, it should be used with caution during pregnancy.

Since cefuroxime is excreted in human milk, caution should be exercised when administering this antibiotic to a nursing mother.

Effects on ability to drive and use machines: Cefuroxime is not known to affect the ability to drive or use machines.

Undesirable effects: Cefuroxime is generally well tolerated. Adverse reactions have been infrequent, generally mild and transient.

Hypersensitivity reactions: Including skin rashes (maculopapular and urticarial), fever and, very rarely, anaphylaxis. As with any antibiotic, prolonged use may lead to overgrowth of non-susceptible organisms, eg, Candida.

Gastro-intestinal disturbance: Including, very rarely, pseudomembranous colitis, which has been reported with most broad spectrum antibiotics.

Haematological: A decrease in haemoglobin concentration, eosinophilia, leucopenia and neutropenia have been observed. Positive Coombs' test have been reported. As with other cephalosporins, thrombocytopenia has been reported rarely.

Hepatic: Transient rises in liver enzymes or serum bilirubin have been observed, particularly in patients with pre-existing liver disease, but there is no evidence of hepatic involvement.

Renal: There may be some variation in the results of biochemical tests or renal function, but these results do not appear to be of clinical significance.

Other: Transient pain may be experienced at the site of intramuscular injection. Occasionally thrombophlebitis may occur at the site of intravenous injection.

Overdose: Overdosage of cephalosporins can lead to cerebral irritation and seizures. With seizures the drug should be discontinued and appropriate anticonvulsive and supportive therapy administered. Serum levels of cefuroxime can be reduced by haemodialysis or peritoneal dialysis.

Pharmacological properties

Pharmacodynamic properties: Cefuroxime (cefuroxime sodium) is a semi-synthetic, broad spectrum cephalosporin antibiotic exerting its bactericidal action by inhibition of cell wall synthesis. This antibiotic is resistant to most beta-lactamases and is active against the following pathogens.

Gram-negative: Haemophilus influenzae, Neisseria spp (including *Neisseria gonorrhoeae*), *Escherichia coli, Klebsiella* spp (including *Klebsiella pneumoniae*), *Enterobacter* spp, *Bordetella pertussis, Salmonella* spp (including *Salmonella typhi* and *Salmonella typhimurium*), *Shigella* spp, *Proteus mirabilis, Proteus rettgeri, Proteus vulgaris, Morganella morganii* (formerly *Proteus morganii*).

Gram-positive: Staphylococcus aureus (including strains resistant to penicillin), *Staphylococcus epidermidis* and certain strains of streptococci, e.g. *Streptococcus pyogenes* and *Streptococcus mitis* (viridans group).

Anaerobic organisms: Clostridium spp, *Bacteroides fragilis.*

Resistant strains: Pseudomonas and *Campylobacter* spp, *Acinetobacter calcoaceticus, Clostridium difficile, Legionella* spp and methicillin-resistant strains of *Staphylococcus aureus* and *Staphylococcus epidermidis.* Some strains of *Streptococcus faecalis, Morganella morganii, Proteus vulgaris, Bacteroides fragilis, Serratia* spp, *Enterobacter* spp and *Citrobacter* spp.

In vitro the activities of cefuroxime and aminoglycoside antibiotics in combination have been shown to be at least additive with occasional evidence of synergy.

Pharmacokinetic properties: The serum half-life after either intramuscular or intravenous administration is approximately 70 minutes. After intramuscular injection the peak serum level occurs after about 45 minutes.

The antibiotic can be found in bone, synovial fluid and aqueous humour above the minimum inhibitory levels for common pathogens. The blood-brain barrier can be passed by cefuroxime when the meninges are inflamed.

Cefuroxime is excreted approximately 50% by glomerular filtration and 50% through the renal tubules. Cefuroxime is almost completely recovered unchanged in the urine within 24 hours, most being excreted within six hours.

Preclinical safety data: There is no experimental evidence of embryopathic or teratogenic effects attributable to cefuroxime.

Pharmaceutical particulars

List of excipients: Each vial contains only the active ingredient, cefuroxime sodium.

Incompatibilities: Cefuroxime should not be mixed in the syringe with aminoglycoside antibiotics.

Shelf life:
Before reconstitution: 18 months when stored below 25°C.

In keeping with good pharmaceutical practice, freshly constituted suspensions or solutions should be used immediately. If this is not practicable then solution may be stored for up to 24 hours under refrigerated conditions (2-8°C).

Special precautions for storage: Protect from light. Before reconstitution store below 25°C. After reconstitution the product may be stored in a refrigerator for up to 24 hours.

Nature and contents of container: Type III flint glass vial, stoppered with halobutyl closures and sealed with aluminium seals that may be combined with a polypropylene cap.

Package quantities:
Vials 250 mg: Single vials
Vials 750 mg: Single vials
Vials 1.5 g: Single vials

Instructions for use/handling:
Intramuscular injection: Add 1 ml of Water for Injections to 250 mg or 3 ml of Water for Injections to 750 mg. Shake gently to produce a suspension.

Intravenous administration: Dissolve cefuroxime in Water for Injections using at least 2 ml for 250 mg, at least 6 ml for 750 mg and at least 15 ml for 1.5 g. For short intravenous infusion, 1.5 g may be dissolved in 50 ml of Water for Injections. Reconstituted solutions may be diluted with:

5% or 10% Dextrose
5% Dextrose containing 0.2%, 0.225%, 0.45% or 0.9% Sodium Chloride Injection
5% Dextrose containing 20 mEq Potassium Chloride
0.9% Sodium Chloride Injection
M/6 Sodium Lactate Injection
Ringer's Injection
Lactated Ringer's Injection
Heparin (10 and 50 units/ml) in 0.9% Sodium Chloride Injection
10 mEq Potassium Chloride in 0.9% Sodium Chloride Injection

These solutions may be given directly into a vein or introduced into the tubing of the giving set if the patient is receiving parenteral fluids.

Marketing authorisation numbers
Cefuroxime Sodium for Injection 250 mg 0006/0318
Cefuroxime Sodium for Injection 750 mg 0006/0332
Cefuroxime Sodium for Injection 1.5 g 0006/0333

Date of approval/revision of SPC 28 January 1997

Legal category POM

CELANCE*

Presentation Tablets (ivory, modified rectangle shaped, scored, marked Lilly 4131) containing 50 micrograms pergolide base.

Tablets (green, modified rectangle shaped, scored, marked Lilly 4133) containing 250 micrograms pergolide base.

Tablets (pink, modified rectangle shaped, scored, marked Lilly 4135) containing 1000 micrograms pergolide base.

Uses Pergolide mesylate is indicated as adjunctive treatment to levodopa in the management of the signs and symptoms of Parkinson's disease. Pergolide mesylate is a dopamine receptor agonist at both D_1 and D_2 receptor sites.

Dosage and administration For oral administration to adults only.

Administration of pergolide mesylate should be initiated with a daily dosage of 50 micrograms for the first 2 days. The dosage should then be gradually increased by 100 or 150 micrograms/day every third day over the next 12 days of therapy. The dosage may then be increased by 250 micrograms/day every third day until an optimal therapeutic dosage is achieved.

Pergolide mesylate is usually administered in divided doses 3 times per day. During dosage titration, the dosage of concurrent *l*-dopa may be cautiously decreased.

In clinical studies, the mean therapeutic daily dosage of pergolide mesylate was 3 mg/day (3000 micrograms/day). The average concurrent daily dosage of *l*-dopa/carbidopa (expressed as *l*-dopa) was approximately 650 mg/day. The efficacy of pergolide mesylate at doses above 5 mg/day (5000 micrograms/day) has not been systematically evaluated.

Children: Safety and effectiveness have not been established.

The major route of excretion is via the kidney.

Contra-indications, warnings, etc
Contra-indication: Hypersensitivity to this drug or other ergot derivatives.

Warnings: Patients should be warned to begin therapy with low doses and to increase dosage in carefully adjusted increments over a period of 3 to 4 weeks (see *Dosage and administration*) to minimise the risk of symptomatic postural and/or sustained hypotension. With gradual dosage titration, tolerance to the hypotension usually develops (but see *Drug interactions*).

In controlled trials, pergolide mesylate with *l*-dopa caused hallucinosis in about 14 per cent of patients, as opposed to 3 per cent taking placebo with *l*-dopa. This was of sufficient severity to cause discontinuation of treatment in about 3 per cent of those enrolled. Tolerance to this untoward effect was not observed.

In the placebo-controlled trial, 2 of 187 patients treated with placebo died, as compared with 1 of 189 patients treated with pergolide mesylate. Of the 2299 patients treated with pergolide mesylate in premarketing studies evaluated in October 1988, 6.2 per cent died while on the drug or shortly after discontinuation. The patient population under evaluation was elderly, ill and at high risk for death. A case-by-case review of the patients who died failed to disclose any unique set of signs, symptoms, or laboratory results that would suggest that treatment with pergolide caused these deaths.

Caution should be exercised when administering to patients prone to cardiac dysrhythmias or with significant underlying cardiac disease.

In a placebo-controlled study, patients taking pergolide mesylate had significantly more episodes of atrial premature contractions (APCs) and sinus tachycardia.

Pergolide should be used with caution in patients with a history of pleuritis, pleural effusion, pleural fibrosis, pericarditis, pericardial effusion, retroperitoneal fibrosis or similar conditions which may have occurred in association with the use of ergot derivatives. There have been rare reports of these conditions in patients receiving pergolide, and in some cases there had been similar events during prior exposure to bromocriptine. Patients with a history of such events should be carefully monitored clinically and with appropriate radiographic and laboratory studies whilst taking pergolide.

Precautions: Use in patients on *l*-dopa may cause and/or exacerbate pre-existing states of confusion and hallucinations (see *Warnings*). Abrupt discontinuation of pergolide mesylate, in patients receiving it chronically as an adjunct to *l*-dopa, may precipitate the onset of hallucinations and confusion; these may occur within a span of several days. Discontinuation of pergolide should be undertaken gradually, even if the patient is to remain on *l*-dopa.

Administration to patients receiving *l*-dopa may cause and/or exacerbate pre–existing dyskinesia.

Patients and their families should be informed of the common adverse consequences of the use of pergolide mesylate and the risk of hypotension.

Patients should be advised to tell their doctor if they become pregnant or intend to become pregnant during therapy. They should also tell their doctor if they are breast feeding.

No specific laboratory tests are essential for the management of patients. Periodic routine evaluation is appropriate.

Drug interactions: Dopamine antagonists, such as the neuroleptics (phenothiazines, butyrophenones, thioxanthines) or metoclopramide, ordinarily should not be administered concurrently with pergolide mesylate (a dopamine agonist); these agents may diminish the effectiveness of pergolide mesylate.

Because pergolide mesylate is approximately 90 per cent associated with plasma proteins, caution should be exercised if it is co-administered with other drugs known to affect protein binding.

There are no studies involving the concomitant administration of pergolide and warfarin. When these two drugs are co-prescribed, careful monitoring of anticoagulation should be performed, with adjustments of dosage as necessary.

Because of the risk of postural and/or sustained hypotension in patients taking pergolide, caution should be exercised if it is co-administered with antihypertensive agents.

Carcinogenesis, mutagenesis and impairment of fertility: Two year carcinogenicity studies in mice and rats used doses up to 340 and 12 times the maximum human oral dose (6 mg or 6000 micrograms/day equivalent to 120 micrograms/kg/day). A low incidence of uterine neoplasms occurred in both rats and mice. Endometrial adenomas and carcinomas were observed in rats. Endometrial sarcomas were observed in mice. These occurrences are probably attributable to the high oestrogen/progesterone ratio, which would occur in rodents as a result of the prolactin-inhibiting action of pergolide mesylate. These endocrine mechanisms are not present in humans. However, there are no human data with pergolide to substantiate this conclusion concerning the lack of potential for human risk.

Mutagenic potential was evaluated in a battery of tests. A weak response was noted in one test but the other three tests were negative. The relevance to humans is unknown.

Impaired fertility was observed in mice at the highest dose (5.6 mg or 5600 micrograms/kg/day). This may be related to depressed prolactin levels.

Pregnancy: In animal studies there was no evidence of harm to the foetus due to pergolide mesylate. There are, however, no adequate and well-controlled studies in pregnant women. In pre-marketing studies there were 33 pregnancies that resulted in healthy babies and 6 pregnancies that resulted in congenital abnormalities, although a causal relationship has not been established. This drug should be used during pregnancy only if clearly needed.

Nursing mothers: It is not known whether pergolide is excreted in human milk. The pharmacological action of pergolide mesylate suggests it may interfere with lactation. A decision should be made whether to discontinue nursing or the drug, taking into account the importance of the drug to the mother.

Side-effects: The following adverse events, which are listed in decreasing order of frequency under body system, were observed during placebo-controlled clinical trials at a frequency of one per cent or greater and at a significantly higher incidence than placebo (P value ≤ 0.05):

Body as a whole: Pain, abdominal pain.

Digestive system: Nausea, dyspepsia.

Nervous system: Dyskinesia, hallucinations, somnolence.

Respiratory system: Rhinitis, dyspnoea. Following market introduction, there have been reports of cases of serosal inflammatory conditions, such as pleuritis, pleural effusion, pleural fibrosis, pericarditis, pericardial effusion and retroperitoneal fibrosis, in patients taking pergolide (see 'Warnings').

Special senses: Diplopia.

Other events that have been reported include insomnia, confusion, dizziness, constipation, diarrhoea, abnormal liver function tests, hypotension, syncope, atrial premature contractions, sinus tachycardia, rash and fever.

The more common events that caused discontinuation were related to the nervous system, primarily hallucinations and confusion.

Rare post-marketing spontaneous reports of neuroleptic malignant syndrome have been received but no clear causal relationship with the drug has been established.

Overdosage: There is no clinical experience with massive overdosage. Overdoses of 60 mg on one day, 19 mg/day for 3 days, or 14 mg/day for 23 days have occurred. Symptoms and signs included vomiting, hypotension, agitation, severe hallucinations, severe involuntary movements and tingling sensations. Another patient who inadvertently received 7 mg, instead of the prescribed 0.7 mg (700 micrograms), experienced palpitations, hypotension and ventricular extrasystoles. The highest daily dose (prescribed for several patients with refractory Parkinson's disease) has exceeded 30 mg.

In animals, manifestations of overdosage include nausea, vomiting, convulsions, decreased blood pressure and CNS stimulation.

Treatment: Symptomatic supportive therapy and cardiac monitoring is recommended.

Arterial blood pressure should be maintained. An antiarrhythmic agent may be necessary. If signs of CNS stimulation are present, a phenothiazine, or other butyrophenone neuroleptic agent, may be indicated.

Activated charcoal may be considered instead of, or in addition to, gastric emptying.

Dialysis or haemoperfusion are unlikely to be of benefit.

Pharmaceutical precautions Store at room temperature.

Legal category POM.

Package quantities
Starter packs of 75 × 50 microgram tablets and 6 × 250 microgram tablets.
Tablets 50 micrograms: Blister packs of 100.
Tablets 250 micrograms: Blister packs of 100.
Tablets 1000 micrograms: Blister packs of 100.

Further information Nil.

Product licence numbers
Tablets 50 micrograms: 0006/0250
Tablets 250 micrograms: 0006/0251
Tablets 1000 micrograms: 0006/0252

CINOBAC*

Presentation Capsules (green and orange, coded 3056) containing 500 mg (1.9 mmol) cinoxacin.

Uses Cinoxacin, a quinolone, has *in vitro* activity against many gram-negative aerobic bacteria, particularly strains of *Enterobacteriaceae*. Cinoxacin inhibits bacterial DNA synthesis, is bactericidal, and is active across the entire urinary pH range.

Cinoxacin is indicated for acute, recurrent and chronic upper and lower urinary tract infections (including cystitis, pyelonephritis or pyelitis and asymptomatic bacteriuria) caused by susceptible micro-organisms.

A single dose of 500 mg, taken at bedtime, for up to 5 months, has been shown to be effective as preventive therapy in women with a history of recurrent urinary tract infections.

Cinoxacin is active against most strains of the following organisms: *Enterobacter* spp. (including *Ent. aerogenes, Ent. cloacae* and *Ent. hafniae), Escherichia coli, Klebsiella* spp., *Proteus mirabilis*, and *Pr. vulgaris*.

Cinoxacin is also active against approximately 50 per cent of strains of *Pr. rettgeri, Providencia* and *Serratia* species.

In vitro susceptibility testing should be performed prior to administration of the drug and, when clinically indicated, during treatment.

Using NCCLS recommended methods for sensitivity testing, the criteria for dilution methods are:

MIC≤16 micrograms/ml: susceptible
MIC=32 micrograms/ml: intermediate
MIC≥64 micrograms/ml: resistant.

Standard cinoxacin powder should give an MIC range of 2.0–8.0 micrograms/ml with *E. coli* ATCC 25922.

For the standard disc test using a 100 microgram cinoxacin disc, zone diameters are:

Zone≥19 mm: susceptible
Zone 15–18 mm: intermediate
Zone≤14 mm: resistant.

Certain strains of *Enterobacteriaceae* exhibit heterogeneity of resistance to cinoxacin by producing isolated colonies within the inhibition zone. The clear inhibition zone should be measured within such isolated colonies.

The 100 microgram disc should give a 26–32 mm zone diameter with *E. coli* ATCC 25922. Other quinolone discs should not be substituted.

Enterococcus species, *Pseudomonas* species and *Staphylococcus* species are resistant.

Cross-resistance with nalidixic acid has been demonstrated. Conventional chromosomal resistance to cinoxacin taken at recommended doses has been reported to emerge in approximately 4 per cent of patients during treatment. However, bacterial resistance to cinoxacin has not been shown to be transferable via R factor.

Dosage and administration The usual adult dose is 1 g daily, administered orally as 500 mg b.d. for seven to fourteen days.

For prophylactic use, a single dose of 500 mg daily, taken at bedtime.

Not recommended for use in children, and growing adolescents, under the age of 18 years.

The elderly: As for adults, unless renal function is impaired (see *Precautions*).

Renal impairment: A reduced dosage must be employed. After an initial dose of 500 mg, use the following maintenance dose schedule:

Renal Function	*Dosage*
Moderate impairment	500 mg once daily
Marked impairment (creatinine clearance <20 ml/min/1.73m²)	Not recommended

Cinoxacin may be taken with or without meals.

Contra-indications, warnings, etc
Contra-indication: Hypersensitivity to cinoxacin or other quinolones.

Warnings: Since cinoxacin, like other quinolones, causes arthropathy in immature animals, its use during pregnancy or for children, and growing adolescents, under 18 years of age is not recommended.

Usage in pregnancy or lactation: Cinoxacin should not be administered during pregnancy or to the nursing mother unless the potential benefit justifies the potential risk to the foetus or infant. Reproduction studies in rats and rabbits, at doses up to 10 times the daily human dose, have revealed no evidence of impaired fertility or harm to the foetus. However, there are no well controlled studies in pregnant women. It is not known whether cinoxacin is excreted in human milk.

Convulsions and abnormal electroencephalograms have been reported with quinolones, although no causal relationship has been established. Convulsions, increased intracranial pressure, toxic psychoses and CNS stimulation (tremors, restlessness, lightheadedness, confusion and hallucinations) have been reported with other quinolones. Cinoxacin should be used with caution in patients with CNS disorders, such as severe cerebral arteriosclerosis, epilepsy, or other factors that predispose to seizures. If such reactions occur discontinue treatment and give appropriate therapy.

Serious and, occasionally, fatal hypersensitivity (anaphylactoid) reactions, some following the first dose, have been reported in patients during quinolone therapy. Some reactions were accompanied by cardiovascular collapse, loss of consciousness, tingling, pharyngeal and facial oedema, dyspnoea, urticaria and itching. Only a few patients had a history of hypersensitivity reactions. If an allergic reaction or skin rash occurs, discontinue the drug. Appropriate supportive therapy is recommended.

Precautions: Since cinoxacin is eliminated primarily by the kidney, dosage should be reduced in patients with reduced renal function (see 'Dosage and Administration'). Administration of cinoxacin is not recommended for patients with severely impaired renal function (creatinine clearance <20 ml/min/1.73 m²). Although crystalluria is not expected to occur with the usually recommended dosages of cinoxacin, patients should be well hydrated and alkalinisation of the urine should be avoided. Patients should be advised to drink fluids liberally.

Moderate to severe phototoxicity reactions have been observed in patients who were exposed to direct sunlight while receiving some quinolones. Patients should be advised to avoid excessive sunlight. Discontinue the drug if phototoxicity occurs.

Since cinoxacin can cause dizziness and lightheadedness, patients should be sure they are not adversely affected before driving, operating machinery, or engaging in other activities requiring mental alertness or co-ordination.

Periodic assessment of renal, hepatic and haematopoietic function is advisable during prolonged therapy.

Drug interactions: Cinoxacin may enhance the effects of oral anticoagulants, such as warfarin. When concomitant administration cannot be avoided, daily coagulation tests are essential.

Elevated plasma levels of theophylline and theophylline-related side-effects have been reported with concomitant quinolone use. Therefore, the monitoring of theophylline plasma levels should be considered, and theophylline dosage adjusted as required.

Quinolones have been shown to reduce the clearance of caffeine and prolong caffeine's half-life.

Antacids or sucralfate interfere with the absorption of some quinolones, resulting in low urine levels. Concomitant administration of quinolones, with products containing iron or multi vitamins containing zinc, may also result in low urine levels.

Elevated cyclosporin serum levels have been reported with the concomitant use of quinolones and cyclosporin.

Seizures have been reported in patients taking another quinolone antimicrobial and fenbufen concurrently.

Side-effects: The most frequently reported adverse events in postmarketing surveillance have been nausea, hypersensitivity reactions, headache and dizziness.

Gastro-intestinal: Nausea, anorexia, vomiting, abdominal cramps, perverse taste and diarrhoea have been reported.

Hypersensitivity: Rash, pruritus, urticaria, oedema, angio-oedema and eosinophilia. Anaphylaxis, anaphylactoid reactions and toxic epidermal necrolysis have been reported rarely. Erythema multiforme and Stevens-Johnson syndrome.

Haematological: Thrombocytopenia has been reported rarely.

Nervous system: Dizziness, headache, insomnia, drowsiness, tingling sensation, perineal burning, photophobia and tinnitus.

Laboratory values: Transient changes in blood urea, AST, ALT, serum creatinine and alkaline phosphatase have been observed occasionally. Reduction in haematocrit/haemoglobin.

Although not observed in clinical studies of cinoxacin involving 1,118 patients, the following side-effects have been reported for drugs in the same class: restlessness, nervousness, change in colour perception, difficulty in focusing, decrease in visual acuity, double vision, weakness, constipation, erythema and bullae, disorientation, agitation, acute anxiety, palpitation, gum soreness, joint stiffness, swelling of extremities, toxic psychoses or, rarely, convulsions.

Overdosage
Signs and symptoms: May include anorexia, nausea, vomiting, epigastric distress and diarrhoea. The severity of epigastric distress and diarrhoea are dose related. Headache, dizziness, insomnia, photophobia, tinnitus and tingling sensation have also been reported.

Treatment: Patients should be kept well hydrated to prevent crystalluria. Symptomatic and supportive therapy is recommended. Activated charcoal should be considered instead of, or in addition to, gastric emptying. Forced diuresis, peritoneal dialysis, haemodialysis, or charcoal haemoperfusion have not been established as beneficial.

Pharmaceutical precautions Store at room temperature (15°–25°C).

Legal category POM.

Package quantity Blister pack of 14.

Further information Nil.

Product licence number 0006/0124.

CYCLOSERINE

Qualitative and quantitative composition Each capsule contains, as active ingredient, 250 mg of cycloserine.

Pharmaceutical form Capsules (red and grey, coded F04) each containing 250 mg Cycloserine BP.

Clinical particulars
Therapeutic indications:

Actions: Cycloserine inhibits cell wall synthesis in susceptible strains of Gram-positive and Gram-negative bacteria and in *Mycobacterium tuberculosis.*

Indications: Cycloserine is indicated in the treatment of active pulmonary and extra-pulmonary tuberculosis (including renal disease) when the organisms are susceptible to this drug and after failure of adequate treatment with the primary medications (streptomycin, isoniazid, rifampicin and ethambutol). Like all anti-tuberculous drugs, cycloserine should be administered in conjunction with other effective chemotherapy and not as the sole therapeutic agent.

Cycloserine may be effective in the treatment of acute urinary tract infections caused by susceptible strains of Gram-positive and Gram-negative bacteria, especially *Klebsiella/Enterobacter* species and *Escherichia coli.* It is generally no more and may be less effective than other antimicrobial agents in the treatment of urinary tract infections caused by bacteria other than mycobacteria. Use of cycloserine in these infections should be considered only when the more conventional therapy has failed and when the organism has been demonstrated to be sensitive to the drug.

Posology and method of administration:
Adults: The usual dosage is 500 mg to 1 g daily in divided doses, monitored by blood level determinations. The initial adult dosage most frequently given is 250 mg twice daily at 12-hour intervals for the first two weeks. A daily dosage of 1 g should not be exceeded.

Children: The usual starting dose is 10 mg/kg/day, then adjusted according to blood levels obtained and therapeutic response.

The elderly: As for adults but reduce dosage if renal function is impaired.

Contra-indications: Cycloserine is contra-indicated in the presence of any of the following: hypersensitivity to cycloserine; epilepsy; depression, severe anxiety or psychosis; severe renal insufficiency; alcohol abuse.

Special warnings and special precautions for use: Administration of cycloserine should be discontinued or the dosage reduced if the patient develops allergic dermatitis or symptoms of central nervous system toxicity, such as convulsions, psychosis, somnolence, depression, confusion, hyper-reflexia, headache, tremor, vertigo, paresis or dysarthria.

Toxicity is usually associated with blood levels of greater than 30 mg/l, which may be the result of high dosage or inadequate renal clearance. The therapeutic index for this drug is low. The risk of convulsions is increased in chronic alcoholics (see below).

Patients should be monitored by haematological, renal excretion, blood level and liver function studies.

Before treatment with cycloserine is begun, cultures should be taken and the susceptibility of the organism to the drug should be established. In tuberculous infections, sensitivity to the other anti-tuberculous agents in the regimen should also be demonstrated.

Blood levels should be determined at least weekly for patients having reduced renal function, for individuals receiving a daily dosage of more than 500 mg, and for those showing signs and symptoms suggestive of toxicity. The dosage should be adjusted to keep the blood level below 30 mg/l.

Anticonvulsant drugs or sedatives may be effective in controlling symptoms of central nervous system toxicity, such as convulsions, anxiety or tremor. Patients receiving more than 500 mg of cycloserine daily should be closely observed for such symptoms. The value of pyridoxine in preventing CNS toxicity from cycloserine has not been proved.

Administration of cycloserine and other anti-tuberculous drugs has been associated in a few instances with vitamin B_{12} and/or folic acid deficiency, megaloblastic anaemia and sideroblastic anaemia. If evidence of anaemia develops during treatment, appropriate investigations and treatment should be carried out.

Interaction with other medicaments and other forms of interaction:
Drug interactions: Concurrent administration of ethionamide has been reported to potentiate neurotoxic side-effects. Alcohol and cycloserine are incompatible, especially during a regimen calling for large doses of the latter. Alcohol increases the possibility and risk of epileptic episodes. Patients receiving cycloserine and isoniazid should be monitored for signs of CNS toxicity, such as dizziness and drowsiness, as these drugs have a combined toxic action on the CNS. Dosage adjustments may be necessary.

Pregnancy and lactation:
Usage in pregnancy: Concentrations in fetal blood approach those found in the serum. A study in 2 generations of rats given doses up to 100 mg/kg/day demonstrated no teratogenic effect in offspring. It is not known whether cycloserine can cause fetal harm when administered to a pregnant woman or can affect reproduction capacity. Cycloserine should be given to a pregnant woman only if clearly needed.

Usage in nursing mothers: Concentrations in the mother's milk approach those found in the serum. A decision should be made whether to discontinue nursing or to discontinue the drug, taking into account the importance of the drug to the mother.

Effects on ability to drive and use machines: None known.

Undesirable effects: Most side-effects occurring during treatment with cycloserine involve the nervous system or are manifestations of drug hypersensitivity. The following side-effects have been observed: nervous system manifestations, which appear to be related to higher dosages of drug, ie, more than 500 mg daily, can be convulsions, drowsiness, somnolence, headache, tremor, dysarthria, vertigo, confusion and disorientation with loss of memory, psychosis, possibly with suicidal tendencies, character changes, hyperirritability, aggression, paresis, hyper-reflexia, paraesthesia, major and minor localised clonic seizures and coma.

Other reported side-effects include allergy, rash, megaloblastic anaemia and elevated serum aminotransferases, especially in patients with pre-existing liver disease.

Sudden development of congestive heart failure, in patients receiving 1 to 1.5 g of cycloserine daily, has been reported.

Overdose:
Signs and symptoms: Acute toxicity can occur if more than 1 g is ingested by an adult. Chronic toxicity is dose related and can occur if more than 500 mg is administered daily. For patients with renal impairment, see *Contra-indications* and *Special warnings and special precautions for use.* Toxicity commonly affects the central nervous system. Effects may include headache, vertigo, confusion, drowsiness, hyper-irritability, paraesthesias, dysarthria and psychosis. Following larger ingestions, paresis, convulsions and coma often occur. Ethanol may increase the risk of seizures.

Treatment: Symptomatic and supportive therapy is recommended. Activated charcoal may be more effective in reducing absorption than emesis or lavage. In adults, many neurotoxic effects can be both treated and prevented with 200-300 mg of pyridoxine daily. Haemodialysis removes cycloserine from the bloodstream but should be reserved for life-threatening toxicity.

Pharmacological properties
Pharmacodynamic properties:
Actions: Cycloserine inhibits cell wall synthesis in susceptible strains of Gram-positive and Gram-negative bacteria and in *Mycobacterium tuberculosis.*

Indications: Cycloserine is indicated in the treatment of active pulmonary and extra-pulmonary tuberculosis (including renal disease) when the organisms are susceptible to this drug and after failure of adequate treatment with the primary medications (streptomycin, isoniazid, rifampicin and ethambutol). Like all anti-tuberculous drugs, cycloserine should be administered in conjunction with other effective chemotherapy and not as the sole therapeutic agent.

Cycloserine may be effective in the treatment of acute urinary tract infections caused by susceptible strains of Gram-positive and Gram-negative bacteria, especially *Klebsiella/Enterobacter* species and *Escherichia coli.* It is generally no more and may be less effective than other antimicrobial agents in the treatment of urinary tract infections caused by bacteria other than mycobacteria. Use of cycloserine in these infections should be considered only when the more conventional therapy has failed and when the organism has been demonstrated to be sensitive to the drug.

Pharmacokinetic properties: Cycloserine is rapidly absorbed from the GI tract after oral administration, giving detectable levels in plasma within an hour. It is widely distributed throughout body fluids and tissues.

There is no appreciable blood-brain barrier, and CSF levels are approximately the same as plasma levels. It is found in the sputum of tuberculous patients and has been detected in pleural and ascitic fluids, bile, amniotic fluid and fetal blood, breast milk, lung and lymph tissues.

Cycloserine is excreted into the urine, levels appearing within half an hour of oral ingestion. Approximately 66 per cent of a dose appears unchanged in the urine in 24 hours. A further 10 per cent is excreted over the next 48 hours. It is not significantly excreted in the faeces. Approximately 35 per cent is metabolised, but the metabolites have not yet been identified.

The half-life of cycloserine is in the range 8-12 hours.

Preclinical safety data: A study in two generations of rats given doses up to 100 mg/kg/day demonstrated no teratogenic effect in offspring.

Pharmaceutical particulars
List of excipients: Talc; liquid paraffin; amaranth; erythrosine; sunset yellow; titanium dioxide; black iron oxide; gelatin.

Incompatibilities: None known.

Shelf-life: Twelve months when stored appropriately.

Special precautions for storage: Keep tightly closed. Protect from moisture. Store below 25°C.

Nature and contents of container: HDPE bottles of 100 capsules.

Instructions for use/handling: For oral administration.

Marketing authorisation number 0006/5045R

Date of approval/revision of SPC 15 September 1995

Legal category POM

DOBUTREX*

Presentation Dobutrex (dobutamine hydrochloride for injection) is available as: Dobutrex Solution: Vials containing 20 ml of sterile solution, for intravenous use only. Each ml contains 12.5 mg dobutamine, 0.24 mg sodium metabisulphite and water for injection.

Uses
Actions: The primary action of dobutamine is to augment cardiac contractility by stimulating the beta-1 receptors of the heart. It is a direct-acting agent.

Indications: Dobutrex is indicated for adults who require inotropic support in the treatment of low output cardiac failure associated with myocardial infarction, open heart surgery, cardiomyopathies, septic shock and cardiogenic shock. Dobutrex can also increase or maintain cardiac output during positive end expiratory pressure (PEEP) ventilation.

Dobutrex may also be used for cardiac stress testing as an alternative to exercise in patients for whom routine exercise testing cannot be satisfactorily performed. This use of dobutamine should only be undertaken in units which already perform exercise stress testing and all normal care and precautions required for such testing are also required when using dobutamine for this purpose.

Dosage and administration For intravenous administration only.

Dobutrex Solution must be further diluted to at least 50 ml prior to administration in an i.v. container with one of the intravenous solutions listed below:

Sodium Chloride Intravenous Infusion BP
5% Glucose Intravenous Infusion BP
5% Glucose + 0.9% Sodium Chloride Intravenous Infusion BP
5% Glucose + 0.45% Sodium Chloride Intravenous Infusion BP
Sodium Lactate Intravenous Infusion BP

If diluting to 250 ml or 500 ml, dilution will give a concentration for administration as follows:

250 ml contains 1,000 micrograms/ml of dobutamine
500 ml contains 500 micrograms/ml of dobutamine

The prepared solution should be used within 24 hours.

Administration: Due to its short half-life, Dobutrex must be administered as a continuous intravenous infusion. After dilution, Dobutrex should be administered intravenously through an intravenous needle or catheter. An i.v. drip chamber or other suitable metering device is essential for controlling the rate of flow in drops per minute.

Recommended dosage for adults and the elderly: Most patients will respond satisfactorily to doses ranging from 2.5 to 10 micrograms/kg/minute. Occasionally, however, a dose as low as 0.5 micrograms/kg/minute will elicit a response. Rarely, a dose as high as 40 micrograms/kg/minute is required.

The rate of administration and the duration of therapy should be adjusted according to the patient's response as determined by heart rate, blood pressure, urine flow, and, if possible, measurement of cardiac output.

Rather than abruptly discontinuing therapy with Dobutrex, it is often advisable to decrease the dosage gradually.

Side-effects, which are dose-related, are infrequent when Dobutrex is administered at rates below 10 micrograms/kg/minute. Rates as high as 40 micrograms/kg/minute have been used occasionally without significant adverse effects.

The final volume administered should be determined by the fluid requirements of the patient. Concentrations as high as 5,000 micrograms/ml have been used in patients on a restricted fluid intake. High concentrations of dobutamine should only be given with an infusion pump, to ensure accurate dosage.

Cardiac stress testing: When used as an alternative to exercise for cardiac stress testing the recommended dose is an incremental increase of 5 micrograms/kg/min from 5 up to 20 micrograms/kg/min, each dose being infused for 8 minutes. Continuous ECG monitoring is essential and the infusion terminated in the event of >3 mm ST segment depression or any ventricular arrhythmia. The infusion should also be terminated if heart rate reaches the age/sex maximum, systolic blood pressure rises above 220 mm Hg or any side-effects occur – see *Side-effects.*

Paediatric use: The safety and efficacy of dobutamine for use in children have not been established.

Contra-indications, warnings, etc
Contra-indication: Previous hypersensitivity to dobutamine.

Warnings: If tachycardia or an undue increase in systolic blood pressure occurs or if an arrhythmia is precipitated, the dose of dobutamine should be reduced or the drug should be discontinued temporarily.

Dobutamine may precipitate or exacerbate ventricular ectopic activity; rarely has it caused ventricular tachycardia or fibrillation. Because dobutamine facilitates atrioventricular conduction, patients with atrial flutter or fibrillation may develop rapid ventricular responses.

Particular care should be exercised when dobutamine is used in patients with acute myocardial infarction because any significant increase in heart rate or excessive increases in arterial pressure that occur may intensify ischaemia and cause anginal pain and ST segment elevation.

Inotropic agents, including dobutamine, do not improve haemodynamics in most patients with mechanical obstruction that hinders either ventricular filling or outflow, or both. Inotropic response may be inadequate in patients with markedly reduced ventricular compliance. Such conditions are present in cardiac tamponade, valvular aortic stenosis, and idiopathic hypertrophic subaortic stenosis.

The use of dobutamine as an alternative to exercise for cardiac stress testing is not recommended for patients with unstable angina, bundle branch block, valvular heart disease, aortic outflow obstruction or any cardiac condition that could make them unsuitable for exercise stress testing.

Usage in pregnancy and lactation: Reproduction studies performed in rats and rabbits have revealed no evidence of harm to the foetus or teratogenic effects due to dobutamine. Animal studies to evaluate effects on fertility have not been conducted. As there are no adequate and well-controlled studies in pregnant women, and as animal reproduction studies are not always predictive of human response, dobutamine should not be used during pregnancy unless the potential benefits outweigh the potential risks to the foetus.

It is not known whether this drug is excreted in human milk, so caution should be exercised. If a mother requires dobutamine treatment, breast feeding should be discontinued for the duration of treatment.

Precautions: During the administration of dobutamine, as with any parenteral catecholamine, heart rate and rhythm, arterial blood pressure, and infusion rate should be monitored closely. When initiating therapy, electrocardiographic monitoring is advisable until a stable response is achieved.

Precipitous decreases in blood pressure (hypotension) have occasionally been described in association with dobutamine therapy. Decreasing the dose or discontinuing the infusion typically results in rapid return of blood pressure to baseline values, but rarely intervention may be required and reversibility may not be immediate.

Dobutamine should be used with caution in the presence of severe hypotension complicating cardiogenic shock (mean arterial pressure less than 70 mm Hg).

Hypovolaemia should be corrected when necessary with whole blood or plasma before dobutamine is administered.

If arterial blood pressure remains low or decreases progressively during administration of dobutamine despite adequate ventricular filling pressure and cardiac output, consideration may be given to the concomitant use of a peripheral vasoconstrictor agent, such as dopamine or noradrenaline.

Dobutrex contains sodium metabisulphite. Sulphites may cause allergic-type reactions, including anaphylactic symptoms and life-threatening or less severe asthmatic episodes in certain susceptible people. Sulphite sensitivity is seen more frequently in asthmatic than in non–asthmatic people.

Drug interactions: The potency of dobutamine may be decreased if the patient is given beta-adrenergic receptor antagonists. In such a case, the unopposed alpha-agonist effects of dobutamine may become apparent, including peripheral vasoconstriction and hypertension. Conversely, alpha-adrenergic blockade may make the beta-1 and beta-2 effects apparent, resulting in tachycardia and vasodilatation.

Side-effects: For cardiovascular effects, see *Warnings* and *Precautions* sections.

Reactions at site of intravenous infusion: Phlebitis has occasionally been reported. Local inflammatory changes have been described following inadvertent infiltration. Isolated cases of cutaneous necrosis have been reported.

The following side-effects have been reported rarely: nausea, headache, anginal pain, non-specific chest pain, palpitations, shortness of breath, and reactions suggestive of hypersensitivity, including rash, fever, eosinophilia and bronchospasm. Isolated cases of thrombocytopenia have been reported.

As with other catecholamines, decreases in serum potassium concentrations have occurred, rarely to hypokalaemic values. Consideration should be given to monitoring serum potassium.

Long-term safety: Infusions for up to 72 hours have revealed no adverse effects other than those seen with shorter infusions. There is evidence that partial tolerance develops with continuous infusions of dobutamine for 72 hours or more; therefore, higher doses may be required to maintain the same effects.

Overdosage: Overdoses of dobutamine have been reported rarely. The symptoms of toxicity may include anorexia, nausea, vomiting, tremor, anxiety, palpitations, headache, shortness of breath and anginal and non–specific chest pain. The positive inotropic and chronotropic effects of dobutamine may cause hypertension, tachyarrhythmias, myocardial ischaemia and ventricular fibrillation. Hypotension may result from vasodilatation.

The duration of action of dobutamine hydrochloride is generally short (half-life, approximately 2 minutes).

Temporarily discontinue dobutamine until the patient's condition stabilises. The patient should be monitored and any appropriate resuscitative measures initiated promptly.

Forced diuresis, peritoneal dialysis, haemodialysis, or charcoal haemoperfusion have not been established as beneficial.

If the product is ingested, unpredictable absorption may occur from the mouth and gastrointestinal tract.

Pharmaceutical precautions
Undiluted vials of Dobutrex Solution: Store below 25°C.

Prepared intravenous solutions are stable for 24 hours at room temperature.

Do not add Dobutrex to 5% Sodium Bicarbonate Intravenous Infusion BP or to any other strongly alkaline solutions. Because of potential physical incompatibilities, it is recommended that dobutamine hydrochloride not be mixed with other drugs in the same solution.

Dobutamine hydrochloride should not be used with other agents or diluents containing both sodium metabisulphite and ethanol.

Solutions containing Dobutrex may turn pink; the colour may intensify with time. This colour change is due to slight oxidation of the drug, but there is no significant loss of potency during the recommended storage period.

Legal category POM.

Package quantity Single 20 ml vials containing 250 mg dobutamine as the hydrochloride salt.

Further information Nil.

Product licence number 0006/0180.

DOLOXENE*

Qualitative and quantitative composition Each capsule contains, as active ingredient, 100 mg Dextropropoxyphene Napsylate BP (approximately equivalent to 65 mg dextropropoxyphene hydrochloride or 60 mg dextropropoxyphene base).

Pharmaceutical form Capsules, opaque pink, coded Lilly H64.

Clinical particulars
Therapeutic indications:
Actions: Dextropropoxyphene is a mild narcotic analgesic structurally related to methadone.

Indications: For the relief of mild to moderate pain.

Posology and method of administration: For oral administration to adults only. The usual dose is one capsule three or four times daily, and should not normally be exceeded. Consideration should be given to a reduced total daily dosage in patients with hepatic or renal impairment.
The elderly: There is evidence of prolonged half-life in the elderly, so reduction in dosage should be considered.

Children: Dextropropoxyphene is not recommended for use in children.

Contra-indications: Hypersensitivity to dextropropoxyphene.

Use in patients who are suicidal or addiction-prone.

Special warnings and special precautions for use:
Warnings: PATIENTS SHOULD BE ADVISED NOT TO EXCEED THE RECOMMENDED DOSE AND TO AVOID ALCOHOL.

Dextropropoxyphene products in excessive doses, either alone or in combination with other CNS depressants, including alcohol, are a major cause of drug-related deaths. Fatalities within the first hour of overdosage are not uncommon and can occur within 15 minutes. Some deaths have occurred as a consequence of the accidental ingestion of excessive quantities of dextropropoxyphene alone, or in combination with other drugs.

Dextropropoxyphene should be prescribed with caution for those patients whose medical condition requires the concomitant administration of sedatives, tranquillisers, muscle relaxants, antidepressants or other CNS-depressant drugs. Patients should be advised of the additive depressant effects of these combinations. Doloxene should also be prescribed with caution in patients who use alcohol in excess.

Drug dependence: Dextropropoxyphene, when taken in higher than recommended doses over long periods of time, can produce drug dependence.

Precautions: Dextropropoxyphene should be administered with caution to patients with hepatic or renal impairment, since higher serum concentrations or delayed elimination may occur.

Interaction with other medicaments and other forms of interaction:
Drug interactions: The CNS-depressant effect of dextropropoxyphene is additive with that of other CNS-depressants, including alcohol.

Dextropropoxyphene may interfere with the metabolism of antidepressants, anticonvulsants and warfarin-like drugs. Severe neurological signs, including coma, have occurred with concomitant use of carbamazepine.

Pregnancy and lactation:
Pregnancy: Safety in pregnancy has not been established relative to possible adverse effects on foetal development. Withdrawal symptoms in neonates have been reported following use during pregnancy. Therefore, dextropropoxyphene should not be used in pregnant women unless, in the judgment of the physician, the potential benefits outweigh the possible hazards.

Nursing mothers: Low levels of dextropropoxyphene have been detected in human milk. In postpartum studies involving nursing mothers who were given dextropropoxyphene, no adverse effects were noted in the infants.

Effects on ability to drive and use machines:
Ambulatory patients: Dextropropoxyphene may impair abilities required for tasks such as driving a car or operating machinery. The patient should be cautioned accordingly.

Undesirable effects: The most frequently reported have been dizziness, sedation, nausea and vomiting. Some of these side-effects may be alleviated if the patient lies down.

Other side-effects include constipation, abdominal pain, rashes, light-headedness, headache, weakness, euphoria, dysphoria, hallucinations and minor visual disturbances.

Dextropropoxyphene therapy has been associated with abnormal liver function tests and, more rarely, with instances of reversible jaundice (including cholestatic jaundice).

Subacute painful myopathy has occurred following chronic dextropropoxyphene overdosage.

Chronic ingestion of dextropropoxyphene in doses exceeding 720 mg per day has caused toxic psychoses and convulsions.

Overdose: Initial consideration should be given to the management of the CNS effects of dextropropoxyphene overdosage. Resuscitative measures should be initiated promptly.

In the acute phase dextropropoxyphene produces symptoms typical of narcosis, with somnolence or coma and respiratory depression, sometimes with convulsions. Blood pressure falls and cardiac performance deteriorates. Cardiac arrhythmias and conduction delay may be present. A combined respiratory-metabolic acidosis occurs, which may be severe if large amounts of salicylates have also been ingested. Death may occur.

Naloxone will reduce the respiratory depression and 0.4-2 mg IV should be administered promptly. (This may be repeated at 2-3 minute intervals, but if there is no response after 10 mg of naloxone the diagnosis should be questioned.) The duration of antagonism may be brief and need repeating for up to 24 hours. Mechanical ventilation, with oxygen, may be required, and PEEP ventilation is desirable if pulmonary oedema is present.

Blood gases, pH and electrolytes should be monitored and electrocardiographic monitoring is essential. Ventricular fibrillation or cardiac arrest may occur. Respiratory acidosis rapidly subsides as ventilation is restored and hypercapnoea eliminated, but lactic acidosis may require IV bicarbonate for prompt correction. In addition to the use of a narcotic antagonist, the patient may require titration with an anti-convulsant to control convulsions. Gastric lavage may be useful and activated charcoal can absorb a significant amount of ingested dextropropoxyphene.

Treatment of dextropropoxyphene overdose in children: See general comments above. Naloxone at 0.01 mg/kg body weight IV should be administered promptly. If there is no response a dose of 0.1 mg/kg IV may be used.

Pharmacological properties
Pharmacodynamic properties: Propoxyphene is a mild centrally acting analgesic agent structurally related to methadone. The potency of propoxyphene hydrochloride is from two-thirds to equal that of codeine. The combination of propoxyphene with a mixture of aspirin and caffeine produces greater analgesia than that produced by either propoxyphene or aspirin and caffeine administered alone.

Pharmacokinetic properties: Equimolar doses of propoxyphene hydrochloride or napsylate provide similar plasma concentrations. Following administration of 65, 130 or 195 mg of propoxyphene hydrochloride, the bioavailability of propoxyphene is equivalent to that of 100, 200 or 300 mg, respectively, of propoxyphene napsylate. Peak plasma concentrations of propoxyphene are reached in two to two and one-half hours. After a 65 mg oral dose of propoxyphene hydrochloride, peak plasma levels of 0.05 to 0.1 mcg/ml are achieved.

Repeated doses of propoxyphene at six-hour intervals lead to increasing plasma concentrations, with a plateau after the ninth dose at 48 hours.

Propoxyphene is metabolised in the liver to yield norpropoxyphene. Propoxyphene has a half-life of six to twelve hours, whereas that of norpropoxyphene is 30 to 36 hours. Norpropoxyphene has substantially less central-nervous-system-depressant effect than propoxyphene but a greater local anaesthetic effect, which is similar to that of amitriptyline and antiarrhythmic agents, such as lignocaine and quinidine.

Preclinical safety data: Animal toxicology studies indicate that, on a molar basis, the napsylate salt of dextropropoxyphene is less toxic than the hydrochloride. This may be due to its relative insolubility and retarded absorption.

Pharmaceutical particulars
List of excipients: Starch; Dimethicone; Gelatin; Titanium dioxide; Red Iron Oxide; Black Edible Printing Ink.

Incompatibilities: Not applicable.

Shelf-life: Two years.

Special precautions for storage: Store below 25°C.

Nature and contents of container: Blister packs of 100 (10 strips of 10 capsules).

Instructions for use/handling: No special instructions.

Marketing authorisation number 0006/5068R

Date of approval/revision of SPC 7 November 1996

Legal category CD (Sch 5), POM

ELDISINE*

WARNING
THIS PRODUCT IS **NOT**
FOR INTRATHECAL USE

Qualitative and quantitative composition

Active Ingredient	*Quantity per ml*
Vindesine Sulphate	*5.0 mg*

Pharmaceutical form A clear glass vial containing a lyophilised plug of white crystalline powder.

Clinical particulars

Therapeutic indications: Eldisine is an anti-neoplastic drug for intravenous use which can be used alone or in combination with other oncolytic drugs. Information available at present suggests that Eldisine as a single agent may be useful for the treatment of: acute lymphoblastic leukaemia of childhood resistant to other drugs; blastic crises of chronic myeloid leukaemia; malignant melanoma unresponsive to other forms of therapy; advanced carcinoma of the breast, unresponsive to appropriate endocrine surgery and/or hormonal therapy.

Posology and method of administration: This preparation is for intravenous use only. It should be administered only by individuals experienced in vindesine administration.

FATAL IF GIVEN INTRATHECALLY.
FOR INTRAVENOUS USE ONLY.
See special warnings in *Special warnings and special precautions for use* for the treatment of patients given intrathecal vindesine sulphate.

Extreme care must be used in calculating and administering the dose of vindesine, since overdosage may have a very serious or fatal outcome.

It is recommended that the drug be administered intravenously in a single rapid bolus injection at weekly intervals. The size of the dose is determined by body surface area. In adults and the elderly, the recommended starting dose is 3 mg/m², and children may be started at 4 mg/m². Thereafter, granulocyte counts should be made prior to each subsequent dose to determine the patient's sensitivity to the drug. Provided there is no granulocytopenia or other toxicity (see 'Undesirable effects') the dosage may be increased in 0.5 mg/m² steps at weekly intervals.

In adults, the maximum total weekly dosage for which data exists is 4 mg/m². The optimum dose of vindesine is that which produces mild to modest granulocytopenia. Sustained granulocyte counts lower than 2,500 cells/mm³ are to be avoided.

Those with decreased marrow function from leukaemia infiltration or replacement will require full doses to attempt to restore marrow function. This must be done under close supervision.

The dose should not be increased after that dose which: (i) reduces the granulocyte count to below 1,500 cells/mm³ or, on rare occasions, (ii) reduces the platelet count to below 100,000/mm³; (iii) causes acute abdominal pain (see *Special warnings and special precautions for use*).

On each of the above occasions there should be full recovery before administering the next dose, which should be reduced from the one causing the adverse reaction. For most patients, however, the weekly dosage will prove to be in the range of 3.0 to 4.0 mg/m² in adults and 4.0 to 5.0 mg/m² in children.

The use of small amounts of vindesine daily for long periods is not advised, even though the resulting total weekly dosage may be similar to that recommended. Little or no added therapeutic advantage has been demonstrated when such regimens have been used, and side-effects are increased. Strict adherence to the recommended dosage schedule is very important.

As vindesine is excreted principally by the liver, it may be necessary to reduce initial doses in the presence of significantly impaired hepatic or biliary function.

The metabolism of vinca alkaloids has been shown to be mediated by hepatic cytochrome P450 isoenzymes in the CYP3A subfamily. This metabolic pathway may be impaired in patients with hepatic dysfunction or who are taking concomitant potent inhibitors of these isoenzymes. (See 'Interaction with other medicaments and other forms of interaction'.)

To prepare a solution containing 1 mg/ml add 5 ml of sterile 0.9% sodium chloride intravenous infusion to the 5 mg of Eldisine in the sterile vial. The drug dissolves rapidly to give a clear solution.

The dose of Eldisine solution (calculated to provide the desired number of milligrams per square metre of the patient's surface area) may be injected either into the tubing of a running intravenous infusion *(compatible infusions are 5% Dextrose Intravenous Infusion BP, Sodium Chloride Intravenous Infusion BP and dextrose/saline infusions)* or directly into a vein.

The latter procedure is readily adaptable to outpatient therapy. In either case, the injection should be completed in 1 to 3 minutes. If care is taken to ensure that the needle is securely within the vein and that no solution containing vindesine is spilled extravascularly, cellulitis and/or phlebitis is unlikely to occur.

Because of the enhanced possibility of thrombosis, it is considered inadvisable to inject a solution into an extremity in which the circulation is impaired, or potentially impaired, by such conditions as compressing or invading neoplasm, phlebitis or varicosity.

Caution

It is extremely important to choose the largest accessible vein and to be certain that the needle is properly positioned in the vein before any vindesine is injected. If leakage into surrounding tissues should occur during intravenous administration it may cause considerable irritation. The injection should be discontinued as soon as leakage occurs, and any remaining portion of the dose should then be introduced into another vein. Local injection of hyaluronidase and the application of moderate heat to the area of leakage help disperse the drug and are thought to minimise discomfort and the possibility of cellulitis.

Contra-indications:

FATAL IF GIVEN INTRATHECALLY.
FOR INTRAVENOUS USE ONLY.
See special warnings in *Special warnings and special precautions for use* for the treatment of patients given intrathecal vindesine sulphate.

Use in patients who have drug-induced severe granulocytopenia (less than 1,500 granulocytes per mm³) or severe thrombocytopenia. Vindesine should not be used in the presence of bacterial infection. Such infections must be brought under control with antiseptics or antibiotics before using vindesine.

Patients with the demyelinating form of Charcot-Marie-Tooth syndrome should not be given vindesine.

Special warnings and special precautions for use: This preparation is for intravenous use only. It should be administered by individuals experienced in the administration of vindesine sulphate. The intrathecal administration of vindesine sulphate usually results in death. Syringes containing this product should be labelled 'FATAL IF GIVEN INTRATHECALLY. FOR INTRAVENOUS USE ONLY'. An auxiliary sticker is provided in the pack with this warning.

Extemporaneously prepared syringes containing this product must be packaged in an overwrap which is labelled "DO NOT REMOVE COVERING UNTIL MOMENT OF INJECTION. FATAL IF GIVEN INTRATHECALLY. FOR INTRAVENOUS USE ONLY".

After inadvertent intrathecal administration of vinca alkaloids, immediate neurosurgical intervention is required in order to prevent ascending paralysis leading to death. In a very small number of patients, life-threatening paralysis and subsequent death was averted but resulted in devastating neurological sequelae, with limited recovery afterwards.

Based on the published management of survival cases involving the related vinca alkaloid vincristine sulphate, if vindesine is mistakenly given by the intrathecal route, the following treatment should be initiated **immediately after the injection**:

1. Removal of as much CSF as is safely possible through the lumbar access.

2. Insertion of an epidural catheter into the subarachnoid space via the intervertebral space above initial lumbar access and CSF irrigation with lactated Ringer's solution. Fresh frozen plasma should be requested and, when available, 25 ml should be added to every 1 litre of lactated Ringer's solution.

3. Insertion of an intraventricular drain or catheter by a neurosurgeon and continuation of CSF irrigation with fluid removal through the lumbar access connected to a closed drainage system. Lactated Ringer's solution should be given by continuous infusion at 150 ml/h, or at a rate of 75 ml/h when fresh frozen plasma has been added as above.

The rate of infusion should be adjusted to maintain a spinal fluid protein level of 150 mg/dl.

The following measures have also been used in addition but may not be essential:

Glutamic acid has been given IV 10 gm over 24 hours, followed by 500 mg tds by mouth for 1 month. Folinic acid has been administered intravenously as a 100 mg bolus and then infused at a rate of 25 mg/h for 24 hours, then bolus doses of 25 mg 6-hourly for 1 week. Pyridoxine has been given at a dose of 50 mg 8-hourly by intravenous infusion over 30 minutes. Their roles in the reduction of neurotoxicity are unclear.

Clinically, the dose-limiting toxicity of vindesine is granulocytopenia, although in general oncolytic activity is obtained at doses causing little or no effect on the granulocytes. Individual patient variation has been observed with respect to the severity of side-effects, including neurotoxicity, granulocytopenia, alopecia, and decrease in bowel motility.

When granulocytopenia occurs, the nadir in the granulocyte count may be expected to occur 3-5 days after the last day of drug administration. Recovery of the granulocyte count is rapid thereafter and is usually complete within 7-10 days after the last dose.

The thrombocyte count is usually either unaffected or increased by weekly therapy with vindesine. However, significant thrombocytopenia has occurred occasionally, particularly when doses are given more frequently than once a week. It is probably more likely to occur when patients are thrombocytopenic (less than 100,000 cells/mm³) prior to therapy with vindesine.

The effect of vindesine upon the red blood cell count and haemoglobin concentration is usually insignificant when other treatment does not complicate the picture. It should be remembered, however, that patients with malignant disease may exhibit anaemia even in the absence of any treatment.

If granulocytopenia with less than 1,000 granulocytes/mm³ occurs following a dose of vindesine, the patient should be watched carefully for evidence of infection until the granulocyte count has returned to a safe level.

While neurotoxicity is not usually dose-limiting, there have been instances in which neurotoxicity has made it necessary to reduce the dosage or temporarily discontinue use of vindesine. Neurotoxicity induced by vindesine is believed to be generally less severe and less progressive in nature than the effects observed with vincristine.

Particular attention should be given to dosage and neurological side-effects if vindesine is administered to patients with pre-existing neuromuscular disease, and also when other drugs with neurotoxic potential are being used. The neurotoxicity associated with vindesine therapy may be additive.

Care should be exercised when vindesine has been the cause of acute abdominal pain, as paralytic ileus may be a significant risk if further doses of vindesine are given, particularly if the dose is increased. Prophylactic measures should be taken to prevent obstipation that may result from a decrease in bowel motility.

Extreme care should be exercised to prevent injection outside the vein. Extravasation during intravenous injection will cause cellulitis and phlebitis. If the amount of extravasation is great, sloughing will occur. Healing of such wounds may require several weeks and be attended by severe pain. The discomfort may persist after healing of the ulcer.

Care must be taken to avoid contamination of the eye with concentrations of vindesine used clinically. If accidental contamination occurs, severe irritation and/or corneal ulceration may result. The eye should be washed immediately and thoroughly with water or saline.

Interaction with other medicaments and other forms of interaction: When chemotherapy is being given in conjunction with radiation therapy through portals which include the liver, the use of vindesine should be delayed until radiation therapy has been completed.

Acute shortness of breath and severe bronchospasm have been reported following the administration of vindesine. These reactions have been encountered most frequently when vindesine was used in combination with mitomycin-C and may be serious when there is pre-existing pulmonary dysfunction. The onset may be within minutes, or several hours after the drug is injected, and may occur up to 2 weeks after a dose of mitomycin-C. Progressive dyspnoea, requiring chronic therapy, may occur. Vindesine should not be re-administered.

The simultaneous oral or intravenous administration of phenytoin and antineoplastic chemotherapy combinations have been reported to have reduced blood levels of the anticonvulsant and to have increased seizure activity. Although the contribution of the vinca alkaloids has not been established, dosage adjustment of phenytoin may need to be made when used in combination with vindesine.

Caution should be exercised in patients concurrently taking drugs shown to inhibit drug metabolism by hepatic cytochrome P450 isoenzyme in the CYP3A subfamily, or in patients with hepatic dysfunction. Concurrent administration of vindesine sulphate with an inhibitor of this metabolic pathway may cause an earlier onset and/or an increased severity of side-effects.

Pregnancy and lactation:

Usage in pregnancy or lactation: The safety of this product for use during pregnancy has not been established. Animal studies with vindesine suggest that teratogenic effects may occur. The benefit-to-risk ratio must be carefully considered before use in pregnant patients. Eldisine should not normally be given to mothers who are breast-feeding.

Effects on ability to drive and use machines: Not applicable.

Undesirable effects: Prior to the use of the drug, patients and/or their parents/guardians should be advised of the possibility of untoward symptoms. Acute toxicity appears to be dose related and is more likely to occur if doses above 4 mg/m² are employed. Granulocytopenia is usually the dose-limiting factor. Neurotoxicity is common and appears to be related to the cumulative total dose given.

The following side-effects have been reported:

Gastro-intestinal: Nausea, vomiting, constipation, stomatitis, vesiculation of the mouth, ileus, diarrhoea, anorexia, abdominal pain, dysphagia, dyspepsia, perforated duodenal ulcer (nausea and vomiting usually may be controlled by anti-emetic agents).

Neurological: Numbness and tingling of hands/feet (paraesthesia), peripheral neuritis, jaw pain, mental depression, loss of deep-tendon reflexes, foot drop, headache, convulsions. Cortical blindness has been reported in patients treated with multiple-agent chemotherapy that has included vindesine. The contribution of vindesine to this reaction is unknown. Treatment with vinca alkaloids has resulted rarely in both vestibular and auditory damage to the eighth cranial nerve. Manifestations include partial or total deafness, which may be temporary or permanent, and difficulties with balance, including dizziness, nystagmus and vertigo. Particular caution is warranted when vindesine sulphate is used in combination with other agents known to be ototoxic, such as the platinum-containing oncolytics.

Haematological: Granulocytopenia, thrombocytopenia, thrombocytosis, mild anaemia.

Pulmonary: See 'Interaction with other medicaments and other forms of interaction'.

Cutaneous: Alopecia from mild to total is the commonest side-effect. Regrowth of hair may occur while still on therapy. Maculopapular rashes, cellulitis with extravasation. Injection site reaction (see 'Posology and method of administration').

Miscellaneous: Generalised musculoskeletal pain, malaise, chills and fevers, asthenia.

Overdose: Side-effects following the use of vindesine are dose related. Therefore, following administration of more than the recommended dose, patients can be expected to experience these effects in an exaggerated fashion.

Supportive care should include: (a) daily blood counts for guidance in transfusion requirement; (b) prevention of the side-effects that result from the syndrome of inappropriate secretion of antidiuretic hormone. This includes restriction of fluid intake and, perhaps, the use of a diuretic drug acting on the loop of Henle and distal tubule function; (c) use of cathartics to prevent ileus; (d) administration of an anticonvulsant; (e) monitoring the patient's cardiovascular system.

The use of folinic acid in addition to the other supportive measures recommended may be considered, although, unlike vincristine, studies have not been conducted to confirm its protective action. Clinical experience of vindesine overdosage is extremely limited, with only one published case.

Pharmacological properties

Pharmacodynamic properties: Vindesine sulphate is an antineoplastic agent derived from vinblastine, like the other vinca alkaloids it causes mitotic arrest in metaphase by binding to microtubular protein.

Pharmacokinetic properties: The pharmacokinetics of vindesine are similar to those of the other vinca alkaloids. After intravenous administration, elimination from the blood is triphasic, the drug is rapidly distributed to body tissues. It is metabolised primarily in the liver and excreted in bile and urine.

Preclinical safety data: Animal studies with vindesine suggest that teratogenic effects may occur.

Pharmaceutical particulars

List of excipients: Mannitol.

Incompatibilities: Eldisine should never be mixed with any other drug.

Shelf-life: 3 years.

Special precautions for storage: Vials of Eldisine should be stored in a refrigerator between 2° and 8°C.

After reconstitution: After a portion of the solution has been removed from a vial, the remainder of the contents of the vial may be stored in a refrigerator for future use for 24 hours without significant loss of potency. When the reconstituted vial of Eldisine is to be stored for more than 24 hours, it is essential to reconstitute with sterile 0.9% sodium chloride intravenous infusion preserved with 2.0% benzyl alcohol. Where preserved diluent is used, the reconstituted solution may be stored in a refrigerator for up to 28 days without significant loss of potency.

Nature and contents of container: A type I glass vial with rubber stopper, aluminium sealing ring and polypropylene cap.

Package quantity: Vials 5 mg. Single vials.

Instructions for use/handling:

Guidelines for the safe handling of antineoplastic agents: Cytotoxic preparations should not be handled by pregnant staff.

Trained personnel should reconstitute the drug. This should be performed in a designated area. The work surface should be covered with disposable plastic-backed absorbent paper.

Adequate protective gloves, masks and clothing should be worn. Precautions should be taken to avoid the drug accidentally coming into contact with the eyes. If accidental contamination occurs, the eye should be washed with water or saline thoroughly and immediately.

Use Luer-lock fittings on all syringes and sets. Large bore needles are recommended to minimise pressure and the possible formation of aerosols. The latter may also be reduced by the use of a venting needle.

Adequate care and precaution should be taken in the disposal of items (syringes, needles, etc.) used to reconstitute cytotoxic drugs.

Special dispensing information: When dispensing vindesine sulphate in other than the original container, eg, a syringe containing a specific dose, it is imperative that it be packaged in an overwrap bearing the statement "DO NOT REMOVE COVER UNTIL MOMENT OF INJECTION. FATAL IF GIVEN INTRATHECALLY. FOR INTRAVENOUS USE ONLY". A syringe containing a specific dose must be labelled, using the auxiliary sticker provided in the pack, with this warning.

Marketing authorisation number PL 0006/0137

Date of approval/revision of SPC September 1998

Legal category POM

EVISTA* ▼

Qualitative and quantitative composition Each film coated tablet contains 60 mg raloxifene hydrochloride, equivalent to 56 mg raloxifene free base.

Pharmaceutical form Film coated tablets. They are presented as elliptically shaped, white tablets which are imprinted with the code 4165.

Clinical particulars

Therapeutic indications: EVISTA is indicated for the prevention of non-traumatic vertebral fractures in postmenopausal women at increased risk of osteoporosis. There are no data on extravertebral fractures. When determining the choice of EVISTA or oestrogen (hormonal replacement therapy) for an individual postmenopausal woman, consideration should be given to menopausal symptoms, effects on breast tissue, and cardiovascular risks and benefits (see 'Pharmacodynamic properties').

Posology and method of administration: The recommended dosage is one tablet daily by oral administration, which may be taken at any time of the day without regard to meals. No dose adjustment is necessary for the elderly. Due to the nature of this disease process, EVISTA is intended for long-term use.

Calcium supplements are advised in women with a low dietary calcium uptake.

Contra-indications: Must not be used in women with child bearing potential.

Active or past history of venous thrombo-embolic events (VTE), including deep vein thrombosis, pulmonary embolism and retinal vein thrombosis.

Hypersensitivity to raloxifene or other ingredients in the tablet.

Hepatic impairment, including cholestasis.

Severe renal impairment.

Unexplained uterine bleeding.

EVISTA should not be used in patients with endometrial or breast cancer, as safety in these patient groups has not been proven.

Special warnings and special precautions for use: Raloxifene is associated with an increased risk for venous thrombo-embolic events that appears to be similar to the reported risk associated with current use of hormone replacement therapy. The risk-benefit balance should be considered in patients at risk of venous thrombo-embolic events of any aetiology. EVISTA should be discontinued in the event of an illness or a condition leading to a prolonged period of immobilisation. Discontinuation should happen as soon as possible in case of the illness, or from three days before the immobilisation occurs. Therapy should not be restarted until the initiating condition has resolved and the patient is fully mobile.

Raloxifene is unlikely to cause endometrial proliferation. Any uterine bleeding during EVISTA therapy is unexpected and should be fully investigated.

Raloxifene is metabolised primarily in the liver. Single doses of raloxifene given to patients with cirrhosis and mild hepatic impairment (Child-Pugh class A) produced plasma concentrations of raloxifene which were approximately 2.5 X the controls. The increase correlated with total bilirubin concentrations. Until safety and efficacy have been evaluated further in patients with hepatic insufficiency, the use of EVISTA is not recommended in this patient population. Serum total bilirubin, gamma-glutamyl transferase, alkaline phosphatase, ALT and AST should be closely monitored during treatment if elevated values are observed.

As there is no experience with co-administration of systemic oestrogens, such use is not recommended.

There is no indication for use of raloxifene in males.

EVISTA is not effective in reducing vasodilatation (hot flushes), or other symptoms of the menopause associated with oestrogen deficiency.

Interaction with other medicinal products and other forms of interaction: Concurrent administration of either calcium carbonate or aluminium and magnesium-hydroxide containing antacids do not affect the systemic exposure of raloxifene.

Co-administration of raloxifene and warfarin does not alter the pharmacokinetics of either compound. However, modest decreases in the prothrombin time have been observed, and if raloxifene is given concurrently with warfarin or other coumarin derivatives, the prothrombin time should be monitored. Effects on prothrombin time may develop over several weeks if EVISTA treatment is started in patients who are already on coumarin anticoagulant therapy.

Raloxifene does not affect the steady-state AUC of digoxin. The C_{max} of digoxin increased by less than 5%.

The influence of concomitant medication on raloxifene plasma concentrations was evaluated in the prevention trials. Frequently co-administered drugs included: paracetamol, non-steroidal anti-inflammatory drugs (such as acetylsalicylic acid, ibuprofen and naproxen), oral antibiotics, H_1 antagonists, H_2 antagonists and benzodiazepines. No clinically relevant effects of the co-administration of the agents on raloxifene plasma concentrations were identified.

In vitro, raloxifene did not interact with the binding of warfarin, phenytoin or tamoxifen.

Raloxifene should not be co-administered with cholestyramine, which significantly reduces the absorption and enterohepatic cycling of raloxifene.

Peak concentrations of raloxifene are reduced with co-administration with ampicillin. Since the overall extent of absorption and the elimination rate of raloxifene are not affected, raloxifene can be concurrently administered with ampicillin.

Raloxifene modestly increases hormone-binding globulin concentrations, including sex steroid binding globulins (SHBG), thyroxine binding globulin (TBG) and corticosteroid binding globulin (CBG), with corresponding increases in total hormone concentrations. These changes do not affect concentrations of free hormones.

Pregnancy and lactation: EVISTA is only for use in postmenopausal women.

EVISTA must not be taken by women of child bearing potential. Raloxifene may cause foetal harm when administered to a pregnant woman. If this drug is used mistakenly during pregnancy or the patient becomes pregnant while taking this drug, the patient should be informed of the potential hazard to the foetus (see 'Preclinical safety data').

It is not known whether raloxifene is excreted in human milk. Its clinical use, therefore, cannot be recommended in lactating women. EVISTA may affect the development of the baby.

Effects on ability to drive and use machines: Raloxifene has no known effect on driving or the ability to use machinery.

Undesirable effects: In studies involving over 2000 women, all undesirable effects were recorded, irrespective of causality. The duration of treatment in these studies ranged from 2 to 24 months.

The majority of undesirable effects have not usually required cessation of therapy.

Adverse reactions

The treatment-emergent events associated with the use of raloxifene that occurred with a significant difference (P <0.05) between raloxifene and placebo treatment are described below.

Across all placebo-controlled clinical trials, venous thrombo-embolic events, including deep vein thrombosis, pulmonary embolism and retinal vein thrombosis, occurred in a frequency of 0.8%. A relative risk of 2.49 (CI 1.23, 5.02) was observed in EVISTA-treated patients compared to placebo. Superficial vein thrombophlebitis occurred in a frequency of less than 1%.

Compared with placebo-treated patients, the occurrence of vasodilatation (hot flushes) was modestly increased in EVISTA patients (24.3% EVISTA and 18.2% placebo). These events were most common in the first 6 months of treatment and seldom occurred *de novo* after that time. Discontinuation rates due to vasodilatation did not differ significantly between EVISTA and placebo groups (1.5% and 2.1%, respectively).

Another adverse reaction observed was leg cramps (5.5% for EVISTA, 1.9% for placebo).

One further change was seen which was not statistically significant (P <0.05), but which did show a significant dose trend. This was of peripheral oedema, which occurred at an incidence of 3.1% in EVISTA-treated patients and 1.9% in placebo-treated women.

Slightly decreased (6-10%) platelet counts have been reported during raloxifene treatment.

Adverse events

Discontinuations of therapy due to any clinical adverse experience occurred in 10.7% of 581 EVISTA-treated patients and 11.1% of 584 placebo-treated patients.

EVISTA (n = 317) was compared with continuous combined (n = 110) hormone replacement therapy (HRT) or cyclic (n = 205) HRT patients in some clinical trials. The incidence of breast symptoms and uterine bleeding in raloxifene-treated women was significantly lower than in women treated with either form of HRT.

Rare cases of moderate increases in AST and/or ALT have been reported where a causal relationship to raloxifene cannot be excluded. A similar frequency of increases was noted among placebo patients.

Overdose: Incidents of overdosage in humans have not been reported. In an 8 week study, a dose of 600 mg per day was safely tolerated. There is no specific antidote for raloxifene hydrochloride.

Pharmacological properties

Pharmacodynamic properties: Pharmaco-therapeutic group: Selective Oestrogen Receptor Modulator (SERM). ATC code: pending.

As a selective oestrogen receptor modulator (SERM), raloxifene has selective agonist or antagonist activities on tissues responsive to oestrogen. It acts as an agonist on bone and partially on cholesterol metabolism (decrease in total and LDL-cholesterol), but not in the hypothalamus or in the uterine or breast tissues.

Raloxifene's biological actions, like those of oestrogen, are mediated through high affinity binding to oestrogen receptors and regulation of gene expression. This binding results in differential expression of multiple oestrogen-regulated genes in different tissues. Recent data suggests that the oestrogen receptor can regulate gene expression by at least two distinct pathways which are ligand-, tissue- and/or gene-specific.

EVISTA is indicated for the prevention of postmenopausal osteoporosis and not for the treatment of menopausal symptoms. In clinical trials, raloxifene did not relieve menopausal symptoms.

a) Skeletal effects

The decrease in oestrogen availability which occurs at menopause, leads to marked increases in bone resorption. Bone loss is particularly rapid for the first 10 years after menopause, when the compensatory increase in bone formation is inadequate to keep up with resorptive losses. Other risk factors which may lead to the development of osteoporosis include early menopause; osteopenia (at least 1 SD below peak bone mass); thin body build; Caucasian or Asian ethnic origin; and a family history of osteoporosis. Replacement therapies generally reverse the excessive resorption of bone. The effects of EVISTA on bone are qualitatively similar to those of oestrogen replacement, but of lesser magnitude.

Based on these risk factors, prevention of osteoporosis with EVISTA is indicated for women within ten years of menopause, with BMD of the spine between 1.0 and 2.5 SD below the mean value of a normal young population, taking into account their high lifetime risk for osteoporotic fractures.

i) Bone Mineral Density (BMD). The efficacy of EVISTA once daily in postmenopausal women aged up to 60 years and with or without a uterus was established over a two-year treatment period. The women were 2 to 8 years postmenopausal. Three trials included 1,764 postmenopausal women who were treated with EVISTA or placebo. In one of these trials, the women had previously undergone hysterectomy. EVISTA produced significant increases in bone density of hip and spine as well as total body mineral mass compared to placebo. This increase was generally a 2% increase in BMD compared to placebo. From a single study, comparative conjugated equine oestrogen figures were 5% (spine) and 3% (hip). In the trials, placebo and treated subjects received supplemental calcium. The percentage of subjects experiencing an increase or decrease in BMD during raloxifene therapy was: for the spine 37% decreased and 63% increased; and for the total hip 29% decreased and 71% increased.

ii) Incidence of fractures. In a two-year interim analysis of a study on 7,705 postmenopausal women with a mean age of 66 years and with osteoporosis or established osteoporosis, EVISTA treatment (60 mg/day) for two years reduced the incidence of vertebral fractures by 42% (RR 0.58, CI 0.36, 0.95; $P = 0.028$) and 34% (RR 0.66, CI 0.51, 0.85; $P = 0.001$), respectively. These figures are in the same range as those reported in observational studies evaluating the anti-fracture efficacy of oestrogen (HRT). In contrast to oestrogen, no data are currently available on the ability of raloxifene to reduce non-vertebral fractures.

iii) Calcium kinetics. EVISTA and oestrogen affect bone remodelling and calcium metabolism similarly. EVISTA was associated with reduced bone resorption and a mean positive shift in calcium balance of 60 mg per day, due primarily to decreased urinary calcium losses. These findings were similar to those observed with oestrogen replacement therapy.

iv) Markers of bone turnover. The bone marker suppression seen demonstrated consistent effects of EVISTA on bone resorption, bone formation and overall bone turnover which is qualitatively similar to that of oestrogen, but of lesser magnitude.

v) Histomorphometry (bone quality). In a study comparing EVISTA with oestrogen, bone from patients treated with either drug was histologically normal, with no evidence of mineralisation defects, woven bone or marrow fibrosis.

These findings consistently demonstrate that the major mechanism of action of raloxifene on bone is reduction of bone resorption.

b) Effects on lipid metabolism and cardiovascular risk

Clinical studies showed that a 60 mg daily dose of EVISTA significantly decreased total cholesterol (3 to 6%) and LDL cholesterol (4 to 10%). HDL cholesterol and triglyceride concentrations did not change significantly. In contrast to oestrogen, no data are yet available to demonstrate benefit of raloxifene on atherosclerotic cardiovascular disease.

The relative risk of venous thrombo-embolic events observed during raloxifene treatment was 2.49 (CI 1.23, 5.02) when compared to placebo, and was 1.0 (CI 0.3, 6.2) when compared to oestrogen or hormonal replacement therapy.

c) Effects on the endometrium

In clinical trials, EVISTA did not stimulate the postmenopausal uterine endometrium. Compared to placebo, raloxifene was not associated with spotting or bleeding or endometrial hyperplasia. Nearly 3,000 transvaginal ultrasound (TVUs) examinations were evaluated from 831 women in all dose groups. Raloxifene-treated women consistently had an endometrial thickness which was indistinguishable from placebo. After 3 years of treatment, at least a 5 mm increase in endometrial thickness, assessed with transvaginal ultrasound, was observed in 1.9% of the 211 women treated with raloxifene 60 mg/day compared to 1.8% of the 219 women who received placebo. There were no differences between the raloxifene and placebo groups with respect to the incidence of reported uterine bleeding.

Endometrial biopsies taken after six months therapy with EVISTA 60 mg daily demonstrated non-proliferative endometrium in all patients. In addition, in a study with 2.5 X the recommended daily dose of EVISTA, there was no evidence of endometrial proliferation and no increase in uterine volume.

After 3 years, raloxifene did not increase the risk of endometrial cancer.

d) Effects on breast tissue

EVISTA does not stimulate breast tissue. Across all placebo-controlled trials, EVISTA was indistinguishable from placebo with regard to frequency and severity of breast symptoms. EVISTA was associated with significantly fewer breast symptoms (swelling, tenderness and breast pain) than reported by patients receiving oestrogens, with or without added progestins.

In clinical trials with EVISTA involving over 12,000 patients, most of whom have been exposed to at least 30 months therapy, the relative risk of newly diagnosed breast cancer was significantly lower (53% reduction, relative risk 0.47, CI 0.28, 0.78) in EVISTA-treated than in placebo-treated postmenopausal women in a combined analysis of several studies. These observations support the conclusion that raloxifene has no intrinsic oestrogen agonist activity in breast tissue. The long-term effect of EVISTA on the risk of breast cancer is unknown.

Pharmacokinetic properties:

Absorption

Raloxifene is absorbed rapidly after oral administration. Approximately 60% of an oral dose is absorbed. Presystemic glucuronidation is extensive. Absolute bioavailability of raloxifene is 2%. The time to reach average maximum plasma concentration and bioavailability are functions of systemic interconversion and enterohepatic cycling of raloxifene and its glucuronide metabolites.

Distribution

Raloxifene is distributed extensively in the body. The volume of distribution is not dose dependent. Raloxifene is strongly bound to plasma proteins (98-99%).

Metabolism

Raloxifene undergoes extensive first pass metabolism to the glucuronide conjugates: raloxifene-4′-glucuronide, raloxifene-6-glucuronide and raloxifene-4′,6-glucuronide. No other metabolites have been detected. Raloxifene comprises less than 1% of the combined concentrations of raloxifene and the glucuronide metabolites. Raloxifene levels are maintained by enterohepatic recycling, giving a plasma half-life of 27.7 hours.

Results from single oral doses of raloxifene predict multiple dose pharmacokinetics. Increasing doses of raloxifene result in slightly less than proportional increase in the area under the plasma time concentration curve (AUC).

Excretion

The majority of a dose of raloxifene and glucuronide metabolites are excreted within 5 days and are found primarily in the faeces, with less than 6% excreted in urine.

Special populations

Renal insufficiency. Less than 6% of the total dose is eliminated in urine. In a population pharmacokinetic study, a 47% decrease in lean body mass adjusted creatinine clearance resulted in a 17% decrease in raloxifene clearance and a 15% decrease in the clearance of raloxifene conjugates.

Hepatic insufficiency. The pharmacokinetics of a single dose of raloxifene in patients with cirrhosis and mild hepatic impairment (Child-Pugh class A) have been compared to that in healthy individuals. Plasma raloxifene concentrations were approximately 2.5-fold higher than in controls and correlated with bilirubin concentrations.

Preclinical safety data: In a 2-year carcinogenicity study in rats, an increase in ovarian tumours of granulosa/theca cell origin was observed in high-dose females (279 mg/kg/day). Systemic exposure (AUC) of raloxifene in this group was approximately 400 times that in postmenopausal women administered a 60 mg dose. In a 21-month carcinogenicity study in mice, there was an increased incidence of testicular interstitial cell tumours and prostatic adenomas and adenocarcinomas in males given 41 or 210 mg/kg, and prostatic leiomyoblastoma in males given 210 mg/kg. In female mice, an increased incidence of ovarian tumours in animals given 9 to 242 mg/kg (0.3 to 32 times the AUC in humans) included benign and malignant tumours of granulosa/theca cell origin and benign tumours of epithelial cell origin. The female rodents in these studies were treated during their reproductive lives, when their ovaries were functional and highly responsive to hormonal stimulation. In contrast to the highly responsive ovaries in this rodent model, the human ovary after menopause is relatively unresponsive to reproductive hormonal stimulation.

Raloxifene was not genotoxic in any of the extensive battery of test systems applied.

The reproductive and developmental effects observed in animals are consistent with the known pharmacological profile of raloxifene. At doses of 0.1 to 10 mg/kg/day in female rats, raloxifene disrupted oestrus cycles of female rats during treatment, but did not delay fertile matings after treatment termination and only marginally reduced litter size, increased gestation length and altered the timing of events in neonatal development. When given during the preimplantation period, raloxifene delayed and disrupted embryo implantation resulting in prolonged gestation and reduced litter size but development of offspring to weaning was not affected. Teratology studies were conducted in rabbits and rats. In rabbits, abortion and a low rate of ventricular septal defects (≥0.1 mg/kg) and hydrocephaly (≥10 mg/kg) were seen. In rats, retardation of foetal development, wavy ribs and kidney cavitation occurred (≥1 mg/kg).

Raloxifene is a potent antioestrogen in the rat uterus and prevented growth of oestrogen-dependent mammary tumours in rats and mice.

Pharmaceutical particulars

List of excipients: Povidone, polysorbate 80, anhydrous lactose, lactose monohydrate, crospovidone, magnesium stearate, titanium dioxide (E171), hypromellose, macrogol 400, carnauba wax, shellac, propylene glycol, indigo carmine (E132).

Incompatibilities: Not applicable.

Shelf-life: 2 years.

Special precautions for storage: Store at room temperature (15-25°C) in a dry place. Do not freeze. Protect from excessive heat and sunlight.

Nature and contents of container: EVISTA tablets are packed either in PVC blisters, Aclar blisters or in high density polyethylene bottles. Blister boxes contain 14, 28 or 84 tablets. Bottles contain 100 tablets.

Marketing authorisation holder

Eli Lilly Nederland BV
Krijtwal 17-23
3432 ZT Nieuwegein
The Netherlands

Marketing authorisation numbers

60 mg X 14 tablets:	EU/1/98/073/001
60 mg X 28 tablets:	EU/1/98/073/002
60 mg X 84 tablets:	EU/1/98/073/003
60 mg X 100 tablets:	EU/1/98/073/004

Date of approval/revision of SPC August 1998

Legal category POM

GEMZAR*

Qualitative and quantitative composition Gemcitabine hydrochloride equivalent to 200 mg gemcitabine.

Gemcitabine hydrochloride equivalent to 1 g gemcitabine.

Gemcitabine (INN) is a pyrimidine analogue.

Pharmaceutical form Vials containing powder for solution for infusion.

Clinical particulars

Therapeutic indications: Gemcitabine is indicated for the palliative treatment of adult patients with locally advanced or metastatic non-small cell lung cancer.

Gemcitabine is indicated for the treatment of adult patients with locally advanced or metastatic adenocarcinoma of the pancreas. Gemcitabine is indicated for patients with 5-FU refractory pancreatic cancer.

Posology and method of administration:

Non-small cell lung cancer

Adults: The recommended dose of gemcitabine is 1,000 mg/m², given by 30 minute intravenous infusion. This should be repeated once weekly for three weeks, followed by a one week rest period. This four week cycle is then repeated. Dosage reduction is applied based upon the amount of toxicity experienced by the patient.

Pancreatic cancer

Adults: The recommended dose of gemcitabine is 1,000 mg/m², given by 30 minute intravenous infusion. This should be repeated once weekly for up to 7 weeks, followed by a week of rest. Subsequent cycles should consist of injections once weekly for 3 consecutive weeks out of every 4 weeks. Dosage reduction is applied based upon the amount of toxicity experienced by the patient.

Patients receiving gemcitabine should be monitored prior to each dose for platelet, leucocyte and granulocyte counts and, if necessary, the dose of gemcitabine may be either reduced or withheld in the presence of haematological toxicity, according to the following scale:

Absolute granulocyte count (× 10⁶/l)		*Platelet count (× 10⁶/l)*	*% of full dose*
>1,000	and	>100,000	100
500-1,000	or	50,000-100,000	75
<500	or	<50,000	hold

Periodic checks of liver and kidney functions, including transaminases and serum creatinine, should also be performed in patients receiving gemcitabine.

Gemcitabine is well tolerated during the infusion, with only a few cases of injection site reaction reported. There have been no reports of injection site necrosis. Gemcitabine can be easily administered on an outpatient basis.

Elderly patients: Gemcitabine has been well tolerated in patients over the age of 65. There is no evidence to suggest that dose adjustments are necessary in the elderly, although gemcitabine clearance and half-life are affected by age.

Children: Gemcitabine has not been studied in children.

Hepatic and renal impairment: Gemcitabine should be used with caution in patients with hepatic insufficiency or with impaired renal function. No studies have been done in patients with significant hepatic or renal impairment.

Radical radiotherapy: Gemcitabine should not be used concurrently with radical radiotherapy (see 'Special Warnings and Special Precautions for Use').

Contra-indications: Gemcitabine is contra-indicated in those patients with a known hypersensitivity to the drug.

Special warnings and special precautions for use:

Warnings: Prolongation of the infusion time and increased dosing frequency have been shown to increase toxicity.

Gemcitabine can suppress bone marrow function as manifested by leucopenia, thrombocytopenia and anaemia. However, myelosuppression is short lived and usually does not result in dose reductions and rarely in discontinuation (see *Posology and method of administration* and *Undesirable effects*).

Gemcitabine should be discontinued at the first signs of any evidence of microangiopathic haemolytic anaemia such as rapidly falling haemoglobin with concomitant thrombocytopenia, elevation of serum bilirubin, serum creatinine, blood urea nitrogen, or LDH, which may indicate development of haemolytic uraemic syndrome (see *Undesirable effects*). Renal failure may not be reversible, even with discontinuation of therapy, and dialysis may be required.

Gemcitabine should not be given with concurrent radical, as opposed to palliative, radiotherapy. In a clinical trial, where gemcitabine, at a dose of 1,000 mg/m² was administered concurrently for up to 6 consecutive weeks with radical thoracic radiation (ie, radiation doses and field sizes for possible cure) to patients with non-small cell lung cancer, significant toxicity in the form of severe, and potentially life-threatening, oesophagitis and pneumonitis was observed, particularly in patients receiving radical radiotherapy over a large field.

Precautions:

General: Patients receiving therapy with gemcitabine must be monitored closely. Laboratory facilities should be available to monitor patient status. Treatment for a patient compromised by drug toxicity may be required.

Laboratory tests: Therapy should be started cautiously in patients with compromised bone marrow function. As with other oncolytics, the possibility of cumulative bone marrow suppression when using combination or sequential chemotherapy should be considered.

Patients receiving gemcitabine should be monitored prior to each dose for platelet, leucocyte and granulocyte counts. Suspension or modification of therapy should be considered when drug-induced marrow depression is detected. Guidelines regarding dose modifications are provided in 'Posology and method of administration' above. Peripheral blood counts may continue to fall after the drug is stopped.

Interaction with other medicaments and other forms of interaction: No interactions have been reported.

Pregnancy and lactation: The safety of this medicinal product for use in human pregnancy has not been established. Evaluation of experimental animal studies has shown reproductive toxicity, eg, birth defects or other effects on the development of the embryo or fetus, the course of gestation or peri and postnatal development. The use of gemcitabine should be avoided in pregnant or nursing women because of the potential hazard to the fetus or infant.

Effects on ability to drive and use machines: Gemcitabine has been reported to cause mild to moderate somnolence. Patients should be cautioned against driving or operating machinery until it is established that they do not become somnolent.

Undesirable effects:

Haematological: Because gemcitabine is a bone marrow suppressant, anaemia, leucopenia and thrombocytopenia can occur as a result of administration of gemcitabine. Myelosuppression is usually mild to moderate, and is more pronounced for the granulocyte count.

Thrombocythaemia is also commonly reported.

Gastro-intestinal: Abnormalities of liver transaminase enzymes occur in about two-thirds of patients, but they are usually mild, non-progressive and rarely necessitate stopping treatment. However, gemcitabine should be used with caution in patients with impaired liver function (see *Posology and method of administration*).

Nausea and nausea accompanied by vomiting are each reported in one-third of patients, respectively. This adverse event requires therapy in about 20% of patients, is rarely dose-limiting, and is easily manageable with standard anti-emetics.

Renal: Mild proteinuria and haematuria are reported in approximately half the patients, but are rarely clinically significant, and are not usually associated with any change in serum creatinine or blood urea nitrogen. However, a few cases of renal failure of uncertain aetiology have been reported, including, in very rare instances, cases of haemolytic uraemic syndrome (signs of microangiopathic haemolytic anaemia such as rapidly falling haemoglobin with concomitant thrombocytopenia, elevation of serum bilirubin, serum creatinine, blood urea nitrogen, or LDH, see 'Special warnings and special precautions for use'). Hence, gemcitabine should be used with caution in patients with impaired renal function.

Allergic: A rash is seen in approximately 25% of patients and is associated with pruritus in about 10% of patients. The rash is usually mild, not dose-limiting, and responds to local therapy. Desquamation, vesiculation and ulceration have been reported rarely. Anaphylaxis has been reported rarely.

Respiratory: Bronchospasm after gemcitabine infusion has been reported in less than 1% of patients. Bronchospasm is usually mild and transient, but parenteral therapy may be required. Gemcitabine should not be administered to patients with a known hypersensitivity to this drug (see 'Contra-indications').

Dyspnoea occurring within hours following gemcitabine injection is reported by approximately 8% of patients. This dyspnoea is usually mild, short-lived, rarely dose-limiting, and usually abates without any specific therapy. The mechanism of this event is unknown and the relationship to gemcitabine is not clear.

Pulmonary effects, sometimes severe (such as pulmonary oedema, interstitial pneumonitis, or adult respiratory distress syndrome [ARDS]), have been reported rarely in association with gemcitabine therapy. The aetiology of these effects is unknown. If such effects develop, consideration should be made to discontinuing gemcitabine. Early use of supportive care measures may help ameliorate the condition.

Other effects: An entity resembling influenza is reported by approximately 20% of patients. This is usually mild, short-lived, and rarely dose-limiting. Fever, headache, back pain, chills, myalgia, asthenia and anorexia are the most commonly reported symptoms. Cough, rhinitis, malaise, sweating and insomnia are also commonly reported. Fever and asthenia are also reported frequently as isolated symptoms. The mechanism of this toxicity is unknown. Reports received indicate that paracetamol may produce symptomatic relief.

Oedema/peripheral oedema is reported by approximately 30% of patients. Some cases of facial oedema have also been reported. Pulmonary oedema was reported infrequently (1%). Oedema/peripheral oedema is usually mild to moderate, rarely dose-limiting, is sometimes reported as painful and is usually reversible after stopping gemcitabine treatment. The mechanism of this toxicity is unknown. It is not associated with any evidence of cardiac, hepatic or renal failure.

The following adverse effects are also commonly reported: alopecia (usually minimal hair loss), 13% of patients; somnolence, 10%; diarrhoea, 8%; oral toxicity (mainly soreness and erythema), 7%; and constipation, 6%.

Radiation toxicity (see *Special warnings and special precautions for use*).

A few cases of hypotension were reported. Cases of myocardial infarction, congestive heart failure and arrhythmia have been reported, but there is no clear evidence that gemcitabine causes cardiac toxicity.

Overdose: There is no antidote for overdosage of gemcitabine. Single doses as high as 5.7 g/m² have been administered by IV infusion over 30 minutes every two weeks with clinically acceptable toxicity. In the event of suspected overdose, the patient should be monitored with appropriate blood counts and should receive supportive therapy, as necessary.

Pharmacological properties

Pharmacodynamic properties:

Cytotoxic activity in cell culture models: Gemcitabine exhibits significant cytotoxicity activity against a variety of cultured murine and human tumour cells. It exhibits cell phase specificity, primarily killing cells undergoing DNA synthesis (S-phase) and under certain conditions blocking the progression of cells through the G1/S-phase boundary. *In vitro* the cytotoxic action of gemcitabine is both concentration and time dependent.

Antitumour activity in preclinical models: In animal tumour models, the antitumour activity of gemcitabine is schedule dependent. When administered daily gemcitabine causes death in animals with minimal antitumour activity. However, when an every third or fourth day dosing schedule is used, gemcitabine can be given at non-lethal doses that have excellent antitumour activity against a broad range of mouse tumours.

Cellular metabolism and mechanisms of action: Gemcitabine (dFdC) is metabolised intracellularly by nucleoside kinases to the active diphosphate (dFdCDP) and triphosphate (dFdCTP) nucleosides. The cytotoxic action of gemcitabine appears to be due to inhibition of DNA synthesis by two actions of dFdCDP and dFdCTP. First, dFdCDP inhibits ribonucleotide reductase which is uniquely responsible for catalysing the reactions that generate the deoxynucleoside triphosphates for DNA synthesis. Inhibition of this enzyme by dFdCDP causes a reduction in the concentrations of deoxynucleosides in general, and especially in that of dCTP. Second, dFdCTP competes with dCTP for incorporation into DNA (self-potentiation). Likewise, a small amount of gemcitabine may also be incorporated into RNA. Thus, the reduction in the intracellular concentration of dCTP potentiates the incorporation of dFdCTP into DNA. DNA polymerase epsilon is essentially unable to remove gemcitabine and repair the growing DNA strands. After gemcitabine is incorporated into DNA, one additional nucleotide is added to the growing DNA strands. After this addition there is essentially a complete inhibition in further DNA synthesis (masked chain termination). After incorporation into DNA, gemcitabine then appears to induce the programmed cellular death process known as apoptosis.

Pharmacokinetic properties:

Gemcitabine pharmacokinetics: The pharmacokinetics of gemcitabine have been examined in 353 patients in seven studies. The 121 women and 232 men ranged in age from 29 to 79 years. Of these patients, approximately 45% had non-small cell lung cancer and 35% were diagnosed with pancreatic cancer. The following pharmacokinetic parameters were obtained for doses ranging from 500 to 2592 mg/m² that were infused from 0.4 to 1.2 hours. Peak plasma concentrations (obtained within 5 minutes of the end of the infusion): 3.2 to 45.5µg/ml.

Volume of distribution of the central compartment: 12.4 l/m² for women and 17.5 l/m² for men (inter-individual variability was 91.9%). Volume of distribution of the peripheral compartment: 47.4 l/m². The volume of the peripheral compartment was not sensitive to gender.

Plasma protein binding: Negligible.

Systemic clearance: Ranged from 29.2 l/hr/m² to 92.2 l/hr/m² depending on gender and age (inter-individual variability was 52.2%). Clearance for women is approximately 25% lower than the values for men. Although rapid, clearance for both men and women appears to decrease with age. For the recommended gemcitabine dose of 1,000 mg/m² given as a 30 minute infusion, lower clearance values for women and men should not necessitate a decrease in the gemcitabine dose.

Urinary excretion: Less than 10% is excreted as unchanged drug.

Renal clearance: 2 to 7 l/hr/m².

Half-life: Ranged from 42 to 94 minutes depending on age and gender. For the recommended dosing schedule, gemcitabine elimination should be virtually complete within 5 to 11 hours of the start of the infusion. Gemcitabine does not accumulate when administered once weekly.

Metabolism: Gemcitabine is rapidly metabolised by cytidine deaminase in the liver, kidney, blood and other tissues.

Intracellular metabolism of gemcitabine produces the gemcitabine mono, di and triphosphates (dFdCMP, dFdCDP and dFdCTP) of which dFdCDP and dFdCTP are considered active. These intracellular metabolites have not been detected in plasma or urine.

The primary metabolite, 2'-deoxy-2',2'-difluorouridine (dFdU), is not active and is found in plasma and urine.

dFdCTP kinetics: This metabolite can be found in peripheral blood mononuclear cells and the information below refers to these cells.

Half-life of terminal elimination: 0.7-12 hours.

Intracellular concentrations increase in proportion to gemcitabine doses of 35-350 mg/m²/30 min, which give steady state concentrations of 0.4-5µg/ml. At gemcitabine plasma concentrations above 5µg/ml, dFdCTP levels do not increase, suggesting that the formation is saturable in these cells. Parent plasma concentrations following a dose of 1,000 mg/m²/30 min are greater than 5µg/ml for approximately 30 minutes after the end of the infusion, and greater than 0.4 µg/ml for an additional hour.

dFdU kinetics

Peak plasma concentrations (3-15 minutes after end of 30 minute infusion, 1,000 mg/m²): 28-52µg/ml.

Trough concentration following once weekly dosing: 0.07-1.12µg/ml, with no apparent accumulation.

Triphasic plasma concentration versus time curve, mean half-life of terminal phase - 65 hours (range 33-84 hr).

Formation of dFdU from parent compound: 91%-98%.

Mean volume of distribution of central compartment: 18 l/m² (range 11-22 l/m²).

Mean steady state volume of distribution (Vss): 150 l/m² (range 96-228 l/m²).

Tissue distribution: Extensive.

Mean apparent clearance: 2.5 l/hr/m² (range 1-4 l/hr/m²).

Urinary excretion: All.

Overall elimination: Amount recovered in one week: 92%-98%, of which 99% is dFdU, 1% of the dose is excreted in faeces.

Preclinical safety data: In repeat dose studies of up to 6 months in duration in mice and dogs, the principal finding was haematopoietic suppression. These effects were related to the cytotoxic properties of the drug and were reversible when treatment was withdrawn. The degree of the effect was schedule and dose-dependent.

Carcinogenesis, mutagenesis, fertility: Cytogenetic damage has been produced by gemcitabine in an *in vivo* assay. Gemcitabine induced forward mutation *in vitro* in a mouse lymphoma (L5178Y) assay. Gemcitabine caused a reversible, dose and schedule dependent hypospermatogenesis in male mice. Although animal studies have shown an effect of gemcitabine on male fertility, no effect has been seen on female fertility. Long-term animal studies have not been conducted to evaluate the carcinogenic potential of gemcitabine.

Pharmaceutical particulars

List of excipients: Mannitol; Sodium Acetate; Hydrochloric Acid; Sodium Hydroxide.

Incompatibilities: Compatibility with other drugs has not been studied.

Shelf-life: 3 years for the lyophilised powder.

Special precautions for storage: Store at room temperature (15 to 25°C).

Solutions of reconstituted gemcitabine, in sterile Sodium Chloride Injection BP, should be kept at controlled room temperature (15 to 25°C). Reconstituted solutions should be used immediately or may be stored for 6 hours if prepared in an appropriately controlled aseptic environment. Solutions should not be refrigerated, as crystallisation may occur.

Nature and contents of container: The product is contained in either 10 ml or 50 ml sterile Type I flint glass vials, which meet the requirements of the PhEur, and are closed with halobutyl rubber stoppers and sealed with aluminium seals with polypropylene caps.

1 vial per pack.

Package quantities:
Vials 200 mg: Single vials
Vials 1 g: Single vials

Instructions for use/handling

Reconstitution: Gemzar has only been shown to be compatible with Sodium Chloride Injection BP. Accordingly, only this diluent should be used for reconstitution. Compatibility with other drugs has not been studied, therefore, it is not recommended to mix Gemzar with other drugs when reconstituted. Due to solubility considerations, the maximum concentration for gemcitabine upon reconstitution is 40 mg/ml. Reconstitution at concentrations greater than 40 mg/ml may result in incomplete dissolution, and should be avoided.

To reconstitute, add at least 5 ml of Sodium Chloride Injection BP to the 200 mg vial or at least 25 ml of Sodium Chloride Injection BP to the 1 g vial. Shake to dissolve. The appropriate amount of drug may be administered as prepared or further diluted with Sodium Chloride Injection BP. Reconstituted solutions should be used immediately or may be stored for 6 hours if prepared in an appropriately controlled aseptic environment.

Parenteral drugs should be inspected visually for particulate matter and discoloration, prior to administration, whenever solution and container permit.

Guidelines for the safe handling of antineoplastic agents: Cytotoxic preparations should not be handled by pregnant staff. Trained personnel should reconstitute the drug. This should be performed in a designated area. The work surface should be covered with disposable plastic-backed absorbent paper.

Adequate protective gloves, masks and clothing should be worn. Precautions should be taken to avoid the drug accidentally coming into contact with the eyes. If accidental contamination occurs, the eye should be washed with water thoroughly and immediately.

Use Luer-lock fittings on all syringes and sets. Large bore needles are recommended to minimise pressure and the possible formation of aerosols. The latter may also be reduced by the use of a venting needle.

Adequate care and precaution should be taken in the disposal of items used to reconstitute Gemzar. Any unused dry product or contaminated materials should be placed in a high risk waste bag. Sharp objects (needles, syringes, vials, etc) should be placed in a suitable rigid container. Personnel concerned with the collection and disposal of this waste should be aware of the hazard involved. Waste material should be destroyed by incineration. Any excess drug solution should be flushed directly into a drain with copious amounts of water.

Marketing authorisation numbers
200 mg vial: 0006/0301
1 g vial: 0006/0302

Date of approval/revision of SPC December 1998.

Legal category POM

GLUCAGON

Qualitative and quantitative composition Vials containing 1 unit (1.09 mg) of glucagon as the hydrochloride.

Pharmaceutical form Parenteral injection. The product is in lyophilised form and is supplied with an accompanying diluting solution.

Clinical particulars

Therapeutic indications:

Indications: Glucagon is useful in counteracting severe hypoglycaemic reactions.

Glucagon is indicated as a diagnostic aid in the radiological examination of the stomach, duodenum, small bowel and colon, when a hypotonic state would be advantageous.

Glucagon is as effective for this examination as the anticholinergic drugs, but it has fewer side-effects. When glucagon is administered concomitantly with an anticholinergic agent, the response is not significantly greater than when either drug is used alone. However, the addition of the anticholinergic agent results in increased side-effects.

Posology and method of administration: The diluent is provided for use only in the preparation of glucagon for *intermittent* parenteral injection and for no other use.

Glucagon should not be used at concentrations greater than 1 unit/ml (1 mg/ml).

Glucagon may be given by subcutaneous, intramuscular or intravenous injection. Administration as a continuous intravenous infusion for long periods is not recommended.

Dosage in the elderly: As for adults.

Directions for the use of glucagon in hypoglycaemia:

1. Dissolve the lyophilised glucagon in the accompanying diluent.
2. For *adults* and children weighing more than 20 kilograms, give 1 unit (1 mg) by subcutaneous, intramuscular or intravenous injection.
3. For *children* weighing less than 20 kilograms, give 0.5 unit (0.5 mg) or a dose equivalent to 20-30 microgram/kilogram.
4. The patient will normally awaken in 15 minutes. If the response is delayed, there is no contra-indication to the administration of 1 or 2 additional doses of glucagon, however, in view of the deleterious effects of cerebral hypoglycaemia and depending on the duration and depth of coma, the use of parenteral glucose *must* be considered.
5. Intravenous glucose *must* be given if the patient fails to respond to glucagon.
6. When the patient responds, give supplementary carbohydrate to restore the liver glycogen and prevent secondary hypoglycaemia.

It is important that the patient be aroused as quickly as possible, because prolonged hypoglycaemic reactions may result in cortical damage. Glucagon or intravenous glucose will awaken the patient sufficiently so that oral carbohydrates may be taken.

Although the patient or family members may use glucagon for the treatment of hypoglycaemia during an emergency, a doctor must still be notified when hypoglycaemic reactions occur so that the treatment regimen may be adjusted if necessary.

Instructions describing the method of using this preparation are included in the vial carton. It is advisable for the patient and family members to become familiar with the technique of preparing Glucagon for Injection before an emergency arises. Patients are instructed to use 1 unit (1 mg) for adults and, if recommended by a doctor, 0.5 unit (0.5 mg) for children weighing less than 20 kilograms.

For use as a diagnostic aid: Dissolve the lyophilised glucagon in the accompanying diluting solution. Glucagon should not be used at concentrations greater than 1 unit/ml (1 mg/ml).

The following doses may be administered for relaxation of the stomach, duodenum and small bowel, depending on the time of onset of action and the duration of effect required for the examination. Since the stomach is less sensitive to the effect of glucagon, 0.5 unit (0.5 mg) IV or 2 units (2 mg) im are recommended.

Dose†	*Route of Adminis-tration*	*Time of Onset of Action*	*Approximate Duration of Effect*
0.25–0.5 units	IV	1 minute	9–17 minutes
1 unit	im	8–10 minutes	12–27 minutes
2 units*	IV	1 minute	22–25 minutes
2 units*	im	4–7 minutes	21–32 minutes

*2-unit (2 mg) doses are associated with a higher incidence of nausea and vomiting than lower doses.
†1 unit equals 1 mg.

For examination of the colon, it is recommended that a 2 unit dose be administered intramuscularly approximately 10 minutes prior to initiation of the procedure. Relaxation of the colon and reduction of discomfort to the patient will allow the radiologist to perform a more satisfactory examination.

Contra-indications: Hypersensitivity to glucagon. Patients with phaeochromocytoma, where glucagon can cause the tumour to release catecholamines, which result in sudden and marked hypertension.

Special warnings and special precautions for use:
Warnings: Glucagon should be administered cautiously to patients with known or suspected insulinoma. In these patients, intravenous administration of glucagon will produce an initial increase in blood

glucose but, because of its insulin-releasing effect, may subsequently cause severe hypoglycaemia. A patient developing symptoms of hypoglycaemia after a dose of glucagon should be given glucose orally, intravenously, or by gavage, whichever is more appropriate.

Exogenous glucagon also stimulates the release of catecholamines. In the presence of phaeochromocytoma, glucagon can cause the tumour to release catecholamines, which results in a sudden and marked increase in blood pressure. Five to 10 mg of phentolamine mesylate may be administered IV in an attempt to control the blood pressure.

Precautions: Glucagon is helpful in hypoglycaemia only if liver glycogen is available. Because glucagon is of little or no help in states of starvation, adrenal insufficiency, or chronic hypoglycaemia, glucose should be considered for the treatment of hypoglycaemia.

Blood glucose determinations should be obtained to follow the patient in hypoglycaemic shock until he is asymptomatic.

Glucagon should be used with caution as a diagnostic aid in diabetic patients.

Interaction with other medicaments and other forms of interaction: Glucagon may enhance the anticoagulant effect of warfarin.

Pregnancy and lactation:
Usage in pregnancy: Animal reproduction studies have revealed no evidence of impaired fertility or foetal harm due to glucagon. However, in the absence of adequate human studies, glucagon should be used during pregnancy only if clearly needed.

Usage in nursing mothers: It is not known whether this drug is excreted in human milk. Although the plasma half-life is only 3 to 6 minutes and it is not active when taken orally, caution should be exercised when glucagon is administered to a nursing woman.

Effects on ability to drive and use machines: Not applicable.

Undesirable effects: Glucagon is relatively free of adverse reactions, except for occasional nausea and vomiting, which may also occur with hypoglycaemia. Diarrhoea and hypokalaemia have rarely been reported, as well as generalised allergic reactions, including urticaria, respiratory distress and hypotension.

Overdose:
Signs and symptoms: Although there is a lack of human experience and glucagon is generally well tolerated, nausea, vomiting, gastric hypotonicity and diarrhoea would be expected. Intravenous glucagon has positive inotropic and chronotropic effects. Increases in blood pressure and pulse might be more severe in patients taking beta-blockers and might require therapy in patients with phaeochromocytoma, insulinomas or coronary artery disease. When large doses (0.5-16 mg/hour by continuous infusion for periods of 5-166 hours) were given to cardiac patients, positive inotropy occurred and side-effects included nausea, vomiting and decreasing serum potassium.

As a polypeptide, glucagon would be rapidly destroyed if ingested.

Treatment: The plasma half-life of glucagon is approximately 3-6 minutes. Symptomatic and supportive therapy might include supplemental potassium for hypokalaemia, or phentolamine if a dramatic increase in blood pressure occurs. Forced diuresis, peritoneal dialysis, haemodialysis, or charcoal haemoperfusion have not been established as beneficial.

Pharmacological properties

Pharmacodynamic properties:
Actions: Glucagon causes an increase in blood glucose concentrations and is used in the treatment of hypoglycaemic states. It is effective in small doses. Glucagon acts only on liver glycogen, converting it to glucose, and is therefore helpful only if liver glycogen is available. It is of little or no help in states of starvation, adrenal insufficiency or chronic hypoglycaemia. The patient with Type I diabetes does not have as great a response in blood glucose levels as does the Type II stable diabetic, therefore, supplementary carbohydrate should be given as soon as possible, especially to juvenile patients.

Parenteral administration of glucagon produces relaxation of the smooth muscle of the stomach, duodenum, small bowel and colon.

Pharmacokinetic properties: The half-life of glucagon in plasma is approximately 3-6 minutes, which is similar to that of insulin.

Preclinical safety data: There are no preclinical data of relevance to the prescriber in addition to that summarised in other sections of the summary of product characteristics.

Pharmaceutical particulars

List of excipients:
Lyophilised product: Lactose

Diluting solution: Glycerin; Phenol; Sodium hydroxide*; Hydrochloric acid*; Water for injection.

*May have been added during manufacture to adjust the pH.

Incompatibilities: Not applicable.

Shelf-life:
Prior to reconstitution: 3 years.
Reconstituted solutions should be used immediately.

Special precautions for storage:
Prior to reconstitution: Store below 25°C.

Nature and contents of container: Glass vial (No. 666), containing 1 unit (1.09 mg) of glucagon as the hydrochloride, accompanied by glass vial (No. 667), containing 1 ml of diluent.

Instructions for use/handling: Crystalline glucagon is a white powder containing less than 0.05% zinc. It is relatively insoluble in water but is soluble at a pH of less than 3 or more than 9.5. Glucagon is stable in lyophilised form at room temperatures.

Use accompanying diluent solution for reconstitution.

After reconstitution, solutions should be used immediately. Glucagon solutions should not be used unless they are clear and of a water-like consistency.

If glucagon is to be given at doses higher than 2 units (2 mg), it should be reconstituted with Sterile Water for Injection, instead of the diluting solution supplied, and used immediately.

Marketing authorisation numbers
Vials 1 unit: 0006/5110
Vials diluting solution: 0006/5112

Date of approval/revision of SPC September 1997

Legal category POM

HUMAJECT* PENS
HUMULIN* PREFILLED INSULIN PENS
HUMAJECT* S (Soluble)
HUMAJECT* I (Isophane)
HUMAJECT* M1 (Mixture 1)
HUMAJECT* M2 (Mixture 2)
HUMAJECT* M3 (Mixture 3)
HUMAJECT* M4 (Mixture 4)

Qualitative and quantitative composition

Active Ingredient	*Quantity per ml*
Human Insulin (recombinant DNA origin)	100IU

Humulin Soluble is a sterile, clear, colourless, aqueous solution of human insulin adjusted to a pH range of 7.0 to 7.8.

Humulin Soluble is a rapidly acting insulin preparation.

Humulin Isophane is a sterile suspension of a white, crystalline precipitate of isophane human insulin in an isotonic phosphate buffer adjusted to a pH range of 6.9 to 7.5.

Humulin Isophane is an intermediate acting insulin preparation.

Humulin Mixture 1, Mixture 2, Mixture 3 and Mixture 4 are sterile suspensions of human insulin in the proportion of 10%, 20%, 30%, 40% and 50% soluble insulin to 90%, 80%, 70%, 60% and 50% isophane insulin, respectively, adjusted to a pH range of 6.9 to 7.5.

Humulin Mixtures are intermediate acting insulin preparations.

Pharmaceutical form A solution or suspension for injection filled into *cartridges* administered via a non-reusable device.

Humaject is a disposable injector containing a 3.0 ml cartridge prefilled with human insulin for parenteral administration.

Clinical particulars

Therapeutic indications: For the treatment of patients with diabetes mellitus who require insulin for the maintenance of glucose homeostasis. Humulin is also indicated for the initial control of diabetes mellitus and diabetes mellitus in pregnancy.

Posology and method of administration: The dosage should be determined by the physician, according to the requirement of the patient.

Humulin Soluble, Humulin Isophane and Mixtures in cartridge presentations should be given by subcutaneous injection but may, although not recommended, also be given by intramuscular injection. These formulations should not be administered intravenously.

Subcutaneous administration should be in the upper arms, thighs, buttocks or abdomen. Use of injection sites should be rotated so that the same site is not used more than approximately once a month.

Care should be taken when injecting any Humulin insulin preparations to ensure that a blood vessel has not been entered. After any insulin injection, the injection site should not be massaged.

Humulin Isophane may be administered in combination with Humulin Soluble (see *Special warnings and special precautions for use - Mixing of insulins*).

Humulin Mixture formulations are ready-made defined mixtures of Humulin Soluble and Humulin Isophane insulin, designed to avoid the need for the patient to mix insulin preparations. A patient's treatment regimen should be based on their individual metabolic requirements.

Contra-indications: Hypoglycaemia.

Hypersensitivity to Humulin or to the formulation excipients.

Under no circumstances should any Humulin formulation, other than Humulin Soluble in vials, be given intravenously.

Special warnings and special precautions for use:
Transferring from other insulins: A small number of patients transferring from insulins of animal origin may require a reduced dosage and/or a change in the ratio of soluble to intermediate preparations, especially if they are very tightly controlled and bordering on hypoglycaemia. The dosage reduction may occur immediately after transfer or be a gradual process lasting for several weeks. There is a risk of hypoglycaemia if insulin requirement is decreased, and both the physician and the patient should be aware of this possibility. The risk can be considered minimal if the daily dosage is less than 40IU. Insulin-resistant patients receiving more than 100IU daily should be referred to hospital for transfer.

A few patients who experienced hypoglycaemic reactions after transfer to human insulin have reported that the early warning symptoms were less pronounced or different from those experienced with their previous animal insulin. Patients whose blood glucose control is greatly improved, eg, by intensified insulin therapy, may lose some or all of the warning symptoms of hypoglycaemia and should be advised accordingly. Other conditions which may make the early warning symptoms of hypoglycaemia different or less pronounced include long duration of diabetes, diabetic nerve disease, or medications such as beta blockers. Uncorrected hypoglycaemic and hyperglycaemic reactions can cause loss of consciousness, coma or death.

Insulin requirements may change significantly in diseases of the adrenal, pituitary or thyroid glands and in the presence of renal or hepatic impairment.

Insulin requirements may be increased during illness or emotional disturbances.

Adjustment of insulin dosage may also be necessary if patients undertake increased physical activity or change their usual diet.

Mixing of insulins: Separate cartridges of Humulin Soluble and Isophane can be used for administration of the correct amount of each formulation.

Interaction with other medicaments and other forms of interaction: The patient should check with their physician when using other medicines in addition to Humulin.

Insulin requirements may be reduced by the concurrent administration of drugs with hypoglycaemic activity, eg, alcohol, monoamine oxidase inhibitors and beta-adrenergic blockers or aspirin.

Insulin requirements may be increased by concurrent administration of drugs, eg, oral contraceptives, corticosteroids or thyroid hormone replacement therapy.

The effects of mixing human insulin with insulins of animal origin have not been studied and this practice is not recommended.

Pregnancy and lactation: It is essential to maintain good control of the insulin treated (insulin-dependent or gestational diabetes) patient throughout pregnancy. Insulin requirements usually fall during the first trimester and increase during the second and third trimesters. Patients with diabetes should be advised to inform their doctors if they are pregnant or are contemplating pregnancy.

Diabetic patients who are lactating may require adjustments in insulin dose and/or diet.

Effects on ability to drive and use machines: Use of the correct therapeutic dose has no known effect on driving or the use of machinery.

Undesirable effects: Lipodystrophy, insulin resistance and hypersensitivity reactions are among the side-effects associated with insulins of animal origin. However, the incidence of such side-effects with Humulin is minimal. In the rare event of a severe allergy to Humulin, treatment is required immediately. A change of insulin or desensitisation may be required.

Hypoglycaemia is the most frequent undesirable effect that a diabetic may suffer. Severe hypoglycaemia may lead to loss of consciousness, and in extreme cases, death.

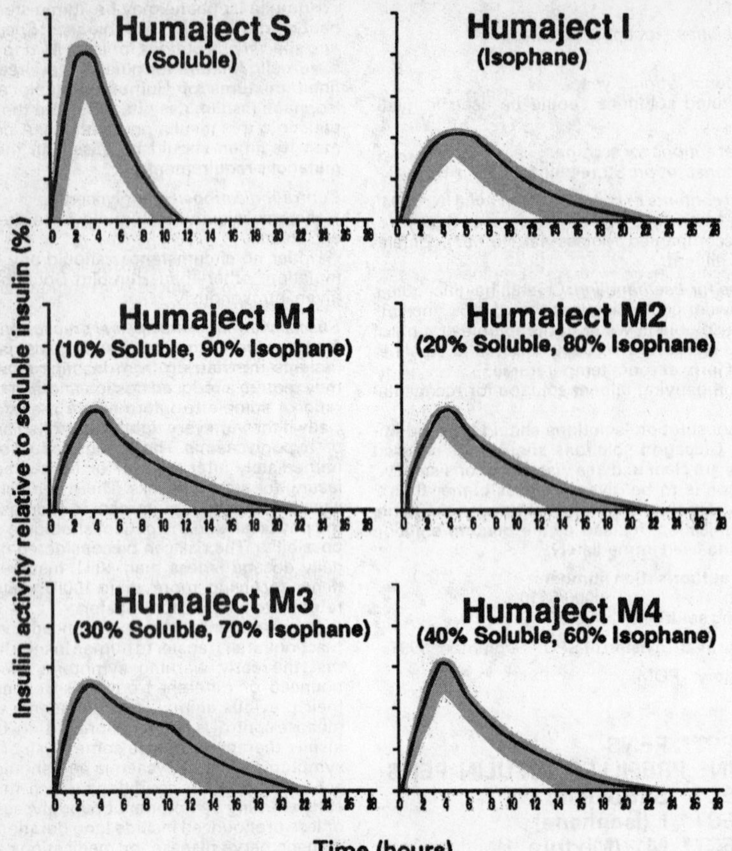

Overdose: Insulin has no specific overdose definitions, because serum glucose concentrations are a result of complex interactions between insulin levels, glucose availability and other metabolic processes. Hypoglycaemia may occur as a result of an excess of insulin relative to food intake and energy expenditure.

Hypoglycaemia may be associated with listlessness, confusion, palpitations, headache, sweating and vomiting.

Mild hypoglycaemic episodes will respond to oral administration of glucose or sugar products.

Correction of moderately severe hypoglycaemia can be accomplished by intramuscular or subcutaneous administration of glucagon, followed by oral carbohydrate when the patient recovers sufficiently. Patients who fail to respond to glucagon must be given glucose solution intravenously.

If the patient is comatose, glucagon should be administered intramuscularly or subcutaneously. However, glucose solution must be given intravenously if glucagon is not available or if the patient fails to respond to glucagon. The patient should be given a meal as soon as consciousness is recovered.

Pharmacological properties

Pharmacodynamic properties: The prime activity of insulin is the regulation of glucose metabolism.

In addition, insulin has several anabolic and anti-catabolic actions on a variety of different tissues. Within muscle tissue this includes increasing glycogen, fatty acid, glycerol and protein synthesis, and amino acid uptake, while decreasing glycogenolysis, glyconeogenesis, ketogenesis, lipolysis, protein catabolism and amino acid output.

The typical activity profile (glucose utilisation curve) following subcutaneous injection is illustrated above by the heavy line. Variations that a patient may experience in timing and/or intensity of insulin activity are illustrated by the shaded area. Individual variability will depend on factors such as size of dose, site of injection temperature and physical activity of the patient.

Pharmacokinetic properties: The pharmacokinetics of insulin do not reflect the metabolic action of that hormone. Therefore, it is more appropriate to examine glucose utilisation curves (as discussed above) when considering the activity of insulin.

Preclinical safety data: Humulin is human insulin produced by recombinant technology. No serious events have been reported in subchronic toxicology studies.

Pharmaceutical particulars

List of excipients:

For Humulin Soluble preparations: Each will contain Human Insulin (recombinant DNA origin) and the following excipients:

(a) *m*-Cresol distilled, 2.5 mg/ml; (b) glycerol; (c) water for injections; (d) hydrochloric acid; and (e) sodium hydroxide.

These are included as:

(a) preservative; (b) tonicity modifier; (c) solvent; (d) pH adjustment; and (e) pH adjustment, respectively.

Hydrochloric acid and/or sodium hydroxide may have been used during manufacture to adjust the pH.

For Humulin Isophane and Mixture preparations: Each will contain Human Insulin (recombinant DNA origin) and the following excipients:

(a) *m*-Cresol distilled, 1.6 mg/ml; (b) glycerol; (c) phenol, 0.65 mg/ml; (d) protamine sulphate; (e) dibasic sodium phosphate; (f) zinc oxide; (g) water for injections; (h) hydrochloric acid; and (i) sodium hydroxide.

These are included as:

(a) preservative; (b) tonicity modifier; (c) preservative; (d) complexes with insulin to prolong its action; (e) buffer; (f) adjust zinc content; (g) solvent; (h) pH adjustment; and (i) pH adjustment, respectively.

Hydrochloric acid and/or sodium hydroxide may have been used during manufacture to adjust the pH.

Incompatibilities: Humulin products should not be mixed with either animal insulins or human insulin preparations produced by other manufacturers.

Shelf-life: The shelf-life for Humulin Soluble, Isophane and Mixture presentations is two years when stored under appropriate conditions.

The in-use shelf-life for all Humaject pens is 28 days.

Special precautions for storage: Humulin preparations should be stored in a refrigerator between 2° and 8°C. They should not be frozen or exposed to excessive heat or sunlight.

When in use the Humaject pens may be kept at room temperature for up to 28 days.

Nature and contents of container:

Humaject pens: The product is filled in cartridges that comply with the requirements of the Ph Eur for Type I flint glass, and sealed with rubber closures consisting of a plunger head at the bottom and a disk seal at the top of the cartridge.

Package quantities: Humaject pens, each containing 3.0 ml Humulin, in packs of 5.

Instructions for use/handling:

(a) Preparing a dose: Humaject containing Humulin Soluble formulation does not require resuspension and should only be used if it is clear, colourless, with no solid particles visible and if it is of water-like appearance.

Humaject containing Humulin Isophane and Mixture formulations should be rolled in the palms of the hands ten times and inverted 180° ten times immediately before use to resuspend the insulin until it appears uniformly cloudy or milky. Do not shake vigorously as this may cause frothing which may interfere with the correct measurement of the dose.

The cartridges should be examined frequently and should not be used if clumps of material are present or if solid white particles stick to the bottom or wall of the cartridge or vial, giving a frosted appearance.

Humulin cartridges are not designed to allow any other insulin to be mixed in the cartridge. Cartridges are not designed to be refilled.

Cartridges: Non-reusable device - Humaject.

Preparing a dose

1. Mixing Insulin Suspensions. Remove pen cap. Roll the pen back and forth in your hands 10 times. Then, turn the pen up and down 10 times until insulin is evenly mixed.

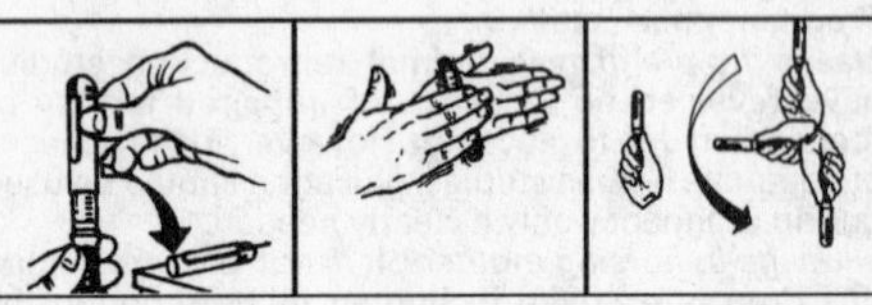

2. Resetting the pen. Before each injection the **star** (★) must appear in the dose window. If the **star** (★) is not in the dose window, while holding the white cylinder firmly, turn the **CLEAR PLASTIC BARREL IN THE DIRECTION OF THE ARROWS.** Turn until the **star** (★) appears in the dose window. (Do **NOT** turn the white dose set/plunger knob to reset to **star** (★).)

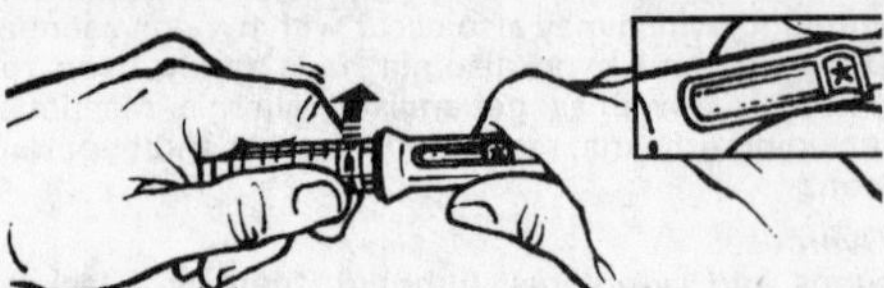

3. Putting on the B-D pen needle. Wipe rubber seal with alcohol. Remove paper tab from needle. Screw capped needle onto the end of the pen until tight.

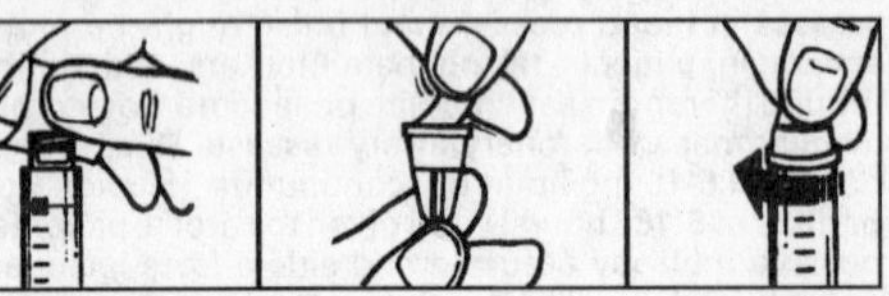

4. Clearing air bubbles.

a) Turn the dose set/plunger knob in direction of the arrow until a '2' shows in the dose display window. You will hear one click.

b) Hold pen upright. Remove outer needle cap and cover.

c) Depress plunger knob to remove any large air bubbles.

A small drop of insulin should appear at the tip of the needle. If insulin does not appear, repeat step a, b and c above.

d) Replace outer needle cap.

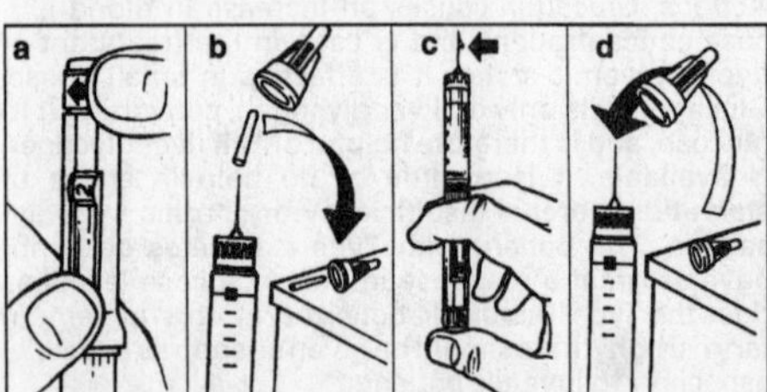

5. Reset Pen so the star (★) appears in the dose window. SEE STEP 2.

6. Setting Your Dose. To set your dose, turn the dose set/plunger knob in the direction of the arrow. Turn until your dose appears in the dose window. Pen will click once for each 2 units dialled. This knob can be moved back and forth to adjust your dose.

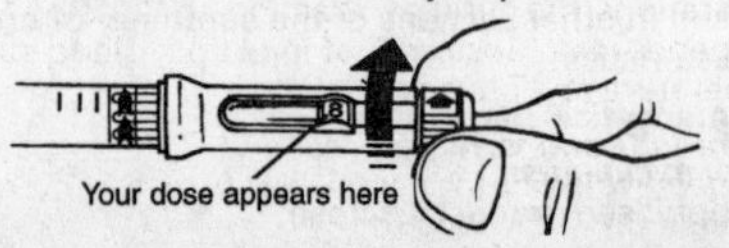

(b) Injecting a dose
Cartridges:

1. Wash your hands.
2. Choose a site for the injection.
3. Clean the skin with an alcohol swab.
4. Remove outer needle cap.
5. Stabilise the skin by spreading it or pinching up a large area. Insert the needle as instructed by your doctor.
6. To inject insulin via a Humaject pen, push the dose knob down with the thumb until a click is heard. Wait 5 seconds.
7. Pull the needle straight out of the skin and apply gentle pressure over the injection site for several seconds. Do not rub the area.
8. Using the outer needle cap, unscrew the needle immediately after injection and dispose of it safely. Removing the needle immediately after injection ensures sterility, prevents leakage and re-entry of air and potential needle clogs.
9. Replace the cap on the pen.

(c) Disposal of used containers and needles:
Do not reuse needles. Dispose of the needle in a responsible manner. Needles and pens must not be shared. Humaject pens can be used until empty, then properly discard or recycle.

Marketing authorisation numbers
Humaject S pen: 0006/0305
Humaject I pen: 0006/0306
Humaject M1 pen:0006/0307
Humaject M2 pen:0006/0308
Humaject M3 pen:0006/0309
Humaject M4 pen:0006/0310

Date of approval/revision of SPC 13 December 1994

Legal category POM

HUMALOG MIX25* ▼

100U/ml suspension for injection in cartridge
100U/ml Pen, suspension for injection

Qualitative and quantitative composition

Active Substance	*Quantity per ml*
Insulin lispro (recombinant DNA origin produced in *E. coli*)	100U

The concentration of insulin lispro is 3.5 mg per ml for the 100U/ml product.

Pharmaceutical form
Humalog Mix25 100U/ml suspension for injection in cartridge
Suspension for injection, in a 3 ml cartridge to be used with a CE marked pen as recommended in the information provided by the device manufacturer.

Humalog Mix25 100U/ml Pen, suspension for injection
Suspension for injection, in a prefilled/disposable pen injector containing a 3 ml cartridge.

Humalog Mix25 is a white, sterile suspension of 25% insulin lispro ([Lys (B28), Pro (B29)] human insulin analogue, rDNA origin) and 75% insulin lispro protamine suspension adjusted to pH 7.0–7.8.

Clinical particulars
Therapeutic indications: Humalog Mix25 is indicated for the treatment of patients with diabetes mellitus who require insulin for the maintenance of normal glucose homeostasis.

Posology and method of administration: The dosage should be determined by the physician, according to the requirement of the patient.

Humalog Mix25 may be given shortly before meals. When necessary, Humalog Mix25 can be given soon after meals. Humalog Mix25 should only be given by subcutaneous injection Under no circumstances should Humalog Mix25 be given intravenously.

Subcutaneous administration should be in the upper arms, thighs, buttocks, or abdomen. Use of injection sites should be rotated so that the same site is not used more than approximately once a month.

Care should be taken when injecting Humalog Mix25 to ensure that a blood vessel has not been entered. After injection, the site of injection should not be massaged.

The rapid onset and early peak of activity of Humalog itself is observed following the subcutaneous administration of Humalog Mix25. This allows Humalog Mix25 to be given very close to mealtime. The duration of action of the insulin lispro protamine suspension (NPL) component of Humalog Mix25 is similar to that of a basal insulin (NPH).

The time course of action of any insulin may vary considerably in different individuals or at different times in the same individual. As with all insulin preparations, the duration of action of Humalog Mix25 is dependent on dose, site of injection, blood supply, temperature and physical activity.

Contra-indications: Hypoglycaemia.

Hypersensitivity to insulin lispro or to any of the excipients.

Special warnings and special precautions for use: Under no circumstances should Humalog Mix25 be given intravenously.

Transferring a patient to another type or brand of insulin should be done under strict medical supervision. Changes in strength, brand (manufacturer), type (regular, NPH, lente, etc), species (animal, human, human insulin analogue) and/or method of manufacture (recombinant DNA versus animal-source insulin) may result in the need for a change in dosage.

Patients taking Humalog Mix25 may require a change in dosage from that used with their usual insulins. If an adjustment is needed, it may occur with the first dose or during the first several weeks or months.

Patients whose blood glucose is greatly improved, eg, by intensified insulin therapy, may lose some or all of the warning symptoms of hypoglycaemia and should be advised accordingly.

A few patients who have experienced hypoglycaemic reactions after transfer from animal-source insulin to human insulin have reported that the early warning symptoms of hypoglycaemia were less pronounced or different from those experienced with their previous insulin. Uncorrected hypoglycaemic or hyperglycaemic reactions can cause loss of consciousness, coma, or death.

The use of dosages which are inadequate or discontinuation of treatment, especially in insulin-dependent diabetics, may lead to hyperglycaemia and diabetic ketoacidosis; conditions which are potentially lethal.

Insulin requirements may be reduced in the presence of renal or hepatic impairment.

Insulin requirements may be increased during illness or emotional disturbances.

Adjustment of dosage may also be necessary if patients undertake increased physical activity or change their usual diet. Exercise taken immediately after a meal may increase the risk of hypoglycaemia.

Administration of insulin lispro to children below 12 years of age should be considered only in case of an expected benefit when compared to regular insulin.

Interaction with other medicaments and other forms of interaction: Insulin requirements may be increased by substances with hyperglycaemic activity, such as oral contraceptives, corticosteroids, or thyroid replacement therapy, danazol, $beta_2$ stimulants (such as ritodrine, salbutamol, terbutaline).

Insulin requirements may be reduced in the presence of substances with hypoglycaemic activity, such as oral hypoglycaemics, salicylates (for example, acetylsalicylic acid), sulpha antibiotics, certain antidepressants, certain angiotensin converting enzyme inhibitors (captopril, enalapril), beta-blockers, octreotide or alcohol.

Mixing Humalog Mix25 with other insulins has not been studied.

The physician should be consulted when using other medications in addition to Humalog Mix25.

Pregnancy and lactation: There is no significant experience with insulin lispro in pregnancy.

It is essential to maintain good control of the insulin-treated (insulin-dependent or gestational diabetes) patient throughout pregnancy. Insulin requirements usually fall during the first trimester and increase during the second and third trimesters. Patients with diabetes should be advised to inform their doctor if they are pregnant or are contemplating pregnancy. Careful monitoring of glucose control, as well as general health, is essential in pregnant patients with diabetes.

Patients with diabetes who are lactating may require adjustments in insulin dose, diet, or both.

Effects on ability to drive and use machines: The patient's ability to concentrate and react may be impaired as a result of hypoglycaemia. This may constitute a risk in situations where these abilities are of special importance (e.g. driving a car or operating machinery).

Patients should be advised to take precautions to avoid hypoglycaemia whilst driving, this is particularly important in those who have reduced or absent awareness of the warning signs of hypoglycaemia or have frequent episodes of hypoglycaemia. The advisability of driving should be considered in these circumstances.

Undesirable effects: Hypoglycaemia is the most frequent undesirable effect of insulin therapy that a patient with diabetes may suffer. Severe hypoglycaemia may lead to loss of consciousness, and in extreme cases, death.

Local allergy in patients occasionally occurs as redness, swelling, and itching at the site of insulin injection. This condition usually resolves in a few days to a few weeks. In some instances, this condition may be related to factors other than insulin, such as irritants in the skin cleansing agent or poor injection technique. Systemic allergy, less common but potentially more serious, is a generalised allergy to insulin. It may cause a rash over the whole body, shortness of breath, wheezing, reduction in blood pressure, fast pulse, or sweating. Severe cases of generalised allergy may be life-threatening.

Lipodystrophy may occur at the injection site.

Overdose: Insulins have no specific overdose definitions because serum glucose concentrations are a result of complex interactions between insulin levels, glucose availability and other metabolic processes. Hypoglycaemia may occur as a result of an excess of insulin activity relative to food intake and energy expenditure.

Hypoglycaemia may be associated with listlessness, confusion, palpitations, headache, sweating and vomiting.

Mild hypoglycaemic episodes will respond to oral administration of glucose or other sugar or saccharated products.

Correction of moderately severe hypoglycaemia can be accomplished by intramuscular or subcutaneous administration of glucagon, followed by oral carbohydrate when the patient recovers sufficiently. Patients who fail to respond to glucagon must be given glucose solution intravenously.

If the patient is comatose, glucagon should be administered intramuscularly or subcutaneously. However, glucose solution must be given intravenously if glucagon is not available or if the patient fails to respond to glucagon. The patient should be given a meal as soon as consciousness is recovered.

Pharmacological properties
Pharmacodynamic properties: Pharmaco-therapeutic group: Humalog Mix25 is a premixed suspension consisting of insulin lispro (fast acting human insulin analogue) and insulin lispro protamine suspension (intermediate acting human insulin analogue). ATC Code: A10A.

The primary activity of insulin lispro is the regulation of glucose metabolism.

In addition, insulins have several anabolic and anti-catabolic actions on a variety of different tissues. Within muscle tissue this includes increasing glycogen, fatty acid, glycerol and protein synthesis and amino acid uptake, while decreasing glycogenolysis, glyconeogenesis, ketogenesis, lipolysis, protein catabolism and amino acid output.

Insulin lispro has a rapid onset of action (approximately 15 minutes), thus allowing it to be given closer to a meal (within zero to 15 minutes of the meal) when compared to regular insulin (30 to 45 minutes before). The rapid onset and early peak of activity of insulin lispro is observed following the subcutaneous administration of Humalog Mix25. NPL has an activity profile that is very similar to that of a basal insulin (NPH) over a period of approximately 15 hours. In the figure below the pharmacodynamics of Humalog Mix25 and NPL are illustrated.

The above representation reflects the relative amount of glucose over time required to maintain the subject's whole blood glucose concentrations near fasting levels and is an indicator of the effect of these insulins on glucose metabolism over time.

Pharmacokinetic properties: The pharmacokinetics of insulin lispro reflect a compound that is rapidly absorbed and achieves peak blood levels 30 to 70 minutes following subcutaneous injection. The pharmacokinetics of insulin lispro protamine suspension are consistent with those of an intermediate acting insulin such as NPH. The pharmacokinetics of Humalog Mix25 are representative of the individual pharmacokinetic properties of the two components. When considering the clinical relevance of these kinetics, it is more appropriate to examine the glucose utilisation curves (as discussed in 'Pharmacodynamic properties').

Preclinical safety data: In *in vitro* tests, including binding to insulin receptor sites and effects on growing cells, insulin lispro behaved in a manner that closely resembled human insulin. Studies also demonstrate that the dissociation of binding to the insulin receptor of insulin lispro is equivalent to human insulin. Acute, one month and twelve month toxicology studies produced no significant toxicity findings.

Pharmaceutical particulars
List of excipients: Each cartridge contains insulin lispro and the following excipients:

Protamine sulphate [0.28 mg/ml], *m*-Cresol distilled [1.76 mg/ml], phenol [0.80 mg/ml], glycerol, dibasic sodium phosphate.$7H_2O$, zinc oxide, water for injections, hydrochloric acid and sodium hydroxide.

Incompatibilities: Mixing Humalog Mix25 with other insulins has not been studied.

Shelf life: Two years.

28 days after first use of the cartridge or Pen (prefilled).

Special precautions for storage: Store at 2°C–8°C. (In a refrigerator.)

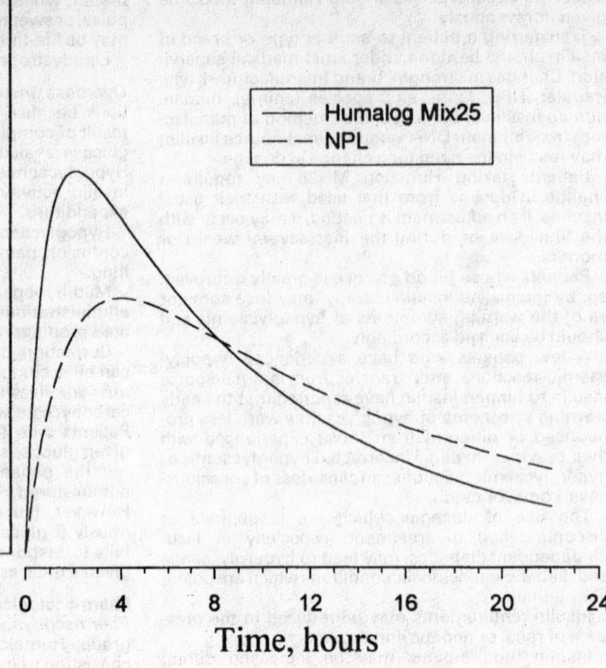

Do not freeze. Do not expose to excessive heat or direct sunlight.

Once in use cartridges and Pens (prefilled) may be used for up to 28 days. Do not use beyond this period.

Humalog Mix25 100U/ml suspension for injection in cartridge

Following insertion in a pen, the cartridge and pen should be stored below 30°C and should not be refrigerated.

Humalog Mix25 100U/ml Pen, suspension for injection

Pens (prefilled) in use should be stored below 30°C and should not be refrigerated.

Nature and contents of container:

Humalog Mix25 100U/ml suspension for injection in cartridge

The suspension is contained in Type I flint glass cartridges, sealed with halobutyl disc seals and plunger heads and secured with aluminium seals. Dimethicone or silicone emulsion may have been used to treat the cartridge plunger and/or the glass cartridge.

Humalog Mix25 100U/ml Pen, suspension for injection

The cartridges are sealed in a disposable pen injector, called the 'Pen'. Needles are not included.

5 X 3 ml Humalog Mix25 cartridges for a 3 ml pen.

5 X 3 ml Humalog Mix25 100U/ml Pens.

Instructions for use/handling, and disposal (if appropriate):

Humalog Mix25 100U/ml suspension for injection in cartridge

(a) Cartridge – Preparing a dose

Cartridges containing Humalog Mix25 should be rotated in the palms of the hands ten times and inverted 180° ten times immediately before use to resuspend the insulin until it appears uniformly cloudy or milky. If not, repeat the above procedure until contents are mixed. Cartridges contain a small glass bead to assist mixing. Do not shake vigorously as this may cause frothing which may interfere with the correct measurement of the dose.

The cartridges should be examined frequently and should not be used if clumps of material are present or if solid white particles stick to the bottom or wall of the cartridge, giving a frosted appearance.

Humalog Mix25 cartridges are not designed to allow any other insulin to be mixed in the cartridge. Cartridges are not designed to be refilled.

The following is a general description. The manufacturer's instructions with each individual pen must be followed for loading the cartridge, attaching the needle and administering the insulin injection.

(b) Cartridge – Injecting a dose

1. Wash your hands.
2. Choose a site for injection.
3. Clean the skin with an alcohol swab.
4. Remove outer needle cap.
5. Stabilise the skin by spreading it or pinching up a large area. Insert the needle as instructed.
6. Press the knob.
7. Pull the needle out and apply gentle pressure over the injection site for several seconds. Do not rub the area.
8. Using the outer needle cap, unscrew the needle and dispose of it safely.
9. Use of injection sites should be rotated so that the same site is not used more than approximately once a month.

Humalog Mix25 100U/ml Pen, suspension for injection

(a) Pen (prefilled) – Preparing a dose

1. Inspect the Humalog Mix25 100U/ml Pen.

The Pen should be rotated in the palms of the hands ten times and inverted 180° ten times immediately before use to resuspend the insulin until it appears uniformly cloudy or milky. If not, repeat the above procedure until contents are mixed. Cartridges contain a small glass bead to assist mixing. Do not shake vigorously as this may cause frothing which may interfere with the correct measurement of the dose.

The cartridges should be examined frequently and should not be used if clumps of material are present or if solid white particles stick to the bottom or wall of the cartridge, giving a frosted appearance.

2. Put on the needle.

Wipe the rubber seal with alcohol. Remove the paper tab from the capped needle. Screw the capped needle clockwise onto the pen until it is tight. Hold the pen with needle pointing up and remove the outer needle cap and inner needle cover.

3. Priming Pen (check insulin flow).

(a) The arrow should be visible in the dose window. If the arrow is not present, turn the dose knob clockwise until the arrow appears and notch is felt or visually aligned.
(b) Pull dose knob out (in direction of the arrow) until a '0' appears in the dose window. A dose cannot be dialled until the dose knob is pulled out.
(c) Turn dose knob clockwise until a '2' appears in the dose window.
(d) Hold the pen with needle pointing up and tap the clear cartridge holder gently with your finger so any air bubbles collect near the top. Depress the injection button fully until you feel or hear a click. You should see a drop of insulin at the tip of the needle. If insulin does not appear, repeat the procedure until insulin appears.
(e) Always prime the pen (check the insulin flow) before each injection. Failure to prime the pen may result in an inaccurate dose.

4. Setting the dose.

(a) Turn the dose knob clockwise until the arrow appears in the dose window and a notch is felt or visually aligned.
(b) Pull the dose knob out (in the direction of the arrow) until a '0' appears in the dose window. A dose cannot be dialled until the dose knob is pulled out.
(c) Turn the dose knob clockwise until the dose appears in the dose window. If too high a dose is dialled, turn the dose knob backward (anti-clockwise) until the correct dose appears in the window. A dose greater than the number of units remaining in the cartridge cannot be dialled.

(b) Pen (prefilled) – Injecting a dose

1. Wash your hands.
2. Choose a site for injection.
3. Clean the skin with an alcohol swab.
4. Remove outer needle cap.
5. Stabilise the skin by spreading it or pinching up a large area. Insert the needle as instructed.
6. Press the injection button down with the thumb (until you hear or feel a click); wait 5 seconds.
7. Pull the needle out and apply gentle pressure over the injection site for several seconds. Do not rub the area.
8. Immediately after an injection, use the outer needle cap to unscrew the needle. Remove the needle from the pen. This will ensure sterility, and prevent leakage, re-entry of air, and potential needle clogs. Do not reuse the needle. Dispose of the needle in a responsible manner. Needles and pens must not be shared.

The pre-filled pen can be used until it is empty. Please properly discard or recycle.

9. Replace the cap on the pen.
10. Use of injection sites should be rotated so that the same site is not used more than approximately once a month.
11. The injection button should be fully depressed before using the pen again.

(c) Mixing insulins

Do not mix insulin in vials with insulin in cartridges.

Marketing authorisation holder: Eli Lilly Nederland BV, Krijtwal 17–23, 3432 ZT Nieuwegein, The Netherlands

Marketing authorisation numbers

Humalog Mix25 100U/ml suspension for injection in cartridge:	EU1/96/007/008
Humalog Mix25 100U/ml Pen, suspension for injection:	EU1/97/042/002

Date of approval/revision of SPC November 1998

Legal category POM

HUMALOG* VIALS AND CARTRIDGES 100U/ML ▼

Qualitative and quantitative composition Humalog is a sterile, clear, colourless, aqueous solution of insulin lispro ([Lys (B28), Pro (B29)] human insulin analog, rDNA origin) adjusted to pH 7.0–7.8. The name insulin lispro is approved by INN, USAN and BAN.

Active ingredient: Insulin lispro (recombinant DNA origin produced in *E. coli*) 100U per ml.

The concentration of insulin lispro is 3.5 mg insulin lispro per ml for the 100U/ml product.

Pharmaceutical forms

Vials: A solution for injection, in a 10 ml vial (100U/ml of insulin lispro) to be used in conjunction with an appropriate syringe (100U markings) for parenteral administration.

Cartridges: A solution for injection, in either 1.5 ml or 3 ml cartridges (100U/ml of insulin lispro) for parenteral subcutaneous administration. To be used with a CE marked pen, as recommended in the information provided by the device manufacturer.

Clinical particulars

Therapeutic indication: For the treatment of patients with diabetes mellitus who require insulin for the maintenance of normal glucose homeostasis. Humalog is also indicated for the initial stabilisation of diabetes mellitus.

Posology and method of administration: The dosage should be determined by the physician, according to the requirement of the patient.

Humalog may be given shortly before meals. When necessary, Humalog can be given soon after meals. Humalog can be given in conjunction with a longer acting human insulin.

Humalog preparations should be given by subcutaneous injection or by continuous subcutaneous infusion pump (see Use of Humalog in an insulin infusion pump), and may, although not recommended, also be given by intramuscular injection.

Subcutaneous administration should be in the upper arms, thighs, buttocks or abdomen. Use of injection sites should be rotated so that the same site is not used more than approximately once a month.

Care should be taken when injecting Humalog to ensure that a blood vessel has not been entered. After injection, the site of injection should not be massaged.

Humalog takes effect rapidly and has a shorter duration of activity (2 to 5 hours) as compared with soluble insulin. This rapid onset of activity allows Humalog to be given very close to mealtime. The time course of action of any insulin may vary considerably in different individuals or at different times in the same individual. As with all insulin preparations, the duration of action of Humalog is dependent on dose, site of injection, blood supply, temperature and physical activity.

Humalog may be administered in conjunction with a longer acting human insulin, on the advice of a physician.

Contra-indications: Hypoglycaemia. Hypersensitivity to insulin lispro or one of its excipients.

Special warnings and special precautions for use: Transferring a patient to another type or brand of insulin should be done under strict medical supervision. Changes in strength, brand (manufacturer), type (soluble, isophane, lente, etc), species (animal, human, human insulin analog) and/or method of manufacture (recombinant DNA versus animal-source insulin) may result in the need for a change in dosage.

Vials: The shorter acting Humalog should be drawn into the syringe first, to prevent contamination of the vial by the longer acting insulin. Mixing of the insulins ahead of time or just before the injection should be on advice of the physician. However, a consistent routine must be followed.

Patients taking Humalog may require a change in dosage from that used with their usual insulins. If an adjustment is needed, it may occur with the first dose or during the first several weeks or months.

Patients whose blood glucose is greatly improved, eg, by intensified insulin therapy, may lose some or all of the warning symptoms of hypoglycaemia and should be advised accordingly.

A few patients who have experienced hypoglycaemic reactions after transfer from animal-source insulin to human insulin have reported that the early warning symptoms of hypoglycaemia were less pronounced or different from those experienced with their previous insulin. Uncorrected hypoglycaemic or hyperglycaemic reactions can cause loss of consciousness, coma or death.

Insulin requirements may be reduced in the presence of renal or hepatic impairment.

Insulin requirements may be increased during illness or emotional disturbances.

Adjustment of dosage may also be necessary if patients undertake increased physical activity or change their usual diet. Exercise taken immediately after a meal may increase the risk of hypoglycaemia.

Administration of insulin lispro to children should be considered only in case of an expected benefit when compared to regular insulin.

Interaction with other medicaments and other forms of interaction: Insulin requirements may be increased by drugs with hyperglycaemic activity, such as oral contraceptives, corticosteroids, or thyroid replacement therapy, danazol, beta 2 stimulants (ritodrine, salbutamol, terbutaline).

Insulin requirements may be reduced in the presence of drugs with hypoglycaemic activity, such as oral hypoglycaemics, salicylates (for example, aspirin), sulpha antibiotics, and certain antidepressants, certain angiotensin converting enzyme inhibitors (captopril, enalapril), beta blockers, octreotide, alcohol.

Humalog should not be mixed with animal insulins.

The physician should be consulted when using other medications in addition to Humalog.

Use in pregnancy and lactation: There is no significant experience with Humalog in pregnancy.

It is essential to maintain good control of the insulin–treated (insulin–dependent or gestational diabetes) patient throughout pregnancy. Insulin requirements usually fall during the first trimester and increase during the second and third trimesters. Patients with diabetes should be advised to inform their doctor if they are pregnant or are contemplating pregnancy. Careful monitoring of glucose control, as well as general health, is essential in pregnant patients with diabetes.

Patients with diabetes who are lactating may require adjustments in insulin dose, diet, or both.

Effects on ability to drive and use machines: The patient's ability to concentrate and react may be impaired as a result of hypoglycaemia. This may constitute a risk in situations where these abilities are of special importance (e.g. driving a car or operating machinery).

Patients should be advised to take precautions to avoid hypoglycaemia whilst driving, this is particularly important in those who have reduced or absent awareness of the warning signs of hypoglycaemia or have frequent episodes of hypoglycaemia. The advisability of driving should be considered in these circumstances.

Undesirable effects: Hypoglycaemia is the most frequent undesirable effect of insulin therapy that a patient with diabetes may suffer. Severe hypoglycaemia may lead to loss of consciousness, and in extreme cases, death.

Local allergy in patients occasionally occurs as redness, swelling, and itching at the site of insulin injection. This condition usually resolves in a few days to a few weeks. In some instances, this condition may be related to factors other than insulin, such as irritants in the skin cleansing agent or poor injection technique. Systemic allergy, less common but potentially more serious, is a generalised allergy to insulin. It may cause rash over the whole body, shortness of breath, wheezing, reduction in blood pressure, fast pulse, or sweating. Severe cases of generalised allergy may be life–threatening.

Lipodystrophy may occur at the injection site.

Overdose: Insulins have no specific overdose definitions because serum glucose concentrations are a result of complex interactions between insulin levels, glucose availability and other metabolic processes. Hypoglycaemia may occur as a result of an excess of insulin or insulin lispro relative to food intake and energy expenditure.

Hypoglycaemia may be associated with listlessness, confusion, palpitations, headache, sweating and vomiting.

Mild hypoglycaemic episodes will respond to oral administration of glucose or other sugar or saccharated products.

Correction of moderately severe hypoglycaemia can be accomplished by intramuscular or subcutaneous administration of glucagon, followed by oral carbohydrate when the patient recovers sufficiently. Patients who fail to respond to glucagon must be given glucose solution intravenously.

If the patient is comatose, glucagon should be administered intramuscularly or subcutaneously. However, glucose solution must be given intravenously if glucagon is not available or if the patient fails to respond to glucagon. The patient should be given a meal as soon as consciousness is recovered.

Pharmacological properties

Pharmacodynamic properties: Pharmaco–therapeutic group: fast acting human insulin analogue.

The primary activity of insulin lispro is the regulation of glucose metabolism.

In addition, insulins have several anabolic and anti-catabolic actions on a variety of different tissues. Within muscle tissue this includes increasing glycogen, fatty acid, glycerol and protein synthesis and amino acid uptake, while decreasing glycogenolysis, glyconeogenesis, ketogenesis, lipolysis, protein catabolism and amino acid output.

Humalog has a rapid onset of action (approximately 15 minutes), thus allowing it to be given closer to a meal (within zero to 15 minutes of the meal) when compared to soluble insulin (30 to 45 minutes before). Humalog takes effect rapidly and has a shorter duration of activity (2 to 5 hours) when compared to soluble insulin. As with all insulin preparations, the time course of Humalog action may vary in different individuals or at different times in the same individual and is dependent on site of injection, blood supply, temperature and physical activity. The typical activity profile following subcutaneous injection is illustrated below. The representation below reflects the relative amount of glucose over time required to maintain subject's whole blood glucose concentrations near fasting levels and is an indicator of the effect of these insulins on glucose metabolism over time.

Pharmacokinetic properties: The pharmacokinetics of Humalog reflect a compound that is rapidly absorbed, and achieves peak blood levels 30 to 70 minutes following subcutaneous injection. When considering the clinical relevance of these kinetics, it is more appropriate to examine the glucose utilisation curves (as discussed in *Pharmacodynamic properties*).

Preclinical safety: In *in vitro* tests, including binding to insulin receptor sites and effects on growing cells, Humalog behaved in a manner that closely resembled human insulin. Studies also demonstrate that the dissociation of binding to the insulin receptor of Humalog is equivalent to human insulin. Acute, one month and twelve month toxicology studies produced no significant toxicity findings.

Pharmaceutical particulars

List of excipients: Each vial or cartridge will contain insulin lispro and the following excipients:

(a) *m*-cresol distilled [3.15 mg/ml]; (b) glycerol; (c) dibasic sodium phosphate.$7H_2O$; (d) zinc oxide; (e) water for injection; (f) hydrochloric acid and (g) sodium hydroxide.

These are included as:

(a) preservative and stabiliser; (b) tonicity modifier; (c) a buffering agent; (d) stabiliser; (e) a vehicle; (f) pH adjustment and (g) pH adjustment, respectively.

Incompatibilities: Humalog preparations should not be mixed with animal insulin preparations.

Shelf life: Two years when stored under appropriate conditions. The in-use shelf life is 28 days.

Special precautions for storage: Humalog preparations should be stored in a refrigerator between 2° and 8°C. They should not be frozen or exposed to excessive heat or sunlight. If refrigeration is not possible, the vial or cartridge being used can be kept at ambient temperature for up to 28 days, below 30°C and away from direct heat and light. Following insertion in a pen, the cartridge and pen should not be refrigerated.

Nature and content of container: The solution is filled aseptically into Type I flint glass vials or cartridges. The glass conforms to PhEur requirements. The vials are then sealed with butyl or halobutyl stoppers. Dimethicone or silicone emulsion may be used to treat the vial stopper. The closures are secured with aluminium seals. The cartridges are sealed with butyl or halobutyl disk seals and plunger heads. Dimethicone or silicone emulsion may be used to treat the cartridge plunger and/or the glass cartridge. The closures are secured with aluminium seals.

Instructions for use/handling:

Humalog Vials

(a) Preparing a dose: Inspect the Humalog. It should be clear and colourless. Do not use Humalog if it appears cloudy, thickened or slightly coloured, or if solid particles are visible.

(a) *Humalog*

1. Wash your hands.
2. If using a new bottle, flip off the plastic protective cap, but **do not remove the stopper.**
3. If the therapeutic regimen requires the injection of basal insulin and Humalog at the same time, the two can be mixed in the syringe. If mixing insulins, refer to the instructions for mixing that follow in Section (b).
4. Draw air into the syringe equal to the prescribed Humalog dose. Wipe the top of the bottle with an alcohol swab. Put the needle through rubber top of the Humalog bottle and inject the air into the bottle.
5. Turn the bottle and syringe upside down. Hold the bottle and syringe firmly in one hand.
6. Making sure the tip of the needle is in the Humalog, withdraw the correct dose into the syringe.
7. Before removing the needle from the bottle, check the syringe for air bubbles that reduce the amount of Humalog in it. If bubbles are present, hold the syringe straight up and tap its side until the bubbles float to the top. Push them out with the plunger and withdraw the correct dose.
8. Remove the needle from the bottle and lay the syringe down so that the needle does not touch anything.

(b) Mixing Humalog with longer-acting human insulins

1. Humalog should be mixed with longer–acting human insulins only on the advice of a doctor.
2. Draw air into the syringe equal to the amount of longer–acting insulin being taken. Insert the needle

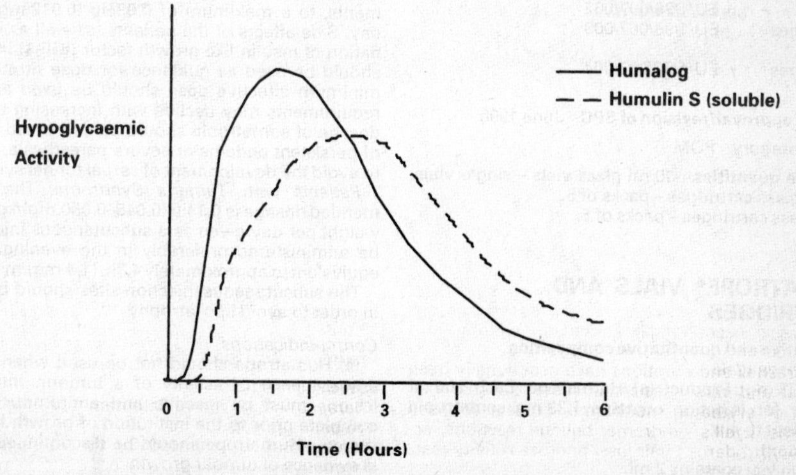

into the longer–acting insulin bottle and inject the air. Withdraw the needle.

3. Now inject air into the Humalog bottle in the same manner, but **do not** withdraw the needle.

4. Turn the bottle and syringe upside down.

5. Making sure the tip of the needle is in the Humalog, withdraw the correct dose of Humalog into the syringe.

6. Before removing the needle from the bottle, check the syringe for air bubbles that reduce the amount of Humalog in it. If bubbles are present, hold the syringe straight up and tap its side until the bubbles float to the top. Push them out with the plunger and withdraw the correct dose.

7. Remove the needle from the bottle of Humalog and insert it into the bottle of the longer–acting insulin. Turn the bottle and syringe upside down. Hold the bottle and syringe firmly in one hand and shake gently. Making sure the tip of the needle is in the insulin, withdraw the dose of longer–acting insulin.

8. Remove the needle and lay the syringe down so that the needle does not touch anything.

(c) Mixing insulins: Do not mix insulins in vials with insulins in cartridges.

Humalog Cartridges

(a) Preparing a dose: Inspect the Humalog. It should be clear and colourless. Do not use Humalog if it appears cloudy, thickened or slightly coloured, or if solid particles are visible.

The following is a general description. The manufacturer's instructions with each individual pen must be followed for loading the cartridge, attaching the needle and administering the insulin injection.

(b) Injecting a dose:

1. Wash your hands.
2. Choose a site for injection.
3. Clean the skin with an alcohol swab.
4. Remove outer needle cap.
5. Stabilise the skin by spreading it or pinching up a large area. Insert the needle as instructed.
6. Press the knob.
7. Pull the needle out and apply gentle pressure over the injection site for several seconds. Do not rub the area.
8. Using the outer needle cap, unscrew the needle and dispose of it safely.
9. Use of injection sites should be rotated so that the same site is not used more than approximately once a month.

(c) Mixing insulins: Do not mix insulins in vials with insulins in cartridges.

(d) Use of Humalog in an insulin infusion pump Minimed and Disetronic insulin infusion pumps may be used to infuse insulin lispro. Read and follow the instructions that accompany the infusion pump. Use the correct reservoir and catheter for the pump. Change the infusion set every 48 hours. Use aseptic technique when inserting the infusion set. In the event of a hypoglycaemic episode, the infusion should be stopped until the episode is resolved. If repeated or severe low blood glucose levels occur, notify your health care professional and consider the need to reduce or stop your insulin infusion. A pump malfunction or obstruction of the infusion set can result in a rapid rise in glucose levels. If an interruption to insulin flow is suspected, follow the instructions in the product literature and, if appropriate, notify your health care professional. When used with an insulin infusion pump, Humalog should not be mixed with any other insulin.

Marketing authorisation holder: Eli Lilly Nederland BV, Krijtwal 17–23, 3432 ZT Nieuwegein, The Netherlands.

Marketing authorisation numbers

Vials:	EU/1/96/007/002
Cartridges 1.5 ml:	EU/1/96/007/003
Cartridges 3.0 ml:	EU/1/96/007/004

Date of approval/revision of SPC June 1998

Legal category POM

Package quantities 10 ml glass vials – single vials. 1.5 ml glass cartridges – packs of 5. 3 ml glass cartridges – packs of 5.

HUMATROPE* VIALS AND CARTRIDGES

Qualitative and quantitative composition

Humatrope Vials

4iu (1.33 mg) Product (a) Humatrope: Each vial of powder for injection contains 1.33 mg somatropin equivalent to 4iu.

(b) Diluent
Each vial contains 2 ml.

16iu (5.33 mg) Product

(a) Humatrope
Each vial of powder for injection contains 5.33 mg somatropin equivalent to 16iu.

(b) Diluent
Each vial contains 8 ml.

Humatrope Cartridges

(a) Humatrope
Three presentations of Humatrope cartridges are available, containing 6 mg, 12 mg or 24 mg of somatropin. Equivalent to 18, 36 or 72iu somatropin, respectively.

(b) Diluent
Each cartridge is supplied in a combination package with an accompanying syringe containing 3.15 ml of diluting solution.

(c) Humatro-Pen II
The pen allows the dose to be dialled in increments of 0.04 ml. The maximum volume that can be administered as a single injection is 0.6 ml. The incremental concentration and maximum injectable dose for each cartridge are shown in the following table.

Cartridge	*Humatrope/ 0.04 ml*	*Maximum injectable dose*
18iu (6 mg)	0.25iu	3.75iu
36iu (12 mg)	0.50iu	7.50iu
72iu (24 mg)	1.00iu	15.00iu

Pharmaceutical form Humatrope is presented as a powder for injection in either vials or cartridges made of Type I glass.

Clinical particulars

Therapeutic indications

Paediatric patients: Humatrope is indicated for the long–term treatment of children who have growth failure due to an inadequate secretion of normal endogenous growth hormone.

Humatrope is also indicated for the treatment of short stature in children with Turner's Syndrome, confirmed by chromosome analysis.

Adult patients: Humatrope is indicated for replacement therapy in adults with pronounced growth hormone deficiency as diagnosed in 2 different dynamic tests for growth hormone deficiency.

Patients must also fulfil the following criteria:

Childhood onset: Patients who were diagnosed as growth hormone deficient during childhood, must be retested and their growth hormone deficiency confirmed before replacement therapy with Humatrope is started.

Adult onset: Patients must have growth hormone deficiency as a result of hypothalamic or pituitary disease and at least one other hormone deficiency diagnosed (except for prolactin) and adequate replacement therapy instituted, before replacement therapy using growth hormone may begin.

Posology and method of administration: Humatrope in vials is administered by subcutaneous or intramuscular injection after reconstitution.

Humatrope in cartridges is administered by subcutaneous injection after reconstitution. The dosage and administration schedule should be personalised for each individual; however, for

Growth hormone deficient paediatric patients: The recommended dosage is 0.07–0.10iu (0.025–0.035 mg)/kg of body weight per day by subcutaneous or intramuscular injection. This is the equivalent to approximately 2.1–3.0iu (0.7–1.0 mg)/m^2 body surface area per day.

Growth hormone deficient adult patients: The recommended dosage at the start of therapy is 0.018iu (0.006 mg)/kg of body weight per day given as a subcutaneous injection. This dose should be gradually increased, according to individual patient requirements, to a maximum of 0.036iu (0.012 mg)/kg per day. Side-effects of the patients, as well as determination of insulin-like growth factor (IGF-1) in serum, should be used as guidance for dose titration. The minimum effective dose should be used and dose requirements may decline with increasing age. The dosage of somatropin should be decreased in cases of persistent oedema or severe paresthesia, in order to avoid the development of carpal tunnel syndrome.

Patients with Turner's Syndrome: The recommended dosage is 0.14iu (0.045–0.050 mg)/kg of body weight per day given as a subcutaneous injection to be administered preferably in the evening. This is equivalent to approximately 4.3iu (1.4 mg)/m^2 per day.

The subcutaneous injection sites should be varied in order to avoid lipo–atrophy.

Contra-indications

(a) Humatrope should not be used when there is any evidence of activity of a tumour. Intracranial lesions must be inactive and antitumour therapy complete prior to the institution of growth hormone therapy. Humatrope should be discontinued if there is evidence of tumour growth.

(b) Humatrope should not be reconstituted with the supplied diluent for patients with a known sensitivity to either *m*–cresol or glycerol.

(c) Humatrope should not be used for growth promotion in children with closed epiphyses.

Special warnings and special precautions for use: (a) Previous paediatric subjects who had been treated with growth hormone during childhood, until final height was attained, should be re-evaluated for growth hormone deficiency after epiphyseal closure before replacement therapy is commenced at the doses recommended for adults.

(b) If sensitivity to the accompanying diluent occurs, the vials may be reconstituted with Sterile Water for Injection. When Humatrope is reconstituted in this manner, use only one reconstituted dose per vial, discard any unused portion. Refrigerate the solution at 2-8°C if it is not to be used immediately after reconstitution. Use the reconstituted dose within 24 hours.

(c) Diagnosis and therapy with Humatrope should be initiated and monitored by physicians who are appropriately qualified and experienced in the diagnosis and management of patients with growth hormone deficiency.

(d) Patients with growth hormone deficiency secondary to an intracranial lesion should be examined frequently for progression or recurrence of the underlying disease process.

(e) In cases of severe or recurrent headache, visual problems, nausea and/or vomiting, a fundoscopy for papilloedema is recommended. If papilloedema is confirmed, a diagnosis of benign intracranial hypertension should be considered and, if appropriate, the growth hormone treatment should be discontinued.

At present there is insufficient evidence to guide clinical decision making in patients with resolved intracranial hypertension. If growth hormone treatment is restarted, careful monitoring for symptoms of intracranial hypertension is necessary.

(f) Patients with endocrine disorders, including growth hormone deficiency, may develop slipped capital epiphyses more frequently. Any child with the onset of a limp during growth hormone therapy should be evaluated.

(g) If injected subcutaneously, the injection sites should be rotated to minimise the risk of lipo-atrophy occurring.

(h) A state of hypothyroidism may develop during somatropin treatment. In patients with (pan)hypopituitarism, standard replacement therapy must be closely monitored.

(i) For paediatric patients, the treatment should be continued until the end of the growth has been reached. It is advisable not to exceed the recommended dosage in view of the potential risks of acromegaly, hyperglycaemia and glucosuria.

(j) After intramuscular injection, hypoglycaemia may appear. Therefore, the recommended dosage should be accurately checked in case of intramuscular injection.

(k) Experience with patients above 60 years is lacking.

(l) Experience with prolonged treatment in adults is lacking.

Interaction with other medicaments and other forms of interaction

(a) Because human growth hormone may induce a state of insulin resistance, patients should be monitored for evidence of glucose intolerance.

(b) Subjects with diabetes mellitus should be carefully monitored during treatment with Humatrope. An adjustment of the insulin dose may be required.

(c) Excessive glucocorticoid therapy will inhibit the growth promoting effect of human growth hormone. Patients with coexisting ACTH deficiency should have their glucocorticoid replacement dose carefully adjusted to avoid an inhibitory effect on growth.

Pregnancy and lactation: Animal reproduction studies have not been conducted with Humatrope. It is not known whether Humatrope can cause foetal harm when administered to a pregnant woman or can affect reproduction capacity. Humatrope should be given to a pregnant woman only if clearly needed.

There have been no studies conducted with Humatrope in nursing mothers. It is not known whether this drug is excreted in human milk. Because many drugs are excreted in human milk, caution should be exercised when Humatrope is administered to a nursing woman.

Effects on the ability to drive and use machines: Humatrope has no known effect on ability to drive or use machines.

Undesirable effects

Paediatric patients: In clinical trials with growth hormone deficient patients, approximately 2% of the patients developed antibodies to growth hormone. In trials in Turner's Syndrome where higher doses were used, up to 8% of patients developed antibodies to growth hormone. The binding capacity of these antibodies was low and growth rate was not affected adversely. Testing for antibodies to growth hormone should be carried out in any patient who fails to respond to therapy.

In clinical studies in which high doses of Humatrope were administered to healthy adult volunteers, the following events occurred infrequently: headache, localised muscle pain, weakness, mild hyperglycaemia and glucosuria.

In studies with growth hormone deficient children, injection site pain was reported infrequently. A mild and transient oedema, which appeared in 2.5% of patients, was observed early during the course of treatment.

Leukaemia has been reported in a small number of children who have been treated with growth hormone of pituitary origin and somatrem and Humatrope. The relationship, if any, between leukaemia and growth hormone therapy is uncertain.

Some rare cases of benign intracranial hypertension have been reported.

Adult patients: Side-effects, possibly related to the biological action or dosage of growth hormone, include: oedema (local and generalised), joint pain and disorder, muscle pain, paraesthesia and hypertension.

In patients with adult onset growth hormone deficiency, oedema, muscle pain, and joint pain and disorder were reported early in therapy and tended to be transient.

Adult patients treated with growth hormone, following diagnosis of growth hormone deficiency in childhood, reported side-effects less frequently than those with adult onset growth hormone deficiency.

Overdose: Acute overdose could lead initially to hypoglycaemia and subsequently to hyperglycaemia. Long-term overdosage could result in signs and symptoms of acromegaly consistent with the known effects of excess human growth hormone.

Pharmacological properties

Pharmacodynamic properties: Humatrope is a polypeptide hormone of recombinant DNA origin. It has 191 amino acid residues and a molecular weight of 22,125 daltons. The amino acid sequence of the product is identical to that of human growth hormone of pituitary origin. Humatrope is synthesised in a strain of *Escherichia coli* that has been modified by the addition of the gene for human growth hormone.

The biological effects of Humatrope are equivalent to human growth hormone of pituitary origin.

The most prominent effect of Humatrope is that it stimulates the growth plates of long bones. Additionally, it promotes cellular protein synthesis and nitrogen retention.

Humatrope stimulates lipid metabolism: it increases plasma fatty acids and HDL-cholesterols and decreases total plasma cholesterol. Humatrope therapy has a beneficial effect on body composition in growth hormone deficient patients, in that body fat stores are reduced and lean body mass is increased. Long-term therapy in growth hormone deficient patients increases bone mineral density.

Humatrope may induce insulin resistance. Large doses of human growth hormone may impair glucose tolerance.

The data available from clinical trials so far in patients with Turner's Syndrome indicate that, while some patients may not respond to this therapy, an increase over predicted height has been observed, the average being 3.3 ± 3.9cm.

Pharmacokinetic properties: The bioavailability of Humatrope is the same whether presented in vials or cartridges. A dose of 100 micrograms/kg to adult male volunteers will give a peak serum level (C_{max}) of about 55ng/ml, a half-life ($t^1/_2$) of nearly four hours and maximal absorption (AUC [0 to ∞]) of about 475ng/hr/ml.

Preclinical safety data: Humatrope is human growth hormone produced by recombinant technology. No serious events have been reported in subchronic toxicology studies. Long-term animal studies for carcinogenicity and impairment of fertility with this human growth hormone (Humatrope) have not been performed. There has been no evidence to date of Humatrope induced mutagenicity.

Pharmaceutical particulars

List of excipients

Humatrope Vials: Humatrope: In addition to somatropin, each vial will contain (a) mannitol, (b) glycine, (c) dibasic sodium phosphate, (d) phosphoric acid and (e) sodium hydroxide if necessary.

These are included respectively as (a) carrier and stabiliser, (b) stabiliser, (c) buffering agent, (d) and (e) adjustment of pH during manufacture if necessary.

Diluent: Each diluent vial will contain (a) glycerol, (b) 3.0 mg/ml *m*-cresol, (c) Water for Injection, (d) hydrochloric acid and (e) sodium hydroxide if necessary.

These are included respectively as (a) tonicity modifier, (b) preservative, (c) solvent, (d) and (e) adjustment of pH during manufacture if necessary.

Humatrope Cartridges: Humatrope: Each cartridge will contain a lyophilised plug composed of somatropin and the following excipients: (a) glycine, (b) mannitol, (c) dibasic sodium phosphate, (d) phosphoric acid and (e) sodium hydroxide if necessary.

These are included respectively as (a) stabiliser, (b) carrier and stabiliser, (c) buffering agent, (d) and (e) adjustment of pH during manufacture if necessary.

Diluent: Each diluent syringe will contain (a) 1.7%, 0.29% and 0.29% glycerol in the 18iu (6 mg), 36iu (12 mg) and 72iu (24 mg) cartridges, respectively; (b) 0.3% *m*-cresol; (c) Water for Injection; (d) hydrochloric acid and (e) sodium hydroxide if necessary.

These are included respectively as (a) tonicity modifier, (b) preservative, (c) solvent, (d) and (e) adjustment of pH during manufacture if necessary.

Incompatibilities: There are no known incompatibilities with Humatrope.

Shelf-life

Humatrope Vials: Before reconstitution: The combination pack of Humatrope and diluent has a shelf-life of 24 months when stored at 2 to 8°C.

After reconstitution: Vials of Humatrope are stable for up to 14 days when reconstituted with diluent for Humatrope and stored at 2 to 8°C.

Humatrope Cartridges: Before reconstitution: Combination pack (cartridge plus diluent syringe): 24 months at 2–8°C.

After reconstitution: Cartridges of Humatrope are stable for up to 28 days when reconstituted with diluent for Humatrope and stored at 2 to 8°C. Daily room temperature exposure should not exceed 30 minutes.

Special precautions for storage: Avoid freezing the diluent and reconstituted drug.

Nature and contents of container

Humatrope Vials: Vials: Humatrope is presented in Type I flint glass vials with rubber stoppers. Humatrope is a white or almost white powder. The presentations are 4iu (1.33 mg) and 16iu (5.33 mg).

Diluent: The diluent is a clear solution and is presented in Type I flint glass with rubber stoppers. Diluent vials contain 2 ml and 8 ml.

Humatrope Cartridges: Cartridges: Humatrope is presented in Type I flint glass cartridges that have been siliconised. The cartridges are fitted with a siliconised rubber plunger and a halobutyl rubber closure, which are secured in place with a plastic lyocap. Humatrope is a white or almost white powder. Humatrope cartridges contain 18iu (6 mg), 36iu (12 mg) or 72iu (24 mg) somatropin.

Diluent: The diluent is a clear solution and is presented in Type I flint glass syringes that have been siliconised. The syringes are fitted with siliconised Teflon faced halobutyl rubber plungers. A diluent syringe contains 3.15 ml formulation, all of which is used to reconstitute one Humatrope cartridge.

Instructions for use/handling

Humatrope Vials: Reconstitution: The diluent should be injected into the vial of Humatrope by aiming the stream of liquid against the glass wall. Following reconstitution, the vial should be swirled with a GENTLE rotary motion until the contents are completely dissolved. DO NOT SHAKE. The resulting solution should be clear, without particulated matter. If the solution is cloudy or contains particulated matter, the contents MUST NOT be injected.

Before and after injection, the septum of the vial should be wiped with alcohol to prevent contamination of the contents by repeated needle insertions.

Sterile disposable syringes and needles should be used for administration of Humatrope. The volume of the syringe should be small enough so that the prescribed dose can be withdrawn from the vial with reasonable accuracy.

Humatrope Cartridges: Reconstitution: Each cartridge of Humatrope should be reconstituted using the accompanying diluent syringe and the diluent connector. To reconstitute, attach the diluent connector to the cartridge and then inject the entire contents of the pre-filled diluent syringe into the cartridge. The diluent connector automatically aims the stream of liquid against the glass wall of the cartridge. Following reconstitution, the cartridge should be gently rocked back and forth until the contents are completely dissolved. DO NOT SHAKE. The resulting solution should be clear, without particulate matter. If the solution is cloudy or contains particulate matter, the contents MUST NOT be injected.

The cartridges have been designed for use only with the Humatro-Pen II. The diluent connector is for single use only. Discard it after use. A sterile needle should be used for each administration of Humatrope.

Marketing authorisation numbers

Vials 4iu:	0006/0237
Vials 16iu:	0006/0263
Cartridges 18iu:	0006/0297
Cartridges 36iu:	0006/0298
Cartridges 72iu:	0006/0299
Diluent:	0006/0254
Diluent (36 and 72iu):	0006/0300

Date of approval/revision of SPC September 1998

Legal category POM

Package quantities Single vials and single cartridges.

HUMULIN* VIALS AND CARTRIDGES
HUMULIN* S (Soluble)
HUMULIN* I (Isophane)
HUMULIN* LENTE
HUMULIN* ZN (Zinc)
HUMULIN* M1 (Mixture 1)
HUMULIN* M2 (Mixture 2)
HUMULIN* M3 (Mixture 3)
HUMULIN* M4 (Mixture 4)
HUMULIN* M5 (Mixture 5)

Qualitative and quantitative composition

Active Ingredient	*Quantity per ml*
Human Insulin (recombinant DNA origin)	100IU

Humulin Soluble is a sterile, clear, colourless, aqueous solution of human insulin adjusted to a pH range of 7.0 to 7.8.

Humulin Soluble is a rapidly acting insulin preparation.

Humulin Isophane is a sterile suspension of a white, crystalline precipitate of isophane human insulin in an isotonic phosphate buffer adjusted to a pH range of 6.9 to 7.5.

Humulin Isophane is an intermediate acting insulin preparation.

Humulin Mixture 1, Mixture 2, Mixture 3, Mixture 4 and Mixture 5 are sterile suspensions of human insulin in the proportion of 10%, 20%, 30%, 40% and 50% soluble insulin to 90%, 80%, 70%, 60% and 50% isophane insulin, respectively, adjusted to a pH range of 6.9 to 7.5.

Humulin Mixtures are intermediate acting insulin preparations.

Humulin Lente is a sterile suspension of human insulin zinc suspension in the proportion of 30% amorphous and 70% crystalline, adjusted to a pH range of 7.0 to 7.8.

Humulin Lente is an intermediate acting insulin preparation.

Humulin Zinc is a sterile, white suspension of crystalline human insulin zinc suspension, adjusted to a pH range of 7.0 to 7.8.

Humulin Zinc is a longer acting insulin preparation.

Pharmaceutical form A solution or suspension for injection filled into:

A. *Cartridges* administered via a reusable device.

The 1.5 ml or 3 ml prefilled cartridge to be used with a CE marked pen, as recommended in the information provided by the device manufacturer. All pen injection delivery systems are designed to deliver insulin by parenteral administration.

B. *Vials*

A 10 ml vial of human insulin for parenteral administration.

Clinical particulars

Therapeutic indications: For the treatment of patients with diabetes mellitus who require insulin for the maintenance of glucose homeostasis. Humulin is also indicated for the initial control of diabetes mellitus and diabetes mellitus in pregnancy.

Posology and method of administration: The dosage should be determined by the physician, according to the requirement of the patient.

Humulin Soluble should be given by subcutaneous injection but may, although not recommended, also be given by intramuscular injection. It may also be administered intravenously.

Humulin Isophane, Mixtures, Lente and Zinc in vials and Humulin Isophane and Mixtures in cartridge presentations should be given by subcutaneous injection but may, although not recommended, also be given by intramuscular injection. These formulations should not be administered intravenously.

Subcutaneous administration should be in the upper arms, thighs, buttocks or abdomen. Use of injection sites should be rotated so that the same site is not used more than approximately once a month.

Care should be taken when injecting any Humulin insulin preparations to ensure that a blood vessel has not been entered. After any insulin injection, the injection site should not be massaged.

Humulin Isophane, Humulin Lente and Humulin Zinc may be administered in combination with Humulin Soluble. (See *Special warnings and special precautions for use - Mixing of insulins.*)

Humulin Mixture formulations are ready-made defined mixtures of Humulin Soluble and Humulin Isophane insulin designed to avoid the need for the patient to mix insulin preparations. A patient's treatment regimen should be based on their individual metabolic requirements.

Contra-indications: Hypoglycaemia.

Hypersensitivity to Humulin or to the formulation excipients.

Under no circumstances should any Humulin formulation, other than Humulin Soluble, be given intravenously.

Special warnings and special precautions for use: *Transferring from other insulins:* A small number of patients transferring from insulins of animal origin may require a reduced dosage and/or a change in the ratio of soluble to intermediate preparations, especially if they are very tightly controlled and bordering on hypoglycaemia. The dosage reduction may occur immediately after transfer or be a gradual process lasting for several weeks. There is a risk of hypoglycaemia if insulin requirement is decreased, and both the physician and the patient should be aware of this possibility. The risk can be considered minimal if the daily dosage is less than 40IU. Insulin-resistant patients receiving more than 100IU daily should be referred to hospital for transfer.

A few patients who experienced hypoglycaemic reactions after transfer to human insulin have reported that the early warning symptoms were less pronounced or different from those experienced with their previous animal insulin. Patients whose blood glucose control is greatly improved, eg, by intensified insulin therapy, may lose some or all of the warning symptoms of hypoglycaemia and should be advised accordingly. Other conditions which may make the early warning symptoms of hypoglycaemia different or less pronounced include long duration of diabetes, diabetic nerve disease, or medications such as beta blockers. Uncorrected hypoglycaemic and hyperglycaemic reactions can cause loss of consciousness, coma or death.

Insulin requirements may change significantly in diseases of the adrenal, pituitary or thyroid glands, and in the presence of renal or hepatic impairment.

Insulin requirements may be increased during illness or emotional disturbances.

Adjustment of insulin dosage may also be necessary if patients undertake increased physical activity or change their usual diet.

Mixing of insulins: The shorter acting insulin should be drawn into the syringe first, to prevent contamination of the vial by the longer acting preparation. It is advisable to inject directly after mixing. However, if a delay is necessary, a consistent routine must be followed.

Alternatively a separate syringe, or separate cartridges of Humulin Soluble and Isophane, can be used for administration of the correct amount of each formulation.

Interactions with other medicaments and other forms of interaction: The patient should check with their physician when using other medicines in addition to Humulin.

Insulin requirements may be reduced by the concurrent administration of drugs with hypoglycaemic activity, e.g. alcohol, monoamine oxidase inhibitors and beta-adrenergic blockers or aspirin.

Insulin requirements may be increased by concurrent administration of drugs, e.g. oral contraceptives, corticosteroids or thyroid hormone replacement therapy.

The effects of mixing human insulin with insulins of animal origin have not been studied and this practice is not recommended.

Pregnancy and lactation: It is essential to maintain good control of the insulin treated (insulin-dependent or gestational diabetes) patient throughout pregnancy. Insulin requirements usually fall during the first trimester and increase during the second and third trimesters. Patients with diabetes should be advised to inform their doctors if they are pregnant or are contemplating pregnancy.

Diabetic patients who are lactating may require adjustments in insulin dose and/or diet.

Effects on ability to drive and use machines: Use of the correct therapeutic dose has no known effect on driving or the use of machinery.

Undesirable effects: Lipodystrophy, insulin resistance and hypersensitivity reactions are among the side-effects associated with insulins of animal origin. However, the incidence of such side-effects with Humulin is minimal. In the rare event of a severe allergy to Humulin, treatment is required immediately. A change of insulin or desensitisation may be required.

Hypoglycaemia is the most frequent undesirable

TIME-ACTION PROFILES

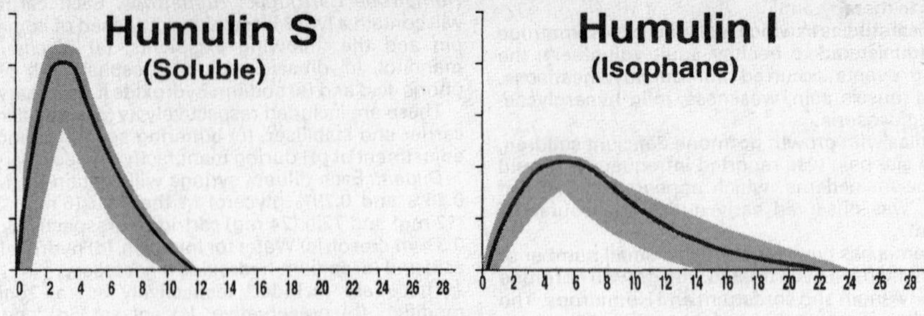

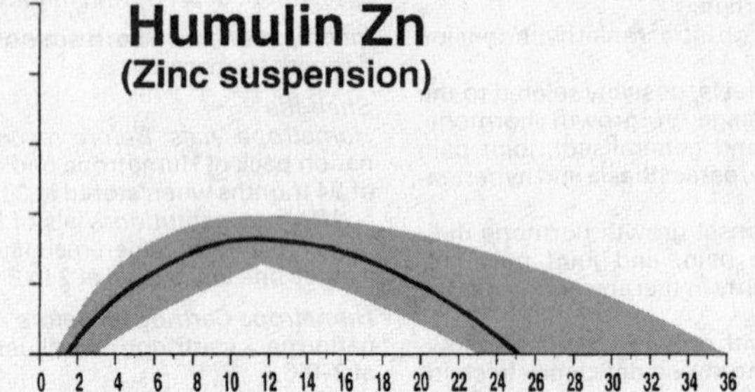

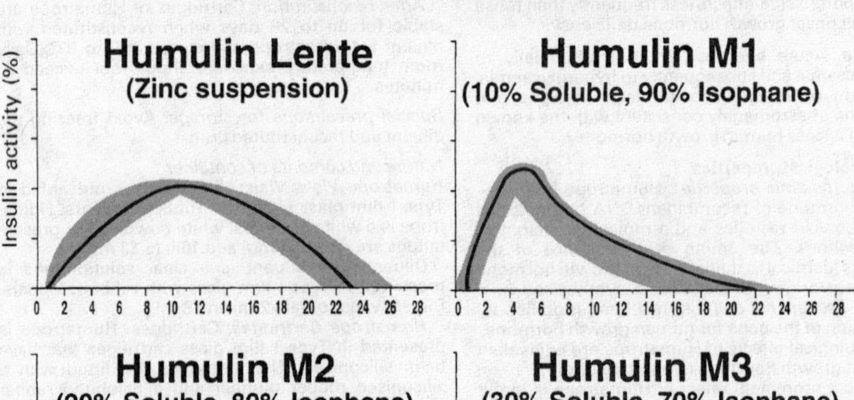

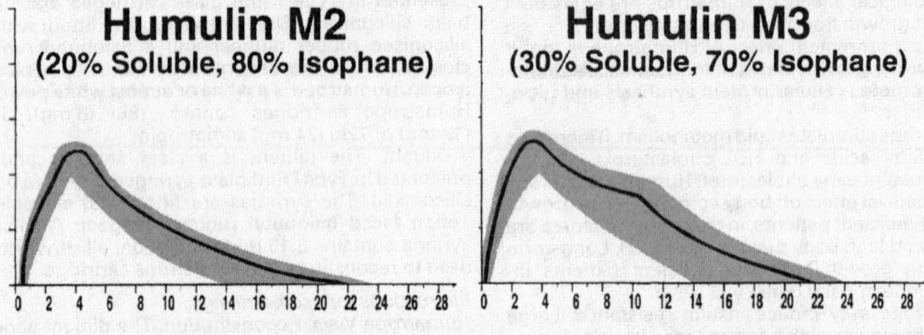

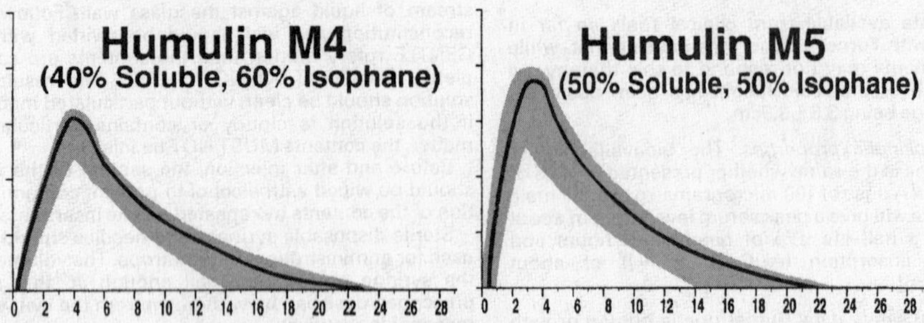

Time (hours)

effect that a diabetic may suffer. Severe hypoglycaemia may lead to loss of consciousness, and in extreme cases, death.

Overdose: Insulin has no specific overdose definitions, because serum glucose concentrations are a result of complex interactions between insulin levels, glucose availability and other metabolic processes. Hypoglycaemia may occur as a result of an excess of insulin relative to food intake and energy expenditure.

Hypoglycaemia may be associated with listlessness, confusion, palpitations, headache, sweating and vomiting.

Mild hypoglycaemic episodes will respond to oral administration of glucose or sugar products.

Correction of moderately severe hypoglycaemia can be accomplished by intramuscular or subcutaneous administration of glucagon, followed by oral carbohydrate when the patient recovers sufficiently. Patients who fail to respond to glucagon must be given glucose solution intravenously.

If the patient is comatose, glucagon should be administered intramuscularly or subcutaneously. However, glucose solution must be given intravenously if glucagon is not available or if the patient fails to respond to glucagon. The patient should be given a meal as soon as consciousness is recovered.

Pharmacological properties

Pharmacodynamic properties: The prime activity of insulin is the regulation of glucose metabolism.

In addition, insulin has several anabolic and anti-catabolic actions on a variety of different tissues. Within muscle tissue this includes increasing glycogen, fatty acid, glycerol and protein synthesis and amino acid uptake, while decreasing glycogenolysis, glyconeogenesis, ketogenesis, lipolysis, protein catabolism and amino acid output.

The typical activity profile (glucose utilisation curve) following subcutaneous injection is illustrated below by the heavy line. Variations that a patient may experience in timing and/or intensity of insulin activity are illustrated by the shaded area. Individual variability will depend on factors such as size of dose, site of injection temperature and physical activity of the patient.

Pharmacokinetic properties: The pharmacokinetics of insulin do not reflect the metabolic action of that hormone. Therefore, it is more appropriate to examine glucose utilisation curves (as discussed above) when considering the activity of insulin.

Preclinical safety data: Humulin is human insulin produced by recombinant technology. No serious events have been reported in subchronic toxicology studies.

Pharmaceutical particulars

List of excipients:
For Humulin Soluble preparations: Each will contain Human Insulin (recombinant DNA origin) and the following excipients:

a. *m*-Cresol distilled, 2.5 mg/ml; b. glycerol; c. water for injections; d. hydrochloric acid; and e. sodium hydroxide.

These are included as:

a. preservative; b. tonicity modifier; c. solvent; d. pH adjustment; and e. pH adjustment, respectively.

Hydrochloric acid and/or sodium hydroxide may have been used during manufacture to adjust the pH.

For Humulin Isophane and Mixture preparations: Each will contain Human Insulin (recombinant DNA origin) and the following excipients:

a. *m*-Cresol distilled, 1.6 mg/ml; b. glycerol; c. phenol, 0.65 mg/ml; d. protamine sulphate; e. dibasic sodium phosphate; f. zinc oxide; g. water for injections; h. hydrochloric acid; and i. sodium hydroxide.

These are included as:

a. preservative; b. tonicity modifier; c. preservative; d. complexes with insulin to prolong its action; e. buffer; f. adjust zinc content; g. solvent; h. pH adjustment; and i. pH adjustment, respectively.

Hydrochloric acid and/or sodium hydroxide may have been used during manufacture to adjust the pH.

For Humulin Lente and Zinc preparations: Each will contain Human Insulin (recombinant DNA origin) and the following excipients:

a. Sodium acetate; b. sodium chloride; c. methyl parahydroxybenzoate, 1 mg/ml; d. water for injections; e. zinc oxide; f. hydrochloric acid; and g. sodium hydroxide.

These are included as:

a. buffering agent; b. tonicity modifier; c. preservative; d. solvent; e. adjust zinc content; f. pH adjustment; and g. pH adjustment, respectively.

Hydrochloric acid and/or sodium hydroxide may have been used during manufacture to adjust the pH.

Incompatibilities: Humulin products should not be mixed with either animal insulins or human insulin preparations produced by other manufacturers.

Shelf-life: The shelf-life for Humulin Soluble, Isophane, Zinc and Mixture presentations is two years when stored under appropriate conditions.

The shelf-life for Humulin Lente is eighteen months.

The in-use shelf-life for all Humulin vials, Humulin Soluble and Mixture 50/50 in 1.5 ml cartridges and all Humulin 3.0 ml cartridges is 28 days.

The in-use shelf-life for Humulin Isophane and Mixtures 10/90, 20/80, 30/70 and 40/60 in 1.5 ml cartridges is 21 days.

Special precautions for storage: Humulin preparations should be stored in a refrigerator between 2° and 8°C. They should not be frozen or exposed to excessive heat or sunlight.

When in use the Humulin vials, Humulin Soluble and 50/50 1.5 ml cartridges and Humulin 3.0 ml cartridges may be kept at room temperature for up to 28 days.

When in use the Humulin Isophane and Mixtures 10/90, 20/80, 30/70 and 40/60 1.5 ml cartridges may be kept at room temperature for up to 21 days.

Nature and contents of container:
Humulin vials: The product is filled in vials that comply with the requirements of the Ph. Eur. for Type I flint glass, stoppered with rubber closures and sealed with aluminium seals combined with a plastic 'flip top'.

Humulin cartridges: The product is filled in cartridges that comply with the requirements of the Ph. Eur. for Type I flint glass, and sealed with rubber closures consisting of a plunger head at the bottom and a disk seal at the top of the cartridge.

Package quantities

10 ml glass vials - single vials.
1.5 ml glass cartridges in packs of 5.
3.0 ml glass cartridges in packs of 5 (Humulin M5 is not available in 3.0 ml cartridges).

Instructions for use/handling:
(a) Preparing a dose: Vials or cartridges containing Humulin Soluble formulation do not require resuspension and should only be used if it is clear, colourless, with no solid particles visible and if it is of water-like appearance.

Vials containing Humulin Isophane, Mixtures, Lente and Zinc formulations should be rotated in the palms of the hands before use to resuspend the insulin. Cartridges containing Humulin Isophane and Mixture formulations should be rolled in the palms of the hands ten times and inverted 180° ten times immediately before use to resuspend the insulin until it appears uniformly cloudy or milky. Do not shake vigorously as this may cause frothing which may interfere with the correct measurement of the dose.

The cartridges and vials should be examined frequently and should not be used if clumps of material are present or if solid white particles stick to the bottom or wall of the cartridge or vial, giving a frosted appearance.

Humulin cartridges are not designed to allow any other insulin to be mixed in the cartridge. Cartridges are not designed to be refilled.

Vials: Prepare your syringe prior to injection, as directed by your doctor or diabetic nurse.

Cartridges: Reusable devices.

The manufacturer's instructions should be followed for loading the cartridge and attaching the needle.

(b) Injecting a dose:
Vials: Inject the correct dose of insulin, as directed by your doctor or diabetic nurse.

Cartridges:

1. Wash your hands.
2. Choose a site for the injection.
3. Clean the skin with an alcohol swab.
4. Remove outer needle cap.
5. Stabilise the skin by spreading it or pinching up a large area. Insert the needle as instructed by your doctor.
6. Inject the insulin according to the instructions of the pen manufacturer.
7. Pull the needle straight out of the skin and apply gentle pressure over the injection site for several seconds. Do not rub the area.
8. Using the outer needle cap, unscrew the needle immediately after injection and dispose of it safely. Removing the needle immediately after injection ensures sterility, prevents leakage and re-entry of air and potential needle clogs.
9. Replace the cap on the pen.

(c) Disposal of used containers and needles
Do not reuse needles. Dispose of the needle in a responsible manner. Needles and pens must not be shared. Vials and cartridges can be used until empty, then properly discard or recycle.

Marketing authorisation numbers

Humulin S vial:	0006/0216
Humulin I vial:	0006/0228
Humulin Lente vial:	0006/0224
Humulin Zn vial:	0006/0226
Humulin M1 vial:	0006/0220
Humulin M2 vial:	0006/0222
Humulin M3 vial:	0006/0233
Humulin M4 vial:	0006/0235
Humulin M5 vial:	0006/0270
Humulin S cartridge:	0006/0242
Humulin I cartridge:	0006/0257
Humulin M1 cartridge:	0006/0258
Humulin M2 cartridge:	0006/0259
Humulin M3 cartridge:	0006/0260
Humulin M4 cartridge:	0006/0261
Humulin M5 cartridge:	0006/0312

Date of approval/revision of SPC 13 March 1998

Legal category POM

KEFADIM*

Qualitative and quantitative composition

	Vial size		
	500 mg	1 g	2 g
Active constituent:			
Ceftazidime pentahydrate	580 mg	1.16 g	2.33 g
equivalent to ceftazidime	500 mg	1.0 g	2.0 g
Other constituents:			
Sodium carbonate	59 mg	118 mg	236 mg

Pharmaceutical form Powder for injection.

Clinical particulars

Therapeutic indications: Kefadim is indicated in the treatment of the following infections when due to susceptible micro-organisms:

Lower respiratory tract infections
Skin and soft tissue infections
Bone and joint infections
Urinary tract infections
Gynaecological infections
Intra-abdominal infections, including peritonitis
Septicaemia
Central nervous system infections, including meningitis. In meningitis, it is recommended that the results of a sensitivity test are known before treatment with ceftazidime as a single agent.

Kefadim may be used alone in cases of confirmed or suspected sepsis. It may also be used concomitantly with other antibiotics, such as aminoglycosides, in severe and life-threatening infections and in the immunocompromised patient.

Posology and method of administration: Ceftazidime may be given intravenously or by deep intramuscular injection into a large muscle mass (such as the upper outer quadrant of the gluteus maximus, or lateral part of the thigh).

The guidelines for dosage of Kefadim are listed in *Table 1*.

Adults and the elderly: The usual dosage range for ceftazidime is 500 mg to 2 g every eight to twelve hours. The dosage and route of administration should be determined by the susceptibility of the causative organisms, the severity of infection, and the condition and renal function of the patient.

In view of the reduced clearance of ceftazidime in acutely ill elderly patients, the daily dosage should not normally exceed 2 g, especially in those over 80 years of age (*Table 2*).

Infants and children over 2 months of age: The dosage range is 50-150 mg/kg/day IV, in three divided doses, with a maximum of 6 g/day. The higher dose should be reserved for immunocompromised children, or children with cystic fibrosis or meningitis.

Neonates and children up to 2 months of age: The dosage range is 25 to 60 mg/kg/day, given as two divided doses. In the neonate, the serum half-life of ceftazidime can be three to four times that in adults.

Dosage in impaired renal function: Ceftazidime is excreted by the kidneys, almost exclusively by glomerular filtration. Therefore, in patients with impaired renal function (GFR <50 ml/min), it is recommended that the dose of ceftazidime should be reduced to compensate for its slower excretion. In patients with suspected renal insufficiency, an initial loading dose of 1 g may be given. An estimate of GFR should be made to determine the appropriate maintenance dose. The recommended dosage is shown in *Table 2*.

Table 1: Recommended Dosage Schedule for Kefadim

	DOSE	FREQUENCY
Adults		
Usual recommended dose	1 g IV or im	q 8 or 12 h
Uncomplicated urinary tract infections	250 mg IV or im	q 12 h
Bone and joint infections	2 g IV	q 12 h
Complicated urinary tract infections	500 mg IV or im	q 8 or 12 h
Uncomplicated pneumonia; mild skin and skin-structure infections	500 mg-1 g IV or im	q 8 h
Serious gynaecological and intra-abdominal infections	2 g IV	q 8 h
Meningitis	2 g IV	q 8 h
Very severe life-threatening infections, especially in immunocompromised patients	2 g IV	q 8 h
Pseudomonal lung infections in patients with cystic fibrosis with normal renal function*	30-50 mg/kg IV to a maximum of 6 g/day	q 8 h
Neonates and children up to 2 months	12.5-30 mg/kg IV	q 12 h
Infants and children (2 months to 12 years of age)	17-50 mg/kg IV to a maximum of 6 g/day†	q 8 h

*Although clinical improvement has been shown, complete eradication of infecting organisms cannot be expected in patients with chronic respiratory disease and cystic fibrosis.

†The higher dose should be reserved for immunocompromised children or children with cystic fibrosis or meningitis.

Table 2: Recommended Maintenance Dosage of Kefadim in Patients with Renal Insufficiency

CREATININE CLEARANCE (ML/MIN)	RECOMMENDED DOSE OF KEFADIM	FREQUENCY
50-31	1 g	q 12 h
30-16	1 g	q 24 h
15-6	500 mg	q 24 h
<5	500 mg	q 48 h

When only serum creatinine is available, the following formula (Cockcroft's equation) may be used to estimate creatinine clearance. The serum creatinine should represent a steady state of renal function:

Males:

$$\text{Creatinine clearance (ml/min)} = \frac{\text{Weight (kg)} \times (140 - \text{age in years})}{72 \times \text{serum creatinine (mg/dl)}}$$

Females:

0.85 x above value

In patients with severe infections who would normally receive 6 g of Kefadim daily, were it not for renal insufficiency, the dose in *Table 2* may be increased by 50% or the dosing frequency increased appropriately. Continued dosage should be determined by further monitoring of creatinine clearance, severity of the infection, and susceptibility of the causative organism. In such patients, it is recommended that ceftazidime serum levels should be monitored and trough levels should not exceed 40 mg/litre.

In children, as for adults, the creatinine clearance should be adjusted for body surface area or lean body mass and the dosing frequency reduced in cases of renal insufficiency.

The serum half-life of ceftazidime during haemodialysis ranges from 3 to 5 hours.

In patients undergoing haemodialysis, a loading dose of 1 g of Kefadim is recommended, followed by 1 g after each haemodialysis period. Kefadim can also be used in patients undergoing intraperitoneal and continuous ambulatory peritoneal dialysis (CAPD). In such patients, a loading dose of 1 g of Kefadim may be given, followed by 500 mg every 24 hours. In addition to intravenous use, Kefadim can be incorporated in the dialysis fluid at a concentration of 250 mg for 2 litres of dialysis fluid.

NOTE: Kefadim should generally be continued for 2 days after the signs and symptoms of infection have disappeared, however, in complicated infections, longer therapy may be required.

Intramuscular administration: Kefadim should be reconstituted with Water for Injections PhEur or 0.5% or 1% Lignocaine Hydrochloride Injection BP. Refer to *Table 3*.

Intravenous administration: For direct intermittent intravenous administration, reconstitute Kefadim with Water for Injections PhEur (see *Table 3*). Slowly inject the solution directly into the vein over a period of 3 to 5 minutes or give through the tubing of a giving set. Ceftazidime is compatible with the most commonly used intravenous fluids (see *Instructions for use/handling*).

For intravenous infusion, reconstitute the 2 g infusion (100 ml) vial with 100 ml Water for Injections PhEur or one of the compatible intravenous fluids. Alternatively, reconstitute the 500 mg, 1 g or 2 g vial and add an appropriate quantity of the resulting solution to an IV container with one of the compatible intravenous fluids.

Intermittent intravenous infusion with a Y-type giving set can be accomplished with compatible solutions. However, during infusion of a solution containing ceftazidime, it is desirable to discontinue the other solution.

Table 3: Preparation of Solutions of Kefadim

	AMOUNT OF DILUENT TO BE ADDED (ML)	APPROXIMATE AVAILABLE VOLUME (ML)	APPROXIMATE CEFTAZIDIME CONCENTRATION (MG/ML)
Intramuscular			
500 mg	1.5	1.8	280
1 g	3.0	3.6	280
Intravenous			
500 mg	5	5.3	100
1 g	10	10.6	100
2 g	10	11.2	180
Infusion (100 ml)			
2 g	100*	100	20

*Note: Addition should be in 2 stages (see *Instructions for reconstitution* below).

When Kefadim is dissolved, carbon dioxide is released and a positive pressure develops. For ease of use, please follow the recommended techniques of reconstitution described below.

Instructions for reconstitution:
For 500 mg im/IV, 1 g im/IV, and 2 g IV vials:

1. Inject the diluent and shake well to dissolve. The vials may contain a vacuum to assist injection of the diluent.
2. Carbon dioxide is released as the antibiotic dissolves, generating pressure within the vial. The solution will become clear within 1 to 2 minutes.
3. Invert the vial and completely depress the syringe plunger prior to insertion.
4. Insert the needle through the vial stopper. Be sure the needle remains within the solution and withdraw contents of the vial in the usual manner. Pressure in the vial may aid withdrawal.
5. The withdrawn solution may contain carbon dioxide bubbles, which should be expelled from the syringe before injection.

For 2 g infusion vials:

1. Inject 10 ml of the diluent and shake to dissolve. The vials may contain a vacuum to assist injection of the diluent.
2. Carbon dioxide is released as the antibiotic dissolves, generating pressure within the vial. The solution will become clear within 1 to 2 minutes.
3. Insert a vent needle to release pressure before adding additional diluent to the vial. Add diluent and then remove the vent needle.
4. Additional pressure that may develop in the vial, especially after storage, should be relieved prior to administration to the patient.

NOTE: To preserve product sterility, it is important that a gas relief needle is *not* inserted through the vial closure before the product has dissolved.

Contra-indications: Ceftazidime is contra-indicated in patients with known hypersensitivity to ceftazidime or cephalosporin antibiotics.

Special warnings and special precautions for use:
Warnings: Before therapy with ceftazidime is instituted, careful inquiry should be made to determine whether the patient has had previous hypersensitivity reactions to ceftazidime, cephalosporins, penicillins, or other drugs. Ceftazidime should be given only with special caution to patients with type 1 or immediate hypersensitivity reactions to penicillin. If an allergic reaction to ceftazidime occurs, discontinue the drug. Serious acute hypersensitivity reactions may require adrenaline, hydrocortisone, antihistamine, or other emergency measures.

Pseudomembranous colitis has been reported with the use of ceftazidime, other cephalosporins and virtually all broad-spectrum antibiotics, therefore, it is important to consider its diagnosis in patients who develop diarrhoea in association with antibiotic use. Such colitis may range in severity from mild to life-threatening. Symptoms can appear during or after treatment.

Mild cases of pseudomembranous colitis usually respond to drug discontinuance alone. In moderate to severe cases, appropriate measures should be taken.

Precautions: Kefadim has not been shown to be nephrotoxic, however, because high and prolonged serum antibiotic concentrations can occur from usual doses in patients with transient or persistent reduction of urinary output because of renal insufficiency, the total daily dosage should be reduced when ceftazidime is administered to such patients to avoid the clinical consequences, eg, seizures due to elevated levels of antibiotics (see *Posology and method of administration*). Continued dosage should be determined by degree of renal impairment, severity of infection and susceptibility of causative organisms.

As with other antibiotics, prolonged use of Kefadim may result in the overgrowth of non-susceptible organisms. Repeated evaluation of the patient's condition is essential. If superinfection occurs during therapy, appropriate measures should be taken.

Kefadim should be used with caution in individuals with a history of gastro-intestinal disease, particularly colitis.

Ceftazidime does not interfere with enzyme-based tests for glycosuria. Slight interference with copper reduction methods (Benedict's, Fehling's, Clinitest) may be observed.

Interaction with other medicaments and other forms of interaction: Nephrotoxicity has been reported following concomitant administration of cephalosporins and aminoglycoside antibiotics or potent diuretics, such as frusemide. Renal function should be carefully monitored, especially if higher dosages of the aminoglycosides are to be administered or if therapy is prolonged, because of the potential nephrotoxicity and ototoxicity of aminoglycoside antibiotics. Nephrotoxicity and ototoxicity were not noted when Kefadim was given alone in clinical trials.

Pregnancy and lactation: Reproduction studies have been performed in mice and rats at doses up to 40 times the human dose and have revealed no evidence of impaired fertility or harm to the foetus due to Kefadim. There are, however, no controlled studies in pregnant women. As animal reproduction studies are not always predictive of human response, this drug should be used during pregnancy only if clearly needed.

Ceftazidime is excreted in human milk in low concentrations and consequently caution should be exercised when ceftazidime is administered to a nursing woman.

Effects on ability to drive and use machines: Not applicable.

Undesirable effects: Clinical trial experience has shown that Kefadim is generally well tolerated. The most common side-effects were local reactions following intravenous injection and allergic and gastro-intestinal reactions.

Local effects: Phlebitis or thrombophlebitis, and inflammation at the site of injection.

Hypersensitivity: Pruritus, rash and fever. Angioedema and anaphylaxis (bronchospasm and/or hypotension) have been reported very rarely.

Gastro-intestinal: Diarrhoea, nausea, vomiting and abdominal pain, pseudomembranous colitis (see *Warnings*). Very rarely, oral thrush.

Central nervous system: Headache, dizziness, paraesthesias and bad taste. There have been reports of neurological sequelae, including tremor, myoclonica, convulsions and encephalopathy, in patients with renal impairment in whom the dose of ceftazidime has not been appropriately reduced.

Miscellaneous: Candidiasis and vaginitis.

Laboratory test changes (usually transient): Eosinophilia, positive Coombs' test without haemolysis, thrombocytosis and slight elevations in one or more hepatic enzymes: AST (SGOT), ALT (SGPT), LDH, GGT and alkaline phosphatase. Transient elevations of blood urea, blood urea nitrogen and/or serum creatinine have been observed occasionally. Transient leucopenia, neutropenia, agranulocytosis, thrombocytopenia and lymphocytosis have been seen very rarely.

Overdose:
Signs and symptoms: Toxic signs and symptoms following an overdose of ceftazidime may include pain, inflammation and phlebitis at the injection site. Overdosage can lead to neurological sequelae, including encephalopathy, convulsions and coma.

The administration of inappropriately large doses of parenteral cephalosporins may cause dizziness, paraesthesias, and headaches. Seizures may occur following overdosage with some cephalosporins, particularly in patients with renal impairment in whom accumulation is likely to occur.

Laboratory abnormalities that may occur after an overdose include elevations in creatinine, BUN, liver enzymes and bilirubin, a positive Coombs' test, thrombocytosis, thrombocytopenia, eosinophilia, leucopenia and prolongation of the prothrombin time.

The subcutaneous median lethal dose in rats and mice ranged from 5.8 to 20 g/kg and the intravenous median lethal dose in rabbits was >2 g/kg.

Treatment: If seizures occur, the drug should be discontinued promptly; anti-convulsant therapy may be administered if clinically indicated. An airway should be established. Cardiac and vital signs monitoring is recommended, along with general symptomatic and supportive measures.

In cases of severe overdosage, especially in a patient with renal failure, combined haemodialysis and haemoperfusion may be considered if response to more conservative therapy fails.

Pharmacological properties

Pharmacodynamic properties: Ceftazidime is a semi-synthetic, beta-lactam antibiotic, for parenteral administration.

In vitro tests demonstrate that ceftazidime is bactericidal. It acts against a wide range of Gram-negative organisms, including strains resistant to gentamicin and other aminoglycosides. It is also active against Gram-positive organisms, and is highly stable to most clinically important beta-lactamases, whether plasmid or chromosomally mediated.

Ceftazidime has been shown to have *in vitro* activity against the following organisms:

Pseudomonas spp. (including *Pseudomonas aeruginosa*); *Klebsiella* spp. (including *Klebsiella pneumoniae*); *Proteus mirabilis* and *Proteus vulgaris*; *Morganella morganii* (formerly *Proteus morganii*); *Providencia* spp. (including *Providencia rettgeri*, formerly *Proteus rettgeri*); *Escherichia coli*; *Enterobacter* spp.; *Citrobacter* spp.; *Serratia* spp.; *Salmonella* spp.; *Shigella* spp.; *Yersinia enterocolitica*; *Pasteurella multocida*; *Acinetobacter* spp.; *Neisseria gonorrhoeae*; *Neisseria meningitidis*; *Haemophilus influenzae* (including ampicillin-resistant strains); *Haemophilus parainfluenzae* (including ampicillin-resistant strains); *Staphylococcus aureus* (methicillin-sensitive strains); *Staphylococcus epidermidis* (methicillin-sensitive strains); *Streptococcus pyogenes*; *Streptococcus* Group B; *Streptococcus pneumoniae*; *Streptococcus* spp.; *Peptococcus* spp.; *Peptostreptococcus* spp.; *Clostridium* spp.; (but not *C. difficile*); *Bacteroides* spp. (but most strains of *B. fragilis* are resistant).

Using the ICS agar dilution method (or its equivalent) for susceptibility testing, the criteria for dilution methods are:

MIC <16 mg/litre:	Susceptible
MIC >16 but <64 mg/litre:	Moderately susceptible (ie, susceptible to high dosage or if infection confined to tissues or fluids [eg, urine] in which high antibiotic levels are attained)
MIC ≥64 mg/litre:	Resistant

and for the standard disc test using a 30 microgram ceftazidime disc, are (zone diameters):

Zone ≥18 mm:	Susceptible
Zone 15-17 mm:	Moderately susceptible
Zone ≤14 mm:	Resistant

Ceftazidime is not active *in vitro* against methicillin-resistant staphylococci; *Streptococcus faecalis* and many other enterococci; *Listeria monocytogenes*; *Campylobacter* spp. or *C. difficile*.

Ceftazidime and the aminoglycosides have been shown to be synergistic *in vitro* against some strains of *P. aeruginosa* and the *Enterobacteriaceae*. Ceftazidime and carbenicillin have also been shown to be synergistic *in vitro* against *P. aeruginosa*.

Pharmacokinetic properties: After intravenous administration of 500 mg or 1 g of ceftazidime, over 5 minutes, to normal adults, mean peak serum concentrations were 45 mg/litre and 90 mg/litre, respectively. Following intravenous infusion of 500 mg, 1 g and 2 g of ceftazidime, over 20 to 30 minutes, to normal adults, mean peak serum concentrations of 42, 69 and 170 mg/litre, respectively, were achieved. The average serum concentrations in these adults, over an 8 hour period, are given in *Table 4*.

Table 4: Ceftazidime Concentrations in Serum

CEFTAZIDIME DOSAGE (IV)	SERUM CONCENTRATIONS (MG/LITRE)				
	0.5h	1h	2h	4h	8h
500 mg	42	25	12	6	2
1 g	60	39	23	11	3
2 g	129	75	42	13	5

Following intramuscular administration of 500 mg and 1 g ceftazidime to normal adults, mean peak serum concentrations at approximately 1 hour were 17 mg/litre and 39 mg/litre, respectively. Serum concentrations remained above 4 mg/litre for 6 and 8 hours after the intramuscular administration of 500 mg and 1 g doses, respectively.

The half-life of ceftazidime was approximately 1.9 hours after intravenous administration and 2 hours after intramuscular administration.

Less than 10% of ceftazidime was protein bound and the degree of protein binding was independent of concentration.

Following multiple intravenous doses of 1 g and 2 g every 8 hours for 10 days, there was no evidence of accumulation of ceftazidime in the serum of individuals with normal renal function.

The presence of hepatic dysfunction had no effect on the pharmacokinetics of ceftazidime in individuals who received 2 g intravenously every 8 hours for 5 days. Therefore, dosage adjustment is not required for patients with hepatic dysfunction, unless renal function is also impaired.

Approximately 80% to 90% of a dose of ceftazidime is excreted unchanged by the kidneys over a 24 hour period. The elimination of ceftazidime by the kidneys resulted in high urinary concentrations.

Concentrations of ceftazidime in excess of the minimum inhibitory levels of common pathogens can be achieved in tissues such as bone, heart, bile, sputum, aqueous humour, synovial, pleural and peritoneal fluids.

Transplacental transfer of the antibiotic readily occurs.

Ceftazidime penetrates the intact blood-brain barrier poorly and low levels are achieved in the CSF in the absence of inflammation. Therapeutic levels of 4 to 20 mg/litre or more are achieved in the CSF when the meninges are inflamed.

Preclinical safety data: Long-term studies in animals have not been performed to evaluate carcinogenic potential. However, a mouse micronucleus test and an Ames test were both negative for mutagenic effects.

Pharmaceutical particulars

List of excipients: Sodium carbonate.

Incompatibilities: Solutions of Kefadim, like those of most beta-lactam antibiotics, should not be added to solutions of aminoglycoside antibiotics because of potential interaction. However, if concurrent therapy with Kefadim and an aminoglycoside is indicated, each of these antibiotics should be administered in different sites.

Precipitation has been reported when vancomycin has been added to ceftazidime in solution. Therefore, it would be prudent to flush giving sets and intravenous lines between administration of these two agents.

Kefadim is less stable in Sodium Bicarbonate Injection than in other intravenous fluids. Sodium Bicarbonate Injection is not recommended as a diluent. Solutions of Kefadim in 5% Dextrose or 0.9% Sodium Chloride Injection are stable for at least 6 hours at room temperature in plastic tubing, drip chambers and volume control devices of common intravenous infusion sets.

Shelf-life:

Unreconstituted vials: 2 years.

Reconstituted vials: It is good practice to reconstitute immediately prior to use. If this is not feasible, Kefadim should be stored in a refrigerator and used within 24 hours. After reconstitution, protection from light is not necessary. The pH of freshly reconstituted solutions ranges from 5.0 to 7.5.

Special precautions for storage:

Unreconstituted vials: Protect from light. Store at room temperature (15°-25°C).

Nature and contents of container: Kefadim is supplied as a sterile dry powder in single-dose flint Type I or III glass vial with a rubber closure and aluminium seal containing 500 mg, 1 g and 2 g ceftazidime (as pentahydrate) with sodium carbonate (118 mg per gram of ceftazidime).

Kefadim is also supplied as a sterile, dry powder, in 100 ml vials, for infusion, containing 2 g ceftazidime.

The total sodium content of the mixture is approximately 54 mg (2.3 mEq) per gram of ceftazidime.

Package quantities:

500 mg/10 ml: Single vials in packs of 10
1 g/20 ml: Single vials in packs of 10
2 g/50 ml: Single vials in packs of 10
2 g/100 ml: Single vials in packs of 1

Instructions for use/handling: Solutions of Kefadim range from light yellow to amber, depending on the diluent and concentration.

Kefadim is compatible with the more commonly used intravenous infusion fluids. Solutions at concentrations between 1 mg/ml and 40 mg/ml in the following infusion fluids may be stored for up to 24 hours at room temperature: 0.9% Sodium Chloride Injection BP; M/6 Sodium Lactate Injection BP; Ringer's Injection USP; Lactated Ringer's Injection USP; 5% Dextrose Injection BP; 0.225% Sodium Chloride and 5% Dextrose Injection BP; 0.45% Sodium Chloride and 5% Dextrose Injection BP; 0.9% Sodium Chloride and 5% Dextrose Injection BP; 10% Dextrose Injection BP; and 10% Invert Sugar in Water for Injection.

At a concentration of 4 mg/ml, Kefadim has been found compatible for 24 hours at room temperature in 0.9% Sodium Chloride Injection or 5% Dextrose Injection when admixed with cefuroxime sodium, 3 mg/ml; heparin, 10u/ml or 50u/ml; or potassium chloride, 10 mEq/l or 40 mEq/l.

Parenteral drug products should be inspected visually and cloudy solutions should be discarded.

Kefadim powder and solutions will darken, depending on storage conditions. However, product potency is not adversely affected if storage conditions and storage periods are observed.

Marketing authorisation numbers

Vials 500 mg:	0006/0239
Vials 1 g:	0006/0240
Vials 2 g:	0006/0241

Date of approval/revision of SPC 26 November 1993

Legal category POM

KEFLEX*

Qualitative and quantitative composition Each tablet contains, as the active ingredient, cephalexin monohydrate equivalent to 250 mg or 500 mg of cephalexin base.

Each capsule contains, as the active ingredient, cephalexin monohydrate equivalent to 250 mg or 500 mg of cephalexin base.

Each bottle, when prepared as directed, contains, as the active ingredient, cephalexin monohydrate equivalent to 125 mg/5 ml or 250 mg/5 ml of cephalexin base.

Pharmaceutical form

Tablets 250 mg: 9.5 mm diameter, peach, marked Lilly U57.

Tablets 500 mg: Pillow-shaped, 16 mm long, scored, peach, marked Lilly U49.

Capsules 250 mg: Green and white, printed Lilly H69.

Capsules 500 mg: Pale green and dark green, printed Lilly H71.

Granules for suspension 125 mg: Pink granules.

Granules for suspension 250 mg: Orange granules.

Clinical particulars

Therapeutic indications: Cephalexin is indicated in the treatment of the following infections due to susceptible micro-organisms:

Respiratory tract infections
Otitis media
Skin and soft tissue infections
Bone and joint infections
Genito-urinary tract infections, including acute prostatitis
Dental infections

Posology and method of administration: Cephalexin is administered orally.

Adults: The adult dosage ranges from 1-4 g daily in divided doses; most infections will respond to a dosage of 500 mg every 8 hours. For skin and soft tissue infections, streptococcal pharyngitis and mild, uncomplicated urinary tract infections, the usual dosage is 250 mg every 6 hours, or 500 mg every 12 hours.

For more severe infections or those caused by less susceptible organisms, larger doses may be needed. If daily doses of cephalexin greater than 4 g are required, parenteral cephalosporins, in appropriate doses, should be considered.

The elderly and patients with impaired renal function: As for adults. Reduce dosage if renal function is markedly impaired (see *Precautions*).

Children: The usual recommended daily dosage for children is 25-50 mg/kg (10-20 mg/lb) in divided doses. For skin and soft tissue infections, streptococcal pharyngitis and mild, uncomplicated urinary tract infections, the total daily dose may be divided and administered every 12 hours. For most infections the following schedule is suggested:

Children under 5 years: 125 mg every 8 hours.

Children 5 years and over: 250 mg every 8 hours.

In severe infections, the dosage may be doubled. In the therapy of otitis media, clinical studies have shown that a dosage of 75 to 100 mg/kg/day in 4 divided doses is required.

In the treatment of beta-haemolytic streptococcal infections, a therapeutic dose should be administered for at least 10 days.

Contra-indications: Cephalexin is contra-indicated in patients with known allergy to the cephalosporin group of antibiotics.

Special warnings and special precautions for use: Before instituting therapy with cephalexin, every effort should be made to determine whether the patient has had previous hypersensitivity reactions to the cephalosporins, penicillins or other drugs. Cephalexin should be given cautiously to penicillin-sensitive patients. There is some clinical and laboratory evidence of partial cross-allergenicity of the penicillins and cephalosporins. Patients have had severe reactions (including anaphylaxis) to both drugs.

Pseudomembranous colitis has been reported with virtually all broad-spectrum antibiotics, including macrolides, semi-synthetic penicillins and cephalosporins. It is important, therefore, to consider its diagnosis in patients who develop diarrhoea in association with the use of antibiotics. Such colitis may range in severity from mild to life-threatening. Mild cases of pseudomembranous colitis usually respond to drug discontinuance alone. In moderate to severe cases, appropriate measures should be taken.

If an allergic reaction to cephalexin occurs, the drug should be discontinued and the patient treated with the appropriate agents.

Prolonged use of cephalexin may result in the overgrowth of non-susceptible organisms. Careful observation of the patient is essential. If superinfection occurs during therapy, appropriate measures should be taken.

Cephalexin should be administered with caution in the presence of markedly impaired renal function. Careful clinical and laboratory studies should be made because safe dosage may be lower than that usually recommended.

Positive direct Coombs' tests have been reported during treatment with the cephalosporin antibiotics. In haematological studies, or in transfusion cross-matching procedures when antiglobulin tests are performed on the minor side, or in Coombs' testing of newborns whose mothers have received cephalosporin antibiotics before parturition, it should be recognised that a positive Coombs' test may be due to the drug.

A false positive reaction for glucose in the urine may occur with Benedict's or Fehling's solutions, or with copper sulphate test tablets.

Interaction with other medicaments and other forms of interaction: None known.

Pregnancy and lactation:
Usage in pregnancy: Although laboratory and clinical studies have shown no evidence of teratogenicity, caution should be exercised when prescribing for the pregnant patient.

Usage in nursing mothers: The excretion of cephalexin in human breast milk increased up to 4 hours following a 500 mg dose. The drug reached a maximum level of 4 micrograms/ml, then decreased gradually and had disappeared 8 hours after administration. Caution should be exercised when cephalexin is administered to a nursing woman.

Effects on ability to drive and use machines: None known.

Undesirable effects:
Gastro-intestinal: Symptoms of pseudomembranous colitis may appear either during or after antibiotic treatment. Nausea and vomiting have been reported rarely. The most frequent side-effect has been diarrhoea. It was very rarely severe enough to warrant cessation of therapy. Dyspepsia and abdominal pain have also occurred. As with some penicillins and some other cephalosporins, transient hepatitis and cholestatic jaundice have been reported rarely.

Hypersensitivity: Allergic reactions have been observed in the form of rash, urticaria, angioedema and, rarely, erythema multiforme, Stevens-Johnson syndrome and toxic epidermal necrolysis. These reactions usually subsided upon discontinuation of the drug, although in some cases supportive therapy may be necessary. Anaphylaxis has also been reported.

Other: These have included genital and anal pruritus, genital candidiasis, vaginitis and vaginal discharge, dizziness, fatigue, headache, agitation, confusion, hallucinations, arthralgia, arthritis and joint disorder. Reversible interstitial nephritis has been reported rarely. Eosinophilia, neutropenia, thrombocytopenia and slight elevations in AST and ALT have been reported.

Overdose: Symptoms of oral overdose may include nausea, vomiting, epigastric distress, diarrhoea and haematuria.

In the event of severe overdosage, general supportive care is recommended, including close clinical and laboratory monitoring of haematological, renal and hepatic functions, and coagulation status until the patient is stable. Forced diuresis, peritoneal dialysis, haemodialysis, or charcoal haemoperfusion have not been established as beneficial for an overdose of cephalexin. It would be extremely unlikely that one of these procedures would be indicated.

Unless 5 to 10 times the normal total daily dose has been ingested, gastro-intestinal decontamination should not be necessary.

There have been reports of haematuria, without impairment of renal function, in children accidentally ingesting more than 3.5 g of cephalexin in a day. Treatment has been supportive (fluids) and no sequelae have been reported.

Pharmacological properties

Pharmacodynamic properties:
Microbiology: In vitro tests demonstrate that the cephalosporins are bactericidal because of their inhibition of cell-wall synthesis.

Cephalexin is active against the following organisms *in vitro:*

Beta-haemolytic streptococci
Staphylococci, including coagulase-positive, coagulase-negative and penicillinase-producing strains.
Streptococcus pneumoniae
Escherichia coli
Proteus mirabilis
Klebsiella species
Haemophilus influenzae
Branhamella catarrhalis

Most strains of enterococci (*Streptococcus faecalis*) and a few strains of staphylococci are resistant to cephalexin. It is not active against most strains of *Enterobacter* species, *Morganella morganii* and *Pr. vulgaris.* It has no activity against *Pseudomonas* or *Herellea* species. When tested by *in vitro* methods, staphylococci exhibit cross-resistance between cephalexin and methicillin-type antibiotics.

Pharmacokinetic properties:
Human pharmacology: Cephalexin is acid stable and may be given without regard to meals. It is rapidly absorbed after oral administration. Following doses of 250 mg, 500 mg and 1 g, average peak serum levels of approximately 9, 18 and 32 mg/l, respectively, were obtained at 1 hour. Measurable levels were present 6 hours after administration. Cephalexin is excreted in the urine by glomerular filtration and tubular secretion. Studies showed that over 90% of the drug was excreted unchanged in the urine within 8 hours. During this period, peak urine concentrations following the 250 mg, 500 mg and 1 g doses were approximately 1000, 2200 and 5000 mg/l, respectively.

Cephalexin is almost completely absorbed from the gastro-intestinal tract, and 75-100% is rapidly excreted in active form in the urine. Absorption is slightly reduced if the drug is administered with food. The half-life is approximately 60 minutes in patients with normal renal function. Haemodialysis and peritoneal dialysis will remove cephalexin from the blood.

Peak blood levels are achieved one hour after administration, and therapeutic levels are maintained for 6-8 hours. Approximately 80% of the active drug is excreted in the urine within 6 hours. No accumulation is seen with dosages above the therapeutic maximum of 4 g/day.

The half-life may be increased in neonates due to their renal immaturity, but there is no accumulation when given at up to 50 mg/kg/day.

Preclinical safety data: The daily oral administration of cephalexin to rats in doses of 250 or 500 mg/kg prior to and during pregnancy, or to rats and mice during the period of organogenesis only, had no adverse effect on fertility, foetal viability, foetal weight, or litter size.

Cephalexin showed no enhanced toxicity in weanling and newborn rats as compared with adult animals.

The oral LD_{50} of cephalexin in rats is 5,000 mg/kg.

Pharmaceutical particulars

List of excipient(s):
The tablets contain the following excipients: Sodium Starch Glycollate Type A; Magnesium Stearate; Povidone; Methylhydroxypropylcellulose; Glycerol; Talc; Titanium Dioxide; Methyl Cellulose; Iron Oxide Yellow; Iron Oxide Red.

The capsules contain the following excipients: Cellulose with Sodium Carboxymethyl Cellulose; Dimethicone; Magnesium Stearate; Patent Blue V; Quinoline Yellow; Titanium Dioxide; Gelatin.

The granules contain the following excipients: Sucrose; Imitation Guarana Flavour; Erythrosine Aluminium Lake (125 mg suspension only); Sunset Yellow (250 mg suspension only).

Incompatibilities: None known.

Shelf-life:
Tablets or capsules: When stored appropriately, 3 years.

Suspension: When stored appropriately,
Unreconstituted product: 2 years (Keflex Suspension 125 mg/5 ml)
3 years (Keflex Suspension 250 mg/5 ml).

Bottles of reconstituted product: 10 days.

Special precautions for storage: Store below 30°C. Keep containers tightly closed.

After mixing, Keflex Suspensions should be stored in a cool place (6°C-15°C) or in a refrigerator (2°C-8°C) and be used within 10 days. Where dilution is unavoidable, Syrup BP should be used after the suspension has been prepared according to the manufacturer's instructions.

Nature and contents of container:
Tablets: The products are filled into HDPE bottles of 100 or 500 tablets, or blister strips of 28 tablets consisting of UPVC with aluminium foil backing. Additionally, the 500 mg product may be packed into blisters of 21 tablets.

Capsules: The products are filled into HDPE bottles of 100 or 500 capsules, or blister strips of 28 capsules consisting of UPVC with aluminium foil backing. Additionally, the 500 mg product may be packed into blisters of 21 capsules.

Suspension: The product is filled into 100 ml HDPE bottles with screw caps.

Package quantities:
Tablets 250 mg: Bottles of 100 and 500, blister packs of 28.

Tablets 500 mg: Bottles of 100 and 500, blister packs of 21 and 28.

Capsules 250 mg: Bottles of 100 and 500, blister packs of 28.

Capsules 500 mg: Bottles of 100 and 500, blister packs of 21 and 28.

Suspension 125 mg/5 ml: Bottles of 100 ml.
Suspension 250 mg/5 ml: Bottles of 100 ml.

Instructions for use/handling: For oral use.
Suspension: To the bottle containing granules, is added a total of 60 ml water in two portions, shaking after each addition until suspended. If dilution is unavoidable, Syrup BP should be used after the suspension has been prepared as described.

Shake well before use.

Marketing authorisation numbers
Tablets: 0006/0073, 5096
Capsules: 0006/0076, 5103
Suspension: 0006/5097, 5098

Date of approval/revision of SPC April 1998

Legal category POM

KEFZOL*

Qualitative and quantitative composition Kefzol is supplied in rubber-stoppered vials containing the equivalent of 500 mg and 1 g cephazolin as the sodium salt.

Pharmaceutical form Powder for injections.

Clinical particulars
Therapeutic indications: Kefzol is indicated in the treatment of the following infections due to susceptible micro-organisms:

Respiratory tract infections
Genito-urinary tract infections
Skin and soft tissue infections
Bone and joint infections
Septicaemia
Endocarditis
Biliary tract infections

Prophylactic use: Perioperative administration of cephazolin may reduce the incidence of postoperative infections in patients undergoing contaminated or potentially contaminated surgical procedures associated with a high risk of infection, or where the occurrence of a postoperative infection could be especially serious.

Cephazolin is active against the following organisms *in vitro:*

Staphylococcus aureus (penicillin-sensitive and penicillin-resistant)
Staphylococcus epidermidis
Group A beta-haemolytic streptococci and other strains of streptococci (many strains of enterococci are resistant)
Streptococcus pneumoniae
Escherichia coli
Klebsiella species
Proteus mirabilis
Haemophilus influenzae
Enterobacter aerogenes

Posology and method of administration: After reconstitution, Kefzol may be administered intramuscularly or intravenously. Kefzol should not be administered intrathecally (see *Precautions*).

Intramuscular administration: Reconstitute with Water for Injections PhEur, 0.9% Sodium Chloride Intravenous Infusion BP, or 5% Dextrose Intravenous Infusion BP, according to Table 1. Shake well until dissolved. Kefzol should be injected into a large muscle mass.

Table 1: Dilution table

Vial Size	*Diluent to be Added*	*Approximate Available Volume*	*Approximate Average Concentration*
500 mg	4.0 ml	4.1 ml	125 mg/ml
500 mg	2.0 ml	2.2 ml	225 mg/ml
1 g*	2.5 ml	3.0 ml	330 mg/ml

*The 1 g vial should be reconstituted only with Water for Injections PhEur.

Intravenous administration: Kefzol may be administered by intravenous injection or by continuous or intermittent infusion. Total daily dosages are the same as for intramuscular injection.

Intermittent intravenous infusion: Kefzol may be administered along with primary intravenous fluid management programmes in a volume control set or in a separate secondary IV bottle. Reconstituted 500 mg or 1 g of Kefzol may be diluted in 50 to 100 ml of Water for Injections PhEur or one of the following intravenous solutions:

0.9% Sodium Chloride Intravenous Infusion BP
5% or 10% Dextrose Intravenous Infusion BP
5% Dextrose in Compound Sodium Lactate Intravenous Infusion BP
0.9% Sodium Chloride and 5% Dextrose Intravenous Infusion BP

0.45% Sodium Chloride and 5% Dextrose Intravenous Infusion BP

Compound Sodium Lactate Intravenous Infusion BP

5% or 10% Invert Sugar in Water for Injections PhEur

Direct intravenous injection: Dilute 500 mg or 1 g of reconstituted Kefzol in a minimum of 10 ml of Water for Injections PhEur and inject solution slowly over a period of three to five minutes. Do not inject in less than 3 minutes. The injection may be made directly into a vein or, for patients receiving the above parenteral fluids, through the tubing.

Dosage: The usual adult dosages are given in Table 2.

Table 2: Usual adult dosage

Type of Infection	*Dose*	*Frequency*
Pneumococcal pneumonia	500 mg	q 12 h
Mild infections caused by susceptible Gram-positive cocci	250 mg to 500 mg	q 8 h
Acute uncomplicated urinary tract infections	1 g	q 12 h
Moderate to severe infections	500 mg to 1 g	q 6 to 8 h
Severe, life-threatening infections (e.g. endocarditis and septicaemia)*	1 g to 1.5 g	q 6 h

*In rare instances, doses up to 12 g cephazolin per day have been used.

In adults with renal impairment, cephazolin is not readily excreted. After a loading dose appropriate to the severity of the infection, the following recommendations (Table 3) may be used as a guide.

In patients undergoing peritoneal dialysis (2 l/h), mean serum levels of cephazolin were approximately 10 and 30 micrograms/ml after 24 hours' instillation of a dialysing solution containing 50 mg/l and 150 mg/l, respectively.

The elderly: As for adults.

Table 3: Dosage of Kefzol in Adults With Reduced Renal Function

Creatinine Clearance (ml/min)	*Serum Creatinine (mg %)*	*Dosage Reduction*
≥55	≤1.5	None
35–54	1.6–3.0	None q 8 + hrs
11–34	3.1–4.5	50% q 12 hrs
≤10	≥4.6	50% q 18–24 hrs

Paediatric dosage: In children, a total daily dosage of 25 to 50 mg/kg of body weight, divided into three or four equal doses, is effective for most mild to moderately severe infections (Table 4). Total daily dosage may be increased to 100 mg/kg of body weight for severe infections.

Table 4: Paediatric Dosage Guide

Weight kg	*25 mg/kg/day Divided into 3 doses*		*25 mg/kg/day Divided into 4 doses*	
	Approximate single dose (q 8 h)	*Volume needed with dilution of 125 mg/ml*	*Approximate single dose (q 6 h)*	*Volume needed with dilution of 125 mg/ml*
4.5	40 mg	0.35 ml	30 mg	0.25 ml
9.0	75 mg	0.6 ml	55 mg	0.45 ml
13.5	115 mg	0.9 ml	85 mg	0.7 ml
18.0	150 mg	1.2 ml	115 mg	0.9 ml
22.5	190 mg	1.5 ml	140 mg	1.1 ml

Weight kg	*50 mg/kg/day Divided into 3 doses*		*50 mg/kg/day Divided into 4 doses*	
	Approximate single dose (q 8 h)	*Volume needed with dilution of 225 mg/ml*	*Approximate single dose (q 6 h)*	*Volume needed with dilution of 225 mg/ml*
4.5	75 mg	0.35 ml	55 mg	0.25 ml
9.0	150 mg	0.7 ml	110 mg	0.5 ml
13.5	225 mg	1.0 ml	170 mg	0.75 ml
18.0	300 mg	1.35 ml	225 mg	1.0 ml
22.5	375 mg	1.7 ml	285 mg	1.25 ml

In children with mild to moderate renal impairment (creatinine clearance of 70-40 ml/min), 60% of the normal daily dose given in divided doses q 12 h should be sufficient. In children with moderate impairment (creatinine clearance of 40-20 ml/min), 25% of the normal daily dose in divided doses q 12 h should be adequate. In children with marked impairment (creatinine clearance of 20-5 ml/min), 10% of the normal daily dose given q 24 h should be sufficient. All dosage recommendations apply after an initial loading dose.

Since safety for use in premature infants and in infants under 1 month of age has not been established, the use of cephazolin in these patients is not recommended.

Prophylactic use: The following doses are recommended for perioperative use:

Adults: 1 g intravenously or intramuscularly one-half to one hour prior to surgical incision, followed by 0.5 to 1 g intravenously or intramuscularly every six to eight hours for 24 hours postoperatively. Additionally, for lengthy operative procedures (e.g. two hours or more), 0.5 to 1 g intravenously or intramuscularly during surgery.

The prophylactic administration of cephazolin should usually be discontinued within a 24 hour period after the surgical procedure. For patients undergoing open-heart surgery or implantation of prosthetic devices, administration may be continued for three to five days.

Contra-indications: Cephazolin is contra-indicated in patients with known allergy to the cephalosporin group of antibiotics.

Special warnings and special precautions for use:
Warnings: Before instituting therapy with cephazolin, every attempt should be made to determine if the patient has had previous hypersensitivity reactions to the cephalosporins, penicillins, or other drugs, in which case this product should be given cautiously. Serious acute hypersensitivity reactions may require epinephrine (adrenaline) and other emergency measures.

There is some evidence of partial cross-allergenicity between the penicillins and the cephalosporins. Patients have been reported to have had severe reactions (including anaphylaxis) to both drugs.

Antibiotics should be administered cautiously to any patient who has demonstrated some form of allergy, particularly to drugs.

Cephalosporins may be absorbed onto the surface of red cell membranes and react with antibodies directed against the drug. This can produce a positive Coombs' test and very rarely a haemolytic anaemia. Cross-reactivity may occur with penicillins for this reaction.

Pseudomembranous colitis has been reported with virtually all broad-spectrum antibiotics, so it is important to consider this diagnosis in patients who develop diarrhoea in association with the use of antibiotics. Severity ranges from mild to life-threatening; mild cases usually respond to drug discontinuance alone. In moderate to severe cases, appropriate measures should be taken.

Precautions: If an allergic reaction to cephazolin occurs, the drug should be discontinued and the patient treated with the usual agents (e.g. epinephrine (adrenaline) or other pressor amines, antihistamines, or corticosteroids).

Broad-spectrum antibiotics should be prescribed with caution in individuals with a history of gastro-intestinal disease, particularly colitis.

Prolonged use of cephazolin may result in the overgrowth of non-susceptible organisms. Careful observation of the patient is essential. If superinfection occurs during therapy, appropriate measures should be taken.

When cephazolin is administered to patients with impaired renal function, the daily dosage should be reduced to avoid toxicity (see *Posology and method of administration).*

The intrathecal administration of Kefzol is not an approved route of administration. There have been reports of severe CNS toxicity, including seizures, when cefazolin was administered in this manner.

Interaction with other medicaments and other forms of interaction: Probenecid may decrease renal tubular secretion of cephalosporins when used concurrently, which results in increased and more prolonged cephalosporin blood levels.

The results of experimental studies in animals given cephalosporins suggest that the concurrent use of potent diuretics, such as furosemide (frusemide) or ethacrynic acid, may increase the risk of renal toxicity.

A false positive reaction for glucose in the urine may occur with Benedict's or Fehling's solutions or with copper sulphate test tablets.

Positive direct and indirect antiglobulin (Coombs') tests have occurred; these may also occur in neonates whose mothers received cephalosporins before delivery.

Pregnancy and lactation:
Usage in pregnancy: Although animal studies have shown no evidence of impaired fertility or teratogenicity, there are no adequate and well-controlled studies in pregnant women. Therefore, caution should be exercised when prescribing for the pregnant patient. When cephazolin has been administered prior to caesarean section, drug levels in cord blood have been approximately one-fourth to one-third of maternal drug levels. The drug appeared to have no adverse effect on the fetus.

Usage in nursing mothers: Caution is required when cephazolin is administered to a nursing woman, as very low concentrations of cephazolin have been found in breast milk.

Usage in neonates: The safety of this product for use in prematures and infants under one month of age has not been established.

Effects on ability to drive and use machines: Not applicable.

Undesirable effects: The following side-effects have been reported:
Gastro-intestinal: Symptoms of pseudomembranous colitis may appear either during or after treatment. Nausea, anorexia, vomiting, diarrhoea and oral candidiasis have been reported.

Hypersensitivity: Drug fever, rash, vulvar pruritus, eosinophilia and anaphylaxis.

Haematological: Neutropenia, leucopenia, thrombocythaemia, and positive direct and indirect Coombs' tests.

Neurological: Convulsions have occasionally been reported, especially after administration of high doses to patients with marked renal impairment.

Renal: Transient rise in blood urea nitrogen levels has been observed without clinical evidence of renal impairment. Interstitial nephritis and other renal disorders have been reported rarely. Most patients experiencing these reactions have been seriously ill and were receiving multiple drug therapies. The role of cephazolin has not been determined.

Hepatic: Transient rises in AST, ALT and ALP levels have been observed rarely. As with some penicillins and some other cephalosporins, transient hepatitis and cholestatic jaundice have been reported rarely.

Other: Pain on intramuscular injection, sometimes with induration, has occurred infrequently. Phlebitis at the site of intravenous injection has been noted. Other side-effects have included genital and anal pruritus, genital candidiasis and vaginitis.

Overdose:
Signs and symptoms: May include pain, inflammation and phlebitis at the injection site.

The administration of inappropriately large doses of parenteral cephalosporins may cause dizziness, paraesthesiae and headaches. Seizures may occur with some cephalosporins, particularly in patients with renal impairment in whom accumulation is likely to occur.

Laboratory abnormalities may include elevations in creatinine, BUN, liver enzymes and bilirubin, a positive Coombs' test, thrombocytosis, thrombocytopenia, eosinophilia, leucopenia and prolongation of prothrombin time.

Treatment: In the event of serious overdosage, general supportive care is recommended, with monitoring of haematological, renal and hepatic functions and coagulation status until the patient is stable. If seizures occur, the drug should be discontinued promptly. Anticonvulsant therapy may be clinically indicated. General supportive therapy is recommended.

In cases of severe overdosage, especially in a patient with renal failure, combined haemodialysis and haemoperfusion may be considered, although supporting data are not available.

Pharmacological properties
Pharmacodynamic properties: Cephazolin is a bactericidal antibiotic which interferes with the final stage of bacterial cell wall synthesis of Gram-negative and Gram-positive bacteria.

Pharmacokinetic properties: Cephazolin is poorly absorbed from the gastro-intestinal tract and is therefore given parenterally. Following 500 mg intramuscularly, peak plasma levels of 30 micrograms/ml are obtained in 1 hour. Cephazolin is 90% bound to plasma proteins. The half-life with normal renal function is 1.8 hours. It is excreted unchanged in the urine, approximately 80% being recoverable in the 24 hours following injection.

Preclinical safety data: There are no preclinical data of relevance to the prescriber in addition to that summarised in other sections of the summary of product characteristics.

Pharmaceutical particulars
List of excipient(s): Not applicable.

Incompatibilities: Extemporaneous mixtures with other antibiotics (including aminoglycosides) are not recommended.

Shelf-life:
Unreconstituted vials: 2 years.

After reconstitution: The reconstituted product should be used immediately, or within 24 hours if stored in a refrigerator (2°–8°C).

Special precautions for storage:
Unreconstituted vials: Protect from light.

Nature and contents of container:
500 mg vials: Glass vials in packs of 10
1 g vials: Glass vials in packs of 10

Instructions for use/handling: Prior to administration, parenteral drug products should be inspected visually for particulate matter and discolouration, whenever solution and container permit.

Marketing authorisation number 0006/0078R

Date of approval/revision of SPC March 1998

Legal category POM

NEBCIN*

Presentation Nebcin is presented in vials in the following strengths:

1 ml vials containing tobramycin sulphate equivalent to 40 mg tobramycin base.

2 ml vials containing tobramycin sulphate equivalent to 80 mg tobramycin base.

2 ml vials containing tobramycin sulphate equivalent to 20 mg tobramycin base.

Also containing 0.5% w/v Phenol BP with sodium bisulphite and Disodium Edetate BP.

Uses Nebcin is indicated for the treatment of the following infections caused by susceptible micro-organisms:

Central nervous system infections, including meningitis, septicaemia and neonatal sepsis.
Gastro-intestinal infections, including peritonitis, and other significant infections such as complicated and recurrent urinary tract infections, including pyelonephritis and cystitis.
Lower respiratory tract infections, including pneumonia, bronchopneumonia and acute bronchitis.
Skin, bone and soft tissue infections, including burns.

Nebcin may be considered in serious staphylococcal infections for which penicillin or other less potentially toxic drugs are contra-indicated and when bacterial susceptibility testing and clinical judgement indicate its use.

Tobramycin is usually active against most strains of the following organisms:

Pseudomonas aeruginosa
Proteus species (indole-positive and indole-negative), including *Pr. mirabilis, Pr. rettgeri* and *Pr. vulgaris*
Morganella morganii
Escherichia coli
Klebsiella-Enterobacter-Serratia species
Citrobacter species
Providencia species
Staphylococci including *Staphylococcus aureus* (coagulase-positive and coagulase-negative).

Most strains of enterococci demonstrate *in vitro* resistance. The combination of penicillin G and tobramycin results in a synergistic bactericidal effect *in vitro* against certain strains of *Enterococcus faecalis* (formerly *Streptococcus faecalis*). However, this combination is not synergistic against other closely related organisms, e.g. *E. faecium* (formerly *S. faecium*). Speciation of enterococci alone cannot be used to predict susceptibility. Susceptibility testing and tests for antibiotic synergism are emphasised.

Cross-resistance between aminoglycosides occurs and depends largely on inactivation by bacterial enzymes.

The combination of tobramycin and carbenicillin is synergistic *in vitro* against most strains of *Ps. aeruginosa.* Other Gram-negative organisms may be affected synergistically by the combination of tobramycin and a cephalosporin.

Dosage and administration Nebcin may be given intramuscularly or intravenously. The patient's pretreatment body weight should be obtained for calculation of correct dosage.

The intramuscular dose is the same as the intravenous dose.

It is recommended that both peak and trough serum levels should be determined whenever possible to ensure the correct dosage is given. Blood levels should always be determined in patients with chronic infections such as cystic fibrosis, or where longer duration of treatment may be necessary, or in patients with decreased renal function.

Patients with normal renal function: Adults: The usual recommended dosage for adults with serious infections is 3 mg/kg/day, administered in three equal doses every eight hours (see Table 1). For life-threatening infections, dosages up to 5 mg/kg/day may be administered in three or four equal doses. The dosage should be reduced to 3 mg/kg/day as soon as clinically indicated. To prevent increased toxicity due to excessive blood levels, dosage should not exceed 5 mg/kg/day unless serum levels are monitored (see 'Warnings' and 'Precautions').

To achieve therapeutic serum levels in patients with cystic fibrosis, it may be necessary to administer up to 8 to 10 mg/kg/day in equally divided doses. Because serum concentrations of tobramycin vary from one patient to another, serum levels should be monitored.

Table 1: Dosage Schedule Guide for Adults with Normal Renal Function (Dosage at 8-hour intervals)

Patient weight (kg)	*Usual dose for serious infections 1 mg/kg q 8 h (total 3 mg/kg/day)*		*Maximum dose for life-threatening infections (reduce as soon as possible) 1.66 mg/kg q 8 h (total 5 mg/kg/day unless monitored)*	
	mg/dose	ml/ dose*	mg/dose	ml/ dose*
120	120	3.0	200	5.0
100	100	2.5	166	4.0
80	80	2.0	133	3.0
60	60	1.5	100	2.5
40	40	1.0	66	1.6

*Applicable to 40 mg/ml product forms.

In adults with normal renal function, mild to moderate infections of the urinary tract have responded to a dosage of 2–3 mg/kg/day administered as a single intramuscular injection.

The elderly: As for adults, but see recommendations for patients with impaired renal function.

Children: The recommended dosage is 6–7.5 mg/kg/day, administered in three or four equally divided doses. In some patients it may be necessary to administer higher doses.

Premature or full-term neonates: Dosages of up to 4 mg/kg/day may be administered in two equal doses every 12 hours, for those between 1.5 and 2.5 kg body weight.

The usual duration of treatment is 7 to 10 days. A longer course of therapy may be necessary in difficult and complicated infections. In such cases, monitoring of renal, auditory and vestibular functions is advised, because neurotoxicity is more likely to occur when treatment is extended for longer than 10 days.

Obese patients: The appropriate dose may be calculated using the patient's estimated lean body weight, plus 40% of the excess, as the weight on which to determine mg/kg.

Patients with impaired renal function: Following a loading dose of 1 mg/kg, subsequent dosage in these patients must be adjusted, either with lower doses administered at eight-hour intervals or with normal doses at prolonged intervals (see Table 2). Both of these regimens are suggested as guides to be used when serum levels of tobramycin cannot be measured directly. They are based on either the creatinine clearance or the serum creatinine of the patient, because these values correlate with the half-life of tobramycin. Neither regimen should be used when dialysis is being performed.

Reduced dosage at eight-hour intervals (Regimen I): An appropriately reduced dosage range can be found in the accompanying table (Table 2) for any patient for whom the blood urea, creatinine clearance or serum creatinine values are known. The choice of dose within the indicated range should be based on the severity of the infection, the sensitivity of the pathogen, and individual patient considerations, especially renal function. An alternative rough guide for determining reduced dosage at eight-hour intervals (for patients whose steady-state serum creatinine values are known) is to divide the normally recommended dose by the patient's serum creatinine value (mg/100 ml).

Normal dosage at prolonged intervals (Regimen II): Recommended intervals between doses are given in the accompanying table (Table 2). As a general rule, the dosage frequency in hours can be determined by multiplying the patient's serum creatinine level (mg/100 ml) by six.

The dosage schedules derived from either method should be used in conjunction with careful clinical and laboratory observations of the patient and should be modified as necessary (see *Warnings*).

Intramuscular administration: Nebcin may be administered by withdrawing the appropriate dose directly from the vial.

Intravenous administration: For intravenous administration, the usual volume of diluent (0.9% Sodium Chloride Intravenous Infusion BP or 5% Dextrose Intravenous Infusion BP) for adult doses is 50–100 ml. For children, the volume of diluent should be proportionately less than for adults. The diluted solution should be infused over a period of 20–60 minutes avoiding admixture with any other drug. Nebcin may be administered slowly by direct intravenous injection or into the tubing of a drip set. When given in this way, serum levels may exceed 12 mg/l for a short time (see *Contra-indications, warnings, etc.*).

Contra-indications, warnings, etc

Contra-indications: Intrathecal administration. Hypersensitivity to any aminoglycoside is a contra-indication to the use of tobramycin because of the known cross-allergenicity of drugs in this class.

Warnings: Nebcin contains sodium bisulphite which may cause allergic-type reactions, including anaphylactic symptoms and life-threatening or less severe asthmatic episodes, in certain susceptible people. The overall prevalence of sulphite sensitivity in the general population is unknown and probably low, but it occurs more frequently in asthmatic patients.

Patients treated with tobramycin should be under close observation because tobramycin and other aminoglycoside antibiotics have an inherent potential for causing nephrotoxicity and ototoxicity.

Both vestibular and auditory ototoxicity can occur. The auditory changes are irreversible, are usually bilateral, and may be partial or total. Eighth cranial nerve impairment may develop in patients with pre-existing renal damage and if tobramycin is administered for longer periods or in higher doses than those recommended. Other manifestations of neurotoxicity may include numbness, skin tingling, muscle twitching and convulsions. The risk of aminoglycoside-induced hearing loss increases with the degree of exposure to either high peak or high trough serum concentrations. Patients who develop cochlear damage may not have symptoms during therapy to warn them of eighth-nerve toxicity, and partial or total irreversible bilateral deafness may continue to develop after the drug has been discontinued. Rarely, nephrotoxicity may not become manifest until the first few days after cessation of therapy. Aminoglycoside-induced nephrotoxicity is usually reversible.

Therefore, renal and eighth cranial nerve function should be closely monitored in patients with known or suspected renal impairment and also in those whose renal function is initially normal but who develop signs of renal dysfunction during therapy. Evidence of impairment in renal, vestibular and/or auditory function requires discontinuation of the drug or dosage adjustment.

Monitoring of renal function is particularly important in elderly patients who may have reduced renal function that may not be evident in the results of routine screening tests, such as blood urea or serum creatinine. A creatinine clearance determination may be more useful.

Serum concentrations should be monitored when feasible, and prolonged concentrations above 12 mg/l should be avoided. Rising trough levels (above 2 mg/l) may indicate tissue accumulation. A useful guideline would be to perform serum level assays after two or three doses, so that the dosage could be adjusted if necessary, and also at three to four day intervals during therapy. In the event of changing renal function, more frequent serum levels should be obtained and the dosage or dosage intervals adjusted according to the guidelines provided in the *Dosage and administration* section. In order to measure the peak level, a serum sample should be drawn about 30 minutes following intravenous infusion or at one hour after intramuscular injection. Trough levels are measured by obtaining serum samples at eight hours or just prior to the next dose of tobramycin.

Urine should be examined for increased excretion of protein, cells and casts. Serum creatinine or creatinine clearance (preferred over blood urea) should be measured periodically. When feasible, it is recommended that serial audiograms be obtained in patients old enough to be tested, particularly high-risk patients.

The risk of toxic reactions is low in patients with normal renal function who do not receive tobramycin in higher doses or for longer periods of time than those recommended.

Patients with reduced renal function, however, are particularly prone to the potential ototoxic and nephrotoxic effects of this drug, so dosage should be adjusted carefully on the basis of regular monitoring of serum drug concentrations and of renal function.

Concurrent and/or sequential use of other potentially neurotoxic and/or nephrotoxic drugs, particularly other aminoglycosides (e.g. amikacin, streptomycin, neomycin, kanamycin, gentamicin and paromomycin), amphotericin B, cephaloridine, viomycin, polymyxin B, colistin, cisplatin and vancomycin, requires careful monitoring. Other factors that may increase patient risk are advanced age and dehydration.

Tobramycin should not be given concurrently with potent diuretics. Some diuretics themselves cause ototoxicity, and intravenously administered diuretics

Table 2. Two maintenance regimens based on renal function and body weight following an initial dose of 1 mg/kg†

Renal function‡					*Regimen I*	*or*	*Regimen II*
					Adjusted doses at 8-hour intervals		*Normal dosage at prolonged intervals*
Blood urea		*Serum creatinine*		*Creatinine clearance*	*Weight*		*Weight/Dose 50–60 kg:60 mg 60–80 kg:80 mg*
mg/100 ml	*mmol/l*	*mg/100 ml*	*mcmol/l*	*ml/min*	*50–60 kg*	*60–80 kg*	
Normal:							
< 42	< 7.0	< 1.3	< 114.9	> 70	60 mg	80 mg	q 8 h
42–74	7.0–12.3	1.4–1.9	123.8–168	69–40	30–60 mg	50–80 mg	q 12 h
75–105	12.5–17.5	2.0–3.3	176.8–291.7	39–20	20–25 mg	30–45 mg	q 18 h
106–140	17.7–23.3	3.4–5.3	300.6–468.5	19–10	10–18 mg	15–24 mg	q 24 h
141–160	23.5–26.7	5.4–7.5	477.4–663	9–5	5–9 mg	7–12 mg	q 36 h
> 160	> 26.7	> 7.6	> 671.8	< 4	2.5–4.5 mg	3.5–6 mg	q 48 h§

†For life-threatening infections, dosages 50% above those normally recommended may be used. The dosages should be reduced as soon as possible when improvement is noted.
‡If used to estimate degree of renal impairment, blood urea and serum creatinine concentrations should reflect a steady state of renal uraemia.
§When dialysis is not being performed.

enhance aminoglycoside toxicity by altering antibiotic concentrations in serum and tissue.

Usage in pregnancy: Aminoglycosides can cause foetal harm when administered to a pregnant woman. Aminoglycoside antibiotics cross the placenta, and there have been several reports of total irreversible bilateral congenital deafness in children whose mothers received streptomycin during pregnancy. Serious side-effects to mother, foetus, or newborn have not been reported in the treatment of pregnant women with other aminoglycosides, but tobramycin should not be administered to the pregnant patient unless the potential benefits clearly outweigh any potential risk. If tobramycin is used during pregnancy or if the patient becomes pregnant whilst taking tobramycin, she should be informed of the potential hazard to the foetus.

Usage in nursing mothers: Tobramycin is excreted in the breast milk and should be avoided in nursing women.

Precautions
Use in neonates: Tobramycin should be used with caution in premature and neonatal infants because of their renal immaturity and the resulting prolongation of serum half-life of the drug.

General: Serum calcium, magnesium, and sodium should be monitored. It is particularly important to monitor serum levels closely in patients with known renal impairment.

In patients with extensive burns, altered pharmacokinetics may result in reduced serum concentrations of aminoglycosides. In such patients treated with tobramycin, measurement of serum concentration is especially recommended as a basis for determination of appropriate dosage.

Aminoglycosides may be absorbed in significant quantities from body surfaces after local irrigation or application and may cause neurotoxicity and nephrotoxicity.

Although not indicated for intraocular and/or subconjunctival use, there have been reports of macular necrosis following this type of injection.

Aminoglycosides should be used with caution in patients with muscular disorders, such as myasthenia gravis or parkinsonism, since these drugs may aggravate muscle weakness because of their potential curare–like effect on neuromuscular function.

Neuromuscular blockade or respiratory paralysis may occur following rapid intravenous administration of many aminoglycosides and have been reported in cats receiving very high doses of tobramycin (40 mg/kg). The possibility of prolonged secondary apnoea should be considered if tobramycin is administered to anaesthetised patients who are also receiving neuromuscular blocking agents such as succinylcholine, tubocurarine or decamethonium, or to patients receiving massive transfusions of citrated blood. If neuromuscular blockade occurs, it may be reversed by the administration of calcium salts.

The inactivation of tobramycin by beta-lactam antibiotics (penicillins or cephalosporins) has been demonstrated *in vitro* and in patients with severe renal impairment. Such inactivation has not been found in patients with normal renal function if the drugs are administered by separate routes.

If overgrowth of non-susceptible organisms occurs, appropriate therapy should be initiated.

Side-effects: Renal function changes, as shown by rising blood urea and serum creatinine and by oliguria, cylindruria and increased proteinuria, have been reported, especially in patients with a history of renal impairment who are treated for longer periods or with higher doses than those recommended. These changes can occur in patients with initially normal renal function.

Side-effects on both vestibular and auditory branches of the eighth cranial nerve have been reported, especially in patients receiving high doses or prolonged therapy, in those given previous courses of therapy with an ototoxin, and in cases of dehydration. Symptoms include dizziness, vertigo, tinnitus, roaring in the ears and hearing loss. Hearing loss is usually irreversible and is manifested initially by diminution of high-tone acuity.

Other reported side-effects, possibly related to tobramycin, include increased AST, ALT, and serum bilirubin; decreased serum calcium, magnesium, sodium and potassium; anaemia, granulocytopenia, thrombocytopenia, leucopenia, leucocytosis and eosinophilia; and fever, rash, exfoliative dermatitis, itching, urticaria, nausea, vomiting, diarrhoea, headache, lethargy, pain at the injection site, mental confusion and disorientation.

Overdosage: Severity of the manifestations of a tobramycin overdose depend on the dose, the patient's renal function, state of hydration, age and whether concurrent medication with similar toxicities is being given. Toxicity may occur in patients treated for more than 10 days, given more than 5 mg/kg/day, children given more than 7.5 mg/kg/day, or patients with reduced renal function whose dose has not been appropriately adjusted.

Nephrotoxicity following the parenteral administration of an aminoglycoside is most closely related to the AUC of serum concentration versus time. Nephrotoxicity is more likely if trough levels fail to fall below 2 mg/l and is also proportional to the average blood concentration. Patients who are elderly, have renal impairment, are receiving other nephrotoxic or ototoxic drugs, or are volume depleted, are at greater risk for developing acute tubular necrosis. Auditory and vestibular toxicities have been associated with aminoglycoside overdose. These toxicities occur in patients treated longer than 10 days, in patients with abnormal renal function, in dehydrated patients, or in patients on other ototoxic drugs. These patients may not have signs or symptoms, or may experience dizziness, tinnitus, vertigo and a loss of high-tone acuity. Signs and symptoms may not occur until long after the drug has been discontinued.

Neuromuscular blockade or respiratory failure may occur following rapid intravenous administration of many aminoglycosides. These reactions and prolonged respiratory paralysis may occur more commonly in patients with myasthenia gravis or Parkinson's disease, or those receiving decamethonium, tubocurarine or succinylcholine. Neuromuscular blockade may be reversed by the administration of calcium salts, but mechanical assistance may be necessary.

Toxicity from ingested tobramycin is unlikely because aminoglycosides are poorly absorbed from an intact gastro-intestinal tract.

Treatment: Resuscitative measures should be initiated promptly if respiratory paralysis occurs. Neuromuscular blockade may be reversed by giving calcium salts. Fluid balance, creatinine clearance and tobramycin plasma levels should be carefully monitored until the tobramycin level falls below 2 mg/l. Haemodialysis or peritoneal dialysis will help remove tobramycin from the blood. Between 25% and 70% of the administered dose may be removed, depending on the duration and type of dialysis employed; haemodialysis is the more effective method.

Pharmaceutical precautions *Undiluted vials:* Store below 25°C. Nebcin should not be physically premixed with other drugs but should be administered separately according to the recommended dose and route.

Prior to administration, parenteral drug products should be inspected visually for particulate matter and discolouration whenever solution and container permit.

Legal category POM.

Package quantity Boxes of 10 rubber-stoppered injection vials.

Further information Nil.

Product licence numbers
40 mg per 1 ml: 0006/0084
10 mg per 1 ml: 0006/0085

NU-SEALS 75*
NU-SEALS 300*

Presentation Enteric sealed tablets of aspirin. Nu-Seals Aspirin is available as 75 mg tablets (coded 75, in red) or as 300 mg tablets (coded 300, in red) of Acetylsalicylic Acid PhEur covered in a special coating, white in colour.

Uses Aspirin has analgesic, antipyretic and anti-inflammatory actions. It also has an antithrombotic action, mediated through inhibition of platelet activation, which has been shown to be useful in secondary prophylaxis following myocardial infarction and in patients with unstable angina or cerebral transient ischaemic attacks.

Nu-Seals Aspirin is indicated wherever high or prolonged dosage of aspirin is required. The special coating resists dissolution in gastric juice, but will dissolve readily in the relatively less acid environment of the duodenum. Owing to the delay that the coating imposes on the release of the active ingredient, Nu-Seals Aspirin is unsuitable for the short-term relief of pain.

Dosage and administration Nu-Seals Aspirin is for oral administration to adults only.

Analgesic, antipyretic and anti-inflammatory actions: 300–900 mg repeated three to four times daily according to clinical needs. In acute rheumatic disorders the dose is in the range of 4–8 g daily, taken in divided doses.

Antithrombotic action: 150 mg at diagnosis and 75 mg daily thereafter. Tablets taken at diagnosis should be chewed in order to gain rapid absorption.

Doses of 300 mg daily have been used with a low incidence of side-effects.

The elderly: Analgesic, antipyretic and anti-inflammatory actions: As for adults. The elderly are more likely to experience gastric side-effects and tinnitus. *Antithrombotic action:* The risk-benefit ratio has not been fully established.

Children: Aspirin should not be given to children, particularly those under 12 years (see *Warnings*).

Contra-indications, warnings, etc
Contra-indications: Hypersensitivity to aspirin. Hypoprothrombinaemia, haemophilia and active peptic ulceration.

Warnings: Aspirin should not be given to children, particularly those under 12 years, unless the expected benefits outweigh the possible risks. Aspirin may be a contributory factor in the causation of Reye's syndrome in some children.

Salicylates should be used with caution in patients with a history of peptic ulceration or coagulation abnormalities. They may also induce gastro-intestinal haemorrhage, occasionally major.

Aspirin should be used with caution in patients with impaired renal function, hepatic function (avoid if severe), or in patients who are dehydrated.

In large doses, salicylates may also decrease insulin requirements.

Usage in pregnancy: Aspirin does not appear to have teratogenic effects. However, prolonged pregnancy and labour, with increased bleeding before and after delivery, decreased birth weight and increased rate of stillbirth were reported with high blood salicylate levels. Aspirin should be avoided during the last 3 months of pregnancy.

Usage in nursing mothers: As aspirin is excreted in breast milk, Nu-Seals should not be taken by patients who are breast-feeding.

Precautions: Salicylates may enhance the effect of anticoagulants, oral hypoglycaemic agents, phenytoin and sodium valproate. They inhibit the uricosuric effect of probenecid and may increase the toxicity of sulphonamides. They may also precipitate bronchospasm or induce attacks of asthma in susceptible subjects.

Patients using enteric-coated aspirin should be advised against ingesting antacids simultaneously, to avoid premature drug release.

Patients with hypertension should be carefully monitored.

Side-effects: Salicylates may induce hypersensitivity, asthma, urate kidney stones, chronic gastro-intestinal blood loss, tinnitus, nausea and vomiting. The special coating of Nu-Seals Aspirin helps to reduce the incidence of side-effects resulting from gastric irritation.

Overdosage: Overdosage produces dizziness, tinnitus, sweating, nausea and vomiting, confusion and hyperventilation. Gross overdosage may lead to CNS depression with coma, cardiovascular collapse and respiratory depression. If overdosage is suspected, the patient should be kept under observation for at least 24 hours, as symptoms and salicylate blood levels may not become apparent for several hours. Treatment of overdosage consists of gastric lavage and forced alkaline diuresis. Haemodialysis may be necessary in severe cases.

Pharmaceutical precautions Store below 25°C. Keep bottles tightly closed.

Legal category P (packs of 28). POM (packs of 56 and 100).

Package quantities Tablets 75 mg: Blister packs of 28 and 56.

Tablets 300 mg: Bottles of 100.

Further information Nil.

Product licence numbers
Tablets 75 mg: 0006/0293
Tablets 300 mg: 0006/5093R

NU-SEALS CARDIO 75* ASPIRIN

Presentation Enteric sealed tablets of aspirin. Nu-Seals Cardio 75 Aspirin is available as 75 mg tablets (coded 75, in red) of Acetylsalicylic Acid PhEur covered in a special coating, white in colour.

Uses Aspirin has an antithrombotic action, mediated through inhibition of platelet activation, which has been shown to be useful in secondary prophylaxis following myocardial infarction and in patients with unstable angina or cerebral transient ischaemic attacks.

Nu-Seals Cardio 75 Aspirin is indicated wherever prolonged dosage of aspirin is required. The special coating resists dissolution in gastric juice, but will dissolve readily in the relatively less acid environment of the duodenum. Owing to the delay that the coating imposes on the release of the active ingredient, Nu-Seals Cardio 75 Aspirin is unsuitable for the short-term relief of pain.

Dosage and administration Nu-Seals Cardio 75 Aspirin is for oral administration to adults only.

Antithrombotic action: 150 mg at diagnosis and 75 mg daily thereafter. Tablets taken at diagnosis should be chewed in order to gain rapid absorption.

The elderly: Antithrombotic action: The risk-benefit ratio has not been fully established.

Children: Aspirin should not be given to children, particularly those under 12 years (see *Warnings*).

Contra-indications, warnings, etc

Contra-indications: Hypersensitivity to aspirin. Hypoprothrombinaemia, haemophilia and active peptic ulceration.

Warnings: Aspirin should not be given to children, particularly those under 12 years, unless the expected benefits outweigh the possible risks. Aspirin may be a contributory factor in the causation of Reye's syndrome in some children.

Salicylates should be used with caution in patients with a history of peptic ulceration or coagulation abnormalities. They may also induce gastro-intestinal haemorrhage, occasionally major.

Aspirin should be used with caution in patients with impaired renal function, hepatic function (avoid if severe), or in patients who are dehydrated.

In large doses, salicylates may also decrease insulin requirements.

Usage in pregnancy: Aspirin does not appear to have teratogenic effects. However, prolonged pregnancy and labour, with increased bleeding before and after delivery, decreased birth weight and increased rate of stillbirth were reported with high blood salicylate levels. Aspirin should be avoided during the last 3 months of pregnancy.

Usage in nursing mothers: As aspirin is excreted in breast milk, Nu-Seals Cardio 75 should not be taken by patients who are breast-feeding.

Precautions: Salicylates may enhance the effect of anticoagulants, oral hypoglycaemic agents, phenytoin and sodium valproate. They inhibit the uricosuric effect of probenecid and may increase the toxicity of sulphonamides. They may also precipitate bronchospasm or induce attacks of asthma in susceptible subjects.

Patients using enteric-coated aspirin should be advised against ingesting antacids simultaneously, to avoid premature drug release.

Patients with hypertension should be carefully monitored.

Side-effects: Salicylates may induce hypersensitivity, asthma, urate kidney stones, chronic gastro-intestinal blood loss, tinnitus, nausea and vomiting. The special coating of Nu-Seals Cardio 75 Aspirin helps to reduce the incidence of side-effects resulting from gastric irritation.

Overdosage: Overdosage produces dizziness, tinnitus, sweating, nausea and vomiting, confusion and hyperventilation. Gross overdosage may lead to CNS depression with coma, cardiovascular collapse and respiratory depression. If overdosage is suspected, the patient should be kept under observation for at least 24 hours, as symptoms and salicylate blood levels may not become apparent for several hours. Treatment of overdosage consists of gastric lavage and forced alkaline diuresis. Haemodialysis may be necessary in severe cases.

Pharmaceutical precautions Store below 25°C.

Legal category P

Package quantities Blister packs of 28 tablets.

Further information Nil.

Product licence number 0006/0293

ONCOVIN*

WARNING
THIS PRODUCT IS **NOT**
FOR INTRATHECAL USE

Presentation

Oncovin Solution: 1 ml vials containing 1 mg Oncovin (Vincristine Sulphate BP) and 100 mg Mannitol BP.

2 ml vials containing 2 mg Oncovin (Vincristine Sulphate BP) and 200 mg Mannitol BP.

The vials also contain 1.8 mg per 1 ml Methyl Hydroxybenzoate PhEur and 0.2 mg per 1 ml Propyl Hydroxybenzoate PhEur as preservatives. Acetic acid and sodium acetate have been added for pH control.

Uses Oncovin is an anti-neoplastic drug for intravenous use.

Information available at present suggests that Oncovin may be useful either alone or in conjunction with other oncolytic drugs for the treatment of:

1. Leukaemias, including acute lymphocytic leukaemia, chronic lymphocytic leukaemia, acute myelogenous leukaemia and blastic crisis of chronic myelogenous leukaemia.
2. Malignant lymphomas, including Hodgkin's disease and non-Hodgkin's lymphomas.
3. Multiple myeloma.
4. Solid tumours, including breast carcinoma, small cell bronchogenic carcinoma, head and neck carcinoma and soft tissue sarcomas.
5. Paediatric solid tumours, including Ewing's sarcoma, embryonal rhabdomyosarcoma, neuroblastoma, Wilms' tumour, retinoblastoma and medulloblastoma.
6. Idiopathic thrombocytopenic purpura. Patients with true ITP refractory to splenectomy and short-term treatment with adrenocortical steroids may respond to vincristine but the drug is not recommended as primary treatment of this disorder. Recommended weekly doses of vincristine given for 3 to 4 weeks have produced permanent remissions in some patients. If patients fail to respond after 3 to 6 doses, it is unlikely that there will be any beneficial results with additional doses.

Dosage and administration *This preparation is for intravenous use only. It should be administered only by individuals experienced in vincristine administration.*

FATAL IF GIVEN INTRATHECALLY.
FOR INTRAVENOUS USE ONLY.
See 'Warnings' section for the treatment of patients given intrathecal vincristine sulphate.

Extreme care must be used in calculating and administering the dose of vincristine, since overdosage may have a very serious or fatal outcome.

The drug is administered intravenously *at weekly intervals.* The recommended dose is 1.4 to 1.5 mg/m², up to a maximum weekly dose of 2 mg.

The dosage must always be adjusted individually because of the narrow range between therapeutic and toxic levels, and individual variations in response.

The elderly: As for adults.

Children: The usual dose is 2 mg/m². For children weighing 10 kg or less, the starting dose should be 0.05 mg/kg, administered once a week.

An increase in the severity of side-effects may be experienced by patients with liver disease sufficient to decrease biliary excretion. A 50 per cent reduction in the dose of vincristine is recommended for patients having a direct serum bilirubin value above 3 mg/100 ml (51 micromol/l).

The metabolism of vinca alkaloids has been shown to be mediated by hepatic cytochrome P450 isoenzymes in the CYP 3A subfamily. This metabolic pathway may be impaired in patients with hepatic dysfunction or who are taking concomitant potent inhibitors of these isoenzymes (see *Precautions*).

Oncovin solution: The concentration of vincristine is 1 mg/ml. Do not add extra fluid to the vial prior to removal of the dose. Withdraw the solution of Oncovin into an accurate dry syringe, measuring the dose carefully. Do not add extra fluid to the vial in an attempt to empty it completely.

The calculated dose of the solution for injection is drawn up into a syringe and injected either directly into a vein or into the tubing of a running intravenous infusion of normal saline or glucose in water, whichever is more suitable for the patient.

Care should be taken to avoid infiltration of subcutaneous tissues. Injection may be completed in about one minute.

Caution: If leakage into surrounding tissue should occur during intravenous administration of vincristine, it may cause considerable irritation. The injection should be discontinued immediately and any remaining portion of the dose should then be introduced into another vein. Local injection of hyaluronidase and the application of moderate heat to the area of leakage help to disperse the drug and are thought to minimise discomfort and the possibility of cellulitis.

Contra-indications, warnings, etc

Contra-indications

FATAL IF GIVEN INTRATHECALLY.
FOR INTRAVENOUS USE ONLY.
See 'Warnings' section for the treatment of patients given intrathecal vincristine sulphate.

Patients with the demyelinating form of Charcot-Marie-Tooth syndrome should not be given vincristine.

Warnings: This preparation is for intravenous use only. It should be administered by individuals experienced in the administration of vincristine sulphate. The intrathecal administration of vincristine sulphate usually results in death. Syringes containing this product should be labelled, using the auxiliary sticker provided, to state 'FATAL IF GIVEN INTRATHECALLY. FOR INTRAVENOUS USE ONLY'.

Extemporaneously prepared syringes containing this product must be packaged in an overwrap which is labelled 'DO NOT REMOVE COVERING UNTIL MOMENT OF INJECTION. FATAL IF GIVEN INTRATHECALLY. FOR INTRAVENOUS USE ONLY'.

After inadvertent intrathecal administration, immediate neurosurgical intervention is required in order to prevent ascending paralysis leading to death. In a very small number of patients, life-threatening paralysis and subsequent death was averted but resulted in devastating neurological sequelae, with limited recovery afterwards.

Based on the published management of these survival cases, if vincristine is mistakenly given by the intrathecal route, the following treatment should be initiated **immediately after the injection**:

1. Removal of as much CSF as is safely possible through the lumbar access.
2. Insertion of an epidural catheter into the subarachnoid space via the intervertebral space above initial lumbar access and CSF irrigation with lactated Ringer's solution. Fresh frozen plasma should be requested and, when available, 25 ml should be added to every 1 litre of lactated Ringer's solution.
3. Insertion of an intraventricular drain or catheter by a neurosurgeon and continuation of CSF irrigation with fluid removal through the lumbar access connected to a closed drainage system. Lactated Ringer's solution should be given by continuous infusion at 150 ml/h, or at a rate of 75 ml/h when fresh frozen plasma has been added as above.

The rate of infusion should be adjusted to maintain a spinal fluid protein level of 150 mg/dl.

The following measures have also been used in addition but may not be essential:

Glutamic acid has been given IV 10 gm over 24 hours, followed by 500 mg tds by mouth for 1 month. Folinic acid has been administered intravenously as a 100 mg bolus and then infused at a rate of 25 mg/h for 24 hours, then bolus doses of 25 mg 6-hourly for 1 week. Pyridoxine has been given at a dose of 50 mg 8-hourly by intravenous infusion over 30 minutes. Their roles in the reduction of neurotoxicity are unclear.

Usage in pregnancy: Caution is necessary with the use of all oncolytic drugs during pregnancy.

Vincristine can cause foetal harm when administered to a pregnant woman, although there are no adequate and well-controlled studies. In several animal species, vincristine can induce teratogenic effects as well as embryolethality with doses that are non-toxic to the pregnant animal. Women of childbearing potential should be advised to avoid becoming pregnant while receiving vincristine. If vincristine is used during pregnancy or if the patient becomes pregnant while receiving this drug she should be informed of the potential hazard to the foetus.

Usage in nursing mothers: It is not known whether Oncovin is excreted in human breast milk. Because of the potential for serious adverse reactions due to Oncovin in nursing infants, a decision should be made whether to discontinue nursing or the drug, taking into account the importance of the drug to the mother.

Precautions: Effective therapy with Oncovin is less likely to be followed by leucopenia than is the case with Velbe (vinblastine sulphate) and other oncolytic agents. A study of the side–effects of Oncovin in all age groups reveals that it is usually neuromuscular rather than bone marrow toxicity that limits dosage. However, because of the possibility of leucopenia, both clinician and patient should remain alert for signs of any complicating infection. Although pre-existing leucopenia does not necessarily contra-indicate the administration of Oncovin, the appearance of leucopenia during treatment warrants careful consideration before giving the next dose.

Acute uric acid nephropathy, which may occur after the administration of oncolytic agents, has also been reported with Oncovin.

If central-nervous-system leukaemia is diagnosed, additional agents may be required, since vincristine does not appear to cross the blood-brain barrier in adequate amounts.

Particular attention should be given to dosage and neurological side-effects if Oncovin is administered to patients with pre-existing neuromuscular disease and also when other drugs with neurotoxic potential are being used.

Acute shortness of breath and severe bronchospasm have been reported following the administration of vinca alkaloids. These reactions have been encountered most frequently when the vinca alkaloid was used in combination with mitomycin-C and may be serious when there is pre-existing pulmonary dysfunction. The onset may be within minutes or several hours after the vinca is injected and may occur up to 2 weeks following the dose of mitomycin. Progressive dyspnoea, requiring chronic therapy, may occur. Vincristine should not be re-administered.

The simultaneous oral or intravenous administration of phenytoin and antineoplastic chemotherapy combinations, that included vincristine sulphate, have been reported to reduce blood levels of the anticonvulsant and to increase seizure activity. Although the contribution of the vinca alkaloids has not been established, dosage adjustment of phenytoin, based on serial blood level monitoring, may need to be made when it is used in combination with vincristine.

Caution should be exercised in patients concurrently taking drugs known to inhibit drug metabolism by hepatic cytochrome P450 isoenzymes in the CYP 3A subfamily, or in patients with hepatic dysfunction. Concurrent administration of vincristine sulphate with itraconazole (a known inhibitor of the metabolic pathway) has been reported to cause an earlier onset and/or an increased severity of neuromuscular side-effects (see 'Adverse reactions'). This interaction is presumed to be related to inhibition of the metabolism of vincristine.

When Oncovin is used in combination with L–asparaginase, it should be given 12 to 24 hours before administration of the enzyme in order to minimise toxicity, since administering L-asparaginase first may reduce hepatic clearance of vincristine.

When chemotherapy is being given in conjunction with radiation therapy through portals which include the liver, the use of vincristine should be delayed until radiation therapy has been completed.

Both *in vivo* and *in vitro* laboratory tests have failed to demonstrate conclusively that this product is mutagenic. Fertility following treatment with vincristine alone for malignant disease has not been studied in humans. Clinical reports of both male and female patients who received multiple-agent chemotherapy that included vincristine indicate that azoospermia and amenorrhoea can occur in postpubertal patients. Recovery occurred many months after completion of chemotherapy in some but not all patients. When the same treatment is administered to prepubertal patients, it is much less likely to cause permanent azoospermia and amenorrhoea.

Patients who received vincristine chemotherapy in combination with anticancer drugs known to be carcinogenic have developed second malignancies. The contributing role of vincristine in this development has not been determined. No evidence of carcinogenicity was found following intraperitoneal administration in rats and mice, although this study was limited.

Care must be taken to avoid contamination of the eye with concentrations of Oncovin used clinically. If accidental contamination occurs, severe irritation (or, if the drug was delivered under pressure, even corneal ulceration) may result. The eye should be washed immediately and thoroughly.

Adverse reactions: Prior to the use of this drug, patients and/or their parents/guardians should be advised of the possibility of untoward symptoms.

In general, adverse reactions are reversible and are related to dosage size and cumulative dosage. The use of small amounts of vincristine daily for long periods is not advised. The most common adverse reaction is alopecia; the most troublesome adverse reactions are neuromuscular in origin.

When single weekly doses of the drug are employed, the adverse reactions of leucopenia, neuritic pain, and constipation are usually of short duration (i.e. less than 7 days). When the dosage is reduced, these reactions may lessen or disappear. They seem to be increased when the calculated amount of drug is given in divided doses. Other adverse reactions, such as alopecia, sensory loss, paraesthesia, difficulty in walking, slapping gait, loss of deep-tendon reflexes and muscle wasting may persist for at least as long as therapy is continued. Generalised sensorimotor dysfunction may become progressively more severe with continued treatment. In most instances, they have disappeared by about the sixth week after discontinuance of treatment, but the neuromuscular difficulties may persist for prolonged periods in some patients. Re-growth of hair may occur while maintenance therapy continues.

The following adverse reactions have been reported:

Neuromuscular (often dose limiting): Neuritic pain, sensory loss, paraesthesiae, difficulty in walking, slapping gait, loss of deep tendon reflexes, muscle wasting, ataxia, paresis, foot drop and cranial nerve palsies, especially ocular palsies and laryngeal nerve paralysis. Jaw pain, pharyngeal pain, parotid gland pain, bone pain, back pain, limb pain and myalgias have been reported; pain in these areas may be severe. Convulsions, frequently with hypertension, have been reported in a few patients receiving vincristine. Several instances of convulsions followed by coma have been reported in children. Transient cortical blindness and optic atrophy with blindness have been reported. Treatment with vinca alkaloids has resulted rarely in both vestibular and auditory damage to the eighth cranial nerve. Manifestations include partial or total deafness, which may be temporary or permanent, and difficulties with balance, including dizziness, nystagmus and vertigo. Particular caution is warranted when vincristine sulphate is used in combination with other agents known to be ototoxic, such as the platinum-containing oncolytics.

Frequently, there appears to be a sequence in the development of neuromuscular side-effects. Initially, one may encounter only sensory impairment and paraesthesiae. With continued treatment, neuritic pain may appear and later, motor difficulties. No reports have yet been made of any agent that can reverse the neuromuscular manifestations of Oncovin.

Haematological: Leucopenia; vincristine does not appear to have any constant or significant effect upon the platelets or the red blood cells, however, anaemia and thrombocytopenia have been reported. If thrombocytopenia is present when treatment with Oncovin is begun, it may actually improve before the appearance of marrow remission.

Gastro-intestinal: Constipation, abdominal cramps, paralytic ileus, diarrhoea, weight loss, nausea, vomiting, oral ulceration, intestinal necrosis and/or perforation, and anorexia have occurred. The constipation which may be encountered responds well to such usual measures as enemas and laxatives. Constipation may take the form of upper colon impaction and the rectum may be found to be empty on physical examination. Colicky abdominal pain, coupled with an empty rectum, may mislead the clinician. A flat film of the abdomen is useful in demonstrating this condition. A routine prophylactic regimen against constipation is recommended for all patients receiving Oncovin. Paralytic ileus may occur, particularly in young children. The ileus will reverse itself upon temporary discontinuance of vincristine and with symptomatic care.

Pulmonary: See under *Precautions.*

Endocrine: Rare occurrences of a syndrome attributable to inappropriate anti-diuretic hormone secretion have been observed in patients treated with vincristine. There is a high urinary sodium excretion in the presence of hyponatraemia; renal or adrenal disease, hypotension, dehydration, azotaemia and clinical oedema are absent. With fluid deprivation, improvement occurs in the hyponatraemia and in the renal loss of sodium.

Genitourinary: Polyuria, dysuria and urinary retention due to bladder atony have occurred. Other drugs known to cause urinary retention (particularly in the elderly) should, if possible, be discontinued for the first few days following administration of vincristine.

Cardiovascular: Hypertension and hypotension have occurred. Chemotherapy combinations which have included vincristine, when given to patients previously treated with mediastinal radiation, have been associated with coronary artery disease and myocardial infarction. Causality has not been established.

Hypersensitivity: Rare cases of allergic-type reactions, such as anaphylaxis, rash and oedema, temporally related to vincristine therapy have been reported in patients receiving vincristine as a part of multi-drug chemotherapy regimens.

Cutaneous: Alopecia, rash.

Other: Fever, headache, injection site reaction (see *Dosage and administration—Caution).*

Overdosage: Side–effects following the use of vincristine are dose related. In children under 13 years of age, death has occurred following doses of vincristine that were 10 times those recommended for therapy. Severe symptoms may occur in this patient group following dosages of 3 to 4 mg/m². Adults can be expected to experience severe symptoms after single doses of 3 mg/m² or more. Therefore, following administration of doses higher than those recommended, patients can be expected to experience side-effects in an exaggerated fashion. Supportive care should include the following: (a) prevention of side-effects resulting from the syndrome of inappropriate antidiuretic hormone secretion (this would include restriction of fluid intake and perhaps the administration of a diuretic affecting the function of Henle's loop and the distal tubule); (b) administration of anticonvulsants; (c) use of enemas or cathartics to prevent ileus (in some instances, decompression of the gastro-intestinal tract may be necessary); (d) monitoring the cardiovascular system; (e) determining daily blood counts for guidance in transfusion requirements.

Folinic acid has been observed to have a protective effect in normal mice which were administered lethal doses of vincristine. Isolated case reports suggest that folinic acid may be helpful in treating humans who have received an overdose. A suggested schedule is to administer 100 mg of folinic acid intravenously every 3 hours for 24 hours and then every 6 hours for at least 48 hours. Theoretical tissue levels of vincristine derived from pharmacokinetic data are predicted to remain significantly elevated for at least 72 hours. Treatment with folinic acid does not eliminate the need for the above-mentioned supportive measures.

Most of an intravenous dose of vincristine is excreted into the bile after rapid tissue binding. Because only very small amounts of the drug appear in dialysate, haemodialysis is not likely to be helpful in cases of overdosage.

Enhanced faecal excretion of parenterally administered vincristine has been demonstrated in dogs pre-treated with cholestyramine. There are no published clinical data on the use of cholestyramine as an antidote in humans.

There are no published clinical data on the consequences of oral ingestion of vincristine. Should oral ingestion occur, the stomach should be evacuated followed by oral administration of activated charcoal and a cathartic.

Pharmaceutical precautions

Special dispensing information: When dispensing vincristine sulphate in other than the original container, it is imperative that it be packaged in an overwrap bearing the statement 'DO NOT REMOVE COVERING UNTIL MOMENT OF INJECTION. FATAL IF GIVEN INTRATHECALLY. FOR INTRAVENOUS USE ONLY'. A syringe containing a specific dose must be labelled, using the auxiliary sticker provided in the pack, with this warning.

Guidelines for the safe handling of antineoplastic agents: Cytotoxic preparations should not be handled by pregnant staff.

Trained personnel should reconstitute the drug. This should be performed in a designated area. The work surface should be covered with disposable plastic-backed absorbent paper.

Adequate protective gloves, masks and clothing should be worn. Precautions should be taken to avoid the drug accidentally coming into contact with the eyes. If accidental contamination occurs, the eye should be washed with water thoroughly and immediately.

Use Luer-lock fittings on all syringes and sets. Large bore needles are recommended to minimise pressure and the possible formation of aerosols. The latter may also be reduced by the use of a venting needle.

Adequate care and precaution should be taken in the disposal of items (syringes, needles, etc.) used to reconstitute cytotoxic drugs.

Oncovin Solution: Store in a refrigerator between 2° and 8°C. Protect from light.

Oncovin should never be mixed with any other drug and should not be diluted in solutions that raise or lower the pH outside the range of 3.5 to 5.5. It should not be mixed with anything other than normal saline or glucose in water.

Whenever solution and container permit, parenteral drug products should be inspected visually for particulate matter and discolouration prior to administration.

Legal category POM.

Package quantities
Vials 1 mg/1 ml: Single vials
Vials 2 mg/2 ml: Single vials

Further information Nil.

Product licence numbers
Vials 1 mg/1 ml: 0006/0169
Vials 2 mg/2 ml: 0006/0169

REOPRO* ▼

Qualitative and quantitative composition Abciximab 2 mg/ml (10 mg/5 ml vial).

Pharmaceutical form Solution for injection.

Clinical particulars

Therapeutic indications: ReoPro is indicated as an adjunct to heparin and aspirin for:

1. Percutaneous Coronary Intervention

The prevention of ischaemic cardiac complications in patients undergoing percutaneous coronary intervention (balloon angioplasty, atherectomy and bail out stent).

2. Unstable Angina

The short-term (1-month) reduction of the risk of myocardial infarction, in patients with unstable angina, not responding to full conventional therapy who have been scheduled for percutaneous coronary intervention.

Posology and method of administration: ReoPro is for intravenous (IV) administration in adults.

Adults: The recommended dose of ReoPro is a 0.25 mg/kg intravenous bolus immediately followed by a 0.125 microgram/kg/min (to a maximum of 10 microgram/min) continuous intravenous infusion.

For the stabilisation of unstable angina patients, the bolus dose followed by the infusion should be started up to 24 hours prior to the possible intervention and concluded 12 hours after the intervention.

For the prevention of ischaemic cardiac complications in patients undergoing percutaneous coronary intervention, and who are not currently receiving a ReoPro infusion, the bolus should be administered 10 to 60 minutes prior to the intervention followed by the infusion for 12 hours.

Administration instructions:

1. Parenteral drug products should be inspected visually for particulate matter prior to administration. Preparations of ReoPro containing visibly opaque particles should NOT be used.

2. Hypersensitivity reactions should be anticipated whenever protein solutions such as ReoPro are administered. Adrenaline, dopamine, theophylline, antihistamines and corticosteroids should be available for immediate use. If symptoms of an allergic reaction or anaphylaxis appear, the infusion should be stopped immediately. Subcutaneous administration of 0.3 to 0.5 ml of aqueous adrenaline (1:1000 dilution), and use of corticosteroids, respiratory assistance and other resuscitative measures are essential.

3. As with all parenteral drug products, aseptic procedures should be used during the administration of ReoPro.

4. Withdraw the necessary amount of ReoPro for the bolus injection into a syringe. Filter the bolus injection using a sterile, non-pyrogenic, low protein-binding 0.2 or 0.22 μm syringe filter (Millipore SLGV025LS or equivalent). The bolus should be administered over one (1) minute.

5. Withdraw the necessary amount of ReoPro for the continuous infusion into a syringe. Inject into an appropriate container of sterile 0.9% saline or 5% dextrose and infuse at the calculated rate via a continuous infusion pump. The continuous infusion should be filtered either upon admixture using a sterile, non-pyrogenic, low protein-binding 0.2 μm or 0.22 μm syringe filter (Millipore SLGV025LS or equivalent) or upon administration using an in-line, sterile, non-pyrogenic, low protein-binding 0.2 μm or 0.22 μm filter (Abbott #4524 or equivalent). Discard the unused portion at the end of the infusion period.

6. Although incompatibilities have not been shown with intravenous infusion fluids or commonly used cardiovascular drugs, it is recommended that ReoPro be administered in a separate intravenous line whenever possible and not mixed with other medications.

7. No incompatibilities have been observed with glass bottles or polyvinyl chloride bags or administration sets.

Contra-indications: ReoPro should not be administered to patients with known sensitivity to abciximab, to any component of the product or to murine monoclonal antibodies.

Because inhibition of platelet aggregation increases the risk of bleeding, ReoPro is contra–indicated in the following clinical situations: active internal bleeding; history of cerebrovascular accident within two years; recent (within two months) intracranial or intraspinal surgery or trauma; recent (within two months) major surgery; intracranial neoplasm, arteriovenous malformation or aneurysm; known bleeding diathesis or severe uncontrolled hypertension; pre–existing thrombocytopenia; vasculitis; hypertensive or diabetic retinopathy; severe hepatic or severe renal failure.

Special warnings and special precautions for use: Careful assessment of risk:benefit should be made in individual patients before commencing therapy with ReoPro. A favourable risk:benefit has not been established in low risk patients >65 years of age.

Requirement for specialist facilities: ReoPro should only be administered in conjunction with extensive specialist medical and nursing care. In addition, there must be availability of laboratory tests of haematology function and facilities for administration of blood products.

Concomitant aspirin and heparin therapy: ReoPro should be used as an adjunct to aspirin and heparin therapy.

Aspirin: Aspirin should be administered orally at a daily dose of approximately but not less than 300 mg.

Heparin: Percutaneous coronary intervention: Heparin bolus pre-PTCA: If a patient's activated clotting time (ACT) is less than 200 seconds prior to the start of the PTCA procedure, an initial bolus of heparin should be given upon gaining arterial access according to the following algorithm:

ACT <150 seconds: administer 70U/kg

ACT 150–199 seconds: administer 50U/kg

The initial heparin bolus dose should not exceed 7,000U.

ACT should be checked a minimum of 2 minutes after the heparin bolus. If the ACT is <200 seconds, additional heparin boluses of 20U/kg may be administered. Should the ACT remain <200 seconds, additional 20U/kg boluses are to be given until an ACT ≥200 seconds is achieved.

Should a situation arise where higher doses of heparin are considered clinically necessary in spite of the possibility of a greater bleeding risk, it is recommended that heparin be carefully titrated using weight–adjusted boluses and that the target ACT not exceed 300 seconds.

Heparin bolus during PTCA: During the PTCA procedure, ACT should be checked every 30 minutes. If ACT is <200 seconds, additional heparin boluses of 20U/kg may be administered. Should the ACT remain <200 seconds, additional 20U/kg boluses may be given until an ACT ≥200 seconds is achieved. ACT should be checked prior to and a minimum of 2 minutes after each heparin bolus.

As an alternative to giving additional boluses as described above, a continuous heparin infusion may be initiated after the initial heparin bolus doses achieve the ACT target ≥200 seconds at a rate of 7U/kg/hour and continued for the duration of the procedure.

Heparin infusion after PTCA: Discontinuation of heparin immediately following completion of the procedure, with removal of the arterial sheath within 6 hours, is *strongly recommended.* In individual patients, if prolonged heparin therapy after PTCA or later sheath removal is used, then an initial infusion rate of 7U/kg/hr is recommended (see Bleeding Precautions: Femoral Artery Sheath Removal). In all circumstances, heparin should be discontinued at least 2 hours prior to arterial sheath removal.

Stabilisation of unstable angina: Anticoagulation should be initiated with heparin to a target APTT of 60–85 seconds. The heparin infusion should be maintained during the ReoPro infusion. Following angioplasty, heparin management is outlined above under *Percutaneous coronary intervention.*

Bleeding precautions:

Femoral artery access site: ReoPro is associated with an increase in bleeding rate particularly at the site of arterial access for femoral artery sheath placement. The following are specific recommendations for access site care:

Femoral artery sheath insertion: When appropriate, place only an arterial sheath for vascular access (avoid venous sheath placement)

Puncture only the anterior wall of the artery or vein when establishing vascular access

The use of a through and through technique to identify the vascular structure is *strongly discouraged*

While femoral artery sheath is in place: Check sheath insertion site and distal pulses of affected leg(s) every 15 minutes for 1 hour, then hourly for 6 hours

Maintain complete bed rest with head of bed ≤30°

Maintain affected leg(s) straight via sheet tuck method or soft restraint

Medicate for back/groin pain as necessary

Educate patient on post-PTCA care via verbal instructions

Femoral artery sheath removal: Heparin should be discontinued at least 2 hours prior to arterial sheath removal

Check APTT or ACT prior to arterial sheath removal: do not remove sheath unless APTT ≤50 seconds or ACT ≤175 seconds

Apply pressure to access site for at least 30 min following sheath removal, using either manual compression or a mechanical device

Apply pressure dressing after haemostasis has been achieved

After femoral artery sheath removal: Check groin for bleeding/haematoma and distal pulses every 15 minutes for the first hour or until stable, then hourly for 6 hours following sheath removal

Continue complete bed rest with head of bed ≤30° and affected leg(s) straight for 6–8 hours following femoral artery sheath removal, 6–8 hours following discontinuation of ReoPro or 4 hours following discontinuation of heparin, whichever is later

Remove pressure dressing prior to ambulation

Continue to medicate for discomfort.

Management of femoral access site bleeding/haematoma formation: In the event of groin bleeding with or without haematoma formation, the following procedures are recommended:

Lower head of bed to 0°

Apply manual pressure/compression device until haemostasis has been achieved

Any haematoma should be measured and monitored for enlargement

Change pressure dressing as needed

If heparin is being given, obtain APTT and adjust heparin as needed

Maintain intravenous access if sheath has been removed

If groin bleed continues or the haematoma expands during ReoPro infusion despite the above measures, the ReoPro infusion should be immediately discontinued and the arterial sheath removed according to the guidelines listed above. After sheath removal intravenous access should be maintained until bleeding is controlled (see Overdose, *Uncontrolled bleeding*).

Potential bleeding sites: Careful attention should be paid to all potential bleeding sites, including arterial and venous puncture sites, catheter insertion sites, cutdown sites, and needle puncture sites.

Retroperitoneal bleeding: ReoPro is associated with an increased risk of retroperitoneal bleeding in association with femoral vascular puncture. The use of venous sheaths should be minimised and only the anterior wall of the artery or vein should be punctured when establishing vascular access (see Bleeding Precautions, *Femoral Artery Access Site*).

GI Bleeding prophylaxis: In order to prevent spontaneous GI bleeding it is recommended that patients are pretreated with H_2–histamine receptor antagonists or liquid antacids. Anti-emetics should be given as needed to prevent vomiting.

General nursing care: Unnecessary arterial and venous punctures, intramuscular injections, routine use of urinary catheters, nasotracheal intubation, nasogastric tubes and automatic blood pressure cuffs should be avoided. When obtaining intravenous access, non–compressible sites (eg, subclavian or jugular veins) should be avoided. Saline or heparin locks should be considered for blood drawing. Vascular puncture sites should be documented and monitored. Gentle care should be provided when removing dressings.

Patient monitoring: Before administration of ReoPro, platelet count, ACT, prothrombin time (PT) and APTT should be measured to identify pre-existing coagulation abnormalities. Haemoglobin and haematocrit measurements should be obtained prior to the ReoPro administration, at 12 hours following the ReoPro bolus injection, and again at 24 hours following the bolus injection. Twelve lead electrocardiograms (ECG) should be obtained prior to the bolus injection of ReoPro, and repeated once the patient has returned to the hospital ward from the catheterisation laboratory, and at 24 hours after the bolus injection of ReoPro. Vital signs (including blood pressure and pulse) should be obtained hourly for the first 4 hours following the ReoPro bolus injection, and then at 6, 12, 18 and 24 hours following the ReoPro bolus injection.

Restoration of platelet function: Transfusion of donor platelets has been shown to restore platelet function following ReoPro administration in animal studies and transfusions of fresh random donor platelets have been given empirically to restore platelet function in humans. In the event of serious uncontrolled bleeding or the need for emergency surgery, ReoPro should be discontinued. In the majority of patients, bleeding time returns to 12 minutes within 12 hours.' A bleeding time should be determined by the Ivy method (see below). If the bleeding time remains greater than 12 minutes, 10 units of platelets may be given. ReoPro may be displaced from endogenous platelet receptors and subsequently bind to platelets which have been transfused. Nevertheless, a single transfusion may be sufficient to reduce receptor blockade to 60% to 70% at which level platelet function is restored. Repeat platelet transfusions may be required to maintain the bleeding time at or below 12 minutes.

Ivy method for determination of bleeding time: Using an automated incision template, make a small incision on the lateral volar surface of the forearm while maintaining 40 mmHg pressure on the arm with a sphygmomanometer cuff. Determine the time for bleeding to stop with a stopwatch. Every 15 to 30 seconds a filter paper should be used to capture the blood from the incision but should not come in contact with the incision.

Use of thrombolytics, anticoagulants and other anti-platelet agents: Because ReoPro inhibits platelet aggregation, caution should be employed when used with other drugs affecting haemostasis such as heparin, oral anticoagulants such as warfarin, thrombolytics and antiplatelet agents other than aspirin, such as dipyridamole, ticlopidine or low molecular weight dextrans (see *Interactions with other medicaments and other forms of interaction*).

Limited data in patients receiving thrombolytics suggest an increase in the risk of bleeding when ReoPro is administered to patients treated with thrombolytics at doses sufficient to produce a systemic fibrinolytic state. If urgent intervention is required for refractory symptoms in a patient receiving ReoPro (or who has received the drug in the previous 48 hours), it is recommended that PTCA be attempted first to salvage the situation. Prior to further surgical interventions, the bleeding time should be determined by the Ivy method (see above) and should be 12 minutes or less. Should PTCA and any other appropriate procedures fail, and should the angiographic appearance suggest that the aetiology is due to thrombosis, consideration may be given to the administration of adjunctive thrombolytic therapy via the intracoronary route. A systemic fibrinolytic state should be avoided if at all possible.

Thrombocytopenia: To reduce the possibility of thrombocytopenia, platelet counts should be monitored prior to treatment, 2 to 4 hours following the bolus dose of ReoPro and at 24 hours. If a patient experiences an acute platelet decrease, additional platelet counts should be determined. These platelet counts should be drawn in three separate tubes containing ethylenediaminetetraacetic acid (EDTA), citrate and heparin, respectively, to exclude pseudothrombocytopenia due to *in vitro* anticoagulant interaction. If true thrombocytopenia is verified, ReoPro should be immediately discontinued and the condition appropriately monitored and treated. A daily platelet count should be obtained until it returns to normal. If a patient's platelet count drops to 60,000 cells/μl, heparin and aspirin should be discontinued. If a patient's platelet count drops below 50,000 cells/μl, platelets should be transfused.

Readministration: There are limited data concerning readministration of ReoPro. Human antichimeric antibody (HACA) appears, generally as a low titre, in approximately 5% to 6% of patients after single administrations of ReoPro (see *Undesirable effects*). Available evidence suggests that human antibodies to other monoclonal antibodies do not cross-react with ReoPro. Readministration of ReoPro to 29 patients known to be HACA-negative has not led to any change in ReoPro pharmacokinetics or to any reduction in antiplatelet potency. Nevertheless, the possibility of allergic or hypersensitivity reactions or diminished benefit cannot be excluded when ReoPro is administered to patients who have previously received monoclonal antibody therapy.

Renal disease and peripheral vascular disease: Benefits may be reduced in patients with renal disease or peripheral vascular disease.

Children or age over 80 years: Children or patients older than 80 years have not been studied.

Interactions with other medicaments and other forms of interaction: ReoPro has been formally studied as an adjunct to heparin and aspirin treatment. In the presence of ReoPro, heparin is associated with an increase in the incidence of bleeding. Limited experience with ReoPro in patients who have received thrombolytics suggests an increase in the risk of bleeding. Although there have been no formal studies of ReoPro with other commonly used cardiovascular drugs, in clinical studies there have been no adverse drug reactions associated with concomitant use of other medications used in the treatment of angina, myocardial infarction or hypertension nor with common intravenous infusion fluids. These medications have included warfarin (before and following but not during PTCA), beta-adrenergic receptor blockers, calcium channel antagonists, angiotensin converting enzyme (ACE) inhibitors, and intravenous and oral nitrates.

Pregnancy and lactation: Animal reproduction studies have not been conducted with ReoPro. It is also not known whether ReoPro can cause foetal harm when administered to a pregnant woman or can affect reproduction capacity. ReoPro should be given to a pregnant woman only if clearly needed.

Breast feeding of infants should be discontinued in nursing mothers since the secretion of abciximab in animal or human breast milk has not been studied.

Effects on ability to drive and use machines: Not applicable.

Undesirable effects: In the EPIC trial, in which a non-weight-adjusted, standard heparin dose regimen was used, the most common complication during ReoPro therapy was bleeding during the first 36 hours. The incidences of major bleeding,[1] minor bleeding[2] and transfusion of blood products were approximately doubled. In patients who had major bleeding, 67% had bleeding associated with the arterial access site in the groin.

In a subsequent clinical trial, EPILOG, using the heparin regimen, sheath removal and femoral access care guidelines outlined in the section *Special warnings and special precautions for use*, the incidence of major bleeding in patients treated with ReoPro (1.8%) was not significantly different from patients receiving placebo (3.1%) and there was no significant increase in the incidence of intracranial haemorrhage. The reduction in major bleeding observed in the EPILOG trial was achieved without loss of efficacy. In the CAPTURE trial, which did not use the low-dose heparin regimen, the incidence of major bleeding not associated with CABG surgery was higher in patients receiving ReoPro (3.8%) than in patients receiving placebo (1.9%).

Although data are limited, ReoPro treatment was not associated with excess major bleeding in patients who underwent CABG surgery. Some patients with prolonged bleeding times received platelet transfusions to correct the bleeding time prior to surgery. See *Bleeding precautions: Restoration of platelet function.*

The total incidence of intracranial haemorrhage and non-haemorrhagic stroke in all three pivotal trials was similar, 7/2225 (0.31%) for placebo patients and 10/3112 (0.32%) for ReoPro treated patients. The incidence of intracranial haemorrhage was 0.13% in placebo patients and 0.19% in ReoPro patients.

The most frequent adverse events are back pain, hypotension, nausea, chest pain, vomiting, headache pain, bradycardia, fever, puncture site pain and thrombocytopenia. Cardiac tamponade and adult respiratory distress syndrome have been reported rarely. Human antichimeric antibody (HACA) appears, generally as a low titre, in approximately 5% to 6% of patients after 2 to 4 weeks. Hypersensitivity or allergic reactions have been observed rarely following treatment with ReoPro. Nevertheless, anaphylaxis may potentially occur at any time during administration (see *Administration instructions*).

[1] Decrease in haemoglobin >5 g/dl.

[2] Spontaneous gross haematuria or haematemesis, or observed blood loss with a haemoglobin decrease >3 g/dl or with a decrease in haemoglobin ≥4 g/dl with no observed blood loss.

Overdose: There has been no experience of adverse events associated with overdosage. However, in the event of acute allergic reactions, thrombocytopenia or uncontrolled bleeding the administration of ReoPro should be immediately discontinued. In the event of thrombocytopenia or uncontrolled bleeding, platelet transfusion is recommended.

Allergic reactions: See Administration Instructions.

Thrombocytopenia: To reduce the possibility of thrombocytopenia, platelet counts should be monitored prior to treatment, 2 to 4 hours following the bolus dose of ReoPro and at 24 hours. If a patient experiences an acute platelet decrease, additional platelet counts should be determined. These platelet counts should be drawn in three separate tubes containing ethylenediaminetetraacetic acid (EDTA), citrate and heparin, respectively, to exclude pseudothrombocytopenia due to *in vitro* anticoagulant interaction. If true thrombocytopenia is verified, ReoPro should be immediately discontinued and the condition appropriately monitored and treated. A daily platelet count should be obtained until it returns to normal. If a patient's platelet count drops to 60,000 cells/μl, heparin and aspirin should be discontinued. If a patient's platelet count drops below 50,000 cells/μl, platelets should be transfused.

Uncontrolled bleeding: (Specific guidelines for access site bleeding are given above under *Bleeding Precautions, Femoral Artery Access Site.*) When considering the need to transfuse patients, the patient's intravascular volume should be assessed. If hypovolaemic, intravascular volume should be adequately restored with crystalloids. In asymptomatic patients, normovolaemic anaemia (haemoglobin 7–10 g/dl) can be well tolerated; transfusion is not indicated unless a deterioration in vital signs is seen or unless the patient develops signs and symptoms. In symptomatic patients (eg, syncope, dyspnoea, postural hypotension, tachycardia), crystalloids should be used to replace intravascular volume. If symptoms persist, the patient should receive transfusions with packed red blood cells or whole blood on a unit-by-unit basis to relieve symptoms; one unit may be sufficient. Transfusion of donor platelets has been shown to restore platelet function following ReoPro administration in animal studies and transfusions of fresh random donor platelets have been given empirically to restore platelet function in humans. In the event of serious uncontrolled bleeding or the need for emergency surgery, ReoPro should be discontinued. In the majority of patients, bleeding time returns to 12 minutes within 12 hours. If the bleeding time remains greater than 12 minutes, 10 units of platelets may be given. ReoPro may be displaced from endogenous platelet receptors and subsequently bind to platelets which have been transfused. Nevertheless, a single transfusion may be sufficient to reduce receptor blockade to 60% to 70% at which level platelet function is restored. Repeat platelet transfusions may be required to maintain the bleeding time at or below 12 minutes.

Pharmacological properties

Pharmacodynamic properties: ReoPro is the Fab fragment of the chimeric monoclonal antibody 7E3. It is directed against the glycoprotein (GP) IIb/IIIa ($\alpha_{IIb}\beta_3$) receptor located on the surface of human platelets. ReoPro inhibits platelet aggregation by preventing the binding of fibrinogen, von Willebrand factor and other adhesive molecules to GPIIb/IIIa receptor sites on activated platelets. ReoPro also binds to the vitronectin ($\alpha_v\beta_3$) receptor found on platelets and endothelial cells. The vitronectin receptor mediates the pro-coagulant properties of platelets and proliferative properties of vessel wall endothelial and smooth muscle cells. Because of its dual specificity, ReoPro more effectively blocks the burst of thrombin generation that follows platelet activation than agents which inhibit GPIIb/IIIa alone.

Intravenous administration in humans of single bolus doses of ReoPro from 0.15 mg/kg to 0.30 mg/kg produced rapid dose-dependent inhibition of platelet function as measured by *ex vivo* platelet aggregation in response to adenosine diphosphate (ADP) or by prolongation of bleeding time. At the two highest doses (0.25 and 0.30 mg/kg) at 2 hours post injection, over 80% of the GPIIb/IIIa receptors were blocked and platelet aggregation in response to 20μM ADP was almost abolished. The median bleeding time increased to over 30 minutes at both doses compared with a baseline value of approximately 5 minutes. The 80% level of receptor blockade was selected as a target for pharmacological efficacy because animal models of severe coronary stenosis have shown that platelet inhibition associated with this degree of blockade prevents platelet thrombosis.

Intravenous administration in humans of a single bolus dose of 0.25 mg/kg followed by a continuous infusion of 10 microgram/min for periods of 12 to 96 hours produced sustained high-grade GPIIb/IIIa receptor blockade (≥80%) and inhibition of platelet function (*ex vivo* platelet aggregation in response to 20μM ADP less than 20% of baseline and bleeding time greater than 30 minutes) for the duration of the infusion in most patients. Equivalent results were obtained when a weight adjusted infusion dose (0.125 microgram/kg/min to a maximum of 10 microgram/min) was used in patients up to 80 kg. Results in patients who received the 0.25 mg/kg bolus followed by a 5 microgram/min infusion for 24 hours showed a similar initial receptor blockade and inhibition of platelet aggregation, but the response was not maintained throughout the infusion period. Although low levels of GPIIb/IIIa receptor blockade are present for more than 10 days following cessation of the infusion, platelet function typically returned to normal over a period of 24 to 48 hours.

In clinical trials, ReoPro has demonstrated marked effects in reducing the thrombotic complications of coronary interventions such as balloon angioplasty, atherectomy and stent placement. These effects were observed within hours of the intervention and sustained for 30 days in the EPIC, EPILOG and CAPTURE trials. In the EPIC trial, which enrolled high-risk angioplasty patients, and in the EPILOG trial, which enrolled low- and high-risk angioplasty patients, the infusion dose was continued for 12 hours after the procedure and the reduction in the composite endpoint of death, MI or repeat intervention was sustained for the period of follow up, 3 years and 6 months, respectively. In the EPIC trial, the reduction in the composite endpoint was derived primarily from the effect on MI and both urgent and non-urgent revascularisations. In the EPILOG trial, the reduction in the composite endpoint was derived primarily from the effect on non-Q-wave MI (identified by cardiac enzyme increases) and urgent revascularisations. In the CAPTURE trial in patients with unstable angina not responding to medical therapy, ReoPro was administered as a bolus plus infusion starting up to 24 hours before the procedure until 1 hour after completion of the procedure. This regimen demonstrated stabilisation of patients prior to angioplasty, as shown for example by a reduction in MIs, and the reduction in thrombotic complications was sustained at the 30-day endpoint but not at 6 months.

Pharmacokinetic properties: Following intravenous bolus administration of ReoPro, free plasma concentrations decrease very rapidly with an initial half-life of less than 10 minutes and a second phase half-life of about 30 minutes, probably related to rapid binding to the platelet GPIIb/IIIa receptors. Platelet function generally recovers over the course of 48 hours, although ReoPro remains in the circulation for 15 days or more in a platelet-bound state. Intravenous administration of a 0.25 mg/kg bolus dose of ReoPro followed by continuous infusion of 10 microgram/min (or a weight adjusted infusion of 0.125 microgram/kg/min to a maximum of 10 microgram/min) produces relatively constant free plasma concentrations throughout the infusion. At the termination of the infusion period, free plasma concentrations fall rapidly for approximately 6 hours then decline at a slower rate.

Preclinical safety data: No remarkable findings.

Pharmaceutical particulars

List of excipients: ReoPro is formulated in a buffered aqueous solution (pH 7.2) containing sodium phosphate, dibasic, dihydrate; sodium phosphate, monobasic, monohydrate; sodium chloride and polysorbate 80. The total sodium content is approximately 3.45 mg/ml. Trace amounts of papain resulting from the production process may be present.

Incompatibilities: No incompatibilities have been shown with intravenous infusion fluids or commonly used cardiovascular drugs. Nevertheless, it is recommended that ReoPro be administered in a separate intravenous line whenever possible and not mixed with other medications.

No incompatibilities have been observed with polyvinyl chloride bags or administration sets.

Shelf-life: Three (3) years at the recommended storage temperature.

ReoPro does not contain a preservative and is for single use only. Unused portions should be discarded. When intended for use by intravenous infusion, ReoPro should be used promptly after dilution.

Special precautions for storage: ReoPro should be stored at 2°C to 8°C. Do not freeze.

Nature and contents of container: ReoPro is supplied in 5 ml (10 mg) glass vials with rubber stoppers and aluminium crimps protected by a plastic cap.

Package quantities: 5 ml glass vials – single vials.

Instructions for use/handling: Do not shake vials. For administration instructions see *Posology and method of administration* section above.

Marketing authorisation holder: Centocor BV, Einsteinweg 101, 2333 CB Leiden, The Netherlands.

Marketing authorisation number 8563/0015

Date of approval/revision of SPC 14 November 1997.

Legal category POM

VANCOCIN* CP INJECTION

Qualitative and quantitative composition

Vial Size	*Quantity of Vancomycin*
10 ml	*250 mg*
10 ml	*500 mg*
20 ml	*1 g*

Pharmaceutical form Injection of vancomycin hydrochloride.

Clinical particulars

Therapeutic indications: Vancomycin is indicated in potentially life-threatening infections which cannot be treated with other effective, less toxic antimicrobial drugs, including the penicillins and cephalosporins.

Vancomycin is useful in the therapy of severe staphylococcal infections in patients who cannot receive or who have failed to respond to the penicillins and cephalosporins, or who have infections with staphylococci resistant to other antibiotics.

Vancomycin is used in the treatment of endocarditis and as prophylaxis against endocarditis in patients at risk from dental or surgical procedures.

Its effectiveness has been documented in other infections due to staphylococci, including osteomyelitis, pneumonia, septicaemia and soft tissue infections.

Vancomycin may be used orally for the treatment of staphylococcal enterocolitis and pseudomembranous colitis due to *Clostridium difficile.* Parenteral administration of vancomycin is not effective for these indications. Intravenous administration may be used concomitantly if required.

Posology and method of administration: For intravenous infusion and oral use only and not for intramuscular administration.

Infusion-related adverse events are related to both concentration and rate of administration of vancomycin.

Concentrations of no more than 5 mg/ml are recommended. In selected patients in need of fluid restriction, a concentration up to 10 mg/ml may be used; use of such higher concentrations may increase the risk of infusion-related events. Infusions should be given over at least 60 minutes. In adults, if doses exceeding 500 mg are used, a rate of infusion of no more than 10 mg/min is recommended. Infusion-related events may occur, however, at any rate or concentration.

Intravenous infusion in patients with normal renal function

Adults: The usual intravenous dose is 500 mg every six hours or 1 g every 12 hours, in Sodium Chloride Intravenous Infusion BP or 5% Dextrose Intravenous Infusion BP. Each dose should be administered at no more than 10 mg/min. Other patient factors, such as age, obesity or pregnancy, may call for modification of the usual daily dose. The majority of patients with infections caused by organisms sensitive to the antibiotic show a therapeutic response within 48-72 hours. The total duration of therapy is determined by the type and severity of the infection and the clinical response of the patient. In staphylococcal endocarditis, treatment for three weeks or longer is recommended.

Pregnancy: It has been reported that significantly increased doses may be required to achieve therapeutic serum concentrations in pregnant patients, but see 'Warnings'.

The elderly: Dosage reduction may be necessary to a greater extent than expected because of decreasing renal function (see below). Monitor auditory function - see 'Warnings' and 'Precautions'.

Children: The usual intravenous dosage is 10 mg/kg per dose given every 6 hours (total daily dosage 40 mg/kg of body weight). Each dose should be administered over a period of at least 60 minutes.

In neonates and young infants, the total daily dosage may be lower. An initial dose of 15 mg/kg is suggested, followed by 10 mg/kg every 12 hours in the first week of life and every 8 hours thereafter until one month of age. Each dose should be administered over 60 minutes. Close monitoring of serum vancomycin concentrations may be warranted in these patients.

Patients with impaired renal function

Dosage adjustments must be made to avoid toxic serum levels. In premature infants and the elderly, greater dosage reductions than expected may be necessary because of decreased renal function. Regular monitoring of serum levels is advised in such patients, as accumulation has been reported, especially after prolonged therapy. Vancomycin serum concentrations may be determined by use of a microbiological assay, radioimmunoassay, fluorescence polarisation immunoassay, fluorescence immunoassay or high-pressure liquid chromatography. The following nomogram, based on creatinine clearance values, is provided:

The nomogram is not valid for functionally anephric patients on dialysis. For such patients, a loading dose of 15 mg/kg body weight should be given to achieve therapeutic serum levels promptly, and the dose required to maintain stable levels is 1.9 mg/kg/24 hours. Since individual maintenance doses of 250 mg to 1 g are convenient, in patients with marked renal impairment a dose may be given every several days rather than on a daily basis. In anuria a dose of 1 g every 7 to 10 days has been recommended.

Preparation of solutions: See 'Instructions for use/handling'.

Measurement of serum concentrations

Following multiple intravenous doses, peak serum concentrations, measured 2 hours after infusion is complete, range from 18-26 mg/l. Trough levels measured immediately prior to the next dose should be 5-10 mg/l. Ototoxicity has been associated with serum drug levels of 80-100 mg/l, but this is rarely seen when serum levels are kept at or below 30 mg/l.

Oral administration

The contents of vials for parenteral administration may be used.

Adults and the elderly: The usual daily dose given is 500 mg in divided doses for 7 to 10 days, although up to 2 g/day have been used in severe cases. The total daily dosage should not exceed 2 g. Each dose may be reconstituted in 30 ml water and either given to the patient to drink, or administered by nasogastric tube.

Children: The usual daily dose is 40 mg/kg in three or four divided doses for 7 to 10 days. The total daily dosage should not exceed 2 g.

Common flavouring syrups may be added to the solution at the time of administration to improve the taste.

Capsules are also available.

Contra-indications: Hypersensitivity to vancomycin.

Special warnings and special precautions for use:

Warnings

Rapid bolus administration (eg, over several minutes) may be associated with exaggerated hypotension, including shock, and, rarely, cardiac arrest. Vancomycin should be infused in a dilute solution over a period of not less than 60 minutes to avoid rapid infusion-related reactions. Stopping the infusion usually results in a prompt cessation of these reactions (see 'Posology and method of administration' and 'Undesirable effects' sections).

Some patients with inflammatory disorders of the intestinal mucosa may have significant systemic absorption of oral vancomycin and, therefore, may be at risk for the development of adverse reactions associated with the parenteral administration of vancomycin. The risk is greater in patients with renal impairment. It should be noted that the total systemic and renal clearances of vancomycin are reduced in the elderly.

Due to its potential ototoxicity and nephrotoxicity, vancomycin should be used with care in patients with renal insufficiency and the dose should be reduced according to the degree of renal impairment. The risk of toxicity is appreciably increased by high blood concentrations or prolonged therapy. Blood levels should be monitored and renal function tests should be performed regularly.

Vancomycin should also be avoided in patients with previous hearing loss. If it is used in such patients, the dose should be regulated, if possible, by periodic determination of the drug level in the blood. Deafness may be preceded by tinnitus. The elderly are more susceptible to auditory damage. Experience with other antibiotics suggests that deafness may be progressive despite cessation of treatment.

Usage in paediatrics: In premature neonates and young infants, it may be appropriate to confirm desired vancomycin serum concentrations. Concomitant administration of vancomycin and anaesthetic agents has been associated with erythema and histamine-like flushing in children.

Usage in the elderly: The natural decrement of glomerular filtration with increasing age may lead to elevated vancomycin serum concentrations if dosage is not adjusted (see 'Posology and method of administration').

Precautions

Clinically significant serum concentrations have been reported in some patients being treated for active *C. difficile*-induced pseudomembranous colitis

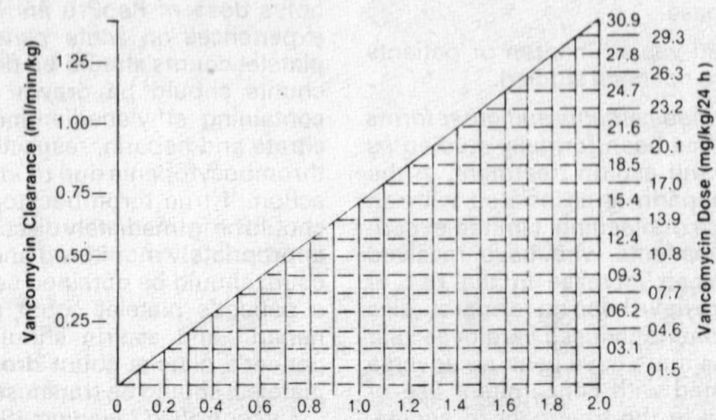

Dosage Nomogram for Vancomycin in Patients with Impaired Renal Function

after multiple oral doses of vancomycin. Therefore, monitoring of serum concentrations may be appropriate in these patients.

Patients with borderline renal function and individuals over the age of 60 should be given serial tests of auditory function and of vancomycin blood levels. All patients receiving the drug should have periodic haematological studies, urine analysis and renal function tests.

Vancomycin is very irritating to tissue, and causes injection site necrosis when injected intramuscularly; it must be infused intravenously. Injection site pain and thrombophlebitis occur in many patients receiving vancomycin and are occasionally severe.

The frequency and severity of thrombophlebitis can be minimised by administering the drug slowly as a dilute solution (2.5 to 5.0 g/l) and by rotating the sites of infusion.

Prolonged use of vancomycin may result in the overgrowth of non-susceptible organisms. Careful observation of the patient is essential. If superinfection occurs during therapy, appropriate measures should be taken. In rare instances, there have been reports of pseudomembranous colitis, due to *C. difficile*, developing in patients who received intravenous vancomycin.

Interaction with other medicaments and other forms of interaction: Concomitant administration of vancomycin and anaesthetic agents has been associated with erythema, histamine-like flushing and anaphylactoid reactions.

There have been reports that the frequency of infusion-related events increases with the concomitant administration of anaesthetic agents. Infusion-related events may be minimised by the administration of vancomycin as a 60-minute infusion prior to anaesthetic induction.

Concurrent or sequential systemic or topical use of other potentially neurotoxic or nephrotoxic drugs, such as amphotericin B, aminoglycosides, bacitracin, polymixin B, colistin, viomycin or cisplatin, when indicated, requires careful monitoring.

Pregnancy and lactation:
Usage in pregnancy: Teratology studies have been performed at 5 times the human dose in rats and 3 times the human dose in rabbits, and have revealed no evidence of harm to the foetus due to vancomycin. In a controlled clinical study, the potential ototoxic and nephrotoxic effects of vancomycin hydrochloride on infants were evaluated when the drug was administered to pregnant women for serious staphylococcal infections complicating intravenous drug abuse. Vancomycin hydrochloride was found in cord blood. No sensorineural hearing loss or nephrotoxicity attributable to vancomycin was noted. One infant, whose mother received vancomycin in the third trimester, experienced conductive hearing loss that was not attributable to vancomycin. Because vancomycin was administered only in the second and third trimesters, it is not known whether it causes foetal harm. Vancomycin should be given in pregnancy only if clearly needed and blood levels should be monitored carefully to minimise the risk of foetal toxicity. It has been reported, however, that pregnant patients may require significantly increased doses of vancomycin to achieve therapeutic serum concentrations.

Usage in nursing mothers: Vancomycin hydrochloride is excreted in human milk. Caution should be exercised when vancomycin is administered to a nursing woman. It is unlikely that a nursing infant can absorb a significant amount of vancomycin from its gastro-intestinal tract.

Effects on ability to drive and use machines: Not applicable.

Undesirable effects:
Infusion-related events: During or soon after rapid infusion of vancomycin, patients may develop anaphylactoid reactions including hypotension, wheezing, dyspnoea, urticaria or pruritus. Rapid infusion may also cause flushing of the upper-body ('red-neck syndrome') or pain and muscle spasm of the chest and back. These reactions usually resolve within 20 minutes but may persist for several hours. In animal studies, hypotension and bradycardia occurred in animals given large doses of vancomycin at high concentrations and rates. Such events are infrequent if vancomycin is given by slow infusion over 60 minutes. In studies of normal volunteers, infusion-related events did not occur when vancomycin was administered at a rate of 10 mg/min or less.

Nephrotoxicity: Rarely, renal failure, principally manifested by increased serum creatinine or blood urea concentrations, have been observed, especially in patients given large doses of intravenously administered vancomycin. Rare cases of interstitial nephritis have been reported. Most occurred in patients who were given aminoglycosides concomitantly or who had pre-existing kidney dysfunction. When vancomycin was discontinued, azotaemia resolved in most patients.

Ototoxicity: Hearing loss associated with intravenously administered vancomycin has been reported. Most of these patients had kidney dysfunction, pre-existing hearing loss, or concomitant treatment with an ototoxic drug. Vertigo, dizziness and tinnitus have been reported rarely.

Haematological: Reversible neutropenia, usually starting one week or more after onset of intravenous therapy or after a total dose of more than 25 g. Neutropenia appears to be promptly reversible when vancomycin is discontinued. Thrombocytopenia has rarely been reported. Reversible agranulocytosis (less than 500 granulocytes per mm^3) has been reported rarely, although causality has not been established.

Miscellaneous: Phlebitis, hypersensitivity reactions, anaphylaxis, nausea, chills, drug fever, eosinophilia, rashes (including exfoliative dermatitis) and rare cases of vasculitis. Vancomycin has been associated with the bullous eruption disorders Stevens-Johnson syndrome, toxic epidermal necrolysis and linear IgA bullous dermatosis. If a bullous disorder is suspected, the drug should be discontinued and specialist dermatological assessment should be carried out.

Overdose: Supportive care is advised, with maintenance of glomerular filtration. Vancomycin is poorly removed from the blood by haemodialysis or peritoneal dialysis. Haemoperfusion with Amberlite resin XAD-4 has been reported to be of limited benefit.

Pharmacological properties

Pharmacodynamic properties: Vancomycin is a glycopeptide antibiotic derived from *Nocardia orientalis* (formerly *Streptomyces orientalis*), and is active against many Gram-positive bacteria, including *Staphylococcus aureus, Staph. epidermidis*, alpha and beta haemolytic streptococci, group D streptococci, corynebacteria and clostridia.

Pharmacokinetic properties: Vancomycin is not significantly absorbed from the normal gastro-intestinal tract and is therefore not effective by the oral route for infections other than staphylococcal enterocolitis and pseudomembranous colitis due to *Clostridium difficile*.

Preclinical safety data: Although no long-term studies in animals have been performed to evaluate carcinogenic potential, no mutagenic potential of vancomycin was found in standard laboratory tests. No definitive fertility studies have been performed.

Pharmaceutical particulars

List of excipients: Vials of Vancocin contain only the active ingredient, vancomycin hydrochloride.

Incompatibilities: Vancomycin solution has a low pH that may cause chemical or physical instability when it is mixed with other compounds.

Shelf-life:

250 mg vial:	2 years
500 mg vial:	3 years
1 g vial:	2 years

Special precautions for storage: Store below 25°C.
After reconstitution: May be stored in a refrigerator (2°-8°C) for 24 hours.

Prior to administration, parenteral drug products should be inspected visually for particulate matter and discolouration whenever solution or container permits.

Solutions of the parenteral powder intended for oral administration may be stored in a refrigerator (2°-8°C) for 96 hours.

Nature and contents of container: Rubber-stoppered 10 ml vials each containing chromatographically purified vancomycin hydrochloride, 250,000iu or 500,000iu, equivalent to 250 mg or 500 mg vancomycin, respectively, as an off-white lyophilised plug.

Rubber-stoppered 20 ml vials containing chromatographically purified vancomycin hydrochloride, 1,000,000iu, equivalent to 1 g vancomycin, as an off-white lyophilised plug.

Package quantities:
Vials 250 mg (250,000iu vancomycin). Single vials.
Vials 500 mg (500,000iu vancomycin). Single vials.
Vials 1 g (1,000,000iu vancomycin). Single vials.

Instructions for use/handling:
Preparation of solution: At the time of use, add 5 ml of Water for Injections PhEur to the 250 mg vial, 10 ml of Water for Injections PhEur to the 500 mg vial, or 20 ml Water for Injections PhEur to the 1 g vial. Vials reconstituted in this manner will give a solution of 50 mg/ml.

FURTHER DILUTION IS REQUIRED. Read instructions which follow:

1. *Intermittent infusion* is the preferred method of administration. Reconstituted solutions containing 250 mg vancomycin must be diluted with at least 50 ml of diluent. Reconstituted solutions containing 500 mg vancomycin must be diluted with at least 100 ml diluent. Reconstituted solutions containing 1 g vancomycin must be diluted with at least 200 ml diluent. Sodium Chloride Intravenous Infusion BP or 5% Dextrose Intravenous Infusion BP are suitable diluents. The desired dose should be given by intravenous infusion over a period of at least 60 minutes. If administered over a shorter period of time or in higher concentrations, there is the possibility of inducing marked hypotension in addition to thrombophlebitis. Rapid administration may also produce flushing and a transient rash over the neck and shoulders.

2. *Continuous infusion* (should be used only when intermittent infusion is not feasible). 1-2 g can be added to a sufficiently large volume of Sodium Chloride Intravenous Infusion BP or 5% Dextrose Intravenous Infusion BP to permit the desired daily dose to be administered slowly by intravenous drip over a 24 hour period.

3. *Oral administration.* The contents of vials for parenteral administration may be used.

Common flavouring syrups may be added to the solution at the time of administration to improve the taste.

Capsules are also available.

Marketing authorisation number PL 0006/5076R

Date of approval/revision of SPC June 1998

Legal category POM

VANCOCIN* MATRIGEL CAPSULES

Qualitative and quantitative composition Matrigel capsules (dark blue and peach, coded Lilly 3125) containing chromatographically purified vancomycin hydrochloride, equivalent to 125 mg vancomycin base.

Matrigel capsules (dark blue and grey, coded Lilly 3126) containing chromatographically purified vancomycin hydrochloride, equivalent to 250 mg vancomycin base.

Pharmaceutical form Capsules.

Clinical particulars

Therapeutic indications: Vancomycin may be used orally for the treatment of staphylococcal enterocolitis and pseudomembranous colitis due to *Clostridium difficile*.

Vancomycin is not significantly absorbed from the normal gastro-intestinal tract and is therefore not effective by the oral route for other types of infection. Intravenous administration may be used concomitantly if required.

Posology and method of administration: For oral administration.

Either the Matrigel capsules or the contents of the 500 mg vial for parenteral administration may be used.

Adults and the elderly: The usual daily dose is 500 mg in divided doses for 7 to 10 days, although up to 2 g/day, in three or four divided doses, have been used in severe cases. The total daily dosage should not exceed 2 g.

Children: The usual daily dose is 40 mg/kg in three or four divided doses for 7 to 10 days. The total daily dosage should not exceed 2 g.

Oral solution: The contents of the 500 mg vial for parenteral administration may be used and either given to the patient to drink or administered by nasogastric tube. Mix thoroughly to dissolve. Common flavouring syrups may be added to the solution at the time of administration to improve the taste.

Contra-indications: Hypersensitivity to vancomycin.

Special warnings and special precautions for use:

Precautions

Clinically significant serum concentrations have been reported in some patients who have taken multiple oral doses of vancomycin for active *C. difficile*-induced pseudomembranous colitis. Therefore, monitoring of serum concentrations may be appropriate in these patients.

Some patients with inflammatory disorders of the intestinal mucosa may have significant systemic absorption of vancomycin and, therefore, may be at risk for the development of adverse reactions associated with the parenteral administration of vancomycin (see package insert accompanying the intravenous preparation). The risk is greater in patients with renal impairment. It should be noted that the total systemic and renal clearances of vancomycin are reduced in the elderly.

Ototoxicity has occurred in patients receiving vancomycin. It may be transient or permanent. It has been reported mostly in patients who have been given excessive intravenous doses, have an underlying hearing loss, or are receiving concomitant therapy with an ototoxic agent such as an aminoglycoside. Serial tests of auditory function may be helpful in order to minimise the risk of ototoxicity.

When treating patients with underlying renal dysfunction or patients receiving concomitant therapy with an aminoglycoside, serial monitoring of renal function should be performed.

Prolonged use of vancomycin may result in the overgrowth of non-susceptible organisms. Careful observation of the patient is essential. If superinfection occurs during therapy, appropriate measures should be taken.

Interaction with other medicaments and other forms of interaction: None known.

Pregnancy and lactation:
Usage in pregnancy: Teratology studies have been performed at 5 times the human dose in rats and 3 times the human dose in rabbits, and have revealed no evidence of harm to the foetus due to vancomycin. In a controlled clinical study, the potential ototoxic and nephrotoxic effects of vancomycin hydrochloride on infants were evaluated when the drug was administered to pregnant women for serious staphylococcal infections complicating intravenous drug abuse. Vancomycin hydrochloride was found in cord blood. No sensorineural hearing loss or nephrotoxicity attributable to vancomycin was noted. One infant, whose mother received vancomycin in the third trimester, experienced conductive hearing loss that was not attributable to vancomycin. Because vancomycin was administered only in the second and third trimesters, it is not known whether it causes foetal harm. Therefore, vancomycin should be given to a pregnant woman only if clearly needed.

Usage in nursing mothers: Vancomycin hydrochloride is excreted in human milk. Caution should be exercised when vancomycin is administered to a nursing woman.

Effects on ability to drive and use machines: None known.

Undesirable effects: Since vancomycin is not usually significantly absorbed from the gastro-intestinal tract, the toxicity encountered with parenteral therapy is unlikely to occur after oral administration (but see 'Precautions').

Nephrotoxicity: Rarely, renal failure, principally manifested by increased serum creatinine or blood urea concentrations, have been observed, especially in patients given large doses of intravenously administered vancomycin. Rare cases of interstitial nephritis have been reported. Most occurred in patients who were given aminoglycosides concomitantly or who had pre-existing kidney dysfunction. When vancomycin was discontinued, azotaemia resolved in most patients.

Ototoxicity: Hearing loss associated with *intravenously* administered vancomycin has been reported. Most of these patients had kidney dysfunction, pre-existing hearing loss, or concomitant treatment with an ototoxic drug. Vertigo, dizziness and tinnitus have been reported rarely.

Haematological: Reversible neutropenia, usually starting one week or more after onset of *intravenous* therapy or after a total dose of more than 25 g. Neutropenia appears to be promptly reversible when vancomycin is discontinued. Thrombocytopenia and reversible agranulocytosis (granulocyte count less than 500/mm^3) have been reported rarely.

Miscellaneous: Hypersensitivity reactions, anaphylaxis, chills, drug fever, eosinophilia, hypotension, wheezing, dyspnoea, urticaria, pruritus, flushing of the upper body ('red neck' syndrome), pain, muscle spasm of the chest and back, nausea and rashes, including exfoliative dermatitis, Stevens-Johnson syndrome, toxic epidermal necrolysis and rare cases of vasculitis.

Overdose:

Treatment of overdosage
Supportive care is advised, with maintenance of glomerular filtration. Vancomycin is poorly removed by dialysis. Haemofiltration and haemoperfusion with Amberlite resin XAD-4 have been reported to be of limited benefit.

Pharmacological properties

Pharmacodynamic properties: Vancomycin is an antibiotic which acts by interfering with bacterial cell wall synthesis. In addition, it also acts by altering bacterial cell-membrane permeability and RNA synthesis. The minimum inhibitory concentration of vancomycin has been reported to range from 0.2 to 0.6 micrograms per ml.

Pharmacokinetic properties: Vancomycin is poorly absorbed from the gastro-intestinal tract. During multiple dosing of 250 mg every 8 hours for 7 doses, faecal concentrations of vancomycin, in volunteers, exceeded 100 mg/kg in the majority of samples. No blood concentrations were detected and urinary recovery did not exceed 0.76%.

Preclinical safety data: There are no preclinical data of relevance to the prescriber in addition to that summarised in other sections of the summary of product characteristics.

Pharmaceutical particulars

List of excipients:
Polyethylene Glycol
Gelatin
Indigo Carmine
Red Iron Oxide
Yellow Iron Oxide (125 mg capsule) or Black Iron Oxide (250 mg capsule)
Titanium Dioxide

Incompatibilities: None known.

Shelf-life: Two years.

Special precautions for storage: Protect from moisture. Store below 25°C.

After reconstitution, solutions of the parenteral powder intended for oral administration may be stored in a refrigerator (2°-8°C) for 96 hours.

Nature and contents of container: Blister packs of 20 capsules (2 strips of 10 capsules).

Instructions for use/handling: This preparation is for oral use only. If parenteral vancomycin therapy is desired, use 'Vancocin' CP Injection (Sterile Vancomycin Hydrochloride BP) and consult literature accompanying that preparation.

The bitter taste of vancomycin can be avoided by the use of the Matrigel capsules. Vancomycin powder should be used when the patient is unable to swallow the capsules.

Marketing authorisation numbers
0006/0193 (125 mg)
0006/0194 (250 mg)

Date of approval/revision of SPC March 1997

Legal category POM

VELBE*

WARNING
THIS PRODUCT IS **NOT**
FOR INTRATHECAL USE

Presentation Vials containing 10 mg Velbe (Vinblastine Sulphate PhEur) in the form of a lyophilised plug.

Uses Velbe is an anti-neoplastic drug for intravenous use.

Information available at present suggests that Velbe may be useful, either alone or in combination with other oncolytic drugs for the treatment of: Hodgkin's disease; non-Hodgkin's lymphoma; carcinoma of the breast; methotrexate-resistant choriocarcinoma; renal cell carcinoma; testicular teratoma and seminoma; histiocytosis X.

Other neoplasms occasionally show a marked response to Velbe, but less frequently than the more susceptible conditions listed above.

Dosage and administration This preparation is for intravenous use only. It should be administered only by individuals experienced in vinblastine administration.

FATAL IF GIVEN INTRATHECALLY.
FOR INTRAVENOUS USE ONLY.
See 'Warnings' section for the treatment of patients given intrathecal vinblastine sulphate.

The recommended dose for adults, the elderly and children is 6 mg/m^2 usually administered no more frequently than once every seven days. For testicular tumours, the dosage may be increased to 0.2 mg/kg administered on each of two consecutive days every three weeks.

As vinblastine is excreted principally by the liver, toxicity may be increased when there is hepatic insufficiency and it may be necessary to reduce initial doses in the presence of significantly impaired hepatic or biliary function. A reduction of 50% in the dose is recommended for patients having a direct serum bilirubin value above 3 mg/100 ml. Since metabolism and excretion are primarily hepatic, no modification is recommended for patients with impaired renal function.

The metabolism of vinca alkaloids has been shown to be mediated by hepatic cytochrome P450 isoenzymes in the CYP 3A subfamily. This metabolic pathway may be impaired in patients with hepatic dysfunction or who are taking concomitant potent inhibitors of these isoenzymes. (See *Precautions.*)

To prepare a solution containing 1 mg/ml, add 10 ml of sterile 0.9% sodium chloride intravenous infusion to the 10 mg vial. The drug dissolves rapidly to give a clear solution.

The dose of Velbe solution may be injected either into the tubing of a running intravenous infusion of sodium chloride 0.9% or directly into a vein. In either case, the injection should be completed in about one minute. If care is taken to ensure that the needle is securely within the vein and that no solution containing vinblastine is spilled extravascularly, cellulitis and/or phlebitis will not occur.

To minimise further the possibility of extravascular spillage, it is suggested that the syringe and needle be rinsed with venous blood before withdrawal. The dose should not be diluted in large volumes of diluent (i.e. 100 to 250 ml) or given intravenously for prolonged periods (ranging from 30 to 60 minutes or more), since this frequently results in irritation of the vein and increases the chance of extravasation.

Because of the enhanced possibility of thrombosis, it is considered inadvisable to inject a solution of Velbe into an extremity in which the circulation is impaired, or potentially impaired, by such conditions as compressing or invading neoplasm, phlebitis or varicosity.

Caution: If leakage into surrounding tissue should occur during intravenous administration of vinblastine, it may cause considerable irritation. The injection should be discontinued immediately and any remaining portion of the dose should then be introduced into another vein. Local injection of hyaluronidase and the application of moderate heat to the area of leakage help disperse the drug and are thought to minimise discomfort and the possibility of cellulitis.

Contra-indications, warnings, etc
Contra-indications

FATAL IF GIVEN INTRATHECALLY.
FOR INTRAVENOUS USE ONLY.
See 'Warnings' section for the treatment of patients given intrathecal vinblastine sulphate.

Vinblastine is contra-indicated in patients who are leucopenic, unless this is the result of the disease being treated. It should not be used in the presence of bacterial infection. Such infections must be brought under control with antiseptics or antibiotics before using vinblastine.

Warnings: This product is for intravenous use only. It should be administered by individuals experienced in the administration of vinblastine sulphate. The intrathecal administration of vinblastine sulphate usually results in death. Syringes containing this product should be labelled 'FATAL IF GIVEN INTRATHECALLY. FOR INTRAVENOUS USE ONLY'. An auxiliary sticker is provided in the pack with this warning.

Extemporaneously prepared syringes containing this product must be packaged in an overwrap which is labelled 'DO NOT REMOVE COVERING UNTIL MOMENT OF INJECTION. FATAL IF GIVEN INTRATHECALLY. FOR INTRAVENOUS USE ONLY'.

After inadvertent intrathecal administration of vinca alkaloids, immediate neurosurgical intervention is required in order to prevent ascending paralysis leading to death. In a very small number of patients, life-threatening paralysis and subsequent death was averted but resulted in devastating neurological sequelae, with limited recovery afterwards.

Based on the published management of survival cases involving the related vinca alkaloid vincristine sulphate, if vinblastine is mistakenly given by the intrathecal route, the following treatment should be initiated **immediately after the injection:**

1. Removal of as much CSF as is safely possible through the lumbar access.
2. Insertion of an epidural catheter into the subarachnoid space via the intervertebral space above initial lumbar access and CSF irrigation with lactated Ringer's solution. Fresh frozen plasma should be requested and, when available, 25 ml should be added to every 1 litre of lactated Ringer's solution.
3. Insertion of an intraventricular drain or catheter by a neurosurgeon and continuation of CSF irrigation with fluid removal through the lumbar access connected to a closed drainage system. Lactated Ringer's solution should be given by continuous infusion at 150 ml/h, or at a rate of 75 ml/h when fresh frozen plasma has been added as above.

The rate of infusion should be adjusted to maintain a spinal fluid protein level of 150 mg/dl.

The following measures have also been used in addition but may not be essential:

Glutamic acid has been given IV 10 gm over 24 hours, followed by 500 mg tds by mouth for 1 month. Folinic acid has been administered intravenously as a 100 mg bolus and then infused at a rate of 25 mg/h for 24 hours, then bolus doses of 25 mg 6-hourly for 1 week. Pyridoxine has been given at a dose of 50 mg 8-hourly by intravenous infusion over 30 minutes. Their roles in the reduction of neurotoxicity are unclear.

Usage in pregnancy: Caution is necessary with the use of all oncolytic drugs during pregnancy. Information on the use of vinblastine during human pregnancy is very limited but vinblastine can cause foetal harm when administered to a pregnant woman. There are no adequate and well-controlled studies in pregnant women. Animal studies with vinblastine suggest that teratogenic effects may occur. Laboratory animals given this drug early in pregnancy suffer resorption of the conceptus; surviving foetuses demonstrate gross deformities.

Women of childbearing potential should be advised to avoid becoming pregnant while receiving vinblastine. If Velbe is used during pregnancy or if the patient becomes pregnant while receiving this drug she should be informed of the potential hazard to the foetus.

Usage in nursing mothers: It is not known whether vinblastine is excreted in human milk. Because of the potential for serious adverse reactions due to Velbe in nursing infants, a decision should be made whether to discontinue nursing or the drug taking into account the importance of the drug to the mother.

Aspermia has been reported in men. Animal studies show metaphase arrest and degenerative changes in germ cells. Amenorrhoea has occurred in some patients treated with vinblastine in combination with other drugs. Recovery of menses was frequent.

Stomatitis and neurological toxicity, although not common or permanent, can be disabling.

Precautions: The dose–limiting factor is myelosuppression. Effective therapy with vinblastine is more likely to be followed by leucopenia than is the case with Oncovin (vincristine sulphate).

In general, the larger the dose employed, the more profound and longer lasting the leucopenia will be. The fact that the granulocyte count returns to normal levels after drug-induced leucopenia is an indication that the granulocyte–producing mechanism is not permanently depressed.

Following therapy with vinblastine, the nadir in the granulocyte count may be expected to occur five to ten days after the last day of drug administration. Recovery of the granulocyte count is fairly rapid thereafter and is usually complete within another seven to fourteen days.

If granulocytopenia with less than 1,000 granulocytes/mm^3 occurs following a dose of vinblastine, the patient should be watched carefully for evidence of infection until the granulocyte count has returned to a safe level. Any infection must be brought under control immediately.

When cachexia or ulcerated areas of the skin surface are present, there may be a more profound granulocytopenic response to the drug; therefore, its use should be avoided in older persons suffering from either of these conditions.

Although the thrombocyte count is not usually significantly lowered by therapy with vinblastine, patients whose bone marrow has been recently impaired by prior therapy with radiation or with other oncolytic drugs may show thrombocytopenia (less than 150,000 platelets/mm^3). When other chemotherapy or radiation has not been employed previously, thrombocyte reduction below the level of 150,000/mm^3 is rarely encountered, even when vinblastine may be causing significant granulocytopenia. Rapid recovery from thrombocytopenia within a few days is the rule.

The effect of vinblastine upon the red blood cell count and haemoglobin is usually insignificant when other treatment does not complicate the picture.

In patients with malignant-cell infiltration of the bone marrow, the granulocyte and platelet counts have sometimes fallen drastically after moderate doses of vinblastine. Further use of the drug in such patients is inadvisable.

When chemotherapy is being given in conjunction with radiation therapy through portals which include the liver, the use of vinblastine should be delayed until radiation therapy has been completed.

Acute shortness of breath and severe bronchospasm have been reported following the administration of the vinca alkaloids. These reactions have been encountered most frequently when the vinca alkaloid was used in combination with mitomycin-C and may be serious when there is pre-existing pulmonary dysfunction. The onset may be within minutes, or several hours after the vinca is injected, and may occur up to 2 weeks following a dose of mitomycin. Progressive dyspnoea, requiring chronic therapy, may occur. Vinblastine should not be re-administered.

The simultaneous oral or intravenous administration of phenytoin and anti-neoplastic chemotherapy combinations, that included vinblastine sulphate, have been reported to reduce blood levels of the anticonvulsant and to increase seizure activity. Although the contribution of the vinca alkaloids has not been established, dosage adjustment of phenytoin, based on serial blood level monitoring, may need to be made when it is used in combination with vinblastine.

Caution should be exercised in patients concurrently taking drugs known to inhibit drug metabolism by hepatic cytochrome P450 isoenzymes in the CYP 3A subfamily, or in patients with hepatic dysfunction. Concurrent administration of vinblastine sulphate with an inhibitor of this metabolic pathway may cause an earlier onset and/or an increased severity of side-effects.

Care must be taken to avoid contamination of the eye with concentrations of Velbe used clinically. If accidental contamination occurs, severe irritation (or, if the drug was delivered under pressure, even corneal ulceration) may result. The eye should be washed with water immediately and thoroughly.

Sperm abnormalities have been noted in mice. Additional studies in mice demonstrated no reduction in fertility of males. Breaks and aberrations were not observed on chromosome analysis of marrow cells from patients treated with vinblastine, although chromosomal changes have been noted in some hamster lung cell *in vitro* tests.

There is no currently available evidence to indicate that vinblastine itself has been carcinogenic in humans although some patients have developed leukaemia following radiation therapy and the administration of vinblastine in combination with alkylating agents.

Adverse reactions: Leucopenia is the most common adverse reaction and is usually the dose-limiting factor.

In general, the incidence of side-effects attending the use of Velbe appears to be related to the size of dosage employed. Symptoms commonly encountered when high doses are employed include constipation, abdominal pain, ileus and myalgia.

The use of small amounts of vinblastine daily for long periods is not advisable, even though the resulting total dosage may be similar to the recommended dosage. Little or no therapeutic advantage has been demonstrated when such regimens have been used and side-effects are increased.

The constipation which may be encountered responds well to such usual measures as enemas and laxatives. Constipation may take the form of upper colon impaction and the rectum may be found to be empty on physical examination. A flat film of the abdomen is useful in demonstrating this condition. A routine prophylactic regimen against constipation is recommended for patients receiving high doses of vinblastine.

The following symptoms may occur after usual doses of vinblastine:

Haematological: Leucopenia, thrombocytopenia, anaemia.

Gastro-intestinal: Nausea, vomiting, constipation, ileus, diarrhoea, anorexia, abdominal pain, rectal bleeding, pharyngitis, haemorrhagic enterocolitis, bleeding from an old peptic ulcer.

Neurological: Numbness, paraesthesiae, peripheral neuritis, mental depression, loss of deep tendon reflexes, headache, convulsions. Treatment with vinca alkaloids has resulted rarely in both vestibular and auditory damage to the eighth cranial nerve. Manifestations include partial or total deafness, which may be temporary or permanent, and difficulties with balance, including dizziness, nystagmus and vertigo. Particular caution is warranted when vinblastine sulphate is used in combination with other agents known to be ototoxic, such as the platinum-containing oncolytics.

Pulmonary: See under 'Precautions'.

Cutaneous: Stomatitis, ulceration of the skin and alopecia. When alopecia develops it is frequently not total and, in some cases, hair regrows while maintenance therapy continues.

Cardiovascular: Hypertension. Cases of unexpected myocardial infarction and cerebrovascular accidents have occurred in patients undergoing combination chemotherapy with vinblastine, bleomycin and cisplatin.

Miscellaneous: Malaise, weakness, dizziness, bone pain, jaw pain, and pain in tumour-containing tissue. Injection site reaction (see *Dosage and administration – Caution*). Syndrome of inappropriate ADH secretion has been reported with higher than recommended doses. Raynaud's phenomenon has occurred when patients are being treated with vinblastine in combination with bleomycin and cisplatin for testicular cancer.

Overdosage: Side-effects following the use of vinblastine are dose related. Therefore, following administration of more than the recommended dose, patients can be expected to experience these effects in an exaggerated fashion. Any dose that results in elimination of platelets and neutrophils from blood and marrow and their precursors from marrow is life-threatening.

Overdoses occurring during prolonged, consecutive day infusions may be more toxic than the same total dose given by rapid i.v. injection.

In addition, neurotoxicity similar to that seen with Oncovin (vincristine sulphate) may be observed.

Supportive care should include: (a) prevention of the side-effects that result from the syndrome of inappropriate secretion of antidiuretic hormone. This includes restriction of fluid intake and perhaps the use of a diuretic acting on the loop of Henle and distal tubule function; (b) administration of an anticonvulsant; (c) prevention and treatment of ileus; (d) monitoring the patient's cardiovascular system; (e) daily blood counts for guidance in transfusion requirement and assessing the risk of infection.

The major effect of excessive doses of vinblastine will be on granulocytopoiesis, and this may be life-threatening.

There is no specific antidote. The use of folinic acid in addition to the other supportive measures recommended may be considered although, unlike vincristine, studies have not been conducted to confirm its protective action.

There is no information regarding the effectiveness of dialysis nor of cholestyramine for the treatment of overdosage.

Vinblastine in the dry state is irregularly and unpredictably absorbed from the gastro-intestinal tract following oral administration. Absorption of the solution has not been studied. If vinblastine is swallowed, activated charcoal in a water slurry may be given by mouth, along with a cathartic. The use of cholestyramine in this situation has not been reported.

Pharmaceutical precautions

Special dispensing information: When dispensing vinblastine sulphate in other than the original container, it is imperative that it be packaged in an overwrap bearing the statement 'DO NOT REMOVE COVERING UNTIL MOMENT OF INJECTION. FATAL IF GIVEN INTRATHECALLY. FOR INTRAVENOUS USE ONLY'. A syringe containing a specific dose must be labelled, using the auxiliary sticker provided in the pack, with this warning.

Guidelines for the safe handling of anti-neoplastic agents: Cytotoxic preparations should not be handled by pregnant staff.

Trained personnel should reconstitute and administer the drug. This should be performed in a designated area. The work surface should be covered with disposable plastic-backed absorbent paper.

Adequate protective gloves, masks and clothing should be worn. Precautions should be taken to avoid the drug accidentally coming into contact with the eyes. If accidental contamination occurs, the eye should be washed with water thoroughly and immediately.

Use Luer-lock fittings on all syringes and sets. Large bore needles are recommended to minimise pressure and the possible formation of aerosols. The latter may also be reduced by the use of a venting needle.

Adequate care and precaution should be taken in the disposal of items (syringes, needles, etc) used to reconstitute cytotoxic drugs.

Vials of Velbe should be stored in a refrigerator between 2°and 8°C.

After reconstitution: After a portion of the solution has been removed from a vial, the remainder of the contents of the vial may be stored in a refrigerator for further use for 24 hours without significant loss of potency. When the reconstituted vial of Velbe is to be stored for more than 24 hours, it is essential to reconstitute with sterile 0.9% sodium chloride intravenous infusion preserved with 2.0% benzyl alcohol. Where preserved diluent is used, the reconstituted solution may be stored in a refrigerator for up to 28 days, without significant loss of potency.

Velbe should never be mixed with any other drug and should not be diluted with solvents that raise or lower the pH from between 3.5 and 5.

Whenever solution and container permit, parenteral drug products should be inspected visually for particulate matter and discolouration prior to administration.

Legal category POM.

Package quantity Vials 10 mg: Single vials.

Further information The presence of this drug or its metabolites in blood or body tissues is not known to interfere with clinical laboratory tests.

Product licence number
Vials 10 mg: 0006/5073

ZYPREXA* ▼

Qualitative and quantitative composition

Each Zyprexa 2.5 mg tablet contains 2.5 mg olanzapine.

Each Zyprexa 5 mg tablet contains 5 mg olanzapine.

Each Zyprexa 7.5 mg tablet contains 7.5 mg olanzapine.

Each Zyprexa 10 mg tablet contains 10 mg olanzapine.

Pharmaceutical form Coated tablets for oral administration.

Zyprexa 2.5 mg tablets are white, coated tablets imprinted with 'LILLY 4112'.

Zyprexa 5 mg tablets are white, coated tablets imprinted with 'LILLY 4115'.

Zyprexa 7.5 mg tablets are white, coated tablets imprinted with 'LILLY 4116'.

Zyprexa 10 mg tablets are white, coated tablets imprinted with 'LILLY 4117'.

Clinical particulars

Therapeutic indications: Olanzapine is indicated for the treatment of schizophrenia.

Olanzapine is effective in maintaining the clinical improvement during continuation therapy in patients who have shown an initial treatment response.

Further information on clinical trials: In a multinational, double-blind, comparative study of schizophrenia, schizoaffective and related disorders, which included 1481 patients with varying degrees of associated depressive symptoms (baseline mean of 16.6 on the Montgomery-Asberg Depression Rating Scale), a prospective secondary analysis of baseline to endpoint mood score change demonstrated a statistically significant improvement ($P = 0.001$) favouring olanzapine (-6.0) versus haloperidol (-3.1).

Posology and method of administration: The recommended starting dose for olanzapine is 10 mg/day, administered as a single daily dose without regard to meals. Daily dosage may subsequently be adjusted on the basis of individual clinical status within the range of 5-20 mg daily. An increase to a dose greater than the routine therapeutic dose of 10 mg/day, ie, to a dose of 15 mg/day or greater, is recommended only after appropriate clinical reassessment.

Children: Olanzapine has not been studied in subjects under 18 years of age.

Elderly patients: A lower starting dose (5 mg/day) is not routinely indicated but should be considered for those 65 and over when clinical factors warrant.

Patients with renal and/or hepatic impairment: A lower starting dose (5 mg) should be considered for such patients. In cases of moderate hepatic insufficiency (cirrhosis, Child-Pugh Class A or B), the starting dose should be 5 mg, and only increased with caution.

Female compared with male patients: The starting dose and dose range need not be routinely altered for female patients relative to male patients.

Non-smoking patients compared with smoking patients: The starting dose and dose range need not be routinely altered for non-smoking patients relative to smoking patients.

When more than one factor is present which might result in slower metabolism (female gender, geriatric age, non-smoking status), consideration should be given to decreasing the starting dose. Dose escalation, when indicated, should be conservative in such patients.

(See also *Interaction with other medicaments and other forms of interaction* and *Pharmacokinetic properties.*)

Contra-indications: Olanzapine is contra-indicated in those patients with a known hypersensitivity to any ingredient of the product. Olanzapine is contra-indicated in patients with known risk of narrow-angle glaucoma.

Special warnings and special precautions for use:
Concomitant illnesses: While olanzapine demonstrated anticholinergic activity *in vitro,* experience during the clinical trials revealed a low incidence of related events. However, as clinical experience with olanzapine in patients with concomitant illness is limited, caution is advised when prescribing for patients with prostatic hypertrophy, or paralytic ileus and related conditions.

Lactose: Olanzapine tablets contain lactose.

Transient, asymptomatic elevations of hepatic transaminases, ALT, AST have been seen occasionally, especially in early treatment. Caution should be exercised in patients with elevated ALT and/or AST, in patients with signs and symptoms of hepatic impairment, in patients with pre-existing conditions associated with limited hepatic functional reserve, and in patients who are being treated with potentially hepatotoxic drugs. In the event of elevated ALT and/or AST during treatment, follow-up should be organised and dose reduction should be considered.

As with other neuroleptic drugs, caution should be exercised in patients with low leucocyte and/or neutrophil counts for any reason, in patients with a history of drug induced bone marrow depression/toxicity, in patients with bone marrow depression caused by concomitant illness, radiation therapy or chemotherapy and in patients with hypereosinophilic conditions or with myeloproliferative disease. Thirty-two patients with clozapine-related neutropenia or agranulocytosis histories received olanzapine without decreases in baseline neutrophil counts.

Neuroleptic malignant syndrome (NMS): NMS is a potentially life-threatening condition associated with antipsychotic medication. Rare cases reported as NMS have also been received in association with olanzapine. Clinical manifestations of NMS are hyperpyrexia, muscle rigidity, altered mental status and evidence of autonomic instability (irregular pulse or blood pressure, tachycardia, diaphoresis and cardiac dysrhythmia). Additional signs may include elevated creatinine phosphokinase, myoglobinuria (rhabdomyolysis), and acute renal failure. If a patient develops signs and symptoms indicative of NMS, or presents with unexplained high fever without additional clinical manifestations of NMS, all antipsychotic drugs, including olanzapine, must be discontinued.

Olanzapine should be used cautiously in patients who have a history of seizures or are subject to factors which may lower the seizure threshold. Seizures have been reported to occur rarely in patients when treated with olanzapine. In most of these cases, a history of seizures or risk factors for seizures were reported.

Tardive dyskinesia: In comparator studies of one year or less duration, olanzapine was associated with a statistically significant lower incidence of treatment emergent dyskinesia. However, the risk of tardive dyskinesia increases with long-term exposure, and therefore if signs or symptoms of tardive dyskinesia appear in a patient on olanzapine, a dose reduction or drug discontinuation should be considered. These symptoms can temporally deteriorate or even arise after discontinuation of treatment.

Given the primary CNS effects of olanzapine, caution should be used when it is taken in combination with other centrally acting drugs and alcohol. As it exhibits *in vitro* dopamine antagonism, olanzapine may antagonise the effects of direct and indirect dopamine agonists.

Postural hypotension was infrequently observed in the elderly in olanzapine clinical trials. As with other antipsychotics, it is recommended that blood pressure is measured periodically in patients over 65 years.

In clinical trials, olanzapine was not associated with a persistent increase in absolute QT intervals. Only 8 of 1685 subjects had increased QTc interval on multiple occasions. However, as with other antipsychotics, caution should be exercised when olanzapine is prescribed with drugs known to increase QTc interval, especially in the elderly.

Interaction with other medicaments and other forms of interaction:
Potential for other drugs to affect olanzapine: Single-doses of antacid (aluminium, magnesium) or cimetidine did not affect the oral bioavailability of olanzapine. However, the concomitant administration of activated charcoal reduced the oral bioavailability of olanzapine by 50 to 60%. The metabolism of olanzapine may be induced by concomitant smoking (the clearance of olanzapine is 33% lower and the terminal elimination half-life is 21% longer in non-smokers compared to smokers) or carbamazepine therapy (clearance is increased 44% and the terminal elimination half-life is reduced by 20% when administered with carbamazepine). Smoking and carbamazepine therapy induce P450-1A2 activity. The pharmacokinetics of theophylline, which is metabolised by P450-1A2, is not altered by olanzapine. The effect of potent inhibitors of P450-1A2 activity on olanzapine pharmacokinetics has not been studied.

Potential for olanzapine to affect other drugs: In clinical trials with single doses of olanzapine, no inhibition of the metabolism of imipramine/desipramine (P450-2D6 or P450-3A/1A2), warfarin (P450-2C9), theophylline (P450-1A2), or diazepam (P450-3A4 and P450-2C19) was evident. Olanzapine showed no interaction when co-administered with lithium or biperiden. The *in vitro* ability of olanzapine to inhibit metabolism by five principal cytochromes has been examined. These studies found inhibitory constants for 3A4 (491μM), 2C9 (751μM), 1A2 (36μM), 2C19 (920μM), 2D6 (89μM), that compared to olanzapine plasma concentrations of approximately 0.2μM, would mean maximum inhibition of these P450 systems by olanzapine would be less than 0.7%. The clinical relevance of these findings is unknown.

Pregnancy and lactation:
Pregnancy: There are no adequate and well-controlled studies in pregnant women. Patients should be advised to notify their physician if they become pregnant or intend to become pregnant during treatment with olanzapine. Nevertheless, because human experience is limited, this drug should be used in pregnancy only if the potential benefit justifies the potential risk to the fetus.

Lactation: Olanzapine was excreted in milk of treated rats during lactation. It is not known if olanzapine is excreted in human milk. Patients should be advised not to breast-feed an infant if they are taking olanzapine.

Effects on ability to drive and use machines: Because olanzapine may cause somnolence, patients should be cautioned about operating hazardous machinery, including motor vehicles.

Undesirable effects:
Frequent (>10%): The only frequent undesirable effects associated with the use of olanzapine in clinical trials were somnolence and weight gain. Weight gain was related to a lower pre-treatment body mass index (BMI) and initial starting dose of 15 mg or greater.

Occasional (1-10%): Occasional undesirable effects associated with the use of olanzapine in clinical trials included dizziness, increased appetite, peripheral oedema, orthostatic hypotension, and mild, transient anticholinergic effects, including constipation and dry mouth.

Transient, asymptomatic elevations of hepatic transaminases, ALT, AST have been seen occasionally, especially in early treatment (see *Special warnings and special precautions for use*).

In active-controlled studies, olanzapine-treated patients had a lower incidence of parkinsonism, akathisia and dystonia compared with titrated doses of haloperidol. In the absence of detailed information on the pre-existing history of individual acute and tardive extrapyramidal movement disorders, it can not be concluded at present that olanzapine produces less tardive dyskinesia and/or other tardive extrapyramidal syndromes.

Rare (<1%): Photosensitivity reaction and rash were reported rarely.

Rare reports of hepatitis have been received.

Seizures have been reported to occur rarely in patients treated with olanzapine. In most of these cases, a history of seizures or risk factors for seizures were reported.

Other findings: Plasma prolactin levels were sometimes elevated, but associated clinical manifestations (eg, gynaecomastia, galactorrhoea and breast enlargement) were rare. In most patients, levels returned to normal ranges without cessation of treatment.

Rare cases reported as Neuroleptic Malignant Syndrome (NMS) have been received in association with olanzapine. (See also *Special warnings and special precautions for use.*)

High creatine phosphokinase levels have been observed in rare cases.

Haematological variations, such as leucopenia and thrombocytopenia, have been occasionally reported.

Overdose: Experience with olanzapine in overdosage is limited. In clinical trials, accidental or intentional acute overdosage of olanzapine was identified in 67 patients. In the patient taking the largest identified amount, 300 mg, the only symptoms reported were drowsiness and slurred speech. In the limited number of patients who were evaluated in hospitals, including the patient taking 300 mg, there were no observations indicating an adverse change in laboratory analytes or ECGs. Vital signs were usually within normal limits following overdoses.

Based on animal data, the predicted symptoms would reflect an exaggeration of the drug's known pharmacological actions. Symptoms may include somnolence, mydriasis, blurred vision, respiratory depression, hypotension and possible extrapyramidal disturbances.

There is no specific antidote to olanzapine; therefore, appropriate supportive measures should be initiated. The possibility of multiple drug involvement should be considered.

In case of acute overdosage, establish and maintain an airway and ensure adequate oxygenation and ventilation. The use of activated charcoal for overdose should be considered because the concomitant administration of activated charcoal was shown to reduce the oral bioavailability of olanzapine by 50 to 60%. Gastric lavage (after intubation, if patient is unconscious) may also be considered. Olanzapine is not substantially removed by haemodialysis.

Hypotension and circulatory collapse should be treated with appropriate measures, such as intravenous fluids and/or sympathomimetic agents such as norepinephrine (do not use epinephrine, dopamine or other sympathomimetic agents with beta-agonist activity since beta stimulation may worsen hypotension in the setting of alpha blockade induced by olanzapine). Cardiovascular monitoring should be considered to detect possible arrhythmias. Close medical supervision and monitoring should continue until the patient recovers.

Pharmacological properties

Pharmacodynamic properties: Pharmacotherapeutic group: Olanzapine is an antipsychotic, ATC code N05A H03 (Diazepines and oxazepines).

Olanzapine is an antipsychotic agent that demonstrates a broad pharmacologic profile across a number of receptor systems.

In preclinical studies, olanzapine exhibited a range of receptor affinities (Ki; <100nM) for serotonin 5HT2A/2C, 5HT3, 5HT6; dopamine D1, D2, D3, D4, D5; cholinergic muscarinic receptors m1-m5; α1 adrenergic; and histamine H1 receptors. Animal behavioural studies with olanzapine indicated 5HT, dopamine, and cholinergic antagonism, consistent with the receptor-binding profile. Olanzapine demonstrated a greater *in vitro* affinity for serotonin 5HT2 than dopamine D2 receptors and greater 5HT2 than D2 activity *in vivo,* models. Electrophysiological studies demonstrated that olanzapine selectively reduced the firing of mesolimbic (A10) dopaminergic neurons, while having little effect on the striatal (A9) pathways involved in motor function. Olanzapine reduced a conditioned avoidance response, a test indicative of antipsychotic activity, at doses below those producing catalepsy, an effect indicative of motor side-effects. Unlike some other antipsychotic agents, olanzapine increases responding in an 'anxiolytic' test.

In a single oral dose (10 mg) Positron Emission Tomography (PET) study in healthy volunteers, olanzapine produced a higher 5HT2A than dopamine D2 receptor occupancy. In addition, a SPECT imaging study in schizophrenic patients revealed that olanzapine-responsive patients had lower striatal D2 occupancy than some other antipsychotic- and risperidone-responsive patients, while being comparable to clozapine-responsive patients.

In two of two placebo and two of three comparator controlled trials with over 2,900 schizophrenic patients presenting with both positive and negative symptoms, olanzapine was associated with statistically significantly greater improvements in negative as well as positive symptoms.

Pharmacokinetic properties: Olanzapine is well absorbed after oral administration, reaching peak plasma concentrations within 5 to 8 hours. The absorption is not affected by food. Absolute oral bioavailability relative to intravenous administration has not been determined.

Olanzapine is metabolised in the liver by conjugative and oxidative pathways. The major circulating metabolite is the 10-N-glucuronide, which does not pass the blood brain barrier. Cytochromes P450-CYP1A2 and P450-CYP2D6 contribute to the formation of the N-desmethyl and 2-hydroxymethyl metabolites, both exhibited significantly less *in vivo* pharmacological activity than olanzapine in animal studies. The predominant pharmacologic activity is from the parent olanzapine. After oral administration, the mean terminal elimination half-life of olanzapine in healthy subjects varied on the basis of age and gender.

In healthy elderly (65 and over) versus non-elderly subjects, the mean elimination half-life was prolonged (51.8 versus 33.8 hr) and the clearance was reduced (17.5 versus 18.2L/hr). The pharmacokinetic variability observed in the elderly is within the range for the non-elderly. In 44 patients with schizophrenia >65 years of age, dosing from 5 to 20 mg/day was not associated with any distinguishing profile of adverse events.

In female versus male subjects the mean elimination half-life was somewhat prolonged (36.7 versus 32.3 hrs) and the clearance was reduced (18.9 versus 27.3L/hr). However, olanzapine (5-20 mg) demonstrated a comparable safety profile in female (n = 467) as in male patients (n = 869).

In renally impaired patients (creatinine clearance <10 ml/min) versus healthy subjects, there was no significant difference in mean elimination half-life (37.7 versus 32.4 hr) or drug clearance (21.2 versus 25.0L/hr). A mass balance study showed that approximately 57% of radiolabeled olanzapine appeared in urine, principally as metabolites.

In smoking subjects with mild hepatic dysfunction, mean elimination half-life (39.3 hr) was prolonged and clearance (18.0L/hr) was reduced analogous to non-smoking healthy subjects (48.8hr and 14.1L/hr, respectively).

In non-smoking versus smoking subjects (males and females) the mean elimination half-life was prolonged (38.6 versus 30.4 hr) and the clearance was reduced (18.6 versus 27.7L/hr).

The plasma clearance of olanzapine is lower in elderly versus young subjects, in females versus males, and in non-smokers versus smokers. However, the magnitude of the impact of age, gender, or smoking on olanzapine clearance and half-life is small in comparison to the overall variability between individuals.

In a study of Caucasians, Japanese and Chinese subjects, there were no differences in the pharmacokinetic parameters among the three populations.

The plasma protein binding of olanzapine was about 93% over the concentration range of about 7 to about 1000ng/ml. Olanzapine is bound predominantly to albumin and α_1-acid-glycoprotein.

Preclinical safety data:
Acute (single-dose) toxicity: Signs of oral toxicity in rodents were characteristic of potent neuroleptic compounds: hypoactivity, coma, tremors, clonic convulsions, salivation, and depressed weight gain. The median lethal doses were approximately 210 (mice) and 175 (rats) mg/kg. Dogs tolerated single oral doses up to 100 mg/kg without mortality. Clinical signs included sedation, ataxia, tremors, increased heart rate, laboured respiration, miosis and anorexia. In monkeys, single oral doses up to 100 mg/kg resulted in prostration and, at higher doses, semi-consciousness.

Repeated-dose toxicity: In studies up to 3 months duration in mice and up to 1 year in rats and dogs, the predominant effects were CNS depression, anticholinergic effects and peripheral haematological disorders. Tolerance developed to the CNS depression. Growth parameters were decreased at high doses. Reversible effects consistent with elevated prolactin in rats included decreased weights of ovaries and uterus and morphologic changes in vaginal epithelium and in mammary gland.

Haematologic toxicity: Effects on haematology parameters were found in each species, including dose-related reductions in circulating leucocytes in mice and non-specific reductions of circulating leucocytes in rats; however, no evidence of bone marrow cytotoxicity was found. Reversible neutropenia, thrombocytopenia, or anaemia developed in a few dogs treated with 8 or 10 mg/kg/day (total olanzapine exposure [AUC] is 12- to 15-fold greater than that of a man given a 12 mg dose). In cytopenic dogs, there were no adverse effects on progenitor and proliferating cells in the bone marrow.

Reproductive toxicity: Olanzapine had no teratogenic effects. Sedation affected mating performance of male rats. Estrous cycles were affected at doses of 1.1 mg/kg (3 times the maximum human dose) and reproduction parameters were influenced in rats given 3 mg/kg (9 times the maximum human dose). In the offspring of rats given olanzapine, delays in fetal development and transient decreases in offspring activity levels were seen.

Mutagenicity: Olanzapine was not mutagenic or clastogenic in a full range of standard tests, which included bacterial mutation tests and *in vitro* and *in vivo* mammalian tests.

Carcinogenicity: Based on the results of studies in mice and rats, it was concluded that olanzapine is not carcinogenic.

Pharmaceutical particulars

List of excipients: Inactive ingredients are carnauba wax (PhEur), colour mixture white (titanium dioxide E171, macrogol, polysorbate 80), crospovidone (PhEur), edible blue ink (contains indigo carmine colour E132), hydroxypropyl cellulose (PhEur), lactose monohydrate (PhEur), magnesium stearate (PhEur), methylhydroxypropylcellulose (PhEur), microcrystalline cellulose (PhEur).

Incompatibilities: None.

Shelf-life: Two years (2.5 mg) when stored under appropriate conditions.

Three years (5 mg, 7.5 mg and 10 mg) when stored under appropriate conditions.

Special precautions for storage: Store at 15°-30°C. Sensitive to light. Keep tablets in the original package, in a dry place.

Nature and contents of container: Blister strips.

Zyprexa 2.5 mg tablets are available in cold-formed aluminium blister strips in cartons of 28 tablets per carton.

Zyprexa 5 mg tablets are available in cold-formed aluminium blister strips in cartons of 28 tablets per carton.

Zyprexa 7.5 mg tablets are available in cold-formed aluminium blister strips in cartons of 56 tablets per carton.

Zyprexa 10 mg tablets are available in cold-formed aluminium blister strips in cartons of 28 or 56 tablets per carton.

Marketing authorisation holder: Eli Lilly Nederland BV, Kritjwal 17-23, 3432 ZT Nieuwegein, The Netherlands

Marketing authorisation numbers

2.5 mg x 28 tablets:	EU/1/96/022/002
5 mg x 28 tablets:	EU/1/96/022/004
7.5 mg x 56 tablets:	EU/1/96/022/006
10 mg x 28 tablets:	EU/1/96/022/009
10 mg x 56 tablets:	EU/1/96/022/010

Date of approval/revision of SPC November 1998.

Legal category POM

**Trade Mark*

Link Pharmaceuticals Ltd
7/8 Sterling Buildings
Carfax
Horsham
West Sussex RH12 1DR

☎ 01403 272451 🖷 01403 272455

COBALIN-H*

Presentation 1 ml ampoules containing a sterile, clear, red solution providing 1000 micrograms hydroxocobalamin per millilitre for injection. Cobalin-H complies with the specification for Hydroxocobalamin Injection BP.

Uses Addisonian pernicious anaemia. Prophylaxis and treatment of other macrocytic anaemias due to B_{12} deficiency. Tobacco amblyopia and Leber's atrophy.

Dosage and administration The following dosages are suitable for children and adults.

Addisonian pernicious anaemia and other macrocytic anaemias without neurological involvement: Initially – 250 micrograms to 1000 micrograms intramuscularly on alternate days for one or two weeks then 250 micrograms weekly until blood count is normal. Maintenance – 1000 micrograms every two or three months.

Addisonian pernicious anaemia and other macrocytic anaemias with neurological involvement: Initially – 1000 micrograms on alternate days as long as improvement continues. Maintenance – 1000 micrograms every two months.

Prophylaxis of macrocytic anaemias associated with Vitamin B_{12} deficiency resulting from gastrectomy, ileal resection, certain malabsorption states and vegetarianism: 1000 micrograms every two or three months.

Tobacco amblyopia and Leber's optic atrophy: Initially – 1000 micrograms daily by intramuscular injection for two weeks then twice weekly as long as improvement is maintained. Maintenance – 1000 micrograms every three months or as required.

Contra-indications, warnings, etc
Contra-indications: Sensitivity to hydroxocobalamin.

Interactions: The serum concentration of hydroxocobalamin may be reduced by concurrent administration of oral contraceptives. Chloramphenicol treated patients may respond poorly to hydroxocobalamin. Vitamin B_{12} assays by microbiological techniques are invalidated by antimetabolites and most antibiotics.

Effects on ability to drive and use machines: None stated.

Other undesirable effects: Allergic hypersensitivity reactions have occurred rarely following the administration of hydroxocobalamin.

Use in pregnancy and lactation: Hydroxocobalamin should not be used to treat megaloblastic anaemia of pregnancy.

Other special warnings and precautions: Should not be given before a megaloblastic marrow has been demonstrated. Regular monitoring of the blood is advisable. Doses of hydroxocobalamin greater than 10 micrograms daily may produce a haematological response in patients with a folate deficiency. Indiscriminate use may mask the exact diagnosis. Cardiac arrhythmias secondary to hypokalaemia have been reported during initial therapy and plasma potassium should therefore be monitored during this period.

Overdose: Treatment is unlikely to be needed in cases of overdosage.

Incompatibilities: None stated.

Pharmaceutical precautions Protect from light. Store below 25°C.

Legal category POM.

Package quantities Boxes of 5 ampoules.

Further information Hydroxocobalamin injection has completely replaced Cyanocobalamin injection and is now the form of Vitamin B_{12} therapy of choice.

Product licence number 12406/0001.

NOZINAN*

Presentation
Injection: Colourless isotonic solution containing 2.5% w/v methotrimeprazine hydrochloride in ampoules of 1 ml. The injection also contains ascorbic acid, sodium sulphite and sodium chloride.

Tablets: Greyish white or cream tablets containing 25 mg methotrimeprazine maleate impressed NOZINAN '25' on one face, with a break line on the reverse.

Uses Methotrimeprazine resembles chlorpromazine and promethazine in the pattern of its pharmacology. It possesses anti-emetic, anti-histamine and anti-adrenaline activity and exhibits a strong sedative effect. Nozinan potentiates the action of other central nervous system depressants but may be given in conjunction with appropriately modified doses of narcotic analgesics in the management of severe pain. Nozinan does not significantly depress respiration and is particularly useful where pulmonary reserve is low.

Nozinan is indicated in the management of severe pain and accompanying anxiety and distress. Nozinan is also indicated in psychiatry as an alternative to Largactil in schizophrenia especially when it is desirable to reduce psychomotor activity.

Kinetics: Maximum serum concentrations are achieved in 2–3 hours depending on route of administration. Excretion is slow, with a half-life of about 30 hours. It is eliminated via urine and faeces.

Dosage and administration Dosage varies with the condition and individual response of the patient.

1. Terminal illness: The usual dose for adults and the elderly is 12.5–25 mg (0.5–1 ml) by intramuscular injection, or by the intravenous route after dilution with an equal volume of normal saline immediately before use. In cases of severe agitation up to 50 mg (2 ml) may be used, repeated every six to eight hours.

Continuous subcutaneous infusion: Nozinan may be administered over a 24 hour period via a syringe driver. The required dose of Nozinan (25–200 mg per day) should be diluted with the calculated volume of normal saline. Diamorphine hydrochloride is compatible with this solution and may be added if greater analgesia is required.

Nozinan tablets 25 mg may be substituted for the injection if oral therapy is more convenient the dosage being 12.5–50 mg 4–8 hourly.

Children: Clinical experience with parenteral methotrimeprazine in children is limited. Where indicated doses of 0.35 mg to 3.0 mg/kg/day by continuous subcutaneous infusion are recommended.

2. Psychiatric conditions: Adults: Ambulant patients: initially the total daily oral dose should not exceed 25–50 mg, usually divided into 3 doses; a larger portion of the dosage may be taken at bedtime to minimise diurnal sedation. The dosage is then gradually increased to the most effective level compatible with sedation and other side-effects.

Bed patients: Initially the total daily oral dosage may be 100–200 mg, usually divided into 3 doses, gradually increased to 1 g daily if necessary. When the patient is stable attempts should be made to reduce the dosage to an adequate maintenance level.

Children: Children are very susceptible to the hypotensive and soporific effects of methotrimeprazine. It is advised that a total daily oral dosage of 1½ tablets should not be exceeded. The average effective daily intake for a 10-year-old is ½ to 1 tablet.

Elderly patients: It is not advised to give methotrimeprazine to ambulant patients over 50 years of age unless the risk of a hypotensive reaction has been assessed.

Contra-indications, warnings, etc Safety in pregnancy has not been established.

There are no absolute contra-indications to the use of Nozinan in terminal care.

The drug should be avoided or used with caution in patients with liver dysfunction or cardiac disease.

Precautions: The hypotensive effects of Nozinan should be taken into account when it is administered to patients with cardiac disease and the elderly or debilitated. Patients receiving large initial doses should be kept in bed.

Nozinan may cause drowsiness, disorientation, confusion or excessive hypotension, which may affect patient's ability to drive or operate machinery. Avoid alcoholic drinks.

Side-effects: Somnolence and asthenia are frequent side effects. Dry mouth is encountered occasionally. Hypotension may occur, especially in elderly patients. A raised ESR may occasionally be encountered. Agranulocytosis has been reported, as have photosensivity and allergic skin reactions. Parkinsonian-like reactions may occur in patients receiving prolonged high dosage. Jaundice is a rare side effect. Other adverse effects common to phenothiazine neuroleptics may be seen.

Interactions: Simultaneous administration of desferrioxamine and prochlorperazine has been observed to induce a transient metabolic encephalopathy characterised by loss of consciousness for 48–72 hours. It is possible that this may occur with Nozinan since it shares many of the pharmacological activities of prochlorperazine. Adrenaline must not be used in patients overdosed with neuroleptics.

Toxicity and treatment of overdosage: Symptoms of methotrimeprazine overdosage include drowsiness or loss of consciousness, hypotension, tachycardia, ECG changes, ventricular arrhythmias and hypothermia. Severe extra-pyramidal dyskinesias may occur.

If the patient is seen sufficiently soon (up to 6 hours) after ingestion of a toxic dose, gastric lavage may be attempted. Pharmacological induction of emesis is unlikely to be of any use. Activated charcoal should be given. There is no specific antidote. Treatment is supportive.

Generalised vasodilatation may result in circulatory collapse; raising the patient's legs may suffice, in severe cases, volume expansion by intravenous fluids may be needed; infusion fluids should be warmed before administration in order not to aggravate hypothermia.

Positive inotropic agents such as dopamine may be tried if fluid replacement is insufficient to correct the circulatory collapse. Peripheral vasoconstrictor agents are not generally recommended; avoid the use of adrenaline.

Ventricular or supraventricular tachy-arrhythmias usually respond to restoration of normal body temperature and correction of circulatory or metabolic disturbances. If persistent or life threatening, appropriate anti-arrhythmic therapy may be considered. Avoid lignocaine and, as far as possible, long acting anti-arrhythmic drugs.

Pronounced central nervous system depression requires airway maintenance or, in extreme circumstances, assisted respiration. Severe dystonic reactions usually respond to procyclidine (5–10 mg) or orphenadrine (20–40 mg) administered intramuscularly or intravenously. Convulsions should be treated with intravenous diazepam.

Neuroleptic malignant syndrome should be treated with cooling. Dantrolene sodium may be tried.

Pharmaceutical precautions Protect from light. Nozinan Injection Solution, on exposure to light, rapidly develops a pink or yellow colouration and any such solution should be discarded. Nozinan Injection Solution is incompatible with alkaline solutions.

Legal category POM.

Package quantities Injection Solution 2.5% Box of 10×1 ml ampoules. Tablets container of 500×25 mg.

Further information Dilutions of Nozinan injection in normal saline, with or without the addition of diamorphine hydrochloride, are stable for 24 hours and may be used in syringe drivers.

Levomepromazine is the recommended International Non-proprietary Name (rINN) and methotrimeprazine is the British Approved Named (BAN) of the active ingredient in Nozinan.

Product licence numbers

Nozinan Injection Solution 2.5%	12406/0006
Nozinan Tablets 25 mg	12406/0007

PABRINEX* INTRAVENOUS HIGH POTENCY PABRINEX* INTRAMUSCULAR HIGH POTENCY

Presentation Pairs of amber glass ampoules of Vitamins B and C Injection BPC for intravenous and intramuscular injection:
I.V. High Potency – 5 ml No. 1+5 ml No. 2 Blue Carton
I.M. High Potency – 5 ml No. 1+2 ml No. 2 Red Carton

Ingredients:

Active ingredient	*Intravenous High Potency Blue carton No. 1*	*No. 2*	*Intramuscular High Potency Red carton No. 1*	*No. 2*
Thiamine Hydrochloride BP (Vitamin B_1)	250 mg		250 mg	
Riboflavin (as Phosphate Sodium BP) (Vitamin B_2)	4 mg		4 mg	
Pyridoxine Hydrochloride BP (Vitamin B_6)	50 mg		50 mg	
Nicotinamide BP		160 mg		160 mg
Ascorbic Acid BP (Vitamin C)		500 mg		500 mg
Anhydrous Glucose BP		1 gm[1]		
Benzyl Alcohol BP			140 mg[2]	
Volume per ampoule	5 ml	5 ml	5 ml	2 ml
Dose volume	10 ml		7 ml	

[1] provides 10% w/v in mixed ampoules
[2] provides 2% w/v in mixed ampoules

Pabrinex Injections are aqueous solutions for intravenous and intramuscular injection and also contain edetic acid and sodium hydroxide as excipients.

Uses Rapid therapy of severe depletion or malabsorption of the water soluble Vitamins B and C, particularly in alcoholism, after acute infections, post operatively and in psychiatric states.

Also used to maintain levels of Vitamins B and C in patients on chronic intermittent haemodialysis.

Dosage and administration
INTRAVENOUS: The preferred method of administration is by drip infusion. The contents of each pair of ampoules should be diluted with 50–100 ml physiological saline or 5% glucose and infused over 15–30 minutes (see *Storage* section for further information).

Alternatively the contents of each pair of ampoules (total 10 ml) are drawn up into a syringe to mix them just before use, then injected slowly, over a period of 10 minutes, into a vein.

NOT FOR INTRAMUSCULAR USE.

INTRAMUSCULAR – The contents of each pair of ampoules (total 7 ml) are drawn up into a syringe to mix them just before use, then injected slowly high into the gluteal muscle, 5 cm below the iliac crest.

NOT FOR INTRAVENOUS USE.

Adult dose (including the elderly): Pabrinex is indicated for rapid therapy of severe vitamin depletion or malabsorption encountered in the following conditions:

Coma or delirium from alcohol, narcotics or barbiturates; collapse following continuous narcosis:	The contents of 2–3 pairs of ampoules INTRAVENOUS HIGH POTENCY (Blue No. 1 and No. 2) injected at intervals of 8 hours or at the discretion of the physician.
Psychosis following narcosis or ECT; toxicity from acute infections:	The contents of one pair of ampoules INTRAVENOUS HIGH POTENCY (Blue No. 1 and No. 2) or INTRAMUSCULAR HIGH POTENCY (Red No. 1 and No. 2) twice daily for up to 7 days.
Haemodialysis:	The contents of one pair of ampoules INTRAVENOUS HIGH POTENCY (Blue No. 1 and No. 2) every two weeks diluted with saline and given at the end of the dialysis.

Children's dose: Pabrinex is rarely indicated for administration to children, but suitable doses are:

Under 6 years	0.25 adult dose
6–10 years	0.33 adult dose
10–14 years	0.50–0.66 adult dose
14 years and over	adult dose

Contra-indications, warnings, etc
Contra-indications: Known hypersensitivity to any of the active constituents.

Interactions: The content of pyridoxine may interfere with the effects of concurrent levodopa therapy.

Effects on ability to drive and use machinery: None known.

Other undesirable effects: Occasionally, hypotension and mild paraesthesia from continued high doses of thiamine; occasionally mild ache at local site of injection.

Use in pregnancy and lactation: No adverse effects at recommended doses when clinically indicated.

Other special warnings and precautions: Repeated injections of preparations containing high concentrations of Vitamin B_1 (thiamine) may give rise to anaphylactic shock. Mild allergic reactions such as sneezing or mild asthma are warning signs that further injections may give rise to anaphylactic shock. Facilities for treating anaphylactic reactions should be available whenever Pabrinex is administered.

Overdosage: Unlikely to occur but if it does, treatment is symptomatic and supportive.

Incompatibilities: If it is necessary to administer Pabrinex I.V. in infusion fluids it is recommended that it be given in Glucose 5% or Sodium Chloride 0.9% by intermittent infusion (i.e. over a short time in a relatively small volume) or by adding via drip tubing.

Pharmaceutical precautions Store blow 25°C protected from light. Do not freeze.

Storage of diluted Pabrinex IVHP: The stability of IVHP Vitamins B and C Injection BPC in intravenous infusion fluids, at room temperature, is as follows:

Intravenous infusion fluid: In the light.
Glucose 5%: 7 hours.
Sodium chloride 0.9%: 7 hours.
Glucose 4.3% with sodium chloride 0.18%: 4 hours.
Glucose 5% with potassium chloride 0.3%: 4 hours.
Sodium lactate M/6: 7 hours.

Although no further specific data are available, the solutions are expected to be stable for longer periods when protected from light. Store diluted solutions at 2–8°C if not used immediately. Do not freeze.

Legal category POM.

Package quantities Packs of 10 pairs of ampoules.

Further information Nil.

Product licence numbers
I.V. High Potency 12406/0003
I.M. High Potency 12406/0004

PIRITON* INJECTION

Presentation Piriton (Chlorpheniramine Maleate BP) is a potent antihistamine. Each 1 ml of Piriton Injection contains Chlorpheniramine Maleate BP 10 mg. It is colourless. Other ingredients: Sodium chloride, Water for Injections.

Uses Piriton Injection is indicated for acute urticaria, control of allergic reactions to insect bites and stings, angioneurotic oedema, drug and serum reactions, desensitisation reactions, hayfever, vasomotor rhinitis, severe pruritus of non-specific origin.

Dosage and Administration The usual dose of Piriton Injection for adults is 10 to 20 mg, but not more than 40 mg should be given per 24 hours. The injection may be subcutaneous, intramuscular or intravenous.

When a rapid effect is desired, as in anaphylactic reactions, the intravenous route is recommended in addition to emergency therapy with adrenaline, corticosteroids, oxygen and supportive therapy as required. In this case Piriton Injection should be injected slowly over a period of one minute, using the smallest adequate syringe. Any drowsiness, giddiness or hypotension which may follow is usually transitory.

In the event of a blood transfusion reaction, a dose of 10 to 20 mg of Piriton should be given by the subcutaneous route. This can be repeated to a total of 40 mg per 24 hours, or oral forms of Piriton may be given until the symptoms subside.

Piriton Injection may be helpful in the prevention of delayed reactions to penicillin and other drugs when given separately by intramuscular injection immediately prior to administration of the other drug. The usual dose is 10 mg.

Piriton Injection cannot, however, be relied on to prevent anaphylactic reactions in patients known to be allergic to a particular drug.

Contra-indications, Warnings, etc

Contra-indications: Piriton Injection is contra-indicated in patients who are hypersensitive to antihistamines or to any of the other ingredients.

The anticholinergic properties of chlorpheniramine are intensified by monoamine oxidase inhibitors (MAOIs). Piriton Injection is therefore contra-indicated in patients who have been treated with MAOIs within the last fourteen days.

Precautions: The anticholinergic properties of chlorpheniramine may cause drowsiness, dizziness, blurred vision and psychomotor impairment, which can seriously hamper patients' ability to drive and use machinery.

Chlorpheniramine, in common with other drugs having anticholinergic effects, should be used with caution in epilepsy; raised intra-ocular pressure including glaucoma; prostatic hypertrophy; severe hypertension or cardiovascular disease; bronchitis; bronchiectasis and asthma; hepatic disease and thyrotoxicosis. Children and the elderly are more likely to experience the neurological anticholinergic effects.

The effects of alcohol may be increased.

Drug interactions: Concurrent use of chlorpheniramine and hypnotics or anxiolytics may potentiate drowsiness. Concurrent use of alcohol may have a similar effect.

Chlorpheniramine inhibits phenytoin metabolism and can lead to phenytoin toxicity.

The anticholinergic effects of chlorpheniramine are intensified by MAOIs (see Contra-indications).

Pregnancy: There is inadequate evidence of safety in human pregnancy. Piriton Injection should only be used during pregnancy when clearly needed and when the potential benefits outweigh the potential unknown risks to the foetus. Use during the third trimester may result in reactions in neonates.

Lactation: It is reasonable to assume that chlorpheniramine maleate may inhibit lactation and may be secreted in breast milk. The use of Piriton preparations in mothers breast feeding their babies requires that the therapeutic benefits of the drug should be weighed against the potential hazards to the mother and baby.

Side-effects: Sedation varying from slight drowsiness to deep sleep. The following may also occasionally occur: inability to concentrate; lassitude; blurred vision; gastro-intestinal disturbances such as anorexia, dyspepsia, nausea, vomiting, diarrhoea and abdominal pain; hepatitis including jaundice; urinary retention; headaches; dry mouth; dizziness; palpitation; tachycardia; arrhythmias; hypotension; chest tightness; thickening of bronchial secretions; haemolytic anaemia and other blood dyscrasias; allergic reactions including exfoliative dermatitis, photosensitivity and urticaria; twitching, muscular weakness and inco-ordination; tinnitus; depression, irritability and nightmares.

Children and the elderly are more likely to experience the neurological anticholinergic effects.

Some patients have reported a stinging or burning sensation at the site of injection. Rapid intravenous injection may cause transitory hypotension or CNS stimulation.

Overdosage: The estimated lethal dose of chlorpheniramine is 25 to 50 mg/kg body weight. Symptoms and signs include sedation, paradoxical stimulation of CNS, toxic psychosis, seizures, apnoea, convulsions, anticholinergic effects, dystonic reactions and cardiovascular collapse including arrhythmias.

Symptomatic and supportive measures should be provided with special attention to cardiac, respiratory, renal and hepatic functions, and fluid and electrolyte balance.

Treat hypotension and arrhythmias vigorously. CNS convulsions may be treated with i.v. diazepam or phenytoin. Haemoperfusion may be used in severe cases.

Pharmaceutical Precautions Piriton Injection should be stored below 25°C and protected from light.

Legal Category POM.

Package Quantities Piriton Injection is supplied in boxes of 5 ampoules.

Further Information Chlorphenamine is the recommended International Non-propriatory Name (rINN) and chlorpheniramine is the British Approved Name (BAN) for the active ingredient in Piriton Injection.

Product Licence Number 12406/0013

SYTRON*

Presentation A clear red mixture with a cherry taste.

Composition: Each 5 ml contains: Sodium ironedetate 190 mg (equivalent to 27.5 mg of iron).

Uses
Action: Sodium ironedetate is not an iron salt as it contains iron in an un-ionised form. In this compound the iron is 'insulated' or 'sequestered' with the sodium salt of ethylenediamine tetra-acetic acid to form a chelate. This accounts for the fact that Sytron is not astringent and does not discolour teeth. Studies using radioactive tracers have shown that iron chelate is split within the gastro-intestinal tract, releasing elemental iron which is absorbed and rendered available for haemoglobin regeneration.

Indications: Iron deficiency anaemia, in paediatrics,

and anaemias complicating rheumatoid arthritis. It is especially suitable in pregnancy when other forms of oral iron are not well tolerated.

Dosage and administration Oral.

Adults: 5 ml increasing gradually to 10 ml three times daily.

Elderly (over 65 years): As for adults.

Children (including premature infants) up to 1 year: 2.5 ml twice daily; somewhat smaller doses should be used initially.

1 to 5 years: 2.5 ml three times daily.

6 to 12 years: 5 ml three times daily.

Contra-indications, warnings, etc

Contra-indications: None known.

Precautions: None known.

Pregnancy: No adverse effects have been reported.

Side effects: Patients have occasionally complained of nausea or mild diarrhoea in the early stages of treatment. In such cases it has been found that if treatment is withdrawn for a short time these symptoms quickly disappear and subsequently the patient will tolerate further doses, which should be on a somewhat reduced scale. Normal individuals have taken Sytron in twice the recommended dosage and some of these have experienced mild diarrhoea. This should be taken into account if dosage is increased much higher than the recommended scale.

Interactions: None known.

Overdose: Initial symptoms of iron overdosage include nausea, vomiting, diarrhoea, abdominal pain, haematemesis, rectal bleeding, lethargy and circulatory collapse. Hyperglycaemia and metabolic acidosis may occur.

Treatment of overdosage:

1. Administer an emetic.
2. Emesis should be followed by gastric lavage with desferrioxamine solution (2 g/l). Desferrioxamine 5 g in 50–100 ml water should be introduced into the stomach following gastric emptying.
3. Keep the patient under constant surveillance to detect possible aspiration of vomitus. Maintain suction apparatus and standby emergency oxygen in case of need.
4. In adults, a drink of mannitol or sorbitol should be given to induce small bowel emptying. Inducing diarrhoea in children may be dangerous and should not be undertaken in young children.
5. Severe poisoning: In the presence of shock and/or coma with high serum iron levels (adults>142 μmol/l, children>90 μmol/l), immediate supportive measures should be introduced. Desferrioxamine should be given by slow I.V. infusion (adults 5 mg/kg/H, children 15 mg/kg/H). The maximum dose is 80 mg/kg/24 H.

   Warning: Hypotension may occur if the infusion rate is too rapid.
6. Less severe poisoning: I.M. desferrioxamine should be administered (adults 50 mg/kg to a maximum of 4 g, children 1 g 4–6 hourly).
7. Serum iron levels should be monitored throughout.

Pharmaceutical precautions Store below 30°C. Recommended diluent: Water. When diluted use within 14 days of preparation.

Legal category P.

Package quantities Bottles of 500 ml.

Further information Sodium feredetate is the recommended International Non-proprietary Name (rINN) and sodium ironedetate is the British Approved Name (BAN) for the active ingredient in Sytron.

Product licence number 12406/0005.

ZOMORPH*

Trade name of the medicinal product

Zomorph 10 mg, 30 mg, 60 mg, 100 mg
Zomorph 200 mg

Qualitative and quantitative composition

- Morphine sulphate BP 10 mg
- Morphine sulphate BP 30 mg
- Morphine sulphate BP 60 mg
- Morphine sulphate BP 100 mg
- Morphine sulphate BP 200 mg

Pharmaceutical form Sustained-release capsules.

Clinical Particulars

Therapeutic indications: Severe chronic pain and/or pain resistant to other analgesics, in particular pain associated with cancer.

Posology and method of administration: Route of administration: orally. As directed by a medical practitioner.

Recommended dosage Adults: Recommended dosage is one capsule twice daily, at 12-hour intervals. *Elderly:* As with all narcotics, a reduction in dosage may be advisable in the elderly, as appropriate. *Children:* Not recommended.

The capsules should not be chewed and should normally be swallowed whole.

The dosage varies according to the severity of pain and the previous analgesic treatments received by the patient.

If the pain persists, or if the patient develops tolerance to morphine, the dosage may be increased by prescribing the 10, 30, 60, 100 and 200 mg capsules in various combinations or alone to obtain the desired relief.

Patients previously treated with immediate-release oral morphine should receive the same daily dose of sustained-release capsules, but in two divided doses at 12-hour intervals.

Patients previously treated with parenteral morphine should be given a sufficiently increased dosage to compensate for any reduction of the analgesic effect associated with oral administration. The dosage should be adjusted to meet the individual requirements of each patient.

For patients who can not swallow the capsules, their contents can be administered directly in semi-solid food (puree, jam, yoghurt) or via gastric or gastrostomy tubes of a diameter of more than 16 F.G. with an open distal end or lateral pores. It is sufficient to rinse the tube with 30 to 50 ml of water.

Contra-indications: Respiratory impairment, acute abdominal syndrome of unknown origin, severely impaired liver function, cranial trauma and raised intracranial pressure, convulsive state, acute alcoholic intoxication and delirium tremens, children, concurrent treatment with MAO (MAO = monoamine oxidase) inhibitors, or within two weeks of their use.

Special warnings and special precautions for use: Caution should be exercised in elderly subjects, in patients with impaired hepatic and/or renal functions, hypothyroidism or hypoadrenalism, in those in a state of shock or with asthma. Urinary retention may occur in patients with urethral or prostatic disease.

Interaction with other medicaments: Serious or fatal accidents have been observed after administration of pethidine in combination with monoamine oxidase inhibitors. It is not known whether this type of reaction may occur with other central analgesics. As a precautionary measure, opioid analgesics should not be administered until 15 days after withdrawal of MAO inhibitor treatment.

When used in conjunction with central nervous system depressants and tricyclic antidepressants, the effects of morphine may be potentiated and there is a risk of overdosage.

Pregnancy and lactation: Since this product rapidly crosses the placental barrier, it should not be used during the second stage of labour or in premature delivery because of the risk of secondary respiratory depression in the newborn infant. If the mother is addicted, a withdrawal syndrome is observed in the newborn infant characterised by: convulsions, irritability, vomiting, increased mortality. As with all drugs, it is not advisable to administer it during pregnancy.

Effects on ability to drive and use machines: Because of the decrease in vigilance induced by this drug, attention is drawn to the possible dangers incurred by drivers of vehicles or machine operators.

Undesirable effects: The most common side effects at usual doses are nausea, constipation, confusion and occasionally vomiting. Other possible effects include: sedation or excitation (particularly in elderly subjects in whom delirium and hallucinations may occur), increased intracranial pressure which may aggravate existing cerebral disorders, increased pressure in the main bile duct and urinary retention in cases of prostatic adenoma or urethral stenosis. Mild respiratory depression occurs even at therapeutic doses. In the event of overdosage it may be severe, serious or even fatal. Physical and psychic dependence may appear after administration of therapeutic doses for periods of 1 to 2 weeks. Some cases of dependence have been observed after only 2 to 3 days.

Withdrawal syndrome: this may occur a few hours after withdrawal of a prolonged treatment, and is maximal between the 36th and 72nd hours.

Overdose: Symptoms include respiratory depression, extreme miosis, hypotension, hypothermia, coma. Treatment is by intravenous injection of naloxone 0.4 mg, repeated every 2 to 3 minutes if necessary, or by an infusion of 2 mg in 500 ml of normal saline or 5% dextrose (0.004 mg/ml).

In subjects dependent on morphine-like drugs, withdrawal symptoms may occur following injection of a high dose of naloxone. It should therefore be injected in gradually increasing doses to such subjects.

Pharmacological and Pharmacokinetic properties

Pharmacological properties: Morphine is an opioid analgesic. It acts mainly on the central nervous system and smooth muscle.

Morphine exerts an analgesic action, and affects psychomotor behaviour: depending on the dose administered, it induces sedation (>1cg) or, in some cases, excitation (<1cg). At high doses, greater than those required to produce analgesia, it induces somnolence and sleep.

Pharmacokinetic properties: Absorption: This is a sustained-release form, which makes possible twice-daily oral administration. Morphine is immediately absorbed from the digestive tract following oral administration. The maximum serum concentrations of morphine are obtained in 2 to 4 hours. *Distribution:* The percentage of binding to plasma proteins after absorption is low (about 34%). There is no clearly defined correlation between the plasma concentration of morphine and the analgesic effect. *Metabolism:* A considerable quantity of morphine is metabolised by the liver to glucuronides, which undergo enterohepatic recirculation. *Excretion:* The product is eliminated essentially in the urine, by glomerular filtration, mainly as glucuronides. A small amount (less than 10%) is eliminated in the faeces.

Pharmaceutical Particulars

List of excipients: Sucrose, maize starch, polyethylene glycol 4000, ethyl-cellulose, cetyl alcohol, sodium lauryl sulphate, dibutyl sebacate, talc, gelatin, iron oxide ink (E172), titanium dioxide (E171)[1]. (The 10 mg capsules also contain quinoline yellow (E104), the 30 mg capsules erythrosine (E127), and the 60 mg capsules sunset yellow (E110)).

[1]The 200 mg capsules do not contain titanium dioxide (E171).

Incompatibilities: Not applicable.

Shelf Life: 36 months.

Special precautions for storage: Store below 25°C in a dry place.

Nature and contents of container: Blister packs (aluminium/PVC). Boxes of 60 capsules.

Instructions for use: Not applicable.

Marketing authorisation numbers

Zomorph 10 mg, 30 mg, 60 mg, 100 mg PL 06934/0006/0007/0008/0009
Zomorph 200 mg PL 06934/0016

Legal category CD (Sch2) POM.

**Trade Mark*

Lipha Pharmaceuticals Limited
Harrier House, High Street
West Drayton
Middlesex UB7 7QG

☎ 01895 452200 　 01895 420605

CAMPRAL EC*

Qualitative and quantitative composition Each tablet contains acamprosate (I.N.N.) calcium 333.0 mg as the active ingredient.

Pharmaceutical form Enteric coated tablets.

Clinical particulars

Therapeutic indications: Campral EC is indicated as therapy to maintain abstinence in alcohol dependent patients. It should be combined with counselling.

Posology and method of administration
Adults: Within the age range 18-65 years:

Subjects weighing 60 kg or more: 2 tablets three times daily with meals (2 tablets morning, noon and night).

Subjects weighing less than 60 kg: 4 tablets divided into three daily doses with meals (2 tablets in the morning, 1 at noon, 1 at night).

The recommended treatment period is one year. Treatment with acamprosate should be initiated as soon as possible after the withdrawal period and should be maintained if the patient relapses.

Children and the elderly: Campral EC should not be administered to children and the elderly.

Contra-indications:
–in patients with a known hypersensitivity to the drug
–in pregnant women and lactating women
–in cases of renal insufficiency (serum creatinine >120 micromol/L)
–in cases with severe hepatic failure (Childs- Pugh Classification C)

Special warnings and precautions for use: Campral EC does not constitute treatment for the withdrawal period. Campral EC does not prevent harmful effects of continuous alcohol abuse. Continued alcohol abuse negates the therapeutic benefit, therefore Campral EC treatment should only be initiated after weaning therapy, once the patient is abstinent from alcohol.

Interactions with other medicaments and other forms of interaction: The concomitant intake of alcohol and Campral EC does not affect the pharmacokinetics of either alcohol or Campral EC. Administering Campral EC with food diminishes the bioavailability of the drug compared with its administration in the fasting state. Pharmacokinetic studies have been completed and show no interaction between acamprosate and diazepam, disulfiram or imipramine. There is no information available on the concomitant administration of Campral EC with diuretics.

Pregnancy and lactation: Although animal studies have not shown any evidence of foetotoxicity or teratogenicity, the safety of Campral EC has not been established in pregnant women. Acamprosate is excreted in the milk of lactating animals and safe use of Campral EC has not been demonstrated in lactating women. Campral EC therefore should not be administered to pregnant or to breast feeding women.

Effects on ability to drive and use machines: Campral EC should not impair the patient's ability to drive or operate machinery.

Undesirable effects: Adverse events associated with Campral EC tend to be mild and transient in nature. They are predominantly gastrointestinal or dermatological. Diarrhoea, and less frequently nausea, vomiting and abdominal pain are the gastrointestinal adverse events. Pruritus is the predominant dermatological adverse event. An occasional maculopapular rash and rare cases of bullous skin reactions have been reported. Fluctuation in libido has been reported by patients receiving Campral EC as well as by patients receiving the placebo.

Overdose: Five cases of overdose associated with Campral EC therapy have been reported in humans, including one patient who ingested 43 g. After gastric lavage all patients had an uneventful recovery. Diarrhoea was observed in two cases. No case of hypercalaemia was reported in the course of these overdoses. However, should this occur, the patients should be treated for acute hypercalcaemia.

Pharmacological properties
Pharmacodynamic properties: Acamprosate calcium (calcium acetylhomotaurinate) has a chemical structure similar to that of amino acid neurotransmitters, such as taurine or gamma-amino-butyric acid (GABA), including an acetylation to permit passage across the blood brain barrier. Acamprosate may act by stimulating GABAergic inhibitory neurotransmission and antagonising excitatory amino-acids, particularly glutamic acid. Animal experimental studies have demonstrated that acamprosate affects alcohol dependence in rats, decreasing the voluntary intake of alcohol without affecting food and total fluid intake.

Pharmacokinetic properties: Acamprosate absorption across the gastrointestinal tract is moderate, slow and sustained and varies substantially from person to person. Oral absorption shows considerable variability and is usually less than 10% of the ingested drug in the first 24 hours. Food reduces the oral absorption of acamprosate. Steady state levels of acamprosate are achieved by the seventh day of dosing. Acamprosate is not protein bound. The drug is excreted in the urine and is not significantly metabolised. There is a linear relationship between creatinine clearance values and total apparent plasma clearance, renal clearance and plasma half-life of acamprosate. The pharmacokinetics of acamprosate are not altered by hepatic dysfunction.

Preclinical safety data: In preclinical studies, signs of toxicity are related to the excessive intake of calcium and not acetylhomotaurine. Disorders of phosphorus/calcium metabolism have been observed including diarrhoea, soft tissue calcification, renal and cardiac lesions. There were no mutagenic or carcinogenic effects, nor any teratogenic or adverse affects on the male or female reproductive systems of animals. Detailed *in vitro* and *in vivo* research on acamprosate to detect genetic and chromosomal mutations has not produced any evidence of potential genetic toxicity.

Pharmaceutical particulars

List of excipients: Crospovidone (Kollidon CL); microcrystalline cellulose (Avicel PH 101); magnesium silicate (Compressil); sodium starch glycolate (Explotab); anhydrous colloidal silica (Aerosil 200); magnesium stearate; anionic copolymer of methacrylic and acrylic acid ethyl ester (Eudragit L30 D); talc; propylene glycol.

Incompatibilities: None known.

Shelf life: 3 years.

Special precautions: None.

Nature and contents of container: Aluminium/PVC sheets of blisters containing 12 tablets. Sheets of blisters are presented in cartons of 84 tablets.

Instructions for use / handling: Not applicable.

Marketing authorisation holder: Lipha S.A., 34 rue Saint Romain, 69379 Lyon Cedex 08, France.

Marketing authorisation number 13466/0001

Date of approval/revision of SPC December 1995.

Legal category POM

GLUCOPHAGE*

Presentation White, film-coated tablets containing Metformin Hydrochloride BP. 500 mg marked GL500; 850 mg marked GL850.

Uses *Indications:* Non-insulin dependent diabetes when diet has failed and especially if the patient is overweight. Glucophage can be given alone as initial therapy, or can be administered in combination with a sulphonylurea.

In insulin-dependent diabetes, Glucophage may be given as an adjuvant to patients whose symptoms are poorly controlled.

Pharmacology: Glucophage is a biguanide oral antihyperglycaemic agent. Its mode of action is thought to be multifactorial and includes delayed uptake of glucose from the gastro-intestinal tract, increased peripheral glucose utilisation mediated by increased insulin sensitivity and inhibition of increased hepatic and renal gluconeogenesis.

Dosage and administration
Adults: Initially, one 850 mg tablet twice a day or one 500 mg tablet three times a day, with or after food. Good diabetic control may be achieved within a few days, but it is not unusual for the full effect to be delayed for up to two weeks. If control is incomplete a cautious increase in dosage to a maximum of 3 g daily is justified. Once control has been obtained it may be possible to reduce the dosage of Glucophage.

Children: Glucophage is not recommended for use.

Elderly: Glucophage is indicated in the elderly, but not when renal function is impaired.

Contra-indications, warnings, etc
Contra-indications: Hypersensitivity to the drug. Diabetic coma and ketoacidosis, impairment of renal function, chronic liver disease, cardiac failure and recent myocardial infarction. History of, or states associated with, lactic acidosis such as shock or pulmonary insufficiency, alcoholism (acute or chronic), and conditions associated with hypoxaemia.

Precautions: Glucophage is excreted by the kidney and regular monitoring of renal function is advised in all diabetics. Intravascular contrast studies with iodinated materials can lead to acute alteration of renal function and have been associated with lactic acidosis in patients receiving Glucophage. Therefore, in patients in whom any such studies are planned, Glucophage should be discontinued at the time of, or prior to the procedure, and withheld for 48 hours subsequent to the procedure and reinstituted only after renal function has been re-evaluated and found to be normal. The use of Glucophage is not advised in conditions which may cause dehydration or in patients suffering from serious infections or trauma.

Patients receiving continuous Glucophage therapy should have an annual estimation of Vitamin B_{12} levels because of reports of decreased Vitamin B_{12} absorption.

During concomitant therapy with a sulphonylurea, blood glucose should be monitored because combined therapy may cause hypoglycaemia. Stabilisation of diabetic patients with Glucophage and insulin should be carried out in hospital because of the possibility of hypoglycaemia until the correct ratio of the two drugs has been obtained.

Reduced renal clearance of Glucophage has been reported during cimetidine therapy, so a dose reduction should be considered. As with a number of drugs, an interaction between Glucophage and anticoagulants is a possibility and dosage of the latter may need adjustment.

Use in pregnancy and lactation: Pregnancy: The use of Glucophage is not advised. Lactation: No information is available.

Adverse reactions: Glucophage is normally well tolerated but gastro-intestinal disturbances sometimes occur. These are usually minor and can often be avoided by taking Glucophage with or after food. Occasionally a temporary lowering of the dose may be needed. It is important that Glucophage treatment is not abandoned at the first sign of intolerance, since this has been found to resolve spontaneously.

Lactic acidosis has been associated with Glucophage but, in the few cases reported, has occurred in patients with contra-indications to therapy. In patients with a metabolic acidosis lacking evidence of ketoacidosis (ketonuria and ketonaemia), lactic acidosis should be suspected and Glucophage therapy stopped. Lactic acidosis is a medical emergency which must be treated in hospital.

Overdosage – Signs and Symptoms: Hypoglycaemia does not occur with Glucophage monotherapy (fifty tablets have been ingested with no untoward effects on blood glucose levels). However, it can occur when Glucophage is given concomitantly with a sulphonylurea, insulin or alcohol.

In excessive dosage, and particularly if there is a possibility of accumulation, lactic acidosis may develop.

Overdosage – Treatment: Intensive supportive therapy is recommended which should be particularly directed at correcting fluid loss and metabolic disturbance.

Pharmaceutical precautions Store below 25°C in a dry place. The shelf-life is 5 years.

Legal category POM.

Package quantities 500 mg: Blister packs of 84 tablets; containers of 500 tablets. 850 mg: Blister packs of 56 tablets; containers of 300 tablets.

Further information Glucophage does not lower blood glucose levels in non-diabetics, and does not cause hypoglycaemia in diabetics when used as monotherapy. Weight loss often occurs during therapy and levels of plasma cholesterol, triglycerides and prebeta-lipoproteins may be lowered. Glucophage has been shown to improve peripheral glucose metabolism.

Product licence numbers
Glucophage 500 mg 3759/0012
Glucophage 850 mg 3759/0013

NITROLINGUAL* PUMP SPRAY

Qualitative and quantitative composition Each metered dose contains 400 micrograms glyceryl trinitrate.

Pharmaceutical form Oromucosal spray.

Clinical particulars

Therapeutic indications: For the treatment and prophylaxis of angina pectoris and the treatment of variant angina.

Posology and method of administration
Adults and the elderly: At the onset of an attack or prior to a precipitating event: one or two 400 microgram metered-doses sprayed under the tongue. It is recommended that no more than three metered-doses are taken at any one time and that there should be a minimum interval of 15 minutes between consecutive treatments.

For the prevention of exercise induced angina or in other precipitating conditions: one or two 400 microgram metered doses sprayed under the tongue immediately prior to the event.

Children: Nitrolingual Pump spray is not recommended for use.

*Administration:*The bottle should be held vertically with the valve head uppermost. If the pump is new, or has not been used for a week or more, the first actuation should be released into the air. The spray orifice should then be placed as close to the mouth as possible. The dose should be sprayed under the tongue and the mouth should be closed immediately after each dose. The spray should not be inhaled. Patients should be instructed to familiarise themselves with the position of the spray orifice, which can be identified by the finger rest on the top of the valve, in order to facilitate orientation for administration at night. During application the patient should rest, ideally in the sitting position.

Contra-indications: Hypersensitivity to nitrates or any constituent of the formulation. Hypotension, hypovolaemia, severe anaemia, cerebral haemorrhage and brain trauma, mitral stenosis and angina caused by hypertrophic obstructive cardiomyopathy.

Special warnings and special precautions for use: Any lack of effect may be an indicator of early myocardial infarction.

As with all glyceryl trinitrate preparations, use in patients with incipient glaucoma should be avoided.

Interaction with other medicaments and other forms of interaction: Tolerance to this drug and cross tolerance to other nitrates may occur. Alcohol may potentiate any hypotensive effect.

Pregnancy and lactation: Nitrolingual Pump spray is not generally recommended and should be used only if its potential benefit justifies any potential risk to the foetus or neonate.

Effects on ability to drive and use machines: Only as a result of hypotension.

Undesirable effects: Headache, dizziness, postural hypotension, flushing, tachycardia and paradoxical bradycardia have been reported.

Overdose
Signs and symptoms: Flushing, severe headache, a feeling of suffocation, hypotension, fainting, restlessness, blurred vision, impairment of respiration, bradycardia and rarely, cyanosis and methaemoglobinaemia may occur. In a few patients there may be a reaction comparable to shock with nausea, vomiting, weakness, sweating and syncope.

Treatment: Recovery often occurs without special treatment. Hypotension may be corrected by elevation of the legs to promote venous return. Methaemoglobinaemia should be treated by intravenous methylene blue.

Symptomatic treatment should be given for respiratory and circulatory defects in more serious cases.

Pharmacological properties

Pharmacodynamic properties: Glyceryl trinitrate relieves angina pectoris by reduction of cardiac work and dilation of the coronary arteries. In this way, not only is there a lessening in arterial oxygen requirement but the amount of oxygenated blood reaching the ischaemic heart is increased.

Pharmacokinetics properties: The pharmacokinetics of glyceryl trinitrate are complex; venous plasma levels of the drug show wide and variable fluctuations and are not predictive of clinical effect. In a human pharmacodynamic study, pharmacological activity had commenced one minute after dosing and was obvious by two minutes.

Pharmaceutical particulars

List of excipients: Fractionated coconut oil, ethanol, medium chain partial glycerides, peppermint oil.

Incompatibilities: None known.

Shelf life: 3 years.

Special precautions for storage: Store below 25°C.

Nature and contents of container: Red plastic coated glass bottle fitted with metering pump. Each bottle contains 4.9, 11.2 or 14.1 g solution (equivalent to about 75, 200 or 250 doses).

Instructions for use/handling: See 'Administration' section.

Marketing authorisation number 03759/0042.

Date of approval/revision of SPC April 1995.

Legal category P

NITRONAL*

Presentation Amber glass 5 ml ampoules and clear glass 50 ml vials filled with a colourless isotonic solution containing 1 mg/ml glyceryl trinitrate.

Excipients: Dextrose, polyethylene glycol 400, water for injections.

Uses
Indications:

1. Unresponsive congestive heart failure, including that secondary to acute myocardial infarction.
2. Refractory unstable angina pectoris and coronary insufficiency, including Prinzmetal's angina.
3. Control of hypertensive episodes and/or myocardial ischaemia during and after cardiac surgery. For the induction of controlled hypotension for surgery.

Pharmacology: Glyceryl trinitrate exerts a spasmolytic action on smooth muscle, particularly in the vascular system. The predominant effect is an increase in venous capacitance resulting in marked diminution of both the left ventricular filling pressure and volume (preload). There is also a reduction in afterload due to moderate dilation of the arteriolar resistance vessels. These haemodynamic changes lower the myocardial oxygen demand. By direct action and through the reduction of myocardial wall tension, glyceryl trinitrate also lowers the resistance to flow in the coronary collateral channels and allows re-distribution of blood flow to ischaemic areas of the myocardium.

Administration of Nitronal by intravenous infusion to patients with congestive heart failure results in a marked improvement in haemodynamics, reduction of elevated left ventricular filling pressure and systolic wall tension, and an increase in the depressed cardiac output. It reduces the imbalance that exists between myocardial oxygen demand and delivery, thereby diminishing myocardial ischaemia and controlling ischaemia-induced ventricular arrhythmias.

Dosage and administration
Dosage: Adults and the Elderly – The dose should be titrated against the individual clinical response.

1. Unresponsive congestive heart failure. The normal dose range is 10–100 micrograms/minute administered as a continuous intravenous infusion with frequent monitoring of blood pressure and heart rate. The infusion should be started at the lower rate and increased cautiously until the desired clinical response is achieved. Other haemodynamic measurements are extremely important in monitoring response to the drug: these may include pulmonary capillary wedge pressure, cardiac output and precordial electrocardiogram depending on the clinical picture.
2. Refractory unstable angina pectoris. An initial infusion rate of 10–15 micrograms/minute is recommended; this may be increased cautiously in increments of 5–10 micrograms until either relief of angina is achieved, headache prevents further increase in dose, or the mean arterial pressure falls by more than 20 mm Hg.
3. Use in surgery. An initial infusion rate of 25 micrograms/minute is recommended; this should be increased gradually until the desired systolic arterial pressure is attained. The usual dose is 25–200 micrograms/minute.

Children: There is no recommended dose for children.

Administration: Nitronal need not be diluted before use but can be diluted with Dextrose Injection BP, Sodium Chloride and Dextrose Injection BP, 0.9% Sodium Chloride Injection BP or other protein-free infusion solution, if required.

The solution, whether or not diluted, should be infused *slowly* (see dosage section) and *not* given by bolus injection.

To ensure a constant infusion rate of glyceryl trinitrate, it is recommended that Nitronal be administered by means of a syringe pump or polyethylene infusion bag with a counter, with a glass or rigid polyethylene syringe and polyethylene tubing. Systems made of polyvinylchloride may adsorb up to 50% of the glyceryl trinitrate from the solution, thus reducing the efficacy of the infusion. If the recommended type of system is unavailable, a 1:10 dilution of Nitronal should be used and the infusion rate modified according to the haemodynamic response of the patient, until the required parameters are attained.

Contra-indications, warnings, etc These are common to all nitrates.

Contra-indications: Hypersensitivity to nitrates. Hypotensive shock, severe anaemia, cerebral haemorrhage, arterial hypoxaemia, uncorrected hypovolaemia and angina caused by hypertrophic obstructive cardiomyopathy.

Precautions: Caution should be exercised in patients with severe liver or renal disease, hypothermia or hypothyroidism. Glyceryl trinitrate may potentiate the action of other hypotensive drugs and the hypotensive and anticholinergic effects of tricyclic anti-depressants; it may also slow the metabolism of morphine-like analgesics.

Pregnancy and lactation: No information is available.

Adverse reactions: Nitronal is generally well tolerated because a minimum dose is administered in unit time. Headache, dizziness, flushing, hypotension and tachycardia may be encountered, particularly if the infusion is administered too rapidly. Nausea, diaphoresis, restlessness, retrosternal discomfort, abdominal pain and paradoxical bradycardia have been reported. These symptoms should be readily reversible on reducing the rate of infusion or, if necessary, discontinuing treatment.

Overdosage – Signs and Symptoms: Vomiting, restlessness, hypotension, syncope, cyanosis, coldness of the skin, impairment of respiration, bradycardia, psychosis and methaemoglobinaemia may occur.

Overdosage – Treatment: The symptoms may be readily reversed by discontinuing treatment; if hypotension persists, raising the foot of the bed and the use of vasoconstrictors such as intravenous methoxamine or phenylephrine is recommended. Methaemaglobinaemia should be treated by intravenous methylene blue. Oxygen and assisted respiration may be required.

Pharmaceutical precautions Store in a cool place away from light. The vial is for single dose use only, and should be stored in the carton until ready for use. The shelf life is 2 years.

The diluted solution should be administered as soon as possible; it is stable for up to 24 hours in the recommended infusion system.

Legal category POM.

Package quantities 10 ampoules; single vials.

Further information Nitronal is free of alcohol, propylene glycol and potassium. Glyceryl trinitrate is also known as nitroglycerin.

Product licence number 3759/0025.

PRAXILENE*

Presentation Pale pink capsules marked PRAXILENE and LIPHA, each containing 100 mg of naftidrofuryl oxalate.

Uses *Indications:* Peripheral vascular disorders – intermittent claudication, night cramps, rest pain, incipient gangrene, trophic ulcers, Raynaud's syndrome, diabetic arteriopathy and acrocyanosis.

Cerebral vascular disorders – cerebral insufficiency and cerebral atherosclerosis, particularly where these manifest themselves as mental deterioration and confusion in the elderly.

Pharmacology: Praxilene has been shown to exert a direct effect on intracellular metabolism. Thus it has been demonstrated in man and animals that it produces an increase of ATP levels and a decrease of lactic acid levels in ischaemic conditions, evidence for an enhancement of cellular oxidative capacity. Furthermore Praxilene is a powerful spasmolytic agent.

Dosage and administration
Adults and the Elderly: Peripheral vascular disorders: one or two 100 mg capsules three times daily for a minimum of three months, or at the discretion of the physician.

Cerebral vascular disorders: one 100 mg capsule three times daily for a minimum of three months, or at the discretion of the physician.

Children: There is no recommended dose.

Contra-indications, warnings, etc
Contra-indications: Hypersensitivity to the drug.

Use in pregnancy and lactation: Pregnancy: There is no, or inadequate, evidence of safety of Praxilene in human pregnancy, but it has been in wide use for many years without apparent ill consequence, animal studies having shown no hazard. If drug therapy is needed in pregnancy, this drug can be used if there is no safer alternative.

Lactation: No information is available.

Adverse reactions: Praxilene is normally well tolerated in the dosage recommended. Occasionally nausea, epigastric pain and rashes have been noted. Rarely, hepatitis has been reported.

Overdosage – Signs and symptoms: Depression of cardiac conduction and convulsions may occur.

Overdosage – Treatment: The stomach should be emptied by gastric lavage and emesis. Activated charcoal may be employed if necessary. Cardiovascular function and respiration should be monitored and, in severe cases, electrical pacemaking or the use of isoprenaline should be considered. Convulsions may be managed by diazepam.

Pharmaceutical precautions Store below 20°C in a dry place away from light. The shelf-life is 3 years.

Legal category POM.

Package quantities Blister pack of 84 capsules (OP); containers of 100 and 500 capsules.

Further information Nil.

Product licence number 3759/0002.

SLO-PHYLLIN 60 mg CAPSULES
SLO-PHYLLIN 125 mg CAPSULES
SLO-PHYLLIN 250 mg CAPSULES

Qualitative and quantitative composition Slo-Phyllin 60 mg capsules each contain theophylline (anhydrous) EP 60 mg

Slo-Phyllin 125 mg capsules each contain theophylline (anhydrous) EP 125 mg

Slo-Phyllin 250 mg capsules each contain theophylline (anhydrous) EP 250 mg

Pharmaceutical form Time release capsule.

Clinical particulars
Therapeutic indications: As a bronchodilator in the symptomatic and prophylactic treatment of asthma and for reversible bronchoconstriction associated with chronic bronchitis and bronchial asthma.

Posology and method of administration
Method of administration: Oral.

Dosage:
Children:
2–6 years (10–20 kg): 60–120 mg twice daily.
6–12 years (20–35 kg) 125–250 mg twice daily.
over 12 years 250-500 mg twice daily.

Adults: 250-500 mg twice daily.

Elderly: There is a tendency for theophylline clearance to decrease with age leading to higher serum levels. A reduction of the adult dosage may therefore be necessary and close monitoring is advised.

Each patient should be titrated to a suitable dosage regimen by clinical assessment. It may also be necessary to measure plasma theophylline levels.

Initially the lowest dosage for each group is recommended. This may be increased gradually if optimal bronchodilator effects are not achieved. The total dosage should not normally exceed 24 mg/kg body weight for children and 13 mg/kg for adults. However the plasma theophylline level measured 4-8 hours after dosing and at least three days after any dosage adjustment, provides a more accurate assessment of the patients' dosage need, especially as significant variations in the rate of drug elimination can occur between individuals. The following table provides a guide:

Plasma level (mcg/ml)	*Result*	*Directions (if clinically indicated)*
Below 10	Too low	Increase dose by 25%
10-20	Correct	Maintain dose
20-25	Too high	Decrease dose by 10%
25-30	Too high	Miss next dose and decrease subsequent doses by 25%
Over 30	Too high	Miss next two doses and decrease subsequent doses by 50%

It is advisable to recheck the plasma level after dose adjustment and every 6-12 months.

It is not possible to ensure bioequivalence between different sustained release theophylline products. Once titrated to an effective dose, patients should not be changed from Slo-Phyllin to another sustained release xanthine preparation without re-titration and clinical assessment.

Contra-indications: Hypersensitivity to theophylline or other xanthines. Concomitant use of theophylline and ephedrine in children.

Special warnings and precautions for use: Smoking and alcohol consumption can increase the clearance of theophylline and a higher dose may be necessary.

Careful monitoring is recommended for patients with congestive heart failure, chronic alcoholism, hepatic dysfunction, or viral infections, as they may have a lower clearance of theophylline, which could lead to higher than normal plasma levels.

Caution should be exercised in patients with peptic ulcers, cardiac arrhythmias, other cardiovascular diseases, hyperthyroidism or hypertension. Slo-Phyllin should not be used concurrently with other preparations containing xanthines derivatives. If it is necessary to administer aminophylline to a patient who is already receiving Slo-Phyllin, plasma theophylline concentration should be monitored.

The use of alternative treatments is advised in patients with a history of seizures, as these may be exacerbated by theophylline.

Interactions with other medicaments and other forms of interaction: Theophylline has been reported to interact with a number of drugs. The following increase clearance and it may therefore be necessary to increase dosage to ensure therapeutic effect: barbiturates, carbamazepine, lithium, phenytoin, rifampicin and sulphinpyrazone.

The following reduce clearance and a reduced dosage may therefore be necessary to avoid side-effects: allopurinol, cimetidine, ciprofloxacin, corticosteroids, diltiazem, erythromycin, frusemide, isoprenaline, oral contraceptives, thiabendazole and verapamil. There is some evidence of an interaction between theophylline and influenza vaccine.

Xanthines can potentiate hypokalaemia resulting from beta$_2$ agonist therapy, steroids, diuretics and hypoxia. Particular caution is advised in severe asthma. It is recommended that serum potassium levels are monitored in such situations.

The concomitant use of theophylline and fluvoxamine should usually be avoided. Where this is not possible, patients should have their theophylline dose halved and plasma theophylline should be monitored closely.

Pregnancy and lactation: Slo-Phyllin is not recommended since theophylline is known to cross the placenta and its safety in pregnancy has not been established.

Theophylline is distributed in breast milk and therefore Slo-Phyllin should be used with caution in nursing mothers.

Effects on ability to drive and use machines: None known.

Undesirable effects: Side effects usually occur when theophylline blood levels exceed 20 micrograms/ml and include gastric irritation, nausea, vomiting, abdominal discomfort, palpitations, a fall in blood pressure, headache, occasional diarrhoea and insomnia. CNS stimulation and diuresis may also occur, especially in children.

Overdose:
Signs and symptoms: Headache, nausea, vomiting, restlessness, hypotension, tachycardia, arrhythmias (usually supraventricular tachyarrhythmias), hypokalaemia, CNS depression, convulsions, dehydration and coma may occur. Massive overdosage may result in cardiac inhibition, circulatory and respiratory failure.

Treatment: The stomach should be emptied by gastric lavage and emesis. Repeated doses of activated charcoal should be considered. Blood glucose, electrolytes, arterial gases and pH should be monitored. Serum theophylline should be measured 4 hours after ingestion and at 4 to 12 hourly intervals thereafter if symptoms are severe. Intensive supportive therapy may be required to maintain respiration and cardiovascular function. Convulsions may be controlled by diazepam. Haemoperfusion may be necessary. Slo-Phyllin is a timed-release capsule and effects may be slow in onset and prolonged.

Pharmacological properties
Pharmacodynamic properties: The mechanism of action of theophylline is unclear although a number of pharmacological actions have been implicated. The principal of these are:–

1) Inhibition of the enzyme phosphodiesterase leading to raised cyclic AMP levels.
2) Antagonism of adenosine receptors.
3) Inhibition of the intracellular release of calcium.
4) Stimulation of catecholamine release
5) Anti-inflammatory action possible involving the inhibition of submucosal action.

Pharmacokinetic properties: Following administration of Slo-Phyllin capsules at an appropriate twice daily dosage, peak levels occur 4-8 hours after dosing, and steady state is achieved in three days.

Pre-clinical safety data: No adverse effects can be predicted from animal toxicology studies other than those documented from human use of theophylline.

Pharmaceutical particulars
Excipients: The inactive ingredients are sucrose, maize starch, refined bleached lac, talc and ethanol. The gelatine capsules contain the following shell colours: Slo-Phyllin 60 mg E171; Slo-Phyllin 125 mg E171 and E172; Slo-Phyllin 250 mg E127 and E132.

Incompatibilities: None stated.

Shelf life: Three years.

Special warnings and precautions for storage: Store in a dry place below 25°C.

Nature and contents of container: PVC/Foil blister packs of 56 tablets.

Plastic container of 100 tablets.

Instructions for use/handling: Patients should be instructed not to chew or suck the capsules or pellets as this destroys the time release properties. However, for those who experience difficulty in swallowing capsules, the contents of a capsule may be sprinkled on to a spoonful of soft food, e.g. yoghurt.

Marketing authorisation holder: Rona Laboratories Ltd., Harrier House, High Street, West Drayton, Middlesex, UB7 7QG, UK.

Marketing Authorisation Number
Slo-Phyllin 60 mg capsules PL 0161/0021
Slo-Phyllin 125 mg capsules PL 0161/0019
Slo-Phyllin 250 mg capsules PL 0161/0020

Date of approval/revision of SPC 28 January 1998

Legal category P

SLOZEM 120 CAPSULES
SLOZEM 180 CAPSULES
SLOZEM 240 CAPSULES

Qualitative and quantitative composition Slozem 120 Capsules each contain 120 mg Diltiazem Hydrochloride USP

Slozem 180 Capsules each contain 180 mg Diltiazem Hydrochloride USP

Slozem 240 Capsules each contain 240 mg Diltiazem Hydrochloride USP

Pharmaceutical form Sustained release capsule.

Clinical particulars
Therapeutic indications: Mild to moderate hypertension. Angina pectoris.

Posology and method of administration:
Adults: 240 mg once daily.

Dosage titration in 60 mg to 120 mg steps at 2-weekly intervals may be required to obtain satisfactory clinical response (usually 240 mg to 360 mg daily will suffice). Dosage should be reduced in the presence of adverse reactions or if the pulse rate falls below 50 per minute.

Elderly and patients with impaired hepatic or renal function: Angina and hypertension: Starting dose 120 mg once daily.

Children: Not recommended.

Contra-indications: In pregnancy and in women of childbearing potential. Slozem depresses atrioventricular node conduction and is therefore contraindicated in patients with marked bradycardia, sick sinus syndrome, uncontrolled heart failure or second or third degree AV block. Hypersensitivity to diltiazem or any of the inactive ingredients.

Special warnings and special precautions for use: Slozem should be used with caution in patients with reduced left ventricular function. Patients with mild bradycardia, and/or having a prolonged PR interval, should be observed closely.

Interaction with other medicaments and other forms of interaction: In common with other calcium antagonists, when Slozem is used with drugs which may induce bradycardia (eg amiodarone and beta-blockers) or with other antihypertensive drugs the possibility of an additive effect should be borne in mind.

Diltiazem has been used safely in combination with beta-blockers, diuretics, ace inhibitors and other antihypertensive agents. It is recommended that patients receiving these combinations should be regularly monitored. Concomitant use with alpha blockers such as Prazosin should be strictly monitored because of the possible marked synergistic hypotensive effect of this combination. Case reports have suggested that blood levels of carbamazepine, cyclosporin, and theophylline may be increased when given concurrently with diltiazem hydrochloride. Care should be exercised in patients taking these drugs. In common with other calcium antagonists diltiazem may cause small increases in plasma levels of digoxin.

In patients taking H_2 receptor antagonists concurrently with diltiazem increased levels of diltiazem may be produced.

Diltiazem hydrochloride treatment has been continued without problem during anaesthesia, but the anesthetist should be informed that the patient is receiving a calcium antagonist.

Pregnancy and lactation: Diltiazem hydrochloride is teratogenic in some animal species. In the absence of adequate evidence of safety in human pregnancy Slozem should not be used in pregnancy or in women of child bearing potential.

Nursing mothers: Diltiazem hydrochloride is excreted in breast milk. One report suggests that concentrations in breast milk reach similar levels to those in serum. If use of Slozem is considered essential, an alternative method of infant feeding should be instituted.

Effects on ability to drive and use of machinery: None known.

Undesirable effects: The following have been reported: Ankle oedema, malaise, headache, hot flushes, gastro-intestinal disturbances and very rarely symptomatic bradycardia, sino-atrial block and atrioventricular block. Rashes and other cutaneous reactions have been reported in association with diltiazem. These reactions are generally mild and resolve on cessation of therapy, however there have been occasional reports of severe vascular skin reactions, and of erythema multiforme. Isolated cases of moderate and transient elevation of liver transaminases have been observed at the start of treatment. Isolated cases of clinical hepatitis have been reported which resolved on cessation of therapy.

The current literature suggests that the effects of vasodilation, particularly ankle oedema, are dose dependent and are more frequent in the elderly.

Overdose

Signs and symptoms: Acute intoxication can lead to severe hypotension, bradycardia, first to third degree atrioventricular block and, on occasions, to cardiac arrest. Hyperglycaemia may require treatment. Onset of symptoms may be delayed for several hours after ingestion and have been described after as little as 900mg diltiazem.

Treatment: Observation in a coronary or intensive care unit is advisable if a substantial overdose has been ingested. Soon after ingestion, gastric lavage followed by 50-100 mg activated charcoal may reduce absorption. Profound hypotension requires plasma expanders, I V calcium gluconate and inotropic agents (eg dopamine, dobutamine or isoprenaline). Symptomatic bradycardia and heart block may respond to atropine, isoprenaline or, if necessary, cardiac pacing. Slozem capsules are extended release capsules and effects may slow in onset and prolonged.

Pharmacological properties

Pharmacodynamic properties: Diltiazem hydrochloride is a calcium antagonist. It selectively reduces calcium entry through voltage-dependent calcium channels into vascular smooth muscle cells and myocardial cells. This lowers the concentration of intracellular calcium which is available to active contractile proteins. In vascular tissue, diltiazem relaxes arterial smooth muscle, reducing systemic peripheral resistance and dilating the coronary arteries. In cardiac muscle diltiazem reduces contractility and slows the heart rate through its negative chronotropic and inotropic actions. Cardiac work and oxygen demand can therefore be reduced and high blood pressure lowered without reflex tachycardia.

Pharmacokinetic properties: Diltiazem is well absorbed from the gastrointestinal tract and is subject to an extensive first-pass effect, giving an absolute bioavailability (compared to intravenous administration) of about 40%.

Diltiazem in plasma is 80-85% protein bound. Plasma levels above 40-50ng/ml are associated with pharmaceutical activity.

Diltiazem is extensively metabolised by the liver, the apparent plasma half-life being on average 3-4.5 hours.

The two major active circulating metabolites, desacetyl-diltiazem and N-monodesmethyl diltiazem possess coronary artery vasodilatory activity equivalent to about 50% of that of diltiazem. Only 0.2 to 4% diltiazem is found unchanged in the urine.

The sustained release pellets in this presentation usually achieve maximum plasma diltiazem levels six to eight hours after dosing and have a plasma elimination half-life of approximately 7 hours, allowing once daily dosing

The bioavailability of diltiazem from the Slozem formulation given once a day is equivalent to that obtained from a conventional release tablet given three times a day, when the same total daily dose is administered.

Data from studies in patients and healthy volunteers have also demonstrated that trough plasma levels (ie 24 hours post dosing) can be maintained within the minimum therapeutic range by appropriate dose titration.

Plasma concentrations in elderly patients and in hepatic failure are in general higher than in young subjects, due to an increase in apparent bioavailability. In renal failure, a reduction in dosage is only necessary as a function of the clinical response

Pharmaceutical particulars

List of excipients: Maize starch, sucrose, povidone, shellac, ethylcellulose, talc, E127, E132, E172 and (180mg and 240mg only) E171.

Shelf life: 3 years.

Special precautions for storage: Store below 30°C in a dry place.

Nature and contents of the container: PVC/PVDC/ Aluminium strips enclosed in a cardboard carton.

Marketing authorisation number

Slozem 120 mg	PL 03759/0043
Slozem 180 mg	PL 03759/0044
Slozem 240 mg	PL 03759/0045

Date of approval/revision of SPC 27 June 1994

Legal category POM

**Trade Mark*

The Liposome Company Ltd
3 Shortlands
Hammersmith International Centre
London W6 8EH

☎ 0181 324 0058   🖷 0181 563 1653

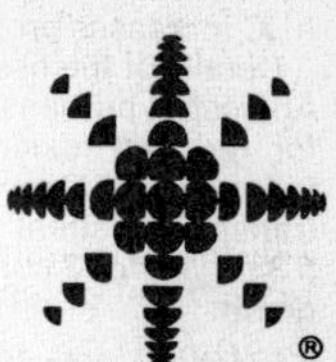

ABELCET*

Qualitative and quantitative composition Abelcet is supplied as a sterile, pyrogen-free suspension in isotonic saline. Each ml of the suspension contains 5.0 mg (5000 IU) of Amphotericin B USP. The full composition is presented in the following table:

Amphotericin B USP	5.0 mg
L-α-Dimyristoylphosphatidylcholine (DMPC)	3.4 mg
L-α-Dimyristoylphosphatidylglycerol (DMPG) (as sodium and ammonium salts)	1.5 mg
Sodium Chloride	9.0 mg
Water for Injection, q.s. ad	1.0 ml

Pharmaceutical form Abelcet is supplied as a suspension containing 5.0 mg amphotericin B per ml, in vials containing 20 ml (100 mg, 100 000 IU of amphotericin B) which must be diluted before intravenous infusion, according to Posology and method of administration section.

Clinical particulars
Clinical indications: Abelcet is indicated for the treatment of severe invasive candidiasis.

Abelcet is also indicated as second line therapy for the treatment of severe systemic fungal infections in patients who have not responded to conventional amphotericin B or other systemic antifungal agents, in those who have renal impairment or other contra-indications to conventional amphotericin B, or in patients who have developed amphotericin B nephrotoxicity. Abelcet treatment is indicated as second line treatment for invasive aspergillosis, cryptococcal meningitis and disseminated cryptococcosis in HIV patients, fusariosis, coccidioidomycosis, zygomycosis and blastomycosis.

Posology and method of administration: Abelcet is a sterile, pyrogen-free suspension to be diluted for intravenous infusion only.

For severe systemic infections treatment is generally recommended at 5.0 mg/kg for at least 14 days. Abelcet should be administered by intravenous infusion at a rate of 2.5 mg/kg/hr. When commencing treatment with Abelcet for the first time it is recommended to administer a test dose immediately prior to the first infusion. The first infusion should be prepared according to the instructions then over a period of 15 minutes approx. 1 mg of the infusion should be administered to the patient. After this amount has been administered the infusion should be stopped and the patient observed carefully for 30 minutes. If the patient shows no signs of hypersensitivity the infusion may be continued. As for use with all amphotericin B products, facilities for cardiopulmonary resuscitation should be readily at hand when administering Abelcet, due to the possible occurrence of anaphylactoid reactions. Abelcet has been administered for as long as 28 months, and cumulative doses have been as high as 73.6 g without significant toxicity.

An in-line filter may be used for intravenous infusion of Abelcet. The mean pore diameter of the filter should be no less than 5.0 microns.

Abelcet may be administered to diabetic patients.

Paediatric use: Systemic fungal infections in children have been treated successfully with Abelcet at doses comparable to the recommended adult dose on a body weight basis.

Adverse events seen in paediatric patients are similar to those seen in adults.

Use in elderly patients: Systemic fungal infections in elderly patients have been treated successfully with Abelcet at doses comparable to the recommended dose on a body weight basis.

Use in neutropenic patients: Abelcet has been used successfully to treat systemic fungal infections in patients who are severely neutropenic as a consequence of haematological malignancy or the use of cytotoxic or immunosuppressive drugs.

Use in patients with renal or liver disease: Systemic fungal infections in patients with renal or liver disease have been treated successfully with Abelcet at doses comparable to the recommended dose on a body weight basis (see special warnings and precautions for further information).

Contra-indications: Abelcet is contra-indicated in patients with known hypersensitivity to any of its constituents, unless in the opinion of the physician the advantages of using Abelcet outweigh the risks of hypersensitivity.

Special warnings and special precautions for use
Renal disease: Since Abelcet is a potentially nephrotoxic drug, monitoring of renal function should be performed before initiating treatment in patients with pre-existing renal disease, and at least once weekly during therapy. Abelcet can be administered to patients during renal dialysis or haemofiltration. Serum potassium and magnesium levels should be monitored regularly.

Liver disease: Patients with concurrent hepatic impairment due to infection, graft-versus-host disease, other liver disease or administration of hepatotoxic drugs have been successfully treated with Abelcet. In cases where serum bilirubin, alkaline phosphatase or serum transaminases increased, factors other than Abelcet were present and possibly accounted for the abnormalities. These factors included infection, hyperalimentation, concomitant hepatotoxic drugs and graft-versus-host disease.

Interactions with other medicaments and other forms of interactions:
Nephrotoxic drugs: Abelcet is a potentially nephrotoxic drug, and particularly close monitoring of renal function is required in patients receiving nephrotoxic drugs concomitantly.

Zidovudine: In dogs, exacerbated myelotoxicity and nephrotoxicity were observed when Abelcet was administered concomitantly with zidovudine. If concomitant treatment with zidovudine is required, renal and haematologic function should be closely monitored.

Cyclosporin: Preliminary data suggest that patients receiving Abelcet concomitantly with high dose cyclosporin experience an increase in serum creatinine. The data also suggest that the increase in serum creatinine is caused by cyclosporin and not Abelcet.

The interaction of Abelcet with other drugs has not been studied to date. Conventional amphotericin B has been reported to interact with antineoplastic agents, corticosteroids and corticotrophin (ACTH), digitalis glycosides and skeletal muscle relaxants.

Leukocyte transfusions: Acute pulmonary toxicity has been reported in patients receiving intravenous amphotericin B and leukocyte transfusions.

Pregnancy and lactation: Conventional amphotericin B has been used successfully to treat systemic fungal infections in pregnant women with no obvious effects on the foetus, but only a small number of cases have been reported. Reproductive toxicity studies of Abelcet in rats and rabbits showed no evidence of embryotoxicity, foetotoxicity or teratogenicity. However, safety for use in pregnant or lactating women has not been established for Abelcet. Therefore, Abelcet should be administered to pregnant or lactating women only for life-threatening disease when the likely benefit exceeds the risk to the mother and foetus.

Effect on ability to drive and use machines: Abelcet is unlikely to affect the ability of an individual to drive or use machines, since adverse reactions are usually infusion-related. However, the clinical condition of patients who require Abelcet generally precludes driving or operating machinery.

Undesirable effects: Adverse reactions that have been reported to occur with conventional amphotericin B may occur with Abelcet. In general, the physician should monitor the patient for any type of adverse event associated with conventional amphotericin B.

Patients in whom significant renal toxicity was observed following conventional amphotericin B frequently did not experience similar effects when Abelcet was substituted. Adverse reactions related to the administration of Abelcet have generally been mild or moderate, and have been most prevalent during the first 2 days of dosing.

Premedication (e.g. paracetamol) may be administered for the prevention of infusion related adverse events. The most common clinical adverse events have been chills, fever, nausea and vomiting, which may occur during the first 2 days of treatment.

Declines in renal function, shown by increased serum creatinine, azotaemia and hypokalaemia, have not typically required discontinuation of treatment. Abnormal liver function tests have been reported with Abelcet and other amphotericin B products. Although other factors such as infection, hyperalimentation, concomitant hepatotoxic drugs and graft-versus-host disease may be contributory, a casual relationship with Abelcet cannot be excluded. Patients with abnormal liver function tests should be carefully monitored and cessation of treatment considered if liver function deteriorates.

Rarely, encephalopathy and peripheral neuropathy have been reported.

Overdose: No instance of toxicity due to overdose with Abelcet has been reported. One paediatric patient received a single dose of 13.1 mg/kg on one occasion, without adverse effects. Should an overdose occur, the patient should be treated as deemed appropriate by the physician.

Pharmacological properties Abelcet consists of the antifungal agent, amphotericin B, complexed to two phospholipids. Amphotericin B is a macrocyclic, polyene, broad-spectrum antifungal antibiotic produced by *Streptomyces nodosus.* The lipophilic moiety of amphotericin B allows molecules of the drug to be complexed in a ribbon-like structure with the phospholipids.

Pharmacodynamic properties
Mechanism of action: Amphotericin B, the active antifungal agent in Abelcet, may be fungistatic or fungicidal, depending on its concentration and on fungal susceptibility. The drug probably acts by binding to ergosterol in the fungal cell membrane causing subsequent membrane damage. As a result, cell contents leak from the fungal cell, and, ultimately, cell death occurs. Binding of the drug to sterols in human cell membranes may result in toxicity, although amphotericin B has greater affinity for fungal ergosterol than for the cholesterol of human cells.

Microbiological activity: Amphotericin B is active against many fungal pathogens *in vitro,* including *Candida* spp., *Cryptococcus neoformans, Aspergillus* spp., *Mucor* spp., *Sporothrix schenckii, Blastomyces dermatitidis, Coccidioides immitis* and *Histoplasma capsulatum.* Most strains are inhibited by amphotericin B concentrations of 0.03–1.0 μg/ml. Amphotericin B has little or no activity against bacteria or viruses. The activity of Abelcet against fungal pathogens *in vitro* is comparable to that of amphotericin B. However, activity of Abelcet *in vitro* may not predict activity in the infected host.

Pharmacokinetic properties: Amphotericin B is complexed to phospholipids in Abelcet. The pharmacokinetic properties of Abelcet and conventional amphotericin B are different. Pharmacokinetic studies in animals showed that, after administration of Abelcet, amphotericin B levels were highest in the liver, spleen and lung. Amphotericin B in Abelcet was rapidly distributed to tissues. The ratio of drug concentrations in tissues to those in blood increased disproportionately with increasing dose, suggesting that elimination of the drug from the tissues was delayed. Peak blood levels of amphotericin B were lower after administration of Abelcet than after administration of equivalent amounts of conventional drug. Administration of conventional amphotericin B resulted in much lower tissue levels than did dosing with Abelcet. However, in dogs, conventional amphotericin B produced 20-fold higher kidney concentrations than did Abelcet given at comparable doses.

The pharmacokinetics of Abelcet in whole blood were determined in patients with mucocutaneous leishmaniasis. Results for mean pharmacokinetic parameters at 5.0 mg/kg/day were as follows:

	Abelcet
Dose: (mg/kg/day)	5.0
Peak blood level C_{max}: (μg/ml)	1.7
Area under time-concentration curve AUC_{0-24}: (μg•hr/ml)	9.5
Clearance: (ml/hr•kg)	211.0
Volume of distribution Vd: (l)	2286.0
Half-life $T_{1/2}$: (hr)	173.4

The rapid clearance and large volume of distribution of Abelcet result in a relatively low AUC and are consistent with preclinical data showing high tissue concentrations. The kinetics of Abelcet are linear, the AUC increases proportionately with dose.

Details of the tissue distribution and metabolism of Abelcet in humans, and the mechanisms responsible for reduced toxicity, are not well understood. The following data are available from necropsy in a heart transplant patient who received Abelcet at a dose of 5.3 mg/kg for 3 consecutive days immediately before death:

Organ	*Abelcet tissue concentration expressed as Amphotericin B content (mg/kg)*
Spleen	290.0
Lung	222.0
Liver	196.0
Kidney	6.9
Lymph node	7.6
Heart	5.0
Brain	1.6

Preclinical safety data: Acute toxicity studies in rodents showed that Abelcet was 10-fold to 20-fold less toxic than conventional amphotericin B. Multiple-dose toxicity studies in dogs lasting 2–4 weeks showed that on a mg/kg basis, Abelcet was 8-fold to 10-fold less nephrotoxic than conventional amphotericin B. This decreased nephrotoxicity was presumably a result of lower drug concentrations in the kidney.

Carcinogenesis, mutagenesis and impairment of fertility: Since conventional amphotericin B first became available, there have been no reports of drug-related carcinogenicity, mutagenicity, teratogenicity or adverse effect on fertility. Abelcet has been shown not to be mutagenic by the *in vivo* mouse micronucleus assay, *in vitro* bacterial and lymphoma mutation assays, and an *in vivo* cytogenetic assay. It has been shown not to be teratogenic in mice and rabbits.

Phospholipids are essential constituents of human cell membranes. The average diet provides several grams of phospholipids each day. There is no evidence that phospholipids, including DMPC and DMPG, are carcinogenic, mutagenic or teratogenic.

Pharmaceutical particulars

List of inactive constituents (excipients): Each ml of Abelcet contains 3.4 mg L-α-dimyristoylphosphatidylcholine (DMPC), 1.5 mg L-α-dimyristoylphosphatidylglycerol (sodium and ammonium salts) (DMPG), 9.0 mg sodium chloride, and Water for Injection, q.s. ad 1.0 ml.

Incompatibilities: Abelcet should not be mixed with other drugs or electrolytes.

Shelf life: Results of stability studies substantiate a shelf life of 24 months at 5°C.

Special precautions for storage: Abelcet should be stored under refrigeration at +2 to +8°C. Do not freeze. Protect from light.

Nature and contents of container: Abelcet is a sterile, pyrogen-free yellow suspension in a single use vial containing 20 ml (100 mg amphotericin B). The vial is sealed with a rubber stopper and aluminium seal. Vials are packaged in cartons of 10 vials.

Instructions for use/handling: Abelcet is a sterile, pyrogen-free suspension to be diluted for intravenous infusion only.

Preparation of the suspension for infusion: ASEPTIC TECHNIQUE MUST BE STRICTLY OBSERVED THROUGHOUT HANDLING OF Abelcet, SINCE NO BACTERIOSTATIC AGENT OR PRESERVATIVE IS PRESENT. Allow the suspension to come to room temperature. Shake gently until there is no evidence of any yellow settlement at the bottom of the vial. Withdraw the appropriate dose of Abelcet from the required number of vials into one or more sterile 20 ml syringes using a 17 to 19 gauge needle. Remove the needle from each syringe filled with Abelcet and replace with the 5 micron filter needle (supplied by B. Braun Medical, Inc.) provided with each vial. Insert the filter needle of the syringe into an IV bag containing 5.0% Dextrose for Injection and empty the content of the syringe into the bag using either manual pressure or an infusion pump. The final infusion concentation should be 1 mg/ml. For paediatric patients and patients with cardiovascular disease the drug may be diluted with 5.0% Dextrose for Injection to a final infusion concentration of 2 mg/ml. Do not use the agent after dilution with 5.0% Dextrose for Injection if there is any evidence of foreign matter. Vials are single use. Unused material should be discarded. The infusion is best administered by means of an infusion pump.

DO NOT DILUTE WITH SALINE SOLUTIONS OR MIX WITH OTHER DRUGS OR ELECTROLYTES. The compatibility of Abelcet with these materials has not been established. An existing intravenous line should be flushed with 5.0% Dextrose for Injection before infusion of Abelcet or a separate infusion line should be used.

The diluted ready for use suspension may be stored under refrigeration (+2 to +8°C) for up to 24 hours prior to use. Shake vigorously before use. Do not store for later use.

Marketing authorisation number 14188/0001.

Date of approval/revision of SPC June 1998.

Legal catetgory POM.

**Trade Mark*

Lorex Synthélabo UK & Ireland Ltd
Foundation Park
Roxborough Way
Maidenhead
Berkshire SL6 3UD
☎ 01628 501200 🗋 01628 501234

Lorex Synthélabo

CYSTRIN* 3 mg TABLETS
CYSTRIN* 5 mg TABLETS

Qualitative and quantitative composition
Oxybutynin hydrochloride 3.0 mg
Oxybutynin hydrochloride 5.0 mg.

Pharmaceutical form Tablet

Clinical particulars
Therapeutic indications: Cystrin is indicated for urinary incontinence, urgency and frequency in unstable bladder conditions due either to idiopathic detrusor instability or neurogenic bladder disorders (detrusor hyperreflexia) in conditions such as spina bifida and multiple sclerosis.

In addition, for children over 5 years of age, oxybutynin may be used in nocturnal enuresis in conjunction with non-drug therapy where this alone, or in conjunction with other drug treatment, has failed.

Posology and method of administration: Children under 5 years of age: Not recommended.

Children over 5 years of age:
Neurogenic bladder disorders: The usual dose is 5 mg twice a day. This may be increased to a maximum of 5 mg three times a day to obtain a clinical response provided that the side effects are tolerated.

Nocturnal enuresis: The usual dose is 5 mg two or three times a day. The last dose should be given before bedtime.

In children the maintenance dose may be achieved by upward titration from an initial dose of 3 mg twice daily.

Adults: The usual dose is 5 mg two or three times a day. This may be increased to a maximum dosage of 5 mg four times a day (20 mg) to obtain a satisfactory clinical response provided that the side effects are tolerated.

Elderly: The elimination half-life may be increased in some elderly patients, therefore, dosage should be individually titrated commencing at 3 mg twice a day. The final dosage will depend on response and tolerance to side-effects. As with other anticholinergic drugs caution should be observed in frail and elderly patients.

Contra-indications: Cystrin is contra-indicated in patients who are hypersensitive to the drug. It is also contra-indicated in patients with a significant degree of bladder outflow obstruction where precipitation of urinary retention may occur.

Cystrin is contra-indicated in myasthenia gravis, glaucoma (since it may raise intra-ocular pressure) and in patients with intestinal atony, severe ulcerative colitis, toxic megacolon and other functional or organic gastrointestinal obstructive disorders.

Special warnings and precautions: Cystrin should be used with caution in the frail elderly and in patients with autonomic neuropathy, hepatic or renal disease.

The symptoms of hyperthyroidism, coronary artery disease, congestive cardiac failure, cardiac arrhythmias, tachycardias and prostatic hypertrophy may be aggravated following administration of Cystrin.

Special care should be taken in patients with hiatus hernia associated with reflux oesophagitis, as anticholinergic drugs can aggravate this condition.

Interaction with other medicaments and other forms of interaction: Care should be taken if other anticholinergic agents are administered together with Cystrin, as potentiation of anticholinergic effects can occur.

Occasional cases of interaction between anticholinergics and phenothiazines, amantidine, butyrophenones, L-dopa, digitalis and tricyclic antidepressants have been reported and care should be taken if Cystrin is administered concurrently with such drugs.

Cystrin by reducing gastro-intestinal motility may affect absorption of other drugs.

Pregnancy and lactation: There is no experience of the use of oxybutynin during pregnancy in humans, however, in foetal toxicity and fertility studies in animals, effects were seen on reproductive processes at dosages associated with maternal toxicity. Cystrin should, therefore, only be prescribed during pregnancy if considered essential. In the absence of animal data on the levels of oxybutynin in milk, Cystrin should not be administered to women who are breast-feeding.

Effects on ability to drive and use machinery: As Cystrin may produce drowsiness or blurred vision, the patient should be cautioned regarding activities requiring mental alertness such as driving, operating machinery or performing hazardous work while taking this drug.

Other undesirable effects: The most frequently reported side effects to oxybutynin are: dry mouth, constipation, blurred vision, nausea, abdominal discomfort, facial flushing and difficulty in micturition. The incidence of facial flushing is more marked in children than adults. The occurrence of these effects may be reduced by lowering the dose. Side effects reported less frequently include: headache, urinary retention, dizziness, drowsiness, skin reactions including rash, angioedema and photosensitivity, diarrhoea, cardiac arrhythmias, excitatory effects on CNS including restlessness, disorientation, hallucinations and convulsions. Children may be more liable to such effects.

Overdose: The symptoms of overdosage with Cystrin progress from an intensification of the usual side-effects of CNS disturbances (from restlessness and excitement to psychotic behaviour), circulatory changes (flushing, fall in blood pressure, circulatory failure etc), respiratory failure, paralysis and coma.

Measures to be taken are: (1) immediate gastric lavage and (2) physostigmine 1.0 to 2.0 mg by slow intravenous injection, repeated as necessary up to a total of 5.0 mg.

Fever should be treated symptomatically with tepid sponging or ice packs.

In pronounced restlessness or excitation, diazepam 10 mg may be given by intravenous injection. Tachycardia may be treated with intravenous propanolol and urinary retention managed by bladder catheterisation.

In the event of progression of the curare-like effect to paralysis of the respiratory muscles, mechanical ventilation will be required.

Pharmacological properties
Pharmacodynamic properties: Oxybutynin hydrochloride is an anticholinergic agent which also exerts a direct antispasmodic effect on smooth muscle. It inhibits bladder contraction and relieves spasm induced by various stimuli; it increases bladder volume, diminishes the frequency of contractions and delays the desire to void in the disturbance of neurogenic bladder. The relaxation of smooth muscle results from the papaverin like effect of the antagonism of the processes distal to the neuromuscular junction in addition to the anticholinergic blocking action of the muscarinic type receptors. In addition oxybutynin hydrochloride has local anaesthetic properties.

Pharmacokinetic properties: Pharmacodynamic reports show oxybutynin to be rapidly absorbed from the gastro-intestinal tract following oral administration with maximum plasma concentrations reached in less than 1 hour subsequently falling bioexponentially with a half-life of between 2 and 3 hours. Maximum effect can be seen within 3–4 hours with some effect still evident after 10 hours.

Repeated oral administration achieved steady state after eight days. Oxybutynin does not appear to accumulate in elderly patients and the pharmacokinetics are similar to those in other adults. Some excretion via the biliary system has been observed in the rabbit and partial first-pass metabolism occurs, the metabolites also appearing to have antimuscarinic properties. The main elimination route is via the kidneys with only 0.3–0.4% of unchanged drug appearing in the urine of the rat after 24 hours and 1% appearing in the urine of the dog after 48 hours. In rats and dogs therefore, oxybutynin appears to be almost completely absorbed.

Preclinical safety data: No additional data available.

Pharmaceutical particulars
List of excipients: Lactose PhEur, Maize starch PhEur, Polyvidone 25000 PhEur, Talc PhEur, Magnesium stearate PhEur, Purified water PhEur.

Film-coating ingredients: Methylhydroxypropylcellulose PhEur, methylhydroxypropylcellulose phthalate PhEur, Ethanol 96% v/v* FDS, Purified water PhEur.

* Finnish Drug Standards.

Incompatibilities: None known.

Shelf life: 3 years.

Special precautions for storage: To be stored in a dry place below 25°C.

Nature and contents of container:
3 mg: 56 tablets in polyethylene container.
5 mg: 84 tablets in polyethylene container.

Instructions for use/handling: No relevance.

Marketing authorisation numbers
Cystrin 3 mg Tablets PL 15819/0039
Cystrin 5 mg Tablets PL 15819/0040

Date of first authorisation May 1998

Date of (partial) revision of the text May 1998

Legal category POM

DICYNENE* 500 TABLETS

Presentation Dicynene 500 Tablets. Each white, scored, capsule-shaped tablet contains 500 mg ethamsylate and is engraved 'D500' one side, with a breakmark on the other.

Mode of action: Dicynene is a non-hormonal agent which reduces capillary exudation and blood loss. Dicynene does not affect the normal coagulation mechanism since administration is without effect on prothrombin time, fibrinolysis, platelet count or function.

Dicynene is thought to act by increasing capillary vascular wall resistance and platelet adhesiveness; in the presence of a vascular lesion, it inhibits the biosynthesis and actions of those prostaglandins which cause platelet disaggregation, vasodilation and increased capillary permeability. It does not have a vasoconstricting action.

Uses Dicynene is used clinically for the short term treatment of blood loss in primary and IUCD-induced menorrhagia.

Dosage and administration The usual dosage is 500 mg four times daily from the start of bleeding until menstruation ceases.

Contra-indications, warnings, etc
Contra-indications: Treatment should only be undertaken following exclusion of other pelvic pathology, in particular the presence of fibroids. Hypersensitivity to ethamsylate.

Warnings: This product contains sulphites which may cause or may exacerbate an anaphylactic reaction. If the patient develops a fever then treatment should be discontinued.

Precautions: In patients receiving Dicynene for menorrhagia the use of the product before onset of bleeding is not recommended.

Use in pregnancy and lactation: Clinical use in pregnancy is not relevant for this indication. Studies in animals have revealed no teratogenic effect of Dicynene, however there is inadequate evidence of safety in human pregnancy.

Dicynene is secreted in breast milk and administration to nursing mothers is not recommended.

Side-effects: Occasional headaches or skin rashes may occur which usually disappear on reduced dosage. A few patients may experience gastro-intestinal disturbances such as nausea, vomiting or diarrhoea; however this may be overcome by administering the dose after food.

Pharmaceutical precautions Dicynene tablets should be stored in a cool, dry place. Dispense in airtight containers offering adequate protection from light and moisture.

Legal category POM.

Package quantities Securitainers: 100 tablets, blister pack of 28 tablets.

Further information Dicynene is fully absorbed when given orally and is excreted unchanged, largely by the urinary route.

Product licence number PL 15819/0013.

Date of last revision of data sheet July 1997.

DICYNENE* INJECTION

Presentation Each clear glass 2 ml ampoule, printed DICYNENE*, contains 250 mg ethamsylate.

Mode of action: Dicynene is a non-hormonal agent which reduces capillary exudation and blood loss. Dicynene does not affect the normal coagulation mechanism since administration is without effect on prothrombin time, fibrinolysis, platelet count or function.

Dicynene is thought to act by increasing capillary vascular wall resistance and platelet adhesiveness; in the presence of a vascular lesion, it inhibits the biosynthesis and actions of those prostaglandins which cause platelet disaggregation, vasodilation and increased capillary permeability. It does not have a vasoconstricting action.

Uses Dicynene injection is used for the prophylaxis and treatment of periventricular haemorrhage in low birth weight infants.

Dosage and administration The normal dosage is 12.5 mg/kg given by intravenous or intramuscular route every six hours.

Contra-indications, warnings, etc
Contra-indications: Hypersensitivity to ethamsylate.

Warnings: This product contains sulphites which may cause or may exacerbate an anaphylactic reaction. If the infant develops a fever then treatment should be stopped.

Precautions: Dicynene Injection is intended for neonatal use only.

Side-effects: In infants, no major side effects have been reported following use in this indication.

In adults side effects such as headache, skin rashes and gastrointestinal disturbances e.g. nausea, vomiting or diarrhoea have been reported rarely following the use of ethamsylate.

Pharmaceutical precautions Dicynene Injection should be stored in a cool place, protected from light. If the contents of the ampoules become coloured they should not be administered.

Dicynene Injection is incompatible with solutions of sodium bicarbonate and compound sodium lactate. When Dicynene Injection is mixed with saline it should be used immediately.

Legal category POM.

Package quantities Boxes containing 10×2 ml ampoules.

Further information Following intravenous administration maximum blood levels of ethamsylate are achieved in 2–3 minutes, while after intramuscular injection, maximum blood levels of ethamsylate are achieved after about one hour. Ethamsylate is excreted unchanged, largely by the urinary route.

Product licence number PL 15819/0014.

Date of last revision of data sheet July 1997.

DITROPAN* ELIXIR

Presentation Clear, colourless elixir. Each 5 ml contains 2.5 mg oxybutynin hydrochloride.

Uses Urinary incontinence, urgency and frequency in the unstable bladder, whether due to neurogenic bladder disorders (detrusor hyperreflexia) in conditions such as multiple sclerosis and spina bifida, or to idiopathic detrusor instability (motor urge incontinence).

Children over 5 years of age: In addition to neurogenic bladder disorders, Ditropan may also be used in nocturnal enuresis in conjunction with non-drug therapy where this alone, or in conjunction with other drug treatment, has failed.

Dosage and administration
Adult: The usual dose is 5 mg (10 ml) two or three times a day. This may be increased to a maximum of 5 mg (10 ml) four times a day to obtain a clinical response provided the side effects are tolerated.

Elderly (including frail elderly): The elimination half-life is increased in the elderly. Therefore, a dose of 2.5 mg (5 ml) twice a day, particularly if the patient is frail, is likely to be adequate. This dose may be titrated upwards to 5 mg (10 ml) two times a day to obtain a clinical response provided the side effects are well tolerated.

Children (under 5 years of age): Not recommended.

Children (over 5 years of age): Neurogenic bladder instability: the usual dose is 2.5 mg (5 ml) twice a day. This dose may be titrated upwards to 5 mg (10 ml) two or three times a day to obtain a clinical response provided the side effects are tolerated. Nocturnal enuresis: the usual dose is 2.5 mg (5 ml) twice a day. This dose may be titrated upwards to 5 mg (10 ml) two or three times a day to obtain a clinical response provided the side effects are tolerated. The last dose should be given before bedtime.

Contra-indications, warnings, etc
Contra-indications: Ditropan is contra-indicated in patients with obstruction of the bowel and in patients with a significant degree of bladder outflow obstruction where urinary retention may be precipitated.

It is also contra-indicated in patients with intestinal atony, severe ulcerative colitis, toxic megacolon, myasthenia gravis or glaucoma.

Precautions: Ditropan should be used with caution in the frail elderly and in patients with autonomic neuropathy, hepatic or renal disease.

The symptoms of hyperthyroidism, coronary artery disease, congestive cardiac failure, cardiac arrhythmias, tachycardias and prostatic hypertrophy may be aggravated following administration of Ditropan.

Special care should be taken in patients with hiatus hernia associated with reflux oesophagitis, as anticholinergic drugs may aggravate this condition.

As Ditropan may produce drowsiness or blurred vision, the patient should be cautioned regarding activities requiring mental alertness such as driving, operating machinery or performing hazardous work while taking this drug.

Pregnancy: There is no evidence as to the safety of Ditropan in human pregnancy nor is there evidence from animal work that it is totally free from hazard. Avoid in pregnancy unless there is no safer alternative.

Lactation: Ditropan has been detected in breast milk and should therefore not be taken by breastfeeding mothers.

Side-effects: The most frequently reported side effects (>1%) to oxybutynin are: dry mouth (about 22%), constipation, blurred vision, nausea, abdominal discomfort, facial flushing and difficulty in micturition. The incidence of facial flushing is more marked in children than adults. The occurrence of these effects may be reduced by lowering the dose. Those side effects reported less frequently include: headache, urinary retention, dizziness, drowsiness, skin reactions including rash, angioedema and photosensitivity, diarrhoea, cardiac arrhythmias, excitatory effects on CNS including restlessness, disorientation, hallucinations and convulsions. Children may be more liable to such effects.

Drug interactions: Care should be taken if other anticholinergic agents are administered together with Ditropan, as potentiation of anticholinergic effects could occur.

Occasional cases of interaction between anticholinergics and phenothiazines, amantidine, butyrophenones, L-dopa, digitalis and tricyclic antidepressants have been reported and care should be taken if Ditropan is administered concurrently with such drugs.

Overdosage: The symptoms of overdosage with Ditropan progress from an intensification of the usual side effects of CNS disturbances (from restlessness and excitement to psychotic behaviour), circulatory changes (flushing, fall in blood pressure, circulatory failure etc), respiratory failure, paralysis and coma.

Measures to be taken are: (1) Immediate gastric lavage, and (2) slow intravenous injection of 1.0 to 2.0 mg of physostigmine, repeated as necessary up to a total of 5 mg.

Fever should be treated symptomatically with tepid sponging or ice packs.

In pronounced restlessness or excitation, diazepam 10 mg may be given by intravenous injections, tachycardia may be treated with intravenous injection of propranolol, and urinary retention can be managed by catheterisation.

In the event of progression of the curare-like effect to the paralysis of the respiratory muscles, mechanical ventilation will be required.

Pharmaceutical precautions Store below 25°C. Protect from light. Discard any remaining medicine 28 days after opening.

Legal category POM.

Package quantities 150 ml bottle contained within a carton with a patient information leaflet.

Further information Oxybutynin has both direct antispasmodic action on the smooth muscle of the bladder detrusor as well as anticholinergic action in blocking the muscarinic effects of acetylcholine on smooth muscle.

These properties cause relaxation of the detrusor muscle of the bladder and in patients with an unstable bladder. Ditropan increases bladder capacity and reduces the incidence of spontaneous contractions of the detrusor muscle.

Ditropan elixir contains 1.3 g sucrose per 5 ml dose.

Product licence number PL 15819/0010.

Date of revision of this leaflet June 1998.

DITROPAN* TABLETS 2.5 mg
DITROPAN* TABLETS 5 mg

Qualitative and quantitative composition Each tablet contains 2.5 mg or 5 mg of oxybutynin hydrochloride as the active ingredient.

Pharmaceutical form
Ditropan tablets 2.5 mg: Pale blue bi-convex oval tablets, marked OXB2.5 on one side.

Ditropan tablets 5 mg: Pale blue circular tablets, with a centre breakline on one side, and marked OXB5 on the reverse.

Clinical particulars
Therapeutic indications: Urinary incontinence, urgency and frequency in the unstable bladder, whether due to neurogenic bladder disorders (detrusor hyperreflexia) in conditions such as multiple sclerosis and spina bifida, or to idiopathic detrusor instability (motor urge incontinence).

Children over 5 years of age: In addition to neurogenic bladder disorders, Ditropan may also be used in nocturnal enuresis in conjunction with non-drug therapy where this alone, or in conjunction with other drug treatment, has failed.

Posology and method of administration
Dosage and administration:
Adults: The usual dose is 5 mg two or three times a day. This may be increased to a maximum of 5 mg four times a day to obtain a clinical response provided that the side effects are tolerated.

Elderly (including frail elderly): The elimination half-life is increased in the elderly. Therefore, a dose of 2.5 mg twice a day, particularly if the patient is frail, is likely to be adequate. This dose may be titrated upwards to 5 mg two times a day to obtain a clinical response provided the side effects are well tolerated.

Children (under 5 years of age): Not recommended.

Children (over 5 years of age): Neurogenic bladder instability: the usual dose is 2.5 mg twice a day. This dose may be titrated upwards to 5 mg two or three times a day to obtain a clinical response provided the side effects are well tolerated. Nocturnal enuresis: the usual dose is 2.5 mg twice a day. This dose may be titrated upwards to 5 mg two or three times a day to obtain a clinical response provided the side effects are tolerated. The last dose should be given before bedtime.

Contra-indications: Ditropan is contra-indicated in patients with obstruction of the bowel and in patients with a significant degree of bladder outflow obstruction where urinary retention may be precipitated.

It is also contra-indicated in patients with intestinal atony, severe ulcerative colitis or toxic megacolon, myasthenia gravis or glaucoma.

Special warnings and precautions for use: Ditropan should be used with caution in the frail elderly and in patients with autonomic neuropathy, hepatic or renal disease.

The symptoms of hyperthyroidism, coronary artery disease, congestive cardiac failure, cardiac arrhythmias, tachycardias and prostatic hypertrophy may be aggravated following administration of Ditropan.

Special care should be taken in patients with hiatus hernia associated with reflux oesophagitis, as anticholinergic drugs may aggravate this condition.

Interactions with other medicaments and other forms of interaction: Care should be taken if other anticholinergic agents are administered together with Ditropan, as potentiation of anticholinergic effects could occur.

Occasional cases of interaction between anticholinergics and phenothiazines, amantidine, butyrophenones, L-dopa, digitalis and tricyclic antidepressants have been reported and care should be taken if Ditropan is administered concurrently with such drugs.

Pregnancy and lactation: There is no evidence as to the safety of Ditropan in human pregnancy nor is there evidence from animal work that it is totally free from hazard. Avoid in pregnancy unless there is no safer alternative.

Ditropan has been detected in breast milk and should therefore not be taken by breast feeding mothers.

Effects on ability to drive and use machines: As Ditropan may produce drowsiness or blurred vision, the patient should be cautioned regarding activities requiring mental alertness such as driving, operating machinery or performing hazardous work while taking this drug.

Undesirable effects: The most frequently reported side effects (>1%) to oxybutynin are: a dry mouth (about 22%), constipation, blurred vision, nausea, abdominal discomfort, facial flushing and difficulty in micturition. The incidence of facial flushing is more marked in children than adults. The occurrence of these effects may be reduced by lowering the dose. Those side effects reported less frequently include: headache, urinary retention, dizziness, drowsiness, skin reactions including rash, angioedema and photosensitivity, diarrhoea, cardiac arrhythmias, excitatory effects on CNS including restlessness, disorientation, hallucinations and convulsions. Children may be more liable to such effects.

Overdosage: The symptoms of overdose with Ditropan progress from an intensification of the usual side effects of CNS disturbances (from restlessness and excitement to psychotic behaviour), circulation changes (flushing, fall in blood pressure, circulatory failure etc), respiratory failure, paralysis and coma.

Measures to be taken are: Immediate gastric lavage, and slow intravenous injection of 1.0 to 2.0 mg of physostigmine, repeated as necessary up to a total of 5 mg.

Fever should be treated symptomatically with tepid sponging or ice packs.

In pronounced restlessness or excitation, diazepam 10 mg may be given by intravenous injection, tachycardia may be treated by intravenous injection of propranolol, and urinary retention can be managed by catheterisation. In the event of progression of the curare-like effect to the paralysis of the respiratory muscles, mechanical ventilation will be required.

Pharmacological properties

Pharmacodynamic properties: Oxybutynin has both direct antispasmodic action on the smooth muscle of the bladder detrusor muscle as well as an anticholinergic action in blocking the muscarinic effects of acetylcholine on smooth muscle. These properties cause relaxation of the detrusor muscle of the bladder in patients with an unstable bladder. Ditropan increases bladder capacity and reduces the incidence of spontaneous contractions of the detrusor muscle.

Pharmacokinetic properties: Oxybutynin is poorly absorbed from the gastrointestinal tract. It is highly bound to plasma proteins, the peak plasma level is reached between 0.5 to 1 hour after administration. The half life is biexponential, the first phase being about 40 minutes and the second about 2–3 hours. The elimination half life may be increased in the elderly, particularly if they are frail.

Oxybutynin and its metabolites are excreted in the faeces and urine. There is no evidence of accumulation.

Preclinical safety data: No data of therapeutic relevance.

Pharmaceutical particulars

List of excipients: Ditropan tablets contain lactose, cellulose, calcium stearate and indigo carmine (E132).

Incompatibilities: None known.

Shelf life: 4 years.

Special precautions for storage: Store at or below 30°C.

Nature and contents of container: Cartons containing 21 or 84 tablets in blister strips.

Instructions for use/handling: No special requirements.

Marketing authorisation number

Ditropan 2.5 mg tablets PL 15819/0008
Ditropan 5 mg tablets PL 15819/0009

Date of first authorisation 01.05.97.

Date of (partial) revision of the text June 1998

DOLMATIL* 200 mg TABLETS
DOLMATIL* 400 mg TABLETS

Qualitative and quantitative composition

Dolmatil 200 mg Tablets: Active ingredient is sulpiride 200 mg. Sulpiride is a benzamide derivative.

Dolmatil 400 mg Tablets: Active ingredient is sulpiride 400 mg. Sulpiride is a benzamide derivative.

Pharmaceutical form

Dolmatil 200 mg Tablets: Plain white round tablet with a transverse breakline on one side and D200 on the other.

Dolmatil 400 mg Tablets: White film coated stick shaped tablet with break bar engraved SLP 400 on one side.

Clinical particulars

Therapeutic indications: Acute and chronic schizophrenia.

Posology and method of administration:

Adults: A starting dose of 400 mg to 800 mg daily, given in two divided doses (morning and early evening) is recommended.

Predominantly positive symptoms (formal thought disorder, hallucinations, delusions, incongruity of affect) respond to higher doses, and a starting dose of at least 400 mg twice daily is recommended, increasing if necessary up to a suggested maximum of 1200 mg twice daily. Increasing the dose beyond this level has not been shown to produce further improvement. Predominantly negative symptoms (flattening of affect, poverty of speech, anergia, apathy), as well as depression, respond to doses below 800 mg daily; therefore, a starting dose of 400 mg twice daily is recommended. Reducing this dose towards 200 mg twice daily will normally increase the alerting effect of Dolmatil.

Patients with mixed positive and negative symptoms, with neither predominating, will normally respond to dosage of 400–600 mg twice daily.

Children: Clinical experience in children under 14 years of age is insufficient to permit specific recommendations.

Elderly: The same dose ranges may be required in the elderly, but should be reduced if there is evidence of renal impairment.

Contra-indications: Phaeochromocytoma and acute porphyria. There are no cardiovascular contra-indications.

Special warnings and special precautions for use: Increased motor agitation has been reported at high dosage in a small number of patients: in aggressive, agitated or excited phases of the disease process, low doses of Dolmatil may aggravate symptoms. Care should be exercised where hypomania is present.

Extrapyramidal reactions, principally akathisia have been reported in a small number of cases. If warranted, reduction in dosage of anti-parkinsonian medication may be necessary.

As with all neuroleptic drugs, the presence of unexplained hyperthermia could indicate the neuroleptic malignant syndrome (NMS). In this event Dolmatil and any associated neuroleptic treatment should be discontinued until the origin of the fever has been determined.

Hepatic reactions have been reported. Although Dolmatil only induces slight EEG modifications, caution is advised in prescribing it for patients with unstable epilepsy. Patients requiring Dolmatil who are receiving anti-convulsant therapy should continue unchanged on the latter medication. Cases of convulsions, sometimes in patients with no previous history, have been reported. Dolmatil has no significant anticholinergic or cardiovascular activity. As with all drugs for which the kidney is the major elimination pathway, the usual precautions should be taken in cases of renal failure.

Interaction with other medicaments and other forms of interaction: While no drug interactions are known, unnecessary polypharmacy should be avoided. As with other psychotropic compounds, sulpiride may increase the effect of antihypertensives and CNS depressants or stimulants.

Pregnancy and lactation: Despite the negative results of teratogenicity studies in animals and the lack of teratogenic effects during widespread clinical use in other countries, Dolmatil should not be considered an exception to the general principle of avoiding drug treatment during pregnancy, particularly during the first 16 weeks, with potential benefits being weighed against possible hazards.

Effects on ability to drive and operate machines: None stated.

Undesirable effects: Dolmatil is very well tolerated and usually only minor side-effects occur, if at all, at the recommended doses.

After over a decade of widespread use in many countries, tardive dyskinesia has occurred rarely. Insomnia has been reported.

Many medicines, including neuroleptics, raise serum prolactin levels, which may be associated with galactorrhoea and amenorrhoea, and less frequently with gynaecomastia. In long-term animal studies with neuroleptic drugs, including sulpiride, an increased incidence of various endocrine tumours (some of which have occasionally been malignant) has been seen in some but not all strains of rats and mice studied. The significance of these findings to man is not known; there is no current evidence of any association between neuroleptic use and tumour risk in man. However, when prescribing neuroleptics to patients with existing mammary neoplasia or a history of this disease, possible risks should be weighed against benefits of therapy.

Overdose: The range of single toxic doses is 1 to 16 g but no death has occurred even at the 16 g dose.

The clinical manifestations of poisoning vary depending upon the size of the dose taken. After single doses of 1 to 3 g restlessness and clouding of consciousness have been reported and (rarely) extra-pyramidal symptoms. Doses of 3 to 7 g may produce a degree of agitation, confusion and extrapyramidal symptoms; more than 7g can cause, in addition, coma and low blood pressure.

The duration of intoxication is generally short, the symptoms disappearing within a few hours. Comas which have occurred after large doses have lasted up to four days. There are no specific complications from overdose. In particular no haematological or hepatic toxicity has been reported.

Overdose may be treated with alkaline osmotic diuresis and, if necessary, anti-parkinsonian drugs. Coma needs appropriate nursing. Emetic drugs are unlikely to be effective in Dolmatil overdosage.

Pharmacological properties

Pharmacodynamic properties: One of the characteristics of Dolmatil is its bimodal activity, as it has both antidepressant and neuroleptic properties. Schizophrenia characterised by a lack of social contact can benefit strikingly. Mood elevation is observed after a few days treatment, followed by disappearance of the florid schizophrenic symptoms. The sedation and lack of effect characteristically associated with classical neuroleptics of the phenothiazine or butyrophenone type are not features of Dolmatil therapy.

Dolmatil is a member of the group of substituted benzamides, which are structurally distinct from the phenothiazines, butyrophenones and thioxanthenes. Current evidence suggests that the actions of Dolmatil hint at an important distinction between different types of dopamine receptors or receptor mechanisms in the brain.

Behaviourally and biochemically, Dolmatil shares with these classical neuroleptics a number of properties indicative of cerebral dopamine receptor antagonism. Essential and intriguing differences include lack of catalepsy at doses active in other behavioural tests, lack of effect in the dopamine sensitive adenylate cyclase systems, lack of effect upon noradrenaline or 5HT turnover, negligible anticholinesterase activity, no effect on muscarinic or GABA receptor binding, and a radical difference in the binding of tritiated sulpiride to striatal preparations in-vitro, compared to ^{3}H-spiperone or ^{3}H-haloperidol. These findings indicate a major differentiation between Dolmatil and classical neuroleptics which lack such specificity.

Pharmacokinetic properties: Peak sulpiride serum levels are reached 3–6 hours after an oral dose. The plasma half-life in man is approximately 8 hours. Approximately 40% sulpiride is bound to plasma proteins. 95% of the compound is excreted in the urine and faeces as unchanged sulpiride.

Preclinical safety data: No further information is available.

Pharmaceutical particulars

List of excipients: Starch, lactose, methylcellulose, magnesium stearate, talc, silica.

Incompatibilities: None known.

Shelf life: 5 years.

Special precautions for storage: Store at or below 25°C.

Nature and contents of container: Cartons containing 100 tablets in blister strips.

Marketing authorisation number

Dolmatil 200 mg: PL 15819/0033.
Dolmatil 400 mg: PL 15819/0034.

Date of approval/revision of SPC 30 June 1998.

Legal category POM.

KERLONE*

Presentation White, biconvex, film-coated tablets engraved KE20 on one side with breakline on reverse. Each tablet contains betaxolol hydrochloride 20 mg.

Uses

Actions: Kerlone (betaxolol hydrochloride) is a beta-adrenoceptor blocking agent which is cardioselective, i.e. acts preferentially on beta$_1$-adrenergic receptors in the heart. It has prolonged activity, permitting once-daily administration which aids patient compliance. Its principal effects are to lower heart rate, especially on exercise, and to lower systolic and diastolic blood pressure in hypertensive subjects. It is devoid of intrinsic sympathomimetic activity and has little membrane stabilising activity. As with other beta-blockers, its mechanism of action in the treatment of hypertension is unclear. Absorption from the gastrointestinal tract is complete and not affected by food. There is little first-pass extraction in the liver. This results in blood levels which vary little within and between subjects and a reproducible bioavailability of 80–90%.

Its long elimination half-life of 16–20 hours results in protection from excessive or inappropriate sympathetic activity throughout the 24 hours after administration of a once daily dose.

Indications: Management of hypertension.

Dosage and administration
Adults: The usual adult dose is one tablet (20 mg) daily. The single daily dose may be increased to two tablets (40 mg) if response is inadequate.

Elderly patients or those with a history of bronchospasm: A starting dose of half tablet (10 mg) daily is recommended.

Impaired renal function: An adjustment of dose is usually unnecessary in patients with renal insufficiency where creatinine clearance is greater than 20 ml/min. However, clinical surveillance is recommended at the start of treatment until steady state blood levels are attained (4 days on average).

For patients on haemo- or peritoneal dialysis the initial recommended dose is 10 mg daily independent of the dialysis schedule.

Hepatic insufficiency: Adjustment of dosage is usually unnecessary in patients with hepatic insufficiency. However, clinical surveillance is recommended at the start of treatment.

Children: Paediatric experience with Kerlone is limited and for this reason it is not currently recommended for use in children.

Most of the reduction of blood pressure is seen during the first 3 hours following the initial dose, permitting an early evaluation of the antihypertensive effect. Little further reduction is seen after seven days of treatment and the response is undiminished in subsequent months. Should an inadequate response be obtained, a further decrease may be achieved by combining Kerlone with another antihypertensive agent such as a diuretic. However, in a large series of controlled clinical trials, 70–80% of patients responded to betaxolol alone.

Patients can be transferred to Kerlone from other anti-hypertensive treatments with the exception of clonidine (see precautions below).

Contra-indications, warnings, etc
Contra-indications: Kerlone is contra-indicated in cardiogenic shock, in patients with uncontrolled congestive cardiac failure and in second or third degree AV block if no pacemaker is present and in patients with marked bradycardia (heart rate less than 50 beats per minute).

Warnings: Concomitant administration of Kerlone and a myocardial depressant or inhibitor of AV conduction, such as the calcium antagonists of the verapamil type, should be carried out only under close supervision, especially in the case of intravenous administration.

Although cardio-selective beta-blockers may have less effect on lung function than non-selective beta-blockers, as with all beta-blockers these should be avoided in patients with wheezing or reversible obstructive airways disease unless there are compelling clinical reasons for their use.

It is recommended that Kerlone treatment is started at the dose of 10 mg daily in such patients. If any increase in airway resistance is provoked, it can be relieved by $beta_2$-mimetics whose effect is not inhibited.

Precautions: Secondary sympathetic hyperactivity has sometimes been reported following discontinuation of treatment with other beta-blockers. Even though Kerlone blood levels decrease slowly, care should be exercised if treatment is withdrawn, especially in patients with ischaemic heart disease.

Patients with a history of cardiac failure, cardiomyopathy, or cardiomegaly should be monitored carefully during treatment with a beta-blocker as sympathetic stimulation may be essential to their circulatory function.

Use with caution where the PR conduction interval is prolonged.

Studies in normal subjects have shown that, unlike non-selective beta-blockers, Kerlone does not inhibit the recovery from insulin-induced hypoglycaemia, nor does it mask the cardiovascular response. Due to its $beta_1$ selectivity, Kerlone is unlikely to interfere with glucose metabolism in insulin-treated diabetics. However, caution is advised when treating such patients.

Anaesthesia: In the event of surgical intervention, the anaesthetist should be advised in advance that the patient is receiving Kerlone. In patients with severe ischaemic heart disease the risk/benefits of continuation of treatment have to be evaluated. If treatment is continued care should be taken when using anaesthetic agents such as ether, cyclopropane and trichloroethylene.

Drug interactions: As with other beta-blockers, use with care in combination with myocardial depressants or drugs which depress AV conduction. If Kerlone and clonidine are given concurrently, clonidine should not be discontinued until several days after withdrawal of the beta-blocker.

Pregnancy: No teratogenic effects have been demonstrated in animal studies but the safety of Kerlone during human pregnancy has not been established. Like other beta-blockers, Kerlone crosses the placental barrier and its use in pregnant women requires that the anticipated benefit be weighed against the possible hazards to the mother and foetus.

Nursing mothers: Kerlone is excreted in human breast milk and the possibility of bradycardic and hypotensive effects on the newborn should therefore be considered if Kerlone is given to nursing mothers.

Side effects: Kerlone is generally well tolerated. The side effects are usually those due to its pharmacological actions and rarely require discontinuation of treatment. Minor side effects include lassitude at the start of treatment, exacerbation of Raynaud's disease or intermittent claudication, and paraesthesia of the extremities. Possible side effects include marked bradycardia and hypotension, AV block, cardiac insufficiency and bronchospasm. There have been reports of rashes and dry eyes associated with the use of all beta-blockers but in most cases the signs and symptoms have cleared when treatment was withdrawn. Nevertheless, the drug should be discontinued if any such reaction is suspected.

Overdosage: Excessive bradycardia can usually be corrected with atropine. If there is no response isoprenaline may be administered with caution. Cardiac failure should be managed with digitalisation and diuretics. Hypotension may be managed with vasopressors such as adrenaline.

Pharmaceutical precautions Store in a dry place below 30°C.

Legal category POM.

Package quantities Pack of 28 tablets (2×14).

Further information Kerlone is unique in having high bioavailability, long blood half-life and high selectivity for cardiac $beta_1$-receptors. Unlike most other cardioselective beta-blockers it has high lipid solubility. This may facilitate rapid arrival of the drug at the receptor, but does not induce an increased incidence of side effects.

These characteristics and the rapidity of response increase patient compliance by virtue of the drug's acceptability, the simple dose regimen and narrow dose range.

The only active metabolite is cardioselective and does not contribute to the clinical effect. Kerlone does not modify the hypoglycaemic response to insulin nor mask the cardiovascular response. It can be used in patients with respiratory disease, and is compatible with most other hypotensive agents.

Product licence number 15819/0011.

MIZOLLEN* ▼

Qualitative and quantitative composition Active ingredient: Mizolastine (INN) 10 mg per tablet.

Excipients: qsp. 1 tablet.

Pharmaceutical form Oblong, white film-coated modified release tablets with a scored line on one side and a mark 'MZI 10' on the reverse side.

Clinical particulars
Therapeutic indications: Mizolastine is a long-acting H_1-antihistamine indicated for the symptomatic relief of seasonal allergic rhinoconjunctivitis (hay fever), perennial allergic rhinoconjunctivitis and urticaria.

Posology and method of administration
Adults, including the elderly, and children 12 years of age and over: The recommended daily dose is one 10 mg tablet.

Contra-indications: Hypersensitivity to mizolastine.

Concomitant administration with macrolide antibiotics or systemic imidazole antifungals.

Significantly impaired hepatic function.

Clinically significant cardiac disease or a history of symptomatic arrhythmias.

Patients with known or suspected QT prolongation or with electrolyte imbalance, in particular hypokalaemia.

Clinically significant bradycardia.

Drugs known to prolong the QT interval, such as Class I and III anti-arrhythmics.

Special warnings and special precautions for use: Mizolastine has a weak potential to prolong the QT interval in a few individuals. The degree of prolongation is modest and has not been associated with cardiac arrhythmias.

The elderly may be particularly susceptible to the sedative effects of mizolastine and the potential effects of the drug on cardiac repolarisation.

Interaction with other medicinal products and other forms of interaction: Although the bioavailability of mizolastine is high and the drug is principally metabolised by glucuronidation, systemically administered ketoconazole and erythromycin moderately increase the plasma concentration of mizolastine and their concurrent use is contra-indicated.

Concurrent use of other potent inhibitors or substrates of hepatic oxidation (cytochrome P450 3A4) with mizolastine should be approached with caution. These would include cimetidine, cyclosporin, and nifedipine.

Alcohol: In studies with mizolastine, no potentiation of the sedation and the alteration in performance caused by alcohol has been observed.

Use during pregnancy and lactation: The safety of mizolastine for use in human pregnancy has not been established. The evaluation of experimental animal studies does not indicate direct or indirect harmful effects with respect to the development of the embryo or foetus, the course of gestation and peri- and post-natal development. However, as with all drugs, mizolastine should be avoided in pregnancy, particularly during the first trimester.

In the absence of information on the levels of mizolastine which may appear in human breast milk after administration, mizolastine is not recommended during lactation.

Effects on ability to drive and use machines: Most patients taking mizolastine may drive or perform tasks requiring concentration. However, in order to identify sensitive people who have unusual reactions to drugs, it is advisable to check the individual response before driving or performing complicated tasks.

Undesirable effects: The following adverse reactions were reported in decreasing order of frequency in mizolastine treated patients: drowsiness and asthenia, often transient in nature, and increased appetite associated with weight gain in some individuals. Dry mouth, diarrhoea, dyspepsia or headache may occur. Isolated cases of hypotension, anxiety and depression, low neutrophil count and raised liver enzymes have been reported rarely. There were reports of bronchospasm and aggravation of asthma but in view of the high frequency of asthma in the patient population being treated, a causal relationship remains uncertain.

Treatment with certain antihistamines has been associated with QT interval prolongation increasing the risk of serious cardiac arrhythmias in susceptible subjects.

Minor changes in blood sugar and electrolytes have been observed rarely. The clinical significance of these changes in otherwise healthy individuals remains unclear. Patients at risk (diabetics, those susceptible to electrolyte imbalance and cardiac arrhythmias) should be monitored periodically.

Overdose: In cases of overdosage, general symptomatic surveillance with cardiac monitoring including QT interval and cardiac rhythm for at least 24 hours is recommended, along with standard measures to remove any unabsorbed drug.

Studies in patients with renal insufficiency suggest that haemodialysis does not increase clearance of the drug.

Pharmacological properties
Pharmacodynamic properties: Mizolastine possesses antihistamine and antiallergic properties due to a specific and selective antagonism of peripheral histamine H_1 receptors. It has also been shown to inhibit histamine release from mast cells (at 0.3 mg/kg orally) and the migration of neutrophils (at 3 mg/kg orally) in animal models of allergic reactions.

In man, histamine-induced wheal and flare studies have shown that mizolastine 10 mg is a rapid, potent (80% inhibition after 4 hrs) and sustained (24 hr) antihistamine. No tachyphylaxis occurred after long-term administration.

In both preclinical and clinical studies, no anticholinergic effect has been demonstrated.

Pharmacokinetic properties: Following oral administration mizolastine is rapidly absorbed. Peak plasma concentration is reached at a median time of 1.5 hours.

Bioavailability is 65% and linear kinetics have been demonstrated.

The mean elimination half-life is 13.0 hours with plasma protein binding of 98.4%.

In hepatic insufficiency the absorption of mizolastine is slower and the distribution phase longer, with a resulting moderate increase in AUC of 50%.

The principal metabolic pathway is glucuronidation of the parent compound. The cytochrome $P_{450}3A4$ enzyme system is involved in one of the additional metabolic pathways with formation of the hydroxylated metabolites of mizolastine. None of the identified metabolites contribute to the pharmacological activity of mizolastine.

An increase in mizolastine plasma levels, observed with systemic ketaconazole and erythromycin, led to concentrations equivalent to those obtained after a 15 to 20 mg dose of mizolastine alone.

In studies carried out in healthy volunteers, no clinically significant interaction has been recorded with food, warfarin, digoxin, theophylline, lorazepam, or diltiazem.

Preclinical safety data: Pharmacological studies in several species have shown an effect on cardiac repolarisation at doses in excess of 10–20 times the therapeutic dose. In conscious dogs, mizolastine has shown pharmacological interactions with ketoconazole at the electrocardiographic level at 70 times the therapeutic dose.

Pharmaceutical particulars
List of excipients:
Core: Hydrogenated castor oil, lactose, microcrystalline cellulose, tartaric acid, polyvidone, anhydrous colloidal silica, magnesium stearate.
Film-coating: Methylhydroxypropyl cellulose, titanium dioxide, propylene glycol.

Incompatibilities: None stated.

Shelf life: 2 years in blisters.

Special precautions for storage: Store in a dry place below 25°C. Tablets should not be taken if they become discoloured.

Nature and contents of container:
Aluminium/PVC blisters Packs of 4* and 30 tablets.
*The 4 tablet pack is a physician's sample.

Instructions for use/handling, and disposal (if appropriate): None stated.

Marketing authorisation number PL 15819/0012

Date of first authorisation/renewal of the authorisation
First authorisation: 20 June 1997.

Date of revision of the text 29 September 1997.

MONIT* TABLETS 20 mg
MONIT* LS TABLETS 10 mg

Qualitative and quantitative composition Each tablet of Monit contains isosorbide mononitrate 20 mg.
Each tablet of Monit LS contains isosorbide mononitrate 10 mg.

Pharmaceutical form Tablet.

Clinical particulars
Therapeutic indications: Monit and Monit LS are indicated in the prophylaxis of angina pectoris.
Monit is indicated as adjunctive therapy in congestive heart failure which does not respond adequately to cardiac glycosides and/or diuretics.

Posology and method of administration: The tablets should be swallowed whole with a little fluid.

Adults: Angina pectoris: Usually one tablet twice or three times daily. Patients already accustomed to prophylactic nitrate therapy (for example with isosorbide dinitrate) may normally be transferred directly to a therapeutic dose of Monit or Monit LS. For patients not receiving prophylactic nitrate therapy, it is recommended that the initial dose should be one Monit LS tablet twice daily. Maintenance dose in individual patients will be between 20 and 120 mg daily. Congestive heart failure: In severe congestive cardiac failure Monit tablets may be taken in doses of 20 mg two to three times daily depending on patients requirements. In this situation optimal individual dose is best determined by continuous haemodynamic monitoring. The use of Monit in severe congestive cardiac failure should be considered adjunctive therapy to more conventional treatment (e.g. cardiac glycosides, diuretics etc).

Elderly: There is no evidence to suggest an adjustment of dosage is necessary. However, caution may be required in elderly patients who are known to be susceptible to the effects of hypotensive medication.

Children: The safety and efficacy of Monit and Monit LS in children has not been established.

Patients with renal or hepatic impairment: No dosage reduction is necessary in patients with renal or hepatic impairment.

Contra-indications: Monit and Monit LS are contra-indicated in patients with a known sensitivity to the drug or to isosorbide dinitrate and in cases of marked low blood pressure, shock and acute myocardial infarction with low left ventricular filling pressure.

Special warnings and special precautions for use: Monit and Monit LS are not indicated for relief of acute anginal attacks. In the event of an acute attack, sublingual or buccal glyceryl trinitrate tablets or spray should be used.

Interaction with other medicaments and other forms of interaction: The hypotensive effects of other drugs may be potentiated.
Beta-adrenoceptor blocking drugs have a different pharmacological action in angina and may have a complementary effect when co-administered with Monit or Monit LS.

Pregnancy and lactation: Animal studies have shown no adverse effects on the foetus, however, since its safety and efficacy during pregnancy and lactation have not been established, Monit, like other drugs should not be administered to pregnant women and nursing mothers unless considered essential. No data are available on the presence of isosorbide-5-mononitrate in breast milk.

Effects on ability to drive and use machines: The effect of isosorbide mononitrate upon an individual's performance of skilled and potentially dangerous tasks such as car driving and the operation of machinery has not been evaluated. However, there have been no published reports of impaired performance of such tasks.

Undesirable effects: A number of nitrate-related adverse effects may occur during treatment, including flushing, headache, dizziness and weakness. The incidence of such effects is normally highest at the commencement of treatment and tends to decline with time. If headache is a problem, a temporary lowering of the dose may be necessary. Nausea and vomiting may occur occasionally. Postural hypotension may occur, especially with high doses. Dry rash and/or exfoliative dermatitis have been described rarely with isosorbide dinitrate and similar reactions might be expected.

Overdose: Overdosage should be treated symptomatically. The stomach should be aspirated to remove any remaining tablets. The main symptom is likely to be hypotension and this may be treated by elevation of the legs to promote venous return. Symptomatic and supportive treatment e.g. plasma expanders and if necessary the careful use of vasopressor agents to counterbalance the hypotensive effects may be necessary.
Methaemoglobinaemia will normally respond to methylene blue infusion.

Pharmacological properties
Pharmacodynamic properties: Isosorbide mononitrate is an active metabolite of isosorbide dinitrate. The predominant action is that of a vasodilator with effects on both veins and arteries.

Pharmacokinetic properties: Isosorbide-5-mononitrate is completely absorbed after oral administration.
The elimination half-life is approximately 5 hours. The volume of distribution is about 0.62 l/kg. The time to maximum plasma level is approximately 1 hour and peak plasma concentration is approximately 500 ng/ml for Monit and 250 ng/ml for Monit LS. In patients with renal failure, the half-life is unchanged, remaining at approximately 5 hours.

Preclinical safety data: Not applicable.

Pharmaceutical particulars
List of excipients: Monit LS Tablets 10 mg: Lactose, microcrystalline cellulose, sodium starch glycollate, povidone 25000, colloidal silicon dioxide, magnesium stearate.
Monit Tablets 20 mg: Anhydrous lactose, colloidal silicon dioxide, magnesium stearate.

Incompatibilities: None known.

Shelf life: 5 years.

Special precautions for storage: Store below 25°C. Protect from moisture.

Nature and contents of container: Monit: PVC (250 micron), aluminium foil (20 micron) blister pack. 56 or 100 tablets.
Monit LS: PVC (250 micron), aluminium foil (20 micron) blister pack. 56 or 100 tablets.

Instructions for use/handling: None.

Marketing authorisation numbers
Monit 15819/0005
Monit LS 15819/0006

Date of approval/revision of SPC October 98

Legal category P.

MONIT* SR TABLETS 40 mg

Qualitative and quantitative composition Isosorbide mononitrate 40 mg.

Pharmaceutical form Slow release, sugar coated tablet.

Clinical particulars
Therapeutic indications: Monit SR is indicated in the prophylaxis of angina pectoris.

Posology and method of administration: The tablets should be swallowed whole without chewing.

Adults: One tablet daily to be taken in the morning.

Elderly: There is no evidence to suggest that an adjustment of dosage is necessary. However, caution may be required in elderly patients who are known to be susceptible to the effects of hypotensive medication.

Children: The safety and efficacy of Monit SR in children has not been established.

Patients with renal or hepatic impairment: No dosage reduction is necessary in patients with renal or hepatic impairment.

Patients who have not previously received nitrates may be started with a low dose which should be increased gradually before introducing Monit SR.

Contra-indications: Monit SR is contra-indicated in patients with a known hypersensitivity to isosorbide mononitrate or isosorbide dinitrate and in cases of marked low blood pressure, shock and acute myocardial infarction with low left ventricular filling pressure.

Special warnings and special precautions for use: Monit SR is not indicated for relief of acute anginal attacks. In the event of an acute attack, sublingual or buccal glyceryl trinitrate tablets or spray should be used.

Interaction with other medicaments and other forms of interaction: The hypotensive effects of other drugs may be potentiated.
Beta-adrenoceptor blocking drugs have a different pharmacological action in angina and may have a complementary effect when co-administered with Monit SR.

Pregnancy and lactation: Animal studies have shown no adverse effects on the foetus, however, since its safety and efficacy during pregnancy and lactation have not been established, Monit SR, like other drugs should not be administered to pregnant women and nursing mothers unless considered essential. No data are available on the presence of isosorbide-5-mononitrate in breast milk.

Effects on ability to drive and use machines: The effect of isosorbide mononitrate upon an individual's performance of skilled and potentially dangerous tasks such as car driving and the operation of machinery has not been evaluated. However, there have been no published reports of impaired performance of such tasks.

Undesirable effects: A number of nitrate-related adverse effects may occur during treatment, including flushing, headache, dizziness and weakness. The incidence of such effects is normally highest at the commencement of treatment and tends to decline with time. If headache is a problem, a temporary reduced dose of isosorbide-5-mononitrate may be necessary. Nausea and vomiting may occur occasionally. Postural hypotension may occur, especially with high doses. Dry rash and/or exfoliative dermatitis have been described rarely with isosorbide dinitrate and similar reactions might be expected.

Overdose: In the event of overdosage with Monit SR the main sign is likely to be hypotension. The stomach should be aspirated to remove any remaining tablets. The patient should be placed in a supine position with the legs elevated to promote venous return. Symptomatic and supportive treatment, e.g. plasma expanders and if necessary the careful use of vasopressor agents to counterbalance the hypotensive effects may be necessary.
Methaemoglobinaemia will normally respond to methylene blue infusion.

Pharmacological properties
Pharmacodynamic properties: Isosorbide-5-mononitrate is an active metabolite of isosorbide dinitrate. The predominant action is that of a vasodilator with effects on both veins and arteries.

Pharmacokinetic properties: Monit SR has been developed to provide a convenient, once daily dosage form of isosorbide-5-mononitrate. It is designed to achieve therapeutic blood concentrations within 30 minutes which persist up to 17 hours. A nitrate free interval of up to 7 hours makes the development of anti-anginal tolerance during chronic therapy unlikely.

Preclinical safety data: Not applicable.

Pharmaceutical particulars
List of excipients: Anhydrous lactose; Hoechst Wax E; povidone 25000; colloidal silicon dioxide; magnesium stearate; Eudragit E12.5; talc; sucrose; kaolin; macrogol; titanium dioxide; liquid glucose.

Incompatibilities: None known.

Shelf life: 36 months.

Special precautions for storage: Store below 25°C. Protect from moisture.

Nature and contents of container: Blister pack 250 micron PVC and 20 micron aluminium foil. 28 tablet pack size.

Instructions for use/handling: None.

Marketing authorisation number 15819/0007

Date of approval/revision of SPC December 1997

Legal category P.

PARAMAX* TABLETS
PARAMAX* SACHETS

Qualitative and quantitative composition
Active ingredients: Paracetamol BP, Metoclopramide Hydrochloride BP.

Quantitative composition: 500 mg paracetamol BP with 5 mg metoclopramide hydrochloride BP (calculated with reference to anhydrous substance).

Pharmaceutical form Tablets and sachets.

Clinical particulars
Therapeutic indications: Paramax is indicated for the symptomatic treatment of migraine.

Posology and method of administration: Paramax should be taken at the first warning of an attack. If symptoms persist, further doses may be taken at four-hourly intervals. Total dosage in any 24-hour period should not exceed the quantity stated.

The dosage recommendations given below should be strictly adhered to if side-effects of the dystonic type are to be avoided. It should be noted that a total daily dosage of metoclopramide, especially for adolescents and young adults, should not normally exceed 0.5 mg/kg body weight.

Usual Recommended Dosage (Tablets or Sachets)

	Initial dose at first warning of attack	*Maximum dosage in any 24-hour period*
Adults (including elderly patients)	2	6
Young adults (12–19 years)	1	3

Young adults and adolescents: Paramax should only be used after careful examination to avoid masking an underlying disorder, e.g. cerebral irritation. In the treatment of this group attention should be given primarily to bodyweight.

Children: A presentation of Paramax suitable for the treatment of children under 12 years of age is not available.

Paramax sachets are emptied into about ⅓ of a glass of water and stirred before taking.

For oral administration only.

Contra-indications: No specific contra-indications stated.

Special warnings and precautions for use: If vomiting persists the patient should be reassessed to exclude the possibility of an underlying disorder, e.g. cerebral irritation.

Care should be exercised in patients being treated with other centrally active drugs e.g. in epilepsy.

Patients should not take Paramax with other paracetamol-containing products.

Care should be exercised in the event of Paramax being prescribed concurrently with a phenothiazine since extra pyramidal symptoms may occur with both products. The action of metoclopramide on the gastrointestinal tract is antagonised by anticholinergics.

Interactions with other medicaments and other forms of interactions: Refer to *Special warnings and precautions for use* for interactions.

Pregnancy and lactation: There is no evidence that metoclopramide or paracetamol by themselves have teratogenic effects. Nevertheless, Paramax should only be used when there are compelling reasons and is not advised during the first trimester.

During lactation, metoclopramide and paracetamol may be found in breast milk.

Effects on ability to drive and use machines: None known (but see *Undesirable effects*).

Undesirable effects: Various extrapyramidal reactions to metoclopramide, usually of the dystonic type, have been reported. The incidence of these reactions may be increased if the metoclopramide dosage exceeds 0.5 mg/kg body weight/day. Reactions include: spasm of the facial muscles, trismus, rhythmic protrusion of the tongue, a bulbar type of speech, spasm of extra-ocular muscles, including oculogyric crises, unnatural positioning of the head and shoulders and opisthotonos. There may be a generalised increase in muscle tone. The majority of reactions occur within 36 hours of starting treatment and the effects usually disappear within 24 hours of withdrawal of the drug. Should treatment of a dystonic reaction be required, a benzodiazepine or an anticholinergic anti-Parkinsonian drug may be used.

Rarely, drowsiness, restlessness and diarrhoea have been reported in patients receiving metoclopramide therapy.

Raised serum prolactin levels have been observed during metoclopramide therapy; this effect is similar to that noted with many other compounds.

Metoclopramide may induce an acute hypertensive response in patients with phaeochromocytoma.

Overdose: Immediate medical advice should be sought in the event of an overdosage, because of the risk of irreversible liver damage. Overdosage should be treated by gastric lavage with appropriate supportive measures. Intravenous N-acetylcysteine or oral methionine if administered within 10 hours of paracetamol overdosage appears to exert a protective effect on the liver.

Pharmacological properties
Pharmacodynamic properties: The mechanism of action of metoclopramide in the gastrointestinal tract remains unclear and current hypotheses have been reviewed by Harrington *et al* (1983). It appears that metoclopramide has both central and local mechanisms of action; at the local level metoclopramide may have a direct effect on gastric muscle, stimulating contractility (Hay, 1975).

The addition of metoclopramide to paracetamol therapy for migraine has the additional benefit of combating the nausea and vomiting which are often experienced by migraine sufferers. The antiemetic activity of metoclopramide is probably mediated, at least in part, by blockade of dopamine receptors in the chemoreceptor trigger zone for vomiting (Harrington *et al* 1983).

Pharmacokinetic properties: Published data concerning the pharmacokinetics of Paramax is limited. In a study involving four healthy volunteers in which plasma paracetamol concentrations were compared following administration of Paramax tablets (1 g paracetamol+10 mg metoclopramide), Panadol tablets (1 g paracetamol) and Solpadeine effervescent tablets (1 g paracetamol+16 mg codeine phosphate+16 mg caffeine), absorption of paracetamol from Paramax tablets was found not to differ significantly from absorption from Panadol or Solpadeine (Dougall *et al*, 1983).

Oral paracetamol is largely absorbed from the small intestine, the rate of absorption depending on the rate of gastric emptying (Heading *et al*, 1973; Clements *et al*, 1978).

Gastric emptying is often severely delayed during migraine attacks (Kreel, 1969); absorption of oral paracetamol has been shown to be delayed and impaired in patients during a migraine attack compared to when the same patients are headache free (Tokala and Neuvonen, 1984).

Preclinical safety data: Paracetamol and metoclopramide hydrochloride are well established drug substances and results of preclinical testing are well documented.

Pharmaceutical particulars
List of excipients:
Paramax tablets: Colloidal silica dioxide, magnesium stearate, microcrystalline cellulose.

Paramax sachets: Sodium carbonate, saccharin sodium, lemon flavour, sodium dihydrogen citrate anhydrous, sodium bicarbonate.

Incompatibilities: None stated.

Shelf life: Shelf life allocation: 5 years.

Do not use after expiry date given on the label.

Special precautions for storage:
Tablets: Protect tablets from light.
Sachets: Store sachets in a dry place.

Nature and contents of container:
Paramax tablets: PVC aluminium blister packs of 42 tablets.

Paramax sachets: Packs of 6 (medical sample) and 42 sachets packed into cartons.

Instructions for use/handling: No special instructions for use.

Marketing authorisation numbers
Paramax tablets PL 15819/0015
Paramax sachets PL 15819/0016

Date of first authorisation 1.9.97

Date of revision of the text April 1998.

PRIADEL*
PRIADEL* 200

Qualitative and quantitative composition Priadel tablets contain 400 mg lithium carbonate. Priadel 200 tablets contain 200 mg lithium carbonate.

Pharmaceutical form
Priadel: White, circular, bi-convex tablets engraved PRIADEL on one side, scored on the other side, in a controlled release formulation.

Priadel 200: White, scored, capsule-shaped tablets engraved P200 on one side, in a controlled release formulation.

Clinical particulars
Therapeutic indications:

1. In the management of acute manic or hypomanic episodes.
2. In the management of episodes of recurrent depressive disorders where treatment with other anti-depressants has been unsuccessful.
3. In the prophylaxis against bipolar affective disorders.
4. Control of aggressive behaviour or intentional self harm.

Posology and method of administration: A simple treatment schedule has been evolved which except for some minor variations should be followed whether using Priadel therapeutically or prophylactically. The minor variations to this schedule depend on the elements of the illness being treated and these are described later.

1. In patients of average weight (70 kg) an initial dose of 400–1,200 mg of Priadel may be given as a single daily dose in the morning or on retiring. Alternatively, the dose may be divided and given morning and evening. The tablets should not be crushed or chewed. When changing between lithium preparations serum lithium levels should first be checked, then Priadel therapy commenced at a daily dose as close as possible to the dose of the other form of lithium. As bioavailability varies from product to product (particularly with regard to retard or slow release preparations) a change of product should be regarded as initiation of new treatment.

2. Four to five days after starting treatment (and never longer than one week) a blood sample should be taken for the estimation of serum lithium level.

3. The objective is to adjust the Priadel dose so as to maintain the serum lithium level permanently within the diurnal range of 0.5–1.5 mmol/l. In practice, the blood sample should be taken between 12 and 24 hours after the previous dose of Priadel. 'Target' serum lithium concentrations at 12 and 24 hours are shown in the table below.

	'Target' serum lithium concentrations (mmol/l)	
	At 12 hours	*At 24 hours*
Once daily dosage	0.7–1.0	0.5–0.8
Twice daily dosage	0.5–0.8	

Both strengths have breaklines, therefore they can be divided accurately to provide dosage requirements as small as 100 mg. Serum lithium levels should be monitored weekly until stabilisation is achieved.

4. Lithium therapy should not be initiated unless adequate facilities for routine monitoring of serum concentrations are available. Following stabilisation of serum lithium levels, the period between subsequent estimations can be increased gradually but should not normally exceed three months. Additional measurements should be made following alteration of dosage, on development of intercurrent disease, signs of manic or depressive relapse, following significant change in sodium or fluid intake, or if signs of lithium toxicity occur.

5. Whilst a high proportion of acutely ill patients may respond within three to seven days of the commencement of Priadel therapy, Priadel should be continued through any recurrence of the affective disturbance. This is important as the full prophylactic effect may not occur for 6 to 12 months after the initiation of therapy.

6. In patients who show a positive response to Priadel therapy, treatment is likely to be long term. Careful clinical appraisal of the patient should be exercised throughout medication (see *Precautions*).

Prophylactic treatment of bipolar affective disorders and control of aggressive behaviour or intentional self harm: It is recommended that the described treatment schedule is followed.

Treatment of acute manic or hypomanic episodes and recurrent depressive disorders: It is likely that a higher than normal Priadel intake may be necessary during an acute phase and divided doses would be required here. Therefore as soon as control of mania or depression is achieved, the serum lithium level should be determined and it may be necessary, dependent on the results, to lower the dose of Priadel and re-stabilise serum lithium levels. In all other details the described treatment schedule is recommended.

Elderly: In elderly patients or those below 50 kg in weight, it is recommended that the starting dose is 400 mg. Elderly patients may be more sensitive to undesirable effects of lithium and also may require lower doses in order to maintain therapeutic serum lithium levels. It follows therefore that long-term patients often require a reduction in dosage over a period of years.

Children and adolescents: Not recommended.

Contra-indications: Cardiac failure. Clinically significant renal impairment. Addison's disease. Untreated hypothyroidism.

Special warnings and precautions for use: When considering Priadel therapy, it is necessary to ascertain whether patients are receiving lithium in any other form. If so, check serum levels before proceeding. It is important to ensure that renal function is normal – if necessary a creatinine clearance test or other renal function test should be performed. Cardiac and thyroid function should be assessed before commencing lithium treatment. Patients should be euthyroid before the initiation of lithium therapy. Renal function, cardiac function and thyroid function should be re-assessed periodically.

Clear instructions regarding the symptoms of impending toxicity should be given by the doctor to all patients receiving long term lithium therapy (see toxic effects). Patients should also be warned to report if polyuria or polydipsia develop. Episodes of nausea and vomiting or other conditions leading to salt/water depletion (including severe dieting) should also be reported.

Elderly patients are particularly liable to lithium toxicity.

Caution should be exercised to ensure that diet and fluid intake are normal thus maintaining a stable electrolyte balance. This may be of special importance in very hot weather or work environment. Infectious diseases including colds, influenza, gastroenteritis and urinary infections may also alter fluid balance and thus affect serum lithium levels. Treatment should be discontinued during any intercurrent infection and should only be reinstituted after the patient's physical health has returned to normal.

Interactions with other medicaments and other forms of interaction: Concurrent use of lithium and diuretics may cause reduced lithium clearance, leading to intoxication. If a diuretic has to be prescribed for a lithium patient, the lithium dosage should first be lowered and the patient re-stabilised with frequent monitoring. Similar precautions should be exercised on diuretic withdrawal. Other drugs affecting electrolyte balance, e.g. steroids, may alter lithium excretion and should be avoided in patients on lithium. If other psychotropic drugs are used they should be initiated at a lower dosage than usual, as their side effects may be potentiated by the use of lithium. This has been shown to be of particular importance for the concurrent use of lithium and haloperidol or flupenthixol.

Concomitant use with NSAIDs can increase serum lithium concentrations, possibly resulting in lithium toxicity. Serum lithium concentrations should be monitored more frequently if NSAID therapy is initiated or discontinued.

There have been isolated reports of possible interactions between lithium and diazepam (resulting in hypothermia), methyldopa, tetracyclines, phenytoin, carbamazepine, indomethacin and other prostaglandin-synthetase inhibitors.

Pregnancy and lactation: Lithium should not be used during pregnancy since there is evidence that the drug may harm the foetus. Because lithium is secreted into breast milk, it is recommended that breast-feeding be discontinued during use.

Should the use of lithium be unavoidable, close monitoring of serum concentrations should be made during pregnancy and parturition.

Babies may show signs of lithium toxicity necessitating fluid therapy in the neonatal period. Babies born with low serum lithium concentrations may have a flaccid appearance which returns to normal without any treatment. Lithium is secreted in breast milk, therefore bottle feeding is recommended.

Effects on ability to drive and use machines: None.

Undesirable effects: Side-effects are less common in patients with plasma lithium concentrations below 1.0 mmol/l. Mild gastrointestinal effects, nausea, vertigo, muscle weakness and a dazed feeling may occur initially, but frequently disappear after stabilisation. Fine hand tremors, polyuria and mild thirst may persist. Weight gain or oedema may present in some patients but should not be treated with diuretics.

Hypercalcaemia, hypermagnesaemia and hyperparathyroidism have been reported. Skin conditions including acne, psoriasis, generalised pustular psoriasis, rashes and leg ulcers have occasionally been reported as being aggravated by lithium treatment.

Long term treatment with lithium may be associated with disturbances of thyroid function, including goitre, hypothyroidism and thyrotoxicosis. Lithium-induced hypothyroidism may be managed successfully with concurrent thyroxine.

Memory impairment may occur during long term use.

Nephrotoxicity: Up to one third of patients on lithium may develop polyuria with a urinary output of up to three litres per day. This is usually due to lithium blocking the effect of ADH and is reversible on lithium withdrawal. However, long term treatment with lithium may also result in permanent changes in kidney histology and impairment of renal function. High serum concentrations of lithium including episodes of acute lithium toxicity may aggravate these changes. The minimum clinically effective dose of lithium should always be used. In patients who develop polyuria or polydipsia, renal function should be monitored, e.g. with measurement of blood urea, serum creatinine and urinary protein levels in addition to the routine serum lithium estimations.

After a period lasting 3–5 years, patients should be carefully assessed to ensure that benefit persists.

Toxic effects: Such effects are indicative of impending lithium intoxication and fall into two groups:

1. Gastro-intestinal: increasing anorexia, diarrhoea and vomiting.
2. Central nervous system: muscle weakness, lack of co-ordination, drowsiness or lethargy progressing to giddiness with ataxia, tinnitus, blurred vision, dysarthria, coarse tremor and muscle twitching.

At blood levels above 2–3 mmol/l there may be a large output of dilute urine, with increasing disorientation, seizures, coma and death.

Patients should be instructed to stop taking their tablets if toxic symptoms appear and to report immediately for a serum lithium estimation.

Overdose: There is no specific antidote to lithium poisoning. In the event of accumulation, lithium should be stopped and serum estimation should be carried out every 6 hours.

Under no circumstances should a diuretic be used. Osmotic diuresis (mannitol or urea infusion) or alkalinisation of the urine (sodium lactate or sodium bicarbonate infusion) should be initiated. If the serum lithium level is over 4.0 mmol/l, if there is a deterioration in the patient's condition, or if the serum lithium concentration is not falling at a rate corresponding to a half-life of under 30 hours, peritoneal or haemodialysis should be instituted promptly. This should be continued until there is no lithium in the serum or dialysis fluid. Serum lithium levels should be monitored for at least a further week to take account of any possible rebound in serum lithium levels as a result of delayed diffusion from body tissues.

Pharmacological properties The mode of action of lithium is still not fully understood. However, lithium modifies the production and turnover of certain neurotransmitters, particularly serotonin, and it may also block dopamine receptors.

It modifies concentrations of some electrolytes, particularly calcium and magnesium, and it may reduce thyroid activity.

Pharmacokinetic properties: Lithium has a half life of about 24 hours although this increases to about 36 hours in the elderly due to a progressive decrease in renal lithium clearance with age. Lithium is 95% eliminated in the urine. Time to peak serum level for controlled release Priadel tablets is about 2 hours and approximately 90% bioavailability would be expected.

Preclinical safety data: Nothing of therapeutic relevance.

Pharmaceutical particulars

List of excipients: Priadel and Priadel 200 contain precirol, mannitol, acacia powder, sodium lauryl sulphate, magnesium stearate, maize starch and primojel. In addition Priadel 200 may contain imwitor.

Incompatibilities: None stated.

Shelf life: Three years.

Special precautions for storage: Store in a cool, dry place.

Nature and contents of container: Pack sizes:

Priadel: Blister packs 100.
Priadel 200: Securitainers 100.

Instructions for use/handling: Not applicable.

Marketing authorisation numbers

Priadel 15819/0025
Priadel 200 15819/0026

Date of approval/revision of SPC December 1997.

Legal category POM.

PRIADEL* LIQUID

Qualitative and quantitative composition A clear, colourless pineapple flavoured, sugar free syrup containing 520 mg lithium citrate equivalent to 200 mg lithium carbonate per 5 ml.

Pharmaceutical form Syrup.

Clinical particulars

Therapeutic indications:

1. Treatment of mania and hypomania.
2. Lithium may also be tried in the treatment of some patients with recurrent bipolar depression, where treatment with other antidepressants has been unsuccessful.
3. Prophylactic treatment of recurrent affective disorders.
4. Control of aggressive or self-mutilating behaviour.

Posology and method of administration: A simple treatment schedule has been evolved which except for some minor variations should be followed whether using Priadel Liquid therapeutically or prophylactically. The minor variations to this schedule depend on the elements of the illness being treated and these are described later.

1. In patients of average weight (70 kg) an initial daily dose of 10–30 ml of Priadel Liquid (equivalent to 400–1200 mg lithium carbonate) should be given in divided doses, ideally twice a day. When changing between lithium preparations serum lithium levels should first be checked, then Priadel Liquid therapy commenced at a daily dose as close as possible to the dose of the other form of lithium. As bioavailability varies from product to product (particularly with regard to slow release preparations) a change of product should be regarded as initiation of new treatment.
2. Four to five days after starting treatment (and never longer than one week) a blood sample should be taken for the estimation of serum lithium level.
3. The objective is to adjust the Priadel Liquid dose so as to maintain the serum lithium level permanently within the diurnal range of 0.5–1.5 mmol/l. In practice, the blood sample should be taken 12 hours after the previous dose of Priadel Liquid. 'Target' serum lithium concentrations at 12 hours should be 0.5–0.8 mmol/l.

   Priadel Liquid is supplied with a 2.5/5 ml double ended spoon to provide dosage adjustments equivalent to 100 mg and 200 mg lithium carbonate respectively. Serum lithium levels should be monitored weekly until stabilisation is achieved.
4. Lithium therapy should not be initiated unless adequate facilities for routine monitoring of serum concentrations are available. Following stabilisation of serum lithium levels, the period between subsequent estimations can be increased gradually but should not normally exceed three months. Additional measurements should be made following alteration of dosage, on development of intercurrent disease, signs of manic or depressive relapse, following significant change in sodium or fluid intake, or if signs of lithium toxicity occur.
5. Whilst a high proportion of acutely ill patients may respond within three to seven days of the commencement of therapy with Priadel Liquid it should be continued through any recurrence of the affective disturbance. This is important as the full prophylactic effect may not occur for 6 to 12 months after the initiation of therapy.
6. In patients who show a positive response to therapy with Priadel Liquid, treatment is likely to be long term. Careful clinical appraisal of the patient should be exercised throughout medication (see *Precautions*).

Prophylactic treatment of recurrent affective disorders: It is recommended that the described treatment schedule is followed.

Treatment of acute mania, hypomania and recurrent bipolar depression: It is likely that a higher than normal Priadel Liquid intake may be necessary during an acute phase. As soon as control of mania or depression is achieved, the serum lithium level should be determined and it may be necessary, dependent on the results, to lower the dose of Priadel Liquid and re-stabilise serum lithium levels.

Use in elderly: In elderly patients or those below 50 kg in weight, it is recommended that the starting dose be 5 ml (equivalent to 200 mg lithium carbonate) taken twice daily. Elderly patients may be more sensitive to undesirable effects of lithium and also may require lower doses in order to maintain normal serum lithium levels. It follows therefore that long term patients often require a reduction in dosage over a period of years.

Use in children and adolescents: Not recommended.

Contra-indications: Renal insufficiency, cardiovascular insufficiency, Addison's disease and untreated hypothyroidism are all contra-indications to lithium therapy.

Special warnings and precautions for use: When considering therapy with Priadel Liquid, it is necessary to ascertain whether patients are receiving lithium in any other form. If so, check serum levels before proceeding. It is important to ensure that renal function is normal – if necessary a creatinine clearance test or other renal function test should be performed. Cardiac and thyroid function should be assessed before commencing lithium treatment. Patients should be euthyroid before the initiation of lithium therapy. Renal function, cardiac function and thyroid function should be reassessed periodically.

Clear instructions regarding the symptoms of impending toxicity should be given by the doctor to all patients receiving long term lithium therapy (see toxic effects). Patients should also be warned to report if polyuria or polydipsia develop.

Episodes of nausea and vomiting or other conditions leading to salt/water depletion (including severe dieting) should also be reported.

Elderly patients are particularly liable to lithium toxicity.

Caution should be exercised to ensure that diet and fluid intake are normal thus maintaining a stable electrolyte balance. This may be of special importance in very hot weather or work environment. Infectious diseases including colds, influenza, gastroenteritis and urinary infections may alter fluid balance and thus affect serum lithium levels. Treatment should be discontinued during any intercurrent infection and should only be reinstituted after the patient's physical health has returned to normal.

Interaction with other medicaments and other forms of interaction: Concurrent use of lithium and diuretics may cause reduced lithium clearance, leading to intoxication. If a diuretic has to be prescribed for a lithium patient, the lithium dosage should first be lowered and the patient restabilised with frequent monitoring. Similar precautions should be exercised on diuretic withdrawal. Other drugs affecting electrolyte balance, e.g. steroids may alter lithium excretion and should be avoided in patients on lithium. If other psychotropic drugs are used they should be initiated at a lower dosage than usual, as their side effects may be potentiated by the use of lithium. This has been shown to be of particular importance for the concurrent use of lithium and haloperidol or flupenthixol.

Concomitant use with NSAIDs can increase serum lithium concentrations, possibly resulting in lithium toxicity. Serum lithium concentrations should be monitored more frequently if NSAID therapy is initiated or discontinued.

There have been isolated reports of possible interactions between lithium and diazepam (resulting in hypothermia), methyldopa, tetracyclines, phenytoin and carbamazepine, indomethacin and other prostaglandin-synthetase inhibitors.

Pregnancy and lactation: There is epidemiological evidence that lithium may be harmful to the foetus in human pregnancy.

Total Number of 'Lithium babies' reported	*Total malformed infants*	*Ebstein's anomaly and other major cardiovascular malformations*
225	25 (11%)	18 (8%)

It is strongly recommended that lithium be discontinued before a planned pregnancy. If it is considered essential to maintain treatment with Priadel Liquid during pregnancy, serum lithium levels should be monitored closely since renal function changes gradually during pregnancy and suddenly at parturition, requiring dosage adjustments. It is recommended that lithium be discontinued shortly before delivery and recommenced a few days post-partum.

Babies may show signs of lithium toxicity necessitating fluid therapy in the neonatal period. Babies born with low serum lithium concentrations may have a flaccid appearance which returns to normal without any treatment. Lithium is secreted in breast milk, therefore bottle feeding is recommended.

Effects on ability to drive and use machines: None stated.

Undesirable effects: Side effects are usually related to serum lithium concentrations and are infrequent at levels below 1.0 mmol/l.

Mild gastrointestinal effects, nausea, vertigo, muscle weakness and a dazed feeling may occur initially, but frequently disappear after stabilisation. Fine hand tremors, polyuria and mild thirst may persist. Weight gain or oedema may be present in some patients but should not be treated with diuretics.

Hypercalcaemia, hypermagnesaemia and hyperparathyroidism have been reported. Skin conditions including acne, psoriasis, generalised pustular psoriasis, rashes and leg ulcers have occasionally been reported as being aggravated by lithium treatment.

Long term treatment with lithium may be associated with disturbances of thyroid function, including goitre, hypothyroidism and thyrotoxicosis. Lithium-induced hypothyroidism may be managed successfully with concurrent thyroxine. Memory impairment may occur during long term use.

Nephrotoxicity: Up to one third of patients on lithium may develop polyuria with a urinary output of up to three litres per day. This is usually due to lithium blocking the effect of ADH and is reversible on lithium withdrawal. However, long term treatment with lithium may also result in permanent changes in kidney histology and impairment of renal function. High serum concentrations of lithium including episodes of acute lithium toxicity may aggravate these changes. The minimum clinically effective dose of lithium should always be used. In patients who develop polyuria or polydipsia, renal function should be monitored, e.g. with measurement of blood urea, serum creatinine and urinary protein levels in addition to the routine serum lithium estimations.

After a period lasting 3–5 years, patients should be carefully assessed to ensure that benefit persists.

Toxic effects: Such effects are indicative of impending lithium intoxication and fall into two groups:

(1) Gastrointestinal: increasing anorexia, diarrhoea and vomiting.

(2) Central nervous system: muscle weakness, lack of coordination, drowsiness or lethargy progressing to giddiness with ataxia, tinnitus, blurred vision, dysarthria, coarse tremor and muscle twitching.

At blood levels above 2–3 mmol/l there may be a large output of dilute urine, with increasing disorientation, seizures, coma and death. Patients should be instructed to stop taking their Priadel Liquid if toxic symptoms appear and to report immediately for a serum lithium estimation.

Overdose: There is no specific antidote to lithium poisoning. In the event of accumulation, lithium should be stopped and serum estimations should be carried out every 6 hours.

Under no circumstances should a diuretic be used. Osmotic diuresis (mannitol or urea infusion) or alkalinisation of the urine (sodium lactate or sodium bicarbonate infusion) should be initiated.

If the serum lithium level is over 4.0 mmol/l, if there is a deterioration in the patient's condition, or if the serum lithium concentration is not falling at a rate corresponding to a half-life of under 30 hours, peritoneal or haemodialysis should be instituted promptly. This should be continued until there is no lithium in the serum or dialysis fluid. Serum lithium levels should be monitored for at least a further week to take account of any possible rebound in serum lithium levels as a result of delayed diffusion from body tissues.

Pharmacological properties

Pharmacodynamic properties: The mode of action of lithium is still not fully understood. However, lithium modifies the production and turnover of certain neurotransmitters, particularly serotonin, and it may also block dopamine receptors.

It modifies concentrations of some electrolytes, particularly calcium and magnesium, and it may reduce thyroid activity.

Pharmacokinetic properties: Lithium has a half-life of about 24 hours although this increases to about 36 hours in the elderly due to a progressive decrease in renal lithium clearance with age. Lithium is 95% eliminated in the urine.

Time to peak serum level for an immediate release product, such as Priadel Liquid, is about 1.5 hours and complete bioavailability would be expected.

Pharmaceutical particulars

List of excipients:

Other ingredients include: Ethanol, keltrol T, saccharin sodium, sorbic acid, citric acid, pineapple flavour, purified water.

Incompatibilities: None known.

Shelf life: Two years.

Special precautions for storage: Store at or below 25°C. Protect from direct sunlight.

Nature and contents of container: Priadel Liquid is supplied in an amber glass bottle fitted with a one-piece polypropylene screw cap. It is available in a pack of 150 ml.

Instructions for use/handling: Dilution of Priadel Liquid is not recommended. There are no special precautions for handling.

Marketing authorisation number PL 15819/0027

Date of first authorisation/renewal of authorisation 1.12.97.

Date of (partial) revision of the text December 1997.

SOLIAN* 50 ▼
SOLIAN* 200 ▼

Qualitative and quantitative composition

50 mg tablet: Active ingredient: Amisulpride (INN) 50 mg per tablet.

200 mg tablet: Active ingredient: Amisulpride (INN) 200 mg per tablet.

Pharmaceutical form Tablet.

Clinical particulars

Therapeutic indications: Solian is indicated for the treatment of acute and chronic schizophrenic disorders, in which positive symptoms (such as delusions, hallucinations, thought disorders) and/or negative symptoms (such as blunted affect, emotional and social withdrawal) are prominent, including patients characterised by predominant negative symptoms.

Posology and method of administration: For acute psychotic episodes, oral doses between 400 mg/d and 800 mg/d are recommended. In individual cases, the daily dose may be increased up to 1200 mg/d. Doses above 1200 mg/d have not been extensively evaluated for safety and therefore should not be used. No specific titration is required when initiating the treatment with Solian. Doses should be adjusted according to individual response.

For patients with mixed positive and negative symptoms, doses should be adjusted to obtain optimal control of positive symptoms.

Maintenance treatment should be established individually with the minimally effective dose.

For patients characterised by predominant negative symptoms, oral doses between 50 mg/d and 300 mg/d are recommended. Doses should be adjusted individually.

Solian can be administered once daily at oral doses up to 300 mg, higher doses should be administered bid.

Elderly: Solian should be used with particular caution because of a possible risk of hypotension or sedation.

Children: Solian is contra-indicated in childen under 15 years of age as its safety has not yet been established.

Renal insufficiency: Solian is eliminated by the renal route. In renal insufficiency, the dose should be reduced to half in patients with creatinine clearance (CR_{CL}) between 30–60 ml/min and to a third in patients with CR_{CL} between 10–30 ml/min.

As there is no experience in patients with severe renal impairment (CR_{CL} < 10 ml/min) particular care is recommended in these patients.

Hepatic insufficiency: Since the drug is weakly metabolised a dosage reduction should not be necessary.

Contra-indications: Hypersensitivity to the active ingredient or to other ingredients of the drug.

Concomitant prolactin-dependent tumours e.g. pituitary gland prolactinomas and breast cancer.

Phaeochromocytoma.

Children under 15 years of age.

Pregnancy or lactation.

Women of childbearing potential unless using adequate contraception.

Special warnings and special precautions for use: As with other neuroleptics, Neuroleptic Malignant Syndrome, characterised by hyperthermia, muscle rigidity, autonomic instability, altered consciousness and elevated CPK, may occur. In the event of hyperthermia, particularly with high daily doses, all antipsychotic drugs including Solian should be discontinued.

Solian is eliminated by the renal route. In cases of severe renal insufficiency, the dose should be decreased and intermittent treatment should be prescribed (see *Posology and method of administration*).

Solian can lower the seizure threshold. Therefore patients with a history of epilepsy should be closely monitored during Solian therapy.

In elderly patients, Solian, like other neuroleptics, should be used with particular caution because of a possible risk of hypotension or sedation.

As with other antidopaminergic agents, caution should be also exercised when prescribing Solian to patients with Parkinson's disease since it may cause worsening of the disease. Solian should be used only if neuroleptic treatment cannot be avoided.

Interaction with other medicaments and other forms of interaction: Solian may enhance the central effects of alcohol.

Caution should be exercised with the concomitant administration of drugs such as: CNS depressants including narcotics, anaesthetics, analgesics, sedative H1 antihistamines, barbiturates, benzodiazepines and other anxiolytic drugs, clonidine and derivatives; antihypertensive drugs and other hypotensive medications; dopamine agonists (e.g. levodopa) since it may attenuate their action.

Pregnancy and lactation:

Pregnancy: In animals, Solian did not show direct reproductive toxicity. A decrease in fertility linked to the pharmacological effects of the drug (prolactin mediated effect) was observed. No teratogenic effects of Solian were noted.

The safety of Solian during human pregnancy has not been established. Therefore, use of the drug is contra-indicated during pregnancy and in women of child bearing potential unless using adequate contraception.

Lactation: It is not known whether Solian is excreted in breast milk, breast-feeding is therefore contra-indicated.

Effects on ability to drive and use machines: Even used as recommended, Solian may affect reaction time so that the ability to drive vehicles or operate machinery can be impaired.

Undesirable effects: The following adverse effects have been observed in controlled clinical trials. It should be noted that in some instances it can be difficult to differentiate adverse events from symptoms of the underlying disease.

Common adverse effects (5–10%): insomnia, anxiety, agitation.

Less common adverse effects (0.1–5%): somnolence, gastrointestinal disorders such as constipation, nausea, vomiting, dry mouth.

In common with other neuroleptics: Solian causes an increase in plasma prolactin levels which is reversible after drug discontinuation. This may result in galactorrhoea, amenorrhoea, gynaecomastia, breast pain, orgasmic dysfunction and impotence.

Weight gain may occur under therapy with Solian.

Acute dystonia (spasm torticolis, oculogyric crisis, trismus) may appear. This is reversible without discontinuation of Solian upon treatment with an antiparkinsonian agent.

Extrapyramidal symptoms may occur: tremor, rigidity, hypokinesia, hypersalivation, akathisia. These symptoms are generally mild at optimal dosages and partially reversible without discontinuation of Solian upon administration of antiparkinsonian medication. The incidence of extrapyramidal symptoms which is dose related, remains very low in the treatment of patients with predominantly negative symptoms with doses of 50–300 mg/day.

Tardive dyskinesia characterised by rhythmic, involuntary movements primarily of the tongue and/or face have been reported, usually after long term administration. Antiparkinsonian medication is ineffective or may induce aggravation of the symptoms.

Hypotension and bradycardia have been reported occasionally as well as an isolated case of QT prolongation.

Allergic reactions and cases of seizures have been reported occasionally.

Rare cases of Neuroleptic Malignant Syndrome have been reported (see *Special warnings and special precautions for use*).

Overdose: Experience with Solian in overdosage is limited. Exaggeration of the known pharmacological effects of the drug have been reported. These include drowsiness and sedation, coma, hypotension and extrapyramidal symptoms.

In cases of acute overdosage, the possibility of multiple drug intake should be considered. Since Solian is weakly dialysed, hemodialysis should not be used to eliminate the drug. There is no specific antidote to Solian. Appropriate supportive measures should therefore be instituted, close supervision of vital functions and cardiac monitoring is recommended until the patient recovers.

If severe extrapyramidal symptoms occur, anticholinergic agents should be administered.

Pharmacological properties

Pharmacodynamic properties: Amisulpride binds selectively with a high affinity to human dopaminergic D_2/D_3 receptor subtypes whereas it is devoid of affinity for D_1, D_4 and D_5 receptor subtypes.

Unlike classical and atypical neuroleptics, amisulpride has no affinity for serotonin, ∞-adrenergic, histamine H_1 and cholinergic receptors. In addition, amisulpride does not bind to sigma sites.

In animal studies, at high doses, amisulpride blocks dopamine receptors located in the limbic structures in preference to those in the striatum. At low doses it preferentially blocks pre-synaptic D_2/D_3 receptors, producing dopamine release responsible for its disinhibitory effects.

This pharmacological profile explains the clinical efficacy of Solian against both negative and positive symptoms of schizophrenia.

Pharmacokinetic properties: In man, amisulpride shows two absorption peaks: one which is attained rapidly, one hour post-dose and a second between 3 and 4 hours after administration. Corresponding plasma concentrations are 39±3 and 54±4 ng/ml after a 50 mg dose.

The volume of distribution is 5.8 l/kg, plasma protein binding is low (16%) and no drug interactions are suspected.

Absolute bioavailability is 48%. Amisulpride is weakly metabolised: two inactive metabolites, accounting for approximately 4% of the dose, have been identified. There is no accumulation of amisulpride and its pharmacokinetics remain unchanged after the administration of repeated doses. The elimination half-life of amisulpride is approximately 12 hours after an oral dose.

Amisulpride is eliminated unchanged in the urine. Fifty percent of an intravenous dose is excreted via the urine, of which 90% is eliminated in the first 24 hours. Renal clearance is in the order of 20 l/h or 330 ml/min.

A carbohydrate rich meal (containing 68% fluids) significantly decreases the AUCs, T_{max} and C_{max} of amisulpride but no changes were seen after a high fat meal. However, the significance of these findings in routine clinical use is not known.

Hepatic insufficiency: since the drug is weakly metabolised a dosage reduction should not be necessary in patients with hepatic insufficiency.

Renal insufficiency: The elimination half-life is unchanged in patients with renal insufficiency while systemic clearance is reduced by a factor of 2.5 to 3. The AUC of amisulpride in mild renal failure increased two-fold and almost ten-fold in moderate renal failure (see *Posology and method of administration*). Experience is however limited and there is no data with doses greater than 50 mg.

Amisulpride is very weakly dialysed.

Limited pharmacokinetic data in elderly subjects (>65 years) show that a 10–30% rise occurs in C_{max}, $T_{1/2}$ and AUC after a single oral dose of 50 mg. No data are available after repeat dosing.

Preclinical safety data: An overall review of the completed safety studies indicates that Solian is devoid of any general, organ-specific, teratogenic, mutagenic or carcinogenic risk. Changes observed in rats and dogs at doses below the maximum tolerated dose are either pharmacological effects or are devoid of major toxicological significance under these conditions. Compared with the maximum recommended dosages in man, maximum tolerated doses are 2 and 7 times greater in the rat (200 mg/kg/d) and dog (120 mg/kg/d) respectively in terms of AUC. No carcinogenic risk, relevant to man, was identified in the rat at up to 1.5 to 4.5 times the expected human AUC.

A mouse carcinogenicity study (120 mg/kg/d) and reproductive studies (160, 300 and 500 mg/kg/d respectively in rat, rabbit and mouse) were performed. The exposure of the animals to amisulpride during these latter studies was not evaluated.

Pharmaceutical particulars

List of excipients: Solian 50 mg and 200 mg tablets: potato starch, lactose monohydrate, methylcellulose, colloidal hydrated silica, magnesium stearate.

Incompatibilities: None known.

Shelf life: Solian 50 and Solian 200: 3 years.

Special precautions for storage: Solian 50 and 200: Store in a dry place below 25°C in its original container.

Nature and contents of container:

Solian 50: PVC/aluminium foil blister packs containing 60 or 90 tablets.

Solian 200: PVC/aluminium foil blister packs containing 60 or 90 tablets.

Instructions for use/handling: No special precautions.

Marketing authorisation numbers

Solian 50 PL 15819/0001
Solian 200 PL 15819/0002

Date of first authorisation/renewal of authorisation 11 August 1997.

Date of (partial) revision of the text August 1997.

STILNOCT* 5 mg
STILNOCT* 10 mg

Qualitative and quantitative composition

Stilnoct 5 mg: Round white film coated tablets containing 5 mg zolpidem hemitartrate.

Stilnoct 10 mg: Oblong, white, scored, film-coated tablets, engraved SN 10, containing 10 mg zolpidem hemitartrate.

Pharmaceutical form Coated tablets for oral administration.

Clinical particulars

Therapeutic indications: The short-term treatment of insomnia in situations where the insomnia is debilitating or is causing severe distress for the patient.

Posology and method of administration: Zolpidem acts rapidly and therefore should be taken immediately before retiring, or in bed. The recommended daily dose for adults is 10 mg. Elderly or debilitated patients may be especially sensitive to the effects of zolpidem therefore a 5 mg dose is recommended. These recommended doses should not be exceeded.

As clearance and metabolism of zolpidem is reduced in hepatic impairment, dosage should begin at 5 mg with particular caution being exercised in elderly patients. In adults (under 65 years) dosage may be increased to 10 mg only where the clinical response is inadequate and the drug is well tolerated.

The duration of treatment should usually vary from a few days to two weeks with a maximum of four weeks including tapering off where clinically appropriate.

As with all hypnotics, long-term use is not recommended and a course of treatment should not exceed four weeks.

Zolpidem should not be used in children.

Contra-indications: Zolpidem is contra-indicated in patients with a hypersensitivity to zolpidem, obstructive sleep apnoea, myasthenia gravis, severe hepatic insufficiency, acute pulmonary insufficiency or respiratory depression. Zolpidem should not be prescribed for children or patients with psychotic illness.

Special warnings and special precautions for use: The cause of insomnia should be identified wherever possible and the underlying factors treated before a hypnotic is prescribed. The failure of insomnia to remit after a 7–14 day course of treatment may indicate the presence of a primary psychiatric or physical disorder which should be evaluated.

Use in depression: As with other sedative/hypnotic drugs, zolpidem should be administered with caution in patients exhibiting symptoms of depression. Suicidal tendencies may be present therefore the least amount of drug that is feasible should be supplied to these patients because of the possibility of intentional overdosage by the patient.

Use in patients with a history of drug or alcohol abuse: Extreme caution should be exercised when prescribing for patients with a history of drug or alcohol abuse. These patients should be under careful surveillance when receiving zolpidem or any other hypnotic, since they are at risk of habituation and psychological dependence.

General information relating to effects seen following administration of benzodiazepines and other hypnotic agents which should be taken into account by the prescribing physician are described below.

Tolerance: Some loss of efficacy to the hypnotic effects of short-acting benzodiazepines and benzodiazepine-like agents may develop after repeated use for a few weeks.

Dependence: Use of benzodiazepines or benzodiazepine-like agents may lead to the development of physical and psychological dependence of these products. The risk of dependence increases with dose and duration of treatment; it is also greater in patients with a history of alcohol or drug abuse. Once physical dependence has developed, abrupt termination of treatment will be accompanied by withdrawal symptoms. These may consist of headaches or muscle pain, extreme anxiety and tension, restlessness, confusion and irritability. In severe cases the following symptoms may occur: derealisation, depersonalisation, hyperacusis, numbness and tingling of the extremities, hypersensitivity to light, noise and physical contact, hallucinations or epileptic seizures.

Rebound insomnia: A transient syndrome whereby the symptoms that led to treatment with a benzodiazepine or benzodiazepine-like agent recur in an enhanced form, may occur on withdrawal of hypnotic treatment. It may be accompanied by other reactions including mood changes, anxiety and restlessness.

It is important that the patient should be aware of the possibility of rebound phenomena, thereby minimising anxiety over such symptoms should they occur when the medicinal product is discontinued. Since the risk of withdrawal phenomena or rebound has been shown to be greater after abrupt discontinuation of treatment, it is recommended that the dosage is decreased gradually where clinically appropriate.

There are indications that, in the case of benzodiazepines and benzodiazepine-like agents with a short duration of action, withdrawal phenomena can become manifest within the dosage interval, especially when the dosage is high.

Amnesia: Benzodiazepines and benzodiazepine-like agents may induce anterograde amnesia. The condition occurs most often several hours after ingesting the product and therefore to reduce the risk patients should ensure that they will be able to have an uninterrupted sleep of 7–8 hours.

Psychiatric and 'paradoxical' reactions: Reactions like restlessness, agitation, irritability, aggressiveness, delusion, rages, nightmares, hallucinations, psychoses, inappropriate behaviour and other adverse behavioural effects are known to occur when using benzodiazepines or benzodiazepine-like agents. Should this occur, use of the product should be discontinued. These reactions are more likely to occur in the elderly.

Interactions with other medicaments and other forms of interaction:

Not recommended: Concomitant intake with alcohol. The sedative effect may be enhanced when the product is used in combination with alcohol. This affects the ability to drive or use machines.

Combination requiring caution: Combination with CNS depressants. Enhancement of the central depressive effect may occur in cases of concomitant use with antipsychotics (neuroleptics), hypnotics, anxiolytics/sedatives, antidepressant agents, narcotic analgesics, antiepileptic drugs, anaesthetics and sedative antihistamines.

In the case of narcotic analgesics enhancement of euphoria may also occur leading to an increase in psychological dependence.

Compounds which inhibit certain hepatic enzymes (particularly cytochrome P450) may enhance the activity of benzodiazepines and benzodiazepine-like agents.

Pregnancy and lactation: Although animal studies

have shown no teratogenic or embryotoxic effects, safety in pregnancy has not been established. As with all drugs zolpidem should be avoided in pregnancy particularly during the first trimester.

If the product is prescribed to a woman of child-bearing potential, she should be warned to contact her physician about stopping the product if she intends to become or suspects that she is pregnant. If, for compelling medical reasons, zolpidem is administered during the late phase of pregnancy, or during labour, effects of the neonate, such as hypothermia, hypotonia and moderate respiratory depression, can be expected due to the pharmacological action of the product. Infants born to mothers who took benzodiazepines or benzodiazepine-like agents chronically during the latter stages of pregnancy may have developed physical dependence and may be at some risk of developing withdrawal symptoms in the postnatal period.

Small quantities of zolpidem appear in breast milk. The use of zolpidem in nursing mothers is, therefore, not recommended.

Effects on ability to drive and use machines: Although studies have shown that during the day following medication with zolpidem, simulated vehicle driving is unaffected, vehicle drivers and machine operators should be warned that, as with other hypnotics, there may be a possible risk of drowsiness the morning after therapy.

Undesirable effects: There is evidence of a dose-relationship for adverse effects associated with zolpidem use, particularly for certain CNS and gastrointestinal events. These occur most frequently in elderly patients.

In clinical trials side effects observed during treatment at doses up to 10 mg included drowsiness, dizziness, diarrhoea, headache, nausea and vertigo.

Daytime drowsiness, dizziness, headache, asthenia, nausea and vomiting occasionally led to withdrawal of treatment in clinical trials of zolpidem.

Memory disturbance (anterograde amnesia), nightmares, nocturnal restlessness, depressive syndrome, episodes of confusion, perceptual disturbances or diplopia, tremor, unsteady gait and falls have been observed very rarely in long-term clinical trials.

Overdose: In reports of overdose with zolpidem alone, impairment of consciousness has ranged from somnolence to light coma. Individuals have fully recovered from zolpidem overdoses up to 400 mg, 40 times the recommended dose.

General symptomatic and supportive measures should be used, along with immediate gastric lavage where appropriate; intravenous fluids should be administered as needed. If there is no advantage in emptying the stomach, activated charcoal should be given to reduce absorption. Sedating drugs should be withheld even if excitation occurs. Use of flumazenil may be considered where serious symptoms are observed.

In the management of overdose with any medicinal product, it should be borne in mind that multiple agents may have been taken.

Pharmacological properties

Pharmacodynamic properties: (GABA-A receptor agonist selective for omega-1-type sub-unit hypnotic agent). Zolpidem is an imidazopyridine which selectively binds the omega-1 receptor subtype (also known as the benzodiazepine-1 subtype) which is the alpha unit of the GABA-A receptor complex. Whereas benzodiazepines non-selectively bind all three omega receptor subtypes, zolpidem preferentially binds the omega-1 subtype. The modulation of the chloride anion channel via this receptor leads to the specific sedative effects demonstrated by zolpidem. These effects are reversed by the benzodiazepine antagonist flumazenil.

In animals: The selective binding of zolpidem to omega-1 receptors may explain the virtual absence at hypnotic doses of myorelaxant and anti-convulsant effects in animals which are normally exhibited by benzodiazepines which are not selective for omega-1 sites.

In humans: The preservation of deep sleep (stages 3 and 4 – slow-wave sleep) may be explained by the selective omega-1 binding by zolpidem. All identified effects of zolpidem are reversed by the benzodiazepine antagonist flumazenil.

Pharmacokinetic properties: Zolpidem has both a rapid absorption and onset of hypnotic action. Bioavailability is 70% following oral administration and demonstrates linear kinetics in the therapeutic dose range. Peak plasma concentration is reached at between 0.5 and 3 hours.

The elimination half-life is short, with a mean of 2.4 hours (0.7–3.5) and a duration of action of up to 6 hours.

Protein binding amounts to 92.5%±0.1%. First pass metabolism by the liver amounts to approximately 35%. Repeated administration has been shown not to modify protein binding indicating a lack of competition between zolpidem and its metabolites for binding sites. The distribution volume in adults is 0.54±0.02 L/kg and decreases to 0.34±0.05 L/kg in the very elderly.

All metabolites are pharmacologically inactive and are eliminated in the urine (56%) and in the faeces (37%).

Zolpidem has been shown in trials to be non-dialysable.

Plasma concentrations in elderly subjects and those with hepatic impairment are increased. In patients with renal insufficiency, whether dialysed or not, there is a moderate reduction in clearance. The other pharmacokinetic parameters are unaffected.

Preclinical safety data: No data of therapeutic relevance.

Pharmaceutical particulars

List of excipients: Tablet core: lactose, microcrystalline cellulose, methylhydroxypropylcellulose, sodium starch glycollate, magnesium stearate. Film coating: methylhydroxypropylcellulose, titanium dioxide (E171), polyoxyethyleneglycol 400.

Incompatibilities: None known.

Shelf life: 3 years.

Special precautions for storage: Store in a dry place below 30°C.

Nature and contents of container: Stilnoct 5 mg: Cartons of 28 tablets in PVC/foil blister strips. Stilnoct 10 mg: Cartons of 4 or 28 tablets in PVC/foil blister strips.

Instructions for use/handling: Please consult the package insert before use. Do not use after the stated expiry date on the carton and blister. Keep out of the reach of children.

Marketing authorisation numbers
Stilnoct 5 mg 15819/0017
Stilnoct 10 mg 15819/0018.

Date of first authorisation/renewal of authorisation
Stilnoct: 5 mg 16.12.93
Stilnoct: 10 mg 16.09.96.

Date of approval/revision of SPC 21 January 1997.

Legal category POM.

TILDIEM* TABLETS 60 mg

Presentation Off-white biconvex tablets, engraved Tildiem 60. Each tablet contains 60 mg of diltiazem hydrochloride in a modified release formulation.

Uses

Mode of action: Tildiem (diltiazem hydrochloride) is a calcium antagonist. It selectively reduces calcium entry through voltage-dependent calcium channels into vascular smooth muscle cells and myocardial cells. This lowers the concentration of intracellular calcium which is available to activate contractile proteins. This action of diltiazem results in dilation of coronary arteries causing an increase in myocardial oxygen supply. It reduces cardiac work by moderating the heart rate and reducing systemic vascular resistance thus reducing oxygen demand.

When Tildiem is given alone or with a beta-blocking agent only slight negative inotropic effects have been reported in patients with preserved ventricular function.

Indication: Angina pectoris.

Dosage and administration

Adults: The usual dose is one tablet (60 mg) three times daily. However, patient responses may vary and dosage requirements can differ significantly between individual patients. If necessary the dosage may be increased to 360 mg/day. Higher doses up to 480 mg/day have been used with benefit in some patients especially in unstable angina. There is no evidence of any decrease in efficacy at these high doses.

Elderly and patients with impaired hepatic or renal function: The recommended starting dose is one tablet (60 mg) twice daily. The heart rate should be measured regularly in these groups of patients and the dose should not be increased if the heart rate falls below 50 beats per minute.

Children: Safety and efficacy in children have not been established.

Contra-indications, warnings, etc

Contra-indications: Tildiem is contra-indicated in pregnancy and in women of child-bearing potential.

Tildiem depresses atrioventricular node conduction and is therefore contra-indicated in patients with marked bradycardia, sick sinus syndrome, left ventricular failure with stasis, or second or third degree AV block except in the presence of a functioning pacemaker.

Tildiem, like any calcium antagonist, should not be administered concurrently with dantrolene infusion because of the risk of ventricular fibrillation.

Warnings and precautions: Tildiem should be used with caution in patients with reduced left ventricular function. Patients with mild bradycardia, first degree AV block or prolonged PR interval should be observed closely.

Drug interactions: In common with other calcium antagonists, when Tildiem is used with drugs which may induce bradycardia or with antiarrhythmic or other antihypertensive drugs the possibility of an additive effect should be borne in mind.

Case reports have suggested that blood levels of carbamazepine, cyclosporin, and theophylline may be increased when given concurrently with diltiazem hydrochloride. Care should be exercised in patients taking these drugs. In common with other calcium antagonists Tildiem may cause small increases in plasma levels of digoxin.

In patients taking H_2 antagonists concurrently with Tildiem there may be increased levels of diltiazem.

Tildiem has been used safely in combination with beta-blockers, diuretics, ACE inhibitors and other antihypertensive agents. It is recommended that patients receiving these combinations should be regularly monitored. Concomitant use of Tildiem with alpha blockers such as prazosin should be strictly monitored because of the possible synergistic hypotensive effect of this combination.

Diltiazem hydrochloride treatment has been continued without problem during anaesthesia, but the anaesthetist should be informed that the patient is receiving a calcium antagonist.

Pregnancy: Diltiazem hydrochloride is teratogenic in some animal species. In the absence of adequate evidence of safety in human pregnancy, Tildiem should not be used in pregnancy or in women of child bearing potential.

Nursing mothers: Diltiazem hydrochloride is excreted in breast milk. One report suggests that concentrations in breast milk reach similar levels to those in serum. If use of Tildiem is considered essential, an alternative method of infant feeding should be instituted.

Adverse effects: Adverse effects are generally mild and transient and are most commonly vasodilatory related events. The following have been described: lower limb oedema, headache, hot flushes/flushing, asthenia/fatigue, palpitations, malaise, minor gastro-intestinal disorders (dyspepsia, abdominal pain, dry mouth) and skin rash. Vasodilatory related events (in particular, oedema) are dose-dependent and appear to be more frequent in elderly subjects.

Rare cases of symptomatic bradycardia, sino-atrial block and atrioventricular block were also recorded.

Experience with diltiazem has shown that skin rashes such as cases of simple erythema, urticaria or occasionally desquamative erythema with or without fever are usually localised and regress when treatment is discontinued. However, erythema multiforme and vasculitis have been reported occasionally.

Isolated cases of moderate and transient elevation of liver transaminases have been observed at the start of treatment. Isolated cases of clinical hepatitis have been reported which resolved on cessation of therapy.

Overdosage: The clinical consequences of overdose can be severe hypotension leading to collapse, and sinus bradycardia which may be accompanied by isorhythmic dissociation and atrioventricular conduction disturbances. Observation in a coronary care unit is advisable. Vasopressors such as adrenaline may be indicated in patients exhibiting profound hypotension. Calcium gluconate may help reverse the effects of calcium entry blockade. Atropine administration and temporary cardiac pacing may be required to manage bradycardia and/or conduction disturbances.

Pharmaceutical precautions Store in a dry place below 30°C (86°F).

Legal category POM.

Package quantities Packs of 90 tablets containing blister strips of 10 tablets.

Further information Diltiazem hydrochloride is effective in angina, protecting the heart against ischaemia, vasodilating coronary arteries and reducing myocardial oxygen requirements. It is well tolerated and does not generally give rise to side effects associated with peripheral vasodilators, nor cause significant myocardial depression.

In pharmacokinetic studies in healthy volunteers, diltiazem was well absorbed. Peak plasma concentrations were reached 3 to 4 hours after dosing. Due to a first pass effect the bioavailability of the Tildiem tablet is about 50%. Mean apparent plasma half life is 5 hours. Diltiazem in plasma is 80–85% protein bound and is poorly dialysed. Diltiazem is extensively metabolised by the liver. The two major active circulating metabolites, desacetyl diltiazem and N-monodemethyl diltiazem possess pharmacological activity equivalent to about 50% of that of diltiazem. Only 0.2 to 4% of diltiazem is found unchanged in the urine.

There is a linear relationship between dose and

plasma concentration. During long-term administration in any one patient plasma concentrations of diltiazem remained constant.

Product licence number 15819/0028.

TILDIEM* LA 200
TILDIEM* LA 300

Qualitative and quantitative composition Each capsule contains a combination of immediate-release and sustained-release pellets with 200 mg or 300 mg diltiazem hydrochloride as the active ingredient.

Pharmaceutical form Opaque capsules for oral administration with a grey body and pink cap (Tildiem LA 200) or white body and yellow cap (Tildiem LA 300).

Clinical particulars
Therapeutic indications: Mild to moderate hypertension and angina pectoris.

Posology and method of administration: Tildiem LA 200 and Tildiem LA 300 are sustained release products for once daily dosing. The capsules should not be chewed but swallowed whole with water, ideally before or during a meal. The dosage requirements may differ in patients with angina or hypertension.

Tildiem (diltiazem hydrochloride) is available in a range of presentations to enable dosage to be adjusted to meet the individual requirements of the patient. Careful titration of the dose should be considered where appropriate, as individual patient response may vary. When changing from one type of Tildiem formulation to another it may be necessary to adjust the dosage until a satisfactory response is obtained. To ensure consistency of response once established, particularly in the sustained release formulations, Tildiem LA 200 and 300 should continue to be prescribed by brand name.

Adults:

Angina and hypertension: the usual starting dose is Tildiem LA 300 once daily. This dose may be increased to 2 capsules of Tildiem LA 200 daily (400 mg), and if clinically indicated a higher dose of one Tildiem LA 300 plus one Tildiem LA 200 capsule (total 500 mg) may be considered.

Elderly and patients with impaired hepatic or renal function: Heart rate should be monitored and if it falls below 50 beats per minute the dose should not be increased. Plasma levels of diltiazem can be increased in this group of patients.

Angina and hypertension: the initial dose should be one Tildiem LA 200 capsule daily. This dose may be increased to one capsule of Tildiem LA 300 daily if clinically indicated.

Children: Safety and efficacy in children have not been established.

Contra-indications: Sick sinus syndrome, 2nd or 3rd degree AV block in patients not fitted with a pacemaker.

Severe bradycardia (less than 50 beats per minute).

Left ventricular failure with pulmonary stasis.

Pregnancy, women of childbearing potential and lactation.

Concurrent use with dantrolene infusion.

Special warnings and special precautions for use: Close observation is necessary in patients with reduced left ventricular function, bradycardia (risk of exacerbation) or with a 1st degree AV block or prolonged PR interval detected on the electrocardiogram (risk of exacerbation and rarely, of complete block). Plasma diltiazem concentrations can be increased in the elderly and patients with renal or hepatic insufficiency. The contraindications and precautions should be carefully observed and close monitoring, particularly of heart rate and the electrocardiogram, should be carried out at the beginning of treatment.

In the case of general anaesthesia, the anaesthetist must be informed that the patient is taking diltiazem.

Interaction with other medicaments and other forms of interaction: Combination contra-indicated for safety reasons: *Dantrolene* (infusion): The combination of a calcium antagonist and dantrolene is potentially dangerous because of the risk of ventricular fibrillation and this combination should not be used.

Combinations requiring caution:

Alpha$_1$-antagonists: Increased hypotensive effect. Concomitant treatment with alpha$_1$ antagonists should be considered only with strict monitoring of blood pressure.

Beta-blockers: Possibility of rhythm disturbances (pronounced bradycardia, sinus arrest), sino-atrial and atrioventricular conduction disturbances and heart failure (synergistic effect). Such a combination must only be used under close clinical and ECG monitoring, particularly at the beginning of treatment.

Digoxin: Increased risk of bradycardia; caution is required when digoxin is combined with diltiazem, particularly in elderly subjects and when high doses are used.

Antiarrhythmic agents: Since diltiazem has antiarrhythmic properties, its concomitant prescription with other antiarrhythmic agents is not recommended due to the risk of increased adverse effects on the heart due to an additive effect. This combination is not without problems and should only be used under close clinical and ECG monitoring.

Nitrate derivatives: Increased hypotensive effects and faintness (additive vasodilating effects). In all patients treated with calcium antagonists, the prescription of nitrate derivatives should only be carried out at gradually increasing doses.

Cyclosporin: Increase in circulating cyclosporin levels. It is recommended that the cyclosporin dose be reduced, renal function be monitored, circulating cyclosporin levels be assayed and that the dose should be adjusted during combined therapy and after its discontinuation.

Carbamazepine: Increase in circulating carbamazepine levels.

Theophylline: Increase in circulating theophylline levels.

H_2 antagonists (cimetidine and ranitidine): Increase in plasma diltiazem concentrations.

Use during pregnancy and lactation: Pregnancy: this drug has been shown to be teratogenic in certain animal species and is therefore contraindicated in pregnancy and in women of child-bearing potential.

Breast feeding: as this drug is excreted in breast milk, breast feeding whilst taking diltiazem should be avoided.

Effects on ability to drive and use machines: No effect reported to date.

Undesirable effects: Adverse effects are generally mild and transient and are most commonly vasodilatory related events. The following have been described: lower limb oedema, headache, hot flushes/flushing, asthenia/fatigue, palpitations, malaise, minor gastrointestinal disorders (dyspepsia, abdominal pain, dry mouth) and skin rash. Vasodilatory related events (in particular oedema) are dose-dependent and appear to be more frequent in the elderly.

Rare cases of symptomatic bradycardia and sinoatrial block and atrioventricular block were also recorded.

Experience with diltiazem has shown that skin rashes such as cases of simple erythema, urticaria, or occasionally desquamative erythema, with or without fever are usually localised and regress when treatment is discontinued.

However, erythema multiforme and vasculitis have been reported occasionally.

Isolated cases of moderate and transient elevation of liver transaminases have been observed at the start of treatment. Isolated cases of clinical hepatitis have been reported which resolved on cessation of therapy.

Overdose: The clinical effects of acute overdose can involve pronounced hypotension leading to collapse, sinus bradycardia with or without isorhythmic dissociation, and atrioventricular conduction disturbances.

Treatment, under hospital supervision, will include gastric lavage, osmotic diuresis. Conduction disturbances may be managed by temporary pacing.

Proposed antidotes: atropine, adrenaline, glucagon or calcium gluconate.

Pharmacological properties Calcium antagonist, antihypertensive agent.

Pharmacodynamic properties: Diltiazem restricts calcium entry into the slow calcium channel of vascular smooth muscle and myocardial muscle fibres in a voltage-dependent manner. By this mechanism, diltiazem reduces the concentration of intracellular calcium in contractile protein.

In animals diltiazem increases coronary blood flow without inducing any coronary steal phenomena. It acts both on small, large and collateral arteries. This vasodilator effect, which is moderate on peripheral systemic arterial territories, can be seen at doses that are not negatively inotropic.

The two major active circulating metabolites, i.e. deacetyl diltiazem and N-monodemethyl diltiazem, possess pharmacological activity in angina corresponding to 10 and 20% respectively of that of the parent compound.

In humans diltiazem increases coronary blood flow by reducing coronary resistance.

Due to its moderate bradycardia-inducing activity and the reduction in systemic arterial resistance, diltiazem reduces cardiac workload.

Tildiem LA does not have a significant myocardial depressant action in man.

Pharmacokinetic particulars: Diltiazem is well absorbed (90%) in healthy volunteers following chronic oral administration. The sustained release capsule provides prolonged absorption of the active constituent, producing steady state plasma concentrations between 2 and 14 hours post-dose, during which time peak plasma levels occur.

Bioavailability of Tildiem LA relative to the Tildiem 60 mg formulation is approximately 80%. The mean apparent plasma half-life is 8 hours.

Diltiazem in plasma is 80 to 85% protein bound and is poorly dialysed. It is extensively metabolised by the liver.

The major circulating metabolites, deacetyl diltiazem and N-monodemethyl diltiazem, possess pharmacological activity equivalent to about 50% that of diltiazem.

Only 0.7 to 5% of diltiazem is found unchanged in the urine.

There is a linear relationship between dose and plasma concentration. During long term administration in any one patient, plasma concentrations of diltiazem remained constant. Mean plasma concentrations in the elderly and patients with renal and hepatic insufficiency are higher than in young subjects.

Preclinical safety data: No data of therapeutic relevance.

Pharmaceutical particulars
List of excipients

Tildiem LA 200: microcrystalline cellulose, acrylic and methacrylic esters copolymer, ethylcellulose, sodium carboxymethylcellulose, diacetylated monoglycerides, magnesium stearate. *In the capsule:* gelatin, black iron oxide (E172), red iron oxide (E172), titanium dioxide (E171).

Tildiem LA 300: microcrystalline cellulose, acrylic and methacrylic esters copolymer, ethylcellulose, sodium carboxymethylcellulose, diacetylated monoglycerides, magnesium stearate. *In the capsule:* gelatin, titanium dioxide (E171), yellow iron oxide (E172).

Incompatibilities: Not applicable.

Shelf life: Three years (Tildiem LA 200). Two years (Tildiem LA 300).

Special precautions for storage: To be stored below 25°C.

Nature and contents of container: 28 capsules, in a PVC/foil blister strip.

Instructions for use: Please consult the package insert before use. Do not use after the stated expiry date on the carton and blister strip. Keep out of the reach of children.

Marketing authorisation numbers
Tildiem LA 200 15819/0032
Tildiem LA 300 15819/0031.

Date of approval/revision of SPC January 1998.

Legal category POM.

TILDIEM RETARD* 90 mg
TILDIEM RETARD* 120 mg

Qualitative and quantitative composition Each tablet contains 90 mg or 120 mg diltiazem hydrochloride as the active ingredient.

Pharmaceutical form Off white biconvex sustained release tablet for oral administration.

Clinical particulars
Therapeutic indications: Mild to moderate hypertension and angina pectoris.

Posology and method of administration: Tildiem Retard tablets should be swallowed with a little water and not chewed.

Patients should be advised that the tablet membrane may pass through the gastro-intestinal tract unchanged.

Tildiem (diltiazem hydrochloride) is available in a range of presentations to enable dosage to be adjusted to meet the individual requirements of the patient. Careful titration of the dose should be considered where appropriate, as individual patient response may vary. When changing from one type of Tildiem formulation to another it may be necessary to adjust the dosage until a satisfactory response is obtained. To ensure consistency of response once established, particularly in the sustained release formulations, Tildiem Retard 90 mg and 120 mg should continue to be prescribed by brand name.

Adults: Angina and hypertension: The usual starting dose is one tablet (90 mg or 120 mg) twice daily. Patient responses may vary and dosage requirements can differ significantly between individual patients. Higher divided doses up to 480 mg/day have been used with benefit in some angina patients especially in unstable angina. Doses of 360 mg/day may be required to provide adequate BP control in hypertensive patients.

Elderly and patients with impaired hepatic or renal function: Heart rate should be monitored in these patients and if it falls below 50 beats per minute the dose should not be increased.

Angina: The recommended starting dose is one

Tildiem 60 mg tablet twice daily. This dose may be increased to one 90 mg or 120 mg Tildiem Retard tablet twice daily.

Hypertension: The starting dose should be one 120 mg Tildiem Retard tablet daily. Dose adjustment to one 90 mg or one 120 mg Tildiem Retard tablet twice daily may be required.

Children: Safety and efficacy in children have not been established.

Contra-indications: Tildiem Retard is contra-indicated in pregnancy and in women of child bearing potential.

Tildiem Retard depresses atrioventricular node conduction and is therefore contraindicated in patients with marked bradycardia, sick sinus syndrome, left ventricular failure with stasis or second or third degree AV block except in the presence of a functioning pacemaker.

Tildiem Retard, like any calcium antagonist, should not be administered concurrently with dantrolene infusion because of the risk of ventricular fibrillation.

Special warnings and special precautions for use: Tildiem Retard should be used with caution in patients with reduced left ventricular function. Patients with mild bradycardia, first degree AV block or a prolonged PR interval should be observed closely. Diltiazem does not affect the glucose or endogenous insulin responses to hypoglycaemia.

Interaction with other medicaments and other forms of interaction: In common with other calcium antagonists, when Tildiem Retard is used with drugs which may induce bradycardia or with other antiarrhythmic or antihypertensive drugs, the possibility of an additive effect should be borne in mind.

Tildiem Retard has been used safely in combination with beta-blockers, diuretics, ace inhibitors and other antihypertensive agents. It is recommended that patients receiving these combinations should be regularly monitored. Particular care should be taken with the combination diltiazem and a beta-blocker. Concomitant use of Tildiem Retard with alpha blockers such as prazosin should be strictly monitored because of the possible synergistic hypotensive effect of this combination.

Case reports have suggested that blood levels of carbamazepine, cyclosporin, and theophylline may be increased when given concurrently with diltiazem hydrochloride. Care should be exercised in patients taking these drugs. In common with other calcium antagonists Tildiem Retard may cause small increases in plasma levels of digoxin.

In patients taking H_2 antagonists concurrently with Tildiem Retard there may be increased levels of diltiazem.

Diltiazem hydrochloride treatment has been continued without problem during anaesthesia, but the anaesthetist should be informed that the patient is receiving a calcium antagonist.

Use during pregnancy and lactation: Diltiazem hydrochloride is teratogenic in some animal species. In the absence of adequate evidence of safety in human pregnancy, Tildiem Retard should not be used in pregnancy or in women of child bearing potential.

Diltiazem hydrochloride is excreted in breast milk. One report suggests that concentrations in breast milk reach similar levels to those in serum. If use of Tildiem Retard is considered essential, an alternative method of infant feeding should be instituted.

Effects on ability to drive and use machines: No effect reported to date.

Undesirable effects: Adverse effects are generally mild and transient and are most commonly vasodilatory related events. The following have been described: lower limb oedema, headache, hot flushes/flushing, asthenia/fatigue, palpitations, malaise, minor gastro-intestinal disorders (dyspepsia, abdominal pain, dry mouth) and skin rash. Vasodilatory related events (in particular oedema) are dose-dependent and appear to be more frequent in elderly subjects.

Rare cases of symptomatic bradycardia, sino-atrial block and atrioventricular block were also recorded.

Experience with diltiazem has shown that skin rashes such as cases of simple erythema, urticaria, or occasionally desquamative erythema, with or without fever are usually localised and regress when treatment is discontinued. However, erythema multiforme and vasculitis have been reported occasionally.

Isolated cases of moderate and transient elevation of liver transaminases have been observed at the start of treatment. Isolated cases of clinical hepatitis have been reported which resolved on cessation of therapy.

Overdose: The clinical consequences of overdose can be severe hypotension leading to collapse, and sinus bradycardia which may be accompanied by isorhythmic dissociation and atrioventricular conduction disturbances. Observation in a coronary care unit is advisable. Vasopressors such as adrenaline may be indicated in patients exhibiting profound hypotension. Calcium gluconate may help reverse the effects of calcium entry blockade. Atropine administration and temporary cardiac pacing may be required to manage bradycardia and/or conduction disturbances.

Pharmacological properties

Pharmacodynamic properties: Tildiem is a calcium antagonist. It restricts the slow channel entry of calcium into the cell and so reduces the liberation of calcium from stores in the sarcoplasmic reticulum. This results in a reduction of the amount of available intracellular calcium reducing myocardial oxygen consumption. It increases exercise capacity and improves all indices of myocardial ischaemia in the angina patient. Tildiem relaxes large and small coronary arteries and relieves the spasm of vasospastic (Prinzmetal's) angina and the response to catecholamines but has little effect on the peripheral vasculature. There is therefore no possibility of reflex tachycardia. A small reduction in heart rate occurs which is accompanied by an increase in cardiac output, improved myocardial perfusion and reduction of ventricular work. In animal studies, Tildiem protects the myocardium against the effects of ischaemia and reduces the damage produced by excessive entry of calcium into the myocardial cell during reperfusion.

Pharmacokinetic particulars: In pharmacokinetic studies in healthy volunteers, diltiazem was well absorbed. Peak plasma concentrations were reached approximately 4 to 8 hours after dosing. Diltiazem in plasma is 80–85% protein bound and is poorly dialysed. Diltiazem is extensively metabolised by the liver. The two major active circulating metabolites, deacetyl diltiazem and N-monodemethyl diltiazem possess pharmacological activity in angina equivalent to about 50% of that of diltiazem. Only 0.2–4% of diltiazem is found unchanged in the urine.

Preclinical safety data: No data of therapeutic relevance.

Pharmaceutical particulars

List of excipients: Tablet core: Sodium dihydrogen citrate, sucrose powdered, povidone, magnesium stearate, polyethylene glycol 6000 powder. Coating: Sucrose powdered, coating polymer, acetate tributyl citrate, castor oil polymerised, sodium bicarbonate, ethyl vanillin, titanium dioxide (E171).

Incompatibilities: Not applicable.

Shelf-life: Two years.

Special precautions for storage: Store in a dry place below 30°C (86°F). Tildiem Retard tablets are coated with a porous polymer membrane which enables the diltiazem to diffuse out of the tablet at a gradual rate. This membrane may pass through the gastro-intestinal tract unchanged. This has no bearing on the efficacy of the product.

Nature and contents of container: 14 or 56 tablets in PVC/foil strips.

Instructions for use/handling: Please consult the package insert before use. Do not use after the stated expiry date on the carton and blister strip. Keep out of the reach of children.

Marketing authorisation numbers
Tildiem Retard 90 mg 15819/0029
Tildiem Retard 120 mg 15819/0030

Date of approval/revision of SPC December 1997.

Legal category POM.

XATRAL*

Qualitative and quantitative composition Each tablet contains 2.5 mg alfuzosin hydrochloride.

Pharmaceutical form White round, film coated tablet for oral administration.

Clinical particulars

Therapeutic indications: Treatment of the functional symptoms of benign prostatic hypertrophy.

Posology and method of administration: Xatral tablets should be swallowed whole. The first dose should be given just before bedtime.

Adults: The usual dose is one tablet three times daily. The dose may be increased to a maximum of 4 tablets (10 mg) per day depending on the clinical response.

Elderly and treated hypertensive patients: As a routine precaution when prescribing alfuzosin to elderly patients (aged over 65 years) and the treated hypertensive patient, the initial dose should be 1 tablet in the morning and 1 tablet in the evening.

Renal insufficiency: In patients with renal insufficiency, as a precaution, it is recommended that the dosing be started at Xatral 2.5 mg twice daily adjusted according to clinical response.

Hepatic insufficiency: In patients with mild to moderate hepatic insufficiency, it is recommended that therapy should commence with a single dose of Xatral 2.5 mg/day to be increased to Xatral 2.5 mg twice daily according to clinical response.

Contra-indications: Hypersensitivity to the product. History of orthostatic hypotension. Combination with other α-blockers. Severe hepatic insufficiency.

Special warnings and special precautions for use:

Warnings: In some subjects, in particular, patients receiving antihypertensive medications, postural hypotension with or without symptoms (dizziness, fatigue, sweating) may develop within a few hours following administration. In such cases, the patient should lie down until the symptoms have completely disappeared.

These effects are transient and do not usually prevent the continuation of treatment after adjustment of the dose. The patient should be warned of the possible occurrence of such events.

Precautions: Treatment should be initiated gradually in patients with hypersensitivity to α_1-blockers. Xatral should be administered carefully to patients being treated with antihypertensives. Blood pressure should be monitored regularly, especially at the beginning of treatment.

In patients with coronary insufficiency specific antianginal therapy should be continued, but if the angina reappears or worsens Xatral should be discontinued.

Interaction with other medicaments and other forms of interaction: Concomitant use with other α_1-receptor blockers should be avoided and antihypertensive agents should be used with caution because of the risk of a hypotensive effect.

The administration of general anaesthetics to patients receiving Xatral could cause profound hypotension. It is recommended that Xatral be withdrawn 24 hours before surgery.

Other forms of interaction: No pharmacodynamic or pharmacokinetic interaction has been observed in healthy volunteers between alfuzosin and the following drugs: warfarin, digoxin, hydrochlorothiazide and atenolol.

Use during pregnancy and lactation: Due to the type of indication this section is not applicable.

Effects on ability to drive and use machines: There are no data available on the effect on driving vehicles. Adverse reactions such as vertigo, dizziness and asthenia may occur. This has to be taken into account when driving vehicles and operating machinery.

Undesirable effects:

Adverse events: The following side-effects have been observed: faintness, vertigo, dizziness or malaise, headache, gastrointestinal disorders (nausea, gastralgia, diarrhoea). The following occurred less frequently: hypotension (postural), syncope, tachycardia, palpitations, chest pain, asthenia, drowsiness, dry mouth, rash, pruritus, flushes and oedema.

Overdosage: In case of overdosage, the patient should be hospitalised, kept in the supine position, and conventional treatment of hypotension should take place.

Alfuzosin is not easily dialysable because of its high degree of protein binding.

Pharmacological properties

Pharmacodynamic properties: Alfuzosin is an orally active quinazoline derivative. It is a selective, peripherally acting antagonist of post synaptic α_1-adrenoceptors.

In vitro pharmacological studies have documented the selectivity of alfuzosin for the alpha$_1$-adrenoreceptor located in the prostate, bladder base and prostatic urethra.

Clinical manifestations of Benign Prostatic Hypertrophy are associated with infra vesical obstruction which is triggered by both anatomical (static) and functional (dynamic) factors. The functional component of obstruction arises from the tension of prostatic smooth muscle which is mediated by α-adrenoceptors. Activation of α_1-adrenoceptors stimulates smooth muscle contraction, thereby increasing the tone of the prostate, prostatic capsule, prostatic urethra and bladder base, and, consequently, increasing the resistance to bladder outflow. This in turn leads to outflow obstruction and possible secondary bladder instability.

Alpha-blockade decreases infra vesical obstruction via a direct action on prostatic smooth muscle.

In vivo, animal studies have shown that alfuzosin decreases urethral pressure and therefore, resistance to the urine flow during micturition. Moreover, alfuzosin inhibits the hypertonic response of the urethra more readily than that of vascular muscle and shows functional uroselectivity in conscious normotensive rats by decreasing urethral pressure at doses that do not affect blood pressure.

In man, alfuzosin improves voiding parameters by reducing urethral tone and bladder outlet resistance, and facilitates bladder emptying.

In placebo controlled studies in BPH patients, alfuzosin:

- significantly increases peak flow rate (Q_{max}) in patients with $Q_{max} \leq 15$ ml/s by a mean of 30%. This improvement is observed from the first dose,
- significantly reduces the detrusor pressure and

increases the volume producing a strong desire to void,
• significantly reduces the residual urine volume.

These favourable urodynamic effects lead to an improvement of lower urinary tract symptoms i.e. filling (irritative) as well as voiding (obstructive) symptoms.

Alfuzosin may cause moderate antihypertensive effects.

Pharmacokinetic particulars: Xatral is well absorbed with a mean bioavailability of 64%, peak plasma levels are generally reached in 0.5–3 hours. Kinetics within the therapeutic range are linear. The kinetic profile is characterised by large interindividual fluctuations in plasma concentrations. The terminal half-life is 3–5 hours. Alfuzosin is 90% protein bound in plasma, 68.2% to human serum albumin and 52.5% to human serum alpha-glycoprotein. It is partially metabolised and excreted mainly in the bile and faeces.

None of the metabolites found in man has any pharmacodynamic activity. The pharmacokinetic profile is not affected by taking Xatral with food.

In subjects over 75 years, absorption is more rapid and peak plasma levels are higher. Bioavailability may be increased and in some patients the volume of distribution is reduced. The elimination half-life does not change.

The volume of distribution and clearance of alfuzosin are increased in renal insufficiency, with or without dialysis, owing to an increase in the free fraction. Chronic renal insufficiency even when severe (creatinine clearance between 15 and 40 mls/min) is not adversely affected by alfuzosin.

In patients with severe hepatic insufficiency, the elimination half-life is prolonged. A two-fold increase in C_{max} values and a three-fold increase in the AUC is observed. Bioavailability is increased compared with healthy volunteers.

The pharmacokinetic profile of alfuzosin is not affected by chronic cardiac insufficiency.

Preclinical safety data: No data of therapeutic relevance.

Pharmaceutical particulars

List of excipients:

Tablet core: Microcrystalline cellulose, lactose, povidone, sodium starch glycollate, magnesium stearate, purified water.

Coating: Methylhydroxypropylcellulose, polyethylene glycol 400, titanium dioxide suspension (E171), purified water.

Major chemical and physical incompatibilities: Not known.

Shelf life: 3 years.

Special precautions for storage: Store in a dry place at or below 30°C.

Nature and contents of containers: Boxes with 60 or 90 tablets in pvc/foil blister strips.

Instructions for use/handling: Please consult insert text before use. Do not use after the stated expiry date on packaging and blisters. Keep out of the reach of children.

Marketing authorisation number PL 15819/0023

Date of first authorisation 1.9.97

Date of (partial) revision of the text April 1998.

XATRAL* SR

Qualitative and quantitative composition Each tablet contains 5 mg alfuzosin hydrochloride.

Pharmaceutical form Sustained release film coated tablets for oral administration.

Clinical particulars

Therapeutic indications: Treatment of the functional symptoms of benign prostatic hypertrophy.

Posology and method of administration: Xatral SR tablets should be swallowed whole. The first dose should be given just before bedtime.

Adults: Dosage is one tablet Xatral SR 5 mg twice daily (morning and evening).

Elderly (over 65 years), treated hypertensive patients, and patients with renal insufficiency: The initial dose should be 1 tablet Xatral SR 5 mg in the evening. If additional efficacy is required and Xatral SR is well tolerated the patient may be given Xatral SR 5 mg, 1 tablet twice daily.

Hepatic insufficiency: In patients with mild to moderate hepatic insufficiency, it is recommended that therapy should commence with a single dose of Xatral 2.5 mg/day to be increased to Xatral 2.5 mg twice daily according to clinical response.

Contra-indications: Hypersensitivity to the product. History of orthostatic hypotension. Combination with other α-blockers. Severe hepatic insufficiency.

Special warnings and special precautions for use:

Warnings: In some subjects, in particular, patients receiving antihypertensive medications, postural hypotension with or without symptoms (dizziness, fatigue, sweating) may develop within a few hours following administration. In such cases, the patient should lie down until the symptoms have completely disappeared.

These effects are transient and do not usually prevent the continuation of treatment after adjustment of the dose. The patient should be warned of the possible occurrence of such events.

Precautions: Treatment should be initiated gradually in patients with hypersensitivity to α_1-blockers. Xatral SR should be administered carefully to patients being treated with antihypertensives. Blood pressure should be monitored regularly, especially at the beginning of treatment.

In patients with coronary insufficiency specific anti-anginal therapy should be continued, but if the angina reappears or worsens Xatral SR should be discontinued.

Interaction with other medicaments and other forms of interaction: Concomitant use with other α_1-receptor blockers should be avoided and antihypertensive agents should be used with caution because of the risk of a hypotensive effect.

The administration of general anaesthetics to patients receiving Xatral SR could cause profound hypotension. It is recommended that Xatral SR be withdrawn 24 hours before surgery.

Other forms of interaction: No pharmacodynamic or pharmacokinetic interaction has been observed in healthy volunteers between alfuzosin and the following drugs: warfarin, digoxin, hydrochlorothiazide and atenolol.

Use during pregnancy and lactation: Due to the type of indication this section is not applicable.

Effects on ability to drive and use machines: There are no data available on the effect on driving vehicles. Adverse reactions such as vertigo, dizziness and asthenia may occur. This has to be taken into account when driving vehicles and operating machinery.

Undesirable effects:

Adverse events: The following side-effects have been observed: faintness, vertigo, dizziness or malaise, headache, gastrointestinal disorders (nausea, gastralgia, diarrhoea). The following occurred less frequently: hypotension (postural), syncope, tachycardia, palpitations, chest pain, asthenia, drowsiness, dry mouth, rash, pruritus, flushes and oedema.

Overdosage: In case of overdosage, the patient should be hospitalised, kept in the supine position, and conventional treatment of hypotension should take place.

Alfuzosin is not easily dialysable because of its high degree of protein binding.

Pharmacological properties

Pharmacodynamic properties: Alfuzosin is an orally active quinazoline derivative. It is a selective, peripherally acting antagonist of postsynaptic α_1-adrenoceptors.

In vitro pharmacological studies have documented the selectivity of alfuzosin for the alpha$_1$-adrenoreceptor located in the prostate, bladder base and prostatic urethra.

Clinical manifestations of Benign Prostatic Hypertrophy are associated with infra vesical obstruction which is triggered by both anatomical (static) and functional (dynamic) factors. The functional component of obstruction arises from the tension of prostatic smooth muscle which is mediated by α-adrenoceptors. Activation of α_1-adrenoceptors stimulates smooth muscle contraction, thereby increasing the tone of the prostate, prostatic capsule, prostatic urethra and bladder base, and, consequently, increasing the resistance to bladder outflow. This in turn leads to outflow obstruction and possible secondary bladder instability.

Alpha-blockade decreases infra vesical obstruction via a direct action on prostatic smooth muscle.

In vivo, animal studies have shown that alfuzosin decreases urethral pressure and therefore, resistance to the urine flow during micturition. Moreover, alfuzosin inhibits the hypertonic response of the urethra more readily than that of vascular muscle and shows functional uroselectivity in conscious normotensive rats by decreasing urethral pressure at doses that do not affect blood pressure.

In man, alfuzosin improves voiding parameters by reducing urethral tone and bladder outlet resistance, and facilitates bladder emptying.

In placebo controlled studies in BPH patients, alfuzosin:

• significantly increases peak flow rate (Q_{max}) in patients with $Q_{max} \leq 15$ ml/s by a mean of 30%. This improvement is observed from the first dose,
• significantly reduces the detrusor pressure and increases the volume producing a strong desire to void,
• significantly reduces the residual urine volume.

This favourable urodynamic effects lead to an improvement of lower urinary tract symptoms i.e. filling (irritative) as well as voiding (obstructive) symptoms.

Alfuzosin may cause moderate antihypertensive effects.

Pharmacokinetic particulars: The peak plasma level is achieved approximately 3 hours post-dose. The elimination half-life of alfuzosin is 8 hours. Bioavailability is decreased by approximately 15% as compared with Xatral 2.5 mg.

Alfuzosin is well-absorbed. The binding to plasma proteins is about 90%.

Alfuzosin is partially metabolised and excreted mainly in the bile and faeces. None of the metabolites found in man has any pharmacodynamic activity. On a normal diet this pharmacokinetic profile is not affected by taking the drug with food.

In subjects over 75 years, absorption is more rapid and the peak levels are higher. Bioavailability may be increased and in some patients the volume of distribution is reduced. The elimination half-life remains unchanged.

The volume of distribution and clearance of alfuzosin is increased in renal insufficiency, with or without dialysis, owing to an increase in the free fraction. Chronic renal insufficiency even when severe (creatinine clearance between 15 and 40 ml/min), is not adversely affected by alfuzosin.

In patients with severe hepatic insufficiency, the elimination half-life is prolonged. A two-fold increase in C_{max} values and a three-fold increase in the AUC is observed. Bioavailability is increased in comparison with that in healthy volunteers. The pharmacokinetic profile of alfuzosin is not affected by chronic cardiac insufficiency.

Preclinical safety data: No data of therapeutic relevance.

Pharmaceutical particulars

List of excipients:

Tablet core: Microcrystalline cellulose, polyvinyl pyrrolidone, calcium hydrogen phosphate dihydrate, magnesium stearate, hydrogenated castor oil.

Coating: Methylhydroxypropylcellulose, propylene glycol, titanium dioxide (E171), iron oxide (E172).

Major chemical and physical incompatibilities: Not known.

Shelf life: 3 years.

Special precautions for storage: Store at room temperature (15–25°C) in its original pack.

Nature and contents of containers: Boxes with 60 tablets in pvc/foil blister strips.

Instructions for use/handling: Please consult insert text before use. Do not use after the stated expiry date on packaging and blisters. Keep out of the reach of children.

Marketing authorisation number PL 15819/0024

Date of first authorisation 1.9.97

Date of (partial) revision of the text April 1998.

**Trade Mark*

LRC Products Limited

London International House
Turnford Place
Broxbourne
Herts EN10 6LN

☎ 01992 451111 🗋 01992 470133

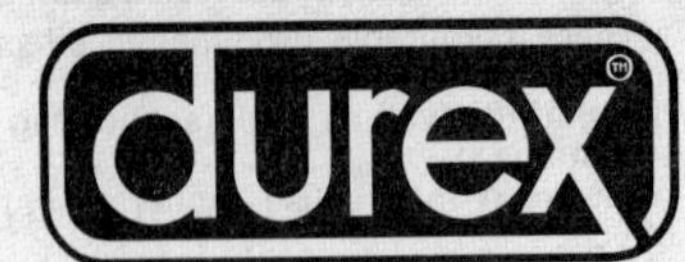

DURAGEL*

Presentation *Duragel:* A colourless unscented gel containing Nonoxynol 9 USP, 2% w/w.

Other constituents: Docusate Sodium BP, Isopropyl Alcohol BP, Propylene Glycol EP, Sodium Hydroxide BP, Carbomer 934P USP, Benzoic Acid EP, Purified Water EP.

Uses Duragel is for use as a spermicidal contraceptive in conjunction with barrier methods of contraception.

Dosage and administration For use only by adult females of child bearing age.

Vaginal diaphragm
At insertion: Two strips (5 cm each) on each side of the diaphragm.At topping up: 1 applicator full (approximately 22 cm strip).

Cervical Cap
At insertion: One 5 ml teaspoonful inside the cap.At topping up: 1 applicator full (approximately 22 cm strip).

All uses: Apply or top up not more than 3 hours before intercourse. Top up between repeated acts of intercourse. Leave in place for at least 6 hours after last intercourse. Do not leave in place for longer than 24 hours.

Contra-indications, warnings, etc
Contra-indications: Hypersensitivity to Nonoxynol 9 or to any component of the preparation. Patients with absent vaginal sensation e.g. paraplegics and quadriplegics.

Undesirable effects: May cause irritation of the vagina or penis.

Use in pregnancy and lactation: There is no evidence from animal and human studies that Nonoxynol 9 is teratogenic. Human epidemiological studies have not shown any firm evidence of adverse effects on the foetus, however some studies have shown that Nonoxynol 9 may be embryotoxic in animals. This product should not be used if pregnancy is suspected or confirmed. Animal studies have detected Nonoxynol 9 in milk after intravaginal administration. Use by lactating women has not been studied.

Other special warnings and precautions: Spermicidal intravaginal preparations are intended for use in conjunction with barrier methods of contraception such as condoms, diaphragms and caps.

Where avoidance of pregnancy is important the choice of contraceptive method should be made in consultation with a doctor or a family planning clinic.

If vaginal or penile irritation occurs discontinue use. If symptoms worsen or continue for more than 48 hours medical advice should be sought.

Overdose: If taken orally the surfactant properties of this preparation may cause gastric irritation. General supportive therapy should be carried out. Hepatic and renal function should be monitored if medically indicated.

Pharmaceutical precautions Store below 30°C. Do not freeze.

Legal category GSL.

Package quantities The product is presented in a collapsible tube containing 100 g. The tubes are supplied in packs of four.

Further information Duragel is suitable for patients requiring extra lubrication in addition to spermicidal action.

Product licence number 2156/5001R

**Trade Mark*

Lundbeck Limited
Sunningdale House
Caldecotte Lake Business Park
Caldecotte, Milton Keynes, MK7 8LF

☎ 01908 649966 🗋 01908 647688

Lundbeck

CIPRAMIL* TABLETS ▼

Qualitative and quantitative composition Tablets of 10, 20 or 40 mg (12.49, 24.98 or 49.96 mg citalopram hydrobromide corresponding to 10, 20 or 40 mg citalopram base).

Pharmaceutical form Tablet.

Clinical particulars
Therapeutic indications: Treatment of depressive illness in the initial phase and as maintenance against potential relapse/recurrence. Cipramil is also indicated in the treatment of panic disorder with or without agoraphobia.

Posology and method of administration
Posology – Treating depression:
Adults: Citalopram should be administered as a single oral dose of 20 mg daily. Dependent on individual patient reponse this may be increased to a maximum of 60 mg daily. The dose may be taken in the morning or evening without regard for food.

Duration of treatment: A treatment period of at least six months is usually necessary to provide adequate maintenance against the potential for relapse.

Treating panic disorder: In common with other pharmacotherapy used in this patient group, a low starting dose is advised to reduce the likelihood of a paradoxical initial anxiogenic effect. A single oral dose of 10 mg daily is recommended for the first week before increasing the dose to 20 mg daily. The dose may be further increased up to a maximum of 60 mg daily dependent on individual patient response; however an optimum dose of 20–30 mg daily was indicated in a clinical study.

Maximum effectiveness of citalopram in treating panic disorder is reached after about 3 months and the response is maintained during continued treatment. Dependent on individual patient response it may be necessary to continue treatment for several months.

Elderly patients: The recommended daily dose is 20 mg. Dependent on individual patient response this may be increased to a maximum of 40 mg daily.

Children: Not recommended, as safety and efficacy have not been established in this population.

Reduced hepatic function: Dosage should be restricted to the lower end of the dose range.

Reduced renal function: Dosage adjustment is not necessary in cases of mild or moderate renal impairment. No information is available in cases of severe renal impairment (creatinine clearance <20 mL/min).

Method of administration: Citalopram tablets are administered as a single daily dose. Citalopram tablets can be taken any time of the day without regard to food intake.

Contra-indications: Hypersensitivity to citalopram. Sumatriptan's serotonergic effects are suspected to be enhanced by SSRIs. Until further evidence is available it is advised not to use citalopram simultaneously with 5-HT agonists e.g. sumatriptan.

Special warnings and special precautions for use: As with other SSRIs, citalopram should not be given to patients receiving Monoamine Oxidase Inhibitors (MAOIs), or for 14 days after their discontinuation. MAOIs should not be introduced for seven days after discontinuation of citalopram. Rarely, the occurrence of 'serotonin syndrome' has been reported in patients receiving SSRIs. A combination of symptoms, possibly including agitation, tremor, myoclonus and hyperthermia, may indicate the development of this condition.

Experience with citalopram has not revealed any clinically relevant interactions with neuroleptics. However, as with other SSRIs, the possibility of a pharmacodynamic interaction cannot be excluded.

Consideration should be given to factors which may affect the disposition of a minor metabolite of citalopram (didemethylcitalopram) since increased levels of this metabolite could theoretically prolong the QTc interval in susceptible individuals. However, in ECG monitoring of 2500 patients in clinical trials, including 277 patients with pre-existing cardiac conditions, no clinically significant changes were noted.

As with most antidepressants, citalopram should be discontinued if the patient enters a manic phase.

There is little clinical experience of concurrent use of citalopram and ECT.

Interactions with other medicaments and other forms of interaction: Monoamine Oxidase Inhibitors (MAOIs) should not be used in combination with SSRIs (see above).

The metabolism of citalopram is only partly dependent on the hepatic cytochrome P450 isozyme CYP2 D6 and, unlike some other SSRIs, citalopram is only a weak inhibitor of this important enzyme system which is involved in the metabolism of many drugs (including antiarrhythmics, neuroleptics, beta-blockers, TCAs and some SSRIs). Protein binding is relatively low (<80%). These properties give citalopram a low potential for clinically significant drug interactions.

There is no pharmacokinetic interaction between lithium and citalopram. However, there have been reports of enhanced serotonergic effects when SSRIs have been given with lithium or tryptophan and therefore the concomitant use of citalopram with these drugs should be undertaken with caution. Routine monitoring of lithium levels need not be adjusted. In a pharmacokinetic study no effect was demonstrated on either citalopram or imipramine levels, although the level of desipramine, the primary metabolite of imipramine, was increased. In animal studies cimetidine had little or no influence on citalopram kinetics.

No pharmacodynamic interactions have been noted in clinical studies in which citalopram has been given concomitantly with benzodiazepines, neuroleptics, analgesics, lithium, alcohol, antihistamines, antihypertensive drugs, beta-blockers and other cardiovascular drugs.

Pregnancy and lactation: Category B1. Animal studies have not shown any evidence of teratogenic potential and citalopram does not affect reproduction or perinatal conditions. Citalopram appears in milk in very low concentrations.

Due to limited human data citalopram should only be used in pregnancy if considered necessary and under the close supervision of a physician. In nursing mothers, caution is recommended as it is not known whether citalopram excreted in milk may affect the infant.

Effects on ability to drive and use machines: Citalopram does not impair intellectual function and psychomotor performance. However, patients who are prescribed psychotropic medication may be expected to have some impairment of general attention and concentration either due to the illness itself, the medication or both and should be cautioned about their ability to drive a car and operate machinery.

Undesirable effects: Adverse effects observed with citalopram are in general mild and transient. They are most prominent during the first one or two weeks of treatment and usually attenuate as the depressive state improves.

The most commonly observed adverse events associated with the use of citalopram and not seen at an equal incidence among placebo-treated patients were: nausea, somnolence, dry mouth, increased sweating and tremor. The incidence of each in excess over placebo is low (<10%).

In comparative clinical trials with tricyclic antidepressants the incidence of adverse events occurring with citalopram was found to be lower in all cases.

Withdrawal reactions have been reported in association with selective serotonin reuptake inhibitors (SSRIs), including cipramil. Common symptoms include dizziness, paraesthesia, headache, anxiety and nausea. Abrupt discontinuation of treatment with cipramil should be avoided. The majority of symptoms experienced on withdrawal of SSRIs are non-serious and self-limiting.

Treatment emergent adverse events reported in clinical trials (N=2985):

Frequent: (≥5–20%) Increased sweating, headache, tremor, dizziness, abnormal accommodation, somnolence, insomnia, agitation, nervousness, nausea, dry mouth, constipation, diarrhoea, palpitation, asthenia.

Less frequent: (1–<5%) Rash, pruritus, paraesthesia, migraine, abnormal vision, taste perversion, sleep disorder, decreased libido, impaired concentration, abnormal dreaming, amnesia, anxiety, increased appetite, anorexia, apathy, impotence, suicide attempt, confusion, yawning, dyspepsia, vomiting, abdominal pain, flatulence, increased salivation, weight decrease, weight increase, postural hypotension, tachycardia, rhinitis, micturition disorder, polyuria, ejaculation failure, female anorgasmia, fatigue.

Rare: (<1%) Myalgia, exrapyramidal disorder, convulsions, tinnitus, euphoria, increased libido, coughing, malaise.

Overdose: Citalopram is given to patients at potential risk of suicide and some reports of attempted suicide have been received. Detail is often lacking regarding precise dose or combination with other drugs and/or alcohol.

Symptoms: Experience from 8 cases considered due to citalopram alone has recorded the following symptoms/signs: somnolence, coma, stiffened expression, episode of grand mal convulsion, sinus tachycardia, occasional nodal rhythm, sweating, nausea, vomiting, cyanosis, hyperventilation. No case was fatal. The clinical picture was inconsistent, no observation being made in more than two individuals.

Six fatalities have been reported. In one overdose was suspected; high post mortem plasma levels were seen although it is not technically possible to interpret these with confidence.

In the remaining five a combination with other drugs had been taken. The clinical syndrome observed prior to death in three of these cases where citalopram was taken with moclobemide was interpreted as that of serotonin syndrome. No clinical details are available on the other two.

Treatment: There is no specific antidote. Treatment is symptomatic and supportive. Gastric lavage should be carried out as soon as possible after oral ingestion. Medical surveillance is advisable.

Pharmacological properties
Pharmacodynamic properties: ATC-code: N 06 AB 04. Biochemical and behavioural studies have shown that citalopram is a potent inhibitor of serotonin (5-HT)-uptake. Tolerance to the inhibition of 5-HT-uptake is not induced by long-term treatment with citalopram.

Citalopram is the most Selective Serotonin Reuptake Inhibitor (SSRI) yet described, with no, or minimal, effect on noradrenaline (NA), dopamine (DA) and gamma aminobutyric acid (GABA) uptake.

In contrast to many tricyclic antidepressants and some of the newer SSRI's, citalopram has no or very low affinity for a series of receptors including 5-HT_{1A}, 5-HT_2, dopamine D_1 and D_2 receptors, alpha1-, alpha2- and beta-adrenoceptors, histamine H_1, muscarine cholinergic, benzodiazepine, and opioid receptors. A series of functional *in vitro* tests in isolated organs as well as functional *in vivo* tests have confirmed the lack of receptor affinity. This absence of effects on receptors could explain why citalopram produces fewer of the traditional side effects such as dry mouth, bladder and gut disturbance, blurred vision, sedation, cardiotoxicity and orthostatic hypotension.

Suppression of rapid eye movement (REM) sleep is considered a predictor of antidepressant activity. Like tricyclic antidepressants, other SSRI's and MAO inhibitors, citalopram suppresses REM-sleep and increases deep slow-wave sleep.

Although citalopram does not bind to opioid receptors it potentiates the anti-nociceptive effect of commonly used opioid analgesics. There was potentiation of d-amphetamine-induced hyperactivity following administration of citalopram.

The main metabolites of citalopram are all SSRIs although their potency and selectivity ratios are lower than those of citalopram. However, the selectivity ratios of the metabolites are higher than those of many of the newer SSRIs. The metabolites do not contribute to the overall antidepressant effect.

In humans citalopram does not impair cognitive (intellectual function) and psychomotor performance and has no or minimal sedative properties, either alone or in combination with alcohol.

Citalopram did not reduce saliva flow in a single dose study in human volunteers and in none of the studies in healthy volunteers did citalopram have significant influence on cardiovascular parameters. Citalopram has no effect on the serum levels of prolactin and growth hormone.

Pharmacokinetic properties

Absorption: Absorption is almost complete and independent of food intake (T_{max} average/mean 3.8 hours). Oral bioavailability is about 80%.

Distribution: The apparent volume of distribution $(V_d)_\beta$ is about 12.3 L/kg. The plasma protein binding is below 80% for citalopram and its main metabolites.

Biotransformation: Citalopram is metabolised to the active demethylcitalopram, didemethylcitalopram, citalopram-N-oxide and an inactive deaminated propionic acid derivative. All the active metabolites are also SSRIs, although weaker than the parent compound. Unchanged citalopram is the predominant compound in plasma.

Elimination: The elimination half-life ($T_{1/2\beta}$) is about 1.5 days and the systemic citalopram plasma clearance (Cl_S) is about 0.33 L/min, and oral plasma clearance (Cl_{oral}) is about 0.41 L/min.

Citalopram is excreted mainly via the liver (85%) and the remainder (15%) via the kidneys. About 12% of the daily dose is excreted in urine as unchanged citalopram. Hepatic (residual) clearance is about 0.35 L/min and renal clearance about 0.068 L/min.

The kinetics is linear. Steady state plasma levels are achieved in 1–2 weeks. Average concentrations of 250 nmol/L (100–500 nmol/L) are achieved at a daily dose of 40 mg. There is no clear relationship between citalopram plasma levels and therapeutic response or side effects.

Elderly patients (≥65 years): Longer half-lives and decreased clearance values due to a reduced rate of metabolism have been demonstrated in elderly patients.

Reduced hepatic function: Citalopram is eliminated more slowly in patients with reduced hepatic function. The half-life of citalopram is about twice as long and steady state citalopram concentrations at a given dose will be about twice as high as in patients with normal liver function.

Reduced renal function: Citalopram is eliminated more slowly in patients with mild to moderate reduction of renal function, without any major impact on the pharmacokinetics of citalopram. At present no information is available for treatment of patients with severely reduced renal function (creatinine clearance <20 mL/min).

Preclinical safety data: Citalopram has low acute toxicity. In chronic toxicity studies there were no findings of concern for the therapeutic use of citalopram. Based on data from reproduction toxicity studies (segment I, II and III) there is no reason to have special concern for the use of citalopram in women of child-bearing potential. Citalopram has no mutagenic or carcinogenic potential.

Pharmaceutical particulars

List of excipients: Maize starch, lactose, microcrystalline-cellulose, copolyvidone, glycerol, croscarmellose sodium type A, magnesium stearate, methylhydroxypropyl-cellulose, macrogol, titanium dioxide.

Incompatibilities: Nil.

Shelf life: 5 years. Each pack has an expiry date.

Special precautions for storage: Store at room temperature (at or below 25°C).

Nature and contents of container: Press through packs (UPVC/PVdC with aluminium closure) containing 28 tablets.

Instructions for use/handling: Nil.

Marketing authorisation numbers
10 mg 0458/0057
20 mg 0458/0058
40 mg 0458/0059

Date of approval/revision of SPC June 1998.

Legal category POM.

CLOPIXOL* ACUPHASE* INJECTION

Qualitative and quantitative composition Zuclopenthixol acetate 5.0% w/v equivalent to 4.526% w/v of zuclopenthixol base.

Pharmaceutical form Oily solution for deep intramuscular injection.

Clinical particulars

Therapeutic indications: For the initial treatment of acute psychoses including mania and exacerbation of chronic psychoses, particularly where a rapid onset of action, and a duration of effect of 2–3 days is desirable.

Posology and method of administration

Dosage

Adults: Dosage should be adjusted according to the severity of the patient's illness. Clopixol Acuphase is administered by deep intramuscular injection, into the upper outer buttock or lateral thigh.

The usual dosage is 50–150 mg (1–3 mL), repeated if necessary after 2 or 3 days. Some patients may need an additional injection between 1 and 2 days after the first injection.

Clopixol Acuphase is not intended for long-term use and duration of treatment should not be more than two weeks. The maximum accumulated dosage in a course should not exceed 400 mg and the number of injections should not exceed four.

Patients with compromised hepatic function should receive half the recommended dosages for normal patients. Where there is reduced renal function, it is not necessary to reduce the dosage but where there is renal failure dosage should be reduced to half the normal dosage.

Elderly: The dosage may need to be reduced in the elderly owing to reduced rates of metabolism and elimination. Maximum dosage per injection should be 100 mg.

Children: Not recommended for children.

Maintenance therapy: Clopixol Acuphase is not intended for long-term use.

A single injection of Clopixol Acuphase has an onset of sedative action shortly after injection and an antipsychotic action persisting for 2 to 3 days. In this period, maintenance treatment with tablets or a longer acting depot neuroleptic can be initiated. The possible side-effects of long-term maintenance treatment with a neuroleptic, including tardive dyskinesia, should be considered.

Maintenance treatment where required can be continued with Clopixol tablets, Clopixol injection or Clopixol Conc. injection, according to the following guidelines:

1. Introduce Clopixol tablets at a dosage of 20–60 mg/day in divided doses, 2 to 3 days after the last injection of Clopixol Acuphase. If necessary increase the tablet dosage by 10–20 mg each day up to a maximum of 150 mg/day.

or

2. Concomitantly with the last injection of Clopixol Acuphase, administer 200–500 mg of Clopixol injection or Clopixol Conc injection by deep intramuscular injection and repeat the Clopixol injection or Clopixol Conc injection at intervals of 2 to 4 weeks. Higher dosages or a shorter interval may be necessary.

Route of administration: Deep intramuscular injection, into the upper outer buttock or lateral thigh.

Contra-indications: Comatose states, including acute alcohol, barbiturate, and opiate intoxication.

Special warnings and special precautions for use: Like other neuroleptics zuclopenthixol acetate should be used with caution in patients with convulsive disorders or advanced hepatic, renal or cardiovascular disease.

Zuclopenthixol is not suitable for patients who do not tolerate oral neuroleptic drugs or for patients suffering from Parkinson's disease.

Interactions with other medicaments and other forms of interaction: Zuclopenthixol enhances the response to alcohol and the effects of barbiturates and other CNS depressants. Potentiation of the effects of general anaesthetics may occur. Zuclopenthixol acetate should not be given concomitantly with guanethidine or similarly acting compounds, since neuroleptics may block the antihypertensive effect of these compounds. Tricyclic antidepressants and neuroleptics mutually inhibit the metabolism of each other. Zuclopenthixol may reduce the effect of levodopa and the effect of adrenergic drugs. Concomitant use of metoclopramide and piperazine increases the risk of extrapyramidal symptoms.

The possibility of interaction with lithium salts should be borne in mind.

Pregnancy and lactation: Animal tests have not revealed any evidence that zuclopenthixol causes an increased incidence of foetal damage. Nevertheless, zuclopenthixol acetate should not be administered during pregnancy or to women of childbearing potential, unless they are taking adequate contraceptive precautions or unless the expected benefit to the patient outweighs the potential risk to the foetus.

Zuclopenthixol is found in very low concentrations in the breast milk of mothers receiving Clopixol treatment. It is recommended that mothers treated with Clopixol Acuphase should not breast feed.

Effects on ability to drive and use machines: The ability to drive a car or operate machinery may be affected and patients should be warned of this risk.

Undesirable effects: The frequency of unwanted effects is in general low and the severity of the symptoms is most often mild. The frequency and severity are most pronounced the day after the first injection and then decrease rapidly.

Extrapyramidal symptoms, including dystonia, rigidity, motor akathisia, hypokinesia and tremor, have been reported. These side effects can be satisfactorily controlled by antiparkinson drugs.

Orthostatic dizziness occurs rarely and only occasionally to a severe degree.

Reduced salivation of a mild degree has been observed.

Overdose: Symptoms: somnolence, coma, extrapyramidal symptoms, convulsions, hypotension, shock, hyper or hypothermia.

Treatment is symptomatic and supportive. Measures aimed at supporting the respiratory and cardiovascular systems should be instituted. Adrenaline (epinephrine) must not be used in these patients. There is no specific antidote.

Pharmacological properties

Pharmacodynamic properties: Zuclopenthixol is a potent neuroleptic of the thioxanthene series with a piperazine side-chain. The antipsychotic effect of neuroleptics is related to their dopamine receptor blocking effect. The thioxanthenes have a high affinity for both the adenylate cyclase coupled dopamine D_1 receptors and for the dopamine D_2 receptors; in the phenothiazine group the affinity for D_1 receptors is much lower than that for D_2 receptors, whereas butyrophenones, diphenylbutylpiperidines and benzamides only have affinity for D_2 receptors.

In the traditional tests for antipsychotic effect, e.g. antagonism of stereotypic behaviour induced by dopamine agonists, the chemical groups of neuroleptics mentioned reveal equal but dosage dependent activity. However, the antistereotypic effect of phenothiazines, butyrophenones, diphenylbutylpiperidines, and benzamindes is strongly counteracted by the anticholinergic drug, scopolamine, while the antisteriotype effect of the thioxanthenes, e.g. zuclopenthixol, is not, or only very slightly, influenced by concomitant treatment with anticholinergics.

Pharmacokinetic properties: By esterification of zuclopenthixol with acetic acid, zuclopenthixol has been converted to a more lipophilic substance, zuclopenthixol acetate. When dissolved in oil and injected intramuscularly this substance diffuses slowly into the surrounding body water, where enzymatic breakdown occurs releasing the active component zuclopenthixol.

Maximum serum concentrations of zuclopenthixol are usually reached 36 hours after an injection, after which the serum levels decline slowly. The average maximum serum level corresponding to the 100 mg dose is 41 ng/mL. Three days after the injection the serum level is about one third of the maximum.

Zuclopenthixol is distrubuted in the body in a similar way to other neuroleptics; with the higher concentrations of drug and metabolites in liver, lungs, intestines and kidneys and lower concentrations in heart, spleen, brain and blood. The apparent volume of distribution is about 20 L/kg and the protein binding about 98%.

Zuclopenthixol crosses the placental barrier in small amounts. Zuclopenthixol is excreted in small amounts with the milk – the ratio milk concentration/serum concentration in women is on average 0.3.

The metabolism of zuclopenthixol proceeds via three main routes – sulphoxidation, side chain N-dealkylation and glucuronic acid conjugation. The metabolites are devoid of psychopharmacolical activity. The excretion proceeds mainly with the faeces but also to some degree with the urine. The systemic clearance is about 0.9 L/min.

The kinetics seem to be linear, since highly significant correlation exist between the dose and the area under the serum concentration curve.

Preclinical safety data: Zuclopenthixol has low acute toxicity and was not mutagenic or carcinogenic in appropriate tests. Local muscle damage is less pronounced with oily solutions of zuclopenthixol (including Clopixol Acuphase) than with aqueous solutions of zuclopenthixol and other neuroleptics.

Pharmaceutical particulars

List of excipients: Thin vegetable oil (derived from coconuts).

Incompatibilities: Zuclopenthixol acetate should not be mixed with other injection fluids.

Shelf life: 2 years as packaged for sale.

Special precautions for storage: Store at or below 25°C. Protect from light.

Nature and contents of container: Clear glass ampoules containing either 1 or 2 mL of zuclopenthixol acetate 5% w/v in thin vegetable oil.

The ampoules are packed in boxes of 5.

Instructions for use/handling: Nil.

Marketing authorisation number 0458/0063.

Date of approval/revision of SPC 14 October 1998.

Legal category POM.

CLOPIXOL* INJECTION
CLOPIXOL* CONC. INJECTION

Presentation *Clopixol Injection* is a sterile, straw-coloured solution of 200 mg/ml (20%) zuclopenthixol decanoate in thin vegetable oil. It is presented in glass ampoules (1 ml).

Clopixol Conc. Injection is a sterile, straw-coloured solution of 500 mg/ml (50%) zuclopenthixol decanoate in thin vegetable oil. It is presented in glass ampoules (1 ml).

Uses The maintenance treatment of schizophrenia and paranoid psychoses.

Dosage and administration
Note: As with all oil based injections it is important to ensure, by aspiration before injection, that inadvertent intravascular entry does not occur.

Adults: Clopixol Injection and Clopixol Conc. Injection are administered by deep intramuscular injection into the upper outer buttock or lateral thigh.

Dosage and dosage interval should be adjusted according to the patients' symptoms and response to treatment.

The usual dosage range of zuclopenthixol decanoate is 200–500 mg every one to four weeks, depending on response, but some patients may require up to 600 mg per week. In patients who have not previously received depot neuroleptics, treatment is usually started with a small dose (e.g. 100 mg) to assess tolerability. An interval of at least one week should be allowed before the second injection is given at a dose consistent with the patients' condition.

Adequate control of severe psychotic symptoms may take up to 4 to 6 months at high enough dosage. Once stabilised lower maintenance doses may be considered, but must be sufficient to prevent relapse.

Injection volumes of greater than 2 ml should be distributed between two injection sites.

When transferring patients from oral to depot neuroleptic treatment, the oral medication should not be discontinued immediately, but gradually withdrawn over a period of several days after administering the first injection.

Elderly: In accordance with standard medical practice initial dosage may need to be reduced to a quarter or half the normal starting dose in the frail or elderly.

Children: Clopixol Injection and Clopixol Conc. Injection are not indicated for children.

Contra-indications, warnings, etc
Contra-indications: Comatose states, including acute alcohol, barbiturates or opiate intoxication.

Warnings and precautions for use: Caution should be exercised in patients having: liver disease; cardiac disease, or arrhythmias; severe respiratory disease; renal failure; epilepsy (and conditions predisposing to epilepsy, e.g. alcohol withdrawal or brain damage); Parkinson's disease; narrow angle glaucoma; prostatic hypertrophy; hypothyroidism; hyperthyroidism; myasthenia gravis; phaeochromocytoma and patients who have shown hypersensitivity to thioxanthenes or other neuroleptics.

The elderly require close supervision because they are especially prone to experience such adverse effects as sedation, hypotension, confusion and temperature changes.

Interactions: In common with other neuroleptics, zuclopenthixol enhances the response to alcohol, and the effects of barbiturates and other CNS depressants, and may potentiate the effects of general anaesthetics. Neuroleptics may antagonise the effects of adrenaline and other sympathomimetic agents, and reverse the antihypertensive effects of guanethidine and similar adrenergic-blocking agents. Neuroleptics may impair the effect of levodopa, adrenergic drugs and anticonvulsants. The metabolism of tricyclic antidepressants may be inhibited and the control of diabetes may be impaired. The effect of anticoagulants may be increased. The anticholinergic effects of atropine may be increased. Anticholinergic effects may be enhanced by antiparkinson drugs and tardive dyskinesia precipitated. Concomitant use of metoclopramide and piperazine increases the risk of extrapyramidal symptoms. Neuroleptics may enhance the cardiac depressant effects of quinidine; the absorption of corticosteroids and digoxin; the hypotensive effect of vasodilator antihypertensive agents such as hydralazine and prolong the action of neuromuscular blocking agents. The possibility of interaction with lithium salts should be borne in mind.

Pregnancy and lactation: As the safety of this drug during pregnancy has not been established, use during pregnancy, especially the first and last trimesters, should be avoided, unless the expected benefit to the patient outweighs the potential risk to the foetus.

Zuclopenthixol is excreted into breast milk. If the use of Clopixol is considered essential, nursing mothers should be advised to stop breast feeding.

The newborn of mothers treated with neuroleptics in late pregnancy, or labour, may show signs of intoxication such as lethargy, tremor and hyperexcitability, and have a low apgar score.

Effects on ability to drive and use machines: Alertness may be impaired, especially at the start of treatment, or following the consumption of alcohol; patients should be warned of this risk and advised not to drive or operate machinery until their susceptibility is known.

Undesirable effects: Drowsiness and sedation may occur but are more often seen with high dosage and at the start of treatment, particularly in the elderly. Other adverse effects include blurring of vision, tachycardia and urinary incontinence and frequency. Dose-related postural hypotension may occur, particularly in the elderly.

Because Clopixol may impair alertness, especially at the start of treatment or following the consumption of alcohol, patients should be warned of this risk and advised not to drive or operate machinery, until their susceptibility is known.

Extrapyramidal reactions in the form of acute dystonias (including oculogyric crisis), parkinsonian rigidity, tremor, akinesia and akathisia have been reported and may occur even at lower dosage in susceptible patients. Such effects would usually be encountered early in treatment, but delayed reactions may also occur. Antiparkinson agents should not be prescribed routinely because of the possible risk of precipitating toxic-confusional states, impairing therapeutic efficacy or causing anticholinergic side-effects. They should only be given if required and their requirement reassessed at regular intervals.

Tardive dyskinesia can occur with neuroleptic treatment. It is more common at high doses for prolonged periods and has been reported at lower dosage for short periods. The risk seems to be greater in the elderly, especially females. It has been reported that fine vermicular movements of the tongue are an early sign. It has been observed occasionally in patients receiving Clopixol. The concurrent use of anticholinergic antiparkinson drugs may exacerbate this effect. The potential irreversibility and seriousness, as well as the unpredictability of the syndrome, requires especially careful assessment of the risk versus benefit, and the lowest possible dosage and duration of treatment consistent with therapeutic efficacy. Short-lived dyskinesia may occur after abrupt withdrawal of the drug.

The neuroleptic malignant syndrome has rarely been reported in patients receiving neuroleptics including zuclopenthixol. This potentially fatal syndrome is characterised by hyperthermia, a fluctuating level of consciousness, muscular rigidity and autonomic dysfunction with pallor, tachycardia, labile blood pressure, sweating and urinary incontinence. Neuroleptic therapy should be discontinued immediately and vigorous symptomatic treatment implemented.

Epileptic fits have occasionally been reported. Confusional states can occur.

The hormonal effects of antipsychotic neuroleptic drugs include hyperprolactinaemia, which may be associated with galactorrhoea, gynaecomastia, oligomenorrhoea or amenorrhoea. Sexual function, including erection and ejaculation may be impaired; but increased libido has also been reported.

ECG changes with prolongation of the QT interval and T-wave changes may occur with moderate to high doses; they are reversible on reducing the dose.

Zuclopenthixol may impair body temperature control, and cases of hyperthermia have occurred rarely. The possible development of hypothermia, particularly in the elderly and hypothyroid, should be borne in mind.

Blood dyscrasias have occasionally been reported. Blood counts should be carried out if a patient develops signs of persistent infection. Jaundice and other liver abnormalities have been reported rarely.

Weight gain and less commonly weight loss have been reported; oedema has occasionally been reported and has been considered to be allergic in origin. Rashes have occurred rarely. Although less likely than with phenothiazines, zuclopenthixol can rarely cause increased susceptibility to sunburn.

Occasional local reactions, such as erythema, swelling or tender fibrous nodules have been reported.

Zuclopenthixol, even in low doses, in susceptible (especially non-psychotic) individuals may unusually cause nausea, dizziness or headache, excitement, agitation, insomnia, or unpleasant subjective feelings of being mentally dulled or slowed down.

Because acute withdrawal symptoms, including nausea, vomiting and insomnia have rarely been described after abrupt cessation of high doses of neuroleptics, gradual withdrawal of Clopixol is advisable. If drugs are withdrawn, recurrence of psychotic symptoms may not become apparent for several weeks or months.

Overdosage: Overdosage may cause somnolence, or even coma, extrapyramidal symptoms, convulsions, hypotension, shock, hyper- or hypothermia. Treatment is symptomatic and supportive, with measures aimed at supporting the respiratory and cardiovascular systems. The following specific measures may be employed if required:

- anticholinergic antiparkinson drugs if extrapyramidal symptoms occur.
- sedation (with benzodiazepines) in the unlikely event of agitation or excitement or convulsions.
- noradrenaline in saline intravenous drip if the patient is in shock. Adrenaline must not be given.

Pharmaceutical precautions The products should be stored at or below 25°C protected from light.

The products may be mixed in the same syringe with other products in the Clopixol Injection range including Clopixol Acuphase Injection (zuclopenthixol acetate 50 mg/ml).

They should not be mixed with any other injection fluids.

Legal category POM.

Package quantities
Clopixol Injection: Boxes of 10 × 200 mg (1 ml) ampoules

Clopixol Conc. Injection: Boxes of 5 × 500 mg (1 ml) ampoules.

Further information Clopixol Injection and Clopixol Conc. Injection contain the decanoic ester of zuclopenthixol in a thin vegetable oil (Viscoleo). The decanoic ester is slowly released from the oil depot and rapidly hydrolysed to release zuclopenthixol. Whereas zuclopenthixol itself is relatively short acting, the decanoic ester in oil provides a predictable slow-release depot preparation.

Product licence numbers
Clopixol Injection: 0458/0017
Clopixol Conc. Injection: 0458/0060

CLOPIXOL* TABLETS

Qualitative and quantitative composition Tablets of 2, 10 or 25 mg (2.36, 11.9 or 29.7 mg zuclopenthixol dihydrochloride equivalent to 2, 10 or 25 mg zuclopenthixol base respectively).

Pharmaceutical form Round, biconvex, pale red, film-coated tablets.

Clinical particulars
Therapeutic indications: The treatment of psychoses, especially schizophrenia.
Posology and method of administration:
Route of administration: Oral.
Adults: The dosage range is 4–150 mg/day in divided doses. The usual initial dose is 20–30 mg/day (sometimes with higher dosage requirements in acute cases), increasing as necessary. The usual maintenance dose is 20–50 mg/day.
Elderly: In accordance with standard medical practice, initial dosage may need to be reduced to a quarter or half the normal starting dose in the frail or elderly.
Children: Not indicated for children.
Contra-indications: Comatose states, including acute alcohol, barbiturate, or opiate intoxication.
Special warnings and special precautions for use: Caution should be exercised in patients having: liver disease; cardiac disease or arrhythmias; severe respiratory disease; renal failure; epilepsy (and conditions predisposing to epilepsy e.g. alcohol withdrawal or brain damage); Parkinson's disease; narrow angle glaucoma; prostatic hypertrophy; hypothyroidism; hyperthyroidism; myasthenia gravis; phaeochromocytoma and patients who have shown hypersensitivity to thioxanthenes or other neuroleptics.

The elderly require close supervision because they are specially prone to experience such adverse effects as sedation, hypotension, confusion and temperature changes.

Interactions with other medicaments and other forms of interaction: In common with other neuroleptics, zuclopenthixol enhances the response to alcohol, and the effects of barbiturates and other CNS depressants, and may potentiate the effects of general anaesthetics. Neuroleptics may antagonise the effects of adrenaline and other sympathomimetic agents, and reverse the antihypertensive effects of guanethidine and similar adrenergic-blocking agents. Neuroleptics may impair the effect of levodopa, adrenergic drugs and anticonvulsants. The metabolism of tricyclic antidepressants may be inhibited and the control of diabetes may be impaired. The effect of anticoagulants may be increased. The anticholinergic effects of atropine may be increased. Anticholinergic effects may be enhanced by antiparkinson drugs and tardive dyskinesia precipitated. Concomitant use of metoclopramide and piperazine increases the risk of extrapyramidal symptoms. Neuroleptics may enhance the cardiac depressant effects of quinidine; the absorption of corticosteroids and digoxin; the hypotensive effect of vasodilator antihypertensive agents such as hydralazine and prolong the action of neuromuscular blocking agents. The possibility of interaction with lithium salts should be borne in mind.

Pregnancy and lactation: As the safety of this drug during pregnancy has not been established, use during pregnancy, especially the first and last trimesters, should be avoided, unless the expected benefit to the patient outweighs the potential risk to the foetus.

Zuclopenthixol is excreted into the breast milk. If the use of Clopixol is considered essential, nursing mothers should be advised to stop breast feeding.

The newborn of mothers treated with neuroleptics in late pregnancy, or labour, may show signs of intoxication such as lethargy, tremor and hyperexcitability, and have a low apgar score.

Effects on ability to drive and use machines: Alertness may be impaired, especially at the start of treatment, or following the consumption of alcohol; patients should be warned of this risk and advised not to drive or operate machinery until their susceptibility is known.

Undesirable effects: Drowsiness and sedation may occur but are more often seen with high dosage and at the start of treatment, particularly in the elderly. Other adverse effects include blurring of vision, tachycardia and urinary incontinence and frequency. Dose-related postural hypotension may occur, particularly in the elderly.

Because Clopixol may impair alertness, especially at the start of treatment or following the consumption of alcohol, patients should be warned of the risk and advised not to drive or operate machinery, until their susceptibility is known.

Extrapyramidal reactions in the form of acute dystonias (including oculogyric crisis), parkinsonian rigidity, tremor, akinesia and akathisia have been reported and may occur even at lower dosage in susceptible patients. Such effects would usually be encountered early in treatment, but delayed reactions may also occur. Antiparkinson agents should not be prescribed routinely because of the possible risk of precipitating toxic-confusional states, impairing therapeutic efficacy or causing anticholinergic side-effects. They should only be given if required and their requirement reassessed at regular intervals.

Tardive dyskinesia can occur with neuroleptic treatment. It is more common at high doses for prolonged periods but has been reported at lower dosage for short periods. The risk seems to be greater in the elderly, especially females. It has been reported that fine vermicular movements of the tongue are an early sign. It has been observed occasionally in patients receiving Clopixol. The concurrent use of anticholinergic antiparkinson drugs may exacerbate this effect. The potential irreversibility and seriousness, as well as the unpredictability of the syndrome, requires especially careful assessment of the risk versus benefit, and the lowest possible dosage and duration of treatment consistent with therapeutic efficacy. Short-lived dyskinesia may occur after abrupt withdrawal of the drug.

The neuroleptic malignant syndrome has rarely been reported in patients receiving neuroleptics, including zuclopenthixol. This potentially fatal syndrome is characterised by hyperthermia, a fluctuating level of consciousness, muscular rigidity and autonomic dysfunction with pallor, tachycardia, labile blood pressure, sweating and urinary incontinence. Neuroleptic therapy should be discontinued immediately and vigorous symptomatic treatment implemented.

Epileptic fits have occasionally been reported. Confusional states can occur.

The hormonal effects of antipsychotic neuroleptic drugs include hyperprolactinaemia, which may be associated with galactorrhoea, gynaecomastia, oligomenorrhoea or amenorrhoea. Sexual function, including erection and ejaculation may be impaired; but increased libido has also been reported.

ECG changes with prolongation of the QT interval and T-wave changes may occur with moderate to high doses; they are reversible on reducing the dose.

Zuclopenthixol may impair body temperature control, and cases of hyperthermia have occurred rarely. The possible development of hypothermia, particularly in the elderly and hypothyroid, should be borne in mind.

Blood dyscrasias have occasionally been reported. Blood counts should be carried out if a patient develops signs of persistent infection. Jaundice and other liver abnormalities have been reported rarely.

Weight gain and less commonly weight loss have been reported; oedema has occasionally been reported and has been considered to be allergic in origin. Rashes have occurred rarely. Although less likely than with phenothiazines, zuclopenthixol can rarely cause increased susceptibility to sunburn.

Zuclopenthixol, even in low doses, in susceptible (especially non-psychotic) individuals may unusually cause nausea, dizziness or headache, excitement, agitation, insomnia, or unpleasant subjective feelings of being mentally dulled or slowed down.

Because acute withdrawal symptoms, including nausea, vomiting and insomnia have rarely been described after abrupt cessation of high doses of neuroleptics, gradual withdrawal of Clopixol is advisable. If drugs are withdrawn, recurrence of psychotic symptoms may not become apparent for several weeks or months.

Overdose: Overdose may cause somnolence, or even coma, extrapyramidal symptoms, convulsions, hypotension, shock, hyper- or hypothermia. Treatment is symptomatic and supportive, with measures aimed at supporting the respiratory and cardiovascular systems. The following specific measures may be employed if required.

- Anitcholinergic antiparkinson drugs if extrapyramidal symptoms occur.
- Sedation (with benzodiazepines) in the unlikely event of agitation or excitement or convulsions.
- Noradrenaline in saline intravenous drip if the patient is in shock. Adrenaline must not be given.
- Gastric lavage should be considered.

Pharmacological properties

Pharmacodynamic properties: The action of zuclopenthixol as with other neuroleptics is mediated through dopamine receptor blockage. Zuclopenthixol has a high affinity for D_1 and D_2 receptors and activity has been demonstrated in standard animal models used to assess neuroleptic action. Serotonergic blocking properties, a high affinity for alpha-adrenoreceptors and slight antihistaminergic properties have been observed.

Pharmacokinetic particulars: Zuclopenthixol given orally in man is relatively quickly absorbed and maximum serum concentrations are reached in 3–6 hours. There is good correlation between the dose of zuclopenthixol and the concentrations achieved in serum. The biological half-life in man is about one day. Zuclopenthixol is distributed in the liver, lungs, intestines and kidney, with somewhat lower concentration in the brain. Small amounts of drug or metabolites cross the placenta and are excreted in milk.

Zuclopenthixol is metabolised by sulphoxidation, N-Dealkylation and glucuronic acid conjugation.

The faecal route of excretion predominates and mostly unchanged zuclopenthixol and N-dealkylated metabolite are excreted in this way.

Preclinical safety data: Nil of relevance.

Pharmaceutical particulars

List of excipients: Potato starch, lactose, microcrystalline cellulose, polyvidone acetate, glycerol, talc, hydrogenated caster oil, magnesium stearate, methylhydroxypropyl cellulose, macrogol, titanium dioxide (E171) and red iron oxide (E172).

Incompatibilities: None known.

Shelf life: Clopixol Tablets 2 mg are stable for two years. Clopixol Tablets 10 mg and 25 mg are stable for 5 years. Each container has an expiry date.

Special precautions for storage: Store in original container, protected from light and moisture, below 25°C.

Nature and contents of container: Grey polypropylene container (with desiccant capsule in 2 mg). Contents: 100 tablets.

Instructions for use handling: Nil.

Marketing authorisation numbers

2 mg tablets 0458/0027
10 mg tablets 0458/0028
25 mg tablets 0458/0029

Date of approval/revison of SPC 15 April 1997.

Legal category POM.

DEPIXOL* INJECTION
DEPIXOL* CONC. INJECTION

Qualitative and quantitative composition

Depixol Injection: 20 mg/mL (2% w/v) cis(Z)-flupenthixol decanoate in thin vegetable oil. Ampoules 1 mL and 2 mL.

Depixol Conc. Injection: 100 mg/mL (10% w/v) cis(Z)-flupenthixol decanoate in thin vegetable oil. Ampoules 0.5 mL and 1 mL Vial 5 mL.

Pharmaceutical form Oily solution for deep intramuscular injection.

Clinical particulars

Therapeutic Indications: The treatment of schizophrenia and other psychoses.

Posology and method of administration: Route of administration: Deep intramuscular injection into the upper outer buttock or lateral thigh. Dosage and dosage interval should be adjusted according to the patient's symptoms and response to treatment.

Note: As with all oil based injections it is important to ensure, by aspiration before injection, that inadvertent intravascular entry does not occur.

Adults: The usual dosage of flupenthixol decanoate lies between 50 mg every 4 weeks and 300 mg every 2 weeks, but some patients may require up to 400 mg weekly. Other patients may be adequately maintained on dosages of 20-40 mg flupenthixol decanoate every 2-4 weeks. In patients who have not previously received depot neuroleptics, treatment is usually started with a small dose (e.g. 20 mg) to assess tolerability. An interval of at least one week should be allowed before the second injection is given at a dose consistent with the patient's condition.

Adequate control of severe psychotic symptoms may take up to 4 to 6 months at high enough dosage. Once stabilised lower maintenance doses may be considered, but must be sufficient to prevent relapse.

The appropriate presentation of Depixol should be selected to achieve an injection volume which does not exceed 2 mL. Volumes greater than 2 mL should be distributed between two injection sites.

When transferring patients from oral to depot neuroleptic treatment, the oral medication should not be discontinued immediately, but gradually withdrawn over a period of several days after administering the first injection.

Elderly: In accordance with standard medical practice, initial dosage may need to be reduced to a quarter or half the normal starting dose in the frail or elderly.

Children: Depixol Injection and Depixol Conc. Injection are not indicated for children.

Contraindications: Comatose states, including alcohol, barbiturate, or opiate poisoning. Not recommended for excitable or agitated patients.

Special warnings and special precautions for use: Caution should be exercised in patients having: liver disease; cardiac disease or arrhythmias; severe respiratory disease; renal failure; epilepsy (and conditions predisposing to epilepsy e.g. alcohol withdrawal or brain damage); Parkinson's disease; narrow angle glaucoma; prostatic hypertrophy; hypothyroidism; hyperthyroidism; myasthenia gravis; phaeochromocytoma and patients who have shown hypersensitivity to thioxanthenes or other neuroleptics.

The elderly require close supervision because they are specially prone to experience such adverse effects as sedation, hypotension, confusion and temperature changes.

Interactions with other medicaments and other forms of interaction: In common with other neuroleptics, flupenthixol enhances the response to alcohol, and the effects of barbiturates and other CNS depressants, and may potentiate the effects of general anaesthetics. Neuroleptics may antagonise the effects of adrenaline and other sympathomimetic agents, and reverse the antihypertensive effects of guanethidine and similar adrenergic-blocking agents. Neuroleptics may impair the effect of levodopa, adrenergic drugs and anticonvulsants. The metabolism of tricyclic antidepressants may be inhibited and the control of diabetes may be impaired. The effect of anticoagulants may be increased. The anticholinergic effects of atropine may be increased. Anticholinergic effects may be enhanced by antiparkinson drugs and tardive dyskinesia precipitated. Concomitant use of metoclopramide and piperazine increases the risk of extrapyramidal symptoms. Neuroleptics may enhance the cardiac depressant effects of quinidine; the absorption of corticosteroids and digoxin; the hypotensive effect of vasodilator antihypertensive agents such as hydralazine and prolong the action of neuromuscular blocking agents. The possibility of interaction with lithium salts should be borne in mind.

Pregnancy and lactation: As the safety of this drug during pregnancy has not been established, use during pregnancy, especially the first and last trimesters, should be avoided, unless the expected benefit to the patient outweighs the potential risk to the foetus.

Flupenthixol is excreted into the breast milk. If the use of Depixol is considered essential, nursing mothers should be advised to stop breast feeding.

The newborn of mothers treated with neuroleptics in late pregnancy, or labour, may show signs of intoxication such as lethargy, tremor and hyperexcitability, and have a low apgar score.

Effects on ability to drive and use machines: Alertness may be impaired, especially at the start of treatment, or following the consumption of alcohol; patients should be warned of this risk and advised not to drive or operate machinery until their susceptibility is known.

Undesirable effects: Drowsiness and sedation are unusual. Sedation, if it occurs, is more often seen with high dosage and at the start of treatment, particularly in the elderly. Other adverse effects include blurring of vision, tachycardia and urinary incontinence and frequency. Dose-related postural hypotension may occur, particularly in the elderly.

Because Depixol may impair alertness, especially at the start of treatment or following the consumption of alcohol, patients should be warned of the risk and advised not to drive or operate machinery, until their susceptibility is known.

Extrapyramidal reactions in the form of acute dystonias (including oculogyric crisis), parkinsonian rigidity, tremor, akinesia and akathisia have been reported and may occur even at lower dosage in susceptible patients. Such effects would usually be encountered early in treatment, but delayed reactions may also occur. Antiparkinson agents should not be prescribed routinely because of the possible risk of precipitating toxic-confusional states, impairing therapeutic efficacy or causing anticholinergic side-effects. They should only be given if required and their requirement reassessed at regular intervals.

Tardive dyskinesia can occur with neuroleptic treatment. It is more common at high doses for prolonged periods but has been reported at lower dosage for short periods. The risk seems to be greater in the elderly, especially females. It has been reported that fine vermicular movements of the tongue are an early sign. It has been observed occasionally in patients receiving Depixol. The concurrent use of anticholinergic antiparkinson drugs may exacerbate this effect. The potential irreversibility and seriousness, as well as the unpredictability of the syndrome, requires especially careful assessment of the risk versus benefit, and the lowest possible dosage and duration of treatment consistent with therapeutic efficacy. Short-lived dyskinesia may occur after abrupt withdrawal of the drug.

The neuroleptic malignant syndrome has rarely been reported in patients receiving neuroleptics, including flupenthixol. This potentially fatal syndrome is characterised by hyperthermia, a fluctuating level of consciousness, muscular rigidity and autonomic dysfunction with pallor, tachycardia, labile blood pressure, sweating and urinary incontinence. Neuroleptic therapy should be discontinued immediately and vigorous symptomatic treatment implemented.

Epileptic fits have occasionally been reported. Confusional states can occur.

The hormonal effects of antipsychotic neuroleptic drugs include hyperprolactinaemia, which may be associated with galactorrhoea, gynaecomastia, oligomenorrhoea or amenorrhoea. Sexual function, including erection and ejaculation may be impaired; but increased libido has also been reported.

ECG changes with prolongation of the QT interval and T-wave changes may occur with moderate to high doses; they are reversible on reducing the dose.

Flupenthixol may impair body temperature control, and cases of hyperthermia have occurred rarely. The possible development of hypothermia, particularly in the elderly and hypothyroid, should be borne in mind.

Blood dyscrasias have occasionally been reported. Blood counts should be carried out if a patient develops signs of persistent infection. Jaundice and other liver abnormalities have been reported rarely.

Weight gain and less commonly weight loss have been reported; oedema has occasionally been reported and has been considered to be allergic in origin. Rashes have occurred rarely. Although less likely than with phenothiazines, flupenthixol can rarely cause increased susceptibility to sunburn.

Occasional local reactions, such as erythema, swelling or tender fibrous nodules have been reported.

Flupenthixol, even in low doses, in susceptible (especially non-psychotic) individuals may unusually cause nausea, dizziness or headache, excitement, agitation, insomnia, or unpleasant subjective feelings of being mentally dulled or slowed down.

Because acute withdrawal symptoms, including nausea, vomiting and insomnia have rarely been described after abrupt cessation of high doses of neuroleptics, gradual withdrawal of Depixol is advisable. If drugs are withdrawn, recurrence of psychotic symptoms may not become apparent for several weeks or months.

Overdose: Overdosage may cause somnolence, or even coma, extrapyramidal symptoms, convulsions, hypotension, shock, hyper-or hypothermia. Treatment is symptomatic and supportive, with measures aimed at supporting the respiratory and cardiovascular systems. The following specific measures may be employed if required.
- anticholinergic antiparkinson drugs if extrapyramidal symptoms occur.
- sedation (with benzodiazepines) in the unlikely event of agitation or excitement or convulsions.
- noradrenaline in saline intravenous drip if the patient is in shock. Adrenaline must not be given.

Pharmacological properties
Pharmacodynamic properties: Flupenthixol is a non-sedating neuroleptic drug of the thioxanthene group. Its primary pharmacological action is dopamine blockade. Flupenthixol has a high affinity for D_1 and D_2 receptors. Depixol Injection contains the deconoic ester of flupenthixol in thin vegetable oil.

Pharmacokinetic properties: After intramuscular injection, the ester is slowly released from the oil depot and is rapidly hydrolysed to release flupenthixol. Flupenthixol is widely distributed in the body and extensively metabolized in the liver. Peak circulating levels occur around 7 days after administration.

Preclinical safety data: Nil of relevance

Pharmaceutical particulars
List of excipients: Thin vegetable oil "Viscoleo" (fractionated coconut oil).

Incompatibilities: This product may be mixed in the same syringe with other products in the Depixol Injection range. It should not be mixed with any other injection fluids.

Shelf-life: Depixol Injection: Ampoules 1 mL and 2 mL : 4 years

Depixol Conc. Injection: Ampoule 0.5 mL: 2 years Ampoule 1 mL: 4 years

Special precautions for storage: Store at or below 25°C. Protect from light.

Nature and contents of container: Depixol Injection: Ampoules containing 1 mL and 2 mL of 20 mg/mL (2% w/v) cis (Z)-flupenthixol decanoate in thin vegetable oil. Pack size = 10 ampoules per box.

Depixol Conc. Injection: Ampoules containing 0.5 mL and 1 mL of 100 mg/mL (10% w/v) cis(Z)-flupenthixol decanoate in thin vegetable oil. Pack size = 10 ampoules per box.

Instructions for use/handling: Nil.

Marketing authorisation number
Depixol Injection PL 0458/0007
Depixol Conc. Injection PL 0458/0015

Date of Approval/Revision of SPC
Depixol Injection 14 October 1998
Depixol Conc. Injection 19 October 1998

Legal category POM

DEPIXOL* LOW VOLUME INJECTION

Qualitative and quantitative composition
200 mg/mL (20% w/v) cis(Z)-flupenthixol decanoate in thin vegetable oil. Ampoules 1 mL.

Pharmaceutical form Oily solution for deep intramuscular injection.

Clinical particulars
Therapeutic indications: The treatment of schizophrenia and other psychoses.

Posology and method of administration: Route of administration: Deep intramuscular injection into the upper outer buttock or lateral thigh. Dosage and dosage interval should be adjusted according to the patient's symptoms and response to treatment.

Note: As with all oil based injections it is important to ensure, by aspiration before injection, that inadvertent intravascular entry does not occur.

Adults: The usual dosage of flupenthixol decanoate lies between 50 mg every 4 weeks and 300 mg every 2 weeks, but some patients may require up to 400 mg weekly. Other patients may be adequately maintained on dosages of 20-40 mg flupenthixol decanoate every 2-4 weeks. In patients who have not previously received depot neuroleptics, treatment is usually started with a small dose (e.g. 20 mg) to assess tolerability. An interval of at least one week should be allowed before the second injection is given at a dose consistent with the patient's condition.

Adequate control of severe psychotic symptoms may take up to 4 to 6 months at high enough dosage. Once stabilised lower maintenance doses may be considered, but must be sufficient to prevent relapse.

The appropriate presentation of Depixol should be selected to achieve an injection volume which does not exceed 2 mL. Volumes greater than 2 mL should be distributed between two injection sites.

When transferring patients from oral to depot neuroleptic treatment, the oral medication should not be discontinued immediately, but gradually withdrawn over a period of several days after administering the first injection.

Elderly: In accordance with standard medical practice, initial dosage may need to be reduced to a quarter or half the normal starting dose in the frail or elderly.

Children: Depixol Low Volume Injection is not indicated for children.

Contra-indications: Comatose states, including alcohol, barbiturate, or opiate poisoning. Not recommended for excitable or agitated patients.

Special warnings and special precautions for use: Caution should be exercised in patients having: liver disease; cardiac disease or arrhythmias; severe respiratory disease; renal failure; epilepsy (and conditions predisposing to epilepsy e.g. alcohol withdrawal or brain damage); Parkinson's disease; narrow angle glaucoma; prostatic hypertrophy; hypothyroidism; hyperthyroidism; myasthenia gravis; phaeochromocytoma and patients who have shown hypersensitivity to thioxanthenes or other neuroleptics.

The elderly require close supervision because they are specially prone to experience such adverse effects as sedation, hypotension, confusion and temperature changes.

Interactions with other medicaments and other forms of interaction: In common with other neuroleptics, flupenthixol enhances the response to alcohol, and the effects of barbiturates and other CNS depressants, and may potentiate the effects of general anaesthetics. Neuroleptics may antagonise the effects of adrenaline and other sympathomimetic agents, and reverse the antihypertensive effects of guanethidine and similar adrenergic-blocking agents. Neuroleptics may impair the effect of levodopa, adrenergic drugs and anticonvulsants. The metabolism of tricyclic antidepressants may be inhibited and the control of diabetes may be impaired. The effect of anticoagulants may be increased. The anticholinergic effects of atropine may be increased. Anticholinergic effects may be enhanced by antiparkinson drugs and tardive dyskinesia precipitated. Concomitant use of metoclopramide and piperazine increases the risk of extrapyramidal symptoms. Neuroleptics may enhance the cardiac depressant effects of quinidine; the absorption of corticosteroids and digoxin; the hypotensive effect of vasodilator antihypertensive agents such as hydralazine and prolong the action of neuromuscular blocking agents. The possibility of interaction with lithium salts should be borne in mind.

Pregnancy and lactation: As the safety of this drug during pregnancy has not been established, use during pregnancy, especially the first and last trimesters, should be avoided, unless the expected benefit to the patient outweighs the potential risk to the foetus.

Flupenthixol is excreted into the breast milk. If the use of Depixol is considered essential, nursing mothers should be advised to stop breast feeding.

The newborn of mothers treated with neuroleptics in late pregnancy, or labour, may show signs of intoxication such as lethargy, tremor and hyperexcitability, and have a low apgar score.

Effects on ability to drive and use machines: Alertness may be impaired, especially at the start of treatment, or following the consumption of alcohol; patients should be warned of this risk and advised not to drive or operate machinery until their susceptibility is known.

Undesirable effects: Drowsiness and sedation are unusual. Sedation, if it occurs, is more often seen with high dosage and at the start of treatment, particularly in the elderly. Other adverse effects include blurring of vision, tachycardia and urinary incontinence and frequency. Dose-related postural hypotension may occur, particularly in the elderly.

Because Depixol may impair alertness, especially at the start of treatment or following the consumption of alcohol, patients should be warned of the risk and advised not to drive or operate machinery, until their susceptibility is known.

Extrapyramidal reactions in the form of acute dystonias (including oculogyric crisis), parkinsonian rigidity, tremor, akinesia and akathisia have been reported and may occur even at lower dosage in susceptible patients. Such effects would usually be encountered early in treatment, but delayed reactions may also occur. Antiparkinson agents should not be prescribed routinely because of the possible risk of precipitating toxic-confusional states, impairing therapeutic efficacy or causing anticholinergic side-effects. They should only be given if required and their requirement reassessed at regular intervals.

Tardive dyskinesia can occur with neuroleptic treatment. It is more common at high doses for prolonged periods but has been reported at lower dosage for short periods. The risk seems to be greater in the elderly, especially females. It has been reported that fine vermicular movements of the tongue are an early sign. It has been observed occasionally in patients receiving Depixol. The concurrent use of anticholinergic antiparkinson drugs may exacerbate this effect. The potential irreversibility and seriousness, as well as the unpredictability of the syndrome, requires especially careful assessment of the risk versus benefit, and the lowest possible dosage and duration of treatment consistent with therapeutic efficacy. Short-lived dyskinesia may occur after abrupt withdrawal of the drug.

The neuroleptic malignant syndrome has rarely been reported in patients receiving neuroleptics, including flupenthixol. This potentially fatal syndrome is characterised by hyperthermia, a fluctuating level of consciousness, muscular rigidity and autonomic dysfunction with pallor, tachycardia, labile blood pressure, sweating and urinary incontinence. Neuroleptic therapy should be discontinued immediately and vigorous symptomatic treatment implemented.

Epileptic fits have occasionally been reported. Confusional states can occur.

The hormonal effects of antipsychotic neuroleptic drugs include hyperprolactinaemia, which may be associated with galactorrhoea, gynaecomastia, oligomenorrhoea or amenorrhoea. Sexual function, including erection and ejaculation may be impaired; but increased libido has also been reported.

ECG changes with prolongation of the QT interval and T-wave changes may occur with moderate to high doses; they are reversible on reducing the dose.

Flupenthixol may impair body temperature control, and cases of hyperthermia have occurred rarely. The possible development of hypothermia, particularly in the elderly and hypothyroid, should be borne in mind.

Blood dyscrasias have occasionally been reported. Blood counts should be carried out if a patient develops signs of persistent infection. Jaundice and other liver abnormalities have been reported rarely.

Weight gain and less commonly weight loss have been reported; oedema has occasionally been reported and has been considered to be allergic in origin. Rashes have occurred rarely. Although less likely than with phenothiazines, flupenthixol can rarely cause increased susceptibility to sunburn.

Occasional local reactions, such as erythema, swelling or tender fibrous nodules have been reported.

Flupenthixol, even in low doses, in susceptible (especially non-psychotic) individuals may unusually cause nausea, dizziness or headache, excitement, agitation, insomnia, or unpleasant subjective feelings of being mentally dulled or slowed down.

Because acute withdrawal symptoms, including nausea, vomiting and insomnia have rarely been described after abrupt cessation of high doses of neuroleptics, gradual withdrawal of Depixol is advisable. If drugs are withdrawn, recurrence of psychotic symptoms may not become apparent for several weeks or months.

Overdose: Overdosage may cause somnolence, or even coma, extrapyramidal symptoms, convulsions, hypotension, shock, hyper- or hypothermia. Treatment is symptomatic and supportive, with measures aimed at supporting the respiratory and cardiovascular systems. The following specific measures may be employed if required.

- anticholinergic antiparkinson drugs if extrapyramidal symptoms occur.
- sedation (with benzodiazepines) in the unlikely event of agitation or excitement or convulsions.
- noradrenaline in saline intravenous drip if the patient is in shock. Adrenaline must not be given.

Pharmacological properties

Pharmacodynamic properties: Cis(Z)-flupenthixol is a neuroleptic of the thioxanthene series.

The antipsychotic effect of neuroleptics is related to their dopamine receptor blocking effect. The thioxanthenes have high affinity for both the adenylate cyclase coupled dopamine D_1 receptors and for the dopamine D_2 receptors; in the phenothiazine group the affinity for D_1 receptors is much lower than that for D_2 receptors, whereas butyrophenones, diphenylbutylpiperidines and benzamides only have affinity for D_2 receptors.

In the traditional tests for antipsychotic effect, eg antagonism of stereotypic behaviour induced by dopamine agonists, the chemical groups of neuroleptics mentioned reveal equal but dosage-dependent activity. However, the antistereotypic effect of phenothiazines, butyrophenones, diphenylbutylpiperidines, and benzamides is strongly counteracted by the anticholinergic drug scopolamine, while the antistereotypic effect of thioxanthenes, eg cis(Z)-flupenthixol is not, or only very slightly, influenced by concomitant treatment with anticholinergics.

Pharmacokinetic properties: By esterification of cis(Z)-flupenthixol with decanoic acid cis(Z)-flupenthixol has been converted to a highly lipophilic substance, cis(Z)-flupenthixol decanoate. When dissolved in oil and injected intramuscularly this substance diffuses slowly into the surrounding body water, where enzymatic breakdown occurs releasing the active component cis(Z)-flupenthixol. The duration of action is 2-4 weeks with maximum serum levels being reached by the end of the first week after injection.

Cis(Z)-flupenthixol is distributed in the body in a similar way to other neuroleptics: with the highest concentrations of drug and metabolites in liver, lungs, intestines and kidneys and lower concentrations in heart, spleen, brain and blood. The apparent volume of distribution is about 14 L/kg and the protein binding >95%.

Cis(Z)-flupenthixol crosses the placental barrier in small amounts; it is also excreted in breast milk in very small amounts.

The metabolism of cis(Z)-flupenthixol proceeds via three main routes–sulphoxidation, side chain N-dealkylation and glucuronic acid conjugation. The metabolites are devoid of psychopharmacological activity. The excretion proceeds mainly with the faeces but also to some degree with the urine system; clearance is about 0.4-0.5 L.min.

Preclinical safety data: Nil of relevance

Pharmaceutical particulars

List of excipients: Thin vegetable oil "Viscoleo" (fractionated coconut oil).

Incompatibilities: This product may be mixed in the same syringe with other products in the Depixol Injection range. It should not be mixed with any other injection fluids.

Shelf-life: Ampoules 1 mL: 2 years

Special precautions for storage: Store below 25°C. Protect from light.

Nature and contents of container: Ampoules containing 1 mL of 200 mg/mL (20% w/v) cis-(Z)-flupenthixol decanoate in thin vegetable oil. Pack size = 5 ampoules per box.

Instructions for use/handling: Nil.

Marketing authorisation number PL 0458/0065

Date of approval/revision of SPC 9 December 1996

Legal category POM

DEPIXOL* TABLETS 3 mg

Qualitative and quantitative composition 3.504 mg flupenthixol dihydrochloride corresponding to 3 mg flupenthixol base.

Pharmaceutical form Round, biconvex, yellow, sugar-coated tablets.

Clinical particulars

Therapeutic indications: The treatment of schizophrenia and other psychoses.

Posology and method of administration:
Route of administration: Oral

Adults: 1–3 tablets twice daily, to a maximum of 18 mg (6 tablets) per day. It is recommended that commencement of treatment and increase in dosage should be carried out under close supervision. As with all neuroleptic drugs, the dose of Depixol should be titrated to the needs of each patient.

Elderly: In accordance with standard medical practice, initial dosage may need to be reduced to a quarter or half the normal starting dose in the frail or elderly.

Children: Not indicated for children.

Contra-indications: Comatose states, including alcohol, barbiturate, or opiate poisoning. Not recommended for excitable or agitated patients.

Special warnings and special precautions for use: Caution should be exercised in patients having: liver disease; cardiac disease or arrhythmias; severe respiratory disease; renal failure; epilepsy (and conditions predisposing to epilepsy, e.g. alcohol withdrawal or brain damage); Parkinson's disease; narrow angle glaucoma; prostatic hypertrophy; hypothyroidism; hyperthyroidism; myasthenia gravis; phaeochromocytoma and patients who have shown hypersensitivity to thioxanthenes or other neuroleptics.

The elderly require close supervision because they are specially prone to experience such adverse effects as sedation, hypotension, confusion and temperature changes.

Interactions with other medicaments and other forms of interaction: In common with other neuroleptics, flupenthixol enhances the response to alcohol, and the effects of barbiturates and other CNS depressants, and may potentiate the effects of general anaesthetics. Neuroleptics may antagonise the effects of adrenaline and other sympathomimetic agents, and reverse the antihypertensive effects of guanethidine and similar adrenergic-blocking agents. Neuroleptics may impair the effect of levodopa, adrenergic drugs and anticonvulsants. The metabolism of tricyclic antidepressants may be inhibited and the control of diabetes may be impaired. The effect of anticoagulants may be increased. The anticholinergic effects of atropine may be increased. Anticholinergic effects may be enhanced by antiparkinson drugs and tardive dyskinesia precipitated. Concomitant use of metoclopramide and piperazine increases the risk of extrapyramidal symptoms. Neuroleptics may enhance the cardiac depressant effects of quinidine; the absorption of corticosteroids and digoxin; the hypotensive effect of vasodilator antihypertensive agents such as hydralazine and prolong the action of neuromuscular blocking agents. The possibility of interaction with lithium salts should be borne in mind. Antacids may impair absorption, as may tea and coffee.

Pregnancy and lactation: As the safety of this drug during pregnancy has not been established, use during pregnancy, especially the first and last trimesters, should be avoided, unless the expected benefit to the patient outweighs the potential risk to the foetus.

Flupenthixol is excreted into the breast milk. If the use of Depixol is considered essential, nursing mothers should be advised to stop breast feeding.

The newborn of mothers treated with neuroleptics in late pregnancy, or labour, may show signs of intoxication such as lethargy, tremor and hyperexcitability, and have a low apgar score.

Effects on ability to drive and use machines: Alertness may be impaired, especially at the start of treatment, or following the consumption of alcohol; patients should be warned of this risk and advised not to drive or operate machinery until their susceptibility is known.

Undesirable effects: Drowsiness and sedation are unusual. Sedation, if it occurs, is more often seen with high dosage and at the start of treatment, particularly in the elderly. Other adverse effects include blurring of vision, tachycardia and urinary incontinence and frequency. Dose-related postural hypotension may occur, particularly in the elderly.

Because Depixol may impair alertness, especially at the start of treatment or following the consumption of alcohol, patients should be warned of this risk and advised not to drive or operate machinery, until their susceptibility is known.

Extrapyramidal reactions in the form of acute dystonias (including oculogyric crisis), parkinsonian rigidity, tremor, akinesia and akathisia have been reported and may occur even at lower dosage in susceptible patients. Such effects would usually be encountered early in treatment, but delayed reactions may also occur. Antiparkinson agents should not be prescribed routinely because of the possible risk of precipitating toxic-confusional states, impairing therapeutic efficacy or causing anticholinergic side-effects. They should only be given if required and their requirement reassessed at regular intervals.

Tardive dyskinesia can occur with neuroleptic treatment. It is more common at high doses for prolonged periods but has been reported at lower dosage for short periods. The risk seems to be greater in the elderly, especially females. It has been reported that fine vermicular movements of the tongue are an early sign. It has been observed occasionally in patients receiving Depixol. The concurrent use of anticholinergic antiparkinson drugs may exacerbate this effect. The potential irreversibility and seriousness, as well as the unpredictability of the syndrome, requires especially careful assessment of the risk versus benefit, and the lowest possible dosage and duration of treatment consistent with therapeutic efficacy. Short-lived dyskinesia may occur after abrupt withdrawal of the drug.

The neuroleptic malignant syndrome has rarely been reported in patients receiving neuroleptics, including flupenthixol. This potentially fatal syndrome is characterised by hyperthermia, a fluctuating level of consciousness, muscular rigidity and autonomic dysfunction with pallor, tachycardia, labile blood pressure, sweating and urinary incontinence. Neuroleptic therapy should be discontinued immediately and vigorous symptomatic treatment implemented.

Epileptic fits have occasionally been reported. Confusional states can occur.

The hormonal effects of antipsychotic neuroleptic drugs include hyperprolactinaemia, which may be associated with galactorrhoea, gynaecomastia, oligomenorrhoea or amenorrhoea. Sexual function, including erection and ejaculation may be impaired; but increased libido has also been reported.

ECG changes with prolongation of the QT interval and T-wave changes may occur with moderate to high doses; they are reversible on reducing the dose.

Flupenthixol may impair body temperature control, and cases of hyperthermia have occurred rarely. The possible development of hypothermia, particularly in the elderly and hypothyroid, should be borne in mind.

Blood dyscrasias have occasionally been reported. Blood counts should be carried out if a patient develops signs of persistent infection. Jaundice and other liver abnormalities have been reported rarely.

Weight gain and less commonly weight loss have been reported; oedema has occasionally been reported and has been considered to be allergic in origin. Rashes have occurred rarely. Although less likely than with phenothiazines, flupenthixol can rarely cause increased susceptibility to sunburn.

Flupenthixol, even in low doses, in susceptible (especially non-psychotic) individuals may unusually cause nausea, dizziness or headache, excitement, agitation, insomnia, or unpleasant subjective feelings of being mentally dulled or slowed down.

Because acute withdrawal symptoms, including nausea, vomiting and insomnia have rarely been described after abrupt cessation of high doses of neuroleptics, gradual withdrawal of Depixol is advisable. If drugs are withdrawn, recurrence of psychotic symptoms may not become apparent for several weeks or months.

Overdose: Overdosage may cause somnolence, or even coma, extrapyramidal symptoms, convulsions,

hypotension, shock, hyper- or hypothermia. Treatment is symptomatic and supportive, with measures aimed at supporting the respiratory and cardiovascular systems. The following specific measures may be employed if required:
- Anticholinergic antiparkinson drugs if extrapyramidal symptoms occur.
- Sedation (with benzodiazepines) in the unlikely event of agitation or excitement or convulsions.
- Noradrenaline in saline intravenous drip if the patient is in shock. Adrenaline must not be given.
- Gastric lavage should be considered.

Pharmacological properties
Pharmacodynamic properties: Flupenthixol is a neuroleptic of the thioxanthene series.

The antipsychotic effect of neuroleptics is believed to be related to their dopamine receptor blocking effect. The thioxanthenes have high affinity for D_1 and D_2 receptors.

Pharmacokinetic particulars: Oral administration to volunteers (8 mg single dose and 1.5 mg/day) and patients (5–60 mg/d) resulted in serum drug concentration curves with a maximum around four hours after administration. Mean biological half-title was about 35 hours in patients. No difference was seen in patients between half-lives estimated after single-dose administration and those estimated after repeated administration. Mean oral bioavailability of flupenthixol varied between 40% and 55%.

Preclinical safety data: Nil of relevance.

Pharmaceutical particulars
List of excipients: Potato starch, lactose, gelatin, talc, magnesium stearate, sucrose and yellow iron oxide (E172).

Incompatibilities: Not applicable.

Shelf-life: Depixol tablets are stable for 5 years. Each container has an expiry date.

Special precautions for storage: Store in original container, protected from light and moisture, below 25°C.

Nature and contents of container: Grey polypropylene container and screw cap. Contents 100 tablets.

Instructions for use/handling: Nil.

Marketing authorisation number 0458/0013.

Date of approval/revision of SPC 28 April 1997.

Legal category POM.

FLUANXOL* TABLETS

Qualitative and quantitative composition
0.5 mg tablets (containing 0.584 mg flupenthixol dihydrochloride equivalent to 0.5 mg flupenthixol base). 1 mg tablets (containing 1.168 mg flupenthixol dihydrochloride equivalent to 1 mg flupenthixol base).

Pharmaceutical form Round, biconvex, red, sugar-coated tablets.

Clinical particulars
Therapeutic indications: Symptomatic treatment of depression (with or without anxiety).

Posology and method of administration: Route of administration: Oral.

Adults: The standard initial dosage is 1 mg as a single morning dose. After one week the dose may be increased to 2 mg if there is inadequate clinical response. Daily dosage of more than 2 mg should be in divided doses up to a maximum of 3 mg daily.

Elderly: The standard initial dosage is 0.5 mg as a single morning dose. After one week, if response is inadequate, dosage may be increased to 1 mg once a day. Caution should be exercised in further increasing the dosage but occasional patients may require up to a maximum of 2 mg a day which should be given in divided doses.

Children: Not recommended for children.
Patients often respond within 2-3 days. If no effect has been observed within one week at maximum dosage the drug should be withdrawn.

Contra-indications: Severe depression requiring ECT or hospitalisation, states of excitement or overactivity, including mania.

Special warnings and special precautions for use: Fluanxol may initially cause drowsiness. Patients should be warned of this possibility if driving or operating machinery.
Recurrence of depressive symptoms on abrupt withdrawal is rare. However, gradual reduction of dosage is advisable. Dependence has not been reported to date.

Interactions with other medicaments and other forms of interaction: The central depressant effect of alcohol may be increased. The anticholinergic effects of atropine and tricyclic antidepressants may be increased and undesirable anticholinergic effects can be enhanced by antiparkinson drugs. Flupenthixol weakly antagonises the action of adrenaline and other sympathomimetic agents and may reverse the blood pressure lowering effects of adrenergic blocking agents such as guanethidine, possibly also clonidine. It may also affect the control of diabetes or the action of anticoagulants.

Pregnancy and lactation: As there is no unequivocal evidence as to the safety of Fluanxol in human pregnancy, use during pregnancy, especially the first and last trimesters, should be avoided. Flupenthixol is excreted in small amounts in breast milk. It is recommended that mothers receiving Fluanxol should not breast feed.

Effects on ability to drive and use machines: Flupenthixol may initially cause drowsiness. Patients should be warned of this possibility if driving or operating machinery.

Undesirable effects: Restlessness or insomnia are occasional side-effects. Others more rarely reported include, dizziness, tremor, visual disturbances, headache, migraine and hyperprolactinaemia. Extrapyramidal symptoms, such as akinesia, may occur rarely at the recommended dose and if they do occur treatment with Fluanxol should be withdrawn. Precipitation of hypomania has been occasionally reported.

Late onset disorders, including tardive dyskinesia, have occasionally been reported in patients receiving flupenthixol but no cases have been confirmed in patients treated with Fluanxol within the recommended dose.

Overdose: Overdosage should be treated by gastric lavage and by parenteral antiparkinson drugs if extrapyramidal symptoms occur.

Pharmacological properties
Pharmacodynamic properties: The precise pharmacological mode of action of flupenthixol has not been determined. It has been postulated that at low dosage flupenthixol binds to presynaptic dopamine receptors causing increased neurotransmitter release. There is evidence that postsynaptic aminergic receptors become down regulated in response to increased levels of neurotransmitter and this is responsible for the observed improvement in depressive symptoms.

Pharmacokinetic properties: Mean oral bioavailability is about 55%. Maximum drug serum concentrations occur about 4 hours after dosing and the biological half-life is about 35 hours. Flupenthixol is widely distributed in the body. Metabolism is by sulphoxidation, N-dealkylation and glucuronic acid conjugation. Excretion is via the urine and faeces.

Preclinical safety data: Nil of relevance.

Pharmaceutical particulars
List of excipients: Potato starch, Lactose, Gelatin, Talc, Magnesium Stearate, Sucrose and Ultralake Ponceau 4R (E124).

Incompatibilities: None known.

Shelf-life: Fluanxol tablets 0.5 mg are stable for 3 years. Fluanxol tablets 1 mg are stable for 5 years. The box is labelled with an expiry date.

Special precautions for storage: None.

Nature and contents of container: PVC/PVdC blister strips of 60 tablets per box.

Instructions for use/handling: Nil.

Marketing authorisation number
Fluanxol tablets 0.5 mg PL 0458/0011R
Fluanxol tablets 1 mg PL 0458/0037

Date of first authorisation/renewal of authorisation
Fluanxol tablets 0.5 mg:23 November 1982 / 25 November 1992
Fluanxol tablets 1 mg:23 September 1982 / 30 November 1992

Date of (partial) revision of the text 20 August 1997

Legal category POM

SERDOLECT* ▼

Qualitative and quantitative composition
Serdolect 4 mg: Sertindole 4 mg
Serdolect 12 mg: Sertindole 12 mg
Serdolect 16 mg: Sertindole 16 mg
Serdolect 20 mg: Sertindole 20 mg

Pharmaceutical form Coated tablets intended for oral administration.

Clinical particulars
Therapeutic indications: Serdolect is indicated for the treatment of schizophrenia.

Serdolect should not be used in emergency situations for urgent relief of symptoms in acutely disturbed patients.

Posology and method of administration: Serdolect is administered orally once daily with or without meals. In patients where sedation is required, a benzodiazepine may be co-administered.

Adults: All patients should be started on Serdolect 4 mg/day. The dose should be increased by 4 mg increments after 4–5 days on each dose to the optimal daily maintenance dosage range of 12–20 mg. Dependent upon individual patient response the dose may be increased to a maximum of 24 mg/day. During maintenance treatment further dose adjustments should be made on the basis of an assessment of the clinical response and should preferably be performed after at least five days of administration of that dose.

Patients' blood pressure should be monitored during the period of dose titration and early follow up on maintenance dose.

A starting dose of 8 mg or a rapid increase in dose carries a significantly increased risk of severe hypotension.

Elderly: A pharmacokinetic study showed no difference between young and elderly subjects, however until further clinical experience is available the product should be used with care.

Slower titration and lower maintenance doses may be appropriate in elderly patients, who potentially have greater sensitivity to cardiovascular effects of sertindole.

Children: The safety and efficacy of Serdolect in children have not been established.

Reduced renal function: Serdolect can be given in usual dosage even to patients with severe renal impairment. The pharmacokinetics of sertindole were not affected by haemodialysis.

Reduced hepatic function: Patients with mild/moderate hepatic impairment require slower titration and a lower maintenance dose.

Retitration of Serdolect in patients previously discontinued: When restarting patients who have had an interval of less than one week without Serdolect, retitration of Serdolect is not required and their maintenance dose can be reintroduced. Otherwise the recommended titration schedule should be followed.

Switching from other antipsychotics: Treatment with Serdolect can be initiated according to the recommended titration schedule concomitantly with either a gradual withdrawal or immediate cessation of other oral antipsychotics. For patients on depot antipsychotics Serdolect is initiated in place of the next depot injection.

Contra-indications: Serdolect is contra-indicated in patients with known prolongation of the QT interval and in patients receiving drugs known to prolong QT interval (e.g. terfenadine and astemizole; thioridazine; a number of antiarrhythmic agents; some antidepressants) and in patients with clinically significant cardiac disease or uncorrected hypokalaemia.

If diuretic treatment is needed, concomitant treatment with a potassium-sparing diuretic is required in order not to affect the potassium balance. Other drugs that may induce hypokalaemia are contra-indicated.

Severe hepatic impairment: Administration of Serdolect is contra-indicated in patients with severe hepatic impairment.

Co-administration of Serdolect with systemic treatment with ketoconazole or itraconazole is contra-indicated (see *Interactions* section).

Known hypersensitivity to sertindole or any of the ingredients in the product.

Serdolect should not be used during pregnancy and lactation (see *Pregnancy and lactation* and *Preclinical safety data*).

Special warnings and precautions
Cardiovascular: Due to the α_1-blocking activity of Serdolect, symptoms of orthostatic hypotension may occur during the initial dose-titration period.

Serdolect lengthens the QT interval in some patients. The risk of QT prolongation is increased in patients receiving concomitant treatment with drugs that prolong the QT interval (see *Contra-indications*) or drugs that inhibit sertindole metabolism. Other risk factors are cardiovascular disease, hypokalaemia, hypomagnesaemia and bradycardia.

Serdolect should be used with caution in patients with known cardiovascular disease, or other conditions that would predispose patients to hypotension.

An ECG should be performed before commencing treatment with Serdolect to establish prospective patients' baseline QT interval.

In clinical trials, QT_{c2} interval (cube root correction of the observed QT interval) prolongation to ≥500 msec was observed in 24 of the 1,446 patients (1.66%). For these 24 patients, the mean (±SD) increase was 26.5 (±7)% to values ranging from 500 msec to 581 msec. This effect did not correlate with plasma concentrations of sertindole and/or its metabolites. Although the effect was observed most often during the first 3–6 weeks of treatment, patients should be monitored by periodic ECGs while receiving Serdolect. If the QT_{c2} interval exceeds 520 msec, the treatment with Serdolect should be discontinued.

Hypokalaemia and hypomagnesaemia should be corrected and maintained within normal range during treatment.

Antipsychotic drugs may inhibit the effects of dopamine agonists. Serdolect should be used cautiously in patients with Parkinson's disease.

Reduced hepatic function: Patients with mild/moderate hepatic dysfunction should be closely observed. Slower titration and a lower maintenance dose are more appropriate.

Diabetic patients: Serdolect may modify insulin and glucose responses in diabetic patients calling for adjustment of antidiabetic therapy.

Tardive dyskinesia: Tardive dyskinesia is thought to be caused by dopamine receptor hypersensitivity in the basal ganglia as a result of chronic receptor blockade by antipsychotics. A low incidence of Extrapyramidal Symptoms on Serdolect (comparable to that of placebo) has been seen in clinical studies. However, long-term treatment with antipsychotic compounds (especially at high dosages) is associated with the risk of tardive dyskinesia. If signs of tardive dyskinesia appear dosage reduction or drug discontinuation should be considered.

Seizures: Serdolect should be used with caution in patients with a history of seizures.

Neuroleptic Malignant Syndrome: A potentially fatal symptom complex sometimes referred to as Neuroleptic Malignant Syndrome (NMS) has been reported in association with antipsychotic drugs. The management of NMS should include immediate discontinuation of antipsychotic drugs.

Interactions with other medicaments and other forms of interaction: Serdolect is extensively metabolised by the CYP2D6 and CYP3A isozymes of the cytochrome P450 system. CYP2D6 is polymorphic in the population and both isozymes can be inhibited by a variety of psychotropic and other drugs.

CYP2D6: The plasma concentration of sertindole is increased by a factor of 2–3 in patients concurrently taking fluoxetine or paroxetine (potent CYP2D6 inhibitors) and a lower maintenance dose of sertindole may be required. Although not investigated, comparable effects are expected for quinidine (potent CYP2D6 inhibitor), which in addition is known to prolong the QT interval (see *Contra-indications*). Other potential CYP2D6 inhibitors (such as sertraline, tricyclic antidepressants, and propranolol) appear not to influence the plasma concentration of sertindole. *In vitro* studies have shown that high concentrations of sertindole and its major metabolites inhibit the activity of CYP2D6. Sertindole is proposed to be a weak inhibitor of CYP2D6 substrates since the dextromethorphan metabolic ratio was only slightly affected during Serdolect treatment.

Substrates of CYP2D6 isozyme include β-blockers, antiarrhythmic agents, some antihypertensives and a large number of neuroleptics and antidepressants. CYP2D6 is markedly inhibited by quinidine, fluoxetine and paroxetine.

CYP3A: Of the interactions detected for CYP3A substrates, none are of sufficient magnitude to be clinically significant. Minor increases (<25%) in sertindole plasma concentrations have been noted for macrolide antibiotics (e.g. erythromycin, CYP3A inhibitor) and calcium channel antagonists (weak CYP3A inhibitors). Ketoconazole and itraconazole are both very strong inhibitors of CYP3A (see *Contra-indications*); however with CYP2D6 poor metabolisers the inhibitory effect could be much larger, since elimination of sertindole by both CYP2D6 and CYP3A would be affected.

Substrates of CYP3A isozyme include immunomodulators, calcium channel blockers and class III antiarrhythmic agents. The most well known inhibitors of CYP3A are cimetidine, many imidazole antifungal agents and macrolide antibiotics.

The metabolism of sertindole is significantly enhanced by agents known to induce CYP isozymes, notably carbamazepine and phenytoin, which can decrease the plasma concentrations of sertindole by a factor of 2 to 3. Reduced antipsychotic efficacy in patients receiving these drugs or other inducing agents may require the dose of Serdolect to be adjusted to the upper dosage range.

Other potent inhibitors of CYP2D6 and CYP3A may increase the AUC and the C_{max} of sertindole. A reduction in the Serdolect dose should be considered for patients taking such drugs.

Pregnancy and lactation: The safety of Serdolect for use during pregnancy has not been established and therefore, Serdolect should not be used during pregnancy. Sertindole was not teratogenic in animal reproduction studies. A peri/postnatal study in rats showed a decrease in offspring fertility at a dose within the therapeutic range for humans (0.2 mg/kg/day) and at higher dosages a decreased pup survival in early lactation period, reduced weight gain and delayed development of pups in doses not clearly free of producing maternal toxicity.

Sertindole is excreted in the milk in rats, however it is not known whether it is excreted in human milk. Therefore, Serdolect should not be used duration lactation. Nursing mothers should not breast feed if they are under treatment with Serdolect.

Effects on ability to drive and use machines: Serdolect is not sedative, however patients should be advised not to drive or operate machinery until their individual susceptibility is known.

Undesirable effects

Side-effects: In clinical trials, adverse events with an incidence greater than 1% associated with the use of Serdolect and significantly different from placebo were (listed in order of decreasing frequency): Rhinitis/nasal congestion, abnormal ejaculation (decreased ejaculatory volume), dizziness, dry mouth, postural hypotension, weight gain, peripheral oedema, dyspnoea, paraesthesia and prolonged QT interval.

Extrapyramidal symptoms (EPS): The incidences of patients treated with Serdolect reporting EPS-related adverse events, were similar to the frequencies occurring in patients receiving placebo. In addition, in placebo-controlled clinical trials, the percentage of Serdolect patients requiring anti-EPS medication was indistinguishable from those receiving placebo.

Decreased ejaculatory volume: Male patients may experience decreased ejaculatory volume. This symptom, which usually occurs within two months of treatment, is generally not associated with decreased libido, erection and orgasm. Patients do produce sperm and should be advised to use appropriate contraceptive measures to avoid unwanted pregnancy. Normal ejaculatory volume generally returns upon discontinuation.

Body weight: As with the use of other antipsychotic drugs, patients should be advised of the potential for weight gain when taking Serdolect.

Convulsions, hyperglycaemia and syncope have been reported rarely. An ECG is desirable to check the QT interval in patients who experience syncope and seizure on Serdolect.

In comparison with control groups, patients on sertindole had a higher frequency of red and white blood cells on microscopy of urine but the clinical significance of this finding is not clear at present.

After long-term treatment (months to years) movement disorders (in particular tardive dyskinesia) may arise either during or after treatment (see *Special warnings and precautions for use*).

Overdose: Experience with Serdolect in acute overdose is limited. Patients taking estimated dosages up to 240 mg have recovered without sequelae. In general, reported signs and symptoms of overdose were somnolence, slurred speech, tachycardia, hypotension and transient prolongation of the QT interval.

Treatment: In case of acute overdose, establishment of an airway and maintenance of adequate oxygenation should be ensured. Cardiovascular monitoring should commence immediately and monitoring of cardiac conduction should be considered to detect possible arrhythmias. Intravenous access should be established, and the administration of activated charcoal with laxative should be considered. The possibility of multiple drug involvement should be considered.

There is no specific antidote to sertindole, and it is not dialysable, therefore appropriate supportive measures should be instituted. Hypotension and circulatory collapse should be treated with appropriate measures such as intravenous fluids. If sympathomimetic agents are used for vascular support, epinephrine and dopamine should not be used, since β-stimulation combined with α_1 antagonism associated with sertindole may worsen hypotension.

If antiarrhythmic therapy is administered, agents such as quinidine, disopyramide, and procainamide carry a theoretical hazard of QT interval-prolonging effects that might be additive to those of sertindole.

In cases of severe extrapyramidal symptoms, anticholinergic medication should be administered. Close medical supervision and monitoring should continue until the patient recovers.

Pharmacological properties

Pharmacodynamic properties: ATC-code: N05A

Serdolect is a limbic selective antipsychotic drug.

It has been proposed that the neuropharmacological profile of sertindole, as an antipsychotic drug, is derived from its selective inhibitory effect on mesolimbic dopaminergic neurons and is due to balanced inhibitory effects on central dopamine D_2 and serotonin $5HT_2$ receptors as well as on α_1-andrenergic receptors.

In animal pharmacology studies, sertindole inhibited spontaneously active dopamine neurons in the mesolimbic ventral tegmental area (VTA) with a selectivity ratio of more than 100 compared to dopamine neurons in substantia nigra pars compacta (SNC). Inhibition of SNC activity is thought to be involved in movement side effects associated with many antipsychotic drugs.

Antipsychotic drugs are known to increase serum prolactin levels through dopamine blockade. Patients receiving Serdolect remained within normal limits both in short-term studies and during long-term treatment (one year).

Sertindole has no effect on muscarinic and histaminic H_1 receptors. This is confirmed by the absence of anticholinergic and sedative effects related to those receptors.

Pharmacokinetic properties: Elimination of sertindole is via hepatic metabolism, with a mean terminal half-life of approximately three days. The clearance of sertindole decreases with multiple dosing to a mean around 14 L/h (females have approximately 20% lower apparent clearance than males, although lean-mass corrected clearances are comparable). Therefore upon multiple dosing, accumulation is greater than predicted from a single dose, due to an increase in the systemic bioavailability. However, at steady state, clearance is dose-independent and concentrations are proportional to dose. There is a moderate intersubject variability in sertindole pharmacokinetics which is due to the polymorphism in the cytochrome P450 2D6 (CYP2D6). Patients who are deficient in this hepatic enzyme have sertindole clearances that are $\frac{1}{2}$ to $\frac{1}{3}$ of those who are CYP2D6 extensive metabolisers. These poor metaboliser patients (up to 10% of the population) will therefore have plasma levels 2–3 times the normal. Sertindole concentration is not predictive of therapeutic effect for an individual patient; thus, dosing individualisation is best achieved by assessment of therapeutic effect and tolerability.

Absorption: Serdolect is well absorbed with a T_{max} of sertindole after oral administration of approximately 10 hours. Different dose strengths are bioequivalent. Food and aluminium-magnesium antacids have no clinically significant effect on the rate or the extent of sertindole absorption.

Distribution: The apparent volume of distribution (V_β/F) of sertindole after multiple dosing is approximately 20 L/kg. Sertindole is about 99.5% bound to plasma proteins, primarily to albumin and α_1-acid glycoprotein. In patients treated with recommended doses, 90% of the measured concentrations are below 140 ng/ml (~320 nmol/L). Sertindole penetrates into red blood cells with a blood/plasma ratio of 1.0. Sertindole readily penetrates the blood-brain and placental barriers.

Metabolism: Two metabolites have been identified in human plasma; dehydrosertindole (oxidation of the imidazolidinone ring) and norsertindole (N-dealkylation). Concentrations of dehydrosertindole and norsertindole are approximately 80% and 40% respectively, of the parent compound at steady state. Sertindole activity is primarily due to the parent drug and the metabolites do not appear to have significant pharmacological effects in humans.

Excretion: Sertindole and its metabolites are eliminated very slowly, with a total recovery of 50–60% of a radiolabelled oral dose, 14 days after administration. Approximately 4% of the dose is excreted into the urine as parent drug plus metabolites of which less than 1% of the dose is parent drug. Faecal excretion is the major route of excretion and accounts for the rest of the parent drug and metabolites.

Preclinical safety data: The acute toxicity of sertindole is low. In chronic toxicity studies in the rat and dog (3–5 times clinical exposure) several effects were observed. These effects are in line with the pharmacological properties of the drug.

Animal reproduction studies have not given evidence of teratogenic effects. Exposure of rats during the last third of pregnancy and during lactation resulted in a decrease in offspring fertility at a dose within the therapeutic range for humans (0.2 mg/kg/day). Mating and fertility were affected in adult male rats at dosages above 0.04 mg/kg/day. The adult fertility impairment, which was reversible, was ascribed to the pharmacological profile of sertindole.

Sertindole was not toxic in a battery of in vitro and in vivo genotoxicity studies. Carcinogenicity studies conducted in the mouse and rat did not indicate any development of tumours relevant to the clinical use of sertindole.

Pharmaceutical particulars

List of excipients: Tablets: Maize starch, lactose monohydrate, hydroxypropylcellulose, microcrystalline-cellulose, croscarmellose sodium, magnesium stearate, macrogol 400, hydroxypropylmethylcellulose and titanium dioxide (E171).

Incompatibilities: None known.

Shelf life: Serdolect tablets have a shelf-life of 24 months.

Special precautions for storage: Store tablets in original pack to protect from light.

Nature and contents of container: Serdolect tablets 4 mg, 12 mg, 16 mg and 20 mg are provided in PVC/PVdC laminate (clear or white) with aluminium foil, inside a carton blackened on the inside, containing 28 or 30 tablets.

Instructions for use/handling: No special precautions.

Marketing authorisation holder: H. Lundbeck A/S, Ottiliavej 9, DK-2500 Copenhagen-Valby, Denmark.

Marketing authorisation numbers

4 mg tablets	13761/0001
12 mg tablets	13761/0003
16 mg tablets	13761/0004
20 mg tablets	13761/0005

Date of approval/revision of SPC 25 October 1996.

Legal category POM.

**Trade Mark*

3M Health Care Limited
Morley Street
Loughborough
Leics LE11 1EP

☎ 01509 611611   🗋 01509 237288

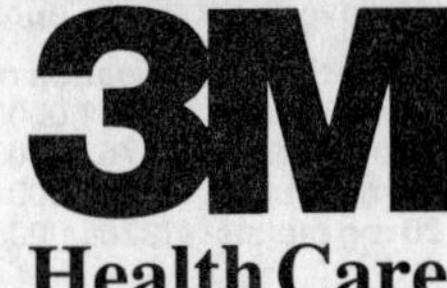

ACUPAN*

Presentation Acupan Tablets: White, film-coated, circular, biconvex tablets, 7 mm in diameter, marked APN on one side. Each tablet contains nefopam hydrochloride 30 mg.

Acupan Injection: Each 2 ml ampoule contains 1 ml of a solution of nefopam hydrochloride 20 mg/ml.

It also contains the following inactive ingredients: Sodium Acid Phosphate PhEur; Sodium Phosphate PhEur; Water for Injections PhEur.

Uses Acupan is indicated for the relief of acute and chronic pain, including: post-operative pain; dental pain; musculo-skeletal pain; acute traumatic pain and cancer pain.

Acupan is a potent and rapidly-acting analgesic. It is totally distinct from other centrally-acting analgesics such as morphine, codeine, pentazocine and propoxyphene.

Unlike the narcotic agents, Acupan has been shown not to cause respiratory depression. There is no evidence from pre-clinical research of habituation occurring with Acupan.

Dosage and administration *Adults: Acupan Tablets:* Dosage may range from 1 to 3 tablets three times daily depending on response. The recommended starting dosage is 2 tablets three times daily.

Acupan Injection: 20 mg (1 ml) intramuscularly repeated if necessary every six hours (see instructions for administration). Onset of effect after intramuscular injection is within 15–20 minutes and peak effect is reached at one to one-and-a-half hours after administration.

Treatment started with Acupan injection may be continued with Acupan Tablets. 60 mg Acupan (2 tablets) is approximately bioequivalent to 20 mg (1 ampoule) given by injection.

Instructions for administration of Acupan Injection: Acupan Injection should always be given with the patient lying down and after injection the patient should remain lying down for 15–20 minutes. The patient should then get up slowly.

Elderly: Elderly patients may require reduced dosage due to slower metabolism. It is strongly recommended that the starting dose does not exceed one tablet three times daily as the elderly appear more susceptible to, in particular, the CNS side-effects of Acupan and some cases of hallucination and confusion have been reported in this age group.

Children: Since Acupan has not been evaluated in children no dosage recommendation can be given for patients under 12 years.

Contra-indications, warnings, etc *Side-effects:* Nausea, nervousness, dry mouth, lightheadedness and urinary retention may occur. Less frequently, vomiting, blurred vision, drowsiness, sweating, insomnia, headache and tachycardia have been reported.

Caution: The side-effects of Acupan may be additive to those of other agents with anticholinergic or sympathomimetic activity.

It should not be used in the treatment of myocardial infarction since there is no clinical experience in this indication.

Hepatic and renal insufficiency may interfere with the metabolism and excretion of nefopam.

Caution should be exercised when nefopam is administered concurrently with tricyclic antidepressants.

Acupan should be used with caution in patients with, or at risk of, urinary retention. Rarely a temporary, harmless pink discolouration has occurred.

Use in pregnancy: There is no evidence as to the drug safety in human pregnancy nor is there evidence from animal work that it is free from hazard. Avoid in pregnancy unless there is no safer treatment.

Contra-indications: Acupan is contra-indicated in patients with a history of convulsive disorders and should not be given to patients taking mono-amine-oxidase (MAO) inhibitors.

Overdosage: The clinical pattern of nefopam toxicity in overdose is on the neurological (convulsions, hallucinations and agitation) and cardiovascular systems (tachycardia with a hyperdynamic circulation). Routine supportive measures should be taken and prompt removal of ingested drug by gastric lavage or induced vomiting with Syrup of Ipecacuanha should be carried out. Oral administration of activated charcoal may help prevent absorption. Convulsions and hallucinations should be controlled (e.g. with intravenously or rectally administered diazepam). Beta-adrenergic blockers may help control the cardiovascular complications.

Pharmaceutical precautions
Acupan tablets: Store below 30°C.
Acupan Injection: Store between 5°C and 30°C. Do not freeze.

Package quantities Acupan Tablets; Packs of 90 tablets (OP).
Acupan Injection; Boxes containing 5×2 ml ampoules filled with 1 ml of solution.

Legal category POM.

Further information Nil.

Product licence numbers
Acupan Tablets 0068/0061
Acupan Injection 0068/0069

AEROBEC* 50 AUTOHALER*

Qualitative and quantitative composition Each actuation delivers beclomethasone dipropionate 50 µg (as propellant solvate) into the mouthpiece of the adapter.

Pharmaceutical form Pressurised aerosol for inhalation therapy.

Clinical particulars
Therapeutic indications: AeroBec 50 Autohaler is indicated for the prophylactic treatment of chronic reversible obstructive airways disease.

Posology and method of administration: The dose should be titrated to the lowest dose at which effective control of asthma is maintained.

Adults: for maintenance: 4 inhalations (200 µg), twice daily or 2 inhalations (100 µg), three or four times daily. In more severe cases a dose of 600–800 µg (12–16 inhalations) daily is recommended, with subsequent reductions. The maximum recommended daily dose of this preparation is 1 mg. In patients receiving doses of 1500 µg or more daily, adrenal suppression may occur.

Children: 1 or 2 inhalations (50–100 µg), two to four times daily.

Elderly: No special dosage recommendations are made for elderly patients.

Contra-indications: Hypersensitivity to beclomethasone is a contra-indication. Caution should be observed in patients with pulmonary tuberculosis.

Special warnings and precautions for use: Patients should be instructed on the proper use of the inhaler. They should be made aware of the prophylactic nature of AeroBec Autohaler therapy and that it should be used regularly at the intervals recommended and not when immediate relief is required.

In patients who have been transferred to inhalation therapy, systemic steroid therapy may need to be re-instated rapidly during periods of stress or where airways obstruction or mucus prevents absorption from the inhalation.

Systemic effects of inhaled corticosteroids may occur, particularly at high doses prescribed for prolonged periods. These effects are much less likely to occur than with oral corticosteroids. Possible systemic effects include adrenal suppression, growth retardation in children and adolescents, decrease in bone mineral density, cataract and glaucoma. It is important therefore that the dose of inhaled steroid is titrated to the lowest dose at which effective control of asthma is maintained.

It is recommended that the height of children receiving prolonged treatment with inhaled corticosteroids is regularly monitored. If growth is slowed, therapy should be reviewed with the aim of reducing the dose of inhaled corticosteroid, if possible, to the lowest dose at which effective control of asthma is maintained. In addition, consideration should be given to referring the patient to a paediatric respiratory specialist.

Prolonged treatment with high doses of inhaled corticosteroids, particularly higher than the recommended doses, may result in clinically significant adrenal suppression. Additional systemic corticosteroid cover should be considered during periods of stress or elective surgery.

Patients who have received systemic steroids for long periods of time or at high doses, or both, need special care and subsequent management when transferred to beclomethasone therapy. Recovery from impaired adrenocortical function, caused by prolonged systemic steroid therapy, is slow. The patient should be in a reasonably stable state before being given AeroBec Autohaler in addition to his usual maintenance dose of systemic steroid. Withdrawal of the systemic steroid should be gradual, starting after about seven days by reducing the daily oral dose by 1 mg prednisolone, or equivalent, at intervals not less than one week. Adrenocortical function should be monitored regularly.

Most patients can be successfully transferred to AeroBec Autohaler with maintenance of good respiratory function, but special care is necessary for the first months after the transfer until the hypothalamic-pituitary-adrenal (HPA) system has sufficiently recovered to enable the patient to cope with emergencies such as trauma, surgery or infections.

Patients who have been transferred to inhalation therapy should carry a warning card indicating that systemic steroid therapy may need to be re-instated without delay during periods of stress. It may be advisable to provide such patients with a supply of oral steroid to use in emergency, for example when the asthma worsens as a result of a chest infection. The dose of AeroBec Autohaler should be increased at this time and then gradually reduced to the maintenance level after the systemic steroid has been discontinued.

Discontinuation of systemic steroids may cause exacerbation of allergic diseases such as atopic eczema and rhinitis. These should be treated as required with antihistamine and topical therapy.

Interactions with other medicaments and other forms of interaction: None known.

Pregnancy and lactation: There is inadequate evidence of safety in human pregnancy. In animals, systemic administration of relatively high doses can cause abnormalities of foetal development including growth retardation and cleft palate. There may therefore be a very small risk of such effects in the human foetus. However, inhalation of beclomethasone dipropionate into the lungs avoids the high level of exposure that occurs with administration by systemic routes.

The use of beclomethasone in pregnancy requires that the possible benefits of the drug be weighed against the possible hazards. The drug has been in widespread use for many years without apparent ill consequence.

It is probable that beclomethasone is excreted in milk. However, given the relatively low doses used by the inhalation route, the levels are likely to be low. In mothers breast feeding their baby the therapeutic benefits of the drug should be weighed against the potential hazards to mother and baby.

Effects on ability to drive and use machines: None.

Undesirable effects: Candidiasis of the throat and mouth may develop in some patients, but this can be treated without discontinuation of beclomethasone therapy. Hoarseness may also occur.

Systemic effects of inhaled corticosteroids may occur particularly at high doses prescribed for prolonged periods. These may include adrenal suppression, growth retardation in children and adolescents, decrease in bone mineral density, cataract and glaucoma.

Overdose: Acute overdosage is unlikely to cause problems. The only harmful effect that follows inhalation of large amounts of the drug over a short time period is suppression of HPA function. Specific emergency action need not be taken. Treatment with AeroBec Autohaler should be continued at the recommended dose to control the asthma; HPA function recovers in a day or two.

If grossly excessive doses of beclomethasone dipropionate were taken over a prolonged period a degree of atrophy of the adrenal cortex could occur in addition to HPA suppression. In this event the patient should be treated as steroid-dependent and transferred to a suitable maintenance dose of a systemic steroid such as prednisolone. Once the condition is stabilised the patient should be returned to AeroBec Autohaler by the method recommended above.

Pharmacological properties

Pharmacodynamic properties: Inhaled beclomethasone dipropionate is now well established in the management of asthma. It is a synthetic glucocorticoid and exerts a topical, anti-inflammatory effect on the lungs, without significant systemic activity.

Pharmacokinetic properties: The beclomethasone dipropionate absorbed directly from the lungs is converted to less active metabolites during its passage through the liver. Peak plasma concentrations are reached 3–5 hours following ingestion. Excretion is via the urine.

Preclinical safety data: Not applicable.

Pharmaceutical particulars

List of excipients: Sorbitan trioleate PhEur, Trichlorofluoromethane (Propellant 11) BP (1988), Dichlorodifluoromethane (Propellant 12) BP (1988), Dichlorotetrafluoroethane (Propellant 114) BP (1988).

Incompatibilties: None known.

Shelf life: 3 years.

Special precautions for storage: Store below 30°C. Avoid storage in direct sunlight or heat. Protect from frost.

Nature and contents of container: 10 ml Aluminium vial closed with a 50 µl metering valve containing 200 doses.

Instruction for use/handling: Pressurised vial. Do not puncture. Do not burn, even when empty.

Marketing authorisation number 0068/0143

Date of first authorisation/renewal of authorisation October 1991

Date of (partial) revision of the text May 1998

AEROBEC* 100 AUTOHALER*

Qualitative and quantitative composition Each actuation delivers beclomethasone dipropionate 100 µg (as propellant solvate) into the mouthpiece of the adapter.

Pharmaceutical form Pressurised aerosol for inhalation therapy.

Clinical particulars

Therapeutic indications: AeroBec 100 Autohaler is indicated for the prophylactic treatment of chronic reversible obstructive airways disease.

Posology and method of administration: The dose should be titrated to the lowest dose at which effective control of asthma is maintained.

Adults: for maintenance: 1 inhalation (100 µg), three or four times daily or 2 inhalations (200 µg), twice daily. In more severe cases a dose of 600–800 µg (6–8 inhalations) daily is recommended, with subsequent reductions. The maximum recommended daily dose of this preparation is 1 mg. In patients receiving doses of 1500 µg or more daily, adrenal suppression may occur.

Children: 1 inhalation (100 µg), two to four times daily.

Elderly: No special dosage recommendations are made for elderly patients.

Contra-indications: Hypersensitivity to beclomethasone is a contra-indication. Caution should be observed in patients with pulmonary tuberculosis.

Special warnings and precautions for use: Patients should be instructed on the proper use of the inhaler. They should be made aware of the prophylactic nature of AeroBec Autohaler therapy and that it should be used regularly at the intervals recommended and not when immediate relief is required.

In patients who have been transferred to inhalation therapy, systemic steroid therapy may need to be reinstated rapidly during periods of stress or where airways obstruction or mucus prevents absorption from the inhalation.

Systemic effects of inhaled corticosteroids may occur, particularly at high doses prescribed for prolonged periods. These effects are much less likely to occur than with oral corticosteroids. Possible systemic effects include adrenal suppression, growth retardation in children and adolescents, decrease in bone mineral density, cataract and glaucoma. It is important therefore that the dose of inhaled steroid is titrated to the lowest dose at which effective control of asthma is maintained.

It is recommended that the height of children receiving prolonged treatment with inhaled corticosteroids is regularly monitored. If growth is slowed, therapy should be reviewed with the aim of reducing the dose of inhaled corticosteroid, if possible, to the lowest dose at which effective control of asthma is maintained. In addition, consideration should be given to referring the patient to a paediatric respiratory specialist.

Prolonged treatment with high doses of inhaled corticosteroids, particularly higher than the recommended doses, may result in clinically significant adrenal suppression. Additional systemic corticosteroid cover should be considered during periods of stress or elective surgery.

Patients who have received systemic steroids for long periods of time or at high doses, or both, need special care and subsequent management when transferred to beclomethasone therapy. Recovery from impaired adrenocortical function, caused by prolonged systemic steroid therapy, is slow. The patient should be in a reasonably stable state before being given AeroBec Autohaler in addition to his usual maintenance dose of systemic steroid. Withdrawal of the systemic steroid should be gradual, starting after about seven days by reducing the daily oral dose by 1 mg prednisolone, or equivalent, at intervals not less than one week. Adrenocortical function should be monitored regularly.

Most patients can be successfully transferred to AeroBec Autohaler with maintenance of good respiratory function, but special care is necessary for the first months after the transfer until the hypothalamic-pituitary-adrenal (HPA) system has sufficiently recovered to enable the patient to cope with emergencies such as trauma, surgery or infections.

Patients who have been transferred to inhalation therapy should carry a warning card indicating that systemic steroid therapy may need to be re-instated without delay during periods of stress. It may be advisable to provide such patients with a supply of oral steroid to use in emergency, for example when the asthma worsens as a result of a chest infection. The dose of AeroBec Autohaler should be increased at this time and then gradually reduced to the maintenance level after the systemic steroid has been discontinued.

Discontinuation of systemic steroids may cause exacerbation of allergic diseases such as atopic eczema and rhinitis. These should be treated as required with antihistamine and topical therapy.

Interactions with other medicaments and other forms of interaction: None known.

Pregnancy and lactation: There is inadequate evidence of safety in human pregnancy. In animals, systemic administration of relatively high doses can cause abnormalities of foetal development including growth retardation and cleft palate. There may therefore be a very small risk of such effects in the human foetus. However, inhalation of beclomethasone dipropionate into the lungs avoids the high level of exposure that occurs with administration by systemic routes.

The use of beclomethasone in pregnancy requires that the possible benefits of the drug be weighed against the possible hazards. The drug has been in widespread use for many years without apparent ill consequence.

It is probable that beclomethasone is excreted in milk. However, given the relatively low doses used by the inhalation route, the levels are likely to be low. In mothers breast feeding their baby the therapeutic benefits of the drug should be weighed against the potential hazards to mother and baby.

Effects on ability to drive and use machines: None.

Undesirable effects: Candidiasis of the throat and mouth may develop in some patients, but this can be treated with discontinuation of beclomethasone therapy. Hoarseness may also occur.

Systemic effects of inhaled corticosteroids may occur particularly at high doses prescribed for prolonged periods. These may include adrenal suppression, growth retardation in children and adolescents, decrease in bone mineral density, cataract and glaucoma.

Overdose: Acute overdosage is unlikely to cause problems. The only harmful effect that follows inhalation of large amounts of the drug over a short time period is suppression of HPA function. Specific emergency action need not be taken. Treatment with AeroBec Autohaler should be continued at the recommended dose to control the asthma; HPA function recovers in a day or two.

If grossly excessive doses of beclomethasone dipropionate were taken over a prolonged period a degree of atrophy of the adrenal cortex could occur in addition to HPA suppression. In this event the patient should be treated as steroid-dependent and transferred to a suitable maintenance dose of a systemic steroid such as prednisolone. Once the condition is stabilised the patient should be returned to AeroBec Autohaler by the method recommended above.

Pharmacological properties

Pharmacodynamic properties: Inhaled beclomethasone dipropionate is now well established in the management of asthma. It is a synthetic glucocorticoid and exerts a topical, anti-inflammatory effect on the lungs, without significant systemic activity.

Pharmacokinetic properties: The beclomethasone dipropionate absorbed directly from the lungs is converted to less active metabolites during its passage through the liver. Peak plasma concentrations are reached 3–5 hours following ingestion. Excretion is via the urine.

Preclinical safety data: Not applicable.

Pharmaceutical particulars

List of excipients: Sorbitan trioleate PhEur, Trichlorofluoromethane (Propellant 11) BP (1988), Dichlorodifluoromethane (Propellant 12) BP (1988), Dichlorotetrafluoroethane (Propellant 114) BP (1988).

Incompatibilities: None known.

Shelf life: 3 years.

Special precautions for storage: Store below 30°C. Avoid storage in direct sunlight or heat. Protect from frost.

Nature and contents of container: 10 ml aluminium vial closed with a 50 µl metering valve containing 200 doses.

Instruction for use/handling: Pressurised vial. Do not puncture. Do not burn, even when empty.

Marketing authorisation number 0068/0145

Date of first authorisation/renewal of authorisation January 1992

Date of last (partial) revision of the text May 1998

AEROBEC* FORTE AUTOHALER*

Qualitative and quantitative composition Each actuation delivers beclomethasone dipropionate 250 µg (as propellant solvate) into the mouthpiece of the adapter.

Pharmaceutical form Pressurised aerosol for inhalation therapy.

Clinical particulars

Therapeutic indications: AeroBec Forte Autohaler is indicated for the prophylactic treatment of chronic reversible obstructive airways disease in those patients who require high doses of beclomethasone to control their symptoms.

Posology and method of administration: The dose should be titrated to the lowest dose at which effective control of asthma is maintained.

Adults: for maintenance: 2 inhalations (500 µg), twice daily or 1 inhalation (250 µg), four times daily, may be increased to 2 inhalations four times daily if necessary.

In patients receiving doses of 1500 µg or more daily, adrenal suppression may occur. The degree of suppression may not always be clinically significant but it is advisable to provide such patients with a supply of oral steroid to use in stressful situations. The risk of adrenal suppression occurring should be balanced against the therapeutic advantages.

Children: AeroBec Forte Autohaler is not recommended for use in children.

Elderly: No special dosage recommendations are made for elderly patients.

Contra-indications: Hypersensitivity to beclomethasone is a contra-indication. Caution should be observed in patients with pulmonary tuberculosis.

Special warnings and precautions for use: Patients should be instructed on the proper use of the inhaler. They should be made aware of the prophylactic nature of AeroBec Autohaler therapy and that it should be used regularly at the intervals recommended and not when immediate relief is required.

In patients who have been transferred to inhalation therapy, systemic steroid therapy may need to be reinstated rapidly during periods of stress or where airways obstruction or mucus prevents absorption from the inhalation.

Systemic effects of inhaled corticosteroids may occur, particularly at high doses prescribed for prolonged periods. These effects are much less likely to occur than with oral corticosteroids. Possible systemic effects include adrenal suppression, growth retardation in adolescents, decrease in bone mineral density, cataract and glaucoma. It is important therefore that the dose of inhaled steroid is titrated to the lowest dose at which effective control of asthma is maintained.

It is recommended that the height of adolescents receiving prolonged treatment with inhaled corticosteroids is regularly monitored. If growth is slowed, therapy should be reviewed with the aim of reducing the dose of inhaled corticosteroid, if possible, to the lowest dose at which effective control of asthma is maintained.

Prolonged treatment with high doses of inhaled corticosteroids, particularly higher than the recommended doses, may result in clinically significant adrenal suppression. Additional systemic corticosteroid cover should be considered during periods of stress or elective surgery.

Patients who have received systemic steroids for long periods of time or at high doses, or both, need special care and subsequent management when transferred to beclomethasone therapy. Recovery from impaired adrenocortical function, caused by prolonged systemic steroid therapy, is slow. The patient should be in a reasonably stable state before being given AeroBec Autohaler in addition to his usual maintenance dose of systemic steroid. Withdrawal of the systemic steroid should be gradual, starting after about seven days by reducing the daily oral dose by 1 mg prednisolone, or equivalent, at intervals not less than one week. Adrenocortical function should be monitored regularly.

Most patients can be successfully transferred to AeroBec Autohaler with maintenance of good respiratory function, but special care is necessary for the first months after the transfer until the hypothalamic-pituitary-adrenal (HPA) system has sufficiently recovered to enable the patient to cope with emergencies such as trauma, surgery or infections.

Patients who have been transferred to inhalation therapy should carry a warning card indicating that systemic steroid therapy may need to be re-instated without delay during periods of stress. It may be advisable to provide such patients with a supply of oral steroid to use in an emergency, for example when the asthma worsens as a result of a chest infection. The dose of AeroBec Autohaler should be increased at this time and then gradually reduced to the maintenance level after the systemic steroid has been discontinued.

Discontinuation of systemic steroids may cause exacerbation of allergic diseases such as atopic eczema and rhinitis. These should be treated as required with antihistamine and topical therapy.

Interactions with other medicaments and other forms of interaction: None known.

Pregnancy and lactation: There is inadequate evidence of safety in human pregnancy. In animals, systemic administration of relatively high doses can cause abnormalities of foetal development including growth retardation and cleft palate. There may therefore be a very small risk of such effects in the human foetus. However, inhalation of beclomethasone dipropionate into the lungs avoids the high level of exposure that occurs with administration by systemic routes.

The use of beclomethasone in pregnancy requires that the possible benefits of the drug be weighed against the possible hazards. The drug has been in widespread use for many years without apparent ill consequence.

It is probable that beclomethasone is excreted in milk. However, given the relatively low doses used by the inhalation route, the levels are likely to be low. In mothers breast feeding their baby the therapeutic benefits of the drug should be weighed against the potential hazards to mother and baby.

Effects on ability to drive and use machines: None.

Undesirable effects: Candidiasis of the throat and mouth may develop in some patients, but this can be treated without discontinuation of beclomethasone therapy. Hoarseness may also occur.

Systemic effects of inhaled corticosteroids may occur particularly at high doses prescribed for prolonged periods. These may include adrenal suppression, growth retardation in adolescents, decrease in bone mineral density, cataract and glaucoma.

Overdose: If grossly excessive doses of beclomethasone dipropionate were taken over a prolonged period a degree of atrophy of the adrenal cortex could occur in addition to HPA suppression. In this event the patient should be treated as steroid-dependent and transferred to a suitable maintenance dose of a systemic steroid such as prednisolone. Once the condition is stabilised the patient should be returned to AeroBec Forte Autohaler by the method recommended above. To guard against unexpected occurrence of adrenal suppression regular tests of adrenal function are advised.

Pharmacological properties

Pharmacodynamic properties: Inhaled beclomethasone dipropionate is now well established in the management of asthma. It is a synthetic glucocorticoid and exerts a topical, anti-inflammatory effect on the lungs, without significant systemic activity.

Pharmacokinetic properties: The beclomethasone dipropionate absorbed directly from the lungs is converted to less active metabolites during its passage through the liver. Peak plasma concentrations are reached 3–5 hours following ingestion. Excretion is via the urine.

Preclinical safety data: Not applicable.

Pharmaceutical particulars

List of excipients: Sorbitan trioleate PhEur, Trichlorofluoromethane (Propellant 11) BP (1988), Dichlorodifluoromethane (Propellant 12) BP (1988), Dichlorotetrafluoroethane (Propellant 114) BP (1988).

Incompatibilities: None known.

Shelf life: 3 years.

Special precautions for storage: Store below 30°C. Avoid storage in direct sunlight or heat. Protect from frost.

Nature and contents of container: 10 ml Aluminium vial closed with a 50 μl metering valve containing 200 doses.

Instruction for use/handling: Pressurised vial. Do not puncture. Do not burn, even when empty.

Marketing authorisation number 0068/0140

Date of first authorisation/renewal of authorisation October 1991

Date of last (partial) revision of the text May 1998

AEROLIN* AUTOHALER*

Qualitative and quantitative composition Each actuation of Aerolin Autohaler delivers Salbutamol Sulphate PhEur equivalent to salbutamol 100 micrograms into the mouthpiece of a breath-actuated adapter.

Pharmaceutical form Aerolin Autohaler is a pressurised aerosol for bronchodilator inhalation therapy.

Clinical particulars

Therapeutic indications: Aerolin Autohaler is indicated in the management of bronchial asthma, for the relief of wheezing and shortness of breath used on an as required basis. Aerolin Autohaler may be used as necessary to relieve attacks of acute dyspnoea and may be used prophylactically before exertion or to prevent exercise-induced asthma.

Aerolin Autohaler may also be used in the treatment of the reversible component of airways obstruction.

Posology and method of administration

Adults: For the relief of wheezing, shortness of breath and attacks of acute dyspnoea in patients with asthma, or reversible airways obstruction associated with chronic bronchitis and emphysema, one or two inhalations may be administered as a single dose.

For prophylaxis of exercise-induced asthma, two inhalations before exercise.

Children: For the relief of wheezing, shortness of breath and attacks of acute dyspnoea in children with asthma, one inhalation increasing to two if necessary may be administered as a single dose.

For prophylaxis of exercise-induced asthma, one inhalation increasing to two if necessary before exercise.

Elderly: No special dosage recommendations are made for elderly patients.

For all patients, the maximum recommended dose should not exceed eight inhalations in 24 hours. With repetitive dosing, inhalations should not usually be repeated more often than every 4 hours.

Contra-indications: Hypersensitivity to salbutamol or any of the inactive ingredients in Aerolin Autohaler.

Aerolin Autohaler is contra-indicated for use in the management of premature labour and threatened abortion.

Special warnings and special precautions for use

Special warnings: Potentially serious hypokalaemia has been reported in patients taking beta-2-agonist therapy. Particular caution is advised in patients with severe asthma. Hypokalaemia may also occur in hypoxic patients and those treated with xanthine derivatives, steroids, diuretics and long-term laxatives. Extra care should therefore be taken if beta-2-agonists are used in these groups of patients and serum potassium levels should be monitored.

Unwanted stimulation of cardiac adrenergic receptors can occur in patients taking beta-2-agonist therapy.

Special precautions for use: The patient should be advised to seek medical advice if the treatment ceases to be effective and/or their asthma seems to be worsening, and not to increase the dose without medical advice.

Administer cautiously to patients with thyrotoxicosis.

Interaction with other medicaments and other forms of interaction: Salbutamol and beta-blockers should not usually be prescribed together.

Hypokalaemia occurring with beta-2-agonist therapy may be exacerbated by treatment with xanthines, steroids, diuretics and long-term laxatives.

Pregnancy and lactation: Aerolin should not be used in pregnancy and lactation unless the expected benefit to the mother is thought to outweigh any risk to the foetus or neonate.

The safe use of inhaled salbutamol during pregnancy has not been established but it has been in widespread use for many years in human beings without apparent ill consequence. In mice and rabbits large doses of salbutamol have been shown to be teratogenic.

It is not known whether salbutamol is distributed into breast milk.

Effects on ability to drive and use machines: None.

Undesirable effects: Mild tremor, headache, palpitations, tachycardia and transient muscle cramps may rarely occur. Potentially serious hypokalaemia has been reported in patients taking beta-2-agonist therapy.

Hypersensitivity reactions and hyperactivity in children have been reported rarely.

As with other inhalation therapy, paradoxical bronchospasm may occur immediately after dosing. In this instance, Aerolin Autohaler should be discontinued immediately and alternative therapy instituted if necessary.

Overdose: Treatment: Asthmatic patients: Monitor biochemical abnormalities, particularly hypokalaemia which should be treated with potassium replacement where necessary. Beta-adrenoceptor antagonists, even beta-1-selective antagonists, are potentially life-threatening and should be avoided.

Non-asthmatic patients: Monitor and correct biochemical abnormalities, particularly hypokalaemia. A non-selective beta-adrenoceptor antagonist (e.g. nadolol, propranolol) will competitively reverse both hypokalaemia and tachycardia (beta-1-selective drugs will be largely ineffective).

Pharmacological properties

Pharmacodynamic properties: Salbutamol is a sympathomimetic agent which has a selective action on beta-2-adrenergic receptors in bronchial smooth muscle.

Pharmacokinetic properties: Salbutamol is readily absorbed from the gastro-intestinal tract, but the systemic absorption of the inhaled drug substance is low. The action of inhaled salbutamol depends on direct stimulation of receptors in the lung. Onset of action is usually within 10 minutes of inhalation and lasts 4–6 hours in most patients.

Salbutamol is subject to first-pass metabolism in the liver; about half is excreted in the urine as an inactive sulphate conjugate. It does not appear to be metabolised in the lung and therefore its fate following inhalation therapy depends on the delivery method used, which determines the proportion of salbutamol inhaled relative to the proportion inadvertently swallowed. It has been suggested that the slightly extended half-life following inhalation may reflect slow removal of active drug from the lungs.

Preclinical safety data: Salbutamol has been in widespread use for many years; there have been no adverse clinical findings with Aerolin Autohaler which might reflect pre-clinical safety issues (see *Pregnancy and lactation*).

Pharmaceutical particulars

List of excipients: The excipients in Aerolin Autohaler are sorbitan trioleate, propellants 11, 12 and 114.

Incompatibilities: None known.

Shelf life: 3 years.

Special precautions for storage: Store below 30°C. Avoid storage in direct sunlight or heat. Protect from frost.

Nature and contents of container: Aerolin Autohaler contains 200 metered doses.

Instructions for use/handling: The patient should read the patient leaflet before use.

As the canister is pressurised, no attempt should be made to puncture it or dispose of it by burning.

Marketing authorisation number PL 0068/0117

Date of first authorisation/renewal of authorisation 27 April 1992/30 September 1997

Date of (partial) revision of the text October 1997

AIROMIR* AUTOHALER*

Qualitative and quantitative composition Each actuation of Airomir Autohaler device delivers Salbutamol Sulphate PhEur equivalent to salbutamol 100 micrograms into the mouthpiece of the adapter.

Pharmaceutical form Airomir Autohaler device is a breath actuated inhaler for bronchodilator inhalation therapy which automatically releases the metered dose of medication during a patient's inhalation through the mouthpiece and overcomes the need for patients to have good manual co-ordination.

Airomir Autohaler device contains a new propellant and does not contain chlorofluorocarbons (CFCs).

Clinical particulars

Therapeutic indications: Airomir Autohaler device is indicated in the management of bronchial asthma, for the relief of wheezing and shortness of breath used on an as required basis. Airomir Autohaler device may be used as necessary to relieve attacks of acute dyspnoea and may be used prophylactically before exertion or to prevent exercise-induced asthma.

Airomir Autohaler device may also be used in the treatment of reversible airways obstruction associated with chronic bronchitis and emphysema.

Posology and method of administration

Adults: For the relief of wheezing, shortness of breath and attacks of acute dyspnoea in patients with asthma, or reversible airways obstruction associated with chronic bronchitis and emphysema, one or two inhalations may be administered as a single dose.

For prophylaxis of exercise-induced asthma, two inhalations before exercise.

Children: For the relief of wheezing, shortness of breath and attacks of acute dyspnoea in children with asthma, one inhalation increasing to two if necessary may be administered as a single dose.

For prophylaxis of exercise-induced asthma, one inhalation increasing to two if necessary before exercise.

Elderly: No special dosage recommendations are made for elderly patients.

For all patients, the maximum recommended dose should not exceed eight inhalations in 24 hours. With repetitive dosing, inhalations should not usually be repeated more often than every 4 hours.

Contra-indications: Hypersensitivity to salbutamol or any of the inactive ingredients in Airomir Autohaler device.

Airomir Autohaler device is contra-indicated for use in the management of premature labour and threatened abortion.

Special warnings and special precautions for use

Special warnings: Potentially serious hypokalaemia has been reported in patients taking beta-2-agonist therapy. Particular caution is advised in patients with severe asthma. Hypokalaemia may also occur in hypoxic patients and those treated with xanthine derivatives, steroids, diuretics and long-term laxatives. Extra care should therefore be taken if beta-2-agonists are used in these groups of patients and serum potassium levels should be monitored.

Unwanted stimulation of cardiac adrenergic receptors can occur in patients taking beta-2-agonist therapy.

Special precautions for use: The patient should be advised to seek medical advice if the treatment ceases to be effective and/or their asthma seems to be worsening, and not to increase the dose without medical advice.

Administer cautiously to patients with thyrotoxicosis.

Interaction with other medicaments and other forms of interaction: Salbutamol and beta-blockers should not usually be prescribed together.

Hypokalaemia occurring with beta-2-agonist therapy may be exacerbated by treatment with xanthines, steroids, diuretics and long-term laxatives.

Because the Airomir Autohaler device contains ethanol there is a theoretical potential for interaction in patients taking disulfiram or metronidazole. The amount of ethanol in the Airomir Autohaler device is small but it may be enough to precipitate a reaction in some sensitive patients.

Pregnancy and lactation

Airomir Autohaler: There is no experience of this product in pregnancy and lactation in humans. An inhalation reproductive study with the Salbutamol Sulphate CFC-Free formulation in rats did not exhibit any teratogenic effects. It should not be used in pregnancy and lactation unless the expected benefit to the mother is thought to outweigh any risk to the foetus or neonate.

Propellant 134a: Studies of propellant 134a administered to pregnant and lactating rats and rabbits have not revealed any special hazard.

Salbutamol: The safe use of inhaled salbutamol during pregnancy has not been established but it has been in widespread use for many years in human beings without apparent ill consequence. In mice and rabbits large doses of salbutamol have been shown to be teratogenic.

It is not known whether salbutamol is distributed into breast milk.

Effects on ability to drive and use machines: None.

Undesirable effects: Nausea and vomiting, dry, sore mouth, dizziness, mild tremor, headache, palpitations, tachycardia and transient muscle cramps may rarely occur. Potentially serious hypokalaemia has been reported in patients taking beta-2-agonist therapy. Hypersensitivity reactions such as angioedema may occur.

Hyperactivity in children has been reported rarely.

No additional adverse effects have been seen with Airomir Autohaler device.

As with other inhalation therapy, paradoxical bronchospasm may occur immediately after dosing. In this instance, Airomir Autohaler device should be discontinued immediately and alternative therapy instituted if necessary. Airomir Autohaler device contains a new propellant and does not contain any chlorofluorocarbons (CFCs). This inhaler has a different feel and taste to CFC containing inhalers that patients may be using or have used in the past.

Overdose: Treatment: Asthmatic patients: Monitor biochemical abnormalities, particularly hypokalaemia which should be treated with potassium replacement where necessary. Beta-adrenoceptor antagonists, even beta-1-selective antagonists, are potentially life-threatening and should be avoided.

Non-asthmatic patients: Monitor and correct biochemical abnormalities, particularly hypokalaemia. A non-selective beta-adrenoceptor antagonist (e.g. nadolol, propranolol) will competitively reverse both hypokalaemia and tachycardia (beta-1-selective drugs will be largely ineffective).

Pharmacological properties

Pharmacodynamic properties: Salbutamol is a sympathomimetic agent which has a selective action on beta-2-adrenergic receptors in bronchial smooth muscle.

Pharmacokinetic properties: Salbutamol is readily absorbed from the gastro-intestinal tract, but the systemic absorption of the inhaled drug substance is low. The action of inhaled salbutamol depends on direct stimulation of receptors in the lung. Onset of action is usually within 10 minutes of inhalation and lasts 4–6 hours in most patients.

Salbutamol is subject to first-pass metabolism in the liver; about half is excreted in the urine as an inactive sulphate conjugate. It does not appear to be metabolised in the lung and therefore its fate following inhalation therapy depends on the delivery method used, which determines the proportion of salbutamol inhaled relative to the proportion inadvertently swallowed. It has been suggested that the slightly extended half-life following inhalation may reflect slow removal of active drug from the lungs.

Preclinical safety data

Propellant 134a: In animal studies propellant 134a has been shown to have no significant pharmacological effects other than at very high exposure concentrations, when narcosis and a relatively weak cardiac sensitising effect were found. The potency of the cardiac sensitisation was less than that of CFC-11 (trichlorofluoromethane).

In studies to detect toxicity, repeated high dose levels of propellant 134a indicated that safety margins based on systemic exposure would be of the order 2200, 1314 and 381 for mouse, rat and dog with respect to humans.

There are no reasons to consider propellant 134a as a potential mutagen, clastogen or carcinogen judged from *in vitro* and *in vivo* studies including long-term administration by inhalation in rodents.

Airomir Autohaler: Safety studies with the Salbutamol Sulphate CFC-Free formulation in rat and dog showed few adverse effects. These occurred at high doses and were consistent with the known effects of salbutamol inhalation.

Pharmaceutical particulars

List of excipients: The excipients in Airomir Autohaler device are Oleic Acid, PhEur; Ethanol, BP; and Propellant 134a.

Airomir Autohaler device contains a new propellant and does not contain chlorofluorocarbons (CFCs).

Incompatibilities: None known.

Shelf life: 2 years.

Special precautions for storage: Airomir Autohaler device should be stored below 30°C; storage in direct sunlight or heat should be avoided. Protect from frost.

Nature and contents of container: Airomir Autohaler device contains 200 metered doses.

Instructions for use/handling: The patient should read the instruction leaflet before use.

As the canister is pressurised, no attempt should be made to puncture or dispose of it by burning.

Marketing authorisation number PL 0068/0178

Date of authorisation/renewal of authorisation August 1997

Date of (partial) revision of the SmPC January 1999

AIROMIR* INHALER

Qualitative and quantitative composition Each actuation of Airomir Inhaler delivers Salbutamol Sulphate PhEur equivalent to salbutamol 100 micrograms into the mouthpiece of the adapter.

Pharmaceutical form Airomir Inhaler is a pressurised aerosol for bronchodilator inhalation therapy.

Airomir Inhaler contains a new propellant and does not contain chlorofluorocarbons (CFCs).

Clinical particulars

Therapeutic indications: Airomir Inhaler is indicated in the management of bronchial asthma, for the relief of wheezing and shortness of breath used on an as required basis. Airomir Inhaler may be used as necessary to relieve attacks of acute dyspnoea and may be used prophylactically before exertion or to prevent exercise-induced asthma.

Airomir Inhaler may also be used in the treatment of reversible airways obstruction associated with chronic bronchitis and emphysema.

Posology and method of administration

Adults: For the relief of wheezing, shortness of breath and attacks of acute dyspnoea in patients with asthma, or reversible airways obstruction associated with chronic bronchitis and emphysema, one or two inhalations may be administered as a single dose.

For prophylaxis of exercise-induced asthma, two inhalations before exercise.

Children: For the relief of wheezing, shortness of breath and attacks of acute dyspnoea in children with asthma, one inhalation increasing to two if necessary may be administered as a single dose.

For prophylaxis of exercise-induced asthma, one inhalation increasing to two if necessary before exercise.

Elderly: No special dosage recommendations are made for elderly patients.

For all patients, the maximum recommended dose should not exceed eight inhalations in 24 hours. With repetitive dosing, inhalations should not usually be repeated more often than every 4 hours.

Contra-indications: Hypersensitivity to salbutamol or any of the inactive ingredients in Airomir Inhaler.

Airomir Inhaler is contra-indicated for use in the management of premature labour and threatened abortion.

Special warnings and special precautions for use

Special warnings: Potentially serious hypokalaemia has been reported in patients taking beta-2-agonist therapy. Particular caution is advised in patients with severe asthma. Hypokalaemia may also occur in hypoxic patients and those treated with xanthine derivatives, steroids, diuretics and long-term laxatives. Extra care should therefore be taken if beta-2-agonists are used in these groups of patients and serum potassium levels should be monitored.

Unwanted stimulation of cardiac adrenergic receptors can occur in patients taking beta-2-agonist therapy.

Special precautions for use: The patient should be advised to seek medical advice if the treatment ceases to be effective and/or their asthma seems to be worsening, and not to increase the dose without medical advice.

Administer cautiously to patients with thyrotoxicosis.

Interaction with other medicaments and other forms of interaction: Salbutamol and beta-blockers should not usually be prescribed together.

Hypokalaemia occurring with beta-2-agonist therapy may be exacerbated by treatment with xanthines, steroids, diuretics and long-term laxatives.

Because Airomir contains ethanol there is a theoretical potential for interaction in patients taking disulfiram or metronidazole. The amount of ethanol in Airomir is small but it may be enough to precipitate a reaction in some sensitive patients.

Pregnancy and lactation

Airomir: There is no experience of this product in pregnancy and lactation in humans. An inhalation reproductive study with Airomir Inhaler in rats did not exhibit any teratogenic effects. It should not be used in pregnancy and lactation unless the expected benefit to the mother is thought to outweigh any risk to the foetus or neonate.

Propellant 134A: Studies of propellant 134a administered to pregnant and lactating rats and rabbits have not revealed any special hazard.

Salbutamol: The safe use of inhaled salbutamol during pregnancy has not been established but it has been in widespread use for many years in human beings without apparent ill consequence. In mice and rabbits large doses of salbutamol have been shown to be teratogenic.

It is not known whether salbutamol is distributed into breast milk.

Effects on ability to drive and use machines: None.

Undesirable effects: Nausea and vomiting, dry, sore mouth, dizziness, mild tremor, headache, palpitations, tachycardia and transient muscle cramps may rarely occur. Potentially serious hypokalaemia has been reported in patients taking beta-2-agonist therapy. Hypersensitivity reactions such as angioedema may occur.

Hyperactivity in children has been reported rarely.

No additional adverse effects have been seen with Airomir Inhaler.

As with other inhalation therapy, paradoxical bronchospasm may occur immediately after dosing. In this instance, Airomir Inhaler should be discontinued immediately and alternative therapy instituted if necessary. Airomir Inhaler contains a new propellant and does not contain any chlorofluorocarbons (CFCs). This inhaler has a different feel and taste to CFC containing inhalers that patients may be using or have used in the past.

Overdose

Treatment: Asthmatic patients: Monitor biochemical abnormalities, particularly hypokalaemia which should be treated with potassium replacement where necessary. Beta-adrenoceptor antagonists, even beta-1-selective antagonists, are potentially life-threatening and should be avoided.

Non-asthmatic patients: Monitor and correct biochemical abnormalities, particularly hypokalaemia. A non-selective beta-adrenoceptor antagonist (e.g. nadolol, propranolol) will competitively reverse both hypokalaemia and tachycardia (beta-1-selective drugs will be largely ineffective).

Pharmacological properties

Pharmacodynamic properties: Salbutamol is a sympathomimetic agent which has a selective action on beta-2-adrenergic receptors in bronchial smooth muscle.

Pharmacokinetic properties: Salbutamol is readily absorbed from the gastro-intestinal tract, but the systemic absorption of the inhaled drug substance is low. The action of inhaled salbutamol depends on direct stimulation of receptors in the lung. Onset of action is usually within 10 minutes of inhalation and lasts 4–6 hours in most patients.

Salbutamol is subject to first-pass metabolism in the liver; about half is excreted in the urine as an inactive sulphate conjugate. It does not appear to be metabolised in the lung and therefore its fate following inhalation therapy depends on the delivery method used, which determines the proportion of salbutamol inhaled relative to the proportion inadvertently swallowed. It has been suggested that the slightly extended half-life following inhalation may reflect slow removal of active drug from the lungs.

Preclinical safety data

Propellant 134a: In animal studies propellant 134a has been shown to have no significant pharmacological effects other than at very high exposure concentrations, when narcosis and a relatively weak cardiac sensitising effect were found. The potency of the cardiac sensitisation was less than that of CFC-11 (trichlorofluoromethane).

In studies to detect toxicity, repeated high dose levels of propellant 134a indicated that safety margins based on systemic exposure would be of the order 2200, 1314 and 381 for mouse, rat and dog with respect to humans.

There are no reasons to consider propellant 134a as a potential mutagen, clastogen or carcinogen judged from *in vitro* and *in vivo* studies including long-term administration by inhalation in rodents.

Airomir: Safety studies with Airomir in rate and dog showed few adverse effects. These occurred at high doses and were consistent with the known effects of salbutamol inhalation.

Pharmaceutical particulars

List of excipients: The excipients in Airomir Inhaler are Oleic Acid PhEur, Ethanol BP and Propellant 134a.

Airomir Inhaler contains a new propellant and does not contain chlorofluorocarbons (CFCs).

Incompatibilities: None known.

Shelf life: 2 years.

Special precautions for storage: Airomir Inhaler should be stored below 30°C; storage in direct sunlight or heat should be avoided. Protect from frost.

Nature and contents of container: Airomir Inhaler contains either 100 or 200 metered doses.

Instructions for use/handling: For patients requiring a spacer device, the Aerochamber has been shown to be compatible with Airomir Inhaler.

The patient should read the instruction leaflet before use.

As the canister is pressurised, no attempt should be made to puncture or dispose of it by burning.

Marketing authorisation number 0068/0165.

Date of approval/revision of SPC February 1995.

Date of partial revision of text September 1998.

Legal category POM.

ALDARA* 5% CREAM

Qualitative and quantitative composition Imiquimod 5 mg per 100 mg cream. Each sachet contains 12.5 mg of imiquimod

Pharmaceutical form Cream.

Clinical particulars

Therapeutic indications: Imiquimod cream is indicated for the topical treatment of external genital and perianal warts (condyloma acuminata) in adult patients.

Posology and method of administration

Posology: Imiquimod cream should be applied 3 times per week (example: Monday, Wednesday, and Friday; or Tuesday, Thursday, and Saturday) prior to normal sleeping hours, and should remain on the skin for 6 to 10 hours. Imiquimod cream treatment should continue until there is clearance of visible genital or perianal warts or for a maximum of 16 weeks per episode of warts, as safety for use longer than 16 weeks has not been established.

Method of administration: Imiquimod cream should be applied in a *thin* layer and rubbed on the clean wart area until the cream vanishes. Imiquimod cream should be applied prior to normal sleeping hours. During the 6 to 10 hour treatment period, showering or bathing should be avoided. After this period imiquimod cream should be removed with mild soap and water. The cream in a single-use sachet is sufficient to cover a wart area of 20 cm^2 (approx. 3 $inches^2$). Sachets are to be used only once.

Hands should be washed carefully before and after application of cream.

Uncircumcised males treating warts under the foreskin should retract the foreskin and wash the area daily (see *Special warnings and special precautions for use*).

Contra-indications: Imiquimod cream is contra-indicated in patients with known hypersensitivity to imiquimod or any of the excipients of the cream.

Special warnings and special precautions for use: There is limited experience in the use of imiquimod cream in the treatment of uncircumcised men with foreskin-associated warts. The safety database in this patient population treated with imiquimod cream three times weekly and carrying out a daily foreskin hygiene routine is less than 100 patients. In other studies, in which a daily foreskin hygiene routine was not followed, there were two cases of severe phimosis and one case of stricture leading to circumcision. Treatment in this patient population is therefore not recommended unless the benefit is felt to outweigh the risk. Early signs of stricture may include local skin reactions (e.g. erosion, ulceration, edema, induration), or increasing difficulty in retracting the foreskin. If these symptoms occur, the treatment should be stopped immediately. Imiquimod cream has not been evaluated for treatment of internal genital warts and is not recommended for treatment of urethral, intra-vaginal, cervical, rectal or intra-anal warts. Imiquimod cream therapy should not be initiated in tissues where open sores or wounds exist until after the area has healed.

Local skin reactions such as erythema, erosion, excoriation, flaking and oedema are common. Other local reactions such as induration, ulceration, scabbing, and vesicles have also been reported. Should an intolerable skin reaction occur, the cream should be removed by washing the area with mild soap and water. Treatment with imiquimod cream can be resumed after the skin reaction has moderated. The use of an occlusive dressing is not recommended with imiquimod cream therapy for genital and perianal warts. Higher than recommended doses may lead to increased local skin reactions. No clinical experience exists with imiquimod cream immediately following treatment with other cutaneously applied drugs for treatment of external genital or perianal warts. Imiquimod cream use is not recommended until the genital or perianal skin has healed after any previous drug or surgical treatment.

Imiquimod cream should be washed from the skin before sexual activity. Imiquimod cream may weaken condoms and diaphragms, therefore concurrent use with imiquimod cream is not recommended. Alternative forms of contraception should be considered.

Imiquimod cream has the potential to exacerbate inflammatory conditions of the skin.

The safety data with imiquimod cream in patients older than 65 years are limited to four patients.

Repeat treatment with imiquimod cream after a recurrence of warts has not been studied, therefore repeat treatment with imiquimod cream is not recommended.

While limited data has shown an increased rate of wart reduction in HIV positive patients, imiquimod cream has not been shown to be as effective in terms of wart clearance in this patient group.

Interaction with other medicinal products and other forms of interaction: Interactions with other medicinal products, including immunosuppressive drugs, have not been studied; such interactions with systemic drugs would be limited by the minimal percutaneous absorption of imiquimod cream.

Use during pregnancy and lactation: In animal teratology (rat and rabbit) and reproductive studies (rat), no teratogenic nor embryo-fetotoxic effects were observed. In the absence of such effects in animals, malformative effects in man are generally considered unlikely to occur. Historically, drugs responsible for malformations in man were teratogenic in well-conducted studies using two animal species.

No information is available on the use of imiquimod cream in human pregnancy or its effect on lactation; it should only be used if the benefits clearly outweigh the potential hazard to the foetus or nursing infant.

Effects on ability to drive and use machines: No studies have been performed.

Undesirable effects: Local skin reactions including erythema, erosion, excoriation, flaking, and oedema were common in controlled clinical trials with imiquimod cream applied three times weekly. Induration, ulceration, scabbing, and vesicles were reported less frequently. Remote site skin reactions, mainly erythema, were also reported in these trials. These reactions were at non-wart sites which may have been in contact with imiquimod cream. Most skin reactions were mild to moderate in severity and resolved within 2 weeks of treatment discontinuation.

In the trials with 3 times a week dosing, the most frequently reported adverse drug reactions judged to be probably or possibly related to imiquimod cream treatment were application site reactions at the wart treatment site. Some systemic adverse reactions, including headache, influenza-like symptoms, and myalgia were also reported by imiquimod cream and placebo cream patients.

Adverse Reaction	*Females*		*Males*	
	Imiquimod cream 5% n=117	*Placebo cream n=103*	*Imiquimod cream 5% n=156*	*Placebo cream n=158*
Application site reaction				
Itching	32%	20%	22%	10%
Burning	26%	12%	9%	5%
Pain	8%	2%	12%	1%
Systemic reactions				
Headache	4%	3%	5%	2%
Influenza-like symptoms	3%	2%	1%	0%
Myalgia	1%	0%	1%	1%

Overdose: When applied topically, systemic overdosage with imiquimod cream is unlikely due to minimal percutaneous absorption. Studies in rabbits reveal a dermal lethal dose of greater that 5 g/kg. Persistent dermal overdosing of imiquimod cream could result in severe local skin reactions.

Following accidental ingestion, nausea, emesis, headache, myalgia and fever could occur after a single dose of 200 mg imiquimod which corresponds to the content of approximately 16 sachets. The most clinically serious adverse event reported following multiple oral doses of ≥200 mg was hypotension which resolved following oral or intravenous fluid administration.

Pharmacological properties

Pharmacodynamic properties: Pharmacotherapeutic group: immunomodulating agents, cytokine ATC code: LO3AX

Imiquimod is an immune response modifier. Saturable binding studies suggest a membrane receptor for imiquimod exists on responding immune cells. Imiquimod has no direct antiviral activity. In animal models imiquimod is effective against viral infections and acts as an antitumor agent principally by induction of alpha interferon and other cytokines. The induction of alpha interferon and other cytokines following imiquimod cream application to genital wart tissue has also been demonstrated in clinical studies.

Pharmacokinetic properties: Less that 0.9% of a topically applied single dose of radiolabeled imiquimod was absorbed through the skin of human subjects. The small amount of drug which was absorbed into the systemic circulation was promptly excreted by both urinary and faecal routes at a mean ratio of approximately 3 to 1. No quantifiable levels (>5 ng/ml) of drug were detected in serum after single or multiple topical doses.

The data defining systemic absorption of imiquimod are limited by the use of bioanalytical method with a 5 ng/mL lower limit of quantitation. Systemic exposure (percutaneous penetration) was calculated from recovery of carbon- 14 from [14C] imiquimod in urine and faeces.

Preclinical safety data: In a four-month rat dermal toxicity study, significantly decreased body weight and increased spleen weight were observed at 0.5 and 2.5 mg/kg; similar effects were not seen in a four month mouse dermal study. Local dermal irritation, especially at higher doses, was observed in both species. Imiquimod is not mutagenic or teratogenic. Dermally applied imiquimod was not carcinogenic in mice.

Pharmaceutical particulars
List of excipients: Isostearic acid, benzyl alcohol, cetyl alcohol, stearyl alcohol, white soft paraffin, polysorbate 60, sorbitan stearate, glycerol, methyl hydroxybenzoate, propyl hydroxybenzoate, xanthan gum, purified water.

Incompatibilities: None known.

Shelf-life: Two years.

Special precautions for storage: Store at or below 25°C.

Nature and content of container: White to slightly yellow cream contained in a single use polyester/aluminium foil sachet. The average fill weight for the single use sachet is not less than 250 mg of imiquimod cream. Imiquimod cream is available in boxes containing 12 single-use sachets.

Instructions for use an handling, and disposal (if appropriate): None.

Marketing authorisation holder: Laboratoires 3M Santé, Boulevard de l'Oise, F-95029 Cergy Pontoise Cedex, France.

Marketing authorisation number EU/1/98/080/001.

Date of first authorisation/renewal of the authorisation September 1998.

Date of revision of the text September 1998.

ALU-CAP* CAPSULES

Presentation Opaque green/red hard gelatin capsule, size 0, marked 3M. Each capsule contains 475 mg Dried Aluminium Hydroxide Gel BP as a white powder.

It also contains the following inactive ingredients: E104; E110; E127; E131.

Uses Alu-Cap is recommended for use as a phosphate-binding agent in the management of renal failure. It may also be used as an antacid.

In the gut, aluminium hydroxide adsorbs phosphate ions. This reduces absorption of phosphate into the body, and thereby reduces serum phosphate levels. In patients with renal failure, the problem of high serum phosphate levels may be partially solved by a diet low in phosphorus. However, a more liberal diet is feasible when a phosphate-binding agent, such as aluminium hydroxide, is used.

Aluminium hydroxide gel is a slow-acting antacid. It is used to provide symptomatic relief in gastric hyperacidity. In addition, the antipeptic and demulcent activity of aluminium hydroxide helps to protect inflamed gastric mucosa against further irritation by gastric secretions.

Dosage and administration *For phosphate-binding: Adults and children:* The dosage must be selected in accordance with individual patient requirements, and may range from 4 to 20 capsules of Alu-Cap daily (approximately 2–10 g dried aluminium hydroxide gel), taken with meals.

As an antacid: Adults: One Alu-Cap four times daily and on retiring. Alu-Cap is not suitable for antacid therapy in children.

Elderly: No special dosage recommendations are made for elderly patients.

Contra-indications, warnings, etc
Side-effects: Aluminium hydroxide is astringent and may cause constipation.

Precautions: Serum phosphate levels should be monitored in all patients receiving phosphate binders, to prevent the development of a phosphate depletion syndrome.

Aluminium hydroxide may form complexes with certain antibiotics (tetracyclines); concomitant administration may result in reduced absorption of the antibiotic.

Pregnancy: There is no evidence of safety of the drug in human pregnancy but it has been in wide use for many years without apparent ill consequence – animal studies having shown no hazard.

Contra-indications: Patients with hypophosphataemia and acute porphyria.

Overdosage: Symptoms and treatment: A single massive dose of aluminium hydroxide is unlikely to have harmful sequelae, as aluminium is not absorbed systemically to any great extent. Gastric lavage should be administered, followed by a mild aperient if required.

Pharmaceutical precautions Store below 30°C.

Legal category P.

Package quantities Bottles of 120 capsules (OP).

Further information Nil.

Product licence number 0068/0052.

CALCISORB* SACHETS

Qualitative and quantitative composition Each sachet of Calcisorb contains 5 g of sodium cellulose phosphate.

Pharmaceutical form Calcisorb is a creamy-white to beige fibrous powder.

Clinical particulars
Therapeutic indications: Calcisorb is used to diminish calcium absorption from the diet in:

(1) the treatment of hypercalciuria and recurrent formation of renal stones;
(2) in osteopetrosis.
It can also be used in:
(3) the treatment of idiopathic hypercalcaemia of infancy;
(4) the treatment of hypercalcaemia in sarcoidosis;
(5) the treatment of vitamin D intoxication.

Calcisorb can also be used as a basis for a test for calcium absorption.

Each 5 g dose will bind approximately 350 mg calcium.

Posology and method of administration
Adults: 15 g daily, divided as three 5 g doses with meals.

Children: 10 g daily, divided as three doses with meals. Growing children should be prescribed Calcisorb only at the discretion of a senior physician and under his direct supervision.

Elderly: No special dosage instructions are required for the elderly.

The required dose should be dispersed in water and taken orally. Alternatively the powder may be sprinkled onto food.

Contra-indications: Renal failure. Congestive heart failure and other conditions in which a low sodium intake is essential.

Special warnings and special precautions for use: Calcisorb should be used in conjunction with a low calcium diet in which dairy products in particular are severely restricted.

During treatment with Calcisorb, restriction of oxalate-rich foods, such as spinach, rhubarb, peanuts, beetroot and chololate may be beneficial. An oral magnesium supplement of 58–87 mg elemental magnesium, twice daily, in patients receiving 10 and 15 g sodium cellulose phosphate daily, respectively, is also recommended. This supplement should be administered at least 1 hour before or 1 hour after Calcisorb.

Interaction with other medicaments and other forms of interaction: Interactions may occur with oral preparations containing calcium or magnesium salts, such as some antacids and laxatives.

Pregnancy and lactation: In view of the absence of data on the effect of cellulose phosphate on calcium levels in pregnant women it is recommended that treatment is discontinued during pregnancy and lactation. No signs of calcium deficiency have been reported during the continuous use of cellulose phosphate for up to 11 years. Therefore, this theoretical hazard in pregnancy is unlikely.

Effects on ability to drive and use machines: None.

Undesirable effects: Side-effects are rare. Isolated cases of diarrhoea have been reported. One patient with mild renal disease developed a moderate magnesium deficiency. This was readily corrected by halving the dose.

Overdose: An overdose of Calcisorb would potentially cause hypocalcaemia. The dose should be reduced. Complete withdrawal of treatment and supplementary calcium may be necessary.

Pharmacological properties
Pharmacodynamic properties: Sodium cellulose phosphate is an ion-exchange compound with a particular affinity for divalent cations. The product binds calcium ions in the lumen of the stomach and intestine and thus prevents hyperabsorption of dietary calcium. Calcium bound by cellulose phosphate is no longer available for absorption and is therefore excreted in the faeces. Each dose of Calcisorb will bind approximately 350 mg calcium.

Pharmacokinetic properties: Calcisorb is not absorbed.

Pharmaceutical particulars
List of excipients: None.

Incompatibilities: None known.

Shelf life: The shelf life expiry date for this product shall not exceed 3 years from the date of its manufacture.

Special precautions for storage: Since cellulose phosphate is an ester, some hydrolysis occurs on storage, the rate increasing with temperature. Calcisorb should therefore be kept in a refrigerator between 2°C and 8°C for long term storage. For short term storage by the patient, i.e. of the order of one month, refrigeration is unnecessary.

Nature and contents of container: Calcisorb is supplied in parchment, foil and polythene sachets. The 5 g sachets are packed in boxes of 90.

Instructions for use/handling: Not applicable.

Marketing authorisation number 0068/5900R.

Date of approval/revision of SPC March 1996.

Legal category P.

DIFFLAM* CREAM

Qualitative and quantitative composition Each tube of Difflam Cream contains Benzydamine Hydrochloride 3% w/w.

Pharmaceutical form Cream.

Clinical particulars
Therapeutic indications: Difflam cream is a topical analgesic and non-steroidal anti-inflammatory agent. It is recommended as a short-term treatment for the relief of symptoms associated with painful inflammatory conditions of the musculo-skeletal system, including:

Acute inflammatory disorders such as myalgia and bursitis.

Traumatic conditions such as sprains, strains, contusions and the after-effects of fractures.

Difflam cream is well absorbed through the skin and has been shown to have anti-inflammatory and local anaesthetic actions.

Posology and method of administration: Difflam cream should be massaged lightly into the affected area. Depending on the size of the site to be treated, 35–85 mm (1–2 g) should be applied three times daily and at the discretion of the doctor, up to six times daily in more severe conditions. It is recommended that treatment be limited to not more than 10 days.

Elderly: No special dosage recommendations are made for elderly patients.

Contra-indications: None.

Special warnings and special precautions for use: To avoid possible irritation, Difflam cream should be kept away from eyes and mucosal surfaces.

Interaction with other medicaments and other forms of interaction: None.

Pregnancy and lactation: There is inadequate evidence of safety of the drug in human pregnancy, but it has been in wide use for many years without apparent ill consequence.

Effects on ability to drive and use machines: None.

Undesirable effects: Photosensitivity reactions have been reported and local skin reactions which have varied from erythema to papular eruption. The skin returned to normal on stopping treatment.

Overdose: Difflam is unlikely to cause adverse systemic effects, even if accidental ingestion should occur. No special measures are required.

Pharmacological properties
Pharmacodynamic properties: Benzydamine exerts an anti-inflammatory and analgesic action by stabilising the cellular membrane and inhibiting prostaglandin synthesis.

Pharmacokinetic properties: Following topical administration, benzydamine is absorbed through intact skin and reaches peak levels between 24–32 hours, amounting to about 20–25% of the plasma levels obtained after the oral administration of the same dose.

About half of the benzydamine is excreted unchanged via the kidney at a rate of 10% of the dose within the first 24 hours. The remainder is metabolised, mostly to N-oxide.

Preclinical safety data: Not applicable.

Pharmaceutical particulars
List of excipients:
'Cutina' MD
Cetyl Alcohol USNF
'Cetiol' V
'Eumulgin' B1
Propylene Glycol PhEur
Perfume, 'Crematest' 0/064060
Methyl Hydroxybenzoate PhEur
Propyl Hydroxybenzoate PhEur
Purified Water PhEur

Incompatibilities: None known.

Shelf life: 3 years.

Special precautions for storage: Store between 5–30°C. Do not freeze.

Nature and contents of container: Collapsible Aluminium tube closed with plastic screwcap *or* Laminate tube closed with plastic screwcap.

Contents: 50 g and 100 g.

Instructions for use/handling: Not applicable.

Marketing authorisation number 0068/0088

Date of first authorisation/renewal of the authorisation 6 March 1980

Date of last (partial) revision of the text June 1995

DIFFLAM* ORAL RINSE

Qualitative and quantitative composition A pleasant tasting, clear, green solution, containing benzydamine hydrochloride 0.15% w/v.

Pharmaceutical form Liquid for use as mouthwash/gargle.

Clinical particulars
Therapeutic indications: Difflam Oral Rinse is a locally acting analgesic and anti-inflammatory treatment for the relief of painful inflammatory conditions of the mouth and throat including:
Traumatic conditions: Pharyngitis following tonsillectomy or the use of a naso-gastric tube.
Inflammatory conditions: Pharyngitis, aphthous ulcers and oral ulceration due to radiation therapy.
Dentistry: For use after dental operations.

Posology and method of administration
Adults: Rinse or gargle with 15 ml (approximately 1 tablespoonful) every 1½ to 3 hours as required for pain relief.

The solution should be expelled from the mouth after use.

Children: Not suitable for children aged 12 years or under.

Elderly: No special dosage recommendations are made for elderly patients.

Difflam Oral Rinse should generally be used undiluted, but if 'stinging' occurs the rinse may be diluted with water.

Uninterrupted treatment should not exceed seven days, unless under medical supervision.

Contra-indications: None.

Special warnings and precautions for use: Difflam Oral Rinse should generally be used undiluted, but if 'stinging' occurs the rinse may be diluted with water.

Avoid contact with eyes.

Interaction with other medicaments and other forms of interaction: None known.

Pregnancy and lactation: There is inadequate evidence of safety of the drug in human pregnancy, but it has been in wide use for many years without apparent ill consequence.

Effects on ability to drive and use machines: Not applicable.

Undesirable effects: Side-effects are minor. Occasionally, oral tissue numbness or 'stinging' sensations may occur.

Overdose: Difflam is unlikely to cause adverse systemic effects, even if accidental ingestion should occur. No special measures are required.

Pharmacological properties
Pharmacodynamic properties: Benzydamine exerts an anti-inflammatory and analgesic effect by stabilising the cellular membrane and inhibiting prostaglandin synthesis.

Pharmacokinetic properties: Oral doses of benzydamine are well absorbed and plasma drug concentrations reach a peak fairly rapidly and then decline with a half-life of about 13 hours. Less than 20% of the drug is bound to plasma proteins.

Although local drug concentrations are relatively large, the systemic absorption of mouthwash-gargle doses of benzydamine is relatively low compared to oral doses. This low absorption should greatly diminish the potential for any systemic drug side-effects when benzydamine is administered by this route. Benzydamine is metabolised primarily by oxidation, conjugation and dealkylation.

Preclinical safety data: Not applicable.

Pharmaceutical particulars
List of excipients:
Ethanol (96% v/v) BP
Glycerol PhEur
Saccharin Sodium BP
Mouthwash flavour, 52 503/T
Polysorbate 20 PhEur
Methyl Hydroxybenzoate PhEur
Quinoline Yellow (E104)
Patent Blue V (E131)
Purified Water PhEur

Incompatibilities: None known.

Shelf life: 3 years.

Special precautions for storage: Do not leave the uncartonned bottle in direct sunlight. Store between 5°C and 30°C. Do not freeze.

Nature and contents of container: Clear glass bottle with screwcap containing 300 ml.

Instructions for use/handling: The solution should be expelled from the mouth after use.

Marketing authorisation number PL 0068/0096

Date of first authorisation/renewal of authorisation
Date of first authorisation 11 June 1981
Date of last renewal 23 December 1991

Date of (partial) revision of the text August 1996

DIFFLAM* SPRAY

Qualitative and quantitative composition Each metered dose pump spray delivers benzydamine hydrochloride 0.15% w/v, approximately 175 microlitres per puff.

Pharmaceutical form Difflam Spray is a metered dose pump throat spray.

Clinical particulars
Therapeutic indications: Difflam Spray is a locally acting analgesic and anti-inflammatory treatment for the throat and mouth.

It is especially useful for the relief of pain in traumatic conditions such as following tonsillectomy or the use of a naso-gastric tube; dental surgery.

Posology and method of administration: For oral administration.

Adults and elderly: 4 to 8 puffs, 1½–3 hourly.

Children (6 to 12): 4 puffs, 1½–3 hourly.

Children under 6: One puff to be administered per 4 kg body weight, up to a maximum of 4 puffs, 1½–3 hourly.

Because of the small amount of drug applied, elderly patients can receive the same dose as adults.

Contra-indications: None.

Special warnings and special precautions for use: Avoid contact with the eyes.

Interaction with other medicaments and other forms of interaction: None known.

Pregnancy and lactation: There is inadequate evidence of safety of the drug in human pregnancy, but it has been in wide use for many years without apparent ill consequence.

Effects on ability to drive and use machines: None.

Undesirable effects: Side-effects are minor. Occasionally, oral tissue numbness or 'stinging' sensations may occur. The stinging has been reported to disappear upon continuation of the treatment, however if it persists it is recommended that treatment be discontinued.

Overdose: Difflam is unlikely to cause adverse systemic effects, even if accidental ingestion should occur. No special measures are required.

Pharmacological properties
Pharmacodynamic properties: Benzydamine exerts an anti-inflammatory and analgesic action by stabilising the cellular membrane and inhibiting prostaglandin synthesis.

Pharmacokinetic properties: Following oral administration, Benzydamine is rapidly absorbed from the gastrointestinal tract and maximum plasma levels reached after 2–4 hours. The most important aspect of the tissue distribution of benzydamine is its tendency to concentrate at the site of inflammation.

About half of the Benzydamine is excreted unchanged via the kidney at a rate of 10% of the dose within the first 24 hours. The remainder is metabolised, mostly to N-Oxide.

Pharmaceutical particulars
List of excipients: The excipients in Difflam Spray include: Glycerol PhEur, Saccharin FU, Sodium Bicarbonate PhEur, Ethanol FU, Methylhydroxybenzoate PhEur, Mouthwash Flavour, Polysorbate 20 PhEur, Purified Water PhEur.

Incompatibilities: None.

Shelf life: The shelf life expiry date for this product shall not exceed 3 years from the date of its manufacture.

Special precautions for storage: Difflam Spray should be stored between 5°C and 30°C, do not freeze.

Nature and contents of container: Difflam Spray is presented in a 30 ml glass bottle with 170 µl valve pump spray and an outer coating of green coloured PVC.

Instructions for use/handling: The patient should read the instruction leaflet before use.

Marketing authorisation number 0068/0112.

Date of approval/revision of SPC August 1996.

Legal category P.

DUROMINE* 15 mg CAPSULES

Qualitative and quantitative composition Phentermine resin complex equivalent to 15 mg phentermine.

Pharmaceutical form Capsules.

Clinical particulars
Therapeutic indications: Adjunctive therapy to diet, in patients with obesity and a body mass index (BMI) of 30 kg/m² or higher who have not responded to an appropriate weight-reducing regimen alone.

Note: short-term efficacy only has been demonstrated with regard to weight reduction. No significant data on changes in morbidity or mortality are yet available.

Posology and method of administration: For oral administration.

Adults: One 15 mg capsule daily at breakfast time.

Evening dosing should be avoided, as this agent may induce nervousness and insomnia.

It is recommended that treatment should be conducted under the care of physicians experienced in the treatment of obesity.

Secondary organic causes of obesity must be excluded by diagnosis before prescribing this agent.

The management of obesity should be undertaken using a global approach which should include dietary, medical and psychotherapeutic methods.

Duration of treatment: The duration of treatment is 4–6 weeks and should not exceed three months.

Children: Duromine is not recommended for children.

Elderly: Duromine is not recommended for the elderly.

Contra-indications:
- Patients sensitive to sympathomimetic agents.
- Pulmonary artery hypertension.
- Severe arterial hypertension.
- Current or past medical history of cardio-vascular or cerebro-vascular disease.
- Current or past medical history of psychiatric disorders including anorexia nervosa and depression.
- Propensity towards drug abuse, known alcoholism.
- Thyrotoxicosis.
- Children below 12 years.
- Women during lactation.

Combination drug therapy with any other centrally acting anorectic agent is contraindicated due to the increased risk of potentially fatal pulmonary artery hypertension.

Special warnings and special precautions for use:
Special warnings: Cases of severe, often fatal pulmonary artery hypertension, have been reported in patients who have received anorectics of the type in this product. An epidemiological study has shown that anorectic intake is a risk factor involved in the development of pulmonary artery hypertension and that use of anorectics is strongly associated with an increased risk for this adverse drug reaction. In view of this rare but serious risk, it must be emphasised that:
- careful compliance with the indication and the duration of treatment is required;
- duration of treatment greater than 3 months and a BMI ≥ 30 kg/m² increase the risk of pulmonary artery hypertension;
- the onset or aggravation of exertional dyspnoea suggests the possibility of occurrence of pulmonary artery hypertension. Under these circumstances, treatment should be immediately discontinued and the patient referred to a specialist unit for investigation.

Special precautions for use: Prolonged treatment may give rise to pharmacological tolerance and drug dependence, and more rarely to severe psychotic disorders in predisposed patients.

Rarely, cases of cardiac and cerebro-vascular accidents have been reported, often following rapid weight loss. Special care should be taken to ensure gradual and controlled weight loss in obese patients, who are subject to a risk of vascular disease. This anorectic agent should not be prescribed in patients with current or a past medical history of cardiovascular or cerebro-vascular disease.

Duromine should be used with caution in patients under treatment with anti-hypertensive agents, since it may cause some loss of blood pressure control, and in patients receiving psychotrophic drugs, including sedatives and sympathomimetic agents.

This anorectic agent should be used with caution in epileptic patients.

Interaction with other medicaments and other forms of interaction: Duromine should not be given to patients under treatment with monoamine-oxidase (MAO) inhibitors, within 2 weeks of stopping such treatment. There may be an interaction with alcohol.

Pregnancy and lactation: Do not use in pregnancy or lactation. There is inadequate evidence of safety in pregnancy and there is no information from animal studies.

Effects on ability to drive and use machines: Patients may be at risk whilst driving or operating machinery.

Undesirable effects: An epidemiological study has shown that anorectic intake is a risk factor involved in the development of pulmonary artery hypertension and that the use of anorectics is strongly associated with an increased risk for this adverse drug reaction. Cases of pulmonary artery hypertension have been reported in patients treated with this agent. Pulmonary artery hypertension is a severe and often fatal disease. The occurrence or aggravation of exertional dyspnoea is usually the first clinical sign and requires treatment discontinuation and investigation in a specialised unit (see *Special warnings*).

CNS effects: The prolonged use of this agent is associated with a risk of pharmocological tolerance, dependence and withdrawal syndrome. The most common adverse reactions which have been described are: psychotic reactions or psychosis, depression, nervousness, agitation, sleep disorders and vertigo. Hallucinations and dizziness may also occur. Convulsions have been reported.

Cardio-vascular effects: The most common reported reactions are tachycardia, palpitations, hypertension, precordial pain. Rarely cases of cardiovascular or cerebro-vascular accidents have been described in patients treated with anorectic agents. In particular stroke, angina, myocardial infarction, cardiac failure and cardiac arrest have been reported. Other side-effects reported are vomiting, dry mouth, facial oedema, rash, headache and urinary frequency.

Overdose: Symptoms: Initially irritability, agitation, disorientation and tremor may occur, followed by cardiac arrhythmias, convulsions, hallucinations and coma.

Treatment: The stomach should be emptied by emesis or stomach tube and washed out with water if the preparation has been ingested within the last three or four hours. Diazepam, preferably by mouth (cautiously by intravenous injection) should be used to control marked excitement and convulsions. Provided renal function is adequate, elimination of phentermine may be assisted by acidification of the urine by agents such as lysine hydrochloride or arginine hydrochloride.

Pharmacological properties

Pharmacodynamic properties: Phentermine is a weak sympathomimetic amine having marked anorexigenic activity. Its appetite suppressant effect is generally considered to be exerted through the hypothalamus, but it is not certain that this is the only effect related to weight loss. In vitro, it has been shown to inhibit phospholipase activity. It may also increase glucose uptake into skeletal muscle, as has been shown with fenfluramine. Phentermine has major effects on the dopaminergic and noradrenergic nervous systems.

Hence in addition to effects upon appetite suppression in the CNS, phentermine may also have peripheral metabolic effects which can help weight loss. The exact mechanisms are not clear.

Pharmacokinetic properties: Phentermine is readily absorbed from the gastro-intestinal tract and approximately 70–80% of all oral dose is excreted unchanged in the urine; the remainder is metabolised in the liver.

Preclinical safety data: Not applicable.

Pharmaceutical particulars

List of excipients: Lactose PhEur, Magnesium Stearate PhEur.

Incompatibilities: None known.

Shelf life: 5 years.

Special precautions for storage: Store below 30°C.

Nature and contents of container: Amber glass bottle with pilfer-proof screw cap.

Instructions for use/handling: Not applicable.

Marketing authorisation number 00068/5055R

Date of approval/revision of SPC January 1997.

Legal category CD(Sch 3), POM.

DUROMINE* 30 mg CAPSULES

Qualitative and quantitative composition Phentermine resin complex equivalent to 30 mg phentermine.

Pharmaceutical form Capsules.

Clinical particulars

Therapeutic indications: Adjunctive therapy to diet, in patients with obesity and a body mass index (BMI) of 30 kg/m² or higher who have not responded to an appropriate weight-reducing regimen alone.

Note: short-term efficacy only has been demonstrated with regard to weight reduction. No significant data on changes in morbidity or mortality are yet available.

Posology and method of administration: For oral administration.

Adults: One 30 mg capsule daily at breakfast time.

Evening dosing should be avoided, as this agent may induce nervousness and insomnia.

It is recommended that treatment should be conducted under the care of physicians experienced in the treatment of obesity.

Secondary organic causes of obesity must be excluded by diagnosis before prescribing this agent.

The management of obesity should be undertaken using a global approach which should include dietary, medical and psychotherapeutic methods.

Duration of treatment: The duration of treatment is 4–6 weeks and should not exceed three months.

Children: Duromine is not recommended for children.

Elderly: Duromine is not recommended for the elderly.

Contra-indications:

- Patients sensitive to sympathomimetic agents.
- Pulmonary artery hypertension.
- Severe arterial hypertension.
- Current or past medical history of cardio-vascular or cerebro-vascular disease.
- Current or past medical history of psychiatric disorders including anorexia nervosa and depression.
- Propensity towards drug abuse, known alcoholism.
- Thyrotoxicosis.
- Children below 12 years.
- Women during lactation.

Combination drug therapy with any other centrally acting anorectic agent is contraindicated due to the increased risk of potentially fatal pulmonary artery hypertension.

Special warnings and special precautions for use:

Special warnings: Cases of severe, often fatal pulmonary artery hypertension, have been reported in patients who have received anorectics of the type in this product. An epidemiological study has shown that anorectic intake is a risk factor involved in the development of pulmonary artery hypertension and that use of anorectics is strongly associated with an increased risk for this adverse drug reaction. In view of this rare but serious risk, it must be emphasised that:

- careful compliance with the indication and the duration of treatment is required;
- duration of treatment greater than 3 months and a BMI≥30 kg/m² increase the risk of pulmonary artery hypertension;
- the onset or aggravation of exertional dyspnoea suggests the possibility of occurrence of pulmonary artery hypertension. Under these circumstances, treatment should be immediately discontinued and the patient referred to a specialist unit for investigation.

Special precautions for use: Prolonged treatment may give rise to pharmacological tolerance and drug dependence, and more rarely to severe psychotic disorders in predisposed patients.

Rarely, cases of cardiac and cerebro-vascular accidents have been reported, often following rapid weight loss. Special care should be taken to ensure gradual and controlled weight loss in obese patients, who are subject to a risk of vascular disease. This anorectic agent should not be prescribed in patients with current or a past medical history of cardio-vascular or cerebro-vascular disease.

Duromine should be used with caution in patients under treatment with anti-hypertensive agents, since it may cause some loss of blood pressure control, and in patients receiving psychotrophic drugs, including sedatives and sympathomimetic agents.

This anorectic agent should be used with caution in epileptic patients.

Interaction with other medicaments and other forms of interaction: Duromine should not be given to patients under treatment with monoamine-oxidase (MAO) inhibitors, within 2 weeks of stopping such treatment. There may be an interaction with alcohol.

Pregnancy and lactation: Do not use in pregnancy or lactation. There is inadequate evidence of safety in pregnancy and there is no information from animal studies.

Effects on ability to drive and use machines: Patients may be at risk whilst driving or operating machinery.

Undesirable effects: An epidemiological study has shown that anorectic intake is a risk factor involved in the development of pulmonary artery hypertension and that the use of anorectics is strongly associated with an increased risk for this adverse drug reaction. Cases of pulmonary artery hypertension have been reported in patients treated with this agent. Pulmonary artery hypertension is a severe and often fatal disease. The occurrence or aggravation of exertional dyspnoea is usually the first clinical sign and requires treatment discontinuation and investigation in a specialised unit (see *Special warnings*).

CNS effects: The prolonged use of this agent is associated with a risk of pharmocological tolerance, dependence and withdrawal syndrome. The most common adverse reactions which have been described are: psychotic reactions or psychosis, depression, nervousness, agitation, sleep disorders and vertigo. Hallucinations and dizziness may also occur. Convulsions have been reported.

Cardio-vascular effects: The most common reported reactions are tachycardia, palpitations, hypertension, precordial pain. Rarely cases of cardiovascular or cerebro-vascular accidents have been described in patients treated with anorectic agents. In particular stroke, angina, myocardial infarction, cardiac failure and cardiac arrest have been reported. Other side-effects reported are vomiting, dry mouth, facial oedema, rash, headache and urinary frequency.

Overdose: Symptoms: Initially irritability, agitation, disorientation and tremor may occur, followed by cardiac arrhythmias, convulsions, hallucinations and coma.

Treatment: The stomach should be emptied by emesis or stomach tube and washed out with water if the preparation has been ingested within the last three or four hours. Diazepam, preferably by mouth (cautiously by intravenous injection) should be used to control marked excitement and convulsions. Provided renal function is adequate, elimination of phentermine may be assisted by acidification of the urine by agents such as lysine hydrochloride or arginine hydrochloride.

Pharmacological properties

Pharmacodynamic properties: Phentermine is a weak sympathomimetic amine having marked anorexigenic activity. Its appetite suppressant effect is generally considered to be exerted through the hypothalamus, but it is not certain that this is the only effect related to weight loss. In vitro, it has been shown to inhibit phospholipase activity. It may also increase glucose uptake into skeletal muscle, as has been shown with fenfluramine. Phentermine has major effects on the dopaminergic and noradrenergic nervous systems.

Hence in addition to effects upon appetite suppression in the CNS, phentermine may also have peripheral metabolic effects which can help weight loss. The exact mechanisms are not clear.

Pharmacokinetic properties: Phentermine is readily absorbed from the gastro-intestinal tract and approximately 70–80% of all oral dose is excreted unchanged in the urine; the remainder is metabolised in the liver.

Preclinical safety data: Not applicable.

Pharmaceutical particulars

List of excipients: Lactose PhEur, Magnesium Stearate PhEur.

Incompatibilities: None known.

Shelf life: 5 years.

Special precautions for storage: Store below 30°C.

Nature and contents of container: Amber glass bottle with pilfer-proof screw cap.

Instructions for use/handling: Not applicable.

Marketing authorisation number 00068/5056R

Date of approval/revision of SPC January 1997.

Legal category CD(Sch 3), POM.

FILAIR* 50 INHALER

Qualitative and quantitative composition Each actuation delivers beclomethasone dipropionate 50 µg (as propellant solvate) into the mouthpiece of the adapter.

Pharmaceutical form Pressurised aerosol for inhalation therapy.

Clinical particulars

Therapeutic indications: Filair 50 Inhaler is indicated for the prophylactic treatment of chronic reversible obstructive airways disease.

Posology and method of administration: The dose should be titrated to the lowest dose at which effective control of asthma is maintained.

Adults: for maintenance: 4 inhalations (200 µg), twice daily or 2 inhalations (100 µg), three or four times daily. In more severe cases a dose of 600–800 µg (12–16 inhalations) daily is recommended, with subsequent reductions. The maximum recommended daily dose of this preparation is 1 mg. In patients receiving doses of 1500 µg or more daily, adrenal suppression may occur.

Children: 1 or 2 inhalations (50–100 µg), two to four times daily.

Elderly: No special dosage recommendations are made for elderly patients.

Contra-indications: Hypersensitivity to beclomethasone is a contra-indication. Caution should be observed in patients with pulmonary tuberculosis.

Special warnings and precautions for use: Patients should be instructed on the proper use of the inhaler. They should be made aware of the prophylactic nature of Filair Inhaler therapy and that it should be used regularly at the intervals recommended and not when immediate relief is required.

In patients who have been transferred to inhalation therapy, systemic steroid therapy may need to be re-instated rapidly during periods of stress or where airways obstruction or mucus prevents absorption from the inhalation.

Systemic effects of inhaled corticosteroids may occur, particularly at high doses prescribed for prolonged periods. These effects are much less likely to occur than with oral corticosteroids. Possible systemic effects include adrenal suppression, growth retardation in children and adolescents, decrease in bone mineral density, cataract and glaucoma. It is important therefore that the dose of inhaled steroid is titrated to the lowest dose at which effective control of asthma is maintained.

It is recommended that the height of children receiving prolonged treatment with inhaled corticosteroids is regularly monitored. If growth is slowed, therapy should be reviewed with the aim of reducing the dose of inhaled corticosteroid, if possible, to the lowest dose at which effective control of asthma is maintained. In addition, consideration should be given to referring the patient to a paediatric respiratory specialist.

Prolonged treatment with high doses of inhaled corticosteroids, particularly higher than the recommended doses, may result in clinically significant adrenal suppression. Additional systemic corticosteroid cover should be considered during periods of stress or elective surgery.

Patients who have received systemic steroids for long periods of time or at high doses, or both, need special care and subsequent management when transferred to beclomethasone therapy. Recovery from impaired adrenocortical function, caused by prolonged systemic steroid therapy, is slow. The patient should be in a reasonably stable state before being given Filair Inhaler in addition to his usual maintenance dose of systemic steroid. Withdrawal of the systemic steroid should be gradual, starting after about seven days by reducing the daily oral dose by 1 mg prednisolone, or equivalent, at intervals not less than one week. Adrenocortical function should be monitored regularly.

Most patients can be successfully transferred to Filair Inhaler with maintenance of good respiratory function, but special care is necessary for the first months after the transfer until the hypothalamic-pituitary-adrenal (HPA) system has sufficiently recovered to enable the patient to cope with emergencies such as trauma, surgery or infections.

Patients who have been transferred to inhalation therapy should carry a warning card indicating that systemic steroid therapy may need to be re-instated without delay during periods of stress. It may be advisable to provide such patients with a supply of oral steroid to use in emergency, for example when the asthma worsens as a result of a chest infection. The dose of Filair Inhaler should be increased at this time and then gradually reduced to the maintenance level after the systemic steroid has been discontinued.

Discontinuation of systemic steroids may cause exacerbation of allergic diseases such as atopic eczema and rhinitis. These should be treated as required with antihistamine and topical therapy.

Interactions with other medicaments and other forms of interaction: None known.

Pregnancy and lactation: There is inadequate evidence of safety in human pregnancy. In animals, systemic administration of relatively high doses can cause abnormalities of foetal development including growth retardation and cleft palate. There may therefore be a very small risk of such effects in the human foetus. However, inhalation of beclomethasone dipropionate into the lungs avoids the high level of exposure that occurs with administration by systemic routes.

The use of beclomethasone in pregnancy requires that the possible benefits of the drug be weighed against the possible hazards. The drug has been in widespread use for many years without apparent ill consequence.

It is probable that beclomethasone is excreted in milk. However, given the relatively low doses used by the inhalation route, the levels are likely to be low. In mothers breast feeding their baby the therapeutic benefits of the drug should be weighed against the potential hazards to mother and baby.

Effects on ability to drive and use machines: None.

Undesirable effects: Candidiasis of the throat and mouth may develop in some patients, but this can be treated without discontinuation of beclomethasone therapy. Hoarseness may also occur.

Systemic effects of inhaled corticosteroids may occur particularly at high doses prescribed for prolonged periods. These may include adrenal suppression, growth retardation in children and adolescents, decrease in bone mineral density, cataract and glaucoma.

Overdose: Acute overdosage is unlikely to cause problems. The only harmful effect that follows inhalation of large amounts of the drug over a short time period is suppression of HPA function. Specific emergency action need not be taken. Treatment with Filair Inhaler should be continued at the recommended dose to control the asthma; HPA function recovers in a day or two.

If grossly excessive doses of beclomethasone dipropionate were taken over a prolonged period a degree of atrophy of the adrenal cortex could occur in addition to HPA suppression. In this event the patient should be treated as steroid-dependent and transferred to a suitable maintenance dose of a systemic steroid such as prednisolone. Once the condition is stabilised the patient should be returned to Filair Inhaler by the method recommended above.

Pharmacological properties

Pharmacodynamic properties: Inhaled beclomethasone dipropionate is now well established in the management of asthma. It is a synthetic glucocorticoid and exerts a topical, anti-inflammatory effect on the lungs, without significant systemic activity.

Pharmacokinetic properties: The beclomethasone dipropionate absorbed directly from the lungs is converted to less active metabolites during its passage through the liver. Peak plasma concentrations are reached 3–5 hours following ingestion. Excretion is via the urine.

Preclinical safety data: Not applicable.

Pharmaceutical particulars *List of excipients:* Sorbitan trioleate PhEur, Trichlorofluoromethane (Propellant 11) BP (1988), Dichlorodifluoromethane (Propellant 12) BP (1988), Dichlorotetrafluoroethane (Propellant 114) BP (1988).

Incompatibilities: None known.

Shelf life: 3 years.

Special precautions for storage: Store below 30°C. Avoid storage in direct sunlight or heat. Protect from frost.

Nature and contents of container: 10 ml Aluminium vial closed with a 50 μl metering valve containing 200 doses.

Instruction for use/handling: Pressurised vial. Do not puncture. Do not burn, even when empty.

Marketing authorisation number 0068/0121

Date of first authorisation/renewal of authorisation October 1991

Date of last (partial) revision of the text May 1998

FILAIR* 100 INHALER

Qualitative and quantitative composition Each actuation delivers beclomethasone dipropionate 100 μg (as propellant solvate) into the mouthpiece of the adapter.

Pharmaceutical form Pressurised aerosol for inhalation therapy.

Clinical particulars

Therapeutic indications: The dose should be titrated to the lowest dose at which effecive control of asthma is maintained.

Filair 100 Inhaler is indicated for the prophylactic treatment of chronic reversible obstructive airways disease.

Posology and method of administration

Adults: for maintenance: 1 inhalation (100 μg), three or four times daily or 2 inhalations (200 μg), twice daily. In more severe cases a dose of 600–800 μg (6–8 inhalations) daily is recommended, with subsequent reductions. The maximum recommended daily dose of this preparation is 1 mg. In patients receiving doses of 1500 μg or more daily, adrenal suppression may occur.

Children: 1 inhalation (100 μg), two to four times daily.

Elderly: No special dosage recommendations are made for elderly patients.

Contra-indications: Hypersensitivity to Filair Inhaler is a contra-indication. Caution should be observed in patients with pulmonary tuberculosis.

Special warnings and precautions for use: Patients should be instructed on the proper use of the inhaler. They should be made aware of the prophylactic nature of Filair 100 Inhaler therapy and that it should be used regularly at the intervals recommended and not when immediate relief is required.

In patients who have been transferred to inhalation therapy, systemic steroid therapy may need to be re-instated rapidly during periods of stress or where airways obstruction or mucus prevents absorption from the inhalation.

Systemic effects of inhaled corticosteroids may occur, particularly at high doses prescribed for prolonged periods. These effects are much less likely to occur than with oral corticosteroids. Possible systemic effects include adrenal suppression, growth retardation in children and adolescents, decrease in bone mineral density, cataract and glaucoma. It is important therefore that the dose of inhaled steroid is titrated to the lowest dose at which effective control of asthma is maintained.

It is recommended that the height of children receiving prolonged treatment with inhaled corticosteroids is regularly monitored. If growth is slowed, therapy should be reviewed with the aim of reducing the dose of inhaled corticosteroid, if possible, to the lowest dose at which effective control of asthma is maintained. In addition, consideration should be given to referring the patient to a paediatric respiratory specialist.

Prolonged treatment with high doses of inhaled corticosteroids, particularly higher than the recommended doses, may result in clinically significant adrenal suppression. Additional systemic corticosteroid cover should be considered during periods of stress or elective surgery.

Patients who have received systemic steroids for long periods of time or at high doses, or both, need special care and subsequent management when transferred to beclomethasone therapy. Recovery from impaired adrenocortical function, caused by prolonged systemic steroid therapy, is slow. The patient should be in a reasonably stable state before being given Filair 100 Inhaler in addition to his usual maintenance dose of systemic steroid. Withdrawal of the systemic steroid should be gradual, starting after about seven days by reducing the daily oral dose by 1 mg prednisolone, or equivalent, at intervals not less than one week. Adrenocortical function should be monitored regularly.

Most patients can be successfully transferred to Filair 100 Inhaler with maintenance of good respiratory function, but special care is necessary for the first months after the transfer until the hypothalamic-pituitary-adrenal (HPA) system has sufficiently recovered to enable the patient to cope with emergencies such as trauma, surgery or infections.

Patients who have been transferred to inhalation therapy should carry a warning card indicating that systemic steroid therapy may need to be re-instated without delay during periods of stress. It may be advisable to provide such patients with a supply of oral steroid to use in emergency, for example when the asthma worsens as a result of a chest infection. The dose of Filair 100 Inhaler should be increased at this time and then gradually reduced to the maintenance level after the systemic steroid has been discontinued.

Discontinuation of systemic steroids may cause exacerbation of allergic diseases such as atopic eczema and rhinitis. These should be treated as required with antihistamine and topical therapy.

Interactions with other medicaments and other forms of interaction: None known.

Pregnancy and lactation: There is inadequate evidence of safety in human pregnancy. In animals, systemic administration of relatively high doses can cause abnormalities of foetal development including growth retardation and cleft palate. There may therefore be a very small risk of such effects in the human foetus. However, inhalation of beclomethasone dipropionate into the lungs avoids the high level of exposure that occurs with administration by systemic routes.

The use of beclomethasone in pregnancy requires that the possible benefits of the drug be weighed against the possible hazards. The drug has been in widespread use for many years without apparent ill consequence.

It is probable that beclomethasone is excreted in milk. However, given the relatively low doses used by the inhalation route, the levels are likely to be low. In mothers breast feeding their baby the therapeutic benefits of the drug should be weighed against the potential hazards to mother and baby.

Effects on ability to drive and use machines: None.

Undesirable effects: Candidiasis of the throat and mouth may develop in some patients, but this can be treated without discontinuation of beclomethasone therapy. Hoarseness may also occur.

Systemic effects of inhaled corticosteroids may occur particularly at high doses prescribed for prolonged periods. These may include adrenal suppression, growth retardation in children and adolescents, decrease in bone mineral density, cataract and glaucoma.

Overdose: Acute overdosage is unlikely to cause problems. The only harmful effect that follows inhalation of large amounts of the drug over a short time period is suppression of HPA function. Specific emergency action need not be taken. Treatment with Filair 100 Inhaler should be continued at the recommended dose to control the asthma; HPA function recovers in a day or two.

If grossly excessive doses of beclomethasone dipropionate were taken over a prolonged period a degree of atrophy of the adrenal cortex could occur in addition to HPA suppression. In this event the patient should be treated as steroid-dependent and transferred to a suitable maintenance dose of a systemic steroid such as prednisolone. Once the condition is stabilised the patient should be returned to Filair 100 Inhaler by the method recommended above.

Pharmacological properties
Pharmacodynamic properties: Inhaled beclomethasone dipropionate is now well established in the management of asthma. It is a synthetic glucocorticoid and exerts a topical, anti-inflammatory effect on the lungs, without significant systemic activity.

Pharmacokinetic properties: The beclomethasone dipropionate absorbed directly from the lungs is converted to less active metabolites during its passage through the liver. Peak plasma concentrations are reached 3–5 hours following ingestion. Excretion is via the urine.

Preclinical safety data: Not applicable.

Pharmaceutical particulars
List of excipients: Sorbitan trioleate PhEur, Trichlorofluoromethane (Propellant 11) BP (1988), Dichlorodifluoromethane (Propellant 12) BP (1988), Dichlorotetrafluoroethane (Propellant 114) BP (1988).

Incompatibilities: None known.

Shelf life: 3 years.

Special precautions for storage: Store below 30°C. Avoid storage in direct sunlight or heat. Protect from frost.

Nature and contents of container: 10 ml Aluminium vial closed with a 50 µl metering valve containing 200 doses.

Instruction for use/handling: Pressurised vial. Do not puncture. Do not burn, even when empty.

Marketing authorisation number 0068/0144

Date of first authorisation/renewal of authorisation January 1992

Date of last (partial) revision of the text May 1998

FILAIR* FORTE INHALER

Qualitative and quantitative composition Each actuation delivers beclomethasone dipropionate 250 µg (as propellant solvate) into the mouthpiece of the adapter.

Pharmaceutical form Pressurised aerosol for inhalation therapy.

Clinical particulars
Therapeutic indications: Filair Forte Inhaler is indicated for the prophylactic treatment of chronic reversible obstructive airways disease in those patients who require high doses of beclomethasone to control their symptoms.

Posology and method of administration: The dose should be titrated to the lowest dose at which effective control of asthma is maintained.

Adults: for maintenance: 2 inhalations (500 µg), twice daily or 1 inhalation (250 µg), four times daily; may be increased to 2 inhalations four times daily if necessary.

In patients receiving doses of 1500 µg or more daily, adrenal suppression may occur. The degree of suppression may not always be clinically significant but it is advisable to provide such patients with a supply of oral steroid to use in stressful situations. The risk of adrenal suppression occurring should be balanced against the therapeutic advantages.

Children: Filair Forte Inhaler is not recommended for use in children.

Elderly: No special dosage recommendations are made for elderly patients.

Contra-indications: Hypersensitivity to beclomethasone is a contra-indication. Caution should be observed in patients with pulmonary tuberculosis.

Special warnings and precautions for use: Patients should be instructed on the proper use of the inhaler. They should be made aware of the prophylactic nature of Filair therapy and that it should be used regularly at the intervals recommended and not when immediate relief is required.

In patients who have been transferred to inhalation therapy, systemic steroid therapy may need to be reinstated rapidly during periods of stress or where airways obstruction or mucus prevents absorption from the inhalation.

Systemic effects of inhaled corticosteroids may occur, particularly at high doses prescribed for prolonged periods. These effects are much less likely to occur than with oral corticosteroids. Possible systemic effects include adrenal suppression, growth retardation in adolescents, decrease in bone mineral density, cataract and glaucoma. It is important therefore that the dose of inhaled steroid is titrated to the lowest dose at which effective control of asthma is maintained.

It is recommended that the height of adolescents receiving prolonged treatment with inhaled corticosteroids is regularly monitored. If growth is slowed, therapy should be reviewed with the aim of reducing the dose of inhaled corticosteroid, if possible, to the lowest dose at which effective control of asthma is maintained.

Prolonged treatment with high doses of inhaled corticosteroids, particularly higher than the recommended doses, may result in clinically significant adrenal suppression. Additional systemic corticosteroid cover should be considered during periods of stress or elective surgery.

Patients who have received systemic steroids for long periods of time or at high doses, or both, need special care and subsequent management when transferred to beclomethasone therapy. Recovery from impaired adrenocortical function, caused by prolonged systemic steroid therapy, is slow. The patient should be in a reasonably stable state before being given Filair Forte Inhaler in addition to his usual maintenance dose of systemic steroid. Withdrawal of the systemic steroid should be gradual, starting after about seven days by reducing the daily oral dose by 1 mg prednisolone, or equivalent, at intervals not less than one week. Adrenocortical function should be monitored regularly.

Most patients can be successfully transferred to Filair Forte Inhaler with maintenance of good respiratory function, but special care is necessary for the first months after the transfer until the hypothalamic-pituitary-adrenal (HPA) system has sufficiently recovered to enable the patient to cope with emergencies such as trauma, surgery or infections.

Patients who have been transferred to inhalation therapy should carry a warning card indicating that systemic steroid therapy may need to be re-instated without delay during periods of stress. It may be advisable to provide such patients with a supply of oral steroid to use in emergency, for example when the asthma worsens as a result of a chest infection. The dose of Filair Forte Inhaler should be increased at this time and then gradually reduced to the maintenance level after the systemic steroid has been discontinued.

Discontinuation of systemic steroids may cause exacerbation of allergic diseases such as atopic eczema and rhinitis. These should be treated as required with antihistamine and topical therapy.

Interactions with other medicaments and other forms of interaction: None known.

Pregnancy and lactation: There is inadequate evidence of safety in human pregnancy. In animals, systemic administration of relatively high doses can cause abnormalities of foetal development including growth retardation and cleft palate. There may therefore be a very small risk of such effects in the human foetus. However, inhalation of beclomethasone dipropionate into the lungs avoids the high level of exposure that occurs with administration by systemic routes.

The use of beclomethasone in pregnancy requires that the possible benefits of the drug be weighed against the possible hazards. The drug has been in widespread use for many years without apparent ill consequence.

It is probable that beclomethasone is excreted in milk. However, given the relatively low doses used by the inhalation route, the levels are likely to be low. In mothers breast feeding their baby the therapeutic benefits of the drug should be weighed against the potential hazards to mother and baby.

Effects on ability to drive and use machines: None.

Undesirable effects: Candidiasis of the throat and mouth may develop in some patients, but this can be treated without discontinuation of beclomethasone therapy. Hoarseness may also occur.

Systemic effects of inhaled corticosteroids may occur particularly at high doses prescribed for prolonged periods. These may include adrenal suppression, growth retardation in adolescents, decrease in bone mineral density, cataract and glaucoma.

Overdose: If grossly excessive doses of beclomethasone dipropionate were taken over a prolonged period a degree of atrophy of the adrenal cortex could occur in addition to HPA suppression. In this event the patient should be treated as steroid-dependent and transferred to a suitable maintenance dose of a systemic steroid such as prednisolone. Once the condition is stabilised the patient should be returned to Filair Forte Inhaler by the method recommended above. To guard against the unexpected occurrence of adrenal suppression regular tests of adrenal function are advised.

Pharmacological properties
Pharmacodynamic properties: Inhaled beclomethasone dipropionate is now well established in the management of asthma. It is a synthetic glucocorticoid and exerts a topical, anti-inflammatory effect on the lungs, without significant systemic activity.

Pharmacokinetic properties: The beclomethasone dipropionate absorbed directly from the lungs is converted to less active metabolites during its passage through the liver. Peak plasma concentrations are reached 3–5 hours following ingestion. Excretion is via the urine.

Preclinical safety data: Not applicable.

Pharmaceutical particulars
List of excipients: Sorbitan trioleate PhEur, Trichlorofluoromethane (Propellant 11) BP (1988), Dichlorodifluoromethane (Propellant 12) BP (1988), Dichlorotetrafluoroethane (Propellant 114) BP (1988).

Incompatibilities: None known.

Shelf life: 3 years.

Special precautions for storage: Store below 30°C. Avoid storage in direct sunlight or heat. Protect from frost.

Nature and contents of container: 10 ml Aluminium vial closed with a 50 µl metering valve containing 200 doses.

Instruction for use/handling: Pressurised vial. Do not puncture. Do not burn, even when empty.

Marketing authorisation number 0068/0139

Date of first authorisation/renewal of authorisation October 1991

Date of last (partial) revision of the text May 1998

HIPREX* TABLETS

Presentation White, oblong tablet with breakline, marked HX on one side and 3M on the other. Each Hiprex tablet contains hexamine hippurate 1 g.

Uses
Hiprex is indicated in the prophylaxis and treatment of urinary tract infections:

1. As maintenance therapy after successful initial treatment of acute infections with antibiotics.
2. As long-term therapy in the prevention of recurrent cystitis.
3. To suppress urinary infection in patients with indwelling catheters and to reduce the incidence of catheter blockage.
4. To provide prophylaxis against the introduction of infection into the urinary tract during instrumental procedures.
5. Asymptomatic bacteriuria.

Hexamine hippurate is readily absorbed from the gastro-intestinal tract and excreted via the kidney.

Plasma concentrations of hexamine hippurate reach a maximum 1–2 hours after a single dose and then decline with a half-life of about 4 hours. Hexamine recovered in the urine corresponds to about 80% of the dose given per 12 hours.

Hiprex is a urinary antibacterial agent with a wide antibacterial spectrum covering both gram-positive and gram-negative organisms. Urinary antibacterial activity can be shown within 30 minutes of administration.

The chemical structure of hexamine hippurate is such that a two-fold antibacterial action is obtained:

1. The slow release of the bactericidal formaldehyde, from the hexamine part, in the urine; acid pH is necessary for this reaction to occur. It is obtained and maintained there by the presence of hippuric acid.
2. The bacteriostatic effect of hippuric acid itself on urinary tract pathogens.

Dosage and administration *Adults:* 1 g twice daily.

In patients with catheters the dosage may be increased to 1 g three times daily.

Children under 6 years: Not recommended.

Children: 6–12 years: 500 mg twice daily.

The tablets may be halved, or they can be crushed and taken with a drink of milk or fruit juice if the patient prefers.

Elderly: No special dosage recommendations.

Contra-indications, warnings, etc *Side-effects:* Occasionally rashes, gastric irritation or irritation of the bladder may occur.

All side-effects are reversible on withdrawal of the drug.

Contra-indications: Severe dehydration, metabolic acidosis, or severe renal failure (creatinine clearance or GFR<10 ml/min.). Hiprex may be used where mild (20–50 ml/min.) to moderate (10 –20 ml/min.) renal insufficiency is present. (If the GFR is not available, the serum creatinine concentration can be used as a guide).

Hiprex should not be administered concurrently with sulphonamides because of the possibility of crystalluria, or with alkalising agents, such as mixture of potassium citrate.

Use in pregnancy: There is inadequate evidence of safety of the drug in human pregnancy but it has been in wide use for many years without apparent ill consequence, animal studies having shown no hazard.

Hexamine is excreted in breast milk but the quantities will be insignificant to the infant. Mothers can therefore breast feed their infants.

Overdosage: Vomiting and haematuria may occur. These can be treated by the use of an anti-emetic and drinking copious quantities of water respectively. Bladder symptoms can be treated by the consumption of copious quantities of water and 2–3 teaspoonfuls of bicarbonate of soda.

Pharmaceutical precautions Store below 30°C.

Legal category P.

Package quantities Bottles of 60 tablets (OP).

Further information Nil.

Product licence number 0068/5003R.

INTRALGIN* GEL

Presentation Intralgin contains Benzocaine BP 2 per cent w/w and salicylamide 5 per cent w/w in an alcoholic vehicle. It contains the following inactive ingredients: Carbopol*; Brij*; Isopropyl Alcohol BP; Strong Ammonia Solution BP. Intralgin is a clear, pleasant-smelling preparation – non-greasy and non-staining.

Uses Intralgin is indicated for the relief of muscle pain from strains, sprains and injuries, and pain associated with fibrositis, lumbago and non-articular rheumatism.

The use of isopropyl alcohol as a vehicle for the medicaments contributes significantly to the action of Intralgin. Isopropyl alcohol because of its penetrative properties facilitates the percutaneous absorption of benzocaine and salicylamide. Vigorous massage is not needed with Intralgin, unlike traditional rubs which rely for effect on erythema or counter-irritation.

Dosage and administration Intralgin Gel should be applied liberally and rubbed gently into the skin until penetration is complete. Vigorous massage is unnecessary.

For more rapid absorption the painful area should be warmed before applying Intralgin.

Children and the elderly: There are no special dosage recommendations for children and elderly patients.

Contra-indications, warnings, etc
Contra-indications: None.

Precautions: If irritation or itching occurs due to hypersensitivity, Intralgin should be discontinued and a soothing cream applied.

Interactions: There are no known interactions with Intralgin therapy.

Side-effects: Local sensitivity reactions to the benzocaine constituent have occasionally been reported.

Overdosage: Not applicable.

Use in pregnancy: There is inadequate evidence of the safety of Intralgin in human pregnancy but it has been in wide use for many years without apparent ill consequence. Excretion in breast milk, if any, is expected to be too low to affect the infant.

Pharmaceutical precautions Store below 25°C. Do not refrigerate or freeze.

Legal category P.

Package quantities Tubes containing 50 g (OP).

Further information For external use only.

Product licence particulars PL 0068/5076R

Date of preparation or last review May 1997

NUELIN* TABLETS

Qualitative and quantitative composition Each Nuelin tablet contains Theophylline PhEur 125 mg.

Pharmaceutical form Tablet.

Clinical particulars
Therapeutic indications: Nuelin is indicated for the prophylaxis and treatment of reversible bronchospasm associated with asthma and chronic obstructive pulmonary disease.

Posology and method of administration
Adults: One tablet three or four times daily, preferably after food; this can be increased to two tablets three or four times daily depending on response.

Elderly: Elderly patients may require lower doses due to reduced theophylline clearance.

Children: 7–12 years (20–35 kg): Half or 1 tablet three or four times daily, preferably after food.

The difficulty of dividing the tablet accurately makes Nuelin unsuitable for use in children under the age of seven.

Nuelin tablets are soluble in water.

Contra-indications: Hypersensitivity to theophylline or other xanthines.

Special warnings and special precautions for use: Use with caution in patients with cardiac arrhythmias, peptic ulcer, hyperthyroidism and severe hypertension.

Smoking and alcohol consumption may increase theophylline clearance and increased doses of theophylline are therefore required. In patients with cardiac failure, hepatic dysfunction/disease and fever the reverse is true and these patients may require a reduced dosage.

Alternative bronchodilator therapy should be used in patients with epilepsy.

It is not recommended that the product be used concurrently with other preparations containing xanthine derivatives.

Xanthines can potentiate hypokalaemia resulting from beta-2-agonist therapy, steroids, diuretics and hypoxia. Particular caution is advised in severe asthma. It is recommended that serum potassium levels are monitored in such situations.

Interaction with other medicaments and other forms of interaction: Cimetidine, allopurinol, corticosteroids, frusemide, isoprenaline, oral contraceptives, thiobendazole, ciprofloxacin, erythromycin or other macrolide antibiotics and the calcium channel blockers, diltiazem and verapamil delay the elimination of theophylline. A reduction of the theophylline dosage is recommended. Phenytoin, carbamazepine, barbiturates, lithium, rifampicin, sulphinpyrazone increase theophylline clearance and therefore the theophylline dosage may need to be increased.

The concomitant use of theophylline and fluvoxamine should usually be avoided. Where this is not possible, patients should have their theophylline dose halved and plasma theophylline should be monitored closely.

Pregnancy and lactation: There is inadequate evidence of safety of the drug in human pregnancy but it has been in wide use for many years without apparent ill consequences; there is evidence of harmful effects in pregnancy in animals. Use in pregnancy only when there is no safer alternative and when the condition itself carries risks for the mother.

Theophylline is excreted in breast milk and has been shown to cause irritability in infants. It is therefore recommended that the mother nurse her infant just prior to taking her next dose, when plasma theophylline levels are expected to be low.

Effects on ability to drive and use machines: No effect.

Undesirable effects: Nausea or other gastric disturbances may occur rarely. Palpitations, headache, CNS stimulation and insomnia have been reported occasionally.

Overdose: Symptoms: Characterised by nausea, vomiting, electrolyte imbalance and gastro-intestinal irritation. Tachycardia and convulsions may also occur.

Treatment: Gastric lavage and general supportive measures (e.g. to maintain circulation, respiration and fluid and electrolyte balance) are recommended. Oral activated charcoal may reduce serum theophylline levels, whilst in severe cases charcoal haemoperfusion may be required.

Pharmacological properties
Pharmacodynamic properties: Theophylline directly relaxes smooth muscle thus acting mainly as a bronchodilator and vasodilator. The drug also possesses other actions typical of the xanthine derivatives; coronary vasodilator, diuretic, cardiac stimulant, cerebral stimulant and skeletal muscle stimulant.

Pharmacokinetic properties: It has been established that the xanthines, which include theophylline, are readily absorbed after oral, rectal or parenteral administration and this fact is well documented in published literature.

Theophylline is excreted in the urine as metabolites, mainly 1,3-dimethyluric acid and 3-methylxanthine and about 10% is excreted unchanged.

Plasma half-lives ranging from 3–9 hours and therapeutic plasma concentrations from about 5–20 μg per ml have been reported.

Pharmaceutical particulars
List of excipients: Lactose Monohydrate PhEur, Sodium carboxymethylcellulose, Magnesium Stearate PhEur.

Incompatibilities: None known.

Shelf life: 3 years.

Special precautions for storage: Store below 30°C in a dry place.

Nature and contents of container: Bottle or blister packs of 90 tablets.

Instructions for use/handling: None.

Marketing authorisation number 0068/0064R

Date of first authorisation/renewal of the authorisation 21 November 1989/25 March 1997

Date of (partial) revision of the text 30 January 1997/31 May 1997

NUELIN* LIQUID

Presentation Clear, light brown, pleasantly flavoured liquid. Each 5 ml dose of Nuelin Liquid contains 60 mg Theophylline Hydrate BP as the sodium glycinate salt. It also contains the following inactive ingredients: sucrose; Sodium Butyl Hydroxybenzoate BP.

Uses Nuelin Liquid is indicated for the prophylaxis and treatment of reversible bronchospasm associated with asthma and chronic obstructive pulmonary disease. Nuelin in tablet form (microcrystalline theophylline 125 mg) is established as a highly effective bronchodilator. Nuelin Liquid is designed to offer comparable relief of bronchospasm with the same low incidence of side-effects, for patients who prefer a liquid presentation. Each 10 ml of Nuelin Liquid approximates to one 125 mg Nuelin tablet.

Dosage and administration *Adults:* 10–20 ml (two to four 5 ml spoonfuls) three or four times daily, preferably after food.

Children: 7–12 years: One-and-a-half or two 5 ml spoonfuls three or four times daily, preferably after food.

2–6 years: One or one-and-a-half 5 ml spoonfuls three or four times daily, preferably after food.

Under 2 years: Nuelin liquid is not recommended for children under 2 years of age.

Elderly: Elderly patients may require lower doses due to reduced theophylline clearance.

Contra-indications, warnings, etc
Contra-indications: Hypersensitivity to theophylline or other xanthines.

Warnings: Xanthines can potentiate hypokalaemia resulting from B_2-agonist therapy, steroids, diuretics and hypoxia. Particular caution is advised in severe asthma. It is recommended that serum potassium levels are monitored in such situations.

Precautions: Use with caution in patients with cardiac arrhythmias, peptic ulcer, hyperthyroidism and severe hypertension.

Smoking and alcohol consumption may increase theophylline clearance and increased doses of theophylline are therefore required. In patients with cardiac failure, hepatic dysfunction/disease and fever the reverse is true and these patients may require a reduced dosage.

Alternative bronchodilator therapy should be used in patients with epilepsy.

It is not recommended that the product be used concurrently with other preparations containing xanthine derivatives.

Interactions: Cimetidine, allopurinol, corticosteroids, frusemide, isoprenaline, oral contraceptives, thiobendazole, ciprofloxacin, erythromycin or other macrolide antibiotics, and the calcium channel blockers, diltiazem and verapamil delay the elimination of theophylline. A reduction of the theophylline dosage is recommended. Phenytoin, carbamazepine, barbiturates, lithium, rifampicin, sulphinpyrazone increase theophylline clearance and therefore the theophylline dosage may need to be increased. The concomitant use of theophylline and fluvoxamine should usually be avoided. Where this is not possible, patients should have their theophylline dose halved and plasma theophylline should be monitored closely.

Also see 'Warnings'.

Side-effects: Nausea or other gastric disturbances may occur rarely. Palpitations, headache, CNS stimulation and insomnia have been reported occasionally.

Overdosage
Symptoms: Characterised by nausea, vomiting, electrolyte imbalance and gastro-intestinal irritation. Tachycardia and convulsions may also occur.

Treatment: Gastric lavage and general supportive measures (e.g. to maintain circulation, respiration and fluid and electrolyte balance) are recommended. Oral activated charcoal may reduce serum theophylline levels, whilst in severe cases charcoal haemoperfusion may be required.

Use in pregnancy: There is inadequate evidence of safety of the drug in human pregnancy but it has been in wide use for many years without apparent ill consequences; there is evidence of harmful effects in pregnancy in animals. Use in pregnancy only when there is no safer alternative and when the condition itself carries risks for the mother.

Theophylline is excreted in breast milk and has been shown to cause irritability in infants. It is therefore recommended that the mother nurse her infant just prior to taking her next dose, when plasma theophylline levels are expected to be low.

Pharmaceutical precautions Store between 5°C and 30°C. Do not freeze.

Legal category P.

Package quantities Bottles of 300 ml (OP).

Further information Each 5 ml spoonful of Nuelin Liquid contains 0.38 mEq sodium (8.7 mg Na).

Product licence number 0068/0084.

NUELIN* SA TABLETS

Presentation Nuelin SA: White, biconvex, round tablets, 9 mm in diameter and marked NLS 175 on one side and 3M on the other.

Each Nuelin SA tablet contains 175 mg anhydrous theophylline in a slow release formulation which gives a particularly smooth release of medicament over a prolonged period. It also contains the following inactive ingredient: lactose.

Nuelin SA-250: White, biconvex, round tablets with breakline, 11 mm in diameter and marked NLS 250 on one side and 3M on the other. Each Nuelin SA-250 tablet contains 250 mg anhydrous theophylline in a slow release formulation. It contains the same inactive ingredients as Nuelin SA.

Uses Nuelin SA and Nuelin SA-250 tablets are indicated for the prophylaxis and treatment of reversible bronchospasm associated with asthma and chronic obstructive pulmonary disease.

Because effective plasma levels are maintained for up to twelve hours from a single dose, less frequent dosing is required than with conventional theophylline preparations.

Dosage and administration *Nuelin SA: Adults:* One tablet twice daily, preferably after food, increasing to two tablets twice daily if necessary.

Children: 6 to 12 years: one tablet twice daily, preferably after food.

Nuelin SA-250: Adults: One tablet twice daily, preferably after food, increasing to two tablets twice daily if necessary.

Children: 6 to 12 years: Half or one tablet twice daily, preferably after food.

Nuelin SA and Nuelin SA-250 tablets are not recommended for children under six years.

Elderly: Elderly patients may require lower dosage due to reduced theophylline clearance.

Nuelin SA tablets should be swallowed whole and not crushed or chewed.

Nuelin SA-250 tablets are scored and may be halved but should not be crushed or chewed.

Contra-indications, warnings, etc

Contra-indications: Hypersensitivity to theophylline or other xanthines.

Warnings: Xanthines can potentiate hypokalaemia resulting from B_2-agonist therapy, steroids, diuretics and hypoxia. Particular caution is advised in severe asthma. It is recommended that serum potassium levels are monitored in such situations.

Precautions: In the case of an acute asthmatic attack in a patient receiving a sustained action theophylline preparation, great caution should be taken when administering intravenous aminophylline. Half the recommended loading dose of aminophylline (generally 6 mg/kg) should be given, i.e. 3 mg/kg, cautiously.

Use with caution in patients with cardiac arrhythmias, peptic ulcer, hyperthyroidism, severe hypertension, acute porphyria, hepatic dysfunction, chronic alcoholism, acute febrile illness and chronic lung disease.

Smoking and alcohol consumption may increase theophylline clearance and increased doses of theophylline are therefore required. In patients with cardiac failure, hepatic dysfunction/disease and fever the reverse is true and these patients may require a reduced dosage.

Alternative bronchodilator therapy should be used in patients with epilepsy.

It is not recommended that the product be used concurrently with other preparations containing xanthine derivatives.

Interactions: Cimetidine, allopurinol, corticosteroids, frusemide, isoprenaline, oral contraceptives, thiobendazole, ciprofloxacin, erythromycin or other macrolide antibiotics, and the calcium channel blockers, diltiazem and verapamil delay the elimination of theophylline. A reduction of the theophylline dosage is recommended. Phenytoin, carbamazepine, barbiturates, lithium, rifampicin, sulphinpyrazone increase theophylline clearance and therefore the theophylline dosage may need to be increased. The concomitant use of theophylline and fluvoxamine should usually be avoided. Where this is not possible, patients should have their theophylline dose halved and plasma theophylline should be monitored closely.

Also see 'Warnings'.

Side-effects: The side-effects commonly associated with xanthine derivatives such as nausea, gastric irritation, palpitations, headache, CNS stimulation and insomnia are much diminished when a sustained action preparation such as Nuelin SA is used. These side-effects are mild and infrequent when the plasma concentration is maintained at less than 20 microgrammes/ml.

Overdosage

Symptoms: Characterised by nausea, vomiting, electrolyte imbalance and gastro-intestinal irritation. Tachycardia and convulsions may also occur.

Treatment: Gastric lavage and general supportive measures (e.g. to maintain circulation, respiration and fluid and electrolyte balance) are recommended. Oral activated charcoal may reduce serum theophylline levels, whilst in severe cases charcoal haemoperfusion may be required.

Use in pregnancy: There is inadequate evidence of safety of the drug in human pregnancy but it has been in wide use for many years without apparent ill consequence; there is evidence of harmful effects in animals. Use in pregnancy only when there is no safer alternative and when the condition itself carries risks for the mother.

Theophylline is excreted in breast milk and has been shown to cause irritability in infants. As it is recommended that the mother nurse her infant just prior to taking her next dose when plasma theophylline levels are expected to be low, a non-sustained release form such as Nuelin is therefore preferable for nursing mothers.

Pharmaceutical precautions Store below 30°C.

Legal category P.

Package quantities Nuelin SA: Packs of 60 tablets (OP).
Nuelin SA-250: Packs of 60 tablets (OP).

Further information Nil.

Product licence numbers
Nuelin SA 0068/0092
Nuelin SA-250 0068/0093

QVAR* 50 AEROSOL
QVAR* 100 AEROSOL
QVAR* 50 AUTOHALER*
QVAR* 100 AUTOHALER*

Qualitative and quantitative composition Each actuation of Qvar aerosol/Autohaler delivers Beclomethasone Dipropionate PhEur 50 micrograms or 100 micrograms ex-valve into the mouthpiece of the actuator.

Phamaceutical form Qvar Autohaler is a breath-actuated inhaler which automatically releases the metered dose of medication during a patient's inhalation through the mouthpiece and overcomes the need for patients to have good manual co-ordination.

Qvar aerosol is recommended for those patients who have demonstrated consistent good technique with co-ordinating actuation and inhalation.

Qvar contains a new propellant and does not contain any chlorofluorocarbons (CFCs).

Qvar contains beclomethasone dipropionate in solution in propellant HFA-134a resulting in an extrafine aerosol. The aerosol droplets are on average much smaller that the beclomethasone dipropionate particles delivered by CFC-suspension formulations or dry powder formulations of beclomethasone dipropionate. The extrafine particle fraction will be 60%±20% of the drug particles ≤ 3.3 microns per shot, ex-actuator.

Radio-labelled deposition studies in patients with mild asthma have demonstrated that the majority of drug (>55% ex-actuator) is deposited in the lung and a small amount (<35% ex-actuator) is deposited in the oropharynx. These delivery characteristics result in equivalent therapeutic effects at lower total daily doses of Qvar, compared with CFC beclomethasone dipropionate formulations.

Clinical particulars

Therapeutic indications: Prophylactic management of mild, moderate or severe asthma.

Posology and method of administration: Qvar is for oral inhalation use only.

NOTE: The recommended total daily dose of Qvar is lower than that for current beclomethasone dipropionate CFC containing products and should be adjusted to the needs of the individual patient.

ADULT STARTING AND MAINTENANCE DOSE: It is important to gain control of asthma symptoms and optimise pulmonary function as soon as possible. When patients' symptoms remain under satisfactory control, the dose should be titrated to the lowest dose at which effective control of asthma is maintained.

To be effective inhaled Qvar must be used on a regular basis even when patients are asymptomatic.

THERAPY IN NEW PATIENTS SHOULD BE INITIATED AT THE FOLLOWING DOSAGES

Mild asthma:	100 to 200 micrograms per day in two divided doses.
Moderate asthma:	200 to 400 micrograms per day in two divided doses.
Severe asthma:	400 to 800 micrograms per day in two divided doses.

TRANSFERRING PATIENTS TO QVAR FROM A CFC-CONTAINING INHALER: The general approach to switching patients to Qvar involves two steps as detailed below. Specific guidance on switching well-controlled and poorly-controlled (symptomatic) patients is given below the table.

Step 1: Consider the dose of CFC containing beclomethasone dipropionate product appropriate to the patient's current condition.

Step 2: Convert the CFC containing beclomethasone dipropionate dose to the Qvar dose according to the table below.

Total Daily Dose (mcg/day)								
CFC–BDP	200–250	300	400–500	600–750	800–1000	1100	1200–1500	1600–2000
QVAR	100	150	200	300	400	500	600	800

1. Dosing in well-controlled patients with asthma.

Patients with well-controlled asthma using beclomethasone dipropionate CFC containing product should be switched to Qvar at a dose in accordance with the table above.

For example:

Patients on 2 puffs twice daily of CFC beclomethasone dipropionate 100 micrograms would change to 2 puffs twice daily of Qvar 50 micrograms.

2. Dosing in poorly-controlled (symptomatic) patients with asthma.

Patients with poorly-controlled asthma may be switched from CFC containing beclomethasone dipropionate products to Qvar at the same microgram for microgram dose up to 800 micrograms daily. Comparative clinical studies have demonstrated that asthma patients achieve equivalent pulmonary function and control of symptoms with Qvar at lower total daily doses than with CFC containing beclomethasone dipropionate products.

Alternatively the patient's current CFC containing beclomethasone dipropionate dose can be doubled and this dose can be converted to the Qvar dose according to the table above.

Patients on budesonide inhalers may be transferred to Qvar as described for CFC containing beclomethasone dipropionate products.

Patients on fluticasone inhalers may be transferred to the same total daily dose of Qvar up to 800 micrograms daily.

Once transferred to Qvar, the dose should be adjusted to meet the needs of the individual patient.

The maximum recommended dose is 800 micrograms per day in divided doses.

The same total daily dose in micrograms from either Qvar 50 or Qvar 100 aerosol provides the same clinical effect.

Patients should be instructed in the proper use of their inhaler, including rinsing out their mouth with water after use. Patients should be advised that Qvar may have a different taste and feel than a CFC inhaler.

Children: There are no data to date on Qvar in children, hence no definitive dosage recommendation can be made.

Special patients groups: No special dosage recommendations are made for elderly or patients with hepatic or renal impairment.

Contra-indications: Hypersensitivity to beclomethasone dipropionate or any other ingredient in Qvar.

Special warnings and special precautions for use: To be effective, Qvar must be used by patients on a regular basis, even when patients do not have asthma symptoms. When symptoms are controlled, maintenance Qvar therapy should be reduced in a stepwise manner to the minimum effective dose. Inhaled steroid treatment should not be stopped abruptly.

Patients with asthma are at risk of acute attacks and should have regular assessments of their asthma control including pulmonary function tests.

Qvar is not indicated for the immediate relief of asthma attacks. Patients therefore need to have relief medication (inhaled short-acting bronchodilator) available for such circumstances.

Qvar is not indicated in the management of status asthmaticus.

Severe asthma exacerbations should be managed in the usual way. Subsequently, it may be necessary to increase the dose of Qvar up to the maximum daily dose. Systemic steroid treatment may be needed and/or an antibiotic, if there is an infection.

Patients should be advised to seek medical attention for review of maintenance Qvar therapy if peak flow falls, symptoms worsen or if the short-acting bronchodilator becomes less effective and increased inhalations are required. This may indicate worsening asthma.

Patients who have received systemic steroids for long periods of time or at high doses, or both, need special care and subsequent management when being transferred to inhaled steroid therapy. Patients should have stable asthma before being given inhaled steroids in addition to the usual maintenance dose of systemic steroid. Withdrawal of systemic steroids should be gradual, starting about seven days after the introduction of Qvar therapy. For daily oral doses of prednisolone of 10 mg or less, dose reduction in 1 mg steps, at intervals of not less than one week is recommended. For patients on daily maintenance doses of oral prednisolone greater that 10 mg, larger weekly reductions in the dose might be acceptable. The dose reduction scheme should be chosen to correlate with the magnitude of the maintenance systemic steroid dose.

Most patients can be successfully transferred to inhaled steroids with maintenance of good respiratory function, but special care is necessary for the first few months after the transfer, until the hypothalamic-pituitary-adrenal (HPA) system has sufficiently recovered to enable the patient to cope with stressful emergencies such as trauma, surgery or serious infections. Patients should, therefore, carry a steroid warning card to indicate the possible need to reinstate systemic steroid therapy rapidly during periods of stress or where airways obstruction or mucus significantly compromises the inhaled route of administration. In addition, it may be advisable to provide such patients with a supply of corticosteriod tablets to use in these circumstances. The dose of inhaled steroids should be increased at this time and then gradually reduced to the maintenance level after the systemic steriod has been discontinued. As recovery from impaired adrenocortical function, caused by prolonged systemic steroid therapy is slow, adrenocortical function should be monitored regularly.

Patients should be advised that they may feel unwell in a non-specific way during systemic steroid withdrawal despite maintenance of, or even improved respiratory function. Patients should be advised to persevere with their inhaled product and to continue withdrawal of systemic steroids, even if feeling unwell, unless there is evidence of HPA axis suppression.

Discontinuation of systemic steroids may also cause exacerbation of allergic diseases such as atopic eczema and rhinitis. These should be treated as required with topical therapy, including corticosteroids and/or antihistamines.

Beclomethasone dipropionate, like other inhaled steroids, is absorbed into the systemic circulation from the lungs. Beclomethasone dipropionate and its metabolites may exert detectable suppression of adrenal function. Within the dose range 100–800 micrograms daily, clinical studies with Qvar have demonstrated mean values for adrenal function and responsiveness within the normal range. However, systemic effects of inhaled corticosteroids may occur, particularly at high doses prescribed for prolonged periods. These effects are much less likely to occur than with oral corticosteroids. Possible systemic effects include adrenal suppression, growth retardation in children and adolescents, decrease in bone mineral density, cataract and glaucoma. It is important, therefore, that the dose of inhaled corticosteroid is titrated to the lowest dose at which effective control of asthma is maintained.

It is recommended that the height of children receiving prolonged treatment with inhaled corticosteroids is regularly monitored. If growth is slowed, therapy should be reviewed with the aim of reducing the dose of inhaled corticosteroid, if possible, to the lowest dose at which effective control of asthma is maintained. In addition, consideration should be given to referring the patient to a paediatric respiratory specialist.

Prolonged treatment with high doses of inhaled corticosteroids, particularly higher than the recommended doses, may result in clinically significant adrenal suppression. Additional systemic corticosteroid cover should be considered during periods of stress or elective surgery.

Like other corticosteroids, caution is necessary in patients with active or latent pulmonary tuberculosis.

Interaction with other medicaments and other forms of interaction: None known.

Pregnancy and lactation

Qvar: There is no experience of this product in pregnancy and lactation in humans, therefore the product should only be used if the expected benefits to the mother are thought to outweigh any potential risk to the foetus or neonate. An inhalation reproductive study with this product in rats did not exhibit any teratogenic effects.

Propellant HFA-134a: Studies of propellant HFA-134a administered to pregnant and lactating rats and rabbits have not revealed any special hazard.

Beclomethasone dipropionate: There is inadequate evidence of safety in human pregnancy. In animals, systemic administration of relatively high doses can cause abnormalities of foetal development including growth retardation and cleft palate. There may therefore be a very small risk of such effects in the human foetus. However, inhalation of beclomethasone dipropionate into the lungs avoids the high level of exposure that occurs with administration by systemic routes.

The use of beclomethasone dipropionate in pregnancy requires that the possible benefits of the drug be weighed against the possible hazards. The drug has been in widespread use for many years without apparent ill consequence.

It is probable that beclomethasone dipropionate is excreted in milk. However, given the relatively low doses used by the inhalation route, the levels are likely to be low. In mothers breast feeding their baby the therapeutic benefits of the drug should be weighed against the potential hazards to mother and baby.

Effects on ability to drive and use machines: None known.

Undesirable effects: When taking Qvar an occasional incidence of hoarseness and/or a rare occurrence of candidiasis of throat and mouth may occur; patients may find it helpful to rinse out their mouth with water after using their inhaler to reduce the risk of candidiasis and hoarseness. Topical anti-fungal therapy can be used for the treatment of candidiasis while continuing treatment with Qvar.

As with other inhaled therapy, paradoxical bronchospasm with wheezing may occur immediately after dosing. Immediate treatment with an inhaled short-acting bronchodilator is required. Qvar should be discontinued immediately and alternate prophylactic therapy introduced.

Systemic effects of inhaled corticosteroids may occur, particularly at high doses prescribed for prolonged periods. These may include adrenal suppression, growth retardation in children and adolescents, decrease in bone mineral density, cataract and glaucoma.

As with other beclomethasone dipropionate products the potential for hypersensitivity reactions including rashes, urticaria, pruritus and erythema, and oedema of the eyes, face, lips and throat should be considered.

For Qvar a rare incidence of nausea has been reported.

Overdose: Acute overdosage is unlikely to cause problems. The only harmful effect that follows inhalation of large amounts of the drug over a short time period is suppression of HPA function. Specific emergency action need not be taken. Treatment with Qvar should be continued at the recommended dose to control the asthma; HPA function recovers in a day or two.

If excessive doses of beclomethasone dipropionate were taken over a prolonged period a degree of atrophy of the adrenal cortex could occur in addition to HPA suppression. In this event the patient should be treated as steroid dependent and transferred to a suitable maintenance dose of a systemic steroid such as prednisolone. Once the condition is stabilised, the patient should be returned to Qvar by the method described above in *Special warnings and special precautions for use.*

Pharmacological properties

Pharmacodynamic properties: Inhaled beclomethasone dipropionate is now well established in the management of asthma. It is a synthetic glucocorticoid and exerts a topical, anti-inflammatory effect on the lungs, with fewer systemic effects than oral corticosteroids.

Comparative clinical studies have demonstrated that asthma patients achieve equivalent pulmonary function and control of symptoms with Qvar at lower total daily doses than CFC containing beclomethasone dipropionate aerosol inhalers.

Pharmacokinetic properties: The pharmacokinetic profile of Qvar shows that the peak serum concentration for total-beclomethasone (BOH) (total of any beclomethasone OH and beclomethasone dipropionate or monopropionate hydrolysed to beclomethasone OH) after single and multiple doses is achieved after 30 minutes. The value at the peak is approximately 2 nanograms/ml after a total daily dose of 800 micrograms and the serum levels after 100, 200 and 400 micrograms are proportional. The principal route of elimination of beclomethasone dipropionate and its several metabolites is in the faeces. Between 10% and 15% of an orally administered dose is excreted in the urine, as both conjugated and free metabolites of the drug.

In both single dose and multiple dose pharmacokinetic studies, a dose of 200 micrograms of Qvar achieved comparable total-BOH levels, as a dose of 400 micrograms of CFC containing beclomethasone dipropionate aerosol. This provided the scientific rationale for investigating lower total daily doses of Qvar to achieve the same clinical effect.

Pharmacodynamic studies in patients with mild asthma given Qvar for 14 days, have shown that there is a linear correlation among urinary free cortisol suppression, dose administered, and serum total-BOH levels obtained. At a daily dose of 800 micrograms Qvar, suppression of urinary free cortisol was comparable with that observed with the same daily dose of CFC containing beclomethasone dipropionate, indicating a wider safety margin, as Qvar is administered at lower doses than the CFC product.

Pharmacokinetic studies with Qvar have not been carried out in any special populations.

Preclinical safety data

Propellant HFA-134a: Statements from CPMP:

1. In animal studies, propellant HFA-134a has been shown to have no significant pharmacological effects other than at very high exposure concentrations, then narcosis and a relatively weak cardiac sensitising effect were found. The potency of the cardiac sensitisation was less than that of CFC-11 (trichlorofluoromethane).

2. In studies to detect toxicity, repeated high dose levels of propellant HFA-134a indicated that safety margins based on systemic exposure would be of the order 2200, 1314 and 381 for mouse, rat and dog with respect to humans.

3. There are no reasons to consider propellant HFA-134a as a potential mutagen, clastogen or carcinogen judged from *in vitro* and *in vivo* studies including long-term administration by inhalation in rodents.

Qvar: Safety studies with this product in rat and dog showed few, if any, adverse effects other than those normally associated with general steroid exposure including lymphoid tissue alterations such as reduction in thymus, adrenal and spleen weights.

Pharmaceutical particulars

List of excipients: Propellant HFA-134a (Norflurane) and ethanol.

Incompatibilities: None known.

Shelf-life: The shelf-life expiry date for this product shall not exceed 2 years from the date of its manufacture.

Special precautions for storage: Qvar should be stored below 30°C. Storage in direct sunlight or heat should be avoided. Protect from frost.

Nature and contents of container: Pressurised canister closed with a metering valve containing 200 actuations.

Instructions for use/handling: The patient should read the instruction leaflet before use.

As the canister is pressurised, no attempt should be made to puncture or dispose of it by burning.

Where a spacer is considered necessary for specific patient needs, Qvar can be used with Aerochamber® holding chamber, as the extrafine particle fraction is maintained.

Qvar delivers a consistent dose:
- whether or not the canister is shaken by the patient.
- without the need for the patient to wait between individual actuations.
- regardless of storage orientation or periods without use of up to 14 days.
- at temperatures as low as –10°C.

Marketing authorisation number

Qvar 50 aerosol	PL0068/0170
Qvar 100 aerosol	PL0068/0171
Qvar 50 Autohaler	PL0068/0172
Qvar 100 Autohaler	PL0068/0173

Date of first authorisation June 1998.

Date of partial revision of text December 1998.

TAMBOCOR* 50 mg TABLETS

Qualitative and quantitative composition Each tablet contains flecainide acetate 50 mg.

Pharmaceutical form Tablet.

Clinical particulars Tambocor is a potent sodium channel blocking agent for the treatment of the conditions listed below:

The effect on the JT interval is insignificant at therapeutic levels.

Therapeutic indications: Tambocor tablets are indicated for:

(a) AV nodal reciprocating tachycardia; arrhythmias associated with Wolff-Parkinson-White Syndrome and similar conditions with accessory pathways.

(b) Paroxysmal atrial fibrillation in patients with

disabling symptoms. Arrhythmias of recent onset will respond more readily.
(c) Symptomatic sustained ventricular tachycardia.
(d) Premature ventricular contractions and/or non-sustained ventricular tachycardia which are causing disabling symptoms, where these are resistant to other therapy or when other treatment has not been tolerated.

Tambocor tablets can be used for the maintenance of normal rhythm following conversion by other means.

Tambocor tablets are for oral administration.

Posology and method of administration: Adults: Supraventricular arrhythmias: The recommended starting dosage is 50 mg twice daily and most patients will be controlled at this dose. If required the dose may be increased to a maximum of 300 mg daily.
Ventricular arrhythmias: The recommended starting dosage is 100 mg twice daily. The maximum daily dose is 400 mg and this is normally reserved for patients of large build or where rapid control of the arrhythmia is required.

After 3–5 days it is recommended that the dosage be progressively adjusted to the lowest level which maintains control of the arrhythmia. It may be possible to reduce dosage during long-term treatment.

Children: Tambocor is not recommended in children under 12, as there is insufficient evidence of its use in this age group.

Elderly patients: The rate of flecainide elimination from plasma may be reduced in elderly people. This should be taken into consideration when making dose adjustments.

Plasma levels: Based on PVC suppression, it appears that plasma levels of 200–1000 ng/ml may be needed to obtain the maximum therapeutic effect. Plasma levels above 700–1000 ng/ml are associated with increased likelihood of adverse experiences.

Dosage in impaired renal function: In patients with significant renal impairment (creatinine clearance of 35 ml/min/1.73 sq. m. or less) the maximum initial dosage should be 100 mg daily (or 50 mg twice daily). When used in such patients, frequent plasma level monitoring is strongly recommended.

It is recommended that treatment with Tambocor should be initiated in hospital.

Contra-indications: Tambocor is contra-indicated in cardiac failure, and in patients with a history of myocardial infarction who have either asymptomatic ventricular ectopics or asymptomatic non-sustained ventricular tachycardia.

It is also contra-indicated in patients with long standing atrial fibrillation in whom there has been no attempt to convert to sinus rhythm, and in patients with haemodynamically significant valvular heart disease.

Unless pacing rescue is available, Tambocor should not be given to patients with sinus node dysfunction, atrial conduction defects, second degree or greater atrio-ventricular block, bundle branch block or distal block.

Special warnings and special precautions for use: Electrolyte disturbances should be corrected before using Tambocor.

Since flecainide elimination from the plasma can be markedly slower in patients with significant hepatic impairment, flecainide should not be used in such patients unless the potential benefits clearly outweigh the risks. Plasma level monitoring is strongly recommended in these circumstances.

Tambocor is known to increase endocardial pacing thresholds – i.e. to decrease endocardial pacing sensitivity. This effect is reversible and is more marked on the acute pacing threshold than on the chronic. Tambocor should thus be used with caution in all patients with permanent pacemakers or temporary pacing electrodes, and should not be administered to patients with existing poor thresholds or non-programmable pacemakers unless suitable pacing rescue is available.

Generally, a doubling of either pulse width or voltage is sufficient to regain capture, but it may be difficult to obtain ventricular thresholds less than 1 Volt at initial implantation in the presence of Tambocor.

The minor negative inotropic effect of flecainide may assume importance in patients predisposed to cardiac failure. Difficulty has been experienced in defibrillating some patients. Most of the cases reported had pre-existing heart disease with cardiac enlargement, a history of myocardial infarction, arterio-sclerotic heart disease and cardiac failure.

Tambocor should be used with caution in patients with acute onset of atrial fibrillation following cardiac surgery.

In a large scale, placebo-controlled clinical trial in post-myocardial infarction patients with asymptomatic ventricular arrhythmia, oral flecainide was associated with a 2.2 fold higher incidence of mortality or non-fatal cardiac arrest as compared with its matching placebo. In that same study, an even higher incidence of mortality was observed in flecainide-treated patients with more than one myocardial infarction. Comparable placebo-controlled clinical trials have not been done to determine if flecainide is associated with higher risk of mortality in other patient groups.

Interaction with other medicaments and other forms of interaction: Use of flecainide with other class 1 anti-arrhythmics is not recommended. Treatment with Tambocor is compatible with use of oral anti-coagulants. Flecainide can cause the plasma digoxin level to rise by about 15%, which is unlikely to be of clinical significance for patients with plasma levels in the therapeutic range. It is recommended that the digoxin plasma level in digitalised patients should be measured not less than six hours after any digoxin dose, before or after administration of flecainide. The possibility of additive negative inotropic effects of beta-blockers and other cardiac depressants with flecainide should be recognised.

Limited data in patients receiving known enzyme inducers (phenytoin, phenobarbital, carbamazepine) indicate only a 30% increase in the rate of flecainide elimination. In healthy subjects receiving cimetidine (1 g daily) for one week, plasma flecainide levels increased by about 30% and the half-life increased by about 10%.

When flecainide is given in the presence of amiodarone, the usual flecainide dosage should be reduced by 50% and the patient monitored closely for adverse effects. Plasma level monitoring is strongly recommended in these circumstances.

Pregnancy and lactation: There is no evidence as to drug safety in human pregnancy. In New Zealand White rabbits high doses of flecainide caused some foetal abnormalities, but these effects were not seen in Dutch Belted rabbits or rats. The relevance of these findings to humans has not been established. Data have shown that flecainide crosses the placenta to the foetus in patients taking flecainide during pregnancy.

Flecainide is excreted in human milk and appears in concentrations which reflect those in maternal blood. The risk of adverse effects to the nursing infant is very small.

Effects on ability to drive and use machines: No effect.

Undesirable effects: Cardiac: Pro-arrhythmic effects occur but are most likely in patients with structural heart disease and/or significant left ventricular impairment.

In patients with atrial flutter the use of Tambocor has been associated with 1:1 AV conduction following initial atrial slowing with resultant ventricular acceleration. This has been seen most commonly following the use of the injection for acute conversion. This effect is usually short lived and abates quickly following cessation of therapy.
Dermatological: A range of allergic skin reactions have been reported including rare but serious reports of urticaria. There have also been isolated cases of photosensitivity.
Immune system: A small number of cases of increases in anti-nuclear antibodies have been reported, with and without systemic inflammatory involvement.
Haematological: Reductions in red blood cells, white blood cells and platelets have been occasionally reported. These changes are usually mild.
Psychiatric: Rarely, hallucinations, depression, confusion and amnesia have been reported.
Gastrointestinal: Occasionally nausea and vomiting.
Hepatic: A number of cases of elevated liver enzymes and jaundice have been reported in association with Tambocor treatment. So far this has always been reversible on stopping treatment.
CNS: Most commonly giddiness, dizziness and lightheadedness which are usually transient. Rare instances of dyskinesia have been reported, which have improved on withdrawal of flecainide therapy. Rare instances of convulsions, and during long term therapy a few cases of peripheral neuropathy, paraesthesia and ataxia have been reported.
Ophthalmological: Visual disturbances, such as double vision and blurring of vision may occur but these are usually transient and disappear upon continuing or reducing the dosage.

Extremely rare cases of corneal deposits and pneumonitis have also been reported.

Overdose: Overdosage with flecainide is a potentially life threatening medical emergency. No specific antidote is known. There is no known way of rapidly removing flecainide from the system, but forced acid diuresis may theoretically be helpful. Neither dialysis nor haemoperfusion is helpful and injections of anticholinergics are not recommended.

Treatment may include therapy with an inotropic agent, intravenous calcium, giving circulatory assistance (e.g. balloon pumping), mechanically assisting respiration, or temporarily inserting a transvenous pacemaker if there are severe conduction disturbances or the patient's left ventricular function is otherwise compromised.

Pharmacological properties
Pharmacodynamic properties: Tambocor is a Class 1 anti-arrhythmic (local anaesthetic) agent.

Tambocor slows conduction through the heart, having its gretest effect on His Bundle conduction. It also acts selectively to increase anterograde and particularly retrograde accessory pathway refractoriness. Its actions may be reflected in the ECG by prolongation of the PR interval and widening of the QRS complex. The effect on the JT interval is insignificant.

Pharmacokinetic properties: Oral administration of flecainide results in extensive absorption, with bioavailability approaching 90 to 95%. Flecainide does not appear to undergo significant hepatic first-pass metabolism. In patients, 200 to 600 mg flecainide daily produced plasma concentrations within the therapeutic range of 200–1000 μg/L. Protein binding of flecainide is within the range 32 to 58%.

Recovery of unchanged flecainide in urine of healthy subjects was approximately 42% of a 200 mg oral dose, whilst the two major metabolites (Meta-O-Dealkylated and Dealkylated Lactam Metabolites) accounted for a further 14% each. The elimination half-life was 12 to 27 hours.

Pre-clinical safety information: Not applicable.

Pharmaceutical particulars
List of excipients: Pregelatinised Starch BP, Croscarmellose Sodium USNF, Microcrystalline cellulose PhEur, Hydrogenated Vegetable Oil USNF, Magnesium Stearate PhEur.

Incompatibilities: None known.

Shelf-life: 5 years.

Special precautions for storage: Store below 30°C.

Nature and contents of container: UPVC/PVDC blister packs containing 60 tablets.

Instructions for use/handling: Not applicable.

Marketing authorisation number 0068/0152

Date of first authorisation/renewal of the authorisation 22 May 1997

Date of last (partial) revision of the text 29 September 1997

TAMBOCOR* 100 mg TABLETS TAMBOCOR* INJECTION

Presentation Tambocor 100 mg tablets: White, circular, biconvex tablets, 8.5 mm in diameter marked '3M' on one side and 'TR100' with a break-line on the other. Each tablet contains flecainide acetate 100 mg.

Tambocor injection: Each ampoule contains 15 ml of a solution of flecainide acetate 10 mg/ml, for intravenous use only.

It also contains the following inactive ingredients: Sodium Acetate PhEur; Glacial Acetic Acid BP.

Uses Tambocor (flecainide) is a potent sodium channel blocking agent for the treatment of the conditions listed below. It is recommended that treatment with Tambocor (flecainide) should be initiated in hospitals.

Tambocor (flecainide) slows conduction through the heart. Its actions may be reflected in the ECG by prolongation of the PR interval and widening of the QRS complex. The effect on the JT interval is insignificant at therapeutic plasma levels.

Indications
Tablets: Tambocor tablets are indicated for:

(a) AV nodal reciprocating tachycardia; arrhythmias associated with Wolff-Parkinson-White Syndrome and similar conditions with accessory pathways.
(b) Paroxysmal atrial fibrillation in patients with disabling symptoms. Arrhythmias of recent onset will respond more readily.
(c) Symptomatic sustained ventricular tachycardia.
(d) Premature ventricular contractions and/or non-sustained ventricular tachycardia which are causing disabling symptoms, where these are resistant to other therapy or when other treatment has not been tolerated.

Tambocor tablets can be used for the maintenance of normal rhythm following conversion by other means.

Injection: Tambocor injection is indicated when rapid control of the following arrhythmias is the main clinical requirement:

(a) Ventricular tachyarrhythmias where these are resistant to other treatment.
(b) AV nodal reciprocating tachycardia; arrhythmias associated with Wolff-Parkinson-White Syndrome and similar conditions with accessory pathways.

(c) Paroxysmal atrial fibrillation in patients with disabling symptoms. Arrhythmias of recent onset will respond more readily.

Dosage and administration

Tablets: Adults:

Supraventricular arrhythmias: The recommended starting dosage is 50 mg twice daily and most patients will be controlled at this dose. If required the dose may be increased to a maximum of 300 mg daily.

Ventricular arrhythmias: The recommended starting dosage is 100 mg twice daily. The maximum daily dose is 400 mg and this is normally reserved for patients of large build or where rapid control of the arrhythmia is required.

After 3–5 days it is recommended that the dosage be progressively adjusted to the lowest level which maintains control of the arrhythmia. It may be possible to reduce dosage during long-term treatment.

Children: Flecainide is not recommended in children under 12, as there is insufficient evidence of its use in this age group.

Elderly patients: The rate of flecainide elimination from plasma may be reduced in elderly people. This should be taken into consideration when making dose adjustments.

Injection:

a) *Bolus injection:* Tambocor injection can be given in an emergency or for rapid effect by a slow injection of 2 mg/kg over not less than ten minutes, or in divided doses. If preferred, the dose may be diluted with 5% glucose and given as a mini-infusion.

Continuous ECG monitoring is recommended in all patients receiving the bolus dose. The injection should be stopped when there is control of the arrhythmia.

It is recommended that Tambocor injection should be administered more slowly to patients in sustained ventricular tachycardia, with careful monitoring of the electrocardiogram. Similar caution should apply to patients with a history of cardiac failure, who may become decompensated during the administration. For such patients it is recommended that the initial dose is given over 30 minutes. The maximum recommended bolus dose is 150 mg.

b) *Intravenous infusion:* When prolonged parenteral administration is required, it is recommended that therapy is initiated by slow injection of 2 mg/kg over 30 minutes and continued by intravenous infusion at the following rates:

First hour: 1.5 mg/kg per hour. *Second and later hours:* 0.1–0.25 mg/kg per hour. It is recommended that the infusion duration should not exceed 24 hours. However, where this is considered necessary, or for patients receiving the upper end of the dose range, plasma level monitoring is strongly recommended. The maximum cumulative dose given in the first 24 hours should not exceed 600 mg. In patients with severe renal impairment (creatinine clearance of less than 35 ml/min/1.73 sq m), each of the above dosage recommendations should be reduced by half.

Transition to oral dosing should be accomplished as soon as possible by stopping the infusion and administering the first required oral dose.

Oral maintenance is then continued as indicated in the relevant oral dosage instructions.

Plasma levels: Based on PVC suppression, it appears that plasma levels of 200–1000 ng/ml may be needed to obtain the maximum therapeutic effect. Plasma levels above 700–1000 ng/ml are associated with increased likelihood of adverse experiences.

Dosage in impaired renal function: In patients with significant renal impairment (creatinine clearance of 35 ml/min/1.73 sq m or less) the maximum initial dosage should be 100 mg daily (or 50 mg twice daily). When used in such patients, frequent plasma level monitoring is strongly recommended.

Contra-indications, warnings, etc

Contra-indications: Flecainide is contra-indicated in cardiac failure, and in patients with a history of myocardial infarction who have either asymptomatic ventricular ectopics or asymptomatic non-sustained ventricular tachycardia.

It is also contraindicated in patients with long standing atrial fibrillation in whom there has been no attempt to convert to sinus rhythm, and in patients with haemodynamically significant valvular heart disease. Unless pacing rescue is available, Flecainide should not be given to patients with sinus node dysfunction, atrial conduction defects, second degree or greater atrio-ventricular block, bundle branch block or distal block.

Precautions: Electrolyte disturbances should be corrected before using flecainide.

Since flecainide elimination from the plasma can be markedly slower in patients with significant hepatic impairment, flecainide should not be used in such patients unless the potential benefits clearly outweigh the risks. Plasma level monitoring is strongly recommended in these circumstances.

Flecainide is known to increase endocardial pacing thresholds – i.e. to decrease endocardial pacing sensitivity. This effect is reversible and is more marked on the acute pacing threshold than on the chronic. Flecainide should thus be used with caution in all patients with permanent pacemakers or temporary pacing electrodes, and should not be administered to patients with existing poor thresholds or non-programmable pacemakers unless suitable pacing rescue is available.

Generally, a doubling of either pulse width or voltage is sufficient to regain capture, but it may be difficult to obtain ventricular thresholds less than 1 Volt at initial implantation in the presence of flecainide.

The minor negative inotropic effect of flecainide may assume importance in patients predisposed to cardiac failure. Difficulty has been experienced in defibrillating some patients. Most of the cases reported had pre-existing heart disease with cardiac enlargement, a history of myocardial infarction, arterio-sclerotic heart disease and cardiac failure.

Flecainide should be used with caution in patients with acute onset of atrial fibrillation following cardiac surgery.

In a large scale, placebo-controlled clinical trial in post-myocardial infarction patients with asymptomatic ventricular arrhythmia, oral flecainide was associated with a 2.2 fold higher incidence of mortality or non-fatal cardiac arrest as compared with its matching placebo. In that same study, an even higher incidence of mortality was observed in flecainide-treated patients with more than one myocardial infarction. Comparable placebo-controlled clinical trials have not been done to determine if flecainide is associated with higher risk of mortality in other patient groups.

Use in Pregnancy and Lactation: There is no evidence as to drug safety in human pregnancy. In New Zealand White rabbits high doses of flecainide caused some foetal abnormalities, but these effects were not seen in Dutch Belted rabbits or rats. The relevance of these findings to humans has not been established. Data have shown that flecainide crosses the placenta to the foetus in patients taking flecainide during pregnancy.

Flecainide is excreted in human milk and appears in concentrations which reflect those in maternal blood. The risk of adverse effects to the nursing infant is very small.

Drug interactions: Use of flecainide with other sodium channel blockers is not recommended. Treatment with flecainide is compatible with use of oral anticoagulants. Flecainide can cause the plasma digoxin level to rise by about 15%, which is unlikely to be of clinical significance for patients with plasma levels in the therapeutic range. It is recommended that the digoxin plasma level in digitalised patients should be measured not less than six hours after any digoxin dose, before or after administration of flecainide. The possibility of additive negative inotropic effects of beta-blockers and other cardiac depressants with flecainide should be recognised.

Limited data in patients receiving known enzyme inducers (phenytoin, phenobarbital, carbamazepine) indicate only a 30% increase in the rate of flecainide elimination. In healthy subjects receiving cimetidine (1 g daily) for one week, plasma flecainide levels increased by about 30% and the half-life increased by about 10%.

When flecainide is given in the presence of amiodarone, the usual flecainide dosage should be reduced by 50% and the patient monitored closely for adverse effects. Plasma level monitoring is strongly recommended in these circumstances.

Side-effects:

Cardiac: Pro-arrhythmic effects occur but are most likely in patients with structural heart disease and/or significant left ventricular impairment.

In patients with atrial flutter the use of flecainide has been associated with 1:1 AV conduction following initial atrial slowing with resultant ventricular acceleration. This has been seen most commonly following the use of the injection for acute conversion. This effect is usually short lived and abates quickly following cessation of therapy.

Dermatological: A range of allergic skin reactions have been reported including rare but serious reports of urticaria. There have been isolated cases of photosensitivity.

Immune system: A small number of cases of increases in anti-nuclear antibodies have been reported, with and without systemic inflammatory involvement.

Haematological: Reductions in red blood cells, white blood cells and platelets have been occasionally reported. These changes are usually mild.

Psychiatric: Rarely, hallucinations, depression, confusion and amnesia have been reported.

Gastrointestinal: Occasionally nausea and vomiting.

Hepatic: A number of cases of elevated liver enzymes and jaundice have been reported in association with flecainide treatment. So far this has always been reversible on stopping treatment.

CNS: Most commonly giddiness, dizziness and light-headedness which are usually transient. Rare instances of dyskinesia have been reported, which have improved on withdrawal of flecainide therapy. Rare instances of convulsions, and during long term therapy a few cases of peripheral neuropathy, paraesthesia and ataxia have been reported.

Opthalmological: Visual disturbances, such as double vision and blurring of vision may occur but these are usually transient and disappear upon continuing or reducing the dosage.

Extremely rare cases of corneal deposits and pneumonitis have also been reported.

Overdosage: Overdosage with flecainide is a potentially life threatening medical emergency. No specific antidote is known. There is no known way of rapidly removing flecainide from the system, but forced acid diuresis may theoretically be helpful. Neither dialysis nor haemoperfusion are helpful and injections of anticholinergics are not recommended.

Treatment may include therapy with an inotropic agent, intravenous calcium, giving circulatory assistance (e.g. balloon pumping), mechanically assisting respiration, or temporarily inserting a transvenous pacemaker if there are severe conduction disturbances or the patient's left ventricular function is otherwise compromised.

Pharmaceutical precautions

Storage: Tambocor tablets should be stored below 30°C. Tambocor injection should be stored between 5°C and 30°C. Do not freeze.

Dilution: When necessary Tambocor injection should be diluted with, or injected into, sterile solutions of 5% glucose. If chloride containing solutions, such as sodium chloride or Ringer's lactate are used, the injection should be added to a volume of not less than 500 ml, otherwise a precipitate will form.

Legal category POM.

Package quantities Tambocor 100 mg Tablets - packs of 60. Tambocor Injection - 5×15 ml ampoules.

Further information Nil.

Product licence numbers

Tambocor 100 mg Tablets PL 0068/0102
Tambocor Injection PL 0068/0101

Date of preparation or last review January 1998

TITRALAC* TABLETS

Presentation White, circular, bi-convex tablets, 11.2 mm in diameter, marked TC on one side and 3M on the other. Each tablet contains Calcium Carbonate BP 420 mg and Glycine BP 180 mg.

Uses Titralac is indicated as a calcium supplement or phosphate binding agent in the management of renal failure.

Dosage and administration

As a calcium supplement: 1 to 4 tablets a day according to patient requirements. The maximum dose should not exceed 12 tablets per day. Each Titralac tablet contains 4.2 mmol (168 mg) calcium.

As a phosphate binder: Starting dose of 6 tablets a day and then titrated up to a maximum of 40 tablets a day by the physician according to the needs of the patient or until undesirable effects are observed such as hypercalcaemia, hypophosphataemia or hypophosphataemic red cell dysfunction. The total daily dose is to be divided between the meals of the day in order to ensure that the tablet is available as a phosphate binder. Each Titralac tablet binds, in vitro, about 340 mg phosphate.

These dosage instructions apply to adults, elderly and children.

Titralac tablets may be chewed, allowed to dissolve in the mouth or swallowed whole as desired.

Contra-indications, warnings, etc

Side-effects: Hypercalcaemia and hypophosphataemia are possible complications of vigorous therapy.

Symptoms of hypercalcaemia include anorexia, nausea, vomiting, constipation, abdominal pain, muscle weakness, thirst, polyuria, drowsiness, confusion, and cardiac arrhythmias leading to cardiac arrest.

Symptoms of hypophosphataemia include weakness, paraesthesia, seizures and coma.

Hypophosphataemic red cell dysfunction impairs effective oxygen delivery to the periphery.

Precautions: Serum phosphate levels should be monitored in all patients receiving phosphate binders, to prevent the development of a phosphate depletion syndrome.

In long-term treatment, serum and urinary calcium levels should be monitored to prevent hypercalcaemia occurring. Serum albumin, magnesium and potassium levels should also be monitored to ensure

Ca++/PO4--- homeostasis, particularly following dialysis.

Sarcoidosis may increase the risk of hypercalcaemia.

Pregnancy and lactation: Epidemiological studies have shown no increase in the teratogenic hazard to the foetus if used in the usual doses recommended for calcium supplementation. The safety of high doses of calcium, however, is not established.

Although some supplemental calcium may be excreted in breast milk, the concentration is not sufficient to produce an adverse effect on the neonate and problems in humans have not been documented.

Contra-indications: Patients with hypophosphataemia, hypercalcaemia or hypercalciuria.

Interactions: Concurrent administration of 1,25-dihydroxycholecalciferol or thiazides increases the risk of hypercalcaemia. There is a risk of digoxin toxicity if hypercalcaemia develops in well-digitalised patients. Corticosteroids may interfere with calcium absorption while calcium interferes with absorption of tetracyclines.

Overdosage: Acute hypercalcaemia may result and this may be aggravated by dehydration. Management of acute hypercalcaemia should be along standard recommendations and should include full hydration, monitoring of other electrolytes, judicious use of frusemide and other symptomatic and supportive measures. ECG monitoring of cardiac rhythm is particularly advisable in patients with renal failure.

Pharmaceutical precautions Store below 30°C.

Legal category GSL.

Package quantities Bottles of 180 tablets (OP).

Further information Nil.

Product licence number 0068/5004R.

ZIDOVAL*

Qualitative and quantitative composition Metronidazole 0.75% w/w

Pharmaceutcial form Vaginal gel

Clinical particulars

Therapeutic indications: Zidoval vaginal gel is indicated for the treatment of bacterial vaginosis (formerly called non-specific vaginitis, Gardnerella vaginalis vaginitis or Haemophilus vaginitis).

Posology and method of administration: For vaginal administration.

Adults and the elderly: One application of Zidoval vaginal gel (5 g) inserted into the vagina once daily, at bedtime, for 5 days. If the patient does not respond to initial therapy it is recommended that appropriate laboratory measures be used to rule out conditions other than bacterial vaginosis before repeating the treatment.

Children: Not recommended for use in children since safety and effectiveness have not been established.

Contra-indications: Zidoval vaginal gel is contra-indicated in patients with a prior history of hypersensitivity to metronidazole, other nitroimidazoles, parabens or any other ingredient of the gel.

Special warnings and special precautions for use: Use during menses is not recommended.

Zidoval vaginal gel affords minimal serum levels of metronidazole compared to oral metronidazole therapy. Although these lower serum levels are less likely to produce the common reactions seen with oral metronidazole, the possibility of these and other reactions cannot be excluded.

In patients with renal failure, there is no accumulation of metronidazole, however the hydroxy and acid metabolites are retained. Haemodialysis removes both metronidazole and the two metabolites.

Although patients with severe hepatic dysfunction metabolise metronidazole slowly leading to retention of metronidazole and its metabolites, a total treatment course of 187.5 mg is unlikely to lead to excessive serum levels.

Known or previously unrecognised candidiasis may present more prominent symptoms during therapy with Zidoval vaginal gel and may require treatment with a candicidal agent.

Metronidazole is a nitroimidazole and should be used with care in patients with evidence of a history of blood dyscrasias. A mild leukopenia has been observed during oral metronidazole administration but no persistent haematological abnormalities attributable to oral metronidazole have been observed in clinical studies. In clinical studies with Zidoval vaginal gel a mild, clinically insignificant leukopenia was observed in some patients but relationship to therapy could not be determined.

Metronidazole may interfere with certain types of determination of serum chemistry values, such as aspartate aminotransferase (AST, SGOT), alanine aminotransferase (ALT, SGPT), lactic dehydrogenase (LDH), triglycerides and hexokinase glucose. Values of zero may be observed.

In patients on intensive or prolonged metronidazole therapy, convulsive seizures and peripheral neuropathy, the latter characterised mainly by numbness or paraesthesia of an extremity, have been reported. These neurological symptoms are unlikely to occur with the low serum levels seen with Zidoval vaginal gel therapy.

Zidoval vaginal gel should be administered with caution in patients with central nervous system diseases.

Interaction with other medicaments and other forms of interaction: Oral metronidazole has been associated with a disulfiram-like reaction. At the low serum levels which result from the use of Zidoval vaginal gel, the possibility of a similar reaction is unlikely although cannot be excluded.

Lithium treatment should be tapered or withdrawn prior to administering metronidazole.

Concomitant administration may lead to lithium retention and the possibility of renal damage.

Oral metronidazole has been reported to potentiate the anticoagulant effect of warfarin and other coumarin anticoagulants, resulting in a prolongation of prothrombin time. This possible drug interaction should be considered when Zidoval vaginal gel is prescribed for patients on this type of anticoagulant therapy.

Pregnancy and lactation: There are no adequate and well-controlled studies with Zidoval vaginal gel in pregnant women. Therefore, this drug should be used during pregnancy only if clearly needed.

In animal studies, oral metronidazole has not been shown to be teratogenic or fetotoxic.

Observations in several hundred pregnancies in women exposed to oral metronidazole during the first trimester have not demonstrated any increased risk of malformation.

A retrospective study of similar sample sizes of women treated with oral metronidazole beyond the first trimester of pregnancy has not demonstrated any fetotoxic effect.

Although metronidazole blood levels are significantly lower than those achieved with oral dosage forms, Zidoval vaginal gel is contra-indicated in lactating women since metronidazole is secreted in milk at concentrations similar to those in serum.

Effects on ability to drive and use machines: None.

Undesirable effects: In clinical trials, adverse experiences reported as possibly related to Zidoval vaginal gel use are primarily genitourinary and gastrointestinal. Genitourinary reports were vaginal candidiasis, vulvovaginal itching/burning/swelling, increased pelvic pressure and abnormal vaginal discharge. Gastrointestinal reports were abdominal cramping or pain, nausea, metallic taste in the mouth, diarrhoea, constipation, decreased appetite; decreased/increased WBC, headache, dizziness, and generalised rash/pruritus.

Post-marketing experience with Zidoval vaginal gel has resulted in very rare reports of the following: vomiting, incoordination, insomnia, flushing, cystitis, incontinence and modification of taste.

Overdose: There is no human experience of overdosage with Zidoval vaginal gel. There is no specific treatment. Metronidazole is readily removed from the plasma by haemodialysis.

Pharmacological properties

Pharmacodynamic properties: Metronidazole is a synthetic antibacterial agent which also possesses amoebicidal activity. The antimicrobial effects result from the disruption of DNA and the inhibition of nucleic acid synthesis. Against susceptible organisms metronidazole is generally bactericidal at concentrations equal to or slightly higher than the minimum inhibitory concentrations. It has been shown to have *in vivo* and clinical activity against:

- anaerobic gram negative bacilli including bacteroides species including the bacteroides fragilis group (B. fragilis, B. distasonis, B. ocatus, B. thetaiotaomicron, B. vulgaris) and fusobacterium species.
- anaerobic gram positive bacilli including clostridium species and susceptible strains of eubacterium.
- anaerobic gram-positive cocci including peptostreptococcus species.

Zidoval vaginal gel has been shown *in vivo* to have clincial activity against the following vaginal pathogens: Gardnerella vaginalis, bacteroides species and Mycoplasma hominis.

Significant increases in lactobacilli are observed in bacterial vaginosis patients following therapy.

Pharmacokinetic properties: Bioavailability studies on the administration of a single 5 g dose of Zidoval vaginal gel into the vagina of 12 normal subjects showed a mean C_{max} serum concentration of 237 nanogram/ml or about 2% of the mean maximum serum concentration of a 500 mg tablet taken orally (mean C_{max} = 12,785 ng/ml). Under normal usage conditions, the formulation therefore affords minimal serum concentrations of metronidazole.

Metronidazole has a large apparent volume of distribution and has the ability to penetrate the blood brain barrier and blood cerebro-spinal fluid barrier at concentrations similar to serum levels.

Metronidazole is metabolised in the liver by side chain oxidation and glucuronide formation and a large portion of the absorbed dose is excreted as metabolites. Both unchanged drug and metabolites are excreted mainly in the urine with about 35–65% of the absorbed dose recovered over 24 hours.

Pre-clinical safety information: In vitro studies have demonstrated that the product is active against target organisms. The toxicity, reproductive toxicity, mutagenicity and carcinogenic potential of metronidazole have been extensively documented in the literature and these data are considered sufficient to characterise the preclinical safety of metronidazole.

Preclinical studies with Zidoval vaginal gel showed an oral LD_{50} in rats of greater than 5 g/kg body weight. In a 21 day vaginal irritation study in rabbits the product was classified as a mild irritant and in an eye irritation study with a single exposure the product was classified as slightly irrtitant.

Sensitisation studies carried out in human volunteers demonstrated that the product did not induce irritation, allergic contact dermatitis, phototoxicity or photoallergic contact dermatitis.

Pharmaceutical particulars

List of excipients: Carbomer (carbopol) 934P, edetate disodium, methyl paraben, propyl paraben, propylene glycol, sodium hydroxide, purified water.

Incompatibilities: None known.

Shelf-life: 3 years.

Special precautions for storage: Store at or below 25°C.

Nature and contents of container: Aluminium tubes with polyethylene screw caps containing 40 g product. The product is packaged with 5 g vaginal applicators.

Instructions for use/handling: Directions for use: Pierce sealed end of tube and screw open end of applicator tightly onto tube of gel. Squeeze tube, filling the applicator with gel. Remove applicator from tube and gently insert applicator into vagina as far as it will comfortably go. Push the plunger to release the gel. Dispose of applicator as instructed.

Apply one applicatorful at bedtime for five consecutive days or as directed by the physician.

Marketing authorisation number 00068/0169

Date of first authorisation/renewal of authorisation 31 January 1997

Date of last (partial) revision of the text July 1998

**Trade Mark*

Manx Pharma
Manx House
Spectrum Business Estate
Bircholt Road
Maidstone
Kent ME15 9YP

☎ 01622 766389 🗋 01622 761435

AVOMINE* TABLETS 25 mg

Qualitative and quantitative composition Promethazine theoclate BP 25 mg.

Pharmaceutical form Tablet.

Clinical particulars

Therapeutic indications: Avomine is a long acting antiemetic, indicated for:
- prevention and treatment of nausea and vomiting, including motion sickness and post operative vomiting.
- vertigo due to Ménière's syndrome, labyrinthitis and other causes.

Posology and method of administration

Motion sickness: Adults: For the prevention on long journeys: one 25 mg tablet each evening at bedtime, starting the day before setting out. The duration of action is such that a second dose in 24 hours is not often necessary.

For the prevention of motion sickness on short journeys: one 25 mg tablet one or two hours before travelling or as soon after as possible.

Treatment of motion sickness: one 25 mg tablet as soon as possible and repeated the same evening followed by a third tablet the following evening.

Nausea and vomiting due to other causes: Adults: One 25 mg tablet at night is often sufficient, but two or three tablets are sometimes necessary. Alternatively, more frequent administration such as 25 mg two or three times a day may be required for some patients. It is often not necessary to give more than four of the 25 mg Avomine tablets in 24 hours.

Children: In the above indications children over 10 years of age may be given the lower adult doses described above. Children between 5 and 10 years may be given half the adult dose.

Elderly: No specific dosage recommendations.

Administration: Oral.

Contra-indications: Avomine should not be used in patients who are in a coma or suffering from CNS depression of any cause. It must not be given to neonates, premature infants or patients hypersensitive to phenothiazines. Avomine should be avoided in patients who have been taking monoamine oxidase inhibitors within the previous 14 days.

Special warnings and special precautions for use: Avomine may thicken or dry lung secretions and impair expectoration, it should therefore be used with caution in patients with asthma, bronchitis or bronchiectasis. Use with care in patients with severe coronary artery disease, narrow angle glaucoma, epilepsy or hepatic and renal insufficiency. Caution should be exercised in patients with bladder neck or pyloroduodenal obstruction. Promethazine may mask the warning signs of ototoxicity caused by ototoxic drugs e.g. salicylates.

It may also delay the early diagnosis of intestinal obstruction or raised intracranial pressure through suppression of vomiting.

Interaction with other medicaments and other forms of interaction: Avomine may enhance the action of any anticholinergic agent, tricyclic antidepressant, sedative or hypnotic. Alcohol should be avoided during treatment.

Avomine may interfere with immunologic urine pregnancy tests to produce false-positive and false-negative results.

Avomine should be discontinued at least 72 hours before any skin tests using allergen extracts as it may inhibit the cutaneous histamine response thus producing false-negative results.

Pregnancy and lactation

Use in pregnancy: There is epidemiological evidence for the safety of promethazine in pregnancy, and animal studies have shown no hazard, nevertheless it should not be used in pregnancy unless the physician considers it essential. The use of Avomine tablets is not recommended in the two weeks prior to delivery in view of the risk of irritability and excitement in the neonate.

Use in lactation: Available evidence suggests that the amount excreted in milk is insignificant. However, there are risks of neonate irritability and excitement.

Effects on ability to drive and use machines: Ambulant patients receiving Avomine for the first time should not be in control of vehicles or machinery for the first few days, until it is established that they are not hypersensitive to the central nervous effects of the drug and do not suffer from disorientation, confusion or dizziness.

Undesirable effects: Side-effects may be seen in a few patients: drowsiness, dizziness, restlessness, headaches, nightmares, tiredness and disorientation. Anticholinergic side-effects such as blurred vision, dry mouth and urinary retention occur occasionally. Newborn and premature infants are susceptible to the anticholinergic effects of promethazine, while other children may display paradoxical hyperexcitability. The elderly are particularly susceptible to the anticholinergic effects and confusion may occur.

Other side-effects include anorexia, gastric irritation, palpitations, hypotension, arrhythmias, extrapyramidal effects, muscle spasms and tic-like movements of the head and face. Anaphylaxis, jaundice and blood dyscrasias including haemolytic anaemia rarely occur. Photosensitive skin reactions have been reported; strong sunlight should be avoided during treatment.

Overdose: Symptoms of severe overdosage are variable. They are characterised in children by various combinations of excitement, ataxia, inco-ordination, athetosis and hallucinations, while adults may become drowsy and lapse into coma. Convulsions may occur in both adults and children; coma or excitement may precede their occurrence. Cardiorespiratory depression is uncommon. If the patient is seen soon enough after ingestion, it should be possible to induce vomiting despite the antiemetic effect of promethazine; alternatively, gastric lavage may be used.

Treatment is otherwise supportive with attention to maintenance of adequate respiratory and circulatory status. Convulsions should be treated with diazepam or other suitable anticonvulsant.

Pharmacological properties Promethazine theoclate is a long acting antihistamine with antiemetic, central sedative and anticholinergic properties.

Pharmacodynamic properties: Promethazine is metabolised in the liver (the major metabolite being the sulphoxide) and slowly excreted in the urine. The drug is highly bound to plasma proteins.

Pharmacokinetic properties: Promethazine is well absorbed after oral administration, peak plasma concentrations occurring in 2–3 hours. It is widely distributed in the body. It enters the brain and crosses the placenta. Phenothiazines pass into the milk at low concentrations.

Pharmaceutical particulars

List of excipients: Lactose, sodium metabisulphite, potato starch, dextrin, cellulose, stearic acid and magnesium stearate.

Incompatibilities: None.

Shelf life: Five years.

Special precautions for storage: Protect from light.

Nature and contents of container

Blister pack of 10×25 mg tablets.
Blister pack of 28×25 mg tablets.
Blister pack of 30×25 mg tablets.
Securitainer or polyethylene bottle of 250×25 mg tablets.

Instructions for use/handling: Not applicable.

Marketing authorisation number 15833/0003.

Date of first authorisation September 1997.

Date of last review November 1997.

*Trade Mark

Martindale Pharmaceuticals

Bampton Road
Harold Hill
Romford, Essex RM3 8UG

☎ 01708 386660 📠 01708 384032

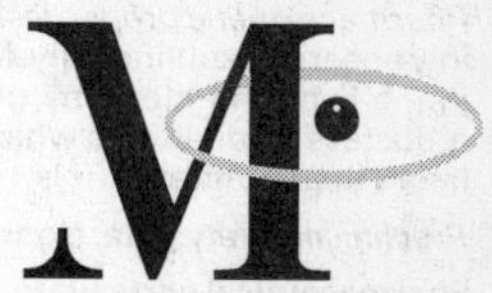

FENTANYL CITRATE INJECTION 50 micrograms/ml

Qualitative and quantitative composition each 2 ml of solution contains 100 micrograms of fentanyl as Fentanyl Citrate BP. Each 10 ml of solution contains 500 micrograms of fentanyl as Fentanyl Citrate BP.

Pharmaceutical form Clear, colourless, sterile solution for injection intended for parenteral administration to human beings.

Clinical particulars

Therapeutic indications: Fentanyl citrate is a narcotic analgesic. In low doses, it is used to provide analgesia during short surgical procedures and as a premedicant. In higher doses it is employed as an analgesic/respiratory depressant in patients who need assisted ventilation. In combination with a neuroleptic drug, fentanyl is employed as part of the technique of neuroleptanalgesia.

Posology and method of administration: Intravenous and Intramuscular routes. Fentanyl Citrate Injection can be administered to both adults and children via the intravenous route according to the following dosage regimen:

	Adults Initial μg	Supplemental μg	Children Initial μg/kg	Supplemental μg/kg
Spontaneous respiration	50-200	50	3-5	1
Assisted ventilation	300-3500	100-200	15	1-3

Doses greater than 200 microgram are solely for use in anaesthesia.

As a premedicament, 1–2 ml may be administered intramuscularly before induction of anaesthesia.

Following intravenous administration in the non-premedicated adult patient, 2 ml fentanyl may be anticipated to provide adequate analgesia for 10–20 minutes in surgical procedures involving low pain intensity. A bolus of 10 ml fentanyl can be expected to provide analgesia for about 1 hour. The analgesia produced is generally adequate for surgery involving moderate pain intensity. Administration of 50 micrograms/kg will provide intense analgesia for some 4 to 6 hours for surgery associated with intense stimulation.

It is important when estimating the required dose to assess the likely degree of surgical stimulation, the effect of premedicant drugs, and the duration of the procedure.

Use in elderly: It is important to reduce the dosage in the elderly.

Contra-indications: Known hypersensitivity to fentanyl citrate; respiratory depression; obstructive airways disease, concurrent administration with monoamine oxidase inhibitors or within 2 weeks of their discontinuation.

Special warnings and precautions for use: In common with other narcotic analgesics, the most common serious adverse reactions with fentanyl are respiratory depression, bradycardia and skeletal muscle rigidity.

As with all narcotic analgesics, care should be observed when administering Fentanyl Citrate Injection to patients with myasthenia gravis.

It is desirable to reduce dosage in the elderly, in hypothyroidism and chronic hepatic disease.

Administration in labour may cause respiratory depression in the new-born infant.

As with all potent opioids, profound analgesia is accompanied by marked respiratory depression, which may persist into or recur in the early post-operative period. It is imperative to ensure that adequate spontaneous breathing has been established and maintained before discharge from the recovery area whenever large doses of infusions of Fentanyl Citrate Injection have been administered. Hyperventilation during anaesthesia may alter the patient's response to CO_2, thus affecting respiration post-operatively. Opioid pre-medication may potentiate or prolong depressant effects of fentanyl citrate.

Repeated use of fentanyl may result in the development of tolerance and dependence.

Interaction with other medicaments and other forms of interaction: If other narcotic or CNS-depressant drugs are used concurrently with fentanyl, the effects of the drugs may be expected to be additive. The pharmacological effects of fentanyl citrate can be reversed by Naloxone.

Pregnancy and lactation: Placental transfer of fentanyl occurs. There has been little usage in human pregnancy but no evidence of teratogenic effects in animals. Administration in labour may cause respiratory depression in the new-born infant. Fentanyl should be used during pregnancy only if the potential benefit justifies the potential risk to the foetus. It is not known whether fentanyl is excreted in human milk. Because many drugs are excreted in human milk, caution should be exercised when administering fentanyl to a nursing mother.

Effects on ability to drive and use machines: Where early discharge (from clinical care) is envisaged, patients should be advised not to drive or to operate machinery.

Undesirable effects: A transient fall in blood pressure may occur following intravenous administration of Fentanyl Citrate Injection.

Significant respiratory depression will occur following administration of fentanyl in doses in excess of 200 micrograms. This and other pharmacological effects of fentanyl can be reversed by naloxone.

Bradycardia may occur due to increased cardiac vagal stimulation; it can be reversed by atropine or glycopyrrolate. Skeletal muscle rigidity (morphine-like effect) may occur and muscle relaxants have been found helpful in such cases. Nausea and vomiting may be troublesome.

Overdose: As with other narcotic analgesics, the possible manifestations of fentanyl overdosage include respiratory depression and hypotension, with circulatory failure and deepening coma.

Intensive supporting therapy may be required to correct respiratory failure and shock. A patent airway must be maintained and assisted respiration may be required. The specific narcotic antagonist naloxone hydrochloride is used to counteract respiratory depression and coma. A dose of 0.4 to 2 mg is given intravenously and may be repeated at intervals of 2 to 3 minutes if necessary, up to 10 mg. The duration of respiratory depression following overdosage with fentanyl may exceed the duration of narcotic antagonist action.

Pharmacological properties

Pharmacodynamic properties: Fentanyl citrate is a potent narcotic analgesic. The principal actions of therapeutic value are analgesia and sedation. When used with a neuroleptic agent it can induce a state of neuroleptanalgesia. As with other narcotic analgesics, fentanyl depresses respiration and this effect increases as the dose is increased.

Following intravenous injection fentanyl has rapid onset of action, although the maximal analgesic and respiratory depressant effect may not occur for several minutes.

Fentanyl Citrate Injection is usually given by the intravenous route, but it may be given intramuscularly as a premedicant.

Pharmacokinetic properties: Fentanyl is a lipid-soluble drug and its pharmacokinetics can be described in terms of a 3 compartment model. following intravenous injection, there is a short distribution phase during which high concentrations of fentanyl are achieved quickly in well perfused tissues such as the lungs, kidneys and brain. The drug is redistributed to other tissues, it accumulates more slowly in skeletal muscle and yet more slowly in fat, from which it is gradually released into the blood. Up to 80% of fentanyl is bound to plasma proteins.

Fentanyl is primarily metabolised in the liver, probably by N-dealkylation, and is excreted mainly in the urine with less than 10% representing the unchanged drug. The terminal half life of fentanyl is 3.7 hours.

Preclinical safety data: No further relevant information other than that which is included in other sections of the Summary of Product Characteristics.

Pharmaceutical particulars

List of excipients: Sodium Chloride BP, Sodium Hydroxide BP, Water for Injections BP

Incompatibilities: Fentanyl citrate is incompatible with thiopentone and methohexitone

Shelf life: Unopened: 3 years (36 months) If only part of an ampoule is used, discard the remaining solution

Special precautions for storage: Store below 25°C. Protect from light.

Nature and contents of container: 2 ml or 10 ml clear glass ampoules, glass type I Ph Eur borosilicate glass, packed in cardboard cartons and contain 10 x 2 ml/10 ml ampoules.

Instructions for use/handling: CD(2), For IV or IM injection. If only part used, discard the remaining solution.

Marketing authorisation number 0156/0038

Marketing authorisation holder: Martindale Pharmaceuticals Limited, Bampton Road, Romford RM3 8UG.

Date of approval/revision of SPC 15 May 1997

Legal category CD (2), POM

GTN 300 mcg

Qualitative and quantitative composition Glyceryl Trinitrate 300 micrograms per tablet + 6.67% overage.

Pharmaceutical form Sublingual tablet.

Clinical particulars

Therapeutic indications: A short acting vasodilator for the prophylaxis and treatment of attacks of angina pectoris.

Posology and method of administration.

Adults and the elderly: One tablet to be allowed to dissolve slowly under the tongue. The treatment may be repeated as necessary.

Children Not recommended for children

Contra-indications: Marked anaemia, closed angle glaucoma, head trauma, cerebral haemorrhage, hypersensitivity to nitrates, hypotensive conditions and hypovolaemia, hypertrophic obstructive cardiomyopathy, aortic stenosis, cardiac tamponade, constrictive pericarditis, mitral stenosis,

Special warnings and special precautions for use: Caution should be exercised in cases of severe hepatic or renal impairment; hypothyroidism, malnutrition, hypothermia or a recent history of myocardial infarction.

Interactions with other medicaments and other forms of interaction: When used with anti-muscarinic, anti-arrhythmic or cyclic antidepressant drugs the effect of Glyceryl Trinitrate may be lost. (due to failure to dissolve under the tongue)

Use in pregnancy and lactation: There is some evidence of hazard in animals when nitrates have been given in pregnancy. Avoid in pregnancy unless there is no safer alternative. Problems in breast feeding have not been documented.

Effect on the ability to drive or operate machines: Dizziness is a known side effect, if affected, patients should not drive or operate machinery.

Undesirable effects: The following side effects have been reported: Throbbing headache, facial flushing, dizziness, postural hypotension and tachycardia.

Overdose:

Symptoms: Vomiting, restlessness, hypotension, cyanosis, methaemoglobinaemia. Severe poisoning may result in bradycardia, respiratory depression and psychosis.

Treatment: Remove any tablet from the mouth and place the patient in a recumbent position with the head down. If recovery is not rapid or in the case of known severe poisoning, the stomach should be emptied to prevent further absorption and general supportive measures, such as oxygen, assisted respiration and plasma expanders employed as necessary.

If methaglobinaemia has occurred it can be treated with Methylene Blue. Intravenous injection of 1–4 mg per kg body weight.

Pharmacological properties

Pharmacodynamic properties: Glyceryl Trinitrate relaxes smooth muscle, including vascular muscle. The precise mechanism of action is not fully understood but it is thought that the cause is a reduction of myocardial oxygen demand.

Pharmacokinetic properties: Glyceryl Trinitrate is rapidly absorbed sublingually. Metabolism occurs mainly in the liver and blood by glutathione-organic nitrate reductase to dinitrates which are less potent vasodilators than trinitrates. T½ is 1 to 4 minutes.

Preclinical safety data: None stated

Pharmaceutical particulars

List of excipients: Mannitol, Acacia, Lactose, Talc, Magnesium Stearate and Stearic Acid.

Incompatibilities: Not applicable.

Shelf life: 24 months. After first opening the product should be used within 8 weeks.

Special precautions for storage and transport: Storage in a dry place below 25°C. Protect from light.

Nature and contents of container: 100 tablets . Glass bottle with aluminium wadded cap.

Instructions for use/handling: After removing a tablet close the cap tightly. Do not transfer the tablets to another bottle. Use within 8 weeks of first opening.

Marketing authorisation holder: Macarthys Laboratories Limited, Bampton Road, Romford RM3 8UG.

Marketing authorisation number 1883/5958R

Date of approval/revision of SPC July 1998

Legal category P.

METHADONE INJECTION BP 1%

Presentation Clear, colourless, glass ampoules of 1 ml, 2 ml, 3.5 ml and 5 ml containing a colourless solution of Methadone Hydrochloride BP 10 mg per ml.

Uses In the treatment of opioid drug addiction (as a narcotic abstinence syndrome suppressant). As an analgesic where the sedative effects of morphine are contra-indicated.

Dosage and route of administration
Adults: In the treatment of opioid drug addiction, by intramuscular or subcutaneous injection. Initially 10–20 mg per day, increasing by 10–20 mg per day until there are no signs of withdrawal or intoxication. The usual dose is 40–60 mg per day. If repeated doses are required the intramuscular route should be used.

The dose is adjusted according to the degree of dependence with the aim of gradual reduction.

As an analgesic, by intramuscular or subcutaneous injection. The dosage is 5–10 mg every 6–8 hours as needed. In prolonged use it should not be administered more than twice daily. If repeated doses are required the intramuscular route should be used.

Elderly: In the case of the elderly or ill patients repeated doses should only be given with extreme caution.

Children: Not recommended for children.

Contra-indications, warnings, etc
Contra-indications: Respiratory depression, obstructive airways disease, concurrent administration with M.A.O. inhibitors or within 2 weeks of discontinuation of treatment with them. Use during an acute asthma attack is not advisable.

Obstetric use not recommended, because in labour the prolonged duration of action increases the risk of neonatal depression.

Methadone is not suitable for children.

Drug interactions:

Alcohol: May induce serious respiratory depression and hypotension.

Cimetidine: Potentiation of opiate action due to displacement of Methadone from protein binding sites.

Rifampicin: Reduced opiate effect due to increased metabolism.

Phenytoin: Potentiation of opiate action due to displacement of Methadone from protein binding sites.

MAOIs: Possible CNS excitation or depression.

Urinary acidifiers: Increases rate of excretion of drug thus decreasing plasma concentration.

CNS depressants: Major and minor tranquillisers, sedatives and tricyclic antidepressants may result in increased CNS depression, respiratory depression and hypotension.

Opioid agonist analgesics: Additive CNS depression, respiratory depression and hypotension.

Naloxone: Antagonizes the analgesic, CNS and respiratory depressant effects of Methadone.

Naltrexone: Administration of Naltrexone to a patient addicted to Methadone will rapidly precipitate long term withdrawal symptoms.

Buprenorphine/Pentazocine: Administration to a patient addicted to Methadone may precipitate withdrawal symptoms.

Effects on the ability to drive or operate machines: This may be severely affected during and after treatment with Methadone. The time after which such activities may be safely resumed is extremely patient dependent and must be decided by the physician.

Other undesirable effects: Nausea, vomiting and dizziness. Methadone has the potential to increase intracranial pressure, particularly in circumstances where it is already raised. It causes pain at the injection site; subcutaneous injection causes local tissue irritation and induration.

In prolonged use as an analgesic it should not be administered more than twice daily to avoid the risk of accumulation and overdosage.

Use in pregnancy and lactation: There is no, or inadequate, evidence of safety in human pregnancy but the drug has been widely used for many years without apparent ill-consequence and animal studies have not shown any hazard.

It should not be used in labour, see *Contra-indications.*

Methadone is excreted in breast milk. This may be permissible during maintenance dosage.

Other special warnings and precautions: In the case of elderly or ill patients, repeated doses should only be given with extreme caution.

The formulation does not contain preservatives or antioxidants and therefore could be administered via the intravenous or intraspinal route. However, this should only be attempted by those with appropriate skill and experience in such administration and is therefore at the discretion of the physician.

Methadone is a drug of addiction and is controlled under the Misuse of Drugs Act 1971 (Schedule 2).

Overdose: Symptoms: Serious overdosage is characterised by respiratory depression, extreme somnolence progressing to stupor or coma, maximally constricted pupils, skeletal muscle flaccidity, cold and clammy skin and sometimes bradycardia and hypotension. In severe overdosage, particularly by the intravenous route, apnea, circulatory collapse, cardiac arrest and death may occur.

Treatment: A patent airway and assisted or controlled ventilation must be assured. Narcotic antagonists may be required, but it should be remembered that Methadone is a long-acting depressant (36 to 48 hours), whereas antagonists act for 1 to 3 hours, so that treatment with the latter must be repeated as needed. An antagonist should not be administered, however, in the absence of clinically significant respiratory or cardiovascular depression. Nalorphine (0.1 mg per kg) or Levallorphan (0.02 mg per kg) should be given intravenously as soon as possible and repeated, if necessary, every 15 minutes. Oxygen, intravenous fluids, vasopressors and other supportive measures should be employed as indicated. In a person physically dependent on narcotics, administration of the usual dose of a narcotic antagonist will precipitate an acute withdrawal syndrome; use of the antagonist in such a person should be avoided if possible but if it must be used to treat serious respiratory depression it should be administered with great care.

Incompatibilities: No major incompatibilities known.

Pharmaceutical precautions Sterile until opened. Protect from light.

Legal category CD (Sch. 2), POM.

Package quantities Boxes of 10.

Further information Nil.

Product licence number 1883/0058.

Product licence holder: Macarthys Laboratories Limited, Bampton Road, Romford RM3 8UG.

METHADONE MIXTURE DTF 1 mg per ml

Presentation A clear, yellow-green mixture containing methadone hydrochloride 1 mg per ml.

The mixture contains sodium methylparaben 0.1%, and sodium propylparaben 0.025% as preservatives.

Contains tartrazine (E102), Green S (E142) and Sunset Yellow (E110).

Uses In the treatment of opioid drug addiction (as a narcotic abstinence syndrome suppressant).

Dosage and administration For oral administration.

Adults: Initially 10–20 mg per day, increasing by 10–20 mg per day until there are no signs of withdrawal or intoxication. The usual dose is 40–60 mg per day.

The dose is adjusted according to the degree of dependence with the aim of gradual reduction.

Elderly: In the case of the elderly or ill patients repeated doses should only be given with extreme caution.

Children: Not recommended for children.

Contra-indications, warnings, etc
Contra-indications: Respiratory depression, obstructive airways disease, concurrent administration with MAO inhibitors or within 2 weeks of discontinuation of treatment with them. Use during an acute asthma attack is not advisable.

Use during labour is not recommended, the prolonged duration of action increases the risk of neonatal depression.

Methadone is not suitable for children.

Drug interactions:

Alcohol: May induce serious respiratory depression and hypotension.

Cimetidine: Potentiation of opiate action due to displacement of methadone from protein binding sites.

Rifampicin: Reduced opiate effect due to increased metabolism.

Phenytoin: Potentiation of opiate action due to displacement of methadone from protein binding sites.

MAOIs: Possible CNS excitation or depression.

Urinary acidifiers: Increases rate of excretion of drug thus decreasing plasma concentration.

CNS depressants: Major and minor tranquillisers, sedatives and tricyclic antidepressants may result in increased CNS depression, respiratory depression and hypotension.

Opioid agonist analgesics: Additive CNS depression, respiratory depression and hypotension.

Naloxone: Antagonises the analgesic, CNS and respiratory depressant effects of methadone.

Naltrexone: Administration of naltrexone to a patient addicted to methadone will rapidly precipitate long term withdrawal symptoms.

Buprenorphine/pentazocine: Administration to a patient addicted to methadone may precipitate withdrawal symptoms.

Effects on the ability to drive or operate machines: This may be severely affected during and after treatment with methadone. The time after which such activities may be safely resumed is extremely patient dependent and must be decided by the physician.

Other undesirable effects: Methadone has the potential to increase intracranial pressure, particularly in circumstances where it is already raised.

Use in pregnancy and lactation: There is no, or inadequate, evidence of safety in human pregnancy but the drug has been widely used for many years without apparent ill-consequence and animal studies have not shown any hazard.

It should not be used during labour, see 'Contra-indications'. Methadone is excreted in breast milk. This may be permissible during maintenance dosage.

Other special warnings and precautions: In the case of elderly or ill patients repeated doses should only be given with extreme caution. Methadone is a drug of addiction and is controlled under the Misuse of Drugs Act 1971 (Schedule 2).

Overdose: Symptoms: Serious overdosage is characterised by respiratory depression, extreme somnolence progressing to stupor or coma, maximally constricted pupils, skeletal muscle flaccidity, cold and clammy skin and sometimes bradycardia and hypotension. In severe overdosage, particularly by the intravenous route, apnea, circulatory collapse, cardiac arrest and death may occur.

Treatment: A patent airway and assisted or controlled ventilation must be assured. Narcotic antagonists may be required, but it should be remembered that Methadone is a long-acting depressant (36 to 48 hours), whereas antagonists act for 1 to 3 hours, so that treatment with the latter must be repeated as needed. An antagonist should not be administered, however, in the absence of clinically significant respiratory or cardiovascular depression. Nalorphine (0.1 mg per kg) or Levallorphan (0.02 mg per kg) should be given intravenously as soon as possible and repeated, if necessary, every 15 minutes. Oxygen, intravenous fluids, vasopressors and other supportive measures should be employed as indicated. In a person physically dependent on narcotics, administration of the usual dose of a narcotic antagonist will precipitate an acute withdrawal syndrome; use of the antagonist in such a person should be avoided if possible but if it must be used to treat serious respiratory depression it should be administered with great care.

Incompatibilities: No major incompatibilities known.

Pharmaceutical precautions None.

Legal category CD (Sch. 2), POM.

Package quantities Amber glass bottles of 30 ml, 50 ml, 100 ml and 500 ml.

Further information Nil.

Product licence number 1883/0018.

Product licence holder: Macarthys Laboratories Limited, Bampton Road, Romford RM3 8UG.

METHADONE MIXTURE DTF (SUGAR FREE) 1 mg in 1 ml

Qualitative and quantitative composition Methadone Hydrochloride BP 0.1% w/v.

Pharmaceutical form Oral solution.

Clinical particulars

Therapeutic indications: In the treatment of Opioid addiction as an abstinence syndrome suppressant.

Posology and method of administration: For oral use only. The dose is adjusted according to the degree of dependence with the aim of gradual reduction.

Adults: Initially 10–20 mg per day, increasing by 10–20 mg daily until there are no signs of withdrawal or intoxication.

The elderly: In the case of the elderly or ill patients, repeated doses should only be given with extreme caution.

Children: Not recommended for use in children.

Contra-indications: Contra-indications are: Respiratory depression, obstructive airways disease, concurrent administration with MAO inhibitors or within 2 weeks of discontinuation of treatment with them. Hypersensitivity to any of the product ingredients. Use during an acute asthma attack is not advisable.

Obstetric use not recommended during labour, as the prolonged duration of action increases the risk of neonatal depression.

Methadone is not suitable for children.

Special warnings and precautions for use: In the case of the elderly or ill patients repeated doses should only be given with extreme caution.

Methadone is a drug of addiction controlled under Schedule 2 of The Misuse of Drugs Act 1971.

Interactions with other medicaments and other forms of interaction:

Alcohol: This may induce serious respiratory depression and hypotension.

Cimetidine: Potentiation of opiate action due to displacement of methadone from protein binding sites.

Rifampicin: Reduced opiate effect due to increased metabolism.

Phenytoin: Potentiation of opiate action due to displacement of Methadone from protein binding sites.

MAOIs: Possible CNS excitation or depression.

Urinary acidifiers: Increases rate of excretion of drug thus decreasing plasma concentration.

CNS depressants: Major and minor tranquillisers, sedatives and tricyclic antidepressants may result in increased CNS depression, respiratory depression and hypotension.

Opioid agonist analgesics: Additive CNS depression, respiratory depression and hypotension.

Naloxone: Antagonises the analgesic, CNS and respiratory depressant effects of Methadone.

Naltrexone: Administration of Naltrexone to a patient addicted to Methadone will rapidly precipitate long term withdrawal symptoms.

Buprenorphine pentazocine: Administration to a patient addicted to Methadone may precipitate withdrawal symptoms.

Pregnancy and lactation: There is no, or inadequate evidence of safety of the drug in human pregnancy but it has been in wide use for a considerable number of years without apparent ill-consequence. Animal studies have not shown any evidence of hazard. It should not be used in labour as the prolonged duration of action increases the risk of neonatal depression. Methadone is excreted in breast milk. This may be permissible during maintenance therapy.

Effects on ability to drive and use machines: The ability to drive or operate machinery may be severely effected during and after treatment with Methadone. The time after which such activity may be safely resumed is extremely patient dependent and must be decided by the physician.

Undesirable effects: Nausea, vomiting and dizziness. Methadone has the potential to increase intracranial pressure, particularly in circumstances where it is already raised.

In prolonged use it should not be administered more than twice daily to avoid the risk of accumulation and overdosage.

Overdose: Symptoms: Serious overdosage is characterised by respiratory depression, extreme somnolence progressing to stupor or coma, maximally constricted pupils, skeletal muscle flaccidity, cold and clammy skin and sometimes bradycardia and hypotension. In severe overdosage, particularly by the intravenous route, apnea, circulatory collapse, cardiac arrest and death may occur.

Treatment: A patent airway and assisted or controlled ventilation must be assured. Narcotic antagonists may be required, but it should be remembered that Methadone is a long-acting depressant (36 to 48 hours), whereas antagonists act for 1 to 3 hours, so that treatment with the latter must be repeated as needed. An antagonist should not be administered, however, in the absence of clinically significant respiratory or cardiovascular depression. Nalorphine (0.1 mg per kg) or levallorphan (0.02 mg per kg) should be given intravenously as soon as possible and repeated, if necessary, every 15 minutes. Oxygen, intravenous fluids, vasopressors and other supportive measures should be employed as indicated. In a person physically dependent on narcotics, administration of the usual dose of a narcotic antagonist will precipitate an acute withdrawal syndrome; use of the antagonist in such a person should be avoided if possible but if it must be used to treat serious respiratory depression it should be administered with great care.

Pharmacological properties

Pharmacodynamic properties: Methadone is a narcotic analgesic in the manner of Morphine but has a less sedative effect.

It acts on the CNS system and smooth muscle. This action is caused by the response of structurally and sterically specific opiate receptor sites in the brain, spinal cord and nervous system.

Methadone depresses the cough and respiratory centres.

In the treatment of opioid addiction the drug of abuse is replaced by methadone. In some situations the use of methadone can reduce or eliminate the effects of other opioids taken during the treatment period. This process is referred to as "narcotic blockade".

Pharmacokinetic properties: Methadone is rapidly absorbed after oral administration.

Protein binding: up to 90% but considerable inter-subject variation. About 15% is bound to immunoglobulin the remainder to albumin.

Distribution in blood: Plasma: Whole blood ratio, about 1:3.

Clearance: Plasma clearance about 2 ml/min/kg.

Volume of distribution: approx. 5L/kg.

Half-life: a) single dose=10–25 hours
b) repeated doses=13–55 hours.

Therapeutic concentration: In plasma, usually in the range 0.05–1.0 μg/ml. During methadone maintenance treatment considerable fluctuations occur day to day.

Dispositions in the body: Widely distributed in the tissues, with higher concentrations in the liver, lungs, and kidneys than in the blood. The main metabolic reaction is N-demethylation resulting in a substance which spontaneously cyclises to form the major metabolites, 2-ethylene-1,5-dimethyl-3,3-diphenylpyrrolidine (EDDP) and 2-ethyl-5-methyl-3,3-diphenyl-1-pyrroline (EMDP), neither of which are active. Hydroxylation to Methadol followed by N-demethylation to Normethadol also occurs to some extent.

Other metabolic reactions occur and there are at least eight known metabolites. In subjects on Methadone maintenance, about 20–60% of a dose is excreted in the urine in 24 hours, with up to about 33% of the dose as unchanged drug and up to about 43% as EDDP; EMDP accounts for about 5 to 10% of the dose. The ratio of EDDP to unchanged Methadone is usually very much higher in the urine of patients on methadone maintenance treatment than in simple overdose cases. Urinary excretion of unchanged drug is pH-dependent, being increased in acid urine. Up to 30% of a dose may be eliminated in the faeces, but this appears to decrease with increasing dosage. About 75% of the total excreted material is unconjugated.

Preclinical safety data: None stated.

Pharmaceutical particulars

List of excipients: Lycasin* 80/55, Potassium Sorbate, Green S, Sunset Yellow, Quinoline Yellow, Hydrochloric Acid and Purified Water.

Incompatibilities: No major incompatibilities known.

Shelf life: 12 months. Use within 28 days of opening.

Special precautions for storage: Store below 25°C.

Nature and contents of container: 30 ml, 50 ml, 100 ml and 500 ml of the oral solution in Amber glass bottles fitted with child-resistant closures. Contact material: Polypropylene.

Instructions for use/handling: None stated.

Marketing authorisation number: 00156/0030.

Marketing authorisation holder: Martindale Pharmaceuticals Limited, Bampton Road, Romford RM3 8UG.

Date of approval/revision of SPC 27 March 1996.

Legal category CD(Sch. 2), POM.

PAMERGAN* P100

Qualitative and quantitative composition Pethidine Hydrochloride BP 5% w/v
Promethazine Hydrochloride BP 2% w/v

Pharmaceutical form Injection.

Clinical particulars

Therapeutic indications:
a. Pre-anaesthetic medication.
b. Obstetric analgesia and amnesia.
c. The management of severe pain.

Posology and method of administration

a. Pre-anaesthetic medication:

Adults and the elderly: 2 ml administered 60–90 minutes before anaesthesia by intramuscular or, if diluted to 10 ml with Water for Injections, by intravenous injection.

Children 12–16 years: 1 ml
8–12 years: 0.75 ml
Under 8 years: Not recommended.
Administered 60–90 minutes before anaesthesia by intramuscular or, if diluted to 10 ml with Water for Injections, by intravenous injection.

b. Obstetric analgesia and amnesia: 1–2 ml when labour is well established, repeated at 4 hourly intervals as required by intramuscular or, if diluted to 10 ml with Water for Injections, by intravenous injection.

c. The management of severe pain: Adults and the elderly: 1–2 ml every 4–6 hours as necessary by intramuscular or, if diluted to 10 ml with Water for Injections, by intravenous injection.

Children: Not recommended.

Contra-indications: Not to be used on patients with severe liver disease, cholecystectomy, biliary colic, increased intracranial pressure, respiratory depression, obstructive airways disease or those taking (or within 2 weeks of taking) any MAOI antidepressant.

Special warnings and special precautions for use: Repeated use may result in dependence of the morphine type.

Administration during labour may cause respiratory depression in the new-born infant.

Pamergan P100 should be given with caution and in reduced doses to patients who are elderly or debilitated or those with head injuries, severe hepatic or renal impairment, biliary tract disorders, hypothyroidism, adreno-cortical insufficiency, shock, prostatic hypertrophy, and supra-ventricular tachycardia.

Caution is also required in patients with acute alcoholism, raised intracranial pressure or convulsive disorders.

Pethidine neurotoxicity may be seen in patients with renal failure, cancer or sickle cell anaemia, during concomitant administration with anticholinergics or during prolonged administration of increasing pethidine doses.

Interactions with other medicaments and other form of interaction: Concurrent use of pethidine with CNS depressants or anaesthetics may potentiate the action of pethidine.

Alcohol potentiates the action of both promethazine and pethidine.

MAOI antidepressants may cause severe CNS excitation and hypertension.

Cimetidine increases the plasma concentration of pethidine.

Hypnotics and anxiolytics are potentiated by both pethidine and promethazine.

The absorption of mexiletine is delayed by pethidine.

Domperidone and metaclopramide have an opposing effect to pethidine on gastro-intestinal activity.

Use in pregnancy and lactation: There is inadequate evidence of safety in human pregnancy, but Pamergan P100 has been widely used for many years without apparent ill consequence. Animal studies have not shown any hazard associated with Pethidine or Promethazine. As with all drugs during pregnancy care should be taken in assessing the risk to benefit ratio.

Pethidine crosses the placental barrier and is excreted in breast milk. This should be taken into account when considering its use in patients during pregnancy or breast feeding.

Administration during labour may cause respiratory depression in the new-born infant.

Problems relating to the use of promethazine during lactation have not been reported however risk/benefit might be considered because of the higher risk of adverse effects of antihistamines on infants especially new born and premature.

Effect on the ability to drive or operate machines: This product will cause drowsiness: patients should not drive or operate machinery.

Undesirable effects: Dizziness, nausea, vomiting, hypertension and respiratory depression. Mild euphoria may occur and CNS excitation has been reported in certain patient groups.

Other side-effects include dryness of the mouth and blurred vision. Occasionally patients may develop a feeling of weakness or syncope accompanied by profuse perspiration.

Overdosage:
Symptoms: Accidental overdose may give rise to respiratory depression, hypotension, convulsions and circulatory collapse.

Treatment: Establish and maintain a patent airway, assisting respiration if necessary. If respiration is severely depressed give a small intravenous dose of Naloxone (Adults: 0.4 mg, Children: 0.005–0.01 mg per kg. Neonates: 0.01 mg per kg.) repeated if necessary at intervals of 2–3 minutes. Hypotension may improve with improved oxygenation but may require treatment with an infusion of plasma or suitable electrolyte solution. Convulsions may need to be treated with a short acting muscle relaxant, intubation and controlled respiration.

Pharmacological properties

Pharmacodynamic properties: Pethidine binds with stereospecific receptors at many sites within the central nervous system (CNS) to alter processes affecting the perception of pain and the emotional response to pain. Although the precise sites and mechanisms of action have not been fully determined, alterations in release of various neurotransmitters from afferent nerves sensitive to painful stimuli may be partially responsible for the analgesic effects. When these medications are used as adjuncts to anaesthesia, analgesic actions may provide dose related protection against haemodynamic responses to surgical stress

Promethazine acts as a CNS depressant possibly by indirect reduction of stimuli to the brain stem reticular system. It may also act as a anti-emetic by inhibition of the medullary chem-receptor trigger zone of the mid brain. In Pamergan P100 the promethazine is present for its ability to prolong the activity of and lower the maintenance requirement of pethidine. It is possible that this is achieved by promethazine stabilising the endoplastic reticulum which will prevent both access of pethidine to and egress of metabolites from the receptor sites.

Pharmacokinetic properties: Pethidine distribution: Rapidly thoughout tissues. Volume of distribution 200–300 Litres.

Crosses placenta and secreted in milk.

Protein binding: High. Half life: 2.4–4 hours.

Metabolism: Hepatic; also intestines. The processes involved are N- Demethylation, hydrolysis, glucuronic acid conjugation and N- Oxidation. The rate of metabolism is decreased in pregnancy and increased in the elderly.

Route of elimination: Renal.

Pethidine is principally metabolised to Norpethidine and only about 5% is eliminated unchanged. Norpethidine is active and toxic (having CNS excitatory activity) and accumulates in patients with impaired renal function.

Promethazine distribution: Volume of distribution about 170 Litres.

Crosses the placenta.

Protein binding: Very high.

Half life: 4 hours.

Metabolism: Subject to extensive first pass metabolism; major reactions appear to be sulphoxidation and glucuronic acid conjugation.

Route of elimination: Renal. Promethazine is principally excreted as the sulphoxide with only about 2% eliminated unchanged.

Pre-clinical safety data: None stated.

Pharmaceutic particulars

List of excipients: Sodium Metabisulphite BP, Sodium Sulphite, Anhydrous BP, Sodium Chloride BP and Water for Injection BP. pH adjustment may be made using either Hydrochloric acid BP or Sodium Hydroxide BP

Incompatibilities: Pamergan P100 has a pH of 5–6 and is incompatible with alkaline products including Thiopentone Sodium.

Shelf life: 36 months.

Special precautions for storage: Protect from light

Nature and contents of container: 2 ml in type 1 colourless neutral glass ampoules. Fusion sealed.

Marketing authorisation number 0156/0020R

Marketing authorisation holder: Martindale Pharmaceuticals Limited, Bampton Road, Romford RM3 8UG.

Date of approval/revision of SPC 27 March 1995

Legal category CD(Sch 2) POM.

TIMOLOL EYE DROPS BP 0.25% w/v and 0.5% w/v

Qualitative and quantitative composition Timolol Maleate PhEur equivalent to 2.5 mg/ml Timolol, Timolol Maleate Ph Eur equivalent to 5.0 mg/ml Timolol.

Pharmaceutical form Ophthalmic solution.

Clinical particulars

Therapeutic indications: Timolol maleate ophthalmic solution is a beta-adrenergic receptor antagonist used topically for the reduction of elevated intra-ocular pressure in various conditions including patients with ocular hypertension; patients with chronic open-angle glaucoma including patients with aphakia; and some patients with secondary glaucoma.

Posology and method of administration

Dosage schedule: Recommended therapy is one drop Timolol Eye Drops 0.25%w/v in the affected eye(s) twice a day. If clinical response is not adequate, dosage may be increased to one drop Timolol Eye Drops 0.5% w/v in the affected eye(s) twice daily. If required, timolol maleate ophthalmic solution may be used with miotics, adrenaline or systemically administered carbonic anhydrous inhibitors.

Intra-ocular pressure should be reassessed approximately four weeks after starting treatment because response to Timolol Eye Drops may take a few weeks to stabilise. Provided that the intra-ocular pressure is maintained at satisfactory levels, many patients can then be placed on once-a-day therapy.

Transfer from other agents: If transferring from another topical beta-blocking agent, its use should be discontinued after a full day of treatment and treatment with Timolol Eye Drops 0.25% w/v started the next day with one drop twice daily in the affected eye(s). As above, if the clinical response is not adequate, the dosage may be increased to one drop of Timolol Eye Drops 0.5% w/v twice daily.

If transferring from a single anti-glaucoma agent which is not a beta-blocker, the agent should be continued and one drop added of the Timolol Eye Drops 0.25% w/v in the affected eye(s) twice daily. On the following day the previous agent should be discontinued and Timolol Eye Drops continued. The dosage may be increased to Timolol Eye Drops 0.5% w/v twice daily if the clinical response is inadequate.

Use in children: Paediatric use is not currently recommended.

Use in the elderly: There has been wide experience with the use of timolol maleate in elderly patients. The dosage recommendations above reflect the clinical data derived from this experience.

Contra-indications: Bronchial asthma, history of bronchial asthma or severe chronic obstructive pulmonary disease, sinus bradycardia, second and third degree AV block, overt cardiac failure, cardiogenic shock, and hypersensitivity to timolol maleate or other beta-blocking agents.

Special warnings and precautions for use: Like other topically applied ophthalmic drugs, timolol maleate ophthalmic solution may be absorbed systemically and adverse reactions seen with systemically administered beta-blockers may occur.

Cardiac failure should be adequately controlled before beginning therapy with timolol maleate ophthalmic solution. Patients with a history of severe cardiac disease should be closely observed for signs of cardiac failure and have their pulse rates checked.

Respiratory and cardiac reactions, including death due to bronchospasm in patients with asthma and, rarely, death associated with cardiac failure, have been reported.

The effect on intra-ocular pressure or the known effects of systemic beta-blockade may be exaggerated when timolol maleate ophthalmic solution is given to patients already receiving an oral beta-blocking agent. The response of these patients should be closely watched.

If timolol maleate ophthalmic solution is used to reduce elevated intra-ocular pressure in angle closure glaucoma it should be used with a miotic and not alone.

There have been reports of skin rashes and/or dry eyes associated with the use of beta-adrenergic receptor blocking drugs. The reported incidence is small and in most cases the symptoms have cleared when treatment was withdrawn. Discontinuation of the drug should be considered if any such reaction is not otherwise explicable. Cessation of therapy involving beta-blockade should be gradual.

Timolol Eye Drops contain benzalkonium chloride as a preservative which may be deposited in soft contact lenses. Therefore, timolol eye drops should not be used while wearing these lenses. The lenses should be removed before application of the drops and not reinserted earlier than 15 minutes after use.

Timolol Eye Drops have generally been well tolerated in glaucoma patients wearing conventional hard contact lenses. Timolol maleate ophthalmic solution has not been studied in patients wearing lenses made of material other than polymethylmethacrylate (PMMA) which is used to make hard contact lenses.

Interaction with other medicaments and other forms of interaction: Although timolol maleate ophthalmic solution alone has little or no effect on pupil size, mydriasis has occasionally been reported when timolol maleate ophthalmic solution is given with adrenaline.

Pregnancy and lactation: Timolol maleate ophthalmic solution has not been studied in human pregnancy. The use of timolol maleate ophthalmic solution requires that the anticipated benefit be weighed against possible hazards. Timolol maleate ophthalmic solution is detectable in human milk. A decision for breast-feeding mothers either to stop taking timolol or stop nursing should be based on the importance of the drug to the mother.

Effects on ability to drive and use machines: Instillation of Timolol Eye Drops may cause transient blurring of vision. Patients should be warned not to drive or operate moving machinery until any blurring of vision after instillation has totally regressed.

Undesirable effects: Timolol maleate ophthalmic solution is usually well tolerated.

Special senses: Signs and symptoms of ocular irritation, including conjunctivitis, blepharitis, keratitis and decreased corneal sensitivity, have been reported. Visual disturbances, including refractive changes (due to withdrawal of miotic therapy in some cases), diplopia and ptosis, can occur.

Cardiovascular: Bradycardia, arrhythmia, hypotension, syncope, heart block, cerebrovascular accident, cerebral ischaemia, congestive heart failure, palpitation and cardiac arrest may occur and are probably the result of systemic absorption.

Respiratory: Bronchospasm (predominantly in patients with pre-existing bronchospastic disease), respiratory failure and dyspnoea have been reported.

Generally: Headache, asthenia, nausea, dizziness, depression and hypersensitivity reactions including localised and generalised rash and urticaria may occasionally occur.

Causal relationship unknown: The following adverse effects have been reported, but a causal relationship to timolol maleate ophthalmic solution has not been established: Aphakic cystoid macular oedema, dry mouth, nasal congestion, anorexia, dyspepsia, CNS effects (eg behavioural change including confusion, hallucinations, anxiety, disorientation, nervousness, somnolence and other psychiatric disturbances), hypertension and retroperitoneal fibrosis.

The adverse reactions seen with oral timolol maleate may occur with timolol maleate ophthalmic solution due to systemic absorption.

Overdose: Overdosage reactions are more likely to follow oral ingestion of timolol maleate than by systemic absorption through its topical use. No specific data on overdosage in humans by either route are available. A study in patients with renal failure suggests that timolol does not readily dialyse. The most common signs and symptoms to be expected following overdosage with a beta-blocker are symptomatic bradycardia, hypotension, bronchospasm and acute cardiac failure. The standard measures to overcome beta-blockade should be undertaken.

Pharmacological properties

Pharmacodynamic properties: Timolol maleate is a non-selective beta-adrenergic antagonist used as an ophthalmic solution for the topical treatment of increased intra-ocular pressure. Timolol maleate has no intrinsic sympathomimetic activity nor membrane-stabilising activity. It is thought that the mode of action is by markedly reducing the production of aqueous humor, probably without any effect on the outflow tract. Timolol maleate ophthalmic solution is effective in a range of concentrations but the usual recommendation is for 0.25% w/v and 0.5% w/v strengths.

Pharmacokinetic properties: Timolol maleate ophthalmic solution lowers intra-ocular pressure within 30-60 minutes of being administered topically, has a maximum IOP-lowering effect 4-5 hours after administration, and the effect persists for 12-14 hours after a single dose. Minute amounts are absorbed systemically; plasma concentrations of up to 1 ng/ml can be detected after single eye drop administration.

Preclinical safety data: None presented

Pharmaceutical particulars

List of excipients: Potassium Dihydrogen Phosphate PhEur, Disodium Hydrogen Phosphate Dodecahydrate PhEur, Benzalkonium Chloride, Purified Water PhEur.

Incompatibilities: None known

Shelf life:
Shelf life of the product as packaged for sale: 3 years (36 months).
Shelf life after first opening the container: 28 days.

Special precautions for storage: Store below 30°C. Protect from light.

Nature and contents of container: A 5 ml low density polyethylene bottle. The dropper insert is made from low density polyethylene and the bottle is closed by a screw cap manufactured from high density polyethylene. The cap is secured by a tamper evident closure.

Instructions for use/handling: Unscrew the cap from the bottle. Pull down the bottom lid of the eye to form a pocket. Place the tip close to the lower eye lid and squeeze the container gently. One drop of solution should fall into the eye.

Marketing authorisation numbers
Timolol Eye Drops 0.25% w/v 0156/0032
Timolol Eye Drops 0.5% w/v 0156/0033

Marketing authorisation holder: Martindale Pharmaceuticals Limited, Bampton Road, Romford RM3 8UG.

Date of approval/revision of SPC September 1997

Legal category POM

** Trade Mark*

medac GmbH
Fehlandtstrasse 3
20354 Hamburg
Germany

☎ 040/3 50 91-0 🗋 040/3 50 91-300

ACLARUBICIN INJECTION 20 mg

Qualitative and quantitative composition Aclarubicin hydrochloride equivalent to aclarubicin 20 mg.

Pharmaceutical form Freeze-dried powder for reconstitution and parenteral administration by injection or infusion.

Clinical particulars
Therapeutic indications: For the treatment of acute non-lymphocytic leukaemia in patients who have relapsed or are resistant or refractory to first line chemotherapy.

Posology and method of administration: Aclarubicin should be administered by intravenous infusion over 30 to 60 minutes.

Dosage in adults including the elderly: The usual initial dosage is 175–300 mg/m² of body surface over 3 to 7 consecutive days, e.g. 80–100 mg/m² on 3 consecutive days or 25 mg/m² daily for 7 consecutive days. Repetition of treatment schedules will be dependent on the patient's haematological profile and the response of the primary disease.

Maintenance dosage should be treatments of 25–100 mg/m² of body surface given as a single infusion every 3 to 4 weeks.

This is a guide to dosage using the drug alone. In combination with other cytotoxic drugs dosage may need to be reduced.

The maximum total dosage given to any individual patient should be decided according to their cardiological status. Most patients treated have received a maximum of 400 mg/m², however, larger doses in some patients have been used without ill consequence.

Dosage in children: Experience suggests that aclarubicin is well tolerated by children at the standard dosage level.

Administration: By parenteral infusion either (i) in a freely flowing iv peripheral line or (ii) in a patent central venous line.

Contra-indications: Severe bone marrow depression.

Special warnings and special precautions for use: Patients receiving aclarubicin require close observation and frequent laboratory monitoring therefore treatment should be carried out by doctors experienced in the use of cytotoxic drugs. Treatment should be carried out at centres where there are adequate laboratory facilities, supportive treatment and facilities for monitoring heart disease readily available.

Therapy should be initiated cautiously in patients with compromised hepatic, renal or cardiac function.

The patient's haematological profile should be taken into account when instituting therapy and monitored during the recovery phase post treatment. Anaemia and thrombocytopenia should be treated with appropriate blood product replacement.

Hyperuricaemia should be avoided (fluid and xanthine oxidase inhibitors) and infections should be treated.

Cardiac function should be monitored by ECG.

Interactions with other medicaments and other forms of interaction: Aclarubicin is a powerful myelosuppressive agent. The concurrent use of other chemotherapeutic drugs with similar actions may be expected to lead to additive myelosuppression and dosage reduction should be considered.

Aclarubicin has been used in combination chemotherapy without signs of interaction with the following drugs: cyclophosphamide, cytarabine, behenoyl cytarabine, 5-fluorouracil, 6-mercaptopurine, methotrexate, 6-thioguanine, prednisolone and vincristine.

Aclarubicin has caused higher myelosuppression in patients previously treated with nitrosourea or mitomycin.

There have been reports of increased toxicity consequent upon irradiation treatment shortly before the administration of anthracyclines. No such reactions have been observed following treatment with aclarubicin but the theoretical risk should be borne in mind.

Pregnancy and lactation: There is no evidence of the drug's safety in human pregnancy. There is evidence from animal work that it is foetotoxic but not teratogenic. Avoid in pregnancy unless there is no safer alternative. If used in pregnancy patients should be warned of the potential risk to the foetus.

Women of childbearing age should take adequate contraceptive precautions.

If the use of aclarubicin is considered essential, nursing mothers should be advised to stop breast feeding.

Effects on ability to drive and use machines: The patient's general condition is likely to be more significant in this consideration than any drug-induced effects.

Undesirable effects:
Haematological: The dose-limiting toxicity of aclarubicin is haematological with myelosuppression seen as leucopenia and thrombocytopenia. The platelet nadir precedes the leucocyte nadir. Myelosuppression is severe at total dosages greater than 300 mg/m². Higher total dosages should be administered in a cyclic schedule including rest periods for recovery of the bone marrow. Myelosuppression is not reduced by dividing a single dose over 2 to 5 days. Thrombocytopenia is at a maximum 1 to 2 weeks after the start of the drug administration with recovery within 2 to 4 weeks. Leucopenia is greatest 2 to 3 weeks after drug administration with recovery within 3 to 4 weeks.

Gastro-intestinal: Nausea and vomiting have been observed in 20–100% (average 60%) of patients depending on dosage and dose schedule used. Single dosages greater than 120 mg/m² given by iv infusion caused nausea and vomiting in all patients.

The same dosage divided over 5 days is better tolerated. A daily dose of up to 30 mg/m² for 7 consecutive days caused nausea and vomiting, (controllable with antiemetics) in about 50% of patients. Bolus injections of more than 50 mg/m² should not be given due to severe gastrointestinal side-effects. Diarrhoea, occasionally haemorrhagic, has been observed in 10–35% (average 26%) of patients. Diarrhoea has been most pronounced after high single dosages or consecutive use of low dosages for more than 10 days. Mucositis/stomatitis has been observed in 15–55% (average 30%) of patients and is also more pronounced at high dosages.

Cardiac: Acute cardiotoxicity during and after drug administration has been associated with ECG changes (including arrhythmia, atrial flutter, flattening or inversion of T waves, sinus tachycardia, ST depression and premature beats) in 10–40% (average 17%) of patients. The frequency of ECG changes is greater with high single doses of aclarubicin. The ECG changes are generally reversible, transient and frequently without clinical signs of cardiotoxocity. ECG QTc prolongation may herald a clinical risk of ventricular fibrillation.

Chronic cardiotoxicity has been observed rarely: in a follow up study of about 1,600 patients congestive heart failure occurred in 5 patients and in 2 patients clinical signs of cardiomyopathy were seen. The risk of cardiotoxicity may be increased in patients previously treated with other cytotoxic agents or irradiation to the thorax.

Alopecia: Mild alopecia has been observed in 1–5% of patients.

Hepatic: Transient and reversible serum transaminase elevation and hepatic dysfunction have been reported in 4–6% of patients.

Other: Phlebitis is rare, occurring in up to 7% of patients. It may be eliminated by dilution of infusion solutions. Allergic reactions (angioedema, urticaria, skin rash, conjunctivitis) have occurred in isolated cases.

After accidental extravasation, aclarubicin caused inflammation and induration, but no tissue necrosis.

Results from some mutagenicity studies with aclarubicin were positive and it showed the capacity to induce chromosomal aberrations. The carcinogenic potential of aclarubicin in man is unknown. The possibility of a carcinogenic effect should be kept in mind when planning long-term therapy.

Overdose: The haematologic profile should be monitored and, in the event of dangerously low haemoglobin, white cell or platelet counts, treatment with appropriate blood products should be carried out as clinically required. Fevers should be investigated and treated properly.

Cardiac function should be monitored and arrhythmias or congestive cardiac failure treated as they appear.

Pharmacological properties
Pharmacodynamic properties: Aclarubicin is a cytotoxic anthracycline antibiotic isolated from a strain of *Streptomyces galileaus*. Like other anthracyclines, aclarubicin is a glycoside but differs from daunorubicin and doxorubicin in having aklavinone as aglycone and in being a trisaccharide.

The cellular uptake is much more rapid and the cellular drug accumulation is significantly higher for aclarubicin than for daunorubicin and doxorubicin. Aclarubicin belongs to Class II anthracyclines which preferentially inhibit RNA synthesis, whereas Class I anthracyclines, daunorubicin and doxorubicin, inhibit RNA and DNA synthesis almost equally. Aclarubicin inhibition of cell progession is greatest for cells in mid G_1 followed by cells in late S and finally by cells in G_2. In contrast to daunorubicin and doxorubicin the cytotoxicity of aclarubicin in vitro is reversible at lower concentrations or after brief exposure to the drug. In vivo antineoplastic activity studies have shown that aclarubicin is more active in repeated daily or intermittent doses than in single dose, i.e. the effect seems to depend more on exposure to aclarubicin over longer periods of time than to high intracellular peak concentration. Aclarubicin induces maturation of human non-lymphocytic leukaemia blasts, unlike doxorubicin, which does not.

Pharmacokinetic properties: After a single iv injection the plasma drug concentration declines rapidly due to the rapid uptake of aclarubicin in the tissues. The initial disposition phases are short ($t_{1/2}$ α=2.6 (range 1.3–5.3) min, $t_{1/2}$ β=23 (range 11–75) min) and are followed by a terminal phase with an elimination half-life $t_{1/2}$ γ=3 (range 1.4–8.5) hours. (The corresponding figures for doxorubicin are: $t_{1/2}$ α=12 (±8) min, $t_{1/2}$ β=3.3 (±2.2) hours and $t_{1/2}$ γ=29.6 (±13.5) hours. Terminal half-lives for daunorubicin and its metabolite daunorubicinol were 18.5 (±4.9) and 26.7 (±12.8) hours.) The disposition half-lives are shorter and aclarubicin is removed more rapidly from plasma than daunorubicin and doxorubicin. Aclarubicin and the principal active metabolite M1 are highly bound to blood cells. The large apparent volume of distribution VD α=1249 (±648) L/m² (mean±sd) indicates that aclarubicin is highly bound to the tissues. The mean plasma total body clearance is 4.03±1.48 L/min/m² (range 1.61–8.83 L/min/m²). No accumulation is seen after repeated daily dosing of 20–40 mg/m² iv over 4–7 days.

An autoradiographic study in rats showed that small amounts of aclarubicin cross the placental barrier, distribution within the foetus is similar to that seen in the dam.

Aclarubicin is rapidly and highly metabolised before excretion. Only 1% or less of the total dose appears unchanged in the urine within 24 hours and only trace amounts are detected in the bile. The metabolic pathway for aclarubicin involves ketoreduction and hydrolysis of the terminal-sugars, reductive glycoside cleavage and glucuronide conjugation to form biologically active glycosides (M1, N1, S1, L1, T1) and inactive aglycones (AKN, C1, E1, F1, F1-acid). M1, N1, S1 and F1 are found in plasma and urine. The other metabolites are found only in urine. M1 and, to a lesser extent, F1 are also found in bile.

In animal experiments active metabolites were found in high concentrations in the lung, spleen and lymph nodes; inactive metabolites were mainly found in the liver, kidneys and intestine.

Following aclarubicin injection the principal active glycoside metabolite M1 appears in plasma within 2–3 minutes and is the major metabolite during the first 2 hours. M1 plasma levels peak at 191±129 minutes after dosing, reaching concentrations of 130±43.8 ng/ml, with a terminal half-life of 13.4 (range 9.6–20.6) hours. The principal inactive aglycone metabolite F1 is detectable from 60 minutes and becomes the major metabolite from 3 hours after dosing. Peak plasma levels of F1, six times those of M1, occurred 18–23 hours after injection and declined slowly with a terminal half-life of 36.1±3 hours, suggesting that it is formed from tissue bound glycosides.

The rate of metabolism is independent of dose in the range 60–150 mg/m² and is unaffected by the rate of administration. There is correlation between plasma concentration of aclarubicin and the side-effects nausea and vomiting. Administration of the drug over a longer period of time by infusion or in divided doses may reduce the frequency of occurrence.

Preclinical safety data: Aclarubicin was non-mutagenic in the Ames test in contrast to daunorubicin and doxorubicin. No immunosuppressive effects were demonstrated for aclarubicin.

Pharmaceutical particulars

List of excipients: Lactose, hydrochloric acid.

Incompatibilities: Aclarubicin is not stable at pH of less than 4.

Aclarubicin should only be reconstituted using 0.9% Sodium Chloride Injection or Water for Injections. Reconstituted aclarubicin should only be added to 0.9% intravenous sodium chloride infusion or to glucose infusion solutions having pH values between 5 and 6.

Exposure of very dilute solutions to light promotes degradation.

Shelf life: Aclarubicin injection 20 mg, in the dry state, has a shelf-life of 3 years when stored at room temperature and protected from light.

Water and saline solutions (reconstituted aclarubicin) should be stored protected from light and should be used within 24 hours if stored below 4°C or within 6 hours if stored at room temperature.

Infusion solutions should be used immediately and protected from sunlight during administration.

Special precautions for storage: Aclarubicin medac injection, dry powder and reconstituted solution, should be stored protected from light.

Nature and contents of container: 10 ml colourless glass vial with butyl rubber stopper and cap of aluminium/polypropylene.

Each vial contains a quantity of freeze dried powder equivalent to 20 mg aclarubicin for reconstitution.

The vials are packed in boxes of 2.

Instructions for use/handling: Preparation of solutions: The vial contents should be reconstituted with 10 ml of 0.9% Sodium Chloride Injection or Water for Injection. The concentration of this reconstituted solution is 2 mg/ml.

To prepare an infusion solution dilute the required volume of reconstituted solution with 200 to 500 ml 0.9% sodium chloride intravenous infusion or, if necessary, 5% glucose intravenous infusion (of pH value between 5 and 6). The final concentration should be 0.2–0.5 mg/ml.

Marketing authorisation number 11587/0004

Date of approval/revison of SPC September 1996.

Legal category POM.

Dacarbazine 100 mg medac
Dacarbazine 200 mg medac
Dacarbazine 500 mg medac
Dacarbazine 1000 mg medac

Qualitative and quantitative composition One single-dose vial of Dacarbazine 100 mg (200 mg) medac with 250 mg (475 mg) sterile dry-powder contains 135 mg (270 mg) dacarbazine citrate, corresponding to 100 mg (200 mg) Dacarbazine as active ingredient.

One single-dose vial of Dacarbazine 500 mg (1000 mg) medac with 1187.5 mg (2375 mg) sterile dry-powder contains 675 mg (1350 mg) dacarbazine citrate, corresponding to 500 mg (1000 mg) Dacarbazine as active ingredient.

Pharmaceutical form

Dacarbazine 100 mg (200 mg) medac: Sterile powder for solution for i.v. injection or infusion.

Dacarbazine 500 mg (1000 mg) medac: Sterile powder for solution for infusion.

Clinical particulars

Therapeutic indications: Dacarbazine is indicated for the treatment of patients with metastasised malignant melanoma.

Further indications for dacarbazine as part of a combination chemotherapy are:

- advanced Hodgkin's disease,
- advanced adult soft tissue sarcomas (except mesothelioma, Kaposi sarcoma).

Posology and method of administration: The use of dacarbazine should be confined to physicians experienced in oncology or hematology respectively.

Dacarbazine is sensitive to light exposure. All reconstituted solutions should be suitably protected from light also during administration (light-resistant infusion set).

Care should be taken of administration of the injection to avoid extravasation into tissues since this will cause local pain and tissue damage. If extravasation occurs, the injection should be discontinued immediately and any remaining portion of the dose should be introduced into another vein.

The following regimes can be used. For further details cf. current scientific literature.

Malignant Melanoma: Dacarbazine can be administered as single agent in doses of 200 to 250 mg/m² body surface area/day as an i.v. injection for 5 days every 3 weeks.

As an alternative to an intravenous bolus injection dacarbazine can be administered as a short-term infusion (over 15–30 minutes).

It is also possible to give 850 mg/m² body surface area on day 1 and then once every 3 weeks as intravenous infusion.

Lymphogranulomatosis (Hodgkin's Disease): Dacarbazine is administered in a daily dose of 375 mg/m² body surface area i.v. every 15 days in combination with doxorubicin, bleomycin and vinblastine (ABVD regimen).

Adult soft-tissue sarcoma: For adult soft tissue sarcomas dacarbazine is given in daily doses of 250 mg/m² body surface area i.v. (days 1-5) in combination with doxorubicin every 3 weeks (ADIC regimen).

During dacarbazine treatment frequent monitoring of blood counts should be conducted as well as monitoring of hepatic and renal function. Since severe gastrointestinal reactions frequently occur, antiemetic and supportive measures are advisable.

Because severe gastrointestinal and hematological disturbances can occur an extremely careful benefit-risk analysis has to be made before every course of therapy with dacarbazine.

Duration of therapy: The treating physician should individually decide about the duration of therapy taking into account the type and stage of the underlying disease, the combination therapy administered and the response to and adverse effects of dacarbazine. In advanced Hodgkin's disease, a usual recommendation is to administer 6 cycles of ABVD combination therapy. In metastasised malignant melanoma and in advanced tissue sarcoma, the duration of treatment depends on the efficacy and tolerability in the individual patient.

Rate of administration: Doses up to 200 mg/m² may be given as a slow intravenous injection. Larger doses (ranging from 200 to 850 mg/m²) should be administered as an i.v. infusion over 15-30 minutes.

It is recommended to test the patency of the vein first with a 5- to 10-ml flush of sodium chloride infusion solution or glucose 5%. The same solutions should be used after infusion to flush any remaining drug from the tubing.

After reconstitution with water for injection without further dilution with sodium chloride infusion solution or glucose 5 %, dacarbazine 100 mg and 200 mg preparations are hypo-osmolar (ca. 100 mOsmol/kg) and should therefore be given by slow intravenous injection e.g. over 1 minute rather than rapid intravenous bolus over a few seconds.

Special populations: Patients with kidney/liver insufficiency:

If there is mild to moderate renal or hepatic insufficiency alone, a dose reduction is not usually required. In patients with combined renal and hepatic impairment elimination of dacarbazine is prolonged. However, no validated recommendations on dose reductions can be given currently.

Elderly patients: As limited experience in elderly patients is available no special instructions for the use in elderly patients can be given.

Contra-indications: Dacarbazine is contra-indicated in patients

- who have a history of hypersensitivity reactions to dacarbazine,
- in pregnant or breastfeeding women,
- in patients with leucopenia and/or thrombocytopenia,
- in patients with severe liver or kidney diseases.

Special warnings and special precautions for use: It is recommended that dacarbazine should only be administered under the supervision of a physician specialised in oncology, having the facilities for regular monitoring of clinical, biochemical and haematological effects, during and after therapy.

If symptoms of a liver or kidney functional disorder or symptoms of a hypersensitivity reaction are observed immediate cessation of therapy is required.

Note: The responsible physician should be aware of a rarely observed severe complication during therapy resulting from liver necrosis due to occlusion of intrahepatic veins. Therefore frequent monitoring of liver size, function and blood counts (especially eosinophils) is required (see *Undesirable effects*).

Long-term therapy can cause cumulative bone marrow toxicity.

The possible bone marrow depression requires careful monitoring of white blood cells, red blood cells and platelet levels. Hemopoetic toxicity may warrant temporary suspension or cessation of therapy.

Extravasation of the drug during i.v. administration may result in tissue damage and severe pain.

Furthermore dacarbazine is a moderate immunosuppressive agent.

Contraceptive measures: Men are advised to take contraceptive measures during and for 6 months after cessation of therapy. Women of child-bearing age must avoid pregnancy during dacarbazine treatment.

Handling of dacarbazine: Dacarbazine should be handled according to standard procedures for cytostatics that have mutagenic, carcinogenic and teratogenic effects.

Interaction with other medicaments and other forms of interaction: In case of previous or concomitant treatment having adverse effects on the bone marrow (particularly cytostatic agents, irradiation) myelotoxic interactions are possible.

Studies to investigate the presence of phenotypic metabolism have not been undertaken but hydroxylation of the parent compound to metabolites with anti-tumour activity has been identified.

Dacarbazine can enhance the effects of methoxypsoralen because of photosensitisation.

Use during pregnancy and lactation: Dacarbazine has been shown to be mutagenic, teratogenic and carcinogenic in animals. It must be assumed that an increased risk for teratogenic effects exists in humans. Therefore dacarbazine must not be used during pregnancy and during breastfeeding (see: *Contra-indications* and *Special warnings and special precautions for use*).

Effects on ability to drive and use machines: Dacarbazine may influence the ability to drive or operate machines because of its central nervous side effects or because of nausea and vomiting.

Undesirable effects: Disturbances of the digestive tract such as anorexia, nausea and vomiting are common and severe. In rare cases diarrhoea has been observed.

Changes in blood counts often observed (decreased red blood cells, white blood cells, platelets) are dose-dependent and delayed, with the nadirs often only occurring after 3 to 4 weeks.

Flu-like symptoms with exhaustion, chills, fever and muscular pain are occasionally observed during or often only days after dacarbazine administration. These disturbances may recur with the next infusion.

In isolated cases liver necrosis due to occlusion of intrahepatic veins has been observed after administration of dacarbazine in monotherapy or in combined treatment modalities. In general the syndrome occurred during the second cycle of therapy. Symptoms included fever, eosinophilia, abdominal pain, enlarged liver, jaundice and shock which worsened rapidly over a few hours or days. As fatal outcome has been described special care has to be taken of frequently monitoring of liver size, function and blood counts (especially eosinophils) (see *Posology and method of administration* and *Special warnings and special precautions for use*).

Venous irritations and some of the systemic adverse reactions are thought to result from formation of photodegradation products.

Impaired renal function with increased blood levels of substances obligatory excreted by urine is rare.

Central nervous side effects such as headaches, impaired vision, confusion, lethargy and convulsions rarely may occur. Facial paraesthesia and flushing may occur shortly after injection.

Allergic reactions of the skin in the form of erythema, maculopapular exanthema or urticaria are observed rarely. Infrequently loss of hair, hyperpigmentation and photosensitivity of the skin may occur. In rare cases anaphylactic reactions have been described.

Inadvertent paravenous injection is expected to cause local pain and necrosis.

Overdose: The primary anticipated complications of overdose are severe bone marrow suppression, eventually bone marrow aplasia which may be delayed by up to two weeks.

Time to occurrence of nadirs of leucocytes and thrombocytes can be 4 weeks. Even if overdosage is only suspected, long-term careful hematologic monitoring is essential. There is no known antidote for dacarbazine overdose. Therefore, special care has to be taken to avoid overdose of this drug.

Pharmacological properties

Pharmacodynamic properties: ATC: L01X X13

Dacarbazine is a cytostatic agent. The antineoplastic effect is due to an inhibition of cell growth which is independent of the cell cycle and due to an inhibition of DNA synthesis. An alkylating effect has also been shown and other cytostatic mechanisms may also be influenced by dacarbazine.

Dacarbazine is considered not to show an antineoplastic effect by itself. However by microsomal N-demethylation it is quickly converted to 5-amino-imidazole-4-carboxamide and a methyl cation, which is responsible for the alkylating effect of the drug.

Pharmacokinetic properties: After intravenous application dacarbazine is quickly distributed into tissue. Plasma protein binding is 5%. Kinetics in plasma are biphasic; the initial (distribution) half life is only 20 minutes, terminal half life is 0.5–3.5 hours.

Dacarbazine is metabolised mainly in the liver by both hydroxylation and demethylation, approx. 20-50% of the drug are excreted unmodified by the kidney via renal tubular secretion.

Preclinical safety data: Because of its pharmacodynamic properties dacarbazine shows mutagenic, carcinogenic and teratogenic effects which are detectable in experimental test systems.

Pharmaceutical particulars
List of excipients: Each vial of Dacarbazine 100 mg (200 mg, 500 mg, 1000 mg) medac contains the excipients citric acid and mannitol.

Incompatibilities: Dacarbazine-solution is chemically incompatible with heparin, hydrocortisone, L-cysteine and sodium hydrogen carbonate.

Shelf life: Vials of dacarbazine should be stored at or below 25°C, protected from light. The shelf-life is 36 months.

Reconstituted solutions should also be protected from light and used immediately.

Special precautions for storage: Store at or below 25 °C, protected from light.

Nature and contents of container: Dacarbazine 100 mg (200 mg) medac is supplied as a sterile powder for solution for injection or infusion in single-dose vials made of amber glass and closed with butyl rubber stoppers. Each carton of Dacarbazine 100 mg (200 mg) medac contains 10 vials.

Dacarbazine 500 mg (1000 mg) medac is supplied as a sterile powder for solution for infusion in single-dose vials made of amber glass and closed with butyl rubber stoppers. Each carton of Dacarbazine 500 mg (1000 mg) medac contains one vial.

Instructions for use, handling and disposal:
Recommendations for the safe handling: Dacarbazine is an antineoplastic agent and, as with other potentially toxic compounds, caution should be exercised when handling it and preparing dacarbazine solutions. The use of gloves is recommended.

If dacarbazine lyophilisate or infusion solution should come into contact with skin, wash immediately and thoroughly with soap and water.

If dacarbazine lyophilisate, or infusion solution should come into contact with mucous membranes, wash immediately and thoroughly with water.

Preparation for the intravenous administration: Dacarbazine-solutions are prepared immediately before use.

Dacarbazine is sensitive to light exposure. During administration, the infusion container and administration set should be protected from exposure to daylight, e.g. by using light-resistant PVC-infusion sets. Normal infusion sets should be wrapped up in e.g. UV-resistant foils.

a) Preparation of Dacarbazine 100 mg (200 mg) medac:

Aseptically transfer the required amount of water for injection (Dacarbazine 100 mg medac: 10 ml; Dacarbazine 200 mg medac: 20 ml) into the vial and shake until a solution is obtained. This freshly prepared solution (dacarbazine: 10 mg/ml*) is administered as a slow injection.

For preparation of Dacarbazine 100 mg (200 mg) medac for i.v. infusion the freshly prepared solution is further diluted with 200-300 ml sodium chloride infusion solution or glucose 5%. This solution is given as a short term infusion over a period between 15–30 minutes.

b) Preparation of Dacarbazine 500 mg (1000 mg) medac:

Aseptically transfer the required amount of 50 ml water for injection into the Dacarbazine 500 mg (1000 mg) medac vial and shake until a solution is obtained⁺. The resulting solution has to be further diluted with 200–300 ml sodium chloride infusion solution or glucose 5%. The obtained infusion solution is ready for i. v. administration (Dacarbazine 500 mg medac: 1.4–2.0 mg/ml; Dacarbazine 1000 mg medac: 2.8–4.0 mg/ml) and should be given within 20–30 minutes.

Disposal: All materials that have been utilised for dilution and administration should be disposed of according to standard procedures (incineration).

* Density of the solution:
ρ = 1.007 mg/ml
⁺ Density of the solution:
ρ = 1.007 mg/ml (Dacarbazine 500 mg medac)
ρ = 1.015 mg/ml (Dacarbazine 1000 mg medac)

Marketing authorisation holder: medac, Gesellschaft für klinische Spezialpräparate mbH, Fehlandtstrasse 3, D-20354 Hamburg.

Marketing authorisation numbers

Dacarbazine 100 mg medac MA-no.:	PL 11587/0008
Dacarbazine 200 mg medac MA-no.:	PL 11587/0009
Dacarbazine 500 mg medac MA-no.:	PL 11587/0010
Dacarbazine 1000 mg medac MA-no.:	PL 11587/0011

Date of first authorisation/renewal of authorisation 28 November 1997.

Date of (partial) revision of text 23 September 1997.

LOMUSTINE 'medac' 40 mg

Presentation Blue gelatin capsules containing 40 mg lomustine.

Active ingredient: 40 mg lomustine (CCNU: 1-(2-chloroethyl)-3-cyclohexyl-1-nitrosourea).

Uses The mechanism of action is believed to be partly as an alkylating agent and partly by inhibition of several other vital enzymatic processes. Cross-resistance with other nitrosoureas is usual but cross-resistance with conventional alkylating agents is unusual.

Indications: As palliative or supplementary treatment, usually in combination with radiotherapy and/or surgery or as part of multiple drug regimens in:

- brain tumours (primary or metastatic);
- lung tumours (especially oat-cell carcinoma);
- Hodgkin's disease (resistant to conventional combination chemotherapy);
- malignant melanoma (metastatic).

Lomustine 'medac' may also be of value as second-line treatment in non-Hodgkin's lymphoma, myelomatosis, gastrointestinal tumours, carcinoma of the kidney, the testis, the ovary, the cervix uteri and the breast.

Dosage and administration
Adults: Lomustine 'medac' is given by mouth. The recommended dose in patients with normally functioning bone marrow receiving Lomustine 'medac' as their only chemotherapy is 120–130 mg/m² as a single dose every six to eight weeks (or as a divided dose over three days, e.g. 40 mg/m²/day). Dosage is reduced if:

(a) Lomustine 'medac' is being given as part of a drug regimen which includes other marrow-depressant drugs, and
(b) in the presence of leucopenia below 3,000/mm³ or thrombocytopenia below 75,000/mm³.

Marrow depression after Lomustine 'medac' is longer sustained than after nitrogen mustards and recover of white cell and platelet counts may not occur for six weeks or more. Blood elements depressed below the above levels should be allowed to recover to 4,000/mm³ (WBC) and 100,000/mm³ (platelets) before repeating Lomustine 'medac' dosage.

Administration to children: Until further data are available administration of Lomustine 'medac' to children with malignancies other than brain tumours should be restricted to specialised centres and exceptional situations. Dosage in children, like that in adults, is based on body surface area (120–130 mg/m² every six to eight weeks, with the same qualifications as apply to adults).

Contra-indications, warnings, etc This product should not normally be administered to patients who are pregnant or to mothers who are breast feeding. Other contra-indications are:

- Previous hypersensitivity to nitrosoureas;
- Previous failure of the tumour to respond to other nitrosoureas;
- Severe bone marrow depression.

Precautions: Patients receiving Lomustine 'medac' chemotherapy should be under the care of doctors experienced in cancer treatment. Blood counts should be carried out before starting the drug and at frequent intervals (preferably weekly) during treatment. Treatment and dosage is governed principally by the haemoglobin, white cell count and platelet count. Liver function should also be assessed periodically.

Interactions: Lomustine 'medac' used in combination with theophylline may potentiate bone marrow toxicity. Cross-resistance with other nitrosoureas is usual, but cross-resistance with conventional alkylating agents is unusual.

Adverse effects:
Haematological: The principal adverse effect is marrow toxicity of a delayed or prolonged nature. Thrombocytopenia appears about four weeks after a dose of Lomustine 'medac' and lasts one to two weeks at a level around 80–100,000/mm³; leucopenia appears after six weeks and persists for one to two weeks at about 4–5,000/mm³. The haematological toxicity may be cumulative, leading to successively lower white cell and platelet counts with successive doses of the drug.

Gastro-intestinal: Nausea and vomiting usually occur four to six hours after a full single dose of Lomustine 'medac' and last for 24–28 hours, followed by anorexia for two to three days. The effects are less troublesome if the six-weekly dose is divided into three doses and given on each of the first three days of the six-week period. Gastrointestinal tolerance is usually good, however, if prophylactic antinauseants are given (e.g. metoclopramide or chlorpromazine). Transient elevation of liver enzymes (SGOT, SGPT, LDH or alkaline phosphatase) are occasionally observed. More rarely patients are troubled by stomatitis.

Other side-effects: Loss of scalp hair has been reported infrequently.

Overdosage: Symptoms of overdosage with Lomustine 'medac' will probably include bone marrow toxicity, haematological toxicity, nausea and vomiting. Overdosage should be treated immediately by gastric lavage. There is no specific antidote. In the event of dangerously low red cell, white cell or platelet counts, cross-matched whole blood should be given as necessary.

Pharmaceutical precautions The capsules should be stored in the original container and protected from light and moisture.

Legal category POM.

The supply of Lomustine 'medac' capsules is restricted to centres with special experience in the chemotherapy of malignant disease. Lomustine 'medac' capsules are available on prescription only.

Package quantities Plastic bottles of 20 capsules each containing 40 mg lomustine.

Further information Nil.

Product licence number 11587/0003.

TREOSULFAN* CAPSULES
TREOSULFAN* INJECTION

Presentation *Capsules:* White opaque capsules each containing 250 mg Treosulfan.

Injection; Infusion bottles containing 1 g or 5 g Treosulfan, a white crystalline powder.

Uses Treosulfan is a bifunctional alkylating agent which has been shown to possess antineoplastic activity in the animal tumour screen and in clinical trials. The activity of Treosulfan is due to the formation of epoxide compounds in vivo.

Indications: For the treatment of all types of ovarian cancer, either supplementary to surgery or palliatively. Some uncontrolled studies have suggested activity in a wider range of neoplasms.

Because of a lack of cross-resistance reported between Treosulfan and other cytotoxic agents Treosulfan may be useful in any neoplasm refractive to conventional therapy.

Treosulfan has been used in combination regimens in conjunction with vincristine, methotrexate, 5-FU and procarbazine.

Dosage and administration *Capsules:* The following dosage regimens have been indicated. All regimens indicate that a total dose of 21–28 g of Treosulfan should be given in the initial 8 weeks of treatment.

Regimen A: 1 g daily, given in four divided doses for four weeks followed by four weeks off therapy.

Regimen B: 1 g daily, given in four divided doses for two weeks, followed by two weeks off therapy.

Regimen C: 1.5 g daily, given in three divided doses for one week only, followed by three weeks off therapy. If no evidence of haematological toxicity at this dose in Regimen C, increase to 2 g daily in four divided doses for one week for the second and subsequent courses.

These cycles should be repeated with the dose being adjusted if necessary, as outlined below, according to the effect on the peripheral blood counts.

The capsules should be swallowed whole and not allowed to disintegrate within the mouth.

Dose modification (All regimens): For excessive haematological toxicity (white blood cell count less than 3,000/microlitre or thrombocyte count less than 100,000/microlitre) a repeat blood count should be made after 1–2 weeks interval and treatment restarted if haematological parameters are satisfactory, reducing dose as follows:

Regimen A: 1 g daily×28 to 0.75 g daily×28 (and to 0.5 g daily×28 if necessary).

Regimen B: 1 g daily×14 to 0.75 g daily×14 (and to 0.5 g daily×14 if necessary).

Regimen C: 2 g daily×7 to 1.5 g daily×7 (and to 1 g daily×7 if necessary).

Present evidence, while not definitive, suggests that Regimens B and C are less myelosuppressive than Regimen A, whilst retaining maximum cytotoxic efficacy.

Injection: 3–8 g/m² i.v. every 1–3 weeks depending on

blood count and concurrent chemotherapy. Single injections of up to 8 g/m² have been given with no serious adverse effects. Doses up to 1.5 g/m² have been given intraperitoneally. Doses up to 3 g/m² treosulfan may be given as a bolus injection. Larger doses should be administered as an i.v. infusion at a rate of 3 g/m² every 5–10 minutes (8 g/m² as a 30 minutes infusion).

Treosulfan Injection 1 g or 5 g is used for intravenous infusion after being dissolved in 20 or 100 ml of water for injection. Once brought into solution the injection should be used immediately.

Treatment should not be given if the white blood cell count is less than 3,000/microlitre or the thrombocyte count less than 100,000/microlitre. A repeat blood count should be made after a weeks interval, when treatment may be restarted if haematological parameters are satisfactory. Lower doses of Treosulfan should be used if other cytotoxic drugs or radiotherapy are being given concurrently. Treatment is initiated as soon as possible after diagnosis.

Care should be taken in administration of the injection to avoid extravasation into tissues since this will cause local pain and tissue damage. If extravasation occurs, the injection should be discontinued immediately and any remaining portion of the dose should be introduced into another vein.

Dosage in the elderly: Treosulfan is renally excreted. Blood counts should be carefully monitored in the elderly and dosage adjusted accordingly.

Children: Not recommended.

Contra-indications, warnings, etc

Contra-indication: Severe and lasting bone marrow depression.

Warning: This product should not normally be administered to patients who are pregnant or to mothers who are breast feeding.

Women of child-bearing age should take adequate contraceptive precautions.

Adverse reactions: The dose-limiting side-effect of treosulfan is a myelosuppression, which is usually reversible. It is manifested by a reduction in leukocytes and platelets and a decrease in haemoglobin.

The leukocytes and platelets usually reach their baseline level after 28 days.

Because the inhibition of bone marrow function is cumulative, the blood count should be monitored at shorter intervals starting with the third course of treatment.

This is especially important if combined with other forms of therapy that suppress bone marrow function such as radiotherapy.

During long-term therapy with oral treosulfan doses eight patients (1.4% of 553 patients) developed an acute non-lymphatic leukaemia.

Skin: Mild alopecia is observed in 16% of the patients and a skin pigmentation in the form of a bronze discoloration in up to 30% of the cases.

The occurrence of urticaria, erythemas, a scleroderma and triggering of a psoriasis have been reported.

Respiratory: In rare cases allergic alveolitis, pneumonia and pulmonary fibrosis have developed.

Gastro-intestinal: Nausea with or without vomiting is observed in approx. 50% of the patients.

Other adverse reactions: In rare cases flu-like complaints, a paraesthesia, haemorrhagic cystitis, Addison's disease and hypoglycaemia have been observed. It cannot be totally ruled out that one case of cardiomyopathy was related to treosulfan.

Due to the possible development of a haemorrhagic cystitis patients are advised to drink more fluids for up to 24 hours after infusion.

During infusion, care must be taken to use a flawless technique, since painful inflammatory reactions may occur as a result of extravasation of treosulfan solution into surrounding tissue.

Overdosage: Although there is no experience of acute overdosage with Treosulfan, nausea, vomiting and gastritis may occur.

Prolonged or excessive therapeutic doses may result in bone marrow depression which has occasionally been irreversible. The drug should be withdrawn, a blood transfusion given and general supportive measures given.

Pharmaceutical precautions As with all cytotoxic substances appropriate precautions should be taken when handling treosulfan.

Guidelines for the safe handling of antineoplastic agents:

1. Trained personnel should reconstitute the drug.
2. This should be performed in a designated area.
3. Adequate protective gloves, masks and clothing should be worn.
4. Precautions should be taken to avoid the drug accidentally coming into contact with the eyes.
5. Cytotoxic preparations should not be handled by staff who may be pregnant.
6. Adequate care and precautions should be taken in the disposal of items (syringes, needles, etc.) used to reconstitute cytotoxic drugs.
7. The work surface should be covered with disposable plastic-backed absorbent paper.
8. Use Luer-lock fittings on all syringes and sets. Large bore needles are recommended to minimize pressure and the possible formation of aerosols. The latter may also be reduced by the use of a venting needle.

Legal category POM.

Package quantities *Capsules:* Amber glass bottles of 100 capsules.

Injection: Boxes of 5×100 ml infusion bottles, each containing 1 g or 5 g Treosulfan, complete with 5 plastic bottle holders.

Further information All centres using Treosulfan have reported noteworthy improvements in the general condition of patients responding to treatment, particularly in regard to reduction or disappearance of ascites. Treosulfan is remarkably well tolerated allowing many patients to become fully ambulatory and return to their normal day to day work.

Product licence numbers

Capsules	11587/0001
Injection	11587/0002

**Trade Mark*

Medeva Pharma Limited

(formerly Evans Medical Ltd)
Medeva House
Regent Park
Kingston Road
Leatherhead
Surrey KT22 7PQ

☎ 01372 364000 📠 01372 364018

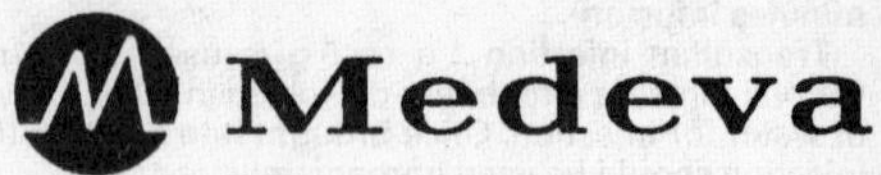

ARILVAX* YELLOW FEVER VACCINE, LIVE BP

Qualitative and quantitative composition The composition in terms of active ingredients is as follows:

Each 0.5 ml dose of reconstituted vaccine contains the equivalent of not less than 1000 mouse LD_{50} units as defined by the World Health Organisation requirements

Pharmaceutical form Stabilised freeze-dried preparation, reconstituted with Water for Injections, BP prior to subcutaneous injection in humans

Clinical particulars

Therapeutic indications: For active immunisation of residents in yellow fever endemic areas. Yellow fever endemic areas are limited to the African and South American continents and Central America.

For active immunisation of travellers to and from such areas.

For the issue of an International Certificate of Vaccination, as required by the national health authorities of certain countries which consider these zones as infected areas (although the 'yellow fever endemic zones' are in fact no longer included in the International Health Regulations). The International Health Regulations define the form of certificate of vaccination to be used which, in the case of primary vaccination, is valid for a period of 10 years from the 10th day after vaccination. In the case of revaccination within 10 years, the certificate is valid at once.

Posology and method of administration:

Children aged 9 months and over, adults and elderly: The dose is 0.5 ml of reconstituted vaccine, given subcutaneously. This dose is the same for persons of all ages.

Children under 9 months of age: Not recommended.

It is good practice to record the title, dose and lot numbers of all vaccines and the dates of administration.

Contra-indications: The vaccine should not be administered to a subject who has experienced a serious reaction (e.g. anaphylaxis) to a previous dose of this vaccine or who is known to be hypersensitive to any component thereof. It is advisable to avoid vaccination during an acute infection. Since the vaccine is prepared in chick embryos and contains small quantities of neomycin and polymyxin, it should not be administered to individuals who are hypersensitive to egg or chick protein or to these antibiotics.

The vaccine should not be given to those with impaired immune responsiveness, whether congenital, idiopathic or as a result of treatment with steroids (with the exception of standard doses of locally-acting, e.g. topical or inhaled, steroids), radiotherapy, cytotoxic drugs or other agents.

The vaccine should not be given to either symptomatic or asymptomatic HIV positive individuals since there is insufficient evidence as to the safety of its use.

Special warnings and precautions for use: The vaccine is not recommended for use in children under the age of 9 months. The decision to vaccinate infants under this age must depend on the anticipated risk of exposure to the disease, since the small number of cases of encephalitis that have been reported, have nearly all occurred in infants under this age.

It is advisable to avoid administration of the vaccine within 6 weeks following the administration of immune globulin on general principles. Similarly, on theoretical grounds it is advisable to avoid the administration of immune globulin within 2 weeks following vaccination. An interval of not less than 3 weeks should normally be allowed to lapse between the administration of any two live vaccines. If time does not permit then they might be given simultaneously at separate sites.

Although anaphylaxis is rare, facilities for its management should always be available during vaccination

Interaction with other medicaments and other forms of interaction: None stated.

Pregnancy and lactation: On theoretical grounds the vaccine should not be administered during pregnancy and lactation.

Effects on ability to drive and use machines: None stated.

Undesirable effects: Severe reactions to the vaccine are extremely rare and include encephalitis and allergic reactions. Occasionally some redness, soreness and swelling may occur at the site of injection, and headache has been reported. Myalgia and low-grade fever may occur a few days after immunisation.

Rare cases of urticaria, bursitis, jaundice and neuritis have been reported in a temporal relationship to vaccination.

Any untoward reactions should be reported to the regulatory authorities and to the manufacturer.

Overdose: Not applicable

Pharmacological particulars

Pharmacodynamic properties: Not applicable

Pharmacokinetic properties: Not applicable

Preclinical safety data: Not applicable

Pharmaceutical particulars

List of excipients: The excipients contained in the preparation are as follows: Polymyxin B sulphate BP, Neomycin sulphate BP, Sorbitol BP, Hydrolysed gelatin HSE*, Sodium chloride PhEur, Disodium hydrogen orthophosphate HSE*, Potassium chloride HSE*, Potassium dihydrogen orthophosphate HSE*, Water for Injections PhEur

Prior to use the vaccine is diluted with Water for Injections BP.

*HSE House specification

Incompatibilities: None stated.

Shelf life:

Vaccine: In filled containers:- 3 years at 2-8°C. After reconstitution:- 1 hour kept cool

Diluent: In filled containers: 3 years at below 25°C

Special precautions for storage: The freeze-dried vaccine should be stored between 2-8°C. Protect from light. Diluent should not be frozen but should be stored below 25°C. After reconstitution the vaccine should be kept cool, protected from light and used within one hour.

Nature and contents of container:

Vaccine: Single Dose: PhEur Type I clear neutral glass vials, 3 ml capacity with grey butyl rubber stopper, aluminium seal and a blue polypropylene flip-off top.

Multi-dose: PhEur Type I clear neutral glass vials, 8 ml capacity with either grey butyl rubber stopper, aluminium seal and a blue polypropylene flip-off top, or red chlorbutyl rubber stopper, aluminium seal and a yellow polypropylene flip-off top.

Diluent : PhEur type I clear neutral glass ampoules, 1 ml or 5 ml.

Instructions for use and handling: The Water for Injections BP supplied should be used for reconstitution using a sterile syringe and needle. The entire contents of the appropriate diluent container are injected into the vaccine vial and gently agitated to ensure reconstitution. The vacuum in the vaccine vial may be broken to facilitate withdrawal of the vaccine solution. After reconstitution, the vaccine should be kept cool and used within one hour.

Contamination with bactericides should be avoided. Use a fresh sterile disposal syringe and needle free from traces of spirit and disinfectant for each injection.

Disposal should be by incineration at a temperature of not less than 1100°C at a registered waste disposal contractor.

Do not attempt to obtain more than the stated number of doses from the vial.

Marketing authorisation numbers

Yellow Fever Vaccine, Live BP	0039/0476
Water for Injections BP	0039/5704

Date of approval/revision of SPC November 1994

Legal category POM

ASMABEC* CLICKHALER* 50, 100, 250

Qualitative and quantitative composition The inhaler contains a powder blend of Beclomethasone Dipropionate with lactose.

The inhaler is available in three strengths: 50, 100 and 250 micrograms of beclomethasone dipropionate in each metered actuation.

Pharmaceutical form Inhalation powder administered from a multidose powder inhaler.

Clinical particulars

Therapeutic Indications: Beclomethasone Dipropionate is indicated for the prophylactic treatment of asthma.

Posology and method of administration: Adults: The usual starting dose is 400 mcg daily, inhaled in 2 to 4 divided doses for maintenance treatment. If necessary dosage may be started at, or increased to, 600 to 800 mcg and subsequently adjusted according to the patient's response. The total daily dose may be administered as two, three or four divided doses.

In patients with severe asthma doses of 1 mg daily (250 mcg four times daily or 500 mcg twice daily) may be used and may be increased to 1.5 to 2 mg daily.

Elderly: as for adults.

Children: 50 or 100 mcg may be inhaled 2 to 4 times daily according to the response.

The 250 mcg inhaler is not suitable for administration to children.

The dose should be titrated to the lowest dose at which effective control of symptoms is achieved.

Contra-indications: Asmabec Clickhaler is contra-indicated in patients with a history of hypersensitivity to any of its components. Special care is necessary in patients with active or quiescent pulmonary tuberculosis.

Special warnings and precautions for use: Patients should be instructed in the proper use of the inhaler. They should also be made aware of the prophylactic nature of therapy with Asmabec Clickhaler and that they should use it regularly, every day, even when they are asymptomatic.

Increasing use of bronchodilators, in particular short-acting inhaled β_2-agonists, to relieve symptoms indicates deterioration of asthma control. If patients find that short-acting relief bronchodilator treatment becomes less effective, or they need more inhalations than usual, medical attention must be sought. In this situation patients should be reassessed and consideration given to the need for increased anti-inflammatory therapy (e.g. higher doses of inhaled corticosteroids or a course of oral corticosteroids). Severe exacerbations of asthma must be treated in the normal way.

Systemic effects of inhaled corticosteroids may occur, particularly at high doses prescribed for prolonged periods. Possible systemic effects include adrenal suppression, growth retardation in children and adolescents, decrease in bone mineral density, cataract and glaucoma. It is important therefore that the dose of inhaled steroids is titrated to the lowest dose at which effective control of symptoms is achieved.

It is recommended that the height of children receiving prolonged treatment with inhaled steroids is regularly monitored. If growth is slowed, therapy should be reviewed with the aim of reducing the dose of inhaled corticosteroid if possible, to the lowest dose at which effective control of symptoms is achieved.

Doses in excess of 1500 micrograms per day may induce adrenal suppression. In such patients the risks of developing adrenal suppression should be balanced against the therapeutic advantages, and precautions should be taken to provide systemic steroid cover in situations of stress or elective surgery.

The transfer to inhaled beclomethasone dipropionate of patients who have been treated with systemic steroids for long periods of time, or at high dose, needs special care and subsequent management as recovery from impaired adrenocortical function is slow. With these patients adrenocortical function should be monitored regularly and their dose of systemic steroid reduced cautiously. Gradual withdrawal of the systemic steroid should commence after about one week. Reductions in dosage, appropriate to the level of maintenance systemic steroid, should be introduced at not less than weekly intervals.

Some patients may feel unwell in a non-specific way during withdrawal of the systemic steroid. They should be encouraged to persevere with the inhaled beclomethasone dipropionate, unless there are objective signs of adrenal insufficiency.

Patients who have been transferred from oral steroids whose adrenocortical function is impaired should carry a steroid warning card indicating that they may need supplementary systemic steroids during periods of stress, eg. worsening asthma attacks, chest infections, major intercurrent illness, surgery, trauma etc.

Replacement of systemic steroid treatment with inhaled therapy sometimes unmasks allergies such as allergic rhinitis or eczema previously controlled by the systemic drug.

Treatment with Asmabec Clickhaler should not be stopped abruptly.

Interactions with other medicaments and other forms of interaction: None known.

Pregnancy and lactation: Pregnancy: There are insufficient data regarding the safety of beclomethasone dipropionate during human pregnancy. Systemic administration of relatively high doses of corticosteroids to pregnant animals can cause abnormalities of foetal development including cleft palate and intra-uterine growth retardation. There may therefore be a very small risk of such effects in the human foetus. Because beclomethasone dipropionate is delivered directly to the lungs by the inhaled route it avoids the high level of exposure that occurs when corticosteroids are given by systemic routes.

The use of beclomethasone dipropionate in pregnancy requires that the possible benefits of the drug be weighed against the possible hazards. It should be noted that the drug has been in widespread use for many years without apparent ill consequence.

Lactation: It is reasonable to assume that beclomethasone dipropionate is secreted in milk, but at the dosages used for direct inhalation there is low potential for significant levels in breast milk.

The use of beclomethasone dipropionate in mothers breast feeding their babies requires that the therapeutic benefits of the drug be weighed against the potential hazards to the mother and baby.

Effects on ability to drive and use machines: None known

Undesirable effects: Candidiasis of the mouth and throat (thrush) may occur in some patients. Patients with high blood levels of *Candida precipitins*, indicating a previous infection, are most likely to develop this complication which can be treated whilst still continuing with Asmabec Clickhaler. Hoarseness may also occur. It may be helpful to rinse out the mouth thoroughly with water immediately after inhalation.

As with other inhalation therapy, the potential for paradoxical bronchospasm should be kept in mind. If it occurs, the preparation should be discontinued immediately and, if necessary, alternative therapy instituted.

Systemic effects of inhaled corticosteroids may occur, particularly at high doses prescribed for prolonged periods. These may include adrenal suppression, growth retardation in children and adolescents, decrease in bone mineral density, cataract and glaucoma.

Overdose: Acute: Inhalation of a large amount of the drug over a short period may lead to temporary suppression of adrenal function. No emergency action is required. Treatment with beclomethasone dipropionate by inhalation should be continued at a dose sufficient to control asthma; adrenal function recovers in a few days and can be verified by measuring plasma cortisol.

Chronic: Use of excessive doses of inhaled beclomethasone dipropionate over a prolonged period may cause adrenal suppression and a degree of atrophy of the adrenal cortex. Transfer to a maintenance dose of a systemic steroid may be required until the condition is stabilised. Treatment with inhaled beclomethasone dipropionate should then be continued at a dose sufficient to control asthma.

Pharmacological properties

Pharmacodynamic properties: Beclomethasone dipropionate is a potent glucocorticoid which has an anti-inflammatory action on the airways following inhalation.

Beclomethasone dipropionate's actions include the following: inhibition of adherence of neutrophils and monocyte-macrophages to endothelial cells, inhibition of activation of plasminogen to plasmin and inhibition of the synthesis of prostaglandins and leukotrienes (via inhibition of phospholipase A_2). It results in a reduction in bronchial hyper-responsiveness and symptoms of asthma.

The maximum beneficial effect may take 1–3 months to achieve. Although inhaled beclomethasone dipropionate has no effect after single dosing on the immediate response to allergen or exercise, there is a protective effect when it is taken regularly over several days.

Pharmacokinetic properties: Absorption from the gastrointestinal tract is slow and bioavailability is low, suggesting that most of the absorbed drug is metabolised during its first passage through the liver. Since the dose of oral beclomethasone dipropionate needed to suppress plasma cortisol is greater than that required by inhalation, this suggests that the portion absorbed from the lungs is mainly responsible for any systemic effects.

Preclinical safety data: Studies in a number of animal species, including rats, rabbits and dogs, have shown no unusual toxicity during acute experiments. The effects of beclomethasone dipropionate in producing signs of glucocorticoid excess during chronic administration by various routes are dose related. Teratogenicity testing has shown cleft palate in mice, as with other glucocorticoids. Beclomethasone dipropionate is non-genotoxic and demonstrates no oncogenic potential in lifetime studies with rats.

Pharmaceutical particulars

List of excipients: Lactose PhEur.

Incompatibilities: None known.

Shelf life: 2 years in unopened foil pouch. 6 months when removed from the foil pouch.

Special precautions for storage: Store in a dry place at room temperature (up to 30°C).

Nature and contents of container: A plastic inhaler device incorporating a specially designed actuator enclosed within an aluminium foil, heat-sealed bag. The number of actuations each device contains are:

50 microgram inhaler – 200 actuations
100 microgram inhaler – 200 actuations
250 microgram inhaler – 100 actuations.

Instructions for use/handling: 1. Remove mouthpiece cover from the inhaler.

2. Shake the inhaler well.

3. Hold the inhaler upright with thumb on the base and finger on the push button. Press the dosing button down firmly–once only.

4. Breathe out as far as is comfortable. Note: do not blow into the device at any time.

5. Place mouthpiece in your mouth. Close lips firmly around it (do not bite it).

6. Breathe in through your mouth steadily and deeply, to draw the medicine into your lungs.

7. Hold your breath, take the inhaler from your mouth and continue holding your breath for about 5 seconds.

8. For the second puff, keep the inhaler upright and repeat steps 2–7.

9. Replace the mouthpiece cover.

Marketing authorisation numbers

50 mcg: 0039/0501
100 mcg: 0039/0502
250 mcg: 0039/0503

Date of approval/revision of the text 30 October 1998

ASMABEC* SPACEHALER* 50 micrograms, 100 micrograms

Qualitative and quantitative composition Asmabec Spacehaler 50 micrograms: Each actuation contains 50 micrograms Beclomethasone Dipropionate BP.

Asmabec Spacehaler 100 micrograms: Each actuation contains 100 micrograms Beclomethasone Dipropionate BP.

Pharmaceutical form Metered-dose inhaler with Spacehaler actuator.

The Spacehaler is a vortex generating actuator which acts to reduce the velocity of the emitted dose. Compared with a standard actuator it decreases the proportion of non-respirable drug particles within the emitted dose cloud whilst achieving a similar respirable fraction.

Clinical particulars

Therapeutic indications:

(i) Treatment of patients whose asthma is becoming worse, and the relief provided by bronchodilators is less effective.

(ii) Treatment of patients with severe asthma who are dependent on systemic corticosteroids or adrenocorticotrophic hormone (ACTH) or its synthetic equivalent.

(iii) Treatment of patients who are inadequately controlled by sodium cromoglycate in addition to bronchodilators.

Posology and method of administration: The dose should be titrated to the lowest dose at which effective control of asthma is maintained.

Adults: The usual starting dose is 200 micrograms twice a day. In more severe cases dosage may be started at, or increased to 600–800 micrograms per day, and subsequently reduced when the patient's asthma has stabilised. The total daily dose may be administered as two, three or four divided doses.

Elderly: There is no need to adjust the dose in elderly patients or in those with hepatic or renal impairment.

Children: 50–100 micrograms should be given two, three or four times daily according to response. Alternatively, 100 or 200 micrograms twice daily may be administered. The usual starting dose is 100 micrograms twice a day.

Contra-indications: Patients with a history of hypersensitivity to any of its components. Special care is necessary in patients with active or quiescent pulmonary tuberculosis.

Special warnings and precautions for use: Patients should be instructed on the proper use of the inhaler to ensure that the drug reaches the target areas within the lungs. They should also be made aware that Asmabec Spacehaler has to be used regularly for optimum benefit. Patients should be made aware of the prophylactic nature of therapy with Asmabec Spacehaler and that it should be taken regularly, even when they are asymptomatic.

The maximum daily intake of Asmabec Spacehaler 50 and 100 micrograms should not exceed 1 mg.

Systemic effects of inhaled corticosteroids may occur, particularly at high doses prescribed for prolonged periods. These effects are much less likely to occur than with oral corticosteroids. Possible systemic effects include adrenal suppression, growth retardation in children and adolescents, decrease in bone mineral density, cataract and glaucoma. It is important therefore that the dose of inhaled corticosteroid is titrated to the lowest dose at which effective control of asthma is maintained.

It is recommended that the height of children receiving prolonged treatment with inhaled corticosteroids is regularly monitored. If growth is slowed, therapy should be reviewed with the aim of reducing the dose of inhaled corticosteroid, if possible, to the lowest dose at which effective control of asthma is maintained. In addition, consideration should be given to referring the patient to a paediatric respiratory specialist.

Prolonged treatment with high doses of inhaled corticosteroids, particularly higher than the recommended doses, may result in clinically significant adrenal suppression. Additional systemic corticosteroid cover should be considered during periods of stress or elective surgery.

Patients inadequately controlled by bronchodilator therapy: The use of Asmabec Spacehaler in patients who have never taken steroids or taken only occasional courses of steroids is straightforward. An improvement in respiratory function is normally obvious within a week. The few patients who do not respond during this period usually have excessive mucus in their bronchi so that the drug is unable to penetrate to its site of action. In such cases, a short course of systemic steroid in relatively high dosage should be given to control secretion of mucus and other inflammatory changes in the lungs. Continuation of treatment with Asmabec Spacehaler usually maintains the improvement achieved, the oral steroid being gradually withdrawn. Exacerbation of asthma caused by infections is usually controlled by appropriate antibiotic treatment, by increasing the dose of inhaled beclomethasone dipropionate and, if necessary, by giving a systemic steroid. Use of a Beta-2-agonist may also be required.

Oral steroid-dependent patients: The transfer of oral steroid-dependent patients to Asmabec Spacehaler and their subsequent management needs special care mainly because recovery from impaired adrenocortical function caused by prolonged systemic steroid therapy is slow. The patient should be in a reasonably stable state before being given Asmabec Spacehaler in addition to his usual maintenance dose of systemic steroid. After about a week, gradual withdrawal of the systemic steroid is started by reducing the daily dose by 1 mg prednisolone, or its equivalent of other corticosteroids, at not less than weekly intervals. Patients treated with systemic steroids for long periods of time or who have received high doses may have adrenocortical suppression. With these patients adrenocortical function should be monitored regularly and their dose of systemic steroid reduced cautiously. Some patients feel unwell during the withdrawal phase despite maintenance or even improvement of respiratory function. They should be encouraged to persevere with the inhaler and withdrawal of systemic steroid continued unless there are objective signs of adrenal insufficiency. Most patients can be successfully transferred to Asmabec Spacehaler with maintenance of good respiratory function, but special care is necessary for the first months after the transfer until the pituitary-adrenal system has sufficiently recovered to enable the patient to cope with emergencies such as trauma, surgery or infections.

Transferred patients whose adrenocortical function is impaired should carry a warning card indicating that they need supplementary systemic steroids during periods of stress, e.g. surgery, chest infection or worsening asthma attacks, but that this can be reduced again after the stress has been resolved. They should also be given a supply of oral steroid to use in emergency, for example when the asthma worsens as a result of a chest infection. The dose of beclomethasone should be increased at this time and then reduced to the maintenance level after the systemic steroid has been discontinued. Replacement of systemic steroid treatment with Asmabec Spacehaler sometimes unmasks allergies such as allergic rhinitis or eczema previously controlled by the systemic drug. These allergies should be symptomatically treated with antihistamine and/or topical preparations.

Interactions with other medicaments and other forms of interaction: None known.

Pregnancy and lactation: Beclomethasone dipropionate should only be used in pregnancy or lactation if the potential benefit outweighs the risk. There is insufficient data regarding safety in human pregnancy. High doses of systemic corticosteroids in pregnant animals can cause abnormalities in foetal development, including cleft palate and intra-uterine growth retardation.

No data regarding excretion of beclomethasone dipropionate in human breast milk is available. However, the dosages recommended for Asmabec Spacehalers suggest a lower potential for transfer to the foetus or infant than with systemic corticosteroids.

Effects on ability to drive and use machines: On the basis of the pharmacodynamic profile, reported adverse drug reactions (ADR) and/or impairment of driving performance related to driving, the medicine is presumed to be safe or unlikely to produce an effect.

Undesirable effects: In some patients hoarseness or throat irritation may occur. Rinsing the mouth and throat with water after each dose to remove residual medication may be helpful.

Paradoxical bronchospasm may occur, in which case use of the inhaler should cease immediately and medical advice should be sought. Alternative therapy should be introduced.

Candidiasis of the mouth and throat (thrush) occurs in some patients; the incidence of which is increased with doses greater than 400 micrograms beclomethasone dipropionate per day. Patients with high blood levels of Candida precipitins, indicating a previous infection, are more likely to develop this complication. Such patients may find it helpful to rinse their mouth with water after using the inhaler. Symptomatic candidiasis can be treated with topical anti-fungal therapy whilst still continuing with Asmabec Spacehaler.

Systemic effects of inhaled corticosteroids may occur, particularly at high doses prescribed for prolonged periods. These may include adrenal suppression, growth retardation in children and adolescents, decrease in bone mineral density, cataract and glaucoma.

Overdose: The acute toxicity of beclomethasone dipropionate is low. The only harmful effect that follows inhalation of large amounts of the drug over a short period is suppression of hypothalamic-pituitary-adrenal (HPA) function. No special emergency action need be taken. Treatment with Asmabec Spacehaler should be continued at the recommended dose to control the asthma; HPA function recovers in a day or two.

Reduction of plasma cortisol levels has been reported in patients who received twice the daily recommended maximum dose of beclomethasone dipropionate. In the unlikely event of excessive intake of beclomethasone dipropionate for weeks or months on end, a degree of adrenocortical atrophy could occur in addition to suppression of HPA function. The patient should be treated as steroid-dependent and transferred to a suitable maintenance dose of a systemic steroid such as prednisolone. Once the patient's condition has stabilised they should be transferred to Asmabec Spacehaler.

To guard against the unexpected event of adrenal suppression, regular tests of adrenal function are advised.

Pharmacological properties
Pharmacodynamic properties: Beclomethasone dipropionate by inhalation has a potent glucocorticoid anti-inflammatory action within the lungs, but at recommended dosage, is without significant systemic activity.

Beclomethasone dipropionate also has vasoconstrictor effects and it inhibits the late responses to antigen challenge.

Pharmacokinetic properties: The pharmacokinetics of beclomethasone dipropionate have not been extensively studied. The currently available chemical methods are not of sufficient sensitivity to measure therapeutically relevant plasma concentrations, particularly those occurring following inhalation.

a) general characteristics of the active substance
- absorption: Beclomethasone dipropionate is readily absorbed from the gastro-intestinal tract. It is also well absorbed from sites of local application.
- distribution: About 25% of an inhaled dose reaches the lungs.

The drug is rapidly distributed to all body tissues. It crosses the placenta and may be excreted in small amounts in breast milk.

- elimination: The drug and its metabolites are excreted chiefly in the faeces via biliary elimination and to a lesser extent in the urine.

b) characteristics in patients
As above.

Preclinical safety data: See Clinical particulars above.

Pharmaceutical particulars
List of excipients: Oleic Acid BP, Trichlorofluoromethane (1988) BP, Dichlorodifluoromethane (1988) BP.

Incompatibilities: None known.

Shelf life: Shelf-life in the product as packaged for sale: 24 months.

Special precautions for storage: Store below 30°C. Protect from frost and direct sunlight. The canister is pressurised, it must not be burnt, punctured or broken even when apparently empty. The therapeutic effect of the medication may decrease when the canister is cold.

Nature and contents of container: The container consists of a seamless aluminium can with a metering dispensing valve crimped to it. The can is inserted into a plastic oral inhalation actuator with a dust cap.

The can is a 19 millilitre nominal capacity aerosol can of deep drawn NS4 aluminium with either a debossed or plain base.

The metering aerosol valves used are 20 mm types, with a nominal 63 microlitre dosing capacity. The valve is composed of metal and rubber components and is assembled into a metal ferrule.

The actuator supports the container during actuation and directs the sprayed aerosol particles into the mouth. The actuator is injection moulded polypropylene which may be plain, printed or embossed with the name of the product. A mouthpiece cover is fitted over the actuator mouthpiece to prevent the ingress of particulates into the mouthpiece cavity between uses.

Instruction for use/handling: Instructions as shown in the leaflet:

1. Remove the cap from the inhaler mouthpiece. Make sure the mouthpiece is clean and clear of fluff and dirt.
2. Hold the inhaler upright, with your thumb on the base and your first finger on the top of the can. Now shake the inhaler gently up and down.
3. Breathe out fully to empty the lungs and then place the mouthpiece firmly between the lips.
4. Now breathe in slowly and deeply. At the same time press the aerosol can with your first finger to fire the aerosol and release the drug.
5. Remove the inhaler from your mouth and hold breath for 10 seconds or as long as is comfortable. Breathe out slowly.
6. If more than one puff is required, wait at least one minute and repeat procedure from step 2. Replace the cap.
7. Your inhaler should be cleaned regularly usually at least once a week. To clean, remove the metal canister from the plastic body and remove the plastic cover from the mouthpiece. Rinse the plastic body and the mouthpiece cover in warm water. Dry thoroughly then replace the canister and mouthpiece cover. Avoid excessive heat. Do not put the metal canister into water.

Important: Do not rush steps 3 and 4. It is important that you start to breathe in as slowly as possible just before operating your inhaler. Practice in the mirror for the first few times. If you see a 'mist' coming from the top of your inhaler or the sides of your mouth, you should start again from step 2.

Marketing authorisation numbers
Asmabec Spacehaler 50 micrograms:
0039/0480
Asmabec Spacehaler 100 micrograms:
0039/0481

Date of approval/revision of the SPC August 1998

Legal Category POM

ASMABEC* SPACEHALER* 250 micrograms

Qualitative and quantitative composition Each actuation contains 250 micrograms Beclomethasone Dipropionate BP.

Pharmaceutical form Metered-dose inhaler with Spacehaler actuator.

The Spacehaler is a vortex generating actuator which acts to reduce the velocity of the emitted dose. Compared with a standard actuator it decreases the proportion of non-respirable drug particles within the emitted dose cloud whilst achieving a similar respirable fraction.

Clinical particulars
Therapeutic indications:

(i) Asmabec Spacehaler 250 micrograms is indicated for those asthmatic patients who have been shown to require high doses (greater than 800–1000 micrograms daily) of Beclomethasone Dipropionate BP to control their symptoms.

(ii) It may also be indicated for those patients whose asthma is no longer controlled by maximum maintenance doses of bronchodilators and Asmabec Spacehaler 50 micrograms or Asmabec Spacehaler 100 micrograms. Some patients with severe asthma require oral corticosteroid therapy in addition to Asmabec Spacehaler 50 micrograms or Asmabec Spacehaler 100 micrograms for the adequate control of their symptoms. Many of these patients may, on transfer to Asmabec Spacehaler 250 micrograms, be able to reduce significantly or eliminate their requirement for additional oral corticosteroids .

Posology and method of administration: The dose should be titrated to the lowest dose at which effective control of asthma is maintained.

Adults: Patients should be given a starting dose of inhaled beclomethasone dipropionate which is appropriate for the severity of their disease. The dose may then be adjusted until control is achieved, or reduced to the minimum effective dose according to individual response.

Patients demonstrating a need for high dose inhaled steroid therapy should start on 1,000 micrograms daily.

The usual maintenance dose is two inhalations (500 micrograms) twice daily, or one inhalation (250 micrograms) four times daily. If necessary, dosage may be increased to two inhalations (500 micrograms) three or four times daily according to response.

Elderly: There is no need to adjust the dose in elderly patients or in those with hepatic or renal impairment.

Children: Asmabec Spacehaler 250 micrograms is not indicated for use in children.

Contra-indications: Patients with a history of hypersensitivity to any of its components. Special care is necessary in patients with active or quiescent pulmonary tuberculosis.

Special warnings and precautions for use: Patients should be instructed on the proper use of the inhaler to ensure that the drug reaches the target areas within the lungs. They should also be made aware that Asmabec Spacehaler 250 micrograms has to be used regularly for optimum benefit. Patients should be made aware of the prophylactic nature of therapy with Asmabec Spacehaler 250 micrograms and that it should be taken regularly, even when they are asymptomatic.

Patients being treated with Asmabec Spacehaler 50 micrograms or Asmabec Spacehaler 100 micrograms may be transferred directly to treatment with Asmabec Spacehaler 250 micrograms.

Increasing use of bronchodilators, in particular short-acting inhaled β_2-agonists, to relieve symptoms indicates deterioration of asthma control. If patients find that short-acting relief bronchodilator treatment becomes less effective, or they need more inhalations than usual, medical attention must be sought. In this situation patients should be reassessed and consideration given to the need for increased anti-inflammatory therapy (e.g. higher doses of inhaled corticosteroids or a course of oral corticosteroids). Severe exacerbation of asthma must be treated in the normal way. Exacerbation of asthma caused by infections is usually controlled by appropriate antibiotic treatment, by increasing the dose of inhaled beclomethasone dipropionate and, if necessary, by giving a systemic steroid. Use of a β_2-agonist may also be required.

Systemic effects of inhaled corticosteroids may occur, particularly at high doses prescribed for prolonged periods. These effects are much less likely to occur than with oral corticosteroids. Possible systemic effects include adrenal suppression, growth retardation in children and adolescents, decrease in bone mineral density, cataract and glaucoma. It is important therefore that the dose of inhaled corticosteroid is titrated to the lowest dose at which effective control of asthma is maintained.

It is recommended that the height of children receiving prolonged treatment with inhaled corticosteroids is regularly monitored. If growth is slowed, therapy should be reviewed with the aim of reducing the dose of inhaled corticosteroid, if possible, to the lowest dose at which effective control of asthma is maintained. In addition, consideration should be given to referring the patient to a paediatric respiratory specialist.

Prolonged treatment with high doses of inhaled corticosteroids, particularly higher than the recommended doses, may result in clinically significant adrenal suppression. Additional systemic corticosteroid cover should be considered during periods of stress or elective surgery.

Patients being treated with oral corticosteroids should be in a stable state before having Asmabec Spacehaler 250 micrograms added to their current therapy. After about a week, gradual withdrawal of the systemic steroid is started by reducing the daily dose by 1 mg prednisolone, or its equivalent of other corticosteroids, at not less than weekly intervals. Patients who have been treated with systemic steroids for long periods of time or at a high dose may have adrenocortical suppression. With these patients adrenocortical function should be monitored regularly and their dose of systemic steroid reduced cautiously. Some patients feel unwell during the withdrawal phase despite maintenance or even improvement of respiratory function. They should be encouraged to persevere with the inhaler and withdrawal of systemic steroid continued unless there are objective signs of adrenal insufficiency. Most patients can be successfully transferred to Asmabec Spacehaler 250 micrograms with maintenance of good respiratory function, but special care is necessary for the first months after the transfer until the pituitary-adrenal system has sufficiently recovered to enable the patient to cope with emergencies such as trauma, surgery or infections. Patients recently transferred from oral steroids to Asmabec Spacehaler 250 micrograms together with those still receiving oral steroids should carry a warning card indicating that they may need to start or increase the dosage of oral steroids during periods of stress, e.g. surgery, chest infection or worsening asthmatic attacks, but that this can be reduced again after the stress has been resolved. A small supply of oral steroids can be given to them for emergency use.

Treatment with Asmabec Spacehaler 250 micrograms should not be stopped abruptly.

Replacement of systemic steroid treatment with Asmabec Spacehaler 250 micrograms sometimes unmasks allergies such as allergic rhinitis or eczema previously controlled by the systemic drug. These allergies should be symptomatically treated with antihistamine and/or topical preparations.

Interactions with other medicaments and other forms of interaction: None known.

Pregnancy and lactation: Beclomethasone dipropionate should only be used in pregnancy or lactation if the potential benefit outweighs the risk. There is insufficient data regarding safety in human pregnancy. High doses of systemic corticosteroids in pregnant animals can cause abnormalities in foetal development, including cleft palate and intra-uterine growth retardation.

No data regarding excretion of beclomethasone dipropionate in human breast milk is available. However, the dosages recommended for Asmabec Spacehalers suggest a lower potential for transfer to the foetus or infant than with systemic corticosteroids.

Effects on ability to drive and use machines: On the basis of the pharmacodynamic profile, reported adverse drug reactions (ADR) and/or impairment of driving performance related to driving, the medicine is presumed to be safe or unlikely to produce an effect.

Undesirable effects: In some patients hoarseness or throat irritation may occur. Rinsing the mouth and throat with water after each dose to remove residual medication may be helpful.

Paradoxical bronchospasm may occur, in which case use of the inhaler should cease immediately and medical advice should be sought. Alternative therapy should be introduced.

Candidiasis of the mouth and throat (thrush) occurs in some patients; the incidence of which is increased with doses greater than 400 micrograms beclomethasone dipropionate per day. Patients with high blood levels of Candida precipitins, indicating a previous infection, are more likely to develop this complication. Such patients may find it helpful to rinse their mouth with water after using the inhaler. Symptomatic candidiasis can be treated with topical anti-fungal therapy whilst still continuing with Asmabec Spacehaler.

Systemic effects of inhaled corticosteroids may occur, particularly at high doses prescribed for prolonged periods. These may include adrenal suppression, growth retardation in children and adolescents, decrease in bone mineral density, cataract and glaucoma.

Overdose: The acute toxicity of beclomethasone dipropionate is low. The only harmful effect that follows inhalation of large amounts of the drug over a short period is suppression of hypothalamic-pituitary-adrenal (HPA) function. No special emergency action need be taken. Treatment with Asmabec Spacehaler should be continued at the recommended dose to control the asthma; HPA function recovers in a day or two.

Reduction of plasma cortisol levels has been reported in patients who received twice the daily recommended maximum dose of beclomethasone dipropionate. In the unlikely event of excessive intake of beclomethasone dipropionate for weeks or months on end, a degree of adrenocortical atrophy could occur in addition to suppression of HPA function. The patient should be treated as steroid-dependent and transferred to a suitable maintenance dose of a systemic steroid such as prednisolone. Once the patient's condition has stabilised he should be transferred to Asmabec Spacehaler 250 micrograms.

To guard against the unexpected event of adrenal suppression, regular tests of adrenal function are advised.

Pharmacological properties

Pharmacodynamic properties: Beclomethasone dipropionate by inhalation has a potent glucocorticoid anti-inflammatory action within the lungs, but at recommended dosage, is without significant systemic activity.

Beclomethasone dipropionate also has vasoconstrictor effects and it inhibits the late responses to antigen challenge.

Pharmacokinetic properties: The pharmacokinetics of beclomethasone dipropionate have not been extensively studied. The currently available chemical methods are not of sufficient sensitivity to measure therapeutically relevant plasma concentrations, particularly those occurring following inhalation.

a) general characteristics of the active substance

– absorption: Beclomethasone dipropionate is readily absorbed from the gastro-intestinal tract. It is also well absorbed from sites of local application.

– distribution: About 25% of an inhaled dose reaches the lungs.

The drug is rapidly distributed to all body tissues. It crosses the placenta and may be excreted in small amounts in breast milk.

– elimination: The drug and its metabolites are excreted chiefly in the faeces via biliary elimination and to a lesser extent in the urine.

b) characteristics in patients

As above.

Preclinical safety data: See Clinical particulars above.

Pharmaceutical particulars

List of excipients: Oleic Acid BP, Trichlorofluoromethane (1988) BP, Dichlorodifluoromethane (1988) BP.

Incompatibilities: None known.

Shelf life: Shelf-life in the product as packaged for sale: 24 months.

Special precautions for storage: Store below 30°C. Protect from frost and direct sunlight. The canister is pressurised, it must not be burnt, punctured or broken even when apparently empty. The therapeutic effect of the medication may decrease when the canister is cold.

Nature and contents of container: The container consists of a seamless aluminium can with a metering dispensing valve crimped to it. The can is inserted into a plastic oral inhalation actuator with a dust cap.

The can is a 19 millilitre nominal capacity aerosol can of deep drawn NS4 aluminium with either a debossed or plain base.

The metering aerosol valves used are 20 mm types, with a nominal 63 microlitre dosing capacity. The valve is composed of metal and rubber components and is assembled into a metal ferrule.

The actuator supports the container during actuation and directs the sprayed aerosol particles into the mouth. The actuator is injection moulded polypropylene which may be plain, printed or embossed with the name of the product. A mouthpiece cover is fitted over the actuator mouthpiece to prevent the ingress of particulates into the mouthpiece cavity between uses.

Instruction for use/handling: Instructions as shown in the leaflet:

1. Remove the cap from the inhaler mouthpiece. Make sure the mouthpiece is clean and clear of fluff and dirt.
2. Hold the inhaler upright, with your thumb on the base and your first finger on the top of the can. Now shake the inhaler gently up and down.
3. Breathe out fully to empty the lungs and then place the mouthpiece firmly between the lips.
4. Now breathe in slowly and deeply. At the same time press the aerosol can with your first finger to fire the aerosol and release the drug.
5. Remove the inhaler from your mouth and hold breath for 10 seconds or as long as is comfortable. Breathe out slowly.
6. If more than one puff is required, wait at least one minute and repeat procedure from step 2. Replace the cap.
7. Your inhaler should be cleaned regularly usually at least once a week. To clean, remove the metal canister from the plastic body and remove the plastic cover from the mouthpiece. Rinse the plastic body and the mouthpiece cover in warm water. Dry thoroughly then replace the canister and mouthpiece cover. Avoid excessive heat. Do not put the metal canister into water.

Important: Do not rush steps 3 and 4. It is important that you start to breathe in as slowly as possible just before operating your inhaler. Practice in the mirror for the first few times. If you see a 'mist' coming from the top of your inhaler or the sides of your mouth, you should start again from step 2.

Marketing authorisation number

Asmabec Spacehaler 250 micrograms 0039/0482

Date of approval/revision of the SPC August 1998

Legal category POM

ASMASAL* CLICKHALER*

Qualitative and quantitative composition Each metered actuation of 3 mg of inhalation powder contains 114 mcg of salbutamol sulphate (95 mcg salbutamol base) and delivers 110 mcg of salbutamol sulphate (90 mcg of salbutamol base).

Pharmaceutical form Inhalation powder administered from a multidose powder inhaler.

Clinical particulars

Therapeutic indications: Asmasal Clickhaler is indicated for the symptomatic treatment of bronchospasm in bronchial asthma and other conditions with associated reversible airways obstruction. Appropriate anti-inflammatory therapy should be considered in line with current practice.

Asmasal Clickhaler may be used when necessary to relieve attacks of acute dyspnoea due to bronchoconstriction.

Asmasal Clickhaler may also be used before exertion to prevent exercise-induced bronchospasm or before exposure to a known unavoidable allergen challenge.

Adults: For the relief of acute bronchospasm and for managing intermittent episodes of asthma, one inhalation may be administered as a single dose; this may be increased to two inhalations if necessary. If the response is inadequate, higher doses than two inhalations can be used. The maximum recommended dose is two inhalations three or four times a day.

To prevent exercise-induced bronchospasm one or two inhalations should be taken 15 minutes before exertion.

One or two inhalations may also be taken before foreseeable contact with allergens.

Elderly: As for adults

Children: One inhalation is the recommended dose for the relief of acute bronchospasm, in the management of episodic asthma or before exercise. If the response is inadequate, higher doses than one inhalation can be used.

On demand use should not exceed four times daily. The bronchodilator effect of each administration of inhaled salbutamol lasts for at least four hours except in patients whose asthma is becoming worse. Such patients should be warned not to increase their usage of the inhaler, but should seek medical advice since treatment with, or an increased dose of an inhaled and/or systemic glucocorticosteroid is indicated.

As there may be adverse effects associated with excessive dosing, the dosage or frequency of administration should only be increased on medical advice.

Contra-indications: Asmasal Clickhaler is contra-indicated in patients with intolerance to this inhaled product.

Special warnings and precautions for use: Bronchodilators should not be the only or main treatment in patients with moderate to severe or unstable asthma. Severe asthma requires regular medical assessment including lung function testing as patients are at risk of severe attacks and even death. Physicians should consider using the maximum recommended dose of inhaled corticosteroid and/or oral corticosteroid therapy in these patients. Increasing use of bronchodilators, in particular short-acting inhaled beta-2-agonists to relieve symptoms, indicates deterioration of asthma control. If patients find that short-acting bronchodilator treatment becomes less effective or they need more inhalations than usual they should be warned by the prescriber of the need for consulting immediately. In this situation, patients should be reassessed and consideration given to the need for increased anti-inflammatory therapy (e.g. higher doses of inhaled corticosteroids or a course of oral corticosteroids).

Salbutamol should be administered cautiously, especially with systemic therapy, to patients suffering from thyrotoxicosis, myocardial insufficiency, hypertension, known aneurysms, decreased glucose tolerance, manifest diabetes, phaeochromocytoma and concomitant use of cardiac glycosides. Caution should also be applied in patients with myocardial ischemia, tachyarrythmias and hypertrophic obstructive cardiomyopathy.

Salbutamol and non-selective beta-blocking drugs such as propranolol, should not usually be prescribed together.

Potentially serious hypokalaemia has resulted from systemic β_2-agonist therapy. Particular caution is advised in acute severe asthma as this effect may be potentiated by concomitant treatment with xanthine derivatives, steroids, diuretics and by hypoxia. It is recommended that serum potassium levels are monitored in such situations.

Interactions with other medicaments and other forms of interaction: Please refer to the precautions listed in *Special warnings and precautions for use* (above).

Patients should be instructed to discontinue salbutamol at least 6 hours before intended anaesthesia with halogenated anaesthetics, wherever possible.

Pregnancy and lactation:

Pregnancy: Administration of salbutamol during pregnancy should only be considered if the expected benefit to the mother is greater than any possible risk to the fetus. As with the majority of drugs there is little published evidence of its safety in the early stages of pregnancy, but in animal studies, there was evidence of some harmful effects in the fetus at very high dose levels.

Lactation: Salbutamol may be secreted in breast milk. It is not known whether salbutamol has a harmful effect on the neonate and so its use should be restricted to situations where it is felt that the expected benefit to the mother is likely to outweigh any potential risk to the neonate.

Effects on ability to drive and use machines: Individual reactions, especially at higher doses, may be such that patients' ability to drive or use machines may be affected, particularly so at the beginning of treatment and in conjunction with alcohol.

The possible side effects of salbutamol such as transient muscle cramps and tremor may necessitate caution when using machines.

Undesirable effects: The side effects are dose dependent and due to the direct mechanism of β_2-agonists.

The drug also causes vasodilation leading to a reflex chronotropic effect and widespread metabolic effects, including hypokalaemia.

Salbutamol may cause mild tremor, headache, slight tachycardia and a feeling of tenseness. These usually disappear with continued treatment.

Oral and pharyngeal irritation can occur.

There have been rare reports of transient muscle cramps.

Hypersensitivity reactions including angioedema and urticaria, bronchospasm, hypotension and collapse have been reported very rarely.

Potentially serious hypokalaemia may result from systemic β_2-agonist therapy. Special precautions should be taken in patients using β_2-agonists with hypokalaemia because of the increased risk of tachycardia and arrhythmias. Hypokalaemia may be potentiated by concomitant therapy with corticosteroids, diuretics and xanthines.

As with other inhalation therapy, the potential for paradoxical bronchospasm should be kept in mind. If it occurs, the preparation should be discontinued immediately and alternative therapy instituted.

Overdose: An overdose should be treated symptomatically.

The preferred antidote for overdosage with salbutamol is a cardioselective beta-blocking agent but beta-blocking drugs should be used with caution in patients with a history of bronchospasm.

If hypokalaemia occurs potassium replacement via the oral route should be given. In patients with severe hypokalaemia intravenous replacement may be necessary.

Pharmacological properties

Pharmacodynamic properties: ATC Code: R03A C02.

Salbutamol is a beta-adrenergic stimulant which has a selective action on bronchial β_2-adrenoceptors and little effect on cardiac β_1-receptors at therapeutic doses. Following inhalation, salbutamol exerts a stimulating action on β_2 receptors on bronchial smooth muscles, and thus ensures rapid bronchodilation which becomes significant within a few minutes and persists for 4 to 6 hours.

The drug also causes vasodilation leading to a reflex chronotropic effect and widespread metabolic effects, including hypokalaemia.

Pharmacokinetic properties: Following treatment with salbutamol by inhalation, only approximately 10% or less of the drug is deposited in the airways and the remainder is swallowed. Pre-systemic metabolism of salbutamol is considerable and occurs primarily in the gastrointestinal tract and by conjugation to form an inactive sulphate ester. The systemic clearance for salbutamol is 30 l/hr. Salbutamol is eliminated both through excretion of unchanged drug in urine and through metabolism mainly via sulphate conjugation. The elimination half-life varies between 3 and 7 hours. Salbutamol is well absorbed from the gastrointestinal tract.

Preclinical safety data: Preclinical data reveal no special hazard for humans based on conventional studies of safety pharmacology, repeated dose toxicity and genotoxicity. Findings concerning teratogenicity in rabbits at high systemic exposure and the induction of benign mesovarian leiomyomas in rats are not considered of clinical concern.

Pharmaceutical particulars

List of excipients: Lactose monohydrate.

Incompatibilities: None known.

Shelf life: 2 years in unopened foil pouch. 6 months when removed from foil pouch.

Special precautions for storage: Store in a dry place at room temperature (up to 30°C).

Nature and contents of container: A plastic inhaler device incorporating an actuating and metering mechanism enclosed within an aluminium foil heat sealed bag. Each device contains 750 mg of powder – sufficient for 200 actuations.

Instructions for use/handling: Instructions for use are included in the patient information leaflet.

1. Remove mouthpiece cover from the inhaler.
2. Shake the inhaler well.
3. Hold the inhaler upright with thumb on the base and finger on the push button. Press the dosing button down firmly–once only.
4. Breathe out as far as is comfortable. Note: do not blow into the device at any time.
5. Place mouthpiece in your mouth. Close lips firmly around it (do not bite it).
6. Breathe in through your mouth steadily and deeply, to draw the medicine into your lungs.
7. Hold your breath, take the inhaler from your mouth and continue holding your breath for about 5 seconds.
8. For the second puff, keep the inhaler upright and repeat steps 2–7.
9. Replace the mouthpiece cover.

Marketing authorisation number 0039/0497

Date of approval/revision of SPC June 1998

Legal Category POM

ASMASAL* SPACEHALER*

Qualitative and quantitative composition Each metered-dose contains 100 micrograms Salbutamol BP.

Pharmaceutical form Metered-dose inhaler with Spacehaler actuator.

The Spacehaler is a vortex generating actuator which acts to reduce the velocity of the emitted dose. Compared with a standard actuator it decreases the proportion of non-respirable drug particles within the emitted dose cloud whilst achieving a similar respirable fraction.

Clinical particulars

Therapeutic indications:

(i) Treatment and prophylaxis of bronchial asthma.
(ii) Treatment of bronchitis and emphysema and conditions associated with reversible airways obstruction.
(iii) Relief of acute dyspnoea associated with reversible airways obstruction.
(iv) Particularly suitable for treatment of bronchospasm and in patients with co-existing heart disease or hypertension.

Posology and method of administration: Each inhalation, as delivered by the metering valve, contains 100 micrograms Salbutamol BP.

Adults:

acute bronchospasm and intermittent episodes of asthma	one or two inhalations as a single dose
chronic maintenance or prophylactic therapy	two inhalations three or four times a day
to prevent exercise–induced bronchospasm	two inhalations should be taken before exercise

Children:

acute bronchospasm, episodic asthma or before exercise	one inhalation
routine maintenance or prophylactic therapy	one inhalation three or four times daily

Elderly:

The dosage is the same as for other adults.

Contra-indications: In spite of the fact that salbutamol has been used intravenously and orally in the management of uncomplicated premature labour, Asmasal Spacehaler is not appropriate for such use.

Salbutamol is contra-indicated in patients with a history of hypersensitivity to any of its components.

Special warnings and precautions for use: Patients with hyperthyroidism or who are especially susceptible to salbutamol should use Asmasal Spacehaler with caution as should those patients suffering from diabetes mellitus, serious cardiovascular disorders or hypertension.

Asthmatic patients whose condition deteriorates despite salbutamol therapy or where a previously effective dose fails to give relief for at least three hours should seek medical advice. Alternative or additional therapy including corticosteroids should be instituted promptly.

Interactions with other medicaments and other forms of interaction: Adverse metabolic effects of high doses of salbutamol may be exacerbated by concomitant administration of high dose of corticosteroids.

Potentially serious hypokalaemia may result from β2-agonist therapy. Particular caution is advised in severe asthma as this effect may be potentiated by concomitant treatment with xanthine derivatives, steroids, diuretics and by hypoxia. It is recommended that serum potassium levels are monitored in such situations.

There is no evidence that adverse interactions occur between cardio-selective betablockers and sympathomimetic bronchodilators. Propranolol and other non-cardioselective beta-adrenoceptor blocking agents antagonise the effects of salbutamol.

Pregnancy and lactation: In spite of the fact that salbutamol has been used intravenously and orally in the management of uncomplicated premature labour, Asmasal Spacehaler is not appropriate for such use.

The existing data regarding the use of inhaled salbutamol during human pregnancy is insufficient to be able to assess possible harmful effects. Similarly little data is known regarding the possible harmful effects for breast-fed babies during lactation. It is therefore advised that salbutamol should be used in pregnancy only after careful consideration by the medical practitioner.

Use during lactation: Salbutamol should be used in lactation only after careful consideration by the medical practitioner.

Effects on ability to drive and use machines: On the basis of the pharmacodynamic profile, reported ADR and/or impairment of driving performance or performance related to driving, the medicine is presumed to be safe or unlikely to produce an effect.

Undesirable effects: Potentially serious hypokalaemia may result from β2-agonist therapy.

Salbutamol in large dosage may cause fine tremor of skeletal muscle (particularly the hands), palpitations and muscle cramps. Slight tachycardia, tenseness, headaches and peripheral vasodilatation have also been reported after large doses but these are less usually associated with the inhalation dosage form.

Overdose: Overdosage may result in skeletal muscle tremor, tachycardia, tenseness, headache and peripheral vasodilatation. Preferred treatment is with cautious use of cardioselective beta-adrenoceptor blocking agents.

Pharmacological properties

Pharmacodynamic properties: Salbutamol is a direct acting sympathomimetic bronchodilator agent with a predominantly beta-adrenergic activity and a selective action on β2-receptors.

Pharmacokinetic properties: Salbutamol is readily absorbed from the gastro-intestinal tract. It is subject to first pass metabolism in the liver; about half is excreted in the urine as an inactive sulphate conjugate following oral administration (the rest being unchanged salbutamol). Salbutamol does not appear to be metabolised in the lung, therefore its behaviour following inhalation depends upon the delivery method used which determines the proportion of inhaled salbutamol relative to the proportion inadvertently swallowed. Spacehaler is considered to reduce buccal deposition and therefore the proportion of drug swallowed, compared with a standard metered dose inhaler.

The plasma half-life has been estimated to range from about two to seven hours.

Preclinical safety data: No preclinical data are available since salbutamol has been used clinically for over 20 years. The safety and efficacy of salbutamol have been proven.

Please see *Clinical Particulars* sections above for further guidance.

Pharmaceutical particulars

List of excipients: Oleic Acid BP, Dichlorodifluoromethane BP 1988, Trichlorofluoromethane BP 1988

Incompatibilities: None known

Shelf life: Thirty-six months

Special precautions for storage: Store below 30°C. Keep away from direct sunlight or heat. Protect from frost. Do not puncture or burn the canister even when it seems empty.

Nature and contents of container: Aerosol for inhalation supplied in a pressurised aluminium container with metering valve crimped in place, containing 80, 200 or 300 metered actuations of Salbutamol BP.

Instructions for use/handling: Instructions as shown in the leaflet:

1. Remove the cap from the inhaler mouthpiece. Make sure the mouthpiece is clean and clear of fluff and dirt.
2. Hold the inhaler upright, with your thumb on the base and your first finger on the top of the can. Now shake the inhaler gently up and down.
3. Breathe out fully to empty the lungs and then place the mouthpiece firmly between the lips.
4. Now breathe in slowly and deeply. At the same time press the aerosol can with your first finger to fire the aerosol and release the drug.
5. Remove the inhaler from your mouth and hold breath for 10 seconds or as long as is comfortable. Breathe out slowly.
6. If more than one puff is required, wait at least one minute and repeat procedure from step 2. Replace the cap.
7. Your inhaler should be cleaned regularly usually at least once a week. To clean, remove the metal canister from the plastic body and remove the plastic cover from the mouthpiece. Rinse the plastic body and the mouthpiece cover in warm water. Dry thoroughly then replace the canister and mouthpiece cover. Avoid excessive heat. Do not put the metal canister into water.

Important: Do not rush steps 3 and 4. It is important that you start to breathe in as slowly as possible just before operating your inhaler. Practice in the mirror for the first few times. If you see a 'mist' coming from the top of your inhaler or the sides of your mouth, you should start again from step 2.

Marketing authorisation number 0039/0479

Date of approval/revision of SPC May 1997

Legal category POM

BETA-CARDONE* TABLETS

Presentation

Beta-Cardone Tablets 200 mg: White, circular, scored tablets engraved Evans/BC20, each containing sotalol hydrochloride 200 mg.

Beta-Cardone Tablets 80 mg: Pink, circular, scored tablets engraved Evans/BC8, each containing sotalol hydrochloride 80 mg.

Beta-Cardone Tablets 40 mg: Green, circular, scored tablets engraved Evans/BC4, each containing sotalol hydrochloride 40 mg.

Uses

Ventricular arrhythmias: Treatment of life-threatening ventricular tachyarrhythmias and symptomatic non-sustained ventricular tachyarrhythmias.

Supraventricular arrhythmias: Prophylaxis of paroxysmal atrial tachycardia, paroxysmal atrial fibrillation, paroxysmal A-V nodal re-entrant tachycardia, paroxysmal A-V re-entrant tachycardia using accessory pathways, and paroxysmal supraventricular tachycardia after cardiac surgery. Maintenance of normal sinus rhythm following conversion of atrial fibrillation or atrial flutter.

Beta-Cardone has both β-adrenoceptor blocking (Vaughan Williams Class II) and cardiac action potential duration prolongation (Vaughan Williams Class III) antiarrhythmic properties. Its action is devoid of intrinsic sympathomimetic and local anaesthetic activity. Its major therapeutic effect is to protect the heart from undesirable sympathetic activity. Beta-Cardone reduces the rate and force of contraction of the heart; cardiac work and oxygen consumption are diminished.

Dosage and administration

Oral administration in adults:

General instructions: When administering Beta-Cardone to a patient for the first time, it is desirable to start with a low dose and gradually increase the dose until the desired response is obtained; as a general rule the heart rate should not be reduced to less than 55 beats per minute.

Before starting treatment or increasing the dose the corrected QT interval should be measured and renal function, electrolyte balance, and concomitant medications assessed. Treatment with Beta-Cardone should be initiated and doses increased in a facility capable of monitoring and assessing cardiac rhythm. The dosage must be individualised and based on the patient's response. Proarrhythmic events can occur not only at initiation of therapy, but also with each upward dosage adjustment.

Treatment with Beta-Cardone should not be discontinued suddenly, especially in patients with ischaemic heart disease (angina pectoris, prior acute myocardial infarction) or hypertension, to prevent exacerbation of the disease (see section 'Abrupt withdrawal' under 'Special warnings').

The following are guidelines for oral administration.

The initial dose is 80 mg, as one or two divided doses. Oral dosage should be adjusted gradually allowing 2–3 days between dosing increments in order to attain steady-state, and to allow monitoring of QT intervals. Most patients respond to 160 to 320 mg per day, in two divided doses.

The dosage should be reduced in renal impairment. Creatinine clearance: 60–30 ml/min: $\frac{1}{2}$ recommended dose. Creatinine clearance 30–10 ml/min: $\frac{1}{4}$ recommended dose.

Administration in children: Beta-Cardone is not intended for administration to children.

Contra-indications, warnings, etc

Contra-indications: Beta-Cardone should not be given to patients with sick sinus syndrome; long QT syndromes, torsades de pointes; symptomatic sinus bradycardia; uncontrolled congestive heart failure; cardiogenic shock; anaesthesia that produces myocardial depression; untreated phaeochromocytoma; hypotension (except due to arrhythmia); Raynaud's phenomenon and severe peripheral circulatory disturbances; chronic obstructive airway disease or bronchial asthma; renal failure (creatinine clearance < 10 ml/min).

Beta-Cardone should not be given to patients suffering from heart block or who may have a history of bronchospasm. In patients with poor cardiac reserve β-blockade can precipitate heart failure; in such cases, Beta-Cardone therapy should not be commenced until the patient has been controlled by therapy (ACE inhibitors, cardiac glycosides or, if necessary, diuretic therapy – see *Interactions*).

Beta-Cardone should not be given to patients suffering from diabetic keto-acidosis or metabolic acidosis; therapy with Beta-Cardone can be commenced or resumed when the metabolic condition has been corrected.

Interactions: In combined therapy, clonidine should not be discontinued until several days after withdrawal of Beta-Cardone. Use with great caution with drugs that also prolong QT interval, e.g. disopyramide, amiodarone, Class I antiarrhythmic agents, calcium antagonists of the verapamil type or tricyclic antidepressants.

Concomitant potassium-depleting diuretics may increase the potential for torsade de pointes.

Proarrhythmic events are more common in patients also receiving digitalis glycosides.

Interactions also occur with phenothiazines, terfenadine, astemizole and diltiazem.

Concomitant use of reserpine, guanethidine, or alpha methyldopa requires close monitoring for evidence of hypotension and/or marked bradycardia, syncope.

Tubocurarin: Neuromuscular blockade is prolonged by beta-blocking agents.

Effects on ability to drive and use machines: Side-effects such as dizziness and fatigue should be taken into account.

Side-effects: The most significant adverse effects are those due to proarrhythmia, including torsades de pointes.

Bradycardia, dyspnoea, chest pain, palpitations, oedema, ECG abnormalities, hypotension, proarrhythmia, syncope, heart failure and presyncope can occur. Nausea/vomiting, diarrhoea, dyspepsia, abdominal pain, flatulence, cramps, fatigue, dizziness, asthenia, lightheadedness, headache, sleep disturbances, depression, paraesthesia, mood changes, anxiety, sexual dysfunction, visual disturbances, taste abnormalities, hearing disturbances and fever have also been reported.

Beta-blockers, even those with apparent cardioselectivity should not be used in patients with asthma or a history of obstructive airways disease unless no alternative treatment is available. In such cases, the risk of inducing bronchospasm should be appreciated and appropriate precautions taken. If bronchospasm should occur after the use of Beta-Cardone it can be treated with $beta_2$-agonist by inhalation e.g. salbutamol (the dose of which may need to be greater than the usual dose in asthma) and, if necessary, intravenous atropine 1 mg.

There have been reports of skin rashes and/or dry eyes associated with the use of β-adrenoceptor-blocking drugs. The reported incidence is small and in most cases the symptoms have cleared when the treatment was withdrawn. Discontinuance of the drug should be considered if any such reaction is not otherwise explicable. Cessation of therapy with a β-blocker should be gradual.

Use in pregnancy and lactation:

Pregnancy: Animal studies with sotalol hydrochloride have shown no evidence of teratogenicity or other harmful effects on the foetus. Nevertheless its use throughout pregnancy should be avoided unless it is absolutely necessary as it crosses the placenta and may cause foetal bradycardia.

Lactation: Infants should not be fed with breast milk from mothers being treated with Beta-Cardone.

Other special warnings and precautions:

Abrupt withdrawal: Patients should be carefully monitored when discontinuing chronically administered sotalol, particularly those with ischaemic heart disease. If possible the dosage should be gradually reduced over a period of 1 to 2 weeks, if necessary at the same time initiating replacement therapy. Hypersensitivity to catecholamines is observed in patients withdrawn from β-blocker therapy. Occasional cases of exacerbation of angina pectoris, arrhythmias and in some cases myocardial infarction have been reported after abrupt discontinuation of therapy. Abrupt discontinuation may unmask latent coronary insufficiency. In addition, hypertension may develop.

Proarrhythmias: Rarely, Beta-Cardone causes aggravation of pre-existing arrhythmias or the provocation of new arrhythmias.

Risk factors for torsades de pointes include prolongation of the QT interval, bradycardia, reduction in serum potassium and magnesium, and history of cardiomegaly or congestive heart failure, sustained ventricular tachycardia.

Proarrhythmic events can occur on initiating therapy and with every upward dose adjustment, The incidence of torsades de pointes is dose dependent.

Caution should be used if the QT_c exceeds 500 msec whilst on therapy. It is advisable to reduce dose or discontinue therapy when the QT_c interval exceeds 550 msec.

Electrolyte disturbances: Beta-Cardone should not be used in patients with hypokalaemia or hypomagnesaemia. Potassium levels should be monitored. In conditions likely to provoke hypokalaemia/hypomagnesaemia, such as persistent diarrhoea, appropriate corrective clinical measures should be taken.

Heart failure: Beta-blockade may precipitate heart failure.

Following myocardial infarction careful monitoring and dose titration are critical during initiation and follow-up of therapy. Sotalol should be avoided in patients with left ventricular ejection fractions ≤40% without serious ventricular arrhythmias.

Thyrotoxicosis: Beta-blockade may mask certain clinical signs of hyperthyroidism.

Treated diabetes: Beta-Cardone, like other β-blocking agents, may reduce or mask the usual pre-hypoglycaemic warning signs. It may be necessary to adjust the dose of anti-diabetic therapy.

General anaesthesia: If desired, Beta-Cardone may be stopped four days prior to surgery under specialist supervision. However, where sudden withdrawal might expose the patient to severe angina or arrhythmias, anaesthesia can proceed provided that the following precautions are taken.

1. Vagal dominance is counteracted by premedication with atropine sulphate (0.25 to 2.0 mg) administered intravenously.
2. Anaesthetic agents such as ether, chloroform, cyclopropane, trichlorethylene, methoxyflurane and enflurane, are not used.

Alcoholism: β-adrenoceptor blocking drugs may precipitate cardiac failure in alcoholic patients.

Upper respiratory infections: In these conditions, patients without a history of airways obstruction may suffer bronchospasm from β-blockade.

The product labelling will bear a statement warning

against use in patients with a history of wheezing or asthma.

Overdosage: Overdosage causes excessive bradycardia and hypotension; to counteract this atropine sulphate (0.25 to 2.0 mg) should be administered intravenously and, if need be, isoprenaline (about 5 micrograms per minute) by slow intravenous injection. In severe overdose, intravenous glucagon may be preferred: an initial bolus dose of 5 to 10 mg in dextrose or saline should be followed by an intravenous infusion of 4 mg/hour or as sufficient to maintain cardiac output. Prolongation of the Q-Tc interval has been reported. Transvenous pacing may be required.

Pharmaceutical precautions Beta-Cardone Tablets should be protected from light.

Legal category POM.

Package quantities
Beta-Cardone 200 mg are available in containers of 30 tablets (OP).
Beta-Cardone 80 mg are available in containers of 100 tablets (OP).
Beta-Cardone 40 mg are available in containers of 100 tablets (OP).

Further information Beta-Cardone is not metabolised and, in the main, is excreted in the urine. After oral administration the plasma half life has been shown to be 17 hours; the lipid solubility is very low.

Product licence numbers

Beta-Cardone Tablets 200 mg	0039/0416
Beta-Cardone Tablets 80 mg	0039/0415
Beta-Cardone Tablets 40 mg	0039/0414

Date of preparation April 1996

BETNELAN* TABLETS

Qualitative and quantitative composition Each tablet contains 500 micrograms (0.5 mg) betamethasone.

Pharmaceutical form Small white tablets engraved 'Betnelan Evans' on one side and scored on the reverse. The product complies with the specification for Betamethasone Tablets BP.

Clinical particulars

Therapeutic indications: Betamethasone is a glucocorticosteroid which is about eight to ten times as active as prednisolone on a weight-for-weight basis.

A wide variety of diseases may sometimes require corticosteroid therapy. Some of the principal indications are:

Bronchial asthma, severe hypersensitivity reactions, anaphylaxis; rheumatoid arthritis, systemic lupus erythematosis, dermatomyositis, mixed connective tissue disease (excluding systemic sclerosis), polyarteritis nodosa; inflammatory skin disorders, including pemphigus vulgaris, bullous pemphigoid and pyoderma gangrenosum; minimal change nephrotic syndrome, acute interstitial nephritis; ulcerative colitis, Crohn's disease; sarcoidosis; rheumatic carditis; haemolytic anaemia (auto-immune), acute and lymphatic leukaemia, malignant lymphoma, multiple myeloma, idiopathic thrombocytopenia purpura; immuno-suppression in transplantation.

Posology and method of administration: The lowest dosage that will produce an acceptable result should be used; when it is possible to reduce the dosage, this must be accomplished in stages. During prolonged therapy, dosage may need to be increased temporarily during periods of stress or in exacerbation of illness (see *Special warnings and precautions for use*).

Adults: The dose used will depend upon the disease, its severity, and the clinical response obtained. The following regimens are for guidance only. Divided dosage is usually employed.

Short-term treatment: 2 to 3 mg daily for the first few days, subsequently reducing the daily dosage by 250 or 500 micrograms (0.25 or 0.5 mg) every two to five days, depending upon the response.

Rheumatoid arthritis: 500 micrograms (0.5 mg) to 2 mg daily. For maintenance therapy the lowest effective dosage is used.

Most other conditions: 1.5 to 5 mg daily for one to three weeks, then reducing to the minimum effective dosage.

Larger doses may be needed for mixed connective tissue diseases and ulcerative colitis.

Children: A proportion of the adult dosage may be used (e.g. 75% at twelve years, 50% at seven years and 25% at one year) but clinical factors must be given due consideration (see *Special warnings and precautions for use*).

Route of administration: Oral.

Contra-indications: Systemic infections, unless specific anti-infective therapy is employed. Hypersensitivity to any component of the tablets.

Special warnings and precautions for use: A Patient Information Leaflet should be supplied with this product.

Undesirable effects may be minimised by using the lowest effective dose for the minimum period, administering the daily requirement as a single morning dose, or as a single morning dose on alternate days whenever possible. Frequent patient review is required to appropriately titrate the dose against disease activity (see *Posology and method of administration*).

Suppression of the inflammatory response and immune function increases the susceptibility to infections and their severity. The clinical presentation may often be atypical and serious infections such as septicaemia and tuberculosis may be masked and may reach an advanced stage before being recognised.

Chickenpox is of particular concern since this normally minor illness may be fatal in immunosuppressed patients. Patients (or parents of children) without a definite history of chickenpox should be advised to avoid close personal contact with chickenpox or herpes zoster and if exposed they should seek urgent medical attention. Passive immunisation with varicella/zoster immunoglobulin (VZIG) is needed by exposed non-immune patients who are receiving systemic corticosteroids or who have used them within the previous 3 months; this should be given within 10 days of exposure to chickenpox. If a diagnosis of chickenpox is confirmed, the illness warrants specialist care and urgent treatment. Corticosteroids should not be stopped and the dose may need to be increased.

Live vaccines should not be given to individuals with impaired immune responsiveness. The antibody response to other vaccines may be diminished.

Adrenal suppression: Adrenal cortical atrophy develops during prolonged therapy and may persist for years after stopping treatment. Withdrawal of corticosteroids after prolonged therapy must therefore always be gradual to avoid acute adrenal insufficiency, being tapered off over weeks or months according to the dose and duration of treatment. During prolonged therapy any intercurrent illness, trauma or surgical procedure will require a temporary increase in dosage; if corticosteroids have been stopped following prolonged therapy they may need to be temporarily re-introduced.

Special precautions: Particular care is required when considering the use of systemic corticosteroids in patients with the following conditions and frequent patient monitoring is necessary.

A. Osteoporosis (post-menopausal females are particularly at risk).
B. Hypertension or congestive heart failure.
C. Existing or previous history of severe affective disorders (especially previous steroid psychosis).
D. Diabetes mellitus (or a family history of diabetes).
E. History of tuberculosis.
F. Glaucoma (or a family history of glaucoma).
G. Previous corticosteroid-induced myopathy.
H. Liver failure – blood levels of corticosteroid may be increased, (as with other drugs which are metabolised in the liver).
I. Renal insufficiency.
J. Epilepsy.
K. Peptic ulceration.

Patients should carry 'steroid treatment' cards which give clear guidance on the precautions to be taken to minimise risk and which provide details of prescriber, drug, dosage and the duration of treatment.

Use in children: Corticosteroids cause dose-related growth retardation in infancy, childhood and adolescence, which may be irreversible. Treatment should be limited to the minimum dosage for the shortest possible time. In order to minimise suppression of the HPA axis and growth retardation, consideration should be given to administration of a single dose on alternate days.

Use in the elderly: The common adverse effects of systemic corticosteroids may be associated with more serious consequences in old age, especially osteoporosis, hypertension, hypokalaemia, diabetes, susceptibility to infection and thinning of the skin. Close clinical supervision is required to avoid life-threatening reactions.

Interactions with other medicaments and other forms of interaction Steroids may reduce the effects of anticholinesterases in myasthenia gravis, cholecystographic X-ray media and non-steroidal anti-inflammatory agents.

Rifampicin, rifabutin, carbamazepine, phenobarbitone, phenytoin, primidone, aminoglutethimide and ephedrine enhance the metabolism of corticosteroids; thus the corticosteroid therapeutic effect may be reduced.

The desired effects of hypoglycaemic agents (including insulin), anti-hypertensives and diuretics are antagonised by corticosteroids, and the hypokalaemic effects of acetazolamide, loop diuretics, thiazide diuretics and carbenoxolone are enhanced.

The efficacy of coumarin anticoagulants may be enhanced by concurrent corticosteroid therapy and close monitoring of the INR or prothrombin time is required to avoid spontaneous bleeding.

The renal clearance of salicylates is increased by corticosteroids and steroid withdrawal may result in salicylate intoxication.

Pregnancy and lactation: Intrauterine growth retardation in the foetus and a small increased risk of cleft palate have been reported. Hypoadrenalism may occur in the neonate. When corticosteroids are essential, however, patients with normal pregnancies may be treated as if they were in the non-gravid state. Patients with pre-eclampsia or fluid retention require close monitoring.

Corticosteroids are excreted in small amounts in breast milk and infants of mothers taking pharmacological doses of steroids should be monitored carefully for signs of adrenal suppression.

Effects on ability to drive and use machine:s None known

Undesirable effects: The incidence of predictable undesirable effects, including hypothalamic-pituitary-adrenal (HPA) axis suppression correlates with the relative potency of the drug, dosage, timing of administration and the duration of treatment (see *Special warnings and precautions for use*).

Endocrine/metabolic: Suppression of the hypothalamic-pituitary-adrenal axis, growth suppression in infancy, childhood and adolescence, menstrual irregularity and amenorrhoea. Cushingoid facies, hirsutism, weight gain, impaired carbohydrate tolerance with increased requirement for antidiabetic therapy. Negative protein and calcium balance. Increased appetite.

Anti-inflammatory and immunosuppressive effects: Increased susceptibility to and severity of infections with suppression of clinical symptoms and signs, opportunistic infections, recurrence of dormant tuberculosis (see *Special warnings and precautions for use*).

Musculoskeletal: Osteoporosis, vertebral and long bone fractures, avascular osteonecrosis, tendon rupture, proximal myopathy.

Fluid and electrolyte disturbance: Sodium and water retention, hypertension, potassium loss, hypokalaemic alkalosis.

Neuropsychiatric: Euphoria, psychological dependence, depression, psychosis, insomnia, and aggravation of schizophrenia. Increased intra-cranial pressure with papilloedema in children (pseudotumour cerebri), usually after treatment withdrawal. Aggravation of epilepsy.

Ophthalmic: Increased intra-ocular pressure, glaucoma, papilloedema, posterior subcapsular cataracts, corneal or scleral thinning, exacerbation of ophthalmic viral or fungal diseases.

Gastrointestinal: Dyspepsia, peptic ulceration with perforation and haemorrhage, acute pancreatitis, candidiasis.

Dermatological: Impaired healing, skin atrophy, bruising, telangiectasia, striae, acne.

General: Hypersensitivity including anaphylaxis, has been reported. Leucocytosis. Thrombo-embolism.

Withdrawal symptoms and signs: Too rapid a reduction of corticosteroid dosage following prolonged treatment can lead to acute adrenal insufficiency, hypotension and death (see *Special warnings and precautions for use*).

A 'withdrawal syndrome' may also occur including; fever, myalgia, arthralgia, rhinitis, conjunctivitis, painful itchy skin nodules and loss of weight.

Overdose: Treatment is unlikely to be needed in cases of acute overdosage.

Pharmacological properties

Pharmacodynamic properties: Betamethasone is a glucocorticoid which is about eight to ten times as active as prednisolone on a weight-for-weight basis.

Pharmacokinetic properties: Corticosteroids are bound to plasma proteins in varying degrees. Corticosteroids are metabolised primarily in the liver and are then excreted by the kidneys.

Pharmaceutical particulars

List of excipients: Lactose, Starch Maize , Gelatin, Magnesium Stearate, Purified Water

Incompatibilities: None known

Shelf life: 3 years

Special precautions for storage: Store below 30°C and protect from light.

Nature and contents of container: Tubular glass vial with a polyurethane snap-plug closure containing 100 tablets

Tamper evident polypropylene container with a polyurethane foam wad and a low density polyethylene lid containing 500 tablets.

Marketing authorisation number 0039/0392

Date of approval/revision of SPC July 1997

Legal category POM

BETNESOL* EYE, EAR AND NOSE DROPS

Qualitative and quantitative composition Betamethasone sodium phosphate BP 0.1% w/v.

Pharmaceutical form A clear and colourless aqueous solution.

Clinical particulars

Therapeutic indications: Short-term treatment of steroid responsive inflammatory conditions of the eye after clinical exclusion of bacterial, viral and fungal infections.

Non-infected inflammatory conditions of the ear or nose.

Posology and method of administration: The frequency of dosing depends on the clinical response. If there is no clinical response within 7 days of treatment, the drops should be discontinued.

Treatment should be the lowest effective dose for the shortest possible time. After more prolonged treatment (over 6 to 8 weeks), the drops should be withdrawn slowly to avoid relapse.

Eyes: 1 or 2 drops instilled into the eye every one or two hours until control is achieved, when the frequency may be reduced.

Ears: 2 or 3 drops instilled into the ear every two or three hours until control is achieved, when the frequency may be reduced.

Nose: 2 or 3 drops instilled into each nostril two or three times daily.

Contra-indications: Bacterial, viral, fungal, tuberculous or purulent conditions of the eye. Use is contra-indicated if glaucoma is present or herpetic keratitis (e.g. dendritic ulcer) is considered a possibility. Use of topical steroids in the latter condition can lead to an extension of the ulcer and marked visual deterioration.

Corticosteroids should not be used in patients with a perforated tympanic membrane.

Hypersensitivity to any component of the preparation.

Special warnings and precautions for use: A patient information leaflet should be supplied with this product.

Topical corticosteroids should never be given for an undiagnosed red eye as inappropriate use is potentially blinding. Ophthalmological treatment with corticosteroid preparations should not be repeated or prolonged without regular review to exclude raised intraocular pressure, cataract formation or unsuspected infections.

Prolonged use may lead to the risk of adrenal suppression in infants.

Interactions with other medicaments and other forms of interaction: Betnesol Drops contain benzalkonium chloride as a preservative and therefore, should not be used to treat patients who wear soft contact lenses.

Pregnancy and lactation: Safety for use in pregnancy and lactation has not been established. There is inadequate evidence of safety in human pregnancy. Topical administration of corticosteroids to pregnant animals can cause abnormalities of foetal development including cleft palate and intrauterine growth retardation. There may therefore be a very small risk of such effects in the human foetus.

Effects on ability to drive and use machines: May cause transient blurring of vision on instillation. Patients should be warned not to drive or operate hazardous machinery unless vision is clear.

Undesirable effects: Hypersensitivity reactions, usually of the delayed type, may occur leading to irritation, burning, stinging, itching and dermatitis.

Topical corticosteroid use may result in increased intraocular pressure leading to optic nerve damage, reduced visual acuity and visual field defects.

Intensive or prolonged use of topical corticosteroids may lead to formation of posterior subcapsular cataracts.

In those diseases causing thinning of the cornea or sclera, corticosteroid therapy may result in thinning of the globe leading to perforation.

Mydriasis, ptosis and epithelial punctate keratitis have also been reported following ophthalmic use of corticosteroids.

Following nasal administration, the most common effects are nasal irritation and dryness, although sneezing, headache, lightheadedness, urticaria, nausea, epistaxis, rebound congestion, bronchial asthma, perforation of the nasal septum and anosmia have also been reported.

Excessive and prolonged intranasal usage above the recommended dose may introduce systemic side effects.

Overdose: Oral ingestion of the contents of one bottle (up to 10 ml) of drops, or one tube (3 g) of ointment is unlikely to lead to any serious adverse effects. Long-term intensive topical use may lead to systemic effects.

Pharmacological particulars

Pharmacodynamic properties: Not applicable.

Pharmacokinetic properties: Not applicable.

Preclinical safety data: None stated.

Pharmaceutical particulars

List of excipients: Benzalkonium chloride solution BP, Disodium hydrogen phosphate anhydrous HSE, Sodium chloride BP, Disodium edetate BP, Sodium hydroxide BP, Phosphoric acid BP, Purified water BP.

Incompatibilities: None known.

Shelf life: Unopened: 24 months, opened: 4 weeks.

Special precautions for storage: Store at a temperature not exceeding 25°C. Avoid freezing. Always replace the bottle back in the carton after use to protect its contents from light. The sterility of the drops is assured until the cap seal is broken.

Nature and contents of container: 5 or 10 ml bottles with nozzle insert moulded in natural low density polyethylene closed with a tamper evident high density polyethylene cap.

Marketing authorisation number 00039/0387

Date of approval/revision of the SPC July 1997

Legal category POM

BETNESOL* EYE OINTMENT

Qualitative and quantitative composition Betamethasone sodium phosphate BP 0.1% w/w

Pharmaceutical form Ointment.

Clinical particulars

Therapeutic indications: Short-term treatment of steroid responsive inflammatory conditions of the eye after clinical exclusion of bacterial, viral and fungal infections.

Posology and method of administration: Adults and children (including the elderly): The frequency of dosing depends on the clinical response. If there is no clinical response within 7 days of treatment, the ointment should be discontinued.

Treatment should be the lowest effective dose for the shortest possible time. After more prolonged treatment (over 6 to 8 weeks), the ointment should be withdrawn slowly to avoid relapse.

An extrusion of the ointment about 1/4 inch long may be introduced beneath the lower lid two or three times daily and/or at night.

Contra-indications: Bacterial, viral, fungal, tuberculous or purulent conditions of the eye. Use is contra-indicated if glaucoma is present, or where herpetic keratitis (e.g. dendritic ulcer) is considered a possibility. Use of topical steroids in the latter condition can lead to an extension of the ulcer and marked visual deterioration.

Hypersensitivity to any component of the preparation.

Special warnings and precautions for use: A patient information leaflet should be supplied with this product.

Topical corticosteroids should never be given for an undiagnosed red eye as inappropriate use is potentially blinding.

Prolonged use may lead to the risk of adrenal suppression in infants.

Treatment with corticosteroid preparations should not be repeated or prolonged without regular review to exclude raised intraocular pressure, cataract formation or unsuspected infections.

Interactions with other medicaments and other forms of interaction: None relevant to topical use.

Pregnancy and lactation: Safety for use in pregnancy and lactation has not been established. There is inadequate evidence of safety in human pregnancy. Topical administration of corticosteroids to pregnant animals can cause abnormalities of foetal development including cleft palate and intrauterine growth retardation. There may therefore be a very small risk of such effects in the human foetus.

Effects on ability to drive and use machines: May cause transient blurring of vision on instillation. Patients should be warned not to drive or operate hazardous machinery unless vision is clear.

Undesirable effects: Hypersensitivity reactions, usually of the delayed type, may occur leading to irritation, burning, stinging, itching and dermatitis.

Topical corticosteroid use may result in increased intraocular pressure leading to optic nerve damage, reduced visual acuity and visual field defects.

Intensive or prolonged use of topical corticosteroids may lead to formation of posterior subcapsular cataracts.

In those diseases causing thinning of the cornea or sclera, corticosteroid therapy may result in thinning of the globe leading to perforation.

Overdose: Oral ingestion of the contents of one tube (3 g) of ointment is unlikely to lead to any serious adverse effects.

Pharmacological particulars

Pharmacodynamic properties: Betamethasone is a glucocorticoid which has topical anti-inflammatory activity.

Pharmacokinetic properties: Not applicable as the ointment is applied topically to the eye.

Preclinical safety data: None stated.

Pharmaceutical particulars

List of excipients: White soft paraffin BP, Liquid paraffin BP.

Incompatibilities: None known.

Shelf life: Unopened: 36 months, opened: 4 weeks.

Special precautions for storage: Store at a temperature below 30°C.

Nature and contents of container: Collapsible aluminium tubes with fine-bore extended nozzle tube fitted with a natural polyethylene cap containing 3 grams of ointment.

Instructions for use/handling: None stated.

Marketing authorisation number 00039/0388

Date of approval/revision of the SPC July 1997

Legal category POM

BETNESOL* INJECTION

Qualitative and quantitative composition Each ampoule of ready-prepared Betnesol Injection contains 4 mg betamethasone as the sodium phosphate ester in 1 ml of sterile aqueous solution. Each ampoule contains 5.3 mg of betamethasone sodium phosphate BP equivalent to 4 mg betamethasone in 1 ml of sterile aqueous solution.

Pharmaceutical form 1 ml ampoules containing a clear colourless to pale yellow solution.

Clinical particulars

Therapeutic indications: Betamethasone is a glucocorticosteroid which is about eight to ten times as active as prednisolone on a weight-for-weight basis. It may be indicated in the following conditions:

Status asthmaticus and acute allergic reactions, including anaphylactic reactions to drugs. Betnesol Injection supplements the action of adrenaline.

Severe shock arising from surgical or accidental trauma or overwhelming infection.

Acute adrenal crisis caused by abnormal stress in Addison's disease, Simmonds' disease, hypopituitarism following adrenalectomy, and when adrenocortical function has been suppressed by prolonged corticosteroid therapy.

Soft tissue lesions such as tennis elbow, tenosynovitis and bursitis.

N.B. Betnesol Injection does not replace other forms of therapy for the treatment of shock and status asthmaticus.

Posology and method of administration: Betnesol Injection may be administered by *slow* intravenous injection, *deep* intramuscular injection or subconjunctival injection. Alternatively, Betnesol Injection may be given by intravenous infusion. Local injections of Betnesol Injection may be used when treating soft tissue lesions (see below).

The incidence of predictable undesirable effects, including hypothalamic-pituitary-adrenal (HPA) axis suppression correlates with the relative potency of the drug, dosage, timing of administration and the duration of treatment (see *Special warnings and precautions for use*).

Systemic therapy in adults: 4 to 20 mg betamethasone (1 to 5 ml) administered by slow intravenous injection over half to one minute. Alternatively, Betnesol Injection may be given by intravenous infusion. The same dose can be given by deep intramuscular injection but the response is likely to be less rapid, especially in shock.

This dose can be repeated three or four times in 24 hours depending upon the condition being treated and the patient's response.

Systemic therapy in children: Infants up to 1 year may be given 1 mg betamethasone intravenously; children aged 1 to 5 years, 2 mg; 6 to 12 years, 4 mg (1 ml). This dose can be repeated three or four times in 24 hours, depending upon the condition being treated and the patient's response.

Other routes: Local injections of 4 to 8 mg Betnesol may be used when treating soft tissue lesions in adults; children may require smaller doses. This dose can be repeated on two or three occasions depending upon the patient's response.

Betnesol Injection has also been administered subconjunctivally as a single injection of 0.5 to 1 ml.

Intrathecal use is not recommended.

Contra-indications: Systemic infections, unless specific anti-infective therapy is employed.

Betnesol Injection contains sodium metabisulphite (0.1% w/v) as a preservative and therefore should not be used to treat patients with known hypersensitivity to bisulphite, metabisulphite or any other component of the injection.

Betnesol Injection should not be injected directly into tendons.

Special warnings and precautions for use: A patient information leaflet should be supplied with this product.

Undesirable effects may be minimised by using the lowest effective dose for the minimum period, and by administering the daily requirement as a single morning dose, or whenever possible as a single morning dose on alternate days. Frequent patient review is required to appropriately titrate the dose against disease activity (see *Posology and method of administration*).

Suppression of the inflammatory response and immune function increases the susceptibility to infections and their severity. The clinical presentation may often be atypical and serious infections such as septicaemia and tuberculosis may be masked and may reach an advanced stage before being recognised.

Chickenpox is of particular concern since this normally minor illness may be fatal in immunosuppressed patients. Patients (or parents of children) without a definite history of chickenpox should be advised to avoid close personal contact with chickenpox or herpes zoster and if exposed they should seek urgent medical attention. Passive immunisation with varicella zoster immunoglobulin (VZIG) is needed by exposed non-immune patients who are receiving systemic corticosteroids or who have used them within the previous 3 months; this should be given within 10 days of exposure to chickenpox. If a diagnosis of chickenpox is confirmed, the illness warrants specialist care and urgent treatment. Corticosteroids should not be stopped and the dose may need to be increased.

Live vaccines should not be given to individuals with impaired immune responsiveness. The antibody response to other vaccines may be diminished.

In the treatment of cerebral oedema due to brain trauma, gastrointestinal bleeding may occur and stool examination may be helpful in diagnosis.

Adrenal suppression: Adrenal cortical atrophy develops during prolonged therapy and may persist for years after stopping treatment. Withdrawal of corticosteroids after prolonged therapy must therefore always be gradual to avoid acute adrenal insufficiency, it should be tapered off over weeks or months according to the dose and duration of treatment. During prolonged therapy any intercurrent illness, trauma or surgical procedure will require a temporary increase in dosage; if corticosteroids have been stopped following prolonged therapy they may need to be temporarily re-introduced.

Special precautions: Particular care is required when considering the use of systemic corticosteroids in patients with the following conditions and frequent patient monitoring is necessary.

A. Osteoporosis (post-menopausal females are particularly at risk).
B. Hypertension or congestive heart failure.
C. Existing or previous history of severe affective disorders (especially previous steroid psychosis).
D. Diabetes mellitus (or a family history of diabetes).
E. History of, or active, tuberculosis.
F. Glaucoma (or a family history of glaucoma).
G. Previous corticosteroid-induced myopathy.
H. Liver failure – blood levels of corticosteroid may be increased, as with other drugs which are metabolised in the liver.
I. Renal insufficiency.
J. Epilepsy.
K. History of, or active, peptic ulceration.
L. Herpes simplex keratitis.
M. Diverticulitis.
N. Thromboembolic tendencies.

Patients should carry 'steroid treatment' cards which give clear guidance on the precautions to be taken to minimise risk and which provide details of prescriber, drug, dosage and the duration of treatment.

Use in children: Corticosteroids cause dose-related growth retardation in infancy, childhood and adolescence, which may be irreversible. Treatment should be limited to the minimum dosage for the shortest possible time. In order to minimise suppression of the HPA axis and growth retardation, consideration should be given to administration of a single dose on alternate days.

Use in the elderly: The common adverse effects of systemic corticosteroids may be associated with more serious consequences in old age, especially osteoporosis, hypertension, hypokalaemia, diabetes, susceptibility to infection and thinning of the skin. Close clinical supervision is required to avoid life-threatening reactions.

Interactions with other medicaments and other forms of interaction: Steroids may reduce the effects of anticholinesterases in myasthenia gravis cholecystographic x-ray media and non-steroidal anti-inflammatory agents.

Rifampicin, rifabutin, carbamazepine, phenobarbitone, phenytoin, primidone, aminoglutethimide and ephedrine enhance the metabolism of corticosteroids and their therapeutic effects may be reduced.

The desired effects of hypoglycaemic agents (including insulin), anti-hypertensives and diuretics are antagonised by corticosteroids, and the hypokalaemic effects of acetazolamide, loop diuretics, thiazide diuretics and carbenoxolone are enhanced.

The efficacy of coumarin anticoagulants may be enhanced by concurrent corticosteroid therapy and close monitoring of the INR or prothrombin time is required to avoid spontaneous bleeding.

The renal clearance of salicylates is increased by corticosteroids and steroid withdrawal may result in salicylate intoxication.

Convulsions have been reported in patients receiving high dose costicosteroids and cyclosporin.

Pregnancy and lactation: Intra-uterine growth retardation in the foetus and a small increased risk of cleft palate have been reported. Hypoadrenalism may occur in the neonate. When corticosteroids are essential however, patients with normal pregnancies may be treated as though they were in the non-gravid state. Patients with pre-eclampsia or fluid retention require close monitoring.

Corticosteroids are excreted in small amounts in breast milk and infants of mothers taking pharmacological doses of steroids should be monitored carefully for signs of adrenal suppression.

Effects on ability to drive and use machines: None known

Undesirable effects: The incidence of predictable undesirable effects, including hypothalamic-pituitary-adrenal (HPA) axis suppression correlates with the relative potency of the drug, dosage, timing of administration and the duration of treatment (see *Special warnings and precautions for use*).

Endocrine/metabolic: Suppression of the hypothalamic-pituitary-adrenal (HPA) axis, growth suppression in infancy, childhood and adolescence, menstrual irregularity and amenorrhoea. Cushingoid facies, hirsutism, weight gain, impaired carbohydrate tolerance with increased requirement for antidiabetic therapy. Negative protein and calcium balance. Increased appetite.

Anti-inflammatory and immunosuppressive effects: Increased susceptibility and severity of infections with suppression of clinical symptoms and signs, opportunistic infections, recurrence of dormant tuberculosis (see *Special warnings and precautions for use*).

Musculoskeletal: Osteoporosis, vertebral and long bone fractures, avascular osteonecrosis, tendon rupture, proximal myopathy.

Fluid and electrolyte disturbance: Sodium and water retention, hypertension, potassium loss, hypokalaemic alkalosis.

Neuropsychiatric: Euphoria, psychological dependence, depression, psychosis, insomnia, and aggravation of schizophrenia. Increased intra-cranial pressure with papilloedema in children (pseudotumour cerebri), usually after treatment withdrawal. Aggravation of epilepsy.

Ophthalmic: Increased intra-ocular pressure, glaucoma, papilloedema, posterior subcapsular cataracts, corneal or scleral thinning, exacerbation of ophthalmic viral or fungal diseases.

Gastrointestinal: Dyspepsia, peptic ulceration with perforation and haemorrhage, acute pancreatitis, candidiasis.

Dermatological: Impaired healing, skin atrophy, bruising, telangiectasia, striae, acne.

General: Hypersensitivity including anaphylaxis, has been reported. Leucocytosis. Thrombo-embolism.

Withdrawal symptoms and signs: Too rapid a reduction of corticosteroid dosage following prolonged treatment can lead to acute adrenal insufficiency, hypotension and death (see *Special warnings and precautions for use*).

A 'withdrawal syndrome' may also occur including; fever, myalgia, arthralgia, rhinitis, conjunctivitis, painful itchy skin nodules and loss of weight.

Overdose: Should overdosage occur, the possibility of adrenal suppression should be minimised by a gradual reduction of dosage over a period of time. The patient may need support during any further trauma.

Pharmacological properties

Pharmacodynamic properties: Betamethasone is a glucocorticoid which is about eight to ten times as active as prednisolone on a weight-for-weight basis.

Pharmacokinetic properties: Corticosteroids are bound to plasma proteins in varying degrees. Corticosteroids are metabolised primarily by the liver and then excreted by the kidneys.

Pharmaceutical particulars

List of excipients Disodium edetate, Sodium metabisulphite, Sodium chloride, Sodium hydroxide/hydrochloric acid, Water for injection.

Incompatibilities: None known

Shelf life: 2 years

Special precautions for storage: Store below 30°C and protect from light.

Nature and contents of container: 1 ml clear neutral glass ampoules in packs of five.

Marketing authorisation number 0039/0391

Date of approval/revision of SPC July 1997

Legal category POM

BETNESOL* TABLETS

Qualitative and quantitative composition Each tablet contains 500 micrograms (0.5 mg) betamethasone as the sodium phosphate ester.

Pharmaceutical form Small, soluble, pink tablets engraved "Betnesol Evans" on one side and scored on the reverse.

The tablets comply with the specification for Betamethasone Sodium Phosphate Tablets BP.

Clinical particulars

Betamethasone is a glucocorticoid which is about eight to ten times as active as prednisolone on a weight-for-weight basis.

Betamethasone sodium phosphate is very soluble in water, and is therefore less likely to cause local gastric irritation than corticosteroids which are only slightly soluble. This is important when high doses are required, as in immuno-suppressive therapy.

Betnesol does not normally cause retention of salt and water and the risk of inducing oedema and hypertension is almost negligible.

Therapeutic indications: A wide variety of diseases may sometimes require corticosteroid therapy. Some of the principal indications are as follows.

Bronchial asthma, severe hypersensitivity reactions, anaphylaxis, rheumatoid arthritis, systemic lupus erythematosus, dermatomyositis, mixed connective tissue disease (excluding systemic sclerosis), polyarteritis nodosa; inflammatory skin disorders, including pemphigus vulgaris, bullous pemphigoid and pyoderma gangrenosum; minimal change nephrotic syndrome, acute interstitial nephritis; ulcerative colitis, Crohn's disease; sarcoidosis; rheumatic carditis; haemolytic anaemia (auto-immune), acute and lymphatic leukaemia, malignant lymphoma, multiple myeloma, idiopathic thrombocytopenic purpura; immunosuppression in transplantation.

Posology and method of administration: Betnesol Tablets are best taken dissolved in water, but they can be swallowed whole without difficulty. The lowest dosage that will produce an acceptable result should be used; when it is possible to reduce the dosage, this must be accomplished by stages. During prolonged therapy, dosage may need to be increased temporarily during periods of stress or in exacerbations of illness (see *Special warnings and precautions for use*).

The dose used will depend on the disease, its severity, and the clinical reponse obtained. The following regimens are for guidance only. Divided dosage is usually employed.

Adults: Short term treatment: 2000–3000 micrograms (4–6 tablets) daily for the first few days, then reducing the daily dose by 250–500 micrograms (½ or 1 tablet) every two to five days, depending upon the response.

Rheumatoid arthritis: 500–2000 micrograms (1–4 tablets) daily. For long-term treatment the lowest effective dosage is used.

Most other conditions: 1500–5000 micrograms (3–10 tablets) daily for one to three weeks, then gradually reducing to the minimum effective dosage. Larger doses may be needed for mixed connective tissue diseases and ulcerative colitis.

Children: A proportion of the adult dosage may be used (e.g. 75% at 12 years, 50% at 7 years and 25% at 1 year).

Route of administration: Oral.

Contra-indications: Systemic infections, unless specific anti-infective therapy is employed. Hypersensitivity to any component of the tablets.

Special warnings and precautions for use: A patient information leaflet should be supplied with this product.

Undesirable effects may be minimised by using the lowest effective dose for the minimum period, and by administering the daily requirement as a single morning dose, or whenever possible as a single morning dose on alternate days. Frequent patient review is required to appropriately titrate the dose against disease activity (see *Posology and method of administration*).

Suppression of the inflammatory response and immune function increases the susceptibility to infections and their severity. The clinical presentation may often be atypical and serious infections such as septicaemia and tuberculosis may be masked and may reach an advanced stage before being recognised.

Chickenpox is of particular concern since this normally minor illness may be fatal in immunosuppressed patients. Patients (or parents of children) without a definite history of chickenpox should be advised to avoid close personal contact with chickenpox or herpes zoster and if exposed they should seek urgent medical attention. Passive immunisation with varicella zoster immunoglobulin (VZIG) is needed by exposed non-immune patients who are receiving systemic corticosteroids or who have used them within the previous 3 months; this should be given within 10 days of exposure to chickenpox. If a diagnosis of chickenpox is confirmed, the illness warrants specialist care and urgent treatment. Corticosteroids should not be stopped and the dose may need to be increased.

Live vaccines should not be given to individuals with impaired immune responsiveness. The antibody response to other vaccines may be diminished.

Adrenal suppression: Adrenal cortical atrophy develops during prolonged therapy and may persist for years after stopping treatment. Withdrawal of corticosteroids after prolonged therapy must therefore always be gradual to avoid acute adrenal insufficiency; and thus should be tapered off over weeks or months according to the dose and duration of treatment. During prolonged therapy any intercurrent illness, trauma or surgical procedure will require a temporary increase in dosage; if corticosteroids have been stopped following prolonged therapy they may need to be temporarily re-introduced.

Special precautions: Particular care is required when considering the use of systemic corticosteroids in patients with the following conditions and frequent patient monitoring is necessary.

A. Osteoporosis (post-menopausal females are particularly at risk).
B. Hypertension or congestive heart failure.
C. Existing or previous history of severe affective disorders (especially previous steroid psychosis).
D. Diabetes mellitus (or a family history of diabetes).
E. History of tuberculosis.
F. Glaucoma (or a family history of glaucoma).
G. Previous corticosteroid-induced myopathy.
H. Liver failure – blood levels of corticosteroid may be increased, (as with other drugs which are metabolised in the liver).
I. Renal insufficiency.
J. Epilepsy.
K. Peptic ulceration.

Patients should carry 'steroid treatment' cards which give clear guidance on the precautions to be taken to minimise risk and which provide details of prescriber, drug, dosage and the duration of treatment.

Use in children: Corticosteroids cause dose-related growth retardation in infancy, childhood and adolescence, which may be irreversible. Treatment should be limited to the minimum dosage for the shortest possible time. In order to minimise suppression of the HPA axis and growth retardation, consideration should be given to administration of a single dose on alternate days.

Use in the elderly: The common adverse effects of systemic corticosteroids may be associated with more serious consequences in old age, especially osteoporosis, hypertension, hypokalaemia, diabetes, susceptibility to infection and thinning of the skin. Close clinical supervision is required to avoid life-threatening reactions.

Interactions with other medicaments and other forms of interaction: Steroids may reduce the effects of anticholinesterases in myasthenia gravis cholecystographic x-ray media and non-steroidal anti-inflammatory agents.

Rifampicin, rifabutin, carbamazepine, phenobarbitone, phenytoin, primidone, aminoglutethimide and ephedrine enhance the metabolism of corticosteroids; thus the corticosteroid therapeutic effect may be reduced.

The desired effects of hypoglycaemic agents (including insulin), anti-hypertensives and diuretics are antagonised by corticosteroids, and the hypokalaemic effects of acetazolamide, loop diuretics, thiazide diuretics and carbenoxolone are enhanced.

The efficacy of coumarin anticoagulants may be enhanced by concurrent corticosteroid therapy and close monitoring of the INR or prothrombin time is required to avoid spontaneous bleeding.

The renal clearance of salicylates is increased by corticosteroids and steroid withdrawal may result in salicylate intoxication.

Pregnancy and lactation: Intra-uterine growth retardation in the foetus and a small increased risk of cleft palate have been reported. Hypoadrenalism may occur in the neonate. When corticosteroids are essential however, patients with normal pregnancies may be treated as though they were in the non-gravid state. Patients with pre-eclampsia or fluid retention require close monitoring.

Corticosteroids are excreted in small amounts in breast milk and infants of mothers taking pharmacological doses of steroids should be monitored carefully for signs of adrenal suppression.

Effects on ability to drive and use machines: None known

Undesirable effects: The incidence of predictable undesirable effects, including hypothalamic-pituitary-adrenal (HPA) axis suppression correlates with the relative potency of the drug, dosage, timing of administration and the duration of treatment (see *Special warnings and precautions for use*).

Endocrine/metabolic: Suppression of the hypothalamic-pituitary-adrenal axis, growth suppression in infancy, childhood and adolescence, menstrual irregularity and amenorrhoea. Cushingoid facies, hirsutism, weight gain, impaired carbohydrate tolerance with increased requirement for antidiabetic therapy. Negative protein and calcium balance. Increased appetite.

Anti-inflammatory and immunosuppressive effects: Increased susceptibility to and severity of infections with suppression of clinical symptoms and signs, opportunistic infections, recurrence of dormant tuberculosis (see *Special warnings and precautions for use*).

Musculoskeletal: Osteoporosis, vertebral and long bone fractures, avascular osteonecrosis, tendon rupture, proximal myopathy.

Fluid and electrolyte disturbance: Sodium and water retention, hypertension, potassium loss, hypokalaemic alkalosis.

Neuropsychiatric: Euphoria, psychological dependence, depression, psychosis, insomnia, and aggravation of schizophrenia. Increased intra-cranial pressure with papilloedema in children (pseudotumour cerebri), usually after treatment withdrawal. Aggravation of epilepsy.

Ophthalmic: Increased intra-ocular pressure, glaucoma, papilloedema, posterior subcapsular cataracts, corneal or scleral thinning, exacerbation of ophthalmic viral or fungal diseases.

Gastrointestinal: Dyspepsia, peptic ulceration with perforation and haemorrhage, acute pancreatitis, candidiasis.

Dermatological: Impaired healing, skin atrophy, bruising, telangiectasia, striae, acne.

General: Hypersensitivity, including anaphylaxis, has been reported. Leucocytosis. Thrombo-embolism.

Withdrawal symptoms and signs: Too rapid a reduction of corticosteroid dosage following prolonged treatment can lead to acute adrenal insufficiency, hypotension and death (see *Special warnings and precautions for use*).

A 'withdrawal syndrome' may also occur including; fever, myalgia, arthralgia, rhinitis, conjunctivitis, painful itchy skin nodules and loss of weight.

Overdose Treatment is unlikely to be needed in cases of acute overdosage.

Pharmacological properties

Pharmacodynamic properties: Betamethasone sodium phosphate is an active corticosteroid with topical anti-inflammatory activity.

Pharmacokinetic properties: The vast majority of corticosteroids, including betamethasone, are absorbed from the gastrointestinal tract.

Corticosteroids are metabolised mainly in the liver but also in the kidney, and are excreted in the urine.

Synthetic corticosteroids, such as prednisolone, have increased potency when compared to the natural corticosteroids, due to their slower metabolism and lower protein-binding affinity.

Pharmaceutical particulars

List of excipients: Sodium Bicarbonate, Sodium Acid Citrate, Saccharin Sodium, Povidone, Erythrosine (E127), Sodium Benzoate.

Incompatibilities: None known

Shelf life: 3 years

Special precautions for storage: Store at a temperature not exceeding 25°C.

Nature and contents of container: The tablets are sealed into individual pockets in an aluminium/polyethylene laminate (30 micron and 38 micron respectively). The tablets are strip packed in cartons of 100.

Marketing authorisation number 0039/0386

Date of approval/revision of SPC July 1997

Legal category POM

BETNESOL-N* EYE, EAR AND NOSE DROPS

Qualitative and quantitative composition

Betamethasone sodium phosphate BP 0.105% w/v (equivalent to 0.1% w/v betamethasone)

Neomycin sulphate BP 0.5% w/v (equivalent to 0.385% w/v neomycin base)

Pharmaceutical form A colourless to pale yellow solution.

Clinical particulars

Therapeutic indications: Eye: Short-term treatment of steroid responsive inflammatory conditions of the eye when prophylactic antibiotic treatment is also required, after excluding the presence of viral and fungal disease. *Ear:* Otitis externa or other steroid responsive conditions where prophylactic antibiotic treatment is also required. *Nose:* Steroid responsive inflammatory conditions where prophylactic antibiotic treatment is also required.

Posology and method of administration: The frequency of dosing depends on the clinical response. If there is no clinical response within 7 days of treatment, the drops should be discontinued.

Treatment should be the lowest effective dose for the shortest possible time. Normally, Betnesol-N Drops should not be given for more than 7 days, unless under expert supervision. After more prolonged treatment (over 6 to 8 weeks), the drops should be withdrawn slowly to avoid relapse.

Eyes: 1 or 2 drops applied to each affected eye up to six times daily depending on clinical response.

Ears: 2 or 3 drops instilled into the ear three or four times daily.

Nose: 2 or 3 drops instilled into each nostril two or three times daily.

Contra-indications: Viral, fungal, tuberculous or purulent conditions of the eye. Fungal infections of the nose or ear. Use is contraindicated if glaucoma is present or herpetic keratitis (e.g. dendritic ulcer) is considered a possibility. Use of topical steroids in the latter condition can lead to an extension of the ulcer and marked visual deterioration.

Otitis externa should not be treated when the eardrum is perforated because of the risk of ototoxicity.

Corticosteroids should not be used in patients with a perforated tympanic membrane.

Hypersensitivity to any component of the preparation.

Betnesol-N Drops contain benzalkonium chloride as a preservative and therefore should not be used as eye drops to treat patients who wear soft contact lenses.

Special warnings and precautions for use: A patient information leaflet should be supplied with this product.

Topical corticosteroids should never be given for an undiagnosed red eye as inappropriate use is potentially blinding.

Treatment with corticosteroid/antibiotic combinations should not be continued for more than 7 days in the absence of any clinical improvement, since prolonged use may lead to occult extension of infection due to the masking effect of the steroid. Prolonged use may also lead to skin sensitisation and the emergence of resistant organisms.

Prolonged use may lead to the risk of adrenal suppression in infants.

Ophthalmological treatment with corticosteroid preparations should not be repeated or prolonged without regular review to exclude raised intraocular pressure, cataract formation or unsuspected infections.

Aminoglycoside antibiotics may cause irreversible, partial or total deafness when given systemically or when applied topically to open wounds or damaged skin. This effect is dose related and is enhanced by renal or hepatic impairment. Although this effect has not been reported following topical ocular use, the possibility should be considered when high dose topical treatment is given to small children or infants.

Interactions with other medicaments and other forms of interaction: None relevant to topical use.

Pregnancy and lactation: Safety for use in pregnancy and lactation has not been established. There is inadequate evidence of safety in human pregnancy. Topical administration of corticosteroids to pregnant animals can cause abnormalities of foetal development including cleft palate and intrauterine growth retardation. There may therefore be a very small risk of such effects in the human foetus.

There is a risk of foetal ototoxicity if aminoglycoside antibiotic preparations are administered during pregnancy.

Effects on ability to drive and use machines: May cause transient blurring of vision on instillation. Patients should be warned not to drive or operate hazardous machinery unless vision is clear.

Undesirable effects: Hypersensitivity reactions, usually of the delayed type, may occur leading to irritation, burning, stinging, itching and dermatitis.

Topical corticosteroid use may result in increased intraocular pressure leading to optic nerve damage, reduced visual acuity and visual field defects.

Intensive or prolonged use of topical corticosteroids may lead to formation of posterior subcapsular cataracts.

In those diseases causing thinning of the cornea or sclera, corticosteroid therapy may result in thinning of the globe leading to perforation.

Mydriasis, ptosis and epithelial punctate keratitis have also been reported following ophthalmic use of corticosteroids.

Following nasal administration, the most common effects are nasal irritation and dryness, although sneezing, headache, lightheadedness, urticaria, nausea, epistaxis, rebound congestion, bronchial asthma, perforation of the nasal septum and anosmia have also been reported.

Overdose: Long-term intensive topical use may lead to systemic effects.

Oral ingestion of the contents of one bottle (up to 10 ml) is unlikely to lead to any serious adverse effects.

Pharmacological particulars
Pharmacodynamic properties: Betamethasone has topical corticosteroid activity. The presence of neomycin should prevent the development of bacterial infection.

Pharmacokinetic properties: Not applicable as the drops are applied topically.

Preclinical safety data: None stated.

Pharmaceutical particulars
List of excipients: Benzalkonium chloride (anhydrous equivalent) BP, Disodium edetate BP, Polyethylene glycol 300 BP, Sodium formate HSE, Anhydrous sodium sulphate BP, Disodium hydrogen phosphate anhydrous HSE, Sodium acid phosphate BP, Sodium hydroxide or BP, Phosphoric acid BP, Purified water BP.

Incompatibilities: None known.

Shelf life: Unopened: 18 months, opened: 4 weeks.

Special precautions for storage: Store at a temperature not exceeding 25°C. Avoid freezing. Always replace the bottle back in the carton after use to protect its contents from light. The sterility of the drops is assured until the cap seal is broken.

Nature and contents of container: 5 and 10 ml bottles with nozzle insert moulded in natural low density polyethylene closed with a tamper evident high density polyethylene cap.

Instructions for use/handling: None stated.

Marketing authorisation number 00039/0389

Date of approval revision of the text July 1997

Legal category POM

BETNESOL-N* EYE OINMENT

Qualitative and quantitative composition
Betamethasone sodium phosphate BP 0.10% w/w
Neomycin sulphate BP 0.50% w/w

Pharmaceutical form Ointment.

Clinical particulars
Therapeutic indications: For the short-term treatment of steroid responsive inflammatory conditions of the eye when prophylactic antibiotic treatment is also required, after excluding the presence of viral and fungal disease.

Posology and method of administration: The frequency of dosing depends on the clinical response. If there is no clinical response within 7 days of treatment, the ointment should be discontinued.

Treatment should be the lowest effective dose for the shortest possible time. Normally, Betnesol-N Ointment should not be given for more than 7 days, unless under expert supervision. After more prolonged treatment (over 6 to 8 weeks), the ointment should be withdrawn slowly to avoid relapse.

An extrusion of the ointment about 1/4 inch long may be introduced beneath the lower lid two or three times daily and/or at night.

Contra-indications: Viral, fungal, tuberculous or purulent conditions of the eye. Use is contraindicated if glaucoma is present or herpetic keratitis (e.g. dendritic ulcer) is considered a possibility. Use of topical steroids in the latter condition can lead to an extension of the ulcer and marked visual deterioration.

Hypersensitivity to any component of the preparation.

Special warnings and precautions for use: A patient information leaflet should be supplied with this product.

Topical corticosteroids should never be given for an undiagnosed red eye as inappropriate use is potentially blinding.

Treatment with corticosteroid/antibiotic combinations should not be continued for more than 7 days in the absence of any clinical improvement, since prolonged use may lead to occult extension of infection due to the masking effect of the steroid. Prolonged use may also lead to skin sensitisation and the emergence of resistant organisms.

Prolonged use may lead to the risk of adrenal suppression in infants.

Treatment with corticosteroid preparations should not be repeated or prolonged without regular review to exclude raised intraocular pressure, cataract formation or unsuspected infections.

Aminoglycoside antibiotics may cause irreversible, partial or total deafness when given systemically or when applied topically to open wounds or damaged skin. This effect is dose related and is enhanced by renal or hepatic impairment. Although this effect has not been reported following topical ocular use, the possibility should be considered when high dose topical treatment is given to small children or infants.

Interactions with other medicaments and other forms of interaction: None relevant to topical use.

Pregnancy and lactation: Safety for use in pregnancy and lactation has not been established. There is inadequate evidence of safety in human pregnancy. Topical administration of corticosteroids to pregnant animals can cause abnormalities of foetal development including cleft palate and intrauterine growth retardation. There may therefore be a very small risk of such effects in the human foetus.

There is a risk of foetal ototoxicity if aminoglycoside antibiotic preparations are administered during pregnancy.

Effects on ability to drive and use machines: May cause transient blurring of vision on instillation. Patients should be warned not to drive or operate hazardous machinery unless vision is clear.

Undesirable effects: Hypersensitivity reactions, usually of the delayed type, may occur leading to irritation, burning, stinging, itching and dermatitis.

Topical corticosteroid use may result in increased intraocular pressure leading to optic nerve damage, reduced visual acuity and visual field defects.

Intensive or prolonged use of topical corticosteroids may lead to formation of posterior subcapsular cataracts.

In those diseases causing thinning of the cornea or sclera, corticosteroid therapy may result in thinning of the globe leading to perforation.

Overdose: Long-term intensive topical use may lead to systemic effects.

Oral ingestion of the contents of one tube (3 g) of ointment is unlikely to lead to any serious adverse effects.

Pharmacological particulars
Pharmacodynamic properties: Betamethasone is a glucocorticoid which has topical anti-inflammatory activity. Neomycin is a broad spectrum aminoglycoside antibiotic.

Pharmacokinetic properties: Not applicable as the ointment is applied topically to the eye.

Preclinical safety data: None stated.

Pharmaceutical particulars
List of excipients: White soft paraffin BP, Liquid paraffin BP.

Incompatibilities: None known.

Shelf life: Unopened: 36 months, opened: 4 weeks.

Special precautions for storage: Store at a temperature not exceeding 25°C. Avoid freezing. Always replace the bottle back in the carton after use to protect its contents from light. The sterility of the ointment is assured until the cap seal is broken.

Nature and contents of container: Collapsible aluminium tubes with fine-bore extended nozzle tube fitted with a natural polyethylene cap containing 3 grams of ointment.

Instructions for use/handling: None stated.

Marketing authorisation number 00039/0390

Date of approval/revision of the SPC July 1997

Legal category POM

BETTAMOUSSE*

Qualitative and quantitative composition Betamethasone 1 mg/g (0.1%) as valerate.

Pharmaceutical form Cutaneous foam.

Clinical particulars
Therapeutic indications: Steroid responsive dermatoses of the scalp, such as psoriasis.

Posology and method of administration: Adults, the elderly and children (over the age of six years): No more than a 'golf-ball' sized amount of mousse (containing approximately 3.5 mg betamethasone), or proportionately less for children, to be massaged into the affected areas of the scalp twice daily (in the morning and evening) until the condition improves. If there is no improvement after 7 days, treatment should be discontinued. Once the condition has improved, application is reduced to once a day and after daily treatment it may be possible to maintain improvement by applying even less frequently. In children over the age of 6 years, this product should not, in general, be used for longer than 5 to 7 days.

Patients should be advised to use the product sparingly.

Contra-indications: Bacterial, fungal, parasitic or viral infections of the scalp unless simultaneous treatment is initiated.

Hypersensitivity to any component of the preparation.

Dermatoses in children under six years of age.

Special warnings and precautions for use: Avoid contact with the eyes, open wounds and mucosae. Do not use near a naked flame.

The least amount of mousse required to control the disease should be used for the shortest possible time. This should minimise the potential for long term side effects. This is particularly the case in children, as adrenal suppression can occur even without its use with an occlusive dressing.

As with other topical corticosteroids, at least monthly clinical review is recommended if treatment is prolonged, and it may be advisable to monitor for signs of systemic activity.

The use of topical corticosteroids in psoriasis requires careful supervision. Glucocorticoids can mask, activate and worsen a skin infection. Development of secondary infection requires appropriate antimicrobial therapy and may necessitate withdrawal of topical corticosteroid therapy. Occlusive treatment should be avoided when there are signs of secondary infection. There is a risk of the development of generalised pustular psoriasis or local or systemic toxicity due to impaired barrier function of the skin.

Tolerance may develop and rebound relapse may occur on withdrawal of treatment.

Interaction with other medicaments and other forms of interaction: Not relevant to topical use.

Pregnancy and lactation: There is inadequate evidence of safety in human pregnancy. Bettamousse should only be used in pregnancy or lactation if the potential benefit outweighs the risk. Topical administration of corticosteroids to pregnant animals can cause abnormalities of foetal development such as cleft palate, but the relevance of this in man is unknown. Reduced placental and birth weight have been recorded in animals and man after long-term treatment.

While betamethasone valerate passes over into the maternal milk, there appears to be little risk of therapeutic doses having an effect on the baby.

Effects on ability to drive and use machines: None known.

Undesirable effects: Prolonged use of large amounts, or treatment of extensive areas can result in sufficient systemic absorption to produce the features of hypercorticism and suppression of the hypothalamic-pituitary-adrenal axis. These effects are more likely to occur in children, and if occlusive dressings are used.

Individual cases of headache, stinging and pruritus have been described. If signs of hypersensitivity appear, application should be stopped immediately.

The following side effects can occur with topical use of steroids:

Less common: 1/100–1/1000. Skin atrophy, stria distensae. Secondary infection. Rosacea-like dermatitis (face). Ecchymoses.

Rare: <1/1000. Hypertrichosis. Hypersensitivity (steroid). Hypo-/hyper-pigmentation. Folliculitis. Telangiectases.

Other side effects include: purpura, acne (especially

during prolonged application). Rarely, perioral dermatitis and systemic activity.

In rare instances, treatment of psoriasis with corticosteroids (or their withdrawal) is thought to have provoked the pustular form of the disease. (See Precautions).

Overdose: Acute overdosage is very unlikely to occur. However, in the case of chronic overdosage or misuse, the features of hypercorticism may appear. In this situation topical steroids should be discontinued under careful clinical supervision, with supportive therapy if appropriate.

Pharmacological properties

Pharmacodynamic properties: Pharmacotherapeutic (ATC) code: DO7AC: Corticosteroids, dermatological preparations, potent (group III).

Betamethasone is a glucocorticosteroid which has topical anti-inflammatory activity.

Pharmacokinetic properties: Under conditions of normal use, topical administration of betamethasone is not associated with clinically significant systemic absorption.

Preclinical safety data: Topical administration of corticosteroids to pregnant animals has been associated with abnormalities of foetal development and growth retardation, although the relevance of this in humans is unknown.

Pharmaceutical particulars

List of excipients: Cetyl alcohol, Stearyl alcohol, Polysorbate 60, Ethanol, Purified Water, Propylene glycol, Citric acid anhydrous, Potassium Citrate, Butane/Propane

Incompatibilities: None known.

Shelf life: Two years.

Special precautions for storage: Store up to 25°C. Do not refrigerate.

Nature and contents of container: Pressurised container. Aluminium EP-lined Cebal can with Precision valve and clear cover cap, with a net weight of 100 g.

Instructions for use/handling: Not applicable.

Marketing authorisation number 0039/0488

Date of approval/revision of text July 1998

Legal category POM

ADSORBED TETANUS VACCINE, BP (CLOSTET*).

Qualitative and quantitative composition The composition in terms of active ingredients is as follows:

Tetanus toxoid not less than 40 IU

Quantities expressed per 0.5 ml dose.

Pharmaceutical form Adsorbed Tetanus Vaccine is a sterile suspension of purified tetanus toxoid, prepared by chemical detoxification of *Clostridium tetani* exotoxin, adsorbed on aluminium hydroxide.

Clinical particulars

Therapeutic indications: For active immunisation against tetanus and for reinforcement of immunity to tetanus.

Primary immunisation against tetanus in infancy is usually carried out by the administration of combined Adsorbed Diphtheria, Tetanus and Pertussis Vaccine (DTPer/Vac/Ads) or Adsorbed Diphtheria and Tetanus Vaccine (CHILD) (DT/Vac/Ads(Child)).

Posology and method of administration: Each dose is 0.5 ml given by deep intramuscular or subcutaneous injection.

The primary course of immunisation against tetanus consists of three doses with an interval of one month between each dose. The intervals between immunisations may be exceeded without the need to repeat the full course of immunisation. Reinforcing doses are given to maintain immunity against tetanus.

Primary course in infants and children under 10 years: Primary immunisation against tetanus may be carried out by the administration of combined Adsorbed Diphtheria, Tetanus and Pertussis Vaccine (DTPer/Vac/Ads), Adsorbed Diphtheria and Tetanus Vaccine (CHILD) (DT/Vac/Ads(Child)) or Adsorbed Tetanus Vaccine (Tet/Vac/Ads) in infancy. Three 0.5 ml doses are given, with a dose at 2, 3 and 4 months of age.

Reinforcing doses in infants and children under 10 years: Children who have received the primary course of immunisation in infancy require reinforcement of immunity against tetanus. This can be achieved by giving one dose (0.5 ml) Adsorbed Diphtheria and Tetanus Vaccine (CHILD) (DT/Vac/Ads(Child)) or Adsorbed Tetanus Vaccine (Tet/Vac/Ads), after at least three years from the last dose of the primary course. The reinforcing dose is commonly given prior to school entry.

Primary course in adults and children over 10 years: Primary immunisation against tetanus consists of three doses separated by intervals of not less than four weeks.

Reinforcing doses in adults and children over 10 years: A reinforcing dose (0.5 ml) of Adsorbed Diphtheria and Tetanus Vaccine for Adults and Adolescents is recommended at 13 to 18 years of age or before leaving school. Teenagers being treated for tetanus prone wounds and who had received their fourth dose of tetanus vaccine approximately ten years earlier, should be given Adsorbed Diphtheria and Tetanus Vaccine for Adults and Adolescents and the school leaving dose omitted. For adults, a single dose of vaccine given at any time after completion of the primary course of three injections can be expected to provide an effective reinforcement of immunity. The administration of a reinforcing dose approximately 10 years after the completion of a primary immunisation course is recommended. Thereafter, a further vaccination at 10 years is thought to provide the potential for lifelong protection. However, this does not preclude the need to consider administration of additional doses in the event of injuries which may give rise to tetanus.

Treatment of patients with tetanus-prone wounds: The following are considered tetanus-prone wounds.

a. Any wound or burn sustained more than six hours before surgical treatment of the wound or burn.
b. Any wound or burn at any interval after injury that shows one or more of the following characteristics:
   i A significant degree of devitalised tissue.
   ii Puncture-type wound.
   iii Contact with soil or manure likely to harbor tetanus organisms.
   iv Clinical evidence of sepsis.

Thorough surgical toilet of the wound is essential whatever the tetanus immunisation history of the patient.

Specific anti-tetanus prophylaxis is as follows:

Immunisation Status	*Type of Wound Clean*	*Type of Wound Tetanus Prone*
Last of 3 dose course, or reinforcing dose within last 10 years	Nil	Nil (A dose of human tetanus immunoglobulin may be given if risk of infection is considered especially high e.g. contamination with stable manure).
Last of 3 dose course or reinforcing dose more than 10 years previously.	A reinforcing dose of adsorbed vaccine.	A reinforcing dose of adsorbed vaccine plus a dose of human tetanus immunoglobulin.
Not immunised or immunisation status not known with certainty.	A full 3 dose course of adsorbed vaccine.	A full 3 dose course of vaccine, plus a dose of tetanus immunoglobulin in a different site.

Reinforcing doses of tetanus vaccine at frequent intervals may provoke hypersensitivity reactions and tetanus vaccine should not be given to any patient who has received a booster dose in the preceding year.

Persons of all ages are susceptible to tetanus unless they have received appropriate immunisation. Rarely, if ever, is natural immunity developed even in persons who have recovered from severe tetanus. Since most tetanus cases follow trivial wounds, all persons should, if possible, be actively immunised against the disease.

Adsorbed Tetanus Vaccine may be administered simultaneously with human tetanus immunoglobulin or tetanus antitoxin but must be given at separate sites. The antibody response of subjects to subsequent doses of vaccine is not significantly impaired by this procedure.

Oral Poliomyelitis Vaccine BP may be given at the same time as Adsorbed Tetanus Vaccine.

Shake well before each dose is withdrawn. It is good practice to record the title, dose and lot numbers of all vaccines and dates of administration.

Contra-indications: Adsorbed tetanus vaccine must not be given intradermally since it may give rise to a persistent skin nodule.

The vaccine should not be administered to a subject who has experienced a serious reaction (e.g. anaphylaxis) to a previous dose of this vaccine or who is known to be hypersensitive to any component thereof.

Adsorbed Tetanus Vaccine should not be given to an individual suffering from an acute febrile illness except in the presence of a tetanus-prone wound.

Tetanus Vaccine should not be given to any patient who has received a booster dose in the preceding year.

Special warnings and special precautions for use: Although anaphylaxis is rare, facilities for its management should always be available during vaccination.

Interactions with other medicaments and other forms of interaction: None known.

Pregnancy and lactation: In countries where the risks of neonatal tetanus are high, tetanus vaccines are widely administered during pregnancy without any apparent significant adverse effect on pregnancy or foetal development.

No relevant information on the immunisation of lactating women is available.

Effects on ability to drive and use machines: None stated.

Undesirable effects: Local reactions of swelling, redness and pain may develop at the injection site and persist for several days. Delays of up to 10 days before symptoms develop are reported. Occasionally these local reactions may be quite marked, with tenderness and swelling of a large area. Local reactions are rare in children, the incidence increases with age and according to the number of previously administered doses of tetanus toxoid containing vaccine. However, reactions may occur after the first dose. Subjects who develop reactions frequently have high titres of circulating antitoxin. Women develop reactions more frequently than men.

General reactions are uncommon but may include rash, arthralgia, lymphadenopathy, faintness, nausea, headache, lethargy, malaise, myalgia and pyrexia. They do not usually persist for more than a few hours. Urticaria, angioneurotic oedema and acute anaphylactic reactions are sometimes seen.

Serum sickness and peripheral neuropathy have been described. Calcifying dermatomyositis has been observed in temporal association with tetanus vaccination.

Persistent nodules at the site of injection may occasionally follow administration of adsorbed vaccines especially if the inoculation is into the superficial layers of subcutaneous tissue.

Any untoward reactions should be reported to the regulatory authorities and to the manufacturer.

Overdose: If overdose or inadvertent administration is suspected, careful observation of the subject may be necessary. There may not be sequelae but subjects should be monitored and appropriate supportive measures should be implemented according to the type of response seen.

Pharmacological properties

Immunisation with Adsorbed tetanus vaccine protects by stimulating the production of antitoxin which provides immunity against the effects of tetanus toxin. The immunogen is prepared by treating a cell free preparation of toxin with formaldehyde and thereby converting it into the inocuous tetanus toxoid. Tetanus toxoid alone is a relatively poor immunogen, and for vaccine use it is adsorbed onto an adjuvant such as aluminium hydroxide.

Pharmaceutical particulars

List of excipients: Each 0.5 ml dose contains: Aluminum hydroxide 1.5 mg, Sodium thimerfonate 0.025 mg, Sodium chloride 4.25 mg, Water for Injections to 0.5 ml.

Incompatibilities: None stated.

Shelf life: Ampoules: 36 months when stored at 2–8°C unopened. Pre-filled syringes: 24 months when stored at 2–8°C unopened.

Special precautions for storage: Store between 2 and 8°C. Protect from light. Do not freeze.

Nature and content of containers: Ampoules: Single dose (0.5 ml) 1 ml clear neutral type 1 glass complying with the PhEur requirements for Containers for Injectables. Pre-filled syringes: Single dose 1 ml Hypack SCF pre-filled syringe containing 0.5 ml vaccine.

Instructions for use/handling: Vaccine which has been frozen should not be used. Disposal should be by incineration at a temperature of not less than 1100°C at a registered waste disposal contractor.

Marketing authorisation number 0039/0444

Date of approval/revision of SPC December 1997

Legal category POM

COCOIS* COCONUT OIL COMPOUND

Presentation Cocois is a presentation of coconut oil compound ointment. It is a buff coloured ointment containing Coal Tar Solution BP 12% w/w, Precipitated Sulphur BP 4% w/w and Salicylic Acid PhEur 2% w/w in a coconut oil emollient base.

Uses Cocois is indicated as a adjunctive treatment of common scaly scalp disorders such as psoriasis, eczema, seborrhoeic dermatitis and dandruff. It has a mild antipruritic and keratolytic action.

Dosage and administration Part the hair and squeeze

a thin ribbon of Cocois onto the affected area(s) of the scalp using the applicator provided. Gently rub in the ointment and leave in contact for approximately 1 hour. Wash out using warm water and a mild shampoo.

For severe scaly scalp conditions, use daily for 3-7 days until improvement has been obtained and then intermittently as necessary.

For less severe conditions such as dandruff, use intermittently as necessary, e.g. once a week.

If symptoms persist after four weeks, consult your doctor.

For children between 6-12 years use under medical supervision only.

Cocois is not recommended for use in children below the age of six years.

Contra-indications, warnings, etc
Contra-indications: Do not use in the presence of acute skin infections of the scalp, acute pustular psoriasis or known sensitivity to any of the ingredients including sulphur and salicylates.

Adverse effects: It has been reported that coal tar may cause skin irritation, folliculitis and rarely, photosensitivity. In the event of such a reaction, discontinue use.

Warnings and precautions: Avoid contact with the eyes and wash the hands immediately after application.

Coal tar may stain bed linen and jewellery. Care should be taken to protect these items during treatment.

Use in pregnancy: There are no data on the use of Cocois in pregnancy.

Pharmaceutical precautions Store between 10°C and 25°C.

Legal category GSL.

Package quantities Tubes of 40 g and 100 g and applicator.

Further information Cocois is based upon a formulation developed at St John's Hospital for Diseases of the Skin, London.

Ingredients: Coal Tar Solution BP 12% w/w, Salicylic Acid PhEur 2% w/w, Precipitated Sulphur BP 4% w/w, Coconut Oil BP, White Soft Paraffin BP, Glycerol PhEur, Cetostearyl Alcohol BP, Liquid Paraffin PhEur, Polyoxyethylene Glycerol Monostearate (Tagat S2), Paraffin Hard BP.

Product licence number 0039/0499

CO-DANTHRUSATE

Presentation
Capsules: Co-danthrusate (Normax) capsules, containing 50 mg danthron and 60 mg docusate sodium. Dark brown capsules, overprinted with the product name 'Normax'.

Suspension: Co-danthrusate (Normax) suspension, containing 50 mg danthron and 60 mg docusate sodium per 5 ml. An orange-yellow suspension with an odour of peppermint.

Uses
Principal action: Danthron is a mild peristaltic stimulant acting on the lower bowel to encourage normal bowel movement without causing irritation. Docusate sodium is a softening agent which prevents excessive colonic dehydration and hardening of stools.

Indications: Constipation in geriatric practice. Analgesic-induced constipation in terminally ill patients over 6 years old. Constipation in cardiac failure and coronary thrombosis (conditions in which defaecation must be free of strain).

Dosage and administration For oral administration only.
Adults (including elderly patients): 1-3 capsules or 5-15 ml suspension at bedtime.

Children (6-12 years): 1 capsule or 5 ml suspension at bedtime.

Prolonged use is not recommended.

Contra-indications, warnings, etc.
Contra-indications: In common with all laxatives, Co-danthrusate is contra-indicated in cases of non-specific abdominal pain and when intestinal obstruction is suspected.

Caution: Danthron is excreted in the urine and metabolised danthron in the faeces. There is evidence that these may cause perineal erythema in patients with urinary and or faecal incontinence. It is recommended therefore that co-danthrusate should be used with caution in all incontinent patients.

Use in pregnancy and lactation: Co-danthrusate should not be used during pregnancy or lactation.

Other special warnings: In experimental animals, danthron has been associated with adenocarcinomas in the bowel and tumours in the liver.

Adverse reactions: The griping often found with other types of laxative is not an appreciable problem with Co-danthrusate. Occasionally, an orange tint in the urine may be observed due to the danthron component.

Overdosage: The patient should be encouraged to drink fluids. An anticholinergic preparation may be used to ease excessive intestinal motility if necessary.

Pharmaceutical precautions
Capsules: Store in a dry place.

Suspension: Store at a temperature not exceeding 25°C and protect from light.

Legal category POM.

Package quantities
Capsules: Capsules in blister packs of 63.
Suspension: 200 ml bottle.

Further information Nil.

Product licence numbers
Co-danthrusate capsules 0039/0380
Co-danthrusate suspension 0039/0381

CORACTEN* SR CAPSULES

Qualitative and quantitative composition Each capsule contains 10 mg or 20 mg Nifedipine USP in sustained release form.

Pharmaceutical form

10 mg: Sustained release capsules with opaque grey body and opaque brownish-pink cap, overprinted in white with 'Coracten' on the body and '10 mg' on the cap, and filled with yellow pellets.

20 mg: Sustained release capsules with opaque brownish-pink body and opaque reddish-brown cap, overprinted in white with 'Coracten' on the body and '20 mg' on the cap, and filled with yellow pellets.

Clinical particulars
Therapeutic indications: Coracten SR Capsules are indicated for the prophylaxis of chronic stable angina pectoris and the treatment of hypertension.

They are also indicated for the treatment of Prinzmetal (variant) angina when diagnosed by a cardiologist.

Posology and method of administration:
Adults only: The recommended starting dose of Coracten SR Capsules is 10 mg every 12 hours swallowed with water with subsequent titration of dosage according to response. The dose may be adjusted to 40 mg every 12 hours.

Children: Coracten SR Capsules are not recommended for use in children.

Elderly: The pharmacokinetics of nifedipine are altered in the elderly so that lower maintenance doses of nifedipine may be required compared to younger patients.

Hepatic impairment: Caution should be exercised in treating patients with hepatic impairment. In these patients the use of one 10 mg Coracten SR Capsule every 12 hours, together with careful monitoring, is suggested when commencing therapy.

Renal impairment: Dosage adjustments are not usually required in patients with renal impairment.

Contra-indications: Coracten SR Capsules are contra-indicated in patients with known hypersensitivity to nifedipine or other dihydropyridines because of the theoretical risk of cross reactivity. They should not be used in women who are or who may become pregnant (see section *Pregnancy and lactation*).

Coracten SR Capsules should not be used in clinically significant aortic stenosis, unstable angina, or during or within one month of a myocardial infarction. They should not be used in patients in cardiogenic shock.

Coracten SR Capsules should not be used for the treatment of acute attacks of angina, or in patients who have had ischaemic pain following its administration previously.

The safety of Coracten SR Capsules in malignant hypertension has not been established.

Coracten SR Capsules should not be used for secondary prevention of myocardial infarction.

Coracten SR Capsules are contra-indicated in patients with acute porphyria.

Coracten SR Capsules should not be administered concomitantly with rifampicin since effective plasma levels of nifedipine may not be achieved owing to enzyme induction.

Special warnings and precautions for use: Nifedipine should be used with caution in patients who are hypotensive; in patients with poor cardiac reserve; in patients with heart failure or significantly impaired left ventricular function as their condition may deteriorate; in diabetic patients as they may require adjustment of their diabetic therapy; and in dialysis patients with malignant hypertension and irreversible renal failure with hypovolaemia, since a significant drop in blood pressure may occur due to the vasodilator effects of nifedipine.

Since nifedipine has no beta-blocking activity, it gives no protection against the dangers of abrupt withdrawal of beta-blocking drugs. Withdrawal of any previously prescribed beta-blockers should be gradual, preferably over 8 to 10 days.

Nifedipine may be used in combination with beta-blockers and other antihypertensive agents, but the possibility of an additive effect resulting in postural hypotension and/or cardiac failure must be borne in mind.

Cardiac ischaemic pain has been reported in a minority of patients within 30 minutes of starting nifedipine treatment; such patients should stop treatment.

Interaction with other medicaments and other forms of interaction: As with other dihydropyridines, nifedipine should not be taken with grapefruit juice because bioavailability is increased.

The simultaneous administration of nifedipine and digoxin may lead to reduced digoxin clearance and hence an increase in the plasma digoxin. Digoxin levels should be monitored and, if necessary, the digoxin dose reduced.

Nifedipine may increase the spectrophotometric values of urinary vanillylmandelic acid falsely. However, HPLC measurements are unaffected.

Coracten SR Capsules should not be administered concomitantly with rifampicin since effective plasma levels of nifedipine may not be achieved owing to enzyme induction (see *Contra-indications*).

Increased plasma levels of nifedipine have been reported during concomitant use of H_2-receptor antagonists (specifically cimetidine), other calcium channel blockers (specifically diltiazem), alcohol and cyclosporin.

Plasma levels of nifedipine are possibly decreased by the concomitant use of antiepileptics.

When used in combination with nifedipine, plasma concentrations of quinidine have been shown to be suppressed regardless of quinidine dosage. The plasma concentrations of phenytoin, theophylline and non-depolarising muscle relaxants (e.g. tubocurarine) are increased when used in combination with nifedipine.

Profound hypotension has been reported with nifedipine and intravenous magnesium sulphate in the treatment of pre-eclampsia.

Pregnancy and lactation:
Pregnancy: Because animal studies show embryotoxicity and teratogenicity, Coracten SR Capsules are contra-indicated during pregnancy (see also *Contra-indications*). Embryotoxicity was noted at 6 to 20 times the maximum recommended dose for Coracten SR Capsules given to rats, mice and rabbits, and teratogenicity was noted in rabbits given 20 times the maximum recommended dose for Coracten SR Capsules.

Lactation: Nifedipine is excreted in breast milk, therefore Coracten SR Capsules are not recommended during lactation.

Effects on ability to drive and use machines: None known.

Undesirable effects: Side-effects are generally transient and mild, and usually occur at the start of treatment only. They include headache, flushing and, usually at higher dosages, nausea, dyspepsia, heartburn, dizziness, lethargy, skin reactions (such as rash, pruritus and urticaria), paraesthesia, hypotension, palpitation, tachycardia, dependent oedema, increased frequency of micturition, eye pain, depression, fever, gingival hyperplasia and telangiectasia.

Other less frequently reported side-effects include myalgia, tremor and visual disturbances. Impotence may occur rarely.

As with other sustained release dihydropyridines, exacerbation of angina pectoris may occur rarely at the start of treatment with sustained release formulations of nifedipine. The occurrence of myocardial infarction has been described although it is not possible to distinguish such an event from the natural course of ischaemic heart disease.

There are reports in older men on long-term therapy of gynaecomastia which usually regresses upon withdrawal of therapy.

Side-effects which may occur in isolated cases are photosensitivity, exfoliative dermatitis, systemic allergic reactions and purpura. Usually, these regress after discontinuation of the drug.

Rare cases of hypersensitivity-type jaundice have been reported. In addition, disturbances of liver function such as intra-hepatic cholestasis may occur. These regress after discontinuation of therapy.

Overdose:
Human experience: Reports of nifedipine overdosage are limited and symptoms are not necessarily dose-related. Severe hypotension due to vasodilation, and

tachycardia or bradycardia are the most likely manifestations of overdose.

Metabolic disturbances include hyperglycaemia, metabolic acidosis and hypo- or hyperkalaemia.

Cardiac effects may include heart block, AV dissociation and asystole, and cardiogenic shock with pulmonary oedema.

Other toxic effects include nausea, vomiting, drowsiness, dizziness, confusion, lethargy, flushing, hypoxia, unconsciousness and coma.

Management of overdose in man: Treatment consists of gastric lavage followed by oral activated charcoal together with supportive and symptomatic measures, principally intravenous fluids to maintain circulating blood volume. If the latter is not sufficient, dopamine or dobutamine may be given. Intravenous calcium gluconate may be considered as an antidote.

Pharmacological particulars

Pharmacodynamic properties: Nifedipine is a potent calcium-channel blocker which, by dilating peripheral arterial smooth muscle, decreases cardiac work and myocardial oxygen requirement. It also dilates coronary arteries, thereby improving myocardial perfusion and reducing coronary artery spasm. In hypertension, it reduces blood pressure but has little or no effect in normotensive subjects. It has no therapeutic antiarrhythmic effect.

Pharmacokinetic properties: Coracten SR Capsules are a sustained release formulation of nifedipine designed to provide less fluctuation and more prolonged nifedipine blood concentrations than standard immediate release preparations.

Nifedipine is highly protein bound. It undergoes hepatic oxidation to inactive metabolites which are excreted in the urine (80%) and faeces (20%).

Preclinical safety data: There are no pre-clinical data of relevance to the prescriber which are additional to that already included in other sections of the SPC.

Pharmaceutical particulars

List of excipients:

Capsule contents: Sucrose PhEur, Maize Starch PhEur, Lactose PhEur, Povidone K30 PhEur, Methacrylic acid copolymer type A (Eudragit L100) NF, Talc PhEur, Purified Water PhEur.

Capsule shells: Gelatin BP, Red iron oxide (E172), Yellow iron oxide (E172), Titanium dioxide (E171) and in Coracten 10 mg tablets only black iron oxide (E172).

Incompatibilities: None known.

Shelf life: 36 months.

Special precautions for storage: Store in original pack at a temperature not exceeding 30°C and protect from light.

Nature and contents of container: Coracten SR Capsules are presented in blister strips packed in cartons containing 60 capsules. The blister strips are formed from PVC with a coating of PVdC backed with aluminium foil.

(Cartons of 10, 15, 30, 56, 100, 150, 250, 500 and 600 capsules are licensed but not marketed.)

Instructions for use and handling: None.

Marketing authorisation numbers
10 mg 0039/0365
20 mg 0039/0367

Date of approval/revision of SPC February 1998

Legal category POM

CORACTEN* XL CAPSULES 30 mg

Qualitative and quantitative composition Each capsule contains 30 mg Nifedipine PhEur in sustained release form.

Pharmaceutical form Prolonged release capsule.

Clinical particulars

Therapeutic indications: Coracten XL Capsules are indicated for the treatment of hypertension and the prophylaxis of chronic stable angina pectoris.

Posology and method of administration: The capsules are for oral administration and should be swallowed whole with a little fluid.

Dosage – Angina pectoris and hypertension: Adults only: Normally treatment is initiated with one 30 mg Coracten XL capsule every 24 hours. Dosage may be titrated to a higher level as clinically warranted. The dose may be adjusted to 90 mg every 24 hours.

Children: Coracten XL capsules are not recommended for use in children.

Elderly: The pharmacokinetics of nifedipine are altered in the elderly so that lower maintenance doses of nifedipine may be required compared to younger patients.

Hepatic impairment: As Coracten XL is a long acting formulation, it should not be administered to patients with hepatic impairment.

Renal impairment: Dosage adjustments are not usually required in patients with renal impairment.

Contra-indications: Coracten XL Capsules are contra-indicated in patients with known hypersensitivity to nifedipine or other dihydropyridines because of the theoretical risk of cross reactivity. They should not be used in nursing mothers and women who are or who may become pregnant (see *Pregnancy and lactation*).

Coracten XL Capsules should not be used in clinically significant aortic stenosis, unstable angina, or during or within one month of a myocardial infarction. They should not be used in patients in cardiogenic shock.

Coracten XL Capsules should not be used for the treatment of acute attacks of angina, or in patients who have had ischaemic pain following its administration previously.

The safety of Coracten XL Capsules in malignant hypertension has not been established.

Coracten XL Capsules should not be used for secondary prevention of myocardial infarction.

Coracten XL Capsules are contra-indicated in patients with acute porphyria.

Coracten XL Capsules should not be administered concomitantly with rifampicin since effective plasma levels of nifedipine may not be achieved owing to enzyme induction.

As Coracten XL is a long acting formulation, it should not be administered to patients with hepatic impairment.

Special warnings and precautions for use: Nifedipine should be used with caution in patients who are hypotensive; in patients with poor cardiac reserve; in patients with heart failure or significantly impaired left ventricular function as their condition may deteriorate; in diabetic patients as they may require adjustment of their diabetic therapy; and in dialysis patients with malignant hypertension and irreversible renal failure with hypovolaemia, since a significant drop in blood pressure may occur due to the vasodilator effects of nifedipine.

Since nifedipine has no beta-blocking activity, it gives no protection against the dangers of abrupt withdrawal of beta-blocking drugs. Withdrawal of any previously prescribed beta-blockers should be gradual, preferably over 8 to 10 days.

Nifedipine may be used in combination with beta-blocking drugs and other antihypertensive agents, but the possibility of an additive effect resulting in postural hypotension should be borne in mind. Nifedipine will not prevent possible rebound effects after cessation of other anti-hypertensive therapy.

Interactions with other medicaments and other forms of interaction: As with other dihydropyridines, nifedipine should not be taken with grapefruit juice because bioavailability is increased.

The simultaneous administration of nifedipine and digoxin may lead to reduced digoxin clearance and hence an increase in the plasma digoxin. Digoxin levels should be monitored and, if necessary, the digoxin dose reduced.

Nifedipine may increase the spectrophotometric values of urinary vanillylmandelic acid falsely. However, HPLC measurements are unaffected.

Coracten XL Capsules should not be administered concomitantly with rifampicin since effective plasma levels of nifedipine may not be achieved owing to enzyme induction (see *Contra-indications*).

Increased plasma levels of nifedipine have been reported during concomitant use of H_2-receptor antagonists (specifically cimetidine), other calcium channel blockers (specifically diltiazem), alcohol and cyclosporin.

Decreased plasma levels of nifedipine have been reported during concomitant use of antibacterials (specifically rifampicin), and probably also antiepileptics.

When used in combination with nifedipine, plasma concentrations of quinidine have been shown to be suppressed regardless of quinidine dosage. The plasma concentrations of phenytoin, theophylline, non-depolarising muscle relaxants (e.g. tubocurarine) and possibly digoxin are increased when used in combination with nifedipine.

Profound hypotension has been reported with nifedipine and intravenous magnesium sulphate in the treatment of pre-eclampsia.

Pregnancy and lactation:

Pregnancy: Because animal studies show embryotoxicity and teratogenicity, nifedipine is contraindicated during pregnancy (see also *Contra-indications*). Embryotoxicity was noted at 6 to 20 times the maximum recommended dose for nifedipine given to rats, mice and rabbits, and teratogenicity was noted in rabbits given 20 times the maximum recommended dose for nifedipine.

Lactation: Nifedipine is secreted in breast milk, therefore, Coracten XL Capsules are not recommended during lactation.

Effects on ability to drive and use machines: None known.

Undesirable effects: Most side-effects are consequences of the vasodilatory effects of nifedipine. They include headache, flushing and, usually at higher dosages, nausea, dyspepsia, heartburn, dizziness, lethargy, skin reactions (rash, urticaria and puritus), paraesthesia, hypotension, palpitation, tachycardia, dependent oedema, increased frequency of micturition, eye pain, depression, allergic hepatitis, fever, gingival hyperplasia and telangiectasia.

Other less frequently reported side-effects include myalgia, tremor and visual disturbances. Impotence may occur rarely. Mood changes may occur rarely. Altered bowel habit may occur occasionally.

As with other sustained release dihydropyridines, exacerbation of angina pectoris may occur rarely at the start of treatment with sustained release formulations of nifedipine. The occurrence of myocardial infarction has been described although it is not possible to distinguish such an event from the natural course of ischaemic heart disease. Ischaemic pain has been reported in a small proportion of patients following the introduction of nifedipine therapy. Although a 'steal' effect has not been demonstrated, patients experiencing this effect should discontinue nifedipine therapy.

There are reports in older men on long-term therapy of gynaecomastia which usually regresses upon withdrawal of therapy.

Side-effects which may occur in isolated cases are photosensitivity, exfoliative dermatitis, systemic allergic reactions and purpura. Usually, these regress after discontinuation of the drug.

Rare cases of hypersensitivity-type jaundice have been reported. In addition, disturbances of liver function such as intra-hepatic cholestasis may occur. These regress after discontinuation of therapy.

Overdose:

Clinical effects: Reports of nifedipine overdosage are limited and symptoms are not necessarily dose-related. Severe hypotension due to vasodilation, and tachycardia and bradycardia are the most likely manifestations of overdose.

Metabolic disturbances include hyperglycaemia, metabolic acidosis and hypo- or hyperkalaemia.

Cardiac effects may include heart block, AV dissociation and asystole, and cardiogenic shock with pulmonary oedema.

Other toxic effects include nausea, vomiting, drowsiness, dizziness, confusion, lethargy, flushing, hypoxia and unconsciousness to the point of coma.

Treatment: As far as treatment is concerned, elimination of nifedipine and the restoration of stable cardiovascular conditions have priority.

After oral ingestion, gastric lavage is indicated, if necessary in combination with irrigation of the small intestine. Ipecacuanha should be given to children.

Elimination must be as complete as possible, including the small intestine, to prevent the otherwise inevitable subsequent absorption of the active substance.

Activated charcoal should be given in 4-hourly doses of 25 g for adults, 10 g for children.

Blood pressure, ECG, central arterial pressure, pulmonary wedge pressure, urea and electrolytes should be monitored.

Hypotension as a result of cardiogenic shock and arterial vasodilation should be treated with elevation of the feet and plasma expanders. If these measures are ineffective, hypotension may be treated with 10% calcium gluconate 10–20 ml intravenously over 5–10 minutes. If the effects are inadequate, the treatment can be continued, with ECG monitoring. In addition, beta-sympathomimetics may be given, e.g. isoprenaline 0.2 mg slowly i.v. or as a continuous infusion of 5 mcg/min. If an insufficient increase in blood pressure is achieved with calcium and isoprenaline, vasoconstricting sympathomimetics such as dopamine or noradrenaline should be administered. The dosage of these drugs should be determined by the patient's response.

Bradycardia may be treated with atropine, beta-sympathomimetics or a temporary cardiac pacemaker, as required.

Additional fluids should be administered with caution to avoid cardiac overload.

Pharmacological properties

Pharmacodynamic properties: Nifedipine is a potent calcium-channel blocker which, by dilating peripheral arterial smooth muscle, decreases cardiac work and myocardial oxygen requirement. It also dilates coronary arteries, thereby improving myocardial perfusion and reducing coronary artery spasm. In hypertension, it reduces blood pressure but has little or no effect in normotensive subjects. It has no therapeutic antiarrhythmic effect.

Pharmacokinetic properties: Coracten XL Capsules are a sustained release formulation of nifedipine designed to provide less fluctuation and more prolonged nifedipine blood concentrations than standard immediate release preparations.

Nifedipine is highly protein bound. It undergoes

hepatic oxidation to inactive metabolites which are excreted in the urine (80%) and faeces (20%).

Preclinical safety data: There are no pre-clinical data of relevance to the prescriber which are additional to that already included in other sections of the Summary of Product Characteristics.

Pharmaceutical particulars

List of excipients:

Capsule contents: Lactose monohydrate PhEur, Microcrystalline Cellulose PhEur, Hydroxylpropyl methylcellulose K100 PhEur, Povidone K30 PhEur, Magnesium Stearate PhEur, Hydroxypropylcellulose PhEur, Ammonio methacrylate copolymer type B USP, Polyethylene Glycol 6000 PhEur, Dibutylphthalate PhEur, Titanium dioxide E171 PhEur, Talc PhEur.

Capsule shells: Yellow iron oxide E172 FrPh, Red iron oxide E172 FrPh, Titanium dioxide E171 PhEur, Gelatin PhEur.

The printing ink is made of shellac, purified water, black iron oxide (E172) with 2-ethoxyethanol, soya lecithin, anitfoam, and IMS *or* with ethyl alcohol, isopropyl alcohol, n-butyl alcohol, propylene glycol, ammonium hydroxide and potassium hydroxide.

Incompatibilities: None known.

Shelf life: 36 months.

Special precautions for storage: Do not store above 25°C. Store in the original package.

Nature and contents of container: Coracten XL Capsules are available in blister strips packed in cartons containing 28, 30, 56 and 60 capsules. The blister strips are formed from PVC with a coating of PVdC backed with aluminium foil.

Instruction for use/handling: None.

Marketing authorisation number 00039/0506

Date of approval of the SPC 7 October 1998

Legal category POM

CORACTEN* XL CAPSULES 60 mg

Qualitative and quantitative composition Each capsule contains 60 mg Nifedipine PhEur in sustained release form.

Pharmaceutical form Prolonged release capsule.

Clinical particulars

Therapeutic indications: Coracten XL Capsules are indicated for the treatment of hypertension and the prophylaxis of chronic stable angina pectoris.

Posology and method of administration: The capsules are for oral administration and should be swallowed whole with a little fluid.

Dosage – Angina pectoris and hypertension: Adults only: Normally treatment is initiated with one 30 mg Coracten XL capsule every 24 hours. Dosage may be titrated to a higher level as clinically warranted. The dose may be adjusted to 90 mg every 24 hours.

Children: Coracten XL capsules are not recommended for use in children.

Elderly: The pharmacokinetics of nifedipine are altered in the elderly so that lower maintenance doses of nifedipine may be required compared to younger patients.

Hepatic impairment: As Coracten XL is a long acting formulation, it should not be administered to patients with hepatic impairment.

Renal impairment: Dosage adjustments are not usually required in patients with renal impairment.

Contra-indications: Coracten XL Capsules are contra-indicated in patients with known hypersensitivity to nifedipine or other dihydropyridines because of the theoretical risk of cross reactivity. They should not be used in nursing mothers and women who are or who may become pregnant (see *Pregnancy and lactation*).

Coracten XL Capsules should not be used in clinically significant aortic stenosis, unstable angina, or during or within one month of a myocardial infarction. They should not be used in patients in cardiogenic shock.

Coracten XL Capsules should not be used for the treatment of acute attacks of angina, or in patients who have had ischaemic pain following its administration previously.

The safety of Coracten XL Capsules in malignant hypertension has not been established.

Coracten XL Capsules should not be used for secondary prevention of myocardial infarction.

Coracten XL Capsules are contra-indicated in patients with acute porphyria.

Coracten XL Capsules should not be administered concomitantly with rifampicin since effective plasma levels of nifedipine may not be achieved owing to enzyme induction.

As Coracten XL is a long acting formulation, it should not be administered to patients with hepatic impairment.

Special warnings and precautions for use: Nifedipine should be used with caution in patients who are hypotensive; in patients with poor cardiac reserve; in patients with heart failure or significantly impaired left ventricular function as their condition may deteriorate; in diabetic patients as they may require adjustment of their diabetic therapy; and in dialysis patients with malignant hypertension and irreversible renal failure with hypovolaemia, since a significant drop in blood pressure may occur due to the vasodilator effects of nifedipine.

Since nifedipine has no beta-blocking activity, it gives no protection against the dangers of abrupt withdrawal of beta-blocking drugs. Withdrawal of any previously prescribed beta-blockers should be gradual, preferably over 8 to 10 days.

Nifedipine may be used in combination with beta-blocking drugs and other antihypertensive agents, but the possibility of an additive effect resulting in postural hypotension should be borne in mind. Nifedipine will not prevent possible rebound effects after cessation of other anti-hypertensive therapy.

Interactions with other medicaments and other forms of interaction: As with other dihydropyridines, nifedipine should not be taken with grapefruit juice because bioavailability is increased.

The simultaneous administration of nifedipine and digoxin may lead to reduced digoxin clearance and hence an increase in the plasma digoxin. Digoxin levels should be monitored and, if necessary, the digoxin dose reduced.

Nifedipine may increase the spectrophotometric values of urinary vanillylmandelic acid falsely. However, HPLC measurements are unaffected.

Coracten XL Capsules should not be administered concomitantly with rifampicin since effective plasma levels of nifedipine may not be achieved owing to enzyme induction (see *Contra-indications*).

Increased plasma levels of nifedipine have been reported during concomitant use of H_2-receptor antagonists (specifically cimetidine), other calcium channel blockers (specifically diltiazem), alcohol and cyclosporin.

Decreased plasma levels of nifedipine have been reported during concomitant use of antibacterials (specifically rifampicin), and probably also antiepileptics.

When used in combination with nifedipine, plasma concentrations of quinidine have been shown to be suppressed regardless of quinidine dosage. The plasma concentrations of phenytoin, theophylline, non-depolarising muscle relaxants (e.g. tubocurarine) and possibly digoxin are increased when used in combination with nifedipine.

Profound hypotension has been reported with nifedipine and intravenous magnesium sulphate in the treatment of pre-eclampsia.

Pregnancy and lactation:

Pregnancy: Because animal studies show embryotoxicity and teratogenicity, nifedipine is contraindicated during pregnancy (see also *Contra-indications*). Embryotoxicity was noted at 6 to 20 times the maximum recommended dose for nifedipine given to rats, mice and rabbits, and teratogenicity was noted in rabbits given 20 times the maximum recommended dose for nifedipine.

Lactation: Nifedipine is secreted in breast milk, therefore, Coracten XL Capsules are not recommended during lactation.

Effects on ability to drive and use machines: None known.

Undesirable effects: Most side-effects are consequences of the vasodilatory effects of nifedipine. They include headache, flushing and, usually at higher dosages, nausea, dyspepsia, heartburn, dizziness, lethargy, skin reactions (rash, urticaria and puritus), paraesthesia, hypotension, palpitation, tachycardia, dependent oedema, increased frequency of micturition, eye pain, depression, allergic hepatitis, fever, gingival hyperplasia and telangiectasia.

Other less frequently reported side-effects include myalgia, tremor and visual disturbances. Impotence may occur rarely. Mood changes may occur rarely. Altered bowel habit may occur occasionally.

As with other sustained release dihydropyridines, exacerbation of angina pectoris may occur rarely at the start of treatment with sustained release formulations of nifedipine. The occurrence of myocardial infarction has been described although it is not possible to distinguish such an event from the natural course of ischaemic heart disease. Ischaemic pain has been reported in a small proportion of patients following the introduction of nifedipine therapy. Although a 'steal' effect has not been demonstrated, patients experiencing this effect should discontinue nifedipine therapy.

There are reports in older men on long-term therapy of gynaecomastia which usually regresses upon withdrawal of therapy.

Side-effects which may occur in isolated cases are photosensitivity, exfoliative dermatitis, systemic allergic reactions and purpura. Usually, these regress after discontinuation of the drug.

Rare cases of hypersensitivity-type jaundice have been reported. In addition, disturbances of liver function such as intra-hepatic cholestasis may occur. These regress after discontinuation of therapy.

Overdose:

Clinical effects: Reports of nifedipine overdosage are limited and symptoms are not necessarily dose-related. Severe hypotension due to vasodilation, and tachycardia and bradycardia are the most likely manifestations of overdose.

Metabolic disturbances include hyperglycaemia, metabolic acidosis and hypo- or hyperkalaemia.

Cardiac effects may include heart block, AV dissociation and asystole, and cardiogenic shock with pulmonary oedema.

Other toxic effects include nausea, vomiting, drowsiness, dizziness, confusion, lethargy, flushing, hypoxia and unconsciousness to the point of coma.

Treatment: As far as treatment is concerned, elimination of nifedipine and the restoration of stable cardiovascular conditions have priority.

After oral ingestion, gastric lavage is indicated, if necessary in combination with irrigation of the small intestine. Ipecacuanha should be given to children.

Elimination must be as complete as possible, including the small intestine, to prevent the otherwise inevitable subsequent absorption of the active substance.

Activated charcoal should be given in 4-hourly doses of 25 g for adults, 10 g for children.

Blood pressure, ECG, central arterial pressure, pulmonary wedge pressure, urea and electrolytes should be monitored.

Hypotension as a result of cardiogenic shock and arterial vasodilation should be treated with elevation of the feet and plasma expanders. If these measures are ineffective, hypotension may be treated with 10% calcium gluconate 10-20 ml intravenously over 5–10 minutes. If the effects are inadequate, the treatment can be continued, with ECG monitoring. In addition, beta-sympathomimetics may be given, e.g. isoprenaline 0.2 mg slowly i.v. or as a continuous infusion of 5 mcg/min. If an insufficient increase in blood pressure is achieved with calcium and isoprenaline, vasoconstricting sympathomimetics such as dopamine or noradrenaline should be administered. The dosage of these drugs should be determined by the patient's response.

Bradycardia may be treated with atropine, beta-sympathomimetics or a temporary cardiac pacemaker, as required.

Additional fluids should be administered with caution to avoid cardiac overload.

Pharmacological properties

Pharmacodynamic properties: Nifedipine is a potent calcium-channel blocker which, by dilating peripheral arterial smooth muscle, decreases cardiac work and myocardial oxygen requirement. It also dilates coronary arteries, thereby improving myocardial perfusion and reducing coronary artery spasm. In hypertension, it reduces blood pressure but has little or no effect in normotensive subjects. It has no therapeutic antiarrhythmic effect.

Pharmacokinetic properties: Coracten XL Capsules are a sustained release formulation of nifedipine designed to provide less fluctuation and more prolonged nifedipine blood concentrations than standard immediate release preparations.

Nifedipine is highly protein bound. It undergoes hepatic oxidation to inactive metabolites which are excreted in the urine (80%) and faeces (20%).

Preclinical safety data: There are no pre-clinical data of relevance to the prescriber which are additional to that already included in other sections of the Summary of Product Characteristics.

Pharmaceutical particulars

List of excipients:

Capsule contents: Lactose monohydrate PhEur, Microcrystalline cellulose PhEur, Hydroxylpropyl methylcellulose K100 PhEur, Povidone K30 PhEur, Magnesium stearate PhEur, Hydroxypropylcellulose PhEur, Ammonio methacrylate copolymer type B USP, Polyethylene glycol 6000 PhEur, Dibutylphthalate PhEur, Titanium dioxide E171 PhEur, Talc PhEur.

Capsule shells: Red iron oxide E172 Fr Ph, Titanium dioxide E171 PhEur, Gelatin PhEur.

The printing ink is made of shellac, purified water, black iron oxide (E172) with 2-ethoxyethanol, soya lecithin, anitfoam, and IMS *or* with ethyl alcohol, isopropyl alcohol, n-butyl alcohol, propylene glycol, ammonium hydroxide and potassium hydroxide.

Incompatibilities: None known.

Shelf life: 36 months.

Special precautions for storage: Do not store above 25°C. Store in the original package.

Nature and contents of container: Coracten XL Capsules are available in blister strips packed in cartons containing 28, 30, 56 and 60 capsules. The blister strips are formed from PVC with a coating of PVdC backed with aluminium foil.

Instruction for use/handling: None.

Marketing authorisation number 00039/0507

Date of first approval of SPC 7 October 1998

Legal category POM

CORLAN* PELLETS

Qualitative and quantitative composition Each pellet contains 2.5 mg Hydrocortisone in the form of the ester hydrocortisone sodium succinate.

Pharmaceutical form Small white pellet engraved 'Corlan Evans' on one side.

Clinical particulars

Therapeutic indications: Local use in previously diagnosed aphthous ulceration of the mouth, whether simple or occuring as a complication in diseases such as sprue, idiopathic steatorrhoea or ulcerative colitis.

Posology and method of administration:

Adults and elderly: Corlan Pellets should not be sucked, but kept in the mouth and allowed to dissolve slowly in close proximity to the ulcers. One pellet should be used in this way four times a day. If the ulcers have not healed after 5 days of treatment (completion of one pack), or if they recur quickly after healing, a doctor should be consulted.

Children under 12 years of age: Children under 12 years old must see a doctor before starting each course of Corlan Pellets.

Contra-indications: Corlan Pellets should not be used in the presence of oral infection unless effective appropriate anti-infective therapy is also employed. Hypersensitivity to any component of the product.

Special warnings and precautions for use: If aphthous ulceration is severe or recurring, serious underlying disease should be excluded.

Interactions with other medicaments and other forms of interaction: None known.

Pregnancy and lactation: There is inadequate evidence of safety in human pregnancy. Topical administration of corticosteroids to pregnant animals can cause abnormalities of foetal development including cleft palate and intra-uterine growth retardation. There may, therefore, be a very small risk of such effects in the human foetus.

Effects on ability to drive and use machines: None known.

Undesirable effects: Corticosteroids may worsen diabetes.

Occasionally, topical therapy may result in an exacerbation of local infection.

Overdose: Treatment is unlikely to be needed in cases of acute overdosage.

Pharmacological particulars

Pharmacodynamic properties: None stated.

Pharmacokinetic properties: None stated.

Preclinical safety data: None stated.

Pharmaceutical particulars

List of excipients: Lactose BP, Acacia BP, Magnesium Stearate BP.

Incompatibilities: None known.

Shelf life: 3 years.

Special precautions for storage: Store below 25°C. Replace cap firmly after use.

Nature and contents of container: Tamper evident polypropylene container with polythene lid containing 20 pellets.

Tubular glass vials with snap-plug closure containing 20 pellets.

Instruction for use/handling: None.

Marketing authorisation number 0039/0397

Date of approval/revision of the SPC September 1997

Legal category POM

CRYSTACIDE* CREAM 1%

Qualitative and quantitative composition

Active ingredient: Hydrogen peroxide 1.0% (w/w). 1 g of cream contains 10 mg of hydrogen peroxide at a concentration of 1%.

Pharmaceutical form Cream.

Clinical particulars

Therapeutic indications: Crystacide cream is intended for topical application for the treatment of primary and secondary superficial skin infections caused by organisms sensitivity to hydrogen peroxide.

Posology and method of administration:

Adults, elderly and children: Crystacide cream is applied 2–3 times daily on the infected skin area. The treatment period should not exceed 3 weeks. A dry film will appear on the skin after application, this can be washed off with water.

Contra-indications: Known hypersensitivity to one or more constiuents of the product.

Special warnings and precautions for use: Contact with the eyes should be avoided.

Interaction with other medicaments and other forms of interaction: Crystacide cream is incompatible with iodine, permanganates and other stronger oxidising agents.

Pregnancy and lactation: Not applicable.

Effects on ability to drive and use machines: Not applicable.

Undesirable effects: Crystacide is generally well tolerated and not associated with any serious side effects. However, a mild sensation of burning may be experienced for a short time after application.

Overdose: Not applicable.

Pharmacological particulars

Pharmacodynamic properties: Hydrogen peroxide is a well-known antiseptic agent, and is effective against a majority of pathogenic micro-organisms.

In vitro pharmacology studies have shown that hydrogen peroxide has both activity against a wide variety of micro-organisms, and is a potent antibacterial agent with effect against Gram-positive as well as Gram-negative bacteria.

In vitro studies have shown that the bactericidal activity of Crystacide cream 1% is equal in effect compared with a 1% aqueous solution of hydrogen peroxide, and the duration of action is longer for the cream.

There are no known pathogenic bacteria or fungi that develop resistance to hydrogen peroxide.

Pharmacokinetic properties: Reports on the rate of absorption, distribution and excretion of hydrogen peroxide after oral administration are sparse. In the absence of stabilising agent, hydrogen peroxide gradually decomposes to oxygen and water. The decomposition is rapid in the presence of the endogenous enzyme catalase or peroxidase.

Preclinical safety data: There are no pre-clinical data of relevance to the prescriber which are additional to that already included in other sections of the SPC.

Pharmaceutical particulars

List of excipients: Glyceryl monolaurate, Glyceryl monomyristate, Polyoxyethylene (100) stearate, Propylene glycol, Citric acid anhydrous, Sodium hydroxide, Sulphuric acid, 1M, Sodium oxalate, Salicylic acid, Disodium edetate, Sodium pyrophosphate, Sodium stannate, Purified water.

Incompatibilities: Iodine, permanganates and other stronger oxidising agents.

Shelf life: The shelf life for Crystacide cream is 2 years from the date of manufacture.

Special precautions for storage: Store below 25°C, in a dry place.

Nature and contents of container: Crystacide cream is filled into polyethylene tubes pigmented with titanium dioxide, and fitted with polypropylene caps. Each tube is subsequently packed in a unit, printed boxboard carton, in pack sizes of 10 g and 25 g. 5 g and 40 g tubes are licensed but not marketed.

Instructions for use and handling: Not applicable.

Product licence holder: Bioglan Laboratories Limited, 5 Hunting Gate, Hitchin, Hertfordshire, SG4 0TJ

Marketing authorisation number 0041/0043

Date of approval/revision of SPC January 1996

Legal category P

CYTAMEN* INJECTION 1000 mcg

Qualitative and quantitative composition Cyanocobalamin BP 1.0 mg.

Pharmaceutical form Solution for injection.

Clinical particulars

Therapeutic indications: Addisonian pernicious anaemia. Prophylaxis and treatment of other macrocytic anaemias associated with vitamin B_{12} deficiency. Schilling test.

Not indicated for treatment of toxic amblyopias – use Neo-Cytamen.

Posology and method of administration: Route of administration: intramuscular.

Adults and Children: *Addisonian pernicious anaemia and other macrocytic anaemias without neurological involvement:* Initially: 250 to 1000 mcg intramuscularly on alternate days for one to two weeks, then 250 mcg weekly until the blood count is normal. Maintenance: 1000 mcg monthly.

Addisonian pernicious anaemia and other macrocytic anaemias with neurological complications: Initially: 1000 mcg intramuscularly on alternate days as long as improvement is occurring. Maintenance: 1000 mcg monthly.

Prophylaxis of macrocytic anaemia associated with vitamin B_{12} deficiency resulting from gastrectomy, some malabsorption syndromes and strict vegetarianism: 250 mcg – 1000 mcg monthly.

Schilling Test: An intramuscular injection of 1000 mcg cyanocobalamin is an essential part of this test.

Contra-indications: Hypersensitivity to cyanocobalamin. Not indicated for treatment of toxic amblyopias– use Neo-Cytamen.

Special warnings and precautions for use: Precautions: The dosage schemes given above are usually satisfactory, but regular examination of the blood is advisable. If megaloblastic anaemia fails to respond to Cytamen, folate metabolism should be investigated. Doses in excess of 10 mcg daily may produce a haematological response in patients with folate deficiency. Indiscriminate administration may mask the true diagnosis. Cardiac arrhythmias secondary to hypokalaemia during initial therapy have been reported. Plasma potassium should therefore be monitored during this period.

Interactions with other medicaments and other forms of interaction: Chloramphenicol-treated patients may respond poorly to Cytamen. Serum concentrations of cyanocobalamin may be lowered by oral contraceptives but this interaction is unlikely to have clinical significance.

Antimetabolites and most antibiotics invalidate vitamin B_{12} assays by microbiological techniques.

Pregnancy and lactation: Cytamen should not be used for the treatment of megaloblastic anaemia of pregnancy unless vitamin B_{12} deficiency has been demonstrated. Cytamen is secreted into breast milk but this is unlikely to harm the infant, and may be beneficial if the mother and infant are vitamin B_{12} deficient.

Effects on ability to drive and use machines: None.

Undesirable effects: Hypersensitivity reactions have been reported including skin reactions (e.g. rash, itching) and exceptionally anaphylaxis. Other symptoms reported include fever, chills, hot flushing, dizziness, malaise, nausea, acneiform and bullous eruptions.

Overdose: Treatment is unlikely to be needed in cases of overdosage.

Pharmacological particulars

Pharmacodynamic properties: Cyanocobalamin is a form of vitamin B_{12}.

Pharmacokinetic properties: Cobalamins are absorbed from the gastro-intestinal tract, but may be irregularly absorbed when given in large therapeutic doses. Absorption is impaired in patients with an absence of intrinsic factor, with a malabsorption syndrome or with a disease or abnormality of the gut, or after gastrectomy.

Preclinical safety data: None stated.

Pharmaceutical particulars

List of excipients: Sodium chloride BP, Acetic acid BP, Water for injection BP.

Incompatibilities: None.

Shelf life: 36 months.

Special precautions for storage: Protect from light.

Nature and contents of container: 1 ml glass ampoules in packs of 5.

Instructions for use/handling: None stated.

Marketing authorisation number 0039/0403

Date of approval/revision of SPC June 1997

Legal category POM

DEXEDRINE* TABLETS 5 mg

Qualitative and quantitative composition Dexamphetamine Sulphate 5 mg.

Pharmaceutical form Tablets for oral administration.

Clinical particulars

Therapeutic indications: Dexedrine is a sympathomimetic amine with central stimulant and anorectic activity. It is indicated in narcolepsy. It is also indicated for children with refractory hyperkinetic states under the supervision of a physician specialising in child psychiatry.

Posology and method of administration:

Adults: In narcolepsy, the usual starting dose is 10 mg Dexedrine a day, given in divided doses. Dosage may be increased if necessary by 10 mg a day at weekly intervals to a suggested maximum of 60 mg a day.

Elderly: Start with 5 mg a day, and increase by increments of 5 mg at weekly intervals.

Children: In hyperkinetic states, the usual starting dosage for children aged 3-5 years is 2.5 mg a day, increased if necessary by 2.5 mg a day at weekly intervals; for children aged 6 years and over, the usual starting dose is 5-10 mg a day increasing if necessary by 5 mg at weekly intervals.

The usual upper limit is 20 mg a day though some older children have needed 40 mg or more for optimal response.

Contra-indications: Do not use in patients known to be intolerant of sympathomimetic amines; during, or for 14 days after treatment with an MAO inhibitor; in those with a history of drug abuse; with symptomatic cardiovascular disease and/or moderate or severe hypertensive disease; in those suffering from hyperthyroidism or hyperexcitability or in those with glaucoma; Gilles de la Tourette syndrome or similar dystonias; porphyria.

Special warnings and precautions for use: Use with caution in patients on guanethidine and patients with mild hypertension or a family history of dystonias. If tics develop, discontinue treatment with dexedrine. Dexamphetamine is likely to reduce the convulsant threshold therefore caution is advised in patients with epilepsy. Height and weight should be carefully monitored in children as growth retardation may occur.

Interaction with other medicaments and other forms of interaction: Adrenoreceptor blocking agents (e.g. propanolol), lithium and α methyltyrosine may antagonise the effects of dexamphetamine. Disulfiram may inhibit metabolism and excretion.

The concurrent use of tricyclic antidepressants may increase the risk of cardiovascular side effects.

Pregnancy and lactation: Dexamphetamine has been thought to produce embroytoxic effects in rodents and retrospective evidence of certain significance in man has suggested a similar possibility. Dexedrine should therefore be avoided in pregnancy, especially during the first trimester.

Dexedrine passes into breast milk.

Effects on ability to drive and use machines: Dexedrine may affect ability to drive or operate machinery.

Undesirable effects: Insomnia, restlessness, irritability, euphoria, tremor, dizziness, headache and other symptoms of over-stimulation have been reported. Also dry mouth, unwanted anorexia and other gastrointestinal symptoms, sweating and cardiovascular effects such as tachycardia, palpitations and minor increases in blood pressure.

There have been isolated reports of cardiomyopathy associated with chronic amphetamine use.

Drug dependence, with consumption of increasing doses to levels many times those recommended, may occur as tolerance develops. At such levels, a psychosis which may be clinically indistinguishable from schizophrenia can occur.

Treatment should be stopped gradually since abrupt cessation may produce extreme fatigue and mental depression.

Intracranial haemorrhages have been reported, presumably precipitated by the hypertensive effect and possibly associated with pre-existing vascular malformation.

A toxic hypermetabolic state, characterised by transient hyperactivity, hyperpyrexia, acidosis and death due to cardiovascular collapse have been reported.

Rhabdomyolysis and renal damage.

Overdose: Symptoms of overdosage include excitement, hallucinations, convulsions leading to coma; tachycardia and cardiac arrhythmias; and respiratory depression.

Treatment consists of the induction of vomiting and/or gastric lavage together with supportive and symptomatic measures. Excessive stimulation or convulsions may be treated with diazepam. Excretion of dexamphetamine may be increased by forced acid diuresis.

Pharmacological particulars

Pharmacodynamic properties: Dexedrine is a sympathomimetic amine with a central stimulant and anorectic activity.

Pharmacokinetic properties: Dexamphetamine is readily absorbed from the gastrointestinal tract. It is resistant to metabolism by monoamine oxidase. It is excreted in the urine as unchanged parent drug together with some hydroxylated metabolites. Elimination is increased in acidic urine. After high doses, elimination in the urine may take several days.

Preclinical safety data: Dexamphetamine has been thought to produce embryotoxic effects in rodents, and retrospective evidence of uncertain significance in man has suggested a similar possibility. Dexedrine should therefore be avoided in pregnancy, especially during the first trimester. Dexedrine passes into breast milk.

Pharmaceutical particulars

List of excipients: Stearic acid BP, Acacia powder EP, Lactose EP, Liquid paraffin EP, Maize starch EP, Sucrose EP, Purified talc EP, Purified water EP.

Incompatibilities: None stated.

Shelf life: 5 years.

Special precautions for storage: No special storage precautions are necessary.

Nature and contents of container: Polypropylene securitainers, amber glass bottles or polythene vials containing 1000 and 100 tablets. Blister packs containing 100 and 28 tablets.

Instructions for use/handling: None.

Marketing authorisation number 0039/0385

Date of approval/revision of SPC September 1997

Legal category CD (Sch 2), POM

DIAMORPHINE HYDROCHLORIDE BP FOR INJECTION

Presentation Ampoules containing 5, 10, 30, 100 and 500 mg of Diamorphine Hydrochloride BP as a white freeze-dried plug. The colour of the plugs in the larger strength ampoules is off-white, and occasionally the integral plug may break up to produce a crystalline powder.

Uses Diamorphine is a powerful narcotic analgesic which is more potent than morphine and more likely to produce euphoria and addiction, but relatively less nausea, constipation and hypotension.

It is readily absorbed after injection and rapidly hydrolysed to 6–monoacetylmorphine in the blood, and then more slowly metabolised to morphine the major active metabolite. Up to 80% of a dose is excreted in the urine in 24 hours, mainly as morphine-3-glucuronide together with about 5 to 7% of the dose as free morphine.

Diamorphine is used to control severe pain, such as that associated with cancer, acute myocardial infarction and in the treatment of acute pulmonary oedema.

Dosage and administration

Administration: The drug may be given by the intramuscular, subcutaneous or intravenous routes, the latter two routes using either bolus injection or infusion.

Its solubility in water is 1 in 1.6, and the small volume of diluent required is of obvious benefit in treating an emaciated patient. Presentations up to 100 mg will readily dissolve in 1 ml of diluent. Because of the bulk of material in the 500 mg ampoule, a minimum of 2 ml of diluent is required to effect solution and it is recommended that the plug be tapped down, thoroughly wetted and the ampoule gently shaken until the plug dissolves.

Dosage: It is important that the dosage be suited to the individual patient, taking into account the properties of the drug, the nature of the pain, the total condition of the patient and previous or concurrent medication.

5, 10, 30, 100 and 500 mg are recommended for:

Cancer: Use of Diamorphine or other narcotic analgesics although very important, should be only one part of the comprehensive approach to total pain control, which ideally should include non-drug measures and psychosocial support. Diamorphine may be used parenterally when oral administration of narcotic analgesics is no longer possible because of the dosage required, impaired absorption, intestinal disorders, nausea and vomiting or difficulty in swallowing.

An initial dosage of 5 to 10 mg every 4 hours may be suitable, but higher doses are reported in the literature (Dover SB. BMJ 1987;294:553-555.). The initial dosage will usually depend on the doses and drugs given previously. Persistent pain is controlled by titrating the dose against the degree of pain, until the smallest dose required to remove the pain is reached. This dose is maintained and the patient's condition continually reassessed, the dose being increased or decreased as necessary. The therapeutic objective must be to control the pain by regular administration of the correct dose when this is determined, and continuous infusion may be preferred to intermittent therapy.

5 mg and 10 mg ampoules are recommended for:

Acute myocardial infarction: A dose of 5 mg may be given by slow intravenous injection (1 mg per minute), followed by 2.5 to 5 mg if necessary.

Acute pulmonary oedema: A dose of 2.5 to 5 mg may be given by slow intravenous injection (1 mg per minute).

Equivalent Doses of Morphine Sulphate by mouth (as oral solution or standard tablets or as modified-release tablets) or of Diamorphine Hydrochloride by Intramuscular Injection or by Subcutaneous Infusion:

These equivalences are approximate only and may need to be adjusted according to response:

ORAL MORPHINE		*PARENTERAL MORPHINE*	
Morphine sulphate oral solution or standard tablets	*Morphine sulphate modified-release tablets*	*Diamorphine hydrochloride by intramuscular injection*	*Diamorphine hydrochloride by subcutaneous infusion*
every 4 hours	**every 12 hours**	**every 4 hours**	**every 24 hours**
5 mg	20 mg	2.5 mg	15 mg
10 mg	30 mg	5 mg	20 mg
15 mg	50 mg	5 mg	30 mg
20 mg	60 mg	7.5 mg	45 mg
30 mg	90 mg	10 mg	60 mg
40 mg	120 mg	15 mg	90 mg
60 mg	180 mg	20 mg	120 mg
80 mg	240 mg	30 mg	180 mg
100 mg	300 mg	40 mg	240 mg
130 mg	400 mg	50 mg	300 mg
160 mg	500 mg	60 mg	360 mg
200 mg	600 mg	70 mg	400 mg

Use in children and the elderly: Mainly because of its respiratory depressant effect, caution should be exercised when giving the drug to the elderly and a reduced dose should be used.

Diamorphine has been used in the treatment of terminally ill children. Diamorphine has been administered in reduced doses to children with neoplastic disease when it becomes difficult to give treatment orally. The starting dose should be selected according to age, size, symptoms and previous analgesic requirements and administered 4 hourly; the dose being titrated according to the degree of pain. If treatment continues for more than 24 hours it may be appropriate to use a syringe driver (Burne R, Hunt A. Palliative Medicine 1987;11:27-30.).

Contra-indications, warnings, etc.

Contra-indications: Respiratory depression, obstructive airways disease and concurrent administration of monoamine oxidase inhibitors or within two weeks of their discontinuation. Biliary colic. Phaeochromocytoma.

Warnings: Administration to patients with head injuries or raised intracranial pressure increases the risk of respiratory depression and further elevation of CSF pressure. The sedation and pupillary changes produced may interfere with accurate monitoring of the patient.

The drug can cause hypotension in patients who already have conditions or drug therapy that interfere with the ability to maintain normal blood pressure.

Concurrent administration of other CNS sedative/hypnotic drugs may have an additive effect necessitating their dosage reduction. Administration of drugs having anti-muscarinic activity (atropine and synthetic anticholinergics) may increase the risk of severe constipation and/or urinary retention.

Precautions: Tolerance and physical dependence on the drug is likely to develop in most patients after a few weeks of treatment, but this does not prevent reduction of dosage or discontinuation when considered necessary, and drug abuse is not normally a problem in patients with severe pain. Caution should be exercised however, in using the drug in patients with a known tendency to, or history of, drug abuse.

Care should be exercised in treating the elderly, debilitated patients, and those with hepatic or renal impairment. It is recommended that a lower than normal initial dose is given to these patients.

Careful consideration should be given before treating patients with myxoedema or hypothyroidism, adrenocortical insufficiency, toxic psychoses, CNS depression, prostatic hypertrophy or urethral stricture, kyphoscoliosis, acute alcoholism and delirium tremens, severe inflammatory bowel disease and severe diarrhoea.

Use in pregnancy: There is no evidence of safety in human pregnancy, therefore, as with all drugs it is not advisable to administer diamorphine during pregnancy. Use during labour is not advisable due to the risk of respiratory depression in the new-born.

There is limited information on diamorphine levels in breast milk and it is, therefore, not advisable for patients on high doses of diamorphine to breast feed.

Side-effects: The most serious hazards of therapy are respiratory depression and arrest, although circulatory depression, shock and cardiac arrest can occur.

The most common side-effects are sedation, nausea and vomiting, constipation and sweating.

Other side-effects include tachycardia, postural hypotension, palpitations, faintness and syncope; euphoria, dysphoria, weakness, insomnia, dizziness, confusional symptoms and occasionally hallucinations; dry mouth, anorexia, cramps, taste alterations; urinary retention, reduced libido or potency; pruritus, urticaria and other skin rashes.

Overdosage: The symptoms of serious overdosage are respiratory depression, stupor or coma, muscle flaccidity, cold clammy skin, constricted pupils and occasionally bradycardia and hypotension.

The specific antidote naloxone is indicated if coma or bradypnoea are present. A dose of 0.4 to 2 mg may be given by SC, IM or IV injection repeated at intervals of 2-3 minutes up to a maximum of 10 mg if respiratory function does not improve. The dosage for children is 10 micrograms per kg body weight. Alternatively naloxone may be given by continuous IV infusion, 2 mg diluted in 500 ml intravenous solution, at a rate adjusted to the patient's response.

Pharmaceutical precautions Diamorphine is incompatible with mineral acids and alkalis. Store below 25°C. Protect from light.

Refer to 'Further information' for pharmaceutical compatibility of diamorphine with continuous infusions or co-administered anti-emetics.

Legal category CD(Sch2), POM.

Package quantities Ampoules of 5, 10, 30 mg in cartons of 5 boxes of 100. Ampoules of 100 mg and 500 mg in cartons of 5.

Further information Diamorphine hydrochloride is compatible with Dextrose and Sodium Chloride intravenous infusions, and an aqueous solution has maximum stability of several days at pH 3.8 to 4.4, the stability reducing as the pH rises. For this reason Dextrose Intravenous Infusion is the preferred diluent, particularly when the drug is administered by a continuous infusion pump over 24 to 48 hours.

The occurrence of nausea and vomiting may require the concurrent administration of an anti-emetic. If given together with diamorphine as a bolus injection, normal infusion or in a continuous infusion pump, hyoscine hydrobromide, metoclopramide and methotrimeprazine are compatible with diamorphine concentrations of up to 50 mg/ml, for at least 24 hours. Haloperidol and cyclizine have also been co-administered with diamorphine hydrochloride, but precipitation may occur when using high concentrations of diamorphine hydrochloride and these antiemetics (data on file). Chlorpromazine and prochlorperazine are also compatible with diamorphine hydrochloride, but are not appropriate for administration via the subcutaneous route.

Product licence numbers

5 mg	0039/5662
10 mg	0039/5663
30 mg	0039/5665
100 mg	0039/0154
500 mg	0039/0163

ADSORBED DIPHTHERIA AND TETANUS VACCINE, BP (CHILD)

Qualitative and quantitative composition The composition in terms of active ingredients is as follows:-

Diphtheria toxoid not less than 30IU
Tetanus toxoid not less than 40IU
Quantities expressed per 0.5 ml dose.

Pharmaceutical form Sterile suspension for deep subcutaneous or intramuscular injection to humans.

Clinical particulars

Therapeutic indications: For active immunisation against diphtheria and tetanus in children under 10 years of age.

Adsorbed Diphtheria and Tetanus Vaccine (CHILD) is used for the primary immunisation of infants and children under 10 years of age against tetanus and diphtheria where the use of Adsorbed Diphtheria, Tetanus and Pertussis Vaccine (DTPer/Vac/Ads) is contra-indicated or not required. It is also given to reinforce immunity in children under 10 years of age immunised in infancy with Adsorbed Diphtheria and Tetanus Vaccine (CHILD), (DT/Vac/Ads(Child)) or Adsorbed Diphtheria, Tetanus and Pertussis Vaccine (DTPer/Vac/Ads).

Posology and method of administration:

Infants and children under 10 years: Each dose is 0.5 ml, given by intramuscular or deep subcutaneous injection. The primary course of immunisation consists of three doses with an interval of at least one month between each dose. The intervals between immunisations may be exceeded without need to repeat the full course of immunisation.

Primary course in infants and children under 10 years: Primary immunisation against diphtheria and tetanus may be carried out by the administration of combined Adsorbed Diphtheria, Tetanus and Pertussis Vaccine (DTPer/Vac/Ads) or Adsorbed Diphtheria and Tetanus Vaccine (CHILD) (DT/Vac/Ads(Child)) in infancy. One 0.5 ml dose is given at 2, 3 and 4 months of age.

Reinforcing doses in children under 10 years: Children who have received the primary course of immunisation in infancy require reinforcement of immunity against diphtheria and tetanus. This can be achieved by giving one dose (0.5 ml) Adsorbed Diphtheria and Tetanus Vaccine (CHILD) (DT/Vac/Ads (Child)), at least three years after the last dose of the primary course. The reinforcing dose is commonly given prior to school entry.

Oral Poliomyelitis Vaccine, BP may be given at the same time as Adsorbed Diphtheria and Tetanus Vaccine (CHILD).

Children aged 10 years and over, adults and elderly: **NOT RECOMMENDED.**

A reinforcing dose (0.5 ml) of either Adsorbed Diphtheria and Tetanus Vaccine for Adults and Adolescents or Adsorbed Tetanus Vaccine may be given at 13-18 years of age or on leaving school. In adults and elderly, reinforcement of immunity to diphtheria and/or tetanus can be achieved by administering one dose (0.5 ml) of either Adsorbed Diphtheria Vaccine for Adults and Adolescents, Adsorbed Diphtheria and Tetanus Vaccine for Adults and Adolescents or Adsorbed Tetanus Vaccine.

Shake well before each dose is withdrawn. It is good practice to record the title, dose and lot numbers of all vaccines and the dates of administration.

Contra-indications: Adsorbed Diphtheria and Tetanus Vaccine (CHILD) must not be given intradermally since it may give rise to a persistent skin nodule.

ADSORBED DIPHTHERIA AND TETANUS VACCINE (CHILD) SHOULD NOT BE ADMINISTERED TO CHILDREN AGED 10 YEARS AND OVER, ADULTS AND ELDERLY.

The vaccine should not be administered to a subject who has experienced a serious reaction (e.g. anaphylaxis) to a previous dose of this vaccine or who is known to be hypersensitive to any component thereof.

It is advisable to avoid vaccination during an acute infection.

Special warnings and special precautions for use: Although anaphylaxis is rare, facilities for its management should always be available during vaccination.

Interactions with other medicaments and other forms of interaction: None stated.

Use during pregnancy and lactation: Accurate information is not available on the safety of Adsorbed Diphtheria and Tetanus Vaccine (CHILD) in pregnancy or on the immunisation of lactating women. The vaccine should not be used in pregnancy or lactation.

Effects on ability to drive or use machines: None stated.

Undesirable effects: Local reactions to diphtheria and tetanus vaccines are uncommon in young children. Local reactions consist of swelling, redness and tenderness at the injection-site and may occasionally be severe.

General reactions consisting of transient fever, malaise and headache occur infrequently. Acute allergic reaction-anaphylaxis, urticaria, pallor, cyanosis and polyradiculoneuritis have been reported very rarely after diphtheria/tetanus vaccines.

Angioneurotic oedema, dyspnoea, serum sickness, peripheral neuropathy, neuropathy and polyneuritis have followed the administration of tetanus vaccine.

Calcifying dermatomyositis has been observed in temporal association with tetanus vaccination.

A small painless nodule may form at the injection-site, but usually disappears without sequelae. Occasionally these nodules persist, especially if the inoculation is introduced into the superficial layers of subcutaneous tissue. Very rarely, circumscribed hypertrichosis and eczema are associated with such nodules.

Transverse myelitis has been reported after simultaneous administration of diphtheria and tetanus vaccine and oral polio vaccine, but a cause and effect relationship has not been established.

Any untoward reactions should be reported to the regulatory authorities and to the manufacturer.

Overdose: If overdosage or inadvertent administration is suspected, careful observation of the subject may be necessary. There may not be any sequelae, but subjects should be monitored and appropriate supportive measures should be implemented, according to the type of response seen.

Pharmacological properties Not applicable.

Pharmaceutical particulars

List of excipients: The excipients contained in the preparation are as follows:- Aluminum hydroxide HSE*, Disodium tetraborate (Sodium borate) BP, Succinic acid HSE*, Sodium chloride PhEur, Thiomersal BP, Water for Injections PhEur.

* HSE house specification.

Incompatibilities: None stated.

Shelf life: In filled containers: 2 years.

Special precautions for storage: Store between 2–8°C. Protect from light. Vials should be stored upright. Do not freeze.

Nature and contents of container: PhEur type 1 clear neutral glass ampoules, 1 ml capacity (0.5 ml fill).

Multidose PhEur type 1 clear neutral glass vials, 8 ml capacity (5 ml fill) with butyl rubber plug with an aluminum collar and pigmented polypropylene flip-off top.

Instructions for use/handling: Vaccine which has been frozen should not be used. Discard any partly used vaccine vials at the end of the vaccination session. Disposal should be by incineration at a temperature not less than 1100°C at a registered waste disposal contractor.

Marketing authorisation number 00039/0467

Date of approval/revision of the text February 1998

Legal category POM

ADSORBED DIPHTHERIA VACCINE, BP (CHILD)

Qualitative and quantitative composition The composition in terms of active ingredients is as follows:-

Diphtheria toxoid not less than 30 IU
Quantities expressed per 0.5 ml dose.

Pharmaceutical form Sterile suspension for deep subcutaneous or intramuscular injection to humans.

Clinical particulars

Therapeutic indications: For active immunisation against diphtheria in children under 10 years of age.

Primary immunisation against diphtheria in infancy is usually carried out by the administration of combined Adsorbed Diphtheria, Tetanus and Pertussis Vaccine (DTPer/Vac/Ads) or Adsorbed Diphtheria and Tetanus Vaccine (CHILD) (DT/Vac/Ads(CHILD)). Primary immunisation against diphtheria alone for children under 10 years of age may be carried out with Adsorbed Diphtheria Vaccine (CHILD) (Dip/Vac/Ads(CHILD)).

Posology and method of administration:

Infants and children under 10 years: Each dose is 0.5 ml, given by intramuscular or deep subcutaneous injection.

The primary course of immunisation consists of three doses with an interval of at least one month between each dose. The intervals between immunisations may be exceeded without the need to repeat the full course of immunisation.

Primary course in infants and children under 10 years: Primary immunisation against diphtheria may be carried out by the administration of combined Adsorbed Diphtheria, Tetanus and Pertussis Vaccine (DTPer/Vac/Ads), Adsorbed Diphtheria and Tetanus Vaccine (CHILD) (DT/Vac/Ads(CHILD)) or Adsorbed Diphtheria Vaccine (CHILD) (Dip/Vac/Ads(CHILD)) in infancy. One 0.5 ml dose is given at 2, 3 and 4 months of age.

Reinforcing doses in children under 10 years: Children who have received the primary course of immunisation in infancy require reinforcement of immunity against diphtheria. This can be achieved by giving one dose (0.5 ml) Adsorbed Diphtheria and Tetanus Vaccine (CHILD) (DT/Vac/Ads(CHILD)) or Adsorbed Diphtheria Vaccine (CHILD) (Dip/Vac/Ads(CHILD)), at least three years after the last dose of the primary course. The reinforcing dose is commonly given prior to school entry.

A reinforcing dose (0.5 ml) of either Adsorbed Diphtheria and Tetanus Vaccine for Adults and Adolescents or Adsorbed Tetanus Vaccine may be given at 13–18 years of age or on leaving school.

Oral Poliomyelitis Vaccine, BP may be given at the same time as Adsorbed Diphtheria Vaccine (CHILD).

Children aged 10 years and over, adults and elderly: **NOT RECOMMENDED.**

Reinforcement of immunity can be achieved by administering one dose (0.5 ml) of Adsorbed Diphtheria Vaccine for Adults and Adolescents. Adsorbed Diphtheria and Tetanus Vaccine for Adults and Adolescents may be used if simultaneous reinforcement of immunity against diphtheria and tetanus is required.

Primary or reinforcing doses are recommended for travellers to epidemic or endemic areas.

Shake well before each dose is withdrawn. It is good practice to record the title, dose and lot numbers of all vaccines and dates of administration.

Contra-indications: Adsorbed Diphtheria Vaccine (CHILD) should not be administered intradermally since it may give rise to a persistent skin nodule.

ADSORBED DIPHTHERIA VACCINE (CHILD) SHOULD NOT BE ADMINISTERED TO CHILDREN AGED 10 YEARS AND OVER, ADULTS OR ELDERLY.

The vaccine should not be administered to a subject who has experienced a serious reaction (e.g. anaphylaxis) to a previous dose of this vaccine or who is known to be hypersensitive to any component thereof.

It is advisable to avoid vaccination during an acute infection.

Special warnings and special precautions for use: Although anaphylaxis is rare, facilities for its management should always be available during vaccination.

Interactions with other medicaments and other forms of interaction: None known.

Pregnancy and lactation: Accurate information is not available on the safety of Adsorbed Diphtheria Vaccine (CHILD) in pregnancy or on the immunisation of lactating women. The vaccine should not be used in pregnancy or lactation.

Effects on ability to drive or use machines: None stated.

Undesirable effects: Reactions may be local or general and they may be more frequent and severe after the second injection. Local reactions are uncommon in children under two years of age. Local reactions consisting of swelling, redness and tenderness at the injection-site may occur and may occasionally be severe.

The incidence and severity of local reactions increases rapidly after the age of 10 years, occurring frequently in adults.

General reactions consisting of transient fever, malaise and headache may occur.

Allergic reactions, urticaria, pallor and dyspnoea have been reported following injection of Adsorbed Diphtheria Vaccine (CHILD).

A small painless nodule may form at the injection-site but usually disappears without sequelae. Occasionally these nodules persist, especially if the inoculation is introduced into the superficial layers of subcutaneous tissue. Very rarely, circumscribed hypertrichosis and eczema are associated with such nodules.

Any untoward reactions should be reported to the regulatory authorities and to the manufacturer.

Overdose: If overdosage or inadvertent administration is suspected, careful observation of the subject may be necessary. There may not be any sequelae, but subjects should be monitored and appropriate supportive measures should be implemented, according to the type of response seen.

Pharmacological properties Not applicable.

Pharmaceutical particulars
List of excipients: The excipients contained in the preparation are as follows:- Aluminium phosphate HSE*, Sodium succinate HSE*, Sodium chloride PhEur, Thiomersal BP, Water for Injections PhEur.

* HSE House specification.

Incompatibilities: None stated.

Shelf life: In filled containers: 2 years.

Special precautions for storage: Store between 2 and 8°C. Protect from light. Do not freeze.

Nature and contents of container: PhEur type 1 clear neutral glass ampoules of 1 ml capacity (0.5 ml fill).

Instructions for use/handling: Vaccine which has been frozen should not be used. Disposal should be by incineration at a temperature not less than 1100°C at a registered waste disposal contractor.

Marketing authorisation number 00039/0466

Date of approval/revision of SPC March 1998

Legal category POM

EUDEMINE* TABLETS

Qualitative and quantitative composition Diazoxide BP 50 mg.

Pharmaceutical form White, sugar coated tablet.

Clinical particulars
Therapeutic indications: Eudemine Tablets are used orally in the treatment of intractable hypoglycaemia.

Diazoxide also causes salt and water retention.

Hypoglycaemia: Eudemine administered orally is indicated for the treatment of intractable hypoglycaemia with severe symptoms from a variety of causes including: idiopathic hypoglycaemia in infancy, leucine-sensitive or unclassified; functional islet cell tumours both malignant and benign if inoperable, extra-pancreatic neoplasms producing hypoglycaemia; glycogen storage disease; hypoglycaemia of unknown origin.

Posology and method of administration:

Hypoglycaemia: In hypoglycaemia, the dosage schedule of Eudemine Tablets is determined according to the clinical needs and the response of the individual patient.

For both adults and children a starting oral dose of 5 mg/kg body weight divided into 2 or 3 equal doses per 24 hours will establish the patient's response and thereafter the dose can be increased until the symptoms and blood glucose level respond satisfactorily. Regular determinations of the blood glucose in the initial days of treatment are essential. The usual maintenance dose is 3–8 mg/kg/day given in two or three divided doses.

Reduced doses may be required in patients with impaired renal function.

In children with leucine-sensitive hypoglycaemia, a dosage range of 15–20 mg/kg/day is suggested.

In adults with benign or malignant islet-cell tumours producing large quantities of insulin, high dosages of up to 1,000 mg per day have been used.

Contra-indications: In the treatment of hypoglycaemia, Eudemine is contraindicated in all cases which are amenable to surgery or other specific therapy.

Hypersensitivity to any component of the preparation or other thiazides.

Special warnings and precautions for use: In the treatment of hypoglycaemia it is necessary that the blood pressure be monitored regularly.

Retention of sodium and water is likely to necessitate therapy with an oral diuretic such as frusemide or ethacrynic acid. The dosage of either of the diuretics mentioned may be up to 1 g daily. It must be appreciated that if diuretics are employed then both the hypotensive and hyperglycaemic activities of diazoxide will be potentiated and it is likely that the dosage of diazoxide will require adjustment downwards. In patients with severe renal failure it is desirable to maintain, with diuretic therapy, urinary volumes in excess of 1 litre daily. Hypokalaemia should be avoided by adequate potassium replacement.

Diazoxide should be used with caution in patients with impaired cardiac reserve, in whom sodium and water retention may precipitate congestive heart failure (see *Undesirable effects*).

Diazoxide should be administered with caution to patients with hyperuricaemia or a history of gout, and it is advisable to monitor serum uric acid concentration.

Whenever Eudemine is given over a prolonged period regular haematological examinations are indicated to exclude changes in white blood cell and platelet counts.

Also in children there should be regular assessment of growth, bone and psychological maturation.

The very rapid, almost complete protein binding of diazoxide requires cautious dosage to be used in patients whose plasma proteins may be lower than normal.

Interactions with other medicaments and other forms of interaction: Drugs potentiated by diazoxide therapy include: oral diuretics, anti-hypertensive agents and anticoagulants.

Phenytoin levels should be monitored as increased dosage may be needed if administered concurrently with diazoxide.

The risk of hyperglycaemia may be increased by concurrent administration of corticosteroids or oestrogen-progestogen combinations.

Pregnancy and lactation: Eudemine Tablets are only to be used in pregnant women when the indicated condition is deemed to put the mother's life at risk.

Side Effects: Prolonged oral therapy of Eudemine during pregnancy has been reported to cause alopecia in the new-born.

Eudemine should not be given to nursing mothers as the safety of diazoxide during lactation has not been established.

Effects on ability to drive and use machines: None known.

Undesirable effects: With oral therapy, nausea is common in the first two or three weeks and may require relief with an anti-nauseant. Prolonged therapy has given rise to reports of hypertrichosis lanuginosa, anorexia and hyperuricaemia.

Extra-pyramidal side-effects have been reported with oral diazoxide. It was found that extra-pyramidal effects such as parkinsonian tremor, cogwheel rigidity and oculogyric crisis could be easily suppressed by intravenous injection of an antiparkinsonian drug such as procyclidine and that they could be prevented by maintenance therapy with such a drug given orally.

Other adverse effects of Eudemine which have been reported are hyperosmolar non-ketotic coma, cardiomegaly, leucopenia, thrombocytopenia, and hirsutism.

Sodium and water retention occur frequently in patients receiving multiple doses of diazoxide, and may precipitate cardiac failure in susceptible patients (e.g. those with impaired cardiac reserve). Symptoms of disturbed cardiac function (tachycardia, arrhythmias), inappropriate hypotension or hyperglycaemia (including ketoacidosis) have also been reported.

Diazoxide may cause gastrointestinal disturbances including nausea, vomiting, abdominal pain, anorexia, diarrhoea, ileus and constipation.

Changes in hepatic and renal function have been observed occasionally, including increased AST, alkaline phosphatase, azotemia, decreased creatinine clearance, reversible nephrotic syndrome, haematuria and albuminuria.

Disorders of blood components (decreased haemoglobin and/or haematocrit, eosinophilia, bleeding) have been reported. Hypogammaglobulinaemia may also occur.

Other reported side effects of diazoxide treatment include: headache, dyspnoea, musculoskeletal pain, hypersensitivity reactions (rash, fever, leucopenia), blurred vision, transient cataracts. Voice changes in children and abnormal facies in children on long term treatment have also been reported.

Overdose: Excessive dosage of Eudemine can result in hyperglycaemia which will respond to insulin and/ or to hypotension which will necessitate maintenance of blood volume with intravenous fluids.

Pharmacological particulars
Pharmacodynamic properties: None stated.

Pharmacokinetic properties: None stated.

Preclinical safety data: None stated.

Pharmaceutical particulars
List of excipients: Lactose BP, Maize starch BP, Maize starch, pre-gelatinised BP, Magnesium stearate BP, Purified water BP, Sugar, mineral water HSE, Gelatin coarse powder 200 bloom BP, Sugar, mineral water HSE, Opaglos AG-7350

Incompatibilities: None stated.

Shelf life: 36 months.

Special precautions for storage: None.

Nature and contents of container: Plastic containers with tamper evident closure containing 100 tablets.

Instructions for use/handling: None stated.

Marketing authorisation number 00039/0412

Date of approval/revision of the SPC November 1997

Legal category POM

FLUVIRIN* [Inactivated Influenza Vaccine (Surface Antigen) PhEur]

Qualitative and quantitative composition Each 0.5 ml contains haemagglutinin and neuraminidase* surface antigens obtained from influenza virus strains prepared in embryonated chicken eggs, inactivated by betapropiolactone, split by Triton N101 (nonoxynol 101) and purified. The strains are in accordance with the WHO recommendation (northern hemisphere) and EU decision, which for the 1998/99 season are:

A/Beijing/262/95 (H1N1)–Like strain (A/Beijing/262/95 X-127)	15 mcg haemagglutinin
A/Sydney/5/97 (H3N2)–Like strain (A/Sydney/5/97 RESVIR-13)	15 mcg haemagglutinin
B/Beijing/184/93–Like strain (B/Harbin/7/94)	15 mcg haemagglutinin

* Quantity varying with haemagglutinin content.

Pharmaceutical form Suspension for injection.

Clinical particulars
Therapeutic indications: Prophylaxis of influenza, especially in those who run an increased risk of associated complications.

Posology and method of administration: Adults and children from 36 months: 0.5 ml.

Children from 6 months to 35 months: Clinical data are limited. Dosages of 0.25 ml or 0.5 ml have been used.

For children who have not previously been infected or vaccinated, a second dose should be given after an interval of at least 4 weeks.

Immunisation should be carried out by intramuscular or deep subcutaneous injection.

When a 0.25 ml dose is indicated, the pre-filled syringe should be held in an upright position and half the volume should be eliminated, the remaining volume should be injected.

Contra-indications: Hypersensitivity to eggs, chicken protein or any constituent of the vaccine. Immunisation should be postponed in patients with febrile illness or acute infection.

Special warnings and special precautions for use: As with all injectable vaccines, appropriate medical treatment and supervision should always be readily available in case of a rare anaphylactic event following the administration of the vaccine.

The vaccine (Fluvirin) should under no circumstances be administered intravascularly.

Antibody response in patients with endogenous or iatrogenic immunosuppression may be insufficient.

Very small quantities of neomycin and polymyxin are used during manufacture. Theoretically the vaccine purification process removes these antibiotics, and no adverse effects have been reported. Nevertheless caution should be exercised in patients known to be hypersensitive to these substances.

Thiomersal is also used in manufacture but is reduced by the purification process to a maximum of 0.005 mg (0.001% w/v). Caution should be exercised in patients known to be hypersensitive to thiomersal.

Interaction with other medicaments and other forms of interaction: The vaccine (Fluvirin) may be given at the same time as other vaccines. Immunisation should be carried out on separate limbs. It should be noted that the adverse reactions may be intensified.

The immunological response may be diminished if the patient is undergoing immunosuppressant treatment.

Following influenza vaccination, false positive results in serology tests using the ELISA method to detect antibodies against HIV1, Hepatitis C and especially HTLV1 have been observed. The Western Blot technique disproves the results. The transient false positive reactions could be due to the IgM response by the vaccine.

Pregnancy and lactation: No relevant animal data are available. In humans, up to now, the data are inadequate to assess teratogenic or fetotoxic risk during pregnancy. In pregnant high risk patients the possible risks of clinical infection should be weighed against the possible risks of vaccination.

The vaccine (Fluvirin) may be used during lactation.

Effects on ability to drive and use machines: The vaccine is unlikely to produce an effect on the ability to drive and use machines.

Undesirable effects: The following reactions are most common:

Local reactions: Redness, swelling, pain, ecchymosis, induration

Systemic reactions: Fever, malaise, shivering, fatigue, headache, sweating, myalgia, arthralgia.

These reactions usually disappear within 1–2 days without treatment.

The following events are observed rarely: Neuralgia, paraesthesia, convulsions, transient thrombocytopenia.

Allergic reactions, in rare cases leading to shock, have been reported.

Vasculitis with transient renal involvement has been reported in very rare cases.

Rarely neurological disorders, such as encephalomyelitis, neuritis and Guillain Barré syndrome have been reported. An increased risk of Guillain Barré syndrome has not been demonstrated with currently used influenza vaccines.

Overdose: Overdosage is unlikely to have any untoward effect.

Pharmacological properties

Pharmacodynamic properties: ATC code : J07B B

Seroprotection is generally obtained within 2 to 3 weeks. The duration of postvaccinal immunity varies but is usually 6–12 months.

Pharmacokinetic properties: Not applicable

Preclinical safety data: Not applicable.

Pharmaceutical particulars

List of excipients: Buffer solution (0.01M): Potassium dihydrogenphosphate, Disodium hydrogenphosphate, Sodium chloride, Water for injection.

Others (trace amounts): Sucrose, Triton N101, Thiomersal, Formaldehyde, Betapropiolactone, Ovalbumin, Neomycin and polymyxin.

Incompatibilities: The vaccine (Fluvirin) should not be mixed with other injection fluids.

Shelf life: The expiry date is indicated on the label and packaging. The shelf-life is 1 year.

Special precautions for storage: This product should be stored at +2°C to +8°C (in a refrigerator). Do not freeze. Protect from light.

Nature and contents of container: 0.5 ml suspension in pre-filled syringe (glass).

Instructions for use/handling: The vaccine should be allowed to reach room temperature before use. Shake before use.

Marketing authorisation number 00039/0505

Date of approval/revision of the SPC June 1998

Legal category POM

INTRADERMAL BCG VACCINE, BP

Qualitative and quantitative composition Each 0.1 ml dose contains:

10 dose vaccine: Bacillus Calmette Guerin (Copenhagen sub-strain 1077) 1.0 to 2.6 x 10^6 viable units.

20 and 50 dose vaccine: Bacillus Calmette Guerin (Copenhagen sub-strain 1077) 0.8 to 2.6 x 10^6 viable units.

Pharmaceutical form Freeze-dried standardised preparation of a sub-strain of Bacillus Calmette-Guerin to be reconstituted with Water for Injections, BP or Sodium Chloride Injection, BP prior to intradermal administration.

Clinical particulars

Therapeutic indications: For active immunisation against tuberculosis. Vaccinated persons normally become Mantoux-positive after eight weeks, but sometimes up to 14 weeks are needed.

Posology and method of administration: The INTRADERMAL inoculation should be given in the arm, over the insertion of the deltoid muscle onto the humerus. Administration in the leg has been associated with more severe reactions in neonates and should be avoided. The administration of INTRADERMAL BCG Vaccine should preferably be carried out with a syringe fitted with a short bevel gauge 25 needle. The use of jet injectors to administer the vaccine is not recommended.

Children aged 3 months and over, adults and elderly: 0.1 ml strictly by **INTRADERMAL** injection (subcutaneous injection must be avoided). A tuberculin skin test must be conducted before BCG immunisation.

Infants under 3 months of age: 0.05 ml strictly by **INTRADERMAL** injection (subcutaneous injection must be avoided).

Reconstitution: The vaccine must not be contaminated with any antiseptic or detergent. Avoid contamination with bactericides. If alcohol is used to swab the rubber stopper of the vial, it must be allowed to evaporate before the stopper is penetrated with the syringe needle.

The vaccine suspension is prepared by adding 1 ml of Water for Injections, BP or Sodium Chloride Injection, BP to the 10 dose vial. When using the 50 dose vial, 5 ml of Sodium Chloride Injection, BP (not Water for Injections, BP) should be added. DO NOT shake as this causes frothing. Allow to stand for one minute, then draw into the syringe twice to ensure homogeneity.

Intradermal injection technique: The vaccine must not be contaminated with any antiseptic or detergent. Avoid contamination with bactericides. If alcohol is used to swab the skin, it must be allowed to evaporate before the vaccine is injected.

The upper arm must be approximately 45° to the body. After cleaning and allowing to dry, the skin should be stretched between thumb and forefinger. The needle should be inserted (bevel upwards) slowly for about 2 mm into the superficial layers of dermis. The needle is almost parallel with the skin surface and should be visible through the epidermis during insertion. A raised, blanched bleb showing tips of hair follicles is a sign of correct injection. If considerable resistance is not felt, the needle should be removed and reinserted.

The injection site is best left uncovered to facilitate healing.

It is good practice to record the title, dose and lot numbers of all vaccines and dates of administration.

Contra-indications: INTRADERMAL BCG VACCINE MUST NOT BE ADMINISTERED USING THE MULTIPLE PUNCTURE TECHNIQUE.

INTRADERMAL BCG Vaccine should NOT be given to persons receiving systemic corticosteroids or immunosuppressive treatment including radiotherapy, those suffering from malignant conditions (e.g. lymphoma, leukaemia, Hodgkin's Disease or other tumours of the reticuloendothelial system), those in whom normal immunological mechanism is impaired (e.g. hypogammaglobulinaemia), those known or suspected to be HIV-positive, including infants born to HIV-positive mothers and persons with pyrexia or generalised infected skin conditions. The effect of INTRADERMAL BCG Vaccine may be exaggerated in these patients and a more generalised infection is possible. Eczema is not a contra-indication, but the vaccine site must be lesion free.

INTRADERMAL BCG Vaccine should not be given to patients who are receiving prophylactic doses of anti-tuberculous drugs.

Tuberculin-positive persons, i.e. those with induration of 5 mm or greater in diameter in the Mantoux test, or those in Heaf grades 2 to 4, do not require the vaccine. Its administration to these persons may result in an accelerated local reaction of larger size than normal.

The vaccine should not be administered to a subject who is known to be hypersensitive to any component of the vaccine.

Special warnings and precautions for use: INTRADERMAL BCG Vaccine may be given concurrently with another live vaccine, including Oral Poliomyelitis Vaccine, BP. An interval of not less than three weeks should normally be allowed to lapse between the administration of any two live vaccines, if they are not given at the same time. However, when INTRADERMAL BCG Vaccine is given to infants, there is no need to delay the primary childhood immunisations which includes polio vaccine.

No further vaccination should be given for at least three months in the arm used for BCG vaccination, because of the risk of regional lymphadenitis.

Although anaphylaxis is rare, facilities for its management should always be available during vaccination.

Infectious mononucleosis, viral infections in general, including those of the upper respiratory tract, live viral vaccines, Hodgkin's disease, sarcoidosis, corticosteroid therapy and immunosuppressing treatment or diseases, including HIV, may suppress the reaction to the tuberculin skin test.

Interaction with other medicaments and other forms of interaction: None known.

Pregnancy and lactation: No reproductive studies have been conducted in animals. There are no data on the use of this vaccine in pregnancy or lactation. Vaccination should be avoided in early pregnancy and if possible delayed until after delivery. The vaccine should not normally be used during lactation unless the benefit outweighs the risk.

Effects on ability to drive and use machines: None known.

Undesirable effects: Normally following intradermal administration of BCG, a local reaction develops at the injection site within two to six weeks. This begins as a small papule which increases in size for a few weeks widening into a circular area up to 7 mm in diameter with scaling, crusting and occasional bruising. The lesion slowly subsides over several months and eventually heals leaving only a small, flat scar. Occasionally an ulcer up to 10 mm in diameter develops.

Rash, fever, local induration, pain and lymphadenopathy may occur.

Occasionally an excessive response to INTRADERMAL BCG Vaccine results in a discharging ulcer. This may be attributable to inadvertent subcutaneous injection or to excessive dosage. The ulcer should be encouraged to dry and abrasion avoided, e.g. by tight clothes. Waterproof dressings should not be used. If the ulcer persists, it can be treated by application of a mild corticosteroid cream and/or a topical antibiotic.

In rare cases of severe local reaction with abscess formation, aspiration may be carried out and anti-tuberculous therapy considered. Enlargement of axillary lymph glands is unlikely except occasionally in young infants.

Anaphylactic reactions have been reported on rare occasions.

Any untoward reactions should be reported to the Regulatory Authorities and to the Marketing Authorisation Holder.

Overdose: If gross overdosage occurs and there is reason to suspect the development of a more generalised infection with BCG, systemic treatment with isoniazid or any other suitable anti-tuberculous drug should be given.

Pharmacological particulars This vaccine is used for active immunisation against tuberculosis, principally for the vaccination of selected groups of the population and of persons likely to be exposed to infection.

The vaccine stimulates production of cell mediated immunity with a specific protective capacity against tuberculosis.

In British schoolchildren efficacy (protection against tuberculosis) is 70-80% with protection lasting at least 15 years.

Pharmaceutical particulars

List of excipients: Before freeze-drying, each vial contains 0.5 to 1.0 ml* (±10%) of freeze-drying medium of the following composition: Dextran 8.3%, Glucose 7.5%, Triton WR 1339 0.025%, Water for Injections, BP 100.0%.

* the amount of freeze-drying medium used is such that the depth of suspension in the vial is suitable for freeze-drying.

Water for Injections, BP (PL00039/5704) and Sodium Chloride Injection, BP (PL00039/5699) are provided as diluents with the vaccine.

Incompatibilities: None known.

Shelf life:

10 dose vaccine: 36 months when stored at 2–8°C unopened. 4 hours after reconstitution.

20 and 50 dose vaccine: 24 months when stored at 2–8°C unopened. 4 hours after reconstitution.

Special precautions for storage: The freeze-dried vaccine should be stored between 2–8°C. Protect from light. Diluent should not be frozen but should be stored below 25°C.

Nature and contents of container:

Size: 3 ml vials (10 and 20 dose), 5 ml vials (50 dose).

Type: Neutral (type 1) amber glass vials complying with the PhEur requirements for containers for injectables.

Seals: Siliconised rubber peg bungs with aluminium overseals and polypropylene flip top caps.

Instructions for use and handling: The vaccine suspension is prepared by adding 1 ml of Water for Injections BP or Sodium Chloride Injection BP to the 10 dose vial. When using the 50 dose vial, 5 ml of Sodium Chloride Injection BP (not Water for Injections BP) should be added. DO NOT shake as this causes frothing. Allow to stand for one minute, then draw into the syringe twice to ensure homogeneity.

After reconstitution the vaccine should be kept cool, protected from light and used in the same session, i.e. within 4 hours. Any reconstituted vaccine remaining at the end of the session (maximum 4 hours) should be discarded.

Disposal should be by incineration at a temperature not less than 1100°C at a registered waste disposal contractor.

Marketing authorisation number 0039/0435

Date of approval/revision of SPC March 1997

Legal category POM

INTRADERMAL BCG VACCINE, BP ISONIAZID RESISTANT

Qualitative and quantitative composition Each 0.1 ml dose contains: Bacillus Calmette-Guerin (Isoniazid resistant sub-strain) 0.8 to 2.6 x 10^6 viable units.

Pharmaceutical form Freeze-dried standardised preparation of an isoniazid resistant sub-strain of Bacillus Calmette-Guerin to be reconstituted with Water for Injections, BP or Sodium Chloride Injection, BP prior to intradermal administration.

Clinical particulars

Therapeutic indications: For active immunisation against tuberculosis in tuberculous contacts while they are receiving prophylactic treatment with isoniazid.

It is well established that BCG vaccination of contacts confers protection against tuberculosis and it is especially useful in this respect for new-born infants of tuberculous mothers or infants born into tuberculous households. However, under such circumstances segregation is necessary until Mantoux testing has shown conversion. This undesirable segregation period of a few weeks can be abolished by giving isoniazid to the infant from birth, but the adoption of this procedure suffers from the disadvantage that concurrent administration of isoniazid interferes with the response to normal BCG vaccine. This can be avoided by the use of an isoniazid resistant BCG vaccine, when administration of isoniazid need only continue until the post-BCG tuberculin test becomes positive.

Posology and method of administration: The **INTRADERMAL** inoculation should be given in the arm, over the insertion of the deltoid muscle onto the humerus. The administration of INTRADERMAL BCG Vaccine, BP Isoniazid Resistant should preferably be carried out with a syringe fitted with a short bevel gauge 25 needle. The use of jet injectors to administer the vaccine is not recommended.

Children aged 3 months and over, adults and elderly: 0.1 ml strictly by **INTRADERMAL** injection (subcutaneous injection must be avoided). A tuberculin skin test must be conducted before BCG immunisation.

Infants under 3 months of age: 0.05 ml strictly by **INTRADERMAL** injection (subcutaneous injection must be avoided).

Reconstitution: The vaccine must not be contaminated with any antiseptic or detergent. Avoid contamination with bactericides. If alcohol is used to swab the rubber stopper of the vial, it must be allowed to evaporate before the stopper is penetrated with the syringe needle.

The vaccine suspension is prepared by adding 1 ml of Water for Injections, BP or Sodium Chloride Injection, BP to the vial. Do NOT shake as this causes frothing. Allow to stand for one minute, then draw into the syringe twice to ensure homogeneity.

Intradermal injection technique: The vaccine must not be contaminated with any antiseptic or detergent. Avoid contamination with bactericides. If alcohol is used to swab the skin, it must be allowed to evaporate before the vaccine is injected.

The upper arm must be approximately 45° to the body. After cleaning and allowing to dry, the skin should be stretched between thumb and forefinger. The needle should be inserted (bevel upwards) slowly for about 2 mm into the superficial layers of dermis. The needle is almost parallel with the skin surface and should be visible through the epidermis during insertion. A raised, blanched bleb showing tips of hair follicles is a sign of correct injection. If considerable resistance is not felt, the needle should be removed and reinserted.

The injection site is best left uncovered to facilitate healing.

It is good practice to record the title, dose and lot numbers of all vaccines and dates of administration.

Contra-indications: INTRADERMAL BCG VACCINE, BP ISONIAZID RESISTANT MUST NOT BE ADMINISTERED BY THE MULTIPLE PUNCTURE TECHNIQUE.

INTRADERMAL BCG Vaccine, BP Isoniazid Resistant should NOT be given to persons receiving systemic corticosteroids or immunosuppressive treatment including radiotherapy, those suffering from malignant conditions (e.g. lymphoma, leukaemia, Hodgkin's Disease or other tumours of the reticuloendothelial system), those in whom normal immunological mechanism is impaired (e.g. hypogammaglobulinaemia), those known or suspected to be HIV-positive, including infants born to HIV positive mothers, and persons with pyrexia or generalised infected skin conditions. The effect of INTRADERMAL BCG Vaccine, BP Isoniazid Resistant may be exaggerated in these patients and a more generalised infection is possible. Eczema is not a contra-indication, but the vaccine site must be lesion free.

Tuberculin-positive persons, i.e. those with induration of 5 mm or greater in diameter in the Mantoux test, or those in Heaf grades 2 to 4, do not require the vaccine. Its administration to these persons may result in an accelerated local reaction of larger size than normal.

The vaccine should not be administered to a subject who is known to be hypersensitive to any component of the vaccine.

Special warnings and precautions for use: INTRADERMAL BCG Vaccine, Isoniazid Resistant, may be given concurrently with another live vaccine, including Oral Poliomyelitis Vaccine, BP.. An interval of not less than three weeks should normally be allowed to lapse between the administration of any two live vaccines, if they are not given at the same time. However, when INTRADERMAL BCG Vaccine, Isoniazid Resistant is given to infants, there is no need to delay primary childhood immunisations which include polio vaccine.

No further vaccination should be given for at least three months in the arm used for BCG vaccination, because of the risk of regional lymphadenitis.

Although anaphylaxis is rare, facilities for its management should always be available during vaccination.

Infectious mononucleosis, viral infections in general, including those of the upper respiratory tract, live viral vaccines, Hodgkin's disease, sarcoidosis, corticosteroid therapy and immunosuppressing treatment or diseases, including HIV, may suppress the reaction to the tuberculin skin test.

Interaction with other medicaments and other forms of interaction: None known.

Pregnancy and lactation: No reproductive studies have been conducted in animals. There are no data on the use of this vaccine in pregnancy or lactation. Vaccination should be avoided in early pregnancy and if possible delayed until after delivery. The vaccine should not normally be used during lactation unless the benefit outweighs the risk.

Effects on ability to drive and use machines: None known.

Undesirable effects: Normally following intradermal administration of BCG, a local reaction develops at the injection site within two to six weeks. This begins as a small papule which increases in size for a few weeks widening into a circular area up to 7 mm in diameter with scaling, crusting and occasional bruising. The lesion slowly subsides over several months and eventually heals leaving only a small, flat scar. Occasionally an ulcer up to 10 mm in diameter develops.

Rash, fever, local induration, pain and lymphadenopathy may occur. Occasionally an excessive response to INTRADERMAL BCG Vaccine, BP Isoniazid Resistant results in a discharging ulcer. This may be attributable to inadvertent subcutaneous injection or to excessive dosage. The ulcer should be encouraged to dry and abrasion avoided, e.g. by tight clothes. Waterproof dressings should not be used. If the ulcer persists, it can be treated by application of a mild corticosteroid cream and/or a topical antibiotic.

In rare cases of severe local reaction with abscess formation, aspiration may be carried out and antituberculous therapy considered. Enlargement of axillary lymph glands is unlikely except occasionally in young infants.

Anaphylactic reactions have been reported on rare occasions with INTRADERMAL BCG Vaccine, BP and PERCUTANEOUS BCG Vaccine, BP.

Any untoward reactions should be reported to the regulatory authorities and to the Marketing Authorisation Holder.

Overdose: Not applicable.

Pharmacological particulars This vaccine is suitable for vaccinating tuberculous contacts while they are receiving prophylactic treatment with isoniazid. The vaccine contains an isoniazid resistant sub-strain of Bacillus Calmette-Guerin prepared by repeated subcultivation in the presence of isoniazid.

The vaccine stimulates production of cell mediated immunity with a specific protective capacity against tuberculosis.

Pharmaceutical particulars

List of excipients: Before freeze-drying, each vial contains 0.5 ml ± (10%)* of freeze-drying medium of the following composition: Dextran 8.3%, Glucose 7.5%, Triton WR 1339 0.025%, Water for Injections, BP 100.0%.

* the amount of freeze-drying medium used is such that the depth of suspension in the vial is suitable for freeze-drying.

Incompatibilities: None known.

Shelf life: 24 months when stored at 2-8°C unopened. 4 hours after reconstitution.

Special precautions for storage: Store between 2 and 8°C. Protect from light.

Nature and contents of container:

Size: 3 ml vial (10 dose).

Type: Neutral (type 1) amber glass vials complying with the PhEur requirements for containers for injectables.

Seals: Siliconised rubber peg bungs with aluminium overseals and polypropylene flip top caps.

Instructions for use and handling: The vaccine suspension is prepared by adding 1 ml of Water for Injections BP or Sodium Chloride Injection BP to the 10 dose vial. Do NOT shake as this causes frothing. Allow to stand for one minute, then draw into the syringe twice to ensure homogeneity.

After reconstitution the vaccine should be kept cool, protected from light and used in the same session, i.e. within 4 hours. Any reconstituted vaccine remaining at the end of the session (maximum 4 hours) should be discarded.

Disposal should be by incineration at a temperature not less than 1100°C at a registered waste disposal contractor.

Marketing authorisation number 0039/0437

Date of approval/revision of SPC January 1997

Legal category POM

INTRADERMAL BCG Vaccine, BP Isoniazid Resistant is not marketed, and is available to the profession on request only.

MICANOL* CREAM 1%
MICANOL* CREAM 3%

Qualitative and quantitative composition Dithranol BP 1.0% or 3.0% w/w

Pharmaceutical form Cream

Clinical particulars

Therapeutic indications: Treatment of sub-acute and chronic psoriasis, including psoriasis of the scalp, by the short contact therapy method.

Posology and method of administration:

Adults including the elderly: Apply Micanol cream only to the affected areas being careful to avoid contact with normal skin. Use only a small amount, rubbing it in gently and thoroughly until it no longer smears.

Micanol cream should be applied once every 24 hours and removed by washing off usually no more than 30 minutes after application. The cream must be washed off using plenty of lukewarm water only. This may be easiest in a bath or shower, particularly if the treated area is extensive.

When removing the cream, it is important that the water is not too hot and soap is not used, as these can damage the Micanol cream base and cause increased staining of the skin. Soap may be used for washing after the Micanol cream has been rinsed off.

The treatment should start with 1% cream on a limited surface. Where the response to dithranol has not been previously established, contact with 1% cream should initially be not greater than 10 minutes. This may gradually be increased to 30 minutes over a period of about seven days depending on the individual response.

After 1-2 weeks patients may progress to Micanol 3% if necessary provided they do not show any sign of skin irritation.

If the skin is irritated, patients should revert to 1% cream. Treatment should be continued until the skin is clear of psoriasis.

For use on the scalp, first wash the hair with shampoo, rinse and then apply Micanol cream while the hair is still damp. Leave in contact for up to 30 minutes and then rinse off using plenty of lukewarm water only. Further shampoo may be used after the cream has been removed.

Micanol 3% cream should always be used under medical supervision.

Micanol cream may cause staining of clothing and bed linen. To remove staining on clothing or bed linen rinse in lukewarm water only (not more than 30°C). To prevent the possibility of discolouration to the bath or shower always rinse with lukewarm water. Should any deposit be left on the surface a suitable cleanser may be used.

Children: There is no evidence of adverse effects in children. However, caution should be exercised and the treatment supervised regularly.

Micanol is not suitable for the treatment of infants and young children.

Contra-indications: Acute pustular psoriasis or presence of inflammation of skin, including folliculitis; erythroderma; hypersensitivity to Dithranol or any other component of Micanol*.

Special warnings and precautions for use: Use with caution if potent steroids have been administered recently. Do not apply to the face and keep away from eyes; if accidentally applied to the eyes, severe conjunctivitis, keratinitis, or corneal opacity may result. If accidental contact occurs, wash with plenty of lukewarm water.

Do not apply to mucous membrane, genitalia or intertriginous skin, do not apply to blistered, raw or oozing area of the skin.

When excessive redness or burning is observed, reduce frequency or concentration, or discontinue application. Such irritation is more likely with higher concentrations.

If sensitivity reactions occur, especially on the normal skin surrounding the plaque site, discontinue use.

Wash hands thoroughly after use.

Interaction with other medicaments and other forms of interaction: Photosensitising medications (concurrent use of these medications with Dithranol may enhance their photosensitising effects).

Propylene glycol containing drugs (Dithranol would be oxidised and inactivated).

Withdrawal of long term steroids in psoriasis may cause a rebound phenomenon. An interval of one or two weeks should therefore be left between stopping long term steroids and starting Micanol treatment. A bland emollient may be used in the intervening period.

Pregnancy and lactation: There is no experimental evidence to support the safety of dithranol in pregnancy. Micanol cream should be given to pregnant women only if clearly needed.

Nursing mothers should not apply Micanol on the breast area, and avoid accidental contamination of the skin or mouth of the baby.

Effects on ability to drive and use machines: None reported and none expected.

Undesirable effects:
Frequent: Perilesional erythema and burning, lesional burning (usually mild or moderate). These reactions usually lessen after one or two weeks of treatment.

Rarely: Allergic reaction (skin rash).

Staining of the treated and surrounding skin may appear. It will disappear within 1 to 2 weeks after the end of treatment.

May temporarily discolour fingernails or grey or white hair, may stain fabrics.

Overdose: Excessive application of the cream and prolonged usage causes burning and deep staining of the skin.

The skin should be rinsed firstly with water only and then washed, never wash at a temperature exceeding 30°C.

Dithranol is a cathartic (laxative) and if accidentally swallowed, should be removed by gastric lavage.

Pharmacological particulars
Pharmacodynamic properties: Dithranol belongs to the family of Hydroxyanthrones, which have been used in the treatment of psoriasis for more than a century.

The therapeutic action of dithranol has been linked to its ability to generate free radicals.

Dithranol has been shown to accumulate in the mitochondria where it induces morphological and functional changes. This affects the cellular energy supply which, in turn, results in inhibition of energy dependent processes such as DNA replication which slows down excessive cell division as seen in psoriasis plaque. Cyclic nucleosides are important in the regulation of epidermal cell division.

The psoriatic hyperproliferative epidermis contains elevated levels of cyclic guanosine monophosphate. As dithranol has been shown to reduce the elevated level of cGMP back to normal, this could represent an additional mechanism of action.

Pharmacokinetic properties:
Absorption and distribution: In vitro studies with human skin showed that more dithranol penetrates into skin with impaired stratum corneum barrier in 30 minutes than into intact skin during 16 hours. The concentration reaches its maximum after 30-60 minutes contact time and remains rather constant thereafter. In intact skin, however, the concentration continues to increase with time.

The highest concentration of unchanged dithranol is found in the horny layer where it can be detected for 24-48 hours, even after the skin has been washed. In deeper dermal layers relatively small amounts of unoxidised dithranol are detected whereas higher concentrations of the dithranol dimer are found.

Metabolism: The unstable dithranol is oxidised to danthron, to dithranol dimer and to further insoluble polymerisation products.

Elimination: There are no studies which indicate that unchanged dithranol is absorbed through the human skin. However, small quantities of oxidation products have been detected in the urine of patients after topical application.

Preclinical safety data: There are no pre-clinical data of relevance to the prescriber which are additional to that already included in other sections of the SPC.

Pharmaceutical particulars
List of excipients: Glyceryl Monolaurate, Glyceryl Monomyristate, Anhydrous Citric Acid PhEur, Sodium Hydroxide PhEur, Purified Water PhEur.

Incompatibilities: Oxidants (like Propylene glycol).

Shelf life: 2 years.

Special precautions for storage: Store below 25°C, in a dry place.

Nature and contents of container: Micanol cream is packed in aluminium tubes lined internally with a protective lacquer and sealed at the nozzle end with an aluminium membrane, and fitted with polypropylene caps.

The tubes are subsequently packed, together with the patient information leaflet, in unit, printed boxboard cartons in a pack size of 50 g. A 5 g tube is licensed but not marketed.

Instructions for use and handling: Micanol may stain fabrics and contact should be avoided if possible. It is especially formulated so that it is easily washed off using lukewarm water only. Do not use very hot water or soap as these may increase the staining of Micanol.

Product licence holder: Bioglan Laboratories Limited, 5 Hunting Gate, Hitchin, Hertfordshire, SG4 0TJ

Marketing authorisation numbers
1% 0041/0041
3% 0041/0042

Date of approval/revision of SPC January 1996

Legal category 1%-P, 3%-POM

MICRALAX* MICRO-ENEMA

Qualitative and quantitative composition Sodium alkylsulphoacetate 0.90% w/v; sodium citrate BP 9.0% w/v.

Pharmaceutical form A colourless viscous liquid.

Clinical particulars
Therapeutic indications: Micralax is indicated whenever an enema is necessary to relieve constipation: in dyschezia, especially in bedridden patients; in geriatrics, paediatrics and obstetrics; and in preparation for X-ray examination, protoscopy and sigmoidoscopy.

Posology and method of administration: Adults and children aged 3 years and over: Administer the contents of one micro-enema rectally, inserting the full length of the nozzle. No lubricant is needed as a drop of the mixture is sufficient.

Contra-indications: Do not use in patients with inflammatory bowel disease.

Special warnings and precautions for use: None.

Interactions with other medicaments and other forms of interaction: None.

Pregnancy and lactation: No special recommendations.

Effects on ability to drive and use machines: None.

Undesirable effects: No side effects have been reported. Excessive use may cause diarrhoea and fluid loss, which should be treated symptomatically.

Overdose: Not applicable.

Pharmacological properties
Pharmacodynamic properties: Micralax combines the action of sodium citrate, a peptidising agent which can displace bound water present in the faeces; sorbitol, which enhances this action, and sodium alkylsulphoacetate, a wetting agent.

Pharmacokinetic properties: Not applicable.

Preclinical safety data: Not applicable.

Pharmaceutical particulars
List of excipients: Sorbitol Solution 70% w/v BP, Glycerin PhEur, Sorbic Acid BP and Purified Water PhEur.

Incompatibilities: None.

Shelf life: 60 months.

Special precautions for storage: Store at a temperature not exceeding 25°C.

Nature and contents of container: Polythene microenema tubes, capped, and with elongated nozzles.

Instruction for use/handling: Micralax usually works within 5 to 15 minutes, so make sure you are near a toilet before using it. Always use a fresh tube of Micralax every time.

1) Lie down on your side with your knees drawn up towards your tummy or, if you prefer, sit on the toilet.
2) Pull or twist the black cap off the tube.
3) If you want to lubricate the nozzle before inserting it, squeeze a drop of liquid out onto the nozzle.
4) Insert the full length of the nozzle into your back passage.
5) Gently squeeze the tube until it is empty.
6) **Keep squeezing** the tube as you pull the nozzle out of your back passage. This is to stop the medicine being drawn back into the tube.
7) Wait for the laxative to work (5–15 minutes)

Marketing authorisation number 0039/0368

Date of approval/revision of SPC May 1996

Legal category P

NEO-CYTAMEN* INJECTION 1000 mcg

Qualitative and quantitative composition Hydroxocobalamin chloride EP 1.27 mg, equivalent to 1 mg hydroxocobalamin.

Pharmaceutical form Solution for injection.

Clinical particulars
Therapeutic indications: Addisonian pernicious anaemia. Prophylaxis and treatment of other macrocytic anaemias associated with vitamin B_{12} deficiency. Tobacco amblyopia and Leber's optic atrophy.

Posology and method of administration: Route of administration: Intramuscular.

Adults and Children: *Addisonian pernicious anaemia and other macrocytic anaemias without neurological involvement:* Initially: 250 to 1000 mcg intramuscularly on alternate days for one to two weeks, then 250 mcg weekly until the blood count is normal. Maintenance: 1000 mcg every two to three months.

Addisonian pernicious anaemia and other macrocytic anaemias with neurological involvement: Initially: 1000 mcg on alternate days as long as improvement is occurring. Maintenance: 1000 mcg every two months.

Prophylaxis of macrocytic anaemia associated with vitamin B_{12} deficiency resulting from gastrectomy, some malabsorption syndromes and strict vegetarianism: 1000 mcg every two to three months.

Tobacco amblyopia and Leber's optic atrophy: initially: 1000 mcg or more daily by intramuscular injection for two weeks. Then twice weekly as long as improvement is occurring. Maintenance: 1000 mcg monthly.

Contra-indications: Hypersensitivity to any ingredient of the preparation.

Special warnings and precautions for use: Precautions: The dosage schemes given above are usually satisfactory, but regular examination of the blood is advisable. If megaloblastic anaemia fails to respond to Neo-Cytamen, folate metabolism should be investigated. Doses in excess of 10 mcg daily may produce a haematological response in patients with folate deficiency. Indiscriminate administration may mask the true diagnosis. Cardiac arrhythmias secondary to hypokalaemia during initial therapy have been reported. Plasma potassium should therefore be monitored during this period.

Interactions with other medicaments and other forms of interaction: Chloramphenicol-treated patients may respond poorly to Neo-Cytamen. Serum concentrations of hydroxocobalamin may be lowered by oral contraceptives but this interaction is unlikely to have clinical significance. Antimetabolites and most antibiotics invalidate vitamin B_{12} assays by microbiological techniques.

Pregnancy and lactation: Neo-Cytamen should not be used for the treatment of megaloblastic anaemia of pregnancy unless vitamin B_{12} deficiency has been demonstrated. Neo-Cytamen is secreted into breast milk but this is unlikely to harm the infant, and may be beneficial if the mother and infant are vitamin B_{12} deficient.

Effects on ability to drive and use machines: None.

Undesirable effects: Hypersensitivity reactions have been reported including skin reactions (e.g. rash, itching) and exceptionally anaphylaxis. Other symptoms reported include fever, chills, hot flushing, dizziness, malaise, nausea, vomiting, diarrhoea, acneiform and bullous eruptions.

Overdose: Treatment is unlikely to be needed in cases of overdosage.

Pharmacological particulars
Pharmacodynamic properties: Neo-Cytamen contains hydroxocobalamin, one of the forms of vitamin B_{12}.

Pharmacokinetic properties: An intramuscular injection of hydroxocobalamin produces higher serum levels than the same dose of cyanocobalamin, and these levels are well maintained.

Preclinical safety data: None stated.

Pharmaceutical particulars
List of excipients: Sodium chloride EP, Acetic acid EP, Water for injection EP

Incompatibilities: None.

Shelf life: 36 months.

Special precautions for storage: Protect from light.

Nature and contents of container: 1 ml glass ampoules in packs of 5.

Instructions for use/handling: None stated.

Marketing authorisation number 0039/0405

Date of approval/revision of the SPC August 1997

Legal category POM

O.P.V. POLIOMYELITIS VACCINE, LIVE (ORAL) BP TRIVALENT (SABIN TYPE)

Qualitative and quantitative composition The vaccine contains live attenuated strains of poliomyelitis virus, types I, II and III at the following levels per dose:

Type I 10^6 $TCID_{50}$
Type II 10^5 $TCID_{50}$
Type III $10^{5.5}$ $TCID_{50}$

$TCID_{50}$–Tissue Culture Infective Dose required to infect 50% of a specific cell culture population.

Pharmaceutical form The attenuated vaccine strain of each type of poliovirus has antibody-inducing characteristics similar to its virulent counterpart. Extensive studies have shown that there is little risk of Sabin attenuated virus reverting to a virulent condition.

The vaccine is a clear pale yellow liquid.

Each dose of OPV, Poliomyelitis Vaccine, Live (Oral) contains up to 6IU polymyxin B sulphate and up to 0.5IU neomycin sulphate. In common with all vaccine derived from Sabin seed it may also contain traces of penicillin and streptomycin.

Clinical particulars
Therapeutic indications: For active immunisation against poliomyelitis.

Posology and method of administration: For oral use only.
Adults and children: The contents of one single dose polythene tube constitutes one dose. The primary course consists of three doses of poliomyelitis vaccine at intervals of not less than four weeks. If there is a known risk of exposure to poliomyelitis in those who have completed a primary course, a single reinforcing dose of OPV, Poliomyelitis Vaccine Live (Oral) is recommended.

Elderly: As for adults.

Administration of the vaccine: Separate a single-dose tube from the strip. The tube should be held by the large tab and shaken down, as with a thermometer, to propel the entire contents to the corrugated end. The tube should be held upright without applying pressure to the tube, and the narrow end removed by twisting the top. Incline tube and shake gently to move the vaccine to the open end.

The contents are then expelled by exerting gentle pressure to the tube just above the surface of the liquid (a small residue of vaccine may remain).

A course of Poliomyelitis Vaccine, Live (Oral) is usually administered simultaneously with Trivax-AD* (DTPer/Vac/Ads)) or Adsorbed Diphtheria and Tetanus Vaccine (CHILD) (DT/Vac/Ads (Child)). Thereafter, it is recommended that all immunised children are given a single reinforcing dose of OPV, Poliomyelitis Vaccine, Live (Oral) at school entry when they receive their reinforcing dose of Diphtheria and Tetanus Vaccine and again at 15-19 years of age or on leaving school.

Adults may be given a single reinforcing dose of OPV, Poliomyelitis Vaccine, Live (Oral) if already immunised or a primary immunisation course if their immunisation histories are uncertain or absent.

OPV, Poliomyelitis Vaccine, Live (Oral) may be administered as early as six weeks of age and the response has been shown to be unaffected by breast-feeding from this age onwards.

If parents or siblings of an infant due for immunisation have never been immunised then, provided there is no contra-indication, it is preferable to immunise them with OPV, Poliomyelitis Vaccine, Live (Oral) at the same time in order to reduce the remote risk of contact paralysis.

Alternatively, two doses of Inactivated Poliomyelitis Vaccine (IPV), one month apart, may be given to the adults before administration of OPV, Poliomyelitis Vaccine, Live (Oral) to the infant.

Administration of oral poliomyelitis vaccine induces circulating antibodies and local antibody responses in the intestine. However, one type of poliovirus in the vaccine may inhibit another from establishing immunity. Thus, when only a single dose of trivalent oral polio vaccine is given successful immunisation against all three types of poliovirus may not occur. Therefore in the primary course the vaccine is administered on at least three occasions to ensure that each type of vaccine poliovirus is given an opportunity of establishing immunity.

It is good practice to record title, dose and lot numbers of all vaccines and the dates of administration.

Contra-indications: The antibiotic content of the vaccine does not normally contra-indicate use except in cases of extreme hypersensitivity, e.g. anaphylaxis following its administration.

No data are available on the co-administration of OPV, Poliomyelitis Vaccine, Live (Oral) and live attenuated Typhoid Vaccine (Ty21a). Concurrent vaccination with OPV, Poliomyelitis Vaccine, live (Oral) and Oral Ty21a is therefore contra-indicated.

The efficacy of the vaccine may be impaired if given while the subject has diarrhoea or vomiting. The vaccine should not be given to those with acute febrile illness or severe chronic illness.

Any patient who has previously experienced a serious reaction to the vaccine or any component thereof should not be re-vaccinated.

Persons residing in the household of susceptible immuno-compromised individuals should not be vaccinated because viable poliomyelitis vaccine virus may be excreted in the faeces of the recipient and be communicated to susceptible persons within the household; IPV should be given.

The vaccine should not be given to those with impaired immune responsiveness, whether congenital, idiopathic or as a result of treatment with steroids (with the exception of locally acting eg topical or inhaled steroids), radiotherapy, cytotoxic drugs or other agents.

The vaccine should not be given either to symptomatic or asymptomatic HIV-positive individuals, since there is insufficient evidence as to the safety of its use.

Special warnings and precautions for use: Although anaphylaxis is rare, facilities for its management should always be available during vaccination.

The vaccine should not be administered on foods containing preservatives, as they may inactivate OPV, Poliomyelitis Vaccine, Live (Oral).

Vaccinees, parents and other household contacts should be made aware of the possible risk of recipient and contact paralysis prior to vaccination.

Any untoward reactions should be reported to the regulatory authorities and to the manufacturer.

Interaction with other medicaments and other forms of interaction: None known.

Pregnancy and lactation: The safety of OPV, Poliomyelitis Vaccine Live (Oral), for use in human pregnancy and breast-feeding has not been established. Therefore, routine vaccination during pregnancy and breast-feeding should be avoided. The benefits of using OPV, a live attenuated poliomyelitis vaccine, during pregnancy and breast-feeding should be weighed against any possible risks.
Effects on ability to drive and use machines: None known.

Undesirable effects: Vaccine-related paralysis in recipients or contacts may occur on very rare occasions.

Overdose: Not applicable.

Pharmacological particulars Not applicable.

Pharmaceutical particulars
List of excipients: The excipients contained in the preparation are as follows: Polymyxin B sulphate PhEur, Neomycin sulphate PhEur, Sucrose PhEur, L-glutamic acid HSE, Human albumin solution (20% w/v) PhEur, Potassium dihydrogen orthophosphate anhydrous HSE, Dipotassium hydrogen orthophosphate anhydrous HSE, Water for Injections PhEur.

Incompatibilities: None known.

Shelf life: 2-8°C: 6 months

Special precautions for storage: The vaccine should be stored between 2 and 8°C until its expiry date.

Nature and contents of container: 2 strips of 5 polyethylene dropper tubes with twist-off ends, each containing one dose.

Instructions for use and handling: Since the vaccine contains live attenuated poliomyelitis virus, care should be taken to avoid transfer of virus to immuno-deficient subjects.

When the vaccine tubes are opened the vaccine should be administered immediately to reduce the risk of contamination with bacteria and moulds which may result in a reduction of vaccine potency.

Caution should be exercised to avoid spillage. All parts of the containers should be subject to disposal by incineration at a temperature not less than 1100°C. If a spoon was used, it should either be incinerated or sterilised in a 0.1% aqueous hypochlorite solution yielding 1000 ppm available chlorine (e.g. 1:10 Milton 1%) and then rinsed thoroughly in water.

Marketing authorisation number 0039/0468

Date of approval/revision of SPC May 1996

Legal category POM

PARVOLEX* INJECTION

Qualitative and quantitative composition Acetylcysteine EP 200 mg/ml.

Pharmaceutical form Sterile solution for intravenous infusion.

Clinical particulars
Therapeutic indications: For the treatment of paracetamol overdosage.

Posology and method of administration: The injection is administered by intravenous infusion.

Adults: An initial dose of 150 mg/kg body weight of acetylcysteine is infused in 200 ml 5% dextrose intravenously over 15 minutes, followed by an intravenous infusion of 50 mg/kg in 500 ml 5% dextrose over the next 4 hours, then 100 mg/kg in 1 litre 5% dextrose over the next 16 hours. (This gives a total dose of 300 mg/kg in 20 hours.)

Children: Children should be treated with the same doses and regimen as adults; however, the quantity of intravenous fluid used should be modified to take into account age and weight, as fluid overload is a potential danger. The National Poisons Centres in the UK have provided the following guidance:

Children weighing 20 kg or more: 150 mg/kg intravenous infusion in 100 ml 5% dextrose over 15 minutes; then 50 mg/kg intravenous infusion in 250 ml 5% dextrose over 4 hours; then 100 mg/kg intravenous infusion in 500 ml 5% dextrose over 16 hours.

Children under 20 kg: Volumes for infusion of the above doses are the responsibility of the prescriber and should be based on the daily maintenance requirements of the child by weight.

Critical times: Acetylcysteine (Parvolex) is very effective in preventing paracetamol-induced hepatotoxicity when administered during the first 8 hours after a paracetamol overdose. When administered after the first 8 hours, the protective effect diminishes progressively as the overdose-treatment interval increases. However, clinical experience indicates that acetylcysteine can still be of benefit when administered up to 24 hours after paracetamol overdose, without any change in its safety profile. It may also be administered after 24 hours in patients at risk of severe liver damage. In general, for patients presenting later than 24 hours after a paracetamol overdose, guidance should be sought from a National Poisons Centre.

Treatment 'nomogram': Plasma paracetamol concentration in relation to time after the overdose is commonly used to determine whether a patient is at risk of hepatotoxicity and should, therefore, receive treatment with an antidote such as acetylcysteine.

For the majority of otherwise healthy patients, a line joining points of 200 mg/l at 4 hours and 30 mg/l at 15 hours on a semilogarithmic plot is used. (Treatment line A – see graph.) This line can be extended to 24 hours after overdose, based on a paracetamol half-life of 4 hours. It is recommended that patients whose plasma paracetamol concentrations fall on or above this line receive acetylcysteine. If there is doubt about the timing of the overdose, consideration should be given to treatment with acetylcysteine.

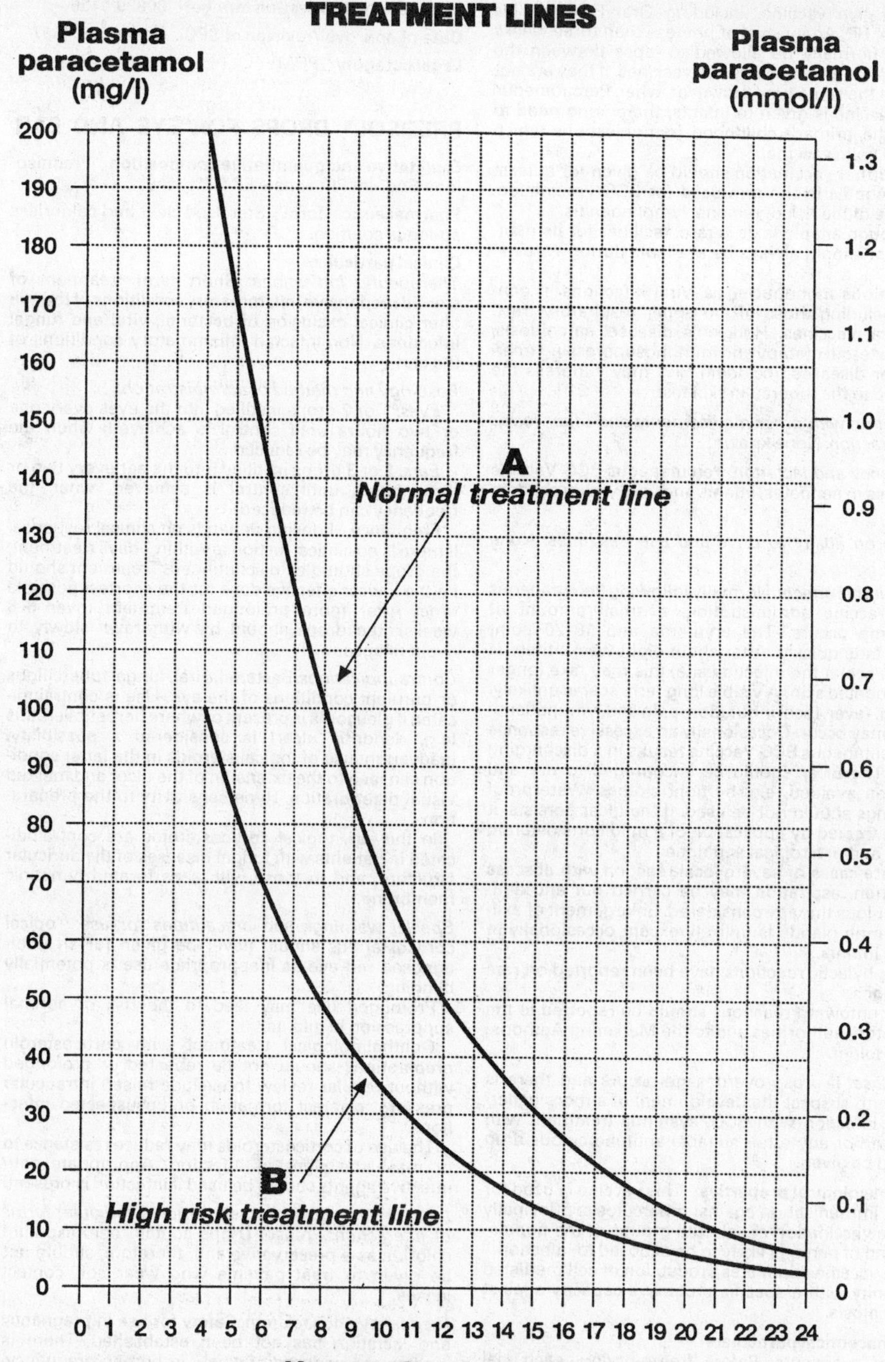

Plasma paracetamol concentrations in relation to time after overdosage as a guide to prognosis. From Guidelines agreed by National Poisons Centres – June 1995
Parvolex is indicated in patients with values on or above the appropriate treatment line.

Patients with induced hepatic microsomal oxidase enzymes (such as chronic alcoholics and patients taking anticonvulsant drugs) are susceptible to paracetamol-induced hepatotoxicity at lower plasma paracetamol concentrations (see *Contra-indications, precautions and warnings*) and should be assessed against treatment line B (see graph).

In patients who have taken staggered overdoses, blood levels are meaningless in relation to the treatment graph. These patients should all be considered for treatment with acetylcysteine.

NB: Blood samples taken less than 4 hours after a paracetamol overdose give unreliable estimates of the serum paracetamol concentration.

Contra-indications: Hypersensitivity to any ingredient in the preparation.

Special warnings and precautions for use:
Precautions: Administer with caution in patients with asthma or a history of bronchospasm.

Liver enzyme-inducing drugs; chronic alcohol abuse: Patients taking drugs that induce liver enzymes, such as some anticonvulsant drugs (e.g. phenytoin, phenobarbitone, primidone and carbamazepam) and rifampicin, and patients who routinely consume alcohol above recommended levels are believed to be at risk of hepatotoxicity from paracetamol poisoning at lower plasma paracetamol concentrations than other patients. It is recommended that such patients whose plasma paracetamol concentrations fall on or above a treatment line joining 100 mg/l at 4 hours after overdose and 15 mg/l at 15 hours after overdose on a semilogarithmic plot (i.e. treatment line B–see graph), be given acetylcysteine.

Other patients predisposed to toxicity: Patients suffering from malnutrition, for example, patients with anorexia or AIDS, may have depleted glutathione reserves. It has been recommended that paracetamol overdose in such patients be treated as for chronic alcohol consumers or patients taking anticonvulsant drugs (treatment line B–see graph).

Interactions with other medicaments and other forms of interaction: There are no known interactions.

Pregnancy and lactation: The safety of acetylcysteine in pregnancy has not been investigated in formal prospective clinical trials. However, clinical experience indicates that use of acetylcysteine in pregnancy for the treatment of paracetamol overdose is effective. Prior to use in pregnancy, the potential risks should be balanced against the potential benefits.

Effects on ability to drive and use machines: There are no known effects on ability to drive and use machines.

Undesirable effects: 'Anaphylactoid' or 'hypersensitivity-like' reactions have been reported. They include nausea/vomiting, injection-site reactions, flushing, itching, rashes/urticaria, angioedema, bronchospasm/respiratory distress, hypotension, and rarely, tachycardia or hypertension. These have usually occurred between 15 and 60 minutes after the start of infusion. In many cases, symptoms have been relieved by stopping the infusion. Occasionally, an antihistamine drug may be necessary. Corticosteroids may occasionally be required. Once an anaphylactoid reaction is under control, the infusion can normally be restarted at the lowest infusion rate (100 mg/kg in 1 litre over 16 hours).

In rare instances, the following side-effects have occurred: coughing, chest tightness or pain, puffy eyes, sweating, malaise, raised temperature, vasodilation, blurred vision, bradycardia, facial or eye pain, syncope, acidosis, thrombocytopenia, respiratory or cardiac arrest, stridor, anxiety, extravasation, arthropathy, arthralgia, deterioration of liver function, generalised seizure, cyanosis, lowered blood urea. Rare instances of fatality have also occurred.

Hypokalaemia and ECG changes have been noted in patients with paracetamol poisoning irrespective of the treatment given. Monitoring of plasma potassium concentration is, therefore, recommended.

If any side-effects to Parvolex (acetylcysteine) develop, advice should be sought from a National Poisons Centre to ensure that the patient receives adequate treatment of the paracetamol overdose.

Overdose: There is a theoretical risk of hepatic encephalopathy. Overdosage of acetylcysteine has been reported to be associated with effects similar to the 'anaphylactoid' reactions noted in *Undesirable effects*, but they may be more severe. General supportive measures should be carried out. Such reactions are managed with antihistamines and steroids in the usual way. There is no specific antidote.

Pharmacological particulars
Pharmacodynamic properties: Acetylcysteine is considered to reduce the hepatic toxicity of NAPQI (n-acetyl-p-benzo-quinoneimine), the highly reactive intermediate metabolite following ingestion of a high dose of paracetamol, by at least two mechanisms. First, acetylcysteine acts as a precursor for the synthesis of glutathione and, therefore, maintains cellular glutathione at a level sufficient to inactivate NAPQI. This is thought to be the main mechanism by which acetylcysteine acts in the early stages of paracetamol toxicity.

Acetylcysteine has been shown to still be effective when infusion is started at up to 12 hours after paracetamol ingestion, when most of the analgesic will have been metabolised to its reactive metabolite. At this stage, acetylcysteine is thought to act by reducing oxidised thiol groups in key enzymes.

When acetylcysteine treatment is begun more than 8 to 10 hours after paracetamol overdose, its efficacy in preventing hepatotoxicity (based on serum indicators) declines progressively with further lengthening of the overdose-treatment interval (the time between paracetamol overdose and start of treatment). However, there is now evidence that it can still be beneficial when given up to 24 hours after overdose. At this late stage of paracetamol hepatotoxicity, acetylcysteine's beneficial effects may be due to its ability to improve systematic haemodynamics and oxygen transport, although the mechanism by which this may occur has yet to be determined.

Pharmacokinetic properties: Following intravenous administration of acetylcysteine using the standard 20-hour intravenous regimen, plasma levels of 300 to 900 mg/l have been reported to occur shortly after the start of the infusion, falling to 11 to 90 mg/l at the end of the infusion period. Elimination half-lives of 2 to 6 hours have been reported after intravenous dosing, with 20 to 30% of the administered dose being recovered unchanged in the urine.

Metabolism appears to be rapid and extensive. There is no information on whether acetylcysteine crosses the blood-brain barrier or the placenta, or whether it is excreted in breast milk.

Preclinical safety data: None stated.

Pharmaceutical particulars
List of excipients: Disodium Edetate EP, Sodium Hydroxide EP, Water for Injections EP.

Incompatibilities: Acetylcysteine is not compatible with rubber or metals, particularly iron, copper and nickel. Silicone rubber and plastic are satisfactory for use with Parvolex.

A change in the colour of the solution to light purple has sometimes been noted and is not thought to indicate significant impairment of safety or efficacy.

Shelf life: 3 years.

Special precautions for storage: Store below 25°C.

Nature and contents of container: Clear, Type I glass, 10 ml snap ring ampoules. 10 x 10 ml ampoules are packed in cartons.

Instruction for use/handling: Acetylcysteine to be

diluted for intravenous infusion using 5% dextrose. The volumes to be used are as directed in *Posology and method of administration.*

Marketing authorisation number 0039/0410

Date of approval/revision of SPC May 1997

Legal category POM

PERCUTANEOUS BCG VACCINE, BP

Qualitative and quantitative composition Each vial contains:

Bacillus Calmette-Guerin (Copenhagen sub-strain 1077)	50 to 250×10^6 viable units

Pharmaceutical form Freeze-dried standardised preparation of a sub-strain of Bacillus Calmette-Guerin to be reconstituted with Water for Injections, BP or Sodium Chloride Injection, BP prior to percutaneous administration.

Clinical particulars

Therapeutic indications: For active immunisation against tuberculosis in neonates, infants and very young children only. Vaccinated persons normally become Mantoux-positive after eight weeks, but sometimes up to 14 weeks are needed.

Posology and method of administration: Percutaneous BCG Vaccine is used with a MULTIPLE PUNCTURE APPARATUS equipped with 18-20 needles giving reliable penetration of the skin to a depth of between 0.62 mm and 0.65 mm for delivery into the mid dermis. The inoculation should be given in the arm, over the insertion of the deltoid muscle onto the humerus. A tuberculin skin test must be conducted before BCG immunisation in children aged 3 months and over.

The multiple puncture apparatus must be properly sterilised each time after use according to the manufacturer's instructions. Alternatively a disposable head may be used each time. Any alcohol should be burnt off before the apparatus is used, which must be allowed to cool before use. Detergents or antiseptics should not be used.

The vaccine must not be contaminated with any antiseptic or detergent. Avoid contamination with bactericides. If alcohol is used to swab the rubber stopper of the vial, it must be allowed to evaporate before the stopper is penetrated with the syringe needle.

The vaccine suspension is prepared by adding 0.3 ml of Water for Injections, BP or 0.3 ml Sodium Chloride Injection, BP to the 10 dose vial. DO NOT shake as this causes frothing. Allow to stand for one minute, then draw into the syringe twice to ensure homogeneity.

The vaccine must not be contaminated with any antiseptic or detergent. Avoid contamination with bactericides. If alcohol is used to swab the skin, it must be allowed to evaporate before the vaccine is injected. Transfer a small amount (about 0.03 ml) of reconstituted vaccine onto the skin using a glass rod, platinum loop or spatula. The treated area of skin is then immediately punctured with the multiple puncture apparatus.

The injection site is best left uncovered to facilitate healing.

It is good practice to record the title, dose and lot numbers of all vaccines and dates of administration.

Contra-indications: **Percutaneous BCG Vaccine MUST NOT BE ADMINISTERED BY INTRADERMAL INJECTION.**

Percutaneous BCG Vaccine should NOT be given to persons receiving systemic corticosteroids or immunosuppressive treatment including radiotherapy, those suffering from malignant conditions (e.g. lymphoma, leukaemia, Hodgkin's Disease or other tumours of the reticuloendothelial system), those in whom normal immunological mechanism is impaired (e.g. hypogammaglobulinaemia), those known or suspected to be HIV-positive, including infants born to HIV-positive mothers and persons with pyrexia or generalised infected skin conditions. The effect of Percutaneous BCG Vaccine may be exaggerated in these patients and a more generalised infection is possible. Eczema is not a contra-indication, but the vaccination site must be lesion free.

Percutaneous BCG Vaccine should not be given to patients who are receiving prophylactic doses of antituberculous drugs.

Tuberculin-positive persons, i.e. those with induration of 5 mm or greater in diameter in the Mantoux test, or those in Heaf grades 2 to 4, do not require the vaccine. Its administration to these persons may result in an accelerated local reaction of larger size than normal.

The vaccine should not be administered to a subject who is known to be hypersensitive to any component of the vaccine.

Special warnings and precautions for use: Percutaneous BCG Vaccine may be given concurrently with another live vaccine, including Oral Poliomyelitis Vaccine, BP. An interval of not less than three weeks should normally be allowed to lapse between the administration of any two live vaccines, if they are not given at the same time. However, when Percutaneous BCG Vaccine is given to infants, there is no need to delay the primary childhood immunisations which include polio vaccine.

No further vaccination should be given for at least three months in the arm used for BCG vaccination, because of the risk of regional lymphadenitis.

Although anaphylaxis is rare, facilities for its management should always be available during vaccination.

Infectious mononucleosis, viral infections in general, including those of the upper respiratory tract, live viral vaccines, Hodgkin's disease, sarcoidosis, corticosteroid therapy and immunosuppressing treatment or diseases, including HIV, may suppress the reaction to the tuberculin skin test.

Interaction with other medicaments and other forms of interaction: None known.

Pregnancy and lactation: Percutaneous BCG Vaccine is for use in neonates, infants and very young children only.

Effects on ability to drive and use machines: None known.

Undesirable effects: Normally following Percutaneous BCG Vaccine administration, a small amount of erythema occurs. The erythema and 18–20 point marks fade quickly. After about eight weeks there is little to see at the injection site; this may take longer in pigmented skin. A visible long term scar is unlikely.

Rash, fever, local induration, pain and lymphadenopathy may occur. Occasionally an excessive response to Percutaneous BCG Vaccine results in a discharging ulcer. The ulcer should be encouraged to dry and abrasion avoided, e.g. by tight clothes. Waterproof dressings should not be used. If the ulcer persists, it can be treated by application of a mild corticosteroid cream and/or a topical antibiotic.

In rare cases of severe local reaction with abscess formation, aspiration may be carried out and antituberculous therapy considered. Enlargement of axillary lymph glands is unlikely except occasionally in young infants.

Anaphylactic reactions have been reported on rare occasions.

Any untoward reactions should be reported to the regulatory authorities and to the Marketing Authorisation Holder.

Overdose: If gross overdosage occurs and there is reason to suspect the development of a more generalised infection with BCG, systemic treatment with isoniazid or any other suitable antituberculous drug should be given.

Pharmacological properties This vaccine is used for active immunisation against tuberculosis; principally for the vaccination of selected groups of the population and of persons likely to be exposed to infection.

The vaccine stimulates production of cell mediated immunity with a specific protective capacity against tuberculosis.

Pharmaceutical particulars

List of excipients: Before freeze-drying, each vial contains 0.5 ml+10%* of freeze-drying medium of the following composition: Glucose 7.5%, Triton WR 1339 0.025%, Water for Injections, BP 100.0%

* the amount of freeze-drying medium used is such that the depth of suspension in the vial is suitable for freeze-drying.

Incompatibilities: None known.

Shelf life: 24 months when stored at 2–8°C unopened. 4 hours after reconstitution.

Special precautions for storage: Store between 2 and 8°C. Protect from light.

Nature and contents of container: SIZE: 3 ml vial (10 dose). TYPE: Neutral (type 1) amber glass vials complying with the PhEur requirements for containers for injectables. SEALS: Siliconised rubber peg bungs with aluminium overseals and polypropylene flip top caps.

Instructions for use/handling: The vaccine suspension is prepared by adding 0.3 ml of Water for Injections, BP or 0.3 ml Sodium Chloride Injection, BP to the 10 dose vial. DO NOT shake as this causes frothing. Allow to stand for one minute, then draw into the syringe twice to ensure homogeneity.

After reconstitution the vaccine should be kept cool, protected from light and used in the same session, i.e. within 4 hours. Any reconstituted vaccine remaining at the end of the session (maximum 4 hours) should be discarded.

Disposal should be by incineration at a temperature not less than 1100°C at a registered waste disposal contractor.

Marketing authorisation number 00039/0436

Date of approval/revision of SPC November 1997

Legal category POM

PREDSOL* DROPS FOR EYE AND EAR

Qualitative and quantitative composition Prednisolone Sodium Phosphate EP 0.5% w/v.

Pharmaceutical form Sterilised clear and colourless aqueous solution.

Clinical particulars

Therapeutic indications: Short term treatment of steroid responsive inflammatory conditions of the eye after clinical exclusion of bacterial, viral and fungal infections. Non-infected inflammatory conditions of the ear.

Posology and method of administration:

Eyes: 1 or 2 drops instilled into the eyes every one or two hours until control is achieved, when the frequency may be reduced.

Ears: 2 or 3 drops instilled into the ear every two or three hours until control is achieved, when the frequency can be reduced.

Frequency of dosing depends on clinical response. If there is no clinical response within 7 days treatment, the drops should be discontinued. Treatment should be the lowest effective dose for the shortest possible time. After more prolonged treatment (over 6–8 weeks), the drops should be withdrawn slowly to avoid relapse.

Contra-indications: Bacterial, viral, fungal tuberculous or purulent conditions of the eye. Use is contraindicated if glaucoma is present or where herpetic keratitis (e.g. dendritic ulcer) is considered a possibility. Inadvertent use of topical steroids in the latter condition can lead to the extension of the ulcer and marked visual deterioration. Hypersensitivity to the preparation.

In the ear, topical corticosteroids are contraindicated in patients with fungal diseases of the auricular structure, and in those with a perforated tympanic membrane.

Special warnings and precautions for use: Topical corticosteroids should never be given for an undiagnosed red eye as inappropriate use is potentially blinding.

Prolonged use may lead to the risk of adrenal suppression in infants.

Ophthalmological treatment with corticosteroid preparations should not be repeated or prolonged without regular review to exclude raised intraocular pressure, cataract formation or unsuspected infections.

The use of corticosteroids may reduce resistance to or mask the signs of infection. Appropriate anti-infective agents should be used if infection is present.

Interactions with other medicaments and other forms of interaction: Predsol Drops contain benzalkonium chloride as a preservative and, therefore, should not be given to treat patients who wear soft contact lenses.

Pregnancy and lactation: Safety for use in pregnancy and lactation has not been established. There is inadequate evidence of safety in human pregnancy. Topical administration of corticosteroids to pregnant animals can cause abnormalities of foetal development including cleft palate and intrauterine growth retardation. There may be a very small risk of such effects in the human foetus.

Effects on ability to drive and use machines: May cause transient blurring of vision on instillation. Warn patients not to drive or operate hazardous machinery unless vision is clear.

Undesirable effects: Hypersensitivity reactions usually of the delayed type may occur leading to irritation, burning, stinging, itching and dermatitis.

Topical corticosteroid use may result in increased intraocular pressure leading to optic nerve damage, reduced visual acuity and visual field defects. Other side effects include mydriasis, ptosis, epithelial punctate keratitis and possible corneal or scleral malacia. Within a few days after discontinuing topical ophthalmic corticosteroid therapy and occasionally during therapy, acute anterior uveitis has occurred in patients (mainly blacks) without pre-existing ocular inflammation or infection.

Intensive or prolonged use of topical corticosteroids may lead to formation of posterior subcapsular cataracts.

In those diseases causing thinning of the cornea or sclera, corticosteroid therapy may result in thinning of the globe leading to perforation.

Overdose: Long term intensive topical use may lead to systemic effects. Oral ingestion of the contents of one bottle (up to 10 ml) is unlikely to lead to any serious adverse effects.

Pharmacological particulars
Pharmacodynamic properties: Not available.

Pharmacokinetic properties: Not applicable.

Preclinical safety data: Not available.

Pharmaceutical particulars
List of excipients: Benzalkonium chloride solution EP, Sodium chloride EP, Sodium acid phosphate EP, Disodium edetate EP, Sodium hydroxide EP, Phosphoric acid EP, Purified water EP.

Incompatibilities: Not known.

Shelf life: 18 months unopened. 4 weeks after first opening.

Special precautions for storage: Store at a temperature not exceeding 25°C. Avoid freezing. Always replace bottle in carton to protect contents from light. Sterility of the drops is assured until cap seal is broken.

Nature and contents of container: Single 5 ml or 10 ml bottle with nozzle insert moulded in natural low density polyethylene closed with a tamper evident high density polyethylene cap.

Instruction for use/handling: Store below 25°C. Protect from light.

Marketing authorisation number 0039/0393

Date of approval/revision of SPC 28 July 1997

Legal category POM

PREDSOL* RETENTION ENEMA

Qualitative and quantitative composition 20 mg prednisolone as the sodium phosphate ester

Pharmaceutical form 100 ml disposable plastic bags, each containing 20 mg prednisolone as the sodium phosphate ester in a buffered solution. The product complies with the specification for Prednisolone Enema BP.

Clinical particulars

Therapeutic indications: Predsol Retention Enema provides local corticosteroid treatment for rectal and rectosigmoidal disease in ulcerative colitis and Crohn's disease.

Posology and method of administration: Adults: 1 enema used nightly, for 2 to 4 weeks. Treatment may be continued in patients showing progressive improvement, but it should not be continued if the response has been inadequate. Some patients may relapse after an interval but are likely to respond equally well to a repeated course of treatment.

The enema is used each night on retiring. It may be warmed before administration by placing the bag in a vessel of warm water for a few minutes. Before use lie in bed on the left side with knees drawn up. Hold the bag with tube upwards and squeeze the base of the tube where it joins the bag. Remove the stopper from the bag, lubricate the nozzle with petroleum jelly and gently insert about half the length of the nozzle into the rectum. The bag should then be squeezed gently until it is emptied, taking a minute or two to do so. The nozzle should then be removed and the whole unit discarded. The patient should then roll over to lie face down for 3 to 5 minutes but may sleep in any comfortable position.

Although Predsol Retention Enema is applied locally, it should be borne in mind that there is likely to be substantial systemic absorption, especially when the bowel is inflamed.

The volume of the enema is considered to be the optimum to ensure maximum coverage of the affected area. However, undesirable effects may be minimised by using for the minimum period.

Frequent patient review is required to monitor therapeutic effect against disease activity.

Children: Predsol Retention Enema is not suitable for use in children.

Route of administration: Rectal.

Contra-indications: Systemic or local infection unless specific anti-infective therapy is employed. Hypersensitivity to any ingredient of the preparation.

Special warnings and precautions for use: Although Predsol Retention Enema is applied locally, it should be borne in mind that there is likely to be substantial systemic absorption, especially when the bowel is inflamed.

The volume of the enema is considered to be the optimum to ensure maximum coverage of the affected area. However, undesirable effects may be minimised by using for the minimum period.

Frequent patient review is required to monitor therapeutic effect against disease activity (see *Posology and method of administration*).

Suppression of the inflammatory response and immune function increases the susceptibility to infections and their severity. The clinical presentation may often be atypical and serious infections such as septicaemia and tuberculosis may be masked and may reach an advanced stage before being recognised.

Chickenpox is of particular concern since this normally minor illness may be fatal in immunosuppressed patients. Patients without a definite history of chickenpox should be advised to avoid close personal contact with chickenpox or herpes zoster and if exposed they should seek urgent medical attention. Passive immunisation with varicella zoster immunoglobulin (VZIG) is needed by exposed non-immune patients who are receiving systemic corticosteroids or who have used them within the previous 3 months; this should be given within 10 days of exposure to chickenpox. If a diagnosis of chickenpox is confirmed, the illness warrants specialist care and urgent treatment. Corticosteroids should not be stopped and the dose may need to be increased.

Live vaccines should not be given to individuals with impaired immune responsiveness. The antibody response to other vaccines may be diminished.

Corticosteroid treatment may reduce the response of the pituitary adrenal axis to stress, and relative insufficiency can persist for up to a year after withdrawal of prolonged therapy. Withdrawal of corticosteroids after prolonged therapy must therefore always be gradual to avoid acute adrenal insufficiency, being tapered off over weeks or months depending on the duration of treatment. During prolonged therapy any intercurrent illness, trauma or surgical procedure will require a temporary increase in dosage. If corticosteroids have been stopped following prolonged therapy they may need to be temporarily re-introduced.

Special precautions: Particular care is required when considering the use of systemic corticosteroids in patients with the following conditions and frequent patient monitoring is necessary.

A. Osteoporosis (post-menopausal females are particularly at risk).
B. Hypertension or congestive heart failure.
C. Existing or previous history of severe affective disorders (especially previous steroid psychosis).
D. Diabetes mellitus (or a family history of diabetes).
E. History of tuberculosis.
F. Glaucoma (or a family history of glaucoma).
G. Previous corticosteroid-induced myopathy.
H. Liver failure – blood levels of corticosteroid may be increased, (as with other drugs which are metabolised in the liver).
I. Renal insufficiency.
J. Epilepsy.
K. Peptic ulceration.

Patients should carry 'steroid treatment' cards which give clear guidance on the precautions to be taken to minimise risk and which provide details of prescriber, drug, dosage and the duration of treatment.

Use in the elderly: The common adverse effects of systemic corticosteroids may be associated with more serious consequences in old age, especially osteoporosis, hypertension, hypokalaemia, diabetes, susceptibility to infection and thinning of the skin. Close clinical supervision is required to avoid life-threatening reactions.

Interactions with other medicaments and other forms of interaction: Systemic absorption of prednisolone should be borne in mind, especially when there is local inflammation. Thus the following interactions are possible.

Rifampicin, rifabutin, carbamazepine, phenobarbitone, phenytoin, primidone, aminoglutethimide enhance the metabolism of corticosteroids and its therapeutic effects may be reduced.

The desired effects of hypoglycaemic agents (including insulin), anti-hypertensives and diuretics are antagonised by corticosteroids, and the hypokalaemic effects of acetazolamide, loop diuretics, thiazide diuretics and carbenoxolone are enhanced.

The efficacy of coumarin anticoagulants may be enhanced by concurrent corticosteroid therapy and close monitoring of the INR or prothrombin time is required to avoid spontaneous bleeding.

The renal clearance of salicylates is increased by corticosteroids and steroid withdrawal may result in salicylate intoxication.

Pregnancy and lactation: Topical administration of corticosteroids to pregnant animals can cause abnormalities of foetal development including cleft palate and intrauterine growth retardation. There may therefore be a very small risk of such effects in the human foetus. Also, hypoadrenalism may occur in the neonate. When corticosteroids are essential however, patients with normal pregnancies may be treated as though they were in the non-gravid state. Patients with pre-eclampsia or fluid retention require close monitoring.

Corticosteroids are excreted in small amounts in breast milk and infants of mothers taking pharmacological doses of steroids should be monitored carefully for signs of adrenal suppression.

Effects on ability to drive and use machines: None known

Undesirable effects: The incidence of predictable undesirable effects, including hypothalamic-pituitary-adrenal (HPA) axis suppression correlates with the relative systemic potency of the drug, dosage, timing of administration and the duration of treatment. (see *Special warnings and precautions for use*).

Endocrine/metabolic: Suppression of the hypothalamic-pituitary-adrenal axis, growth suppression in infancy, childhood and adolescence, menstrual irregularity and amenorrhoea. Cushingoid facies, hirsutism, weight gain, impaired carbohydrate tolerance with increased requirement for antidiabetic therapy. Negative protein and calcium balance. Increased appetite.

Anti-inflammatory and immunosuppressive effects: Increased susceptibility and severity of infections with suppression of clinical symptoms and signs, opportunistic infections, recurrence of dormant tuberculosis (see 'Other Special Warnings and Precautions').

Musculoskeletal: Osteoporosis, vertebral and long bone fractures, avascular osteonecrosis, tendon rupture, proximal myopathy.

Fluid and electrolyte disturbance: Sodium and water retention, hypertension, potassium loss, hypokalaemic alkalosis.

Neuropsychiatric: Euphoria, psychological dependence, depression, insomnia, and aggravation of schizophrenia. Increased intra-cranial pressure with papilloedema in children (pseudotumour cerebri), usually after treatment withdrawal. Aggravation of epilepsy.

Ophthalmic: Increased intra-ocular pressure, glaucoma, papilloedema, posterior subcapsular cataracts, corneal or scleral thinning, exacerbation of ophthalmic viral or fungal diseases.

Gastrointestinal: Dyspepsia, peptic ulceration with perforation and haemorrhage, acute pancreatitis, candidiasis.

Dermatological: Impaired healing, skin atrophy, bruising, telangiectasia, striae, acne.

General: Hypersensitivity including anaphylaxis, has been reported. Leucocytosis. Thrombo-embolism.

Withdrawal symptoms and signs: Too rapid a reduction of corticosteroid dosage following prolonged treatment can lead to acute adrenal insufficiency, hypotension and in severe cases this could be fatal.

A 'withdrawal syndrome' may also occur including; fever, myalgia, arthralgia, rhinitis, conjunctivitis, painful itchy skin nodules and loss of weight.

Overdose Treatment is unlikely to be needed in cases of acute overdosage.

Pharmacological properties Not applicable

Pharmaceutical particulars
List of excipients: E214, E216, E218, Butyl 4-hydroxybenzoate, Disodium Edetate, Sodium Acid Phosphate, Disodium Hydrogen Phosphate Anhydrous, Sodium Hydroxide, Purified Water.

Incompatibilities: None known.

Shelf life: 2 years

Special precautions for storage: Store below 25°C and protect from light.

Nature and contents of container: Boxes of seven 100 ml disposable bags (instructions to patients enclosed).

Marketing authorisation number 0039/0396

Date of approval/revision of SPC June 1997

Legal category POM

PREDSOL SUPPOSITORIES

Qualitative and quantitative composition 5 mg prednisolone as the sodium phosphate ester.

Pharmaceutical form Suppositories.

Clinical particulars
Therapeutic indications: Prednisolone is a glucocorticosteroid which is about four times as potent as hydrocortisone on a weight for weight basis.

Predsol Suppositories are indicated for the treatment of haemorrhagic and granular proctitis and the anal complications of Crohn's disease.

Posology and method of administration:
Adults and children: 1 suppository inserted at night and one in the morning after defaecation. When the response is good, treatment is usually continued for some months. If symptoms recur later, treatment should be resumed.

Contra-indications: Systemic or local infection unless specific anti-infective therapy is employed. Hypersensitivity to any ingredient.

Special warnings and precautions for use: Although

Predsol Suppositories are applied locally, it should be borne in mind that substantial systemic absorption is a possibility, especially when the bowel is inflamed.

Undesirable effects may be minimised by using the minimum period.

Frequent patient review is required to monitor therapeutic effect against disease activity.

Suppression of the inflammatory response and immune function increases the susceptibility of infections and their severity. The clinical presentation may often be atypical and serious infections such as septicaemia and tuberculosis may be masked and may reach an advanced stage before being recognised.

Chickenpox is of particular concern since this normally minor illness may be fatal in immunosuppressed patients. Patients without a definite history of chickenpox should be advised to avoid close personal contact with chickenpox or herpes zoster and if exposed they should seek urgent medical attention. Passive immunisation with varicella zoster immunoglobulin (VZIG) is needed by exposed non-immune patients who are receiving systemic corticosteroids or who have used them within the previous 3 months; this should be given within 10 days of exposure to chickenpox. If a diagnosis of chickenpox is confirmed, the illness warrants specialist care and urgent treatment. Corticosteroids should not be stopped and the dose may need to be increased.

Live vaccines should not be given to individuals with impaired immune responsiveness. The antibody response to other vaccines may be diminished.

Corticosteroid treatment may reduce the response of the pituitary adrenal axis to stress, and relative insufficiency can persist for up to a year after withdrawal of prolonged therapy. Withdrawal of corticosteroids after prolonged therapy must therefore always be gradual to avoid acute adrenal insufficiency, being tapered off over weeks or months according to the dose and duration of treatment. During prolonged therapy any intercurrent illness, trauma or surgical procedure will require a temporary increase in dosage; if corticosteroids have been stopped following prolonged therapy they may need to be temporarily re-introduced.

Special precautions: Particular care is required when considering the use of systemic corticosteroids in patients with the following conditions and frequent patient monitoring is necessary.

A. Osteoporosis (post-menopausal females are particularly at risk).
B. Hypertension or congestive heart failure.
C. Existing or previous history of severe affective disorders (especially previous steroid psychosis).
D. Diabetes mellitus (or a family history of diabetes).
E. History of tuberculosis.
F. Glaucoma (or a family history of glaucoma).
G. Previous corticosteroid-induced myopathy.
H. Liver failure–blood levels of corticosteroid may be increased (as with other drugs which are metabolised in the liver).
I. Renal insufficiency.
J. Epilepsy.
K. Peptic ulceration.

Patients should carry 'steroid treatment' cards which give clear guidance on the precautions to be taken to minimise risk and which provide details of prescriber, drug, dosage and the duration of treatment.

Use in the elderly: The common adverse effects of systemic corticosteroids may be associated with more serious consequences in old age, especially osteoporosis, hypertension, hypokalaemia, diabetes, susceptibility to infection and thinning of the skin. Close clinical supervision is required to avoid life-threatening reactions.

Interaction with other medicaments and other forms of interaction: Systemic absorption of prednisolone should be borne in mind, especially when there is local inflammation. Thus the following interactions are possible.

Rifampicin, rifabutin carbamazepine, phenobarbitone, phenytoin, primidone, aminoglutethimide enhance the metabolism of corticosteroids and its therapeutic effects may be reduced.

The desired effects of hypoglycaemic agents (including insulin), anti-hypertensives and diuretics are antagonised by corticosteroids, and the hypokalaemic effects of acetazolamide, loop diuretics, thiazide diuretics and carbenoxolone are enhanced.

The efficacy of coumarin anticoagulants may be enhanced by concurrent corticosteroid therapy and close monitoring of the INR or prothrombin time is required to avoid spontaneous bleeding.

The renal clearance of salicylates is increased by corticosteroids and steroid withdrawal may result in salicylate intoxication.

Pregnancy and lactation: There is inadequate evidence of safety in human pregnancy. Topical administration of corticosteroids to pregnant animals can cause abnormalities of foetal development including cleft palate and intrauterine growth retardation. There may therefore be a very small risk of such effects in the human foetus. Also, hypoadrenalism may occur in the neonate. When corticosteroids are essential however, patients with normal pregnancies may be treated as though they were in the non-gravid state. Patients with pre-eclampsia or fluid retention require close monitoring.

Corticosteroids are excreted in small amounts in breast milk and infants of mothers taking pharmacological doses of steroids should be monitored carefully for signs of adrenal suppression.

Effects on ability to drive and use machines: None known.

Undesirable effects: The incidence of predictable undesirable effects, including hypothalamic-pituitary-adrenal (HPA) axis suppression correlates with the relative systemic potency of the drug, dosage, timing of administration and the duration of treatment. (See *Special warnings and precautions for use.*)

Endocrine/metabolic: Suppression of the hypothalamic-pituitary-adrenal axis, growth suppression in infancy, childhood and adolescence, menstrual irregularity and amenorrhoea. Cushingoid facies, hirsutism, weight gain, impaired carbohydrate tolerance with increased requirement for antidiabetic therapy. Negative protein and calcium balance. Increased appetite.

Anti-inflammatory and immunosuppressive effects: Increased susceptibility and severity of infections with suppression of clinical symptoms and signs, opportunistic infections, recurrence of dormant tuberculosis (see *Special warnings and precautions for use*).

Musculoskeletal: Osteoporosis, vertebral and long bone fractures, avascular osteonecrosis, tendon rupture, proximal myopathy.

Fluid and electrolyte disturbance: Sodium and water retention, hypertension, potassium loss, hypokalaemic alkalosis.

Neuropsychiatric: Euphoria, psychological dependence, depression, insomnia, and aggravation of schizophrenia. Increased intra-cranial pressure with papilloedema in children (pseudotumour cerebri), usually after treatment withdrawal. Aggravation of epilepsy.

Ophthalmic: Increased intra-ocular pressure, glaucoma, papilloedema, posterior subcapsular cataracts, corneal or scleral thinning, exacerbation of ophthalmic viral or fungal diseases.

Gastrointestinal: Dyspepsia, peptic ulceration with perforation and haemorrhage, acute pancreatitis, candidiasis.

Dermatological: Impaired healing, skin atrophy, bruising, telangiectasia, striae, acne.

General: Hypersensitivity including anaphylaxis, has been reported. Leucocytosis. Thrombo-embolism.

Withdrawal symptoms and signs: Too rapid a reduction of corticosteroid dosage following prolonged treatment can lead to acute adrenal insufficiency, hypotension and in severe cases this could be fatal (see *Other Special Warnings and Precautions*).

A 'withdrawal syndrome' may also occur including fever, myalgia, arthralgia, rhinitis, conjunctivitis, painful itchy skin nodules and loss of weight.

Overdose: Treatment is unlikely to be needed in cases of acute overdosage.

Pharmacological particulars

Pharmacodynamic properties: Prednisolone sodium phosphate is an active corticosteroid with topical anti-inflammatory activity.

Pharmacokinetic properties: Corticosteroids are metabolised mainly in the liver but also in the kidney and are excreted in the urine.

Synthetic corticosteroids such as prednisolone have increased potency when compared with the natural corticosteroids, due to their slower metabolism and lower protein-binding affinity.

Preclinical safety data: None stated.

Pharmaceutical particulars

List of excipients: Witepsol H15.

Incompatibilities: None known.

Shelf life: 2 years.

Special precautions for storage: Store below 25°C.

Nature and contents of container: Fin sealed plastic cavities moulded from 100 micron non-toxic PVC. Each cartoned plastic mould contains 10 suppositories (2 strips of 5 suppositories).

Marketing authorisation number 0039/0395

Date of approval/revision of SPC May 1997

Legal category POM

PREDSOL-N* DROPS FOR EYE AND EAR

Qualitative and quantitative composition
Prednisolone Sodium Phosphate EP 0.5% w/v.
Neomycin Sulphate EP 0.5% w/v.

Pharmaceutical form Solution.

Clinical particulars
Therapeutic indications:

Eye: For the short-term treatment of steroid responsive conditions of the eye when prophylactic antibiotic treatment is also required, after excluding the presence of fungal and viral disease.

Ear: Otitis externa or other steroid responsive conditions where prophylactic antibiotic treatment is also required.

Posology and method of administration: Frequency of dosing depends on clinical response. If there is no clinical response within 7 days treatment, the drops should be discontinued.

Treatment should be the lowest effective dose for the shortest possible time. Normally, do not give for more than 7 days, unless under expert supervision. After more prolonged treatment (over 6-8 weeks), the drops should be withdrawn slowly to avoid relapse.

Eye: 1 or 2 drops applied to each affected eye up to six times daily depending upon clinical response.

Ear: 2 or 3 drops instilled into each ear three or four times daily.

Contra-indications: Viral, fungal, tuberculous or purulent conditions of the eye. Use is contraindicated if glaucoma is present or herpetic keratitis (e.g. dendritic ulcer) is considered a possibility. Use of topical steroids in the latter condition can lead to extension of the ulcer and marked visual deterioration. Otitis externa should not be treated when the eardrum is perforated because of the risk of ototoxicity. Hypersensitivity to the preparation.

Special warnings and precautions for use: Topical corticosteroids should never be given for an undiagnosed red eye as inappropriate use is potentially blinding.

Treatment with corticosteroid/antibiotic combinations should not be continued for more than 7 days in the absence of any clinical improvement, since prolonged use may lead to occult extension of infection due to the masking effect of the steroid. Prolonged use may also lead to skin sensitisation and the emergence of resistant organisms.

Prolonged use may lead to the risk of adrenal suppression in infants.

Ophthalmological treatment with corticosteroid preparations should not be repeated or prolonged without regular review to exclude raised intraocular pressure, cataract formation or unsuspected infections.

Aminoglycoside antibiotics may cause irreversible, partial or total deafness when given systemically or when applied topically to open wounds or damaged skin. This effect is dose related and is enhanced by renal or hepatic impairment. Although this effect has not been reported following topical ocular use, the possibility should be considered when high dose topical treatment is given to small children or infants.

Interactions with other medicaments and other forms of interaction: Predsol-N Drops contain benzalkonium chloride as a preservative and, therefore, should not be used to treat patients who wear soft contact lenses.

Pregnancy and lactation: Safety for use in pregnancy and lactation has not been established. There is inadequate evidence of safety in human pregnancy. Topical administration of corticosteroids to pregnant animals can cause abnormalities of foetal development including cleft palate and intrauterine growth retardation. There may, therefore, be a very small risk of such effects in the human foetus. There is a risk of foetal ototoxicity if aminoglycoside antibiotic preparations are administered during pregnancy.

Effects on ability to drive and use machines: May cause transient blurring of vision on instillation. Warn patients not to drive or operate hazardous machinery unless vision is clear.

Undesirable effects: Hypersensitivity reactions, usually of the delayed type, may occur leading to irritation, burning, stinging, itching, dermatitis, contact conjunctivitis and erythema.

Topical corticosteroid use may result in increased intraocular pressure leading to optic nerve damage, reduced visual acuity and visual field defects.

Intensive or prolonged use of topical corticosteroids may lead to formation of posterior subcapsular cataracts.

In those diseases causing thinning of the cornea or sclera, corticosteroid therapy may result in thinning of the globe leading to perforation.

Other side effects include mydriasis, ptosis, epithelial punctate keratitis and possible corneal or scleral malacia. Within a few days after discontinuing topical ophthalmic corticosteroid therapy and occasionally during therapy, acute anterior uveitis has occurred in patients (mainly blacks) without pre-existing ocular inflammation or infection.

Overdose: Long term intensive topical use may lead to systemic effects. Oral ingestion of the contents of one bottle (up to 10 ml) is unlikely to lead to any serious adverse effects.

Pharmacological particulars
Pharmacodynamic properties: Prednisolone has topical corticosteroid activity. The presence of neomycin should prevent the development of bacterial infection.

Pharmacokinetic properties: Not applicable as the drops are applied topically.

Preclinical safety data: Not available.

Pharmaceutical particulars
List of excipients: Benzalkonium Chloride EP, Disodium Edetate EP, Polyethylene Glycol 300 EP, Sodium Formate EP, Anhydrous Sodium Sulphate EP, Disodium Hydrogen Phosphate Anhydrous HSE, Sodium Acid Phosphate EP, Sodium Hydroxide EP, Phosphoric Acid EP, Purified Water EP.

Incompatibilities: None known.

Shelf life: 18 months unopened. 4 weeks after first opening.

Special precautions for storage: Store below 25°C. Avoid freezing. Always replace bottle in carton to protect contents from light. Sterility of the drops is assured until cap seal is broken.

Nature and contents of container: Single 5 ml or 10 ml bottle with nozzle insert moulded in natural, low density polyethylene closed with a tamper evident high density polyethylene cap.

Instruction for use/handling: None.

Marketing authorisation number 0039/0394

Date of approval/revision of SPC August 1997

Legal category POM

PREGADAY* TABLETS

Qualitative and quantitative composition Each tablet contains Ferrous Fumarate EP 322.00 mg and Folic Acid EP 0.35 mg.

Pharmaceutical form Film-coated tablet.

Clinical particulars
Therapeutic indications: There is evidence that a daily intake of 100 mg of elemental iron in the ferrous form is adequate to prevent development of iron deficiency in expectant mothers. If a mild iron deficiency is present when Pregaday administration is started, this will be corrected by increased absorption of iron.

The daily folate requirement rises steeply during the final trimester of pregnancy, and evidence of maternal depletion may be found. To ensure normal tissue folate levels in the mother after delivery a daily supplement of about 300 micrograms is required during the second and third trimester of pregnancy. This does not obscure the blood picture of addisonian pernicious anaemia.

Pregaday Tablets are indicated during the second and third trimester of pregnancy for prophylaxis against iron deficiency and megaloblastic anaemia of pregnancy. Pregaday Tablets are not intended as a treatment for established megaloblastic anaemia.

Posology and method of administration: Adults: It is usual to begin therapy with Pregaday Tablets about the thirteenth week of pregnancy (see precautions) either as routine prophylaxis or selectively if the haemoglobin concentration is less than 11 g/100 ml (less than 75% normal).

One tablet should be taken daily by mouth.

Children: Not applicable.

Contra-indications: Known hypersensitivity to the product, Vitamin B_{12} deficiency, paroxysmal nocturnal haemoglobinuria, haemosiderosis, haemochromatosis, active peptic ulcer, repeated blood transfusion, regional enteritis and ulcerative colitis.

Pregaday must not be used in the treatment of anaemias other than those due to iron deficiency.

Special warnings and precautions for use: Some post-gastrectomy patients show poor absorption of iron. Care is needed when treating iron deficiency anaemia in patients with treated or controlled peptic ulceration. Caution should be exercised when administering folic acid to patients who may have folate dependent tumours.

Since anaemia due to combined iron and vitamin B_{12} or folate deficiencies may be microcytic in type, patients with microcytic anaemia resistant to therapy with iron alone should be screened for vitamin B_{12} or folate deficiency.

Pregaday tablets should be kept out of the reach of children.

Interactions with other medicaments and other forms of interaction: Iron reduces the absorption of penicillamine. Iron compounds impair the bioavailability of fluoroquinolones, levodopa, carbidopa, thyroxine and bisphosphonates.

Absorption of both iron and antibiotic may be reduced if Pregaday is given with tetracycline.

Absorption of both iron and zinc are reduced if taken concomitantly.

Concurrent administration of antacids may reduce absorption of iron. Co-trimoxazole, chloramphenicol, sulphasalazine, aminopterin, methotrexate, pyrimethamine or sulphonamides may interfere with folate metabolism.

Serum levels of anticonvulsant drugs may be reduced by administration of folate.

Oral chloramphenicol delays plasma iron clearance, incorporation of iron into red blood cells and interferes with erythropoiesis.

Some inhibition of iron absorption may occur if it is taken with cholestyramine, trientine, tea, eggs or milk.

Administration of oral iron may increase blood pressure in patients receiving methyldopa.

Coffee may be a factor in reducing iron bioavailability.

Neomycin may alter the absorption of iron.

Pregnancy and lactation: Administration of Pregaday Tablets during the first trimester of pregnancy may be undesirable.

A minority of pregnant women are not protected by physiological doses of folic acid. The development of anaemia despite prophylaxis with Pregaday Tablets calls for investigation.

Effects on ability to drive and use machines: None.

Undesirable effects: Gastro-intestinal disorders have been reported including gastro-intestinal discomfort, anorexia, nausea, vomiting, constipation, diarrhoea. Darkening of the stools may occur.

Rarely allergic reactions may occur.

Overdose: Acute overdose of oral iron requires emergency treatment. In young children 200–250 mg/kg ferrous fumarate is considered to be extremely dangerous.

Symptoms and signs of abdominal pain, vomiting and diarrhoea appear within 60 minutes. Cardiovascular collapse with coma may follow. Some improvement may occur after this phase which, in some patients, is followed by recovery. In others, after about 16 hours, deterioration may occur involving diffuse vascular congestion, pulmonary oedema, convulsions, anuria, hypothermia, severe shock, metabolic acidosis, coagulation abnormalities and hypoglycaemia.

Vomiting should be induced immediately, followed as soon as possible by parenteral injection of desferrioxamine mesylate, and then gastric lavage. In the meantime, it is helpful to give milk and/or 5% sodium bicarbonate solution by mouth.

Dissolve 2 g desferrioxamine mesylate in 2 to 3 ml of water for injections and give intramuscularly. A solution of 5 g desferrioxamine in 50 to 100 ml of fluid may be left in the stomach. If desferrioxamine is not available, leave 300 ml of 1% to 5% sodium bicarbonate in the stomach. Fluid replacement is essential.

Recovery may be complicated by long-term sequelae such as hepatic necrosis, pyloric stenosis or acute toxic encephalitis which may lead to CNS damage.

Pharmacological particulars
Pharmacodynamic properties: There is evidence that a daily dose of 100 mg of elemental iron in the ferrous form is adequate to prevent development of iron deficiency in expectant mothers. If a mild iron deficiency is present when Pregaday administration is started, this will be corrected by increased absorption of iron. The daily folate requirement rises steeply during the final trimester of pregnancy, and evidence of maternal depletion may be found. To ensure normal tissue folate levels in the mother after delivery a daily supplement of about 300 micrograms is required during the second and third trimester of pregnancy. This does not obscure the blood picture of addisonian pernicious anaemia.

Pharmacokinetic properties: Iron is absorbed chiefly in the duodenum and jejunum, absorption being aided by the acid secretion of the stomach and being more readily effected when the iron is in the ferrous state.

Folic acid is absorbed mainly from the proximal part of the small intestine. Folate polyglutamates are considered to be de-conjugated to monoglutamates during absorption. Folic acid rapidly appears in the blood, where it is extensively bound to plasma proteins. The amounts of folic acid absorbed from normal diets are rapidly distributed in body tissues and about 4 to 5 micrograms is excreted in the urine daily. When larger amounts are absorbed, a high proportion is metabolised in the liver to other active forms of folate and a proportion is stored as reduced and methylated folate. Larger amounts of folate are rapidly excreted in the urine.

Preclinical safety data: Not stated.

Pharmaceutical particulars
List of excipients: The tablet cores also contain maize starch EP, sodium lauryl sulphate EP, gelatin EP and liquid paraffin EP. The film coat contains **either** hydroxypropylmethyl cellulose EP (E464), acetylated monoglyceride and Opaspray pink **or** hydroxypropylmethyl cellulose EP (E464), propylene glycol EP and Opaspray pink.

Opaspray pink contains hydroxypropyl cellulose (E463), red iron oxide(E172) and titanium dioxide (E171).

Incompatibilities: None.

Shelf life: 36 months.

Special precautions for storage: Protect from light, store below 25°C.

Nature and contents of container: Cartons containing two calendar blister packs of 14 tablets prepared from PVdC coated opaque 250 micron PVC film and 20 micron tempered aluminium foil.

Instruction for use/handling: Not applicable.

Marketing authorisation number 0039/0398

Date of approval/revision of the SPC November 1997

Legal category POM

RUBILIN* RUBELLA VACCINE, LIVE BP

Qualitative and quantitative composition The composition in terms of active ingredient is as follows:

Each 0.5 ml dose of reconstituted vaccine contains not less than 1000 $CCID_{50}$ live attenuated virus (Wistar RA 27/3).

Pharmaceutical form Freeze-dried preparation, reconstituted with Water for Injections BP prior to intramuscular or deep subcutaneous injection to humans.

The reconstituted vaccine may vary in colour from pale straw to pink.

Clinical particulars
Therapeutic indications: For active immunisation against rubella.

It is recommended that all girls between the ages of 10 and 14 and seronegative non-pregnant women of child-bearing age, should be vaccinated. The latter group should be advised not to become pregnant within 3 months of vaccination. Because clinical diagnosis without laboratory tests is unreliable a past history of rubella is not a reliable guide to immune status.

One dose of vaccine will produce a seroconversion rate of over 95% in vaccinees.

Posology and method of administration:
Children, adults and elderly: One 0.5 ml dose of reconstituted vaccine is given by intramuscular or deep subcutaneous injection. The freeze-dried plug should be reconstituted by slowly adding the 0.5 ml Water for Injections BP provided, immediately prior to use.

Contra-indications: The vaccine must not be given to pregnant women and pregnancy should be avoided for three months after vaccination.

The vaccine should not be administered to a subject who has experienced a serious reaction (e.g. anaphylaxis) to a previous dose of this vaccine or who is known to be hypersensitive to any component thereof. The vaccine contains a small amount of neomycin and polymyxin and should not be given to individuals known to be hypersensitive to either of them.

The vaccine should not be given to subjects suffering from a febrile illness.

The vaccine should not be given to those suffering from malignant conditions (e.g. lymphoma, leukaemia, Hodgkin's Disease), impaired immunological mechanism (e.g. hypogammaglobulinaemia) or impaired immune responsiveness, whether congenital, idiopathic or as a result of treatment with steroids (with the exception of standard doses of locally acting, e.g. topical or inhaled, steroids), radiotherapy, cytotoxic drugs or other agents.

Special warnings and precautions for use: Although anaphylaxis is rare, facilities for its management should always be available during vaccination.

The vaccine may depress tuberculin skin sensitivity for 4 weeks or longer.

The vaccine virus is not transmitted and there is no risk to pregnant women from contact with vaccinees.

After vaccination, women must ensure they do not conceive in the following three months until the theoretical risk of congenital abnormality is significantly reduced.

The vaccine should not be given to infants under

one year of age as there may be interference from persisting maternal antibodies.

An interval of not less than 3 weeks should normally be allowed to lapse between the administration of any two live vaccines. If time does not permit they may be given simultaneously at separate sites. A 3 week interval should be allowed between the administration of Rubella Vaccine and BCG.

Rubella Vaccine should not be given within three months of an injection of immunoglobulin. The vaccine should not normally be given within 3 months of a transfusion of blood or plasma. If these have been used near the time of vaccination, the presence of antibodies should be checked at a later date.

Do not attempt to obtain more than the stated number of doses from the vial. It is good practice to record the title, dose and lot numbers of all vaccines and dates of administration

Interaction with other medicaments and other forms of interaction: The vaccine is inactivated by alcohol and if this is used to clean the skin prior to vaccination, it must be allowed to evaporate before the vaccine is given. Avoid contamination with bactericides. Use only sterile disposable syringes and needles which are free from traces of disinfectants or spirits. Use a fresh needle and syringe for each injection.

Pregnancy and lactation: There is a possibility that live attenuated virus administered during pregnancy could infect and damage the foetus, producing congenital abnormalities. Therefore, pregnant women must not be vaccinated. After vaccination women must ensure they do not conceive in the following 3 months until the theoretical risk of congenital abnormality returns to baseline.

Effects on ability to drive and use machines: Not applicable.

Undesirable effects: Fever, malaise, headache, sore throat, lymphadenopathy, rash, arthralgia and arthritis may occur. Such symptoms commence between one and three weeks after vaccination, and are usually mild and self limiting. Induration, pain and erythema at the injection site may occur. Joint symptoms are more common in adult females than in children and adolescents. Neurological symptoms have been reported on rare occasions. Thrombocytopenia has occasionally been reported after vaccination.

Any untoward reactions should be reported to the regulatory authorities and to the manufacturer

Overdose: If overdosage or inadvertant administration is suspected, careful observation of the subject may be necessary. There may not be any sequelae, but subjects should be monitored and appropriate supportive measures should be implemented, according to the type of response seen.

Pharmacological particulars Not applicable

Pharmaceutical particulars

List of excipients: The excipients contained in the preparation are as follows: Polymyxin BP, Neomycin BP, 199 Medium HSE, Sucrose BP, Sorbitol BP, Glutamic Acid (L) sodium salt HSE, Potassium dihydrogen phosphate HSE, Dipotassium hydrogen phosphate HSE, Peptone (Proteose) HSE, Water for Injections HSE.

Incompatibilities: None stated.

Shelf life:

2 to 8°C: 24 months

Special precautions for storage: Store between 2 and 8°C. Do not freeze. Protect from light. Use the reconstituted vaccine within one hour after which time any remaining vaccine should be discarded.

Nature and contents of container: The vaccine is supplied as single dose vials in packs of 1 with siliconised rubber bungs, aluminium overseals and polypropylene flip off tops. Each vial contains freeze-dried powder for reconstitution of one dose of vaccine with 0.5 ml of Water for Injections. Each 0.5 ml Water for Injections is supplied in a glass ampoule.

Instructions for use and handling: After reconstitution with supplied Water for Injections, the vaccine should be administered immediately to reduce the risk of contamination with bacteria and moulds which may result in a reduction of vaccine potency.

Disposal should be by incineration at a temperature of not less than 1100°C at a registered waste disposal contractor.

Marketing authorisation number 0039/0349

Date of approval/revision of SPC May 1998

Legal category POM

STREPTOMYCIN SULPHATE BP STERILE POWDER

Qualitative and quantitative composition Each vial contains 1.342 g Streptomycin Sulphate Sterile BP (equivalent to 1 g Streptomycin base).

Pharmaceutical form A white sterile powder for preparation of Streptomycin Sulphate Injection BP, intended for intramuscular injection.

Clinical particulars

Therapeutic indications: Streptomycin may be used in the treatment of tuberculosis and other serious infections resistant to alternative antibiotics.

Posology and method of administration:

Monitoring advice: Serum levels should be monitored, especially if there is renal impairment. Dosages may need to be adjusted to avoid toxicity. In general, peak levels should not exceed 40 mcg/ml and trough levels 3 mcg/ml. In the elderly, the trough may need to be even lower (1 mcg/ml).

Route of administration: By deep intramuscular injection.

The injection should be given deeply into muscle and the site changed for each injection.

A 1 g dose is usually dissolved in 2 or 3 ml of Water for Injections. (The displacement volume of 1 g is approximately 0.75 ml). Use of a sterile disposable membrane filter of 0.45 micron pore size is convenient to ensure clarity of the solution.

Tuberculosis: Streptomycin is always given together with other antituberculosis drugs. It can be given on a daily basis or three times a week if intermittent treatment is more appropriate.

Adults under 40 years of age AND bodyweight greater than 50 kg: 1 g daily or intermittently.

Elderly and adults over 40 years of age OR bodyweight less than 50 kg: 0.5-0.75 g per day if given daily; 0.75 g per day if given intermittently. (See also monitoring advice).

Children: 15-20 mg/kg bodyweight (up to 1 g maximum) daily or intermittently.

Renal impairment: Dosages may need to be adjusted (see monitoring advice).

Streptomycin treatment should usually continue for the initial 2 month treatment phase and may be included in the subsequent continuation phase. Treatment should be supervised by a specialist physician.

Non-tuberculous infections:

Adults: Usually 1 g per day for 3-7 days.

Elderly: The adult dosage may require some adjustment (see monitoring advice).

Children: Up to 40 mg/kg bodyweight (up to 1 g maximum) daily for 3-7 days. Divided doses are often used.

Note: in urinary-tract infections the urine should be kept alkaline as aminoglycosides are inhibited by acidic environments.

Maximum tolerated daily dose and maximum dose for an entire course of therapy: Side-effects increase after a cumulative dose of 100 g, which should only be exceeded in exceptional circumstances.

In tuberculosis treatment: Intramuscular dosages of 2 g daily (divided) for 6 weeks and 1 g twice daily for up to 8 weeks have been administered.

In non-tuberculous treatment: Intramuscular dosage of 2.4 g daily (divided) for up to 14 days has been administered.

Contra-indications: Streptomycin is contra-indicated in patients with known hypersensitivity to the drug; in patients with diseases of the ear, particularly suppurative otitis media and labyrinthine disturbances; in pregnancy; in patients with myasthenia gravis and in patients with impaired renal function, unless the dosage is adjusted (see *Posology and method of administration*).

Special warnings and precautions for use: Intrathecal administration of streptomycin is not recommended.

Renally impaired and elderly patients should have dosages adjusted and plasma concentrations monitored as indicated under *Posology and method of administration.*

Skin sensitisation may occur in persons handling the antibiotic and care should be taken to avoid contact with the substance. Use of rubber gloves is recommended.

Interactions with other medicaments and other forms of interaction: Streptomycin should not be given with potentially ototoxic diuretics (e.g. frusemide and ethacrynic acid); if concurrent use is unavoidable administration of the aminoglycoside and of the diuretic should be separated by as long a period as practicable.

Concurrent use with other nephrotoxic drugs, including other aminoglycosides, vancomycin and some of the cephalosporins, should be avoided as they increase the risk of toxicity.

Streptomycin and benzylpenicillin act synergistically against *Streptococcus faecalis.* They should not be given together unless the preparation is freshly made because the combination rapidly becomes less active on storage.

Pregnancy and lactation:

Pregnancy: Streptomycin is contra-indicated during pregnancy as it crosses the placenta and can cause foetal eighth nerve damage.

Lactation: The drug enters breast milk but the exact significance is unknown. However, the risk of possible sensitisation should be borne in mind.

Effects on ability to drive and use machines: None known.

Undesirable effects: The main adverse effect is ototoxicity: some impairment of vestibular function (less often of auditory function) can occur, particularly with prolonged or intensive therapy, in the presence of renal dysfunction and in the elderly and neonate. Reported symptoms include giddiness, vertigo, tinnitus, ataxia and deafness, which is sometimes irreversible.

Paraesthesia in and around the mouth is not uncommon after intramuscular injection and other neurological symptoms, including peripheral neuropathies, optic neuritis and scotoma have occasionally occurred.

Nephrotoxicity can also occur; evidence of minor renal tubular dysfunction, such as urinary casts and minor degrees of albuminuria are common, but severe renal damage (proximal tubular necrosis) is rare.

Cutaneous and generalised hypersensitivity reactions, such as rash and fever, are common. (Note precautions (*Special warnings and precautions for use*) for persons handling the drug.) Occasional allergic-type reactions, rarely severe and often responding to antihistamine treatment. Severe exfoliative dermatitis and anaphylactic shock have been reported.

Aplastic anaemia and agranulocytosis have also been rarely reported.

Overdose

Human experience: Acute haemolytic anaemia and renal failure have been reported following repeated injection of streptomycin for 15 years.

Management of overdose in man: Streptomycin can be removed from the body by haemodialysis.

Pharmacological particulars

Pharmacodynamic properties: Streptomycin is an aminoglycoside antibiotic which is active against *Mycobacterium tuberculosis.* It is not active against *Pseudomonas aeruginosa.* Resistance develops fairly rapidly in many organisms, limiting its use.

Pharmacokinetic properties: Oral absorption of streptomycin is poor (0-40%) and it is thus administered parenterally. Following parenteral administration, approximately 50-60% of the dose is excreted unchanged in the urine within 24 hours. The plasma half life is approximately 2.5 hours, increasing to approximately 100 hours when blood urea nitrogen concentrations are in the range of 100-150 mg per 100 ml. A small proportion of the dose (about 1%) is excreted in the bile, this proportion falling when there is chronic hepatic dysfunction. Approximately 20% of the dose cannot be accounted for by urinary excretion but no metabolites have yet been identified.

Preclinical safety data: There are no pre-clinical data of relevance to the prescriber which are additional to that already included in other sections of the Summary of Product Characteristics.

Pharmaceutical particulars

List of excipients: None.

Incompatibilities: Streptomycin is incompatible with acids and alkalis.

Shelf life: Dry powder: 4 years.

Special precautions for storage: Dry powder: Store at a temperature not exceeding 25°C.

Nature and contents of container: Streptomycin Sulphate BP Sterile Powder is presented in glass vials which are packaged in cartons containing 10 vials.

Instructions for use/handling: Sterile solutions of streptomycin should be used as soon as possible after reconstitution.

Note: skin sensitisation can occur in persons handling the drug and care should be taken to avoid contact with the substance. Use of rubber gloves is recommended.

Marketing authorisation number 0039/6002R

Date of approval/revision of SPC April 1996

Legal category POM.

ADSORBED TETANUS VACCINE, BP

Qualitative and quantitative composition The composition in terms of active ingredient is as follows:-

Tetanus toxoid not less than 40 IU
Quantities expressed per 0.5 ml dose.

Pharmaceutical form Sterile suspension for deep subcutaneous or intramuscular injection to humans.

Clinical particulars
Therapeutic indications: For active immunisation against tetanus.

Primary immunisation against tetanus in infancy is usually carried out by administration of combined Adsorbed Diphtheria, Tetanus and Pertussis Vaccine (DTPer/Vac/Ads) or Adsorbed Diphtheria and Tetanus Vaccine (CHILD) (DT/Vac/Ads(Child)).

Posology and method of administration:
Children, adults and elderly: Each dose is 0.5 ml given by deep intramuscular or subcutaneous injection.

The primary course of immunisation against tetanus consists of three doses with an interval of one month between each dose. The intervals between immunisations may be exceeded without the need to repeat the full course of immunisation. Reinforcing doses are given to maintain immunity against tetanus.

Primary course in infants and children under 10 years: Primary immunisation against tetanus may be carried out by the administration of combined Adsorbed Diphtheria, Tetanus and Pertussis Vaccine (DTPer/Vac/Ads), Adsorbed Diphtheria and Tetanus Vaccine (CHILD) (DT/Vac/Ads(Child)) or Adsorbed Tetanus Vaccine (Tet/Vac/Ads) in infancy. Three 0.5 ml doses are given, with a dose at 2, 3 and 4 months of age.

Reinforcing doses in children under 10 years: Children who have received the primary course of immunisation in infancy require reinforcement of immunity against tetanus. This can be achieved by giving one dose (0.5 ml) Adsorbed Diphtheria and Tetanus Vaccine (CHILD) (DT/Vac/Ads(Child)) or Adsorbed Tetanus Vaccine (Tet/Vac/Ads), after at least three years from the last dose of the primary course. The reinforcing dose is commonly given prior to school entry.

Primary course in adults and children over 10 years: Primary immunisation against tetanus consists of three doses separated by intervals of not less than four weeks.

Reinforcing doses in adults and children over 10 years: A reinforcing dose (0.5 ml) of Adsorbed Diphtheria and Tetanus Vaccine for Adults and Adolescents is recommended at 13 to 18 years of age or before leaving school. Teenagers being treated for tetanus prone wounds and who had received their fourth dose of tetanus vaccine approximately ten years earlier, should be given Tetanus Vaccine for Adults and Adolescents and the school leaving dose omitted. For adults, a single dose of vaccine given at any time after completion of the primary course of three injections can be expected to provide an effective reinforcement of immunity. The administration of a reinforcing dose approximately 10 years after the completion of a primary immunisation course is recommended. Thereafter, a further vaccination at 10 years is thought to provide the potential for lifelong protection. However, this does not preclude the need to consider administration of additional doses in the event of injuries which may give rise to tetanus.

Treatment of patients with tetanus-prone wounds: The following are considered tetanus-prone wounds.

a. Any wound or burn sustained more than six hours before surgical treatment of the wound or burn.
b. Any wound or burn at any interval after injury that shows one or more of the following characteristics:
   i A significant degree of devitalised tissue.
   ii Puncture-type wound.
   iii Contact with soil or manure likely to harbour tetanus organisms.
   iv Clinical evidence of sepsis.

Thorough surgical toilet of the wound is essential whatever the tetanus immunisation history of the patient.

Specific anti-tetanus prophylaxis is as follows:

Immunisation Status	*Type of Wound*	*Type of Wound*
	Clean	*Tetanus Prone*
Last of 3 dose course, or reinforcing dose within last 10 years	Nil	Nil (A dose of human tetanus immunoglobulin may be given if risk of infection is considered especially high e.g. contamination with stable manure).
Last of 3 dose course or reinforcing dose more than 10 years previously.	A reinforcing dose of adsorbed vaccine.	A reinforcing dose of adsorbed vaccine plus a dose of human tetanus immunoglobulin.
Not immunised or immunisation status not known with certainty.	A full 3 dose course of adsorbed vaccine.	A full 3 dose course of vaccine, plus a dose of tetanus immunoglobulin in a different site.

Reinforcing doses of tetanus vaccine at frequent intervals may provoke hypersensitivity reactions and tetanus vaccine should not be given to any patient who has received a booster dose in the preceding year.

Persons of all ages are susceptible to tetanus unless they have received appropriate immunisation. Rarely, if ever, is natural immunity developed even in persons who have recovered from severe tetanus. Since most tetanus cases follow trivial wounds, all persons should, if possible, be actively immunised against the disease.

Adsorbed Tetanus Vaccine may be administered simultaneously with human tetanus immunoglobulin or tetanus antitoxin but must be given at separate sites. The antibody response of subjects to subsequent doses of vaccine is not significantly impaired by this procedure.

Oral Poliomyelitis Vaccine BP may be given at the same time as Adsorbed Tetanus Vaccine.

Shake well before each dose is withdrawn. It is good practice to record the title, dose and lot numbers of all vaccines and dates of administration.

Contra-indications: Adsorbed Tetanus Vaccine must not be given intradermally since it may give rise to a persistent skin nodule.

The vaccine should not be administered to a subject who has experienced a serious reaction (e.g. anaphylaxis) to a previous dose of this vaccine or who is known to be hypersensitive to any component thereof.

Adsorbed Tetanus Vaccine should not be given to an individual suffering from an acute febrile illness except in the presence of a tetanus-prone wound.

Tetanus vaccine should not be given to any patient who has received a booster dose in the preceding year.

Special warnings and special precautions for use: Although anaphylaxis is rare, facilities for its management should always be available during vaccination.

Interactions with other medicaments and other forms of interaction: None known.

Pregnancy and lactation: In countries where the risks of neonatal tetanus are high, tetanus vaccines are widely administered during pregnancy without any apparent significant adverse effect on pregnancy or foetal development.

No information on the immunisation of lactating women is available.

Effects on ability to drive or use machines: None stated.

Undesirable effects: Local reactions consisting of swelling, redness and pain may develop at the injection site and persist for several days. Delays of up to 10 days before symptoms develop are reported. Occasionally these local reactions may be quite marked, with tenderness and swelling of a large area. Local reactions are rare in children, the incidence increases with age and according to the number of previously administered doses of tetanus toxoid containing vaccine. However, reactions may occur after the first dose. Subjects who develop reactions frequently have high titres of circulating antitoxin. Women develop reactions more frequently than men.

General reactions are uncommon but may include rash, arthralgia, lymphadenopathy, faintness, nausea, headache, lethargy, malaise, myalgia and pyrexia. They do not usually persist for more than a few hours. Urticaria, angioneurotic oedema and acute anaphylactic reactions are sometimes seen.

Serum sickness and peripheral neuropathy have been described. Calcifying dermatomyositis has been observed in temporal association with tetanus vaccination.

Persistent nodules at the site of injection may occasionally follow administration of adsorbed vaccines especially if the inoculation is into the superficial layers of subcutaneous tissue.

Any untoward reactions should be reported to the regulatory authorities and to the manufacturer.

Overdose: If overdosage or inadvertent administration is suspected, careful observation of the subject may be necessary. There may not be sequelae but subjects should be monitored and appropriate supportive measures should be implemented according to the type of response seen.

Pharmacological properties Not applicable.

Pharmaceutical particulars
List of excipients: The excipients contained in the preparation are as follows:- Aluminium hydroxide HSE*, Disodium Tetraborate, (Sodium borate) BP, Succinic acid HSE*, Sodium chloride PhEur, Thiomersal BP, Water for Injections PhEur.
* HSE house specification.

Incompatibilities: None stated.

Shelf life: In filled containers: 2 years.

Special precautions for storage: Store between 2–8°C. Protect from light. Do not freeze. Vials should be stored upright.

Nature and contents of container: PhEur type 1 clear neutral glass ampoules, 1 ml capacity (0.5 ml fill).

Multidose PhEur type 1 clear neutral glass vials, 8 ml capacity (5 ml fill), with red butyl rubber plug with an aluminium collar and blue polypropylene flip-off top.

Instructions for use/handling: Vaccine which has been frozen should not be used. Discard partly used vials at the end of the vaccination session. Disposal should be by incineration at a temperature of not less than 1100°C at a registered waste disposal contractor.

Marketing authorisation number 00039/0473

Date of Approval/revision of SPC December 1997

Legal category POM

TRANDATE* INJECTION

Presentation Trandate Injection: 20 ml ampoules each containing 100 mg (5 mg/ml) labetalol hydrochloride in an aqueous colourless solution. Labetalol hydrochloride is 2-hydroxy-5-[1-hydroxy-2-(1-methyl-3-phenyl-propylamino) ethyl] benzamide hydrochloride.

Uses
Indications: Trandate Injection is indicated when rapid control of blood pressure is essential in severely hypertensive patients including severe hypertension of pregnancy and for use in anaesthesia where a hypotensive technique is indicated.

It is also indicated in hypertensive episodes following acute myocardial infarction.

Mode of action: Trandate lowers the blood pressure primarily by blocking alpha-adrenoceptors in peripheral arterioles and thereby reducing the peripheral resistance.

Concurrent beta-blockade protects the heart from reflex sympathetic drive normally induced by peripheral vasodilatation. Cardiac output is not significantly reduced at rest or after moderate exercise. Increases in systolic pressure during exercise are, however, reduced after Trandate, corresponding changes in diastolic pressure are essentially normal. All these effects would be expected to benefit hypertensive patients.

Dosage and administration
Adults: Trandate Injection is intended for intravenous use in hospitalised patients. The plasma concentrations achieved after intravenous doses of Trandate in severe hypertension are substantially greater than those following oral administration of the drug and provide the greater degree of blockade of alpha-adrenoceptors necessary to control the more severe disease. Patients should, therefore, always receive the drug whilst in the supine or left lateral position. Raising the patient into the upright position, within three hours of intravenous Trandate administration, should be avoided since excessive postural hypotension may occur.

Bolus Injection: If it is essential to reduce the blood pressure quickly, as for example, in hypertensive encephalopathy, a dose of 50 mg of Trandate should be given by intravenous injection over a period of at least one minute. If necessary, doses of 50 mg may be repeated at five minute intervals until a satisfactory response occurs. The total dose should not exceed 200 mg. After bolus injection, the maximum effect usually occurs within five minutes and the effective duration of action is usually about six hours but may be as long as eighteen hours.

Intravenous Infusion: An alternative method of administering Trandate is intravenous infusion of a solution made by diluting the contents of two ampoules (200 mg) to 200 ml with Sodium Chloride and Dextrose Injection BP or 5% Dextrose Intravenous Infusion BP. The resultant infusion solution contains 1 mg/ml of Trandate. It should be administered using a paediatric giving set fitted with a 50 ml graduated burette to facilitate dosage.

In the hypertensions of pregnancy: The infusion can be started at the rate of 20 mg per hour and this dose may be doubled every thirty minutes until a satisfactory reduction in blood pressure has been obtained or a dosage of 160 mg per hour is reached. Occasionally, higher doses may be necessary.

In hypertensive episodes following acute myocardial infarction: Infusion should be commenced at 15 mg per hour and gradually increased to a maximum of 120 mg per hour depending on the control of blood pressure.

In hypertension due to other causes: The rate of infusion of Trandate should be about 2 mg (2 ml of infusion solution) per minute, until a satisfactory response is obtained; the infusion should then be stopped. The effective dose is usually in the range of 50-200 mg, depending on the severity of the hypertension. For most patients it is unnecessary to administer more than 200 mg but larger doses may be required especially in patients with phaeochromocytoma. The rate of infusion may be adjusted according to the response, at the discretion of the physician. The blood pressure and pulse rate should be monitored throughout the infusion.

It is desirable to monitor the heart rate after injection and during infusion. In most patients, there is a small decrease in the heart rate; severe bradycardia is unusual but may be controlled by injecting atropine 1-2 mg intravenously. Respiratory function should be observed particularly in patients with any known impairment.

Once the blood pressure has been adequately reduced, maintenance therapy with Trandate Tablets should be instituted with a starting dose of one 100 mg tablet twice daily. (See Trandate Tablets Data Sheet for further details). Trandate Injection has been administered to patients with uncontrolled hypertension already receiving other hypotensive agents, including beta-blocking drugs, without adverse effects.

In hypotensive anaesthesia: Induction should be with standard agents (e.g. sodium thiopentone) and anaesthesia maintained with nitrous oxide and oxygen with or without halothane. The recommended starting dose of Trandate Injection is 10-20 mg intravenously depending on the age and condition of the patient. Patients for whom halothane is contra-indicated usually require a higher initial dose of Trandate (25-30 mg). If satisfactory hypotension is not achieved after five minutes, increments of 5-10 mg should be given until the desired level of blood pressure is attained.

Halothane and Trandate act synergistically therefore the halothane concentration should not exceed 1 to 1.5% as profound falls in blood pressure may be precipitated.

Following Trandate Injection the blood pressure can be quickly and easily adjusted by altering the halothane concentration and/or adjusting table tilt. The mean duration of hypotension following 20-25 mg of Trandate is fifty minutes.

Hypotension induced by Trandate Injection is readily reversed by atropine 0.6 mg and discontinuation of halothane.

Tubocurarine and pancuronium may be used when assisted or controlled ventilation is required. IPPV may further increase the hypotension resulting from Trandate Injection and/or halothane.

Children: Safety and efficacy have not been established.

Contra-indications, warnings, etc

Contra-indications: History of wheezing or asthma, hypersensitivity to labetalol, second or third degree heart block, cardiogenic shock and other conditions associated with severe and prolonged hypotension or severe bradycardia. Uncontrolled, incipient or digitalis-refractory heart failure.

Where peripheral vasoconstriction suggests low cardiac output, the use of Trandate Injection to control hypertensive episodes following acute myocardial infarction is contra-indicated.

Precautions: There have been rare reports of severe hepatocellular injury with labetalol therapy. The hepatic injury is usually reversible and has occurred after both short and long term treatment. Appropriate laboratory testing should be done at the first sign or symptom of liver dysfunction.

If there is laboratory evidence of liver injury or the patient is jaundiced, labetalol therapy should be stopped and not re-started.

Where cardiac reserve is poor, control with a cardiac glycoside and a diuretic should be obtained prior to the cautious use of Trandate Injection.

Beta-blockers, even those with apparent cardioselectivity, should not be used in patients with a history of obstructive airways disease unless no alternative treatment is available. In such cases, the risk of inducing bronchospasm should be appreciated and appropriate precautions taken. If bronchospasm should occur after the use of Trandate, it can be treated with a β_2-agonist by inhalation e.g. salbutamol (the dose of which may need to be greater than the usual dose in asthma) and if necessary intravenous atropine 1 mg. It is not necessary to discontinue Trandate therapy in patients requiring anaesthesia but they should be given intravenous atropine prior to induction; the effect of halothane on blood pressure may be enhanced by Trandate. During anaesthesia Trandate may mask the compensatory physiological responses to sudden haemorrhage (tachycardia and vasoconstriction). Close attention must therefore be paid to blood loss and the blood volume maintained.

Care should be taken in the concomitant use of labetalol and either Class I antiarrhythmic agents or calcium antagonists of the verapamil type.

Risk of anaphylactic reaction: While taking beta-blockers, patients with a history of severe anaphylactic reaction to a variety of allergens may be more reactive to repeated challenge, either accidental, diagnostic or therapeutic. Such patients may be unresponsive to the usual doses of adrenaline used to treat allergic reaction.

Pregnancy: Although no teratogenic effects have been demonstrated in animals, Trandate should only be used during the first trimester of pregnancy if the potential benefit outweighs the potential risk. Trandate crosses the placental barrier and the possibility of the consequences of alpha- and beta-adrenoceptor blockade in the fetus and neonate should be borne in mind.

Perinatal and neonatal distress (bradycardia, hypotension, respiratory depression, hypoglycaemia, hypothermia) has been rarely reported. Sometimes these symptoms developed a day or two after birth. Response to supportive measures (e.g. intravenous fluids and glucose) is usually prompt but with severe pre-eclampsia, particularly after prolonged intravenous labetalol, recovery may be slower. This may be related to diminished liver metabolism in premature babies. Intra-uterine and neonatal deaths have been reported but other drugs (e.g. vasodilators, respiratory depressants) and the effects of pre-eclampsia, intra-uterine growth retardation and prematurity were implicated.

Such clinical experience warns against unduly prolonging high dose labetalol and delaying delivery and against co-administration of hydralazine.

Trandate is excreted in breast milk. No adverse effects in breast feeding infants have been reported.

Side-effects: Trandate Injection is usually well tolerated. Excessive postural hypotension may occur if patients are allowed to assume the upright position within three hours of receiving Trandate Injection.

There have been a few reports of nasal congestion and rare reports of hypersensitivity: rash, pruritus, angioedema and dyspnoea.

There are rare reports of raised liver function tests, jaundice (both hepatocellular and cholestatic), hepatitis and hepatic necrosis. The signs and symptoms are usually reversible on withdrawal of the drug. There are reports of bradycardia and heart block.

Overdosage: Profound cardiovascular effects are to be expected e.g. excessive, posture-sensitive hypotension and sometimes bradycardia. Patients should be laid supine with legs raised. Use a cardiac glycoside and a diuretic in cardiac failure; for bronchospasm, administer a β_2-agonist per aerosol. Intravenous atropine 0.25 to 3 mg should be given to relieve bradycardia. Intravenous noradrenaline 5 to 10 micrograms initially, repeated according to response, may be preferable to isoprenaline to improve the circulation. Alternatively, noradrenaline may be infused at a rate of 5 micrograms per minute until the response is satisfactory.

In severe overdose, intravenous glucagon may be preferred: an initial bolus dose of 5 to 10 mg in dextrose or saline should be followed by an intravenous infusion of 5 mg/hour or as sufficient to maintain cardiac output. Transvenous pacing may be required.

Oliguric renal failure has been reported after massive overdosage of labetalol orally. In one case, the use of dopamine to increase the blood pressure may have aggravated the renal failure.

Haemodialysis removes less than 1% labetalol hydrochloride from the circulation.

Pharmaceutical precautions Protect from light.

Trandate Injection has been shown to be incompatible with Sodium Bicarbonate Injection BP 4.2% w/v.

Legal category POM.

Package quantities Trandate Injection 20 ml ampoules: Boxes of 5.

Further information Trandate does not adversely affect renal function and is a particularly suitable drug for use in hypertensive patients with renal disease. The metabolites of Trandate are excreted in the faeces as well as in the urine and so the drug is unlikely to accumulate in the body even in renal failure.

The plasma half-life of Trandate is about 4 hours. Only about 50% of Trandate in blood is protein bound.

Trandate fluoresces in alkaline solution at an excitation wavelength of 334nm and a fluorescence wavelength of 412nm and may therefore interfere with the assays of certain fluorescent substances.

The presence of labetalol metabolites in the urine may result in falsely elevated levels of urinary catecholamines, metanephrine, normetanephrine, and vanillylmandelic acid (VMA) when measured by fluorimetric or photometric methods. In screening patients suspected of having a phaeochromocytoma and being treated with Trandate a specific method, such as a high performance liquid chromatographic assay with solid phase extraction (e.g. J. Chromatogr. 385, 241, 1987) should be employed in determining levels of catecholamines.

Product licence number 0039/0492

TRANDATE* TABLETS

Presentation Trandate Tablets: Circular, orange-coloured, film-coated, biconvex tablets marked TRANDATE and the strength in milligrams on one face.

Trandate Tablets 50 mg: each containing labetalol hydrochloride 50 mg.

Trandate Tablets 100 mg: each containing labetalol hydrochloride 100 mg.

Trandate Tablets 200 mg: each containing labetalol hydrochloride 200 mg.

Trandate Tablets 400 mg: each containing labetalol hydrochloride 400 mg.

Labetalol hydrochloride is 2 hydroxy-5[1-hydroxy-2(1-methyl-3-phenyl-propylamino) ethyl] benzamide hydrochloride.

Uses

Indications: Trandate Tablets are indicated in mild, moderate and severe hypertension including the hypertensions of pregnancy, when oral therapy is desirable. Trandate Tablets are also indicated in angina pectoris with existing hypertension.

Mode of action: Trandate lowers blood pressure by blocking peripheral arteriolar alpha-adrenoceptors, thus reducing peripheral resistance and by concurrent beta-blockade, protects the heart from reflex sympathetic drive that would otherwise occur. Cardiac output is not significantly reduced at rest or after moderate exercise. Increases in systolic blood pressure during exercise are reduced but corresponding changes in diastolic pressure are essentially normal.

In patients with anginal pectoris coexisting with hypertension, the reduced peripheral resistance decreases myocardial afterload and oxygen demand. All these effects would be expected to benefit hypertensive patients and those with coexisting angina.

Dosage and administration Trandate Tablets should be taken with food.

Adults: Hypertension: Treatment should start with 100 mg twice daily. In patients already being treated with antihypertensives and in those of low body weight this may be sufficient to control blood pressure. In others, increase in dosage of 100 mg twice daily should be made at fortnightly intervals. Many patients' blood pressure is controlled by 200 mg twice daily and up to 800 mg daily may be given as a twice daily regimen. In severe, refractory hypertension, daily doses up to 2400 mg have been given. Such doses should be divided into a three or four times a day regimen.

Elderly: In elderly patients, an initial dose of 50 mg twice daily is recommended. This has provided satisfactory control in some cases.

In hypertensions of pregnancy: The initial dosage of 100 mg twice daily may be increased if necessary, at weekly intervals by 100 mg twice daily. During the second and third trimesters, the severity of the hypertension may require further dose titration to a three times daily regimen, ranging from 100 mg tds to 400 mg tds. A total daily dose of 2400 mg should not be exceeded.

Hospital in-patients with severe hypertension, particularly of pregnancy, may have daily increases in dosage.

General: If rapid reduction of blood pressure is necessary, see the data sheet for Trandate Injection. If long-term control of hypertension following the use of Trandate Injection is required, oral therapy with Trandate Tablets should start with 100 mg twice daily.

Additive hypotensive effects may be expected if Trandate Tablets are administered together with other antihypertensives, e.g. diuretics, methyldopa etc. When transferring patients from such agents. Trandate Tablets should be introduced with a dosage of 100 mg twice daily and the previous therapy gradually decreased. Abrupt withdrawal of clonidine or beta-blocking agents is undesirable.

Angina coexisting with hypertension: In patients with angina pectoris coexisting with hypertension, the dose of Trandate will be that required to control the hypertension.

Children: Safety and efficacy in children have not been established.

Contra-indications, warnings, etc

Contra-indications: Trandate Tablets are contra-indicated in history of wheezing or asthma, second or third degree heart block, cardiogenic shock, other conditions associated with severe and prolonged hypotension or severe bradycardia and uncontrolled, incipient or digitalis-refractory heart failure.

Labetalol is contra-indicated for patients known to have a hypersensitivity to the drug.

Warnings: There have been reports of skin rashes and/or dry eyes associated with the use of beta-adrenoceptor blocking drugs. The reported incidence is small and in most cases the symptoms have cleared when the treatment was withdrawn. Gradual discontinuance of the drug should be considered if any such reaction is not otherwise explicable.

There have been rare reports of severe hepatocellular injury with labetalol therapy. The hepatic injury is usually reversible and has occurred after both short-term and long-term treatment. Appropriate laboratory testing should be done at the first sign or symptom of liver dysfunction. If there is laboratory evidence of liver injury or the patient is jaundiced, labetalol should be stopped and not re-started.

Precautions: Special care should be taken with patients whose cardiac reserve is poor and heart failure should be controlled with a cardiac glycoside and a diuretic before starting Trandate therapy.

Beta-blockers, even those with apparent cardioselectivity, should not be used in patients with a history of obstructive airways disease unless no alternative treatment is available. In such cases, the risk of inducing bronchospasm should be appreciated and appropriate precautions taken. If bronchospasm should occur after the use of Trandate, it can be treated with a β_2-agonist by inhalation e.g. salbutamol (the dose of which may need to be greater than the usual dose in asthma) and, if necessary, intravenous atropine 1 mg.

Trandate Tablets need not be discontinued prior to anaesthesia but patients should receive intravenous atropine prior to induction. Trandate may enhance the hypotensive effect of halothane. Care should be taken if labetalol is used concomitantly with either Class I anti-arrhythmic agents or calcium antagonists of the verapamil type.

Patients, particularly those with ischaemic heart disease, should not interrupt/discontinue abruptly Trandate therapy.

Risk of anaphylactic reaction: While taking beta-blockers, patients with a history of severe anaphylactic reaction to a variety of allergens may be more reactive to repeated challenge, either accidental, diagnostic or therapeutic. Such patients may be unresponsive to the usual doses of adrenaline used to treat allergic reaction.

Pregnancy: Although not teratogenic effects have been demonstrated in animals, Trandate should only be used during the first trimester of pregnancy if the potential benefit outweighs the potential risk. Trandate crosses the placental barrier and the possibility of the consequences of alpha- and beta-adrenoceptor blockade in the fetus and neonate should be borne in mind.

Perinatal and neonatal distress (bradycardia, hypotension, respiratory depression, hypoglycaemia, hypothermia) has been rarely reported. Sometimes these symptoms developed a day or two after birth. Response to supportive measures (e.g. intravenous fluids and glucose) is usually prompt but with severe pre-eclampsia, particularly after prolonged intravenous labetalol, recovery may be slower. This may be related to diminished liver metabolism in premature babies. Intra-uterine and neonatal deaths have been reported but other drugs (e.g. vasodilators, respiratory depressants) and the effects of pre-eclampsia, intra-uterine growth retardation and prematurity were implicated. Such clinical experience warns against unduly prolonging high dose labetalol and delaying delivery and against co-administration of hydralazine.

Trandate is excreted in breast milk. No adverse effects in breast feeding infants have been reported.

Side-effects: Most side-effects are transient and occur during the first few weeks of treatment. They include headache, tiredness, dizziness, depressed mood, lethargy, nasal congestion, sweating, and rarely, ankle oedema. Postural hypotension is uncommon except at very high doses or if the initial dose is too high or doses are increased too rapidly. A tingling sensation in the scalp, usually transient, also may occur in a few patients early in treatment. Tremor has been reported in the treatment of hypertensions of pregnancy. Acute retention of urine, difficulty in micturition, ejaculatory failure, epigastric pain, nausea and vomiting have been reported. There have been rare reports of positive anti-nuclear antibodies unassociated with disease as well as rare cases of systemic lupus erythematosus and very rarely drug fever.

There have been very rare reports of toxic myopathy. Rare reports of hypersensitivity: rash, pruritus, angioedema and dyspnoea. A reversible lichenoid rash has occurred rarely. Blurred vision, eye irritation and cramps have been reported but were not necessarily related to Trandate. There are rare reports of raised liver function tests, jaundice (both hepatocellular and cholestatic), hepatitis and hepatic necrosis. The signs and symptoms are usually reversible on withdrawal of the drug. There are rare reports of bradycardia and heart block.

Drug interactions: Concomitant use of tricyclic antidepressants may increase the incidence of tremor. Cimetidine may increase the bioavailability of labetalol and care is required in the oral dosing of the latter.

Overdosage: Profound cardiovascular effects are to be expected e.g. excessive, posture-sensitive hypotension and sometimes bradycardia. Patients should be laid supine with the legs raised. Gastric lavage or induced emesis is warranted for a few hours after ingestion; use a cardiac glycoside and a diuretic in cardiac failure; for bronchospasm, administer a β_2-agonist per aerosol. Intravenous atropine 0.25 to 3 mg should be given to relieve bradycardia. Intravenous noradrenaline 5 to 10 micrograms initially, repeated according to response, may be preferable to isoprenaline to improve the circulation. Alternatively, noradrenaline may be infused at a rate of 5 micrograms per minute until the response is satisfactory.

In severe overdose, intravenous glucagon may be preferred: an initial bolus dose of 5 to 10 mg in dextrose or saline should be followed by an intravenous infusion of 5 mg/hour or as sufficient to maintain cardiac output. Transvenous pacing may be required.

Oliguric renal failure has been reported after massive overdosage of labetalol orally. In one case, the use of dopamine to increase the blood pressure may have aggravated the renal failure.

Haemodialysis removes less than 1% labetalol hydrochloride from the circulation.

Pharmaceutical precautions No special storage precautions are required.

Legal category POM.

Package quantities Trandate Tablets 100 mg and 200 mg are available in containers of 250; Trandate Tablets 400 mg in containers of 56 (OP) and 250; Trandate Tablets 50 mg, 100 mg and 200 mg are also available in calendar blister packs of 56 tablets (OP).

Further information Trandate does not adversely affect renal function and is particularly suitable for use in hypertensive patients with renal disease. Its metabolites are excreted in faeces as well as urine and the drug is unlikely to accumulate in the body even in renal failure.

The plasma half-life of Trandate is about 4 hours. Only 50% of labetalol in the blood is protein bound. It fluoresces in alkaline solution at an excitation wavelength of 334nm and a fluorescence wavelength of 412nm and may therefore interfere with the assays of certain fluorescent substances including catecholamines.

The presence of labetalol metabolites in the urine may result in falsely elevated levels of urinary catecholamines, metanephrine, normetanephrine, and vanillylmandelic acid (VMA) when measured by fluorimetric or photometric methods. In screening patients suspected of having a phaeochromocytoma and being treated with Trandate a specific method, such as a high performance liquid chromatographic assay with solid phase extraction (e.g. J. Chromatogr. 385, 241, 1987) should be employed in determining levels of catecholamines.

Product licence numbers

Trandate Tablets 50 mg	0039/0493
Trandate Tablets 100 mg	0039/0494
Trandate Tablets 200 mg	0039/0495
Trandate Tablets 400 mg	0039/0496

TRIVAX-AD*

Adsorbed Diphtheria, Tetanus and Pertussis Vaccine, BP

Qualitative and quantitative composition The composition in terms of active ingredients is as follows:-

Diphtheria toxoid	not less than 30IU
Tetanus toxoid	not less than 60IU
Bordetella pertussis	not more than 20,000 million chemically killed organisms with a potency of not less than 4IU

Quantities expressed per 0.5 ml dose.

Pharmaceutical form Sterile suspension for deep subcutaneous or intramuscular injection to humans.

Clinical particulars

Therapeutic indications: For active immunisation against diphtheria, tetanus and whooping cough in infants and children under 10 years of age.

Posology and method of administration:

Children aged 10 years and over, adults and elderly: **NOT RECOMMENDED.**

Children under 10 years of age: Each dose is 0.5 ml, given by intramuscular or deep subcutaneous injection. The primary course of immunisation consists of three doses with an interval of at least one month between each dose. The intervals between immunisations may be exceeded without the need to repeat the full course of immunisation.

The primary course should start at 2 months of age, with an interval of at least one month between each dose.

When Adsorbed Diphtheria and Tetanus Vaccine (CHILD) has been administered at the start of a primary course, Adsorbed Diphtheria, Tetanus and Pertussis Vaccine may be administered for subsequent doses. Once three doses of Adsorbed Diphtheria and Tetanus Vaccine (CHILD) have been administered, monovalent pertussis vaccine may be given at monthly intervals to complete the course.

A single dose of Adsorbed Diphtheria, Tetanus and Pertussis Vaccine is recommended as the initial dose of a primary pertussis vaccination course for children who require simultaneous reinforcement of immunity to diphtheria and tetanus. Vaccination against pertussis should be completed using monovalent pertussis vaccine.

Reinforcing doses: Children who have received the primary course of Adsorbed Diphtheria, Tetanus and Pertussis Vaccine do not require further immunisation against pertussis. Reinforcement of immunity against diphtheria and tetanus is necessary. This can be achieved by giving one dose (0.5 ml) Adsorbed Diphtheria and Tetanus Vaccine (CHILD) after at least three years from the last dose of the primary course. The reinforcing dose is commonly given prior to school entry. A reinforcing dose (0.5 ml) of either Adsorbed Diphtheria and Tetanus Vaccine for Adults and Adolescents or Adsorbed Tetanus Vaccine may be given at 13 to 18 years of age or on leaving school.

Shake well before withdrawing a dose. It is good practice to record title, dose and lot numbers of all vaccines and dates of administration.

Contra-indications: Current acute febrile illness (eg temperature above 39.5°C).

Progressive degenerative neurological disorder.

Severe local reaction to previous dose of the vaccine or one of its components–an area of erythema, swelling and induration involving most of the antero-lateral thigh or a major part of the circumference of the upper arm.

Severe general reaction to a previous dose of the vaccine or one of its components–for example:

(a) Prolonged inconsolable crying or screaming for over 3 hours.
(b) A convulsion or temperature >40.5°C occurring within 72 hours for which no other cause was found.
(c) Hypotonia–hyporesponsive episode occurring within 72 hours.
(d) Severe, acute neurological illness occurring within 72 hours.
(e) Immediate allergic reaction (severe or anaphylactic) to a previous dose of Diphtheria, Tetanus or Pertussis Vaccine.

Any child exhibiting a severe local or significant general reaction to a previous dose of a pertussis-containing vaccine should not be given a further dose of pertussis-containing vaccine. However, protection against diphtheria and tetanus is advisable and can be accomplished by giving Adsorbed Diphtheria and Tetanus Vaccine (CHILD).

The vaccine should not be injected intradermally.

ADSORBED DIPHTHERIA, TETANUS AND PERTUSSIS VACCINE SHOULD NOT BE ADMINISTERED TO CHILDREN AGED 10 YEARS AND OVER, ADULTS AND ELDERLY.

Special warnings and special precautions for use: When there is a family or personal history of febrile convulsions, there is an increased risk of these occurring after pertussis immunisation. In such children, immunisation is recommended but advice on prevention of fever should be given at the time of immunisation.

In a recent British study, children with a personal or family history of epilepsy were immunised with pertussis vaccine without any significant adverse events. These childrens' developmental progress has been normal. In children with a close family history (first degree relatives) of idiopathic epilepsy there may be a risk of developing this condition irrespective of vaccination. Immunisation is recommended for these children. Children whose epilepsy is well controlled may receive pertussis vaccine.

Advice on the prevention of fever should be given.

When there is still an evolving neurological problem, immunisation should be deferred until the condition is stable. When there has been a documented history of cerebral damage in the neonatal period, immunisation should be carried out unless there is evidence of an evolving neurological abnormality. A personal or family history of allergy is not a contraindication to immunisation with pertussis nor are stable neurological conditions such as cerebral palsy or spina bifida. Where there is doubt, appropriate advice should be sought from a consultant paediatrician, district (Health Board) Immunisation co-ordinator or a consultant in communicable disease control rather than withholding the vaccine. HIV positive individuals may receive pertussis vaccine in the absence of contraindications.

Although anaphylaxis is rare, facilities for its management should always be available during vaccination.

Antipyretic measures may be indicated in those who experience a febrile convulsion following vaccination.

Use of Adsorbed Diphtheria, Tetanus and Pertussis Vaccine in individuals aged 10 years and over may be associated with severe hypersensitivity reactions.

Interaction with other medicaments and other forms of interaction: None stated.

Pregnancy and lactation: No reproductive studies have been conducted in animals since simultaneous vaccination against diphtheria, tetanus and pertussis in adults is uncommon. There is no accurate information on the safety of this vaccine in pregnancy therefore this vaccine should not be used in pregnancy or during lactation.

Effects on ability to drive and use machines: Not applicable.

Undesirable effects: Local reactions, particularly erythema at the site of injection, are commonly seen during the 24 hours following vaccination. They normally subside without treatment. A nodule may be found at the site of injection, especially if the inoculation is introduced into the superficial layers of subcutaneous tissue.

A transient rise in temperature, restlessness, irritability, crying or loss of appetite may sometimes occur a few hours after vaccination, but does not generally call for treatment. Systemic reactions such as headache, malaise and somnolence have been reported. Allergic manifestations including pallor, dyspnoea and collapse have been observed rarely.

Neurological events have occasionally been observed following the administration of pertussis-containing vaccines. The events reported do not appear to constitute a single, identifiable clinical syndrome but include isolated febrile convulsions, infantile spasms, episodes of persistent screaming and severe encephalopathy resulting in permanent brain damage or death. These events cannot be distinguished from those occurring in unvaccinated children of similar age.

In the absence of a common, identifiable pathological mechanism, it is not possible to produce a reliable estimate of the incidence of neurological events attributable to pertussis vaccination *per se*.

An increased incidence of reactions may occur due to failure to shake the container and re-suspend the vaccine before withdrawing a dose, to inadvertent intravenous administration, or to an over-rapid injection.

Since combined diphtheria, tetanus and pertussis vaccines are widely used in a population in which sudden illnesses of undefined origin are not uncommon, intercurrent illness bearing a temporal but not a causal relationship to vaccination may be expected.

Any untoward reactions should be reported to the regulatory authorities and to the manufacturer.

Overdose: If overdosage or inadvertent administration is suspected, careful observation of the subject may be necessary. Prophylactic treatment with appropriate anti-pyretics may be advisable in certain circumstances to reduce the incidence of fever. There may not be any sequelae, but subjects should be monitored and appropriate supportive measures should be implemented according to the type of response seen.

Pharmacological properties Not applicable.

Pharmaceutical particulars

List of excipients: The excipients contained in the preparation are as follows:- Aluminium hydroxide HSE*, Disodium tetraborate, (Sodium borate) BP, Succinic acid HSE*, Sodium chloride PhEur, Thiomersal BP, Water for Injections PhEur.

* HSE House specification

Incompatibilities: None stated.

Shelf life: In filled containers: 2 years

Special precautions for storage: Store between 2 and 8°C. Protect from light. Do not freeze.

Nature and contents of container: PhEur type 1 clear neutral glass ampoules, 1 ml capacity (0.5 ml fill).

Instructions for use/handling: Vaccine which has been frozen should not be used. Disposal should be by incineration at a temperature not less than 1100°C at a registered waste disposal contractor.

Marketing authorisation number 00039/0474

Date of approval/revision of the SPC December 1997

Legal category POM

TUBERCULIN PPD 10 units/ml

Qualitative and quantitative composition Tuberculin PPD BP 10 units/ml.

Pharmaceutical form Sterile aqueous solution for intradermal injection containing Tuberculin PPD BP prepared from human strains of *Mycobacterium tuberculosis.*

Clinical particulars

Therapeutic indications: As an intradermal diagnostic test for hypersensitivity to Tubercle bacilli. **FOR USE WITH MANTOUX TEST ONLY.**

A tuberculin skin test must be conducted prior to BCG vaccination in all subjects with the exception of infants aged under three months of age.

Posology and method of administration: MANTOUX TEST: Dose: 0.1 ml by **INTRADERMAL INJECTION**. The inoculation should preferably be carried out with a syringe fitted with a short bevel gauge 25 or 26 needle. A separate syringe and needle must be used for each subject to prevent cross-infection.

The test is performed on the flexor surface of the left forearm at the junction of the upper third with the lower two-thirds. The site is cleaned if visible dirty with spirit and allowed to dry. Using a disposable syringe and needle, a dose (0.1 ml) of the appropriate tuberculin dilution is administered **intradermally** so that a bleb is produced, typically of 7 mm diameter.

Routinely one dose (0.1 ml) of **100 units per ml** Tuberculin PPD (equivalent to 10 units) is given. If there is any doubt about interpretation of the area of induration produced, a second dose (0.1 ml) of **1000 units per ml** Tuberculin PPD (equivalent to 100 units) may be given 3 days later. If that reading is negative, the patient is normally assessed as tuberculin negative. If a second tuberculin test is necessary, it should be carried out on the other arm. Repeat testing at one site may alter the reactivity either by hypo- or more often hypersensitising the skin and changed response may reflect local changes in sensitivity only.

If there is concern that a person may be hypersensitive to tuberculin, or in whom tuberculosis is suspected, a dose (0.1 ml) of **10 units per ml** Tuberculin PPD (equivalent to 1 unit) or even less should be given.

A positive reaction is characterised by an area of 5 mm or greater of palpable induration, which may sometimes be surrounded by erythema. The results should be read after 72 hours, but usually a valid reading can be obtained up to 96 hours. Tuberculin positive subjects should not be given BCG vaccine.

Control Solution for Mantoux Test may be used at the same time but at a different site, to assess an individual patient's response to the vehicle used.

Contra-indications: Tuberculin testing should not be carried out within three weeks of receiving a live viral vaccine.

Special warnings and precautions for use: Caution should be exercised in giving tuberculin to persons who have, or are suspected of having active tuberculosis. The reaction to the tuberculin skin test may be suppressed by the following factors: ultra-violet light treatment, corticosteroid therapy, immunosuppressive diseases, including HIV, sarcoidosis, Hodgkin's disease, live viral vaccines, glandular fever and viral infections in general, including those of the upper respiratory tract. Sensitivity to tuberculin may also be reduced in the elderly or malnourished.

Subjects who have a negative test but who may have had a upper respiratory tract or other viral infection at the time of testing should be retested 2-3 weeks after clinical recovery before being given BCG.

The potency of the Tuberculin PPD may be affected if it is diluted with diluents which differ in composition from the vehicle used in its preparation. Where it is necessary to dilute, Control Solution for Mantoux Test should be used.

Use contents of the ampoule as soon as possible and within 1 hour of opening provided adequate aseptic precautions are taken. Care should be taken to avoid contamination of the ampoule contents.

Interaction with other medicaments and other forms of interaction: None stated.

Pregnancy and lactation: Vaccination with BCG vaccines (INTRADERMAL, INTRADERMAL Isoniazid Resistant and PERCUTANEOUS) should be avoided during early pregnancy and if possible delayed until after delivery. Similarly, use of the tuberculin skin test should be avoided during pregnancy unless subsequent immunisation with BCG vaccine is considered appropriate should the skin test reading be negative.

Effects on ability to drive and use machines: No specific warning.

Undesirable effects: Nausea, headache, malaise and rash have occasionally been reported after tuberculin skin testing.

Immediate local reactions have been reported following tuberculin testing and these reactions were more common in atopic subjects. Rarely vesicular or ulcerating local reactions, regional adenopathy and fever may occur. Use of a dry dressing may be appropriate with local reactions of this severity.

Lymphangitis and anaphylactic reactions have been reported very rarely.

Tuberculin PPD can cause a severe local reaction in some individuals if the solution is allowed to come into contact with open cuts, the eyes or the mouth. The affected area should be washed with copious quantities of water followed, if necessary, by a topical corticosteroid.

Overdose: There is limited information available regarding the effects of overdosage.

Inadvertant subcutaneous or intramuscular injection of Tuberculin dilutions may result in tissue damage and scarring at the injection site. There may be systemic symptoms such as fever, nausea and malaise. A dry dressing may be appropriate for a serious local reaction. Systemic upset shoul be treated symptomatically if necessary.

Pharmacological particulars When the Tuberculin protein is injected into the skin a delayed hypersensitivity reaction is induced in persons previously sensitised by micro-organisms of the same species. The active fraction which is predominantly protein is isolated by precipitation.

Pharmaceutical particulars

List of excipients: Tween/Phosphate Buffered Diluent: Polysorbate 80 (Tween 80) 0.005% v/v, Potassium dihydrogen phosphate 0.138% w/v, Disodium hydrogen phosphate 0.724% w/v, Sodium chloride 0.457% w/v, Water for injection 100.000% v/v.

Incompatibilities: Control Solution for Mantoux Test should not be used with Tuberculins other than those manufactured by Medeva Pharma Limited.

Shelf life: Tuberculin PPD 10 u/ml shelf life is 12 months when stored unopened. Use contents of the ampoule at once and within one hour provided adequate aseptic precautions are taken.

Special precautions for storage: Store between 2°C and 8°C. Do not freeze. Protect from light. Disposal should be by incineration at a temperature not less than 1100°C at a registered waste disposal contractor.

Nature and contents of containers: Sealed labelled neutral glass ampoules contained within printed cardboard carton and held in position by divided plastic tray.

Instructions for use/handling: Use contents of ampoule as soon as possible and within 1 hour of opening provided adequate aseptic precautions are taken. Care should be taken to avoid contamination of the ampoule contents.

Marketing authorisation number 00039/0442

Date of approval/revision of SPC September 1997

Legal category POM

TUBERCULIN PPD 100 units/ml

Qualitative and quantitative composition Tuberculin PPD BP 100 units/ml.

Pharmaceutical form Sterile aqueous solution for intradermal injection containing Tuberculin PPD BP prepared from human strains of *Mycobacterium tuberculosis.*

Clinical particulars

Therapeutic indications: As an intradermal diagnostic test for hypersensitivity to Tubercle bacilli. **FOR USE WITH MANTOUX TEST ONLY.**

A tuberculin skin test must be conducted prior to BCG vaccination in all subjects with the exception of infants aged under three months of age.

Posology and method of administration: MANTOUX TEST: *Dose:* 0.1 ml by **INTRADERMAL INJECTION**. The inoculation should preferably be carried out with a syringe fitted with a short bevel gauge 25 or 26 needle. A separate syringe and needle must be used for each subject to prevent cross-infection.

The test is performed on the flexor surface of the left forearm at the junction of the upper third with the lower two-thirds. The site is cleaned if visible dirty with spirit and allowed to dry. Using a disposable syringe and needle, a dose (0.1 ml) of the appropriate tuberculin dilution is administered **intradermally** so that a bleb is produced, typically of 7 mm diameter.

Routinely one dose (0.1 ml) of **100 units per ml** Tuberculin PPD (equivalent to 10 units) is given. If there is any doubt about interpretation of the area of induration produced, a second dose (0.1 ml) of **1000 units per ml** Tuberculin PPD (equivalent to 100 units) may be given 3 days later. If that reading is negative, the patient is normally assessed as tuberculin negative. If a second tuberculin test is necessary, it should be carried out on the other arm. Repeat testing at one site may alter the reactivity either by hypo- or more often hypersensitising the skin and changed response may reflect local changes in sensitivity only.

If there is concern that a person may be hypersensitive to tuberculin, or in whom tuberculosis is suspected, a dose (0.1 ml) of **10 units per ml** Tuberculin PPD (equivalent to 1 unit) or even less should be given.

A positive reaction is characterised by an area of 5 mm or greater of palpable induration, which may sometimes be surrounded by erythema. The results should be read after 72 hours, but usually a valid reading can be obtained up to 96 hours. Tuberculin positive subjects should not be given BCG vaccine.

Control Solution for Mantoux Test may be used at the same time but at a different site, to assess an individual patient's response to the vehicle used.

Contra-indications: Tuberculin testing should not be carried out within three weeks of receiving a live viral vaccine.

Special warnings and precautions for use: Caution should be exercised in giving tuberculin to persons who have, or are suspected of having active tuberculosis. The reaction to the tuberculin skin test may be suppressed by the following factors: ultra-violet light treatment, corticosteroid therapy, immunosuppressive diseases, including HIV, sarcoidosis, Hodgkin's disease, live viral vaccines, glandular fever and viral infections in general, including those of the upper respiratory tract. Sensitivity to tuberculin may also be reduced in the elderly or malnourished.

Subjects who have a negative test but who may have had a upper respiratory tract or other viral infection at the time of testing should be retested 2-3 weeks after clinical recovery before being given BCG.

The potency of the Tuberculin PPD may be affected if it is diluted with diluents which differ in composition from the vehicle used in its preparation. Where it is necessary to dilute, Control Solution for Mantoux Test should be used.

Use contents of the ampoule as soon as possible and within 1 hour of opening provided adequate aseptic precautions are taken. Care should be taken to avoid contamination of the ampoule contents.

Interaction with other medicaments and other forms of interaction: None stated.

Pregnancy and lactation: Vaccination with BCG vaccines (INTRADERMAL, INTRADERMAL Isoniazid Resistant and PERCUTANEOUS) should be avoided during early pregnancy and if possible delayed until after delivery. Similarly, use of the tuberculin skin test should be avoided during pregnancy unless subsequent immunisation with BCG vaccine is considered appropriate should the skin test reading be negative.

Effects on ability to drive and use machines: No specific warning.

Undesirable effects: Nausea, headache, malaise and rash have occasionally been reported after tuberculin skin testing.

Immediate local reactions have been reported following tuberculin testing and these reactions were more common in atopic subjects. Rarely vesicular or ulcerating local reactions, regional adenopathy and fever may occur. Use of a dry dressing may be appropriate with local reactions of this severity.

Lymphangitis and anaphylactic reactions have been reported very rarely.

Tuberculin PPD can cause a severe local reaction in some individuals if the solution is allowed to come into contact with open cuts, the eyes or the mouth. The affected area should be washed with copious quantities of water followed, if necessary, by a topical corticosteroid.

Overdose: There is limited information available regarding the effects of overdosage.

Inadvertant subcutaneous or intramuscular injection of Tuberculin dilutions may result in tissue damage and scarring at the injection site. There may be systemic symptoms such as fever, nausea and malaise. A dry dressing may be appropriate for a serious local reaction. Systemic upset shoul be treated symptomatically if necessary.

Pharmacological particulars When the Tuberculin protein is injected into the skin a delayed hypersensitivity reaction is induced in persons previously sensitised by micro-organisms of the same species. The active fraction which is predominantly protein is isolated by precipitation.

Pharmaceutical particulars
List of excipients: Tween/Phosphate Buffered Diluent: Polysorbate 80 (Tween 80) 0.005% v/v, Potassium dihydrogen phosphate 0.138% w/v, Disodium hydrogen phosphate 0.724% w/v, Sodium chloride 0.457% w/v, Water for injection 100.000% v/v

Incompatibilities: Control Solution for Mantoux Test should not be used with Tuberculins other than those manufactured by Medeva Pharma Limited.

Shelf life: Tuberculin PPD 100 u/ml shelf life is 12 months when stored unopened. Use contents of the ampoule at once and within one hour provided adequate aseptic precautions are taken.

Special precautions for storage: Store between 2°C and 8°C. Do not freeze. Protect from light. Disposal should be by incineration at a temperature not less than 1100°C at a registered waste disposal contractor.

Nature and contents of container: Sealed labelled neutral glass ampoules contained within printed cardboard carton and held in position by divided plastic tray.

Instructions for use/handling: Use contents of ampoule as soon as possible and within 1 hour of opening provided adequate aseptic precautions are taken. Care should be taken to avoid contamination of the ampoule contents.

Marketing authorisation number 00039/0441

Date of approval/revision of SPC September 1997

Legal category POM

TUBERCULIN PPD 1000 units/ml

Qualitative and quantitative composition Tuberculin PPD BP 1000 units/ml.

Pharmaceutical form Sterile aqueous solution for intradermal injection containing Tuberculin PPD BP prepared from human strains of *Mycobacterium tuberculosis.*

Clinical particulars
Therapeutic indications: As an intradermal diagnostic test for hypersensitivity to Tubercle bacilli. **FOR USE WITH MANTOUX TEST ONLY.**

A tuberculin skin test must be conducted prior to BCG vaccination in all subjects with the exception of infants aged under three months of age.

Posology and method of administration: MANTOUX TEST: *Dose:* 0.1 ml by **INTRADERMAL INJECTION.** The inoculation should preferably be carried out with a syringe fitted with a short bevel gauge 25 or 26 needle. A separate syringe and needle must be used for each subject to prevent cross-infection.

The test is performed on the flexor surface of the left forearm at the junction of the upper third with the lower two-thirds. The site is cleaned if visible dirty with spirit and allowed to dry. Using a disposable syringe and needle, a dose (0.1 ml) of the appropriate tuberculin dilution is administered **intradermally** so that a bleb is produced, typically of 7 mm diameter.

Routinely one dose (0.1 ml) of **100 units per ml** Tuberculin PPD (equivalent to 10 units) is given. If there is any doubt about interpretation of the area of induration produced, a second dose (0.1 ml) of **1000 units per ml** Tuberculin PPD (equivalent to 100 units) may be given 3 days later. If that reading is negative, the patient is normally assessed as tuberculin negative. If a second tuberculin test is necessary, it should be carried out on the other arm. Repeat testing at one site may alter the reactivity either by hypo- or more often hypersensitising the skin and changed response may reflect local changes in sensitivity only.

If there is concern that a person may be hypersensitive to tuberculin, or in whom tuberculosis is suspected, a dose (0.1 ml) of **10 units per ml** Tuberculin PPD (equivalent to 1 unit) or even less should be given.

A positive reaction is characterised by an area of 5 mm or greater of palpable induration, which may sometimes be surrounded by erythema. The results should be read after 72 hours, but usually a valid reading can be obtained up to 96 hours. Tuberculin positive subjects should not be given BCG vaccine.

Control Solution for Mantoux Test may be used at the same time but at a different site, to assess an individual patient's response to the vehicle used.

Contra-indications: Tuberculin testing should not be carried out within three weeks of receiving a live viral vaccine.

Special warnings and precautions for use: Caution should be exercised in giving tuberculin to persons who have, or are suspected of having active tuberculosis. The reaction to the tuberculin skin test may be suppressed by the following factors: ultra-violet light treatment, corticosteroid therapy, immunosuppressive diseases, including HIV, sarcoidosis, Hodgkin's disease, live viral vaccines, glandular fever and viral infections in general, including those of the upper respiratory tract. Sensitivity to tuberculin may also be reduced in the elderly or malnourished.

Subjects who have a negative test but who may have had a upper respiratory tract or other viral infection at the time of testing should be retested 2–3 weeks after clinical recovery before being given BCG.

The potency of the Tuberculin PPD may be affected if it is diluted with diluents which differ in composition from the vehicle used in its preparation. Where it is necessary to dilute, Control Solution for Mantoux Test should be used.

Use contents of the ampoule as soon as possible and within 1 hour of opening provided adequate aseptic precautions are taken. Care should be taken to avoid contamination of the ampoule contents.

Interaction with other medicaments and other forms of interaction: None stated.

Pregnancy and lactation: Vaccination with BCG vaccines (INTRADERMAL, INTRADERMAL Isoniazid Resistant and PERCUTANEOUS) should be avoided during early pregnancy and if possible delayed until after delivery. Similarly, use of the tuberculin skin test should be avoided during pregnancy unless subsequent immunisation with BCG vaccine is considered appropriate should the skin test reading be negative.

Effects on ability to drive and use machines: No specific warning.

Undesirable effects: Nausea, headache, malaise and rash have occasionally been reported after tuberculin skin testing.

Immediate local reactions have been reported following tuberculin testing and these reactions were more common in atopic subjects. Rarely vesicular or ulcerating local reactions, regional adenopathy and fever may occur. Use of a dry dressing may be appropriate with local reactions of this severity.

Lymphangitis and anaphylactic reactions have been reported very rarely.

Tuberculin PPD can cause a severe local reaction in some individuals if the solution is allowed to come into contact with open cuts, the eyes or the mouth. The affected area should be washed with copious quantities of water followed, if necessary, by a topical corticosteroid.

Overdose: There is limited information available regarding the effects of overdosage.

Inadvertant subcutaneous or intramuscular injection of Tuberculin dilutions may result in tissue damage and scarring at the injection site. There may be systemic symptoms such as fever, nausea and malaise. A dry dressing may be appropriate for a serious local reaction. Systemic upset shoul be treated symptomatically if necessary.

Pharmacological particulars When the Tuberculin protein is injected into the skin a delayed hypersensitivity reaction is induced in persons previously sensitised by micro-organisms of the same species. The active fraction which is predominantly protein is isolated by precipitation.

Pharmaceutical particulars
List of excipients: Tween/Phosphate Buffered Diluent: Polysorbate 80 (Tween 80) 0.005% v/v, Potassium dihydrogen phosphate 0.138% w/v, Disodium hydrogen phosphate 0.724% w/v, Sodium chloride 0.457% w/v, Water for injection 100.000% v/v.

Incompatibilities: Control Solution for Mantoux Test should not be used with Tuberculins other than those manufactured by Medeva Pharma Limited.

Shelf life: Tuberculin PPD 1000 u/ml shelf life is 12 months when stored unopened. Use contents of the ampoule at once and within one hour provided adequate aseptic precautions are taken.

Special precautions for storage: Store between 2°C and 8°C. Do not freeze. Protect from light. Disposal should be by incineration at a temperature not less than 1100°C at a registered waste disposal contractor.

Nature and contents of containers: Sealed labelled neutral glass ampoules contained within printed cardboard carton and held in position by divided plastic tray.

Instructions for use/handling: Use contents of ampoule as soon as possible and within 1 hour of opening provided adequate aseptic precautions are taken. Care should be taken to avoid contamination of the ampoule contents.

Marketing authorisation number 00039/0440

Date of approval/revision of SPC September 1997

Legal category POM

TUBERCULIN PPD 100,000 units/ml

Qualitative and quantitative composition Tuberculin PPD BP 100,000 units/ml.

Pharmaceutical form Sterile aqueous solutions for

percutaneous injection containing Tuberculin PPD BP prepared from human strains of *Mycobacterium tuberculosis.*

Clinical particulars

Therapeutic indications: As an percutaneous diagnostic test for hypersensitivity to Tubercle bacilli. **FOR USE WITH A HEAF MULTIPLE PUNCTURE APPARATUS ONLY.**

A tuberculin skin test must be conducted prior to BCG vaccination in all subjects with the exception of infants aged under three months of age.

Posology and method of administration: HEAF TEST: The following preparation is used; **100,000 UNITS PER ML.**

The recommended site for testing is on the flexor surface of the left forearm at the junction of the upper third with the lower two thirds, avoiding any eczematous areas. Cleansing the skin is only necessary if it is visibly dirty, in which case spirit should be used but must be allowed to dry completely before the test.

Tuberculin 100,000 units/ml should be withdrawn from the ampoule by needle and syringe and after detaching the needle, a small quantity of solution should be dropped directy from the syringe onto the skin at the standard test site. Sufficient tuberculin should be used to disperse over an area of skin just greater than the diameter of the perforated head of the unit. (Note that the head of the disposable head is wider than the standard gun). The head of the apparatus should be used to disperse the tuberculin.

If using the disposable head apparatus, check that the correct head is being used. Apply the apparatus firmly and evenly to the tuberculin covered skin and press on the handle until a click occurs, indicating that the needles have been fired. Do not press further after this, but remove the apparatus from the skin, remove the disposable head from the handle by holding the outer rim and discard the head into a 'sharps' bin. **If using the single use device,** press firmly on the top (purple) firing arm. After firing, an audible click is heard as the needles retract. **If using the conventional gun,** check that the gun is at the correct setting. The puncture depth of the needles should be adjusted to give 1 mm for children under two years of age or 2 mm for children aged two years and over and adults. The end plate should then be applied firmly and evenly to the area of skin covered by the tuberculin and pressure applied to the handle until the clicking firing mechanism operates. Do not apply further pressure after this and withdraw the apparatus. It is very important that the conventional gun is properly sterilised after each application.

Wipe off any excess tuberculin from the skin and observe the presence of **six** puncture marks. If these are not present, the test has not been adequately applied. The arm may be wetted and washed normally but perfumes and other cosmetics should be avoided.

The test should be read between 3 and 10 days. The reaction is graded 0–4 according to the degree of induration produced.

Grade 0	no induration at the puncture sites.
Grade 1	discrete induration at 4 or more needle sites.
Grade 2	induration around each needle site merging with the next, forming a ring of induration but with a clear centre.
Grade 3	the centre of the reaction becomes filled with induration to form one uniform circle of induration 5–10 mm wide.
Grade 4	solid induration over 10 mm wide. Vesiculation or ulceration may also occur.

Grades 0 and 1 are regarded as negative. Grades 2 to 4 are regarded as positive. Tuberculin positive subjects should not be given BCG vaccine.

Contraindications: Tuberculin testing should not be carried out within three weeks of receiving a live viral vaccine.

Special warnings and precautions for use: Caution should be exercised in giving tuberculin to persons who have, or are suspected of having active tuberculosis. The reaction to the tuberculin skin test may be suppressed by the following factors: ultra-violet light treatment, corticosteroid therapy, immunosuppressive diseases, including HIV, sarcoidosis, Hodgkin's disease, live viral vaccines, glandular fever and viral infections in general, including those of the upper respiratory tract. Sensitivity to tuberculin may also be reduced in the elderly and malnourished.

Subjects who have a negative test but who may have had a upper respiratory tract or other viral infection at the time of testing should be retested 2–3 weeks after clinical recovery before being given BCG.

The potency of the Tuberculin PPD may be affected if it is diluted with diluents which differ in composition from the vehicle used in its preparation. Where it is necessary to dilute, Control Solution for Mantoux Test should be used. The conventional Heaf multiple puncture apparatus should be checked at regular intervals to ensure the needles are sufficiently sharp to penetrate the skin.

Use contents of the ampoule as soon as possible and within 1 hour of opening provided adequate aseptic precautions are taken. Care should be taken to avoid contamination of the ampoule contents.

Interaction with other medicaments and other forms of interaction: None stated.

Pregnancy and lactation: Vaccination with BCG vaccines (INTRADERMAL, INTRADERMAL Isoniazid Resistant and PERCUTANEOUS) should be avoided during early pregnancy and if possible delayed until after delivery. Similarly, use of the tuberculin skin test should be avoided during pregnancy unless subsequent immunisation with BCG vaccine is considered appropriate should the skin test reading be negative.

Effects on ability to drive and use machines: No specific warning.

Undesirable effects: Nausea, headache, malaise and rash have occasionally been reported after tuberculin skin testing.

Immediate local reactions have been reported following tuberculin testing and these reactions were more common in atopic subjects. Rarely vesicular or ulcerating local reactions, regional adenopathy and fever may occur. Use of a dry dressing may be appropriate with local reactions of this severity.

Lymphangitis and anaphylactic reactions have been reported very rarely.

Tuberculin PPD can cause a severe local reaction in some individuals if the solution is allowed to come into contact with open cuts, the eyes or the mouth. The affected area should be washed with copious quantities of water followed, if necessary, by a topical corticosteroid.

Overdose: There is limited information available regarding the effects of overdosage.

Inadvertant intradermal injection of Tuberculin 100,000 units/ml intended for use in the Heaf Test may result in tissue damage and scarring at the injection site. There may be systemic symptoms such as fever, nausea and malaise. A dry dressing may be approprate for a serious local reaction. Systemic upset should be treated symptomatically if necessary.

Pharmacological particulars When the Tuberculin protein is injected into the skin a delayed hypersensitivity reaction is induced in persons previously sensitised by micro-organisms of the same species. The active fraction which is predominantly protein is isolated by precipitation.

Pharmaceutical particulars

List of excipients: Tween/Phosphate Buffered Diluent: Glycerol 20.00% v/v, Phenol 0.25% w/v, Polysorbate 80 (Tween 80) 0.005% v/v, Potassium dihydrogen phosphate 0.138% w/v, Disodium hydrogen phosphate 0.724% w/v, Sodium chloride 0.457% w/v, Water for injection 100.000% v/v.

Incompatibilities: None stated.

Shelf life: Tuberculin PPD 100,000 units/ml shelf life is 24 months when stored unopened. Use contents of the ampoule at once and within one hour provided adequate aseptic precautions are taken.

Special precautions for storage: Store between 2°C and 8°C. Do not freeze. Protect from light.

Disposal should be by incineration at a temperature not less than 1100°C at a registered waste disposal contractor.

Nature and contents of container: Sealed labelled neutral glass ampoules contained within printed cardboard carton and held in position by divided plastic tray.

Instructions for use/handling: Use contents of ampoule as soon as possible and within 1 hour of opening provided adequate aseptic precautions are taken. Care should be taken to avoid contamination of the ampoule contents.

Marketing authorisation number 00039/0439

Date of approval/revision of the SPC September 1997

Legal category POM

**Trade Mark*

Merck Pharmaceuticals
(A Division of Merck Ltd)
Harrier House
High Street
West Drayton
Middlesex UB7 7QG
☎ 01895 452200 Fax 01895 452296

MERCK

EMCOR*
EMCOR LS

Presentation Emcor LS tablets, containing 5 mg bisoprolol fumarate (2:1) are heart-shaped, pale yellow and film-coated. Emcor tablets, containing 10 mg bisoprolol fumarate (2:1) are heart-shaped, pale orange and film-coated. Both tablets are scored.

Uses
(i) Management of hypertension
(ii) Management of angina pectoris

Mode of action: Bisoprolol is a potent, highly β_1-selective-adrenoreceptor blocking agent devoid of intrinsic sympathomimetic activity and without relevant membrane stabilising activity.

As with other β_1-blocking agents, the mode of action in hypertension is not clear but it is known that bisoprolol markedly depresses plasma renin activity.

In patients with angina, the blockade of β_1-receptors reduces heart action and thus reduces oxygen demand. Hence bisoprolol is effective in eliminating or reducing the symptoms.

Pharmacokinetics: Bisoprolol is absorbed almost completely from the gastrointestinal tract. Together with the very small first pass effect in the liver, this results in a high bioavailability of approximately 90%. The drug is cleared equally by the liver and kidney.

The plasma elimination half-life (10–12 hours) provides 24 hours efficacy following a once daily dosage. About 95% of the drug substance is excreted through the kidney, half of this is as unchanged bisoprolol. There are no active metabolites in man.

Dosage and administration

Adults: The usual dose is 10 mg once daily with a maximum recommended dose of 20 mg per day. In some patients 5 mg per day may be adequate. In patients with final stage impairment of renal (creatinine clearance <20 ml/min) or liver function, the dose should not exceed 10 mg bisoprolol once daily.

Experience of the use of bisoprolol in renal dialysis patients is limited, however, there is no evidence that the dosage regimen needs to be altered.

Elderly: No dosage adjustment is normally required but 5 mg per day may be adequate in some patients; as for other adults, dosage may have to be reduced in cases of severe renal or hepatic dysfunction.

Children: There is no paediatric experience with bisoprolol, therefore its use cannot be recommended for children.

Contra-indications, warnings, etc

Contra-indications: As with other β_1-adrenoceptor antagonists, bisoprolol should not be used in cases of untreated cardiac failure, cardiogenic shock, sinoatrial block, second or third degree AV block, marked bradycardia (heart rate less than 50 beats/min), extreme hypotension, or severe asthma.

Precautions: Use with care in patients with a prolonged PR conduction interval, poor cardiac reserve and peripheral circulatory disturbances, such as Raynaud's phenomenon.

In patients with ischaemic heart disease, treatment should not be withdrawn abruptly.

Although bisoprolol is a highly selective β_1-adrenoceptor blocking agent, it should be used with caution in patients with chronic obstructive airways diseases or a family history of asthma. In some asthmatic patients some increase in airways resistance may occur, this may be regarded as a signal to discontinue therapy. This bronchospasm can usually be reversed by commonly used bronchodilators such as salbutamol.

Due to the low affinity of bisoprolol for β_2-receptors, the drug does not appear to have a hypoglycaemic effect. However, it should be used with caution in diabetic patients since the symptoms of hypoglycaemia (in particular, tachycardia) may be masked.

Pregnancy: No teratogenic effects have been demonstrated in animal studies, but the safety of bisoprolol during human pregnancy has not been established. Like other β-blockers, the benefits of use during pregnancy should be weighed against the possible hazard to mother and foetus. β-blockers administered in late pregnancy may cause bradycardia or hypotension in the foetus/neonate. Studies in animals suggest that no clinically relevant levels of bisoprolol reach the milk. However, as in pregnancy, caution should be exercised for use during lactation.

Drug interactions: Bisoprolol may potentiate the effect of other concurrently administered antihypertensive drugs. Concomitant treatment with reserpine, α-methyldopa and clonidine may cause an exaggerated decrease in heart rate. In particular, if clonidine is to be discontinued, this should not be done until bisoprolol treatment has been discontinued for several days.

Bisoprolol should also be used with care when myocardial depressants, inhibitors of AV conduction such as calcium antagonists of the verapamil and diltiazem type, or class I antidysrhythmic agents such as disopyramide are used concurrently.

The intravenous administration of calcium antagonists and antiarrythmic agents is not recommended during bisoprolol therapy.

The concurrent use of rifampicin can reduce the elimination half-life of bisoprolol, although an increase in dose is generally not necessary. The effects of insulin or oral hypoglycaemic agents may be potentiated when used concurrently with bisoprolol.

Anaesthesia: Prior to anaesthesia, the anaesthetist should be informed if the patient is taking bisoprolol. In cases of severe ischaemic heart disease the risk/benefit of continuing treatment should be evaluated. Care should be taken when using either cyclopropane or trichloroethylene.

Side-effects: Bisoprolol is usually well tolerated. The reported side effects are generally attributable to its pharmacological actions and include lassitude, fatigue, dizziness, mild headache, muscle and joint ache, perspiration, aggravation of intermittent claudication or Raynaud's disease and parasthaesia and coldness of the extremities, bronchospasm, oedema and occasional GI side-effects such as nausea, vomiting and diarrhoea. Occasionally a marked decrease in blood pressure, and pulse rate or a disturbance of AV conduction, skin rashes and dry eyes may be observed. Sleep disturbances including vivid dreams of the type noted with other β-blockers have rarely been reported.

Overdosage: In the case of overdosage or a precipitous drop in pulse rate and/or blood pressure, treatment with bisoprolol must be discontinued. If necessary, the following antidotes should be administered alone or consecutively: intravenous atropine 0.5–2.0 mg, intravenous orciprenaline 0.5 mg by slow intravenous injection; also glucagon may be given at a dose level of 1 to 5 mg.

Pharmaceutical precautions No special requirement.

Legal category POM.

Package quantities Calendar blister packs of 28 tablets. Strips of 14 tablets, two strips in each carton.

Further information Bisoprolol is effective in hypertension and angina pectoris for at least 24 hours following a single oral dose. The high bioavailability and the dual pathway of clearance lead to predictable blood levels. Patient compliance is increased by the reliable and simple administration regimen.

Product licence numbers
Emcor LS 0493/0126
Emcor 0493/0127

EMFLEX* CAPSULES

Qualitative and quantitative composition Each capsule contains Acemetacin 60 mg.

Pharmaceutical form Gelatine capsule.

Clinical particulars

Therapeutic indications: Rheumatoid arthritis, osteoarthritis, low back pain, and post-operative pain and inflammation.

Posology and method of administration: The recommended starting dose is 120 mg/day in divided doses, increasing to 180 mg/day in divided doses, depending on patient response.

For the treatment of elderly patients, adjustment of dosage is not normally required. However, non-steroidal anti-inflammatory drugs should be used with particular care in older patients who may be more prone to adverse reactions.

Emflex should be taken with food, milk or an antacid to reduce the possibility of gastro-intestinal disturbance.

Contra-indications: Active peptic ulcer; history of recurrent ulceration; known hypersensitivity to acemetacin or indomethacin. Patients who have experienced asthma attacks, urticaria or acute rhinitis resulting from treatment with aspirin or non-steroidal anti-inflammatory drugs. Patients with nasal polyps associated with angioneurotic oedema. Safety in children is not established.

Special warnings and special precautions for use: As rare instances of peptic ulceration have been reported administration should be closely supervised in patients with a history of upper gastrointestinal disease. Treatment should be discontinued if peptic ulceration or gastrointestinal bleeding occurs.

Inhibition of platelet aggregation may occur.

Aggravation of psychiatric disorders, epilepsy or parkinsonism may occur.

Signs and symptoms of infection may be masked.

Emflex should be used with caution in patients with reduced renal blood flow where renal perfusion may be maintained by prostaglandins. In patients at particular risk – renal or hepatic dysfunction, congestive heart failure, electrolyte or fluid imbalance, sepsis, concomitant use of nephrotoxic drugs – the dose should be kept as low as possible and renal function should be monitored.

Patients receiving long-term treatment should be periodically screened for renal and hepatic function and blood counts. Borderline elevation of renal and hepatic function test parameters may occur. If this persists or worsens, treatment should be stopped.

Eye changes may occur in chronic rheumatoid disease and patients should receive periodic ophthalmological examinations and therapy discontinued if changes occur.

Hyperkalaemia has been reported with use of indomethacin and this should be considered when administration with potassium sparing diuretics is proposed.

Interactions with other medicaments and other forms of interaction: Emflex is highly protein bound and it may therefore be necessary to modify the dosage of other highly protein bound drugs e.g. anti-coagulants. As there is a possibility of either a pharmacokinetic or pharmacodynamic interaction with aspirin or other salicylates, diflusinal, probenecid, lithium, triamterene, ACE inhibitors, haloperidol and methotrexate, patients receiving such combinations should be carefully monitored and dosages adjusted as necessary. Non-steroidal anti-inflammatory drugs may reduce the anti-hypertensive effects of beta-blockers, although clinical studies showed no propensity for Emflex to antagonise the effects of propranolol. Likewise the reduction of diuretic effects of thiazides and frusemide may occur with non-steroidal anti-inflammatory drugs and this should be borne in mind when treating patients with compromised cardiac function or hypertension.

Pregnancy and lactation: The safety of this product for use in human pregnancy and lactation has not been established. Animal reproduction studies do not provide reassurance regarding the lack of reproductive toxicity/ teratogenicity. Due to maternal toxicity, the studies were conducted at doses below the therapeutic dose or a very low multiple of the therapeutic dose. It should not therefore be used in pregnancy or lactation in women of childbearing age unless they are taking adequate contraceptive precautions.

Effects on ability to drive and use machines: The ability to drive a car or operate machinery may be affected.

Undesirable effects: The following side effects have been either reported with Emflex or could possibly occur as they are common to a number of NSAIDs:
Gastro-intestinal: Gastro-intestinal discomfort/pain, anorexia, nausea, vomiting, indigestion, diarrhoea and constipation, peptic ulceration, gastrointestinal perforation and haemorrhage.

Central nervous system: Symptoms most frequently encountered are headache, dizziness, vertigo and insomnia. Rarely, confusion, depressed mood, irritability.

Hepatic: Occasional elevation of liver function test parameters without overt clinical symptomology. Very rarely, symptoms of cholestasis.

Cardiovascular/renal: Rarely, oedema, chest pain, palpitations, blood urea elevation. NSAIDs have been reported to cause nephrotoxicity in various forms and their use can lead to interstitial nephritis, nephrotic syndrome and renal failure.

Dermatological/hypersensitivity: Pruritus, urticaria, erythema, skin rash, alopecia, angio-neurotic oedema and excessive sweating have been reported.

Haematological: Rarely, thrombocytopenia, leucopenia and reduced haemoglobin levels. Very rarely, reversible agranulocytosis, bone marrow depression.

Ocular/auditory: Infrequently, tinnitus, blurred vision and rarely, eye pain.

Overdose: Symptomatic and supportive therapy is indicated. If ingestion is recent, vomiting should be induced or gastric lavage should be performed. Progress should be followed for several days as gastrointestinal ulceration and haemorrhage have been reported with overdosage of other NSAIDs. Antacids may be helpful.

Pharmacological properties
Pharmacodynamic properties: Acemetacin is a glycolic acid ester of indomethacin and the pharmacological activity resulting from acemetacin administration in man is derived from the presence of both acemetacin and indomethacin. The precise pharmacological mode of action of acemetacin is not known. However, unlike other NSAIDs, acemetacin is only a relatively weak inhibitor of prostaglandin synthetase. Prostaglandins are known to have an antisecretory and cytoprotective effect on the gastric mucosa. Acemetacin shows activity in many of the established in vitro tests of anti-inflammatory activity, including inhibition of the release of a number of mediators of inflammation.

Pharmacokinetic properties: Acemetacin is well absorbed after oral administration. Its major metabolite is indomethacin which, after repeated administration, is present at levels in excess of those of acemetacin. Acemetacin is bound to plasma protein to a slightly lesser extent than indomethacin and has a relatively short plasma elimination half-life. It is eliminated by both hepatic and renal mechanisms. The pharmacokinetics appear to be linear at recommended therapeutic doses, unaffected by moderate renal or hepatic impairment, and unchanged in the elderly.

Preclinical safety data: Emflex Capsules show similar toxicity to other non-steroidal anti-inflammatory drugs.

Pharmaceutical particulars
List of excipients: Lactose, magnesium stearate, silicon dioxide, talc, gelatine, sodium dodecylsulphate, ferric III oxide, ferric oxide hydrate, titanium dioxide.

Incompatibilities: None known.

Shelf life: 5 years.

Special warnings and precautions: Store below 25°C.

Nature and contents of container: White polypropylene bottles with polypropylene screw caps containing 90 capsules. PVC/PVDC foil blister packs in cartons: Four different pack sizes of 90, 30, 10, and 6 capsules

Instructions for use/handling: To be taken with food.

Marketing authorisation number 0493/0141

Date of approval/revision of SPC March 1996.

Legal category POM

FEMSEVEN 50
FEMSEVEN 75
FEMSEVEN 100

Qualitative and quantitative composition FemSeven 50 contains 1.5 mg estradiol hemihydrate delivering 50 micrograms of estradiol in 24 hours. FemSeven 75 contains 2.25 mg estradiol hemihydrate delivering 75 micrograms of estradiol in 24 hours. FemSeven 100 contains 3.0 mg estradiol hemihydrate delivering 100 micrograms of estradiol in 24 hours.

Pharmaceutical form Transdermal patch (patch sizes of 15 cm², 22.5 cm² and 30 cm² active surface area for FemSeven 50, FemSeven 75 and 100 respectively).

Clinical particulars
Therapeutic indications: Hormone replacement therapy for the symptomatic relief of menopausal symptoms including:

- Vasomotor symptoms such as sweating and flushing.
- Other symptoms related to oestrogen deficiency, e.g. urogenital atrophy, urinary urgency, sleeping disorders and mood swings.

Hormone replacement therapy is also indicated for the:

- Prevention of postmenopausal bone loss in women considered at risk of developing fractures. Epidemiological studies have suggested that there are a number of risk factors associated with accelerated postmenopausal bone loss such as early menopause, a family history of osteoporosis, prolonged exposure to corticosteroid therapy, small and thin skeletal frame and excessive cigarette smoking.

Posology and method of administration:
Adults and the elderly: The patch should be applied once each week on a continuous basis, i.e. each patch is replaced with a new one after 7 days.
Therapy normally should be started with FemSeven 50 (delivering 50 micrograms of estradiol in 24 hours). If the prescribed dose does not eliminate the menopausal symptoms the dose should be adjusted by using FemSeven 75 or FemSeven 100 after the first few months. A maximum dose of 100 micrograms estradiol per day should not be exceeded. If there are persistent signs of overdose, such as breast tenderness, the dose should be reduced accordingly. In women with an intact uterus the addition of a progestogen for at least 10 days per cycle is essential.

Consecutive new patches should be applied to different sites. It is recommended that sites are chosen below the waist where little wrinkling of the skin occurs e.g., buttock, hip or abdomen. The patch must not be applied on or near the breasts. The patch should be applied to clean, dry, healthy and intact skin. The patch should be applied to the skin as soon as it is removed from its wrapping. The patch is applied by removing both parts of the protective liner and then holding it in contact with the skin for at least 30 seconds (warmth is essential to ensure maximal adhesive strength). Should part or all of a patch detach prematurely (before 7 days) it should be removed and a new patch applied. (To aid compliance it is recommended the patient then continues to change the patch on their usual day.)

Children: Not indicated.
Contra-indications: FemSeven patches are contra-indicated in:

- Known or suspected pregnancy or lactation.
- History of, known or suspected cancer of the breast.
- Known or suspected oestrogen-dependent neoplasia.
- Undiagnosed abnormal genital bleeding.
- Severe forms of endometriosis.
- Acute or chronic liver disease, severe liver disease or history of liver disease where the liver function tests have failed to return to normal. Rotor syndrome or Dubin-Johnson syndrome.
- Active deep venous thrombosis, thromboembolic disorders, or a history of confirmed venous thromboembolism.
- Severe renal disease.
- Known hypersensitivity to components of this product.

Special warnings and special precautions for use: Prior to commencing oestrogen replacement therapy, it is recommended that the patient should have a complete medical which includes a gynaecological examination and a family history taken. Periodically they should be given a thorough physical and gynaecological examination.

At the present time there is suggestive evidence of an overall change in the relative risk of breast cancer in post-menopausal women receiving hormone replacement therapy. A careful appraisal of the risk/benefit ratio should be undertaken before treating for longer than 5 years. Regular breast examinations should be carried out.

There is no indication from published studies that the risk of myocardial infarction and stroke is increased with oestrogen replacement therapy at the current recommended low dosage in apparently normal women.

Epidemiological studies have suggested that hormone replacement therapy (HRT) is associated with an increased relative risk of developing venous thromboembolism (VTE) i.e. deep vein thrombosis or pulmonary embolism. The studies find a 2-3 fold increase for users compared with non-users which for healthy women amounts to a low risk of one extra case of VTE each year for every 5000 patients taking HRT.

Generally recognised risk factors for VTE include a personal or family history and severe obesity (Body Mass Index > 30 kg/m²). In women with these factors the benefits of treatment with HRT need to be carefully weighed against risks.
If venous thromboembolism develops after initiating therapy the drug should be discontinued.

Patients with a history or a known risk of thromboembolic diseases (e.g. blood coagulation disorders, immobilisation, severe varicose veins, certain malignant diseases, certain cardiac diseases) should not be treated with oestrogens unless the benefit of the treatment outweighs the increased risk for thrombosis.

Similar caution should be exercised in patients with a history of endometriosis.

Close monitoring of patients with epilepsy, diabetes, hypertension, mild to moderate liver or renal disease, benign breast diseases, porphyria, otosclerosis, uterine fibroids and hypophyseal tumours or a significant family history of breast cancer is recommended.

If jaundice, migraine-like headaches, visual disturbances or a significant increase in blood pressure develop after initiating therapy, the medication should be discontinued while the cause is investigated.

The risk of VTE may be temporarily increased with prolonged immobilisation, major trauma or major surgery. In women on HRT, scrupulous attention should be given to prophylactic measures to prevent VTE following surgery. Where prolonged immobilisation is liable to follow elective surgery, particularly abdominal or orthopaedic surgery to the lower limbs, consideration should be given to temporarily stopping HRT 4 weeks earlier, if this is possible.

Hormone replacement therapy for 5 or more years has been shown in epidemiological studies to reduce fracture frequency by up to 50%, however, data showing benefit extending beyond 10 years is limited at present. A careful review of benefit versus risk is necessary in patients treated longer than 5 to 10 years.

The patch is not a contraceptive nor will it restore fertility. If it is administered together with a progestogen to women with an intact uterus of child bearing potential they should be advised to adhere to non-hormonal contraceptive methods. Repeated breakthrough bleeding should be investigated, including an endometrial biopsy.

The use of oestrogens may influence the results of certain endocrine and liver function tests.

Interaction with other medicaments and other forms of interaction: Liver enzyme inducing drugs, e.g. barbiturates, carbamazepine, rifampicin, phenylbutazone, meprobamate, and hydantoins, may impair the activity of oestrogens. Whether this is as relevant with transdermally administered formulations which do not suffer first pass metabolism is unknown.

Pregnancy and lactation: Accidental use during pregnancy or lactation is unlikely to have adverse effects, because only physiological levels of estradiol are achieved with the transdermal patch. There are no reports of risk for embryonic or foetal malformation.

Effects on ability to drive and use of machinery: There is no evidence from the clinical data available on oestrogen therapy to suggest that FemSeven patches should have any effect on a patient's ability to drive or operate machinery.

Undesirable effects: The following side effects have been reported:

Skin: Transient erythema and irritation at the site of application with or without pruritus. This usually disappears 2–3 days after patch removal and is similar to the effect sometimes observed after occlusion of the skin with sticking plasters.

Urogenital tract: Breakthrough bleeding.

Unopposed oestrogen treatment may cause hyperplasia of the endometrium, when given to women with an intact uterus, unless regular therapy with a progestogen takes place.

Endocrine system: Breast tenderness.

Gastro-intestinal tract: Nausea, abdominal cramps, bloating.
Central nervous system: Headache, migraine, dizziness.
Cardiovascular system: Rarely: venous thromboembolic disorders, and increase in blood pressure.

Miscellaneous: Leg cramps (not related to thromboembolic disease and usually transient lasting 3–6 weeks, if symptoms persist the dose of oestrogen should be reduced). Rarely: Oedema and/or weight changes.

Overdose: The mode of administration makes significant overdose unlikely; removal of the patches is all that is required should it occur.

Pharmacological properties
Pharmacodynamic properties: Estradiol, produced by

the female from the menarche through to the menopause predominantly by the ovarian follicle, is the most active oestrogen at receptor level. After the menopause, when the functions of the ovaries cease, only a small amount of estradiol continues to be produced in the body, by the liver and adipose tissue from oestrone.

In many women, the loss of ovarian estradiol leads to vasomotor and thermoregulatory instability (hot flushes), sleep disturbances, as well as increasing atrophy of mucosa and other tissues of the urogenital system. In a large proportion of women, osteoporosis especially of the spinal column develops after the menopause as a result of the oestrogen deficiency. These disorders can be largely avoided by oestrogen substitution.

Administration of exogenous oestrogens to postmenopausal women has been shown to decrease the potentially atherogenic low density lipoproteins (LDLs) and increase the cholesterol scavenging high density lipoproteins (HDLs). This produces an alteration in the HDL to LDL ratio and as seen in observational studies, an improvement of the lipid profile can be a factor contributing to the beneficial effect of oestrogens on the risk of coronary disease in postmenopausal women. This effect on lipids of HRT may vary with the gestagen used. In addition oestrogens have been shown to favourably affect the relative activity of osteoblasts and osteoclasts. This has been demonstrated in epidemiological studies to reduce the amount of bone loss in post-menopausal women. A number of factors are believed to be related to postmenopausal osteoporosis including early menopause, family history of osteoporosis, recent prolonged corticosteroid therapy, excessive cigarette consumption and a small, thin frame.

If a patient is at risk of osteoporosis consideration should be given to oestrogen replacement therapy. Therapy may be commenced at any convenient time, but for maximal effect therapy should be started as soon as possible after the menopause.

Pharmacokinetic properties: FemSeven patches deliver therapeutic estradiol levels within 3 hours of application and maintains these throughout the application interval (7 days). After removal of the patch, estradiol levels return to baseline values within 24 hours.

By transdermal administration, there is no hepatic first-pass effect and the estradiol reaches the bloodstream directly in unchanged form and in physiological amounts. With the use of FemSeven patches the estradiol concentrations are raised to values similar to those of the early to middle follicular phase.

Preclinical safety data: No adverse effects can be predicted from animal toxicology studies other than those documented from human use of estradiol.

Pharmaceutical particulars

List of excipients: Backing layer: Transparent polyethylene terephthalate (PET) foil.
Adhesive matrix: Styrene-isoprene-styrene block copolymer, glycerine esters of completely hydrogenated resins.

Incompatibilities: None known.

Shelf life: 2 years.

Special precautions for storage: Do not store above 30°C.

Nature and contents of the container: The container (primary packaging) consists of a sealed laminated sachet. This comprises layers of food grade paper/polyethylene/aluminium/ethylene copolymer.
Package sizes: Cartons of 4 and 12 patches.

Instructions for use/handling: After removal from the laminated sachet, peel off the two part protective liner. Try to avoid touching the adhesive. Stick the adhesive side down to the upper left or right buttock on a clean and dry area of skin. Hold the applied patch to the skin with the palm of the hand for at least 30 seconds, in order to ensure optimal adhesion to the skin.
Recommended application sites are clean, dry and intact areas of skin on the trunk below the waistline. The patches should not be applied on or near the breasts. After removal the used patch should be folded and disposed of with the normal household solid waste.

Marketing authorisation numbers
FemSeven 50 PL 11648/0021
FemSeven 75 PL 11648/0023
FemSeven 100 PL 11648/0024

Date of approval/revision of SPC October 1998

Legal Category POM

GAMANIL*

Qualitative and quantitative composition Lofepramine hydrochloride 76.10 mg, equivalent to lofepramine 70 mg.

Pharmacetical form Oral tablet.

Clinical particulars

Therapeutic indications: In the treatment of symptoms of depressive illness.

Posology and method of administration:
Route of administration: Oral.
Recommended dosage: The usual dose is 70mg twice daily (140mg) or three times daily (210mg) depending upon patient response.
Children: Not recommended
Elderly: May respond to lower doses in some cases

Contra-indications: Lofepramine should not be used in patients hypersensitive to dibenzazepines, in mania, severe liver impairment and/or severe renal impairment, heart block, cardiac arrythmias, or during the recovery phase following a myocardial infarction.

Special warnings and precautions for use: Lofepramine should be used with caution in patients with cardiovascular disease, impaired liver or renal function, narrow angle glaucoma, symptoms suggestive of prostatic hypertrophy, a history of epilepsy or recent convulsions, hyperthyroidism, blood dyscrasias or porphyria.

Interactions with other medicaments and other forms of interaction: Lofepramine should not be administered with or within 2 weeks of cessation of therapy with monoamine oxidase inhibitors. It should be introduced cautiously using a low initial dose. Lofepramine should not be given with sympathomimetic agents, central nervous depressants including alcohol or thyroid hormone therapy since its effects may be potentiated. Lofepramine may decrease the antihypertensive effects of adrenergic neurone-blocking drugs; it is therefore advisable to review this form of antihypertensive therapy during treatment. Anaesthetics given during tricyclic antidepressant therapy may increase the risk of arrhythmias and hypotension. If surgery is necessary, the anaesthetist should be informed that a patient is being so treated. Barbiturates may increase the rate of metabolism.

Pregnancy and lactation: The safety of lofepramine for use during pregnancy has not been established and there is evidence of harmful effects in pregnancy in animals when high doses are given. Lofepramine has been shown to be excreted in breast milk. The administration of lofepramine in pregnancy and during breast feeding therefore is not advised unless there are compelling medical reasons.

Effects on ability to drive and use machines: As with other antidepressants, ability to drive a car and operate machinery may be affected. Therefore caution should be exercised initially until the individual reaction to treatment is known.

Undesirable effects: The following side effects have been reported with lofepramine:
Cardiovascular: hypotension, tachycardia
CNS & Neuromuscular: dizziness, drowsiness, agitation, confusion, headache, malaise, paraesthesia and rarely hypomania and convulsions.
Anticholinergic: dryness of mouth, constipation, disturbances of accommodation, urinary hesitancy, urinary retention, sweating and tremor.
Allergic: skin rash, allergic skin reactions, "photosensitivity reactions".
Gastrointestinal: nausea, vomiting.
Endocrine: rarely, inappropriate secretion of antidiuretic hormone, interference with sexual function.
Haematological/biochemical: rarely, bone marrow depression including isolated reports of: agranulocytosis, eosinophilia, granulocytopenia, leucopenia, pancytopenia, thrombocytopenia.

Increases in liver enzymes, sometimes progressing to clinical hepatitis and jaundice, have been reported in some patients, usually occurring within the first 3 months of starting therapy.

The following adverse effects have been encountered in patients under treatment with tricyclic antidepressants and should therefore be considered as theoretical hazards of lofepramine even in the absence of substantiation: psychotic manifestations, including mania and paranoid delusions may be exacerbated during treatment with tricyclic antidepressants; withdrawal symptoms may occur on abrupt cessation of therapy and include insomnia, irritability and excessive perspiration; adverse effects such as withdrawal symptoms, respiratory depression and agitation have been reported in neonates whose mothers have taken tricylic antidepressants during the last trimester of pregnancy.

Overdose: The treatment of overdosage is symptomatic and supportive. It should include immediate gastric lavage and routine close monitoring of cardiac function. reports of overdosage with 0.7-6.72g have shown no serious sequelae directly attributable to lofepramine.

Pharmacological properties

Pharmacodynamic properties: Lofepramine is a tricyclic antidepressant. It exerts its therapeutic effect by blocking the uptake of noradrenaline by the nerve cell thus increasing the amine in the synaptic cleft and hence the effect on the receptors. There is evidence to suggest that serotonin may also be involved. Other pharmacological effects are due to anti-cholinergic activity, but less sedation is observed than with other tricyclics.

Pharmacokinetic properties: Lofepramine is a tertiary amine, similar in structure to imipramine but with improved lipophilicity and lower base strength. It is readily absorbed when given orally. From the plasma it is distributed throughout the body notably to the brain, lungs, liver and kidney. It is metabolised in the liver by cleavage of the p-chlorophenacyl group from the lofepramine molecule leaving desmethylimipramine (DMI).

The latter is pharmacologically active. The p-chlorobenzoyl portion is mainly metabolised to p-chlorobenzoic acid which is then conjugated with glycine. The conjugate is excreted mostly in the urine. DMI has been found excreted in the faeces. In a study of protein binding capability it has been found that lofepramine is up to 99% protein bound.

Preclinical safety data: N/A

List of excipients: Lactose, Corn starch, L(+) ascorbic acid, Talcum, Glycerol, Glycerol monostearate, Ethylene dinitriletetra acetic acid disodium salt (dihydrate) [titriplex III], Dimethicone, Silicone dioxide, Hydroxypropyl methyl cellulose, Coating, 1,2-Propanediol, Hydroxypropyl methyl cellulose, Ponceau 4R aluminium lake E124, Talc, Titanium dioxide, Indigotine lake E132.

Incompatabiilities: None.

Shelf life: 3 years.

Special precautions for storage: Protect from light and moisture.

Nature and contents of container: 1. PVDC/Al foil blister calendar packs containing 56 tablets
2. Polypropylene containers containing 250 tablets.
3. Amber glass bottles containing 56 tablets.

Instruction for use/handling: None.

Marketing Authorisation Number 0493/0060

Date of approval/revision of SPC December 1998

Legal Category POM

GASTROMIRO*

Qualitative and quantitative composition Active component Iopamidol (INN) 612.4 mg per ml (61.24% w/v).

Pharmaceutical form Gastromiro is an aqueous solution for oral or rectal administration (enema)

Clinical particulars

Therapeutic indications: All forms of radiological investigations of gastrointestinal tract, in particular:

Paediatric radiology of the gastro-intestinal tract (GIT) where there is the possibility of:

spill into the respiratory tract, for example in:
swallowing disorders
oesophageal obstruction with a foreign body, atresia or stricture
tracheo-oesophageal fistula.

- spill into the mediastinum, pleura, peritoneum or retroperitoneal tissues, for example due to perforation of the GIT.
- Inspissation of fluid, for example in:

Meconium ileus equivalent.
Intussusception.
Colonic obstruction.
Hirschsprung's disease.

Adult radiology of the gastro-intestinal tract, such as:

- Suspected upper gastro-intestinal perforation for example in:

Oesophagogastrectomy, endoscopy, partial gastrectomy, pneumonectomy, ingestion of foreign body, duodenal ulceration, small bowel resection, Whipples procedure and blunt abdominal trauma.

- Computer Tomography (CT) of the abdominal and pelvic regions, for example:

Suspicion of expanding lesions of pancreas, liver and gall bladder.

Space occupying metastatic lesions originating from prostate or recto-sigmoidal region in post-surgical staging of cancer.

Posology and method of administration:
Adults:
Radiology of gastro-intestinal tract:
Oral: 40-100 ml undiluted
Rectal: 200 ml of a 50% dilution, up to 1000 ml of a 2% dilution
Computer tomography:
Oral: Abdominal CT: 100 ml of a 17% dilution, up to 600 ml of a 3% dilution.
Rectal–Pelvic CT: 500-700 ml of a 3% dilution

Infants and children:
Radiology of gastro-intestinal tract:
Oral: 10-100 ml undiluted or, for use in infants 20-200 ml of up to a 50% dilution to provide isotonic contrast medium
Rectal: 200 ml of 50-60% dilution

Elderly: Dosage as for adults.
Dilution of Gastromiro should be carried out using sterile water. Any unused solution should be discarded after 6 hours.

Contra-indications: Proven or suspected hypersensitivity to iodine containing preparations of this type. It must not be used for parenteral administration.

Special warnings and precautions for use: Disturbances in water or electrolyte balance must first be corrected. This product is formulated for gastro-intestinal use only and should not be used parenterally.

Care should also be exercised in patients with severe functional impairment of the liver, kidney or myocardium, severe systemic disease and in myelomatosis. In such patients adequate hydration should be maintained and parameters of hepatic and renal function, especially urinary output should be monitored after the procedure.

Patients with hepato-renal insufficiency should not be examined unless benefits clearly outweigh risks and re-examination should be delayed for 5-7 days.

In patients with a history of adverse reactions during similar investigations additional caution should be exercised and the procedure should only be carried out if benefits clearly outweigh any risks.

X-ray examination of women should be conducted as far as possible during the pre-ovulation phase of the menstrual cycle. This product may interfere with tests of thyroid function.

Interactions with other medicaments and other forms of interaction: None known.

Pregnancy and lactation: The safety of iopamidol during pregnancy and lactation has not been demonstrated clinically. Due, however, to the extremely low absorption of iopamidol from the gastro-intestinal tract it is unlikely that a foetus could be exposed to significant levels. In animal experiments iopamidol is neither teratogenic nor foetotoxic. Similarly, during lactation breast fed infants are unlikely to be exposed to significant levels of iopamidol. However, the product should not be used during pregnancy or when breast feeding unless considered essential.

Effects on ability to drive and use machines: None known.

Undesirable effects: Systemic effects are rare since Gastromiro is only poorly absorbed from the alimentary tract. Owing to slight hypertonicity Gastromiro may occasionally cause diarrhoea in infants and children.

Overdose: The contrast agent is not absorbed from the gastrointestinal tract, therefore any systemic accumulation of the contrast medium following overdosage will not occur. Any treatment should be symptomatic.

Pharmacological properties

Pharmacodynamic properties: Iopamidol is a contrast medium belonging to the new generation of non-ionic compounds whose solubility is due to the presence of hydrophilic substituents in the molecule. This results in a solution of low osmolality when compared with ionic media.

Iopamidol has been shown to be effective as an X-ray contrast medium in neuroradiology, angiography, venography, arthrography, urography, cerebral angiography, and left ventriculography, coronary arteriography, and investigations of the gastrointestinal tract. Its toxicity, particularly cardiac and CNS toxicity, is less than that of ionic contrast media.

Pharmacokinetic properties: Serum iopamidol concentration curves conform to an open two compartment pharmacokinetic model with first order elimination. Iopamidol is very poorly absorbed (about 1-2%) after oral or rectal administration.

Distribution volume is equivalent to extracellular fluid.

Following parenteral administration elimination is almost completely through the kidneys. Less than 1% of the administered dose has been recovered in the faeces up to seventy two hours after dosing. Renal elimination is rapid and up to half the administered dose may be recovered in the urine within the first two hours of dosing.

There is no evidence of biotransformation.
Serum protein binding is negligible.

Preclinical safety data: In animals, Gastromiro was well tolerated after repeated oral administration. After 4 weeks adminstration of Gastromiro equivalent to 9 gl/kg day, i.e. about 20 times higher than the recommended clinical dose, no severe symptoms of sub-acute intoxication were observed in rats. Following intraperitoneal injection of Gastromiro in rats, iopamidol was rapidly cleared and almost totally eliminated by the renal route within the first 24 hours.

The intraperitoneal acute toxicity was relatively low. Necroscopic examination revealed no irritant effects on the peritoneal membrane. Gastromiro also showed good local tolerability after both local intratracheal installation and systemic administration. It therefore offers a good margin of safety for examination in which there is the risk of an accidental inspiration of the diagnostic medium.

Pharmaceutical particulars

List of Excipients Quantity per ml:
Orange flavour 2.2 mg
Sodium cyclamate 1.5 mg
Red Curaçao flavour 1.1 mg
Disodium edetate dihydrate 0.3 mg
Sodium saccharinate 0.176 mg
Citric acid monohydrate 0.055 mg
Water for injections

Incompatibilities: No incompatibility studies have been performed: other drugs should not be mixed with Gastromiro.

Shelf life: Three years.

Special warnings and precautions: Protect from light.

Nature and contents of container: The containers are amber glass bottles (Type III) with aluminium screw caps, guarantee seals, and elastomer inserts.
Boxes of 1 bottle 20 ml
Boxes of 1 bottle 50 ml
Boxes of 1 bottle 100 ml

Instructions for use / handling: Gastromiro is formulated for gastro-intestinal use only and should not be administered parenterally.

The dosage of Gastromiro should be adjusted according to age, total weight, the segment of the digestive tract to be examined and the X-ray procedure.

The bottle once opened has to be used immediately. Solutions not used in one examination session must be discarded.

Gastromiro formulation is a colourless to pale yellow solution containing undissolved solids. Discard in case of discolouration.

Marketing authorisation number 0493/01139

Date of approval/revision of SPC 9 January 1996.

Legal category POM

IOMERON

Qualitative and quantitative composition
Iomeron 150 contains 30.62% w/v iomeprol equivalent to 15% iodine or 150 mg iodine/ml.
Iomeron 200 contains 40.82% w/v iomeprol equivalent to 20% iodine or 200 mg iodine/ml.
Iomeron 250 contains 51.03% w/v iomeprol equivalent to 25% iodine or 250 mg iodine/ml.
Iomeron 300 contains 61.24% w/v iomeprol equivalent to 30% iodine or 300 mg iodine/ml.
Iomeron 350 contains 71.44% w/v iomeprol equivalent to 35% iodine or 350 mg iodine/ml.
Iomeron 400 contains 81.65% w/v iomeprol equivalent to 40% iodine or 400 mg iodine/ml.

Pharmaceutical form Solution for parenteral administration.

Clinical particulars
Therapeutic indications: X-ray contrast medium. For indications see table overleaf.

Posology and method of administration:
† repeat as necessary
‡ according to body size and age
Peripheral arteriography: adults 10–90 ml†; children ‡
Venography: adults 10–100 ml†, max 250 ml
– 10–50 ml upper extremity
– 50–100 ml lower extremity
Aortography: adults 50–80 ml; children ‡
Angiocardiography and left ventriculography: adults 30–80 ml max 250 ml; children ‡
Cerebral arteriography: adults 5–12 ml†; children 3–7 ml or ‡
Coronary arteriography: adults 4-10 ml per artery†
Visceral arteriography: adults 5–50 ml† or according to type of examination; max 250 ml; children ‡
Digital subtraction angiography:
Intra arterial:
cerebral: adults 6–10 ml per artery†
visceral: adults 2–20 ml per artery†
aorta 25–50 ml†
both 250 ml max
peripheral: adults 5–10 ml per artery†, max 250 ml
Intravenous: adults 30–60 ml†, max 250 ml
Computed tomography:
brain: adults 50–150 ml; children‡
body: adults 40–150 ml, max 250 ml; children‡
Urography:
Infusion: adults 250 ml
Intravenous: adults 50–150 ml
neonates 3–4.8 ml/kg
babies 2.5–4 ml/kg
children 1–2.5 ml/kg or †
Arthrography: adults 1–10 ml
ERCP: adults 12–30 ml
Dacryocystography: adults 3–8 ml
Sialography: adults 1–3 ml
Fistulography: adults 1–50 ml
Galactography: adults 0.2–1.5 ml
Hysterosalpingography: adults 8–20 ml
Cavernosography: adults 40–250 ml
In elderly patients the lowest effective dose should be used.

Contra-indications: Proven or suspected hypersensitivity to iodine containing preparations of this type.

Special warnings and precautions for use: A positive history of allergy, asthma or untoward reaction during previous similar investigations indicates a need for extra caution since, as with other contrast media, this product may provoke anaphylaxis or other manifestations of allergy with nausea, vomiting, dyspnoea, erythema, urticaria and hypotension. The benefits should clearly outweigh the risks in such patients and appropriate resuscitative measures should be immediately available. The primary treatments are as follows:

Effect	*Major Symptoms*	*Primary Treatment*
Vasomotor effect	warmth	reassurance
	nausea/ vomiting	
Cutaneous	scattered hives	H_1-antihistamines
	severe urticaria	H_2-antihistamines
Bronchospastic	wheezing	oxygen
		β_2 agonist inhalers
Anaphylactoid reaction	angioedema	oxygen
	urticaria	iv fluids
	bronchospasm	adrenergics
	hypotension	(iv epinephrine)
		β_2 agonist inhalers
		antihistamines (H_1 and H_2 antagonist)
		corticosteroids
Hypotensive vagal reaction	hypotension	iv fluids
	bradycardia	iv atropine

From Bush WH The Contrast Media Manual
Katzburg RW Ed. Williams and Wilkins
Baltimore 1992 Chapter 2 p23

Any severe disorders of water and electrolyte balance must be corrected prior to administration. Adequate hydration must be ensured particularly in patients with multiple myeloma, diabetes mellitus, polyuria, oliguria and hyperuricaemia; also in babies, small children and the elderly. Rehydration prior to use of iomeprol is recommended in patients with sickle cell disease.

Care should be taken in severe cardiac disease particularly heart failure and coronary artery disease. Reactions may include pulmonary oedema, haemodynamic changes, ischaemic ECG changes and arrhythmias.

In severe, chronic hypertension the risk of renal damage following administration of a contrast medium is increased. In these cases the risks associated with the catheterization procedure are increased. Care should be taken in renal impairment and diabetes. In these patients it is important to maintain hydration in order to minimise deterioration in renal function.

A combination of severe hepatic and renal impairment delays excretion of the contrast medium therefore such patients should not be examined unless absolutely necessary.

The product should be used with caution in patients with hyperthyroidism or goitre. Use may interfere with thyroid function tests.

Particular care is needed in patients with acute cerebral infarction, acute intracranial haemorrhage and any conditions involving damage to the blood brain barrier, brain oedema or acute demyelination. Convulsive seizures are more likely in patients with intracranial tumours or metastases or with a history of epilepsy.

Neurological symptoms related to cerebrovascular diseases, intracranial tumours/metastases or degenerative or inflammatory pathologies may be exacerbated.

There is an increased risk of transient neurological complications in patients with symptomatic cerebrovascular disease eg stroke, transient ischaemic attacks. Cerebral ischaemic phenomena may be caused by intravascular injection.

In acute and chronic alcoholism the increase in

Iomeron: Indications for use

Indication	*Iomeron* 150	200	250	300	350	400
peripheral arteriography				✓	✓	✓
venography			✓	✓	✓	
aortography					✓	✓
angiocardiography and left ventriculography				✓	✓	✓
cerebral arteriography			✓	✓		
coronary arteriography					✓	✓
visceral arteriography				✓	✓	✓
digital subtraction angiography						
Intra-arterial						
cerebral	✓	✓				
visceral	✓	✓	✓	✓		
peripheral	✓	✓	✓	✓		
Intravenous			✓	✓	✓	✓
computed tomography enhancement						
brain	✓	✓	✓	✓	✓	
body	✓	✓	✓	✓	✓	✓
urography						
infusion	✓					
intravenous			✓	✓	✓	✓
ERCP (endoscopic retrograde cholangiopancreatography)				✓		
arthrography		✓		✓	✓	
dacryocystography				✓	✓	✓
sialography				✓	✓	✓
fistulography				✓	✓	✓
galactography				✓	✓	✓
hysterosalpingography		✓				
cavernosography	✓	✓	✓			

	Iomeron 150	*Iomeron 200*	*Iomeron 250*	*Iomeron 300*	*Iomeron 350*	*Iomeron 400*
50 ml			✓	✓	✓	✓
75 ml		✓		✓	✓	✓
100 ml	✓			✓	✓	✓
150 ml			✓			
200 ml				✓	✓	✓
250 ml						✓

blood brain barrier permeability facilitates the passage of the contrast medium into cerebral tissue possibly leading to CNS disorders. There is a possibility of a reduced seizure threshold in alcoholics. In patients with a drug addiction there is also the possibility of a reduced seizure threshold.

Patients with phaeochromocytoma may develop severe, occasionally uncontrollable hypertensive crises during intravascular administration. Premedication with an alpha blocker is recommended in these patients. Pronounced excitement, anxiety and pain can cause side effects or intensify reaction to the contrast medium. A sedative may be given.

Since, on rare occasions, delayed reactions can occur, driving or operating machinery is not advisable for the first 24 hours after the procedure. Anticonvulsant therapy should not be discontinued. A normal diet should be maintained until the patient refrains from eating 2 hours before the procedure.

Non ionic contrast media have less anticoagulant activity in vitro than ionic media. Meticulous attention should therefore be paid to angiographic technique. Non ionic media should not be allowed to remain in contact with blood in a syringe, and intravascular catheters should be flushed frequently to minimise the risk of clotting which, rarely, has led to serious thromboembolic complications.

The presence of renal damage in diabetic patients is one of the factors predisposing to renal impairment following contrast media administration. This may precipitate lactic acidosis in patients who are taking metformin. As a precaution, metformin should be stopped 48 hours prior to examination and reinstated only after control of renal function has been regained.

Intravascular administration should be performed if possible with the patient lying down. The patient should be kept in this position and closely observed for at least 30 minutes after the procedure since the majority of severe incidents occur within this time.

Children: Infants up to 1 year, especially the newborn, are particularly susceptible to electrolyte imbalance and haemodynamic alterations. Care should be taken regarding the dosage used.

Elderly: There is special risk of reactions involving the circulatory system such that myocardial ischaemia, major arrhythmias and extrasystoles are more likely to occur. A combination of neurological disturbances and vascular pathologies present a serious complication. The probability of acute renal insufficiencies is higher in these people.

Interaction with other medicaments and other forms of interaction: Use of the product may interfere with tests for thyroid function. Vasopressor agents should not be administered prior to iomeprol.

Pregnancy and lactation: Animal studies have not indicated any harmful effects with respect to the course of pregnancy or on the health of the unborn or neonate. The safety of iomeprol in human pregnancy however has not been established. Therefore avoid in pregnancy unless there is no safer alternative.

No human data exist concerning the excretion of iomeprol in breast milk. Animal studies have demonstrated that the excretion of iomeprol in breast milk is similar to that of other contrast agents and that these compounds are only minimally absorbed by the gastrointestinal tract of the young. Adverse effects on the nursing infant are therefore unlikely to occur.

Effects on ability to drive and use machines: Driving or operating machinery is not advisable for the first 24 hours following the procedure in case of delayed reaction.

Undesirable effects: Common reactions are pain at the site of injection, sensations of heat and a disturbance of the taste sensation.

The product may occasionally provoke the following mild to moderate effects: generalised transient pain sensation, chills, fever, asthenia, dizziness, fainting, nausea, vomiting, sweating, pallor, dyspnoea, moderate hypotension, generalised and localised flushing, widespread erythema, oedema, agitation, headache, laryngeal oedema and nasal congestion, rashes accompanied by itching. Symptoms related to CNS disturbances are usually mild and short lived.

More severe effects involve the cardiovascular system. These are peripheral vasodilation with pronounced hypotension, hypertension, tachycardia or bradycardia, cyanosis, dyspnoea and circulatory collapse. More severe neurological effects can occur but only as a result of pre-existing pathologies.

A transient renal failure may arise, particularly in patients with a pre existing impairment of renal function. Haemorrhage and oedema may arise at the site of injection.

Overdose: The effects of overdose on the pulmonary and cardiovascular systems may become life-threatening. Treatment consists of support of the vital functions and prompt use of symptomatic therapy. Iomeprol does not bind to plasma or serum proteins and is therefore dialyzable.

Pharmacological properties

Pharmacodynamic properties: Iomeprol is a low osmolality, non-ionic organic molecule with radio-opacity conferred by an iodine content of 49% of the molecular weight. It is formulated for use as an intravascular/intracavitary contrast medium in concentrations of up to 400 mg iodine per ml. Even at this concentration the low viscosity allows delivery of high doses through thin catheters.

Pharmacokinetic properties: The pharmacokinetics of intravascularly administered iomeprol are similar to those of other iodinated contrast media and conform to a two-compartment model with a rapid distribution and a slower elimination phase. In healthy subjects, the mean distribution and elimination half-lives of iomeprol were 0.37 hours and 1.83 hours respectively.

Distribution volume is similar to that of extra cellular fluid. There is no significant serum protein binding and iomeprol is not metabolized.

Elimination is almost exclusively through the kidneys (90% of the dose recovered in the urine within 96 hours of its administration) and is rapid (50% of an intravascularly administered dose within 2 hours).

Preclinical safety data: There are no preclinical data of relevance which are additional to those included in other sections of the SPC.

Pharmaceutical particulars

List of excipients: trometamol, hydrochloric acid, water for injections

Incompatibilities: No other drug should be mixed with the contrast medium.

Shelf life: Five years. Solutions not used in one examination session must be discarded.

Special precautions for storage: Store below 30°C. Protect from light.

Nature and contents of container: Colourless Type 1 glass bottles with rubber/aluminium cap (see table above).

Instructions for use/handling: Not relevant.

Marketing authorisation number 11648/0005-0010

Date of approval/revision of SPC December 1998

Legal category POM

MULTIBIONTA* INFUSION

Presentation A 10 ml ampoule of an aqueous solution containing:

Active ingredients:

Vitamin A as palmitate PhEur	10,000 iu
Thiamine hydrochloride PhEur	50 mg
Riboflavin sodium phosphate BP	10 mg
Nicotinamide BP	100 mg
Pantothenol INN	25 mg
Pyridoxine hydrochloride PhEur	15 mg
Vitamin C	500 mg
Alpha tocopheryl acetate PhEur	5 mg

Inactive ingredients: Polysorbate 80, propylene glycol, glycerol 85%, benzyl alcohol, DL-α-tocopherol, trometamol.

Uses Intravenous infusions of vitamins should only be considered when oral intake is impossible or inadequate.

Infants: Multibionta for infusion is indicated as part of a total parenteral feeding regimen in young children in the following conditions.

1. Protracted diarrhoea unresponsive to dietary treatment.
2. Renal failure.

In older children and adults:

1. Obstructing lesions of the gastro-intestinal tract.
2. Massive bowel resection.
3. Extensive burns.
4. Major trauma and severe infections.
5. Acute states of inflammatory bowel disease.
6. Severe uncontrolled malabsorptive states with undernutrition.
7. Disorders of swallowing as might occur in poliomyelitis, tetanus or following severe trauma.
8. Prolonged coma.

Dosage and administration The exact requirements of intravenously administered vitamins (particularly in sick infants) are not known. For adults 10 ml of Multibionta in an average daily dose should be added to a full infusion bottle containing not less than 250 ml of the infusion. For small children 2 ml per litre of the infusion fluid is adequate; alternatively the dose can be calculated as 0.15 ml/kilogram/24 hours. However, if preferred, the adult dose may be used with complete safety.

There is no preparation which contains all the essential vitamins in recommended amounts. It is, therefore, suggested that the following are given during prolonged intravenous nutrition in the dosage indicated.

Folic acid	0.1–0.5 mg/day
Vitamin B_{12}	100 micrograms/month
Vitamin D	300 Units/day (administered IM as calciferol. 1 ml contains 300,000 Units)
Vitamin K	3 mg twice weekly
Choline chloride	500 mg/day (normally present in adequate amounts as cholinephosphatides in fat emulsions)

Their compatibility with the carrier intravenous infusion should always be checked with the pharmacy before addition.

Additional information: The miscibility of 10 ml of Multibionta has been tested and it was found to be compatible with amino-acid solutions, carbohydrate solutions such as glucose at various concentrations, and fat solutions.

Although Multibionta is compatible with many infusion fluids, it is best introduced into separate normal saline or dextrose-saline mixtures.

Contra-indications, warnings, etc Rarely, intravenous thiamine may act as an allergen.

Multibionta must not be used in neonates, especially in immature preterm babies, because of the benzyl alcohol content.

Multibionta should only be given in pregnancy if there are compelling reasons because of the possible embryotoxic effect of propylene glycol.

In order to minimise possible loss of active substance in a mixture (masked incompatibility), it is recommended that solutions to which Multibionta is added should not be kept for longer than six hours. Amino-acid solutions or dextran solutions containing Multibionta should not be kept longer than one hour.

A mixture should be discarded if visible turbidity or crystallisation appear in the infusion solution.

Especial care should be taken to avoid exposure of a plastic bag or giving set containing Multibionta to direct sunlight.

Pharmaceutical precautions Should be stored at a temperature not exceeding 8°C.

Legal category POM.

Package quantities 10 ml ampoules in packs of 3.

Further information Nil.

Product licence number 0493/0076.

NIOPAM

Qualitative and quantitative composition
Niopam 150 contains 30.62% w/v iopamidol equivalent to 150 mg iodine/ml
Niopam 200 contains 40.8% w/v iopamidol equivalent to 200 mg iodine/ml
Niopam 300 contains 61.2% w/v iopamidol equivalent to 300 mg iodine/ml
Niopam 340 contains 69.4% w/v iopamidol equivalent to 340 mg iodine/ml
Niopam 370 contains 75.5% w/v iopamidol equivalent to 370 mg iodine/ml

Pharmaceutical form Solution for injection.

Clinical particulars
Therapeutic indications: X-ray contrast medium for use in lumbar and thoraco-cervical myelography, cerebral angiography, peripheral arteriography and venography, angiocardiography, digital subtraction angiography, left ventriculography and coronary arteriography, aortography, selective visceral angiography, computer tomography enhancement, urography, arthrography in accordance with the table:

Posology and method of administration
Method of administration: In accordance with the table:

Intra-arterial
Intravenous
Intraventricular
Intra-articular

Contra-indications: Use in patients with proven or suspected hypersensitivity to iodine containing preparations of this type.

Special warnings and special precautions for use: A positive history of allergy, asthma or untoward reaction during previous similar investigations indicates a need for extra caution; the benefit should clearly outweigh the risk in such patients. Appropriate resuscitative measures should be immediately available.

Care should be exercised in carrying out radiographic procedures with contrast media in patients with severe functional impairment of the liver or myocardium, severe systemic disease and in myelomatosis. In the latter condition patients should not be exposed to dehydration; similarly abnormalities of fluid or electrolyte balance should be corrected prior to use.

Care should also be exercised in patients with moderate to severe impairment of renal function (as reflected by a raised blood urea) or in diabetes. Substantial deterioration in renal function is minimised if the patient is well hydrated. Renal function parameters should be monitored after the procedure in these patients.

Patients with severe hepato-renal insufficiency should not be examined unless absolutely indicated. Re-examination should be delayed for 5-7 days.

Special care should be exercised when this product

NIOPAM – Recommended Dosage Schedule

Procedure	*Niopam product and dosage*		
Lumbar Myelography	Niopam 200 Niopam 300	Adults	10–15 ml 5–10 ml
Thoraco-Cervical Myelography	Niopam 200 Niopam 300	Adults	5–15 ml 5–10 ml
Cerebral Angiography	Niopam 300	Adults Children	5–10 ml † 5–7 ml ‡
Peripheral Arteriography	Niopam 300 Niopam 340 Niopam 370	Adults Children	20–50 ml † ‡
Venography	Niopam 300	Adults Children	20–50 ml ‡
Angiocardiography & Left Ventriculography	Niopam 340 Niopam 370	Adults Children	30–80 ml ‡
Coronary Arteriography	Niopam 340 Niopam 370	Adults	4–8 ml per artery †
Aortography-retrograde	Niopam 340 Niopam 370	Adults	30–80 ml
Selective Renal Arteriography	Niopam 340 Niopam 370	Adults Children	5–10 ml ‡
Selective Visceral Angiography: Hepatic Coeliac Superior Mesenteric Inferior Mesenteric	Niopam 340	Adults	30–70 ml 40–70 ml 25–70 ml 5–30 ml
Hepatic Coeliac Superior Mesenteric and inferior Mesenteric	Niopam 370	Adults	30–70 ml 40–70 ml 5–30 ml
		Children	‡
Digital Subtraction Angiography Intra-arterial injection	Niopam 150	Adults Children	1–40 ml 0.5–0.75 ml/kg
Intra-venous injection	Niopam 340 Niopam 370	Adults Children	30–50 ml 0.5–0.75 ml/kg ‡
Left ventriculography	Niopam 340 Niopam 370	Adults	25 ml
	Niopam 150	Children	1.0–1.5 ml/kg
and selective coronary arteriography by intra-arterial DSA	Niopam 340 Niopam 370	Adults	2–5 ml
Computer Tomography Enhancement	Niopam 200 Niopam 300 Niopam 340	Adults	Brain Scanning 50–100 ml Whole Body Scanning 40–100 ml
Intravenous Urography	Niopam 300 Niopam 340 Niopam 370	Adults	40–80 ml In severe renal failure the usual high dose methods should be employed (up to 1.5 ml/kg)
		Children	1–2.5 ml/kg or ‡
Arthrography	Niopam 300 Niopam 340	Adults	1–10 ml According to joint being examined

† Repeat as necessary
‡ According to body size and age.
Elderly: dosage as for adults.

is injected into the right heart or pulmonary artery in patients with pulmonary hypertension. Right heart angiography should be carried out only when absolutely indicated.

In patients who are known epileptics or have a history of epilepsy, anticonvulsant therapy should be maintained before and following myelographic procedures. In some instances, anticonvulsant therapy may be increased for 48 hours before the examination.

Non-ionic contrast media have less anti-coagulant activity in-vitro than ionic media. Meticulous attention should therefore be paid to angiographic technique. Non-ionic media should not be allowed to remain in contact with blood in the syringe and intravascular catheters should be flushed frequently, to minimise the risk of clotting, which rarely has led to serious thromboembolic complications after procedures.

Niopam should be used with caution in patients with hyperthyroidism. It is possible that hyperthyroidism may recur in patients previously treated for Graves' disease.

The presence of renal damage in diabetic patients is one of the factors predisposing to renal impairment following contrast media administration. This may precipitate lactic acidosis in patients who are taking metformin. As a precaution, metformin should be stopped 48 hours prior to the examination and reinstated only after the control of renal function has been regained.

Interactions with other medicaments and other forms of interaction: Use of the product may interfere with tests for thyroid function.

Pregnancy and lactation: X-ray examination of women should if possible be conducted during the pre-ovulation phase of the menstrual cycle and should be avoided during pregnancy; also, since it has not been demonstrated that Niopam is safe for use in pregnant women, it should be administered only if the procedure is considered essential by the physician.

Effects on ability to drive and use machines: Not applicable.

Undesirable effects: As with all other contrast media this product may provoke anaphylaxis or other manifestations of allergy; e.g. nausea, vomiting, dyspnoea, erythema, urticaria and hypotension. Other frequently occurring effects are normally mild and include headache, nausea, vomiting, heat sensation, dyspnoea and hypotension. Skin rashes may occur in some patients.

During intracardiac and/or coronary arteriography, ventricular arrhythmias may infrequently occur.

Following use in myelography, water soluble non-ionic contrast media have been reported to cause neurological side effects. These include rare cases of seizures, transient confusion or transient motor or sensory dysfunction. Meningism and meningitis have also been reported. The possibilityof an infective meningitis should be considered. Headaches, dizziness, nausea and vomiting may occasionally occur.

Overdose: Not known

Pharmacological properties

Pharmacodynamic properties: Iopamidol is contrast medium belonging to the new generation of non-ionic compounds whose solubility is due to the presence of hydrophilic substitutes in the molecule. This results in a solution of low osmolality when compared with ionic media.

Iopamidol has been shown to be effective as an X-ray contrast medium in neuroradiology, angiography, venography, arthrography, urography, cerebral angiography and left ventriculography and coronary arteriography. Its toxicity, particularly cardiac and CNS toxicity, are less than those of ionic contrast media.

Pharmacokinetic properties: The pharmacokinetics of iopamidol conform to an open two compartment pharmacokinetic model with first order elimination.

Distribution volume is equivalent to extracellular fluid.

Elimination is almost completely through the kidneys. Less that 1% of the administered dose has been recovered in the faeces up to 72 hours after dosing. Elimination is rapid; up to half the administered dose may be recovered in the urine in the first two hours of dosing.

There is no evidence of biotransformation.

Serum protein binding is negligible.

Preclinical safety data: No adverse effects can be predicted from animal toxicology studies other than those documented from human use of iopamidol.

Pharmaceutical particulars

List of excipients: The other constituents are trometamol, hydrochloric acid and edetate calcium disodium.

Incompatibilities: No other drug should be mixed with the contrast medium.

Shelf life: 5 years.

Special precautions for storage: Protect from light.

Nature and contents of container: 10, 20 ml clear, colourless (type 1 EP) glass ampoules.
30 ml clear, colourless (type 1 EP) glass vials with rubber closures and aluminium caps. 50, 70, 100, 200 and 250 ml clear, colourless (type 1 EP) glass bottles with rubber closures and aluminium caps.

Instructions for use/handling: Discard if the solution is not clear of particulate matter.

Marketing authorisation number
Niopam 150 PL 0493/0119
Niopam 200 PL 0493/0065
Niopam 300 PL 0493/0066
Niopam 340 PL 0493/0131
Niopam 370 PL 0493/0067

Date of approval/revision of SPC August 1998

Legal category POM

NUTRIZYM* GR

Presentation Hard gelatin capsules with opaque olive green cap and orange body each containing Pancreatin BP 300 mg with not less than the following activities:

Lipase 10,000 BP-U
Protease 650 BP-U
Amylase 10,000 BP-U

Uses Fibrocystic disease of the pancreas, chronic pancreatitis, steatorrhoea and other pancreatic deficiency states.

Dosage and administration

Adults: 1–2 capsules with meals. In severe cases dosage may be increased.

Children: 1–2 capsules to be taken with meals and further capsules may be taken according to the degree of exocrine sufficiency.

Colonic damage has been reported in patients with cystic fibrosis taking in excess of 10,000 units of lipase/kg/day. The dose of Nutrizym GR should usually not exceed this dose.

Capsules should be swallowed whole with water. Where swallowing of capsules proves to be difficult, the capsule may be opened and the pellets sprinkled on soft foods which do not require chewing. When Nutrizym GR is mixed with foods in this way, the resulting mixture should not be allowed to stand for more than one hour prior to use.

Contra-indications, warnings, etc

Contra-indications: Known hypersensitivity to active ingredient (porcine pancreatin).

Precautions: Hyperuricaemia and hyperuricosuria have been reported to occur in cystic fibrosis patients; pancreatin extracts contain a very small amount of purine which might, in high doses, contribute to this condition.

Patients who are taking or have been given in excess of 10,000 units of lipase/kg/day are at risk of developing colon damage. Abdominal symptoms (not usually experienced by the patient) or changes in abdominal symptoms should be reviewed to exclude the possibility of colonic damage – especially if the patient is taking in excess of 10,000 units of lipase/kg/day.

Use in pregnancy: Safety in pregnancy has not been established.

Side-effects: Very rarely hypersensitivity reactions may occur. As with any pancreatin extract, high doses may cause buccal and perianal irritation, in rare cases amounting to inflammation.

Stricture of the ileo-caecum and large bowel and colitis have been reported in children with cystic fibrosis taking pancreatic enzymes.

Pharmaceutical precautions Store below 25°C in tightly closed containers.

Legal category P.

Package quantities Containers of 100 capsules.

Further information Each Nutrizym GR capsule contains enteric coated pellets of pancreatin extract thus giving maximum enzymatic activity in the gastro-intestinal tract.

Product licence number 0493/0121.

NUTRIZYM 10

Qualitative and quantitative composition Each capsule contains Pancreatin BP 155 mg with not less than the following activities. Lipase 10,000 BP Units, Protease 500 BP Units and Amylase 9000 BP Units.

Pharmaceutical form Hard gelatin capsule containing enteric coated pancreatin minitablets for oral administration.

Clinical particulars

Therapeutic indications: For the symptomatic relief of pancreatic exocrine insufficiency such as in fibrocystic disease of the pancreas and chronic pancreatitis.

Posology and method of administration: Adults (including the elderly) and children: 1-2 capsules with meals and 1 capsule with snacks.

Since the individual response to pancreatin supplements is variable, the number of capsules taken may need to be titrated to the individual according to symptoms and at the discretion of the physician. Dose increase, if required should be added slowly with careful monitoring of response and symptomatology. Colonic damage has been reported in patients with cystic fibrosis taking in excess of 10,000 units of lipase/kg/day. The dose of Nutrizym 10 should usually not exceed this dose.

Capsules should be swallowed whole with water. Where swallowing of capsules proves to be difficult, the minitablets may be removed and taken with water or mixed with a small amount of soft food and swallowed immediately without chewing.

Adequate patient hydration should be ensured at all times whilst treating with Nutrizym 10.

Contra-indications: Known hypersensitivity to the active ingredient (porcine pancreatin) or any of the excipients.

Special warnings and precautions for use: Hyperuricaemia and hyperuricosuria have been reported to occur in cystic fibrosis patients; pancreatin extracts contain a small amount of purine which might, in high doses, contribute to this condition.

Interactions with other medicaments and other forms of interaction: None known.

Pregnancy and lactation: Safety has not been established and animal toxicological studies are lacking, therefore the use of Nutrizym 10 capsules is not recommended.

Effects on ability to drive and use machines: Not known.

Undesirable effects: Hypersensitivity reactions may occur. As with any pancreatin extract, high doses may cause buccal and perianal irritation, in some cases resulting in inflammation.

Stricture of the ileo-caecum and large bowel, and colitis have been reported in children with cystic fibrosis taking pancreatic enzymes. Abdominal symptoms (those not usually experienced by the patient) or changes in abdominal symptoms should be reviewed to exclude the possibility of colonic damage–especially if the patient is taking in excess of 10,000 units of lipase/kg/day.

Overdose: Inappropriately large doses could result in abdominal discomfort, nausea, vomiting and perianal irritation or inflammation.

Pharmacological properties

Pharmacodynamic properties: The active ingredient is a preparation of porcine pancreas with lipase, amylase and protease activity. Lipase enzymes hydrolyse fats to glycerol and fatty acids. Amylase converts starch into dextrins and sugars and protease enzymes change proteins into proteoses and derived substances.

Pharmacokinetic properties: The active ingredient of Nutrizym 10 is pancreatin which is a substance involved in the digestive process. During the enzymatic degradation of food substances the enzymes themselves are degraded. Any breakdown products are those that would be expected to appear following normal digestion.

Preclinical safety data: Preclinical data are not available.

Pharmaceutical particulars

List of excipients: uncoated minitablets: Castor Oil (hydrogenated), Silicon dioxide, colloidal, Magnesium stearate, Sodium carboxymethylcellulose, Microcrystalline cellulose.

Minitablet coating: Simethicone emulsion, Methacrylic acid copolymer, type C (Eudragit L30D), Talc, Triethyl citrate.

Gelatin capsules: Titanium dioxide, Iron oxide, red, Iron oxide, yellow, Gelatin.

Incompatibilities: Not known.

Shelf life: Two years.

Special precautions for storage: Store below 25°C in tightly close containers.

Nature and contents of container: Polyethylene or polypropylene containers with polyethylene tamper evident closures containing 100 capsules.

Instructions for use/handling: Not relevant.

Marketing authorisation number PL0493/0158.

Date of approval/revision of SPC October 1997.

Legal category P

NUTRIZYM 22 ▼

Qualitative and quantitative composition Each capsule contains Pancreatin BP 340 mg with not less than the following activities. Lipase 22,000 BP Units, Protease 1,100 BP Units and Amylase 19,800 BP Units.

Pharmaceutical form Hard gelatin capsule containing enteric coated pancreatin minitablets for oral administration.

Clinical particulars

Therapeutic indications: For the symptomatic relief of pancreatic exocrine insufficiency such as in fibrocystic disease of the pancreas and chronic pancreatitis.

Posology and method of administration: Adults (including the elderly) and children: 1-2 capsules with meals and 1 capsule with snacks.

Since the individual response to pancreatin supplements is variable, the number of capsules taken may need to be titrated to the individual according to symptoms and at the discretion of the physician. Dose increase, if required should be added slowly with careful monitoring of response and symptomatology. Colonic damage has been reported in patients with cystic fibrosis taking in excess of 10,000 units of lipase/kg/day. The dose of Nutrizym 22 should usually not exceed this dose.

Where a patient is already receiving a lower unit dose enteric coated pancreatic supplement, then Nutrizym 22 may be substituted at 1/2 of the number of capsules normally consumed with the previous preparation.

Capsules should be swallowed whole with water. Where swallowing of capsules proves to be difficult, the minitablets may be removed and taken with water or mixed with a small amount of soft food and swallowed immediately without chewing.

Adequate patient hydration should be ensured at all times whilst treating with Nutrizym 22.

Contra-indications: In children aged 15 years and under with cystic fibrosis. Known hypersensitivity to the active ingredient (porcine pancreatin) or any of the excipients.

Special warnings and special precautions for use: Hyperuricaemia and hyperuricosuria have been reported to occur in cystic fibrosis patients; pancreatin extracts contain a small amount of purine which might, in high doses, contribute to this condition.

Interactions with other medicaments and other forms of interaction: None known.

Pregnancy and lactation: Safety has not been established and animal toxicological studies are lacking, therefore the use of Nutrizym 22 capsules is not recommended.

Effects on ability to drive and use machines: Not known.

Undesirable effects: Hypersensitivity reactions may occur. As with any pancreatin extract, high doses may cause buccal and perianal irritation, in some cases resulting in inflammation.

Stricture of the ileo-caecum and large bowel, and colitis have been reported in children with cystic fibrosis taking pancreatic enzymes. Abdominal symptoms (those not usually experienced by the patient) or changes in abdominal symptoms should be reviewed to exclude the possibility of colonic damage–especially if the patient is taking in excess of 10,000 units of lipase/kg/day.

Overdose: Inappropriately large doses could result in abdominal discomfort, nausea, vomiting and perianal irritation or inflammation.

Pharmacological properties

Pharmacodynamic properties: The active ingredient is a preparation of porcine pancreas with lipase, amylase and protease activity. Lipase enzymes hydrolyse fats to glycerol and fatty acids. Amylase converts starch into dextrins and sugars and protease enzymes change proteins into proteoses and derived substances.

Pharmacokinetic properties: The active ingredient of Nutrizym 22 is pancreatin which is a substance involved in the digestive process. During the enzymatic degradation of food substances the enzymes themselves are degraded. Any breakdown products are those that would be expected to appear following normal digestion.

Preclinical safety data: Preclinical data are not available.

Pharmaceutical particulars

List of excipients: Uncoated minitablets: Castor Oil (hydrogenated), Silicon dioxide, colloidal, Magnesium stearate, Sodium carboxymethylcellulose, Microcrystalline cellulose.

Minitablet coating: Simethicone emulsion, Methacrylic acid copolymer, type C (Eudragit L30D), Talc, Triethyl citrate.

Gelatin capsules: Titanium dioxide, Iron oxide, red, Iron oxide, yellow, Gelatin.

Incompatibilities: Not known.

Shelf life: Two years.

Special precautions for storage: Store below 25°C in tightly close containers.

Nature and contents of container: Polyethylene or polypropylene containers with polyethylene tamper evident closures containing 100 capsules.

Instructions for use/handling: Not relevant.

Market authorisation number PL0493/0158.

Date of approval/revision of SPC October 1997.

Legal category POM.

OPTIMAX* ▼

Presentation Optimax Tablets: White capsule shaped tablets, Optimax engraved on one side with a break line on the reverse. Each tablet contains 500 mg L-tryptophan.

Uses Optimax should only be used by hospital specialists in patients who have had severe and disabling depressive illness continuously for more than 2 years, only after an adequate trial of standard antidepressant drug treatments, and only as an adjunct to other antidepressant medication.

Prior to supply of Optimax, the prescriber and patient must be registered with the Optimax Information and Clinical Support (OPTICS) Unit, Merck Pharmaceuticals (see Further Information).

Dosage and administration

Adults: The usual dose is two tablets, three times daily; for some patients up to 6 g L-tryptophan may be required. A lower dose may be appropriate in the elderly, especially where there is evidence of renal or hepatic impairment.

Children: Not recommended.

Contra-indications, warnings, etc

Contra-indications: Patients with a previous history of eosinophilia myalgia syndrome (EMS) following the use of L-tryptophan. This syndrome which is a multisystem disorder, is characterised by raised eosinophils ($>1.0\times10^9/1$), and severe myalgia in the absence of either an infectious or neoplastic cause.

Warnings: Eosinophilia Myalgia Syndrome (EMS) has been reported in association with the use of oral L-tryptophan – containing products. It is a multisystem disorder which is usually reversible but rarely, fatal. Various investigations have not as yet identified the aetiological factors precisely.

It is recommended therefore, that patients who are receiving L-tryptophan should be kept under close and regular surveillance with particular attention to monitoring eosinophil levels, haematological changes and muscle symptomatology. If the patient develops any of the symptoms of EMS, treatment with L-tryptophan should be stopped and the symptoms investigated further.

The possible interaction between L-tryptophan and 5HT reuptake inhibitors could lead to the 'serotonin syndrome' characterised by a combination of agitation, restlessness and gastro-intestinal symptoms including diarrhoea. Combinations with 5HT reuptake inhibitors should only be used with care (see Interactions).

Safety in pregnancy or lactation has not been established.

Precautions: Caution should be exercised with patients who may have experienced some, but not all of the symptoms of EMS after taking L-tryptophan. Treatment with L-tryptophan should be withheld and the symptoms investigated until the possibility of EMS can be excluded. These symptoms have been reported to include eosinophilia, arthralgia or myalgia, fever, dyspnoea, neuropathy, peripheral oedema, and skin lesions which can include sclerosis or papular and urticarial lesions.

Drug interactions: Where L-tryptophan is combined with an MAO Inhibitor the side effects of the latter may be enhanced. Use of L-tryptophan in combination with a 5-HT reuptake inhibitor has the potential for increasing the severity of the adverse effects of the latter and could lead to serotonin syndrome (see Warnings).

In patients taking L-tryptophan in conjunction with phenothiazines or benzodiazepines there have been isolated reports of sexual disinhibition.

Adverse effects: L-tryptophan may produce drowsiness. Patients who drive or operate machinery should be warned of the possible hazard.

In some patients, L-tryptophan may cause a slight feeling of nausea which usually disappears within 2 or 3 days. Such nausea can be minimised by giving L-tryptophan after food. Other adverse reactions include headache and lightheadedness.

Overdosage: Drowsiness and vomiting may occur; supportive measures should be employed.

Pharmaceutical precautions Store in a cool dry place.

Legal category POM.

Package quantities Containers of 84.

Further information Optimax can only be supplied once the prescriber and patient have been registered with the Optimax Information and Clinical Support (OPTICS) Unit. Following supply of the product, the prescriber will be contacted and asked to provide particular information relating to therapy. Further contact will be made at 3 months, and 6 monthly thereafter. All orders for Optimax will be dealt with through the OPTICS Unit. Ordering and other information is available from the OPTICS Unit, Merck Pharmaceuticals, Harrier House, High Street, West Drayton, Middlesex UB7 7QG.Tel: 0345 626902. Fax: 01895 452297.

Product licence number 0493/5900

OSTRAM* 1.2 g

Qualitative and quantitative composition Tricalcium phosphate PhEur, 3.30 g; corresponding to elemental calcium, 1.20 g.

Pharmaceutical form Powder for reconstitution to oral suspension.

Clinical particulars

Therapeutic indications:

- Calcium supplement for the treatment of osteoporosis (post-menopausal, senile, under corticosteroid therapy) treament of calcium deficiencies during growth, pregnancy and lactation.
- Calcium supplement as an adjunct to conventional therapy in the arrest or slowing down of bone demineralisation in osteoporosis (post-menopausal, senile, under corticosteroid therapy).
- Therapeutic supplementation in calcium deficiency during growth, pregnancy and lactation.

Posology and method of administration: 1 sachet a day.

Pour the contents of the sachet into about half a glass of water and stir until a homogeneous suspension is obtained. Drink without delay.

Contra-indications:

- Hypercalciuria, calcium lithiasis, calcification of tissues, chronic renal insufficiency, prolonged immobilisation accompanied by hypercalciuria and/or hypercalcaemia.
- Hypersensitivity to one of the constituents.

Special warnings and special precautions for use: None stated.

Interaction with other mecidaments and other forms of interaction: In cases of treatment with oral tetracyclines the dose of Ostram 1.2 g should be taken at least three hours later, in order to avoid possible interference with the absorption of tetracyclines.

Thiazide diuretics reduce urinary calcium excretion so the risk of hypercalcaemia should be considered.

Pregnancy and lactation: The likelihood of hypercalcaemia is increased in pregnant women in whom calcium and vitamin D are co-administered. Epidemiological studies with calcium have shown no increase in the teratogenic hazard to the foetus if used in the doses recommended.

Although supplemental calcium may be excreted in breast milk, the concentration is unlikely to be sufficient to produce any adverse effect on the neonate.

Effect on ability to drive and use machines: None.

Undesirable effects: None stated.

Overdose: Symptoms: Thirst, polyuria, nausea, vomiting, dehydration, arterial hypertension, vascular disorders, constipation.

Treatment: Stop all administration of calcium and vitamin D, rehydrate and depending on the gravity of the intoxication, use diuretics, corticosteroids, calcitonin, and peritoneal dialysis alone or in association.

Pharmacological properties

Pharmacodynamic properties: Calcium is predominantly (98%) involved in the formation of teeth and bone. The remainder is distributed between the soft tissues and body fluids where it plays an important physiological role in the form of ionised calcium. It is a constituent of cell membrane and is involved in regulation of cellular permeability. It is also an essential element for the function of nervous, muscular and glandular tissues.

Calcium is commonly used at this dosage in the prevention or the curative treatment of osteoporosis, alone, or in addition with oestrogens or sodium fluoride. The tolerance test performed with Ostram 1.2 g has shown very good clinical and biological tolerance.

Pharmacokinetic properties: Calcium is essentially absorbed by the duodenum exclusively in ionised form and distributed into all body fluids. About 50% of the plasma calcium is present in ionised form, 5-10% combined with diffusible anions and the remainder protein bound. Ionised serum calcium undergoes continuous exchange with bony and extracellular calcium.

Calcium is eliminated via the faeces, urine and sweat and is secreted into milk.

Ostram 1.2 g intestinal absorption test had been performed on 19 healthy adult volunteers. The signigicant increase in urine calcium and serum calcium bears evidence of good intestinal absorption of this salt. The magnitude of the modifications of serum phosphorus and urine phosphate remains moderate.

Preclinical safety data: No adverse effects can be predicted from animal toxicology studies other than those already documented from human use.

Pharmaceutical particulars

List of excipients: Sodium carboxymethylcellulose; Saccharin sodium; Natural lime flavouring (essential oil of lemon, essential oil of lime, citral, citronellal, vegetable gum, maltodextrin, sorbitol).

Incompatibilities: None stated.

Shelf life: 2 years.

Special precautions for storage: None.

Nature and contents of container: Sachets of paper/polyethylene/aluminium complex, packed in boxes of 30 sachets.

Instruction for use/handling: Pour the contents of the sachet into about half a glass of water and stir until a homogeneous suspension is obtained.

Marketing authorisation number PL11648/0029.

Date of first approval/revision of SPC August 1998.

Legal category P.

**Trade Mark*

Merck Sharp & Dohme Limited
Hertford Road
Hoddesdon
Hertfordshire EN11 9BU

☎ 01992 467272 🖷 01992 451066

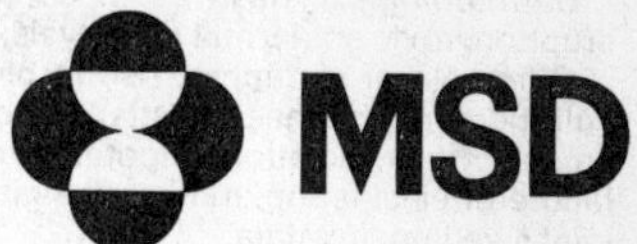

ALDOMET*

Presentation Yellow, film-coated tablets containing Methyldopa PhEur equivalent to the following amounts of anhydrous methyldopa: 125 mg (marked 'ALDOMET MSD 135'), 250 mg (marked 'ALDOMET MSD 401'), or 500 mg (marked 'ALDOMET MSD 516').

Injection, ampoules containing 50 mg Methyldopate Hydrochloride BP per millilitre, as a colourless solution. The injection contains sodium metabisulphite as preservative.

Uses Hypertension. Aldomet Injection is indicated for hypertension when parenteral medication is required. Treatment of acute hypertensive crises may be initiated with Aldomet Injection when an immediate effect is not necessary.

Mode of action: The antihypertensive effect of methyldopa is probably due to its metabolism to alpha-methylnoradrenaline, which lowers arterial pressure by stimulation of central inhibitory alpha-adrenergic receptors, false neurotransmission, and/or reduction of plasma renin activity.

Dosage and administration *Oral therapy – Adults: Initial dosage:* Usually 250 mg two or three times a day, for two days.

Adjustment: Usually adjusted at intervals of not less than two days, until an adequate response is obtained. The maximum recommended daily dosage is 3 g.

Many patients experience sedation for two or three days when therapy with Aldomet is started or when the dose is increased. When increasing the dosage, therefore, it may be desirable to increase the evening dose first.

General considerations: Methyldopa is largely excreted by the kidney, and patients with impaired renal function may respond to smaller doses.

Withdrawal of Aldomet is followed by return of hypertension, usually within 48 hours. This is not complicated generally by an overshoot of blood pressure.

Therapy with Aldomet may be initiated in most patients already on treatment with other antihypertensive agents by terminating these antihypertensive medications gradually if required (see manufacturer's recommendations on stopping these drugs). Following such previous antihypertensive therapy, Aldomet should be limited to an initial dose of not more than 500 mg daily and increased as required at intervals of not less than two days.

A thiazide may be added at any time during methyldopa therapy and is recommended if therapy has not been started with a thiazide or if effective control of blood pressure cannot be maintained on 2.0 g of methyldopa daily.

Aldomet may also be used concomitantly with the combination of amiloride hydrochloride and hydrochlorothiazide (such as Moduretic*) or beta-blocking agents, such as timolol maleate (Blocadren*).

When methyldopa is given to patients on other antihypertensives the dose of these agents may need to be adjusted to effect a smooth transition.

Oral therapy – Children: Initial dosage is based on 10 mg/kg of body weight daily in 2–4 oral doses. The daily dosage then is increased or decreased until an adequate response is achieved. The maximum dosage is 65 mg/kg or 3.0 g daily, whichever is less.

Intravenous therapy: Aldomet Injection is for intravenous use only, it must not be given intramuscularly or subcutaneously. An effective dose will produce a fall in blood pressure that may begin in 4 to 6 hours and be maintained for 10 to 16 hours.

The required dose of Aldomet Injection should be added to 100 ml of 5% Dextrose Injection BP. Alternatively, Aldomet may be given with 5% dextrose infusion solution BP at a concentration of 100 mg to each 10 ml solution. This intravenous infusion should be given slowly over a period of 30 to 60 minutes.

When practicable, oral therapy with Aldomet may be substituted, starting with the same dosage as that being used by the parenteral route.

Usual adult dosage: 250–500 mg six-hourly. In severe cases, up to 1 g six-hourly may be needed, and this is the maximum recommended dosage. If there is renal impairment, lower dosages should suffice.

Children's dosage: The recommended intravenous dosage for children is 20–40 mg/kg of body weight daily in divided doses every six hours. The maximum dosage is 65 mg/kg or 3.0 g daily, whichever is less. If there is renal impairment, lower dosages should suffice.

Use in the elderly: The initial dose in elderly patients should be kept as low as possible, not exceeding 250 mg daily; an appropriate starting dose in the elderly would be 125 mg b.d. increasing slowly as required, but not to exceed a maximum daily dosage of 2 g.

Contra-indications, warnings, etc

Contra-indications: Active hepatic disease, such as acute hepatitis and active cirrhosis; hypersensitivity (including hepatic disorders associated with previous methyldopa therapy), depression.

Aldomet is not recommended for the treatment of phaeochromocytoma (see 'Precautions').

Precautions: Acquired haemolytic anaemia has occurred rarely; should symptoms suggest anaemia, haemoglobin and/or haematocrit determinations should be made. If anaemia is confirmed, tests should be done for haemolysis. If haemolytic anaemia is present, Aldomet should be discontinued. Stopping therapy, with or without giving a corticosteroid, has usually brought prompt remission. Rarely, however, deaths have occurred.

Some patients on continued therapy with methyldopa develop a positive direct Coombs test. From the reports of different investigators, the incidence averages between 10% and 20%. A positive Coombs test rarely develops in the first six months of therapy, and if it has not developed within 12 months, it is unlikely to do so later on continuing therapy. Development is also dose-related, the lowest incidence occurring in patients receiving 1 g or less of methyldopa per day. The test becomes negative usually within weeks or months of stopping methyldopa.

Prior knowledge of a positive Coombs reaction will aid in evaluating a cross-match for transfusion. If a patient with a positive Coombs reaction shows an incompatible minor cross-match, an indirect Coombs test should be performed. If this is negative, transfusion with blood compatible in the major cross-match may be carried out. If positive, the advisability of transfusion should be determined by a haematologist.

Reversible leucopenia, with primary effect on granulocytes has been reported rarely. The granulocyte count returned to normal on discontinuing therapy. Reversible thrombocytopenia has occurred rarely.

Occasionally, fever has occurred within the first three weeks of therapy, sometimes associated with eosinophilia or abnormalities in liver function tests. Jaundice, with or without fever, also may occur. Its onset is usually within the first two or three months of therapy. In some patients the findings are consistent with those of cholestasis. Rare cases of fatal hepatic necrosis have been reported. Liver biopsy, performed in several patients with liver dysfunction, showed a microscopic focal necrosis compatible with drug hypersensitivity. Liver function tests and a total and differential white blood cell count are advisable before therapy and at intervals during the first six weeks to twelve weeks of therapy, or whenever an unexplained fever occurs. Should fever, abnormality in liver function, or jaundice occur, therapy should be withdrawn. If related to methyldopa, the temperature and abnormalities in liver function will then return to normal. Methyldopa should not be used again in these patients. Methyldopa should be used with caution in patients with a history of previous liver disease or dysfunction.

The antihypertensive effect of Aldomet may be diminished by sympathomimetics, phenothiazines, tricyclic antidepressants and MAOIs.

A paradoxical pressor response has been reported with Aldomet Injection.

Patients may require reduced doses of anaesthetics when on methyldopa. If hypotension does occur during anaesthesia, it can usually be controlled by vasopressors. The adrenergic receptors remain sensitive during treatment with methyldopa.

Dialysis removes methyldopa; therefore, hypertension may recur after this procedure.

Rarely, involuntary choreoathetotic movements have been observed during therapy with methyldopa in patients with severe bilateral cerebrovascular disease. Should these movements occur, therapy should be discontinued.

Aldomet should be used with extreme caution in patients, or in near relatives of patients, with hepatic porphyria.

The preservatives in Aldomet Injection have been reported to cause hypersensitivity. Sodium metabisulphite in particular is associated with circulatory collapse, and depression of the central nervous system in certain susceptible individuals with allergic tendencies.

Interference with laboratory tests: Methyldopa may interfere with the measurement of urinary uric acid by the phosphotungstate method, serum creatinine by the alkaline picrate method, and AST (SGOT) by colorimetric method. Interference with spectrophotometric methods for AST (SGOT) analysis has not been reported.

As methyldopa fluoresces at the same wavelengths as catecholamines, spuriously high amounts of urinary catecholamines may be reported interfering with a diagnosis of phaeochromocytoma.

It is important to recognise this phenomenon before a patient with a possible phaeochromocytoma is subjected to surgery. Methyldopa does not interfere with measurements of VMA (vanillylmandelic acid) by those methods which convert VMA to vanillin.

Rarely, when urine is exposed to air after voiding, it may darken because of breakdown of methyldopa or its metabolites.

Pregnancy and breast-feeding mothers: Aldomet has been used under close medical supervision for the treatment of hypertension during pregnancy. There was no clinical evidence that Aldomet caused fetal abnormalities or affected the neonate.

Methyldopa crosses the placental barrier and appears in cord blood and breast milk.

Although no obvious teratogenic effects have been reported, the possibility of fetal injury cannot be excluded and the use of the drug in women who are, or may become, pregnant or who are breast-feeding their newborn infant requires that anticipated benefits be weighed against possible risks.

Drug interactions: When methyldopa and lithium are given concomitantly the patient should be monitored carefully for symptoms of lithium toxicity.

When methyldopa is used with other antihypertensive drugs, potentiation of antihypertensive action may occur. The progress of patients should be carefully followed to detect side reactions or manifestations of drug idiosyncrasy.

Side-effects: Sedation, usually transient, may occur during the initial period of therapy or whenever the dose is increased. If affected, patients should not attempt to drive, or operate machinery. Headache, asthenia or weakness may be noted as early and transient symptoms.

The following reactions have been reported:

Central nervous system: Sedation (usually transient), headache, asthenia or weakness, paraesthesiae, parkinsonism, Bell's palsy, involuntary choreoathetotic movements. Psychic disturbances including nightmares, impaired mental acuity and reversible mild psychoses or depression. Dizziness, light-headedness, and symptoms of cerebrovascular insufficiency (may be due to lowering of blood pressure).

Cardiovascular: Bradycardia, prolonged carotid sinus hypersensitivity, aggravation of angina pectoris. Orthostatic hypotension (decrease daily dosage). Oedema (and weight gain) usually relieved by use of a diuretic. (Discontinue methyldopa if oedema progresses or signs of heart failure appear.)

Gastro-intestinal: Nausea, vomiting, distension, constipation, flatus, diarrhoea, colitis, mild dryness of mouth, sore or 'black' tongue, pancreatitis, sialadenitis.

Hepatic: Liver disorders including hepatitis, jaundice, abnormal liver function tests.

Haematological: Positive Coombs test, haemolytic anaemia, bone marrow depression, leucopenia, granulocytopenia, thrombocytopenia. Positive tests for antinuclear antibody, LE cells, and rheumatoid factor.

Allergic: Drug-related fever and lupus-like syndrome, myocarditis, pericarditis.

Dermatological: Rash as in eczema or lichenoid eruption, toxic epidermal necrolysis.

Other: Nasal stuffiness, rise in blood urea, breast enlargement, gynaecomastia, hyperprolactinaemia, amenorrhoea, lactation, impotence, decreased libido, failure of ejaculation, mild arthralgia with or without joint swelling, myalgia.

Overdosage: Acute overdosage may produce acute hypotension with other responses attributable to brain and gastro-intestinal malfunction (excessive sedation, weakness, bradycardia, dizziness, light-headedness, constipation, distension, flatus, diarrhoea, nausea, and vomiting). If ingestion is recent, emesis may be induced or gastric lavage performed. There is no specific antidote. Methyldopa is dialysable. Treatment is symptomatic. Infusions may be helpful to promote urinary excretion. Special attention should be directed towards cardiac rate and output, blood volume, electrolyte balance, paralytic ileus, urinary function and cerebral activity. Administration of sympathomimetic agents may be indicated. When chronic overdosage is suspected, Aldomet should be discontinued.

The plasma half-life of methyldopa is 105 minutes. Peak plasma levels were reached about two hours after oral ingestion.

Pharmaceutical precautions Keep containers well closed and store the tablets below 25°C, protected from light. The injection should also be protected from freezing. Only 5% dextrose should be used as diluent for the injection.

Legal category POM.

Package quantities *Tablets 125 mg:* Packs of 60.
Tablets 250 mg: Packs of 60.
Tablets 500 mg: Packs of 30.
Injection: Ampoules of 5 ml.

Further information Aldomet reduces both supine and standing blood pressure. Symptomatic postural hypotension, exercise hypotension and diurnal blood pressure variations rarely occur. By adjustment of dosage, morning hypotension can be prevented without sacrificing control of afternoon blood pressure.

Methyldopa has no direct effect on cardiac function and usually does not reduce glomerular filtration rate, renal blood flow or filtration fraction. Cardiac output usually is maintained without cardiac acceleration. In some patients, the heart rate is slowed.

Because of its relative freedom from adverse effects on kidney function, methyldopa can be of benefit in the control of high blood pressure, even in the presence of renal impairment. It may help arrest or retard the progression of renal function impairment and damage due to sustained elevation of blood pressure.

Normal or elevated plasma renin activity may decrease in course of methyldopa therapy.

Product licence numbers

Tablets 125 mg	0025/0098
Tablets 250 mg	0025/0099
Tablets 500 mg	0025/0100
Injection	0025/5003

ARAMINE*

Presentation A clear, colourless solution containing, in each millilitre, Metaraminol Tartrate BP equivalent to 10 mg metaraminol. Aramine also contains methylhydroxybenzoate, propylhydroxybenzoate and sodium bisulphite as preservatives; with the solution made isotonic by the inclusion of sodium chloride.

Uses Sympathomimetic amine (vasopressor agent). For the treatment of acute hypotension due to loss of vasoconstrictor tone as may occur during spinal anaesthesia, and as an adjunct to accepted remedial procedures (e.g. tilting of patient and attention to fluid volumes). (See 'Precautions'.)

The pressor effect of a single dose of Aramine lasts from about twenty minutes up to one hour. Its onset is around one or two minutes after direct intravenous injection.

Dosage and administration Aramine Injection may be given intravenously either directly or by infusion. Because the maximum effect is not immediately apparent, allow at least ten minutes before increasing the dose. Since the vasopressor effect tapers off when therapy is stopped, be prepared to restart promptly if the blood pressure falls too rapidly. Patients with coexistent shock and acidosis may show poor response.

Direct intravenous injection is recommended only in grave emergencies. *Particular care should be taken to use the correct dose.*

Intravenous infusion (for adjunctive treatment of hypotension): 15–100 mg (1.5–10 ml) in 500 ml of Sodium Chloride Injection BP or 5% Dextrose Injection BP, adjusting the rate of infusion to maintain the blood pressure at the desired level. Higher concentrations of Aramine 150–500 mg per 500 ml of infusion fluid, have been used. If the patient needs additional saline or dextrose at a rate of flow that would provide an excessive dose of Aramine when used as recommended, the volume of infusion fluid should be increased accordingly. Aramine may also be added to *less* than 500 ml of infusion fluid if a smaller volume is desired.

Aramine is physically and chemically compatible with Injection Sodium Chloride BP, 5% Injection Dextrose BP, Ringer's Injection USP, Lactated Ringer's Injection USP, Dextran 70 Injection.

When Aramine is mixed with an infusion solution, sterile precautions should be observed. Mixtures should be used within 24 hours since infusion solutions do not contain preservatives.

Direct intravenous injection (to be employed only in grave emergencies, when immediate action is necessary to save life): 0.5–5 mg (0.05–0.5 ml), followed by an infusion of 15–100 mg (1.5–10 ml) in 500 ml of infusion liquid. *Particular care should be taken to use the correct dose when injecting undiluted Aramine.*

Children: Aramine should not be used in children.

Use in the elderly: The dosage may not require modification for elderly patients; however geriatric patients may be more sensitive to sympathomimetic agents, therefore particular caution should be taken in this age group.

Contra-indications, warnings, etc
Contra-indications: Concurrent use with cyclopropane or halothane anaesthesia, unless clinical circumstances demand it. Hypersensitivity to any component of Aramine including sulphites. Children.

Precautions: Each preservative in Aramine has been reported to cause hypersensitivity. Sodium bisulphite in particular is associated with circulatory or respiratory collapse, and depression of the CNS in certain susceptible individuals, particularly in those with asthma.

Caution should be exercised to avoid excessive blood pressure changes since response to treatment with Aramine is very variable and the ensuing control of the blood pressure may prove difficult.

Rapidly induced hypertensive responses have been reported to cause acute pulmonary oedema, cardiac arrhythmias and arrest. Aramine should be used with caution in patients with cirrhosis; electrolyte levels should be adequately restored if a diuresis ensues. A fatal ventricular arrhythmia was reported in a patient with Laënnec's cirrhosis while receiving metaraminol tartrate. In several instances, ventricular extrasystoles that appeared during infusion of Aramine promptly subsided when the rate of flow was reduced.

With the prolonged action of Aramine, a cumulative effect is possible. An excessive vasopressor response may cause a prolonged elevation of blood pressure, even after discontinuation of therapy.

Aramine should be used with caution in cases of heart disease, hypertension, thyroid disease or diabetes mellitus because of its vasoconstrictor action.

Sympathomimetic amines may provoke a relapse in patients with a history of malaria.

When vasopressor amines are used for long periods, the resulting vasoconstriction may prevent adequate expansion of circulating volume and may cause perpetuation of the shock state. There is evidence that plasma volume may be reduced in all types of shock, and that the measurement of central venous pressure is useful in assessing the adequacy of the circulating blood volume. Blood, or plasma-volume expanders, should therefore be employed when the principal reason for hypotension or shock is decreased circulating volume.

In choosing the site for injection, it is important to avoid those areas generally recognised as being unsuitable for the use of any pressor agent and to discontinue the infusion immediately if infiltration or thrombosis occurs. Although the urgent nature of the patient's condition may force the choice of an unsuitable injection site, the preferred areas of injection should be used when possible. The larger veins of the antecubital fossa or thigh are preferred to the veins in the ankle or dorsum of the hand, particularly in patients with peripheral vascular disease, diabetes mellitus, Buerger's disease or conditions with coexistent hypercoagulability.

Accidental spillage of Aramine on the skin can cause dermatitic reactions linked to the presence of the agent's preservatives.

Pregnancy: There are no well-controlled studies in pregnant women. Aramine should be used during pregnancy only if the potential benefit justifies the potential risk to the fetus.

Breast-feeding mothers: It is not known whether Aramine is secreted in human milk. Because many drugs are secreted in human milk, caution should be exercised if Aramine is given to a breast-feeding mother.

Drug interactions: Aramine should be used with caution in digitalised patients since the combination of digitalis and sympathomimetic amines is capable of causing ectopic arrhythmic activity.

Monoamine oxidase inhibitors have been reported to potentiate the action of sympathomimetic amines. The pressor effect of Aramine is decreased but not reversed by alpha-adrenergic blocking agents.

Side effects: Sympathomimetic amines, including Aramine, may cause sinus or ventricular tachycardia, or other arrhythmias, especially in patients with myocardial infarction.

Abscess formation, tissue necrosis, and sloughing rarely may follow the use of Aramine.

Overdosage: Aramine acts rapidly. Its major therapeutic effects are complete within an hour of parenteral administration. Overdosage may result in severe hypertension accompanied by headache, constricting sensation in the chest, nausea, vomiting, euphoria, diaphoresis, pulmonary oedema, tachycardia, bradycardia, sinus arrhythmia, atrial or ventricular arrhythmias, myocardial infarction, cardiac arrest or convulsions.

If the drug has been ingested, induce emesis or perform gastric lavage. If Aramine has been administered by subcutaneous or intramuscular injection, local ice packs may be applied to delay absorption. Intravenous infusion should be stopped immediately, but reinstated if hypotension occurs. If needed, an alpha-adrenergic blocking agent such as phenoxybenzamine may be used to reduce hypertension. Intravenous beta-adrenergic blocking agents may also be useful for reducing hypertension and may have a beneficial effect on cardiac arrhythmia, if present. Parenteral diazepam may be given for convulsions.

Pharmaceutical precautions Store below 25°C, protected from light and from freezing. Aramine is physically and chemically compatible with Injection Sodium Chloride BP, 5% Injection Dextrose BP, Ringer's Injection USP, Lactated Ringer's Injection USP, Dextran 70 Injection. The ampoule may be autoclaved.

Legal category POM.

Package quantities Ampoules of 1 ml.

Further information Aramine is a potent sympathomimetic amine which increases the force of myocardial contractions as well as having a peripheral vasoconstrictor action. It increases both systolic and diastolic blood pressures.

Renal, coronary, and cerebral blood flow are a function of perfusion pressure and regional resistance. In most instances of cardiogenic shock, the beneficial effect of sympathomimetic amines is attributable to their positive inotropic effect. In patients with insufficient or failing vasoconstriction, there is additional advantage to the peripheral action of Aramine, but in most patients with shock, vasoconstriction is adequate and any further increase is unnecessary. Therefore, blood flow to vital organs may decrease with Aramine if the regional resistance increases excessively.

The pressor effect of Aramine is decreased but not reversed by alpha-adrenergic blocking agents. Primary or secondary fall in blood pressure and tachyphylactic response to repeated use are uncommon.

Product licence number 10 mg/ml injection 0025/5020.

BENEMID* TABLETS 500 mg

Qualitative and quantitative composition Benemid contains 500 mg of the active ingredient, Probenecid PhEur.

Pharmaceutical form Benemid is supplied as white, half-scored tablets marked 'MSD 501'.

Clinical particulars
Therapeutic indications: Probenecid is a uricosuric and renal tubular blocking agent designed for maintenance treatment of gout and gouty arthritis. It inhibits the reabsorption of urate ions in the renal tubules, thus increasing urinary excretion of uric acid and decreasing serum uric acid levels. This action is reversible upon withdrawal of the drug and is demonstrable in normal individuals as well as in patients under treatment. Effective uricosuria reduces the miscible urate pool, retards the deposition of urates, and promotes reabsorption of urate deposits. Also selectively inhibits the urinary excretion of β-lactam antibiotics (other than cephaloridine) and p-aminosalicylic acid.

Gout and other forms of hyperuricaemia: Benemid is an effective uricosuric agent for the treatment of hyperuricaemia in gout and gouty arthritis. Time is required to achieve clinical results with Benemid despite the marked uricosuric activity of Benemid. Although acute attacks may occur in the early stages of therapy, as therapy is continued these attacks should become less frequent and less intense. Benemid may also be given prophylactically, to treat the asymptomatic hyperuricaemia that often occurs in 'gouty' families, in an attempt to forestall the development of acute gouty attacks and urate deposition in tissues.

Benemid may be used to control the hyperuricaemia induced or aggravated by diuretics employed in oedema and hypertension.

Beta-lactam antibiotic therapy: Benemid is indicated as an adjunctive therapy with β-lactam antibiotics (other than cephaloridine) and p-aminosalicylic acid. Benemid interferes with the renal tubular excretion of these substances and thus elevates and prolongs the plasma levels by whatever route the antibiotics are given. A twofold to fourfold increase in plasma concentration has been demonstrated for: penicillin G or V; the synthetic penicillins, ampicillin, methicillin, oxacillin, cloxacillin, carbenicillin, and nafcillin; the cephamycin, cefoxitin sodium; and the cephalosporins, cephalothin, cephalexin, and cephaloglycin.

Adjunctive therapy of this type is particularly useful when treating severe or resistant infections, such as gonorrhoea, subacute bacterial endocarditis, staphylococcal osteomyelitis, staphylococcal septicaemia, and meningitis due to Gram-positive organisms.

Posology and method of administration

Uricosuric therapy: The usual adult dosage is ½ tablet (250 mg) twice a day for one week, followed thereafter by 1 tablet (500 mg) twice a day.

Some degree of renal impairment is common in patients with gout; therefore, a daily dosage of 2 tablets (1 g) may be adequate in many patients. If, however, symptoms of gouty arthritis remain uncontrolled or the 24-hour urate excretion is not above 700 mg, the daily dosage may be increased by 1 tablet (500 mg) every four weeks within tolerance [usually not more than 4 tablets (2 g) a day]. Benemid may not be effective in chronic renal insufficiency, particularly when the glomerular filtration rate is 30 ml/min or less.

Gastric intolerance may be indicative of overdosage, and may be corrected by reducing the dosage without losing the therapeutic response.

Benemid should be continued at a dosage that will maintain a normal serum uric acid level. When acute attacks have been absent for at least six months and serum uric acid levels remain within normal limits, dosage of Benemid may be reduced by 1 tablet (500 mg) every six months to the minimum effective dosage. The maintenance dosage should not be reduced to the point where serum uric acid levels tend to rise.

Gonorrhoea: For uncomplicated gonorrhoea in men or women, a single dose of 2 tablets (1 g) with adequate doses of either oral ampicillin or intramuscular aqueous procaine penicillin G, or cefoxitin. If oral ampicillin is used, Benemid should be given simultaneously; if a parenteral antibiotic is administered, Benemid should be given at least 30 minutes before the injection.

β-lactam antibiotic therapy (general): Adults: 4 tablets (2 g) a day in divided doses. Elderly patients with suspected renal impairment should be given a reduced dosage. Benemid should not be given concurrently with a β-lactam antibiotic in known cases of renal impairment.

Children over 2 years: 25 mg per kg bodyweight (or 0.7 g/m² body surface) initially, followed by 40 mg per kg (or 1.2 g/m²) a day in divided doses every six hours. For children weighing more than 50 kg, the adult dosage is recommended.

Use in the elderly: As with all drugs which are primarily renally excreted, care should be taken in the elderly whose renal function may be impaired.

Contra-indications: Known hypersensitivity to any component of this product. History of blood dyscrasias. Uric acid kidney stones. Children under 2 years old. Therapy with Benemid should not be started until an acute gouty attack has subsided. Salicylates are contra-indicated in patients taking Benemid.

Special warnings and precautions for use: Benemid should be used with caution in patients with a history of peptic ulcer.

If hypersensitivity reactions appear during therapy, the drug should be withdrawn.

Haematuria, renal colic, costovertebral pain and the formation of urate stones associated with the use of probenecid in gouty patients may be prevented by a liberal fluid intake and enough sodium bicarbonate (3–7.5 g daily) or potassium citrate (7.5 g daily) to keep the urine alkaline. When alkali is given, the acid-base balance of the patient should be carefully monitored.

Alkalisation of urine is recommended until the serum uric acid level returns to normal tophaceous deposits disappear, i.e. during the period when urinary excretion of urates is at a high level. After the miscible pool of uric acid decreases to normal (about 1 g) and deposited urates are reabsorbed and eliminated, alkalisation of the urine probably is unnecessary, since the urinary urate concentration is lower and less likely to cause crystallisation.

Exacerbation of gout during therapy with Benemid may occur; if so, a full therapeutic dosage of colchicine, indomethacin, or other appropriate therapy should be given.

Interaction with other medicaments and other forms of interaction: The use of acetylsalicylic acid is contra-indicated because it antagonises the uricosuric action of probenecid. If patients on Benemid require a mild analgesic, paracetamol is preferred.

Since probenecid decreases the renal excretion of conjugated sulphonamides, plasma concentrations of the latter should be determined from time to time when a sulphonamide and probenecid are given together for prolonged periods. Probenecid may prolong or enhance the action of oral sulphonylureas and thereby increase the risk of hypoglycaemia.

Benemid increases the mean plasma elimination half-life of a number of other drugs which can lead to increased peak plasma concentrations. These drugs include paracetamol, naproxen, indomethacin, ketoprofen, meclofenamate, lorazepam, and rifampicin acyclovir, ganciclovir and zidovudine. The clinical significance of this effect is not known; however, adjustment in the usual dosage of these drugs may be required.

Caution should be used if Benemid is administered simultaneously with methotrexate, as Benemid has been reported to decrease the tubular secretion of methotrexate and potentiate toxicity. If Benemid is given with methotrexate, the dosage of methotrexate should be reduced and serum levels may need to be monitored.

The uricosuric action of Benemid is antagonised by pyrazinamide.

Because of the mechanism of action, Benemid is not recommended in conjunction with a beta-lactam antibiotic in the presence of known renal impairment.

In addition to the effect of Benemid on the excretion of uric acid and β-lactam antibiotics (other than cephaloridine), Benemid decreases the urinary excretion of ρ-aminosalicylic acid (PAS), ρ-aminohippuric acid (PAH), phenolsulphonylphthalein (PSP), pantothenic acid, 17-ketosteroids, indomethacin, and sodium iodomethamate and related iodinated organic acids. Benemid decreases both hepatic and renal excretion of sulphobromophthalein (BSP). The renal tubular reabsorption of phosphorus is inhibited in hypoparathyroid, but not in euparathyroid, individuals.

Benemid does not affect the excretion of streptomycin, chloramphenicol, chlortetracycline, oxytetracycline, or neomycin. The effects on the excretion of cephaloridine are not clinically significant.

Pregnancy and lactation

Use in pregnancy: Probenecid crosses the placental barrier and appears in cord blood. Its use in women of childbearing age requires that the anticipated benefit be weighed against possible hazards.

Use in breast-feeding: It is not known whether this drug is excreted in human milk. Because many drugs are excreted in human milk, caution should be exercised when Benemid is administered to a breast-feeding mother.

Effects on ability to drive and use machines: Benemid may cause dizziness in some patients. If patients experience dizziness, they should be instructed not to drive and to avoid operating machinery or performing other hazardous activities requiring alertness.

Undesirable effects: Headache, gastro-intestinal symptoms (e.g. anorexia, nausea, vomiting), frequency of micturition, hypersensitivity reactions (including anaphylaxis, dermatitis, pruritus, urticaria, and fever and Stevens Johnson syndrome), sore gums, flushing, alopecia, dizziness, anaemia and haemolytic anaemia (in some cases associated with genetic deficiency of glucose-6-phosphate dehydrogenase in red blood cells) have occurred. Toxic epidermal necrolysis has been reported rarely after combination therapy of colchicine and probenecid. The nephrotic syndrome, leucopenia, hepatic necrosis, and aplastic anaemia occur rarely. In gouty patients, exacerbation of gout, and uric acid stones with or without haematuria, renal colic, or costovertebral pain, have been seen.

Laboratory tests: A reducing substance may appear in the urine of patients receiving Benemid. This may give a false-positive Benedict's test, but the substance disappears when therapy is discontinued.

Falsely high readings for theophylline have been reported in an *in vitro* study using the Schack and Waxler technique, when therapeutic concentrations of theophylline and Benemid were added to human plasma.

Overdosage: No specific antidote is available. The usual measures to remove unabsorbed material from the gastro-intestinal tract, clinical monitoring, and supportive therapy should be employed. If signs of CNS excitation are present, a short-acting barbiturate or intravenous diazepam should be given parenterally. Adrenaline should be given for anaphylactoid reactions. For less severe hypersensitivity reactions, antihistamines or corticosteroids may be given.

The plasma half-life of probenecid is between six to twelve hours; between 85 to 95% of the drug is bound to plasma proteins.

Pharmacological properties

Pharmacodynamic properties: Probenecid increases the excretion of urate in the urine by inhibiting its reabsorption in the renal tubule. It also decreases the excretion of penicillin and other beta-lactam antibiotics (therapy raising and prolonging plasma levels) by inhibiting their secretion in the renal tubule.

Pharmacokinetic properties: Probenecid is completely absorbed on oral administration. Peak plasma levels are reached in two to four hours. Plasma half life varies from less than five hours to more than eight hours, depending on the dose. Between 85% and 95% is bound to plasma albumin. It is partially metabolised to the glucuronide and hydroxylated, carboxylated, and N-depropylated metabolites. Unchanged drug and its metabolites are excreted in the urine.

Preclinical safety data: No evidence of mutagenicity was observed in a microbial mutagenicity test using mutant strains of salmonella typhimurium with or without rat or hamster liver metabolic activation. No genetic damage was noted in a chromosome aberration study in CHO cells. Variable results were obtained in a sister chromatid exchange (SCE) text in CHO cells. One trial caused a dose-related increase in SCEs; a second trial was negative, and a third trial had significant increases at the lowest and highest doses tested (but not the intermediate doses).

In a 23 month carcinogenic study in mice, a significant increase in the incidence of heptocellular carcinomas and adenomas was observed at a dose of 400 mg/kg/day (10 times the maximum recommended human dose) in the females. These changes were not observed in male mice or rats of either sex that received the same dose, or in mice of either sex at a dose of 100 mg/kg/day (2.5 times the maximum recommended human dose).

The oral LD_{50} of probenecid is 1.7 g/kg and 1.6 g/kg in the mouse and rat respectively.

Pharmaceutical particulars

List of excipients: Calcium Stearate PhEur, Gelatin PhEur, Magnesium Carbonate, Heavy PhEur, Maize Starch PhEur.

Incompatibilities: None.

Shelf life: 60 months.

Special precautions for storage: Store below 25°C.

Nature and contents of container: High density, polyethylene bottles with cap-to-cap pilfer evident closures containing 60 tablets.

Instruction for use/handling: None.

Marketing authorisation number 0025/5021R.

Date of approval/revision of SPC February 1998.

Legal category POM.

BLOCADREN*

Presentation Light blue, half-scored tablets, marked 'MSD 136' on one side and scored on the other, containing 10 mg Timolol Maleate BP.

Uses Beta-adrenergic-receptor blocking agent. For the treatment of essential hypertension and in angina pectoris due to ischaemic heart disease.

Blocadren is also indicated for the long-term prevention of myocardial infarction and cardiac death (including sudden death) in those who have survived the acute phase of a myocardial infarction.

Prophylactic treatment of common and classic migraine.

Dosage and administration

Hypertension: The initial dosage is 10 mg a day in a single or divided dosage. Depending on the response of the patient, increases in dosage may be made gradually to a maximum of 60 mg daily. Daily dosages above 20 mg should be given on a divided dose schedule.

Use with Moduretic (amiloride hydrochloride 5 mg and hydrochlorothiazide 50 mg):* Studies have shown that Blocadren can be administered once daily when used concomitantly with Moduretic. The majority of patients will respond to a regimen of 10 or 20 mg of Blocadren once a day and 1 tablet of Moduretic.

Use with other antihypertensives: Blocadren may be used with thiazides, hydralazine, or methyldopa. Dosage adjustments are usually required.

For concomitant use with catecholamine-depleting

drugs such as reserpine or guanethidine, see 'Precautions'.

Angina: Therapy should be initiated with 5 mg two or three times a day. Dosage increases may be necessary, depending on the symptomatic response, pulse rate, and blood pressure. The first increase should not exceed 10 mg a day in divided doses, and subsequent increases should not exceed 15 mg a day in divided doses. There should be an interval of at least three days between increases in dosage.

The usual dosage range is 15 to 45 mg a day. The majority of patients respond to a dosage in the range of 35 to 45 mg a day.

Preventive use in ischaemic heart disease: For long-term preventive use in patients who have survived the acute phase of myocardial infarction, the maintenance dose is 10 mg twice daily. Therapy should be initiated with 5 mg twice daily and the patient observed carefully. If no adverse reaction occurs, the dosage should then be increased after 2 days to 10 mg twice daily. In the studies evaluating Blocadren following myocardial infarction, treatment was begun 7 to 28 days after the acute phase.

Migraine: The recommended dosage in the prophylactic treatment of common and classic migraine is 10 to 20 mg administered once-a-day.

Paediatric use: not established (see 'Precautions').

Use in the elderly: Initial dosage should be 5 mg b.d. Dosage may be increased cautiously depending on clinical response. *For the preventive use in ischaemic heart disease:* The dosage should be increased to 10 mg b.d. after the second day of treatment.

Contra-indications, warnings, etc
Contra-indications: Bronchospasm (including bronchial asthma), history of bronchospasm, severe chronic obstructive pulmonary disease; sinus bradycardia; atrioventricular block; overt heart failure (see 'Precautions'); right ventricular failure secondary to pulmonary hypertension; significant cardiomegaly; cardiogenic shock; hypersensitivity to this product. The packaging carries the warning: do not take this medicine if you have a history of wheezing or asthma.

See also 'Use in pregnancy and breast-feeding mothers', under 'Precautions'.

Precautions: Congestive heart failure: Blocadren may be given cautiously to patients with a history of cardiac failure who are well compensated, usually with digitalis or diuretics. Both digitalis and timolol maleate slow AV conduction. If cardiac failure persists, Blocadren should be withdrawn.

In patients without history of cardiac failure: At the first sign or symptom of cardiac failure, patients receiving Blocadren should be digitalised and/or given a diuretic, and the response closely observed. If cardiac failure still continues, Blocadren should be withdrawn.

Thyrotoxicosis: Beta-adrenergic blockade may mask certain clinical signs (e.g. tachycardia) of hyperthyroidism. Patients suspected of developing thyrotoxicosis should be managed carefully to avoid abrupt withdrawal of Blocadren which might precipitate a thyroid storm.

Exacerbation of ischaemic heart disease following abrupt withdrawal: Hypersensitivity to catecholamines has been seen in patients withdrawn from beta-blocker therapy; exacerbation of angina and, in some cases, myocardial infarction has occurred after *abrupt* withdrawal of such therapy. When discontinuing chronically administered Blocadren, particularly in patients with ischaemic heart disease, the dosage should be gradually reduced over one to two weeks and the patient carefully monitored. If angina markedly worsens or acute coronary insufficiency develops, Blocadren should be reinstated promptly, at least temporarily, and other appropriate measures taken. Patients should be warned against interruption or discontinuation of Blocadren without the physician's advice. Because coronary artery disease is both common and may be unrecognised, it may be prudent not to discontinue Blocadren abruptly, even when only treating hypertension.

Major surgery: Because beta-adrenergic-receptor blockade impairs the heart's response to beta-adrenergic mediated reflex stimuli, some patients on beta-adrenergic receptor blocking agents have shown protracted severe hypotension during anaesthesia. Difficulty in restarting and maintaining the heartbeat has also been reported.

Some authorities now recommend gradual withdrawal of beta-adrenergic-receptor blocking agents from anginal patients before elective surgery. If necessary during surgery, the effects of Blocadren may be reversed by sufficient doses of such agonists as isoprenaline, dopamine, dobutamine or noradrenaline (see 'Overdosage').

Diabetes mellitus: Blocadren should be administered with caution to patients liable to spontaneous hypoglycaemia, or to diabetic patients (especially those with labile diabetes) who are receiving insulin or oral hypoglycaemic agents. Beta-adrenergic receptor blocking agents may mask the premonitory signs and symptoms of acute hypoglycaemia.

Impaired hepatic or renal function: Since Blocadren is partially metabolised in the liver and excreted mainly by the kidney, dosage reduction may be necessary when hepatic and/or renal insufficiency is present.

In the presence of marked renal failure: Although the pharmacokinetics of Blocadren are not greatly altered by renal impairment, marked hypotensive responses have been seen in patients with marked renal impairment undergoing dialysis after 20 mg doses. Dosing in such patients should, therefore, be especially cautious.

Musculoskeletal: Beta-blockers have been reported to induce myasthenic symptoms such as diplopia, ptosis and generalised weakness. Timolol has been reported rarely to increase muscle weakness in some patients with myasthenic symptoms.

Cerebrovascular insufficiency: As an agent affecting both pulse and blood pressure, Blocadren should be used cautiously in patients with cerebrovascular insufficiency. Signs or symptoms suggesting reduced cerebral blood flow should prompt consideration of withdrawing therapy with Blocadren.

General: There have been reports of skin rashes and/or dry eyes associated with the use of beta-adrenoceptor-blocking drugs. The reported incidence is small and in most cases the symptoms have cleared when treatment was withdrawn. Discontinuation of the drug should be considered if any such reaction is not otherwise explicable. Cessation of therapy involving beta-blockade should be gradual.

Paediatric use: Safety and efficacy in children has not been established.

Use in pregnancy and breast-feeding mothers: There are no adequate and well-controlled studies in pregnant women. Blocadren should only be used if the potential benefit justifies the risk to the fetus.

Timolol is detectable in human milk. Because of the potential for serious adverse reactions in breast-feeding babies, a decision to discontinue breast-feeding, or Blocadren, should be made taking into account the importance of the drug to the mother.

Risk from anaphylactic reaction: While taking beta-blockers, patients with a history of atopy or a history of severe anaphylactic reaction to a variety of allergens, may be more reactive to repeated challenge with such allergens, either accidental, diagnostic or therapeutic. Such patients may be unresponsive to the usual doses of adrenaline used to treat anaphylactic reactions.

Drug interactions: Close observation of the patient is recommended when Blocadren is administered to patients on catecholamine-depleting drugs such as reserpine, because of possible additive effects and the production of hypotension and/or marked bradycardia, which may produce vertigo, syncope, or postural hypotension.

Attenuation of the antihypertensive effect of beta-blockers by NSAIDs has been reported. Patients treated with both agents should be monitored to confirm that the desired therapeutic effect has been obtained.

Oral calcium antagonists may be combined with Blocadren only when heart function is normal. The potential exists for hypotension, AV conduction disturbances, and left ventricular failure to occur in patients receiving a beta-blocking agent when an oral calcium antagonist is added to the treatment regimen. The nature of any cardiovascular adverse effect tends to depend on the type of calcium antagonist used. Dihydropyridine derivatives, such as nifedipine, may lead to hypotension, whereas verapamil or diltiazem have a greater propensity to lead to AV conduction disturbances or left ventricular failure when used with a beta-blocker. Intravenous calcium antagonists and Blocadren should only be used together with caution.

Concomitant use of beta-blockers and digitalis with either diltiazem or verapamil may further prolong the AV conduction time.

Side-effects: Blocadren is usually well tolerated. Most adverse reactions have been mild and transient. *General:* Asthenia, fatigue, headache, chest pain, extremity pain, decreased exercise tolerance, weight loss. *Cardiovascular:* Bradycardia, cardiac arrest, cerebral vascular accident, palpitation, arrhythmia, sinoatrial block, AV block (2nd or 3rd degree), syncope, hypotension, oedema, pulmonary oedema, cardiac failure, Raynaud's phenomenon, cold extremities, claudication, worsening of arterial insufficiency or angina pectoris, vasodilatation. *Digestive:* Dyspepsia, nausea, vomiting, diarrhoea, hepatomegaly. *Endocrine:* Hyperglycaemia, hypoglycaemia. *Integumentary:* Rash, pruritus, skin irritation, increased pigmentation, sweating, exfoliative dermatitis (one case). *Musculoskeletal:* Arthralgia. *Nervous system:* Dizziness, vertigo, paraesthesiae, local weakness. *Psychiatric:* Nervousness, diminished concentration, hallucinations, nightmares, increased dreaming, insomnia, depression, somnolence, decreased libido. *Haematological:* Non-thrombocytopenic purpura. *Respiratory:* Dyspnoea, bronchial spasm, rales, cough. *Special senses:* Tinnitus, visual disturbances, diplopia, ptosis, eye irritation, dry eyes. *Urogenital:* Impotence, micturition difficulties. *Clinical laboratory tests:* Changes in clinical laboratory tests are rare. Slight increases in blood urea, serum potassium and serum uric acid, and slight decreases in haemoglobin and haematocrit occurred, but were not progressive or associated with clinical manifestations.

Overdosage: No specific data are available in humans. A study in patients with renal failure suggests that Blocadren does not readily dialyse.

The most common signs and symptoms to be expected following overdosage with a beta-adrenergic-receptor blocking agent are symptomatic bradycardia, hypotension, bronchospasm, acute cardiac failure, and heart block. If overdosage occurs, the following measures are suggested. In all cases therapy with Blocadren should be stopped, and the patient closely observed.

1. Gastric lavage.
2. Symptomatic bradycardia: atropine sulphate, 0.25 to 2 mg intravenously, should be used to induce vagal blockade. If bradycardia persists, intravenous isoprenaline hydrochloride should be administered cautiously. In refractory cases, the use of a cardiac pacemaker may be considered.
3. Hypotension: a sympathomimetic pressor agent such as dopamine, dobutamine or noradrenaline should be used. In refractory cases, the use of glucagon has been reported to be useful.
4. Bronchospasm: isoprenaline hydrochloride should be used. Additional therapy with aminophylline may be considered.
5. Acute cardiac failure: conventional therapy with digitalis, diuretics, and oxygen should be instituted immediately. In refractory cases, the use of intravenous aminophylline is suggested. This may be followed, if necessary, by glucagon which has been reported useful.
6. Heart block: isoprenaline hydrochloride or a pacemaker should be used.

Timolol is rapidly and nearly completely absorbed following ingestion. Plasma half-life is approximately four hours.

Pharmaceutical precautions Store in a cool place below 25°C, protected from light.

Legal category POM.

Package quantities PVC blister packs of 60 tablets.

Further information Blocadren reduces blood pressure without acute hypotensive episodes in most patients with essential hypertension. The exact mechanism of action is still unknown. Blocadren does not usually affect normal blood pressure.

Blocadren effectively delays or prevents the development of anginal pain in most patients. It acts by modifying the cardiac response to stress or exercise.

Blocadren has been shown to be highly effective in reducing the incidence of cardiac death, including sudden death, and of reinfarction in patients who have survived the acute phase of a myocardial infarction.

Product licence number 0025/0091.

CLINORIL*

Qualitative and quantitative composition Clinoril 100 mg Tablets contain 100 mg of sulindac PhEur.

Clinoril 200 mg Tablets contain 200 mg of sulindac PhEur.

Pharmaceutical form Brilliant yellow, hexagonal-shaped tablets, with one side scored. The 200 mg tablets are marked 'MSD 942' and the 100 mg tablets are marked 'MSD 943'.

Clinical particulars
Therapeutic indications: Clinoril is a non-steroidal, analgesic/anti-inflammatory agent with antipyretic properties.

Indicated in osteoarthritis, rheumatoid arthritis, ankylosing spondylitis, acute gouty arthritis, peri-articular disorders such as bursitis, tendinitis, and tenosynovitis.

Posology and method of administration: The dosage should be taken twice a day and adjusted to the severity of the disease.

The usual dosage is 400 mg a day. However, the dosage may be lowered depending on the response. Doses above 400 mg per day are not recommended.

In the treatment of acute gouty arthritis, therapy for seven days is usually adequate.

In peri-articular disorders, treatment should be limited to seven to ten days.

Clinoril should be adminstered with fluids or food.

Children: The use of Clinoril in children is contra-indicated.

Use in the elderly: The dosage does not require modification for the elderly patient.

Contra-indications: Hypersensitivity to any component of this product.

Clinoril should not be used in patients in whom acute asthmatic attacks, urticaria, or rhinitis have been precipitated by aspirin or other non-steroidal anti-inflammatory agents.

The drug should not be administered to patients with active gastro-intestinal bleeding.

The use of Clinoril should be avoided in patients with active peptic ulcer.

Since paediatric indications and dosage have not yet been established, Clinoril should not be given to children.

Special warnings and precautions for use

Platelet aggregation: Clinoril has less effect on platelet function and bleeding time than aspirin; however, since Clinoril is an inhibitor of platelet function, patients who may be adversely affected should be carefully observed when 'Clinoril' is administered.

Gastro-intestinal effects: Clinoril should be used with caution in patients having a history of gastro-intestinal haemorrhage or ulcers.

Hypersensitivity syndrome: A potentially life-threatening, apparent hypersensitivity syndrome has been reported. In cases where the syndrome is suspected, therapy should be discontinued immediately, and not recontinued. This syndrome may include constitutional symptoms (fever, chills, diaphoresis, flushing), cutaneous findings (rash or other dermatological reactions, see *Undesirable effects*), conjunctivitis, involvement of major organs (changes in liver-function tests, hepatic failure, jaundice, pancreatitis, pneumonitis with or without pleural effusion, leucopenia, leucocytosis, eosinophilia, disseminated intravascular coagulation, anaemia, renal impairment, including renal failure), and other less specific findings (adenitis, arthralgia, arthritis, myalgia, fatigue, malaise, hypotension, chest pain, tachycardia).

Infections: Non-steroidal anti-inflammatory drugs, including Clinoril, may mask the usual signs and symptoms of infection; therefore, the physician must be continually on the alert for this and should use the drug with extra care in the presence of existing infection.

Ocular effects: Because of reports of adverse eye findings with agents of this class it is recommended that patients who develop eye complaints during treatment with Clinoril have ophthalmological evaluations.

Cardiovascular effects: Peripheral oedema has been observed in some patients taking Clinoril. Therefore, as with other drugs in this class, Clinoril should be used with caution in patients with compromised cardiac function, hypertension, or other conditions predisposed to fluid retention.

Hepatic effects: A patient with signs and/or symptoms suggesting liver dysfunction, or in whom an abnormal liver-function test has occurred, should be evaluated for evidence of a more severe hepatic reaction while on therapy. Significant elevations of AST (SGOT) and ALT (SGPT) (three times higher than normal) were seen in less than 1% of patients in controlled clinical trials.

Poor liver function may alter the blood levels of circulating metabolites of Clinoril. Patients with liver dysfunction on Clinoril should be monitored closely; daily dosage reduction may be required.

Cases of hepatitis, jaundice, or both, with or without fever, may occur within the first three months of therapy. In some patients, the findings are consistent with those of cholestatic hepatitis.

Fever or other evidence of hypersensitivity, including abnormalities in one or more liver function tests and skin reactions, have occurred during therapy. Some fatalities have occurred.

Whenever a patient develops unexplained fever, rash or other dermatological reactions, or constitutional symptoms, Clinoril should be permanently stopped and liver function investigated. Fever and abnormal liver function are reversible.

Renal effects: As with other non-steroidal anti-inflammatory drugs, there have been reports of acute interstitial nephritis with haematuria, proteinuria, and occasionally, nephrotic syndrome in patients receiving sulindac.

In patients with reduced renal blood flow where renal prostaglandins play a major role in maintaining renal perfusion, administration of a non-steroidal anti-inflammatory agent may precipitate overt renal decompensation. Patients at greatest risk of this reaction are those with renal or hepatic dysfunction, diabetes mellitus, advanced age, extracellular volume depletion, congestive heart failure, sepsis, or concomitant use of any nephrotoxic drug. A non-steroidal anti-inflammatory drug should be given with caution and renal function should be monitored in any patient who may have reduced renal reserve. Discontinuation of non-steroidal anti-inflammatory therapy is usually followed by recovery to the pre-treatment state.

Since Clinoril is eliminated primarily by the kidneys, patients with significantly impaired renal function should be closely monitored; a lower daily dosage should be used to avoid excessive drug accumulation.

Sulindac metabolites have been reported rarely as the major, or a minor, component in renal stones in association with other calculus components. Clinoril should be used with caution in patients with a history of renal lithiasis and they should be kept well hydrated while receiving Clinoril. In patients with renal functional impairment, since the major route of excretion of the drug is via the kidney, the dosage may need to be reduced.

Interaction with other medicaments and other forms of interaction: Dimethyl sulphoxide: Dimethyl sulphoxide should not be used with Clinoril. Concomitant use has been reported to reduce plasma levels of the active metabolite of Clinoril, and also cause peripheral neuropathy.

Methotrexate: Caution should be used if Clinoril is administered concomitantly with methotrexate. Non-steroidal anti-inflammatory drugs have been reported to decrease the tubular secretion of methotrexate and potentiate the toxicity.

Cyclosporin: Administration of non-steroidal anti-inflammatory drugs concomitantly with cyclosporin has been associated with an increase in cyclosporin-induced toxicity, possibly due to the decreased synthesis of renal prostacyclin. NSAIDs should be used with caution in patients taking cyclosporin, and renal function should be monitored carefully.

Oral anticoagulants and hypoglycaemic agents: Although sulindac and its sulphide metabolite are highly bound to protein, studies (in which Clinoril was given at a dose of 400 mg daily) have shown no clinically significant interaction with oral anticoagulants or oral hypoglycaemic agents. However, patients should be monitored carefully until it is certain that no change in their anticoagulant or hypoglycaemic dose is required.

Aspirin: Concomitant administration with aspirin in normal volunteers significantly depressed plasma levels of the active sulphide metabolite. Clinical study of the combination showed an increase in GI side effects with no improvement in the therapeutic response to Clinoril. The combination is not recommended.

Diflunisal: Concomitant administration with diflunisal in normal volunteers reduced the plasma level of active sulphide metabolite by approximately one-third.

Other NSAIDs: The concomitant use of Clinoril with other NSAIDs is not recommended due to the increased possibility of gastro-intestinal toxicity, with little or no increase in efficacy.

Probenecid: Probenecid given concomitantly with sulindac had only a slight effect on plasma sulphide levels, while plasma levels of sulindac and sulphone were increased. Sulindac was shown to produce a modest reduction in the uricosuric action of probenecid which probably is not usually significant.

Dextropropoxyphene hydrochloride/paracetamol: Neither dextropropoxyphene hydrochloride nor paracetamol had any effect on the plasma levels of sulindac or its sulphide metabolite.

Antacids: In a drug interaction study, an antacid (magnesium and aluminium hydroxides in suspension) was administered with Clinoril with no significant difference in absorption.

Antihypertensive agents: In contrast to most other non-steroidal anti-inflammatory drugs, Clinoril does not reduce the antihypertensive effect of thiazides and a variety of other agents used to treat mild to moderate hypertension. However, the blood pressure of patients taking Clinoril with antihypertensive agents should be closely monitored.

Pregnancy and lactation

Use in pregnancy: Clinoril should be used during the first two trimesters of pregnancy only if the potential benefit justifies the potential risk to the fetus.

The known effects of drugs of this class on the human fetus during the third trimester of pregnancy include: constriction of the ductus arteriosus prenatally, tricuspid incompetence, and pulmonary hypertension; non-closure of the ductus arteriosus postnatally which may be resistant to medical management; myocardial degenerative changes, platelet dysfunction with resultant bleeding, intracranial bleeding, renal dysfunction or failure, renal injury/dysgenesis which may result in prolonged or permanent renal failure, oligohydramnios, gastro-intestinal bleeding or perforation and increased risk of necrotising enterocolitis. Use of Clinoril during the third trimester of pregnancy is not recommended.

Use in breast-feeding: It is not known whether sulindac is excreted in human milk. Because other drugs of this class are excreted in human milk, a decision should be made whether to discontinue breast-feeding or discontinue the drug, taking into account the importance of the drug to the mother.

Effects on ability to drive and use machines: Clinoril may cause dizziness in some people. Patients taking the product should not drive or operate machinery unless it has been shown not to interfere with their physical or mental ability.

Undesirable effects: Clinoril is generally well tolerated. Those side-effects experienced are usually mild and may often respond to a reduction in dosage.

Side effects reported frequently

Gastro-intestinal: The most frequent types of side effects occurring with Clinoril are gastro-intestinal; these include gastro-intestinal pain, dyspepsia, nausea with or without vomiting, diarrhoea, constipation, flatulence, anorexia, and gastro-intestinal cramps.

Dermatological: Rash, pruritus.

Central nervous system: Dizziness, headache, nervousness.

Special senses: Tinnitus.

Miscellaneous: Oedema.

Side effects reported less frequently:

The following side effects were reported less frequently. The probability exists of a causal relationship between Clinoril and these side effects:

Gastro-intestinal: Stomatitis, gastritis or gastroenteritis. Peptic ulcer, colitis, as well as gastro-intestinal bleeding and gastro-intestinal perforations have been reported rarely. Fatalities have occurred. Liver-function test abnormalities, jaundice sometimes with fever, cholestasis, hepatitis, hepatic failure, pancreatitis, ageusia, glossitis, and intestinal strictures (diaphragms).

It has also been reported that a probable sulindac metabolite has been found in biliary sludge in patients with symptoms of cholecystitis who underwent a cholecystectomy.

Dermatological: Sore or dry mucous membranes, alopecia, photosensitivity, erythema multiforme, toxic epidermal necrolysis, Stevens-Johnson syndrome, exfoliative dermatitis.

Cardiovascular: Congestive heart failure, especially in patients with marginal cardiac function; palpitation, hypertension.

Haematological: Thrombocytopenia; ecchymosis; purpura; leucopenia; agranulocytosis; neutropenia; bone-marrow depression, including aplastic anaemia; haemolytic anaemia, increased prothrombin time in patients on oral anticoagulants.

Genito-urinary: Urine discoloration, dysuria, vaginal bleeding, haematuria, proteinuria, crystalluria, renal impairment including renal failure, interstitial nephritis, nephrotic syndrome.

Nervous system: Vertigo, somnolence, insomnia, sweating, asthenia, paraesthesia, convulsions, syncope, depression, psychic disturbances including acute psychosis, aseptic meningitis.

Metabolic: hyperkalaemia.

Musculoskeletal: Muscle weakness.

Special senses: Visual disturbances including blurred vision, decreased hearing, metallic or bitter taste.

Respiratory: Epistaxis.

Hypersensitivity reactions: Anaphylaxis and angioneurotic oedema. Bronchial spasm, dyspnoea, hypersensitivity vasculitis, hypersensitivity syndrome (see *Special warnings and precautions for use*).

Causal relationship unknown: Other reactions have been reported in clinical trials or since the drug was marketed, but occurred under circumstances where a causal relationship could not be established. However, in these rarely reported events, that possibility cannot be excluded. Therefore, these observations are listed to serve as alerting information to physicians.

Cardiovascular: Arrhythmia.

Metabolic: Hyperglycaemia.

Nervous system: Neuritis.

Special senses: Disturbances of the retina and its vasculature.

Miscellaneous: Gynaecomastia.

Rarely, occurrences of fulminant necrotising fasciitis, particularly in association with Group A β-haemolytic streptococcus, has been described in persons treated with non-steroidal anti-inflammatory agents, sometimes with fatal outcome (see *Special warnings and precautions for use*).

Overdose: Cases of overdosage have been reported and, rarely, fatalities have occurred. The following signs and symptoms may be observed following overdosage: stupor, coma, diminished urine output and hypotension. In isolated cases patients have received up to 600 mg a day without adverse consequences being reported.

In the event of acute overdosage, if ingestion is recent, the stomach should be emptied by inducing vomiting or by gastric lavage, and the patient carefully observed and given symptomatic and supportive treatment.

Animal studies show that absorption is decreased by the prompt administration of activated charcoal, and excretion is enhanced by alkalinisation of the urine.

The readiness of sulindac and its metabolites to dialyse is unknown at present. But because they are highly bound to plasma proteins, dialysis is not likely to be effective.

The mean half-life of sulindac is 7.8 hours while the mean half-life of the active sulphide metabolite is 16.4 hours.

Pharmacological properties

Pharmacodynamic properties: Clinoril is a non-steroidal, antirheumatic agent with anti-inflammatory analgesic and antipyretic properties. It is not a salicylate, propionic acid, pyrazolone or corticosteroid.

Prostaglandin synthetase inhibition has been hypothesised to be the mechanism of action of non-steroidal anti-inflammatory agents. Following absorption, sulindac undergoes two major biotransformations: reversible reduction to the sulphide metabolite, and irreversible oxidation to the inactive sulphone metabolite. The sulphide metabolite is a potent inhibitor of prostaglandin synthesis and available evidence indicates that the biological activity of Clinoril resides with the sulphide metabolite, thus the sulphoxide form (sulindac) is a prodrug.

Pharmacokinetic properties: Sulindac is approximately 90% absorbed in man after oral administration. The peak plasma concentrations of the biologically active sulphide metabolite are achieved in about two hours when sulindac is administered in the fasting state; and in about three to four hours when sulindac is administered with food. The mean half-life of sulindac is 7.8 hours, while the mean half-life of the sulphide metabolite is 16.4 hours. Sustained plasma levels of the sulphide metabolite are consistent with a prolonged anti-inflammatory action.

Sulindac and its sulphone metabolite undergo extensive enterohepatic circulation relative to the sulphide metabolite. The enterohepatic circulation together with the reversible metabolism are probably major contributors to sustained plasma levels of the active drug.

The primary route of excretion in man is via the urine as both sulindac and its sulphone metabolite and glucoronide conjugates. Approximately 50% of an oral dose is excreted in the urine, with the conjugated sulphone metabolite accounting for the major portion. Approximately 25% of an oral dose is found in the faeces, primarily as the sulphone and sulphide metabolutes.

The bioavailability of sulindac and the active metabolite from the oral liquid is greater than 90% of that of the tablet.

Preclinical safety data: No relevant information.

Pharmaceutical particulars

List of excipients: Cellulose microcrystalline PhEur, pregelatinised maize starch BP, magnesium stearate PhEur, and purified water PhEur. (An alternative method of manufacture uses maize starch PhEur instead of pregelatinised maize starch BP.)

Incompatibilities: None known.

Shelf life: 60 months.

Special precautions for storage: Keep container well closed, stored in a dry place, below 25°C, protected from light.

Nature and contents of container: Blister packs containing 60 tablets.

Instructions for use/handling: None.

Marketing authorisation number

100 mg, PL 0025/0121
200 mg, PL 0025/0122

Date of first authorisation/renewal of authorisation

Clinoril 100 mg Tablets first granted 5 January 1997. Last renewed 17 June 1997.
Clinoril 200 mg Tablets first granted 5 January 1997. Last renewed 17 June 1997.

Date of revision of the text July 1997.

Legal category POM

COGENTIN* TABLETS
COGENTIN* INJECTION

Qualitative and quantitative composition Each tablet of Cogentin contains 2 mg of Benztropine Mesylate BP.

Each sterile injection of Cogentin contains 0.1% w/v Benztropine Mesylate BP.

Pharmaceutical form Cogentin Tablets are supplied as white, quarter-scored tablets, marked 'MSD 60'.

Cogentin Injection is supplied as a colourless, sterile solution for injection.

Clinical particulars

Therapeutic indications: Cogentin is an anti-parkinsonian agent with powerful anticholinergic effects.

It is indicated for symptomatic treatment of all types of 'classical' parkinsonism including arteriosclerotic, post-encephalitic, and idiopathic parkinsonism, and of extrapyramidal reactions induced by phenothiazines or reserpine.

Cogentin is particularly effective in the relief of rigidity and tremor. Among other symptoms which it can ameliorate are: sialorrhoea, drooling, mask-like facies, oculogyric crises, speech and writing difficulties, gait disturbances, dysphagia, and pain and insomnia due to muscle spasm and cramps.

Cogentin often is helpful in patients who have become unresponsive to other agents. Therapy is directed toward control of disturbing symptoms to permit the patient maximum integration of function with minimum discomfort. In non-drug-induced parkinsonism, partial control of symptoms is usually achieved.

Cogentin Injection is only to be used in an emergency or when a patient is unable to swallow tablets.

Posology and method of administration: As Cogentin is cumulative in action, treatment should begin with a low dosage, which can be increased by amounts of 0.5 mg at intervals of five to six days, to the smallest dosage necessary for optimal relief without excessive side-effects. Maximum dosage, 6 mg a day.

Cogentin Injection may be used intramuscularly or intravenously in emergencies, or for patients unable to swallow tablets. (As there is no significant difference in time of onset of effect between intramuscular and intravenous administration, the intravenous route is not usually necessary.)

In emergencies, 1–2 ml (1–2 mg) of Cogentin Injection will normally provide quick relief. If signs of parkinsonism begin to return, the dose can be repeated.

'Classical' parkinsonism: Usual dosage: 1–2 mg a day, with a range of 0.5–6 mg a day. Dosage must be adjusted on an individual basis, taking into consideration the age and weight of the patient, and the type of parkinsonism. Older patients, thin patients and those with arteriosclerotic parkinsonism usually cannot tolerate large dosages. Most patients with post-encephalitic parkinsonism need and indeed tolerate fairly large dosages. Patients with a poor mental outlook may respond poorly. In arteriosclerotic and idiopathic parkinsonism, therapy may be initiated with a single daily dose of 0.5–1 mg at bedtime. This dosage will be adequate in some patients, whereas 4–6 mg a day may be required by others. In post-encephalitic parkinsonism, therapy may be initiated in most patients with 2 mg a day in one or more doses. In highly sensitive individuals, therapy may be initiated with 0.5 mg at bedtime, and increased as necessary.

Some patients obtain greatest relief by taking the entire dose at bedtime; others react more favourably to divided dosage, two to four times a day. One dose a day frequently is sufficient; divided doses may be unnecessary or even undesirable.

Drug-induced parkinsonism: Usual dosage range: 1–4 mg once or twice a day.

Acute dystonic reactions: 1–2 ml (1–2 mg) by intravenous injection followed usually by 1–2 mg orally twice a day.

Extrapyramidal reactions appearing soon after starting phenothiazine or reserpine therapy are likely to be temporary, and are usually controlled in one or two days by 1–2 mg of Cogentin orally two or three times a day. Cogentin should be withdrawn after one or two weeks to determine if it is still needed. It can be reinstated if necessary.

Certain extrapyramidal reactions which develop slowly (e.g. tardive dyskinesia) do not usually respond to Cogentin.

Paediatric use: Use with caution in children over 3 years old (see *Contra-indications*).

Use in the elderly: As with younger patients, dosage should be the smallest possible for optimum relief of symptoms. Initial dosage should be 0.5–1 mg preferably at night, increasing until optimum effect is seen. Older patients usually cannot tolerate large doses.

Contra-indications: Because of the atropine-like side effects, Cogentin is contra-indicated in children under 3 years old and should be used with caution in older children. Cogentin is contra-indicated in patients who are hypersensitive to this product.

Special warnings and special precautions for use: Continued supervision of patients is recommended as Cogentin has a cumulative action. Patients with a tendency towards tachycardia and those with prostatic hypertrophy, should be closely observed.

Patients with mental disorders should be carefully supervised when Cogentin is used to control drug-induced extrapyramidal reactions, especially when therapy is started or the dosage of Cogentin is increased. Intensification of mental symptoms may occasionally occur. Cogentin should be temporarily withdrawn if the reactions are severe.

Cogentin has anticholinergic effects, and glaucoma is a possibility. Although Cogentin does not appear to have any adverse effect on simple glaucoma, its use is probably not advisable in narrow-angle glaucoma. It may cause anhidrosis; this should be borne in mind, particularly in hot weather, especially when given concomitantly with other atropine-like drugs to the chronically ill, alcoholics, or patients with a central nervous system disease and those who do manual labour in a hot environment. Cogentin should be used cautiously in patients with or prone to abnormalities of sweating. If there is evidence of anhidrosis, the possibility of hyperthermia should be considered. Dosage should be decreased as necessary to maintain body heat equilibrium by the action of perspiration. Severe anhidrosis and fatal hyperthermia have occurred.

Interaction with other medicaments and other forms of interaction: Extra care should be taken when Cogentin is given concomitantly with phenothiazines, haloperidol or other drugs with anticholinergic or antidopaminergic activity. Patients should be advised to report gastro-intestinal complaints, fever or heat intolerance promptly. Paralytic ileus, sometimes fatal, has occurred in patients taking anticholinergic-type anti-parkinsonian drugs, including Cogentin, in combination with phenothiazines and/or tricyclic antidepressants.

Tardive dyskinesia may appear in some patients on long-term therapy with phenothiazines or related agents, or after discontinuation of such therapy. Anti-parkinsonian agents do not usually alleviate symptoms of tardive dyskinesia, and in some cases may aggravate or unmask them. Cogentin is not recommended in tardive dyskinesia.

Pregnancy and lactation: It is not known whether Cogentin can cause foetal harm when administered to a pregnant woman or can affect reproductive capacity. Cogentin should be given to a pregnant woman only if clearly needed.

Breast-feeding mothers: It is not known whether this drug is excreted in human milk. Because many drugs are excreted in human milk, caution should be exercised when Cogentin is administered to a breast-feeding mother.

Effects on ability to drive and use machines: Cogentin may impair the mental alertness and physical ability required for the performance of such hazardous tasks as driving a car or operating machinery.

Undesirable effects: Side-effects, most of which are anticholinergic or antihistaminic in nature are listed below by body system in order of decreasing severity.

Cardiovascular: Tachycardia.

Digestive: Constipation, dry mouth, nausea, vomiting.

If dry mouth is so severe that there is difficulty in swallowing or speaking, or loss of appetite and weight occur, reduce dosage, or discontinue the drug temporarily.

Slight reduction in dosage may control nausea and still give sufficient relief of symptoms. Vomiting may be controlled by temporary discontinuation, followed by resumption at a lower dosage.

Nervous system: Toxic psychosis, including confusion, disorientation, memory impairment, visual hallucinations; exacerbation of pre-existing psychotic symptoms; nervousness; depression; listlessness; numbness of fingers.

Special senses: Blurred vision, dilated pupils.

Urogenital: Urinary retention, dysuria.

Metabolic/immune and skin: Occasionally, an allergic reaction, e.g., skin rash, develops. If this cannot be controlled by dosage reduction, the medication should be discontinued.

Other: Heat stroke, hyperthermia, fever.

Overdosage: Symptoms may be any of those seen in atropine poisoning or antihistamine overdosage: CNS depression, preceded or followed by stimulation; confusion; nervousness; listlessness; intensification of mental symptoms or toxic psychosis in patients with mental illness being treated with neuroleptic drugs (e.g. phenothiazines); hallucinations (especially visual); dizziness; muscle weakness; ataxia; dry mouth; mydriasis; blurred vision; palpitations; tachycardia; nausea; vomiting; dysuria; numbness of fingers; dysphagia, allergic reactions, e.g. skin rash; headache; hot, dry, flushed skin; delirium; coma; shock; convulsions; respiratory arrest; anhidrosis; hyperthermia; glaucoma; constipation.

Physostigmine salicylate (1–2 mg, subcutaneously or intravenously) is reported to reverse symptoms of anticholinergic intoxication. A second injection may be given after two hours if needed. Otherwise, treatment is symptomatic and supportive.

If ingestion is recent, emesis should be induced or gastric lavage performed. A short-acting barbiturate may be used for CNS excitement, but with caution to avoid subsequent depression. Supportive care for CNS depression may be required (such convulsant stimulants as picrotoxin, leptazol or bemegride should be avoided). In severe respiratory depression, artificial respiration may be required. Also needed may be a local miotic for mydriasis and cycloplegia, ice bags or other cold applications and alcohol sponges for hyperpyrexia, a vasopressor and fluids for circulatory collapse, and a darkened room for photophobia.

Data on the metabolism of benztropine maleate are not available at present; but a death was recorded 1½ hours after ingestion.

Pharmacological properties
Pharmacodynamic properties: Anticholinergic drugs exert their anti-parkinsonian effect by correcting the relating cholinergic excess which is thought to occur in parkinsonism as a result of dopamine deficiency.

The deficiency of dopamine in the striatum of patients with parkinsonism intensifies the excitatory effects of the cholinergic system within the striatum. Anticholinergics aid such patients by blunting this component of the nigrostriated pathway.

Pharmacokinetic properties: Following i.m. injection, the clinical effects of benztropine are apparent within 10 minutes and the maximal effect is seen within 30 minutes.

Benztropine has a cumulative effect and a prolonged duration of action when compared with other anticholinergic agents used in the treatment of Parkinson's disease such as trihexyphenidyl. In patients on long-term maintenance therapy, it may take up to seven days before all evidence of drug-related effects have ceased.

Preclinical safety data: No relevant information.

Pharmaceutical particulars
List of excipients:

Cogentin Tablets: Calcium hydrogen phosphate PhEur, cellulose powder PhEur, lactose PhEur, magnesium stearate PhEur E572, and maize starch PhEur.

Cogentin Injection: Sodium chloride PhEur, and water for injection PhEur.

Incompatibilities: None known.

Shelf life: 60 months.

Special precautions for storage: Congentin Tablets: Store below 25°C.

Cogentin Injection: Store below 25°C, protected from light and freezing.

Nature and contents of container: Congentin Tablets: Polypropylene bottles of 500 or 60.

Congentin Injection: Type I glass ampoules of 2 ml.

Instructions for use/handling: None.

Marketing authorisation numbers Cogentin Tablet: PL 0025/5023R
Cogentin Injection PL 0025/5024R.

Date of first authorisation/renewal of authorisation Reviewed licence: 25 September 1986.
Renewal: 12 December 1996.

Date of (partial) revision of the text December 1997.

Legal category POM.

CONCORDIN*

Presentation Concordin-5, salmon-red, film-coated tablets, marked 'MSD 26', containing 5 mg Protriptyline Hydrochloride BP.

Concordin-10, white, film-coated tablets, marked 'MSD 47', containing 10 mg Protriptyline Hydrochloride BP.

Uses Symptoms of depressive illness.

Concordin may be used successfully in depression that is a manifestation of psychosis or neurosis, whether endogenous or reactive. Endogenous depression is more likely to respond. Concordin is especially recommended in apathetic, withdrawn patients, because it promptly relieves anergia, and it lacks sedative activity.

The following 'target' symptoms of depression may be expected to respond well to Concordin: depressed mood; excessive crying; apathy; withdrawal; psychomotor retardation; loss of interest; fatigue; lassitude; feelings of guilt; anorexia; headache; functional somatic complaints (e.g. gastro-intestinal symptoms).

Dosage and administration Dosage should be adjusted for each patient, bearing in mind the cyclic nature and variable severity of depression, the danger of relapse, and the possibility of spontaneous remission.

Adults: Dosage range, 15–60 mg. Usual starting dosage, 30–40 mg a day, divided into 3 or 4 doses. Any increase in dosage should be made gradually, and added to the morning dose first. If insomnia is present, the last dose should be given no later than mid-afternoon. When a satisfactory response is noted, the dosage should be reduced to the smallest amount necessary to maintain relief. Maintenance therapy should be continued for at least three months after satisfactory improvement. If relapse occurs, Concordin may be reinstated.

If the dosage required for adequate antidepressant effect produces overstimulation, concurrent use of a tranquilliser will provide effective control. Overstimulation is unlikely if the dosage of Concordin is kept below 20 mg a day.

Therapy may be usefully initiated with a tranquilliser and preventive supervision in suicidal patients, because these patients usually have a high level of anxiety, and Concordin may relieve anergia before recovery from depression is complete.

Children: Concordin is not recommended for children under 16 years old.

Elderly patients: Initially 5 mg three times a day. These patients may not tolerate higher doses as well as other patients. If the elderly receive more than 20 mg a day, they should be observed for effects on the cardiovascular system.

Contra-indications, warnings, etc
Contra-indications: Hypersensitivity to any component of this product. Concurrent use with a monoamine oxidase inhibitor. Hyperpyretic crises, severe convulsions, and deaths have occurred when tricyclic antidepressants and MAOIs have been given simultaneously (see also 'Precautions'); the acute recovery phase after recent myocardial infarction; known sensitivity to protriptyline. Any degree of heart block or other cardiac arrhythmias, mania, marked agitation, severe liver disease, during breast feeding. For 'Use in pregnancy', see 'Precautions'.

Precautions: Protriptyline should be used with caution in patients with a history of epilepsy, impaired liver function, a tendency to urinary retention, prostatic hypertrophy, or increased intra-ocular pressure.

Concordin should be used cautiously in elderly patients and patients with cardiovascular disorders. Such patients should be closely observed because of the tendency of protriptyline to produce tachycardia, hypotension, arrhythmias, and prolongation of the conduction time. The elderly are particularly liable to experience agitation and confusion. Myocardial infarction and stroke have occurred with drugs of this class.

Protriptyline may impair abilities needed for performing hazardous tasks, such as driving a vehicle or operating machinery.

In patients who may use alcohol excessively, potentiation may increase the danger inherent in any suicide attempt or overdosage.

Psychotic symtoms may be aggravated when Concodin is used in schizophrenic patients. Manic depressive patients may shift towards the manic phase. Paranoid delusions, with or without hostility, may be exaggerated. In any of these circumstances, it may be advisable to reduce the dosage, or to use a major tranquilliser concurrently.

Concordin may aggravate anxiety or agitation in over-active or agitated patients.

The possibility of suicide in depressed patients remains during treatment until significant remission has occurred; suicidal patients should not have access to large quantities of Concordin tablets and should be carefully supervised.

The natural course of depression often is of many months' duration. It is appropriate, therefore, to continue maintenance therapy for three months or longer to lessen the possibility of relapse.

Discontinue the drug several days before elective surgery if possible.

Drug interactions: A minimum of 14 days should elapse between discontinuing a monoamine oxidase inhibitor and introducing Concordin, which should then be started cautiously, with gradual increases in dosage until optimum response is achieved.

Protriptyline may block the antihypertensive effect of guanethidine, debrisoquine, bethanidine, and possibly clonidine or similar compounds. Review all antihypertensive therapy during treatment.

Protriptyline should not be given with sympathomimetic agents such as ephedrine, isoprenaline, noradrenaline, phenylephrine, and phenylpropanolamine.

Protriptyline may enhance the response to alcohol and the effects of barbiturates and other CNS depressants.

Cimetidine is reported to reduce hepatic metabolism of certain tricyclic antidepressants.

Concurrent administration of Concordin may increase the hazards of electroconvulsive therapy. Such combined treatment should be limited to those for whom it is essential.

Anaesthetics given during tricyclic antidepressant therapy may increase the risk of arrhythmias and hypotension. If surgery is necessary, the anaesthetist should be informed that the patient is receiving protriptyline.

On rare occasions, hyperthyroid patients or those receiving thyroid medication may develop arrhythmias when protriptyline is given.

Use in pregnancy and lactation: Safe use in pregnancy and lactation has not been established. Avoid during pregnancy, especially during the first and last trimesters. Use in pregnant women, breast-feeding mothers or women who may become pregnant requires that possible benefits be weighed against possible hazards to the mother and child.

There is no evidence as to drug safety in human pregnancy, nor is there evidence from animal work that it is free from hazard.

Side-effects: Some of the adverse reactions below have not been specifically reported for Concordin, but are included because of the similar pharmacological properties of the tricyclic group of antidepressants. Concordin is more likely to aggravate anxiety and agitation and to produce such cardiovascular reactions as tachycardia and hypotension.

As improvement may not occur during the first two to four weeks of treatment, patients should be closely monitored during this period.

Cardiovascular: Hypotension (particularly orthostatic hypotension), hypertension, tachycardia, palpitation, myocardial infarction, arrhythmias, heart block, stroke.

Psychiatric: Confusional states (especially in the elderly) with hallucinations, disorientation, delusions, anxiety, restlessness, agitation; insomnia, panic, and nightmares; hypomania; exacerbation of psychosis.

Neurological: Numbness, tingling and paraesthesiae of extremities; incoordination, ataxia, tremors, peripheral neuropathy; extrapyramidal symptoms; seizures; alteration in EEG patterns, tinnitus, drowsiness, dizziness, weakness and fatigue; headache.

Anticholinergic: Dry mouth and rarely associated sublingual adenitis; blurred vision, disturbance of accommodation, mydriasis; constipation, paralytic ileus; hyperpyrexia; urinary retention, delayed micturition, dilatation of the urinary tract.

Allergic: Skin rash, petechiae, urticaria, itching, oedema (generally, or of face and tongue), drug fever. Some rashes have been associated with photosensitisation. In view of this, patients should avoid excessive exposure to sunlight, including sunbathing.

Haematological: Bone-marrow depression; agranulocytosis; leucopenia; eosinophilia; purpura; thrombocytopenia.

Gastro-intestinal: Nausea and vomiting, anorexia, epigastric distress, diarrhoea, peculiar taste, stomatitis, abdominal cramps, black tongue.

Endocrine: Gynaecomastia in the male; breast enlargement and galactorrhoea in the female; increased or decreased libido, impotence; testicular swelling; elevation or depression of blood sugar levels; syndrome of inappropriate ADH secretion.

Other: Jaundice (simulating obstructive); altered liver function; weight gain or loss; perspiration; flushing; urinary frequency; nocturia; parotid swelling; alopecia.

Withdrawal symptoms: Though not indicative of addiction, abrupt cessation of treatment after prolonged therapy may produce nausea, insomnia, irritability, excessive perspiration, headache and malaise.

Gradual dosage reduction has been reported to produce, within two weeks, transient symptoms including irritability, restlessness, and dream and sleep disturbance. These symptoms are not indicative of addiction. Rare instances have been reported of mania or hypomania occurring within 2–7 days following cessation of chronic therapy with tricyclic antidepressants.

Withdrawal symptoms in neonates whose mothers receive tricyclic antidepressants during the third trimester have also been reported.

Overdosage: High doses may cause temporary confusion, disturbed concentration, or transient visual hallucinations. Overdosage may cause drowsiness; hypothermia; tachycardia and other arrhythmic abnormalities, for example bundle branch block; ECG evidence of impaired conduction; congestive heart failure; dilated pupils; convulsions; severe hypotension; stupor; and coma. Other symptoms may be agitation, hyperactive reflexes, muscle rigidity, vomiting, and hyperpyrexia, or any of those listed under 'Side-effects'.

Experience in the management of overdosage with protriptyline is limited. All patients suspected of having taken an overdosage should be admitted to a hospital as soon as possible. Treatment is symptomatic and supportive. If ingestion is recent, empty the stomach as quickly as possible by emesis followed by gastric lavage upon arrival at the hospital. Following gastric lavage, activated charcoal may be administered; 20 to 30 g of activated charcoal may be given every four to six hours during the first 24 to 48 hours after ingestion. An ECG should be taken and close monitoring of cardiac function instituted if there is any sign of abnormality. Maintain an open airway and adequate fluid intake; regulate body temperature.

Anticonvulsants may be given to control convulsions.

Dialysis is of no value because of low plasma concentrations of the drug.

The intravenous administration of 1–3 mg of physostigmine salicylate is reported to reverse the symptoms of tricyclic antidepressant poisoning in humans. Because physostigmine is rapidly metabolised, the dosage of physostigmine should be repeated as required, particularly if life-threatening signs such as arrhythmias, convulsions, and deep coma recur or persist after the initial dosage of physostigmine. Because physostigmine itself may be toxic, it is not recommended for routine use.

Standard measures should be used to manage circulatory shock and metabolic acidosis. Cardiac arrhythmias may be treated with neostigmine, pyridostigmine, or propranolol. Should cardiac failure occur, the use of digitalis should be considered. Close monitoring of cardiac function for not less than five days is advisable.

Protriptyline has been estimated to have a very prolonged half-life ranging from 55 to 198 hours, which may be further prolonged in overdosage.

Pharmaceutical precautions Store below 25°C, protected from light.

Legal category POM.

Package quantities
5 mg: Blister packs of 30.
10 mg: Blister packs of 30.

Further information Concordin is a member of the tricyclic group of antidepressants. Concordin is not a monoamine oxidase inhibitor, and dietary restrictions are not necessary. Concordin has not produced addiction or habituation.

Concordin has a rapid onset of effect, which can be of particular importance where there is a risk of suicide. It is advisable, however, to administer a tranquilliser and to ensure preventative supervision when starting Concordin in suicidal patients since they usually have a high level of anxiety, and especially because Concordin may relieve the anergia before there is complete recovery from the depressed state.

When Concordin has to be used in conjunction with ECT, the total number of shock treatments required may be reduced.

Product licence numbers
5 mg 0025/5004
10 mg 0025/5005

COSMEGEN* LYOVAC* (dactinomycin MSD)

Qualitative and quantitative composition Cosmegen Lyovac is supplied as a yellow, lyophilised powder, in a vial containing 500 micrograms dactinomycin with 20 mg of mannitol.

Pharmaceutical form Lyophilised powder for reconstitution and injection.

Clinical particulars
Therapeutic indications: Dactinomycin is a cytotoxic, antineoplastic antibiotic with immunosuppressant properties.

Recommended only in the treatment, under appropriate supervision, of hospitalised patients with Wilms' tumour, rhabdomyosarcoma, and carcinoma of the testis or uterus. All other indications for dactinomycin are as yet experimental (e.g. Ewing's sarcoma, osteogenic sarcoma).

Wilms' tumour: The neoplasm responding most frequently to Cosmegen is Wilms' tumour. With low doses of both dactinomycin and radiotherapy, temporary objective improvement may be as good as, and may last longer than, that obtained with higher doses of each given alone.

Rhabdomyosarcoma: Temporary regression of the tumour and beneficial subjective results have occurred with dactinomycin in rhabdomyosarcoma, which, like most soft-tissue sarcomas, is comparatively radioresistant.

Carcinoma of the testis and uterus: The sequential use of dactinomycin and methotrexate, along with meticulous monitoring of human chorionic gonadotrophin levels until normal, has resulted in survival in the majority of women with metastatic choriocarcinoma.

Sequential therapy is used if there is:
(1) stability in gonadotrophin titres following two successive courses of an agent.
(2) rising gonadotrophin titres during treatment.
(3) severe toxicity preventing adequate therapy.

In patients with non-metastatic choriocarcinoma, dactinomycin or methotrexate or both have been used successfully with or without surgery.

Cosmegen has been beneficial as a single agent in the treatment of metastatic non-seminomatous testicular carcinoma.

Other neoplasms: Dactinomycin has been given intravenously or by regional perfusion, alone or with other antineoplastic compounds or with X-ray therapy, in the palliative treatment of Ewing's sarcoma and sarcoma botryoides. For non-metastatic Ewing's sarcoma, promising results were obtained when dactinomycin (45 micrograms/m²) and cyclophosphamide (1,200 mg/m²) were given sequentially and with radiotherapy over an 18-month period. Those with metastatic disease remain the subject of continued investigation with a more aggressive chemotherapeutic regimen employed initially.

Temporary objective improvement and relief of pain and discomfort have followed the use of dactinomycin, usually in conjunction with radiotherapy for sarcoma botryoides. This palliative effect ranges from transitory inhibition of tumour growth to a considerable but temporary regression in tumour size.

Cosmegen and radiation therapy: Much evidence suggests that Cosmegen potentiates the effects of X-ray therapy. The converse also appears likely: that Cosmegen may be more effective when radiation therapy is given concurrently.

With combined Cosmegen and radiation therapy, the normal skin, as well as the buccal and pharyngeal mucosa, shows early erythema. When given with dactinomycin, a smaller than usual X-ray dose causes erythema and vesiculation, which progresses more rapidly through the stages of tanning and desquamation.

Healing may occur in four to six weeks rather than in two to three months. Erythema from previous X-ray therapy may be reactivated by the administration of Cosmegen alone, especially when the interval between the two forms of therapy is brief. This potentiation of radiation effects represents a special problem when the irradiation treatment area includes the mucous membrane. When irradiation is directed towards the nasopharynx, the combination may produce severe oropharyngeal mucositis.

Severe reactions may ensue if high doses of both Cosmegen and radiation therapy are used, or if the patient is particularly sensitive to such combined therapy.

Because of this potentiating effect, Cosmegen may be tried in radiosensitive tumours not responding to doses of X-ray therapy that can be tolerated. Objective improvement in tumour size and activity may be observed when lower, better tolerated doses of both types of therapy are employed.

Isolation-perfusion technique: Cosmegen, alone or with other antineoplastic agents, has also been given by the isolation-perfusion technique, either as palliative treatment or as an adjunct to resection of a tumour. Some tumours that are considered resistant to chemotherapy and radiation therapy may respond when the drug is given by the perfusion technique. Neoplasms in which dactinomycin has been tried by this technique include various types of sarcoma, carcinoma and adenocarcinoma.

In some instances, tumours regressed, pain was relieved for variable periods, and surgery made possible. On other occasions, however, the outcome has been less favourable. Nevertheless, in selected cases, Cosmegen given by the perfusion technique may provide more effective palliation than when given systemically.

Posology and method of administration: Toxic reactions due to Cosmegen are frequent and may be severe, thus limiting the amount that may be given in many cases. However, the severity of toxicity varies markedly and is only partly dependent on the dosage used.

Cosmegen must be given only in short courses.

Intravenous use: The dosage of Cosmegen will vary with the tolerance of the patient, the size and location of the neoplasm, and the use of other forms of therapy. It may be necessary to reduce the usual dosage suggested below when other chemotherapy or X-ray therapy is used concurrently or has been employed previously.

The dosage of Cosmegen is calculated in micrograms. The dosage for adults or children should not exceed 15 micrograms per kg or 400–600 micrograms per square metre of body surface daily, intravenously, for five days. Calculation of the dosage for obese or oedematous patients should be on the basis of surface area in an effort to relate dosage to lean body mass.

Adults: Usually 500 micrograms a day for a maximum of five days, given intravenously.

Children: 15 micrograms per kg bodyweight a day for a maximum of five days, given intravenously. Alternatively, a total dosage of 2,500 micrograms per square metre of body surface is given intravenously over a one-week period.

Cosmegen should not normally be given to infants under the age of 12 months.

In both adults and children, a second course may be given, but not until at least three weeks have elapsed, and all evidence of toxicity has disappeared.

Isolation-perfusion technique: Administration by the isolation-perfusion technique offers certain advantages, provided leakage of the drug through the general circulation into other areas of the body is minimal. By this technique, dactinomycin is in continuous contact with the tumour for the duration of treatment. The dose may be increased well above that used by the systemic route, usually without adding to the danger of toxic effects. If the agent is confined to an isolated part, it should not interfere with the patient's defence mechanisms. Systemic absorption of toxic products from neoplastic tissue can be minimised by removing the perfusate when the procedure is finished.

The dosage schedules and the technique itself vary from one investigator to another, and the published literature should, therefore, be consulted for details. In general the following doses are suggested:

For a lower extremity or pelvis – 50 micrograms per kg bodyweight.

For an upper extremity – 35 micrograms per kg bodyweight.

It may be advisable to use lower doses in obese patients, or when previous chemotherapy or radiation therapy has been employed.

Use in the elderly: The general considerations already outlined also apply to elderly patients.

When reconstituted, the solution of dactinomycin can be added to an infusion solution of 5% dextrose injection or sodium chloride injection, either directly or into the tubing of a running intravenous infusion.

Since dactinomycin is extremely corrosive to soft tissue, precautions for materials of this nature should be observed. To avoid extravasation, the calculated dose of Cosmegen should be given through the tubing of a running intravenous infusion, so that when administration is completed, the tubing can be flushed immediately to avoid damage to the vein.

If extravasation occurs, stop the infusion and disconnect the i.v. administration set, but leave the cannula or needle *in situ*. Attempt to aspirate the extravasated drug via the cannula or needle, inject antidote if desired, and remove the cannula or needle. Elevate the limb and apply a cold compress for 45 minutes. There is no generally accepted antidote for local use, but the following have been used with some success:

Sodium thiosulphate 25% (1.6 ml+3 ml of Water for Injection).

Sodium thiosulphate 10% (4 ml+6 ml of Water for Injection).

Ascorbic acid injection (50 mg/ml) (1 ml).

In severe cases, debridement may become necessary.

Partial removal of dactinomycin from intravenous solutions by cellulose ester membrane filters used in some intravenous in-line filters has been reported.

If Cosmegen is to be injected directly into the vein without the use of an infusion, the 'two-needle' technique should be used. The calculated dose should be reconstituted and withdrawn from the vial with one sterile needle; direct injection into the vein should then be performed with another sterile needle.

Although reconstituted Cosmegen is chemically stable, the product does not contain a preservative and accidental microbial contamination might result. Any unused portion of the solution should be discarded.

Contra-indications: If Cosmegen is given at or about the time of infection with chickenpox or herpes zoster, a severe generalised disease, which may be fatal, can occur.

Special warnings and precautions for use: Cosmegen should be administered only under the supervision of a physician who is experienced in the use of a cancer chemotherapeutic agent.

Cosmegen is highly toxic and both powder and solution must be handled and administered with care. This drug is extremely corrosive to soft tissue. If extravasation occurs during intravenous use, severe damage to soft tissue will occur.

Cosmegen, like all antineoplastic agents, is a toxic drug, and very careful and frequent observation of the patient for adverse reactions is necessary. These reactions may involve any tissue of the body. The possibility of an anaphylactic reaction should be borne in mind.

An increased incidence of gastro-intestinal toxicity and bone marrow depression has been reported when dactinomycin was given with X-ray therapy.

Particular caution is necessary when administering dactinomycin within two months of irradiation for the treatment of right-sided Wilms' tumour, since hepatomegaly and elevated AST (SGOT) levels have been seen.

Nausea and vomiting due to dactinomycin make it necessary to give Cosmegen intermittently. It is extremely important to observe the patient daily for toxic side effects when combined therapy is employed, since a full course of therapy is occasionally not tolerated. If stomatitis, diarrhoea or severe haemopoietic depression appear during therapy, these drugs should be discontinued until the patient has recovered.

Recent reports indicate an increased incidence of secondary primary tumours following treatment with radiation and antineoplastic agents, such as dactinomycin. Multi-modal therapy creates the need for careful, long-term observation of cancer survivors.

Dactinomycin can affect male fertility adversely.

Laboratory tests: A variety of abnormalities of renal, hepatic and bone-marrow function have been reported in patients with neoplastic disease receiving dactinomycin. It is advisable to make frequent checks of renal, hepatic and bone-marrow functions.

Interaction with other medicaments and other forms of interaction: Much evidence suggests that Cosmegen potentiates the effects of X-ray therapy. The converse also appears likely: that Cosmegen may be more effective when radiation therapy is given concurrently. See *Cosmegen and radiation therapy.*

It has been reported that dactinomycin may interfere with bio-assay procedures for the determination of antibacterial drug levels.

Pregnancy and lactation: Dactinomycin has been shown to be teratogenic in animals and should not normally be given to pregnant women.

Dactinomycin should not be administered to mothers who are breast-feeding.

Use in children: As there is a greater frequency of toxic effects of dactinomycin in infants, Cosmegen should not normally be given to children less than 12 months old.

Effects on ability to drive and use machines: There are no data available. The potential side effects, fatigue and lethargy, should be taken into account.

Side effects: Toxic effects (except nausea and vomiting) do not usually become apparent until two to four days after a course of therapy is stopped, and may not reach a maximum before one to two weeks have elapsed. Deaths have been reported. However, side effects are usually reversible on discontinuing therapy, they include the following:

General: malaise, fatigue, lethargy, fever, myalgia, proctitis, hypocalcaemia.

Oral: cheilitis, dysphagia, oesophagitis, ulcerative stomatitis, pharyngitis.

Gastro-intestinal: anorexia, nausea, vomiting, abdominal pain, diarrhoea, gastro-intestinal ulceration, liver toxicity including ascites, hepatomegaly, hepatitis and liver-function test abnormalities. Nausea and vomiting, which occur early during the first few hours after administration, may be alleviated by giving anti-emetics.

Haematological: anaemia (even to the point of aplastic anaemia, agranulocytosis, leucopenia, thrombocytopenia, pancytopenia, reticulocytopenia). Platelet and white blood-cell counts should be done daily to detect severe haemopoietic depression. If either count shows a marked decrease, dactinomycin should be withheld to allow marrow recovery. This often takes up to three weeks.

Dermatological: alopecia, skin eruptions, acne, flare-up of erythema or increased pigmentation of previously irradiated skin.

Soft tissues: dactinomycin is extremely corrosive to soft tissues. If extravasation occurs during intravenous use, severe damage to soft tissues will occur. In at least one instance this has led to contracture of the arms.

Side effects relating especially to the isolation-perfusion technique: Complications of the perfusion technique are related mainly to the amount of drug that escapes into the systemic circulation and may consist of haemopoietic depression, increased susceptibility of infection, absorption of toxic products from massive destruction of neoplastic tissue, impaired wound healing and superficial ulceration of the gastric mucosa. Other side effects may include oedema of the extremity involved, damage to the soft tissues of the perfused area, and potentially venous thrombosis.

Overdosage: In the event of overdosage, dactinomycin therapy should be withdrawn immediately. Limited information is available on overdosage in humans. Manifestations of overdose have included nausea, vomiting, diarrhoea, stomatitis, gastro-intestinal ulceration, severe haemopoietic depression, acute renal failure and death. Treatment should be symptomatic and supportive. There is no known antidote. It is advisable to check renal, hepatic and bone-marrow functions frequently.

Pharmacological properties

Pharmacodynamic properties: Mode of action: Cosmegen inhibits the proliferation of cells by forming a stable complex with DNA and interfering with DNA-dependent RNA synthesis.

Generally, the actinomycins exert an inhibitory effect on Gram-positive and Gram-negative bacteria and on some fungi. However, the toxic properties of the actinomycins (including dactinomycin) in relation to antibacterial activity are such as to preclude their use as antibiotics in the treatment of infectious diseases.

Because the actinomycins are cytotoxic, they have an antineoplastic effect which has been demonstrated in experimental animals with various types of tumour implant. This cytotoxic action is the basis for their use in the palliative treatment of certain types of cancer.

Pharmacokinetic properties: Results of a study in patients with malignant melanoma indicate that dactinomycin (^{3}H actinomycin D) is minimally metabolised, is concentrated in nucleated cells and does not penetrate the blood brain barrier. Approximately 30% of the dose was recovered in urine and faeces in one week. The terminal plasma half-life for radioactivity was approximately 36 hours.

Preclinical safety data: The international Agency on Research on Cancer has judged that dactinomycin is a positive carcinogen in animals. Local sarcomas were produced in mice and rats after repeated subcutaneous or intraperitoneal injection. Mesenchymal tumours occurred in male F344 rats given intraperitoneal injections of 0.05 mg/kg, two to five times per week for 18 weeks. The first tumour appeared at 23 weeks.

Dactinomycin has been shown to be mutagenic in a number of test systems *in vitro* and *in vivo*, including human fibroblasts and leucocytes, and HELA cells. DNA damage and cytogenetic effects have been demonstrated in the mouse and the rat.

Adequate fertility studies have not been reported.

Impairment of fertility: Cosmegen has been shown to cause malformations and embryotoxicity in the rat, rabbit and hamster when given in doses of 50–100 mcg/kg intravenously (three to seven times the maximum recommended human dose).

Pharmaceutical particulars

List of excipients: Mannitol EP.

Incompatibilities: Use of water containing preservatives (benzyl alcohol or parabens) to reconstitute Cosmegen for injection results in the formation of a precipitate.

Shelf life: The shelf life is 60 months.

Special precautions for storage: Cosmegen Lyovac should be stored below 25°C, protected from light. Avoid freezing.

Nature and contents of container: Glass vials containing 500 micrograms dactinomycin with 20 mg mannitol.

Instructions for use/handling:

Reconstitution and administration: Cosmegen is reconstituted by adding 1.1 ml of Water for Injections BP without preservative to the vial. For injection, 1.0 ml of the reconstituted solution, which will contain 500 micrograms of dactinomycin, is withdrawn into the syringe. Only Water for Injections BP (which does not contain preservatives) should be used. Other injection fluids may cause precipitation. Cosmegen should be inspected for particulate matter and discolouration, whenever possible. The reconstituted solution is clear and gold-coloured.

It is recommended that Cosmegen is reconstituted only by trained personnel wearing protective gloves. A designated area should be set aside for this purpose and the work surface covered with disposable plastic-backed absorbent paper.

Luer-lock fittings on all syringes and sets are recommended, and use of large-bore needles or a venting needle will help to minimise back pressure and the possible formation of aerosols. Accidental splashing on to the skin or eye should be treated immediately with copious irrigation of isotonic saline or water. Pregnant staff should not handle Cosmegen.

Adequate care should be taken in the disposal of equipment after contact with Cosmegen.

Disposal of unwanted Cosmegen:

(a) Unwanted made-up solution and open empty vials: Treatment with a solution of 5% trisodium phosphate for 30 minutes has been shown to destroy dactinomycin. Approximately twice the volume of trisodium phosphate solution as made-up dactinomycin solution is considered adequate. After such treatment, vials and solution are safe for disposal by normal laboratory procedures.

(b) Unopened vials: Incinerate at high temperature (982°–1204°C [1800°–2200°F]). Allow incinerator to cool. Scrape off the residue and re-incinerate it.

Product licence number 0025/5075R.

Date of first authorisation/renewal of authorisation
Renewal date: 12 January 1991.
Approval date: 27 March 1996.

Date of revision of the text N/A.

Legal category POM.

COSOPT* ▼

Qualitative and quantitative composition Each millilitre contains 22.26 mg dorzolamide hydrochloride corresponding to 20 mg dorzolamide and 6.83 mg of timolol maleate corresponding to 5 mg timolol.

Pharmaceutical form Eye drops, solution.

Clinical particulars

Therapeutic indications: Cosopt is indicated in the treatment of elevated intraocular pressure (IOP) in patients with open-angle glaucoma, or pseudoexfoliative glaucoma when topical beta-blocker monotherapy is not sufficient.

Posology and method of administration: The dose of one drop of Cosopt in the (conjunctival sac of the) affected eye(s) two times daily.

If another ophthalmic agent is being used, Cosopt and the other agent should be administered at least ten minutes apart.

Contra-indications: Cosopt is contra-indicated in patients with:

- reactive airway disease, including bronchial asthma or a history of bronchial asthma, or severe chronic obstructive pulmonary disease
- sinus bradycardia, second- or third-degree atrioventricular block, overt cardiac failure, cardiogenic shock
- severe renal impairment (CrCl<30 ml/min) or hyperchloraemic acidosis
- hypersensitivity to any component of this product.

The above are based on the components and are not unique to the combination.

Special warnings and precautions for use: Cardiovascular/respiratory reactions: As with other topically-applied ophthalmic agents, this drug may be absorbed systemically. The timolol component is a beta-blocker. Therefore, the same types of adverse reactions found with systemic administration of beta-blockers may occur with topical administration, including worsening of Prinzmetal's angina, worsening of severe peripheral and central circulatory disorders, and hypotension.

Because of the timolol maleate component, cardiac failure should be adequately controlled before beginning therapy with Cosopt. In patients with a history of severe cardiac disease, signs of cardiac failure should be watched for and pulse rates should be checked.

Respiratory reactions and cardiac reactions, including death due to bronchospasm in patients with asthma and rarely death in association with cardiac failure, have been reported following administration of timolol maleate.

Hepatic impairment: Cosopt has not been studied in patients with hepatic impairment and therefore should be used with caution in such patients.

Immunology and hypersensitivity: As with other topically-applied ophthalmic agents, this drug may be absorbed systemically. The dorzolamide component is a sulphonamide. Therefore the same types of adverse reactions found with systemic administration of sulphonamides may occur with topical administration. If signs of serious reactions or hypersensitivity occur, discontinue use of this preparation.

In clinical studies, local ocular adverse effects, primarily conjunctivitis and lid reactions, were reported with chronic administration of dorzolamide hydrochloride ophthalmic solution. Some of these reactions had the clinical appearance and course of an allergic-type reaction that resolved upon discontinuation of drug therapy. Similar reactions have been reported with Cosopt. If such reactions are observed, discontinuation of treatment with Cosopt should be considered.

While taking β-blockers, patients with a history of atopy or a history of severe anaphylactic reaction to a variety of allergens may be more reactive to accidental, diagnostic, or therapeutic repeated challenge with such allergens. Such patients may be unresponsive to the usual doses of epinephrine (adrenaline) used to treat anaphylactic reactions.

Concomitant therapy: There is a potential for an additive effect on the known systemic effects of carbonic anhydrase inhibition in patients receiving oral and topical carbonic anhydrase inhibitors concomitantly. The concomitant administration of Cosopt and oral carbonic anhydrase inhibitors has not been studied and is not recommended.

Patients who are already receiving a beta-adrenergic blocking agent systemically and who are given Cosopt should be observed for a potential additive effect either on the intraocular pressure or on the known systemic effects of beta-blockade. The use of two topical beta-adrenergic blocking agents is not recommended.

Withdrawal of therapy: Severe prolonged hypotension has been observed in some patients after administration of systemic beta-blockers during anaesthesia. Therefore, a gradual discontinuation of Cosopt is recommended prior to scheduled surgery.

As with systemic beta-blockers, if discontinuation of ophthalmic timolol is needed in patients with coronary heart disease, therapy should be withdrawn gradually.

Additional effects of beta-blockade: Therapy with beta-blockers may mask certain symptoms of hypoglycaemia in patients with diabetes mellitus or hypoglycaemia.

Therapy with beta-blockers may mask certain symptoms of hyperthyroidism. Abrupt withdrawal of beta-blocker therapy may precipitate a worsening of symptoms.

Therapy with beta-blockers may aggravate symptoms of myasthenia gravis.

Additional effects of carbonic anhydrase inhibition: Therapy with oral anhydrase inhibitors has been associated with urolithiasis as a result of acid-base disturbances, especially in patients with a prior history of renal calculi. Although no acid-base disturbances have been observed with Cosopt, urolithiasis has been reported infrequently. Because Cosopt contains a topical carbonic anhydrase inhibitor that is absorbed systemically, patients with a prior history of renal calculi may be at increased risk of urolithiasis while using Cosopt.

Other: The management of patients with acute angle-closure glaucoma requires therapeutic interventions in addition to ocular hypotensive agents. Cosopt has not been studied in patients with acute angle-closure glaucoma.

Choroidal detachment has been reported with administration of aqueous suppressant therapy (e.g. timolol, acetazolamide) after filtration procedures.

As with the use of other antiglaucoma drugs, diminished responsiveness to ophthalmic timolol maleate after prolonged therapy has been reported in some patients. However, in clinical studies in which 164 patients have been followed for at least three years, no significant difference in mean intraocular pressure has been observed after initial stabilisation.

Contact lens use: Cosopt contains the preservative benzalkonium chloride, which may be deposited in soft cotact lenses; therefore, Cosopt should not be administered while wearing these lenses. The lenses should be removed before application of the drops and not be reinserted earlier than 15 minutes after use.

Paediatric use: Safety and effectiveness in children have not been established.

Interaction with other medicaments and other forms of interaction: Specific drug interaction studies have not been performed with Cosopt.

In clinical studies, Cosopt was used concomitantly with the following systemic medications without evidence of adverse interactions: ACE-inhibitors, calcium channel blockers, diuretics, non-steroidal anti-inflammatory drugs including aspirin, and hormones (e.g. oestrogen, insulin, thyroxine).

However, the potential exists for additive effects and production of hypotension and/or marked bradycardia when timolol maleate ophthalmic solution is administered together with oral calcium channel blockers, catecholamine-depleting drugs or beta-adrenergic blocking agents, antiarrhythmics (including amiodarone), digitalis glycosides, parasympathomimetics, narcotics and monoamine oxidase (MAO) inhibitors.

Potentiated systemic beta-blockade (e.g. decreased heart rate) has been reported during combined treatment with quinidine and timolol, possibly because quinidine inhibits the metabolism of timolol via the P-450 enzyme, CYP2D6.

The dorzolamide component of Cosopt is a carbonic anhydrase inhibitor and although administered topically, is absorbed systemically. In clinical studies, dorzolamide hydrochloride ophthalmic solution was not associated with acid-base disturbances. However, these disturbances have been reported with oral carbonic anhydrase inhibitors and have in some instances, resulted in drug interactions (e.g. toxicity associated with high-dose salicylate therapy). Therefore, the potential for such drug interactions should be considered in patients receiving Cosopt.

Although Cosopt alone has little or no effect on pupil size, mydriasis resulting from concomitant use of ophthalmic timolol maleate and epinephrine (adrenaline) has been reported occasionally.

Beta-blockers may increase the hypoglycaemic effects of antidiabetic agents.

Pregnancy and lactation

Use during pregnancy: No studies were performed in pregnant women. In rabbits given maternotoxic doses of dorzolamide associated with metabolic acidosis, malformations of the vertebral bodies were observed. Cosopt should not be used during pregnancy.

Use during lactation: It is not known whether dorzolamide is excreted in human milk. In lactating rats receiving dorzolamide, decreases in the body weight gain of offspring were observed. Timolol does appear in human milk. Cosopt should not be used during lactation.

Effects on ability to drive and use machines: Possible side effects such as blurred vision may affect some patients' ability to drive and/or operate machinery.

Undesirable effects: In clinical studies, no adverse experiences specific to Cosopt have been observed; adverse experiences have been limited to those that were reported previously with dorzolamide hydrochloride and/or timolol maleate. In general, common adverse experiences were mild and did not cause discontinuation.

During clinical studies, 1,035 patients were treated with Cosopt. Approximately 2.4% of all patients discontinued therapy with Cosopt because of local ocular adverse reactions, approximately 1.2% of all patients discontinued because of local adverse reactions suggestive of allergy or hypersensitivity (such as lid inflammation and conjunctivitis).

The most frequently reported drug-related adverse effects were: ocular burning and stinging (10.7%), taste perversion (5.8%), corneal erosion (2.0%), conjunctival injection (1.8%), blurred vision (1.4%), tearing (1.4%), and ocular itching (1.0%). Urolithiasis was reported (0.9%).

Additional side effects that have been seen with one of the components and may be potential side effects of Cosopt are:

Dorzolamide hydrochloride ophthalmic solution

- *Ocular:* eyelid inflammation, eyelid irritation, irritation including redness, pain, iridocyclitis, transient myopia (which resolved upon discontinuation)
- *Nervous system:* headache, asthenia/fatigue, dizziness, paraesthesia
- *Hypersensitivity:* signs and symptoms of systemic allergic reactions including angioderma, urticaria, pruritus, shortness of breath, rarely bronchospasm
- *Body as a whole:* rash, nausea
- *Skin:* contact dermatitis.

Timolol maleate ophthalmic solution

- *Special senses:* signs and symptoms of ocular irritation including blepharitis, keratitis, decreased corneal sensitivity, and dry eyes; visual disturbances including refractive changes (due to withdrawal of miotic therapy in some cases), diplopia, ptosis, choroidal detachment (following filtration surgery), tinnitus.
- *Cardiovascular:* bradycardia, arrhythmia, hypotension, syncope, heart block, cerebrovascular accident, cerebral ischaemia, congestive heart failure, palpitation, cardiac arrest, oedema, claudication, Raynaud's phenomenon, cold hands and feet
- *Respiratory:* bronchospasm (predominantly in patients with pre-existing bronchospastic disease), respratory failure, dyspnoea, cough
- *Body as a whole:* headache, asthenia, fatigue, chest pain
- *Integumentary:* alopecia, psoriasiform rash or exacerbation of psoriasis
- *Hypersensitivity:* signs and symptoms of allergic reactions including angiodema, urticaria, localised and generalised rash
- *Nervous system/psychiatric:* dizziness, depression, insomnia, nightmares, memory loss, increase in signs and symptoms of myasthenia gravis, paraesthesia
- *Digestive:* nausea, diarrhoea, dyspepsia, dry mouth
- *Urogenital:* decreased libido, Peyronie's disease
- *Immunologic:* systemic lupus erythematosus.

Laboratory findings: Cosopt was not associated with clinically meaningful electrolyte disturbances in clinical studies.

Overdose: No data are available in humans in regard to overdosage by accidental or deliberate ingestion of Cosopt.

There have been reports of inadvertent overdosage with timolol maleate ophthalmic solution resulting in systemic effects similar to those seen with systemic beta-adrenergic blocking agents such as dizziness, headache, shortness of breath, bradycardia, bronchospasm, and cardiac arrest. The most common signs and symptoms to be expected with overdosage of dorzolamide are electrolyte imbalance, development of an acidotic state, and possibly central nervous system effects.

Treatment should be symptomatic and supportive. Serum electrolyte levels (particularly potassium) and blood pH levels should be monitored. Studies have shown that timolol does not dialyse readily.

Pharmacological properties

Pharmacotherapeutic group: S01E D51: (Ophthalmological – Beta-Blocking Agents – Timolol – Combinations).

Pharmacodynamic properties: Mechanism of action: Cosopt is comprised of two components: dorzolamide hydrochloride and timolol maleate. Each of these two components decreases elevated intraocular pressure by reducing aqueous humour secretion, but does so by a different mechanism of action.

Dorzolamide hydrochloride is a potent inhibitor of human carbonic anhydrase II. Inhibition of carbonic anhydrase in the ciliary processes of the eye decreases aqueous humour secretion, presumably by slowing the formation of bicarbonate ions with subsequent reduction in sodium and fluid transport. Timolol maleate is a non-selective beta-adrenergic receptor blocking agent. The precise mechanism of action of timolol maleate in lowering intraocular pressure is not clearly established at this time, although a fluoroscein study and tonography studies indicate that the predominant action may be related to reduced aqueous formation. However, in some studies a slight increase in outflow facility was also observed. The combined effect of these two agents results in additional intraocular pressure reduction compared to either component administered alone.

Following topical administration, Cosopt reduces elevated intraocular pressure, whether or not associated with glaucoma. Elevated intraocular pressure is a major risk factor in the pathogenesis of optic nerve damage and glaucomatous visual field loss. Cosopt reduces intraocular pressure without the common side effects of miotics such as night blindness, accomodative spasm and pupillary constriction.

Pharmacodynamic effects: Clinical effects: Clinical studies of up to 15 months duration were conducted to compare he IOP-lowering effect of Cosopt b.i.d. (dosed morning and bedtime) to individually- and concomitantly-administered 0.5% timolol and 2.0% dorzolamide in patients with glaucoma or ocular hypertension for whom concomitant therapy was considered appropriate in the trials. This included both untreated patients and patients inadequately controlled with timolol monotherapy. The majority of patients were treated with topical beta-blocker monotherapy prior to study enrolment. In an analysis of the combined studies, the IOP-lowering effect of Cosopt b.i.d. was greater than that of monotherapy with either 2% dorzolamide t.i.d. or 0.5% timolol b.i.d. The IOP-lowering effect of Cosopt b.i.d. was equivalent to that of concomitant therapy with dorzolamide b.i.d. and timolol b.i.d. The IOP-lowering effect of Cosopt b.i.d. was demonstrated when measured at various time points throughout the day and this effect was maintained during long-term administration.

Pharmacokinetic properties: Dorzolamide hydrochloride: Unlike oral carbonic anhydrase inhibitors, topical administration of dorzolamide hydrochloride allows for the drug to exert its effects directly in the eye at substantially lower doses and therefore with less systemic exposure. In clinical trials, this resulted in a reduction in IOP without the acid-base disturbances or alteratios in electrolytes characteristic of oral carbonic anhydrase inhibitors.

When topically applied, dorzolamide reaches the systemic circulation. To assess the potential for systemic carbonic anhydrase inhibition following topical administration, drug and metabolite concentrations in red blood cells (RBCs) and plasma and carbonic anhydrase inhibition in RBCs were measured. Dorzolamide accumulates in RBCs during chronic dosing as a result of selective binding to CA-II while extremely low concentrations of free drug in plasma are maintained. The parent drug forms a single N-desethyl metabolite that inhibits CA-II less potently than the parent drug but also inhibits a less active isoenzyme (CA-I). The metabolite also accumulates in RBCs where it binds primarily to CA-I. Dorzolamide binds moderately to plasma proteins (approximately 33%). Dorzolamide is primarily excreted unchanged in the urine; the metabolte is also excreted in urine. After dosing ends, dorzolamide washes out of RBCs non-linearly, resulting in a rapid decline of drug concentration initially, followed by a slower elimination phase with a half-life of about four months.

When dorzolamide was given orally to simulate the maximum systemic exposure after long term topical ocular administration, steady state was reached within 13 weeks. At steady state, there was virtually no free drug or metabolite in plasma; CA inhibition in RBCs was less than that anticipated to be necessary for a pharmacological effect on renal function or respiration. Similar pharmacokinetic results were observed after chronic, topical administation of dorzolamide hydrochloride. However, some elderly patients with renal impairment (estimated CrCl 30–60 millilitre/min) had higher metabolite concentrations in RBCs, but no meaningful differences in carbonic anhydrase inhibition and no clinically significant systemic side effects were directly attributable to this finding.

Timolol maleate: In a study of plasma drug concentration in six subjects, the systemic exposure to timolol was determined following twice-daily topical administration of timolol maleate ophthalmic solution 0.5%. The mean peak plasma concentration following morning dosage was 0.46 ng/millilitre and following afternoon dosing was 0.35 ng/millilitre.

Preclinical safety data: The ocular and systemic safety profile of the individual components is well established. Furthermore, no adverse ocular effects were seen in animals treated topically with dorzolamide hydrochloride and timolol maleate ophthalmic solution or with concomitantly-administered dorzolamide hydrochloride and timolol maleate. *In vitro* and *in vivo* studies with each of the components did not reveal a mutagenic potential. Therefore, no significant risk of human safety is expected with therapeutic doses of Cosopt.

Pharmaceutical particulars

List of excipients: Hydroxyethylcellulose, mannitol, sodium citrate, sodium hydroxide (to adjust pH), and water for injection. Benzalkonium chloride (0.0075%) is added as preservative.

Incompatibilities: None known.

Shelf life: The shelf life is 24 months.

Cosopt should be used no longer than 4 weeks after first opening the container.

Special precautions for storage: Protect from light.

Cosopt should be used no longer than 4 weeks after first opening the container.

Nature and contents of container: The 5 ml ALP container consists of an oval, translucent, low-density polyethylene bottle with a controlled-drop tip and a yellow-coloured polypropylene cap. The tip and cap are covered with a translucent, tamper-evident, disposable overcap.

Cosopt is available in the following packaging configurations.

1×5 ml (single 5-ml container).

Instructions for use/handling: Patients should be instructed to avoid allowing the tip of the dispensing container to contact the eye or surrounding structures.

Patients should also be instructed that ocular solutions, if handled improperly, can become contaminated by common bacteria known to cause ocular infections. Serious damage to the eye and subsequent loss of vision may result from using contaminated solutions.

Marketing authorisation number PL 0025/0373.

Date of first authorisation/renewal of authorisation 4 August 1998.

Date of revision of the text N/A.

Legal category POM.

COZAAR* TABLETS 50 mg COZAAR* HALF STRENGTH TABLETS 25 mg

Qualitative and quantitative composition The active ingredient in Cozaar is losartan. Each Cozaar 50 mg Tablet contains 45.8 mg of losartan, present as 50 mg of losartan potassium.

Each Cozaar Half Strength Tablet contains 22.9 mg of losartan, present as 25 mg of losartan potassium.

Pharmaceutical form Cozaar is supplied as white, film-coated tablets with a single score line on one side and '952' on the other.

Cozaar Half Strength is supplied as white, film-coated tablets marked '951' on one side and plain on the other.

Clinical particulars

Therapeutic indications: Cozaar is indicated for the treatment of hypertension.

Posology and method of administration: The starting and maintenance dose is 50 mg once daily for most patients. The maximal antihypertensive effect is attained 3–6 weeks after initiation of therapy. Some patients may receive an additional benefit by increasing the dose to 100 mg once daily.

Use in the elderly: Patients up to 75 years: No initial dosage adjustment is necessary for this group of patients.

Patients over 75 years: Presently there is limited clinical experience in this group; a lower starting dose of 25 mg once daily is recommended.

Use in renal impairment: No initial dosage adjustment is necessary in patients with mild renal impairment (i.e. creatinine clearance 20–50 ml/min). For patients with moderate to severe renal impairment (i.e. creatinine clearance <20 ml/min) or patients on dialysis, a lower starting dose of 25 mg once daily is recommended.

Use in patients with intravascular volume depletion: For the very small proportion of patients who have intravascular volume depletion (e.g. those treated with high-dose diuretics), a starting dose of 25 mg once daily is recommended (see *Special warnings and special precautions for use*).

Use in hepatic impairment: A lower dose should be considered for patients with a history of hepatic impairment (see *Special warnings and special precautions for use*).

Cozaar may be administered with other antihypertensive agents.

Cozaar may be administered with or without food.

Contra-indications: Cozaar is contra-indicated in pregnancy (see *Pregnancy and lactation*) and in patients who are hypersensitive to any component of this product.

Special warnings and special precautions for use: In patients who are intravascularly volume depleted (e.g. those treated with high-dose diuretics), symptomatic hypotension may occur. These conditions should be corrected prior to administration of Cozaar, or a lower starting dose should be used (see *Posology and method of administration*).

Based on pharmacokinetic data which demonstrate significantly increased plasma concentrations of losartan in cirrhotic patients, a lower dose should be considered for patients with a history of hepatic impairment (see *Posology and method of administration* and *Pharmacological properties, Pharmacokinetic properties*).

As a consequence of inhibiting the renin-angiotensin-aldosterone system, changes in renal function including renal failure have been reported (in particular, in patients whose renal function is dependent on the renin-angiotensin-aldosterone system such as those with severe cardiac insufficiency or pre-existing renal dysfunction).

As with other drugs that affect the renin-angiotensin-aldosterone system, increases in blood urea and serum creatinine have also been reported in patients with bilateral renal artery stenosis or stenosis of the artery to a solitary kidney, these changes in renal function may be reversible upon discontinuation of therapy.

Cozaar should not be used with potassium-sparing diuretics.

Interaction with other medicaments and other forms of interaction: No drug interactions of clinical significance have been identified. Compounds which have been studied in clinical pharmacokinetic trials include hydrochlorothiazide, digoxin, warfarin, cimetidine, ketoconazole and and phenobarbital (phenobarbitone).

Pregnancy and lactation

Use in pregnancy: Although there is no experience with the use of Cozaar in pregnant women, animal studies with losartan potassium have demonstrated foetal and neonatal injury and death, the mechanism of which is believed to be pharmacologically mediated through effects on the renin-angiotensin-aldosterone system.

In humans, fetal renal perfusion, which is dependent upon the development of the renin-angiotensin-aldosterone system, begins in the second trimester; thus risk to the foetus increases if Cozaar is administered during the second or third trimesters of pregnancy.

When used in pregnancy during the second and third trimesters, drugs that act directly on the renin-angiotensin-aldosterone system can cause injury and even death in the developing foetus. Cozaar should not be used in pregnancy, and if pregnancy is detected Cozaar should be discontinued as soon as possible.

Use during lactation: It is not known whether losartan is excreted in human milk. However, significant levels of losartan and the active metabolite were shown to be present in rat milk. Because of the potential for adverse effects on the nursing infant, a decision should be made whether to discontinue breast-feeding or discontinue the drug, taking into account the importance of the drug to the mother.

Effects on ability to drive and use machines: There are no data to suggest that Cozaar affects the ability to drive and use machines.

Undesirable effects: Side effects have usually been mild and transient in nature and have not required discontinuation of therapy. The overall incidence of side effects reported with Cozaar was comparable to placebo.

In controlled clinical trials for essential hypertension, dizziness was the only side effect reported as drug related that occurred with an incidence greater than placebo in 1% or more of patients treated with Cozaar. In addition, dose-related orthostatic effects were seen in less than 1% of patients. Rarely, rash was reported, although the incidence in controlled clinical trials was less than placebo.

The following adverse reactions have been reported in post-marketing experience:

Hypersensitivity: Angioedema (involving swelling of the face, lips, pharynx and/or tongue) has been reported rarely in patients treated with losartan.

Gastro-intestinal: Diarrhoea, liver function abnormalities.

Musculoskeletal: Myalgia.

Nervous system/psychiatric: Migraine.

Skin: Urticaria, pruritus.

Laboratory test findings: In controlled clinical trials, clinically important changes in standard laboratory parameters were rarely associated with administration of Cozaar. Hyperkalaemia (serum potassium >5.5 mmol/l) occurred in 1.5% of patients. Serum potassium should be monitored, particularly in the elderly and patients with renal impairment. Elevations of ALT occurred rarely and usually resolved upon discontinuation of therapy.

Overdose: Significant lethality was observed in mice and rats after oral administration of 1000 mg/kg (3000 mg/m^2) and 2000 mg/kg (11,800 mg/m^2) (500 and 1000 times† the maximum recommended daily human dose), respectively.

Limited data are available in regard to overdosage in humans. The most likely manifestation of overdosage would be hypotension and tachycardia; bradycardia could occur from parasympathetic (vagal) stimulation. If symptomatic hypotension should occur, supportive treatment should be instituted.

Neither losartan nor the active metabolite can be removed by haemodialysis.

† Based on a patient weight of 50 kg.

Pharmacological properties

Pharmacodynamic properties: Losartan is an oral, specific angiotensin-II receptor (type AT_1) antagonist. Angiotensin II binds to the AT_1 receptor found in many tissues (e.g. vascular smooth muscle, adrenal gland, kidneys, and the heart) and elicits several important biological actions, including vasoconstriction and the release of aldosterone. Angiotensin II also stimulates smooth-muscle proliferation. Based on binding and pharmacological bioassays, it binds selectively to the AT_1 receptor. *In vitro* and *in vivo*, both losartan and its pharmacologically active carboxylic acid metabolite (E-3174) block all physiologically relevant actions of angiotensin II, regardless of the source or route of synthesis.

During losartan administration, removal of angiotensin-II negative feedback on renin secretion leads to increased plasma renin activity. Increases in plasma renin activity lead to increases in angiotensin II in plasma. Even with these increases, antihypertensive activity and suppression of plasma aldosterone concentration are maintained, indicating effective angiotensin-II receptor blockade.

Losartan binds selectively to the AT_1 receptor and does not bind to or block other hormone receptors or ion channels important in cardiovascular regulation. Furthermore, losartan does not inhibit ACE (kininase II), the enzyme that degrades bradykinin. Consequently, effects not directly related to blocking the AT_1 receptor, such as the potentiation of bradykinin-mediated effects, the generation of oedema (losartan 1.7%, placebo 1.9%) or fatigue (losartan 3.8%, placebo 3.9%), are not associated with losartan.

Losartan has been shown to block responses to angiotensin I and angiotensin II without affecting responses to bradykinin, a finding which is consistent with the specific mechanism of action of Losartan. In contrast, ACE inhibitors have been shown to block responses to angiotensin I and enhance responses to bradykinin without altering the response to angiotensin II, thus providing a pharmacodynamic distinction between losartan and ACE inhibitors.

A study was carried out which was specifically designed to assess the incidence of cough in patients treated with Cozaar as compared to patients treated with ACE inhibitors. In this study and in the controlled clinical trials for hypertension, the incidence of cough reported by patients receiving Cozaar or an agent not associated with ACE-inhibitor-induced cough (hydrochlorothiazide or placebo) was similar and was significantly less than in patients treated with an ACE inhibitor. In addition, in an overall analysis of 16 double-blind clinical trials in 4,131 patients, the incidence of spontaneously reported cough in patients treated with Cozaar was similar (3.1%) to that of patients treated with placebo (2.6%) or hydrochlorothiazide (4.1%), whereas the incidence with ACE inhibitors was 8.8%.

In non-diabetic hypertensive patients with proteinuria, the administration of losartan potassium significantly reduces proteinuria, fractional excretion of albumin and IgG. Losartan maintains glomerular filtration rate and reduces filtration fraction. Generally, losartan causes a decrease in serum uric acid (usually <24 μmol) which was persistent in chronic therapy.

Losartan has no effect on autonomic reflexes and no sustained effect on plasma noradrenaline.

Losartan potassium administered in doses of up to 150 mg once daily did not cause clinically important changes in fasting triglycerides, total cholesterol or HDL cholesterol in patients with hypertension. The same doses of losartan had no effect on fasting glucose levels.

In clinical studies, once-daily administration of 50 mg Cozaar to patients with mild to moderate essential hypertension produced statistically significant reductions in systolic and diastolic blood pressure; the antihypertensive effect was maintained in clinical studies for up to one year. Measurement of blood pressure at trough (24 hours post-dose) relative to peak (5–6 hours post-dose) demonstrated relatively smooth blood pressure reduction over 24 hours. The antihypertensive effect paralleled the natural diurnal rhythms. Blood pressure reduction at the end of the dosing interval was approximately 70–80% of the effect seen 5–6 hours post-dose. Discontinuation of losartan in hypertensive patients did not result in an abrupt rebound of blood pressure. Despite the significant decrease in blood pressure, administration of Cozaar had no clinically significant effect on heart rate.

The antihypertensive effect of Cozaar 50 mg is

similar to once-daily administration of enalapril 20 mg. The antihypertensive effect of once-daily administration of Cozaar 50–100 mg is comparable to once-daily administration of atenolol 50–100 mg. The effect of administration of Cozaar 50–100 mg once daily also is equivalent to felodipine extended-release 5–10 mg in older hypertensives (≥65 years) after 12 weeks of therapy.

Although Cozaar is antihypertensive in all races, as with other drugs that affect the renin-angiotensin-aldosterone system, black hypertensive patients have a smaller average response to losartan monotherapy than non-black patients.

If Cozaar is given together with thiazide-type diuretics, the blood-pressure-lowering effects are approximately additive.

Pharmacokinetic properties

Absorption: Following oral administration, losartan is well absorbed and undergoes first-pass metabolism, forming an active carboxylic acid metabolite and other inactive metabolites. The systemic bioavailability of losartan tablets is approximately 33%. Mean peak concentrations of losartan and its active metabolite are reached in 1 hour and in 3–4 hours, respectively. There was no clinically significant effect on the plasma concentration profile of losartan when the drug was administered with a standardised meal.

Distribution: Both losartan and its active metabolite are ≥99% bound to plasma proteins, primarily albumin. The volume of distribution of losartan is 34 litres. Studies in rats indicate that losartan crosses the blood-brain barrier poorly, if at all.

Biotransformation: About 14% of an intravenously or orally-administered dose of losartan is converted to its active metabolite. Following oral and intravenous administration of ^{14}C-labelled losartan potassium, circulating plasma radioactivity primarily is attributed to losartan and its active metabolite.

In addition to the active metabolite, inactive metabolites are formed, including two major metabolites formed by hydroxylation of the butyl side chain and a minor metabolite, an N-2 tetrazole glucuronide.

Elimination: Plasma clearance of losartan and its active metabolite is about 600 ml/min and 50 ml/min, respectively. Renal clearance of losartan and its active metabolite is about 74 ml/min and 26 ml/min, respectively. When losartan is administered orally, about 4% of the dose is excreted unchanged in the urine, and about 6% of the dose is excreted in the urine as active metabolite. The pharmacokinetics of losartan and its active metabolite are linear with oral losartan potassium doses up to 200 mg.

Following oral administration, plasma concentrations of losartan and its active metabolite decline polyexponentially with a terminal half-life of about 2 hours and 6–9 hours, respectively. During once-daily dosing with 100 mg, neither losartan nor its active metabolite accumulates significantly in plasma.

Both biliary and urinary excretion contribute to the elimination of losartan and its metabolites. Following an oral dose of ^{14}C-labelled losartan in man, about 35% of radioactivity is recovered in the urine and 58% in the faeces.

Characteristics in patients: Following oral administration in patients with mild to moderate alcoholic cirrhosis of the liver, plasma concentrations of losartan and its active metabolite were, respectively, 5-fold and 1.7-fold greater than those seen in young male volunteers.

Plasma concentrations of losartan are not altered in patients with creatinine clearance above 10 ml/min. Compared to patients with normal renal function, the AUC for losartan is approximately 2-fold greater in haemodialysis patients. Plasma concentrations of the active metabolite are not altered in patients with renal impairment or in haemodialysis patients. Neither losartan nor the active metabolite can be removed by haemodialysis.

Preclinical safety data: The toxic potential of losartan potassium was evaluated in a series of repeated dose oral toxicity studies of up to three months in monkeys and up to one year in rats and dogs. There were no findings that would preclude administration at the therapeutic dosage level.

Losartan potassium was not carcinogenic when administered at maximum tolerated dosage levels to rats and mice for 105 and 92 weeks, respectively. These maximum tolerated dosage levels provided respective margins of systemic exposure for losartan and its pharmacologically active metabolite over that achieved in humans treated with 50 mg of losartan of approximately 270- and 150-fold in rats and 45- and 27-fold in mice.

There was no evidence of direct genotoxicity in studies conducted with losartan potassium or its primary pharmacologically active metabolite (E-3174).

Fertility and reproductive performance were not affected in studies with male and female rats given oral doses of losartan potassium up to approximately 150 and 300 mg/kg/day, respectively. These dosages provide respective margins of systemic exposure for losartan and its pharmacologically active metabolite of approximately 150/125-fold in male rats and 300/170-fold in female rats over that achieved in man at the recommended daily dose.

Losartan potassium has been shown to produce adverse effects in rat foetuses and neonates. The effects include decreased bodyweight, mortality and/or renal toxicity. In addition, significant levels of losartan and its active metabolite were shown to be present in rat milk. Based on pharmacokinetic assessments, these findings are attributed to drug exposure in late gestation and during lactation.

Pharmaceutical particulars

List of excipients: Cozaar and Cozaar Half Strength Tablets contain the following inactive ingredients: Hydroxypropyl Cellulose PhEur; Hydroxypropyl Methylcellulose PhEur; Lactose PhEur; Magnesium Stearate PhEur; Microcrystalline Cellulose PhEur; Pregelatinised Starch BP; Titanium Dioxide PhEur.

Cozaar 50 mg also contains Carnauba Wax PhEur.

Cozaar 50 mg also contains 4.24 mg (0.108 mmol) of potassium.

Cozaar Half Strength 25 mg also contains 2.12 mg (0.054 mmol) of potassium.

Incompatibilities: None.

Shelf life: 24 months.

Special precautions for storage: Store in a dry place at temperatures below 30°C (86°F).

Nature and contents of container: White, opaque PVC/PE/PVDC blisters with aluminium foil lidding. 50 mg tablets: Pack of 28 tablets. 25 mg tablets: Pack of 7 tablets.

Instructions for use/handling: None.

Marketing authorisation numbers

50 mg tablet 0025/0324
25 mg tablet 0025/0336

Date of approval/revision of SPC September 1997.

Legal category POM.

COZAAR*-COMP 

Qualitative and quantitative composition The active ingredients in Cozaar-Comp are losartan and hydrochlorothiazide. Each Cozaar-Comp Tablet contains 45.8 mg of losartan, present as 50 mg losartan potassium, and 12.5 mg of hydrochlorothiazide PhEur.

Pharmaceutical form Cozaar-Comp is supplied as oval, yellow, film-coated tablets '717' on one side and plain on the other.

Clinical particulars

Therapeutic indications: For the treatment of hypertension in patients whose blood pressure has been stabilised on losartan and hydrochlorothiazide given separately in the same proportion.

Posology and method of administration: The usual starting and maintenance dose is 1 tablet once daily for most patients. For patients who do not respond adequately, the dosage may be increased to 2 tablets once daily. The maximum dose is 2 tablets once daily. In general, the antihypertensive effect is attained within three weeks after initiation of therapy.

Use in the elderly: Patients up to 75 years: No initial dosage adjustment is necessary for elderly patients.

Patients over 75 years: Presently there is limited clinical experience in this group. Cozaar-Comp can be initiated if the patient has already been stabilised on Cozaar. (In this age group initiation with Cozaar Half Strength is recommended.)

Use in renal impairment: No initial dosage adjustment is necessary in patients with mild renal impairment (i.e. creatinine clearance 20–50 ml/min). Cozaar-Comp is not recommended for patients with moderate to severe renal impairment (i.e. creatinine clearance <20 ml/min) or patients on dialysis.

Use in patients with intravascular volume depletion: Cozaar-Comp should not be initiated in patients who are intravascularly volume depleted (e.g. those treated with high-dose diuretics).

Use in hepatic impairment: Cozaar-Comp is not recommended for patients with hepatic impairment.

Comcomitant therapy: Cozaar-Comp may be administered with other antihypertensive agents.

Cozaar-Comp may be administered with or without food.

Use in children: Safety and efficacy in children have not been established.

Contra-indications: Cozaar-Comp is contra-indicated in pregnancy (see *Pregnancy and lactation*), in patients who are hypersensitive to any component of this product, in patients with anuria, and in patients who are hypersensitive to other sulphonamide-derived drugs.

Special warnings and special precautions for use: Losartan and hydrochlorothiazide combination tablet: Hepatic and renal impairment: Cozaar-Comp is not recommended for patients with hepatic impairment or moderate to severe renal impairment (creatinine clearance <20 ml/min) (see *Posology and method of administration*).

Losartan:

Effects on renal function: As a consequence of inhibiting the renin-angiotensin-aldosterone system, changes in renal function, including renal failure, have been reported (in particular, in patients whose renal function is dependent on the renin-angiotensin-aldosterone system, such as those with severe cardiac insufficiency or pre-existing renal dysfunction).

As with other drugs that affect the renin-angiotensin-aldosterone system, increases in blood urea and serum creatinine have also been reported in patients with bilateral renal artery stenosis or stenosis of the artery to a solitary kidney; these changes in renal function may be reversible upon discotinuation of therapy.

Hydrochlorothiazide:

Hypotension and electrolyte/fluid imbalance: As with all antihypertensive therapy, symptomatic hypotension may occur in some patients. This was rarely seen in uncomplicated hypertensive patients, but was more likely in the presence of fluid or electrolyte imbalance. Periodic determination of serum electrolytes should be performed at appropriate intervals, as in any patients receiving diuretics.

Metabolic and endocrine effects: Thiazide therapy may impair glucose tolerance. Dosage adjustment of antidiabetic agents, including insulin, may be required (see *Interaction with other medicaments and other forms of interaction*).

Thiazides may decrease urinary calcium excretion and may cause intermittent and slight elevation of serum calcium. Marked hypercalcaemia may be evidence of hidden hyperparathyroidism. Thiazides should be discontinued before carrying out tests for parathyroid function.

Increases in cholesterol and triglyceride levels may be associated with thiazide diuretic therapy.

Thiazide therapy may precipitate hyperuricaemia and/or gout in certain patients. Because losartan decreases uric acid, losartan in combination with hydrochlorothiazide attenuates the diuretic-induced hyperuricaemia.

Other: In patients receiving thiazides, hypersensitivity reactions may occur with or without a history of allergy or bronchial asthma. Exacerbation or activation of systemic lupus erythematosus has been reported with the use of thiazides.

Cozaar-Comp should not be used with potassium-sparing diuretics, without appropriate serum potassium monitoring.

Interaction with other medicaments and other forms of interaction:

Losartan: No drug interactions of clinical significance have been identified. Compounds which have been studied in clinical pharmacokinetic trials include hydrochlorothiazide, digoxin, warfarin, cimetidine, and phenobarbital (phenobarbitone) (see *Hydrochlorothiazide: alcohol, barbiturates, or narcotics* below).

Hydrochlorothiazide: When given concurrently, the following drugs may interact with thiazide diuretics:

Alcohol, barbiturates, or narcotics – potentiation of orthostatic hypotension may occur.

Antidiabetic drugs (oral agents and insulin) – dosage adjustment of the antidiabetic drug may be required.

Other antihypertensive drugs – there may be an additive effect.

Cholestyramine and colestipol resins – absorption of hydrochlorothiazide is impaired in the presence of anionic exchange resins. Single doses of either cholestyramine or colestipol resins bind the hydrochlorothiazide and reduce its absorption from the gastro-intestinal tract by up to 85% and 43%, respectively.

Corticosteroids, ACTH – there may be intensified electrolyte depletion, particularly hypokalaemia.

Pressor amines (e.g. adrenaline) – possible decreased response to pressor amines, but not sufficient to preclude their use.

Skeletal muscle relaxants, non-depolarising (e.g. tubocurarine) – possible increased responsiveness to the muscle relaxant.

Lithium – diuretic agents reduce the renal clearance of lithium and add a high risk of lithium toxicity. Therefore, concomitant use is not recommended. Refer to the prescribing information for lithium preparations before use of such preparations.

Non-steroidal anti-inflammatory drugs – in some patients, the administration of a non-steroidal anti-inflammatory agent can reduce the diuretic, natriuretic, and antihypertensive effects of diuretics.

Drug/laboratory test interactions: Because of their effects on calcium metabolism, thiazides may interfere with tests for parathyroid function (see *Special warnings and special precautions for use*).

Pregnancy and lactation:

Use during pregnancy: Although there is no experience with the use of Cozaar-Comp in pregnant women, animal studies with losartan potassium have demonstrated foetal and neonatal injury and death, the mechanism of which is believed to be pharmacologically mediated through effects on the renin-angiotensin system.

In humans, foetal renal perfusion, which is dependent upon the development of the renin-angiotensin system, begins in the second trimester; thus, risk to the foetus increases if Cozaar-Comp is administered during the second or third trimesters of pregnancy.

Thiazides cross the placental barrier and appear in cord blood. The routine use of diuretics in otherwise healthy pregnant women is not recommended and exposes mother and foetus to unnecessary hazard, including foetal or neonatal jaundice, thrombocytopenia and possibly other adverse reactions which have occurred in the adult. Diuretics do not prevent development of toxaemia of pregnancy and there is no satisfactory evidence that they are useful in the treatment of toxaemia.

When used in pregnancy during the second and third trimesters, drugs that act directly on the renin-angiotensin system can cause injury and even death to the developing foetus. When pregnancy is detected, Cozaar-Comp should be discontinued as soon as possible.

Use during lactation: It is not known whether losartan is excreted in human milk. Significant levels of losartan and the active metabolite were shown to be present in rat milk. Thiazides appear in human milk. Because of the potential for adverse effects on the breast-feeding infant, a decision should be made whether to discontinue breast-feeding or discontinue the drug, taking into account the importance of the drug to the mother.

Effects on ability to drive and use machines: There are no data to suggest that Cozaar-Comp affects the ability to drive and use machines.

Undesirable effects: In clinical trials with the combination tablet of losartan and hydrochlorothiazide, no adverse experiences peculiar to this combination drug have been observed. Adverse experiences have been limited to those that were reported previously with losartan potassium and/or hydrochlorothiazide. The overall incidence of adverse experiences reported with the combination was comparable to placebo. The percentage of discontinuations of therapy was also comparable to placebo. For the most part, adverse experiences have been mild and transient in nature and have not required discontinuation of therapy.

In controlled clinical trials for essential hypertension, dizziness was the only adverse experience reported as drug related that occurred with an incidence greater than placebo in 1% or more of patients treated with losartan potassium-hydrochlorothiazide.

The following adverse reactions have been reported in post-marketing experience:

Hypersensitivity: Angioedema (involving swelling of the face, lips, and/or tongue) has been reported rarely in patients treated with losartan.

Gastro-intestinal: Diarrhoea.

Additional side-effects that have been seen with one of the individual components and may be potential side effects with Cozaar-Comp are the following:

Losartan: Dose-related orthostatic effects liver function abnormalities, myalgia, migraine, rash, pruritis, urticaria.

Hydrochlorothiazide: Anorexia, gastric irritation, nausea, vomiting, cramping, diarrhoea, constipation, jaundice (intrahepatic cholestatic jaundice), pancreatitis, sialadenitis, vertigo, paraesthesiae, headache, xanthopsia, leucopenia, agranulocytosis, thrombocytopenia, aplastic anaemia, haemolytic anaemia, purpura, photosensitivity, fever, urticaria, necrotising angiitis (vasculitis, cutaneous vasculitis), respiratory distress (including pneumonitis and pulmonary oedema), anaphylactic reactions, toxic epidermal necrolysis, hyperglycaemia, glycosuria, hyperuricaemia, electrolyte imbalance (including hyponatraemia and hypokalaemia), renal dysfunction, interstitial nephritis, renal failure, muscle spasm, weakness, restlessness, transient blurred vision.

Laboratory test findings: In controlled clinical trials, clinically important changes in standard laboratory parameters were rarely associated with administration of Cozaar-Comp. Hyperkalaemia (serum potassium >5.5 mmol/l) occurred in 0.7% of patients, but in these trials discontinuation of Cozaar-Comp due to hyperkalaemia was not necessary. Serum potassium should be monitored, particularly in the elderly and patients with renal impairment. Elevations of ALT occurred rarely and usually resolved upon discontinuation of therapy.

Overdosage: No specific information is available on the treatment of overdosage with Cozaar-Comp. Treatment is symptomatic and supportive. Therapy with Cozaar-Comp should be discontinued and the patient observed closely. Suggested measures include induction of emesis if ingestion is recent, and correction of dehydration, electrolyte imbalance, hepatic coma, and hypotension by established procedures.

Losartan: Limited data are available in regard to overdosage in humans. The most likely manifestation of overdosage would be hypotension and tachycardia; bradycardia could occur from parasympathetic (vagal) stimulation. If symptomatic hypotension should occur, supportive treatment should be instituted.

Neither losartan nor the active metabolite can be removed by haemodialysis.

Hydrochlorothiazide: The most common signs and symptoms observed are those caused by electrolyte depletion (hypokalaemia, hypochloraemia, hyponatraemia) and dehydration resulting from excessive diuresis. If digitalis has also been administered, hypokalaemia may accentuate cardiac arrhythmias.

The degree to which hydrochlorothiazide is removed by haemodialysis has not been established.

Pharmacological properties

Pharmacodynamic properties:

Losartan and hydrochlorothiazide combination tablet: The components of Cozaar-Comp have been shown to have an additive effect on blood-pressure reduction, reducing blood pressure to a greater degree than either component alone. This effect is thought to be a result of the complimentary actions of both components. Further, as a result of its diuretic effect, hydrochlorothiazide increases plasma-renin activity, increases aldosterone secretion, decreases serum potassium, and increases the levels of angiotensin II. Administration of losartan blocks all the physiologically relevant actions of angiotensin II and through inhibition of aldosterone could tend to attenuate the potassium loss associated with the diuretic.

Losartan has been shown to have a mild and transient uricosuric effect. Hydrochlorothiazide has been shown to cause modest increases in uric acid; the combination of losartan and hydrochlorothiazide tends to attenuate the diuretic-induced hyperuricaemia.

The antihypertensive effect of Cozaar-Comp is sustained for a 24-hour period. In clinical studies of at least one year's duration, the antihypertensive effect was maintained with continued therapy. Despite the significant decrease in blood pressure, administration of Cozaar-Comp had no clinically significant effect on heart rate. In clinical trials, after 12 weeks of therapy with losartan 50 mg/hydrochlorothiazide 12.5 mg, trough sitting diastolic blood pressure was reduced by an average of up to 13.2 mm Hg.

Cozaar-Comp is effective in reducing blood pressure in males and females, blacks and non-blacks, and in younger (<65 years) and older (≥65 years) patients and is effective in all degrees of hypertension.

Losartan: Losartan is an oral, specific angiotensin-II receptor (type AT_1) antagonist. Angiotensin II binds to the AT_1 receptor found in many tissues (e.g. vascular smooth muscle, adrenal gland, kidneys, and the heart) and elicits several important biological actions, including vasoconstriction and the release of aldosterone. Angiotensin II also stimulates smooth-muscle proliferation. Based on binding and pharmacological bioassays, angiotensin II binds selectively to the AT_1 receptor. *In vitro* and *in vivo*, both losartan and its pharmacologically active carboxylic acid metabolite (E-3174) block all physiologically relevant actions of angiotensin II, regardless of the source or route of synthesis.

During losartan administration, removal of angiotensin-II negative feedback on renin secretion leads to increased plasma-renin activity. Increases in plasma-renin activity lead to increases in angiotensin II in plasma. Even with these increases, antihypertensive activity and suppression of plasma-aldosterone concentration are maintained, indicating effective angiotensin-II receptor blockade.

Losartan binds selectively to the AT_1 receptor and does not bind to or block other hormone receptors or ion channels important in cardiovascular regulation. Furthermore, losartan does not inhibit ACE (kininase II), the enzyme that degrades bradykinin. Consequently, effects not directly related to blocking the AT_1 receptor, such as the potentiation of bradykinin-mediated effects or the generation of oedema (losartan 1.7%, placebo 1.9%), are not associated with losartan.

Losartan has been shown to block responses to angiotensin I and angiotensin II without affecting responses to bradykinin, a finding which is consistent with the specific mechanism of action of losartan. In contrast, ACE inhibitors have been shown to block responses to angiotensin I and enhance responses to bradykinin without altering the response to angiotensin II, thus providing a pharmacodynamic distinction between losartan and ACE inhibitors.

A study was carried out which was specifically designed to assess the incidence of cough in patients treated with losartan as compared to patients treated with ACE inhibitors. In this study, the incidence of cough reported by patients receiving losartan or hydrochlorothiazide was similar and was significantly less than in patients treated with an ACE inhibitor. In addition, in an overall analysis of 16 double-blind clinical trials in 4,131 patients, the incidence of spontaneously reported cough in patients treated with losartan was similar (3.1%) to that of patients treated with placebo (2.6%) or hydrochlorothiazide (4.1%), whereas the incidence with ACE inhibitors was 8.8%.

In non-diabetic hypertensive patients with proteinuria, the administration of losartan potassium significantly reduces proteinuria, fractional excretion of albumin and IgG. Losartan maintains glomerular filtration rate and reduces filtration fraction. Generally, losartan causes a decrease in serum uric acid (usually <24 μmol/l) which was persistent in chronic therapy.

Losartan has no effect on autonomic reflexes and no sustained effect on plasma noradrenaline.

In clinical studies, once-daily administration of losartan to patients with mild to moderate essential hypertension produced statistically significant reductions in systolic and diastolic blood pressure; in clinical studies of up to one year the antihypertensive effect was maintained. Measurement of blood pressure at trough (24 hours post-dose) relative to peak (5–6 hours post-dose) demonstrated relatively smooth blood pressure reduction over 24 hours. The antihypertensive effect paralleled the natural diurnal rhythms. Blood-pressure reduction at the end of the dosing interval was approximately 70–80% of the effect seen 5–6 hours post-dose. Discontinuation of losartan in hypertensive patients did not result in an abrupt rebound of blood pressure. Despite the significant decrease in blood pressure, administration of losartan had no clinically significant effect on heart rate.

The antihypertensive effect of losartan 50 mg is similar to once-daily administration of enalapril 20 mg. The antihypertensive effect of once-daily administration of losartan 50–100 mg is comparable to once-daily administration of atenolol 50–100 mg. The effect of administration of losartan 50–100 mg once daily also is equivalent to felodipine extended-release 5–10 mg in older hypertensives (≥65 years) after 12 weeks of therapy.

Losartan is equally effective in males and females and in younger (<65 years) and older (≥65 years) hypertensives. Although losartan is antihypertensive in all races, as with other drugs that affect the renin-angiotensin system, black hypertensive patients have a smaller average response to losartan monotherapy than non-black patients.

When given together with thiazide-type diuretics, the blood-pressure lowering effects of losartan are approximately additive.

Hydrochlorothiazide: The mechanism of the antihypertensive effect of thiazides is unknown. Thiazides do not usually affect normal blood pressure.

Hydrochlorothiazide is a diuretic and antihypertensive. It affects the distal renal tubular mechanism of electrolyte reabsorption. Hydrochlorothiazide increases excretion of sodium and chloride in approximately equivalent amounts. Natriuresis may be accompanied by some loss of potassium and bicarbonate.

After oral use, diuresis begins within 2 hours, peaks in about 4 hours and lasts about 6 to 12 hours.

Pharmacokinetic properties:

Absorption – Losartan: Following oral administration, losartan is well absorbed and undergoes first-pass metabolism, forming an active carboxylic acid metabolite and other inactive metabolites. The systemic bioavailability of losartan tablets is approximately 33%. Mean peak concentrations of losartan and its active metabolite are reached in 1 hour and in 3–4 hours, respectively. There was no clinically significant effect on the plasma-concentration profile of losartan when the drug was administered with a standardised meal.

Distribution – Losartan: Both losartan and its active metabolite are ≥99% bound to plasma proteins, primarily albumin. The volume of distribution of losartan is 34 litres. Studies in rats indicate that losartan crosses the blood-brain barrier poorly, if at all.

Hydrochlorothiazide: Hydrochlorothiazide crosses the placental but not the blood-brain barrier and is excreted in breast milk.

Biotransformation – Losartan: About 14% of an intravenously or orally administered dose of losartan is converted to its active metabolite. Following oral and intravenous administration of ^{14}C-labelled losartan potassium, circulating plasma radioactivity primarily is attributed to losartan and its active metabolite. Minimal conversion of losartan to its active metabolite was seen in about 1% of individuals studied.

In addition to the active metabolite, inactive metabolites are formed, including two major metabolites formed by hydroxylation of the butyl side chain and a minor metabolite, an N-2 tetrazole glucuronide.

Elimination – Losartan: Plasma clearance of losartan and its active metabolite is about 600 ml/min and 50 ml/min, respectively. Renal clearance of losartan and its active metabolite is abot 74 ml/min and 26 ml/min, respectively. When losartan is administered orally, about 4% of the dose is excreted unchanged in the urine, and about 6% of the dose is excreted in the urine as active metabolite. The pharmacokinetics of losartan and its active metabolite are linear with oral losartan potassium doses up to 200 mg.

Following oral administration, plasma concentrations of losartan and its active metabolite decline polyexponentially with a terminal half-life of about 2 hours and 6–9 hours, respectively. During once-daily dosing with 100 mg, neither losartan nor its active metabolite accumulates significantly in plasma.

Both biliary and urinary excretion contribute to the elimination of losartan and its metabolites. Following an oral dose of ^{14}C-labelled losartan in man, about 35% of radioactivity is recovered in the urine and 58% in the faeces.

Hydrochlorothiazide: Hydrochlorothiazide is not metabolised but is eliminated rapidly by the kidney. When plasma levels have been followed for at least 24 hours, the plasma half-life has been observed to vary between 5.6 and 14.8 hours. At least 61% of the oral dose is eliminated unchanged within 24 hours.

Characteristics in patients – Losartan and hydrochlorothiazide combination tablet: The plasma concentrations of losartan and its active metabolite and the absorption of hydrochlorothiazide in elderly hypertensives are not significantly different from those in young hypertensives.

Losartan: Following oral administration in patients with mild to moderate alcoholic cirrhosis of the liver, plasma concentrations of losartan and its active metabolite were, respectively, fivefold and 1.7-fold greater than those seen in young male volunteers.

Neither losartan nor the active metabolite can be removed by haemodialysis.

Preclinical safety data: The toxic potential of losartan potassium and hydrochlorothiazide was evaluated in repeated-dose oral toxicity studies for up to six months in rats and dogs. There were no findings that would preclude administration to man at the therapeutic dosage level.

There was no evidence of direct genotoxicity in studies conducted with the losartan and hydrochlorothiazide combination.

Losartan potassium and hydrochlorothiazide administration had no effect on the reproductive performance or fertility in male rats at dosage levels of up to 135 mg/kg/day losartan in combination with 33.75 mg/kg/day hydrochlorothiazide. These dosage levels provided respective plasma concentrations (AUC) for losartan, the active metabolite and hydrochlorothiazide that were approximately 260-, 120-, and 50-fold greater than those achieved in man with 50 mg losartan potassium in combination with 12.5 mg hydrochlorothiazide. In female rats, however, the co-administration of losartan potassium and hydrochlorothiazide (10/2.5 mg/kg/day) induced a slight but statistically significant decrease in fecundity and fertility indices. Compared to plasma concentrations in man (see above) these dosage levels provided respective increases in plasma concentration (AUC) for losartan, the active metabolite, and hydrochlorothiazide of approximately 15-, 4-, and 5-fold.

There was no evidence of teratogenicity in rats or rabbits treated with losartan potassium and hydrochlorothiazide combination. Foetal toxicity in rats, as evidenced by a slight increase in supernumerary ribs in the F_1 generation, was observed when females were treated prior to and throughout gestation. As observed in studies with losartan alone, adverse foetal and neonatal effects, including decreased bodyweight, mortality and/or renal toxicity, also occurred when pregnant rats were treated with losartan potassium and hydrochlorothiazide combination during late gestation and/or lactation.

Pharmaceutical particulars

List of excipients: Each Cozaar-Comp Tablet contains the following inactive ingredients: Hydroxypropylcellulose PhEur; Methylhydroxypropylcellulose PhEur; Lactose Monohydrate PhEur; Magnesium Stearate PhEur; Microcrystalline Cellulose PhEur; Pregelatinised Maize Starch BP; Titanium Dioxide PhEur; Quinoline yellow aluminium lake E104; Carnauba Wax PhEur.

Cozaar-Comp also contains 4.24 mg (0.108 mmol) of potassium.

Incompatibilities: None.

Shelf life: 24 months.

Special precautions for storage: Store in a dry place at temperatures below 30°C (86°F).

Nature and contents of container: White, opaque PVC/PE/PVDC blisters with aluminium foil lidding. Available in blister calendar packs of 28 tablets.

Instructions for use/handling: None.

Marketing authorisation number 0025/0338.

Date of approval/revision of SPC January 1998.

Legal category POM.

CRIXIVAN* ▼

Qualitative and quantitative composition Crixivan 200 mg Capsules contain 250 mg of indinavir sulphate corresponding to 200 mg of indinavir.

Crixivan 400 mg Capsules contain 500 mg of indinavir sulphate corresponding to 400 mg of indinavir.

Pharmaceutical form Capsules.

Clinical particulars

Therapeutic indications: Crixivan is indicated in combination with antiretroviral nucleoside analogues for the treatment of HIV-1 infected adult patients.

Posology and method of administration: The recommended dosage of Crixivan is 800 mg orally every 8 hours.

Crixivan should be used in combination with other antiretroviral agents (i.e. nucleoside analogues).

The capsules should be swallowed whole.

Since Crixivan must be taken at intervals of 8 hours, a schedule convenient for the patient should be developed. For optimal absorption, Crixivan should be administered without food but with water 1 hour before or 2 hours after a meal. Alternatively, Crixivan may be administered with a low-fat, light meal.

To ensure adequate hydration, it is recommended that the patient drinks at least 1.5 litres of liquids during the course of 24 hours.

Due to an increase in the plasma concentrations of rifabutin and a decrease in the plasma concentrations of indinavir, a dosage reduction of rifabutin to half the standard dose (consult manufacturer's package circular for rifabutin) and a dosage increase of Crixivan to 1000–1200 mg every 8 hours are suggested when rifabutin is co-administered with Crixivan. This dose regimen has not been confirmed in clinical studies and could result in a clinically significant increase in the plasma concentrations of rifabutin.

Due to an increase in the plasma concentrations of indinavir, a dosage reduction of Crixivan to 600 mg every 8 hours should be considered when administering ketoconazole concurrently.

In patients with mild-to-moderate hepatic insufficiency due to cirrhosis, the dosage of Crixivan should be reduced to 600 mg every 8 hours.

Medical management in patients with one or more episodes of nephrolithiasis must include adequate hydration and may include temporary interruption of therapy (e.g. 1–3 days) during the acute episode of nephrolithiasis or discontinuation of therapy.

Contra-indications: Clinically significant hypersensitivity to any component of this product.

Indinavir should not be administered concurrently with drugs with narrow therapeutic windows and which are substrates of CYP3A4. Co-administration may result in competitive inhibition of the metabolism of these drugs and create the potential for serious and/or life-threatening adverse events such as cardiac arrhythmias (e.g. terfenadine, astemizole, cisapride) prolonged sedation or respiratory depression (e.g. alprazolam, triazolam, midazolam).

Indinavir should not be administered concurrently with rifampicin because co-administration results in 90% reduction in indinavir plasma concentrations.

Special warnings and special precautions for use: Nephrolithias has occurred with Crixivan. In some cases, nephrolithiasis has been associated with renal insufficiency or acute renal failure; in the majority of these cases, renal insufficiency and acute renal failure were reversible. If signs and symptoms of nephrolithiasis, including flank pain with or without haematuria (including microscopic haematuria), occur, temporary interruption of therapy (e.g. 1–3 days) during the acute episode of nephrolithiasis or discontinuation of therapy may be considered. Adequate hydration is recommended in all patients on Crixivan (see *Posology and method of administration* and *Undesirable effects, Post-marketing experience*).

Drug interactions: Indinavir should be used cautiously with other drugs that are potent inducers of CYP3A4. Co-administration may result in decreased plasma concentrations of indinavir and as a consequence an increased risk for suboptimal treatment and facilitation of development of resistance (see *Interaction with other medicinal products and other forms of interaction*).

Acute haemolytic anaemia: Acute haemolytic anaemia has been reported which in some cases was severe and progressed rapidly. Once diagnosis is apparent, appropriate measures for the treatment of haemolytic anaemia should be instituted which may include discontinuation of Crixivan.

Hyperglycaemia: New onset diabetes mellitus, hyperglycaemia or exacerbation of existing diabetes mellitus has been reported in patients receiving protase inhibitors. In some of these the hyperglycaemia was severe and in some cases also associated with ketoacidosis. Many patients had confounding medical conditions, some of which required therapy with agents that have been associated with the development of diabetes mellitus or hyperglycaemia.

Patients with coexisting conditions: There have been reports of increased bleeding, including spontaneous skin haematomas and haemarthroses, in haemophiliac patients type A and B treated with protease inhibitors. In some patients additional factor VIII was given. In more than a half of the reported cases, treatment with protease inhibitors was continued or reintroduced if treatment had been discontinued. A causal relationship has been evoked, although the mechanism of action has not been elucidated. Haemophiliac patients should therefore be made aware of the possibility of increased bleeding.

Patients with mild to moderate hepatic insufficiency due to cirrhosis will require a dosage reduction of Crixivan due to decreased metabolism of indinavir (see *Posology and method of administration*). Patients with severe hepatic impairment have not been studied. In the absence of such studies, caution should be exercised as increased levels of indinavir may occur.

Safety in patients with impaired renal function has not been studied; however, less than 20% of indinavir is excreted in the urine as unchanged drug or metabolites.

Other: In clinical trials, the majority of investigated patients were Caucasian males.

Safety and effectiveness in children have not been established.

In clinical trials, patients treated with rifampicin, rifabutin, or chronically with acyclovir were excluded. However, patients treated intermittently with acyclovir were not excluded from the clinical trials.

Each 200 mg capsule contains 74 mg lactose (anhydrous). Each 400 mg capsule contains 149 mg lactose (anhydrous). These quantities are probably not sufficient to induce specific symptoms of intolerance.

Interaction with other medicinal products and other forms of interaction: Specific drug interaction studies were performed with indinavir and the following drugs: zidovudine, zidovudine/lamivudine, stavudine, trimethoprim/sulphamethoxazole, fluconazole, isoniazid, clarithromycin, quinidine, cimetidine, and an oral contraceptive (norethindrone/ethinyl oestradiol 1/35). No clinically significant interactions were observed with these drugs. Clinically significant interactions with other drugs are described below.

A formal interaction study has not been performed between Crixivan and warfarin. Combined treatment could result in increased levels of warfarin.

Rifabutin: The co-administration of indinavir 800 mg q8h with rifabutin either 300 mg once daily or 150 mg once daily was evaluated in two separate clinical studies. The results of these studies showed a decrease in indinavir AUC (34% and 33%, respectively, vs indinavir 800 mg q8h alone) and an increase in rifabutin AUC (173% and 55%, respectively, vs rifabutin 300 mg once daily alone). This increase in rifabutin plasma concentrations is likely related to inhibition of CYP3A4-mediated metabolism of rifabutin by indinavir. A dosage increase of idinavir and a dosage reduction of rifabutin are necessary when indinavir and rifabutin are co-administered (see *Posology and method of administration*).

Ketoconazole: Administration of a 400 mg dose of ketoconazole, a potent inhibitor of CYP3A4, with a 400 mg dose of indinavir, resulted in a 62% increase in the AUC of indinavir, which is clinically significant, and a 14% increase in the C_{max} of indinavir. A dosage reduction of indinavir to 600 mg every 8 hours should be considered when indinavir and ketoconazole are co-administered.

Other: A formal drug-interaction study between indinavir and methadone has not been performed. Concomitant use may result in increased plasma concentrations of methadone. The clinical relevance of this is unknown.

A formal drug-interaction study between indinavir and itraconazole has not been performed. Because itraconazole is a potent inhibitor of CYP3A4, concomitant use could result in clinically significant increases in plasma concentrations of indinavir and this combination should be avoided.

Concomitant use of other drugs that are inducers of CYP3A4, such as phenobarbital, phenytoin, dexamethasone and carbamazepine, may reduce indinavir plasma concentrations.

The efficacy and safety of indinavir in combination with other protease inhibitors have not been established. Co-administration with ritonavir is likely to result in significant increases in plasma concentrations of indinavir.

A formal drug-interaction study between indinavir and didanosine has not been performed. However, a normal (acidic) gastric pH may be necessary for optimum absorption of indinavir whereas acid rapidly degrades didanosine which is formulated with buffering agents to increase pH. Indinavir and didanosine should be administered at least one hour apart on an empty stomach (consult the manufacturer's prescribing information for didanosine). Antiretroviral activity was unaltered when didanosine was administered three hours after treatment with indinavir in one clinical study.

For optimal absorption, indinavir should be administered with water 1 hour before or 2 hours after a meal. Alternatively, indinavir may be taken with a low-fat light meal. Ingestion of indinavir with a meal high in calories, fat and protein reduces the absorption of indinavir.

Use during pregnancy and lactation:

Use during pregnancy: Crixivan has not been studied in pregnant women. Until additional data become available, Crixivan should be used during pregnancy only if the potential benefit justifies the potential risk to the foetus.

Hyperbilirubinaemia, reported predominantly as elevated indirect bilirubin, has occurred in 10% of patients during treatment with Crixivan. Because it is unknown whether indinavir will exacerbate physiological hyperbilirubinaemia in neonates, careful consideration must be given to the use of Crixivan in pregnant women at the time of delivery (see *Undesirable effects*).

In rhesus monkeys, administration of indinavir to neonates caused a mild exacerbation of the transient physiologic hyperbilirubinemia seen in this species after birth. Administration of indinavir to pregnant Rhesus monkeys during the third trimester did not cause a similar exacerbation in neonates; however, only limited placental transfer of indinavir occurred.

Developmental toxicity studies performed in rats, rabbits and dogs (at doses which produced systemic exposures comparable to or slightly greater than human exposure) and revealed no evidence of teratogenicity. No external or visceral changes were observed in rats, however, increases in the incidence of supernumerary ribs and of cervical ribs were seen. No external, visceral, or skeletal changes were observed in rabbits or dogs. In rats and rabbits, no effects on embryonic/foetal survival or foetal weights were observed. In dogs, a slight increase in resorptions was seen; however, all foetuses in drug-treated animals were viable, and the incidence of live foetuses in drug-treated animals was comparable to that in controls.

Use during lactation: Health experts recommend that HIV-infected women should not breast-feed their infants under any circumstances in order to avoid transmission of HIV. It is not known whether indinavir is excreted in human milk. However, indinavir was shown to be present in rat milk and excretion in rat milk was also manifested as decreased pup weight gain during lactation. Until more data become available, mothers should be instructed to discontinue breast-feeding during treatment.

Effects on ability to drive and use machines: There are no data to suggest that indinavir affects the ability to drive and use machines. However, patients should be informed that dizziness and blurred vision have been reported during treatment with indinavir.

Undesirable effects: In controlled clinical trials conducted worldwide, indinavir was administered alone or in combination with other antiretroviral agents (zidovudine, didanosine, stavudine, and/or lamivudine) to approximately 2,000 patients, the majority of whom were Caucasian males (15% females).

Indinavir did not alter the type, frequency, or severity of known major adverse effects associated with the use of zidovudine, didanosine, or lamivudine.

Clinical adverse experiences reported by the investigators as possibly, probably, or definitely drug related in ≥5% of patients treated with Crixivan alone or in combination (n=309) for 24 weeks are listed below. Many of these adverse experiences were also identified as common pre-existing or frequently occurring medical conditions in this population. These adverse experiences were: nausea (35.3%), headache (25.2%), diarrhoea (24.6%), asthenia/fatigue (24.3%), rash (19.1%), taste perversion (19.1%), dry skin (16.2%), abdominal pain (14.6%), vomiting (11.0%), dizziness (10.7%), dyspepsia (10.7%), flatulence (7.8%), insomnia (7.4%), pruritus (7.4%), hypaesthesia (7.1%), dry mouth (6.8%), dysuria (6.5%), acid regurgitation (6.5%), paraesthesia (5.2%), and myalgia (5.2%). With the exception of dry skin, rash, and taste perversion, the incidence of clinical adverse experiences was similar or higher among patients treated with antiretroviral nucleoside analogue controls than among patients treated with Crixivan alone or in combination. This overall safety profile remained similar for 107 patients treated with Crixivan alone or in combination for up to 48 weeks.

Nephrolithiasis, including flank pain with or without haematuria (including microscopic haematuria), has been reported in approximately 4% (79/2205) of patients receiving Crixivan in clinical trials. In general, these events were not associated with renal dysfunction and resolved with hydration and temporary interruption of therapy (e.g. 1–3 days).

Laboratory test findings: The laboratory abnormalities reported by the investigators as possibly, probably, or definitely drug related in ≥10% of patients treated with Crixivan alone or in combination were: increases in MCV, ALT, AST, indirect bilirubin, total serum bilirubin; a decrease in neutrophils; haematuria, proteinuria, crystalluria.

Isolated asymptomatic hyperbilirubinaemia (total bilirubin ≥2.5 mg/dl, 43 mcmol/l), reported predominantly as elevated indirect bilirubin and rarely associated with elevations in ALT, AST, or alkaline phosphatase, has occurred in approximately 10% of patients treated with Crixivan alone or in combination with other antiretroviral agents. Most patients continued treatment with Crixivan without dosage reduction and bilirubin values gradually declined toward baseline. Hyperbilirubinaemia occurred more frequently at doses exceeding 2.4 g/day compared to doses less than 2.4 g/day.

Post-marketing experience: The following additional adverse reactions have been reported in post-marketing experience:

Body as a whole/site unspecified: abdominal distension; redistribution/accumulation of body fat in areas such as the back of the neck, abdomen and retroperitoneum.

Digestive system: liver function abnormalities; hepatitis including rare reports of hepatic failure (see *Special warnings and special precautions for use*).

Endocrine/Metabolic: new onset of diabetes mellitus or hyperglycaemia, or exacerbation of pre-existing diabetes mellitus (see *Special warnings and special precautions for use*).

Haematological: increased spontaneous bleeding in patients with haemophilia; acute haemolytic anaemia (see *Special warnings and special precautions for use*).

Hypersensitivity: anaphylactoid reactions.

Skin and skin appendage: rash including erythema multiforme and Stevens Johnson syndrome; hyperpigmentation; alopecia; urticaria.

Urogenital system: nephrolithiasis, in some cases with renal insufficiency or acute renal failure; (see *Special warnings and precautions for use*) interstitial nephritis.

Laboratory test findings: The following additional laboratory abnormalities have been reported:

Increased serum triglycerides.

Overdose: There have been reports of human overdosage with Crixivan. The most commonly reported symptons were gastro-intestinal (e.g. nausea, vomiting diarrhoea) and renal (e.g. nephrolithiasis flank pain, haematuria).

It is not known whether indinavir is dialysable by peritoneal or haemodialysis.

Pharmacological properties

Pharmacodynamic properties: Pharmacotherapeutic group: protease inhibitor, ATC code JO5AE02.

Mechanism of action: Indinavir inhibits recombinant HIV-1 and HIV-2 protease with an approximate tenfold selectivity for HIV-1 over HIV-2 proteinase. Indinavir binds reversibly to the protease active site and inhibits competitively the enzyme, thereby preventing cleavage of the viral precursor polyproteins that occurs during maturation of the newly formed viral particle. The resulting immature particles are non-infectious and are incapable of establishing new cycles of infection. Indinavir did not significantly inhibit the eukaryotic proteases human renin, human cathepsin D, human elastase, and human factor Xa.

Microbiology: Indinavir at concentrations of 50 to 100 nM mediated 95% inhibition (IC_{95}) of viral spread (relative to an untreated virus-infected control) in human T-lymphoid cell cultures and primary human monocytes/macrophages infected with HIV-1 variants LAI, MN, RF, and a macrophage-tropic variant SF-162, respectively. Indinavir at concentrations of 25 to 100 nM mediated 95% inhibition of viral spread in cultures of mitogen-activated human peripheral blood mononuclear cells infected with diverse, primary clinical isolates of HIV-1, including isolates resistant to zidovudine and non-nucleoside reverse transcriptase inhibitors. Synergistic antiretroviral activity was observed when human T-lymphoid cells infected with the LAI variant of HIV-1 were incubated with indinavir and either zidovudine, didanosine, or a non-nucleoside reverse transcriptase inhibitor.

Drug resistance: Loss of suppression of viral RNA levels occurred in some patients; however, CD4 cell counts were often sustained above pretreatment levels. When loss of viral RNA suppression occurred, it was typically associated with replacement of circulating susceptible virus with resistant viral variants. Resistance was correlated with the accumulation of mutations in the viral genome that resulted in the expression of amino-acid substitutions in the viral protease.

At least eleven HIV-1 protease amino-acid residue positions, at which substitutions are associated with resistance, have been identified. No single substitution was capable of engendering measurable resistance to the inhibitor. In general, higher levels of resistance result from the co-expression of greater numbers of substitutions at the eleven identified positions. Substitutions at these positions appeared to accumulate sequentially, probably as the result of ongoing viral replication.

It should be noted that the decrease in suppression of viral RNA levels was seen more frequently when therapy with Crixivan was initiated at doses lower than the recommended oral dose of 2.4 g/day. **Therefore, therapy with Crixivan should be initiated at the recommended dose to increase suppression of viral replication and therefore inhibit the emergence of resistant virus.**

The concomitant use of indinavir with nucleoside analogues (to which the patient is naive) may lessen the risk of the development of resistance to both indinavir and the nucleoside analogues. In one comparative trial, combination therapy with nucleoside analogues (triple therapy with zidovudine plus didanosine) conferred protection against the selection of virus expressing at least one resistance-associated amino-acid substitution to both indinavir (from 13/24 to 2/20 at therapy week 24) and to the nucleoside analogues (from 10/16 to 0/20 at therapy week 24).

Combination treatment with Crixivan is preferred because of the concern about the emergence of resistance.

Cross-resistance: HIV-1 patient isolates with reduced susceptibility to indinavir expressed varying patterns and degrees of cross-resistance to a series of diverse HIV protease inhibitors, including ritonavir and saquinavir. Complete cross-resistance was noted between indinavir and ritonavir; however, cross-resistance to saquinavir varied among isolates. Many of the protease amino-acid substitutions reported to be associated with resistance to ritonavir and saquinavir were also associated with resistance to indinavir.

Pharmacodynamic effects: Treatment with indinavir alone or in combination with other antiretroviral agents (i.e. nucleoside analogues) has so far been documented to reduce viral load and increase CD4 lymphocytes in patients with CD4 cell counts below 500 cells/mm^3.

In zidovudine experienced patients, indinavir, zidovudine and lamivudine in combination compared with lamivudine added to zidovudine reduced the probability of AIDS defined illness or death (ADID) at 48 weeks from 13% to 7%. Similarly, in antiretroviral naive patients, indinavir with and without zidovudine compared with zidovudine alone reduced the probability of ADID at 48 weeks from 15% with zidovudine alone to approximately 6% with indinavir alone or in combination with zidovudine.

Effects on viral load were consistently more pronounced in patients treated with indinavir in combination with nucleoside analogues, but the proportion of patients with serum viral RNA below the limit of quantification (500 copies/ml) varied betwen studies, at week 24 from 40% to more than 80%. This proportion tends to remain stable over prolonged periods to follow-up. Similarly, effects on CD4 cell count tend to be more pronounced in patients treated with indinavir in combination with nucleoside analogues compared with indinavir alone. Within studies, this effect is sustained also after prolonged periods of follow-up.

Pharmacokinetic properties:

Absorption: Indinavir is rapidly absorbed in the fasted state with a time to peak plasma concentration of 0.8 hours±0.3 hours (mean±S.D.). A greater than dose-proportional increase in indinavir plasma concentrations was observed over the 200–800 mg dose range. Between 800-mg and 1000-mg dose levels, the deviation from dose-proportionality is less pronounced. As a result of the short half-life, 1.8±0.4 hours, only a minimal increase in plasma concentrations occurred after multiple dosing. The bioavailability of a single 800 mg dose of indinavir was approximately 65% (90% CI, 58–72%).

Administration of indinavir with a meal high in calories, fat, and protein resulted in a blunted and reduced absorption with an approximate 80% reduction in AUC and an 86% reduction in C_{max}. Administration with light meals (e.g. dry toast with jam or fruit conserve, apple juice, and coffee with skimmed or fat-free milk and sugar or corn flakes, skimmed or fat-free milk and sugar) resulted in plasma concentrations comparable to the corresponding fasted values.

Distribution: Indinavir was not highly bound to human plasma proteins (39% unbound).

There are no data concerning the penetration of indinavir into the central nervous system in humans.

Biotransformation: Seven major metabolites were identified and the metabolic pathways were identified as glucuronidation at the pyridine nitrogen, pyridine-N-oxidation with and without 3′-hydroxylation on the indane ring, 3′-hydroxylation of indane, p-hydroxylation of phenylmethyl moiety, and N-depyridomethylation with and without the 3′-hydroxylation. *In vitro* studies with human liver microsomes indicated that CYP3A4 is the only P450 isozyme that plays a major role in the oxidative metabolism of indinavir. Analysis of plasma and urine samples from subjects who received indinavir indicated that indinavir metabolites had little proteinase inhibitory activity.

Elimination: Over the 200–1000 mg dose range administered in both volunteers and HIV-infected patients, there was a slightly greater than dose-proportional increase in urinary recovery of indinavir. Renal clearance (116 ml/min) of indinavir is concentration-independent over the clinical dose range. Less than 20% of indinavir is excreted renally. Mean urinary excretion of unchanged drug following single dose administration in the fasted state was 10.4% following a 700-mg dose, and 12.0% following a 1000-mg dose. Indinavir was rapidly eliminated with a half-life of 1.8 hours.

Characteristics in patients: Pharmacokinetics of indinavir do not appear to be affected by gender or by race.

Patients with mild-to-moderate hepatic insufficiency and clinical evidence of cirrhosis had evidence of decreased metabolism of indinavir resulting in approximately 60% higher mean AUC following a 400-mg dose. The mean half-life of indinavir increased to approximately 2.8 hours.

At steady state following a dosage regimen of 800 mg every 8 hours, HIV-seropositive patients in one study achieved AUC values of 28,713 nM h, peak plasma concentrations of 11,144 nM and plasma concentrations at 8 hours post dose of 211 nM.

Preclinical safety data: Crystals have been seen in the urine of rats, one monkey, and one dog. The crystals have not been associated with drug-induced renal injury. An increase in thyroidal weight and thyroidal follicular-cell hyperplasia, due to an increase in thyroxine clearance, was seen in rats treated with indinavir at doses ≥160 mg/kg/day. An increase in hepatic weight occurred in rats treated with indinavir at doses ≥40 mg/kg/day and was accompanied by hepatocellular hypertrophy at doses ≥320 mg/kg/day.

The maximum non-lethal oral dose of indinavir was at least 5000 mg/kg in rats and mice, the highest dose tested in acute toxicity studies.

Studies in rats indicated that uptake into brain tissue was limited, distribution into and out of the lymphatic system was rapid, and excretion into the milk of lactating rats was extensive. Distribution of indinavir across the placental barrier was significant in rats, but limited in rabbits.

Mutagenicity: Indinavir did not have any mutagenic or genotoxic activity in studies with or without metabolic activation.

Carcinogenicity: No carcinogenicity was noted in mice at the maximum tolerated dose, which corresponded to a systemic exposure approx. 2 to 3 times higher than the clinical exposure. In rats, at similar exposure levels, an increased incidence of thyroid adenomas was seen, probably related to an increase of TSH secondary to an increase in thyroxine clearance. The relevance of the findings to humans is likely limited.

Pharmaceutical particulars

List of excipients: each capsule contains the inactive ingredients anhydrous lactose and magnesium stearate. The capsule shell contains the excipients gelatine, titanium dioxide, silicon dioxide, and sodium lauryl sulphate. The 200-mg capsules are printed with printing ink containing titanium dioxide (E 171) and indigo carmine (E 132). The 400-mg capsules are printed with printing ink containing titanium dioxide (E 171), indigo carmine (E 132) and iron oxide (E 172).

The 200 mg capsules are white opaque and coded 'Crixivan 200 mg' in blue.

The 400 mg capsules are white opaque and coded 'Crixivan 400 mg' in green.

Incompatibilities: Not applicable.

Shelf life: The shelf life is 18 months.

Special precautions for storage: Sensitive to moisture. Store in a well-closed container.

Nature and contents of container: Crixivan 200 mg is supplied in HDPE bottles with a polypropylene cap and a foil induction cap containing 360 capsules.

Crixivan 400 mg is supplied in HDPE bottles with a polypropylene cap and a foil induction cap containing 180 capsules or 90 capsules.

The containers contain desiccant canisters that should remain in the bottle. Patients should be advised not to swallow desiccant.

Marketing authorisation numbers

Crixivan 200 mg, 180 capsules EU/1/96/024/001
Crixivan 200 mg, 270 capsules EU/1/96/024/002
Crixivan 200 mg, 360 capsules EU/1/96/024/003
Crixivan 400 mg, 90 capsules EU/1/96/024/004
Crixivan 400 mg, 180 capsules EU/1/96/024/005

Date of approval/revision of SPC May 1998.

Legal category POM.

DECADRON* INJECTION

Qualitative and quantitative composition Dexamethoasone sodium phosphate BP equivalent to 4 mg dexamethasone phosphate or approximately 3.3 mg dexamethasone in each millilitre.

Pharmaceutical form Clear, colourless, sterile solution in a vial.

Clinical particulars

Therapeutic indications: Corticosteroid.

For use in certain endocrine and non-endocrine disorders responsive to corticosteroid therapy.

Systemic administration: Decadron Injection is recommended for systemic administration by intravenous or intramuscular injection when oral therapy is not feasible or desirable in the following conditions.

Endocrine disorders: Primary or secondary adrenocortical insufficiency (hydrocortisone or cortisone is the first choice, but synthetic analogues may be used with mineralocorticoids where applicable and, in infancy, mineralocorticoid supplementation is particularly important.)

Non-endocrine disorders: Decadron Injection may be used in the treatment of non-endocrine corticosteroid responsive conditions including:

Allergy and anaphylaxis: Angioneurotic oedema and anaphylaxis.

Gastro-intestinal: Crohn's disease and ulcerative colitis.

Infection (with appropriate chemotherapy): Miliary tuberculosis and endotoxic shock.

Neurological disorders: Raised intracranial pressure secondary to cerebral tumours and infantile spasms.

Respiratory: Bronchial asthma and aspiration pneumonitis.

Skin disorders: Toxic epidermal necrolysis.

Shock: Adjunctive treatment where high pharmacological doses are needed. Treatment is an adjunct to, and not a substitute for, specific and supportive measures the patient may require. Dexamethasone has been shown to be beneficial when used in the early treatment of shock, but it may not influence overall survival.

Local administration

Decadron Injection is suitable for intra-articular or soft-tissue injection as adjunctive therapy for short-term administration in:

Soft-tissue disorders such as carpal tunnel syndrome and tenosynovitis.

Intra-articular disorders such as rheumatoid arthritis and osteoarthritis with an inflammatory component.

Decadron Injection may be injected intralesionally in selected skin disorders such as cystic acne vulgaris, localised lichen simplex, and keloids.

Posoloioy and method of administration: Decadron Injection can be given without mixing or dilution, but if preferred, can be added without loss of potency to sodium chloride injection or dextrose injection and given by intravenous drip. The infusion mixture must be used within 24 hours, and the usual aseptic techniques for injections should be observed.

Solutions used for intravenous administration or further dilution of this product should be preservative-free when used in the neonate, especially the premature infant.

All dosage recommendations are given in units of dexamethasone phosphate.

Intravenous and intramuscular injection:

General considerations: Dosage must be individualised on the basis of the disease and the reponse of the patient. In order to minimise side effects, the lowest possible dosage adequate to control the disease process should be used (see *Undesirable effects*).

Usually the parenteral dosage ranges are one-third to one-half the oral dose, given every 12 hours.

The usual initial dosage is 0.5 mg–20 mg (0.125 ml–5 ml) a day. In situations of less severity, lower doses will generally suffice. However, in certain overwhelming, acute, life-threatening situations, administration in dosages exceeding the usual dosages may be justified. In these circumstances, the slower rate of absorption by intramuscular administration should be recognised.

Both the dose in the evening, which is useful in alleviating morning stiffness, and the divided dosage regimen are associated with greater suppression of the hypothalamo-pituitary-adrenal axis. After a favourable response is noted, the proper maintenance dosage should be determined by decreasing the initial dosage by small amounts at appropriate intervals to the lowest dosage which will maintain an adequate clinical response. Chronic dosage should preferably not exceed 500 micrograms dexamethasone daily. Close monitoring of drug dosage is needed.

To avoid hypoadrenalism and/or a relapse of the underlying disease, it may be necessary to withdraw the drug gradually (see *Special warnings and special precautions for use*).

Whenever possible, the intravenous route should be used for the initial dose and for as many subsequent doses as are given while the patient is in shock (because of the irregular rate of absorption of any medicament administered by any other route in such patients). When the blood pressure responds, use the intramuscular route until oral therapy can be substituted. For the comfort of the patient, not more than 2 ml should be injected intramuscularly at any one site.

In emergencies, the usual dose of Decadron Injection by intravenous or intramuscular injection is 4 mg–20 mg (1 ml–5 ml) (in shock use only the i.v. route). This dose may be repeated until adequate response is noted.

After initial improvement, single doses of 2 mg–4 mg (0.5 ml–1 ml) repeated as necessary, should be sufficient. The total daily dosage usually need not exceed 80 mg (20 ml), even in severe conditions.

When constant maximal effect is desired, dosage must be repeated at three-hour or four-hour intervals, or maintained by slow intravenous drip.

Intravenous and intramuscular injections are advised in acute illness. When the acute stage has passed, oral steroid therapy should be substituted as soon as feasible.

Shock (of haemorrhagic, traumatic or surgical origin): Usually 2 mg–6 mg/kg body weight as a single intravenous injection. This may be repeated in two to six hours if shock persists. Alternatively, this may be followed immediately by the same dose in an intravenous infusion. Therapy with Decadron Injection is an adjunct to, and not a replacement for, conventional therapy.

Administration of these high doses should be continued only until the patient's condition has stabilised and usually no longer than 48–72 hours.

Cerebral oedema: Associated with primary or metastatic brain tumour, pre-operative preparation of patients with increased intracranial pressure secondary to brain tumour: initially 10 mg (2.5 ml) intravenously, followed by 4 mg (1 ml) intramuscularly every six hours until symptoms of cerebral oedema subside. Response is usually noted within 12–24 hours; dosage may be reduced after two to four days and gradually discontinued over five to seven days.

High doses of Decadron Injection are recommended for initiating short-term intensive therapy for acute life-threatening cerebral oedema. Following the high-loading dose schedule of the first day of therapy, the dose is scaled down over the seven- to ten-day period of intensive therapy and subsequently reduced to zero over the next seven to ten days. When maintenance therapy is required, substitute oral Decadron as soon as possible (see table below).

Palliative management of recurrent or inoperable brain tumours: Maintenance therapy should be determined for each patient; 2 mg (0.5 ml) two or three times a day may be effective.

The smallest dosage necessary to control cerebral oedema should be used.

Suggested high dose schedule in cerebral oedema:

Adults:	
Initial Dose	50 mg i.v.
1st day	8 mg i.v. every 2 hours
2nd day	8 mg i.v. every 2 hours
3rd day	8 mg i.v. every 2 hours
4th day	4 mg i.v. every 2 hours
5th–8th days	4 mg i.v. every 4 hours
Thereafter	decrease by daily reduction of 4 mg
Children (35 kg and over):	
Initial Dose	25 mg i.v.
1st day	4 mg i.v. every 2 hours
2nd day	4 mg i.v. every 2 hours
3rd day	4 mg i.v. every 2 hours
4th day	4 mg i.v. every 4 hours
5th–8th days	4 mg i.v. every 6 hours
Thereafter	decrease by daily reduction of 2 mg
Children (below 35 kg):	
Initial Dose	20 mg i.v.
1st day	4 mg i.v. every 3 hours
2nd day	4 mg i.v. every 3 hours
3rd day	4 mg i.v. every 3 hours
4th day	4 mg i.v. every 6 hours
5th–8th days	2 mg i.v. every 6 hours
Thereafter	decrease by daily reduction of 1 mg

Dual therapy: In acute self-limiting allergic disorders or acute exacerbations of chronic allergic disorders, the following schedule combining oral and parenteral therapy is suggested:

First day	Decadron Injection, 4 mg–8 mg (1 ml–2 ml) intramuscularly
Second day	Two 500 microgram Decadron Tablets twice a day
Third day	Two 500 microgram Decadron Tablets twice a day
Fourth day	One 500 microgram Decadron Tablet twice a day
Fifth day	One 500 microgram Decadron Tablet twice a day
Sixth day	One 500 microgram Decadron Tablet
Seventh day	One 500 microgram Decadron Tablet
Eighth day	Reassessment day

(For information on Decadron Tablets, see separate Summary of Product Characteristcs.)

Intrasynovial, intralesional, and soft-tissue injection: In general, these injections are employed when only one or two joints or areas are affected.

Some of the usual single doses are:

Site of injection	*Amount of dexamethasone phosphate*
Large joints (e.g. knee)	2–4 mg (0.5–1 ml)
Small joints (e.g. interphalangeal, temporomandibular)	0.8–1 mg (0.2–0.25 ml)
Bursae	2–3 mg (0.5–0.75 ml)
Tendon sheaths*	0.4–1 mg (0.1–0.25 ml)
Soft-tissue infiltration	2–6 mg (0.5–1.5 ml)
Ganglia	1–2 mg (0.25–0.5 ml)

* Injection should be made into the tendon sheath, and not directly into the tendon.

Frequency of injection: once every three to five days to once every two to three weeks, depending on response.

Use in children: Dosage should be limited to a single dose on alternate days to lessen retardation of growth and minimise suppression of the hypothalamo-pituitary-adrenal axis.

Use in the elderly: Treatment of elderly patients, particularly if long term, should be planned bearing in mind the more serious consequences of the common side effects of corticosteroids in old age, especially osteoporosis, diabetes, hypertension, hypokalaemia, susceptibility to infection and thinning of the skin. Close clinical supervision is required to avoid life-threatening reactions (see *Undesirable effects*).

Contra-indications: Systemic fungal infection; systemic infection unless specific anti-infective therapy is employed; hypersensitivity to sulphites or any other component of this medication. Administration of live virus vaccines (see *Special warnings and special precautions for use*).

Special warnings and special precautions for use: Frequent intra-articular injections over a prolonged period may lead to joint destruction with bone necrosis. Intra-articular injection of corticosteroid may produce systemic adverse reactions including adrenal suppression.

Undesirable effects may be minimised by using the lowest effective dose for the minimum period. Frequent patient review is required to appropriately titrate the dose against disease activity. Where reduction in dosage is possible, the reduction should be gradual (see *Posology and method of administration*).

Decadron Injection contains sodium bisulphite, a sulphite that may cause allergic-type reactions, including anaphylactic symptoms and life-threatening or less severe asthmatic episodes in certain susceptible people. The overall prevalence of sulphite sensitivity in the general population is unknown and probably low. Sulphite sensitivity is seen more frequently in asthmatic than in non-asthmatic people.

Corticosteroids may exacerbate systemic fungal infections and, therefore, should not be used in the presence of such infections, unless they are needed to control drug reactions due to amphotericin. Moreover, there have been cases reported in which, concomitant use of amphotericin and hydrocortisone, was followed by cardiac enlargement and congestive failure.

Average and large doses of hydrocortisone or cortisone can cause elevation of blood pressure, retention of salt and water, and increased excretion of potassium, but these effects are less likely to occur with synthetic derivatives, except when used in large doses. Dietary salt restriction and potassium supplementation may be necessary. All corticosteroids increase calcium excretion.

The slower rate of absorption by intramuscular administration should be recognised.

In patients on corticosteroid therapy subjected to unusual stress (e.g. intercurrent illness, trauma, or surgical procedures), dosage should be increased before, during and after the stressful situation. Drug-induced secondary adrenocortical insufficiency may result from too rapid withdrawal of corticosteroids and may be minimised by gradual dosage reduction, being tapered off over weeks and months, depending on the dose and duration of treatment, but may persist for up to a year after discontinuation of therapy. In any stressful situation during that period, therefore, corticosteroid therapy should be reinstated. If the patient is already receiving corticosteroids, the current dosage may have to be temporarily increased. Salt and/or a mineralocorticoid should be given concurrently, since mineralocorticoid secretion may be impaired.

Stopping corticosteroids after prolonged therapy may cause withdrawal symptoms, including fever, myalgia, arthralgia, and malaise. This may occur in patients even without evidence of adrenal insufficiency.

In patients who have received more than physiological doses of systemic cortcosteroids (approximately 1 mg dexamethasone) for greater than three weeks, withdrawal should not be abrupt. How dose reduction should be carried out depends largely on whether the disease is likely to relapse as the dose of systemic corticosteroids is reduced. Clinical assessment of disease activity may be needed during withdrawal. If the disease is unlikely to relapse on withdrawal of systemic corticosteroids but there is uncertainty about hypothalmic-pituitary adrenal (HPA) suppression, the dose of systemic corticosteroids ***may*** be reduced rapidly to physiological doses. Once a daily dose of 1 mg dexamethasone is reached, dose reduction should be slower to allow the HPA-axis to recover.

Abrupt withdrawal of systemic corticosteroid treatment, which has continued up to three weeks is appropriate if it is considered that the disease is unlikely to relapse. Abrupt withdrawal of doses of up to 6 mg daily of dexamethasone for three weeks is unlikely to lead to clinically relevant HPA-axis suppression, in the majority of patients. In the following patient groups, gradual withdrawal of systemic corticosteroid therapy should be ***considered*** even after courses lasting three weeks or less:

- patients who have had repeated courses of systemic corticosteroids, particularly if taken for greater than three weeks,
- when a short course has been prescribed within one year of cessation of long-term therapy (months or years),
- patients who may have reasons for adrenocortical insufficiency other than exogenous corticosteroid therapy,
- patients receiving doses of systemic corticosteroid greater than 6 mg daily of dexamethasone,
- patients repeatedly taking doses in the evening.

Patients should carry 'steroid treatment' cards, which give clear guidance on the precautions to be taken to minimise risk and which provide details of prescriber, drug, dosage and the duration of treatment.

Because anaphylactoid reactions have occurred, rarely, in patients receiving parenteral corticosteroid therapy, appropriate precautions should be taken prior to administration, especially when the patient has a history of allergy to any drug.

Administration of live virus vaccines is contra-indicated in individuals receiving immunosuppressive doses of corticosteroids. If inactivated viral or bacterial vaccines are administered to individuals receiving immunosuppressive doses of corticosteroids, the expected serum antibody response may not be obtained. However, immunisation procedures may be undertaken in patients who are receiving corticosteroids as replacement therapy, e.g. for Addison's disease.

Literature reports suggest an apparent association between use of corticosteroids and left ventricular free wall rupture after a recent myocardial infarction; therefore, therapy with corticosteroids should be used with great caution in these patients.

The use of Decadron Injection in active tuberculosis should be restricted to those cases of fulminating or disseminated tuberculosis in which the corticosteroid is used for the management of the disease in conjunction with an appropriate antituberculosis regimen. If the corticosteroids are indicated in patients with latent tuberculosis or tuberculin reactivity, close observation is necessary as reactivation may occur. During prolonged corticosteroid therapy, these patients should receive prophylactic chemotherapy.

Corticosteroids may mask some signs of infection, and new infections may appear during their use. Suppression of the inflammatory response and immune function increases the susceptibility to infections and their severity. The clinical presentation may often be atypical, and serious infections such as septicaemia and tuberculosis may be masked and reach an advanced stage before being recognised. There may be decreased resistance, and inability to localise infection.

A report shows that the use of corticosteroids in cerebral malaria is associated with a prolonged coma and an increased incidence of pneumonia and gastro-intestinal bleeding.

Chickenpox is of particular concern, since this normally minor illness may be fatal in immunosuppressed patients. Patients (or parents of children) without a definite history of chickenpox should be advised to avoid close personal contact with chickenpox or herpes zoster, and if exposed they should seek urgent medical attention. Passive immunisation with varicella/zoster immunoglobulin (VZIG) is needed by exposed non-immune patients who are receiving systemic corticosteroids or who have used them within the previous three months; this should be given within ten days of exposure to chickenpox.

If a diagnosis of chickenpox is confirmed, the illness warrants specialist care and urgent treatment. Corticosteroids should not be stopped and the dose may need to be increased.

Measles can have a more serious or even fatal course in immunosuppressed patients. In such children or adults particular care should be taken to avoid exposure to measles. If exposed, prophylaxis with intramuscular pooled immunoglobulin (IG) may be indicated. Exposed patients should be advised to seek medical advice without delay.

Corticosteroids may activate latent amoebiasis or strongyloidiasis or exacerbate active disease. Therefore, it is recommended that latent or active amoebiasis and strongyloidiasis be ruled out, before initiating corticosteroid therapy in any patient at risk of, or with symptoms of either condition.

Prolonged use of corticosteroids may produce posterior subcapsular cataracts, glaucoma with possible damage to the optic nerves, and may enhance the establishment of secondary ocular infections due to fungi or viruses. Corticosteroids may increase or decrease motility and number of spermatozoa.

Special precautions: Particular care is required when considering the use of systemic corticosteroids in patients with the following conditions, and frequent patient monitoring is necessary: renal insufficiency, hypertension, diabetes or in those with a family history of diabetes, congestive heart failure, osteoporosis, previous steroid myopathy, glaucoma (or family history of glaucoma), myasthenia gravis, non-specific ulcerative colitis, diverticulitis, fresh intestinal anastomoses, active or latent peptic ulcer, existing or previous history of severe affective disorders (especially previous steroid psychosis), liver failure, and epilepsy. Signs of peritoneal irritation following gastro-intestinal perforation in patients receiving large doses of corticosteroids may be minimal or absent. Fat embolism has been reported as a possible complication of hypercortisonism.

There is an enhanced effect of corticosteroids in patients with hypothyroidism and in those with cirrhosis.

Corticosteroids should be used cautiously in patients with ocular herpes simplex because of possible corneal perforation.

Local steroid injection should be undertaken in an aseptic environment to reduce the particular risk of bacterial infection. Injection of a steroid into an infected site should be avoided.

Appropriate examination of joint fluid is necessary to exclude a septic process.

A marked increase in pain accompanied by local swelling, further restriction of joint motion, fever, and malaise are suggestive of septic arthritis. If this complication occurs and the diagnosis of sepsis is confirmed, appropriate antimicrobial therapy should be instituted.

Patients should understand the great importance of not over-using joints that are still diseased, despite symptomatic improvement.

Corticosteroids should not be injected into unstable joints.

Frequent intra-articular injections have been reported to cause development of Charcot-like arthropathies.

Children: Corticosteroids cause growth retardation in infancy, childhood and adolescence, which may be irreversible. Treatment should be limited to the minimum dosage for the shortest possible time. In order to minimise suppression of the hypothalamo-pituitary-adrenal axis and growth retardation, treatment should be limited, where possible, to a single dose on alternate days.

Growth and development of infants and children on prolonged corticosteroid therapy should be carefully monitored.

Interactions with other medicaments and other forms of interaction: Aspirin should be used cautiously in conjunction with corticosteroids in hypoprothrombinaemia.

The renal clearance of salicylates is increased by corticosteroids and therefore salicylate dosage should be reduced along with steroid withdrawal.

As phenytoin, barbiturates, ephedrine, rifabutin, carbamazepine, rifampicin, and aminoglutethimide may enhance the metabolic clearance of corticosteroids, resulting in decreased blood levels and reduced physiological activity, the dosage may have to be adjusted. These interactions may interfere with dexamethasone suppression tests, which should be interpreted with caution during administration of these drugs.

False-negative results in the dexamethasone suppression test in patients being treated with indomethacin have been reported.

The efficacy of coumarin anticoagulants may be changed by concurrent corticosteroid treatment. The prothrombin time should be checked frequently in patients who are receiving corticosteroids and coumarin anticoagulants at the same time, in order to avoid spontaneous bleeding.

The desired effects of hypoglycaemic agents (including insulin), are antagonised by corticosteroids.

When corticosteroids are administered concomitantly with potassium-depleting diuretics, patients should be observed closely for development of hypokalaemia.

Corticosteroids may affect the nitrobluetetrazolium test for bacterial infection and produce false-negative results.

Pregnancy and lactation: The ability of corticosteroids to cross the placenta varies between individual drugs, however, dexamethasone readily crosses the placenta.

Administration of corticosteroids to pregnant animals can cause abnormalities of foetal development including cleft palate, intra-uterine growth retardation and effects on brain growth and development. There is no evidence that corticosteroids result in an increased incidence of cogenital abnormalities, such as cleft palate/lip in man. However, when administered for prolonged periods or repeatedly during pregnancy, corticosteroids may increase the risk of intra-uterine growth retardation. Hypoadrenalism may, in theory, occur in the neonate following prenatal exposure to corticosteroids but usually resolves spontaneously following birth and is rarely clinically important. As with all drugs, corticosteroids should only be prescribed when the benefits to the mother and child outweigh the risks. When corticosteroids are essential however, patients with normal pregnancies may be treated as though they were in the non-gravid state.

Corticosteroids may pass into breast milk, although no data are available for dexamethoasone. Infants of mothers taking high doses of systemic corticosteroids for prolonged periods may have a degree of adrenal supression.

Effects on ability to drive and use machines: None reported.

Undesirable effects: The incidence of predictable undesirable effects, including hypothalamic-pituitary-adrenal suppression, correlates with the relative potency of the drug, dosage, timing of administration and the duration of treatment (see *Special warnings and special precautions for use*).

Fluid and electrolyte disturbances: Sodium retention, fluid retention, congestive heart failure in susceptible patients, potassium loss, hypokalaemic alkalosis, hypertension, increased calcium excretion (see *Special warnings and special precautions for use*).

Musculoskeletal: Muscle weakness, steroid myopathy, loss of muscle mass, osteoporosis (especially in post-menopausal females), vertebral compression fractures, aseptic necrosis of femoral and humeral heads, pathological fracture of long bones, tendon rupture, and post-injection flare (following intra-articular use).

Gastro-intestinal: Peptic ulcer with possible perforation and haemorrhage, perforation of the small and large bowel, particularly in patients with inflammatory bowel disease, pancreatitis, abdominal distension, ulcerative oesophagitis, dyspepsia, oesophageal candidiasis.

Dermatological: Impaired wound healing, thin fragile skin, petechiae and ecchymoses, erythema, striae, telangiectasia, acne, increased sweating, possible suppression of skin tests, burning or tingling especially in the perineal area (after intravenous injection), other cutaneous reactions such as allergic dermatitis, urticaria, angioneurotic oedema, and hypo- or hyperpigmentation.

Neurological: Convulsions, increased intracranial pressure with papilloedema (pseudotumour cerebri) usually after treatment, vertigo, headache, psychic disturbances (e.g. euphoria, psychological dependence, depression, insomnia).

Endocrine: Menstrual irregularities, amenorrhoea, development of Cushingoid state, suppression of growth in children and adolescents, secondary adrenocortical and pituitary unresponsiveness (particularly in times of stress, as in trauma, surgery or illness), decreased carbohydrate tolerance, manifestations of latent diabetes mellitus, increased requirements for insulin or oral hypoglycaemic agents in diabetes, hirsutism.

Anti-inflammatory and immunosuppressive effects: Increased susceptibility and severity of infections with suppression of clinical symptoms and signs. Opportunistic infections, recurrence of dormant tuberculosis (see *Special warnings and special precautions for use*).

Ophthalmic: Posterior subcapsular cataracts, increased intra-ocular pressure, papilloedema, corneal or scleral thinning, exacerbation of ophthalmic viral disease, glaucoma, exophthalmos, rare instances of blindness associated with intra-lesional therapy around the face and head, retinopathy of prematurity.

Metabolic: Negative nitrogen balance due to protein catabolism. Negative calcium balance.

Cardiovascular: Myocardial rupture following recent myocardial infarction (see *Special warnings and special precautions for use*). Hypertrophic cardiomyopathy in low birth-weight infants.

Other: Hypersensitivity, including anaphylaxis has been reported, leucocytosis, thrombo-embolism, weight gain, increased appetite, nausea, malaise, hiccups, and sterile abscess.

Withdrawal symptoms and signs: Too rapid a reduction of corticosteroid dosage following prolonged treatment can lead to acute adrenal insufficiency, hypotension, and death (see *Special warnings and special precautions for use*).

In some instances, withdrawal symptoms may simulate a clinical relapse of the disease for which the patient has been undergoing treatment.

Overdosage: Reports of acute toxicity and/or deaths following overdosage with glucocorticoids are rare. No antidote is available. Treatment is probably not indicated for reactions due to chronic poisoning, unless the patient has a condition that would render a patient unusually susceptible to ill effects from corticosteroids. In this case, symptomatic treatment should be instituted as necessary.

Anaphylactic and hypersensitivity reactions may be treated with adrenaline, positive-pressure artificial respiration and aminophylline. The patient should be kept warm and quiet.

The biological half-life of dexamethasone in plasma is about 190 minutes.

Pharmacological properties

Pharmacodynamic properties: Dexamethasone possesses the actions and effects of other basic glucocorticoids and is among the most active members of its class.

Glucocorticoids are adrenocortical steroids, both naturally occurring and synthetic, which are readily absorbed from the gastro-intestinal tract. They cause profound and varied metabolic effects and in addition, they modify the body's immune responses to diverse stimuli. Naturally-occurring glucocorticoids (hydrocortisone and cortisone), which also have salt-retaining properties, are used primarily for their potent anti-inflammatory effects in disorders of many organ systems.

Dexamethasone has predominant glucocorticoid activity with little propensity to promote renal retention of sodium and water. Therefore it does not offer complete replacement therapy and must be supplemented with salt or desoxycorticosterone.

Pharmacokinetic properties: The biological half-life of dexamethasone in plasma is about 190 minutes.

Binding of dexamethasone to plasma proteins is less than for most other corticosteroids and is estimated to be about 77%.

Up to 65% of a dose is excreted in the urine in 24 hours, the rate of excretion being increased following concomitant administration of phenytoin.

The more potent halogenated corticosteroids such as dexamethasone, appear to cross the placental barrier with minimal inactivation.

Preclinical safety data: Not relevant.

Pharmaceutical particulars

List of excipients: Creatinine, methyl hydroxybenzoate PhEur, propyl hydroxybenzoate PhEur, sodium citrate PhEur, sodium metabisulphate PhEur, sodium hydroxide PhEur, water for injections PhEur.

Incompatibilities: None.

Shelf life: 36 months.

Special precautions for storage: Store below 25°C protected from light. Do not freeze.

Nature and content of the container: Type I clear glass vial with grey butyl rubber stopper and roll-on aluminium collars containing 2 ml.

Instructions for use and handling: Decadron Injection is sensitive to heat and should not be autoclaved to sterilise the outside of the vial. Only sodium chloride injection or dextrose injection should be used as diluent. Any infusion mixture must be used within 24 hours.

Decadron Injection is ready for immediate use. An adequate dose is contained in a small volume of vehicle, and small-bore needles can be used wherever appropriate.

Product licence number PL 0026/5045R.

Date of first authorisation/renewal 31 July 1987.

Date last renewed 24 November 1997.

Date of (partial) revision of text April 1998.

Legal category POM.

DECADRON* INJECTION SHOCK-PAK

Qualitative and quantitative composition The active ingredient in Decadron Injection Schock-Pak is dexamethasone sodium phosphate equivalent to 20 mg of dexamethasone per ml.

Pharmaceutical form Sterile solution in a vial.

Clinical particulars

Therapeutic indications: Corticosteroid.

Only for the adjunctive treatment of shock where massive doses of corticosteroids are needed: severe shock of haemorrhagic, traumatic, or surgical origin. It is an adjunct to, and not a substitute for, specific or supportive measures that the patient may require, e.g. restoration of circulating blood volume, correction of fluid and electrolyte balance, oxygen, and surgical measures.

Posology and method of administration: Decadron Injection Shock-Pak is for administration by the intravenous route only.

Intravenous injection in shock: Decadron Injection Shock-Pak can be used without mixing or diluting. Injection should be made slowly.

The usual dosage by intravenous injection is 2–6 mg/kg bodyweight given as a single intravenous injection. This may be repeated in two to six hours, if shock persists. As an alternative, the initial intravenous injection may be followed immediately by an intravenous infusion containing the same dose. (Although Decadron Injection Shock-Pak was not primarily designed for intravenous infusion, it can be added to sodium chloride injection, or to dextrose injection, and administered by intravenous drip without loss of potency. When the Shock-Pak is added to an infusion solution, the mixture must be used within 24 hours, as infusion solutions do not contain preservatives.)

Solutions used for intravenous administration or further dilution of this product should be preservative-free when used in the neonate, especially the premature infant.

These dosages are large in comparison with the usual recommended dosages of dexamethasone sodium phosphate. They are, however, for emergency use in acute conditions needing massive doses of corticosteroid, and reflect the tendency in current medical practice to use such high doses in the treatment of shock.

Therapy with Decadron Injection Shock-Pak is an adjunct to, and not a replacement for, conventional therapy. Administration of high doses of corticosteroids should be continued only until the patient's condition has stabilised, and usually no longer than 48–72 hours. Prolonged therapy at such high doses should be avoided to prevent possible complications, such as adrenal suppression or gastro-intestinal ulceration.

Use in the elderly: These dosage recommendations apply to all adults, including the elderly.

Contra-indications: Systemic fungal infections; hypersensitivity to sulphites or to any other component of this product. Administration of live virus vaccines.

Special warnings and special precautions for use: Decadron Injection Shock-Pak contains sodium bisulphite, a sulphite that may cause allergic-type reactions, including anaphylactic symptoms and life-threatening or less severe asthmatic episodes in certain susceptible people. The overall prevalence of sulphite sensitivity in the general population is unknown and probably low. Sulphite sensitivity is seen more frequently in asthmatic than in non-asthmatic people.

Decadron Injection Shock-Pak is for adjunctive use in the treatment of shock, and therapy must be accompanied by the usual standard measures employed in its management.

The pronounced hormonal effects associated with prolonged corticosteroid therapy will probably not be seen when this injection is used for short-term adjunctive therapy in shock.

Because rare instances of anaphylactic reactions have occurred in patients receiving parenteral corticosteroid therapy, appropriate precautionary measures should be taken prior to administration, especially when the patient has a history of allergy to any drug.

Administration of live virus vaccines is contra-indicated in individuals receiving immunosuppressive doses of corticosteroids. If inactivated viral or bacterial vaccines are administered to individuals receiving immunosuppressive doses of corticosteroids, the expected serum antibody response may not be obtained.

Literature reports suggest an apparent association

between use of corticosteroids and left ventricular free wall rupture after a recent myocardial infarction; therefore, therapy with corticosteroids should be used with great caution in these patients.

Chickenpox is of particular concern, since this normally minor illness may be fatal in immunosuppressed patients. Patients (or parents of children) without a definite history of chickenpox should be advised to avoid close personal contact with chickenpox or herpes zoster, and if exposed they should seek urgent medical attention. Passive immunisation with varicella/zoster immunoglobulin (VZIG) is needed by exposed non-immune patients who are receiving systemic corticosteroids or who have used them within the previous three months; this should be given within 10 days of exposure to chickenpox. **If a diagnosis of chickenpox is confirmed, the illness warrants specialist care and urgent treatment. Corticosteroids should not be stopped and the dose may need to be increased.**

Measles can have a more serious or even fatal course in immunosuppressed patients. In such children or adults, particular care should be taken to avoid exposure to measles. If exposed, prophylaxis with intramuscular pooled immunoglobulin (IG) may be indicated. Exposed patients should be advised to seek medical advice without delay.

Precautions for prolonged corticosteroid therapy: The following precautions are listed for Decadron Injection and should be considered for any dexamethasone preparation.

Undesirable effects may be minimised by using the lowest effective dose for the minimum period. Frequent patient review is required to appropriately titrate the dose against disease activity. When reduction in dosage is possible, the reduction should be gradual.

Corticosteroids may exacerbate systemic fungal infections and, therefore, should not be used in the presence of such infections unless they are needed to control drug reactions due to amphotericin. Moreover, there have been cases reported in which concomitant use of amphotericin and hydrocortisone was followed by cardiac enlargement and congestive failure.

Average and large doses of hydrocortisone or cortisone can cause elevation of blood pressure, retention of salt and water, and increased excretion of potassium, but these effects are less likely to occur with synthetic derivatives, except when used in large doses. Dietary salt restriction and potassium supplementation may be necessary. All corticosteroids increase calcium excretion.

In patients on corticosteroid therapy subjected to unusual stress (e.g. intercurrent illness, trauma, or surgical procedures), dosage should be increased before, during and after the stressful situation. Drug-induced secondary adrenocortical insufficiency may result from too rapid withdrawal of corticosteroids and may be minimised by gradual dosage reduction, being tapered off over weeks and months depending on the dose and duration of treatment, but may persist for up to a year after discontinuation of therapy. In any stressful situation during that period, therefore, corticosteroid therapy should be reinstated. If the patient is already receiving corticosteroids, the current dosage may have to be temporarily increased. Salt and/or a mineralocorticoid should be given concurrently, since mineralocorticoid secretion may be impaired.

Stopping corticosteroids after prolonged therapy may cause withdrawal symptoms, including fever, myalgia, arthralgia, and malaise. This may occur in patients even without evidence of adrenal insufficiency.

In patients who have received more than physiological doses of systemic corticosteroids (approximately 1 mg dexamethasone) for greater than three weeks, withdrawal should not be abrupt. How dose reduction should be carried out depends largely on whether the disease is likely to relapse as the dose of systemic corticosteroids is reduced. Clinical assessment of disease activity may be needed during withdrawal. If the disease is unlikely to relapse on withdrawal of systemic corticosteroids but there is uncertainty about hypothalamic-pituitary adrenal (HPA) suppression, the dose of systemic corticosteroids ***may*** be reduced rapidly to physiological doses. Once a daily dose of 1 mg dexamethasone is reached, dose reduction should be slower to allow the HPA-axis to recover.

Abrupt withdrawal of systemic corticosteroid treatment, which has continued up to three weeks is appropriate if it is considered that the disease is unlikely to relapse. Abrupt withdrawal of doses of up to 6 mg daily of dexamethasone for three weeks is unlikely to lead to clinically relevant HPA-axis suppression, in the majority of patients. In the following patient groups, gradual withdrawal of systemic corticosteroid therapy should be ***considered*** evey after courses lasting three weeks or less:

- patients who have had repeated courses of systemic corticosteroids, particularly if taken for greater than three weeks,
- when a short course has been prescribed within one year of cessation of long-term therapy (months or years),
- patients who may have reasons for adrenocortical insufficiency other than exogenous corticosteroid therapy,
- patients receiving doses of systemic corticosteroid greater than 6 mg daily of dexamethasone,
- patients repeatedly taking does in the evening.

Patients should carry 'steroid treatment' cards, which give clear guidance on the precautions to be taken to minimise risk and which provide details of prescriber, drug, dosage and the duration of treatment.

The use of Decadron Injection in active tuberculosis should be restricted to those cases of fulminating or disseminated tuberculosis in which the corticosteroid is used for the management of the disease in conjunction with an appropriate antituberculosis regimen. If the corticosteroids are indicated in patients with latent tuberculosis or tuberculin reactivity, close observation is necessary as reactivation may occur. During prolonged corticosteroid therapy, these patients should receive prophylactic chemotherapy.

Corticosteroids may mask some signs of infection, and new infections may appear during their use. Suppression of the inflammatory response and immune function increases the susceptibility to infections and their severity. The clinical presentation may often be atypical, and serious infections such as septicaemia and tuberculosis may be masked and reach an advanced stage before being recognised. There may be decreased resistance, and inability to localise infection.

A report shows that the use of corticosteroids in cerebral malaria is associated with a prolonged coma and an increased incidence of pneumonia and gastrointestinal bleeding.

Corticosteroids may activate latent amoebiasis or strongyloidiasis or exacerbate active disease. Therefore, it is recommended that latent or active amoebiasis and strongyloidiasis be ruled out before initiating corticosteroid therapy in any patient at risk of or with symptoms of either condition.

Prolonged use of corticosteroids may produce posterior subcapsular cataracts, glaucoma with possible damage to the optic nerves, and may enhance the establishment of secondary ocular infections due to fungi or viruses. Corticosteroids may increase or decrease motility and number of spermatozoa.

Special precautions: Particular care is required when considering the use of systemic corticosteroids in patients with the following conditions, and frequent patient monitoring is necessary: renal insufficiency, hypertension, diabetes or in those with a family history of diabetes, congestive heart failure, osteoporosis, previous steroid myopathy, glaucoma (or family history of glaucoma), myasthenia gravis, non-specific ulcerative colitis, diverticulitis, fresh intestinal anastomoses, active or latent peptic ulcer, existing or previous history of severe affective disorders (especially previous steroid psychosis), liver failure, and epilepsy. Signs of peritoneal irritation following gastro-intestinal perforation in patients receiving large doses of corticosteroids may be minimal or absent. Fat embolism has been reported as a possible complication of hypercortisonism.

There is an enhanced effect of corticosteroids in patients with hypothyroidism and in those with cirrhosis.

Corticosteroids should be used cautiously in patients with ocular herpes simplex because of possible corneal perforation.

Children: Corticosteroids cause growth retardation in infancy, childhood and adolescence, which may be irreversible. Treatment should be limited to the minimum dosage for the shortest possible time. In order to minimise suppression of the hypothalamo-pituitary-adrenal axis and growth retardation, treatment should be limited, where possible, to a single dose on alternate days.

Growth and development of infants and children on prolonged corticosteroid therapy should be carefully monitored.

Interactions with other medicaments and other forms of interaction: Aspirin should be used cautiously in conjunction with corticosteroids in hypoprothrombinaemia.

As phenytoin, barbiturates, ephedrine, rifabutin, carbamazepine, rifampicin, and aminoglutethimide may enhance the metabolic clearance of corticosteroids, resulting in decreased blood levels and reduced physiological activity, the dosage may have to be adjusted. These interactions may interfere with dexamethasone suppression tests, which should be interpreted with caution during administration of these drugs.

False-negative results in the dexamethasone suppression test in patients being treated with indomethacin have been reported.

The efficacy of coumarin anticoagulants may be changed by concurrent corticosteroid treatment. The prothrombin time should be checked frequently in patients who are receiving corticosteroids and coumarin anticoagulants at the same time, in order to avoid spontaneous bleeding.

When corticosteroids are administered concomitantly with potassium-depleting diuretics, patients should be observed closely for development of hypokalaemia.

Corticosteroids may affect the nitrobluetetrazolium test for bacterial infection and produce false-negative results.

Pregnancy and lactation: The ability of corticosteroids to cross the placenta varies between individual drugs, however, dexamethasone readily crosses the placenta.

Administration of corticosteroids to pregnant animals can cause abnormalities of foetal development including cleft palate, intra-uterine growth retardation and effects on brain growth and development. There is no evidence that corticosteroids result in an increased incidence of congenital abnormalities, such as cleft palate/lip in man. However, when administered for prolonged periods or repeatedly during pregnancy, corticosteroids may increase the risk of intra-uterine growth retardation. Hypoadrenalism may, in theory, occur in the neonate following prenatal exposure to corticosteroids but usually resolves spontaneously following birth and is rarely clinically important. As with all drugs, corticosteroids should only be prescribed when the benefits to the mother and child outweigh the risks. When corticosteroids are esential however, patients with normal pregnancies may be treated as though they were in the non-gravid state.

Corticosteroids may pass into breast milk, although no data are available for dexamethasone. Infants of mothers taking high doses of systemic corticosteroids for prolonged periods may have a degree of adrenal suppression.

Effects on ability to drive and use machines: None reported.

Undesirable effects: Although adverse reactions associated with short-term corticosteroid therapy in high doses are uncommon, peptic ulceration may occur. Some patients have reported transitory burning or tingling sensations, often in the perineal area, when intravenous injections of large doses of dexamethasone sodium phosphate were given. The usual aseptic techniques governing injections should be observed.

The following side effects reported with Decadron Injection should be regarded as potential side effects for any dexamethasone preparation.

Fluid and electrolyte disturbances: Sodium retention, fluid retention, congestive heart failure in susceptible patients, potassium loss, hypokalaemic alkalosis, hypertension, increased calcium excretion (see *Special warnings and special precautions for use*).

Musculoskeletal: Muscle weakness, steroid myopathy, loss of muscle mass, osteoporosis (especially in post-menopausal females), vertebral compression fractures, aseptic necrosis of femoral and humeral heads, pathological fracture of long bones, tendon rupture, and post-injection flare (following intra-articular use).

Gastro-intestinal: Peptic ulcer with possible perforation and haemorrhage, perforation of the small and large bowel, particularly in patients with inflammatory bowel disease, pancreatitis, abdominal distension, ulcerative oesophagitis, dyspepsia, oesophageal candidiasis.

Dermatological: Impaired wound healing, thin fragile skin, petechiae and ecchymoses, erythema, striae, telangiectasia, acne, increased sweating, possible suppression of skin tests, burning or tingling especially in the perineal area (after intravenous injection), other cutaneous reactions such as allergic dermatitis, urticaria, angioneurotic oedema, and hypo- or hyperpigmentation.

Neurological: Convulsions, increased intracranial pressure with papilloedema (pseudotumour cerebri) usually after treatment, vertigo, headache, psychic disturbances (e.g. euphoria, psychological dependence, depression, insomnia).

Endocrine: Menstrual irregularities, amenorrhoea, development of Cushingoid state, suppression of growth in children and adolescents, secondary adrenocortical and pituitary unresponsiveness (particularly in times of stress, as in trauma, surgery or illness), decreased carbohydrate tolerance, manifestations of latent diabetes mellitus, increased requirements for insulin or oral hypoglycaemic agents in diabetes, hirsutism.

Anti-inflammatory and immunosuppressive effects: Increased susceptibility and severity of infections with suppression of clinical symptoms and signs. Opportunistic infections, recurrence of dormant tuberculosis (see *Special warnings and special precautions for use*).

Ophthalmic: Posterior subcapsular cataracts, increased intra-ocular pressure, papilloedema, corneal or scleral thinning, exacerbation of ophthalmic viral disease, glaucoma, exophthalmos, rare instances of blindness associated with intra-lesional therapy around the face and head, retinopathy of prematurity.

Metabolic: Negative nitrogen balance due to protein catabolism. Negative calcium balance.

Cardiovascular: Myocardial rupture following recent myocardial infarction (see *Special warnings and special precautions for use*). Hypertrophic cardiomyopathy in low birth-weight infants.

Other: Hypersensitivity, including anaphylaxis has been reported, leucocytosis, thrombo-embolism, weight gain, increased appetite, nausea, malaise, hiccups, and sterile abscess.

Overdosage: Reports of acute toxicity and/or deaths following overdosage with glucocorticoids are rare. No antidote is available. Treatment is probably not indicated for reactions due to chronic poisoning unless the patient has a condition that would render a patient unusually susceptible to ill effects from corticosteroids. In this case, symptomatic treatment should be instituted as necessary.

Anaphylactic and hypersensitivity reactions may be treated with adrenaline, positive-pressure artificial respiration and aminophylline. The patient should be kept warm and quiet.

The biological half-life of dexamethasone in plasma is about 190 minutes.

Pharmacological properties

Pharmacodynamic properties: Dexamethasone possesses the actions and effects of other basic glucocorticoids and is among the most active members of its class.

Glucocorticoids are adrenocortical steroids, both naturally occurring and synthetic, which are readily absorbed from the gastro-intestinal tract. They cause profound and varied metabolic effects and in addition, they modify the body's immune responses to diverse stimuli.

Naturally-occurring glucocorticoids (hydrocortisone and cortisone), which also have salt-retaining properties, are used primarily for their potent anti-inflammatory effects in disorders of many organ systems.

Dexamethasone has predominant glucocorticoid activity with little propensity to promote renal retention of sodium and water. Therefore it does not offer complete replacement therapy and must be supplemented with salt or desoxycorticosterone.

Pharmacokinetic properties: The biological half-life of dexamethasone in plasma is about 190 minutes.

Binding of dexamethasone to plasma proteins is less than for most other corticosteroids and is estimated to be about 77%.

Up to 65% of a dose is excreted in the urine in 24 hours, the rate of excretion being increased following concomitant administration of phenytoin.

The more potent halogenated corticosteroids such as dexamethasone, appear to cross the placental barrier with minimal inactivation.

Preclinical data: Not relevant.

Pharmaceutical particulars

List of excipients: Creatinine, disodium edetate PhEur, methyl hydroxybenzoate PhEur, propyl hydroxybenzoate PhEur, sodium citrate PhEur, sodium metabisulphite PhEur, sodium hydroxide PhEur, water for injections PhEur.

Incompatibilities: None.

Shelf life: 36 months.

Special precautions for storage: Store below 25°C, protected from light.

Nature and contents of the container: Type I 5 ml clear glass vials with grey butyl rubber stopper and roll-on aluminium collar seals containing 1 ml.

Instructions for use/handling: Decadron Injection Shock-Pak is sensitive to heat and should not be autoclaved to sterilise the outside of the vial. It should be stored below 25°C and protected from light.

Only sodium chloride injection or dextrose injection should be used as diluents for infusion. Any infusion mixture must be used within 24 hours.

Marketing authorisation number PL 0025/0077R.

Date of first authorisation/renewal 26 July 1987. Last renewed 5 January 1998.

Date of revision of text April 1998.

DECADRON* TABLETS

Qualitative and quantitative composition Each tablet of Decadron contains 500 micrograms dexamethasone PhEur.

Pharmaceutical form Decadron is supplied as a round, white, half-scored tablet, marked 'MSD 41'.

Clinical particulars

Therapeutic indications: Decadron is indicated as a treatment for certain endocrine and non-endocrine disorders, in certain cases of cerebral oedema, and for diagnostic testing of adrenocortical hyperfunction.

Endocrine disorders: Primary or secondary adrenocortical insufficiency, congenital adrenal hyperplasia.

Non-endocrine disorders: Dexamethasone may be used in the treatment of non-endocrine corticosteroid responsive conditions including:

Allergy and anaphylaxis: Angioneurotic oedema, anaphylaxis.

Arteritis collagenosis: Polymyalgia rheumatica, polyarteritis nodosa.

Blood disorders: Haemolytic anaemia, leukaemia, myeloma.

Cardiovascular disorders: Post-myocardial infarction syndrome.

Gastro-intestinal: Crohn's disease, ulcerative colitis.

Hypercalcaemia: Sarcoidosis.

Infections (with appropriate chemotherapy): Miliary tuberculosis.

Muscular disorders: Polymyositis.

Neurological disorders: Raised intra-cranial pressure secondary to cerebral tumours.

Ocular disorders: Anterior and posterior uveitis, optic neuritis.

Renal disorders: Lupus nephritis.

Respiratory disease: Bronchial asthma, aspiration pneumonitis.

Rheumatic disorders: Rheumatoid arthritis.

Skin disorders: Pemphigus vulgaris.

Posology and method of administration: General considerations: Dosage must be individualised on the basis of the disease and the response of the patient. In order to minimise side effects, the lowest possible dosage adequate to control the disease process should be used (see *Undesirable effects*).

The initial dosage varies from 0.5 to 9 mg a day depending on the disease being treated. In more severe diseases, doses higher than 9 mg may be required. The initial dosage should be maintained or adjusted until the patient's response is satisfactory. Both the dose in the evening, which is useful in alleviating morning stiffness, and the divided dosage regimen are associated with greater suppression of the hypothalamo-pituitary-adrenal axis. If satisfactory clinical response does not occur after a reasonable period of time, discontinue Decadron Tablets and transfer the patient to other therapy.

After a favourable initial response, the proper maintenance dosage should be determined by decreasing the initial dosage in small amounts to the lowest dosage that maintains an adequate clinical response. Chronic dosage should preferably not exceed 1.5 mg dexamethasone daily.

Patients should be monitored for signs that might require dosage adjustment, including changes in clinical status resulting from remissions or exacerbations of the disease, individual drug responsiveness, and the effect of stress (e.g. surgery, infection, trauma). During stress it may be necessary to increase dosage temporarily.

To avoid hypoadrenalism and/or a relapse of the underlying disease, it may be necessary to withdraw the drug gradually (see *Special warnings and special precautions for use*).

The following equivalents facilitate changing to Decadron from other glucocorticoids.

Milligram for milligram, dexamethasone is approximately equivalent to betamethasone, 4 to 6 times more potent than methylprednisolone and triamcinolone, 6 to 8 times more potent than prednisone and prednisolone, 25 to 30 times more potent than hydrocortisone, and about 35 times more potent than cortisone.

In acute, self-limiting allergic disorders or acute exacerbations of chronic allergic disorders, the following dosage schedule combining parenteral and oral therapy is suggested.

First day	Decadron Injection, 4 mg or 8 mg (1 ml or 2 ml) intramuscularly
Second day	Two 500 microgram Decadron Tablets twice a day
Third day	Two 500 microgram Decadron Tablets twice a day
Fourth day	One 500 microgram Decadron Tablet twice a day
Fifth day	One 500 microgram Decadron Tablet twice a day
Sixth day	One 500 microgram Decadron Tablet
Seventh day	One 500 microgram Decadron Tablet
Eighth day	Reassessment day

This schedule is designed to ensure adequate therapy during acute episodes while minimising the risk of overdosage in chronic cases.

Dexamethasone suppression tests:

1. *Tests for Cushing's syndrome:* 2 milligram Decadron is given orally at 11 p.m., then blood is drawn for plasma cortisol determination at 8 a.m. the following morning.

For greater accuracy, 500 microgram Decadron is given orally every 6 hours for 48 hours. Plasma cortisol is measured at 8 a.m. on the third morning. Twenty-four-hour urine collections are made for determination of 17-hydroxycorticosteroid excretion.

2. *Test to distinguish Cushing's syndrome caused by pituitary ACTH excess from the syndrome induced by other causes:* 2 milligram Decadron is given orally every 6 hours for 48 hours. Plasma cortisol is measured at 8 a.m. on the morning following the last dose. Twenty-four-hour urine collections are made for determination of 17-hydroxycorticosteroid excretion.

Use in children: Dosage should be limited to a single dose on alternate days to lessen retardation of growth and minimise suppression of hypothalamo-pituitary-adrenal axis.

Use in the elderly: Treatment of elderly patients, particularly if long term, should be planned bearing in mind the more serious consequences of the common side effects of corticosteroids in old age, especially osteoporosis, diabetes, hypertension, hypokalaemia, susceptibility to infection and thinning of the skin. Close clinical supervision is required to avoid life-threatening reactions (see *Undesirable effects*).

Contra-indications: Systemic fungal infections; systemic infection unless specific anti-infective therapy is employed; hypersensitivity to any component of the drug. Administration of live virus vaccines (see *Special warnings and special precautions for use*).

Special warnings and special precautions for use: Undesirable effects may be minimised by using the lowest effective dose for the minimum period and when appropriate by administering the daily requirement as a single morning dose or whenever possible as a single morning dose on alternative days. Frequent patient review is required to appropriately titrate the dose against disease activity. When reduction in dosage is possible, the reduction should be gradual (see *Posology and method of administration*).

Corticosteroids may exacerbate systemic fungal infections and should not be used in the presence of such infections unless they are needed to control drug reactions due to amphotericin. Moreover, there have been cases reported in which concomitant use of amphotericin and hydrocortisone was followed by cardiac enlargement and heart failure.

Reports in the literature suggest an apparent association between use of corticosteroids and left ventricular free-wall rupture after a recent myocardial infarction; therefore, corticosteroids should be used with great caution in these patients.

A report shows that the use of corticosteroids in cerebral malaria is associated with a prolonged coma and an increased incidence of pneumonia and gastro-intestinal bleeding.

Average and large doses of hydrocortisone or cortisone can cause elevation of blood pressure, retention of salt and water, and increased excretion of potassium, but these effects are less likely to occur with synthetic derivatives, except when used in large doses. Dietary salt restriction and potassium supplementation may be necessary. All corticosteroids increase calcium excretion.

In patients on corticosteroid therapy subjected to unusual stress (e.g. intercurrent illness, trauma, or surgical procedure), dosage should be increased before, during and after the stressful situation. Drug-induced secondary adrenocortical insufficiency may result from too rapid withdrawal of corticosteroids and may be minimised by gradual dosage reduction, being tapered off over weeks and/or months depending on the dose and duration of treatment, but may persist for up to a year after discontinuation of therapy. In any stressful situation during that period, therefore, corticosteroid therapy should be reinstated. If the patient is already receiving corticosteroids, the current dosage may have to be temporarily increased. Salt and/or a mineralocorticoid should be given concurrently, since mineralocorticoid secretion may be impaired.

Stopping corticosteroids after prolonged therapy may cause withdrawal symptoms including fever, myalgia, arthralgia, and malaise. This may occur in patients even without evidence of adrenal insufficiency.

In patients who have received more than physiological doses of systemic cortcosteroids (approximately 1 mg dexamethasone) for greater than three weeks, withdrawal should not be abrupt. How dose reduction should be carried out depends largely on whether the disease is likely to relapse as the dose of systemic corticosteroids is reduced. Clinical assessment of disease activity may be needed during withdrawal. If the disease is unlikely to relapse on withdrawal of systemic corticosteroids but there is uncertainty about hypothalmic-pituitary adrenal (HPA) suppression, the dose of systemic corticosteroins ***may*** be reduced rapidly to physiological doses. Once a daily dose of 1 mg dexamethasone is reached, dose reduction should be slower to allow the HPA-axis to recover.

Abrupt withdrawal of systemic corticosteroid treatment, which has continued up to three weeks is appropriate if it is considered that the disease is unlikely to relapse. Abrupt withdrawal of doses of up to 6 mg daily of dexamethasone for three weeks is unlikely to lead to clinically relevant HPA-axis suppression, in the majority of patients. In the following patient groups, gradual withdrawal of systemic corticosteroid therapy should be ***considered*** even after courses lasting three weeks or less:

- Patients who have had repeated courses of systemic corticosteroids, particularly if taken for greater than three weeks.
- When a short course has been prescribed within one year of cessation of long-term therapy (months or years).
- Patients who may have reasons for adrenocortical insufficiency other than exogenous corticosteroid therapy.
- Patients receiving doses of systemic corticosteroid greater than 6 mg daily of dexamethasone.
- Patients repeatedly taking doses in the evening.

Patients should carry 'steroid treatment' cards, which give clear guidance on the precautions to be taken to minimise risk, and which provide details of prescriber, drug, dosage and the duration of treatment.

Administration of live virus vaccines is contraindicated in individuals receiving immunosuppressive doses of corticosteroids. If inactivated viral or bacterial vaccines are administered to individuals receiving immunosuppressive doses of corticosteroids, the expected serum antibody response may not be obtained. However, immunisation procedures may be undertaken in patients who are receiving corticosteroids as replacement therapy, e.g. for Addison's disease.

The use of Decadron Tablets in active tuberculosis should be restricted to those cases of fulminating or disseminated tuberculosis in which the corticosteroid is used for the management of the disease in conjunction with an appropriate antituberculous regimen. If corticosteroids are indicated in patients with latent tuberculosis or tuberculin reactivity, close observation of the disease is necessary as reactivation may occur. During prolonged corticosteroid therapy, these patients should receive prophylactic chemotherapy.

There is an enhanced effect of corticosteroids in patients with hypothyroidism and in those with cirrhosis.

Corticosteroids may mask some signs of infection, and new infections may appear during their use. Suppression of the inflammatory response and immune function increases the susceptibility to infections and their severity. The clinical presentation may often be atypical, and serious infections such as septicaemia and tuberculosis may be masked and reach an advanced stage before being recognised. There may be decreased resistance and inability to localise infection in patients on corticosteroids.

Chickenpox is of particular concern, since this normally minor illness may be fatal in immunosuppressed patients. Patients (or parents of children) without a definite history of chickenpox should be advised to avoid close personal contact with chickenpox or herpes zoster, and if exposed they should seek urgent medical attention. Passive immunisation with varicella/zoster immunoglobulin (VZIG) is needed by exposed non-immune patients who are receiving systemic corticosteroids or who have used them within the previous three months; this should be given within ten days of exposure to chickenpox. **If a diagnosis of chickenpox is confirmed, the illness warrants specialist care and urgent treatment. Corticosteroids should not be stopped and the dose may need to be increased.**

Measles can have a more serious or even fatal course in immunosuppressed patients. In such children or adults particular care should be taken to avoid exposure to measles. If exposed, prophylaxis with intramuscular pooled immunoglobulin (IG) may be indicated. Exposed patients should be advised to seek medical advice without delay.

Corticosteroids may activate latent amoebiasis or strongyloidiasis or exacerbate active disease. Therefore, it is recommended that latent or active amoebiasis and strongyloidiasis be ruled out before initiating corticosteroid therapy in any patient at risk of or with symptoms suggestive of either condition.

Prolonged use of corticosteroids may produce subcapsular cataracts, glaucoma with possible damage to the optic nerves, and may enhance the establishment of secondary ocular infections due to fungi or viruses. Steroids may increase or decrease the motility and number of spermatozoa.

Special precautions: Particular care is required when considering the use of systemic corticosteroids in patients with the following conditions, and frequent patient monitoring is necessary: renal insufficiency, hypertension, diabetes or in those with a family history of diabetes, congestive heart failure, osteoporosis, previous steroid myopathy, glaucoma (or family history of glaucoma), myasthenia gravis, non-specific ulcerative colitis, diverticulitis, fresh intestinal anastomosis, active or latent peptic ulcer, existing or previous history of severe affective disorders (especially previous steroid psychosis), liver failure, and epilepsy. Signs of peritoneal irritation following gastro-intestinal perforation in patients receiving large doses of corticosteroids may be minimal or absent. Fat embolism has been reported as a possible complication of hypercortisonism.

Corticosteroids should be used cautiously in patients with ocular herpes simplex, because of possible corneal perforation.

Children: Corticosteroids cause growth retardation in infancy, childhood and adolescence, which may be irreversible. Treatment should be limited to the minimum dosage for the shortest possible time. In order to minimise suppression of the hypothalamo-pituitary-adrenal axis and growth retardation, treatment should be limited, where possible, to a single dose on alternate days.

Growth and development of infants and children on prolonged corticosteroid therapy should be carefully monitored.

Interaction with other medicaments and other forms of interaction: Aspirin should be used cautiously in conjunction with corticosteroids in hypoprothrombinaemia.

The renal clearance of salicylates is increased by corticosteroids and, therefore, salicylate dosage should be reduced along with steroid withdrawal.

As phenytoin, barbiturates, ephedrine, rifabutin, carbamazepine, rifampicin, and aminoglutethimide may enhance the metabolic clearance of corticosteroids, resulting in decreased blood levels and reduced physiological activity, the dosage of Decadron may have to be adjusted. These interactions may interfere with dexamethasone-suppression tests which should be interpreted with caution during administration of these drugs.

False-negative results in the dexamethasone suppression test in patients being treated with indomethacin have been reported.

The efficacy of coumarin anticoagulants may be changed by concurrent corticosteroids treatment. The prothrombin time should be checked frequently in patients who are receiving corticosteroids and coumarin anticoagulants at the same time, in order to avoid spontaneous bleeding.

The desired effects of hypoglycaemic agents (including insulin) are antagonised by corticosteroids.

When corticosteroids are administered concomitantly with potassium-depleting diuretics, patients should be observed closely for development of hypokalaemia.

Corticosteroids may affect the nitrobluetetrazolium test for bacterial infection and produce false-negative results.

Pregnancy and lactation: The ability of corticosteroids to cross the placenta varies between individual drugs, however, dexamethasone readily crosses the placenta.

Administration of corticosteroids to pregnant animals can cause abnormalities of foetal development including cleft palate, intra-uterine growth retardation and effects on brain growth and development. There is no evidence that corticosteroids result in an increased incidence of congenital abnormalities, such as cleft palate/lip in man. However, when administered for prolonged periods or repeatedly during pregnancy, corticosteroids may increase the risk of intra-uterine growth retardation. Hypoadrenalism may, in theory, occur in the neonate following prenatal exposure to corticosteroids but usually resolves spontaneously following birth and is rarely clinically important. As with all drugs, corticosteroids should only be prescribed when the benefits to the mother and child outweigh the risks. When corticosteroids are essential however, patients with normal pregnancies may be treated as though they were in the non-gravid state.

Corticosteroids may pass into breast milk, although no data are available for dexamethasone. Infants of mothers taking high doses of systemic corticosteroids for prolonged periods may have a degree of adrenal suppression.

Effects on ability to drive and use machines: None reported.

Undesirable effects: The incidence of predictable undesirable effects, including hypothalamic-pituitary-adrenal suppression, correlates with the relative potency of the drug, dosage, timing of administration and the duration of treatment (see *Special warnings and special precautions for use*).

Fluid and electrolyte disturbances: Sodium retention, fluid retention, congestive heart failure in susceptible patients, potassium loss, hypokalaemic alkalosis, hypertension, increased calcium excretion (see *Special warnings and special precautions for use*).

Musculoskeletal effects: Muscle weakness, steroid myopathy, loss of muscle mass, osteoporosis (especially in post-menopausal females), vertebral compression fractures, aseptic necrosis of femoral and humeral heads, pathological fracture of long bones, tendon rupture.

Gastro-intestinal: Peptic ulcer with possible perforation and haemorrhage, perforation of the small and large bowel particularly in patients with inflammatory bowel disease, pancreatitis, abdominal distension, ulcerative oesophagitis, dyspepsia, oesophageal candidiasis.

Dermatological: Impaired wound healing, thin fragile skin, petechiae and ecchymoses, erythema, striae, telangiectasia, acne, increased sweating, suppressed reaction to skin tests, other cutaneous reactions such as allergic dermatitis, urticaria, angioneurotic oedema.

Neurological: Convulsions, vertigo, headache. Increased intracranial pressure with papilloedema (pseudotumour cerebri) may occur usually after treatment, psychic disturbances, (e.g. euphoria, psychological dependence, depression, insomnia).

Endocrine: Menstrual irregularities, amenorrhoea, development of Cushingoid state, suppression of growth in children and adolescents, secondary adrenocortical and pituitary unresponsiveness (particularly in times of stress as in trauma, surgery or illness), decreased carbohydrate tolerance, manifestations of latent diabetes mellitus, increased requirements for insulin or oral hypoglycaemic agents in diabetics, hirsutism.

Anti-inflammatory and immunosuppressive effects: Increased susceptibility and severity of infections with suppression of clinical symptoms and signs. Opportunistic infections, recurrence of dormant tuberculosis (see *Special warnings and special precautions for use*).

Ophthalmic: Posterior subcapsular cataracts, increased intra-ocular pressure, papilloedema, corneal or scleral thinning, exacerbation of ophthalmic viral disease, glaucoma, exophthalmos.

Metabolic: Negative nitrogen balance due to protein catabolism. Negative calcium balance.

Cardiovascular: Myocardial rupture following recent myocardial infarction (see *Special warnings and special precautions for use*).

Other: Hypersensitivity including anaphylaxis has been reported, leucocytosis, thrombo-embolism, weight gain, increased appetite, nausea, malaise, hiccups.

Withdrawal symptoms and signs: Too rapid a reduction of corticosteroid dosage following prolonged treatment can lead to acute adrenal insufficiency, hypotension, and death (see *Special warnings and special precautions for use*).

In some instances, withdrawal symptoms may simulate a clinical relapse of the disease for which the patient has been undergoing treatment.

Overdosage: Reports of acute toxicity and/or deaths following overdosage with glucocorticoids are rare. No antidote is available. Treatment is probably not indicated for reactions due to chronic poisoning unless the patient has a condition that would render him unusually susceptible to ill effects from corticosteroids. In this case, the stomach should be emptied and symptomatic treatment should be instituted as necessary.

Anaphylactic and hypersensitivity reactions may be treated with epinephrine (adrenaline), positive-pressure artificial respiration and aminophylline. The patient should be kept warm and quiet.

The biological half-life of dexamethasone in plasma is about 190 minutes.

Pharmacological properties

Pharmacodynamic properties: Dexamethasone is a glucocorticoid. It possesses the actions and effects of other basic glucocorticoids, and is among the most active members. Glucocorticoids are adrenocortical steroids, both naturally occurring and synthetic, which are readily absorbed from the gastro-intestinal tract. They cause profound and varied metabolic effects and in addition they modify the body's immune responses to diverse stimuli.

Naturally occurring glucocorticoids (hydrocortisone and cortisone), which also have salt-retaining properties, are used as replacement therapy in adrenocortical deficiency states. Their synthetic analogs, including dexamethasone, are used primarily for their potent anti-inflammatory effects in disorders of many organ systems.

Pharmacokinetic properties: Dexamethasone is readily absorbed from the gastro-intestinal tract.

Its biological half-life in plasma is about 190 minutes.

Binding of dexamethasone to plasma proteins is less than for most other corticosteroids and is estimated to be about 77%.

Up to 65% of a dose is excreted in the urine in 24 hours, the rate of excretion being increased following concomitant administration of phenytoin.

The more potent halogenated corticosteroids such as dexamethasone, appear to cross the placental barrier with minimal inactivation.

Dexamethasone has predominant glucocorticoid activity with little propensity to promote renal retention of sodium and water. Therefore, it does not offer complete replacement therapy, and must be supplemented with salt and/or deoxycorticosterone. Cortisone and hydrocortisone also act predominately as glucocorticoids, although their mineralcorticoid action is greater than that of dexamethasone. Their use in patients with total adrenocortical insufficiency also may require supplemental salt, deoxycorticsone, or both.

Preclinical safety data: No relevant information.

Pharmaceutical particulars

List of excipients: Calcium hydrogen phosphate E341, lactose PhEur, magnesium stearate E572, maize starch PhEur, purified water PhEur.

Incompatibilities: None reported.

Shelf life: Five years.

Special precautions for storage: Store in a dry place below 25°C.

Nature and contents of container: Opaque PVC blister lidded with aluminium foil, containing 30 tablets.

Instructions for use/handling: None.

Marketing authorisation number: PL 0025/5046R.

Date of first authorisation/renewal of authorisation 11 February 1987/9 June 1997.

Date of revision of text April 1998.

Legal category POM.

DEMSER*

Presentation Available as, two-tone blue, opaque capsules, marked 'MSD 690', and 'DEMSER', containing 250 mg metirosine.

Uses The treatment of phaeochromocytoma during: pre-operative preparation of patients for surgery; management of patients when surgery is contra-indicated; prolonged treatment of patients with phaeochromocytoma.

Demser is not recommended for the control of essential hypertension.

Dosage and administration *Adults and children over 12 years of age:* Initially, 1 capsule (250 mg) four times a day. This may be increased by 1 or 2 capsules (250 or 500 mg) daily to a maximum of 4 g daily in divided doses. When used pre-operatively, the optimum dosage should be given for at least five to seven days before surgery.

The optimum dosage range is usually between 8 and 12 capsules (2 to 3 g) a day, titrated by monitoring clinical symptoms and catecholamine excretion. In patients who are hypertensive, dosage should be adjusted to lower blood pressure and control symptoms; in patients whose blood pressure is normal, adjust dosage until the urinary excretion of catecholamines and/or vanillylmandelic acid is reduced by 50% or more.

It is recommended that an alpha-adrenergic blocking agent such as phenoxybenzamine be added if control with Demser is not adequate.

The use of Demser in children under twelve years of age has been limited, and a dosage recommendation cannot be made.

Use in the elderly: These dosage recommendations apply to all adults, including the elderly.

Contra-indications, warnings, etc

Contra-indications: Hypersensitivity.

Warnings: When Demser is used pre-operatively, especially in combination with alpha-adrenoceptor blocking agents, blood volume must be maintained during and after surgery to avoid hypotension and decreased perfusion of vital organs. During surgery, life-threatening arrhythmias may occur requiring treatment with a beta-blocker or lignocaine. Blood pressure and ECG should be monitored continuously throughout surgery.

Demser does not eliminate the danger of arrhythmias or hypertensive crises occurring during manipulation of the tumour and additional alpha-blockade may be necessary.

Precautions: Crystalluria and urolithiasis have occurred in dogs; and crystalluria has been seen in a few patients. To minimise the risk, fluid intake should be sufficient to maintain a urine volume of 2,000 ml or more daily. Urine should be examined routinely, and if metirosine crystals (needles or rods) are seen, fluid intake should be increased. If crystalluria persists, the dosage of Demser should be reduced or discontinued.

Caution should be observed in administering Demser to patients receiving phenothiazines or haloperidol because the extrapyramidal effects of these drugs can be expected to be potentiated by inhibition of catecholamine synthesis; this has been documented to date only for haloperidol.

No evidence of adverse effects on hepatic, haematological or other functions (except for a few instances of increased AST) has been seen during clinical trials. However, total experience in man is limited to approximately 300 patients, and few patients have been studied long-term. Therefore, suitable laboratory tests should be carried out periodically in patients on prolonged therapy, particularly those with impaired hepatic or renal function.

Demser may cause spurious increases in urinary catecholamine measurements.

Breast-feeding mothers: It is not known whether Demser is excreted in human milk. Mothers who need Demser should stop breast-feeding.

Pregnancy: Demser is not recommended for use in pregnant patients. Complete reproduction studies have not been performed in animals to determine whether Demser affects fertility in males or females, has teratogenic potential, or has other adverse effects on the fetus. There are no well-controlled studies of Demser in pregnant women. The use of Demser in pregnant women should be avoided, if possible, but may be appropriate when anticipated benefits outweigh the potential risks.

Adverse reactions: The most common adverse reaction to Demser is moderate to severe sedation, which has been observed in almost all patients. It occurs at both low and high dosages. Sedative effects begin within the first 24 hours of therapy, are maximal after two to three days, and tend to wane during the next few days. Sedation usually is not obvious after one week unless the dosage is increased, but at dosages greater than 2,000 mg/day some degree of sedation or fatigue may persist.

When receiving Demser, patients should be warned about engaging in activities requiring mental alertness and motor co-ordination, such as driving a motor vehicle or operating machinery. Demser may have additive effects with alcohol and other CNS depressants, e.g. hypnotics, sedatives, tranquillisers, anti-anxiety agents.

In most patients who experience sedation, temporary changes in sleep pattern occur following withdrawal of the drug. Changes consist of insomnia that may last for two or three days and feelings of increased alertness and ambition. Even patients who do not experience sedation while on Demser may report symptoms of psychic stimulation when the drug is discontinued.

Extrapyramidal signs such as drooling, speech difficulty and tremor have been reported in approximately 10% of patients, occasionally with trismus and frank parkinsonism.

Anxiety, depression, hallucinations, disorientation and confusion have occurred but may disappear on reduction of the dosage.

Diarrhoea occurs in about 10% of patients, and may be severe. Infrequently, slight swelling of the breast, galactorrhoea, nasal stuffiness, decreased salivation, dry mouth, headache, nausea, vomiting, abdominal pain, and impotence or failure of ejaculation may occur. Crystalluria transient dysuria and haematuria have been seen in a few patients. Eosinophilia, increased AST levels, peripheral oedema, and hypersensitivity such as urticaria and pharyngeal oedema has been reported rarely.

Overdosage: Signs of metirosine overdosage include the CNS effects seen at therapeutic dosages such as fatigue, anxiety or agitated depression, neuromuscular effects, diarrhoea, and decreased salivation. At therapeutic levels, reduction of dose or cessation of treatment usually results in the disappearance of these symptoms.

Since there is little clinical experience, the treatment of overdosage has not been identified. There is no antidote.

Metirosine is well-absorbed from the gastro-intestinal tract. Maximal biochemical effect is usually seen within two or three days.

Pharmaceutical precautions Store in a cool place, protected from light.

Legal category POM.

Package quantities Bottles of 100.

Further information Nil.

Product licence number 0025/0132.

DOLOBID* 250 mg tablets
DOLOBID* 500 mg tablets

Qualitative and quantitative composition Dolobid 250 mg tablets contains 250 mg of the active ingredient, diflunisal BP.

Dolobid 500 mg tablets contains 500 mg of the active ingredient, diflunisal BP.

Pharmaceutical form

Dolobid 250 mg tablets are supplied as peach-coloured, capsule-shaped, film-coated tablets, marked 'MSD 675'.

Dolobid 500 mg tablets are supplied as orange-coloured, film-coated tablets, marked 'MSD 697'.

Clinical particulars

Therapeutic indications: Dolobid is indicated in the relief of pain.

Dolobid is also indicated in the relief of pain and inflammation associated with osteoarthritis and rheumatoid arthritis.

Dolobid is also indicated in the relief of pain and associated symptoms of primary dysmenorrhoea.

Posology and method of administration: Tablets should be swallowed whole, not crushed or chewed.

It is prudent to start at the bottom end of the dose range. In certain cases, it will be necessary to start with a high initial dose, as described in the dosage recommendations below.

For relief of pain: An initial dose of 1000 mg, followed by 500 mg every 12 hours, is recommended for most patients. Following the initial dose some patients may require 500 mg every eight hours.

Maintenance doses higher than 1500 mg a day are not recommended.

For osteoarthritis and rheumatoid arthritis: The recommended dosage range is 500 mg to 1000 mg per day. Dolobid may be administered once or twice a day.

Dosage should be adjusted to the nature and intensity of the pain being treated.

For dysmenorrhoea: The recommended dosage is 1000 mg at the onset of cramps or bleeding, followed by 500 mg every 12 hours for as long as symptoms last, usually a maximum of five days.

Use in children: Dolobid is not recommended for children.

Use in the elderly: The dosage does not require modification for elderly patients.

Contra-indications: Hypersensitivity to any component of this product.

In patients who have previously experienced acute asthmatic attacks, urticaria, or rhinitis precipitated by aspirin or non-steroidal anti-inflammatory agents.

The drug should not be administered to patients with active gastro-intestinal bleeding.

NSAIDs, including Dolobid, should not be given to patients with active peptic ulceration.

Dolobid is contra-indicated in pregnancy and lactation (see *Pregnancy and lactation*).

Special warnings and precautions for use: Although Dolobid has less effect on platelet function and bleeding time than aspirin, it does inhibit platelet function at higher doses; patients who may be adversely affected should be carefully observed.

Because of reports of adverse eye findings with agents of this class, if eye complaints develop during treatment with Dolobid they should be fully examined.

Dolobid should be used with caution in patients having a history of gastro-intestinal haemorrhage or ulcers. Fatalities have occurred, rarely.

In patients with a history of peptic-ulcer disease and in the elderly, NSAIDs should be given only after other forms of treatment have been carefully considered.

Dolobid should be used with caution in patients suffering from, or with a previous history of bronchial asthma.

Although there have been no known reports associated with the use of Dolobid to date, acetylsalicylic acid has been associated with Reye's syndrome. Because diflunisal is a compound related to salicylic acid, the possibility of an association with Reye's syndrome cannot be excluded.

As with other NSAIDs, Dolobid should be used with caution in patients with reduced renal blood flow, since renal prostaglandins play a supportive role in the maintenance of renal perfusion.

The dosage of Dolobid may need to be reduced in patients with renal functional impairment since the major route of excretion is via the kidney. In patients with severe renal impairment, the drug should not be used.

In rats and dogs, high oral doses of diflunisal (50 to 200 mg/kg/day), as with aspirin, produced similar pathological changes (gastro-intestinal ulceration and renal papillary oedema). These dosages are approximately 3 to 12 times the maximum dosages recommended in man.

Peripheral oedema has been observed in some patients taking Dolobid. Therefore, as with other drugs in this class, Dolobid should be used with caution in patients with compromised cardiac function, hypertension, or other conditions predisposing to fluid retention.

A potentially life-threatening apparent hypersensitivity syndrome has been reported. This multisystem syndrome includes constitutional symptoms, (fever, chills), and cutaneous findings (see *Dermatological* under *Side-effects*). It may also include involvement of major organs (changes in liver function), jaundice, leucopenia, thrombocytopenia, eosinophilia, disseminated intravascular coagulation, renal impairment (including renal failure); and less specific findings (adenitis, arthralgia, myalgia, arthritis, malaise, anorexia, disorientation).

Laboratory tests: AST (SGOT) and ALT (SGPT) levels rose significantly by three times the upper limit of normal in less than 1% of patients in controlled clinical trials of non-steroidal anti-inflammatory drugs.

A patient on Dolobid with signs or symptoms suggesting liver disease, or in whom abnormal liver function tests have occurred, should be evaluated for evidence of a more severe hepatic reaction. If abnormal liver tests persist or worsen, if signs or symptoms of liver disease develop, or if systemic manifestations such as eosinophilia or rash occur, Dolobid should be discontinued.

Interaction with other medicaments and other forms of interaction: Indomethacin: The combined use of indomethacin and Dolobid has been associated with fatal gastro-intestinal haemorrhage. The combination should not be used. Co-administration of Dolobid with indomethacin increases the plasma level of indomethacin by about 30 to 35% with a concomitant decrease in renal clearance of indomethacin and its conjugate.

Other NSAIDs: the concomitant use of Dolobid with other NSAIDs is not recommended due to the increased possibility of gastro-intestinal toxicity, with little or no increase in efficacy.

Aspirin: Co-administration of aspirin causes approximately a 15% decrease in plasma levels of Dolobid.

Codeine: Co-administration with Dolobid improves the analgesic efficacy of either drug taken alone.

Methotrexate: Caution should be used if Dolobid is administered concomitantly with methotrexate. Non-steroidal anti-inflammatory drugs have been reported to decrease the tubular secretion of methotrexate and potentiate the toxicity.

Cyclosporin: Administration of non-steroidal anti-inflammatory drugs concomitantly with cyclosporin has been associated with an increase in cyclosporin-induced toxicity, possibly due to decreased synthesis of renal prostacyclin. Non-steroidal anti-inflammatory drugs should be used with caution in patients taking cyclosporin, and renal function should be monitored carefully.

Oral anticoagulant drugs: The concomitant administration of Dolobid and warfarin or nicoumalone resulted in prolongation of prothrombin time in normal volunteers. This may occur because diflunisal competitively displaces coumarins from protein binding sites. Accordingly, prothrombin time should be monitored during, and for several days after, the concomitant drug administration of Dolobid and oral anticoagulants. The dosage of oral anticoagulants may require adjustment.

Antihypertensives: The antihypertensive effects of some antihypertensive agents including ACE inhibitors, beta-blocking agents and diuretics, may be reduced when used concomitantly with NSAIDs. Caution should therefore be exercised when considering the addition of NSAID therapy to the regimen of a patient taking antihypertensives therapy.

Cardiac glycosides: An increase in serum-digoxin concentration has been reported with concomitant use of aspirin, indomethacin and other NSAIDs. Therefore when concomitant digoxin and NSAID therapy is initiated or discontinued, serum-digoxin levels should be closely monitored.

Lithium: Concomitant use of indomethacin with lithium, produced a clinically relevant elevation of plasma lithium and reduction in renal lithium clearance in psychatric patients and normal subjects with steady-state plasma lithium concentrations. This effect has been attributed to inhibition of prostaglandin synthesis and the potential exists for a similar effect with other NSAIDs.

As a consequence, when an NSAID and lithium are given concomitantly, the patient should be observed carefully for signs of lithium toxicity. In addition the frequency of monitoring serum lithium concentrations should be increased at the outset of such combination therapy.

Corticosteroids: The risk of gastro-intestinal bleeding and ulceration associated with NSAIDs is increased when used with corticosteroids.

Mifepristone: NSAIDs and aspirin should be avoided until at least 8 to 12 days after administration of mifepristone.

Quinolone antibiotics: There have been reports that 4-quinolones may induce convulsions, in patients with or without a history of convulsions. Taking NSAIDs at the same time may also induce them.

Tolbutamide: No significant changes occurred in the plasma levels of tolbutamide or in the fasting blood sugar levels of diabetic patients who also took Dolobid.

Hydrochlorothiazide: Co-administration increases the plasma levels of hydrochlorothiazide by 25 to 35% with a concomitant decrease in renal clearance of the diuretic. This change is not clinically important. Dolobid counteracts the hyperuricaemic effect of hydrochlorothiazide.

Frusemide: Co-administration did not affect the diuretic activity of frusemide in normal volunteers, but its hyperuricaemic activity was decreased by Dolobid.

Antacids: The clinical effect of occasional doses of antacid is insignificant, but this becomes significant when antacids are used continuously. Co-administration of aluminium hydroxide suspension significantly decreases the absorption of Dolobid by approximately 40%.

Paracetamol: Co-administration significantly increased the plasma levels of paracetamol by approximately 50%, but the plasma levels of Dolobid were unaffected.

Other non-steroidal, anti-inflammatory agents: No clinical data on the safety and efficacy of concomitant administration are available. No recommendations can be made. However, normal volunteers given sulindac and Dolobid showed substantial but not statistically significant lower levels of the active sulphide metabolite of sulindac. Normal volunteers given naproxen and Dolobid showed no changes in plasma levels of either drug, but a significant decrease in urinary excretion of naproxen and its glucuronide metabolite.

Gold salts: In clinical studies of patients with rheumatoid arthritis, Dolobid added to the regimen of gold salts usually resulted in additional symptomatic relief.

Drug/laboratory test interactions: Serum salicylate assays: caution should be used in interpreting the results of serum salicylate assays when diflunisal is present. Because of the cross-reactivity between the two compounds, salicylate levels have been found to be falsely elevated with some assay methods.

Pregnancy and lactation: Dolobid should not be given to pregnant women, since the safety for this use has not been established. Breast-feeding mothers should not take Dolobid, or should stop breast-feeding.

Effects on ability to drive and use machines: None stated.

Side effects: 3% to 9% incidence: Gastro-intestinal: gastro-intestinal pain, dyspepsia, diarrhoea, nausea. *Dermatological:* rash. *Central nervous system:* headache.

1% to 3% incidence: Gastro-intestinal: vomiting, constipation, flatulence. *Central nervous system/Psychiatric:* dizziness, somnolence, insomnia. *Special senses:* tinnitus. *Miscellaneous:* fatigue.

Less than 1% incidence: Gastro-intestinal: peptic ulcer, gastro-intestinal perforation and bleeding, anorexia, jaundice, cholestasis, liver-function abnormality, hepatitis, gastritis. *Dermatological:* pruritus, sweating, dry mucous membranes, stomatitis, photosensitivity, urticaria, erythema multiforme and Stevens-Johnson syndrome, toxic epidermal necrolysis, exfoliative dermatitis. *Genito-urinary:* dysuria, renal impairment including renal failure, interstitial nephritis, haematuria. *Central nervous system/Psychiatric:* vertigo, light-headedness, paraesthesiae, nervousness, depression, hallucinations, confusion. *Haematological:* thrombocytopenia, agranulocytosis, haemolytic anaemia. *Special senses:* transient visual disturbances including blurred vision. *Miscellaneous:* asthenia, oedema. *Hypersensitivity reactions:* acute anaphylactic reaction with bronchospasm, angioedema, hypersensitivity vasculitis, hypersensitivity syndrome (see *Special warnings and precautions for use*).

Side-effects – causal relationship unknown: Other reactions have been reported in clinical trials or since the drug was marketed, but occurred under circumstances where a causal relationship could not be established. However, in these rarely reported events, that possibility cannot be excluded. Therefore, the following observations are listed to serve as alerting information to physicians.

Respiratory: Dyspnoea. *Cardiovascular:* Palpitations, syncope. *Musculoskeletal:* Muscle cramps. *Miscellaneous:* Chest pain. *Genito-rinary:* Nephrotic syndrome.

Overdose: Cases of overdosage have occurred and fatalities have been reported. The most common signs and symptoms observed with overdosage were drowsiness, vomiting, nausea, diarrhoea, hyperventilation, tachycardia, sweating, tinnitus, disorientation, stupor, and coma. Diminished urine output and cardiorespiratory arrest have also been reported. The lowest dose of Dolobid alone at which death was reported was 15 g; death has been reported from a mixed drug overdose that included 7.5 g Dolobid.

In the event of recent overdosage, the stomach should be emptied by inducing vomiting or gastric lavage, and the patient observed carefully and given symptomatic and supportive treatment.

To facilitate urinary elimination of the drug, attempt to maintain renal function. Because of the high degree of protein binding, haemodialysis is not recommended.

The initial plasma half-life following single oral doses of diflunisal seems to be dose dependent, ranging from approximately 7.5 hours for a 250 mg dose to 11 hours for a 500 mg dose.

Pharmacological properties

Pharmacodynamic properties: Dolobid in man has been shown to possess analgesic activity lasting up to 12 hours or more. In clinical trials, Dolobid produced highly effective levels of analgesia when administered twice a day.

As an inhibitor of prostaglandin synthetase, Dolobid has a dose related effect on platelet function. In normal volunteers given Dolobid twice a day for 8 days at doses within the recommended range 500–1000 mg daily, 500 mg daily had no effect on platelet function and 1000 mg daily had a slight effect. However, at 2000 mg daily, which exceeds the maximum recommended dosage, Dolobid inhibited platelet function. In contrast to aspirin, these effects of Dolobid were reversible.

A loading dose of 1000 mg provides faster onset of pain relief, shorter time to peak analgesic effect, and greater peak analgesic effects than an initial 500 mg dose.

Dolobid at 1000 mg twice daily (NOTE: exceeds the recommended dosage) causes a statistically significant increase in faecal blood loss, but this increase was only one-half as large as that associated with aspirin 1300 mg twice daily.

Pharmacokinetic properties: Dolobid is rapidly and completely absorbed following oral administration with peak plasma concentrations occurring between 2 and 3 hours. The drug is excreted in the urine as two soluble glucuronide conjugates accounting for about 90% of the administered dose. Little or no diflunisal is excreted in the faeces. As diflunisal is excreted primarily by the kidney, the greater the degree of renal impairment, the slower the plasma disappearance rate of the drug and its glucuronides. Diflunisal appears in human milk in concentrations of 2–7% of those in plasma. More than 90% of diflunisal in plasma is bound to proteins.

The plasma half-life of diflunisal is 8–12 hours. Because of this long half-life and non-linear pharmacokinetics, several days are required for diflunisal plasma levels to reach steady-state following multiple doses. For this reason, an initial loading dose is necessary to shorten the time to reach steady-state levels, and 2–3 days of observation are necessary for evaluating changes in treatment regimens if a loading dose is not used.

Preclinical safety data: No relevant information.

Pharmaceutical particulars

List of excipients: Dolobid 250 mg and 500 mg tablets contain the following inactive ingredients: Cellulose; microcrystalline PhEur; Hydroxypropylcellulose PhEur; Magnesium stearate PhEur; Pregelatinised maize starch BP; Sunset yellow aluminium lake E110 EEC; Talc PhEur; Titanium dioxide PhEur; Methylhydroxypropylcellulose PhEur.

Dolobid 250 mg tablets also contains carnauba wax PhEur.

Incompatibilities: None.

Shelf life: PVC blister packs of 60 tablets: 36 months.

Special precautions for storage: Store below 25°C, protected from light.

Nature and contents of container: Dolobid 250 mg tablets are available in:

Packs of 60 tablets containing six PVC blister strips of 10 tablets, to give a total of 60 tablets.

Dolobid 500 mg tablets are available in:

Packs of 60 tablets containing six PVC blister strips of 10 tablets, to give a total of 60 tablets.

Instructions for use/handling: None.

Product licence numbers

250 mg tablets: 0025/0128.
500 mg tablets: 0025/0146.

Date of first authorisation/renewal of authorisation PL 0025/0128 (250 mg): granted 29 September 1977, renewed 15 May 1998.

PL 0025/0146 (500 mg): granted 23 April 1980, renewed 21 May 1998.

Date of revision of the text May 1998.

Legal category POM.

EDECRIN* INJECTION (ethacrynic acid)

Qualitative and quantitative composition Intravenous injection vials containing sodium ethacrynate equivalent to 50 mg ethacrynic acid, as a dry lyophilised powder.

Pharmaceutical form Lyophilised powder for injection.

Clinical particulars

Therapeutic indications: Diuretic.

Edecrin is indicated when urgent and potent diuresis is essential. It is particularly recommended in oedema associated with: Congestive heart failure; pulmonary oedema; renal oedema; hepatic cirrhosis with ascites; ascites due to malignancy; oedema due to other causes, including idiopathic oedema and lymphoedema.

Edecrin Injection is not recommended for children.

Posology and method of administration: Dosage should be carefully regulated to prevent a more rapid or substantial diuresis than necessary. Daily weighing of the patient and, where possible, serum electrolyte determinations will greatly contribute to the success of treatment.

Edecrin Injection is intended for intravenous injection when oral treatment is impractical or when urgent diuresis is essential, as in acute pulmonary oedema.

Usual adult intravenous dose: 0.5–1 mg/kg of bodyweight. The dosage for an average-sized adult is 50 mg. Usually only one dose is necessary; however, if a second dose is required, it should be given at a new injection site to avoid thrombophlebitis.

Single intravenous doses of up to 100 mg have been used in critical situations.

The solution may be given slowly through the tubing of a running infusion, or by direct intravenous injection over several minutes.

Edecrin Injection should not be mixed with whole blood or blood derivatives. If it is desired to administer it at the same time as a blood transfusion, it should be given independently.

Children: As paediatric experience with Edecrin Injection is limited, it is not recommended for children.

Use in the elderly: The general considerations on adjustment of dosage to meet individual needs apply equally to elderly patients (see *Special warnings and special precautions for use*).

Contra-indications: Anuria. Infants (under 2 years). For 'Use in pregnancy' and 'Use in breast-feeding mothers', see *Pregnancy and lactation.* Hypersensitivity to this product.

Special warnings and special precautions for use: The effects of Edecrin on electrolytes are based on its renal pharmacology and are usually dose related.

To minimise the possibility of profound electrolyte and water loss, therapy should be initiated with a low dosage and this carefully adjusted as necessary; intermittent dosage should be used where possible and the patient weighed regularly throughout treatment. If diuresis is excessive, Edecrin should be withdrawn until homeostasis is restored.

Frequent serum electrolyte, alkali reserve and blood urea determinations should be made early in therapy, and periodically thereafter while active diuresis is taking place. Any electrolyte abnormality should be corrected or the drug temporarily withdrawn.

If increasing electrolyte imbalance, uraemia and/or oliguria occur during treatment of severe progressive renal disease, the diuretic should be discontinued.

Inclusion of potassium supplements or potassium-sparing agents is often advisable, especially during the treatment of cirrhotic or nephrotic patients and patients receiving digitalis.

Although treatment with Edecrin generally allows patients greater freedom with their salt intake, cirrhotic patients should usually have their salt moderately restricted while on therapy.

Edecrin should be given with caution to patients with advanced cirrhosis of the liver, particularly those with a history of episodes of electrolyte imbalance or hepatic encephalopathy. Edecrin may precipitate hepatic coma and death.

When metabolic alkalosis may be anticipated (e.g. in cirrhosis with ascites), a potassium-conserving agent or potassium chloride may mitigate or prevent hypokalaemia.

Loop diuretics may cause hypomagnesaemia.

Too vigorous a diuresis may induce an acute hypotensive episode. In elderly cardiac patients, severe diuresis may cause a rapid contraction of plasma volume, which should be avoided to prevent possible thrombo-embolic episodes.

Weakness, muscle cramps, paraesthesiae, thirst, anorexia, and signs of hyponatraemia, hypokalaemia and/or hypochloraemic alkalosis may follow vigorous or excessive diuresis or be accentuated by rigid salt restriction. Rarely, tetany has been reported following vigorous diuresis. Adequate salt intake and potassium chloride supplements are often necessary.

A few patients have had a sudden onset of profuse watery diarrhoea. If this occurs and other causes are eliminated, Edecrin should be discontinued and not re-administered.

Edecrin should be used cautiously in critically ill patients, particularly (1) those patients with severe myocardial disease who have been receiving digitalis; they may develop acute hypokalaemia with fatal arrhythmias. (2) Patients with severely decompensated hepatic cirrhosis with ascites (with or without accompanying encephalopathy) who are in electrolyte imbalance may undergo further deterioration of the electrolyte defect. A number of possible drug-related deaths have occurred among such patients.

Edecrin has little or no effect on glomerular filtration rate or renal blood flow, except immediately after a pronounced reduction in plasma volume following rapid diuresis. An increase in blood urea may occur, although transient it may usually be readily reversed by discontinuing Edecrin.

Edecrin may potentiate the effect of carbonic anhydrase inhibitors, increasing sodium and potassium excretion. If Edecrin is given to patients already receiving a carbonic anhydrase inhibitor, the initial dose and increments should be only 25 mg.

Interaction with other medicaments and other forms of interaction:

Antihypertensive agents may require adjustment of dosage with concurrent use. Orthostatic hypotension may occur in patients on antihypertensive agents when given Edecrin.

Antibiotics: The concurrent use of such drugs as aminoglycosides with Edecrin should be avoided because of the risk of increasing their ototoxic potential.

Warfarin: Several drugs, including Edecrin, have been shown to displace warfarin from plasma protein. In patients receiving both types of drug, a reduction in the dosage of the anticoagulant may therefore be required.

Lithium: Lithium should generally not be given to patients receiving diuretics, since the risk of lithium toxicity is very high in such patients.

Corticosteroids: Edecrin may increase the risk of gastric haemorrhage associated with corticosteroid treatment.

Pregnancy and lactation: As clinical experience is limited, Edecrin is not recommended in pregnant patients. The routine use of diuretics in otherwise healthy pregnant women with or without mild oedema is not indicated because they may be associated with hypovolaemia, increased blood viscosity and decreased placental perfusion. If administration in confirmed or suspected pregnancy is considered, the benefits of therapy should be weighed against the possible hazard to the foetus.

Use in breast-feeding mothers: Edecrin is contra-indicated in breast-feeding mothers. If its use is deemed essential, the patient should stop breast-feeding.

Effects on ability to drive and use machines: None known.

Undesirable effects:

Gastro-intestinal: Anorexia, malaise, abdominal discomfort or pain, dysphagia, nausea, vomiting, and diarrhoea. A few patients have had profuse, watery diarrhoea, gastro-intestinal bleeding, and acute pancreatitis.

Metabolic: Reversible hyperuricaemia, decreased urinary urate excretion and hyperglycaemia may occur. Acute gout may be precipitated. Rarely, acute symptomatic hypoglycaemia with convulsions, jaundice and abnormal liver-function tests have been reported.

Haematological: Agranulocytosis, severe neutropenia, thrombocytopenia and Henoch-Schönlein purpura have been reported rarely.

Special senses: Deafness, tinnitus and vertigo with a sense of fullness in the ears, and blurred vision have occurred.

Central nervous system: Fatigue, apprehension and confusion.

Other: Skin rash, headache, fever, rigors, and haematuria.

Edecrin Injection has occasionally caused local irritation and pain due to extravasation of injected fluid.

Overdosage: Treatment should be symptomatic and supportive; no specific antidote is available. Dehydration, electrolyte imbalance, hepatic coma and hypotension should be corrected by standard methods. If respiration is impaired, oxygen or artificial respiration should be given.

The drug is fairly rapidly absorbed after ingestion with a plasma half-life of 30 minutes to one hour. Ethacrynic acid is bound to plasma proteins: haemodialysis is unlikely to be effective.

Pharmacological properties

Pharmacodynamic properties: Ethacrynic acid acts by reducing resorption of sodium and chloride in the proximal renal tubule, in the ascending loop of Henle and, to a lesser extent, in the distal renal tubules; distal tubular potassium secretion is also decreased to a variable degree. Urinary pH is decreased, bicarbonate excretion is diminished, ammonium excretion is increased, and serum uric acid levels may be increased. The intense initial enhancement of sodium and chloride may diminish on prolonged use, but potassium and hydrogen-ion losses may be increased.

Pharmacokinetic properties: Following intravenous injection, about one-third of the dose is excreted by the liver and about two-thirds by the kidney. the drug recovered from the urine is about equally divided into three fractions: the parent compound, a cysteine adduct, and an unstable metabolite of undetermined nature. Ethacrynic acid is secreted by the organic-acid secretory mechanism of the proximal tubule. The net rate of urinary secretion is also dependent on urinary pH. Thus, ethacrynic acid probably normally undergoes substantial back diffusion.

The half-life for elimination of ethacrynic acid is approximately 0.5 to 1.0 hours.

Preclinical safety data: Ethacrynic acid has acute toxicity in mice, with an oral LD_{50} of about 600 mg/kg and an intravenous LD_{50} of about 200 mg/kg when given in solution as the sodium salt. The compound is somewhat less toxic for the rat, the oral LD_{50} for weanling and adult male and female rats being of the order of 1000 to 1200 mg/kg. The acute oral LD_{50} for rabbits and guinea pigs was about 450 mg/kg.

In oral chronic studies, rats, which are largely unresponsive to the saluretic effects of ethacrynic acid, tolerated oral doses up to about 80 mg/kg day in the diet for 18 months, although one rat on the middle dose (15 mg/kg/day) had small ulcers in the glandular portion of the stomach, which were considered incidental to treatment. No other histomorphological changes due to treatment were found in other tissues in either of the oral toxicity studies.

Dogs tolerated 10 to 15 mg/kg/day in divided doses for one year. A greater degree of tolerance, 30 mg/kg/day as single daily doses, was achieved in this species by adding sodium chloride to the drinking water. There were no haematological, biochemical, or histomorphological changes observed in the chronic studies, except those secondarily related to its saluretic-diuretic action.

When 10 mg/kg/day (as single daily doses) or larger doses (divided or single without saline) were given, some animals showed marked electrolyte imbalance and dehydration. Reproduction studies on ethacrynic acid in the mouse, rat, rabbit, and dog revealed no drug-related changes in the reproductive capacity or foetal developments in these species.

Pharmaceutical particulars

List of excipients: Edecrin Injection contains the following ingredient: Mannitol PhEur.

Incompatibilities: None known.

Shelf life: 24 months.

Special precautions for storage: Store in tightly closed container, protected from light, at 25°C; (the product is stable between 15°C and 30°C). After reconstitution can be stored up to 24 hours at 2–8°C.

Nature and contents of container: Nominal 50 ml clear glass vials with red rubber stoppers and roll-on aluminium collar seals with plastic 'flip-off' tops.

Pack size: Single vials containing 50 mg ethacrynic acid.

Instructions for use/handling: Edecrin Injection is reconstituted by adding 50 ml of 5% dextrose injection or of isotonic saline to the vial (some 5% dextrose injection solutions have a pH below 5. If such a preparation is used as diluent, the resulting solution may be cloudy. The use of such a solution is not recommended.)

The solution may be given slowly through the tubing of a running infusion, or by direct intravenous injection over several minutes.

Edecrin Injection should not be mixed with whole blood or blood derivatives. If it is desired to administer it at the same time as a blood transfusion, it should be given independently.

Marketing authorisation number PL 0025/5007R.

Date of first authorisation/renewal of authorisation 20 November 1987.

30 December 1997.

Date of revision of the text February 1998.

Legal category POM.

FOSAMAX* ▼

Qualitative and quantitative composition Each tablet of Fosamax contains 13.05 mg of alendronate sodium, which is the molar equivalent to 10 mg of alendronic acid.

Pharmaceutical form Fosamax is supplied as round white tablets, with convex faces, marked with an embossed bone symbol and Fosamax on one side, and an embossed bone symbol and 'MSD 936' on the other.

Clinical particulars

Therapeutic indications: Fosamax is indicated for the treatment of osteoporosis in post-menopausal women.

Posology and method of administration: The recommended dosage is 10 mg once a day.

To permit adequate absorption of Fosamax: Fosamax must be taken at least 30 minutes before the first food, beverage, or medication of the day with plain water only. Other beverages (including mineral water), food and some medications are likely to reduce the absorption of Fosamax (see 'Interaction with other medicaments and other forms of interaction').

To facilitate delivery to the stomach and thus reduce the potential for local and oesophageal irritation/adverse experiences (see 'Special warnings and special precautions for use'): Fosamax should only be swallowed upon rising for the day with a full glass of water (not less than 200 ml or 7 fl. oz.).

Patients should not chew or suck the tablets.

Patients should not lie down for at least 30 minutes after taking Fosamax.

Patients should not lie down until after their first food of the day, which should be at least 30 minutes after taking the tablet.

Fosamax should not be taken at bedtime or before rising for the day.

All patients with osteoporosis should have adequate dietary calcium (see 'Special warnings and special precautions for use').

Use in the elderly: In clinical studies there was no age-related difference in the efficacy or safety profiles of Fosamax. Therefore no dosage adjustment is necessary for the elderly.

Use in renal impairment: No dosage adjustment is necessary for patients with mild renal impairment where GFR is greater than 35 ml/min. Fosamax is not recommended for patients with mild renal impairment where GFR is 20–35 ml/min, or for patients with moderate to severe renal impairment (GFR <20 ml/min).

Use in children: Fosamax has not been studied in children and should not be given to them.

Contra-indications: Abnormalities of the oesophagus and other factors which delay oesophageal emptying, such as stricture or achalasia.

Inability to stand or sit upright for at least 30 minutes.

Hypersensitivity to any component of this product.

Hypocalcaemia (see 'Special warnings and special precautions for use').

Special warnings and special precautions for use: Fosamax can cause local irritation of the upper gastro-intestinal mucosa. Because there is a potential for worsening of the underlying disease, caution should be used when Fosamax is given to patients with active upper gastro-intestinal problems, such as dysphagia, oesophageal disease, gastritis, duodenitis, or ulcers (see 'Contra-indications').

Oesophageal reactions (sometimes severe and requiring hospitalisation), such as oesophagitis, oesophageal ulcers and oesophageal erosions, have been reported in patients receiving Fosamax. Physicians should therefore be alert to any signs or symptoms signalling a possible oesophageal reaction, and patients should be instructed to discontinue Fosamax and seek medical attention if they develop symptoms of oesophageal irritation such as dysphagia, pain on swallowing, retrosternal pain, or new or worsening heartburn.

In order to reduce potential for oesophageal adverse reactions, and to facilitate delivery to the stomach, patients should be instructed to swallow Fosamax with a full glass of water and not lie down for at least 30 minutes and until after their first food of the day (see 'Posology and method of administration'). Patients should be specifically instructed not to take the tablets at bedtime or before rising for the day. Patients should not chew or suck the tablets because of a potential for oropharyngeal ulceration.

While no increased risk was observed in extensive clinical trials, there have been rare (post-marketing) reports of gastric and duodenal ulcers, some severe and with complications. However, a causal relationship has not been established.

Fosamax is not recommended for patients with mild renal impairment where GFR is 20–35 ml/min, or for patients with moderate to severe renal impairment (see 'Posology and method of administration').

Causes of osteoporosis other than oestrogen deficiency and ageing should be considered. Hypocalcaemia must be corrected before initiating therapy with Fosamax (see *Contra-indications*). Other disturbances of mineral metabolism (such as vitamin D deficiency) should also be effectively treated.

Interaction with other medicaments and other forms of interaction: If taken at the same time, it is likely that calcium supplements, antacids, and some oral medications will interfere with absorption of Fosamax. Therefore, patients must wait at least 30 minutes after taking Fosamax before taking any other oral medication.

No other drug interations of clinical significance are anticipated. A small number of patients in the clinical trials received oestrogen (intravaginal, transdermal, or oral) while taking Fosamax. No adverse experiences attributable to their concomitant use were identified.

Although specific interaction studies were not performed, Fosamax was used concomitantly in post-menopausal osteoporosis studies with a wide range of commonly prescribed drugs without evidence of clinical adverse interactions. However, the incidence of upper gastro-intestinal adverse events associated with non-steroidal anti-inflammatory drugs and aspirin appears to be greater with concomitant administration of Fosamax.

Pregnancy and lactation

Use during pregnancy: Fosamax has not been studied in pregnant women and should not be given to them.

In developmental toxicity studies in animals, there were no adverse effects at doses up to 25 mg/kg/day in rats and 35 mg/kg/day in rabbits.

Use during lactation: Fosamax has not been studied in breast-feeding women and should not be given to them.

Effects on ability to drive and use machines: There are no data to suggest that Fosamax affects the ability to drive or use machines.

Undesirable effects:

Clinical studies: Side-effects, which usually were mild, generally did not require discontinuation of therapy.

In two large, three-year studies of virtually identical design, with a total of 994 post-menopausal women (Fosamax: N=597, placebo: N=397) the overall safety profiles of Fosamax 10 mg/day and placebo were similar. Adverse experiences reported by the investigators as possibly, probably or definitely drug related in ≥1% of patients treated with 'Fosamax' 10 mg/day and at a greater incidence than in patients given placebo are presented in the following table:

	FOSAMAX 10 mg/day (n=196) %	Placebo (n=397) %
Gastro-intestinal		
abdominal pain	6.6	4.8
dyspepsia	3.6	3.5
constipation	3.1	1.8
diarrhoea	3.1	1.8
flatulence	2.6	0.5
oesophageal ulcer	1.5	0.0
dysphagia	1.0	0.0
abdominal distension	1.0	0.8
Musculoskeletal		
musculoskeletal (bone, muscle or joint) pain	4.1	2.5
Neurological		
headache	2.6	1.5

Rarely, rash and erythema have occurred.

Post-marketing experience: In addition to the adverse experiences reported during clinical studies and listed above under *Clinical studies*, the following adverse experiences have been reported during post-marketing use.

Uncommon (>0.1% and <1%) – Gastro-intestinal: nausea, vomiting, oesophagitis, oesophageal erosions, and as previously noted in clinical trials, oesophageal ulcers (see *Special warnings and special precautions for use* and *Posology and method of administration*).

Rare (≥0.01% and <0.1%) – Body as a whole: hypersensitivity reactions including urticaria and rarely angioedema. *Gastro-intestinal:* oropharyngeal ulceration; gastric or duodenal ulcers, some severe and with complications although a causal relationship has not been established (see *Special warnings and special precautions for use* and *Posology and method of administration*).

Laboratory test findings: In clinical studies, asymptomatic, mild and transient decreases in serum calcium and phosphate were observed in approximately 18% and 10%, respectively, of patients taking Fosamax versus approximately 12% and 3% of those taking placebo. However, the incidences of decreases in serum calcium to <8.0 mg/dl (<2.0 mmol/l) and serum phosphate to ≤2.0 mgP/dl (≤0.65 mmol/l) were similar in both treatment groups.

Overdose: Significant lethality after single oral doses was seen in female rats and mice at 552 mg/kg (3256 mg/m²) and 966 mg/kg (2898 mg/m²) (equivalent to human oral doses* of 27,600 and 48,300 mg), respectively. In males, these values were slightly higher, 626 and 1280 mg/kg, respectively. There was no lethality in dogs at oral doses up to 200 mg/kg (4000 mg/m²) (equivalent to human oral dose* of 10,000 mg).

* Based on a patient weight of 50 kg.

No specific information is available on the treatment of overdosage with Fosamax. Hypocalcaemia, hypophosphataemia and upper gastro-intestinal adverse events, such as upset stomach, heartburn, oesophagitis, gastritis, or ulcer, may result from oral overdosage. Milk or antacids should be given to bind alendronate. Owing to the risk of oesophageal irritation, vomiting should not be induced and the patient should remain fully upright.

Pharmacological properties

Pharmacodynamic properties: Alendronate is an aminobisphosphonate that in animal studies, localises preferentially to sites of bone resorption, specifically under osteoclasts and inhibits osteoclastic bone resorption with no direct effect on bone formation.

Since bone formation and bone resorption are coupled, bone formation is also reduced but less so than bone resorption, leading to progressive gains in bone mass. During exposure to alendronate, normal bone is formed that incorporates alendronate into its matrix where it is pharmacologically inactive.

Evidence from animal models confirms the selective nature of alendronate's activity. In growing rats, the doses causing inhibition of bone resorption were significantly lower than those leading to inhibition of mineralisation.

Osteoporosis in post-menopausal women: Osteoporosis is characterised by low bone mass and a consequent increased risk of fracture, most commonly of the spine, hip, and wrist. It occurs in both males and females but is most common among women following the menopause, when bone turnover increases and the rate of bone resorption exceeds that of bone formation, leading to loss of bone mass.

Daily oral doses of alendronate in post-menopausal women produced biochemical changes indicative of dose-dependent inhibition of bone resorption, including decreases in urinary calcium and urinary markers of bone collagen degradation (such as hydroxyproline, deoxypyridinoline, and cross-linked N-telopeptides of type I collagen). These biochemical changes returned towards baseline values as early as three weeks following the discontinuation of alendronate, despite the long retention of alendronate in the skeleton.

In long-term (two or three-year studies), Fosamax 10 mg/day reduced urinary excretion of markers of bone resorption, including deoxypyridinoline and cross-linked N-telopeptides of Type I collagen, by approximately 50–60% to reach levels similar to those seen in healthy premenopausal women. The decrease in the rate of bone resorption indicated by these markers was evident as early as one month and at three to six months reached a plateau that was maintained for the entire duration of treatment with Fosamax. In addition, the markers of bone formation, osteocalcin and total serum alkaline phosphatase were also reduced by approximately 50% and 25–30%, respectively, to reach a plateau after 6 to 12 months.

Effects on bone mineral density: The efficacy of Fosamax 10 mg once daily in post-menopausal women with osteoporosis was demonstrated in four clinical studies of two or three years' duration. In patients receiving Fosamax 10 mg/day, the mean increases in bone-mineral density (BMD) of the lumbar spine, femoral neck, and trochanter at three years for the pooled data from the two largest studies of virtually identical design were 8.82%, 5.90% and 7.81% relative to placebo.

These increases were highly significant relative both to baseline and placebo at each measurement site in each study. Total body BMD also increased significantly in both studies, indicating that the increases in bone mass of the lumbar spine and hip did not occur at the expense of the other skeletal sites. Increases in BMD were evident as early as three months and continued throughout the entire three years of treatment with no evidence of a plateau. Thus Fosamax reverses the progression of osteoporosis.

Fosamax is equally effective in older (≥65 years) and younger (≤65 years) patients.

In patients with post-menopausal osteoporosis

treated with Fosamax for one or two years the effects of treatment withdrawal were assessed. Following discontinuation, neither further increases in bone mass nor accelerated bone loss was observed.

Effect on fracture incidence: Analysis of the data pooled across doses at three years from the two largest treatment studies revealed a statistically significant and clinically meaningful 48% reduction in the proportion of patients treated with Fosamax experiencing one or more vertebral fractures (3.2%) relative to those treated with placebo (6.2%). Furthermore, of patients who sustained any vertebral fracture, those treated with Fosamax experienced less height loss (5.9 mm vs. 23.3 mm) due to a reduction in both the number and severity of fractures.

Additionally, analysis of the data pooled across doses of ≥2.5 mg from five studies of two or three years' duration including the two largest treatment studies revealed a significant 29% reduction in non-vertebral fracture incidence (Fosamax 9.0% vs. Placebo 12.6%).

Bone Histology: Bone histology in 270 post-menopausal patients with osteoporosis treated with Fosamax at doses ranging from 1 to 20 mg/day for one, two or three years revealed normal mineralisation and structure, as well as the expected decrease in bone turnover relative to placebo. These data, together with the normal bone histology and increased bone strength observed in ovariectomised rats and baboons exposed to long-term alendronate treatment, indicate that bone formed during therapy with Fosamax is of normal quality.

Pharmacokinetic properties

Absorption: Relative to an intravenous (IV) reference dose, the oral bioavailability of alendronate was 0.7% for doses ranging from 5 to 40 mg when administered after an overnight fast and two hours before a standardised breakfast. Bioavailability was decreased similarly to an estimated 0.46% and 0.39% when alendronate was administered one hour or half an hour before a standardised breakfast. In the two largest controlled studies (see 'Pharmacodynamic properties') that demonstrated efficacy, Fosamax 10 mg/day was administered one hour before the first food or beverage of the day. Therefore, bioavailability and therapeutic response should be similar to that seen in the studies if Fosamax is taken as directed (see 'Posology and method of administration').

Bioavailability was negligible whether alendronate was administered with, or up to two hours after, a standardised breakfast. Concomitant administration of alendronate with coffee or orange juice reduced bioavailability by approximately 60%.

Distribution: Studies in rats show that alendronate transiently distributes to soft tissues following 1 mg/kg i.v. administration but is then rapidly redistributed to bone or excreted in the urine. The mean steady-state volume of distribution, exclusive of bone, is at least 28 litres in humans. Concentrations of drug in plasma following therapeutic oral doses are too low for analytical detection (<5 ng/ml). Protein binding in human plasma is approximately 78%.

Biotransformation: There is no evidence that alendronate is metabolised in animals or humans.

Elimination: Following a single i.v. dose of [^{14}C]alendronate, approximately 50% of the radioactivity was excreted in the urine within 72 hours and little or no radioactivity was recovered in the faeces. Following a single 10 mg i.v. dose, the renal clearance of alendronate was 71 ml/min, and systemic clearance did not exceed 200 ml/min. Plasma concentrations fell by more than 95% within 6 hours following i.v. administration. The terminal half-life in humans is estimated to exceed 10 years, reflecting release of alendronate from the skeleton. Alendronate is not excreted through the acidic or basic transport systems of the kidney in rats, and thus it is not anticipated to interfere with the excretion of other drugs by those systems in humans.

Characteristics in patients: Preclinical studies show that the drug that is not deposited in bone is rapidly excreted in the urine. No evidence of saturation of bone uptake was found after chronic dosing with cumulative i.v. doses up to 35 mg/kg in animals. Although no clinical information is available, it is likely that, as in animals, elimination of alendronate via the kidney will be reduced in patients with impaired renal function. Therefore, somewhat greater accumulation of alendronate in bone might be expected in patients with impaired renal function (see 'Posology and method of administration').

Preclinical safety data: In test animal species the main target organs for toxicity were kidneys and gastrointestinal tract. Renal toxicity was seen only at doses >2 mg/kg/day orally (ten times the recommended dose) and was evident only on histological examination as small widely scattered foci or nephritis, with no evidence of effect on renal function. The gastrointestinal toxicity, seen in rodents only, occurred at doses >2.5 mg/kg/day and appears to be due to a direct effect on the mucosa. There is no additional relevant information.

Pharmaceutical particulars

List of excipients: Microcrystalline Cellulose PhEur, Anhydrous Lactose USNF, Croscarmellose Sodium USNF, and Magnesium Stearate PhEur.

Incompatibilities: None known.

Shelf life: 24 months.

Special precautions for storage: Store at temperatures below 30°C.

Nature and contents of container: Blister packs of opaque PVC lidded with aluminium foil. Pack size: 28 tablets.

Instructions for use/handling: None.

Marketing authorisation number 0025/0326.

Date of approval/revision of SPC August 1997.

Legal category POM.

HYDROCORTONE* TABLETS

Presentation White, quarter-scored tablets, marked 'MSD 619', containing 10 mg hydrocortisone. White, half-scored tablets, marked 'MSD 625', containing 20 mg hydrocortisone.

Uses Corticosteroid.

For use as replacement therapy in primary, secondary, or acute adrenocortical insufficiency.

Pre-operatively, and during serious trauma or illness in patients with known adrenal insufficiency or doubtful adrenocortical reserve.

Dosage and administration Dosage must be individualised according to the response of the individual patient. The lowest possible dosage should be used.

Patients should be observed closely for signs that might require dosage adjustment, including changes in clinical status resulting from remissions or exacerbations of the disease, individual drug responsiveness, and the effect of stress (e.g. surgery, infection, trauma). During stress it may be necessary to increase the dosage temporarily.

To avoid hypoadrenalism and/or a relapse of the underlying disease, it may be necessary to withdraw the drug gradually (see *Precautions*).

In chronic adrenocortical insufficiency, a dosage of 10–20 mg a day or occasionally more is recommended, together with 4–6 g of sodium chloride or 1–3 mg of deoxycorticosterone acetate. When immediate support is mandatory, one of the soluble adrenocortical hormone preparations (e.g. Decadron* Injection, dexamethasone sodium phosphate, MSD), which may be effective within minutes after parenteral administration, can be life-saving.

Use in children: In chronic adrenocortical insufficiency, the dosage should be approximately 0.4 to 0.8 mg/kg/day in two or three divided doses, adjusted to the needs of the individual child.

Use in the elderly: Treatment of elderly patients, particularly if long term, should be planned bearing in mind the more serious consequences of the common side effects of corticosteroids in old age, especially osteoporosis, diabetes, hypertension, susceptibility to infection and thinning of the skin.

Contra-indications, warnings, etc

Contra-indications: Systemic fungal infections. Hypersensitivity to any component of this product.

Precautions: The lowest possible dosage of corticosteroid should be used and when reduction in dosage is possible, the reduction should be gradual.

Corticosteroids may exacerbate systemic fungal infections and therefore should not be used in the presence of such infections unless they are needed to control drug reactions due to amphotericin. Moreover, there have been cases reported in which concomitant use of amphotericin and hydrocortisone was followed by cardiac enlargement and congestive heart failure.

Literature reports suggest an apparent association between use of corticosteroids and left ventricular free wall rupture after a recent myocardial infarction; therefore, therapy with corticosteroids should be used with great caution in these patients.

Average and large dosages of hydrocortisone or cortisone can cause elevation of blood pressure, salt and water retention, and increase excretion of potassium. These effects are less likely to occur with the synthetic derivatives except when used in large doses. Dietary salt restriction and potassium supplementation may be necessary. All corticosteroids increase calcium excretion.

A report shows that the use of corticosteroids in cerebral malaria is associated with a prolonged coma and an increased incidence of pneumonia and gastro-intestinal bleeding.

Drug-induced secondary adrenocortical insufficiency may result from too rapid a withdrawal of corticosteroids and may be minimised by gradual reduction of dosage. This type of relative insufficiency may persist for months after discontinuation of therapy; therefore, in any situation of stress occurring during that period, corticosteroid therapy should be reinstated. If the patient is receiving steroids already, the dosage may have to be increased. Since mineralocorticoid secretion may be impaired, salt and/or a mineralocorticoid should be administered concurrently.

Stopping corticosteroids after prolonged therapy may cause withdrawal symptoms including fever, myalgia, arthralgia, and malaise.

In patients who have received more than physiological doses of systemic corticosteroids (approximately 30 mg hydrocortisone) for greater than three weeks, withdrawal should not be abrupt. How dose reduction should be carried out depends largely on whether the disease is likely to relapse as the dose of systemic corticosteroids is reduced. Clinical assessment of disease activity may be needed during withdrawal. If the disease is unlikely to relapse on withdrawal of systemic corticosteroids but there is uncertainty about hypothalamic-pituitary adrenal (HPA) suppression, the dose of systemic corticosteroid ***may*** be reduced rapidly to physiological doses. Once a daily dose of 30 mg hydrocortisone is reached, dose reduction should be slower to allow the HPA-axis to recover.

Abrupt withdrawal of systemic corticosteroid treatment, which has continued up to three weeks is appropriate if it is considered that the disease is unlikely to relapse. Abrupt withdrawal of doses of up to 160 mg hydrocortisone for three weeks is unlikely to lead to clinically relevant HPA-axis suppression, in the majority of patients. In the following patient groups, gradual withdrawal of systemic corticosteroid therapy should be ***considered*** even after courses lasting three weeks or less.

- Patients who have had repeated courses of systemic corticosteroids, particularly if taken for greater than three weeks,
- When a short course has been prescribed within one year of cessation of long-term therapy (months or years),
- Patients who may have reasons for adrenocortical insufficiency other than exogenous corticosteroid therapy.
- Patients receiving doses of systemic corticosteroid greater than 160 mg hydrocortisone,
- Patients repeatedly taking doses in the evening.

If corticosteroids are indicated in patients with latent tuberculosis or tuberculin reactivity, close observation is necessary as reactivation may occur. During prolonged corticosteroid therapy, these patients should receive prophylactic chemotherapy.

The use of Hydrocortone Tablets in active tuberculosis should be restricted to those cases of fulminating or disseminated tuberculosis.

Corticosteroids should be used with caution in renal insufficiency, hypertension, diabetes or in those with a family history of diabetes, congestive heart failure, osteoporosis, previous steroid myopathy, glaucoma (or family history), myasthenia gravis, non-specific ulcerative colitis, diverticulitis, fresh intestinal anastomoses, active or latent peptic ulcer. Signs of peritoneal irritation following gastro-intestinal perforation in patients receiving large doses of corticosteroids may be minimal or absent. Fat embolism has been reported as a possible complication of hypercortisonism.

There is an enhanced effect of corticosteroids in patients with hypothyroidism and in those with cirrhosis.

Corticosteroids may mask some signs of infection, and new infections may appear during their use. There may be decreased resistance and inability to localise infection in patients on corticosteroids. Corticosteroids may affect the nitrobluetetrazolium test for bacterial infection and produce false negative results.

Corticosteroids may activate latent amoebiasis. Therefore, it is recommended that latent or active amoebiasis be excluded before initiating corticosteroid therapy in any patient who has either spent time in the tropics, or has unexplained diarrhoea.

Prolonged use of corticosteroids may produce posterior subcapsular cataracts, glaucoma with possible damage to the optic nerves, and may enhance the establishment of secondary ocular infections due to fungi and viruses.

Corticosteroids should be used cautiously in patients with ocular herpes simplex because of possible corneal perforation.

Corticosteroids may increase or decrease motility and number of spermatozoa.

Drug interactions: Aspirin should be used cautiously in conjunction with corticosteroids in hypoprothrombinaemia.

Phenytoin, ephedrine, rifabutin, carbamazepine, barbiturates, rifampicin and aminoglutethimide may enhance the metabolic clearance of corticosteroids, resulting in decreased blood levels and lessened physiological activity, thus requiring adjustment in corticosteroid dosage.

The prothrombin time should be checked frequently in patients who are receiving corticosteroids and coumarin anticoagulants at the same time because of reports of altered response to these anticoagulants. Studies have shown that the usual effect produced by adding corticosteroids is inhibition of reponse to coumarins, although there have been some conflicting reports of potentiation not substantiated by studies.

When corticosteroids are administered concomitantly with potassium-depleting diuretics, patients should be observed closely for development of hypokalaemia.

Children: Corticosteroids cause growth retardation in infancy, childhood and adolescence. Treatment should be limited to the minimum dosage in order to minimise suppression of the hypothalamo-pituitary-adrenal axis and growth retardation.

Growth and development of infants and children on prolonged corticosteroid therapy should be carefully monitored.

Use in pregnancy and lactation: The ability of corticosteroids to cross the placenta varies between individual drugs, however, hydrocortisone readily crosses the placenta.

Administration of corticosteroids to pregnant animals can cause abnormalities of foetal development including cleft palate, intra-uterine growth retardation and effects on brain growth and development. There is no evidence that corticosteroids result in an increased incidence of congenital abnormalities, such as cleft palate/lip in man. However, when administered for prolonged periods or repeatedly during pregnancy, corticosteroids may increase the risk of intra-uterine growth retardation. Hypoadrenalism may, in theory, occur in the neonate following prenatal exposure to corticosteroids but usually resolves spontaneously following birth and is rarely clinically important. As with all drugs, corticosteroids should only be prescribed when the benefits to the mother and child outweigh the risks. When corticosteroids are essential however, patients with normal pregnancies may be treated as though they were in the non-gravid state.

Corticosteroids are excreted in breast milk, although no data are available for hydrocortisone. Infants of mothers taking high doses of systemic corticosteroids for prolonged periods may have a degree of adrenal suppression.

Side-effects: Fluid and electrolyte disturbances: Sodium retention, fluid retention, congestive heart failure in susceptible patients, potassium loss, hypokalaemic alkalosis, hypertension, increased calcium excretion.

Musculoskeletal effects: Muscle weakness, steroid myopathy, loss of muscle mass, osteoporosis (especially in post-menopausal females), vertebral compression fractures, aseptic necrosis of femoral and humeral heads, pathological fracture of long bones, tendon rupture.

Gastro-intestinal: Peptic ulcer with possible perforation and haemorrhage, perforation of the small and large bowel particularly in patients with inflammatory bowel disease, pancreatitis, abdominal distension, ulcerative oesophagitis, dyspepsia, oesophageal candidiasis.

Dermatological: Impaired wound healing, thin fragile skin, petechiae, and ecchymoses, erythema, striae, telangiectasia, acne, increased sweating, may suppress reactions to skin tests, other cutaneous reactions such as allergic dermatitis, urticaria, angioneurotic oedema.

Neurological: Convulsions, increased intracranial pressure with papilloedema (pseudotumour cerebri) usually after treatment, vertigo, headache. Psychic disturbances.

Endocrine: Menstrual irregularities, amenorrhoea, development of Cushingoid state, suppression of growth in children, secondary adrenocortical and pituitary unresponsiveness (particularly in times of stress, as in trauma, surgery, or illness), decreased carbohydrate tolerance, manifestations of latent diabetes mellitus, increased requirements for insulin or oral hypoglycaemic agents in diabetics, hirsutism.

Ophthalmic: Posterior subcapsular cataracts, increased intra-ocular pressure, papilloedema, corneal or scleral thinning, exacerbation of ophthalmic viral disease, glaucoma, exophthalmos.

Metabolic: Negative nitrogen balance due to protein catabolism.

Cardiovascular: Myocardial rupture following recent myocardial infarction (see 'Precautions').

Other: Hypersensitivity, leucocytosis, thrombo-embolism, weight gain, increased appetite, nausea, malaise.

Overdosage: Reports of acute toxicity and/or deaths following overdosage with glucocorticoids are rare. No antidote is available. Treatment is probably not indicated for reactions due to chronic poisoning unless the patient has a condition that would render him unusually susceptible to ill effects from corticosteroids. In this case, symptomatic treatment should be instituted as necessary.

Anaphylactic and hypersensitivity reactions may be treated with adrenaline, positive-pressure artificial respiration and aminophylline. The patient should be kept warm and quiet.

The biological half-life of hydrocortisone is about 100 minutes.

Pharmaceutical precautions Keep container well closed, store in a cool place, below 25°C, protected from light.

Legal category POM.

Package quantities *10 mg:* Packs of 30. *20 mg:* Packs of 30.

Further information Nil.

Product licence numbers
10 mg 0025/5053
20 mg 0025/5054

HYDROSALURIC*

Presentation White, half-scored tablets, marked 'MSD 42', containing 25 mg Hydrochlorothiazide BP.

White, half-scored tablets, marked 'MSD 105', containing 50 mg Hydrochlorothiazide BP.

Uses Thiazide diuretic and antihypertensive.

Oedema associated with congestive heart failure, hepatic cirrhosis, premenstrual tension and oedema due to various forms of renal dysfunction (i.e. the nephrotic syndrome, acute glomerulonephritis, chronic renal failure). Hypertension, either alone or as an adjunct to other antihypertensive drugs.

Dosage and administration Dosage should be determined on an individual basis, and the lowest dosage necessary to achieve the desired result should be used.

Adults – for oedema: Usually 25–100 mg a day given in a single dose or in two divided doses. Many patients respond to intermittent therapy; for example, every other day, or three to five days a week. Intermittent therapy is less likely to produce excessive diuretic response with resulting undesirable electrolyte imbalance. The maximum recommended daily dose is 100 mg.

In oedema accompanying premenstrual tension: 25–50 mg once or twice a day, from the first morning of symptoms until the onset of the menses.

Adults – for control of hypertension: Usual starting dosage, 25 mg a day as a single or divided dose. In some patients, a starting dose of 12.5 mg, alone or with another antihypertensive, may be sufficient. Dosage should be adjusted to response, but should not exceed 50 mg a day.

Thiazides may add to the action of other antihypertensives. If HydroSaluric is used with other antihypertensive agents, it may be necessary to reduce the dosage of such agents so as to prevent an excessive drop in blood pressure.

Infants and children: Usually 2.5 mg per kg bodyweight a day, given in two doses. Infants under 6 months may need up to 3.5 mg per kg a day, in two doses. Infants up to 2 years of age may be given 12.5–37.5 mg of HydroSaluric a day in two doses. Children from 2 to 12 years of age may be given 37.5–100 mg a day in two doses. Dosage should be based on bodyweight.

Uses in the elderly: Particular caution is needed in the elderly because of their susceptibility to electrolyte imbalance; the dosage should be carefully adjusted according to renal function and clinical response. If lower dosage is required, 25 mg tablets are available.

Contra-indications, warnings, etc

Contra-indications: Anuria, hypersensitivity to any component of this product or to other sulphonamide-derived drugs, severe renal or hepatic failure, Addison's disease, hypercalcaemia, concurrent lithium therapy. See 'Use in pregnancy' and 'Use in breast-feeding mothers', under 'Precautions'.

Precautions: Patients should be carefully monitored for signs of fluid and electrolyte imbalance (hyponatraemia, hypochloraemic alkalosis, hypokalaemia and hypomagnesaemia). It is particularly important to make serum and urine electrolyte determinations when the patient is vomiting excessively or receiving parenteral fluids. Warning signs or symptoms of fluid and electrolyte imbalance include: dryness of mouth, thirst, weakness, lethargy, drowsiness, restlessness, seizures, confusion, muscle pains or cramps, muscle fatigue, hypotension, oliguria, tachycardia, and gastro-intestinal disturbances such as nausea and vomiting.

Hypokalaemia may develop, especially with brisk diuresis, when severe cirrhosis is present, or after prolonged therapy. Hypokalaemia can sensitise or exaggerate the response of the heart to the toxic effects of digitalis (e.g. increased ventricular irritability).

Sensitivity reactions may occur in patients with or without history of allergy or bronchial asthma.

Hypokalaemia may be avoided or treated in the adult by concurrent use of amiloride hydrochloride (Midamor*), a potassium-conserving agent. It may also be avoided by giving potassium chloride or foods with a high potassium content. (Note that symptoms and signs which might indicate ulceration or obstruction of the small bowel in patients taking tablets or capsules containing potassium salts are indications for stopping treatment with such preparations immediately.)

Diuretic-induced hyponatraemia is usually mild and asymptomatic. Dilutional hyponatraemia may occur in oedematous patients in hot weather; and, except in rare instances when hyponatraemia is life-threatening, appropriate therapy is water restriction rather than administration of salt.

Thiazides may decrease serum Protein Bound Iodine levels without signs of thyroid disturbances.

Thiazides may decrease urinary calcium excretion, and may also cause intermittent and slight elevation of serum calcium in the absence of known disorders of calcium metabolism. Thiazides should be discontinued before carrying out tests for parathyroid function.

When creatinine clearance falls below 30 ml/min, thiazide diuretics become ineffective.

Uraemia may be precipitated or increased by chlorothiazide. Cumulative effects of the drug may develop in patients with impaired renal function. If increasing uraemia and oliguria occur during treatment of renal disease, HydroSaluric should be discontinued.

Thiazides should be used with caution in patients with impaired hepatic function or progressive liver disease, since minor alterations of fluid and electrolyte balance may precipitate hepatic coma.

Hyperuricaemia may occur, or gout may be precipitated, in certain patients receiving thiazide therapy.

Thiazide therapy may impair glucose tolerance.

Increases in cholesterol and triglyceride levels may be associated with thiazide diuretic therapy.

The possibility of exacerbation or activation of systemic lupus erythematosus has been reported.

Latent diabetes may become manifest during thiazide administration.

Use in pregnancy: Thiazides cross the placental barrier and appear in cord blood. The use of HydroSaluric when pregnancy is present or suspected requires, therefore, that the benefits of the drug be weighed against possible hazards to the fetus. These hazards include fetal or neonatal jaundice, thrombocytopenia, and possibly other adverse reactions which have occurred in the adult. The routine use of diuretics in otherwise healthy pregnant women with or without mild oedema is not recommended, because their use may be associated with hypovolaemia, increased blood viscosity and decreased placental perfusion.

Use in breast-feeding mothers: Thiazides appear in breast milk. If use of the drug is deemed essential, the patient should stop breast-feeding.

Drug interactions: Alcohol, barbiturates or narcotics: Co-administration may potentiate orthostatic hypotension. *Oral and parenteral antidiabetic drugs* may require adjustment of dosage with concurrent use. *Other antihypertensive drugs* may have an additive effect. Discontinuation of diuretic therapy 2–3 days before the initiation of treatment with an ACE inhibitor may reduce the likelihood of first-dose hypotension. The antihypertensive effect of the drug may be enhanced in the post-sympathectomy patient. *Cholestyramine and colestipol resin:* Absorption of hydrochlorothiazide is impaired in the presence of anionic exchange resins. Single doses of either cholestyramine or colestipol resins bind hydrochlorothiazide and reduce its absorption from the gastro-intestinal tract by up to 85% and 43%, respectively. *Corticosteroids or ACTH* may intensify any thiazide-induced electrolyte depletion, particularly hypokalaemia. *Pressor amines such as adrenaline* may show decreased arterial responsiveness when used with HydroSaluric, but this reaction is not enough to preclude their therapeutic usefulness. *Non-depolarising muscle relaxants such as tubocurarine* may possibly interact with HydroSaluric to increase muscle relaxation. *Non-steroidal anti-inflammatory drugs* may attenuate the diuretic and antihypertensive effect of diuretics.

Drug/laboratory tests: Because thiazides may affect calcium metabolism, HydroSaluric may interfere with tests for parathyroid function.

Side-effects

Gastro-intestinal system: Anorexia, gastric irritation, nausea, vomiting, cramps, diarrhoea, constipation, jaundice (intrahepatic cholestatic jaundice), pancreatitis, salivary gland inflammation.

Central nervous system: Dizziness, vertigo, paraesthesiae, headache, yellow vision.

Haematological: Leucopenia, agranulocytosis, thrombocytopenia, aplastic anaemia, haemolytic anaemia.

Cardiovascular: Hypotension, including orthostatic hypotension.

Hypersensitivity: Purpura, photosensitivity, rash, urticaria, necrotising angiitis (vasculitis, cutaneous vasculitis), fever, respiratory distress including pneumonitis and pulmonary oedema, anaphylactic reactions, toxic epidermal necrolysis.

Metabolic: Hyperglycaemia, glycosuria, hyperuricaemia, electrolyte imbalance including hyponatraemia and hypokalaemia.

Renal: Renal dysfunction, interstitial nephritis, renal failure.

Other: Muscle spasm, weakness, restlessness, transient blurred vision, impotence.

Whenever side-effects are moderate to severe, thiazide dosage should be reduced or therapy withdrawn.

Overdosage: The most common signs and symptoms observed are those caused by electrolyte depletion (hypokalaemia, hypochloraemia, hyponatraemia) and dehydration resulting from excessive diuresis. If digitalis has also been administered, hypokalaemia may accentuate cardiac arrhythmias.

In the event of overdosage, symptomatic and supportive measures should be employed. If ingestion is recent, emesis should be induced or gastric lavage performed. Dehydration, electrolyte imbalance, hepatic coma and hypotension should be corrected by established methods. If required, give oxygen or artificial respiration for respiratory impairment.

Pharmaceutical precautions Keep container tightly closed; store in a cool place, protected from light.

Legal category POM.

Package quantities 25 mg: Packs of 30.
50 mg: Packs of 30.

Further information Diuresis begins within two hours following administration, is at a peak after four hours and persists for six to twelve hours. No rigid dietary salt restriction required.

The plasma half-life of hydrochlorothiazide is 5.6 hours with a subsequently longer terminal phase. The biological half-life is 14.8 hours when the plasma level can be followed for at least 24 hours.

Product licence numbers
25 mg tablet 0025/5009R
50 mg tablet 0025/5010R

INDOCID*

Presentation Ivory, opaque capsules containing 25 mg or 50 mg Indomethacin PhEur, marked 'MSD 25' and 'MSD 50' respectively.

Opaque ivory headed, transparent blue based, sustained release capsules carrying white and blue pellets containing 75 mg indomethacin, marked 'INDOCID R 693'. The 75 mg of indomethacin provides 25 mg of free indomethacin for immediate dissolution, and 50 mg of time-release coated pellets.

A fruit-flavoured suspension containing in each 5 ml, 25 mg Indomethacin PhEur.

Polyethylene glycol suppositories containing 100 mg Indomethacin PhEur.

Uses Non-steroidal anti-inflammatory agent indicated for the active stages of rheumatoid arthritis, osteoarthritis, ankylosing spondylitis, degenerative joint disease of the hip, acute musculoskeletal disorders, low-back pain, and acute gouty arthritis.

Also indicated in inflammation, pain and oedema following orthopaedic procedures; and the treatment of pain and associated symptoms of primary dysmenorrhoea.

Indocid Suppositories may be used where night pain and morning stiffness are prominent. One suppository at bedtime will frequently give relief from pain and stiffness for 13 to 16 hours after administration.

Indocid-R: Indocid-R may be substituted for all the indications of Indocid except acute gouty arthritis, as clinical evidence is not currently available for this dosage form in this condition.

Dosage and administration The dosage of Indocid should be carefully adjusted to suit the needs of the individual patient.

Oral therapy: In order to reduce the possibility of gastro-intestinal disturbances, *Indocid/Indocid-R Capsules and Suspension should always be taken with food or an antacid.* (Note, however, that Indocid Suspension should not be mixed with an antacid, but should be taken separately, because indomethacin is unstable in an alkaline medium.) Indocid Suspension should not be diluted.

In chronic conditions, starting therapy with a low dosage, increasing this gradually as necessary, and continuing a trial of therapy for an adequate period (in some cases, up to one month) will give the best results with a minimum of unwanted reactions. The recommended oral dosage range is 50–200 mg daily in divided doses. Paediatric dosage not established.

Dosage in dysmenorrhoea: Up to 75 mg a day, starting with onset of cramps or bleeding, and continuing for as long as the symptoms usually last.

Dosage in acute gouty arthritis: 150–200 mg daily in divided doses until all symptoms and signs subside.

Adult dosage for suppositories: 1 suppository to be inserted once or twice a day. One should be used at bedtime. If another is necessary, it should be used in the morning.

Dosage for Indocid-R: The sustained-release capsule may be given once or, where necessary, twice a day depending on patient needs and response.

Use in the elderly: Indocid should be used with particular care in older patients who are more prone to adverse reactions.

Contra-indications, warnings, etc

Contra-indications: Active peptic ulcer; a recurrent history of gastro-intestinal lesions; in patients who have nasal polyps associated with angioneurotic oedema, who show sensitivity to Indocid, or who have experienced acute asthmatic attacks, urticaria or rhinitis as a result of therapy with aspirin or other non-steroidal anti-inflammatory drugs. Safety for use in children has not been established. Indocid Suppositories are contra-indicated in patients with a history of proctitis or recent rectal bleeding.

Use in pregnancy: Indocid should be used during the first two trimesters of pregnancy only if the potential benefit justifies the potential risk to the fetus.

The known effects of indomethacin and other drugs of this class on the human fetus during the third trimester of pregnancy include: constriction of the ductus arteriosus prenatally, tricuspid incompetence, and pulmonary hypertension; non-closure of the ductus arteriosus postnatally which may be resistant to medical management; myocardial degenerative changes, platelet dysfunction with resultant bleeding, intracranial bleeding, renal dysfunction or failure, renal injury/dysgenesis which may result in prolonged or permanent renal failure, oligohydramnios, gastro-intestinal bleeding or perforation and increased risk of necrotising enterocolitis. Use of Indocid during the third trimester of pregnancy is not recommended.

Use in breast-feeding mothers
Administration of Indocid is not recommended in breast-feeding mothers. Indomethacin is excreted in breast milk.

Precautions: Headache, sometimes accompanied by dizziness and lightheadedness, may occur, usually early in treatment. Starting therapy with a low dosage and increasing it gradually will usually minimise the incidence of headache. These symptoms frequently disappear on continuing therapy or reducing the dosage, but if headache persists despite dosage reduction, Indocid should be withdrawn. Patients should be warned that they may experience dizziness and, if they do, should not drive a car or undertake potentially dangerous activities needing alertness.

Indocid should be used cautiously in patients with a history of bronchial asthma and in patients with psychiatric disorders, epilepsy, or parkinsonism, as it may tend to aggravate these disorders.

Gastro-intestinal disturbances may be minimised by giving Indocid orally with food or an antacid. They usually disappear on reducing the dosage; if not, the risks of continuing therapy should be weighed against the possible benefits. If gastro-intestinal bleeding does occur, Indocid should immediately be discontinued.

Single or multiple ulcerations, including perforation and haemorrhage of the oesophagus, stomach, duodenum or small or large intestine have been reported to occur with Indocid. Fatalities have been reported in some instances. Rarely, intestinal ulceration has been associated with stenosis and obstruction.

Gastro-intestinal bleeding without obvious ulcer formation and perforation of pre-existing sigmoid lesions (diverticulum, carcinoma, etc.) have occurred. Increased abdominal pain in ulcerative colitis patients or the development of ulcerative colitis and regional ileitis have been reported to occur rarely.

Fluid retention and peripheral oedema have been observed in some patients taking Indocid. It should therefore be used with caution in patients with cardiac dysfunction, hypertension or other conditions predisposing to fluid retention.

Tenesmus and irritation of the rectal mucosa have been reported occasionally with Indocid Suppositories.

Indocid may mask the signs and symptoms of infection. Indocid should be used with caution in patients with existing, but controlled infection.

In patients with rheumatoid arthritis, eye changes may occur which may be related to the underlying disease or to the therapy. Therefore, in chronic rheumatoid disease, ophthalmological examinations at periodic intervals are recommended. Discontinue therapy if eye changes are observed.

Patients should be periodically observed to allow early detection of any unwanted effects on peripheral blood (anaemia), liver function or gastro-intestinal tract.

Indocid can inhibit platelet aggregation. This effect usually disappears within 24 hours of discontinuing Indocid. Bleeding time is prolonged (but within normal range) in normal adults. Because this effect may be exaggerated in patients with underlying haemostatic defects, Indocid should be used cautiously in patients with coagulation defects.

As with other non-steroidal anti-inflammatory drugs, there have been reports of acute interstitial nephritis with haematuria, proteinuria, and occasionally nephrotic syndrome, in patients receiving long-term administration of indomethacin.

In patients with reduced renal blood flow where renal prostaglandins play a major role in maintaining renal perfusion, administration of a non-steroidal anti-inflammatory agent may precipitate overt renal decompensation. Patients at greatest risk of this reaction are those with renal or hepatic dysfunction, diabetes mellitus, advanced age, extracellular volume depletion, congestive heart failure, sepsis, or concomitant use of any nephrotoxic drug. A non-steroidal anti-inflammatory drug should be given with caution and renal function should be monitored in any patient who may have reduced renal reserve. Discontinuation of non-steroidal anti-inflammatory therapy is usually followed by recovery to the pretreatment state.

Increases in plasma potassium concentration, including hyperkalaemia, have been reported, even in some patients without renal impairment. In patients with normal renal function, these effects have been attributed to a hyporeninaemic-hypoaldosteronism state (see 'Drug interactions').

Since Indocid is eliminated primarily by the kidneys, patients with significantly impaired renal function should be closely monitored; a lower daily dosage should be used to avoid excessive drug accumulation.

Laboratory tests: Borderline elevations of one or more liver tests may occur, and significant elevations of ALT (SGPT) or AST (SGOT) have been seen in less than 1% of patients receiving therapy with non-steroidal anti-inflammatory drugs in controlled clinical trials. If abnormal liver tests persist or worsen, if clinical signs and symptoms consistent with liver disease develop or if systemic manifestations such as rash or eosinophilia occur, Indocid should be stopped.

False negative results in the dexamethasone suppression test (DST) in patients being treated with Indocid have been reported. Thus, results of this test should be used with caution in these patients.

Drug interactions: Aspirin: The use of Indocid with aspirin or other salicylates is not recommended. Controlled clinical studies have shown no enhanced therapeutic effect, and one study showed a significant increase in the incidence of gastro-intestinal side effects. A study in normal volunteers showed that chronic administration of 3.6 g aspirin with indomethacin lowered the indomethacin blood levels by approximately 20%.

Diflunisal: Co-administration of diflunisal with Indocid increases the plasma level of indomethacin by about a third with a concomitant decrease in renal clearance. Fatal gastro-intestinal haemorrhage has occurred. The combination should not be used.

Other NSAIDs: the concomitant use of Indocid with other NSAIDs is not recommended due to the increased possibility of gastro-intestinal toxicity, with little or no increase in efficacy.

Anticoagulants: Although clinical studies suggest that Indocid does not influence the hypoprothrombinaemia induced by anticoagulants, patients also receiving anticoagulants should be closely observed for alterations of the prothrombin time.

Probenecid: Co-administration of probenecid may increase plasma levels of indomethacin.

Methotrexate: Caution should be exercised with simultaneous use of Indocid with methotrexate. Indocid has been reported to decrease the tubular secretion of methotrexate and to potentiate toxicity.

Cyclosporin: Administration of non-steroidal anti-inflammatory drugs concomitantly with cyclosporin has been associated with an increase in cyclosporin-induced toxicity, possibly due to decreased synthesis of renal prostacyclin. NSAIDs should be used with caution in patients taking cyclosporin and renal function should be monitored carefully.

Lithium: Indomethacin 50 mg three times a day produced a clinically relevant elevation of plasma lithium and reduction in renal lithium clearance in psychiatric patients and normal subjects with steady state plasma lithium concentrations. This effect has been attributed to inhibition of prostaglandin synthesis. As a consequence, when indomethacin and lithium are given concomitantly, the patient should be observed carefully for signs of lithium toxicity.

In addition, the frequency of monitoring serum lithium concentrations should be increased at the outset of such combination drug treatment.

Diuretics: In some patients, the administration of Indocid can reduce the diuretic and antihypertensive effects of loop, potassium-sparing, and thiazide diuretics. Therefore, when Indocid and diuretics are used concomitantly, the patient shoud be observed closely to determine if the desired effect of the diuretic is obtained.

Indocid reduces basal plasma renin activity (PRA), as well as those elevations of PRA induced by frusemide administration, or salt or volume depletion. These facts should be considered when evaluating plasma renin activity in hypertensive patients.

It has been reported that the addition of triamterene to a maintenance schedule of Indocid resulted in reversible acute renal failure in two of four healthy volunteers. Indocid and triamterene should not be administered together.

Indocid and potassium-sparing diuretics each may be associated with increased plasma potassium levels. The potential effects of Indocid and potassium-sparing diuretics on potassium kinetics and renal function should be considered when these agents are administered concurrently.

Most of the above effects concerning diuretics have been attributed, at least in part, to mechanisms involving inhibition of prostaglandin synthesis by Indocid.

Digoxin: Indocid given concomitantly with digoxin has been reported to increase the serum concentration and prolong the half life of digoxin. Therefore when 'Indocid' and digoxin are used concomitantly serum digoxin levels should be closely monitored.

Antihypertensive medications: Coadministration of Indocid and some antihypertensive agents may attenuate acutely the hypotensive effect of the latter, due partly to indomethacin's inhibition of prostaglandin synthesis. Therefore caution should be exercised when considering the addition of Indocid to the regimen of a patient taking any of the following antihypertensive agents: alpha-adrenergic blocking agents, ACE inhibitors, beta-adrenergic blocking agents, diuretics or hydralazine.

Phenylpropanolamine: Hypertensive crises have been reported due to oral phenylpropanolamine alone and rarely to phenylpropanolamine given with Indocid. This additive effect is probably due partly to indomethacin's inhibition of prostaglandin synthesis. Caution should be exercised when Indocid and phenylpropanolamine are administered concomitantly.

Corticosteroids: the risk of gastro-intestinal bleeding and ulceration associated with NSAIDs is increased when used with corticosteroids.

Mifepristone: NSAIDs and aspirin should be avoided until at least 8 to 12 days after administration of mifepristone.

Quinolones antibiotics: there have been reports that 4-quinolones may induce convulsions, in patients with or without history of convulsions; taking NSAIDs at the same time may also induce them.

Warnings and adverse reactions: CNS reactions – headaches, dizziness, lightheadedness, depression, vertigo, and fatigue (including malaise and listlessness). Reactions reported infrequently include mental confusion, anxiety, syncope, drowsiness, convulsions, coma, peripheral neuropathy, muscle weakness, involuntary muscle movements, insomnia, psychiatric disturbances such as depersonalisation; and, rarely, paraesthesiae, dysarthria, aggravation of epilepsy and parkinsonism. These are often transient and disappear frequently with continued or with reduced dosage. However, occasionally, severe reactions require stopping therapy.

Gastro-intestinal – the more frequent reactions are nausea, anorexia, vomiting, epigastric distress, abdominal pain, constipation, and diarrhoea. Others which may develop are ulceration (single or multiple) of oesophagus, stomach, duodenum or small or large intestine including perforation and haemorrhage with a few fatalities having been reported; gastro-intestinal tract bleeding without obvious ulcer formation; increased abdominal pain when used in patients with pre-existing ulcerative colitis. Reactions occurring infrequently are stomatitis; gastritis; flatulence; bleeding from the sigmoid colon (occult or from a diverticulum); perforation of pre-existing sigmoid lesions (diverticulae and carcinoma).

Rarely, intestinal strictures (diaphragms) and intestinal ulceration followed by stenosis and obstruction have been reported. With suppositories, tenesmus and irritation of the rectal mucosa have occasionally been reported. Other gastro-intestinal side effects which may or may not be caused by indomethacin include ulcerative colitis and regional ileitis.

Hepatic – rarely, hepatitis and jaundice (some fatalities reported).

Cardiovascular/renal – oedema, increased blood pressure, tachycardia, chest pain, arrhythmia, palpitation, hypotension, congestive heart failure, blood urea elevation, and haematuria (all infrequent).

Dermatological/hypersensitivity – pruritus, urticaria, angioneurotic oedema, angiitis, erythema nodosum, skin rash, exfoliative dermatitis, Stevens-Johnson syndrome, erythema multiforme, toxic epidermal necrolysis, loss of hair, rapid fall in blood pressure resembling a shock-like state, acute anaphylaxis, acute respiratory distress including sudden dyspnoea, asthma and pulmonary oedema (all infrequent). Bronchospasm may be precipitated in patients suffering from, or with a history of, bronchial asthma or allergic disease.

Haematological – infrequently, blood dyscrasias may occur, including leucopenia, petechiae or ecchymosis, purpura, aplastic or haemolytic anaemia, agranulocytosis, bone-marrow depression, disseminated intravascular coagulation, and particularly thrombocytopenia. Because some patients may develop anaemia secondary to obvious or occult gastro-intestinal bleeding, appropriate blood determinations are recommended.

Ocular – infrequently, blurred vision, diplopia, and orbital and peri-orbital pain. Corneal deposits and retinal disturbances, including those of the macula, have been reported in patients with rheumatoid arthritis on prolonged therapy, but similar changes may also be expected in patients with rheumatoid arthritis who have not received indomethacin.

Aural – tinnitus, hearing disturbances (rarely deafness).

Genito-urinary – proteinuria, nephrotic syndrome, interstitial nephritis, and renal insufficiency including renal failure (all rare).

Miscellaneous – vaginal bleeding, hyperglycaemia, glycosuria, hyperkalaemia, flushing and sweating, epistaxis, breast changes including enlargement and tenderness, gynaecomastia, and ulcerative stomatitis (all rare).

The following adverse reactions have been associated with use of Indocid Suppositories: tenesmus; proctitis; rectal bleeding, burning, pain, discomfort, and itching.

Overdosage: The following symptoms may be observed following overdosage: nausea, vomiting, intense headache, dizziness, mental confusion, disorientation, or lethargy. There have been reports of paraesthesiae, numbness, and convulsions.

Treatment is symptomatic and supportive. The stomach should be emptied as quickly as possible if the ingestion is recent.

If vomiting has not occurred spontaneously, the patient should be induced to vomit with syrup of ipecac. If the patient is unable to vomit, gastric lavage should be performed. Once the stomach has been emptied, 25 or 50 g of activated charcoal may be given. Depending on the condition of the patient, close medical observation and nursing care may be required. The patient should be followed for several days because gastro-intestinal ulceration and haemorrhage have been reported as adverse reactions of indomethacin. Use of antacids may be helpful.

The plasma elimination of indomethacin is biphasic with the half-life of the terminal plasma half-life phase between 2.6 and 11.2 hours.

Pharmaceutical precautions Store in a dry place below 25°C.

Indocid/Indocid-R Capsules and Suspension should always be taken with food or an antacid. (Note, however, that Indocid Suspension should not be mixed with an antacid but should be taken separately because indomethacin is unstable in an alkaline medium.) Indocid Suspension should not be diluted.

Legal category POM.

Package quantities *Capsules:* 25 mg, packs of 90; 50 mg, packs of 90; 75 mg, packs of 30.
Suppositories: Boxes of 10.
Suspension: Bottles of 200 ml.

Further information Nil.

Product licence numbers

25 mg	0025/0111
50 mg	0025/0112
75 mg	0025/0125
Suppositories	0025/0062
Suspension	0025/0120

INDOCID* PDA

Qualitative and quantitative composition Indocid PDA contains indomethacin sodium trihydrate equivalent to 1.0 mg indomethacin PhEur.

Pharmaceutical form Indocid PDA is available in vials containing a sterile, off-white to yellow lyophilised mass of indomethacin sodium trihydrate.

Clinical particulars

Therapeutic indications: Indocid PDA is indicated for the closure of patent ductus arteriosus in premature babies.

Posology and method of administration: For intravenous use only.

A course of therapy is defined as three intravenous doses of Indocid PDA given at 12- to 24-hour intervals, with careful attention to urinary output.

If anuria or marked oliguria (urinary output of 0.6 ml/kg/hour) is evident at the time of the scheduled second or third dose, Indocid PDA must not be given until laboratory studies indicate that renal function has returned to normal.

Dosage recommendations depend closely on the age of the infant:

	Dosage (mg/kg)		
Age at 1st dose	*1st*	*2nd*	*3rd*
Less than 48 hours	0.2	0.1	0.1
2–7 days	0.2	0.2	0.2
Over 7 days	0.2	0.25	0.25

If the ductus arteriosus is closed or significantly reduced in size 48 hours after the first course of therapy, no further treatment is necessary. If the ductus arteriosus reopens, a second course of therapy may be given.

If the condition is unchanged after the second course of therapy, surgery may then be necessary. If severe adverse reactions occur, stop the treatment.

Contra-indications: Indocid PDA is contra-indicated in infants with established or suspected untreated infection; infants who are bleeding, especially with active intracranial haemorrhage or gastro-intestinal bleeding; infants with congenital heart disease in whom patency of the ductus arteriosus is necessary for satisfactory pulmonary or systemic blood flow (e.g. pulmonary atresia, severe tetralogy of Fallot, severe coarctation of the aorta); infants with thrombocytopenia; infants with coagulation defects; infants with known or suspected necrotising enterocolitis; infants with significant impairment of renal function.

Special warnings and special precautions for use:

General: Indocid may mask the usual signs and symptoms of infection. The drug must therefore be used cautiously in the presence of existing controlled infection.

Because severe hepatic reactions have been reported in adults on prolonged therapy with oral indomethacin, Indocid PDA should be discontinued if signs and symptoms consistent with liver disease develop in the neonate.

Indocid PDA may inhibit platelet aggregation. Premature babies should be observed for signs of bleeding.

Indocid PDA should be administered carefully to avoid extravasation and resultant irritation to tissues.

Gastro-intestinal effects: Clinical results indicate that major gastro-intestinal bleeding was no more common in those babies receiving indomethacin than those receiving placebo. However, minor gastro-intestinal bleeding (i.e. chemical detection of blood in the stool) was more common in infants treated with indomethacin. Severe gastro-intestinal effects have been reported in adults treated for prolonged periods with oral indomethacin.

CNS reactions: Prematurity *per se* is associated with an increased incidence of spontaneous intraventricular haemorrhage. Because indomethacin may inhibit platelet aggregation, the potential for intraventricular bleeding may be increased.

Renal effects: Indocid PDA may cause significant reduction in urine output (50% or more) with elevated blood urea and creatinine, and reduced GFR and creatinine clearance. In most babies, these effects are transient and disappear when therapy with Indocid PDA is stopped. However, because adequate renal function can depend on renal prostaglandin synthesis, Indocid PDA may precipitate renal insufficiency including acute renal failure. This is most likely in babies with conditions such as extracellular volume depletion from any cause, congestive heart failure, sepsis, or hepatic dysfunction or who are undergoing therapy with nephrotoxic drugs which may affect renal function.

Whenever a significant suppression of urine volume occurs with treatment, treatment with Indocid PDA must stop until urine output returns to normal.

Indocid PDA may suppress water excretion in premature babies to a greater extent than the excretion of sodium. This may result in hyponatraemia. Renal function and plasma electrolytes should be monitored.

Interaction with other medicaments and other forms of interaction: The half-life of digitalis in premature babies with patent ductus arteriosus and with cardiac failure is often prolonged by indomethacin. When both drugs are used concomitantly, frequent monitoring of ECG and serum digitalis may help prevention or early detection of digitalis toxicity.

In a study of premature infants treated with Indocid

PDA and also receiving gentamicin or amikacin, both peak and trough levels of these aminoglycosides were significantly elevated.

Indocid may reduce the diuretic effect of frusemide.

Pregnancy and lactation: Not applicable.

Effects on ability to drive and use machines: Not applicable.

Undesirable effects:

Haemorrhagic: gross or microscopic bleeding into the gastro-intestinal tract; oozing from the skin after needle puncture; pulmonary haemorrhage; and disseminated intravascular coagulopathy.

Renal: renal dysfunction including one or more of the following: reduced urinary output; reduced urine sodium, chloride or potassium, urine osmolality, free water clearance, or glomerular filtration rate; uraemia; transient oliguria; and hypercreatinaemia.

Gastro-intestinal: vomiting; abdominal distension; melaena; transient ileus; and localised perforations of the small and/or large intestine.

Metabolic: hypersensitivity; hyponatraemia; elevated plasma potassium; elevated blood urea; hypoglycaemia.

Cardiovascular: pulmonary hypertension, intracranial bleeding.

Coagulation: decreased platelet aggregation.

General: weight gain (fluid retention); and exacerbation of infection.

See Summary of Product Characteristics for Indocid (indomethacin) for additional information concerning side-effects reported in the treatment of inflammatory and other conditions in patients of two years of age and older.

Causal relationship unknown: Although the following reactions have been reported in babies, a definite causal relationship has not been established.

Cardiovascular: bradycardia.

Respiratory: apnoea; exacerbation of pre-existing pulmonary infection.

Haematological: disseminated intravascular coagulation.

Metabolic: acidosis, alkalosis.

Gastro-intestinal: necrotising enterocolitis.

Ophthalmic: retrolental fibroplasia.

Overdosage: It is recommended that Indocid PDA should be administered only in a neonatal intensive-care unit.

Dosage is critical. The following signs and symptoms have occurred in individuals (not necessarily in premature infants) following an overdose of oral indomethacin: nausea, vomiting, intense headache, dizziness, mental confusion, disorientation, lethargy, paraesthesiae, numbness, and convulsions. There are no specific measures to treat acute overdosage with Indocid PDA. The patient should be monitored for several days because gastro-intestinal ulceration and haemorrhage have been reported as adverse reactions of indomethacin. Any complications occurring in the gastro-intestinal, renal and central nervous systems should be treated symptomatically and supportively.

Plasma half-life of intravenous indomethacin was inversely variable to the post-natal age and weight of the baby. In one study, a mean plasma half-life in babies less than a week old averaged 20 hours, while older babies showed a 12-hour average. Grouping the same babies by weight, the mean plasma half-life seen in babies under 1,000 g was 21 hours, in heavier babies the half-life was reduced to an average of 15 hours.

Pharmacological properties

Pharmacodynamic properties: Although the exact mechanism of action through which indomethacin causes closure of patent ductus arteriosus is not known, it is believed to be through inhibition of prostaglandin synthesis. Indomethacin has been shown to be a potent inhibitor of prostaglandin synthesis, both *in vitro* and *in vivo.* In human newborns with certain congenital heart malformations, PGE 1 dilates the ductus arteriosus. In foetal and newborn lambs, E type prostaglandins have also been shown to maintain the patency of the ductus; as in human newborns, indomethacin causes its constriction.

Studies in healthy young animals and in premature infants with patent ductus ateriosus indicated that, after the first dose of intravenous indomethacin, there was a transient reduction in cerebral blood flow velocity and cerebral blood flow. Similar decreases in mesenteric blood flow and velocity have been observed. The clinical significance of these effects have not been established.

Pharmacokinetic properties: The disposition of indomethacin following intravenous administration in preterm neonates with patent ductus arteriosus has not been extensively evaluated. Even though the plasma half-life of indomethacin was variable among premature infants, it was shown to vary inversely with post-natal age and weight. In one study of 28 evaluable infants, the plasma half-life in those infants less than 7 days old averaged 20 hours, and in infants older than 7 days, the mean plasma half-life was 12 hours. Grouping the infants by weight, the mean plasma half-life in those weighing less than 1,000 g was 21 hours, and in those weighing more than 1,000 g was 15 hours.

Preclinical safety data: No relevant information.

Pharmaceutical particulars

List of excipients: Water for injection PhEur.

Incompatibilities: None reported.

Shelf life: 36 months.

Special precautions for storage: The vial may be shipped and stored below 25°C. Intravenous solution should be prepared just prior to use and any unused portion remaining in the opened vial should be discarded.

When reconstituted, Indocid PDA is acceptable for use only when clear and free from particulate matter.

Further dilution with intravenous infusion solutions is not recommended. Indocid PDA is not buffered, and reconstitution at pH levels below 6 may cause precipitation of insoluble indomethacin.

Nature and contents of container: Available in cartons of three Type I glass vials each containing 1 ml.

Instructions for use/handling: The solution should be prepared only with 1 to 2 ml 0.9% Sodium Chloride Injection BP or Water for Injections PhEur. Preparations containing dextrose must not be used.

Preservatives should be carefully avoided at every stage because of the risk of toxicity in the newborn; any unused portion remaining in the opened vial should be discarded.

A fresh solution should be prepared just prior to each administration according to the dilution table below:

Amount of diluent used for each vial	*Concentration achieved*
1 ml	0.1 mg/0.1 ml
2 ml	0.05 mg/0.1 ml

While the optimal rate of injection has not been established, published literature suggests an infusion rate over 20–30 minutes.

Further dilution with intravenous infusion solutions is not recommended.

Marketing authorisation number 0025/0201

Date of approval/revision of SPC October 1998.

Legal category POM.

INNOVACE*

Qualitative and quantitative composition There are four strengths of Innovace Tablets available, each containing 2.5 mg, 5 mg, 10 mg and 20 mg of the active ingredient enalapril maleate.

Pharmaceutical form

2.5 mg–White, round tablets, marked 'INNOVACE'.

5 mg–White, half-scored, triangular tablets, marked 'INNOVACE'.

10 mg–Red, triangular tablets, marked 'INNOVACE'.

20 mg–Peach-coloured, triangular tablets, marked 'INNOVACE'.

Clinical particulars

Therapeutic indications:

Treatment of hypertension: All grades of essential hypertension and renovascular hypertension.

Treatment of heart failure: In heart failure, Innovace should be used as an adjunctive therapy with non-potassium-sparing diuretics and, where appropriate, digitalis. Innovace has been shown to improve symptoms, retard the progression of the disease, and reduce mortality and hospitalisation.

Prevention of symptomatic heart failure: When used in asymptomatic patients with left ventricular dysfunction, Innovace retards the development of symptomatic heart failure, and reduces hospitalisation for heart failure.

Prevention of coronary ischaemic events in patients with left ventricular dysfunction: Innovace reduces the incidence of myocardial infarction and reduces hospitalisation for unstable angina pectoris.

Posology and method of administration: The maximum daily dose is 40 mg.

The absorption of Innovace is not affected by food.

Essential and renovascular hypertension: Treatment should be initiated with 5 mg once a day. Where concomitant therapy is a diuretic, the recommended initial dose of Innovace is 2.5 mg (see *With concomitant diuretic therapy*). The dose should be titrated to give optimum control of blood pressure. The usual maintenance dose is 10–20 mg given once daily. In severe hypertension, the dosage may be increased incrementally to a maximum of 40 mg once daily.

The dosage of other antihypertensive agents being used together with Innovace may need to be adjusted. Where Innovace replaces a beta-blocking drug in the therapeutic regime, the beta-blocking agent should not be discontinued abruptly; the dosage should be titrated down after commencing therapy with Innovace.

With concomitant diuretic therapy: The recommended initial dose of Innovace is 2.5 mg. Symptomatic hypotension can occur following the initial dose of Innovace; this is more likely when Innovace is added to previous diuretic therapy. Caution is recommended, therefore, since these patients may be volume- or salt-depleted. If possible, the diuretic therapy should be discontinued for 2–3 days prior to initiation of therapy with Innovace.

Innovace minimises the development of thiazide-induced hypokalaemia and hyperuricaemia.

Use in the elderly (over 65 years): The starting dose should be 2.5 mg. Innovace is effective in the treatment of hypertension in the elderly. Some elderly patients may be more responsive to Innovace than younger patients.

The dose should be titrated according to need for the control of blood pressure.

Heart failure/Asymptomatic left ventricular dysfunction: The recommended starting dose in patients with symptomatic heart failure or asymptomatic left ventricular dysfunction is 2.5 mg once daily initiated under close medical supervision. For patients with severe heart failure, therapy should be initiated in hospital. Evidence of systolic left ventricular dysfunction should be obtained by relevant techniques (e.g. radionuclide ventriculography or echocardiography or equivalent) prior to initiation of preventive treatment; however, a repeated measurement may not be necessary in patients with one or more myocardial infarctions and documented reduction in cardiac function.

Following initiation of therapy, the dose should be titrated gradually to the usual maintenance dose of 20 mg, given as a single dose or two divided doses, according to the tolerability of the patient. In patients with symptomatic heart failure, this dosage schedule has been shown to improve survival.

The dose titration of Innovace may be performed over a two- to four-week period or more rapidly if indicated by the presence of residual signs and symptoms of heart failure. Blood pressure and renal function should be monitored closely both before and during treatment with Innovace. Serum potassium should also be monitored.

Some patients, other than those with severe heart failure, are considered to be at higher risk when started on an ACE inhibitor and are recommended for initiation of therapy in hospital. Research data have shown such patients to be: those on multiple or high-dose diuretics (e.g. >80 mg frusemide); patients with hypovolaemia; hyponatraemia (serum sodium <130 mmol/l); pre-existing hypotension (systolic blood pressure <90 mm Hg); patients with unstable cardiac failure; renal impairment (serum creatinine >150 μ mol/l); those on high-dose vasodilator therapy; patients aged 70 years or over (see *Special warnings and special precautions for use*).

In order to decrease the possibility of symptomatic hypotension, patients on previous high-dose diuretics should have the diuretic dose reduced before introducing Innovace. The appearance of hypotension after the initial dose of Innovace does not preclude subsequent careful dose titration with the drug, following effective treatment of the hypotension.

Use in impaired renal function: (see *Special warnings and special precautions for use*) Innovace is excreted by the kidney. It should be used with caution in patients with renal impairment. The recommended starting dose is 2.5 mg. The dose should be titrated against the response, and should be kept as low as possible to maintain adequate control of blood pressure or heart failure.

Innovace is dialysable. Dialysis patients may be given the usual dose of Innovace on dialysis days (see *Haemodialysis patients*). On the days when patients are not on dialysis the dosage should be tailored to the blood-pressure response.

Children: The paediatric use of Innovace has not been studied.

Contra-indications:

Pregnancy: (see *Pregnancy and lactation*).

Hypersensitivity to the product or any of the components, and in patients with a history of angioneurotic oedema relating to previous treatment with an ACE inhibitor.

Special warnings and special precautions for use:

Pretreatment assessment of renal function: Evaluation of the patient should include assessment of renal function prior to initiation of therapy, and during treatment where appropriate.

Symptomatic hypotension was seen rarely in uncomplicated hypertensive patients. In hypertensive patients receiving Innovace, hypotension is more likely to occur if the patient has been volume-depleted, e.g. by diuretic therapy, dietary salt restriction, dialysis, diarrhoea or vomiting. In patients with heart failure, with or without associated renal insufficiency, symptomatic hypotension has been observed. This is most likely to occur in those patients with more severe degrees of heart failure, as reflected by the use of high doses of loop diuretics, hyponatraemia or functional renal impairment (see *Posology and method of administration* for management of these patients).

Similar considerations may apply to patients with ischaemic heart or cerebrovascular disease in whom an excessive fall in blood pressure could result in a myocardial infarction or cerebrovascular accident.

If hypotension develops, the patient should be placed in a supine position. Volume repletion with oral fluids or intravenous normal saline may be required. Intravenous atropine may be necessary if there is associated bradycardia. A transient hypotensive response is not a contra-indication to further doses, which can usually be given without difficulty once the blood pressure has increased after volume expansion.

In some patients with heart failure who have normal or low blood pressure, additional lowering of systemic blood pressure may occur with Innovace. This effect is anticipated, and usually is not a reason to discontinue treatment. If such hypotension becomes symptomatic, a reduction of dose and/or discontinuation of the diuretic and/or Innovace may become necessary.

Impaired renal function: Innovace should be used with caution in patients with renal insufficiency as they may require reduced or less frequent doses (see *Posology and method of administration*).

Close monitoring of renal function before and during therapy should be performed as deemed appropriate in those with renal insufficiency. In the majority, renal function will not alter, or may improve.

Renal failure has been reported in association with Innovace and has been mainly in patients with severe heart failure or underlying renal disease, including renal artery stenosis. If recognised promptly and treated appropriately, renal failure when associated with therapy with Innovace is usually reversible.

Some hypertensive patients, with no apparent pre-existing renal disease, have developed increases in blood urea and creatinine when Innovace has been given concurrently with a diuretic. Dosage reduction of Innovace and/or discontinuation of the diuretic may be required. This situation should raise the possibility of underlying renal artery stenosis (see comment below).

Renovascular hypertension: Innovace can be used when surgery is not indicated, or prior to surgery. In some patients with bilateral renal artery stenosis or stenosis of the artery to a solitary kidney, increases of blood urea and creatinine, reversible upon discontinuation of therapy, have been seen. This is especially likely in patients treated with diuretics and/or those with renal insufficiency.

Angioneurotic oedema has been reported with angiotensin-converting enzyme inhibitors, including Innovace. This may occur at any time during treatment. In such cases, Innovace should be discontinued immediately and appropriate monitoring should be instituted to ensure complete resolution of symptoms prior to dismissing the patient. Where swelling is confined to the face, lips and mouth the condition will usually resolve without further treatment, although antihistamines may be useful in relieving symptoms. These patients should be monitored carefully until the swelling has resolved. However, where there is involvement of the tongue, glottis or larynx, likely to cause airways obstruction, appropriate therapy such as subcutaneous adrenaline (0.5 ml, 1:1000) should be administered promptly.

Patients with a history of angioedema unrelated to ACE-inhibitor therapy may be at increased risk of angioedema while receiving an ACE inhibitor (see also *Contra-indications*).

Other hypersensitivity reactions including urticaria have been reported.

Anaphylactic reactions during hymenoptera desensitisation: Rarely, patients receiving ACE inhibitors during desensitisation with hymenoptera venom (e.g. Bee or Wasp venom) have experienced life-threatening anaphylactoid reactions. These reactions were avoided by temporarily withholding ACE-inhibitor therapy prior to each desensitisation.

Haemodialysis patients: A high incidence of anaphylactoid reactions have been reported in patients dialysed with high-flux membranes and treated concomitantly with an ACE inhibitor. This combination should therefore be avoided.

Anaphylactoid reactions during LDL apheresis: Rarely, patients receiving ACE inhibitors during low-density lipoprotein (LDL) apheresis with dextran sulphate have experienced life-threatening anaphylactoid reactions. These reactions were avoided by temporarily withholding ACE-inhibitor therapy prior to each apheresis.

Cough: Cough has been reported with the use of ACE inhibitors. Characteristically, the cough is non-productive, persistent and resolves after discontinuation of therapy. ACE-inhibitor-induced cough should be considered as part of the differential diagnosis of cough.

Surgery/anesthesia: In patients undergoing major surgery or during anesthesia with agents that produce hypotension, Innovace blocks angiotensin-II formation secondary to compensatory renin release. This may lead to hypotension which can be corrected by volume expansion.

General: Where Innovace has been used as a single agent in hypertension, Afro-Caribbean patients may show a reduced therapeutic response.

Innovace should not be used in patients with aortic stenosis or outflow tract obstruction.

Interaction with other medicaments and other forms of interaction:

Drug interactions: Combination with other antihypertensive agents such as beta-blockers, methyldopa, calcium antagonists, and diuretics may increase the antihypertensive efficacy. Adrenergic-blocking drugs should only be combined with Innovace under careful supervision. Concomitant propranolol may reduce the bioavailability of Innovace, but this does not appear to be of any clinical significance.

Concomitant therapy with lithium may increase the serum lithium concentration.

Plasma potassium usually remains within normal limits, although cases of hyperkalaemia have been reported. If Innovace is given with a potassium-losing diuretic, the likelihood of diuretic-induced hypokalaemia may be lessened. Innovace may elevate plasma potassium levels in patients with renal failure. Potassium supplements, potassium-sparing diuretics and potassium-containing salt substitutes are not recommended, particularly in patients with impaired renal function, since they may lead to significant increases in plasma potassium. However, if the concomitant use of these agents is deemed appropriate, they should be used with caution and with frequent monitoring of plasma potassium.

Epidemiological studies have suggested that concomitant administration of ACE inhibitors and antidiabetic medicines (insulins, oral hypoglycaemic agents) may cause an increased blood-glucose-lowering effect with risk of hypoglycaemia. This phenomenon appeared to be more likely to occur during the first weeks of combined treatment and in patients with renal impairment. Long-term controlled clinical trials with enalapril have not confirmed these findings, and do not preclude the use of enalapril in diabetic patients. It is advised however, that these patients be monitored.

Narcotic drugs/antipsychotics: Postural hypotension may occur with ACE inhibitors.

Allopurinol, cytostatic or immunosuppressive agents, systemic corticosteroids or procainamide: Concomitant administration with ACE inhibitors may lead to an increased risk for leucopenia.

Non-steroidal anti-inflammatory drugs: The administration of a non-steroidal anti-inflammatory agent may reduce the antihypertensive effect of an ACE inhibitor. However, in a clinical pharmacology study indomethacin or sulindac was administered to hypertensive patients receiving Innovace and there was no evidence of a blunting of the antihypertensive action of Innovace. Furthermore, it has been described that NSAIDs and ACE inhibitors exert an additive effect on the increase in serum potassium, whereas renal function may decrease. These effects are in principle reversible, and occur especially in patients with compromised renal function.

Antacids: induce decreased bioavailability of ACE inhibitors.

Sympathomimetics: may reduce the antihypertensive effects of ACE inhibitors; patients should be carefully monitored to confirm that the desired effect is being obtained.

Alcohol: enhances the hypotensive effect with ACE inhibitors.

Cyclosporin: increase in the risk of hyperkalaemia with ACE inhibitors.

Pregnancy and lactation:

Use in pregnancy: Innovace has been shown to be fetotoxic in rabbits during middle and late pregnancy.

Foetal exposure in humans during the second and third trimesters of pregnancy has been associated with foetal and neonatal morbidity and mortality.

ACE inhibitors in human pregnancy have been associated with oligohydramnios which may result in limb contractures, craniofacial deformations and hypoplastic lung development. Hypotension, renal failure, hyperkalaemia and skull hypoplasia have occurred in the newborn. These adverse effects to the embryo and foetus do not appear to have resulted from intra-uterine ACE-inhibitor exposure limited to the first trimester.

Because of these findings, Innovace is contra-indicated in pregnancy. When pregnancy is detected, treatment with Innovace should be discontinued as soon as possible.

Use during lactation: Enalapril and enalaprilat are secreted in human milk; caution should be exercised if Innovace is given to breast-feeding mothers.

Effects on ability to drive and use machines: There are no data to suggest that Innovace affects the ability to drive and use machines.

Undesirable effects: Severe hypotension and renal failure have occurred in association with therapy with Innovace. These appear to occur in certain specific sub-groups (see *Special warnings and special precautions for use*).

Other adverse reactions: Dizziness and headaches are the most commonly reported side effects. Less frequently, fatigue, asthenia, hypotension, orthostatic hypotension, syncope, nausea, diarrhoea, muscle cramps, rash, and cough have been reported. Even less frequently, renal dysfunction, renal failure, and oliguria have been reported.

Rarely reported side effects include:

Cardiovascular: myocardial infarction or cerebrovascular accident, possibly secondary to severe hypotension in high-risk patients (see *Special warnings and special precautions for use*), chest pain, palpitations, rhythm disturbances, angina pectoris.

Gastro-intestinal: ileus, pancreatitis, hepatic failure, hepatitis–either hepatocellular or cholestatic, jaundice, abdominal pain, vomiting, dyspepsia, constipation, anorexia, stomatitis.

Nervous system/psychiatric: depression, confusion, somnolence, insomnia, nervousness, paraesthesiae, vertigo.

Respiratory: pulmonary infiltrates, bronchospasm, asthma, dyspnoea, rhinorrhoea, sore throat, and hoarseness.

Skin: diaphoresis, erythema multiforme, exfoliative dermatitis, Stevens-Johnson syndrome, toxic epidermal necrolysis, pemphigus, pruritus, urticaria, alopecia.

Other: impotence, flushing, taste alteration, tinnitus, glossitis, blurred vision.

A complex of symptoms has been reported which may include fever, serositis, vasculitis, myalgia/myositis, arthralgia/arthritis, a positive ANA, elevated ESR, eosinophilia, and leucocytosis. Rash, photosensitivity or other dermatological manifestations may occur.

Hypersensitivity/angioneurotic oedema: angioneurotic oedema of the face, extremities, lips, tongue, glottis and/or larynx has been reported rarely (see *Special warnings and special precautions for use*).

Laboratory test findings: Increases in blood urea and plasma creatinine, reversible on discontinuation of Innovace, are most likely in the presence of severe heart failure or bilateral renal artery stenosis, especially in patients with renal insufficiency (see *Special warnings and special precautions for use*). However, increases in blood urea and plasma creatinine may occur without evidence of pre-existing renal impairment, especially in patients taking diuretics. In this event, undiagnosed renal artery stenosis should be suspected. Dosage reduction of Innovace and/or discontinuation of the diuretic should be considered.

Hyperkalaemia and hyponatraemia have also been reported in a few cases (for further information see *Interaction with other medicaments and other forms of interaction, Plasma potassium*).

Decreases in haemoglobin and haematocrit as well as elevation of liver enzymes and/or serum bilirubin have been reported in a few patients, and are usually reversible upon discontinuation of Innovace.

Decreases in platelets and white cell count, and rare cases of neutropenia, thrombocytopenia, bone-marrow depression, and agranulocytosis have been reported, but a causal relationship to Innovace has not been established.

Overdose: Limited data are available for overdosage in humans. The most prominent features of overdosage reported to date are marked hypotension, beginning some six hours after ingestion of tablets, concomitant with blockade of the renin-angiotensin-aldosterone system, and stupor. Serum enalaprilat levels 100 times and 200 times higher than usually seen after therapeutic doses have been reported after ingestion of 300 mg and 440 mg of enalapril, respectively.

The recommended treatment of overdosage is intravenous infusion of normal saline solution. If ingestion is recent, induce emesis. Innovace can be removed from the general circulation by haemodialysis.

Pharmacological properties

Pharmacodynamic properties: Innovace is the maleate

salt of enalapril, a derivative of two amino acids; L-alanine and L-proline. Angiotensin-converting enzyme (ACE) is a peptidyl dipeptidase which catalyses the conversion of angiotensin I to the pressor substance angiotensin II. After absorption Innovace is hydrolysed to enalaprilat which inhibits ACE. Inhibition of ACE results in decreased plasma renin activity (due to removal of negative feedback of renin release) and decreased aldosterone secretion.

ACE is identical to kinase II, and may therefore block the degradation of bradykinin. The possible role of this mechanism in the therapeutic effects of enalapril has not yet been elucidated.

While the mechanism through which Innovace lowers blood pressure is believed to be primarily suppression of the renin-angiotensin-aldosterone system, which plays a major role in the regulation of blood pressure, Innovace is anthypertensive even in patients with low-renin hypertension.

Pharmacokinetic properties: Innovace is rapidly absorbed, with peak serum concentrations of enalapril occurring within one hour. Based on urinary recovery, the extent of absorption of enalapril from Innovace is approximately 60%.

Following absorption, Innovace is rapidly and extensively hydrolysed to enalaprilat. Peak serum concentrations of enalaprilat occur 3 to 4 hours after an oral dose of Innovace. Excretion of Innovace is primarily renal. The principal components in urine are enalaprilat, accounting for about 40% of the dose and intact enalapril. In subjects with normal renal function, steady state serum concentrations of enalaprilat were achieved by the fourth day of administration. The effective half-life for accumulation of enalaprilat following multiple doses of Innovace is 11 hours. Accumulation may occur, however in patients with severely impaired renal function, and the dosage of enalapril should be adjusted accordingly. The absorption of Innovace is not influenced by the presence of food in the gastro-intestinal tract. The extent of absorption and hydrolysis of enalapril are similar for the various doses in the recommended therapeutic range.

Preclinical safety data: No relevant information.

Pharmaceutical particulars

List of excipients: All Innovace Tablets contain the following inactive ingredients: Lactose PhEur; Magnesium Stearate PhEur; Maize Starch PhEur; Pregelatinised Maize Starch BP; Sodium Bicarbonate PhEur. In addition the red 10 mg tablets contain red iron oxide E172 and the peach-coloured 20 mg tablets containing red iron oxide E172 and yellow iron oxide E172.

Incompatibilities: None.

Shelf life: 36 months.

Special precautions for storage: Store in a dry place below 25°C.

Nature and contents of container: Innovace Tablets are available in calendar packs of 28

Instructions for use/handling: None.

Marketing authorisation numbers

2.5 mg tablet	0025/0220
5 mg tablet	0025/0194
10 mg tablet	0025/0195
20 mg tablet	0025/0196

Date of approval/revision of SPC April 1997

Legal category POM

INNOVACE* MELT

Qualitative and quantitative composition Innovace Melt contains 2.5 mg, 5 mg, 10 mg and 20 mg of the active ingredient enalapril maleate.

Pharmaceutical form

Innovace Melt is a rapidly dissolving freeze-dried wafer (oral lyophilisate).

Clinical particulars

Therapeutic indications:

Treatment of hypertension: All grades of essential hypertension and renovascular hypertension.

Treatment of heart failure: In heart failure, Innovace should be used as an adjunctive therapy with non-potassium-sparing diuretics and, where appropriate, digitalis. Innovace has been shown to improve symptoms, retard the progression of the disease, and reduce mortality and hospitalisation.

Prevention of symptomatic heart failure: When used in asymptomatic patients with left ventricular dysfunction, Innovace retards the development of symptomatic heart failure, and reduces hospitalisation for heart failure.

Prevention of coronary ischaemic events in patients with left ventricular dysfunction: Innovace reduces the incidence of myocardial infarction and reduces hospitalisation for unstable angina pectoris.

Posology and method of administration: Innovace Melt: Patients should be instructed to open the blister pack by peeling the foil with dry hands. Patients should place the wafer on the tongue. The wafer will rapidly dissolve and be swallowed with the patient's saliva. No water is needed for taking the wafer.

The maximum daily dose is 40 mg.

The absorption of Innovace is not affected by food.

Essential and renovascular hypertension: Treatment should be initiated with 5 mg once a day. Where concomitant therapy is a diuretic, the recommended initial dose of Innovace is 2.5 mg (see *With concomitant diuretic therapy*). The dose should be titrated to give optimum control of blood pressure. The usual maintenance dose is 10–20 mg given once daily. In severe hypertension, the dosage may be increased incrementally to a maximum of 40 mg once daily.

The dosage of other antihypertensive agents being used together with Innovace may need to be adjusted. Where Innovace replaces a beta-blocking drug in the therapeutic regime, the beta-blocking agent should not be discontinued abruptly; the dosage should be titrated down after commencing therapy with Innovace.

With concomitant diuretic therapy: The recommended initial dose of Innovace is 2.5 mg. Symptomatic hypotension can occur following the initial dose of Innovace; this is more likely when Innovace is added to previous diuretic therapy. Caution is recommended, therefore, since these patients may be volume- or salt-depleted. If possible, the diuretic therapy should be discontinued for 2–3 days prior to initiation of therapy with Innovace.

Innovace minimises the development of thiazide-induced hypokalaemia and hyperuricaemia.

Use in the elderly (over 65 years): The starting dose should be 2.5 mg. Innovace is effective in the treatment of hypertension in the elderly. Some elderly patients may be more responsive to Innovace than younger patients.

The dose should be titrated according to need for the control of blood pressure.

Heart failure/Asymptomatic left ventricular dysfunction: The recommended starting dose in patients with symptomatic heart failure or asymptomatic left ventricular dysfunction is 2.5 mg once daily initiated under close medical supervision. For patients with severe heart failure, therapy should be initiated in hospital. Evidence of systolic left ventricular dysfunction should be obtained by relevant techniques (e.g. radionuclide ventriculography or echocardiography or equivalent) prior to initiation of preventive treatment; however, a repeated measurement may not be necessary in patients with one or more myocardial infarctions and documented reduction in cardiac function.

Following initiation of therapy, the dose should be titrated gradually to the usual maintenance dose of 20 mg, given as a single dose or two divided doses, according to the tolerability of the patient. In patients with symptomatic heart failure, this dosage schedule has been shown to improve survival.

The dose titration of Innovace may be performed over a two- to four-week period or more rapidly if indicated by the presence of residual signs and symptoms of heart failure. Blood pressure and renal function should be monitored closely both before and during treatment with Innovace. Serum potassium should also be monitored.

Some patients, other than those with severe heart failure, are considered to be at higher risk when started on an ACE inhibitor and are recommended for initiation of therapy in hospital. Research data have shown such patients to be: those on multiple or high-dose diuretics (e.g. >80 mg frusemide); patients with hypovolaemia; hyponatraemia (serum sodium <130 mmol/l); pre-existing hypotension (systolic blood pressure <90 mm Hg); patients with unstable cardiac failure; renal impairment (serum creatinine >150 μmol/l); those on high-dose vasodilator therapy; patients aged 70 years or over (see *Special warnings and special precautions for use*).

In order to decrease the possibility of symptomatic hypotension, patients on previous high-dose diuretics should have the diuretic dose reduced before introducing Innovace. The appearance of hypotension after the initial dose of Innovace does not preclude subsequent careful dose titration with the drug, following effective treatment of the hypotension.

Use in impaired renal function: (see *Special warnings and special precautions for use*) Innovace is excreted by the kidney. It should be used with caution in patients with renal impairment. The recommended starting dose is 2.5 mg. The dose should be titrated against the response, and should be kept as low as possible to maintain adequate control of blood pressure or heart failure.

Innovace is dialysable. Dialysis patients may be given the usual dose of Innovace on dialysis days (see *Haemodialysis patients*). On the days when patients are not on dialysis the dosage should be tailored to the blood-pressure response.

Children: The paediatric use of Innovace has not been studied.

Contra-indications:

Pregnancy: (see *Pregnancy and lactation*).

Hypersensitivity to the product or any of the components, and in patients with a history of angioneurotic oedema relating to previous treatment with an ACE inhibitor.

Special warnings and special precautions for use:

Pretreatment assessment of renal function: Evaluation of the patient should include assessment of renal function prior to initiation of therapy, and during treatment where appropriate.

Symptomatic hypotension was seen rarely in uncomplicated hypertensive patients. In hypertensive patients receiving Innovace, hypotension is more likely to occur if the patient has been volume-depleted, e.g. by diuretic therapy, dietary salt restriction, dialysis, diarrhoea or vomiting. In patients with heart failure, with or without associated renal insufficiency, symptomatic hypotension has been observed. This is most likely to occur in those patients with more severe degrees of heart failure, as reflected by the use of high doses of loop diuretics, hyponatraemia or functional renal impairment (see *Posology and method of administration* for management of these patients).

Similar considerations may apply to patients with ischaemic heart or cerebrovascular disease in whom an excessive fall in blood pressure could result in a myocardial infarction or cerebrovascular accident.

If hypotension develops, the patient should be placed in a supine position. Volume repletion with oral fluids or intravenous normal saline may be required. Intravenous atropine may be necessary if there is associated bradycardia. A transient hypotensive response is not a contra-indication to further doses, which can usually be given without difficulty once the blood pressure has increased after volume expansion.

In some patients with heart failure who have normal or low blood pressure, additional lowering of systemic blood pressure may occur with Innovace. This effect is anticipated, and usually is not a reason to discontinue treatment. If such hypotension becomes symptomatic, a reduction of dose and/or discontinuation of the diuretic and/or Innovace may become necessary.

Impaired renal function: Innovace should be used with caution in patients with renal insufficiency as they may require reduced or less frequent doses (see *Posology and method of administration*).

Close monitoring of renal function before and during therapy should be performed as deemed appropriate in those with renal insufficiency. In the majority, renal function will not alter, or may improve.

Renal failure has been reported in association with Innovace and has been mainly in patients with severe heart failure or underlying renal disease, including renal artery stenosis. If recognised promptly and treated appropriately, renal failure when associated with therapy with Innovace is usually reversible.

Some hypertensive patients, with no apparent pre-existing renal disease, have developed increases in blood urea and creatinine when Innovace has been given concurrently with a diuretic. Dosage reduction of Innovace and/or discontinuation of the diuretic may be required. This situation should raise the possibility of underlying renal artery stenosis (see comment below).

Renovascular hypertension: Innovace can be used when surgery is not indicated, or prior to surgery. In some patients with bilateral renal artery stenosis or stenosis of the artery to a solitary kidney, increases of blood urea and creatinine, reversible upon discontinuation of therapy, have been seen. This is especially likely in patients treated with diuretics and/or those with renal insufficiency.

Angioneurotic oedema has been reported with angiotensin-converting enzyme inhibitors, including Innovace. This may occur at any time during treatment. In such cases, Innovace should be discontinued immediately and appropriate monitoring should be instituted to ensure complete resolution of symptoms prior to dismissing the patient. Where swelling is confined to the face, lips and mouth the condition will usually resolve without further treatment, although antihistamines may be useful in relieving symptoms. These patients should be monitored carefully until the swelling has resolved. However, where there is involvement of the tongue, glottis or larynx, likely to cause airways obstruction, appropriate therapy such as subcutaneous adrenaline (0.5 ml, 1:1000) should be administered promptly.

Patients with a history of angioedema unrelated to ACE-inhibitor therapy may be at increased risk of angioedema while receiving an ACE inhibitor (see also *Contra-indications*).

Other hypersensitivity reactions including urticaria have been reported.

Anaphylactic reactions during hymenoptera desensitisation: Rarely, patients receiving ACE inhibitors during desensitisation with hymenoptera venom (e.g. Bee or Wasp venom) have experienced life-threatening anaphylactoid reactions. These reactions were avoided by temporarily withholding ACE-inhibitor therapy prior to each desensitisation.

Haemodialysis patients: A high incidence of anaphylactoid reactions have been reported in patients dialysed with high-flux membranes and treated concomitantly with an ACE inhibitor. This combination should therefore be avoided.

Anaphylactoid reactions during LDL apheresis: Rarely, patients receiving ACE inhibitors during low-density lipoprotein (LDL) apheresis with dextran sulphate have experienced life-threatening anaphylactoid reactions. These reactions were avoided by temporarily withholding ACE-inhibitor therapy prior to each apheresis.

Cough: Cough has been reported with the use of ACE inhibitors. Characteristically, the cough is non-productive, persistent and resolves after discontinuation of therapy. ACE-inhibitor-induced cough should be considered as part of the differential diagnosis of cough.

Surgery/anesthesia: In patients undergoing major surgery or during anesthesia with agents that produce hypotension, Innovace blocks angiotensin-II formation secondary to compensatory renin release. This may lead to hypotension which can be corrected by volume expansion.

General: Where Innovace has been used as a single agent in hypertension, Afro-Caribbean patients may show a reduced therapeutic response.

Innovace should not be used in patients with aortic stenosis or outflow tract obstruction.

Interaction with other medicaments and other forms of interaction:

Drug interactions: Combination with other antihypertensive agents such as beta-blockers, methyldopa, calcium antagonists, and diuretics may increase the antihypertensive efficacy. Adrenergic-blocking drugs should only be combined with Innovace under careful supervision. Concomitant propranolol may reduce the bioavailability of Innovace, but this does not appear to be of any clinical significance.

Concomitant therapy with lithium may increase the serum lithium concentration.

Plasma potassium usually remains within normal limits, although cases of hyperkalaemia have been reported. If Innovace is given with a potassium-losing diuretic, the likelihood of diuretic-induced hypokalaemia may be lessened. Innovace may elevate plasma potassium levels in patients with renal failure. Potassium supplements, potassium-sparing diuretics and potassium-containing salt substitutes are not recommended, particularly in patients with impaired renal function, since they may lead to significant increases in plasma potassium. However, if the concomitant use of these agents is deemed appropriate, they should be used with caution and with frequent monitoring of plasma potassium.

Epidemiological studies have suggested that concomitant administration of ACE inhibitors and antidiabetic medicines (insulins, oral hypoglycaemic agents) may cause an increased blood-glucose-lowering effect with risk of hypoglycaemia. This phenomenon appeared to be more likely to occur during the first weeks of combined treatment and in patients with renal impairment. Long-term controlled clinical trials with enalapril have not confirmed these findings and do not preclude the use of enalapril in diabetic patients. It is advised, however, that these patients be monitored.

Narcotic drugs/antipsychotics: Postural hypotension may occur with ACE inhibitors.

Allopurinol, cytostatic or immunosuppressive agents, systemic corticosteroids or procainamide: Concomitant administration with ACE inhibitors may lead to an increased risk for leucopenia.

Non-steroidal anti-inflammatory drugs: The administration of a non-steroidal anti-inflammatory agent may reduce the antihypertensive effect of an ACE inhibitor. However, in a clinical pharmacology study indomethacin or sulindac was administered to hypertensive patients receiving Innovace and there was no evidence of a blunting of the antihypertensive action of Innovace. Furthermore, it has been described that NSAIDs and ACE inhibitors exert an additive effect on the increase in serum potassium, whereas renal function may decrease. These effects are in principle reversible, and occur especially in patients with compromised renal function.

Antacids: Induce decreased bioavailability of ACE inhibitors.

Sympathomimetics: May reduce the antihypertensive effects of ACE inhibitors; patients should be carefully monitored to confirm that the desired effect is being obtained.

Alcohol: Enhances the hypotensive effect with ACE inhibitors.

Cyclosporin: Increases in the risk of hyperkalaemia with ACE inhibitors.

Pregnancy and lactation:

Use in pregnancy: Innovace has been shown to be fetotoxic in rabbits during middle and late pregnancy.

Foetal exposure in humans during the second and third trimesters of pregnancy has been associated with foetal and neonatal morbidity and mortality.

ACE inhibitors in human pregnancy have been associated with oligohydramnios which may result in limb contractures, craniofacial deformations and hypoplastic lung development. Hypotension, renal failure, hyperkalaemia and skull hypoplasia have occurred in the newborn. These adverse effects to the embryo and foetus do not appear to have resulted from intra-uterine ACE-inhibitor exposure limited to the first trimester.

Because of these findings, Innovace is contraindicated in pregnancy. When pregnancy is detected, treatment with Innovace should be discontinued as soon as possible.

Use during lactation: Enalapril and enalaprilat are secreted in human milk; caution should be exercised if Innovace is given to breast-feeding mothers.

Effects on ability to drive and use machines: There are no data to suggest that Innovace affects the ability to drive and use machines.

Undesirable effects: Severe hypotension and renal failure have occurred in association with therapy with Innovace. These appear to occur in certain specific sub-groups (see *Special warnings and special precautions for use*).

Other adverse reactions: Dizziness and headaches are the most commonly reported side effects. Less frequently, fatigue, asthenia, hypotension, orthostatic hypotension, syncope, nausea, diarrhoea, muscle cramps, rash, and cough have been reported. Even less frequently, renal dysfunction, renal failure, and oliguria have been reported.

Rarely reported side effects include:

Cardiovascular: myocardial infarction or cerebrovascular accident, possibly secondary to severe hypotension in high-risk patients (see *Special warnings and special precautions for use*), chest pain, palpitations, rhythm disturbances, angina pectoris.

Gastro-intestinal: ileus, pancreatitis, hepatic failure, hepatitis – either hepatocellular or cholestatic, jaundice, abdominal pain, vomiting, dyspepsia, constipation, anorexia, stomatitis.

Nervous system/psychiatric: depression, confusion, somnolence, insomnia, nervousness, paraesthesiae, vertigo.

Respiratory: pulmonary infiltrates, bronchospasm, asthma, dyspnoea, rhinorrhoea, sore throat, and hoarseness.

Skin: diaphoresis, erythema multiforme, exfoliative dermatitis, Stevens-Johnson syndrome, toxic epidermal necrolysis, pemphigus, pruritus, urticaria, alopecia.

Other: impotence, flushing, taste alteration, tinnitus, glossitis, blurred vision.

A complex of symptoms has been reported which may include fever, serositis, vasculitis, myalgia/myositis, arthralgia/arthritis, a positive ANA, elevated ESR, eosinophilia, and leucocytosis. Rash, photosensitivity or other dermatological manifestations may occur.

Hypersensitivity/angioneurotic oedema: angioneurotic oedema of the face, extremities, lips, tongue, glottis and/or larynx has been reported rarely (see *Special warnings and special precautions for use*).

Laboratory test findings: Increases in blood urea and plasma creatinine, reversible on discontinuation of Innovace, are most likely in the presence of severe heart failure or bilateral renal artery stenosis, especially in patients with renal insufficiency (see *Special warnings and special precautions for use*). However, increases in blood urea and plasma creatinine may occur without evidence of pre-existing renal impairment, especially in patients taking diuretics. In this event, undiagnosed renal artery stenosis should be suspected. Dosage reduction of Innovace and/or discontinuation of the diuretic should be considered.

Hyperkalaemia and hyponatraemia have also been reported in a few cases (for further information see *Interaction with other medicaments and other forms of interaction, plasma potassium*).

Decreases in haemoglobin and haematocrit as well as elevation of liver enzymes and/or serum bilirubin have been reported in a few patients, and are usually reversible upon discontinuation of Innovace.

Decreases in platelets and white cell count, and rare cases of neutropenia, thrombocytopenia, bone-marrow depression, and agranulocytosis have been reported, but a causal relationship to Innovace has not been established.

Overdosage: Limited data are available for overdosage in humans. The most prominent features of overdosage reported to date are marked hypotension, beginning some six hours after ingestion of tablets, concomitant with blockade of the renin-angiotensin-aldosterone system, and stupor. Serum enalaprilat levels 100 times and 200 times higher than usually seen after therapeutic doses have been reported after ingestion of 300 mg and 440 mg of enalapril, respectively.

The recommended treatment of overdosage is intravenous infusion of normal saline solution. If ingestion is recent, induce emesis. Innovace can be removed from the general circulation by haemodialysis.

Pharmacological properties

Pharmacodynamic properties: Innovace is the maleate salt of enalapril, a derivative of two amino acids; L-alanine and L-proline. Angiotensin-converting enzyme (ACE) is a peptidyl dipeptidase which catalyses the conversion of angiotensin I to the pressor substance angiotensin II. After absorption, enalapril is hydrolysed to enalaprilat which inhibits ACE. Inhibition of ACE results in decreased plasma renin activity (due to removal of negative feedback of renin release) and decreased aldosterone secretion.

ACE is identical to kinase II, and may therefore block the degradation of bradykinin. The possible role of this mechanism in the therapeutic effects of enalapril has not yet been elucidated.

While the mechanism through which enalapril lowers blood pressure is believed to be primarily suppression of the renin-angiotensin-aldosterone system, which plays a major role in the regulation of blood pressure, enalapril is antihypertensive even in patients with low-renin hypertension.

Pharmacokinetic properties: Oral enalapril is rapidly absorbed, with peak serum concentrations of enalapril occurring within one hour. Based on urinary recovery, the extent of absorption of enalapril from Innovace Melt is approximately 60%.

Following absorption, oral enalapril is rapidly and extensively hydrolysed to enalaprilat. Peak serum concentrations of enalaprilat occur about 4 hours after an oral dose of Innovace Melt. Excretion of enalaprit is primarily renal. The principal components in urine are enalaprilat, accounting for about 40% of the dose, and intact enalapril. In subjects with normal renal function, steady state serum concentrations of enalaprilat were achieved by the fourth day of administration of oral enalapril. The effective half-life for accumulation of enalaprilat following multiple doses of oral enalapril is 11 hours. Accumulation may occur, however, in patients with severely impaired renal function, and the dosage of enalapril should be adjusted accordingly. The absorption of enalapril is not influenced by the presence of food in the gastrointestinal tract. The extent of absorption and hydrolysis of enalapril are similar for the various doses in the recommended therapeutic range.

Preclinical safety data: No relevant information.

Pharmaceutical particulars

List of excipients: Innovace Melt contains the following inactive ingredients: gelatin PhEur, mannitol E421, peppermint flavour, sodium hydroxide PhEur.

Innovace Melt also contains aspartame PhEur. The equivalent amount of phenylalanine in each 2.5 mg wafer is 1.4 mg; in each 5 mg wafer is 2.8 mg; in each 10 mg wafer is 5.6 mg; and in each 20 mg wafer is 11.2 mg.

Incompatibilities: None.

Shelf life: 24 months.

Special precautions for storage: Store below 25°C.

Nature and contents of container: Each wafer is supplied in an all-aluminium-foil blister with peelable aluminium foil lidding. The wafers are available in strips of 10 with 3 strips (30 wafers) in each pack.

Instructions for use/handling:

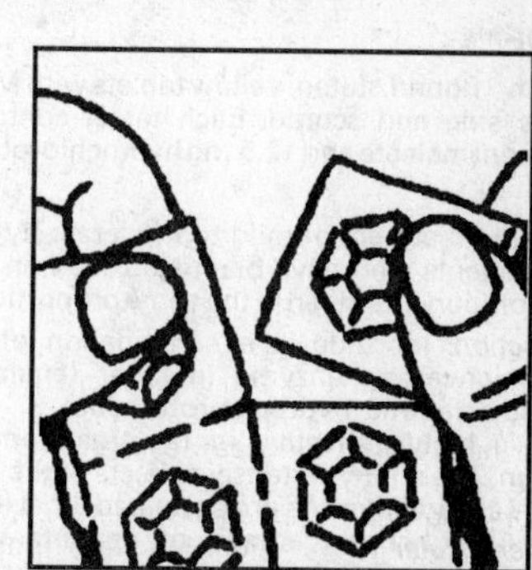

Fig. 1: The patient should be instructed to open the blister pack with dry hands.

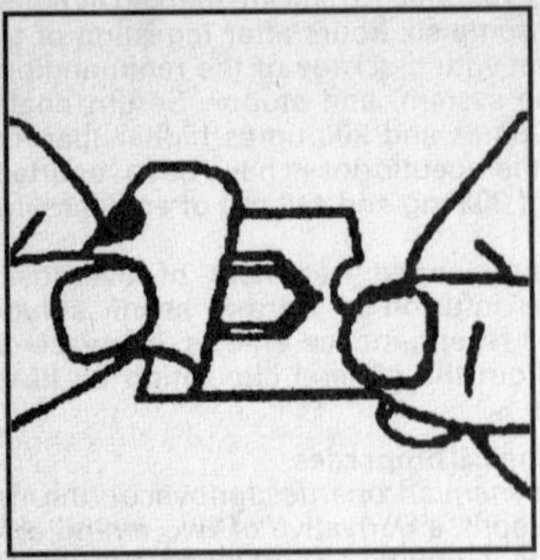

Fig. 2: The patient should peel away the aluminium foil from the blister.

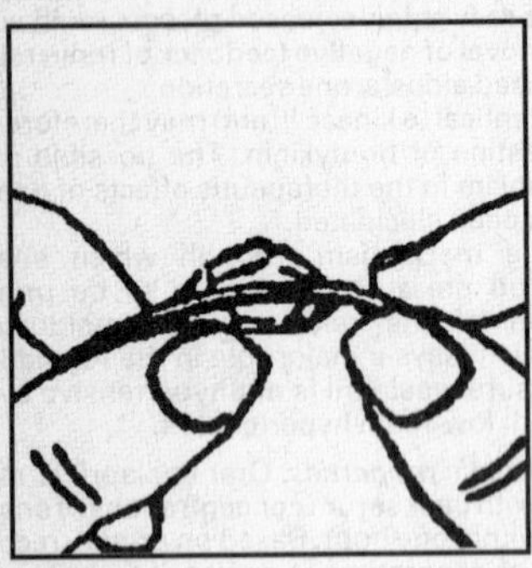

Fig. 3: To remove the wafer, push the bottom of the blister and the wafer will pop out. The patient should not attempt to push the wafer out of the blister before peeling away the aluminium foil as the wafer may break.

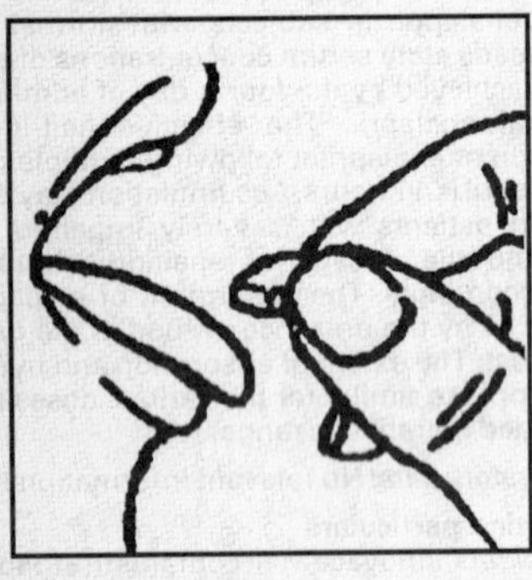

Fig 4: The patient should place the wafer on the tongue. The wafer will dissolve rapidly and be swallowed with the patient's saliva. No water is needed for taking the wafer.

Product licence numbers

2.5 mg wafer	PL 0025/0346
5 mg wafer	PL 0025/0347
10 mg wafer	PL 0025/0348
20 mg wafer	PL 0025/0349

Date of first authorisation/renewal of authorisation May 1997.

Date of revision of the text May 1997.

Legal category POM

INNOZIDE*

Presentation Round, fluted, yellow tablets with MSD 718 on one side and scored. Each tablet contains 20 mg enalapril maleate and 12.5 mg hydrochlorothiazide.

Uses For the treatment of mild to moderate hypertension in patients who have been stabilised on the individual components given in the same proportions.

Mode of action: Innozide is a combination of an angiotensin-converting enzyme inhibitor (enalapril maleate) and a diuretic (hydrochlorothiazide).

Innozide is highly effective in the treatment of hypertension. The antihypertensive effects of the two components are additive and are sustained for at least 24 hours. A higher percentage of patients with hypertension respond satisfactorily to Innozide than to either component administered alone.

Enalaprilat, the active metabolite of enalapril maleate, is a highly specific, long-acting, non-sulphydryl angiotensin-converting enzyme inhibitor. Enalapril maleate modulates a specific physiological mechanism, the renin-angiotensin-aldosterone system, which plays a major role in the regulation of blood pressure.

Hydrochlorothiazide is a diuretic and antihypertensive agent. Use of this agent alone results in increased renin secretion. Although enalapril maleate alone is antihypertensive, concomitant administration with hydrochlorothiazide results in a greater reduction in blood pressure. Enalapril maleate attenuates the potassium loss associated with hydrochlorothiazide.

Dosage and administration The dosage of Innozide should be determined primarily by the experience with the enalapril maleate component.

Adults

Essential hypertension: The usual dosage is one tablet, taken once daily. If necessary, the dosage may be increased to two tablets, taken once daily.

Prior diuretic therapy: Symptomatic hypotension may occur following the initial dose of Innozide; this is more likely in patients who are volume and/or salt depleted as a result of prior diuretic therapy. The diuretic therapy should be discontinued for 2–3 days prior to initiation of therapy with Innozide.

Dosage in renal insufficiency: Thiazides may not be appropriate diuretics for use in patients with renal impairment and are ineffective at creatinine clearance values of 30 ml/min or below (i.e. moderate or severe renal insufficiency).

In patients with creatinine clearance of >30 and <80 ml/min, Innozide should be used only after titration of the individual components.

Use in the elderly: In clinical studies the efficacy and tolerability of enalapril maleate and hydrochlorothiazide, administered concomitantly, were similar in both elderly and younger hypertensive patients.

Paediatric use: Safety and effectiveness in children have not been established.

Contra-indications, warnings, etc

Contra-indications: Innozide is contra-indicated in patients with anuria.

Innozide is contra-indicated in patients who are hypersensitive to any component of the product and in patients with a history of angioneurotic oedema relating to previous treatment with an angiotensin-converting enzyme inhibitor.

Innozide is contra-indicated in patients who are hypersensitive to other sulphonamide-derived drugs.

Innozide is contra-indicated in pregnancy. ACE inhibitors have been shown to be foetotoxic in rabbits during middle and late pregnancy. Effects of exposure of the foetus to ACE inhibitors during the first trimester of human pregnancy are unknown. Foetal exposure during the second and third trimesters of pregnancy has been associated with foetal and neonatal morbidity and mortality. ACE inhibitors in human pregnancy have been associated with oligohydramnios. Hypotension and renal failure have occurred in the newborn.

See also 'Breast-feeding mothers' under 'Precautions'.

Precautions

Hypotension and electrolyte/fluid imbalance: As with all antihypertensive therapy, symptomatic hypotension may occur in some patients. This was rarely seen in uncomplicated hypertensive patients but is more likely in the presence of fluid or electrolyte imbalance, e.g. volume depletion, hyponatraemia, hypochloraemic alkalosis, hypomagnesaemia or hypokalaemia which may occur from prior diuretic therapy, dietary salt restriction, dialysis, or during intercurrent diarrhoea or vomiting. Periodic determination of serum electrolytes should be performed at appropriate intervals in such patients.

Particular consideration should be given when therapy is administered to patients with ischaemic heart or cerebrovascular disease because an excessive fall in blood pressure could result in a myocardial infarction or cerebrovascular accident.

If hypotension occurs, the patient should be placed in the supine position and, if necessary, should receive an intravenous infusion of normal saline. A transient hypotensive response is not a contra-indication to further doses. Following restoration of effective blood volume and pressure, reinstitution of therapy at reduced dosage may be possible; or either of the components may be used appropriately alone.

Renal function impairment: Thiazides may not be appropriate diuretics for use in patients with renal impairment and are ineffective at creatinine clearance values of 30 ml/min or below (i.e. moderate or severe renal insufficiency).

Innozide should not be administered to patients with renal insufficiency (creatinine clearance ≤80 ml/min) until titration of the individual components has shown the need for the doses present in the combination tablet.

Some hypertensive patients with no apparent pre-existing renal disease have developed usually minor and transient increases in blood urea and serum creatinine when enalapril maleate has been given concomitantly with a diuretic. If this occurs during therapy with Innozide, the combination should be discontinued. Reinstitution of therapy at reduced dosage may be possible, or either of the components may be used appropriately alone.

In some patients, with bilateral renal artery stenosis or stenosis in the artery to a solitary kidney, increases in blood urea and serum creatinine, reversible upon discontinuation of therapy, have been seen with angiotensin-converting enzyme (ACE) inhibitors.

Haemodialysis patients: A high incidence of anaphylactoid reactions has been reported in patients dialysed with high-flux membranes and treated concomitantly with an ACE inhibitor. This combination should therefore be avoided.

Anaphylactic reactions during LDL apheresis: Rarely, patients receiving ACE inhibitors during low-density lipoprotein (LDL) apheresis with dextran sulphate have experienced life-threatening anaphylactoid reactions. These reactions were avoided by temporarily withholding ACE-inhibitor therapy prior to each apheresis.

Hepatic disease: Thiazides should be used with caution in patients with impaired hepatic function or progressive liver disease, since minor alterations of fluid and electrolyte balance may precipitate hepatic coma.

Surgery/anaesthesia: In patients undergoing major surgery or during anaesthesia with agents that produce hypotension, enalaprilat blocks angiotensin-II formation secondary to compensatory renin release. If hypotension occurs and is considered to be due to this mechanism, it can be corrected by volume expansion.

Metabolic and endocrine effects: Thiazide therapy may impair glucose tolerance. Dosage adjustment of antidiabetic agents, including insulin, may be required.

Thiazides may decrease urinary calcium excretion and may cause intermittent and slight elevation of serum calcium. Marked hypercalcaemia may be evidence of hidden hyperparathyroidism. Thiazides should be discontinued before carrying out tests for parathyroid function.

Increases in cholesterol and triglyceride levels may be associated with thiazide diuretic therapy; however, at the 12.5 mg dose contained in Innozide, minimal or no effect was reported.

Thiazide therapy may precipitate hyperuricaemia and/or gout in certain patients. However, enalapril may increase urinary uric acid and thus may attenuate the hyperuricaemic effect of hydrochlorothiazide.

Hypersensitivity/angioneurotic oedema: Angioneurotic oedema of the face, extremities, lips, tongue, glottis and/or larynx has been reported rarely in patients treated with angiotensin-converting enzyme inhibitors, including enalapril maleate. This may occur any time during treatment. In such cases, enalapril maleate should be discontinued promptly and appropriate monitoring should be carried out to ensure complete resolution of symptoms before dismissing the patient.

In those instances where swelling has been confined to the face and lips the condition generally resolved without treatment, although antihistamines have been useful in relieving symptoms.

Angioneurotic oedema associated with laryngeal oedema may be fatal. Where there is involvement of the tongue, glottis or larynx, likely to cause airway obstruction, appropriate therapy such as subcutaneous adrenaline solution 1:1000 (0.3 ml to 0.5 ml) should be administered promptly.

Patients with a history of angioedema unrelated to ACE-inhibitor therapy may be at increased risk of angioedema while receiving an ACE inhibitor. (See also: 'Contra-indications').

In patients receiving thiazides, sensitivity reactions may occur with or without a history of allergy or bronchial asthma. Exacerbation or activation of systemic lupus erythematosus has been reported with the use of thiazides.

Anaphylactoid reactions during Hymenoptera desensitisation: Rarely, patients receiving ACE inhibitors during desensitisation with hymenoptera venom (e.g. Bee or Wasp venom) have experienced life-threatening anaphylactoid reactions. These reactions were avoided by temporarily withholding ACE-inhibitor therapy prior to each desensitisation.

Cough: Cough has been reported with the use of ACE inhibitors. Characteristically, the cough is non-productive, persistent and resolves after discontinuation of therapy. ACE inhibitor-induced cough should be considered as part of the differential diagnosis of cough.

Breast-feeding mothers: Enalapril, enalaprilat and

thiazides appear in human milk. If use of Innozide is deemed essential, breast-feeding should stop.

Drug Interactions

Serum potassium: The potassium-losing effect of thiazide diuretics is usually attenuated by the effect of enalapril maleate. Serum potassium usually remains within normal limits, although in clinical trials with enalapril maleate hyperkalaemia did occur in a few cases.

The use of potassium supplements, potassium-sparing agents or potassium-containing salt substitutes, particularly in patients with impaired renal function, may lead to a significant increase in serum potassium. If concomitant use of 'Innozide' and any of these agents is deemed appropriate, they should be used with caution and with frequent monitoring of serum potassium.

Lithium: Lithium generally should not be given with diuretics or ACE inhibitors (ACE-I). Diuretic agents and ACE-I reduce the renal clearance of lithium and add a high risk of lithium toxicity. Refer to the prescribing information for lithium preparations before use of such preparations.

Non-depolarising muscle relaxants: Thiazides may increase the responsiveness to tubocurarine.

Other agents: The combination of enalapril maleate with beta-adrenergic blocking agents, methyldopa, or calcium entry blockers has been shown to improve the efficacy of lowering the blood pressure.

Ganglionic-blocking agents or adrenergic-blocking agents, combined with enalapril, should only be administered under careful observation of the patient.

When administered concurrently, the following drugs may interact with thiazide diuretics:

Alcohol, barbiturates, narcotics or phenothiazines: Potentiation of orthostatic hypotension may occur.

Antidiabetic drugs (oral agents and insulin): Dosage adjustment of the antidiabetic drug may be required.

Corticosteroids, ACTH: Intensified electrolyte depletion, particularly hypokalaemia.

Pressor amines (e.g. adrenaline): Possible decreased response to pressor amines but not sufficient to preclude their use.

Non-steroidal anti-inflammatory drugs: In some patients, the administration of non-steroidal anti-inflammatory agent can reduce the diuretic, natriuretic, and antihypertensive effects of diuretics.

Side-effects: Innozide is usually well tolerated. In clinical studies, side effects have usually been mild and transient, and in most instances have not required interruption of therapy.

The most common clinical side-effects were dizziness and fatigue, which generally responded to dosage reduction and seldom required discontinuation of therapy.

Other side-effects (1–2%) were: Muscle cramps, nausea, asthenia, orthostatic effects including hypotension, headache, cough, and impotence.

Less common side-effects which occurred either during controlled trials or during marketed use include:

Cardiovascular: Syncope, non-orthostatic hypotension, palpitation, tachycardia, chest pain.

Gastro-intestinal: Pancreatitis, diarrhoea, vomiting, dyspepsia, abdominal pain, flatulence, constipation. Pancreatitis has been reported rarely with enalapril and with hydrochlorothiazide and, therefore, is a potential side-effect of Innozide.

Nervous system/psychiatric: Insomnia, somnolence, paraesthesia, vertigo, nervousness.

Respiratory: Dyspnoea.

Skin: Stevens–Johnson syndrome, rash, pruritis, diaphoresis.

Other: Renal dysfunction, renal failure, decreased libido, dry mouth, gout, tinnitus, arthralgia.

A symptom complex has been reported which may include fever, serositis, vasculitis, myalgia/myositis, arthralgia/arthritis, a positive ANA, elevated ESR, eosinophilia and leucocytosis. Rash, photosensitivity or other dermatological manifestations may occur.

Hypersensitivity/angioneurotic oedema: Angioneurotic oedema of the face, extremities, lips, tongue, glottis and/or larynx has been reported rarely (see 'Precautions').

Side-effects due to individual components: Additional side-effects that have been seen with one of the individual components and may be potential side-effects with Innozide are the following:

Enalapril maleate: Ileus, hepatic failure, hepatitis – either hepatocellular or cholestatic jaundice, depression, confusion, pulmonary infiltrates, bronchospasm/asthma, rhythm disturbances, angina pectoris, myocardial infarction or cerebrovascular accident, rhinorrhoea, photosensitivity, alopecia, flushing, taste alteration, anorexia, blurred vision, urticaria, stomatitis, glossitis, oliguria, toxic epidermal necrolysis, erythema multiforme, exfoliative dermatitis, pemphigus.

Hydrochlorothiazide: Anorexia, gastric irritation, constipation, jaundice (intrahepatic cholestatic jaundice), sialoadenitis, vertigo, xanthopsia, leucopenia, agranulocytosis, thrombocytopenia, aplastic anaemia, haemolytic anaemia, purpura, photosensitivity, fever, urticaria, necrotising angiitis (vasculitis), respiratory distress (including pneumonitis and pulmonary oedema), anaphylactic reaction, glycosuria, electrolyte imbalance including hyponatraemia, restlessness, muscle spasm, transient blurred vision.

Laboratory test findings: Clinically important changes in standard laboratory parameters were rarely associated with administration of 'Innozide'. Occasional hyperglycaemia, hyperuricaemia and hyper- or hypokalaemia have been noted. Increases in blood urea and serum creatinine, and elevations of liver enzymes and/or serum bilirubin have been seen. Decreases in haemoglobin and haematocrit have been reported in hypertensive patients treated with Innozide. These are usually reversible upon discontinuation of Innozide.

Decreases in platelets and white cell count, and rare cases of neutropenia, thrombocytopenia and bone marrow depression have been reported, but a causal relationship to 'Innozide' has not been established.

Hyponatraemia has occurred with enalapril and may be a potential finding with 'Innozide'.

Overdosage: No specific information is available on the treatment of overdosage with 'Innozide'. Treatment is symptomatic and supportive. Therapy with 'Innozide' should be discontinued and the patient observed closely. Suggested measures include induction of emesis and/or gastric lavage, and correction of dehydration, electrolyte imbalance and hypotension by established procedures.

Enalapril maleate: The most prominent feature of overdosage reported to date is marked hypotension, beginning some six hours after ingestion of tablets, concomitant with blockade of the renin-angiotensin system, and stupor. Serum enelaprilat levels 100 times and 200 times higher than usually seen after therapeutic doses have been reported after ingestion of 300 mg and 440 mg of enalapril maleate respectively.

Enalaprilat may be removed from the general circulation by haemodialysis.

Hydrochlorothiazide: The most common signs and symptoms observed are those caused by electrolyte depletion (hypokalaemia, hypochloraemia, hyponatraemia) and dehydration resulting from excessive diuresis. If digitalis has also been administered, hypokalaemia may accentuate cardiac arrhythmias.

Pharmaceutical precautions Store in a dry place below 25°C.

Legal category POM.

Package quantities Calendar pack of 28 tablets.

Further information Nil.

Product licence number 0025/0249.

MAXALT* 5 mg TABLETS ▼
MAXALT* 10 mg TABLETS ▼
MAXALT* MELT 10 mg ORAL LYOPHILISATES ▼

Qualitative and quantitative composition Each 5 mg tablet contains 5 mg of rizatriptan (corresponding to 7.265 mg of the benzoate salt).

Each 10 mg tablet contains 10 mg of rizatriptan (corresponding to 14.53 mg of the benzoate salt).

Each 10 mg oral lyophilisate contains 10 mg of rizatriptan (corresponding to 14.53 mg of the benzoate salt).

Pharmaceutical form Tablets.
Oral lyophilisates.

Clinical particulars

Therapeutic indications: Acute treatment of the headache phase of migraine attacks, with or without aura.

Posology and method of administration: General: Maxalt should not be used prophylactically.

The oral tablets should be swallowed whole with liquid. Maxalt Melt oral lyophilisates need not be taken with liquid.

The oral lyophilisate is packaged in a blister within an outer aluminium sachet. Patients should be instructed not to remove the blister from the outer sachet until just prior to dosing. The blister pack should then be peeled open with dry hands and the oral lyophilisate placed on the tongue, where it will dissolve and be swallowed with the saliva.

The oral lyophilisate can be used in situations in which liquids are not available, or to avoid the nausea and vomiting that may accompany the ingestion of tablets with liquids. However the onset of effect may be delayed due to slower absorption of rizatriptan.

Adults 18 years of age and older: The recommended dose is 10 mg.

Redosing: Doses should be separated by at least two hours, no more than two doses should be taken in any 24-hour period.

- *for headache recurrence within 24 hours:* if headache returns after relief of the initial attack, one further dose may be taken. The above dosing limits should be observed.
- *after non-response:* the effectiveness of a second dose for treatment of the same attack, when an initial dose is ineffective, has not been examined in controlled trials. Therefore, if a patient does not respond to the first dose, a second dose should not be taken for the same attack.

Clinical studies have shown that patients who do not respond to treatment of an attack are still likely to respond to treatment for subsequent attacks.

Some patients should receive the lower (5 mg) dose of Maxalt, in particular the following patient groups:

- patients on propranolol. Administration of rizatriptan should be separated by at least two hours from administration of propranolol. (See *Interaction with other medicaments and other forms of interaction.*)
- patients with mild or moderate renal insufficiency,
- patients with mild to moderate hepatic insufficiency.

Doses should be separated by at lest two hours; no more than two doses should be taken in any 24-hour period.

Paediatric patients: Safety and effectiveness of rizatriptan in paediatric patients have not been evaluated; therefore, Maxalt is not recommended for use in paediatric patients under 18 years of age.

Patients older than 65 years: The safety and effectiveness of rizatriptan in patients older than 65 years have not been systematically evaluated.

Contra-indications: Hypersensitivity to rizatriptan or any of the ingredients.

Concurrent administration of monoamine oxidase (MAO) inhibitors or use within two weeks of discontinuation of MAO inhibitor therapy. (See *Interaction with other medicaments and other forms of interaction.*)

Maxalt is contra-indicated in patients with severe hepatic or severe renal insufficiency.

Maxalt is contra-indicated in patients with previous cerebrovascular accident (CVA) or transient ischaemic attack (TIA).

Moderately severe or severe hypertension, or untreated mild hypertension.

Established coronary artery disease, including ischaemic heart disease (angia pectoris, history of myocardial infarction, or documented silent ischaemia), signs and symptoms of ischaemic heart disease, or Prinzmetal's angina.

Peripheral vascular disease.

Concomitant use of rizatriptan and ergotamine, ergot derivatives (including methysergide), or other 5-$HT_{1B/1D}$ receptor agonists.

Special warnings and special precautions for use: Maxalt should only be administered to patients in whom a clear diagnosis of migraine has been established. Maxalt should not be administered to patients with basilar or hemiplegic migraine.

Maxalt should not be used to treat 'atypical' headaches, i.e. those that might be associated with potentially serious medical conditions (e.g. CVA, ruptured aneurysm) in which cerebrovascular vasoconstriction could be harmful.

As with other 5-$HT_{1B/1D}$ receptor agonists, rizatriptan should not be given, without prior evaluation, to patients in whom unrecognised cardiac disease is likely or to patients at risk for coronary artery disease (CAD) [e.g. patients with hypertension, diabetics, smokers, men over 40 years of age, post-menopausal women, patients with bundle branch block, and those with a strong family history for CAD]. Those in whom CAD is established should not be given Maxalt. (See *Contra-indications.*)

If symptoms consistent with ischaemic heart disease occur, appropriate evaluation should be carried out.

Other 5-$HT_{1B/1D}$ agonists, (e.g. sumatriptan) should not be used concomitantly with Maxalt.

It is advised to wait at least six hours following use of rizatriptan before administering ergotamine-type medications (e.g. ergotamine, dihydro-ergotamine or methysergide). At least 24 hours should elapse after the administration of an ergotamine-containing preparation before rizatriptan is given. Although additive vasospastic effects were not observed in a clinical pharmacology study in which 16 healthy males received oral rizatriptan and parenteral ergotamine, such additive effects are theoretically possible (see *Contra-indications*).

The quantity of lactose in each tablet (30.25 mg in the 5 mg tablet and 60.50 mg in the 10 mg tablet) is probably not sufficient to induce specific symptoms of lactose intolerance.

Phenylketonurics: Phenylketonuric patients should

be informed that Maxalt Melt oral lyophilisates contain phenylalanine (a component of aspartame). Each 10 mg oral lyophilisates contains 2.10 mg phenylalanine.

The potential for interaction should be considered when rizatriptan is administered to patients taking CYP 2D6 substrates (see *Interaction with other medicaments and other forms of interaction*).

Interaction with other medicaments and other forms of interaction: Monoamine oxidase inhibitors: Rizatriptan is principally metabolised via monoamine oxidase, 'A' subtype (MAO-A). Plasma concentrations of rizatriptan and its active N-monodesmethyl metabolite were increased by concomitant administration of a selective, reversible MAO-A inhibitor. Similar or greater effects are expected with non-selective, irreversible MAO inhibitors. Administration of 'Maxalt' to patients taking inhibitors of MAO is contra-indicated. (See *Contra-indications*.)

Beta-blockers: Plasma concentrations of rizatriptan may be increased by concomitant administration of propranolol. This increase is most probably due to first-pass metabolic interaction between the two drugs, since MAO-A plays a role in the metabolism of both rizatriptan and propranolol. This interaction leads to a mean increase in AUC and C_{max} of 70–80%. In patients receiving propranolol, the 5 mg dose of Maxalt should be used. (See *Posology and method of administration*.)

In drug-interaction study, nadolol and metoprolol did not alter plasma concentrations of rizatriptan. In *in-vitro* studies with human liver microsomes, timolol and atenolol did not alter the metabolism of rizatriptan.

Selective serotonin-reuptake inhibitors (SSRIs): No pharmacodynamic or pharmacokinetic interactions were observed when rizatriptan was administered with paroxetine. However the theoretical possibility regarding the occurrence of a serotonin syndrome (weakness, hyper-reflexia, co-ordination disturbances) in case of concomitant treatment with SSRIs cannot be ruled out.

Rizatriptan inhibits cytochrome P450 2D6 (CYP 2D6) *in vitro* at concentrations (i.e. K_i) approximately 10-fold greater than C_{max} in patients. Clinical interaction data are not available. The potential for interaction should be considered when rizatriptan is administered to patients taking CYP 2D6 substrates.

Food: Tablets: The absorption of rizatriptan is delayed by approximately one hour when administered together with food. Therefore, onset of effect may be delayed when rizatriptan is administered in the fed state. (See *Pharmacokinetic properties, Absorption*.)

Food: Oral lyophilisate: The effect of food on the absorption of rizatriptan from the oral lyophilisate has not been studied. For the rizatriptan tablets, T_{max} is delayed by approximately one hour when the tablets are administered in the fed state. A further delay in the absorption of rizatriptan may occur when the oral lyophilisate is administered after meals. (See *Pharmacokinetic properties, Absorption*.)

Pregnancy and lactation

Use during pregnancy: The safety of rizatriptan for the use in human pregnancy has not been established. Animal studies do not indicate harmful effects at dose levels that exceed therapeutic dose levels with respect to the development of the embryo or foetus, or the course of gestation, parturition and post-natal development.

Because animal reproductive and developmental studies are not always predictive of human response, Maxalt should be used during pregnancy only if clearly needed.

Use during lactation: Studies in rats indicated that very high milk transfer of rizatriptan occurred. Transient, very slight decreases in pre-weaning pup body weights were observed only when the mother's systemic exposure was well in excess of the maximum exposure level for humans. No data exist in humans.

Therefore, caution should be exercised when administering rizatriptan to women who are breast-feeding. Infant exposure should be minimised by avoiding breast-feeding for 24 hours after treatment.

Effects on ability to drive and use machines: Migraine or treatment with Maxalt may cause somnolence in some patients. Dizziness has also been reported in some patients receiving Maxalt. Patients should, therefore, evaluate their ability to perform complex tasks during migraine attacks and after administration of Maxalt.

Undesirable effects: Maxalt (as the tablet and oral lyophilisates formulation) was evaluated in over 3,600 patients for up to one year in controlled clinical studies. The most common side effects were dizziness, somnolence, and asthenia/fatigue.

Additional side effects in patients taking one or more doses of Maxalt 5 mg or 10 mg during acute (incidence ≥1% and greater than placebo) or long-term (incidence ≥1%) clinical trials included, in decreasing order of frequency within body systems:

Body as a whole: pain in abdomen or chest;
Cardiovascular: palpitation, tachycardia;
Digestive: nausea, vomiting, dry mouth, diarrhoea, dyspepsia, thirst;
Musculoskeletal: neck pain, stiffness, regional heaviness, regional tightness, muscle weakness;
Nervous system: headache, paraesthesia, decreased mental acuity, insomnia, hypesthesia, tremor, ataxia, nervousness, vertigo, disorientation;
Respiratory: pharyngeal discomfort, dyspnoea;
Skin: flushing, pruritus, sweating, urticaria;
Special senses: blurred vision;
Urogenital: hot flushes/ flashes.

Syncope and hypertension occurred rarely (≤0.1% of patients).

Overdose: Rizatriptan 40 mg (administered as either a single tablet dose or as two doses with a two-hour interdose interval) was generally well tolerated in over 300 patients; dizziness and somnolence were the most common drug-related adverse effects.

In a clinical pharmacology study in which 12 subjects received rizatriptan, at total cumulative doses of 80 mg (given within four hours), two subjects experienced syncope and/or bradycardia. One subject, a female aged 29 years, developed vomiting, bradycardia, and dizziness beginning three hours after receiving a total of 80 mg rizatriptan (administered over two hours). A third degree AV block, responsive to atropine, was observed an hour after the onset of the other symptoms. The second subject, a 25 year-old male, experienced transient dizziness, syncope, incontinence, and a five-second systolic pause (on ECG monitor) immediately after a painful venipuncture. The venipuncture occurred two hours after the subject had received a total of 80 mg rizatriptan (administered over four hours).

In addition, based on the pharmacology of rizatriptan, hypertension or other more serious cardiovascular symptoms could occur after overdosage. Gastro-intestinal decontamination (e.g. gastric lavage followed by activated charcoal), should be considered in patients suspected of an overdose with Maxalt. Clinical and electrocardiographic monitoring should be continued for at least 12 hours, even if clinical symptoms are not observed.

The effects of haemo- or peritoneal dialysis on serum concentrations of rizatriptan are unknown.

Pharmacological properties

Pharmacodynamic properties:

Mechanism of action: ATC-code: N02C C.

Rizatriptan binds selectively with high affinity to human $5\text{-}HT_{1B}$ and $5\text{-}HT_{1D}$ receptors and has little or no effect or pharmacoogical activity at $5\text{-}HT_2$ or $5\text{-}HT_3$ adrenergic $alpha_1$, $alpha_2$ or beta; D_1, D_2 dopaminergic, histamic H_i; muscarinic; or benzodiazepine receptors.

The therapeutic activity of rizatriptan in treating migraine headache may be attributed to its agonist effects at $5\text{-}HT_{1B}$ and $5\text{-}HT_{1D}$ receptors on the extracerebral intracranial blood vessels that are thought to become dilated during an attack and on the trigeminal sensory nerves that innervate them. Activation of these $5\text{-}HT_{1B}$ and $5\text{-}HT_{1D}$ receptors may result in constriction of pain-producing intracranial blood vessels and inhibition of neuropeptide release that leads to decreased inflammation in sensitive tissues and reduced central trigeminal pain signal transmission.

Pharmacodynamic effects: Tablets: The efficacy of Maxalt Tablets in the acute treatment of migraine attacks was established in four multicentre, placebo-controlled trials that included over 2000 patients who received Maxalt 5 or 10 mg for up to one year. Headache relief occurred as early as 30 minutes following dosing, and response rates (i.e. reduction of moderate or severe headache pain to no or mild pain), two hours after treatment were 67–77% with the 10 mg tablet, 60–63% with the 5 mg tablet, and 23–40% with placebo. Although patients who did not respond to initial treatment with Maxalt were not redosed for the same attack, they were still likely to respond to treatment for a subsequent attack. Maxalt reduced the functional disability and relieved the nausea, photophobia, and phonophobia associated with migraine attacks.

Oral lyophilisates: In a placebo-controlled trial of Maxalt Melt oral lyophilisates, the efficacy of the oral lyophilisate formulation was comparable to that observed in similarly designed trials of Maxalt tablets. Onset of the effect occurred as early as 60 minutes following dosing. By two hours post-dosing, relief rates in patients treated with Maxalt Melt oral lyophilisates were approximately 66%, compared to 47% in the placebo group. Maxalt Melt oral lyophilisates also relieved the disability, nausea, photophobia, and phonophobia which accompanied the migraine episodes.

Maxalt Melt oral lyophilisates enables migraine patients to treat their migraine attacks without having to swallow liquids. This may allow patients to administer their medication earlier, for example, when liquids are not available, and to avoid possible worsening of GI symptoms by swallowing liquids.

Pharmacokinetic properties: Absorption: Rizatriptan is rapidly and completely absorbed following oral administration.

Tablets: The mean oral bioavailability of the tablet approximately 40–45%, and mean peak plasma concentrations (C_{max}) are reached in approximately 1–1.5 hours (T_{max}). Administration of an oral tablet dose with a high-fat breakfast had no effect on the extent of rizatriptan absorption, but absorption was delayed for approximately one hour.

Oral lyophilisates: The mean oral bioavailability of the oral lyophilisate is approximately 40–45%, and mean peak plasma concentrations (C_{max}) are reached in approximately 1.6–2.5 hours (T_{max}). The time to maximum plasma concentration following administration of rizatriptan as the oral lyophilisate formulation is delayed by 30–60 minutes relative to the tablet.

Distribution: Rizatriptan is minimally bound (14%) to plasma proteins. The volume of distribution is approximately 140 litres in male subjects, and 110 litres in female subjects.

Biotransformation: The primary route of rizatriptan metabolism is via oxidative deamination by monoamine oxidase-A (MAO-A) to the indole acetic acid metabolite, which is not pharmacologically active. N-monodesmethyl-rizatriptan, a metabolite with activity similar to that of parent compound at the $5\text{-}HT_{1B/1D}$ receptor, is formed to a minor degree, but does not contribute significantly to the pharmacodynamic activity of rizatriptan. Plasma concentrations of N-monodesmethyl-rizatriptan are approximately 14% of those of parent compound, and it is eliminated at a similar rate. Other minor metabolites include the N-oxide, the 6-hydroxy compound, and the sulphate conjugate of the 6-hydroxy metabolite. None of these minor metabolites is pharmacologically active. Following oral administration of ^{14}C-labelled rizatriptan, rizatriptan accounts for about 17% of circulating plasma radioactivity.

Elimination: Following intravenous administration, AUC in men increases proportionally and in women near-proportionally with the dose over a dose range of 10–60 mcg/kg. Following oral administration, AUC increases near-proportionally with the dose over a dose range of 2.5–10 mg. The plasma half-life of rizatriptan in males and females averages 2–3 hours. The plasma clearance of rizatriptan averages about 1000–1500 ml/min in males and about 900–1100 ml/min in females; about 20–30% of this is renal clearance. Following an oral dose of ^{14}C-labelled rizatriptan, about 80% of the radioactivity is excreted in urine, and about 10% of the dose is excreted in faeces. This shows that the metabolites are excreted primarily via the kidneys.

Consistent with its first pass metabolism, approximately 14% of an oral dose is excreted in urine as unchanged rizatriptan while 51% is excreted as indole acetic acid metabolite. No more than 1% is excreted in urine as the active N-monodesmethyl metabolite.

If rizatriptan is administered according to the maximum dosage regimen, no drug accumulation in the plasma occurs from day to day.

Characteristics in patients: The following data are based on studies with the oral tablet formulation.

Patients with a migraine attack: A migraine attack does not affect the pharmacokinetics of rizatriptan.

Gender: The AUC of rizatriptan (10 mg orally) was about 25% lower in males as compared to females, C_{max} was 11% lower, and T_{max} occurred at approximately the same time. This apparent pharmacokinetic difference was of no clinical significance.

Elderly: The plasma concentrations of rizatriptan observed in elderly subjects (age range 65 to 77 years) after tablet administration were similar to those observed in young adults.

Hepatic impairment (Child-Pugh's score 5–6): Following oral tablet administration in patients with hepatic impairment caused by mild alcoholic cirrhosis of the liver, plasma concentrations of rizatriptan were similar to those seen in young male and female subjects. A significant increase in AUC (50%) and C_{max} (25%) was observed in patients with moderate hepatic impairment (Child-Pugh's score 7). Pharmacokinetics were not studied in patients with Child-Pugh's score >7 (severe hepatic impairment).

Renal impairment: In patients with renal impairment (creatinine clearance 10–60 ml/min/1.73 m²), the AUC of rizatriptan after tablet administration was not significantly different from that in healthy subjects. In haemodialysis patients (creatinine clearance <10 ml/min/1.73 m²), the AUC for rizatriptan was approximately 44% greater than that in patients with normal renal function. The maximal plasma concentration of rizatriptan in patients with all degrees of renal impairment was similar to that in healthy subjects.

Preclinical safety data: Preclinical data indicate no risk for humans based on conventional studies of repeat dose toxicity, genotoxicity, carcinogenic potential, reproductive and developmental toxicity, safety pharmacology, and pharmacokinetics and metabolism.

Pharmaceutical particulars
List of excipients: Each compressed tablet contains the following inactive ingredients: lactose monohydrate, microcrystalline cellulose, pregelatinised corn starch, ferric oxide (Red) E172, and magnesium stearate.

Each oral lyophilisate contains the following inactive ingredients: gelatin, mannitol, glycine, aspartame, and peppermint flavour.

Incompatibilities: None.

Shelf life: 24 months.

Special precautions for storage: Do not store above 30°C.

Nature and contents of container: 5 mg tablets: All aluminium blister push through, packs with 6 tablets.

10 mg tablets: All aluminium blister push through, packs with 3 or 6 tablets.

10 mg oral lyophilisates: PVC/PVDC blister with one oral lyophilisate within an aluminium sachet. Packs with 3 or 6 oral lyophilisates.

Instructions for use/handling: Tablets: None.

Oral lyophilisates: The oral lyophilisate is packaged in a blister within an outer aluminium sachet. Patients should be instructed not to remove the blister from the outer sachet until just prior to dosing. The blister pack should then be peeled open with dry hands and the oral lyophilisate placed on the tongue, where it will dissolve and be swallowed with the saliva.

Marketing authorisation numbers

Tablet 5 mg	PL 0025/0369
Tablet 10 mg	PL 0025/0370
Oral lyophilisate 10 mg	PL 0025/0372

Date of first authorisation/renewal of authorisation 24 June 198.

Date of revision of the text N/A.

Legal category POM.

MEFOXIN* INJECTION

Presentation In vials containing 1 g or 2 g of cefoxitin as the sodium salt. Each gram of cefoxitin contains approximately 2.3 mEq sodium.

Uses Mefoxin is indicated for the treatment of the following infections caused by sensitive bacteria: peritonitis and other intra-abdominal and intrapelvic infections; gonorrhoea; female genital tract infections; septicaemia; urinary tract infections; respiratory tract infections; bone and joint infections; and skin and soft-tissue infections.

Mefoxin is a broad-spectrum bactericidal antibiotic indicated for the treatment of infections caused by susceptible strains of Gram-positive and Gram-negative pathogens both aerobic and anaerobic.

Mefoxin has been clinically effective not only in infections due to antibiotic-sensitive organisms, but also in infections due to organisms resistant to one or more of the following antibacterial agents: penicillin, ampicillin, carbenicillin, tetracyclines, erythromycin, chloramphenicol, cephalosporins, kanamycin, gentamicin, tobramycin, and sulphamethoxazole-trimethoprim.

Many Gram-negative pathogens are resistant to penicillins and cephalosporins through the action of the beta-lactamases which are produced by these pathogens. Mefoxin is remarkably stable in the presence of these bacterial beta-lactamases, both penicillinases and cephalosporinases. Hence, the clinical efficacy of Mefoxin extends to many infections caused by such pathogens.

Mefoxin is indicated for the treatment of mixed infections caused by susceptible strains of aerobic and anaerobic bacteria. The majority of these mixed infections are associated with contamination by faecal flora as well as flora originating from the vagina, skin, and mouth. In these mixed infections, *Bacteroides fragilis* is the most commonly encountered anaerobic pathogen and is usually resistant to aminoglycosides, cephalosporins, and virtually all penicillins. However, *Bacteroides fragilis* is usually susceptible to Mefoxin.

Mefoxin is indicated for adjunctive therapy in the surgical treatment of infections, including abscesses, infection complicating hollow visceral perforations, cutaneous infections, and infections of serous surfaces, whether caused by aerobes, mixed aerobes and anaerobes, or anaerobes.

Clinical experience has demonstrated that Mefoxin can be administered to patients who are also receiving carbenicillin, kanamycin, gentamicin, tobramycin, or amikacin (see 'Precautions' and 'Dosage and administration').

Prophylaxis: Mefoxin is indicated for the prevention of certain post-operative infections in patients undergoing contaminated or potentially contaminated surgical procedures or where the occurrence of post-operative infection could be especially serious.

Microbiology: Mefoxin is active *in vitro* against: Aerobic bacteria: *Gram-positive cocci* including: *Staphylococci:* (including coagulase-positive, coagulase-negative, and penicillinase-producing strains); Group A beta-haemolytic streptococci (*Streptococcus pyogenes*); Group B beta-haemolytic streptococci (*Streptococcus agalactiae*); *Streptococcus pneumoniae* (*Diplococcus pneumoniae*); other streptococci (except group D streptococci including enterococci, most strains of which are resistant, e.g. *Streptococcus faecalis*), *Gram-negative cocci* including: *Neisseria gonorrhoea* (including penicillinase-producing strains); *Neisseria meningitidis. Gram-negative rods (facultative anaerobes)* including: *Escherichia coli; Klebsiella pneumoniae;* Klebsiella spp.; *Proteus mirabilis. Proteus* (indole-positive); *Morganella morganii* (formerly *Proteus morganii*); *Proteus vulgaris; Haemophilus influenzae; Serratia marcescens; Providencia* spp.; *Providencia rettgeri* (formerly *Proteus rettgeri*); *Salmonella* spp. and *Shigella* spp.

Anaerobic bacteria: *Gram-positive cocci* including: *Peptococcus* spp.; *Peptostreptococcus* spp.; Microaerophilic *streptococcus. Gram-positive rods* including: *Clostridium perfringens; Clostridium* spp.; *Eubacterium* spp.; *Propionibacterium acnes. Gram-negative cocci* including: *Veillonella* spp. *Gram-negative rods* including: *Bacteroides fragilis; Bacteroides melaninogenicus; Bacteroides* spp. (including both penicillin-susceptible and penicillin-resistant strains); *Fusobacterium* spp.

Mefoxin is active against some strains of the following bacteria: *Acinetobacter calcoaceticus var. anitratum* (*Herellea vaginicola*); *Acinetobacter calcoaceticus* var. *lwoffi* (*Mima polymorpha*); *Alcaligenes faecalis; Citrobacter* spp. and *Flavo-bacterium* spp.; *Enterobacter* spp.

Mefoxin is not active against *Pseudomonas* spp., most strains of enterococci, many strains of *Enterobacter cloacae*, and methicillin-resistant staphylococci, and *Listeria monocytogenes.*

Human pharmacology: Mefoxin administered parenterally, produces high serum and urine concentrations. It is excreted virtually unchanged as active Mefoxin by the kidneys, and has a mean terminal serum half-life of approximately one hour. Mefoxin passes rapidly into body fluids such as pleural, bile, and ascitic fluids. Probenecid slows tubular excretion and increases and prolongs blood levels.

Intravenous: Peak serum concentrations of Mefoxin following 1 g infused intravenously over 3 minutes was 125 micrograms/ml, infused over 30 minutes was 72 micrograms/ml, and infused over 120 minutes was 25 micrograms/ml. Following 2 g infused intravenously over 3 minutes, peak serum concentration was 221 micrograms/ml. In a number of studies using 0.5 g, 1 g, or 2 g intravenous doses of Mefoxin mean total urinary recovery ranged from 77% to 99% of the cefoxitin dose.

Intramuscular: When Mefoxin was reconstituted for intramuscular injection with 0.5% or 1% lidocaine (lignocaine) hydrochloride, the lidocaine (lignocaine) had no effect on the absorption or elimination of Mefoxin.

Intramuscular injections of 1 g of Mefoxin in 0.5% lidocaine (lignocaine) hydrochloride solution produced a peak serum concentration of 30 micrograms/ml at 20 minutes. Approximately 85% of an intramuscular dose is excreted by the kidneys in the first six hours; this results in high urine levels (e.g. >3,000 micrograms/ml between one and two hours after a 1 g dose).

Dosage and administration Mefoxin may be administered intravenously or intramuscularly. (See reconstitution directions for each route below.) Dosage and route of administration should be determined by severity of infection, susceptibility of the causative organisms, and condition of the patient.

Therapy may be started while awaiting the results of susceptibility testing.

Adults Dosage: The usual dosage is 1 g or 2 g of Mefoxin every eight hours. (See 'Usual adult dosage' chart.)

Usual adult dosage

Type of infection	*Dose (g)*	*Frequency (hrs)*	*Total daily dosage*
Uncomplicated	1	Every 8 (occasionally every 6)	3 g (4 g)
Moderately severe or severe	2	Every 8 (occasionally every 6)	6 g (8 g)
Infections generally needing antibiotics in higher dosage	3 (2)	Every 6 (every 4)	12 g

In adults with renal insufficiency, an initial loading dose of 1 g to 2 g may be given. After a loading dose, the following recommendations for *maintenance dosage* may be used as a guide.

Maintenance dosage of Mefoxin in adults with reduced renal function

Renal function	Creatinine clearance (ml/min)	Dose (g)	Frequency (hrs)
Mild impairment	50–30	1–2	Every 8–12
Moderate impairment	29–10	1–2	Every 12–24
Severe impairment	9–5	0.5–1	Every 12–24
Essentially no function	<5	0.5–1	Every 24–48

In the patients undergoing haemodialysis, the loading dose of 1–2 g should be given after each haemodialysis, and the maintenance dose should be given as indicated in the chart giving 'Maintenance dosage of Mefoxin in adults with reduced renal function'.

Uncomplicated urinary tract infections: In uncomplicated urinary tract infections due to susceptible organisms, 1 g intramuscularly twice a day for ten days has been shown to be effective.

Uncomplicated gonorrhoea: For single dose therapy of uncomplicated gonorrhoea, including that caused by penicillinase-producing strains, the recommended dose is 2 g of Mefoxin intramuscularly given with 1 g of probenecid by mouth (at the same time or up to one hour before).

Neonates, infants and children:

*Neonates**	
0–1 week of age	20–40 mg/kg every 12 hours
1–4 weeks of age	20–40 mg/kg every 8 hours
*Infants**	20–40 mg/kg every 6 hours or every 8 hours
Children	20–40 mg/kg every 6 hours or every 8 hours

*Clinical data are insufficient to recommend use of the intramuscular formulation in infants less than 3 months of age.

In severe infections, the total daily dosage may be increased to 200 mg/kg, but not to exceed 12 g per day.

Mefoxin is not recommended for the therapy of meningitis. If meningitis is suspected an appropriate antibiotic should be used.

In children with renal insufficiency dosage frequency should be reduced as indicated for adults.

Prophylactic administration to adults: 2 g administered intramuscularly or intravenously just prior to surgery (½–1 hour before initial incision), then 2 g every 6 hours. Prophylactic therapy should not usually be given for more than 24 hours.

Prophylactic administration for neonates, infants and children: In infants and children, 30–40 mg/kg doses may be given at the same times as designated for adults. However, in neonates, 30–40 mg/kg doses may be given ½ to 1 hour before initial incision and the second and third dose may be given every 8–12 hours.

Clinical data are insufficient to recommend use of the intramuscular formulation in infants less than 3 months of age.

Obstetric and gynaecological surgery: For patients undergoing caesarean section, a single 2 g dose is administered intravenously as soon as the cord is clamped. If necessary, a second and third dose of 2 g may be administered intravenously 4 hours and 8 hours after the first dose.

In gynaecological surgical procedures, a single prophylactic dose of 2 g intravenously or intramuscularly has been effective given ½ to 1 hour before surgery.

In prolonged or heavily contaminated cases, additional 2 g doses may be given at 6-hour intervals. Prophylactic therapy does not ordinarily extend beyond 24 hours.

Intravenous administration: Reconstitute Mefoxin with Water for Injections BP: 1 g is soluble in 2 ml. Although Mefoxin is very soluble, for intravenous use it is preferable to add 10 ml of Water for Injections BP to the 1 g vial or to the 2 g vial. Shake to dissolve and then withdraw entire contents of vial into syringe.

Solutions of Mefoxin range from clear to light amber in colour. The pH of freshly reconstituted solutions usually ranges from 4.2 to 7.0.

For direct intravenous injection, Mefoxin may be slowly injected into the vein over a period of three to five minutes or may be given through the tubing when the patient is receiving parenteral solutions.

An intermittent intravenous infusion of Mefoxin may be employed when large amounts of fluid are to be given. However, during infusion of the solution containing Mefoxin, it may be advisable temporarily to discontinue administration of any other infusion solution at the same site (by using an appropriate IV infusion set).

A solution of Mefoxin may also be given by continuous intravenous infusion (see below for compatibility and stability).

Intramuscular administration ONLY: Reconstitute Mefoxin 1 g with 2 ml of Water for Injections BP, or 0.5% or 1% lidocaine (lignocaine) hydrochloride (without adrenaline) solution. Mefoxin is given by deep injection into a large muscle mass. Avoid injection into a blood vessel.

Note: Some patients may be hypersensitive to lidocaine (lignocaine).

Preparation of solution: The following table is provided for convenience in reconstituting Mefoxin for both intravenous and intramuscular administration.

Strength	*Amount of diluent to be added (ml*)*	*Approximate final volume (ml)*	*Approximate average concentration (mg/ml)*
1 gram vial	2 (Intramuscular)	2.5	400
1 gram vial	10 (IV)	10.5	95
2 gram vial	10 or 20 (IV)	11 or 21	180 or 95

* Shake to dissolve and let stand until clear.

Compatibility and stability: A solution of Mefoxin in Water for Injections BP may be added to the following solutions: 0.9% Sodium Chloride Injection BP, 5% or 10% Dextrose Injection BP, Dextrose and Sodium Chloride Injection BP (5%/0.9%, 5%/0.45%, or 5%/0.2%). Lactated Ringer's Injection USP, 5% Dextrose Injection in 0.02% sodium bicarbonate solution, 5% Dextrose in Lactated Ringer's Injection, 5% or 10% invert sugar in water, 10% invert sugar in saline solution, 5% Sodium Bicarbonate Injection BP, M/6 Sodium Lactate Injection BP, insulin (in normal saline or 10% invert sugar), heparin (100 units/ml and 0.1 units/ml), mannitol (2.5%, 5% and 10%).

Mefoxin has been shown to be chemically and visually compatible with aminoglycosides such as amikacin, gentamicin, kanamycin, and tobramycin mixed in 200 ml of 0.9% sodium chloride or 5% dextrose in water.

Use in the elderly: The dosage should be determined by the severity of the infection, the susceptibility of the causative organisms, the patient's clinical condition and renal function.

Contra-indications, warnings, etc

Contra-indications: Mefoxin is contra-indicated in persons who have shown hypersensitivity to cefoxitin. In the absence of clinical experience, Mefoxin should not be administered to patients who have shown hypersensitivity to cephalosporins.

Precautions: There is some clinical and laboratory evidence of partial cross-allergenicity between cephamycins and other beta-lactam antibiotics, penicillins, and cephalosporins. Severe reactions (including anaphylaxis) have been reported with most beta-lactam antibiotics.

Before therapy with Mefoxin, careful inquiry should be made concerning previous hypersensitivity reactions to beta-lactam antibiotics. Mefoxin should be given cautiously to penicillin-allergic patients.

Any patient who has demonstrated some form of allergy, particularly to drugs, should receive antibiotics cautiously. If an allergic reaction to Mefoxin occurs, the drug should be discontinued.

Pseudomembranous colitis, reported with virtually all antibiotics, can range from mild to life threatening in severity. Antibiotics should be prescribed with caution in patients with a history of gastro-intestinal disease, particularly colitis. Treatment-related diarrhoea should always be considered as a pointer to this diagnosis. While studies indicate that a toxin of *Clostridium difficile* is one of the primary causes of antibiotic-related colitis, other causes should be considered.

The total daily dosage should be reduced when Mefoxin is administered to patients with transient or persistent reduction of urinary output due to renal insufficiency (see 'Dosage and administration') because high and prolonged serum antibiotic concentrations can occur from usual doses.

Interference with laboratory tests: A false-positive reaction to glucose in the urine may occur with reducing substances but not with the use of specific glucose oxidase methods.

Using the Jaffe technique, falsely high creatinine values in serum may occur if Mefoxin serum concentrations exceed 100 mcg/ml. Serum samples from patients treated with Mefoxin should not be analysed for creatinine if withdrawn within two hours of drug administration.

High concentration of cefoxitin in the urine may interfere with the measurement of 17-hydroxy-corticosteroids by the Porter-Silber reaction to give slight, falsely increased results.

Use in pregnancy: Use of the drug in women of childbearing potential requires that the anticipated benefits be weighed against possible hazards. Reproductive and teratogenic studies have been performed in mice and rats and have revealed no evidence of impaired fertility or harm to the foetus due to Mefoxin. There are no controlled studies with Mefoxin in pregnant women.

Nursing mothers: Mefoxin is excreted in human milk. Caution should be exercised if use is indicated.

Side-effects: Mefoxin is generally well tolerated. Side-effects have usually been mild and transient and treatment rarely needs to be stopped. The most common side effects have been local reactions following intravenous or intramuscular injection.

Local reactions: Thrombophlebitis has occurred with intravenous administration. Pain, induration and tenderness after intramuscular injections have been reported.

Allergic: Rash (including exfoliative dermatitis and toxic epidermal necrolysis), urticaria, pruritus, eosinophilia, fever and other allergic reactions (including anaphylaxis, interstitial nephritis and angioedema) have been reported.

Cardiovascular: Hypotension.

Gastro-intestinal: Diarrhoea, including pseudomembraneous colitis can appear during or after antibiotic treatment. Nausea and vomiting have been reported rarely.

Blood: Eosinophilia, leucopenia including granulocytopenia, neutropenia, anaemia including haemolytic anaemia, thrombocytopenia and bone-marrow depression have been reported. Some individuals, particularly those with azotaemia, may develop positive direct Coombs tests during therapy with Mefoxin.

Musculoskeletal: Worsening myasthenia gravis (single case).

Liver function: Transient elevations in AST (SGOT), ALT (SGPT), serum LDH, serum alkaline phosphatase and jaundice have been reported.

Kidney function: Elevations in serum creatinine and/or blood urea levels have been observed. Acute renal failure has been reported rarely. The role of Mefoxin in changes in renal function tests is difficult to assess, since factors predisposing to pre-renal azotaemia or to impaired renal function usually have been present.

Overdosage: No specific information is available on the treatment of overdose with Mefoxin.

After injection, cefoxitin has a half-life between 45 and 60 minutes with a 70% binding to plasma proteins.

The parenteral dose of Mefoxin is carefully controlled by the physician and no case of overdosage has been recorded. No known antidote is available.

Pharmaceutical precautions Mefoxin may be reconstituted with Water for Injections BP, Water for Injections BP preserved with parabens or benzyl alcohol, 0.9% Sodium Chloride Injection BP, 5% Dextrose Injection BP, or 0.5% and 1.0% lidocaine (lignocaine) hydrochloride (preserved in parabens). When reconstituting Mefoxin for neonates, Water for Injections must be preservative free.

Mefoxin, as reconstituted above, maintains satisfactory potency for 24 hours at room temperature, for one week under refrigeration (below 5°C) and for at least 30 weeks in the frozen state and will maintain potency after thawing for at least 24 hours at room temperature.

In keeping with good clinical and pharmaceutical practice, 'Mefoxin' should be administered as a freshly prepared solution. If circumstances make this impracticable, reconstituted material, should be used on the same day and stored at 2°C to 8°C before use.

Note: Mefoxin in the dry state should be stored below 30°C. The dry material as well as solutions tend to darken, depending on storage conditions; product potency, however, is not adversely affected.

Legal category POM.

Package quantities Sterile Mefoxin is supplied in vials containing 1 g or 2 g of cefoxitin as the sodium salt, both strengths available in packs of 5 vials.

Further information Nil.

Product licence numbers
1 g 0025/0130
2 g 0025/0131

MINTEZOL*

Presentation Orange-coloured chewable tablets, marked 'MSD 907', containing 500 mg Thiabendazole BP.

Uses Anthelmintic.

Mintezol is indicated as primary treatment against Strongyloidiasis; Cutaneous larva migrans (creeping eruption); Dracunculiasis (guinea worm); Visceral larva migrans.

Mintezol is indicated as secondary treatment against Enterobiasis (threadworm) when the infestation is mixed with a primary indication.

Mintezol can relieve the symptoms and fever of trichinosis during the invasion stage.

Mintezol is indicated (a) when specific therapy is unavailable, (b) when other therapy cannot be used or (c) as additive therapy against *Necator americanus* and *Ancylostoma duodenale* (hookworm); *Trichuriasis* (whipworm); *Ascariasis* (large roundworm).

Dosage and administration Dosage depends on the body weight of the patient and is independent of the condition being treated. Usually, 2 doses are given each day. For patients weighing less than 60 kg (132 lb), each dose is based on 25 mg thiabendazole per kg body weight. For patients weighing 60 kg or more, each dose is 1.5 g thiabendazole. The maximum daily dosage for adults weighing 60 kg or more is 3 g.

Mintezol should be taken with meals and chewed before swallowing. Dietary restrictions, complementary medications and cleansing enemas are not necessary.

The table below relates dosage to body weight:

Patient's weight		*Dose (twice daily)*
kg	*lb*	*Tablets (500 mg thiabendazole)*
10	22	½
20	44	1
30	66	1½
40	88	2
50	110	2½
60 (or more)	132 (or more)	3

Clinical experience, as well as safety experience in children weighing less than 15 kg has been limited.

Duration of therapy depends on the particular nematode infestation, and is as follows:

Strongyloidiasis, ascariasis, uncinariasis and trichuriasis: 2 doses a day for two successive days. Alternatively, a single dose of 50 mg/kg may be given, but a higher incidence of side-effects would be expected.

Cutaneous larva migrans: 2 doses a day for two successive days. If active lesions are still present two days after completion of this therapy, a second similar course is recommended.

Visceral larva migrans: 2 doses a day for 7 successive days. (Safety and efficacy data on this duration of treatment are limited.)

Trichinosis: 2 doses a day for two to four successive days, according to the response of the patient. The optimum dosage in trichinosis has not yet been established.

Dracunculiasis: 50–100 mg/kg in two equally divided doses for one day. The lower dosage for patients with 1 or 2 visible worms; the higher dosage for patients with multiple infection (3 or more worms). In massive infections (10 worms or more), a second dose of 50 mg/kg can be given five to eight days after treatment, if required.

Further considerations: In certain patients, 2 doses a day may lead to a higher incidence of side-effects. In these circumstances, 25 mg per kg body weight may be given after the largest meal on the first day and repeated 24 hours later after a similar meal on the second day.

For mass treatment, a single dose of 50 mg/kg after the evening meal is highly effective and most convenient, though a higher incidence of side-effects may be expected.

Use in the elderly: Since CNS and hepatic side effects have been reported to occur and since excretion is primarily renal, use with caution in elderly patients who have renal, hepatic or CNS dysfunction. As with younger patients, the dosage should be calculated on the basis of body weight.

Use in children: Clinical experience, as well as safety experience with thiabendazole treatment in children weighing less than 15 kg has been limited.

Contra-indications, warnings, etc

Contra-indication: Hypersensitivity to any component of this product.

Precautions: If any hypersensitivity reactions occur, therapy should be discontinued immediately and not resumed. Erythema multiforme, including fatal cases of Stevens-Johnson syndrome, has been associated with thiabendazole therapy.

Mintezol may impair alertness in some patients, who should avoid driving, operating machinery, or other activities made hazardous by diminished alertness.

Ideally, anaemic, dehydrated or malnourished patients should be given supportive therapy before starting treatment with Mintezol. Liver and renal function should be carefully monitored in patients with disorders of these organs.

Mintezol is not suitable for the treatment of mixed infections with ascaris because it may cause these worms to migrate.

Mintezol should not be used prophylactically.

Pregnancy and the nursing mother: Mintezol should

not be used during pregnancy or lactation. Reports have suggested that thiabendazole is teratogenic in mice, although reproduction studies in generations of rabbits, rats, sheep, cattle and pigs have shown no fetal abnormalities attributable to the drug. Nevertheless, Mintezol should not be used in women of childbearing potential unless pregnancy has been excluded.

Drug interactions: Thiabendazole may compete with other drugs, such as theophylline, for sites of metabolism in the liver and thus elevate the serum levels of such drugs to potentially toxic levels. Therefore, when the concomitant use of thiabendazole and xanthine derivatives is anticipated, it may be necessary to monitor blood levels and/or reduce the dosage of such compounds. Such concomitant use should only be made under careful medical supervision.

Side-effects: The most common are anorexia, nausea, vomiting and dizziness. Diarrhoea, epigastric distress, pruritus, weariness, giddiness, headache and drowsiness occur less often.

Rare side-effects are tinnitus, collapse, abnormal sensation in the eyes, blurring of vision, reduced vision, hyperirritability, numbness, hyperglycaemia, yellow vision (in isolated cases these ocular effects persisted for prolonged intervals), enuresis, hypotension, jaundice, transient leucopenia, perianal rash, crystalluria, haematuria, convulsions, psychic disturbances, drying of mucous membranes (mouth, eyes etc.), intrahepatic cholestasis and parenchymal liver damage (in isolated cases liver damage has been severe and irreversible). The appearance of live ascaris in the mouth and nose has been reported on rare occasions.

Hypersensitivity reactions include fever, facial flush, chills, conjunctival injection, angioneurotic oedema, anaphylaxis, skin rashes, erythema multiforme including Stevens-Johnson syndrome, and lymphadenopathy.

Some patients excrete a metabolite which imparts a characteristic odour to their urine, similar to that which occurs after eating asparagus.

Laboratory test findings: Rarely a transient rise in cephalin flocculation and aspartate transferase (AST) has occurred in patients receiving Mintezol.

Overdosage: The stomach should be emptied promptly either by inducing emesis, if necessary, or by gastric lavage. Toxic disturbances of the GI and CNS systems can be expected and these should be treated symptomatically and supportively. There is no known antidote.

Thiabendazole is readily absorbed from the GI tract with a peak plasma level reached in 1 to 2 hours.

Pharmaceutical precautions Store in a dry place below 25°C. Protect from light.

Legal category POM.

Package quantities *Tablets:* Packs of 6.

Further information Nil.

Product licence number 0025/5031R.

MODUCREN*

Presentation Blue, square, half-scored tablets, marked 'MSD 17', containing 25 mg hydrochlorothiazide, 2.5 mg amiloride hydrochloride, and 10 mg timolol maleate.

Uses Mild to moderate hypertension.

Dosage and administration 1 to 2 tablets once a day.

Use in the elderly: Moducren has been shown to be as well tolerated in the elderly as in younger patients. The recommended starting dose is one tablet daily.

Children: Because the safety and efficacy of Moducren has not been established in children, it is not recommended for paediatric use.

Contra-indications, warnings, etc

Contra-indications: Patients with bronchial asthma or with a history of bronchial asthma, severe chronic obstructive pulmonary disease, sinus bradycardia, second- or third-degree AV block, overt cardiac failure, right ventricular failure secondary to pulmonary hypertension, significant cardiomegaly, and cardiogenic shock. Hyperkalaemia (plasma potassium over 5.5 mmol/l). Anuria, acute and chronic renal insufficiency, severe progressive renal disease and diabetic nephropathy. Patients with blood urea over 10 mmol/l or serum creatinine over 130 mmol/l or diabetes mellitus should not receive Moducren without careful and frequent serum urea and serum electrolyte monitoring.

Anaesthetic agents causing myocardial depression, hypersensitivity to any component of Moducren or other sulphonamide-derived drugs. Use with other potassium-conserving agents. Use with potassium supplements or potassium-rich food except in severe and/or refractory cases of hypokalaemia when careful monitoring of the serum potassium level is necessary.

See also 'Pregnancy', 'Breast-feeding mothers' and 'Children', under 'precautions'.

Precautions:

Congestive cardiac failure: care should be exercised before and during treatment of patients with cardiomegaly or history of cardiac failure. *Cardiac arrhythmias:* patients at risk of congestive heart failure should be carefully observed for bradycardia, AV block and respiratory distress. If congestive cardiac failure persists, Moducren should be withdrawn. Beta-adrenergic blocking agents should be used with caution in patients with cerebrovascular insufficiency. If signs or symptoms suggesting reduced cerebral blood flow are observed, consideration should be given to discontinuing these agents. *Exacerbation of ischaemic heart disease following abrupt withdrawal:* Exacerbation of angina and, in some cases, myocardial infarction have occurred after abrupt withdrawal of beta-blocker therapy. Therefore, it is recommended that if Moducren is to be withdrawn, dosage should be gradually reduced. *Elective or emergency surgery:* Moducren should also be gradually withdrawn prior to elective surgery of anginal patients. Agonists such as isoprenaline, dopamine, dobutamine or noradrenaline may be used to counter the effects of beta-blockade in emergency surgery. *Renal and hepatic disease and electrolyte disturbances:* Moducren should be used with caution in patients with renal or hepatic disease and in those patients in whom fluid and electrolyte balance is critical. When creatinine clearance falls below 30 ml/min, thiazide diuretics are ineffective. Azotaemia may be precipitated or increased by hydrochlorothiazide. Cumulative effects of the drug may develop in patients with impaired renal function. If increasing azotaemia and oliguria occur during treatment of renal disease, the diuretic should be discontinued. *Metabolic or respiratory acidosis:* acid-base balance should be monitored frequently in severely ill patients at risk of respiratory or metabolic acidosis. *Electrolyte and fluid balance:* serum and urine electrolyte determinations should be made in patients vomiting excessively or receiving parenteral fluids. Dilutional hyponatraemia may occur in oedematous patients in hot weather which calls for appropriate therapy; hypochloraemia requires specific treatment only under exceptional circumstances. Hyponatraemia, hypochloraemic alkalosis, hypokalaemia, hyperkalaemia or hypomagnesaemia may occur. If hyperkalaemia occurs, Moducren should be discontinued immediately and, if necessary, active measures taken to reduce the plasma potassium level. The degree of thiazide-induced hypomagnesaemia is reduced. *Diabetes mellitus, hypoglycaemia:* Moducren should be given with caution to diabetic patients and to patients subject to spontaneous hypoglycaemia as the symptoms and signs of acute hypoglycaemia may be masked. To minimise the risk of hyperkalaemia in diabetic or suspected diabetic patients, the status of renal function should be known before initiating therapy with Moducren. Therapy should be discontinued for at least three days prior to glucose tolerance testing. Thiazide therapy may impair glucose tolerance. Dosage adjustment of antidiabetic agents, including insulin, may be required. *Skin and sensitivity reactions:* there have been reports of skin rashes and/or dry eyes associated with the use of beta-adrenergic blocking drugs. The reported incidence is small and in most cases the symptoms have cleared when treatment was withdrawn. Discontinuation of the drug should be considered if any such reaction is not otherwise explicable. Withdrawal should be gradual. Sensitivity reactions to Moducren may occur with or without a history of allergy or bronchial asthma. Possible exacerbation or activation of systemic lupus erythematosus reactions have been reported with thiazide diuretics. *Metabolic and endocrine:* beta-adrenergic blocking agents may mask the signs of hyperthyroidism. Patients suspected of developing thyrotoxicosis should be managed carefully to avoid abrupt withdrawal of beta blockade which might precipitate a thyroid storm. Hypercalcaemia and hypophosphataemia have also been reported with thiazide diuretics. Moducren should be discontinued in patients prior to testing for parathyroid function. Increases in cholesterol and triglyceride levels may be associated with thiazide diuretic therapy. Hyperuricaemia or acute gout may be precipitated in some patients. *Musculoskeletal:* beta-blockers have been reported to induce myasthenic symptoms such as diplopia, ptosis, and generalised weakness.

Drug interactions: Moducren may potentiate other antihypertensive agents, such as reserpine or guanethidine. The antihypertensive effect of beta-blockers may be reduced by NSAIDs. NSAIDs may reduce the diuretic, natriuretic and antihypertensive effects of diuretics. Its effect may be enhanced in the post-sympathectomy patient.

Oral calcium antagonists may be combined with Moducren only when heart function is normal. When the heart function is impaired, combination of beta-blockers with dihydropyridine derivatives such as nifedipine may lead to hypotension; and combination with verapamil or diltiazem may cause AV conduction disturbances or left ventricular failure. Intravenous calcium antagonists and Moducren should only be used together with caution. Concomitant beta-blockers and digitalis with either diltiazem or verapamil may further prolong the AV conduction time.

When Moducren (which contains amiloride HCl) is administered concomitantly with an angiotensin-converting enzyme inhibitor, the risk of hyperkalaemia may be increased. Therefore, if concomitant use of these agents is indicated because of demonstrated hypokalaemia, they should be used with caution and with frequent monitoring of serum potassium.

When given concomitantly, the following drugs may interact with thiazide diuretics.

Alcohol, barbiturates, or narcotics: Co-administration may potentiate orthostatic hypotension. *Oral and parenteral antidiabetic drugs* may require adjustment of dosage with concurrent use.

Corticosteroids or ACTH may intensify any thiazide-induced electrolyte depletion, particularly hypokalaemia. *Pressor amines such as adrenaline* may show decreased arterial responsiveness when used with Moducren, but this reaction is not enough to preclude their therapeutic usefulness. *Non-depolarising muscle relaxants such as tubocurarine* may possibly interact with Moducren to increase muscle relaxation. *Lithium* should not generally be given with diuretics, because they reduce its renal clearance and add a high risk of lithium toxicity. *Drug/laboratory test interactions:* because thiazides may affect calcium metabolism, Moducren may interfere with tests for parathyroid function (see 'Precautions').

Breast-feeding mothers: Thiazides appear in breast milk, but it is not known whether timolol maleate or amiloride are also excreted. If the use of Moducren is deemed essential, the mother should stop breast-feeding.

Pregnancy: Moducren is not recommended for use during pregnancy. The use of any drug in women of child-bearing age requires that the anticipated benefit be weighed against possible hazards, which include fetal or neonatal jaundice, thrombocytopenia, and possibly other adverse reactions which have occurred in the adult.

Side effects: Moducren is usually well tolerated with significant side effects only infrequently reported.

Most common side-effects are dizziness, asthenia, fatigue, and bradycardia. Other clinical adverse reactions are: *Body as a whole:* Asthenia, fatigue, headache. *Cardiovascular:* Bradycardia, peripheral vascular disorder (cold extremities), hypotension, syncope, arrhythmia, angina pectoris. *Respiratory:* Dyspnoea, wheezing. *Digestive:* Nausea, dyspepsia, constipation, diarrhoea, vomiting, GI pain, anorexia, thirst, dry mouth, stomatitis. *Urogenital:* Impotence. *Nervous:* Dizziness, vertigo, paraesthesiae, tremors. *Integumentary:* Sweating. *Musculoskeletal:* Muscle cramps. *Psychiatric:* Insomnia, nervousness, depression, somnolence, abnormal dreaming, sleep disturbance. *Special senses:* Visual disturbances.

Side-effects that have been reported with the individual components may be considered as potential adverse effects of Moducren.

Amiloride-related effects

Digestive: abnormal liver function, activation of probable pre-existing peptic ulcer, jaundice. *Integumentary:* dry mouth, alopecia. *Haematological:* aplastic anaemia, neutropenia. *Cardiovascular:* one patient with partial heart block developed complete heart block, palpitation. *Psychiatric:* decreased libido. *Respiratory:* cough. *Special senses:* tinnitus, increased intra-ocular pressure. *Urogenital:* polyuria, urinary frequency, bladder spasm.

Hydrochlorothiazide-related effects

Body as a whole: Anaphylactic reaction, fever. *Cardiovascular:* Necrotising angiitis (vasculitis, cutaneous vasculitis). *Digestive:* Jaundice (intrahepatic cholestatic jaundice), pancreatitis, cramping, gastric irritation. *Integumentary:* Photosensitivity. *Endocrine/metabolic:* Glycosuria, hypoglycaemia, hyperglycaemia, hyperuricaemia, sialadenitis, urticaria. *Psychiatric:* Restlessness. *Renal:* Renal dysfunction, interstitial nephritis, renal failure. *Respiratory:* Respiratory distresses including pneumonitis, pulmonary oedema. *Special senses:* Transient blurred vision, xanthopsia. *Haematological:* Agranulocytosis, aplastic anaemia, haemolytic anaemia, leucopenia, purpura, thrombocytopenia.

Timolol maleate-related effects.

Body as a whole: chest pain, extremity pain, decreased exercise tolerance, weight loss. *Cardiovascular:* cardiac arrest, cerebral vascular accident, palpitation, second- or third-degree AV block, sino-atrial block, oedema and pulmonary oedema, cardiac failure, Raynaud's phenomenon, claudication, worsening of arterial insufficiency and angina pectoris, vasodilatation. *Digestive:* diarrhoea, hepatomegaly. *Endocrine:* hypoglycaemia, hyperglycaemia. *Integumentary:* rash, pruritus, skin irritation, increased pigmentation, exfoliative dermatitis (one case). *Musculoskeletal:* arthralgia. *Nervous system:* local weakness. *Psychiatric:* diminished concentration, hallucinations, decreased libido. *Haematological:* non-thrombocytopenic purpura. *Respiratory:* bronchial spasm, rales, cough. *Special senses:* tinnitus, visual disturbances, diplopia, ptosis, eye irritation, dry eyes. *Urogenital:* micturition difficulties.

Clinical laboratory tests: Clinically important changes in standard laboratory tests associated with timolol maleate are rare. Slight increases in blood urea, serum potassium and serum uric acid, and slight decreases in haemoglobin and haematocrit occurred but were not progressive or associated with clinical manifestations.

Overdosage: No specific data are available regarding symptoms or the treatment of overdosage with Moducren and no antidote is available. Little is known about dialysability of its components; a study of patients with renal failure showed that timolol did not readily dialyse. Treatment is symptomatic and supportive.

Therapy with Moducren should be stopped and emesis and/or gastric lavage induced.

Hydrochlorothiazide and amiloride hydrochloride: The signs and symptoms most likely are dehydration and electrolyte imbalance. If hyperkalaemia occurs, active measures should be taken to reduce plasma potassium levels.

Timolol maleate: The most common signs and symptoms to be expected following overdosage with a beta-blocker are symptomatic bradycardia, hypotension, bronchospasm, acute cardiac failure, and heart block.

If overdosage occurs, the following measures are recommended:

1. *Gastric lavage*
2. *For symptomatic bradycardia:* Atropine sulphate, 0.25 to 2 mg intravenously, should be used to induce vagal blockade. If bradycardia persists, intravenous isoprenaline hydrochloride should be administered cautiously. In refractory cases, the use of a transvenous cardiac pacemaker may be considered.
3. *For hypotension:* A sympathomimetic pressor agent such as dopamine, dobutamine or noradrenaline should be used. In refractory cases, the use of glucagon has been reported to be useful.
4. *For bronchospasm:* Isoprenaline hydrochloride should be used. Additional therapy with aminophylline may be considered.
5. *For acute cardiac failure:* Conventional therapy with digitalis, diuretics, and oxygen should be instituted immediately. In refractory cases, the use of intravenous aminophylline is suggested. This may be followed, if necessary, by glucagon which has been reported useful.
6. *For heart block:* Isoprenaline hydrochloride or a transvenous cardiac pacemaker should be used.

The components of Moducren have, respectively, plasma half-lives of: Hydrochlorothiazide at 5.6 hours with a longer terminal phase; amiloride at about 6–9.5 hours; and timolol at about four hours.

Pharmaceutical precautions Store in a dry place below 25°C, protected from light.

Legal category POM.

Package quantities Calendar packs of 28 tablets.

Further information The combination of amiloride with hydrochlorothiazide has been shown to cause less magnesium excretion than either the thiazides or loop diuretics alone.

Similar dosage schedules and similar bioavailability rationalise the combination of hydrochlorothiazide (a saluretic), timolol maleate (a beta-adrenergic receptor blocking agent), and amiloride hydrochloride (a potassium-conserving agent) for the treatment of hypertension.

Product licence number 0025/0141.

PEPCID*

Presentation Brown, round-cornered square tablets, marked 'PEPCID' on one face with '40' on the other, containing 40 mg famotidine.

Beige, round-cornered square tablets, marked 'PEPCID' on one face with '20' on the other, containing 20 mg famotidine.

Uses
Indications: Duodenal ulcer.

Prevention of relapses of duodenal ulceration.

Benign gastric ulcer.

Hypersecretory conditions such as Zollinger-Ellison syndrome.

Treatment of gastro-oesophageal reflux disease.

Prevention of relapse of symptoms and erosions or ulcerations associated with gastro-oesophageal reflux disease.

Mode of action: Pepcid is a highly specific and potent competitive H_2-receptor antagonist. It has a rapid onset of action. Although the plasma half-life of famotidine in patients is approximately 3.0 hours, Pepcid has a long duration of action, and a single 40 mg dose has been shown to reduce gastric acid secretion for at least 10 hours.

Pepcid reduces the acid and pepsin content, as well as the volume of basal, nocturnal and stimulated gastric secretion.

Dosage and administration It is unnecessary to time the dose in relation to meals; bioavailability is not clinically affected by food in the stomach. In all cases the clinical response of the patient should be taken into consideration

In benign gastric and duodenal ulceration, the dose of Pepcid is one 40 mg tablet at night.

Duodenal ulcer: The recommended initial dose is one 40 mg tablet of Pepcid at night. Treatment should continue for four to eight weeks. In most patients, healing occurs on this regimen within four weeks. In those patients whose ulcers have not healed completely after four weeks, a further four-week period of treatment is recommended.

Maintenance therapy: For preventing the recurrence of duodenal ulceration, the reduced dose of 20 mg of Pepcid at night is recommended. This 20 mg maintenance dose has been continued effectively in clinical studies of 12 months duration.

Benign gastric ulcer: The recommended dose is one 40 mg tablet of Pepcid at night. Treatment should continue for four to eight weeks unless endoscopy reveals earlier healing.

Zollinger-Ellison syndrome: Patients without prior antisecretory therapy should be started on 20 mg of Pepcid every six hours. Dosage should then be adjusted to individual response: doses up to 800 mg daily have been used up to one year without the development of significant adverse effects or tachyphylaxis. Patients who have been receiving another H_2 antagonist may be switched directly to Pepcid at a dose higher than that recommended for new cases. This starting dose will depend on the severity of the condition and the last dose of H_2 antagonist previously used.

Gastro-oesophageal reflux disease: The recommended dosage for the symptomatic relief of gastro-oesophageal reflux disease is 20 mg of famotidine twice daily, which may be given for six to twelve weeks. Most patients experience improvement after two weeks.

Where gastro-oesophageal reflux disease is associated with the presence of oesophageal erosion or ulceration, the recommended dosage is 40 mg of famotidine, twice daily, which may be given for six to twelve weeks.

Maintenance therapy: For the prevention of recurrence of symptoms and erosions or ulcerations associated with gastro-oesophageal reflux disease, the recommended dosage is 20 mg of famotidine twice daily.

Use in the elderly: The recommended dosage in most elderly patients is the same as in younger patients for all indications (see above). No change in the incidence or type of drug-related side-effects were seen in treated elderly patients.

Use in impaired renal function: Since Pepcid is excreted primarily by the kidney, caution should be observed in patients with impaired renal function. The dose should be reduced to 20 mg *nocte* if creatinine clearance falls below 10 ml/min.

Paediatric use: The efficacy and safety of Pepcid in children have not been established.

Contra-indications, warnings, etc
Contra-indications: Hypersensitivity to any component of this product.

Precautions
Gastric carcinoma: Gastric malignancy should be excluded prior to initiation of therapy of gastric ulcer with Pepcid. Symptomatic response of gastric ulcer to therapy with Pepcid does not preclude the presence of gastric malignancy.

Impaired renal function: Since Pepcid is primarily excreted via the kidney, caution should be exercised when treating patients with impaired renal function.

The dose should be reduced to 20 mg *nocte* when creatinine clearance falls below 10 ml/min.

Pregnancy: Pepcid is not recommended for use in pregnancy, and should be prescribed only if clearly needed. Before a decision is made to use Pepcid during pregnancy, the physician should weigh the potential benefits from the drug against the possible risks involved.

Breast-feeding mothers: Pepcid is secreted in human milk, therefore breast-feeding mothers should either stop breast-feeding or stop taking the drug.

Drug interactions: No clinically important drug interactions have been identified. Pepcid does not interact with the cytochrome P450-linked drug metabolising enzyme system. Compounds metabolised by this system which have been tested in man have included warfarin, theophylline, phenytoin, diazepam, propranolol, aminopyrine and phenazone. Indocyanine green as an index of hepatic blood flow and/or hepatic drug extraction has been tested and no significant effects have been found.

Side-effects: In controlled studies, Pepcid has been shown to be generally well tolerated.

Headache, dizziness, constipation, and diarrhoea have been reported rarely. Other side effects reported even less frequently included dry mouth, nausea and/or vomiting, abdominal discomfort or distension, anorexia, fatigue, rash, pruritus and urticaria, liver enzyme abnormalities, cholestatic jaundice, anaphylaxis, angioedema, arthralgia, muscle cramps, reversible psychic disturbances including depression, anxiety disorders, agitation, confusion and hallucinations. Toxic epidermal necrolysis has been reported very rarely with H_2-receptor antagonists. Pancytopenia, leucopenia, and isolated cases of worsening of existing hepatic disease have been reported; however, a causal relationship to therapy with Pepcid has not been established. No clinically significant increase in endocrine or gonadal function has been reported.

Gynaecomastia has been reported rarely. In most cases that were followed up, it was reversible on discontinuing treatment.

Overdosage: There is no experience to date with overdosage.

The usual measures to remove unabsorbed material from the gastro-intestinal tract, clinical monitoring, and supportive therapy only should be employed.

Patients with Zollinger-Ellison syndrome have tolerated a dosage of 800 mg daily for more than a year without the development of significant adverse effects.

Pharmaceutical precautions Store in a dry place below 25°C.

Legal category POM.

Package quantities Calendar packs of 28 tablets.

Further information Pepcid is a chemically novel competitive H_2-receptor antagonist with a guanidinothiazole ring. Pepcid is rapidly absorbed, with dose-related peak plasma concentrations reached in one to three hours. When used as recommended, there was no accumulation effect with repeated doses.

In clinical studies, a single dose of Pepcid at night relieved the pain associated with peptic ulcer, usually within a week, and suppressed gastric secretion.

Studies in animals and human volunteers have not shown anti-androgenic effects.

Product licence numbers
20 mg tablets 0025/0215
40 mg tablets 0025/0216

PERIACTIN*

Presentation White, half-scored tablets, marked 'MSD 62', containing Cyproheptadine Hydrochloride PhEur equivalent to 4 mg anhydrous cyproheptadine hydrochloride.

Uses Periactin is a serotonin and histamine antagonist with anticholinergic and sedative properties.

In allergy and pruritus: Periactin has a wide range of anti-allergic and antipruritic activity, and can be used successfully in treatment of acute and chronic allergic and pruritic conditions, such as: dermatitis, including neurodermatitis and neurodermatitis circumscripta; eczema; eczematoid dermatitis; dermatographism; mild, local allergic reactions to insect bites; hay fever and other seasonal rhinitis; perennial allergic and vasomotor rhinitis; allergic conjunctivitis due to inhalant allergens and foods; urticaria; angioneurotic oedema; drug and serum reactions; anogenital pruritus; pruritus of chickenpox.

Periactin is indicated as adjunctive therapy to adrenaline and other standard measures for the relief of anaphylactic reactions after the acute manifestations have been controlled.

In migraine headache: Periactin has been reported to have beneficial effects in a significant number of patients having vascular types of headache. Many patients who have responded inadequately to all other agents have reported amelioration of symptoms with Periactin. The characteristic headache and feeling of malaise may disappear within an hour or two of the first dose.

Dosage and administration There is no recommended dosage for children under 2 years old.

Periactin is not recommended for elderly debilitated patients.

In allergy and pruritus: Dosage must be determined on an individual basis. The effect of a single dose usually lasts for four to six hours. For continuous effective relief, the daily requirement should be given in divided doses, usually three times a day, or as often as necessary, to provide continuous relief.

Adults: The therapeutic range is 4–20 mg a day, most patients requiring 12–16 mg a day. It is recommended that dosage be initiated with 4 mg three times a day and then adjusted according to the weight and response of the patient.

Maximum: 32 mg a day.

Children aged 7–14 years: Usually 4 mg two or three times a day, according to the patient's weight and response. If an additional dose is required it should be given at bedtime. Maximum 16 mg a day.

Children aged 2–6 years: Initially 2 mg two or three times a day, adjusted according to the patient's weight and response. If an additional dose is required it should be given at bedtime. Maximum 12 mg a day.

In vascular headache and migraine: For both prophylactic and therapeutic use at an initial dose of 4 mg repeated if necessary after half an hour. Patients who respond usually obtain relief with 8 mg, and this dose should not be exceeded within a 4- to 6-hour period.

Maintenance: 4 mg every four to six hours.

Use in the elderly: Periactin should not be used in elderly, debilitated patients. Elderly patients are more likely to experience dizziness, sedation, and hypotension.

Contra-indications, warnings, etc
Contra-indications: Therapy of an acute asthmatic attack; newborn or premature infants; breast-feeding mothers; known sensitivity to cyproheptadine hydrochloride or drugs with similar chemical structure; concurrent use with monoamine oxidase inhibitors; glaucoma; stenosing peptic ulcer; symptomatic prostatic hypertrophy; bladder neck obstruction; pyloroduodenal obstruction; elderly, debilitated patients; predisposition to urinary retention.

Precautions: Antihistamines should not be used to treat lower respiratory tract symptoms including those of acute asthma.

The safety and efficacy of Periactin is not established in children under 2 years old.

Antihistamines may diminish mental alertness; conversely, particularly in the young child, they may occasionally produce excitation.

Patients should be warned against engaging in activities requiring motor co-ordination and mental alertness such as driving a car or operating machinery.

Rarely, prolonged therapy with antihistamines may cause blood dyscrasias.

Because Periactin has an atropine-like action, it should be used cautiously in patients with a history of bronchial asthma, increased intra-ocular pressure, hyperthyroidism, cardiovascular disease, or hypertension.

Drug interactions: MAO inhibitors prolong and intensify the anticholinergic effects of antihistamines.

Antihistamines may have additive effects with alcohol and other CNS depressants, e.g. hypnotics, sedatives, tranquillisers and anti-anxiety agents.

Pregnancy and breast-feeding mothers: The use of any drug in pregnancy or in women of child-bearing age requires that the potential benefit of the drug should be weighed against possible hazards to the embryo or fetus. It is not known whether Periactin is excreted in human milk, and because of the potential for serious adverse reactions in breast-feeding infants from Periactin, a decision should be made whether to discontinue breast-feeding or to discontinue the drug, taking into account the importance of the drug to the mother (see 'Contra-indications').

Side-effects: The side-effects that appear frequently are drowsiness and somnolence. Many patients who initially complain of drowsiness may no longer do so after the first three to four days of continuous administration. Side-effects reported with antihistamines are:

Central nervous system: Sedation, sleepiness (often transient), dizziness, disturbed co-ordination, confusion, restlessness, excitation, nervousness, tremor, irritability, insomnia, parasthesiae, neuritis, convulsions, euphoria, hallucinations, hysteria, faintness.

Integumentary: Allergic manifestations of rash and oedema, excessive perspiration, urticaria, photosensitivity.

Special senses: Acute labyrinthitis, blurred vision, diplopia, vertigo, tinnitus.

Cardiovascular: Hypotension, palpitation, tachycardia, extrasystoles, anaphylactic shock.

Haematological: Haemolytic anaemia, leucopenia, agranulocytosis, thrombocytopenia.

Digestive system: Dryness of mouth, epigastric distress, anorexia, nausea, vomiting, diarrhoea, constipation, jaundice.

Genito-urinary: Frequency and difficulty of micturition, urinary retention, early menses.

Respiratory: Dryness of the nose and throat, thickening of bronchial secretions, tightness of chest and wheezing, nasal stuffiness.

Miscellaneous: Fatigue, rigors, headache.

Overdosage: Antihistamine overdosage may vary from CNS depression or stimulation to convulsions and death, especially in infants and children. Atropine-like and GI symptoms may occur.

If vomiting has not occurred spontaneously, it should be induced in the conscious patient with syrup of ipecac. If the patient cannot vomit, gastric lavage with isotonic or half isotonic saline is indicated followed by activated charcoal. Precautions against aspiration must be taken, especially in infants and children.

Life-threatening CNS signs and symptoms should be treated appropriately.

Saline cathartics usefully draw water into the bowel by osmosis to dilute bowel content rapidly.

Central stimulants must not be used, but vasopressors may be used to counteract hypotension.

Pharmaceutical precautions Periactin should be stored below 25°C, protected from light.

Legal category P.

Package quantities Packs of 30 tablets.

Further information Nil.

Product licence number 0025/5017.

PRIMAXIN*

Presentation
For intravenous infusion: Vials containing sterile powders of:

250 mg imipenem (as the monohydrate) with 250 mg cilastatin (as the sodium salt) named Primaxin IV 250 mg.

500 mg imipenem (as the monohydrate) with 500 mg cilastatin (as the sodium salt) named Primaxin IV 500 mg.

Monovial presentation: A monovial of 500 mg imipenem (as the monohydrate) with 500 mg cilastatin (as the sodium salt), named 'Primaxin' IV 500 mg Monovial. The monovial has a built-in transfer needle to allow constitution of the product directly into an infusion bag.

For intramuscular administration: Vials containing sterile powders of:

500 mg imipenem (as the monohydrate) with 500 mg cilastatin (as the sodium salt), named Primaxin IM 500 mg.

Uses Broad-spectrum beta-lactam antibiotic.

Primaxin contains imipenem, a member of a new class of beta-lactam antibiotics – the thienamycins; and cilastatin sodium, a specific enzyme-inhibitor, that blocks the metabolism of imipenem in the kidney and substantially increases the concentration of unchanged imipenem in the urinary tract.

Primaxin is bactericidal against an unusually wide-spectrum of Gram-positive, Gram-negative, aerobic and anaerobic pathogens. Primaxin is useful for treating single, and polymicrobic infections, and initiating therapy prior to identification of the causative organisms.

Primaxin is indicated for the treatment of the following infections due to susceptible organisms:

Primaxin IV	*Primaxin IM*
Lower respiratory tract infections	Lower respiratory tract infections (except those caused by *Pseudomonas aeruginosa)*
Intra-abdominal infections	Intra-abdominal infections
Genito-urinary infections	Genito-urinary infections
Gynaecological infections	Gynaecological infections
Septicaemia	Not indicated
Bone and joint infections	Bone and joint infections (there is limited experience in patients with these infections)
Skin and soft tissue infections	Skin and soft tissue infections

Note: Primaxin is not indicated against central nervous system infections.

Primaxin is indicated against mixed infections caused by susceptible aerobic and anaerobic bacteria. The majority of these infections are associated with contamination by faecal flora, or flora originating from the vagina, skin, and mouth. In these mixed infections, Primaxin is usually effective against *Bacteroides fragilis* sp., the most commonly encountered anaerobic pathogen, that is usually resistant to the aminoglycosides, cephalosporins and penicillins.

Prophylaxis: Primaxin IV is also indicated for the prevention of certain post-operative infections in patients undergoing contaminated or potentially contaminated surgical procedures or where the occurrence of post-operative infection could be especially serious.

Mode of action: Imipenem is a potent inhibitor of bacterial cell wall synthesis and is highly reactive towards penicillin-binding protein. Imipenem is more potent in its bactericidal effect than other antibiotics studied. Imipenem also provides excellent stability to degradative bacterial beta-lactamases. Imipenem is therefore active against a high percentage of organisms resistant to other beta-lactam antibiotics.

Cilastatin sodium is a competitive, reversible, and specific inhibitor of dehydropeptidase-I, the renal enzyme which metabolises and inactivates imipenem. Cilastatin sodium is devoid of intrinsic antibacterial activity itself and does not affect the antibacterial activity of imipenem.

Bacteriology: Primaxin has a unique anti-bacterial spectrum. Against Gram-negative species, it shares the spectrum of the newer cephalosporins and penicillins; against Gram-positive species Primaxin exerts the high bacterial potency previously only associated with narrow-spectrum beta-lactam antibiotics and the first-generation cephalosporins.

The antibiotic spectrum of Primaxin is broader than other antibiotics studied and includes virtually all clinically significant pathogenic genera.

Organisms against which Primaxin is usually active *in vitro* include:

Gram-negative aerobes: *Escherichia coli; Proteus mirabilis; Proteus vulgaris; Proteus* spp.; *Morganella morganii* (formerly *Proteus morganii*); *Providencia rettgeri* (formerly *Proteus rettgeri*); *Providencia stuartii; Providencia* spp; *Hafnia alvei; Serratia marcescens; Serratia liquefaciens; Serratia* spp.; *Klebsiella oxytoca; Klebsiella pneumoniae; Klebsiella* spp.; *Enterobacter aerogenes; Enterobacter agglomerans; Enterobacter cloacae; Enterobacter* spp.; *Citrobacter freundii; Citrobacter diversus; Citrobacter* spp.; *Campylobacter* spp.; *Salmonella typhi; Salmonella* spp.; *Shigella* spp.; *Pseudomonas aeruginosa; Pseudomonas fluorescens; Pseudomonas* spp.†; *Acinetobacter* spp. (formerly *Mima-Herellea*); *Haemophilus influenzae* (including beta-lactamase-producing strains); *Haemophilus parainfluenzae; Neisseria gonorrhoeae* (including penicillinase-producing strains); *Moraxella* spp.; *Pasteurella multocida; Aeromonas hydrophila; Yersinia* spp. (formerly *Pasteurella*); *Yersinia enterocolitica; Achromobacter* spp.; *Gardnerella* spp.

†*Xanthomonas maltophilia* and some strains of *Pseudomonas cepacia* are generally not sensitive to Primaxin.

Gram-positive aerobes: Streptococcus Group A (*S. pyogenes*); Streptococcus Group B (*S. agalactiae*); Streptococcus Group C; Enterococcus including *Enterococcus faecalis*; Streptococcus Group D; Streptococcus Group G; *Streptococcus pneumoniae; Viridans streptococci* (including alpha and gamma haemolytic strains); *Staphylococcus aureus* (including penicillinase-producing strains); *Staphylococcus epidermidis* (including penicillinase-producing strains); *Erysipelothrix rhusiopathiae.*

Some methicillin-resistant staphylococci and some group D streptococci are not sensitive to Primaxin.

Microaerophilic streptococcus

Gram-negative anaerobes: *Bacteroides fragilis; Bacteroides vulgatus; Bacteroides melaninogenicus; Bacteroides asaccharolyticus; Bacteroides distasonis; Bacteroides ovatus; Bacteroides thetaiotaomicron; Bacteroides* spp.; *Fusobacterium nucleatum; Fusobacterium necrophorum; Fusobacterium* spp.; *Veillonella* spp.

Gram-positive anaerobes: *Actinomyces* spp.; *Clostridium perfringens; Clostridium* spp.; *Eubacterium* spp.; *Peptococcus* spp.; *Peptostreptococcus* spp.; *Propionibacterium* spp. including *P. acnes.*

In vitro tests show that imipenem acts synergistically with aminoglycoside antibiotics against some isolates of *Pseudomonas aeruginosa.*

Dosage and administration The total daily dosage and route of administration of Primaxin should be based on the type or severity of infection, consideration of degree of susceptibility of the pathogen(s), renal function and bodyweight. Doses cited are based on a bodyweight of 70 kg. The total daily requirement should be given in equally divided doses.

The dosage recommendations that follow specify the amounts of imipenem to be given. An equivalent amount of cilastatin is provided with this. One vial of Primaxin IV 250 mg therefore provides the equivalents of 250 mg anhydrous imipenem and 250 mg cilastatin;

similarly one vial of Primaxin IV or IM 500 mg, provides the equivalents of 500 mg anhydrous imipenem and 500 mg cilastatin.

Use in the elderly: Age does not usually affect the tolerability and efficacy of Primaxin. The dosage should be determined by the severity of the infection, the susceptibility of the causative organism(s), the patient's clinical condition, and renal function.

INTRAVENOUS ADMINISTRATION: This formulation should not be used intramuscularly. The dosage of Primaxin IV should be determined by the severity of the infection, the antibiotic susceptibility of the causative organism(s) and the condition of the patient.

Note: All recommended doses refer to the imipenem fraction of Primaxin.

Adults (based on 70 kg bodyweight): The usual adult daily dosage is 1–2 g of Primaxin administered in 3–4 equally divided doses (see chart below). In infections due to less sensitive organisms, the daily dose of Primaxin may be increased to a maximum dose of 50 mg/kg/day (or not exceeding 4 g daily).

Usual adult intravenous dosage

Each 250 mg or 500 mg dose should be given by intravenous infusion over 20–30 minutes. Each 1000 mg dose should be infused over 40–60 minutes. In patients who develop nausea during infusion, the infusion rate may be slowed.

Severity of infection	*I.V. administration*		
	Dose	*Dosage interval*	*Total daily dose*
Mild	250 mg	6 hours	1.0 g
Moderate	500 mg	8 hours	1.5 g
Severe – fully susceptible	500 mg	6 hours	2.0 g
Severe and/or life-threatening infections due to less sensitive organisms (primarily some strains of *P. aeruginosa*)	1000 mg	8 hours	3.0 g
	1000 mg	6 hours	4.0 g

Primaxin has been used successfully as monotherapy in immunocompromised cancer patients for confirmed or suspected infections such as sepsis.

Prophylactic use: For prophylaxis against post-surgical infections in adults, 1 g of Primaxin should be given intravenously on induction of anaesthesia and 1 g three hours later. For high-risk (i.e. colorectal) surgery, two additional 0.5 g doses can be given at 8 and 16 hours after induction.

In patients with renal insufficiency: As in patients with normal renal function, dosing is based on the severity of the infection. The maximum dosage for patients with various degrees of renal functional impairment is shown in the following Table. Doses cited are based on a bodyweight of 70 kg. Proportionate reduction in dose administered should be made for patients with lower bodyweight.

Maximum dosage in relation to renal function

Renal function	*Creatinine clearance (ml/min)*	*Dose (mg)*	*Dosage interval (hrs)*	*Maximum total daily dose† (g)*
Mild impairment	31–70	500	6–8	1.5–2
Moderate impairment	21–30	500	8–12	1–1.5
Severe‡ impairment	0–20	250–500	12	0.5–1.0

†The higher dose should be reserved for infections caused by less susceptible organisms.
‡Patients with creatinine clearance of 6–20 ml/min should be treated with 250 mg (or 3.5 mg/kg, whichever is lower) every 12 hours for most pathogens. When the 500 mg dose is used in these patients, there may be an increased risk of convulsions.

Patients with a creatinine clearance of ≤5 ml/min should not receive Primaxin IV unless haemodialysis is started within 48 hours.

Primaxin is cleared by haemodialysis. The patient should receive Primaxin IV immediately after haemodialysis and at 12-hourly intervals thereafter. Dialysis patients, especially those with background CNS disease, should be carefully monitored; patients on haemodialysis should only receive Primaxin IV when the benefit outweighs the potential risk of convulsions (see 'Precautions').

There are currently inadequate data to recommend the use of Primaxin IV for patients on peritoneal dialysis.

Paediatric dosage

Age	*Dose*	*Dosage interval*	*Total daily dose*
3 months of age and older (less than 40 kg bodyweight)	15 mg/kg	6 hours	60 mg/kg

Children over 40 kg bodyweight should receive adult doses.

The maximum daily dose should not exceed 2 g.

Clinical data are insufficient to recommend an optimal dose for children under 3 months of age or infants and children with impaired renal function.

Primaxin IV is not recommended for the therapy of meningitis. If meningitis is suspected an appropriate antibiotic should be used.

Primaxin IV may be used in children with sepsis as long as they are not suspected of having meningitis.

Preparation of solution: The following table is provided for convenience in reconstituting Primaxin IV for intravenous infusion.

Amount of Primaxin (mg)	*Volume of diluent added (ml)†*	*Approximate concentration of imipenem (mg/ml)*
Primaxin IV 500 mg	100	5
Primaxin IV 250 mg	50	5

†Shake to dissolve to a colourless or yellow solution. Variation of colour within this range does not affect potency.

Compatibility and stability: In keeping with good clinical and pharmaceutical practice, Primaxin IV should be administered as a freshly prepared solution. On the few occasions where changing circumstances make this impracticable, reconstituted Primaxin IV retains satisfactory potency for 3 hours at room temperature (up to 25°C) or 24 hours in a refrigerator (below 4°C) when prepared in any of the following diluents: 0.9% Sodium Chloride Injection; 5% Dextrose and 0.9% Sodium Chloride; 5% Dextrose and 0.225% Sodium Chloride; 5% Mannitol; 2.5% Mannitol.

Primaxin IV is chemically incompatible with lactate and should not be reconstituted with diluents containing lactate. Primaxin IV can, however, be administered into an IV tubing through which a lactate solution is being infused.

Primaxin IV should not be mixed with, or physically added to, other antibiotics.

Addition of Primaxin IV Injection in a Monovial to an infusion solution

Step 1 EXAMINE
Examine the vial for any foreign material in the powder and make sure the tamper-evident seal between the cap and the vial is intact.

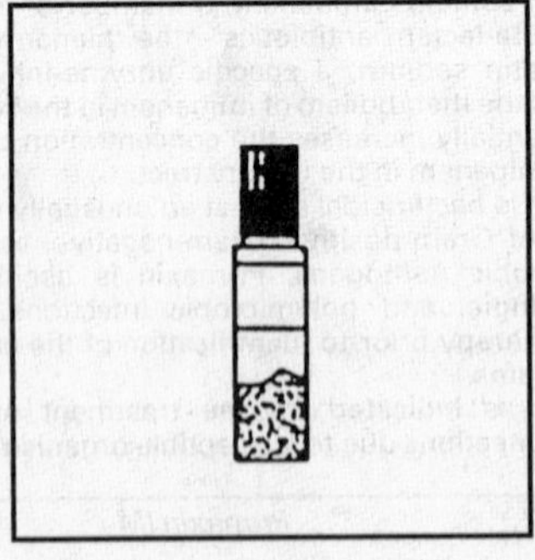

Step 2 REMOVE CAP
Remove the cap by first twisting it and pulling it up to break the tamper-evident seal.

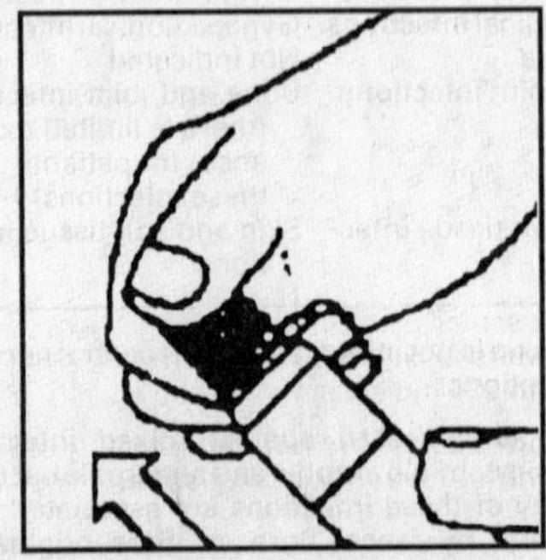

Step 3 CONNECT
Insert the needle into the infusion-bag connector. *Push* the needle-holder and vial together ntil they 'click' into place. Ensure the *additive* part is used.

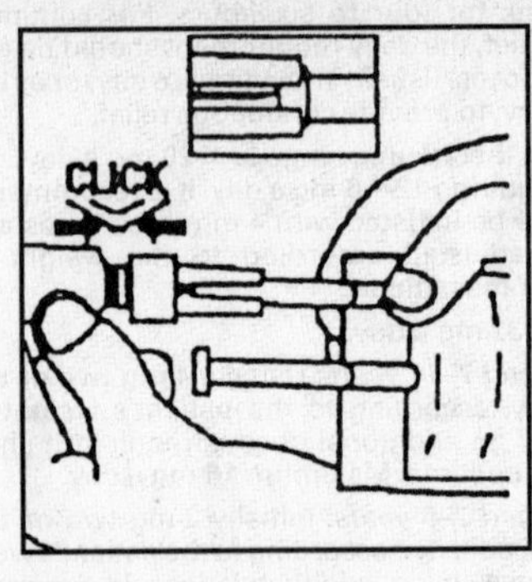

Step 4 MIX
Hold the vial in an upright position. *Squeeze* the infusion bag several times to transfer the diluent into the vial. Shake the vial to reconstitute the substance.

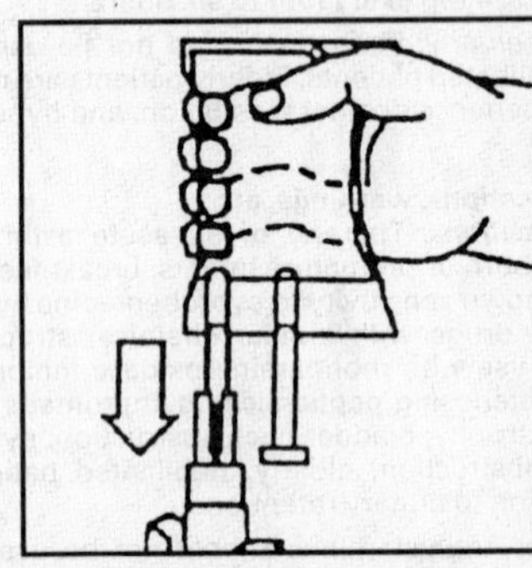

Step 5 TRANSFER
Now reverse the connected IV assembly, holding the vial upside down. Squeeze the infusion bag several times. This will create an over-pressure in the vial, allowing the contents of the vial to be transferred back into the infusion bag. Repeat steps 4 and 5 until the vial is completely empty.

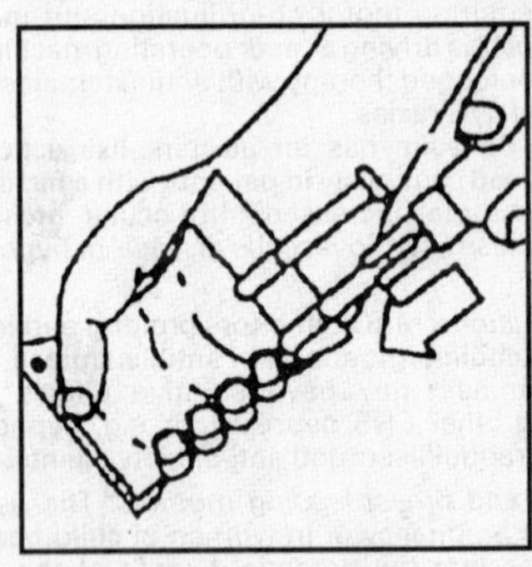

Step 6 IDENTIFY
Fill out the peel-off label on the vial and *affix* it to the infusion bag for proper identification.

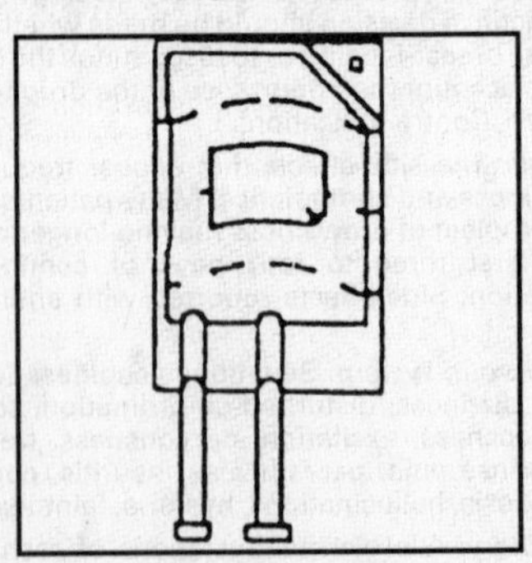

INTRAMUSCULAR ADMINISTRATION: This formulation is for intramuscular use only and should not be administered intravenously.

Note: All recommended doses refer to the imipenem fraction of Primaxin.

Adults: A single 500 mg dose of the intramuscular formulation may be used for the treatment of urethritis or cervicitis due to non-penicillinase-producing *Neisseria gonorrhoea.*

The intramuscular formulation may be used as an alternative to the intravenous formulation in the treatment of mild and moderate infections.

Primaxin IM should be given by deep intramuscular injection into a large muscle mass (such as the gluteal muscle or lateral part of the thigh).

Usual adult intramuscular dose

	IM administration		
Type or severity of infection	*Dose of imipenem*	*Dosage interval*	*Total daily dose*
Gonococcal urethritis/cervicitis	500 mg	single dose	0.5 g
Mild infections	500 mg	12 hours	1.0 g
Moderate infections	750 mg	12 hours	1.5 g

In infants and children: The safety and efficacy of the intramuscular formulation have not been studied in the paediatric group.

In patients with renal insufficiency: The safety and efficacy of the intramuscular formulation have not been studied in patients with renal insufficiency.

Preparation of intramuscular suspension: The following table is provided for convenience in reconstituting Primaxin IM with 1% lidocaine (lignocaine) solution for intramuscular use.

Strength	*Volume of 1% lidocaine (lignocaine) solution to be added (ml†)*	*Final volume (ml)*
Primaxin IM 500 mg	2	2.8

†Shake to prepare a white to light-tan-coloured suspension. Variation of colour within this range does not affect potency. Use immediately after making up. Lidocaine (Lignocaine) should not be used if patients are known or suspected to be hypersensitive to local anaesthetics of the amide type or in patients with severe shock or heart block.

Contra-indications, warnings, etc

Contra-indication: Hypersensitivity to this product.

Warning: There is some clinical and laboratory evidence of partial cross-allergenicity between Primaxin and the other beta-lactam antibiotics, penicillins and cephalosporins. Severe reactions (including anaphylaxis) have been reported with most beta-lactam antibiotics. Before initiating therapy with Primaxin, careful inquiry should be made concerning previous hypersensitivity reactions to beta-lactam antibiotics. If an allergic reaction to Primaxin occurs, the drug should be discontinued and appropriate measures undertaken.

Precautions: Pseudomembranous colitis, reported with virtually all antibiotics, can range from mild to life-threatening in severity. Primaxin should be prescribed with caution in patients with a history of gastro-intestinal disease, particularly colitis. Treatment-related diarrhoea should always be considered as a pointer to this diagnosis. While studies indicate that a toxin of *Clostridium difficile* is one of the primary causes of antibiotic-associated colitis, other causes should be considered.

Use in pregnancy and lactation: Pregnant monkeys showed evidence of maternal and foetal toxicity with bolus injections at doses equivalent to twice the human dose.

The use of Primaxin in pregnant women has not been studied and Primaxin should therefore not be given in pregnancy unless the anticipated benefit to the mother outweighs the possible risk to the foetus.

It is not known whether Primaxin is excreted in human milk. Because many drugs are excreted by this route, the breast feeding mother should not receive Primaxin. If the use of Primaxin is deemed essential, the mother should stop breast feeding.

Paediatric use: Primaxin IV: Efficacy and tolerability in infants under three months of age have yet to be established; therefore, Primaxin is not recommended for use below this age.

Primaxin IM: Tolerability and efficacy of 'Primaxin' IM have not yet been studied in the paediatric group; therefore, at present, Primaxin IM is not recommended for use in this group.

Central nervous system: Patients with CNS disorders and/or compromised renal function (accumulation of Primaxin may occur) have shown CNS side effects, especially when recommended dosages based on body weight and renal function were exceeded. Hence it is recommended that the dosage schedules of Primaxin should be strictly adhered to, and established anticonvulsant therapy continued.

If focal tremors, myoclonus or convulsions occur, the patient should be evaluated neurologically and placed on anticonvulsant therapy if not already instituted. If these symptoms still continue, the dosage should be reduced, or Primaxin withdrawn completely.

Drug interactions: There are no data on adverse drug interactions. However, concomitant probenecid has been shown to double the plasma level and half-life of cilastatin, but with no effect on its urinary recovery.

Concomitant probenecid showed only minimal increases in plasma level and half-life of imipenem, with urinary recovery of active imipenem decreased to approximately 60% of the administered dose.

Use in patients with renal insufficiency: Primaxin IV: Patients with creatinine clearances of ≤5 ml/min should not receive Primaxin IV unless haemodialysis is instituted within 48 hours. For patients on haemodialysis, Primaxin IV is only recommended when the benefit outweighs the potential risk of convulsions.

Primaxin IM: Safety and efficacy of Primaxin IM have not yet been studied in patients with renal insufficiency, therefore, at present, Primaxin IM is not recommended for use in this group.

Side-effects: Primaxin is generally well tolerated. Side-effects rarely require cessation of therapy and are generally mild and transient; serious side-effects are rare.

Local reactions: Erythema, local pain and induration, thrombophlebitis.

Allergic: Rash, pruritus, urticaria, toxic epidermal necrolysis (rarely), fever, anaphylactic reactions.

Gastro-intestinal: Nausea, vomiting, diarrhoea. Pseudomembranous colitis has been reported.

Blood: Eosinophilia, leucopenia, neutropenia including agranulocytosis, thrombocytopenia, thrombocytosis decreased haemoglobin, and hepatitis (rarely). A positive direct Coombs test may develop.

Liver function: Mild increases in serum transaminases, bilirubin and/or serum alkaline phosphatase have been reported.

Renal function: Oliguria/anuria, polyuria, acute renal failure (rarely). The role of Primaxin in changes in renal function is difficult to assess, since factors predisposing to pre-renal uraemia or to impaired renal function usually have been present. Elevated serum creatinine and blood urea have been seen. A harmless reddish urine discoloration, not to be confused with haematuria, has been seen in children.

Central nervous system: Myoclonic activity, psychic disturbances, confusional states or convulsions have been reported.

Special senses: Taste perversion.

Other reported reactions with an unknown causal relationship

Gastro-intestinal: Haemorrhagic colitis, gastro-enteritis, abdominal pain, glossitis, tongue papillar hypertrophy, heartburn, pharyngeal pain, increased salivation.

Central nervous system: Dizziness, somnolence, encephalopathy, paraesthesiae, vertigo, headache.

Special senses: Transient hearing loss in patients with impaired hearing, tinnitus.

Respiratory: Chest discomfort, dyspnoea, hyperventilation, thoracic spine pain.

Cardiovascular: Hypotension, palpitations, tachycardia.

Skin: Erythema multiforme, facial oedema, flushing, cyanosis hyperhidrosis, skin texture changes, candidiasis, pruritus vulvae.

Body as a whole: Polyarthralgia, asthenia/weakness.

Treatment of overdosage: No information is available at present.

Pharmaceutical precautions Vials of dry Primaxin should be stored below 25°C protected from light until immediately before use. They should not be frozen, or exposed to temperatures above 50°C.

Legal category POM.

Package quantities *For intravenous use:* Single 50-ml vial containing sterile powders of 250 mg imipenem (as the monohydrate) with 250 mg cilastatin (as the sodium salt).

Single 100-ml vial containing sterile powders of 500 mg imipenem (as the monohydrate) with 500 mg cilastatin (as the sodium salt).

Monovial presentation: Single 20-ml vial with transfer needle containing 500 mg imipenem (as the monohydrate) with 500 mg cilastatin (as the sodium salt).

For intramuscular use: Single 13-ml vial containing sterile powders of 500 mg imipenem (as the monohydrate) with 500 mg cilastatin (as the sodium salt).

Further information *The differences between intramuscular and intravenous administration should be recognised.*

Intramuscular use has a 75% bioavailability of intravenous infusion. Effective absorption from the intramuscular site is longer; plasma levels of a single 500 mg or 750 mg dose of imipenem remained above 2 mcg/ml for at least six to eight hours. This is above the MIC_{90} of such pathogens as *Serratia* spp., *Acinetobacter* spp., *Bacteroides fragilis* and all Gram-positive cocci except enterococci. Alternatively, intravenous infusion offers peak plasma levels from single 250, 500 and 1000 mg doses of 17, 39 and 66 mcg/ml, respectively. The plasma levels of these doses decline below 1 microgram/ml or less in four to six hours.

Approximately 70% of the antibiotic administered intravenously was recovered intact from the urine in 10 hours. Concentrations exceeded 10 micrograms/ml for up to eight hours after a single intravenous dose of 500 mg Primaxin. However, intramuscular administration of a single dose of 500 mg or 750 mg of the antibiotic gave urine levels above 10 micrograms/ml for 12 hours with a total urinary recovery of 50% of the dose.

No accumulation of imipenem is seen in patients with normal kidney function in either plasma or urine at any of the dosage regimens recommended.

Product licence numbers

Primaxin for intravenous administration:
250 mg 0025/0228
500 mg 0025/0229

Primaxin for intramuscular administration: 500 mg 0025/0230.

PROSCAR*

Qualitative and quantitative composition Each tablet cotains 5 mg finasteride.

Pharmaceutical form Blue-coloured, apple-shaped, film-coated tablets marked 'Proscar' on one side and 'MSD 72' on the other.

Clinical particulars

Therapeutic indications: Proscar is indicated for the treatment and control of benign prostatic hyperplasia (BPH) in patients with an enlarged prostate to:

- cause regression of the enlarged prostate, improve urinary flow, and improve the symptoms associated with BPH.
- reduce the incidence of acute urinary retention and the need for surgery including transurethral resection of the prostate (TURP) and prostatectomy.

Posology and method of administration: The recommended adult dose is one 5 mg tablet daily, with or without food.

Although early improvement may be seen, treatment for at least six months may be necessary to assess whether a beneficial response has been achieved. Thereafter treatment should be continued long term.

No dosage adjustment is required in the elderly or in patients with varying degrees of renal insufficiency (creatinine clearances as low as 9 ml/min).

There are no data available in patients with hepatic insufficiency.

Proscar is contra-indicated in children.

Contra-indications: Hypersensitivity to any component of this product; women who are or may become pregnant; children.

Special warnings and special precautions for use

General: Patients with large residual urine volume and/or severely diminished urinary flow should be carefully monitored for obstructive uropathy.

Effects on prostate-specific antigen (PSA) and prostate cancer detection: No clinical benefit has yet been demonstrated in patients with prostate cancer treated with "Proscar'. Digital rectal examination, as well as other evaluations for prostate cancer, should be carried out on patients with BPH prior to initiating therapy with Proscar and periodically thereafter. Generally, when PSA assays are performed a baseline PSA > 10 ng/ml (Hybritech) prompts further evaluation and consideration of biopsy; for PSA levels between 4 and 10 ng/ml, further evaluation is advisable.
There is considerable overlap in PSA levels among men with and without prostate cancer. Therefore, in men with BPH, PSA values within the normal reference range do not rule out prostate cancer regardless of treatment with Proscar. A baseline PSA <4 ng/ml does not exclude prostate cancer.

Proscar causes a decrease in serum PSA concentrations by approximately 50% in patients with BPH even in the presence of prostate cancer. This decrease in serum PSA levels in patients with BPH treated with Proscar should be cosidered when evaluating PSA data and does not rule out concomitant prostate cancer. This decrease is predictable over the entire range of PSA values, although it may vary in individual patients. In patients treated with Proscar for six months or more, PSA values should be doubled for comparison with normal ranges in untreated men. This adjustment preserves the sensitivity and specificity of the PSA assay and maintains its ability to detect prostate cancer.

Any sustained increase in PSA levels of patients treated with finasteride should be carefully evaluated, including consideration of non-compliance to therapy with Proscar.

Interaction with other medicaments and other forms of interaction: No clinically important drug interactions have been identified. Proscar does not appear to significantly affect the cytochrome P450-linked drug metabolising enzyme system. Compounds which have been tested in man include propranolol, digoxin, glibenclamide, warfarin, theophylline, and antipyrine and no clinically meaningful interactions were found.

Other concomitant therapy: Although specific interaction studies were not performed in clinical studies, Proscar was used concomitantly with ACE inhibitors, alpha-blockers, beta-blockers, calcium channel blockers, cardiac nitrates, diuretics, H_2 antagonists, HMG-CoA reductase inhibitors, non-steroidal anti-inflammatory drugs (NSAIDs) including aspirin and paracetamol, quinolones and benzodiazepines without evidence of clinically significant adverse interactions.

Pregnancy and lactation

Pregnancy: Proscar is contra-indicated in women who are or may become pregnant.

Because of the ability of Type II 5 alpha-reductase inhibitors to inhibit conversion of testosterone to dihydrotestosterone, these drugs, including finasteride, may cause abnormalities of the external genitalia of a male foetus when administered to a pregnant woman.

In animal developmental studies, dose-dependent development of hypospadias were observed in the male offspring of pregnant rats given finasteride at doses ranging from 100 μg/kg/day to 100 mg/kg/day, at an incidence of 3.6% to 100%. Additionally, pregnant rats produced male offspring with decreased prostatic and seminal vesicular weights, delayed preputial separation, transient nipple development and decreased anogenital distance, when given finasteride at doses below the recommended human dose. The critical period during which these effects can be induced has been defined in rats as days 16–17 of gestation.

The changes described above are expected pharmacological effects of Type II 5 alpha-reductase inhibitors. Many of the changes, such as hypospadias, observed in male rats exposed *in utero* to finasteride are similar to those reported in male infants with a genetic deficiency of Type II 5 alpha reductase. It is for these reasons that Proscar is contra-indicated in women who are or may become pregnant.

No effects were seen in female offspring exposed *in utero* to any dose of finasteride.

Exposure to finasteride – risk to male foetus: Women should not handle crushed or broken tablets of Proscar when they are or may become pregnant because of the possibility of absorption of finasteride and the subsequent potential risk to a male foetus (see *Pregnancy*). Proscar tabets are coated and will prevent contact with the active ingredient during normal handling, provided that the tablets have not been broken or crushed.

Small amounts of finasteride have been recovered from the semen in subjects receiving Proscar 5 mg/day. It is not known whether a male foetus may be adversely affected if his mother is exposed to the semen of a patient being treated with finasteride. Therefore, when the patient's sexual partner is or may become pregnant, the patient should either avoid exposure of his partner to semen (e.g. by use of a condom) or discontinue Proscar.

Lactation: Proscar is not indicated for use in women. It is not known whether finasteride is excreted in human milk.

Effects on ability to drive and use machines: None reported.

Undesirable effects: Proscar is well tolerated. In controlled clinical studies where patients received 5 mg of finasteride over periods of up to four years, the following adverse reactions were considered possibly, probably or definitely drug-related and occurred with a frequency greater than placebo and greater than or equal to 1%: impotence, decreased libido, ejaculation disorder, decreased volume of ejaculate, breast enlargement, breast tenderness and rash. There was no evidence of increased adverse experiences with increased duration of treatment with Proscar and the incidence of new drug-related sexual adverse experiences decreased with duration of treatment.

The following adverse experiences have been reported in post-marketing experience: hypersensitivity reactions, including lip swelling.

Laboratory test findings: Serum PSA concentration is correlated with patient age and prostatic volume, and prostatic volume is correlated with patient age. When PSA laboratory determinations are evaluated, consideration should be given to the fact that PSA levels generally decrease in patients treated with Proscar. In most patients, a rapid decrease in PSA is seen within the first months of therapy, after which time PSA levels stabilise to a new baseline. The post-treatment baseline approximates half of the pre-treatment value. Therefore, in typical patients treated with Proscar for six months or more, PSA values should be doubled for comparison to normal ranges in untreated men.

For clinical interpretation see *Special warnings and special precautions for use, Effects on prostate-specific antigen (PSA) and prostate cancer detection.*

No other difference was observed in patients treated with placebo or Proscar in standard laboratory tests.

Overdose: No specific treatment of overdosage with Proscar is recommended. Patients have received single doses of Proscar up to 400 mg and multiple doses of Proscar up to 80 mg/day for up to three months without any adverse effects.

Pharmacological properties

Pharmacodynamic properties: Finasteride is a competitive inhibitor of human 5 alpha reductase, an intracellular enzyme which metabolises testosterone into the more potent androgen, dihydrotestosterone (DHT). In benign prostatic hyperplasia (BPH), enlargement of the prostate gland is dependent upon the conversion of testosterone to DHT within the prostate. Proscar is highly effective in reducing circulating and intraprostatic DHT. Finasteride has no affinity for the androgen receptor.

In clinical studies of patients with moderate to severe symptoms of BPH, and enlarged prostate on digital rectal examination and low residual urinary volumes, Proscar reduced the incidence of acute retention of urine from 7/100 to 3/100 over four years and the need for surgery (TURP or prostatectomy) from 10/100 to 5/100. These reductions were associated with a 2-point improvement in QUASI-AUA symptom score (range 0–34), a sustained regression in prostate volume of approximately 20% and a sustained increase in urinary flow rate.

Pharmacokinetic properties: After an oral dose of ^{14}C-finasteride in man, 39% of the dose was excreted in the urine in the form of metabolites (virtually no unchanged drug was excreted in the urine), and 57% of total dose was excreted in the faeces. Two metabolites have been identified which possess only a small fraction of the 5 alpha-reductase activity of finasteride.

The oral bioavailability of finasteride is approximately 80%, relative to an intravenous reference dose, and is unaffected by food. Maximum plasma concentrations are reached approximately two hours after dosing and the absorption is complete within 6–8 hours. Protein binding is approximately 93%. Plasma clearance and the volume of distribution are approximately 165 ml/min and 76 l, respectively.

In the elderly, the elimination rate of finasteride is somewhat decreased. Half-life is prolonged from a mean half-life of approximately 6 hours in men aged 18–60 years to 8 hours in men aged more than 70 years. This is of no clinical significance and does not warrant a reduction in dosage.

In patients with chronic renal impairment, whose creatinine clearance ranged from 9–55 ml/min, the disposition of a single dose of ^{14}C-finasteride was not different from that in healthy volunteers. Protein binding also did not differ in patients with renal impairment. A portion of the metabolites which normally is excreted renally was excreted in the faeces. It therefore appears that faecal excretion increases commensurate to the decrease in urinary excretion of metabolites. Dosage adjustment in non-dialysed patients with renal impairment is not necessary.

There are not data available in patients with hepatic insufficiency.

Finasteride has been found to cross the blood-brain barrier. Small amounts of finasteride have been recovered in the seminal fluid of treated patients.

Preclinical safety data: No further information provided.

Pharmaceutical particulars

List of excipients: Cellulose, Microcrystalline PhEur; Docusate Sodium BP; Lactose PhEur; Magnesium Stearate PhEur; Pregelatinised Maize Starch BP; Sodium Starch Glycollate BP; Yellow Iron Oxide EEC; Hydroxypropylcellulose PhEur; Indigo Carmine Aluminium Lake EEC; Methylhydroxypropylcellulose PhEur; Talc PhEur; Titanium Dioxide PhEur.

Incompatibilities: None reported.

Shelf life: Two years.

Special precautions for storage: Protect from light. Keep container closed. Store below 25°C.

Nature and contents of container: Opaque PVC/PE/PVDC blisters lidded with aluminium foil; packs of 28 tablets.

Instructions for use/handling: Women should not handle crushed or broken Proscar Tablets when they are or may become pregnant (see *Contra-indications, Pregnancy and lactation, Exposure to finasteride – risk to male foetus*).

Marketing authorisation number 0025/0279.

Date of first authorisation/renewal of authorisation July 1997.

Date of approval/revision of SPC October 1998.

Legal category POM.

SALURIC*

Qualitative and quantitative composition Each tablet of Saluric contains 500 mg chlorothiazide PhEur.

Pharmaceutical form Saluric is supplied as white, half-scored tablets, marked 'MSD 432'.

Clinical particulars

Therapeutic indications: Saluric is a thiazide diuretic and antihypertensive.

Saluric is indicated for oedema associated with congestive heart failure, hepatic cirrhosis, premenstrual tension, and in oedema due to various forms of renal dysfunction (i.e. nephrotic syndrome, acute glomerulonephritis and chronic renal failure). Saluric can be used to treat hypertension, either alone or as an adjunct to other antihypertensive drugs.

Posology and method of administration: Dosage should be determined on an individual basis, and the lowest dosage necessary to achieve the desired result should be used.

Adults – for oedema: Usually ½–2 tablets (250–1000 mg) a day given in a single dose or in two divided doses. Many patients respond to intermittent therapy: every other day, or three to five consecutive days a week. Intermittent therapy is less likely to produce excessive diuretic response with resulting electrolyte imbalance. The maximum recommended daily dose is 2 tablets (1000 mg).

In oedema accompanying premenstrual tension: ½–1 tablet (250–500 mg) once or twice a day, from the first morning of symptoms until the onset of the menses.

Adults – for control of hypertension: The usual starting dose is ½ tablet (250 mg) a day as a single or divided dose.

In some patients, a ¼ tablet (125 mg), alone or with another antihypertensive, may be sufficient to initiate therapy. Dosage should be adjusted to response, but should not exceed 1 tablet (500 mg) a day.

Thiazides may add to the action of other antihypertensives. If Saluric is added to therapy with other antihypertensive agents, dosage reduction of such agents may be necessary to prevent an excessive drop in blood pressure.

Infants and children: Usually 25 mg per kg bodyweight a day, given in two doses. Infants under six months may need up to 35 mg per kg a day, in two doses.

On this basis, infants up to two years of age may be given 125–375 mg of Saluric daily in two doses. Children from 2 to 12 years of age may be given 375 mg to 1.0 g daily in two doses. Dosage in both age groups should be based on bodyweight.

Use in the elderly: Particular caution is needed in the elderly because of their susceptibility to electrolyte imbalance; the dosage should be carefully adjusted according to renal function and clinical response.

Contra-indications: Anuria, known hypersensitivity to this product or to other sulphonamide-derived drugs, severe renal or hepatic failure, Addison's disease, hypercalcaemia, concurrent lithium therapy. See *Use in pregnancy* and *Use in lactation* under *Special warnings and special precautions for use.*

Special warnings and special precautions for use: Patients should be carefully monitored for signs of fluid and electrolyte imbalance (hyponatraemia, hypochloraemic alkalosis, hypokalaemia and hypomagnesaemia). It is particularly important to make serum and urine electrolyte determinations when the patient is vomiting excessively or receiving parenteral fluids. Warning signs or symptoms of fluid and electrolyte imbalance include: dryness of mouth, thirst, weakness, lethargy, drowsiness, restlessness, seizures, confusion, muscle pains or cramps, muscular fatigue, hypotension, oliguria, tachycardia, and gastro-intestinal disturbances such as nausea and vomiting.

Hypokalaemia may develop, especially with brisk diuresis, when severe cirrhosis is present, or after prolonged therapy. Hypokalaemia can sensitise or exaggerate the response of the heart to the toxic effects of digitalis (e.g. increased ventricular irritability).

Sensitivity reactions may occur in patients with or without history of allergy or bronchial asthma.

Hypokalaemia may be avoided or treated in the adult by concurrent use of amiloride hydrochloride (Midamor*), a potassium-conserving agent. It may also be avoided by giving potassium chloride or foods with a high potassium content. (Note that symptoms and signs which might indicate ulceration or obstruction of the small bowel in patients taking tablets or capsules containing potassium salts are indications for stopping treatment with such preparations immediately.)

Diuretic-induced hyponatraemia is usually mild and asymptomatic. Dilutional hyponatraemia may occur in oedematous patients in hot weather; and, except in rare instances when hyponatraemia is life-threatening, appropriate therapy is water restriction rather than administration of salt.

Thiazides may decrease serum Protein Bound Iodine levels without signs of thyroid disturbances.

Thiazides may decrease urinary calcium excretion, and may also cause intermittent and slight elevation of serum calcium in the absence of known disorders of calcium metabolism. Thiazides should be discontinued before carrying out tests for parathyroid function.

When creatinine clearance falls below 30 ml/min, thiazide diuretics become ineffective.

Uraemia may be precipitated or increased by Saluric. Cumulative effects of chlorothiazide may develop in patients with impaired renal function. If increasing uraemia and oliguria occur during treatment of renal disease, Saluric should be discontinued.

Thiazides should be used with caution in patients with impaired hepatic function or progressive liver disease, since minor alterations of fluid and electrolyte balance may precipitate hepatic coma.

Hyperuricaemia may occur, or gout may be precipitated, in certain patients receiving thiazide therapy.

Thiazide therapy may impair glucose tolerance.

Increases in cholesterol and triglyceride levels may be associated with thiazide diuretic therapy.

The possibility of exacerbation or activation of systemic lupus erythematosus has been reported.

Latent diabetes may become manifest during thiazide administration.

Interaction with other medicaments and other forms of interaction: Alcohol, barbiturates or narcotics: Co-administration may potentiate orthostatic hypotension.

Oral and parenteral antidiabetic drugs may require adjustment of dosage with concurrent use. *Other antihypertensive drugs* may have an additive effect. Discontinuation of diuretic therapy 2–3 days before the initiation of treatment with an ACE-inhibitor may reduce the likelihood of first-dose hypotension. The antihypertensive effect of the drug may be enhanced in the post-sympathectomy patient. *Cholestyramine and colestipol resins:* Both cholestyramine and colestipol resins have the potential of binding thiazide diuretics and reducing diuretic absorption from the gastro-intestinal tract. *Corticosteroids or ACTH* may intensify any thiazide-induced electrolyte depletion, particularly hypokalaemia. *Pressor amines such as adrenaline* may show decreased arterial responsiveness when used with Saluric, but this reaction is not enough to preclude their therapeutic usefulness. *Non-depolarising muscle relaxants such as tubocurarine* may possibly interact with Saluric to increase muscle relaxation. *Non-steroidal anti-inflammatory drugs* may attenuate the diuretic and antihypertensive effect of diuretics.

Drug/laboratory tests: Because thiazides may affect calcium metabolism, Saluric may interfere with tests for parathyroid function.

Pregnancy and lactation

Use in pregnmancy: Thiazides cross the placental barrier and appear in the cord blood. The use of Saluric when pregnancy is present or suspected, requires that the benefits of the drug be weighed against the possible hazards to the fetus. These hazards include fetal or neonatal jaundice, thrombocytopenia, and possibly other adverse reactions which have occurred in the adult. The routine use of diuretics in otherwise healthy, pregnant women with or without mild oedema is not recommended, because their use may be associated with hypovolaemia, increased blood viscosity and decreased placental perfusion.

Use in lactation: Thiazides appear in breast milk. If use of the drug is deemed essential, the patient should stop breast-feeding.

Effects on ability to drive and use machines: There are no data to suggest that Saluric affects the ability to drive or use machines.

Undesirable effects: The following side-effects have been reported with chlorothiazide or other thiazide diuretics:

Gastro-intestinal system: Anorexia, gastric irritation, nausea, vomiting, cramps, diarrhoea, constipation, jaundice (intrahepatic cholestatic jaundice), pancreatitis, salivary gland inflammation.

Central nervous system: Dizziness, vertigo, paraesthesiae, headache, yellow vision.

Haematological: Leucopenia, agranulocytosis, thrombocytopenia, aplastic anaemia, haemolytic anaemia.

Cardiovascular: Hypotension, including orthostatic hypotension.

Hypersensitivity: Purpura, photosensitivity, rash, urticaria, necrotising angiitis (vasculitis, cutaneous vasculitis), fever, respiratory distress including pneumonitis and pulmonary oedema, anaphylactic reactions, toxic epidermal necrolysis.

Metabolic: Hyperglycaemia, glycosuria, hyperuricaemia, electrolyte imbalance including hyponatraemia and hypokalaemia.

Renal: Renal dysfunction, interstitial nephritis, renal failure.

Other: Muscle spasm, weakness, restlessness, transient blurred vision, impotence.

Overdosage: The most common signs and symptoms observed are those caused by electrolyte depletion (hypokalaemia, hypochloraemia, hyponatraemia) and dehydration resulting from excessive diuresis. If digitalis has also been administered, hypokalaemia may accentuate cardiac arrhythmias.

In the event of overdosage, symptomatic and supportive measures should be employed. If ingestion is recent, emesis should be induced or gastric lavage performed. Dehydration, electrolyte imbalance, hepatic coma, and hypotension should be corrected by established procedures. If required, give oxygen or artificial respiration for respiratory impairment.

Pharmacological properties

Pharmacodynamic properties: Chlorothiazide is an orally effective diuretic and antihypertensive agent – the first in the thiazide class. It interferes with the distal renal tubular mechanism of electrolyte reabsorption and increases the excretion of sodium and chloride in approximately equivalent amounts. Natriuresis may be accompanied by some loss of potassium, magnesium, and bicarbonate. While chlorothiazide is predominately a saluretic agent, *in vitro* studies have shown that it has a carbonic anhyrase inhibitory action which seems to be relatively specific for the renal tubular mechanism. It does not appear to be concentrated in erythrocytes or the brain in sufficient amounts to influence the activity of carbonic anhydrase in those tissues.

Pharmacokinetic properties: Chlorothiazide is not metabolised but is rapidly eliminated by the kidney. The plasma half life of chlorothiazide is 45–120 minutes. After oral doses, 20–24% is excreted unchanged in the urine. Chlorothiazide crosses the placenta but not the blood-brain barrier and is excreted in breast milk.

Preclinical safety data: No additional relevant information.

Pharmaceutical particulars

List of excipients: Magnesium stearate PhEur, maize starch PhEur and purified water PhEur.

Incompatibilities: None known.

Shelf life: 60 months.

Special precautions for storage: Store in a dry place below 25°C.

Nature of content of container: Opaque HDPE or amber glass bottles with green opaque HDPE cap-to-cap tamper-evident closures.

Pack size: 100 tablets.

Instructions for use/handling: None.

Marketing authorisation number PL 0025/5019R.

Date of first authorisation/renewal of authorisation Licence first granted 30 October 1986.
Licence last renewed 30 October 1996.

Date of (partial) revision of text June 1996.

Legal category POM.

SINGULAIR* PAEDIATRIC 5 mg CHEWABLE TABLETS ▼ SINGULAIR* 10 mg TABLETS ▼

Qualitative and quantitative composition 5 mg chewable tablet: 5.2 mg montelukast sodium, which is equivalent to 5 mg montelukast acid.

10 mg film-coated tablet: 10.4 mg montelukast sodium, which is equivalent to 10 mg of montelukast acid.

Pharmaceutical form 5 mg strength: Pink, round, biconvex chewable tablet (diameter 9.5 mm), with 'SINGULAIR' engraved on one side and 'MSD 275' on the other.

10 mg strength: Beige, rounded square film-coated tablet (size 7.9 mm by 7.9 mm) with 'SINGULAIR' engraved on one side and 'MSD 117' on the other.

Clinical particulars

Therapeutic indications: Singulair is indicated in the treatment of asthma as add-on therapy in those patients with mild to moderate persistent asthma who are inadequately controlled on inhaled corticosteroids and in whom 'as needed' short-acting β-agonists provide inadequate clinical control of asthma.

Singulair is also indicated in the prophylaxis of asthma in which the predominant component is exercise-induced bronchoconstriction.

No specific safety issues have been identified but experience in the paediatric population is limited (see *Undesirable effects*).

Posology and method of administration: The dosage for adults 15 years of age and older is one 10 mg tablet daily to be taken at bedtime with or without food.

The dosage for paediatric patients 6–14 years of age is one 5 mg chewable tablet daily to be taken at bedtime. If taken in connection with food, Singulair should be taken 1 hour before or 2 hours after food. No dosage adjustment within this age group is necessary. There are no data on safety and efficacy in children below 6 years of age.

General recommendations: The therapeutic effect of Singulair on parameters of asthma control occurs within one day. Patients should be advised to continue taking Singulair even if their asthma is under control, as well as during periods of worsening asthma.

No dosage adjustment is necessary for the elderly, or for patients with renal insufficiency, or mild to moderate hepatic impairment. There are no data on patients with severe hepatic impairment. The dosage is the same for both male and female patients.

Therapy with Singulair in relation to other treatments for asthma: Singulair can be added to a patient's existing treatment regimen.

β-agonist therapy: Singulair can be added to the treatment regimen of patients who are not adequately controlled on 'as needed' short-acting β-agonist. When a clinical response is evident (usually after the first dose), the patient may be able to decrease the use of 'as-needed' short-acting β-agonist.

Inhaled corticosteroids: Treatment with Singulair can be used as add-on therapy in patients when other agents, such as inhaled corticosteroids provide inadequate clinical control. Singulair should not be substituted for inhaled corticosteoids (see *Special warnings and special precautions for use*).

Contra-indications: Hypersensitivity to any component of this product.

Special warnings and special precautions for use: Patients should be advised never to use oral tablets of Singulair to treat acute asthma attacks and to keep their usual appropriate rescue medication for this purpose readily available. If an acute attack occurs, a short-acting inhaled β-agonist should be used. Patients should seek their doctor's advice as soon as possible if they need more inhalations of short-acting β-agonists than usual.

Singulair should not be substituted for inhaled or oral corticosteroids.

There are no data demonstrating that oral corticosteroids can be reduced when Singulair is given concomitantly. In addition, reduction of the oral corticosteroid dose may, in some patients, unmask underlying conditions (e.g. allergic rhinitis, eczema, eosinophilic conditions) controlled by the administration of oral corticosteroids. Reduction in the dose of oral corticosteroids should be considered only when necessary and with caution. The possibility that leukotriene receptor antagonists may be associated with the emergence of Churg-Strauss syndrome cannot be excluded. However, a detailed search of the montelukast clinical trials database has not revealed any cases of this syndrome or any evidence that this syndrome is associated with Singulair.

Treatment with Singulair does not alter the need for patients with aspirin-sensitive asthma to avoid taking aspirin and other non steroidal anti-inflammatory drugs.

Experience in the paediatric population is limited (see *Undesirable effects*).

5 mg chewable tablets contain aspartame which is a source of phenylalanine (0.842 mg phenylalanine per 5 mg chewable tablet).

Interaction with other medicaments and other forms of interaction: Singulair may be administered with other therapies routinely used in the prophylaxis and chronic treatment of asthma. In drug-interactions studies, the recommended clinical dose of montelukast did not have clinically important effects on the pharmacokinetics of the following drugs: theophylline, prednisone, predisolone, oral contraceptives (ethinyl estradiol/norethindrone 35/1), terfenadine, digoxin and warfarin.

The area under the plasma concentration curve (AUC) for montelukast was decreased approximately 40% in subjects with co-administration of phenobarbitone. Since montelukast is metabolised by CYP 3A4, caution should be exercised, particularly in children, when Singulair is co-administered with inducers of CYP 3A4, such as phenytoin, phenobarbitone and rifampicin.

Pregnancy and lactation: In pregnant rabbits and pregnant rats, montelukast did not affect fertility or reproductive performance nor was montelukast teratogenic at systemic exposures of >24-fold and

>69-fold the systemic exposure observed at the intended clinical dosage in humans, respectively. Montelukast has been shown to cross the placental barrier and is excreted in breast milk of animals. Since there are no controlled studies in pregnant or nursing women, Singulair should not be used during pregnancy or in nursing mothers unless it is considered to be clearly essential.

Effects of ability to drive and use machines: There is no evidence that Singulair affects the ability to drive and use machines.

Undesirble effects: Singulair has been generally well tolerated. Side effects, which usually were mild, generally did not require discontinuation of therapy.

Singulair 10 mg: Singulair 10 mg film-coated tablets have been evaluated in approximately 2,600 adult patients 15 years of age and older in clinical studies. In two similarly designed, 12-week placebo-controlled clinical trials, only abdominal pain and headache were reported as drug-related in ≥1% of patients treated with Singulair and at a greater incidence than in patients treated with placebo. The incidences of these events were not significantly different in the two treatment groups.

Although a causal relationship with montelukast was not established, the following adverse events were reported in ≥1% of patients and at an incidence greater than in placebo in clinical trials (% in Montelukast-treated patients, % placebo, respectively);

Body as a whole: asthenia/fatigue (1.8%, 1.2%), fever (1.5%, 0.9%), abdominal pain (2.9%, 2.5%), trauma (1.0%, 0.8%);

Digestive system disorders: diarrhoea (3.1%, 3.1%), dyspepsia (2.1%, 1.1%), infectious gastro-enteritis (1.5%, 0.5%), dental pain (1.7%, 1.0%);

Nervous system/psychiatric: dizziness (1.9%, 1.4%), headache (18.4%, 18.1%), insomnia (1.3%, 1.3%);

Respiratory system disorders: nasal congestion (1.6%, 1.3%), cough (2.7%, 2.4%), influenza (4.2%, 3.9%);

Skin/skin appendages disorder: rash (1.6%, 1.2%).

With prolonged treatment in clinical trials with a limited number of patients for up to 2 years, the adverse experience profile did not change.

Singulair Paediatric: Singulair Paediatric 5 mg chewable tablets have also been evaluated in approximately 320 paediatric patients 6 to 14 years of age. Long-term experience (more than one year) in this population is limited to 121. In an 8-week, placebo-controlled clinical trial, only headache was reported as drug-related in ≥1% of patients treated with Singulair and at a greater incidence than in patients treated with placebo. The incidence was not significantly different in the two treatment groups.

Although a causal relationship with montelukast was not established the following adverse events were reported in ≥3% of paediatric patients and at an incidence greater than in placebo in clinical trials (% in montelukast-treated patients, % placebo, respectively);

Body as a whole: fever (7.5%, 3.7%);

Digestive system disorders: diarrhoea (3.0%, 0.7%), nausea (4.0%, 3.7%);

Respiratory system disorders: influenza (8.5%, 4.4%), pharyngitis (13.9%, 12.6%), sinusitis (5.5%, 1.5%).

With prolonged treatment in clinical trials with a limited number of patients for up to 6 months, the adverse experience profile did not change.

Overdosage: No deaths occurred following a single oral administration of montelukast sodium at doses up to 5000 mg/kg in mice and rats, (15,000 mg/m^2 and 30,000 mg/m^2 in mice and rats, respectively) the maximum dose tested. This dose is equivalent to 25,000 times the recommended daily adult human dose (based on an adult patient weight of 50 kg).

No specific information is available on the treatment of overdosage with Singulair. In chronic asthma studies, Singulair has been administered at doses up to 200 mg/day to patients for 22 weeks and in short-term studies, up to 900 mg/day to patients for approximately one week without clinically important adverse experiences.

It is not known whether montelukast is dialysable by peritoneal- or haemo-dialysis.

Pharmacological properties

Pharmacodynamic properties: ATC Code: RO3D CO3.

The cysteinyl leukotrienes (LTC_4, LTD_4, LTE_4), are potent inflammatory eicosanoids released from various cells including mast cells and eosinophils. These important pro-asthmatic mediators bind to cysteinyl leukotriene receptors (CysLT) found in the human airway and cause airway actions, including bronchoconstriction, mucous secretion, vascular permeability, and eosinophil recruitment.

Montelukast is an orally active compound which binds with high affinity and selectivity to the $CysLT_1$ receptor. In clinical studies, montelukast inhibits bronchoconstriction due to inhaled LTD_4 at doses as low as 5 mg. Bronchodilation was observed within 2 hours of oral administration. The bronchodilation effect caused by a β-agonist was additive to that caused by montelukast. Treatment with Singulair inhibited both early- and late-phase bronchconstriction due to antigen challenge. Singulair, compared with placebo, decreased peripheral blood eosinophils in adult and paediatric patients. In a separate study, treatment with Singulair significantly decreased eosinophils in the airways (as measured in sputum) and in peripheral blood while improving clinical asthma control.

In studies in adults, Singulair 10 mg once daily, compared with placebo, demonstrated significant improvements in morning FEV_1 (10.4% vs 2.7% change from baseline), AM peak expiratory flow rate (PEFR) (24.5 L/min vs 3.3 L/min change from baseline), and significant decrease in total β-agonist use (–26.1% vs –4.6% change from baseline). Improvement in patient-reported daytime and night-time asthma symptoms scores was significantly better than placebo.

Studies in adults demonstrated the ability of Singulair to add to the clinical effect of inhaled corticosteroid (% change from baseline for inhaled beclomethasone plus montelukast vs beclomethasone, respectively for FEV_1: 5.43% vs 1.04%; β-agonist use: –8.7% vs 2.64%). Compared with inhaled beclomethasone (200 µg twice daily with a spacer device), Singulair demonstrated a more rapid initial response, although over the 12-week study, beclomethasone provided a greater average treatment effect (% change from baseline for montelukast vs beclomethasone, respectively for FEV_1: 7.49% vs 13.3%; β-agonist use: –28.28% vs –43.89%). However, compared with beclomethasone, a high percentage of patients treated with Singulair achieved similar clinical reponses (e.g. 50% of patients treated with beclomethasone achieved an improvement in FEV_1 of approximately 11% or more over baseline while approximately 42% of patients treated with Singulair achieved the same response).

In an 8-week study in paediatric patients, Singulair 5 mg once daily, compared with placebo, significantly improved respiratory function (FEV_1 8.71% vs 4.16% change from baseline; AM PEFR 27.9 L/min vs 17.8 L/min change from baseline) and decreased 'as needed' β-agonist use (–11.7% vs +8.2% change from baseline).

Significant reduction of exercise-induced bronchoconstriction (EIB) was demonstrated in a 12-week study in adults (maximal fall in FEV_1 22.23% for montelukast vs 32.40% for placebo; time to recovery to within 5% of baseline FEV_1 44.22 min vs 60.64 min). The effect was consistent throughout the 12-week study period. Reduction in EIB was also demonstrated in a short term study in paediatric patients (maximal fall in FEV_1 18.27% vs 26.11%; time to recovery to within 5% of baseline FEV_1 17.76 min vs 27.98 min). The effect in both studies was demonstrated at the end of the once-daily dosing interval.

In aspirin-sensitive asthmatic patients receiving concomitant inhaled and/or oral corticosteroids, treatment with Singulair, compared with placebo resulted in significant improvements in asthma control (FEV_1 8.55% vs –1.74% change from baseline and decrease in total β-agonist use –27.78% vs 2.09% change from baseline).

Pharmacokinetic properties: Absorption: Montelukast is rapidly absorbed following oral administration. For the 10 mg film-coated tablet, the mean peak plasma concentration (C_{max}) is achieved 3 hours (T_{max}) after administraiton in adults in the fasted state. The mean oral bioavailability is 64%. The oral bioavailability and C_{max} are not influenced by a standard meal. Safety and efficacy were demonstrated in clinical trials where the 10 mg film-coated tablet was administered without regard to the timing of food ingestion.

For the 5 mg chewable tablet, the C_{max} is achieved in 2 hours after administration in adults in the fasted state. The mean oral bioavailability is 73% and is decreased to 63% by a standard meal.

Distribution: Montelukast is more than 99% bound to plasma proteins. The steady-state volume of distribution of montelukast averages 8–11 litres. Studies in rats with radiolabelled montelukast indicate minimal distribution across the blood-brain barrier. In addition, concentrations of radiolabelled material at 24 hours post-dose were minimal in all other tissues.

Biotransformation: Montelukast is extensively metabolised. In studies with therapeutic doses, plasma concentrations of metabolites of montelukast are undetectable at steady state in adults and children.

In vitro studies using human liver microsomes indicate that cytochromes P450 3A4, 2A6 and 2C9 are involved in the metabolism of montelukast. Based on further *in vitro* results in human liver microsomes, therapeutic plasma concentrations of montelukast do not inhibit cytochromes P450 3A4, 2C9, 1A2, 2A6, 2C19 or 2D6. The contribution of metabolites to the therapeutic effect of montelukast is minimal.

Elimination: The plasma clearance of montelukast averages 45 ml/min in healthy adults. Following an oral dose of radiolabelled montelukast, 86% of the radioactivity was recovered in 5-day faecal collections and <0.2% was recovered in urine. Coupled with estimates of montelukast oral bioavailability, this indicates that montelukast and its metabolites are excreted almost exclusively via the bile.

Characteristics in patients: No dosage adjustment is necessary for the elderly, or mild to moderate hepatic insufficiency. Studies in patients with renal impairment have not been undertaken. Because montelukast and its metabolites are eliminated by the biliary route, no dose adjustment is anticipated to be necessary in patients with renal impairment. There are no data on the pharmacokinetics of montelukast in patients with severe hepatic insufficiency (Child-Pugh score >9).

With high doses of montelukast (20- and 60-fold the recommended adult dose), a decrease in plasma theophylline concentration was observed. This effect was not seen at the recommended dose of 10 mg once daily.

Preclinical safety data: In animal toxicity studies, minor serum biochemical alterations in ALT, glucose, phosphorus and triglycerides were observed which were transient in nature. The signs of toxicity in animals were increased excretion of saliva, gastro-intestinal symptoms, loose stools and ion imbalance. These occurred at dosages which provided >17-fold the systemic exposure seen at the clinical dosage. In monkeys, the adverse effects appeared at doses from 150 mg/kg/day (>232-fold the systemic exposure seen at the clinical dose). In animal studies, montelukast did not affect fertility or reproductive performace at systemic exposure exceeding the clinical systemic exposure by greater than 24-fold. A slight decrease in pup body weight was noted in the female fertility study in rats at 200 mg/kg/day (>69-fold the clinical systemic exposure). In studies in rabbits, a higher incidence of incomplete ossification, compared with concurrent control animals, was seen at systemic exposure >24-fold the clinical systemic exposure seen at the clinical dose. No abnormalities were seen in rats.

Montelukast was determined not to be phototoxic in mice for UVA, UVB or visible light spectra at doses up to 500 mg/kg/day (approximately >200-fold based on systemic exposure).

Montelukast was neither mutagenic in *in vitro* and *in vivo* tests nor tumorigenic in *in vivo* tests in rodent species.

Pharmaceutical particulars

List of excipients: 5 mg chewable tablet:

Mannitol (E421), microcrystalline cellulose (E460), hydroxypropyl cellulose, red ferric oxide (E172) (colouring agent) croscarmellose sodium, cherry flavour, apartame (E951) and magnesium stearate (E572).

10 mg film-coated tablet:

Microsrystalline cellulose (E460), lactose monohydrate (89.3 mg), croscarmellose sodium, hydroxypropyl cellulose, and magnesium stearate (E572).

Film coating: hypromellose, hydroxypropyl cellulose, titanium dioxide (E171) (colouring agent), red and yellow ferric oxide (E172) (colouring agent) and carnauba wax.

Incompatibilities: None.

Shelf life: 5 mg chewable tablet: 2 years.

10 mg film-coated tablet: 2 years.

Special precautions for storage: Store below 30°C, protected from moisture and light.

Nature and contents of container: Polyamide/PVC/aluminium blister pack enclosed in a cardboard carton containing 28 tablets.

Instructions for use/handling: No particulars.

Marketing authorisation numbers

5 mg Chewable Tablet: PL 0025/0357
10 mg Tablet: PL 0025/0358

Date of first authorisation/renewal of authorisation 15 January 1998.

Date of (partial) revision of text N/A.

Legal catgegory POM.

SODIUM PARA-AMINOHIPPURATE

Presentation A clear, colourless to slightly yellow solution for intravenous injection, containing in each 10 ml of sterile solution 2 g sodium para-aminohippurate. Inactive ingredient: Sodium Hydroxide BP.

Uses As a diagnostic agent for the estimation of effective renal plasma flow (RPF). In research procedures, for the measurement of the functional capacity of the renal tubular secretory mechanism (Tm_{PAH}).

Dosage and administration For intravenous use only.

For the measurement of RPF, the concentration of sodium para-aminohippurate in the plasma is maintained at 2 mg per 100 ml. As a research procedure for the measurement of Tm_{PAH}, the plasma level of sodium para-aminohippurate must be sufficient to saturate the capacity of the tubular secretory cells. Concentrations of from 40 to 60 mg per 100 ml are necessary.

Contra-indications, warnings, etc
Contra-indication
Hypersensitivity to this product or its components.

Precautions: Intravenous solutions must be administered with caution in patients with low cardiac reserve, since a rapid increase in plasma volume can precipitate congestive heart failure.

For measurement of RPF, small doses of sodium para-aminohippurate are used. However, in research procedures for Tm_{PAH} determinations high plasma levels are required to saturate the capacity of the tubular cells. During these procedures the intravenous administration of sodium para-aminohippurate solutions should be carried out slowly and with caution. The patient should be continuously observed for any adverse reactions.

Renal clearance measurement of sodium para-aminohippurate cannot be made with any significant accuracy in patients receiving sulphonamides, procaine or thiazolesulphone. These compounds interfere with chemical colour development essential to the analytical procedures.

Probenecid depresses tubular secretion of certain weak acids such as sodium para-aminohippurate; therefore, patients receiving probenecid will have erroneously low RPF and Tm_{PAH} values. Clearance is also affected by penicillins and salicylates.

Pregnancy and lactation: Animal reproduction studies have not been conducted with sodium para-aminohippurate. It is also not known whether sodium para-aminohippurate can cause fetal harm when administered to a pregnant woman or can affect reproduction capacity. Sodium Para-aminohippurate should be given to a pregnant woman only if clearly needed.

It is not known whether this drug is excreted in human milk. Because many drugs are excreted in human milk, caution should be exercised when Sodium Para-aminohippurate is administered to a breast-feeding woman.

Side-effects: Vasomotor disturbances, flushing, tingling, nausea, vomiting, cramps. Patients may have a sensation of warmth or the desire to defaecate or urinate during or shortly after the administration of a primary dose.

Overdosage: The dose is carefully controlled by experiment; no data are available on the symptoms of overdosage. No antidote is available.

The biological half-life of sodium para-aminohippurate is 10.2 minutes.

Pharmaceutical precautions No special requirements.

Legal category POM.

Package quantities Vials of 10 ml.

Further information Methods of calculating renal function are to be found in the package leaflet.

Product licence number 0025/5080.

TIMOPTOL*

Presentation Clear, colourless to light yellow, sterile eye drops containing Timolol Maleate PhEur equivalent to 0.25% and 0.5% w/v solution of timolol. Each concentration is presented in:

Metered-dose Ocumeter* Dispensers containing 5 ml Ophthalmic Solution Timoptol with preservative.

Uses Timoptol Ophthalmic Solution is a beta-adrenoreceptor blocking agent used topically in the reduction of elevated intra-ocular pressure in various conditions including the following: patients with ocular hypertension; patients with chronic open-angle glaucoma including aphakic patients; some patients with secondary glaucoma.

Dosage and administration Recommended therapy is one drop 0.25% solution in the affected eye twice a day.

If clinical response is not adequate, dosage may be changed to one drop 0.5% solution in each affected eye twice a day. If needed, Timoptol may be used with other agent(s) for lowering intra-ocular pressure. The use of two topical beta-adrenergic blocking agents is not recommended (see *Precautions*).

Intra-ocular pressure should be reassessed approximately four weeks after starting treatment because response to Timoptol may take a few weeks to stabilise.

Provided that the intra-ocular pressure is maintained at satisfactory levels, many patients can then be placed on once-a-day therapy.

Transfer from other agents: When another topical beta-blocking agent is being used, discontinue its use after a full day of therapy and start treatment with Timoptol the next day with one drop of 0.25% Timoptol in each affected eye twice a day. The dosage may be increased to one drop of 0.5% solution in each affected eye twice a day if the response is not adequate.

When transferring a patient from a single anti-glaucoma agent other than a topical beta-blocking agent, continue the agent and add one drop of 0.25% Timoptol in each affected eye twice a day. On the following day, discontinue the previous agent completely, and continue with Timoptol. If a higher dosage of Timoptol is required, substitute one drop of 0.5% solution in each affected eye twice a day (see 'Further information').

Paediatric use is not currently recommended.

Use in the elderly: There has been wide experience with the use of timolol maleate in elderly patients. The dosage recommendations above reflect the clinical data derived from this experience.

Contra-indications, warnings, etc
Contra-indications: Bronchial asthma, history of bronchial asthma, or severe chronic obstructive pulmonary disease; sinus bradycardia, second and third degree AV block, overt cardiac failure, cardiogenic shock; and hypersensitivity to this product or other beta-blocking agents.

Precautions: Like other topically applied ophthalmic drugs, Timoptol may be absorbed systemically and adverse reactions seen with oral beta-blockers may occur.

Cardiac failure should be adequately controlled before beginning therapy with Timoptol. Patients with a history of severe cardiac disease should be watched for signs of cardiac failure and have their pulse rates checked.

Respiratory and cardiac reactions, including death due to bronchospasm in patients with asthma and, rarely, death associated with cardiac failure have been reported.

The effect on intra-ocular pressure or the known effects of systemic beta-blockade may be exaggerated when Timoptol is given to patients already receiving a systemic beta-blocking agent. The response of these patients should be closely observed. The use of two two topical beta-adrenergic blocking agents is not recommended.

There have been reports of skin rashes and/or dry eyes associated with the use of beta-adrenoreceptor blocking drugs. The reported incidence is small and in most cases the symptoms have cleared when treatment was withdrawn. Discontinuation of the drug should be considered if any such reaction is not otherwise explicable. Cessation of therapy involving beta-blockade should be gradual.

Choroidal detachment has been reported with administration of aqueous suppresant therapy (e.g. timolol, acetazolamide) after filtration procedures.

The Ocumeter Dispenser of Timoptol contains benzalkonium chloride as a preservative which may be deposited in soft contact lenses; therefore, Timoptol should not be used while wearing these lenses. The lenses should be removed before application of the drops and not reinserted earlier than 15 minutes after use.

Timoptol has been generally well tolerated in glaucoma patients wearing conventional hard contact lenses. Timoptol has not been studied in patients wearing lenses made with material other than polymethylmethacrylate (PMMA), which is used to make hard contact lenses.

In patients with angle-closure glaucoma, the immediate objective of treatment is to reopen the angle. This requires constricting the pupil with a miotic. Timoptol has little or no effect on the pupil. When Timoptol is used to reduce elevated intraocular pressure in angle closure glaucoma it should be used with a miotic and not alone.

Patients should be instructed to avoid allowing the tip of the dispensing container to contact the eye or surrounding structures.

Patients should also be instructed that ocular solutions, if handled improperly, can become contaminated by common bacteria known to cause ocular infections. Serious damage to the eye and subsequent loss of vision may result from using contaminated solutions.

Patients should also be advised that if they develop an intercurrent ocular condition (e.g. trauma, ocular surgery or infection), they should immediately seek their physician's advice concerning the continued use of the present multidose container.

There have been reports of bacterial keratitis associated with the use of multiple dose containers of topical ophthalmic products. These containers had been inadvertently contaminated by patients who, in most cases, had a concurrent corneal disease or disruption of the ocular epithelial surface.

Risk from anaphylactic reaction: While taking beta-blockers, patients with a history of atopy or a history of severe anaphylactic reaction to a variety of allergens may be more reactive to repeated challenge with such allergens, either accidental, diagnostic or therapeutic. Such patients may be unresponsive to the usual doses of adrenaline used to treat anaphylactic reactions.

Drug interactions: Although Timoptol alone has little or no effect on pupil size, mydriasis has occasionally been reported when Timoptol is given with adrenaline.

Potentiated systemic beta-blockade (e.g. decreased heart rate) has been reported during combined treatment with quinidine and timolol, possibly because quinidine inhibits the metabolism of timolol via the P-450 enzyme, CYP2D6.

Close observation of the patient is recommended when a beta-blocker is administered to patients receiving catecholamine-depleting drugs such as reserpine, because of possible additive effects and the production of hypotension and/or marked bradycardia, which may produce vertigo, syncope, or postural hypotension.

Timoptol may potentially add to the effects of oral calcium antagonists, rauwolfia alkaloids or beta-blockers to induce hypotension and/or marked bradycardia.

Oral calcium antagonists may be used in combination with beta-adrenergic blocking agents when heart function is normal, but should be avoided in patients with impaired cardiac function.

The potential exists for hypotension, AV conduction disturbances and left ventricular failure to occur in patients receiving a beta-blocking agent when an oral calcium entry blocker is added to the treatment regimen. The nature of any cardiovascular adverse effect tends to depend on the type of calcium blocker used. Dihydropyridine derivatives, such as nifedipine, may lead to hypotension, whereas verapamil or diltiazem have a greater propensity to lead to AV conduction disturbances or left ventricular failure when used with a beta-blocker.

Intravenous calcium entry blockers should be used with caution in patients receiving beta-adrenergic blocking agents.

The concomitant use of beta-adrenergic blocking agents and digitalis with either diltiazem or verapamil may have additive effects in prolonging AV conduction time.

Breast-feeding mothers: Timoptol is detectable in human milk. A decision for breast-feeding mothers either to stop taking Timoptol or stop nursing should be based on the importance of the drug to the mother.

Use in pregnancy: Timoptol has not been studied in human pregnancy. The use of Timoptol requires that the anticipated benefit be weighed against possible hazards.

Side-effects: Timoptol is usually well tolerated.

Special senses: Signs and symptoms of ocular irritation, including burning and stinging, conjunctivitis, blepharitis, keratitis, decreased corneal sensitivity and dry eyes. Tinnitus, visual disturbances, including refractive changes (due to withdrawal of miotic therapy in some cases), diplopia, and ptosis and choroidal detachment following filtration surgery (see *Precautions*).

Cardiovascular: Bradycardia, arrhythmia, hypotension, syncope, heart block, cerebrovascular accident, cerebral ischaemia, congestive heart failure, palpitation, cardiac arrest, oedema, claudication, Raynaud's phenomenon, cold hands and feet.

Respiratory: Bronchospasm (predominantly in patients with pre-existing bronchospastic disease), respiratory failure, dyspnoea, cough.

Body as a whole: Headache, asthenia, fatigue, chest pain.

Integumentary: Alopecia, psoriasiform rash or exacerbation of psoriasis.

Hypersensitivity: Signs and symptoms of allergic reactions including angioedema, urticaria, localised and generalised rash.

Nervous system/psychiatric: Dizziness, depression, insomnia, nightmares, memory loss, increase in signs and symptoms of myasthenia gravis, paresthesia.

Digestive: Nausea, diarrhoea, dyspepsia, dry mouth.

Urogential: Decreased libido, Peyronie's disease.

Immunologic: Systemic lupus erythematosus.

Causal relationship unknown: The following adverse effects have been reported, but a causal relationship to Timoptol has not been established; aphakic cystoid macular oedema, nasal congestion, anorexia, CNS effects (e.g. behavioural changes including confusion, hallucinations, anxiety, disorientation, nervousness, somnolence, and other psychiatric disturbances), hypertension, retroperitoneal fibrosis and pseudopemphigoid.

The adverse reactions seen with systemic timolol maleate may occur with Timoptol.

Potential side effects: The following additional side effects have been reported in clinical experiences with systemic timolol maleate, and may be considered potential effects of ophthalmic timolol maleate:

Body as a whole: extremity pain, decreased exercise tolerance.

Cardiovascular: AV block (2nd or 3rd degree),

sinoatrial block, pulmonary oedema, worsening of arterial insufficiency, worsening of angina pectoris, vasodilation.

Digestive: vomiting.

Endocrine: hyperglycemia, hypoglycemia.

Integumentary: pruritus, sweating, exfoliative dermatitis.

Musculoskeletal: arthralgia.

Nervous system: vertigo, local weakness.

Psychiatric: diminished concentration, increased dreaming.

Haematologic: nonthrombocytopenic purpura.

Respiratory: rales.

Urogenital: impotence, micturition difficulties.

Overdosage: There have been reports of inadvertent overdosage with Timoptol resulting in systemic effects, similar to those seen with systemic beta-adrenergic blocking agents, such as dizziness, headache, shortness of breath, bradycardia, bronchospasm, and cardiac arrest (see also *Side effects*). If overdosage occurs, the following measures should be considered:

1. Gastric lavage, if ingested. Studies have shown that timolol does not dialyse readily.
2. Symptomatic bradycardia: Atropine sulphate, 0.25 to 2 mg intravenously, should be used to induce vagal blockade. If bradycardia persists, intravenous isoprenaline hydrochloride should be administered cautiously. In refractory cases, the use of a cardiac pacemaker may be considered.
3. Hypotension: A sympathomimetic pressor agent such as dopamine, dobutamine or noradrenaline should be used. In refractory cases, the use of glucagon has been reported to be useful.
4. Bronchospasm: Isoprenaline hydrochloride should be used. Additional therapy with aminophylline may be considered.
5. Acute cardiac failure: Conventional therapy with digitalis, diuretics, and oxygen should be instituted immediately. In refractory cases, the use of intravenous aminophylline is suggested. This may be followed, if necessary, by glucagon which has been reported useful.
6. Heart block (second or third degree): Isoprenaline hydrochloride or a pacemaker should be used.

Pharmaceutical precautions Timoptol is stable at room temperature. Protect from light. Timoptol Metered-dose should be discarded one month after first opening.

Legal category POM.

Package quantities Both the 0.25% and 0.5% w/v solution are presented in:
Special metered-dose Ocumeter* Dispensers, each containing 5 ml.

Further information Unlike miotics, Timoptol reduces IOP with little or no effect on accommodation or pupil size. In patients with cataracts, the inability to see around lenticular opacities when the pupil is constricted is avoided. When changing patients from miotics to Timoptol a refraction might be necessary when these effects of the miotic have passed.

Diminished response after prolonged therapy with Timoptol has been reported in some patients.

Product licence numbers

0.25% Ophthalmic Solution 5 ml Ocumeter	0025/0134
0.5% Ophthalmic Solution 5 ml Ocumeter	0025/0135

TIMOPTOL* OPHTHALMIC SOLUTION UNIT DOSE

Qualitative and quantitative composition Timoptol Ophthalmic Solution Unit Dose 0.25% contains timolol maleate PhEur equivalent to 0.25% w/v solution of timolol without preservative.

Timoptol Ophthalmic Solution Unit Dose 0.5% contains timolol maleate PhEur equivalent to 0.5% w/v solution of timolol without preservative.

Pharmaceutical form Clear, colourless to light yellow, sterile eye drops.

Clinical particulars

Therapeutic indications: Timoptol Ophthalmic Solution is a beta-adrenoreceptor blocking agent used topically in the reduction of elevated intra-ocular pressure in various conditions including the following: patients with ocular hypertension; patients with chronic open-angle glaucoma including aphakic patients; some patients with secondary glaucoma.

Posology and method of administration: Recommended therapy is one drop 0.25% solution in the affected eye twice a day.

If clinical response is not adequate, dosage may be changed to one drop 0.5% solution in each affected eye twice a day. If needed, Timoptol may be used with other agent(s) for lowering intra-ocular pressure. The use of two topical beta-adrenergic blocking agents is not recommended (see *Special warnings and special precautions for use*).

Intra-ocular pressure should be reassessed approximately four weeks after starting treatment because response to Timoptol may take a few weeks to stabilise.

Provided that the intra-ocular pressure is maintained at satisfactory levels, many patients can then be placed on once-a-day therapy.

Transfer from other agents: When another topical beta-blocking agent is being used, discontinue its use after a full day of therapy and start treatment with Timoptol the next day with one drop of 0.25% Timoptol in each affected eye twice a day. The dosage may be increased to one drop of 0.5% solution in each affected eye twice a day if the response is not adequate.

When transferring a patient from a single anti-glaucoma agent other than a topical beta-blocking agent, continue the agent and add one drop of 0.25% Timoptol in each affected eye twice a day. On the following day, discontinue the previous agent completely, and continue with Timoptol. If a higher dosage of Timoptol is required, substitute one drop of 0.5% solution in each affected eye twice a day.

Timoptol Unit dose: The Unit-dose Dispenser of Timoptol is free from preservative and should be used for patients who may be sensitive to the preservative benzalkonium chloride, or when use of a preservative-free topical medication is advisable.

Timoptol Unit-dose is a sterile solution. The solution from one individual unit is to be used immediately after opening for administration to one or both eyes. Since sterility cannot be maintained after the individual unit is opened, the remaining contents should be discarded immediately after administration.

Paediatric use: Is not currently recommended.

Use in the elderly: There has been wide experience with the use of timolol maleate in elderly patients. The dosage recommendations above reflect the clinical data derived from this experience.

Contra-indications: Bronchial asthma, history of bronchial asthma, or severe chronic obstructive pulmonary disease; sinus bradycardia, second- and third-degree AV block, overt cardiac failure, cardiogenic shock; and hypersensitivity to this product or other beta-blocking agents.

Special warnings and special precautions for use: Like other topically applied ophthalmic drugs, Timoptol may be absorbed systemically and adverse reactions seen with oral beta-blockers may occur.

Cardiac failure should be adequately controlled before beginning therapy with Timoptol. Patients with a history of severe cardiac disease should be watched for signs of cardiac failure and have their pulse rates checked.

Respiratory and cardiac reactions, including death due to bronchospasm in patients with asthma and, rarely, death associated with cardiac failure have been reported.

The effect on intra-ocular pressure or the known effects of systemic beta-blockade may be exaggerated when Timoptol is given to patients already receiving a systemic beta-blocking agent. The response of these patients should be closely observed. The use of two topical beta-adrenergic blocking agents is not recommended.

There have been reports of skin rashes and/or dry eyes associated with the use of beta-adrenoreceptor blocking drugs. The reported incidence is small and in most cases the symptoms have cleared when treatment was withdrawn. Discontinuation of the drug should be considered if any such reaction is not otherwise explicable. Cessation of therapy involving beta-blockade should be gradual.

Choroidal detachment has been reported with administration of aqueous suppressant therapy (e.g. timolol, acetazolamide) after filtration procedures.

Timoptol has been generally well tolerated in glaucoma patients wearing conventional hard contact lenses. Timoptol has not been studied in patients wearing lenses made with material other than polymethylmethacrylate (PMMA), which is used to make hard contact lenses.

The Unit-dose Dispenser of Timoptol is free from preservative and should, therefore, be discarded after single use to one or both eyes.

In patients with angle-closure glaucoma, the immediate objective of treatment is to reopen the angle. This requires constricting the pupil with a miotic. Timoptol has little or no effect on the pupil. When Timoptol is used to reduce elevated intra-ocular pressure in angle-closure glaucoma it should be used with a miotic and not alone.

Patients should be advised that if they develop an intercurrent ocular condition (e.g. trauma, ocular surgery or infection), they should immediately seek their physician's advice concerning the continued use of the present multidose container (see *Instructions for use/handling*).

There have been reports of bacterial keratitis associated with the use of multiple dose containers of topical ophthalmic products. These containers had been inadvertently contaminated by patients who, in most cases, had a concurrent corneal disease or disruption of the ocular epithelial surface.

Risk from anaphylactic reaction: While taking beta-blockers, patients with a history of atopy or a history of severe anaphylactic reaction to a variety of allergens may be more reactive to repeated challenge with such allergens, either accidental, diagnostic or therapeutic. Such patients may be unresponsive to the usual doses of adrenaline used to treat anaphylactic reactions.

Interactions with other medicaments and other forms of interaction: Although Timoptol alone has little or no effect on pupil size, mydriasis has occasionally been reported when Timoptol is given with adrenaline.

Potentiated systemic beta-blockade (e.g. decreased heart rate) has been reported during combined treatment with quinidine and timolol, possibly because quinidine inhibits the metabolism of timolol via the P-450 enzyme, CYP2D6.

Timoptol may potentially add to the effects of oral calcium antagonists, rauwolfia alkaloids or beta-blockers to induce hypotension and/or marked bradycardia.

Close observation of the patient is recommended when a beta-blocker is administered to patients receiving catecholamine-depleting drugs such as reserpine, because of possible additive effects and the production of hypotension and/or marked bradycardia, which may produce vertigo, syncope, or postural hypotension.

Oral calcium antagonists may be used in combination with beta-adrenergic blocking agents when heart function is normal, but should be avoided in patients with impaired cardiac function.

The potential exists for hypotension, AV conduction disturbances and left ventricular failure to occur in patients receiving a beta-blocking agent when an oral calcium entry blocker is added to the treatment regimen. The nature of any cardiovascular adverse effect tends to depend on the type of calcium blocker used. Dihydropyridine derivatives, such as nifedipine, may lead to hypotension, whereas verapamil or diltiazem have a greater propensity to lead to AV conduction disturbances or left ventricular failure when used with a beta-blocker.

Intravenous calcium entry blockers should be used with caution in patients receiving beta-adrenergic blocking agents.

The concomitant use of beta-adrenergic blocking agents and digitalis with either diltiazem or verapamil may have additive effects in prolonging AV conduction time.

Pregnancy and lactation

Use in pregnancy: Timoptol has not been studied in human pregnancy. The use of Timoptol requires that the anticipated benefit be weighed against possible hazards.

Breast-feeding mothers: Timoptol is detectable in human milk. A decision for breast-feeding mothers either to stop taking Timoptol or stop nursing should be based on the importance of the drug to the mother.

Effects on the ability to drive and use machines: Possible side effects such as dizziness and visual disturbances may affect some patients' ability to drive or operate machinery.

Undesirable effects: Side effects: Timoptol is usually well tolerated. The following adverse reactions have been reported with ocular administration of this or other timolol maleate formulations, either in clinical trials or since the drug has been marketed.

Special senses: Signs and symptoms of ocular irritation, including burning and stinging, conjunctivitis, blepharitis, keratitis, dry eyes, and decreased corneal sensitivity. Tinnitus, visual disturbances, including refractive changes (due to withdrawal of miotic therapy in some cases), diplopia, and ptosis and choroidal detachment following filtration surgery (see *Special warnings and special precautions for use*).

Cardiovascular: Bradycardia, arrhythmia, hypotension, syncope, heart block, cerebrovascular accident, cerebral ischaemia, congestive heart failure, palpitation, cardiac arrest, oedema, claudication, Raynaud's phenomenon, cold hands and feet.

Respiratory: Bronchospasm (predominantly in patients with pre-existing bronchospastic disease), respiratory failure, dyspnoea, cough.

Body as a whole: Headache, asthenia, fatigue, chest pain.

Integumentary: Alopecia, psoriasiform rash or exacerbation of psoriasis.

Hypersensitivity: Signs and symptoms of allergic reactions including angioedema, urticaria, localised and generalised rash.

Nervous system/psychiatric: Dizziness, depression, insomnia, nightmares, memory loss, increase in signs and symptoms of myasthenia gravis, paresthesia.

Digestive: Nausea, diarrhoea, dyspepsia, dry mouth.

Urogenital: Decreased libido, Peyronie's disease.

Immunologic: Systemic lupus erythematosus.

Causal relationship unknown: The following adverse effects have been reported, but a causal relationship to Timoptol has not been established: aphakic cystoid macular oedema, nasal congestion, anorexia, CNS effects (e.g. behavioural changes including confusion, hallucinations, anxiety, disorientation, nervousness, somnolence, and other psychiatric disturbances), hypertension, and retroperitoneal fibrosis and pseudopemphigoid.

The adverse reactions seen with oral timolol maleate may occur with Timoptol.

Potential side effects: The following additional side effects have been reported in clinical experiences with systemic timolol maleate, and may be considered potential effects of ophthalmic timolol maleate:

Body as a whole: extremity pain, decreased exercise tolerance.

Cardiovascular: AV block (2nd or 3rd degree), sinoatrial block, pulmonary oedema, worsening of arterial insufficiency, worsening of angina pectoris, vasodilation.

Digestive: vomiting.

Endocrine: hyperglycemia, hypoglycemia.

Integumentary: pruritus, sweating, exfoliative dermatitis.

Musculoskeletal: arthralgia.

Nervous system: vertigo, local weakness.

Psychiatric: diminished concentration, increased dreaming.

Haematologic: nonthrombocytopenic purpura.

Respiratory: rales.

Urogenital: impotence, micturition difficulties.

Overdosage: There have been reports of inadvertent overdosage with Timoptol resulting in systemic effects, similar to those seen with systemic beta-adrenergic blocking agents, such as dizziness, headache, shortness of breath, bradycardia, bronchospasm, and cardiac arrest (see also *Side effects*).

If overdosage occurs, the following measures should be considered:

1. Gastric lavage, if ingested. Studies have shown that timolol does not dialyse readily.
2. Symptomatic bradycardia: Atropine sulphate, 0.25 to 2 mg intravenously, should be used to induce vagal blockade. If bradycardia persists, intravenous isoprenaline hydrochloride should be administered cautiously. In refractory cases, the use of a cardiac pacemaker may be considered.
3. Hypotension: A sympathomimetic pressor agent such as dopamine, dobutamine or noradrenaline should be used. In refractory cases, the use of glucagon has been reported to be useful.
4. Bronchospasm: Isoprenaline hydrochloride should be used. Additional therapy with aminophylline may be considered.
5. Acute cardiac failure: Conventional therapy with digitalis, diuretics, and oxygen should be instituted immediately. In refractory cases, the use of intravenous aminophylline is suggested. This may be followed, if necessary, by glucagon which has been reported useful.
6. Heart block (second- or third-degree): Isoprenaline hydrochloride or a pacemaker should be used.

Pharmacological properties

Pharmacodynamic properties: Timolol maleate is a non selective beta-adrenergic receptor blocking agent that does not have significant intrinsic sympathomimetic, direct myocardial depressant, or local anaesthetic activity. Timolol maleate combines reversibly with the beta-adrenergic receptor, and this inhibits the usual biologic response that would occur with stimulation of that receptor. This specific competitive antagonism blocks stimulation of the beta-adrenergic stimulating (agonist) activity, whether these originate from an endogenous or exogenous source. Reversal of this blockade can be accomplished by increasing the concentration of the agonist which will restore the usual biological response.

Unlike miotics, Timoptol reduces IOP with little or no effect on accommodation or pupil size. In patients with cataracts, the inability to see around lenticular opacities when the pupil is constricted is avoided. When changing patients from miotics to Timoptol a refraction might be necessary when the effects of the miotic have passed.

Diminished response after prolonged therapy with Timoptol has been reported in some patients.

Pharmacokinetic properties: The onset of reduction in intra-ocular pressure can be detected within one-half hour after a single dose. The maximum effect occurs in one or two hours; significant lowering of IOP can be maintained for as long as 24 hours with a single dose.

Preclinical safety data: No adverse ocular effects were observed in rabbits and dogs administered Timoptol topically in studies lasting one and two years, respectively. The oral LD_{50} of the drug is 1190 and 900 mg/kg in female mice and female rats, respectively.

Carcinogenesis, mutagenesis, impairment of fertility: In a two-year oral study of timolol maleate in rats there was a statistically significant ($p \leq 0.05$) increase in the incidence of adrenal pheochromocytomas in male rats administered 300 mg/kg/day (300 times the maximum recommended human oral dose.) Similar differences were not observed in rats administered oral doses equivalent to 25 or 100 times the maximum recommended human oral dose.

In a lifetime oral study in mice, there were statistically significant ($p \leq 0.05$) increases in the incidence of benign and malignant pulmonary tumours, benign uterine polyps and mammary adenocarcinoma in female mice at 500 mg/kg/day (500 times the maximum recommended human dose), but not at 5 or 50 mg/kg/day. In a subsequent study in female mice, in which post-mortem examinations were limited to uterus and lungs, a statistically significant increase in the incidence of pulmonary tumours was again observed at 500 mg/kg/day.

The increased occurrence of mammary adenocarcinoma was associated with elevations in serum prolactin which occurred in female mice administered timolol at 500 mg/kg/day, but not at doses of 5 or 50 mg/kg/day. An increased incidence of mammary adenocarcinomas in rodents has been associated with administration of several other therapeutic agents which elevate serum prolactin, but no correlation between serum prolactin levels and mammary tumors has been established in man. Furthermore, in adult human female subjects who received oral dosages of up to 60 mg of timolol maleate, the maximum recommended human oral dosage, there were no clinically meaningful changes in serum prolactin.

Timolol maleate was devoid of mutagenic potential when evaluated *in vivo* (mouse) in the micronucleus test and cytogenetic assay (doses up to 800 mg/kg) and *in vitro* in a neoplastic cell transformation assay (up to 100 mcg/ml). In Ames tests the highest concentrations of timolol employed, 5000 or 10,000 mcg/plate, were associated with statistically significant ($p \leq 0.05$) elevations of revertants observed with tester strain TA1OO (in seven replicate assays) but not in the remaining three strains. In the assays with tester strain TA1OO, no consistent dose-response relationship was observed, nor did the ratio of test to control revertants reach 2. A ratio of 2 is usually considered the criterion for a positive Ames test.

Reproduction and fertility studies in rats showed no adverse effect on male or female fertility at doses up to 150 times the maximum recommended human oral dose.

Pharmaceutical particulars

List of excipients: Timoptol Ophthalmic Solution Unit Dose contains the following inactive ingredients:

Disodium phosphate dihydrate PhEur; Sodium dihydrogen phosphate dihydrate PhEur; Sodium hydroxide PhEur.

Incompatibilities: None known.

Shelf life: 36 months.

Timoptol Ophthalmic Solution Unit Dose should be used immediately after opening and any remaining contents should be discarded immediately after administration.

Special precautions for storage: Store below 25°C and protect from light.

Nature and content of the container: Both the 0.25% and the 0.5% w/v solutions are presented in:

Unit-dose Dispensers, available in cartons of 30 unit doses.

Instructions for use/handling: Patients should be instructed to avoid allowing the tip of the dispensing container to contact the eye or surrounding structures.

Patients should also be instructed that ocular solutions, if handled improperly, can become contaminated by common bacteria known to cause ocular infections. Serious damage to the eye and subsequent loss of vision may result from using contaminated solutions.

Marketing authorisation numbers

0.25% Ophthalmic Solution, 0.20 ml Unit Dose, 0025/0210

0.5% Ophthalmic Solution, 0.20 ml Unit Dose, 0025/0211

Date of first authorisation/renewal

0.25% Ophthalmic Solution Unit Dose

Granted: 17 March 1992

Last renewed: 21 March 1997

0.5% Ophthalmic Solution Unit Dose

Granted: 17 March 1992

Last renewed: 21 March 1997

Date of (partial) revision of text June 1998.

Legal category POM.

TIMOPTOL*-LA ▼

Qualitative and quantitative composition Each millilitre of 0.25% w/v solution contains an amount of Timolol Maleate PhEur equivalent to 2.5 mg/ml timolol.

Each millilitre of 0.5% w/v solution contains an amount of Timolol Maleate PhEur equivalent to 5 mg/ml timolol.

Pharmaceutical form Sterile ophthalmic gel-forming solution.

Clinical particulars

Therapeutic indications: A beta-adrenoreceptor blocker used topically in the reduction of elevated intra-ocular pressure in various conditions including the following: patients with ocular hypertension; patients with chronic open-angle glaucoma including aphakic patients; some patients with secondary glaucoma.

Posology and method of administration: Invert the closed container and shake once before each use. It is not necessary to shake the container more than once.

Recommended therapy is one drop 0.25% solution in each affected eye once a day.

If clinical response is not adequate, dosage may be changed to one drop 0.5% solution in each affected eye once a day.

If needed, Timoptol-LA may be used with other agent(s) for lowering intra-ocular pressure. Other topically applied medication should be administered no less than 10 minutes before Timoptol-LA. The use of two topical beta-adrenergic blocking agents is not recommended (see *Special warnings and special precautions for use*).

Intra-ocular pressure should be reassessed approximately four weeks after starting treatment because response to Timoptol-LA may take a few weeks to stabilise.

Transfer from other agents: When transferring a patient from Timoptol to Timoptol-LA, discontinue Timoptol after a full day of therapy, starting treatment with the same concentration of Timoptol-LA on the following day.

When another topical beta-blocking agent is being used, discontinue its use after a full day of therapy and start treatment with Timoptol-LA the next day with one drop of 0.25% Timoptol-LA in each affected eye once a day. The dosage may be increased to one drop of 0.5% solution in each affected eye once a day if the response is not adequate.

When transferring a patient from a single anti-glaucoma agent other than a topical beta-blocking agent, continue the agent and add one drop of 0.25% Timoptol-LA in each affected eye once a day. On the following day, discontinue the previous agent completely, and continue with Timoptol-LA. If a higher dosage of Timoptol-LA is required, substitute one drop of 0.5% solution in each affected eye once a day (see 'Pharmacodynamic properties').

Paediatric use is not currently indicated.

Use in the elderly: There has been wide-experience with the use of timolol maleate in elderly patients. The dosage recommendations given above reflect the clinical data derived from this experience.

Contra-indications: Bronchial asthma, history of bronchial asthma or severe chronic obstructive pulmonary disease; sinus bradycardia, second- or third-degree AV block, overt cardiac failure, cardiogenic shock; and hypersensitivity to any component of this product or other beta-blocking agents. Timoptol-LA should not be used in patients wearing contact lenses as it has not been studied in these patients.

Special warnings and special precautions for use: Like other topically applied ophthalmic drugs, this drug may be absorbed systemically and adverse reactions seen with oral beta-blockers may occur.

Cardiac failure should be adequately controlled before beginning therapy with Timoptol LA. Patients with a history of severe cardiac disease should be watched for signs of cardiac failure and have their pulse rates monitored.

Respiratory and cardiac reactions, including death due to bronchospasm in patients with asthma and, rarely, death associated with cardiac failure, are potential complications of therapy with Timoptol-LA.

The effect on intra-ocular pressure or the known effects of systemic beta-blockade may be exaggerated when Timoptol-LA is given to patients already receiving a systemic beta-blocking agent. The response of these patients should be closely observed. The use of two topical beta-adrenergic blocking agents is not recommended.

There have been reports of skin rashes and/or dry eyes associated with the use of beta-adrenoreceptor blocking drugs. The reported incidence is small and in most cases the symptoms have cleared when treatment was withdrawn. Discontinuation of the drug should be considered if any such reaction is not otherwise explicable. Cessation of therapy involving beta-blockade should be gradual.

The dispenser of Timoptol-LA contains benzododecinium bromide as a preservative. In a clinical study, the time required to eliminate 50% of the gellan solution from the eye was up to 30 minutes.

In patients with angle-closure glaucoma, the immediate objective of treatment is to reopen the angle. This requires constricting the pupil with a miotic. Timoptol-LA has little or no effect on the pupil. When Timoptol-LA is used to reduce elevated intra-ocular pressure in angle-closure glaucoma it should be used with a miotic and not alone.

Choroidal detachment has been reported with administration of aqueous suppresant therapy (e.g. timolol, acetazolamide) after filtration procedures.

Transient blurred vision following instillation may occur, generally lasting from 30 seconds to 5 minutes, and in rare cases up to 30 minutes or longer. Blurred vision and potenial visual disturbances may impair the ability to perform hazardous tasks such as operating machinery or driving a motor vehicle.

Patients should be advised that if they develop an intercurrent ocular condition (e.g. trauma, ocular surgery or infection), they should immediately seek their physician's advice concerning the continued use of the present multidose container (see *Instructions for use/handling*).

There have been reports of bacterial keratitis associated with the use of multiple dose containers of topical ophthalmic products. These containers had been inadvertently contaminated by patients who, in most cases, had a concurrent corneal disease or a disruption of the ocular epithelial surface.

Risk from anaphylactic reactions: While taking beta-blockers, patients with a history of atopy or a history of severe anaphylactic reaction to a variety of allergens may be more reactive to repeated challenge with such allergens, either accidental, diagnostic, or therapeutic. Such patients may be unresponsive to the usual doses of adrenaline used to treat anaphylactic reactions.

Interactions with other medicaments and other forms of interaction: Although Timoptol alone has little or no effect on pupil size, mydriasis has occasionally been reported when Timoptol is given with adrenaline. The potential for mydriasis exists from concomitant therapy with Timoptol-LA and adrenaline.

Close observation of the patient is recommended when a beta-blocker is administered to patients receiving catecholamine-depleting drugs such as reserpine, because of possible additive effects and the production of hypotension and/or marked bradycardia, which may produce vertigo, syncope, or postural hypotension.

The potential exists for hypotension, atrioventricular (AV) conduction disturbances and left ventricular failure to occur in patients receiving a beta-blocking agent when an oral calcium-channel blocker is added to the treatment regimen. The nature of any cardiovascular adverse effect tends to depend on the type of calcium-channel blocker used. Dihydropyridine derivatives, such as nifedipine, may lead to hypotension, whereas verapamil or diltiazem have a greater propensity to lead to AV conduction disturbances or left ventricular failure when used with a beta-blocker.

The concomitant use of beta-adrenergic blocking agents and digitalis with either diltiazem or verapamil may have additive effects in prolonging AV conduction time.

Oral calcium-channel antagonists may be used in combination with beta-adrenergic blocking agents when heart function is normal, but should be avoided in patients with impaired cardiac function.

Intravenous calcium-channel blockers should be used with caution in patients receiving beta-adrenergic blocking agents.

Potentiated systemic beta-blockade (e.g. decreased heart rate) has been reported during combined treatment with quinidine and timolol, possibly because quinidine inhibits the metabolism of timolol via the P-450 enzyme, CYP2D6.

Pregnancy and lactation

Use in pregnancy: Timoptol-LA has not been studied in human pregnancy. The use of Timoptol-LA requires that the anticipated benefit be weighed against possible hazards.

Breast-feeding mothers: Timolol is detectable in human milk. Because of the potential for adverse reactions to Timoptol-LA in infants, a decison should be made whether to discontinue nursing or to discontinue the drug, taking into account the importance of the drug to the mother.

Effects on the ability to drive and use machines: Transient blurred vision following instillation may occur, generally lasting from 30 seconds to 5 minutes, and in rare cases, up to 30 minutes or longer. Blurred vision and potential visual disturbances may impair the ability to perform hazardous tasks such as operating machinery or driving a motor vehicle.

Undesirable effects

Side-effects: Timopotol-LA is usually well tolerated. The most frequent drug-related complaint in clinical studies was transient blurred vision (6.0%), lasting from 30 seconds to 5 minutes following instillation.

The following possibly, probably, or definitely drug-related adverse reactions occurred with frequency of at least 1% in parallel active treatment controlled clinical trials:

Ocular: Burning and stinging, discharge, foreign body sensation, itching.

The following side-effects reported with Timoptol, either in clinical trials or since the drug has been marketed, are potential side effects of Timoptol-LA.

Special senses: Signs and symptoms of ocular irritation, including conjunctivitis, blepharitis, keratitis, decreased corneal sensitivity and dry eyes. Tinnitus, visual disturbances, including refractive changes (due to withdrawal of miotic therapy in some cases), diplopia, and ptosis. Choroidal detachment following filtration surgery (see *Special warnings and special precautions for use*).

Cardiovascular: Bradycardia, arrhythmia, hypotension, syncope, heart block, cerebrovascular accident, cerebral ischaemia, congestive heart failure, palpitation, cardiac arrest, oedema, claudication, Raynaud's phenomenon, cold hands and feet.

Respiratory: Bronchospasm (predominantly in patients with pre-existing bronchospastic disease), respiratory failure, dyspnoea, cough.

Body as a whole: Headache, asthenia, fatigue, chest pain.

Integumentary: Alopecia, psoriasiform rash or exacerbation of psoriasis.

Hypersensitivity: Signs and symptoms of allergic reactions including angioedema, urticaria, localised and generalised rash.

Nervous system/psychiatric: Dizziness, depression, insomnia, nightmares, memory loss, paresthesia.

Neuromuscular: Increase in signs and symptoms of myasthenia gravis.

Digestive: Nausea, diarrhoea, dyspepsia, dry mouth.

Urogenital: Decreased libido, Peyronie's disease.

Immunonologic: Systemic lupus erythematosus.

Causal relationship unknown: The following adverse effects have been reported but a causal relationship to therapy with timolol maleate has not been established: aphakic cystoid macular oedema, nasal congestion, anorexia, CNS effects (e.g. behavioural changes including confusion, hallucinations, anxiety, disorientation, nervousness, somnolence, and other psychic disturbances), hypertension, retroperitoneal fibrosis and pseudopemphigoid.

Potential side-effects associated with systemic administration of timolol: The following additional side effects have been reported in clinical experiences with systemic timolol maleate, and may be considered potential effects of ophthalmic timolol maleate:

Body as a whole: Extremity pain, decreased exercise tolerance.

Cardiovascular: AV block (second- or third-degree), sino-atrial block, pulmonary oedema, worsening of arterial insufficiency, worsening of angina pectoris, vasodilatation.

Digestive: Vomiting.

Endocrine: Hyperglycaemia, hypoglycaemia.

Integumentary: Pruritus, sweating, exfoliative dermatitis.

Musculoskeletal: Arthralgia.

Nervous system: Vertigo, local weakness.

Psychiatric: Diminished concentration, increased dreaming.

Haematological: Non-thrombocytopenic purpura.

Respiratory: Rales.

Urogenital: Impotence, micturition difficulties.

Overdosage: There have been reports of inadvertent overdosage with Timoptol resulting in systemic effects similar to those seen with systemic beta-adrenergic blocking agents such as dizziness, headache, shortness of breath, bradycardia, bronchospasm, and cardiac arrest (see also *Side effects*). If overdosage occurs, the following measures should be considered:

1. Symptomatic bradycardia: atropine sulphate, 0.25 to 2 mg intravenously, should be used to induce vagal blockade. If bradycardia persists, intravenous isoprenaline hydrochloride should be administered cautiously. In refractory cases, the use of a cardiac pacemaker may be considered.

2. Hypotension: a sympathomimetic pressor agent such as dopamine, dobutamine or noradrenaline should be used. In refractory cases, the use of glucagon has been reported to be useful.

3. Bronchospasm: isoprenaline hydrochloride should be used. Additional therapy with aminophylline may be considered.

4. Acute cardiac failure: conventional therapy with digitalis, diuretics, and oxygen should be instituted immediately. In refractory cases, the use of intravenous aminophylline is suggested. This may be followed, if necessary, by glucagon, which has been reported useful.

5. Heart block (second- or third-degree): isoprenaline hydrochloride or a pacemaker should be used.

Timolol does not dialyse readily.

Pharmacological properties

Pharmacodynamic properties

Pharmacotherapeutic group: Beta-adrenergic receptor blocking agent.

Mechanism of action: The precise mechanism of action of timolol maleate in lowering intra-ocular pressure is not clearly established. A fluorescein study and tonography studies indicate that the predominant action may be related to reduced aqueous formation. However, in some studies a slight increase in outflow facility was also observed.

Timoptol-LA is a new ophthalmic formulation comprising timolol maleate and a new delivery vehicle. Gellan solution contains a highly purified anionic heteropolysaccharide derived from gellan gum. Aqueous solutions of gellan gum form a clear transparent gel at low polymer concentrations in the presence of cations. When Timoptol-LA contacts the precorneal tear film, it becomes a gel. Gellan gum increases the contact time of the drug with the eye.

Pharmacodynamics: In parallel active treatment controlled, double-masked, multiclinic studies in patients with untreated elevated intra-ocular pressure of greater than 22 mm Hg in one or both eyes, 0.25% and 0.5% Timoptol-LA administered once daily had an intra-ocular pressure-lowering effect equivalent to the same concentration of Timoptol administered twice daily (see table below).

For the five independent comparative studies listed in the table below, the entrance criterion was an intraocular pressure of greater than 22 mm Hg in one or both eyes after a washout period of one week for most antiglaucoma medications and up to three weeks for ophthalmic beta-adrenergic antagonists. The dosage used was one drop of Timoptol-LA in each affected eye once daily versus one drop of Timoptol in each affected eye twice daily.

Mean change in intra-ocular pressure (mm Hg) from baseline at trough (immediately before the morning dose) for the final week of the double-masked study

Concentration	*Timoptol-LA (n)*	*Timoptol (n)*	*Week*
0.25%	−5.8 (94)	−5.9 (96)	12
0.25%	−6.0 (74)	−5.9 (73)	12
0.50%	−8.3 (110)*	−8.2 (111)*	12
0.50%	−5.6 (189)	−6.3 (94)	24
0.50%	−6.4 (212)	−6.1 (109)	24

* The baseline intra-ocular pressure was elevated in comparison to the other studies due to the higher intra-ocular pressure of patients with pseudoexfoliative glaucoma.

Onset of action of timolol maleate is usually rapid, occurring approximately 20 minutes after topical application to the eye.

Maximum reduction of intra-ocular pressure occurs in two to four hours with Timoptol-LA. Significant lowering of intra-ocular pressure has been maintained for 24 hours with both 0.25% and 0.5% Timoptol-LA.

As compared with 0.5% Timoptol administered twice daily, in three clinical studies 0.5% Timoptol-LA administered once daily reduced mean heart rate less and produced bradycardia less frequently (see 'Special warnings and special precautions for use'). At trough (24 hours post-dose Timoptol-LA, 12 hours post-dose Timoptol), the mean reduction in heart rate was 0.8 beats/minute for Timoptol-LA and 3.6 beats/minute for Timoptol, whereas at two hours post-dose, the mean reduction was comparable (3.8 beats/minute for Timoptol-LA and 5 beats/minute for Timoptol).

Timolol maleate is a non-selective beta-adrenergic receptor blocking agent that does not have significant intrinsic sympathomimetic, direct myocardial depressant, or local anaesthetic (membrane-stabilising) activity.

Unlike miotics, timolol maleate reduces intra-ocular pressure with little or no effect on accommodation or pupil size. Thus, changes in visual acuity due to increased accommodation are uncommon, and the dim or blurred vision and night blindness produced by miotics are not evident. In addition, in patients with cataracts the inability to see around lenticular opacities when the pupil is constricted by miotics is avoided. When changing patients from miotics to Timoptol-LA, refraction may be necessary after the effects of the miotic have passed.

As with other antiglaucoma drugs, diminished responsiveness to timolol maleate after prolonged therapy has been reported in some patients. However, in clinical studies of Timoptol in which 164 patients were followed for at least three years, no significant difference in mean intra-ocular pressure was observed after initial stabilisation. This indicates that the intra-ocular pressure-lowering effects of timolol maleate is well maintained.

Pharmacokinetic properties: Onset of action of timolol maleate is usually rapid, occurring approximately 20 minutes after topical application to the eye.

Maximum reduction of intra-ocular pressure occurs in two to four hours with Timoptol-LA. Significant lowering of intra-ocular pressure has been maintained for 24 hours with both 0.25% and 0.5% Timoptol-LA. In a study of plasma timolol concentrations, the systemic exposure to timolol was less when normal healthy volunteers received 0.5% Timoptol-LA once daily than when they received 0.5% Timoptol twice daily.

Preclinical safety data: No adverse ocular effects were observed in monkeys and rabbits administered Timoptol-LA topically in studies lasting 12 months and one month, respectively. The oral LD_{50} of timolol is 1,190 and 900 mg/kg in female mice and female rats, respectively. The oral LD_{50} of gellan gum is greater than 5,000 mg/kg in rats.

In a two-year oral study of timolol maleate in rats there was a statistically significant ($p \leq 0.05$) increase in the incidence of adrenal phaeochromocytomas in male rats administered 300 mg/kg/day (300 times the maximum recommended human oral dose*). Similar differences were not observed in rats administered oral doses equivalent to 25 or 100 times the maximum recommended human oral dose.

* The maximum recommended daily oral dose of timolol is 60 mg. One drop of 0.5% Timoptol-LA contains about 1/300 of this dose, which is about 0.2 mg.

In a lifetime oral study in mice, there were statistically significant ($p \leq 0.05$) increases in the incidence of benign and malignant pulmonary tumours, benign uterine polyps and mammary adrenocarcinoma in female mice at 500 mg/kg/day (500 times the maximum recommended human dose), but not at 5 or 50 mg/kg/day. In a subsequent study in female mice, in which post-mortem examinations were limited to uterus and lungs, a statistically significant increase in the incidence of pulmonary tumours was again observed at 500 mg/kg/day.

The increased occurrence of mammary adenocarcinoma was associated with elevations in serum prolactin which occurred in female mice administered timolol at 500 mg/kg/day, but not at doses of 5 or 50 mg/kg/day. An increased incidence of mammary adenocarcinomas in rodents has been associated with administration of several other therapeutic agents which elevate serum prolactin, but no correlation between serum prolactin levels and mammary tumours has been established in man. Furthermore, in adult human female subjects who received oral dosages of up to 60 mg of timolol maleate, the maximum recommended human oral dosage, there were no clinically meaningful changes in serum prolactin.

In oral studies of gellan gum administered to rats for up to 105 weeks at concentrations up to 5% of their diet and to mice for 96–98 weeks at concentrations up to 3% of their diet, no overt signs of toxicity and no increase in the incidence of tumours was observed.

Timolol maleate was devoid of mutagenic potential when evaluated *in vivo* (mouse) in the micronucleus test and cytogenetic assay (doses up to 800 mg/kg) and *in vitro* in a neoplastic cell-transformation assay (up to 100 mcg/ml). In Ames tests the highest concentrations of timolol employed, 5,000 or 10,000 mcg/plate, were associated with statistically significant elevations ($p \leq 0.05$) of revertants observed with tester strain TAIOO (in seven replicate assays), but not in the remaining three strains. In the assays with tester strain TAIOO, no consistent dose-response relationship was observed, nor did the ratio of test to control revertants reach 2. A ratio of 2 is usually considered the criterion for a positive Ames test.

Gellan gum was devoid of mutagenic potential when evaluated *in vivo* (mouse) in micronucleus assay using doses up to 450 mg/kg. In addition, gellan gum in concentrations up to 20 mg/ml was not detectably mutagenic in the following *in-vitro* assays: (1) unscheduled DNA synthesis in rat hepatocytes assay, (2) V-79 mammalian cell mutagenesis assay, and (3) chromosomal aberrations in Chinese hamster ovary cells assay.

In Ames tests, gellan gum (in concentrations up to 1,000 mcg/plate, which is its limit of solubility) did not induce a twofold or greater increase in revertants relative to the solvent control. It is therefore not detectably mutagenic.

Pharmaceutical particulars

List of excipients: Gellan gum, Trometamol PhEur, Mannitol PhEur, and Purified Water PhEur. Benzododecinium bromide (0.012%) is added as preservative.

Incompatibilities: None known.

Shelf life: 'Use not later than' date is printed on the package. The shelf life is 24 months. After opening the shelf life is 4 weeks.

Special precautions for storage: Store at or below 25°C. Avoid freezing. Protect from light.

Nature and contents of the container: Flexible-walled vials with controlled drop-size tips made from translucent low-density polyethylene activated by pressing once on the sides, closed by light-blue polypropylene caps (0.25%) or dark-blue polypropylene caps (0.5%).

Each metered-dose dispenser contains 2.5 ml Timoptol-LA-Ophthalmic gel-forming solution 0.25% or 0.5%.

Instructions for use/handling: Invert the container and shake once before each use.

It is not necessary to shake the container more than once.

Discard 4 weeks after opening.

Patients should be instructed to avoid allowing the tip of the dispensing container to contact the eye or surrounding structures.

Patients should also be instructed that ocular solutions, if handled improperly, can become contaminated by common bacteria known to cause ocular infections. Serious damage to the eye and subsequent loss of vision may result from using contaminated solutions.

Marketing authorisation numbers

0.25% 0025/0310
0.5% 0025/0311

Date of revision of SPC June 1998.

Legal category POM.

TRUSOPT*

Qualitative and quantitative composition Trusopt Sterile Ophthalmic Solution is supplied as an isotonic, buffered, slightly viscous, aqueous solution of dorzolamide hydrochloride. Each ml of Trusopt 2% contains 20 mg dorzolamide (22.3 mg of dorzolamide hydrochloride).

Pharmaceutical form Ophthalmic solution.

Clinical particulars

Therapeutic indications: Trusopt Ophthalmic Solution is indicated:

- as adjunctive therapy to beta-blockers
- as monotherapy in patients unresponsive to beta-blockers or in patients in whom beta-blockers are contra-indicated in the treatment of elevated intra-ocular pressure in:
  - ocular hypertension
  - open-angle glaucoma
  - pseudo-exfoliative glaucoma.

Posology and method of administration: When used as monotherapy, the dose is one drop of Trusopt Ophthalmic Solution in the conjunctival sac of the affected eye(s) three times daily.

When used as adjunctive therapy with an ophthalmic beta-blocker, the dose is one drop of Trusopt in the affected eye(s) twice daily.

When substituting Trusopt for another ophthalmic antiglaucoma agent, discontinue the other agent after proper dosing on one day, and start Trusopt on the next day.

If more than one topical ophthalmic drug is being used, the drugs should be administered at least 10 minutes apart.

Contra-indications: Trusopt is contra-indicated in patients who are hypersensitive to any component of this product.

Trusopt has not been studied in patients with severe renal impairment (CrCl <30 ml/min) or in patients with hyperchloraemic acidosis. Because Trusopt and its metabolites are excreted predominantly by the kidney, Trusopt is therefore contra-indicated in such patients.

Special warnings and special precautions for use: Trusopt has not been studied in patients with hepatic impairment and should therefore be used with caution in such patients.

The management of patients with acute angle-closure glaucoma requires therapeutic interventions in addition to ocular hypotensive agents. Trusopt has not been studied in patients with acute angle-closure glaucoma.

Trusopt is a sulphonamide and, although administered topically, is absorbed systemically. Therefore, the same types of adverse reactions that are attributable to sulphonamides may occur with topical administration. If signs of serious reactions or hypersensitivity occur, discontinue the use of this preparation.

In clinical studies, local ocular adverse effects, primarily conjunctivitis and lid reactions, were reported with chronic administration of Trusopt. Some of these reactions had the clinical appearance and course of an allergic-type reaction that resolved upon discontinuation of drug therapy. If such reactions are observed, discontinuation of treatment with Trusopt should be considered.

There is a potential for an additive effect on the known systemic effects of carbonic anhydrase inhibition in patients receiving an oral carbonic anhydrase inhibitor and Trusopt. The concomitant administration of Trusopt and oral carbonic anhydrase inhibitors has not been studied and is not recommended.

Safety and effectiveness in children has not been established.

Trusopt has not been studied in patients wearing contact lenses. The preservative in Trusopt Ophthalmic Solution, benzalkonium chloride, may be absorbed by soft contact lenses. Trusopt should not be administered while wearing soft contact lenses.

Interaction with other medicaments and other forms of interaction: Specific drug interaction studies have not been performed with Trusopt Ophthalmic Solution. In clinical studies, Trusopt was used concomitantly with the following medications without evidence of adverse interactions: timolol ophthalmic solution, betaxolol ophthalmic solution, and systemic medications including ACE inhibitors, calcium-channel blockers, diuretics, non-steroidal anti-inflammatory drugs including aspirin, and hormones (e.g. oestrogen, insulin, thyroxine). Association between Trusopt and miotics and adrenergic agonists has not been fully evaluated during glaucoma therapy.

Trusopt is a carbonic anhydrase inhibitor and, although administered topically, is absorbed systemically. In clinical studies, Trusopt was not associated with acid-base disturbances. However, these disturbances have been reported with oral carbonic anhydrase inhibitors and have, in some instances, resulted in drug interactions (e.g. toxicity associated with high-dose salicylate therapy). Therefore, the potential for such drug interactions should be considered in patients receiving Trusopt.

Pregnancy and lactation

Pregnancy: No studies were performed in pregnant women. Trusopt should not be used during pregnancy. In rabbits given maternotoxic doses associated with metabolic acidosis, malformations of the vertebral bodies were observed.

Breast-feeding: There are no data showing whether the drug is excreted in human milk. Trusopt should not be used during lactation. In lactating rats, decreases in the body weight gain of offspring were observed.

Effects on ability to drive and operate machinery: Possible side-effects such as dizziness and visual disturbances may affect the ability to drive and use machines.

Undesirable effects: The following adverse events have been reported either during clinical trials or during post-marketing experience:

Ocular: Burning and stinging, blurred vision, eye itching, tearing, conjunctivitis, eyelid inflammation, eyelid irritation, irritation including redness, pain, superficial punctate keratitis, iridocyclitis, transient myopia (which resolved upon discontinuation of therapy).

Nervous system: Headache, asthenia/fatigue, dizziness, paraesthesia.

Hypersensitivity: Signs and symptoms of systemic allergic reactions including angioedema, urticaria, pruritus, shortness of breath, rarely bronchospasm.

Body as whole: Rash, nausea, bitter taste, urolithiasis.

Laboratory findings: Trusopt was not associated with clinically meaningful electrolyte disturbances.

Overdose: No data are available in humans in regard to overdosage by accidental or deliberate ingestion.

Treatment should be symptomatic and supportive. Electrolyte imbalance, development of an acidotic state, and possible central nervous system effects may occur. Serum electrolyte levels (particularly potassium) and blood pH levels should be monitored.

The oral LD_{50} of the drug is 1,320 mg/kg (3,960 mg/m²) in mice and 1,927 mg/kg (11,369 mg/m²) in female rats.

Pharmacological properties

Pharmacodynamic properties

Mechanism of action: Carbonic anhydrase (CA) is an enzyme found in many tissues of the body, including the eye. In humans, carbonic anhydrase exists as a number of isoenzymes, the most active being carbonic anhydrase II (CA-II) found primarily in red blood cells (RBCs) but also in other tissues. Inhibition of carbonic anhydrase in the ciliary processes of the eye decreases aqueous humour secretion. The result is a reduction in intra-ocular pressure (IOP).

Trusopt Ophthalmic Solution contains dorzolamide hydrochloride, a potent inhibitor of human carbonic anhydrase II. Following topical ocular administration, Trusopt reduces elevated intra-ocular pressure, whether or not associated with glaucoma. Elevated intra-ocular pressure is a major risk factor in the pathogenesis of optic-nerve damage and glaucomatous visual-field loss. Trusopt does not cause pupillary constriction and reduces intra-ocular pressure without side effects such as night blindness and accommodative spasm. Trusopt has minimal or no effect on pulse rate or blood pressure.

Topically applied beta-adrenergic blocking agents also reduce IOP by decreasing aqueous humour secretion but by a different mechanism of action.

Studies have shown that when Trusopt is added to a topical beta-blocker additional reduction in IOP is observed; this finding is consistent with the reported additive effects of beta-blockers and oral carbonic anhydrase inhibitors.

Pharmacodynamic effects: Clinical effects: In patients with glaucoma or ocular hypertension, the efficacy of Trusopt given t.d.s. as monotherapy (baseline IOP ≥23 mm Hg) or given b.d. as adjunctive therapy while receiving ophthalmic beta-blockers (baseline IOP ≥22 mm Hg) was demonstrated in large-scale clinical studies of up to one-year duration. The IOP-lowering effect of Trusopt as monotherapy and as adjunctive therapy was demonstrated throughout the day and this effect was maintained during long-term administration. Efficacy during long-term monotherapy was similar to betaxolol and slightly less than timolol. When used as adjunctive therapy to ophthalmic beta-blockers, Trusopt demonstrated additional IOP lowering similar to pilocarpine 2% q.d.s.

Pharmacokinetic properties: Unlike oral carbonic anhydrase inhibitors, topical administration of dorzolamide hydrochloride allows for the drug to exert its effects directly in the eye at substantially lower doses and therefore with less systemic exposure. In clinical trials, this resulted in a reduction in IOP without the acid-base disturbances or alterations in electrolytes characteristic of oral carbonic anhydrase inhibitors.

When topically applied, dorzolamide reaches the systemic circulation. To assess the potential for systemic carbonic anhydrase inhibition following topical administration, drug and metabolite concentrations in RBCs and plasma and carbonic anhydrase inhibitions in RBCs were measured. Dorzolamide accumulates in RBCs during chronic dosing as a result of selective binding to CA-II while extremely low concentrations of free drug in plasma are maintained. The parent drug forms a single N-desethyl metabolite that inhibits CA-II less potently than the parent drug but also inhibits a less active isoenzyme (CA-I). The metabolite also accumulates in RBCs where it binds primarily to CA-I. Dorzolamide binds moderately to plasma proteins (approximately 33%). Dorzolamide is primarily excreted unchanged in the urine; the metabolite is also excreted in urine. After dosing ends, dorzolamide washes out of RBCs non-linearly, resulting in a rapid decline of drug concentration initially, followed by a slower elimination phase with a half-life of about 4 months.

When dorzolamide was given orally to simulate the maximum systemic exposure after long-term topical occular administration, steady state was reached within 13 weeks. At steady state, there was virtually no free drug or metabolite in plasma; CA inhibition in RBCs was less than that anticipated to be necessary for a pharmacological effect on renal function or respiration. Similar pharmacokinetic results were observed after chronic, topical administration of Trusopt. However, some elderly patients with renal impairment (estimated CrCl 30–60 ml/min) had higher metabolite concentrations in RBCs but no meaningful differences in carbonic anhydrase inhibition, and no clinically significant systemic side effects were directly attributable to this finding.

Preclinical safety data: The main findings in animal studies with dorzolamide hydrochloride administered orally were related to the pharmacological effects of systemic carbonic anhydrase inhibition. Some of these findings were species-specific and/or were a result of metabolic acidosis.

In clinical studies, patients did not develop signs of metabolic acidosis or serum electrolyte changes which are indicative to systemic CA inhibition. Therefore, it is not expected that the effects noted in animal studies would be observed in patients receiving therapeutic doses of Trusopt.

Pharmaceutical particulars

List of excipients: Hydroxyethylcellulose, mannitol, sodium citrate, sodium hydroxide (to adjust pH), and water for injection. Benzalkonium chloride 0.0075% is added as preservative.

Incompatibilities: None known.

Shelf life: The shelf life is 24 months.

Trusopt should be used no longer than 4 weeks after first opening the container.

Special precautions for storage: Store Trusopt Ophthalmic Solution below 30°C. Protect from light.

Nature and contents of container: The 5 ml ALP vial consists of an oval, translucent, low-density polyethylene container with a metered dropper tip and an orange-coloured polypropylene cap. The tip and orange cap are covered with a translucent tamper-evident, disposable overcap.

Instructions for use/handling: Patients should be instructed to avoid allowing the tip of the dispensing container to contact the eye or surrounding structures.

Patients should also be instructed that ocular solutions, if handled improperly, can become contaminated by common bacteria known to cause ocular infections. Serious damage to the eye and subsequent loss of vision may result from using contaminated solutions.

Marketing authorisation number 0025/0323.

Date of approval/revision of SPC November 1997.

Legal category POM.

TRYPTIZOL*

Presentation Blue, film-coated tablets, marked 'MSD 23', containing 10 mg Amitriptyline Hydrochloride BP; yellow, film-coated tablets, marked 'MSD 45', containing 25 mg; and brown, film-coated tablets, marked 'MSD 102', containing 50 mg.

Injection, a colourless solution containing per ml 10 mg amitriptyline hydrochloride.

Uses Symptoms of depression (especially where sedation is required); also effective in nocturnal enuresis where organic pathology is excluded.

Dosage and administration *Depression.*

Oral therapy: Therapy should be started with a low dosage and increased gradually, according to the clinical response and any evidence of intolerance.

Adults – initial dosage: Usually 75 mg a day in divided doses (or a single dose at night). If necessary, this may be increased to a total of 150 mg a day, the additional doses being given in the late afternoon and/or at bedtime.

The sedative effect is usually rapidly apparent. The antidepressant activity may be seen within three or four days or may take up to 30 days to develop adequately.

Adults – maintenance dosage: Usually 50–100 mg a day. For maintenance therapy, the total dosage may be given in a single dose preferably in the evening or at bedtime. When satisfactory improvement has been reached, dosage should be reduced to the lowest amount that will maintain relief of symptoms. Maintenance therapy should be continued for three months or longer to lessen the chances of relapse.

Parenteral therapy: Parenteral use of amitriptyline should be restricted to patients for whom oral therapy is inappropriate or difficult. Substitute oral therapy as soon as possible: 10–20 mg (1–2 ml) four times a day. The dosage should not exceed that for oral therapy and should always be given in divided doses, intramuscularly or intravenously.

Children: Due to lack of clinical experience, Tryptizol is not recommended for the treatment of *depression* in children under 16 years of age.

Enuresis: Children aged 6–10 years may receive 10–20 mg a day, while those aged 11–16 years may need 25–50 mg a day. The recommended dosage must not be exceeded. Treatment should not exceed three months.

Most patients who respond, do so in the first few days of therapy.

Plasma levels: Because of the wide variation in the absorption and distribution of tricyclic antidepressants in body fluids, dosage should be adjusted to clinical response and not based on plasma levels. However, plasma levels may be used as a guide to toxicity or to non-compliance.

Elderly patients: In general, lower dosages are recommended for these patients and an initial dosage of 10–25 mg t.d.s. is recommended, which should be increased slowly. A daily dosage of 50 mg may be satisfactory in elderly patients who may not tolerate higher dosages. The required dosage may be administered either as divided doses or as a single dose preferably in the evening or at bedtime.

Contra-indications, warnings, etc

Contra-indications: Co-administration with monoamine oxidase inhibitors; prior sensitisation to amitriptyline; during the recovery phase after myocardial infarction; arrhythmias, particularly heartblock of any degree; mania; severe liver disease; lactation; children under 6 years of age. See also 'Use in pregnancy' under 'Precautions'.

Precautions: General: Tryptizol should be used with caution in patients with a history of epilepsy, in patients with impaired liver function and, because of its atropine-like action, in patients with a history of urinary retention, prostatic hypertrophy, narrow-angle glaucoma, or increased intra-ocular pressure. In patients with narrow-angle glaucoma, even average doses may precipitate an attack of glaucoma.

There has been a report of fatal dysarrhythmia occurring as late as 56 hours after amytriptyline overdose.

If possible, discontinue Tryptizol several days before surgery. But if emergency surgery is unavoidable, the anaesthetist should be informed that the patient is being treated with Tryptizol, because anaesthesia may increase the risk of hypotension and arrhythmias.

Hyperpyrexia has been reported when tricyclic antidepressants are administered with anticholinergic agents or with neuroleptic drugs, particularly during hot weather.

Tryptizol may impair alertness in some patients and activities made hazardous by diminished alertness (e.g. driving a car) should be avoided.

Elderly patients are particularly liable to experience adverse reactions: especially agitation, confusion, and postural hypotension.

Cardiovascular/endocrine disorders: Patients with cardiovascular disorders, hyperthyroid patients, and those receiving thyroid medication or anticholinergic agents should be closely supervised and the dosage of all medications carefully adjusted.

Central nervous system disorders: When Tryptizol is used for the depressive component of schizophrenia, psychotic symptoms may be aggravated. In manic-depressives, a shift towards the manic phase may occur; paranoid delusions, with or without associated hostility, may be aggravated. In such cases, a major tranquilliser should be given concurrently, or the dosage of Tryptizol reduced.

The risk of suicide remains during treatment of depressed patients and until significant remission occurs. Such patients require careful supervision.

Use in Children: Behavioural changes have been observed in children receiving tricyclics for the treatment of enuresis.

Use in pregnancy: The safety of Tryptizol for use during pregnancy has not been established. Tryptizol is not recommended during pregnancy, especially during the first and third trimesters unless there are compelling reasons, and in these patients the benefits should be weighed against possible hazards to the foetus, child, or mother. Clinical experience of the use of Tryptizol in pregnancy has been limited. Animal studies have shown harmful effects at exceptionally high doses.

Breast-feeding mothers: Amitriptyline is detectable in breast milk. Because of the potential for serious adverse reactions in infants from amitriptyline, a decision should be made whether to discontinue breast-feeding or discontinue the drug.

Drug interactions: Other antidepressant drugs: The concurrent use of antidepressants having varying modes of action should be made only with due recognition of their possible potentiation and with a thorough knowledge of their respective pharmacologies. Monoamine oxidase inhibitors can potentiate the effects of tricyclic antidepressants such as Tryptizol, and hyperpyretic crises, severe convulsions, and fatalities have occurred. A minimum of 14 days should elapse between discontinuing an MAOI and starting Tryptizol, which should be introduced cautiously and dosage increased gradually.

Guanethidine: Tryptizol may block the antihypertensive action of guanethidine, debrisoquine, bethanidine, and possibly clonidine. It would be advisable to review all antihypertensive therapy during treatment with tricyclic antidepressants.

Anticholinergic agents/sympathomimetic drugs: Amitriptyline should not be given with sympathomimetic agents such as adrenaline, ephedrine, isoprenaline, noradrenaline, phenylephrine, and phenylpropanolamine.

Paralytic ileus may occur in patients taking tricyclic antidepressants in combination with drugs having an anticholinergic action.

Central nervous system depressants: Tryptizol may enhance the response to alcohol, barbiturates, and other CNS depressants. In turn, barbiturates may decrease, and methylphenidate may increase, the antidepressant action of amitriptyline. Caution is advised if patients receive large doses of ethchlorvynol concurrently. Transient delirium has been reported in patients treated with 1 g ethchlorvynol and 75 mg to 150 mg of Tryptizol.

Disulfiram: Delirium has been reported in patients taking amitriptyline with disulfiram.

Cimetidine: Cimetidine is reported to reduce hepatic metabolism of certain tricyclic antidepressants.

Electroconvulsive therapy: Concurrent administration with ECT may increase the hazards of treatment, and should be limited to patients for whom it is deemed essential.

Warnings and adverse effects: In general, Tryptizol is well tolerated. The side effects given below are essentially a combined list of all those of the tricyclic group of antidepressants. Some of them have not been reported with Tryptizol, but are included because of the similar pharmacologies of the group members. As the antidepressant effects of Tryptizol may not become apparent for the first 2–4 weeks of therapy, patients should be closely monitored during this period.

Cardiovascular reactions: hypotension, syncope, postural hypotension, hypertension, tachycardia, palpitations, myocardial infarction, arrhythmias, heart block, stroke, non-specific ECG changes and changes in AV conduction. Arrhythmias and severe hypotension are likely to occur with high dosage or overdosage.

CNS and neuromuscular: confusional states, disturbed concentration, disorientation, delusions, hallucinations, hypomania, excitement, anxiety, restlessness, drowsiness, insomnia, nightmares, numbness, tingling, and paraesthesiae of the extremities, peripheral neuropathy, incoordination, ataxia, tremors, coma, convulsions, alteration of the EEG, extrapyramidal symptoms, including abnormal involuntary movements and tardive dyskinesia, dysarthria, tinnitus.

Anticholinergic: dry mouth, blurred vision, mydriasis, disturbance of accommodation, increased intraocular pressure, constipation, paralytic ileus, hyperpyrexia, urinary retention, urinary tract dilatation.

Allergic: skin rash, urticaria, photosensitisation, oedema of face and tongue.

Haematological: bone-marrow depression including agranulocytosis, leucopenia, eosinophilia, purpura, thrombocytopenia.

Gastro-intestinal: nausea, epigastric distress, vomiting, anorexia, stomatitis, unpleasant taste, diarrhoea, parotid swelling, black tongue, rarely hepatitis (including altered liver function and jaundice).

Endocrine: testicular swelling, gynaecomastia; breast enlargement, galactorrhoea, increased or decreased libido, impotence, interference with sexual function, elevation or lowering of blood sugar levels, syndrome of inappropriate ADH (antidiuretic hormone) secretion.

Other reactions: dizziness, weakness, fatigue, headache, weight loss, oedema, increased perspiration, urinary frequency, alopecia, increased appetite and weight gain (may be a drug reaction or due to relief of the depression). Abrupt withdrawal after prolonged administration has caused nausea, headache and malaise. Reports have associated gradual withdrawal with transient symptoms including irritability, restlessness, as well as dream and sleep disturbances during the first two weeks of dosage reduction. These symptoms are not indicative of addiction.

Adverse reactions such as withdrawal symptoms, respiratory depression and agitation have been reported in neonates whose mothers had taken tricyclic anti-depressants in the last trimester of pregnancy.

Mania or hypomania has been reported rarely within 2–7 days of stopping chronic therapy with tricyclic antidepressants.

Side effects in enuresis: Dosages used in enuresis are low compared with those used in depression, and side effects are therefore less frequent. The most common are drowsiness and anticholinergic effects. The only other side effects, reported infrequently at these dosages, have been mild sweating and itching.

The recommended dosage must not be exceeded.

Side effects—causal relationship unknown: The following additional side-effects have been reported; however, a causal relationship to therapy with amitriptyline has not been established: lupus-like syndrome (migratory arthritis, positive ANA and rheumatoid factor).

Overdosage: High dosage may cause temporary confusion, disturbed concentration, or transient visual hallucinations. Overdosage may cause drowsiness; hypothermia; tachycardia and other arrhythmic abnormalities such as bundle branch block; ECG evidence of impaired conduction; congestive heart failure; dilated pupils; disorders of ocular motility, convulsions; severe hypotension; stupor, coma and polyradiculoneuropathy, constipation. Other symptoms may be agitation, hyperactive reflexes, muscle rigidity, vomiting, hyperpyrexia, or any of those listed as adverse effects.

All persons suspected of having taken an overdosage should be admitted to hospital as soon as possible. Treatment is symptomatic and supportive. The stomach should be emptied as quickly as possible by emesis, followed by gastric lavage upon arrival at hospital. Following lavage, activated charcoal may be given during the first 24–48 hours at a dosage of 20–30 g every four to six hours. An ECG should be taken and close monitoring of cardiac function instituted if there is any sign of abnormality. An open airway and an adequate fluid intake should be maintained, and body temperature regulated.

Intravenous physostigmine salicylate, 1–3 mg, has been reported to reverse the symptoms of tricyclic antidepressant poisoning. Because physostigmine is rapidly metabolised, the dosage of physostigmine should be repeated as required, particularly if life-threatening signs such as arrhythmias, convulsions, and deep coma recur or persist after the initial dose of physostigmine. Because physostigmine itself may be toxic, it is not recommended for routine use.

Standard measures should be used to manage circulatory shock and metabolic acidosis. Cardiac arrhythmias may be treated with neostigmine, pyridostigmine or propranolol. Should cardiac failure occur, use of digitalis should be considered. Close monitoring of cardiac function for not less than five days is advisable.

If convulsions occur, they should be treated with paraldehyde, diazepam or an inhalation anaesthetic. Barbiturates should not be used because Tryptizol increases their CNS-depressant action.

Dialysis is of no value because of low plasma concentrations of amitriptyline. Since overdosage is often deliberate, patients may attempt suicide by other means during the recovery phase. Deaths by deliberate or accidental overdosage have occurred with this class of medicament.

Pharmaceutical precautions Keep containers well closed and store below 25°C, protected from light. The injection should also be protected from freezing.

Legal category POM.

Package quantities
Tablets 10 mg: Blister packs of 30.
Tablets 25 mg: Blister packs of 30.
Tablets 50 mg: Blister packs of 30.
Injection: Vials of 10 ml.

Further information Tryptizol is a member of the tricyclic group of antidepressants. Its mode of action in man is not known, but it is not a monoamine oxidase inhibitor (special dietary restrictions are not necessary), and it does not act primarily by stimulating the CNS.

Product licence numbers

Tablets 10 mg	0025/0093
Tablets 25 mg	0025/0094
Tablets 50 mg	0025/0095
Injection	0025/5036

UTINOR* TABLETS 400 mg

Qualitative and quantitative composition Utinor contains 400 mg of the active ingredient, norfloxacin USP.

Pharmaceutical form Utinor is supplied as off-white oval tablets marked 'MSD 705'.

Clinical particulars
Therapeutic indications: Broad-spectrum, bactericidal agent indicated for the treatment of:

Upper and lower, complicated and uncomplicated, acute and chronic urinary tract infections. These infections include cystitis, pyelitis, pyelonephritis, chronic prostatitis and those urinary infections associated with urological surgery, neurogenic bladder or nephrolithiasis caused by bacteria susceptible to Utinor.

Posology and method of administration: Utinor should be taken with a glass of water at least one hour before or two hours after a meal or milk ingestion.

Susceptibility of the causative organism to Utinor should be tested. However, therapy may be initiated before obtaining the results of these tests.

Diagnosis	*Dosage*	*Therapy duration*
Uncomplicated lower urinary tract infections (e.g. cystitis)†	400 mg twice daily	3 days
Urinary tract infections	400 mg twice daily	7–10 days
Chronic relapsing urinary tract infection‡	400 mg twice daily	up to 12 weeks

†Trials in over 600 patients have demonstrated the efficacy and tolerability of Utinor in the three-day treatment of uncomplicated urinary tract infections.
‡If adequate suppression is obtained within the first four weeks of therapy, the dose of Utinor may be reduced to 400 mg daily.

Patients with renal impairment: Utinor is suitable for the treatment of patients with renal impairment. In studies involving patients whose creatinine clearance was less than 30 ml/min/1.73 m², but who did not require haemodialysis, the plasma half-life of norfloxacin was approximately eight hours. Clinical studies showed there was no difference in the mean half-life of norfloxacin in patients with a creatinine clearance of less than 10 ml/min/1.73 m², compared to patients with creatinine clearance of 10–30 ml/min/1.73 m². Hence, for these patients, the recommended dose is one 400 mg tablet once daily. At this dosage, concentrations in appropriate body tissues or fluids exceed the MICs for most pathogens sensitive to norfloxacin.

Use in the elderly: Pharmacokinetic studies have shown no appreciable changes when compared to younger patients, apart from a slight prolongation of half-life. In the absence of renal impairment, no adjustment of dosage is necessary. Limited clinical studies have shown Utinor to be well tolerated.

Contra-indications: Hypersensitivity to any component of this product or any chemically related quinolone antibacterials.

Utinor is contra-indicated in prepubertal children and growing adolescents.

Special warnings and precautions for use: Convulsions have been reported rarely with norfloxacin, although a causal relationship has not been established.

As with other drugs in this class, Utinor should not be used in patients with a history of convulsions or known factors that predispose to seizures unless there is an overwhelming clinical need.

Tendinitis and/or tendon rupture, particularly affecting the Achilles tendon, may occur with quinolone antibiotics. Such reactions have been observed, particularly in older patients and in those treated concurrently with corticosteroids. At the first sign of pain or inflammation, patients should discontinue Utinor and rest the affected limbs.

Photosensitivity reactions have been observed in patients who are exposed to excessive sunlight while receiving some members of this drug class. Excessive sunlight should be avoided. Therapy should be discontinued if photosensitivity occurs.

Rarely, haemolytic reactions have been reported in patients with latent or actual defects in glucose-6-phosphate dehydrogenase activity who take quinolone antibacterial agents, including norfloxacin (see *Undesirable effects*).

Use in children: As with other quinolones, Utinor has been shown to cause arthropathy in immature animals. The safety of Utinor in children has not been adequately explored and therefore the use of Utinor in prepubertal children or growing adolescents is contra-indicated.

Interaction with other medicaments and other forms of interaction: Co-administration of probenecid does not affect serum concentrations of norfloxacin, but urinary excretion of the drug diminishes.

As with other organic acid antibacterials, antagonism has been demonstrated *in vitro* between Utinor and nitrofurantoin.

Elevated plasma levels of theophylline have been reported with concomitant quinolone use. There have been rare reports of theophylline-related side effects in patients on concomitant therapy with norfloxacin and theophylline. Therefore, monitoring of theophylline plasma levels should be considered and dosage of theophylline adjusted as required.

Elevated serum levels of cyclosporin have been reported with concomitant use of norfloxacin. Cyclosporin serum levels should be monitored and appropriate cyclosporin dosage adjustments made when these drugs are used concomitantly.

Quinolones, including norfloxacin, may enhance the effects of the anticoagulant warfarin, or its derivatives, by displacing significant amounts from serum albumin-binding sites. When concomitant administration of these products cannot be avoided, measurements of prothrombin time or other suitable coagulation tests should be carried out.

Multivitamins, products containing iron or zinc, antacids or sucralfate should not be administered concomitantly with, or within two hours of, the administration of norfloxacin because they may interfere with absorption, resulting in lower serum and urine levels of norfloxacin.

Some quinolones, including norfloxacin, have also been shown to interfere with the metabolism of caffeine. This may lead to reduced clearance of caffeine and a prolongation of its plasma half-life.

Animal data have shown that quinolones in combination with fenbufen can lead to convulsions. Therefore, concomitant administration of quinolones and fenbufen should be avoided.

Pregnancy and lactation: There is no evidence from animal studies that norfloxacin has any teratogenic or mutagenic effects. Embryotoxicity secondary to maternotoxicity was observed after large doses in rabbits. Embryonic losses were observed in cynomolgus monkeys without any teratogenic effects. The relevance of these findings for humans is uncertain.

The safe use of Utinor in pregnant women has not been established; however, as with other quinolones, norfloxacin has been shown to cause arthropathy in immature animals and therefore its use during pregnancy is not recommended.

It is not known whether Utinor is excreted in human milk; administration to breast-feeding mothers is thus not recommended.

Effects on ability to drive and use machines: There are side-effets associated with this product that may affect some patients' ability to drive or operate machinery (see *Undesirable effects*).

Undesirable effects: The overall incidence of drug-related side effects reported during clinical trials was approximately 3%.

The most common side effects have been gastrointestinal, neuropsychiatric and skin reactions, and include nausea, headache, dizziness, rash, heartburn, abdominal pain/cramps, and diarrhoea.

Less commonly, other side effects such as anorexia, sleep disturbances, depression, anxiety/nervousness, irritability, euphoria, disorientation, hallucination, tinnitus, and epiphora have been reported.

Abnormal laboratory side effects observed during clinical trials included: leucopenia, elevation of ALAT (SGPT), ASAT (SGOT), eosinophilia, neutropenia, thrombocytopenia.

With more widespread use the following additional side effects have been reported:

Hypersensitivity reactions: Hypersensitivity reactions including anaphylaxis, interstitial nephritis, angioedema, vasculitis, urticaria, arthritis, myalgia, arthralgia.

Skin: Photosensitivity, Stevens-Johnson syndrome, toxic epidermal necrolysis, exfoliative dermatitis, erythema multiforme, pruritus.

Gastro-intestinal: Pseudomembranous colitis, pancreatitis (rare), hepatitis, including elevated liver-function tests.

Musculoskeletal: Tendinitis, tendon rupture, possible exacerbation of myasthenia gravis.

Nervous system/psychiatric: Polyneuropathy including Guillaine-Barré syndrome, confusion, paraesthesia, psychic disturbances including psychotic reactions.

Haematological: Haemolytic anaemia, sometimes associated with glucose-6-phosphate dehydrogenase deficiency.

Genito-urinary: Vaginal candidiasis.

Overdose: No information is available at present.

In the event of recent acute overdosage, the stomach should be emptied by induced vomiting or by gastric lavage and the patient carefully observed and given symptomatic and supportive treatment. Adequate hydration must be maintained.

Pharmacological properties

Pharmacodynamic properties: Norfloxacin inhibits bacterial deoxyribonucleic acid synthesis and is bactericidal. At the molecular level, three specific events were attributed to norfloxacin in *Escherichia coli* cells:

1. Inhibition of the ATP-dependent DNA supercoiling reaction catalysed by DNA gyrase
2. Inhibition of the relaxation of supercoiled DNA
3. Promotion of double-stranded DNA breakage.

Spontaneous mutation resistance to norfloxacin has occurred rarely, and resistance of the organism during therapy has developed in less than 1% of patients treated.

Bacteriology: Utinor has a broad spectrum of antibacterial activity against Gram-positive and Gram-negative aerobic pathogens. The fluorine atom at the 6 position provides increased potency against Gram-negative organisms and the piperazine moiety at the 7 position is responsible for the anti-pseudomonal activity.

Utinor is active *in vitro* against the following bacteria:

Bacteria found in urinary tract infections:

Enterobacteriaceae – Citrobacter spp, *Citrobacter diversus, Citrobacter freundii, Edwardsiella tarda, Enterobacter* spp, *Enterobacter agglomerans, Enterobacter aerogenes, Enterobacter cloacae, Escherichia coli, Hafnia alvei, Klebsiella* spp, *Klebsiella oxytoca, Klebsiella pneumoniae, Morganella morganii, Proteus* spp (indole positive), *Proteus mirabilis, Proteus vulgaris, Providencia* spp, *Providencia rettgeri, Providencia stuartii, Serratia* spp, *Serratia marcescens.*

Pseudomonadaceae – Pseudomonas aeruginosa, Pseudomonas cepacia, Pseudomonas fluorescens, Pseudomonas stutzeri.

Other – Flavobacterium spp.

Gram-positive cocci – Enterococci faecalis, Group G steptococci, Staphylococcus spp, *Staphylococcus* Coag. negative, *Staphylococcus aureus* (including penicillinase-producing and most methicillin-resistant strains), *Staphylococcus epidermidis, Staphylococcus saprophyticus, Streptococcus agalactiae, Viridans group streptococci*

In addition, Utinor is active against *Bacillus cereus, Neiserria gonorrhoea, Ureaplasma urealyticum, Haemophilus influenzae* and *Haemophilus ducreyi.*

Utinor is not active against anaerobes, including *Actinomyces* spp, *Fusobacterium* spp, *Bacteroides* spp, and *Clostridium* spp, other than *C. perfringens.*

There is no cross-resistance between norfloxacin and structurally unrelated antibacterial agents such as penicillins, cephalosporins, tetracyclines, macrolides, aminocyclitols and sulphonamides, 2,4 diaminopyrimidines, or combinations thereof (e.g. co-trimoxazole).

Pharmacokinetic properties: Norfloxacin is rapidly absorbed following oral administration. In healthy volunteers, at least 30–40% of an oral dose of norfloxacin is absorbed. This results in a serum concentration of 1.5 mcg/ml being attained approximately 1 hour after administration of a 400 mg dose. Mean serum half-life is 3 to 4 hours, and is independent of dose.

The following are mean concentrations of norfloxacin in various fluids and tissues measured 1 to 4 hours post-dose after the two 400 mg doses, unless otherwise indicated:

Renal parenchyma	7.3 mcg/g
Prostate	2.5 mcg/g
Seminal fluid	2.7 mcg/ml
Testicle	1.6 mcg/g
Uterus/cervix	3.0 mcg/g
Vagina	4.3 mcg/g
Fallopian tube	1.9 mcg/g
Bile	6.9 mcg/ml (after 2×200 mg doses).

Norfloxacin is eliminated through metabolism, biliary excretion and renal excretion. After a single 400 mg dose of norfloxacin, mean antimicrobial activities equivalent to 278, 773 and 82 mcg of norfloxacin/g of faeces were obtained at 12, 24 and 48 hours, respectively.

Renal excretion occurs by both glomerular filtration and net tubular secretion, as evidenced by the high rate of renal clearance (approximately 275 ml/min). After a single 400 mg dose, urinary concentrations reach a value of 200 or more mcg/ml in healthy volunteers and remain above 30 mcg/ml for at least 12 hours. In the first 24 hours, 33–48% of the drug is recovered in the urine.

Norfloxacin exists in the urine as norfloxacin and six active metabolites of lesser antimicrobial potency. The parent compound accounts for over 70% of total excretion. The bactericidal potency of norfloxacin is not affected by the pH of urine.

Protein binding is less than 15%.

Preclinical safety data: Norfloxacin, when administered to 3- to 5-month-old dogs at doses four or more times the usual human dose, produced blister formation and eventual erosion of the articular cartilage of the weight-bearing joints. Similar changes have been produced by other structurally related drugs. Dogs six months or older were not susceptible to these changes.

Teratology studies in mice and rats and fertility studies in mice at oral doses of 30 to 50 times the usual dose for humans did not reveal teratogenic or fetal toxic effects. Embryotoxicity was observed in rabbits at does of 100 mg/kg/day. This was secondary to maternal toxicity and it is a non-specific antimicrobial effect in the rabbit due to an unusual sensitivity to antibiotic-induced changes in the gut microflora.

Although the drug was not teratogenic in cynomolgus monkeys at several times the therapeutic human dosage, an increased percentage of embryonic losses was observed.

Pharmaceutical particulars

List of excipients: Utinor contains the following inactive ingredients: Croscarmellose sodium USNF; Magnesium stearate PhEur; Microcrystalline cellulose PhEur; Hydroxypropylcellulose PhEur; Hypromellose PhEur; Titanium dioxide PhEur; Carnauba wax PhEur.

Incompatibilities: None.

Shelf life: 36 months shelf life for blister packs.

Special precautions for storage: Store in a cool, dry place protected from light.

Nature and contents of container: Utinor is available as blister packs of 6 and 14 tablets.

Instruction for use/handling: None.

Marketing authorisation number PL 0025/0254

Date of first authorisation/renewal of authorisation Authorisation first granted 3 August 1990. Licence renewed 15 April 1996.

Date of revision of text October 1997.

ZINAMIDE*

Qualitative and quantitative composition Each tablet of Zinamide contains 500 mg of pyrazinamide PhEur.

Pharmaceutical form White tablets, with one side scored and the other side marked 'MSD 504'.

Clinical particulars

Therapeutic indications: Zinamide is indicated in patients with active tuberculosis caused by *Mycobacterium tuberculosis.* Zinamide is not active against the atypical mycobacteria. Zinamide should only be given in combination with other antituberculous agents.

Posology and method of administration:

Usual adult dosage: 20–35 mg/kg a day divided into three or four doses; the maximum daily dosage is 3 g regardless of body weight. Zinamide should be administered with at least one other effective antituberculous drug. The use of Zinamide in combination therapy does not modify the accepted dosages of other antituberculous agents.

Paediatric use has not been established (see *Special warnings and special precautions for use*).

Use in the elderly: The general considerations outlined above should also apply to elderly patients.

Contra-indications: Zinamide is contra-indicated in patients hypersensitive to any component of this product; in patients with hepatic disease; and in those with hyperuricaemia and/or gouty arthritis.

Zinamide is contra-indicated in breast-feeding mothers (see *Pregnancy and lactation*).

Special warnings and special precautions for use: Zinamide should only be used when close daily observation of the patient is possible, and when laboratory facilities are available for performing frequent liver-function tests and blood uric acid determinations. Pre-treatment examinations should include *in vitro* sensitivity tests of recent cultures of *M. tuberculosis* from the patient as measured against the usual antituberculous drugs.

Liver-function tests, especially aspartate transferase (AST) and alanine transferase (ALT) determinations, should be carried out prior to therapy, and then every two to four weeks during therapy. Therapy with Zinamide should be withdrawn and not reinstated if signs of hepatocellular damage occur.

Reduction in the size and/or frequency of dose is recommended for patients with renal insufficiency.

If hyperuricaemia accompanied by an acute gouty arthritis occurs, therapy should be discontinued and not reinstated. Close monitoring is advised to detect any increasing difficulty in the management of patients with a history of gout or diabetes mellitus.

Children: The safety of Zinamide for use in children has not been established. Because of its potential toxicity, the use of Zinamide in children should be avoided unless it is considered crucial.

Interaction with other medicaments and other forms of interaction: None known.

Pregnancy and lactation:

Use during pregnancy: There have been no well-controlled studies in pregnant women. Zinamide should only be used if the potential benefit justifies the risk to the foetus.

Use during lactation: Zinamide is contra-indicated in breast-feeding mothers. If its use is deemed essential, the patient should stop breast-feeding.

Effects on ability to drive and use machines: There are no data to suggest that Zinamide affects the ability to drive or use machines.

Undesirable effects: A hepatic reaction is the most common side-effect of Zinamide. This varies from a symptomless abnormality of hepatic cell function, detectable only by laboratory tests, through a mild syndrome of fever, anorexia, malaise, liver tenderness, hepatomegaly and spleenomegaly, to more serious reactions such as clinical jaundice, and rare cases of progressive fulminating acute yellow atrophy and death.

Other side-effects – active gout, sideroblastic anaemia, arthralgias, anorexia, nausea and vomiting, dysuria, malaise, fever, urticaria, aggravation of peptic ulcer.

Overdose: Liver toxicity and hyperuricaemia may occur with overdosage.

The stomach should be emptied by gastric lavage if necessary.

There is no specific antidote. General supportive measures should be employed. Liver function should be monitored closely, and a high-carbohydrate, low-fat diet employed. Care should be taken to avoid exposure of the patient to other potential hepatotoxic agents, including alcohol. Benzodiazepines may be given if there is evidence of central nervous system stimulation.

Probenecid may be given for hyperuricaemia.

The plasma half-life of pyrazinamide is about nine to ten hours.

Pharmacological properties

Pharmacodynamic properties: Pyrazinamide exhibits tuberculostatic activity *in vitro* only at slightly acidic pH. The growth of tubercle bacilli within monocytes *in vitro* is completely inhibited by pyrazinamide at a concentration of 12.5 mcg/ml.

Pyrazinamide is active only at an acid pH, and it is therefore active mainly on the tubercle bacilli located within the cell. It is these bacteria which are probably responsible for microbial persistence and thus for relapses after chemotherapy has stopped.

Pyrazinamide has low bacterial activity compared with isoniazide. It is thought that when these are used in combination, isoniazide is the key bactericidal drug, whilst pyrazinamide has a sterilising role, acting on a special bacterial population inhibited by the acid environment inside the macrophage or the walls of tuberculous cavities.

Pharmacokinetic properties: Pyrazinamide is readily absorbed from the gastrointestinal tract. Peak concentrations occur about 2 hours after an oral dose and have been reported to be 33 mcg per ml after 1.5 g and 59 mcg per ml after 3 g.

Serum concentrations then decline, with a plasma half-life of about 9–10 hours.

About 30% of the dose is excreted in the urine as pyrazinoic acid and 4% as unchanged pyrazinamide within 24 hours.

Preclinical safety data: No relevant information.

Pharmaceutical particulars

List of excipients: Lactose PhEur, maize starch PhEur, magnesium stearate PhEur, silicon dioxide USNF, and purified water PhEur.

Incompatibilities: None known.

Shelf life: 60 months.

Special precautions for storage: Store at temperatures below 25°C.

Nature and contents of container: Blister packs cotaining 60 tablets.

Instructions for use/handling: None.

Marketing authorisation number 0025/5038R

Date of approval/revision of SPC January 1998.

Legal category POM.

ZOCOR*

Qualitative and quantitative composition Simvastatin 10 mg/20 mg/40 mg.

Pharmaceutical form Zocor is supplied as oval-shaped, film-coated tablets. The peach-coloured oval-shaped tablets marked 'Zocor 10' contain 10 mg simvastatin. The tan-coloured tablets marked 'Zocor 20' contain 20 mg simvastatin. The brick-red-coloured tablets marked 'MSD 749' contain 40 mg simvastatin.

Clinical particulars

Therapeutic indications

Coronary heart disease: In patients with coronary heart disease with a plasma cholesterol level of 5.5 mmol/l or greater, Zocor is indicated to:

- reduce the risk of mortality;
- reduce the risk of coronary death and non-fatal myocardial infarction;
- reduce the risk for undergoing myocardial revascularisation procedures (coronary artery bypass grafting and percutaneous transluminal coronary angioplasty); and
- slow the progression of coronary atherosclerosis, including reducing the development of new lesions and new total occlusions.

Hyperlipidaemia: Zocor is indicated as an adjunct to diet for reduction of elevated total cholesterol, LDL-cholesterol, apolipoprotein B and triglycerides in patients with primary hypercholesterolaemia, heterozygous familial hypercholesterolaemia or combined (mixed) hyperlipidaemia when response to diet and other non-pharmacological meaures is inadequate. Zocor also raises HDL-cholesterol and therefore lowers the LDL/HDL and total cholesterol/HDL ratios.

As with any cholesterol-lowering therapy other modifiable risk factors should also be considered when treatment is started.

Posology and method of administration: Route of administration is oral.

The patient should be placed on a standard cholesterol-lowering diet before receiving Zocor and should continue on this diet during treatment with Zocor.

Hyperlipidaemia: The recommended dose is 10 mg once daily taken in the evening. The dose range is 10 to 40 mg a day in single doses taken at night. A marked response to Zocor is seen within two weeks and the maximum therapeutic response occurs within four to six weeks. The response is maintained during continuation of therapy. When therapy with Zocor is stopped, total cholesterol has been shown to return to pretreatment levels. Adjustment of dosage, if required, should be made at intervals of not less than four weeks, depending on the patient's individual response.

If LDL-cholesterol levels fall below 1.94 mmol/l or total serum cholesterol levels fall below 3.6 mmol/l, consideration should be given to reducing the dose of Zocor.

Coronary heart disease: Patients with coronary heart disease can be treated with a starting dose of 20 mg/day given as a single dose in the evening. Adjustment of dosage, if required, should be made as specified above (see *Posology and method of administation, Hyperlipidaemia*).

Concomitant therapy: Zocor is effective alone or in combination with bile-acid sequestrants. In patients taking immunosuppressive drugs concomitantly with Zocor, the maximum recommended dosage is 10 mg/day (see *Special warnings and special precautions for use, Muscle effects*).

Dosage in renal insufficiency: Because Zocor does not undergo significant renal excretion, modification of dosage should not be necessary in patients with moderate renal insufficiency.

In patients with severe renal insufficiency (creatinine clearance <30 ml/min), dosages above 10 mg/day should be carefully considered and, if deemed necessary, implemented cautiously.

Use in the elderly: Although experience in elderly patients is limited, efficacy using standard doses appears similar to that seen in the population as a whole. There is no apparent increase in the frequency of clinical or laboratory adverse findings.

Children: Studies to show safety and effectiveness in children have not been carried out.

Contra-indications: Hypersensitivity to this product; active liver disease or unexplained persistent elevations of serum transaminases; concomitant therapy with the tetralol class calcium channel blocker mibefradil (see *Special warnings and special precautions for use*); porphyria; pregnancy and breast-feeding (see also *Special warnings and special precautions for use*); women of childbearing potential unless adequately protected by non-hormonal methods.

Special warnings and special precautions for use

Muscle effects: Simvastatin and other inhibitors of HMG-CoA reductase occasionally cause myopathy, which is manifested as muscle pain or weakness associated with grossly elevated creatine phosphokinase (CPK) (>10X the upper limit of normal [ULN]). Rhabdomyolysis, with or without acute renal failure secondary to myoglobinuria, has been reported rarely.

Myopathy caused by drug interactions: The incidence and severity of myopathy are increased by concomitant administation of HMG-CoA reductase inhibitors with drugs that can cause myopathy when given alone, such as gemfibrozil and other fibrates, and lipid-lowering doses (≥1 g/day) of niacin (nicotinic acid).

In addition, the risk of myopathy appears to be increased by high levels of HMG-CoA reductase inhibitory activity in plasma. Simvastatin and other HMG-CoA reductase inhibitors are metabolised by the cytochrome P450 isoform 3A4. Certain drugs that have a significant inhibitory effect at therapeutic doses on this metabolic pathway can substantially raise the plasma levels of HMG-CoA reductase inhibitors and thus increase the risk of myopathy. These include cyclosporin, the tetralol-class calcium channel blocker mibefradil, itraconazole, ketoconazole and other antifungal azoles, the macrolide antibiotics erythomycin and clarithromycin, and the antidepressant nefazodone.

Reducing the risk of myopathy:

1. General measures
   Patients starting therapy with simvastatin should be advised of the risk of myopathy and told to report promptly unexplained muscle pain, tenderness or weakness. A CPK level above 10x ULN in a patient with unexplained muscle symptoms indicates myopathy. Simvastatin therapy should be discontinued if myopathy is diagnosed or suspected. In most cases, when patients were promptly discontinued from treatment, muscle symptoms and CPK increases resolved.
   Of the patients with rhabdomyolysis, many had complicated medical histories. Some had pre-existing renal insufficiency, usually as a consequence of long-standing diabetes. In such patients, dose escalation requires caution. Also, as there are no known adverse consequences of brief interruption of therapy, treatment with simvastatin should be stopped a few days before elective major surgery and when any major acute medical or surgical condition supervenes.
2. Measures to reduce the risk of myopathy caused by drug interactions (see above).
   Physicians contemplating combined therapy with simvastatin and any of the interacting drugs should weigh the potential benefits and risks, and should carefully monitor patients for any signs and symptoms of muscle pain, tenderness, or weakness, particularly during the initial months of therapy and during any periods of upward dosage titration of either drug. Periodic CPK determinations may be considered in such situations, but here is no assurance that such monitoring will prevent myopathy.

The combined use of simvastatin with fibrates or niacin should be avoided unless the benefit of further alteration in lipid levels is likely to outweigh the increased risk of this drug combination. Combinations of fibrates or niacin with low doses of simvastatin have been used without myopathy in small, short-term clinical trials with careful monitoring. Addition of these drugs to HMG-CoA reductase inhibitors typically provides little additional reduction in LDL-cholesterol, but further reductions of triglycerides and further increases in HDL cholesterol may be obtained. If one of these drugs must be used with simvastatin, clinical experience suggests that the risk of myopathy is less with niacin than with the fibrates.

In patients taking concomitant cyclosporin, fibrates or niacin, the dose of simvastatin should generally not exceed 10 mg (see *Posology and method of administration, Concomitant therapy*), as the risk of myopathy increases substantially at higher doses. Interruption of simvastatin therapy during a course of treatment with systemic antifungal azole or a macrolide antibiotic should be considered. The use of mibefradil together with simvastatin is contra-indicated. Concomitant use with other medicines labelled as having a potent inhibitory effect on cytochrome P450 3A4 at therapeutic doses should be avoided unless the benefits of combined therapy outweigh the increased risk.

Homozygous familial hypercholesterolaemia: In patients with the homozygous form of familial hypercholesterolaemia, in whom there is a complete absence of LDL receptors, therapy with Zocor is unlikely to result in clinical benefit.

Hypertriglyceridaemia: Although Zocor has a triglyceride lowering effect, it is not indicated where hypertriglyceridaemia is the abnormality of most concern (i.e. hyperlipidaemia types I, IV and V).

Hepatic effects: Minor asymptomatic transient rises in serum transaminase may occur soon after initiation of therapy with simvastatin which do not require the drug to be discontinued. There is no evidence that these changes are due to hypersensitivity to Zocor.

In the Scandinavian Simvastatin Survival Study (see *Pharmacodynamic properties*) the number of patients with one or more transaminase elevation to >3 times the upper limit of normal, over the course of the study, was not significantly different between the simvastatin and placebo groups (14 [0.7%] vs 12 [0.6%]), the number of patients with single elevations of SGPT (ALT) to 3 times the upper limit of normal was significantly higher in the simvastatin group in the first year of the study (20 vs 8, p=0.023), but not thereafter.

Elevated transaminases resulted in the discontinuation of 8 patients from therapy in the simvastatin group (n=2,221) and 5 in the placebo group (n=2,223). All of the patients in this study received a starting dose of 20 mg of simvastatin; 37% were titrated to 40 mg.

It is recommended that liver-function tests be performed before treatment begins, and periodically thereafter (e.g. twice a year) for the first year of treatment or until one year after the last elevation in dose in all patients. Special attention should be paid to patients who develop elevated serum transaminase levels, and in these patients measurements should be repeated promptly and then performed more frequently. If the transaminase levels show evidence of progression, particularly if they rise to three times the upper limit of normal and are persistent, the drug should be discontinued.

The drug should be used with caution in patients who consume substantial quantities of alcohol and/or have a past history of liver disease. Active liver diseases or unexplained transaminase elevations are contra-indications to the use of simvastatin.

Ophthalmic examination: In the absence of any drug therapy, an increase in the prevalence of lens opacities with time is expected as a result of ageing. Current long-term data from clinical trials do not indicate an adverse effect of simvastatin on the human lens.

Paediatric use: Safety and effectiveness in children have not been established. Zocor is not recommended for paediatric use at this time.

Interactions with other medicaments and other forms of interaction: The risk of rhabdomyolysis is increased by the concomitant use of Zocor with drugs that have an inhibitory effect on cytochrome P450 3A4 at therapeutic doses (such as cyclosporin, mibefradil, itraconazole, ketoconazole, erythromycin, clarithromycin and nefazodone), or with fibric acid derivatives or niacin (see *Special warnings and special precautions for use, Muscle Effects*).

Phenazone: is a model for drugs metabolised by the microsomal hepatic enzyme system (cytochrome P450 system). Zocor had little or no detectable effect on the pharmacokinetics of phenazone in hypercholesterolaemic patients.

Propranolol: In normal volunteers, there was no clinically significant pharmacokinetic or pharmacodynamic interaction with concomitant administration of single doses of Zocor and propranolol.

Digoxin: Concomitant administration of Zocor and digoxin resulted in a slight elevation (less than 0.3 ng/ml) in drug concentrations (as measured by a digoxin radio-immuno-assay) in plasma compared to concomitant administration of placebo and digoxin.

Coumarin derivatives: In two clinical studies, one in normal volunteers and the other in hypercholesterolaemic patients, simvastatin 20–40 mg/day modestly potentiated the effect of coumarin anticoagulants: the prothrombin time, reported as International Normalised Ratio (INR), increased from a baseline of 1.7 to 1.8 and from 2.6 to 3.4 in the volunteer and patient studies, respectively. In patients taking coumarin anticoagulants, prothrombin time should be determined before starting simvastatin and frequently enough during early therapy to ensure that no significant alteration of prothrombin time occurs. Once a stable prothrombin time has been documented, prothrombin times can be monitored at the intervals usually recommended for patients on coumarin anticoagulants. If the dose of simvastatin is changed, the same procedure should be repeated. Simvastatin therapy has not been associated with bleeding or with changes in prothrombin time in patients not taking anticoagulants.

Fibric-acid derivatives: (see *Special warnings and special precautions for use, Muscle effects*).

Other concomitant therapy: In clinical studies, Zocor was used concomitantly with ACE inhibitors, beta-blockers, calcium antagonists, diuretics, and non-steroidal anti-inflammatory drugs (NSAIDs) without evidence of clinically significant adverse interactions.

Caution should be exercised in the concomitant use of Zocor with immunosuppressant therapy, itraconazole or nicotinic acid (see *Special warnings and special precautions for use, Muscle effects*).

Pregnancy and lactation

Pregnancy: Zocor is contra-indicated in pregnancy.

Atherosclerosis is a chronic process and the discontinuation of lipid-lowering drugs during pregnancy should have little impact on the outcome of long-term therapy of primary hyperlipidaemia. Moreover, cholesterol and other products of the cholesterol biosynthesis pathway are essential components for foetal development, including synthesis of steroids and cell membranes. Because of the ability of inhibitors of HMG-CoA reductase such as Zocor to decrease the synthesis of cholesterol and possibly other products of the cholesterol biosynthesis pathway, Zocor is contra-indicated for use in pregnancy and women of child bearing potential unless such patients are highly unlikely to conceive or such patients are adequately protected by non-hormonal methods. An interval of one month should elapse between the end of therapy with Zocor and planned conception. If the patient becomes pregnant while taking this drug Zocor should be discontinued immediately and the patient apprised of the potential hazard to the foetus.

The active metabolite of simvastatin was shown to produce foetal malformations in the offspring of pregnant rats. A few reports have been received of congenital anomalies in infants whose mothers were treated during pregnancy with HMG-CoA reductase inhibitors.

In a review of approximately 100 prospectively followed pregnancies in women exposed to Zocor or another structurally related HMG-CoA reductase inhibitor, the incidences of congenital anomalies, spontaneous abortions and foetal death/stillbirths did not exceed what would be expected in the general population. As safety in pregnant women has not been established and there is no apparent benefit to therapy with Zocor during pregnancy, treatment should be immediately discontinued as soon as pregnancy is recognised.

Breast-feeding mothers: It is not known whether simvastatin or its metabolites are excreted in human milk. Zocor should be avoided during lactation.

Effects on the ability to drive and use machines: Not applicable.

Undesirable effects: Zocor is generally well tolerated; for the most part, side effects have been usually mild and transient in nature. Less than 2% of patients on Zocor were discontinued from controlled clinical studies due to side effects attributable to Zocor.

In the pre-marketing controlled clinical studies, adverse effects occurring with a frequency of 1% or more and considered by the investigator as possibly, probably or definitely drug-related were: abdominal pain, constipation, and flatulence. Other side effects occurring in 0.5–0.9% of patients were asthenia and headache. Myopathy has been reported rarely.

In the Scandinavian Simvastatin Survival Study (4S) involving 4,444 patients treated with Zocor 20–40 mg/day (n=2,221) or placebo (n=2,223), the safety and tolerability profiles were comparable between groups over the median 5.4 years of the study.

The following additional side effects were reported either in long-term extension studies or in marketed use: nausea, diarrhoea, rash, dyspepsia, pruritus, alopecia, dizziness, muscle cramps, myalgia, pancreatitis, paraesthesia, peripheral neuropathy, vomiting, and anaemia. Rarely, rhabdomyolysis and hepatitis/jaundice occurred. An apparent hypersensitivity syndrome has been reported rarely which has included some of the following features: angioedema, lupus-like syndrome, polymyalgia rheumatica, vasculitis, thrombocytopenia, eosinophilia, ESR increased, arthritis, arthralgia, urticaria, photosensitivity, fever, flushing, dyspnoea, and malaise.

Laboratory test findings: Marked and persistent increases of serum transaminases have been reported infrequently. Elevated alkaline phosphatase and γ-glutamyl transpeptidase have been reported.

Liver-function test abnormalities have generally been mild and transient. Increases in serum creatinine phosphokinase (CPK) levels derived from skeletal muscle have been reported (see *Special warnings and special precautions for use*).

Side effects – causal relationship unknown: The following side effects have been reported; however, a causal relationship to therapy with Zocor has not been established: depression, erythema multiforme, including Stevens-Johnson syndrome, leucopenia, and purpura.

Overdosage: A few cases of overdosage have been reported; no patient had any specific symptoms, and all patients recovered without sequelae. The maximum dosage taken was 450 mg. General measures should be adopted.

The maximum plasma concentration of inhibitors occurred within 1.3 to 2.4 hours of administration.

Pharmacological properties

Pharmacodynamic properties: The involvement of LDL cholesterol in atherogenesis has been well documented in clinical and pathological studies, as well as in many animal experiments. Epidemiological studies have established that high LDL cholesterol and low HDL (high-density lipoprotein) cholesterol are both risk factors for coronary heart disease.

The value of drug- and/or diet-induced reduction in plasma cholesterol levels has long been controversial, but recently the beneficial effect of reduction of LDL cholesterol on morbidity and mortality due to coronary heart disease has been established. The Lipid Research Clinics – Coronary Primary Prevention Trial (LRC–CPPT) demonstrated in a seven-year, double-blind, placebo-controlled study that lowering LDL cholesterol with diet and cholestyramine decreased the combined rate of coronary heart disease death plus non-fatal myocardial infarction.

Zocor has been shown to reduce both normal and elevated LDL-cholesterol concentrations. LDL is formed from VLDL and is catabolised predominantly by the high affinity LDL receptor. The mechanism of the LDL-lowering effect of Zocor may involve both reduction of VLDL-cholesterol concentration and induction of the LDL receptor, leading to reduced production and increased catabolism of LDL cholesterol. Apolipoprotein B also falls substantially during treatment with Zocor. Since each LDL particle contains one molecule of apolipoprotein B, and since little apolipoprotein B is found in other lipoproteins, this strongly suggests that Zocor does not merely cause cholesterol to be lost from LDL but also reduces the concentration of circulating LDL particles. In addition, Zocor increases HDL cholesterol and reduces plasma triglycerides. As a result of these changes the ratios of total to HDL cholesterol and LDL to HDL cholesterol are reduced.

In the Scandinavian Simvastatin Survival Study (4S), the effect on total mortality of therapy with Zocor for a median of 5.4 years was assessed in 4,444 patients with coronary heart disease (CHD) and baseline total cholesterol 5.5 to 8.0 mmol/l. In this multicentre, randomised, double-blind, placebo-controlled study, Zocor reduced the risk of death by 30%, of CHD death by 42%, and of having a hospital-verified non-fatal myocardial infarction by 37%. Furthermore, Zocor reduced the risk for undergoing myocardial revascularisation procedures (coronary artery by-pass grafting or percutaneous transluminal coronary angioplasty) by 37%.

In a *post hoc* analysis performed on fatal plus non-fatal cerebrovascular events (stroke and transient ischaemic attacks), there were 75 patients with such events in the Zocor group and 102 in the placebo group (risk reduction 28%, p=0.033). Prospective trials are needed to confirm this result.

In a multicentre, placebo-controlled clinical trial in 404 patients using quantitative coronary angiography, Zocor slowed the progression of coronary atherosclerosis and reduced the development of both new lesions and new total occlusions, whereas coronary atherosclerosis lesions steadily worsened over four years in patients receiving standard care.

Zocor is a specific inhibitor of HMG-CoA reductase, the enzyme which catalyses the conversion of HMG-CoA to mevalonate. However, at therapeutic doses, the enzyme is not completely blocked, thereby allowing biologically necessary amounts of mevalonate to be available. Because the conversion of HMG-CoA to mevalonate is an early step in the biosynthetic pathway of cholesterol, therapy with Zocor would not be expected to cause an accumulation of potentially toxic sterols. In addition, HMG-CoA is metabolised readily back to acetyl CoA, which participates in many biosynthetic processes in the body.

Pharmacokinetic properties: Simvastatin is an inactive lactone which is readily hydrolysed *in vivo* to the corresponding β-hydroxyacid, L-654,969, a potent inhibitor of HMG-CoA reductase. Inhibition of HMG-CoA reductase is the basis for an assay in pharmacokinetic studies of the β-hydroxyacid metabolites (active inhibitors) and, following base hydrolysis, active plus latent inhibitors (total inhibitors). Both are measured in plasma following administration of simvastatin.

In a disposition study with ^{14}C-labelled simvastatin, 100 mg (20 uCi) of drug was administered as capsules (5×20 mg), and blood, urine, and faeces collected. Thirteen per cent of the radioactivity was recovered in the urine and 60% in faeces. The latter represents absorbed drug equivalents excreted in bile as well as any unabsorbed drug. Less than 0.5% of the dose was recovered in urine as HMG-CoA reductase inhibitors. In plasma, the inhibitors account for 14% and 28% (active and total inhibitors) of the AUC of total radioactivity, indicating that the majority of chemical species present were inactive or weak inhibitors.

The major metabolites of simvastatin present in human plasma are L-654,969 and four additional active metabolites. Both simvastatin and L-654,969 are highly bound to human plasma proteins (>94%). The availability of L-654,969 to the systemic circulation following an oral dose of simvastatin was estimated using an i.v. reference dose of L-654,969; the value was found to be less than 5% of the dose. By analogy to the dog model, simvastatin is well absorbed and undergoes extensive first-pass extraction in the liver, its primary site of action, with subsequent excretion of drug equivalents in the bile. Consequently, availability of active drug to the general circulation is low.

In dose-proportionality studies, utilising doses of simvastatin of 5, 10, 20, 60, 90 and 120 mg, there was no substantial deviation from linearity of AUC of inhibitors in the general circulation with an increase in dose. Relative to the fasting state, the plasma profile of inhibitors was not affected when simvastatin was administered immediately before a test meal.

The pharmacokinetics of single and multiple doses of simvastatin showed that no accumulation of drug occurred after multiple dosing. In all of the above pharmacokinetic studies, the maximum plasma concentration of inhibitors occurred 1.3 to 2.4 hours post-dose.

Preclinical safety data: The oral LD_{50} of simvastatin in mice is approximately 3.8 g/kg and in rats approximately 5 g/kg.

Administration of high dosage levels of simvastatin and related analogues to a variety of animal species has revealed a spectrum of changes in several tissues. These changes were not unexpected in view of the large doses used, the potency of these drugs in inhibiting mevalonate synthesis, and the essential role of the target enzyme in maintenance of cellular homeostasis. Extensive data generated on several of these changes indicate that they represent an exaggeration of the biochemical effect of these drugs at the high end of the dose-response curve. Thus, morphological changes in the livers of rats, squamous epithelial hyperplasia of the forestomach of rats and mice, and hepatotoxicity in rabbits have all been shown to be directly related to inhibition of HMG-CoA reductase.

Cataracts have been detected at high dosage levels in dog studies with simvastatin, although at a very low incidence. While there is no clear correlation between the magnitude of serum lipid-lowering and the development of cataracts, a consistent relationship has been observed between high serum levels of drug and cataract development with simvastatin and related HMG-CoA reductase inhibitors.

Serum levels (expressed as total inhibitors) in dogs receiving the minimally cataractogenic dose of simvastatin of 50 mg/kg/day are 21 times higher than those in man receiving the maximally anticipated therapeutic dose of 0.8 mg/kg (based on a 50 kg man).

Elevated serum transaminases have been observed in dogs receiving simvastatin. These occur either as chronic low-level elevations or as transient enzyme spikes in approximately 10–40% of the dogs receiving this drug. None of the dogs experiencing these transaminase elevations demonstrated any symptoms of illness; and none of the transaminase elevations have progressed to levels associated with frank hepatic necrosis, despite continued drug administration. No histopathological changes have been identified in the liver of any dogs receiving simvastatin.

Testicular degeneration has been seen in two dog safety studies with simvastatin. Special studies designed to further define the nature of these changes have not met with success, since the effects are poorly reproducible and unrelated to dose, serum cholesterol levels, or duration of treatment. Simvastatin has been administered for up to 2 years to dogs at a dose of 50 mg/kg/day without any testicular effects.

Skeletal muscle necrosis was seen in one study in rats given 90 mg/kg b.d., but this was a lethal dosage in rats.

Genetic toxicology and carcinogenicity: An extensive battery of *in vitro* and *in vivo* genetic toxicity tests have been conducted on both simvastatin and the corresponding open acid L-654,969. These include assays for microbial mutagenesis, mammalian cell mutagenesis, single stranded DNA breakage, and tests for chromosome aberrations. The results of these studies provided no evidence of an interaction between simvastatin or L-654,969 with genetic material at the highest soluble non-cytotoxic concentration tests in *in vitro* assay systems or at maximally tolerated doses tested *in vivo*.

Initial carcinogenicity studies conducted in rats and mice with simvastatin employed doses ranging from 1 mg/kg/day to 25 mg/kg/day. No evidence of a treatment-related incidence of tumour types was found in mice in any tissue. A statistically significant ($p \leq 0.05$) increase in the incidence of thyroid follicular cell adenomas was observed in female rats receiving 25 mg/kg of simvastatin per day (31 times the maximum recommended human dose). This benign tumour type was limited to female rats; no similar changes were seen in male rats or in female rats at lower dosages (up to 5 mg/kg/day). These tumours are a secondary effect reflective of a simvastatin-mediated enhancement of thyroid hormone clearance in the female rat. No other statistically significant increased incidence of tumour types was identified in any tissues in rats receiving simvastatin.

Data from both of these studies indicated that squamous epithelial hyperplasia of the forestomach occurred at all dosage levels. These gastric changes are confined to an anatomical structure which is not found in man. Moreover, identical cells found in other locations (e.g. oesophagus and anorectal junction of the rat, mouse and dog) are unaffected.

Results of a 73-week carcinogenicity study in mice receiving simvastatin doses up to 400 mg/kg/day (500 times the maximum recommended human dose, based on a 50 kg person) exhibited increased incidences of hepatocellular adenomas and carcinomas, pulmonary adenomas and Harderian gland adenomas. A no-effect dose of 25 mg/kg/day (31 times the maximum recommended human dose) was established in this study and from the results of the initial 92-week carcinogenicity study in mice.

Results of an additional 106-week carcinogenicity study in rats receiving simvastatin doses ranging from 50 mg/kg/day to 100 mg/kg/day (62.5 to 125 times the maximum recommended human dose) exhibited a treatment-related increase in the incidence of hepatocellular neoplasms. The no-effect dose remains at 25 mg/kg/day (31 times the maximum recommended human dose) as established in the initial carcinogenicity study. An increase in the incidence of thyroid hyperplastic lesions was also observed; however, this is consistent with the previous finding that this is a species-specific response and has no implications for man.

Pharmaceutical particulars

List of excipients: Each simvastatin tablet strength contains the following excipients: Ascorbic Acid PhEur, Butylated Hydroxyanisole PhEur, Citric Acid Monohydrate PhEur, Lactose PhEur, Magnesium Stearate PhEur, Microcrystalline Cellulose PhEur, Pregelatinised Maize Starch PhEur, Hydroxypropylcellulose PhEur, Methylhydroxypropylcellulose PhEur, Talc PhEur, Titanium Dioxide PhEur.

The 10 mg and 20 mg simvastatin tablets contain Yellow iron oxide E172 and Red iron oxide E172.

The 40 mg simvastatin tablet contains Red iron oxide E172.

Incompatibilities: None known.

Shelf life: The shelf life is 24 months.

Special precautions for storage: Tablets should be stored below 25°C in a dry place.

Nature and content of container: Blister packs of opacified PVC lidded with aluminium foil containing 28 tablets.

Instructions for use/handling: Not applicable.

Marketing authorisation numbers

10 mg Tablet	0025/0241
20 mg Tablet	0025/0242
40 mg Tablet	0025/0243

Date of first authorisation/renewal
Licence first granted April 1989.
Last renewed August 1995.

Date of (partial) revision of text June 1998.

Legal category POM.

**Trade Mark*

Monmouth Pharmaceuticals Limited

3 & 4 Huxley Road
The Surrey Research Park
Guildford GU2 5RE

☎ 01483 565299 🗋 01483 563658

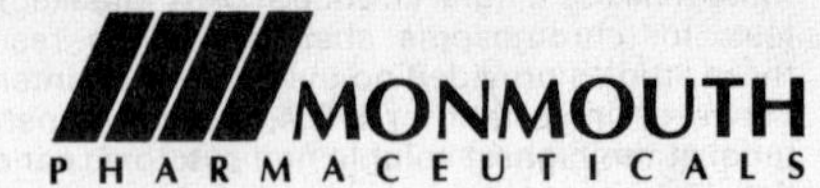

BARATOL* TABLETS 25 mg
BARATOL* TABLETS 50 mg

Quantitative and qualitative composition Each 25 mg tablet contains Indoramin Hydrochloride 27.63 mg (equivalent to 25 mg of indoramin base). Each 50 mg tablet contains Indoramin Hydrochloride 55.25 mg (equivalent to 50 mg of indoramin base).

Pharmaceutical form Baratol tablets are round, film coated with shallow convex faces. The 25 mg tablets are blue and marked 'MPL 020' on one face and '25' on the other. The 50 mg tablets are green and marked 'MPL 021' on one face and '50' on the other.

Clinical particulars
Therapeutic indications: Treatment of all grades of essential hypertension and conditions for which alpha blockade is indicated.

Posology and method of administration:

Route of administration: The tablet is taken orally.

Adults: Dose range: 50 mg–200 mg daily.

Initial dose: 25 mg twice daily for all patients.

Dose titration: The dose of Baratol should be titrated as necessary to control blood pressure to a maximum of 200 mg daily in two or three divided doses. The daily dose may be increased by the progressive addition of 25 mg or 50 mg. This may be done at intervals of two weeks. Many patients may be stabilised with doses up to 100 mg daily, especially those already being treated with diuretics. When unequal doses are used, the largest dose should be given at night in order to avoid day time sedation.

Elderly: Initial dose: 25 mg twice daily.
Clearance of indoramin may be affected in the elderly. A reduced dose and/or frequency of dosing may be sufficient for effective control of blood pressure in some elderly patients.

Children: Baratol is not recommended for children.

Combination with other anti-hypertensive agents: The anti-hypertensive effect of Baratol is enhanced by concomitant administration of a thiazide diuretic or a β-adrenoceptor blocking drug.
When Baratol is used in combination with other anti-hypertensive agents, the dose of Baratol should be titrated in the same way as when it is used alone.

Contra-indications: Baratol is contraindicated in patients:
- Who are currently receiving monoamine oxidase inhibitors.
- With established heart failure.

Special warnings and precautions for use: Drowsiness is sometimes seen in the initial stages of treatment with Baratol or when dosage is increased too rapidly. Patients should be warned not to drive or operate machinery until it is established that they do not become drowsy while taking Baratol.
Incipient cardiac failure should be controlled with diuretics and digitalis before treatment with Baratol.
Caution should be observed in prescribing Baratol for patients with hepatic or renal insufficiency.
A few cases of extrapyramidal disorders have been reported in patients treated with Baratol. Caution should be observed in prescribing Baratol in patients with Parkinson's Disease.
In animals and in the one reported overdose in humans, convulsions have occurred. Due consideration should be given and great caution exercised in the use of Baratol in patients with epilepsy.
Caution should be observed in prescribing Baratol for patients with a history of depression.
Clearence of indoramin may be affected in the elderly. A reduced dose and/or frequency of dosing may be sufficient for effective control of blood pressure.

Interaction with other medicaments and other forms of interaction: The ingestion of ethanol has been shown to increase both the rate and the extent of absorption of Baratol, and patients should be cautioned to avoid the ingestion of alcohol or other central nervous system depressants.

Pregnancy and lactation: Animal experiments indicate no teratogenic effects but Baratol Tablets should not be prescribed for pregnant women unless considered essential by the physician.
There is no data available on the excretion of Baratol in human milk but the drug should not be administered during lactation unless in the judgement of the physician such administration is clinically justifiable.

Effects on ability to drive and use machines: Baratol may cause drowsiness. See *Special warnings and precautions for use.*

Undesirable effects: Sedation occurs in some patients but it is rarely intolerable and is usually overcome by a modest reduction in dosage. Less commonly, dry mouth, nasal congestion, weight gain, dizziness, failure of ejaculation and depression have also been noted.

Overdose: The information available at present of the effects of acute overdosage in humans with Baratol is limited to one case. Effects seen in this case included deep sedation leading to coma, hypotension and fits. Results of animal work suggest that hypothermia may occur.
The suggested therapy is along the following lines:
- Recent ingestion of large numbers of tablets would require gastric lavage or a dose of Ipecacuanha to remove any of the product still in the stomach of the conscious patient.
- Ventilation should be monitored and assisted if necessary.
- Circulatory support and control of hypotension should be maintained.
- If convulsions occur, diazepam may be tried.
- Temperature should be closely monitored. If hypothermia occurs, rewarming should be carried out very slowly to avoid possible convulsions.

Pharmacological properties
Pharmacodynamic properties: Baratol is an α-adrenoceptor blocking agent which acts selectively and competitively on post-synaptic α_1-adrenoceptors, causing a decrease in peripheral resistance.

Pharmacokinetic properties: Baratol tablets are rapidly absorbed and have a half-life of about 5 hours. There is little accumulation during long-term treatment. When three volunteers and four hypertensive patients were treated with radiolabelled indoramin at dose of 40–60 mg daily for up to 3 days, plasma concentrations reached a peak 1–2 hours after administration of single doses. Over 90% of plasma indoramin was protein bound. After 2 or 3 days, 35% of the radioactivity was excreted in the urine and 46% in the faeces. Extensive first pass metabolism was suggested.

Preclinical safety data: None applicable.

Pharmaceutical particulars
List of excipients: Amberlite; Avicel; Lactose; Magnesium Stearate.
Coating: Hydroxypropylmethyl Cellulose; Polyethylene Glycol; Opaspray pigment.

Incompatibilities: Not applicable.

Shelf life: 36 months.

Special precautions for storage: Store below 25°C and protect from light.

Nature and contents of container: Pack size of 100 in amber glass bottles with suitable closures, aluminium/polyethylene foil strip or securitainers.

Instructions for use/handling: None.

Marketing authorisation numbers
Baratol Tablets 25 mg: PL 10536/0015
Baratol Tablets 50 mg: PL 10536/0016

Date of first authorisation/renewal of authorisation
23 April 1993.

Date of (partial) revision of the text March 1998.

Legal category POM.

CELEVAC* TABLETS

Presentation Pink tablets, with breakline on one face and Celevac on the other, containing 500 mg Methylcellulose BP.

Uses *Action:* Methylcellulose is a hydrophilic colloid which absorbs water to swell to a soft gel of uniform consistency.
Indications:
1. In the control of colostomy, ileostomy and diarrhoea.
2. In the management of diverticular disease.
3. In the management of simple constipation.
4. As an aid to appetite control and as an aid in the management of obesity.

Dosage and administration
1. *Colostomy and ileostomy control and for diarrhoea:* 3–6 tablets twice daily with the minimum of liquid. Liquids should be avoided for 30 minutes before and after each dose. Dosage should be adjusted to give stools the required consistency.

2. *Diverticular disease:* 3–6 tablets twice daily, adjusted according to the degree of constipation, diarrhoea or spastic pain.

3. *Simple constipation:* 3–6 tablets twice daily, to be taken with at least 300 ml of liquid. The dose may be reduced as normal bowel function is restored.

4. *Appetite control and obesity:* 3 tablets, with at least 300 ml of warm liquid, half an hour before each meal, and between meals when hunger pangs are severe.

No specific information on the use of this product in the elderly is available. Clinical trials have included patients over 65 years and no adverse reactions specific to this age group have been reported.

Contra-indications, warnings, etc Celevac should not be used in cases where the physician believes there is a pathological cause for the diarrhoea which would render the condition unsuitable for symptomatic medical treatment, e.g. infective bowel disease and imminent or threatened bowel obstruction. Bowel obstruction is a rare complication of treatment with any bulk-forming hydrophilic colloid.
Although Celevac has been in wide general use for many years there is no evidence of ill-consequence during human pregnancy.
Medicines should not be used in pregnancy, especially the first trimester, unless the expected benefit is thought to outweigh any possible risk to the foetus.

Overdosage: Methylcellulose is not absorbed. The features to be expected would be abdominal distension which may be followed by intestinal obstruction.
Gastric lavage should be employed where appropriate. The patient should be observed and fluids given. If obstruction develops, appropriate measures such as rectal washout must be taken.

Pharmaceutical precautions Protect from heat and moisture.

Legal category GSL.

Package quantities Tablet pack of 112 (OP).

Further information Methylcellulose is a hydrophilic colloid which bonds loosely with H_2O and with H_2S, thus acting as a bulking agent and a deodorising agent. In diverticular disease its use has been associated with a fall in intracolonic pressures as well as relief of symptoms.
Inactive ingredients include lactose.

Product licence number 10536/0017.

EMINASE*

Presentation Eminase is presented as a white to off-white sterile, freeze-dried solid in vials containing 30 Units of anistreplase.
Its chemical name is p-anisoylated (human) lys-plasminogen-streptokinase activator complex (APSAC). The approved name is anistreplase.
The potency of Eminase is measured using a reference standard which is specific for Eminase and is not comparable with units used for other thrombolytic agents.
Eminase includes the following inactive ingredients as solubilisers and stabilisers: aminocaproic acid, human albumin, lysine hydrochloride, mannitol, p-amidinophenyl-p'-anisate hydrochloride.

Uses
Indication: Eminase is indicated in the treatment of acute myocardial infarction to establish reperfusion, to preserve left ventricular function, to limit infarct size and to reduce mortality.
Clinical studies have shown that Eminase significantly reduces 30 day and 1 year mortality, limits infarct size and preserves left ventricular function.

Action: Eminase is a thrombolytic enzyme complex in which the catalytic centre of the activator complex is temporarily masked by an anisoyl group.
Eminase binds to fibrin strongly: this assists both its initial uptake and retention within the thrombus.
After intravenous injection, deacylation proceeds immediately with formation of the enzymatically active lys-plasminogen-streptokinase activator complex. Deacylation of Eminase proceeds in a controlled and sustained manner, resulting in a long plasma half-life which allows progressive clot uptake. This ensures sustained activation which may be useful in facilitating a low rate of early reocclusion.
The generation of lys-plasminogen-streptokinase activator complex within the thrombus converts fibrin-bound plasminogen to plasmin. The plasmin then dissolves the fibrin of the thrombus. The enzymatic efficiency of lys-plasminogen-streptokinase activator complex is enhanced by clot fibrin, ensuring efficient thrombolysis.

Dosage and administration
Dosage
Adults: Eminase is given as a single 30 Unit dose as a 4 to 5 minute intravenous injection.
Elderly: As above. See *Precautions.*
Thrombolytic therapy should be administered as soon as possible after the onset of symptoms and preferably within 6 hours. The ease of administration of Eminase should facilitate early treatment of the patient with acute myocardial infarction, for whom time is critical.

Preparation: Eminase should be reconstituted by dissolving the contents of a 30 Unit vial in 5 ml Water for Injections BP. (5 ml Sodium Chloride Injection BP [0.9% w/v] is a suitable alternative.) To avoid foaming, the diluent should be directed against the wall of the vial and the powder dissolved by gently swirling. AVOID SHAKING. Eminase dissolves immediately to give a clear or slightly turbid, colourless to pale yellow solution.
NO OTHER MEDICATION SHOULD BE ADDED TO THE VIAL OR SYRINGE CONTAINING EMINASE.

Administration: Eminase should be given by slow intravenous injection over 4 to 5 minutes.
The reconstituted solution should be administered as soon as possible. If unused after 30 minutes the solution must be discarded.
Discoloured solutions should not be used.
RECONSTITUTED SOLUTION MUST NOT BE ADMINISTERED BY INTRAMUSCULAR INJECTION OR ADDED TO INFUSION FLUIDS.

Anticoagulation: The use of anticoagulants or antiplatelet drugs following administration of Eminase has not been shown to be of unequivocal benefit. In clinical studies a majority of patients treated with Eminase received heparin therapy 4 to 6 hours after Eminase during their hospital stay, followed by oral anticoagulation as appropriate.
Following Eminase, there is a decrease in plasma fibrinogen and plasminogen concentrations and an increase in fibrin degradation products. Values have generally returned to normal within 24 to 48 hours of therapy.

Contra-indications, warnings, etc
Contra-indications: Since all thrombolytic therapies increase the risk of bleeding, Eminase is contra-indicated in the following situations:
- After surgery or major trauma within the previous 10 days.
- Recent neurosurgical procedure (previous 2 months).
- Recent traumatic cardio-pulmonary resuscitation.
- In patients with active gastro-intestinal bleeding or other internal bleeding (within the previous 6 months), e.g. active peptic ulcer.
- History of cerebrovascular accident.
- In patients with known bleeding diathesis.
- In patients with severe, uncontrolled hypertension.
- In patients with known intracranial neoplasm, or aneurysm.
- In women with heavy vaginal bleeding.

Eminase should not be administered to patients who have experienced severe allergic reactions to this product or streptokinase.
Precautions: The most common complication associated with Eminase therapy is bleeding.
Patients with any condition in which bleeding constitutes a significant hazard, or which would be particularly difficult to manage because of its location, should be monitored carefully. The risks of Eminase therapy may be increased in such patients and should be weighed against the anticipated benefits.
Venepuncture and other invasive procedures should be kept to a minimum in order to reduce the risk of bleeding. In patients undergoing cardiac catheterisation the sheath should not be removed until 24 hours after dosing.
In the following conditions the risks associated with thrombolytic therapy may be increased and should be weighed against the anticipated benefits: haemorrhagic retinopathy, coagulation defects and treatment with anticoagulants.
Patients with evidence of intramural ventricular thrombus or thrombus within abdominal aneurysms should be treated with caution as there is a risk of dissolution of clot with subsequent embolisation. This risk should be considered against the benefits of Eminase therapy.
Accelerated idioventricular rhythm may be associated with reperfusion of the coronary artery. Other arrhythmias (such as sinus bradycardia, ventricular tachycardia and ventricular fibrillation) may occur. These are not different from those often seen in the course of acute myocardial infarction and should be managed with standard measures.
Experience is limited in patients over 70 years of age and the benefits of Eminase should be balanced against risk in this group.
Because of the increased likelihood of resistance due to anti-streptokinase antibody, Eminase may not be effective if administered more than 5 days after prior Eminase or streptokinase therapy, particularly between 5 days and 12 months. Furthermore, increased anti-streptokinase antibody levels after Eminase or streptokinase may also increase the risk of allergic reactions following readministration.
Rapid injection of Eminase has been followed, in some patients, by a precipitate but transient fall in blood pressure. Eminase should be given by slow intravenous injection over 4 to 5 minutes.

Use in pregnancy and lactation: There is no evidence as to the drug safety in human pregnancy nor is there evidence from animal work that it is free from hazard. Avoid in pregnancy unless there is no safer alternative.
There is no information regarding the use of Eminase in lactating mothers.

Drug interactions: The interaction of Eminase and other drugs has not been formally studied.

Side-effects
Early reactions: Bradycardia and/or occasionally ventricular arrhythmias (including ventricular fibrillation) can occur, as in the course of acute myocardial infarction. Flushing and transient hypotension (usually within the first hour) as well as fever and nausea/vomiting (usually within 6 to 24 hours) have been reported but such reactions are generally not severe.
Allergic reactions including bronchoconstriction and anaphylaxis have been reported but are uncommon and usually reversible. Vasculitis generally manifest as a purpuric rash has occasionally been reported. All patients recovered spontaneously without sequelae.
Transient back pain immediately following administration of Eminase has been reported rarely.

Other reactions: The most common complication associated with thrombolytic therapy is bleeding, most frequently from arterial and venous puncture sites. Haemoptysis, haematuria, haematemesis and melaena have been reported occasionally. Cerebrovascular accidents have been reported but the incidence is low and there has usually been a predisposing factor.
Careful patient selection with due regard to risk factors and contra-indications can reduce the likelihood of haemorrhage.

Guillain-Barré syndrome has been rarely reported after streptokinase treatment.

Treatment of reactions: Local bleeding can be controlled with pressure. In cases of severe uncontrolled bleeding, if the haematocrit has fallen significantly, transfusion with packed cells or whole blood may be necessary. Cryoprecipitate or purified clotting factor concentrates may also be used to correct the haemostatic deficiency. Tranexamic acid (10 mg/kg body weight given by slow intravenous injection) or aprotinin (see manufacturer's literature) will competitively inhibit the fibrinolytic action of Eminase.
Mild to moderate allergic reactions may be treated, if required, with an antihistamine. Severe anaphylactic reactions should be treated with adrenaline, corticosteroids and antihistamines as appropriate. Corticosteroids may be given prophylactically, if desired.

Treatment of overdosage: see under *Treatment of reactions.*

Pharmaceutical precautions
Stability and storage: Eminase must be stored at 2–8°C (not frozen) and must not be used after the expiry date printed on the pack and vial. The IV Injection Pack, which includes Water for Injections, must not be frozen. Eminase vials must not be stored at room temperature. If a vial of Eminase is removed from the refrigerator in anticipation of being used, but is then not used, the vial can be returned to the refrigerator provided the material has not been reconstituted and is returned within 2 to 3 hours.
Reconstituted solution should be administered as soon as possible. If unused after 30 minutes the solution must be discarded.

Compatibility: No other medication should be added to the vial or syringe containing Eminase.

Legal category POM.

Package quantities
Vials of Eminase 30 Units, boxed singly.
IV Injection Pack: 1 vial Eminase 30 Units, a 5 ml ampoule of Water for Injections BP, a 5 ml disposable syringe and needle.
Each pack contains instructions for use.

Further information Eminase belongs to a new class of thrombolytic agents designed for use in the treatment of acute myocardial infarction. Eminase can be given as a single, slow intravenous injection, over 4 to 5 minutes, unlike other thrombolytic agents which require intravenous infusions of various degrees of complexity. The ease of administration of Eminase facilitates early treatment of the patient with acute myocardial infarction, for whom time is critical.
The fibrinolytic mean half-life of Eminase is 94 minutes (range of 70 to 120 minutes).
At the recommended dose of 30 Units injected intravenously in patients with acute myocardial infarction of less than 6 hours' duration, patency of coronary arteries has occurred in 70–80% of patients.
The incidence of early reocclusion with Eminase is low and is less than 10% in reported studies.
Clinical studies have shown that reperfusion with Eminase preserves myocardial function and improves patient survival.
Randomised controlled studies have demonstrated that treatment with Eminase reduces mortality for at least 1 year when administered within 6 hours after the onset of symptoms of acute myocardial infarction.
It is recommended that antiarrhythmic therapy for bradycardia, ventricular tachycardia and ventricular fibrillation be available when infusions of Eminase are administered as would normally be required in the early phase of acute myocardial infarction.

Product licence numbers

Eminase 30 Unit vial	0038/0353.
Water for Injections BP	10536/0039.

HRF*

Presentation HRF (gonadorelin hydrochloride) is a synthetic decapeptide that has a chemical composition and structure identical to the naturally-occurring luteinizing hormone-releasing hormone (LH-RH) isolated from porcine or ovine hypothalami, in a freeze-dried form. HRF is available as a 100 microgram vial also containing 100 mg lactose. An ampoule of sterile diluent is supplied which contains 2% benzyl alcohol and water for injection.

Uses HRF as a single injection is indicated for evaluating the functional capacity and response of the gonadotropes of the anterior pituitary. The LH response is used in testing patients with suspected gonadotropin deficiency, whether due to the hypothalamus alone or in combination with anterior pituitary failure. HRF is also indicated for evaluating residual gonadotropic function of the pituitary following removal of a pituitary tumour or surgery and/or irradiation.

Dosage and administration *Adults:* 100 micrograms dose, subcutaneously or intravenously. In females for whom the phase of the menstrual cycle can be established, the test should be performed in early follicular phase (days 1–7).

Test methodology: To determine the status of the gonadotropin secretory capacity of the anterior pituitary, a test procedure requiring seven venous blood samples for LH is recommended.
Procedure
1. Venous blood samples should be drawn at −15 minutes and immediately prior to HRF administration. The LH baseline is obtained by averaging the LH values of the two samples.
2. Administer a bolus of HRF subcutaneously or intravenously.
3. Draw venous blood samples at 15, 30, 45, 60 and 120 minutes after administration.
4. Blood samples should be handled as recommended by the laboratory that will determine the LH content. It must be emphasised that the reliability of the test is directly related to the inter-assay and intra-assay reliability of the laboratory performing the assay.

Interpretation of test results: Interpretation of the LH

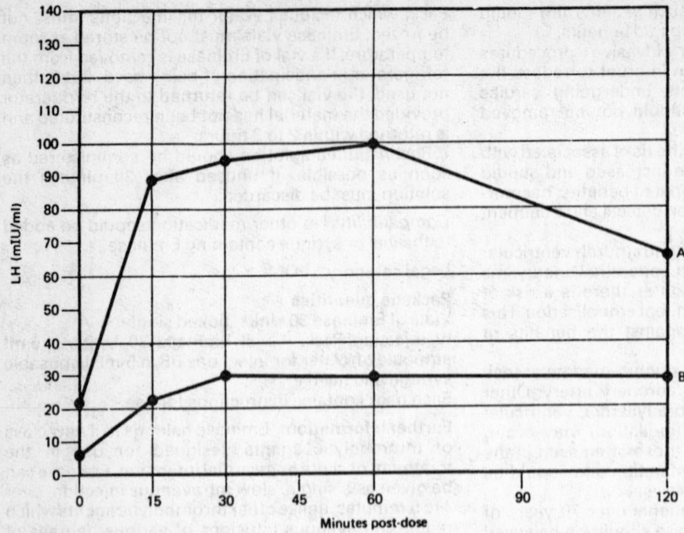

Figure 1. **Normal male LH response after HRF 100 micrograms subcutaneous administration 10th and 90th percentiles.**

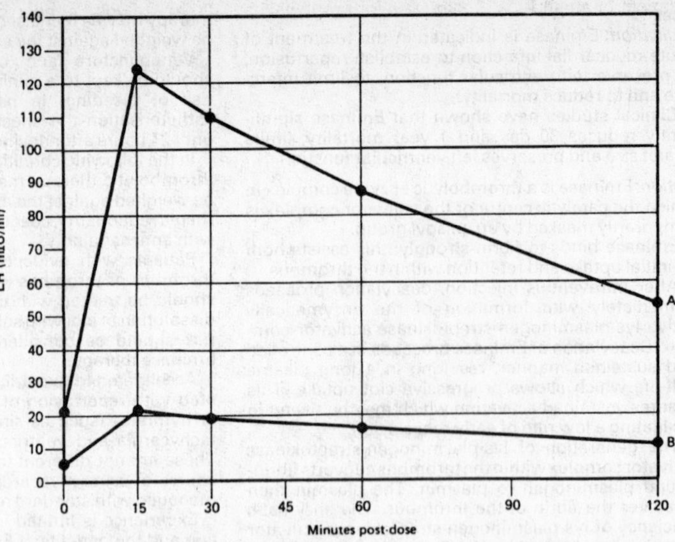

Figure 2. **Normal male LH response after HRF 100 micrograms intravenous administration 10th and 90th percentiles.**

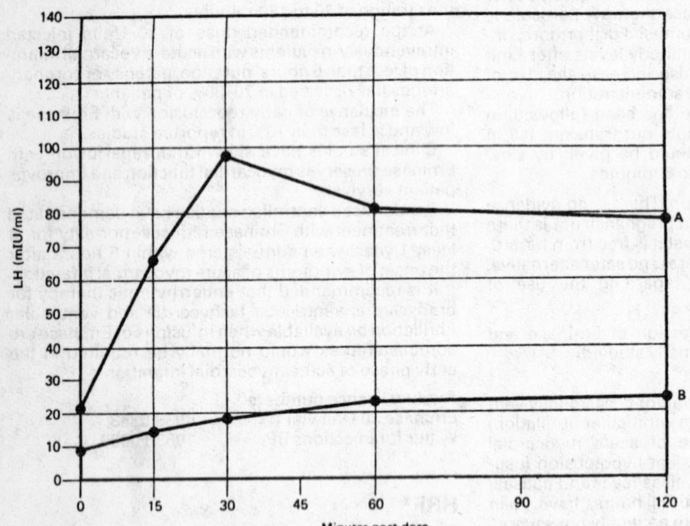

Figure 3. **Normal female LH response after HRF 100 micrograms subcutaneous administration 10th and 90th percentiles.**

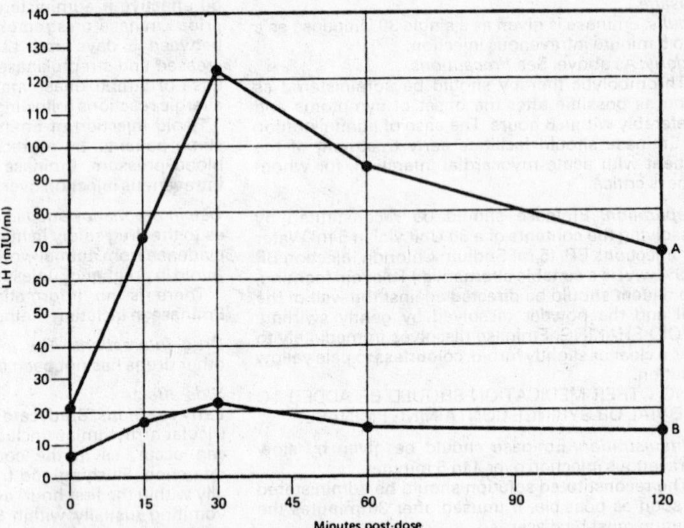

Figure 4. **Normal female LH response after HRF 100 micrograms intravenous administration 10th and 90th percentiles.**

response to HRF requires an understanding of the hypothalamic-pituitary physiology, knowledge of the clinical status of the individual patient, and familiarity with the normal ranges and the standards used in the laboratory performing the LH assays.

Figures 1–4 represent the LH response curves after HRF administration in normal subjects. The normal LH response curves were established between the 10th percentile (B line) and 90th percentile (A line) of all LH responses in normal subjects analysed from the results of clinical studies. Individual patient responses should be plotted on the appropriate curve. A subnormal response in patients is defined as three or more LH values which fall below the B line of the normal LH response curve.

In cases where there is a blunted or borderline response, the HRF test should be repeated.

The HRF test complements the clinical assessment of patients with a variety of endocrine disorders involving the hypothalamic-pituitary axis. In cases where there is a normal response, it indicates the presence of functional pituitary gonadotropes. The single injection test does not determine the pathophysiological cause for the subnormal response and does not measure pituitary gonadotropic reserve.

Contra-indications, warnings, etc

Contra-indications: Hypersensitivity to HRF or any of the components. Known or suspected pregnancy. Do not use in children under one year of age as diluent contains 2% benzyl alcohol.

Precautions: Although allergic and hypersensitivity reactions have been observed with other polypeptide hormones, to date no such reactions have been encountered following the administration of a single 100 micrograms dose of HRF used for diagnostic purposes. Rare instances of hypersensitivity reactions have been reported (see Side Effects). Therefore, patients treated by intermittent pulsatile therapy in whom re-administration is considered, particularly by the intravenous route, should be carefully observed. Administration during the follicular phase of a normal cycle may result in premature ovulation and appropriate measures are advised to prevent an unwanted pregnancy in these circumstances.

Drug interactions: The HRF test should be conducted in the absence of other drugs which directly affect the pituitary secretion of the gonadotrophins. These would include a variety of preparations which contain androgens, oestrogens, progestins, or glucocorticoids. The gonadotropin levels may be transiently elevated by spironolactone, minimally elevated by levodopa, and suppressed by oral contraceptives and digoxin. The response to HRF may be blunted by phenothiazines and dopamine antagonists which cause a rise in prolactin.

Side-effects: Systemic complaints such as headaches, nausea, lightheadedness, abdominal discomfort and flushing have been reported rarely following administration of HRF. Local swelling, occasionally with pain and pruritus at the injection site may occur if HRF is administered subcutaneously. Local and generalised skin rash have been noted after chronic subcutaneous administration.

Thrombophlebitis with septicaemia, mild and severe, has been reported in isolated cases at the site of intravenous injection. Rare instances of hypersensitivity reaction (bronchospasm, tachycardia, flushing, urticaria, swelling, itching and redness of face, eyelids and lips, induration at injection site) have been reported following multiple-dose administration of large doses. Antibody formation has also been reported rarely after chronic administration of large doses.

Overdosage: HRF has been administered parenterally in doses up to 3 mg bd for 28 days without any signs or symptoms of overdosage. In case of overdosage or idiosyncrasy, symptomatic treatment should be administered as required.

Pharmaceutical precautions Both the lyophilised powder vial and diluent ampoule have a shelf life of 4 years. Store at room temperature (approximately 25°C). Preparation for single injection administration: Reconstitute 100 micrograms vial with 1.0 ml of the accompanying sterile diluent of 2% benzyl alcohol. Prepare solution immediately before use. After reconstitution, refrigerate and use within 1 day. Discard unused reconstituted solution and diluent.

Legal category POM.

Package quantities Packs comprise a vial containing 100 micrograms freeze-dried material and a 5 ml ampoule of sterile diluent (OP).

Further information Nil.

Product licence number
HRF 100 micrograms 10536/0013

ISORDIL* TABLETS 5 mg
ISORDIL* TABLETS 10 mg
ISORDIL* TABLETS 30 mg

Quantative and qualitative composition Each 5 mg, 10 mg and 30 mg tablet contains diluted isosorbide dinitrate (equivalent to 5 mg, 10 mg and 30 mg isosorbide dinitrate respectively – diluent is lactose).

Pharmaceutical form Tablet.

Clinical particulars

Therapeutic indications: For the prophylactic treatment of angina (classic effort associated angina, chronic stable angina, vasospastic angina, variant angina, and angina decubitus): acute and chronic congestive heart failure including that associated with myocardial infarction as adjunctive therapy.

The 5 mg sublingual tablets are also used for the

treatment of an attack of angina and for prophylaxis in situations likely to provoke attacks.

Posology and method of administration: The 5 mg tablet is taken sublingually.

The 10 mg and 30 mg tablets are taken orally.

Adults:

Angina pectoris: Acute attack or prophylactically in situations likely to provoke attacks: one or two 5 mg Isordil Tablets sublingually every 2 hours or as required.

10 mg and 30 mg tablets: Prophylaxis: 40 to 120 mg daily in divided doses or as required. In selected cases, daily doses of up to 240 mg Isordil have been administered without undue adverse effects.

In order to obtain maximal therapeutic effect it is important that the dosages of sublingual and oral forms of Isordil be individualised in accordance with patient needs, response and tolerance.

Congestive heart failure: Acute and chronic, including after myocardial infarction: Sublingual Isordil 5 mg to 15 mg every 2–3 hours or as needed. The 10 mg or 30 mg tablets of Isordil may be administered in doses of 10 to 60 mg four times daily or as needed.

The therapeutic uses of Isordil in selected cases of acute and chronic congestive heart failure should be considered as an adjunct to the more conventional modes of therapy such as cardiac glycosides, diuretics and other vasodilators. In refractory cases Isordil may be used alone or concomitantly with other vasodilators. Haemodynamic monitoring of the patient under treatment is desirable and optimal dose regimens should be determined for individual cases depending on these results. Isordil therapy should begin with the lowest effective dose, based on assessment of the severity of heart failure and then adjusted as necessary.

In both acute and chronic failure Isordil should be administered initially in the sublingual form to stabilise the patients' symptoms and determine the magnitude of haemodynamic response, and then in the oral form for maintenance therapy.

Use in children: Isordil is not recommended for children.

Use in the elderly: There are no special dosage requirements for elderly patients, but as with all medicines, the lowest effective dose should be used.

Contra-indications: Hypersensitivity to this drug.

Special warnings and precautions for use: Tolerance to this drug and cross tolerance to other nitrates may occur; withdrawal restores the original sensitivity. In congestive heart failure, as a rule, pulmonary capillary pressure should not be allowed to fall below 15 mmHg or systolic blood pressure below normal physiological range in normal or hypertensive patients. In patients with hypotension in the range of 90–100 mmHg of systolic pressure there should be no fall at all. As with other vasodilators in sensitive patients Isordil may cause paradoxical side effects which may increase ischaemia and may even lead to extension of myocardial damage and advanced congestive heart failure. Treatment should therefore be discontinued.

Interaction with other medicaments and other forms of interaction: This drug can act as a physiological antagonist to noradrenaline, acetylcholine, histamine and many other agents.

Pregnancy and lactation: This product has not been studied in human pregnancy. The use of Isordil requires that the anticipated benefit be weighed against possible hazard.

Lactation – it is not known whether Isordil is excreted in human milk. It is unlikely that a nursing woman would require Isordil but the decision depends on the condition of the patient and caution should be exercised.

Effects on ability to drive and use machines: None known.

Undesirable effects: Cutaneous vasodilatation with flushing. Headache is common and in some patients may be severe and persistent. Analgesics have been useful in some cases. Transient episodes of dizziness and weakness and other signs of cerebral ischaemia associated with postural hypotension may occur. An occasional individual exhibits a marked sensitivity to the hypotensive effects of nitrates and severe responses (nausea, vomiting, weakness, restlessness, pallor, perspiration and collapse) can occur, even with the usual therapeutic dose. Alcohol may enhance this effect. Drug rash and/or exfoliative dermatitis may occasionally occur.

Overdose: The main manifestation is hypotension. In such an event, the drug should be withheld and the patient carefully monitored. Passive exercise and elevation of the legs of the recumbent patient will promote venous return. In life threatening situations administration of vasopressors should be considered. The LD_{50} of isosorbide dinitrate in rodents is of the order of 1000 mg/kg.

Pharmacological properties

Pharmacodynamic properties: Isosorbide dinitrate is a vasodilator, causing relaxation of smooth muscle of blood vessels. Vasodilation occurs in coronary arteries and collaterals, peripheral arterioles, the venous system and major vascular beds. The subsequent reductions in peripheral resistance and venous return unload the heart and so lower oxygen demand. Dilatation of coronary arteries and improved myocardial perfusion increases the supply of oxygen.

Pharmacokinetic properties: The anti-anginal effects of sublingual Isordil generally occur within 2–5 minutes after administration and last for 1–2 hours. The haemodynamic effects of the oral tablets are observed within 20–60 minutes and last for 4–6 hours.

The major route of metabolism of isosorbide dinitrate in man is by enzymatic denitration followed by formulation of glucuronides. The half-life is approximately 45 minutes. The primary initial metabolites, isosorbide-2-mononitrate and isosorbide-5-mononitrate have longer half-lives (2–5 hours).

Preclinical safety data: None given.

Pharmaceutical particulars

List of excipients: Isordil Tablets 5 mg contain Anhydrous Lactose, Dried Maize Starch, Magnesium Stearate, Powdered Cellulose (Solka Flock), Colloidal Anydrous Silica and E127.

Isordil Tablets 10 mg and 30 mg contain Anhydrous Lactose, Microcrystalline Cellulose and Magnesium Stearate.

Incompatibilities: Not applicable.

Shelf life: Isordil Tablets 5 mg and 10 mg: 36 months. Isordil Tablets 30 mg: 60 months.

Special precautions for storage: None.

Nature and contents of container: Isordil Tablets 5 mg: Securitainers (with secondary packaging as appropriate) containing 100 tablets.

Isordil Tablets 10 mg: Securitainers (with secondary packaging as appropriate) containing 112 tablets.

Isordil Tablets 30 mg: Securitainers (with secondary packaging as appropriate) containing 112 tablets.

Instructions for use/handling: None given.

Marketing authorisation numbers

Isordil Tablets 5 mg: 10536/0009
Isordil Tablets 10 mg: 10536/0010
Isordil Tablets 30 mg: 10536/0011

Date of first authorisation

Isordil Tablets 5 mg: 31 March 1993
Isordil Tablets 10 mg and 30 mg: 29 January 1993

Date of partial revision of SPC September 1997.

Legal category P.

ISORDIL* TEMBIDS* CAPSULES 40 mg

Quantitative and qualitative composition Each capsule contains diluted isosorbide dinitrate (equivalent to 40 mg isosorbide dinitrate – diluent is lactose).

Pharmaceutical form Capsule.

Clinical particulars

Therapeutic indications: For the prophylactic treatment of angina (classic effort associated angina, chronic stable angina, vasospastic angina, variant angina and angina decubitus).

Posology and method of administration:

Adults: For oral administration – one capsule 2 or 3 times a day. In selected cases, daily doses of up to 240 mg Isordil have been administered. Capsules should be swallowed without chewing.

Use in children: Isordil is not recommended for children.

Use in the elderly: There are no special dosage requirements for elderly patients, but as with all medicines, the lowest effective dose should be used.

Contraindications: Idiosincrasy to this drug.

Special warnings and precautions for use: Tolerance to this drug and cross-tolerance to other nitrates may occur; withdrawal restores the original sensitivity. In congestive heart failure, as a rule, pulmonary capillary pressure should not be allowed to fall below 15 mm Hg, or systolic blood pressure below normal physiological range in normal or hypertensive patients. In patients with hypotension in the range 90–100 mm Hg of systolic pressure, there should be no fall at all. As with other vasodilators in sensitive patients, Isordil may cause paradoxical side effects which may increase ischaemia and may even lead to extension of myocardial damage and advanced congestive heart failure.

Interaction with other medicaments and other forms of interaction: This drug can act as a physiological antagonist to noradrenaline, acetylcholine, histamine and many other agents.

Pregnancy and lactation: The product has not been studied in human pregnancy. The use of Isordil requires that the anticipated benefit be weighed against possible hazard.

Lactation – it is not known whether Isordil is excreted in human milk. Since many drugs are excreted in human milk, caution should be exercised if Isordil is administered to a nursing woman.

Effects on ability to drive and use machines: None known.

Undesirable effects: Cutaneous vasodilation with flushing. Headache is common and in some patients may be severe and persistent. Analgesics have been useful in some cases. Transient episodes of dizziness and weakness and other signs of cerebral ischaemia associated with postural hypotension may occur. An occasional individual exhibits a marked sensitivity to the hypotensive effects of nitrates and severe responses (nausea, vomiting, weakness, restlessness, pallor, perspiration and collapse) can occur, even with the usual therapeutic dose. Alcohol may enhance this effect. Drug rash and/or exfoliative dermatitis may occasionally occur.

As with other vasodilators in sensitive patients, Isordil may cause paradoxical side effects which may increase ischaemia and may even lead to extension of myocardial damage and advanced congestive heart failure. Treatments should therefore be discontinued.

Overdose: The main manifestation is hypotension. In such an event, the drug should be withheld and the patient carefully monitored. Passive exercise and elevation of the legs of the recumbent patient will promote venous return. In life threatening situations administration of vasopressors should be considered. The LD_{50} of isosorbide dinitrate in rodents is of the order of 1000 mg/kg.

Pharmacological properties

Pharmacodynamic properties: Isosorbide dinitrate is a vasodilator, causing relaxation of smooth muscle of blood vessels. Vasodilation occurs in coronary arteries and collaterals, peripheral arterioles, the venous system and major vascular beds.

The subsequent reductions in peripheral resistance and venous return unload the heart and so lower oxygen demand. Dilatation of coronary arteries and improved myocardial perfusion increases the supply of oxygen.

Pharmacokinetic properties: The major route of metabolism of isosorbide dinitrate in man is by enzymatic denitration followed by formulation of glucuronides. The half-life is approximately 45 minutes. The primary initial metabolites, isosorbide-2-mononitrate and isosorbide-5-mononitrate have longer half-lives (2–5 hours).

The pharmacological activity and bioavailability of Isordil Tembids capsules was evaluated by digital plethysmography. The capsules demonstrated statistically significant activity versus placebo for 12 hours post drug.

Preclinical safety drug: None given.

Pharmaceutical particulars

List of excipients: Isordil Tembids Capsules 40 mg contain Acacia, Talc, Sucrose, Povidone, Calcium Stearate, Shellac Solution, Lactose, Gelatin, FD & C Blue (E132), Titanium Dioxide (E171).

Incompatibilities: Not applicable.

Shelf life: 60 months.

Special precautions for storage: None.

Nature and contents of container: Securitainers (with secondary packaging as appropriate) containing 56 capsules.

Instructions for use/handling: None given.

Marketing authorisation number PL 10536/0012.

Date of first authorisation 17 May 1993.

Date of partial revision of SPC September 1997.

Legal category P.

LODINE*
LODINE* SR

Presentation

Lodine capsules containing etodolac 200 mg are hard gelatin capsules with an opaque dark grey body and light grey cap, printed with two red bands and 'Lodine 200'.

Lodine capsules containing etodolac 300 mg are hard gelatin capsules with an opaque light grey body and cap, printed with two red bands and 'Lodine 300'.

Lodine tablets contain etodolac 200 mg and are brown, oval biconvex film coated tablets, printed 'WYETH' or 'LODINE' and '200'.

Lodine SR tablets contain etodolac 600 mg in a sustained release formulation and are capsular, oval shaped light grey film coated tablets, impressed on one side with Lodine SR600.

Uses Lodine (etodolac) is indicated for acute or long-term use in rheumatoid arthritis and osteoarthritis.

Dosage and administration
Adults: Lodine Capsules 200 mg, 300 mg and Lodine Tablets 200 mg – The recommended dosage for Lodine is 400 mg to 600 mg daily in two divided doses or administered as a single daily dose.

Lodine SR Tablets 600 mg: One tablet daily, swallowed whole with a tumblerful of water. If a lower dose is sufficient, conventional Lodine capsules or tablets may be used. The safety of doses in excess of 600 mg per day has not been established. No occurrence of tolerance or tachyphylaxis has been reported.

Elderly: No change in initial dosage is generally required in the elderly (see *Precautions*).

Children: Not recommended.

Contra-indications, warnings, etc
Contra-indications:
1. Lodine should not be used in patients who have previously shown hypersensitivity to it.
2. Lodine should not be used in patients with active peptic ulceration or a history of peptic ulcer disease (including gastrointestinal haemorrhage due to another non-steroidal anti-inflammatory drug).
3. Due to possible cross-reactivity, Lodine should not be administered to patients who experience asthma, rhinitis or urticaria during therapy with aspirin or other non-steroidal anti-inflammatory drugs.

Pregnancy: Drugs which inhibit prostaglandin biosynthesis may cause dystocia and delayed parturition as evidenced by studies in pregnant animals. Some inhibitors of prostaglandin biosynthesis have been shown to interfere with the closure of the ductus arteriosus. Safety in human pregnancy has not been established and Lodine should not be used during pregnancy. Safety of Lodine use during lactation has not been established and as such its use in nursing mothers should be avoided.

Precautions:
1. Although non-steroidal anti-inflammatory drugs do not have the same direct effects on platelets as does aspirin, all drugs which inhibit the biosynthesis of prostaglandins may interfere, to some extent, with platelet function. Patients receiving Lodine who may be adversely affected by such actions should be carefully observed.
2. In patients with renal, cardiac or hepatic impairment especially those taking diuretics, caution is required since the use of NSAIDs may result in deterioration of renal function. The dose should be kept as low as possible and renal function should be monitored. However, impairment of renal or hepatic functions due to other causes may alter drug metabolism; patients receiving concomitant long term therapy, especially the elderly, should be observed for potential side effects and their drug doses adjusted as needed, or the drug discontinued.
3. Serious gastrointestinal adverse effects such as bleeding, ulceration and perforation can occur at any time with or without warning symptoms in patients treated with NSAIDs. If any sign of gastrointestinal bleeding occurs, Lodine should be stopped immediately.
4. Patients on long-term treatment with Lodine should be regularly reviewed as a precautionary measure e.g. for changes in renal function, haematological parameters, or hepatic function.
5. Lodine should be used with caution in patients with fluid retention, hypertension or heart failure.

Drug interactions:
1. Since Lodine is extensively protein-bound, it may be necessary to modify the dosage of other highly protein-bound drugs.
The concomitant administration of warfarin and Lodine should not require a dosage adjustment of either drug, however it has rarely led to prolonged prothrombin times, therefore caution should be exercised when Lodine is administered with warfarin.
2. Concomitant use of cyclosporin, digoxin, or lithium with NSAIDs may cause an increase in serum levels of these compounds and associated toxicities.
3. Bilirubin tests can give a false positive result due to the presence of phenolic metabolites of Lodine in the urine.

Side-effects:
1. Reported side effects include nausea, epigastric pain, diarrhoea, indigestion, heartburn, flatulence, abdominal pain, constipation, vomiting, ulcerative stomatitis, dyspepsia, gastritis, haematemesis, melaena, rectal bleeding, colitis, vasculitis, headaches, dizziness, abnormal vision, pyrexia, drowsiness, tinnitus, rash, pruritus, fatigue, depression, insomnia, confusion, paraesthesia, tremor, weakness/malaise, dyspnoea, oedema, palpitations, bilirubinuria, hepatic function abnormalities and jaundice, urinary frequency, dysuria, angioedema, anaphylactoid reaction, photosensitivity, urticaria and Stevens-Johnson syndrome.
2. More serious adverse reactions which may occasionally occur are gastro-intestinal ulceration and peptic ulceration.
3. NSAIDs have been reported to cause nephrotoxicity in various forms and their use can lead to interstitial nephritis, nephrotic syndrome and renal failure. There have been reports of nephritis and renal failure with etodolac.
4. Occasionally blood disorders have been reported including: thrombocytopenia, neutropenia, agranulocytosis and anaemia.

Overdosage: The standard practices of gastric lavage, activated charcoal administration and general supportive therapy should be undertaken.

Pharmaceutical precautions Store at room temperature – below 25°C.

Legal category POM

Package quantities
Lodine 200 mg capsules: Securitainers of 60.
Lodine 300 mg capsules: Cartons containing 60 capsules, (blisters of 10).
Lodine 200 mg tablets: White HDPE bottles of 60.
Lodine SR 600 mg tablets: Cartons containing 30 tablets, (blisters of 10).

Further information All non-steroidal anti-inflammatory drugs (NSAIDs) have been shown to inhibit the formation of prostaglandins. It is this action which is primarily responsible both for their therapeutic effects and some of their side-effects. The inhibition of prostaglandin synthesis observed with etodolac differs from that of other NSAIDs. In an animal model at an established anti-inflammatory dose, cytoprotective PGE concentrations in the gastric mucosa have been shown to be reduced to a lesser degree and for a shorter period with eotdolac than with other NSAIDs

This finding is consistent with subsequent in-vitro studies which have found etodolac to be selective for induced cyclo-oxygenase 2 (COX-2, associated with inflammation) over COX-1 (cytoprotective). Furthermore, studies in human cell models have confirmed that etodolac is selective for the inhibition of COX-2. The clinical benefit of preferential COX-2 inhibition over COX-1 has yet to be proven.

Product licence numbers

Lodine Capsules 200 mg	0011/0144
Lodine Capsules 300 mg	0011/0145
Lodine Tablets 200 mg	0011/0148
Lodine SR Tablets 600 mg	0011/0197

Product licence holder: Wyeth Laboratories, Huntercombe Lane South, Taplow, Maidenhead.

MAXOLON*

Qualitative and quantitative composition
Maxolon Tablets 5 mg: Each tablet contains Metoclopramide Hydrochloride BP equivalent to 5 mg of the anhydrous substance.

Maxolon Tablets 10 mg: Each tablet contains Metoclopramide Hydrochloride BP equivalent to 10 mg of the anhydrous substance.

Maxolon Syrup: The syrup contains Metoclopramide Hydrochloride BP equivalent to 1 mg/ml of the anhydrous substance.

Maxolon Paediatric Liquid: The liquid contains Metoclopramide Hydrochloride BP equivalent to 1 mg/ml of the anhydrous substance.

Maxolon Injection: Each 2 ml ampoule contains Metoclopramide Hydrochloride BP equivalent to 10 mg of the anhydrous substance.

Pharmaceutical form
Maxolon Tablets 5 mg: White to ivory-white circular tablets.

Maxolon Tablets 10 mg: White uncoated tablets scored and engraved Maxolon.

Maxolon Syrup and Paediatric Liquid: Clear colourless lemon-lime solution for oral administration.

Maxolon Injection: Clear colourless solution for intramuscular or intravenous administration.

Clinical particulars
Therapeutic indications: Adults (20 years and over):
Digestive disorders: Maxolon restores normal coordination and tone to the upper digestive tract. Maxolon relieves the symptoms of gastro-duodenal dysfunction including: dyspepsia, heartburn, flatulence, sickness, regurgitation of bile, pain. These symptoms may be associated with such conditions as: peptic ulcer, duodenitis, reflux oesophagitis, hiatus hernia, gastritis, cholelithiasis and post-cholecystectomy dyspepsia.

Nausea and vomiting: Maxolon is indicated for the treatment of the nausea and vomiting associated with: gastro-intestinal disorders, cyclical vomiting, intolerance to cytotoxic drugs, congestive heart failure, deep x-ray or cobalt therapy, post-anaesthetic vomiting.

Migraine: Maxolon relieves symptoms of nausea and vomiting, and overcomes gastric stasis associated with attacks of migraine. This improvement in gastric emptying assists the absorption of concurrently administered oral anti-migraine therapy (e.g. paracetamol) which may otherwise be impaired in such patients.

Post-operative conditions: Post-operative gastric hypotonia, post-vagotomy syndrome. Maxolon promotes normal gastric emptying and restores motility in vagotomised patients, and where post-operative symptoms suggest gastro-duodenal dysfunction.

Diagnostic procedures: Radiology, Duodenal intubation. Maxolon speeds up the passage of a barium meal by decreasing gastric emptying time, co-ordinating peristalsis and dilating the duodenal bulb. Maxolon also facilitates duodenal intubation procedures.

Young adults and children: The use of Maxolon in patients under 20 years should be restricted to the following:

Severe intractable vomiting of known cause, vomiting associated with radiotherapy and intolerance to cytotoxic drugs, as an aid to gastro-intestinal intubation, and as part of the premedication before surgical procedures.

Posology and method of administration:

Route of administration
Oral: The dosage recommendations given below should be strictly adhered to if side effects of the dystonic type are to be avoided. It should be noted that total daily dosage of Maxolon, especially for children and young adults, should not normally exceed 0.5 mg/kg body weight.

In patients with clinically significant degrees of renal or hepatic impairment, therapy should be at reduced dosage. Metoclopramide is metabolised in the liver and the predominant route of elimination of metoclopramide and its metabolites is via the kidney.

Injection: Maxolon injection may be administered either intramuscularly or by slow intravenous injection (1-2 minutes).

Otherwise as for oral dosage.

Medical indications:
Adults 20 years and over: 10 mg three times daily. For patients of less than 60 kg see below.

Elderly patients: As for adults. To avoid adverse reactions adhere strictly to dosage recommendations and where prolonged therapy is considered necessary, patients should be regularly reviewed.

Young adults and children: Maxolon should only be used after careful examination to avoid masking an underlying disorder, e.g. cerebral irritation. In the treatment of this group attention should be given primarily to body weight and treatment should commence at the lower dosage where stated.

Young adults:	15-19 years, 60 kg and over	10 mg three times daily
	30-59 kg	5 mg three times daily
Children:	9-14 years, 30 kg and over	5 mg three times daily
	5-9 years, 20-29 kg	2½ mg three times daily
	3-5 years, 15-19 kg	2 mg two to three times daily
	1-3 years, 10-14 kg	1 mg two to three times daily
	Under 1 year, up to 10 kg	1 mg twice daily

Tablets should not be used in children under the age of 15. Maxolon Injection or an oral liquid presentation should be used in the younger age groups; more accurate dosage is facilitated by the use of the Paediatric Liquid.

Diagnostic indications: A single dose of Maxolon may be given 5-10 minutes before the examination subject to body weight consideration,(see above); the following dosages are recommended.

Adults:	20 years and over	10-20 mg
Young adults:	15-19 years	10 mg
Children:	9-14 years	5 mg
	5-9 years	2½ mg
	3-5 years	2 mg
	Under 3 years	1 mg

Maxolon Injection or an oral liquid presentation should be used in the younger age groups; more accurate dosage is facilitated by the use of the Paediatric liquid.

Contra-indications: No absolute contra-indications to the use of Maxolon.

Special warnings and special precautions for use: Precautions: If vomiting persists the patient should be reassessed to exclude the possibility of an underlying disorder e.g. cerebral irritation.

Care should be exercised in patients being treated with other centrally active drugs e.g. in epilepsy.

Since extrapyramidal symptoms may occur with both metoclopramide and neuroleptics such as the phenothiazines, particular care should be exercised in the event of these drugs being prescribed concurrently.

The neuroleptic malignant syndrome has been reported with metoclopramide in combination with neuroleptics as well as with metoclopramide monotherapy *(see side effects)*.

Special care should be taken in cases of severe renal insufficiency (see also under dosage and administration).

Following operations such as pyloroplasty or gut anastomosis metoclopramide therapy should be withheld for three or four days as vigorous muscular contractions may not help healing.

Metoclopramide may induce an acute hypertensive response in patients with phaeochromocytoma.

Interaction with other medicaments and other forms of interaction: The action of Maxolon on the gastro-intestinal tract is antagonised by anticholinergics. The absorption of any concurrently administered oral medication may be modified by the effect of Maxolon on gastric motility.

Pregnancy and lactation: Animal tests in several mammalian species and clinical experience have not indicated a teratogenic effect. Nevertheless Maxolon should only be used when there are compelling reasons and is not advised during the first trimester.

During lactation metoclopramide is found in breast milk.

Effects on ability to drive and use machines: None but see below.

Undesirable effects: Various extrapyramidal reactions to Maxolon, usually of the dystonic type, have been reported. The incidence of dystonic reactions, particularly in children and young adults, is increased if daily dosages higher than 0.5 mg per kg body weight are administered. Dystonic reactions include: spasm of the facial muscles, trismus, rhythmic protrusion of the tongue, a bulbar type of speech, spasm of extra-ocular muscles including oculogyric crises, unnatural positioning of the head and shoulders and opisthotonos. There may be a generalised increase in muscle tone. The majority of reactions occur within 36 hours of starting treatment and the effects usually disappear within 24 hours of withdrawal of the drug. Should treatment of a dystonic reaction be required an anticholinergic anti-Parkinsonian drug, or a benzodiazepine may be used.

Very rare occurrences of the neuroleptic malignant syndrome have been reported. This syndrome is potentially fatal and comprises hyperpyrexia, altered consciousness, muscle rigidity, autonomic instability and elevated levels of creatine phosphokinase (CPK) and must be treated urgently (recognised treatments include dantrolene and bromocriptine). Metoclopramide should be stopped immediately if this syndrome occurs.

Tardive dyskinesia has been reported during prolonged treatment in a small number of mainly elderly patients. Patients on prolonged treatment should be regularly reviewed.

Rarely, drowsiness, restlessness, confusion and diarrhoea have been reported in patients receiving metoclopramide therapy. Depression has been reported extremely rarely.

Raised serum prolactin levels have been observed during metoclopramide therapy: this effect is similar to that noted with many other compounds.

Extremely rarely cases of red cell disorders such as methaemoglobinaemia and sulphaemoglobinaemia have been reported, particularly at high doses of metoclopramide. If this occurs the drug should be withdrawn. Methaemoglobinaemia may be treated using methylene blue.

For intravenous use: There have been very rare reports of abnormalities of cardiac conduction (such as bradycardia and heart block) in association with intravenous metoclopramide.

Overdose: In cases of overdosage, acute dystonic reactions have occurred. Overdosage should be treated by gastric lavage with appropriate supportive measures. For treatment of a dystonic reaction see *Side effects.* Very rarely AV block has been observed with Maxolon Injection.

Pharmacological properties

Pharmacodynamic properties: The action of metoclopramide is closely associated with parasympathetic nervous control of the upper gastro-intestinal tract, where it has the effect of encouraging normal peristaltic action. This provides for a fundamental approach to the control of those conditions where disturbed gastro-intestinal motility is a common underlying factor.

Pharmacokinetic properties: Metoclopramide is metabolised in the liver and the predominant route of elimination of metoclopramide and its metabolites is via the kidney.

Preclinical safety data: No additional data available.

Pharmaceutical particulars

List of excipients: Maxolon Tablets 5 mg and 10 mg: Maize starch (dried), colloidal silicon dioxide, magnesium stearate, pregelatinised maize starch, lactose.

Maxolon Syrup and Paediatric Liquid: Hydroxyethylcellulose, methyl parahydroxybenzoate, propyl parahydroxybenzoate, saccharin sodium, citric acid monohydrate, soluble lemon oil, No.1 lime flavour, purified water.

Maxolon Injection: Sodium chloride, sodium metabisulphite, water for injection.

Incompatibilities: Not applicable.

Shelf life: Maxolon Tablets 10 mg and Injection: Sixty months.

Maxolon Tablets 5 mg and Syrup: Thirtysix months.

Maxolon Paediatric Liquid: Thirtysix months. The liquid should be used within 14 days of opening.

Special precautions for storage: Maxolon Tablets 5 mg: Store at or below 25°C.

Maxolon Tablets 10 mg: None. Maxolon Syrup and Paediatric Liquid: Protect from light. Maxolon Injection: If ampoules are removed from their carton, they should be stored away from light. If inadvertent exposure occurs, ampoules showing discolouration must be discarded.

Nature and contents of container:
Maxolon Tablets 5 mg: PVC (250 microns)/PVDC (60 gsm) blister (84 tablets) backed with aluminium foil (20 microns). The underside of the foil is coated with vinyl based lacquer.
Maxolon Tablets 10 mg: Plastic recloseable containers packed into carton of 100 or 500 tablets. PVC blister (300 microns) of 84 tablets backed with aluminium foil (20 microns). The underside of the foil is coated with vinyl based lacquer.
Maxolon Syrup: Amber glass bottles of 200 ml.
Maxolon Paediatric Liquid: Amber glass bottles with pipette administration device of 15 ml liquid.
Maxolon Injection: Clear glass 2 ml ampoules (PhEur, Type I neutral glass) in packs of 12 ampoules.

Instructions for use/handling:
Maxolon Tablets 5 mg, 10 mg, Syrup, Paediatric Liquid: None.
Maxolon Injection: Protect from light.

Marketing authorisation numbers
Maxolon Tablets 10 mg: 10536/0031
Maxolon Syrup: 10536/0032
Maxolon Paediatric Liquid: 10536/0033
Maxolon Injection: 10536/0034
Maxolon Tablets 5 mg: 10536/0037

Date of approval/revision of SPC April 1998

Legal category POM.

MAXOLON* HIGH DOSE

Qualitative and quantitative composition Each 20 ml ampoule contains Metoclopramide Hydrochloride BP equivalent to 100 mg of the anhydrous substance.

Pharmaceutical form Clear colourless solution for intravenous infusion.

Clinical particulars

Therapeutic indications: Maxolon High Dose is indicated for the treatment of nausea and vomiting associated with intolerance to cytotoxic drugs.

Posology and method of administration: Maxolon High Dose is administered by IV infusion, suitably diluted. The recommended method of administration is by continuous infusion which allows steady serum levels of metaclopramide to be maintained.

Continuous infusion (recommended method): Maxolon High Dose is given by IV infusion as a loading dose followed by a continuous infusion to maintain a metoclopramide serum concentration of 0.85 microgram–1.0 microgram/ml. The loading dose should be given before starting cytotoxic chemotherapy.

	Maxolon High Dose	*Volume of Diluent*	*IV Infusion Time*
Loading dose	2-4 mg/kg body weight	50-100 ml	15-20 minutes
Maintenance dose	3-5 mg/kg body weight	500 ml	8-12 hours

Total dosage in any 24 hour period should not normally exceed 10 mg/kg body weight. Where cisplatin is to be used the loading dose of Maxolon High Dose should be at least 3 mg/kg body weight and the maintenance dose at least 4 mg/kg body weight.

Intermittent Infusion (alternative regimen): Maxolon High Dose can be given by intermittent IV infusion suitably diluted. The initial dose should be given before starting cytotoxic chemotherapy.

	Maxolon High Dose	*Volume of Diluent*	*IV Infusion Time*
Initial dose	Up to 2 mg/kg body weight	at least 50 ml	at least 15 minutes
Repeat doses at 2 hourly intervals	Up to 2 mg/kg body weight	at least 50 ml	at least 15 minutes

Total dosage in any 24 hour period should not normally exceed 10 mg/kg body weight.

Abnormal renal or liver function: In patients with clinically significant degrees of renal or hepatic impairment, therapy should be at reduced dosage. Metoclopramide is metabolised in the liver and the predominant route of elimination of metoclopramide and its metabolites is via the kidney.

Compatibility with cytotoxic agents: Maxolon High Dose is compatible with a number of cytotoxic drugs; however it should not be mixed in solution with therapeutic agents other than those stated. Maxolon High Dose is compatible with cisplatin, cyclophosphamide and doxorubicin hydrochloride and is stable over the concentration ranges listed below for 24 hours at room temperature when protected from light.

40-200 ml cisplatin (1 mg/ml) per 100 mg/20 ml of Maxolon High Dose in 1 litre of sodium chloride 0.9%.

Up to 40 mg doxorubicin hydrochloride (powder) per 100 mg/20 ml of Maxolon High Dose.

Up to 4 g cyclophosphamide (1 g/50 ml) per 100 mg/20 ml of Maxolon High Dose.

Compatibility with morphine/diamorphine: Maxolon High Dose is compatible with morphine hydrochloride and diamorphine hydrochloride and is stable over the concentration ranges listed below for 48 hours at room temperature under normal fluorescent lighting. Up to 100 mg of morphine hydrochloride per 100 mg/20 ml of Maxolon High Dose. Up to 50 mg of diamorphine hydrochloride per 100 mg/20 ml of Maxolon High Dose. Maxolon High Dose 100 mg/20 ml also remains stable for 48 hours at room temperature with 100 mg of morphine hydrochloride, or 50 mg diamorphine hydrochloride, when diluted 1 in 10 with sodium chloride 0.9%.

Stability in intravenous fluids: Ideally intravenous solutions should be prepared at the time of infusion.

However, Maxolon High Dose has been shown to be stable for at least 48 hours at room temperature in the following solutions when administered in a PVC infusion bag (e.g. Viaflex[R] Travenol).

Sodium chloride intravenous infusion BP (0.9% w/v), Glucose intravenous infusion BP (5% w/v), Sodium chloride and glucose intravenous infusion BP (sodium chloride 0.18% w/v; glucose 4% w/v), Compound sodium lactate intravenous infusion BP (ringer-lactate solution; Hartmann's solution).

Note: preparation must be under appropriate aseptic conditions if the above extended storage periods are required. The high dose ampoule presentation is not suitable for multidose use.

Contra-indications: No absolute contraindications to the use of Maxolon.

Special warnings and special precautions for use: Other special warnings and precautions: Precautions: Care should be exercised in patients being treated with other centrally active drugs e.g. in epilepsy.

Since extrapyramidal symptoms may occur with both metoclopramide and neuroleptics such as the phenothiazines, particular care should be exercised in the event of these drugs being prescribed concurrently.

The neuroleptic malignant syndrome has been reported with metoclopramide in combination with neuroleptics as well as with metoclopramide monotherapy (see undesirable side effects).

Following operations such as pyloroplasty or gut anastomosis metoclopramide therapy should be withheld for three or four days as vigorous muscular contractions may not help healing.

Metoclopramide may induce an acute hypertensive response in patients with phaeochromocytoma.

Interaction with other medicaments and other forms of interaction: The action of Maxolon on the gastro-intestinal tract is antagonised by anticholinergics. The absorption of any concurrently administered oral medication may be modified by the effect of Maxolon on gastric motility.

Pregnancy and lactation: Animal tests in several mammalian species and clinical experience have not

indicated a teratogenic effect. Nevertheless Maxolon should only be used when there are compelling reasons and is not advised during the first trimester.
During lactation metoclopramide is found in breast milk.

Effects on ability to drive and use machines: None but see *'Undesirable effects'.*

Undesirable effects: When given at high dose in association with cancer chemotherapy, Maxolon has been found to be well tolerated with few adverse events. Various extrapyramidal reactions to Maxolon, usually of the dystonic type, have been reported. Studies of Maxolon given in doses up to 10 mg/kg body weight/day by IV infusion report an incidence of extrapyramidal reactions of less than 10%. The incidence of such reactions may be increased in the younger patient. Reactions to Maxolon have included spasm of the facial muscles, trismus, rhythmic protrusion of the tongue, a bulbar type of speech, spasm of extra-ocular muscles including oculogyric crises, unnatural positioning of the head and shoulders and opisthotonos. There may be a generalised increase in muscle tone. The majority of reactions occur within 36 hours of starting treatment and the effects usually disappear within 24 hours of withdrawal of the drug. Should treatment of a dystonic reaction be required an anticholinergic anti-Parkinsonian drug, or a benzodiazepine may be used.
Very rare occurrences of the neuroleptic malignant syndrome have been reported. This syndrome is potentially fatal and comprises hyperpyrexia, altered consciousness, muscle rigidity, autonomic instability and elevated levels of creatine phosphokinase (CPK) and must be treated urgently (recognised treatments include dantrolene and bromocriptine). Metoclopramide should be stopped immediately if these syndrome occurs.
There have been very rare reports of abnormalities of cardiac conduction (such as bradycardia and heart block) in association with intravenous metoclopramide.
Mild drowsiness, confusion and diarrhoea have been noted. Depression has been reported extremely rarely.
Raised serum prolactin levels have been observed during metoclopramide therapy: this effect is similar to that noted with many other compounds.
Extremely rarely cases of red cell disorders such as methaemoglobinaemia and sulphaemoglobinaemia have been reported, particularly at high doses of metoclopramide. If this occurs the drug should be withdrawn. Methaemoglobinaemia may be treated using methylene blue.

Overdose: In cases of overdosage, acute dystonic reactions have occurred. Very rarely AV block has been observed. For treatment of a dystonic reaction see *'Undesirable effects'.*

Pharmacological properties
Pharmacodynamic properties: Maxolon High Dose is indicated for the treatment of nausea and vomiting associated with intolerance to cytotoxic drugs. It is specially formulated to ensure compatibility in solution with cisplatin.
Maxolon exerts a three-fold anti-emetic action: by inhibiting central dopamine receptors Maxolon raises the threshold of the chemoreceptor trigger zone, and reduces the reaction of the adjacent vomiting centre to centrally-acting emetics. Maxolon decreases the sensitivity of the visceral afferent nerves to the vomiting centre, reducing the effect of locally-acting emetics and irritant substances. In the upper gastro-intestinal tract Maxolon promotes normal gastric emptying and it may thus abolish gastric stasis which is part of the vomiting reflex.
Maxolon High Dose is not intended for use in the wider range of indications for which Maxolon at standard dose is indicated.

Pharmacokinetic properties: Based on current literature, a metoclopramide concentration range of about 0.85 microgram/ml would appear desirable for the control of cytotoxic drug induced emesis. Such plasma concentrations may be achieved by the administration of a loading dose of 2-4 mg/kg infused over 15-30 minutes prior to cytotoxic drug therapy followed by a maintenance continuous infusion of 3-5 mg/kg over 8-12 hours.
Metoclopramide is metabolised in the liver and the predominant route of elimination of metoclopramide and its metabolites is via the kidney. In patients with clinically significant degrees of renal or hepatic impairment, therapy should be at reduced dosage.

Preclinical safety data: No additional data available.

Pharmaceutical particulars
List of excipients: Sodium chloride, water for injections.

Incompatibilities: Not applicable.

Shelf life: Thirty six months.

Special precautions for storage: If ampoules are removed from their carton, they should be stored away from light. If inadvertent exposure occurs, ampoules showing discolouration must be discarded.

Nature and contents of container: Clear glass 20 ml ampoules (PhEur Type I neutral glass) packed in boxes of 10.

Instructions for use/handling: Protect from light.

Marketing authorisation number 10536/0035

Date of approval/revision of SPC April 1998

Legal category POM.

MAXOLON* SR

Qualitative and quantitative composition Each capsule contains Metoclopramide Hydrochloride BP equivalent to 15 mg of the anhydrous substance.

Pharmaceutical form Colourless, transparent capsules, overprinted 'Maxolon SR 15', containing white sustained release microgranules.

Maxolon SR does not contain tartrazine or any other azo dyes.

Clinical particulars
Therapeutic indications: Digestive disorders: Maxolon SR restores normal co-ordination and tone to the upper digestive tract. Maxolon SR relieves symptoms of gastro-duodenal dysfunction. Including: dyspepsia, heartburn, flatulence, sickness, pain, regurgitation of bile. These symptoms may be associated with such conditions as: reflux oesophagitis, hiatus hernia, gastritis, duodenitis, peptic ulcer, cholelithiasis and post-cholecystectomy dyspepsia.
Nausea and vomiting: Maxolon SR is indicated for the treatment of the nausea and vomiting associated with gastro-intestinal disorders and intolerance to cytotoxic drugs.

Posology and method of administration: Adults: In adults 20 years and over: 1 capsule (15 mg) twice daily, swallowed whole. Total daily dosage of Maxolon SR should not normally exceed 0.5 mg/kg body weight.
Elderly: As for adults. To avoid adverse reactions adhere strictly to dosage recommendations and where prolonged therapy is considered necessary, patients should be regularly reviewed.
The interval between doses many need to be extended in patients with clinically significant degrees of renal or hepatic impairment. The predominant route of elimination is via the kidney.
Children and young adults: A presentation of Maxolon SR suitable for patients under 20 years of age is not available.
Note: Presentations suitable for patients of low body weight are described on the separate Maxolon data sheet.

Contra-indications: Maxolon SR is contra-indicated in patients under 20 years since the dose level cannot be reduced.

Special warnings and special precautions for use: Precautions: If vomiting persists the patient should be reassessed to exclude the possibility of an underlying disorder e.g. cerebral irritation.
Care should be exercised in patients being treated with other centrally active drugs e.g. epilepsy.
Since extrapyramidal symptoms may occur with both metoclopramide and neuroleptics such as the phenothiazines, particular care should be exercised in the event of these drugs being prescribed concurrently.
The neuroleptic malignant syndrome has been reported with metoclopramide in combination with neuroleptics as well as with metoclopramide monotherapy (see side effects).
Special care should be taken in cases of severe renal insufficiency (see Posology).
Following operations such as pyloroplasty or gut anastomosis metoclopramide therapy should be withheld for three or four days as vigorous muscular contractions may not help healing.
Metoclopramide may induce an acute hypertensive response in patients with phaeochromocytoma.

Interaction with other medicaments and other forms of interaction: The action of metoclopramide on gastro-intestinal tract is antagonised by anticholinergics. The absorption of any concurrently administered oral medication may be modified by the effect of metoclopramide on motility. See also under *Special warnings.*

Pregnancy and lactation: Animal tests in several mammalian species and clinical experience have not indicated a teratogenic effect. Nevertheless Maxolon SR should only be used when there are compelling reasons and is not advised during the first trimester.
During lactation metoclopramide is found in breast milk.

Effects on ability to drive and use machines: None but see *Undesirable effects.*

Undesirable effects: Various extrapyramidal reactions to metoclopramide, usually of the dystonic type, have been reported. The incidence of these reactions may be increased if daily dosages higher than 0.5 mg per kg body weight are administered. Dystonic reactions include: spasm of the facial muscles, trismus, rhythmic protrusion of the tongue, a bulbar type of speech, spasm of extra-ocular muscles including oculogyric crises, unnatural positioning of the head and shoulders and opisthotonos. There may be a generalised increase in muscle tone. The majority of reactions occur within 36 hours of starting treatment and the effects usually disappear within 24 hours of withdrawal of the drug. Should treatment of a dystonic reaction be required an anticholinergic anti-Parkinsonian drug, or a benzodiazepine may be used.
Very rare occurrences of the neuroleptic malignant syndrome have been reported. This syndrome is potentially fatal and comprises hyperpyrexia, altered consciousness, muscle rigidity, autonomic instability and elevated levels of creatine phosphokinase (CPK) and must be treated urgently (recognised treatments include dantrolene and bromocriptine).
Tardive dyskinesia has been reported during prolonged treatment in a small number of mainly elderly patients. Patients on prolonged treatment should be regularly reviewed.
Rarely, drowsiness, restlessness, confusion and diarrhoea have been reported in patients receiving metoclopramide therapy. Depression has been reported extremely rarely.
Raised serum prolactin levels have been observed during metoclopramide therapy: this effect is similar to that noted with many other compounds.
Extremely rarely cases of red cell disorders such as methaemoglobinaemia and sulphaemoglobinaemia have been reported, particularly at high doses of metoclopramide. If this occurs the drug should be withdrawn. Methaemoglobinaemia may be treated using methylene blue.

Overdose: In cases of overdosage, acute dystonic reactions have occurred. Overdosage should be treated by gastric lavage with appropriate supportive measures. For treatment of a dystonic reaction see Undesirable effects.

Pharmacological properties
Pharmacodynamic properties: The action of metoclopramide is closely associated with parasympathetic nervous control of the upper gastro-intestinal tract, where it has the effect of encouraging normal peristaltic action. This provides for a fundamental approach to the control of those conditions where disturbed gastro-intestinal motility is a common underlying factor.

Pharmacokinetic properties: The following pharmacokinetic parameters for Maxolon SR after a single administration have been established.

C_{max} 102.5 nmol/litre; T_{max} 4.5 hours; AUC 1514.25 nmol.hr/litre; $t_{1/2}$ (elim) 7.04 hours; C12 hrs 54.75 nmol/litre

On repeated administration the following parameters have been established.

C_{max} 188 nmol/l; C_{min} 109 nmol/l

Preclinical safety data: No relevant information available.

Pharmaceutical particulars
List of excipients: Sucrose; maize starch; dibutyl phthalate; talc; polymethacrylates; gelatin; black iron oxide.

Incompatibilities: Not applicable.

Shelf life: See *Nature and contents of container.*

Special precautions for storage: Protect from direct light.

Nature and contents of container: All pack sizes (8*, 14* or 56 capsules) are available in the following packaging:
PVC blister (300 microns) backed with aluminium foil (20 microns)*. The underside of the foil is coated with vinyl based lacquer. Shelf life 24 months.
PVC (200 microns)/PVDC (60 gsm) blister*.
Polypropylene containers with polyethylene caps. Shelf life 36 months.
*Not available.

Instructions for use/handling: None.

Marketing authorisation number 10536/0030

Date of approval/revision of SPC April 1998

Legal category POM.

MEPTID* INJECTION 100 mg/ml

Quantitative and qualitative composition Each ampoule contains 100 mg of meptazinol base as meptazinol hydrochloride.

Pharmaceutical form Solution for injection.

Clinical particulars
Therapeutic indications: For the treatment of moderate to severe pain, including post-operative pain, obsteric pain and the pain of renal colic.

Posology and method of administration:
Adults: Intramuscular dosage: 75–100 mg Meptid. The injection may be repeated 2–4 hourly as required. For obstetric pain a dose of 100–150 mg should be used according to weight. This dose should approximate 2 mg/kg.

Intravenous dosage: 50–100 mg Meptid by slow intravenous injection. The injection may be repeated 2–4 hourly as required. If vomiting occurs, a suitable antiemetic should be given.

Epidural/intrathecal use: This formulation is not suitable for these routes.

Elderly: The adult dosage schedule may be used in the elderly.

Children: Meptid Injection has not been evaluated for use in children.

Contra-indications: None known, except for individuals with known sensitivity to the product.

Special warnings and precautions for use: Caution should be observed in treating patients with hepatic or renal insufficiency.

Clinical studies have indicated absence of clinically significant respiratory depression but caution should be exercised in patients already severely compromised.

Safety for use in myocardial infarction has not been established.

Meptid Injection is a useful analgesic in labour, but in accordance with general medical principles, it should not be given in other stages of pregnancy unless considered essential by the physician. There is no evidence from animal reproductive studies to anticipate a teratogenic risk.

Meptid should be used cautiously in patients with head injuries, as other drugs of this class have the potential to elevate cerebrospinal fluid pressure and to obscure the clinical course of such patients.

Interaction with other medicaments and other forms of interaction: None known.

Pregnancy and lactation: Meptid Injection is a useful analgesic in labour, but in accordance with general medical principles, it should not be given in other stages of pregnancy unless considered essential by the physician. There is no evidence from animal reproductive studies to anticipate a teratogenic risk. Meptid should not be given to lactating women unless considered essential by the physician.

Effects on ability to drive and use machines: Since dizziness and occasionally drowsiness have been reported, patients should be cautioned against driving or operating machinery until it is established that they do not become dizzy or drowsy while taking meptazinol.

Undesirable effects: The most commonly reported adverse reactions after treatment with meptazinol are nausea, vomiting, dizziness, diarrhoea and increased sweating, abdominal pain, rash, vertigo, headache, somnolence and dyspepsia.

Overdose: Overdose with Meptid Injection has not been reported. Large doses, including seven times the recommended therapeutic dose, have been given in balanced and total intravenous anaesthesia without significant respiratory depressant effects. In the event of cardiovascular and respiratory collapse, normal resuscitative procedures should be employed. Respiratory depression caused by overdosage with meptazinol may be reversed in part with therapeutic doses of Naloxone.

Pharmacological properties
Pharmacodynamic properties: Meptid (meptazinol) is a centrally acting analgesic belonging to the hexahydroazepine series, which has demonstrated mixed agonist and antagonist activity at opioid receptors.

Receptor binding studies have shown that although meptazinol displays only a low affinity for δ and κ opioid receptor sites, it has a somewhat higher affinity for the subpopulation of μ sites. Theses binding sites also display a high affinity for the endogenous opioid peptides, and are thought to be responsible for, among other things, analgesia, but not for the mediation of respiratory depression.

A component of its analgesic action is also attributable, in mice at least, to an effect on central cholinergic transmission. In this respect it differs from all conventional analgesic drugs which have been examined.

Pharmacokinetic properties: After intramuscular administration, meptazinol is rapidly absorbed and peak plasma levels are reached within 30 minutes. The plasma half-life is approximately 2 hours. The peak analgesic effect is seen within 30–60 minutes and lasts about 3–4 hours. After intravenous administration, the onset of action is immediate, occurring within minutes, and lasts a minimum of one hour.

The major route of metabolism is via the glucuronidation pathway and excretion occurs mainly in the urine.

Preclinical safety data: None given.

Pharmaceutical particulars
List of excipients: Glucose, water for injections.

Incompatibilities: Meptid Injection should not be mixed with other drugs in the same infusion solution or in the same syringe. Meptid Injection is an acidic solution of the hydrochloride salt of meptazinol and is therefore pharmaceutically incompatible with injection solutions known to be strongly basic (for example thiopentone) as precipitation of the meptazinol base may occur.

Shelf life: 36 months.

Special precautions for storage: Store below 25°C.

Nature and contents of container: 1 ml clear glass ampoules. The glass complies with the requirements of the European Pharmacopoeia Type I. The ampoules are packed in cartons of 10.

Instructions for use/handling: None given.

Marketing authorisation number PL 10536/0008

Date of first authorisation 16 December 1992

Date of partial revision of SPC July 1997.

Legal category POM.

MEPTID* TABLETS 200 mg

Quantitative and qualitative composition Each tablet contains 200 mg of meptazinol base as meptazinol hydrochloride.

Pharmaceutical form Orange film coated tablets. The tablets are engraved 'MPL023' on one side.

Clinical particulars
Therapeutic indications: For the short term treatment of moderate pain.

Posology and method of administration:
Adults: 200 mg 3–6 hourly as required. Usually one tablet 4 hourly.

Elderly: The adult dosage schedule may be used in the elderly.

Children: Meptid Tablets have not been evaluated for use in children.

Contraindications: None known, except for individuals with known sensitivity to the product.

Special warnings and precautions for use: Caution should be observed in treating patients with hepatic or renal insufficiency. Clinical studies have indicated absence of clinically significant respiratory depression but caution should be exercised in patients already severely compromised.

Safety for use in myocardial infarction has not yet been established. Meptid should be used cautiously in patients with head injuries as other drugs of this class have the potential to elevate cerebrospinal fluid pressure and to obscure the clinical course of some patients.

Interaction with other medicaments and other forms of interaction: None known.

Pregnancy and lactation: In accordance with general medical principles, Meptid Tablets should not be given to pregnant or lactating women unless considered essential by the physician. There is no evidence from animal reproductive studies to anticipate a teratogenic risk.

Effects on ability to drive and use machines: Since dizziness and occasionally drowsiness have been reported, patients should be cautioned against driving or operating machinery until it is established that they do not become dizzy or drowsy whilst taking meptazinol.

Undesirable effects: The most commonly reported adverse reactions after treatment with meptazinol are nausea, vomiting, dizziness, diarrhoea and increased sweating, abdominal pain, rash, vertigo, headache, somnolence and dyspepsia.

Overdose: Meptid Tablets are subject to hepatic first pass metabolism which prevents systemic concentrations of the drug reaching levels achieved by parental administration. In the unlikely event of overdose producing respiratory depression, naloxone is the treatment of choice. Recommended treatment includes gastric lavage, supportive therapy and naloxone if required.

Pharmacological properties
Pharmacodynamic properties: Meptid (meptazinol) is a centrally acting analgesic belonging to the hexahydroazepine series, which has demonstrated mixed agonist and antagonist activity at opioid receptors.

Receptor binding studies have shown that although meptazinol displays only a low affinity for δ and κ opioid receptor sites, it has a somewhat higher affinity for the subpopulation of μ sites. These binding sites also display a high affinity for the endogenous opioid peptides, and are thought to be responsible for, among other things, analgesia, but not for the mediation of respiratory depression. A component of its analgesic action is also attributable, in mice at least, to an effect on central cholinergic transmission. In this respect it differs from all conventional analgesic drugs which have been examined.

Pharmacokinetic properties: After oral administration, meptazinol is rapidly absorbed and peak plasma levels are reached within 90 minutes. The plasma elimination half-life is variable (1.4–4 hours). The peak analgesic effect is seen within 30–60 minutes and lasts about 3–4 hours.

The drug is rapidly metabolised to the glucuronide, and mostly excreted in the urine.

Preclinical safety data: None given.

Pharmaceutical particulars
List of excipients: Avicel, Amberlite, and Magnesium Stearate. The coating contains hydroxypropylmethyl cellulose, polyethylene glycol and opaspray pigment.

Incompatibilities: Not applicable.

Shelf life: 36 months.

Special precautions for storage: None.

Nature and contents of container: Cartons containing PVC blister packs of 112 tablets.

Instructions for use/handling: None given.

Marketing authorisation number PL 10536/0007

Date of first authorisation 17 December 1992

Date of partial revision of SPC July 1997.

Legal category POM

MINTEC*

Qualitative and quantitative composition Each capsule contains 0.2 ml Peppermint Oil BP

Pharmaceutical form Enteric coated, soft gelatin capsule. Oral, size no. 4, one half green, the other half ivory.

Clinical particulars
Therapeutic indications: Symptomatic relief of irritable bowel or spastic colon syndrome.

Posology and method of administration: Adults and elderly: one capsule orally three times a day, preferably before meals with a small quantity of water, but not immediately after food. The capsules must not be broken or chewed. When symptoms are more severe, the dose may be increased to two capsules three times a day. Mintec should be taken until symptoms resolve, but may be continued for up to 2 to 3 months.

Children: Not recommended for children.

Contra-indications: None known.

Special warnings and special precautions for use: In patients with pre-existing heartburn, symptoms may be exacerbated.

Interaction with other medicaments and other forms of interaction: None known.

Pregnancy and lactation: The usual precautions concerning the administration of any drug during pregnancy should be observed.

Effects on ability to drive and use machines: None known.

Undesirable effects: Heartburn, and rarely allergic reactions including erythematous skin rash, bradycardia, muscle tremor and ataxia.

Overdose: Treatment consists of gastric lavage, together with symptomatic and supportive measures.

Pharmacological properties
Pharmacodynamic properties: Mintec (peppermint oil) is an aromatic carminative which acts locally to relax gastro-intestinal smooth muscle and relieve gastro-intestinal flatulence and colic. The enteric coating of the capsules is designed to delay release of the peppermint oil beyond the stomach and upper small bowel.

Pharmacokinetic properties: An open cross-over study was conducted in eight healthy volunteers, to compare the excretion pattern of menthol (the major constituent of peppermint oil) from peppermint oil contained in enteric coated soft gelatin capsules ('Mintec'), and similar, uncoated capsules. In each leg of the study, each volunteer received 0.4 ml of peppermint oil as two capsules of one of the preparations. The excretion of the oil in the urine (as the glucuronide) was followed over a 24 hour period. 'Mintec' capsules significantly delayed the rate of excretion of menthol compared with the non-coated capsules. The maximum amounts of menthol were excreted within 0 to 2 hours following administration of uncoated capsules and between 2 to 4 hours following 'Mintec' administration. There were no significant differences between treatments in terms of the maximum or total amounts of menthol excreted over the 24 hour post-dose period.

Preclinical safety data: No additional data available.

Pharmaceutical particulars

List of excipients: Capsule shell: Gelatin, glycerol, titanium dioxide (E171), chlorophyll KK (E141). Enteric coat: Hydroxypropylmethyl cellulose phthalate, dibutyl phthalate.

Incompatibilities: Not applicable.

Shelf life: Thirty months.

Special precautions for storage: Store at a temperature not exceeding 25°. Protect from light.

Nature and contents of container: Aluminium/PVC/PVDC blister strips in packs of 3 (sample), 12, 25 and 84.

Instructions for use/handling: None.

Marketing authorisation number 10536/0036

Date of approval/revision of SPC May 1998

Legal category GSL.

TOPICYCLINE*

Qualitative and quantitative composition One bottle of powder containing 154 mg of Tetracycline Hydrochloride PhEur.

One bottle containing 70 ml of diluent for use only with Topicycline Powder (PL 10536/0025). Once reconstituted, Topicycline contains tetracycline hydrochloride 2.2 mg per ml.

Pharmaceutical form Topicycline is presented in two separate bottles as a yellow powder and as a diluent which must be combined prior to topical application.

Clinical particulars

Therapeutic indications: For the treatment of acne vulgaris

Posology and method of administration: Topicycline is first prepared by the Pharmacist according to the manufacturer's instructions.

Once reconstituted, Topicycline is applied topically, twice daily. It should be applied generously to the entire affected area, not just to the individual lesions, until the skin is thoroughly wet.

The average amount of Topicycline delivered to the skin by application to the face and neck twice a day is approximately 1.3 ml/day. This quantity of the medication contains approximately 2.9 mg of tetracycline hydrochloride. Twice-daily use of Topicycline on other acne-involved areas, in addition to the face and neck, has resulted in an average application of about 2.2 ml/day, or 4.8 mg of tetracycline hydrochloride.

Contra-indications: In patients who have shown hypersensitivity to any of its ingredients or to any of the other tetracyclines.

Special warnings and special precautions for use: Topicycline is for external use only, and care should be taken to keep it out of eyes, nose and other mucosal surfaces. Liver damage from Topicycline is highly unlikely because of the low levels of systemic absorption, however the warnings and precautions associated with the use of oral tetracyclines should be considered before prescribing to patients with renal impairment.

Interaction with other medicaments and other forms of interaction: None.

Pregnancy and lactation: Reproduction studies in rats and rabbits have revealed no evidence of impaired fertility or harm to the foetus from Topicycline. There are no data on the use of this product in pregnant women. It is not known whether tetracycline or any other component of Topicycline, administered in this topical form, is secreted in human milk. Because many drugs are secreted in human milk, caution should be exercised if Topicycline is administered to nursing mothers.

Effects on ability to drive and use machines: None.

Undesirable effects: Some patients may experience stinging or tingling sensations, skin rashes and skin discolouration at the site of application. The stinging or tingling reaction normally occurs for no more than a few minutes, does not occur on every application and often diminishes with continued use.

Topicycline may leave a faint yellow colour on the skin which could result in the staining of clothing and bed linen. This can be avoided by advising the patient to wash lightly the affected area one hour *after* applying Topicycline.

Overdose: Not applicable.

Pharmacological properties

Pharmacodynamic properties: Topicycline is a topical antibiotic preparation containing the active ingredient tetracycline hydrochloride. It has a broad spectrum of antimicrobial activity against both gram positive and gram negative pathogenic bacteria and it is mainly bacteriostatic.

In this topical preparation, Topicycline delivers tetracycline hydrochloride to the pilosebaceous apparatus and the adjacent tissues. Topicycline reduces the inflammatory acne lesions but its mode of action is not fully understood.

Pharmacokinetic properties: Very small amounts of tetracycline hydrochloride are absorbed systemically after application of Topicycline to the skin, compared with oral dosing. The serum level of tetracycline resulting from the use of Topicycline is less than 0.1 microgram/ml which is less than 7% of the level associated with an oral therapeutic dose of 500 mg/day.

Preclinical safety data: Not applicable.

Pharmaceutical particulars

List of excipients: The powder also contains 4-epitetracycline hydrochloride and sodium bisulphite (E223). The diluent contains n-decyl methyl sulphoxide and citric acid (E330) in 70 ml of a 40% ethanol solution.

Incompatibilities: None.

Shelf life: Shelf life of unreconstituted product is 24 months. Shelf life of reconstituted product is 8 weeks.

Special precautions for storage: Store at or below 25°.

Nature and contents of container: A single carton containing a plastic bottle and cap with an applicator and overcap supplied for the reconstituted product. On reconstitution of active powder (PL 10536/0025) and diluent (PL 10536/0026), the pack size is 70 ml.

Instructions for use/handling: At the time of dispensing the entire contents of the diluent–containing bottle are poured into the bottle containing the powder. The resultant mixture is then shaken well. Any unused material should be discarded.

Marketing authorisation numbers
Topicycline Powder 10536/0025
Diluent for Topicycline Powder 10536/0026

Date of approval/revision of SPC 9 December, 1995

Legal category POM.

**Trade Mark*

Napp Pharmaceuticals Limited
Cambridge Science Park
Milton Road
Cambridge CB4 0GW

☎ 01223 424444 🗋 01223 424441

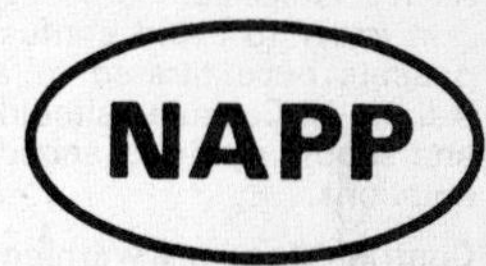

ADIZEM*-SR CAPSULES 90, 120, 180 mg
ADIZEM-SR TABLETS 120 mg

Presentation
Adizem-SR Capsules 90 mg are size 3 capsules with opaque white caps and bodies with "90 mg" printed in black on the caps and bodies. Each capsule contains 90 mg of Diltiazem Hydrochloride PhEur in a controlled release formulation.

Adizem-SR Capsules 120 mg are size 3 capsules with opaque brown caps and opaque white bodies with "120 mg" printed in black on the caps and bodies. Each capsule contains 120 mg of Diltiazem Hydrochloride PhEur in a controlled release formulation.

Adizem-SR Capsules 180 mg are size 2 capsules with opaque pale brown caps and opaque white bodies with "180 mg" printed in black on the caps and bodies. Each capsule contains 180 mg of Diltiazem Hydrochloride PhEur in a controlled release formulation.

Adizem-SR Tablets 120 mg are white, film coated, capsule shaped tablets marked with DL/120 on one side, scoreline on the other. Each tablet contains 120 mg of Diltiazem Hydrochloride PhEur in a controlled release formulation.

Uses
Actions: Diltiazem is a calcium antagonist. It restricts the slow channel entry of calcium ions into the cell and so reduces the liberation of calcium from stores in the sarcoplasmic reticulum. This results in a reduction in the amount of available intracellular calcium and consequently a (1) reduction of myocardial oxygen consumption (2) dilation of small and large coronary arteries (3) mild peripheral vasodilation (4) negative dromotropic effects (5) a slight reduction or no change in heart rate due to the negative chronotropic effects of diltiazem counteracting the reflex increase in heart rate that occurs as a result of peripheral vasodilation.

The antihypertensive effect is due to the reduction in peripheral vascular resistance.

The antianginal effect is due to a reduction in peripheral resistance, thereby decreasing the afterload, whilst a reduction in the vasomotor tone of the coronary circulation maintains the coronary blood flow. Cardiac contractility and ventricular ejection fraction are unchanged. Diltiazem increases exercise capacity and improves indices of myocardial ischaemia in the angina patient. Diltiazem relieves the spasm of vasospastic (Prinzmetal's) angina.

Indications: For the management of angina pectoris and treatment of mild to moderate hypertension.

Dosage and administration Dosage may be taken with or without food, and should be swallowed whole and not chewed.

Angina
Adults: The usual initial dose is 90 mg, 12-hourly. Dosage may be increased gradually to 120 mg, 12-hourly or 180 mg, 12-hourly if required. Patients' responses may vary and dosage requirements can differ significantly between individual patients.

Elderly and patients with renal and hepatic dysfunction: In the elderly, dosage should commence at one Adizem-60 Tablet 12-hourly and the dose carefully titrated as required.

Hypertension
Adults: The usual dose is one Adizem-SR 120 mg Tablet or Capsule 12-hourly. Patients may benefit by titrating from a lower total daily dose.

Elderly and patients with renal and hepatic dysfunction: The starting dose should be one Adizem-60 Tablet 12-hourly, increasing to one Adizem-SR 90 mg Capsule 12-hourly and then to one Adizem-SR 120 mg Tablet or Capsule 12-hourly if clinically indicated.

Children: The Adizem preparations are not recommended for children. Safety and efficacy in children have not been established.

Contra-indications, warnings, etc
Contra-indications: Pregnancy and in women of child bearing capacity. Patients with bradycardia (less than 50 bpm), second or third degree heart block, sick sinus syndrome, decompensated cardiac failure, patients with left ventricular dysfunction following myocardial infarction. Concurrent use with dantrolene infusion is contra-indicated because of the risk of ventricular fibrillation.

Warnings and precautions: The product should be used with caution in patients with reduced left ventricular function. Patients with mild bradycardia, first-degree atrioventricular block or prolonged PR interval should be observed closely.

Drug interactions: Due consideration should be given to the possibility of an additive effect when diltiazem is prescribed with drugs which may induce bradycardia or other anti-arrhythmic drugs.

Diltiazem hydrochloride has been used safely in combination with beta-blockers, diuretics, ACE-inhibitors and other anti-hypertensive agents. It is recommended that patients receiving these combinations should be regularly monitored. Concomitant use with alpha-blockers such as prazosin should be strictly monitored because of the possible synergistic hypotensive effect of this combination. Patients with pre-existing conduction defects should not receive the combination of diltiazem and beta-blockers.

Case reports have suggested that blood levels of carbamazepine, cyclosporin and theophylline may be increased when given concurrently with diltiazem hydrochloride. Care should be exercised in patients taking these drugs. In common with other calcium antagonists diltiazem hydrochloride may cause small increases in plasma levels of digoxin.

Concurrent use with H_2-antagonists may increase serum levels of diltiazem.

Treatment with diltiazem has been continued without problem during anaesthesia, but the anaesthetist should be made aware of the treatment regimen.

Use in pregnancy and lactation: Diltiazem hydrochloride is contra-indicated in pregnant women or women of child bearing capacity, and is not recommended in nursing mothers.

Side-effects: Diltiazem is generally well tolerated. Occasional undesirable effects are nausea, headache, oedema of the legs, flushing, hypotension, fatigue, gastrointestinal disturbance and gingival hyperplasia which disappear on cessation of treatment. Serious skin reactions such as exfoliative dermatitis and allergic skin reactions, such as angioneurotic oedema, erythema multiforme and vasculitis have been reported. Diltiazem may cause depression of atrioventricular nodal conduction and bradycardia. Isolated cases of moderate and transient increased liver transaminases have been observed at the start of treatment. Isolated cases of clinical hepatitis have been reported, which resolved when diltiazem was withdrawn.

Overdosage: The clinical symptoms of acute intoxication may include pronounced hypotension or even collapse, sinus bradycardia with or without atrioventricular conduction defects.

The patient should be closely monitored in hospital to exclude arrhythmias or atrioventricular conduction defects. Gastric lavage and osmotic diuresis should be undertaken when considered appropriate. Symptomatic bradycardia and high grade atrioventricular block may respond to atropine, isoprenaline or occasionally temporary cardiac pacing.

Hypotension may require correction with plasma volume expanders, intravenous calcium gluconate and positive inotropic agents.

The formulations are controlled release systems which will continue to release diltiazem for some hours.

Pharmaceutical precautions Store in a dry place at less than 30°C.

Legal category POM.

Package quantities
Capsules 90, 120, 180 mg: Blister packs containing 56 capsules.
Tablets 120 mg: Blister packs containing 56 tablets.

Further information
Transferability: In order to avoid confusion it is suggested that patients once titrated to an effective dose using any of the ADIZEM preparations should remain on this treatment and should not be changed between different presentations.

Product licence numbers
Adizem-SR Capsules 90 mg 0337/0221
Adizem-SR Capsules 120 mg 0337/0222
Adizem-SR Tablets 120 mg 0337/0137
Adizem-SR Capsules 180 mg 0337/0223

ADIZEM*-XL CAPSULES 120, 180, 240 and 300 mg

Presentation
Adizem-XL Capsules 120 mg are size 3 hard gelatin capsules with pale pink bodies and navy blue caps, marked "DCR 120". Each capsule contains 120 mg Diltiazem Hydrochloride PhEur in a controlled release formulation.

Adizem-XL Capsules 180 mg are size 2 hard gelatin capsules with dark pink bodies and royal blue caps, marked "DCR 180". Each capsule contains 180 mg Diltiazem Hydrochloride PhEur in a controlled release formulation.

Adizem-XL Capsules 240 mg are size 1 hard gelatin capsules with dark red bodies and blue caps, marked "DCR 240". Each capsule contains 240 mg Diltiazem Hydrochloride PhEur in a controlled release formulation.

Adizem-XL Capsules 300 mg are size 0 hard gelatin capsules with maroon bodies and pale blue caps, marked "DCR 300". Each capsule contains 300 mg Diltiazem Hydrochloride PhEur in a controlled release formulation.

Uses
Actions: Diltiazem is a calcium antagonist. It restricts the slow channel entry of calcium ions into the cell and so reduces the liberation of calcium from stores in the sarcoplasmic reticulum. This results in a reduction in the amount of available intracellular calcium and consequently a (1) reduction of myocardial oxygen consumption (2) dilation of small and large coronary arteries (3) mild peripheral vasodilation (4) negative dromotropic effects (5) a slight reduction or no change in heart rate due to the negative chronotropic effects of diltiazem counteracting the reflex increase in heart rate that occurs as a result of peripheral vasodilation.

The antihypertensive effect is due to the reduction in peripheral vascular resistance.

The antianginal effect is due to reduction in the peripheral resistance, thereby decreasing the afterload, whilst a reduction in the vasomotor tone of the coronary circulation maintains the coronary blood flow. Cardiac contractility and ventricular ejection fraction are unchanged. Diltiazem increases exercise capacity and improves indices of myocardial ischaemia in the angina patient. Diltiazem relieves the spasm of vasospastic (Prinzmetal's) angina.

Indications: Management of angina pectoris and treatment of mild to moderate hypertension.

Dosage and administration Dosage requirements may differ between patients with angina and patients with hypertension. In addition, individual patients' responses may vary, necessitating careful titration. This range of capsule strengths facilitates titration to the optimal dose.

The capsules should be swallowed whole and not chewed.

Adults: For patients new to diltiazem therapy, the usual starting dose is one 240 mg capsule daily.

Patients currently receiving a total daily dose of 180 mg diltiazem (as 90 mg bd or 60 mg tid) and transferring to Adizem-XL Capsules, should be given the 240 mg capsule (od). A patient receiving 240 mg/day of diltiazem (as 120 mg bd) should commence treatment on the 240 mg capsule (od), titrating to the 300 mg capsule (od) if required.

Elderly and patients with impaired hepatic and renal function: For patients new to diltiazem therapy, the usual starting dose is one 120 mg capsule daily. If necessary the dose may be gradually increased, but careful monitoring of this group of patients is advised.

Elderly patients transferring to Adizem-XL Capsules should receive the same total daily dose, titrating upwards as required.

Children: Adizem-XL Capsules are not recommended for children. Safety and efficacy in children have not been established.

In order to avoid confusion it is suggested that patients once titrated to an effective dose using Adizem-XL Capsules, should remain on this treatment and should not be changed between different presentations.

Contra-indications, warnings, etc
Contra-indications: Pregnancy and in women of child bearing capacity. Patients with bradycardia (less than 50 bpm), second or third degree heart block, sick sinus syndrome, decompensated cardiac failure, patients with left ventricular dysfunction following myocardial infarction. Concurrent use with dantrolene infusion is contra-indicated because of the risk of ventricular fibrillation.

Warnings and precautions: The product should be used with caution in patients with reduced left ventricular function. Patients with mild bradycardia, first degree atrioventricular block or prolonged PR interval should be observed closely. Diltiazem is considered unsafe in patients with acute porphyria.

Drug interactions: Due consideration should be given to the possibility of an additive effect when diltiazem is prescribed with drugs which may induce bradycardia or other anti-arrhythmic drugs.

Diltiazem hydrochloride has been used safely in combination with beta-blockers, diuretics, ACE-inhibitors and other anti-hypertensive agents. It is recommended that patients receiving these combinations should be regularly monitored. Concomitant use with alpha-blockers such as prazosin should be strictly monitored because of the possible synergistic hypotensive effect of this combination. Patients with pre-existing conduction defects should not receive the combination of diltiazem and beta-blockers.

Case reports have suggested that blood levels of carbamazepine, cyclosporin and theophylline may be increased when given concurrently with diltiazem hydrochloride. Care should be exercised in patients taking these drugs. In common with other calcium antagonists diltiazem hydrochloride may cause small increases in plasma levels of digoxin.

Concurrent use with H_2-antagonists may increase serum levels of diltiazem.

Treatment with diltiazem has been continued without problem during anaesthesia, but the anaesthetist should be made aware of the treatment regimen.

Use in pregnancy and lactation: Diltiazem hydrochloride is contra-indicated in pregnant women or women of child bearing potential, and is not recommended in nursing mothers.

Side-effects: Diltiazem is generally well tolerated. Occasional undesirable effects are nausea, headache, oedema of the legs, flushing, hypotension, fatigue, gastrointestinal disturbance and gingival hyperplasia which disappear on cessation of treatment. Serious skin reactions such as exfoliative dermatitis and allergic skin reactions, such as angioneurotic oedema, erythema multiforme and vasculitis have been reported. Diltiazem may cause depression of atrioventricular nodal conduction and bradycardia. Isolated cases of moderate and transient increased liver transaminases have been observed at the start of treatment. Isolated cases of clinical hepatitis have been reported, which resolved when diltiazem was withdrawn.

Overdosage: The clinical symptoms of acute intoxication may include pronounced hypotension or even collapse and sinus bradycardia with or without atrioventricular conduction defects.

The patient should be closely monitored in hospital to exclude arrhythmias or atrioventricular conduction defects. Gastric lavage and osmotic diuresis should be undertaken when considered appropriate. Symptomatic bradycardia and high grade atrioventricular block may respond to atropine, isoprenaline or occasionally temporary cardiac pacing.

Hypotension may require correction with plasma volume expanders, intravenous calcium gluconate and positive inotropic agents. The formulations employ a controlled release system which will continue to release diltiazem for some hours.

Pharmaceutical precautions Store at or below 25°C.

Legal category POM.

Package quantities Blister packs containing 28 capsules.

Further information An oral dose of diltiazem is almost completely absorbed. Despite this, diltiazem has a low bioavailability owing to extensive first pass metabolism. This process is saturable at higher doses of the drug, resulting in a non-linear accumulation and higher blood concentrations at steady state than would be anticipated from those following a single dose. Adizem-XL Capsules reduce the degree of saturation by presenting diltiazem in a retarded fashion therefore eliminating the high peak concentrations of the absorption phase. This allows the capsule to be administered once daily.

In pharmacokinetic studies in healthy volunteers, diltiazem was well absorbed. The controlled release capsules provided prolonged absorption of the drug, producing peak steady state plasma concentrations between 4 and 14 hours post-dose. The availability of diltiazem from Adizem-XL Capsules 120 mg (od) relative to a modified release 60 mg diltiazem preparation (bd) was approximately 79% at steady state. Similarly, the availability of diltiazem from the 240 mg capsule (od) relative to Adizem-SR Tablets 120 mg (bd) was approximately 78%. The extent of absorption of diltiazem was not affected when Adizem-XL Capsules were co-administered with a high-fat meal.

Product licence numbers
Adizem-XL Capsules 120 mg 0337/0217
Adizem-XL Capsules 180 mg 0337/0218
Adizem-XL Capsules 240 mg 0337/0219
Adizem-XL Capsules 300 mg 0337/0220

CODAFEN CONTINUS* TABLETS

Qualitative and quantitative composition
Ibuprofen BP 300 mg
Codeine Phosphate BP 20 mg

Pharmaceutical form Bi-layer tablets containing ibuprofen 300 mg in a controlled release layer and codeine phosphate 20 mg in a normal release layer.

Clinical particulars
Therapeutic indications: Relief of pain in osteoarthritis, rheumatoid arthritis, ankylosing spondylitis and sero-negative arthropathies; inflammatory disorders such as bursitis, capsulitis of the shoulder, tendinitis, tenosynovitis; relief of severe pain in such clinical conditions as post-episiotomy pain, dental extraction pain, post-operative pain, dysmenorrhoea, migraine, sprains, strains and low back pain.

Posology and method of administration:
Route of Administration: Oral.

Adults: The starting dose is two tablets taken twelve hourly. This may be increased to three tablets twelve hourly.

Children under 12 years: Not recommended.

Elderly: No special dosage modifications are required for elderly patients, unless renal or hepatic function is impaired, in which case dosage should be assessed individually.

Contra-indications: Respiratory depression; hypersensitivity to codeine, ibuprofen, aspirin or other NSAIDS; history of, or active, peptic ulceration; chronic constipation.

Special warnings and special precautions for use: CODAFEN CONTINUS tablets should be used with caution in patients with gastro-intestinal disease. If given to patients receiving anti-coagulant therapy prothrombin time should be monitored daily for the first few days of combined treatment.

CODAFEN CONTINUS tablets should be used with caution in those with hypotension, hypothyroidism, hepatic and/or renal impairment (GFR <20 ml.min^{-1}).

CODAFEN CONTINUS tablets should be given with care to patients with a history of heart failure or hypertension since oedema has been reported in association with ibuprofen administration.

NSAIDs have been reported to cause nephrotoxicity in various forms: interstitial nephritis, nephrotic syndrome and renal failure. In patients with renal, cardiac or hepatic impairment, caution is required since the use of NSAIDs may result in the deterioration of renal function. The dose should be kept as low as possible and renal function should be monitored in these patients.

The tablets should be used with caution in patients with raised intracranial pressure or head injury. Bronchospasm may be precipitated in patients suffering from or with a history of bronchial asthma or allergic disease. The possibility of cross-sensitivity with aspirin and other non-steroidal anti-inflammatory agents should be considered.

Interaction with other medicaments and other forms of interaction: Care should be exercised in patients taking monamine oxidase inhibitors, thiazide diuretics, oral anticoagulants, antihypertensives, cardiac glycosides, lithium, methotrexate, cyclosporin, mifepristone, other NSAIDs, corticosteroids, quinolone antibiotics.

Pregnancy and lactation: Whilst no teratogenic effects have been demonstrated in animal toxicology studies, the use of CODAFEN CONTINUS tablets during pregnancy should, if possible, be avoided. Congenital abnormalities have been reported in association with ibuprofen administration in man; however, these are low in frequency and do not appear to follow any discernible pattern. In view of the known effects of NSAIDs on the foetal cardiovascular system (closure of ductus arteriosis), use in late pregnancy should be avoided.

Ibuprofen and codeine are both excreted in breast milk.

Effects on ability to drive and use machines: Patients may become dizzy or sedated with CODAFEN CONTINUS tablets. If affected, patients should not drive or operate machinery.

Undesirable effects:
Ibuprofen: Epidemiological data indicate that of the most widely-used oral, non-aspirin NSAIDs, ibuprofen presents the lowest risk of upper gastrointestinal toxicity. The most commonly-observed gastrointestinal effects are nausea, vomiting, diarrhoea, dyspepsia, abdominal pain, melaena, haematemesis, ulcerative stomatitis and gastrointestinal haemorrhage. Less frequently, gastritis, duodenal ulcer, gastric ulcer and gastrointestinal perforation have been observed.

Oedema has been reported in association with ibuprofen treatment.

Other adverse events reported less commonly for which causality has not necessarily been established include: nephrotoxicity including interstitial nephritis, nephrotic syndrome and renal failure; abnormal liver function, hepatitis and jaundice; visual disturbances, optic neuritis, headaches, paraesthesia, depression, confusion, hallucinations, tinnitus, vertigo, dizziness, malaise, fatigue and drowsiness, thrombocytopenia, neutropenia, agranulocytosis, aplastic anaemia and haemolytic anaemia, photosensitivity.

Codeine: Adverse events occurring with codeine include constipation, respiratory depression, cough suppression, nausea and drowsiness.

Overdose: Symptoms of overdose with ibuprofen may include the following; headache, vomiting, drowsiness, loss of consciousness and hypotension. Nausea and vomiting are prominent features of codeine overdose. Respiratory depression may also occur with a large codeine overdose.

The stomach should be emptied.

Symptoms should be treated on appearance and any imbalance in electrolyte levels should be corrected. Monitoring of potassium levels should be considered.

If severe CNS depression has occurred artificial respiration, oxygen and parenteral naloxone may be needed. The physician should be aware that the tablets in the intestine may release ibuprofen for a period of hours.

Pharmacological properties
Pharmacodynamic properties: Ibuprofen is a non-steroidal anti-inflammatory drug with potent analgesic properties. It inhibits prostaglandin synthetase and therefore the synthesis of prostaglandins which are known to be involved in the sensitisation of pain receptors and the inflammatory process.

Codeine is a narcotic analgesic and acts at opioid/opiate receptors in the CNS, particularly μ receptors which mediate analgesia.

The combination of ibuprofen and codeine in this formulation provides optimum pain relief, with a clinically demonstrated synergistic effect between the two ingredients.

Ibuprofen also provides anti-inflammatory activity.

Pharmacokinetic properties: CODAFEN CONTINUS tablets provide immediate release of codeine to achieve rapid pain relief whilst allowing controlled release of ibuprofen to achieve continuous relief from pain and inflammation.

The plasma half-life for ibuprofen is 2 hours whilst that for codeine is 2.5–3 hours. Both drugs are metabolised by the liver and excreted mainly in the urine.

Pre-clinical safety data: There are no pre-clinical data of relevance to the prescriber which are additional to that already included in other sections of the SPC.

Pharmaceutical particulars
List of excipients:
Microcrystalline cellulose Ph Eur
Lactose (anhydrous) NF
Hydroxyethylcellulose Ph Eur
Hydroxypropylmethylcellulose Ph Eur
Ponceau 4 R (E124)
Cetostearyl alcohol BP
Purified talc BP
Pregelatinised maize starch BP
Povidone (K30) BP

Incompatibilities: None known.

Shelf-life: Three years.

Special precautions for storage: Store below 25°C.

Nature and contents of container: Polypropylene containers with polyethylene lids, containing 10, 28, 56 or 112 tablets.

PVdC coated PVC/aluminium blister packs, containing 28 or 56 tablets.

Instructions for use/handling: None.

Marketing authorisation number PL 0337/0146

Date of first authorisation/renewal of authorisation 1 November 1991

Date of (partial) revision of the text September 1997

Legal category POM

CO-DANTHRAMER SUSPENSIONS (Codalax) AND CAPSULES STRONG CO-DANTHRAMER SUSPENSIONS (Codalax Forte) AND CAPSULES

Presentation Co-danthramer Suspension and Strong Co-danthramer Suspension are peach flavoured, orange liquids. Each 5 ml spoonful of Co-danthramer Suspension contains: Poloxamer 188 BP, 200 mg and Danthron BP, 25 mg. Each 5 ml spoonful of Strong Co-danthramer Suspension contains: Poloxamer 188 BP, 1000 mg and Danthron BP, 75 mg.

Co-danthramer Capsules have light brown bodies, opaque orange caps and are marked CX and NAPP. Each capsule contains: Poloxamer 188 BP, 200 mg and Danthron BP, 25 mg. Strong Co-danthramer Capsules have light brown bodies, opaque green caps and are marked CXF and NAPP. Each capsule contains: Poloxamer 188 BP, 500 mg and Danthron BP, 37.5 mg.

Uses
Action: As a lubricant, faecal softener and laxative for oral administration. Danthron is a hydroquinone compound that acts on the nerve endings of the myenteric plexus to stimulate the muscle of the large intestine. It acts between 6 and 12 hours after administration.

Poloxamer 188 increases the penetration of water into faecal material thus preventing the faecal mass from drying and hardening excessively. The surface activity of poloxamer improves the penetration of water and thereby lubricates the contents of the distal colon.

Indications: The use of these products is strictly limited to:

Constipation in geriatric practice.

The prophylaxis of analgesic-induced constipation in terminally ill cancer patients.

Analgesic-induced constipation in the terminally ill, in all age groups.

Constipation in cardiac failure and coronary thrombosis, conditions in which defaecation must be free of strain.

Dosage and administration
Co-danthramer Suspension and Capsules:
Adults: One or two 5 ml spoonfuls *or* one or two capsules at bedtime.
Children: Half to one 5 ml spoonful *or* one capsule at bedtime.

Strong Co-danthramer Suspension and Capsules:
Adults: One 5 ml spoonful *or* one or two capsules at bedtime.
Children: Not recommended for children under 12 years.

Please note that *one* 5 ml spoonful of Strong Co-danthramer Suspension is equivalent to *two* Strong Co-danthramer Capsules.

Contra-indications, warnings, etc
Contra-indications: In common with other gastrointestinal evacuants Co-danthramer preparations should not be given when acute or painful conditions of the abdomen are present, or the cause of constipation is suspected to be intestinal inflammation or obstruction. Pregnancy and lactation.

Caution: Co-danthramer preparations may cause staining of the buttocks in incontinent and/or bedridden patients. This may lead to superficial sloughing of the skin. Therefore, these products should not be given to infants in nappies and should be used with caution in all incontinent patients.

Use in pregnancy and lactation: As there is inadequate evidence of the safety of these products in pregnancy and lactation, Co-danthramer preparations are contra-indicated.

Special warning: Oral administration of danthron has been reported to cause liver or intestinal tumours in rats and mice. There is no sound evidence to conclude a no-effect dose and therefore there may be a risk of such effects in humans. The use of Co-danthramer preparations should be restricted to the licensed indications.

Side-effects: Danthron may cause temporary harmless pink or red colouring of the urine and perianal skin. With prolonged high dosage the mucosa of the large intestine may become coloured.

Overdosage: Patients should be given plenty of fluids. An anticholinergic preparation such as atropine sulphate may be given to offset the excessive intestinal motility.

Pharmaceutical precautions Suspensions: Store in a cool place, away from stong light. Capsules: Store at or below 30°C.

Suspension diluents: Tragacanth Mucilage BP or Syrup BP should be used if diluents are required.

N.B. It is not possible to dilute Strong Co-danthramer Suspension to obtain Co-danthramer Suspension since the proportions of the two active ingredients are different.

Legal category POM.

Package quantities
Co-danthramer Suspension: Bottles of 300 ml and 1 litre.
Strong Co-danthramer Suspension: Bottles of 300 ml.
Co-danthramer Capsules: Blister packs of 60 capsules.
Strong Co-danthramer Capsules: Blister packs of 60 capsules.

Further information Nil.

Product licence numbers

Co-Danthramer Suspension	12724/0001
Strong Co-Danthramer Suspension	12724/0002
Co-danthramer Capsules	0337/0248
Strong Co-danthramer Capsules	0337/0249.

DHC CONTINUS* TABLETS

Qualitative and quantitative composition Dihydrocodeine Tartrate BP 60 mg, 90 mg, 120 mg.

Pharmaceutical form Controlled release tablet.

Clinical particulars
Therapeutic indications: For the relief of severe pain in cancer and other chronic conditions.

Posology and method of administration:
Route of administration: Oral.
Adults and children over 12 years: 60 mg–120 mg every 12 hours.
Elderly: Dosage should be reduced.
Children 12 years or under: Not recommended.

Contra-indications: Respiratory depression, obstructive airways disease. As dihydrocodeine may cause the release of histamine, it should not be given during an asthma attack and should be given with caution to asthmatics.

Special warnings and special precautions for use: Dosage should be reduced in the elderly, in hypothyroidism, chronic hepatic disease and renal insufficiency. Opioid analgesics should be avoided in those patients with raised intracranial pressure or head injury.

Interaction with other medicaments and other forms of interaction: Alcohol should be avoided whilst under treatment with dihydrocodeine. Dihydrocodeine should be used with caution in patients taking monoamine oxidase inhibitors.

Pregnancy and lactation: There is little published evidence on safety in human pregnancy but dihydrocodeine has been used for many years without apparent ill effects. Dihydrocodeine has not been reported to be excreted in breast milk. However, it is advisable that dihydrocodeine only be administered to breast-feeding mothers if considered essential.

Effects on ability to drive and use machines: Dihydrocodeine may cause drowsiness and, if affected, patients should not drive or operate machinery.

Undesirable effects: Constipation, nausea, vomiting, headache, vertigo and urinary retention can occur.

Overdose: Conservative management is recommended and should include gastric lavage. Severe respiratory depression can be treated with naloxone hydrochloride 0.8 mg intravenously, repeated as required at 2–3 minute intervals.

Pharmacological properties
Pharmacodynamic properties: Dihydrocodeine is a semisynthetic narcotic analgesic with a potency between morphine and codeine. It acts on opioid receptors in the brain to reduce the patient's perception of pain and improve the psychological reaction to pain by reducing the associated anxiety.

Pharmacokinetic properties: Dihydrocodeine is well absorbed from the gastrointestinal tract following administration of DHC Continus tablets and plasma levels are maintained throughout the twelve hour dosing interval.

Like other phenanthrene derivatives, dihydrocodeine is mainly metabolised in the liver with the resultant metabolites being excreted mainly in the urine. Metabolism of dihydrocodeine includes o-demethylation, n-demethylation and 6-keto reduction.

Preclinical safety data: There are no preclinical data of relevance to the prescriber which are additional to that already included in other sections of the SPC.

Pharmaceutical particulars
List of excipients: Lactose (anhydrous) USNF; Hydroxyethylcellulose PhEur; Cetostearyl Alcohol BP; Magnesium Stearate BP; Purified Talc BP; Purified Water PhEur.

Incompatibilities: None known.

Shelf life: Three years.

Special precautions for storage: Store at or below 25°C.

Nature and contents of container: Polypropylene containers with polyethylene lids containing 56 tablets.

Instructions for use/handling: None stated.

Marketing authorisation numbers

60 mg	0337/0115
90 mg	0337/0140
120 mg	0337/0141

Date of approval/revision of SPC November 1996

Legal category POM.

FLEXIN* -25, -50, -75 CONTINUS* TABLETS

Qualitative and quantitative composition
FLEXIN-25 CONTINUS tablets contain Indomethacin BP 25 mg
FLEXIN-50 CONTINUS tablets contain Indomethacin BP 50 mg
FLEXIN-75 CONTINUS tablets contain Indomethacin BP 75 mg

Pharmaceutical form FLEXIN-25 CONTINUS tablets are controlled release, smooth, green, capsule shaped tablets embossed with "IC" and "25" on one side.

FLEXIN-50 CONTINUS tablets are controlled release, smooth, red, capsule shaped tablets embossed with "IC" and "50" on one side.

FLEXIN-75 CONTINUS tablets are controlled release, smooth, bright yellow, capsule shaped tablets embossed with "IC" and "75" on one side.

Clinical particulars
Therapeutic indications: For the treatment of rheumatoid arthritis; osteoarthritis; ankylosing spondylitis; degenerative joint disease of the hip; painful musculoskeletal disorders; low back pain; gout and any severe periarticular disorders such as bursitis, tendinitis, synovitis, tenosynovitis and capsulitis. Also indicated in inflammation, pain and oedema following orthopaedic procedures and treatment of pain and associated symptoms of primary dysmenorrhoea.

Posology and method of administration
Route of administration: Oral.

FLEXIN CONTINUS tablets should always be given with food, milk or an antacid.

The recommended dosage of the tablets is 25–200 mg daily taken once or twice a day depending on the patients' need and response. In dysmenorrhoea, up to 75 mg daily can be taken, starting with the onset of cramps or bleeding and continuing for as long as the symptoms usually last.

The elderly: As for adults but particular care should be taken in older patients who are more prone to adverse reactions.

Children: A paediatric dose has not been established.

Contra-indications: Contra-indicated in children and pregnant and lactating women; active peptic ulcer; a history of recurrent gastro-intestinal lesions; sensitivity to indomethacin, aspirin or other non-steroidal anti-inflammatory drugs.

Special warnings and special precautions for use: FLEXIN CONTINUS tablets should be used with caution in patients with hepatic or renal dysfunction. Hepatitis and jaundice have been reported rarely with indomethacin.

In common with other anti-inflammatory analgesic antipyretic agents, indomethacin may mask the signs and symptoms of infectious disease.

FLEXIN CONTINUS tablets should be used cautiously in patients with psychiatric disorders, epilepsy or Parkinsonism as indomethacin may tend to aggravate these disorders. FLEXIN CONTINUS tablets should be used with caution in patients with coagulation defects. Indomethacin can inhibit platelet aggregation. The effect usually disappears within 24 hours of discontinuing therapy.

In patients with renal, cardiac or hepatic impairment, caution is required since the use of NSAIDs may result in deterioration of renal function. The dose should be kept as low as possible and renal function should be monitored.

FLEXIN CONTINUS tablets should be used with caution in patients suffering from, or with a history of, bronchial asthma.
Concomitant use of more than one NSAID should be avoided.

Interaction with other medicaments and other forms of interaction: Aspirin may decrease and diflunisal and probenecid may increase plasma levels of indomethacin. The antihypertensive effect of beta-blockers and the diuretic and antihypertensive effect of thiazides and frusemide may be reduced by FLEXIN CONTINUS tablets. Plasma lithium levels in patients with steady state concentrations may be increased by FLEXIN CONTINUS tablets. Indomethacin may reduce the tubular secretion and therefore potentiate the toxicity of methotrexate.

There is an increased risk of gastro-intestinal bleeding when corticosteroids are administered concomitantly with NSAIDs.

Treatment with FLEXIN CONTINUS tablets should not be started until 8 - 12 days after mifepristone administration.

Caution should be exercised in patients taking anticoagulants, cardiac glycosides, quinolone antibiotics and other NSAIDs.

NSAIDs should be used with caution in patients taking cyclosporin and renal function should be monitored carefully.

Pregnancy and lactation: It is not known whether indomethacin is safe to use in pregnant and lactating women and should not be given to such patients.

Effects on ability to drive and use machines: If patients become dizzy following administration of FLEXIN CONTINUS tablets, they should not drive or operate machinery.

Undesirable effects: The most common side-effects are headache, dizziness and dyspepsia. If headache persists even after dosage reduction, indomethacin should be withdrawn.

Other CNS side-effects which may occur include mental confusion, depression, convulsions, coma, depersonalisation and tinnitus. These are often transient and disappear with time or on reduction of dosage.

Gastro-intestinal disorders which occur most frequently are nausea, vomiting, epigastric distress, abdominal pain and diarrhoea. Giving indomethacin with food or milk lowers the incidence of these side-effects. Ulceration of the oesophagus, stomach or duodenum may also occur, accompanied by haemorrhage and perforation. Gastro-intestinal bleeding without obvious ulceration may also occur. If this happens indomethacin treatment should be discontinued. Use of FLEXIN CONTINUS tablets will minimise these GI effects.

Blood dyscrasias, particularly thrombocytopenia, have been reported. Blurred vision and orbital and peri-orbital pain are seen infrequently. Corneal deposits and retinal disturbances have been reported in some patients with rheumatoid arthritis on prolonged therapy with indomethacin, and ophthalmic examinations are desirable in patients given prolonged treatment. Oedema, increased blood pressure, haematuria and anorexia occur infrequently.

Hypersensitivity reactions include pruritus, urticaria, angiitis, erythema nodosum. Skin rash and hair loss may also occur.

Acute respiratory distress including sudden dyspnoea and asthma have been reported on rare occasions. Bronchospasm may be precipitated in patients suffering from, or with a previous history of, bronchial asthma or allergic disease.

NSAIDs have been reported to cause nephrotoxicity in various forms and their use can lead to interstitial nephritis, nephrotic syndrome and renal failure.

Overdose: Gastric lavage should be given if FLEXIN CONTINUS tablets are still considered part of the stomach contents. Otherwise supportive therapy is required and a watch should be kept for gastro-intestinal bleeding for several days. Antacids may be useful.

Pharmacological properties

Pharmacodynamic properties: Indomethacin is a non steroidal anti-inflammatory drug which has analgesic, antipyretic and anti-inflammatory activity. The exact mechanisms have not been clearly established but many actions appear to be associated principally with inhibition of prostaglandin synthesis both peripherally and centrally. Indomethacin inhibits the synthesis of prostaglandins in body tissues by inhibiting cyclo-oxygenase, an enzyme that catalyses the formation of prostaglandin precursors (endoperoxides) from arachidonic acid. Indomethacin inhibits the migration of leukocytes into inflammatory sites and lysosomal enzyme release from polymorphonuclear leukocytes and may increase levels of cyclic AMP which may play a role in the anti-inflammatory response.

Pharmacokinetic properties: Following administration of FLEXIN CONTINUS tablets, peak plasma levels of indomethacin are achieved after approximately four hours. FLEXIN CONTINUS tablets should be taken with food or milk.

Concomitant ingestion of food may delay peak absorption. However, the amount of indomethacin absorbed is not reduced. In therapeutic concentrations, indomethacin is approximately 90% bound to plasma proteins. Peak indomethacin concentrations in synovial fluid occur 1.5 hours after peak serum concentrations and are approximately 20% of those in the serum. Indomethacin crosses the blood-brain barrier in small amounts and appears to freely cross the placenta.

Indomethacin is metabolised in the liver to its glucuronide conjugate and to desmethyl, desbenzoyl and desmethyl-desbenzoyl metabolites and their glucuronides. A portion of the drug is also N-deacylated by a non microsomal system.

Indomethacin and its conjugates undergo entero-hepatic circulation. About 40% is excreted in the faeces after biliary secretion as indomethacin and its unconjugated demethylated metabolites. About 60% is excreted in the urine in 48 hours, 30% of this being indomethacin and its glucuronide derivative and the balance consisting of the metabolites and their glucuronides. A two compartmental open model with correction for biliary recycling can be used to describe the disposition of indomethacin.

Pre-clinical safety data: There are no pre-clinical data of relevance to the prescriber which are additional to that already included in other sections of the SPC.

Pharmaceutical particulars

List of excipients:

Lactose, Anhydrous USP
Hydroxyethylcellulose Ph Eur
Cetostearyl Alcohol BP
Talc BP
Magnesium Stearate BP

Film coat

FLEXIN-25 CONTINUS tablets:
Opadry OY-S-8828 containing Hypromellose (5 cps) PhEur, Propylene Glycol BP, Titanium Dioxide (E171), Quinoline yellow aluminium lake (E104), FD&C yellow No. 6 aluminium lake (E110), Patent Blue V aluminium lake (E131).

FLEXIN-50 CONTINUS tablets:
Opadry OY-S-7603 containing Hypromellose (5 cps) PhEur, Propylene Glycol BP, Purified Glycol BP, Iron oxide yellow (E172), Erythrosine aluminium lake (E127).

FLEXIN-75 CONTINUS tablets:
Opadry OY-S-7900 containing Hypromellose Ph Eur, Macrogol 400 Ph Eur, Quinoline yellow E104, Titanium dioxide (E171).

Incompatibilities: None

Shelf-life: Three years.

Special precautions for storage: Store at or below 25°C.

Nature and contents of container: Polypropylene container with polyethylene lid, containing 56 tablets (FLEXIN-25 CONTINUS tablets) or 28 tablets (FLEXIN-50 and FLEXIN-75 CONTINUS tablets).

Instructions for use/handling: None.

Marketing authorisation number PL 0337/0144, 0145, 0128

Date of first authorisation/renewal of authorisation
FLEXIN-25, FLEXIN-50 CONTINUS tablets:
29 April 1991/29 May 1996
FLEXIN-75 CONTINUS tablets:
6 October 1992/14 January 1998

Date of (partial) revision of the text February 1998

Legal category POM

GASTROBID* CONTINUS* TABLETS 15 mg

Qualitative and quantitative composition GASTROBID CONTINUS tablets contain Metoclopramide Hydrochloride B.P. in a controlled release formulation.

Pharmaceutical form GASTROBID CONTINUS tablets are smooth, white biconvex tablets embossed with the NAPP logo on one side and 15 mg on the other.

Clinical particulars

Therapeutic indications: To relieve symptoms of gastro-duodenal dysfunction, including heartburn, dyspepsia, nausea and vomiting associated with such conditions as reflex oesophagitis, gastritis, duodenitis and hiatus hernia.

For the treatment of nausea and vomiting associated with cytostatic and cytotoxic drugs.

Posology and method of administration:
Route of administration: Oral.
Dosage and administration:
Adults over 20 years only: The usual dose for GASTROBID CONTINUS tablets is one tablet (15 mg) morning and evening.
Elderly: As for adults.
Children: Contraindicated.

Contra-indications: GASTROBID CONTINUS tablets are contra-indicated in patients under 20 years, since dosage titration is not possible; epilepsy, phaeochromocytoma.

Special warnings and special precautions for use: Following operations such as pyloroplasty or gut anastomosis, therapy with GASTROBID CONTINUS tablets should be withheld for three or four days as vigorous muscular contractions may impair healing. To avoid adverse reactions adhere strictly to dosage recommendations and where prolonged therapy is considered necessary patients should be regularly reviewed.

Interaction with other medicaments and other forms of interaction: GASTROBID CONTINUS tablets should not be given during, or within 15 days of completing treatment with monoamine oxidase inhibitors, nor with tricyclic antidepressants or sympathomimetic drugs. It is also recommended that combination with neuroleptics (synergy of central effect) and derivatives of anticholinergic drugs (neutralisation of effect) be avoided. Special care should be taken if GASTROBID CONTINUS tablets are administered concomitantly with other medicines. For example, the presence of metoclopramide may decrease gastric absorption of digoxin and increase the intestinal absorption of paracetamol.

Pregnancy and lactation: Although animal tests in several mammalian species have shown no teratogenic effects, treatment with GASTROBID CONTINUS tablets is not advised during the first trimester of pregnancy. Metoclopramide is excreted in breast milk and should not be given to the nursing mother.

Effects on ability to drive and use machines: Metoclopramide may cause drowsiness and if affected, patients should not drive or operate machinery.

Undesirable effects: The following side-effects have occasionally been reported with metoclopramide therapy: drowsiness, lethargy, dizziness and headache. More rarely, various extrapyramidal reactions, usually of the dystonic type, have been reported. These include spasm of the facial muscles, trismus, rhythmic protrusion of the tongue, a bulbar type of speech, spasm of extra-ocular muscles including oculogyric crises, unnatural positioning of the head and shoulders and opisthotonos. These have been shown to be more common in young adults, particularly females aged 12–19. Parkinsonian reactions are significantly more common in the elderly. Tardive dyskinesa has been reported during prolonged treatment with metoclopramide in a small number of mainly elderly patients. Insomnia, diarrhoea and flatulence have also been reported.

Cases of neuroleptic malignant syndrome, an idiosyncratic response characterised by hyperthermia, muscle rigidity, altered consciousness including coma and elevated CPK have been reported with metoclopramide.

The majority of reactions occur within 36 hours of starting treatment and the effects are reversible, usually disappearing within 24 hours of stopping treatment.

Raised serum prolactin levels have been observed during metoclopramide therapy; this effect is similar to that noted with many other compounds. Metoclopramide may induce an acute hypertensive response in patients with phaeochromocytoma.

Overdose: Gastric lavage and intensive supportive therapy should be initiated. Should treatment of a dystonic reaction be required, an anticholinergic antiparkinsonian drug, or a benzodiazepine may be used. The physician should be aware that tablets remaining in the intestine will continue to release metoclopramide hydrochloride for a period of hours.

Pharmacological properties

Pharmacodynamic properties: Metoclopramide is a benzamide derivative which acts peripherally to enhance cholinergic action at muscarinic synapses and in the central nervous system to antagonise dopamine.

Pharmacokinetic properties: The drug is presented in a controlled release formulation. After absorption, metoclopramide undergoes significant first-pass hepatic metabolism. It is excreted in the urine as unchanged drug and metabolites in both free and conjugated form.

Pre-clinical safety data: There are no pre-clinical data of relevance to the prescriber which are additional to that already included in other sections of the SPC.

Pharmaceutical particulars

List of excipients:
Lactose Anhydrous BP
Hydroxyethylcellulose BP
Cetostearyl Alcohol BP
Magnesium Stearate Ph Eur
Purified Talc Ph Eur
Purified Water Ph Eur

Incompatibilities: None known.

Shelf-life: Three years.

Special precautions for storage: Store at or below 25°C.

Nature and contents of container: PVdC coated PVC/aluminium backed blisters containing either 28 or 56 tablets.

Instructions for use/handling: None stated.

Marketing authorisation number PL 0337/0106.

Date of first authorisation/renewal of the authorisation 7 November 1986/12 June 1998.

Date of (partial) revision of the text December 1996.

Legal category POM

MST* CONTINUS* TABLETS 5 mg, 10 mg, 15 mg, 30 mg, 60 mg, 100 mg, 200 mg

Qualitative and quantitative composition Tablets containing Morphine Sulphate BP 5 mg, 10 mg, 15 mg, 30 mg, 60 mg, 100 mg, 200 mg.

Pharmaceutical form Modified release, film-coated, biconvex tablets marked with the NAPP logo on one side and the strength of the preparation on the other.
MST CONTINUS tablets 5 mg are white.
MST CONTINUS tablets 10 mg are golden brown.
MST CONTINUS tablets 15 mg are green.
MST CONTINUS tablets 30 mg are purple.
MST CONTINUS tablets 60 mg are orange.
MST CONTINUS tablets 100 mg are grey.
MST CONTINUS tablets 200 mg are teal green.

Clinical particulars
Therapeutic indications: For the prolonged relief of severe and intractable pain. MST CONTINUS tablets 5 mg, 10 mg, 15 mg and 30 mg are additionally indicated for the relief of post-operative pain.

Posology and method of administration
Route of administration: Oral.
MST CONTINUS tablets should be swallowed whole and not chewed.
MST CONTINUS tablets should be used at 12-hourly intervals. The dosage is dependent upon the severity of the pain, the patient's age and previous history of analgesic requirements.
Adults: A patient presenting with severe pain, uncontrolled by weaker opioids (e.g. dihydrocodeine) should normally be started on 30 mg 12-hourly. Patients previously on normal release oral morphine should be given the same total daily dose as MST CONTINUS tablets but in divided doses at 12-hourly intervals.
Increasing severity of pain will require an increased dosage of the tablets. Higher doses should be made, where possible in 30-50% increments as required. The correct dosage for any individual patient is that which is sufficient to control pain with no, or tolerable, side effects for a full 12 hours. It is recommended that the 200 mg strength is reserved for patients who have already been titrated to a stable analgesic dose using lower strengths of morphine or other opioid preparations.
Patients receiving MST CONTINUS tablets in place of parenteral morphine should be given a sufficiently increased dosage to compensate for any reduction in analgesic effects associated with oral administration. Usually such increased requirement is of the order of 100%. In such patients individual dose adjustments are required.
Children: For children with severe cancer pain, a starting dose in the range of 0.2 to 0.8 mg morphine per kg bodyweight 12-hourly is recommended. Doses should then be titrated as for adults.
Post-operative pain: MST CONTINUS tablets are not recommended in the first 24 hours post-operatively or until normal bowel function has returned; thereafter it is suggested that the following dosage schedule be observed at the physician's discretion:
(a) MST CONTINUS tablets 20 mg 12-hourly to patients under 70 kg
(b) MST CONTINUS tablets 30 mg 12-hourly to patients over 70 kg
(c) Elderly–a reduction in dosage may be advisable in the elderly
(d) Children–not recommended.
Supplemental parenteral morphine may be given if required but with careful attention to the total dosages of morphine, and bearing in mind the prolonged effects of morphine in this controlled release formulation.

Contra-indications: Respiratory depression, head injury, paralytic ileus, 'acute abdomen', delayed gastric emptying, obstructive airways disease, known morphine sensitivity, acute hepatic disease, concurrent administration of monoamine oxidase inhibitors or within two weeks of discontinuation of their use. Children under one year of age.
Not recommended for pre-operative use or for the first 24 hours post-operatively.

Special warnings and precautions for use: As with all narcotics a reduction in dosage may be advisable in the elderly, in hypothyroidism and in patients with significantly impaired renal or hepatic function. Use with caution in opiate dependent patients and in patients with raised intracranial pressure, hypotension with hypovolaemia, diseases of the biliary tract, pancreatitis, inflammatory bowel disorders, prostatic hypertrophy and adrenocortical insufficiency.
Should paralytic ileus be suspected or occur during use, MST CONTINUS tablets should be discontinued immediately. As with all morphine preparations, patients who are to undergo cordotomy or other pain relieving surgical procedures should not receive MST CONTINUS tablets for 24 hours prior to surgery. If further treatment with MST CONTINUS tablets is then indicated, the dosage should be adjusted to the new post-operative requirement.
As with all oral morphine preparations, MST CONTINUS tablets should be used with caution post-operatively and following abdominal surgery, as morphine impairs intestinal motility and should not be used until the physician is assured of normal bowel function.
It is not possible to ensure bioequivalence between different brands of controlled release morphine products. Therefore, it should be emphasised that patients, once titrated to an effective dose, should not be changed from MST CONTINUS preparations to other slow, sustained or controlled release morphine or other potent narcotic analgesic preparations without retitration and clinical assessment.

Interactions with other medicaments and other forms of interaction: Morphine potentiates the effects of tranquillisers, anaesthetics, hypnotics, sedatives, alcohol, muscle relaxants and antihypertensives. Cimetidine inhibits the metabolism of morphine. Monoamine oxidase inhibitors are known to interact with narcotic analgesics producing CNS excitation or depression with hyper- or hypotensive crisis.

Pregnancy and lactation: MST CONTINUS tablets are not recommended during pregnancy and labour due to the risk of neonatal respiratory depression. Administration to nursing mothers is not recommended as morphine is excreted in breast milk. Withdrawal symptoms may be observed in the newborn of mothers undergoing chronic treatment.

Effects on ability to drive and use machines: Morphine may modify the patient's reactions to a varying extent depending on the dosage and susceptibility. If affected, patients should not drive or operate machinery.

Undesirable effects: In normal doses, the commonest side effects of morphine are nausea, vomiting, constipation and drowsiness. With chronic therapy, nausea and vomiting are unusual with MST CONTINUS tablets but should they occur the tablets can be readily combined with an anti-emetic if required. Constipation may be treated with appropriate laxatives. Dry mouth, sweating, vertigo, headache, disorientation, facial flushing, mood changes, palpitations, hallucinations, bronchospasm and colic may occur in a few patients. Micturition may be difficult and there may be biliary or ureteric spasm. Overdose may produce respiratory depression. Rarely, clinically relevant reductions in blood pressure and heart rate have been observed. Morphine has histamine-releasing effects which may be responsible in part for reactions such as urticaria and pruritus.
The effects of morphine have led to its abuse and dependence may develop with regular, inappropriate use. This is not a major concern in the treatment of patients with severe pain.

Overdose: Signs of morphine toxicity and overdosage are pin-point pupils, respiratory depression and hypotension. Circulatory failure and deepening coma may occur in more severe cases.

Treatment of morphine overdosage
Primary attention should be given to the establishment of a patent airway and institution of assisted or controlled ventilation.
In the case of massive overdosage, administer naloxone 0.8 mg intravenously. Repeat at 2-3 minute intervals as necessary, or by an infusion of 2 mg in 500 ml of normal saline or 5% dextrose (0.004 mg/ml).
The infusion should be run at a rate related to the previous bolus doses administered and should be in accordance with the patient's response. However, because the duration of action of naloxone is relatively short, the patient must be carefully monitored until spontaneous respiration is reliably re-established. MST CONTINUS tablets will continue to release and add to the morphine load for up to 12 hours after administration and the management of morphine overdosage should be modified accordingly.
For less severe overdosage, administer naloxone 0.2 mg intravenously followed by increments of 0.1 mg every 2 minutes if required.
Naloxone should not be administered in the absence of clinically significant respiratory or circulatory depression secondary to morphine overdosage. Naloxone should be administered cautiously to persons who are known, or suspected, to be physically dependent on morphine. In such cases, an abrupt or complete reversal of opioid effects may precipitate an acute withdrawal syndrome.
Gastric contents may need to be emptied as this can be useful in removing unabsorbed drug, particularly when a modified release formulation has been taken.

Pharmacological properties
Pharmacodynamic properties: Morphine acts as an agonist at opiate receptors in the CNS, particularly mu and, to a lesser extent, kappa receptors. Mu receptors are thought to mediate supraspinal analgesia, respiratory depression and euphoria, and kappa receptors, spinal analgesia, miosis and sedation. Morphine also has a direct action on the bowel wall nerve plexus, causing constipation.

Pharmacokinetic properties: Morphine is well absorbed from MST CONTINUS tablets and, in general, peak plasma concentrations are achieved 1-5 hours following administration. The availability is complete when compared to an equivalent dose of immediate release oral solution. Morphine is subject to a significant first-pass effect which results in a lower bioavailability when compared to an equivalent intravenous dose.
The major metabolic transformation of morphine is glucuronidation to morphine-3-glucuronide and morphine-6-glucuronide which then undergo renal excretion. These metabolites are excreted in bile and may be subject to hydrolysis and subsequent re-absorption.
Patients are titrated to appropriate pain control using the wide range of strengths of MST CONTINUS tablets. Consequently, there is a large inter-patient variation in required dosage, the minimum dosage being 5 mg 12-hourly, and a dose of 5.6 g 12-hourly has been recorded.

Pre-clinical safety data: There are no pre-clinical data of relevance to the prescriber which are additional to that already included in other sections of the SPC.

Pharmaceutical particulars
List of excipients:
Tablet core
Hydroxyethylcellulose PhEur
Purified Water PhEur
Cetostearyl Alcohol BP
Magnesium Stearate PhEur
Purified Talc PhEur
Lactose Anhydrous NF (except for 100 mg and 200 mg tablets)
Hypromellose (E464)
Polyethylene glycol
Titanium dioxide (E171)
The following tablets have the colourants listed below:
10 mg–Iron oxide (E172)
15 mg–Iron oxide (E172), patent blue V (E131), quinoline yellow (E104), indigo carmine (E132)
30 mg–Erythrosine (E127), indigo carmine (E132), sunset yellow (E110)
60 mg–Erythrosine (E127), quinoline yellow (E104), sunset yellow (E110)
100 mg–Iron oxide (E172), indigo carmine (E132)
200 mg–Patent blue V (E131), quinoline yellow (E104).

Incompatibilities: None stated.

Shelf-life: Five years.

Special precautions for storage: MST CONTINUS tablets should be stored at or below 25°C.

Nature and contents of container: Aluminium foil-backed PVdC/PVC blister packs. Pack size 60 tablets.

Instruction for use/handling: None.

Marketing authorisation numbers PL 0337/0179, 0055, 0180, 0059, 0087, 0088, 0149.

Date of first authorisation/renewal of authorisation:
MST CONTINUS tablets 5 mg and 15 mg–26 February 1992
MST CONTINUS tablets 10 mg–26 July 1979/31 May 1996
MST CONTINUS tablets 30 mg–16 March 1982/30 January 1995
MST CONTINUS tablets 60 mg, 100 mg–26 April 1983/28 March 1995
MST CONTINUS tablets 200 mg–8 January 1991/11 June 1996

Date of (partial) revision of the text October 1997

Legal category CD (Sch. 2) POM

MST* CONTINUS* SUSPENSION

Qualitative and quantitative composition Morphine equivalent to Morphine Sulphate BP 20, 30, 60, 100 and 200 mg.

Pharmaceutical form Modified release granules for oral suspension.

Clinical particulars
Therapeutic indications: For the prolonged relief of severe and intractable pain.

Posology and method of administration
Route of administration: Oral.

20, 30 & 60 mg strengths: The contents of one sachet should be mixed with at least 10 ml water or sprinkled on to soft food, for example yogurt.

100 mg strength: The contents of one sachet should be mixed with at least 20 ml water or sprinkled on to soft food, for example yogurt.

200 mg strength: The contents of one sachet should be mixed with at least 30 ml water or sprinkled on to soft food, for example yogurt.

MST Continus suspension should be used at 12-hourly intervals. The dosage is dependent upon the severity of the pain, the patient's age and previous history of analgesic requirements.

Adults: A patient presenting with severe pain, uncontrolled by weaker opioids (eg dihydrocodeine) should normally be started on 30 mg 12 hourly. Patients previously on normal release oral morphine should be given the same total daily dose as MST Continus suspension but in divided doses at 12-hourly intervals.

Increasing severity of pain will require an increased dosage of the suspension. Higher doses should be made, where possible in 30–50% increments as required. The correct dosage for any individual patient is that which is sufficient to control pain with no, or tolerable, side effects for a full 12 hours. It is recommended that the 200 mg strength is reserved for patients who have already been titrated to a stable analgesic dose using lower strengths of morphine or other opioid preparations.

Patients receiving MST Continus Suspension in place of parenteral morphine should be given a sufficiently increased dosage to compensate for any reduction in analgesic effects associated with oral administration. Usually such increased requirement is of the order of 100%. In such patients individual dose adjustments are required.

Children: The use of MST Continus suspension in children has not been extensively evaluated. For children with severe cancer pain, a starting dose in the range of 0.2 to 0.8 mg morphine per kg bodyweight 12 hourly is recommended. Doses should then be titrated as for adults.

Post-operative pain: MST Continus suspension is not recommended in the first 24 hours post-operatively or until normal bowel function has returned; thereafter it is suggested that the following dosage schedule be observed at the physician's discretion:

(a) MST Continus suspension 20 mg 12 hourly to patients under 70 kg.
(b) MST Continus suspension 30 mg 12 hourly to patients over 70 kg.
(c) Elderly – a reduction in dosage may be advisable in the elderly
(d) Children – not recommended

Supplemental parenteral morphine may be given if required but with careful attention to the total dosage of morphine, and bearing in mind the prolonged effects of morphine in this controlled release formulation.

Contra-indications: Respiratory depression, head injury, paralytic ileus, 'acute abdomen', delayed gastric emptying, obstructive airways disease, known morphine sensitivity, acute hepatic disease, concurrent administration of monoamine oxidase inhibitors or within two weeks of discontinuation of their use. Children under one year of age. Pre-operative administration of MST Continus suspension is not recommended.

Special warnings and special precautions for use: As with all narcotics a reduction in dosage may be advisable in the elderly, in hypothyroidism and in patients with significantly impaired renal or hepatic function. Use with caution in opiate dependent patients and in patients with raised intracranial pressure, hypotension with hypovolaemia, diseases of the biliary tract, pancreatitis, inflammatory bowel disorders, prostatic hypertrophy and adrenocortical insufficiency.

Should paralytic ileus be suspected or occur during use, MST Continus suspension should be discontinued immediately. As with all morphine preparations, patients who are to undergo cordotomy or other pain relieving surgical procedures should not receive MST Continus suspension for 24 hours prior to surgery. If further treatment with MST Continus suspension is then indicated, the dosage should be adjusted to the new post-operative requirement.

As with all oral morphine preparations, MST Continus suspension should be used with caution post-operatively, and following abdominal surgery as morphine impairs intestinal motility and should not be used until the physician is assured of normal bowel function.

It is not possible to ensure bio-equivalence between different brands of controlled release morphine products. Therefore, it should be emphasised that patients, once titrated to an effective dose, should not be changed from MST Continus preparations to other slow, sustained or controlled release morphine or other potent narcotic analgesic preparations without retitration and clinical assessment.

Interactions with other medicaments and other forms of interaction: Morphine potentiates the effects of tranquillisers, anaesthetics, hypnotics, sedatives, alcohol, muscle relaxants and antihypertensives. Concurrent administration of antacids may result in a more rapid release of morphine than otherwise expected; dosing should therefore be separated by a minimum of two hours. Cimetidine inhibits the metabolism of morphine. Monoamine oxidase inhibitors are known to interact with narcotic analgesics producing CNS excitation or depression with hyper- or hypotensive crisis.

Pregnancy and lactation: MST Continus Suspension is not recommended during pregnancy and labour due to the risk of neonatal respiratory depression. Administration to nursing mothers is not recommended as morphine is excreted in breast milk. Withdrawal symptoms may be observed in the newborn of mothers undergoing chronic treatment.

Effects on ability to drive and use machines: Morphine may modify the patient's reactions to a varying extent depending on the dosage and susceptibility. If affected, patients should not drive or operate machinery.

Undesirable effects: In normal doses, the commonest side effects of morphine are nausea, vomiting, constipation and drowsiness. With chronic therapy, nausea and vomiting are unusual with MST Continus suspensions but should they occur the suspensions can be readily combined with an anti-emetic if required. Constipation may be treated with appropriate laxatives. Dry mouth, sweating, vertigo, headache, disorientation, facial flushing, mood changes, palpitations, hallucinations, bronchospasm and colic may occur in a few patients. Micturition may be difficult and there may be biliary or ureteric spasm. Overdose may produce respiratory depression. Rarely, clinically relevant reductions in blood pressure and heart rate have been observed. Morphine has histamine releasing effects which may be responsible in part for reactions such as urticaria and pruritus.

The effects of morphine have led to its abuse and dependence may develop with regular, inappropriate use. This is not a major concern in the treatment of patients with severe pain.

Overdosage: Signs of morphine toxicity and overdosage are pin-point pupils, respiratory depression and hypotension. Circulatory failure and deepening coma may occur in more severe cases.

Treatment of morphine overdosage: Primary attention should be given to the establishment of a patent airway and institution of assisted or controlled ventilation.

In the case of massive overdosage, administer naloxone 0.8 mg intravenously. Repeat at 2–3 minute intervals as necessary, or by an infusion of 2 mg in 500 ml of normal saline or 5% dextrose (0.004 mg/ml).

The infusion should be run at a rate related to the previous bolus doses administered and should be in accordance with the patient's response. However, because the duration of action of naloxone is relatively short, the patient must be carefly monitored until spontaneous respiration is reliably re-established. MST Continus suspension will continue to release and add to the morphine load for up to 12 hours after administration and the management of morphine overdosage should be modified accordingly.

For less severe overdosage, administer naloxone 0.2 mg intravenously followed by increments of 0.1 mg every 2 minutes if required.

Naloxone should not be administered in the absence of clinical significant respiratory or circulatory depression secondary to morphine overdosage. Naloxone should be administered cautiously to persons who are known, or suspected, to be physically dependent on morphine. In such cases, an abrupt or complete reversal of opioid effects may precipitate an acute withdrawal syndrome.

Gastric contents may need to be emptied as this can be useful in removing unabsorbed drug, particularly when a modified release formulation has been taken.

Pharmacological properties
Pharmacodynamic properties: Morphine acts as an agonist at opiate receptors in the CNS particularly Mu and to a lesser extent Kappa receptors. Mu receptors are thought to mediate supraspinal analgesia, respiratory depression and euphoria, and Kappa receptors, spinal analgesia, miosis and sedation. Morphine also has a direct action on the bowel wall nerve plexuses causing constipation.

Pharmacokinetic properties: Morphine is bound to a cationic exchange resin and drug release is effected when morphine is displaced by ions in the gastrointestinal tract. Morphine is well absorbed and adequate plasma morphine levels are achieved following the recommended dosage regimen. However, first pass metabolism occurs in the liver. In a single dose study in healthy volunteers, the systemic availability of morphine from MST Continus suspension 30 mg was equivalent to that from an immediate release solution 30 mg (mean 91%, 95% CI 81–102%) and from MST Continus tablet 30 mg (mean 101%, 95% CI 93–109%). The suspension provided a retarded plasma profile which was comparable to that of the MST Continus tablet.

Preclinical data: There are no pre-clinical data of relevance to the prescriber which are additional to that already included in other sections of the SPC.

Pharmaceutical particulars
List of excipients: Dowex 50WX8 100–200 mesh cationic exchange resin; xylitol; xanthan gum; raspberry flavour; Ponceau 4R (E 124).

Incompatibilities: None known.

Shelf life: Two years.

Special precautions for storage: Store at or below 25°C.

Nature and contents of container: Pack type: Surlyn lined, laminated aluminium foil sachets coated with polyethylene and clay coated Kraft paper.

Pack size: Boxboard cartons of 10, 20, 30, 60 sachets or medical sample packs of up to 14 sachets.

Instructions for use/handling: The contents of the sachet should be added to water or sprinkled onto soft food, e.g. yogurt (see *Posology and method of administration*).

Marketing authorisation numbers 0337/0165, 0166, 0225–0227.

Date of approval/revision of SPC February 1997.

Legal category CD (Sch 2) POM.

MXL* CAPSULES

Qualitative and quantitative composition Capsules containing Morphine Sulphate BP 30 mg, 60 mg, 90 mg, 120 mg, 150 mg, 200 mg.

Pharmaceutical form Modified release, hard gelatin capsules containing white to off white multiparticulates.

MXL capsules 30 mg are size 4, light blue capsules marked MS OD30.

MXL capsules 60 mg are size 3, brown capsules marked MS OD60.

MXL capsules 90 mg are size 2, pink capsules marked MS OD90.

MXL capsules 120 mg are size 1, olive capsules marked MS OD120.

MXL capsules 150 mg are size 1, blue capsules marked MS OD150.

MXL capsules 200 mg are size 0, rust capsules marked MS OD200.

Clinical particulars
Therapeutic indications: The prolonged relief of severe and intractable pain.

Posology and method of administration:
Route of administration: Oral.

The capsules may be swallowed whole or opened and the contents sprinkled on to soft cold food. The capsules and contents should not be crushed or chewed. MXL capsules should be used at 24-hourly intervals. The dosage is dependent upon the severity of the pain, the patient's age and previous history of analgesic requirements.

Adults and elderly: Patients presenting with severe uncontrolled pain, who are not currently receiving opioids, should have their dose requirements calculated through the use of immediate release morphine, where possible, before conversion to MXL capsules.

Patients presenting in pain, who are currently receiving weaker opioids should be started on:

(a) 60 mg MXL capsule once-daily if they weigh over 70 kg.

(b) 30 mg MXL capsule once-daily if they weigh under 70 kg, are frail or elderly.

Increasing severity of pain will require an increased dosage of MXL capsules using 30 mg, 60 mg, 90 mg, 120 mg, 150 mg or 200 mg alone or in combination to achieve pain relief. Higher doses should be made, where appropriate in 30%–50% increments as required. The correct dosage for any individual patient is that which controls the pain with no or tolerable side effects for a full 24 hours.

Patients receiving MXL capsules in place of parenteral morphine should be given a sufficiently increased dosage to compensate for any reduction in analgesic effects associated with oral administration. Usually such increased requirement is of the order of 100%. In such patients individual dose adjustments are required.

Children aged 1 year and above: The use of MXL capsules in children has not been extensively evaluated. For severe and intractable pain in cancer a starting dose in the range of 0.4 to 1.6 mg morphine per kg bodyweight daily is recommended. Doses should be titrated in the normal way as for adults.

Contra-indications: Respiratory depression, head injury, paralytic ileus, acute abdomen, delayed gastric emptying, obstructive airways disease, known morphine sensitivity, acute hepatic disease, concurrent administration of monoamine oxidase inhibitors (MAOIs) or within two weeks of discontinuation of their use. Not recommended during pregnancy or for pre-operative use or for the first 24 hours post-operatively. Children under one year of age.

Special warnings and special precautions for use: As with all narcotics, a reduction in dosage may be advisable in the elderly, in hypothyroidism, in renal and chronic hepatic disease. Use with caution in patients with convulsive disorders, raised intracranial pressure, hypotension with hypovolaemia, opioid dependent patients, diseases of the biliary tract, pancreatitis, inflammatory bowel disorders, prostatic hypertrophy and adrenocortical insufficiency. MXL capsules should not be used where there is a possibility of paralytic ileus occurring. Should paralytic ileus be suspected or occur during use, MXL capsules should be discontinued immediately. As with all morphine preparations, patients who are to undergo cordotomy or other pain relieving surgical procedures should not receive MXL capsules for 24 hours prior to surgery. If further treatment with MXL capsules is then indicated the dosage should be adjusted to the new post-operative requirement.

It is not possible to ensure bio-equivalence between different brands of controlled release morphine products. Therefore, it should be emphasised that patients, once titrated to an effective dose should not be changed from MXL capsules to other slow, sustained or controlled release morphine or other potent narcotic analgesic preparations without retitration and clinical assessment.

Interaction with other medicaments and other forms of interaction: Monoamine oxidase inhibitors have been reported to react with narcotic analgesics, producing CNS excitation or depression with hyper- or hypotensive crisis. Morphine potentiates the effects of tranquillisers, anaesthetics, hypnotics and sedatives, alcohol, muscle relaxants and antihypertensives. Cimetidine inhibits the metabolism of morphine. Mixed agonist/antagonist opioid analgesics (e.g. buprenorphine, nalbuphine, pentazocine) should not be administered to a patient who has received a course of therapy with a pure opioid agonist analgesic.

Pregnancy and lactation: MXL capsules are not recommended for use in pregnancy and labour due to the risk of neonatal respiratory depression. Administration to nursing mothers is not recommended as morphine is excreted in breast milk. Withdrawal symptoms may be observed in the newborn of mothers undergoing chronic treatment.

Effects on ability to drive and use machines: Morphine may modify the patient's reactions to a varying extent depending on the dosage and individual susceptibility. If affected, patients should not drive or operate machinery.

Undesirable effects: In normal doses, the commonest side effects of morphine are nausea, vomiting, constipation and drowsiness. With chronic therapy, nausea and vomiting are unusual with MXL capsules but should they occur the capsules can be readily combined with an anti-emetic if required. Constipation may be treated with appropriate laxatives. Dry mouth, sweating, vertigo, headache, disorientation, facial flushing, mood changes, palpitations, hallucinations, bronchospasm and colic may occur in a few patients. Micturition may be difficult and there may be biliary or ureteric spasm. Overdose may produce respiratory depression. Rarely, clinically relevant reductions in blood pressure and heart rate have been observed. Morphine has histamine releasing effects which may be responsible in part for reactions such as urticaria and pruritus.

The effects of morphine have led to its abuse and dependence may develop with regular, inappropriate use. This is not a major concern in the treatment of patients with severe pain.

Overdose: Signs of morphine toxicity and overdosage are pin-point pupils, respiratory depression and hypotension. Circulatory failure and deepening coma may occur in more severe cases.

Treatment of morphine overdosage: Primary attention should be given to the establishment of a patent airway and institution of assisted or controlled ventilation.

In the case of massive overdosage, administer naloxone 0.8 mg intravenously. Repeat at 2–3 minute intervals as necessary, or by an infusion of 2 mg in 500 ml of normal saline or 5% dextrose (0.004 mg/ml).

The infusion should be run at a rate related to the previous bolus doses administered and should be in accordance with the patient's response. However, because the duration of action of naloxone is relatively short, the patient must be carefully monitored until spontaneous respiration is reliably re-established. MXL capsules will continue to release and add to the morphine load for up to 24 hours after administration and the management of morphine overdosage should be modified accordingly.

For less severe overdosage, administer naloxone 0.2 mg intravenously followed by increments of 0.1 mg every 2 minutes if required.

Naloxone should not be administered in the absence of clinically significant respiratory or circulatory depression secondary to morphine overdosage. Naloxone should be administered cautiously to persons who are known, or suspected, to be physically dependent on morphine. In such cases, an abrupt or complete reversal of opioid effects may precipitate an acute withdrawal syndrome.

Gastric contents may need to be emptied as this can be useful in removing unabsorbed drug, particularly when a modified release formulation has been taken.

Pharmacological properties

Pharmacodynamic properties: Morphine acts as an agonist at opiate receptors in the CNS particularly mu and to a lesser extent kappa receptors. mu receptors are thought to mediate supraspinal analgesia, respiratory depression and euphoria and kappa receptors, spinal analgesia, miosis and sedation. Morphine has also a direct action on the bowel wall nerve plexuses causing constipation.

Pharmacokinetic properties: Morphine is well absorbed from the capsules and, in general, peak plasma concentrations are achieved 2–6 hours following administration. The availability is complete when compared to an immediate release oral solution or MST Continus tablets. The pharmacokinetics of morphine are linear across a very wide dose range. Morphine is subject to a significant first-pass effect which results in a lower bioavailability when compared to an equivalent intravenous or intramuscular dose.

The major metabolic transformation of morphine is glucuronidation to morphine-3-glucuronide and morphine-6-glucuronide which then undergo renal excretion. These metabolites are excreted in bile and may be subject to hydrolysis and subsequent reabsorption.

Because of the high inter-patient variation in morphine pharmacokinetics, and in analgesic requirements, the daily dosage in individual patients must be titrated to achieve appropriate pain control. Daily doses of up to 11.2 g have been recorded from twelve-hourly MST Continus tablets. For this reason the capsules have been formulated in strengths of 30 mg, 60 mg, 90 mg, 120 mg, 150 mg and 200 mg.

Pre-clinical safety data: There are no pre-clinical data of relevance to the prescriber which are additional to that already included in other sections of the SPC.

Pharmaceutical particulars

List of excipients: Hydrogenated Vegetable Oil BP; Macrogol 6000 PhEur; Talc PhEur; Magnesium Stearate PhEur.

Capsule shells: Gelatin (containing sodium dodecylsulphate). The following colours are also present:

30 mg: indigo carmine (E132); titanium dioxide (E171)
60 mg: indigo carmine (E132); titanium dioxide (E171); iron oxide (E172)
90 mg: erythrosine (E127); titanium dioxide (E171); iron oxide (E172)
120 mg: indigo carmine (E132); titanium dioxide (E171); iron oxide (E172)
150 mg: erythrosine (E127); indigo carmine (E132); titanium dioxide (E171); iron oxide (E172)
200 mg: titanium dioxide (E171); iron oxide (E172)

Printing ink: Shellac DAB 10, iron oxide, black (E172), soya lecithin, dimethylpolysiloxane.

Incompatibilities: None known.

Shelf life: 3 years.

Special precautions for storage: Store at or below 25°C.

Nature and contents of container: Polypropylene containers with polyethylene caps, containing 28 or 30 capsules.

PVDC (≥40 gsm) coated PVC (250 μm) blister strip with aluminium backing foil. The blister strips will be enclosed in a cardboard box. Each box will contain 28 or 30 capsules.

Instructions for use/handling: None.

Marketing authorisation numbers 0337/0259–0264

Date of (partial) revision of the text September 1998

Legal category CD (Sch 2), POM.

NARPHEN* TABLETS

Qualitative and quantitative composition Phenazocine Hydrobromide BP 5 mg.

Pharmaceutical form White, round, biconvex tablets marked with N on one side and 5 on the other.

Clinical particulars

Therapeutic indications: Narphen is a powerful analgesic for the relief of severe pain. Pain relief usually occurs within 20 minutes and lasts for five to six hours. Narphen is indicated for acute and chronic pain, including pre- and post-operative pain, and for obstetric analgesia. Narphen is particularly suitable for the treatment of intractable pain such as that of carcinoma as it produces minimal sedation.

In treating biliary or pancreatic pain, constriction of the Sphincter of Oddi is undesirable and the low spasmogenic activity of Narphen may be advantageous.

Posology and method of administration:
Route of administration: Orally/sublingually.

Adults and elderly: One tablet every four to six hours; up to 20 mg may be given in a single dose if necessary.

Children: A paediatric dosage has not been established.

Contra-indications: Narphen is contra-indicated in coma, convulsive disorders, delirium tremens, myxoedema, alcoholism, respiratory depression and obstructive airways disease.

Special warnings and special precautions for use: It is wise to reduce dosage in the elderly and in hypothyroidism or chronic hepatic disease.

Care is required in the presence of renal insufficiency.

Interaction with other medicaments and other forms of interaction: Narphen should not be given concurrently with monoamine oxidase inhibitors, nor within two weeks of discontinuation of treatment with them.

Care is required with concurrent administration of other narcotic analgesics, sedatives/hypnotics or anaesthetics.

Pregnancy and lactation: Although there is insufficient evidence of the safety of this drug in human pregnancy, animal studies have not shown any hazard. Nevertheless the use of phenazocine during pregnancy is not recommended.

Administration in labour may cause respiratory depression in the new-born infant.

Effects on ability to drive and use machines: Initially some patients may experience a feeling of light-headedness or dizziness, which soon passes, but if affected the patient should not attempt to drive or operate machinery.

Undesirable effects: Nausea and vomiting may be troublesome although emetic symptoms and constipation are less than with other narcotic analgesics. If nausea and vomiting occur phenazocine can be readily combined with an anti-emetic. Pruritus and occasionally dryness of the mouth and sweating have occurred. Hypotension is rare. As with other narcotics respiratory depression, tolerance and dependence may occur.

Overdose: Naloxone may be used as an antidote to overdosage or to antagonise any respiratory depression that may occur.

Pharmacological properties

Pharmacodynamic properties: Phenazocine is a synthetic morphine-like compound with agonist activity on mu opioid receptors. There is speculation that phenazocine may also possess some antagonist activity.

The knowledge of the pharmacological similarities between phenazocine and morphine has permitted the long and safe clinical use of Narphen.

Phenazocine produces only minimal sedation, and euphoria, and low spasmogenic activity on the Sphincter of Oddi.

Naloxone may be used as an antidote to overdosage or to antagonise any respiratory depression that may occur.

Pharmacokinetic properties: There are no data on the pharmacokinetics of phenazocine. It is considered unnecessary to provide such data as phenazocine is used in the treatment of severe pain, particularly in patients who are terminally ill. The interpretation of pain relief is subjective and therefore cannot be clearly related to specific blood levels.

Preclinical safety data: There are no preclinical data of relevance to the prescriber which are additional to that already included in other sections of the SPC.

Pharmaceutical particulars

List of excipients: Lactose PhEur, Maize Starch PhEur, Magnesium Stearate PhEur.

Incompatibilities: None known.

Shelf life: 42 months.

Special precautions for storage: Store at or below 25°C.

Nature and contents of container: Polypropylene securitainer with polyethylene lid (pack sizes 25, 28, 100, 112 tablets).

Instructions for use/handling: None stated.

Marketing authorisation number 0337/0198

Date of approval/revision of SPC November 1996

Legal category CD (Sch 2), POM.

PALLADONE* CAPSULES

Qualitative and quantitative composition Palladone capsules contain Hydromorphone Hydrochloride USP 1.3 mg or 2.6 mg.

Pharmaceutical form Palladone capsules 1.3 mg are orange/clear capsules marked HNR 1.3.

Palladone capsules 2.6 mg are red/clear capsules marked HNR 2.6.

Clinical particulars

Therapeutic indications: For the relief of severe pain in cancer.

Posology and method of administration

Route of administration: The capsules can be swallowed whole or opened and their contents sprinkled on to cold soft food.

Dosage

Adults and children over 12 years: Palladone capsules should be used at 4-hourly intervals. The dosage is dependent upon the severity of the pain and the patient's previous history of analgesic requirements. 1.3 mg of hydromorphone has an efficacy approximately equivalent to 10 mg of morphine given orally. A patient presenting with severe pain should normally be started on a dosage of one Palladone capsule 4-hourly. Increasing severity of pain will require increased dosage of hydromorphone to achieve the desired relief.

Elderly and patients with renal impairment: The elderly and patients with renal impairment should be dose titrated with Palladone capsules in order to achieve adequate analgesia. It should be noted, however, that these patients may require a lower dosage to achieve adequate analgesia.

Patients with hepatic impairment: Contra-indicated.

Children under 12 years: Not recommended.

Contra-indications: Respiratory depression, pregnancy, coma, acute abdomen, hepatic impairment, known hydromorphone sensitivity, concurrent administration of monoamine oxidase inhibitors or within 2 weeks of discontinuation of their use. Hydromorphone should be avoided in patients with raised intracranial pressure or head injury, and also in patients with convulsive disorders or acute alcoholism.

Special warnings and special precautions for use: As with all narcotics, a reduction in dosage may be advised in the elderly, in hypothyroidism, in chronic obstructive airways disease, in renal or adrenocortical insufficiency, prostatic hypertrophy, shock or reduced respiratory reserve. Palladone capsules are not recommended in the first 24 hours post-operatively. After this time they should be used with caution, particularly following abdominal surgery.

Palladone capsules should not be used where there is the possibility of paralytic ileus occurring. Should paralytic ileus be suspected or occur during use, Palladone capsules should be discontinued immediately.

Patients about to undergo cordotomy or other pain-relieving surgical procedures should not receive Palladone capsules for 4 hours prior to surgery. If further treatment with Palladone capsules is indicated, the dosage should be adjusted to the new post-operative requirement.

Interaction with other medicaments and other forms of interaction: Hydromorphone potentiates the effects of tranquillisers, anaesthetics, hypnotics and sedatives.

Pregnancy and lactation: Palladone capsules are not recommended in pregnancy or in the breast-feeding mother as there are insufficient animal or human data to justify such use.

Effects on ability to drive and use machines: Hydromorphone may cause drowsiness and patients should not drive or operate machinery if affected.

Undesirable effects: Hydromorphone may cause constipation, nausea and vomiting. Constipation may be treated with appropriate laxatives. When nausea and vomiting are troublesome, Palladone capsules can be readily combined with anti-emetics. Tolerance and dependence may occur.

Overdose: Signs of hydromorphone toxicity and overdosage are pin-point pupils, respiratory depression and hypotension. Circulatory failure and deepening coma may occur in more severe cases.

Treatment of overdosage: Primary attention should be given to the establishment of a patent airway and institution of assisted or controlled ventilation.

In the case of massive overdosage, administer naloxone 0.8 mg intravenously. Repeat at 2–3 minute intervals as necessary, or by an infusion of 2 mg in 500 ml of normal saline or 5% dextrose (0.004 mg/ml).

The infusion should be run at a rate related to the previous bolus doses administered and should be in accordance with the patient's response. However, because the duration of action of naloxone is relatively short, the patient must be carefully monitored until spontaneous respiration is reliably re-established.

For less severe overdosage, administer naloxone 0.2 mg intravenously followed by increments of 0.1 mg every 2 minutes if required.

Naloxone should not be administered in the absence of clinically significant respiratory or circulatory depression secondary to hydromorphone overdosage. Naloxone should be administered cautiously to persons who are known, or suspected, to be physically dependent on hydromorphone. In such cases, an abrupt or complete reversal of opioid effects may precipitate an acute withdrawal syndrome.

Gastric contents may need to be emptied as this can be useful in removing unabsorbed drug.

Pharmacological properties

Pharmacodynamic properties: Like morphine, hydromorphone is an agonist of mu receptors. The pharmacological actions of hydromorphone and morphine do not differ significantly. The oral analgesic potency ratio of hydromorphone to morphine is approximately 5–10: 1. Hydromorphone and related opioids produce their major effects on the central nervous system and bowel. The effects are diverse and include analgesia, drowsiness, changes in mood, respiratory depression, decreased gastrointestinal motility, nausea, vomiting, and alteration of the endocrine and autonomic nervous system.

Pharmacokinetic properties: Hydromorphone is absorbed from the gastrointestinal tract and undergoes pre-systemic elimination resulting in an oral bioavailability of about 50%. It is metabolised and excreted in the urine mainly as conjugated hydromorphone, dihydroisomorphine and dihydromorphine.

Preclinical safety data: There are no preclinical data of relevance to the prescriber which are additional to that already included in other sections of the SPC.

Pharmaceutical particulars

List of excipients: Microcrystalline Cellulose PhEur, Lactose (anhydrous) USNF.

Capsule shells: Gelatin PhEur, erythrosine (E127), iron oxide (E172), titanium dioxide (E171), sodium dodecylsulphate DAB.

Incompatibilities: None known.

Shelf life: Two years.

Special precautions for storage: Store at or below 25°C. Protect from moisture.

Nature and contents of container: PVdC coated PVC blisters with aluminium backing foil containing 30, 56 or 60 capsules.

Instructions for use/handling: None stated.

Marketing authorisation numbers

Palladone capsules 1.3 mg 0337/0238
Palladone capsules 2.6 mg 0337/0239

Date of approval/revision of SPC January 1997

Legal category CD (Sch 2), POM.

PALLADONE-SR* CAPSULES

Qualitative and quantitative composition The capsules contain Hydromorphone Hydrochloride USP 2 mg, 4 mg, 8 mg, 16 mg, 24 mg.

Pharmaceutical form Hard gelatin capsule containing spherical controlled release pellets.

Palladone-SR capsules 2 mg are yellow/clear capsules marked HCR 2.

Palladone-SR capsules 4 mg are pale blue/clear capsules marked HCR 4.

Palladone-SR capsules 8 mg are pink/clear capsules marked HCR 8.

Palladone-SR capsules 16 mg are brown/clear capsules marked HCR 16.

Palladone-SR capsules 24 mg are dark blue/clear capsules marked HCR 24.

Clinical particulars

Therapeutic indications: For the relief of severe pain in cancer.

Posology and method of administration

Route of administration: The capsules can be swallowed whole or opened and their contents sprinkled on to cold soft food.

Dosage

Adults and children over 12 years: Palladone-SR capsules should be used at 12-hourly intervals. The dosage is dependent upon the severity of the pain and the patient's previous history of analgesic requirements. 4 mg of hydromorphone has an efficacy approximately equivalent to 30 mg of morphine sulphate given orally. A patient presenting with severe pain should normally be started on a dosage of 4 mg Palladone-SR capsules 12-hourly. Increasing severity of pain will require increased dosage of hydromorphone to achieve the desired relief.

Elderly and patients with renal impairment: The elderly and patients with renal impairment should be dose titrated with Palladone-SR capsules in order to achieve adequate analgesia. It should be noted, however, that these patients may require a lower dosage to achieve adequate analgesia.

Patients with hepatic impairment: Contra-indicated.

Children under 12 years: Not recommended.

Contra-indications: Respiratory depression, pregnancy, coma, acute abdomen, hepatic impairment, known hydromorphone sensitivity, concurrent administration of monoamine oxidase inhibitors or within 2 weeks of discontinuation of their use. Use of Palladone-SR capsules should be avoided in patients with raised intracranial pressure or head injury, and also in patients with convulsive disorders or acute alcoholism.

Pre-operative administration of Palladone-SR capsules is not recommended and is not an approved indication.

Special warnings and special precautions for use: As with all narcotics, a reduction in dosage may be advised in the elderly, in hypothyroidism, in chronic obstructive airways disease, in renal or adrenocortical insufficiency, prostatic hypertrophy, shock or reduced respiratory reserve. Palladone-SR capsules are not recommended in the first 24 hours post-operatively. After this time they should be used with caution, particularly following abdominal surgery.

Palladone-SR capsules should not be used where there is the possibility of paralytic ileus occurring. Should paralytic ileus be suspected or occur during use, Palladone-SR capsules should be discontinued.

Patients about to undergo cordotomy or other pain relieving surgical procedures should not receive Palladone-SR capsules for 24 hours prior to surgery. If further treatment with Palladone-SR capsules is indicated, then the dosage should be adjusted to the new post-operative requirement.

Interaction with other medicaments and other forms of interaction: Hydromorphone potentiates the effects of tranquillisers, anaesthetics, hypnotics and sedatives.

Pregnancy and lactation: Palladone-SR capsules are not recommended in pregnancy or in the breast-feeding mother as there are insufficient animal or human data to justify such use.

Effects on ability to drive and use machines: Hydromorphone may cause drowsiness and patients should not drive or operate machinery if affected.

Undesirable effects: Hydromorphone may cause constipation, nausea and vomiting. Constipation may be treated with appropriate laxatives. When nausea and vomiting are troublesome, Palladone-SR capsules can be readily combined with antiemetics. Tolerance and dependence may occur.

Overdose: Signs of hydromorphone toxicity and overdosage are pin-point pupils, respiratory depression and hypotension. Circulatory failure and deepening coma may occur in more severe cases.

Treatment of overdosage: Primary attention should be given to the establishment of a patent airway and institution of assisted or controlled ventilation.

In the case of massive overdosage, administer naloxone 0.8 mg intravenously. Repeat at 2–3 minute intervals as necessary, or by an infusion of 2 mg in 500 ml of normal saline or 5% dextrose (0.004 mg/ml).

The infusion should be run at a rate related to the previous bolus doses administered and should be in accordance with the patient's response. However, because the duration of action of naloxone is relatively short, the patient must be carefully monitored until spontaneous respiration is reliably re-established. Palladone-SR capsules will continue to release and add to the hydromorphone load for up to 12 hours after administration, and the management of the overdosage should be modified accordingly.

For less severe overdosage, administer naloxone 0.2 mg intravenously followed by increments of 0.1 mg every 2 minutes if required.

Naloxone should not be administered in the absence of clinically significant respiratory or circulatory depression secondary to hydromorphone overdosage. Naloxone should be administered cautiously to persons who are known, or suspected, to be physically dependent on hydromorphone. In such cases, an abrupt or complete reversal of opioid effects may precipitate an acute withdrawal syndrome.

Gastric contents may need to be emptied as this can be useful in removing unabsorbed drug, particularly when a modified release formulation has been taken.

Pharmacological properties
Pharmacodynamic properties: Like morphine, hydromorphone is an agonist of mu receptors. The pharmacological actions of hydromorphone and morphine do not differ significantly. The oral analgesic potency ratio of hydromorphone to morphine is approximately 5–10:1. Hydromorphone and related opioids produce their major effects on the central nervous system and bowel. The effects are diverse and include analgesia, drowsiness, changes in mood, respiratory depression, decreased gastrointestinal motility, nausea, vomiting and alteration of the endocrine and autonomic nervous system.

Pharmacokinetic properties: Hydromorphone is absorbed from the gastrointestinal tract and undergoes pre-systemic elimination resulting in an oral bioavailability of about 50%. It is metabolised and excreted in the urine mainly as conjugated hydromorphone and with smaller amounts of unchanged hydromorphone, dihydroisomorphine and dihydromorphine. Palladone-SR capsules have been formulated to produce therapeutic plasma levels following 12-hourly dosing.

Preclinical safety data: There are no preclinical data of relevance to the prescriber which are additional to that already included in other sections of the SPC.

Pharmaceutical particulars
List of excipients: Microcrystalline Cellulose PhEur; Hydroxypropylmethylcellulose (15 cps) PhEur; Purified Water PhEur; Ethylcellulose (N10) USNF; Colloidal Anhydrous Silica PhEur; Dibutyl Sebacate USNF; Methanol BP (1973), Dichloromethane.

Capsule shells: Gelatin PhEur; Sodium Dodecylsulphate DAB.

The following colours are included in the capsule shells: 2 mg (E104, E171), 4 mg (E127, E132, E171), 8 mg (E127, E171), 16 mg (E171, E172), 24 mg (E132, E171).

Incompatibilities: None known.

Shelf life: Eighteen months.

Special precautions for storage: Store at or below 25°C.

Nature and contents of container:
PCdC/PVC blister packs with aluminium backing foil containing 56 capsules.

Instructions for use/handling: None stated.

Marketing authorisation numbers

Palladone-SR capsules 2 mg	0337/0246
Palladone-SR capsules 4 mg	0337/0242
Palladone-SR capsules 8 mg	0337/0243
Palladone-SR capsules 16 mg	0337/0244
Palladone-SR capsules 24 mg	0337/0245

Date of (partial) revision of the text May 1998

Legal category CD (Sch 2), POM.

PHYLLOCONTIN* PAEDIATRIC CONTINUS TABLETS 100 mg PHYLLOCONTIN* CONTINUS TABLETS 225 mg PHYLLOCONTIN* FORTE CONTINUS TABLETS 350 mg

Qualitative and quantitative composition Modified release tablets containing 100 mg, 225 mg and 350 mg of Aminophylline Hydrate PhEur.

Pharmaceutical form
PHYLLOCONTIN Paediatric CONTINUS tablets 100 mg are mottled peach tablets with the Napp logo on one side and SA/2 on the other.

PHYLLOCONTIN CONTINUS tablets 225 mg are pale yellow, film-coated tablets with the Napp logo on one side and SA on the other.

PHYLLOCONTIN Forte CONTINUS tablets 350 mg are pale yellow, film-coated tablets with the Napp logo on one side and SA 350 on the other.

Clinical particulars
Therapeutic indications: For the treatment and prophylaxis of bronchospasm associated with asthma, chronic obstructive pulmonary disease and chronic bronchitis. Also indicated in adults for the treatment of left ventricular and congestive cardiac failure.

Posology and method of administration
Route of administration: Oral.

Tablets should be swallowed whole and not chewed.

Children: The maintenance dose (expressed as mg aminophylline) is 12 mg/kg twice daily adjusted to the nearest 100 mg. It is recommended that half the maintenance dose be given for the first week of therapy if the patient has not previously been receiving xanthine preparations.

Some children with chronic asthma require and tolerate much higher doses (13-20 mg/kg twice daily). Lower doses (based on the usual adult dose) may be required by adolescents. Not recommended for children under 3 years of age.

Adults: The usual dose is two PHYLLOCONTIN CONTINUS tablets 225 mg twice-daily following an initial week of therapy on one tablet twice-daily.

The elderly: The dose should be adjusted following the response to the initial week of therapy on one tablet twice-daily.

Dose titration: Patients vary in their response to xanthines and it may be necessary to titrate dosage individually. Steady state theophylline levels are generally attained 3-4 days after dose adjustment. If a satisfactory clinical response is not achieved, serum theophylline should be measured 4-6 hours after the last dose. Based on serum theophylline assay results dosage should be titrated using the following as a guide:

Peak serum theophylline level	*Dosage adjustment to nearest 125 mg*
<10 micrograms/ml	Increase total daily dose by half.
10–15 micrograms/ml	Increase total daily dose by one quarter if symptoms persist.
16–20 micrograms/ml	No adjustment required.
21–25 micrograms/ml	Decrease dose by one quarter.
26–30 micrograms/ml	Miss next dose and decrease maintenance by one half.

Contra-indications Should not be given concomitantly with ephedrine in children.

Special warnings and special precautions for use: A reduction of dosage may be necessary in the elderly patient.

The hypokalaemia resulting from beta agonist therapy, steroids, diuretics and hypoxia may be potentiated by xanthines. Particular care is advised in patients suffering from severe asthma who require hospitalisation. It is recommended that serum potassium levels are monitored in such situations.

Alternative treatment is advised for patients with a history of seizure activity.

Interaction with other medicaments and other forms of interaction: The following increase clearance and it may therefore be necessary to increase dosage to ensure a therapeutic effect: aminoglutethimide, carbamazepine, moracizine, phenytoin, rifampicin, sulphinpyrazone and barbiturates. Smoking and alcohol consumption can also increase clearance of theophylline.

The following reduce clearance and a reduced dosage may therefore be necessary to avoid side-effects: allopurinol, carbimazole, cimetidine, ciprofloxacin, clarithromycin, diltiazem, disulfiram, erythromycin, fluconazole, interferon, isoniazid, isoprenaline, methotrexate, mexiletine, nizatidine, norfloxacin, oxpentifylline, propafenone, propranolol, ofloxacin, thiabendazole, verapamil, viloxazine hydrochloride and oral contraceptives. The concomitant use of theophylline and fluvoxamine should usually be avoided. Where this is not possible, patients should have their theophylline dose halved and plasma theophylline should be monitored closely.

Factors such as viral infections, liver disease and heart failure also reduce theophylline clearance. There are conflicting reports concerning the potentiation of theophylline by influenza vaccine and physicians should be aware that interaction may occur. A reduction of dosage may be necessary in elderly patients. Thyroid disease or associated treatment may alter theophylline plasma levels. There is also a pharmacological interaction with adenosine, benzodiazepines, halothane, lomustine and lithium and these drugs should be used with caution.

Theophylline may decrease steady state phenytoin levels.

Pregnancy and lactation: Safety in human pregnancy has not been established but it has been in use for many years without apparent ill consequence. Theophylline crosses the placental barrier and is secreted in breast milk. Use of theophylline during the third trimester, or during breast feeding, may be associated with irritability in the infant. Use in pregnancy only when there is no safe alternative, or when the disease itself carries risk for the mother or child.

Effects on ability to drive and use machines: No known effects.

Undesirable effects: The risk of side-effects usually associated with theophylline and xanthine derivatives such as nausea, gastric irritation, headache and CNS stimulation is significantly reduced when PHYLLOCONTIN CONTINUS tablet preparations are given.

Overdose: Empty stomach contents. Monitor electrocardiogram and maintain fluid balance. Oral activated medical charcoal has been found to reduce high theophylline blood levels. In severe poisoning, employ charcoal-column haemoperfusion. Treat symptoms on appearance. The physician should be aware that tablets in the intestine will continue to release theophylline for a period of hours.

In the event of hypokalaemia, potassium chloride should be given by slow intravenous infusion. Repeated measurements of plasma potassium should be made.

Pharmacological properties
Pharmacodynamic properties: Aminophylline (theophylline) is a bronchodilator. In addition it affects the function of a number of cells involved in the inflammatory processes associated with asthma and chronic obstructive airways disease. Of most importance may be enhanced suppressor, T-lymphocyte activity and reduction of eosinophil and neutrophil function. These actions may contribute to an anti-inflammatory prophylactic activity in asthma and chronic obstructive airways disease. Theophylline stimulates the myocardium and produces a diminution of venous pressure in congestive heart failure leading to marked increase in cardiac output.

Pharmacokinetic properties: Aminophylline (theophylline) is well absorbed from PHYLLOCONTIN CONTINUS tablets and at least 60% may be bound to plasma proteins. The main urinary metabolites are 1,3 dimethyl uric acid and 3-methylxanthine. About 10% is excreted unchanged.

Pre-clinical safety data: There are no pre-clinical data of relevance to the prescriber which are additional to that already included in other sections of the SPC.

Pharmaceutical particulars
List of excipients: All PHYLLOCONTIN CONTINUS tablets contain:
Hydroxyethylcellulose
Povidone [K25]
Cetostearyl Alcohol
Purified Talc
Magnesium Stearate
PHYLLOCONTIN Paediatric CONTINUS tablets 100 mg also contain Saccharin Sodium and Annatto No. 6 (E160).

PHYLLOCONTIN CONTINUS tablets 225 mg and PHYLLOCONTIN Forte CONTINUS tablets 350 mg also contain Hypromellose (E464), Polyethylene Glycol 400, Industrial Methylated Spirit, Titanium Dioxide (E171), and Iron Oxide (E172).

Incompatibilities: Not applicable.

Shelf-life: Three years.

Special precautions for storage: Store at or below 25°C.

Nature and contents of container: PHYLLOCONTIN Paediatric CONTINUS tablets and PHYLLOCONTIN Forte CONTINUS tablets are available in polypropylene containers containing 56 tablets.

PHYLLOCONTIN CONTINUS tablets 225 mg are available in PVC blister packs containing 56 tablets and polypropylene containers containing 1000 tablets.

Instructions for use/handling: None.

Marketing authorisation number
PHYLLOCONTIN Paediatric CONTINUS tablets 100 mg–PL 0337/0040

PHYLLOCONTIN CONTINUS tablets 225 mg–PL 0337/0026R

PHYLLOCONTIN Forte CONTINUS tablets 350 mg–PL 0337/0090

Date of first authorisation/renewal of the authorisation
PHYLLOCONTIN Paediatric CONTINUS tablets 100 mg–26 January 1977/30 June 1997

PHYLLOCONTIN CONTINUS tablets 225 mg–7 July 1989/7 January 1998

PHYLLOCONTIN Forte CONTINUS tablets 350 mg–17 August 1983/30 March 1994

Date of preparation/last revision March 1998

Legal category P

REMEDEINE* EFFERVESCENT and REMEDEINE FORTE* EFFERVESCENT TABLETS

Qualitative and quantitative composition Remedeine Effervescent Tablets contain Dihydrocodeine Tartrate BP 20 mg, Paracetamol PhEur 250 mg, Paracetamol (direct compression containing gelatin) 260 mg.

Remedeine Forte Effervescent Tablets contain Dihydrocodeine Tartrate BP 30 mg, Paracetamol PhEur 250 mg, Paracetamol (direct compression containing gelatin) 260 mg.

Pharmaceutical form Effervescent tablet

Clinical particulars

Therapeutic indications: For the treatment of severe pain. REMEDEINE FORTE Effervescent Tablets are for the treatment of severe pain, where there is a higher analgesic requirement (higher than REMEDEINE Effervescent Tablets 500/20 mg).

Posology and method of administration:

Route of administration: Oral.

Dosage and administration: The tablets should be taken during or after meals. The tablets should be dissolved in water.

Adults and children over 12 years: One or two tablets every four to six hours. Do not exceed eight tablets in any 24 hour period.

Children under 12 years: Not recommended.

Elderly: One tablet every four to six hours increasing to two tablets every four to six hours if required and tolerated. Do not exceed eight tablets in any 24 hour period.

Contra-indications: Respiratory depression, obstructive airways disease, hypersensitivity to paracetamol, dihydrocodeine or other tablet constituents.

Special warnings and special precautions for use: REMEDEINE effervescent tablets and REMEDEINE FORTE effervescent tablets should be given with caution to patients with allergic disorders and should not be given during an attack of asthma. Caution should also be observed if there is marked impairment of liver function, advanced kidney disease and in chronic alcoholics.

Do not exceed the recommended dose.

Patients should be advised not to take other paracetamol-containing products simultaneously.

Dosage should be reduced in the elderly, in hypothyroidism and in chronic hepatic disease. An overdose can cause hepatic necrosis.

Dihydrocodeine should be used with caution in patients taking monoamine oxidase inhibitors and should be avoided in those patients with raised intracranial pressure or head injury.

Use with caution in patients with prostatic hypertrophy since dihydrocodeine may cause urinary retention.

In patients already habituated to a drug such as pethidine, the substitution of dihydrocodeine in equianalgesic doses has led to the appearance of abstinence symptoms. This suggests that dihydrocodeine, despite its effectiveness as an analgesic, has a low addiction potential. Nevertheless, when dihydrocodeine is prescribed for chronic use the physician should take care to avoid any unnecessary increase in dosage especially where there is a previous history of drug dependence or abuse.

REMEDEINE effervescent tablets and REMEDEINE FORTE effervescent tablets contain approximately 350 mg of sodium. This should be taken into account in patients requiring sodium restriction.

Interaction with other medicaments and other forms of interaction: Additive CNS depression may occur with alcohol, and other CNS depressants such as anxiolytics, anti-depressants, hypnotics and anti-psychotics. The rate of absorption of paracetamol may be increased by metoclopramide or domperidone and absorption of paracetamol may be reduced by cholestyramine.

The anti-coagulant effect of warfarin and other coumarins may be enhanced by prolonged regular use of paracetamol with increased risk of bleeding.

Pregnancy and lactation: Epidemiological studies in human pregnancy have shown no effects due to paracetamol or dihydrocodeine. However, both drugs should be avoided during pregnancy unless considered essential by the physician.

Paracetamol is excreted in breast milk but not in a clinically significant amount. Available published data do not contraindicate breast feeding.

Effects on ability to drive and use machines: Dihydrocodeine may cause drowsiness and, if affected, patients should not drive or operate machinery.

Undesirable effects: Constipation, if it occurs, is readily treated with a mild laxative.

Other side effects of dihydrocodeine which may occur in a few patients, are nausea, vomiting, headache, vertigo, giddiness, urinary retention, pruritus, sedation, dysphoria, hallucinations and allergic reactions including skin rashes.

Adverse effects of paracetamol are rare but hypersensitivity reactions including skin rashes, blood dyscrasias, acute pancreatitis have been reported.

Overdose: Symptoms of paracetamol overdosage in the first 24 hours are pallor, nausea, vomiting, anorexia and abdominal pain. Liver damage may become apparent 12 to 48 hours after ingestion. Abnormalities of glucose metabolism and metabolic acidosis may occur. In severe poisoning, hepatic failure may progress to encephalopathy, coma and death. Acute renal failure with acute tubular necrosis may develop even in the absence of severe liver damage. Cardiac arrhythmias have been reported.

Liver damage is likely in adults who have taken 10 g or more of paracetamol. It is considered that excess quantities of a toxic metabolite (usually adequately detoxified by glutathione when normal doses of paracetamol are ingested), become irreversibly bound to liver tissue.

Immediate treatment is essential in the management of paracetamol overdose. Despite a lack of significant early symptoms, patients should be referred to hospital urgently for immediate medical attention and any patient who has ingested around 7.5 g or more of paracetamol in the preceding 4 hours should undergo gastric lavage. Administration of oral methionine or intravenous N-acetylcysteine which may have a beneficial effect up to at least 48 hours after the overdose, may be required. General supportive measures must be available.

Severe respiratory depression due to dihydrocodeine can be treated with naloxone hydrochloride 0.8 to 2 mg intravenously, repeated as required at 2 or 3 minute intervals.

Pharmacological properties

Pharmacodynamic properties: Paracetamol is an effective analgesic possessing a remarkably low level of side effects. Its broad clinical utility has been extensively reported, and it now largely replaces aspirin for routine use. Paracetamol is well tolerated; having a bland effect on gastric mucosa, unlike aspirin, it neither exacerbates symptoms of peptic ulcer nor precipitates bleeding. Dihydrocodeine tartrate has been widely used for a number of years as a powerful analgesic.

In addition the compound exhibits well-defined anti-tussive activity.

Fortifying paracetamol with dihydrocodeine tartrate provides an effective combination of drugs for the treatment of severe pain.

Pharmacokinetic properties: Dihydrocodeine is well absorbed from the gastrointestinal tract. Like other phenanthrene derivatives, dihydrocodeine is mainly metabolised in the liver with the resultant metabolites being excreted mainly in the urine. Metabolism of dihydrocodeine includes o-demethylation, n-demethylation and 6-keto reduction.

Paracetamol is readily absorbed from the gastrointestinal tract with peak plasma concentrations occurring 30 minutes to 2 hours after ingestion. It is metabolised in the liver and excreted in the urine mainly as the glucuronide and sulphate conjugates.

Pre-clinical data: There are no pre-clinical data of relevance to the prescriber which are additional to that already included in other sections of the SPC.

Pharmaceutical particulars

List of excipients: Citric Acid PhEur (anhydrous, added as Citric Acid Monohydrate); Sodium Hydrogen Carbonate PhEur; Sodium Carbonate (anhydrous) PhEur; Sodium Benzoate PhEur; Sucrose PhEur; Saccharin Sodium PhEur; Gelatin PhEur.

Incompatibilities: None known.

Shelf life: 24 months.

Special precautions for storage: Store at or below 25°C.

Nature and contents of container:

1. Blister packs: 43 μm soft tempered aluminium foil coated with 25 μm nylon on the outside and 25 μm polyethylene on the inside.
2. Aluminium foil strip packs: 30 μm soft tempered aluminium foil and 38 μm polyethylene on the inside.

Pack sizes: 2, 4, 12, 24, 56, 60, 100, 112 tablets.

Instructions for use/handling: None stated.

Marketing authorisation numbers

Remedeine Effervescent tablets	0337/0257
Remedeine Forte Effervescent tablets	0337/0258

Date of (partial) revision of the text November 1997

Legal category POM.

REMEDEINE* and REMEDEINE FORTE* TABLETS

Qualitative and quantitative composition REMEDEINE tablets contain Paracetamol 500 mg and Dihydrocodeine Tartrate BP 20 mg.

REMEDEINE FORTE tablets contain Paracetamol 500 mg and Dihydrocodeine Tartrate BP 30 mg.

Pharmaceutical form White to off-white, circular, flat-faced tablets with a bevelled edge.

REMEDEINE tablets are engraved PD/20 on one side.

REMEDEINE FORTE tablets are engraved PD/30 on one side.

Clinical particulars

Therapeutic indications: For the treatment of severe pain.

Posology and method of administration

Route of administration: Oral

REMEDEINE/REMEDEINE FORTE tablets should, if possible, be taken during or after meals.

Adults and children over 12 years: 1 or 2 tablets every four to six hours.

Do not exceed eight tablets in any 24-hour period.

Children under 12 years: Not recommended.

Elderly: One tablet every 4–6 hours increasing to two tablets every 4–6 hours if required and tolerated. Caution should be exercised when increasing the dose in the elderly.

Contra-indications: Respiratory depression, obstructive airways disease, hypersensitivity to paracetamol, dihydrocodeine or other tablet constituents.

Special warnings and special precautions for use: REMEDEINE/REMEDEINE FORTE tablets should be given with caution in patients with allergic disorders and should not be given during an attack of asthma. Caution should also be observed if there is marked impairment of liver function, advanced kidney disease and in chronic alcoholics.

Do not exceed the recommended dose.

Patients should be advised not to take other paracetamol-containing products concurrently.

Dosage should be reduced in the elderly, hypothyroidism and in chronic hepatic disease. An overdose can cause hepatic necrosis.

Dihydrocodeine should be used with caution in patients taking monoamine oxidase inhibitors and should be avoided in those patients with raised intracranial pressure or head injury.

Use with caution in patients with prostatic hypertrophy since dihydrocodeine may cause urinary retention.

In patients already habituated to a drug such as pethidine, the substitution of dihydrocodeine in equianalgesic doses has led to the appearance of abstinence symptoms. This suggests that dihydrocodeine, despite its effectiveness as an analgesic, has a low addiction potential. Nevertheless, when dihydrocodeine is prescribed for chronic use the physician should take care to avoid any unnecessary increase in dosage especially when there is a previous history of drug dependence or abuse.

Interaction with other medicaments and other forms of interaction: Additive CNS depression may occur with alcohol, and other CNS depressants such as anxiolytics, anti-depressants, hypnotics and anti-psychotics. The rate of absorption of paracetamol may be increased by metoclopramide or domperidone and absorption of paracetamol may be reduced by cholestyramine.

The anti-coagulant effect of warfarin and other coumarins may be enhanced by prolonged regular use of paracetamol with increased risk of bleeding.

Pregnancy and lactation: Epidemiological studies in human pregnancy have shown no effects due to paracetamol or dihydrocodeine. However, both drugs should be avoided during pregnancy unless considered essential by the physician.

Paracetamol is excreted in breast milk but not in a clinically significant amount. Available published data do not contraindicate breast feeding.

Effects on ability to drive and use machines: Dihydrocodeine may cause drowsiness and, if affected, patients should not drive or operate machinery.

Undesirable effects: Constipation, if it occurs, is readily treated with a mild laxative.

Other side-effects of dihydrocodeine which may occur in a few patients, are nausea, vomiting, headache, vertigo, giddiness, urinary retention, pruritus, sedation, dysphoria, hallucinations and allergic reactions including skin rashes.

Adverse effects of paracetamol are rare but hypersensitivity reactions including skin rash, blood dyscrasias, acute pancreatitis have been reported.

Overdose: Symptoms of paracetamol overdosage in the first 24 hours are pallor, nausea, vomiting, anorexia and abdominal pain. Liver damage may become apparent 12 to 48 hours after ingestion. Abnormalities of glucose metabolism and metabolic acidosis may occur. In severe poisoning, hepatic failure may progress to encephalopathy, coma and death. Acute renal failure with acute tubular necrosis may develop even in the absence of severe liver damage. Cardiac arrhythmias have been reported.

Liver damage is likely in adults who have taken 10 g or more of paracetamol. It is considered that excess quantities of a toxic metabolite (usually adequately detoxified by glutathione when normal doses of paracetamol are ingested), become irreversibly bound to liver tissue.

Immediate treatment is essential in the management of paracetamol overdose. Despite a lack of significant early symptoms, patients should be referred to hospital urgently for immediate medical attention and any patient who has ingested around 7.5 g or more of paracetamol in the preceding 4 hours should undergo gastric lavage. Administration of oral methionine or intravenous N-acetylcysteine which may have a beneficial effect up to at least 48 hours after the overdose, may be required. General supportive measures must be available.

Severe respiratory depression due to dihydrocodeine can be treated with naloxone hydrochloride 0.8 to 2 mg intravenously, repeated as required at 2 or 3 minute intervals.

Pharmacological properties

Pharmacodynamic properties: Paracetamol is an effective analgesic possessing a remarkably low level of side effects. Its broad clinical utility has been extensively reported, and it now largely replaces aspirin for routine use. Paracetamol is well tolerated; having a bland effect on gastric mucosa, unlike aspirin, it neither exacerbates symptoms of peptic ulcer nor precipitates bleeding. Dihydrocodeine tartrate has been widely used for a number of years as a powerful analgesic.

In addition the compound exhibits well-defined anti-tussive activity.

Fortifying paracetamol with dihydrocodeine tartrate provides an effective combination of drugs for the treatment of severe pain.

Pharmacokinetic properties: Dihydrocodeine is well absorbed from the gastrointestinal tract. Like other phenanthrene derivatives, dihydrocodeine is mainly metabolised in the liver with the resultant metabolites being excreted mainly in the urine. Metabolism of dihydrocodeine includes 0-demethylation, N-demethylation and 6-keto reduction.

Paracetamol is readily absorbed from the gastrointestinal tract with peak plasma concentrations occurring 30 minutes to 2 hours after ingestion. It is metabolised in the liver and excreted in the urine as the glucuronide and sulphate conjugates.

Pre-clinical safety data: There are no pre-clinical data of relevance to the prescriber which are additional to that already included in other sections of the SPC.

Pharmaceutical particulars

List of excipients:
Magnesium Stearate PhEur
Starch Maize Special PhEur

Incompatibilities: None known.

Shelf-life: Three years.

Special precautions for storage: Store at or below 30°C protected from moisture.

Nature and contents of container: REMEDEINE Tablets are available in plastic tamper-evident containers of 112 tablets.

REMEDEINE FORTE tablets are available in plastic tamper-evident containers of 56 tablets.

Instructions for use/handling: None.

Marketing authorisation number PL 0337/0192, 0193.

Date of first authorisation/renewal of authorisation 20 November 1991/14 January 1998.

Date of (partial) revision of the text January 1998.

Legal category POM.

SEVREDOL* TABLETS 10 mg, 20 mg, 50 mg

Qualitative and quantitative composition Morphine Sulphate BP 10 mg, 20 mg, 50 mg.

Pharmaceutical form

10 mg: Blue film-coated capsule shaped, biconvex tablet with a score line on one side. 'IR' is marked on the left side and '10' on the right.

20 mg: Pink film-coated capsule shaped, biconvex tablet, with a score line on one side. 'IR' is marked on the left side and '20' on the right.

50 mg: Pale green film-coated capsule shaped, biconvex tablet, with a score line on one side. 'IR' is marked on the left side and '50' on the right.

Clinical particulars

Therapeutic indications: Sevredol tablets are indicated for the relief of severe pain.

Posology and method of administration

Route of administration: Oral.

Adults and children over 12 years: The dosage of Sevredol tablets is dependent on the severity of pain and the patient's previous history of analgesic requirements. One tablet to be taken every four hours or as directed by a physician. Increasing severity of pain or tolerance to morphine will require increased dosage of Sevredol tablets using 10 mg, 20 mg or 50 mg alone or in combination to achieve the desired relief.

Patients receiving Sevredol tablets in place of parenteral morphine should be given a sufficiently increased dosage to compensate for any reduction in analgesic effects associated with oral administration. Usually such increased requirement is of the order of 100 per cent. In such patients individual dose adjustments are required.

Elderly: A reduction in adult dosage may be advisable.

Children 3–12 years of age: Only Sevredol 10 mg tablets are suitable for children.
3–5 years – 5 mg, 4-hourly.
6–12 years – 5–10 mg, 4-hourly.

Contra-indications: Respiratory depression, head injury, obstructive airways disease, paralytic ileus, acute abdomen, delayed gastric emptying, known morphine sensitivity, acute hepatic disease, concurrent administration of monoamine oxidase inhibitors or within two weeks of discontinuation of their use. Not recommended during pregnancy.

Not recommended for children below 3 years of age.

Special warnings and special precautions for use: Sevredol tablets should not be used where there is a possibility of paralytic ileus occurring. Should paralytic ileus be suspected or occur during use, Sevredol tablets should be discontinued immediately. Patients who are about to undergo cordotomy or other pain relieving procedures should not receive Sevredol tablets 4 hours prior to surgery. A reduction in dosage may be advisable in hypothyroidism, and in renal and chronic hepatic disease. Sevredol tablets should be used with caution post-operatively particularly following abdominal surgery.

Use with caution in opiate dependent patients and in patients with raised intracranial pressure, hypotension with hypovolaemia, diseases of the biliary tract, pancreatitis, inflammatory bowel disorders, prostatic hypertrophy and adrenocortical insufficiency, acute alcoholism, and in patients with convulsive disorders.

Interaction with other medicaments and other forms of interaction: Monoamine oxidase inhibitors are known to interact with narcotic analgesics producing CNS excitation or depression with hyper- or hypotensive crisis. Morphine potentiates the effects of tranquilisers, anaesthetics, hypnotics, sedatives, alcohol, muscle relaxants and antihypertensives. Cimetidine inhibits the metabolism of morphine.

Pregnancy and lactation: Not recommended.

Effects on ability to drive and use machines: Treatment with Sevredol tablets may cause sedation and it is not recommended that patients drive or use machines if they experience drowsiness.

Undesirable effects: In normal doses, the commonest side effects of morphine are nausea, vomiting, constipation and drowsiness. With chronic therapy, nausea and vomiting are unusual with Sevredol tablets but should they occur the tablets can be readily combined with an anti-emetic if required. Constipation may be treated with appropriate laxatives. Dry mouth, sweating, vertigo, headache, disorientation, facial flushing, mood changes, palpitations, hallucinaitons, bronchospasm and colic may occur in a few patients. Micturition may be difficult and there may be biliary or ureteric spasm. Overdosage may produce respiratory depression. Rarely, clinically relevant reductions in blood pressure and heart rate have been observed. Morphine has histamine releasing effects which may be responsible in part for reactions such as urticaria and pruritus.

The effects of morphine have led to its abuse and dependence may develop with regular, inappropriate use. This is not a major concern in the treatment of patients with severe pain.

Overdose: Signs of morphine toxicity and overdosage are pin-point pupils, respiratory depression and hypotension. Circulatory failure and deepening coma may occur in more severe cases.

Treatment of morphine overdosage: Primary attention should be given to the establishment of a patent airway and institution of assisted or controlled ventilation.

In the case of massive overdosage, administer naloxone 0.8 mg intravenously. Repeat at 2–3 minute intervals as necessary, or by an infusion of 2 mg in 500 ml of normal saline or 5% dextrose (0.004 mg/ml).

The infusion should be run at a rate related to the previous bolus doses administered and should be in accordance with the patient's response. However, because the duration of action of naloxone is relatively short, the patient must be carefully monitored until spontaneous respiration is reliably re-established.

For less severe overdosage, administer naloxone 0.2 mg intravenously followed by increments of 0.1 mg every 2 minutes if required.

Naloxone should not be administered in the absence of clinically significant respiratory or circulatory depression secondary to morphine overdosage. Naloxone should be administered cautiously to persons who are known, or suspected, to be physically dependent on morphine. In such cases, an abrupt or complete reversal of opioid effects may precipitate an acute withdrawal syndrome.

Gastric contents may need to be emptied as this can be useful in removing unabsorbed drug.

Pharmacological properties

Pharmacodynamic properties: Morphine acts as an agonist at opiate receptors in the CNS particularly mu and to a lesser extent kappa receptors. Mu receptors are thought to mediate supraspinal analgesia, respiratory depression, and euphoria, and kappa receptors, spinal analgesia, miosis and sedation. Morphine also has a direct action on the bowel wall nerve causing constipation.

Pharmacokinetic properties: Morphine is well absorbed from Sevredol tablets, however first pass metabolism does occur. Apart from the liver, metabolism also occurs in the kidney and intestinal mucosa. The major urinary metabolite is morphine-3-glucuronide but morphine 6-glucuronide is also formed. The half life for morphine in the plasma is approximately 2.5–3.0 hours.

Pre-clinical safety data: There are no pre-clinical data of relevance to the prescriber which are additional to that already included in other sections of the SPC.

Pharmaceutical particulars

List of excipients:

Tablet core: Lactose (anhydrous) NF; Pregelatinised Maize Starch BP; Povidone K25 BP; Purified Water PhEur; Magnesium Stearate BP; Purified Talc BP.

Film coat

10 mg tablet: Opaspray M-1F-4448 blue containing hydroxypropylmethyl cellulose E464, titanium dioxide E171, polyethylene glycol 400, Patent Blue V E131, industrial methylated spirit.

20 mg tablet: Opaspray M-1-15503 pink containing hydroxypropylmethyl cellulose E464, titanium dioxide E171, erythrosine E127, Sunset yellow E110, industrial methylated spirit.

50 mg tablet: Opadry 0Y-21037 green containing hydroxypropylmethyl cellulose E464, titanium dioxide E171, quinoline yellow E104, indigo carmine E132, iron oxide E172, polyethylene glycol 400.

Incompatibilities: None stated.

Shelf life: 3 years.

Special precautions for storage: Store at or below 30°C.

Nature and contents of container: PVdC coated PVC blister packs and polypropylene containers with polyethylene lids containing 56 and 112 tablets.

Medical sample packs containing up to 24 tablets are also available.

Instructions for use/handling: None.

Marketing authorisation numbers

Sevredol tablets 10 mg	0337/0142
Sevredol tablets 20 mg	0337/0143
Sevredol tablets 50 mg	0337/0265

Date of approval/revision of SPC June 1997.

Legal category CD (Sch 2), POM.

UNIPHYLLIN CONTINUS TABLETS 200, 300 and 400 mg

Qualitative and quantitative composition Tablets containing 200, 300 or 400 mg of Theophylline BP.

Pharmaceutical form

200 mg	Capsule shaped, white, modified-release tablet with a scoreline on one side and U200 on the other.
300 mg	Capsule shaped, white, modified-release tablet with a scoreline on one side and U300 on the other.
400 mg	Capsule shaped, white, modified-release tablet with UNIPHYLLIN on one side and the Napp logo and U400 on either side of a scoreline on the reverse.

Clinical particulars

Therapeutic indications: For the treatment and prophylaxis of bronchospasm associated with asthma, chronic obstructive pulmonary disease and chronic bronchitis. Also indicated for the treatment of left ventricular and congestive cardiac failure.

Posology and method of administration

Route of administration: Oral.

The tablets should be swallowed whole and not chewed.

Children: The maintenance dose is 9 mg/kg twice daily. Some children with chronic asthma require and tolerate much higher doses (10–16 mg/kg twice daily). Lower dosages (based on usual adult dose) may be required by adolescents.

Adults: The usual maintenance dose for elderly patients or those less than 70 kg body weight is 300 mg 12-hourly following an initial week of therapy on 200 mg 12-hourly.

The usual maintenance dose for patients of 70 kg

body weight or over is 400 mg 12-hourly following an initial week of therapy on 200 or 300 mg 12-hourly.

The elderly: The dose should be adjusted following the response to the initial week of therapy.

It may be appropriate to administer a larger evening or morning dose in some patients, in order to achieve optimum therapeutic effect when symptoms are most severe e.g. at the time of the 'morning dip' in lung function.

In patients whose night time or day time symptoms persist despite other therapy and who are not currently receiving theophylline, then the total daily requirement of UNIPHYLLIN CONTINUS tablets (as specified above) may be added to their treatment regimen as either a single evening or morning dose.

Dose titration: Patients vary in their response to xanthines and it may be necessary to titrate their dose individually.

Contra-indications: Should not be given concomitantly with ephedrine in children.

Special warnings and special precautions for use: A reduction of dosage may be necessary in the elderly patient.

The hypokalaemia resulting from beta agonist therapy, steroids, diuretics and hypoxia may be potentiated by xanthines. Particular care is advised in patients suffering from severe asthma who require hospitalisation. It is recommended that serum potassium levels are monitored in such situations.

Alternative treatment is advised for patients with a history of seizure activity.

Interaction with other medicaments and other forms of interaction: The following increase clearance and it may therefore be necessary to increase dosage to ensure a therapeutic effect: aminoglutethimide, carbamazepine, moracizine, phenytoin, rifampicin, sulphinpyrazone and barbiturates. Smoking and alcohol consumption can also increase clearance of theophylline.

The following reduce clearance and a reduced dosage may therefore be necessary to avoid side-effects: allopurinol, carbimazole, cimetidine, ciprofloxacin, clarithromycin, diltiazem, disulfiram, erythromycin, fluconazole, interferon, isoniazid, isoprenaline, methotrexate, mexiletine, nizatidine, norfloxacin, oxpentifylline, propafenone, propranolol, ofloxacin, thiabendazole, verapamil, viloxazine hydrochloride and oral contraceptives. The concomitant use of theophylline and fluvoxamine should usually be avoided. Where this is not possible, patients should have their theophylline dose halved and plasma theophylline should be monitored closely.

Factors such as viral infections, liver disease and heart failure also reduce theophylline clearance. There are conflicting reports concerning the potentiation of theophylline by influenza vaccine and physicians should be aware that interaction may occur. A reduction in dosage may also be necessary in elderly patients. Thyroid disease or associated treatment may alter theophylline plasma levels. There is also a pharmacological interaction with adenosine, benzodiazepines, halothane, lomustine and lithium and these drugs should be used with caution.

Theophylline may decrease steady state phenytoin levels.

Pregnancy and lactation: Safety in human pregnancy has not been established but it has been in use for many years without apparent ill consequence. Theophylline crosses the placental barrier and is secreted in breast milk. Use of theophylline during the third trimester, or during breast feeding, may be associated with irritability in the infant. Use in pregnancy only when there is no safe alternative, or when the disease itself carries risk for the mother or child.

Effects on ability to drive and use machines: No known effects.

Undesirable effects: The risk of side-effects usually associated with theophylline and xanthine derivatives such as nausea, gastric irritation, headache and CNS stimulation is significantly reduced when UNIPHYLLIN CONTINUS tablet preparations are given.

Overdose: Empty stomach contents. Monitor electrocardiogram and maintain fluid balance. Oral activated medical charcoal has been found to reduce high theophylline blood levels. In severe poisoning, employ charcoal-column haemoperfusion. Treat symptoms on appearance. The physician should be aware that tablets in the intestine will continue to release theophylline for a period of hours.

In the event of hypokalaemia, potassium chloride should be given by slow intravenous infusion. Repeated measurements of plasma potassium should be made.

Pharmacological properties

Pharmacodynamic properties: Theophylline is a bronchodilator. In addition it affects the function of a number of cells involved in the inflammatory processes associated with asthma and chronic obstructive airways disease. Of most importance may be enhanced suppressor, T-lymphocyte activity and reduction of eosinophil and neutrophil function. These actions may contribute to an anti-inflammatory prophylactic activity in asthma and chronic obstructive airways disease. Theophylline stimulates the myocardium and produces a diminution of venous pressure in congestive heart failure leading to marked increase in cardiac output.

Pharmacokinetic properties: Theophylline is well absorbed from UNIPHYLLIN CONTINUS tablets and at least 60% may be bound to plasma proteins. The main urinary metabolites are 1,3 dimethyl uric acid and 3-methylxanthine. About 10% is excreted unchanged.

Pre-clinical safety data: There are no pre-clinical data of relevance to the prescriber which are additional to that already included in other sections of the SPC.

Pharmaceutical particulars

List of excipients:
Hydroxyethylcellulose
Povidone (K25)
Cetostearyl Alcohol
Macrogol 6000
Purified Talc
Magnesium Stearate

Incompatibilities: Not applicable.

Shelf-life: Three years.

Special precautions for storage: Store at or below 25°C.

Nature and contents of container: Blister packs consisting of aluminium foil sealed to 250 µm PVC with a PVdC coating of at least 40 gsm thickness, containing 8 or 56 tablets.

Instructions for use/handling: None.

Marketing authorisation number
200 mg–PL 0337/0057
300 mg–PL 0337/0129
400 mg–PL 0337/0074

Date of first authorisation/renewal of the authorisation
200 mg–23 August 1979/7 January 1998
300 mg–16 January 1994/22 February 1998
400 mg–29 October 1982/30 June 1997

Date of preparation/last revision June 1998

Legal category P

ZANIDIP TABLETS

Qualitative and quantitative composition Each film-coated tablet contains as active ingredient: lercanidipine 9.4 mg (present as 10 mg of lercanidipine hydrochloride).

Pharmaceutical form Film-coated tablets.

Clinical particulars

Therapeutic indications: ZANIDIP is indicated for the treatment of mild to moderate essential hypertension.

Posology and method of administration: The recommended dosage is 10 mg orally once a day at least 15 minutes before meals; the dose may be increased to 20 mg depending on the individual patient's response.

Dose titration should be gradual, because it may take about 2 weeks before the maximal antihypertensive effect is apparent.

Some individuals, not adequately controlled on a single antihypertensive agent, may benefit from the addition of ZANIDIP to therapy with a beta-adrenoceptor blocking drug (atenolol), a diuretic (hydrochlorothiazide) or an angiotensin converting enzyme inhibitor (captopril or enalapril).

Since the dose-response curve is steep with a plateau at doses between 20-30 mg, it is unlikely that efficacy will be improved by higher doses; whereas side effects may increase.

Use in the elderly: although the pharmacokinetic data and clinical experience suggest that no adjustment of the daily dosage is required, special care should be exercised when initiating treatment in the elderly.

Use in children: since there is no clinical experience in patients under the age of 18 years, use in children is not currently recommended.

Use in renal or hepatic dysfunction: special care should be exercised when treatment is commenced in patients with mild to moderate renal or hepatic dysfunction. Although the usually recommended dose schedule may be tolerated by these subgroups, an increase in dose to 20 mg daily must be approached with caution.

ZANIDIP is not recommended for use in patients with severe hepatic dysfunction or in patients with severe renal dysfunction (creatinine clearance <10 ml/min).

Contra-indications: Hypersensitivity to any dihydropyridine or any ingredient of the preparation. Lercanidipine is also contraindicated during pregnancy and during lactation, in women of child-bearing potential unless effective contraception is used, patients with left ventricular outflow tract obstruction, untreated congestive cardiac failure, unstable angina pectoris, severe renal or hepatic dysfunctions or within 1 month of a myocardial infarction.

Special warnings and precautions for use: Special care should be exercised when ZANIDIP is used in patients with sick sinus syndrome (if a pacemaker is not in situ). Although haemodynamic controlled studies revealed no impairment of ventricular function, care is also required in patients with LV dysfunction. It has been suggested that some short-acting dihydropyridines may be associated with increased cardiovascular risk in patients with ischaemic heart disease. Although ZANIDIP is long-acting caution is required in such patients.

The amount of lactose per tablet (30 mg) is probably too small to give rise to significant symptoms in patients with lactose intolerance.

Interactions with other medicaments and other forms of interaction: ZANIDIP has been safely administered with diuretics and ACE inhibitors. It may also be administered safely with beta-adrenoceptor blocking drugs which are eliminated unchanged such as atenolol. Caution should, however, be exercised when combining ZANIDIP with beta-adrenoceptor blocking drugs which are metabolised in the liver (such as propranolol and metoprolol) as there is a risk of increased hypotensive effect.

Co-administration of ZANIDIP in patients chronically treated with cardiac glycosides showed no evidence of pharmacokinetic interaction; patients on concomitant digoxin treatment should nevertheless be closely monitored clinically for signs of digoxin toxicity.

Concomitant administration of cimetidine 800 mg daily does not cause significant modifications in plasma levels of lercanidipine, but at higher doses caution is required since the bioavailability and the hypotensive effect of lercanidipine may be increased.

The interaction potential of lercanidipine has not been fully characterised. As for other dihydropyridines, the main metabolic pathway for lercanidipine most probably involves the enzyme CYP 3A4 (see "Pharmacokinetic properties").

Until further evidence is available, great caution should be exercised when ZANIDIP is co-prescribed with:

- inhibitors (e.g. ketoconazole, itraconazole, erythromycin, and fluoxetine)
- inducers (e.g. phenytoin, carbamazepine and rifampicin) or
- other substrates (e.g. terfenadine, astemizole, cyclosporin, class III antiarrhythmic drugs such as amiodarone, quinidine, some benzodiazepines such as diazepam and midazolam, propranolol and metoprolol) of cytochrome P450 3A4.

Co-administration of ZANIDIP with anticonvulsants should be approached with caution. The antihypertensive effect of ZANIDIP may be reduced and blood pressure should be monitored more frequently than usual.

Dihydropyridines appear to be particularly sensitive to inhibition of metabolism by grapefruit juice, with a consequent rise in their systemic availability and increased hypotensive effect.

Alcohol should be avoided since it may potentiate the effect of vasodilating antihypertensive drugs.

Pregnancy and lactation: Data for lercanidipine provide no evidence of a teratogenic effect in the rat and the rabbit and reproductive performance in the rat was unimpaired. Nevertheless, since there is no clinical experience with lercanidipine in pregnancy and lactation, and other dihydropyridine compounds have been found teratogenic in animals, ZANIDIP should not be administered during pregnancy or to women with child-bearing potential unless effective contraception is used. Because of high lipophilicity of lercanidipine, distribution in milk may be expected. Therefore, it should not be administered to nursing mothers.

Effects on ability to drive and use machines: Clinical experience with lercanidipine indicates that it is unlikely to impair a patient's ability to drive or use machinery. However, caution should be exercised because dizziness, asthenia, fatigue and rarely somnolence may occur.

Undesirable effects: Treatment with ZANIDIP is generally well tolerated. In controlled clinical trials the most commonly observed side effects were related to the vasodilatory properties of ZANIDIP: flushing, peripheral oedema, palpitation, tachycardia, headache, dizziness, asthenia. Other adverse experiences which were not clearly drug related and which occurred in less than 1% of patients were: fatigue, gastrointestinal disturbances such as dyspepsia, nausea, vomiting, epigastric pain and diarrhoea, polyuria, rash, somnolence and myalgia. Hypotension may occur in rare cases. Although not observed in the clinical trials, gingival hyperplasia may rarely occur as reported following the use of other dihydropyridines. There were reports of isolated and reversible increases in serum levels of hepatic transaminases; no other clinically significant pattern of laboratory test abnormalities related to ZANIDIP has been observed. Lercanidipine does not appear to influence adversely blood sugar or serum lipid levels.

Some dihydropyridines may rarely lead to precordial pain or angina pectoris. Very rarely patients with pre-existing angina pectoris may experience increased frequency, duration or severity of these attacks. Isolated cases of myocardial infarction may be observed.

Overdose: There is no experience with ZANIDIP overdosage. As with other dihydropyridines, overdosage might be expected to cause excessive peripheral vasodilation with marked hypotension and reflex tachycardia. In case of severe hypotension, bradycardia and unconsciousness, cardiovascular support could be helpful, with intravenous atropine for bradycardia.

In view of the prolonged pharmacological effect of lercanidipine, it is essential that the cardiovascular status of patients who take an overdose is monitored for 24 hours at least. There is no information on the value of dialysis. Since the drug is highly lipophilic, it is most probable that plasma levels are no guide to the duration of the period of risk and dialysis may not be effective.

Pharmacological properties

Pharmacodynamic properties: Lercanidipine is a calcium antagonist of the dihydropyridine group and inhibits the transmembrane influx of calcium into cardiac and smooth muscle. The mechanism of its antihypertensive action is due to a direct relaxant effect on vascular smooth muscle thus lowering total peripheral resistance. Despite its short pharmacokinetic plasma half-life, lercanidipine is endowed with a prolonged antihypertensive activity because of its high membrane partition coefficient, and is devoid of negative inotropic effects due to its high vascular selectivity.

Since the vasodilatation induced by ZANIDIP is gradual in onset, acute hypotension with reflex tachycardia has rarely been observed in hypertensive patients.

As for other asymmetric 1,4-dihydropyridines, the antihypertensive activity of lercanidipine is mainly due to its (S)-enantiomer.

In addition to the clinical studies conducted to support the therapeutic indications, a further small uncontrolled but randomised study of patients with severe hypertension (mean ± SD diastolic blood pressure of 114.5 ± 3.7 mmHg) showed that blood pressure was normalised in 40% of the 25 patients on 20 mg once daily dose and in 56% of 25 patients on 10 mg twice daily doses of ZANIDIP. In a double-blind, randomised, controlled study versus placebo in patients with isolated systolic hypertension ZANIDIP was efficacious in lowering systolic blood pressure from mean initial values of 172.6 ± 5.6 mmHg to 140.2 ± 8.7 mmHg.

Pharmacokinetic properties: ZANIDIP is completely absorbed after 10-20 mg oral administration and peak plasma levels, 3.30 ng/ml ± 2.09 SD and 7.66 ng/ml ± 5.90 SD respectively, occur about 1.5-3 hours after dosing.

Distribution from plasma to tissues and organs is rapid and extensive. The degree of serum protein binding of lercanidipine exceeds 98%. Since plasma protein levels are reduced in patients with severe renal or hepatic dysfunction, the free fraction of the drug may be increased.

Elimination occurs essentially by biotransformation; the absolute bioavailability of orally administered ZANIDIP is low as a consequence of high first pass metabolism.

The pharmacokinetic half-life is 2-5 hours but the therapeutic activity lasts for 24 hours because of its high binding to lipid membrane. No accumulation was seen upon repeated administration.

Formal studies identifying the cytochrome P450 isozyme responsible for the metabolism of lercanidipine have not been carried out. ZANIDIP is extensively metabolised most likely by CYP 3A4; no parent drug is found in the urine or the faeces. It is predominantly converted to inactive metabolites and about 50% of the dose is excreted in the urine.

Oral administration of ZANIDIP leads to plasma levels of lercanidipine not directly proportional to dosage (non-linear kinetics). After 10, 20 or 40 mg, peak plasma concentrations observed were in the ratio 1:3:8 and areas under plasma concentration-time curves in the ratio 1:4:18, suggesting a progressive saturation of first pass metabolism. Accordingly, availability increases with dosage elevation.

The two enantiomers of lercanidipine show a similar plasma level profile: the time to peak plasma concentration is the same, the peak plasma concentration and AUC are, on average, 1.2-fold higher for the (S)-enantiomer and the elimination half-lives of the two enantiomers are essentially the same. No *in vivo* interconversion of enantiomers is observed.

Oral availability of lercanidipine increases 4-fold when ZANIDIP is ingested up to 2 hours after a high fat meal. Accordingly, ZANIDIP should be taken before meals.

In elderly patients and in patients with mild to moderate renal dysfunction or mild to moderate hepatic impairment the pharmacokinetic behaviour of lercanidipine was shown to be similar to that observed in the general patient population; patients with severe renal dysfunction or dialysis-dependent patients showed higher levels (about 70%) of the drug. In patients with moderate to severe hepatic impairment, the systemic bioavailability of lercanidipine is likely to be increased since the drug is normally metabolised extensively in the liver.

Preclinical safety data: Safety pharmacological studies in animals have shown no effects on the autonomic nervous system, the central nervous system or on gastrointestinal function at antihypertensive doses.

The relevant effects which have been observed in long-term studies in rats and dogs were related, directly or indirectly, to the known effects of high doses of Ca-antagonists, predominantly reflecting exaggerated pharmacodynamic activity.

Lercanidipine was not genotoxic and showed no evidence of carcinogenic hazard.

Fertility and general reproductive performance in rats were unaffected by treatment with lercanidipine.

There was no evidence of any teratogenic effect in rats and rabbits; however, in rats, lercanidipine at high dose levels induced pre- and post- implantation losses and delay in foetal development.

Lercanidipine hydrochloride, when administered at high dose (12 mg/kg/day) during labour, induced dystocia.

The distribution of lercanidipine and/or its metabolites in pregnant animals and their excretion in breast milk have not been investigated.

Metabolites have not been evaluated separately in toxicity studies.

Pharmaceutical particulars

List of excipients: The tablet core excipients are: lactose monohydrate, microcrystalline cellulose, sodium starch glycolate, polyvinylpyrrolidone, magnesium stearate.

The film coating contains: methylhydroxypropylcellulose, talc, titanium dioxide (E171), macrogol 6000, ferric oxide (E172).

Incompatibilities: None known.

Shelf life: Three years.

Special precautions for storage: None.

Nature and contents of container: Aluminium/opaque PVC blisters.

Packs of 14, 28, 35, 50 and 100 tablets.

Instruction for use/handling: None.

Administrative data

Marketing authorisation holder: RECORDATI Industria Chimica e Farmaceutica SpA, Via Matteo Civitali, 1–20148 Milan, ITALY

Marketing authorisation number 04595/0005 (UK)

Date of first authorisation/renewal of authorisation 22 March 1996 (UK)

Date of (partial) revision of the text 19 November 1996

Legal category POM

**Trade Mark*

Newport Pharmaceuticals Limited

Frans Maas House
Swords Business Park
Swords
Co. Dublin
Ireland

☎ 00353 1 890 3011 🗋 00353 1 890 3016

IMUNOVIR*

Qualitative and quantitative composition Each tablet contains 500 mg inosine pranobex.

Pharmaceutical form Tablet.

Clinical Particulars

Therapeutic indications: Imunovir tablets are indicated in the management of:

(a) Mucocutaneous infections due to herpes simplex (type I and/or type II)
(b) Genital warts as adjunctive therapy to podophyllin or carbon dioxide laser
(c) Subacute sclerosing panencephalitis (SSPE).

Posology and Method of Administration

Adults: Mucocutaneous herpes simplex: 1 g q.d.s. (4 g daily), for 7–14 days.

Genital warts: 1 g t.d.s. (3 g daily), for 14–28 days as adjunctive therapy to podophyllin or carbon dioxide laser.

Subacute sclerosing panencephalitis (SSPE): 50–100 mg/kg daily, in divided doses every 4 hours.

Children: No information is available in children.

Elderly: No dosage alterations are necessary in the elderly.

Contra-indications: There are no known contra-indications to therapy with this drug.

Special warnings and precautions for use: As the inosine component of Imunovir is metabolished to uric acid, it should be used with caution in patients with renal impairment, a history of gout or hyperuricaemia.

Interactions with other medicaments and other forms of interaction: None known.

Pregnancy and lactation: Although animal tests have shown no teratogenic effect, the use of Imunovir in women where pregnancy is suspected or confirmed should be avoided.

Effects on ability to drive and use machines: Not applicable.

Undesirable effects: Side effects are rare and usually of a transitory nature. The only commonly associated adverse effects occurring during treatment with Imunovir are elevated serum and urinary concentrations of uric acid. These return to normal once treatment is withdrawn.

Overdose: There has been no experience of overdosage with Imunovir. However, serious adverse effects apart from increased levels of uric acid in the body seem unlikely in view of the animal toxicity studies. Treatment should be restricted to symptomatic and supportive measures.

Pharmacological properties

Pharmacodynamic properties: Imunovir is an agent demonstrating anti-viral activity and possessing immunopotentiating action in viral diseases.

Pharmacokinetic properties: Following a single oral dose of inosine pranobex, peak plasma conditions of inosine occur after 1 hour. However, 2 hours after administration, plasma concentrations decrease to undetectable amounts. Inosine pranobex has a very short plasma half-life of 50 minutes following an oral dose. The major excretion product of the inosine moiety is uric acid, while the p-acetamidobenzoic acid and N,N-dimethylamino-2-propanol components are excreted in the urine as glucuronidated and oxidised products, respectively, as well as being excreted unchanged.

Preclinical safety data: There is no preclinical data of relevance to the prescriber which is additional to that included in other sections of the SPC.

Pharmaceutical particulars

List of excipients: Povidone, starch modified, stearic acid, magnesium stearate, microcrystalline cellulose.

Incompatibilities: None are known.

Shelf life: 36 months.

Special precautions for storage: Store below 25°C.

Nature and contents of container: 8, 56, 100 and 500 tablets in glass bottles.

(Only the 100 pack size is available in the UK at present).

Instructions for use/handling: None.

Marketing authorisation holder
Newport Pharmaceuticals Limited, Frans Maas House, Swords Business Park, Swords, Co. Dublin, Ireland.

Marketing authorisation number PL 17232/0001.

Date of first authorisation/renewal of authorisation 15/11/98.

Date of (partial) revision of the text 15/05/97.

Promoter and Distributor in the UK: Ardern Healthcare Ltd., Pipers Brook Farm, Eastham, Tenbury Wells, Worcestershire WR15 8NP Ph: (01584) 781 777.

**Trade Mark*

Nexstar Pharmaceuticals Ltd

The Quorum
Barnwell Road
Cambridge CB5 8RE

☎ 01223 571400   🖷 01223 507047

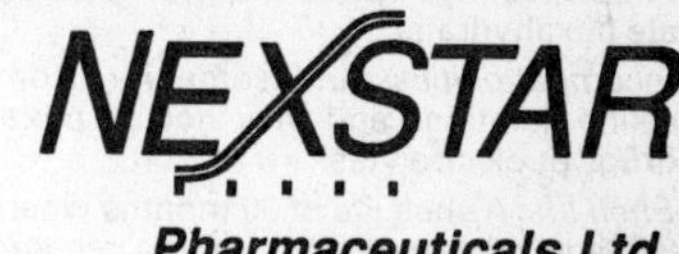

AMBISOME*

Qualitative and quantitative composition
AmBisome is a sterile lyophilized product for intravenous infusion. Each vial contains 50 mg of Amphotericin BP (50,000 units) encapsulated in liposomes consisting of approximately 213 mg hydrogenated soy phosphatidylcholine, 52 mg Cholesterol USNF, 84 mg distearoylphosphatidylglycerol, 0.64 mg alpha tocopherol, PhEur, together with 900 mg Sucrose BP, PhEur and 27 mg disodium succinate hexahydrate.

Amphotericin B has a molecular weight of 924.10 and is represented by the formula and structure shown below:

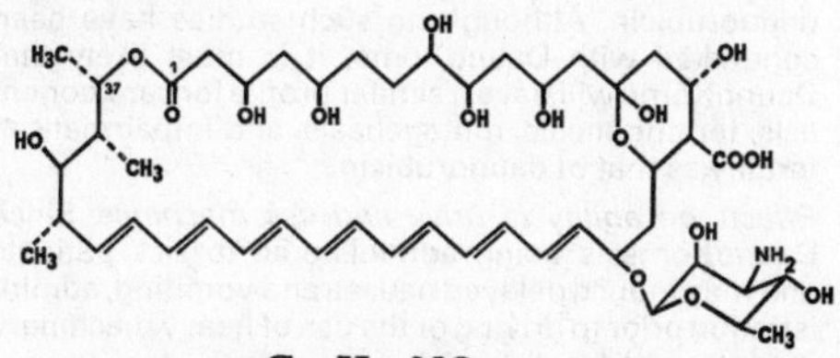

$C_{47}H_{73}NO_{17}$

Pharmaceutical form AmBisome is a sterile, lyophilized product for intravenous infusion. After reconstitution, the product is an injectable intended to be administered by intravenous infusion.

Clinical particulars
Therapeutic indications: AmBisome is indicated in:

- the treatment of severe systemic and/or deep mycoses where toxicity (particularly nephrotoxicity) precludes the use of conventional amphotericin B in effective dosages.
- the treatment of visceral leishmaniasis in immunocompetent patients including both adults and children.
- the empirical treatment of presumed fungal infections in febrile neutropenic patients, where the fever has failed to respond to broad spectrum antibiotics and appropriate investigations have failed to define a bacterial or viral cause

Infections successfully treated with AmBisome include: disseminated candidiasis, aspergillosis, mucormycosis, chronic mycetoma, cryptococcal meningitis and visceral leishmaniasis.

This drug should not be used to treat the common clinically inapparent forms of fungal disease which show only positive skin or serologic tests.

Posology and method of administration: AmBisome should be administered by intravenous infusion over a 30–60 minute period. The recommended concentration for intravenous infusion is 0.20 mg/ml to 2.00 mg/ml amphotericin as AmBisome. AmBisome therapy has been administered for as long as three months, with a cumulative dose of 16.8 g of amphotericin as AmBisome without significant toxicity.

Treatment of mycoses: Therapy is usually instituted at a daily dose of 1.0 mg/kg of body weight, and increased stepwise to 3.0 mg/kg, as required. Data are presently insufficient to define total dosage requirements and duration of treatment necessary for resolution of *mycoses.* However, a cumulative dose of 1.0–3.0 g of amphotericin as AmBisome over 3–4 weeks has been typical. Dosage of amphotericin as AmBisome must be adjusted to the specific requirements of each patient.

Treatment of visceral leishmaniasis: A total dose of 21.0–30.0 mg/kg given over 10–21 days may be used in the treatment of *visceral leishmaniasis.* Particulars as to the optimal dosage and the eventual development of resistance are as yet incomplete. The product should be administered under strict medical supervision.

Empirical treatment of febrile neutropenia: The recommended daily dose is 3 mg/kg body weight per day. Treatment should be continued until the recorded temperature is normalised for 3 consecutive days. In any event, treatment should be discontinued after a maximum of 42 days.

Paediatric patients: Both systemic fungal infections in children and presumed fungal infections in children with febrile neutropenia have been successfully treated with AmBisome, without reports of unusual adverse events. Paediatric patients have received AmBisome at doses comparable to those used in adults on a per kilogram body weight basis.

Elderly patients: No specific dosage recommendations or precautions.

Contra-indications: AmBisome is contra-indicated in those patients who have shown hypersensitivity to any of its constituents unless, in the opinion of the physician, the condition requiring treatment is life-threatening and amenable only to AmBisome therapy.

Special warnings and special precautions for use: AmBisome has been shown to be substantially less toxic than conventional amphotericin; however, adverse events may still occur. In particular, caution should be exercised when prolonged therapy is required. Laboratory evaluation of renal, hepatic and haematopoietic function should be performed regularly, and at least once weekly. Levels of serum potassium and magnesium should be monitored regularly. Particular attention should be paid to patients receiving concomitant therapy with nephrotoxic drugs. Renal function should be closely monitored in these patients.

Although the frequencies of severe allergic or anaphylactic reactions after AmBisome are rare, administration of a test dose is still advisable before a new course of treatment. For this purpose a small amount of an AmBisome infusion (e.g. 1 mg) can be administered for about 10 minutes, the infusion stopped and the patient observed carefully for the next 30 minutes. If there have been no severe allergic or anaphylactic reactions the infusion of AmBisome dose can be continued.

In the treatment of diabetic patients: It should be noted that AmBisome contains approximately 900 mg of sucrose in each vial.

In the treatment of renal dialysis patients: The administration of AmBisome should commence *only* when dialysis is completed.

Drug interactions with other medicaments and other forms of interaction: Although interactions of AmBisome with other drugs have not been observed to date, patients requiring concomitant drug therapy should be monitored closely. Conventional amphotericin has been reported to interact with the following drugs: antineoplastic agents, corticosteroids and corticotropin (ACTH), digitalis glycosides and skeletal muscle relaxants.

No evidence of benefit from the use of flucytosine with AmBisome has been observed. Whilst synergy between amphotericin and flucytosine has been reported, amphotericin may enhance the toxicity of flucytosine by increasing its cellular uptake and impeding its renal excretion.

Pregnancy and lactation: No reproductive toxicity studies have been conducted with AmBisome in pregnant women. Systemic fungal infections have been successfully treated in pregnant women with conventional amphotericin without obvious effect on the foetus, but the number of cases reported have been small. Safety for use in pregnant women has not been established with AmBisome. Therefore, AmBisome should only be used during pregnancy if the possible benefits to be derived outweigh the potential risks involved. Breast feeding should be discontinued during treatment.

Effects on ability to drive and use machines: The effects of AmBisome on the ability to drive and/or use machines has not been investigated.

Undesirable effects: Generally, patients who experienced significant acute toxicity with conventional amphotericin did not experience acute toxicity when AmBisome was substituted.

Patients who developed renal dysfunction, while receiving conventional amphotericin, improved or stabilised when AmBisome was substituted, even when doses were increased. Transient decreases in renal function (hypokalaemia, azotaemia, increased serum creatinine, and renal tubular acidosis) were reported, but did not require discontinuation of AmBisome treatment.

No significant changes in hepatic or haematopoietic function have been observed. However, the possibility of haemolysis must be considered, as it has been associated with the use of conventional amphotericin B. In general, the clinician should monitor the patient for any type of adverse event associated with the use of amphotericin.

Mild headache, nausea, vomiting and lumbar pain have been rarely reported.

Reduction of the infusion rate may lessen the infusion related toxicity.

Phlebitis and thrombophlebitis at infusion sites have not been observed.

Rash and anaphylactic reactions have been reported rarely.

Overdose: If overdosage should occur, cease administration immediately. Carefully monitor renal function.

Pharmacological properties
Pharmacodynamic properties: Amphotericin is a macrocyclic, polyene antifungal antibiotic produced by *Streptomyces nodosus.*

Liposomes are closed, spherical vesicles formed from a variety of amphiphilic substances such as phospholipids. Phospholipids arrange themselves into membrane bilayers when exposed to aqueous solutions. The lipophilic moiety of amphotericin allows the drug to be integrated into the lipid bilayer of the liposomes.

Amphotericin is fungistatic or fungicidal depending on the concentration attained in body fluids and the susceptibility of the fungus. The drug probably acts by binding to sterols in the fungal cell membrane, with a resultant change in membrane permeability, allowing leakage of a variety of small molecules. Mammalian cell membranes also contain sterols, and it has been suggested that the damage to human cells and fungal cells caused by amphotericin B may share common mechanisms.

Microbiology: Amphotericin, the antifungal component of AmBisome, shows a high order of *in vitro* activity against many species of fungi. Most strains of *Histoplasma capsulatum, Coccidioides immitis, Candida* spp., *Blastomyces dermatitidis, Rhodotorula, Cryptococcus neoformans, Sporothrix schenkii, Mucor mucedo* and *Aspergillus fumigatus,* are inhibited by concentrations of amphotericin ranging from 0.03 to 1.0 mcg/ml *in vitro.* Amphotericin has minimal or no effect on bacteria and viruses.

Pharmacokinetic properties: Pharmacokinetic data from animal studies demonstrated that higher peak plasma levels and greater total area under the curve values for amphotericin were achieved after AmBisome administration, as compared to conventional amphotericin. Higher levels of amphotericin were achieved in hepatic and splenic tissues with AmBisome in biodistribution studies in mice and rats. However, in rats amphotericin levels in renal tissue were 5 to 6 fold lower for a given dose of AmBisome, compared to conventional drug after repeated administration for 28 days. For other organs, tissue levels of amphotericin were similar, following dosing with AmBisome or with the conventional drug.

The following table shows the results of human studies with AmBisome at doses of 2.0, 3.0 and 4.0 mg/kg/day. Some variability of the data in patients has been observed.

	2.0 mg/kg	*3.0 mg/kg*	*4.0 mg/kg*
Distribution half-life (hrs)	1.70	1.82	1.30
Elimination half-life (hrs)	8.33	6.76	8.57
AUC (mcg-hr/ml)	84.80	158.00	283.30
Clearance (L/hr)	1.30	1.27	0.97
Volume of Distribution (L)	15.70	12.40	11.90

These values were determined by pooling serum data at each dose level, generating a curve fit and calculating the pharmacokinetic parameters from that curve.

Detailed human tissue distribution and possible metabolic pathways of conventional amphotericin are not fully understood, and have not been established for AmBisome.

Pharmaceutical particulars
List of excipients: 213 mg hydrogenated soy phospha-

tidylcholine, 52 mg cholesterol USNF, 84 mg distearoylphosphatidylglycerol, 0.64 mg alpha tocopherol PhEur, 900 mg sucrose PhEur, 27 mg disodium succinate hexahydrate.

Incompatibilities: AmBisome is incompatible with saline solutions and may not be mixed with other drugs or electrolytes.

Shelf life: A shelf life of 30 months when stored at 2°–8°C and protected from light is recommended. The reconstituted product concentrate may be stored for up to 24 hours at 2°–8°C following reconstitution with water. When diluted with 5% dextrose, AmBisome may be stored for up to 6 hours.

Special precautions for storage:

Storage: Unopened vials of lyophilized material must be stored under refrigeration at 2°–8°C (36°–46°F). Protect against exposure to light. Do not freeze.

Storage precautions of reconstituted product concentrate: The reconstituted product concentrate may be stored for up to 24 hours at 2°–8° C (36°–46° F) following reconstitution with water. Protect against exposure to light. Do not freeze.

Storage precautions of the reconstituted, diluted with 5% dextrose product: Protect against exposure to light. Do not freeze. Infusion of AmBisome should commence within 6 hours of dilution with 5% Dextrose.

DO NOT STORE partially used vials for future patient use.

Nature and contents of container: AmBisome is presented in 30 ml, sterile, Type I glass vials. The closure consists of West 4416/50 gray butyl rubber stoppers and aluminium ring seals fitted with removable plastic caps. Single-dose vials are packed in ten per carton with 10 filters.

Instructions for use/handling: READ THIS ENTIRE SECTION CAREFULLY BEFORE BEGINNING RECONSTITUTION.

AmBisome must be reconstituted by suitably trained staff.

AmBisome must be reconstituted using Sterile Water for Injection (**without a bacteriostatic agent**).

Vials of AmBisome containing 50 mg of Amphotericin are prepared as follows:

1. Add 12 ml of Sterile Water for Injection to each AmBisome vial, to yield a preparation containing 4 mg/ml amphotericin.
2. SHAKE VIALS VIGOROUSLY for at least 15 seconds to completely disperse the AmBisome.
3. Calculate the amount of reconstituted (4 mg/ml) AmBisome to be further diluted.
4. The infusion solution is obtained by dilution of the reconstituted AmBisome with between one (1) and nineteen (19) parts 5% Dextrose Injection by volume, to give a final concentration in the recommended range of 2.00 mg/ml to 0.20 mg/ml amphotericin as AmBisome.
5. Withdraw the calculated volume of reconstituted AmBisome into a sterile syringe. Using the 5-micron filter provided, instill the AmBisome preparation into a sterile container with the correct amount of 5% Dextrose Injection.

Do not reconstitute the lyophilized powder/cake with saline or add saline to the reconstituted concentrate, or mix with other drugs. Use only Water for Injection to reconstitute the powder/cake. Use only 5% Dextrose Injection to dilute the reconstituted product to the appropriate concentration for infusion.

Aseptic technique must be strictly observed in all handling, since no preservative or bacteriostatic agent is present in AmBisome, or in the materials specified for reconstitution and dilution. The use of any solution other than those recommended, or the presence of a bacteriostatic agent (e.g. benzyl alcohol) in the solution, may cause precipitation of AmBisome. Do not use material if there is any evidence of precipitation of foreign matter.

An in-line membrane filter may be used for intravenous infusion of AmBisome. However, **the mean pore diameter of the filter should not be less than 1.0 micron.**

Note: **AmBisome is not physically compatible with saline solutions and should not be mixed with other drugs or electrolytes. An existing intravenous line must be flushed with 5% Dextrose Injection prior to infusion of AmBisome. If this is not feasible, AmBisome should be administered through a separate line.**

Marketing authorisation number 16807/0001.

Marketing authorisation holder: NeXstar Pharmaceuticals International Ltd

Date of approval/revision of SPC August 13, 1998.

Legal category POM.

DAUNOXOME* ▼

Qualitative and quantitative composition Each 50 ml vial contains 50 mg Daunorubicin PhEur, encapsulated in liposomes consisting of approximately 753 mg distearoylphosphatidylcholine and 180 mg cholesterol USNF and 7 mg citric acid PhEur, suspended in a buffer of 2,125 mg sucrose PhEur, 94 mg glycine BP, and 7 mg calcium chloride PhEur, q.s. to approximately 25 ml with Water for Injection PhEur. The liposomes are small unilamellar vesicles with mean diameter of about 45 nm. The active ingredient is daunorubicin, an anthracycline antibiotic with antineoplastic activity originally obtained from *Streptomyces peucetius.* Daunorubicin has a four-ring anthracycline moiety linked by a glycosidic bond to daunosamin, an amino sugar. Daunorubicin is currently isolated from *Streptomyces coeruleorubidus* and is described by the following chemical name:

(8S, 10S)-8-acetyl-10-[(3-amino-2, 3, 6-trideoxy-α-L-lyxo-hexopyranosyl)oxy]-6, 8, 11-trihydroxy-1-methoxy-7, 8, 9, 10-tetrahydronaphthacene-5, 12-dione

Daunorubicin has a molecular weight of 527.5 and is represented by the formula $C_{27}H_{29}NO_{10}$.

Pharmaceutical form Each vial contains a sterile, pyrogen-free, preservative-free liposomal emulsion. This emulsion is red and clear to slightly opalescent in appearance. The product is an injectable intended to be administered by intravenous infusion.

Clinical particulars

Therapeutic indications: DaunoXome is indicated for the treatment of advanced HIV-related Kaposi's sarcoma.

Posology and method of administration: Dosage of DaunoXome must be adjusted for each patient. Therapy should be instituted at 40 mg/m² every two weeks. Therapy should be continued as long as disease control can be maintained.

DaunoXome should be diluted with 5% Dextrose Injection (D5W) before administration. The recommended concentration after dilution is between 0.2 mg and 1 mg daunorubicin/ml of solution. DaunoXome should be administered intravenously over a 30–60 minute period and within six hours of dilution with D5W.

Myelosuppression is a known reaction to DaunoXome therapy. The colony stimulating factor G-CSF has been used to manage patients whose absolute neutrophil count (ANC) fell below 1000/mm³.

Safety and effectiveness in children and the elderly has not been established.

Contra-indications: DaunoXome is a bone marrow suppressant. Suppression may occur in patients given therapeutic doses of this drug. Combination of DaunoXome with other cancer chemotherapeutic agents which suppress blood counts is contra-indicated. Therapy with DaunoXome is contra-indicated in patients who have had a serious hypersensitivity reaction to previous doses of DaunoXome or to any of its constituents unless the benefit from such treatment warrants the risk.

Special warnings and precautions for use: Conventional daunorubicin has been associated with cardiomyopathy and congestive heart failure. Although no such side-effects have been observed in the clinical use of DaunoXome, there must be a presumption that this is possible. As such, cardiac function should be evaluated in each patient, by means of history, physical examination and appropriate measurements of cardiac ejection fraction as indicated.

Also, it is recommended to give special attention to patients who received cumulative doses of daunorubicin equal to or in excess of 400 mg/m². These patients should undergo four weekly monitoring of the cardiac function by echo cardiography. Conventional daunorubicin has also been associated with local tissue necrosis at the site of drug infiltrations. No such local necrosis has been observed with DaunoXome. Nonetheless, care should be taken to ensure that there is no extravasation of drug when DaunoXome is administered.

Aseptic technique must be strictly observed in all handling, since no preservative or bacteriostatic agent is present in DaunoXome or in the materials recommended for dilution.

Caution: The only fluid which may be mixed with DaunoXome is D5W; DaunoXome should not be mixed with saline, bacteriostatic agents such as benzyl alcohol, or any other solution.

An in-line filter is not recommended for the intravenous infusion of DaunoXome. However, if such a filter is used, the mean pore diameter of the filter should not be less than 5 μm.

All parenteral drug products should be inspected visually for particulate matter prior to administration, wherever solution and container permit.

Procedures for proper handling and disposal of anticancer drugs should be followed.

Interactions with other medicaments and other forms of interaction: No interactions between DaunoXome and other drugs have been observed to date. DaunoXome has been safely administered during antiretroviral therapy with zidovudine (AZT), dideoxycytidene (ddC, zalcitabine), and dideoxyinosine (ddI, didanosine) and with the colony stimulating factor G-CSF. Although interaction of DaunoXome with other drugs has not been observed, patients requiring concomitant drug therapy should be monitored closely. During preparation and administration DaunoXome should not be mixed with saline; aggregation of the liposomes may result.

So far no safety information is available on the combination of DaunoXome with other cancer chemotherapeutic agents which suppress blood counts. Concomitant use of DaunoXome and parenteral nutritional lipid solutions or other liposomal products should be avoided.

Pregnancy and lactation: Safety for use of DaunoXome in pregnant and lactating women has not been established. Since it is not known if the administration of DaunoXome during pregnancy can cause fetal harm, DaunoXome should only be used during pregnancy if the possible benefits to be derived outweigh the potential risks involved. Breast feeding should be discontinued during treatment.

Daunorubicin, the active component of DaunoXome, has been shown to impair fertility and to have teratogenic effects in experimental animals, and there is also positive evidence of human fetal risk. Daunorubicin is also mutagenic both *in vitro* and *in vivo*, and carcinogenic *in vivo.* A high incidence of mammary tumours was observed in rats treated with daunorubicin. Although no such studies have been conducted with DaunoXome, it is most likely that DaunoXome will have a similar profile for carcinogenesis, teratogenesis, mutagenesis, and impairment of fertility as that of daunorubicin.

Effects on ability to drive and use machines: Since DaunoXome is being administered to sick patients and may induce delayed nausea and vomiting, administration prior to driving or the use of heavy machinery is contra-indicated.

Undesirable effects: Conventional daunorubicin has been associated with cardiomyopathy and congestive heart failure. Although no such side-effects have been observed in the clinical use of DaunoXome, there must be a presumption that this is possible. As such, cardiac function should be evaluated in each patient, including history, physical examination, and appropriate measures of cardiac ejection fraction as indicated.

Conventional daunorubicin has also been associated with local tissue necrosis at the site of drug infiltrations. No such local necrosis has been observed with DaunoXome. Nonetheless, care should be taken to ensure that there is no infiltration of drug when DaunoXome is administered intravenously.

The primary toxicity of DaunoXome is myelosuppresion and, as such, close patient observation and frequent monitoring of the blood cell counts is mandated. In patients with malignancies or with HIV infection, the immune system is already compromised, and the use of a cytotoxic agent decreasing the white blood cell count may cause further immunosuppression and make the patient more susceptible to intercurrent or opportunistic infections.

Back pain, flushing, and chest tightness were occasionally reported during the clinical trials. This syndrome may occur during a patient's initial infusion and may also occur in patients who have previously been exposed to DaunoXome without incident. This combination of symptoms does not always appear to be dose related, and generally occurs during the first ten minutes of the infusion. The etiology is unclear. The symptoms usually subside when the infusion is slowed or halted, and acetaminophen (paracetamol) may be used for analgesia. Other allergic or immune reactions may also be seen, and have been reported to be associated with hypotension. Anaphylactic reactions have been reported in rare cases.

Various other minor reactions, such as headache, fatigue, chills, mucositis, lightheadedness, nausea and vomiting, have also been reported.

Overdose: No experience exists for an overdose with this medication. The primary anticipated toxicity from such an overdose would be myelosuppression, and under these circumstances bone marrow function should be carefully monitored with appropriate therapy for any severe side-effects.

Pharmacological properties

Pharmacodynamic properties: DaunoXome is a liposomal preparation of daunorubicin formulated to maximise the selectivity of daunorubicin for solid tumours *in situ.* This tumour selectivity has been demonstrated for transplanted tumours in animal models. While in the circulation, the DaunoXome formulation protects the entrapped daunorubicin from chemical and enzymatic degradation, minimises protein binding, and generally decreases uptake by normal tissues, as well as by the non-reticuloendothelial system. The specific mechanism by which DaunoXome is able to deliver daunorubicin to solid tumours *in situ* is not known. However, it is believed to be a function of increased permeability of the tumour neovasculature to some particulates in the size range of DaunoXome. Thus, by a decrease in distribution and uptake of normal tissues and binding to plasma proteins and by selective extravasation in tumour neovasculature, the pharmacokinetics of daunorubicin are favourably shifted towards an accumulation of DaunoXome in tumour tissue. Once within the tumour environment, DaunoXome vesicles enter the tumour cells intact. Daunorubicin is then released over time in the cytoplasm, where it is able to exert its antineoplastic activity over a longer period.

Pharmacokinetic properties: DaunoXome has a pharmacokinetic profile significantly different from that of conventional daunorubicin. DaunoXome was administered intravenously over approximately 30 minutes as a single dose of 10, 20, 40, 60 or 80 mg/m². Plasma pharmacokinetic profiles for most patients demonstrated monoexponential declines, although biexponential or Michaelis-Menton (saturation) kinetics occurred in some instances. Peak plasma levels at 40 mg/m² ranged from 14.8 to 22.0 micrograms/ml with a mean peak plasma level of 18.0 micrograms/ml. The mean terminal half-life at this dose was 4.0 hours and mean total body clearance was 10.5 ml/minute. This resulted in a mean area under the plasma curve of 120 micrograms.hr/ml. Metabolism of DaunoXome appeared not to be significant at lower doses. At 60 mg/m² and above, three metabolites were observed, although they have not yet been identified.

DaunoXome's pharmacokinetic parameters were also compared to published values for conventional daunorubicin. At 80 mg/m², peak plasma levels ranged from 33.4 to 52.3 micrograms/ml for DaunoXome compared to 0.40 micrograms/ml for conventional drug. At this dose, DaunoXome plasma levels decline monoexponentially with a terminal half-life of 5.2 hours versus an initial half-life of 0.77 hours and a final half-life of 55.4 hours for conventional daunorubicin. Mean clearance for DaunoXome is 6.6 ml/min versus 223 ml/minute for daunorubicin. When combined, these parameters indicate that DaunoXome produces a 36-fold increase in mean area under the plasma curve compared to conventional drug (375.3 versus 10.33 micrograms.hr/ml).

Preclinical safety data: Animal studies with tumour models in mice have demonstrated that DaunoXome can increase daunorubicin tumour exposure ten-fold (in terms of area under the tumour concentration vs. time curve, AUC) when compared with equivalent doses of conventional (free) drug. The rate of drug accumulation in tumour tissues, however, appears to be slower for DaunoXome than for conventional daunorubicin. This difference is thought to be due to a slow diffusion process by which DaunoXome extravasates through the tumour neovasculature into the extracellular space while free drug, in contrast, is able to rapidly equilibrate from the circulation to both normal and neoplastic tissues. Since tumour accumulation of DaunoXome-delivered daunorubicin is a gradual process, it is important that DaunoXome remains in the circulation at high levels for prolonged periods. This has been shown to occur in animal studies where plasma AUC values for daunorubicin were approximately 200-fold greater for DaunoXome than for conventional drug. In contrast to tumour tissue, however, AUC values for normal tissues were only moderately elevated in DaunoXome-treated animals, relative to conventional daunorubicin. Exclusive of reticuloendothelial tissues (liver and spleen, AUC values increased by 110% and 60%, respectively) and brain tissue (AUC value increased by 3.5 fold) AUC increases ranged from 10% for heart and lungs to 30% for kidney and small intestines.

Pharmaceutical particulars

List of excipients: Liposome: 753 mg distearoylphosphatidylcholine; 180 mg cholesterol USNF; 7 mg citric acid PhEur. *Buffer:* 2,125 mg sucrose PhEur; 94 mg glycine BP; 7 mg calcium chloride PhEur, q.s. to approximately 25 ml with Water for Injection PhEur.

Incompatibilities: To date, no incompatibilities of DaunoXome with other drugs have been reported. However, it is known that the active component daunorubicin is physically incompatible with heparin sodium and with dexamethasone phosphate when directly admixed. A precipitate is produced with either drug. Additionally, because of the chemical instability of the glycosidic bond of daunorubicin, admixture into a highly alkaline media (pH >8.0) is not recommended.

DaunoXome should not be mixed with saline; aggregation of the liposomes may result.

Admixtures containing bacteriostatic agents such as benzyl alcohol or other detergent-like molecules should be avoided as well because such compounds can rupture the bilayer wall of the liposomes causing premature leakage of the active drug.

Shelf life: An expiry period of 40 weeks, when stored at 2°-8°C, is recommended. The product should be used within six hours of dilution in 5% dextrose as DaunoXome does not contain a preservative or bacteriostatic agent.

Special precautions for storage: Store at 2°-8°C. Do not freeze. Protect against exposure to light. Do not store partially used vials for future patient use. Vials are for single use only.

Nature and contents of container: DaunoXome is presented in 50-ml, sterile, Type I glass vials. The closure consists of West 4416/50 gray butyl rubber and aluminium ring seals fitted with removable plastic caps. Each single-dose vial is packed in a white chipboard carton. Included in each carton are directions for use.

Instruction for use/handling

Use aseptic technique: Aseptic technique must be strictly observed in all handling, since no preservative or bacteriostatic agent is present in DaunoXome or in the materials recommended for dilution.

Withdraw the calculated volume of DaunoXome into a sterile syringe. Instil the DaunoXome preparation into a sterile container with the correct amount of 5% Dextrose Injection (D5W) and administer within six hours. The recommended concentration after dilution is between 0.2 mg and 1 mg daunorubicin/ml of solution. Infuse over a 30–60 minute period. As with all parenteral drug products, inspect the solution visually for particulate matter prior to administration.

Caution: The only fluid which may be mixed with DaunoXome is D5W; DaunoXome should not be mixed with saline, bacteriostatic agents such as benzyl alcohol, or any other solution.

An in-line filter is not recommended for the intravenous infusion of DaunoXome. However, if such a filter is used, the mean pore diameter of the filter should not be less than 5 μm.

Procedures for proper handling and disposal of anticancer drugs should be followed.

Marketing authorisation number 11972/0002.

Date of approval/revision of SPC February 1997.

Legal category POM.

**Trade Mark*

Norgine Limited

Chaplin House
Widewater Place
Moorhall Road
Harefield
Middlesex UB9 6NS

☎ 01895 826600 🗋 01895 825865

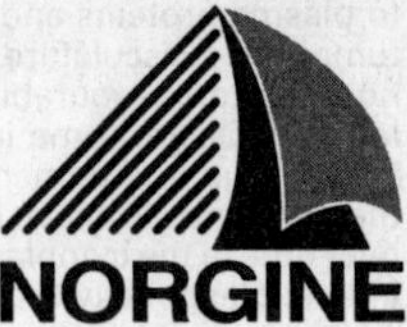

ALVERCOL*

Qualitative and quantitative composition The active ingredients are 62% Sterculia BP and 0.5% alverine citrate.

Pharmaceutical form Beige granules for oral administration.

Clinical particulars
Therapeutic indications: The treatment of hypertonic disorders of the colon and irritable bowel syndrome.

Posology and method of administration
Adults (including the elderly): 1-2 heaped 5 ml spoonfuls, once or twice daily after meals.

Children: (6-12 years): a reduced amount may be given at the discretion of the doctor.

The granules should be placed dry on the tongue and, without chewing or crushing, swallowed immediately with plenty of water or a cool drink.

Contra-indications: Intestinal obstruction, faecal impaction, and total atony of the colon.

Special warnings and special precautions for use: Patients should be advised to maintain an adequate fluid intake and to avoid taking Alvercol immediately before going to bed (especially if they are elderly).

Interaction with other medicaments and other forms of interaction: None known.

Pregnancy and lactation
Pregnancy: No teratogenic effects have been reported, but caution should be exercised during the first trimester.

Lactation: There is no evidence to suggest that Alvercol is unsuitable for use.

Effects on the ability to drive and use machines: None known.

Undesirable effects: Occasionally mild abdominal distension may occur. Oesophageal obstruction is possible if the product is not adequately washed down with fluid.

Overdose: Intestinal obstruction is possible in overdosage, particularly in combination with inadequate fluid intake. Management is as for intestinal obstruction from other causes. Alverine in overdosage can produce hypotension and atropine-like toxic effects, which should be treated as for atropine poisoning.

Pharmacological properties
Pharmacodynamic properties: Sterculia is insoluble in water and has no known pharmacological actions. Its pharmacodynamic properties are attributable entirely to the mechanical consequences of the expansion of the bulk and water content, and softening of the consistency of the colonic contents. Alverine citrate is a spasmolytic which acts selectively on the smooth muscle of the alimentary tract and uterus.

Pharmacokinetic properties: Sterculia is pharmacokinetically inert, having no significant absorption, metabolism or excretion. With only a change in physical state, resulting from the absorption or adsorption of water, it is evacuated in the faeces. Alverine is a prodrug and is rapidly converted *in vivo* to metabolites which are excreted by the kidney.

Preclinical safety data: There are no preclinical data of relevance to the prescriber.

Pharmaceutical particulars
List of excipients: Sucrose BP; Talc USP; Sodium Bicarbonate PhEur; Paraffin Wax; Titanium Dioxide BP; Flavourings: Anethole; Caramel (E150).

The sugar provides 7.5 calories (1.9 g carbohydrate) per heaped 5 ml spoonful, and the sodium content is 0.8 mmol. Alvercol is gluten free.

Incompatibilities: None known.

Shelf life: The shelf life is 4 years.

Special precautions for storage: Store in a dry place below 25°C.

Nature and contents of container: Lined box of 200 g and 500 g containing beige granules.

Instructions for use/handling: None.

Marketing authorisation number 00322/5009

Date of approval/revision of SPC December 1994.

Legal category P

CAMCOLIT* 250

Qualitative and quantitative composition The active ingredient is Lithium Carbonate BP; 250 mg/tablet.

Pharmaceutical form White film, coated tablets, engraved 'CAMCOLIT' around one face and having a breakline on the reverse. For oral administration.

Clinical particulars
Therapeutic indications: The treatment and prophylaxis of mania, manic-depressive illness and recurrent depression, and the treatment of aggressive or self mutilating behaviour.

Posology and method of administration: Regular monitoring of plasma lithium concentration is always obligatory when lithium is used; lithium therapy should not be initiated unless adequate facilities for routine monitoring of plasma concentrations are available. On initiation of therapy plasma concentrations should be measured weekly until stabilisation is achieved, then weekly for one month and at monthly intervals thereafter. Additional measurements should be made if signs of lithium toxicity occur, on dosage alteration, development of significant intercurrent disease, signs of manic or depressive relapse and if significant change in sodium or fluid intake occurs. More frequent monitoring is required if patients are receiving any drug treatment that affects renal clearance of lithium eg diuretics and NSAID. As bioavailability may vary between formulations, should a change of preparation be made, blood levels should be monitored weekly until restabilisation is achieved.

Acute mania: Treatment should be initiated in hospital where regular monitoring of plasma lithium levels can be conducted. The dosage of Camcolit should be adjusted to produce a plasma lithium level between 0.6 and 1.0 mmol/l 12 hours after the last dose. The required plasma lithium level may be achieved in one of two ways but, whichever is adopted, regular estimations must be carried out to ensure maintenance of levels within the therapeutic range. For consistent results it is essential that the blood samples for plasma lithium estimations are taken 12 hours after the last dose of lithium.

1. 1,000-1,500 mg of lithium carbonate are administered daily for the first five days. A blood sample for plasma lithium estimation is taken 12 hours after the last dose on the fifth day, and the dosage of Camcolit is adjusted to keep the plasma lithium level within the therapeutic range. Subsequently, regular plasma lithium estimations must be carried out and, where necessary, the dosage of Camcolit adjusted accordingly. The precise initial dose of lithium should be decided in the light of the age and weight of the patient; young patients often require a dose higher than average and older patients a lower dose.

2. A lithium clearance test is carried out and the initial dosage calculated from the results. Even when the initial dosage is calculated in this way, it is still desirable that plasma lithium levels should be determined at weekly intervals during the first three weeks of treatment, and any necessary adjustments to dosage made as a result of the levels actually obtained.

Most of the above applies in the treatment of hypomania as well as mania, but the patient (if not too ill) can be started on treatment as an outpatient provided that facilities for regular plasma lithium monitoring are available, and assays are initiated within one week.

Prophylaxis of recurrent affective disorders: (Including unipolar mania unipolar depressions and bipolar manic-depressive illness): A low dose of 300-400 mg of lithium carbonate can be administered daily for the first seven days. A blood sample for plasma lithium estimation is then taken 12 hours after the last dose , and the dosage of Camcolit is adjusted to keep the plasma lithium level within the range of 0.4-0.8 mmol/l. Toxic symptoms are usually associated with concentrations exceeding 1.5 mmol/l.

Use in elderly: As for prophylaxis above, but 12 hour lithium levels should be kept in the range of 0.4-0.7 mmol/l as toxic symptoms are likely with plasma concentrations above 1.0 mmol/l.

Use in children: Not recommended.

Contra-indications: Patients with renal disease, cardiovascular disease, Addison's disease or those breast feeding.

Special warnings and special precautions for use: Pretreatment and periodic routine clinical monitoring is essential. This should include assessment of renal function, urine analysis, assessment of thyroid function and cardiac function, especially in patients with cardiovascular disease.

Patients should be euthyroid before initiation of lithium therapy.

Clear instructions regarding the symptoms of impending toxicity should be given by the doctor to all patients receiving long-term lithium therapy.

Patients should also be warned to report if polyuria or polydipsia develop. Episodes of nausea and vomiting or other conditions leading to salt/water depletion (including severe dieting) should also be reported. Patients should be advised to maintain their usual salt and fluid intake.

Elderly patients are particularly liable to lithium toxicity.

Interactions with other medicaments and other forms of interaction: Lower doses of lithium may be required during diuretic therapy as lithium clearance is reduced.

Serum lithium concentrations may increase during concomitant therapy with non-steroidal anti-inflammatory drugs or tetracycline, possibly resulting in lithium toxicity. Serum lithium concentrations therefore should be monitored more frequently if NSAID or tetracycline therapy is initiated or discontinued.

Raised plasma levels of ADH may occur during treatment.

Symptoms of nephrogenic diabetes insipidus are particularly prevalent in patients receiving concurrent treatment with tricyclic or tetracyclic anti-depressants.

Pregnancy and lactation: Pregnancy: There is epidemiological evidence to suggest that the drug may be harmful during human pregnancy. Should the use of lithium be unavoidable, close monitoring of serum concentrations should be made throughout pregnancy and parturition.

Lactation: Infants of mothers on lithium should be bottle fed as lithium is present in the breast milk.

Effects on the ability to drive and use machines: None known.

Undesirable effects: Long term treatment with lithium may result in permanent changes in the kidney and impairment of renal function. High serum concentrations of lithium, including episodes of acute lithium toxicity may enhance these changes. The minimum clinically effective dose of lithium should always be used. Patients should only be maintained on lithium after 3-5 years if, on assessment, benefit persists.

Renal function should be routinely monitored in patients with polyuria and polydipsia.

Side effects are usually related to serum lithium concentrations and are infrequent at levels below 1.0 mmol/l.

Mild gastro-intestinal effects, nausea, vertigo, muscle weakness and a dazed feeling may occur, but frequently disappear after stabilisation. Fine hand tremors, polyuria and mild thirst may persist. Some studies suggest that the tremor can be controlled by relatively small doses of propranolol.

Long term treatment with lithium is frequently associated with disturbances of thyroid function including goitre and hypothyroidism. These can be controlled by administration of small doses of thyroxine (0.05-0.2 mg daily) concomitantly with lithium. Thyrotoxicosis has also been reported.

Mild cognitive impairment may occur during long term use.

Hypercalcaemia, hypermagnesaemia, hyperparathyroidism and an increase in antinuclear antibodies have also been reported.

Exacerbation of psoriasis may occur.

Overdose: Appearance or aggravation of gastro-intestinal symptoms, muscle weakness, lack of co-ordination, drowsiness or lethargy may be early signs of intoxication. With increasing toxicity, ataxia, giddiness, tinnitus, blurred vision, coarse tremor, muscle twitching and a large output of dilute urine may be seen. At blood levels above 2-3 mmol/l, increasing disorientation, seizures, coma and death may occur.

There is no antidote to lithium poisoning. In the event, lithium treatment should be stopped immediately and serum lithium levels estimated every 6 hours. When ingestion is recent, gastric lavage should be carried out, together with general supportive measures. Special attention must be given to the maintenance of fluid and electrolyte balance, and also adequate renal function. Sodium-depleting diuretics should not be used in any circumstances. Forced alkaline diuresis may be used. If the serum lithium level is above 4.0 mmol/l, or if there is a deterioration in the patient's condition, or if the serum lithium concentration is not falling at a rate equivalent to a half-life of less than 30 hours, peritoneal dialysis or haemodialysis should be instituted promptly. This should be continued until the serum and dialysis fluid are free of lithium. Serum lithium levels should be monitored for at least another 7 days thereafter, as a rebound rise is possible due to delayed diffusion from the tissues.

Pharmacological properties

Pharmacodynamic properties: The precise mechanism of action of lithium as a mood-stabilising agent remains unknown, although many cellular actions of lithium have been characterised.

Pharmacokinetic properties

The pharmacokinetics of lithium are extremely well documented. A single oral dose of CAMCOLIT 250 gives a peak plasma level approximately 2-3 hours later, with the level at 24 hours being approximately 40% of peak levels.

Preclinical safety data

There is no preclinical data of relevance to the prescriber.

Pharmaceutical particulars

List of excipients

Maize Starch Ph Eur
Magnesium Stearate Ph Eur
Pregelatinised Maize Starch BP
Hydroxypropylmethyl Cellulose 2910 USP
Polyethylene Glycol 400 USNF

Incompatibilities: See *Interactions with other medicaments and other forms of interaction* and *Undesirable effects* above.

Shelf life: The shelf life is 5 years.

Special precautions for storage: Store below 25°C.

Nature and contents of container: Polypropylene containers of 100 or 1000 tablet capacity, and for hospital use only, screw-cap amber glass bottles of 50 or 100 tablet capacity.

Instructions for use/handling: None.

Marketing authorisation holder: Norgine Limited, Chaplin House, Widewater Place, Moorhall Road, Harefield, Uxbridge, Middlesex UB9 6NS, UK.

Marketing authorisation number PL 00322/5900R.

Date of first authorisation/renewal of authorisation
25th November 1981 27th February 1992

Date of revision of text July 1998.

Legal category POM.

CAMCOLIT* 400

The product may also be sold as LITHONATE.

Qualitative and quantitative composition The active ingredient is Lithium Carbonate BP; 400 mg/tablet.

Pharmaceutical form White film coated tablets, engraved 'CAMCOLIT-S' around one face and having a breakline on the reverse. The tablet is a controlled release formulation. If sold as LITHONATE the tablets are engraved on one side 'LIT 400'.

For oral administration.

Clinical particulars

Therapeutic indications: The treatment and prophylaxis of mania, manic-depressive illness and recurrent depression, and the treatment of aggressive or self mutilating behaviour.

Posology and method of administration: Regular monitoring of plasma lithium concentration is always obligatory when lithium is used; lithium therapy should not be initiated unless adequate facilities for routine monitoring of plasma concentrations are available. On initiation of therapy plasma concentrations should be measured weekly until stabilisation is achieved, then weekly for one month and at monthly intervals thereafter. Additional measurements should be made if signs of lithium toxicity occur, on dosage alteration, development of significant intercurrent disease, signs of manic or depressive relapse and if significant change in sodium or fluid intake occurs. More frequent monitoring is required if patients are receiving any drug treatment that affects renal clearance of lithium e.g. diuretics and NSAID. As bioavailability may vary between formulations, should a change of preparation be made, blood levels should be monitored weekly until restabilisation is achieved.

Acute mania: Treatment should be initiated in hospital where regular monitoring of plasma lithium levels can be conducted. The dosage of Camcolit should be adjusted to produce a plasma lithium level between 0.6 and 1.0 mmol/l 12 hours after the last dose. The required plasma lithium level may be achieved in one of two ways but, whichever is adopted, regular estimations must be carried out to ensure maintenance of levels within the therapeutic range. For consistent results it is essential that the blood samples for plasma lithium estimations are taken 12 hours after the last dose of lithium.

1. 1,000–1,500 mg of lithium carbonate are administered daily for the first five days. A blood sample for plasma lithium estimation is taken 12 hours after the last dose on the fifth day, and the dosage of Camcolit is adjusted to keep the plasma lithium level within the therapeutic range. Subsequently, regular plasma lithium estimations must be carried out and, where necessary, the dosage of Camcolit adjusted accordingly. The precise initial dose of lithium should be decided in the light of the age and weight of the patient; young patients often require a dose higher than average and older patients a lower dose.

2. A lithium clearance test is carried out and the initial dosage calculated from the results. Even when the initial dosage is calculated in this way, it is still desirable that plasma lithium levels should be determined at weekly intervals during the first three weeks of treatment, and any necessary adjustments to dosage made as a result of the levels actually obtained.

Most of the above applies in the treatment of hypomania as well as mania, but the patient (if not too ill) can be started on treatment as an outpatient provided that facilities for regular plasma lithium monitoring are available, and assays are initiated within one week.

Prophylaxis of recurrent affective disorders: (Including unipolar mania and unipolar depressions and bipolar manic-depressive illness): A low dose of 300–400 mg of lithium carbonate can be administered daily for the first seven days. A blood sample for plasma lithium estimation is then taken 12 hours after the last dose, and the dosage of Camcolit is adjusted to keep the plasma lithium level within the range of 0.4–0.8 mmol/l. Toxic symptoms are usually associated with concentrations exceeding 1.5 mmol/l.

Use in elderly: As for prophylaxis above, but 12 hour lithium levels should be kept in the range of 0.4–0.7 mmol/l as toxic symptoms are likely with plasma concentrations above 1.0 mmol/l.

Use in children: Not recommended.

Contra-indications: Patients with renal disease, cardiovascular disease, Addison's disease or those breast feeding.

Special warnings and special precautions for use: Pre-treatment and periodic routine clinical monitoring is essential. This should include assessment of renal function, urine analysis, assessment of thyroid function and cardiac function, especially in patients with cardiovascular disease.

Patients should be euthyroid before initiation of lithium therapy.

Clear instructions regarding the symptoms of impending toxicity should be given by the doctor to all patients receiving long-term lithium therapy. Patients should also be warned to report if polyuria or polydipsia develop. Episodes of nausea and vomiting or other conditions leading to salt/water depletion (including severe dieting) should also be reported. Patients should be advised to maintain their usual salt and fluid intake.

Elderly patients are particularly liable to lithium toxicity.

Interactions with other medicaments and other forms of interaction: Lower doses of lithium may be required during diuretic therapy as lithium clearance is reduced.

Serum lithium concentrations may increase during concomitant therapy with non-steroidal anti-inflammatory drugs or tetracycline, possibly resulting in lithium toxicity. Serum lithium concentrations therefore should be monitored more frequently if NSAID or tetracycline therapy is initiated or discontinued.

Raised plasma levels of ADH may occur during treatment.

Symptoms of nephrogenic diabetes insipidus are particularly prevalent in patients receiving concurrent treatment with tricyclic or tetracyclic anti-depressants.

Pregnancy and lactation: Pregnancy: There is epidemiological evidence to suggest that the drug may be harmful during human pregnancy. Should the use of lithium be unavoidable, close monitoring of serum concentrations should be made throughout pregnancy and parturition.

Lactation: Infants of mothers on lithium should be bottle fed as lithium is present in the breast milk.

Effects on the ability to drive and use machines: None known.

Undesirable effects: Long term treatment with lithium may result in permanent changes in the kidney and impairment of renal function. High serum concentrations of lithium, including episodes of acute lithium toxicity may enhance these changes. The minimum clinically effective dose of lithium should always be used. Patients should only be maintained on lithium after 3–5 years if, on assessment, benefit persists.

Renal function should be routinely monitored in patients with polyuria and polydipsia. Side effects are usually related to serum lithium concentrations and are infrequent at levels below 1.0 mmol/l.

Mild gastro-intestinal effects, nausea, vertigo, muscle weakness and a dazed feeling may occur, but frequently disappear after stabilisation. Fine hand tremors, polyuria and mild thirst may persist. Some studies suggest that the tremor can be controlled by relatively small doses of propranolol.

Long term treatment with lithium is frequently associated with disturbances of thyroid function including goitre and hypothyroidism. These can be controlled by administration of small doses of thyroxine (0.05–0.2 mg daily) concomitantly with lithium. Thyrotoxicosis has also been reported.

Mild cognitive impairment may occur during long term use.

Hypercalcaemia, hypermagnesaemia, hyperparathyroidism and an increase in antinuclear antibodies have also been reported.

Exacerbation of psoriasis may occur.

Overdose: Appearance or aggravation of gastro-intestinal symptoms, muscle weakness, lack of co-ordination, drowsiness or lethargy may be early signs of intoxication. With increasing toxicity, ataxia, giddiness, tinnitus, blurred vision, coarse tremor, muscle twitching and a large output of dilute urine may be seen. At blood levels above 2–3 mmol/l, increasing disorientation, seizures, coma and death may occur.

There is no antidote to lithium poisoning. In the event, lithium treatment should be stopped immediately and serum lithium levels estimated every 6 hours. When ingestion is recent, gastric lavage should be carried out, together with general supportive measures. Special attention must be given to the maintenance of fluid and electrolyte balance, and also adequate renal function. Sodium-depleting diuretics should not be used in any circumstances. Forced alkaline diuresis may be used. If the serum lithium level is above 4.0 mmol/l, or if there is a deterioration in the patient's condition, or if the serum lithium concentration is not falling at a rate equivalent to a half-life of less than 30 hours, peritoneal dialysis or haemodialysis should be instituted promptly. This should be continued until the serum and dialysis fluid are free of lithium. Serum lithium levels should be monitored for at least another 7 days thereafter, as a rebound rise is possible due to delayed diffusion from the tissues.

Pharmacological properties

Pharmacodynamic properties: The precise mechanism of action of lithium as a mood-stabilising agent remains unknown, although many cellular actions of lithium have been characterised.

Pharmacokinetic properties: The pharmacokinetics of lithium are extremely well documented. A single oral dose of CAMCOLIT 400 gives a peak plasma level approximately 3–4 hours later, with the level at 24 hours being approximately 40% of peak levels.

Preclinical safety data: There is no preclinical data of relevance to the prescriber.

Pharmaceutical particulars

List of excipients

Maize Starch PhEur
Acacia PhEur
Magnesium Stearate PhEur
Sodium Lauryl Sulphate PhEur
Hydroxypropylmethyl Cellulose 2910 USP
Polyethylene Glycol 400 USNF
Opaspray M-1-7111B

Incompatibilities: See *Interactions with other medicaments and other forms of interaction* and *Undesirable effects* above.

Shelf life: The shelf life is 3 years.

Special precautions for storage: Store in a cool dry place below 25°C.

Nature and contents of container: Polypropylene containers of 100 or 500 tablet capacity, and for hospital use only, screw-cap amber glass bottles of 50 or 100 tablet capacity.

Instructions for use/handling: None.

Marketing authorisation number PL 00322/0015

Date of first authorisation/renewal of authorisation 2 March 1977/2 March 1992

Date of revision of text November 1998

Legal category POM

DESTOLIT

Qualitative and quantitative composition Each tablet contains 150 mg ursodeoxycholic acid.

Pharmaceutical form Tablet.

Clinical particulars *Therapeutic indications:* Destolit is indicated for the dissolution of radiolucent (ie non-radio opaque) cholesterol gallstones in patients with a functioning gallbladder

Posology and method of administration: The daily dose for most patients is 3 or 4 tablets of 150 mg according to body weight. This dose should be divided into 2 administrations after meals, with one administration always to be taken after the evening meal.

A daily dose of about 8 to 10 mg/kg will produce cholesterol desaturation of bile in the majority of cases. The measurement of the lithogenic index on bile-rich duodenal drainage fluid after 4-6 weeks of therapy may be useful for determining the minimal effective dose. The lowest effective dose has been found to be 4 mg/kg.

The duration of treatment required to achieve gallstone dissolution will usually not be extended beyond 2 years and should be monitored by regular cholecystograms. Treatment should be continued for 3-4 months after the radiological disappearance of the gallstones.

Any temporary discontinuation of treatment, if prolonged for 3-4 weeks, will allow the bile to return to a state of supersaturation and will extend the total time required for litholysis. In some cases stones may recur after successful treatment.

For oral administration

Contra-indications: Active gastric or duodenal ulcers are contra-indications, as are hepatic and intestinal conditions interfering with the enterohepatic circulation of bile acids (ileal resection and stoma, regional ileitis, extra and intra-hepatic cholestasis, severe, acute, and chronic liver diseases). A product of this class has been found to be carcinogenic in animals. The relevance of these findings to the clinical use of ursodeoxycholic acid has not been established.

Special warnings and precautions for use: Excessive dietary intake of calories and cholesterol should be avoided; a low cholesterol diet will probably improve the effectiveness of Destolit tablets.

Interactions with other medicaments and other forms of interaction: It is also recommended that drugs known to increase cholesterol elimination in bile, such as oestrogenic hormones, oral contraceptive agents and certain blood cholesterol lowering agents should also not be prescribed concomitantly

Pregnancy and lactation: In common with all drugs, it is advised that ursodeoxycholic acid should not be given during the first trimester of pregnancy. (In the rabbit, embryotoxicity has been observed, but this has not been seen in the rat). Treatment in women of child-bearing age should only be undertaken if measures to prevent pregnancy are used. Non-hormonal contraceptive measures are recommended. In cases of conception during treatment, therapy should be discontinued.

Effects on ability to drive and use machines: None known.

Undesirable effects: Destolit is normally well tolerated. Diarrhoea has been found to occur only occasionally. No significant alterations have so far been observed in liver function.

Overdose: It is unlikely that overdosage will cause serious adverse effects. Diarrhoea may occur and it is recommended that liver function tests be monitored. Ion-exchange resins may be useful to bind bile acids in the intestines

Pharmacological Properties
Pharmacodynamic properties: Ursodeoxycholic acid is a gallstone dissolving agent which acts by reducing the content of cholesterol in bile. This may be due either to a reduction in hepatic cholesterol synthesis or reduced absorption of cholesterol or both.

Pharmacokinetic properties: Intestinal absorption after an oral dose of UDCA is high, with a first-pass clearance of about 50 to 60%. Studies show that passive diffusion occurs, whereupon the drug enters the enterohepatic circulation and is subject to an efficient hepatic extraction mechanism. The "spillover" into the systemic blood supply is therefore minimal. Plasma levels are not clinically important but may be useful in estimating patient compliance; they reach maximum concentrations at about 60 minutes after ingestion with another peak recorded at 3 hours.

Ursodeoxycholic acid is rapidly conjugated with glycine and taurine in the liver. Microbial biotransformation of the drug and its metabolites occurs when they leave the enterohepatic circulation and is responsible for high levels of faecal lithocholic and 7-ketolithocholic acids during ursodeoxycholic acid therapy. Intestinal flora also hydrolyse conjugated drug back to the parent compound and interconvert ursodeoxycholic and chenodeoxycholic acids

Preclinical safety data: None applicable.

Pharmaceutical Particulars
List of excipients: Lactose, pregelatinised maize starch, acacia gum, talc, magnesium stearate, purifed water.

Incompatibilities: None known.

Shelf life: 3 years.

Special precautions for storage: None.

Nature and contents of container: Blister pack of 60 tablets.

Instruction for use/handling: None.

Marketing authorisation number PL 00322/0076.

Date of first authorisation/renewal of authorisation 4 December 1997.

Date of (partial) revision of the text September 1997.

Legal category POM.

KAMILLOSAN*

Presentation Light brown ointment containing Chamomile extracts 10.5% (standardised to provide 0.01% L-α bisabolol) in a base containing lanolin. Kamillosan also contains beeswax, maize oil and mixed esters of p-hydroxy-benzoic acid.

Uses Prophylaxis and treatment of sore nipples in nursing mothers, nappy rash, nappy chafe and chapped hands.

Dosage and administration Ointment for topical application.

Sore nipples: Apply after breastfeeding.

Nappy chafe and nappy rash: Apply at every nappy change.

Other conditions: Apply twice daily as necessary.

Contra-indications, warnings, etc
Contra-indications: None known.

Precautions: None known.

Use in pregnancy: There is no evidence to suggest that Kamillosan should not be used during pregnancy or lactation.

Side-effects: None reported.

Overdosage: There are no known symptoms of overdosage.

Pharmaceutical precautions Store in a cool, dry place below 25°C.

Legal category GSL.

Package quantities Tubes of 30 g.

Further information Breast pads may be worn to prevent staining of clothing by the ointment.

Product licence number 0322/5914

KLEAN-PREP*

Qualitative and quantitative composition Each sachet of Klean-Prep contains the following active ingredients:

Polyethylene Glycol 3350 USNF	59.000 g
Anhydrous Sodium Sulphate PhEur	5.685 g
Sodium Bicarbonate PhEur	1.685 g
Sodium Chloride PhEur	1.465 g
Potassium Chloride PhEur	0.7425 g

The content of electrolyte ions per sachet when made up to one litre of water is as follows:

Sodium	125 mM
Sulphate	40 mM
Chloride	35 mM
Bicarbonate	20 mM
Potassium	10 mM

Pharmaceutical form A whitish powder which, when dissolved in water, gives a clear, colourless solution for oral administration.

Clinical particulars
Therapeutic indications: For colonic lavage prior to diagnostic examination or surgical procedures requiring a clean colon, e.g. colonoscopy, barium enema or colonic resection.

Posology and method of administration
Adults: Each sachet should be dissolved in 1 litre of water. The usual dose is up to 4 sachets taken at a rate of 250 ml every 10 to 15 minutes until the total volume is consumed or rectal effluent is clear, or as directed by the physician.

The solutions from all 4 sachets should be drunk within 4 to 6 hours. Alternatively, administration may be divided, for example, taking 2 sachets during the evening before the examination, and the remaining 2 sachets on the morning of the examination.

If administration is by nasogastric tube, the usual rate should be 20 to 30 ml/minute.

Children: There is no recommended dosage for children.

Renal patients: No dosage adjustment need be made.

Contra-indications: Use in patients with known or suspected gastrointestinal obstruction or perforation, ileus, gastric retention, acute intestinal or gastric ulceration, toxic colitis or toxic megacolon.

Special warnings and special precautions for use: No solid food should be eaten for at least 2 hours before taking Klean-Prep. The product should only be administered with caution to patients with impaired gag reflex, reflux oesophagitis or those with diminished levels of consciousness and patients with ulcerative colitis.

Unconscious, semi-conscious patients or patients prone to aspiration or regurgitation should be observed during administration especially if this is via the nasogastric route.

Interaction with other medicaments and other forms of interaction: Oral medication taken within one hour of administration of Klean-Prep may be flushed from the gastro-intestinal tract and not absorbed.

Pregnancy and lactation: The preparation should only be used during pregnancy and lactation if considered essential by the physician. There is no experience of use during pregnancy. The purpose and mechanisms of use should be borne in mind if the physician is considering administration.

Effects on the ability to drive and use machines: There is no known effect on the ability to drive and use machines.

Undesirable effects: Nausea, abdominal fullness and bloating may be experienced. Should distension or pain arise, the rate of administration should be slowed down or temporarily stopped until symptoms subside. Abdominal cramps, vomiting and anal irritation occur less frequently.

These effects normally subside rapidly. Urticaria and allergic reactions have been reported rarely.

Overdose: In case of gross accidental overdosage, where diarrhoea is severe, conservative measures are usually sufficient; generous amounts of fluid, especially fruit juices, should be given.

Pharmacological properties
Pharmacodynamic properties: Polyethylene glycol 3350 exerts its effects by virtue of its osmotic effect in the gut, which induces a laxative effect. The electrolytes also present in the formulation ensure that there is virtually no net gain or loss of sodium, potassium or water, and thus no dehydration.

Pharmacokinetic properties: Polyethylene glycol 3350 is unchanged along the gut. It is virtually unabsorbed from the gastro-intestinal tract and has no known pharmacological activity. Any polyethylene glycol 3350 that is absorbed is excreted via the urine.

Preclinical safety data: Preclinical studies provide evidence that polyethylene glycol 3350 has no significant systemic toxicity potential.

Pharmaceutical particulars
List of excipients: Vanilla flavour; aspartame.

Incompatibilities: None are known.

Shelf life: Sachets: 2 years. Solution: 24 hours.

Special precautions for storage: Sachets: Store in a dry place below 25°C.

Nature and contents of container: Sachets containing 69 gm white powder, in boxes of 4 sachets.

Instructions of use/handling: The solution should be used within 24 hours.

Marketing authorisation number 00322/0068

Date of approval/revision of SPC March 1997

Legal category P

MOVICOL*

Qualitative and quantitative composition Each sachet of MOVICOL contains the following active ingredients:

Polyethylene Glycol 3350 USP	13.125 g
Sodium Chloride PhEur	350.7 mg
Sodium Bicarbonate PhEur	178.5 mg
Potassium Chloride PhEur	46.6 mg

The content of electrolyte ions per sachet when made up to 125 ml of solution is as follows:

Sodium	65 mmol/l
Chloride	53 mmol/l
Potassium	5.4 mmol/l
Bicarbonate	17 mmol/l

Pharmaceutical form Powder for oral solution.

Clinical particulars
Therapeutic indications: For the treatment of chronic constipation. MOVICOL is also effective in resolving faecal impaction, defined as refractory constipation with faecal loading of the rectum and/or colon confirmed by physical examination of the abdomen and rectum.

Posology and method of administration:
Chronic constipation: As for all laxatives, prolonged use is not recommended. A course of treatment for constipation with MOVICOL does not normally exceed two weeks, although this can be repeated if required.
Adults: 2 or 3 sachets daily in divided doses.
Elderly: Initially 1 sachet per day is recommended.
Children: Not recommended.

Faecal impaction: A course of treatment for faecal impaction with MOVICOL does not normally exceed 3 days.
Adults including the elderly: 8 sachets daily, all of which should be consumed within a 6 hour period.
Children: Not recommended.
Patients with impaired cardiovascular function: For the treatment of faecal impaction the dose should be divided so that no more than two sachets are taken in any one hour.
Patients with renal insufficiency: No dosage change is necessary for treatment of either constipation or faecal impaction.

Administration: Each sachet should be dissolved in 125 ml water. For use in faecal impaction 8 sachets may be dissolved in 1 litre water.

Contra-indications: Intestinal perforation or obstruction due to structural or functional disorder of the gut wall, ileus, severe inflammatory conditions of the intestinal tract, such as Crohn's disease and ulcerative colitis and toxic megacolon.
Known hypersensitivity to polyethylene glycol.

Special warnings and special precautions for use: Mild adverse drug reactions are possible as indicated in Section 4.8. If patients develop any symptoms indicating shifts of fluid/electrolytes (e.g. oedema, shortness of breath, increasing fatigue, dehydration, cardiac failure) MOVICOL should be stopped immediately and electrolytes measured, and any abnormality should be treated appropriately.

Interaction with other medicaments and other forms of interaction: No clinical interactions with other medicaments have been reported. Polyethylene glycol raises the solubility of drugs that are soluble in alcohol and relatively insoluble in water. There is therefore a theoretical possibility that the absorption of such drugs could be transiently reduced.

Pregnancy and lactation: There is no experience of the use of MOVICOL during pregnancy and lactation and it should only be used if considered essential by the physician.

Effects on the ability to drive and use machines: There is no effect on the ability to drive and use machines.

Undesirable effects: Abdominal distension and pain, borborygmi and nausea, attributable to the expansion of the contents of the intestinal tract can occur. Allergic reactions are a possibility.

Overdose: Severe pain or distension can be treated by nasogastric aspiration. Extensive fluid loss by diarrhoea or vomiting may require correction of electrolyte disturbances.

Pharmacological properties
Pharmacodynamic properties: Polyethylene glycol 3350 acts by virtue of its osmotic action in the gut, which induces a laxative effect. The electrolytes also present in the formulation ensure that there is virtually no net gain or loss of sodium, potassium or water. The laxative action of polyethylene glycol 3350 has a time course which will vary according to the severity of the constipation or faecal impaction being treated.
For the indication of faecal impaction controlled comparative studies have not been performed with other treatments (e.g. enemas). In a non-comparative study in 27 adult patients, MOVICOL cleared the faecal impaction in 12/27 (44%) after 1 day's treatment; 23/27 (85%) after 2 days' treatment and 24/27 (89%) at the end of 3 days.

Pharmacokinetic properties: Polyethylene glycol 3350 is unchanged along the gut. It is virtually unabsorbed from the gastro-intestinal tract and has no known pharmacological activity. Any polyethylene glycol 3350 that is absorbed is excreted via the urine.

Preclinical safety data: Preclinical studies provide evidence that polyethylene glycol 3350 has no significant systemic toxicity potential, although no tests of its effects on reproduction or genotoxicity have been conducted.

Pharmaceutical particulars
List of excipients: Acesulfame K (E950); Lime and Lemon Flavour.

Incompatibilities: None are known.

Shelf life: The shelf life of the sachets is 3 years.

Special precautions for storage: Sachet: Store below 25°C
Solution: Store Refrigerated (2-8°C) and covered. Discard any solution not used within 6 hours.

Nature and contents of container: 13.8 g sachets contained in boxes of 8 or 20 sachets.

Instruction of use/handling: None.

Marketing authorisation number PL 00322/0070.

Date of first authorisation December 1995.

Date of revision of text December 1997.

Legal Category P.

NORGALAX*

Presentation Ready-to-use, disposable micro-enema of 10 g liquid containing Docusate Sodium USP 120 mg.

Uses Norgalax is indicated for symptomatic treatment of constipation, whenever an enema is required, and for the preparation of the colon and rectum for endoscopic examination. Norgalax is usually effective in 5 to 20 minutes.

Dosage and administration For rectal administration.

Adults, elderly and children over 12: One enema is usually sufficient.

Children under 12: Not recommended.

Remove the protective cap, insert the nozzle into the rectum, squeezing gently until the tube is empty. No additional lubricant is needed as a drop of the mixture is sufficient.

Contra-indications, warnings, etc
Contra-indications: Haemorrhoids, anal fissures, rectocolitis bleeding, abdominal pain, intestinal obstruction, nausea, vomiting and inflammatory bowel disease.

Use in pregnancy and lactation: Norgalax may be used in pregnancy and lactation.

Interactions: Norgalax may increase the resorption of medicines and is not be used in combination with hepatotoxic agents.

Side-effects: Anal or rectal burning and pain, usually short lasting, diarrhoea, congestion of the rectal mucosa, rectal bleeding may occur occasionally. Hepatotoxicity has been described, especially when used in association with other laxatives. As with all laxatives, Norgalax should not be administered chronically. Prolonged use can precipitate the onset of an atonic non-functioning colon and hypokalaemia.

Overdosage: Excessive use will lead to excessive purgation, which should be treated symptomatically.

Pharmaceutical precautions Store in a cool place, below 25°C.

Legal category P.

Package quantities Boxes of 6.

Further information Norgalax utilises docusate sodium as a faecal softening agent. It is an anionic surfactant which acts by increasing the penetration of fluid into the faeces.

Product licence number 0322/0065.

NORMACOL*

Qualitative and quantitative composition The active ingredient is Sterculia BP 62% w/w.

Pharmaceutical form Oral granules.

Clinical particulars
Therapeutic indications: The treatment of constipation, particularly simple or idiopathic constipation and constipation during pregnancy.
Management of colostomies and ileostomies.
The 'High Residue Diet' management of diverticular disease of the colon and other conditions requiring a high fibre regimen.
The initiation and maintenance of bowel action after rectal and anal surgery.
Administration after ingestion of sharp foreign bodies to provide a coating and reduce the possibility of intestinal damage during transit.

Posology and method of administration:
Adults: 1 or 2 sachets or 1-2 heaped 5 ml spoonfuls, once or twice daily after meals.
Elderly: As adult dose.
Children: (6-12 years): one half the above amount.
The granules should be placed dry on the tongue and without chewing or crushing, swallowed immediately with plenty of water or a cool drink Prior to drinking they may also be sprinkled onto and taken with soft food such as yoghurt.

Contra-indications: Intestinal obstruction, faecal impaction, and total atony of the colon.

Special warnings and special precautions for use: Not to be taken immediately before retiring, especially in the elderly. Adequate fluid should be maintained. Caution should be exercised in cases of ulcerative colitis. Not to be taken for more than 4 days if there has been no movement of the bowels.

Interaction with other medicaments and other forms of interaction: None known.

Pregnancy and lactation: NORMACOL may be recommended during pregnancy or lactation.

Effects on the ability to drive and use machines: None known.

Undesirable effects: Occasionally mild abdominal distension may occur. Oesophageal obstruction is possible if the product is taken in overdosage or if it is not adequately washed down with fluid.

Overdose: Intestinal obstruction is possible in overdosage particularly in combination with inadequate fluid intake. Management is as for intestinal obstruction from other causes.

Pharmacological properties
Pharmacodynamic properties: Sterculia acts in the colon by forming a soft bulky stool and inducing a laxative effect.

Pharmacokinetic properties: Sterculia is not absorbed or digested in the gastrointestinal tract and its laxative action is normally effective within 12 hours of oral administration.

Preclinical safety data: There is no evidence that Sterculia has a significant systemic toxicity potential.

Pharmaceutical particulars
List of excipients: Sodium Bicarbonate BP
Sucrose BP
Talc USP
Paraffin wax
Titanium Dioxide BP
Vanillin BP

Incompatibilities: None known.

Shelf life: The shelf life is 3 years.

Special precautions for storage: Store in a dry place below 25°C.

Nature and contents of container: Sachet containing 7 g of white granules in boxes of 60 sachets.
Lined box of 500 g of white granules.

Instruction for use/handling: None.

Marketing authorisation number PL 0322/5010R.

Date of first authorisation January 1991.

Date of revision of text September 1997.

Legal category GSL.

NORMACOL* PLUS

Presentation Brown, coated granules containing:

Sterculia BP	62%
Frangula BPC 1949	8%

The coating of the granules also contains sucrose and colouring including azo dye. The product is gluten-free.

Uses Treatment of constipation, particularly hypotonic or slow transit constipation resistant to bulk alone.

The initiation and maintenance of bowel action after rectal surgery and after haemorrhoidectomy.

Dosage and administration Granules for oral administration.

Adults (including the elderly): 1 or 2 sachets or 1–2 heaped 5 ml spoonfuls once or twice daily after meals.

Children (6–12 years): A reduced amount may be given at the discretion of the physician.

The granules should be placed dry on the tongue and, without chewing or crushing, swallowed immediately with plenty of liquid (water or a cool drink). Prior to drinking they may also be sprinkled onto and taken with soft foods such as yoghurt.

Contra-indications, warnings, etc
Contra-indications: Intestinal obstruction, faecal impaction, and total atony of the colon.

Precautions: Not to be taken immediately before retiring to bed, especially in the elderly. Adequate fluid intake should be maintained. Caution should be exercised in cases of ulcerative colitis. Not to be taken for more than 4 days if there has been no movement of the bowels.

Use in pregnancy: No teratogenic effects have been reported, but caution should be exercised during the first trimester of pregnancy.

Use during lactation: There is no evidence to suggest that Normacol Plus is unsuitable for use during lactation, though Normacol (sterculia alone) is available, if preferred.

Side-effects: Abdominal distension. Intestinal obstruction is possible if the product is taken in overdosage or is not adequately washed down with fluid.

Overdosage: Intestinal obstruction is possible in overdosage particularly in combination with inadequate fluid intake. Management is as for intestinal obstruction from other causes.

Pharmaceutical precautions Store in a dry place below 25°C.

Legal category GSL.

Package quantities Packs of 60 sachets, each sachet containing 7 g of granules, or packs of 500 g.

Further information Normacol Plus is likely to take about 12 hours to exert its effect. Each 7 g sachet of granules contains 1.72 g of available carbohydrate, equivalent to 6.75 kcal.

Product licence number 0322/5011.

POSALFILIN* OINTMENT

Qualitative and quantitative composition Each 10 g tube of Posalfilin Ointment contains 20% w/w Podophyllum Resin BP and 25% w/w Salicylic Acid BP.

Pharmaceutical form Dark brown ointment.

Clinical particulars
Therapeutic indications: For the treatment of plantar warts.

Posology and method of administration
Adults (including the elderly) and children: A corn ring should be placed around the wart, cutting the ring to fit if necessary. A minimal amount of ointment should be applied to the exposed wart, taking care to avoid normal skin. The wart and corn ring should be covered with a plaster and the treatment repeated daily. When the wart appears soft and spongy, it should be left exposed and allowed to drop off. If the wart remains, the procedure should be repeated.

Contra-indications: Use in pregnancy and breastfeeding mothers. Patients with peripheral neuropathy, diabetes mellitus or peripheral vascular insufficiency.

Special warnings and special precautions for use: Misapplication of Posalfilin Ointment to healthy skin may cause inflammation, desquamation or necrosis. Treatment should be suspended if such inflammation occurs. If applied to delicate areas of skin such as in the ano-genital area, the skin may be seriously damaged, depending on the amount applied.

Interaction with other medicaments and other forms of interaction: None known.

Pregnancy and lactation: Contra-indicated in pregnancy and breastfeeding mothers.

Effects on the ability to drive and use machines: There is no effect on the ability to drive and use machines.

Undesirable effects: Posalfilin Ointment does not normally cause side effects when used as directed.

Overdose: Over-application can cause cutaneous necrosis and should be treated as a caustic burn.

Pharmacological properties
Pharmacodynamic properties: The salicylic acid macerates the horny layer covering the wart and allows the podophyllum to penetrate the wart where it has a specific cytotoxic effect on the nuclei of the hyperplastic cells.

Pharmacokinetic properties: Not applicable, as Posalfilin Ointment applied topically directly to the wart.

Preclinical safety data: There are no preclinical data of relevance to the prescriber which are additional to that already included in other sections of the SPC.

Pharmaceutical particulars
List of excipients: Yellow Soft Paraffin BP; Liquid Paraffin BP.

Incompatibilities: None known.

Shelf life: The shelf life is 4 years.

Special precautions for storage: Store below 25°C.

Nature and contents of container: Aluminium tube containing 10 g of ointment.

Instruction of use/handling: None.

Marketing authorisation number 00322/5901R

Date of approval/revision of SPC July 1996.

Legal category P

PYRALVEX*

Qualitative and quantitative composition Pyralvex contains the following active ingredients in each 1 ml of solution: Rhubarb extract 50 mg (equivalent to 5 mg anthraquinone glycosides) and Salicylic Acid BP 10 mg.

Pharmaceutical form Oromucosal solution.

Clinical particulars
Therapeutic indications: For the symptomatic relief of pain associated with recurrent mouth ulcers and denture irritation.

Posology and method of administration
Adults (including the elderly): To be applied to the inflamed oral mucosa (after removing any dentures) three or four times daily using the brush provided.

Children: Not recommended below the age of 12 years.

Contra-indications: None known.

Special warnings and special precautions for use: Each bottle of Pyralvex should be used by only one person.

Interaction with other medicaments and other forms of interaction: None known.

Pregnancy and lactation: There is no evidence to suggest that Pyralvex should not be used during pregnancy or lactation.

Effects on the ability to drive and use machines: None.

Undesirable effects: None known.

Overdose: Not applicable.

Pharmacological properties
Pharmacodynamic properties: Pharmacological studies have shown that the active ingredients of Pyralvex display anti-inflammatory, analgesic and anti-microbial properties, which are the basis of its clinical efficacy.

Pharmacokinetic properties: Systemic availability of Pyralvex is unlikely to be significant, owing to the low levels of ingredients administered.

Preclinical safety data: Preclinical studies indicate that at clinically effective doses, the ingredients in Pyralvex are unlikely to have any potential for toxic effects.

Pharmaceutical particulars
List of excipients: Ethanol BP; Water.

Incompatibilities: None known.

Shelf life: The shelf life is 3 years.

Special precautions for storage: Store below 25°C.

Nature and contents of container: An amber glass bottle with brush applicator containing 10 ml of solution.

Instructions of use/handling: Avoid rinsing of the mouth or eating for 15 minutes after application. Any discolouration which may occur will disappear during normal cleaning of the teeth.

Marketing authorisation number 00322/5013

Date of approval/revision of SPC October 1996.

Legal category P

SOMNITE* SUSPENSION (Nitrazepam Mixture)

Presentation An off-white, translucent, thixotropic suspension with a cherry flavour. Each 5 ml spoonful contains Nitrazepam BP 2.5 mg. The suspension also contains sucrose and mixed esters of p-hydroxybenzoic acid.

Uses Short term treatment of insomnia where daytime sedation is acceptable. Benzodiazepines should be used to treat insomnia only when it is severe, disabling, or subjecting the individual to extreme distress. An underlying cause for insomnia should be sought before deciding upon the use of benzodiazepines for symptomatic relief.

Dosage and administration Suspension for oral administration. *Adults:* 5 mg (two 5 ml spoonfuls) before retiring. This dose may, if necessary, be increased to 10 mg (four 5 ml spoonfuls).

Elderly patients: 2.5 mg (one 5 ml spoonful) before retiring. This dose may, if necessary, be increased to 5 mg (two 5 ml spoonfuls).

Children: Not recommended.

The lowest dose which can control the symptoms should be used. It should not be continued beyond four weeks. Long term chronic use is not recommended. Treatment should always be tapered off gradually. Patients who have taken benzodiazepines for a long time may require a longer period during which doses are reduced. When a benzodiazepine is used as a hypnotic, treatment should, if possible, be intermittent.

Contra-indications, warnings, etc
Contra-indications: Known sensitivity to benzodiazepines. Acute pulmonary insufficiency.

Precautions: Chronic pulmonary insufficiency. In chronic renal or hepatic disease. In labour. High single doses or repeated low doses have been reported to produce hypotonia, poor sucking and hypothermia in the neonate and irregularities in the foetal heart. Avoid if possible in lactation. The concurrent use of other CNS depressant drugs should be avoided. Benzodiazepines should not be used alone to treat depression or anxiety associated with depression. Suicide may be precipitated in such patients. They should not be used for phobic or obsessional states. They should not be used for the treatment of chronic psychosis. In cases of loss or bereavement, psychological adjustment may be inhibited by benzodiazepines. Disinhibiting effects may be manifested in various ways. Suicide may be precipitated in patients who are depressed, and aggressive behaviour towards self and others may be precipitated. Extreme caution should therefore be used in prescribing benzodiazepines in patients with personality disorders.

Pregnancy and lactation: If the product is prescribed to a woman of childbearing potential, she should be warned to contact her physician regarding discontinuance of the product if she intends to become or suspects that she is pregnant.

If, for compelling medical reasons, the product is administered during the late phase of pregnancy, or during labour at high doses, effects on the neonate, such as hypothermia, hypotonia and moderate respiratory depression, can be expected, due to the pharmacological action of the compound.

Moreover, infants born to mothers who took benzodiazepines chronically during the latter stages of pregnancy may have developed physical dependence and may be at some risk for developing withdrawal symptoms in the postnatal period.

Since benzodiazepines are found in the breast milk, benzodiazepines should not be given to breast feeding mothers.

Side-effects: Common adverse effects include drowsiness, sedation, blurring of vision, unsteadiness and ataxia. These effects occur following single as well as repeated dosage and may persist well into the following day. Performance at skilled tasks and alertness may be impaired. Patients should be warned of this hazard and advised not to drive or operate machinery during treatment. These effects are potentiated by alcohol. The elderly are particularly liable to experience these symptoms together with confusion especially if organic brain symptoms are present. See also Dependence Potential and Withdrawal Symptoms below.

Abnormal psychological reactions to benzodiazepines have been reported. Behavioural adverse effects include paradoxical aggressive outbursts, excitement, confusion, and the uncovering of depression with suicidal tendencies.

Other rare adverse effects including hypotension, gastrointestinal and visual disturbances, skin rashes, urinary retention, headache, vertigo, changes in libido; blood dyscrasias and jaundice have also been reported.

Dependence potential and withdrawal symptoms: In general the dependence potential of benzodiazepines is low but this increases when high dosages are attained, especially when given over long periods. This is particularly so in patients with a history of alcoholism, drug abuse or in patients with marked personality disorders. Regular monitoring of treatment in such patients is essential and routine repeat prescriptions should be avoided.

Treatment in all patients should be withdrawn

gradually. Withdrawal from benzodiazepines may be associated with physiological and psychological symptoms of withdrawal including depression, nervousness, rebound insomnia, irritability, sweating and diarrhoea. Withdrawal symptoms occur with benzodiazepines following normal therapeutic doses given for short periods of time.

Abrupt withdrawal following excessive dosage may produce confusion, toxic psychosis, convulsions or a condition resembling delirium tremens.

Overdosage: The primary symptoms of overdosage are drowsiness, dizziness, ataxia and slurred speech. Treatment is symptomatic but gastric lavage may be useful if performed soon after ingestion.

Pharmaceutical precautions Somnite suspension should be stored in a cool place, protected from light. Avoid freezing.

Legal category CD (Sch 4) POM.

Package quantities Bottles of 150 ml

Further information Nil.

Product licence number 0322/0039.

SPASMONAL* 60 mg

Qualitative and quantitative composition Each capsule contains 60 mg alverine citrate.

Pharmaceutical form An opaque size 3 capsule with a grey cap marked SP60 and blue body marked with a logo.

Clinical particulars
Therapeutic indications: The relief of smooth muscle spasm, in conditions such as irritable bowel syndrome, painful diverticular disease of the colon and primary dysmenorrhoea.

Posology and method of administration: Recommended dose and dosage schedules:

Adults (including the elderly): 1or 2 capsules one to three times daily.

Children below the age of 12 years: not recommended.

Contra-indications: Paralytic ileus or known hypersensitivity to any of the ingredients.

Special warnings and special precautions for use: None.

Interaction with other medicaments and other forms of interaction: None stated.

Pregnancy and lactation: Although no teratogenic effects have been reported, use during pregnancy or lactation is not recommended as evidence of safety in preclinical studies is limited.

Effects on the ability to drive and use machines: None.

Undesirable effects: Possible side effects may include nausea, headache, dizziness, itching, rash, and allergic reactions.

Overdose: Can produce hypotension and atropine-like toxic effects. Management is as for atropine poisoning with supportive therapy for hypotension.

Pharmacological properties
Pharmacodynamic properties: Alverine citrate is a spasmolytic which has a specific action on the smooth muscle of the alimentary tract and uterus, without affecting the heart, blood vessels and tracheal muscle at therapeutic doses.

Pharmacokinetic properties: After oral administration, alverine is rapidly converted to its primary active metabolite, which is then further converted to two secondary metabolites. There is a high renal clearance of all metabolites indicating that they are eliminated by active renal secretion. The peak plasma level of the most active metabolite occurs between 1 and 1½ hours after oral dosing.

Preclinical safety data: Preclinical studies provide evidence that alverine citrate has no significant systemic toxicity potential at the proposed dosage.

Pharmaceutical particulars
List of excipients:
Maize Starch BP
Magnesium Stearate BP
Capsule Shell:
Gelatin, E132, E171, E172

Incompatibilities: None stated.

Shelf life: 3 years.

Special precautions for storage: Store in a dry place below 25°C.

Nature and contents of container: Plastic containers of 20 or 100 capsules; foil/UPVC blister packs containing 3, 10, 12, 20, 90 or 100 capsules.

Instruction for use/handling: None.

Marketing authorisation number PL 00322/5014R.

Date of first authorisation/renewal of the authorisation 12th July 1990.

Date of revision of text June 1998.

Legal category P.

SPASMONAL* Forte 120 mg ▼

Qualitative and quantitative composition Each capsule contains 120 mg alverine citrate.

Pharmaceutical form An opaque, size 1 capsule with a grey cap and blue body, marked 'SP120'.

Clinical particulars
Therapeutic indications: The relief of smooth muscle spasm, in conditions such as irritable bowel syndrome, painful diverticular disease of the colon and primary dysmenorrhoea.

Posology and method of administration: Recommended dose and dosage schedules:

Adults (including the elderly): 1 capsule one to three times daily.

Children below the age of 12 years: not recommended.

Contra-indications: Paralytic ileus or known hypersensitivity to any of the ingredients.

Special warnings and special precautions for use None.

Interaction with other medicaments and other forms of interaction: None stated.

Pregnancy and lactation: Although no teratogenic effects have been reported, use during pregnancy or lactation is not recommended as evidence of safety in preclinical studies is limited.

Effects on the ability to drive and use machines: None.

Undesirable effects: Possible side effects may include nausea, headache, dizziness, itching, rash, and allergic reactions, including anaphylaxis.

Overdose: Can produce hypotension and atropine-like toxic effects. Management is as for atropine poisoning with supportive therapy for hypotension.

Pharmacological properties
Pharmacodynamic properties: Alverine citrate is a spasmolytic which has a specific action on the smooth muscle of the alimentary tract and uterus, without affecting the heart, blood vessels and tracheal muscle at therapeutic doses.

Pharmacokinetic properties: After oral administration, alverine is rapidly converted to its primary active metabolite, which is then further converted to two secondary metabolites. There is a high renal clearance of all metabolites indicating that they are eliminated by active renal secretion. The peak plasma level of the most active metabolite occurs between 1 and 1½ hours after oral dosing.

Preclinical safety data: Preclinical studies provide evidence that alverine citrate has no significant systemic toxicity potential at the proposed dosage.

Pharmaceutical particulars
List of excipients:
Maize Starch BP
Magnesium Stearate BP
Capsule Shell:
Gelatin, E132, E171, E172

Incompatibilities: None stated.

Shelf life: 3 years.

Special precautions for storage: Store in a dry place below 25°C.

Nature and contents of container: A box of aluminium foil/UPVC blister strips containing 60 capsules, in strips of 10 capsules.

Instruction for use/handling: None.

Marketing authorisation number PL 00322/0075.

Date of first authorisation/renewal of the authorisation October 9th, 1997.

Legal category P.

WAXSOL* EAR DROPS

Qualitative and quantitative composition Waxsol Ear Drops contain the following active ingredient: Docusate Sodium BP 0.5% w/v.

Pharmaceutical form Ear drops.

Clinical particulars
Therapeutic indications: Waxsol Ear Drops are indicated as an aid in the removal of ear wax.

Posology and method of administration: Recommended dose and dosage schedules:

Adults (including the elderly): The application of ear drops sufficient to fill the affected ear on not more than two consecutive nights, prior to attending syringing if this is necessary.

Children: As for adult dose.

Contra-indications: Perforation of the ear drum or inflammation of the ear.

Special warnings and special precautions for use: If pain or inflammation is experienced, treatment should be discontinued.

Interaction with other medicaments and other forms of interaction: None known.

Pregnancy and lactation: There is no evidence to suggest that Waxsol Ear Drops should not be used during pregnancy and lactation.

Effects on ability to drive and use machines: None known.

Undesirable effects: Rarely, transient stinging or irritation may occur.

Overdose: None known.

Pharmacological properties The so-called 'wax' which often obstructs the external auditory meatus of the ear contains less than 50% of fatty matter derived from secretions of the sebaceous ceruminous glands. The majority of the wax consists of desquamated epithelium, foreign matter and shed hairs. This non-fatty material forms a matrix holding together the granules of fatty matter to form the ceruminous mass.

The addition of oils or solvents binds the mass more firmly together, but aqueous solutions, if they are able to penetrate the matrix, cause a disintegration of the ceruminous mass.

Waxsol Ear Drops, because of their low surface tension and miscibility, rapidly penetrate the dry matrix of the ceruminous mass, reducing the solid material to a semi-solid debris. This can be syringed away readily, or in less severe or chronic cases, is ejected by normal physiological processes.

Pharmaceutical particulars
List of excipients: Glycerine BP; Phenonip (solution of esters of 4-hydroxybenzoic acid in phenoxetol); water.

Incompatibilities: None known.

Shelf life: The shelf life is 3 years.

Special precautions for storage: Store below 25°C.

Nature and contents of container: Amber glass bottle of 10 ml capacity with a dropper applicator.

Instructions for use/handling: The dropper applicator must be filled before dripping Waxsol Ear Drops into the affected ear.

Marketing authorisation number 00322/5016.

Date of approval/revision of SPC June 1995.

Legal category P.

*Trade Mark

Novartis Consumer Health
Wimblehurst Road
Horsham
West Sussex RH12 5AB
☎ 01403 210211 🗋 01403 323939

NOVARTIS

EURAX* CREAM

Qualitative and quantitative composition Crotamiton BP 10% w/w.

Pharmaceutical form Topical cream.

Clinical particulars
Therapeutic indications: (1) For the relief of itching and skin irritation caused by, for example sunburn, dry eczema, itchy dermatitis, allergic rashes, hives, nettle rash, chickenpox, insect bites and stings, heat rashes and personal itching.
(2) The treatment of scabies.

Posology and method of administration: For cutaneous use.

Recommended dose and dosage schedules
PRURITUS: Adults (including the elderly) and children: Apply to the affected area 2–3 times daily. Eurax will provide relief from irritation for 6–10 hours after each application. Eurax can be used in children. There are no special dosage recommendations in the elderly.

SCABIES: Adults (including the elderly): After the patient has taken a warm bath, the skin should be well dried and Eurax rubbed into the entire body surface (excluding the face and scalp) until no traces of the preparation remain visible on the surface. The application should be repeated once daily, preferably in the evening, for a total of 3–5 days. Depending on the response, special attention should be paid to sites that are particularly susceptible to infestation by the mites (e.g. interdigital spaces, wrists, axillae and genitalia). Areas where there is pus formation should be covered with a dressing impregnated with Eurax. While the treatment is in progress the patient may take a bath shortly before the next application. After completion of the treatment, a cleansing bath should be taken followed by a change of bed linen and underclothing.

Children: Application as described for adults but in children under 3 years of age Eurax should not be applied more than once a day.

Contra-indications: Acute exudative dermatoses. Hypersensitivity to any of the ingredients. Eurax should not be used in or around the eyes since contact with the eyelids may give rise to conjunctival inflammation.

Special warnings and special precautions for use: Eurax can be used for children; consult your doctor before use on children under 3 years of age.

For external use only.

Do not use in or around the eyes, on broken skin, for weeping skin conditions or if you are sensitive to any of the ingredients.

Keep all medicines out of the reach of children.

Consult your doctor or pharmacist before using Eurax if you are pregnant or breast feeding, or suffering from genital itching.

If symptoms persist consult your doctor.

Interactions with other medicaments and other forms of interaction: None.

Pregnancy and lactation: There is no experience to judge the safety of Eurax in pregnancy, therefore Eurax is not recommended during pregnancy, especially in the first three months. It is not known whether the active substance passes into breast milk. Nursing mothers should avoid applying Eurax in the area of the nipples.

Effect on ability to drive and use machines: None.

Undesirable effects: Occasionally irritation of the skin or contact allergy may occur. In such cases the preparation should be discontinued.

Overdose: Eurax is for application to the skin only. Following accidental ingestion, nausea, vomiting and irritation of the buccal, oesophageal and gastric mucosa have been reported. If accidental ingestion of large quantities occurs, there is no specific antidote and general measures to eliminate the drug and reduce its absorption should be undertaken. Symptomatic treatment should be administered as appropriate. A risk of methaemoglobinaemia exists, which may be treated with methylene blue.

Pharmacological properties
Pharmacodynamic properties: Eurax has a symptomatic action on pruritus and is an acaricide.

Pharmacokinetic properties: Eurax penetrates rapidly into human skin. Low but measurable concentrations of crotamiton are found in plasma, with a maximum level after 4–10 hours, declining rapidly thereafter.

Preclinical safety data: Eurax cream administered dermally once daily under occlusive dressing for 3 months to rabbits was tolerated at doses of up to 250 mg/kg without signs of toxicity, apart from transient skin irritation. No sensitising or photo-sensitising potential has been observed in animal studies. Crotamiton does not induce mutations in bacteria nor chromosomal damage in mammalian cells. Studies to detect a possible effect on fertility and reproductive behaviour also gave negative results.

Pharmaceutical particulars
List of excipients: Methyl hydroxybenzoate, phenylethyl alcohol, glycerol, triethanolamine, sodium lauryl sulphate, ethylene glycol monostearate, stearyl alcohol, strong ammonia solution, stearic acid, hard paraffin, white beeswax, perfume, purified water.

Incompatibilities: None.

Shelf life: 5 years.

Special precautions for storage: Protect from heat.

Nature and contents of container: Internally lacquered aluminium tube, with a screw cap, in a cardboard carton. Pack sizes 30 g, 100 g.

Instructions for use/handling: Medicines should be kept out of the reach of children.

Marketing authorisation number 0030/0092.

Date of approval/revision of SPC September 1997.

Legal category GSL.

EURAX* LOTION

Qualitative and quantitative composition Crotamiton BP 10% w/w.

Pharmaceutical form Topical emulsion.

Clinical particulars
Therapeutic indications: (1) For the relief of itching and skin irritation caused by, for example sunburn, dry eczema, itchy dermatitis, allergic rashes, hives, nettle rash, chickenpox, insect bites and stings, heat rashes and personal itching.
(2) The treatment of scabies.

Posology and method of administration: For cutaneous use.

Recommended dose and dosage schedules
PRURITUS: Adults (including the elderly) and children: Apply to the affected area 2–3 times daily. Eurax will provide relief from irritation for 6–10 hours after each application. Eurax can be used in children. There are no special dosage recommendations in the elderly.

SCABIES: Adults (including the elderly): After the patient has taken a warm bath, the skin should be well dried and Eurax rubbed into the entire body surface (excluding the face and scalp) until no traces of the preparation remain visible on the surface. The application should be repeated once daily, preferably in the evening, for a total of 3–5 days. Depending on the response, special attention should be paid to sites that are particularly susceptible to infestation by the mites (e.g. interdigital spaces, wrists, axillae and genitalia). Areas where there is pus formation should be covered with a dressing impregnated with Eurax. While the treatment is in progress the patient may take a bath shortly before the next application. After completion of the treatment, a cleansing bath should be taken followed by a change of bed linen and underclothing.

Children: Application as described for adults but in children under 3 years of age Eurax should not be applied more than once a day.

Contra-indications: Acute exudative dermatoses. Hypersensitivity to any of the ingredients. Eurax should not be used in or around the eyes since contact with the eyelids may give rise to conjunctival inflammation.

Special warnings and special precautions for use: Eurax can be used for children; consult your doctor before use on children under 3 years of age.

For external use only.

Do not use in or around the eyes, on broken skin, for weeping skin conditions or if you are sensitive to any of the ingredients.

Keep all medicines out of the reach of children.

Consult your doctor or pharmacist before using Eurax if you are pregnant or breast feeding, or suffering from genital itching.

If symptoms persist consult your doctor.

Interactions with other medicaments and other forms of interaction: None.

Pregnancy and lactation: There is no experience to judge the safety of Eurax in pregnancy, therefore Eurax is not recommended during pregnancy, especially in the first three months. It is not known whether the active substance passes into breast milk. Nursing mothers should avoid applying Eurax in the area of the nipples.

Effect on ability to drive and use machines: None.

Undesirable effects: Occasionally irritation of the skin or contact allergy may occur. In such cases the preparation should be discontinued.

Overdose: Eurax is for application to the skin only. Following accidental ingestion, nausea, vomiting and irritation of the buccal, oesophageal and gastric mucosa have been reported. If accidental ingestion of large quantities occurs, there is no specific antidote and general measures to eliminate the drug and reduce its absorption should be undertaken. Symptomatic treatment should be administered as appropriate. A risk of methaemoglobinaemia exists, which may be treated with methylene blue.

Pharmacological properties
Pharmacodynamic properties: Eurax has a symptomatic action on pruritus and is an acaricide.

Pharmacokinetic properties: Eurax penetrates rapidly into human skin. Low but measurable concentrations of crotamiton are found in plasma, with a maximum level after 4–10 hours, declining rapidly thereafter.

Preclinical safety data: Eurax cream administered dermally once daily under occlusive dressing for 3 months to rabbits was tolerated at doses of up to 250 mg/kg without signs of toxicity, apart from transient skin irritation. No sensitising or photo-sensitising potential has been observed in animal studies. Crotamiton does not induce mutations in bacteria nor chromosomal damage in mammalian cells. Studies to detect a possible effect on fertility and reproductive behaviour also gave negative results.

Pharmaceutical particulars
List of excipients: Glyceryl monostearate, cetomacrogol, cetyl alcohol, stearyl alcohol, sodium cetostearyl sulphate, 2-octyl dodecanol, sorbic acid, citric acid, phenylethyl alcohol, propylene glycol, perfume, purified water.

Incompatibilities: None.

Shelf life: 5 years.

Special precautions for storage: Protect from heat.

Nature and contents of container: Amber glass bottle with wadless polypropylene cap in cardboard carton. Pack size 100 ml.

Instructions for use/handling: Medicines should be kept out of the reach of children.

Marketing authorisation number 0030/0095.

Date of approval/revision of SPC September 1997.

Legal category GSL.

EURAX* HYDROCORTISONE CREAM

Qualitative and quantitative composition
Active ingredients: Crotamiton BP 10.0% w/w, Hydrocortisone PhEur BP 0.25% w/w.

Pharmaceutical form Cream.

Clinical particulars
Therapeutic indications: Eczema and dermatitis of all types including atopic eczema, photodermatitis, otitis externa, primary irritant and allergic dermatitis, intertrigo, prurigo nodularis, seborrhoeic dermatitis and insect bite reactions.

Route of administration: Topical.

Posology and method of administration
Adults: A thin layer of Eurax Hydrocortisone Cream should be applied to the affected area 2–3 times a day. Occlusive dressings should not be used. Treatment

should be limited to 10–14 days or up to 7 days if applied to the face.

Use in the elderly: Clinical evidence would indicate that no special dosage regime is necessary.

Use in children: Eurax Hydrocortisone should be used with caution in infants and for not more than 7 days. Eurax Hydrocortisone should not be applied more than once a day to large areas of the body surface in young children.

Contra-indications: Hypersensitivity to any component of the formulation. Bacterial, viral or fungal infections of the skin. Acute exudative dermatoses. Application to ulcerated areas.

Special warnings and special precautions for use: Eurax Hydrocortisone should be used with caution in infants and for not more than 7 days; long-term continuous topical therapy should be avoided since this can lead to adrenal suppression even without occlusion.

Eurax Hydrocortisone should not be allowed to come into contact with the conjunctiva and mucous membranes.

Interactions with other medicaments and other forms of interaction: None known.

Pregnancy and lactation: There is inadequate evidence of safety in human pregnancy. Topical administration of corticosteroids to pregnant animals can cause abnormalities of foetal development, including cleft palate and intra-uterine growth retardation. There may therefore be a very small risk of such effects in the human foetus.

It is not known whether the active substances of Eurax Hydrocortisone and/or their metabolite(s) pass into the breast milk after topical administration. Use in lactating mothers should only be at the doctor's discretion.

Effect on ability to drive and use machines: None known.

Undesirable effects: Occasionally at the site of application signs of irritation such as a burning sensation, itching, contact dermatitis/contact allergy may occur. Treatment should be discontinued if patients experience severe irritation or sensitisation.

Overdose: Eurax Hydrocortisone is for application to the skin only. If accidental ingestion of large quantities occurs, there is no specific antidote and general measures to eliminate the drug and reduce its absorption should be undertaken. Symptomatic treatment should be administered as appropriate.

Pharmacological properties

Pharmacodynamic properties: Eurax Hydrocortisone combines the antipruritic action of crotamiton with the anti-inflammatory and anti-allergic properties of hydrocortisone.

Pharmacokinetic properties: No pharmacokinetic data on Eurax Hydrocortisone Cream are available.

Preclinical safety data: Not applicable.

Pharmaceutical particulars

List of excipients (qualitative):

Stearyl alcohol	Propylene glycol
White soft paraffin	Methyl hydroxybenzoate
Polyoxy 40 stearate	Perfume
Propyl hydroxybenzoate	Purified water

Incompatibilities: None known.

Shelf life: 60 months.

Special precautions for storage: Protect from heat.

Nature of container and closure: Collapsible aluminium tube. Pack size: 30 g.

Instructions for use/handling: Medicines should be kept out of the reach of children.

Marketing authorisation number 0030/0094.

Date of revision of summary of product characteristics 1 September 1997.

Legal Category POM.

LACTITOL*

Presentation Lactitol is a white, crystalline, slightly sweet tasting powder composed of lactitol monohydrate. There are no other ingredients.

Uses

Mode of action: Lactitol is a disaccharide derivative consisting of galactose and sorbitol which is only minimally absorbed and is not hydrolysed by the disaccharidases of the gastrointestinal tract and thus reaches the colon unchanged. In the colon it is broken down to short chain organic acids, mainly acetic, propionic and butyric acid, by the intestinal flora, in particular by the bacteroides and lactobacilli, thus acidifying the contents of the colon. The effect of this acidification is to reduce the absorption of ammonia. It also seems that the above-mentioned bacteria prefer Lactitol to amino acids: an in-vitro faecal incubation study has shown that the presence of Lactitol reduces the production of ammonia by bacteria.

The transformation of Lactitol into low molecular weight organic acids results in an increase in osmotic pressure in the colon, thereby causing an increase in the stool water content and stool volume, which explains the laxative effect.

Lactitol produces its effect in the lumen of the colon, where it is virtually 100% bioavailable. It is absorbed only in minimal amounts. Up to 2% can be found unchanged in the urine.

Indications: Constipation. Acute and chronic portal systemic encephalopathy.

Dosage and administration For oral administration. It can be mixed with hot or cold beverages, cereals, puddings, etc. Due to variations in individual patient response the dosage will require adjustment to obtain one daily bowel movement in constipated patients and two daily bowel movements in patients with portal systemic encephalopathy.

Constipation: Lactitol should be given in a single daily dose, in the morning or in the evening, at meal times, mixed with food or drink. The choice between morning or evening intake should be left to the patient, according to the individual response: the laxative effect has been found mostly to occur within a few hours after intake.

Patients should be informed that in some cases the first laxative response may be delayed until the second or third day of administration. Patients should be advised to maintain an adequate daily fluid intake.

Adults (including the elderly): The initial daily dosage should be 20 g (two 10 g sachets) taken in a single dose with the morning or evening meal. After a few days, a daily dose of 10 g (one sachet) may be sufficient for many patients.

Children: The mean dosage is 0.25 g/kg body weight daily, e.g.:

1 to 6 years old:	$\frac{1}{4}$ to $\frac{1}{2}$ sachet daily	(2.5 to 5 g).
6 to 12 years old:	$\frac{1}{2}$ to 1 sachet daily	(5 to 10 g).
12 to 16 years old:	1 to 2 sachets daily	(10 to 20 g).

In all cases dosage should be individually adjusted to obtain one daily bowel movement.

Portal systemic encephalopathy: The dosage should be adjusted according to the severity of the patient's disease and their individual response. The initial recommended dose is 0.5 to 0.7 g/kg body weight daily, divided into three daily doses with meals. The dosage should then be adjusted to produce two soft bowel movements daily.

To obtain a 40% solution for administration by nasogastric tube if required, in patients with acute portal systemic encephalopathy proceed as follows: add 200 g of lactitol monohydrate to 200 ml of hot distilled water, stirring continuously. When dissolved, complete to a final volume of 500 ml with cold distilled water. This solution can be given by nasogastric tube at a dosage of 1 to 2 ml/kg body weight daily (corresponding to 0.4 to 0.8 g/kg). Unused solution should be disposed of in the normal manner.

Contra-indications, warnings, etc

Contra-indications: In common with other laxatives, Lactitol should not be used in patients with intestinal obstruction, where an underlying organic lesion of the gastrointestinal tract is suspected, or in cases of unexplained abdominal pain or bleeding. Faecal impaction should be treated by alternative methods prior to using Lactitol.

Lactitol is not recommended for use in patients with galactosaemia.

Precautions: To avoid disturbances of electrolyte balance which may occur as a result of overdose-induced diarrhoea, the doctor should try, from the beginning of the treatment, to determine the optimal dosage (see 'Dosage and Administration') to achieve one daily bowel movement in constipated patients and two daily bowel movements in cirrhotic patients.

Elderly or debilitated patients receiving long-term treatment with Lactitol should have their serum electrolytes monitored regularly.

As for all laxatives, pre-existing fluid or electrolyte imbalance should be corrected before starting treatment with Lactitol.

Following treatment with Lactitol, hydrogen may accumulate in the bowel. Patients who need to undergo electrocauterisation procedures should therefore have a thorough bowel cleansing with a non-fermentable solution.

Patients who complain of nausea should be advised to take Lactitol with a meal.

Lactitol is not recommended in cases of ileostomy or colostomy.

Prolonged use of laxatives without interruption should be avoided.

All cases of chronic constipation should first be treated by a fibre-rich diet, intake of liquids or physical activity.

Interactions: Antacids and neomycin, as they can neutralise the stool acidifying effect of Lactitol, should not be given simultaneously with Lactitol to cirrhotic patients with portal systemic encephalopathy. Antacids and neomycin do not alter the laxative effect in constipated patients.

Like all laxatives, Lactitol may increase the potassium loss caused by other drugs e.g. thiazide diuretics, corticosteroids, carbenoxolone, amphotericin B. Potassium deficiency may enhance the risk of toxic effects of glycosides in patients receiving concomitant therapy.

Lactitol monohydrate has a calorific value of 2 kcal/g (8.5 KJ/g) and has no effect on blood glucose levels. It can therefore be given to diabetic patients.

Use in pregnancy and lactation: At present there is inadequate evidence of safety in human pregnancy. Therefore, it is recommended that, during the first trimester of pregnancy, Lactitol should only be used if there is no safer alternative.

Although the passage of Lactitol into breast milk has not been studied, it appears unlikely to have any clinical relevance since it is only minimally absorbed.

Side-effects: At the start of treatment Lactitol may produce abdominal discomfort such as meteorism and flatulence, pain, cramps or sensation of fullness. In clinical trials these untoward effects were observed in about 25% of adult patients and 35% of elderly patients. Such effects tend to diminish or disappear after a few days of regular intake of Lactitol. Occasionally, nausea, borborygmi or anal pruritus have been reported as well as vomiting in rare cases. Because of inter-individual variation, some patients may experience diarrhoea at the recommended dosage. A reduction in dosage will overcome this.

Overdosage: Doses of up to 72 g/day in portal systemic encephalopathy and up to 40 g/day in constipation have been tolerated in some patients. The sign of overdosage is diarrhoea, which can be stopped by decreasing the dosage. It may also result in an alteration of serum electrolytes which may need correcting.

Pharmaceutical precautions No special precautions.

Package quantities Sachets: packs of 10 sachets, each sachet containing 10 g of lactitol monohydrate powder.

Further information Nil.

Product licence number 0030/0062.

Legal Category P.

LOCORTEN* VIOFORM* EAR DROPS

Qualitative and quantitative composition

Active ingredients: Flumethasone Pivalate 0.02% w/v, Clioquinol BP 1.0% w/v.

Pharmaceutical form Ear drops.

Clinical particulars

Therapeutic indications: Inflammatory conditions of the external ear where a secondary infection is suspected. Otorrhoea.

Route of administration: Topical.

Posology and method of administration: Instil 2 or 3 drops twice daily directly into the auditory canal of the affected ear. Treatment should be limited to 7–10 days.

If there is little improvement after 7 days treatment with Locorten Vioform, appropriate microbiological investigations should be carried out and local or systemic antibiotic treatment given.

Use in the elderly: There is no evidence to suggest that dosage should be different in the elderly.

Use in children: Locorten Vioform Ear Drops are contra-indicated in children below the age of two years.

Contra-indications: Hypersensitivity to any component of the formulation or iodine. Primary bacterial, viral or fungal infections of the outer ear. Perforation of the tympanic membrane. Use in children below the age of two years.

Special warnings and precautions for use: Long-term continuous topical therapy should be avoided since this can lead to adrenal suppression.

Topical application of clioquinol-containing preparations may lead to a marked increase in protein-bound iodine (PBI). The results of thyroid function tests, such as PBI, radioactive iodine and butanol extractable iodine, may be affected. However, other thyroid function tests, such as the T3 resin sponge test or T4 determination, are unaffected.

The ferric chloride test of phenylketonuria may yield a false-positive result when clioquinol is present in the urine. Locorten Vioform should not be allowed to come into contact with the conjunctiva.

Interactions with other medicaments and other forms of interaction: None known via this topical route.

Pregnancy and lactation: There is inadequate evidence

of safety in human pregnancy. Topical administration of corticosteroids to pregnant animals can cause abnormalities of foetal development, including cleft palate and intra-uterine growth retardation. There may, therefore, be a very small risk of such effects in the human foetus.

It is not known whether the active substances of Locorten Vioform and/or their metabolite(s) pass into breast milk after topical administration. Use in lactating mothers should only be at the doctor's discretion.

Effect on ability to drive and use machines: None known.

Undesirable effects: Locorten Vioform is generally well tolerated, but occasionally at the site of application, there may be signs of irritation such as a burning sensation, itching, or skin rash. Hypersensitivity reactions may also occasionally occur. Treatment should be discontinued if patients experience severe irritation or sensitisation.

Locorten Vioform may cause hair discoloration.

Overdose: Locorten Vioform is for topical (external) use only. If accidental ingestion of large quantities occurs, there is no specific antidote and general measures to eliminate the drug and reduce its absorption should be undertaken. Symptomatic treatment should be administered as appropriate.

Pharmacological properties

Pharmacodynamic properties: Locorten Vioform Ear Drops combine the anti-fungal and anti-bacterial properties of clioquinol with the anti-inflammatory activity of flumethasone pivalate.

Pharmacokinetic properties: No pharmacokinetic data on Locorten Vioform Ear Drops are available.

Preclinical safety data: Not applicable.

Pharmaceutical particulars

List of excipients: Polyethylene Glycol.

Incompatibilities: None known.

Shelf life: 60 months.

Special precautions for storage: None.

Nature of container and closure: Plastic dropper bottle.

Instructions for use/handling: Medicines should be kept out of the reach of children.

Marketing authorisation number 0030/0049.

Date of revision of SPC 3 February 1997.

Legal category POM.

NICOTINELL* FRUIT 4 mg and NICOTINELL* MINT 4 mg

Qualitative and quantitative composition Nicotine 4 mg per gum, in a resin complex, available in a fruit or mint flavour.

Pharmaceutical form Chewing gum.

Clinical particulars

Therapeutic indications: Nicotinell treatment is indicated for the relief of nicotine withdrawal symptoms, in nicotine dependency as an aid to smoking cessation. Nicotinell 4 mg gum is for use when severe withdrawal of symptoms are experienced.

Posology and method of administration:

Adults and elderly: Users should stop smoking completely during treatment with Nicotinell gum. One piece of Nicotinell gum to be chewed when the user feels the urge to smoke.

Normally, 8–12 pieces per day, up to a maximum of 15 pieces per day.

The characteristics of chewing gum as a pharmaceutical form are such that individually different nicotine levels can result in the blood. Therefore, dosage frequency should be adjusted according to individual requirements within the stated maximum limit.

Directions for use:

1. One piece of gum should be chewed until the taste becomes strong.
2. The chewing gum should be rested between the gum and cheek.
3. When the taste fades, chewing should commence again.
4. The chewing routine should be repeated for 30 minutes.

After three months, the user should gradually cut down the number of pieces chewed each day until they have stopped using the product.

Children: Not to be used by children.

Concomitant use of acidic beverages such as coffee or soda may interfere with the buccal absorption of nicotine. Acidic beverages should be avoided for 15 minutes prior to chewing the gum.

Contra-indications: Nicotinell gum should not be used by non-smokers or people under 18 years of age. Furthermore, people should not use the gum and smoke concomitantly.

Use is contra-indicated during pregnancy and lactation, acute myocardial infarction, unstable or worsening angina pectoris, severe cardiac arrhythmias, and recent cerebrovascular accident.

Special warnings and precautions for use: Swallowed nicotine may exacerbate symptoms in subjects suffering from active oesophagitis, oral or pharyngeal inflammation, gastritis or peptic ulcer.

Use with caution in patients with hypertension, stable angina pectoris, cerebrovascular disease, occlusive peripheral arterial disease, heart failure, hyperthyroidism, diabetes mellitus, and renal or hepatic impairment.

Counselling may help smokers to quit.

Doses of nicotine that are tolerated by adult smokers during treatment may produce severe symptoms of poisoning in small children and may prove fatal (please see *Overdose*).

Interactions with other medicaments and other forms of interaction:

Drug interactions: No information is available on interactions between Nicotinell gum and other drugs.

Smoking cessation: This is different in the case of smoking where interactions with other medications may occur due to a multitude of other substances contained in the smoke. Presumably due to the polycyclic aromatic hydrocarbons contained in the smoke, the metabolism of different medicinal products may be speeded up by enzyme induction: e.g. caffeine, theophylline, paracetamol, phenazone, phenylbutazone, pentazocine, lidocaine, benzodiazepines, imipramine, warfarin, oestrogen and vitamin B12.

Upon smoking cessation it may be expected that the hitherto increased metabolism of these medicinal products is slowed down or normalised. Unaltered dosage of the products may result in an increase in their blood concentration.

Therefore when prescribing Nicotinell a possible dose adjustment should be considered in patients treated with the above mentioned medicinal products.

Other reported effects of smoking include reduction of the analgesic effects of propoxyphene, reduced diuretic response to frusemide, change in the pharmacological effect of propranolol and altered responder rates in ulcer healing with H_2-antagonists.

Smoking and nicotine may raise the blood levels of cortisol and catecholamines. Dose adjustment of nifedipine, adrenergic agonists or adrenergic antagonists may be necessary.

Increased subcutaneous absorption of insulin which occurs upon smoking cessation may necessitate a reduction in insulin dose.

Pregnancy and lactation: In common with medical advice on stopping smoking in these situations, Nicotinell gum is contra-indicated in pregnant women and during breast feeding.

Reproductive toxicity studies with nicotine in several animal studies have demonstrated non-specific retardation of foetal growth. Studies in rats produced evidence of decreased fertility, prolonged pregnancy, and behavioural disorders in the offspring. In mice the offspring of animals exposed to very high doses of nicotine showed skeletal defects in the peripheral parts of the limbs.

Overall, there are no clear cut grounds for believing that nicotine at the concentrations reached by treatment with nicotine gum has any teratogenic potential and/or inhibitory effects on fertility.

Effects on ability to drive and use machines: Smoking cessation can cause behavioural changes. There is no evidence of any risks associated with driving or operating machinery when the gum is used following the recommended dose.

Undesirable effects: In principle, Nicotinell gum can cause adverse reactions similar to those associated with nicotine administered by smoking.

Nicotine from gum may sometimes cause a slight irritation of the throat and increase salivation at the start of treatment. Excessive swallowing of dissolved nicotine may, at first, cause hiccuping. Those with a tendency to indigestion may suffer initially from minor indigestion or heartburn. Slower chewing will usually overcome this problem. Excessive consumption of gum by subjects who have not been in the habit of inhaling tobacco smoke could possibly lead to nausea, faintness or headaches.

Overdose: In overdose, symptoms corresponding to heavy smoking may be seen.

The acute lethal oral dose of nicotine is about 0.5–0.75 mg per kg bodyweight, corresponding in an adult to 40–60 mg. Even small quantities of nicotine are dangerous in children, and may result in severe symptoms of poisoning which may prove fatal. If poisoning is suspected in a child, a doctor must be consulted immediately.

Overdose with Nicotinell gum may only occur if many pieces are chewed simultaneously. Risk of overdose is small as nausea or vomiting usually occurs at an early stage. Risk of poisoning by swallowing the gum is small. Since the release of nicotine from the gum is slow, very little nicotine is absorbed from the stomach and intestine, and if any is, it will be inactivated in the liver.

General symptoms of nicotine poisoning include: weakness, perspiration, salivation, throat burn, nausea, vomiting, diarrhoea, abdominal pain, hearing and visual disturbances, headache, tachycardia and cardiac arrhythmia, dyspnoea, prostration, circulatory collapse, coma and terminal convulsions.

Treatment of overdosage: In the event of overdosage, vomiting should be induced with syrup of ipecacuanha or gastric lavage carried out (wide bore tube). A suspension of activated charcoal should then be passed through the tube and left in the stomach. Artificial respiration with oxygen should be instituted if needed and continued for as long as necessary. Other therapy, including treatment of shock, is purely symptomatic.

Pharmacological properties

Pharmacodynamic properties: Nicotine gum mimics the pharmacological effects of nicotine from smoking, and may therefore be used to help provide relief from nicotine withdrawal symptoms. In addition to effects on the central nervous system, nicotine produces haemodynamic effects such as increased heart rate and systolic blood pressure.

Pharmacokinetic properties: When the gum is chewed, nicotine is steadily released into the mouth and is rapidly absorbed through the buccal mucosa. A proportion, by the swallowing of nicotine containing saliva, reaches the stomach and intestine where it is inactivated.

The peak plasma concentration of the 2 mg gum after a single dose is approximately 4.8 nanograms per ml and following steady state administration is approximately 14 nanograms per ml (average plasma concentration of nicotine when smoking a cigarette is 15–30 nanograms per ml). For a chewing gum of 4 mg it has been calculated that a maximum plasma concentration of approximately 10 ng/ml is reached after approximately 30 minutes.

Nicotine is eliminated mainly via hepatic metabolism; small amounts of nicotine are eliminated in unchanged form via the kidneys. The plasma half-life is approximately three hours. Nicotine crosses the blood-brain barrier, the placenta and is detectable in breast milk.

Pre-clinical safety data: No animal studies have been undertaken on Nicotinell Chewing Gum.

The toxicity of nicotine as a constituent of tobacco has been well documented. Acute toxic effects include convulsions, cardiac insufficiency, and paralysis of the respiratory system.

At high doses in cats and dogs, nicotine has been shown to potentiate histamine-induced peptic ulcer.

Nicotine has no genotoxic activity in most of the mutagenicity test systems. The well-known carcinogenicity of tobacco smoking is mainly caused by pyrolysis products. Application of nicotine chewing gum, however, avoids the high temperature required for the formation of these carcinogenic products.

All excipients used in Nicotinell Chewing Gum are of food grade.

Pharmaceutical particulars

List of excipients: Gum base, calcium carbonate, sorbitol, glycerin, sodium carbonate, sodium bicarbonate, amberlite, menthol, butylated hydroxytoluene, acesulfame potassium, saccharin, sodium saccharin, talc, carnauba wax.

Nicotinell Fruit 4 mg contains fruit flavouring and Nicotinell Mint 4 mg contains peppermint and eucalyptus.

Nicotinell gum is sugar-free.

Incompatibilities: Not applicable.

Shelf life: 18 months.

Special precautions for storage: Store below 25°C.

Nature and contents of container: The chewing gum is packed in PVC/aluminium blister packs each containing 12 pieces of gum. The blisters are packed in boxes containing 12 and 48 pieces of gum.

Instructions for use/handling: Medicines should be kept out of the reach of children.

Marketing authorisation numbers
0030/0111 Nicotinell Fruit 4 mg.
0030/0113 Nicotinell Mint 4 mg.

Date of (partial) revision of the text 18 June 1998.

Legal category P.

NICOTINELL* FRUIT 2 mg/ NICOTINELL* MINT 2 mg

Qualitative and quantitative composition Nicotine 2 mg per gum, in a resin complex, available in a fruit or mint flavour.

Pharmaceutical form Chewing gum.

Clinical particulars

Therapeutic indications: Nicotinell treatment is indicated for the relief of nicotine withdrawal symptoms, in nicotine dependency as an aid to smoking cessation.

Posology and method of administration:

Adults and elderly: Users should stop smoking completely during treatment with Nicotinell gum. One piece of Nicotinell gum to be chewed when the user feels the urge to smoke.

Normally, 8–12 pieces per day, up to a maximum of 25 pieces per day.

The characteristics of chewing gum as a pharmaceutical form are such that individually different nicotine levels can result in the blood. Therefore, dosage frequency should be adjusted according to individual requirements within the stated maximum limit.

Directions for use:

1. One piece of gum should be chewed until the taste becomes strong.
2. The chewing gum should be rested between the gum and cheek.
3. When the taste fades, chewing should commence again.
4. The chewing routine should be repeated for 30 minutes.

After three months, the user should gradually cut down the number of pieces chewed each day until they have stopped using the product.

Children: Not to be used by children.

Concomitant use of acidic beverages such as coffee or soda may interfere with the buccal absorption of nicotine. Acidic beverages should be avoided for 15 minutes prior to chewing the gum.

Contra-indications: Nicotinell gum should not be used by non-smokers, or people under 18 years of age. Furthermore, people should not use the gum and smoke concomitantly.

Use is contra-indicated during pregnancy and lactation, acute myocardial infarction, unstable or worsening angina pectoris, severe cardiac arrhythmias, and recent cerebrovascular accident.

Special warnings and precautions for use: Swallowed nicotine may exacerbate symptoms in subjects suffering from active oesophagitis, oral or pharyngeal inflammation, gastritis or peptic ulcer.

Use with caution in patients with hypertension, stable angina pectoris, cerebrovascular disease, occlusive peripheral arterial disease, heart failure, hyperthyroidism, diabetes mellitus, and renal or hepatic impairment.

Counselling may help smokers to quit.

Doses of nicotine that are tolerated by adult smokers during treatment may produce severe symptoms of poisoning in small children and may prove fatal (please see *Overdose*).

Interactions with other medicaments and other forms of interaction:

Drug interactions: No information is available on interactions between Nicotinell gum and other drugs.

Smoking cessation: This is different in the case of smoking where interactions with other medications may occur due to a multitude of other substances contained in the smoke. Presumably due to the polycyclic aromatic hydrocarbons contained in the smoke, the metabolism of different medicinal products may be speeded up by enzyme induction: e.g. caffeine, theophylline, paracetamol, phenazone, phenylbutazone, pentazocine, lidocaine, benzodiazepines, imipramine, warfarin, oestrogen and vitamin B12.

Upon smoking cessation it may be expected that the hitherto increased metabolism of these medicinal products is slowed down or normalised. Unaltered dosage of the products may result in an increase in their blood concentration.

Therefore when prescribing Nicotinell a possible dose adjustment should be considered in patients treated with the above mentioned medicinal products.

Other reported effects of smoking include a reduction of the analgesic effects of propoxyphene, reduced diuretic response to frusemide, change in the pharmacological effect of propranolol and altered responder rates in ulcer healing with H_2-antagonists.

Smoking and nicotine may raise the blood levels of cortisol and catecholamines. Dose adjustment of nifedipine, adrenergic agonists or adrenergic antagonists may be necessary.

Increased subcutaneous absorption of insulin which occurs upon smoking cessation may necessitate a reduction in insulin dose.

Pregnancy and lactation: In common with medical advice on stopping smoking in these situations, Nicotinell gum is contra-indicated in pregnant women and during breast feeding.

Reproductive toxicity studies with nicotine in several animal studies have demonstrated non-specific retardation of foetal growth. Studies in rats produced evidence of decreased fertility, prolonged pregnancy, and behavioural disorders in the offspring. In mice the offspring of animals exposed to very high doses of nicotine showed skeletal defects in the peripheral parts of the limbs.

Overall, there are no clear cut grounds for believing that nicotine at the concentrations reached by treatment with nicotine gum has any teratogenic potential and/or inhibitory effects on fertility.

Effects on ability to drive and use machines: Smoking cessation can cause behavioural changes. There is no evidence of any risks associated with driving or operating machinery when the gum is used following the recommended dose.

Undesirable effects: In principle, Nicotinell gum can cause adverse reactions similar to those associated with nicotine administered by smoking.

Nicotine from gum may sometimes cause a slight irritation of the throat and increase salivation at the start of treatment. Excessive swallowing of dissolved nicotine may, at first, cause hiccuping. Those with a tendency to indigestion may suffer initially from minor indigestion or heartburn. Slower chewing will usually overcome this problem. Excessive consumption of gum by subjects who have not been in the habit of inhaling tobacco smoke could possibly lead to nausea, faintness or headaches.

Overdose: In overdose, symptoms corresponding to heavy smoking may be seen.

The acute lethal oral dose of nicotine is about 0.5–0.75 mg per kg bodyweight, corresponding in an adult of 40–60 mg. Even small quantities of nicotine are dangerous in children, and may result in severe symptoms of poisoning which may prove fatal. If poisoning is suspected in a child, a doctor must be consulted immediately.

Overdose with Nicotinell gum may only occur if many pieces are chewed simultaneously. Risk of overdose is small as nausea or vomiting usually occurs at an early stage. Risk of poisoning by swallowing the gum is small. Since the release of nicotine from the gum is slow, very little nicotine is absorbed from the stomach and intestine, and if any is, it will be inactivated in the liver.

General symptoms of nicotine poisoning include: weakness, perspiration, salivation, throat burn, nausea, vomiting, diarrhoea, abdominal pain, hearing and visual disturbances, headache, tachycardia and cardiac arrhythmia, dyspnoea, prostration, circulatory collapse, coma and terminal convulsions.

Treatment of overdosage: In the event of overdosage, vomiting should be induced with syrup of ipecacuanha or gastric lavage carried out (wide bore tube). A suspension of activated charcoal should then be passed through the tube and left in the stomach. Artificial respiration with oxygen should be instituted if needed and continued for as long as necessary. Other therapy, including treatment of shock, is purely symptomatic.

Pharmacological properties

Pharmacodynamic properties: Nicotine gum mimics the pharmacological effects of nicotine from smoking, and may therefore be used to help provide relief from nicotine withdrawal symptoms. In addition to effects on the central nervous system, nicotine produces haemodynamic effects such as increased heart rate and systolic blood pressure.

Pharmacokinetic properties: When the gum is chewed, nicotine is steadily released into the mouth and is rapidly absorbed through the buccal mucosa. A proportion, by the swallowing of nicotine containing saliva, reaches the stomach and intestine where it is inactivated.

The peak plasma concentration of the 2 mg gum after a single dose is approximately 4.8 nanograms per ml and following steady state administration is approximately 14 nanograms per ml (average plasma concentration of nicotine when smoking a cigarette is 15–30 nanograms per ml). For a chewing gum of 4 mg it has been calculated that a maximum plasma concentration of approximately 10 ng/ml is reached after approximately 30 minutes.

Nicotine is eliminated mainly via hepatic metabolism; small amounts of nicotine are eliminated in unchanged form via the kidneys. The plasma half-life is approximately three hours. Nicotine crosses the blood-brain barrier, the placenta and is detectable in breast milk.

Pre-clinical safety data: No animal studies have been undertaken on Nicotinell Chewing Gum.

The toxicity of nicotine as a constituent of tobacco has been well documented. Acute toxic effects include convulsions, cardiac insufficiency, and paralysis of the respiratory system.

At high doses in cats and dogs, nicotine has been shown to potentiate histamine-induced peptic ulcer.

Nicotine has no genotoxic activity in most of the mutagenicity test systems. The well-known carcinogenicity of tobacco smoking is mainly caused by pyrolysis products. Application of nicotine chewing gum, however, avoids the high temperature required for the formation of these carcinogenic products.

All excipients used in Nicotinell Chewing Gum are of food grade.

Pharmaceutical particulars

List of excipients: Gum base, calcium carbonate, sorbitol, glycerin, sodium carbonate, sodium bicarbonate, amberlite, menthol, butylated hydroxytoluene, acesulfame potassium, saccharin, sodium saccharin, talc, carnauba wax.

Nicotinell Fruit 2 mg contains fruit flavouring and Nicotinell Mint 2 mg contains peppermint and eucalyptus.

Nicotinell gum is sugar-free.

Incompatibilities: Not applicable.

Shelf life: 2 years.

Special precautions for storage: Store below 25°C.

Nature and contents of container: The chewing gum is packed in PVC/aluminium blister packs each containing 12 pieces of gum. The blisters are packed in boxes containing 12, 48 and 96 pieces of gum.

Instructions for use/handling: Medicines should be kept out of the reach of children.

Marketing authorisation numbers
0030/0110 (Nicotinell Fruit 2 mg).
0030/0112 (Nicotinell Mint 2 mg).

Date of (partial) revision of the text 18 June 1998.

Legal category P.

NICOTINELL TTS* 10
NICOTINELL TTS* 20
NICOTINELL TTS* 30

Qualitative and quantitative composition Each Nicotinell TTS 10 patch contains S(-)-nicotine 17.5 mg; each Nicotinell TTS 20 patch contains S(-)-nicotine 35 mg; each Nicotinell TTS 30 patch contains S(-)-nicotine 52.5 mg.

Pharmaceutical form Transdermal patch.

Nicotinell is a transdermal therapeutic system, consisting of a round, flat, matrix-type self-adhesive, yellowish-ochre coloured patch. It is protected by a rectangular metallic release liner backing to be discarded before application.

Nicotinell TTS 10 has a drug releasing area of 10 cm^2 and is printed CG CWC on the patch surface. Nicotinell TTS 20 has a drug releasing area of 20 cm^2 and is printed CG FEF on the patch surface. Nicotinell TTS 30 has a drug releasing area of 30 cm^2 and is printed CG EME on the patch surface.

Clinical particulars

Therapeutic indications: The treatment of nicotine dependence, as an aid to smoking cessation.

Route of administration: Transdermal.

Posology and method of administration:

Adults: Users should stop smoking completely during treatment with Nicotinell TTS.

For individuals smoking 20 cigarettes or more a day, it is recommended that treatment be started with Nicotinell TTS 30 once daily, applied to a dry non-hairy area of the skin on the trunk or upper arm. Those smoking less than this are recommended to start with Nicotinell TTS 20.

Sizes of 30 cm^2, 20 cm^2 and 10 cm^2 are available to permit gradual withdrawal of nicotine replacement, using treatment periods of 3–4 weeks (for each size). The size of patch may be adjusted according to individual response, maintaining or increasing the dose if abstinence is not achieved or if withdrawal symptoms are experienced. Total treatment periods of more than 3 months and daily doses above 30 cm^2 have not been evaluated. The treatment is designed to be used continuously for 3 months but not beyond. However, if abstinence is not achieved at the end of the 3 month treatment period, further treatments may be recommended following a re-evaluation of the patient's motivation by the doctor.

The dosage must not be adjusted by cutting a patch.

Nicotinell TTS should be used as soon as it has been removed from the child-resistant pouch. Following removal of the metallic backing, the Nicotinell TTS patch should be applied to the skin and held in position for 10–20 seconds with the palm of the hand. Each patch should be removed after 24 hours and disposed of safely (see 'Warnings'). A different site of application should be chosen each day and several days should be allowed to elapse before a new patch is applied to the same area of skin.

Children: Safety and efficacy in individuals under 18 years of age have not been established. Nicotinell TTS is contra-indicated in children.

Elderly: Experience in the use of Nicotinell TTS in smokers over the age of 65 years is limited. Nicotinell TTS does not appear to pose safety problems in this age group.

Potential for abuse and dependence: Transdermal nicotine is likely to have a very low abuse potential because of its slow onset of action, low fluctuations in blood concentrations, inability to produce high blood concentrations of nicotine, and the infrequent (once daily) use. Moreover, gradual weaning from Nicotinell TTS is instituted within the treatment schedule, and the risk of dependence after therapy is minimal. The effects of abrupt withdrawal from Nicotinell TTS are likely to be similar to those observed with tobacco withdrawal from comparable nicotine concentrations.

Contra-indications: Nicotinell TTS should not be administered to non-smokers, occasional smokers or children. The system is also contra-indicated during pregnancy and breast-feeding (see 'Use in Pregnancy and Lactation'), and in acute myocardial infarction, unstable or worsening angina pectoris, severe cardiac arrhythmias, recent cerebrovascular accident, diseases of the skin which may complicate patch therapy, and known hypersensitivity to nicotine or any of the components of the patch.

Special warnings and precautions for use
Warnings: Nicotine is a toxic drug and milligram doses are potentially fatal if rapidly absorbed. Treatment with Nicotinell TTS should be discontinued if symptoms of nicotine overdosage appear. Mild intoxication produces nausea, vomiting, abdominal pain, diarrhoea, headache, sweating and pallor (see 'Overdosage').

Doses of nicotine that are tolerated by adult smokers during treatment can produce severe symptoms of poisoning in small children and may prove fatal. Both before and after use, Nicotinell TTS contains a significant amount of nicotine. Subjects must be cautioned that the patches must not be handled casually or left where they might be inadvertently misused or consumed by children. Used patches must be disposed of with care by folding them in half with the adhesive sides inwards, and ensuring that they do not fall into the hands of children under any circumstances.

Precautions: Users should stop smoking completely during therapy with Nicotinell TTS. They should be informed that if they continue to smoke while using Nicotinell TTS, they may experience increased adverse effects due to the hazards of smoking, including cardiovascular effects.

In subjects with the conditions listed below, Nicotinell TTS should only be used following a careful risk-benefit assessment, and only in cases where subjects have found it impossible to stop smoking without use of Nicotinell TTS: hypertension, stable angina pectoris, cerebrovascular disease, occlusive peripheral arterial disease, heart failure, hyperthyroidism, diabetes mellitus, renal or hepatic impairment and peptic ulcer.

Discontinuation of treatment may be advisable in cases of severe or persistent skin reactions.

Contact sensitisation was reported in a few patients using transdermal nicotine in clinical trials. Patients who develop contact sensitisation to nicotine should be cautioned that a severe reaction could occur from smoking or exposure to other nicotine containing products.

Interactions with other medicaments and other forms of interaction: No information is available on interactions between Nicotinell TTS and other drugs.

Cessation of smoking, with or without nicotine replacement, may alter the individual's response to concomitant medication and may require adjustment of dose. Smoking is thought to increase the metabolism through enzyme induction and thus to lower the blood concentrations of drugs such as antipyrine, caffeine, oestrogens, desmethyldiazepam, imipramine, lignocaine, oxazepam, pentazocine, phenacetin, theophylline, and warfarin. Cessation of smoking may result in increased concentrations of these drugs.

Other reported effects of smoking include reduced analgesic efficacy of propoxyphene, reduced diuretic response to frusemide and reduced pharmacological response to propranolol, as well as reduced rates of ulcer healing with H_2-antagonists.

Both smoking and nicotine can increase levels of circulating cortisol and catecholamines. Dosages of nifedipine, adrenergic agonists, or adrenergic blocking agents may need to be adjusted.

Pregnancy and lactation: In common with medical advice on stopping smoking in these situations, Nicotinell TTS is contra-indicated in pregnant women and during breast-feeding.

Teratogenicity studies with nicotine in several animal species have demonstrated non-specific retardation of foetal growth. Studies in pregnant rats have indicated the presence of behavioural disorders in the offspring, and in the mouse the unborn offspring of animals treated with approximately 120 times the human transdermal dose showed skeletal defects in the peripheral parts of the limbs. Embryo implantation in rats and rabbits may be inhibited or delayed by nicotine. Overall, there are no clear cut grounds for believing that nicotine at the concentrations reached by treatment with Nicotinell TTS has any teratogenic potential and/or inhibitory effects on fertility.

Effects on ability to drive and use machines: When Nicotinell TTS is used as recommended, there are minimal risks for driving vehicles or operating machinery.

Undesirable effects: In principle, Nicotinell TTS can cause adverse reactions similar to those associated with nicotine administered by smoking. Since the maximum plasma concentrations of nicotine that are produced by Nicotinell TTS are lower than those produced by smoking and fluctuate less, nicotine-related adverse reactions occurring during treatment with Nicotinell TTS can be expected to be less marked than during smoking.

Some of the symptoms listed below are hard to differentiate from recognised tobacco withdrawal symptoms when comparison with placebo is made. The placebo used contained about 13% of the nicotine of a matching Nicotinell TTS (to match colour and odour for blinding purposes).

The main unwanted effect of Nicotinell TTS is application site reaction. This led to premature discontinuation of Nicotinell TTS in about 6% of clinical trial participants. Skin reactions consisted of erythema or pruritus at the patch site.

Oedema, burning sensation, blisters, rash, or pinching sensation at the application site were also noted. The majority of these reactions were mild. Most of the skin reactions resolved within 48 hours, but in more severe cases the erythema and infiltration lasted from 1 to 3 weeks. The time of onset of important skin reactions was between 3 and 8 weeks from the start of therapy. In isolated cases the skin reactions extended beyond the application sites. Isolated cases of urticaria, angioneurotic oedema and dyspnoea were reported.

The following are the adverse events/withdrawal symptoms most commonly reported in three double-blind clinical trials *irrespective of causal association to study drug.*

	Nicotinell TTS (N=401)	*Placebo (N=391)*
Application site reaction	34.9%	17.6%
Headache	29.7%	29.2%
Cold and flu-like symptoms	12.0%	8.4%
Dysmenorrhoea (% of female subjects)	6.6%	8.8%
Insomnia	6.5%	5.4%
Nausea	6.2%	4.6%
Myalgia	6.0%	4.1%
Dizziness	6.0%	5.9%

Other unwanted experiences reported (irrespective of causal association with Nicotinell TTS) with an incidence of 1%–5.9% and more frequently than placebo, included: abdominal pain, vomiting, dyspepsia, allergy, motor dysfunction, chest pain, vivid dreams, blood pressure changes, generalised rash, somnolence, impaired concentration and fatigue.

Overdose: The toxicity of nicotine cannot be directly compared with that of smoking, because tobacco smoke contains additional toxic substances (e.g. carbon monoxide and tar).

Chronic smokers can tolerate doses of nicotine that, in a non-smoker, would be more toxic, because of the development of tolerance.

Application of several Nicotinell TTS patches could result in serious overdosage. Slower absorption after cutaneous exposure to nicotine favours the development of tolerance to toxic effects.

Rapid systemic delivery of nicotine from Nicotinell TTS would not be expected on chewing and swallowing, owing to the slow release of nicotine from the patch and first-pass metabolism.

Acute toxic effects: Signs and symptoms of overdosage would be the same as those of acute nicotine poisoning. In non-smoking children and adults, these include pallor, sweating, nausea, salivation, vomiting, abdominal cramps, diarrhoea, headache, dizziness, hearing and vision disturbances, tremor, mental confusion, muscle weakness, convulsions, prostration, absence of neurological reaction, and respiratory failure. Lethal doses may produce convulsions, and death follows as a result of peripheral or central respiratory paralysis, or, less frequently, cardiac failure.

The acute lethal oral dose of nicotine in non-smoking adults is approximately 60 mg.

Management: If the patient shows signs of overdosage, Nicotinell TTS should be removed immediately. The skin surface may be washed with water and dried (no soap should be used). The skin will continue to deliver nicotine into the blood stream for several hours after removal of the system, possibly because of a depot of nicotine in the skin.

Other treatment measures for acute nicotine poisoning include artificial respiration in the case of respiratory paralysis, maintaining normal body temperature, and treatment for hypotension and cardiovascular collapse.

Each Nicotinell TTS patch is sealed in a child-resistant sachet and the product must be kept out of the reach of children at all times (see 'Warnings'). Even doses of nicotine which are tolerated by adults during treatment with Nicotinell TTS could produce severe symptoms of poisoning in small children following accidental application, and may prove fatal.

Pharmacological properties

Pharmacodynamic properties: S(-)-nicotine is the most pharmacologically active form of nicotine, the major alkaloid of tobacco. S(-)-nicotine acts primarily on cholinergic receptors of the nicotinic type in the peripheral and central nervous system.

For many effects, low doses of S(-)-nicotine have a stimulant action, and high doses a depressant effect. Intermittent administration of S(-)-nicotine affects neurohormonal pathways, and results in the release of acetylcholine, noradrenaline, dopamine, serotonin, vasopressin, beta-endorphin, growth hormone, cortisol and ACTH. These neuroregulators may be involved in the reported behavioural and subjective effects of smoking.

Nicotine replacement is an established therapy as an aid to smoking cessation. Nicotinell TTS provides for a convenient once daily administration by exploiting the fact that S(-)-nicotine is readily absorbed through the skin into the systemic circulation. Placebo-controlled, double-blind studies have shown that nicotine replacement with Nicotinell TTS produces smoking abstinence rates statistically significantly better than placebo, with or without group support. There was also a strong trend towards reduction of withdrawal symptoms.

Application of Nicotinell TTS 20 to smokers abstinent overnight resulted in small increases in mean heart rate and systolic blood pressure and a decrease in stroke volume. The effects were smaller in magnitude than those produced by cigarette smoking.

Pharmacokinetic properties: Following single application of Nicotinell TTS to the skin of healthy abstinent smokers there is an initial 1–2 hours delay followed by a progressive rise in nicotine plasma concentrations, with a plateau attained at about 8–10 hours after application.

In the majority of subjects the area under the plasma concentration curve (AUC 0–24 hours) varies approximately in proportion to the drug releasing area of the patch. Nicotinell TTS is designed to deliver approximately 0.7 mg/cm²/24 hours. In comparison with an i.v. infusion, 76.8% of the nicotine released from Nicotinell TTS is systemically available. Steady state plasma concentrations after repeated daily administration are within the range observed during moderate cigarette smoking.

Absorption of nicotine over 24 hours varies by a factor of two between different individuals; however within-individual variability is small indicating consistent performance of the transdermal system.

S(-)-nicotine is distributed widely in the body with a volume of distribution of approximately 180 litres. It crosses the blood-brain barrier, placenta and is detectable in breast milk. Plasma protein binding is only 5%. Total plasma clearance of nicotine ranges from 0.92 to 2.43 litres/min. It is eliminated mainly via hepatic metabolism. Only small amounts of nicotine are eliminated in unchanged form via the kidneys, a process which is pH dependent, being negligible under alkaline conditions.

Preclinical safety data: No additional data.

Pharmaceutical particulars

List of excipients:
- Pad
- Polyester film
- Acrylate esters vinylacetate co-polymers
- Fractionated coconut oil
- Methacrylic acid esters co-polymers.

Incompatibilities: None known.

Shelf life: 24 months.

Special precautions for storage: Store below 25°C.

Nature and contents of container: Heat-seal paper/aluminium/polyamide/polyacrylnitrile pouches (child-resistant) enclosed in a cardboard carton.

Pack sizes:
Nicotinell TTS 10, 20: 7 patches.
Nicotinell TTS 30: 7 and 21 patches.

Instructions for use/handling: Keep all medicines out of the reach of children.

Marketing authorisation numbers

Nicotinell TTS 10: 00030/0107
Nicotinell TTS 20: 00030/0108
Nicotinell TTS 30: 00030/0109

Date of (partial) revision of the text 22 September 1997.

Legal category P.

OTRIVINE*

Presentation Clear, colourless, odourless solutions, Otrivine Adult Formula Nasal Drops and Spray contain 0.1% w/v Xylometazoline Hydrochloride BP. Otrivine Children's Formula Nasal Drops contain 0.05% w/v Xylometazoline Hydrochloride BP. Otrivine also contains sodium acid phosphate, sodium phosphate, sodium chloride, disodium edetate, benzalkonium chloride, and purified water.

Uses
Mode of action: Otrivine is a sympathomimetic agent with marked alpha-adrenergic activity, and is intended for use in the nose. It constricts the nasal blood vessels, thereby decongesting the mucosa of the nose and neighbouring regions of the pharynx. This enables patients suffering from colds to breathe more easily through the nose. The effect of Otrivine begins within a few minutes and persists for several hours. Otrivine is generally well tolerated and does not impair the function of ciliated epithelium.

Pharmacokinetics: Systemic absorption may occur following nasal application of xylometazoline hydrochloride solutions. It is not used systemically.

Indications: For the symptomatic relief of nasal congestion, perennial and allergic rhinitis (including hay fever), sinusitis.

Dosage and administration
Adults: 2 or 3 drops of Otrivine Adult Formula Nasal Drops or one application of Otrivine Formula Nasal Spray in each nostril, two or three times daily.

N.B. The Otrivine Adult Formula Nasal Drops and Spray should not be used for children under the age of 12 years.

Children under 12: 1 or 2 drops of the Otrivine Children's Formula Nasal Drops in each nostril once or twice daily. Not to be used in infants less than 3 months.

Contra-indications, warnings, etc
Contra-indications: Patients with trans-sphenoidal hypophysectomy or surgery exposing the dura mater. Known hypersensitivity to Otrivine.

Warnings: Each Otrvine pack should be used by one person only to prevent any cross-infection.

Precautions: Patients are advised not to take decongestants for more than seven consecutive days. Otrivine, like other preparations belonging to the same class of active substances, should be used only with caution in patients showing a strong reaction to sympathomimetic agents as evidenced by signs of insomnia, dizziness, etc.

Side-effects: The following side-effects have occasionally been encountered: a burning sensation in the nose and throat, local irritation, nausea, headache, and dryness of the nasal mucosa. Systemic cardiovascular effects have occurred, and this should be kept in mind when giving Otrivine to people with cardiovascular disease.

Pregnancy and lactation: No foetal toxicity or fertility studies have been carried out in animals. In view of its potential systemic vasoconstrictor effect, it is advisable to take the precaution of not using Otrivine during pregnancy.

Drug interactions: No drug interactions have been reported.

Overdosage: No cases of overdosage in adults have yet been reported. In rare instances of accidental poisoning in children, the clinical picture has been marked chiefly by signs such as acceleration and irregularity of the pulse, elevated blood pressure, drowsiness, respiratory depression or irregularity. There is no specific treatment and appropriate supportive treatment should be initiated.

Pharmaceutical precautions Protect from heat. For reasons of hygiene, do not use the bottle more than 28 days after opening it.

Package quantities
Otrivine Adult Formula Nasal Drops 10 ml (OP).
Otrivine Adult Formula Nasal Spray 10 ml (OP).
Otrivine Children's Formula Nasal Drops 10 ml (OP).

Further information May be prescribed under the NHS Pharmaceutical Services as Xylometazoline Hydrochloride.

Product licence numbers

Otrivine Adult Formula Nasal Drops	0030/0115
Otrivine Adult Formula Nasal Spray	0030/0116
Otrivine Children's Formula Nasal Drops	0030/0114

Legal category GSL.

PAROVEN* CAPSULES

Qualitative and quantitative composition Oxerutins 250 mg.

Pharmaceutical form Capsules.

Clinical particulars
Therapeutic indications: Relief of symptoms of oedema associated with chronic venous insufficiency.

Posology and method of administration:
Adults and elderly: 2 capsules (500 mg) twice daily.
Children: not recommended for children under 12 years.

Contra-indications: Hypersensitivity to any of the ingredients.

Special warnings and special precautions for use: Treatment of leg oedema due to cardiac, renal or hepatic disease should be directed to the underlying cause; Paroven should not be used in these conditions. If leg pain and swelling do not improve, or get worse, the patient should consult their doctor.

Interactions with other medicaments and other forms of interaction: None reported. Oxerutins have been shown not to interact with warfarin anticoagulants.

Pregnancy and lactation: Clinical trials and animal studies have shown no increase in teratogenic (or other) hazard to the foetus if used in the recommended dosage during pregnancy. However, in keeping with current medical opinion, Paroven should not be used during the first trimester of pregnancy.

In animal studies traces of oxerutins and/or their metabolites have been found in breast milk, but the levels are not considered to be of clinical relevance. The use of Paroven in lactating women is therefore at the physician's discretion.

Effect on ability to drive and use machines: None known.

Undesirable effects: Occasionally, mild adverse reactions (skin allergies, minor gastrointestinal disturbances, headaches and flushes) have been reported. They disappear rapidly on stopping treatment.

Overdose: No cases of overdosage with symptoms have been reported. No specific antidotes are known.

Pharmacological properties
Pharmacodynamic properties: Oxerutins has uniquely useful therapeutic actions in the microcirculation and particularly in the post-capillary venous segment. Oxerutins reduces capillary leakage and hence oedema formation.

Pharmacokinetic properties: Not all conventional pharmacokinetic parameters are available due to technical difficulties. Oxerutins is absorbed from the gastrointestinal tract of mammals. Its metabolism is, in part, determined by the degree of hydroxyethylation of the aromatic ring systems of the constituent rutoside derivatives. Biliary excretion plays a major role in elimination in the animal species studied. It is, however, not clear if this route of elimination is equally important in man since quantitative data in humans are not available. The same applies to enterohepatic recycling.

Preclinical safety data: Not applicable.

Pharmaceutical particulars
List of excipients: Polyethylene glycol, gelatin, titanium dioxide E171, yellow iron oxide E172, black iron oxide E172.

Incompatibilities: None.

Shelf life: 60 months.

Special precautions for storage: Protect from moisture.

Nature and contents of container: Blister pack composed of PVC blisters sealed with aluminium foil. Pack sizes: 120 capsules.

Instructions for use/handling: Medicines should be kept out of the reach of children.

Marketing authorisation number 0030/5002R.

Date of approval/revision of SPC July 1997.

Legal category P.

PROFLEX* CREAM

Qualitative and quantitative composition Ibuprofen BP 5% w/w.

Pharmaceutical form Cream.

Clinical particulars
Therapeutic indications: Topical analgesic and anti-inflammatory treatment for the fast relief of the symptoms of rheumatic pain, muscular aches and pains, backache, lumbago, fibrositis, pains or swellings such as strains, sprains, and sports injuries.

Route of administration: Topical.

Posology and method of administration:
Adults and elderly: 4–10 cm (1½–4 inches) of cream (50–125 mg ibuprofen) 3–4 times daily, massaged into the skin over a large area at the affected site.

A period of at least 4 hours should be left between each application.

Children: Not recommended for children under 12 years.

Contra-indications: Hypersensitivity to any of the constituents. Hypersensitivity to aspirin or other non-steroidal anti-inflammatory drugs including provocation or exacerbation of asthma, rhinitis, or urticaria.

Special warnings and precautions for use: Keep away from inflamed or broken skin, lips and near the eyes. Discontinue if rash develops. Wash hands after use.

Interactions with other medicaments and other forms of interaction: Concurrent aspirin or other NSAIDs may result in an increased incidence of adverse reactions.

Pregnancy and lactation: Whilst no teratogenic effects have been demonstrated in animal experiments, ibuprofen should be avoided during pregnancy. The onset of labour may be delayed and duration of labour may be increased. Ibuprofen appears in breast milk in very low concentration and is unlikely to affect the breast-fed infant adversely.

Effect on ability to drive and use machines: Proflex Cream will not impair the ability to drive and the ability to use machines.

Undesirable effects: Skin reactions are most frequently reported.
Skin: Application site reactions, rashes, pruritus, urticaria.
Gastro-intestinal: Abdominal pain, dyspepsia.
Respiratory: Bronchospasm may be precipitated in patients suffering from or with a previous history of bronchial asthma or allergic disease.

Overdose: Overdosage with a topical presentation of ibuprofen is unlikely. Symptoms of ibuprofen overdose include headache, vomiting, drowsiness and hypotension. Correction of severe electrolyte abnormalities should be considered.

Pharmacological properties
Pharmacodynamic properties: Ibuprofen is a phenylpropionic acid derivative which has analgesic anti-inflammatory and anti-pyretic actions.

Pharmacokinetic properties: Percutaneous absorption approximately 5% that of oral ibuprofen.
C_{max}=0.64 mcg/ml (higher concentrations achieved locally)
T_{max}=2.00 h

Preclinical safety data: Not applicable.

Pharmaceutical particulars
List of excipients: Fractionated coconut oil; Arlacel 165 (glyceryl stearate); Arlatone 983S (polyoxyethylene fatty acid ester); propylene glycol; sodium methyl hydroxybenzoate; Keltrol F (xanthan gum); purified water.

Incompatibilities: None stated.

Shelf life: 36 months.

Special precautions for storage: Store in a cool place.

Nature and contents of container: Internally lacquered aluminium tube. Contents 100 g.

Instructions for use/handling: Keep all medicines out of the reach of children. For external use only. Wash hands after use.

Marketing authorisation number 0030/0052.

Date of approval/revision of SPC 18 March 1997.

Legal category P.

VIOFORM* HYDROCORTISONE CREAM
VIOFORM* HYDROCORTISONE OINTMENT

Qualitative and quantitative composition Both pharmaceutical forms contain: Clioquinol BP 3% w/w, Hydrocortisone PhEur 1% w/w.

Pharmaceutical form Cream and ointment.

Clinical particulars
Therapeutic indications: Exudative and secondarily infected eczema and dermatitis, including atopic eczema, primary irritant dermatitis, allergic and seborrhoeic dermatitis, infected insect bite reactions, genital or perianal intertrigo.

Posology and method of administration: Vioform-Hydrocortisone is indicated for external application only.

The preparation should be applied sparingly to the affected area, 1–3 times daily. Treatment should be limited to 7 days. Occlusive dressings should not be used.

If there is little improvement after 7 days treatment with Vioform-Hydrocortisone, the appropriate microbiological investigations should be carried out and local or systemic antibiotic treatment given.

Use in the elderly: There is no evidence to suggest that dosage should be different in the elderly.

Use in children: Vioform-Hydrocortisone is contra-indicated in children below the age of two years.

Contra-indications: Hypersensitivity to any component of the formulation or iodine. Primary bacterial, viral or fungal infections of the skin. Secondary infections due to yeasts. Application to ulcerated areas. Use in children below the age of two years.

Special warnings and special precautions for use: Long-term continuous topical therapy should be avoided since this can lead to adrenal suppression even without occlusion.

Application to relatively large and/or eroded areas of skin, use of occlusive dressings, and treatment for longer than one week, should be avoided, because this may lead to a marked increase in protein-bound iodine (PBI). Thyroid function tests such as PBI, radioactive iodine and butanol extractable iodine, may be affected, consequently it is advisable that such tests are not performed within one month of discontinuing treatment. However, other thyroid function tests, such as the T3 resin sponge test or T4 determination are unaffected.

The ferric chloride test for phenylketonuria may yield a false-positive result when clioquinol is present in the urine.

Vioform-Hydrocortisone should be used with caution in patients suffering from hepatic and/or renal failure.

Vioform-Hydrocortisone should not be allowed to come into contact with the conjunctiva.

Interactions with other medicaments and other forms of interaction: None known.

Pregnancy and lactation: There is inadequate evidence of safety in human pregnancy. Topical administration of corticosteroids to pregnant animals can cause abnormalities of foetal development, including cleft palate and intra-uterine growth retardation. There may, therefore, be a very small risk of such effects in the human foetus.

It is not known whether the active substances of Vioform-Hydrocortisone and/or their metabolite(s) pass into the breast milk after topical administration. Use in lactating mothers should only be at the doctor's discretion.

Effects on ability to drive and use machines: None known.

Undesirable effects: Vioform-Hydrocortisone is usually well tolerated but occasionally, at the site of application, there may be signs of irritation, such as a burning sensation, itching or skin rash. Hypersensitivity reactions may also occasionally occur. Treatment should be discontinued if patients experience severe irritation or sensitisation.

Vioform-Hydrocortisone may cause hair discoloration.

Overdose: Vioform-Hydrocortisone is for topical (external) use only. If accidental ingestion of large quantities occurs, there is no specific antidote and general measures to eliminate the drug and reduce its absorption should be undertaken. Symptomatic treatment should be administered as appropriate.

Pharmacological properties

Pharmacodynamic properties: Vioform-Hydrocortisone combines the anti-fungal and anti-bacterial properties of clioquinol with the anti-inflammatory, anti-allergic and anti-pruritic effects of hydrocortisone.

Pharmacokinetic properties: Following topical application of Vioform-Hydrocortisone, clioquinol has been shown to be absorbed to an extent of about 2% to 3%, as judged by the urinary excretion. Clioquinol is excreted in the urine mainly in glucuronide form and to a smaller extent as sulphate, whereas unchanged clioquinol is found in traces only.

Preclinical safety data: Not applicable.

Pharmaceutical particulars

List of excipients:

Cream:	Glycerol
	Sodium lauryl sulphate
	2-Phenoxyethanol
	Cetostearyl alcohol
	Cetyl palmitate
	White soft paraffin
	Purified water
Ointment:	Light liquid paraffin
	Soft white paraffin

Incompatibilities: None.

Shelf life: 60 months.

Special precautions for storage: Protect from heat.

Nature of container and closure: Collapsible aluminium tube.

Pack size: 30 g.

Instructions for use/handling: Medicines should be kept out of the reach of children.

Marketing authorisation numbers

Vioform Hydrocortisone Cream	0030/0050
Vioform Hydrocortisone Ointment	0030/0051

Date of revision of SPC 3 February 1997

Legal category POM.

**Trade Mark*

Novartis Pharmaceuticals UK Ltd
Frimley Business Park
Frimley
Camberley
Surrey GU16 5SG
☎ 01276 698370 🗋 01276 698449

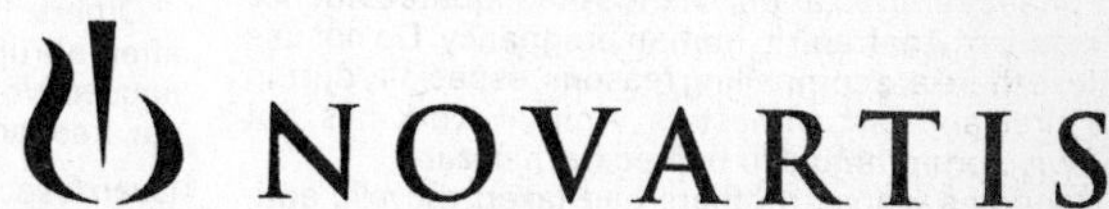

ANAFRANIL AMPOULES

Qualitative and quantitative composition Chemical name: 3-chloro-5-[3-(dimethylamino)-propyl] 10, 11-dihydro-5H-dibenz [b, f] azepine hydrochloride (= clomipramin.hydrochloric).

Each ampoule contains 25 mg clomipramine hydrochloride BP in 2 ml.

Pharmaceutical form Ampoule.

Clinical particulars

Therapeutic indications: Symptoms of depressive illness especially where sedation is required. Obsessional and phobic states. Adjunctive treatment of cataplexy associated with narcolepsy.

Posology and method of administration

Intramuscular administration: Commence with 1–2 ampoules of 25 mg daily, then increase the dosage by 1 ampoule daily until the patient is receiving 4–6 ampoules a day. Once improvement has occurred, the number of injections should be gradually reduced while at the same time switching the patient to oral treatment (maintenance doses).

Intravenous infusion: administration and dosage: Any standard giving set may be used but a cannula or fine needle with a flange which can be strapped in position should be chosen. Anafranil ampoules may be diluted with either physiological saline or 5% Dextrose BP. The required dose of Anafranil should be introduced into the infusion fluid with a sterile syringe and the contents should be agitated to ensure even distribution of the drug before infusion is commenced into a forearm vein.

In the first instance a small dose of Anafranil (25 mg or 50 mg) should be diluted in 250–500 ml of infusion fluid and infused over a period of 1.5–3 hours to assess tolerability. If satisfactory, the dose may be increased by 25 mg daily until an optimum therapeutic dose has been achieved. At the same time the volume of fluid may be reduced (to a minimum of 125 ml) and the duration of infusion decreased (to a minimum of 45 minutes). The normal therapeutic dose will be in the region of 100 mg but higher doses may be required in more severe depressions or in obsessional and phobic states.

Length of treatment: Infusions should be given only to patients who are unable to take the drug orally. Oral therapy should be substituted once therapy has started to be effective, usually after 7–10 days.

Changeover to oral therapy: it is advisable to give double the maximum intravenous dosage orally until the patient's response is assured. Thereafter, a suitable maintenance dose, if considered necessary, can be selected.

Monitoring during treatment: During the course of infusion, patients should be monitored carefully for adverse effects. Particular attention should be paid to blood pressure recording, especially if there are any changes of position after conclusion of the infusion, as hypotension may occur. Patients often feel drowsy during treatment and not infrequently fall asleep.

Elderly: The initial dose should be 10 mg/day, which may be increased with caution under close supervision to an optimum level of 30–50 mg daily, which should be reached after about 10 days and then maintained until the end of treatment.

Children: Not recommended.

Obsessional/phobic states (oral or parenteral treatment): The maintenance dosage of Anafranil is generally higher than that used in depression. It is recommended that the dose be built up to 100–150 mg Anafranil daily, according to the severity of the condition. This should be attained gradually over a period of 2 weeks starting with 1×25 mg Anafranil daily. In elderly patients and those sensitive to tricyclic antidepressants a starting dose of 1×10 mg Anafranil daily is recommended. Again where a higher dosage is required, the SR 75 mg formulation may be preferable.

Contra-indications: Known hypersensitivity to clomipramine, or any of the excipients or cross-sensitivity to tricyclic antidepressants of the dibenzazepine group. Recent myocardial infarction. Any degree of heart block or other cardiac arrhythmias. Mania, severe liver disease, narrow angle glaucoma. Retention of urine. Anafranil should not be given in combination or within 3 weeks before or after treatment with a MAO inhibitor (see *Drug Interactions*). The concomitant treatment with selective, reversible MAO-A inhibitors, such as moclobemide, is also contra-indicated.

Special warnings and special precautions for use: As improvement in depression may not occur for the first two to four weeks treatment, patients should be closely monitored during this period.

Tricyclic antidepressants are known to lower the convulsion threshold and Anafranil should therefore be used with extreme caution in patients with epilepsy and other predisposing factors, e.g. brain damage of varying aetiology, concomitant use of neuroleptics, withdrawal from alcohol or drugs with anticonvulsive properties (e.g. benzodiazepines). It appears that the occurence of seizures is dose dependent, therefore the recommended total daily dose of Anafranil should not be exceeded.

Caution is called for when giving tricyclic antidepressants to patients with tumours of the adrenal medulla (e.g. phaeochromocytoma, neuroblastoma), in whom they may provoke hypertensive crises.

Concomitant treatment of Anafranil and electroconvulsive therapy should only be resorted to under careful supervision.

Elderly patients are particularly liable to experience adverse effects, especially agitation, confusion, and postural hypotension.

Many patients with panic disorders experience intensified anxiety symptoms at the start of the treatment with antidepressants. This paradoxical initial increase in anxiety is most pronounced during the first few days of treatment and generally subsides within two weeks.

Isolated cases of anaphylactic shock have been reported. Caution is called for when administering Anafranil intravenously.

Precautions: Before initiating treatment it is advisable to check the patient's blood pressure, because individuals with hypotension or a labile circulation may react to the drug with a fall in blood pressure.

Although changes in the white blood cell count have been reported with Anafranil only in isolated cases, periodic blood cell counts and monitoring for symptoms such as fever and sore throat are called for, particularly during the first few months of therapy. They are also recommended during prolonged therapy.

It is advisable to monitor cardiac and hepatic function during long-term therapy with Anafranil. In patients with liver disease, periodic monitoring of hepatic enzyme levels is recommended.

Caution is indicated in patients with hyperthyroidism or during concomitant treatment with thyroid preparations since aggravation of unwanted cardiac effects may occur.

Because of its anticholinergic properties, Anafranil should be used with caution in patients with a history of increased intra-ocular pressure, narrow angle glaucoma or urinary retention (e.g. diseases of the prostate).

An increase in dental caries has been reported during long-term treatment with tricyclic antidepressants. Regular dental check-ups are therefore advisable during long-term treatment.

Caution is called for in patients with chronic constipation. Tricyclic antidepressants may cause paralytic ileus, particularly in the elderly and in bedridden patients.

Decreased lacrimation and accumulation of mucoid secretions due to the anticholinergic properties of tricyclic antidepressants may cause damage to the corneal epithelium in patients with contact lenses.

Risk of suicide is inherent to severe depression and may persist until significant remission occurs. Patients posing a high suicide risk require close initial supervision.

Activation of psychosis has occasionally been observed in schizophrenic patients receiving tricyclic antidepressants. Hypomanic or manic episodes have also been reported during a depressive phase in patients with cyclic affective disorders receiving treatment with a tricyclic antidepressant. In such cases it may be necessary to reduce the dosage of Anafranil or to withdraw it and administer an antipsychotic agent. After such episodes have subsided, low dose therapy with Anafranil may be resumed if required.

Anafranil may cause anxiety, feelings of unrest, and hyperexcitation in agitated patients and patients with accompanying schizophrenic symptoms.

In predisposed and elderly patients, Anafranil may, particularly at night, provoke pharmacogenic (delirious) psychoses, which disappear without treatment within a few days of withdrawing the drug.

Before general or local anaesthesia, the anaesthetist should be aware that the patient has been receiving Anafranil and of the possible interactions (see *Interactions with other medicaments and other forms of interaction*).

Abrupt withdrawal should be avoided because of possible adverse reactions (see *Undesirable effects*).

Interactions with other medicaments and other forms of interaction

MAO inhibitors: Do not give Anafranil for at least 3 weeks after discontinuation of treatment with MAO inhibitors (there is a risk of severe symptoms such as hypertensive crisis, hyperpyrexia, myoclonus, agitation, seizures, delirium and coma). The same applies when giving a MAO inhibitor after previous treatment with Anafranil. In both instances the treatment should initially be given in small gradually increasing doses and its effects monitored. There is evidence to suggest that Anafranil may be given as little as 24 hours after a reversible MAO-A inhibitor such as moclobemide, but the 3 week wash-out period must be observed if the MAO-A inhibitor is used after Anafranil.

Selective serotonin reuptake inhibitors: Co-medication may lead to additive effects on the serotonin system. Fluoxetine and fluvoxamine may also increase plasma concentrations of clomipramine, with corresponding effects.

CNS depressants: Tricyclic antidepressants may potentiate the effects of alcohol and other central depressant substances (e.g. barbiturates, benzodiazepines, or general anaesthetics).

Neuroleptics: Comedication may result in increased plasma levels of tricyclic antidepressants, a lowered convulsion threshold, and seizures. Combination with thioridazine may produce severe cardiac arrhythmias.

Anticoagulants: Tricyclic antidepressants may potentiate the anticoagulant effect of coumarin drugs by inhibiting their metabolism by the liver. Careful monitoring of plasma prothrombin is therefore advised.

Anticholinergic agents: Tricyclic antidepressants may potentiate the effects of these drugs (e.g. phenothiazine, antiparkinsonian agents, antihistamines, atropine, biperiden) on the eye, central nervous system, bowel and bladder.

Adrenergic neurone blockers: Anafranil may diminish or abolish the antihypertensive effects of guanethidine, betanidine, reserpine, clonidine and alphamethyldopa. Patients requiring comedication for hypertension should therefore be given antihypertensives of a different type (e.g. diuretics, vasodilators, or beta-blockers).

Sympathomimetic drugs: Anafranil may potentiate the cardiovascular effects of adrenaline, ephedrine, isoprenaline, noradrenaline, phenylephrine, and phenylpropanolamine (e.g. as contained in local and general anaesthetic preparations and nasal decongestants).

Quinidine: Tricyclic antidepressants should not be employed in combination with antiarrhythmic agents of the quinidine type.

Liver-enzyme inducers: Drugs which activate the hepatic mono-oxygenase enzyme system (e.g. barbiturates, carbamazepine, phenytoin, nicotine and oral contraceptives) may accelerate the metabolism and lower the plasma concentrations of clomipramine, resulting in decreased efficacy. Plasma levels of phenytoin and carbamazepine may increase, with corresponding adverse effects. It may be necessary to adjust the dosage of these drugs.

Cimetidine, methylphenidate and estrogens: these

drugs increase plasma concentrations of tricyclic antidepressants, whose dosage should therefore be reduced.

Pregnancy and lactation: There is inadequate evidence of safety of Anafranil in human pregnancy. Do not use unless there are compelling reasons, especially during the first and last trimesters. Animal work has not shown clomipramine to be free from hazard.

Neonates whose mothers had taken tricyclic antidepressants up until delivery have developed dyspnoea, lethargy, colic, irritability, hypotension or hypertension, tremor or spasms, during the first few hours or days. Anafranil should – if this is at all justifiable – be withdrawn at least 7 weeks before the calculated date of confinement.

The active substance of Anafranil passes into the breast milk in small quantities. Therefore nursing mothers should be advised to withdraw the medication or cease breast-feeding.

Effects on ability to drive and use machinery: Patients receiving Anafranil should be warned that blurred vision, drowsiness and other CNS symptoms (see *Undesirable effects*) may occur in which case they should not drive, operate machinery or do anything else which may require alertness or quick actions. Patients should also be warned that consumption of alcohol or other drugs may potentiate these effects (see *Interactions with other medicaments and other forms of interaction*).

Undesirable effects: Unwanted effects are usually mild and transient, disappearing under continued treatment or with a reduction in the dosage. They do not always correlate with plasma drug levels or dose. It is often difficult to distinguish certain undesirable effects from symptoms of depression such as fatigue, sleep disturbances, agitation, anxiety, constipation and dry mouth.

If severe neurological or psychiatric reactions occur, Anafranil should be withdrawn.

Elderly patients are particularly sensitive to anticholinergic, neurological, psychiatric, or cardiovascular effects. Their ability to metabolise and eliminate drugs may be reduced, leading to a risk of elevated plasma concentrations at therapeutic doses.

The following side-effects, although not necessarily observed with Anafranil, have occured with tricyclic antidepressants.

Frequency estimate: frequent > 10%, occasional > 1–10%, rare >0.001–1%, isolated cases <0.001%.

Anticholinergic effects: Frequently: dryness of the mouth, sweating, constipation, disorders of visual accommodation and blurred vision, disturbances of micturition.

Occasionally: hot flushes, mydriasis.

Isolated cases: of glaucoma.

Central nervous system:

Psychiatric effects: Frequently: drowsiness, transient fatigue, feelings of unrest, increased appetite.

Occasionally: confusion accompanied by disorientation and hallucinations (particularly in geriatric patients and patients suffering from Parkinson's disease), anxiety states, agitation, sleep disturbances, mania, hypomania, aggressiveness, impaired memory, yawning, depersonalisation, insomnia, nightmares, aggravated depression, impaired concentration.

Isolated cases of activation of psychotic symptoms.

Neurological effects: Frequently: dizziness, tremor, headache, myoclonus.

Occasionally: delirium, speech disorders, paraesthesia, muscle weakness, muscle hypertonia.

Rarely: convulsions, ataxia.

Isolated cases: EEG changes, hyperpyrexia.

Cardiovascular system: Occasionally: postural hypotension, sinus tachycardia, and clinically irrelevant ECG changes in patients of normal cardiac status (e.g. T and ST changes), palpitations.

Rarely: arrhythmias, increased blood pressure.

Isolated cases: conduction disorders (e.g. widening of QRS complex, PQ changes, bundle-branch block).

Gastro-intestinal tract: Frequently: nausea.

Occasionally: vomiting, abdominal disorders, diarrhoea, anorexia.

Hepatic effects: Rarely: elevated transaminases.

Isolated cases: hepatitis with or without jaundice.

Skin: Occasionally: allergic skin reactions (skin rash, urticaria), photosensitivity, pruritus.

Isolated cases: local reactions after intravenous injections (thrombophlebitis, lymphangitis, burning sensation, and allergic skin reactions), oedema (local or generalised), hair loss.

Endocrine system and metabolism: Frequently: weight gain, disturbances of libido and potency.

Occasionally: galactorrhoea, breast enlargement.

Isolated cases: SIADH (inappropriate antidiuretic hormone secretion syndrome).

Hypersensitivity: Isolated cases: allergic alveolitis (pneumonitis) with or without eosinophilia, systemic anaphylactic/anaphylactoid reactions including hypotension.

Blood: Isolated cases: leucopenia, agranulocytosis, thrombocytopenia, eosinophilia, and purpura.

Sense organs: Occasionally: taste disturbances, tinnitus.

Others: The following symptoms occasionally occur after abrupt withdrawal or reduction of the dose: nausea, vomiting, abdominal pain, diarrhoea, insomnia, headache, nervousness and anxiety.

Overdose: The signs and symptoms of overdose with Anafranil are similar to those reported with other tricyclic antidepressants. Cardiac abnormalities and neurological disturbances are the main complications. In children accidental ingestion of any amount should be regarded as serious and potentially fatal.

Signs and symptoms: Symptoms generally appear within 4 hours of ingestion and reach maximum severity after 24 hours. Owing to delayed absorption (anticholinergic effect), long half-life, and enterohepatic recycling of the drug, the patient may be at risk for up to 4–6 days.

The following signs and symptoms may be seen:

Central nervous system: drowsiness, stupor, coma, ataxia, restlessness, agitation, enhanced reflexes, muscular rigidity and choreoathetoid movements, convulsions.

Cardiovascular system: hypotension, tachycardia, arrhythmias, conduction disorders, shock, heart failure; in very rare cases cardiac arrest.

Respiratory depression, cyanosis, vomiting, fever, mydriasis, sweating and oliguria or anuria may also occur.

Treatment: There is no specific antidote, and treatment is essentially symptomatic and supportive.

Anyone suspected of receiving an overdose of Anafranil, particularly children, should be hospitalised and kept under close surveillance for at least 72 hours.

Perform gastric lavage or induce vomiting as soon as possible if the patient is alert. If the patient has impaired consciousness, secure the airway with a cuffed endotracheal tube before beginning lavage, and do not induce vomiting. These measures are recommended for up to 12 hours or even longer after the overdose, since the anticholinergic effect of the drug may delay gastric emptying. Administration of activated charcoal may help to reduce drug absorption.

Treatment of symptoms is based on modern methods of intensive care, with continuous monitoring of cardiac function, blood gases, and electrolytes and, if necessary, emergency measures such as:

- anticonvulsive therapy
- artificial respiration,
- insertion of a temporary cardiac pacemaker,
- plasma expander, dopamine or dobutamine administered by intravenous drip,
- resuscitation.

Since it has been reported that physostigmine may cause severe bradycardia, asystole and seizures, its use is not recommended in cases of overdosage with Anafranil. Haemodialysis or peritoneal dialysis are ineffective because of the low plasma concentrations of clomipramine.

Pharmacological particulars

Pharmacodynamic properties: Clomipramine is a tricyclic antidepressant and its pharmacological action includes alpha-adrenolytic, anticholinergic, antihistaminic and 5-HT receptor blocking properties. The therapeutic activity of Anafranil is thought to be based on its ability to inhibit the neuronal re-uptake of noradrenaline and 5-HT. Inhibition of the latter is the dominant component.

Pharmacokinetic properties:

Absorption: The active substance is completely absorbed following oral administration and intramuscular injection.

The systemic bioavailability of unchanged clomipramine is reduced by 50% by 'first-pass' metabolism to desmethylclomipramine (an active metabolite). The bioavailability of clomipramine is not markedly affected by the ingestion of food but the onset of absorption and therefore the time to peak may be delayed. Coated tablets and sustained release tablets are bioequivalent with respect to amount absorbed.

During oral administration of constant daily doses of Anafranil the steady state plasma concentrations of clomipramine and desmethylclomipramine (active metabolite) and the ratio between these concentrations show a high variability between patients, e.g. 75 mg Anafranil daily produces steady state concentrations of clomipramine ranging from about 20 to 175 ng/ml. Levels of desmethylclomipramine follow a similar pattern but are 40–85% higher.

Following repeated intravenous or intramuscular administration of 50–150 mg Anafranil daily, steady-state plasma concentrations are attained in the second week of treatment. These range from <15 to 447 ng/ml for clomipramine and from <15 to 669 ng/ml for desmethylclomipramine.

Distribution: Clomipramine is 97.6% bound to plasma proteins. The apparent volume of distribution is about 12–17 L/kg bodyweight. Concentrations in cerebrospinal fluid are about 2% of the plasma concentration.

Biotransformation: The major route of transformation of clomipramine is demethylation to desmethylclomipramine. In addition, clomipramine and desmethylclomipramine are hydroxylated to 8-hydroxy-clomipramine and 8-hydroxy-desmethylclomipramine but little is known about their activity *in vivo*. The hydroxylation of clomipramine and desmethylclomipramine is under genetic control similar to that of debrisoquine. In poor metabolisers of debrisoquine this may lead to high concentrations of desmethylclomipramine; concentrations of clomipramine are less significantly influenced.

Elimination: Oral clomipramine is eliminated from the blood with a mean half-life of 21 hours (range 12–36 h), and desmethylclomipramine with a half-life of 36 hours.

After intramuscular and intravenous administration, clomipramine is eliminated from plasma with a mean terminal half-life of 25 hours (range 20–40 h) and 18 hours respectively.

About two-thirds of a single dose of clomipramine is excreted in the form of water-soluble conjugates in the urine, and approximately one-third in the faeces. The quantity of unchanged clomipramine and desmethylclomipramine excreted in the urine amounts to about 2% and 0.5% of the administered dose respectively.

Characteristics in patients: In elderly patients, plasma clomipramine concentrations may be higher for a given dose than would be expected in younger patients because of reduced metabolic clearance.

The effects of hepatic and renal impairment on the pharmacokinetics of clomipramine have not been determined.

Preclinical safety data: None stated.

Pharmaceutical particulars

List of excipients: Glycerine and water.

Incompatibilities: None.

Shelf life: 60 months.

Special precautions for storage: Protect from light. Discard any unused portion.

Nature and contents of container: Ampoules of clear glass containing 25 mg clomipramine hydrochloride BP in 2 ml available in pack size of 10.

Instructions for use/handling: None.

Marketing authorisation holder: Novartis Pharmaceuticals UK Limited, Trading as Geigy Pharmaceuticals, Frimley Business Park, Frimley, Camberley, Surrey GU16 5SG.

Marketing authorisation number PL 00101/0437

Date of first authorisation/renewal of authorisation Date of grant: 4 July 1997.

Date of (partial) revision of the text 18 August 1998.

ANAFRANIL 75 mg SR TABLETS

Qualitative and quantitative composition Chemical name: 3-chloro-5-[3-(dimethylamino)-propyl] 10, 11-dihydro-5H-dibenz[b, f] azepine hydrochloride (= clomipramin.hydrochloric).

Each tablet contains 75 mg clomipramine hydrochloride BP.

Pharmaceutical form Slow release, film coated tablets.

Clinical particulars

Therapeutic indications: Antidepressant: Symptoms of depressive illness especially where sedation is required. Obsessional and phobic states. Adjunctive treatment of cataplexy associated with narcolepsy.

Posology and method of administration

Adults: Oral – 10 mg/day initially, increasing gradually to 30–150 mg/day, if required, in divided doses throughout the day or as a single dose at bedtime. Many patients will be adequately maintained on 30–50 mg/day. Higher doses may be needed in some patients, particularly those suffering from obsessional or phobic disorders. In severe cases this dosage can be increased up to a maximum of 250 mg per day. Once a distinct improvement has set in, the daily dosage may be adjusted to a maintenance level averaging either 2–4 capsules of 25 mg or 1 tablet of 75 mg. Where a higher dose is required, the 75 mg SR formulation may be preferable.

Elderly: The initial dose should be 10 mg/day, which may be increased with caution under close supervision to an optimum level of 30–75 mg daily, which should be reached after about 10 days and then maintained until the end of treatment.

Children: Not recommended.

Obsessional/phobic states: The maintenance dosage of Anafranil is generally higher than that used in depression. It is recommended that the dose be built up to 100–150 mg Anafranil daily, according to the severity of the condition. This should be attained gradually over a period of 2 weeks starting with 1 x 25 mg Anafranil daily. In elderly patients and those sensitive to tricyclic antidepressants a starting dose of 1 x 10 mg Anafranil daily is recommended. Again where a higher dose is required, the SR 75 formulation may be preferable.

Adjunctive treatment of cataplexy associated with narcolepsy: (Oral treatment): 10–75 mg daily. It is suggested that treatment is commenced with 10 mg Anafranil daily and gradually increased until a satisfactory response occurs. Control of cataplexy should be achieved within 24 hours of reaching the optimal dose. Where necessary, therapy may be combined with capsules and syrup up to the maximum dose of 75 mg per day.

Contra-indications: Known hypersensitivity to clomipramine or any of the excipients, or cross-sensitivity to tricyclic antidepressants of the dibenzazepine group. Recent myocardial infarction. Any degree of heart block or other cardiac arrhythmias. Mania, severe liver disease, narrow angle glaucoma. Retention of urine, Anafranil should not be given in combination or with or within 3 weeks before or after treatment with a MAO inhibitor (see *Interactions with other medicaments and other forms of interaction*).

The concomitant treatment with selective, reversible MAO-A inhibitors, such as moclobamide, is also contra-indicated.

Special warnings and special precautions for use

Warnings: As improvement in depression may not occur for the first two to four weeks treatment, patients should be closely monitored during this period.

Tricyclic antidepressants are known to lower the convulsion threshold and Anafranil should therefore be used with extreme caution in patients with epilepsy and/or other predisposing factors, e.g. brain damage of varying aetiology, concomitant use of neuroleptics, withdrawal from alcohol or drugs with anticonvulsive properties (e.g. benzodiazepines). It appears that the occurence of seizures is dose dependent, therefore the recommended total daily dose of Anafranil should not be exceeded.

Caution is called for when giving tricyclic antidepressants to patients with tumours of the adrenal medulla (e.g. phaeochromocytoma, neuroblastoma), in whom they may provoke hypertensive crises.

Concomitant treatment of Anafranil and electroconvulsive therapy should only be resorted to under careful supervision.

Elderly patients are particularly liable to experience adverse effects, especially agitation, confusion, and postural hypotension.

Many patients with panic disorders experience intensified anxiety symptoms at the start of the treatment with antidepressants. This paradoxical initial increase in anxiety is most pronounced during the first few days of treatment and generally subsides within two weeks.

Precautions: Before initiating treatment it is advisable to check the patient's blood pressure, because individuals with hypotension or a labile circulation may react to the drug with a fall in blood pressure.

Caution is indicated in patients with hyperthyroidism or during concomitant treatment with thyroid preparations since aggravation of unwanted cardiac effects may occur.

Although changes in the white blood cell count have been reported with Anafranil only in isolated cases, periodic blood cell counts and monitoring for symptoms such as fever and sore throat are called for, particularly during the first few months of therapy. They are also recommended during prolonged therapy.

It is advisable to monitor cardiac and hepatic function during long-term therapy with Anafranil. In patients with liver disease, periodic monitoring of hepatic enzyme levels is recommended.

Because of its anticholinergic properties, Anafranil should be used with caution in patients with a history of increased intra-ocular pressure, narrow angle glaucoma or urinary retention (e.g. disease of the prostate).

An increase in dental caries has been reported during long-term treatment with tricyclic antidepressants. Regular dental check-ups are therefore advisable during long-term treatment.

Caution is called for in patients with chronic constipation. Tricyclic antidepressants may cause paralytic ileus, particularly in the elderly and in bedridden patients.

Decreased lacrimation and accumulation of mucoid secretions due to the anticholinergic properties of tricyclic antidepressants may cause damage to the corneal epithelium in patients with contact lenses.

Risk of suicide is inherent to severe depression and may persist until significant remission occurs. Patients posing a high suicide risk require close initial supervision.

Activation of psychosis has occasionally been observed in schizophrenic patients receiving tricyclic antidepressants. Hypomanic or manic episodes have also been reported during a depressive phase in patients with cyclic affective disorders receiving treatment with a tricyclic antidepressant. In such cases it may be necessary to reduce the dosage of Anafranil or to withdraw it and administer an antipsychotic agent. After such episodes have subsided, low dose therapy with Anafranil may be resumed if required.

Anafranil may cause anxiety, feelings of unrest, and hyperexcitation in agitated patients and patients with accompanying schizophrenic symptoms.

In predisposed and elderly patients, Anafranil may, particularly at night, provoke pharmacogenic (delirious) psychoses, which disappear without treatment within a few days of withdrawing the drug.

Before general or local anaesthesia, the anaesthetist should be aware that the patient has been receiving Anafranil and of the possible interactions (see *Interactions with other medicaments and other forms of interaction*).

Abrupt withdrawal should be avoided because of possible adverse reactions (see *Undesirable effects*).

Interactions with other medicaments and other forms of interaction

MAO inhibitors: Do not give Anafranil for at least 3 weeks after discontinuation of treatment with MAO inhibitors (there is a risk of severe symptoms such as hypertensive crisis, hyperpyrexia, myoclonus, agitation, seizures, delirium and coma). The same applies when giving a MAO inhibitor after previous treatment with Anafranil. In both instances the treatment should initially be given in small gradually increasing doses and its effects monitored. There is evidence to suggest that Anafranil may be given as little as 24 hours after a reversible MAO-A inhibitor such as moclobamide, but the 3 week wash-out period must be observed if the MAO-A inhibitor is used after Anafranil.

Selective serotonin reuptake inhibitors (SSRI): Comedication may lead to additive effects on the serotonergic system. Fluoxetine and fluvoxamine may also increase plasma concentrations of imipramine, with corresponding effects.

CNS depressants: Tricyclic antidepressants may potentiate the effects of alcohol and other central depressant substances (e.g. barbiturates, benzodiazepines, or general anaesthetics).

Neuroleptics: Comedication may result in increased plasma levels of tricyclic antidepressants, a lowered convulsion threshold and seizures. Combination with thioridazine may produce severe cardiac arrhythmias.

Anticoagulants: Tricyclic antidepressants may potentiate the anticoagulant effect of coumarin drugs due to their inhibition of hepatic metabolism of the anticoagulants. Careful monitoring of plasma prothrombin is therefore advised.

Anticholinergic agents: Tricyclic antidepressants may potentiate the effects of these drugs (e.g. phenothiazine, antiparkinsonian agents, antihistamines, atropine, biperiden) on the eye, central nervous system, bowel and bladder.

Adrenergic neurone blockers: Anafranil may diminish or abolish the antihypertensive effects of guanethidine, betanidine, reserpine, clonidine and alphamethyldopa. Patients requiring comedication for hypertension should therefore be given antihypertensives of a different type (e.g. diuretics, vasodilators, or beta-blockers).

Sympathomimetic drugs: Anafranil may potentiate the cardiovascular effects of adrenaline, ephedrine, isoprenaline, noradrenaline, phenylephrine, and phenylpropanolamine (e.g. as contained in local and general anaesthetic preparations and nasal decongestants).

Quinidine: Tricyclic antidepressants should not be employed in combination with anti-arrhythmic agents of the quinidine type.

Liver-enzyme inducers: Drugs which activate the hepatic mono-oxygenase enzyme system (e.g. carbamazepine, barbiturates, phenytoin, nicotine and oral contraceptives) may accelerate the metabolism and lower the plasma concentrations of clomipramine, resulting in decreased efficacy. Plasma levels of phenytoin and carbamazepine may increase, with corresponding adverse effects. It may be necessary to adjust the dosage of these drugs.

Cimetidine, methylphenidate and estrogens: these drugs increase plasma concentrations of tricyclic antidepressants, whose dosage should therefore be reduced.

Pregnancy and lactation: There is inadequate evidence of safety of Anafranil in human pregnancy. Do not use, especially during the first and last trimesters unless there are compelling reasons. Animal work has not shown clomipramine to be free from hazard.

Neonates whose mothers had taken tricyclic antidepressants up until delivery have developed dyspnoea, lethargy, colic, irritability, hypotension or hypertension, tremor or spasms, during the first few hours or days. Anafranil should – if this is at all justifiable – be withdrawn at least 7 weeks before the calculated date of confinement.

The active substance of Anafranil passes into the breast milk in small quantities. Therefore nursing mothers should be advised to withdraw the medication or cease breast-feeding.

Effects on ability to drive and use machinery: Patients receiving Anafranil should be warned that blurred vision, drowsiness and other CNS symptoms (see *Undesirable effects*) may occur in which case they should not drive, operate machinery or do anything else which may require altertness or quick actions. Patients should also be warned that alcohol or other drugs may potentiate these effects (see *Interactions with other medicaments and other forms of interaction*).

Undesirable effects: Unwanted effects are usually mild and transient, disappearing under continued treatment or with a reduction in the dosage. They do not always correlate with plasma drug levels or dose. It is often difficult to distinguish certain undesirable effects from symptoms of depression such as fatigue, sleep disturbances, agitation, anxiety, constipation and dry mouth.

If severe neurological or psychiatric reactions occur, Anafranil should be withdrawn.

Elderly patients are particularly sensitive to anticholinergic, neurological, psychiatric, or cardiovascular effects. Their ability to metabolise and eliminate drugs may be reduced, leading to a risk of elevated plasma concentrations at therapeutic doses.

The following side effects, although not necessarily observed with Anafranil, have occured with tricyclic antidepressants.

Frequency estimate: frequent > 10%, occasional > 1–10%, rare > 0.001–1%, isolated cases < 0.001%.

Anticholinergic effects: Frequently: dryness of the mouth, sweating, constipation, disorders of visual accommodation and blurred vision, disturbances of micturition. Occasionally: hot flushes, mydriasis. Isolated cases of glaucoma.

Central nervous system – psychic effects: Frequently: drowsiness, transient fatigue, feelings of unrest, increased appetite.

Occasionally: confusion accompanied by disorientation and hallucinations (particularly in geriatric patients and patients suffering from Parkinson's disease), anxiety states, agitation, sleep disturbances, mania, hypomania, aggressiveness, impaired memory, yawning, depersonalisation, insomnia, nightmares, aggravated depression, impaired concentration. Isolated cases of activation of psychotic symptoms.

Neurological effects: Frequently: dizziness, tremor, headache, myoclonus. Occasionally: delirium, speech disorders, paraesthesia, muscle weakness, muscle hypertonia. Rarely: convulsions, ataxia. Isolated cases of ECG changes, hyperpyrexia.

Cardiovascular system: Occasionally: postural hypotension, sinus tachycardia, and clinically irrelevant ECG changes in patients of normal cardiac status (e.g. T and ST changes), palpitations. Rarely: arrhythmias, increased blood pressure. Isolated cases of conduction disorders (e.g. widening of QRS complex, PQ changes, bundle-branch block).

Gastro-intestinal tract: Frequently: nausea. Occasionally: vomiting, abdominal disorders, diarrhoea, anorexia.

Hepatic effects: Rarely: elevated transaminases. Isolated cases of hepatitis with or without jaundice.

Skin: Occasionally: allergic skin reactions (skin rash, urticaria), photosensitivity, pruritus. Isolated cases of local reactions after intravenous injections (thrombophlebitis, lymphangitis, burning sensation and allergic skin reactions), oedema (local or generalised), hair loss.

Endocrine system and metabolism: Frequently: weight gain, disturbances of libido and potency. Occasionally: galactorrhoea, breast enlargement. Isolated cases of SIADH (inappropriate antidiuretic hormone secretion syndrome).

Hypersensitivity: Isolated cases of allergic alveolitis (pneumonitis) with or without eosinophilia, systemic anaphylactic/anaphylactoid reactions including hypotension.

Sense organs: Occasionally: taste disturbances, tinnitus.

Blood: Isolated cases: leucopenia, agranulocytosis, thrombocytopenia, eosinophilia and purpura.

Others: The following symptoms occasionally occur after abrupt withdrawal or reduction of the dose: nausea, vomiting, abdominal pain, diarrhoea, insomnia, headache, nervousness and anxiety.

Overdose: The signs and symptoms of overdose with Anafranil are similar to those reported with other tricyclic antidepressants. Cardiac abnormalities and neurological disturbances are the main complications. In children accidental ingestion of any amount should be regarded as serious and potentially fatal.

Signs and symptoms: Symptoms generally appear within 4 hours of ingestion and reach maximum severity after 24 hours. Owing to delayed absorption (anticholinergic effect), long half-life, and enterohepatic recycling of the drug, the patient may be at risk for up to 4–6 days.

The following signs and symptoms may be seen:

Central nervous system: drowsiness, stupor, coma, ataxia, restlessness, agitation, enhanced reflexes, muscular rigidity and choreoathetoid movements, convulsions

Cardiovascular system: hypotension, tachycardia, arrhythmias, conduction disorders, shock, heart failure; in very rare cases cardiac arrest

Respiratory depression, cyanosis, vomiting, fever, mydriasis, sweating and oliguria or anuria may also occur.

Treatment: There is no specific antidote, and treatment is essentially symptomatic and supportive.

Anyone suspected of receiving an overdose of Anafranil, particularly children, should be hospitalised and kept under close surveillance for at least 72 hours.

Perform gastric lavage or induce vomiting as soon as possible if the patient is alert. If the patient has impaired consciousness, secure the airway with a cuffed endotracheal tube before beginning lavage, and do not induce vomiting. These measures are recommended for up to 12 hours or even longer after the overdose, since the anticholinergic effect of the drug may delay gastric emptying.

Administration of activated charcoal may help to reduce drug absorption.

Treatment of symptoms is based on modern methods of intensive care, with continuous monitoring of cardiac function, blood gases, and electrolytes; and, if necessary, emergency measures such as:

- anticonvulsive therapy,
- artificial respiration,
- insertion of a temporary cardiac pacemaker,
- plasma expander, dopamine or dobutamine administered by intravenous drip,
- resuscitation.

Since it has been reported that physostigmine may cause severe bradycardia, asystole and seizures, its use is not recommended in cases of overdosage with Anafranil. Haemodialysis or peritoneal dialysis are ineffective because of the low plasma concentrations of clomipramine.

Pharmacological particulars

Pharmacodynamic properties: Clomipramine is a tricyclic antidepressant and its pharmacological action includes alpha-adrenolytic, anticholinergic, antihistaminic and 5-HT receptor blocking properties. The therapeutic activity of Anafranil is thought to be based on its ability to inhibit the neuronal re-uptake of noradrenaline and 5-HT. Inhibition of the latter is the dominant component.

Pharmacokinetic properties:

Absorption: The active substance is completely absorbed following oral administration and intramuscular injection.

The systemic bioavailability of unchanged clomipramine is reduced by 50% by 'first-pass' metabolism to desmethylclomipramine (an active metabolite). The bioavailability of clomipramine is not markedly affected by the ingestion of food but the onset of absorption and therefore the time to peak may be delayed. Coated tablets and sustained release tablets are bioequivalent with respect to amount absorbed.

During oral administration of constant daily doses of Anafranil the steady state plasma concentration of clomipramine and desmethylclomipramine (active metabolite) and the ratio between these concentrations show a high variability between patients, e.g. 75 mg Anafranil daily produces steady state concentrations of clomipramine ranging from about 20 to 175 ng/ml. Levels of desmethylclomipramine follow a similar pattern but are 40–85% higher.

Distribution: Clomipramine is 97.6% bound to plasma proteins. The apparent volume of distribution is about 12–17 L/kg bodyweight. Concentrations in cerebrospinal fluid are about 2% of the plasma concentration.

Biotransformation: The major route of transformation of clomipramine is demethylation to desmethylclomipramine. In addition, clomipramine and desmethylclomipramine are hydroxylated to 8-hydroxy-clomipramine and 8-hydroxy-desmethylclomipramine but little is known about their activity *in vivo.* The hydroxylation of clomipramine and desmethylclomipramine is under genetic control similar to that of debrisoquine. In poor metabolisers of debrisoquine this may lead to high concentrations of desmethylclomipramine; concentrations of clomipramine are less significantly influenced.

Elimination: Clomipramine is eliminated from the blood with a mean half-life of 21 hours (range 12–36 h), and desmethylclomipramine with a half-life of 36 hours.

About two-thirds of a single dose of clomipramine is excreted in the form of water-soluble conjugates in the urine, and approximately one-third in the faeces. The quantity of unchanged clomipramine and desmethylclomipramine excreted in the urine amounts to about 2% and 0.5% of the administered dose respectively.

Characteristics in patients: In elderly patients, plasma clomipramine concentrations may be higher for a given dose than would be expected in younger patients because of reduced metabolic clearance.

The effects of hepatic and renal impairment on the pharmacokinetics of clomipramine have not been determined.

Preclinical safety data: None stated.

Pharmaceutical particulars

List of excipients: Colloidal silicon dioxide (Aerosil 200), calcium hydrogen phosphate, Eudrogit E 30D (dry substance), calcium stearate. The coating constituents are hydroxypropylmethylcellulose 3CPS (2910), red iron oxide (E172), polyethoxylated castor oil (cremophor RH40), purified talc special, titanium dioxide (E171) and purified water.

Incompatibilities: None.

Shelf life: 60 months.

Special precautions for storage: Protect from moisture.

Nature and contents of container: The tablets are dull greyish-red film coated, round, slightly convex with bevelled edges, imprinted 'Geigy' on one face and GD on the other, and come in PVC blister packs of 28.

Instructions for use/handling: None.

Marketing authorisation holder: Novartis Pharmaceuticals UK Limited, Trading as Geigy Pharmaceuticals, Frimley Business Park, Frimley, Camberley, Surrey GU16 5SG.

Marketing authorisation number PL 00101/0436

Date of first authorisation/renewal of authorisation 17 July 1997.

Date of (partial) revision of the text 6 October 1997.

ANTURAN* Tablets 100 mg

Qualitative and quantitative composition The active ingredient is 1,2-Diphenyl-3,5-dioxo-4-(2-phenylsulphinylethyl)-pyrazolidine (=sulphinpyrazone BP). Each coated tablet contains 100 mg sulphinpyrazone.

Pharmaceutical form Coated tablets.

Clinical particulars

Therapeutic indications: Chronic, including tophaceous gout; recurrent gouty arthritis; hyperuricaemia.

Posology and method of administration: Anturan is administered orally in tablet form with meals or milk.

Adults: 100–200 mg daily increasing gradually (over the first two or three weeks) to 600 mg daily (rarely 800 mg), and maintained until the serum urate level has fallen within the normal range. Subsequent dosage should be reduced, to the lowest level which maintains serum urate within the normal range. Maintenance dose may be as low as 200 mg daily. Reduced dose required in renal impairment. Not to be used in severe renal impairment.

Children: Paediatric usage not established.

Contra-indications: Acute attacks of gout. Treatment with Anturan should not be initiated during an acute attack of gout.

Gastric and duodenal ulcer (overt or case-history).

Known hypersensitivity to sulphinpyrazone and other pyrazolone derivatives. Sulphinpyrazone is contra-indicated in patients in whom attacks of asthma, urticaria, or acute rhinitis are precipitated by acetylsalicylic acid or by other drugs with prostaglandin-synthetase inhibiting activity.

Severe parenchymal lesions of the liver or kidneys (also in the case history). Porphyria. Blood dyscrasias (also in the case history). Haemorrhagic diatheses (e.g. blood coagulation disorders).

In the treatment of chronic gout salicylates antagonise the action of Anturan and should not be given concurrently.

Special warnings and precautions for use

Warnings: During the early stages of treatment in patients with hyperuricaemia or gout, acute attacks of gout may be precipitated. To help prevent episodes of urolithiasis or renal colic, ensure adequate fluid intake and alkalinisation of the urine during initial stages of therapy.

Since Anturan may cause salt and water retention, caution is called for in patients with overt or latent heart failure.

For the early detection of a haematological abnormality, careful clinical supervision and full blood count should be done before and at regular intervals during treatment.

Precautions: Use with caution in patients with impaired renal function.

In patients with an elevated plasma uric acid level and/or with a history of nephrolithiasis or renal colic, and also when resuming treatment after interruption of the medication, a cautious incremental dosage schedule should be adopted. As with any form of long-term uricosuric medication, renal function tests should be performed regularly, particularly in cases where there is pre-existing evidence of renal failure.

Interactions with other medicaments and other types of interactions: Since Anturan may potentiate the action of coumarin-type anticoagulants, frequent estimation of prothrombin time should be undertaken when these drugs are given concurrently, and the dosage of anticoagulant adjusted accordingly.

Anturan may also potentiate the action of other plasma protein binding drugs such as hypoglycaemic agents and sulphonamides, which may necessitate a modification in dosage.

Penicillins (e.g. penicillin G): Inhibition of tubular secretion may raise the plasma concentrations of penicillins.

Theophylline: Activation of microsomal liver enzymes and resultant acceleration of metabolism lowers the plasma concentration of theophylline.

Phenytoin: Displacement of phenytoin from its plasma protein-binding sites as well as inhibition of microsomal liver enzymes delays the metabolism of phenytoin, thus prolonging its half-life and raising its plasma concentration.

Substances affecting haemostasis: Such substances, e.g. non-steroidal antirheumatic drugs, may exert a synergistic effect on the blood coagulation system and thus increase the risk of haemorrhage.

Pregnancy and lactation: Anturan should be used with caution in pregnant women, weighing the potential risk against the possible benefits.

It is not known whether the active substance of Anturan and/or its metabolite(s) pass into breast milk. For safety reasons mothers should refrain from taking the drug.

Effects on ability to drive or use machines: None known.

Undesirable effects:

Gastro-intestinal tract: Frequent: mild transient gastro-intestinal upsets, such as nausea, vomiting, diarrhoea.

In isolated cases: gastro-intestinal bleeding and ulcers.

Urogenital system: Rare: acute renal failure (mostly reversible), especially with high initial dosages.

In isolated cases: salt and water retention.

Skin: Rare: allergic skin reactions (e.g. drug rash, urticaria).

Blood: In isolated cases: leucopenia, thrombocytopenia, agranulocytosis, aplastic anaemia.

Liver: In isolated cases: hepatic dysfunction (increase in transaminases and alkaline phosphatase), jaundice, and hepatitis.

Overdose:

Signs and symptoms: Nausea, vomiting, abdominal pains, diarrhoea, hypotension, cardiac arrhythmias, hyperventilation, respiratory disorders, impairment of consciousness, coma, epileptic seizures, oliguria or anuria, acute renal failure, renal colic.

Treatment: Immediate treatment consists of forced emesis to recover undigested tablets. This is followed by gastric lavage preferably with mild alkaline solution such as sodium bicarbonate solution and supportive therapy as indicated.

Note that forced diuresis is of no value.

Pharmacological properties

Pharmacodynamic properties

Mode of action: Anturan lowers serum urate levels by blocking tubular reabsorption, thereby increasing renal excretion of uric acid. As a result of increased excretion, serum urate deposits are mobilised and tophi are no longer formed.

Pharmacokinetic properties: After oral administration the active substance is absorbed rapidly and almost completely (>85%).

Following a single oral dose of 100 mg or 200 mg sulphinpyrazone, peak plasma concentrations of 5–6 mcg/ml or 13–22 mcg/ml, respectively, are attained after 1–2 hours. Sulphinpyrazone has a half-life of 2–4 hours.

Following repeated administration of sulphinpyrazone in a dosage of 400 mg bid for 23 days, a significant decrease in the AUC values and an increase in the drug's clearance was observed as compared with the values recorded after a single dose. After multiple dosing with 400 mg bid, the mean steady-state concentration of sulphinpyrazone amounts to 5.1 mcg/ml, which corresponds to only half of the calculated value after a single dose (9.6 mcg/ml). The reason for this is an increase in total clearance brought about by the fact that the drug induces its own metabolism.

Sulphinpyrazone is metabolised by reduction to the sulphide and by oxidation to the sulphone and to hydroxy-compounds. The sulphide metabolite inhibits platelet aggregation *in vitro* about 12 times more strongly than sulphinpyrazone itself. In comparison with sulphinpyrazone the plasma concentrations of the sulphide metabolite are low. Peak sulphide concentrations are reached approx. 19 hours after administration of a single dose.

Preclinical safety data: Animal experimental findings indicate that Anturan is neither mutagenic nor carcinogenic or teratogenic.

Pharmaceutical particulars
List of excipients: All coated tablets contain lactose, maize starch, aerosil 200, magnesium stearate, gelatin, sodium starch glycollate, sucrose, talc, povidone, titanium dioxide (E171), polyethylene glycol, avicel and yellow iron oxide (E172).

Incompatibilities: None known.

Shelf life: Five years.

Special precautions for storage: Protect from moisture and store below 25°C.
Medicines should be kept out of reach of children.

Nature and contents of container: Containers of 84 tablets.

Instructions for use/handling: None.

Marketing authorisation holder: Novartis Pharmaceuticals UK Limited, Trading as Geigy Pharmaceuticals, Frimley Business Park, Frimley, Camberley, Surrey GU16 5SG.

Marketing authorisation number PL 00101/0515.

Date of first authorisation 10 April 1998.

Date of revision of the text 26 May 1998.

ANTURAN* Tablets 200 mg

Presentation The active ingredient, sulphinpyrazone BP is presented as light yellow, sugar coated, round, biconvex, approximately 10.6 mm diameter, printed GEIGY on one side, each containing 200 mg.
The tablets also contain lactose and sucrose.

Uses
Indications: Chronic, including tophaceous, gout; recurrent gouty arthritis; hyperuricaemia.

Mode of action: Anturan lowers serum urate levels by blocking tubular reabsorption, thereby increasing renal excretion of uric acid. As a result of increased excretion, serum urate deposits are mobilised and tophi are no longer formed.

Pharmacokinetics: After oral administration the active substance is absorbed rapidly and almost completely (> 85%).
Following a single oral dose of 100 mg or 200 mg, sulphinpyrazone, peak plasma concentrations of 5-6μg/ml or 13-22μg/ml, respectively, are attained after 1-2 hours. Sulphinpyrazone has a half-life of 2-4 hours.
Following repeated administration of sulphinpyrazone in a dosage of 400 mg bid for 23 days, a significant decrease in the AUC values and an increase in the drug's clearance was observed as compared with the values recorded after a single dose. After multiple dosing with 400 mg bid, the mean steady-state concentration of sulphinpyrazone amounts to 5.1μg/ml, which corresponds to only half of the calculated value after a single dose (9.6μg/ml). The reason for this is an increase in total clearance brought about by the fact that the drug induces its own metabolism.
Sulphinpyrazone is metabolised by reduction to the sulphide and by oxidation to the sulphone and to hydroxy-compounds. The sulphide metabolite inhibits platelet aggregation *in vitro* about 12 times more strongly than sulphinpyrazone itself. In comparison with sulphinpyrazone the plasma concentrations of the sulphide metabolite are low. Peak sulphide concentrations are reached approx. 19 hours after administration of a single dose.

Dosage and administration Anturan is administered orally in tablet form with meals or milk.

Hyperuricaemia
Adults: 100-200 mg daily increasing gradually (over the first two or three weeks) to 600 mg daily (rarely 800 mg), and maintained until the serum urate level has fallen within the normal range. Subsequent dosage should be reduced, to the lowest level which maintains serum urate within the normal range. Maintenance dose may be as low as 200 mg daily. Reduced dose required in renal impairment. Not to be used in severe renal impairment.

Children: Paediatric usage not established.

Contra-indications, warnings, etc
Contra-indications: Acute attacks of gout. Treatment with Anturan should not be initiated during an acute attack of gout.
Gastric and duodenal ulcer (overt or case-history).
Known hypersensitivity to sulphinpyrazone and other pyrazolone derivatives. Sulphinpyrazone is contra-indicated in patients in whom attacks of asthma, urticaria, or acute rhinitis are precipitated by acetylsalicylic acid or by other drugs with prostaglandin-synthetase inhibiting activity.
Severe parenchymal lesions of the liver or kidneys (also in the case history). Porphyria. Blood dyscrasias (also in the case history). Haemorrhagic diatheses (e.g. blood coagulation disorders).
In the treatment of chronic gout salicylates antagonise the action of Anturan and should not be given concurrently.

Warnings: During the early stages of treatment in patients with hyperuricaemia or gout, acute attacks of gout may be precipitated. To help prevent episodes of urolithiasis or renal colic, ensure adequate fluid intake and alkalinisation of the urine during initial stages of therapy.
Since Anturan may cause salt and water retention, caution is called for in patients with overt or latent heart failure.
For the early detection of a haematological abnormality, careful clinical supervision and full blood count should be done before and at regular intervals during treatment.

Precautions: Use with caution in patients with impaired renal function.

In patients with an elevated plasma uric acid level and/or with a history of nephrolithiasis or renal colic, and also when resuming treatment after interruption of the medication, a cautious incremental dosage schedule should be adopted. As with any form of long-term uricosuric medication, renal function tests should be performed regularly, particularly in cases where there is pre-existing evidence of renal failure.

Use during pregnancy and lactation: Anturan should be used with caution in pregnant women, weighing the potential risk against the possible benefits.
It is not known whether the active substance of Anturan and/or its metabolite(s) pass into breast milk. For safety reasons mothers should refrain from taking the drug.

Drug interactions: Since Anturan may potentiate the action of coumarin-type anticoagulants, frequent estimation of prothrombin time should be undertaken when these drugs are given concurrently, and the dosage of anticoagulant adjusted accordingly.
Anturan may also potentiate the action of other plasma protein binding drugs such as hypoglycaemic agents and sulphonamides, which may necessitate a modification in dosage.
Penicillins (e.g. penicillin G): Inhibition of tubular secretion may raise the plasma concentrations of penicillins.
Theophylline: Activation of microsomal liver enzymes and resultant acceleration of metabolism lowers the plasma concentration of theophylline.
Phenytoin: Displacement of phenytoin from its plasma protein-binding sites as well as inhibition of microsomal liver enzymes delays the metabolism of phenytoin, thus prolonging its half-life and raising its plasma concentration.
Substances affecting haemostasis: Such substances, e.g. non-steroidal antirheumatic drugs, may exert a synergistic effect on the blood coagulation system and thus increase the risk of haemorrhage.

Side effects:
Gastro-intestinal tract: Frequent: mild transient gastro-intestinal upsets, such as nausea, vomiting, diarrhoea. In isolated cases: gastro-intestinal bleeding and ulcers.
Urogenital system: Rare: acute renal failure (mostly reversible), especially with high initial dosages. In isolated cases: salt and water retention.
Skin: Rare: allergic skin reactions (e.g. drug rash, urticaria).
Blood: In isolated cases: leucopenia, thrombocytopenia, agranulocytosis, aplastic anaemia.
Liver: In isolated cases: hepatic dysfunction (increase in transaminases and alkaline phosphatase), jaundice, and hepatitis.

Overdosage: There is no antidote to Anturan.
Signs and symptoms: Nausea, vomiting, abdominal pains, diarrhoea, hypotension, cardiac arrhythmias, hyperventilation, respiratory disorders, impairment of consciousness, coma, epileptic seizures, oliguria or anuria, acute renal failure, renal colic.
Treatment: Immediate treatment consists of forced emesis to recover undigested tablets. This is followed by gastric lavage preferably with mild alkaline solution such as sodium bicarbonate solution and supportive therapy as indicated.
Note that forced diuresis is of no value.

Pharmaceutical precautions
Storage: Protect from moisture and store below 25°C.

Legal category POM.

Package quantities
Containers of 84 tablets.

Product licence number PL 00101/0516

Product licence holder: Novartis Pharmaceuticals UK Limited, trading as Geigy Pharmaceuticals.

Date of last revision 26 May 1998.

AREDIA* DRY POWDER

Qualitative and quantitative composition The active ingredient is disodium 3-amino-1-hydroxypropylidene-1, 1-bisphosphonate pentahydrate (pamidronate disodium).
One vial contains 15 mg, 30 mg or 90 mg of sterile, lyophilised pamidronate disodium. An ampoule containing 5 mL sterile water for injections is supplied with each 15 mg vial, and a 10 mL ampoule with each 30 mg or 90 mg vial.

Pharmaceutical form Powder in vials together with ampoules of water for reconstitution.

Clinical particulars
Therapeutic indications: Treatment of conditions associated with increased osteoclast activity:
- Tumour-induced hypercalcaemia
- Osteolytic lesions and bone pain in patients with bone metastases associated with breast cancer or multiple myeloma
- Paget's disease of bone.

Posology and method of administration: Aredia must never be given as a bolus injection (see 'Warnings'). The reconstituted solution of Aredia from powder in vials should be diluted in a calcium-free infusion solution (0.9% w/v Sodium Chloride Intravenous Infusion BP is recommended) and infused slowly.
The infusion rate should never exceed 60 mg/hour (1 mg/min), and the concentration of Aredia in the infusion solution should not exceed 60 mg/250 ml. In patients with established or suspected renal impairment (e.g. those with tumour-induced hypercalcaemia or multiple myeloma) it is recommended that the infusion rate does not exceed 20 mg/h (see also 'Renal Impairment'). In order to minimise local reactions at the infusion site, the cannula should be inserted carefully into a relatively large vein.
Until further experience is gained, Aredia is only recommended for use in adult patients.

Tumour-induced hypercalcaemia: It is recommended that patients be rehydrated with 0.9% w/v sodium chloride solution before or during treatment.
The total dose of Aredia to be used for a treatment course depends on the patient's initial serum calcium levels. The following guidelines are derived from clinical data on uncorrected calcium values. However, doses within the ranges given are also applicable for calcium values corrected for serum protein or albumin in rehydrated patients.

Initial serum calcium (mmol/L)	*(mg %)*	*Recommended total dose (mg)*
up to 3.0	up to 12.0	15–30
3.0–3.5	12.0–14.0	30–60
3.5–4.0	14.0–16.0	60–90
> 4.0	> 16.0	90

The total dose of Aredia may be administered either in a single infusion or in multiple infusions over 2–4 consecutive days. The maximum dose per treatment course is 90 mg for both initial and repeated courses.
A significant decrease in serum calcium is generally observed 24–48 hours after administration of Aredia, and normalisation is usually achieved within 3 to 7 days. If normocalcaemia is not achieved within this time, a further dose may be given. The duration of the response may vary from patient to patient, and treatment can be repeated whenever hypercalcaemia recurs. Clinical experience to date suggests that Aredia may become less effective as the number of treatments increases.

Osteolytic lesions and bone pain in multiple myeloma: The recommended dose is 90 mg every 4 weeks.
Osteolytic lesions and bone pain in bone metastases associated with breast cancer.
The recommended dose is 90 mg every 4 weeks. This dose may also be administered at 3 weekly intervals to coincide with chemotherapy if desired.

Paget's disease of bone: The recommended treatment course consists of a total dose of 180 mg administered in unit doses of either 30 mg once a week for 6 consecutive weeks, or 60 mg every other week over 6 weeks. Experience to date suggests that any mild and transient unwanted effects (see 'Side-effects') tend to occur after the first dose. For this reason if unit doses of 60 mg are used it is recommended that treatment be started with an initial additional dose of 30 mg (i.e. total dose 210 mg). Each dose of 30 or 60 mg should be diluted in 125 or 250 ml 0.9% w/v Sodium Chloride Intravenous Infusion BP respectively, and the infusion rate should not exceed 60 mg/hour (1 mg/min). This regimen or increased dose levels according to disease severity, up to a maximum total dose of 360 mg (in divided doses of 60 mg) can be repeated every 6 months until remission of disease is achieved, and if relapse occurs.

Renal impairment: Pharmacokinetic studies indicate that no dose adjustment is necessary in patients with any degree of renal impairment. However, until further experience is gained a maximum infusion rate of 20 mg/h is recommended in renally impaired patients.

Contra-indications: Known hypersensitivity to Aredia or to other bisphosphonates.

Special warnings and special precautions for use: Warnings: Aredia should not be given as a bolus injection, but should always be diluted and given as a slow intravenous infusion (see 'Posology and method of administration').

Aredia should not be given with other bisphosphonates because their combined effects have not been investigated.

Convulsions have been precipitated in some patients with tumour-induced hypercalcaemia due to the electrolyte changes associated with this condition and its effective treatment.

Precautions: Serum electrolytes, calcium and phosphate should be monitored following initiation of therapy with Aredia. Patients who have undergone thyroid surgery may be particularly susceptible to develop hypocalcaemia due to relative hypoparathyroidism.

Patients receiving frequent infusions of Aredia over a prolonged period of time, especially those with pre-existing renal disease or a predisposition to renal impairment (e.g. patients with multiple myeloma and/or tumour-induced hypercalcaemia), should have periodic evaluations of standard laboratory and clinical parameters of renal function as deterioration of renal function (including renal failure) has been reported following long-term treatment with Aredia in patients with multiple myeloma. However, underlying disease progression and/or concomitant complications were also present and therefore a causal relationship with Aredia is unproven.

There is very little experience of the use of Aredia in patients receiving haemodialysis.

In patients with cardiac disease, especially in the elderly, additional saline overload may precipitate cardiac failure (left ventricular failure or congestive heart failure). Fever (influenza-like symptoms) may also contribute to this deterioration.

Pagetic patients at risk of calcium or Vitamin D deficiency (e.g. through malabsorption or lack of exposure to sunlight) should take oral supplements of both during Aredia therapy to minimise the potential risk of hypocalcaemia.

Interactions with other drugs and other types of interactions: Aredia has been administered concomitantly with commonly used anticancer agents without interactions occurring.

Aredia has been used in combination with calcitonin in patients with severe hypercalcaemia, resulting in a synergistic effect producing a more rapid fall in serum calcium.

Since pamidronate binds to bone, it could in theory interfere with bone scintigraphy examinations.

Pregnancy and lactation: In animal experiments, pamidronate showed no teratogenic potential and did not affect general reproductive performance or fertility. In rats, prolonged parturition and reduced survival rate of pups were probably caused by a decrease in maternal serum calcium levels. In pregnant rats, pamidronate has been shown to cross the placental barrier and accumulate in fetal bone in a manner similar to that observed in adult animals.

There is insufficient clinical experience to support the use of Aredia in pregnant women. Therefore, Aredia should not be administered during pregnancy except in cases of life-threatening hypercalcaemia.

A study in lactating rats has shown that pamidronate will pass into the milk. Mothers treated with Aredia should therefore not breast-feed their infants.

Ability to drive or use machines: Patients should be warned that in rare cases somnolence and/or dizziness may occur following Aredia infusion, in which case they should not drive, operate potentially dangerous machinery, or engage in other activities that may be hazardous because of decreased alertness.

Undesirable effects: Adverse reactions to Aredia are usually mild and transient. The most common adverse reactions are asymptomatic hypocalcaemia and fever (an increase in body temperature of 1–2°C), typically occurring within the first 48 hours of infusion. Fever usually resolves spontaneously and does not require treatment. Symptomatic hypocalcaemia is rare.

Frequency estimate: frequent >10%, occasional >1–10%, rare >0.001–1%, isolated cases <0.001%.

Body as a whole: Frequent: fever and influenza-like symptoms sometimes accompanied by malaise, rigor, fatigue, and flushes.

Local reactions: Occasional: reactions at the infusion site: pain, redness, swelling, induration, phlebitis, thrombophlebitis.

Musculoskeletal system: Occasional: transient bone pain, arthralgia, myalgia, generalised pain. Rare: muscle cramps.

Gastrointestinal tract: Occasional: nausea, vomiting. Rare: anorexia, abdominal pain, diarrhoea, constipation, dyspepsia. Isolated cases: gastritis.

Central nervous system: Occasional: headache. Rare: symptomatic hypocalcaemia (paraesthesia, tetany), agitation, confusion, dizziness, insomnia, somnolence, lethargy. Isolated cases: seizures, visual hallucinations.

Blood: Occasional: lymphocytopenia. Rare: anaemia, leukopenia. Isolated cases: thrombocytopenia.

Cardiovascular system: Rare: hypotension, hypertension.

Renal system: Isolated cases: haematuria, acute renal failure, deterioration of pre-existing renal disease.

Skin: Rare: rash, pruritus.

Special senses: Isolated cases: conjunctivitis, uveitis (iritis, iridocyclitis), scleritis, episcleritis, xanthopsia.

Others: Rare: allergic reactions including anaphylactoid reactions, bronchospasm/dyspnoea, Quincke's (angioneurotic) oedema. Very rare: anaphylactic shock. Isolated cases: reactivation of herpes simplex and herpes zoster.

Biochemical changes: Frequent: hypocalcaemia, hypophosphataemia. Occasional: hypomagnesaemia. Rare: hyperkalaemia, hypokalaemia, hypernatraemia. Isolated cases: abnormal liver function tests, increase in serum creatinine and urea.

Many of these undesirable effects may have been related to the underlying disease.

Overdose: Patients who have received doses higher than those recommended should be carefully monitored. In the event of clinically significant hypocalcaemia with paraesthesia, tetany and hypotension, reversal may be achieved with an infusion of calcium gluconate.

Pharmacological properties

Pharmacodynamic properties: Pamidronate disodium, the active substance of Aredia, is a potent inhibitor of osteoclastic bone resorption. It binds strongly to hydroxyapatite crystals and inhibits the formation and dissolution of these crystals in vitro. Inhibition of osteoclastic bone resorption in vivo may be at least partly due to binding of the drug to the bone mineral.

Pamidronate suppresses the accession of osteoclast precursors onto the bone. However, the local and direct anti-resorptive effect of bone-bound bisphosphonate appears to be the predominant mode of action in vitro and in vivo.

Experimental studies have demonstrated that pamidronate inhibits tumour-induced osteolysis when given prior to or at the time of inoculation or transplantation with tumour cells. Biochemical changes reflecting the inhibitory effect of Aredia on tumour-induced hypercalcaemia, are characterised by a decrease in serum calcium and phosphate and secondarily by decreases in urinary excretion of calcium, phosphate, and hydroxyproline.

Hypercalcaemia can lead to a depletion in the volume of extracellular fluid and a reduction in the glomerular filtration rate (GFR). By controlling hypercalcaemia, Aredia improves GFR and lowers elevated serum creatinine levels in most patients.

Clinical trials in patients with breast cancer and predominantly lytic bone metastases or with multiple myeloma showed that Aredia prevented or delayed skeletal-related events (hypercalcaemia, fractures, radiation therapy, surgery to bone, spinal cord compression) and decreased bone pain.

Paget's disease of bone, which is characterised by local areas of increased bone resorption and formation with qualitative changes in bone remodelling, responds well to treatment with Aredia. Clinical and biochemical remission of the disease has been demonstrated by bone scintigraphy, decreases in urinary hydroxyproline and serum alkaline phosphatase, and by symptomatic improvement.

Pharmacokinetic properties:

General characteristics: Pamidronate has a strong affinity for calcified tissues, and total elimination of pamidronate from the body is not observed within the time-frame of experimental studies. Calcified tissues are therefore regarded as site of 'apparent elimination'.

Absorption: Pamidronate disodium is given by intravenous infusion. By definition, absorption is complete at the end of the infusion.

Distribution: Plasma concentrations of pamidronate rise rapidly after the start of an infusion and fall rapidly when the infusion is stopped. The apparent half-life in plasma is about 0.8 hours. Apparent steady-state concentrations are therefore achieved with infusions of more than about 2–3 hours' duration. Peak plasma pamidronate concentrations of about 10 nmol/mL are achieved after an intravenous infusion of 60 mg given over 1 hour, and the apparent plasma clearance is about 180 mL/min.

In animals and in man, a similar percentage of the dose is retained in the body after each dose of pamidronate disodium. Thus the accumulation of pamidronate in bone is not capacity-limited, and is dependent solely on the total cumulative dose administered.

The percentage of circulating pamidronate bound to plasma proteins is relatively low (about 54%), and increases when calcium concentrations are pathologically elevated.

Elimination: Pamidronate does not appear to be eliminated by biotransformation. After an intravenous infusion, about 20–55% of the dose is recovered in the urine within 72 hours as unchanged pamidronate. Within the time-frame of experimental studies the remaining fraction of the dose is retained in the body. The percentage of the dose retained in the body is independent of both the dose (range 15–180 mg) and the infusion rate (range 1.25–60 mg/h). From the urinary elimination of pamidronate, two decay phases, with apparent half-lives of about 1.6 and 27 hours, can be observed. The apparent renal clearance is about 54 mL/min, and there is a tendency for the renal clearance to correlate with creatinine clearance.

Characteristics in patients: Hepatic and metabolic clearance of pamidronate are insignificant. Impairment of liver function is therefore not expected to influence the pharmacokinetics of Aredia. Aredia thus displays little potential for drug-drug interactions both at the metabolic level and at the level of protein binding (see above).

Preclinical safety data: The toxicity of pamidronate is characterised by direct (cytotoxic) effects on organs with a copious blood supply, particularly the kidneys following i.v. exposure. The compound is not mutagenic and does not appear to have carcinogenic potential.

Pharmaceutical particulars

List of excipients: Mannitol, phosphoric acid.

Incompatibilities: Pamidronate will form complexes with divalent cations and should not be added to calcium-containing intravenous solutions.

Shelf-life: 3 years.

Special precautions for storage: Protect vials from heat (store below 30°C). Reconstituted solutions that have been further diluted with one of the recommended diluents for intravenous infusion should be used immediately. Discard the unused portion.

Nature and contents of container: Colourless glass vials of 10 mL, with closures made from a butyl rubber derivative.

Instructions for use/handling: Powder in vials should be first dissolved in sterile water for injection, i.e. 15 mg in 5 mL, and 30 mg or 90 mg in 10 mL. The sterile water for injection is available in ampoules which are supplied together with vials. The pH of the reconstituted solution is 6.0–7.0. The reconstituted solution should be further diluted with a calcium-free infusion solution (0.9% w/v Sodium Chloride Intravenous Infusion BP is recommended) before administration. It is important that the powder be completely dissolved before the reconstituted solution is withdrawn for dilution.

Market authorisation holder: Novartis Pharmaceuticals UK Ltd, trading as Ciba Laboratories.

Marketing authorisation numbers

Aredia Dry Powder 15 mg 00101/0518
Aredia Dry Powder 30 mg 00101/0519
Aredia Dry Powder 90 mg 00101/0521
Water for Injections PhEur 00101/0479

Date of approval/revision of SPC December 1997.

Legal category POM.

BUTACOTE* Enteric Coated Tablets 100 mg

Qualitative and quantitative composition The active ingredient is 1,2-diphenyl-3,5-dioxo-4-n-butyl-pyrazolidine (phenylbutazone).

One enteric-coated tablet contains 100 mg phenylbutazone PhEur.

Pharmaceutical form Gastro-resistant tablets which are pale blue coloured, sugar-coated, enteric, biconvex tablets, approximately 7.8 mm in diameter, and imprinted GEIGY on one side and DM on the other.

Clinical particulars

Therapeutic indications: Ankylosing spondylitis. Butacote should only be used where other therapies have been found unsuitable.

Posology and method of administration: The dosage selected should be as low as possible, and duration of treatment should be as short as possible; when long term treatment is unavoidable, special precautions should be taken (see *Precautions*) and the dosage should be adjusted to the needs of each patient taking account of the patient's age and general condition.

Butacote tablets should be swallowed whole with a meal together with liquid.

Adults: For the initial 48 hours 400–600 mg daily in divided doses. Thereafter, reduce to the minimum amount necessary, usually 200–300 mg daily in divided doses.

Elderly: In the elderly, always use the minimum effective dose (see *Precautions*).

Children: Not recommended for children under 14 years.

Contra-indications: Butacote is contra-indicated in patients with an active peptic ulcer or a history, however remote, of peptic ulcer, gastro-intestinal haemorrhage, patients with symptoms or a history of inflammatory bowel disease with or without ulceration, blood dyscrasia. Haemorrhagic diathesis (thrombocytopenia, disorders of blood coagulation), severe cardiac, hepatic, renal or pulmonary insufficiency, oedema or hypertension where there is danger of cardiac decompensation, thyroid disease, salivary gland disorder, Sjögren's syndrome and previous adverse reactions to pyrazoles.

Like other non-steroidal anti-inflammatory agents, Butacote is also contra-indicated in asthmatic patients in whom attacks of asthma, urticaria, or acute rhinitis are precipitated by acetylsalicylic acid or by other drugs with prostaglandin synthetase inhibiting activity.

There is not enough experience with the use of Butacote in pregnant women.

Special warnings and special precautions for use

Precautions: Like all potent drugs, Butacote should be used only under close medical supervision.

In elderly patients, who are generally more prone to side-effects, particular caution should be execised.

Serious gastro-intestinal reactions such as bleeding, ulceration and perforation can occur at any time, with or without warning symptoms, in patients treated with non-steroidal anti-inflammatory drugs. Although minor upper gastrointestinal symptoms such as dyspepsia are common, usually developing early in therapy, physicians should watch for ulceration and bleeding in patients treated with non-steroidal anti-inflammatory drugs, even in the absence of previous gastro-intestinal tract symptoms. If any of the symptoms or signs suggestive of gastro-intestinal toxicity occur, Butacote should be discontinued immediately.

As blood dyscrasias may occur suddenly after a small dose or insidiously after prolonged therapy, particularly in the elderly, blood counts should be monitored before and regularly during therapy, if it is anticipated that treatment may continue for more than one week. If significant changes occur, e.g. decrease in leucocyte and/or platelet count or in the haematocrit, the drug should be withdrawn. Therapy should also be stopped if symptoms suggestive of these complications arise (e.g. bruising, fever, sore throat, rash, mouth ulceration), and patients should be advised accordingly.

NSAIDs should be given with care to patients with a history of heart failure or hypertension since oedema and sodium retention have been reported in association with phenylbutazone administration (see *Undesirable effects*).

Severe hepatic reactions including jaundice and hepatitis have been reported with Butacote, as with other non-steroidal anti-inflammatory drugs. If abnormal liver tests persist or worsen, or clinical signs and symptoms consistent with liver disease develop, the drug should be discontinued.

Patients with impaired renal function should be closely monitored. Overt renal failure may be precipitated due to the inhibition of prostaglandin synthesis.

Granulocytopenia or aplastic anaemia have to be excluded in patients with stomatitis before treatment with Butacote is started, because stomatitis might be an indication of pre-existing haematological abnormality of this type.

If Butacote is given for more than one week, liver function tests, kidney function tests, and blood counts should be performed periodically. In case of significant changes, the drug should be withdrawn.

Use of acetylsalicylic acid and other NSAIDs should be avoided in patients receiving therapy with Butacote, since concomitant administration of these drugs may increase the risk of serious gastrointestinal adverse reactions.

Butacote should not be given to patients on oral anticoagulant therapy because of an increased risk of bleeding. Patients being treated with oral antidiabetics should not receive Butacote owing to possible occurrence of serious hypoglycaemia.

Like other drugs that inhibit prostaglandin synthetase activity, NSAIDs can precipitate acute attacks of asthma in patients suffering from, or with a previous history of, bronchial asthma.

Interaction with other medicaments and other forms of interaction: By competitively displacing them from their serum-protein binding sites, phenylbutazone may increase the activity and duration of effect of other drugs, e.g. other anti-inflammatory agents, oral anticoagulants, oral antidiabetic drugs, phenytoin, and sulphonamides. Phenylbutazone may also accelerate the metabolism of dicoumarol, digitoxin, and cortisone by inducing hepatic microsomal enzymes. Conversely, it may inhibit the metabolic degradation of phenytoin and potentiate the effect of insulin. In patients previously treated with drugs which activate the hepatic microsomal enzyme system, e.g. barbiturates, chlorpheniramine, rifampicin, promethazine, and corticosteroids (e.g. prednisone), the elimination half-life of phenylbutazone is shortened. When phenylbutazone is given together with methylphenidate, the serum concentration of the metabolite oxyphenbutazone rises and the elimination half-life of phenylbutazone is prolonged.

During concomitant administration of anabolic steroids and phenylbutazone, the serum concentration of the metabolite oxyphenbutazone rises.

Since phenylbutazone may potentiate the effect of methotrexate, caution is indicated in cases where the two drugs are given concomitantly. Concomitant administration of cholestyramine reduces the enteral absorption of phenylbutazone. Phenylbutazone displaces thyroid hormone from its serum protein-binding sites and may thus make it more difficult to interpret tests of thyroid function.

When given together with lithium preparations, phenylbutazone causes increased tubular reabsorption of lithium, thereby raising the latter's serum concentration.

Concomitant administration of Butacote with aspirin, other NSAIDs or corticosteroids increases the risk of serious gastrointestinal adverse reactions.

When given concomitantly, Butacote and misoprostol may induce adverse symptoms related to the central nervous system, such as dizziness, headache and transient diplopia.

Butacote may potentiate the effects of alcohol on the central nervous system.

Concomitant use of NSAIDs with antihypertensive drugs (i.e. beta-blockers, angiotensin converting enzyme (ACE) inhibitors, diuretics) may cause a decrease in their antihypertensive effect via inhibition of vasodilatory prostaglandin synthesis.

Cases of nephrotoxicity have been reported in patients receiving concomitant cyclosporin and NSAIDs. This might be mediated through combined renal antiprostaglandin effects of both the NSAID and cyclosporin.

Convulsions may occur in patients, with or without previous history of epilepsy or convulsions, due to an interaction between quinolones and NSAIDs. Therefore, caution should be exercised when considering the use of a quinolone in patients who are already receiving an NSAID.

NSAIDs may exacerbate cardiac failure and an increase in plasma cardiac glycoside levels may occur when renal function is affected.

NSAIDs should not be used for 8–12 days after mifepristone administration, NSAIDs can reduce the effects of mifepristone.

Pregnancy and lactation: Butacote may appear in cord blood and should not be used during pregnancy. If other drugs have been tried and found ineffective, Butacote may be used, but only if the benefits to the mother justify the potential risk to the foetus (e.g. premature closure of ductus arteriosus). Since phenylbutazone passes into breast milk, albeit in small quantities, nursing mothers taking Butacote should not breast feed their infants.

Effects on ability to drive and use machines: Patients receiving treatment with Butacote should be warned that drowsiness or dizziness may occur, in which case they should not drive, operate potentially dangerous machinery, or engage in other activities that may become hazardous because of decreased alertness. Concomitant ingestion of alcohol may potentiate these effects.

Undesirable effects

Gastro-intestinal tract: Frequent: nausea, gastritis.

Occasional: gastro-intestinal discomfort, heartburn, epigastric pain, peptic ulcer, diarrhoea.

Rare: Vomiting, gastro-intestinal bleeding (haematemesis and/or melaena), bleeding or perforation of peptic ulcer.

Isolated cases: Pancreatitis, oesophagitis, oesophageal ulcer, benign stricture of the oesophagus, exacerbation of inflammatory bowel disease, including Crohn's disease with bleeding, ulceration or perforation, small bowel obstruction, constipation.

Body as a whole: Frequent: oedema, water retention.

Skin: Occasional: rash.

Rare: urticaria, pruritus, purpura, exfoliative dermatitis.

Isolated cases: bullous eruptions, fixed drug eruptions, erythema multiforme, Stevens-Johnson syndrome, toxic epidermal necrolysis (Lyell's syndrome), photosensitivity, erythema nodosum, precipitation of generalised pustula psoriasis.

Others: Occasional: stomatitis.

Rare: salivary gland enlargement, dry mouth.

Endocrine system: Occasional: goitre, lowering of plasma thyroid hormone concentration.

Isolated cases: hypothyroidism.

Nervous system: Rare: dizziness, headache.

Isolated cases: peripheral neuropathy, confusional states, excitation.

Blood and lymph: Rare: anaemia due to occult gastrointestinal blood loss, haemolytic anaemia, thrombocytopenia, agranulocytosis, leucopenia, pancytopenia, bone marrow depression, aplastic anaemia.

Liver: Rare: increase in serum transaminases, hepatitis with or without jaundice.

Isolated cases: fulminant hepatitis.

Kidneys: Rare: impaired renal function, acute renal failure, haematuria, proteinuria.

Isolated cases: acute tubular necrosis, acute interstitial nephritis, nephrotic syndrome, glomerulonephritis, papillary necrosis, ureteral obstruction with uric acid crystal formation.

Cardiovascular system: Rare: congestive heart failure, pulmonary oedema.

Isolated cases: hypertension, myocarditis, pericarditis.

Hypersensitivity: Isolated cases: anaphylactic/anaphylactoid reactions with and without shock, angioedema, serum sickness, lymphadenopathy, vasculitis, systemic lupus erythematosus-like syndrome, eosinophilic pulmonary infiltrates, fever.

Respiratory tract: Isolated cases: exacerbation of bronchial asthma.

Isolated occurrences of an 'acute pulmonary syndrome' marked by dyspnoea, fever, shadows in radiographs of the lungs and sometimes also by eosinophilia – have been reported. Although a causal relationship has not been proven, the drug should be withdrawn at first signs of this potentially serious syndrome, for the treatment of which corticosteroids and supportive cardiotherapy may be necessary.

Special senses: Isolated cases: blurred vision, retinal haemorrhage, hearing loss.

Overdose

Signs and symptoms: Where the recommended dosage has been appreciably exceeded, the following are the signs and symptoms liable to be encountered: Nausea, vomiting, abdominal pain, diarrhoea, gastro-intestinal bleeding, peptic ulceration.

Hyperpyrexia, restlessness, dizziness, somnolence, agitation, convulsions, coma.

Alkalosis, acidosis, electrolyte disturbances, oedema.

Tachycardia, hyperventilation, respiratory arrest, cyanosis, hypotension, electrocardiographic abnormalities, cardiac arrest.

Acute renal failure.

Abnormal liver function test, jaundice, hepatic failure.

Anaemia, leucopenia, thrombocytopenia, hypoprothrombinaemia.

Treatment: Evacuation of the stomach (induction of vomiting, gastric lavage), and activated charcoal. If necessary, saline purgatives, artificial respiration, measures to support the circulation, anticonvulsants (e.g. diazepam i.v.). Forced diuresis and haemodialysis are considered to be ineffective in removing the drug. Haemoperfusion may be useful.

Pharmacological properties

Pharmacodynamic properties: Therapeutic/pharmacological group: non-steroidal anti-inflammatory agent. A pyrazolone derivative.

Pharmacokinetic properties: Phenylbutazone, the active substance of Butacote is rapidly and completely absorbed from the gastrointestinal tract. At therapeutic plasma concentrations, phenylbutazone is 98–99% plasma bound, exclusively to albumin. It is extensively metabolised in the liver and less than 1% is excreted unchanged in the urine. It inhibits the metabolism of several drugs, but it can also act as an inducer of liver enzymes (see *Interaction with other medicaments and other forms of interaction*). The drug forms the active metabolite oxyphenbutazone. The mean plasma elimination half life of phenylbutazone is about 75 hours, with wide inter- and intra-individual variations.

Preclinical safety data: In a 2-year carcinogenicity study in mice and rats a small increase in the incidence of neoplasms in the liver or kidney was seen. The incidence of liver tumours in male mice might be a response to rodent-specific hepatotropic effects, including liver-enzyme induction. The clinical significance of these findings is not clear.

Pharmaceutical particulars

List of excipients: Silica aerogel, gelatin, maize starch, sodium carboxymethyl starch, magnesium stearate, stearic acid, microcrystalline cellulose, polyethylene glycol, sucrose, talc, polyvidone, titanium dioxide, cellulose acetate phthalate, diethyl phthalate, colourings – E132, E127, E171, E172.

Incompatibilities: None known.

Shelf life: 5 years.

Special precautions for storage: Store below 25°C. Protect from moisture.

Keep all medicines out of reach of children.

Nature and contents of container: The tablets are packed in a securitainer or child resistant/tamper evident loose fill pack of 100 tablets.

Instructions for use/handling: There are no specific instructions for use/handling.

Marketing authorisation holder: Novartis Pharmaceuticals UK Limited, Trading as Geigy Pharmaceuticals, Frimley Business Park, Frimley, Camberley, Surrey GU16 5SG.

Marketing authorisation number PL 00101/0522.

Date of first authorisation/renewal of authorisation 30.1.98.

Date of revision of the text April 1998.

CLIMAGEST 1 mg*

Qualitative and quantitative composition Sixteen tablets each containing 1 mg oestradiol valerate USP, 12 tablets each containing 1 mg oestradiol valerate USP and 1 mg norethisterone PhEur.

Pharmaceutical form Film-coated tablet.

Clinical particulars

Therapeutic indications: Hormone replacement therapy for the treatment of menopausal symptoms.

Posology and method of administration: Treatment commences with one grey-blue tablet daily for the first 16 days followed by one white tablet daily for the next 12 days, as directed on the 28 day calendar pack. Women not menstruating may start therapy at any time. However, if the patient is menstruating regularly it is advised that the patient starts therapy on the first day of bleeding. Menstrual bleeding during initial Climagest therapy may be irregular. Pregnancy should be excluded before starting therapy.

Climagest may be taken continuously by women with an intact uterus as it provides both oestrogen and progestogen to reduce endometrial hyperstimulation.

Use in elderly: Climagest should only be used in the elderly for the indications listed.

Use in children: Climagest should not be used in children.

Contra-indications: Known or suspected pregnancy. History of, known or suspected cancer of the breast. Known or suspected oestrogen-dependent neoplasia. Undiagnosed abnormal genital bleeding. Active thrombophlebitis or thromboembolic disorders. Severe cardiac, hepatic or renal disease. Known hypersensitivity to one of the ingredients.

Special warnings and special precautions for use: A thorough gynaecological and physical examination is advised before and periodically during treatment with Climagest.

At present there is suggestive evidence of a slight increase in the relative risk of carcinoma of the breast with hormone replacement therapy used for longer than five years. Regular breast examinations and mammography where appropriate, should be carried out in women on HRT. Breast status should also be closely monitored in women with a history of, or known, breast nodules, or fibrocystic disease.

Some conditions can deteriorate on hormone replacement therapy and it is essential that patients with these conditions should be closely monitored, including otosclerosis, migraine, multiple sclerosis, epilepsy, diabetes, hypertension, asthma, hypercalcaemia, porphyria, uterine fibroids and tetany.

Patients with mild chronic liver disease should have their liver function checked every 8–12 weeks. Patients with cardiac or renal dysfunction, cholelithiasis, Dubin-Johnson syndrome or Rotor syndrome should also be closely monitored.

If migrainous or frequent unusually severe headaches occur for the first time, or any other symptoms that are possible prodromata of vascular occlusion occur, treatment should be suspended pending further investigation.

If jaundice, hepatitis, itching of the whole body, an increase in epileptic seizures or a significant rise in blood-pressure occur, treatment should be stopped immediately. Consider discontinuation of treatment when impending surgery, trauma or illness is considered to entail a risk of thrombosis.

Some epidemiological evidence suggests that the use of hormone replacement therapy (HRT) is associated with an increased risk of developing deep vein thrombosis (DVT) or pulmonary embolism (PE). The relative risk is about 2–3.6% for healthy women which would represent one additional case of venous thromboembolism (VTE) among 5000 women treated with HRT during a year.

Women with severe varicose veins, severe obesity (Body Mass Index >30 kg/m^2), or those undergoing immobilisation for 3 weeks or more, trauma or surgery requiring bed rest, are generally considered to be at increased risk of VTE. These women and those with a positive family history and women with a history of thromboembolic disorders during pregnancy or in association with oestrogen use should be given careful consideration before receiving HRT. If venous thromboembolism develops after initiating therapy, the drug should be discontinued.

Irregular bleeding during tablet taking is common during the first few months of therapy. If this persists an endometrial assessment including biopsy should be carried out. Patients with known or symptomatic endometriosis should be closely monitored.

As Climagest is not an oral contraceptive adequate non-hormonal measures should be taken to exclude pregnancy.

Interactions with other medicaments and other forms of interaction: Preparations which induce microsomal liver enzymes such as barbiturates, rifampicin, phenytoin and carbamazepine may accelerate the metabolism of oestrogen/progestogens and may reduce their efficacy.

Pregnancy and lactation: Climagest should not be used in pregnant or nursing women.

Effects on ability to drive and use machinery: No adverse effects on the ability to drive or operate machines have been recorded.

Undesirable effects: A number of side-effects have been reported during treatment: Dyspepsia, flatulence, nausea, vomiting, abdominal pain and bloating, weight gain, breast tension and pain, palpitations, increased libido, headaches, dizziness, vertigo, epistaxis, biliary stasis, hypertension, urticaria and other rashes, thrombophlebitis, mucous vaginal discharge, general pruritus, oedema, alopecia, depressive mood and decrease in glucose tolerance.

Overdose: There have been no reports of ill-effects from overdosage. There are no specific antidotes and further treatment should be symptomatic.

Pharmacological particulars

Pharmacodynamic properties: Oestradiol valerate is used in oestrogen deficiency states. Treatment with oestrogens relieves menopausal vasomotor symptoms. Oestrogens cross the placenta.

Norethisterone is a progestogen added to prevent endometrial hyperplasia and increased risk of endometrial carcinoma which can be induced by unopposed oestrogen use.

Pharmacokinetic properties: Oestradiol valerate, like most natural oestrogens, is readily and fully absorbed from the GI tract, is 50% bound to plasma proteins and is rapidly metabolised in the liver to oestriol and oestrone. When given orally in doses of 1–2 mg, peak levels of oestradiol are generally observed 3–6 hours after ingestion, but by 24 hours (range 6–48 hours) concentrations have returned to baseline (i.e. pretreatment concentrations).

Oestradiol undergoes first-pass effect in the liver. There is some enterohepatic recycling. It is excreted via the kidney in the urine as water soluble esters (sulphate and glucuronide) together with a small proportion of unchanged oestradiol. Other metabolites have been identified.

Norethisterone is absorbed from the GI tract and its effects last for at least 24 hours. When a dose of 1 mg is given, there are wide variations in serum norethisterone levels at any particular time point after doing (100–1700 pg/mL). Norethisterone undergoes first pass effects with a resulting loss of 36% of the dose. When injected, it is detectable in the plasma after 2 days and it is not completely excreted in the urine after 5 days. There are large inter-subject variations in elimination half-life and bioavailability. The most important metabolites are several isomers of 5α-dihydronorethisterone and tetrahydro-norethisterone which are excreted mainly as glucuronides.

Preclinical safety data: The toxicity profiles of oestradiol valerate and norethisterone are well known and reveal no risk human health risk.

Pharmaceutical particulars

List of excipients: Lactose, maize starch, povidone, talc, magnesium stearate, hydroxypropylmethyl cellulose, propylene glycol, FD & C blue no. 2 lake (E132), Opaspray blue M-1-6516, Opaspray white M-1-7-111B, purified water.

Incompatibilities: Not applicable.

Shelf life: 36 months as packaged for sale.

Special precautions for storage: Store the tablets below 25°C, in a dry place. Do not refrigerate. Protect from light.

Nature and contents of container: Blister strips of aluminium foil/UPVC (20 μm/250 μm), in cardboard cartons, each blister contains 28 tablets and cartons will contain 1 or 3 blisters.

Instructions for use/handling: There are no special instructions for handling.

Marketing authorisation holder: Novartis Pharmaceuticals UK Limited, Trading as Sandoz Pharmaceuticals, Frimley Business Park, Frimley, Camberley, Surrey GU16 5SG.

Marketing authorisation number PL 0101/0328.

Date of first authorisation/renewal of authorisation 18 September 1997.

Date of (partial) revision of the text September 1997.

CLIMAGEST 2 mg*

Qualitative and quantitative composition Sixteen tablets each containing 2 mg oestradiol valerate USP, 12 tablets each containing 2 mg oestradiol valerate USP and 2 mg norethisterone PhEur.

Pharmaceutical form Tablets for oral administration.

Clinical particulars

Therapeutic indications: Hormone replacement therapy for the treatment of menopausal symptoms.

Posology and method of administration: Treatment commences with one blue tablet daily for the first 16 days followed by one yellow tablet daily for the next 12 days, as directed on the 28 day calendar pack. Women not menstruating may start therapy at any time. However, if the patient is menstruating regularly it is advised that the patient starts therapy on the first day of bleeding. Menstrual bleeding during initial Climagest therapy may be irregular. Pregnancy should be excluded before starting therapy.

Climagest may be taken continuously by women with an intact uterus as it provides both oestrogen and progestogen to reduce endometrial hyperstimulation.

Use in elderly: Climagest should only be used in the elderly for the indications listed.

Use in children: Climagest should not be used in children.

Contra-indications: Known or suspected pregnancy. History of, known or suspected cancer of the breast. Known or suspected oestrogen-dependent neoplasia. Undiagnosed abnormal genital bleeding. Active thrombophlebitis or thromboembolic disorders. Severe cardiac, hepatic or renal disease. Known hypersensitivity to one of the ingredients.

Special warnings and special precautions for use: A thorough gynaecological and physical examination is advised before and periodically during treatment with Climagest.

At present there is suggestive evidence of a slight increase in the relative risk of carcinoma of the breast with hormone replacement therapy used for longer than five years. Regular breast examinations should be carried out in women on HRT and mammography where appropriate. Breast status should also be closely monitored in women with a history of, or known, breast nodules, or fibrocystic disease.

Some conditions can deteriorate on hormone replacement therapy and it is essential that patients with these conditions should be closely monitored, including otosclerosis, migraine, multiple sclerosis, epilepsy, diabetes, hypertension, asthma, hypercalcaemia, porphyria, uterine fibroids and tetany.

Patients with mild chronic liver disease should have their liver function checked every 8–12 weeks. Patients with cardiac or renal dysfunction, cholelithiasis, Dubin-Johnson syndrome or Rotor syndrome should be closely monitored.

If migrainous or frequent unusually severe headaches occur for the first time, or any other symptoms that are possible prodromata of vascular occlusion occur, treatment should be suspended pending further investigation.

If jaundice, hepatitis, itching of the whole body, an increase in epileptic seizures or a significant rise in blood-pressure occur, treatment should be stopped immediately. Consider discontinuation of treatment when impending surgery, trauma or illness is considered to entail a risk of thrombosis.

Caution should be exercised in patients with a history or increased risk of thromboembolic disorders including myocardial infarction, stroke, pulmonary embolism and thrombophlebitis.

Irregular bleeding during tablet taking is common during the first few months of therapy. If this persists an endometrial assessment including biopsy should be carried out. Patients with known or symptomatic endometriosis should be closely monitored.

As Climagest is not an oral contraceptive adequate non-hormonal measures should be taken to exclude pregnancy.

Interactions with other medicaments and other forms of interaction: Preparations which induce microsomal liver enzymes such as barbiturates, rifampicin, phenytoin and carbamazepine may accelerate the metabolism of oestrogen/progestogens and may reduce their efficacy.

Pregnancy and lactation: Climagest should not be used in pregnant or nursing women.

Effects on ability to drive and use machinery: No adverse effects on the ability to drive or operate machines have been recorded.

Undesirable effects: A number of side-effects have been reported during treatment. They are dyspepsia, flatulence, nausea, vomiting, abdominal pain and bloating, weight gain, breast tension and pain, palpitations, changes in libido, headaches, dizziness, vertigo, epistaxis, biliary stasis, hypertension, urticaria and other rashes, thrombophlebitis, mucous vaginal discharge, general pruritus, oedema, alopecia, depressive mood and decrease in glucose tolerance.

Overdose: No reports of ill-effects from overdosage have been reported. There are no specific antidotes for overdosage and if further treatment is required it should be symptomatic.

Pharmacological particulars
Pharmacodynamic properties: Oestradiol valerate is used in oestrogen deficiency states. Treatment with oestrogens relieves menopausal vasomotor symptoms. Oestrogens cross the placenta.

Norethisterone is a progestogen added to prevent endometrial hyperplasia and increased risk of endometrial carcinoma which can be induced by unopposed oestrogen use.

Pharmacokinetic properties: Oestradiol valerate, like most natural oestrogens, is readily and fully absorbed from the GI tract, is 50% bound to plasma proteins and is rapidly metabolised in the liver to oestriol and oestrone. When given orally in doses of 1–2 mg, peak levels of oestradiol are generally observed 3–6 hours after ingestion, but by 24 hours (range 6–48 hours) concentrations have returned to baseline (i.e. pre-treatment concentrations).

Oestradiol undergoes first-pass effect in the liver. There is some enterohepatic recycling. It is excreted via the kidney in the urine as water soluble esters (sulphate and glucuronide) together with a small proportion of unchanged oestradiol. Other metabolites have been identified.

Norethisterone is absorbed from the GI tract and its effects last for at least 24 hours. When a dose of 1 mg is given, there are wide variations in serum norethisterone levels at any particular time point after doing (100–1700 pg/mL). Norethisterone undergoes first pass effects with a resulting loss of 36% of the dose. When injected, it is detectable in the plasma after 2 days and it is not completely excreted in the urine after 5 days. There are large inter-subject variations in elimination half-life and bioavailability. The most important metabolites are several isomers of 5α-dihydronorethisterone and tetrahydro-norethisterone which are excreted mainly as glucuronides.

Preclinical safety data: The toxicity profiles of oestradiol valerate and norethisterone are well known and reveal no human health risk.

Pharmaceutical particulars
List of excipients: Lactose, maize starch, povidone, talc, magnesium stearate, hydroxypropylmethyl cellulose, propylene glycol, FD & C blue no. 2 lake (E132), Opaspray blue M-1-6517, iron oxide yellow (E172), Opaspray yellow M-1-8462, purified water.

Incompatibilities: Not applicable.

Shelf life: 36 months as packaged for sale.

Special precautions for storage: Store the tablets below 25°C, in a dry place. Do not refrigerate. Protect from light.

Nature and contents of container: Blister strips of aluminium foil/UPVC (20 μm/250 μm), in cardboard cartons, each blister contains 28 tablets and cartons will contain 1 or 3 strips.

Instructions for use/handling: There are no special instructions for handling.

Marketing authorisation holder: Novartis Pharmaceuticals UK Limited, Trading as Sandoz Pharmaceuticals, Frimley Business Park, Frimley, Camberley, Surrey GU16 5SG.

Marketing authorisation number PL 0101/0366.

Date of first authorisation/renewal of authorisation 12 May 1993.

Date of (partial) revision of the text September 1997.

CLIMAVAL 1 mg

Qualitative and quantitative composition One tablet of Climaval 1 mg contains 1 mg oestradiol valerate.

Pharmaceutical form Film-coated tablet.

Clinical particulars
Therapeutic indications: Hormone replacement therapy for the treatment of menopausal symptoms in hysterectomised women.

Posology and method of administration: 1 mg to 2 mg daily. Dosage may be adjusted according to severity of symptoms or clinical response. Climaval may be taken continuously in hysterectomised patients. The lowest dose compatible with the control of symptoms should always be used.

Use in children: Not to be used in children.

Use in the elderly: In the elderly, Climaval should only be used for the control of post-menopausal symptoms.

Contra-indications: History of, known or suspected cancer of the breast. Known or suspected oestrogen-dependent neoplasia. Undiagnosed abnormal genital bleeding or endometriosis. Severe cardiac, liver or renal disease. Active thrombophlebitis or thrombo-embolic disorders. Known hypersensitivity to one of the ingredients.

Special warnings and special precautions for use: A thorough gynaecological and physical examination is advised before and periodically during treatment with Climaval.

Some conditions can deteriorate on hormone replacement therapy and it is essential that patients with these conditions should be closely monitored, including multiple sclerosis, epilepsy, diabetes, hypertension, porphyria tetany, migraine, asthma, hypercalcaemia, otosclerosis and uterine fibroids.

Patients with mild chronic liver disease should have their liver function checked every 8–12 weeks. Patients with cardiac or renal dysfunction, cholelithiasis, Dubin-Johnson syndrome or Rotor syndrome should also be closely monitored.

If migrainous or frequent unusually severe headaches occur for the first time, or any other symptoms that are possible prodromata of vascular occlusion occur, treatment should be suspended pending further investigation.

If trauma, illness or impending surgery is considered to entail a risk of thrombosis, consideration should be given to discontinuing treatment. Treatment should be stopped at once if jaundice, hepatitis, itching of the whole body or an increase in epileptic seizures occur, or if there is a significant rise in blood pressure.

At present there is suggestive evidence of a slight increase in the relative risk of carcinoma of the breast with hormone replacement therapy used for longer than five years. Regular breast examinations and mammography where appropriate, should be carried out in women on HRT.

Breast status should also be closely monitored in women with a history of, or known, breast nodules, or fibrocystic disease.

Caution should be exercised in patients with a history or increased risk of thromboembolic disorders including myocardial infarction, stroke, pulmonary embolism and thrombophlebitis.

Interactions with other medicaments and other forms of interaction: There are no recorded interactions with other medicaments.

Pregnancy and lactation: Climaval 1 mg is indicated only in hysterectomised women.

Effects on ability to drive and use machinery: No adverse effects on the ability to drive or operate machines have been recorded.

Undesirable effects: The following have been reported during treatment: Dyspepsia, flatulence, nausea, vomiting, abdominal pain and bloating, weight gain, breast tension and pain, palpitations, cardiac symptoms, increased libido, headaches, dizziness, vertigo, epistaxis, biliary stasis, hypertension, urticaria and other rashes, thrombophlebitis, mucous vaginal discharge, general pruritus, oedema, alopecia, depressive mood and decrease in glucose tolerance.

Overdose: There have been no reports of ill-effects from overdose. There are no specific antidotes, and further treatment should be symptomatic.

Pharmacological particulars
Pharmacodynamic properties: Oestradiol valerate is used in oestrogen deficiency states.

After the menopause the protective effects which endogenous oestrogens appear to have on the female cardiovascular system are lost, therefore the risk of women developing cardiovascular disease rises to become similar to that of men. Studies have shown that the oral administration of oestradiol valerate to post-menopausal women decreases low density lipoprotein cholesterol (LDL-C) and also increases high density lipoprotein cholesterol (HDL-C). Such changes are recognised as potentially offering protection from the development of coronary artery disease.

Pharmacokinetic properties: Oestradiol valerate, like most natural oestrogens, is readily and fully absorbed from the GI tract, is 50% bound to plasma proteins and is rapidly metabolised in the liver to oestriol and oestrone. When given orally in doses of 1–2 mg, peak levels of oestradiol are generally observed 3–6 hours after ingestion, but by 24 hours (range 6–48 hours) concentrations have returned to baseline (i.e. pre-treatment concentrations). The average half-life of oestradiol in plasma is about one hour.

Oestradiol undergoes first-pass effect in the liver. There is some enterohepatic recycling. It is excreted via the kidney in the urine as sulphate and glucuronide esters together with a small proportion of unchanged oestradiol. Other metabolites have been identified.

Preclinical safety data: Oestradiol valerate is a well established pharmaceutical active and is the subject of a pharmacopoeial monograph (USP). No specific preclinical studies have therefore been performed.

Pharmaceutical particulars
List of excipients: Lactose, maize starch, FD & C blue no. 2 lake (E132), povidone (grade 30), purified water, talc (sterilised, white), magnesium stearate, hydroxypropylmethyl cellulose, propylene glycol, Opaspray blue M-1-6517.

Incompatibilities: No incompatibilities have been described.

Shelf life: 36 months in blister packs.

Special precautions for storage: Store the tablets below 25°C, in a dry place, protected from light.

Nature and contents of container: Blister strips of 28 tablets packed in cardboard cartons. Two sizes are available; cartons containing one blister strip or three blister strips.

Blister consists of 20 μm layer of aluminium foil on a 250 μm UPVC blister.

Instructions for use/handling: The pack was designed to help patients take the tablets correctly. The arrows on the foil should be followed and the tablets taken on the days shown.

Marketing authorisation holder: Novartis Pharmaceuticals UK Limited, Trading as Sandoz Pharmaceuticals, Frimley Business Park, Frimley, Camberley, Surrey GU16 5SG.

Marketing authorisation number PL 0101/0307.

Date of first authorisation/renewal of authorisation 25 March 1997.

Date of (partial) revision of the text September 1997.

CLIMAVAL 2 mg

Qualitative and quantitative composition One tablet of Climaval 2 mg contains 2 mg oestradiol valerate.

Pharmaceutical form Film-coated tablet.

Clinical particulars
Therapeutic indications: Hormone replacement therapy for the treatment of menopausal symptoms in hysterectomised women.

Posology and method of administration: 1 mg to 2 mg daily. Dosage may be adjusted according to severity of symptoms or clinical response. Climaval may be taken continuously in hysterectomised patients. The lowest dose compatible with the control of symptoms should always be used.

Use in children: Not to be used in children.

Use in the elderly: In the elderly, Climaval should only be used for the control of post-menopausal symptoms.

Contra-indications: History of, known or suspected cancer of the breast. Known or suspected oestrogen-dependent neoplasia. Undiagnosed abnormal genital bleeding or endometriosis. Severe cardiac, liver or renal disease. Active thrombophlebitis or thrombo-embolic disorders. Known hypersensitivity to one of the ingredients.

Special warnings and special precautions for use: A thorough gynaecological and physical examination is advised before and periodically during treatment with Climaval.

Some conditions can deteriorate on hormone replacement therapy and it is essential that patients with these conditions should be closely monitored, including multiple sclerosis, epilepsy, diabetes, hypertension, porphyria, tetany, migraine, asthma, hypercalcaemia, otosclerosis and uterine fibroids.

Patients with mild chronic liver disease should have their liver function checked every 8–12 weeks. Patients with cardiac or renal dysfunction, cholelithiasis, Dubin-Johnson syndrome or Rotor syndrome should also be closely monitored.

If migrainous or frequent unusually severe headaches occur for the first time, or any other symptoms that are possible prodromata of vascular occlusion occur, treatment should be suspended pending further investigation.

If trauma, illness or impending surgery is considered to entail a risk of thrombosis, consideration should be given to discontinuing treatment. Treatment should be stopped at once if jaundice, hepatitis, itching of the whole body or an increase in epileptic seizures occur, or if there is a significant rise in blood pressure.

At present there is suggestive evidence of a slight increase in the relative risk of carcinoma of the breast with hormone replacement therapy used for longer than five years. Regular breast examinations and mammography where appropriate, should be carried out in women on HRT.

Breast status should also be closely monitored in

women with a history of, or known, breast nodules, or fibrocystic disease.

Caution should be exercised in patients with a history or increased risk of thromboembolic disorders including myocardial infarction, stroke, pulmonary embolism and thrombophlebitis.

Interactions with other medicaments and other forms of interaction: There are no recorded interactions with other medicaments.

Pregnancy and lactation: Climaval 2 mg is indicated only in hysterectomised women.

Effects on ability to drive and use machinery: No adverse effects on the ability to drive or operate machines have been recorded.

Undesirable effects: A number of side effects have been reported during treatment: Dyspepsia, flatulence, nausea, vomiting, abdominal pain and bloating, weight gain, breast tension and pain, palpitations, cardiac symptoms, increased libido, headaches, dizziness, vertigo, epistaxis, biliary stasis, hypertension, urticaria and other rashes, thrombophlebitis, mucous vaginal discharge, general pruritus, oedema, alopecia, depressive mood and decrease in glucose tolerance.

Overdose: There have been no reports of ill-effects from overdose. There are no specific antidotes, and further treatment should be symptomatic.

Pharmacological particulars

Pharmacodynamic properties: Oestradiol valerate is used in oestrogen deficiency states.

After the menopause the protective effects which endogenous oestrogens appear to have on the female cardiovascular system are lost, therefore the risk of women developing cardiovascular disease rises to become similar to that of men. Studies have shown that the oral administration of oestradiol valerate to post-menopausal women decreases low density lipoprotein cholesterol (LDL-C) and also increases high density lipoprotein cholesterol (HDL-C). Such changes are recognised as potentially offering protection from the development of coronary artery disease.

Pharmacokinetic properties: Oestradiol valerate, like most natural oestrogens, is readily and fully absorbed from the GI tract, is 50% bound to plasma proteins and is rapidly metabolised in the liver to oestriol and oestrone. When given orally in doses of 1–2 mg, peak levels of oestradiol are generally observed 3–6 hours after ingestion, but by 24 hours (range 6–48 hours) concentrations have returned to baseline (i.e. pre-treatment concentrations). The average half-life of oestradiol in plasma is about one hour.

Oestradiol undergoes first-pass effect in the liver. There is some enterohepatic recycling. It is excreted via the kidney in the urine as sulphate and glucuronide esters together with a small proportion of unchanged oestradiol. Other metabolites have been identified.

Preclinical safety data: Oestradiol valerate is a well established pharmaceutical active and is the subject of a pharmacopoeial monograph (USP). No specific preclinical studies have therefore been performed.

Pharmaceutical particulars

List of excipients: Lactose, maize starch, FD & C blue no. 2 lake (E132), povidone (grade 30), purified water, talc (sterilised, white), magnesium stearate, hydroxypropylmethyl cellulose, propylene glycol, Opaspray blue M-1-6517.

Incompatibilities: No incompatibilities have been described.

Shelf life: 36 months in blister packs.

Special precautions for storage: Store the tablets below 25°C, in a dry place, protected from light.

Nature and contents of container: Blister strips of 28 tablets packed in cardboard cartons. Two sizes are available; cartons containing one blister strip or three blister strips.

Blister consists of 20 μm layer of aluminium foil on a 250 μm UPVC blister.

Instructions for use/handling: The pack was designed to help patients take the tablets correctly. The arrows on the foil should be followed and the tablets taken on the days shown.

Marketing authorisation holder: Novartis Pharmaceuticals UK Limited, Trading as Sandoz Pharmaceuticals, Frimley Business Park, Frimley, Camberley, Surrey GU16 5SG.

Marketing authorisation number PL 0101/0308.

Date of first authorisation/renewal of authorisation 25 March 1997.

Date of (partial) revision of the text September 1997.

CLIMESSE

Qualitative and quantitative composition 28 tablets each containing 2 mg oestradiol valerate USP and 0.7 mg norethisterone PhEur.

Pharmaceutical form Film-coated tablet.

Clinical particulars

Therapeutic indications: Hormone replacement therapy for the treatment of menopausal symptoms.

Prevention of bone mass loss in post-menopausal women at high risk of developing fractures.

Posology and method of administration: One tablet to be taken daily, as directed on the 28 day calendar pack. Climesse should be taken continuously without a break between packs.

It is recommended that Climesse should not be taken by women until at least 12 months after their last natural menstrual bleed. Irregular bleeding during tablet taking may occur during the first few months of therapy but is usually transient, and amenorrhoea will develop in a majority of women. Amenorrhoea is most likely to occur in women who are more than 2 years post-menopausal but may also be achieved before that in a significant proportion of women. After 3–4 months treatment, some women may experience continued unacceptable bleeding and in these cases Climesse should be discontinued. If bleeding subsides within three weeks then no further investigation is needed.

Bleeding after a period of amenorrhoea or heavy bleeding after a period of light bleeding may occur. Any doubt as to the cause of bleeding is a reason for endometrial evaluation, including some form of endometrial biopsy.

Pregnancy should be excluded before starting therapy.

Changing from sequential hormone replacement therapy: Patients changing from a sequential hormone replacement therapy preparation to Climesse should do so at the end of the oestrogen plus progestogen phase of the sequential therapy, without a tablet free interval. Climesse should normally be used only in women more than 12 months post-menopausal. When changing from sequential therapy menopausal status may not be known, and in some women endogenous oestrogens may still be produced. This could result in unpredictable bleeding patterns.

Use in the elderly: Climesse should only be used in the elderly for the indications listed.

Use in children: Climesse should not be used in children.

Contra-indications: Known or suspected pregnancy. History of, known or suspected cancer of the breast. Known or suspected oestrogen-dependent neoplasia. Undiagnosed abnormal genital bleeding. Active thrombophlebitis or thromboembolic disorders. Severe cardiac, hepatic or renal disease. Known hypersensitivity to one of the ingredients.

Special warnings and special precautions for use: A thorough gynaecological and physical examination is advised before and periodically during treatment with Climesse.

At the present time there is suggestive evidence of a slight increase in the relative risk of carcinoma of the breast with hormone replacement therapy used for longer than five years. Regular breast examinations should be carried out in women on HRT and mammography where appropriate. Breast status should also be closely monitored in women with a history of, or known, breast nodules, or fibrocystic disease, or with a family history of breast cancer.

Some conditions can deteriorate on hormone replacement therapy and it is essential that patients with these conditions should be closely monitored, including otosclerosis, migraine, multiple sclerosis, epilepsy, diabetes, hypertension, asthma, hypercalcaemia, porphyria, systemic lupus erythematosus, uterine fibroids and tetany.

Patients with mild chronic liver disease should have their liver function checked every 8–12 weeks. Patients with cardiac or renal dysfunction, cholelithiasis, Dubin-Johnson syndrome or Rotor syndrome should also be closely monitored.

If migrainous or frequent unusually severe headaches occur for the first time, or any other symptoms that are possible prodromata of vascular occlusion occur, treatment should be suspended pending further investigation.

If jaundice, hepatitis, itching of the whole body, an increase in epileptic seizures or a significant rise in blood pressure occur, treatment should be stopped immediately. Consider discontinuation of treatment when trauma, illness or impending surgery is considered to entail a risk of thrombosis.

Some epidemiological evidence suggests that the use of hormone replacement therapy (HRT) is associated with an increased risk of developing deep vein thrombosis (DVT) or pulmonary embolism (PE). The relative risk is about 2–3.6 for healthy women, which would represent one additional case of venous thromboembolism (VTE) among 5000 women treated with HRT during a year.

Women with severe varicose veins, severe obesity (Body Mass Index >30 kg/m²), or those undergoing immobilisation for 3 weeks or more, trauma or surgery requiring bed rest, are generally considered to be at increased risk of VTE. These women and those with positive family history and women with a history of thromboembolic disorders during pregnancy or in association with oestrogen use should be given careful considerations before receiving HRT. If venous thromboembolism develops after initiating the drug should be discontinued.

Climesse is designed to prevent stimulation of the endometrium in postmenopausal women, usually resulting in amenorrhoea. Irregular bleeding may occur in the first few months of therapy but this will usually settle completely. A certain proportion of women, particularly those closer to the menopause, may fail to develop amenorrhoea and for these women an alternative form of hormone replacement therapy may be more suitable. Certain conditions may predispose to persistent irregular bleeding, such as uterine polyps and fibroids and this may warrant further investigation. As for all postmenopausal bleeding, appropriate investigations, including endometrial assessment should be carried out in all women who experience prolonged bleeding or who begin to bleed after initiation of therapy following a period of amenorrhoea.

Premenopausal women should not receive Climesse therapy because it may inhibit ovulation, disturb cycle regularity and result in unpredictable bleeding patterns. Climesse is not intended to be an oral contraceptive and should not be used to prevent pregnancy.

Interactions with other medicaments and other forms of interaction: Preparations which induce hepatic microsomal liver enzymes such as barbiturates, rifampicin, phenytoin and carbamazepine may accelerate the metabolism of oestrogens/progestogens and may reduce their efficacy.

Pregnancy and lactation: Climesse should not be used in pregnant or nursing women.

Effects on ability to drive and use machinery: No adverse effects on the ability to drive or operate machines have been recorded.

Undesirable effects

Urogenital tract: During the first few months of therapy, irregular bleeding or spotting may occur; this is usually transient. Mucous vaginal discharge, dysmenorrhoea.

Central nervous system: Headaches, dizziness, vertigo, fatigue, irritability, depressive mood, changes in libido.

Cardiovascular system: Hypertension, palpitations, thrombophlebitis, oedema, epistaxis.

Gastrointestinal tract: Dyspepsia, flatulence, nausea, vomiting, abdominal pain and bloating, biliary stasis.

Skin and appendages: General pruritus, urticaria and other rashes, acne, alopecia.

Endocrine system: Breast tension and pain, enlargement of the breast, decrease in glucose tolerance.

Miscellaneous: Weight gain, leg cramps.

Overdose: No reports of ill-effects from overdosage have been reported. There are no specific antidotes for overdosage and if further treatment is required it should be symptomatic.

Pharmacological particulars

Pharmacodynamic properties: Oestradiol valerate is used in oestrogen deficiency states. Treatment with oestrogens relieves menopausal vasomotor symptoms. Oestrogens cross the placenta.

Norethisterone is a progestogen added to prevent endometrial hyperplasia and increased risk of endometrial carcinoma which can be induced by unopposed oestrogen use.

Pharmacokinetic properties: Oestradiol valerate, like most natural oestrogens is readily and fully absorbed from the GI tract is 50% bound to plasma proteins and is rapidly metabolised in the liver to oestriol and oestrone. When given orally in doses of 1–2 mg, peak levels of oestradiol are generally observed 3–6 hours after ingestion, but by 24 hours (range 6–48 hours) concentrations have returned to baseline (i.e. pre-treatment concentrations).

Oestradiol undergoes first-pass effect in the liver. There is some enterohepatic recycling. It is excreted via the kidney in the urine as water soluble esters (sulphate and glucoronide) together with a small proportion of unchanged oestradiol. Other metabolites have been identified.

Norethisterone is absorbed from the GI tract and its effects last for at least 24 hours. When a dose of 1 mg is given, there are wide variations in serum norethisterone levels at any particular time point after dosing (100–1700 pg/mL). Norethisterone undergoes first pass effect with a resulting loss of 36% of the dose. When injected, it is detectable in the plasma after 2 days and is not completely excreted in the urine after 5 days. There are large inter-subject variations in elimination half-life and bioavailability. The most important metabolites are several isomers of 5-adihydronorethisterone and of tetrahydronorethisterone which are excreted mainly as glucuronides.

Preclinical safety data: The toxicity profiles of oestradiol valerate and norethisterone are well known and reveal no human health risk.

Pharmaceutical particulars

List of excipients: Lactose, maize starch, povidine, purified water, talc, magnesium stearate, hydroxypropylmethyl cellulose, propylene glycol, iron oxide red (E172), titanium dioxide (E171), purified water.

Incompatibilities: Not applicable.

Shelf life: 36 months as packaged for sale.

Special precautions for storage: Store the tablets below 25°C, in a dry place. Do not refrigerate. Protect from light.

Nature and contents of container: Blister strips of aluminium foil/UPVC (20 μm/250 μm), in cardboard cartons. Each blister contains 28 tablets and cartons will contain 1 or 3 blisters.

Instructions for use/handling: There are no special instructions for handling.

Marketing authorisation holder: Novartis Pharmaceuticals UK Limited, Trading as Sandoz Pharmaceuticals, Frimley Business Park, Frimley, Camberley, Surrey GU16 5SG.

Marketing authorisation number PL 0101/0396.

Date of first authorisation/renewal of authorisation 27 October 1995.

Date of (partial) revision of the text September 1997.

CLOZARIL 25 mg
CLOZARIL 100 mg

Qualitative and quantitative composition
Each tablet contains 25 mg or 100 mg clozapine.

Pharmaceutical form Tablet.

Clinical particulars

Therapeutic indications: The indication of treatment-resistant schizophrenic patients, i.e. patients who are unresponsive to, or intolerant of, conventional neuroleptics.

Non-responsiveness is defined as a lack of satisfactory clinical improvement despite the use of adequate doses of at least two marketed neuroleptics prescribed for adequate durations.

Intolerance is defined as the impossibility to achieve adequate benefit with conventional neuroleptic drugs because of severe and untreatable neurological adverse reactions (extrapyramidal symptoms or tardive dyskinesia).

Posology and method of administration

Dosage and administration: Initiation of Clozaril treatment must be in hospital in-patients and is restricted to those patients with a white blood cell count >3.5×10⁹/l and a normal differential blood count. *The use of Clozaril is restricted to patients who are registered with the Clozaril patient monitoring service.*

The dosage must be adjusted individually. For each patient the lowest effective dose should be used.

Adults

Initial dose: 12.5 mg (one half of a 25 mg tablet) once or twice on the first day, followed by one or two 25 mg tablets on the second day. If well tolerated, the daily dose may then be increased slowly in increments of 25 mg to 50 mg in order to achieve a dose level of up to 300 mg/day within 2 to 3 weeks. Thereafter, if required, the daily dose may be further increased in increments of 50 to 100 mg at half-weekly or, preferably, weekly intervals.

Therapeutic dose range: in most patients, antipsychotic efficacy can be expected with 200 to 450 mg/day in divided doses. The total daily dose may be divided unevenly, with the larger portion at bedtime.

Maximum dose: a few patients may require larger doses to obtain maximum therapeutic benefit. Judicious increments (not exceeding 100 mg per increment) are permissible up to a maximum dose of 900 mg/day. Adverse reactions may increase at doses over 450 mg/day, in particular seizures.

Maintenance dose: after achieving maximum therapeutic benefit, many patients can be maintained on lower doses. Careful downward titration to the level of 150–300 mg/day given individual doses is recommended. At daily doses not exceeding 200 mg, a single administration in the evening may be appropriate.

Ending therapy: if termination of Clozaril therapy is planned, a gradual reduction in dose is recommended over at least a 1 to 2 week period. If abrupt discontinuation is necessary the patient should be carefully observed, particularly in view of the return of psychotic symptoms.

Restarting therapy (providing the patient has not ceased therapy due to a haematological abnormality – see Precautions): in patients for whom the interval since the last dose of Clozaril exceeds 2 days, treatment should be re-initiated with 12.5 mg (one half of a 25 mg tablet) given once or twice on the first day. If this dose is well tolerated, it may be feasible to titrate the dose to the therapeutic level more quickly than is recommended for initial treatment. However, if patients have previously experienced respiratory or cardiac arrest with initial dosing, and were then able to be successfully titrated to a therapeutic dose, re-titration should be done with extreme caution.

Switching from a previous neuroleptic to Clozaril: it is generally recommended that Clozaril should not be used in combination with other neuroleptics, including depot preparations, which may have a myelosuppressive effect. When Clozaril treatment is to be initiated in a patient who is on oral neuroleptic therapy, it is recommended that the other neuroleptic be discontinued by tapering the dosage downwards, before Clozaril therapy is initiated as described above.

Children: Not recommended.

Use in the elderly: In elderly patients it is recommended to initiate treatment at a particularly low dose (12.5 mg given once on the first day) and to restrict subsequent dose increments to 25 mg/day.

Other special patient groups: Patients with a history of epilepsy should be closely monitored during Clozaril therapy since dose-related convulsions have been reported. Therefore in patients with a history of seizures, as well as those suffering from cardiovascular, renal or hepatic disorders, the initial dose should be 12.5 mg given once on the first day, and dosage increase should be slow and in small increments.

Method of administration: Oral.

Contra-indications: Allergy to one or more of the constituents of the formulation.

Patients with a history of drug-induced neutropenia/agranulocytosis, or with myeloproliferative disorders, must not be treated with Clozaril.

Other contra-indications are uncontrolled epilepsy, alcoholic and toxic psychoses, drug intoxication, comatose conditions, circulatory collapse and/or CNS depression of any cause and severe renal or cardiac failure. Patients with active liver disease associated with nausea, anorexia or jaundice. Progressive liver disease or hepatic failure are also contra-indicated.

Special warnings and special precautions for use

Precautions: Clozaril can cause agranulocytosis – the following precautionary measures are mandatory: Before starting Clozaril treatment, a white blood cell count and differential count must be performed. Generally, only patients with normal findings may receive the drug.

During Clozaril treatment the white blood cell count and differential count must be monitored weekly for the first 18 weeks and at least at 2 week intervals for the first year of therapy. After the patient has been on treatment for 1 year with stable neutrophil counts over that period, then the frequency of monitoring may be changed to 4 week intervals. Monitoring must continue throughout treatment and for 4 weeks after complete discontinuation of Clozaril.

Particular attention should be paid to the white blood cell count and the neutrophil count if any, flu-like complaints or other symptoms develop which might suggest infection. Each time Clozaril is prescribed the patients should be reminded to contact the treating physician immediately if any kind of infection begins to develop.

An immediate differential blood count must be obtained when any symptoms or signs of infection develop.

If the white blood cell count falls below 3.0×10⁹/l and/or the absolute neutrophil count drops below 1.5×10⁹/l Clozaril must be withdrawn at once and the patient closely monitored. The patient must not be re-exposed to Clozaril.

In the event of an infection or a routine white blood cell count between 3.0 and 3.5×10⁹/l and/or a neutrophil count between 1.5 and 2.0×10⁹/l, the patient should be re-evaluated immediately with respect to the white blood cell count and the differential count. Should there be a decline in either, Clozaril must be withdrawn at once. If the blood cell count remains the same or increases, treatment with Clozaril may continue provided that the leucocytosis and granulocytosis are checked at least twice weekly until it is certain that the patient has a stable leucocyte count within the range 3.0 to 3.5×10⁹/l or higher. If Clozaril has been withdrawn and a further fall of the white blood cell count below 1.0×10⁹/l occurs and/or the neutrophils decrease below 0.5×10⁹/l, the patient should be referred immediately to a unit experienced in the management of febrile neutropenia.

If possible, the patient should be referred to a specialised haematological unit, where protective isolation and the administration of broad spectrum antibiotics and GM-CSF (granulocyte-macrophage colony stimulating factor) or G-CSF (granulocyte colony stimulating factor) should be considered. Due to the myelotoxic potential of some antibiotics, careful consideration should be given to the antibiotics chosen. It is recommended that the colony stimulating factor therapy be discontinued when the neutrophil count has returned to a level above 1.0×10⁹/l.

Clozaril lowers the seizure threshold – see *Dosage and administration – Other special patient groups.*

Clozaril has anticholinergic activity therefore, careful supervision is indicated in the presence of prostatic enlargement, narrow-angle glaucoma and paralytic ileus.

Patient with pre-existing liver disorders may receive Clozaril but need regular liver function test monitoring. Patients who develop symptoms of possible liver dysfunction such as nausea, vomiting and/or anorexia during Clozaril treatment should have their liver function tests performed immediately. If the elevation is clinically relevant or if the patient is jaundiced Clozaril should be immediately discontinued. It may be resumed (see *Restarting therapy*) only when the liver function tests have returned to normal values. In such cases liver function should be closely monitored after the re-introduction of the drug (see *Undesirable effects*).

Orthostatic hypotension with or without syncope, can occur with Clozaril treatment. Rarely collapse can be profound and may be accompanied by cardiac and/or respiratory arrest. Such events are more likely to occur during initial titration in association with rapid dose escalation; on very rare occasions they have occurred after the first dose. Therefore, patients commencing Clozaril treatment require close medical supervision.

During Clozaril therapy, patients may experience transient temperature elevations above 38°C, with the peak incidence within the first 3 weeks of treatment. This fever is generally benign. Occasionally, it may be associated with an increase or decrease in the white blood cell count. Patients with fever should be carefully evaluated to rule out the possibility of an underlying infection or the development of agranulocytosis. In the presence of high fever, the possibility of Neuroleptic Malignant Syndrome (NMS) must be considered.

Since Clozaril may cause sedation and weight gain, thereby increasing the risk of thromboembolism, immobilisation of patients should be avoided.

Warning: Clozaril can cause agranulocytosis. A fatality rate of up to 1 in 300 has been estimated when Clozaril was used prior to recognition of the risk of agranulocytosis and the need for routine blood monitoring. Since that time careful monitoring of patients has been demonstrated to be effective in markedly reducing the risk of fatality.

Because of the risk associated with Clozaril therapy its use is limited to treatment-resistant schizophrenic patients (see *indications*):

1. Who have normal leucocyte findings (white blood cell count and differential blood count), and

2. In whom regular leucoctye counts can be performed weekly during the first 18 weeks and at least every 2 weeks for the first year of therapy. After the patient has been on treatment for 1 year with stable neutrophil counts over that period, then the frequency of monitoring may be changed to 4 week intervals. Monitoring must continue throughout treatment and for 4 weeks after complete discontinuation of Clozaril.

The patient must be under the supervision of a specialist and supply of Clozaril is restricted to hospital and retail pharmacies registered with the Clozaril Patient Monitoring Service.

Prescribing physicians must register themselves, their patients and a nominated pharmacist with the Clozaril Patient Monitoring Service. This service provides for the required leucocyte counts as well as a drug supply audit so that Clozaril treatment is promptly withdrawn from any patient who develops abnormal leucocyte findings.

Each time Clozaril is prescribed, patients should be reminded to contact the treating physician immediately if any kind of infection begins to develop. Particular attention should be paid to flu-like complaints or other symptoms which might suggest infection, such as fever or sore throat.

Interaction with other medicaments and other forms of interaction: Clozaril should not be used concurrently with drugs associated with a substantial potential to depress bone marrow function, such as co-trimoxazole, chloramphenicol, sulphonamides, pyrazolone analgesics, phenylbutazone, penicillamine, carbamazepine or cytotoxic agents. Concomitant use of long-acting depot antipsychotics (which have myelosuppressive potential) is not recommended because these medicaments cannot be rapidly removed from the body in situations where this may be required e.g. Neutropenia.

Concomitant use of Clozaril and lithium or other centrally-acting agents may increase the risk of development of neuroleptic malignant syndrome.

Clozaril may enhance the central effects of alcohol,

MAO inhibitors, CNS depressants including narcotics, benzodiazepines and antihistamines. Caution is advised with patients who are receiving (or have recently received) benzodiazepines or any other psychotropic drug, as these patients may have an increased risk of circulatory collapse which, on rare occasions, can be profound and may lead to cardiac and/or respiratory arrest. Because of the possibility of additive effects, caution in the concomitant administration of drugs with anticholinergic, hypotensive or respiratory depressant effects is essential.

Since Clozaril is highly bound to plasma proteins, the administration of Clozaril to a patient taking another drug which is highly bound to protein (e.g. Warfarin) may cause an increase in plasma concentrations of this drug, potentially resulting in adverse effects. Conversely, adverse effects may result from displacement of protein-bound clozapine by other highly protein-bound drugs.

The metabolism of clozapine is mediated mainly by cytochrome P450 1A2 and probably to a minor extent by cytochrome P450 2D6. The concomitant administration of drugs which possess affinity to one or both of these enzymes may result in an increase in the plasma levels of clozapine and/or the co-administered drug.

However, with tricyclic antidepressants, phenothiazines and type 1c antiarrhythmics, which are known to bind to cytochrome P450 2D6, no clinically relevant interactions with clozapine have been observed thus far. On theoretical grounds, however, it is possible that the plasma levels of such drugs are increased by clozapine, so that it may be appropriate to use them at doses lower than usually prescribed.

Administration of cimetidine concomitantly with high-dose Clozaril therapy was associated with increased plasma clozapine levels and the occurrence of adverse effects.

Elevated serum levels of clozapine have been reported in patients receiving drug in combination with fluoxetine (up to 2 fold) or fluvoxamine (up to 10 fold).

Drugs known to increase the activities of cytochrome P450 enzymes may decrease the plasma levels of clozapine. Discontinuation of the concomitant administration of carbamazepine resulted in an increase of the clozapine plasma levels. The concomitant use of phenytoin has been found to decrease the clozapine plasma concentration, resulting in reduced effectiveness of a previously effective Clozaril dose.

Owing to its noradrenolytic action, Clozaril may reduce the blood pressure increasing effect of noradrenaline or other predominantly alpha-adrenergic agents and reverse the pressor effect of adrenaline.

Pregnancy and lactation: The safe use of Clozaril in pregnancy has not been established and its use is not recommended. A return to normal menstrual cycling may occur as a result of switching from conventional neuroleptics to Clozaril, therefore adequate contraceptive measures must be ensured in women of child bearing potential. Animal studies suggest that Clozaril is excreted in breast milk; therefore, mothers receiving Clozaril must not breast-feed.

Effects on ability to drive and to use machines: Drowsiness may occur, especially at the beginning of therapy. Owing to its sedative action, Clozaril may impair the reactions of the patients, e.g. when driving vehicles or operating machinery. Clozaril should be administered with caution to patients who participate in activities requiring complete mental alertness.

Undesirable effects: Neutropenia leading to agranulocytosis is a risk of Clozaril treatment. This reaction, although generally reversible, can prove fatal. The majority of cases occur in the first 18 weeks of treatment. Because immediate withdrawal of the drug is required to prevent the development of life-threatening agranulocytosis, monitoring of the white blood cell count is mandatory (see *Warning* and *Precautions*).

Patients on Clozaril may develop unexplained leucocytosis, including eosinophilia, especially in the initial weeks of treatment. Isolated cases of various types of leukaemia have been reported in patients treated with Clozaril. However, there is no evidence to suggest a causal relationship between the drug and any type of leukaemia. The reported occurrence rate is in the range of the background incidence of these diseases in the general population. Isolated cases of thrombocytopenia have been reported but no causal relationship has been established.

Central nervous system: Fatigue, drowsiness and sedation are among the most common side-effects observed. Dizziness or headache may also occur.

Clozaril lowers the seizure threshold in a dose-dependent manner and may cause EEG changes, including the occurrence of spike and wave complexes. Myoclonic jerks or convulsions may, therefore, be precipitated in individuals who have epileptogenic potential but no previous history of epilepsy. In this case Clozaril treatment should be suspended for 24 hours and then resumed at a lower dose. It may be possible to control the problem by reducing the dosage and if necessary, raising it again very gradually. Anticonvulsant treatment may be considered but carbamazepine should be avoided because of its potential to depress bone marrow function and, with other anticonvulsant drugs, the possibility of a pharmacokinetic interaction should be considered.

Valproic acid was found to cause only non-significant increases in clozapine blood levels and to be well tolerated in the majority of patients receiving it in combination with Clozaril. In rare cases Clozaril may cause confusion, restlessness, agitation and delirium.

Extrapyramidal symptoms are limited mainly to tremor, akathisia and rigidity and if such effects occur, they tend to be mild and transient. Very rarely, tardive dyskinesia has been reported in patients on Clozaril. Some patients in whom tardive dyskinesia developed with other neuroleptics have improved on Clozaril.

There have been several reported cases of Neuroleptic Malignant Syndrome (NMS) in patients receiving Clozaril either alone or in combination with lithium or other CNS-active agents.

Autonomic nervous system: Dry mouth, disturbances of accommodation and disturbances in sweating and temperature regulation have been reported. Hypersalivation is a common side effect.

Cardiovascular system: Tachycardia and/or postural hypotension, with or without syncope, may occur, especially in the initial weeks of treatment. Less commonly, hypertension may also occur. In rare cases profound circulatory collapse has been reported. ECG changes may occur and isolated cases of cardiac arrhythmias, pericarditis and myocarditis (with or without eosinophilia) have been reported, some of which have been fatal. Myocarditis can be difficult to diagnose as symptoms may be non-specific. Heart failure, arrhythmia or symptoms mimicking myocardial infarction or pericarditis may, however, be presenting features. Confirmation of diagnosis may not be possible but if suspicion is high, Clozaril medication should be stopped.

Rare cases of thromboembolism have been reported.

Respiratory system: In isolated cases, with or without circulatory collapse, respiratory depression or arrest has occurred. Rarely, aspiration of ingested food may occur in patients presenting with dysphagia or as a consequence of acute overdosage.

Gastro-intestinal system: Clozaril has been reported to cause nausea and vomiting. Constipation may occur, probably due to the anticholinergic properties of the compound. This is usually mild, however, on occasions more severe and sometimes fatal complications have been reported, including gastrointestinal obstruction and paralytic ileus. Patients receiving clozapine should be monitored for constipation and laxatives prescribed as required. Particular care is indicated in patients who are receiving concomitant medications known to cause constipation (especially those with anticholinergic properties such as some neuroleptics, antidepressants and antiparkinsonians), have a history of colonic disease, or have a history of lower abdominal surgery as these may exacerbate the situation. The importance of recognising and treating constipation cannot be over emphasised.

Asymptomatic elevations in liver enzymes occur commonly particularly in the first three months of treatment and usually resolve without the need to interrupt Clozaril treatment. Rarely hepatitis and cholestatic jaundice may occur. Very rarely fulminant hepatic necrosis has been reported. If jaundice develops, Clozaril should be discontinued (see *Precautions*).

As a rare event, Clozaril treatment may be associated with dysphagia, a possible cause of aspiration. Parotid gland enlargement has also been reported rarely.

In rare cases, acute pancreatitis has been reported.

Genito-urinary system: Urinary incontinence, urinary retention and, in a few cases, priapism have been reported. Isolated cases of acute interstitial nephritis have been reported in association with Clozaril.

Miscellaneous: Benign hyperthermia may occur, especially in the initial weeks of treatment. Isolated reports of skin reactions have been received.

Clozaril has not been associated with elevated prolactin levels.

Sudden unexplained deaths are known to occur among psychiatric patients who receive antipsychotic medication as well as those who do not. Isolated cases of such deaths have been reported in patients receiving Clozaril.

On rare occasions, hyperglycaemia has been reported in patients on Clozaril treatment. Rarely, increases in CPK values have occurred.

With prolonged treatment considerable weight gain has been observed in some patients.

Overdose: In cases of acute intentional or accidental Clozaril overdosage, for which information on the outcome is available to date, the mortality is about 12%. Most of the fatalities were associated with cardiac failure or pneumonia caused by aspiration and occurred at doses above 2000 mg. There have been reports of patients recovering from an overdose in excess of 10,000 mg. However, in a few adult individuals, primarily those not previously exposed to Clozaril, the ingestion of doses as low as 400 mg led to life-threatening comatose conditions and, in one case, to death. In young children, the intake of 50 to 200 mg resulted in strong sedation or coma without being lethal.

Signs and symptoms: drowsiness, lethargy, coma, areflexia, confusion, hallucinations, agitation, delirium, extrapyramidal symptoms, hyper-reflexia, convulsions, hypersalivation, mydriasis, blurred vision, thermolability, tachycardia, hypotension, collapse, cardiac arrhythmias, aspiration pneumonia, dyspnoea, respiratory depression or failure.

Treatment: gastric lavage and/or the administration of activated charcoal within the first 6 hours post ingestion (peritoneal dialysis and haemodialysis are not very effective). Symptomatic treatment under continuous cardiac monitoring, surveillance of respiration, monitoring of electrolytes and acid-base balance. The use of adrenaline should be avoided in the treatment of hypotension because of the possibility of a 'reverse adrenaline' effect. Close medical supervision is necessary for at least five days because of the possibility of delayed reactions.

Pharmacological properties

Pharmacodynamic properties: Clozaril is an antipsychotic agent which differs from conventional neuroleptics.

In pharmacological experiments, it does not induce catalepsy or inhibit apomorphine- or amphetamine-induced steroptyped behaviour. It has weak dopamine receptor-blocking activity at both D_1, D_2, D_3 and D_5 receptors, but shows high potency for the D_4 receptor, in addition to potent noradrenolytic, anticholinergic, antihistaminic and arousal reaction inhibiting effects. It has also been shown to possess antiserotoninergic properties.

Clinically, Clozaril produces rapid and marked sedation, and exerts strong antipsychotic effects. In particular, the antipsychotic effects have been demonstrated in schizophrenic patients resistant to other drug treatment. In such cases, Clozaril has proven effective in relieving both positive and negative schizophrenic symptoms, with over half showing clinically relevant improvement.

Pharmacokinetic properties: The absorption of orally administered Clozaril is 90–95%; the rate or extent of absorption is not influenced by food.

Clozapine the active ingredient of Clozaril, is subject to a moderate first-pass metabolism, resulting in an absolute bioavailability of 50–60%. In steady-state conditions, when given twice daily, peak blood levels occur on average at 2.1 hours (range: 0.4–4.2 hr). The volume of distribution is 1.6 L/kg. Clozapine is 95% bound to plasma proteins. Its elimination is biphasic with a mean terminal half-life of 12 hours (range: 6–26 hr). After single doses of 75 mg the mean terminal half-life was 7.9 hours; it increased to 14.2 hours when steady-state conditions were reached by administering daily doses of 75 mg for at least 7 days. Dosage increases from 37.5 to 75 and 150 mg given twice daily were found to result during steady-state in linearly dose-proportional increases in the area under the plasma concentration/time curve (AUC), as well as in the peak and minimum plasma concentrations.

Clozapine is almost completely metabolised before excretion. Of the main metabolites only the desmethyl metabolite was found to be active. Its pharmacological actions resemble those of clozapine, but are considerably weaker and of short duration. Only trace amounts of unchanged drug are detected in the urine and faeces, approximately 50% of the administered dose being excreted as metabolites in the urine and 30% in the faeces.

Preclinical safety data: There are no pre-clinical data of relevance to the prescriber which are additional to that already included in other sections of the SmPC.

Pharmaceutical particulars

List of excipients: Magnesium stearate, colloidal anhydrous silica, talc, polyvinylpyrrolidone, maize starch, lactose.

Incompatibilities: None.

Shelf life: 4 years.

Special precautions for storage: None.

Nature and contents of container: PVC/PVDC blister packs in a cardboard carton containing 28 or 84 tablets.

Instructions for use/handling: None.

Marketing authorisation holder: Norvatis Pharmaceuticals UK Limited, Trading as Sandoz Pharmaceuticals, Frimley Business Park, Frimley, Camberley, Surrey GU16 5SG.

Marketing authorisation number

Clozaril 25 mg Tablets: PL 0101/0228

Clozaril 100 mg Tablets: PL 0101/0229.

Date of first authorisation/renewal of authorisation Date Present Licence Granted: 22.12.89
Date of last renewal: 15.2.95.

Date of (partial) revision of the text 9 September 1998.

DESFERAL*

Presentation A sterile, lyophilised powder available in vials containing 500 mg of Desferrioxamine Mesylate PhEur.

Uses

Indications: Iron overload–Acute iron poisoning; primary and secondary haemochromatosis including thalassaemia and transfusional haemosiderosis; in patients in whom concomitant disorders (eg severe anaemia, hypoproteinaemia, renal or cardiac failure) preclude phlebotomy; and for the diagnosis of iron storage disease and certain anaemias.

Aluminium overload–in patients on maintenance dialysis for end stage renal failure where preventative measures (eg reverse osmosis) have failed and with proven aluminium-related bone disease and/or anaemia, dialysis encephalopathy; and for diagnosis of aluminium overload.

Mode of action: Desferal is a chelating agent for trivalent iron and aluminium ions; the resulting chelates (ferrioxamine and aluminoxamine) are stable and non-toxic. Neither chelate undergoes significant intestinal absorption, and any formed systemically as a result of parenteral administration is rapidly excreted via the kidneys without deleterious effects. Desferal takes up iron either free or bound to ferritin and haemosiderin. Similarly it mobilises and chelates tissue bound aluminium. It does not remove iron from haemin containing substances including haemoglobin and transferrin. Since both ferrioxamine and aluminoxamine are completely excreted, Desferal promotes the excretion of iron and aluminium in urine and faeces thus reducing pathological iron or aluminium deposits in the organs and tissues.

Pharmacokinetics: Desferrioxamine mesylate is rapidly absorbed following intramuscular or subcutaneous administration. In healthy volunteers peak plasma concentrations of desferrioxamine (15.5μmol/l, 8.7μg/ml) and ferrioxamine (3.7μmol/l, 2.3μg/ml) were observed at 30 minutes and 1 hour respectively, following an injection (10 mg/kg) of desferrioxamine. It is only poorly absorbed from the gastrointestinal tract in the presence of intact mucosa.

Serum protein binding of desferrioxamine is less than 10% *in vitro*.

In healthy subjects elimination is biphasic, first phase half-lives for desferrioxamine and ferrioxamine are 1 hour and 2.4 hours, respectively. In the second phase both compounds have a half-life of 6 hours. Of the injected dose 22% appears in the urine as desferrioxamine and 1% as ferrioxamine, after 6 hours.

In patients with haemochromatosis peak plasma levels of 7.0μmol/l (3.9μg/ml) were measured for desferrioxamine, and 15.7μmol/l (9.6μg/ml) for ferrioxamine, 1 hour after intramuscular injection of 10 mg/kg desferrioxamine. These patients eliminated desferrioxamine and ferrioxamine with half-lives of 5.6 and 4.6 hours, respectively. Six hours after the injection 17% of the dose was excreted in the urine as desferrioxamine and 12% as ferrioxamine.

In patients dialysed for renal failure who received 40 mg/kg desferrioxamine infused i.v. within 1 hour, the plasma concentration at the end of the infusion was 152μmol/l (85.2μg/ml) when the infusion was given between dialysis sessions. Plasma concentrations of desferrioxamine were between 13% and 27% lower when the infusion was administered during dialysis. Concentrations of ferrioxamine were in all cases approx. 7.0μmol/l (4.3μg/ml) with concomitant aluminoxamine levels of 2-3μmol/l (1.2-1.8μg/ml). After the infusion was discontinued, the plasma concentration of desferrioxamine decreased rapidly with a half-life of 20 minutes. A smaller fraction of the dose was eliminated with a longer half-life of 14 hours. Plasma concentrations of aluminoxamine continued to increase for up to 48 hours post-infusion and reached values of approx. 7μmol/l (4μg/ml). Following dialysis the plasma concentration of aluminoxamine fell to 2.2μmol/l (1.3μg/ml), indicating that the aluminoxamine complex is dialysable.

During peritoneal dialysis desferrioxamine is absorbed if administered in the dialysis fluid.

Dosage and administration Desferal may be administered parenterally or orally (for acute iron poisoning only).

Preparation: For parenteral administration: The drug should preferably be employed in the form of a 10% solution, eg by dissolving the contents of one vial (500 mg) in 5 ml of water for injection. When administered subcutaneously the needle should not be inserted too close to the dermis. The 10% Desferal solution can be diluted with routinely employed infusion solutions (saline, dextrose or dextrose-saline), although these should not be used as solvent for the dry substance. Dissolved Desferal can also be added to dialysis fluid and given intraperitoneally to patients on continuous ambulatory peritoneal dialysis (CAPD) or continuous cyclic peritoneal dialysis (CCPD).

Only clear pale yellow Desferal solutions should be used. Opaque, cloudy or discoloured solutions should be discarded. Heparin is pharmaceutically incompatible with Desferal solutions.

For oral administration: 5-10 g Desferal should be dissolved in 50-100 ml of water.

Treatment: Acute iron poisoning:

Adults and children: Desferal may be administered both orally and parenterally. It is important to initiate treatment as soon as possible.

Gastric lavage should be carried out as quickly as possible using, if readily available, 1% sodium bicarbonate solution. This should be followed by oral administration of Desferal which will chelate any iron remaining in the stomach and prevent any further absorption. Further measures, eg. sodium bicarbonate, sedatives, oxygen etc., may be given as necessary.

Patients with–

- serum iron levels >500 μg/dl (89.5 μmol/l), or
- serum iron levels >350 μg/dl (62.6μmol/l) with evidence of free iron, or
- with signs and symptoms of acute iron poisoning,

should be given Desferal either intramuscularly or intravenously to eliminate iron that has already been absorbed. The dosage and route of administration should be adapted to the severity of the poisoning.

Dosage: The normal dose is 2 g for an adult and 1 g for a child, administered as a single intramuscular dose.

If the patient is hypotensive or in shock, the intravenous route of administration is recommended. Initially the maximum rate of i.v. administration should be 15 mg/kg/h. It should be reduced after 4-6 hours so that the total dose does not exceed 80 mg/kg/24 hours. However, in the absence of adverse effects much larger doses may be tolerated.

Therapy should be continued until serum iron levels are less than the total iron binding capacity.

The effectiveness of treatment is dependent on an adequate urine output in order that the iron complex (ferrioxamine) is excreted from the body. Therefore, if oliguria or anuria develop, peritoneal dialysis or haemodialysis may become necessary to remove ferrioxamine.

It should be noted that the serum iron level may rise sharply when the iron is released from the tissues.

Theoretically 100 mg Desferal can chelate 8.5 mg of ferric iron.

Primary and secondary haemochromatosis including thalassaemia, in patients in whom concomitant disorders (e.g. severe anaemia, hypoproteinaemia) preclude phlebotomy: The main aim of therapy in younger patients is to achieve an iron balance and prevent haemosiderosis, whilst in the older patient a negative iron balance is desirable in order to slowly deplete the increased iron stores and to prevent the toxic effects of iron.

Adults and children: Desferal therapy should be commenced after the first 10–15 blood transfusions, or when serum ferritin levels reach 1,000ng/ml. The dose and mode of administration should be individually adapted according to the degree of iron overload.

Dose: The lowest effective dose should be used. The average daily dose will probably lie between 20 and 60 mg/kg. Patients with serum ferritin levels of <2,000ng/ml should require about 25 mg/kg/day, and those with levels between 2,000 and 3,000ng/ml about 35 mg/kg/day. Higher doses should only be employed if the benefit for the patient outweighs the risk of unwanted effects.

To assess the chelation therapy, 24 hour urinary iron excretion should initially be monitored daily. Starting with a dose of 500 mg daily the dose should be raised until a plateau of iron excretion is reached. Once the appropriate dose has been established, urinary iron excretion rates can be assessed at intervals of a few weeks.

Mode of administration: Slow subcutaneous infusions by means of a portable, light-weight, infusion pump over a period of 8-12 hours is effective and particularly convenient for ambulant patients. It may be possible to achieve a further increase in iron excretion by infusing the same daily dose over a 24 hour period. Patients should be treated 4-7 times a week depending on the degree of iron overload.

As intramuscular injections are less effective they should be given only when subcutaneous infusions are not appropriate.

Desferal can be administered by intravenous infusion during blood transfusion.

Continuous intravenous infusion is recommended for patients incapable of continuing subcutaneous infusions and in those who have cardiac problems secondary to iron overload. Implanted intravenous systems can be used when intensive chelation is carried out at home

Diagnosis of iron storage disease and certain anaemias: The Desferal test for iron overload is based on the principle that normal subjects do not excrete more than a fraction of a milligram of iron in their urine daily, and that a standard intramuscular injection of 500 mg of Desferal will not increase this above 1 mg (18 μmol). In iron storage diseases, however, the increase may be well over 1.5 mg (27μmol). It should be borne in mind that the test only yields reliable results when renal function is normal.

Desferal is administered as a 500 mg intramuscular injection. Urine is then collected for a period of 6 hours and its iron content determined. Excretion of 1-1.5 mg (18-27μmol) of iron during this 6-hour period is suggestive of iron overload; values greater than 1.5 mg (27μmol) can be regarded as pathological.

Use in the elderly: No special dosage regime is necessary but concurrent renal insufficiency should be taken into account.

Treatment for aluminium overload in patients with end-stage renal failure: Patients should receive Desferal if:

- they have symptoms or evidence of organ impairment due to aluminium overload
- they are asymptomatic but their serum aluminium levels are consistently above 60ng/ml and associated with a positive Desferal test (see below), particularly if a bone biopsy provides evidence of aluminium-related bone disease

Adults and children: Patients on maintenance haemodialysis or haemofiltration: 5 mg/kg once a week administered during the last hour of a dialysis as a slow intravenous infusion (to reduce loss of free drug in the dialysate).

Four weeks after the completion of a 3 month course of Desferal treatment a Desferal infusion test should be performed, followed by a second test 1 month later. Serum aluminium increases above baseline of less than 75ng/ml measured in 2 successive infusion tests indicate that further Desferal treatment is not necessary.

Patients on CAPD or CCPD: 5 mg/kg once a week prior to the final exchange of the day. Desferal may be administered i.v. (by slow infusion), i.m., s.c. or intraperitoneally; the intraperitoneal route is recommended for these patients.

Diagnosis of aluminium overload in patients with end-stage renal failure: A Desferal infusion test is recommended in patients with serum aluminium levels > 60ng/ml associated with serum ferritin levels > 100ng/ml.

Serum aluminium values should be determined from blood samples taken:

- immediately before a haemodialysis session (baseline); 5 mg/kg should then be administered as a slow intravenous infusion during the last hour of the dialysis
- at the start of the next haemodialysis session

An increase in serum aluminium above baseline of more than 150ng/ml is suggestive of aluminium overload. It should be noted that a negative test does not completely exclude the possibility of aluminium overload.

Theoretically 100 mg Desferal can bind 4.1 mg Al^{+++}.

Contra-indications, warnings and precautions

Contra-indications: Hypersensitivity to desferrioxamine mesylate unless the patient can be desensitised.

Warnings and precautions: Desferal should be used with caution in patients with renal impairment since the metal complexes are excreted via the kidneys. In these patients, dialysis will increase the elimination of chelated iron and aluminium.

Used alone Desferal may exacerbate neurological impairment in patients with aluminium-related encephalopathy. This deterioration (manifest as seizures) is probably related to an acute increase in brain aluminium secondary to elevated circulating levels. Pretreatment with clonazepam has been shown to afford protection against such impairment.

Treatment with Desferal by the intravenous route should only be administered in the form of *slow* infusions. If an intramuscular injection is accidentally given intravenously, this may lead to circulatory collapse.

Desferal should not be administered s.c. in concentrations and/or doses higher than those recommended as otherwise local irritation at the site of administration may occur more frequently.

Patients suffering from iron overload are particularly susceptible to infection. There have been reports of Desferal promoting some infections such as *Yersinia enterocolitica* and *Y.pseudotuberculosis*. If patients develop fever with pharyngitis, diffuse abdominal pain or enteritis/enterocolitis, Desferal therapy should be stopped, and appropriate treatment with antibiotics should be instituted. Desferal therapy may be resumed once the infection has cleared.

In patients undergoing haemodialysis while receiving Desferal, there have been rare reports of severe fungal infection (i.e. cases of mucormycosis). If any characteristic signs or symptoms occur Desferal treatment should be discontinued, mycological tests carried out and appropriate treatment immediately instituted. Mucormycosis has been reported to occur in dialysis patients not receiving Desferal, thus no causal link with the use of the drug has been established.

Disturbances of vision and hearing have been reported during prolonged Desferal therapy. In particular this has occurred in patients on higher than recommended therapy or in patients with low serum ferritin levels. Therefore, ophthalmological and audiological tests should be carried out both prior to the institution of long-term therapy with Desferal and at 3-monthly intervals during treatment. A detailed ophthalmological assessment is recommended (visual field measurements, funduscopy, colour vision testing using pseudoisochromatic plates and the Farnsworth D-15 colour test, slit lamp investigation, visual evoked potential studies).

If disturbances of vision or hearing do occur, treatment with Desferal should be stopped. Such disturbances may be reversible. If Desferal therapy is re-instituted later at a lower dosage, close monitoring of ophthalmological/ auditory function should be carried out with due regard to the risk-benefit ratio.

The use of inappropriately high doses of Desferal in patients with low ferritin levels has also been associated with growth retardation; dose reduction has been found to restore the growth rate to pretreatment levels in some cases. Three monthly checks on body weight and height are recommended in children.

Patients experiencing CNS effects such as dizziness or impaired vision or hearing should be warned against driving or operating machinery.

Use in pregnancy and lactation: Desferal has caused teratogenic effects in animals when given during pregnancy, particularly in the first trimester.

In rabbits, desferrioxamine caused skeletal malformations. However, these teratogenic effects in the foetuses were observed at doses which were toxic to the mother. In mice and rats desferrioxamine appears to be free of teratogenic activity.

Malformations have not occurred in children borne by patients reported to have received Desferal during pregnancy.

It is not known whether Desferal is excreted into the breast milk.

Desferal should not be given to pregnant or lactating women unless in the judgement of the physician, the expected benefits to the mother outweigh the potential risk to the child. This particularly applies to the first trimester.

Drug interactions: Oral administration of vitamin C (up to a maximum of 200 mg daily, given in divided doses) may serve to enhance excretion of the iron complex in response to Desferal; larger doses of vitamin C fail to produce an additional effect. Monitoring of cardiac function is indicated during such combined therapy. Vitamin C should be given only if the patient is receiving Desferal regularly, and should not be administered within the first month of Desferal therapy. In patients with severe chronic iron-storage disease undergoing combined treatment with Desferal and high doses of vitamin C (more than 500 mg daily) impairment of cardiac function has been encountered; this proved reversible when the vitamin C was withdrawn. Vitamin C supplements should not therefore be given to patients with cardiac failure.

Desferal should not be used in combination with prochlorperazine (a phenothiazine derivative) since prolonged unconsciousness may result.

Gallium^{67} imaging results may be distorted because of the rapid urinary excretion of Desferal-bound radiolabel. Discontinuation of Desferal 48 hours prior to scintigraphy is advised.

There is evidence that aluminium intoxication causes reduced erythropoiesis. In dialysed patients with aluminium and/or iron overload treated with desferrioxamine and erythropoietin some dosage adjustment of the latter may be necessary. Regular monitoring of iron stores should also be carried out.

Side-effects: The following unwanted effects have been reported:

Local reactions: Frequent: pain, swelling, induration, erythema, burning, pruritus, wheals; rash at the injection/infusion site, occasionally accompanied by fever, chills and malaise

Allergy: Rare: anaphylactic/anaphylactoid reactions with or without shock, angioedema

Special senses: Rare: blurred vision, decreased visual acuity, loss of vision, impairment of colour vision, night blindness, visual field defects, scotoma, retinopathy (pigmentary degeneration of the retina), optic neuritis, cataracts, corneal opacities; tinnitus; hearing loss (including high-frequency sensorineural hearing loss).

Skin: Rare: generalised rash, pruritus, urticaria.

Endocrine system: Rare: growth retardation.

Pulmonary system: Isolated cases: adult respiratory distress syndrome (with dyspnoea, cyanosis and interstitial pulmonary infiltrates; following excessively high i.v. doses of Desferal).

Central nervous system: Rare: neurological disturbances, dizziness, convulsions, exacerbation of neurological impairment in aluminium-related encephalopathy. Isolated cases: precipitation of dialysis dementia, peripheral sensory neuropathy, paraesthesia

Gastrointestinal system: Rare: nausea, vomiting, diarrhoea, abdominal cramps.

Renal system: Isolated cases: impaired renal function.

Liver: Rare: impaired hepatic function.

Cardiovascular system: Rare: hypotension.

Haematological system: Isolated cases: blood dyscrasias (e.g. thrombocytopenia).

Other: Rare: leg cramps. Isolated cases: malaise, bone pain.

Some of the side-effects mentioned above must be considered as signs and symptoms of the underlying disease. Excretion of iron complex during treatment with Desferal causes reddish-brown discolouration of the urine.

Overdosage: Desferal is usually administered parenterally and acute poisoning is unlikely to occur.

Signs and symptoms: Tachycardia, hypotension and gastrointestinal symptoms have occasionally occurred in patients who received an overdose of Desferal. Accidental administration of Desferal by the i.v. route may be associated with acute but transient loss of vision, aphasia, agitation, headache, nausea, bradycardia and hypotension.

Treatment: There is no specific antidote to Desferal but signs and symptoms may be eliminated by reducing the dosage and Desferal is dialysable. Appropriate supportive therapy should be instituted.

Pharmaceutical precautions

Storage: Desferal should be stored below 25°C.

Dilution: The reconstituted solution should be stored at room temperature (23°C or below) and used within 24 hours.

Legal category POM.

Package quantities Packs of 10 vials containing 500 mg Desferal.

Further information Nil.

Product licence number 00101/0523

DIOVAN* ▼

Qualitative and quantitative composition Active substance: (*S*)-N-valeryl-N-{[2'-(1H-tetrazol-5-yl)biphenyl-4-yl]methyl}-valine (INN=valsartan). One capsule contains 40 mg, 80 mg or 160 mg valsartan.

Pharmaceutical form Capsules.

Appearance:

40 mg: Light grey cap and body, marked CG HBH in black ink on the cap.

80 mg: Light grey cap and flesh opaque body, marked CG FZF in black ink on the cap.

160 mg: Dark grey cap and flesh opaque body, marked CG GOG in white ink on the cap.

Clinical particulars

Therapeutic indications: Treatment of hypertension.

Posology and method of administration: The recommended dose of Diovan is 80 mg once daily for most patients. The antihypertensive effect is substantially present within 2 weeks and maximal effects are seen after 4 weeks. In some patients whose blood pressure is not adequately controlled, the dose can either be increased to 160 mg, or a greater decrease in BP may be achieved by adding in a thiazide diuretic.

Diovan may also be administered with other antihypertensive agents.

Use in patients over 75 years: A lower starting dose of 40 mg once daily is recommended.

Use in renal impairment: No initial dose adjustment is required in patients with mild renal impairment (i.e. creatinine clearance 20–50 ml/min). For patients with moderate to severe renal impairment (i.e. creatinine less than 20 ml/min) or patients on dialysis, a lower starting dose of 40 mg once daily is recommended.

Use in patients with intravascular volume depletion: For those patients who have intravascular volume depletion (e.g. those treated with high dose diuretics who are unable to have their dose of diuretic reduced) a starting dose of 40 mg is recommended.

Use in patients with mild to moderate hepatic impairment: Treatment should commence at a dose of 40 mg once daily. A daily dose of 80 mg should not be exceeded. Patients with severe hepatic impairment, cirrhosis or biliary obstruction should not use Diovan (see *Contra-indications*).

Use in children: The safety and efficacy of Diovan have not been established in children.

Contra-indications: Hypersensitivity to any of the components of Diovan.

Pregnancy (see *Pregnancy and lactation*).

Severe hepatic impairment, cirrhosis, biliary obstruction.

Special warnings and precautions for use:

Sodium and/or volume depleted patients—In severely sodium-depleted and/or volume-depleted patients, such as those receiving high doses of diuretics, symptomatic hypotension may occur in rare cases after initiation of therapy with Diovan. For those patients whose diuretic dose cannot be reduced in order to correct their sodium and/or volume depletion a starting dose of 40 mg is recommended.

Renal artery stenosis—Short-term administration of Diovan to twelve patients with renovascular hypertension secondary to unilateral renal artery stenosis did not induce any significant changes in renal haemodynamics, serum creatinine, or blood urea nitrogen (BUN). However, since other drugs that affect the renin-angiotensin-aldosterone system may increase blood urea and serum creatinine in patients with bilateral or unilateral renal artery stenosis, monitoring is recommended as a safety measure.

Hepatic impairment—Based on pharmacokinetic data which demonstrate significantly increased plasma concentrations of valsartan in mild to moderately hepatically impaired patients, a lower dose is recommended (see *Posology and method of administration*). In these patients the dose of 80 mg should not be exceeded. Patients with severe hepatic impairment, cirrhosis or biliary obstruction are contra-indicated from using Diovan (see *Contra-indications*).

Interaction with other medicaments and other forms of interaction: Compounds which have been studied in clinical trials include cimetidine, warfarin, furosemide, digoxin, atenolol, indomethacin, hydrochlorothiazide, amlodipine, glibenclamide. Used together with cimetidine, the systemic exposure of valsartan may be marginally increased. A combination with glibenclamide may cause a decrease in the systemic exposure to valsartan.

As Diovan is not metabolised to a significant extent, clinically relevant drug-drug interactions in the form of metabolic induction or inhibition of the cytochrome P450 system are not expected with valsartan. Although valsartan is highly bound to plasma proteins, *in vitro* studies have not shown any interaction at this level with a range of molecules which are also highly protein-bound, such as diclofenac, furosemide, and warfarin.

Concomitant use of potassium-sparing diuretics (e.g. spironolactone, triamterene, amiloride), potassium supplements, or salt substitutes containing potassium may lead to increases in serum potassium. Comedication is not advisable.

Pregnancy and lactation: Although there is no experience with Diovan in pregnant women, in utero exposure to angiotensin converting enzyme (ACE) inhibitors given to pregnant women during the second and third trimesters has been reported to cause injury and death to the developing fetus. Thus, as for any drug that also acts directly on the renin-angiotensin-aldosterone system (RAAS), Diovan should not be used during pregnancy. If pregnancy is detected during therapy, Diovan should be discontinued as soon as possible.

It is not known whether valsartan is excreted in human milk. Valsartan was excreted in the milk of lactating rats. Thus, it is not advisable to use Diovan in lactating mothers.

Effects in ability to drive and use machines: As with other antihypertensive agents, it is advisable to exercise caution when driving or operating machinery.

Undesirable effects: In general, Diovan has a side-effect profile comparable to placebo; adverse experiences have been mild and transient in nature.

In placebo controlled clinical trials of essential hypertension in 3204 patients, side effects that were reported whether or not drug related with an incidence greater than placebo in patients treated with Diovan were:

Body as a whole: Occasionally: Fatigue.

Respiratory system: Rarely: Epistaxis. There was one isolated case of angioedema.

[Frequency estimates are as follows: frequently, >10%; occasionally, 1–10%; rarely, 0.001–1%].

Laboratory findings: In controlled clinical trials, clinically significant changes in laboratory parameters were rarely seen in patients taking Diovan.

In rare cases, Diovan was associated with decreases

in haemoglobin and haematocrit; neutropenia was observed occasionally.

Occasional elevations of liver function tests occurred in Diovan treated patients but no more frequently than in patients taking placebo.

Occasional elevation of serum potassium was seen but rarely was this of clinical significance and no patient discontinued for hyperkalaemia. Serum potassium should be monitored in renally impaired or elderly patients if they are also taking potassium supplements.

Occasional minor elevations of creatinine and bilirubin were also seen in controlled trials.

Overdose: Although there is no experience of overdosage with Diovan, the major sign that might be expected is marked hypotension. If the ingestion is recent, vomiting should be induced. Otherwise, the usual treatment would be intravenous infusion of normal saline solution.

Valsartan is unlikely to be removed by haemodialysis.

Pharmacological properties

Pharmacodynamic properties: The active hormone of the RAAS is angiotensin II, which is formed from angiotensin I through ACE. Angiotensin II binds to specific receptors located in the cell membranes of various tissues. It has a wide variety of physiological effects, including in particular both direct and indirect involvement in the regulation of blood pressure. As a potent vasoconstrictor, angiotensin II exerts a direct pressor response. In addition it promotes sodium retention and stimulation of aldosterone secretion.

Diovan (valsartan) is an orally active, potent, and specific angiotensin II (Ang II) receptor antagonist. It acts selectively on the AT_1 receptor subtype, which is responsible for the known actions of angiotensin II. The AT_2 subtype is unrelated to cardiovascular effects. Valsartan does not exhibit any partial agonist activity at the AT_1 receptor and has much (about 20,000 fold) greater affinity for the AT_1 receptor than for the AT_2 receptor.

Valsartan does not inhibit ACE, also known as kininase II, which converts Ang I to Ang II and degrades bradykinin. Since there is no effect on ACE and no potentiation of bradykinin or substance P, angiotensin II antagonists are unlikely to be associated with cough. In clinical trials where valsartan was compared with an ACE inhibitor, the incidence of dry cough was significantly ($P<0.05$) less in patients treated with valsartan than in those treated with an ACE inhibitor (2.6% versus 7.9% respectively). In a clinical trial of patients with a history of dry cough during ACE inhibitor therapy, 19.5% of trial subjects receiving valsartan and 19.0% of those receiving a thiazide diuretic experienced cough compared to 68.5% of those treated with an ACE inhibitor ($P<0.05$). Valsartan does not bind to or block other hormone receptors or ion channels known to be important in cardiovascular regulation.

Administration of Diovan to patients with hypertension results in reduction of blood pressure without affecting pulse rate.

In most patients, after administration of a single oral dose, onset of antihypertensive activity occurs within 2 hours, and the peak reduction of blood pressure is achieved within 4–6 hours. The antihypertensive effect persists over 24 hours after dosing. During repeated dosing, the maximum reduction in blood pressure with any dose is generally attained within 2–4 weeks and is sustained during long-term therapy. Combined with hydrochlorothiazide, a significant additional reduction in blood pressure is achieved.

Abrupt withdrawal of Diovan has not been associated with rebound hypertension or other adverse clinical events.

In multiple dose studies in hypertensive patients valsartan had no notable effects on total cholesterol, fasting triglycerides, fasting serum glucose, or uric acid.

Pharmacokinetic properties: Absorption of valsartan after oral administration is rapid, although the amount absorbed varies widely. Mean absolute bioavailability for Diovan is 23%. Valsartan shows multi-exponential decay kinetics ($t_{1/2}\ \alpha<1$ h and $t_{1/2}\ \beta$ about 9 h).

The pharmacokinetics of valsartan are linear in the dose range tested. There is no change in the kinetics of valsartan on repeated administration, and little accumulation when dosed once daily. Plasma concentrations were observed to be similar in males and females.

Valsartan is highly bound to serum protein (94–97%), mainly serum albumin. Steady-state volume of distribution is low (about 17 L). Plasma clearance is relatively slow (about 2 L/h) when compared with hepatic blood flow (about 30 L/h). After oral dosing, 83% is excreted in the faeces and 13% in the urine, mainly as unchanged compound.

When Diovan is given with food, the area under the plasma concentration curve (AUC) of valsartan is reduced by 48%, although from about 8 h post dosing plasma valsartan concentrations are similar for the fed and fasted group. This reduction in AUC, however, is not accompanied by a clinically significant reduction in the therapeutic effect, and Diovan can therefore be given either with or without food.

Special populations:

Elderly: A somewhat higher systemic exposure to valsartan was observed in some elderly subjects compared with young subjects; and a lower starting dose (40 mg) is recommended for the elderly.

Impaired renal function: As expected for a compound where renal clearance accounts for only 30% of total plasma clearance, no correlation was seen between renal function and systemic exposure to valsartan. Dose adjustment is therefore not required in patients with mild renal impairment (creatinine clearance 20–50 ml/min). Limited data are available in patients with moderate-severe impairment of renal function and a starting dose of 40 mg is recommended for these patients. No studies have been performed in patients undergoing dialysis. However, valsartan is highly bound to plasma protein and is unlikely to be removed by dialysis.

Hepatic impairment: In a pharmacokinetics trial in patients with mild to moderate hepatic dysfunction, exposure to valsartan was increased approximately 2-fold compared with healthy volunteers.

Preclinical safety data: In a variety of preclinical safety studies conducted in several animal species, there was no evidence of systemic or target organ toxicity, apart from fetotoxicity. Offspring from rats given 600 mg/kg during the last trimester and during lactation showed a slightly reduced survival rate and a slight developmental delay (see *Pregnancy and lactation*). The main preclinical safety findings are attributed to the pharmacological action of the compound, and have not been demonstrated to have any clinical significance.

There was no evidence of mutagenicity, clastogenicity or carcinogenicity.

Pharmaceutical particulars

List of excipients: Microcrystalline cellulose, polyvidone, sodium lauryl sulfate, crospovidone, magnesium stearate.

Incompatibilities: None known.

Shelf life: 3 years.

Special precautions for storage: Protect from moisture and heat, store below 30°C.

Nature and contents of container: PVC/PE/PVDC blister packs.

80 mg and 160 mg capsules are supplied in packs of 7 or 28.

40 mg capsules are supplied in packs of 7 capsules.

Instructions for use/handling: No specific instructions for use/handling.

Marketing authorisation holder: Novartis Pharmaceuticals UK Ltd, trading as Ciba Laboratories.

Marketing authorisation numbers

40 mg 00101/0524
80 mg 00101/0525
160 mg 00101/0526

Date of approval/revision of SPC October 1997.

Legal category POM.

ESTRACOMBI TTS*

Estracombi TTS is a combination of Estraderm TTS 50 and Estragest TTS transdermal patches.

Qualitative and quantitative composition

Active substances: Estra-1,3,5(10)-triene-3, 17β-diol (estradiol) and 17-Hydroxy-19-nor-17α-pregn-4-en-20-yn-3-one-acetate (norethisterone acetate).

One package of Estracombi TTS comprises 4 Estraderm TTS 50 patches and 4 Estragest TTS (0.25/50) patches.

One Estraderm TTS 50 transdermal patch contains 4 mg estradiol PhEur. One Estragest TTS (0.25/50) transdermal patch contains 10 mg estradiol PhEur and 30 mg norethisterone acetate PhEur.

Pharmaceutical form

Estraderm TTS 50 is a thin, round, multilayer, transparent, transdermal patch, i.e. an adhesive patch for application to an area of intact skin.

Estragest TTS (0.25/50) is a thin, goggle-shaped, multilayer transparent transdermal patch, with two separate drug reservoir chambers, i.e. an adhesive patch for application to an area of intact skin.

Clinical particulars

Therapeutic indications: Hormone replacement therapy for patients with an intact uterus with disorders due to natural or surgically induced menopause, which may include, for example, vasomotor symptoms (hot flushes and nocturnal sweating), urogenital conditions such as atrophic vaginitis/vulvitis, and/or atrophic urethritis and trigonitis, sleep disturbances as well as accompanying mood changes.

Prevention of postmenopausal osteoporosis in women considered at risk of developing fractures. Epidemiological studies suggest a number of risk factors may contribute to postmenopausal osteoporosis, including:

- early menopause (either natural or surgically induced)
- family history of osteoporosis
- recent prolonged corticosteroid therapy
- a small, thin frame
- excessive cigarette consumption.

If several risk factors are present consideration should be given to hormone replacement therapy. Bone mineral density measurements may help to confirm the presence of low bone mass. For maximum prophylactic benefit treatment should commence as soon as possible after the menopause.

Posology and method of administration: Estracombi TTS provides continuous oestrogen and sequential progestogen therapy to women with an intact uterus.

One treatment cycle of Estracombi TTS consists of 4 patches of transdermal estradiol followed by 4 patches of transdermal estradiol and norethisterone acetate. Therapy is started with transdermal estradiol (Estraderm TTS 50) which should be applied twice weekly for 2 weeks, i.e. the patch should be changed once every 3 to 4 days. For the following 2 weeks, one transdermal estradiol plus norethisterone acetate patch (Estragest TTS) is applied twice weekly. The next treatment cycle should be started immediately after the removal of the last Estragest TTS patch.

Each fresh patch should be applied to a slightly different site. Recommended application sites are clean, dry and intact areas of skin on the trunk below the waistline. The site selected should be one at which little wrinkling of the skin occurs during movement of the body, e.g. buttock, hip, abdomen. Experience to date has shown that less irritation of the skin occurs on the buttocks than at other sites of application, and this site is preferred by patients. It is therefore recommended to apply Estracombi TTS to the buttock. Estracombi TTS should NOT be applied on or near the breasts.

Estracombi TTS incorporates a combined oestrogen and progestogen patch to induce withdrawal bleeding, thereby minimising the risk of endometrial hyperplasia and carcinoma which can occur with unopposed estrogen therapy. Most patients will bleed towards the end of progestogen therapy. The first transdermal patch of the new cycle should be applied irrespective of the duration of bleeding. It is important that the patches be used in the correct sequence (i.e. 2 weeks Estraderm TTS 50 followed by 2 weeks Estragest TTS each cycle) to ensure regular cyclic bleeding.

For most postmenopausal women Estracombi TTS therapy may be started at any convenient time. However, if the patient is still menstruating commencement within 5 days of the onset of bleeding is recommended.

Some breakthrough bleeding or spotting may be seen until therapy has become established. Some effects, usually of estrogenic origin, e.g. breast discomfort, water retention or bloating, are often observed at the start of treatment, especially in patients receiving hormone replacement therapy for the first time. However, if symptoms persist for more than 6 weeks, treatment should be reconsidered.

The transdermal patch should not be exposed to sunlight.

The use of creams, oils or lotions should be avoided since these may reduce patch adhesion.

Children: Estracombi TTS is not indicated.

Contra-indications: Known or suspected cancer of the breast, genital tract, endometrium or other estrogen-dependent neoplasia; severe hepatic, renal or cardiac disease; undiagnosed vaginal bleeding; porphyria, active deep vein thrombosis, thromboembolic disorders or a history of confirmed venous thromboembolism Dubin-Johnson syndrome; Rotor syndrome; known hypersensitivity to the components of the patch, pregnancy and lactation.

Special warnings and special precautions for use: Before commencing any oestrogen replacement therapy it is recommended that the patient should have a thorough general medical and gynaecological examination to rule out endometrial abnormalities and breast cancer. In patients receiving prolonged treatment these examinations, including endometrial assessment where necessary, should be repeated at regular intervals (e.g. every 6 to 12 months).

In all cases of undiagnosed persistent or irregular vaginal bleeding, adequate diagnostic measures, including endometrial sampling when indicated should be undertaken to rule out abnormality and the treatment should be re-evaluated.

Contact sensitisation is known to occur with all topical applications. Although it is extremely rare, patients who develop contact sensitisation to any of the components of the patch should be warned that a severe hypersensitivity reaction may occur with continuing exposure to the causative agent.

At the present time there is some evidence which suggests a slight increase in the relative risk of breast cancer in postmenopausal women receiving long-term hormone replacement therapy. A careful appraisal of the risk/benefit ratio should be undertaken before treating for longer than 5 years.

It is recommended to avoid giving to women previously treated for breast cancer. Women on this therapy, in particular those with a family history of breast cancer (first degree relatives) or any other breast condition associated with an increased risk of breast cancer should have regular breast examinations, including mammography, and should be instructed in breast self examination.

Caution is advised in patients with a history of estrogen related jaundice and pruritis. If cholestatic jaundice develops during treatment, the treatment should be stopped and appropriate investigations carried out. Although observations to date suggest that estrogens, including transdermal estradiol do not impair carbohydrate metabolism diabetic patients should be monitored during initiation of therapy until further information is available. Pre-existing uterine leiomyomas or fibroids may become enlarged during estrogen therapy. Women with endometriosis should be carefully monitored.

Epidemiological studies have suggested that hormone replacement therapy is associated with an increased relative risk of developing venous thromboembolism (VTE) i.e. deep vein thrombosis or pulmonary embolism. The studies find a 2–3 fold increase for users compared with non-users which for healthy women amounts to a low risk of one extra case of VTE each year for every 5000 patients taking HRT.

Generally recognised risk factors for VTE include a personal or family history and severe obesity (Body Mass Index >30 kg/m²). In women with these factors the benefits of treatment with HRT need to be carefully weighed against the risks. There is consensus about the possible role of varicose veins in VTE.

The risk of VTE may be temporarily increased with prolonged immobilisation, major trauma or major surgery. In women on HRT scrupulous attention should be given to prophylactic measures to prevent VTE following surgery. Where prolonged immobilisation is liable to follow elective surgery, particularly abdominal or orthopaedic surgery to the lower limbs, consideration should be given to temporarily stopping HRT four weeks earlier, if this is possible.

If venous thromboembolism develops after initiating therapy the drug should be discontinued.

The following conditions may deteriorate on HRT: Hypertension, asthma, heart failure, disorders of renal or hepatic function, migraine or epilepsy. It is essential that affected patients be kept under surveillance and HRT be stopped if there is an increase in epileptic seizures. If worsening of any of the above mentioned conditions is diagnosed or suspected during HRT the benefits and risks of HRT should be reassessed on an individual case.

Women with familial hypertriglyceridaemia need special surveillance. Lipid lowering measures are recommended additionally before HRT is started. Estracombi TTS is not a contraceptive.

Interaction with other medicaments and other forms of interaction: Preparations inducing microsomal liver enzymes e.g. barbiturates, hydantoins, carbamazepine, meprobamate, phenylbutazone, antibiotics (including rifampicin) and activated charcoal, may impair the activity of estrogens and progestogens (irregular bleeding and recurrence of symptoms may occur).

The extent of interference with transdermally administered estradiol and norethisterone acetate is not known; these problems should be minimised by the transdermal route of administration which avoids any first pass hepatic metabolism.

Pregnancy and lactation: Estracombi TTS is not indicated.

Effects on ability to drive and use machines: None stated.

Undesirable effects:
Frequency estimates: Very common ≥10%; common >1% to <10%; uncommon ≥0.1% to <1%; rare ≥0.01%; very rare <0.01%.
Skin: Very common: Transient erythema and irritation at site of application with or without pruritus. This usually disappears 3-4 days after patch removal and is similar to the effect observed after occlusion of the skin with household medical adhesive plasters.

Very rare: Allergic contact dermatitis, reversible post-inflammatory pigmentation; generalised pruritus and exanthema.

Urogenital tract: Very common: Breakthrough bleeding, spotting.

Common: Heavy, sometimes prolonged bleeding, dysmenorrhoea, pre-menstrual syndrome-like symptoms; endometrial hyperplasia (incidence similar to that reported for other opposed HRT regimes). Amenorrhoea may occur during treatment.

Endocrine system: Very common: Breast discomfort.

Gastro-intestinal tract: Common: Nausea, abdominal cramps, bloating.

Very rare: Asymptomatic impaired liver function, cholestatic jaundice.

Central nervous system: Common: Headache, migraine.

Rare: Dizziness.

Cardiovascular system: Very rare: Thromboembolic disorders, exacerbation of varicose veins, increase in blood pressure.

Miscellaneous: Rare: Oedema and/or weight changes.

Common: Leg cramps (not related to thromboembolic disease and usually transient lasting 3-6 weeks; if symptoms persist treatment should be reviewed).

Very rare: Anaphylactoid reactions (history of previous allergy or allergic disorders in some cases).

Overdose: Due to the mode of administration overdosage is unlikely.

Signs and symptoms: Signs of acute oestrogen overdosage may be either one of, or a combination of breast discomfort, fluid retention and bloating, or nausea.

Signs of progestogen overdosage may be nausea, vomiting, breast enlargement and vaginal bleeding.

Treatment: Overdosage can if necessary be reversed by removal of the patch.

Pharmacological properties
Pharmacodynamic properties
Estradiol: Estrogen substitution effectively prevents the symptomatic, metabolic and trophic changes due to loss of ovarian function associated with the menopause.

The patch formulation (transdermal therapeutic system, TTS) delivers hormone into the bloodstream via intact skin. Estraderm TTS and Estragest TTS are both designed to deliver estradiol at a low rate over several days.

Studies of bone mineral content have shown Estracombi TTS to be effective in the prevention of progressive bone loss following the menopause.

Adverse effects on lipid and non-lipid mediated markers of cardiovascular disease may contribute to the increased incidence of cardiovascular disease seen in women post-menopause.

An improved lipid profile may be one factor contributing to the beneficial effect of estrogen replacement therapy on the risk of coronary heart disease in postmenopausal women.

Studies have indicated beneficial effects of Estraderm TTS with progestogen on serum total cholesterol, low density lipoprotein (LDL), triglyceride and high density lipoprotein (HDL) levels. There have been few long-term studies of the effect of Estraderm TTS alone on these measurements and the results are thus less conclusive although generally favourable. Studies of Estraderm TTS incorporating progestogen treatment have demonstrated effects on arterial tone which may have a beneficial effect on cardiovascular risk, and have not shown deleterious effects on blood pressure, coagulation and insulin resistance.

Epidemiological studies indicate that a useful reduction in fracture frequency of approx. 50% is achieved with 5 to 6 years oestrogen therapy.

Norethisterone acetate: With Estragest TTS progestogen is added for the last 14 days in each cycle in order to prevent endometrial hyperstimulation. A regular cyclic bleed can be expected to start on day 24–26 of treatment.

Pharmacokinetic properties
Estradiol: Within four hours of application of the first Estraderm TTS 50 patch plasma estradiol levels reach the therapeutic range, and these are maintained throughout the dose interval (for up to four days).

After removal of the last patch plasma oestrogen levels return to baseline values in less than 24 hours, and urinary oestrogen conjugates within 2–3 days.

Mean plasma concentrations of estradiol are similar during both phases of the treatment (i.e. transdermal estradiol alone with Estraderm TTS 50, or transdermal estradiol plus norethisterone acetate with Estragest TTS).

Absorption rates of estradiol from both Estraderm TTS 50 and Estragest TTS may vary between individual patients.

Norethisterone acetate: Norethisterone acetate is metabolised to the active progestogen, norethisterone, which reaches plasma levels of 0.5–1.0 ng/ml within 2 days after Estragest TTS application. These levels are maintained throughout the dose interval and are sufficient to prevent endometrial hyperstimulation. After removal of the transdermal patch, levels of norethisterone return to baseline within 2 days. The absorption rate of norethisterone acetate may vary between individual patients.

Preclinical safety data: None relevant.

Pharmaceutical particulars
List of excipients: The patches contain ethanol, hydroxypropylcellulose, polyethylene terephthalate, ethylenevinylacetate copolymer, liquid paraffin, polyisobutylene, silicone-coating (on the inner side of the protective release liner which is removed before patch application).

Incompatibilities: None known.

Shelf life: 2 years.

Special precautions for storage: Store below 25°C.

Nature and contents of container: Cartons containing four transdermal estradiol (marked CG EFE), and four transdermal estradiol and norethisterone acetate patches (marked CG FNF), each individually sealed in a protective pouch (sufficient for one month's treatment).

A three monthly pack containing twelve transdermal estradiol and twelve transdermal estradiol and norethisterone acetate patches each individually sealed in a protective pouch is also available.

Instructions for use/handling: None stated

Marketing authorisation holder: Novartis Pharmaceuticals UK Limited, Trading as Ciba Laboratories, Frimley Business Park, Frimley, Camberley, Surrey GU16 5SG.

Marketing authorisation number PL 00101/0485.

Date of first authorisation/renewal of authorisation 12 September 1997.

Date of (partial) revision of the text July 1998.

ESTRADERM MX 25*
ESTRADERM MX 50*
ESTRADERM MX 100*

Qualitative and quantitative composition The active ingredient is Estra-1, 3,5(10)-triene-3,17β-diol (estradiol).

Patches contain 0.75, 1.5 and 3.0 mg estradiol PhEur corresponding to surface areas of 11, 22 and 44 cm² respectively.

Pharmaceutical form Estraderm MX is a square-shaped, self-adhesive, transparent, transdermal patch for application to the skin surface. Each patch comprises an impermeable polyester backing film, an adhesive matrix containing estradiol and an oversized protective liner which is removed prior to application of the patch to the skin. Estraderm MX releases estradiol into the circulation via intact skin at a low rate for up to 4 days.

Cross section:

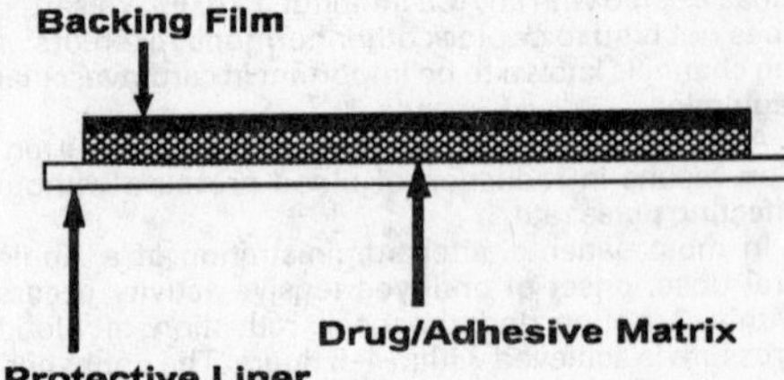

Dosage strength	*Estraderm MX 25*
Nominal rate of estradiol release	25 mcg/day
Estradiol content	0.75 mg
Drug-releasing area	11 cm²
Imprint (on backing film)	CG GRG

Dosage strength	*Estraderm MX 50*
Nominal rate of estradiol release	50 mcg/day
Estradiol content	1.5 mg
Drug-releasing area	22 cm²
Imprint (on backing film)	CG GSG

Dosage strength	*Estraderm MX 100*
Nominal rate of estradiol release	100 mcg/day
Estradiol content	3.0 mg
Drug-releasing area	44 cm²
Imprint (on backing film)	CG GTG

Clinical particulars
Therapeutic indications: Estrogen replacement therapy for patients with disorders due to natural or surgically induced menopause which may include, e.g. vasomotor symptoms (hot flushes and nocturnal sweating), urogenital conditions such as atrophic vaginitis/vulvitis, and/or atrophic urethritis and trigonitis, sleep disturbances as well as accompanying mood changes.

Prevention of postmenopausal osteoporosis in women considered at risk of developing fractures. Epidemiological studies suggest a number of risk factors may contribute to postmenopausal osteoporosis, including:

- early menopause (either natural or surgically induced)
- family history of osteoporosis
- recent prolonged corticosteroid therapy
- a small, thin frame
- excessive cigarette consumption

If several risk factors are present, consideration should be given to hormone replacement therapy. Bone mineral density measurements may help to confirm the presence of low bone mass. For maximum prophylactic benefit treatment should commence as soon as possible after the menopause.

Estrogen therapy must not be used in patients with an intact uterus unless an appropriate dose of progestogen is administered for twelve days per month.

Posology and method of administration:
Menopausal symptoms: Therapy should be initiated with one Estraderm MX 50 and the dose adjusted after the first treatment month depending on efficacy and signs of overdosage. Effects usually of estrogenic origin, e.g. breast discomfort, water retention or bloating, are often observed at the start of treatment especially in patients receiving hormone replacement therapy for the first time, however, if symptoms persist for more than six weeks the dose should be reduced. For maintenance therapy the lowest effective dose should be used; a maximum dose of 100 micrograms per day should not be exceeded. Unopposed estrogen therapy should not be used unless the patient has had a hysterectomy.

Postmenopausal osteoporosis: Estraderm MX 50 is recommended as an effective bone-sparing dose. Estraderm MX 100 is not recommended as the risk/benefit of the higher dose in osteoporosis has not been assessed in clinical studies. However, it may be used if necessary to control concurrent menopausal symptoms. Estraderm MX 25 is not recommended as it has been shown to slow down but not completely halt the rate of bone loss.

Where a progestogen is considered necessary, the appropriate dose should be administered for 12 days per month. If the estrogen is adequately combined with a progestogen withdrawal bleeding occurs, in a way similar to normal menstrual bleeding. Breakthrough bleeding or spotting may be seen until therapy has become established. Signs of breakthrough bleeding early in the cycle should be investigated.

Estraderm MX is not indicated in children

Administration: Estraderm MX should be applied immediately after removal of the protective liner (see Figs.), to an area of clean, dry, and intact skin on the trunk below the waistline. The site chosen should be one at which little wrinkling of skin occurs during movement of the body, e.g. buttock. Estraderm MX should NOT be applied on or near the breasts.

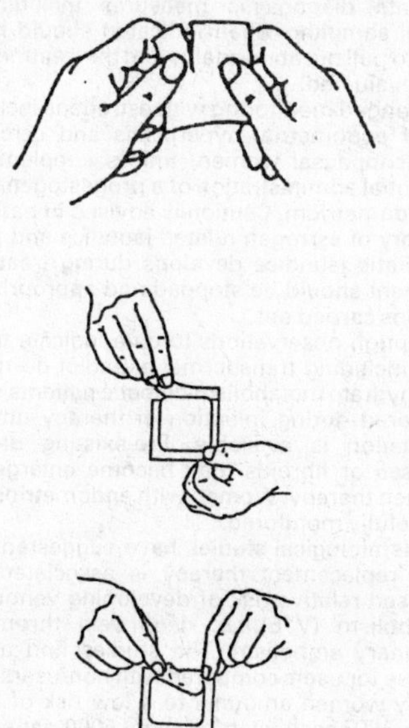

Estraderm MX should be applied twice weekly on a continuous basis, each used patch being removed after 3–4 days and a fresh transdermal patch applied to a slightly different site. The patch should not be exposed to sunlight.

Contra-indications: Known or suspected cancer of the breast, genital tract, endometrium or other estrogen-dependent neoplasia, severe hepatic, renal or cardiac disease, undiagnosed vaginal bleeding, active deep vein thrombosis, thromboembolic disorders, or a history of confirmed thromboembolism, Dubin-Johnson syndrome, Rotor syndrome, known hypersensitivity to the components of the patch, pregnancy and lactation.

Special warnings and special precautions for use: Before commencing any estrogen replacement therapy it is recommended that the patient should have a thorough physical and gynaecological examination to rule out endometrial abnormalities and breast cancer. This should be repeated at regular intervals including monitoring of the endometrium if thought necessary.

In all cases of undiagnosed persistent or irregular vaginal bleeding, adequate diagnostic measures, including endometrial sampling when indicated should be undertaken to rule out abnormality and the treatment should be re-evaluated.

Prolonged monotherapy with estrogens increases the risk of endometrial hyperplasia and carcinoma in postmenopausal women unless supplemented by sequential administration of a progestogen to protect the endometrium.

Contact sensitisation is known to occur with all topical applications. Although it is extremely rare, patients who develop contact sensitisation to any of the components of the patch should be warned that a severe hypersensitivity reaction may occur with continuing exposure to the causative agent.

At the present time there is some evidence which suggests a slight increase in the relative risk of breast cancer in postmenopausal women receiving long-term hormone replacement therapy. A careful appraisal of the risk/benefit ratio should be undertaken before treating for longer than 5 years.

It is recommended to avoid giving estrogens to women previously treated for breast cancer. Women on this therapy, in particular those with a family history of breast cancer (first degree relatives) or any other breast condition associated with an increased risk of breast cancer should have regular breast examinations, including mammography, and should be instructed in breast self examination.

The following conditions may deteriorate on HRT: hypertension, asthma, heart failure, disorders of renal or hepatic function, migraine or epilepsy. It is essential that affected patients are kept under surveillance and HRT be stopped if there is an increase in epileptic seizures. If worsening of any of the above mentioned conditions is diagnosed or suspected during HRT, the benefits and risks of HRT should be reassessed based on the individual case.

Caution is advised in patients with a history of estrogen related jaundice and pruritis. If cholestatic jaundice develops during treatment the treatment should be stopped and appropriate investigations carried out. Although observations to date suggest that estrogens, including transdermal estradiol, do not impair carbohydrate metabolism, diabetic patients should be monitored during initiation of therapy until further information is available. Preexisting uterine leiomyomas or fibroids may become enlarged during estrogen therapy. Women with endometriosis should be carefully monitored.

Epidemiological studies have suggested that hormone replacement therapy is associated with an increased relative risk of developing venous thromboembolism (VTE) i.e. deep vein thrombosis or pulmonary embolism. The studies find a 2–3 fold increase for users compared with non-users which for healthy women amounts to a low risk of one extra case of VTE each year for every 5000 patients taking HRT.

Generally recognised risk factors for VTE include a personal or family history and severe obesity (Body Mass Index >30 kg/m²). In women with these factors the benefits of treatment with HRT need to be carefully weighed against the risks. There is no consensus about the possible role of varicose veins in VTE.

The risk of VTE may be temporarily increased with prolonged immobilisation, major trauma or major surgery. In women on HRT scrupulous attention should be given to prophylactic measures to prevent VTE following surgery. Where prolonged immobilisation is liable to follow elective surgery, particularly abdominal or orthopaedic surgery to the lower limbs, consideration should be given to temporarily stopping HRT four weeks earlier, if this is possible.

If venous thromboembolism develops after initiating therapy drug should be discontinued.

Women with familial hypertriglyceridaemia need special surveillance. Lipid lowering measures are recommended additionally, before HRT is started.

Interaction with other medicaments and other forms of interaction: Preparations inducing microsomal liver enzymes, e.g. barbiturates, hydantoins, anticonvulsants, meprobamate, phenylbutazone; antibiotics and activated charcoal, may impair the activity of estrogens (irregular bleeding and recurrence of symptoms may occur).

The extent of interference with transdermally administered estradiol is not known; these problems should be minimised by the transdermal route of administration which avoids any first pass hepatic metabolism.

Pregnancy and lactation: Estraderm MX should not be used during pregnancy and lactation.

Effects on ability to drive and use machines: None known.

Undesirable effects: Frequency estimates are as follows: frequently >10%; occasionally 1–10%; rarely 0.001–1%; isolated cases <0.001%.

The following systemic effects have been reported for Estraderm TTS, which is bioequivalent to Estraderm MX:

Skin: Frequently: transient erythema and irritation with or without pruritus. Isolated cases: allergic contact dermatitis, reversible post inflammatory pigmentation, generalised pruritus and exanthema.

Urogenital tract: Frequently: breakthrough bleeding (usually a sign of estrogen overdosage).

Endocrine system: Frequently: breast discomfort.

Gastrointestinal tract: Occasionally: nausea, abdominal cramps, bloating. Isolated cases: asymptomatic impaired liver function, cholestatic jaundice.

Central nervous system: Occasionally: headache, migraine. Rarely: dizziness.

Cardiovascular system: Isolated cases: thromboembolic disorders, exacerbation of varicose veins, increase in blood pressure.

Miscellaneous: Rarely: oedema and/or weight changes. Occasionally: leg cramps (not related to thromboembolic disease and usually transient lasting 3–6 weeks; if symptoms persist the dose of estrogen should be reduced).

Overdose: This is not likely due to the mode of administration.

Signs and symptoms: See *Dosage.*

Treatment: Overdosage can if necessary be reversed by removal of the patch.

Pharmacological properties

Pharmacodynamic properties: Like all steroid hormones, estrogens exert their metabolic effects intracellularly. In the cells of target organs estrogens interact with specific receptors to form a complex which stimulates both DNA and protein synthesis. Such receptors have been identified in various organs, e.g. the hypothalamus, pituitary, vagina, urethra, breast and liver, and in osteoblasts.

Estradiol, which in women from the menarche to the menopause is produced mainly by the ovarian follicles, is the most active estrogen at the receptor level. After the menopause, when the ovaries have ceased to function, only small amounts of estradiol are still produced from aromatisation of androstenedione and to a lesser extent of testosterone by the aromatase enzyme, yielding estrone and estradiol, respectively. Estrone is further transformed to estradiol by the enzyme 17β-hydroxysteroid dehydrogenase. Both enzymes are found in fat, liver and muscle tissue.

In many women, the cessation of ovarian estradiol production results in vasomotor and thermoregulatory instability (hot flushes), sleep disturbances, and progressive atrophy of the urogenital system. These disorders can be largely eliminated by means of estrogen replacement therapy. Owing to the accelerated loss of bone substance induced by postmenopausal estrogen deficiency many women develop osteoporosis, particularly of the vertebral column, hip and wrist. This can be prevented by estrogen replacement therapy, preferably initiated early in the menopause. Epidemiological studies indicate that a useful reduction in fracture frequency of approx. 50% is achieved with 5 to 6 years estrogen therapy.

Transdermal therapy with Estraderm MX delivers the physiological estrogen estradiol in unchanged form into the bloodstream via intact skin. Estraderm MX raises estradiol concentrations to levels similar to those found in the early to mid-follicular phase and maintains them over the application period of 3–4 days. The estradiol/estrone ratio is restored to premenopausal levels.

The following pharmacodynamic effects have been reported for Estraderm TTS, which is bioequivalent to Estraderm MX:

Estraderm TTS treatment for 28 days did not result in changes in circulating levels of fibrinopeptide A, high molecular weight fibrinogen, or antithrombin III. There were no changes in concentrations either of circulating renin substrate or of the sex-hormone-binding, thyroxine-binding and cortisol-binding globulins.

After only a few weeks treatment Estraderm TTS has been shown to elicit a dose-dependent reduction in urinary excretion of calcium and hydroxyproline which is indicative of a slowing down of the rate of bone loss.

Adverse effects on lipid and non-lipid mediated markers of cardiovascular disease may contribute to the increased incidence of cardiovascular disease seen in women post-menopause. An improved lipid profile may be one factor contributing to the beneficial effect of estrogen replacement therapy on the risk of coronary heart disease in postmenopausal women. Studies have indicated beneficial effects of Estraderm TTS with progestogen on serum total cholesterol, low density lipoprotein (LDL), triglyceride and high density lipoprotein (HDL) levels. There have been few long-term studies of the effect of Estraderm TTS alone on these measurements and the results are thus less conclusive although generally favourable. Studies of Estraderm TTS incorporating progestogen treatment have demonstrated effects on arterial tone which may have a beneficial effect on cardiovascular risk, and have not shown deleterious effects on blood pressure, coagulation and insulin resistance.

Regardless of the route of administration, the estrogen doses required to relieve menopausal symptoms and conserve bone mass are also a potent stimulus for endometrial mitosis and proliferation. Unopposed estrogens increase the incidence of endometrial hyperplasia and the risk of endometrial carcinoma. Following 1 year of unopposed estrogen therapy endometrial hyperplasia has been found in up to 57% of biopsies. Endometrial hyperplasia is also possible as a result of unopposed transdermal estrogen therapy. A high rate of endometrial hyperplasia has been observed with the higher doses of Estraderm TTS.

Pharmacokinetic properties: Within 8 hours after application of Estraderm MX 25, 50 and 100 steady-state plasma estradiol concentrations are reached and remain stable throughout the dose interval (up to 4 days). The average increase in estradiol concentration over baseline reached with Estraderm MX 50 is 37 pg/ml. The estradiol/estrone ratio increases from a postmenopausal value of 0.3 to a value of 1.3, similar to the physiological ratio observed before menopause in women with normally functioning ovaries. Following 12 weeks treatment with Estraderm MX 50 the average increase in estradiol concentration over baseline was 36 pg/ml, indicating an absence of estradiol accumulation.

Absorption rates may vary between individual patients. However, the plasma estradiol levels achieved with different sized transdermal patches have been shown to be proportional to the drug-releasing area of the dosage form.

After removal of the last transdermal patch, plasma estradiol levels return to baseline values in less than 24 hours.

Estradiol: The plasma elimination half-life of estradiol is approx. 1 hour. The metabolic plasma clearance ranges from 650 to 900 l/(day×m²). Estradiol is mainly metabolised in the liver. Its most important metabolites are estriol and estrone and their conjugates (glucuronides, sulphates); these are far less active than estradiol.

The bulk of the conjugates are excreted in urine. Estrogen metabolites are also subject to enterohepatic circulation.

Preclinical safety data: At low physiological doses of estradiol (similar to those delivered by Estraderm MX), the potential for neoplasia is negligible in experimental animals. Most of the documented effects of exogenously administered estradiol in animal studies have been consequences of the administration of higher doses and are consistent with an exaggerated pharmacological response (most notably the promotion of tumours in estrogen-responsive tissues). However, long term unopposed treatment with physiological doses of estradiol may potentially lead to hyperplastic changes in estrogen-dependent reproductive organs like the uterus.

Some dermal irritation associated with the patch has been observed in the rabbit.

Pharmaceutical particulars

List of excipients: Acrylate, methacrylate, isopropyl palmitate, polyethylene terephthalate, ethylene-vinylacetate copolymer, silicone–coating (on the inner side of the protective release liner which is removed before patch application).

Incompatibilities: None known.

Shelf life: 2 years.

Special precautions for storage: Store below 25°C.

Keep out of the reach of children both before and after use.

Nature and contents of container: Two, eight or twenty four Estraderm MX pouches are placed in an appropriately sized carton which comprises the finished product (a 'starter pack', one or three month's treatment respectively). Each transdermal patch is individually heat sealed in a paper/aluminium/polyacrylonitrile pouch.

Instructions for use/handling: See *Posology and method of administration.* Exposure of Estraderm MX patches to ultra-violet light results in degradation of estradiol. Patches should not be exposed to sunlight. They should be applied immediately after removal from the pouch to skin sites covered by clothing.

Marketing authorisation holder: Novartis Pharmaceuticals UK Ltd, Trading as Ciba Laboratories, Frimley Business Park, Frimley, Camberley, Surrey GU16 5SG.

Marketing authorisation numbers

Estraderm MX 25: PL 0101/0486
Estraderm MX 50: PL 0101/0487
Estraderm MX 100: PL 0101/0488

Date of first authorisation/renewal of authorisation The first authorisation was granted 27 September 1995.

Date of (partial) revision of the text July 1998.

ESTRADERM TTS*

Presentation Estraderm TTS is a self-adhesive, transparent, transdermal therapeutic system (patch), containing a drug reservoir of 17β-estradiol PhEur. It is available in three sizes: Estraderm TTS 25, with an absorption rate of approx. 25 micrograms estradiol/24 hours (active surface area 5cm², estradiol content 2 mg); Estraderm TTS 50, with an absorption rate of approx. 50 micrograms estradiol/24 hours (active surface area 10cm², estradiol content 4 mg); Estraderm TTS 100, with an absorption rate of approx. 100 micrograms estradiol/24 hours (active surface area 20cm², estradiol content 8 mg).

Patches also contain: ethanol, hydroxypropylcellulose, polyethylene terephthalate, ethylenevinylacetate copolymer, liquid paraffin, polyisobutylene, silicone-coating (on the inner side of the protective release liner which is removed before patch application).

Uses

Indications: Estrogen replacement therapy for patients with disorders due to natural or surgically induced menopause which may include for example vasomotor symptoms (hot flushes and nocturnal sweating), urogenital conditions such as atrophic vaginitis/vulvitis, and/or atrophic urethritis and trigonitis. Sleep disturbances, as well as accompanying mood changes.

Prevention of postmenopausal osteoporosis in women considered at risk of developing fractures. Epidemiological studies suggest a number of risk factors may contribute to postmenopausal osteoporosis, including:

- early menopause (either natural or surgically induced)
- family history of osteoporosis
- recent prolonged corticosteroid therapy
- a small, thin frame
- excessive cigarette consumption

If several risk factors are present consideration should be given to hormone replacement therapy. Bone mineral density measurements may help to confirm the presence of low bone mass. For maximum prophylactic benefit treatment should commence as soon as possible after the menopause.

Estrogen therapy must not be used in patients with an intact uterus unless an appropriate dose of progestogen is administered for twelve days per month.

Mode of action: Estrogen substitution effectively prevents the characteristic symptomatic, metabolic and trophic changes associated with loss of ovarian function due to natural or surgical menopause.

The patch formulation (transdermal therapeutic system, TTS) delivers hormone into the bloodstream via intact skin. Estraderm TTS is designed to deliver 17β-estradiol at a low rate over several days.

Pharmacokinetics: Within four hours after application of the first system, plasma estradiol levels reach the therapeutic range and these are maintained throughout the dose interval (for up to four days).

After removal of the last system plasma estrogen levels return to baseline values in less than 24 hours and urinary estrogen conjugates within 2-3 days.

Absorption rate may vary between individual patients. However, the plasma estradiol levels achieved with different sized systems have been shown to be proportional to the drug-releasing area of the dosage form.

Dosage and administration

Adults and elderly: Menopausal symptoms–Therapy should be initiated with one Estraderm TTS 50 and the dose adjusted after the first treatment month depending on efficacy and signs of overdosage. Effects usually of estrogenic origin eg breast discomfort, water retention or bloating are often observed at the start of treatment especially in patients receiving hormone replacement therapy for the first time, however, if symptoms persist for more than six weeks the dose should be reduced. For maintenance therapy the lowest effective dose should be used; a maximum dose of 100 micrograms per day should not be exceeded. Unopposed estrogen therapy should not be used unless the patient has had a hysterectomy. *Postmenopausal osteoporosis:* Estraderm TTS 50 is recommended as an effective bone-sparing dose. Estraderm TTS 100 is not recommended as the risk/benefit of the higher dose in osteoporosis has not been assessed in clinical studies. However, it may be used if necessary to control concurrent menopausal symptoms. Estraderm TTS 25 is not recommended as it has been shown to slow down but not completely halt the rate of bone loss.

Where a progestogen is considered necessary, the appropriate dose should be administered for 12 days per month. If the estrogen is adequately combined with a progestogen withdrawal bleeding occurs, in a way similar to normal menstrual bleeding. Breakthrough bleeding or spotting may be seen until therapy has become established. Signs of breakthrough bleeding early in the cycle should be investigated.

Estraderm TTS should be applied twice weekly on a continuous basis, each used system being removed after 3-4 days and a fresh system applied to a slightly different site. Recommended application sites are clean, dry and intact areas of skin on the trunk below the waistline. The site selected should be one at which little wrinkling of the skin occurs during movement of the body, eg buttock, hip, abdomen. Experience to date has shown that less irritation of the skin occurs on the buttocks than on other sites of application. It is therefore advisable to apply Estraderm TTS to the buttock. Estraderm TTS should **NOT** be applied on or near the breasts.

The system should not be exposed to sunlight.

Children: Estraderm TTS is not indicated in children.

Use in pregnancy and lactation: Estraderm TTS is not indicated.

Contra-indications, warnings, etc

Contra-indications: Known or suspected cancer of the breast, genital tract, endometrium or other estrogen-dependent neoplasia. Severe hepatic, renal or cardiac disease. Undiagnosed vaginal bleeding, porphyria. Active deep vein thrombosis or thromboembolic disorders or a history of confirmed venous thromboembolism, Dubin-Johnson syndrome. Rotor syndrome, known hypersensitivity to the components of the patch, pregnancy and lactation.

Precautions and warnings: Contact sensitisation is known to occur with all topical applications. Although it is extremely rare, patients who develop contact sensitisation to any of the components of the patch should be warned that a severe hypersensitivity reaction may occur with continuing exposure to the causative agent.

Before commencing any estrogen therapy it is recommended that the patient should have a thorough physical and gynaecological examination to rule out endometrial abnormalities and breast cancer. This should be repeated regularly including monitoring of the endometrial if thought necessary. In all cases of undiagnosed persistent or irregular vaginal bleeding adequate diagnosatic measures including endometrial sampling when indicated should be undertaken to pull out abnormality and the treatment should be re-evaluated.

Prolonged monitoring with estrogens including the risk of endometrial hyperplasia and carcinoma in postmenopausal women, unless supplemented by sequential administration of a progestogen to protect the endometrium. Caution is advised in patients with a history of estrogen related jaundice and pruritis. If cholestatic jaundice develops during treatment the treatment should be stopped and appropriate investigations carried out.

Although observations to date indicate that estrogens, including transdermal estradiol do not impair carbohydrate metabolism diabetic patients should be monitored during initiation of therapy until further information is available. Pre-existing uterine leiomyoses or fibroids may become enlarged during estrogen therapy. Women with endometriosis should be carefully monitored.

Epidemiological studies have suggested that hormone replacement therapy is associated with an increased relative risk of developing venous thromboembolism (VTE) i.e. deep vein thrombosis or pulmonary embolism. The studies find a 2–3 fold increase for users compared with non-users which for healthy women amounts to a low risk of one extra case of VTE each year for every 5000 patients taking HRT.

Generally recognised risk factors for VTE include a personal or family history and severe obesity (Body Mass Index >30 kg/m²). In women with those factors the benefits of treatment with HRT need to be carefully weighed against the risks. There is no consensus about the possible role of varicose veins in VTE.

The risk of VTE may be temporarily increased with prolonged immobilisation. Major trauma or major surgery. In women on HRT scrupulous attention should be given to prophylactic measures to prevent VTE following surgery. Where prolonged immobilisation is liable to follow elective surgery, particularly abdominal or orthopaedic surgery to the lower limbs, consideration should be given to temporarily stopping HRT four weeks earlier, if this is possible.

If venous thromboembolism develops after initiating therapy the drug should be discontinued.

The following conditions may deteriorate on HRT: hypertension, asthma, heart failure, disorders of renal or hepatic function, migraine or epilepsy. It is essential that affected patients are kept under surveillance and HRT be stopped if there is an increase in epileptic seizures. If worsening of any of the above mentioned conditions is diagnosed or suspected during HRT, the benefits and risks of HRT should be reassessed based on the individual case.

Women with familial hyperglyceridaemia need special surveillance. Lipid lowering measures are recommended additionally, before HRT is started.

At the present time there is some evidence which suggests a slight increase in the relative risk of breast cancer in postmenopausal women receiving long-term hormone replacement therapy. A careful appraisal of the risk/benefit ratio should be undertaken before treating for longer than 5 years.

Women on this therapy, in particular those with fibrocystic disease of the breast, or with a family history of breast cancer (first degree relatives) should have regular breast examinations, including mammography, and should be instructed in breast self examination.

Drug interactions: Preparations inducing microsomal liver enzymes, eg barbiturates, hydantoins, anticonvulsants (including carbamazepine), meprobamate, phenylbutazone; antibiotics (including rifampicin) and activated charcoal, may impair the activity of estrogens (irregular bleeding and recurrence of symptoms may occur).

The extent of interference with transdermally administered estradiol is not known; these problems should be minimised by the transdermal route of administration which avoids any first pass hepatic metabolism.

Side-effects:
Skin: Frequently: transient erythema and irritation at the site of application with or without pruritus. This usually disappears 3-4 days after patch removal and is similar to the effect sometimes observed after occlusion of the skin with household medical adhesive plasters. Very infrequently: local swelling, papules/vesicles and scaling have been reported, which also resolved spontaneously and did not result in permanent skin damage. Isolated cases: Allergic contact dermatitis, reversible post-inflammatory pigmentation; generalised pruritus and exanthema

Urogenital tract: Frequently: breakthrough bleeding (usually a sign of estrogen overdosage, see 'Dosage and administration').

Endocrine system: Frequently: breast discomfort

Gastrointestinal tract: Occasionally: nausea, abdominal cramps, bloating. Isolated cases: asymptomatic impaired liver function, cholestatic jaundice.

Central nervous system: Occasionally: headache, migraine. Rarely: dizziness.

Cardiovascular system: Isolated cases: thromboembolic disorders, exacerbation of varicose veins, increase in blood pressure.

Miscellaneous: Occasionally: leg cramps (not related to thromboembolic disease and usually transient lasting 3-6 weeks, if symptoms persist the dose of estrogen should be reduced). Rarely: Oedema and/or weight changes. Isolated cases: Anaphylactoid reactions (history of previous allergy or allergic disorders in some cases)

Overdosage: This is not likely due to the mode of administration.

Signs and symptoms: (see *Dosage and administration*).

Treatment: Overdosage can if necessary be reversed by removal of the patch(es).

Pharmaceutical precautions Store below 25°C.

Shelf life: 24 months.

Legal category POM.

Package quantities Cartons containing eight Estraderm TTS patches, each individually sealed in a protective pouch (sufficient for one month's treatment). A three-monthly pack containing twenty-four Estraderm TTS patches, each individually sealed in a protective pouch is also available.

Further information Adverse effects on lipid and non-lipid mediated markers of cardiovascular disease may contribute to the increased incidence of cardiovascular disease seen in women post-menopause.

An improved lipid profile may be one factor contributing to the beneficial effect of estrogen replacement therapy on the risk of coronary heart disease in postmenopausal women. Studies have indicated beneficial effects of Estraderm TTS with progestogen on serum total cholesterol, low density lipoprotein (LDL), triglyceride and high density lipoprotein (HDL) levels. There have been few long-term studies of the effect of Estraderm TTS alone on these measurements and the results are thus less conclusive although generally favourable. Studies of Estraderm TTS incorporating progestogen treatment have demonstrated effects on arterial tone which may have a beneficial effect on cardiovascular risk, and have not shown deleterious effects on blood pressure, coagulation and insulin resistance.

Epidemiological studies indicate that a useful reduction in fracture frequency of approx. 50% is achieved with 5 to 6 years estrogen therapy.

Marketing authorisation holder: Novartis Pharmaceuticals UK Ltd, Trading as Ciba Laboratories.

Date of last revision July 1998.

Product licence numbers
Estraderm TTS 25: 00101/0489
Estraderm TTS 50: 00101/0490
Estraderm TTS 100: 00101/0491

ESTRAPAK* 50

Qualitative and quantitative composition The active ingredients are estra-1,3,5 (10)-triene-3, 17β-diol (estradiol) and 17β-hydroxy-19-nor-17∞ pren-4-en 20-yn-3-one acetate (norethisterone acetate). One pack of Estrapak contains: 8 Estraderm TTS 50 patches (each containing 4 mg estradiol PhEur) and 12 tablets containing 1 mg norethisterone acetate (NETA PhEur) each.

The transdermal patch (Estraderm TTS 50) has a drug releasing area of 10 cm². It is imprinted on the backing side with CG EFE.

Pharmaceutical form Estrapak 50 is made up of transdermal patches (transdermal therapeutic systems, TTS, Estraderm TTS 50) and norethisterone acetate tablets for oral use.

Estraderm TTS 50 is a thin, multilayer, transparent, transdermal therapeutic system. It is a patch for application to an area of intact skin. The drug reservoir is sealed between a backing film and a release-controlling membrane which limits the rate at which estradiol are continuously released across the adhesive layer to the skin. The active substance of the patch penetrates the skin ahd passes directly into the bloodstream.

Clinical particulars
Therapeutic indications: Hormone replacement therapy for patients with an intact uterus with disorders due to natural or surgically induced menopause, which may include, for example, vasomotor symptoms (hot flushes and nocturnal sweating), urogenital conditions such as atrophic vaginitis/ vulvitis, and/or atrophic urethritis and trigonitis, sleep disturbances as well as accompanying mood changes.

Prevention of post menopausal osteoporosis in women considered at risk of developing fractures. Epidemiological studies suggest a number of risk factors may contribute to postmenopausal osteoporosis, including:

- early menopause (either natural or surgically induced)
- family history of osteoporosis
- recent prolonged corticosteroid therapy
- a small, thin frame
- excessive cigarette consumption.

If several risk factors are present, consideration should be given to hormone replacement therapy. Bone mineral density measurements may help to confirm the presence of low bone mass. For maximum prophylactic benefit treatment should commence as soon as possible after the menopause.

Posology and method of administration
Adults and elderly: In women with an intact uterus for whom hormone replacement therapy is required, Estrapak 50 should be administered in preference to unopposed estrogen therapy.

Estrapak 50 contains estrogen and a progestogen to induce withdrawal bleeding, thereby avoiding endometrial hyperstimulation. Most patients will bleed towards the end of progestogen therapy. The median duration of bleeding is 7 days.

Transdermal estrogen administration is continued without a break in therapy; an oral progestogen is given for 12 days during each month of estrogen replacement.

The transdermal estrogen patch should be applied twice weekly on a continuous basis, each used patch being removed after 3–4 days and a fresh patch applied to a slightly different site. Recommended application sites are clean, dry and intact areas of skin on the trunk below the waistline. The estrogen patches should not be applied on or near the breasts. One norethisterone acetate tablet should be taken by mouth daily for days 15–26 of each 28 days of estrogen replacement therapy.

For most postmenopausal women Estrapak 50 therapy may be started at any convenient time. However, if the patient is still menstruating commencement within 5 days of onset of bleeding is recommended. Some breakthrough bleeding or spotting may be seen until therapy has become established.

Children: Estrapak 50 is not indicated in children.

Contra-indications: Known or suspected cancer of the breast, genital tract, endometrium or other estrogen-dependent neoplasia; severe hepatic, renal or cardiac disease; undiagnosed vaginal bleeding; porphryia, active deep vein thrombosis or thromboembolic disorders or a documented history of these conditons; Dubin-Johnson syndrome; Rotor syndrome; known hypersensitivity to the components of the patch; pregnancy and lactation.

Special warnings and special precautions for use: Before commencing any oestrogen replacement therapy it is recommended that the patient should have a thorough physical and gynaecological examination to rule out endometrial abnormalities and breast cancer. This should be repeated at regular intervals including monitoring of the endometrium if thought necessary.

In all cases of undiagnosed persistent or irregular vaginal bleeding, adequate diagnostic measures, including endometrial sampling when indicated should be undertaken to rule out abnormality and the treatment should be re-evaluated.

Contact sensitisation is known to occur with all topical applications. Although it is extremely rare, patients who develop contact sensitisation to any of the components of the patch should be warned that a severe hypersensitivity reaction may occur with continuing exposure to the causative agent.

At the present time there is some evidence which suggests a slight increase in the relative risk of breast cancer in postmenopausal women receiving long-term hormone replacement therapy. A careful appraisal of the risk/benefit ratio should be undertaken before treating for longer than 5 years.

It is recommended to avoid giving women previously treated for breast cancer. Women on this therapy, in particular those with a family history of breast cancer (first degree relatives) or any other breast condition associated with an increased risk of breast cancer should have regular breast examinations, including mammography, and should be instructed in breast self examination.

Caution is advised in patients with a history of estrogen related jaundice and pruritis. If cholestatic jaundice develops during treatment, the treatment should be stopped and appropriate investigations carried out. Although observations to date suggest that estrogens, including transdermal estradiol do not impair carbohydrate metabolism diabetic patients should be monitored during initiation of therapy until further information is available. Pre-existing uterine leiomyomas or fibroids may become enlarged during estrogen therapy. Women with endometriosis should be carefully monitored.

Epidemiological studies have suggested that hormone replacement therapy is associated with an increased relative risk of developing venous thromboembolism (VTE), i.e. deep vein thrombosis or pulmonary embolism. The studies find a 2–3 fold increase for users compared with non-users which for healthy women amounts to a low risk of one extra case of VTE each year for every 5000 patients taking HRT.

Generally recognised risk factors for VTE include a personal or family history and severe obesity (Body Mass Index >30 kg/m²). In women with these factors the benefits of treatment with HRT need to be carefully weighed against the risks. There is no consensus about the possible role of varicose veins in VTE.

The risk of VTE may be temporarily increased with prolonged immobilisation, major trauma or major surgery. In women on HRT scrupulous attention should be given to prophylactic measures to prevent VTE following surgery. Where prolonged immobilisation is liable to follow elective surgery, particularly abdominal or orthopaedic surgery to the lower limbs, consideration should be given to temporarily stopping HRT four weeks earlier, if this is possible.

If venous thromboembolism develops after initiating therapy the drug should be discontinued.

The following conditions may deteriorate on HRT: Hypertension, asthma, heart failure, disorders of renal or hepatic function, migraine or epilepsy. It is essential that affected patients be kept under surveillance and HRT be stopped if there is an increase in epileptic seizures. If worsening of any of the above mentioned conditions is diagnosed or suspected during HRT the benefits and risks of HRT should be reassessed on an individual case.

Women with familial hypertriglyceridaemia need special surveillance. Lipid lowering measures are recommended additionally before HRT is started.

Estrapak 50 is not an oral contraceptive.

Interactions with other medicaments and other forms of interaction: Preparations inducing microsomal liver enzymes, e.g. barbiturates, hydantoins, carbamazepine, meprobamate, phenylbutazone; antibiotics (including rifampicin) and activated charcoal, may impair the activity of estrogens and progestogens (irregular bleeding and reoccurrence of symptoms may occur).

The extent of interference with transdermally administered estradiol is not known. Rifampicin deceases the half life of norethisterone by 50%. Antiepileptics may increase the binding of progestogen to the binding protein SHBG, thereby reducing the free progestogen concentration. Oral steroids increase the half life of prednisolone and theophylline.

Pregnancy and lactation: Estrapak 50 should not be used during pregnancy and lactation.

Effects on ability to drive and use machinery: Not known.

Undesirable effects: Ferquency estimates: very common ≥10%; common ≥1% to <10%; uncommon ≥0.1% to <1%; rare ≥0.01% to <0.1%; very rare <0.01%.

Skin: Very common: Transient erythema and irritation at site of application with or without pruritus. This usually disappears 3–4 days after patch removal and is similar to the effect observed after occlusion of the skin with household medical adhesive plasters.

Very rare: Allergic contact dermatitis, reversible post-inflammatory pigmentation, generalised pruritus and exanthema.

Urogenital tract: Very common: Breakthrough bleeding, spotting. Common: Heavy, sometimes prolonged bleeding, dysmenorrhoea, pre-menstrual syndrome-like symptoms; endometrial hyperplasia (incidence similar to that reported for other opposed HRT regimes). Amenorrhoea may occur during treatment.

Endocrine system: Very common: Breast discomfort.

Gastrointestinal tract: Common: Nausea, abdominal cramps, bloating.

Very rare: Asymptomatic impaired liver function, cholestatic jaundice.

Central nervous system: Common: Headache. Rare: Dizziness.

Cardiovascular system: Very rare: Thromboembolic disorders, exacerbation of varicose veins, increase in blood pressure.

Miscellaneous: Rare: Oedema and/or weight changes.

Common: Leg cramps (not related to thromboembolic disease and usually transient lasting 3–6 weeks, if symptoms persist treatment should be reviewed).

Very rare: Anaphylactoid reactions (history of previous allergy or allergic disorders in some cases).

Overdose: This is not likely due to the mode of administration.

Signs and symptoms: Signs of estrogen overdosage may be either one of, or a combination of, breast discomfort, fluid retention and bloating, or nausea.

Signs of progestogen overdosage may be nausea, vomiting, breast enlargment and vaginal bleeding.

Treatment: Oestrogen overdosage can if necessary be reversed by removal of the patch. There is no specific antidote for progestogen overdose and treatment should be symptomatic. Gastric lavage may be employed if the overdosage is large and the patient is seen sufficiently early (within 4 hours).

Pharmacological particulars

Pharmacodynamic properties

Estradiol: Estrogen substitution effectively prevents the characteristic symptomatic metabolic and trophic changes associated with loss of ovarian function due to the menopause.

The patch formulation (transdermal therapeutic system, TTS) delivers hormone into the bloodstream via intact skin. Estraderm TTS is designed to deliver estradiol at a low rate over several days.

Adverse effects on lipid and non-lipid mediated markers of cardiovascular disease may contribute to the increased incidence of cardiovascular disease seen in women post-menopause.

An improved lipid profile may be one factor contributing to the beneficial effect of estrogen replacement therapy on the risk of coronary heart disease in postmenopausal women. Studies have indicated beneficial effects of Estraderm TTS with progestogen on serum total cholesterol, low density lipoprotein (LDL), triglyceride and high density lipoprotein (HDL) levels. There have been few long-term studies of the effect of Estraderm TTS alone on these measurements and the results are thus less conclusive although generally favourable. Studies of Estraderm TTS incorporating progestogen treatment have demonstrated effects on arterial tone which may have a beneficial effect on cardiovascular risk, and have not shown deleterious effects on blood pressure, coagulation and insulin resistance.

Epidemiological studies that a useful reduction in fracture frequency of approx. 50% is achieved with 5 to 6 years estrogen therapy.

Norethisterone acetate: An oral progestogen is included for 12 days in each cycle in order to prevent endometrial hyperstimulation. A withdrawal bleed can be expected to start on day 24–26 of treatment.

Pharmacokinetic properties

Estradiol: Within four hours after application of the first transdermal estrogen patch, plasma estradiol levels reach the therapeutic range and these are maintained throughout the dose interval (for up to four days).

After removal of the last patch, plasma estradiol levels return to baseline values in less that 24 hours and urinary estrogen conjugates within 2–3 days.

Absorption rates may vary between individual patients.

Norethisterone acetate: Norethisterone acetate is rapidly absorbed from the gastrointestinal tract and converted to norethisterone, which has a half-life of 7.5–8 hours.

Preclinical safety date: None relevant.

Pharmaceutical particulars

List of excipients: Estraderm TTS 50; Ethanol, hydroxypropylcellulose, polyethylene terephthalate, ethylenevinylacetate copolymer, liquid paraffin, polyisobutylene, silicone coating (on the inner side of the protective release liner which is removed before application of the patch).

Norethisterone Acetate tablets: Lactose, magnesium stearate, maize starch, polyvinylpyrrolidone, hydroxypropyl methylcellulose, glyceryl polyoxyethylene glycol stearate, talc, red iron oxide (E172) and titanium oxide (E171).

Incompatibilities: None known.

Shelf life: The shelf life for Estraderm TTS 50 patches is 24 months. The shelf life for norethisterone tablets is 60 months. The shelf life of the packaged product is determined by the unexpired shelf life of the patch or tablet (whichever is the shorter) at the time of assembly.

Special precautions for storage: Store below 25°C.

Nature and contents of container: Cartons containing 8 transdermal estrogen patches (each individually sealed in a protective pouch) and 12 norethisterone acetate tablets (in a blister pack). A three monthly pack is also available containing 24 transdermal estrogen patches (each individually sealed in a protective pouch) and 36 norethisterone acetate tablets (in a blister pack).

Instructions for use/handling: None stated.

Marketing authorisation holder: Novartis Pharmaceuticals UK Limited, trading as Ciba Laboratories, Frimley Business Park, Frimley, Camberley, Surrey GU16 5SG.

Marketing authorisation number PL00101/0492.

Date of first authorisation/renewal of authorisation 12 September 1997.

Date of (partial) revision of the text July 1998.

EXELON 1.5 mg Hard Capsules
EXELON 3 mg Hard Capsules
EXELON 4.5 mg Hard Capsules
EXELON 6 mg Hard Capsules

Qualitative and quantitative composition Each capsule contains rivastigmine hydrogen tartrate corresponding to rivastigmine 1.5 mg, 3 mg, 4.5 mg or 6 mg.

Pharmaceutical form Capsule, hard.

Clinical particulars

Therapeutic indications: Symptomatic treatment of mild to moderately severe Alzheimer's dementia.

Posology and method of administration

Administration: Rivastigmine should be administered twice a day, with morning and evening meals. The capsules should be swallowed whole.

Initial dose: 1.5 mg twice a day.

Dose titration: The recommended starting dose is 1.5 mg twice a day. If this dose is well tolerated after a minimum of two weeks of treatment, the dose may be increased to 3 mg twice a day. Subsequent increases to 4.5 mg and then 6 mg twice a day should also be based on good tolerability of the current dose and may be considered after a minimum of two weeks of treatment at that dose level.

If adverse effects (e.g. nausea, vomiting, abdominal pain or loss of appetite) or weight decrease are observed during treatment, these may respond to omitting one or more doses. If adverse effects persist, the daily dose should be temporarily reduced to the previous well-tolerated dose.

Maintenance dose: The effective dose is 3 to 6 mg twice a day; to achieve maximum therapeutic benefit patients should be maintained on their highest well-tolerated dose. The recommended maximum daily dose is 6 mg twice a day.

Maintenance treatment can be continued for as long as a therapeutic benefit for the patient exists. Therefore, the clinical benefit of rivastigmine should be reassessed on a regular basis, especially for patients treated at doses less than 3 mg twice a day. Discontinuation should be considered when evidence of a therapeutic effect is no longer present. Individual response to rivastigmine cannot be predicted.

Treatment effect has not been studied in placebo-controlled trials beyond 6 months.

Renal and hepatic impairment: Due to increased exposure in renal and mild to moderate hepatic impairment, dosing recommendations to titrate according to individual tolerability should be closely followed.

Children: Rivastigmine is not recommended for use in children.

Contraindications: The use of this medicinal product is contraindicated in patients with

- known hypersensitivity to rivastigmine, other carbamate derivatives or to any excipients used in the formulation,
- severe liver impairment, as it has not been studied in this population.

Special warnings and special precautions for use: Treatment should be initiated and supervised by a physician experienced in the diagnosis and treatment of Alzheimer's dementia. Diagnosis should be made according to current guidelines. Therapy with rivastigmine should only be started if a caregiver is available who will regularly monitor drug intake by the patient.

The use of rivastigmine in patients with severe Alzheimer's dementia, other types of dementia or other types of memory impairment (e.g. age-related cognitive decline) has not been investigated.

Gastrointestinal disorders such as nausea and vomiting may occur particularly when initiating treatment and/or increasing the dose. These adverse events occur more commonly in women. Patients with Alzheimer's disease lose weight. Cholinesterase inhibitors, including rivastigmine, have been associated with weight loss in these patients. During therapy patients' weight should be monitored.

As with other cholinomimetics, care must be taken when using rivastigmine in patients with sick sinus syndrome or conduction defects (sino-atrial block, atrio-ventricular block).

As with other cholinergic drugs, rivastigmine may cause increased gastric acid secretions. Although rivastigmine did not show an increased incidence of ulcers relative to placebo, care should be exercised in treating patients with active gastric or duodenal ulcers or patients predisposed to these conditions.

Cholinesterase inhibitors should be prescribed with care to patients with a history of asthma or obstructive pulmonary disease.

Cholinomimetics may induce or exacerbate urinary obstruction and seizures. Although this has not been observed with rivastigmine caution is recommended in treating patients predisposed to such diseases.

Interaction with other medicinal products and other forms of interaction: As a cholinesterase inhibitor, rivastigmine may exaggerate the effects of succinylcholine-type muscle relaxants during anaesthesia.

In view of its pharmacodynamic effects, rivastigmine should not be given concomitantly with other cholinomimetic drugs and might interfere with the activity of anticholinergic medications.

No pharmacokinetic interaction was observed between rivastigmine and digoxin, warfarin, diazepam or fluoxetine in studies in healthy volunteers. The increase in prothrombin time induced by warfarin is not affected by administration of rivastigmine. No untoward effects on cardiac conduction were observed following concomitant administration of digoxin and rivastigmine.

According to its metabolism, metabolic drug interactions appear unlikely, although rivastigmine may inhibit the butyrylcholinesterase mediated metabolism of other drugs.

Pregnancy and lactation

Pregnancy: No effects on fertility or embryofoetal development were observed in rats and rabbits, except at doses related to maternal toxicity. In peri/postnatal studies in rats, an increased gestation time was observed. The safety of rivastigmine in human pregnancy has not been established and it should only be given to pregnant women if the potential benefit outweighs the potential risk for the foetus.

Lactation: In animals, rivastigmine is excreted into milk. It is not known if rivastigmine is excreted into human milk. Therefore, women on rivastigmine should not breastfeed.

Effects on ability to drive and use machines: Alzheimer's disease may cause gradual impairment of driving performance or compromise the ability to use machinery. Furthermore, rivastigmine can induce dizziness and somnolence, mainly when initiating treatment or increasing the dose. Therefore, the ability of Alzheimer patients on rivastigmine to continue driving or operating complex machines should be routinely evaluated by the treating physician.

Undesirable effects: The most common adverse effects (incidence ≥5% and twice the frequency of placebo) were asthenia, anorexia, dizziness, nausea, somnolence and vomiting. Female patients were found to be more susceptible to nausea, vomiting, loss of appetite and weight loss.

Other common adverse effects (incidence ≥5% and ≥placebo) were abdominal pain, accidental trauma, agitation, confusion, depression, diarrhoea, dyspepsia, headache, insomnia, upper respiratory tract infection and urinary tract infection.

Other common side-effects were: increased sweating, malaise, weight loss and tremor.

Rare cases of angina pectoris, gastrointestinal haemorrhage and syncope were observed.

No notable abnormalities in laboratory values were observed.

Overdose

Symptoms: Most cases of accidental overdosage have not been associated with any clinical signs or symptoms and almost all of the patients concerned continued rivastigmine treatment. Where symptoms have occurred, they have included nausea, vomiting and diarrhoea. In the majority of these events, no therapeutic intervention was required. Ingestion of 46 mg occurred in one case; folowing conservative management the patient fully recovered within 24 hours.

Treatment: As rivastigmine has a plasma half-life of about 1 hour and a duration of acetylcholinesterase inhibition of about 9 hours, it is recommended that in cases of asymptomatic overdose, no further dose of rivastigmine should be administered for the next 24 hours. In overdose accompanied by severe nausea and vomiting, the use of anti-emetics should be considered. Symptomatic treatment for other adverse events should be given as necessary.

In massive overdose, atropine can be used. An initial dose of 0.03 mg/kg intravenous atropine sulphate is recommended, with subsequent doses based on clinical response. Use of scopolamine as an antidote is not recommended.

Pharmacological properties

Pharmacodynamic properties: Pharmacotherapeutic group: acetylcholinesterase inhibitor; ACT-code: N07AA.

Rivastigmine is an acetylcholinesterase inhibitor of the carbamate type, thought to facilitate cholinergic neurotransmission by slowing the degradation of acetylcholine released by functionally intact cholinergic neurones. Thus, rivastigmine may have an ameliorative effect on cholinergic-mediated cognitive deficits associated with Alzheimer's disease.

Rivastigmine interacts with its target enzyme by forming a covalently bound complex that temporarily inactivates the enzyme. In man, an oral 3 mg dose decreases acetylcholinesterase activity in CSF by approximately 40% within the first 1.5 hours after administration. Activity of the enzyme returns to baseline levels about 9 hours after the maximum inhibitory effect has been achieved. In patients with Alzheimer's disease, inhibition of acetylcholinesterase in CSF by rivastigmine was dose-dependent up to 6 mg given twice-daily, the highest dose tested.

Clinical studies: The efficacy of Exelon has been established through the use of three independent, domain specific, assessment tools which were assessed at periodic intervals during 6 month treatment periods. These include the ADAS-Cog (a performance based measure of cognition), the CIBIC-Plus (a comprehensive global assessment of the patient by the physician incorporating caregiver input), and the PDS (a caregiver-rated assessment of the activities of daily living including personal hygiene, feeding, dressing, household chores such as shopping, retention of ability to orient oneself to surroundings as well as involvement in activities relating to finances, etc.).

The results for clinically-relevant responders pooled from two flexible dose studies out of the three pivotal 26-week multicentre studies in patients with mild-to-moderately severe Alzheimer's dementia, are provided in the Table. Clinically relevant improvement in these studies was defined a priori as at least 4-point improvement on the ADAS-Cog, improvement on the CIBIC-Plus, or at least a 10% improvement on the PDS.

In addition, a post-hoc definition of response is provided in the same table. The secondary definition of response required a 4-point or greater improvement on the ADAS-Cog, no worsening on the CIBIC-Plus, and no worsening on the PDS. The mean actual daily dose for responders in the 6–12 mg group, corresponding to this definition, was 9.3 mg. It is important to note that the scales used in this indication vary and direct comparisons of results for different therapeutic agents are not valid.

Pharmacokinetic properties

Absorption: Rivastigmine is rapidly and completely absorbed. Peak plasma concentrations are reached in approximately 1 hour. As a consequence of the drug's interaction with its target enzyme, the increase in bioavailability is about 1.5-fold greater than that

Response measure	*Patients with clinically significant response (%)*			
	Intent to treat		*Last observation carried forward*	
	Rivastigmine 6–12 mg N=473	*Placebo N=472*	*Rivastigmine 6–12 mg N=379*	*Placebo N=444*
ADAS-Cog: improvement of at least 4 points	21***	12	25***	12
CIBIC-Plus: improvement	29***	18	32***	19
PDS: improvement of at least 10%	26***	17	30***	18
At least 4 point improvement on ADAS-Cog with no worsening on CIBIC-Plus and PDS	10*	6	12**	6

* $p<0.05$. ** $p<0.01$. *** $p<0.001$.

expected from the increase in dose. Absolute bioavailability after a 3 mg dose is about 36%±13%. Administration of rivastigmine with food delays absorption (t_{max}) by 90 min and lowers C_{max} and increases AUC by approximately 30%.

Distribution: Rivastigmine is weakly bound to plasma proteins (approximately 40%). It readily crosses the blood brain barrier and has an apparent volume of distribution in the range of 1.8–2.7 l/kg.

Metabolism: Rivastigmine is rapidly and extensively metabolised (half-life in plasma approximately 1 hour), primarily via cholinesterase-mediated hydrolysis to the decarbamylated metabolite. *In vitro*, this metabolite shows minimal inhibition of acetylcholinesterase (<10%). Based on evidence from *in vitro* and animal studies, the major cytochrome P450 isoenzymes are minimally involved in rivastigmine metabolism. Total plasma clearance of rivastigmine was approximately 130 l/h after a 0.2 mg intravenous dose and decreased to 70 l/h after a 2.7 mg intravenous dose.

Excretion: Unchanged rivastigmine is not found in the urine; renal excretion of the metabolites is the major route of elimination. Following administration of 14C-rivastigmine, renal elimination was rapid and essentially complete (>90%) within 24 hours. Less than 1% of the administered dose is excreted in the faeces. There is no accumulation of rivastigmine or the decarbamylated metabolite in patients with Alzheimer's disease.

Elderly subjects: While bioavailability of rivastigmine is greater in elderly than in young healthy volunteers, studies in Alzheimer patients aged between 50 and 92 years showed no change in bioavailability with age.

Subjects with hepatic impairment: The C_{max} of rivastigmine was approximately 60% higher and the AUC of rivastigmine was more than twice as high in subjects with mild to moderate hepatic impairment compared to healthy subjects.

Subjects with renal impairment: C_{max} and AUC of rivastigmine were more than twice as high in subjects with moderate renal impairment compared with healthy subjects; however there were no changes in C_{max} and AUC of rivastigmine in subjects with severe renal impairment.

Preclinical safety data: Repeated-dose toxicity studies in rats, mice and dogs revealed only effects associated with an exaggerated pharmacological action. No target organ toxicity was observed. No safety margins to human exposure were achieved in the animal studies due to the sensitivity of the animal models used.

Rivastigmine was not mutagenic in a standard battery of *in vitro* and *in vivo* tests, except in a chromosomal aberration test in human peripheral lymphocytes at a dose 104 times the maximum clinical exposure. The *in vivo* micronucleus test was negative.

No evidence of carcinogenicity was found in studies in mice and rats at maximum tolerated dose, although the exposure to rivastigmine and its metabolites was lower than the human exposure. When normalised to body surface area, the exposure to rivastigmine and its metabolites was approximately equivalent to the maximum recommended human dose of 12 mg/day; however, when compared to the maximum human dose, a multiple of approximately 6-fold was achieved in animals.

In animals, rivastigmine crosses the placenta and is excreted into milk. Oral studies in pregnant rats and rabbits gave no indication of teratogenic potential on the part of rivastigmine.

Pharmaceutical particulars

List of excipients: Gelatin; magnesium stearate; methylhydroxypropylcellulose; microcrystalline cellulose; silica, colloidal anhydrous; yellow iron oxide (E172); red iron oxide (E172) and titanium dioxide (E171).

Incompatibilities: Not applicable.

Shelf-life: 24 months.

Special precautions for storage: Store below 30°C.

Nature and content of container: Blister with 14 capsules; clear PVC tray with blue lidding foil. Each box contains 2 or 4 blisters.

Instructions for use/handling: Not applicable.

Marketing authorisation holder: Novartis Europharm Limited, Wimblehurst Road, Horsham, West Sussex RH12 4AB.

Marketing authorisation numbers

1.5 mg×28 capsules:	EU/1/98/066/001
1.5 mg×56 capsules:	EU/1/98/066/002
3 mg×28 capsules:	EU/1/98/066/004
3 mg×56 capsules:	EU/1/98/066/005
4.5 mg×28 capsules:	EU/1/98/066/007
4.5 mg×56 capsules:	EU/1/98/066/008
6 mg×28 capsules:	EU/1/98/066/010
6 mg×56 capsules:	EU/1/98/066/011

Date of first authorisation/renewal of the authorisation 12 May 1998.

FEMARA*

Qualitative and quantitative composition Active substance: 4,4'-[(1H-1,2,4-triazol-1-yl)-methylene]bis-benzonitrile (INN/USAN=letrozole). Each coated tablet contains 2.5 mg letrozole.

Pharmaceutical form Coated tablets.

Clinical particulars

Therapeutic indications: Treatment of advanced breast cancer in post-menopausal women in whom tamoxifen or other anti-oestrogen therapy has failed.

Posology and method of administration:

Adult and elderly patients: The recommended dose of Femara is 2.5 mg once daily. Treatment with Femara should continue until tumour progression is evident. No dose adjustment is required for elderly patients.

Children: Not recommended for use in children.

Patients with hepatic and/or renal impairment: No dosage adjustment is required for patients with mild to moderate hepatic impairment (Child-Pugh grade A and B) or renal impairment (creatinine clearance ≥10 mL/min) (see *Pharmacokinetic properties*).

Contra-indications: Hypersensitivity to the active substance or to any of the excipients. Pre-menopausal, pregnant or lactating women; patients with severe hepatic impairment (Child-Pugh grade C).

Special warnings and special precautions for use: Femara is not recommended for use in children as efficacy and safety in this patient group have not been assessed in clinical studies. There are no efficacy data to support the use of Femara in men with breast cancer.

Femara has not been investigated in patients with creatinine clearance <10 mL/min. As letrozole is weakly bound to plasma proteins (see *Pharmacokinetic properties*), it is anticipated that it could be removed from circulation by dialysis. The potential risk/benefit to such patients should be carefully considered before administration of Femara.

Interaction with other medicaments and other forms of interaction: Clinical interaction studies with cimetidine and warfarin indicated that the co-administration of Femara with these drugs does not result in clinically significant drug interactions, even though cimetidine is a known inhibitor of one of the cytochrome P450 isoenzymes capable of metabolising letrozole *in vitro* (see also *Metabolism and elimination*).

Additionally, in a large clinical trial there was no evidence of clinically relevant interaction in patients receiving other commonly prescribed drugs (e.g. benzodiazepines; barbiturates; NSAIDs such as diclofenac sodium, ibuprofen; paracetamol; furosemide; omeprazole).

There is no clinical experience to date on the use of Femara in combination with other anti-cancer agents.

Pregnancy and lactation: There is no experience of the use of Femara in human pregnancy or lactation. Femara is contra-indicated during pregnancy, lactation and in pre-menopausal women.

Embryotoxicity and foetotoxicity were seen in pregnant rats following oral administration of Femara, and there was an increase in the incidence of foetal malformation among the animals treated. However, it is not known whether this was an indirect consequence of the pharmcological activity of Femara (inhibition of oestrogen biosynthesis) or a direct drug effect.

Ability to drive and use machines: Femara is unlikely to impair the ability of patients to drive or to operate machinery. However, fatigue and dizziness have been observed with the use of Femara. Patients should be advised that their physical and/or mental abilities required for operating machinery or driving a car may be impaired.

Undesirable effects: In clinical trials, adverse experiences were generally mild to moderate and rarely severe enough to require discontinuation of treatment. Many can be attributed to either the underlying disease or the normal pharmacological consequences of oestrogen deprivation (e.g. hot flushes, hair thinning).

Most frequently reported (>5%) adverse events (% patients) irrespective of trial drug relationship

	Comparative clinical trial		*All trials*
	Femara 2.5 mg	*Megestrol acetate 160 mg*	*Femara 2.5 mg*
musculoskeletal pain	27.0	30.2	19.3
arthralgia	13.2	7.9	8.4
headache	12.6	9.0	8.9
fatigue	10.9	11.1	6.6
nausea	10.9	9.0	12.4
dyspnoea	9.2	16.4	6.8
peripheral oedema	8.6	7.9	—
coughing	8.0	7.4	5.8
constipation	7.5	8.5	5.6
vomiting	7.5	5.3	7.1
chest pain	6.9	7.4	5.3
viral infection	6.9	6.3	6.1
diarrhoea	6.3	2.6	5.6
hot flushes	5.7	3.7	5.3
rash	5.7	3.2	—
abdominal pain	5.7	8.5	5.6
dyspepsia	5.2	5.8	—
anorexia	5.2	4.8	—
dizziness	3.4	6.9	—
weight increase	2.3	8.5	—
pruritus	1.7	5.3	—

Overdose: There is no clinical experience of overdosage. In animal studies, Femara exhibits only a slight degree of acute toxicity. In clinical trials, the highest single and multiple dose tested in healthy volunteers was 30 mg and 5 mg, respectively, the latter also being the highest dose tested in post-menopausal breast cancer patients. Each of these doses was well tolerated. There is no clinical evidence for a particular dose of Femara resulting in life-threatening symptoms.

There is no specific antidote to Femara. Since Femara is not highly protein bound, dialysis may be helpful. Emesis may be induced if the patient is alert. In general, supportive care and frequent monitoring of vital signs is appropriate.

Pharmacological properties

Pharmacodynamic properties:

Pharmacotherapeutic group: Non-steroidal aromatase inhibitor (inhibitor of oestrogen biosynthesis); anti-neoplastic agent.

Pharmacodynamic effects: The elimination of oestrogen-mediated stimulatory effects is a prerequisite for tumour response in cases where the growth of tumour tissue depends on the presence of oestrogens. In post-menopausal women, oestrogens are mainly derived from the action of the aromatase enzyme, which converts adrenal androgens – primarily androstenedione and testosterone – to oestrone (El) and oestradiol (E2). The suppression of oestrogen biosynthesis in peripheral tissues and the cancer tissue itself can therefore be achieved by specifically inhibiting the aromatase enzyme.

Letrozole is a non-steroidal aromatase inhibitor. It inhibits the aromatase enzyme by competitively binding to the haem of the cytochrome P450 subunit of the enzyme, resulting in a reduction of oestrogen biosynthesis in all tissues.

In healthy post-menopausal women, single doses of 0.1, 0.5, and 2.5 mg letrozole suppress serum oestrone and oestradiol by 75–78% and 78% from baseline respectively. Maximum suppression is achieved in 48–78 h.

In post-menopausal patients with advanced breast cancer, daily doses of 0.1 to 5 mg suppress plasma concentration of oestradiol, oestrone, and oestrone sulphate by 75–95% from baseline in all patients treated. With doses of 0.5 mg and higher, many values of oestrone and oestrone sulphate are below the limit of detection in the assays, indicating that higher oestrogen suppression is achieved with these doses. Oestrogen suppression was maintained throughout treatment in all these patients.

Letrozole is highly specific in inhibiting aromatase activity. Impairment of adrenal steroidogenesis has not been observed.

No clinically relevant changes were found in the plasma concentrations of cortisol, aldosterone, 11-deoxycortisol, 17-hydroxy-progesterone, and ACTH or in plasma renin activity among post-menopausal patients treated with a daily dose of letrozole 0.1 to 5 mg. The ACTH stimulation test performed after 6 and 12 weeks of treatment with daily doses of 0.1, 0.25, 0.5, 1, 2.5, and 5 mg did not indicate any attenuation of aldosterone or cortisol production. Thus, glucocorticoid and mineralocorticoid supplementation is not necessary.

No changes were noted in plasma concentrations of androgens (androstenedione and testosterone) among healthy post-menopausal women after 0.1, 0.5, and 2.5 mg single doses of letrozole or in plasma concentrations of androstenedione among post-menopausal patients treated with daily doses of 0.1 to 5 mg, indicating that the blockade of oestrogen biosynthesis does not lead to accumulation of androgenic precursors. Plasma levels of LH and FSH are not affected by letrozole in patients, nor is thyroid function as evaluated by TSH, T4 and T3 uptake.

Pharmacokinetic properties:

Absorption: Letrozole is rapidly and completely absorbed from the gastrointestinal tract (mean absolute bioavailability: 99.9%). Food slightly decreases the rate of absorption (median t_{max}: 1 hour fasted versus 2 hours fed; and mean C_{max}: 129±20.3 nmol/L fasted versus 98.7±18.6 nmol/L fed) but the extent of absorption (AUC) is not changed. The minor effect on the absorption rate is not considered to be of clinical relevance and therefore letrozole may be taken without regard to mealtimes.

Distribution: Plasma protein binding of letrozole is approximately 60%, mainly to albumin (55%). The concentration of letrozole in erythrocytes is about 80% of that in plasma. After administration of 2.5 mg ^{14}C-labelled letrozole, approximately 82% of the radioactivity in plasma was unchanged compound. Systemic exposure to metabolites is therefore low. Letrozole is rapidly and extensively distributed to tissues. Its apparent volume of distribution at steady state is about 1.87±0.47 L/kg.

Metabolism and elimination: Metabolic clearance to a pharmacologically inactive carbinol metabolite is the major elimination pathway of letrozole (CL_m=2.1 L/h) but is relatively slow when compared to hepatic blood flow (about 90 L/h). The cytochrome P450 isoenzymes 3A4 and 2A6 were found to be capable of converting letrozole to this metabolite *in vitro*, but their individual contributions to letrozole clearance *in vivo* have not been established. In an interaction study co-administration with cimetidine, which is known to inhibit only the 3A4 isoenzyme, did not result in a decrease in letrozole clearance suggesting that *in vivo* the 2A6 isoenzyme plays an important part in total clearance. In this study a slight decrease in AUC and increase in C_{max} were observed. Formation of minor unidentified metabolites and direct renal and faecal excretion play only a minor role in the overall elimination of letrozole. Within 2 weeks after administration of 2.5 mg ^{14}C-labelled letrozole to healthy post-menopausal volunteers, 88.2±7.6% of the radioactivity was recovered in urine and 3.8±0.9% in faeces. At least 75% of the radioactivity recovered in urine up to 216 hours (84.7±7.8% of the dose) was attributed to the glucuronide of the carbinol metabolite, about 9% to two unidentified metabolites, and 6% to unchanged letrozole.

The apparent terminal elimination half-life in plasma is about 2 days. After daily administration of 2.5 mg steady-state levels are reached within 2 to 6 weeks. Plasma concentrations at steady state are approximately 7 times higher than concentrations measured after a single dose of 2.5 mg while they are 1.5 to 2 times higher than the steady-state values predicted from the concentrations measured after a single dose, indicating a slight non-linearity in the pharmacokinetics of letrozole upon daily administration of 2.5 mg. Since steady-state levels are maintained over time, it can be concluded that no continuous accumulation of letrozole occurs.

Age had no effect on the pharmacokinetics of letrozole.

Special populations: In a study involving volunteers with varying degrees of renal function (24 hours creatinine clearance 9–116 mL/min) no effect on the pharmacokinetics of letrozole or the urinary excretion of the glucuronide of its carbinol metabolite was found after a single dose of 2.5 mg. The C_{max}, AUC and half-life of the metabolite have not been determined. In a similar study involving subjects with varying degrees of hepatic function, the mean AUC values of the volunteers with moderate hepatic impairment was 37% higher than in normal subjects, but still within the range seen in subjects without impaired function.

Preclinical safety data: Femara showed a low degree of acute toxicity in rodents exposed to up to 2000 mg/kg. In dogs Femara caused signs of moderate toxicity at 100 mg/kg.

In repeated-dose toxicity studies in rats and dogs up to 12 months, the main findings can be attributed to the pharmacological action of the compound. Effects on the liver (increased weight, hepatocellular hypertrophy, fatty changes) were observed, mainly at high dose levels. Increased incidences of hepatic vacuolation (both sexes, high dose) and necrosis (intermediate and high dose females) were also noted in rats treated for 104 weeks in a carcinogenicity study. They may have been associated with the endocrine effects and hepatic enzyme-inducing properties of Femara. However, a direct drug effect cannot be ruled out.

In a 104-week mouse carcinogenicity study, dermal and systemic inflammation occurred, particularly at the highest dose of 60 mg/kg, leading to increased mortality at this dose level. Again it is not known whether these findings were an indirect consequence of the pharmacological activity of Femara (i.e. linked to long-term oestrogen deprivation) or a direct drug effect.

Both *in vitro* and *in vivo* investigations on Femara's mutagenic potential revealed no indication of any genotoxicity.

In the carcinogenicity studies no treatment-related tumours were noted in male animals. In female animals, treatment-related changes in genital tract tumours (a reduced incidence of benign and malignant mammary tumours in rats, an increased incidence of benign ovarian stromal tumours in mice) were secondary to the pharmacological effect of the compound.

Pharmaceutical particulars

List of excipients: Silica aerogel, cellulose, lactose, magnesium stearate, maize starch, sodium carboxymethyl starch, hydroxypropyl methylcellulose, polyethylene glycol, talc, titanium dioxide, iron oxide yellow.

Incompatibilities: None known.

Shelf life: Two years.

Special precautions for storage: Protect from heat, store below 30°C.

Nature and contents of container: PVC/PE/PVDC blister packs of 14 or 28 tablets.

Instructions for use/handling: No specific instructions for use/handling.

Marketing authorisation holder: Novartis Pharmaceuticals UK Limited, trading as Ciba Laboratories, Frimley Business Park, Frimley, Camberley, Surrey GU16 5SG.

Marketing authorisation number 00101/0493.

Date of approval/revision of SPC November 1996.

Date of (partial) revision of the text December 1997.

Legal category POM.

FORADIL* 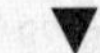

Qualitative and quantitative composition Active substance: (±)-2'-hydroxy-5'-[(RS)-1-hydroxy-2-[[(RS)-p-methoxy-a methylphenethyl]-amino] ethyl] formanilide fumarate dihydrate (= eformoterol fumarate).

One capsule contains 12 micrograms eformoterol fumarate.

Pharmaceutical form Inhalation powder in capsules.

Clinical particulars

Therapeutic indications: The treatment of reversible airways obstruction (including nocturnal asthma and prevention of exercise induced bronchospasm) in patients requiring long-term regular bronchodilator therapy. Such patients should normally also be receiving regular and adequate doses of inhaled anti-inflammatory agents (e.g. corticosteroids and/or sodium cromoglycate) or oral corticosteroids.

Posology and method of administration:

For use in adults (including the elderly):

Regular maintenance therapy: One inhalation capsule (12 micrograms) to be inhaled twice daily. For more severe cases two inhalation capsules twice daily. This dosing regimen provides symptomatic relief throughout day and night.

Foradil should be taken twice daily. The maximum daily dose is 24 micrograms b.d. (4 capsules).

Although Foradil has a rapid onset of action, current asthma management guidelines recommend that long-acting inhaled bronchodilators should be used for maintenance bronchodilator therapy. They further recommend that in the event of an acute attack, a β-agonist with a short duration of action should be used.

In accordance with the current management guidelines, long-acting β2-agonists may be added to the treatment regimen in patients experiencing problems with high dose inhaled steroids. Alternatively, where regular symptomatic treatment of asthma is required in addition to inhaled steroids, then long-acting β2-agonists can be used. Patients should be advised not to stop or change their steroid therapy when Foradil is introduced.

If the symptoms persist or worsen, or if the recommended dose of Foradil fails to control symptoms (maintain effective relief), this is usually an indication of a worsening of the underlying condition.

Children under 18 years: Foradil inhalation capsules are not recommended in children, because of the limited clinical experience with this patient group.

Renal and hepatic impairment: There is no theoretical reason to suggest that Foradil dosage requires adjustment in patients with renal or hepatic impairment, however no clinical data have been generated to support its use in these groups.

Contra-indications: Hypersensitivity to eformoterol fumarate or lactose.

Special warnings and special precautions for use:
Anti-inflammatory therapy: In general, asthmatic patients who require regular therapy with a β2-agonist should also receive regular and adequate doses of an inhaled anti-inflammatory agent (e.g. corticosteroids, and/or sodium cromoglycate) or oral corticosteroids. Whenever Foradil is prescribed, patients should be evaluated for the adequacy of the anti-inflammatory therapy they receive. Patients must be advised to continue taking anti-inflammatory therapy unchanged after the introduction of Foradil, even when the symptoms improve. Should symptoms persist, or should the number of doses of Foradil required to control symptoms increase, this usually indicates a worsening of the underlying condition and warrants a reassessment of asthma therapy by a physician.

Concomitant conditions: Special care and supervision, with particular emphasis on dosage limits, is required in patients receiving Foradil when the following conditions may exist:

Ischaemic heart disease, cardiac arrhythmias, especially third degree atrioventricular block, severe cardiac decompensation, idiopathic subvalvular aortic stenosis, hypertrophic obstructive cardiomyopathy, thyrotoxicosis, known or suspected prolongation of the QT interval (QTc > 0.44 sec.; see *Interaction with other medicaments and other forms of interaction*).

Due to the hyperglycaemic effect of β2-stimulants, additional blood glucose controls are recommended in diabetic patients.

Hypokalaemia: Potentially serious hypokalaemia may result from β2-agonist therapy. Particular caution is advised in severe asthma as this effect may be potentiated by hypoxia and concomitant treatment (see *Interaction with other medicaments and other forms of interaction*). It is recommended that serum potassium levels be monitored in such situations.

Paradoxical bronchospasm: As with other inhalation therapy, the potential for paradoxical bronchospasm should be kept in mind. If it occurs, the preparation should be discontinued immediately and alternative therapy substituted.

Interaction with other medicaments and other forms of interaction: There are no clinical data to support the advice given below, but from consideration of first principles one might expect the following interactions:

Drugs such as quinidine, disopyramide, procainamide, phenothiazines, antihistamines and tricyclic antidepressants may be associated with QT-interval prolongation and an increased risk of ventricular arrhythmia (see *Contra-indications*).

Concomitant administration of other sympathomimetic agents may potentiate the undesirable effects of Foradil.

Administration of Foradil to patients being treated with monoamine oxidase inhibitors or tricyclic antidepressants should be performed with caution, since the action of β2-adrenergic stimulants on the cardiovascular system may be potentiated.

Concomitant treatment with xanthine derivatives, steroids, or diuretics may potentiate a possible hypokalaemic effect of β2-agonists. Hypokalaemia may increase susceptibility to cardiac arrhythmias in patients treated with digitalis (see *Special warnings and special precautions for use*).

β-adrenergic blockers may weaken or antagonise the effect of Foradil. Therefore, Foradil should not be given together with β-adrenergic blockers (including eye drops) unless there are compelling reasons for their use.

Pregnancy and lactation: There were no teratogenic effects revealed in animal tests. However, until further experience is gained, Foradil is not recommended for use during pregnancy (particularly at the end of pregnancy or during labour) unless there is no more established alternative. As with any medicine, use during pregnancy should only be considered if the expected benefit to the mother is greater than any risk to the foetus. The substance has been detected in the milk of lactating rats, but it is not known whether eformoterol passes into human breast milk, therefore mothers using Foradil should refrain from breast feeding their infants.

Effects on ability to drive and use machines: Foradil is unlikely to have any effect on the ability to drive and operate machinery.

Undesirable effects: Frequency estimate: Frequent=>10%, occasional=>1%-10%, rare=>0.001%-1%, isolated cases=<0.001%

Musculoskeletal system: *Occasional:* Tremor. *Rare:* Muscle cramps, myalgia.

Cardiovascular system: *Occasional:* Palpitations. *Rare:* Tachycardia.

Central nervous system: *Occasional:* Headache. *Rare:* Agitation, dizziness, anxiety, nervousness, insomnia.

Respiratory tract: *Rare:* Aggravated bronchospasm.

Local irritation: *Rare:* Oropharyngeal irritation.

Others: *Isolated cases:* Pruritus, conjunctival irritation and eyelid oedema, taste disturbance, exanthema, nausea

Overdose:
Symptoms: There is no clinical experience to date on the management of overdose, however, an overdosage of Foradil would be likely to lead to effects that are typical of β2-adrenergic agonists: nausea, vomiting, headache, tremor, somnolence, palpitations, tachycardia, ventricular arrhythmias, metabolic acidosis, hypokalaemia, hyperglycaemia.

Treatment: Supportive and symptomatic treatment is indicated. Serious cases should be hospitalised.

Use of cardioselective beta-blockers may be considered, but only subject to extreme caution since the use of β-adrenergic blocker medication may provoke bronchospasm.

Serum potassium should be monitored.

Pharmacological properties
Pharmacodynamic properties: Eformoterol is a potent selective β2-adrenergic stimulant. It exerts a bronchodilator effect in patients with reversible airways obstruction. The effect sets in rapidly (within 1-3 minutes) and is still significant 12 hours after inhalation.

In man, Foradil has been shown to be effective in preventing bronchospasm induced by exercise and methacholine.

Pharmacokinetic properties:
Absorption: As reported for other inhaled drugs, it is likely that about 90% of eformoterol administered from an inhaler will be swallowed and then absorbed from the gastrointestinal tract. This means that the pharmacokinetic characteristics of the oral formulation largely apply also to the inhalation powder.

Oral doses of up to 300 micrograms eformoterol fumarate are readily absorbed from the gastrointestinal tract. Peak plasma concentrations of the unchanged substance are reached 0.5–1 hour after administration. The absorption of an oral 80 micrograms dose is 65% or more.

The pharmacokinetics of eformoterol appear linear in the range of oral doses investigated, i.e. 20–300 micrograms. Repeated oral administration of 40–160 micrograms daily does not lead to significant accumulation of the drug.

Following inhalation of therapeutic doses, eformoterol cannot be detected in the plasma using current analytical methods. However, analysis of urinary excretion rates suggests that inhaled eformoterol is rapidly absorbed. The maximum excretion rate after administration of 12–96 micrograms is reached within 1–2 hours of inhalation.

Cumulative urinary excretion of eformoterol after administration of the inhalation powder (12–24 micrograms) and two different aerosol formulations (12–96 micrograms) showed the amount of eformoterol available in the circulation to increase in proportion to the dose.

Distribution: The plasma protein binding of eformoterol is 61-64% (34% primarily to albumin). There is no saturation of binding sites in the concentration range reached with therapeutic doses.

Biotransformation: Eformoterol is eliminated primarily by metabolism, direct glucuronidation being the major pathway of biotransformation. O-demethylation followed by glucuronidation is another pathway.

Elimination: Elimination of eformoterol from the circulation seems to be polyphasic; the apparent half-life depends on the time interval considered. On the basis of plasma or blood concentrations up to 6, 8 or 12 hours after oral administration, an elimination half-life of about 2-3 hours was determined. From urinary excretion rates between 3 and 16 hours after inhalation, a half-life of about 5 hours was calculated.

The drug and its metabolites are completely eliminated from the body; about two-thirds of an oral dose appear in the urine and one-third in the faeces. After inhalation about 6-9% of the dose on average is excreted unchanged in the urine. Renal clearance of eformoterol is 150 mL/min.

Preclinical safety data:
Mutagenicity: Mutagenicity tests covering a broad range of experimental endpoints have been conducted. No genotoxic effects were found in any of the *in vitro* or *in vivo* tests performed.

Carcinogenicity: Two-year studies in rats and mice did not show any carcinogenic potential.

Male mice treated at very high dose levels showed a slightly higher incidence of benign adrenal subcapsular cell tumours, which are considered to reflect alterations in the physiological ageing process.

Two studies in rats, covering different dose ranges, showed an increase in mesovarial leiomyomas. These benign neoplasms are typically associated with long-term treatment of rats at high doses of β2-adrenergic drugs. Increased incidences of ovarian cysts and benign granulosa/theca cell tumours were also seen; β-agonists are known to have effects on the ovary in rats in which are very likely specific to rodents. A few other tumour types noted in the first study using the higher doses were within the incidences of the historical control population, and were not seen in the lower-dose experiment.

None of the tumour incidences were increased to a statistically significant extent at the lowest dose of the second study, a dose leading to a systemic exposure 10 times higher than that expected from the maximum recommended dose of eformoterol.

On the basis of these findings and the absence of a mutagenic potential, it is concluded that use of eformoterol at therapeutic doses not present a carcinogenic risk.

Reproduction toxicity: Animal tests showed no teratogenic effects; after oral administration, eformoterol was excreted in the milk of lactating rats.

Pharmaceutical particulars
List of excipients: Lactose EP/USP NF/JP (150 mesh).

Incompatibilities: None known.

Shelf life: 3 years in PVC/PE/PVDC blisters

Special precautions for storage: In PVC/PE/PVdC blisters: protect from heat and moisture (store below 25°C).

Nature and contents of container: Blister calendar packs of 14 or 56 capsules, with an inhaler device in each pack.

Instructions for use/handling: To ensure proper administration of the drug, the patient should be shown how to use the inhaler by a physician or other health professional.

It is important for the patient to understand that the gelatin capsule may very occasionally break up and small pieces of gelatin might reach the mouth or throat after inhalation. The patient may be reassured that gelatin is harmless and will soften in the mouth and can be swallowed. The tendency for the capsule to break up is minimised by not piercing the capsule more than once.

The capsules should be removed from the blister strip **only** immediately before use.

Marketing authorisation holder: Novartis Pharmaceuticals UK Limited, trading as Geigy Pharmaceuticals.

Marketing authorisation number 00101/0494

Date of revision of SPC December 1997

Legal category POM

HYDERGINE*

Presentation *1·5 mg Tablets:* Hydergine 1.5 mg is available as white, flat, bevel-edged tablets, scored on one side, with HYDERGINE 1.5 engraved on the other, and of 240 mg weight, 9 mm diameter and 2.9 mm thickness. Each tablet contains 1.5 mg Co-dergocrine Mesylate BP.

4·5 mg Tablets: Hydergine 4.5 mg is available as white, round, biconvex tablets coded HYDERGINE on one side with 4.5 engraved on the other, and of 240 mg weight and 9 mm diameter. Each tablet contains 4.5 mg Co-dergocrine Mesylate BP.

Uses *Indications:* As an adjunct in the management of elderly patients with mild to moderate dementia.

Dosage and administration 1.5 mg three times a day or a once daily dosage of 4.5 mg.

Hydergine should be taken before meals.

The effect of Hydergine is not immediate: alleviation of symptoms is usually gradual and may not be apparent for two to three weeks. Continuing improvement may be expected for at least three months.

Contra-indications, warnings, etc
Contra-indications: Known hypersensitivity to the drug.

Precautions: Caution should be exercised in the administration of Hydergine to patients with severe bradycardia.

There are no known drug interactions involving Hydergine.

Overdosage: Symptoms might include nausea, vomiting, nasal stuffiness, flushing of the face, headache, hypotension and collapse. Treatment should be directed to the elimination of the drug from the gastrointestinal tract by gastric lavage, followed by the administration of activated charcoal. General supportive measures should be applied with particular reference to the cardiovascular system.

Side-effects: Side-effects are infrequent following administration of Hydergine and even relatively large doses are well tolerated. Minor side-effects including gastro-intestinal disturbances, flushes, rashes, nasal stuffiness, abdominal cramps, headaches, dizziness and postural hypotension in hypotensive patients have on occasion been reported.

Pharmaceutical precautions Protect from light.

Legal category POM.

Package quantities *1.5 mg Tablets:* Blister pack of 100.
4.5 mg Tablets: Calendar pack of 28.

Further information Double-blind studies have shown that improvement occurs with all the symptoms listed in the Sandoz Clinical Assessment-Geriatric (SCAG) scale except for hostility; significant improvement can be expected for nine of the symptoms, namely confusion, impairment of recent memory, disorientation, anxiety, depression, emotional lability, irritability, unsociability and the overall impression of the patient.

Product licence numbers

1.5 mg Tablets	0101/0042R
4.5 mg Tablets	0101/0117

Product licence holder: Novartis Pharmaceuticals UK Ltd, trading as Sandoz Pharmaceuticals, Frimley Business Park, Frimley, Camberley Surrey GU16 5SG.

LACTULOSE SOLUTION BP

Qualitative and quantitative composition Lactulose BP 67.0% w/v.

Pharmaceutical form Solution.

Clinical particulars
Therapeutic indications: A. Chronic constipation.
B. Chronic portal-systemic encephalopathy.

Posology and method of administration:
Adults: Initially: 15–30 ml daily for first 2–3 days (45 ml may be given in obstinate cases).

Maintenance: 10–15 ml daily or according to the need of the patient.

Children: Initially: 10–25 ml daily for first 2–3 days.

Maintenance: 5–15 ml daily or according to the need of the patient.

Dosage does not appear to be related to the age or weight of the child and should be adjusted to produce the required response.

Chronic portal-systemic encephalopathy: Initially 30–50 ml three times daily according to the requirements of the patient for adequate acidification of the colonic contents.

Use in the elderly: No evidence exists that elderly patients require different dosages or show different side-effects from younger patients.

Contra-indications: In common with other preparations used for the treatment of constipation, LACTULOSE SOLUTION should not be used in patients with gastrointestinal obstruction. LACTULOSE SOLUTION should not be given to patients with galactosaemia or lactose intolerance.

Special warnings and precautions for use: Not applicable.

Interaction with other medicaments and other forms of interaction: There are no known drug interactions involving LACTULOSE.

Pregnancy and lactation: LACTULOSE SOLUTION should be used with caution during the first trimester of pregnancy.

Effects on ability to drive and to use machines: There is no evidence that LACTULOSE affects driving ability.

Undesirable effects: Side-effects rarely occur after the administration of LACTULOSE SOLUTION. Mild transient effects such as abdominal distension or cramps and flatulence, which subside after the initial stages of treatment, have occasionally been reported. High doses may provoke nausea in some patients. This can be minimised by administration with water, fruit juice or with meals.

Overdose: No cases of intoxication due to deliberate or accidental overdosage with LACTULOSE SOLUTION have been reported to the company.

Pharmacological properties
Pharmacodynamic properties: The active principle of LACTULOSE SOLUTION, lactulose, is neither broken down nor absorbed in the stomach and small intestine. In the colon it acts as a substrate for and promotes the growth of naturally occurring glycolytic microorganisms, and is broken down to lactic acid. The pH of the intestinal contents is lowered, the growth of acidophilic flora is promoted and the putrefactive micro-organisms are suppressed. This reduces the formation of ammonia and amines and their absorption from the gut, thus leading to a fall in blood ammonia levels (responsible for hepatic encephalopathy). By normalising the intestinal flora LACTULOSE SOLUTION ensures the passage of normal stools, without excessive peristalsis.

Pharmacokinetic properties: Not applicable.

Preclinical safety data: There are no pre-clinical data of relevance to the prescriber which are additional to those already included in other sections of the Summary of Product Characteristics.

Pharmaceutical particulars
List of excipients: Other sugars (lactose, galactose, tagatose and other ketoses), demineralised water.

Incompatibilities: Not applicable.

Shelf life: 36 months.

Special precautions for storage: Store below 25°C.

Nature and contents of container: Amber glass bottles, plastic bottles (HDPE), PET bottles with polythene closure (polythene wad faced with PP, PVDC or PET lining), containing 200 ml, 300 ml, 500 ml or 1 L of LACTULOSE SOLUTION.

Instructions for use/handling: Not applicable.

Marketing authorisation holder: Novartis Pharmaceuticals UK Limited, trading as Sandoz Pharmaceuticals, Frimley Business Park, Frimley, Camberley, Surrey GU16 5SG.

Marketing authorisation number PL 0101/0076.

Date of first authorisation/renewal of the authorisation 2nd September 1974.

Date of (partial) revision of the text 14 March 1997.

LAMISIL* CREAM

Qualitative and quantitative composition Terbinafine hydrochloride 1.0% w/w.

Pharmaceutical form White, smooth or almost smooth glossy cream.

Clinical particulars
Therapeutic indications: Fungal infections of the skin caused by *Trichophyton* (e.g. *T. rubrum, T. mentagrophytes, T. verrucosum, T. violaceum*), *Microsporum canis* and *Epidermophyton floccosum.*

Yeast infections of the skin, principally those caused by the genus *Candida* (e.g. *C. albicans*).

Pityriasis (tinea) versicolor due to *Pityrosporum orbiculare* (also known as *Malassezia furfur*).

Posology and method of administration: Lamisil can be applied once or twice daily. Cleanse and dry the affected areas thoroughly before application of Lamisil. Apply the cream to the affected skin and surrounding area in a thin layer and rub in lightly. In the case of intertriginous infections (submammary, interdigital, intergluteal, inguinal) the application may be covered with a gauze strip, especially at night.

The likely durations of treatment are as follows:

Tinea corporis, cruris:	1 to 2 weeks
Tinea pedis:	1 week
Cutaneous candidiasis:	2 weeks
Pityriasis versicolor:	2 weeks

Relief of clinical symptoms usually occurs within a few days. Irregular use or premature discontinuation of treatment carries the risk of recurrence. If there are no signs of improvement after two weeks, the diagnosis should be verified.

Children: The experience with topical Lamisil in children is still limited and its use cannot therefore be recommended.

Use in the elderly: There is no evidence to suggest that elderly patients require different dosages or experience side-effects different to those of younger patients.

Method of administration: Via the topical route.

Contra-indications: Hypersensitivity to terbinafine or any of the excipients contained in the cream.

Special warnings and precautions for use: Lamisil Cream is for external use only. Contact with the eyes should be avoided.

Interaction with other medicaments and other forms of interaction: There are no known drug interactions with Lamisil Cream.

Pregnancy and lactation: Foetal toxicity and fertility studies in animals suggest no adverse effects.

There is no clinical experience with Lamisil Cream in pregnant women, therefore, unless the potential benefits outweigh any potential risks, Lamisil Cream should not be administered during pregnancy.

Terbinafine is excreted in breast milk and therefore mothers should not receive Lamisil whilst breastfeeding.

Effects on ability to drive and to use machines: None known.

Undesirable effects: Redness, itching or stinging occasionally occur at the site of application; however, treatment rarely has to be discontinued for this reason. This must be distinguished from allergic reactions which are rare but require discontinuation.

Overdose: No case of ingestion of Lamisil Cream has been reported to the company. However, if accidental ingestion of Lamisil Cream occurs, an appropriate method of gastric emptying may be used if considered appropriate.

Pharmacological properties
Pharmacodynamic properties: Terbinafine is an allylamine which has a broad spectrum of antifungal activity. At low concentrations terbinafine is fungicidal against dermatophytes, moulds and certain dimorphic fungi. The activity versus yeasts is fungicidal or fungistatic depending on the species.

Terbinafine interferes specifically with fungal sterol biosynthesis at an early step. This leads to a deficiency in ergosterol and to an intracellular accumulation of squalene, resulting in fungal cell death. Terbinafine acts by inhibition of squalene epoxidase in the fungal cell membrane.

The enzyme squalene epoxidase is not linked to the cytochrome P450 system. Terbinafine does not influence the metabolism of hormones or other drugs.

Pharmacokinetic properties: Less than 5% of the dose is absorbed after topical application to humans; systemic exposure is therefore very slight.

Pharmaceutical particulars
List of excipients: Sodium hydroxide, benzyl alcohol, sorbitan monostearate, cetyl palmitate, cetyl alcohol, stearyl alcohol, polysorbate 60, isopropyl myristate, demineralised water.

Incompatibilities: None known.

Shelf life: Aluminium tube: 5 years.

Special precautions for storage: None.

Nature and contents of container: Aluminium tube with membrane, with an interior coating of phenolepoxy based lacquer, closed with a polypropylene cap, containing 15 g or 30 g Lamisil Cream.

Instruction for use/handling: Not applicable.

Marketing authorisation holder: Novartis Pharmaceuticals UK Limited, trading as Sandoz Pharmaceuticals.

Marketing authorisation number 0101/0305.

Date of approval/revision of SPC 3 March 1997.

Legal category POM.

LAMISIL* TABLETS 250 mg

Qualitative and quantitative composition Each tablet contains 281.25 mg terbinafine hydrochloride, equivalent to 250 mg terbinafine.

Pharmaceutical form Tablets for oral administration.

Clinical particulars
Therapeutic indications: Fungal infections of the skin and nails caused by *Trichophyton* (e.g. *T. rubrum, T. mentagrophytes, T. verrucosum, T. violaceum*), *Microsporum canis* and *Epidermophyton floccosum.*

1. Oral Lamisil is indicated in the treatment of ringworm (tinea corporis, tinea cruris and tinea pedis) where oral therapy is considered appropriate due to the site, severity or extent of the infection.
2. Oral Lamisil is indicated in the treatment of onychomycosis.

Posology and method of administration:
Adults: 125 mg b.d. or 250 mg o.d. The duration of treatment varies according to the indication and the severity of the infection.

Skin infections:
Likely durations of treatment are as follows:

Tinea pedia (interdigital, plantar/ moccasin type):	2 to 6 weeks
Tinea corporis:	4 weeks
Tinea cruris:	2 to 4 weeks

Onychomycosis: The duration of treatment for most patients is between 6 weeks and 3 months. Treatment periods of less than 3 months can be anticipated in patients with fingernail infection, toenail infection other than of the big toe, or patients of younger age. In the treatment of toenail infections, 3 months is usually sufficient although a few patients may require treatment of 6 months or longer. Poor nail outgrowth during the first weeks of treatment may enable identification of those patients in whom longer therapy is required.

Complete resolution of the signs and symptoms of infection may not occur until several weeks after mycological cure.

Children: A review of safety experience with oral Lamisil in children, which includes 314 patients involved in the UK Lamisil Post Marketing Surveillance study, has shown that the adverse event profile in children is similar to that seen in adults. No evidence of any new, unusual or more severe reactions to those seen in the adult population have been noted. However, as data is still limited its use is not recommended.

Use in the elderly: There is no evidence to suggest that elderly patients require different dosages or experience side-effects different to those of younger patients. The possibility of impairment of liver or kidney function should be considered in this age group (see *Precautions*).

Method of administration: Via the oral route.

Contra-indications: Hypersensitivity to Lamisil.

Special warnings and precautions for use: Rarely, cases of cholestasis and hepatitis have been reported, these usually occur within two months of starting treatment. If patients develop symptoms of liver dysfunction such as pruritis, anorexia, nausea, vomiting, fatigue, abdominal pain or dark urine, treatment should be immediately discontinued.

Patients with a known history of liver disease or pre-existing stable chronic liver dysfunction are not known to be at greater risk but should be carefully monitored. Patients with pre-existing, stable, chronic liver dysfunction or impaired renal function (creatinine clearance less than 50 ml/minute or serum creatinine of more than 300 µmol/l) should receive half the normal dose (see also *Undesirable effects*).

Interaction with other medicaments and other forms of interaction: Based on studies undertaken in-vitro and in healthy volunteers, terbinafine shows negligible potential to inhibit or induce the clearance of drugs that are metabolised via the cytochrome P450 system (e.g. cyclosporin, tolbutamide, oral contraceptives). However, some cases of menstrual disturbance (breakthrough bleeding and irregular cycle) have been reported in patients taking Lamisil concomitantly with oral contraceptives. The plasma clearance of terbinafine may however be accelerated by drugs which induce metabolism (such as rifampicin) and may be inhibited by drugs which inhibit cytochrome P450 (such as cimetidine). Where coadministration of such agents is necessary the dosage of Lamisil may need to be adjusted accordingly.

Pregnancy and lactation: Foetal toxicity and fertility studies in animals suggest no adverse effects.

There is no clinical experience with Lamisil in pregnant women, therefore, unless the potential benefits outweigh any potential risks, Lamisil should not be administered during pregnancy.

Terbinafine is excreted in breast milk and therefore mothers should not receive Lamisil treatment whilst breast-feeding.

Effects on ability to drive and to use machines: None.

Undesirable effects: Side effects are generally mild to moderate, and transient. The most common are gastrointestinal symptoms (dyspepsia, fullness, loss of appetite, nausea, mild abdominal pain, diarrhoea), allergic skin reactions (rash, urticaria) and headache. Paraesthesia, hypoaesthesia, dizziness, malaise and fatigue have also been reported rarely.

Musculo-skeletal disorders including arthralgia and myalgia have been reported. These may occur as part of a hypersensitivity reaction in association with allergic skin reactions.

Rare cases of serious skin reactions (e.g. Stevens-Johnson syndrome, toxic epidermal necrolysis, photosensitivity and angioneurotic oedema) have been reported. If progressive skin rash occurs, Lamisil treatment should be discontinued.

Taste loss and taste disturbance have been reported in approximately 0.6% of patients treated with Lamisil. This usually resolves slowly on drug discontinuation.

Rare cases of serious hepatic dysfunction, including jaundice, cholestasis and hepatitis have been reported. If hepatic dysfunction develops, treatment with Lamisil should be discontinued (see also *Precautions*).

Haematological disorders such as neutropenia, thrombocytopenia and agranulocytosis have been reported very rarely.

Overdose: Based on the observed adverse effects in man, the main symptoms of an acute overdosage are likely to be gastrointestinal, e.g. nausea or vomiting.

Pharmacological properties

Pharmacodynamic properties: Terbinafine is an allylamine which has a broad spectrum of antifungal activity. At low concentrations terbinafine is fungicidal against dermatophytes, moulds and certain dimorphic fungi. The activity versus yeasts is fungicidal or fungistatic depending on the species.

Terbinafine interferes specificlaly with fungal sterol biosynthesis at an early step. This leads to a deficiency in ergosterol and to an intracellular accumulation of squalene, resulting in fungal cell death. Terbinafine acts by inhibition of squalene epoxidase in the fungal cell membrane.

The enzyme squalene epoxidase is not linked to the cytochrome P450 system. Terbinafine does not influence the metabolism of hormones or other drugs.

When given orally, the drug concentrates in skin at levels associated with fungicidal activity.

Pharmacokinetic properties: A single oral dose of 250 mg terbinafine results in mean peak plasma concentrations of 0.97 mcg/ml within 2 hours after administration. The absorption half-life is 0.8 hours and the distribution half life is 4.6 hours. Terbinafine binds strongly to plasma proteins. It rapidly diffuses through the dermis and concentrates in the lipophilic stratum corneum.

Terbinafine is also secreted in sebum, thus achieving high concentrations in hair follicles, hair and sebum rich skins. There is also evidence that terbinafine is distributed into the nail plate within the first few weeks of commencing therapy. Biotransformation results in metabolites with no antifungal activity, which are excreted predominantly in the urine. The elimination half-life is 17 hours. There is no evidence of accumulation.

No age-dependent changes in pharmacokinetics have been observed but the elimination rate may be reduced in patients with renal or hepatic impairment, resulting in higher blood levels of terbinafine.

The bioavailability of Lamisil is unaffected by food.

Pharmaceutical particulars

List of excipients: Magnesium stearate, colloidal anhydrous silica, hydroxy propyl methylcellulose, sodium carboxy methyl starch, microcystalline cellulose.

Incompatibilities: None known.

Shelf life: 5 years.

Special precautions for storage: Protect from light.

Nature and contents of container: PVC/PVDC blister pack, containing 14 or 28 tablets.

Instructions for use/handling: Not applicable.

Marketing authorisation holder: Novartis Pharmaceuticals UK Limited, trading as Sandoz Pharmaceuticals.

Marketing authorisation number 0101/0304.

Date of first authorisation/renewal of authorisation
Date present licence granted: 12 December 1995.

Date of approval/revision of SPC 18 April 1997.

Legal category POM.

LENTARON* I.M. DEPOT

Presentation Vials of clear glass containing formestane 250 mg as a white or slightly yellowish sterile lyophilised cake, together with ampoules of clear glass containing 2 ml of 0.9% Sodium Chloride PhEur sterile aqueous suspension medium.

Lentaron vials also contain polyethylene glycol, soybean lecithin, and vitamin E.

Uses

Indication: Treatment of advanced breast cancer in women with natural or artificially induced postmenopausal status.

Mode of action: Lentaron is a potent and highly specific competitive inhibitor of the aromatase enzyme which is responsible for the conversion of androgens to oestrogens. The anti-tumour effects are mediated via the primary endocrine effect of oestrogen deprivation. Clinical studies indicate that the response rate, as with other endocrine therapies, is higher in patients in whom the receptor status of the tumour tissue is positive than in those patients in whom this parameter is negative.

Injection of 250 mg Lentaron i.m. depot results in a clinically significant reduction of oestrogen biosynthesis. Plasma oestradiol and oestrone are suppressed in parallel.

Lentaron does not affect the plasma levels of androstenedione, testosterone or dihydrotestosterone. Levels of sex-steroid hormone binding globulin (SHBG) were decreased slightly in clinical studies, but this effect was not of statistical significance. However, no clinical androgenic effects have been observed.

No clinically relevant changes in plasma levels of cortisol, 11-desoxycortisol, 17-hydroxy-progesterone or dehydroepiandrosterone sulphate have been observed during treatment. Glucocorticoid supplements are therefore not necessary.

Pharmacokinetics: Intramuscular injection of Lentaron gives rise to the formation of a depot characterised by slow release of formestane into the systemic circulation. After single i.m. doses of 250 mg in postmenopausal breast cancer patients, maximum plasma concentrations are reached within 30-48 hours. After a relatively rapid decline between 2-4 days, the active substance is eliminated from plasma with an apparent half-life of about 5-6 days. Levels of formestane are still measurable in the plasma at 14 days, but are undetectable after 2 months.

Steady-state plasma levels are reached after the fourth dose, and accumulation does not occur after repeated dosing.

Formestane has not been shown to influence its own metabolism and 82-86% of the circulating formestane is bound to plasma protein.

An assessment of the extent of the systemic uptake (or of the absolute bioavailability) is not possible due to the poor solubility of formestane in aqueous media. Assuming that plasma is the sole carrier of systemically available formestane, a preliminary estimate of the systemic uptake, which is based on hepatic clearance, is about 20-25% of the i.m. dose in 14 days.

As shown in oral studies, the major circulating and urinary metabolite of formestane is its pharmacologically inactive glucuronide.

Dosage and administration

Dosage:,The recommended dosage is 250 mg i.m. fortnightly. Lentaron should be administered by deep i.m. intragluteal injection high into the upper outer quadrant. The alternate buttock should be chosen for each subsequent injection. Lentaron should be given until further tumour progression is evident.

The contents of the vial should be reconstituted under aseptic conditions into an aqueous microcrystalline suspension by injecting 2 ml of 0.9% Sodium Chloride PhEur sterile aqueous suspension medium provided. Gentle shaking facilitates dispersal of the drug. It is recommended that the suspension is prepared freshly before use and allowed to come to room temperature before injection.

Hepatic and renal impairment: No specific studies have been performed in such patients. Conjugation appears to be a major route of elimination for Lentaron and its metabolites, and less than 1% of the dose is excreted unchanged in the urine. Impairment of either hepatic or renal function is therefore not expected to require dose adjustment. Lentaron has been used without problem in patients with mild impairment of renal function (creatinine clearance not less than 20 ml/min).

Elderly: There is no evidence to suggest that dosage requirements are different in the elderly.

Children: Not applicable.

Contra-Indications, warnings and precautions.

Contra-indications: Lentaron is contra-indicated in women with pre-menopausal endocrine status and during pregnancy and lactation. Lentaron should not be given to patients with known hypersensitivity to the active substance, polyethylene glycol, soybean lecithin or Vitamin E.

Precautions: Care should be taken to inject the drug deep intramuscularly; intravascular injection must be avoided. Rapid venous uptake of the drug following intravascular injection has led to symptoms of bitter taste, feeling hot, tachycardia, breathlessness or dizziness immediately after administration. Care should also be taken to avoid injection into or near the sciatic nerve. The risks associated with improper injection include pain and temporary nerve trauma. There is the theoretical risk of severe or permanent damage if the nerve is injured directly. No injection should be given in an area where resistance is felt or where there is inflammation from a previous injection.

As with all i.m. injections, caution should be observed in patients taking anticoagulants owing to the risk of haematoma or bleeding at the injection site.

As occasional lethargy, drowsiness or dizziness have been reported, caution should be observed when driving or using machinery.

No studies have been performed in diabetic patients. Blood glucose should therefore be monitored as a precautionary measure.

Use in pregnancy and lactation: There is no experience of the use of Lentaron in human pregnancy or lactation. Lentaron is contra-indicated during pregnancy, lactation and in women of pre-menopausal endocrine status (see **'Contra-indications'**).

Drug interactions: No information is available at present on the use of Lentaron in combination with other anti-cancer agents.

Increased growth of facial hair was observed in a single patient concomitantly treated with phenytoin.

Side-effects: In clinical trials, adverse events were generally mild or moderate. All reactions resolved without permanent consequence. Local intolerability was the most frequent adverse reaction. Many of the adverse events which have been observed can be classified as being due to the pharmacological consequences of oestrogen deprivation (e.g. hot flushes). The following adverse events have been observed:

Local adverse events:

Skin and appendages: Frequent: itching, pain, irritation, burning sensation, indolent or painful lump, granuloma at the injection site. Occasional: sterile abscess, inflammation at the injection site. Rare: haematoma at the injection site.

General adverse events:

Skin and appendages: Occasional: rash, pruritus, exanthema. Rare: facial hypertrichosis, alopecia.

Nervous system: Rare: lethargy, drowsiness, emotional lability, headache, dizziness.

Vascular system: Rare: oedema of the lower leg, thrombophlebitis.

Endocrine system: Occasional: hot flushes.

Urogenital system: Rare: vaginal spotting or bleeding, pelvic cramps, colpitis.

Digestive system: Occasional: nausea, vomiting. Rare: constipation, diarrhoea.

Musculoskeletal system: Rare: muscle cramps, arthralgia, exacerbation of bone pain.

Respiratory system: Rare: sore throat.

Others: Rare: faintness due to vasovagal reaction, giddiness immediately following injection, anaphylactoid reaction (rash, nausea, vertigo, chest pain and tachycardia, fatigue).

Overdosage: There is no experience of accidental overdosage with Lentaron. In clinical trials, doses up to 1000 mg per week led only to an increased frequency of local adverse reactions.

Pharmaceutical precautions Lentaron vials should be stored below 25°C. The reconstituted suspension is stable for 24 hours in the refrigerator; (2–8°); after this period the suspension should be discarded.

Lentaron should not be mixed with any other medication for injection.

Legal category POM.

Package quantities Packs containing one vial of Lentaron i.m. depot 250 mg and one ampoule of Sodium Chloride PhEur 0.9% w/v sterile aqueous suspension medium.

Further information Nil.

Product licence numbers
Lentaron i.m. depot 250 mg 00101/0528
Sodium Chloride PhEur 0.9% w/v sterile aqueous suspension medium 2 ml 00101/0529

Product licence holder: Novartis Pharmaceuticals UK Limited, trading as Ciba Laboratories.

Date of last revision Dec 1997.

LESCOL* ▼

Qualitative and quantitative composition One capsule containing 21.06 mg/42.12 mg fluvastatin sodium corresponding to 20 mg/40 mg fluvastatin free acid.

Pharmaceutical form Capsules for oral administration.

Clinical particulars

Therapeutic indications: The therapeutic indication for Lescol is in the treatment of primary hypercholesterolaemia (with a cholesterol level in excess of 6.5 mmol/l) in patients who do not adequately respond to dietary control.

Lescol is also indicated to slow the progression of coronary atherosclerosis in patients with primary hypercholesterolaemia and concomitant coronary heart disease who do not adequately respond to dietary control.

Posology and method of administration: Prior to initiating Lescol, secondary causes of hypercholesterolaemia should be excluded, and the patient placed on a standard cholesterol-lowering diet. Dietary therapy should be continued during treatment.

An initial starting dose of 20–40 mg once daily in the evening should be used. Since the maximal reduction in LDL-C at a given dose can be seen within four weeks, this dose should be adjusted at monthly intervals to achieve the desired effect up to 40 mg twice daily. Most patients will however require a dose of 20 to 40 mg daily. In a study in patients with primary hypercholesterolaemia and concomitant coronary heart disease 40 mg daily slowed the progression of coronary atherosclerosis. The therapeutic effect of Lescol is maintained with prolonged administration.

For patients requiring a daily dose of 40 mg twice daily, a calendar pack of 56 Lescol Capsules 40 mg is available containing morning and evening doses in marked blister strips.

Lescol is efficacious in monotherapy or in combination with bile acid sequestrants. When Lescol is used in combination with cholestyramine or other resins, it should be administered at least four hours after the resin to avoid a significant interaction due to binding of the drug to the resin. Minimal data exist to support the efficacy and safety of Lescol in combination with nicotinic acid or fibrates.

Since Lescol is cleared by the liver, with less than 6% of the administered dose excreted into the urine, dose adjustments for mild or moderate renal impairment (creatinine <160 μmol/l) are not necessary.

Use in the elderly: There is no evidence of reduced tolerability or altered dosage requirements in elderly patients.

Use in children: As there is no experience with the use of Lescol in individuals less than 18 years of age, its use is contra-indicated in this group.

Contra-indications:

Known hypersensitivity to any component of Lescol.

Patients with severe renal impairment (creatinine ≥160 μmol/l).

Patients with active liver disease, hepatic impairment, or unexplained, persistent elevations in serum transaminases.

Individuals under 18 years of age.

Special warnings and special precautions for use: HMG-CoA reductase inhibitors, including Lescol, are unlikely to be of benefit in patients with rare homozygous familial hypercholesterolaemia.

Although no hypersensitivity reactions have been reported with Lescol during clinical trials, these have occurred rarely with other HMG-CoA reductase inhibitors.

As with other lipid-lowering drugs, it is recommended that liver function tests be performed before the initiation of treatment and periodically thereafter in all patients. Should an increase in aspartate aminotransferase (AST) or alanine aminotransferase (ALT) exceed 3 times the upper limit of normal and persist, therapy should be discontinued. In very rare cases, possibly drug-related hepatitis was observed that resolved upon discontinuation of treatment.

Caution should be exercised when Lescol is administered to patients with a history of liver disease or heavy alcohol ingestion.

Since fluvastatin is eliminated primarily via the biliary route and is subject to significant pre-systemic metabolism, the potential exists for drug accumulation in patients with hepatic insufficiency.

Skeletal muscle: Myopathy including myositis and rhabdomyolysis has been reported in patients receiving other HMG-CoA reductase inhibitors. With Lescol such cases have been reported very rarely. In patients with unexplained diffuse myalgias, muscle tenderness or weakness, and marked elevation of creatinine phosphokinase (CPK) values (greater than 10 times the upper limit of normal), myopathy should be considered. Patients should be advised to report promptly unexplained muscle pain, tenderness, or weakness, particularly if accompanied by malaise or fever. Lescol therapy should be discontinued if markedly elevated CPK levels occur or myopathy is diagnosed or suspected.

The risk of myopathy is known to be increased in patients receiving immunosuppressive drugs (including cyclosporin), gemfibrozil, nicotinic acid or erythromycin together with other HMG-CoA reductase inhibitors. However, myopathy has not been observed in clinical trials involving small numbers of patients who were treated with Lescol for short periods together with nicotinic acid, its derivatives, fibrates or cyclosporin. Minimal data exist to support the efficacy or safety of Lescol in combination with nicotinic acid, its derivatives, fibrates or cyclosporin. Lescol should be used with caution in patients receiving such concomitant medication.

Interactions with other medicaments and other forms of interaction:

Food: Although AUC and C_{max} were lowered and t_{max} prolonged when Lescol was taken with food, there was no apparent difference in the lipid-lowering effects whether Lescol was taken with food or not.

Immunosuppressive drugs (including cyclosporin), gemfibrozil, nicotinic acid, erythromycin: Lescol has been safely administered concomitantly with nicotinic acid, gemfibrozil, bezafibrate and cyclosproin (at doses up to 40 mg Lescol) in clinical trials involving small numbers of patients for short periods (see *Special warnings and special precautions for use*).

Antipyrine: Administration of Lescol does not influence the metabolism and excretion of antipyrine. As antipyrine is a model for drugs metabolised by the microsomal hepatic enzyme systems, interactions with other drugs metabolised by these systems are not expected.

Nicotinic acid/propranolol: Concomitant administration of Lescol with nicotinic acid or propranolol has no effect on the bioavailability of Lescol.

Bile-acid sequestering agents: Administration of Lescol 4 hours after cholestyramine results in a clinically significant additive effect compared with that achieved with either drug alone. Lescol should be administered at least 4 hours after the resin (e.g. cholestyramine) to avoid a significant interaction due to drug binding to the resin.

Digoxin: Concomitant administration of Lescol with digoxin has no effect on digoxin plasma concentrations.

Cimetidine/ranitidine/omeprazole: Concomitant administration of Lescol with cimetidine, ranitidine or omeprazole results in an increase in the bioavailability of Lescol, which, however, is of no clinical relevance.

Rifampicin: Administration of Lescol to subjects pre-treated with rifampicin resulted in a reduction of the bioavailability of Lescol by about 50%.

Warfarin/salicylic acid/glibenclamide: In vitro protein binding studies demonstrated no interaction at therapeutic concentrations.

In vitro findings have shown a potential effect of fluvastatin on the activity of P_{450} CYP2C subfamily, indicating the theoretical possibility of an interaction with drugs also metabolised by this sub-family such as warfarin, sulphonylureas, diclofenac and phenytoin if co-administered with fluvastatin, although the clinical significance of this is unknown. However, an *in vivo* study with warfarin as representative of the drugs metabolised through this P_{450} enzyme sub-family, has shown that fluvastatin had no effect on prothrombin times or warfarin blood levels.

Bleeding and/or increased prothrombin times have, however, been reported very rarely in patients on Lescol receiving concomitant coumarin derivatives.

Other concomitant therapy: In clinical studies in which Lescol was used concomitantly with angiotensin converting enzyme (ACE) inhibitors, beta-blockers, calcium channel blockers, oral sulphonylureas, salicylic acid, H_2-blockers and non-steroidal anti-inflammatory drugs (NSAIDs), no clinically significant adverse interactions occurred.

Pregnancy and lactation: Animal studies have indicated that fluvastatin is devoid of embryotoxic and teratogenic potential. However, since HMG-CoA reductase inhibitors decrease the synthesis of cholesterol and possibly of other biologically active substances derived from cholesterol, they may cause fetal harm when administered to pregnant women. Therefore, HMG-CoA reductase inhibitors are contra-indicated during pregnancy, and in women of child-bearing potential, not taking adequate contraceptive precautions. If a patient becomes pregnant while taking this class of drug, therapy should be discontinued. As small amounts of fluvastatin have been found in rat milk, Lescol is contra-indicated in nursing mothers.

Effects on ability to drive and use machines: No data exist on the effects of Lescol on the ability to drive and use machines.

Undesirable effects: Adverse events, both clinical and biochemical, are usually mild and transient. In placebo controlled trials, events occurring with a frequency of 1% or more (over that with placebo) were: dyspepsia, nausea, abdominal pain, headache and insomnia. The only adverse events with an incidence of ≥1% that can be clearly attributed to Lescol treatment are minor gastrointestinal symptoms.

For a discussion of the very rarely occurring myopathies see *Special warnings and special precautions for use – skeletal muscle.*

Biochemical abnormalities of liver function have been associated with HMG-CoA reductase inhibitors and other lipid lowering agents. Confirmed elevations of transaminase levels to more than 3 times the upper limit of normal developed in a small number of patients (less than or equal to 1%). The majority of these abnormal biochemical findings were asymptomatic and resolved or improved towards pre-treatment values after discontinuation of treatment.

Overdosage: The experience with overdoses of Lescol is very limited. Should an accidental overdosage occur, administration of activated charcoal is recommended. In the case of a very recent oral intake gastric lavage may be considered. Treatment should be symptomatic.

Pharmacological properties

Pharmacodynamic properties: Lescol, a hydrophilic, fully synthetic cholesterol-lowering agent, is a competitive inhibitor of HMG-CoA reductase, which is responsible for the conversion of HMG-CoA to mevalonate, a precursor of sterols, including cholesterol. Lescol exerts its main effect in the liver. The inhibition of cholesterol biosynthesis reduces the cholesterol in hepatic cells, which stimulates the synthesis of LDL receptors and thereby increases the uptake of LDL particles. The ultimate result of these mechanisms is a reduction of the plasma cholesterol concentration.

A variety of clinical studies has demonstrated that elevated levels of total cholesterol (total-C), LDL-C and apolipoprotein B (a membrane transport complex for LDL-C) promote human atherosclerosis. Similarly, decreased levels of high density lipoprotein cholesterol (HDL-C) and its transport complex, apolipoprotein A, are associated with the development of atherosclerosis. Epidemiologic investigations have established that cardiovascular morbidity and mortality vary directly with the level of total-C and LDL-C and inversely with the level of HDL-C. In multicentre clinical trials, those pharmacologic and/or non-pharmacologic interventions that simultaneously lowered LDL-C and increased HDL-C reduced the rate of cardiovascular events (both fatal and non-fatal myocardial infarctions). The overall cholesterol profile is improved with the principal effects being the reduction of total-C and LDL-C. Lescol also produces a moderate reduction in triglycerides and a moderate increase in HDL-C.

Pharmacokinetic properties: Lescol is a racemate of the two erythro enantiomers of which one exerts the pharmacological activity. Lescol is absorbed rapidly and completely (98%) following oral administration to fasted volunteers. In a fed state, the drug is absorbed at a reduced rate. Fluvastatin exerts its main effect in the liver, which is also the main organ for its metabolism. The absolute bioavailability assessed from systemic blood concentrations is 24%. The apparent volume of distribution (V_zf) for the drug is 330 L. More than 98% of the circulating drug is bound to plasma proteins, and this binding is unaffected by drug concentration.

The major circulating blood components are fluvastatin and the pharmacologically inactive N-desisopropyl-propionic acid metabolite. The hydroxylated metabolites have pharmacological activity but do not circulate systemically.

Following administration of ^{3}H-fluvastatin to healthy volunteers, excretion of radioactivity is about 6% in the urine and 93% in the faeces, and fluvastatin accounts for less than 2% of the total radioactivity excreted. The plasma clearance (CL/f) for fluvastatin in man is calculated to be 1.8±0.8 L/min. Steady-state plasma concentrations show no evidence of fluvastatin accumulation following administration of 40 mg daily. Following oral administration of 40 mg of Lescol, the terminal disposition half-life for fluvastatin is 2.3±0.9 hours.

Food: Although AUC and C_{max} were lowered and t_{max} prolonged when Lescol was taken with food, there was no apparent difference in the lipid-lowering effect whether Lescol was taken with food or not.

Plasma concentrations of fluvastatin do not vary as a function of either age or gender in the general population.

Preclinical safety data: The safety of fluvastatin was extensively investigated in toxicity studies in rats, dogs, monkeys, mice and hamsters. A variety of changes were identified that are common to HMG-CoA reductase inhibitors, viz. hyperplasia and hyperkeratosis of the rodent non-glandular stomach, cataracts in dogs, myopathy in rodents, mild liver changes in most laboratory animals with gall bladder changes in dog, monkey and hamster, thyroid weight increases in the rat and testicular degeneration in the hamster. Fluvastatin is devoid of the CNS vascular and degenerative changes recorded in dogs with other members of this class of compound.

A carcinogenicity study was performed in rats at dose levels of 6, 9 and 18 mg/kg a day (escalated to 24 mg/kg a day after 1 year) to establish a clear maximum tolerated dose. These treatment levels yielded plasma drug levels approximately 9, 13 and 26 to 35 times the mean human plasma drug concentration after a 40-mg oral dose. A low incidence of forestomach squamous papillomas and one carcinoma of the forestomach was observed at the 24 mg/kg a day dose level. In addition, an increased incidence of thyroid follicular cell adenomas and carcinomas was recorded in male rats treated with 18 to 24 mg/kg a day.

The forestomach neoplasms observed in rats and mice reflect chronic hyperplasia caused by direct contact exposure to fluvastatin rather than a genotoxic effect of the drug. The increased incidence of thyroid follicular cell neoplasms in male rats given fluvastatin appears to be consistent with species-specific findings with other HMG-CoA reductase inhibitors. In contrast to other HMG-CoA reductase inhibitors, no treatment-related increases in the incidences of hepatic adenomas or carcinomas were observed.

The carcinogenicity study conducted in mice at dose levels of 0.3, 15 and 30 mg/kg a day revealed, as in rats, a statistically significant increase in forestomach squamous cell papillomas in males and females at 30 mg/kg a day and in females at 15 mg/kg a day. These treatment levels yielded plasma drug levels approximately 0.2, 10 and 21 times the mean human plasma drug concentration after a 40-mg oral dose.

No evidence of mutagenicity was observed *in vitro*, with or without rat-liver metabolic activation, in the following studies: microbial mutagen tests using mutant strains of *Salmonella typhimurium* or *Escherichia coli*; malignant transformation assay in BALB/3T3 cells; unscheduled DNA synthesis in rat primary hepatocytes; chromosomal aberrations in V79 Chinese hamster cells; HGPRT V79 Chinese hamster cells. In addition, there was no evidence of mutagenicity *in vivo* in either a rat or mouse micronucleus test.

In a study in rats at dose levels in females of 0.6, 2 and 6 mg/kg a day and in males of 2, 10 and 20 mg/kg a day, fluvastatin had no adverse effects on the fertility or reproductive performance. Teratology studies in rats and rabbits showed maternal toxicity at high dose levels, but there was no evidence of embryotoxic or teratogenic potential. A study in which female rats were dosed at 12 and 24 mg/kg a day during late gestation until weaning of the pups resulted in maternal mortality at or near term and post partum accompanied by fetal and neonatal lethality. No effects on the pregnant females or fetuses occurred at the low dose level of 2 mg/kg a day.

A second study at levels of 2, 6, 12 and 24 mg/kg a day during late gestation and early lactation showed similar effects at 6 mg/kg a day and above caused by cardiotoxicity. In a third study, pregnant rats were administered 12 or 24 mg/kg a day during late gestation until weaning of pups with or without the presence of concurrent supplementation with mevalonic acid, a derivative of HMG-CoA that is essential for cholesterol biosynthesis. The concurrent administration of mevalonic acid completely prevented the cardiotoxicity and the maternal and neonatal mortality. Therefore, the maternal and neonatal lethality observed with fluvastatin reflects its exaggerated pharmacologic effect during pregnancy.

Pharmaceutical particulars

List of excipients: Magnesium stearate; sodium hydrogen carbonate; talc; cellulose microcrystalline, fine powder; cellulose microcrystalline, granular powder; maize starch, physically modified; calcium carbonate; purified water; titanium dioxide E171; iron oxide red E172; iron oxide yellow E172; gelatin.

Incompatibilities: None.

Shelf life: On the basis of the results obtained so far, a shelf life of 3 years in temperate, hot or tropical climate is proposed.

Special precautions for storage: Store below 25°C.

Nature and contents of container: Alu/alu blister consisting of an aluminium coating foil and an aluminium covering foil.

For 20 mg capsules, capsules are No 3 size hard gelatine capsules with a strong reddish brown opaque cap with a Sandoz triangle imprinted in white, and a pale yellow opaque body with XU 20 mg imprinted in red.

For 40 mg capsules, capsules are No 1 size hard gelatine capsules with a strong reddish brown opaque cap with a Sandoz triangle imprinted in white, and a moderate orange yellow body with XU 40 mg imprinted in red.

Both the 20 mg and 40 mg capsules are contained in calendar packs of 28 capsules. The 40 mg capsules are also available in calendar packs of 56 capsules for 40 mg twice daily dosing.

Instructions for use/handling: None.

Marketing authorisation holder: Novartis Pharmaceuticals UK Limited, trading as Sandoz Pharmaceuticals.

Marketing authorisation numbers
20 mg capsules 0101/0360
40 mg capsules 0101/0361

Date of approval/revision of SPC April 1998.

Legal category POM.

LEUCOMAX* ▼

Presentation Leucomax contains molgramostim, a recombinant human granulocyte macrophage-colony stimulating factor (rHuGM-GSF), non-glycosylated with isoleucine at position 100.

Molgramostim is a water-soluble, non-glycosylated protein produced by recombinant techniques. Its activity is expressed in International Units (IU) with 1 million IU corresponding to approximately 90 mcg of molgramostim protein. Each vial of Leucomax contains the labelled quantity of molgramostim in million IU.

Uses Leucomax is indicated for reduction of risk of infection and to allow better adherence to the chemotherapeutic regimen, by decreasing the severity of cytotoxic chemotherapy-induced neutropenia (see *Precautions, Laboratory tests*).

Leucomax is also indicated for the acceleration of myeloid recovery in patients following autologous or syngeneic bone marrow transplantation. Leucomax has not been shown to improve overall survival or increase time to relapse.

Leucomax is also indicated as adjuvant therapy in ganciclovir (DHPG)-induced neutropenia in patients with AIDS-related cytomegalovirus (CMV) retinitis in order to maintain recommended DHPG dosage.

Dosage and administration Leucomax must be reconstituted before administration (see under *Pharmaceutical Precautions – Technical instructions*). Leucomax dosing regimens vary according to the indication for therapy. The maximum daily dose should not exceed 0.11×10^6 IU/kg/day (10 mcg/kg). The recommended dosage regimens are:

Cancer chemotherapy: 0.06–0.11×10^6 IU/kg/day (5 to 10 mcg/kg/day) administered subcutaneously. Treatment should be initiated 24 hours after the last dose of chemotherapy and continued for 7 to 10 days. Dosing may be initiated at 0.06×10^6 IU/kg/day (5 mcg/kg/day).

Bone marrow transplantation (BMT): 0.11×10^6 IU/kg/day (10 mcg/kg/day) administered by intravenous infusion over 4 to 6 hours, beginning the day after BMT. Continue until the absolute neutrophil count (ANC) is $\geq 1 \times 10^9$/l. The maximum duration of treatment is 30 days.

AIDS-related CMV retinitis as adjuvant therapy to ganciclovir (DHPG): 0.06×10^6 IU/kg (5 mcg/kg) once daily by subcutaneous injection. After the fifth Leucomax dose has been administered the dose may be titrated to maintain the ANC and the WBC count at the desired levels, usually $\geq 1 \times 10^9$/l and $< 20 \times 10^9$/l respectively.

Use in children: The safety of Leucomax has been demonstrated in a limited number of patients below the age of 18 years.

Use in the elderly: There are no apparent differences in safety of Leucomax in elderly patients.

Contra-indications, warnings, etc

Contra-indications: Leucomax is contra-indicated in patients with a history of hypersensitivity to molgramostim or any component of the injectable formulation.

Leucomax should not be used in patients with myeloid malignancies.

Precautions: Leucomax should be used under the supervision of a physician experienced in the treatment of oncologic and haematopoietic disorders or infectious diseases.

The first dose of Leucomax should be administered under medical supervision.

Acute severe, life threatening hypersensitivity reactions, including anaphylaxis, angioedema or bronchoconstriction have occurred in patients receiving Leucomax. If such reactions occur Leucomax should be withdrawn immediately and not re-introduced.

Leucomax has been associated infrequently with pleurisy, or pleural effusion. Pericarditis occurred in 2% (21/1098) and pericardial effusion in <2% (16/1098). If such reactions occur Leucomax should be withdrawn. Patients with pre-existing pulmonary disease may be predisposed to decreased pulmonary function and dyspnoea, and should be monitored closely when being treated with Leucomax.

In clinical trials, adverse events reported with initiation of dosing were mostly mild to moderate in severity and included rigors, dyspnoea, fever, nausea, vomiting, non-specific chest pain, asthenia, hypotension or flushing. These symptoms, which infrequently required withdrawal of Leucomax, were managed symptomatically.

In a few isolated instances, autoimmune disease developed or was exacerbated during rHuGM-CSF therapy. Therefore when administering Leucomax to patients with a history of, or predisposition to autoimmune disease, this should be considered.

Laboratory tests–Standard haematologic tests (full blood count with differential white cell count and platelet count) should be performed and serum albumin levels monitored during therapy with Leucomax.

Because of the potential of receiving higher doses of chemotherapy (ie full doses on the prescribed schedule), the patients may be at greater risk of thrombocytopenia and anaemia as consequences of increased chemotherapy doses. Regular monitoring of the platelet count and haematocrit is recommended.

Drug interactions: Since dosing with Leucomax has been associated with a decrease in serum albumin, drugs that are highly bound to serum albumin may require dosage adjustment.

Use in pregnancy and lactation: Safety of Leucomax for use in human pregnancy has not been established. Animal studies have shown reproductive toxicity. In primate models, administration of molgramostim was associated with foetal death and spontaneous abortion at doses of 0.07 and 0.11×10^6 IU/kg/day (6 and 10 mcg/kg/day).

In the absence of clinical data in pregnancy, the therapeutic benefit to the patient must be weighed against potential risks to the progress of pregnancy.

It is not known whether Leucomax is excreted in human milk. However, because of the potential for adverse effects in infants, nursing is not recommended in women receiving Leucomax.

Side-effects: Since many of the undesirable events reported during Leucomax clinical trials are often associated with underlying or concurrent disease or their treatment, the causal relationship of many of these events to Leucomax cannot be definitively determined. Most adverse reactions were mild to moderate in severity. Rarely were they severe or life threatening.

The most frequently reported undesirable effects across all indications were fever, nausea, dyspnoea, diarrhoea, rash, rigors, injection site reaction (with s.c administration), vomiting, fatigue, anorexia, musculoskeletal pain and asthenia.

Less frequently reported events include: non-specific chest pain, stomatitis, headache, increased sweating, abdominal pain, pruritus, dizziness, peripheral oedema, paraesthesia and myalgia.

Serious reactions, which occurred rarely in clinical trials, include: anaphylaxis, bronchospasm, cardiac failure, capillary leak syndrome, cerebrovascular disorders, confusion, convulsions, hypotension, cardiac rhythm abnormalities, intracranial hypertension, pericardial effusion, pericarditis, pleural effusion, pulmonary oedema and syncope.

Laboratory findings – in all patient groups the most frequently occurring changes in laboratory values were decreased platelet count, decreased haemoglobin level, decreased serum albumin level and an increase in eosinophils (absolute count and percent). The causal relationship of these changes to Leucomax cannot be determined definitively.

The frequency of antibodies that bind to molgramostim, measured by enzyme-linked immunosorbent assay (ELISA) and bioassay, was determined to be 1% post treatment. No loss of activity of Leucomax was evident in these patients.

Overdosage: Overdosing has not been reported with Leucomax. As for any pharmacologically active compound, symptomatic treatment with frequent monitoring of vital signs and close observation of the patient is indicated if severe reactions occur.

Pharmaceutical precautions Leucomax sterile powder should be stored at 2°C to 8°C and protected from light.

Following reconstitution with sterile water for injection Leucomax solution can be used for 24 hours when refrigerated at 2°C to 8°C. Unused Leucomax solution should be discarded.

Technical instructions

Reconstitution of Leucomax: Add 1.0 ml of diluent (sterile water for injection) to the vial of Leucomax. Agitate the vial gently to dissolve the powder completely. This provides the labelled amount of Leucomax as an isotonic solution, which may be used for subcutaneous administration. When diluted further in accordance with the instructions below, Leucomax may be administered intravenously.

Dilution for i.v. administration: **Dilution instructions must be followed carefully to avoid loss of molgramostim as a result of adsorption to the infusion system.**

Reconstitute each of the required number of vials of lyophilised powder to the appropriate strength of molgramostim with 1 ml of sterile water for injection. The reconstituted molgramostim solution may be further diluted in 25 ml, 50 ml or 100 ml infusion bags or bottles of either normal saline solution or 5% dextrose in water. The number and the strength of lyophilised powder vials required must be such that the above infusion admixture solution contains a final concentration of molgramostim of *not less than* 0.08×10^6 *IU (7 mcg) per ml.* The resulting infusion solution is stable for 24 hours when stored in a refrigerator.

Leucomax infusion solution is compatible with the following infusion sets: Travenol 2C0001 and C0334, Intrafix air, Infusionsgerat R, 87 Plus, Souplix, Steriflex, Intrafix Air Euroklappe-ISO, Soluset and Linfosol sets. **Significant adsorption of Leucomax has been observed in a Port-A-Cath (Pharmacia) system, and its use is not recommended.**

For i.v. administration, the use of an in-line, low protein binding 0.2 or 0.22 micrometer filter is recommended. The reconstituted solution is colourless to light yellow and should be inspected visually for discolouration and particulate matter prior to administration.

Legal category POM.

Package quantities Leucomax sterile lyophilised powder is supplied in Type 1 glass vials with butyl or halobutyl rubber closures and aluminium seal in the following strengths:

1.67×10^6 IU/vial (150 mcg/vial)
3.33×10^6 IU/vial (300 mcg/vial)
4.44×10^6 IU/vial (400 mcg/vial)

Further information The excipients contained in Leucomax are mannitol, citric acid, dibasic sodium phosphate, polyethylene glycol and human albumin.

Molgramostim has an elimination half-life of one to two hours following intravenous administration and two to three hours following subcutaneous administration.

Product licence numbers
1.67×10^6 IU/vial (150 micrograms/vial) 0201/0150
3.33×10^6 IU/vial (300 micrograms/vial) 0201/0181
4.44×10^6 IU/vial (400 micrograms/vial) 0201/0151

Product licence holder: Schering-Plough Ltd, Schering-Plough House, Welwyn Garden City, Hertfordshire AL7 1TW.

Date of last revision September 1994.

LIORESAL*

Presentation Lioresal tablets each containing 10 mg Baclofen PhEur; circular, flat, white to faintly yellowish tablets, uncoated, with bevelled edges, having the monogram CG on one side and the letters KJ and a break line on the other.

Lioresal liquid containing 5 mg/5 ml baclofen Ph.Eur; clear, very slightly yellow solution with a raspberry flavour.

Uses

Indications: Lioresal is indicated for the relief of spasticity of voluntary muscle resulting from such disorders as: multiple sclerosis, other spinal lesions, e.g. tumours of the spinal cord, syringomyelia, motor neurone disease, transverse myelitis, traumatic partial section of the cord.

Lioresal is also indicated in adults and children for the relief of spasticity of voluntary muscle arising from eg. cerebrovascular accidents, cerebral palsy, meningitis, traumatic head injury.

Patient selection is important when initiating Lioresal therapy; it is likely to be of most benefit in patients whose spasticity constitutes a handicap to activities and/or physiotherapy. Treatment should not be commenced until the spastic state has become stabilised.

Mode of action: Lioresal is an antispastic agent acting at the spinal level. A gamma-aminobutyric acid (GABA) derivative, Lioresal is chemically unrelated to other antispastic agents.

Lioresal depresses monosynaptic and polysynaptic reflex transmission, probably by stimulating the $GABA_B$-receptors, this stimulation in turn inhibiting the release of the excitatory amino acids glutamate and aspartate. Neuromuscular transmission is unaffected by Lioresal.

The major benefits of Lioresal stem from its ability to reduce painful flexor spasms and spontaneous clonus thereby facilitating the mobility of the patient, increasing his independence and helping rehabilitation.

Lioresal also exerts an antinociceptive effect. General well being is often improved and sedation is less often a problem than with centrally acting drugs.

Pharmacokinetics: Lioresal (baclofen) is rapidly and completely absorbed from the gastro-intestinal tract. Following oral administration of single doses (10-30 mg) peak plasma concentrations are recorded after 0.5 to 1.5 hours and areas under the serum concentration curves are proportional to the dose.

In cerebrospinal fluid active substance concentrations are approximately 8.5 times lower than in the plasma.

The plasma elimination half-life of baclofen averages 3 to 4 hours. The serum protein binding rate is approximately 30%.

Baclofen is eliminated largely in unchanged form. Within 72 hours, about 75% of the dose is excreted via the kidneys with about 5% of this amount as metabolites.

Dosage and administration Lioresal is given orally in either tablet or liquid form. These two formulations are bioequivalent. The liquid may be particularly suitable for children or those adults who are unable to take tablets. Dosage titration can be more precisely managed with the liquid.

Before starting treatment with Lioresal it is prudent to realistically assess the overall extent of clinical improvement that the patient may be expected to achieve. Careful titration of dosage is essential (particularly in the elderly) until the patient is stabilised. If too high a dose is initiated or if the dosage is increased too rapidly side effects may occur. This is particularly relevant if the patient is ambulant in order to minimise muscle weakness in the unaffected limbs or where spasticity is necessary for support.

Adults: The following gradually increasing dosage regimen is suggested, but should be adjusted to suit individual patient requirements.

5 mg three times a day for three days
10 mg three times a day for three days
15 mg three times a day for three days
20 mg three times a day for three days

Satisfactory control of symptoms is usually obtained with doses of up to 60 mg daily, but a careful adjustment is often necessary to meet the requirements of each individual patient. The dose may be increased more slowly if required, but a maximum daily dose of more than 100 mg is not advised unless the patient is in hospital under careful medical supervision. Small frequent dosage may prove better in some cases than larger spaced doses. Also some patients benefit from the use of Lioresal only at night to counteract painful flexor spasm. Similarly a single dose given approximately 1 hour prior to performance of specific tasks such as washing, dressing, shaving, physiotherapy, will often improve mobility.

Once the maximum recommended dose has been reached, if the therapeutic effect is not apparent within 6 weeks a decision whether to continue with Lioresal should be taken.

Elderly: Elderly patients may be more susceptible to side effects, particularly in the early stages of introducing Lioresal. Small doses should therefore be used at the start of treatment, the dose being titrated gradually against the response, under careful supervision. There is no evidence that the eventual average maximum dose differs from that in younger patients.

Children: A dosage range of 0.75-2 mg/kg body weight should be used. In children over 10 years of age however, a maximum daily dosage of 2.5 mg/kg body weight may be given. Treatment is usually started with 2.5 mg given 4 times daily. The dosage should be cautiously raised at about 3 day intervals, until it becomes sufficient for the child's individual requirements. The recommended daily dosages for maintenance therapy are as follows:

Children aged, 12 months–2 years : 10-20 mg;
2 years–6 years : 20-30 mg;
6 years–10 years : 30-60 mg

Patients with impaired renal function: In patients with impaired renal function or undergoing chronic haemodialysis, a particularly low dosage of Lioresal should be selected ie. approx. 5 mg daily.

Patients with spastic states of cerebral origin: Unwanted effects are more likely to occur in these patients. It is therefore recommended that a very cautious dosage schedule be adopted and that patients be kept under appropriate surveillance.

Contra-indications, warnings, etc

Contra-indications: Hypersensitivity to baclofen, peptic ulceration.

Precautions: Psychotic disorders, schizophrenia or confusional states may be exacerbated by treatment with Lioresal. Patients suffering from these conditions should therefore be treated cautiously and kept under close surveillance.

Lioresal may also exacerbate epileptic manifestations but can be employed provided appropriate supervision and adequate anticonvulsive therapy are maintained. Lioresal should be used with extreme care in patients already receiving antihypertensive therapy, (see Interactions).

Lioresal should be used with caution in patients suffering from cerebrovascular accidents or from respiratory, hepatic or renal impairment.

Since under treatment with Lioresal neurogenic disturbances affecting emptying of the bladder may show an improvement, whereas in patients with preexisting sphincter hypertonia acute retention of urine may occur, the drug should be used with caution in such patients.

Anxiety and confusional states, hallucinations, psychotic, manic or paranoid states, convulsions (status epilepticus), tachycardia and as rebound phenomenon temporary aggravation of spasticity have been reported with abrupt withdrawal of Lioresal, especially after long term medication. Treatment should, always (unless serious adverse effects occur) therefore, be gradually discontinued by successively reducing the dosage over a period of about 1-2 weeks.

The patients reactions may be adversely affected by Lioresal induced sedation or decreased alertness, patients should therefore exercise due caution. Operating equipment or machinery may be hazardous.

Since in rare instances elevated SGOT, alkaline phosphatase and glucose levels in serum have been recorded, appropriate laboratory tests should be performed in patients with liver diseases or diabetes mellitus in order to ensure that no drug induced changes in these underlying diseases have occurred.

Use in pregnancy and lactation: Baclofen increases the incidence of omphaloceles (ventral hernias) in the foetuses of rats at high doses. No teratogenic effects have been noted in mice or rabbits.

A dose related increase in the incidence of ovarian cysts, and a less marked increase in enlarged and/or haemorrhagic adrenals have been observed in female rats treated for 2 years. The clinical relevance of these findings is not known.

During pregnancy, especially in the first 3 months, Lioresal should only be employed if its use is of vital necessity. The benefits of the treatment for the mother must be carefully weighed against the possible risks for the child. Baclofen crosses the placental barrier.

In mothers taking Lioresal in therapeutic doses, the active substance passes into the breast milk, but in quantities so small that no undesirable effects on the infant are to be expected.

Interactions: Where Lioresal is taken concomitantly with other drugs acting on the CNS or with alcohol, increased sedation may occur.

Lioresal may produce severe aggravation of hyperkinetic symptoms in patients receiving Lithium.

Pretreatment with Lioresal may prolong the duration of Fentanyl induced analgesia.

During concurrent treatment with tricyclic antidepressants, the effect of Lioresal may be potentiated, resulting in pronounced muscular hypotonia.

Since concomitant treatment with Lioresal and antihypertensives is likely to increase the fall in blood pressure, the dosage of antihypertensive medication should be adjusted accordingly.

Drugs which may produce renal insufficiency eg. ibuprofen, may reduce baclofen excretion leading to toxic effects.

In patients with Parkinson's disease receiving treatment with Lioresal and levodopa plus carbidopa, there have been reports of mental confusion, hallucinations and agitation.

Side-effects: Unwanted effects occur mainly at the start of treatment, if the dosage is raised too rapidly, if large doses are employed, or in elderly patients. They are often transitory and can be attenuated or eliminated by reducing the dosage; they are seldom severe enough to necessitate withdrawal of the medication.

Central nervous system: Particularly at the start of treatment, unwanted effects such as daytime sedation, drowsiness, and nausea may frequently occur. Also occasionally encountered are dryness of the mouth, respiratory depression, light-headedness, lassitude, exhaustion, mental confusion, dizziness, retching, vomiting, headache, and insomnia.

Should nausea persist following a reduction in dosage, it is recommended that Lioresal be ingested with food or a milk beverage.

Neurological and/or psychiatric manifestations which have occasionally or rarely been reported include: euphoria, depressive states, paraesthesiae, myalgia, muscular weakness, ataxia, tremor, nystagmus, accommodation disorders, hallucinations and nightmares. It is often difficult to distinguish between these manifestations and those of the disease under treatment. Lowering of the convulsion threshold and attacks of convulsions may possibly occur, particularly in epileptic patients.

Gastro-intestinal tract: Occasionally, mild gastro-intestinal disturbances (constipation, diarrhoea).

Cardiovascular system: Occasionally, hypotension, respiratory or cardiovascular depression.

Urogenital system: Occasionally or rarely, dysuria, frequency of micturition, enuresis. It is often difficult to distinguish between these manifestations and those of the diseases under treatment.

Miscellaneous unwanted effects: In rare or isolated cases visual disturbances, alterations in the taste sensation, hyperhidrosis, skin rash, deterioration in liver function tests.

Certain patients have shown increased spasticity as a paradoxical reaction to the medication.

An undesirable degree of muscular hypotonia–making it more difficult for patients to walk or fend for themselves–may occur and can usually be relieved by re-adjusting the dosage (ie. by reducing the doses given during the day and possibly increasing the evening dose).

Overdosage

Symptoms: Prominent features are signs of central nervous depression: drowsiness, impairment of consciousness, respiratory depression, coma. Also liable to occur are: confusion, hallucinations, agitation, accommodation disorders, absent pupillary reflex; generalised muscular hypotonia, myoclonia, hyporeflexia or areflexia; convulsions; peripheral vasodilatation, hypotension, bradycardia; hypothermia; nausea, vomiting, diarrhoea, hypersalivation; elevated LDH, SGOT and AP values.

A deterioration in the condition may occur if various substances or drugs acting on the central nervous system (eg. alcohol, diazepam, tricyclic antidepressants) have been taken at the same time.

Treatment: No specific antidote is known.

Elimination of the drug from the gastro-intestinal tract (induction of vomiting, gastric lavage; comatose patients should be intubated prior to gastric lavage), administration of activated charcoal; if necessary, saline aperient; in respiratory depression, administration of artificial respiration, also measures in support of cardiovascular functions. Since the drug is excreted chiefly via the kidneys, generous quantities of fluid should be given, possibly together with a diuretic. In the event of convulsions diazepam should be administered cautiously i.v.

Pharmaceutical precautions Lioresal tablets should be protected from heat (store below 25°C) and moisture.

Lioresal liquid should be protected from light and heat (store below 25°C) and should not be refrigerated.

Dilution: Lioresal liquid may be diluted with Purified Water BP and stored at room temperature for up to 14 days.

Legal category POM

Package quantities
Tablets 10 mg: Securitainers of 84
Liquid 5 mg/5 ml: Bottles of 300 ml with child proof closures.

Further information Lioresal liquid contains no sucrose and is therefore suitable for diabetics and children.

Product licence numbers
Tablets 10 mg 00101/0504
Liquid 5 mg/5 ml 00101/0503

LIORESAL* INTRATHECAL

Qualitative and quantitative composition
Active substance: b-(Aminomethyl)-p-chlorohydrocinnamic acid (=baclofen), a racemic mixture of the R, (–) and S, (+) isomers.

One ampoule of 1 ml contains 50 micrograms baclofen, (50 micrograms/ml).

One ampoule of 20 ml contains 10 mg baclofen (500 micrograms/ml).

One ampoule of 5 ml contains 10 mg baclofen (2000 micrograms/ml).

Pharmaceutical form Solutions for intrathecal injection and intrathecal infusion.

Clinical particulars
Therapeutic indications: Lioresal Intrathecal is indicated in patients with severe chronic spasticity of spinal or cerebral origin (associated with injury, multiple sclerosis, cerebral palsy) who are unresponsive to oral baclofen or other orally administered antispastic agents and/or those patients who experience unacceptable side-effects at effective oral doses.

Lioresal Intrathecal is not recommended for use in patients under 18 years of age with spasticity of spinal origin due to limited clinical experience in this age group.

In patients with spasticity due to head injury a delay of at least one year before treatment with Lioresal Intrathecal is recommended, to allow the symptoms of spasticity to stabilise.

Lioresal Intrathecal may be considered as an alternative to ablative neurosurgical procedures.

Posology and method of administration
Adults, Children and the Elderly: Lioresal Intrathecal 50 micrograms/1 ml is intended for administration in single bolus test injections via a lumbar puncture or intrathecal catheter. Lioresal Intrathecal 10 mg/20 ml and 10 mg/5 ml have been developed specifically for use with implantable pumps.

Individual titration of dosage is essential due to a high interindividual variability in response. Each patient must undergo an initial screening phase to determine the response to test bolus doses followed by a dose-titration phase to determine the optimum dose schedule for maintenance therapy with an appropriate implanted delivery system.

Respiratory function should be monitored and appropriate resuscitation facilities should be available during the introduction of treatment with Lioresal Intrathecal. Intrathecal administration using an implanted delivery system should only be undertaken by physicians with appropriate knowledge and experience. Specific instructions for using the implantable pump should be obtained from the pump manufacturers. Only pumps constructed of material known to be compatible with the product and incorporating an in-line bacterial retentive filter should be used.

Screening phase: Prior to initiation of a chronic infusion, the patient's response to intrathecal bolus doses administered via a catheter or lumbar puncture must be assessed. Low concentration ampoules containing 50 micrograms baclofen in 1 ml are available for the purpose. Patients should be infection-free prior to screening, as the presence of a systemic infection may prevent an accurate assessment of the response.

The usual initial test dose in adults is 25 or 50 micrograms, increasing step-wise by 25 microgram increments at intervals of not less than 24 hours until a response of approximately 4 to 8 hours duration is observed. The recommended initial test dose in children (patients under 18 years) is 25 micrograms. Each dose should be given **slowly** (over at least one minute). In order to be considered a responder the patient must demonstrate a significant decrease in muscle tone and/or frequency and/or severity of muscle spasms.

The variability in sensitivity to intrathecal baclofen between patients is emphasised. Signs of severe overdose (coma) have been observed in an adult after a single test dose of 25 micrograms. It is recommended that the initial test dose is administered with resuscitative equipment on hand.

Patients who do not respond to a 100 micrograms test dose should not be given further dose increments or considered for continuous intrathecal infusion.

Monitoring of respiratory and cardiac function is essential during this phase, especially in patients with cardiopulmonary disease and respiratory muscle weakness or those being treated with benzodiazepine-type preparations or opiates, who are at higher risk of respiratory depression.

Dose-titration phase: Once the patient's responsiveness to Lioresal Intrathecal has been established, an intrathecal infusion may be introduced. Lioresal Intrathecal is most often administered using an infusion pump which is implanted in the chest wall or abdominal wall tissues. Implantation of pumps should only be performed in experienced centres to minimise risks during the perioperative phase.

Infection may increase the risk of surgical complications and complicate attempts to adjust the dose.

The initial total daily infused dose is determined by doubling the bolus dose which gave a significant response in the initial screening phase and administering it over a 24 hour period. However, if a prolonged effect (i.e. lasting more than 12 hours) is observed during screening the starting dose should be the unchanged screening dose delivered over 24 hours. No dose increases should be attempted during the first 24 hours.

After the initial 24 hour period dosage should be adjusted slowly to achieve the desired clinical effect. If a programmable pump is used the dose should be increased only once every 24 hours; for non-programmable multi-dose reservoir pumps, intervals of 48 hours between dose adjustments are recommended. In either case increments should be limited as follows to avoid possible overdosage:

Patients with spasticity of spinal origin:
10–30% of the previous daily dose
Patients with spasticity of cerebral origin:
5–15% of the previous daily dose.

If the dose has been significantly increased without apparent clinical effect, pump function and catheter patency should be investigated.

There is limited clinical experience using doses greater than 1000 micrograms/day.

It is important that patients are monitored closely in an appropriately equipped and staffed environment during screening and immediately following pump implantation. Resuscitative equipment should be available for immediate use in case of life-threatening adverse reactions.

Maintenance therapy: The clinical goal is to maintain as normal a muscle tone as possible, and to minimise the frequency and severity of spasms without inducing intolerable side effects. The lowest dose producing an adequate response should be used. The retention of some spasticity is desirable to avoid a sensation of 'paralysis' on the part of the patient. In addition, a degree of muscle tone and occasional spasms may help support circulatory function and possibly prevent the formation of deep vein thrombosis.

In patients with spasticity of spinal origin, maintenance dosing for long-term continuous infusions of intrathecal baclofen has been found to range from 12 to 2003 micrograms/day, with most patients being adequately maintained on 300 to 800 micrograms/day.

In patients with spasticity of cerebral origin, maintenance dosage has been found to range from 22 to 1400 micrograms/day, with a mean daily dosage of 276 micrograms per day at 12 months and 307 micrograms per day at 24 months Paediatric patients under the age of 12 will generally require lower doses; maintenance dosage has been found to range from 24 to 1199 micrograms per day (mean daily dose of 274 micrograms per day).

Delivery specifications: Lioresal Intrathecal ampoules of 20 ml containing 500 micrograms/ml and 5 ml containing 2 mg (2000 micrograms)/ml are intended for use with infusion pumps. The concentration to be used depends on the dose requirements and size of pump reservoir. Use of the more concentrated solution obviates the need for frequent re-filling in patients with high dosage requirements.

Delivery regimen: Lioresal Intrathecal is most often administered in a continuous infusion mode immediately following implant. After the patient has stabilised with regard to daily dose and functional status, and provided the pump allows it, a more complex mode of delivery may be started to optimise control of spasticity at different times of the day. For example, patients who have increased spasm at night may require a 20% increase in their hourly infusion rate. Changes in flow rate should be programmed to start two hours before the desired onset of clinical effect.

Most patients require gradual dose increases to maintain optimum response during chronic therapy due to decreased responsiveness or disease progression. In patients with spasticity of spinal origin the daily dose may be increased gradually by 10–30% to maintain adequate symptom control. Where the spasticity is of cerebral origin any increase in dose should be limited to 20% (range: 5–20%). In both cases the daily dose may also be reduced by 10–20% if patients suffer side effects.

A sudden requirement for substantial dose escalation is indicative of a catheter complication (i.e. a kink or dislodgement) or pump malfunction.

In order to prevent excessive weakness the dosage of Lioresal Intrathecal should be adjusted with caution whenever spasticity is required to maintain function.

During long-term treatment approximately 5% of patients become refractory to increasing doses. There is insufficient clinical experience on which to base firm recommendations for tolerance management. However, sensitivity to baclofen may be restored by switching for 10 to 14 days to intrathecal preservative-free morphine sulphate treatment. Lioresal Intrathecal should be resumed at the initial continuous infusion dose followed by re-titration to avoid overdose; this should be performed in a hospital unit. Caution should be exercised when switching from Lioresal Intrathecal to morphine and vice versa (see *Interactions*).

Contra-indications: Known hypersensitivity to baclofen.

The drug should not be administered by any route other than intrathecal.

Special warnings and special precautions for use: Intrathecal baclofen therapy is valuable but hazardous. Careful pre-operative assessment is mandatory.

The patient must be given adequate information regarding the risks of this mode of treatment, and be physically and psychologically able to cope with the pump. It is essential that the responsible physicians and all those involved in the care of the patient receive adequate instruction on the signs and symptoms of overdose, procedures to be followed in the event of an overdose and the proper home care of the pump and insertion site.

Reservoir refilling: Reservoir refilling must be performed by trained and qualified personnel in accordance with the instructions provided by the pump manufacturer. Refills should be timed to avoid excessive depletion of the reservoir.

When refilling the pump, care should be taken to avoid discharging the contents of the catheter into the intrathecal space.

Strict asepsis is required to avoid microbial contamination and infection.

Extreme caution must be taken when filling a pump equipped with an injection port that allows direct access to the intrathecal catheter as a direct injection into the catheter through the access port could cause a life-threatening overdose.

Precautions in paediatric patients: Children should be of sufficient body mass to accommodate the implantable pump for chronic infusion. There is very limited clinical experience of the use of Lioresal Intrathecal in children under six. The safety of Lioresal Intrathecal in children under four has not yet been established.

Precautions in special patient populations: In patients with abnormal CSF flow the circulation of drug and hence antispastic activity may be inadequate.

Psychotic disorders, schizophrenia, confusional states or Parkinson's disease may be exacerbated by treatment with oral Lioresal. Patients suffering from these conditions should therefore be treated cautiously and kept under close surveillance.

Special attention should be given to patients known to suffer from epilepsy as seizures have been occasionally reported during overdose with, and withdrawal from, Lioresal Intrathecal, as well as in patients maintained on therapeutic doses.

Lioresal Intrathecal should be used with caution in patients with a history of autonomic dysreflexia. The presence of nociceptive stimuli or abrupt withdrawal of Lioresal Intrathecal may precipitate an autonomic dysreflexic episode.

Lioresal should be used with caution in patients with cerebrovascular or respiratory insufficiency.

An effect of Lioresal Intrathecal on underlying, non-CNS related diseases is unlikely because its systemic availability is substantially lower than after oral administration. Observations after oral baclofen therapy suggest that caution should be exercised in patients with a history of peptic ulcers, pre-existing sphincter hypertonia and impaired renal function.

In rare cases elevated SGOT, alkaline phosphatase and glucose levels in the serum have been recorded when using oral Lioresal.

Several patients over the age of 65 years have been treated with intrathecal baclofen without specific problems, and as doses are individually titrated there are unlikely to be any specific problems in elderly patients.

Treatment withdrawal: Except in overdose-related emergencies or where serious adverse effects occur, treatment should always be discontinued gradually with successive reductions in dosage. Sudden cessation of treatment, especially after doses exceeding the normal dose range, may result in a hyperactive state with rapid uncontrolled spasms and increased rigidity to intolerable levels lasting for several days.

Confusional states, hallucinations, psychotic, manic or paranoid states, convulsions (status epilepticus), and – as a rebound phenomenon – temporary aggravation of spasticity have been reported upon the abrupt withdrawal of oral Lioresal, especially after long-term treatment.

Interaction with other medicaments and other forms of interaction: The co-administration of other intrathecal agents with Lioresal Intrathecal is not recommended.

An attempt should be made to reduce or discontinue concomitant oral antispastic medications, preferably before initiating baclofen infusion. However, abrupt reduction or discontinuation during chronic intrathecal baclofen therapy should be avoided.

There is inadequate experience with Lioresal Intrathecal in combination with systemic medications to be able to predict specific drug–drug interactions, although it is suggested that the lower plasma baclofen levels produced by intrathecal administration should reduce the potential for interactions. Experience with oral baclofen would suggest that:

- There may be increased sedation where Lioresal is taken concomitantly with other drugs acting on the CNS or with alcohol.
- During concurrent treatment with tricyclic antidepressants, the effect of Lioresal may be potentiated, resulting in muscular hypotonia.
- Since concomitant treatment with Lioresal and antihypertensives is likely to increase the fall in blood pressure, it may be necessary to reduce the dosage of antihypertensive medication.
- In patients with Parkinson's disease receiving treatment with Lioresal and levodopa plus carbidopa, mental confusion, hallucinations and agitation may occur.

The combined use of morphine and intrathecal baclofen has been responsible for hypotension in one patient; the potential for this combination to cause dyspnoea or CNS symptoms cannot be excluded.

Pregnancy and lactation: There are no adequate and well-controlled studies in pregnant women. Oral baclofen increases the incidence of omphaloceles (ventral hernias) in the foetuses of rats at high doses. No teratogenic effects have been noted in mice or rabbits.

A dose related increase in the incidence of ovarian cysts, and a less marked increase in enlarged and/or haemorrhagic adrenals have been observed in female rats treated for 2 years. The clinical relevance of these findings is not known.

Lioresal Intrathecal should not be used during pregnancy unless the potential benefit is judged to outweigh the potential risk to the foetus. Baclofen crosses the placental barrier.

In mothers taking oral Lioresal in therapeutic doses the active substance passes into the breast milk, but in quantities so small that no undesirable effects on the infant are to be expected. It is not known whether detectable levels of drug are present in the breast milk of nursing mothers receiving Lioresal Intrathecal.

Effects on ability to drive and use machines: Drowsiness has been reported in some patients receiving intrathecal baclofen, and patients should be advised to exercise due caution. Operating equipment or machinery may be hazardous.

Undesirable effects: A causal link between the following observed events and the administration of baclofen cannot be reliably assessed in many cases, since many of the adverse events reported are known to occur in association with the underlying conditions being treated. Nonetheless, some of the more commonly reported reactions – drowsiness/somnolence, dizziness, headache, nausea, hypotension, hypotonia – appear to be drug-related.

Some of the adverse events listed below have been reported in patients with spasticity of spinal origin but could also occur in patients with spasticity of cerebral origin. Adverse events that are more frequent in either population are indicated below.

Frequency estimate: very common ≥10%, common ≥1% to <10%, uncommon ≥0.1% to <1%, rare ≥0.01% to <0.1%, very rare <0.01%.

Adverse events associated with the delivery system (e.g. catheter dislocation, pocket infection, meningitis, overdose due to wrong manipulation of the device) are not included here.

Central nervous system: Very common: drowsiness/somnolence.

Common: sedation, dizziness/lightheadedness, seizures, headache, paraesthesiae, accommodation disorders/blurred vision/double vision, slurred speech, lethargy, asthenia, respiratory depression, insomnia, confusion/disorientation, anxiety/agitation, depression.

Uncommon: hypothermia, nystagmus, dysphagia, ataxia, impaired memory, suicidal ideation and attempt, euphoria, dysphoria, hallucinations, paranoia

(Seizures and headache occur more often in patients with spasticity of cerebral origin than in patients with spasticity of spinal origin.)

Cardiovascular system: Common: hypotension.

Uncommon: hypertension, bradycardia, deep vein thrombosis, skin flushing, paleness.

Musculoskeletal system: Very common: muscular hypotonia.

Common: muscular hypertonia.

Gastro-intestinal tract: Common: nausea/vomiting, constipation, dry mouth, diarrhoea, decreased appetite, increased salivation.

Uncommon: dehydration, ileus, decreased taste.

(Nausea and vomiting occur more often in patients with spasticity of cerebral origin than in patients with spasticity of spinal origin.)

Respiratory system: Common: dyspnoea, bradypnoea, pneumonia.

Genitourinary system: Common: urinary incontinence, urinary retention, sexual dysfunction.

(Urinary retention occurs more often in patients with spasticity of cerebral origin than in patients with spasticity of spinal origin.)

Skin and appendages: Common: urticaria/pruritis, facial or peripheral oedema.

Uncommon: alopecia diaphoresis.

Miscellaneous: Common: pain, fever/chills.

Overdose: Special attention should be given to recognising the signs and symptoms of overdosage at all times, but especially during the initial 'screening' and 'dose titration' phases and also during the reintroduction of Lioresal Intrathecal after an interruption of therapy.

Signs of overdose may appear suddenly or (more usually) insidiously.

Symptoms of overdose: excessive muscular hypotonia, drowsiness, lightheadedness, dizziness, somnolence, seizures, loss of consciousness, excessive salivation, nausea and vomiting.

Respiratory depression, apnoea and coma result from serious overdosage. Seizures may occur with increasing dosage or, more commonly, during recovery from an overdose. Serious overdose may occur through the inadvertent delivery of the catheter contents, errors in pump programming, excessively rapid dose increases or concomitant treatment with oral baclofen. Possible pump malfunction should also be investigated.

Treatment: There is no specific antidote for treating overdosages of intrathecal baclofen. Any instructions provided by the pump manufacturer should be followed, and the following steps should generally be undertaken:

- Where a programmable continuous infusion pump is used, further delivery of baclofen should be halted immediately by removal of residual drug solution from the reservoir.
- If it is possible to do so without surgical intervention, the intrathecal catheter should be disconnected from the pump as soon as possible, and infusion fluid allowed to drain back together with some CSF (up to 30–40 ml is suggested).
- Patients with respiratory depression should be intubated if necessary, and ventilated artificially if required. Cardiovascular functions should be supported and in the event of convulsions, i.v. diazepam cautiously administered.

Anecdotal reports suggest that intravenous physostigmine may assist in the reversal of central side-effects (notably drowsiness and respiratory depression), but its use has been associated with the induction of seizures, bradycardia and cardiac conduction disturbances, and it should not be used in cases of severe overdose. In such cases intubation and ventilation are essential. In adults a total dose of 1–2 mg physostigmine may be tried intravenously over 5–10 minutes. Patients should be monitored closely during this time. Repeated doses of 1 mg may be administered at 30–60 minute intervals in an attempt to maintain adequate respiration in the absence of facilities for respiratory support.

In children a dose of 0.02 mg/kg physostigmine may be administered i.v. at a rate not exceeding 0.5 mg per minute. This dose may be repeated at 5 to 10 minute intervals until a therapeutic effect is obtained or a total dose of 2 mg has been administered.

Pharmacological properties

Pharmacodynamic properties: Antispastic with a spinal site of attack.

Baclofen depresses both monosynaptic and polysynaptic reflex transmission in the spinal cord by stimulating the $GABA_B$ receptors. Baclofen is a chemical analogue of the inhibitory neurotransmitter gamma-aminobutyric acid (GABA).

Neuromuscular transmission is not affected by baclofen. Baclofen exerts an antinociceptive effect. In neurological diseases associated with spasm of the skeletal muscles, the clinical effects of Lioresal take the form of a beneficial action on reflex muscle contractions and of marked relief from painful spasm, automatism, and clonus. Lioresal improves the patient's mobility, makes it easier for him/her to manage without aid, and facilitates physiotherapy.

Consequent important gains include improved ambulation, prevention and healing of decubitus ulcers, and better sleep patterns due to elimination of painful muscle spasms. In addition, patients experience improvement in bladder and sphincter function and catheterisation is made easier, all representing significant improvements in the patient's quality of life. Baclofen has been shown to have general CNS depressant properties, causing sedation, somnolence, and respiratory and cardiovascular depression.

Baclofen, when introduced directly into the intrathecal space, permits effective treatment of spasticity with doses at least 100 times smaller than those for oral administration.

Intrathecal bolus: The onset of action is generally half an hour to one hour after administration of a single intrathecal dose. Peak spasmolytic effect is seen at approximately 4 hours after dosing, the effect lasting 4 to 8 hours. Onset, peak response, and duration of action may vary with individual patients depending on the dose and severity of symptoms and the method and speed of drug administration.

Continuous infusion: Baclofen's antispastic action is first seen at 6 to 8 hours after initiation of continuous infusion. Maximum efficacy is observed within 24 to 48 hours.

Pharmacokinetic properties: The following kinetic parameters have to be interpreted in the light of intrathecal administration coupled with slow CSF circulation.

Absorption: Direct infusion into the spinal subarachnoid space by-passes absorption processes and allows exposure to the receptor sites in the dorsal horn of the spinal cord.

Distribution: After single intrathecal bolus injection/short-term infusion the volume of distribution, calculated from CSF levels, ranges from 22 to 157 ml.

With continuous intrathecal infusion daily doses of 50 to 1200 micrograms result in lumbar CSF concentrations of baclofen as high as 130 to 1240 ng/ml at steady state. According to the half-life measured in the CSF, CSF steady-state concentrations will be reached within 1–2 days. No paediatric data are available.

During intrathecal infusion the plasma concentrations do not exceed 5 ng/ml (10 ng/ml in paediatric patients), confirming that baclofen passes only slowly across the blood-brain barrier.

Elimination: The elimination half-life in the CSF after single intrathecal bolus injection/short-term infusion of 50 to 136 micrograms baclofen ranges from 1 to 5 hours. Elimination half-life of baclofen after having reached steady-state in the CSF has not been determined.

After both single bolus injection and chronic lumbar subarachnoid infusion using an implantable pump system, the mean CSF clearance was about 30 ml/h.

At steady-state conditions during continuous intrathecal infusion, a baclofen concentration gradient is built up in the range between 1.8:1 and 8.7:1 (mean: 4:1) from lumbar to cisternal CSF. This is of clinical importance insofar as spasticity in the lower extremities can be effectively treated with little effect on the upper limbs and with fewer CNS adverse reactions due to effects on the brain centres.

Preclinical safety data: Subacute and subchronic studies with continuous intrathecal baclofen infusion in two species (rat, dog) revealed no signs of local irritation or inflammation on histological examination.

A 2-year rat study (oral administration) showed that baclofen is not carcinogenic. In the same study a dose-related increase in incidence of ovarian cysts and a less marked increase in enlarged and/or haemorrhagic adrenal glands was observed.

Ovarian cysts have been found by palpation in about 5% of the multiple sclerosis patients who were treated with oral Lioresal for up to one year. In most cases these cysts disappeared spontaneously while patients continued to receive the drug. Ovarian cysts are known to occur spontaneously in a proportion of the normal female population.

Mutagenicity assays *in vitro* and *in vivo* showed no evidence of mutagenic effects.

Pharmaceutical particulars

List of excipients: Sodium chloride; water for injection.

Incompatibilities: If alternative baclofen concentrations are required, Lioresal Intrathecal may be diluted under aseptic conditions with sterile preservative-free sodium chloride for injections. The ampoules should not be mixed with other solutions for injection or infusion (dextrose has proved to be incompatible due to a chemical reaction with baclofen).

The compatibility of Lioresal Intrathecal with the components of the infusion pump (including the chemical stability of baclofen in the reservoir) and the presence of an in-line bacterial retentive filter should be confirmed with the pump manufacturer prior to use.

Shelf life

Lioresal Intrathecal 50 micrograms/1 ml: 3 years
Lioresal Intrathecal 10 mg/20 ml: 5 years
Lioresal Intrathecal 10 mg/5 ml: 3 years

Special precautions for storage: Protect from heat (store below 30°C).

Medicines should be kept out of the reach of children.

Nature and content of container: Colourless glass ampoules, glass type I, according to PhEur.

Instructions for use/handling: Each ampoule is intended for single use only, and any unused solution should be discarded. Ampoules should not be either frozen or autoclaved.

Marketing authorisation holder: Novartis Pharmaceuticals UK Limited, trading as Ciba Laboratories, Frimley Business Park, Frimley, Camberley, Surrey GU16 5SG.

Marketing authorisation number

Lioresal Intrathecal 50 micrograms/1 ml: PL 00101/0500
Lioresal Intrathecal 10 mg/20 ml: PL 00101/0501
Lioresal Intrathecal 10 mg/5 ml: PL 00101/0502

Date of revision 6 July 1998.

LOPRESOR TABLETS 100 mg
LOPRESOR TABLETS 50 mg

Qualitative and quantitative composition Each tablet contains 100 mg metroprolol tartrate BP.

Each tablet contains 50 mg metroprolol tartrate BP.

Pharmaceutical form Film coated tablet.

Clinical particulars

Therapeutic indications: Hypertension and angina pectoris, cardiac arrhythmias, especially supraventricular tachyarrhythmias. Adjunct to treatment of thyrotoxicosis. Early intervention with Lopresor in acute myocardial infarction reduces infarct size and the incidence of ventricular fibrillation. Pain relief may also decrease the need for opiate analgesics. Lopresor has been shown to reduce mortality when administered to patients with acute myocardial infarction. Prophylaxis of migraine.

Posology and method of administration: Lopresor tablets should be administered orally and swallowed unchewed. The dose must always be adjusted to the individual requirements of the patient but should not exceed 400 mg/day. The following are guidelines:

Adults: Hypertension: Initially a dose of 100 mg per day should be prescribed either as single or divided doses.

Depending upon the response the dosage may be increased by 100 mg per day at weekly intervals to 200 mg daily given in single or divided doses. Over the dosage range most patients may be expected to respond rapidly and satisfactorily. A further reduction in blood pressure may be achieved if Lopresor is used in conjunction with an antihypertensive diuretic or other hypotensive agent.

Lopresor may be administered with benefit both to previously untreated patients with hypertension and to those in whom the response to previous therapy is inadequate. In the latter type of patient the previous therapy may be continued and Lopresor added into the regime with adjustment of the previous therapy if necessary.

Angina pectoris: 50–100 mg twice or three times daily.

In general a significant improvement in exercise tolerance and reduction of anginal attacks may be expected with a dose of 50-100 mg twice daily.

Cardiac arrhythmias: A dosage of 50 mg two or three times daily is usually sufficient. If necessary the dose can be increased up to 300 mg per day administered in divided doses.

Hyperthyroidism: 50 mg four times daily. The dosage should be progressively reduced as euthyroid state is slowly achieved.

Myocardial infarction: Early intervention: 50 mg every 6 hours for 48 hours, preferably within 12 hours of the onset of chest pain.

Maintenance: the usual maintenance dose is 200 mg daily given in divided doses. The treatment should be continued for at least 3 months.

Prophylaxis of migraine: 100–200 mg daily, given in divided doses (morning and evening).

Elderly: There is no evidence to suggest that dosage requirements are different in otherwise healthy elderly patients. However, caution is indicated in elderly patients as an excessively pronounced decrease in blood pressure or pulse rate may cause the blood supply to vital organs to fall to inadequate levels.

In patients with significant hepatic dysfunction the lower dosage recommendations will be more appropriate.

Children: Not recommended.

Contra-indications: Known hypersensitivity to metoprolol and related derivatives, severe asthma, atrioventricular block of second or third degree, uncontrolled heart failure, clinically relevant sinus bradycardia, sick-sinus syndrome, severe peripheral arterial disease, cardiogenic shock. Metoprolol is also contra-indicated when myocardial infarction is complicated by significant bradycardia, first degree heart block, systolic hypotension (less than 100 mmHg) and/or severe heart failure.

Special warnings and precautions for use: A warning stating 'Do not take this medicine if you have a history of wheezing or asthma' will appear on the label.

Metoprolol may aggravate bradycardia, symptoms of peripheral arterial circulatory disorders and anaphylactic shock. If the patient develops increasing bradycardia, Lopresor should be given in lower doses or gradually withdrawn.

Abrupt cessation of therapy with a beta-blocker should be avoided. When possible, Lopresor should be withdrawn gradually over a period of 10 days, the doses diminishing to 25 mg for the last 6 days. During its withdrawal the patient should be kept under close surveillance.

Although cardioselective beta-blockers may have less effect on lung function than non-selective beta-blockers, as with all beta-blockers these should be avoided in patients with reversible obstructive airway disease unless there are compelling clinical reasons for their use. Therapy with a beta$_2$-stimulant may become necessary or current therapy require adjustment.

Lopresor may be administered when heart failure has been controlled.

Digitalisation and/or diuretic therapy should also be considered for patients with a history of heart failure or patients who are known to have a poor cardiac reserve.

Lopresor may mask some of the symptoms of thyrotoxicosis and of hypoglycaemia by inhibition of sympathetic nerve functions.

In labile and insulin-dependent diabetes it may be necessary to adjust the hypoglycaemic therapy.

In patients with a phaeochromocytoma, an alpha-blocker should be given concomitantly.

In patients with significant hepatic dysfunction it may be necessary to adjust the dosage because metoprolol undergoes biotransformation in the liver.

The administration of adrenaline to patients undergoing beta-blockade can result in an increase in blood pressure and bradycardia although this is less likely to occur with beta$_1$-selective drugs.

Lopresor should be given cautiously to patients with metabolic acidosis.

Lopresor therapy should be brought to the attention of the anaesthetist prior to general anaesthesia. In a patient under beta-blockade, the anaesthetic selected should be one exhibiting as little negative inotropic activity as possible (halothane/nitrous oxide).

Interaction with other medicaments and other forms of interaction: The effects of metoprolol and other antihypertensive drugs on blood pressure are usually additive, and care should be taken to avoid hypotension. As with all beta-blockers particular action is called for when metoprolol is administered together with prazosin for the first time. However, combinations of antihypertensive drugs may often be used with benefit to improve control of hypertension.

Metoprolol can reduce myocardial contractility and impair intracardiac conduction. Care should be exercised when drugs with similar activity, e.g. anti-arrhythmic agents, general anaesthetics, are given concurrently. Like all other beta-blockers, metoprolol should not be given in combination with verapamil since this may cause bradycardia, hypotension and asystole.

Care should also be exercised when beta-blockers are given in combination with sympathetic ganglion blocking agents, other beta-blockers (also in the form of eye drops) or MAO inhibitors.

If combination treatment with clonidine is to be discontinued, metoprolol should be withdrawn several days before clonidine.

As beta-blockers may affect the peripheral circulation, care should be exercised when drugs with similar activity, e.g. ergotamine, are given concurrently.

Metoprolol will antagonise the beta$_1$ effects of sympathomimetic agents but should have little influence on the bronchodilator effects of beta$_2$-agonists at normal therapeutic doses.

Enzyme inducing agents (e.g. rifampicin) may reduce plasma concentrations of metoprolol, whereas enzyme inhibitors (e.g. cimetidine) may increase plasma concentrations.

During concomitant ingestion of alcohol and metoprolol the concentration of blood alcohol may reach higher levels and may decrease more slowly.

Metoprolol may impair the elimination of lignocaine.

Indomethacin may reduce the antihypertensive effect of beta-blockers.

Nitroglycerin may enhance the hypotensive effect of Lopresor.

Pregnancy and lactation: Lopresor should not be used in pregnancy or lactation unless it is considered that the benefit outweighs the possible risk to the foetus/infant. Metoprolol has, however, been used in pregnancy associated hypertension under close supervision after 20 weeks gestation. Although the drug crosses the placental barrier and is present in cord blood no evidence of foetal abnormalities have been reported. Animal experiments have shown neither teratogenic potential nor other adverse events on the embryo and/or foetus relevant to the safety assessment of the product.

The amount of metoprolol ingested via breast milk seems to be negligible with regard to its beta-blocking effects if the mother is treated in doses within the therapeutic range.

If Lopresor is used during pregnancy and lactation special attention should be paid to the foetus, neonate and breast-fed infant for undesirable effects of the drug's beta-blocking action (e.g. bradycardia, hypoglycaemia).

Effects on ability to drive and use machinery: As with all beta-blockers, metoprolol may affect patient's ability to drive and operate machinery. Patients should be warned accordingly.

Undesirable effects

Central and peripheral nervous system: Occasionally: fatigue, dizziness, headache.

Rarely: paraesthesiae, muscle cramps, depression, decreased mental alertness, somnolence or insomnia, nightmares. In isolated cases: personality disorder, hallucinations.

Cardiovascular system: Occasionally: bradycardia, postural disorders (occasionally with syncope).

Rarely: heart failure, cardiac arrhythmias, oedema, palpitation, Raynaud's Phenomenon.

In isolated cases: disturbances of cardiac conduction, precordial pain, gangrene in patients with preexisting severe peripheral circulatory disorders.

Gastro-intestinal tract: Occasionally: nausea and vomiting, abdominal pain.

Rarely: diarrhoea or constipation.

In isolated cases: dryness of the mouth, liver function test abnormalities.

Skin and appendages: Rarely: skin rash (in the form of urticaria, psoriasiform and dystrophic skin lesions), occurrence of antinuclear antibodies (not associated with SLE).

In isolated cases: photosensitivity, increased sweating, loss of hair.

Respiratory tract: Occasionally: exertional dyspnoea.

Rarely: bronchospasm, also in patients without a history of obstructive lung disease.

In isolated cases: rhinitis.

Endocrine system and metabolism: In isolated cases: weight gain.

Urogenital system: There are isolated reports on disturbances of libido and potency.

Sense organs: In isolated cases: disturbances of vision, dry and/or irritated eyes, tinnitus, in doses exceeding those recommended loss of hearing.

Blood: In isolated cases: thrombocytopenia.

Other organ systems: In isolated cases: arthritis.

The reported incidence of skin rashes and/or dry eyes associated with the use of beta-blockers is small and in most cases the symptoms have cleared when treatment was withdrawn. Discontinuation of the drug should be considered if any such reaction is not otherwise explicable.

Overdosage: Signs: In more severe cases an overdosage of metoprolol may lead to severe hypotension, sinus bradycardia, atrioventricular block, heart failure, cardiogenic shock, cardiac arrest, bronchospasm, impairment of consciousness, coma, nausea, vomiting, cyanosis, hypoglycaemia and occasionally hyperkalaemia. The first manifestations usually appear 20 minutes to 2 hours after drug ingestion.

Treatment: Treatment should include close monitoring of cardiovascular, respiratory and renal functions, and blood glucose and electrolytes. Further absorption may be prevented by induction of vomiting, gastric lavage or administration of activated charcoal if ingestion is recent. Cardiovascular complications should be treated symptomatically which may require the use of sympathomimetic agents (e.g. noradrenaline, metaraminol), atropine or inotropic agents (e.g. dopamine, dobutamine). Temporary pacing may be required for AV block. Glucagon can reverse the effects of excessive beta-blockade given in a dose of 1–10 mg intravenously. Intravenous $beta_2$-stimulants may be required to relieve bronchospasm. Metoprolol cannot be effectively removed by haemodialysis.

Pharmacological particulars

Pharmacodynamic properties: Lopresor is a cardioselective beta-adrenergic blocking agent. It has a relatively greater blocking effect on $beta_1$-receptors (i.e. those mediating adrenergic stimulation of heart rate and contractility and release of free fatty acids from fat stores) than on $beta_2$-receptors which are chiefly involved in broncho and vasodilation.

Pharmacokinetic properties: Metoprolol is well absorbed after oral administration, peak plasma concentrations occurring 1.5–2 hours after dosing. The bioavailability of a single dose is approximately 50%, increasing to approximately 70% during repeated administration. The bioavailability also increases if metoprolol is given with food

Elimination is mainly by hepatic metabolism and the average elimination half-life is 3.5 hours (range 1 to 9 hours). Rates of metabolism vary between individuals, with poor metabolisers (approximately 10%) showing higher plasma concentrations and slower elimination than extensive metabolisers. Within individuals, however, plasma concentrations are stable and reproducible.

Because of variation in rates of metabolism, the dose of metoprolol should always be adjusted to the individual requirements of the patient. As the therapeutic response, adverse effects and relative cardioselectivity are related to plasma concentration, poor metabolisers may require lower than normal doses. Dosage adjustment is not routinely required in the elderly or in patients with renal failure, but dosage may need to be reduced in patients with significant hepatic dysfunction when metoprolol elimination may be impaired.

Preclinical safety data: There are no further data of relevance to the prescriber which are additional to those already included in other sections.

Pharmaceutical particulars

List of excipients: Avicel PH101, povidone, Aerosil 200, sodium starch glycollate, magnesium stearate, hydroxypropylmethylcellulose, polysorbate 80, purified special talc, (50 mg tablets) red iron oxide (E172), (100 mg tablets) dispersed blue (E132), titanium dioxide (E171).

Incompatibilities: None known.

Shelf life: 60 months.

Special precautions for storage: Protect from moisture.

Nature and contents of container: 56 Tablets in an Al/PVC (PVdC) blister pack.

Instructions for use/handling: Not applicable.

Marketing authorisation holder: Novartis Pharmaceuticals UK Limited, Trading as Geigy Pharmaceuticals, Wimblehurst Road, Horsham, West Sussex RH12 5AB.

Marketing authorisation numbers

Lopresor Tablets 50 mg: PL 00101/0418
Lopresor Tablets 100 mg: PL 00101/0419

Date of first authorisation/renewal of authorisation

Lopresor Tablets 50 mg: April 1998.
Lopresor Tablets 100 mg: April 1998.

LOPRESOR SR*

Qualitative and quantitative composition The active ingredient is di-[(±)-1-(isopropylamino)-3-[p-(2-methoxyethyl)phenoxy]-2-propanol] L(+)-tartrate (metoprolol tartrate).

One coated slow release tablet contains 200 mg metoprolol tartrate.

Pharmaceutical form Film coated tablets.

Clinical particulars

Therapeutic indications: For the treatment of hypertension, angina pectoris, prophylaxis of migraine.

Posology and method of administration: Lopresor SR Tablets should be swallowed unchewed.

The dose must always be adjusted to the individual requirements of the patient but should not exceed 400 mg/day. The following are guidelines:

Adults:

Hypertension: One Lopresor SR Tablet should be given in the morning. Most patients may be expected to respond satisfactorily within 14 days. Further antihypertensive effect may be achieved by the addition of a diuretic or a vasodilator.

Lopresor SR may be administered with benefit to both previously untreated patients with hypertension and to those in whom the response to previous therapy is inadequate. In the latter type of patient therapy may be continued and Lopresor SR added into the regime with adjustment of previous therapy if necessary.

Angina pectoris: Initially, one Lopresor SR Tablet daily. The dose may be increased to two tablets once daily if required. In general, a significant improvement in exercise tolerance and a reduction of anginal attacks may be expected with a dose of one Lopresor SR Tablet daily.

Prophylaxis of migraine: One tablet daily given in the morning.

Elderly: There is no evidence to suggest that dosage requirements are different in otherwise healthy elderly patients. However, caution is indicated in elderly patients as an excessive decrease in blood pressure or pulse rate may cause the blood supply to vital organs to fall to inadequate levels.

In patients with significant hepatic dysfunction the lower dosage recommendations will be more appropriate.

Children: Not recommended.

Contra-indications: Known sensitivity to metoprolol and related derivatives, severe asthma, atrioventricular block of second or third degree, uncontrolled heart failure, clinically relevant sinus bradycardia, sick-sinus syndrome, severe peripheral arterial disease, cardiogenic shock. Metoprolol is also contra-indicated when myocardial infarction is complicated by significant bradycardia, first degree heart block, systolic hypotension (less than 100 mmHg) and/or severe heart failure.

Special warnings and precautions for use:

Warnings: None.

Precautions: Metoprolol may aggravate bracycardia, symptoms of peripheral arterial circulatory disorders and anaphylactic shock. If the patient develops increasing bradycardia, Lopresor should be given in lower doses or gradually withdrawn.

Abrupt cessation of therapy with a beta-blocker should be avoided. When possible, Lopresor SR should be withdrawn gradually over a period of 10 days, the doses diminishing to 25 mg for the last 6 days. During its withdrawal the patient should be kept under close surveillance.

Although cardioselective beta-blockers may have less effect on lung function than non selective beta-blockers, as with all beta-blockers these should be avoided in patients with reversible obstructive airways disease unless there are compelling clinical reasons for their use. Therapy with a $beta_2$-stimulant may become necessary or current therapy require adjustment.

Lopresor SR may be administered when heart failure has been controlled. Digitalisation and/or diuretic therapy should also be considered for patients with a history of heart failure or patients known to have a poor cardiac reserve.

Lopresor SR may mask some of the symptoms of thyrotoxicosis and of hypoglycaemia by inhibition of sympathetic nerve functions.

In labile and insulin-dependent diabetes it may be necessary to adjust the hypoglycaemic therapy.

In patients with a phaeochromocytoma, an alpha-blocker should be given concomitantly.

In patients with significant hepatic dysfunction it may be necessary to adjust the dosage because metoprolol undergoes biotransformation in the liver.

The administration of adrenaline to patients undergoing beta-blockade can result in an increase in blood pressure and bradycardia, although this is less likely to occur with $beta_1$-selective drugs.

Lopresor SR should be given cautiously to patients with metabolic acidosis.

Lopresor SR therapy should be brought to the attention of the anaesthetist prior to general anaesthesia. In a patient under beta-blockade, the anaesthetic selected should be one exhibiting as little negative inotropic activity as possible (halothane/nitrous oxide).

Interactions with other drugs and other types of interactions:

Drug interactions: The effects of metoprolol and other antihypertensive drugs on blood pressure are usually additive, and care should be taken to avoid hypotension. As with all beta-blockers, particular caution is called for when metoprolol is administered together with prazosin for the first time. However, combinations of antihypertensive drugs may often be used with benefit to improve control of hypertension.

Metoprolol can reduce myocardial contractility and impair intracardiac conduction. Care should be exercised when drugs with similar activity e.g. antiarrhythmic agents, general anaesthetics, are given concurrently. Like all other beta-blockers, metoprolol should not be given in combination with verapamil since this may cause bradycardia, hypotension and asystole.

Care should also be exercised when beta-blockers are given in combination with sympathetic ganglion blocking agents, other beta-blockers (also in the form of eye drops) or MAO inhibitors.

If combination treatment with clonidine is to be discontinued metoprolol should be withdrawn several days before clonidine.

As beta-blockers may affect the peripheral circulation, care should be exercised when drugs with similar activity, e.g. ergotamine, are given concurrently.

Metoprolol will antagonise the $beta_1$ effects of

sympathomimetic agents, but should have little influence on the bronchodilator effects of beta$_2$-agonists at normal therapeutic doses.

Enzyme inducing agents (e.g. rifampicin) may reduce plasma concentration of metoprolol, whereas enzyme inhibitors (e.g. cimetidine) may increase plasma concentrations.

During concomitant ingestion of alcohol and metoprolol the concentration of blood alcohol may reach higher levels and may decrease more slowly.

Metoprolol may impair the elimination of lignocaine.

Indomethacin may reduce the antihypertensive effect of beta-blockers.

Nitroglycerin may enhance the hypotensive effect of Lopresor SR.

Pregnancy and lactation: Lopresor SR should not be used in pregnancy or lactation unless it is considered that the benefit outweighs the possible risk to the foetus/infant. Metoprolol has, however, been used in pregnancy associated hypertension under close supervision after 20 weeks gestation. Although the drug crosses the placental barrier and is present in cord blood no evidence of foetal abnormalities have been reported. The amount of metoprolol ingested via breast milk seems to be negligible with regard to its beta-blocking effects if the mother is treated in doses within the therapeutic range.

If Lopresor SR is used during pregnancy and lactation special attention should be paid to the foetus, neonate and breast-fed infant for undesirable effects of the drug's beta-blocking action (e.g. bradycardia, hypoglycaemia).

Effects on ability to drive or use machines: As with all beta-blockers, metoprolol may affect patients ability to drive and operate machinery. Patients should be warned accordingly.

Undesirable effects: Frequency estimate: frequent, 10%; occasional, 1–10%; rare, 0.001–1%; isolated cases, 0.001%.

Central and peripheral nervous system: Occasionally: Fatigue, dizziness, headache. *Rarely:* Paraesthesiae, muscle cramps, depression, decreased mental alertness, somnolence or insomnia, nightmares. *In isolated cases:* Personality disorder, hallucinations.

Cardiovascular system: Occasionally: Bradycardia, postural disorders (occasionally with syncope). *Rarely:* Heart failure, cardiac arrhythmias, oedema, palpitation, Raynaud's phenomenon. *In isolated cases:* Disturbances of cardiac conduction, precordial pain, gangrene in patients with pre-existing severe peripheral circulatory disorders.

Gastro-intestinal tract: Occasionally: Nausea and vomiting, abdominal pain. *Rarely:* Diarrhoea or constipation. *In isolated cases:* Dryness of the mouth, liver function test abnormalities, hepatitis.

Skin and appendages: Rarely: Skin rash (in the form of urticaria, psoriasiform and dystrophic skin lesions), occurrence of antinuclear antibodies (not associated with SLE). *In isolated cases:* Photosensitivity, increase sweating, loss of hair.

Respiratory tract: Occasionally: Exertional dyspnoea. *Rarely:* Bronchospasm, also in patients without a history of obstructive lung disease. *In isolated cases:* Rhinitis.

Endocrine system and metabolism: In isolated cases: Weight gain.

Urogenital system: There are isolated reports on disturbances of libido and potency.

Sense organs: In isolated cases: Disturbances of vision, dry and/or irritated eyes, tinnitus, in doses exceeding those recommended loss of hearing.

Blood: In isolated cases: Thrombocytopenia.

Other organ systems: In isolated cases: Arthritis.

The reported incidence of skin rashes and/or dry eyes associated with the use of beta-blockers is small and in most cases the symptoms have cleared when treatment was withdrawn. Discontinuation of the drug should be considered if any such reaction is not otherwise explicable.

Overdose:

Signs: In more severe cases an overdosage of metoprolol may lead to severe hypotension, sinus bradycardia, atrioventricular block, heart failure, cardiogenic shock, cardiac arrest, bronchospasm, impairment of consciousness, coma, nausea, vomiting, cyanosis, hypoglycaemia and occasionally hyperkalaemia. The first manifestations usually appear 20 minutes to 2 hours after drug ingestion.

Treatment: Treatment should include close monitoring of cardiovascular, respiratory and renal functions, and blood glucose and electrolytes. Further absorption may be prevented by induction of vomiting, gastric lavage or administration of activated charcoal if ingestion is recent. Cardiovascular complications should be treated symptomatically which may require the use of sympathomimetic agents (e.g. noradrenaline, metaraminol), atropine or inotropic agents (e.g. dopamine, dobutamine). Temporary pacing may be required for AV block. Glucagon can reverse the effects of excessive beta-blockage given in a dose of 1–10 mg intravenously. Intravenous beta$_2$-stimulants may be required to relieve bronchospam. Metoprolol cannot be effectively removed by haemodialysis.

Pharmacological properties

Pharmacodynamic properties:

Pharmacotherapeutic group: Lopresor SR is a cardioselective beta-adrenergic receptor blocking agent.

Mechanism of action: It has a relatively greater blocking effect on beta$_1$-receptors (i.e. those mediating adrenergic stimulation of heart rate and contractility and release of free fatty acids from fat stores) than on beta$_2$-receptors, which are chiefly involved in broncho- and vasodilation.

Pharmacokinetic properties:

Absorption: Lopresor SR is well absorbed after oral administration, peak plasma concentrations occurring 4–5 hours after dosing. The bioavailability of a single dose is approximately 50%, increasing to approximately 70% during repeated administration. The bioavailability also increases if metoprolol is given with food.

Biotransformation: Rates of metabolism vary between individuals, with poor metabolisers (approximately 10%) showing higher plasma concentrations and slower elimination than extensive metabolisers. Within individuals, however, plasma concentrations are stable and reproducible.

Elimination: Elimination is mainly by hepatic metabolism and the average elimination half-life is 3.5 hours (range 1 to 9 hours).

Characteristics in patients: Because of variation in rates of metabolism, the dose of metoprolol should always be adjusted to the individual requirements of the patient. As the therapeutic response, adverse effects and relative cardioselectivity are related to plasma concentration, poor metabolisers may require lower than normal doses. Dosage adjustment is not routinely required in the elderly or in patients with renal failure, but dosage may need to be reduced in patients with significant hepatic dysfunction when metoprolol elimination may be impaired.

Preclinical safety data: Animal experiments have shown neither teratogenic potential nor other adverse events on the embryo and/or foetus relevant to the safety assessment of the product.

Pharmaceutical particulars

List of excipients: The coated tablets contain silicon dioxide, microcystalline cellulose, calcium phosphate, polyacrylic/methacrylic copolymer, magnesium stearate, stearic acid, hydroxypropylmethylcellulose, glyceryl palmitostearate, talc, titanium dioxide, polysorbate, and yellow iron oxide.

Incompatibilities: None known.

Shelf-life: Five years.

Special precautions for storage: No special recommendations. Medicines should be kept out of reach of children.

Nature and contents of container: The tablets are pale yellow, capsule shaped, biconvex, film coated tablets, one face imprinted CG/CG, the other face with the letters CDC/CDC and packed in PVC/PVdC/foil bubble packs of 28 tablets.

Instruction for use/handling: None.

Marketing authorisation holder: Novartis Pharmaceuticals UK Limited, trading as Geigy Pharmaceuticals.

Marketing authorisation number 00101/0420.

Date of approval/revision of SPC 5 July 1997.

Legal category POM.

LUDIOMIL*

Qualitative and quantitative composition The active ingredient is 1-(3-methylaminopropyl)-dibenzo[b,e] bicyclo[2.2.2]octadiene hydrochloride (maprotiline hydrochloride INN).

One coated tablet contains 10 mg, 25 mg, 50 mg, or 75 mg maprotiline hydrochloride.

Pharmaceutical form Coated tablets.

Clinical particulars

Therapeutic indications: Symptoms of depressive illness, especially where sedation is required.

Posology and method of administration: Ludiomil tablets should be swallowed with sufficient liquid. The dose should be gradually increased to achieve a therapeutic effect with the lowest possible dose. This is particularly important for elderly patients with an unstable autonomic nervous system as these patients show a more marked response to Ludiomil than younger patients. A daily dosage of 150 mg should not be exceeded.

Adults: The usual dose range is 25–75 mg daily which may be given either in one dose or in three divided doses.

For moderate or severe depression, treatment should start with 75 mg daily, increasing step-wise, if necessary, to a maximum of 150 mg daily. Initially the patient should be closely monitored and dosage adjusted after 1 to 2 weeks according to response. Once a distinct improvement has set in the daily dosage may be adjusted to a maintenance level, i.e. the lowest dose that maintains the improvement.

Use in the elderly: It may be advisable in elderly patients, or those who may be sensitive to this type of drug, to start treatment with lower doses such as 30 mg once a day or 10 mg three times a day. This should then be adjusted in a stepwise fashion over one or two weeks up to 25 mg tid or 75 mg once a day, depending on the patient's response. In the majority of cases, half the normal dose should be sufficient.

Use in children: Not recommended.

Contra-indications: Ludiomil is contra-indicated in: patients who are known or suspected to have epilepsy or have a lowered convulsion threshold, recent myocardial infarction, the presence of defects in bundle-branch conduction, narrow angle glaucoma, retention of urine (e.g. prostatic disease), severe liver or renal disease, mania.

Concurrent use in patients receiving or within 14 days of cessation of therapy with monoamine oxidase inhibitors.

Known hypersensitivity to maprotiline or any of the excipients, or cross-sensitivity to tricyclic antidepressants.

Acute poisoning with alcohol, hypnotics, or psychotropic drugs.

Special warnings and precautions for use:

Warnings: In some patients, improvement may not occur for 2–3 weeks.

There have been rare reports of seizures occurring in patients without a history of seizures who were treated with therapeutic doses of Ludiomil. In some cases, other confounding factors were present such as concomitant medications known to lower the seizure threshold. The risk of seizures may be increased in comedication with phenothiazines (see Interactions), with benzodiazepines that are withdrawn abruptly, or when the recommended dosage of Ludiomil is rapidly exceeded.

While a causal relationship has not been established, the risk of seizures may be reduced by:

- initiating therapy at a low dosage,
- maintaining the initial dosage for two weeks and then raising it gradually in small increments,
- keeping the maintenance dosage at a minimally effective level,
- cautious alteration or avoidance of co-medication with drugs that lower the seizure threshold (e.g. phenothiazines),
- avoidance of rapid tapering of benzodiazepines.

Tricyclic and tetracyclic antidepressants have been reported to produce cardiac arrhythmias, sinus tachycardia and prolongation of conduction time. Caution is indicated in elderly patients and patients with cardiovascular disease, including a history of myocardial infarction, arrhythmias and/or ischaemic heart disease. Monitoring of cardiac function, including ECG, is indicated in such patients, especially during long-term treatment. Regular measurements of blood pressure are called for in patients susceptible to postural hypotension.

Activation of psychosis has occasionally been observed in schizophrenic patients receiving tricyclic antidepressants and must be considered a risk with Ludiomil. Similarly, hypomanic or manic episodes have been reported in patients with cyclic effective disorders while under treatment with a tricyclic antidepressant during a depressive phase. In such cases it may be necessary to reduce the dosage of Ludiomil or to withdraw the drug and administer an antipsychotic agent.

Precautions: The possibility of suicide in depressed patients is inherent in their illness and may persist until significant remission occurs. There are reports that antidepressants can, in rare instances, exacerbate suicidal tendencies. One study where Ludiomil was given as prophylactic treatment for unipolar depression suggested an increase in suicidal behaviour in the treated group. Therefore, patients must be carefully supervised during all phases of treatment with Ludiomil and prescriptions should be written for the smallest number of tablets consistent with good patient management.

In predisposed and elderly patients, tricyclic antidepressants may provoke pharmacogenic (delirious) psychoses, especially at night; these disappear without treatment within a few days of withdrawing the drug.

The elderly are particularly liable to experience side effects, especially agitation, confusion and postural hypotension. The initial dosage should therefore be increased with caution and the patients kept under close supervision (see *Dosage*).

Concomitant treatment with electroconvulsive therapy should be carried out only under careful supervision.

Abrupt withdrawal or dose reduction should be avoided because of possible adverse reactions (see *Side effects*).

Although reductions in the white blood cell count have been reported with Ludiomil only in isolated cases, periodic blood cell counts and monitoring for symptoms such as fever and sore throat are called for, particularly during the first few months of therapy.

During long-term treatment it is advisable to monitor hepatic and renal function.

Caution is also called for when treating patients with hyperthyroidism, or when administering thyroid hormone preparations, in view of the possibility of an increase in unwanted cardiac effects.

Because of its anticholinergic properties, Ludiomil should be used with caution in patients with a history of increased intra-ocular pressure, chronic severe constipation or a history of urinary retention (see *Contra-indications*).

Caution is called for in patients with chronic constipation. Tricyclic antidepressants may cause paralytic ileus, particularly in the elderly and bedridden patients.

An increase in dental caries has been reported in long-term treatment with antidepressants. Regular dental inspections are therefore advisable during long-term therapy.

Decreased lacrimation and relative accumulation of mucoid secretion associated with the anticholinergic properties of tricyclic antidepressants may cause damage to the corneal epithelium in patients who wear contact lenses.

Before general or local anaesthesia, inform the anaesthetist that the patient has been receiving Ludiomil. It is safer to continue treatment than to risk the potential disruption due to discontinuation of the drug before surgery.

Interactions with other drugs and other types of interactions: Concomitant treatment with Ludiomil and major tranquillisers may give rise to elevated concentrations of maprotiline in the serum, to lowering of the convulsion threshold and to seizures. Combination with thioridazine may produce severe cardiac arrythmia.

The following drug interactions, although not necessarily reported with Ludiomil, have been reported with tri/tetracyclic antidepressants.

Monoamine oxidase inhibitors (MAO): Do not give Ludiomil for at least 14 days after discontinuation of treatment with MAO inhibitors (there is a risk of severe interactions such as hyperpyrexia, tremor, delirium and possibly death). The same applies with giving a MAO inhibitor after previous treatment with Ludiomil. In both instances, the treatment should initially be given in small gradually increasing doses and its effects monitored.

Selective serotonin reuptake inhibitors (SSRI): Comedication may lead to additive effects on the serotonergic system. Fluvoxetine and fluvoxamine may also increase plasma concentrations of imipramine, with corresponding adverse effects.

Central nervous system depressants: Tricyclic antidepressants may potentiate the effects of alcohol and other central depressant substances (e.g. barbiturates, benzodiazepines or general anaesthetics).

Neuroleptics: concomitant use of these agents may cause an increase in plasma levels of maprotiline, a lowered convulsion threshold and seizures. Combination with thioridazine may produce severe cardiac arrhythmias.

Anticoagulants: Tricyclic antidepressants may potentiate the anticoagulant effect of coumarin drugs by inhibiting their metabolism by the liver. Careful monitoring of plasma prothrombin is therefore advised.

Anticholinergic agents: The effects of anticholinergic agents (e.g. phenothiazines, antiparkinsonian agents, atropine, biperiden, antihistamines) on the eye, central nervous system, bowel and bladder, may be potentiated.

Adrenergic neuronblockers: Diminution or abolition of the antihypertensive effects of drugs such as guanethidine, bethanidine, reserpine, clonidine and alpha-methyldopa, may occur. Patients requiring comedication for hypertension should therefore be given antihypertensives of a different type (e.g. diuretics, vasodilators or β-blockers).

Plasma concentrations of maprotiline may rise when the drug is given concomitantly with β-blockers that undergo substantial biotransformation, e.g. propranolol. In such cases, monitor plasma levels and adjust the dosage accordingly. Sudden withdrawal of Ludiomil can also result in serious hypotension.

Sympathomimetic drugs: Ludiomil may potentiate the cardiovascular effects of adrenaline, ephedrine, isoprenaline, noradrenaline, phenylephrine and phenylpropanolamine (e.g. as contained in local and general anaesthetic preparations and nasal decongestants). Close supervision (blood pressure, cardiac rhythm) and careful dosage adjustment are therefore required.

Quinidine: Tricyclic antidepressants should not be employed in combination with anti-arrhythmic agents of the quinidine type.

Liver-enzyme inducers: Drugs which activate the hepatic mono-oxygenase enzyme system (e.g. carbamazepine, barbiturates, phenytoin, nicotine and oral contraceptives) may accelerate the metabolism and lower the plasma concentrations of maprotiline, resulting in decreased efficacy. Plasma levels of phenytoin and carbamazepine may increase, with corresponding adverse effects. It may be necessary to adjust the dosage of these drugs.

Cimetidine: It is known that administration of cimetidine together with tricyclic antidepressants may lead to a rise in the latter's serum concentration and may cause unwanted effects (e.g. very severe dryness of the mouth, disturbances of vision).

Neuroleptics and methylphenidate may also increase plasma levels of Ludiomil.

Oral sulfonylureas or insulin: Comedication with antidiabetic agents may potentiate their hypoglycaemic effect. Diabetic patients should monitor their blood glucose when treatment with Ludiomil is initiated or discontinued.

Pregnancy and lactation: Use of Ludiomil during pregnancy should be avoided unless it is essential and there is no safer alternative.

As a general rule no drugs should be taken during the first 3 months of pregnancy, and the benefits and risks of taking drugs should be carefully considered throughout the whole of pregnancy.

Experience with Ludiomil in pregnancy is limited. Isolated cases suggesting a possible association between Ludiomil and adverse effects on the foetus have been reported. There is no evidence as to drug safety in human pregnancy; nor is there evidence that it is free from hazard.

Withdrawal symptoms in neonates whose mothers received tri/tetracyclic antidepressants during the third trimester have been reported.

Should use of Ludiomil during pregnancy be unavoidable Ludiomil should be withdrawn at least 7 weeks before the expected date of delivery, provided the clinical status of the patient permits, to prevent possible symptoms such as dyspnoea, lethargy, irritability, tachycardia, hypotonia, convulsions, jitters and hypothermia in the new-born.

Maprotiline passes into breast milk. After repeated administration of 150 mg daily for 5 days, the concentration measured in the breast milk exceeds that in the blood by a factor of 1.3–1.5. Nursing mothers should be advised to cease breast-feeding, although reports available so far have shown no adverse effects on the infant.

Effects on ability to drive or use machines: Patients receiving Ludiomil should be warned that blurred vision, drowsiness and other CNS symptoms (see *Side-effects*) may occur, in which case they should not drive, operate machinery or do anything else which may require alertness or quick actions. Patients should also be warned that consumption of alcohol or other drugs may potentiate these effects (see *Interactions*).

Undesirable effects: Side-effects: Various unwanted effects of Ludiomil are of a mild and transient nature and usually disappear in the further course of treatment or following a decrease in the dosage. Convulsions have been reported as occurring in patients both with and without a history of epilepsy. The rare occurrence of convulsions may increase at higher doses. Skin rashes are not uncommon, an incidence of 3% has been reported.

Elderly patients are particularly sensitive to adverse anticholinergic, neurological, psychiatric or cardiovascular reactions. Their ability to metabolise and eliminate drugs may be reduced, leading to a risk of elevated plasma concentrations at therapeutic doses.

The following adverse effects, although not necessarily reported with Ludiomil, have occurred with tri/tetracyclic antidepressants.

Frequency estimate: frequent >10%, occasional >1–10%, rare >0.001–1%, isolated cases <0.001%.

Central nervous system: Psychiatric: Frequent: drowsiness, fatigue. Occasional: increased appetite, restlessness, daytime sedation, anxiety, agitation, mania, hypomania, aggressiveness, impaired memory, sleep disturbances, insomnia, nightmares, aggravated depression, impaired concentration. Rare: delirium, hallucinations (particularly in geriatric patients), nervousness. Isolated cases: activation of psychotic symptoms, depersonalisation, fine tremor, myoclonus.

Neurological: Frequent: light-headedness, headache. Occasional: dizziness, dysarthria, muscle weakness, paraesthesiae (numbness, tingling). Rare: convulsions, ataxia, akathisia. Isolated cases: EEG changes, dyskinesia, inco-ordination, falls.

Anticholinergic effects: Frequent: dryness of the mouth. Occasional: constipation, sweating, hot flushes, blurred vision, disorders of visual accommodation, disturbances of micturition. Isolated cases: stomatitis, dental caries.

Cardiovascular system: Occasional: sinus tachycardia, postural hypotension, clinically irrelevant ECG changes (e.g. ST and T changes) in patients of normal cardiac status. Rare: arrhythmias, increased blood pressure. Isolated cases: conduction disorders (e.g. widening of QRS complex, bundle-branch block, PQ changes), syncope.

Gastro-intestinal tract: Occasional: nausea, vomiting; abdominal disorders. Rare: diarrhoea, elevated liver enzymes (transaminases, alkaline phosphatase). Isolated cases: hepatitis with or without jaundice.

Skin: Occasional: allergic skin reactions (rash, urticaria), sometimes with fever; photosensitivity. Isolated cases: itching, purpura, oedema (local or generalised), cutaneous vasculitis, alopecia, erythema multiforme.

Endocrine system and metabolism: Occasional: weight gain, disturbances of libido and potency. Isolated cases: enlarged mammary glands, galactorrhoea, SIADH (inappropriate antidiuretic hormone secretion syndrome).

Respiratory tract: Isolated cases: allergic alveolitis with or without eosinophilia, bronchospasm.

Blood: Isolated cases: leucopenia, agranulocytosis, eosinophilia, thrombocytopenia.

Sense organs: Isolated cases of tinnitus, taste disturbances, nasal congestion.

Miscellaneous: Withdrawal symptoms: Although not indicative of addiction, the following symptoms occasionally occur after abrupt cessation of therapy or reduction of the dose: nausea, vomiting, abdominal pain, diarrhoea, insomnia, headache, nervousness, anxiety, worsening of underlying depression or recurrence of depressed mood.

Overdose: The signs and symptoms of overdose with Ludiomil are similar to those reported with tricyclic antidepressants. Cardiac abnormalities and neurological disturbances are the main complications. In children accidental ingestion of any amount should be regarded as serious and potentially fatal.

Signs and symptoms: Symptoms generally appear within 4 hours of ingestion and reach a maximum severity at 24 hours. Due to delayed absorption (anticholinergic effect), long half-life and enterohepatic recycling, the patient may remain at risk for up to 4–6 days.

The following signs and symptoms may be seen.

Central nervous system: Drowsiness, stupor, coma, ataxia, restlessness, agitation, enhanced reflexes, muscular rigidity, choreo-athetotic movements, convulsions.

Cardiovascular system: Hypotension, tachycardia, arrhythmias, conduction disorders, shock, heart failure, in very rare cases, cadiac arrest. In addition, respiratory depression, cyanosis, vomiting, fever, midriasis, sweating and oliguria or anuria may occur.

Treatment: There is no specific antidote and treatment is essentially symptomatic and supportive.

Anyone suspected of receiving an overdose of Ludiomil, particularly children, should be hospitalised and kept under close surveillance for at least 72 hours.

Perform gastric lavage or induce vomiting as soon as possible if the patient is alert. If the patient has impaired consciousness, secure the airway with a cuffed endotracheal tube before beginning lavage, and do not induce vomiting. These measures are recommended for up to 12 hours or even longer after the overdose, since the anticholinergic effect of the drug may delay gastric emptying. Administration of activated charcoal may help to reduce drug absorption.

Treatment of symptoms is based on modern methods of intensive care, with continuous monitoring of cardiac function, blood gases, and electrolytes, and if necessary emergency measures such as:

- anticonvulsive therapy
- artificial respiration
- insertion of a temporary cardiac pacemaker
- plasma expander, dopamine or dobutamine administered by intravenous drip
- resuscitation.

Since it has been reported that physostigmine may cause severe bradycardia, asystole, and seizures, its use is not recommended in cases of overdosage with Ludiomil. Haemodialysis or peritoneal dialysis are ineffective because of the low plasma concentrations of maprotiline.

Pharmacological properties

Pharmacodynamic properties: Mode of action: Maprotiline is a tetracyclic antidepressant which shares basic therapeutic properties with the tricyclic antidepressants but differs from them structurally and pharmacologically. It has a potent and selective inhibitory effect on the re-uptake of noradrenalin. Maprotiline has a weak affinity for the central alpha$_1$-adrenoceptors but exerts little inhibitory effect on re-uptake of serotonin. It displays marked antihistaminic activity and a moderate anticholinergic effect.

Pharmacokinetic properties:

Absorption: Maprotiline is completely absorbed from Ludiomil film coated tablets, peak levels in the blood occurring within 8 hours. Steady state concentrations in the blood are attained during the second week of treatment and they are linearly proportional to dose but tend to be higher in elderly patients.

Distribution: The protein binding rate is 88–89%, independent of the patient's age or disease. The partition coefficient between blood and plasma is 1.7 and the apparent volume of distribution is 23–27 litres/kg. Concentrations in the cerebrospinal fluid are 2–13% of those in serum.

Biotransformation: Maprotiline hydrochloride is extensively metabolised; only 2–4% of the dose is excreted unchanged in the urine. The principal metabolite is the pharmacologically active desmethyl derivative. There are also several hydroxylated or methoxylated metabolites, which are excreted by the kidneys as conjugates.

Elimination: Maprotiline is eliminated from blood with a mean half-life of 43 hours. The mean systemic clearance ranges between 510 and 570 ml/min. Within 21 days, about two thirds of a single dose is excreted in the urine (predominantly as unchanged drug and conjugated metabolites) and 30% in the faeces.

Impairment of renal function does not affect maprotiline elimination half life provided that hepatic function is normal.

Characteristics in patients: In patients over 60 years of age: The steady-state concentrations for a given dose are higher and the elimination half-life longer than in younger patients. The dose should be halved.

Preclinical safety data: Animal experiments showed no teratogenic or mutagenic effects and no evidence of impaired fertility or harm to the foetus.

Pharmaceutical particulars

List of excipients: All coated tablets contain lactose, wheat starch, calcium phosphate, magnesium stearate, stearic acid, talc, hydroxypropyl methylcellulose, titanium dioxide, polysorbate 80, aerosil 200, yellow iron oxide.

Coated tablets of 25 mg, 50 mg and 75 mg also contain red iron oxide.

Incompatibilities: None known.

Shelf life: Five years.

Special precautions for storage: No special recommendations. Medicines should be kept out of reach of children.

Nature and contents of container: All tablets are packed in PVC/foil bubble packs of 28 tablets.

Instructions for use/handling: None.

Market authorisation holder: Novartis Pharmaceuticals (UK) Ltd, Trading as Ciba Laboratories, Frimley Business Park, Frimley, Camberley, Surrey GU16 5SG.

Marketing authorisation numbers

10 mg 00101/0505
25 mg 00101/0506
50 mg 00101/0507
75 mg 00101/0508

Date of approval/revision of SPL 1 December 1997.

Legal category POM.

MELLERIL* SUSPENSION

Qualitative and quantitative composition

Melleril Suspension 0.5%: Thioridazine base USP 25 mg/5 ml.

Melleril Suspension 2%: Thioridazine base USP 100 mg/5 ml.

Pharmaceutical form Opaque, grey/white viscous liquid.

Clinical particulars

Therapeutic indications:

Adults: Schizophrenia: treatment of symptoms and prevention of relapse.

Mania and hypomania.

As an adjunct to the short-term management of anxiety, moderate to severe psychomotor agitation, excitement, violent or dangerously impulsive behaviour. Agitation and restlessness in the elderly.

Children: Behaviour disorders and epilepsy – only where there are severe mental or behavioural problems such as senseless hyperactivity, aggressiveness, temper tantrums, self injury or mutilation, or agitation.

Posology and method of administration: Oral administration.

Adults: Daily dose range in terms of the hydrochloride†:

Schizophrenia, mania, hypomania: 150–600 mg.

For acute schizophrenia, an initial loading dose of 200 mg may be given. In hospitalised, resistant patients under specialist supervision, up to 800 mg daily may be administered for not more than 4 weeks.

Psychomotor agitation, excitement, violent or dangerously impulsive behaviour: 75–200 mg.

Anxiety, agitation and restlessness in the elderly: 30–100 mg.

There may be great variability in individual response and dosage requirements. In underweight patients, or in those suffering from kidney or liver disease, lower initial doses and more gradual increases are indicated.

Use in the elderly: In elderly patients lower initial doses and more gradual increases are indicated.

Children:

1 to 5 years of age: 1 mg/kg bodyweight.

5 years and over: Usually 75–150 mg/day. In severe cases up to 300 mg/day may be used.

Melleril suspension contains Thioridazine base. To convert from hydrochloride to base, multiply by 0.91.

As might be expected the *in vitro* dissolution profiles of the suspension and tablets differ; bioequivalence of the liquid and solid dose formulations should not therefore be assumed.

Contra-indications: Comatose states, severe depression of the CNS or a history of blood dyscrasia or severe cardiovascular disease. Phenothiazines can cause sleep apnoea and because of a possible correlation with sudden infant death syndrome, Melleril should not be given to children below one year of age.

Special warnings and precautions for use: Melleril should be used with caution in patients with cardiac arrhythmias, cardiac disease, severe respiratory disease, renal failure, Parkinson's disease, a personal or family history of narrow angle glaucoma, in prostatic hypertrophy, myasthenia gravis, epilepsy, phaeochromocytoma and in patients who have shown hypersensitivity to other phenothiazines. In patients with liver disease, regular monitoring of liver function is essential. Regular blood counts should be carried out during the first three to four months of treatment or if any clinical signs of blood dyscrasias appear. Phenothiazines generally may affect temperature regulation and decrease serum thyroxine concentrations, although this is very unlikely with Melleril.

Acute withdrawal symptoms including nausea, vomiting and insomnia have rarely been described after abrupt cessation of high dose Melleril. Gradual withdrawal is advisable. Drug withdrawal in children may lead to rapid clinical relapse and neurological symptoms, although this is less common with Melleril than with other antipsychotics.

Interaction with other medicaments and other forms of interaction: Melleril may enhance the central nervous system depression produced by other CNS depressant drugs including alcohol, hypnotics, sedatives or narcotic analgesics. In common with other phenothiazines, Melleril antagonises the action of adrenaline and other sympathomimetic agents, and may reverse the blood pressure lowering effects of adrenergic-blocking agents such as guanethidine and clonidine. Phenylpropanolamine has been reported to interact with phenothiazines and cause ventricular arrythmias. Melleril may affect the metabolism of tricyclic antidepressants, phenytoin and other anticonvulsants. It may also impair the antiparkinsonian effects of levodopa; it may possibly affect the control of diabetes or the action of anticoagulants. It may enhance the cardiac depressant effects of quinidine. Antacids should not be used within two hours of taking phenothiazines. Undesirable anticholinergic effects can be enhanced by anticholinergic drugs. Neurotoxicity resulting from combination with lithium has been reported rarely.

Pregnancy and lactation: Do not use during pregnancy unless there are compelling reasons. There is inadequate evidence for safety of the drug in human pregnancy, and there is some evidence of harmful effects in a few, but not all, animal studies. The newborn of mothers treated with Melleril in late pregnancy may show signs of intoxication such as excessive sleepiness, tremor and hyperactivity.

Do not use during lactation. If the use of Melleril is considered essential, breast feeding should be discontinued.

Effects on ability to drive and to use machines: Phenothiazines should be administered with caution to patients who participate in activities requiring complete mental alertness. They may impair the reactions of the patient e.g. when driving vehicles or operating machinery.

Undesirable effects: Common side-effects, particularly with higher dosage and at the start of treatment, include drowsiness, sedation, dry mouth and nasal stuffiness. Dose-related postural hypotension may occur, particularly in the elderly. Other dose-related anticholinergic-type side-effects including blurring of vision, tachycardia, constipation and urinary hesitancy or retention.

Even in low dosage, in susceptible (especially non-psychotic) individuals, Melleril may cause feelings of being mentally dulled or slowed down, nausea, dizziness, headache or paradoxical effects of excitement, agitation or insomnia. Confusional states or epileptic fits can occur.

At higher dose levels, as with other phenothiazines, ECG changes such as prolongation of the Q-T interval, flattening of the T-wave and the appearance of U-waves have been reported. These changes are more likely to occur in the presence of a low potassium blood level. Like all phenothiazines, Melleril may induce arrhythmias.

Pigmentary retinopathy has been observed in a small number of patients receiving long-term therapy with daily doses above the recommended maximum of 600 mg and has been seen rarely in patients taking less. It is characterised by decreased visual acuity, chromatopsia (usually brown-tinted vision) and impairment of dark adaption; progressive loss of vision may occur. Fundoscopic examination discloses deposits of pigment. The patient should be told of the importance of reporting any change in vision. If prolonged high-dose treatment is envisaged full ophthalmic examinations should be carried out at appropriate intervals.

The possibility of pigmentary retinopathy, together with the possibility of cardiotoxic reactions, emphasises the need not to increase doses beyond the recommended maximum daily dose of 600 mg. Extrapyramidal reactions may occur but are uncommon within the recommended dosage range; antiparkinsonian agents are therefore rarely required and should be prescribed with caution.

Whenever an antipsychotic agent is used, the possible risk of development of tardive dyskinesia should be considered, and the patient monitored for early signs. With Melleril the risk is less than with other phenothiazines, and tardive dyskinesia tends to be seen particularly with prolonged treatment at high doses. The potential seriousness and unpredictability of tardive dyskinesia and the fact that it has occasionally been reported to occur when neuroleptic antipsychotic drugs have been prescribed for relatively short periods in low dosage means that the prescribing of such agents requires especially careful assessment of risks versus benefit. Tardive dyskinesia can be precipitated or aggravated by antiparkinsonian drugs. Short-lived dyskinesias may occur after abrupt drug withdrawal.

Antipsychotic drugs such as Melleril may cause hyperprolactinaemia resulting in galactorrhoea and oligo- and amenorrhoea. Sexual function, including erection and ejaculation may be impaired. Weight gain is occasionally seen with Melleril and oedema has been reported. These effects may be prevented by reduction in dosage.

Blood dyscrasias have been reported: transient leucopenia can occur and agranulocytosis has been reported very rarely, most commonly in the first three months of treatment, but occasionally later. Blood counts should be performed if a patient develops signs of persistent infection.

Melleril very rarely may cause a photosensitivity reaction. The critical dose for this to occur is 400 to 600 mg daily. Other rare side-effects include skin rashes, altered seizure control, jaundice, hepatitis and liver dysfunction.

Long-term usage at doses above the recommended maximum may rarely cause increased melanin pigmentation of the skin, which may be irreversible. Although not reported with Melleril, phenothiazines have been reported to cause raised serum cholesterol, rarely hyperglycaemia, faecal impaction, severe paralytic ileus or megacolon.

Sudden and unexplained death, apparently due to arrhythmia or cardiac arrest, has been reported in patients treated with tricyclic neuroleptic agents including Melleril.

In isolated cases, neuroleptic malignant syndrome (muscular rigidity, hyperthermia, altered mental status, autonomic instability) a condition necessitating immediate discontinuation of the drug and appropriate symptomatic treatment, has been observed.

Overdose: Acute overdosage of Melleril usually gives rise to coma with shallow breathing, hypotension and absence of reflexes. Motor restlessness, hyperflexia, cardiac arrhythmias and epileptiform convulsions may occur. Treatment should be directed to the elimination of the ingested material by emesis and gastric lavage. General supportive measures should be applied with particular reference to the cardiovascular and respiratory systems.

Acute hypotension should be treated with plasma expanders. If treatment with a vasopressor (*not* adrenaline) proves necessary (as it might in resistant cases) careful monitoring of the patient, particularly of cardiac function, is indicated. Attention should be paid to symptoms of metabolic acidosis and delayed cardiac effects.

Pharmacological properties

Pharmacodynamic properties: Melleril exhibits the

same general pharmacological properties as the other members of the phenothiazine class of compounds. However, probably, as a result of more selective dopaminergic-blocking action in the limbic forebrain region rather than the nigrostriatal region Melleril has been shown to exhibit less extrapyramidal side-effects compared to the other major tranquillisers.

Pharmacokinetic properties: Melleril is rapidly and completely absorbed from the gastrointestinal tract. Maximum plasma concentrations are reached 2–4 hours after ingestion. The average systemic bioavailability is approximately 60%. The relative distribution volume is about 10 l/kg. Protein binding is high (more than 95%). Thioridazine is metabolised in the liver; some of the metabolites (e.g. thioridazine sulforidazine) possess pharmacodynamic properties similar to those of the parent compound. Excretion is mainly with the faeces (50%), but also via the kidney (less than 4% as unchanged drug, about 30% as metabolites). Plasma elimination half-life is approximately 10 hours. Thioridazine crosses the placenta, and passes into breast milk.

Preclinical safety data: Thioridazine was examined for genotoxicity in Ames tests and *in vivo* examinations such as the micronucleus test in mice, cytogenetic analysis in Chinese hamster bone marrow cells and the dominant lethal test in mice. The results of these tests gave no indications that thioridazine has mutagenic potential.

Fertility and carcinogenicity studies were not performed.

Pharmaceutical particulars

List of excipients: Buttermint, polysorbate 80, sodium hydroxide, carbomer, sugar granulated No 1, purified water.

Incompatibilities: None.

Shelf life: 48 months.

Special precautions for storage: Protect from light and heat.

Nature and contents of container: Amber glass bottle with a child resistant, tamper evident closure composed of polypropylene or polyethylene outer, a polypropylene or polyethylene inner with a wad faced with PP, PVDC or PET lining in pack sizes of either 1000 ml, 500 ml or 300 ml.

Instruction for use/handling: None.

Marketing authorisation holder: Novartis Pharmaceuticals UK Ltd, Trading as Sandoz Pharmaceuticals.

Marketing authorisation numbers

Suspension 0.5% 0101/0052R
Suspension 2.0% 0101/0053R

Date of approval/revision of SPC October 1997.

Legal category POM.

MELLERIL* SYRUP
MELLERIL* TABLETS

Qualitative and quantitative composition

Syrup: Thioridazine Hydrochloride PhEur 27.5 mg/5 ml.

Tablets
Thioridazine Hydrochloride PhEur 10 mg.
Thioridazine Hydrochloride PhEur 25 mg.
Thioridazine Hydrochloride PhEur 50 mg.
Thioridazine Hydrochloride PhEur 100 mg.

Pharmaceutical form

Syrup: Clear, pale brown syrup with the odour of spearmint/anise.

Tablets: White film coated tablets with a bevel edge, embossed MEL on one side with the strength on the other. Dimensions are as follows:
10 mg Tablets: 6.3 mm in diameter, 2.7 mm thick and weigh 82 mg.
25 mg Tablets: 7.3 mm in diameter, 3.4 mm thick and weigh 143 mg.
50 mg Tablets: 8.3 mm in diameter, 3.7 mm thick and weigh 204 mg.
100 mg Tablets: 9.3 mm in diameter, 3.8 mm thick and weigh 245 mg.

Clinical particulars

Therapeutic indications:

Adults: Schizophrenia: treatment of symptoms and prevention of relapse.

Mania and hypomania.

As an adjunct to the short-term management of anxiety, moderate to severe psychomotor agitation, excitement, violent or dangerously impulsive behaviour.

Agitation and restlessness in the elderly.

Children: Behaviour disorders and epilepsy – only where there are severe mental or behavioural problems such as senseless hyperactivity, aggressiveness, temper trantrums, self injury or mutilation, or agitation.

Posology and method of administration: Oral administration.

Adults: Daily dose range in terms of the hydrochloride. Schizophrenia, mania, hypomania: 150–600 mg.

For acute schizophrenia, an initial loading dose of 200 mg may be given. In hospitalised, resistant patients under specialist supervision, up to 800 mg daily may be administered for not more than 4 weeks.

Psychomotor agitation, excitement, violent or dangerously impulsive behaviour: 75–200 mg.

Anxiety, agitation and restlessness in the elderly: 30–100 mg.

There may be great variability in individual response and dosage requirements. In underweight patients, or in those suffering from kidney or liver disease, lower initial doses and more gradual increases are indicated.

Use in the elderly: In elderly patients lower initial doses and more gradual increases are indicated.

Children:
Syrup:
1 to 5 years of age: 1 mg/kg bodyweight.
5 years and over. Usually 75–150 mg/day. In severe cases up to 300 mg/day may be used.

MELLERIL syrup may be diluted with water, Sorbitol solution (70%) or preservative free syrup BP.

Tablets:
0 to 1 year of age: Not recommended, see *Contra-indications.*
1 to 5 years of age: 10 mg tablet: 1 mg/kg/body weight. The 25 mg, 50 mg and 100 mg tablets are not suitable for children.
5 years and over: Usually 75–150 mg/day. In severe cases up to 300 mg/day may be used.

Contra-indications: Comatose states, severe depression of the CNS or a history of blood dyscrasia or severe cardiovascular disease. Phenothiazines can cause sleep apnoea and because of a possible correlation with sudden infant death syndrome, MELLERIL should not be given to children below one year of age.

Special warnings and precautions for use: MELLERIL should be used with caution in patients with cardiac arrhythmias, cardiac disease, severe respiratory disease, renal failure, Parkinson's disease, a personal or family history of narrow angle glaucoma, in prostatic hypertrophy, myasthenia gravis, epilepsy, phaeochromocytoma and in patients who have shown hypersensitivity to other phenothiazines. In patients with liver disease, regular monitoring of liver function is essential. Regular blood counts should be carried out during the first three to four months of treatment or if any clinical signs of blood dyscrasias appear. Phenothiazines generally may affect temperature regulation and decrease serum thyroxine concentrations, although this is very unlikely with MELLERIL.

Acute withdrawal symptoms including nausea, vomiting and insomnia have rarely been described after abrupt cessation of high dose MELLERIL. Gradual withdrawal is advisable. Drug withdrawal in children may lead to rapid clinical relapse and neurological symptoms, although this is less common with MELLERIL than with other antipsychotics.

Interaction with other medicaments and other forms of interaction: MELLERIL may enhance the central nervous system depression produced by other CNS depressant drugs including alcohol, hypnotics, sedatives or narcotic analgesics. In common with other phenothiazines, MELLERIL antagonists the action of adrenaline and other sympathomimetic agents, and may reverse the blood pressure lowering effects of adrenergic-blocking agents such as guanethidine and clonidine. Phenylpropanolamine has been reported to interact with phenothiazines and cause ventricular arrythmias. MELLERIL may affect the metabolism of tricyclic antidepressants, phenytoin and other anticonvulsants. It may also impair the antiparkinsonian effects of levodopa; it may possibly affect the control of diabetes or the action of anticoagulants. It may enhance the cardiac depressant effects of quinidine. Antacids should not be used within two hours of taking phenothiazines. Undesirable anticholinergic effects can be enhanced by anticholinergic drugs. Neurotoxicity resulting from combination with lithium has been reported rarely.

Pregnancy and lactation: Do not use during pregnancy unless there are compelling reasons. There is inadequate evidence for safety of the drug in human pregnancy, and there is some evidence of harmful effects in a few, but not all, animal studies. The newborn of mothers treated with MELLERIL in late pregnancy may show signs of intoxication such as excessive sleepiness, tremor and hyperactivity.

Do not use during lactation. If the use of MELLERIL is considered essential, breast feeding should be discontinued.

Effects on ability to drive and to use machines: Phenothiazines should be administered with caution to patients who participate in activities requiring complete mental alertness. They may impair the reactions of the patient e.g. when driving vehicles or operating machinery.

Undesirable effects: Common side-effects, particularly with higher dosage and at the start of treatment, include drowsiness, sedation, dry mouth and nasal stuffiness. Dose-related postural hypotension may occur, particularly in the elderly. Other dose-related anticholinergic-type side-effects including blurring of vision, tachycardia, constipation and urinary hesitancy or retention.

Even in low dosage, in susceptible (especially non-psychotic) individuals, MELLERIL may cause feelings of being mentally dulled or slowed down, nausea, dizziness, headache or paradoxical effects of excitement, agitation or insomnia. Confusional states or epileptic fits can occur.

At higher dose levels, as with other phenothiazines, ECG changes such as prolongation of the Q-T interval, flattening of the T-wave and the appearance of U-waves have been reported. These changes are more likely to occur in the presence of a low potassium blood level. Like all phenothiazines, MELLERIL may induce arrhythmias.

Pigmentary retinopathy has been observed in a small number of patients receiving long-term therapy with daily doses above the recommended maximum of 600 mg and has been seen rarely in patients taking less. It is characterised by decreased visual acuity, chromatopsia (usually brown-tinted vision) and impairment of dark adaption; progressive loss of vision may occur. Fundoscopic examination discloses deposits of pigment. The patient should be told of the importance of reporting any change in vision. If prolonged high-dose treatment is envisaged full ophthalmic examination should be carried out at appropriate intervals.

The possibility of pigmentary retinopathy, together with the possibility of cardiotoxic reactions, emphasises the need not to increase doses beyond the recommended maximum daily dose of 600 mg. Extrapyramidal reactions may occur but are uncommon within the recommended dosage range; antiparkinsonian agents are therefore rarely required and should be prescribed with caution.

Whenever an antipsychotic agent is used, the possible risk of development of tardive dyskinesia should be considered, and the patient monitored for early signs. With MELLERIL the risk is less than with other phenothiazines, and tardive dyskinesia tends to be seen particularly with prolonged treatment at high doses. The potential seriousness and unpredictability of tardive dyskinesia and the fact that it has occasionally been reported to occur when neuroleptic antipsychotic drugs have been prescribed for relatively short periods in low dosage means that the prescribing of such agents requires especially careful assessment of risks versus benefit. Tardive dyskinesia can be precipitated or aggravated by antiparkinsonian drugs. Short-lived dyskinesias may occur after abrupt drug withdrawal.

Antipsychotic drugs such as MELLERIL may cause hyperprolactinaemia resulting in galactorrhoea and oligo- and amenorrhoea. Sexual function, including erection and ejaculation may be impaired. Weight gain is occasionally seen with MELLERIL and oedema has been reported. These effects may be prevented by reduction in dosage.

Blood dyscrasias have been reported: transient leucopenia can occur and agranulocytosis has been reported very rarely, most commonly in the first three months of treatment, but occasionally later. Blood counts should be performed if a patient develops signs of persistent infection.

MELLERIL very rarely may cause a photosensitivity reaction. The critical dose for this to occur is 400 to 600 mg daily. Other rare side-effects include skin rashes, altered seizure control, jaundice, hepatitis and liver dysfunction.

Long-term usage at doses above the recommended maximum may rarely cause increased melanin pigmentation of the skin, which may be irreversible. Although not reported with MELLERIL, phenothiazines have been reported to cause raised serum cholesterol, rarely hyperglycaemia, faecal impaction, severe paralytic ileus or megacolon.

Sudden and unexplained death, apparently due to arrhythmia or cardiac arrest, has been reported in patients treated with tricyclic neuroleptic agents including MELLERIL.

In isolated cases, neuroleptic malignant syndrome (muscular rigidity, hyperthermia, altered mental status, autonomic instability) a condition necessitating immediate discontinuation of the drug and appropriate symptomatic treatment, has been observed.

Overdose: Acute overdosage of MELLERIL usually gives rise to coma with shallow breathing, hypotension and absence of reflexes. Motor restlessness, hyperflexia, cardiac arrhythmias and epileptiform convulsions may occur. Treatment should be directed to the elimination of the ingested material by emesis and gastric lavage. General supportive measures should be applied with particular reference to the cardiovascular and respiratory systems.

Acute hypotension should be treated with plasma expanders. If treatment with a vasopressor (*not* adrenaline) proves necessary (as it might in resistant cases) careful monitoring of the patient, particularly of cardiac function, is indicated. Attention should be paid to symptoms of metabolic acidosis and delayed cardiac effects.

Pharmacological properties

Pharmacodynamic properties: MELLERIL exhibits the same general pharmacological properties as the other members of the phenothiazine class of compounds. However, probably as a result of more selective dopaminergic-blocking action in the limbic forebrain region rather than the nigrostriatal region MELLERIL has been shown to exhibit less extrapyramidal side-effects compared to the other major tranquillisers.

Pharmacokinetic properties: MELLERIL is rapidly and completely absorbed from the gastrointestinal tract. Maximum plasma concentrations are reached 2–4 hours after ingestion. The average systemic bioavailability is approximately 60%. The relative distribution volume is about 10 l/kg. Protein binding is high (more than 95%). Thioridazine is metabolised in the liver; some of the metabolites (e.g. thioridazine sulforidazine) possess pharmacodynamic properties similar to those of the parent compound. Excretion is mainly with the faeces (50%), but also via the kidney (less than 4% as unchanged drug, about 30% as metabolites). Plasma elimination half-life is approximately 10 hours. Thioridazine crosses the placenta, and passes into breast milk.

Preclinical safety data: Thioridazine was examined for genotoxicity in Ames tests and *in vivo* examinations such as the micronucleus test in mice, cytogenetic analysis in Chinese hamster bone marrow cells and the dominant lethal test in mice. The results of these tests gave no indications that thioridazine has mutagenic potential.

Fertility and carcinogenicity studies were not performed.

Pharmaceutical particulars

List of excipients:

Syrup: Caramel 16398, menthol, ascorbic acid, spearmint essence, essence of anise, monopropylene glycol, ethyl alcohol, glycerol, polyvinylpyrrolidone, liquid glucose, sorbitol syrup (70%), sugar granulated No. 1, purified water.

Tablets: Collidal anhydrous silica, magnesium stearate, talc, polyvinylpyrrolidone, maize starch, lactose. The film coating constituents are hydroxypropyl methylcellulose, polyethylene glycol, titanium dioxide, carnuba wax.

Incompatibilities: None.

Shelf life: Syrup: 36 months. *Tablets:* 36 months (polypropylene securitainer). 60 months (opaque white PVC/PVdC blister strips).

Special precautions for storage: Syrup: Protect from light; shake bottle before use. Diluted syrup should be used within 14 days of preparation. *Tablets:* Protect from direct light.

Nature and contents of container: Syrup: Amber glass bottle with a polyethylene closure (polythene wad faced with PP, PVDC or PET lining). *Tablets:* Opaque white PVC/PVDC blister strip or polypropylene securitainers.

Instructions for use/handling: None.

Marketing authorisation holder Novartis Pharmaceuticals UK Ltd, Trading as Sandoz Pharmaceuticals.

Marketing authorisation numbers

Syrup	0101/5034R
Tablets	
10 mg	0101/5033R
25 mg	0101/5053R
50 mg	0101/5054R
100 mg	0101/5055R

Date of approval/revision of SPC May 1997.

Legal category POM.

METROGEL*

Qualitative and quantitative composition Metronidazole BP 0.75%.

Pharmaceutical form Aqueous gel for cutaneous use.

Clinical particulars

Therapeutic indications: For the treatment of acute inflammatory exacerbations of rosacea.

For the deodorisation of the smell associated with malodorous fungating tumours.

Posology and method of administration: For the treatment of rosacea.

Adults and elderly: Apply to the affected skin of the face in a thin film twice daily for a period of eight to nine weeks. Thereafter, further applications may be necessary depending on the severity of the condition.

Children: Not recommended.

For the deodorisation of malodorous fungating tumours.

Adults and elderly: Clean the wound thoroughly. Apply the gel over the complete area and cover with a non-adherent dressing. Use once or twice daily as necessary.

Children: Not recommended.

Contra-indications: In patients known to be hypersensitive to metronidazole or bronopol.

Special warnings and precautions for use: Avoid contact with the eyes. If contact occurs the gel should be washed out carefully with water.

Interaction with other medicaments and other forms of interaction: The following statement takes into account the possibility that metronidazole may be absorbed after topical application. However, there is evidence to suggest that the systemic absorption of metronidazole following the topical administration of Metrogel is slight. A disulfiram-like reaction has been reported in a small number of patients taking oral metronidazole and alcohol concomitantly.

Pregnancy and lactation: The safety of metronidazole in pregnancy and lactation has not been adequately established. The gel should therefore not be used in these circumstances unless the physician considers it essential. Medication should be stopped if pregnancy occurs.

Effects on ability to drive and use machines: None.

Undesirable effects: Dryness of the skin may be experienced after application.

Overdose: Overdosage is extremely unlikely. If necessary, medication should be removed by washing with warm water.

Pharmacological properties

Pharmacodynamic properties: The aetiology of rosacea is unknown although a variety of hypotheses have been reported.

Pharmacokinetic properties: The systemic concentration of Metronidazole following the topical administration of 1 g of a 0.75% metronidazole gel to 10 patients with rosacea ranged from 25 ng/ml (limit of detection), to 66 ng/ml with a mean C_{max} of 40.6 ng/ml.

The corresponding mean C_{max} following the oral administration of a solution containing 30 mg of metronidazole was 850 ng/ml (equivalent to 212 ng/ml if dose corrected). The mean T_{max} for the topical formulation was 6.0 hours compared to 0.97 hours for the oral solution.

Preclinical safety data: Metronidazole is a well established pharmaceutical active ingredient and to the subject of pharmacopoeial monograph in both the BP and PhEur.

Pharmaceutical particulars

List of excipients:

Bronopol	BP
Hydroxybenzoic acid esters	HSE
Hydroxyethylcellulose	HSE
Propylene glycol	PhEur
Phosphoric acid	PhEur
Purified water	PhEur

Incompatibilities: None known.

Shelf life: 2 years.

Special precautions for storage: Store between 15°C and 25°C in a dry place.

Nature and contents of container: Tube: Internally lacquered, membrane sealed aluminium.

Cap: Low density polyethylene.

Pack sizes available: 5 g (sample size), and 40 g.

Instructions for use/handling: There are no special instructions for use/handling.

Marketing authorisation holder: Galderma UK Limited, Leywood House, Woodside Road, Amersham, Buckinghamshire, HP6 6AA.

Marketing authorisation number PL 10590/0035

Date of first authorisation/renewal of authorisation 27 February 1998.

Date of (partial) revision of the text March 1997.

MIACALCIC* AMPOULES MIACALCIC* MULTIDOSE VIALS

Qualitative and quantitative composition

Ampoules: Salcatonin BP 50 IU/ml and 100 IU/ml.

Multidose vials: Salcatonin BP 200 IU/ml.

Pharmaceutical form Clear, colourless parenteral solution.

Clinical particulars

Therapeutic indications:

Hypercalcaemic crisis: Due to tumoral osteolysis secondary to breast, lung, kidney and other malignancies.

Due to osteolysis induced by myeloma.

Due to primary hyperparathyroidism.

Short term treatment of chronic hypercalcaemia: Paget's disease of bone (osteitis deformans), particularly in cases with:

- bone pain;
- neurological complications;
- increased bone turnover reflected in elevated alkaline phosphatase and hydroxyproline excretion;
- progressive extension of bone lesions;
- incomplete or repeated fractures.

Pain associated with advanced metastatic bone cancer:

Short term use in post menopausal osteoporosis: Studies based on total blood calcium determinators have indicated that Miacalcic may be effective in the prevention of progressive loss of bone mass in the treatment of post-menopausal osteoporosis.

Posology and method of administration: Miacalcic may be administered subcutaneously, intramuscularly or by intravenous injection.

The solution provided in multidose vials contains phenol (5 mg/ml) as a preservative and is not suitable for intravenous bolus injection.

The 50 IU/ml or 100 IU/ml ampoules can be used for intravenous infusion, which is the most effective method of administration and should always be used in emergencies or severe cases. However, there is a loss of potency of approximately 20% when Miacalcic is diluted. This should be taken into account when calculating dosage 5–10 IU (0.50–0.1 ml) Miacalcic per kg body weight daily, by slow intravenous infusion in 500 ml physiological saline over at least six hours.

Short term treatment of chronic hypercalcaemia: 5–10 IU per kg body weight daily by subcutaneous or intramuscular injection as a single dose or in two divided doses. If the volume for injection exceeds 2 ml intramuscular injection is preferable and multiple sites of injection should be used.

Treatment should be adjusted according to the patient's response and should not exceed three months; the definitive treatment should be for the underlying cause.

Paget's disease: 100 IU (1 ml) daily by subcutaneous or intramuscular injection. In some cases the injections may be given only every second day. In particular after improvement of the objective and subjective symptoms, an injection of 50 IU per day may be sufficient. Clinical improvement is usually seen within 3 months, but may occasionally be delayed for as long as a year.

Treatment should be limited to one course of 6 months followed by a treatment free period. A new treatment course of 6 months can be resumed in the case of biochemical relapse.

Pain associated with advanced metastatic bone cancer: 200 IU, depending on tolerability, up to 4 times in 24 hours by either the subcutaneous or intramuscular route has been shown to be effective in some patients and to permit reduction in the dose of concomitantly administered analgesics. Relief of pain may last for one week or longer. Treatment may be repeated at the discretion of the physician.

Postmenopausal osteoporosis: 100 IU daily by subcutaneous or intramuscular injection. Patients should also receive supplementary calcium (equivalent to 600 mg elemental calcium daily) and if necessary, vitamin D (400 units daily). An adequate diet is also essential.

Use in children: There is very little experience with use in children. The recommended adult dose should be reduced according to the child's lower body weight.

Miacalcic should be given to children for periods not more than a few weeks, unless physicians conclude that longer treatment is indicated on compelling grounds. Careful surveillance of bone growth is recommended.

Use in elderly: There is no evidence to suggest that elderly patients require different dosages or show different side-effects from younger patients. However, elderly patients should be supervised as factors sometimes associated with ageing such as poor diet or impaired renal function, may affect tolerance and may required dosage reduction.

Contra-indications: Hypersensitivity see *Precautions.*

Special warnings and precautions for use: Treatment with Miacalcic markedly reduces serum alkaline phosphatase and urinary hydroxyproline excretion, often to normal levels. In rare cases alkaline phosphatase and hydroxyproline excretion levels may rise after an initial fall; the physician must then judge from the clinical picture whether treatment should be continued. Disorders of bone metabolism may recur one or several months after treatment has been discontinued, necessitating a new course of Miacalcic.

Miacalcic is excreted mainly via the kidneys, therefore dosage adjustment may be required in patients with impaired renal function. Antibodies to salmon calcitonin may develop in a few patients following prolonged therapy. Clinical efficacy, however, is usually not affected. Escape phenomena are sometimes observed following prolonged use, but this is not necessarily related to the development of antibodies. Therapeutic response to Miacalcic may be restored after an interruption of treatment.

Interaction with other medicaments and other forms of interaction: Following injections of calcitonin, serum calcium levels may be transiently lowered but usually stay within normal values. This effect is noted most frequently on initiation of therapy where bone turnover is abnormally high, but diminishes as osteoclastic activity is reduced with Miacalcic. This phenomenon does not usually give rise to complications. It is theoretically possible that dosage adjustments may be required in patients receiving concurrent cardiac glycosides as their effect might be modified by changes in cellular electrolyte concentrations.

Pregnancy and lactation: Salmon calcitonin has been shown to cause decrease in foetal birth weight in rabbits when given in doses of 14–56 times the dose recommended for human use. Since calcitonin does not cross the placental barrier, this finding may be due to metabolic effects of calcitonin on the pregnant animal. Studies have not been carried out in pregnant women. Whenever possible, treatment should be avoided in women of child-bearing potential. Calcitonin has been shown to inhibit lactation in animals and should not be administered to nursing mothers.

Effects on ability to drive and to use machines: None known.

Other undesirable side-effects: Nausea and occasional vomiting, slight facial flushing accompanied by a sensation of heat.

Occasional irritation at injection site, skin rash, diarrhoea and dizziness have occurred. Effects are usually dose dependent and occur more frequently after intravenous than after subcutaneous or intramuscular administration. They usually subside spontaneously and a temporary reduction in dosage is only necessary in exceptional cases.

Anti-emetics may be used if necessary during treatment.

Hypersensitivity reactions may occur (see *Precautions*).

As Miacalcic is a polypeptide, local or general hypersensitivity reactions are a possibility in rare cases. Symptoms may include local effects at the injection site or generalised skin reactions. Isolated anaphylactic-type reactions resulting in tachycardia, dyspnoea, hypotension and collapse have been reported. If any symptoms observed can definitely be ascribed to the drug, the treatment should be stopped.

In patients with a history of allergic reactions a skin sensitivity test is advisable before starting treatment. A 1:100 dilution in physiological saline may be used.

Overdosage: No serious consequences due to overdosage have yet been reported. Treatment would be symptomatic.

Pharmacological properties

Pharmacodynamic properties: Calcitonin is a major regulating factor in mineral and skeletal metabolism; it interferes with the action of parathyroid hormone in the maintenance of skeletal mass, by acting both on bone and on calcium homeostasis. It markedly reduces the removal of calcium from bone in conditions with a greatly increased rate of resorption and formation such as Paget's disease and malignant osteolysis. Osteoclast activity is inhibited and osteoblast formation and activity seem to be stimulated. Calcitonin inhibits osteolysis, thus lowering the abnormally increased serum calcium. Additionally, it increases the urinary excretion of calcium, phosphorus and sodium by reducing their tubular re-uptake. Serum calcium is not reduced below the normal range.

Calcitonin reduces gastric and exocrine pancreatic secretion without influencing gastrointestinal motility. Clinical experience demonstrates that Miacalcic possesses analgesic activity. Investigations have shown specific salmon calcitonin binding sites in some areas of the central nervous system.

All calcitonin structures show 32 amino-acids in a single chain, the sequence of which differs from species to species. Due to its greater affinity to receptor binding sites than synthetic calcitonins from mammalian species, including the synthetic human calcitonin, Miacalcic is clinically more potent and longer acting.

Pharmacokinetic properties: Pharmacokinetic studies indicate the bioavailability after intramuscular or subcutaneous injection to be about 70%. Maximum plasma concentrations are obtained within one hour. Elimination half-life of 70 to 90 minutes. Miacalcic and its metabolites are excreted up to 95% by the kidney, percentage of parent drug being about 2%. The apparent volume of distribution is 0.15–0.3 litre/kg and the protein binding is 30–40%.

Pre-clinical safety data: No relevant pre-clinical safety data are available. Miacalcic has been marketed for many years.

Pharmaceutical particulars

List of excipients:

50 IU/ml and 100 IU/ml ampoules: Glacial acetic acid, sodium acetate trihydrate, sodium chloride, water for injection.

400 IU/2 ml multidose vials: Glacial acetic acid, sodium acetate trihydrate, sodium chloride, phenol, water for injection.

Incompatibilities: None.

Shelf life: 50 IU/ml and 100 IU/ml ampoules – 60 months. 400 IU/2 ml multidose vials – 36 months, 1 month after initial use.

Special precautions for storage: Store in a refrigerator (2–8°C). Do not freeze. Allow to reach room temperature before subcutaneous or intramuscular use.

The multidose vial can be stored at room temperature once started. Its unused portion of contents must be discarded one month after initial use.

Nature and contents of container: Ampoules: glass ampoule – uncoloured.

Multidose vial: glass vial – uncoloured, with rubber stopper.

Instructions for use/handling: Allow to reach room temperature before intramuscular or subcutaneous use. Solutions for infusions should be prepared immediately before use and glass or hard plastic containers should not be used.

Marketing authorisation holders: Novartis Pharmaceuticals Ltd, Trading as Sandoz Pharmaceuticals.

Marketing authorisation numbers

50 IU ampoule	0101/0202
100 IU ampoule	0101/0095
400 IU multidose vial	0101/0203

Date of approval/revision of SPC May 1996.

Legal category POM.

NAVISPARE TABLETS*

Qualitative and quantitative composition 6-Chloro-3-(cyclopentylmethyl)-3,4-dihydro-2H-1,2,4-benzothiadiazine-7-sulfonamide 1,1-dioxide (Cyclopenthiazide BP) 0.25 mg.

N-amindino-3,5-diamino-6-chloropyrazine-2-carboxamide hydrochloride dihydrate (Amiloride Hydrochloride PhEur) 2.5 mg.

Pharmaceutical form Coated tablets.

Clinical particulars

Therapeutic indications: For the treatment of mild to moderate hypertension.

Posology and method of administration

Adults: Usually 1 or 2 Navispare tablets taken once a day in the morning.

Elderly: Although no special dosage regime is necessary in the elderly, particular caution should be exercised in the elderly, since they are more susceptible to electrolyte imbalances.

Children: Navispare is not suitable for use in children.

Contra-indications: Hypersensitivity to cyclopenthiazide or other sulphonamide derivatives; Addison's disease; hyperkalaemia; in the presence of other potassium conserving agents or potassium supplements; anuria; severe renal and hepatic failure; diabetic nephropathy; concurrent lithium therapy; refractory hypokalaemia and hyponatraemia; hypercalcaemia; symptomatic hyperuricaemia.

Special warnings and special precautions for use

Warnings: None known.

Precautions: Diabetes mellitus: Hyperkalaemia has occurred in diabetic patients receiving amiloride hydrochloride, especially those with chronic renal disease or pre-renal azotaemia. The status of renal function should therefore be determined before use in a known or suspected diabetic patient. Navispare should be discontinued for at least three days before a glucose tolerance test.

Prolonged doses may bring about a decrease in glucose tolerance and precipitate a diabetic condition. In known diabetics the addition of a thiazide to the treatment regime may alter their antidiabetic requirement.

Metabolic or respiratory acidosis: Potassium conserving therapy should be initiated with caution in patients in whom metabolic or respiratory acidosis may occur, e.g. patients with cardiopulmonary disease or decompensated diabetes. Shifts in acid-base balance of extracellular potassium and the development of acidosis may be associated with rapid increase in plasma potassium.

Electrolyte considerations: In patients with renal impairment, a rise in blood urea can occur. In such cases, either the dose should be reduced or the treatment interrupted temporarily. Thiazides may precipitate an attack of gout in patients predisposed to this condition.

The elderly, especially those suffering from chronic disease and patients with hepatic cirrhosis are more susceptible to a lack of electrolyte and fluid balance homeostasis. During treatment with thiazides hyponatraemia accompanied by neurological symptoms has been observed in isolated cases. In the elderly and patients with hepatic cirrhosis, the serum electrolytes should be monitored at more frequent intervals.

Patients receiving relatively high doses of thiazides may develop hypomagnesaemia accompanied by signs and symptoms such as nervousness, muscle spasms and cardiac arrhythmias.

Miscellaneous: In patients with hyperlipidaemia, the serum lipids should be regularly monitored. In the event of a rise in serum lipids, withdrawal of the thiazide medication should be considered.

Lupus erythematosus may possibly become activated under treatment with thiazides.

Interaction with other medicaments and other forms of interaction: The concomitant administration of thiazides with other antihypertensive agents (e.g. beta-blockers, vasodilators, calcium antagonists) may necessitate adjustment of the dosage of those drugs.

The concomitant administration of potassium-sparing agents such as amiloride and ACE inhibitors may increase serum potassium levels and is not to be recommended. However, if the concomitant use of these agents is deemed appropriate, they should be used with caution and with frequent monitoring of plasma potassium.

NSAIDs may attenuate the antihypertensive effect of thiazide diuretics.

Thiazide containing drugs may increase the responsiveness to tubocurarine.

Orthostatic hypotension may occur and may be potentiated by alcohol, barbiturates and narcotics.

Pregnancy and lactation: Diuretics are best avoided for the management of oedema or hypertension in pregnancy as their use may be associated with hypovolaemia, increased blood viscosity and reduced placental perfusion. There is inadequate evidence of safety in human pregnancy and there have been reports of foetal bone marrow depression, thrombocytopenia, and foetal and neonatal jaundice reported with the use of thiazide diuretics.

As cyclopenthiazide passes into breast milk, Navispare should be avoided in mothers who wish to breast-feed. It is not known whether amiloride hydrochloride passes into breast milk.

Effects on ability to drive and use machines: None stated.

Undesirable effects: Navispare is generally well tolerated. Reported side effects of the combination include rare cases of dizziness, headache, light-headedness, tiredness, nausea and vomiting, discomfort/pain in the chest. However, the following side effects of cyclopenthiazide and amiloride as single agents have been reported.

Cyclopenthiazide:

Skin: Occasional: allergic urticaria (nettle rash) and other forms of skin rash.

Rare: photosensitisation. Isolated cases: necrotising vasculitis.

Gastro-intestinal tract: Occasional: loss of appetite, mild nausea, vomiting.

Rare: gastrospasm, diarrhoea or possibly constipation. Isolated cases: pancreatitis.

Central nervous system: Rare: headache, muzziness, dizziness, sleep disturbances, depression and paraesthesiae.

Blood: Rare: thrombocytopenia, sometimes with purpura. In isolated cases: leucopenia, agranulocytosis, anaemia and bone marrow depression.

Electrolytes: Frequent: hypokalaemia. Occasional: hyponatraemia, hypomagnesaemia.

Rare: hypercalcaemia. If hypercalcaemia occurs, further diagnostic clarification is necessary (e.g. possibility of hyperparathyroidism).

In isolated cases: hypochloraemic alkalosis.

Liver: Rare: intrahepatic cholestasis or jaundice.

Miscellaneous: Occasional impotence.

Metabolic: Occasional: hyperuricaemia. Rare: hyperglycaemia, glycosuria. Gout or diabetes may be precipitated or aggravated. Increased blood lipid levels in response to higher doses.

Cardiovascular system: Occasional: postural hypotension, which may be aggravated by alcohol, anaesthetics, or sedatives. Rare: cardiac arrhythmias.

Amiloride:

Gastro-intestinal tract: Rare: anorexia, nausea, vomiting, abdominal pain.

In isolated cases: diarrhoea, constipation, GI bleeding, jaundice, thirst, dyspepsia, heartburn, flatulence.

Central nervous system: Rare: dizziness, paraesthesiae, tremors, mental confusion.

In isolated cases: encephalopathy, nervousness, insomnia, decreased libido, depression, somnolence, vertigo.

Cardiovascular system: Rare: palpitation. In isolated cases: angina pectoris, orthostatic hypotension, arrhythmias.

Respiratory: Rare: cough, dyspnoea.

Urogenital: Rare: frequency of micturition. In isolated cases: impotence, polyuria, dysuria.

Musculoskeletal: Rare: joint pain. In isolated cases: muscle cramps.

Skin and appendages: Rare: pruritus, rash, alopecia. In isolated cases: dryness of mouth.

Overdose:

Signs and symptoms: In cases of overdosage the following signs and symptoms may occur. Dizziness, nausea, somnolence, hypovolaemia, hypotension and electrolyte disturbances associated with cardiac arrhythmias and muscle spasms.

Treatment: Emesis should be induced or gastric lavage performed. Intravenous fluid and electrolyte replacement may be indicated.

Pharmacological properties

Pharmacodynamic properties: Mode of action: Cyclopenthiazide is a benzothiadiazine (thiazide) diuretic.

Cyclopenthiazide is a thiazide diuretic which exerts diuretic effect by inhibiting the reabsorption of sodium chloride and water probably at the distal renal tubule.

Amiloride hydrochloride is a mild potassium-sparing diuretic, belonging to the pyrazine carboxamide class, which acts mainly on the distal part of the renal tubule. It increases the excretion of sodium and chloride and reduces the excretion of potassium.

Pharmacokinetic properties: The lipophilic thiazides – such as cyclopenthiazide – attain higher concentration in the cells and thus have a larger distribution volume than the hydrophilic derivatives. Their protein binding rate is also greater, amounting to approximately 92%. They therefore exert a more prolonged action than the more hydrophilic thiazides.

Amiloride is completely absorbed from the GI tract; peak serum concentrations are achieved about 3 and 4 hours after oral administration. It is excreted unchanged in the urine and has been estimated to have a serum half life of about 6 hours.

Preclinical safety data: Cyclopenthiazide: In reproduction toxicity studies with mice, rats and rabbits, no teratogenic effects were observed.

Pharmaceutical particulars

List of excipients: The coated tablets contain lactose, wheat starch, polyvinylpyrrolidone (K90), stearic acid, talc, sodium starch glycollate, titanium dioxide (E171), yellow iron oxide (E172), polyethoxylated hydrogenated castor oil, hydroxypropylmethylcellulose and water.

Incompatibilities: None known.

Shelf life: Three years.

Special precautions for storage: Protect from moisture. Store below 25°C.

Medicines should be kept out of reach of children.

Nature and contents of container: All tablets are packed in PVC/PVDC packs of 28 tablets.

Instructions for use/handling: None.

Marketing authorisation holder: Novartis Pharmaceuticals UK Limited, Trading as Ciba Laboratories, Frimley Business Park, Frimley, Camberley, Surrey GU16 5SG.

Marketing authorisation number PL 0101/0424.

Date of first authorisation/renewal of authorisation 16 May 1997.

Date of (partial) revision of the text January 1998.

NAVOBAN AMPOULES 2 mg/2 ml

Qualitative and quantitative composition 2 mg/2 mL ampoules. Uncoloured glass ampoules containing clear, colourless or very faintly brown-yellow solution. Each ampoule contains 2.26 mg of tropisetron hydrochloride (corresponding to 2 mg of tropisetron base) in 2 ml.

Pharmaceutical form Glass ampoules containing an aqueous solution for intravenous administration.

Clinical particulars

Therapeutic indications: Treatment of post-operative nausea and vomiting.

Prevention of post-operative nausea and vomiting in patients at high risk of developing post-operative nausea and vomiting.

Posology and method of administration: Navoban is recommended as a single 2 mg dose given intravenously either as an infusion (diluted in a common infusion fluid such as normal saline, Ringer's solution, glucose 5% or fructose 5%) administered over 15 minutes, or as a slow injection (not less than 30 seconds).

In the case of treatment of postoperative nausea and vomiting, Navoban has been shown to be effective when given within two hours of the end of anaesthesia prior to patients being moved from the operating theatre recovery area.

In the case of prevention of post-operative nausea and vomiting, Navoban should be administered shortly before the induction of anaesthesia.

Contra-indications: Hypersensitivity to tropisetron or other 5-HT_3 receptor antagonists. Navoban must not be given to pregnant women, unless termination of early pregnancy is part of the surgical procedure.

Special warnings and precautions for use

Use in poor metabolisers of sparteine/debrisoquine: In patients belonging to this group (about 8% of the Caucasian population), the elimination half-life of tropisetron is prolonged (4 to 5 times longer than in extensive metabolisers), however, studies indicate that for 7 day courses in patients with poor metabolism the usual of 2 mg does not need to be reduced.

Use in patients with impaired hepatic or renal function: No change in the pharmacokinetics of tropisetron occurs in patients with acute hepatitis or fatty liver disease. In contrast, patients with liver cirrhosis or impaired kidney function may have plasma concentrations up to 50% higher than those found in healthy volunteers belonging to the group of extensive metabolisers of sparteine/debrisoquine. Nevertheless, no dosage reduction is necessary in such patients when the recommended 2 mg dose is given.

Use in children: Navoban is not recommended for use in children.

Use in the elderly: There is no evidence that elderly patients require different dosages or experience side effects different from those in younger patients.

Interaction with other medicaments and other forms of interactions: Concomitant administration of Navoban with therapeutic agents known to induce hepatic metabolic enzymes (e.g. rifampicin, phenobarbital) results in lower plasma concentrations of tropisetron and, therefore requires an increase in dosage in extensive metabolisers (but not in poor metabolisers). The effects of cytochrome P450 enzyme inhibitors such as cimetidine on tropisetron plasma levels are negligible and do not require dose adjustment.

Pregnancy and lactation: Navoban must not be given to pregnant women, unless termination of early pregnancy is part of the surgical procedure. There is no experience with Navoban in human pregnancy. In animal studies no teratogenic effects occurred at doses which were not toxic to the dams, but effects on female reproductive capacity were observed.

Nursing mothers: In the rat, after administration of radiolabelled tropisetron, radioactivity was excreted in the milk. Breast-feeding patients should not be given Navoban.

Effects on ability to drive and use machines: No data exist on the effect of this drug on the ability to drive. The occurrence of dizziness and fatigue as side effects should be taken into account.

Not relevant in the context of general anaesthesia.

Undesirable effects: The undesirable effects are transient at the recommended dose. Most frequently reported at the recommended 2 mg dose was headache, whereas at higher doses constipation and, less frequently, dizziness, fatigue and gastrointestinal disorders such as abdominal pain and diarrhoea were observed as well.

As with other 5-HT_3 receptor antagonists, hypersensitivity reactions ('type I-reactions') with one or more of the following symptoms have rarely been observed: facial flushing and/or generalised urticaria, chest tightness, dyspnoea, acute bronchospasm, hypotension.

In very rare instances when Navoban has been used to prevent chemotherapy induced nausea and vomiting, collapse, syncope or cardiovascular arrest have been reported, the relationship to Navoban has not been established and these effects may have been caused by the concomitant therapy or the underlying disease.

Overdose: At very high repeated doses (100 mg for 5 days), visual hallucinations have been observed. In patients with pre-existing hypertension, an increase in blood pressure has been observed at cumulative doses of 27 to 80 mg Navoban.

Symptomatic treatment with frequent monitoring of vital signs and close observation of the patient is indicated.

Pharmacological properties

Pharmacodynamic properties: Tropisetron is a highly potent and selective competitive antagonist of the 5-HT_3 receptor, a subclass of serotonin receptors located on peripheral neurons and within the CNS. Surgery and treatment with certain substances, including some chemotherapeutic agents, may trigger the release of serotonin (5-HT) from enterochromaffin-like cells in the visceral mucosa and initiate the emesis reflex and its accompanying feeling of nausea. Tropisetron selectively blocks the excitation of the presynaptic 5-HT_3 receptors of the peripheral neurons in this reflex, and may exert additional direct actions within the CNS on 5-HT_3 receptors mediating the actions of vagal input to the area postrema. These effects are considered to be the underlying mechanism of action of the anti-emetic effect of tropisetron.

Pharmacokinetic properties: Absorption of Navoban from the gastrointestinal tract is rapid (mean half-life of about 20 minutes) and extensive (more than 95%). The peak plasma concentration is attained within 3 hours.

Tropisetron is 71% bound to plasma proteins (particularly α_1-glycoproteins) in a non-specific manner. The volume of distribution in adults is 400 to 600 L.

The metabolism of tropisetron occurs by hydroxylation at the 5, 6, or 7 position of its indole ring, followed by a conjugation reaction to form the glucuronide or sulphate and excretion in the urine or bile (urine to faeces ratio 5:1). The metabolites have a greatly reduced potency for the 5-HT_3 receptor and do not contribute to the pharmacological action of the drug. The metabolism of tropisetron is linked to the genetically determined sparteine/debrisoquine polymorphism. About 8% of the Caucasian population are known to be poor metabolisers for the sparteine/debrisoquine pathway.

The elimination half-life (β-phase) is about 8 hours in extensive metabolisers; in poor metabolisers this could be extended to 45 hours (see *Special warnings and precautions for use*). The total clearance of tropisetron is about 1 L/min, with the renal clearance contributing approx. 10%. In patients who are poor metabolisers, the total clearance is reduced to 0.1 to 0.2 L/min although the renal clearance remains unchanged. This reduction in non-renal clearance results in an approximately 4 to 5-fold longer elimination half-life and in 5 to 7-fold higher AUC values. C_{max} and volume of distribution are not different when compared to extensive metabolisers. In poor metabolisers, a greater proportion of unchanged tropisetron is excreted in the urine than in extensive metabolisers.

Preclinical safety data: In several *in vitro* and *in vivo* tests, Navoban has been shown to have no mutagenic potential, however in a long term study in male mice at doses of 300 mg/kg per day (300 times the human daily dose) an increased incidence of hepatocellular adenomas was observed.

Pharmaceutical particulars

List of excipients: Acetic acid, glacial EP; sodium acetate trihydrate EP; sodium chloride EP; water for injection EP.

Incompatabilities: Navoban glass ampoules contain a 1 mg/ml aqueous solution to be used for i.v. administration. Ampoule solutions are compatible with the following solutions for injection: glucose 5% (w/v); Ringer's solution; sodium chloride 0.9% (w/v) and fructose 5% (w/v), in concentrations of 5 mg in 100 ml solution. Diluents other than those listed should not be used. The diluted solutions are physically and chemically stable for at least 24 hours. However, considering the risk of microbial contamination during the preparation of the infusion, the solution must be used within 8 hours of preparation. The solutions are also compatible with the usual types of containers (glass, PVC) and their infusion sets.

Shelf life: 5 years.

Special precautions for storage: No special precautions.

Nature and contents of the container: Navoban Ampoules 2 mg/2 ml are made of uncoloured glass, and are coded with two blue colour rings. They are available in packs of one and packs of five.

Instructions for use/handling: None.

Marketing authorisation holder: Novartis Pharmaceuticals UK Ltd, Trading as 'Sandoz Pharmaceuticals', Frimley Business Park, Frimley, Camberley, Surrey GU16 5SG.

Marketing authorisation number PL 00101/0413.

Date of first authorisation/renewal of authorisation

Date of (partial) revision of the text May 1997.

NAVOBAN AMPOULES 5 mg/5 ml

Qualitative and quantitative composition Uncoloured glass ampoules containing clear, colourless or very faintly brown-yellow solution. Each ampoule contains 5.64 mg of tropisetron hydrochloride (corresponding to 5 mg of tropisetron base) in 5 ml.

Pharmaceutical form Glass ampoules containing an aqueous solution for intravenous administration.

Clinical particulars
Therapeutic indications: Prevention of cancer chemotherapy-induced nausea and vomiting.

Posology and method of administration: Adults: Navoban is recommended as six-day courses of 5 mg per day.

On day one, shortly before chemotherapy commences, 5 mg Navoban should be given by intravenous administration as a slow injection or as an injection into a running infusion. For intravenous administration, one Navoban ampoule should be diluted in 100 ml of sodium chloride 0.9% w/v (physiological saline). Alternatively, diluents are Ringer's solution, glucose 5% and fructose 5%; diluents other than those specified should not be used.

On days two to six, one Navoban capsule 5 mg should be taken with water each morning upon rising at least one hour before food.

Children: Navoban is not recommended.

Elderly: There is no evidence that a special dosing schedule is needed in this patient group. 5 mg Navoban daily for six days is recommended.

Poor metabolisers of sparteine/debrisoquine: In patients belonging to this group (about 8% of the Caucasian population) the elimination half-life of tropisetron is prolonged (4–5 times longer than in extensive metabolisers). However, no dosage reduction is necessary in such patients. The recommended dosage is, therefore, 5 mg daily for 6 successive days.

Patients with impaired hepatic or renal function: No change in pharmacokinetics of tropisetron occurs in patients with acute hepatitis or fatty liver disease. In contrast, patients with liver cirrhosis or impaired kidney function may have plasma concentrations up to 50% higher than those found in healthy volunteers belonging to the group of extensive metabolisers of sparteine/debrisoquine. Nevertheless, no dosage reduction is necessary in such patients when the recommended 6-day courses of 5 mg Navoban per day are given.

Use in patients with uncontrolled hypertension: In patients with uncontrolled hypertension, it is important not to exceed the recommended daily dose since higher dosages, particularly when administered after intravenous prehydration therapy, have been reported to aggravate this condition.

Method of administration: Intravenous.

Contra-indications: Hypersensitivity to tropisetron or other 5-HT_3 receptor antagonists. Navoban must not be given to pregnant women.

Special warnings and precautions for use: In patients with uncontrolled hypertension, it is important not to exceed the recommended daily dose since higher doses, particularly when administered after intravenous prehydration therapy, have been reported to aggravate this condition.

In several *in vitro* and *in vivo* tests, Navoban has been shown to have no mutagenic potential, but in a long term study in male mice at doses of 30 mg/kg per day (300 times the human daily dose) an increased incidence of hepatocellular adenomas was observed.

Interaction with other medicaments and other forms of interaction: Concomitant administration of Navoban with therapeutic agents known to induce hepatic enzymes may result in lower tropisetron plasma concentrations, particularly in extensive metabolisers. Conversely the effects of the agents which characteristically inhibit these enzyme systems may lead to enhanced plasma concentrations. Such changes are unlikely to be of practical importance provided the dosage regime of 5 mg daily for six days is followed.

Pregnancy and lactation: Navoban must not be given to pregnant women. There is no experience with Navoban in human pregnancy. In animal studies, no teratogenic effects occurred at doses which were not toxic to the dams, but effects on reproductive capacity were observed. Therefore, women should not try to conceive when on Navoban therapy.

It has not been established whether tropisetron is excreted into human milk. Patients taking Navoban should not therefore breast-feed.

Effects on ability to drive and use machinery: Patients should be cautioned against driving or operating machinery until it is established that they do not become dizzy or drowsy whilst receiving Navoban.

Undesirable effects: The most frequently reported adverse reactions are headache, constipation, dizziness, fatigue and gastrointestinal disorders such as abdominal pain and diarrhoea. In very rare incidences, collapse, syncope, bradycardia or cardiovascular arrest have been reported with Navoban. However, as with other 5-HT_3 receptor antagonists, the relationship to Navoban has not been established. Some of these reactions could be attributed to concomitant chemotherapy or the underlying disease. As with other 5-HT_3 receptor antagonists, hypersensitivity reactions (Type I reactions) with one or more of the following symptoms have rarely been observed: Facial flushing and/or generalised urticaria, chest tightness, dyspnoea, acute bronchospasm, hypotension.

Overdose: At very high repeated doses, visual hallucinations and in patients with pre-existing hypertension, an increase in blood pressure may have been observed. Seizure threshold may also be lowered in susceptible patients. Symptomatic treatment with frequent monitoring of vital signs and close observation of the patient is indicated.

Pharmacological properties
Pharmacodynamic properties: Navoban is a highly potent and selective competitive antagonist of the 5-HT_3 receptor, a subclass of serotonin receptors located on peripheral neurons and within the CNS. Certain substances, including some chemotherapeutic agents are believed to trigger the release of serotonin (5-HT) from enterochromaffin-like cells in the visceral mucosa and initiate the emesis reflex and its accompanying feeling of nausea. Navoban selectively blocks the excitation of the pre-synaptic 5-HT_3 receptors of the peripheral neurons in this reflex, and may exert additional direct actions within the CNS on 5-HT_3 receptors mediating the actions of vagal input to the area postrema.

Navoban has a 24-hour duration of action which allows once-a-day administration.

In studies where Navoban has been administered over multiple chemotherapy cycles, treatment has remained effectve. Navoban prevents nausea and vomiting induced by cancer chemotherapy without causing extrapyramidal side effects.

Pharmacokinetic properties: Absorption of Navoban from the gastrointestinal tract is rapid (mean half-life of about 20 minutes) and extensive (more than 95%). The peak plasma concentration is attained within 3 hours. Owing to a saturable metabolic pathway. The absolute bioavailability is dose-dependent. Tropisetron is 71% bound to plasma protein in a non-specific manner. Volume of distribution is 400–600 L.

The metabolism of tropisetron is linked to the genetically determined sparteine/debrisoquine pathway.

The elimination half-life (β-phase) is about 8 hours in extensive metabolisers and 30 hours after i.v. administration or 42 hours after oral administration in poor metabolisers. In extensive metabolisers, about 8% of tropisetron is excreted in the urine as unchanged drug, 70% as metabolites; 15% is excreted in the faeces, almost entirely as metabolites. The metabolites of tropisetron do not contribute to its pharmacological action. In poor metabolisers, a greater proportion of unchanged tropisetron is excreted in the urine than in extensive metabolisers.

Preclinical safety data: In several *in vitro* and *in vivo* tests, Navoban has been shown to have no mutagenic potential, but in the long term study in male mice at doses of 30 mg/kg per day (300 times the human daily dose) an increased incidence of hepatocellular adenomas was observed.

Pharmaceutical particulars
List of excipients: Acetic acid, glacial (EP), Sodium acetate trihydrate (EP), Sodium chloride (EP), Water for injection (EP).

Incompatibilities: None.

Shelf life: 60 months.

Special precautions for storage: No special precautions (see *Instructions for use/handling*).

Nature and contents of container: Clear glass 5 ml ampoule with a rupture ring in pack sizes of 1 and 10 ampoules.

Instructions for use/handling: Ampoule solution may be diluted with specified diluents (see *Posology and method of administration* for diluents). Diluted solution should be used immediately or stored between 2–8°C for no more than 24 hours.

Marketing authorisation holder: Novartis Pharmaceuticals UK Ltd, Trading as Sandoz Pharmaceuticals, Frimley Business Park, Frimley, Camberley, Surrey GU16 5SG.

Marketing authorisation number 00101/0344.

Date of first authorisation/renewal of authorisation 28 October 1992/28 October 2002.

Date of (partial) revision of the text January 1998.

NAVOBAN CAPSULES 5 mg

Qualitative and quantitative composition Opaque yellow and white, hard gelatin capsule, 16 mm in length and 6 mm in diameter. Each capsule contains 5 mg tropisetron base (equivalent to tropisetron hydrochloride 5.64 mg) and is marked with Navoban 5 mg in red print.

Pharmaceutical form Hard gelatin capsule for oral administration.

Clinical particulars
Therapeutic indications: Prevention of cancer chemotherapy-induced nausea and vomiting.

Posology and method of administration: Adults: Navoban is recommended as six-day courses of 5 mg per day.

On day one, shortly before chemotherapy commences, 5 mg Navoban should be given by intravenous administration as a slow injection or as an injection into a running infusion. For intravenous administration, one Navoban ampoule should be diluted in 100 ml of sodium chloride 0.9% w/v (physiological saline). Alternatively, diluents are Ringer's solution, glucose 5% and fructose 5%; diluents other than those specified should not be used.

On days two to six, one Navoban capsule 5 mg should be taken with water each morning upon rising at least one hour before food.

Children: Navoban is not recommended.

Elderly: There is no evidence that a special dosing schedule is needed in this patient group 5 mg Navoban daily for six days is recommended.

Poor metabolisers of sparteine/debrisoquine: In patients belonging to this group (about 8% of the Caucasian population) the elimination half-life of tropisetron is prolonged (4–5 times longer than in extensive metabolisers). However, no dosage reduction is necessary in such patients. The recommended dosage is, therefore, 5 mg daily for 6 successive days.

Patients with impaired hepatic or renal function: No change in pharmacokinetics of tropisetron occurs in patients with acute hepatitis or fatty liver disease. In contrast, patients with liver cirrhosis or impaired kidney function may have plasma concentrations up to 50% higher than those found in healthy volunteers belonging to the group of extensive metabolisers of sparteine/debrisoquine. Nevertheless, no dosage reduction is necessary in such patients when the recommended 6-day courses of 5 mg Navoban per day are given.

Use in patients with uncontrolled hypertension: In patients with uncontrolled hypertension, it is important not to exceed the recommended daily dose since higher dosages, particularly when administered after intravenous prehydration therapy, have been reported to aggravate this condition.

Method of administration: Oral.

Contra-indications: Hypersensitivity to tropisetron or other 5-HT_3 receptor antagonists. Navoban must not be given to pregnant women.

Special warnings and special precautions for use: In patients with uncontrolled hypertension, it is important not to exceed the recommended daily dose since higher doses, particularly when administered after intravenous prehydration therapy have been reported to aggravate this condition.

In several *in vitro* and *in vivo* tests, Navoban has been shown to have no mutagenic potential, but in a long term study in male mice at doses of 30 mg/kg per day (300 times the human daily dose) an increased incidence of hepatocellular adenomas was observed.

Interaction with other medicaments and other forms of interaction: Concomitant administration of Navoban with therapeutic agents known to induce hepatic enzymes may result in lower tropisetron plasma concentrations, particularly in extensive metabolisers. Conversely the effects of the agents wh'ch characteristically inhibit these enzyme systems may lead to enhanced plasma concentrations. Such changes are unlikely to be of practical importance provided the dosage regime of 5 mg daily for six days is followed. Ingestion of the capsule with food has no relevant influence on the bioavailability but may slightly delay the absorption of Navoban.

Pregnancy and lactation: Navoban must not be given to pregnant women. There is no experience with Navoban in human pregnancy. In animal studies, no teratogenic effects occurred at doses which were not toxic to the dams, but effects on reproductive capacity were observed. Therefore, women should not try to conceive when on Navoban therapy.

It is not known whether tropisetron is excreted into human milk. Patients taking Navoban should not therefore breast-feed.

Effects on ability to drive and use machinery: Patients should be cautioned against driving or operating machinery until it is established that they do not become dizzy or drowsy whilst receiving Navoban.

Undesirable effects: The most frequently reported adverse reactions are headache, constipation, dizziness, fatigue and gastrointestinal disorders such as abdominal pain and diarrhoea. In very rare incidences, collapse, syncope, bradycardia or cardiovascular arrest have been reported with Navoban. However, as with other 5-HT_3 receptor antagonists, the relationship to Navoban has not been established. Some of these reactions could be attributed to concomitant chemotherapy or the underlying disease. As with other 5-HT_3 receptor antagonists, hypersensitivity reactions (Type I reactions) with one or more of the following symptoms have rarely been observed: Facial flushing and/or generalised urticaria, chest tightness, dyspnoea, acute bronchospasm, hypotension.

Overdose: At very high repeated doses, visual hallucinations and in patients with pre-existing hypertension, an increase in blood pressure may have been observed. Seizure threshold may also be lowered in susceptible patients. Symptomatic treatment with frequent monitoring of vital signs and close observation of the patient is indicated.

Pharmacological properties

Pharmacodynamic properties: Navoban is a highly potent and selective competitive antagonist of the 5-HT_3 receptor, a subclass of serotonin receptors located on peripheral neurons and within the CNS. Certain substances, including some chemotherapeutic agents are believed to trigger the release of serotonin (5-HT) from enterochromaffin-like cells in the visceral mucosa and initiate the emesis reflex and its accompanying feeling of nausea. Navoban selectively blocks the excitation of the pre-synaptic 5-HT_3 receptors of the peripheral neurons in this reflex, and may exert additional direct actions within the CNS on 5-HT_3 receptors mediating the actions of vagal input to the area postrema.

Navoban has a 24 hour duration of action which allows once-a-day administration.

In studies where Navoban has been administered over multiple chemotherapy cycles, treatment has remained effective. Navoban prevents nausea and vomiting induced by cancer chemotherapy without causing extrapyramidal side effects.

Pharmacokinetic properties: Absorption of Navoban from the gastro-intestinal tract is rapid (mean half-life of about 20 minutes) and extensive (more than 95%). The peak plasma concentration is attained within 3 hours. Owing to a saturable metabolic pathway. The absolute bioavailability is dose-dependent. Tropisetron is 71% bound to plasma protein in a non-specific manner. Volume of distribution is 400–600 L.

The metabolism of tropisetron is linked to the genetically determined sparteine/debrisoquine pathway.

The elimination half-life (β-phase) is about 8 hours in extensive metabolisers, and 30 hours after i.v. administration or 42 hours after oral administration in poor metabolisers. In extensive metabolisers, about 8% of tropisetron is excreted in the urine as unchanged drug, 70% as metabolites; 15% is excreted in the faeces, almost entirely as metabolites. The metabolites of tropisetron do not contribute to its pharmacological action. In poor metabolisers, a greater proportion of unchanged tropisetron is excreted in the urine than in extensive metabolisers.

Preclinical safety data: In several *in vitro* and *in vivo* tests, Navoban has been shown to have no mutagenic potential, but in the long term study in male mice at doses of 30 mg/kg per day (300 times the human daily dose) an increased incidence of hepatocellular adenomas was observed.

Pharmaceutical particulars

List of excipients:

Contents: Silica, colloidal anhydrous EP, Magnesium stearate EP, Maize starch EP, Lactose EP.

Shell: Iron oxide, yellow (E172) EEC, Titanium dioxide (E171) EP, Gelatin EP.

Imprint: Shellac BPC, Iron oxide, red (E172) EEC.

Incompatabilities: None.

Shelf life: 60 months.

Special precautions for storage: Store in a dry place below 25°C.

Nature and contents of container: Navoban 5 mg Capsules are available commercially in PVC/PVDC blister strips containing 5 capsules in boxes of 1 or 10 blisters. Capsules are number 3 size hard gelatin capsules with an opaque yellow upper part with a Sandoz triangle imprinted in red, and an opaque white lower part with Navoban (or the code EA in NL and B) and the dose strength of 5 mg imprinted in red.

Instructions for use/handling: For oral administration.

Marketing authorisation holder: Novartis Pharmaceuticals UK Ltd, Trading as Sandoz Pharmaceuticals, Frimley Business Park, Frimley, Camberley, Surrey GU16 5SG.

Marketing authorisation number 00101/0345.

Date of first authorisation/renewal of authorisation 28 October 1992.

Date of (partial) revision of the text July 1997.

NEORAL*

Qualitative and quantitative composition Neoral Soft Gelatin Capsules containing 10, 25, 50, or 100 mg cyclosporin.

Neoral Oral Solution containing 100 mg cyclosporin/mL.

Pharmaceutical form Neoral Soft Gelatin Capsules and Neoral Oral Solution are for oral administration.

Neoral is an improved pharmaceutical form of the active ingredient cyclosporin. Neoral is a pre-concentrate formulation of cyclosporin which undergoes a microemulsification process in the presence of water, either in the form of a beverage or in the form of the gastrointestinal fluid. Neoral reduces the intra-patient variability of pharmacokinetic parameters, with a more consistent absorption profile and less influence of concomitant food intake and the presence of bile. In pharmacokinetic and clinical studies it has been demonstrated that the correlation between trough concentration (C_{min}) and total exposure (AUC) is significantly stronger when cyclosporin is given as Neoral than when it is given as Sandimmun*. Neoral therefore allows greater predictability and consistency of cyclosporin exposure.

Clinical particulars

Therapeutic indications:

Transplantation indications: Organ transplantation: Prevention of graft rejection following kidney, liver, heart, combined heart-lung, lung or pancreas transplants.

Treatment of transplant rejection in patients previously receiving other immunosuppressive agents.

Bone marrow transplantation: Prevention of graft rejection following bone marrow transplantation and prophylaxis of graft-versus-host disease (GVHD).

Treatment of established graft-versus-host disease (GVHD).

Non-transplantation indications:

Psoriasis: Neoral Soft Gelatin Capsules and Neoral Oral Solution are indicated in patients with severe psoriasis in whom conventional therapy is ineffective or inappropriate.

Atopic dermatitis: Neoral Soft Gelatin Capsules and Neoral Oral Solution are indicated for the short term treatment (8 weeks) of patients with severe atopic dermatitis in whom conventional therapy is ineffective or inappropriate.

Rheumatoid arthritis: Neoral Soft Gelatin Capsules and Neoral Oral Solution are indicated for the treatment of severe, active rheumatoid arthritis in patients in whom classical, slow-acting anti-rheumatic agents are inappropriate or ineffective.

Nephrotic syndrome: Neoral Soft Gelatin Capsules and Neoral Oral Solution are indicated for the treatment of steroid dependent or steroid resistant nephrotic syndrome (associated with adverse prognostic features) due to minimal change glomerulonephritis, focal segmental glomerulosclerosis or membranous glomerulonephritis in both adults and children.

Posology and method of administration: Following initiation of treatment with Neoral, due to the different bioavailabilities of the different oral cyclosporin formulations, patients should not be transferred to any other oral formulation of cyclosporin without appropriate monitoring of cyclosporin blood concentrations, serum creatinine levels and blood pressure. This does not apply to the conversion between Neoral Soft Gelatin Capsules and Neoral Oral Solution as these two forms are bioequivalent.

Due to the differences in bioavailability between different oral fomulations of cyclosporin, it is important that prescribers, pharmacists, and patients be aware that substitution of Neoral with any other oral formulation of cyclosporin is not recommended as this may lead to alterations in cyclosporin blood levels. For this reason it may be appropriate to prescribe by brand.

Dosage:

Transplantation indications – Organ transplantation: Treatment with Neoral Soft Gelatin Capsules or Neoral Oral Solution should be initiated within 12 hours before transplantation at a dose of 10 to 15 mg/kg body weight given in two divided doses.

As a general rule, treatment should continue at a dose of 10 to 15 mg/kg per day given in two divided doses for one to two weeks post-operatively. Dosage should then be gradually reduced until a maintenance dose of about 2 to 6 mg/kg per day is reached. This total daily dose should be given in two divided doses. Dosage should be adjusted by monitoring cyclosporin trough levels and kidney function (see *Precautions*).

When Neoral is given with other immunosuppressants (e.g. with corticosteroids or as part of a triple or quadruple drug therapy), lower doses (e.g. 3 to 6 mg/kg per day given orally in two divided doses) may be used for the initial treatment. For trough level monitoring, whole blood is preferred, measured by a specific analytical method. Target trough concentration ranges depend on organ type, time after transplantation and immunosuppressive regimen.

The use of Sandimmun Concentrate for Intravenous Infusion is recommended in organ transplant patients who are unable to take Neoral Soft Gelatin Capsules or Neoral Oral Solution (e.g. shortly after surgery) or in whom the absorption of Neoral might be impaired during episodes of gastrointestinal disturbances. It is recommended, however, that patients be transferred to Neoral therapy as soon as the given circumstances allow (please refer to Sandimmun data sheet/SmPC for prescribing information on Sandimmun Concentrate for I.V. Infusion).

Bone marrow transplantation/prevention and treatment of graft-versus-host-disease (GVHD): Sandimmun Concentrate for Intravenous Infusion is usually preferred for initiation of therapy, although Neoral Soft Gelatin Capsules or Neoral Oral Solution may be used (please refer to Sandimmun data sheet/SmPC for prescribing information on Sandimmun Concentrate for I.V. Infusion).

Treatment should continue using Neoral Soft Gelatin Capsules or Neoral Oral Solution at a dosage of 12.5 mg/kg per day, given in two divided doses, for at least three and preferably six months before tailing off to zero. In some cases it may not be possible to withdraw Neoral until a year after bone marrow transplantation. Higher doses of Neoral or the use of Sandimmun Concentrate for Intravenous Infusion may be necessary in the presence of gastro-intestinal disturbances which might decrease absorption.

If Neoral Soft Gelatin Capsules or Neoral Oral Solution are used to initiate therapy, the recommended dose is 12.5 to 15 mg/kg per day, given in two divided doses, starting on the day before transplantation.

If GVHD develops after Neoral is withdrawn it should respond to reinstitution of therapy. Low doses of Neoral should be used for mild, chronic GVHD.

Non-transplantation indications:

Psoriasis (refer also to *Additional precautions in psoriasis and atopic dermatitis* section)*:* Due to the variability of this condition, treatment must be individualised. To induce remission, the recommended initial dose of Neoral is 2.5 mg/kg a day given orally in two divided doses. If there is no improvement after 1 month, the daily dose may be gradually increased, but should not exceed 5 mg/kg. Treatment should be discontinued if sufficient response is not achieved within 6 weeks on a daily basis of 5 mg/kg per day, or if the effective dose is not compatible with the safety guidelines given below (see *Precautions*). Initial doses of 5 mg/kg per day of Neoral are justified in patients whose condition requires rapid improvement. For *maintenance treatment,* Neoral dosage must be individually titrated to the lowest effective level, and the dosage should not exceed 5 mg/kg a day, given orally in two divided doses.

Some clinical data are available which provide evidence that once satisfactory response is achieved, Neoral may be discontinued and subsequent relapse managed with re-introduction of Neoral at the previous effective dose. In some patients continuous maintenance therapy may be necessary.

Atopic dermatitis (refer also to *Additional precautions in atopic dermatitis* section)*:* The recommended dose range for Neoral is 2.5–5 mg/kg per day given orally in two divided doses for a maximum of 8 weeks. If a starting dose of 2.5 mg/kg per day does not achieve a good initial response within 2 weeks the dose may be rapidly increased to a maximum of 5 mg/kg per day. In very severe cases rapid and adequate control of disease is more likely with a starting dose of 5 mg/kg per day, given orally in two divided doses.

Rheumatoid arthritis (refer also to *Additional precautions in rheumatoid arthritis* section)*:* It is recommended that initiation of Neoral therapy should take place over a period of 12 weeks. For the first 6 weeks of treatment, the recommended dose is 2.5 mg/kg per day, given orally in two divided doses. If the clinical effect is considered insufficient, the daily dose may be increased gradually as tolerability permits, but should not exceed 4 mg/kg per day.

If, after 3 months of treatment at the maximum permitted or tolerable dose the response is considered inadequate, treatment should be discontinued.

For maintenance treatment the dose has to be titrated individually according to tolerability.

Neoral can be given in combination with low-dose corticosteroids. Pharmacodynamic interactions can occur between cyclosporin and NSAIDs and therefore this combination should be used with care (see *Additional precautions in rheumatoid arthritis* section and *Interactions* section).

Long-term data on the use of cyclosporin in the treatment of rheumatoid arthritis are still limited. Therefore, it is recommended that patients are re-evaluated after 6 months of maintenance treatment and therapy only continued if the benefits of treatment outweigh the risks.

Nephrotic syndrome (refer also to *Additional precautions in nephrotic syndrome* section)*:* To induce remission, the recommended dose is 5 mg/kg per day given orally in two divided doses for adults and 6 mg/kg per day given orally in two divided doses for children if, with the exception of proteinuria, renal function is normal. In patients with impaired renal function, the initial dose should not exceed 2.5 mg/kg per day orally.

In focal segmental glomerulosclerosis, the combination of Neoral and low dose corticosteroids may be of benefit.

In the absence of efficacy after 3 months treatment for minimal change glomerulonephritis and focal segmental glomerulosclerosis or 6 months treatment for membranous glomerulonephritis, Neoral therapy should be discontinued.

For maintenance treatment the maximum recommended dose is 5 mg/kg per day orally in adults or 6 mg/kg per day orally in children. The doses need to be slowly reduced individually according to efficacy (proteinuria) and safety (primarily serum creatinine), to the lowest effective level.

Long term data of cyclosporin in the treatment of nephrotic syndrome are limited. However, in clinical trials patients have received treatment for 1 to 2 years. Long term treatment may be considered if there has been a significant reduction in proteinuria with preservation of creatine clearance and provided adequate precautions are taken (see *Additional precautions in nephrotic syndrome* section).

Conversion of transplant patients from Sandimmun Soft Gelatin Capsules or Oral Solution to Neoral: Cyclosporin absorption from Sandimmun oral formulations is highly variable and the relationship between Sandimmun dose and cyclosporin exposure (AUC) is non-linear. In contrast, with Neoral the absorption of cyclosporin is less variable and the correlation between cyclosporin trough concentrations and exposure is much stronger than with Sandimmun.

For converting patients from Sandimmun to Neoral an initial mg for mg conversion from Sandimmun to Neoral is recommended with subsequent dose titration if required. Available data confirm that following this initial mg for mg conversion comparable trough concentrations of cyclosporin in whole blood are achieved, maintaining adequate immunosuppression. In many patients, higher peak concentrations (C_{max}) and an increased exposure to the drug (AUC) may occur. No additional adverse events, including renal dysfunction, however, were observed due to these changes in pharmacokinetic parameters during long term treatment. In a small percentage of patients, these changes may be more marked and of clinical significance. Their magnitude depends largely on the individual ability to absorb cyclosporin from the originally used Sandimmun. In these patients, dose reduction should be undertaken to achieve the appropriate trough concentration range.

Long term clinical data in renal transplant patients have demonstrated that a large proportion of patients previously on Sandimmun therapy can be maintained at the same dose of Neoral as with Sandimmun.

All patients should be monitored according to the following recommendations:

(a) Preconversion (i.e. on Sandimmun): Measure cyclosporin trough concentration, serum creatinine and blood pressure.
(b) Day 1: Convert the patient to the same daily dose of Neoral as was previously used with oral Sandimmun (i.e. on a mg to mg basis).
(c) Day 4–7 post conversion: Follow-up visit to measure cyclosporin trough concentration, serum creatinine and blood pressure.
(d) Subsequent follow-up: Depending on the findings on review at day 4–7, subsequent follow-up visits may need to be arranged (e.g. week 2 and week 4) in the first 2 month period after conversion to Neoral. During these visits, cyclosporin trough concentrations, serum creatinine and blood pressure should be measured and, dependent on these measurements, the dose of Neoral adjusted accordingly.

Further information on conversion can be obtained via the Neoral Helpline (01276 698494).

Conversion of non-transplant (i.e. psoriasis, atopic dermatitis, rheumatoid arthritis, nephrotic syndrome) patients from Sandimmun Soft Gelatin Capsules or Oral Solution to Neoral: Cyclosporin absorption from Sandimmun oral formulations is highly variable and the relationship between Sandimmun dose and cyclosporin exposure (AUC) is non-linear. In contrast, with Neoral the absorption of cyclosporin is less variable.

With equivalent doses following conversion from Sandimmun to Neoral, higher peak concentrations (C_{max}) and an increased exposure to the drug may occur. In a small percentage of patients, these changes may be more marked and of clinical significance. Their magnitude depends largely on the individual ability to absorb cyclosporin from the originally used Sandimmun. Therefore, the clinical status of each patient should be assessed prior to initiating Neoral therapy.

It is recommended that where any potential loss of efficacy results in considerable risk to the patients (e.g. rheumatoid arthritis), conversion from Sandimmun to Neoral is on a mg for mg basis. In other patients, the lowest recommended starting dose of Neoral is recommended initially with appropriate dose titration according to clinical response, serum creatinine and blood pressure levels.

All patients converting on a mg for mg basis should be monitored according to the following recommendations:

(a) Preconversion (i.e. on Sandimmun): Measure serum creatinine and blood pressure.
(b) Day 1: Start the patient with the same daily dose of Neoral as was previously used with oral Sandimmun (i.e. on a mg for mg basis).
(c) Week 2: Measure serum creatinine and blood pressure and consider reducing the dose of Neoral if either parameter significantly exceeds the preconversion level.
(d) Week 4: Measure serum creatinine and blood pressure and consider reducing the dose of Neoral if either parameter significantly exceeds the preconversion level.
(e) Week 8: Measure serum creatinine blood pressure and consider reducing the dose of Neoral if either parameter significantly exceeds the preconversion level.

If on more than one measurement, the serum creatinine increases more than 30% above the pre-Sandimmun baseline the dose of Neoral should be decreased (see *Additional precautions for psoriasis, atopic dermatitis, rheumatoid arthritis* and *nephrotic syndrome* sections).

Administration: The total daily dosage of Neoral Soft Gelatin Capsules or Neoral Oral Solution should always be given in two divided doses. Neoral Soft Gelatin Capsules should be taken with a mouthful of water and should then be swallowed whole.

Neoral Oral Solution should be diluted immediately before being taken. For improved taste the solution can be diluted with orange juice or squash or apple juice. However, it may also be taken with water if preferred. It should be stirred well.

Neoral Oral Solution has a characteristic taste which is distinct to that of Sandimmun Oral Solution.

The measuring device should not come into contact with the diluent. The measuring device should not be rinsed with water, alcohol or any other liquid. If it is necessary to clean the measuring device, the outside should be wiped with a dry tissue.

Owing to its possible interference with the P450-dependent enzyme system, grapefruit or grapefruit juice should not be ingested for 1 hour prior to dose administration, and grapefruit juice should not be used as a diluent for the Oral Solution.

Use in the elderly: There is currently no experience with Neoral in the elderly. However, no particular problems have been reported following the use of cyclosporin at the recommended dose. However, factors sometimes associated with ageing, in particular impaired renal function, make careful supervision essential and may necessitate dosage adjustment.

Use in children: There is currently no experience with Neoral in young children. However, transplant recipients from three months of age have received cyclosporin at the recommended dosage with no particular problems although at dosages above the upper end of the recommended range children seem to be more susceptible to fluid retention, convulsions and hypertension. This responds to dosage reduction.

Contra-indications: Known hypersensitivity to cyclosporin. Neoral is contra-indicated in psoriatic and atopic dermatitis patients with abnormal renal function, uncontrolled hypertension, uncontrolled infections or any kind of malignancy other than of the skin (see *Precautions* section). Neoral is contra-indicated in rheumatoid arthritis patients with abnormal renal function, uncontrolled hypertension, uncontrolled infections or any kind of malignancy. Neoral should not be used to treat rheumatoid arthritis in patients under the age or 18 years. Neoral is contra-indicated in nephrotic syndrome patients with uncontrolled hypertension, uncontrolled infections, or any kind of malignancy.

Special warnings and special precautions for use:

Precautions: Cyclosporin can impair renal function. Close monitoring of serum creatinine and urea is required and dosage adjustment may be necessary. Increases in serum creatinine and urea occurring during the first few weeks of cyclosporin therapy are generally dose-dependent and reversible and usually respond to dosage reduction. During long-term treatment, some patients may develop structural changes in the kidney (e.g. interstitial fibrosis) which, in renal transplant recipients, must be distinguished from chronic rejection.

Cyclosporin may also affect liver function and dosage adjustment, based on the results of bilirubin and liver enzyme monitoring, may be necessary.

Since cyclosporin occasionally causes hyperkalaemia or may aggravate pre-existing hyperkalaemia, monitoring of serum potassium is recommended, especially in patients with marked renal dysfunction. Patients receiving cyclosporin should avoid a high dietary potassium intake (see also *Interactions*).

Caution is required in treating patients with hyperuricaemia.

Cyclosporin should preferably not be administered with other immunosuppressive agents except corticosteroids. However, some transplant centres use cyclosporin together with azathioprine and corticosteroids, or other immunosuppressive agents (all in low doses) with the aim of reducing the risk of cyclosporin-induced renal dysfunction or renal structural changes. When cyclosporin is used with other immunosuppressive agents, there is a risk of over-immunosuppression, which can lead to increased susceptibility to infection and to possible development of lymphoma.

There are differences in bioavailability between different oral formulations of cyclosporin however, Neoral Soft Gelatin Capsules are bioequivalent to Neoral Oral Solution.

Regular monitoring of blood pressure is required during treatment with cyclosporin. If hypertension develops, appropriate anti-hypertensive treatment must be instituted.

Cyclosporin can induce a reversible increase in blood lipids. It is, therefore, advisable to perform lipid determinations before treatment and thereafter as appropriate.

Additional precautions in psoriasis and atopic dermatitis: Careful dermatological and physical examinations, including measurements of blood pressure and renal function on at least two occasions prior to starting therapy should be performed to establish an accurate baseline status.

Development of malignancies (particularly of the skin) have been reported in psoriatic patients treated with cyclosporin as well as during treatment with conventional therapy. A search for all forms of pre-existing tumours, including those of the skin and cervix should be carried out. Skin lesions which are not typical for psoriasis should be biopsied before starting Neoral treatment to exclude skin cancers, mycosis fungoides or other pre-malignant disorders. Patients with malignant or pre-malignant alterations of the skin should be treated with Neoral only after appropriate treatment of such lesions and only if no other option for successful therapy exists.

Because of the possibility of renal dysfunction or renal structural changes, serum creatinine should be measured at two weekly intervals during the first three months of therapy. Thereafter, if creatinine remains stable, measurements should be made at monthly intervals. If serum creatinine increases and remains increased to more than 30% above baseline at more than one measurement, Neoral dosage must be reduced by 25 to 50%. These recommendations apply even if the patient's values still lie within the laboratory's normal range. If dosage reduction is not successful within one month, Neoral treatment should be discontinued.

In atopic dermatitis patients serum creatinine should be measured at two weekly intervals throughout the treatment period.

If hypertension develops which cannot be controlled by Neoral dosage reduction or appropriate antihypertensive therapy, discontinuation of Neoral is recommended.

Neoral treatment and its monitoring should be carried out under the supervision of a dermatologist experienced in the management of severe skin diseases.

In view of the potential risk of skin malignancy, patients on Neoral should be warned to avoid excessive unprotected sun exposure and should not receive concomitant therapeutic ultraviolet B irradiation or PUVA photochemotherapy.

Additional precautions in atopic dermatitis: Active herpes simplex infections should be allowed to clear before initiating treatment with Neoral but are not necessarily a reason for drug withdrawal if they occur during treatment unless infection is severe.

Skin infections with *Staphylococcus aureus* are not an absolute contra-indication for Neoral therapy but should be controlled with appropriate antibacterial agents. Oral erythromycin, known to have the potential to increase the blood concentration of cyclosporin (see *Interactions*) should be avoided or, if there is no alternative, its concomitant use must be accompanied by close monitoring of the blood levels of cyclosporin.

There is currently no experience with Neoral in children with atopic dermatitis. Its use in patients under 16 years of age cannot, therefore, be recommended.

Additional precautions in rheumatoid arthritis: Since cyclosporin can impair renal function, a reliable baseline level of serum creatinine should be established by at least two measurements prior to treatment, and serum creatinine should be monitored at 2 weekly intervals during the first 3 months of therapy. Thereafter, measurements can be made every 4 weeks, but more frequent checks are necessary when the Neoral dose is increased or concomitant treatment with a non-steroidal anti-inflammatory drug is initiated or its dosage increased. Because the pharmacodynamic interaction between cyclosporin and NSAIDs may adversely affect renal function, caution should be exercised if NSAID therapy is to be continued.

If the serum creatinine remains increased by more than 30% above creatinine levels recorded before starting cyclosporin therapy at more than one measurement, the dosage of Neoral should be reduced. If the serum creatinine increases by more than 50%, a dosage reduction by 50% is mandatory. These recommendations apply even if the patient's values still lie within the laboratory normal range. If dosage reduction is not successful in reducing levels within one month, Neoral treatment should be discontinued.

Discontinuation of the drug may also become necessary if hypertension developing during Neoral therapy cannot be controlled by appropriate anti-hypertensive therapy.

The combination of non-steroidal anti-inflammatory drugs and cyclosporin should be used with caution in patients with rheumatoid arthritis and should be accompanied by particularly close monitoring of renal function as detailed above.

As hepatotoxicity is a potential side effect of non-steroidal anti-inflammatory drugs, regular monitoring of hepatic function is advised when Neoral is co-administered with these drugs in rheumatoid arthritis patients.

The use of cyclosporin therapy for the treatment of patients with rheumatoid arthritis requires careful monitoring and follow-up. Neoral should only be used provided that the necessary expertise and adequate equipment, laboratory and supportive medical resources are available.

Patients with rheumatoid arthiritis have an increased incidence of malignancies compared to the general population. Use of disease modifying drugs increases the risk of malignancy further. The use of cyclosporin in the treatment of rheumatoid arthritis has not been shown to increase the incidence of malignancies more than other disease-modifying drugs.

Additional precautions in nephrotic syndrome: Development of malignancies (including Hodgkin's lymphoma) has occasionally been reported in nephrotic syndrome patients treated with cyclosporin, as well as during treatment with other immunosuppressive agents. However, malignancy may be related to the pathogenesis of the disease.

Since cyclosporin can impair renal function, it is necessary to assess renal function frequently and if the serum creatinine remains increased by more than 30% above baseline at more than one measurement, to reduce the dosage of Neoral by 25–50%. Patients with abnormal baseline renal function are at higher risk. They should initially be treated with 2.5 mg/kg per day orally and must be monitored very carefully.

In some patients it may be difficult to detect Neoral-induced renal dysfunction because of changes in renal function related to the underlying renal disease. If Neoral is indicated for more than one year in the long-term management, then renal biopsies should be performed at 1 yearly intervals to assess the progression of the renal disease and the extent of any Neoral-associated changes in the renal morphology that may co-exist.

The use of Neoral therapy for the treatment of patients with nephrotic syndrome requires careful monitoring and follow-up. Neoral should only be used provided that the necessary expertise and adequate equipment, laboratory and supporting medical resources are available.

Interactions with other medicaments and other forms of interactions: Care should be taken when using cyclosporin in combination with systemic antibiotics or other compounds known to have nephrotoxic effects e.g. aminoglycosides, amphotericin B, ciprofloxacin, melphalan and trimethoprim.

Various agents are known to either increase or decrease the plasma or whole blood concentrations of cyclosporin by competitive inhibition or induction of hepatic enzymes involved in the metabolism and excretion of cyclosporin, in particular cytochrome P450. Agents known to increase plasma or whole blood concentrations of cyclosporin include clarithromycin ketoconazole, erythromycin, oral contraceptives, danazol and some calcium channel blockers including diltiazem, nicardipine and verapamil. Doxycycline, fluconazole, itraconazole, propafenone and lipid solutions are also suspected of having the same effect. Agents known to decrease plasma or whole blood cyclosporin concentrations include phenytoin, carbamazepine, barbiturates and rifampicin. Sulphadiazine is also suspected of having the same effect.

In transplant patients, frequent measurement of cyclosporin and, if necessary, cyclosporin dosage adjustment is required, particularly during the introduction or withdrawal of co-administered drug. In non-transplant patients, the relationship between blood level and clinical effect is less well established. If drugs known to increase cyclosporin levels are given concomitantly, frequent assessment of renal function and careful monitoring for cyclosporin related side-effects may be more appropriate than blood level measurement.

Intraveneous (but not oral) administration of sulphadimidine and trimethoprim has also resulted in a marked reduction of plasma or whole blood levels of cyclosporin. Concomitant administration of such drugs with cyclosporin should, therefore, be avoided. Where combined administration is unavoidable, careful monitoring of cyclosporin blood levels and appropriate adjustment of cyclosporin dosage are essential.

In addition, it has been noted that cyclosporin reduces the clearance of prednisolone and, conversely, high-dose therapy with methylprednisolone can increase the blood concentration of cyclosporin.

As non-steroidal anti-inflammatory drugs alone can have an adverse effect on renal function, addition of these drugs to cyclosporin therapy or an increase in their dosages, should initially be accompanied by particularly close monitoring of renal function.

Cyclosporin given in combination with diclofenac causes an increase in plasma concentration of diclofenac. Diclofenac dosages should, therefore, be reduced by approximately half when given with cyclosporin. There have been reports of pharmacokinetic interactions between cyclosporin with other non-steroidal anti-inflammatory drugs, but there are insufficient data available to clarify their significance. However, a lack of pharmacokinetic interaction has been demonstrated between aspirin and cyclosporin.

Some studies have shown that various NSAIDs interact pharmacodynamically with cyclosporin to affect renal function. An analysis of clinical trials of cyclosporin and non-steroidal anti-inflammatory drugs suggest that plasma creatinine is not higher in patients if they receive concomitant NSAID therapy. The combination of these drugs, however, should be used with care.

Administration of cyclosporin may enhance the potential of the HMG-CoA reductase inhibitor lovastatin to induce rhabdomyolysis. The potential for interaction with other drugs in this class should be considered.

Muscular toxicity, including muscle pains and weakness, have also been reported in patients receiving colchicine concurrently with cyclosporin.

The concurrent administration of nifedipine and cyclosporin has resulted in an increased rate of gingival hyperplasia when compared with that for cyclosporin alone. It is recommended that nifedipine should be avoided in patients who develop gingival hypertrophy during therapy with cyclosporin. Where there is a risk of hyperkalaemia, potassium-sparing diuretics should be avoided and care should be taken when prescribing potassium supplements or potassium containing medications.

Since cyclosporin occasionally causes hyperkalaemia or may aggravate pre-existing hyperkalaemia, monitoring of serum potassium is recommended, especially in patients with marked renal dysfunction. Patients receiving cyclosporin should avoid a high dietary potassium intake.

During treatment with cyclosporin, vaccination may be less effective, and the use of live attenuated vaccines should be avoided.

Pregnancy and lactation: Cyclosporin is not teratogenic in animals. There is currently no clinical experience with Neoral and experience with Sandimmun is still limited. However, data available from organ transplant recipients indicate that, compared with traditional therapy, cyclosporin treatment imposes no increased risk of adverse effects on the course and outcome of pregnancy. However, there are no adequate and well controlled studies in pregnant women, therefore cyclosporin should be used during pregnancy only if the potential benefit justifies the potential risk to the foetus.

Cyclosporin passes into breast milk. Mothers receiving treatment with cyclosporin should not, therefore, breast-feed their infants.

Effects on ability to drive and use machines: No data exists on the effects of Neoral on the ability to drive and use machines.

Undesirable effects: The following side-effects have been observed with cyclosporin treatment. They are usually dose dependent and responsive to dose reduction.

A frequent and potentially serious complication is a dose-dependent and reversible increase in serum creatinine and urea during the first few weeks of therapy. Less frequently, renal structural changes (e.g. interstitial fibrosis) may develop during long-term treatment. Impairment of renal function may necessitate dosage reduction or, in patients treated for psoriasis, discontinuation of cyclosporin therapy (see *Precautions*).

Apart from impaired renal function, the most frequently observed side-effects include hypertrichosis, tremor, hypertension (particularly in heart transplant patients) hepatic dysfunction, fatigue, gingival hypertrophy, gastrointestinal disturbances (abdominal pain, anorexia, nausea, vomiting, diarrhoea) and burning sensations of the hands and feet (usually during the first week of treatment).

Occasionally, headaches, rashes of possible allergic origin, mild anaemia, hyperkalaemia, hyperuricaemia, gout, hypomagnesaemia, hypercholesterolaemia, weight increase, oedema, pancreatitis, neuropathy, confusion, paraesthesia, convulsions, reversible dysmenorrhoea or amenorrhoea may develop.

Muscle weakness, muscle cramps, or myopathy have been reported.

Especially in liver transplant patients, signs of encephalopathy, vision and movement disturbances, and impaired consciousness are described. Whether these alterations are caused by cyclosporin, or are a consequence of the underlying disease, or other conditions, remains to be established.

On rare occasions, a syndrome of thrombocytopenia, in some patients in combination with micro-angiopathic haemolytic anaemia and renal failure (haemolytic uraemic syndrome) has been observed.

Gynaecomastia has been rarely reported, occasionally in patients receiving concomitant spironolactone.

Malignancies and lymphoproliferative disorders have developed, but their incidence and distribution were found to be similar to those in patients on conventional immunosuppressive therapy. Where lymphoproliferative disorders have developed in patients with psoriasis, they have been responsive to prompt drug discontinuation.

In a few cases, colitis has developed after treatment with cyclosporin.

Overdose: No experience of acute overdosage with Neoral is available and little experience is available with regards to overdosage with Sandimmun. Symptomatic treatment and general supportive measures should be followed in all cases of overdosage. Forced emesis could be of value within the first few hours after intake. Signs of nephrotoxicity might occur which should be expected to resolve following drug withdrawal. Cyclosporin is not dialysable to any great extent nor is it well cleared by charcoal haemoperfusion. Hypertension and convulsions have been reported in some patients receiving cyclosporin therapy at doses above the recommended range and in others with high trough blood levels of cyclosporin. This might, therefore, be expected as a feature of overdosage.

Pharmacological properties

Pharmacodynamic properties: Cyclosporin is a cyclic polypeptide consisting of 11 amino acids. It is a potent immunosuppressive agent which prolongs survival of allogeneic transplants involving skin, heart, kidney, pancreas, cornea, bone marrow, small intestine and lung in animals.

Successful solid organ and bone marrow allogeneic transplants have been performed in man, using cyclosporin to prevent and treat rejection and GVHD. Marked beneficial effects of cyclosporin therapy have also been shown in partients with severe psoriasis, atopic dermatitis and rheumatoid arthritis, conditions that may be considered to have an immunological mechanism.

Studies in animals suggest that cyclosporin inhibits the development of cell mediated reactions. It appears to block the resting lymphocytes in the G_0 or early G_1 phase of the cell cycle, and also inhibits lymphokine production and release, including interleukin 2 (T cell growth factor, TCGF). The available evidence suggests that cyclosporin acts specifically and reversibly on lymphocytes. It does not depress haemopoiesis and has no effect on the function of phagocytic cells.

Pharmacokinetic properties: Neoral is an improved pharmaceutical form of the active ingredient cyclosporin. Neoral is a pre-concentrate formulation of cyclosporin which undergoes a microemulsification process in the presence of water, either in the form of a beverage or in the form of the gastrointestinal fluid. Neoral reduces the intra-patient variability of pharmacokinetic parameters, with a more consistent absorption profile and less influence of concomitant food intake and the presence of bile. In pharmacokinetic and clinical studies it has been demonstrated that the correlation between trough concentration (C_{min}) and total exposure (AUC) is significantly stronger when cyclosporin is given as Neoral than when it is given as Sandimmun. Neoral, therefore, allows greater predictability and consistency of cyclosporin exposure.

The data available indicate that following a 1:1 conversion from Sandimmun Soft Gelatin Capsules and Sandimmun Oral Solution to Neoral, trough concentrations in whole blood are comparable, thereby remaining in the desired therapeutic trough level range. Compared to oral administration of Sandimmun (with which peak blood concentrations are achieved within 1 to 6 hours), Neoral is more quickly absorbed (resulting in a 1 hour earlier mean t_{max} and a 59% higher mean C_{max}) and exhibits, on average, a 29% higher bioavailability. In a clinical trial involving maintained renal transplant patients the correlation (r^2) between trough concentration (C_{min}) and exposure (AUC) was good (0.8).

Cyclosporin is extensively biotransformed to approximately 15 metabolites. There is no single major metabolic pathway. Elimination is primarily biliary, with only 6% of the oral dose excreted in the urine, only 0.1% is excreted in the urine as unchanged drug.

There is a high variability in the data reported on the terminal half-life of cyclosporin depending on the assay applied and the target population. The terminal half-life ranged from 6.3 hours in healthy volunteers to 20.4 hours in patients with severe liver disease.

Preclinical safety data: Cyclosporin gave no evidence of mutagenic or teratogenic effects in appropriate test systems. Only at dose levels toxic to dams were adverse effects seen in reproduction studies in rats. At toxic doses (rats at 30 mg/kg and rabbits at 100 mg/kg a day orally), cyclosporin was embryo- and fetotoxic as indicated by increased pre-natal and post-natal mortality and reduced fetal weight together with related skeletal retardation. In the well-tolerated dose range (rats up to 17 mg/kg and rabbits up to 30 mg/kg a day orally), cyclosporin proved to be without any embryolethal or teratogenic effects.

Carcinogenicity studies were carried out in male and female rats and mice. In the 78-week mouse study, at doses of 1, 4, and 16 mg/kg a day, evidence of a statistically significant trend was found for lymphocytic lymphomas in females, and the incidence of hepatocellular carcinomas in mid-dose males significantly exceeded the control value. In the 24-month rat study conducted at 0.5, 2, and 8 mg/kg a day, pancreatic islet cell adenomas significantly exceeded the control rate at the low dose level. The hepatocellular carcinomas and pancreatic islet cell adenomas were not dose related. No impairment in fertility was demonstrated in studies in male and female rats.

Cyclosporin has not been found to be mutagenic/genotoxic in the Ames test, the V79-HGPRT test, the micronucleus test in mice and Chinese hamsters, the chromosome-aberration tests in Chinese hamster bone marrow, the mouse dominant lethal assay, and the DNA repair test in sperm from treated mice. A study analysing sister chromatid exchange (SCE) induction by cyclosporin using human lymphocytes *in vitro* gave indication of a positive effect (i.e. induction of SCE) at high concentrations in this system.

An increased incidence of malignancy is a recognised complication of immunosuppression in recipients of organ transplants. The most common forms of neoplasms are non-Hodgkin's lymphoma and carcinomas of the skin. The risk of malignancies during cyclosporin treatment is higher than in the normal, healthy population, but similar to that in patients receiving other immunosuppressive therapies. It has been reported that reduction or discontinuance of immunosuppression may cause lesions to regress.

Pharmaceutical particulars

List of excipients:

Soft gelatin capsules: DL-α-tocopherol, absolute ethanol, propylene glycol, corn oil mono-di-triglycerides, polyoxyl 40 hydrogenated castor oil.

Capsule shell: Iron oxide black (25 mg and 100 mg capsules), titanium dioxide, glycerol 85% propylene glycol, gelatin.

Solution: DL-α-tocopherol, absolute ethanol, propylene glycol, corn oil mono-di-triglycerides, polyoxyl 40 hydrogenated castor oil.

Incompatibilities: None known.

Shelf life: Soft gelatin capsules and solution 36 months.

Special precautions for storage: Neoral Soft Gelatin Capsules should be stored below 25°C.

Neoral Soft Gelatin Capsules should be left in the blister pack until required for use. When a blister is opened, a characteristic smell is noticeable.

Neoral Oral Solution should be stored below 30°C (preferably not below 15°C, as it contains oily components of natural origin which tend to solidify at low temperatures). A jelly-like formation may occur below 20°C which is, however, reversible at temperatures up to 30°C. Minor flakes or a slight sediment may still be observed. These phenomena do not affect the efficacy and safety of the product, and the dosing by means of the measuring device remains accurate.

Nature and contents of container: Neoral Soft Gelatin Capsules are available in 6×5 blister packs of double-sided aluminium consisting of an aluminium bottom foil and an aluminium covering foil.

Neoral Oral Solution is available in 50 ml amber glass bottles with an aluminium cap and rubber stopper. A dispenser set is also provided.

Instructions for use/handling: Initial use of Neoral Oral Solution:

1. Flip off plastic cap and bend right back.
2. Tear off whole of cap and sealing ring.
3. Remove black stopper from bottle and dispose of carefully.
4. Push tube unit firmly into neck of bottle.
5. Insert syringe into stopper.
6. Draw up prescribed volume of solution.
7. Expel any *large* bubbles by depressing and withdrawing plunger a few times before removing syringe containing prescribed dose from bottle. The presence of a few tiny bubbles is of no importance and will not affect the dose in any way.
8. After use, wipe syringe *on outside only* with a *dry* tissue and replace in its case. Dispose of the tissue carefully. White stopper and tube should remain in bottle. Close bottle with cap provided.

Subsequent use: Commence at point 5.

Marketing authorisation holder: Novartis Pharmaceuticals UK Limited, trading as Sandoz Pharmaceuticals.

Marketing authorisation numbers

Neoral Soft Gelatin Capsules	10 mg	0101/0483
	25 mg	0101/0387
	50 mg	0101/0388
	100 mg	0101/0389
Neoral Oral Solution		0101/0390

Date of approval/revision of SPC April 1998.

Legal category POM.

NORPROLAC*

Qualitative and quantitative composition Quinagolide as the hydrochloride, 25 mcg, 50 mcg, 75 mcg or 150 mcg.

Pharmaceutical form Tablet for oral administration.

Clinical particulars

Therapeutic indications: Hyperprolactinaemia (idiopathic or originating from a prolactin-secreting pituitary microadenoma or macroadenoma).

Posology and method of administration: Since dopaminergic stimulation may lead to symptoms of orthostatic hypotension, the dosage of Norprolac should be initiated gradually with the aid of the 'starter pack', and given only at bedtime.

Adults: The optimal dose must be titrated individually on the basis of the prolactin-lowering effect and tolerability.

With the 'starter pack', treatment begins with 25 mcg/day for the first 3 days, followed by 50 mcg/day for a further 3 days. From day 7 onwards, the recommended dose is 75 mcg/day.

If necessary, the daily dose may then be increased stepwise until the optimal individual response is attained. The usual maintenance dosage is 75 to 150 mcg/day.

Daily doses of 300 mcg or higher doses are required in less than one-third of patients. In such cases, the daily dosage may be increased in steps of 75 to 150 mcg at intervals not shorter than 4 weeks until satisfactory therapeutic effectiveness is achieved or reduced tolerability, requiring the discontinuation of treatment, occurs.

Elderly: Experience with the use of Norprolac in elderly patients is not available.

Children: Experience with the use of Norprolac in children is not available.

Method of administration: Norprolac should be taken once a day with some food at bedtime.

Contra-indications: Hypersensitivity to the drug. Impaired hepatic or renal function. For procedure during pregnancy, see *Pregnancy and lactation.*

Special warnings and precautions for use: Fertility may be restored by treatment with Norprolac. Women of child-bearing age who do not wish to conceive should therefore be advised to practice a reliable method of contraception.

Since orthostatic hypotension may result in syncope, it is recommended to check blood pressure both lying and standing during the first days of therapy and following dosage increases.

In a few cases, including patients with no previous history of mental illness, treatment with Norprolac has been associated with the occurrence of acute psychosis, usually reversible upon discontinuation. Particular caution is required in patients who have had psychotic episodes in their previous history.

To date no data is available with the use of Norprolac in patients with impaired renal or hepatic function (see *Contra-indications*).

Norprolac should be kept out of the reach of children.

Interactions with other medicaments and other forms of interaction: No interactions between Norprolac and other drugs have so far been reported. On theoretical grounds, a reduction of the prolactin-lowering effect could be expected when drugs (e.g. neuroleptic agents) with strong dopamine antagonistic properties are used concomitantly. As the potency of Norprolac for 5-HT_1 and 5-HT_2 receptors is some 100 times lower than that for D_2 receptors, an interaction between Norprolac and 5-HT_{1a} receptors is unlikely. However, care should be taken when using these medicaments concomitantly.

The tolerability of Norprolac may be reduced by alcohol.

Pregnancy and lactation

Pregnancy: Animal data provide no evidence that Norprolac has any embryotoxic or teratogenic potential, but experience in pregnant women is still limited. In patients wishing to conceive, Norprolac should be discontinued when pregnancy is confirmed, unless there is a medical reason for continuing therapy. No increased incidence of abortion has been observed following withdrawal of the drug at this point.

If pregnancy occurs in the presence of a pituitary adenoma and Norprolac treatment has been stopped, close supervision throughout pregnancy is essential.

Lactation: Breast-feeding is usually not possible since Norprolac suppresses lactation. If lactation should continue during treatment, breast-feeding cannot be recommended because it is not known whether quinagolide passes into human breast milk.

Effects on ability to drive and to use machines: Since, especially during the first days of treatment, hypotensive reactions may occasionally occur and result in reduced alertness, patients should be cautious when driving a vehicle or operating machinery.

Undesirable effects: The adverse reactions reported with the use of Norprolac are characteristic for dopamine receptor agonist therapy. They are usually not sufficiently serious to require discontinuation of treatment and tend to disappear when treatment is continued.

The most frequent side effects (>10%) are nausea, vomiting, headache, dizziness and fatigue. They occur predominantly during the first few days of the initial treatment or, as a mostly transient event, following dosage increase. If necessary, nausea and vomiting may be prevented by the intake of a peripheral dopaminergic antagonist, such as domperidone, for a few days, at least 1 hour before the ingestion of Norprolac.

Less frequent side effects (1 to 10%) include anorexia, abdominal pain, constipation or diarrhoea, insomnia, oedema, flushing, nasal congestion and hypotension. Orthostatic hypotension may result in faintness or syncope (see *Special warnings and special precautions for use*).

In a few isolated cases, treatment with Norprolac has been associated with the occurrence of acute psychosis, reversible upon discontinuation.

Overdose:

Symptoms: Acute overdosage with Norprolac tablets has not been reported. It would be expected to cause severe nausea, vomiting, headache, dizziness, drowsiness, hypotension and possibly collapse. Hallucinations could also occur.

Treatment: Should be symptomatic.

Pharmacological properties

Pharmacodynamic properties: Quinagolide, the active ingredient of Norprolac, is a selective dopamine D_2-receptor agonist not belonging to the chemical classes of ergot or ergoline compounds. Owing to its dopaminergic action, the drug exerts a strong inhibitory effect on the secretion of the anterior pituitary hormone prolactin, but does not reduce normal levels of other pituitary hormones. In some patients the reduction of prolactin secretion may be accompanied by short-lasting, small increases in plasma growth hormone levels, the clinical significance of which is unknown.

As a specific inhibitor of prolactin secretion with a prolonged duration of action, Norprolac has been shown to be effective and suitable for once-a-day oral treatment of patients presenting with hyperprolactinaemia and its clinical manifestations such as galactorrhoea, oligomenorrhoea, amenorrhoea, infertility and reduced libido.

Pharmacokinetic properties: After oral administration of radiolabelled drug, quinagolide is rapidly and well absorbed. Plasma concentration values obtained by a non-selective radio-immunoassay (RIA), measuring quinagolide together with some of it metabolites, were close to the limit of quantification and gave no reliable information.

The apparent volume of distribution of quinagolide after single oral administration of radiolabelled compound was calculated to be approx. 100 L. For the parent drug, a terminal half-life of 11.5 hours has been calculated under single dose conditions, and of 17 hours at steady state.

Quinagolide is extensively metabolised during its first pass. Studies performed with ^{3}H-labelled quinagolide revealed that more than 95% of the drug is excreted as metabolites. About equal amounts of total radioactivity are found in faeces and urine.

In blood, quinagolide and its N-desethyl analogue are the biologically active but minor components. Their inactive sulphate or glucuronide conjugates represent the major circulating metabolites. In urine, the main metabolites are the glucuronide and sulphate conjugates of quinagolide and the N-desethyl, N,N-didesethyl analogues. In the faeces the unconjugated forms of the three components are found.

The protein binding of quinagolide is approximately 90% and is non-specific.

The results, obtained in pharmacodynamic studies, indicate that with the recommended therapeutic dosage a clinically significant prolactin-lowering effect occurs within 2 hours after ingestion, reaches a maximum within 4 to 6 hours and is maintained for about 24 hours.

A definite dose-response relationship could be established for the duration, but not for the magnitude, of the prolactin-lowering effect which, with a single oral dose of 50 mcg was close to maximum. Higher doses did not result in a considerably greater effect but prolonged its duration.

Preclinical safety data:

Acute toxicity: The LD_{50} of quinagolide was determined for several species after single oral administration: mice 357 to >500 mg/kg; rats >500 mg/kg; rabbits >150 mg/kg.

Chronic toxicity: Decreased cholesterol levels of treated female rats suggest that quinagolide influences lipid metabolism. Since similar observations have been made with other dopaminergic drugs, a causal relationship with low prolactin levels is assumed. In several chronic studies with rats, enlarged ovaries resulting from an increased number of corpora lutea and, additionally, hydrometra and endometritis were observed. These changes were reversible and reflect the pharmacodynamic effect of quinagolide: suppression of prolactin secretion inhibits luteolysis in rats and thus influences the normal sexual cycle. In humans, however, prolactin is not involved in luteolysis.

Carcinogenic and mutagenic potential: In comprehensive in vitro and in vivo mutagenic studies there was no evidence of a mutagenic effect.

The changes which were observed in carcinogenicity studies reflect the pharmacodynamic activity of quinagolide. The drug modulates the prolactin level as well as, specially in male rats, the level of luteinising hormone and, in female rodents, the ratio of progesterone to oestrogen.

Long-term studies with high doses of quinagolide revealed Leydig cell tumours in rats and mesenchymal uterine tumours in mice. The incidence of Leydig cell tumours in a carcinogenicity study in rats was increased even at low doses (0.01 mg/kg). These results were without relevance for the therapeutic application in humans since there are fundamental differences between humans and rodents in the regulation of the endocrine system.

Reproductive toxicity: Animals studies in rats and rabbits showed no evidence for embryotoxic or teratogenic effects. The prolactin inhibiting effect led to a decrease of milk production in rats, which was associated with an increased loss of rat pups. Possible post-natal effects of exposure during fetal development (2nd and 3rd trimester) and effects on female fertility are not sufficiently investigated.

Pharmaceutical particulars

List of excipients: Iron oxide, red; indigotin lake; silica, colloidal anhydrous; magnesium stearate; methylhydroxypropylcellulose; maize starch; cellulose, microcrystalline; lactose.

Incompatibilities: Not applicable.

Shelf life: The shelf life is 3 years. The expiry date is printed on the box. On the blister the expiry date is marked with the letters EXP.

Special precautions for storage: The expiry date refers to original unopened boxes, which were stored under the correct conditions, i.e. between 15 and 30°C. No special warning with respect to light sensitivity or humidity is necessary because the tablets are protected by the packaging.

Nature and contents of container: The 'starter pack' (Norprolac 25/50) consists of 3 tablets of 25 mcg and 3 tablets of 50 mcg. These tablets are packed in an aluminium PVC/PVDC blister which is sealed in a moisture-proof aluminium bag.

The 75 mcg and 150 mcg tablets are in packs of 30 tablets (3 × 10 tablets in aluminium blisters).

Instructions for special handling: None.

Marketing authorisation holder: Novartis Pharmaceuticals UK Limited, trading as Sandoz Pharmaceuticals.

Marketing authorisation numbers

25 mcg 0101/0380
50 mcg 0101/0381
75 mcg 0101/0382
150 mcg 0101/0383

Date of approval/revision of SPC March 1997.

Legal category POM.

ORIMETEN TABLETS 250 mg

Qualitative and quantitative composition The active ingredient is 2-(p-Aminophenyl)-2-ethylglutarimide (aminoglutethimide).

Each tablet contains 250 mg aminoglutethimide INN.

Pharmaceutical form Tablets.

Clinical particulars

Therapeutic indications: Advanced carcinoma of the breast in post-menopausal or oophorectomised women (especially where the tumours are oestrogen-sensitive), including in particular patients who have previously responded to endocrine therapy or have painful bony metastases.

Advanced carcinoma of the prostate as palliative treatment. Subjective improvement and pain relief have been noted in up to 50% of patients.

Cushing's syndrome due to malignant disease, e.g. adrenocortical carcinoma or ectopic ACTH syndrome, in place of or in conjunction with surgery.

Posology and method of administration: Orimeten tablets should be administered orally.

Administration of Orimeten in small, gradually increasing doses substantially improves tolerability.

Adults: Advanced carcinoma of the breast and of the prostate: The initial dose of one tablet daily, should be increased each week by one tablet per day to the maximum tolerated dose, not exceeding 1000 mg daily e.g. Week 1–250 mg once daily, Week 2–250 mg twice daily, Week 3–250 mg three times daily, Week 4–250 mg four times daily.

In some patients with breast cancer a dose of 250 mg twice daily has proved sufficient.

In the majority of patients treated for carcinoma of the prostate the effective dose has not exceeded 750 mg daily.

Supplementary therapy: Orimeten should be employed in combination with glucocorticoid in order to offset the decrease in endogenous corticosteroid biosynthesis which Orimeten may provoke. Hydrocortisone, 30 mg daily (preferably 20 mg in the morning plus 10 mg in the afternoon or evening) or cortisone acetate in daily doses of 37.5 mg (25 mg in the morning and 12.5 mg in the afternoon) are suitable for supplementary therapy. Orimeten accelerates the metabolism of dexamethasone (or other synthetic corticosteroids) to a variable extent, therefore individual titration to a relatively high dose (up to 3 mg daily) may be required if this glucocorticoid is used.

Cushing's syndrome: Initially 250 mg daily, increasing gradually according to response up to 1 g daily in divided doses. In some cases, especially ectopic ACTH syndrome, higher dosages (of up to 1.5–2 g daily) may occasionally prove necessary to achieve adequate suppression.

Supplementary therapy: When treating Cushing's syndrome, the plasma cortisol levels should be determined regularly and the dosage of aminoglutethimide adjusted accordingly. Substitution therapy with corticosteroids occasionally proves necessary.

Children: Safety and efficacy have not been established in children.

Elderly: There is no evidence to suggest that dosage should be different in the elderly.

Contra-indications: History of severe hypersensitivity reactions to aminoglutethimide or glutethimide. Pregnancy and lactation. Porphyria.

Special warnings and special precautions for use: Orimeten may cause adrenal hypofunction, especially under conditions of stress, such as surgery, trauma, or acute illness. Patients should be carefully monitored and given hydrocortisone as recommended in the dosage section. If inhibition of aldosterone synthesis leads to hyponatraemia, hypotension, or dizziness, a mineralocorticoid, e.g. fludrocortisone (0.1–0.15 mg daily or every other day) should be given in addition. Patients should be warned of the possibility of hypotension and its symptoms.

The patients blood pressure, plasma electrolytes, blood counts and thyroid function should be checked during treatment with Orimeten. Particularly during the first 2–3 months of treatment when blood counts should be carried out once every 2–3 weeks. If blood dyscrasias develop, Orimeten should be withdrawn. In the event of hypothyroidism, substitution therapy with thyroxine must be instituted; such therapy, however, very seldom proves necessary because the decrease in thyroxine provoked by Orimeten is usually offset by a reactive rise in TSH.

Patients frequently develop a skin rash at the start of treatment; if this does not disappear within 10 days, Orimeten should be temporarily withdrawn and/or the corticosteroid dosage increased.

In a long-term rat carcinogenicity study an increased incidence in benign and malignant neoplasms of the adrenal cortex and the thyroid gland was noted in both sexes in one or more of the treated groups. These findings are not unexpected in view of the known pharmacodynamic properties of aminoglutethimide. The relevance of these findings in humans is not known.

Interaction with other medicaments and other forms of interaction: By inducing hepatic enzymes, Orimeten increases its own metabolism and also that of several drugs including synthetic glucocorticoids such as dexamethasone, warfarin and other oral anticoagulants, theophylline, medroxyprogesterone and oral antidiabetics. If necessary, the dosage of these drugs may have to be raised.

Concomitant therapy with diuretics may lead to hyponatraemia.

The effects of Orimeten may be potentiated if it is taken in combination with alcohol.

Pregnancy and lactation: Since foetal abnormalities and an increase in foetal deaths and resorption have been observed in animals and there have been cases of pseudohermaphroditism in newborn infants of women treated with Orimeten, the possible presence of a pregnancy must be excluded before prescribing Orimeten for women of child-bearing age (see *Contra-indications*). During treatment, such women should employ non-hormonal contraceptives.

No mutagenic potential was observed with Orimeten in standard *in vitro* and *in vivo* mutagenicity tests.

Effects on ability to drive and use machines: Patients should be warned that drowsiness may occur, in which case they should not drive, operate potentially dangerous machinery, or engage in other activities that may become hazardous because of decreased alertness.

Undesirable effects: Frequency estimate: frequent >10%, occasional >1%–<10%, rare >0.001%–<1%, isolated cases <0.001%.

Central nervous system: Frequent: drowsiness, lethargy. These are commonly observed at the beginning of treatment and generally abate after about 6 weeks. Occasional: dizziness (vertigo). Rare: ataxia, headache, depression. Isolated cases: insomnia, confusion.

Skin and appendages: Frequent: rash, sometimes accompanied by fever. This commonly occurs within the first 2 weeks of starting treatment and usually resolves spontaneously despite continued treatment. Rare: pruritus, urticaria. Isolated cases: exfoliative dermatitis, Stevens–Johnson syndrome

Gastrointestinal system: Occasional: nausea. Rare: diarrhoea, vomiting, constipation, anorexia.

Systemic: Rare: fever, sweating.

Liver: Isolated cases: hepatitis (cholestatic type, associated with itching and skin rash), jaundice.

Endocrine system: Rare: adrenal insufficiency (hyponatraemia, hypotension, dizziness, hypoglycaemia). Isolated cases: hypothyroidism, inappropriate ADH secretion, masculinisation and hirsutism in females.

Kidney: Isolated cases: renal function abnormalities.

Cardiovascular system: Rare: hypotension.

Haematological system: Rare: agranulocytosis, leucopenia, thrombocytopenia. Isolated cases: pancytopenia, anaemia.

Allergy: Isolated cases: allergic/anaphylactic reactions, allergic alveolitis (eosinophilic pulmonary infiltrates). Where such alveolitis is suspected, Orimeten should be withdrawn immediately.

Laboratory abnormalities: Rare: increased gamma-glutamyl transferase (gamma-GT). This is due to the enzyme-inducing effect of Orimeten and is usually not a sign of liver damage. Hyponatraemia, hyperkalaemia, hypoglycaemia. Isolated cases: hypercholesterolaemia.

Adverse reactions due to glucocorticoid replacement therapy: Isolated cases: Cushingoid symptoms (moon face, weight gain, oedema), arterial hypertension, hyperglycaemia, muscle cramps.

Overdose: Following an overdosage of Orimeten, signs and symptoms may appear which are caused by its effects both on the adrenal cortex and on the central nervous system, e.g. hypotension, drowsiness, lethargy, dizziness, ataxia, coma, electrolyte disturbances, respiratory depression and hypoventilation.

The signs and symptoms of acute overdosage with Orimeten may be aggravated or modified if alcohol, hypnotics, tranquillisers, or tricyclic antidepressants have been taken at the same time.

The following countermeasures should be taken:

Removal of the tablets ingested; intravenous administration of a glucocorticoid such as hydrocortisone; measures to increase plasma volume; administration of oxygen; intravenous treatment with vasoactive drugs, e.g. noradrenaline; if necessary, artificial respiration. Haemoperfusion may be considered.

Pharmacological properties

Pharmacodynamic properties: Aminoglutethimide inhibits the enzyme aromatase which converts androgens to oestrogens, and thus effects a reduction in oestrogen biosynthesis. In post-menopausal (or oophorectomised) women, oestrogens are derived primarily from extra-glandular (non-ovarian) aromatisation of adrenal precursors. Oestrogens are important in maintaining the growth of hormone dependent breast cancer. Treatment designed to lower circulating levels of oestrogens, results in tumour regression in patients with oestrogen receptor-positive tumours. In many cases of carcinoma of the breast, metastases or recurring tumours diminish in size, or even disappear during treatment with Orimeten. Such remission may be maintained for several years. Patients with soft tissue and bone metastases show the highest response rates, and some patients experience marked subjective relief from bone pain.

Orimeten also inhibits several other Cytochrome P450 mediated hydroxylation steps in the adrenal cortex, including conversion of cholesterol to 5 pregnenolone. Orimeten thus reduces the production of glucocorticoids and mineralocorticoids from the adrenal cortex, and reduces excessive plasma cortisol in patients with adrenocortical hyperfunction, such as Cushing's syndrome.

A decrease in adrenal secretion of cortisol leads to a reflex rise in adrenocorticotrophic hormone (ACTH) which will overcome the cortisol-lowering effect of Orimeten. This compensatory increase in ACTH secretion can be suppressed by the simultaneous administration of glucocorticoid.

The mode of action of Orimeten in prostatic carcinoma is not fully understood. Patients may benefit from marked relief of bone pain. Objective tumour regression has also been seen in some patients.

Pharmacokinetic properties: Orimeten is well absorbed and has a systemic availability of 92–98%. Peak plasma concentrations are attained within 1–4 hours. Mean steady state plasma concentrations vary between patients, but are proportional over the dose range 125–1000 mg/day. The drug is 21–25% bound to plasma proteins and during long term therapy the steady state elimination half-life averages 9 hours. Approximately 50% of the dose at steady state is excreted unchanged in the urine, and up to 25% in the form of N-hydroxylamino-glutethimide. Between 90% and 97% of the total dose is recovered in the urine. No reports of impaired metabolism or excretion of aminoglutethimide due to renal or hepatic dysfunction have been reported.

Preclinical safety data: No mutagenic potential was observed with Orimiten in standard *in vitro* and *in vivo* mutagenicity tests.

Pharmaceutical particulars

List of excipients: The tablets also contain silica aerogel, hydroxypropyl methylcellulose, magnesium stearate, maize starch and talc.

Incompatibilities: None known.

Shelf life: 5 years.

Special precautions for storage: Store below 30°C and protect from light and moisture.

Nature and contents of container: The tablets are white to yellowish white, round with slightly convex faces and slightly bevelled edges, printed 'CG' on one side and 'GG' with a score on the other and are contained in a blister pack of 56 tablets.

Instructions for use/handling: There is no specific instruction for use/handling.

Marketing authorisation holder: Novartis Pharmaceuticals UK Limited, trading as Ciba Laboratories, Frimley Business Park, Frimley, Camberley, Surrey GU16 5SG.

Marketing authorisation number PL 00101/0531.

Date of first authorisation/renewal of authorisation 17 November 1997.

Date of (partial) revision of the text December 1997.

PARLODEL*

Presentations

1 mg tablets: White, round, flat, bevel-edged Bromocriptine Mesylate Tablets PhEur, impressed PARLODEL 1 on one side and scored on the reverse. The tablets are 8 mm in diameter, with a nominal weight of 180 mg, and provide the equivalent of 1 mg bromocriptine base.

2.5 mg tablets: White, round, flat, bevel-edged Bromocriptine Mesylate Tablets PhEur, impressed PARLODEL 2.5 on one side and scored on the reverse. The tablets are 7 mm in diameter, with a nominal weight of 140 mg, and provide the equivalent of 2.5 mg bromocriptine base.

5 mg capsules: Opaque, hard gelatin Bromocriptine Mesylate Capsules PhEur. The capsules are size 3, upper part powder blue, lower part white, printed PARLODEL 5 in red and provide the equivalent of 5 mg bromocriptine base.

10 mg capsules: Opaque, hard gelatin Bromocriptine Mesylate Capsules PhEur. The capsules are size 1, white, printed PARLODEL 10 in red and provide the equivalent of 10 mg bromocriptine base.

Uses *Principal action:* Parlodel is a dopaminergic-receptor stimulant or dopamine agonist. This pharmacological action is manifest in normal individuals and those with hyperprolactinaemic states by an inhibition of the secretion of prolactin by the pituitary; in many acromegalic patients a lowering of elevated circulating growth hormone levels results.

In patients with prolactin secreting adenomas there is radiological evidence to indicate tumour regression in some cases.

Because of its dopaminergic activity Parlodel is also effective in idiopathic Parkinson's disease, which is characterised by a specific nigro-striatal dopamine deficiency.

Indications: The inhibition or suppression of puerperal lactation for medical reasons. Parlodel is not recommended for the routine suppression of lactation, or for the relief of symptoms of postpartum pain and engorgement, which can be adequately treated with simple analgesics and breast support.

The treatment of hyperprolactinaemia in men and women with hypogonadism and/or galactorrhoea.

The treatment of hyperprolactinaemic infertility. Parlodel has been used successfully in the treatment of a number of infertile women who do not have demonstrable hyperprolactinaemia.

In a number of specialized units, patients who have been shown to have prolactin secreting adenomas have been treated successfully with Parlodel. In particular Parlodel can be considered as a first choice of treatment in patients with macroadenomas and as an alternative to the surgical procedure, transsphenoidal hypophysectomy, in patients with microadenomas.

The treatment of cyclical benign breast disease/cyclical pronounced mastalgia.

Cyclical menstrual disorders have also responded to Parlodel, particularly breast symptomatology, but in the premenstrual syndrome there is also some evidence that other symptoms, such as headache, mood changes and bloatedness, may be alleviated.

Parlodel has been used in a number of specialized units, as an adjunct to surgery and/or radiotherapy, to reduce circulating growth hormone levels in the management of acromegalic patients.

In the treatment of idiopathic Parkinson's disease, Parlodel has been used both alone and in combination with levodopa in the management of previously untreated patients and those disabled by 'on-off' phenomena. Parlodel has been used with occasional benefit in patients who do not respond to, or are unable to tolerate, levodopa and those whose response to levodopa is declining.

Dosage and administration Parlodel should always be taken during a meal.

A number of disparate conditions are amenable to treatment with Parlodel and, for this reason, the recommended dosage regimens are variable. In most indications, irrespective of the final dosage, the optimum response with the minimum of side-effects is best achieved by gradual introduction of Parlodel. The following scheme is suggested:

Initially 1 mg to 1.25 mg at bedtime, increasing after 2 to 3 days to 2 mg to 2.5 mg at bedtime. Dosage may then be increased by 1 mg to 2.5 mg at 2 to 3 day intervals, until a dosage of 2.5 mg twice daily is achieved. Further dosage increments, if necessary, should be added in a similar manner.

Prevention of lactation: 2.5 mg on the day of delivery, followed by 2.5 mg twice daily for 14 days. Gradual introduction of Parlodel is not necessary in this indication.

Suppression of lactation: 2.5 mg on the first day, increasing after 2 to 3 days to 2.5 mg twice daily for 14 days. Gradual introduction of Parlodel is not necessary in this indication.

Hypogonadism/galactorrhoea syndromes/infertility: Introduce Parlodel gradually according to the suggested scheme. Most patients with hyperprolactinaemia have responded to 7.5 mg daily, in divided doses, but doses of up to 30 mg daily have been used. In infertile patients without demonstrably elevated serum prolactin levels, the usual dosage is 2.5 mg twice daily.

Prolactinomas: Introduce Parlodel gradually according to the suggested scheme. Dosage may then be increased by 2.5 mg daily at 2 to 3 day intervals as follows: 2.5 mg eight-hourly, 2.5 mg six-hourly, 5 mg six-hourly. Patients have responded to doses of up to 30 mg daily.

Cyclical benign breast disease/cyclical pronounced mastalgia/cyclical menstrual disorders: Introduce Parlodel gradually, according to the suggested scheme, until the recommended dosage of 2.5 mg twice daily is reached.

Acromegaly: Introduce Parlodel gradually, according to the suggested scheme. Dosage may then be increased by 2.5 mg daily at 2 to 3 day intervals as follows: 2.5 mg eight-hourly, 2.5 mg six-hourly, 5 mg six-hourly.

Parkinson's disease: Introduce Parlodel gradually, as follows: Week 1: 1 mg to 1.25 mg at bed time. Week 2: 2 mg to 2.5 mg at bed time. Week 3: 2.5 mg twice daily. Week 4: 2.5 mg three times daily. Thereafter, take three times a day increasing by 2.5 mg every 3 to 14 days depending on the patient's response. Continue until the optimum dose is reached. This will usually be between 10 and 40 mg daily. In patients already receiving levodopa the dosage of this drug may be gradually decreased, while the dosage of Parlodel is increased until the optimum balance is determined.

Use in children: Administration of Parlodel is not appropriate for children less than 15 years old.

Use in the elderly: There is no clinical evidence that Parlodel poses a special risk to the elderly.

Contra-indications, warnings, etc

Contra-indications: Hypersensitivity to bromocriptine or other ergot alkaloids. Toxaemia of pregnancy, hypertension postpartum and in the puerperium. For procedure during pregnancy see *Use in pregnancy*.

Precautions: Parlodel should not be used in the postpartum or puerperium in women with high blood pressure, coronary artery disease or symptoms and/or a history of serious mental disorders (see 'Side-effects'). In postpartum women receiving Parlodel, blood pressure should be carefully monitored, especially during the first days of therapy. Particular caution is required in patients who are on concomitant therapy with, or have recently been treated with, drugs that can alter blood pressure. Although there is no conclusive evidence of an interaction between Parlodel and other ergot alkaloids, a concomitant course of these medications during the puerperium is not recommended. If hypertension, unremitting headache, or any signs of CNS toxicity develop, treatment should be discontinued immediately.

Hyperprolactinaemia may be idiopathic, drug-induced, or due to hypothalamic or pituitary disease. The possibility that hyperprolactinaemic patients may have a pituitary tumour should be recognised and complete investigation at specialized units to identify such patients is advisable. Parlodel will effectively lower prolactin levels in patients with pituitary tumours but does not obviate the necessity for radiotherapy or surgical intervention where appropriate in acromegaly.

In women suffering from prolactin-related fertility disorders, treatment with Parlodel results in ovulation. Patients who do not wish to conceive should be advised to practice a reliable method of contraception. Oral contraceptives have, however, been reported to increase serum prolactin levels. When women of child-bearing age are treated with Parlodel for conditions not associated with hyperprolactinaemia the lowest effective dose should be used. This is in order to avoid suppression of prolactin to below normal levels, with consequent impairment of luteal function.

Gynaecological assessment, preferably including cervical and endometrial cytology, is recommended for women receiving Parlodel for extensive periods. Six-monthly assessment is suggested for post-menopausal women and annual assessment for women with regular menstruation.

Hypotensive reactions may be disturbing in some patients during the first few days of treatment and particular care should be exercised when driving vehicles or operating machinery.

Tolerance to Parlodel may be reduced by alcohol.

The concomitant use of erythromycin may increase bromocriptine plasma levels.

In acromegalic patients, whilst Parlodel may effectively lower growth hormone levels, treatment to limit expansion of the tumour is also indicated. Acromegalic patients should be carefully assessed for peptic ulceration prior to treatment with Parlodel and advised to report gastro-intestinal side-effects promptly, as gastro-intestinal bleeding has been reported, though the connection with treatment is not proven.

Caution is required where Parlodel is being given in high doses to patients with a history of psychotic disorders or severe cardiovascular disease.

Among parkinsonian patients on long-term, high-dose Parlodel treatment, pleural effusions have been observed. Patients with unexplained pleuro-pulmonary signs or symptoms should be examined thoroughly and discontinuation of Parlodel therapy should be contemplated.

In a few patients treated for more than a year, with daily doses greater than 30 mg, retroperitoneal fibrosis has been reported. Patients on long-term, high-dose therapy should therefore be observed for manifestations of retroperitoneal fibrosis (e.g. back pain, oedema of the lower limbs or impaired kidney function) so that retroperitoneal fibrosis may be detected at an early stage. Parlodel should be withdrawn if fibrotic changes in the retroperitoneum are diagnosed or suspected.

Use in pregnancy: If pregnancy occurs it is generally advisable to withdraw Parlodel after the first missed menstrual period.

Rapid expansion of pituitary tumours sometimes occurs during pregnancy and this may also occur in patients who have been able to conceive as a result of Parlodel therapy. As a precautionary measure, patients should be monitored to detect signs of pituitary enlargement so that Parlodel may be reintroduced if necessary. Based on the outcome of more than 2,000 pregnancies, the use of Parlodel to restore fertility has not been associated with an increased risk of abortion, premature delivery, multiple pregnancy or malformation in infants. Because this accumulated evidence suggests a lack of teratogenic or embryopathic effect in humans, maintenance of Parlodel treatment during pregnancy may be considered where there is a large tumour or evidence of expansion.

Overdosage: Overdosage with Parlodel is likely to result in vomiting and other symptoms which could be due to over-stimulation of dopaminergic receptors and might include confusion, hallucinations and hypotension. General supportive measures should be undertaken to remove any unabsorbed material and maintain blood pressure if necessary.

Side-effects: Nausea is the most commonly occurring side-effect. Postural hypotension, dizziness, headache, vomiting, and mild constipation have also occasionally been reported. The occurrence of side-effects is minimised by taking Parlodel during a meal and by gradual introduction of the dose. If side-effects do occur, a reduction of dosage, followed in a few days by a more gradual increase, will ameliorate the symptoms.

Episodes of reversible pallor of the fingers and toes induced by cold have occasionally been reported to occur during prolonged treatment, particularly in patients previously exhibiting Raynaud's phenomenon. Drowsiness, and less frequently, confusion, psychomotor excitation, hallucinations, dyskinesia, dry mouth and leg cramps have been reported during high-dose treatment of Parkinson's disease with Parlodel. All these side-effects are dose-dependent and can usually be controlled by a reduction in dosage and a more gradual implementation of dosage increments.

In extremely rare cases (in post partum women treated with Parlodel for the prevention of lactation) serious adverse events including hypertension, myocardial infarction, seizures, stroke, or mental disorders, have been reported although the causal relationship is uncertain. In some patients the occurrence of seizures or stroke was preceded by severe headache and/or transient visual disturbances.

Pharmaceutical precautions Protect from light.

Legal category POM.

Package quantities 1 mg Tablets: Containers of 100.
2.5 mg Tablets: Blister pack of 30 and containers of 100.
5 mg Capsules: Containers of 100.
10 mg Capsules: Containers of 100.

Further information Nil.

Product licence numbers

1 mg Tablets	0101/0176
2.5 mg Tablets	0101/0061
5 mg Capsules	0101/0131
10 mg Capsules	0101/0108

Product licence holder: Novartis Pharmaceuticals UK Ltd, trading as Sandoz Pharmaceuticals.

Date of last revision: May 1997.

PRESCAL*

Presentation The active ingredient, isradipine, is presented as: 2.5 mg yellow, flat circular angled scored tablets (designed to be easily divided), 6 mm diameter, marked NM on one face and CIBA on the other.

Uses

Indication: Prescal is recommended for the treatment of essential hypertension.

Mode of action: Isradipine is a dihydropyridine calcium antagonist with a higher affinity for calcium channels in arterial smooth muscle than for those in the myocardium. Thus it produces vasodilation of peripheral, coronary, and cerebral arteries without notably depressing cardiac function. As a result of the vasodilation of peripheral arteries, the arterial blood pressure is lowered; the attending after-load reduction improves myocardial contractility and increases cardiac output, while myocardial oxygen consumption decreases. In animal studies isradipine has been observed to exert a cardioprotective effect against ischaemic injury without cardiodepression.

Pharmacokinetics: Following oral administration of Prescal, isradipine is almost completely absorbed (90-95%) from the gastrointestinal tract and undergoes extensive first pass metabolism resulting in a bioavailability of about 15-24%. Single oral doses are detectable in the plasma within 20 minutes and peak plasma concentrations are reached approximately 2 hours after intake. Isradipine is approximately 95% bound to plasma proteins.

No clear correlation between renal function and pharmacokinetic parameters has been found; both an increase and decrease in bioavailability has been observed in patients with impaired renal function. The bioavailability of isradipine was increased in elderly patients with impaired liver function.

Dosage and administration Prescal can be administered with or without food.

The recommended dosage is 2.5 mg twice a day (i.e about every 12 hours). Treatment for 3-4 weeks is required for the maximum effect to develop. If blood pressure is not adequately controlled after this period patients may require a dosage of 5 mg twice a day, or if more appropriate, the addition of a low dose of another antihypertensive agent i.e. thiazide diuretic or beta-blocker. Exceptionally, some patients may require up to 10 mg twice a day. Prescal can also be added to an ongoing regimen of other antihypertensive agents.

Use in the elderly and patients with impaired hepatic or renal function: In elderly patients, or where hepatic or renal function is impaired, a more suitable starting dose is 1.25 mg twice a day for hypertension. However, the dosage may be increased according to the requirements of the individual patient. Once daily maintenance treatment with 2.5 mg or 5 mg may be sufficient in some hypertensive patients.

Use in children: The efficacy and safety of Prescal has not been established in children and is therefore not recommended in these patients.

Contra-indications, warnings, etc

Contra-indications: Patients with a previous allergic reaction to isradipine and other dihydropyridines because of the theoretical risk of cross-reactivity.

Dihydropyridines, including Prescal tablets, should be discontinued in patients who develop cardiogenic shock. They should also not be used in patients with symptomatic or tight aortic stenosis, and during or within one month of myocardial infarction.

Dihydropyridines including Prescal tablets should not be used for the prevention of secondary myocardial infarctions and they have not been approved for the treatment of hypertensive crisis.

Precautions: As for other calcium antagonists Prescal does not give protection against the danger of abrupt beta-blocker withdrawal. Beta-blockers should therefore be withdrawn gradually, preferably over 8–10 days.

Caution should be taken when treating patients with documented or strongly suspected sick sinus syndrome who are not fitted with a pacemaker.

Prescal should be used with caution in patients with poor cardiac reserve.

Care is recommended when treating patients with a low systolic blood pressure.

There is no evidence that Prescal interferes with glucose metabolism, however, diabetic patients should be initially monitored in accordance with good clinical practice.

Use in pregnancy and lactation: Although some dihydropyridine compounds have been found to be teratogenic in animals, animal data in the rat and rabbit on isradipine provide no evidence for a teratogenic or embryotoxic effect. There is insufficient experience of the drug in pregnant women to justify its use during pregnancy, unless the potential benefit to the mother is expected to outweigh any potential risk to the offspring. Pre-natal observations in animals suggest that high doses of isradipine may cause prolongation of labour.

Animal data indicate that small quantities of isradipine may be excreted in the breast milk. Therefore breast-feeding should not be undertaken by mothers treated with Prescal.

Drug interactions: The bioavailability of isradipine is not affected by co-administration of food, however the lag time to absorption and time to peak plasma concentration may be delayed by about one hour.

The pharmacokinetics of isradipine is not modified by the concomitant administration of digoxin, propranolol, or hydrochlorothiazide. Nor are the kinetics of digoxin or hydrochlorothiazide altered by the concomitant administration of Prescal. However, Prescal increases the bioavailability of propranolol, but this does not appear to be of any clinical significance. Isradipine is non-specifically bound to proteins. Enzyme inducing anticonvulsants may be associated with reduced levels of isradipine. As with other dihydropyridines, Prescal should not be taken with grapefruit juice because bioavailability may be increased.

Concurrent administration of cimetidine, an inhibitor of the cytochrome P450 system, results in an increase of about 50% in the bioavailability of Prescal whereas concomitant administration of rifampicin, an inducer of the cytochrome P450 system, greatly reduces the plasma concentrations of Prescal. Therefore, when Prescal is administered together with other drugs which alter the activity of the cytochrome P450 system, patients should be monitored carefully and doses of these drugs altered accordingly.

Side-effects: Clinical studies indicate that Prescal is well tolerated with an overall incidence of adverse events similar to that of placebo when used in doses up to 2.5 mg twice a day. Generally side effects are mild, dose dependent and tend to disappear or decrease in intensity as treatment is continued. Discontinuation of therapy is generally not required. Those side effects mentioned most often are related to the vasodilating properties of Prescal: headache, flushing, dizziness, tachycardia and palpitation, and localised peripheral oedema of non-cardiac origin; hypotension is uncommon and there have been no reports of orthostatic hypotension.

Non-specific side-effects are rare and include: weight gain, fatigue, abdominal discomfort, and skin rash.

Elevations of serum transaminases have been observed on very rare occasions; these changes were reversible both spontaneously and on following Prescal withdrawal.

As with other dihydropyridines, aggravation of underlying angina has been reported in a small number of individuals especially after starting treatment. This is more likely to happen in patients with symptomatic ischaemic heart disease. Prescal should be discontinued under medical supervision in patients who develop unstable angina.

Overdosage

Symptoms: Available data on calcium antagonists suggest that overdosage would result in marked and prolonged systemic hypotension requiring cardiovascular support, with monitoring of cardiac and respiratory functions and attention to possible cerebral ischaemia (elevation of the lower extremities) and to circulating blood volume (intravenous fluid or plasma volume expanders).

Management: In cases of severe hypotension, vasoconstrictors could be beneficial provided there is no contra-indication to their use. Intravenous calcium may help to reverse the effect of calcium entry blockade. Animal data suggest the risk for cardiodepression with Prescal should be minimal, but depression of the sinus node may occur in which case temporary pacemaker treatment may be useful.

Since isradipine is bound to plasma proteins to a very large extent, dialysis cannot be expected to be of benefit.

Pharmaceutical precautions The tablets should be protected from light.

Legal category POM

Package quantities Boxes of 56 tablets consisting of 2 blister strips each containing 28 tablets.

Further information Prescal is effective in both Negroid and Caucasian hypertensive patients, requiring no alteration of dose. Additionally, no potential deleterious first dose effects have been observed.

In asthmatic patients a single dose of isradipine has been found to blunt the bronchospastic response to exercise.

In patients with congestive heart failure, single oral doses of Prescal improved cardiac performance in terms of increasing cardiac output and decreasing pulmonary capillary venous pressure.

Prescal has not been shown to be arrhythmogenic and does not depress the atrioventricular node.

Product licence number 00101/0537

Product licence holder: Novartis Pharmaceuticals UK Limited, trading as Ciba Laboratories.

Date of revision of text: 11.12.97.

REGULOSE*

Presentation Regulose is a clear, almost colourless to brownish-yellow plum flavoured syrup. Each 5 ml spoonful contains 3.33 g lactulose and 1.33 g of other sugars (lactose, galactose, tagatose and other keto-sugars).

Uses

Principal action: Lactulose prevents the formation of hard stools and encourages normal bowel movement. Unlike traditional laxative preparations which act either on the innervation or musculature of the intestine or by bulk stimulus, lactulose provides a natural substrate for the saccharolytic bacterial flora in the colon.

Lactulose is a disaccharide which is not hydrolysed in the small intestine. Therefore it cannot be absorbed and is transported to the colon with water to retain the osmotic balance. In the colon, several species of bacteria can hydrolyse lactulose to the monosaccharides galactose and fructose.

By encouraging this normal metabolic activity of the bacteria, the osmotic pressure of the colonic contents is doubled and more water is drawn into the bowel.

Further metabolism of the monosaccharides leads to the production of acetic and lactic acids and the subsequent lowering of colonic pH. This acidification of the colonic contents is considered to be the main reason for the effectiveness of lactulose solution. In chronic portal-systemic encephalopathy it may be associated with the decrease in the relative concentration of free ammonia, the major agent involved in the cerebral disturbance.

Indications: Chronic constipation. Chronic portal-systemic encephalopathy.

Dosage and administration

Chronic constipation: Because lactulose acts naturally to encourage the normal activity of the bowel, it may be two or three days before the full benefit of the treatment is obtained. It is important, therefore, to follow the dosage regimen set out below.

Adults

Initially: Three to six 5 ml spoonfuls for the first two to three days of treatment. (Nine spoonfuls may be given in obstinate cases).

Maintenance: Two to three 5 ml spoonfuls daily or according to the needs of the patient.

Children

Initially: Two to five 5 ml spoonfuls for the first two to three days of treatment.

Maintenance: One to three 5 ml spoonfuls daily or according to the needs of the patient.

Chronic portal-systemic encephalopathy: Six to ten 5 ml spoonfuls three times daily according to the requirements of the patient, for adequate acidification of the colonic contents.

Use in the elderly: No evidence exists that elderly patients require different dosages or show different side-effects from younger patients.

Contra-indications, warnings, etc

Contra-indications: In common with other preparations used for the treatment of constipation, Regulose should not be used in patients with gastrointestinal obstruction. Regulose should not be given to patients with galactosaemia or lactose intolerance.

Precautions: Regulose should be used with caution during the first trimester of pregnancy. There are no known drug interactions involving Regulose. There is no evidence that Regulose affects driving ability.

Overdosage: No cases of intoxication due to deliberate or accidental overdosage with Regulose have been reported to the company.

Side-effects: Side-effects rarely occur after the administration of Regulose. Mild transient effects such as abdominal distension or cramps and flatulence, which subside after the initial stages of treatment, have occasionally been reported.

High doses may provoke nausea in some patients. This can be minimised by administration with water, fruit juice, or with meals.

Pharmaceutical precautions Regulose should be stored below 25°C. Dilution is not recommended.

Legal category P.

Package quantities Bottles of 200 ml, 300 ml and 500 ml.

Further information Nil.

Marketing licence holder: Novartis Pharmaceuticals UK Ltd, trading as Sandoz Pharmaceuticals.

Product licence number 0101/0363

Date of last revision: March 1997.

RIMACTANE*

Qualitative and quantitative composition The active ingredient is 3-(4-Methyl-1-piperazinyliminomethyl)rifamycin SV.

One capsule contains 150 mg or 300 mg Rifampicin PhEur.

The syrup contains 100 mg Rifampicin BP in every 5 mls.

Pharmaceutical form Capsules and syrup.

Clinical particulars

Therapeutic indications: Rimactane is a major drug in the management of tuberculosis (all forms) and certain opportunistic mycobacterial infections. It is effective in cases resistant to other anti-tuberculosis agents and shows no cross-resistance outside the rifampycin group of drugs. In the treatment of tuberculosis Rimactane must always be combined with other anti-tuberculosis agents. It is effective in combination with isoniazid, streptomycin, pyrazinamide, ethambutol and the majority of second line drugs.

Rimactane is also indicated for the chemoprophylaxis of meningococcal meningitis.

Posology and method of administration

For the management of tuberculosis and certain opportunistic mycobacterial infections: Rimactane must always be given in association with other anti-tuberculosis drugs, to prevent emergence of resistant strains.

Use in adults: 450–600 mg daily as a single dose (based on approximately 10 mg per kg body weight). Those patients 50 kg (8 stone) and over should take 600 mg rifampicin daily, whilst patients under 50 kg should take 450 mg).

The following chemotherapeutic agents are employed today as combined therapy for tuberculosis; rifampicin (Rimactane) (RMP), isoniazid (INH), pyrazinamide (PZA), ethambutol (EMB), streptomycin (STM).

The dosages recommended by the Centres for Disease Control and Prevention are given in the table.

For the treatment of sputum-positive pulmonary tuberculosis, preference is given to the following regimens: (for dosage information please refer to the text above for Rimactane and to the table for other components of the treatment).

Continuous therapy:

Daily for a total of 9 months:

Initial phase for 2 months:	RMP + INH + PZA + EMB or STM
Continuation phase for 7 months:	RMP + INH

A total duration of 9 months is recommended for tuberculosis with HIV infection and for tuberculous meningitis, disseminated tuberculosis, or spinal involvement with neurological complications.

Daily for a total of 6 months:

Initial phase for 2 months:	RMP + INH + PZA + EMB or STM
Continuation phase for 4 months:	RMP + INH

Partially intermittent therapy:

Total duration 6 months:

Initial phase for 2 months:	RMP + INH + PZA + EMB or STM
Continuation phase for 4 months:	RMP + INH twice or 3 times a week

Fully intermittent therapy:

Total duration 6 months:	RMP + INH + PZA + EMB or STM 3 times a week

In the case of all regimens administered twice or three times weekly, the patient should be monitored with directly observed therapy (i.e. administration of tablets under supervision). The same applies for relapses and treatment failures.

Use in children: Up to 20 mg per kg body weight daily to a maximum of 600 mg as a single dose.

Use in premature and new-born infants: 10 mg/kg once daily. Premature and new-born infants should be treated only in cases of emergency and with extreme caution since their liver enzyme system may not be fully developed.

Use in elderly: No special dosage regime is necessary but concurrent hepatic insufficiency should be taken into account (see *Pharmacokinetics*).

For the chemoprophylaxis of meningococcal meningitis: Note: Rimactane should not be used to treat overt meningococcal meningitis.

Use in adults: 600 mg twice daily (12 hourly) for 2 days.

Use in children (aged 1-12 years): 10 mg/kg twice daily (12 hourly) for 2 days. Children at the lower end of this age range may metabolise rifampicin more rapidly and produce significantly lower serum levels than new-borns or adults. In such cases doses up to 15 mg/kg 12 hourly may be required.

Use in infants (up to 1 year): 5 mg/kg twice daily (12 hourly) for 2 days.

Use in the elderly: There is no evidence to suggest that dose adjustments are necessary.

This prophylactic administration should be started as soon as possible. It is recommended that Rimactane is only given for 2 days in this indication since resistance to this class of antibacterial agent may develop.

Contra-indications: Hypersensitivity to rifamycins or other excipients of the capsules or syrup.

Special warnings and precautions for use:

Warnings: Patients receiving Rimactane for the chemoprophylaxis of meningococcal meningitis should be kept under close surveillance. Special attention should be paid to signs of overt infection.

Rimactane should not be used to treat an overt meningococcal infection.

To prevent the emergence of resistant bacteria, Rimactane must always be combined with other antibiotics/chemotherapeutic agents when used to treat infections.

Intermittent therapy: The 'flu syndrome' (see *Side effects*) is chiefly encountered during intermittent therapy and may be a prelude to serious complications such as thrombocytopenia, purpura, haemolytic anaemia, dyspnoea and asthma-like attacks, shock and renal failure. In the event of its onset, therefore, one should consider the possibility of switching to daily medication. Such a switch must always be made where the 'flu syndrome' assumes a relatively severe form and if the aforementioned serious complications occur, the medication must be withdrawn at once and never reinstituted.

When changing over from intermittent to daily therapy, an incremental dosage must be employed, starting with approx. 75–150 mg on the first day. The desired therapeutic dose should be reached within 3–4 days. During this time the patient's renal function should be closely monitored. Corticosteroids may prove useful in attenuating possible immunopathological reactions.

Resumption of therapy after its interruption: since severe reactions such as shock and renal failure may occur in rare cases upon resumption of therapy, incremental dosing under close surveillance is mandatory (see *Intermittent therapy*).

Precautions: In the treatment of tuberculosis rifampicin should be given under the supervision of a respiratory or other suitably qualified physician.

As Rimactane is excreted principally by the biliary tract, caution should be exercised in treating patients with hepatic disorders.

All tuberculosis patients should have pretreatment measurement of liver function.

If a patient has no evidence of pre-existing liver disease and normal pretreatment liver function, liver function tests need only be repeated if fever, vomiting, jaundice or other deterioration in the patients condition occurs.

In patients with or likely to have liver function abnormalities including those with chronic liver disease, chronic alcoholism, the elderly and the undernourished, the benefit of combined treatment with rifampicin must be weighed against the possible risks. This applies particularly to combination of isoniazid and/or pyrazinamide with rifampicin. In the presence of severely impaired liver function or jaundice the dosage may have to be reduced.

Regular monitoring of liver function is required in patients with chronic liver disease throughout treatment with rifampicin. Weekly testing for two weeks followed by tests every two weeks for the next six weeks is recommended initially. Blood counts and liver function tests should also be performed periodically during prolonged treatment.

Rifampicin should be withdrawn if clinically significant changes in hepatic function occur. The need for other forms of antituberculous therapy and a different regimen should be considered. Urgent advice should be obtained from a specialist in the management of

Combined therapy for tuberculosis: Dosages recommended by the Centres for Disease Control and Prevention

Drug	*Daily mg/kg Children*	*Adults*	*max. mg*	*Twice a week mg/kg Children*	*Adults*	*max. mg*	*3 times a week mg/kg Children*	*Adults*	*max. mg*
RMP	10–20	10	600	10–20	10	600	10–20	10	600
INH	10–20	5	300	20–40	15	900	20–40	15	900
PZA	15–30	15–30	2,000	50–70	50–70	4,000	50–70	50–70	3,000
EMB	15–25	5–25	2,500	50	50	2,500	25–30	25–30	2,500
STM	20–30	15	1,000	25–30	25–30	1,500	25–30	25–30	1,000

tuberculosis. If rifampicin is reintroduced after liver function has returned to normal, liver function should be monitored daily until the maintenance dose has been established. This should be followed by weekly testing for two weeks and then testing every two weeks for the next six weeks. Liver function should be monitored periodically thereafter.

Owing to its enzyme-inducing effect, rifampicin must be employed with extreme caution in patients with porphyria, because activation of delta-aminolaevulinic acid synthetase may lead to an acute manifestation of the porphyria.

To preclude all possibility of pregnancy during treatment with Rimactane, non-hormonal means of contraception must be employed (see *Interactions*).

Interactions with other medicaments and other types of interactions: Antacids, opiates, and anticholinergic drugs and ketoconazole reduce the bioavailability of rifampicin when given concomitantly by mouth. The same applies to PAS preparations containing bentonite. To avoid this interaction, rifampicin must be administered a few hours before these preparations.

Rifampicin is a potent inducer of liver enzymes which may increase the metabolism of concomitantly administered drugs such as those listed below. The activity of the following drugs may be impaired and their dosage must be reassessed during and after treatment with Rifampicin.

Oral anticoagulants; oral antidiabetic agents, digitalis preparations, antiarrhythmic agents (disopyramide, quinidine, mexiletine, tocainide, lorcainide, propafenone), methadone (withdrawal signs may set in), hydantoins (phenytoin); hexobarbital, nortriptyline, benzodiazepines, corticosteroids (Addison patients may develop a crisis; exacerbation of pemphigus may occur; treatment for corticoid-dependent asthma patients may become more difficult or impossible); sex hormones (menstrual disorders may appear); oral contraceptives (their effect can no longer be relied upon); theophyllines, dapsone, chloramphenicol, azole antifungal agents (ketoconazole; itraconazole), cyclosporin A; azathioprine (transplants may be rejected); beta blockers, calcium-channel blockers (nifedipine, verapamil); enalapril, cimetidine.

Although concurrent use of isoniazid, pyrazinamide and rifampicin is common and therapeutically valuable, hepatic toxicity may be increased.

Rifampicin can delay the biliary excretion of contrast media employed to X-ray the gall bladder.

Microbiological techniques for assaying folic acid and vitamin B_{12} in the serum are unsuitable for use during treatment with Rimactane.

Pregnancy and lactation: In studies of over 300 women exposed to rifampicin during pregnancy, no significant increase in the rate of malformations in their offspring, over and above the background level was observed. Rimactane should not be given during pregnancy unless the potential benefit justifies the potential risk to the foetus.

Administration of Rimactane during the last few weeks of pregnancy can cause post-natal haemorrhage in the mother and new-born infant. This may necessitate treatment with vitamin K preparations.

Rifampicin passes into the breast milk but no adverse effects on breast-fed infants have been observed. Therefore nursing mothers may continue to breast-feed their infants.

Effects on ability to drive or use machines: None known.

Undesirable effects: Rifampicin may cause reddish discolouration of body fluids and occasionally other body secretions, e.g. urine, sputum, lacrimal fluid, faeces, saliva, sweat. It may permanently discolour soft contact-lenses.

Unwanted effects which may occur during continuous daily or intermittent therapy.

Frequency estimates: frequent>10%, occasional>1–10%, rare>0.001%–1%, isolated cases<0.001%.

Skin and appendages: Occasionally: flushing, itching with or without skin rash, and reddening of the eyes. Isolated cases: severe signs and symptoms, such as exudative conjunctivitis or generalised hypersensitivity reactions involving the skin, e.g. exfoliative dermatitis, Lyell's syndrome and pemphigoid reactions.

Gastro-intestinal tract: Occasionally: anorexia, nausea, abdominal pains, gaseous distension; rarely: vomiting or diarrhoea; isolated occurrences of erosive gastritis and pseudomembranous colitis.

Hepatic: Frequently: an asymptomatic increase in liver enzymes; rarely: hepatitis or jaundice; here account should also be taken of the liver toxicity of chemotherapeutic agents, e.g. isoniazid or pyrazinamide, employed in combination with rifampicin. Induction of porphyria in isolated cases.

Central and peripheral nervous system: Occasionally: tiredness, drowsiness, headache, light-headedness, dizziness; rarely: ataxia, mental confusion. Isolated cases: muscular weakness, visual disturbances.

Blood: Isolated occurrences of transient leucopenia; eosinophilia; thrombocytopenia and thrombocytopenic purpura are encountered more frequently under intermittent therapy than on continuous daily treatment, during which they occur only in isolated cases.

Endocrine: In rare instances disturbances in the menstrual cycle (in extreme cases amenorrhoea); induction of a crisis in Addison patients (see *Interactions*).

Unwanted effects chiefly occurring during intermittent therapy or upon resumption of treatment after temporary interruption: In patients taking rifampicin other than on a daily basis or in those resuming treatment with the drug after a temporary interruption, an influenza-like syndrome ('flu syndrome') may occur, this being very probably of immunopathological origin. It is characterised by fever, shivering, and possibly headache, dizziness and musculoskeletal pain. In rare cases the 'flu syndrome' may be followed by thrombocytopenia, purpura, dyspnoea, asthma-like attacks, haemolytic anaemia, shock and acute renal failure. These serious complications may, however, also set in suddenly with no preceding 'flu syndrome', chiefly when treatment is resumed after a temporary interruption or when rifampicin is given only once a week in high doses (25 mg/kg or more). When Rimactane is administered in lower doses (600 mg) 2–3 times a week, the syndrome is encountered less frequently, its incidence then being comparable to that observed during daily medication.

Overdose:

Signs and symptoms: Nausea, vomiting, abdominal pains; enlargement of the liver, jaundice, elevated liver enzyme levels, possibly acute pulmonary oedema, lethargy, clouding of consciousness, convulsions.

Treatment: Gastric lavage together with instillation of an activated charcoal suspension via a stomach tube; general supportive measures to maintain vital functions; forced diureses; haemodialysis; in the presence of severe liver damage, cholecystotomy if necessary. Bear in mind that other drugs used in combination with Rimactane may also have been taken in an overdosage and necessitate additional specific measures.

Pharmacological properties

Pharmacodynamic properties:

Pharmacotherapeutic group: Rifampicin is a rifamycin antibiotic.

Mechanisms of action: Rimactane exerts, both *in vitro* and *in vivo* bactericidal effects on *Mycobacterium tuberculosis.* It also exhibits variable activity against other atypical species of Mycobacterium.

In vivo it exerts its bactericidal effect not only on micro-organisms in the extracellular spaces but also on those located intracellularly. Rifampicin has a potent sterilising effect.

Rifampicin inhibits the DNA-dependent RNA polymerase of sensitive bacterial strains, but without affecting the corresponding mammalian enzyme.

Since relatively rapid 'one-step' selection of resistant bacteria occurs with rifampicin, the drug must not be employed as monotherapy to treat overt infections. Bacteria resistant to rifampicin display no cross-resistance to other antibiotics with the exception of the rifamycins.

Pharmacokinetic properties:

Absorption: Rifampicin is rapidly and completely absorbed. Following a single dose taken on an empty stomach (600 mg) the peak serum concentrations (approx. 10 mcg/ml) are observed after about 2 hours. Ingestion with food may adversely affect the absorption of rifampicin.

Distribution: The apparent distribution volume is 1.6 L/kg in adults and 1.1 L/kg in children. Binding to serum proteins amounts to 84%–91%.

Rifampicin penetrates rapidly into various body fluids and tissues, including bone tissue. Rifampicin crosses the blood/brain barrier in the case of inflamed meninges only, but concentrations in the cerebrospinal fluid may remain above the MIC for *Mycobacterium tuberculosis* for up to two months with continuous therapy of 600 mg/day orally.

Rifampicin crosses the human placenta and is secreted in human breast milk. However, it is estimated that a breast-fed infant would receive no more than 1% of the usual therapeutic dose.

Biotransformation: Rifampicin is metabolised in the liver, the principal metabolite being 25-O-deacetylrifampicin, which is microbiologically active and, like rifampicin, subject to enterohepatic circulation. Rifampicin induces its own metabolism.

Elimination: The plasma elimination half-life of rifampicin increases with increasing doses and amounts to 2.5 h, 3–4 h and about 5 h after single doses of 300 mg, 600 mg and 900 mg respectively. After a few days of repeated daily administration, the bioavailability of rifampicin diminishes, and the half-life value following repeated doses of 600 mg falls to 1–2 hours.

Owing to its enzyme-inducing effect in the liver, rifampicin accelerates its own metabolism, with the result that its systemic clearance, which amounts to approx. 6 L/h after the first dose, rises to approx. 9 L/h after repeated dosing.

Although the bulk of the drug is eliminated in the bile, 80% of the quantity excreted being accounted for by the deacetylrifampicin metabolite, rifampicin also appears in the urine. In a dosage range of 150–900 mg, 4–18% of a dose is excreted dose-dependently in the urine in unchanged form.

Characteristics in patients: In elderly patients, renal clearance is reduced, but, owing to the large scale on which the drug is eliminated via the liver, the plasma concentrations are similar to those in young patients.

With impaired renal function, the elimination half-life becomes prolonged only at doses exceeding 600 mg daily. Provided that hepatic excretory function is normal, the dosage in patients with impaired renal function does not need to be reduced below 600 mg daily. Rifampicin is eliminated by peritoneal or haemodialysis. Dosage adjustment is not necessary during dialysis. Because rifampicin is dialysable it is recommended that the drug should not be administered until after the period of dialysis is complete.

In patients with severe hepatic dysfunction the dosage may have to be adjusted as plasma concentrations are raised and half-life prolonged.

Preclinical safety data: There is limited evidence as to the carcinogenic potential of rifampicin in animals. In female mice of a strain known to be susceptible to hepatomas, a significant increase in such tumours was observed after 1 year of treatment with rifampicin in quantities equivalent to 2–10 times the maximum clinical doses.

In mice of another strain treated for 1 year, and in rats treated for 2 years, no significant increase was noted in the incidence of any type of tumour. Studies with various mammalian models, as well as with bacteria, yielded no evidence that rifampicin has a mutagenic effect.

In daily doses of 150–250 mg/kg, rifampicin proved teratogenic in mice and rats, insofar as an increased occurrence of spina bifida and cleft palate was observed. In rabbits it had no teratogenic effect. In all three animal species, unspecific embryotoxic effects occurred after doses>150 mg/kg.

Pharmaceutical particulars

List of excipients: The capsules contain calcium stearate, lactose, titanium dioxide (E171), iron oxide red (E172) and gelatin. 300 mg capsules also contain iron oxide yellow (E172) and iron oxide black (E172).

The syrup contains zanthan gum, methyl hydroxybenzoate (E218), propyl hydroxybenzoate (E216), sucrose, potassium sorbate (E202), saccharin, sodium metabisulphite (E223), raspberry flavour, antifoam AF (dimethylpolysiloxane and silica).

Incompatibilities: None known.

Shelf-life: Capsules: Four years. Syrup: Three years.

Special precautions for storage: Capsules: Protect from moisture and heat (store below 30°C). Syrup: Store below 25°C.

Medicines should be kept out of reach of children.

Nature and contents of container: The capsules are opaque, two-piece, hard gelatine capsule size 2, reddish-brown in colour, marked with the monogram CG on each half and the code JZ 150, and come in PVC/PVdC blister packs of 56.

The syrup is an opaque, red-coloured suspension having the odour and taste of raspberry and is contained in a glass bottle with a child resistant clicloc cap.

Instructions for use/handling: None.

Marketing authorisation holder: Novartis Pharmaceuticals UK Ltd, trading as Ciba Laboratories.

Marketing authorisation numbers

Capsules 150 mg	00101/0445
Capsules 300 mg	00101/0446
Syrup	00101/0448

Date of approval/revision of SPC 6 September 1997.

Legal category POM.

RIMACTANE* INFUSION

Qualitative and quantitative composition The active ingredient is 3-[[(4-Methyl-1-piperazinyl)-imino]-methyl]-rifamycin SV natrium (=rifampicin sodium) equivalent to rifampicin 300 mg.

One vial contains 308.2 mg rifampicin sodium salt, equivalent to 300 mg Rifampicin BP.

Pharmaceutical form Vial.

Clinical particulars

Therapeutic indications: Rimactane is a major drug in the management of tuberculosis (all forms) and certain opportunistic mycobacterial infections. It is effective in cases resistant to other anti-tuberculous agents and shows no cross-resistance outside the rifampycin group of drugs. In the treatment of tuberculosis Rimactane must always be combined with other anti-tuberculosis agents. It is effective in combination with isoniazid, streptomycin, pyrazinamide, ethambutol and the majority of second line drugs.

Rimactane infusion is indicated in patients with all forms of tuberculosis who are unable to tolerate oral therapy, e.g. post-operative or comatose patients or patients in whom gastro-intestinal absorption is impaired.

Posology and method of administration

For the management of tuberculosis and certain opportunistic mycobacterial infections: Rimactane must always be given in association with other anti-tuberculosis drugs, to prevent emergence of resistant strains.

Use in adults: 450–600 mg daily as a single dose (based on approximately 10 mg per kg body weight). A daily dose of 600 mg given in an intravenous infusion over two to three hours has been found to be effective and well tolerated for the majority of adult patients. Serum levels following this regimen are similar to those obtained following oral administration. Lower doses are recommended for small or frail patients. (Patients 50 kg (8 stone) and over should take 600 mg rifampicin daily, whilst patients under 50 kg should take 450 mg).

The chemotherapeutic agents usually employed today as combined therapy for tuberculosis are rifampicin (Rimactane) (RMP), isoniazid (INH), pyrazinamide (PZA), ethambutol (EMB), streptomycin (STM).

The dosages recommended by the Centres for Disease Control and Prevention are as follows (see Table):

For the treatment of sputum-positive pulmonary tuberculosis, preference is given to the following regimens: (for dosage information please refer to the text above for Rimactane and to the table for other components of the treatment).

Continuous therapy:

Daily for a total of 9 months:

Initial phase for 2 months: RMP + INH + PZA + EMB or STM

Continuation phase for 7 months: RMP + INH

A total duration of 9 months is recommended for tuberculosis with HIV infection and for tuberculous meningitis, disseminated tuberculosis, or spinal involvement with neurological complications.

Daily for a total of 6 months:

Initial phase for 2 months: RMP + INH + PZA + EMB or STM

Continuation phase for 4 months: RMP + INH

Partially intermittent therapy:

Total duration 6 months:

Initial phase for 2 months: RMP + INH + PZA + EMB or STM

Continuation phase for 4 months: RMP + INH twice or 3 times a week

Fully intermittent therapy:

Total duration 6 months: RMP + INH + PZA + EMB or STM 3 times a week

In the case of all regimens administered twice or three times weekly, the patient should be monitored with directly observed therapy (i.e. administration of tablets under supervision). The same applies for relapses and treatment failures.

Use in children: Paediatric usage has not yet been established. However, the following regimen is suggested. In tuberculosis, a single daily dose of up to 20 mg/kg body weight daily is recommended, although total daily dose should not usually exceed 600 mg.

Use in premature and new-born infants: 10 mg/kg once daily. Premature and new-born infants should be treated only in cases of emergency and with extreme caution since their liver enzyme system may not be fully developed.

Use in elderly: No special dosage regime is necessary but concurrent hepatic insufficiency should be taken into account (see *Pharmacokinetics*).

Transfer to oral therapy: When patients are able to accept oral medication, they should be transferred to Rimactane capsules or syrup. Oral dosage would be expected to be the same as that used with the infusion (see oral Rimactane data sheet).

Contra-indications: Hypersensitivity to rifamycins or other excipients of the infusion.

Special warnings and precautions for use:

Warning: To prevent the emergence of resistant bacteria, Rimactane must always be combined with other antibiotics/chemotherapeutic agents when used to treat infections.

There have been isolated reports of hypersensitivity reactions affecting the face and hands of nursing staff preparing and applying infusions. Care should be taken to avoid contact with rifampicin.

Intermittent therapy: The 'flu syndrome' (see *Side effects*) is chiefly encountered during intermittent therapy and may be a prelude to serious complications such as thrombocytopenia, purpura, haemolytic anaemia, dyspnoea and asthma-like attacks, shock and renal failure. In the event of its onset, therefore, one should consider the possibility of switching to daily medication. Such a switch must always be made where the 'flu syndrome' assumes a relatively severe form and if the aforementioned serious complications occur, the medication must be withdrawn at once and never reinstituted.

When changing over from intermittent to daily therapy, an incremental dosage must be employed, starting with approx. 75–150 mg on the first day. The desired therapeutic dose should be reached within 3–4 days. During this time the patient's renal function should be closely monitored. Corticosteroids may prove useful in attenuating possible immuno-pathological reactions.

Resumption of therapy after its interruption: since severe reactions such as shock and renal failure may occur in rare cases upon resumption of therapy, incremental dosing under close surveillance is mandatory (see 'intermittent therapy').

Precautions: In the treatment of tuberculosis rifampicin should be given under the supervision of a respiratory or other suitably qualified physician.

As Rimactane is excreted principally by the biliary tract, caution should be exercised in treating patients with hepatic disorders.

All tuberculosis patients should have pretreatment measurement of liver function.

If a patient has no evidence of pre-existing liver disease and normal pretreatment liver function, liver function tests need only be repeated if fever, vomiting, jaundice or other deterioration in the patients condition occurs.

In patients with or likely to have liver function abnormalities including those with chronic liver disease, chronic alcoholism, the elderly and the under-nourished, the benefit of combined treatment with rifampicin must be weighed against the possible risks. This applies particularly to combination of isoniazid and/or pyrazinamide with rifampicin. In the presence of severely impaired liver function or jaundice the dosage may have to be reduced.

Regular monitoring of liver function is required in patients with chronic liver disease throughout treatment with rifampicin. Weekly testing for two weeks followed by tests every two weeks for the next six weeks is recommended initially. Blood counts and liver function tests should also be performed periodically during prolonged treatment.

Rifampicin should be withdrawn if clinically significant changes in hepatic function occur. The need for other forms of antituberculous therapy and a different regimen should be considered. Urgent advice should be obtained from a specialist in the management of tuberculosis. If rifampicin is reintroduced after liver function has returned to normal, liver function should be monitored daily until the maintenance dose has been established. This should be followed by weekly testing for two weeks and then testing every two weeks for the next six weeks. Liver function should be monitored periodically thereafter.

Owing to its enzyme-inducing effect, rifampicin must be employed with extreme caution in patients with porphyria, because activation of delta-aminolaevulinic acid synthetase may lead to an acute manifestation of the porphyria.

To preclude all possibility of pregnancy during treatment with Rimactane, non-hormonal means of contraception must be employed (see *Interactions*).

Interactions with other drugs and other types of interactions: Antacids, opiates, and anticholinergic drugs and ketoconazole reduce the bioavailability of rifampicin when given concomitantly by mouth. The same applies to PAS preparations containing bentonite. To avoid this interaction, rifampicin must be administered a few hours before these preparations.

Rifampicin is a potent inducer of liver enzymes which may increase the metabolism of concomitantly administered drugs such as those listed below. The activity of the following drugs may be impaired and their dosage must be reassessed during and after treatment with Rifampicin.

Oral anticoagulants; oral antidiabetic agents, digitalis preparations, antiarrhythmic agents (disopyramide, quinidine, mexiletine, tocainide, lorcainide, propafenone), methadone (withdrawal signs may set in), hydantoins (phenytoin); hexobarbital, nortriptyline, benzodiazepines, corticosteroids (Addison patients may develop a crisis; exacerbation of pemphigus may occur; treatment for corticoid-dependent asthma patients may become more difficult or impossible); sex hormones (menstrual disorders may appear); oral contraceptives (their effect can no longer be relied upon); theophyllines, dapsone, chloramphenicol, azole antifungal agents (ketoconazole; itraconazole), cyclosporin A; azathioprine (transplants may be rejected); beta blockers, calcium-channel blockers (nifedipine, verapamil); enalapril, cimetidine.

Although concurrent use of isoniazid, pyrazinamide and rifampicin is common and therapeutically valuable, hepatic toxicity may be increased.

Rifampicin can delay the biliary excretion of contrast media employed to X-ray the gall bladder.

Microbiological techniques for assaying folic acid and vitamin B_{12} in the serum are unsuitable for use during treatment with Rimactane.

Pregnancy and lactation: In studies of over 300 women exposed to rifampicin during pregnancy, no significant increase in the rate of malformations in their offspring, over and above the background level was observed. Rimactane should not be given during pregnancy unless the potential benefit justifies the potential risk to the foetus.

Administration of Rimactane during the last few weeks of pregnancy can cause post-natal haemorrhage in the mother and new-born infant. This may necessitate treatment with vitamin K preparations.

Rifampicin passes into the breast milk but no adverse effects on breast-fed infants have been observed. Therefore nursing mothers may continue to breast-feed their infants.

Effects on ability to drive or use machines: None known.

Undesirable effects:

Effects relating to intravenous administration: During prolonged (more than 30 days) administration i.v., local thrombophlebitis occasionally occurs. Nursing staff preparing and applying infusions may develop hypersensitivity reactions to the hands and face.

Rifampicin may cause reddish discolouration of body fluids and occasionally other body secretions, e.g. urine, sputum, lacrimal fluid, faeces, saliva, sweat. It may permanently discolour soft contact-lenses.

Unwanted effects which may occur during continuous daily or intermittent therapy.

Frequency estimates: frequent>10%, occasional>1–10%, rare>0.001%–1%, isolated cases<0.001%.

Skin and appendages: Occasionally: flushing, itching with or without skin rash, and reddening of the eyes. Isolated cases: severe signs and symptoms, such as exudative conjunctivitis or generalised hypersensitivity reactions involving the skin, e.g. exfoliative dermatitis, Lyell's syndrome and pemphigoid reactions.

Gastro-intestinal tract: Occasionally: anorexia, nausea, abdominal pains, gaseous distension; rarely: vomiting or diarrhoea; isolated occurrences of erosive gastritis and pseudomembranous colitis.

Hepatic: Frequently: an asymptomatic increase in liver enzymes; rarely: hepatitis or jaundice; here account should also be taken of the liver toxicity of chemotherapeutic agents, e.g. isoniazid or pyrazinamide, employed in combination with rifampicin. Induction of porphyria in isolated cases.

Central and peripheral nervous system: Occasionally: tiredness, drowsiness, headache, light-headedness, dizziness; rarely: ataxia, mental confusion. Isolated cases: muscular weakness, visual disturbances.

Blood: Isolated occurrences of transient leucopenia; eosinophilia; thrombocytopenia and thrombocytopenic purpura are encountered more frequently under intermittent therapy than on continuous daily treatment, during which they occur only in isolated cases.

Endocrine: In rare instances disturbances in the menstrual cycle (in extreme cases amenorrhoea); induction of a crisis in Addison patients (see *Interactions*).

Unwanted effects chiefly occurring during intermittent therapy or upon resumption of treatment after temporary interruption: In patients taking rifampicin

Drug	*Daily mg/kg Children*	*Adults*	*max. mg*	*Twice a week mg/kg Children*	*Adults*	*max. mg*	*3 times a week mg/kg Children*	*Adults*	*max. mg*
RMP	10–20	10	600	10–20	10	600	10–20	10	600
INH	10–20	5	300	20–40	15	900	20–40	15	900
PZA	15–30	15–30	2,000	50–70	50–70	4,000	50–70	50–70	3,000
EMB	15–25	5–25	2,500	50	50	2,500	25–30	25–30	2,500
STM	20–30	15	1,000	25–30	25–30	1,500	25–30	25–30	1,000

other than on a daily basis or in those resuming treatment with the drug after a temporary interruption, an influenza-like syndrome ('flu syndrome') may occur, this being very probably of immunopathological origin. It is characterised by fever, shivering, and possibly headache, dizziness and musculoskeletal pain. In rare cases the 'flu syndrome' may be followed by thrombocytopenia, purpura, dyspnoea, asthma-like attacks, haemolytic anaemia, shock and acute renal failure. These serious complications may, however, also set in suddenly with no preceding 'flu syndrome', chiefly when treatment is resumed after a temporary interruption or when rifampicin is given only once a week in high doses (25 mg/kg or more). When Rimactane is administered in lower doses (600 mg) 2–3 times a week, the syndrome is encountered less frequently, its incidence then being comparable to that observed during daily medication.

Overdose:

Signs and symptoms: Nausea, vomiting, abdominal pains; enlargement of the liver, jaundice, elevated liver enzyme levels, possibly acute pulmonary oedema, lethargy, clouding of consciousness, convulsions.

Treatment: General supportive measures to maintain vital functions; forced diureses; haemodialysis; in the presence of severe liver damage, cholecystotomy if necessary. Bear in mind that other drugs used in combination with Rimactane may also have been taken in an overdosage and necessitate additional specific measures.

Pharmacological properties

Pharmacodynamic properties:

Pharmacotherapeutic group: Rifampicin is a rifamycin antibiotic.

Mechanisms of action: Rimactane exerts, both *in vitro* and *in vivo* bactericidal effects on *Mycobacterium tuberculosis*. It also exhibits variable activity against other atypical species of Mycobacterium.

In vivo it exerts its bactericidal effect not only on micro-organisms in the extracellular spaces but also on those located intracellularly. Rifampicin has a potent sterilising effect.

Rifampicin inhibits the DNA-dependent RNA polymerase of sensitive bacterial strains, but without affecting the corresponding mammalian enzyme.

Since relatively rapid 'one-step' selection of resistant bacteria occurs with rifampicin, the drug must not be employed as monotherapy to treat overt infections. Bacteria resistant to rifampicin display no cross-resistance to other antibiotics with the exception of the rifamycins.

Pharmacokinetic properties:

Absorption: An intravenous drip infusion of rifampicin (600 mg) lasting 3 hours produces peak plasma concentrations of approx. 10 mcg/ml. The plasma profiles are similar to those obtained following the administration of the same dose in capsules.

Distribution: The apparent distribution volume is 1.6 L/kg in adults and 1.1 L/kg in children. Binding to serum proteins amounts to 84%–91%.

Rifampicin penetrates rapidly into various body fluids and tissues, including bone tissue. Rifampicin crosses the blood/brain barrier in the case of inflamed meninges only, but concentrations in the cerebrospinal fluid may remain above the MIC for *Mycobacterium tuberculosis* for up to two months with continuous therapy of 600 mg/day orally.

Rifampicin crosses the human placenta and is secreted in human breast milk. However, it is estimated that a breast-fed infant would receive no more than 1% of the usual therapeutic dose.

Biotransformation: Rifampicin is metabolised in the liver, the principal metabolite being 25-O-deacetyl-rifampicin, which is microbiologically active and, like rifampicin, subject to enterohepatic circulation.

Rifampicin induces its own metabolism.

Elimination/excretion: The plasma elimination half-life of rifampicin increases with increasing doses and amounts to 2.5 h, 3–4 h and about 5 h after single doses of 300 mg, 600 mg and 900 mg respectively.

After a few days of repeated daily administration, the bioavailabilty of rifampicin diminishes, and the half-life value following repeated doses of 600 mg falls to 1–2 hours.

Owing to its enzyme-inducing effect in the liver, rifampicin accelerates its own metabolism, with the result that its systemic clearance, which amounts to approx. 6 L/h after the first dose, rises to approx. 9 L/h after repeated dosing.

Although the bulk of the drug is eliminated in the bile, 80% of the quantity excreted being accounted for by the deacetylrifampicin metabolite, rifampicin also appears in the urine. In a dosage range of 150–900 mg, 4–18% of a dose is excreted dose-dependently in the urine in unchanged form.

Characteristics in patients: In elderly patients, renal clearance is reduced, but, owing to the large scale on which the drug is eliminated via the liver, the plasma concentrations are similar to those in young patients.

With impaired renal function, the elimination half-life becomes prolonged only at doses exceeding 600 mg daily. Provided that hepatic excretory function is normal, the dosage in patients with impaired renal function does not need to be reduced below 600 mg daily.

Rifampicin is eliminated by peritoneal or haemodialysis. Dosage adjustment is not necessary during dialysis. Because rifampicin is dialysable it is recommended that the drug should not be administered until after the period of dialysis is complete.

In patients with severe hepatic dysfunction the dosage may have to be adjusted as plasma concentrations are raised and half-life prolonged.

Preclinical safety data: There is limited evidence as to the carcinogenic potential of rifampicin in animals. In female mice of a strain known to be susceptible to hepatomas, a significant increase in such tumours was observed after 1 year of treatment with rifampicin in quantities equivalent to 2–10 times the maximum clinical doses.

In mice of another strain treated for 1 year, and in rats treated for 2 years, no significant increase was noted in the incidence of any type of tumour. Studies with various mammalian models, as well as with bacteria, yielded no evidence that rifampicin has a mutagenic effect.

In daily doses of 150–250 mg/kg, rifampicin proved teratogenic in mice and rats, insofar as an increased occurrence of spina bifida and cleft palate was observed. In rabbits it had no teratogenic effect. In all three animal species, unspecific embryotoxic effects occurred after doses>150 mg/kg.

Pharmaceutical particulars

List of excipients: The vials also contain sodium formaldehyde sulphoxylate (pyrogen free).

Incompatibilities: Rimactane infusion is incompatible with the following infusion solutions: sodium bicarbonate 5%, Ringer's solution (acetate) plus glucose, Perfudex and sodium lactate 0.167M.

Rimactane infusion diluted in glucose or saline is not compatible with: cephamandole, tetracycline, rolitetracycline, doxycyline.

Rimactane infusion should not be mixed with other drugs if there is a possibility that precipitation may occur; concurrent intravenous therapy should be administered via a different site of injection.

Shelf-life: Three years.

Special precautions for storage: Protect from light and heat (store below 30°C).

The reconstituted solution should be stored in a refrigerator (2–8°C) and used within 24 hours.

Medicines should be kept out of reach of children.

Nature and contents of containers: Colourless glass vials of 300 mg.

Instructions for use/handling:

Preparation of infusion: (see *Warnings*). Rimactane infusion is prepared for use by aseptically adding 5 ml Water for Injections PhEur to the vial of dry rifampicin powder and shaking vigorously and continuously for 30–60 seconds.

When the powder has completely dissolved, the solution should be immediately diluted in 250 ml of 5% glucose solution or other suitable infusion fluid (see *Pharmaceutical particulars*). Freshly prepared solutions must be used within 6 hours. It is recommended that the infusion be administered over a period of 2–3 hours.

Care should be taken to avoid contact with rifampicin.

Compatibility: Rimactane infusion is compatible with the following infusion solutions: NaCl 0.9%, Ringer's solution (lactate or acetate), dextrose 5% or 10%, mannitol 10% or 20%, sodium bicarbonate 1.4%, Macrodex with saline solution, Macrodex with glucose solution, Rheomacrodex and Fructose 5% and 10%.

Marketing authorisation holder: Novartis Pharmaceuticals UK Ltd, trading as Ciba Laboratories.

Marketing authorisation number PL 00101/0447.

Date of revision of the text 6 September 1997.

Legal category POM.

RIMACTAZID*

Qualitative and quantitative composition The active ingredient for rifampicin is 3-[[(4-Methyl-1-piperazinyl)-imino]-methyl]-rifamycin SV.

The active ingredient for isoniazid is isonicotonic acid hydrazide.

One tablet contains 150 mg or 300 mg rifampicin PhEur and 100 mg or 150 mg Isoniazid PhEur.

Pharmaceutical form Coated tablets.

Clinical particulars

Therapeutic indications: Rimactane and isoniazid are both major drugs in the management of tuberculosis and in certain opportunist mycobacterial infections. Rifampicin is effective in cases resistant to other anti-tuberculous agents and shows no cross-resistance outside the rifamycin group of drugs. Rimactazid must always be used in combination with other anti-tuberculosis agents, e.g. streptomycin, pyrazinamide, ethambutol and the majority of second-line drugs.

Posology and method of administration: Rimactazid should be given as a single dose, preferably on an empty stomach, at least 30 minutes before breakfast to ensure a high peak serum concentration.

Adults:

Continuous therapy	
Body weight less than 50 kg:	3 tablets Rimactazid 150 (=450 mg Rifampicin +300 mg INH) once daily
Body weight 50 kg or more:	2 tablets Rimactazid 300 (=600 mg Rifampicin +300 mg INH) once daily
Intermittent therapy	
Body weight less than 50 kg:	3 tablets Rimactazid 150 (=450 mg Rifampicin +300 mg INH) twice or 3 times weekly
Body weight 50 kg or more:	2 tablets Rimactazid 300 (=600 mg Rifampicin +300 mg INH) twice or 3 times weekly

Rimactazid has to be supplemented with 150 mg isoniazid for every 10 kg body weight above 20 kg (i.e. body weight 60 kg: 150×4=600 mg additional isoniazid needed). To a maximum of 900 mg daily.

The chemotherapeutic agents usually employed today as combined therapy for tuberculosis are rifampicin (Rimactane) (RMP), isoniazid (INH), pyrazinamide (PZA), ethambutol (EMB), streptomycin (STM).

The dosages recommended by the Centres for Disease Control and Prevention are as follows (see Table below):

For the treatment of sputum-positive pulmonary tuberculosis, preference is given to the following regimens: (for dosages information please refer to the text above for rifampicin and isoniazid, and to the table for advice on the other components of the treatment).

Continuous therapy:	
Daily for a total of 9 months:	
Initial phase for 2 months:	RMP + INH + PZA + EMB or STM
Continuation phase for 7 months:	RMP + INH

A total duration of 9 months is recommended for tuberculosis with HIV infection and for tuberculous meningitis, disseminated tuberculosis, or spinal involvement with neurological complications.

Daily for a total of 6 months:	
Initial phase for 2 months:	RMP + INH + PZA + EMB or STM
Continuation phase for 4 months:	RMP + INH
Partially intermittent therapy:	
Total duration 6 months:	
Initial phase for 2 months:	RMP + INH + PZA + EMB or STM daily
Continuation phase for 4 months:	RMP + INH twice or 3 times a week
Fully intermittent therapy:	
Total duration 6 months:	RMP + INH + PZA + EMB or STM 3 times a week

In the case of all regimens administered twice or three times weekly, the patient should be monitored with directly observed therapy (i.e. administration of tablets under supervision). The same applies for relapses and treatment failures.

Use in children: The ratios of Rimactane and isoniazid present in Rimactazid 150 and 300 make it difficult for both components to be administered in a dosage suitable for children. Rimactazid tablets are therefore not recommended for paediatric use.

Use in elderly: No special dosage regime is necessary but concurrent hepatic insufficiency should be taken into account (see *Pharmacokinetics*).

Contra-indications: Known hypersensitivity to rifampicin and/or to isoniazid, a history of drug induced hepatitis, acute liver diseases regardless of their origin, peripheral neuritis.

Special warnings and precautions for use:

Warnings: Intermittent therapy, resumption of therapy after its interruption – The presence of rifampicin means that, if treatment with Rimactazid is withdrawn for a while and then resumed again, or if the medication is not taken regularly, potentially serious side effects can occur (see under rifampicin in *Undesirable effects*). For this reason, both temporary interruption of treatment and non-compliance should if possible be avoided. Where temporary withdrawal of the medication is unavoidable, the two components rifampicin and INH should be administered separately

Drug	Daily mg/kg	max. mg	Twice a week mg/kg	max. mg	3 times a week mg/kg	max. mg
RMP	10	600	10	600	10	600
INH	5	300	15	900	15	900
PZA	15–30	2,000	50–70	4,000	50–70	3,000
EMB	5–25	2,500	50	2,500	25–30	2,500
STM	15	1,000	25–30	1,500	25–30	1,000

when resuming the treatment, because rifampicin should then be given in an incremental dosage. A start should be made with approx. 75–150 mg rifampicin on the first day, and the desired therapeutic dose should be reached within 3–4 days. During this time the patient's renal function should be close monitored. Corticosteroids may prove useful in attenuating possible immunopathological reactions. Isoniazid should be given in its normal dosage from the first day onwards.

If severe acute hypersensitivity reactions set in, such as thrombocytopenia, purpura, haemolytic anaemia, dyspnoea and asthmas-like attacks, shock, or renal failure (these being side effects which rifampicin may provoke in exceptional cases), Rimactazid should be withdrawn at once. Patients developing such complications should never again be treated with rifampicin.

If other signs of hypersensitivity appear, such as fever or skin reactions, Rimactazid should be withdrawn. For safety reasons, treatment should not be continued with rifampicin. Where isoniazid is considered essential, treatment should be resumed in low doses and under strict surveillance.

Precautions: In the treatment of tuberculosis rifampicin should be given under the supervision of a respiratory or other suitably qualified physician.

As rifampicin and isoniazid are metabolised in the liver, patients with impaired liver function should be treated with caution.

All tuberculosis patients should have pretreatment measurement of liver function.

If a patient has no evidence of pre-existing liver disease and normal pretreatment liver function, liver function tests need only be repeated if fever, vomiting, jaundice or other deterioration in the patients condition occurs.

The occurrence of liver function abnormalities is more common when rifampicin and isoniazid are used in combination and special care is therefore required in patients with pre-existing liver impairment or malnourished patients.

In patients with chronic liver disease, as well as in chronic alcoholics and undernourished patients, the therapeutic benefits of treatment with Rimactazid must be weighed against the possible risks. If the treatment is considered necessary, the dosage of both components must be correspondingly reduced. In such cases it is only possible to adapt the dosage by administering rifampicin and isoniazid separately.

Regular monitoring of liver function is required in patients with chronic liver disease throughout treatment with Rimactazid. Weekly testing for two weeks followed by tests every two weeks for the next six weeks is recommended initially. Blood counts and liver function tests should also be performed periodically during prolonged treatment. Any deterioration in liver function in these patients is an indication for stopping treatment

Rimactazid should be withdrawn if clinically significant changes in hepatic function occur. The need for other forms of antituberculous therapy and a different regimen should be considered. Urgent advice should be obtained from a specialist in the management of tuberculosis. If rifampicin or isoniazid are reintroduced after liver function has returned to normal, liver function should be monitored daily until the maintenance dose has been established. This should be followed by weekly testing for two weeks and then testing every two weeks for the next six weeks. Liver function should be monitored periodically thereafter.

Owing to its enzyme-inducing effect, rifampicin must be employed with extreme caution in patients with porphyria, because activation of delta-aminolaevulinic acid synthetase may lead to an acute manifestation of the porphyria.

To preclude all possibility of pregnancy during treatment with rifampicin, additional non-hormonal means of contraception must be employed (see *Interactions*).

Owing to the neurotoxic action of isoniazid, patients suffering from convulsive disorders must be kept under special observation during treatment with Rimactazid.

Pyridoxine may be useful in preventing the occurrence of peripheral neuritis and should be given in a dose of 10 mg daily from the start of treatment with Rimactazid.

Patients should abstain from alcohol while under treatment with Rimactazid.

Interactions with other drugs and other types of interactions:
Rifampicin: Antacids, opiates, and anticholinergic drugs and ketoconazole reduce the bioavailability of rifampicin when given concomitantly by mouth. The same applies to PAS preparations containing bentonite. To avoid this interaction, rifampicin must be administered a few hours before these preparations.

Rifampicin is a potent inducer of liver enzymes which may increase the metabolism of concomitantly administered drugs such as those listed below. The activity of the following drugs may be impaired and their dosage must be reassessed during and after treatment with Rifampicin.

Oral anticoagulants; oral antidiabetic agents, digitalis preparations, antiarrhythmic agents (disopyramide, quinidine, mexiletine, tocainide, lorcainide, propafenone), methadone (withdrawal signs may set in), hydantoins (phenytoin); hexobarbital, nortriptyline, benzodiazepines, corticosteroids (Addison patients may develop a crisis; exacerbation of pemphigus may occur; treatment for corticoid-dependent asthma patients may become more difficult or impossible); sex hormones (menstrual disorders may appear); oral contraceptives (their effect can no longer be relied upon); theophyllines, dapsone, chloramphenicol, azole antifungal agents (ketoconazole; itraconazole), cyclosporin A; azathioprine (transplants may be rejected); beta blockers, calcium-channel blockers (nifedipine, verapamil); enalapril, cimetidine.

Although concurrent use of isoniazid, pyrazinamide and rifampicin is common and therapeutically valuable, hepatic toxicity may be increased.

Rifampicin can delay the biliary excretion of contrast media employed to X-ray the gall bladder.

Microbiological techniques for assaying folic acid and vitamin B_{12} in the serum are unsuitable for use during treatment with Rimactane.

Isoniazid: The absorption of isoniazid is reduced by antacids. Isoniazid retards the metabolism of various concomitantly administered drugs, including hydantoins (phenytoin), carbamazepine, primidone, and valproic acid. The dosages of these drugs may have to be reduced. It is not advisable to administer disulfiram concomitantly with isoniazid as this may lead to mental disturbances, the mechanism of this interaction is not known.

Concomitant use of halothane and isoniazid (and possibly rifampicin) may increase the risk of hepatotoxic reactions.

As alcohol tolerance is decreased under isoniazid, the consumption of alcoholic beverages should be avoided. The metabolism of isoniazid is increased in chronic alcoholics.

Pregnancy and lactation:
Rifampicin: In studies of over 300 women exposed to rifampicin during pregnancy, no significant increase in the rate of malformations in their offspring, over and above the background level was observed. Rimactane should not be given during pregnancy unless the potential benefit justifies the potential risk to the foetus.

Administration of Rimactane during the last few weeks of pregnancy can cause post-natal haemorrhage in the mother and new-born infant. This may necessitate treatment with vitamin K preparations.

Isoniazid: Isoniazid, besides having weak direct genotoxic activity, is a promutagen in the sense that the formation of the toxic metabolites, hydrazine and acetylhydrazine, is the first step in metabolic activation. In lymphocytes of patients treated with isoniazid no chromosomal alterations could be detected whereas in a study comparing the effects of combination treatment an increased frequency of chromosomal alterations was observed.

Nevertheless isoniazid has been found to entail relatively little risk during pregnancy in humans. Congenital malformations have not been observed to be any greater than those expected for the normal population. Since it is theoretically possible that the drug might exert neurotoxic effects on the child, it is recommended that the mother should take pyridoxine during her pregnancy.

Rimactazid should not be given during pregnancy unless the potential benefit justifies the potential risk to the foetus.

Although rifampicin and isoniazid pass into the breast milk, no adverse effects on breast-fed infants have been observed. It is therefore not absolutely necessary to wean the infant. However, in view of the theoretical possibility of neurotoxic effects due to isoniazid, beast-fed infants should be kept under careful surveillance. Prophylactic administration of pyridoxine to mother and child is recommended.

Effects on ability to drive or use machines: Doses of 10 mg/kg or greater, of isoniazid may produce adverse reactions of the nervous system, e.g. peripheral neuropathy and thus impair the patients ability to drive or operate machinery.

Undesirable effects: Rifampicin may cause reddish discolouration of body fluids and occasionally other body secretions, e.g. urine, sputum, lacrimal fluid, faeces, saliva, sweat. It may permanently discolour soft contact-lenses.

Unwanted effects which may occur during continuous daily or intermittent therapy.

Frequency estimates: frequent>10%, occasional>1–10%, rare>0.001–1%, isolated cases<0.001%.

Associated with Rifampicin:
Skin and appendages: Occasionally: flushing, itching with or without skin rash, and reddening of the eyes. Isolated cases: severe signs and symptoms, such as exudative conjunctivitis or generalised hypersensitivity reactions involving the skin, e.g. exfoliative dermatitis, Lyell's syndrome and pemphigoid reactions.

Gastro-intestinal tract: Occasionally: anorexia, nausea, abdominal pains, gaseous distension; rarely: vomiting or diarrhoea; isolated occurrences of erosive gastritis and pseudomembranous colitis.

Hepatic: Frequently: an asymptomatic increase in liver enzymes; rarely: hepatitis or jaundice; here account should also be taken of the liver toxicity of chemotherapeutic agents, e.g. isoniazid or pyrazinamide, employed in combination with rifampicin. Induction of porphyria in isolated cases.

Central and peripheral nervous system: Occasionally: tiredness, drowsiness, headache, light-headedness, dizziness; rarely: ataxia, mental confusion. Isolated cases: muscular weakness, visual disturbances.

Blood: Isolated occurrences of transient leucopenia; eosinophilia; thrombocytopenia and thrombocytopenic purpura are encountered more frequently under intermittent therapy than on continuous daily treatment, during which they occur only in isolated cases.

Endocrine: Rarely: disturbances in the menstrual cycle (in extreme cases amenorrhoea); induction of a crisis in Addison patients (see *Interactions*).

Unwanted effects chiefly occurring during intermittent therapy or upon resumption of treatment after temporary interruption: In patients taking rifampicin other than on a daily basis or in those resuming treatment with the drug after a temporary interruption, an influenza-like syndrome ('flu syndrome') may occur, this being very probably of immunopathological origin. It is characterised by fever, shivering, and possibly headache, dizziness and musculoskeletal pain. In rare cases the 'flu syndrome' may be followed by thrombocytopenia, purpura, dyspnoea, asthma-like attacks, haemolytic anaemia, shock and acute renal failure. These serious complications may, however, also set in suddenly with no preceding 'flu syndrome', chiefly when treatment is resumed after a temporary interruption or when rifampicin is given only once a week in high doses (25 mg/kg or more). When Rimactane is administered in lower doses (600 mg) 2–3 times a week, the syndrome is encountered less frequently, its incidence then being comparable to that observed during daily medication.

Associated with Isoniazid:
Central nervous system: Frequently: peripheral neuropathy (dose dependent and more common in undernourished patients, alcoholics and diabetes). Rarely: damage to the optic nerve, convulsions, psychoses, dizziness, light-headedness, headache. Isolated cases: toxic encephalopathy. High doses may increase seizure frequency in epileptics.

Gastro-intestinal: Occasionally: nausea, vomiting, epigastric distress.

Hepatic: Frequently: disburbances of liver function (usually transient). Rarely: hepatitis. Isolated cases: severe hepatitis. The incidence of hepatitis increases with the patient's age.

Blood: Isolated cases: agranulocytosis, eosinophilia, thrombocytopenia, anaemia (haemolytic, hypoplastic).

Allergic and miscellaneous reactions: Occasional: drug rash, fever. Rarely: dryness of the mouth, heartburn, disorders of micturition, rheumatic syndrome, lupus erythematosus-like signs and symptoms, pellagra. Isolated cases: gynaecomastia, vasculitis.

Overdose:
Signs and symptoms: Rifampicin: Nausea, vomiting, abdominal pains; enlargement of the liver, jaundice, elevated liver enzyme levels, possibly acute pulmonary oedema, lethargy, clouding of consciousness, convulsions.

Isoniazid: In mild poisoning – ataxia, symptoms of polyneuritis, disturbed articulation, vertigo. In severe poisoning – hallucinations, epileptiform tonic-clonic attacks, respiratory depression, coma, severe metabolic acidosis, hyperglycaemia, acetonuria.

Treatment:: General supportive measures to maintain vital functions; intravenous administration of anti-convulsants and pyridoxine in large doses; control of metabolic acidosis, gastric lavage together with instillation of an activated charcoal suspension via a stomach tube; forced diuresis; haemodialysis, in the presence of severe liver damage, cholecystotomy if necessary.

Pharmacological properties

Pharmacodynamic properties:

Pharmacotherapeutic group: Rifampicin is a rifamycin antibiotic and isoniazid is a specific antituberculous agent.

Mechanism of action: Rifampicin exerts, both *in vitro* and *in vivo* bactericidal effects on *Mycobacterium tuberculosis.* It also exhibits variable activity against other atypical species of Mycobacterium.

In vivo it exerts its bactericidal effect not only on micro-organisms in the extracellular spaces but also on those located intracellularly. Rifampicin has a potent sterilising effect.

Rifampicin inhibits the DNA-dependent RNA polymerase of sensitive bacterial strains, but without affecting the corresponding mammalian enzyme.

Isoniazid exerts a strong bactericidal effect mainly on rapidly growing populations of *Mycobacterium tuberculosis.* Its mechanism of action is probably based chiefly on inhibition of mycolic acid synthesis, mycolic acid being an important constituent of the mycobacterial cell wall.

Pharmacokinetic properties:

Absorption: An oral administration of the fixed combination on an empty stomach, the two active substances are well absorbed.

Rifampicin, following a single dose of 600 mg, reaches mean peak plasma concentrations of 9.4 mcg/mL after 2–3 hours.

Isoniazid, following a single dose of 300 mg, reaches mean peak plasma concentrations of 6.1 mcg/mL after 0.5–2 hours. However, plasma concentrations vary interindividually, depending on the acetylator status of the patient.

Concomitant intake of food reduces the absorption of both active components.

Distribution: Rifampicin: The apparent distribution volume is 1.6 L/kg in adults and 1.1 L/kg in children. Binding to serum proteins amounts to 84%–91%.

Isoniazid: The apparent distribution volume is 0.61 L/kg. Isoniazid is not appreciably bound to serum proteins.

Rifampicin and isoniazid penetrate rapidly into various body fluids and tissues, including bone tissue (rifampicin) and cerebrospinal fluid, in therapeutically active concentrations.

Rifampicin crosses the blood/brain barrier in the case of inflamed meninges only, but concentrations in the cerebrospinal fluid may remain above the MIC for *Mycobacterium tuberculosis* for up to two months with continuous therapy of 600 mg/day orally.

Rifampicin and isoniazid cross the human placenta and are secreted in human breast milk.

Isoniazid attains the highest levels, but it is estimated that a breast-fed infant would receive no more than 20%, and in the case of *rifampicin* less than 1% of the usual therapeutic dose.

Biotransformation: Rifampicin is metabolised in the liver, the principal metabolite being 25-O-deacetyl-rifampicin, which is microbiologically active and, like rifampicin, subject to enterohepatic circulation. Rifampicin induces its own metabolism.

Isoniazid is acetylated and hydrolysed in the liver. Acetylation is the most important metabolic pathway and is subject to genetic predisposition (fast and slow acetylators).

Elimination/excretion: Rifampicin: The plasma elimination half-life of rifampicin increases with increasing doses and amounts to 2.5 h, 3–4 h and about 5 h after single doses of 300 mg, 600 mg and 900 mg respectively. After a few days of repeated daily administration, the bioavailabilty of rifampicin diminishes, and the half-life value following repeated doses of 600 mg falls to 1–2 hours.

Owing to its enzyme-inducing effect in the liver, rifampicin accelerates its own metabolism, with the result that its systemic clearance, which amounts to approx. 6 L/h after the first dose, rises to approx. 9 L/h after repeated dosing.

Although the bulk of the drug is eliminated in the bile, 80% of the quantity excreted being accounted for by the deacetylrifampicin metabolite, rifampicin also appears in the urine.

In a dosage range of 150–900 mg, 4–18% of a dose is excreted dose-dependently in the urine in unchanged form.

Isoniazid: The plasma elimination half-life is 0.6–1.8 hours in fast acetylators and 1.8–6.7 hours in slow acetylators.

Within 24 hours 75–95% of the dose administered is excreted in the urine, mainly as metabolites. N-cetylisoniazid is eliminated in the urine together with other metabolites. The quantity appearing in the urine as unchanged isoniazid is equivalent to 12% of the dose in fast acetylators and to 27% in slow acetylators.

Characteristics in patients: Rifampicin: In elderly patients, plasma concentrations are similar to those in young patients.

With impaired renal function, the elimination half-life becomes prolonged only at doses exceeding 600 mg daily. Provided that hepatic excretory function is normal, the dosage in patients with impaired renal function does not need to be reduced below 600 mg daily.

Rifampicin is eliminated by peritoneal or haemodialysis. Dosage adjustment is not necessary during dialysis. Because rifampicin is dialysable it is recommended that the drug should not be administered until after the period of dialysis is complete.

In patients with impaired liver function, the plasma concentrations are raised and the elimination half-life prolonged. In the presence of severe hepatic dysfunction the dosage may have to be adjusted accordingly.

Isoniazid: Elderly patients: In fast acetylators, old age has no significant influence on the rate at which the drug is eliminated. However, clearance and elimination half-life vary significantly in elderly slow acetylators, so that it might be necessary to adjust the dosage accordingly.

In slow acetylators with severely impaired renal function, accumulation of isoniazid may occur. In such cases, the serum concentration of isoniazid should be monitored and, if necessary, the dosage reduced.

In the presence of impaired liver function the elimination half-life of isoniazid is prolonged. To avoid unwanted effects it may therefore be necessary to adapt the dosage accordingly.

Preclinical safety data: Rifampicin: There is limited evidence as to the carcinogenic potential of rifampicin in animals. In female mice of a strain known to be susceptible to hepatomas, a significant increase in such tumours was observed after 1 year of treatment with rifampicin in quantities equivalent to 2–10 times the maximum clinical doses.

In mice of another strain treated for 1 year, and in rats treated for 2 years, no significant increase was noted in the incidence of any type of tumour. Studies with various mammalian models, as well as with bacteria, yielded no evidence that rifampicin has a mutagenic effect.

In daily doses of 150–250 mg/kg, rifampicin proved teratogenic in mice and rats, insofar as an increased occurrence of spina bifida and cleft palate was observed. In rabbits it had no teratogenic effect. In all three animal species, unspecific embryotoxic effects occurred after doses >150 mg/kg.

Isoniazid: Teratogenic effects have been noted in animal models. Limited evidence shows that isoniazid produces lung tumours in mice after various modes of administration. Available evidence of human exposure has not suggested that isoniazid is carcinogenic in man at doses applicable to the treatment and prophylaxis of tuberculosis.

Pharmaceutical particulars

List of excipients: The tablets contain calcium stearate, sodium lauryl sulphate, talc, maize starch, sodium carboxymethylcellulose, talc, hydroxypropyl methylcellulose, povidone, titanium dioxide, microcrystalline cellulose, polyethylene glycol, polyvinylpyrrolidone, sugar (sucrose), red iron oxide (E172), yellow iron oxide (E172) (300 mg only) and water.

Incompatibilities: None known.

Shelf life: Three years.

Special precautions for storage: Protect from moisture and heat (store below 25°C).

Medicines should be kept out of reach of children.

Nature and contents of containers: Rimactazid 150 tablets are round, pale red, sugar-coated tablets, printed CG on one side and EI on the other side in brown ink, and are packed in PVC/PVdC blister packs of 84.

Rimactazid 300 tablets are round, reddish-orange, sugar-coated tablets, printed CG on one side and DH on the other side in brown ink, and are packed in PVC/PVdC blister packs of 56.

Instructions for use/handling: None.

Marketing authorisation holder: Novartis Pharmaceuticals UK Limited, trading as Ciba Laboratories.

Marketing authorisation numbers

150 mg tablet 00101/0449
300 mg tablet 00101/0450

Date of revision of the text 6 September 1997.

Legal category POM.

RITALIN*

Qualitative and quantitative composition The active ingredient is Methylphenidate (INN for α-Phenyl-2-piperidineacetic acid methyl ester hydrochloride.

One tablet contains 10 mg methylphenidate hydrochloride.

Pharmaceutical form Tablets.

Clinical particulars

Therapeutic indications: Ritalin is indicated as a part of a comprehensive treatment programme for attention-deficit hyperactivity disorder (ADHD) where remedial measures alone prove insufficient. Treatment must be under the supervision of a specialist in childhood behavioural disorders. Diagnosis should be made according to DSM-IV criteria or the guidelines in ICD-10.

Additional information on the safe use of the product: ADHD is also known as attention-deficit disorder (ADD). Other terms used to describe this behavioural syndrome include: hyperkinetic disorder, minimal brain damage, minimal brain dysfunction in children, minor cerebral dysfunction and psycho-organic syndrome of children.

A part of a comprehensive treatment programme, typically includes psychological, educational and social measures and is aimed at stabilising children with a behavioural syndrome characterised by symptoms which may include chronic history of short attention span, distractibility, emotional lability, impulsivity, moderate to severe hyperactivity, minor neurological signs and abnormal EEG. Learning may or may not be impaired.

Ritalin treatment is not indicated in all children with this syndrome and the decision to use the drug must be based on a very thorough assessment of the severity of the child's symptoms.

Posology and method of administration:

Adults: Not applicable.

Elderly: Not applicable.

Children: (over 6 years). Begin with 5 mg once or twice daily (e.g. at breakfast and lunch), increasing the dose and frequency of administration if necessary by weekly increments of 5–10 mg in the daily dose. Doses above 60 mg daily are not recommended. The total daily dose should be administered in divided doses. Ritalin is not indicated in children less than 6 years of age.

If the effect of the drug wears off too early in the evening, disturbed behaviour and/or inability to go to sleep may recur. A small evening dose may help to solve this problem.

Note: If improvement of symptoms is not observed after appropriate dosage adjustment over a one-month period, the drug should be discontinued. Ritalin should be discontinued periodically to assess the child's condition. Drug treatment is usually discontinued during or after puberty.

Contra-indications: The presence of marked anxiety, agitation or tension is a contra-indication to the use of Ritalin as it may aggravate these symptoms.

Ritalin is also contra-indicated in patients with motor tics, tics in siblings, or a family history or diagnosis of Tourette's syndrome.

It is also contra-indicated in patients with hyperthyroidism, severe angina pectoris, cardiac arrhythmias, glaucoma, thyrotoxicosis, or known sensitivity to methylphenidate or to any of the excipients in Ritalin.

Special warnings and precautions for use:

Warnings: Ritalin should not be used in children under 6 years of age, since safety and efficacy in this age group have not been established.

Ritalin should not be used to treat severe exogenous or endogenous depression.

Clinical experience suggests that Ritalin may exacerbate symptoms of behavioural disturbance and thought disorder in psychotic children.

Available clinical evidence indicates that treatment during childhood does not increase the likelihood of addiction in later life.

Chronic abuse of Ritalin can lead to marked tolerance and psychological dependence with varying degrees of abnormal behaviour. Frank psychotic episodes may occur, especially with parenteral abuse.

Precautions: Treatment with Ritalin is not indicated in all cases of Attention-Deficit-Hyperactivity disorders, and should be considered only after detailed history-taking and evaluation. The decision to prescribe Ritalin should depend on an assessment of the severity of symptoms and their appropriateness to the child's age and not simply on the presence of one or more abnormal behavioural characteristics. Where these symptoms are associated with acute stress reactions, treatment with Ritalin is usually not indicated.

Moderately reduced weight gain and slight growth retardation have been reported with the long-term use of stimulants in children, although a causal relationship has not been confirmed. Careful monitoring of growth is recommended during extended treatment with Ritalin.

Blood pressure should be monitored at appropriate intervals in all patients taking Ritalin, especially those with hypertension.

Caution is called for in emotionally unstable patients, such as those with a history of drug dependence or alcoholism, because such patients may increase the dosage on their own initiative.

Ritalin should be used with caution in patients with epilepsy as clinical experience has shown that it can cause an increase in seizure frequency in a small number of such patients. If seizure frequency increases, Ritalin should be discontinued.

The long-term safety and efficacy profiles of Ritalin are not fully known. Patients requiring long-term therapy should therefore be carefully monitored and complete and differential blood counts and a platelet count performed periodically.

Careful supervision is required during drug withdrawal, since this may unmask depression as well as chronic over-activity. Some patients may require long-term follow-up.

Interactions with other medicaments and other forms of interaction: Human pharmacological studies have shown that Ritalin may inhibit the metabolism of coumarin anticoagulants, some anticonvulsants (e.g. phenobarbitone, phenytoin, primidone), phenylbutazone and tricyclic antidepressants. The dosage of these drugs may have to be reduced. Ritalin should be used cautiously in patients being treated with pressor agents and MAO inhibitors.

Ritalin may reduce the antihypertensive effects of guanethidine.

Alcohol may exacerbate the adverse CNS effect of psychoactive drugs, including Ritalin. It is therefore advisable for patients to abstain from alcohol during treatment.

Pregnancy and lactation: There is no evidence of risk to the foetus but experience during pregnancy is limited. In animal studies, Ritalin did not affect the reproductive performance or fertility and had no embryotoxic, foetotoxic or teratogenic effects at about 2–5 times the therapeutic dose in humans. Ritalin should not be given to pregnant women unless the potential benefit outweighs the risk to the foetus.

It is not known whether the active substance of Ritalin and/or its metabolites passes into breast milk, but for safety reasons breast-feeding mothers should not use Ritalin.

Effects on ability to drive or use machines: Ritalin may cause dizziness and drowsiness. It is therefore advisable to exercise caution when driving, operating machinery, or engaging in other potentially hazardous activities.

Undesirable effects: Frequency estimate: very common ≥10%; common ≥1% to <10%; uncommon ≥0.1% to <1%; rare ≥0.01% to <0.1%; very rare <0.01%.

Nervousness and insomnia are very common adverse reactions occurring at the beginning of treatment, but can usually be controlled by reducing the dosage and/or omitting the afternoon or evening dose.

Decreased appetite is also common but usually transient.

Central and peripheral nervous system: Common: Headache, drowsiness, dizziness, dyskinesia. *Rare:* Difficulties in visual accommodation, and blurred vision. *Very rare:* Hyperactivity, convulsions, muscle cramps, choreo-athetoid movements, tics or exacerbation of existing tics, and Tourette's syndrome, toxic psychosis (sometimes with visual and tactile hallucinations), transient depressed mood, cerebral arteritis and/or occlusion.

Very rare reports of poorly documented neuroleptic malignant syndrome (NMS) have been received. In most of these reports patients were also receiving other medications. It is uncertain what role Ritalin played in these cases.

Gastro-intestinal tract: Common: Abdominal pain, nausea and vomiting These usually occur at the beginning of treatment and may be alleviated by concomitant food intake. Dry mouth. *Very rare:* Abnormal liver function, ranging from transaminase elevation to hepatic coma.

Cardiovascular system: Common: Tachycardia, palpitations, arrhythmias, changes in blood pressure and heart rate (usually an increase). *Rare:* Angina pectoris.

Skin and appendages: Common: Rash, pruritus, urticaria, fever, arthralgia, scalp hair loss. *Very rare:* Thrombocytopenic purpura, exfoliative dermatitis and erythema multiforme.

Blood: Very rare: Leucopenia, thrombocytopenia and anaemia.

Miscellaneous: Rare: Moderately reduced weight gain and slight growth retardation during prolonged use in children.

Overdose: Signs and symptoms: Acute overdose, mainly due to overstimulation of the central and sympathetic nervous systems, may result in vomiting, agitation, tremors, hyperreflexia, muscle twitching, convulsions (may be followed by coma), euphoria, confusion, hallucinations, delirium, sweating, flushing, headache, hyperpyrexia, tachycardia, palpitations, cardiac arrhythmias, hypertension, mydriasis and dryness of mucous membrane.

Treatment: There is no specific antidote to Ritalin overdosage.

Management consists of appropriate supportive measures, preventing self-injury and protecting the patient from external stimuli that would aggravate over-stimulation already present. If the signs and symptoms are not too severe and the patient is conscious, gastric contents may be evacuated by induction of vomiting or gastric lavage. In the presence of severe intoxication, a carefully titrated dose of a short-acting barbiturate should be given before performing gastric lavage.

Intensive care must be provided to maintain adequate circulation and respiratory exchange; external cooling procedures may be required to reduce hyperpyrexia.

Efficacy of peritoneal dialysis or extracorporeal haemodialysis for overdose of Ritalin has not been established.

Pharmacological properties

Pharmacodynamic properties: Mode of action: Ritalin is a mild CNS stimulant with more prominent effects on mental than on motor activities. Its mode of action in man is not completely understood but its effects are thought to be due to cortical stimulation and possibly to stimulation of the reticular activating system.

The mechanism by which Ritalin exerts its mental and behavioural effects in children is not clearly established, nor is there conclusive evidence showing how these effects relate to the condition of the central nervous system.

Pharmacokinetic properties: Absorption: The active substance methylphenidate hydrochloride is rapidly and almost completely absorbed from the tablets. Owing to extensive first-pass metabolism its systemic availability amounts to only 30% (11–51%) of the dose. Ingestion together with food accelerates its absorption, but has no influence on the amount absorbed. Peak plasma concentrations of approximately 40 nmol/litres (11 ng/ml) are attained, on average, 1–2 hours after administration of 0.30 mg/kg. The peak plasma concentrations, however, show considerable intersubject variability. The area under the plasma concentration curve (AUC), as well as the peak plasma concentration (C_{max}), are proportional to the dose.

Distribution: In the blood, methylphenidate and its metabolites become distributed in the plasma (57%) and the erythrocytes (43%). Methylphenidate and its metabolites have a low plasma protein-building rate (10–33%). The apparent distribution volume has been calculated as 13.1 litres/kg.

Biotransformation: Biotransformation of methylphenidate is rapid and extensive. Peak plasma concentrations of 2-phenyl-2-piperidyl acetic acid (PPAA) are attained approximately 2 hours after administration of methylphenidate and are 30–50 times higher than those of the unchanged substance. The half-life of PPAA is roughly twice as long as that of methylphenidate, and the mean systemic clearance is 0.17 litres/h/kg. Only small amounts of hydroxylated metabolites (e.g. hydroxymethlphenidate and hydroxyritalinic acid) are detectable. Therapeutic activity seems to be principally due to the parent compound.

Elimination: Methylphenidate is eliminated from the plasma with a mean half-life of 2 hours, and the calculated mean systemic clearance is 10 litres/h/kg. Within 48–96 hours 78–97% of the dose administered is excreted in the urine and 1–3% in the faeces in the form of metabolites. Unchanged methylphenidate appears in the urine only in small quantities (<1%). The bulk of the dose is excreted in the urine as PPAA (60–86%).

Characteristics in patients: There are no apparent differences in the pharmacokinetic behaviour of methylphenidate in hyperactive children and healthy adult volunteers.

Elimination data from patients with normal renal function suggest that renal excretion of the unchanged methylphenidate would hardly be diminished at all in the presence of impaired renal function. However, renal excretion of PPAA may be reduced.

Preclinical safety data: In a lifetime carcinogenicity study carried out in mice, methylphenidate caused an increase in hepatocellular adenomas and, in males only, an increase in hepatoblastomas, at a daily dose of approximately 60 mg/kg/day. This is considerably higher than the recommended human dose on a mg/kg basis. Hepatoblastoma is a relatively rare rodent malignant tumour type. There was no increase in total malignant hepatic tumours. The mouse strain used is sensitive to the development of hepatic tumours, and the significance of these results to humans is unknown.

Similar studies in rats showed no evidence of carcinogenicity.

Sister chromatid exchange and chromosome aberrations were elevated in an *in vitro* test on cultured ovary cells of Chinese hamster. In two further *in vitro* tests (Ames reverse mutation test, mouse lymphoma forward mutation test) no mutagenic effects were observed.

In an *in vivo* study of the effect of methylphenidate on mouse bone marrow cells (micronucleus test), in which doses up to 250 mg/kg were tested, there was no evidence of clastogenic or aneugenic effects.

In the general population, the risk of hepatoblastoma is greatest in children under 4 years of age, for whom Ritalin treatment is not recommended. The estimated incidence is 1 per 10 million in children aged 5 to 9 years, and falls thereafter. There is no indication that the incidence is higher in patients exposed to Ritalin.

Pharmaceutical particulars

List of excipients: The tablets also contain calcium phosphate tribasic special, lactose, wheat starch, gelatin, magnesium stearate and talc.

Incompatibilities: None known.

Shelf life: Two years.

Special precautions for storage: Protect from moisture and store below 30°C.

Medicines should be kept out of reach of children.

Nature and contents of container: The tablets are available in blister packs of 30 tablets.

Instruction for use/handling: None.

Marketing authorisation holder: Novartis Pharmaceuticals UK Limited, trading as Ciba Laboratories, Frimley Business Park, Frimley, Camberley, Surrey GU16 5SG.

Marketing authorisation number PL 00101/0539.

Date of first authorisation 31 October 1997.

Date of revision of the text 2 April 1998.

Legal category CD (Sch 2) POM.

SANDIMMUN Concentrate for Infusion 50 mg/ml

Qualitative and quantitative composition Cyclosporin 50 mg in 1 ml.

Pharmaceutical form Clear, brown yellow, oily solution.

Clinical particulars

Therapeutic indications

Organ transplantation: Prevention of graft rejection following kidney, liver, heart, combined heart-lung, lung or pancreas transplant.

Treatment of transplant rejection in patients previously receiving other immunosuppressive agents.

Bone marrow transplantation: Prevention of graft rejection following bone marrow transplantation and prophylaxis of graft-versus-host disease (GVHD).

Treatment of established graft-versus-host disease (GVHD).

Posology and method of administration

Organ transplantation: Initially, a single oral dose of 10–15 mg/kg body weight, should be given 4–12 hours before transplantation. As a general rule, treatment should continue at a dose of 10–15 mg/kg/day for 1–2 weeks post-operatively. Dosage should then be gradually reduced until a maintenance dose of 2–6 mg/kg/day is reached. Dosage should be adjusted by monitoring cyclosporin blood levels and kidney function. When Sandimmun is given with other immunosuppressants (e.g. with corticosteroids or as part of a triple or quadruple drug therapy) lower doses (e.g. 3–6 mg/kg/day orally initially) may be used.

The use of the Concentrate for intravenous infusion is recommended in organ transplant patients who are unable to take Sandimmun orally (e.g. shortly after surgery) or in whom the absorption of the oral forms might be impaired during episodes of gastrointestinal disturbances. In such cases the intravenous dose is one third of the recommended oral dose. It is recommended, however, that patients are transferred to oral therapy as soon as the given circumstances allow.

Bone marrow transplantation/prevention and treatment of graft-versus-host disease (GVHD): Sandimmun Concentrate for intravenous infusion is usually preferred for initiation of therapy, although the oral forms may be used. The recommended dosage by the intravenous route is 3–5 mg/kg/day, starting on the day before transplantation and continuing during the immediate post-transplant period of up to two weeks until oral maintenance therapy begins.

Treatment with Sandimmun should continue using the oral forms at a dosage of 12.5 mg/kg/day for at least three and preferably six months before tailing off to zero. In some cases higher oral doses or the use of i.v. therapy may be necessary in the presence of gastrointestinal disturbances which might decrease absorption. If oral treatment is used to initiate therapy the recommended dose is 12.5–15 mg/kg/day starting on the day before transplantation.

If GVHD develops after Sandimmun is withdrawn it should respond to reinstitution of therapy. Low doses should be used for mild, chronic GVHD.

Intravenous administration: When Sandimmun is administered by the intravenous route, the intravenous dose is one third of the recommended oral dose.

Sandimmun Concentrate should be diluted 1:20 to 1:100 with normal saline or 5% glucose before use and given by slow intravenous infusion over 2–6 hours.

Use in the elderly: Experience in the elderly is limited but no particular problems have been reported following the use of the drug at the recommended dose. However, factors sometimes associated with ageing, in particular impaired renal function, make careful supervision essential and may necessitate dosage adjustment.

Use in children: Experience with Sandimmun in young children is still limited. Transplant recipients from three months of age have received the drug at the recommended dosage with no particular problems although at dosages above the upper end of the recommended range, children seem to be more susceptible to fluid retention, convulsions and hypertension. This responds to dosage reduction.

Contra-indications: Known hypersensitivity to cyclosporin.

Sandimmun Concentrate for intravenous infusion should not be used in patients known to be hypersensitive to polyethoxylated castor oils.

Special warnings and special precautions for use: Sandimmun can impair renal function. Close monitoring of serum creatinine and urea is required and dosage adjustment may be necessary. Increases in serum creatinine and urea occurring during the first few weeks of Sandimmun therapy are generally dose-dependent and reversible and usually respond to dosage reduction. During long-term treatment, some patients may develop structural changes in the kidney (e.g. interstitial fibrosis) which, in renal transplant recipients, must be distinguished from chronic rejection.

Sandimmun may also affect liver function and dosage adjustment, based on the results of bilirubin and liver enzyme monitoring, may be necessary.

Regular monitoring of blood pressure is required during Sandimmun therapy. If hypertension develops, appropriate antihypertensive treatment must be instituted.

Since Sandimmun occasionally causes hyperkalaemia or may aggravate pre-existing hyperkalaemia, monitoring of serum potassium is recommended, especially in patients with marked renal dysfunction. Patients receiving Sandimmun should avoid a high dietary potassium intake.

Caution is required in treating patients with hyperuricaemia because Sandimmun can aggravate this condition (see *Undesirable effects*).

Sandimmun should preferably not be administered with other immunosuppressive agents except corticosteroids. However, some transplant centres use Sandimmun together with azathioprine and corticosteroids or other immunosuppressive agents (all in low doses) with the aim of reducing the risk of Sandimmun-induced renal dysfunction or renal structural changes. When Sandimmun is used with other immunosuppressive agents, there is a risk of over-immunosuppression, which can lead to increased susceptibility to infection and to possible development of lymphoma.

In Sandimmun treated renal transplant recipients, a machine perfusion time of more than 24 hours and a reanastomosis time of more than 45 minutes can have a significant effect on graft function. Both factors appear to increase the incidence of acute tubular necrosis.

The concentrate for intravenous infusion contains polyethoxylated castor oil, which has been reported to cause anaphylactoid reactions. These reactions consist of flushing of face and upper thorax, acute respiratory distress with dyspnoea and wheezing, blood pressure changes and tachycardia. Special caution is therefore necessary in patients who have previously received intravenous injections or intravenous infusions containing polyethoxylated castor oil, or in patients with an allergic predisposition.

Thus patients receiving Sandimmun i.v. should be under continuous observation for at least the first 30 minutes following start of the infusion and at frequent intervals thereafter. If anaphylaxis occurs, the infusion should be discontinued and the patient managed in accordance with common clinical practice.

Sandimmun can induce a reversible increase in blood lipids. It is therefore advisable to perform lipid determinations before treatment and thereafter as appropriate.

Interactions with other medicaments and other forms of interaction: Care should be taken when using Sandimmun in combination with systemic antibiotics or compounds known to have nephrotoxic effects, e.g. aminoglycosides, amphotericin B, ciprofloxacin, melphalan and trimethoprim.

Various agents are known to either increase or decrease the plasma or whole blood concentrations of cyclosporin by competitive inhibition or hepatic enzymes involved in the metabolism and excretion of Sandimmun, in particular cytochrome P450.

Agents known to increase plasma or whole blood concentrations include clarithromycin, ketoconazole, erythromycin, oral contraceptives, danazol, and some calcium channel blockers including diltiazem, nicardipine and verapamil, whereas doxycycline, fluconazole, itraconazole, propafenone and lipid solutions are suspected to have the same effect. Agents known to decrease plasma or whole blood cyclosporin concentrations include phenytoin, carbamazepine, barbiturates and rifampicin, whereas sulphadiazine is suspected to have the same effect.

In transplant patients, frequent measurement of cyclosporin levels and, if necessary, Sandimmun dosage adjustment is required, particularly during the introduction or withdrawal of the co-administered drug.

Intravenous (but not oral) administration of sulphadimidine and trimethoprim has also resulted in a marked reduction of plasma or whole blood levels. Concomitant administration of such drugs with Sandimmun should, therefore, be avoided. Where combined administration is unavoidable, careful monitoring of cyclosporin blood levels and adjustment of Sandimmun dosage are essential.

In addition, it has been noted that Sandimmun reduces the clearance of prednisolone and, conversely, high-dose therapy with methylprednisolone can increase the blood concentration of cyclosporin.

As non-steroidal anti-inflammatory drugs alone can have an adverse effect on renal function, addition of these drugs to Sandimmun therapy or an increase in their dosage should initially be accompanied by particularly close monitoring of renal function.

Sandimmun, given in combination with diclofenac, causes an increase in plasma concentration of diclofenac. Diclofenac dosages should, therefore, be reduced by approximately half when given with Sandimmun. There have been reports of pharmacokinetic interactions with other non-steroidal anti-inflammatory drugs, but there are insufficient data available to clarify their significance. However, a lack of pharmacokinetic interaction has been demonstrated between aspirin and Sandimmun. Some studies have shown that various NSAIDs interact pharmacodynamically with Sandimmun to affect renal function. An analysis of clinical trials of Sandimmun and non-steroidal anti-inflammatory drugs suggests that plasma creatinine is not higher in patients if they receive concomitant NSAID therapy. The combination of these drugs, however, should be used with care.

Sandimmun may enhance the potential of the HMG-CoA reductase inhibitor lovastatin to induce rhabdomyolysis. The potential for interaction with other drugs in this class should be considered.

Muscular toxicity, including muscle pains and weakness, have also been reported in patients receiving colchicine concurrently with Sandimmun.

The concurrent administration of nifedipine and Sandimmun has resulted in an increased rate of gingival hyperplasia when compared with that for Sandimmun alone.

Where there is a risk of hyperkalaemia, potassium-sparing diuretics should be avoided and care should be taken when prescribing potassium supplements or potassium-containing medications.

The concomitant intake of grapefruit juice has been reported to increase the bioavailability of cyclosporin.

During treatment with Sandimmun, vaccination may be less effective, and the use of live attenuated vaccines should be avoided.

Pregnancy and lactation: Cyclosporin is not teratogenic in animals. As the safety of Sandimmun in human pregnancy has not been fully established it should only be used in pregnancy if the benefit outweighs any potential risks.

Cyclosporin passes into the breast milk and mothers receiving treatment with Sandimmun should not, therefore, breast feed their infants.

Effects on ability to drive and use machinery: Not applicable.

Undesirable effects: Side-effects are usually dose dependent and responsive to dose reduction.

A frequent and potentially serious complication is a dose-dependent and reversible increase in serum creatinine and urea during the first few weeks of Sandimmun therapy. Less frequently, renal structural changes (e.g. interstitial fibrosis) may develop during long-term treatment. Impairment of renal function may necessitate dosage reduction.

Apart from impaired renal function, the most frequently observed side-effects include hypertrichosis, tremor, hypertension (particularly in heart transplant patients) hepatic dysfunction, fatigue, gingival hypertrophy, gastrointestinal disturbances (anorexia, nausea, vomiting, diarrhoea) and burning sensations of the hands and feet (usually during the first week of treatment).

Occasionally headaches, rashes of possible allergic origin, mild anaemia, hyperkalaemia, hyperuricaemia, gout, hypomagnesaemia, hypercholesterolaemia, weight increase, oedema, pancreatitis, neuropathy, confusion, paraesthesia, convulsions, reversible dysmenorrhoea or amenorrhoea may develop.

Muscle weakness, muscle cramps, or myopathy have also been reported.

Especially in liver transplant patients, signs of encephalopathy, vision and movement disturbances, and impaired consciousness are described. Whether these alterations are caused by Sandimmun, or are a consequence of the underlying disease or other conditions, remains to be established.

On rare occasions, a syndrome of thrombocytopenia, in some patients in combination with microangiopathic haemolytic anaemia and renal failure (haemolytic uraemic syndrome) has been observed.

Gynaecomastia has been rarely reported, occasionally in patients receiving concomitant spironolactone.

Malignancies and lymphoproliferative disorders have developed, but their incidence and distribution were found to be similar to those in patients on conventional immunosuppressive therapy.

In a few cases, colitis has developed after treatment with Sandimmun.

Overdose: Little experience is available with overdosage. Symptomatic treatment and general supportive measures should be followed in all cases of overdosage.

Signs of nephrotoxicity might occur which would be expected to resolve following drug withdrawal. Sandimmun is not dialysable to any great extent nor is it well cleared by charcoal haemoperfusion. Hypertension and convulsions have been reported in some patients receiving Sandimmun therapy at doses above the recommended range and in others with high trough blood levels of cyclosporin. This might, therefore, be expected as a feature of overdosage.

Pharmacological properties

Pharmacodynamic properties: Cyclosporin A is a cyclic undecapeptide with immunosuppressant properties. Studies suggest that cyclosporin A inhibits the development of cell-mediated reactions, including allograft immunity, delayed cutaneous hypersensitivity, experimental allergic encephalomyelitis, Freund's adjuvant arthritis, graft-versus-host disease and also T-cell dependent antibody production. It also inhibits lymphokine production and release, including interleukin 2 or T-cell growth factor (TCGF). Cyclosporin appears to block the resting lymphocytes in the G_0 or G_1 phase of the cell cycle.

All available evidence suggests that cyclosporin acts specifically and reversibly on lymphocytes. Unlike cytostatic agents it does not depress haemopoeisis and has no effect on the function of phagocytic cells.

Pharmacokinetic properties: Sandimmun Concentrate for intravenous infusion has been shown to be bioequivalent to Sandimmun oral solution.

Absolute bioavailability is 25–50% at steady state and peak blood concentrations are achieved within 1–6 hours.

Cyclosporin A is distributed largely outside the blood volume. Within blood, 33–47% is present in plasma, 4–9% in lymphocytes, 5–12% in granulocytes and 41–58% in erythocytes. In plasma, approximately 90% is bound to protein, mainly lipoproteins.

Cyclosporin is extensively biotransformed to approximately 15 metabolites, there being no single major metabolic pathway. Elimination is primarily biliary, with only 6% of the oral dose excreted in the urine; only 0.1% is excreted in the urine as unchanged drug. The terminal elimination half-life from blood is approximately 19 hours, irrespective of the dose or route of administration.

Preclinical safety data: None stated.

Pharmaceutical particulars

List of excipients: Absolute ethanol and polyethoxylated castor oil.

Incompatibilities: The polyethoxylated castor oil contained in the concentrate for intravenous infusion can cause phthalate stripping from PVC.

Shelf life: 4 years.

Special precautions for storage: Store below 30°C.

Nature and contents of container: Sandimmun Concentrate for infusion is available in 1 ml and 5 ml uncoloured glass ampoules.

Instructions for use/handling: Not stated.

Marketing authorisation holder: Novartis Pharmaceuticals UK Limited, trading as Sandoz Pharmaceuticals,

Frimley Business Park, Frimley, Camberley, Surrey GU16 5SG.

Marketing authorisation number PL 00101/0153.

Date of first authorisation/renewal of authorisation 17 February 1983.

Date of (partial) revision of the text 18 February 1998.

SANDOCAL*
CALCIUM-SANDOZ*

Presentation
Sandocal 400: White, round, flat-faced, effervescent tablets with a slightly rough surface, weighing 2.92 g, 25 mm diameter and 4.35 mm thick, citrus flavoured. Each effervescent tablet contains 930.8 mg calcium lactate gluconate and 700 mg calcium carbonate and provides 400 mg calcium (10 mmol: 20 mEq Ca^{++}), and 1.189 g anhydrous citric acid.
Sandocal 1000: White, round, flat-faced effervescent tablets with a slightly rough surface, weighing 7.30 g, 33 mm diameter and 6.4 mm thick, citrus flavoured. Each effervescent tablet contains 2.327 g calcium lactate gluconate, 1.75 g calcium carbonate and provides 1 g calcium (25 mmol: 50 mEq Ca^{++}), 2.973 g anhydrous citric acid.

Uses
Principal action: Calcium is an essential body electrolyte. It is involved in the maintenance of normal muscle and nerve function, is essential for normal cardiac function and is essential to blood coagulation. There is a dynamic equilibrium between the calcium in blood and that in the skeleton. Homeostasis is mainly regulated by parathyroid hormone, by calcitonin and by vitamin D.
Indications
1. As an adjunct to conventional therapy in the arrest or slowing down of bone demineralisation in osteoporosis.
2. In the arrest or slowing down of bone demineralisation in osteoporosis where other effective treatment is contra-indicated.
3. As a supplemental source of calcium in the correction of dietary deficiencies or when normal requirements are high.

Signs of hypocalcaemia may occur when the serum calcium concentration falls below 2.25 mmol per litre (or 4.5 mEq per litre). Symptoms may include paraesthesia, laryngospasm, muscle cramps, increased muscle excitability leading to tetany, prolongation of the Q-T interval on the ECG, convulsions and mental changes (e.g. anxiety, depression, delusions). Also ectodermal changes including loss of hair, grooved and brittle fingernails, defects of dental enamel and fungal infections, typically generalised candidiasis.

Dosage and administration In health the concentration of calcium in serum is maintained close to 2.5 mmol per litre (normal range 2.25–2.75 mmol or 4.5–5.5 mEq per litre). Treatment or therapeutic supplementation should aim to restore or maintain this level.
Effervescent tablets must be dissolved in ⅓ to ½ a tumblerful of water.

Indication	*Daily Dose Sandocal 400*	*Sandocal 1000*
Adults		
Osteoporosis	3–4	1–2
Therapeutic supplement (dose dependent upon severity)	1–4	1–2
Children		
Calcium deficiency	1–2	1
Dietary supplementation	1	—

Use in the elderly: No evidence exists that tolerance of Sandocal 400 or Sandocal 1000 is directly affected by advanced age; however, elderly patients should be supervised as factors sometimes associated with ageing, such as poor diet or impaired renal function, may indirectly affect tolerance and may require dosage reduction.

Contra-indications, warnings, etc
Contra-indications: Hypercalcaemia (e.g. in hyperparathyroidism, vitamin D overdosage, decalcifying tumours such as plasmocytoma, severe renal failure, bone metastases), severe hypercalciuria, and renal calculi.
Precautions: In mild hypercalciuria (exceeding 300 mg (7.5 mmol)/24 hours) or renal failure, or where there is evidence of stone formation in the urinary tract, adequate checks must be kept on urinary calcium excretion; if necessary the dosage should be reduced or calcium therapy discontinued. High vitamin D intake should be avoided during calcium therapy, unless especially indicated.
Thiazide diuretics reduce urinary calcium excretion so the risk of hypercalcaemia should be considered.
Oral calcium supplementation is aimed at restoring normal serum calcium levels. Although it is extremely unlikely that high enough levels will be achieved to adversely affect digitalised patients, this theoretical possibility should be considered.
Oral calcium administration may reduce the absorption of oral tetracycline or fluoride preparations. An interval of 3 hours should be observed if the two are to be given.
Use in pregnancy and lactation: The likelihood of hypercalcaemia is increased in pregnant women in whom calcium and vitamin D are co-administered. Epidemiological studies with calcium have shown no increase in the teratogenic hazard to the foetus if used in the doses recommended. Although supplemental calcium may be excreted in breast milk, the concentration is unlikely to be sufficient to produce any adverse effect on the neonate.
Side-effects: Mild gastrointestinal disturbances have occurred rarely (e.g. constipation, diarrhoea). Although hypercalcaemia would not be expected in patients unless their renal function were impaired, the following symptoms could indicate the possibility of hypercalcaemia: nausea, vomiting, anorexia, constipation, abdominal pain, bone pain, thirst, polyuria, muscle weakness, drowsiness or confusion.
Overdosage: The amount of calcium absorbed following overdosage with Sandocal 400 or Sandocal 1000 will depend on the individual's calcium status. Deliberate overdosage is unlikely with effervescent preparations and acute overdosage has not been reported. It might cause gastrointestinal disturbances but would not be expected to cause hypercalcaemia except in patients treated with excessive doses of vitamin D. Treatment should be aimed at lowering serum calcium levels, e.g. administration of oral phosphates.

Pharmaceutical precautions Sandocal 400 and Sandocal 1000 tablets must be stored below 30°C. Protect from humidity.

Legal category P.

Package quantities
Sandocal 400 Effervescent Tablets: Boxes of 100 (5 tubes of 20).
Sandocal 1000 Effervescent Tablets: Boxes of 30 (3 tubes of 10).

Further information Sandocal 400 and Sandocal 1000 contain aspartame as an artificial sweetener, so that the preparations are free from sucrose. There is no added sodium or potassium in the tablets.

Product licence numbers
Sandocal 400 0101/5043R
Sandocal 1000 0101/0205
Product licence holders: Novartis Pharmaceuticals UK Ltd, trading as Sandoz Pharmaceuticals.

Date of last revision August 1998.

SANDOGLOBULIN 1 g
SANDOGLOBULIN 3 g
SANDOGLOBULIN 6 g
SANDOGLOBULIN 12 g

Qualitative and quantitative composition
Active ingredients: Human normal immunoglobulin for intravenous administration PhEur.
Quantitative composition: Unmodified immunoglobulin G (IgG) of human origin, supplied in units of 1 g (1.1 g/bottle), 3 g (3.1 g/bottle), 6 g (6.1 g/bottle) and 12 g (12.1 g/bottle). At least 96% of the total protein is IgG (at least 90% of it as monomers and dimers), the remainder consisting of IgG fragments, albumin, small amounts of IgA (max 40 mg in 1 g protein, 120 mg in 3 g protein, 240 mg in 6 g protein and 480 mg in 12 g protein) and polymeric IgG and traces of IgM. The distribution of the IgG subclasses closely resembles that in normal human plasma. Sucrose is added as a stabiliser, and the preparation also contains traces of sodium chloride (see *List of excipients*).

Pharmaceutical form Lyophilisate for reconstitution in a suitable solvent for parenteral use (see *Method of administration*) prior to i.v. infusion.

Clinical particulars
Therapeutic indications
Replacement therapy: Primary immunodeficiency syndromes:
– congenital agammaglobulinaemia and hypogammaglobulinaemia
– common variable immunodeficiency
– severe combined immunodeficiencies.

Secondary hypogammaglobulinaemia in patients with chronic lymphocytic leukaemia and multiple myeloma with recurrent bacterial infections.
Children with congenital AIDS who have repeated bacterial infections.
Immunomodulatory effect: Idiopathic thrombocytopenic purpura (ITP), in adults or children at high risk of bleeding or prior to surgery to correct the platelet count.
Allogeneic bone marrow transplantation.
Kawasaki disease.
Posology and method of administration
Posology: The dose and dosage regimen is dependent on the indication (replacement or immunomodulation) and on the *in vivo* half life in individual patients.
Because of this, the dosage may need to be individualised for each patient. The following dosage regimens are given as a guideline.
Replacement therapy in primary immunodeficiencies: The dosage regimen should achieve a trough level of IgG (measured before the next infusion) of at least 4–6 g/L. Three to six months are required after the initiation of therapy for equilibration to occur. The recommended starting dose is 0.4–0.8 g/kg depending on the circumstances (e.g. active infection) followed by 0.2 g/kg every three weeks.
The dose required to achieve a trough level of 6 g/L is of the order of 0.2–0.8 g/kg/month. The dosage interval when steady state has been reached varies from 2–4 weekly.
Trough levels should be measured in order to adjust the dose and dosage interval.
Replacement therapy in secondary immunodeficiencies (including children with AIDS): The recommended dose is 0.2–0.4 g/kg every three to four weeks.
Idiopathic thrombocytopenic purpura: For the treatment of an acute episode, 0.8–1 g/kg on day one, repeated on day three if necessary, or 0.4 g/kg daily for two to five days. The treatment can be repeated if relapse occurs.
Kawasaki disease: 1.6–2.0 g/kg should be administered in divided doses over two to five days or 2 g/kg as a single dose. Patients should receive concomitant treatment with aspirin.
Allogeneic bone marrow transplantation: Intravenous immunoglobulin treatment may be used as part of the conditioning regimen and after the transplant. The regimen should be individualised. A starting dose of 0.5 g/kg/week is recommended.
Method of administration: Depending on the patient's requirements, the lyophilisate can be dissolved in sodium chloride 0.9% w/v, water for injection or dextrose 5%. The concentration of Sandoglobulin in any of these solutions for i.v. infusion may range from 3 to 12%, according to the volume used. It should be noted that a 3% solution of Sandoglobulin in water for injection is hypotonic (192 mOsm/kg).
Patients being treated with Sandoglobulin for the first time should be given a 3% infusion at an initial rate of 0.5 to 1.0 ml/min (approximately 10 to 20 drops/min for adult infusion sets). If no adverse reactions occur within the first 15 minutes, the rate may be gradually increased to a maximum of 2.5 ml/min (approximately 50 drops/min for adult infusion sets).
In patients receiving Sandoglobulin regularly and tolerating it well, higher concentrations (up to a maximum of 12%) may be used, but the infusion should always start at a low rate and close monitoring of the patient is required when the rate is gradually increased.
Contra-indications: Hypersensitivity to human immunoglobulins, especially in patients with IgA deficiency known to have antibodies to IgA.
Special warnings and precautions for use: Patients with agammaglobulinaemia or severe hypogammaglobulinaemia who have never received immunoglobulin replacement therapy or whose time from last treatment is greater than 8 weeks, may be at risk of suffering from anaphylactoid reactions, occasionally leading to shock, when receiving i.v. immunoglobulin by rapid i.v. infusion. In such patients, rapid infusion must be avoided; vital signs should be monitored continuously and careful surveillance of the patient is required throughout the infusion. Adrenaline and a parenteral corticosteroid preparation should be available in case of possible anaphylactoid reaction (see *Undesirable effects*).
Very rarely, i.v. immunoglobulin may cause a precipitous fall in blood pressure associated with the clinical signs of anaphylaxis, even in patients in whom previous administration of immunoglobulin preparations was well tolerated.
As with other i.v. immunoglobulin preparations, transient increases in creatinine levels including a few cases of acute renal failure have been reported after Sandoglobulin administration, especially in elderly patients with pre-existing diabetes or impairment of renal function. All patients presented with multiple risk factors and the majority received >0.4 g/kg/day. The renal impairment was transient (5 to 12 days) and was noted 2–5 days after the infusion. In the majority

of cases, the dysfunction is mild, but occasionally supportive therapy may be required. In patients with the above mentioned conditions, serum creatinine should be monitored for 3 days after the infusion.

A few cases of usually mild haemolysis have been reported after infusion of Sandoglobulin as well as with other i.v. immunoglobulin preparations. They were attributed to transfer of blood-type antibodies and appeared to be promoted by concomitant blood transfusion.

Aseptic meningeal irritation with transient alteration of cerebrospinal fluid has been reported after the infusion of Sandoglobulin as well as with other i.v. immunoglobulin preparations, primarily in patients presenting with idiopathic thrombocytopenic purpura and receiving high i.v. immunoglobulin doses. Discontinuation has resulted in remission within several days.

Patients naive to immunoglobulin G usually experience a higher frequency of minor events than those well maintained on regular therapy.

Patients should be observed for at least 20 minutes after administration.

The *Instructions for use/handling* should be carefully followed. Shaking the bottle resulting in foaming must be avoided. The reconstituted product should be inspected visually for particulate matter. The solution should be used only if it is clear. Once prepared, it should be infused without delay. Partially used bottles should be discarded.

Interaction with other medicaments and other forms of interaction: Sandoglobulin should not be mixed with any other drug and should always be given through a separate infusion line.

Live attenuated vaccines: The effectiveness of an active immunisation can be reduced by simultaneous treatment with i.v. immunoglobulin. Immunoglobulin administration may impair the efficacy of live-attenuated virus vaccines such as measles, rubella, mumps and varicella. Impairment usually lasts from 6 weeks to 3 months. Where doses of immunoglobulin above 0.4 g/kg are given, this period may be as long as 1 year.

Interference with serological testing: After the administration of immunoglobulin, the transitory rise of the passively transferred antibodies into the patient's blood may result in misleading positive results in serological testing.

Pregnancy and lactation: No animal reproduction studies with Sandoglobulin have been performed and experience in pregnant women is limited. Although no adverse effects on the foetus or on reproduction capacity have been reported, Sandoglobulin should be given to pregnant women only if clearly needed.

Being normal constituents of human plasma, the proteins contained in Sandoglobulin are likely to be excreted into breast milk without having an adverse effect on the breast-fed infant. They may contribute to the transfer of protective antibodies to the neonate.

Effects on ability to drive and use machines: There is no evidence that Sandoglobulin affects the patient's ability to drive or operate machinery.

Undesirable effects: If the contra-indications, precautions for use and recommendations for dosage and administration are observed (see corresponding sections), serious adverse reactions to Sandoglobulin are rare. They are more likely to occur with the first infusion than with subsequent administrations (either shortly after its initiation or often within the next 30 to 60 min) and may be of the anaphylactoid type.

Less serious reactions, observed with a frequency of 1–3% during or after the infusion, include headache, hyperthermia, nausea and rarely (<1%), vomiting, abdominal pain, diarrhoea, fatigue, malaise, dizziness, chills, sweating, cyanosis, dyspnoea, feeling of tightness or pain in the chest, back pain, myalgia, rigor, flushing or pallor, hypertension, hypotension and tachycardia. Most of these effects are related to the rate of infusion and may be relieved by reducing the rate or temporarily stopping the infusion.

Severe hypotension, circulatory collapse and loss of consciousness are very rare events. If such reactions occur, the infusion should be discontinued until the symptoms have subsided and therapy with adrenaline, corticosteroids, an antihistamine and i.v. fluid may be indicated. As with other i.v. immunoglobulin preparations, transient increases in creatinine levels, haemolysis and aseptic meningeal irritation have been reported in a few patients (see *Special warnings and precautions for use*).

When medicinal products prepared from human blood or plasma are administered, infectious diseases due to the transmission of infective agents cannot be totally excluded. This also applies to pathogens of hitherto unknown nature.

To reduce the risk of transmission of infective agents, selection of donors and donations by suitable means is performed, plasma pools are tested, and removal/inactivation procedures are included in the production process.

The inactivation procedures may be of limited value against non-enveloped viruses.

Overdose: No case of overdosage of Sandoglobulin has ever been reported; should it occur, no serious effects would be expected.

Pharmacological properties

Pharmacodynamic properties: Pharmacotherapeutic group ATC code: J06BA02 – Immunoglobulins, normal human, for intravascular administration.

Sandoglobulin is a polyvalent human immunoglobulin for i.v. infusion, possessing a broad spectrum of opsonic and neutralising antibodies against bacteria, viruses and other pathogens. In patients with primary or secondary immunodeficiency syndromes, Sandoglobulin replaces missing IgG antibodies, thereby reducing the risk of infection. In some other disorders of immune function e.g. idiopathic thrombocytopenic purpura and Kawasaki disease, the mechanism of action responsible for the beneficial effects of Sandoglobulin is not fully understood.

Pharmacokinetic properties: Being administered by i.v. infusion, 100% of the Sandoglobulin dose is immediately available in the patient's circulation. Thereafter, distribution between plasma and the extravascular compartment takes place and reaches equilibrium within approximately 7 days. The antibodies present in Sandoglobulin possess the same pharmacokinetic characteristics as those of endogenous IgG. The biological half life of i.v. immunoglobulin is 21 days on average in subjects with normal IgG serum levels, whereas in patients with primary hypogammaglobulinaemia or agammaglobulinaemia treated with Sandoglobulin, the average half life of total IgG was found to be 32 days. There are, however, considerable interindividual variations which may be important in determining the individual dosage regimen. IgG and IgG-complexes are broken down in cells of the reticuloendothelial system.

Preclinical safety data: Sandoglobulin is prepared from plasma obtained from non-remunerated healthy donors who must – as far as can be ascertained from their medical history, after clinical examination and laboratory tests on their blood – be free from detectable agents of infection transmissible by transfusion of blood or blood derivatives. In particular, tests for hepatitis B surface antigen (HBsAg), antibodies directed to human immunodeficiency virus type 1 (HIV-1), HIV-2, or hepatitis C virus (HCV) and elevated alanine aminotransferase (ALAT) are carried out by accredited methods and must give negative results. In addition, the testing for HBsAg, HIV-1 and -2 and HCV antibodies is repeated on the plasma pools.

The cold ethanol fractionation is carried out according to the Kistler-Nitschmann process.

Virus removal and inactiviation steps are included in the production process of Sandoglobulin. The fractionation procedure by which Sandoglobulin is prepared from plasma includes several steps validated for removal of enveloped and non-enveloped viruses. It was also shown that the treatment at pH4 in the presence of trace amounts of pepsin used in the manufacturing of Sandoglobulin represents a dedicated virus inactivation step for enveloped viruses. Overall viral clearance by elimination and inactivation has been documented for a variety of model viruses. Whilst these measures minimise the risk of transmission of infective agents, they do not completely eliminate all risk associated with the administration of medicinal products prepared from human blood or plasma.

Sandoglobulin given by i.v. infusion to laboratory animals in doses several times the therapeutic doses in man did not exert any toxic effects. However, toxicological testing in animals is of little predictive value for human use since:

(a) the fluid volume associated with single administration of a high dose results in circulatory overloading,

(b) repeated administration is impracticable because of the formation of antibodies against the heterologous proteins.

Being normal constituents of the human body, the proteins contained in i.v. immunoglobulin preparations can be considered to be non-toxic in man. The broad clinical use of Sandoglobulin and other immunoglobulin preparations over more than 10 years has not yet revealed any toxic, mutagenic or tumorigenic potential.

Pharmaceutical particulars

List of excipients

	1 g	3 g	6 g	12 g
sucrose PhEur (g/bottle)	1.67	5.0	10.0	20.0
NaCl PhEur (g per g protein)	0.02	0.06	0.12	0.24

Sandoglobulin contains no preservatives.

Incompatibilities: Nothing other than sodium chloride 0.9% w/v (physiological saline), water for injection or 5% dextrose should be used to reconstitute Sandoglobulin. Sandoglobulin should not be mixed with any other pharmaceutical product. Sandoglobulin should always be given through a separate infusion line.

Shelf life: 4 years.

Special precautions for storage: Store at temperatures not exceeding 25°C. Do not freeze. Protect from light. Do not use after the expiry date.

Nature and contents of container: Sandoglobulin is filled in DIN infusion bottles, glass type II, surface tested.

Sandoglobulin 1 g:	50 ml bottle
Sandoglobulin 3 g:	100 ml bottle
Sandoglobulin 6 g:	250 ml bottle
Sandoglobulin 12 g:	250 ml bottle

Instructions for use/handling: Each package contains a detailed health professional information leaflet describing dissolution of the lyophilisate. Reconstituted products should be inspected visually for particulate matter and discolouration prior to administration. Products which are not clear or have a sediment shall not be used.

Marketing authorisation number

Sandoglobulin 1 g	PL 0101/0353
Sandoglobulin 3 g	PL 0101/0354
Sandoglobulin 6 g	PL 0101/0355
Sandoglobulin 12 g	PL 0101/0356

Date of first authorisation/renewal or authorisation

PL 0101/0353	10 February 1998
PL 0101/0354	10 February 1998
PL 0101/0355	10 February 1998
PL 0101/0356	13 February 1998

Date of (partial) revision of text January 1998.

Legal category POM.

SANDOSTATIN AMPOULES 0.05 mg/ml
SANDOSTATIN AMPOULES 0.1 mg/ml
SANDOSTATIN AMPOULES 0.5 mg/ml
SANDOSTATIN MULTIDOSE VIALS 1 mg/5 ml

Qualitative and quantitative composition

0.05 mg octreotide (INN) per ml
0.1 mg octreotide (INN) per ml
0.5 mg octreotide (INN) per ml
0.2 mg octreotide (INN) per ml

Pharmaceutical form Sandostatin Ampoules 0.05 mg/ml, 0.1 mg/ml and 0.5 mg/ml: 1 ml ampoules containing clear colourless solution.

Sandostatin Multidose vials 1 mg/5 ml: 5 ml vial containing clear colourless solution.

Clinical particulars

Therapeutic indications

GEP tumours: For the relief of symptoms associated with gastroenteropancreatic endocrine tumours including:

- carcinoid tumours with features of carcinoid syndrome.
- VIPomas
- Glucagonomas.

Sandostatin is not antitumour therapy and is not curative in these patients.

Acromegaly: For symptomatic control and reduction of growth hormone and somatomedin C plasma levels in patients with acromegaly:

- in short term treatment, prior to pituitary surgery, or
- in long term treatment in those who are inadequately controlled by pituitary surgery, dopamine agonist treatment, radiotherapy, or in the interim period until radiotherapy becomes effective.

Sandostatin is indicated for acromegalic patients for whom surgery is inappropriate.

Evidence from short term studies demonstrate that tumour size is reduced in some patients (prior to surgery); further tumour shrinkage however cannot be expected as a feature of continued long term treatment.

Prevention of complications following pancreatic surgery. Route of administration: Subcutaneous or intravenous injection.

Posology and method of administration

For the treatment of GEP tumours: Initially 50 micrograms once or twice daily by s.c. injection. Depending on response, dosage can be gradually increased to 200 micrograms three times daily. Under exceptional circumstances higher doses may be required. Maintenance doses are variable.

The recommended route of administration is subcutaneous. However, in instances where a rapid response is required, e.g. carcinoid crises, the initial recommended dose of Sandostatin may be administered by the intravenous route, diluted and given as a bolus, whilst monitoring the cardiac rhythm.

In carcinoid tumours, if there is no beneficial effect within a week, continued therapy is not recommended.

For short term treatment of acromegalic patients prior to intervention therapy: 100–200 micrograms three times daily by s.c. injection.

If no relevant reduction of growth hormone levels and no improvement of clinical symptoms have been achieved within three months of starting treatment, therapy should be discontinued.

For the prevention of complications following pancreatic surgery: 0.1 mg three times daily by subcutaneous injection for 7 consecutive days, starting on the day of operation at least one hour before laparotomy.

Use in patients with impaired renal function: Impaired renal function did not affect the total exposure (AUC; area under the curve) to octreotide when administered s.c. therefore, no dose adjustment of Sandostatin is necessary.

Use in patients with impaired hepatic function: In a study with Sandostatin administered s.c. and i.v. it was shown that the elimination capacity may be reduced in patients with liver cirrhosis, but not in patients with fatty liver disease. Due to the wide therapeutic window of octreotide, no dose adjustment of Sandostatin is necessary in patients with liver cirrhosis.

Use in the elderly: In elderly patients treated with Sandostatin, there is no evidence of reduced tolerability or altered dosage requirements.

Use in children: Experience with Sandostatin in children is very limited.

Contra-indications: Hypersensitivity to the drug.

Special warnings and precautions for use: Sudden escape of gastroenteropancreatic endocrine tumours from symptomatic control by Sandostatin may occur infrequently, with rapid recurrence of severe symptoms.

Sandostatin may increase the depth and duration of hypoglycaemia in patients with insulinoma. This is because it is relatively more potent in inhibiting growth hormone and glucagon secretion than in inhibiting insulin and because its duration of insulin inhibition is shorter. If Sandostatin is given to a patient with insulinoma, close observation is necessary on introduction of therapy and at each change of dosage. Marked fluctuations of blood glucose may be reduced by more frequent administration of Sandostatin.

Sandostatin may reduce insulin or oral hypoglycaemic requirements in patients with diabetes mellitus.

Thyroid function should be monitored in patients receiving long-term Sandostatin therapy.

Sandostatin exerts an inhibiting effect on gallbladder motility, bile acid secretion and bile flow and there is an acknowledged association with the development of gallstones. In some studies, an incidence of up to 20% has been reported. Therefore ultrasound examination of the gallbladder is recommended before treatment is initiated and at six to twelve month intervals thereafter. If gallstones do occur, they are usually asymptomatic; symptomatic stones should be treated in the normal manner with due attention to abrupt withdrawal of the drug.

Interactions with other medicaments and other forms of interaction: Sandostatin has been reported to reduce the intestinal absorption of cyclosporin and to delay that of cimetidine.

Pregnancy and lactation: Experience with Sandostatin in pregnant or nursing women is not available. Studies in animals showed transient growth retardation of offspring, possibly consequent upon the specific endocrine profiles of the species tested, but there was no evidence of foetotoxic, teratogenic or other reproduction effects. Nevertheless, Sandostatin should not be given during pregnancy except in compelling circumstances.

Women receiving treatment with Sandostatin should not breast feed their infants.

Effects on ability to drive and use machines: None known.

Undesirable effects: The main side-effects are local and gastrointestinal.

Local reactions include pain, a sensation of stinging, tingling or burning at the site of injection, with redness and swelling. They rarely last more than fifteen minutes. Local discomfort may be reduced by allowing the solution to reach room temperature before injection.

Gastrointestinal side-effects include anorexia, nausea, vomiting, abdominal pain, abdominal bloating, flatulence, loose stools, diarrhoea and steatorrhoea. Although measured faecal fat excretion may increase, there is no evidence to date that long-term treatment with Sandostatin has led to nutritional deficiency due to malabsorption. In rare instances, gastrointestinal side-effects may resemble acute intestinal obstruction with progressive abdominal distention, severe epigastric pain, abdominal tenderness and guarding. Occurrence of gastrointestinal side-effects may be reduced by avoiding meals around the time of Sandostatin administration, that is, by injecting between meals or on retiring to bed.

Because of its inhibitory action on insulin release, Sandostatin may impair postprandial glucose tolerance. In rare instances, with chronic administration, a state of persistent hyperglycaemia may be induced. Hypoglycaemia has also been observed. Rarely, hair loss has been reported in patients receiving Sandostatin treatment.

There have been isolated reports of hepatic dysfunctions associated with Sandostatin administration. These consist of acute hepatitis, without cholestasis, where transaminase values have normalised on withdrawal of Sandostatin, or slow development of hyperbilirubinaemia in association with elevation of alkaline phosphatase, gamma-glutamyl transferase and, to a lesser extent, transaminases.

Formation of gallstones has been reported in patients on long term Sandostatin treatment and there have been isolated cases of biliary colic following the abrupt withdrawal of the drug in acromegalic patients in whom biliary sludge or gallstones had developed.

Overdose: No life-threatening reactions have been reported after acute overdosage. The maximum single dose so far given to an adult has been 1 mg by intravenous bolus injection. The observed signs and symptoms were a brief drop in heart rate, facial flushing, abdominal cramps, diarrhoea, an empty feeling in the stomach and nausea, which resolved within 24 hours of drug administration.

One patient has been reported to have received an accidental overdosage of Sandostatin by continuous infusion (250 micrograms per hour for forty-eight hours instead of 25 micrograms per hour). He experienced no side-effects.

The management of overdosage is symptomatic.

Pharmacological properties
Pharmacodynamic properties: Sandostatin is a synthetic octapeptide analogue of naturally occurring somatostatin with similar pharmacological effects, but with a longer duration of action. It inhibits the secretion of peptides of the gastroenteropancreatic endocrine system and of growth hormone.

In animals, Sandostatin is a more potent inhibitor of growth hormone, glucagon and insulin release than somatostatin with greater selectivity for growth hormone and glucagon suppression.

In normal healthy subjects Sandostatin inhibits the release of growth hormone stimulated by arginine, exercise and insulin-induced hypoglycaemia; postprandial release of insulin, glucagon, gastrin other peptides of the gastroenteropancreatic system; arginine-stimulated release of insulin and glucagon and thyrotropin-releasing hormone-stimulated release of thyroid stimulating hormone.

For patients undergoing pancreatic surgery, the peri and post-operative administration of Sandostatin reduces the incidence of typical post-operative complications (e.g. pancreatic fistula, abscess and subsequent sepsis, post-operative acute pancreatitis).

Pharmacokinetic properties: After subcutaneous injection, Sandostatin is rapidly and completely absorbed. Peak plasma concentrations are reached within 30 minutes. The elimination half-life after subcutaneous administrations is 100 minutes. After intravenous injection the elimination is biphasic with half-lives of 10 and 90 minutes respectively. The volume of distribution is 0.27 L/kg and the total body clearance 160 ml/min. Plasma protein binding amounts to 65%. The amount of Sandostatin bound to blood cells is negligible.

Preclinical safety data: No relevant preclinical safety data are available.

Pharmaceutical particulars
List of excipients: Lactic acid, mannitol, sodium hydrogen carbonate, water for injections. Sandostatin Multidose vials 1 mg/5 ml also contain phenol.

Incompatibilities: None known.

Shelf life: Sandostatin Ampoules 0.05 mg/ml, 0.1 mg/ml and 0.5 mg/ml: 3 years.

Sandostatin Multidose vials 1 mg/5 ml: 3 years unopened. Opened vials may be stored for 2 weeks at room temperature for day to day use.

Special precautions for storage: For prolonged storage Sandostatin Ampoules and Multidose vials should be stored between 2°C and 8°C. For day to day use they may be stored at room temperature for up to two weeks. Protect from light.

Nature and contents of container: Sandostatin Ampoules 0.05 mg/ml, 0.1 mg/ml and 0.5 mg/ml: 1 ml ampoule of uncoloured glass containing clear colourless solution. Boxes of 5 ampoules.

Sandostatin Multidose vials 1 mg/5 ml: 1 ml vial of uncoloured glass containing clear colourless solution. Boxes of 1 vial.

Instruction for use/handling: For i.v. use Sandostatin should be diluted with normal saline to a ratio of not less than 1:1 and not more than 1:9. Dilution of Sandostatin with glucose solution is not recommended.

If Sandostatin has been diluted, the prepared solution may be kept at room temperature but should be administered within 8 hours of preparation.

To reduce local discomfort, let the solution reach room temperature before injection. Avoid multiple injections at short intervals at the same site.

Sandostatin Multidose vials 1 mg/5 ml only: To prevent contamination, it is recommended to puncture the cap of the vial not more than 10 times.

Marketing authorisation holder: Novartis Pharmaceuticals UK Limited, trading as Sandoz Pharmaceuticals, Frimley Business Park, Frimley, Camberley, Surrey GU16 5SG.

Marketing authorisation number

Sandostatin Ampoules 0.05 mg/ml	PL 00101/0212
Sandostatin Ampoules 0.1 mg/ml	PL 00101/0213
Sandostatin Ampoules 0.5 mg/ml	PL 00101/0214
Sandostatin Multidose vials 1 mg/ml	PL 00101/0300

Date of first authorisation/renewal of authorisation
Sandostatin Ampoules 0.05 mg/ml, 0.1 mg/ml and 0.5 mg/ml:

First authorised:	3 April 1989
Renewal of authorisation:	12 August 1994

Sandostatin Multidose vials 1 mg/5 ml:

First authorised:	20 October 1990
Renewal of authorisation:	12 September 1995

Date of (partial) revision of the text 22 December 1998.

Legal category POM.

SANDOSTATIN LAR*

Qualitative and quantitative composition One vial containing: Microspheres for suspension for injection.

Active: Octreotide† free peptide, 10, 20 or 30 mg (present as octreotide acetate) 4.65% of nominal fill weight.

Other: Poly(DL-lactide-co-glycolide) 78.35% of nominal fill weight. Sterlile mannitol 17.0% of nominal fill weight.

Each vial is filled with an overage of microspheres which ensures the correct dosage can be administered.

One injection set containing: 1 plastic 5 ml syringe and 2 needles [40 mm (1.5 inch), 20 gauge].

† INN rec.

Pharmaceutical form Sandostatin LAR is a long-acting depot injection form of octreotide. Microspheres to be suspended in a vehicle immediately prior to i.m. injection.

Clinical particulars
Therapeutic indications: Treatment of patients with acromegaly who are adequately controlled on s.c. treatment with Sandostatin; in whom surgery, radiotherapy or dopamine agonist treatment is inappropriate or ineffective, or in the interim period until radiotherapy becomes fully effective.

GEP tumours: For the relief of symptoms associated with gastroenteropancreatic tumours including:

- Carcinoid tumours with features of carcinoid syndrome
- VIPomas
- Glucagonomas

in patients whose symptoms are adequately controlled on s.c. treatment with Sandostatin. Sandostatin is not antitumour therapy and is not curative in these patients.

Posology and method of administration: Sandostatin LAR may only be administered by deep intragluteal injection. The site of repeat intragluteal injections should be alternated between the left and right gluteal muscle (see *Instructions for use/handling*).

Acromegaly: After adequate control has been established with s.c. Sandostatin, treatment should be started with 20 mg Sandostatin LAR intramuscularly at 4-week intervals for 3 months. Treatment with Sandostatin LAR can be started on the day after the last dose of s.c. Sandostatin. Subsequent dosage adjustment should be based on serum growth hormone (GH) and insulin-like growth factor I (IGF 1)/somatomedin C concentrations and clinical symptoms.

For patients in whom clinical symptoms and biochemical parameters (GH; IGF 1) are not fully controlled (GH concentrations still above 2.5 mcg/L), the dose may be increased to 30 mg every 4 weeks.

For patients whose GH concentrations are consistently below 1 mcg/L, whose IGF 1 serum concentrations have normalised, and in whom most reversible signs/symptoms of acromegaly have disappeared after 3 months of treatment with 20 mg, the dose may be reduced to 10 mg every 4 weeks. However, in this group of patients serum GH and IGF 1 concentrations, and clinical signs/symptoms should be monitored particularly closely.

Gastroenteropancreatic tumours: After adequate control has been established with Sandostatin s.c., treatment should be started with 20 mg Sandostatin LAR intramuscularly at 4-week intervals. Treatment with Sandostatin s.c. should be continued at the previously effective dosage for 2 weeks after the first injection of Sandostatin LAR. Response should be assessed after 3 months of treatment.

For patients in whom symptoms are only partially controlled after 3 months of treatment, the dose may be increased to 30 mg Sandostatin LAR every 4 weeks.

For patients in whom symptoms and biological markers are well controlled after 3 months of treatment, the dose may be reduced to 10 mg Sandostatin LAR every 4 weeks.

For days when symptoms associated with gastroenteropancreatic tumours may increase during treatment with Sandostatin LAR, additional administration of s.c. Sandostatin is recommended at the dose used prior to the Sandostatin LAR treatment.

Use in patients with impaired renal function: Impaired renal function did not affect the total exposure (AUC; area under the curve) to octreotide when administered s.c. as Sandostatin. Therefore, no dose adjustment of Sandostatin LAR is necessary.

Use in patients with impaired hepatic function: In a study with Sandostatin administered s.c. and i.v. it was shown that the elimination capacity may be reduced in patients with liver cirrhosis, but not in patients with fatty liver disease. Due to the wide therapeutic window of octreotide no adjustment of Sandostatin LAR is necessary in patients with liver cirrhosis.

Use in elderly patients: In a study with Sandostatin administered s.c., no dose adjustment was necessary in patients ≥65 years of age. Therefore, no dose adjustment is necessary in this group with Sandostatin LAR.

Use in children: There is very limited experience with use of Sandostatin LAR in children.

Contra-indications: Hypersensitivity to octreotide or any components of the formulation.

Special warnings and precautions for use: As GH-secreting pituitary tumours may sometimes expand, causing serious complications (e.g. visual field defects), it is essential that all patients be carefully monitored. If evidence of tumour expansion appears, alternative procedures are advisable.

Development of gallstones has been reported in 10 to 20% of long-term recipients of s.c. Sandostatin. Long term exposure to Sandostatin LAR of patients with acromegaly or gastroenteropancreatic tumours suggests that treatment with Sandostatin LAR does not increase the incidence of gallstone formation, compared with s.c. treatment. Ultrasonic examination of the gallbladder before and at about 6 monthly intervals during Sandostatin LAR therapy is however recommended. If gallstones do occur, they are usually asymptomatic; symptomatic stones should be treated either by dissolution therapy with bile acids or by surgery.

In patients with concomitant diabetes mellitus, Sandostatin LAR may impair insulin secretion. It is therefore recommended to monitor glucose tolerance and antidiabetic treatment.

In patients with insulinomas, octreotide, because of its greater relative potency in inhibiting the secretion of GH and glucagon than that of insulin, and because of the shorter duration of the inhibitory action on insulin, may increase the depth and prolong the duration of hypoglycaemia. These patients should be closely monitored.

Interactions with other medicaments and other forms of interaction: Ocreotide has been found to reduce the intestinal absorption of cyclosporin and to delay that of cimetidine.

Concomitant administration of octreotide and bromocriptine increases the bioavailability of bromocriptine.

Pregnancy and lactation: Experience with octreotide in pregnant or nursing women is not available and they should therefore be given the drug only under compelling circumstances.

Effects on ability to drive and use machines: No data exist on the effects of Sandostatin LAR on the ability to drive and use machines.

Undesirable effects: Local injection site reactions to Sandostatin LAR may occur, and are usually mild and of short duration. They include local pain and, rarely, swelling and rash.

Gastrointestinal side-effects include anorexia, nausea, vomiting, crampy abdominal pain, abdominal bloating, flatulence, loose stools, diarrhoea and steatorrhoea. Although measured faecal fat excretion may increase, there is no evidence to date that long-term treatment with octreotide has led to nutritional deficiency due to malabsorption. In rare instances, gastrointestinal side-effects may resemble acute intestinal obstruction with progressive abdominal distention, severe epigastric pain, abdominal tenderness and guarding.

Prolonged use of Sandostatin LAR may result in gallstone formation (see *Special warnings and precautions for use*).

Because of its inhibitory action on growth hormone, glucagon and insulin release, Sandostatin LAR may affect glucose regulation. Post-prandial gluclose tolerance may be impaired. As reported for patients treated with s.c. Sandostatin, in some instances a state of persistent hyperglycaemia may be induced as a result of chronic administration. Hypoglycaemia has also been observed. Rarely, transient hair loss has been reported in patients receiving Sandostatin LAR treatment.

In rare instances, acute pancreatitis has been reported within the first hours or days of s.c. Sandostatin treatment. In addition, cholelithiasis-induced pancreatitis has been reported for patients on long-term s.c. Sandostatin treatment.

There have been isolated reports of hepatic dysfunctions associated with s.c. Sandostatin administration. These concern:

- acute hepatitis without cholestasis, where there has been normalisation of transaminase values on withdrawal of s.c. Sandostatin
- the slow development of hyperbilirubinaemia in association with elevation of alkaline phosphatase, γ-glutamyl transferase and, to a lesser extent, transaminases.

Overdose: To date no data are available on overdosage with Sandostatin LAR. However, no unexpected adverse events have been reported with doses up to 90 mg Sandostatin LAR administered to cancer patients every 2 weeks. The signs and symptoms observed after a single dose of 1.0 mg octreotide given as an i.v. bolus injection to an adult patient were a brief drop in heart rate, facial flushing, abdominal cramps, diarrhoea, an empty feeling in the stomach and nausea, all of which resolved within 24 hours of drug administration.

The management of overdosage is symptomatic.

Pharmacological properties

Pharmacodynamic properties: Octreotide is a synthetic octapeptide derivative of naturally occurring somatostatin with similar pharmacological effects, but with a considerably prolonged duration of action. It inhibits pathologically increased secretion of GH and of peptides and serotonin produced within the gastroenteropancreatic (GEP) endocrine system.

In animals, octreotide is a more potent inhibitor of GH, glucagon and insulin release than somatostatin with greater selectivity for GH and glucagon suppression.

In healthy subjects octreotide, like somatostatin, has been shown to inhibit:

- release of GH stimulated by arginine, exercise and insulin-induced hypoglycaemia;
- post-prandial release of insulin, glucagon, gastrin, other peptides of the GEP system; arginine-stimulated release of insulin and glucagon;
- thyrotropin-releasing hormone (TRH)-stimulated release of thyroid-stimulating hormone (TSH).

Unlike somatostatin, octreotide inhibits GH preferentially over insulin and its administration is not followed by rebound hypersecretion of hormones (i.e. GH in patients with acromegaly).

In patients with acromegaly, Sandostatin LAR, a galenical formulation of octreotide suitable for repeated administration at intervals of 4 weeks, delivers consistent and therapeutic octreotide serum concentrations thus consistently lowering GH and normalising IGF 1 serum concentrations in the majority of patients. In most patients, Sandostatin LAR markedly reduces the clinical symptoms of the disease, such as headache, perspiration, paresthesia, fatigue, osteoarthralgia and carpal tunnel syndrome. In individual patients with GH-secreting pituitary adenoma, Sandostatin LAR was reported to lead to shrinkage of the tumour mass.

For patients with functional tumours of the gastroenteropancreatic endocrine system, treatment with Sandostatin LAR provides continuous control of symptoms related to the underlying disease. The effect of octreotide in different types of gastroenteropancreatic tumours are as follows:

Carcinoid tumours: Administration of octreotide may result in improvement of symptoms, particularly of flushing and diarrhoea. In many cases, this is accompanied by a falling plasma serotonin and reduced urinary excretion of 5-hydroxyindole acetic acid.

VIPomas: The biochemical characteristics of these tumours is overproduction of vasoactive intestinal peptide (VIP). In most cases, administration of octreotide results in alleviation of the severe secretory diarrhoea typical of the condition, with consequent improvement in quality of life. This is accompanied by an improvement in associated electrolyte abnormalities, e.g. hypokalaemia, enabling enteral and parenteral fluid and electrolyte supplementation to be withdrawn. Clinical improvement is usually accompanied by a reduction in plasma VIP levels, which may fall into the normal reference range.

Glucagonomas: Administration of octreotide results in most cases in substantial improvement of the necrolytic migratory rash which is characteristic of the condition. The effect of octreotide on the state of mild diabetes mellitus which frequently occurs is not marked and, in general, does not result in a reduction of requirements for insulin or oral hypoglycaemic agents. Octreotide produces improvement of diarrhoea, and hence weight gain, in those patients affected. Although administration of octreotide often leads to an immediate reduction in plasma glucagon levels, this decrease is generally not maintained over a prolonged period of administration, despite continued symptomatic improvement.

Pharmacokinetic properties: After single i.m. injections of Sandostatin LAR, the octreotide concentration reaches a transient initial peak within 1 hour after administration, followed by a progressive decrease to a low undetectable octreotide level within 24 hours. After this peak on day 1, octreotide remains at subtherapeutic levels in the majority of the patients for the following 7 days. Thereafter, octreotide concentrations increase again, reach plateau concentrations at around day 14 and remain relatively constant during the following 3 to 4 weeks. The peak level during day 1 is lower than levels during the plateau phase, and no more than 0.5% of the total drug release occurs during day 1. After about day 42, the octreotide concentration decreases slowly, concomitant with the terminal degradation phase of the polymer matrix of the dosage form.

In patients with acromegaly, mean plateau octreotide concentrations after single doses of 10 mg, 20 mg and 30 mg of Sandostatin LAR amount to 358 ng/L, 926 ng/L and 1710 ng/L, respectively. Steady-state serum octreotide concentrations, reached after 3 injections at 4-week intervals, are higher by a factor of approximately 1.6 to 1.8 and amount to 1557 ng/L, and 2384 ng/L after multiple injections of 20 mg and 30 mg of Sandostatin LAR, respectively.

In patients with carcinoid tumours, the mean (and median) steady-state serum concentrations of octreotide after multiple injections of 10 mg, 20 mg and 30 mg of Sandostatin LAR given at 4-week intervals also increase linearly with dose and were 1231 (894) ng/L, 2620 (2270) ng/L, and 3928 (3010) ng/L respectively.

No accumulation of octreotide beyond that expected from overlapping release profiles occured over a duration of up to 28 monthly injections of Sandostatin LAR.

The pharmacokinetic profile of octreotide after injection of Sandostatin LAR reflects the release profile from the polymer matrix and its biodegradation. Once released into the systemic circulation, octreotide distributes according to its known pharmacokinetic properties, as described for s.c. administration. The volume of distribution of octreotide at steady state is 0.27 L/kg and the total body clearance is 160 ml/min. Plasma protein binding amounts to 65% and essentially no drug is bound to blood cells.

Preclinical safety data

Acute toxicity: Acute toxicity studies of octreotide in mice revealed LD_{50} values of 72 mg/kg by the i.v. route and of 470 mg/kg by the s.c. route. The acute i.v. LD_{50} value of octreotide in rats was determined at 18 mg/kg. Octreotide acetate was well tolerated by dogs receiving up to 1 mg/kg body weight by i.v. bolus injection.

Repeated dose toxicity: In a repeat dose study performed in rats by i.m. injection of 2.5 mg Sandostatin LAR in 50 mg microspheres every 4 weeks for 21 weeks, with necropsy at 26 weeks, no drug-related necropsy findings were observed. The only histopathological findings considered to be of significance were at the injection site in treated and control animals, where the microspheres had provoked a reversible granulomatous myositis. After a single i.m. injection of Sandostatin LAR in rats and rabbits, biodegradation of microspheres was complete by day 75 after injection in both species.

Mutagenicity: Sandostatin administered s.c. and/or its metabolites were devoid of mutagenic potential when investigated *in vitro* in validated bacterial and mammalian cell test systems. Increased frequencies of chromosomal changes were observed in V79 Chinese hamster cells *in vitro*, albeit at high and cytotoxic concentrations only. Chromosomal aberrations were however not increased in human lymphocytes incubated with octreotide acetate *in vitro. In vivo*, no clastogenic activity was observed in the bone marrow of mice treated with octreotide i.v. (micronucleus test) and no evidence of genotoxicity was obtained in male mice using a DNA repair assay of sperm heads. The microspheres were devoid of mutagenic potential when tested in a validated *in vitro* bacterial assay.

Carcinogenicity/chronic toxicity: In studies of rats in which s.c. Sandostatin at daily doses up to 1.25 mg/kg body weight were administered, fibrosarcomas were observed, predominantly in a number of male animals, at the s.c. injection site after 52, 104 and 113/116 weeks. Local tumours occurred also in the control rats, however development of these tumours was attributed to disordered fibroplasia produced by sustained irritant effects at the injection sites, enhanced by the acidic lactic acid/mannitol vehicle. This non-specific tissue reaction appeared to be particular to rats. Neoplastic lesions were observed neither in mice receiving daily s.c. injections of Sandostatin at doses up to 2 mg/kg for 98 weeks, nor in dogs which were treated with daily s.c. doses of the drug for 52 weeks.

The 116-week carcinogenicity study in rats with s.c. Sandostatin also revealed uterine endometrial adenocarcinomas, their incidence reaching statistical significance at the highest s.c. dose level of 1.25 mg/kg per day. The finding was associated with an increased incidence of endometritis, a decreased number of ovarian corpora lutea, a reduction in mammary adenomas and the presence of uterine glandular and luminal dilation, suggesting a state of hormonal imbalance. The available information clearly indicates that the findings of endocrine-mediated tumours in rats are species-specific and are not relevant for the use of the drug in humans.

Reproduction toxicity: Fertility as well as pre-, peri- and post-natal studies in female rats revealed no adverse effects on reproductive performance and development of the offspring, when s.c. doses up to 1 mg/kg body weight per day were administered. Some retardation of the physiological growth noted in pups was transient and attributable to GH inhibition brought about by excessve pharmacodynamic activity.

Pharmaceutical particulars

List of excipients: Vial: Poly (DL-lactide-co-glycolide); mannitol.

Ampoule: Carboxymethylcellulose, sodium; mannitol; water for injection.

Incompatibilities: Sandostatin LAR microspheres for injection is to be used as a single dose container, without any dilution with other products. Therefore, no compatibility data with other products have been generated.

Shelf life: 18 months.

Special precautions for storage: Store at 2°C to 8°C, protect from light. Sandostatin LAR can remain at room temperature on the day of injection. However, the suspension must only be prepared immediately prior to i.m. injection.

Nature and contents of container: The microspheres are packaged in 5 ml glass vials (Type I, PhEur), with a PTFE-faced rubber stopper and sealed with an aluminium flip-off seal.

Instructions for use/handling

Instructions for i.m. injection of Sandostatin LAR for deep intragluteal injection only: Remove the cap from vial containing Sandostatin LAR. Assure that the powder is settled at the botom of the vial by lightly tapping the vial. Open one ampoule containing the vehicle. If the ampoule breaks on opening, discard it and use the reserve ampoule supplied.

For all Sandostatin LAR doses, attach one of the supplied needles to the supplied 5 ml syringe.

Draw the entire contents of one ampoule into the syringe and adjust for 2 ml delivery. Insert needle through centre of rubber stopper of the Sandostatin LAR vial.

Without disturbing the Sandostatin LAR powder, gently inject the vehicle into the vial by running the vehicle down the inside wall of the vial. Withdraw any excess air present in the vial.

Do not disturb the vial until the vehicle has wetted the Sandostatin LAR powder for suspension. Once complete wetting (approximately 2–5 minutes) has occurred, the vial should be moderately swirled until a uniform suspension is achieved. Do not vigorously shake the vial.

Immediately draw 2 ml of air into the syringe and insert the needle through the rubber stopper. Inject the 2 ml of air into the vial and then, with the bevel down and the vial tipped at approximately 45 degree angle, slowly draw the entire contents of the vial containing the suspension into the syringe. Immediately change the needle (supplied). Gently invert the syringe as needed to maintain a uniform suspension. Eliminate air from syringe and disinfect the injection site. Insert needle into right or left gluteus and draw back to ensure that no blood vessel has been penetrated. Immediately inject i.m. by deep intragluteal injection.

Sandostatin LAR must be given only by intragluteal injection, never i.v. If a blood vessel has been penetrated, select another injection site.

Marketing authorisation holder: Novartis Pharmaceuticals UK Limited, trading as Sandoz Pharmaceuticals, Frimley Business Park, Frimley, Camberley, Surrey GU16 5SG.

Marketing authorisation number

Sandostatin LAR 10 mg:	PL 0101/0511
Sandostatin LAR 20 mg:	PL 0101/0512
Sandostatin LAR 30 mg:	PL 0101/0513
Diluent for Sandostatin LAR:	PL 0101/0514

Date of first authorisation/renewal of authorisation 29 April 1998.

Date of (partial) revision of the text 26 June 1998.

SANOMIGRAN* TABLETS 1.5 mg
SANOMIGRAN* TABLETS 0.5 mg
SANOMIGRAN* ELIXIR 0.25 mg/5ml

Qualitative and quantitative composition The active ingredient is: 4-(1-methyl-4-piperidylidene)-9,10-dihydro-4H-benzo-[4,5]cyclohepta [1,2-b] thiophene hydrogen maleate (=pizotifen hydrogen malate).

1.5 mg tablets: Each tablet contains 2.175 mg pizotifen hydrogen malate BP.

0.5 mg tablets: Each tablet contains 0.725 mg pizotifen hydrogen malate BP.

Elixir: The syrup contains 0.365 mg of pizotifen hydrogen malate BP in every 5 mls.

Pharmaceutical form Coated tablets. Syrup.

Clinical particulars

Therapeutic indications: Prophylactic treatment of recurrent vascular headaches, including classical migraine, common migraine and cluster headache (periodic migrainous neuralgia).

Posology and method of administration

Adults: Usually 1.5 mg daily. This may be taken as a single dose at night or in three divided doses. Dosage should be adjusted to individual patient requirements up to a maximum of 4.5 mg daily. Up to 3 mg may be given as a single dose.

Children: 1.5 mg Tablets: Use of 1.5 mg Sanomigran Tablets is not recommended. The appropriate paediatric doses may be given using the 0.5 mg Sanomigran Tablets or Sanomigran Elixir.

0.5 mg Tablets and Elixir: Up to 1.5 mg daily, usually as a divided dose, although up to 1 mg has been given as a single dose at night.

Use in the elderly: Clinical work with Sanomigran has not shown that elderly patients require different dosages from younger patients.

Method of administration: Oral.

Contra-indications: Hypersensitivity to the drug.

Special warnings and precautions: Although the anticholinergic activity of Sanomigran is relatively weak, caution is required in the presence of closed angle glaucoma and in patients with a predisposition to urinary retention. Dosage adjustment may be necessary in patients with kidney insufficiency.

Sanomigran Elixir does not contain sucrose nor tartrazine. The sweetening agent in Sanomigran Elixir is Lycasin 80155 (hydrogenated glucose syrup) at a concentration of 4 mg in 5 ml. Lycasin contains 45% readily absorbable carbohydrate. This should be considered if prescribing the drug for diabetic patients.

Interactions with other medicaments and other forms of interaction: The central effects of sedatives, hypnotics, antihistamines (including certain common cold preparations) and alcohol may be enhanced by Sanomigran.

Pregnancy and lactation: As clinical data with Sanomigran in pregnancy are very limited it should only be administered under compelling circumstances.

Although the concentrations of Sanomigran measured in the milk of treated mothers are not likely to affect the infant, its use in nursing mothers is not recommended.

Effects on ability to drive and use machinery: Patients should be cautioned about the possibility of drowsiness and informed of its significance in the driving of vehicles and the operation of machinery.

Undesirable effects: The most commonly occurring side-effects are drowsiness and an increased appetite which may lead to an increase in body weight. Other side-effects such as dizziness, dry mouth, nausea and constipation have been reported infrequently. Rare instances of depression have occurred. In children CNS stimulation may occur.

Overdose: Symptoms of overdosage may include drowsiness, dizziness, hypotension, dryness of the mouth, confusion, excitatory states (in children), ataxia, nausea, vomiting, dyspnoea, cyanosis, tachycardia, convulsions (particularly in children), coma and respiratory paralysis. Treatment should be directed to the elimination of the drug by gastric lavage and diuresis. Severe hypotension must be corrected (CAVE: adrenaline may produce paradoxical effects). Convulsions may be treated with short-acting barbiturates or benzodiazepines. General surveillance measures are indicated.

Pharmacological properties

Pharmacodynamic properties: Pharmacodynamic studies demonstrate pizotifen to have powerful anti-serotonin and anti-tryptaminic properties, marked anti-histamic effects and some antagonistic activity against kinins. It also possesses weak anti-cholinergic effects and sedative properties.

Pizotifin also possesses appetite-stimulating properties.

The prophylactic effect of Sanomigran in migraine is associated with its ability to modify the humoral mechanisms of headache.

It inhibits the permeability-increasing effect of serotonin and histamine on the affected cranial vessels, thereby checking the transudation of plasmakinin so that the pain threshold of the receptors is maintained at 'normal' levels. In the sequence of events leading to migraine attack, depletion of plasma serotonin contributes to loss of tone in the extracranial vessels. Pizotifen inhibits serotonin re-uptake by the platelets, thus maintaining plasma serotonin and preventing the loss of tone and passive distension of the extracranial arteries.

Pharmacokinetic properties: The absorption of pizotifen is fast (absorption half-life 0.5 to 0.8 hours) and nearly complete (80%). The substance is metabolised with a half-life of about one hour. The main metabolite (n-glucuronide) is eliminated with a half life of approximately 23 hours. Protein binding amounts to 91% and distribution volume to 485 litres. Less than 1% of the administered dose is excreted unchanged in the urine, whereas 55% is excreted as metabolites.

Preclinical safety data: There are no pre-clinical data of relevance to the prescriber which are additional to that already included in other sections of the SPC.

Pharmaceutical particulars

List of excipients: 0.5 mg Tablets and 1.5 mg Tablets: The tablets contain lactose, maize starch, polyvinylpyrrolidone, magnesium stearate, talc (acid washed). The coating constituents are sugar (granulated no. 2), talc, gum acacia, titanium dioxide, iron oxide yellow, carnauba wax, printing wax, colloidal anhydrous silica and purified water.

Syrup: The syrup contains raspberry flavour 50969, maraschino flavour, methyl hydroxybenzoate, propyl hydroxybenzoate, citric acid (anhydrous), disodium phosphate (anhydrous), Lycasin 80/55, ethyl alcohol and purified water.

Incompatibilities: None.

Shelf life: 0.5 mg Tablets, 1.5 mg Tablets and Syrup: 60 months.

Special precautions for storage: 0.5 mg Tablets and 1.5 mg Tablets: Protect from direct light. Syrup: None.

Nature and contents of container: 0.5 mg Tablets: The tablets are ivory, circular biconvex opaque printed SMG on one side and come in PVD/PVdC opaque blister packs containing 60 tablets.

1.5 mg Tablets: The tablets are ivory, circular, biconvex printed SMG 1.5 on one side and come in PVDC opaque blister packs containing 28 tablets.

Syrup: The syrup is clear, colourless liquid, with a fruity odour and taste and comes in amber glass bottles with a polypropylene closure (polythene wad faced with PP, PVDC or PET lining) in a 300 ml pack size.

Instructions for use/handling: None.

Marketing authorisation holder: Novartis Pharmaceuticals UK Limited, trading as Sandoz Pharmaceuticals, Frimley Business Park, Frimley, Camberley, Surrey GU16 5SG.

Marketing authorisation number

0.5 mg tablets:	PL 00101/0036
1.5 mg tablets:	PL 00101/0129
Elixir:	PL 00101/0163

Date of first authorisation/renewal of authorisation

0.5 mg tablets:	15/03/74
1.5 mg tablets:	28/04/81
Syrup:	06/06/83

Date of (partial) revision of the text

0.5 mg tablets:	May 1998
1.5 mg tablets:	September 1997
Elixir:	May 1998.

SCOPODERM TTS

Qualitative and quantitative composition Each patch contains 1.5 mg hyoscine USP.

Pharmaceutical form Scopoderm TTS is a transdermal therapeutic system. Each patch is a flat system of laminates, sealed around the edge, containing a clear oily filling. The system is a thin circular disc, tan coloured and fitted with a transparent, hexagonal protective liner which projects over the edge of the disc. Viewed through the liner, the system appears silver in colour. Each system has a contact surface area measuring 2.5 cm^2 and hyoscine content of 1.5 mg. The average amount of hyoscine absorbed from each system in 72 hours is 1 mg.

Clinical particulars

Therapeutic indications: For the prevention of symptoms of motion sickness such as nausea, vomiting and vertigo.

Posology and method of administration

Route of administration: Transdermal.

Dosage and administration: Adults: To achieve the optimum protective effect, one system should be applied about 5-6 hours before embarking on a journey (or on the evening before). The system should be placed onto a clean, dry, hairless area of skin behind the ear, taking care to avoid any cuts or irritation. One system can provide protection for up to 72 hours. Should protection be required for longer periods of time, a fresh system should be placed behind the other ear after 72 hours. (No more than one system should be used at a time). Conversely, if protection is only required for shorter periods of time, the system should be removed at the end of the journey.

Patients should wash their hands thoroughly after handling the system. In addition, after removal of the system, the site of application should also be washed. These precautions are necessary to minimise any chance of hyoscine accidentally being transferred to the eyes (see *Undesirable effects*).

Limited contact with water (i.e. during bathing or swimming), should not affect the system, although it should be kept as dry as possible.

If the Scopoderm TTS becomes accidentally detached, it should be replaced by a fresh system.

Use in elderly: Scopoderm TTS may be used in the elderly (see dosage recommendations for adults) although the elderly may be more prone to suffer from the side-effects of hyoscine (see *Special warnings and precautions for use*).

Use in children: Scopoderm TTS can be used in children aged 10 years or over (see dosage recommendations for adults). Insufficient data are available to recommend the use of Scopoderm TTS for younger children.

Contra-indications: Scopoderm TTS is contra-indicated in patients with glaucoma or with a history of the condition, and in patients with known hypersensitivity to hyoscine.

Special warnings and precautions for use: Scopoderm TTS should be used with caution in patients with pyloric stenosis, those who have bladder outflow obstruction, or in patients with intestinal obstruction.

Patients should not consume alcohol whilst using Scopoderm TTS.

Scopoderm TTS should also be used with caution in elderly patients, and in patients with impaired hepatic or renal function.

In rare cases, confusional states and visual hallucinations may occur. In such cases, Scopoderm TTS should be removed immediately. If severe symptoms persist, appropriate therapeutic measures should be taken (see *Overdose*).

Idiosyncratic reactions may occur with ordinary therapeutic doses of hyoscine.

In isolated cases an increase in seizure frequency in epileptic patients has been reported.

Care should be taken after removal of the system as side-effects may persist for up to 24 hours or longer.

Interactions with other medicaments and other forms of interaction: Scopoderm TTS should be used with caution in patients being treated with drugs that act on the central nervous system (including acohol) or drugs with anticholinergic properties.

Pregnancy and lactation: Teratogenic studies have been performed in pregnant rats and rabbits with hyoscine administered by daily intravenous injection. No adverse effects were noted in rats. In rabbits, the drug had a marginal embryotoxic effect at a high dose (at drug plasma levels approximately 100 times those observed in humans using Scopoderm TTS).

Scopoderm TTS should only be used during pregnancy if the expected benefits to the mother outweigh the potential risks to the foetus.

It is not known if hyoscine passes into the breast milk. Therefore, nursing mothers should refrain from breast feeding their infants whilst using Scopoderm TTS.

Effects on ability to drive and use machines: Scopoderm TTS may cause drowsiness, dizziness, confusion or visual disturbance in certain individuals. Patients using the system must not drive, operate machinery, pilot an aircraft, dive or engage in any other activities in which such symptoms could be dangerous (see *Undesirable effects*).

Undesirable effects: The following side-effects may occur:

Eyes: In isolated cases papillary dilatation may precipitate acute glaucoma, particularly narrow angle glaucoma (see *Contra-indications*). Occasional: irritation of the eyelids. If traces of hyoscine on the hands enter the eyes, transient cycloplegia and pupillary dilatation (occasionally unilateral) frequently occur.

Mouth: Frequent: transient dryness of the mouth.

Central nervous system: Occasional: drowsiness. Rare: impairment of memory and concentration, restlessness, dizziness, disorientation, confusion and visual hallucinations (see *Special warnings and precautions for use*).

Skin: Occasional: local irritation. In isolated cases: a generalised skin rash.

Urogenital system: Rare: disturbances of micturition (i.e. urine retention).

Side-effects after removal of Scopoderm TTS: Rare: unwanted effects, including headache, nausea, vomiting and disturbance of balance, occurring after removal of the system. These symptoms have occurred most often in patients who have used the system for several days. In such cases, patients should not drive or engage in other activities requiring concentration (see *Special warnings and precautions for use*).

Overdose:

Symptoms: Initially, restlessness, excitation and confusion may be observed. In response to higher doses, delirium, hallucinations and convulsions set in. At very high doses, coma and respiratory paralysis may occur.

Treatment: If symptoms of overdosage occur, the system(s) should be removed immediately. Physostigmine is the most effective antidote. Depending on the severity of poisoning, physostigmine should be given by slow intravenous injection in doses of 1–4 mg (0.5 mg in children). Repeated injections may be necessary since physostigmine is rapidly metabolised. Diazepam may be used to counter excitation and convulsions although at higher doses it may cause respiratory depression. In severe cases, artificial respiration may be necessary. If hyperthermia occurs, immediate action should be taken to dissipate heat.

Pharmacological properties

Pharmacodynamic properties: The transdermal therapeutic system (TTS) is a novel form of drug delivery designed to achieve a continuous release of hyoscine through the intact skin to the systemic circulation for up to 72 hours.

Hyoscine has anticholinergic properties. It acts as a competitive antagonist to acetylcholine and other parasympathomimetic agents. Its mechanism of action in the central nervous system in preventing motion sickness has yet to be elucidated. Hyoscine produces classical symptoms of parasympathetic blockade.

Pharmacokinetic properties: Following Scopoderm TTS administration, measurement of the urinary excretion has shown the equilibrium between absorption and elimination to be reached within about 6 hours. Steady plasma concentrations of hyoscine in the range of 0.17–0.33 nmol/litre are produced. Provided the system is not removed, this equilibrium is maintained and plasma hyoscine levels are within this therapeutic range for up to 72 hours.

After removal of Scopoderm TTS, the plasma concentration diminishes slowly to approximately one third over the following 24 hours because hyoscine in the skin continues to enter the blood stream.

Preclinical safety data: None stated.

Pharmaceutical particulars

List of excipients

Drug reservoir: Light mineral oil, polyisobutylene (1.200.000), polyisobutylene (35.000).

Backing film: Pigmented MDPE/AL/PET/HS film (vapour coated aluminised polyester with outer coating of pigmented medium density polyethylene (MDPE) and a heat sealable inner coating. Thickness 0.0686 mm.

Release controlling membrane: Polypropylene film. Thickness 0.0254 mm.

Adhesive (to skin): Light mineral oil, polyisobutylene (1.200.000), polyisobutylene (35.000).

Release liner (discarded before use): Silicone/polyester film. Thickness 0.0762 mm.

Incompatibilities: None stated.

Shelf life: 24 months.

Special precautions for storage: Store below 25°C. Do not freeze.

Nature and contents of container: Scopoderm TTS – Individually packed into sealed paper laminated aluminium foil pouches. Outer cardboard carton containing two patches.

Instructions for use/handling: Patients should wash their hands thoroughly after handling the system. In addition, after removal of the system, the site of application should also be washed. These precautions are necessary to minimise any chance of hyoscine accidentally being transferred to the eyes (see *Undesirable effects*).

Marketing authorisation holder: Novartis Pharmaceuticals UK Limited, trading as Ciba Laboratories, Frimley Business Park, Frimley, Camberley, Surrey GU16 5SG.

Marketing authorisation number PL 00101/0541.

Date of first authorisation/renewal of authorisation 17 November 1997.

Date of (partial) revision of the text 21 October 1998.

SLOW-FE*

Presentation A circular, biconvex, greenish-white tablet, impressed with the letters CG 503 on one side and plain on the other side. The tablets have a thin, transparent film coat and contain 160 mg of dried ferrous sulphate in a special slow-release wax core (equivalent to approx. 50 mg elemental iron). The tablets also contain lactose.

Uses

Indication: As a haematinic for the treatment of, or for the prophylaxis of iron deficiency anaemia, including that associated with post-gastrectomy and other malabsorption syndromes.

Mode of action: Slow-Fe (Ferrous Sulphate in a slow release preparation) provides a source of iron which is an essential constituent of the body. It is necessary for haemoglobin formation and for the oxidative processes of living tissues. Insufficient iron in the body results in iron deficiency anaemia which may be treatable with an iron supplement such as Slow-Fe.

Pharmacokinetics: Iron is a dietary requirement, about 5%–10% of the iron ingested with food is absorbed. Absorption is increased in conditions of deficiency and decreased when body stores are overloaded. Apart from haemorrhage iron is lost from the body in: urine, hair, nails, skin and sweat. In healthy men and non-menstruating women absorption of 1 mg/day is required, in menstruating women this rises to 2 mg/day and in pregnancy/lactation 3 mg/day is required.

In therapy haemoglobin levels return to normal after about 10 weeks. Three to six months are required to replenish body stores.

There is no significant difference between the absorption of iron from ferrous sulphate tablets and from Slow-Fe in healthy persons, in anaemia, following gastrectomy, or in coeliac disease.

Dosage and administration

Adults: For prophylaxis, one tablet daily. For the treatment of iron deficiency anaemia, two tablets daily.

Children: For treatment, one tablet daily for children over the age of six years.

The tablets should be swallowed whole with fluid and may be taken at any time of the day.

Contra-indications, warnings, etc

Contra-indications: Known hypersensitivity to ferrous sulphate.

Iron therapy is contra-indicated in the presence of haemochromatosis, haemosiderosis and haemolytic anaemia.

Precautions: As with all iron preparations, Slow-Fe should be used with care in patients with known or suspected gastro-intestinal strictures or diverticulae.

Pregnancy and lactation: Slow-Fe can be used in the iron deficiency anaemia of pregnancy, with or without additional folic acid as appropriate.

Drug interactions: Concurrent administration of antacids may reduce absorption of iron preparations. Iron chelates with tetracyclines and absorption of both agents may be impaired. Iron may reduce the absorption of penicillamine and zinc salts.

Side-effects: As with all iron containing preparations gastro-intestinal side effects such as abdominal discomfort, nausea, vomiting, constipation, diarrhoea and dark stools may occur.

Overdosage:

Symptoms: Include abdominal pain, nausea and vomiting, diarrhoea and haematemesis.

Treatment: Gastric lavage or emesis should be carried out immediately. To chelate excess free iron in the gastro-intestinal tract, 5 g desferrioxamine dissolved in 50 ml water should be introduced into the stomach. To chelate excess free iron in the blood, desferrioxamine may be given parenterally; depending on the patients condition, 1 g desferrioxamine given every three hours intramuscularly may be appropriate.

Pharmaceutical precautions Tablets should be protected from moisture.

Legal category P

Package quantities The tablets are available form-packed in quantities of 28.

Further information The precision release principle of Slow-Fe ensures that the iron is released evenly over a period of 1 to 2 hours. Complete release therefore normally occurs before the tablet has left the duodenum or upper jejunum, and maximum iron absorption can take place.

The incidence of side-effects would appear to be lower than with plain ferrous sulphate.

Product licence holder: Novartis Pharmaceuticals UK Limited, trading as Ciba Laboratories.

Product licence number 00101/0509

Date of last revision September 1997.

SLOW-FE* FOLIC

Presentation A circular biconvex yellowish-white tablet impressed with the monogram CIBA on one side and the letters TP on the other. The tablets have a thin transparent film-coat and contain 160 mg dried ferrous sulphate U.S.P (equivalent to 50 mg elemental iron) in a special slow-release core and 0.4 mg Folic Acid BP. The tablets also contain lactose.

Uses

Indications: Slow-Fe Folic is indicated throughout pregnancy for prophylaxis of iron and folic acid deficiency. Slow-Fe Folic is designed to minimise the problems of gastro-intestinal disturbance associated with most oral iron preparations, and contains 0.4 mg of folic acid, a daily supplement which prevents the occurrence of megaloblastic anaemia due to folate deficiency.

Mode of action: Slow-Fe Folic incorporates iron (as ferrous sulphate) and folic acid in a slow release preparation. Both are essential constituents of the body. Iron is necessary for haemoglobin formation and for the oxidative processes of the tissues. Folic acid undergoes reduction in the body to tetrahydrofolate which is a co-enzyme for various metabolic processes including DNA synthesis. Deficiency of iron causes microcytic hypochromic anaemia; deficiency of folic acid leads to megaloblastic anaemia. Epidemiological work has shown that folic acid deficiency in pregnancy is associated with an increased risk of neural tube defect. A supplement of folic acid given from the time of conception to the 12th week of pregnancy may reduce this risk. In the absence of supplementation of dietary iron and folic acid during pregnancy anaemia is likely to occur. Slow-Fe Folic can be used for prophylaxis of anaemia of pregnancy.

Pharmacokinetics: Both iron and folic acid are obtained in the diet. Iron absorption is increased in conditions of deficiency and decreased when body stores are overloaded. In healthy men and non-menstruating women absorption of 1 mg/day is required. This rises to >3 mg/day in pregnancy. Folic acid is absorbed mainly from the proximal small intestine and circulates bound to plasma proteins. 4-5μg is excreted daily in urine. A high proportion is stored in the liver; folic acid undergoes enterohepatic circulation.

A combination of iron and folic acid acts more effectively against the anaemia of pregnancy than either substance alone.

Dosage and administration

Adults: The product is intended for oral administration, one tablet to be taken daily throughout pregnancy. In the case of a multiple pregnancy the dosage should be increased to two tablets daily. The tablets should be swallowed whole and for preference taken after food.

Use in children: Not indicated.

Use in the elderly: Not indicated.

Contra-indications, warnings, etc

Contra-indications: Iron therapy is contra-indicated in the presence of haemochromatosis, haemosiderosis and haemolytic anaemia. Hypersensitivity to the active ingredient.

Precautions: In epileptic patients who have become folate deficient (for instance during phenytoin treatment) folic acid supplementation can result in decreased anticonvulsant serum concentrations, which (unless the anticonvulsant dosage is adjusted) can lead to loss of seizure control.

Use in pregnancy and lactation: Slow-Fe Folic is indicated throughout pregnancy for prophylaxis of iron and folic acid deficiency.

Drug interactions: Concurrent administration of antacids may reduce absorption of iron preparations. Iron chelates with tetracyclines and absorption of both agents may be impaired. Iron may reduce the absorption of penicillamine and zinc salts.

Side-effects: Slow-Fe Folic is particularly well tolerated although gastro-intestinal side effects such as nausea, vomiting, constipation or diarrhoea may occur infrequently. On very rare occasions, skin rashes have been reported.

Overdosage:

Symptoms: Symptoms include abdominal pain, nausea and vomiting, diarrhoea and haematemesis.

Treatment: Gastric lavage or emesis should be carried out immediately. To chelate excess free iron in the gastro-intestinal tract, 5 g desferrioxamine dissolved in 50 ml water should be introduced into the stomach. To chelate excess free iron in the blood, desferrioxamine may be given parenterally; depending on the patient's condition, 1 g desferrioxamine given every 3 hours intramuscularly may be appropriate.

Pharmaceutical precautions Tablets should be protected from moisture.

Legal category Slow-Fe Folic is not subject to poisons regulations but it is recommended for use only under medical supervision.

Package quantities Slow-Fe Folic tablets are available form-packed in quantities of 28.

Further information The precision-release principle of Slow-Fe Folic ensures that the iron is released evenly over a period of 1½ to 2 hours. Complete release therefore occurs before the tablet has left the duodenum or upper jejunum, and maximum iron absorption can take place. This avoids wastage, and associated side effects, whilst producing an effective haematinic response from a relatively low dose of iron.

The incidence of side effects is comparable with placebo levels and considerably lower than with plain ferrous sulphate.

Product licence holder: Novartis Pharmaceuticals UK Limited, trading as Ciba Laboratories.

Product licence number 00101/0510

Date of last revision December 1997.

SLOW-TRASICOR*

Presentation Slow-Trasicor tablets each containing 160 mg oxprenolol hydrochloride PhEur in a special sustained release formulation. Circular, slightly biconvex, white film-coated tablets, having the monogram CIBA impressed on one side and Slow-Trasicor on the other.

The tablets also contain lactose, silicon dioxide, calcium stearate, methacrylic acid copolymer, glyceryl palmitostearate, hydroxypropylmethylcellulose, magnesium stearate, polysorbate, talc and titanium dioxide.

Uses

Indications: Hypertension: As monotherapy or for use in combination with other antihypertensives, e.g. with a diuretic, peripheral vasodilator, calcium channel blocker or ACE inhibitor.

Angina pectoris: For long-term prophylactic use (if necessary nitrates should be employed for alleviating acute attacks).

Mode of action: Oxprenolol, the active substance of Trasicor, is a non-selective, lipophilic beta-blocker exerting a sympatholytic effect and displaying mild to modest partial agonistic activity (PAA), also known as intrinsic sympathomimetic activity (ISA).

Drugs like oxprenolol with PAA cause comparatively less slowing of the resting heart rate and a less marked negative-inotropic effect than those without PAA. The risk of substantial bradycardia at rest and heart failure is lessened.

The antiarrhythmic effect of oxprenolol is primarily due to suppression of the arrhythmogenic sympathetic influence of catecholamines. Evidence that increased sympathetic stimulation predisposes to many arrhythmias is strong. This is supported by the increased incidence of arrhythmias in man in situations associated with high sympathetic drive or myocardial sensitisation to catecholamines e.g. exercise, emotional stress, phaeochromocytoma, trauma, myocardial ischaemia, anaesthesia, hyperthyroidism.

Oxprenolol decreases cardiac impulse formation in the sinus node with resultant slowing of the sinus rate; it slightly prolongs the sino-atrial conduction time; both the atrio-ventricular (AV) conduction time and the AV node refractory periods are lengthened.

Some β-blockers such as oxprenolol possess a membrane stabilising activity (MSA) on the cardiac action potential, also known as 'quinidine-like' or 'local anaesthetic' action, a property that tends to result in greater cardiac depression than is seen with β-blockers which do not have this pharmacological characteristic. However, at normal therapeutic doses, this property is probably clinically irrelevant and it only becomes manifest after overdose.

In coronary artery disease, oxprenolol is beneficial in increasing exercise tolerance and decreasing the frequency and severity of anginal attacks.

Emotional stress and anxiety states the symptoms of which are largely caused by increased sympathetic drive are alleviated by the sympatholytic effect of oxprenolol.

The exact way in which β-blockers exert their antihypertensive action is still not fully understood. Various modes of action have been postulated. During chronic therapy the antihypertensive effect of β-blockers is associated with a decline in peripheral resistance.

Oxprenolol is effective in lowering elevated supine, standing and exercise blood pressure; postural hypotension is unlikely to occur.

Pharmacokinetics:

Absorption: Oxprenolol is rapidly and completely absorbed from the sustained release tablets, regardless of whether or not they are taken together with food. Peak plasma concentrations are attained after an average of approximately 3 hours.

During treatment with the sustained release forms, prolongation of the absorption phase enables therapeutically active plasma concentrations to be maintained over a longer period than when the same doses are given in conventional dosage forms and avoids high peak drug concentrations in the plasma.

Biotransformation: Oxprenolol is subject to first-pass metabolism. Its systemic bioavailability is 20–70%.

Distribution: Oxprenolol has a plasma-protein binding rate of approx. 80% and a calculated distribution volume of 1.2 L/kg.

Oxprenolol crosses the placental barrier. The concentration in the breast milk is equivalent to approx. 30% of that in the plasma.

Elimination: Oxprenolol has an elimination half-life of 1–2 hours. Oxprenolol is extensively metabolised, direct O-glucuronidation being the major metabolic pathway and oxidative reactions minor ones. Oxprenolol is excreted chiefly in the urine (almost exclusively in the form of inactive metabolites). The drug is not likely to accumulate.

Characteristics in patients: Age has no effect on the pharmacokinetics of oxprenolol.

In patients with acute or chronic inflammatory diseases an increase in the plasma levels of oxprenolol has been observed. The plasma levels may also increase in the presence of severe hepatic insufficiency associated with a reduced metabolism.

Impaired renal function generally leads to an increase in the blood levels of oxprenolol, but the concentrations measured remain within – although at the upper limit of – the concentration range recorded in subjects with healthy kidneys. In addition, in patients with renal failure the apparent elimination half-life for unchanged, i.e. active, oxprenolol is comparable with the corresponding half-life values determined in subjects with no renal disease. Hence, there is no need to readjust the dosage in the presence of impaired renal function.

Dosage and administration The dosage should be individualised. Before raising the dosage, the heart rate at rest should always be checked. If it is 50–55 beats/min, the dosage should not be increased, see *Contra-indications*. The tablets should be swallowed with liquid.

If the maximum recommended dose is insufficient to produce the desired response, appropriate combined therapy should be considered.

When discontinuing prolonged treatment with a beta-blocker, the medication should not be interrupted abruptly, but withdrawn gradually.

The sustained-release formulation provides a longer pharmacological action from a given dose, thus allowing once daily administration. When the dose is raised to more than one Trasicor sustained-release tablet, it is usual for this to continue to be given once daily.

The sustained-release tablets should be swallowed whole with liquid. Oxprenolol is only gradually released from the sustained-release tablet, extending the duration of effect. The occurrence of high peak concentrations in the plasma is thus avoided.

Elderly: No special dosage regime is necessary but concurrent hepatic insufficiency should be taken into account.

Children: No adequate experience has been acquired on the use of Slow-Trasicor in children.

Adults:

Hypertension: 160 mg once daily. If necessary, the dosage can be raised to 320 mg.

Angina pectoris: 160 mg once daily. If necessary, the dosage can be raised to 320 mg.

Contra-indications, warnings, etc

Contra-indications: Slow-Trasicor is contra-indicated in patients with:

Hypersensitivity to oxprenolol and related derivatives, cross-sensitivity to other β-blockers or to any of the excipients
Cardiogenic shock
Second or third degree atrioventricular block

Uncontrolled heart failure
Sick-sinus syndrome
Bradycardia (<45–50 bpm)
Hypotension
Untreated phaeochromocytoma
Severe peripheral arterial circulatory disturbances
History of bronchospasms and broncial asthma
Prinzmetal's angina (variant angina pectoris)
Use of anaesthetics which are known to have a negative inotropic effect
Metabolic acidosis

Warnings: Patients receiving oxprenolol should be warned that dizziness, fatigue or visual disturbances (see *Side-effects*) may occur, in which case they should not drive, operate machinery or do anything else requiring alertness, particularly if they also consume alcohol.

Precautions: Owing to the risk of bronchoconstriction, non-selective beta-blockers such as Slow-Trasicor should be used with particular caution in patients with chronic obstructive lung disease (see *Contra-indications*).

As β-blockers increase the AV conduction time, beta-blockers should only be given with caution to patients with first degree AV block.

Beta-blockers should not be used in patients with untreated congestive heart failure. This condition should first be stabilised.

If the patient develops increasing bradycardia less than 50–55 beats per minute at rest and the patient experiences symptoms related to bradycardia, the dosage should be reduced or gradually withdrawn (see *Contra-indications*).

β-blockers are liable to affect carbohydrate metabolism. Diabetic patients, especially those dependent on insulin, should be warned that β-blockers can mask the symptoms of hypoglycaemia (e.g. tachycardia) (see *Drug interactions*). Hypoglycaemia, producing loss of consciousness in some cases, may occur in non-diabetic individuals who are taking β-blockers, particularly those who undergo prolonged fasting or severe exercise. The concurrent use of β-blockers and anti-diabetic medication should always be monitored to confirm that diabetic control is well maintained.

β-blockers may mask certain clinical signs (e.g. tachycardia) of hyperthyroidism and the patients should be carefully monitored.

Beta-blockers may reduce liver function and thus affect the metabolism of other drugs. Like many beta-blockers oxprenolol undergoes substantial first-pass hepatic metabolism. In the presence of liver cirrhosis the bioavailability of oxprenolol may be increased leading to higher plasma concentrations (see *Pharmacokinetics*). Patients with severe renal failure might be more susceptible to the effects of antihypertensive drugs due to haemodynamic effects. Careful monitoring is advisable (see *Pharmacokinetics*).

In patients with peripheral circulatory disorders (e.g. Raynaud's disease or syndrome, intermittent claudication), beta-blockers should be used with great caution as aggravation of these disorders may occur (see *Contra-indications*).

In patients with phaeochromocytoma a β-blocker should only be given together with an α-blocker (see *Contra-indications*).

Owing to the danger of cardiac arrest, a calcium antagonist of the verapamil type must not be administered intravenously to a patient already receiving treatment with a β-blocker. Furthermore, since β-blockers may potentiate the negative-inotropic and dromotropic effects of calcium antagonists, like verapamil or diltiazem, any oral comedication (e.g. in angina pectoris) requires close clinical control (see also *Drug interactions*).

Anaphylactic reactions precipitated by other agents may be particularly severe in patients taking beta-blockers, especially non-selective drugs, and may require higher than normal doses of adrenaline for treatment. Whenever possible, β-blockers should be discontinued in patients who are at increased risk for anaphylaxis.

Especially in patients with ischaemic heart disease, treatment should not be discontinued suddenly. The dosage should gradually be reduced, i.e. over 1–3 weeks, if necessary, at the same time initiating alternative therapy, to prevent exacerbation of angina pectoris.

If a patient receiving oxprenolol requires anaesthesia, the anaesthetist should be informed of the use of the medication prior to the use of general anaesthetic to permit him to take the necessary precautions. The anaesthetic selected should be one exhibiting as little inotropic activity as possible, e.g. halothane/nitrous oxide. If, on the other hand, inhibition of sympathetic tone during the operation is regarded as undesirable, the β-blocker should be withdrawn gradually at least 48 hours prior to surgery.

The full development of the 'oculomucocutaneous syndrome', as previously described with practolol has not been reported with oxprenolol. However, some features of this syndrome have been noted such as dry eyes alone or occasionally associated with skin rash. In most cases the symptoms cleared after withdrawal of the treatment. Discontinuation of oxprenolol should be considered, and a switch to another antihypertensive drug might be advisable, see advice on discontinuation above.

Use in pregnancy and lactation: As in the case of any form of drug therapy, oxprenolol should be employed with caution during pregnancy, especially in the first 3 months.

β-blockers may reduce placental perfusion, which may result in intrauterine foetal death, immature and premature deliveries. Use the lowest possible dose. If possible, discontinue beta-blocker therapy at least 2 to 3 days prior to delivery to avoid the effects on uterine contractility and possible adverse effects, especially bradycardia and hypoglycaemia, in the foetus and neonate.

Oxprenolol is excreted into breast milk (see *Pharmacokinetic properties*) and although the estimated daily infant dose derived from breast-feeding is likely to be very low, breast feeding is not recommended.

Drug interactions:

Calcium channel blockers: e.g. verapamil, dilitiazem: potentiation of bradycardia, myocardial depression and hypotension; particularly after intravenous administration of verapamil in patients taking oral β-blockers, the possibility of hypotension and cardiac arrhythmia cannot be excluded (see *Warnings* and *Precautions*).

Class I anti-arrhythmic drugs and amiodarone: Drugs like disopyramide, quinidine and amiodarone may increase atrial-conduction time and induce negative inotropic effect when administered concomitantly with beta-blockers.

Sympathomimetic drugs: Non-cardioselective beta-blockers such as oxprenolol enhance the pressor response to sympathomimetic drugs such as adrenaline, noradrenaline, isoprenaline, ephedrine and phenylephrine (e.g. local anaesthetics in dentistry, nasal and ocular drops), resulting in hypertension and bradycardia.

Clonidine: When clonidine is used in conjunction with non-selective beta-blockers, such as oxprenolol, treatment with clonidine should be continued for some time after β-blocker has been discontinued to reduce the danger of rebound hypertension.

Catecholamine-deleting drugs: e.g. guanethidine, reserpine, may have an additive effect when administered concomitantly with beta-blockers. Patients should be closely observed for hypotension.

Beta-blockers may modify blood glucose concentrations in patients being treated with insulin and oral antidiabetic drugs and may alter the response to hypoglycaemia by prolonging the recovery (blood glucose rise) from hypoglycaemia, causing hypotension and blocking tachycardia. In diabetic patients receiving β-blockers hypoglycaemic episodes may not result in the expected tachycardia but hypoglycaemia-induced sweating will occur and may even be intensified and prolonged (see *Warnings* and *Precautions*).

Non-steroidal anti-inflammatory drugs (NSAIDs): Non-steroidal anti-inflammatory drugs (NSAIDs) can reduce the hypotensive effect of beta-blockade.

Cimetidine: Hepatic metabolism of beta-blockers may be reduced, resulting in increased plasma levels of β-blocker and prolonged serum half-life. Marked bradycardia may occur.

Ergot alkaloids: Concomitant administration with beta-blockers may enhance the vasoconstrictive action of ergot alkaloids.

Anaesthetic drugs: β-blockers and certain anaesthetics (e.g. halothane) are additive in their cardiodepressant effect. However, continuation of beta-blockers reduces the risk of arrhythmia during anaesthesia (see *Warnings* and *Precautions*).

Digitalis glycosides: Beta-blockers and digitalis glycosides may be additive in their depressant effect on myocardial conduction, particularly through the atrioventricular node, resulting in bradycardia or heart block.

Lidocaine: Concomitant administration with beta-blockers may increase lidocaine blood concentrations and potential toxicity; patients should be closely monitored for increased lidocaine effects.

Alcohol and beta-blocker effects on the central nervous system have been observed to be additive and it is possible that symptoms such as dizziness may be exaggerated if alcohol and Trasicor are taken together (see also *Warnings*).

Side-effects: Frequency estimate: *very common* >10%, *common* >1%–<10%, *uncommon* >0.1%–<1%, *rare* >0.01%–<0.1%, *very rare* <0.01%.

Central nervous system: Common: fatigue, dizziness, headache, mental depression. *Uncommon:* sleep disturbances, nightmares. Rare: hallucinations, exertional tiredness.

Cardiovascular system: Common: hypotension, heart failure, peripheral vascular disorders (e.g. cold extremities, paraesthesia). *Uncommon:* bradycardia, disturbance of cardiac conduction. *Rare:* Raynaud-like symptoms.

Gastro-intestinal tract: Very common: dry mouth, constipation. *Common:* nausea. *Uncommon:* diarrhoea, vomiting, flatulence..

Skin and appendages: Uncommon: Allergic skin rash (e.g. urticarial, psoriasiform, eczematous, lichenoid). *Rare:* worsening of psoriasis.

Respiratory system: Common: dyspnoea, bronchoconstriction (see *Precautions* and *Contra-indications*).

Sense organs: Uncommon: visual disturbances ('blurred vision', 'vision abnormal'). *Rare:* dry eyes, keratoconjunctivitis.

Others: disturbances of libido and potency. Very rare: thrombocytopenia.

Overdosage:

Signs and symptoms: Poisoning due to an overdosage of β-blocker may lead to pronounced hypotension, bradycardia, hypoglycaemia, heart failure, cardiogenic shock, conduction abnormalities (first or second degree block, complete heart block, asystole), or even cardiac arrest. In addition, dyspnoea, bronchospasm, vomiting, impairment of consciousness, and also generalised convulsions may occur.

The manifestations of poisoning with beta-blockers are dependent on the pharmacological properties of the ingested drug. Although the onset of action is rapid, effects of massive overdose may persist for several days despite declining plasma levels. Watch carefully for cardiovascular or respiratory deterioration in an intensive care setting, particularly in the early hours. Observe mild overdose cases for at least 4 hours for the development of signs of poisoning.

Treatment: Patients who are seen soon after potentially life-threatening overdosage (within 4 hours) should be treated by gastric lavage and activated charcoal.

Treatment of symptoms is based on modern methods of intensive care, with continuous monitoring of cardiac function, blood gases, and electrolytes, and if necessary, emergency measures such as artificial respiration, resuscitation or cardiac pacemaker.

Significant bradycardia should be treated initially with atropine. Large doses of isoprenaline may be necessary for control of heart rate and hypotension. Glucagon has positive chronotropic and inotropic effects on the heart that are independent of interactions with beta-adrenergic receptors and it represents a useful alternative treatment for hypotension and heart failure.

For seizures, diazepam has been effective and is the drug of choice.

For bronchospasms, aminophylline, salbutamol or terbutaline (β_2 agonist) are effective bronchodilator drugs. Monitor the patient for dysrhythmias during and after administration.

Patients who recover should be observed for signs of β-blocker withdrawal phenomenon (see *Warnings* and *Precautions*).

Pharmaceutical precautions No special storage requirements.

Legal category POM.

Package quantities Cartons of 28 Slow-Trasicor tablets consisting of two reminder calendar foils of 14 (each carton of 28 represents 2-4 weeks treatment, depending on whether the dosage is one or two tablets daily).

Further information Nil.

Product licence number 00101/0429.

Product licence holder: Novartis Pharmaceuticals UK Limited, trading as Ciba Laboratories.

Date of revision of text 05.07.97.

TAVEGIL*

Presentation

Tablets: White, uncoated, round tablets, 7 mm in diameter, with bevelled edges, branded TAVEGIL on one side with a single break line on the other. Each tablet contains 1.34 mg clemastine hydrogen fumarate (equivalent to 1 mg clemastine base).

Elixir: A clear, colourless liquid with an odour of peaches. Each 5 ml spoonful contains 670 micrograms (0.67 mg) clemastine hydrogen fumarate (equivalent to 500 micrograms (0.5 mg) clemastine base).

Uses *Principal action:* Tavegil is a potent, specific antihistamine which is innately long-acting.

Indications: Allergic rhinitis, including hay fever and perennial rhinitis, vasomotor rhinitis. Allergic dermatoses, including pruritus, atopic eczema and contact dermatitis. Urticaria. Angioneurotic oedema. Drug allergy.

Dosage and administration
Adults: 1 mg clemastine base (one tablet or two 5 ml spoonfuls of elixir) night and morning.

In individual cases the dose may be increased to 6 mg clemastine base daily if necessary (six tablets or twelve 5 ml spoonfuls of elixir).

Children:

1 to 3 years:	250 micrograms to 500 micrograms clemastine base night and morning.
3 to 6 years:	500 micrograms clemastine base night and morning.
6 to 12 years:	500 micrograms to 1000 micrograms (1 mg) clemastine base night and morning.

For doses less than 500 micrograms Tavegil Elixir may be diluted. For dilution details see 'Pharmaceutical precautions'.

Use in the elderly: No evidence exists that elderly patients require different dosages or show different side-effects from younger patients.

Contra-indications, warnings, etc
Contra-indications: Tavegil is contra-indicated in patients with a known hypersensitivity to clemastine or other arylalkylamine antihistamines.

Tavegil should not be given to children below one year of age.

Precautions: Patients should be warned not to take charge of vehicles or machinery until the effect of Tavegil treatment on the individual is known. Tavegil may potentiate the effects of sedatives, hypnotics, monoamine-oxidase inhibitors and alcohol. Patients should be advised to avoid alcoholic drinks.

Antihistamines should be used with caution in patients with narrow-angle glaucoma, stenosing peptic ulcer, pyloroduodenal obstruction, prostatic hypertrophy with urinary retention and bladder neck obstruction.

Use in pregnancy and lactation: Tavegil should not be given during pregnancy and breast feeding unless it is strictly indicated.

Side-effects: Drowsiness, fatigue, occasionally CNS stimulation has been reported, particularly in children. Very occasional miscellaneous side-effects such as weakness, dizziness, dry mouth, headache, palpitations, gastro-intestinal disturbance, heartburn and skin rash have occurred. In general, these adverse effects can be controlled by a diminution of dosage.

Overdosage: May give rise to confusion, nausea and vomiting. Treatment should be directed to the removal of ingested material by induced emesis or gastric lavage as appropriate. Routine supportive measures are indicated to combat respiratory depression and hypotension.

Pharmaceutical precautions Store both the tablets and elixir below 25°C. Tavegil Elixir may be diluted with Syrup BP or Sorbitol Syrup (70%). The diluted elixir should be used within 14 days.

Legal category P.

Package quantities *Tavegil Tablets:* Blister pack of 60 (OP).

Tavegil Elixir: Bottles of 150 ml.

Further information Tavegil Elixir is sucrose free and is suitable for diabetic patients. It has an approximate calorific value of 11 kcals per 5 ml spoonful.

Product licence numbers

Tavegil Tablets	0101/0033
Tavegil Elixir	0101/0058

Product licence holder: Novartis Pharmaceuticals UK Limited, trading as Sandoz Pharmaceuticals.

Date of last revision May 1997.

TEGRETOL* CHEWTABS 100 mg and 200 mg
TEGRETOL TABLETS 100 mg, 200 mg and 400 mg

Qualitative and quantitative composition The active ingredient is 5-Carbamoyl-5-H-dibenz(b,f)azepine.

Each chewtab contains 100 mg or 200 mg carbamazepine PhEur and each tablet contains 100 mg, 200 mg or 400 mg carbamazepine PhEur.

Pharmaceutical forms The 100 mg chewable tablets are pale orange, square shaped tablets, with a pronounced orange odour, embossed with 'T' on one side and impressed with Tegretol 100 on the other.

The 200 mg chewable tablets are pale orange, square shaped tablets, with a pronounced orange odour, embossed with 'T' on one side and impressed with Tegretol 200 on the other.

The 100 mg tablets are white, round, flat, uncoated tablets with bevelled edges, having a breakline on one face and impressed 'TEGRETOL 100' on the other.

The 200 mg tablets are white, round, flat, uncoated tablets with bevelled edges, having a breakline on one face and impressed 'TEGRETOL 200' on the other.

The 400 mg tablets are white, flat rod-shaped tablets with bevelled edges. One side bears the imprint 'CG/CG', the other 'TEGR/ETOL' and both sides are scored.

Clinical particulars
Therapeutic indications: Epilepsy – generalised tonic-clinic and partial siezures.

Note: Tegretol is not usually effective in absences (petit mal). Moreover, anecdotal evidence suggests that seizure exacerbation may occur in patients with atypical absences.

The paroxysmal pain of trigeminal neuralgia.

For the prophylaxis of manic-depressive psychosis in patients unresponsive to lithium therapy.

Posology and method of administration: Tegretol is given orally, usually in two or three divided doses. Tegretol may be taken during, after or between meals, with a little liquid e.g. a glass of water.

The chewtabs should be chewed before swallowing, preferably with a little liquid to wash down possible remnants of the tablets.

The chewtabs are particularly suitable for children and adults who have difficulty in swallowing tablets.

Epilepsy: Adults: It is advised that with all formulations of Tegretol, a gradually increasing dosage scheme is used and this should be adjusted to suit the needs of the individual patient. It may be helpful to monitor the plasma concentration of carbamazepine to establish the optimum dose (see *Pharmacokinetics, Precautions* and *Interactions*).

Tegretol should be taken in a number of divided doses although initially 100–200 mg once or twice daily is recommended. This may be followed by a slow increase until the best response is obtained, often 800–1,200 mg daily. In some instances, 1,600 mg or even 2,000 mg daily may be necessary.

Elderly: There is no evidence to suggest that dosage requirements are different in the elderly but it is recommended that the intitial dose be small.

Children: It is advised that with all formulations of Tegretol, a gradually increasing dosage scheme is used and this should be adjusted to suit the needs of the individual patient. It may be helpful to monitor the plasma concentration of carbamazepine to establish the optimum dose (see *Pharmacokinetics, Precautions* and *Interactions*).

Usual dosage 10–20 mg/kg bodyweight daily taken in several divided doses. Tegretol tablets are not recommended for very young children.

1–5 years: 2–4×100 mg per day, where appropriate (Tegretol Chewtabs 100 mg and 200 mg only)

5–10 years: 2–3×200 mg tablets per day, to be taken in divided doses.

10–15 years: 3–5×200 mg tablets per day, to be taken in several divided doses.

Wherever possible, anti-epileptic agents should be prescribed as the sole anti-epileptic agent but if used in polytherapy the same incremental dosage pattern is advised.

Trigeminal neuralgia: The individual dosage requirements of Tegretol vary considerably. It is recommended that the initial dose be small but in some patients a high dose early in treatment may be required. In elderly patients, an initial dose of 100 mg twice daily is recommended.

The dose may be increased gradually until a satisfactory clinical response is obtained, which in some instances necessitates 1,600 mg Tegretol daily. It has been found that in the majority of patients a dosage of 200 mg three or four times a day is sufficient to maintain a pain-free state. When the pain goes into remission the dose may be gradually reduced and Tegretol discontinued in the absence of recurrence.

For the prophylaxis of manic depressive psychosis in patients unresponsive to lithium therapy: Initial starting dose of 400 mg daily, in divided doses, increasing gradually until symptoms are controlled or a total of 1,600 mg given in divided doses is reached. The usual dosage range is 400–600 mg daily, given in divided doses.

Contra-indications: Previous drug sensitivity to carbamazepine or structurally related drugs, e.g. tricyclic antidepressants. Because Tegretol depresses AV-conduction, it is inadvisable to administer this drug to patients with atrioventricular conduction abnormalities. Patients with a history of previous bone marrow depression or a history of intermittent porphyria. On theoretical grounds i.e. a structural relationship to tricyclic anti-depressants, the use of Tegretol is not recommended in combination with monoamine oxidase inhibitors (MAOIs); before administering Tegretol, MAOIs should be discontinued for a minimum of 2 weeks, or longer if the clinical situation permits.

Special warnings and special precautions for use
Warnings: Agranulocytosis and aplastic anaemia have been associated with Tegretol; however, due to the very low incidence of these diseases, meaningful risk estimates for Tegretol are difficult to obtain. The overall risk in the general untreated population has been estimated at 4.7 persons per million per year for agranulocytosis and 2.0 persons per million per year for aplastic anaemia.

Blood counts, platelet count and serum biochemistry including electrolytes and indices of hepatic function should be checked before commencing treatment with Tegretol. Blood counts should be performed before and periodically during treatment. Clinical monitoring is of primary importance during the whole treatment.

Patients and their relatives should be informed on how to recognise early toxic signs and symptoms indicative of a potential haematological problem, or of dermatological or hepatic reactions. If reactions such as fever, sore throat, rash, ulcers in the mouth, easy bruising, petechial or purpuric haemorrhage appear, the patient should be advised to consult his physician immediately.

Non-progressive or fluctuating asymptomatic leucopenia, which occurs in about 10% of treated patients does not generally call for withdrawal of Tegretol. However, treatment with Tegretol should be discontinued if the patient develops leucopenia which is severe, progressive or accompanied by clinical manifestations, e.g. fever or sore throat. Tegretol should be discontinued if any evidence of significant bone marrow depression appears.

Liver function tests should also be performed before commencing treatment and periodically thereafter, particularly in patients with a history of liver disease and in elderly patients.

Some liver function tests in patients receiving carbamazepine may be found to be abnormal, particularly gamma glutamyl transferase. This is probably due to hepatic enzyme induction. Enzyme induction may also produce modest elevations in alkaline phosphatase. These enhancements of hepatic metabolising capacity are not an indication for the withdrawal of carbamazepine.

Severe hepatic reactions to carbamazepine occur very rarely. The development of signs and symptoms of liver dysfunction or active liver disease should be urgently evaluated and treatment with Tegretol suspended pending the outcome of the evaluation.

Mild skin reactions, e.g. isolated macular or maculopapular exanthemata, are mostly transient and not hazardous, and they usually disappear within a few days. However, the patient should be kept under close surveillance and a worsening rash or accompanying symptoms are an indication for the immediate withdrawal of Tegretol. Severe skin reactions e.g. Stevens-Johnson syndrome, Lyell's syndrome (toxic epidermal necrolysis), also necessitate immediate withdrawal.

If treatment with Tegretol has to be withdrawn abruptly, the changeover to another anti-epileptic drug should if necessary be effected under the cover of a suitable drug, e.g. i.v. or rectal benzodiazepines, or i.v. phenytoin.

The induction of hepatic enzymes by carbamazepine may reduce the activity of the hormones contained in the combined oral contraceptive pill. This may appear clinically as breakthrough bleeding or spotting. Patients taking Tegretol and requiring oral contraception should receive a preparation containing not less than 50 mcg oestrogen or use of some alternative non-hormonal method of contraception should be considered.

Although correlations between dosages and plasma levels of carbamazepine, and between plasma levels and clinical efficacy or tolerability are rather tenuous, serum level monitoring of carbamazepine may prove useful during stabilisation, for optimum seizure control and in particular situations, e.g. pregnancy, for verification of compliance, in suspected toxicity and when carbamazepine is used in polytherapy.

In rats treated with carbamazepine for two years, the incidence of tumours of the liver was found to be increased. There is, however, no evidence to indicate that this observation has any significant bearing on the therapeutic use of the drug.

Precautions: Tegretol should be prescribed only after a critical benefit-risk appraisal and under close monitoring in patients with a history of cardiac, hepatic or renal damage, adverse haematological reactions to other drugs, or interrupted courses of therapy with Tegretol.

Baseline and periodic complete urinalysis and BUN determinations are recommended.

Tegretol has shown mild anticholinergic activity; patients with glaucoma should therefore be warned and advised regarding possible hazards.

The possibility of activation of a latent psychosis, and in elderly patients the possibility of agitation or confusion, especially when high doses of Tegretol are administered, should be borne in mind.

Interaction with other medicaments and other forms of interaction: Induction of hepatic enzymes in response to Tegretol may increase the metabolism and reduce the effectiveness of certain other drugs that are metabolised in the liver including: clobazam, clonazepam, ethosuximide, primidone, valproic acid, alprazolam, corticosteroids, hormonal contraceptive agents, cyclosporin, digoxin, doxycycline, felodipine, haloperidol, imipramine, methadone, theophylline, warfarin. The concurrent administration of carbamazepine has been reported to both raise and lower phenytoin levels and in rare instances mephenytoin plasma levels have been reported to increase.

Certain drugs have been shown to increase carbamazepine serum levels: macrolide antibiotics (erythromycin), isoniazid, calcium antagonists (verapamil, diltiazem), dextropropoxyphene, viloxazine, fluoxetine, cimetidine, acetazolamide, danazol, possibly desipramine and nicotinamide (only in adults and at high doses). Since raised carbamazepine levels may produce signs of overdosage (e.g. dizziness, drowsiness, ataxia, diplopia), the dosage of Tegretol should be adjusted accordingly.

Concomitant use of carbamazepine and isoniazid has been reported to increase isoniazid hepatotoxicity.

The combination of lithium and carbamazepine may cause enhanced neurotoxicity in spite of lithium plasma concentrations being within the therapeutic range.

Combined use of carbamazepine with metoclopramide or major tranquillisers, e.g. haloperidol, thioridazine, may also result in an increase in neurological side-effects.

Plasma levels of carbamazepine may be reduced by phenobarbitone, phenytoin, primidone, theophylline, also possibly clonazepam, and valproic acid (the data on the latter two compounds are contradictory).

Valproic acid, valpromide and primidone have been reported to increase the degree of conversion of carbamazepine to the active metabolite carbamazepine-10,11-epoxide.

Concomitant medication with Tegretol and some diuretics (hydrochlorothiazide, frusemide) may lead to symptomatic hyponatraemia.

Carbamazepine may antagonise the effects of non-depolarising muscle relaxants (e.g. pancuronium); their dosage may need to be raised and patients monitored closely for unexpectedly rapid recovery from neuromuscular blockade.

Isotretinoin has been reported to alter unpredictably the bioavailability and/or clearance of carbamazepine and carbamazepine-10,11-epoxide; carbamazepine plasma concentrations should be monitored.

Alcohol may exacerbate the CNS side-effects of psychoactive drugs including Tegretol; it is therefore advised that patients abstain from alcohol during treatment.

Pregnancy and lactation: If pregnancy occurs in a woman receiving Tegretol or if the use of Tegretol is considered necessary during pregnancy the need to control seizures in the mother should be carefully weighed against the possible risk to the foetus. This is particularly important during the first three months of pregnancy. Minimum effective doses should be given and monitoring of plasma levels is recommended.

In women of childbearing age Tegretol should be administered as monotherapy, whenever possible.

Cases of developmental disorders and malformations, including spina bifida, have been reported in association with carbamazepine. However, offspring of mothers with untreated epilepsy are known to be prone to an increased incidence of development disorders and conclusive evidence that carbamazepine given alone increases the risk further is not available. Patients should be counselled regarding the possibility of an increased risk of malformations and given the opportunity of antenatal screening.

In animals (mice, rats and rabbits) oral administration of carbamazepine during organogenesis led to increased embryo mortality at a daily dose which caused maternal toxicity (above 200 mg/kg b.w. daily i.e. 20 times the usual human dosage). No evidence of a teratogenic effect was observed in the three species studied but in one study using mice carbamazepine (40–240 mg/kg b.w. daily orally) caused defects in 4.7% of exposed foetuses compared with 1.3% in controls.

Anti-epileptic drugs may contribute to folic acid deficiency, a possible contributory cause of foetal abnormality. Folic acid supplementation is recommended before and during pregnancy.

Bleeding disorders in the new-born caused by anti-epileptic agents have been reported. As a precaution, Vitamin K1 should be administered as a preventive measure in the last weeks of pregnancy and to the new-born.

Carbamazepine passes into the breast milk in concentrations of about 25–60% of the plasma level. This is not believed to present a significant hazard to the infant, which is likely to receive at most 10% of an appropriate therapeutic dose of carbamazepine for an infant with epilepsy. As with all drugs, the benefits of breast-feeding should be weighed against the remote possibility of an adverse effect occurring in the infant. There is one report of a severe skin (hypersensitivity) reaction in a breast-fed baby.

Effects on ability to drive and use machines: The patient's reactions, e.g. as a road user, may be impaired by Tegretol, especially in the early stages of treatment. Patients should be warned of the possible hazard when driving or operating machinery.

Undesirable effects: Provided a gradually increasing dosage scheme is followed, Tegretol is generally well tolerated but side effects may occur particularly at the start of treatment, or if the initial dose is too high. Dizziness, headache, ataxia, drowsiness, fatigue, diplopia, nausea or vomiting may be symptoms of carbamazepine overdosage and usually abate within a few days either spontaneously or after a transient dosage reduction. It is advisable to monitor the plasma levels and divide the daily dosage into smaller (i.e. 3–4) fractional doses.

Central nervous system: Neurological: Frequent: Dizziness, ataxia, drowsiness, fatigue. Occasional: Headache, diplopia, accommodation disorders (blurred vision). Rare: Abnormal involuntary movements (tremor, asterixis, orofacial dyskinesia, choreoathetotic disorders, dystonia, tics), nystagmus. Isolated cases: Oculomotor disturbances, speech disorders (e.g. dysarthria or slurred speech), peripheral neuritis, paraesthesiae, muscle weakness, and paretic symptoms.

Psychiatric: Isolated cases: Hallucinations (visual or acoustic), depression, loss of appetite, restlessness, aggressive behaviour, agitation, confusion, activation of psychosis.

Skin and appendages: Occasional or frequent: Allergic skin reactions, urticaria, which may be severe. Rare: Exfoliative dermatitis and erythroderma, Stevens-Johnson syndrome, systemic lupus erythematosus-like syndrome. Isolated cases: Toxic epidermal necrolysis, photosensitivity, erythema multiforme and nodosum, alterations in skin pigmentation, purpura, pruritus, acne, sweating, hair loss, hirsutism.

Blood: Occasional or frequent: Leucopenia. Occasional: Eosinophilia, thrombocytopenia. Rare: Leucocytosis. Isolated cases: Agranulocytosis, aplastic anaemia, pure red cell aplasia, megaloblastic anaemia, acute intermittent porphyria, reticulocytosis, folic acid deficiency, and possibly haemolytic anaemia.

Liver: Frequent: Elevated gamma-GT (due to hepatic enzyme induction), usually not clinically relevant. Occasional: Elevated alkaline phosphatase, rarely transaminases. Rare: Jaundice, hepatitis of cholestatic, parenchymal (hepatocellular), or mixed type. Isolated cases: Granulomatous hepatitis.

Gastro-intestinal tract: Occasional or frequent: Nausea, vomiting. Occasional: Dryness of the mouth. Rare: Diarrhoea or constipation. Isolated cases: Abdominal pain, glossitis, stomatitis.

Hypersensitivity reactions: Rare: A delayed multi-organ hypersensitivity disorder (of serum sickness type) with fever, skin rashes, vasculitis, lymphadenopathy, disorders mimicking lymphoma, arthralgia, leucopenia, eosinophilia, hepato-splenomegaly and abnormal liver function tests, occurring in various combinations. Other organs may also be affected (e.g. lungs, kidneys, pancreas, myocardium). Isolated cases: Aseptic meningitis, with myoclonus and peripheral eosinophilia, anaphylactic reaction.

Treatment must be discontinued immediately if such hypersensitivity reactions occur.

Cardiovascular system: Rare: Disturbances of cardiac conduction. Isolated cases: Bradycardia, arrhythmias, AV-block with syncope, collapse, congestive heart failure, hypertension or hypotension, aggravation of coronary artery disease, thrombophlebitis, thrombo-embolism.

Endocrine system and metabolism: Occasional: Hyponatraemia, fluid retention, oedema, weight gain, and reduced plasma osmolality due to an antidiuretic hormone (ADH)-like effect, leading in isolated cases to water intoxication accompanied by lethargy, vomiting, headache, mental confusion, neurological abnormalities. Isolated cases: Gynaecomastia or galactorrhoea. Impaired male fertility and/or abnormal spermatogenesis. Loss of libido/impotence. Abnormal thyroid function tests: decreased L-thyroxine (FT4, T4, T3) and increased TSH, usually without clinical manifestations. Disturbances of bone metabolism (decrease in plasma calcium and 25-OH-cholecalciferol), leading to osteomalacia. Elevated levels of cholesterol, including HDL cholesterol, and triglycerides.

Renal: Isolated cases: Interstitial nephritis and renal failure. Signs of renal dysfunction including albuminuria, haematuria, oliguria and elevated BUN/azotaemia, urinary frequency, urinary retention.

Sense organs: Isolated cases: Taste disturbances; lens opacities, conjunctivitis, tinnitus, hyperacusis.

Musculoskeletal system: Isolated cases: Arthralgia, muscle pain or cramp.

Respiratory tract: Isolated cases: Pulmonary hypersensitivity characterised by dyspnoea, pneumonitis or pneumonia.

Overdosage

Signs and symptoms: The presenting signs and symptoms of overdosage involve the central nervous, cardiovascular or respiratory systems.

Central nervous system: CNS depression; disorientation, somnolence, agitation, hallucination, coma; blurred vision, slurred speech, dysarthria, nystagmus, ataxia, dyskinesia, initially hyperreflexia, later hyporeflexia; convulsions, psychomotor disturbances, myoclonus, hypothermia.

Respiratory system: Respiratory depression, pulmonary oedema.

Cardiovascular system: Tachycardia, changes in blood pressure (hypotension and at times hypertension), cardiac arrhythmias, conduction disturbance with widening of QRS complex; syncope.

Gastro-intestinal system: Vomiting, delayed gastric emptying, reduced bowel motility.

Renal function: Retention of urine, oliguria or anuria; fluid retention, water intoxication due to ADH-like effect of carbamazepine.

Laboratory findings: Hyponatraemia, possibly metabolic acidosis, possibly hyperglycaemia, increased muscle creatinine phosphokinase.

Treatment: There is no specific antidote.

Management according to the patient's clinical condition. Possible admission to hospital. Measurement of the plasma level to confirm carbamazepine poisoning and to ascertain the size of the overdose. Evacuation of the stomach, gastric lavage, and administration of activated charcoal. Supportive medical care in an intensive care unit with cardiac monitoring and careful correction of electrolyte imbalance, if required.

Special recommendations:

Hypotension: Administer dopamine or dobutamine i.v.

Disturbances of cardiac rhythm: To be managed on an individual basis.

Convulsions: Administer a benzodiazepine (e.g. diazepam) or another anticonvulsant, e.g. phenobarbitone (with caution because of increased respiratory depression) or paraldehyde.

Hyponatraemia (water intoxication): fluid restriction and slow careful NaCl 0.9% infusion i.v. These measures may be useful in preventing brain damage.

Charcoal haemoperfusion has been recommended. Forced diuresis, haemodialysis, and peritoneal dialysis have been reported not to be effective.

Relapse and aggravation of symptomatology on the 2nd and 3rd day after overdose, due to delayed absorption, should be anticipated.

Pharmacological properties

Pharmacodynamic properties: Mode of action: Carbamazepine is a dibenzazepine derivative with anti-epileptic, neurotropic and psychotropic properties.

The mechanism of action of carbamazepine has only been partially elucidated. It is conceivable that blockade of voltage-sensitive sodium channels may be one or even the main primary effect of carbamazepine.

Pharmacokinetic properties: Absorption: Carbamazepine is almost completely absorbed but the rate of absorption from the tablets is slow and may vary amongst the various formulations and between patients. Peak plasma concentrations of the unchanged active substance after administration of single doses of Tegretol tablets: chewable tablets are attained at 6 hours and conventional tablets are attained at 12 hours.

The bioavailability of Tegretol in various oral formulations has been shown to lie between 85–100%. Bioavailability is unaffected by food.

Distribution: The concentration of unchanged substance in the CSF and saliva represents the unbound portion in plasma i.e. 20–30% of total plasma concentration, breast milk 25–60% of total plasma concentration. Carbamazepine crosses the placental barrier. Apparent volume of distribution 0.8–1.5 L/kg.

Serum protein binding: 70–80%.

Biotransformation: Carbamazepine is extensively metabolised in the liver, mainly by oxidative pathways and the greater part is excreted as the inactive glucuronide with up to 40% as metabolites, of which only carbamazepine epoxide is pharmacologically active. This may constitute up to 30% of the circulating active material originating as carbamazepine; in particular polytherapy is an important factor in augmenting epoxide levels. The inactive 10,11-diol represents the final stage of carbamazepine biotransformation. Only about 3% of pharmacologically active material (unchanged plus epoxide) is excreted.

In advanced hepatic disease carbamazepine metabolism may be impaired.

Elimination: The elimination half-life of unchanged drug in the plasma averages approximately 36 hours following a single dose, whereas after repeated administration, which leads to auto-induction of hepatic enzymes, it averages only 16–24 hours, depending on the duration of the medication. In patients receiving co-medication with other enzyme-inducing drugs (phenytoin, phenobarbitone) half-life values averaging 9–10 hours have been observed. The therapeutic plasma concentration range of carbamazepine at steady state is usually between 4–12 mcg/ml (17–50 μmol/l).

Characteristics in patients: The pharmacokinetics of carbamazepine are unaltered in the elderly but its metabolism may be affected by hepatic dysfunction (see above). In children the relatively high rate of metabolism of the drug may require higher doses (in mg/kg b.w.) of carbamazepine to maintain therapeutic concentrations.

Preclinical safety data: None relevant.

Pharmaceutical particulars

List of excipients: Each chewtab contains crospovidone, red iron oxide, yellow iron oxide, magnesium stearate, orange flavour 51.941/AP, sorbitol, stearic acid.

Each uncoated tablet contains aerosil 200 standard, avicel PH 102, nymcel ZSB-10 and magnesium stearate.

Incompatibilities: None known.

Shelf life:
Tegretol Chewtabs 100 mg and 200 mg: Five years
Tegretol Tablets 100 mg, 200 mg and 400 mg: Five years

Special precautions for storage:
Tegretol Chewtabs 100 mg and 200 mg: Protect from heat (store below 30°C).
Tegretol Tablets 100 mg and 200 mg: There are no special precautions for storage.
Tegretol Tablets 400 mg: Protect from moisture.

Nature and contents of container: Tegretol Chewtabs 100 mg and 200 mg come in aluminium blister packs of 56.
Tegretol Tablets 100 mg and 200 mg come in PVC/PVdC blister packs of 84 tablets, and containers of 50 and 500 tablets (100 mg only).
Tegretol Tablets 400 mg comes in PVC blister packs of 56.

Instructions for use/handling: None.

Marketing authorisation holder: Novartis Pharmaceuticals UK Limited: Trading as Geigy Pharmaceuticals, Frimley Business Park, Frimley, Camberley, Surrey GU16 5SG.

Marketing authorisation number

Tegretol Chewtabs 100 mg:	PL 00101/0454
Tegretol Chewtabs 200 mg:	PL 00101/0455
Tegretol Tablets 100 mg:	PL 00101/0461
Tegretol Tablets 200 mg:	PL 00101/0462
Tegretol Tablets 400 mg:	PL 00101/0463

Date of first authorisation 4 July 1997.

Date of (partial) revision of the text 21.11.97.

Legl category POM.

TEGRETOL LIQUID 100 mg/5 ml

Qualitative and quantitative composition The active ingredient is 5-Carbamoyl-5-H-dibenz(b,f)azepine.

The liquid contains 100 mg carbamazepine PhEur in each 5 ml.

Pharmaceutical form Oral liquid.

Clinical particulars

Therapeutic indications: Epilepsy – generalised tonic-clonic and partial seizures.

Note: Tegretol is not usually effective in absences (petit mal). Moreover, anecdotal evidence suggests that seizure exacerbation may occur in patients with atypical absences.

The paroxysmal pain of trigeminal neuralgia.

For the prophylaxis of manic-depressive psychosis in patients unresponsive to lithium therapy.

Posology and method of administration: Tegretol Liquid is given orally, usually in two or three divided doses.

Tegretol Liquid (the liquid should be shaken before use) may be taken during, after or between meals.

Since a given dose of Tegretol Liquid will produce higher peak levels than the same dose in tablet form, it is advisable to start with low doses of the liquid and to increase them slowly so as to avoid adverse effects on the central nervous system such as dizziness and lethargy.

When switching a patient from tablets to liquid the same overall dose may be used but in smaller, more frequent, doses.

Epilepsy: Adults: It is advised that with all formulations of Tegretol, a gradually increasing dosage scheme is used and this should be adjusted to suit the needs of the individual patient. It may be helpful to monitor the plasma concentration of carbamazepine to establish the optimum dose (see *Pharmacokinetics, Precautions* and *Interactions*).

Tegretol should be taken in a number of divided doses although initially 100–200 mg once or twice daily is recommended. This may be followed by a slow increase until the best response is obtained, often 800–1,200 mg daily. In some instances, 1,600 mg or even 2,000 mg daily may be necessary.

Elderly: There is no evidence to suggest that dosage requirements are different in the elderly but it is recommended that the intitial dose be small.

Children: It is advised that with all formulations of Tegretol, a gradually increasing dosage scheme is used and this should be adjusted to suit the needs of the individual patient. It may be helpful to monitor the plasma concentration of carbamazepine to establish the optimum dose (see *Pharmacokinetics, Precautions* and *Interactions*).

Usual dosage 10–20 mg/kg bodyweight daily taken in several divided doses.

Age up to 1 year:	5–10 ml liquid per day.
1–5 years:	10–20 ml liquid per day.
5–10 years:	20–30 ml liquid per day to be taken in divided doses.
10–15 years:	30–50 ml liquid per day to be taken in several divided doses.

Wherever possible, anti-epileptic agents should be prescribed as the sole anti-epileptic agent but if used in polytherapy, the same incremental dosage pattern is advised.

Trigeminal neuralgia: The individual dosage requirements of Tegretol vary considerably. It is recommended that the initial dose be small but in some patients a high dose early in treatment may be required. In elderly patients, an initial dose of 100 mg twice daily is recommended.

The dose may be increased gradually until a satisfactory clinical response is obtained, which in some instances necessitates 1,600 mg Tegretol daily. It has been found that in the majority of patients a dosage of 200 mg three or four times a day is sufficient to maintain a pain-free state. When the pain goes into remission the dose may be gradually reduced and Tegretol discontinued in the absence of recurrence.

For the prophylaxis of manic depressive psychosis in patients unresponsive to lithium therapy: Initial starting dose of 100–200 mg daily, in divided doses, increasing gradually until symptoms are controlled or a total of 1,600 mg given in divided doses is reached. The usual dosage range is 400–600 mg daily, given in divided doses.

Contra-indications: Previous drug sensitivity to carbamazepine or structurally related drugs, e.g. tricyclic antidepressants. Because Tegretol depresses AV-conduction, it is inadvisable to administer this drug to patients with atrioventricular conduction abnormalities. Patients with a history of previous bone marrow depression or a history of intermittent porphyria. On theoretical grounds, i.e. a structural relationship to tricyclic antidepressants, the use of Tegretol is not recommended in combination with monoamine oxidase inhibitors (MAOIs); before administering Tegretol, MAOIs should be discontinued for a minimum of 2 weeks, or longer if the clinical situation permits.

Special warnings and special precautions for use

Warnings: Agranulocytosis and aplastic anaemia have been associated with Tegretol; however, due to the very low incidence of these diseases, meaningful risk estimates for Tegretol are difficult to obtain. The overall risk in the general untreated population has been estimated at 4.7 persons per million per year for agranulocytosis and 2.0 persons per million per year for aplastic anaemia.

Blood counts, platelet count and serum biochemistry including electrolytes and indices of hepatic function should be checked before commencing treatment with Tegretol. Blood counts should be performed before and periodically during treatment. Clinical monitoring is of primary importance during the whole treatment.

Patients and their relatives should be informed on how to recognise early toxic signs and symptoms indicative of a potential haematological problem, or of dermatological or hepatic reactions. If reactions such as fever, sore throat, rash, ulcers in the mouth, easy bruising, petechial or purpuric haemorrhage appear, the patient should be advised to consult his physician immediately.

Non-progressive or fluctuating asymptomatic leucopenia, which occurs in about 10% of treated patients does not generally call for withdrawal of Tegretol. However, treatment with Tegretol should be discontinued if the patient develops leucopenia which is severe, progressive or accompanied by clinical manifestations, e.g. fever or sore throat. Tegretol should be discontinued if any evidence of significant bone marrow depression appears.

Liver function tests should also be performed before commencing treatment and periodically thereafter, particularly in patients with a history of liver disease and in elderly patients.

Some liver function tests in patients receiving carbamazepine may be found to be abnormal, particularly gamma glutamyl transferase. This is probably due to hepatic enzyme induction. Enzyme induction may also produce modest elevations in alkaline phosphatase. These enhancements of hepatic metabolising capacity are not an indication for the withdrawal of carbamazepine.

Severe hepatic reactions to carbamazepine occur very rarely. The development of signs and symptoms of liver dysfunction or active liver disease should be urgently evaluated and treatment with Tegretol suspended pending the outcome of the evaluation.

Mild skin reactions, e.g. isolated macular or maculopapular exanthemata, are mostly transient and not hazardous, and they usually disappear within a few days. However, the patient should be kept under close surveillance and a worsening rash or accompanying symptoms are an indication for the immediate withdrawal of Tegretol. Severe skin reactions e.g. Stevens-Johnson syndrome, Lyell's syndrome (toxic epidermal necrolysis), also necessitate immediate withdrawal.

If treatment with Tegretol has to be withdrawn abruptly, the changeover to another anti-epileptic drug should if necessary be effected under the cover of a suitable drug, e.g. i.v. or rectal benzodiazepines, or i.v. phenytoin.

The induction of hepatic enzymes by carbamazepine may reduce the activity of the hormones contained in the combined oral contraceptive pill. This may appear clinically as breakthrough bleeding or spotting. Patients taking Tegretol and requiring oral contraception should receive a preparation containing not less than 50 mcg oestrogen or use of some alternative non-hormonal method of contraception should be considered.

Although correlations between dosages and plasma levels of carbamazepine, and between plasma levels and clinical efficacy or tolerability are rather tenuous, serum level monitoring of carbamazepine may prove useful during stabilisation, for optimum seizure control and in particular situations, e.g. pregnancy, for verification of compliance, in suspected toxicity and when carbamazepine is used in polytherapy.

In rats treated with carbamazepine for two years, the incidence of tumours of the liver was found to be increased. There is, however, no evidence to indicate that this observation has any significant bearing on the therapeutic use of the drug.

Precautions: Tegretol should be prescribed only after a critical benefit-risk appraisal and under close monitoring in patients with a history of cardiac, hepatic or renal damage, adverse haematological reactions to other drugs, or interrupted courses of therapy with Tegretol.

Baseline and periodic complete urinalysis and BUN determinations are recommended.

Tegretol has shown mild anticholinergic activity; patients with glaucoma should therefore be warned and advised regarding possible hazards.

The possibility of activation of a latent psychosis, and in elderly patients the possibility of agitation or confusion, especially when high doses of Tegretol are administered, should be borne in mind.

Interaction with other medicaments and other forms of interaction: Induction of hepatic enzymes in response to Tegretol may increase the metabolism and reduce the effectiveness of certain other drugs that are metabolised in the liver including: clobazam, clonazepam, ethosuximide, primidone, valproic acid, alprazolam, corticosteroids, hormonal contraceptive agents, cyclosporin, digoxin, doxycycline, felodipine, haloperidol, imipramine, methadone, theophylline, warfarin. The concurrent administration of carbamazepine has been reported to both raise and lower phenytoin levels and in rare instances mephenytoin plasma levels have been reported to increase.

Certain drugs have been shown to increase carbamazepine serum levels: macrolide antibiotics (erythromycin), isoniazid, calcium antagonists (verapamil, diltiazem), dextropropoxyphene, viloxazine, fluoxetine, cimetidine, acetazolamide, danazol, possibly desipramine and nicotinamide (only in adults and at high doses). Since raised carbamazepine levels may produce signs of overdosage (e.g. dizziness, drowsiness, ataxia, diplopia), the dosage of Tegretol should be adjusted accordingly.

Concomitant use of carbamazepine and isoniazid has been reported to increase isoniazid hepatotoxicity.

The combination of lithium and carbamazepine may cause enhanced neurotoxicity in spite of lithium plasma concentrations being within the therapeutic range.

Combined use of carbamazepine with metoclopramide or major tranquillisers, e.g. haloperidol, thioridazine, may also result in an increase in neurological side-effects.

Plasma levels of carbamazepine may be reduced by phenobarbitone, phenytoin, primidone, theophylline, also possibly clonazepam, and valproic acid (the data on the latter two compounds are contradictory).

Valproic acid, valpromide and primidone have been reported to increase the degree of conversion of carbamazepine to the active metabolite carbamazepine-10,11-epoxide.

Concomitant medication with Tegretol and some diuretics (hydrochlorothiazide, frusemide) may lead to symptomatic hyponatraemia.

Carbamazepine may antagonise the effects of non-depolarising muscle relaxants (e.g. pancuronium); their dosage may need to be raised and patients monitored closely for unexpectedly rapid recovery from neuromuscular blockade.

Isotretinoin has been reported to alter the bioavailability and/or clearance of carbamazepine and carbamazepine-10,11-epoxide; carbamazepine plasma concentrations should be monitored.

Alcohol may exacerbate the CNS side-effects of psychoactive drugs including Tegretol; it is therefore advised that patients abstain from alcohol during treatment.

Pregnancy and lactation: If pregnancy occurs in a woman receiving Tegretol or if the use of Tegretol is considered necessary during pregnancy the need to control seizures in the mother should be carefully weighed against the possible risk to the foetus. This is particularly important during the first three months of pregnancy. Minimum effective doses should be given and monitoring of plasma levels is recommended.

In women of childbearing age, Tegretol should be administered as monotherapy wherever possible.

Cases of developmental disorders and malformations, including spina bifida, have been reported in association with carbamazepine. However, offspring of mothers with untreated epilepsy are known to be prone to an increased incidence of development disorders and conclusive evidence that carbamazepine given alone, increases the risk further is not available. Patients should be counselled regarding the possibility of an increased risk of malformations and given the opportunity of antenatal screening.

In animals (mice, rats and rabbits) oral administration of carbamazepine during organogenesis led to increased embryo mortality at a daily dose which caused maternal toxicity (above 200 mg/kg b.w. daily, i.e. 20 times the usual human dosage). No evidence of a teratogenic effect was observed in the three species studied but in one study using mice, carbamazepine (40–240 mg/kg b.w. daily orally) caused defects in 4.7% of exposed foetuses compared with 1.3% in controls.

Anti-epileptic drugs may contribute to folic acid deficiency, a possible contributory cause of foetal abnormality. Folic acid supplementation is recommended before and during pregnancy.

Bleeding disorders in the new-born caused by anti-epileptic agents have been reported. As a precaution, vitamin K1 should be administered as a preventive measure in the last weeks of pregnancy and to the newborn.

Carbamazepine passes into the breast milk in concentrations of about 25–60% of the plasma level. This is not believed to present a significant hazard to the infant, which is likely to receive at most 10% of an appropriate therapeutic dose of carbamazepine for an infant with epilepsy. As with all drugs, the benefits of breast-feeding should be weighed against the remote possibility of an adverse effect occurring in the infant. There is one report of a severe skin (hypersensitivity) reaction in a breast-fed baby.

Effects on ability to drive and use machinery: The patient's reactions, e.g. as a road user, may be impaired by Tegretol, especially in the early stages of treatment. Patients should be warned of the possible hazard when driving or operating machinery.

Undesirable effects: Provided a gradually increasing dosage scheme is followed, Tegretol is generally well tolerated but side effects may occur particularly at the start of treatment, or if the initial dose is too high. Dizziness, headache, ataxia, drowsiness, fatigue, diplopia, nausea or vomiting may be symptoms of carbamazepine overdosage and usually abate within a few days either spontaneously or after a transient dosage reduction. It is advisable to monitor the plasma levels and divide the daily dosage into smaller (i.e. 3-4) fractional doses.

Central nervous system: Neurological: Frequent: Dizziness, ataxia, drowsiness, fatigue. Occasional: Headache, diplopia, accommodation disorders (blurred vision). Rare: Abnormal involuntary movements (tremor, asterixis, orofacial dyskinesia, choreoathethotic disorders, dystonia, tics), nystagmus. Isolated cases: Oculomotor disturbances, speech disorders (e.g. dysarthria or slurred speech), peripheral neuritis, paraesthesiae, muscle weakness, and paretic symptoms.

Psychiatric: Isolated cases: Hallucinations (visual or acoustic), depression, loss of appetite, restlessness, aggressive behaviour, agitation, confusion, activation or psychosis.

Skin and appendages: Occasional or frequent: Allergic skin reactions, urticaria, which may be severe. Rare: Exfoliative dermatitis and erythroderma, Stevens-Johnson syndrome, systemic lupus erythematosus-like syndrome. Isolated cases: Toxic epidermal necrolysis, photosensitivity, erythema multiforme and nodosum, alterations in skin pigmentation, purpura, pruritus, acne, sweating, hair loss, hirsutism.

Blood: Occasional or frequent: Leucopenia. Occasional: Eosinophilia, thrombocytopenia. Rare: Leucocytosis. Isolated cases: Agranulocytosis, aplastic anaemia, pure red cell aplasia, megaloblastic anaemia, acute intermittent porphyria, reticulocytosis, folic acid deficiency, and possibly haemolytic anaemia.

Liver: Frequent: Elevated gamma-GT (due to hepatic enzyme induction), usually not clinically relevant. Occasional: Elevated alkaline phosphatase, rarely transaminases. Rare: Jaundice, hepatitis of cholestatic, parenchymal (hepatocellular) or mixed type. Isolated cases: Granulomatous hepatitis.

Gastro-intestinal tract: Occasional or frequent: Nausea, vomiting. Occasional: Dryness of the mouth. Rare: Diarrhoea or constipation. Isolated cases: Abdominal pain, glossitis, stomatitis.

Hypersensitivity reactions: Rare: A delayed multi-organ hypersensitivity disorder (of serum sickness type) with fever, skin rashes, vasculitis, lymphadenopathy, disorders mimicking lymphoma, arthralgia, leucopenia, eosinophilia, hepatosplenomegaly and abnormal liver function tests, occurring in various combinations. Other organs may also be affected (e.g. lungs, kidneys, pancreas, myocardium). Isolated cases: Aseptic meningitis, with myoclonus and peripheral eosinophilia, anaphylactic reaction.

Treatment must be discontinued immediately if such hypersensitivity reactions occur.

Cardiovascular system: Rare: Disturbances of cardiac conduction. Isolated cases: Bradycardia, arrhythmias, AV-block with syncope, collapse, congestive heart failure, hypertension or hypotension, aggravation of coronary artery disease, thrombophlebitis, thrombo-embolism.

Endocrine system and metabolism: Occasional: Hyponatraemia, fluid retention, oedema, weight gain, and reduced plasma osmolality due to an antidiuretic hormone (ADH)-like effect, leading in isolated cases to water intoxication accompanied by lethargy, vomiting, headache, mental confusion, neurological abnormalities. Isolated cases: Gynaecomastia or galactorrhoea. Impaired male fertility and/or abnormal spermatogenesis. Loss of libido/impotence. Abnormal thyroid function tests: decreased L-thyroxine (FT4, T4, T3) and increased TSH, usually without clinical manifestations. Disturbances of bone metabolism (decrease in plasma calcium and 25-OH-cholecalciferol), leading to osteomalacia. Elevated levels of cholesterol, including HDL cholesterol, and triglycerides.

Renal: Isolated cases: Interstitial nephritis and renal failure, signs of renal dysfunction including albuminuria, haematuria, oliguria and elevated bun/azotaemia, urinary frequency, urinary retention.

Sense organs: Isolated cases: Taste disturbances; lens opacities, conjunctivitis, tinnitus, hyperacusis.

Musculoskeletal system: Isolated cases: Arthralgia, muscle pain or cramp.

Respiratory tract: Isolated cases: Pulmonary hypersensitivity characterised by dyspnoea, pneumonitis or pneumonia.

Overdose

Signs and symptoms: The presenting signs and symptoms of overdosage involve the central nervous, cardiovascular or respiratory systems. Central nervous system: CNS depression; disorientation, somnolence, agitation, hallucination, coma; blurred vision, slurred speech, dysarthria, nystagmus, ataxia, dyskinesia, initially hyperreflexia, later hyporeflexia; convulsions, psychomotor disturbances, myoclonus, hypothermia.

Respiratory system: Respiratory depression, pulmonary oedema.

Cardiovascular system: Tachycardia, changes in blood pressure (hypotension and at times hypertension), cardiac arrhythmias, conduction disturbance with widening of QRS complex; syncope.

Gastro-intestinal system: Vomiting, delayed gastric emptying, reduced bowel motility.

Renal function: Retention of urine, oliguria or anuria; fluid retention, water intoxication due to ADH-like effect of carbamazepine.

Laboratory findings: Hyponatraemia, possibly metabolic acidosis, possibly hyperglycaemia, increased muscle creatinine phosphokinase.

Treatment: There is no specific antidote. Management according to the patient's clinical condition. Possible admission to hospital. Measurement of the plasma level to confirm carbamazepine poisoning and to ascertain the size of the overdose. Evacuation of the stomach, gastric lavage, and administration of activated charcoal. Supportive medical care in an intensive care unit with cardiac monitoring and careful correction of electrolyte imbalance, if required.

Special recommendations: Hypotension: Administer dopamine or dobutamine i.v.

Disturbances of cardiac rhythm: To be managed on an individual basis.

Convulsions: Administer a benzodiazepine (e.g. diazepam) or another anticonvulsant, e.g. phenobarbitone (with caution because of increased respiratory depression) or paraldehyde.

Hyponatraemia (water intoxication): Fluid restriction and slow careful NaCl 0.9% infusion i.v. These measures may be useful in preventing brain damage.

Charcoal haemoperfusion has been recommended. Forced diuresis, haemodialysis, and peritoneal dialysis have been reported not to be effective.

Relapse and aggravation of symptomatology on the 2nd and 3rd day after overdose, due to delayed absorption, should be anticipated.

Pharmacological properties

Pharmacodynamic properties: Mode of action: Carbamazepine is a dibenzazepine derivative with anti-epileptic, neurotropic and psychotropic properties.

The mechanism of action of carbamazepine has only been partially elucidated. It is conceivable that blockade of voltage-sensitive sodium channels may be one or even the main primary effect of carbamazepine.

Pharmacokinetic properties: Absorption: Carbamazepine is almost completely absorbed but the rate of absorption from the tablets is slow and may vary amongst the various formulations and between patients. Peak plasma concentrations of the unchanged active substance after administration of single doses of Tegretol syrup are attained at 2 hours.

The bioavailability of Tegretol in various oral formulations has been shown to lie between 85–100%. Bioavailability is unaffected by food.

Distribution: The concentration of unchanged substance in the CSF and saliva represents the unbound portion in plasma, i.e. 20–30% of total plasma concentration, breast milk 25–60% of total plasma concentration. Carbamazepine crosses the placental barrier. Apparent volume of distribution 0.8–1.5 L/kg.

Serum protein binding: 70–80%.

Biotransformation: Carbamazepine is extensively metabolised in the liver, mainly by oxidative pathways and the greater part is excreted as the inactive glucuronide with up to 40% as metabolites, of which only carbamazepine epoxide is pharmacologically active. This may constitute up to 30% of the circulating active material originating as carbamazepine; in particular polytherapy is an important factor in augmenting epoxide levels. The inactive 10,11-diol represents the final stage of carbamazepine biotransformation. Only about 3% of pharmacologically active material (unchanged plus epoxide) is excreted.

In advanced hepatic disease carbamazepine metabolism may be impaired.

Elimination: The elimination half-life of unchanged drug in the plasma averages approximately 36 hours following a single dose, whereas after repeated administration, which leads to auto-induction of hepatic enzymes, it averages only 16–24 hours, depending on the duration of the medication. In patients receiving co-medication with other enzyme-inducing drugs (phenytoin, phenobarbitone) half-life values averaging 9–10 hours have been observed. The therapeutic plasma concentration range of carbamazepine at steady state is usually between 4–12 mcg/ml (17–50 μmol/l).

Characteristics in patients: The pharmacokinetics of carbamazepine are unaltered in the elderly but its metabolism may be affected by hepatic dysfunction (see above). In children the relatively high rate of metabolism of the drug may require higher doses (in mg/kg b.w.) of carbamazepine to maintain therapeutic concentrations.

Preclinical safety data: None relevant.

Pharmaceutical particulars

List of excipients: Cremophor S9, Avicel RC581, sorbitol solution 70%, saccharin sodium, Natrosol 250 g, methyl hydroxybenzoate, propyl hydroxybenzoate, sorbic acid, propylene glycol, caramel flavour 52.929A (E150), purified water.

Incompatibilities: None known.

Shelf life: Five years.

Special precautions for storage: Protect from heat (store below 25°C). Keep container tightly closed.

Nature and contents of container: Tegretol Liquid is a white suspension. It comes in a 300 ml amber glass bottle with either a conventional cap, child resistant/tamper evident cap, tamper evident cap or child resistant cap.

Instructions for use/handling: None.

Marketing authorisation holder: Novartis Pharmaceuticals UK Limited: Trading as Geigy Pharmaceuticals, Frimley Business Park, Frimley, Camberley, Surrey GU16 5SG.

Marketing authorisation number PL 00101/0456.

Date of first authorisation 4 July 1997.

Date of (partial) revision of the text 14.01.98.

Legal category POM.

TEGRETOL RETARD TABLETS 200 mg and 400 mg

Qualitative and quantitative composition The active ingredient is 5-Carbamoyl-5-H-dibenz(b,f)azepine.

Each coated tablet contains 200 mg or 400 mg carbamazepine PhEur.

Pharmaceutical form The 200 mg tablets are beige-orange, oval, slightly biconvex, coated tablets with a score on each side. One side bears the imprint 'H/C', the other 'C/G'.

The 400 mg tablets are brownish-orange, oval, slightly biconvex coated tablets with a score on each side. One side bears the imprint 'ENE/ENE', the other 'C/G'.

Clinical particulars

Therapeutic indications: Epilepsy – generalised tonic-clonic and partial seizures. Tegretol Retard is indicated in newly diagnosed patients with epilepsy and in those patients who are uncontrolled or unable to tolerate their current anti-convulsant therapy.

Note: Carbamazepine is not usually effective in absences (petit mal). Moreover, anecdotal evidence suggests that seizure exacerbation may occur in patients with atypical absences.

The paroxysmal pain of trigeminal neuralgia.

For the prophylaxis of manic-depressive psychoses in patients unresponsive to lithium therapy.

Posology and method of administration: Tegretol Retard is given orally, generally in the same total daily dose as conventional Tegretol dosage forms but usually in two divided doses. In a few patients when changing from other oral dosage forms of Tegretol to Tegretol Retard the total daily dose may need to be increased, particularly when it is used in polytherapy. When starting treatment with Tegretol Retard in monotherapy, 100–200 mg once or twice daily is recommended. This may be followed by a slow increase in dosage until the best response is obtained, often 800–1,200 mg daily. In some instances, 1,600 mg or even 2,000 mg daily may be necessary.

Tegretol Retard (either the whole or half divisible tablet as prescribed), should *not* be chewed but should be swallowed with a little liquid, before, during or between meals. The divisible tablet presentation enables flexibility of dosing to be achieved.

Epilepsy: Adults: It is advised that with all formulations of Tegretol, a gradually increasing dosage scheme is used and this should be adjusted to suit the needs of the individual patient. It may be helpful to monitor the plasma concentration of carbamazepine to establish the optimum dose (see *Pharmacokinetics, Precautions* and *Interactions*).

Elderly: There is no evidence to suggest that dosage requirements are different in the elderly but it is recommended that the intitial dose be small.

Children: It is advised that with all formulations of Tegretol, a gradually increasing dosage scheme is used and this should be adjusted to suit the needs of the individual patient. It may be helpful to monitor the plasma concentration of carbamazepine to establish the optimum dose (see *Pharmacokinetics, Precautions* and *Interactions*).

Usual dosage 10–20 mg/kg bodyweight daily in several divided doses.

Age		
	up to 5 years:	Tegretol Retard Tablets are not recommended
	5–10 years:	400–600 mg daily
	10–15 years:	600–1,000 mg

Wherever possible, Tegretol Retard should be used as the sole drug anti-epileptic agent but if used in polytherapy, the same incremental dosage pattern is advised.

Trigeminal neuralgia: The individual dosage requirements of Tegretol vary considerably. It is recommended that the initial dose be small but in some patients a high dose early in treatment may be required. In elderly patients, an initial dose of 100 mg twice daily is recommended.

The dose may be increased gradually until a satisfactory clinical response is obtained, which in some instances necessitates 1,600 mg Tegretol daily. It has been found that in the majority of patients a dosage of 200 mg three or four times a day is sufficient to maintain a pain-free state. When pain goes into remission the dose may be gradually reduced and Tegretol discontinued in the absence of recurrence.

For the prophylaxis of manic depressive psychosis in patients unresponsive to lithium therapy: Initial starting dose of 400 mg daily, in divided doses, increasing gradually until symptoms are controlled or a total of 1,600 mg given in divided doses is reached. The usual dosage range is 400–600 mg daily, given in divided doses.

Contra-indications: Previous drug sensitivity to carbamazepine or structurally related drugs, e.g. tricyclic antidepressants. Because Tegretol depresses AV-conduction, it is inadvisable to administer this drug to patients with atrioventricular conduction abnormalities. Patients with a history of previous bone marrow depression or a history of intermittent porphyria. On theoretical grounds, i.e. a structural relationship to tricyclic antidepressants, the use of Tegretol is not recommended in combination with monoamine oxidase inhibitors (MAOIs); before administering Tegretol, MAOIs should be discontinued for a minimum of 2 weeks, or longer if the clinical situation permits.

Special warnings and special precautions for use:

Warnings: Agranulocytosis and aplastic anaemia have been associated with Tegretol; however, due to the very low incidence of these diseases, meaningful risk estimates for Tegretol are difficult to obtain. The overall risk in the general untreated population has been estimated at 4.7 persons per million per year for agranulocytosis and 2.0 persons per million per year for aplastic anaemia.

Blood counts, platelet count and serum biochemistry including electrolytes and indices of hepatic function should be checked before commencing treatment with Tegretol. Blood counts should be performed before and periodically during treatment. Clinical monitoring is of primary importance during the whole treatment.

Patients and their relatives should be informed on how to recognise early toxic signs and symptoms indicative of a potential haematological problem, or of dermatological or hepatic reactions. If reactions such as fever, sore throat, rash, ulcers in the mouth, easy bruising, petechial or purpuric haemorrhage appear, the patient should be advised to consult his physician immediately.

Non-progressive or fluctuating asymptomatic leucopenia, which occurs in about 10% of treated patients does not generally call for withdrawal of Tegretol. However, treatment with Tegretol should be discontinued if the patient develops leucopenia which is severe, progressive or accompanied by clinical manifestations, e.g. fever or sore throat. Tegretol should be discontinued if any evidence of significant bone marrow depression appears.

Liver function tests should also be performed before commencing treatment and periodically thereafter, particularly in patients with a history of liver disease and in elderly patients.

Some liver function tests in patients receiving carbamazepine may be found to be abnormal, particularly gamma glutamyl transferase. This is probably due to hepatic enzyme induction. Enzyme induction may also produce modest elevations in alkaline phosphatase. These enhancements of hepatic metabolising capacity are not an indication for the withdrawal of carbamazepine.

Severe hepatic reactions to carbamazepine occur very rarely. The development of signs and symptoms of liver dysfunction or active liver disease should be urgently evaluated and treatment with Tegretol suspended pending the outcome of the evaluation.

Mild skin reactions, e.g. isolated macular or maculopapular exanthemata, are mostly transient and not hazardous, and they usually disappear within a few days. However, the patient should be kept under close surveillance and a worsening rash or accompanying symptoms are an indication for the immediate withdrawal of Tegretol. Severe skin reactions, e.g. Stevens-Johnson syndrome and Lyell's syndrome (toxic epidermal necrolysis), also necessitate immediate withdrawal.

If treatment with Tegretol has to be withdrawn abruptly, the changeover to another anti-epileptic drug should if necessary be effected under the cover of a suitable drug, e.g. i.v. or rectal benzodiazepines, or i.v. phenytoin.

The induction of hepatic enzymes by carbamazepine may reduce the activity of the hormones contained in the combined oral contraceptive pill. This may appear clinically as breakthrough bleeding or spotting. Patients taking Tegretol and requiring oral contraception should receive a preparation containing not less than 50 mcg oestrogen or use of some alternative non-hormonal method of contraception should be considered.

Although correlations between dosages and plasma levels of carbamazepine, and between plasma levels and clinical efficacy or tolerability are rather tenuous, serum level monitoring of carbamazepine may prove useful during stabilisation, for optimum seizure control and in particular situations, e.g. pregnancy, for verification of compliance, in suspected toxicity and when carbamazepine is used in polytherapy.

In rats treated with carbamazepine for two years, the incidence of tumours of the liver was found to be increased. There is, however, no evidence to indicate that this observation has any significant bearing on the therapeutic use of the drug.

Precautions: Tegretol should be prescribed only after a critical benefit-risk appraisal and under close monitoring in patients with a history of cardiac, hepatic or renal damage, adverse haematological reactions to other drugs, or interrupted courses of therapy with Tegretol.

Baseline and periodic complete urinalysis and BUN determinations are recommended.

Tegretol has shown mild anticholinergic activity; patients with glaucoma should therefore be warned and advised regarding possible hazards.

The possibility of activation of a latent psychosis, and in elderly patients the possibility of agitation or confusion, especially when high doses of Tegretol are administered, should be borne in mind.

Interaction with other medicaments and other forms of interaction: Induction of hepatic enzymes in response to Tegretol may increase the metabolism and reduce the effectiveness of certain other drugs that are metabolised in the liver including: clobazam, clonazepam, ethosuximide, primidone, valproic acid, alprazolam, corticosteroids, hormonal contraceptive agents, cyclosporin, digoxin, doxycycline, felodipine, haloperidol, imipramine, methadone, theophylline, warfarin. The concurrent administration of carbamazepine has been reported to both raise and lower phenytoin levels and in rare instances mephenytoin plasma levels have been reported to increase.

Certain drugs have been shown to increase carbamazepine serum levels: macrolide antibiotics (erythromycin), isoniazid, calcium antagonists (verapamil, diltiazem), dextropropoxyphene, viloxazine, fluoxetine, cimetidine, acetazolamide, danazol, possibly desipramine and nicotinamide (only in adults and at high doses). Since raised carbamazepine levels may produce signs of overdosage (e.g. dizziness, drowsiness, ataxia, diplopia), the dosage of Tegretol should be adjusted accordingly.

Concomitant use of carbamazepine and isoniazid has been reported to increase isoniazid hepatotoxicity.

The combination of lithium and carbamazepine may cause enhanced neurotoxicity in spite of lithium plasma concentrations being within the therapeutic range.

Combined use of carbamazepine with metoclopramide or major tranquillisers, e.g. haloperidol, thioridazine, may also result in an increase in neurological side-effects.

Plasma levels of carbamazepine may be reduced by phenobarbitone, phenytoin, primidone, theophylline, also possibly clonazepam, and valproic acid (the data on the latter two compounds are contradictory).

Valproic acid, valpromide and primidone have been reported to increase the degree of conversion of carbamazepine to the active metabolite carbamazepine-10,11-epoxide.

Concomitant medication with Tegretol and some diuretics (hydrochlorothiazide, frusemide) may lead to symptomatic hyponatraemia.

Carbamazepine may antagonise the effects of non-depolarising muscle relaxants (e.g. pancuronium); their dosage may need to be raised and patients monitored closely for unexpectedly rapid recovery from neuromuscular blockade.

Isotretinoin has been reported to alter the bioavailability and/or clearance of carbamazepine and carbamazepine-10,11-epoxide; carbamazepine plasma concentrations should be monitored.

Alcohol may exacerbate the CNS side-effects of psychoactive drugs including Tegretol; it is therefore advised that patients abstain from alcohol during treatment.

Pregnancy and lactation: If pregnancy occurs in a woman receiving Tegretol or if the use of Tegretol is considered necessary during pregnancy the need to control seizures in the mother should be carefully weighed against the possible risk to the foetus. This is particularly important during the first three months of pregnancy. Minimum effective doses should be given and monitoring of plasma levels is recommended.

In women of childbearing age, Tegretol should be administered as monotherapy, wherever possible.

Cases of developmental disorders and malformations, including spina bifida, have been reported in association with carbamazepine. However, offspring of mothers with untreated epilepsy are known to be prone to an increased incidence of development disorders and conclusive evidence that carbamazepine given alone, increases the risk further is not available. Patients should be counselled regarding the possibility of an increased risk of malformations and given the opportunity of antenatal screening.

In animals (mice, rats and rabbits) oral administration of carbamazepine during organogenesis led to increased embryo mortality at a daily dose which caused maternal toxicity (above 200 mg/kg b.w. daily, i.e. 20 times the usual human dosage). No evidence of a teratogenic effect was observed in the three species studied but in one study using mice carbamazepine (40–240 mg/kg b.w. daily orally) caused defects in 4.7% of exposed foetuses compared with 1.3% in controls.

Anti-epileptic drugs may contribute to folic acid deficiency, a possible contributory cause of foetal abnormality. Folic acid supplementation is recommended before and during pregnancy.

Bleeding disorders in the new-born caused by anti-epileptic agents have been reported. As a precaution, vitamin K1 should be administered as a preventive measure in the last weeks of pregnancy and to the newborn.

Carbamazepine passes into the breast milk in concentrations of about 25–60% of the plasma level. This is not believed to present a significant hazard to the infant, which is likely to receive at most 10% of an appropriate therapeutic dose of carbamazepine for an infant with epilepsy. As with all drugs, the benefits of breast-feeding should be weighed against the remote possibility of an adverse effect occurring in the infant. There is one report of a severe skin (hypersensitivity) reaction in a breast-fed baby.

Effects on ability to drive and use machinery: The patient's reactions, e.g. as a road user, may be impaired by Tegretol, especially in the early stages of treatment. Patients should be warned of the possible hazard when driving or operating machinery.

Undesirable effects: Provided a gradually increasing dosage scheme is followed, Tegretol is generally well tolerated but side effects may occur particularly at the start of treatment, or if the initial dose is too high. Dizziness, headache, ataxia, drowsiness, fatigue, diplopia, nausea or vomiting may be symptoms of carbamazepine overdosage and usually abate within a few days either spontaneously or after a transient dosage reduction. It is advisable to monitor the plasma levels and divide the daily dosage into smaller (i.e. 3–4) fractional doses.

Central nervous system: Neurological: Frequent: Dizziness, ataxia, drowsiness, fatigue.

Occasional: Headache, diplopia, accommodation disorders (blurred vision).

Rare: Abnormal involuntary movements (tremor, asterixis, orofacial dyskinesia, choreoathethotic disorders, dystonia, tics), nystagmus.

Isolated cases: Oculomotor disturbances, speech disorders (e.g. dysarthria or slurred speech), peripheral neuritis, paraesthesiae, muscle weakness, and paretic symptoms.

Psychiatric: Isolated cases: Hallucinations (visual or acoustic), depression, loss of appetite, restlessness, aggressive behaviour, agitation, confusion, activation or psychosis.

Skin and appendages: Occasional or frequent: Allergic skin reactions, urticaria, which may be severe. Rare: Exfoliative dermatitis and erythroderma, Stevens-Johnson syndrome, systemic lupus erythematosus-like syndrome.

Isolated cases: Toxic epidermal necrolysis, photosensitivity, erythema multiforme and nodosum, alterations in skin pigmentation, purpura, pruritus, acne, sweating, hair loss, hirsutism.

Blood: Occasional or frequent: Leucopenia. Occasional: Eosinophilia, thrombocytopenia. Rare: Leucocytosis. Isolated cases: Agranulocytosis, aplastic anaemia, pure red cell aplasia, megaloblastic anaemia, acute intermittent porphyria, reticulocytosis, folic acid deficiency, and possibly haemolytic anaemia.

Liver: Frequent: Elevated gamma-GT (due to hepatic enzyme induction), usually not clinically relevant. Occasional: Elevated alkaline phosphatase, rarely transaminases. Rare: Jaundice, hepatitis of cholestatic, parenchymal (hepatocellular), or mixed type. Isolated cases: Granulomatous hepatitis.

Gastro-intestinal tract: Occasional or frequent: Nausea, vomiting. Occasional: Dryness of the mouth, Rare: Diarrhoea or constipation. Isolated cases: Abdominal pain, glossitis, stomatitis.

Hypersensitivity reactions: Rare: A delayed multi-organ hypersensitivity disorder (of serum sickness type) with fever, skin rashes, vasculitis, lymphadenopathy, disorders mimicking lymphoma, arthralgia, leucopenia, eosinophilia, hepatosplenomegaly and abnormal liver function tests, occurring in various combinations. Other organs may also be affected (e.g. lungs, kidneys, pancreas, myocardium). Isolated cases: Aseptic meningitis, with myoclonus and peripheral eosinophilia, anaphylactic reaction.

Treatment must be discontinued immediately if such hypersensitivity reactions occur.

Cardiovascular system: Rare: Disturbances of cardiac conduction. Isolated cases: Bradycardia, arrhythmias, AV-block with syncope, collapse, congestive heart failure, hypertension or hypotension, aggravation of coronary artery disease, thrombophlebitis, thrombo-embolism.

Endocrine system and metabolism: Occasional: Hyponatraemia, fluid retention, oedema, weight gain, and reduced plasma osmolality due to an antidiuretic hormone (ADH)-like effect, leading in isolated cases to water intoxication accompanied by lethargy, vomiting, headache, mental confusion, neurological abnormalities. Isolated cases: Gynaecomastia or galactorrhoea. Impaired male fertility and/or abnormal spermatogenesis. Loss of libido/impotence. Abnormal thyroid function tests: decreased L-thyroxine (FT4, T4, T3) and increased TSH, usually without clinical manifestations. Disturbances of bone metabolism (decrease in plasma calcium and 25-OH-cholecalciferol), leading to osteomalacia. Elevated levels of cholesterol, including HDL cholesterol, and triglycerides.

Renal: Isolated cases: Interstitial nephritis and renal failure, signs of renal dysfunction including albuminuria, haematuria, oliguria and elevated bun/azotaemia, urinary frequency, urinary retention.

Sense organs: Isolated cases: Taste disturbances; lens opacities, conjunctivitis, tinnitus, hyperacusis.

Musculoskeletal system: Isolated cases: Arthralgia, muscle pain or cramp.

Respiratory tract: Isolated cases: Pulmonary hypersensitivity characterised by dyspnoea, pneumonitis or pneumonia.

Overdose

Signs and symptoms: The presenting signs and symptoms of overdosage involve the central nervous, cardiovascular or respiratory systems.

Central nervous system: CNS depression; disorientation, somnolence, agitation, hallucination, coma; blurred vision, slurred speech, dysarthria, nystagmus, ataxia, dyskinesia, initially hyperreflexia, later hyporeflexia; convulsions, psychomotor disturbances, myoclonus, hypothermia.

Respiratory system: Respiratory depression, pulmonary oedema.

Cardiovascular system: Tachycardia, changes in blood pressure (hypotension and at times hypertension), cardiac arrhythmias, conduction disturbance with widening of QRS complex; syncope.

Gastro-intestinal system: Vomiting, delayed gastric emptying, reduced bowel motility.

Renal function: Retention of urine, oliguria or anuria; fluid retention, water intoxication due to ADH-like effect of carbamazepine.

Laboratory findings: Hyponatraemia, possibly metabolic acidosis, possibly hyperglycaemia, increased muscle creatinine phosphokinase.

Treatment: There is no specific antidote. Management according to the patient's clinical condition. Possible admission to hospital. Measurement of the plasma level to confirm carbamazepine poisoning and to ascertain the size of the overdose. Evacuation of the stomach, gastric lavage and administration of activated charcoal. Supportive medical care in an intensive care unit with cardiac monitoring and careful correction of electrolyte imbalance, if required.

Special recommendations: Hypotension: Administer dopamine or dobutamine i.v.

Disturbances of cardiac rhythm: To be managed on an individual basis.

Convulsions: Administer a benzodiazepine (e.g. diazepam) or another anticonvulsant, e.g. phenobarbitone (with caution because of increased respiratory depression) or paraldehyde.

Hyponatraemia (water intoxication): Fluid restriction and slow careful NaCl 0.9% infusion i.v. These measures may be useful in preventing brain damage.

Charcoal haemoperfusion has been recommended. Forced diuresis, haemodialysis and peritoneal dialysis have been reported not to be effective.

Relapse and aggravation of symptomatology on the 2nd and 3rd day after overdose, due to delayed absorption, should be anticipated.

Pharmacological properties

Pharmacodynamic properties: Mode of action: Carbamazepine is a dibenzazepine derivative with anti-epileptic, neurotropic and psychotropic properties.

The mechanism of action of carbamazepine has only been partially elucidated. It is conceivable that blockade of voltage-sensitive sodium channels may be one or even the main primary effect of carbamazepine.

Pharmacokinetic properties: Absorption: Carbamazepine is almost completely absorbed but the rate of absorption from the tablets is slow and may vary amongst the various formulations and between patients. Peak concentrations of active substance in the plasma are attained within 24 hours of administration of single dose of Tegretol Retard tablets.

The retard formulation shows about 15% lower bioavailability than standard preparations due mainly to the considerable reduction in peak plasma levels occasioned by controlled release of the same dosage of carbamazepine. Plasma concentrations show less fluctuation but auto-induction of carbamazepine occurs as with standard carbamazepine preparations.

The bioavailability of Tegretol in various oral formulations has been shown to lie between 85–100%. Bioavailability is unaffected by food.

Distribution: The concentration of unchanged substance in the CSF and saliva represents the unbound portion in plasma, i.e. 20–30% of total plasma concentration, breast milk 25–60% of total plasma concentration. Carbamazepine crosses the placental barrier. Apparent volume of distribution 0.8–1.5 L/kg.

Serum protein binding: 70–80%.

Biotransformation: Carbamazepine is extensively metabolised in the liver, mainly by oxidative pathways and the greater part is excreted as the inactive glucuronide with up to 40% as metabolites, of which only carbamazepine epoxide is pharmacologically active. This may constitute up to 30% of the circulating active material originating as carbamazepine; in particular polytherapy is an important factor in augmenting epoxide levels. The inactive 10,11-diol represents the final stage of carbamazepine biotransformation. Only about 3% of pharmacologically active material (unchanged plus epoxide) is excreted.

In advanced hepatic disease carbamazepine metabolism may be impaired.

Elimination: The elimination half-life of unchanged drug in the plasma averages approximately 36 hours following a single dose, whereas after repeated administration, which leads to auto-induction of hepatic enzymes, it averages only 16–24 hours, depending on the duration of the medication. In patients receiving co-medication with other enzyme-inducing drugs (phenytoin, phenobarbitone) half-life values averaging 9–10 hours have been observed. The therapeutic plasma concentration range of carbamazepine at steady state is usually between 4–12 mcg/ml (17–50 μmol/l).

Characteristics in patients: The pharmacokinetics of carbamazepine are unaltered in the elderly but its metabolism may be affected by hepatic dysfunction (see above). In children the relatively high rate of metabolism of the drug may require higher doses (in mg/kg b.w.) of carbamazepine to maintain therapeutic concentrations.

Preclinical safety data: None relevant.

Pharmaceutical particulars

List of excipients: Each 200 mg and 400 mg tablet contains colloidal silicon dioxide, ethylcellulose pseudolatex, microcrystalline cellulose, ethyl acrylate/methyl methacrylate copolymer, magnesium stearate, croscarmellose sodium type A, talc, hydroxypropylmethylcellulose, glyceryl polyoxyethylene glycol stearate, red iron oxide (E.172), yellow iron oxide (E.172) and titanium dioxide (E.171).

Incompatibilities: None known.

Shelf life: Three years.

Special precautions for storage: Store below 25°C and protect from moisture.

Nature and contents of container: Tegretol Retard Tablets 200 mg and 400 mg come in PVC/PCTFE (PVC 190–270 micron; PCTFE 15–25 micron; aluminium foil 26–34 micron) or PCV/PE/PVdC (PVC 190–270 micron; PE 20–40 micron; PVdC 32–59 micron; aluminium foil 26–34 micron) blister packs of 56 tablets.

Instructions for use/handling: None.

Marketing authorisation holder: Novartis Pharmaceuticals UK Limited, Trading as Geigy Pharmaceuticals, Frimley Business Park, Frimley, Camberley, Surrey GU16 5SG.

Marketing authorisation numbers

Tegretol Retard Tablets 200 mg: PL 00101/0457
Tegretol Retard Tablets 400 mg: PL 00101/0458

Date of first authorisation 4 July 1997.

Date of (partial) revision of the text 23.01.98.

Legal category POM.

TEGRETOL SUPPOSITORIES 125 mg and 250 mg

Qualitative and quantitative composition The active ingredient is 5-Carbamoyl-5-H-dibenz(b,f)azepine.

Each suppository contains 125 mg or 250 mg carbamazepine PhEur.

Pharmaceutical form White to practically white, torpedo-shaped suppositories.

Clinical particulars

Therapeutic indications: Epilepsy – generalised tonic-clonic and partial seizures.

Note: Tegretol is not usually effective in absences (petit mal). Moreover, anecdotal evidence suggests that seizure exacerbation may occur in patients with atypical absences.

No clinical data are available on the use of Tegretol Suppositories in indications other than epilepsy.

Posology and method of administration: Epilepsy in Adults, Elderly and Children: 125 mg and 250 mg suppositories are available for short-term use as replacement therapy (maximum period recommended: 7 days) in patients for whom oral treatment is temporarily not possible, for example in post-operative or unconscious subjects.

When switching from oral formulations to suppositories the dosage should be increased by approximately 25% (the 125 and 250 mg suppositories correspond to 100 and 200 mg tablets respectively).

The final dose adjustment should always depend on the clinical response in the individual patient (plasma level monitoring is recommended). Tegretol Suppositories have been shown to provide plasma levels which are well within the therapeutic range (see *Pharmacokinetics*).

Where suppositories are used the maximum daily dose is limited to 1,000 mg (250 mg qid at 6 hour intervals, see *Pharmacokinetics*).

Route of administration: Rectal.

Contra-indications: Previous drug sensitivity to carbamazepine or structurally related drugs, e.g. tricyclic antidepressants. Because Tegretol depresses AV-conduction, it is inadvisable to administer this drug to patients with atrioventricular conduction abnormalities. Patients with a history of previous bone marrow depression or a history of intermittent porphyria. On theoretical grounds, i.e. a structural relationship to tricyclic antidepressants, the use of Tegretol is not recommended in combination with monoamine oxidase inhibitors (MAOIs); before administering Tegretol, MAOIs should be discontinued for a minimum of 2 weeks, or longer if the clinical situation permits.

Special warnings and special precautions for use

Warnings: Agranulocytosis and aplastic anaemia have been associated with Tegretol; however, due to the very low incidence of these diseases, meaningful risk estimates for Tegretol are difficult to obtain. The overall risk in the general untreated population has been estimated at 4.7 persons per million per year for agranulocytosis and 2.0 persons per million per year for aplastic anaemia.

Blood counts, platelet count and serum biochemistry including electrolytes and indices of hepatic function should be checked before commencing treatment with Tegretol. Blood counts should be performed before and periodically during treatment. Clinical monitoring is of primary importance during the whole treatment.

Patients and their relatives should be informed on how to recognise early toxic signs and symptoms indicative of a potential haematological problem, or of dermatological or hepatic reactions. If reactions such as fever, sore throat, rash, ulcers in the mouth, easy bruising, petechial or purpuric haemorrhage appear, the patient should be advised to consult his physician immediately.

Non-progressive or fluctuating asymptomatic leucopenia, which occurs in about 10% of treated patients does not generally call for withdrawal of Tegretol. However, treatment with Tegretol should be discontinued if the patient develops leucopenia which is severe, progressive or accompanied by clinical manifestations, e.g. fever or sore throat. Tegretol should be discontinued if any evidence of significant bone marrow depression appears.

Liver function tests should also be performed before commencing treatment and periodically thereafter, particularly in patients with a history of liver disease and in elderly patients.

Some liver function tests in patients receiving carbamazepine may be found to be abnormal, particularly gamma glutamyl transferase. This is probably due to hepatic enzyme induction. Enzyme induction may also produce modest elevations in alkaline phosphatase. These enhancements of hepatic metabolising capacity are not an indication for the withdrawal of carbamazepine.

Severe hepatic reactions to carbamazepine occur very rarely. The development of signs and symptoms of liver dysfunction or active liver disease should be urgently evaluated and treatment with Tegretol suspended pending the outcome of the evaluation.

Mild skin reactions, e.g. isolated macular or maculopapular exanthemata, are mostly transient and not hazardous, and they usually disappear within a few days. However, the patient should be kept under close surveillance and a worsening rash or accompanying symptoms are an indication for the immediate withdrawal of Tegretol. Severe skin reactions, e.g. Stevens-Johnson syndrome, Lyell's syndrome (toxic epidermal necrolysis), also necessitate immediate withdrawal.

If treatment with Tegretol has to be withdrawn abruptly, the changeover to another anti-epileptic drug should if necessary be effected under the cover of a suitable drug, e.g. i.v. or rectal benzodiazepines, or i.v. phenytoin.

The induction of hepatic enzymes by carbamazepine may reduce the activity of the hormones contained in the combined oral contraceptive pill. This may appear clinically as breakthrough bleeding or spotting. Patients taking Tegretol and requiring oral contraception should receive a preparation containing not less than 50 mcg oestrogen or use of some alternative non-hormonal method of contraception should be considered.

Although correlations between dosages and plasma levels of carbamazepine, and between plasma levels and clinical efficacy or tolerability are rather tenuous, serum level monitoring of carbamazepine may prove useful during stabilisation, for optimum seizure control and in particular situations, e.g. pregnancy, for verification of compliance, in suspected toxicity and when carbamazepine is used in polytherapy.

In rats treated with carbamazepine for two years, the incidence of tumours of the liver was found to be increased. There is, however, no evidence to indicate that this observation has any significant bearing on the therapeutic use of the drug.

Precautions: Tegretol should be prescribed only after a critical benefit-risk appraisal and under close monitoring in patients with a history of cardiac, hepatic or renal damage, adverse haematological reactions to other drugs, or interrupted courses of therapy with Tegretol.

Baseline and periodic complete urinalysis and BUN determinations are recommended.

Tegretol has shown mild anticholinergic activity; patients with glaucoma should therefore be warned and advised regarding possible hazards.

The possibility of activation of a latent psychosis, and in elderly patients the possibility of agitation or confusion, especially when high doses of Tegretol are administered, should be borne in mind.

Interaction with other medicaments and other forms of interaction: Induction of hepatic enzymes in response to Tegretol may increase the metabolism and reduce the effectiveness of certain other drugs that are metabolised in the liver including: clobazam, clonazepam, ethosuximide, primidone, valproic acid, alprazolam, corticosteroids, hormonal contraceptive agents, cyclosporin, digoxin, doxycycline, felodipine, haloperidol, imipramine, methadone, theophylline, warfarin. The concurrent administration of carbamazepine has been reported to both raise and lower phenytoin levels and in rare instances mephenytoin plasma levels have been reported to increase.

Certain drugs have been shown to increase carbamazepine serum levels: macrolide antibiotics (erythromycin), isoniazid, calcium antagonists (verapamil, diltiazem), dextropropoxyphene, viloxazine, fluoxetine, cimetidine, acetazolamide, danazol, possibly desipramine and nicotinamide (only in adults and at high doses). Since raised carbamazepine levels may produce signs of overdosage (e.g. dizziness, drowsiness, ataxia, diplopia), the dosage of Tegretol should be adjusted accordingly.

Concomitant use of carbamazepine and isoniazid has been reported to increase isoniazid hepatotoxicity.

The combination of lithium and carbamazepine may cause enhanced neurotoxicity in spite of lithium plasma concentrations being within the therapeutic range.

Combined use of carbamazepine with metoclopramide or major tranquillisers, e.g. haloperidol, thioridazine may also result in an increase in neurological side-effects.

Plasma levels of carbamazepine may be reduced by phenobarbitone, phenytoin, primidone, theophylline, also possibly clonazepam, and valproic acid (the data on the latter two compounds are contradictory).

Valproic acid, valpromide and primidone have been reported to increase the degree of conversion of carbamazepine to the active metabolite carbamazepine-10,11-epoxide.

Concomitant medication with Tegretol and some diuretics (hydrochlorothiazide, frusemide) may lead to symptomatic hyponatraemia.

Carbamazepine may antagonise the effects of non-depolarising muscle relaxants (e.g. pancuronium); their dosage may need to be raised and patients monitored closely for unexpectedly rapid recovery from neuromuscular blockade.

Isotretinoin has been reported to alter the bioavailability and/or clearance of carbamazepine and carbamazepine-10,11-epoxide; carbamazepine plasma concentrations should be monitored.

Alcohol may exacerbate the CNS side-effects of psychoactive drugs including Tegretol; it is therefore advised that patients abstain from alcohol during treatment.

Pregnancy and lactation: If pregnancy occurs in a woman receiving Tegretol or if the use of Tegretol is considered necessary during pregnancy the need to control seizures in the mother should be carefully weighed against the possible risk to the foetus. This is particularly important during the first three months of pregnancy. Minimum effective doses should be given and monitoring of plasma levels is recommended.

In women of childbearing age, Tegretol should be administered as monotherapy wherever possible.

Cases of developmental disorders and malformations, including spina bifida, have been reported in association with carbamazepine. However, offspring of mothers with untreated epilepsy are known to be prone to an increased incidence of development disorders and conclusive evidence that carbamazepine given alone, increases the risk further is not available. Patients should be counselled regarding the possibility of an increased risk of malformations and given the opportunity of antenatal screening.

In animals (mice, rats and rabbits) oral administration of carbamazepine during organogenesis led to increased embryo mortality at a daily dose which caused maternal toxicity (above 200 mg/kg b.w. daily, i.e. 20 times the usual human dosage). No evidence of a teratogenic effect was observed in the three species studied but in one study using mice carbamazepine (40–240 mg/kg b.w. daily orally) caused defects in 4.7% of exposed foetuses compared with 1.3% in controls.

Anti-epileptic drugs may contribute to folic acid deficiency, a possible contributory cause of foetal abnormality. Folic acid supplementation is recommended before and during pregnancy.

Bleeding disorders in the newborn caused by anti-epileptic agents have been reported. As a precaution, vitamin K_1 should be administered as a preventive measure in the last weeks of pregnancy and to the newborn.

Carbamazepine passes into the breast milk in concentrations of about 25–60% of the plasma level. This is not believed to present a significant hazard to the infant, which is likely to receive at most 10% of an appropriate therapeutic dose of carbamazepine for an infant with epilepsy. As with all drugs, the benefits of breast-feeding should be weighed against the remote possibility of an adverse effect occurring in the infant. There is one report of a severe skin (hypersensitivity) reaction in a breast-fed baby.

Effects on ability to drive and use machinery: The patient's reactions, e.g. as a road user, may be impaired by Tegretol, especially in the early stages of treatment. Patients should be warned of the possible hazard when driving or operating machinery.

Undesirable effects: Provided a gradually increasing dosage scheme is followed, Tegretol is generally well tolerated but side effects may occur particularly at the start of treatment, or if the initial dose is too high. Dizziness, headache, ataxia, drowsiness, fatigue, diplopia, nausea or vomiting may be symptoms of carbamazepine overdosage and usually abate within a few days either spontaneously or after a transient dosage reduction. It is advisable to monitor the plasma levels and divide the daily dosage into smaller (i.e. 3-4) fractional doses.

Central nervous system: Neurological: Frequent: Dizziness, ataxia, drowsiness, fatigue. Occasional: Headache, diplopia, accommodation disorders (blurred vision). Rare: Abnormal involuntary movements (tremor, asterixis, orofacial dyskinesia, choreoathethotic disorders, dystonia, tics), nystagmus. Isolated cases: Oculomotor disturbances, speech disorders (e.g. dysarthria or slurred speech), peripheral neuritis, paraesthesiae, muscle weakness and paretic symptoms.

Psychiatric: Isolated cases: Hallucinations (visual or acoustic), depression, loss of appetite, restlessness, aggressive behaviour, agitation, confusion, activation or psychosis.

Skin and appendages: Occasional or frequent: Allergic skin reactions, urticaria, which may be severe. Rare: Exfoliative dermatitis and erythroderma, Stevens-Johnson syndrome, systemic lupus erythematosus-like syndrome. Isolated cases: Toxic epidermal necrolysis, photosensitivity, erythema multiforme and nodosum, alterations in skin pigmentation, purpura, pruritus, acne, sweating, hair loss, hirsutism.

Blood: Occasional or frequent: Leucopenia. Occasional: Eosinophilia, thrombocytopenia. Rare: Leucocytosis. Isolated cases: Agranulocytosis, aplastic anaemia, pure red cell aplasia, megaloblastic anaemia, acute intermittent porphyria, reticulocytosis, folic acid deficiency, and possible haemolytic anaemia.

Liver: Frequent: Elevated gamma-GT (due to hepatic enzyme induction), usually not clinically relevant. Occasional: Elevated alkaline phosphatase, rarely transaminases. Rare: Jaundice, hepatitis of cholestatic, parenchymal (hepatocellular) or mixed type. Isolated cases: Granulomatous hepatitis.

Gastro-intestinal tract: Occasional or frequent: Nausea, vomiting. Occasional: Dryness of the mouth. Rare: Diarrhoea or constipation. Isolated cases: Abdominal pain, glossitis, stomatitis.

With suppositories occasional rectal irritation may occur.

Hypersensitivity reactions: Rare: A delayed multi-organ hypersensitivity disorder (of serum sickness type) with fever, skin rashes, vasculitis, lymphadenopathy, disorders mimicking lymphoma, arthralgia, leucopenia, eosinophilia, hepatosplenomegaly and abnormal liver function tests, occurring in various combinations. Other organs may also be affected (e.g. lungs, kidneys, pancreas, myocardium). Isolated cases: Aseptic meningitis, with myoclonus and peripheral eosinophilia, anaphylactic reaction.

Treatment must be discontinued immediately if such hypersensitivity reactions occur.

Cardiovascular system: Rare: Disturbances of cardiac conduction. Isolated cases: Bradycardia, arrhythmias, AV-block with syncope, collapse, congestive heart failure, hypertension or hypotension, aggravation of coronary artery disease, thrombophlebitis, thrombo-embolism.

Endocrine system and metabolism: Occasional: Hyponatraemia, fluid retention, oedema, weight gain, and reduced plasma osmolality due to an antidiuretic hormone (ADH)-like effect, leading in isolated cases to water intoxication accompanied by lethargy, vomiting, headache, mental confusion, neurological abnormalities. Isolated cases: Gynaecomastia or galactorrhoea. Impaired male fertility and/or abnormal spermatogenesis. Loss of libido/impotence. Abnormal thyroid function tests: decreased L-thyroxine (FT_4, T_4, T_3) and increased TSH, usually without clinical manifestations. Disturbances of bone metabolism (decrease in plasma calcium and 25-OH-cholecalciferol), leading to osteomalacia. Elevated levels of cholesterol, including HDL cholesterol, and triglycerides.

Renal: Isolated cases: Interstitial nephritis and renal failure, signs of renal dysfunction including albuminuria, haematuria, oliguria and elevated bun/azotaemia, urinary frequency, urinary retention.

Sense organs: Isolated cases: Taste disturbances; lens opacities, conjunctivitis, tinnitus, hyperacusis.

Musculoskeletal system: Isolated cases: Arthralgia, muscle pain or cramp.

Respiratory tract: Isolated cases: Pulmonary hypersensitivity characterised by dyspnoea, pneumonitis or pneumonia.

Overdose

Signs and symptoms: The presenting signs and symptoms of overdosage involve the central nervous, cardiovascular or respiratory systems.

Central nervous system: CNS depression; disorientation, somnolence, agitation, hallucination, coma; blurred vision, slurred speech, dysarthria, nystagmus, ataxia, dyskinesia, initially hyperreflexia, later hyporeflexia; convulsions, psychomotor disturbances, myoclonus, hypothermia.

Respiratory system: Respiratory depression, pulmonary oedema.

Cardiovascular system: Tachycardia, changes in blood pressure (hypotension and at times hypertension), cardiac arrhythmias, conduction disturbance with widening of QRS complex; syncope.

Gastro-intestinal system: Vomiting, delayed gastric emptying, reduced bowel motility.

Renal function: Retention of urine, oliguria or anuria; fluid retention, water intoxication due to ADH-like effect of carbamazepine.

Laboratory findings: Hyponatraemia, possibly metabolic acidosis, possibly hyperglycaemia, increased muscle creatinine phosphokinase.

Treatment: There is no specific antidote. Management according to the patient's clinical condition. Possible admission to hospital. Measurement of the plasma level to confirm carbamazepine poisoning and to ascertain the size of the overdose. Evacuation of the stomach, gastric lavage and administration of activated charcoal. Supportive medical care in an intensive care unit with cardiac monitoring and careful correction of electrolyte imbalance, if required.

Special recommendations: Hypotension: Administer dopamine or dobutamine i.v.

Disturbances of cardiac rhythm: To be managed on an individual basis.

Convulsions: Administer a benzodiazepine (e.g. diazepam) or another anticonvulsant, e.g. phenobarbitone (with caution because of increased respiratory depression) or paraldehyde.

Hyponatraemia (water intoxication): Fluid restriction and slow careful NaCl 0.9% infusion i.v. These measures may be useful in preventing brain damage.

Charcoal haemoperfusion has been recommended. Forced diuresis, haemodialysis and peritoneal dialysis have been reported not to be effective.

Relapse and aggravation of symptomatology on the 2nd and 3rd day after overdose, due to delayed absorption, should be anticipated.

Pharmacological properties

Pharmacodynamic properties: Mode of action: Carbamazepine is a dibenzazepine derivative with antiepileptic, neurotropic and psychotropic properties.

The mechanism of action of carbamazepine has only been partially elucidated. It is conceivable that blockade of voltage-sensitive sodium channels may be one or even the main primary effect of carbamazepine.

Pharmacokinetic properties: Absorption: The elimination half-life of unchanged drug in the plasma averages approximately 36 hours following a single dose, whereas after repeated administration, which leads to auto-induction of hepatic enzymes, it averages only 16–24 hours, depending on the duration of the medication. In patients receiving co-medication with other enzyme-inducing drugs (phenytoin, phenobarbitone) half-life values averaging 9–10 hours have been observed. The therapeutic plasma concentration range of carbamazepine at steady state is usually between 4–12 mcg/ml (17–50 μmol/l).

The bioavailability of Tegretol in various oral formulations has been shown to lie between 85–100%. Bioavailability is unaffected by food regardless of dosage form.

As measured by AUC calculations the total bioavailability of carbamazepine from Tegretol suppositories is approximately 25% less than from oral formulations. For doses up to 300 mg approximately 75% of the total amount absorbed reaches the general circulation within 6 hours of application. For these reasons the maximum recommended daily dose is limited to 250 mg qid (1,000 mg per day), the equivalent to 800 mg per day orally. Clinical trials have shown that when Tegretol suppositories are substituted for oral dosage forms plasma levels within the range 5–8 mcg/ml (19–34 μmol/l) are reached. It should be possible, therefore, to maintain therapeutically effective plasma levels in most patients.

Serum protein binding: 70–80%.

Distribution: The concentration of unchanged substance in the CSF and saliva represents the unbound portion in plasma, i.e. 20–30% of total plasma concentration, breast milk 25–60% of total plasma concentration. Carbamazepine crosses the placental barrier. Apparent volume of distribution 0.8–1.5 L/kg.

Metabolism: Carbamazepine is extensively metabolised in the liver, mainly by oxidative pathways and the greater part is excreted as the inactive glucuronide with up to 40% as metabolites, of which only carbamazepine epoxide is pharmacologically active. This may constitute up to 30% of the circulating active material originating as carbamazepine; in particular polytherapy is an important factor in augmenting epoxide levels. The inactive 10,11-diol represents the final stage of carbamazepine biotransformation. Only about 3% of pharmacologically active material (unchanged plus epoxide) is excreted. In advanced hepatic disease carbamazepine metabolism may be impaired.

Characteristics in patients: The pharmacokinetics of carbamazepine are unaltered in the elderly but its metabolism may be affected by hepatic dysfunction (see above). In children the relatively high rate of metabolism of the drug may require higher doses (in mg/kg b.w.) of carbamazepine to maintain therapeutic concentrations.

Preclinical safety data: None relevant.

Pharmaceutical particulars

List of excipients: Each suppository contains hydroxypropylmethylcellulose and suppository mass 15.

Incompatibilities: None known.

Shelf life: Three years.

Special precautions for storage: Protect from heat (store below 30°C).

Nature and contents of container: Tegretol Suppositories 125 mg and 250 mg are sealed in polyethylene laminated aluminium foil and come in packs of 5.

Instructions for use/handling: None.

Marketing authorisation holder: Novartis Pharmaceuticals UK Limited, Trading as Geigy Pharmaceuticals, Frimley Business Park, Frimley, Camberley, Surrey GU16 5SG.

Marketing authorisation numbers

Tegretol Suppositories 125 mg:	PL 00101/0459
Tegretol Suppositories 250 mg:	PL 00101/0460

Date of first authorisation/renewal of authorisation 4 July 1997.

Date of (partial) revision of the text 12.01.98.

Legal category POM.

TOFRANIL*

Qualitative and quantitative composition The active ingredient is N-(γ-dimethylaminopropyl)-iminodibenzyl hydrochloride (imipramine hydrochloride).

One coated tablet contains 25 mg imipramine hydrochloride.

The syrup contains 25 mg imipramine base (equivalent to 25 mg imipramine hydrochloride) in every 5 mls.

Pharmaceutical form Coated tablets. Syrup.

Clinical particulars

Therapeutic indications: Symptoms of depressive illness. Relief of nocturnal enuresis in children.

Posology and method of administration

Depression: Adults: 1 x 25 mg up to three times daily, increasing stepwise to 150-200 mg. This should be reached by the end of the first week and maintained until definite improvement has occurred. The subsequent maintenance dose should be individually determined by gradually reducing the dosage, usually to about 50-100 mg daily.

In patients in hospital, i.e. severe cases, the dose may be increased to 100 mg three times daily until a distinct improvement is seen. Again the subsequent maintenance dose should be determined individually by reducing the dosage, usually to about 100 mg daily.

Elderly patients: Patients over 60 years of age may respond to lower doses of Tofranil than those recommended above. Treatment should be initiated with 10 mg daily, gradually increasing to 30-50 mg daily. The optimum dose should be reached after about 10 days and then continued until the end of treatment.

Children: (for nocturnal enuresis only). Not for use in children under 6 years.

6–7 years (weight 20-25 kg or 44-55lbs) 25 mg

8–11 years (weight 25-35 kg or 55-77lbs) 25–50 mg

Over 11 years (weight 35-54 kg or 77-119lbs) 50–75 mg

A daily dosage of 2.5 mg/kg should not be exceeded in children. The dose should be taken just before bedtime. The maximum period of treatment should not exceed three months and withdrawal should be gradual. Should a relapse occur, a further course of treatment should not be started until a full physical examination has been made.

Contra-indications: Known hypersensitivity to imipramine, any of the excipients or cross-sensitivity to other tricyclic antidepressants of the dibenzazepine group. Recent myocardial infarction. Any degree of heart block or other cardiac arrhythmias, mania, severe liver disease, narrow angle glaucoma. Infants and children under 6 years old. Retention of urine. Concurrent use in patients receiving, or within 3 weeks of cessation of therapy with, monoamine oxidase inhibitors. Concomitant treatment with selective, reversible MAO-A inhibitors such as moclobemide, is also contra-indicated.

Special warnings and precautions for use

Warnings: As improvement in depression may not occur for the first two to four weeks treatment, patients should be closely monitored during this period.

Precautions: Tricyclic antidepressants are known to lower the convulsion threshold and Tofranil should therefore be used with extreme caution in patients with epilepsy and other predisposing factors, e.g. brain damage of varying aetiology, concomitant use of neuroleptics, withdrawal from alcohol or drugs with anticonvulsive properties (e.g. benzodiazepines). It appears that the occurrence of seizures is dose dependent.

Concomitant treatment of Tofranil and electroconvulsive therapy should only be resorted to under careful supervision.

Caution is called for when giving tricyclic antidepressants to patients with severe renal disease.

Caution is called for when giving tricyclic antidepressants to patients with tumours of the adrenal medulla (e.g. phaeochromocytoma, neuroblastoma), in whom they may provoke hypertensive crises.

Many patients with panic disorders experience intensified anxiety symptoms at the start of the treatment with antidepressants. This paradoxical initial increase in anxiety is most pronounced during the first few days of treatment and generally subsides within two weeks.

Caution is indicated in patients with hyperthyroidism or during concomitant treatment with thyroid preparations, since aggravation of unwanted cardiac effects may occur.

Before initiating treatment it is advisable to check the patient's blood pressure, because individuals with hypotension or a labile circulation may react to the drug with a fall in blood pressure.

Althought changes in the white blood cell count have been reported with Tofranil only in isolated cases, periodic blood cell counts and monitoring for symptoms such as fever and sore throat are called for, particularly during the first few months of therapy.

Periodic monitoring of hepatic enzyme levels is recommended in patients with liver disease.

In elderly patients monitoring of cardiac function is indicated.

Because of its anticholinergic properties, Tofranil should be used with caution in patients with a history of increased intra-ocular pressure, narrow angle glaucoma, or urinary retention (e.g. diseases of the prostate).

Caution is called for in patients with chronic constipation. Tricyclic antidepressants may cause paralytic ileus, particularly in the elderly and bedridden patients.

Before general or local anaesthesia, the anaesthetist should be aware that the patient has been receiving Tofranil. Anaesthetics given during tri/tetracyclic antidepressant therapy may increase the risk of arrhythmias and hypotension (see interactions).

An increase in dental caries has been reported during long-term treatment with tricyclic antidepressants. Regular dental check-ups are therefore advisable during long-term treatment.

Decreased lacrimation and accumulation of mucoid secretions due to the anticholinergic properties of tricyclic antidepressants may cause damage to the corneal epithelium in patients with contact lenses.

Risk of suicide is inherent to severe depression and may persist until significant remission occurs. Patients posing a high suicide risk require close supervision.

Tofranil may cause anxiety, feelings of unrest, and hyperexcitation in agitated patients and patients with accompanying schizophrenic symptoms.

Activation of psychosis has occasionally been observed in schizophrenic patients receiving tricyclic antidepressants. Hypomanic or manic episodes have also been reported during a depressive phase in patients with cyclic affective disorders receiving treatment with a tricyclic antidepressant. In such cases it may be necessary to reduce the dosage of Tofranil or to withdraw it and administer an antipsychotic agent. After such episodes have subsided, low dose therapy with Tofranil may be resumed if required.

In predisposed and elderly patients, Tofranil may, particularly at night, provoke pharmacogenic (delirious) psychoses, which disappear without treatment within a few days of withdrawing the drug. Agitation, confusion and postural hypotension may occur.

Abrupt withdrawal should be avoided because of possible adverse reactions (see side effects).

Behavioural changes may occur in children receiving Tofranil for treatment of nocturnal enuresis.

Interactions with other drugs and other types of interactions

MAO inhibitors: Do not give Tofranil for at least 3 weeks after discontinuation of treatment with MAO inhibitors (there is a risk of severe symptoms such as hypertensive crisis, hyperpyrexia, myoclonus, agitation, seizures, dilirium and coma). The same applies when giving a MAO inhibitor after previous treatment with Tofranil. In both instances Tofranil or the MAO inhibitor should initially be given in small, gradually increasing doses and its effects monitored. There is evidence to suggest that tricyclic antidepressants may be given as little as 24 hours after a reversible MAO inhibitor such as moclobemide, but the 3 week washout period must be observed if the MAO inhibitor is given after a tricyclic antidepressant has been used.

Selective serotonin reuptake inhibitors: Co-medication may lead to additive effects on the serotonergic system. Fluvoxetine and fluvoxamine may also increase plasma concentrations of imipramine, with corresponding adverse effects, resulting in increased plasma levels of tricyclic antidepressants, a lowered convulsion threshold and seizures.

CNS depressants: Tricyclic antidepressants may also increase the effect of alcohol and central depressant drugs (eg barbiturates, benzodiazepines or general anaesthetics).

Alprazolam and disulfiram: It may be necessary to reduce the dosage of imipramine if it is administered concomitantly with aprazolam or disulfiram.

Neuroleptics: Co-medication may result in increased plasma levels of tricyclic antidepressants, a lowered convulsion threshold and seizures. Combination with thioridazine may produce severe cardiac arrhythmias.

Adrenergic neurone blockers: Tofranil may diminish or abolish the antihypertensive effects of guanethidine, betanidine, reserpine, clonidine and α-methyldopa. Patients requiring co-medication for hypertension should therefore be given antihypertensives of a different type (e.g. diuretics, vasodilators, or β-blockers).

Anticoagulants: Tricyclic antidepressants may potentiate the anti-coagulant effect of coumarin drugs by inhibiting hepatic metabolism of these anticoagulants. Careful monitoring of plasma prothrombin is therefore advised.

Anticholinergic agents: Tricyclic antidepressants may potentiate the effects of these drugs (e.g. phenothiazine, antiparkinsonian agents, antihistamines, atropine, biperiden) on the eye, central nervous system, bowel and bladder.

Sympathomimetic drugs: Tofranil may potentiate the cardiovascular effects of adrenaline, ephedrine, isoprenaline, noradrenaline, phenylephrine and phenylpropanolamine (e.g. as contained in local anaesthetic preparations and nasal decongestants).

Quinidine: Tricyclic antidepressants should not be employed in combination with anti-arrhythmic agents of the quinidine type.

Liver enzyme inducers: Drugs which activate the hepatic mono-oxygenase enzyme system (e.g. barbiturates, carbamazepine, phenytoin, nicotine, and oral contraceptives) may accelerate the metabolism and lower plasma concentrations of imipramine, resulting in decreased efficacy. Plasma levels of phenytoin and carbamazepine may increase, with corresponding adverse effects. It may be necessary to adjust the dosage of these drugs.

Cimetidine, methylphenidate: These drugs may increase the plasma concentrations of tricyclic antidepressants, whose dosage should therefore be reduced.

Oestrogens: There is evidence that oestrogens can sometimes paradoxically reduce the effects of Tofranil yet at the same time cause Tofranil toxicity.

Pregnancy and lactation: There is no evidence of the safety of the drug in human pregnancy. There have been isolated reports of a possible connection between the use of tricyclic antidepressants and adverse effects (developmental disorders) on the foetus, treatment with Tofranil should be avoided during pregnancy, unless the anticipated benefits justify the potential risk to the foetus.

Neonates whose mothers had taken Tofranil up until delivery have developed dyspnoea, lethargy, colic, irritability, hypotension or hypertension, tremor or spasms, during the first few hours or days. Tofranil should if possible be gradually withdrawn at least 7 weeks before the calculated date of confinement.

The active substance of Tofranil and its metabolite, desmethylimipramine, pass into the breast milk in small quantities. Tofranil should be gradually withdrawn or the mother advised to cease breast-feeding.

Effects on ability to drive or use machines: Patients receiving Tofranil should be warned that blurred vision, drowsiness and other CNS symptoms (see side effects) may occur, in which case they should not drive, operate machinery, or do anything which may require alertness or quick actions. Patients should also be warned that alcohol or other drugs may potentiate these effects (see Interactions).

Undesirable effects: If severe neurological or psychiatric reactions occur, Tofranil should be withdrawn.

Elderly patients are particularly sensitive to anticholinergic, neurological, psychiatric, or cardiovascular effects. Their ability to metabolise and eliminate drugs may be reduced, leading to a risk of elevated plasma concentrations at therapeutic doses.

The following side-effects, although not necessarily observed with Tofranil, have occured with tricyclic antidepressants.

(The following frequency estimates are used: frequent > 10%, occasional >1-10%, rare >0.001-1%, isolated cases < 0.001%)

Central nervous system:

Psychiatric effects: Occasionally fatigue, drowsiness, restlessness, delirium confusion, disorientation and hallucinations (particularly in geriatric patients and those suffering from Parkinsons's disease), increased anxiety, agitation, sleep disturbances, swings from depression to hypomania or mania. Rare: activation of psychotic symptoms. Isolated cases: aggresiveness.

Neurological effects: Frequently: tremor. Occasionally: paraesthesiae, headache, dizziness. Rarely, epileptic seizures. Isolated cases of EEG changes, myoclonus, weakness, extrapyramidal symptoms, ataxia, speech disorders, drug fever.

Cardiovascular system: Frequently sinus tachycardia and clinically irrelevant ECG changes (T and ST changes) in patients of normal cardiac status, postural hypotension.

Occasionally arrhythmias, conduction disorders (widening of QRS complex and PR interval, bundle-branch block), palpitations.

Isolated cases of increased blood pressure, cardiac decompensation, peripheral vasospastic reactions.

Anticholinergic effects: Frequently: dry mouth, sweating, constipation, disorders of visual accomodation, blurred vision, hot flushes. Occasionally: disturbances of micturition. Isolated cases of mydriasis, glaucoma, paralytic ileus.

Gastro-intestinal tract: Occasionally nausea, vomiting, anorexia. Isolated cases of stomatitis, tongue lesions, abdominal disorders.

Hepatic effects: Occasionaliy: elevated transaminases. Isolated cases of hepatitis with or without jaundice.

Skin: Occasionally: allergic skin reactions (skin rash, urticaria). Isolated cases of oedema (local or generalised), photosensitivity, pruritus, petechiae, hair loss.

Endocrine system and metabolism: Frequently weight gain. Occasionally disturbances of libido and potency. Isolated cases of enlarged mammary glands, galactorrhoea, SIADH (syndrome of inappropriate antidiuretic hormone secretion), increase or decrease in blood sugar, weight loss.

Hypersensitivity: Isolated cases of allergic alveolitis (pneumonitis) with or without eosinophilia, systemic anaphylactic/anaphylactoid reactions including hypotension.

Blood: Isolated cases of eosinophilia, leucopenia, agranulocytosis, thrombocytopenia and purpura.

Sense organs: Tinnitus.

Miscellaneous: Occasional withdrawal symptoms following abrupt discontinuation of treatment : nausea, vomiting, abdominal pain, diarrhoea, insomnia, headache, nervousness and anxiety.

Overdose: The signs and symptoms of overdose with Tofranil are similar to those reported with other tricyclic antidepressants. Cardiac abnormalities and neurological disturbances are the main complications. In children accidental ingestion of any amount should be regarded as serious and potentially fatal.

Signs and symptoms: Symptoms generally appear within 4 hours of ingestion and reach a maximum severity after 24 hours. Owing to delayed absorption (increased anticholinergic effect due to overdose), long half-life and enterohepatic recycling of the drug, the patient may be at risk for up to 4-6 days.

The following may be encountered :

Central nervous system : drowsiness, stupor, coma, ataxia, restlessness, agitation, enhanced reflexes, muscular rigidity, athetoid and choreiform movements, convulsions.

Cardiovascular System: Hypotension, tachycardia, arrhythmia, conduction disorders, heart failure; in very rare cases, cardiac arrest.

In addition, respiratory depression, cyanosis, shock, vomiting, fever, hydriasis, sweating and oliguria or anuria may occur.

Treatment: There is no specific antidote and treatment is essentially symptomatic and supportive

Anyone suspected of receiving an overdose of Tofranil, particularly children, should be admitted to hospital and kept under close surveillance for at least 72 hours.

Perform gastric lavage or induce vomiting as soon as possible if the patient is fully conscious. If the patient has impaired consciousness, secure the airway with a cuffed endotracheal tube before beginning lavage, and do not induce vomiting. These measures are recommended for up to 12 hours or even longer after the overdose, since the anticholinergic effect of the drug may delay gastric emptying. Administration of activated charcoal may help reduce drug absorption.

Treatment of symptoms is based on modern methods of intensive care, with continuous monitoring of cardiac function, blood gases and electrolytes, and if necessary emergency measures such as:

- anticonvulsive therapy,
- artificial respiration,
- insertion of a temporary cardiac pacemaker,
- plasma expander, dopamine or dobutamine administered by intravenous drip,
- resuscitation.

Since it has been reported that physostigmine may cause severe bradycardia, asystole and seizures, its use is not recommended in cases of overdosage with Tofranil. Haemodialysis or peritoneal dialysis are ineffective because of the low plasma concentrations of Tofranil.

Pharmacological properties

Pharmacodynamic properties: Pharmacotherapeutic group: Tricyclic antidepressant. Noradrenaline (NA) and serotonin (5HT) re-uptake inhibitor.

Mechanism of action: Imipramine is a tricyclic antidepressant and has several pharmacological actions including alpha-adrenolytic, anti-histaminic, anticholinergic and 5HT-receptor blocking properties. However, the main therapeutic activity is believed to be inhibition of the neuronal re-uptake of noradrenaline and 5HT. Imipramine is a so-called 'mixed' re-uptake blocker, i.e.it inhibits the reuptake of NA and 5HT to about the same extent.

Pharmacokinetic properties

Absorption: Imipramine is absorbed quickly and completely following oral administration. The intake of food has no effect on its absorption and bioavailability. During its first passage through the liver, orally administered imipramine becomes partly converted to desmethylimipramine, a metabolite which also exhibits antidepressant activity.

During oral administration of 50 mg 3 times daily for 10 days, the mean steady-state plasma concentrations of imipramine and desmethylimipramine were 33-85ng/ml and 43-109ng/ml respectively. Owing to lower clearance in the plasma, resulting in increased systemic availability, elderly patients require lower doses of imipramine than patients in intermediate age groups. Renal impairment is not expected to have any influence on the kinetics of unchanged imipramine and its desmethyl metabolite since both are excreted only in small amounts by the kidneys.

Distribution: About 86% of imipramine binds to plasma proteins. Concentrations of imipramine in the cerebrospinal fluid and the plasma are highly correlated. The mean distribution volume is about 21L/kg.

Imipramine and its metabolite desmethylimipramine both pass into breast milk in concentrations similar to those found in the plasma.

Biotransformation: Imipramine is extensively metabolised in the liver. It is cleared mainly by demethylation and to a lesser extent by hydroxylation. Both metabolic pathways are under genetic control.

Elimination: Imipramine is eliminated from the blood with a mean half-life of about 19 hours. About 80% is excreted in the urine and about 20% in the faeces, mainly in the form of inactive metabolites. Urinary excretion of unchanged imipramine and of the active metabolite desmethylimipramine is about

5% and 6%, respectively. Only small quantities of these are excreted in the faeces.

Characteristics in patients: Owing to reduced metabolic clearance, plasma concentrations of imipramine are higher in elderly patients than in younger patients.

In children the mean clearance and elimination half-life does not differ significantly from adult controls but the between-patient variability is high.

In patients with severe renal impairment, no change occurs in renal excretion of imipramine and its biologically active unconjugated metabolites. However steady-state plasma concentrations of the conjugated metabolites, which are considered to be biologically inactive are elevated. The clinical significance of this finding is not known.

Preclinical safety data: Imipramine has no mutagenic or carcinogenic potential. Studies in four species (mouse, rat, rabbit and monkey) led to the conclusion that orally administered imipramine has no teratogenic potential. Experiments with high doses of parenterally administered imipramine resulted mainly in severe maternal and embryotoxic effects, they were thus inconclusive with regard to teratogenic effects.

Pharmaceutical particulars

List of excipients: Coated tablets of 25 mg contain glycerol, lactose, magnesium stearate, maize starch, stearic acid, silicon dioxide, hydroxypropyl methylcellulose, microcrystalline cellulose, titanium dioxide, red iron oxide, polyethylene glycol, povidone, sucrose, talc.

The syrup contains tragacanth, sucrose, methyl hydroxybenzoate, propyl hydroxybenzoate, sorbitol, titanium dioxide, cream flavour (Cornish C9014) and water.

Incompatibilities: None known.

Shelf-life: Coated tablets of 25 mg: Five years.

Syrup: Four years

Special precautions for storage: Coated tablets of 25 mg: Protect from moisture.

Syrup: Store below 25°C. Keep containers tightly closed.

Medicines should be kept out of reach of children.

Nature and contents of container: Tablets 25 mg: Red-brown, sugar coated, round biconvex tablets, 5.5 mm in diameter imprinted GEIGY on one side–packed in PVC/foil bubble packs of 84 tablets.

Syrup 25 mg/5 ml: White, viscous syrup contained in a glass bottle with a child resistant clic-loc cap.

Instruction for use/handling: None.

Marketing authorisation holder: Novartis Pharmaceuticals UK Ltd, Trading as Geigy Pharmaceuticals.

Marketing authorisation numbers

Tablets 25 mg 00101/0547
Syrup 25 mg/5 ml 00101/0545

Date of approval/revision of SPC 11 December 1997

Legal category POM

TRANSIDERM-NITRO* 5 and 10

Presentation Transiderm-Nitro is a transdermal drug delivery system, comprising a self-adhesive, pink coloured patch, containing a drug reservoir of glyceryl trinitrate.

For each Transiderm-Nitro 5, the average amount of glyceryl trinitrate absorbed per patch in 24 hours is 5 mg. Each patch has a contact surface measuring 10cm², and a glyceryl trinitrate content of 25 mg.

For Transiderm-Nitro 10, the average amount of glyceryl trinitrate absorbed per patch in 24 hours is 10 mg. Each patch has a contact surface measuring 20cm², and a glyceryl trinitrate content of 50 mg.

Uses

Indications: Prophylactic treatment of attacks of angina pectoris, as monotherapy or in combination with other anti-anginal agents.

Transiderm-Nitro 5 only: Prophylactic treatment of phlebitis and extravasation secondary to venous cannulation for intravenous fluid and drug administration when the duration of treatment is expected to last for 2 days or longer.

Mode of action: Nitroglycerin relaxes smooth muscle. It acts chiefly on systemic veins and large coronary arteries, with more predominant effects on the former. In angina pectoris the fundamental mechanism of action of nitroglycerin is based on an increase in venous capacitance leading to a decreased return of blood to the heart. Owing to this, preload and hence filling volume diminishes, resulting in a decreased myocardial oxygen requirement at rest and especially during exercise.

In the coronary arterial circulation nitroglycerin dilates extramural conductance and small resistance vessels. It appears to cause redistribution of coronary blood flow to the ischaemic subendocardium by selectively dilating large epicardial vessels and also relaxes vasospasm.

Nitroglycerin dilates the arteriolar vascular bed, as a result of which afterload and left ventricular systolic wall tension decrease, leading to a reduction in myocardial oxygen consumption.

Pharmacokinetics: Following single application, plasma concentrations of nitroglycerin reach a plateau within 2 hours, which is maintained throughout the day until patch removal. The height of this plateau is directly proportional to the size of the system's drug-releasing area.

The same plasma levels are attained regardless of whether the system is applied to the skin of the upper arm, pelvis or chest. Upon removal of Transiderm-Nitro the plasma level falls rapidly. After repeated application of Transiderm-Nitro no cumulation occurs.

Dosage and administration

Adults:

Angina: Treatment should be initiated with one Transiderm-Nitro 5 patch daily. If a higher dosage is required a Transiderm-Nitro 10 patch may be substituted. The dosage may be increased to a maximum of two Transiderm-Nitro 10 patches daily in resistant cases. Transiderm-Nitro may be given either continuously, or intermittently with a patch-off period of 8-12 hours, usually at night, during each 24 hour period. Development of tolerance or attenuation of therapeutic effect commonly occurs with prolonged or frequent administration of all long-acting nitrates. Recent evidence suggests that intermittent therapy with Transiderm-Nitro may reduce the incidence of tolerance.

Prior to the use of intermittent therapy, the clinical benefits to the patient should be weighed against the risks of angina in the patch-free interval. In patients considered to be at risk, concomitant anti-anginal therapy should be implemented (see *Precautions*).

It is recommended that the patch is applied to the lateral chest wall. The replacement patch should be applied to a new area of skin. Allow several days to elapse before applying a fresh patch to the same area of skin.

If acute attacks of angina pectoris occur, rapidly acting nitrates may be required.

Phlebitis and extravasation: One Transiderm-Nitro 5 patch is to be applied distal to the site of intravenous cannulation at the time of venepuncture. The patch should be removed after 3-4 days and a new replacement patch applied to a different area of skin. Treatment with Transiderm-Nitro should be discontinued once intravenous therapy has stopped.

Use in the elderly: No specific information on use in the elderly is available, however, no evidence exists to suggest that an alteration in dosage is required.

Use in children: There is insufficient knowledge of the effects of Transiderm-Nitro in children and therefore recommendations for its use cannot be made.

Contra-indications, warnings, etc

Contra-indications: Transiderm-Nitro should not be prescribed to patients hypersensitive to nitrates. Severe hypotension. Increased intracranial pressure. Myocardial insufficiency due to obstruction (e.g. in the presence of aortic or mitral stenosis or of constrictive pericarditis).

Precautions: In recent myocardial infarction or acute heart failure, Transiderm-Nitro should be employed only under careful surveillance.

As with all anti-anginal nitrate preparations, withdrawal of long-term treatment should be gradual, by replacement with decreasing doses of long-acting oral nitrates.

The system should be removed before cardioversion or DC defibrillation is attempted. This is to avoid the possibility of arcing between the patch and the electrodes. Also the system should be removed before diathermy treatment.

Caution should be exercised in patients with arterial hypoxaemia due to severe anaemia because, in such patients the biotransformation of nitroglycerin is reduced. Similarly, caution is called for in patients with hypoxaemia and a ventilation/perfusion imbalance due to lung disease or ischaemic heart failure.

Postural hypotension has been reported rarely following initiation of treatment with Transiderm-Nitro and care is advised when driving or operating machinery.

Nitrate therapy may aggravate the angina caused by hypertrophic cardiomyopathy.

The possibility of increased frequency of angina during patch-off periods should be considered. In such cases, the use of concomitant anti-anginal therapy is desirable.

If tolerance to nitroglycerin patches develops, the effect of sublingual nitroglycerin on exercise tolerance may be partially diminished.

Pregnancy and lactation: As with all drugs, Transiderm-Nitro should not be prescribed during pregnancy, particularly during the first trimester, unless there are compelling reasons for doing so.

It is not known whether the active substance passes into the breast milk. The benefits for the mother must be weighed against the risks for the child.

Drug interactions: Concomitant treatment with other vasodilators, calcium antagonists, ACE inhibitors, beta-blockers, diuretics, antihypertensives, tricyclic antidepressants and major tranquillisers, as well as the consumption of alcohol, may potentiate the blood pressure lowering effects of Transiderm-Nitro.

Concurrent administration of Transiderm-Nitro with dihydroergotamine may increase the bioavailability of dihydroergotamine and lead to coronary vasoconstriction.

The possibility that the ingestion of acetylsalicylic acid and non-steroidal anti-inflammatory drugs might diminish the therapeutic response to Transiderm-Nitro cannot be excluded.

Side effects:

Central nervous system: Like other preparations, Transiderm-Nitro may give rise to headache, which is due to cerebral vasodilation and is dose-dependant. Such headaches, however, may regress after a few days despite continuation of the therapy. If they do not disappear, they should be treated with mild analgesics. In cases where headaches are unresponsive to treatment, the dosage of nitroglycerin should be reduced or use of the product discontinued.

Skin: Reddening of the skin, with or without local itching or burning sensation, as well as allergic contact dermatitis may occasionally occur. Upon removal of the patch, any slight reddening of the skin will usually disappear within a few hours. The application site should be changed on patch replacement to prevent local irritation.

Cardiovascular: Facial flushing, faintness, dizziness or lightheadedness, and postural hypotension, which may be associated with reflex-induced tachycardia, have been reported rarely. Reflex tachycardia can be controlled by concomitant treatment with a beta-blocker.

Gastro-intestinal: Rarely nausea, vomiting.

Treatment of overdosage:

Signs: High doses of glyceryl trinitrate are known to cause pronounced systemic side effects, eg a marked fall in blood pressure and reflex tachycardia resulting in collapse and syncope. Methemoglobinaemia has also been reported following accidental overdosage of nitroglycerin. However, with Transiderm-Nitro, the release membrane will reduce the likelihood of overdosage occurring.

Management: In contrast to long acting oral nitrate preparations, the effect of Transiderm-Nitro can be rapidly terminated simply by removing the system. Any fall in blood pressure or signs of collapse that may occur, may be managed by general resuscitative measures.

Pharmaceutical precautions Store below 25°C.

Legal category P

Package quantities Boxes of 28 patches.

Further information Transiderm-Nitro gives a controlled release of glyceryl trinitrate over at least 24 hours, and thereby avoids high peaks of blood levels, minimising the incidence of side-effects.

Although glyceryl trinitrate is volatile, resulting, in the case of most products, in a loss of the drug after relatively short storage, the design of the Transiderm-Nitro patch ensures that the dosage to the patient is maintained even after 2 years storage.

Product licence numbers

Transiderm-Nitro 5 00101/0464
Transiderm-Nitro 10 00101/0465

Product licence holder: Novartis Pharmaceuticals UK Limited, trading as Ciba Laboratories.

Date of revision of text 06.09.97.

TRASICOR*

Presentation Trasicor tablets each containing 20 mg oxprenolol hydrochloride PhEur. Circular, flat, white film-coated tablets with bevelled edges having the monogram CIBA impressed on one side and Trasicor 20 on the other.

Trasicor tablets each containing 40 mg oxprenolol hydrochloride PhEur. Circular, flat, white film-coated tablets with bevelled edges having the monogram CIBA impressed on one side and Trasicor 40 on the other.

Trasicor tablets each containing 80 mg oxprenolol hydrochloride PhEur. Circular, flat, pale-yellow film-coated tablets with bevelled edges having the monogram CIBA impressed on one side and Trasicor 80 on the other.

All strengths of Trasicor tablets contain: calcium phosphate, hydroxypropyl-methylcellulose, magnesium stearate, talc, and titanium dioxide.

In addition: 20 mg and 40 mg tablets contain: polyvinylpyrrolidone, sucrose, wheat starch and vinylpyrrolidone-vinylacetate copolymer.

80 mg tablets contain: maize starch, polyvinylpyrrolidone, silicon dioxide, sodium starch glycollate (sodium carboxymethyl starch), polysorbate and yellow iron oxide.

Uses

Indications: Angina pectoris: for long-term prophylactic use (if necessary nitrates should be employed for alleviating acute attacks).

Hypertension: as monotherapy or for use in combination with other antihypertensives, e.g. with a diuretic, peripheral vasodilator, calcium channel blocker or ace inhibitor.

Disburbances of cardiac rhythm: especially supraventricular tachycardia, atrial fibrillation and digitalis-induced arrhythmias, ventricular tachycardia.

Short-term relief of functional cardiovascular disorders due to adrenergic hyperactivity: such as cardiac neurosis, hyperkinetic heart syndrome and anxiety-induced cardiovascular disorders.

Mode of action: Oxprenolol, the active substance of Trasicor, is a non-selective, lipophilic beta-blocker exerting a sympatholytic effect and displaying mild to modest partial agonistic activity (PAA), also known as intrinsic sympathomimetic activity (ISA).

Drugs like oxprenolol with PAA cause comparatively less slowing of the resting heart rate and a less marked negative-inotropic effect than those without PAA. The risk of substantial bradycardia at rest and heart failure is lessened.

The antiarrhythmic effect of oxprenolol is primarily due to suppression of the arrhythmogenic sympathetic influence of catecholamines. Evidence that increased sympathetic stimulation predisposes to many arrhythmias is strong. This is supported by the increased incidence of arrhythmias in man in situations associated with high sympathetic drive or myocardial sensitisation to catecholamines e.g. exercise, emotional stress, phaeochromocytoma, trauma, myocardial ischaemia, anaesthesia, hyperthyroidism.

Oxprenolol decreases cardiac impulse formation in the sinus node with resultant slowing of the sinus rate; it slightly prolongs the sino-atrial conduction time; both the atrio-ventricular (AV) conduction time and the AV node refractory periods are lengthened.

Some β-blockers such as oxprenolol possess a membrane stabilising activity (MSA) on the cardiac action potential, also known as 'quinidine-like' or 'local anaesthetic' action, a property that tends to result in greater cardiac depression than is seen with β-blockers which do not have this pharmacological characteristic. However, at normal therapeutic doses, this property is probably clinically irrelevant and it only becomes manifest after overdose.

In coronary artery disease, oxprenolol is beneficial in increasing exercise tolerance and decreasing the frequency and severity of anginal attacks.

Emotional stress and anxiety states, the symptoms of which are largely caused by increased sympathetic drive, are alleviated by the sympatholytic effect of oxprenolol.

The exact way in which β-blockers exert their antihypertensive action is still not fully understood. Various modes of action have been postulated. During chronic therapy the antihypertensive effect of β-blockers is associated with a decline in peripheral resistance.

Oxprenolol is effective in lowering elevated supine, standing and exercise blood pressure; postural hypotension is unlikely to occur.

Pharmacokinetics: Absorption: Oral oxprenolol is rapidly and completely absorbed. Food has no significant effect on absorption. Peak plasma concentrations are achieved approximately 1 hour after drug administration.

Biotransformation: Oxprenolol is subject to a first-pass metabolism. Its systemic bioavailability is 20–70%.

Distribution: Oxprenolol has a plasma protein binding rate of approximately 80% and a calculated distribution volume of 1.2 l/kg.

Oxprenolol crosses the placental barrier. The concentration in the breast milk is equivalent to approx. 30% of that in the plasma.

Elimination: Oxprenolol has an elimination half-life of 1-2 hours. Oxprenolol is extensively metabolised, direct O-glucuronidation being the major metabolic pathway and oxidative reactions minor ones. Oxprenolol is excreted chiefly in the urine (almost entirely in the form of inactive metabolites). The drug is not likely to accumulate.

Characteristics in patients: Age has no effect on the pharmacokinetics of oxprenolol.

In patients with acute or chronic inflammatory diseases, an increase in the plasma levels of oxprenolol has been observed. The plasma levels may also increase in the presence of severe hepatic insufficiency associated with a reduced metabolism.

Impaired renal function generally leads to an increase in the blood levels of oxprenolol, but the concentrations measured remain within – although at the upper limit of – the concentration range recorded in subjects with healthy kidneys. In addition, in patients with renal failure the apparent elimination half-life for unchanged, i.e. active, oxprenolol is comparable with the corresponding half-life values determined in subjects with no renal disease. Hence, there is no need to readjust the dosage in the presence of impaired renal function.

Dosage and administration The dosage should be individualised. Before raising the dosage, the heart rate at rest should always be checked. If it is 50-55 beats/min, the dosage should not be increased, see *Contra-indications.* The tablets should be swallowed with liquid.

If the maximum recommended dose is insufficient to produce the desired response appropriate combined therapy should be considered.

When discontinuing prolonged treatment with a beta-blocker, the medication should not be interrupted abruptly, but withdrawn gradually.

Higher doses using conventional Trasicor tablets may be administered in two or more divided doses.

Elderly: no special dosage regime is necessary but concurrent hepatic insufficiency should be taken into account.

Children: no adequate experience has been acquired on the use of Trasicor in children.

Hypertension: 80-160 mg total daily dose, given in 2 to 3 doses. If necessary, the dosage can be raised to 320 mg.

Angina pectoris: 80–160 mg total daily dose, given in 2 to 3 doses. If necessary, the dosage can be raised to 320 mg.

Disturbances of cardiac rhythm: 40–240 mg total daily dose given in 2 to 3 doses. The maximum dose recommended is 240 mg/day.

Short-term relief of functional cardiovascular disorders due to adrenergic hyperactivity, e.g. short-term relief of sympathomimetic symptoms of anxiety: 40–80 mg daily, given in 1 or 2 doses, is usually sufficient.

Contra-indications, warnings, etc

Contra-indications: Trasicor is contra-indicated in patients with:

- Hypersensitivity to oxprenolol and related derivatives, cross-sensitivity to other β-blockers or to any of the excipients
- Cardiogenic shock
- Second or third degree atrioventricular block
- Uncontrolled heart failure
- Sick-sinus syndrome
- Bradycardia (<45–50 bpm)
- Hypotension
- Untreated phaeochromocytoma
- Severe peripheral arterial circulatory disturbances
- History of bronchospasm and broncial asthma
- Prinzmetal's angina (variant angina pectoris)
- Use of anaesthetics which are known to have a negative inotropic effect
- Metabolic acidosis

Warnings: Patients receiving oxprenolol should be warned that dizziness, fatigue or visual disturbances (see *Side effects*) may occur, in which case they should not drive, operate machinery or do anything else requiring alertness, particularly if they also consume alcohol.

Precautions: Owing to the risk of bronchoconstriction, non-selective beta-blockers such as Trasicor should be used with particular caution in patients with chronic bronchitis or emphysema (see *Contra-indications*).

As β-blockers increase the AV conduction time, beta-blockers should only be given with caution to patients with first degree AV block.

Beta-blockers should not be used in patients with untreated congestive heart failure. This condition should first be stabilised.

If the patient develops increasing bradycardia less than 50–55 beats per minute at rest and the patient experiences symptoms related to bradycardia, the dosage should be reduced or gradually withdrawn (see *Contra-indications*).

β-blockers are liable to affect carbohydrate metabolism. Diabetic patients, especially those dependent on insulin, should be warned that β-blockers can mask the symptoms of hypoglycaemia (e.g. tachycardia) (see *Drug interactions*). Hypoglycaemia, producing loss of consciousness in some cases, may occur in non-diabetic individuals who are taking β-blockers, particularly those who undergo prolonged fasting or severe exercise. The concurrent use of β-blockers and anti-diabetic medication should always be monitored to confirm that diabetic control is well maintained.

β-blockers may mask certain clinical signs (e.g. tachycardia) of hyperthyroidism and the patients should be carefully monitored.

Beta-blockers may reduce liver function and thus affect the metabolism of other drugs. Like many beta-blockers, oxprenolol undergoes substantial first-pass hepatic metabolism. In the presence of liver cirrhosis the bioavailability of oxprenolol may be increased leading to higher plasma concentrations (see *Pharmacokinetic properties*). Patients with severe renal failure might be more susceptible to the effects of antihypertensive drugs due to haemodynamic effects. Careful monitoring is advisable (see *Pharmacokinetic properties*).

In patients with peripheral circulatory disorders (e.g. Raynaud's disease or syndrome, intermittent claudication), beta-blockers should be used with great caution as aggravation of these disorders may occur (see *Contra-indications*).

In patients with phaeochromocytoma a β-blocker should only be given with an α-blocker (see *Contra-indications*).

Owing to the danger of cardiac arrest, a calcium antagonist of the verapamil type must not be administered intravenously to a patient already receiving treatment with a β-blocker. Furthermore, since β-blockers may potentiate the negative-inotropic and dromotropic effects of Ca-antagonists, like verapamil or diltiazem, any oral co-medication (e.g. in angina pectoris) requires close clinical control (see also *Drug interactions*).

Anaphylactic reactions precipitated by other agents may be particularly severe in patients taking beta-blockers, especially non-selective drugs, and may require higher than normal doses of adrenaline for treatment. Whenever possible, β-blockers should be discontinued in patients who are at increased risk for anaphylaxis.

Especially in patients with ischaemic heart disease, treatment should not be discontinued suddenly. The dosage should gradually be reduced, i.e. over 1–3 weeks, if necessary, at the same time initiating alternative therapy to prevent exacerbation of angina pectoris.

If a patient receiving oxprenolol requires anaesthesia, the anesthetist should be informed of the use of the medication prior to the use of a general anaesthetic to permit him to take the necessary precautions. The anaesthetic selected should be one exhibiting as little negative inotropic activity as possible, e.g. halothane/nitrous oxide. If, on the other hand, inhibition of sympathetic tone during the operation is regarded as undesirable, the β-blocker should be withdrawn gradually at least 48 hours prior to surgery.

The full development of the 'oculomucocutaneous syndrome', as previously described with practolol has not been reported with oxprenolol. However, some features of this syndrome have been noted, such as dry eyes alone or occasionally associated with skin rash. In most cases the symptoms cleared after withdrawal of the treatment. Discontinuation of oxprenolol should be considered, and a switch to another antihypertensive drug might be advisable, see advice on discontinuation above.

Use in pregnancy and lactation: As in the case of any form of drug therapy, oxprenolol should be employed with caution during pregnancy, especially in the first 3 months.

β-blockers may reduce placental perfusion, which may result in intrauterine foetal death, immature and premature deliveries. Use the lowest possible dose. If possible, discontinue beta-blocker therapy at least 2 to 3 days prior to delivery to avoid the effects on uterine contractility and possible adverse effects, especially bradycardia and hypoglycaemia, in the foetus and neonate.

Oxprenolol is excreted into breast milk (see *Pharmacokinetic properties*) and although the esimated daily infant dose derived from breast-feeding is likely to be very low, breast feeding is not recommended.

Drug interactions:

Calcium channel blockers: e.g. Verapamil, diltiazem: Potentiation of bradycardia, myocardial depression and hypotension; particularly after intravenous administration of verapamil in patients taking oral β-blockers, the possibility of hypotension and cardiac arrhythmia cannot be excluded (see *Warnings* and *Precautions*).

Class 1 anti-arrhythmic drugs and amiodarone: Drugs like disopyramide, quinidine and amiodarone may increase atrial-conduction time and induce negative isotropic effect when administered concomitantly with beta-blockers.

Sympathomimetic drugs: Non-cardioselective beta-blockers such as oxprenolol enhance the pressor response to sympathomimetic drugs such as adrenaline, noradrenaline, isoprenaline, ephedrine and phenylphrine (e.g. local anaesthetics in dentistry, nasal and ocular drops), resulting in hypertension and bradycardia.

Clonidine: When clonidine is used in conjunction with non-selective beta-blockers, such as oxprenolol, treatment with clonidine should be continued for some time after β-blocker has been discontinued to reduce the danger of rebound hypertension.

Catecholamine-depleting drugs: e.g. guanethidine, reserpine, may have an additive effect when administered concomitantly with beta-blockers. Patients should be closely observed for hypotension.

Beta-blockers may modify blood glucose concentrations in patients being treated with insulin and oral antidiabetic drugs and may alter the response to hypoglycaemia by prolonging the recovery (blood glucose rise) from hypoglycaemia, causing hypotension and blocking tachycardia. In diabetic patients receiving β-blockers hypoglycaemic episodes may not result in the expected tachycardia but hypoglycaemia-induced sweating will occur and may even be intensified and prolonged (see *Warnings* and *Precautions*).

Non-steroidal anti-inflammatory drugs (NSAIDs): NSAIDs can reduce the hypotensive effect of betablockade.

Cimetidine: Hepatic metabolism of beta-blockers may be reduced resulting in increased plasma levels of β-blocker and prolonged serum half-life. Marked bradycardia may occur.

Ergot alkaloids: Concomitant administration with beta-blockers may enhance the vasoconstrictive action of ergot alkaloids.

Anaesthetic drugs: β-blockers and certain anaesthetics (e.g. halothane) are additive in their cardiodepressant effect. However, continuation of betablockers reduces the risk of arrhythmia during anaesthesia (see *Warnings* and *Precautions*).

Digitalis glycosides: Beta-blockers and digitalis glycosides may be additive in their depressant effect on myocardial conduction, particularly through the atrioventricular node, resulting in bradycardia or heart block.

Lidocaine: Concomitant administration with betablockers may increase lidocaine blood concentrations and potential toxicity; patients should be closely monitored for increased lidocaine effects.

Alcohol and beta-blocker effects on the central nervous system have been observed to be additive and it is possible that symptoms such as dizziness may be exaggerated if alcohol and Trasicor are taken together (see also *Warnings*).

Side-effects: Frequency estimate: Very common >10%, common >1%–10%, uncommon >0.1%–1%, rare >0.01%–0.1%, very rare <0.01%.

Central nervous system: Common: fatigue, dizziness, headache, mental depression. Uncommon: sleep disturbances, nightmares. Rare: hallucinations, exertional tiredness.

Cardiovascular system: Common: hypotension, heart failure, peripheral vascular disorders (e.g. cold extremities, paraesthesia). Uncommon: bradycardia, disturbance of cardiac conduction. Rare: Raynaud-like symptoms.

Gastro-intestinal tract: Very common: dry mouth, constipation. Common: nausea. Uncommon: diarrhoea, vomiting, flatulence.

Skin and appendages: Uncommon: allergic skin rash (e.g. urticarial, psoriasiform, eczematous, lichenoid). Rare: worsening of psoriasis.

Respiratory system: Common: dyspnoea, bronchoconstriction (see *Precautions* and *Contra-indications*).

Sense organs: Uncommon: visual disturbances ('blurred vision', 'vision abnormal'). Rare: dry eyes, keratoconjunctivitis.

Others: disturbances of libido and potency. Very rare: thrombocytopenia.

Overdosage: Signs and symptoms: Poisoning due to an overdosage of β-blocker may lead to pronounced hypotension, bradycardia, hypoglycaemia, heart failure, cardiogenic shock, conduction abnormalities (first or second degree block, complete heart block, asystole), or even cardiac arrest. In addition, dyspnoea, bronchospasm, vomiting, impairment of consciousness, and also generalised convulsions may occur.

The manifestations of poisoning with beta-blockers are dependent on the pharmacological properties of the ingested drug. Although the onset of action is rapid, effects of massive overdose may persist for several days despite declining plasma levels. Watch carefully for cardiovascular or respiratory deterioration in an intensive care setting, particularly in the early hours. Observe mild overdose cases for at least 4 hours for the development of signs of poisoning.

Treatment: Patients who are seen soon after potentially life-threatening overdosage (within 4 hours) should be treated by gastric lavage and activated charcoal.

Treatment of symptoms is based on modern methods of intensive care, with continuous monitoring of cardiac function, blood gases, and electrolytes, and if necessary, emergency measures such as artificial respiration, resuscitation or cardiac pacemaker.

Significant bradycardia should be treated initially with atropine. Large doses of isoprenaline may be necessary for control of heart rate and hypotension. Glucagon has positive chronotropic and inotropic effects on the heart that are independent of interactions with beta-adrenergic receptors and it represents a useful alternative treatment for hypotension and heart failure.

For seizures, diazepam has been effective and is the drug of choice.

For bronchospasm, aminophylline, salbutamol or terbutaline (β_2 agonist) are effective bronchodilator drugs. Monitor the patient for dysrhythmias during and after administration.

Patients who recover should be observed for signs of β-blocker withdrawal phenomenon (see *Special warnings and precautions*).

Pharmaceutical precautions The tablets should be protected from moisture.

Legal category POM.

Package quantities
Tablets 20 mg: Blister packs of 56.
Tablets 40 mg: Blister packs of 56.
Tablets 80 mg: Blister packs of 56.

Further information Nil.

Product licence numbers

Tablets 20 mg	00101/0430
Tablets 40 mg	00101/0431
Tablets 80 mg	00101/0432

Product licence holder: Novartis Pharmaceuticals UK Limited, trading as Ciba Laboratories.

Date of revision of text 05/07/97.

TRASIDREX*

Presentation Trasidrex tablets each contain 160 mg oxprenolol hydrochloride PhEur in a sustained release core and 0.25 mg cyclopenthiazide BP in the coat. The tablets are circular, with a pinkish-red sugar coat, and are printed CIBA on one side and TRASIDREX on the other, both words in black.

Trasidrex tablets also contain sucrose.

Uses
Indications: Hypertension.

Mode of action: Trasidrex contains two components which have different sites of action and whose antihypertensive effects are mutually complimentary.

Oxprenolol – Oxprenolol, one of the active substances of Trasidrex, is a non-selective, lipophilic β-blocker exerting a sympatholytic effect and displaying mild to moderate partial agonist activity (PAA), also known as intrinsic sympathomimetic activity (ISA).

The exact way in which β-blockers exert their antihypertensive action is still not fully understood. Various modes of action have been postulated. In the long run the antihypertensive effect of β-blockers always parallels a decline in peripheral vascular resistance.

Oxprenolol is effective in lowering elevated supine, standing and exertional blood pressure; substantial hypotensive reactions are less likely to occur. Emotional stress and anxiety states which are largely caused by increased sympathetic drive are alleviated by the sympatholytic effect of oxprenolol.

Cyclopenthiazide– Cyclopenthiazide, one of the two active substances of Trasidrex, is a benzothiadiazine (thiazide) diuretic.

Thiazide diuretics act primarily on the distal renal tubule (early convoluted part), inhibiting NaCl reabsorption (by antagonising the Na^+Cl^- co-transporter), and promoting Ca^{++} reabsorption (by an unknown mechanism). Increased delivery of Na^+ and water to the cortical collecting tubule and/or the higher flow rate lead to more secretion and excretion of K^+ and H^+.

In healthy volunteers or in patients with oedema, diuresis is already enhanced after administration of a single dose of 0.125 mg of cyclopenthiazide. The resulting increase in urinary excretion of sodium and chloride and the less marked increase in kaliuresis are dose dependent. The diuretic/natriuretic effect appears within 1–3 hours after oral administration of cyclopenthiazide, reaches its maximum after 6–9 hours, and subsides within 24 hours.

Thiazide-induced diuresis initially leads to decreases in plasma volume, cardiac output, and systemic blood pressure. The renin-angiotensin-aldosterone system may become activated. The hypotensive effect is maintained during continued administration, probably owing to a fall in total peripheral vascular resistance; cardiac output returns to pretreatment values, plasma volume remains slightly reduced, and plasma renin activity may be elevated.

During chronic administration, the antihypertensive effect of cyclopenthiazide is dose dependent.

Like other diuretics, cyclopenthiazide given as monotherapy achieves blood pressure control in about 40–50% of patients with mild to moderate hypertension.

Combination with oxprenolol potentiates the blood-pressure-lowering effect, making it possible to achieve a further decrease in blood pressure in a large proportion of patients who have failed to respond adequately to monotherapy.

Pharmacokinetics: The active substances of Trasidrex show the same pharmacokinetic behaviour in the fixed combination as following simultaneous administration of Slow-Trasicor and Navidrex.

Oxprenolol – general characteristics:

Absorption: In the gastrointestinal tract, oxprenolol is completely absorbed from the sustained-release tablets, regardless of whether or not they are taken together with food. Peak plasma concentrations are reached after an average of approx. 3 hours.

During treatment with sustained-release forms, prolongation of the absorption phase enables therapeutically active plasma concentrations to be maintained over a longer period of time than when the same doses are given in conventional dosage forms and avoids high peak drug concentrations in the plasma.

After the active substance has been absorbed, the insoluble matrix of the tablet is excreted in a softened form in the faeces.

Oxprenolol is subject to a first-pass effect. Its systemic bioavailability amounts to 20–70%.

Distribution: Oxprenolol has a plasma-protein binding rate of approx. 80% and a calculated distribution volume of 1.2 L/kg.

Oxprenolol crosses the placental barrier. The concentration in the breast milk is equivalent to approx. 30% of that in the plasma.

Elimination (biotransformation and excretion): Oxprenolol has an elimination half-life of 1–2 hours.

Oxprenolol is extensively metabolised, direct O-glucuronidation being the major metabolic pathway and oxidative reactions minor ones. Oxprenolol is excreted chiefly in the urine (almost exclusively in the form of inactive metabolites). Oxprenolol is not likely to accumulate.

Characteristics in patients: Age has no effect on the pharmacokinetics of oxprenolol.

In patients with acute or chronic inflammatory diseases an increase in the plasma levels of oxprenolol has been observed.

The plasma levels may also increase in the presence of severe hepatic insufficiency associated with a reduced metabolic rate.

Impaired renal function generally leads to an increase in the blood levels of oxprenolol, but the concentrations measured remain within – although at the upper limit of – the concentration range recorded in subjects with healthy kidneys. In addition, in patients with renal failure the apparent elimination half-life for unchanged, i.e. active oxprenolol is comparable with the corresponding half-life values determined in subjects with no renal disease. Hence there is no need to readjust the dosage in the presence of impaired renal function.

Cyclopenthiazide – general characteristics: After oral administration of single doses of 0.5 mg or 1 mg cyclopenthiazide, peak plasma levels of about 3 and 7 ng/mL respectively were reached after an average of 3–4 hours. Twelve hours after administration of 1 mg cyclopenthiazide, plasma concentrations fall to about 25% of the peak concentrations. Thiazide diuretics cross the placental barrier and also pass into the breast milk.

Lipophilic thiazides also have a higher protein-binding rate, that of cyclopenthiazide amounting to approx. 92%. They therefore exert a more prolonged action than the more hydrophilic thiazides.

In humans receiving cyclopenthiazide, the drug can be detected in the urine 24 hours after administration of 0.5 mg, for instance, concentrations in the urine are about 400 ng/mL.

Characteristics in patients: In patients with impaired renal function thiazides accumulate and uraemia may become more marked. Thiazide diuretics (including cyclopenthiazide) lose their diuretic effect when creatinine clearance is <30 mL/min (or at serum creatinine levels of >2.5 mg/100 mL).

Dosage and administration The dosage should be individualised. The sustained release tablets should be swallowed whole with liquid. When discontinuing prolonged treatment with a β-blocker, the medication should not be stopped abruptly, but withdrawn gradually. The physician may wish to switch to products containing the individual components of Trasidrex, i.e. conventional oxprenolol and cyclopenthiazide tablets to facilitate a stepwise reduction in dose.

Adults: In mild to moderate hypertension the recommended dosage is 1 tablet daily in the morning. Depending on the response it may be necessary to raise the dosage to two tablets daily. This should be done after an interval of about 1 week, because the antihypertensive effect often only sets in slowly after 1–2 weeks. In resistant cases, treatment in combination with other antihypertensives can be given, e.g. with a peripheral vasodilator, calcium channel blocker, or ACE inhibitor (see *Interaction with other medicaments*).

Children: Adequate experience of the use of Trasidrex in children has not been acquired.

Elderly: No special dosage regime is necessary but concurrent hepatic insufficiency and susceptibility to electrolyte imbalances should be taken into account. The lowest effective dosage should be used.

Contra-indications, warnings, etc. Hypersensitivity to oxprenolol, cyclopenthiazide and related derivatives or to any of the excipients, or cross sensitivity to other β-blockers.

Oxprenolol:
- Cardiogenic shock.
- Heart failure refractory to treatment.
- Atrioventricular block of second or third degree.
- Sick sinus syndrome.
- Bradycardia (<45–50 beats/min).
- Hypotension.
- Severe peripheral arterial circulatory disturbances.
- Bronchial asthma and history of bronchospasm.
- Prinzmetal's angina (variant angina pectoris).
- Untreated phaeochromocytoma.
- Metabolic acidosis.
- Use of anaesthetics with a negative inotropic effect.

Cyclopenthiazide:
- Anuria.
- Renal failure.
- Hepatic failure.
- Refractory hyponatraemia and hypercalcaemia.
- Refractory hypokalaemia and conditions involving increased potassium loss, e.g. salt-losing nephropathies and prerenal (cardiogenic) impairment of kidney function.
- Untreated Addison's disease.
- Symptomatic hyperuricaemia (history of gout or uric acid calculi).
- Concomitant treatment with Lithium.
- Hypertension during pregnancy.

Warnings: Trasidrex should be used with caution in patients with renal disease or with impaired hepatic function (see *Contra-indications* and *Precautions*).

Patients receiving Trasidrex should be warned that dizziness, fatigue or visual disturbances (see *Side effects*) may occur, in which case they should not drive, operate machinery, or do anything else requiring alertness, particularly if they also consume alcohol.

Precautions:
Oxprenolol: Owing to the danger of cardiac arrest, a calcium antagonist of the verapamil type must not be administered intravenously to a patient already receiving treatment with a β-blocker (see *Drug interactions*).

Owing to the risk of bronchoconstriction, non-selective β-blockers such as oxprenolol should be used with caution in patients with chronic bronchitis or emphysema.

Due to the negative effect on AV conduction time, β-blockers should only be given with caution to patients with AV block of first degree (see *Contra-indications*).

β-blockers should not be used in patients with untreated congestive heart failure (see *Contra-indications*). This condition should first be stabilised.

If the patient develops increasing bradycardia (<50–55 beats/min at rest) and experiences related symptoms, the dosage should be reduced or gradually withdrawn (see *Contra-indications*).

β-blockers may mask certain clinical signs of hyperthyroidism (e.g. tachycardia), and the patients should be carefully monitored.

β-blockers may reduce liver function and thus affect the metabolism of other drugs. Like many β-blockers, oxprenolol undergoes substantial first-pass hepatic metabolism. In the presence of liver cirrhosis the bioavailability of oxprenolol may be increased leading to higher plasma concentrations (see *Pharmacokinetic properties*).

In patients with peripheral circulatory disorders (e.g. Raynaud's disease or syndrome, intermittent claudication), β-blockers should be used with great caution as aggravation of these disorders may occur (see *Contra-indications*).

In patients with phaeochromocytoma a β-blocker should only be given with an α-blocker, see *Contra-indications*.

Anaphylactic reactions precipitated by other agents may be particularly severe in patients taking β-blockers, require higher than normal doses of adrenaline. Whenever possible, β-blockers should be avoided (replaced by other antihypertensive drugs) in patients who are at increased risk for anaphylaxis.

In patients with ischaemic heart disease, treatment should not be discontinued suddenly. The dosage should be gradually reduced, i.e. over 1–3 weeks, if necessary at the same time initiating alternative therapy, to prevent exacerbation of angina pectoris.

If a patient receiving oxprenolol requires anaesthesia, the anesthetist should be informed of the use of the medication prior to the use of a general anaesthetic to permit him to take the necessary precautions. The anaesthetic selected should be one exhibiting as little negative inotropic activity as possible, e.g. halothane/nitrous oxide. If, on the other hand, inhibition of sympathetic tone during the operation is regarded as undesirable, the β-blocker should be withdrawn gradually at least 48 hours prior to surgery.

The full development of the 'oculomucocutaneous syndrome', as previously described with practolol, has not been reported with oxprenolol. However, some features of this syndrome have been noted, such as dry eyes alone or occasionally associated with skin rash. In most cases the symptoms cleared after withdrawal of treatment. Discontinuation of oxprenolol should be considered and a switch to another antihypertensive drug might be advisable.

Cyclopenthiazide: Electrolytes: all patients receiving thiazide therapy should be observed for clinical signs of fluid or electrolyte unbalance, namely dose dependent hyponatraemia, hypochloremic alkalosis and hypokalaemia. Since the excretion of electrolytes is increased during thiazide treatment, an excessively strict low-salt diet should be avoided.

Periodic serum electrolyte determinations should be carried out, especially in digitalised patients, in the elderly, especially in those suffering from chronic diseases, in patients with liver cirrhosis, who are more susceptible to regulatory disorders affecting the electrolytes and fluid balance, and in patients with oedema due to nephrotic syndrome.

Serum potassium concentrations should be checked initially and 3–4 weeks after the start of therapy. Unless the potassium balance is disturbed by other factors (e.g. vomiting, diarrhoea, change in renal function, malnutrition, liver cirrhosis, hyperaldosteronism, treatment with ACTH or corticosteroids) controls should be carried out every 4–6 months.

Hypokalaemia may be avoided or treated by the use of potassium supplements and/or foods with a high potassium content.

Oral potassium supplementation (e.g. KCl) may be considered in patients receiving digitalis and diuretics, particularly if their plasma potassium concentrations are <3.0 mmol/L. If oral potassium supplementation is not well tolerated, Trasidrex may be combined with a potassium sparing diuretic e.g. amiloride.

Combined treatment consisting of Trasidrex and a potassium salt or a potassium-sparing diuretic must be avoided in patients also receiving ACE inhibitors.

If hypokalaemia is acocmpanied by clinical signs (e.g. muscular weakness, paresis, or ECG changes), Trasidrex should be discontinued.

During treatment with thiazides, hyponatraemia accompanied by neurological symptoms (nausea, asthenia, progressive disorientation, apathy) has been observed in isolated cases.

Patients receiving relatively high doses of thiazides may develop hypomagnesaemia accompanied by signs and symptoms such as irritability, muscle cramps, and cardiac arrhythmias.

Metabolic effects: Like other diuretics, thiazides may raise serum uric acid levels, but attacks of gout are rarely observed during chronic treatment.

Small and partly reversible increases in plasma concentrations of total cholesterol, triglycerides or low-density lipoprotein cholesterol were reported in patients during long-term treatment with thiazides and thiazide-like diuretics. The clinical relevance of these findings is not clear.

Calcium excretion is decreased by thiazides. Pathological changes in the parathyroid gland associated with hypercalcaemia and hypophosphataemia have been observed in a few patients on prolonged thiazide therapy. If hypercalcaemia occurs, further diagnostic clarification is necessary. The usual complications of hyperparathyroidism, e.g. renal lithiasis, bone resorption, and peptic ulceration, have not been observed.

Others: Lupus erythematosus may become activated under treatment with thiazides.

Oxprenolol and cyclopenthiazide
Diabetes/glucose tolerance: β-blockers as well as thiazide diuretics are liable to affect carbohydrate metabolism. Diabetic patients, especially those dependent on insulin, should be warned that β-blockers can mask the signs of hypoglycaemia (e.g. tachycardia) (see *Drug interactions*). Hypoglycaemia, producing loss of consciousness in some cases, may occur in non-diabetic individuals who are taking β-blockers, particularly those who undergo prolonged fasting or strenuous exercise.

Although glucose tolerance may be adversely affected, diabetes mellitus very seldom occurs under treatment.

The concurrent use of β-blockers, thiazide diuretics and antidiabetic medication should always be monitored to confirm that glycaemic control is well maintained (see *Drug interactions*).

Renal function: In patients with renal impairment, the elimination half-life for unchanged oxprenolol is not expected to be significantly different from the subjects with normal renal function, but thiazides accumulate and uraemia may become more marked.

Creatinine clearance, urea and electrolytes should be monitored in patients with renal impairment since they might be more susceptible to the effects of antihypertensive drugs. At creatinine clearance levels of <30 mL/min (or at serum creatinine levels of greater than 2.5 mg/100 mL=221 mmol/l), thiazides no longer exert an adequate diuretic effect.

The antihypertensive effect of ACE inhibitors is potentiated by diuretics that increase plasma renin activity. A cautious dosage schedule should therefore be adopted when an ACE inhibitor is added to a diuretic agent.

As with all antihypertensive agents, a cautious dosage schedule is indicated in patients with severe coronary or cerebral arteriosclerosis.

Use in pregnancy and lactation: Trasidrex should not be given during pregnancy unless there are no safer alternatives. If used, as in the case of any form of drug therapy, Trasidrex should be employed with caution, especially in the first 3 months.

β-blockers may reduce placental perfusion, which may result in intrauterine foetal death, immature and premature deliveries. Use the lowest possible dose. If possible, discontinue β-blocker therapy at least 2–3 days prior to delivery to avoid the effects of uterine contractility and possible adverse effects, especially bradycardia and hypoglycaemia, in the foetus and neonate.

Cyclopenthiazide must not be used to treat hypertension during pregnancy (see *Contra-indications*). There have been reports of foetal bone marrow depression, thrombocytopenia, and foetal and neonatal jaundice associated with the use of thiazide diuretics. Other adverse reactions associated with use in adults may also occur.

Oxprenolol and cyclopenthiazide pass into breast milk (see *Pharmacokinetic properties*) and although the estimated daily infant dose derived from breast feeding is likely to be very low, breast feeding is not recommended.

Trasidrex may also suppress lactation.

Drug interactions: The antihypertensive effect of Trasidrex is enhanced by concomitant treatment with other antihypertensives.

In addition, the following interactions may occur with the individual components.

Oxprenolol: Alcohol and β-blocker effects on the central nervous system have been observed to be additive and it is possible that symptoms such as dizziness may be exaggerated if alcohol and Trasidrex are taken together (see also *Effects on ability to use machines*).

Oxprenolol and cyclopenthiazide:
Antidiabetics: Trasidrex may modify blood glucose concentrations in patients being treated with insulin and oral antidiabetic drugs, and may alter the response to hypoglycaemia by prolonging the recovery (blood glucose rise) from hypoglycaemia, reversing hypotension, and blocking tachycardia. In diabetic patients receiving Trasidrex hypoglycaemic episodes may not result in the expected tachycardia, but hypoglycaemia-induced sweating will occur, and may even be intensified and prolonged (see *Warnings* and *Precautions*).

Hyperglycaemia may also occur with thiazide diuretics. Thus latent diabetes mellitus may become manifest during Trasidrex therapy.

During concurrent therapy with antidiabetics a close watch should therefore be kept on carbohydrate metabolism, and the dosage of hypoglycaemic medication may have to be readjusted (see *Warnings* and *Precautions*).

Non-steroidal anti-inflammatory drugs (NSAIDs): NSAIDs such as indomethacin can reduce the hypotensive effect of Trasidrex and there have been isolated reports of a deterioration in renal function in predisposed patients.

Calcium channel blockers: Calcium channel blockers such as verapamil and diltiazem may protentiate bradycardia, myocardial depression, and hypotension induced by Trasidrex, particularly after intravenous administration of verapamil, the possibility of hypotension, cardiac arrhythmia and cardiac arrest cannot be excluded (see *Warnings* and *Precautions*).

Catecholamine-depleting drugs: Catecholamine-depleting drugs, such as guanethidine or monoamine oxidase inhibitors may have an additive effect when administered concomitantly with β-blockers such as oxprenolol and with thiazide diuretics. Patients should be closely observed for hypotension.

Digitalis glycosides: β-blockers and digitalis glycosides may be additive in their depressant effect on myocardial conduction, particularly at the atrioventricular node, resulting in bradycardia or heart block.

Thiazide induced hypokalaemia or hypomagnesaemia may also favour the onset of digitalis-induced cardiac arrhythmias (see *Warnings* and *Precautions*).

In addition, the following interactions may occur with the individual components:

Oxprenolol: Class I anti-arrhythmic drugs and amiodarone.

Drugs such as disopyramide, quinidine and amiodarone may have a potentiating effect on atrial conduction time and induce negative isotropic effect when administered concomitantly with β-blockers.

Sympathomimetic drugs: Non-cardioselective β-blockers such as oxprenolol may enhance the pressor response to sympathomimetic drugs such as adrenaline, noradrenaline, isoprenaline, ephedrine, and phenylephrine (e.g. local anaesthetics in dentistry, nasal and ocular drops), resulting in hypertension and bradycardia.

Clonidine: When clonidine is used in conjunction with a non-selective β-blocker, such as oxprenolol, treatment with clonidine should be continued for some time after the β-blocker has been discontinued to reduce the danger of rebound hypertension.

Cimetidine: Hepatic metabolism of β-blockers may be reduced by cimetidine, resulting in increased plasma concentrations and prolonged serum half-life. Marked bradycardia may occur.

Ergot alkaloids: Concomitant administration with β-blockers may enhance the vasoconstrictive action of ergot alkaloids.

Anaesthetic agents: Beta-blockers and certain inhaled anaesthetics may be additive in their cardiodepressant effect. However, continued use of β-blockers during anaesthesia reduces the risk of cardiac arrhythmias and hypertension (see *Warnings* and *Precautions*).

Lignocaine: Concomitant administration with β-blockers may increase blood lidocaine concentrations and potential toxicity; patients should be closely monitored for increased lidocaine effects.

Cyclopenthiazide:

Lithium: Diuretics raise the blood level of lithium. Where lithium has produced polyuria, diuretics may exert a paradoxical antidiuretic effect (see *Contra-indications*)

Curare derivatives and antihypertensive drugs: Thiazides potentiate the action of curare derivatives and antihypertensive drugs (e.g. methyldopa, β-blockers, vasodilators, ACE inhibitors).

Potassium lowering drugs (such as corticosteroids, ACTH, amphotericin B, carbenoxolone): These drugs may increase the hypokalaemic effect of thiazides.

Allopurinol: Co-administration of thiazide diuretics may increase the incidence of hypersensitivity reactions to allopurinol.

Amantadine: Co-administration of thiazide diuretics may increase the risk of adverse effects caused by amantadine.

Antineoplastic agents (e.g. cyclophosphamide, methotrexate): Concomitant use of thiazide diuretics may reduce renal excretion of cytotoxic agents and potentiate their myelosuppressive effects.

Anticholinergics (e.g. atropine, biperiden): The bioavailability of thiazide-type diuretics may be increased by anticholinergic agents, apparently owing to a decrease in gastrointestinal motility and stomach-emptying rate.

Cholestyramine: Absorption of thiazide diuretics is decreased by cholestyramine. A decrease in the pharmacological effect of thiazides may be expected.

Vitamin D: Thiazide diuretics may reduce urinary calcium excretion caused by vitamin D, while vitamin D may potentiate the increase in serum calcium caused by thiazides.

Cyclosporin: Concomitant use of thiazide-type diuretics and cyclosporin may increase the risk of hyperuricaemia and gout-type complications.

Calcium salts: Concomitant use of thiazide-type diuretics and calcium salts may cause hypercalcaemia by increasing tubular calcium reabsorption.

Diazoxide: Thiazide diuretics may enhance the hyperglycaemia effect of diazoxide.

Methyldopa: There have been reports in the literature of haemolytic anaemia occurring when a thiazide diuretic and methyldopa were administered concomitantly.

Alcohol, barbiturates or narcotics: may potentiate orthostatic hypotension induced by cyclopenthiazide.

Side-effects: Frequency estimate: very common 10%, common 1% to >10%, uncommon 0.1% to <1%, rare 0.01% to <0.1%, very rare <0.01%.

Central nervous system – Common: fatigue, dizziness, headache, mental depression, sleep disturbances, nightmares.

Rare: hallucinations, exertional tiredness.

Uncommon: paresthesias.

Cardiovascular system – Common: postural hypotension which can be aggravated by alcohol, anaesthetics or sedatives, heart failure, peripheral vascular disorders (peripheral coldness).

Uncommon: bradycardia, disturbances of cardiac conduction.

Rare: Raynaud-like symptoms, cardiac arrhythmia.

Gastronintestinal tract – Very common: dry mouth, constipation.

Common: nausea, vomiting, flatulence, loss of appetite.

Uncommon: diarrhoea.

Very rare: pancreatitis, abdominal distress.

Skin and appendages – Common: allergic skin rash, urticaria.

Rare: worsening of psoriasis, photosensitivity.

Very rare: necrotising vasculitis and toxic epidermal necrolysis, cutaneous lupus erythematosus like-lesions, and reactivation of cutaneous lupus erythematosus.

Respiratory system – Common: dyspnoea, bronchospasm.

Sense organs – Uncommon: visual disturbances.

Very rare: dry eyes, keratoconjunctivitis.

Blood – Very rare: thrombocytopenia sometimes with purpura, leucopenia, agranulocytosis, bone marrow depression and haemolytic anaemia.

Liver – Rare: intrahepatic cholestasis or jaundice.

Electrolytes and metabolic disorders – Very common: mainly with higher doses, hypokalaemia and rise in serum lipids.

Common: hyponatraemia, hypomagnesaemia, and hyperuricaemia.

Rare: hypercalcaemia, hyperglycaemia, glycosuria and worsening of diabetic metabolic status.

Very rare, hypochloraemic alkalosis.

Other effects: Common: disturbances of libido and potency.

Very rare: hypersensitivity reactions – respiratory distress including pneumonitis and pulmonary oedema.

Overdosage:

Signs and symptoms:

Oxprenolol – Poisoning due to an overdose of a β-blocker may lead to pronounced hypotension, bradycardia, conduction abnormalities (first or second degree block, complete heart block, asystole), or even cardiac arrest; heart failure, cardiogenic shock, hypoglycaemia, in addition, dyspnoea, bronchospasm, vomiting, impairment of consciousness, and also generalised convulsions may occur.

The manifestations of poisoning with β-blockers are dependent on the pharmacological properties of the ingested drug. Although the onset of action is rapid, effects of massive overdose may persist for several days despite declining plasma levels. Watch carefully for cardiovascular or respiratory deterioration in an intensive care setting, particularly in the early hours. Observe mild overdose cases for at least 4 hours for the development of signs of poisoning.

Cyclopenthiazide – Additional symptoms due to overdosage with cyclopenthiazide are nausea, dizziness, somnolence, hypovolaemia, electrolyte disturbances associated with cardiac arrhythmias and muscles spasms.

Treatment: Patients who are seen soon after potentially life-threatening overdosage (within 4 hours) should be treated by gastric lavage and activated charcoal.

Treatment of symptoms is based on modern methods of intensive care, with continuous monitoring of cardiac function, blood gases, electrolytes, and if necessary intravenous fluid and electrolyte replacement, and emergency measures such as artificial respiration, resuscitation or cardiac pacemaker.

Significant bradycardia should be treated initially with atropine. Large doses of isoprenaline may be necessary for control of heart rate and hypotension. Glucagon has positive chronotropic and inotropic effect on the heart that are independent of interactions with β-adrenergic receptors, and it represents a useful alternative treatment for hypotension and heart failure.

For the treatment of seizures, diazepam has been effective and is the drug of choice.

For the treatment of bronchospasm, β_2-agonists (such as salbutamol or terbutaline) or aminophylline are effective bronchodilator drugs. Monitor the patient for dysrhythmias during and after administration.

Patients who recover should be observed for signs of β-blocker withdrawal phenomenon (see *Warnings* and *Precautions*).

Pharmaceutical precautions Protect from heat, light and moisture. Store below 25°C.

Legal category POM.

Package quantities Cartons of 28 tablets consisting of two reminder calendar foils of 14 tablets (each carton of 28 represents 2–4 weeks' treatment depending on whether dosage is one or two tablets daily).

Further information Nil.

Product licence number 00101/0434.

Product licence holder: Novartis Pharmaceuticals UK Limited, trading as Ciba Laboratories.

Date of revision of text 05.07.97.

VISKALDIX* TABLETS

Qualitative and quantitative composition Each tablet contains 10 mg pindolol and 5 mg clopamide.

Pharmaceutical form Tablet.

Clinical particulars

Therapeutic indications: Mild to moderate hypertension.

Posology and method of administration

Adults: One tablet daily in the morning. If blood pressure is not satisfactorily lowered after 2 to 3 weeks then two tablets daily as a single dose in the morning. Maximum dose of three tablets daily, if required.

Children: There is no experience with Viskaldix in children.

Use in the elderly: There is no evidence that the dosage or tolerability of Viskaldix is directly affected by advanced age. However, because of the diuretic component, such patients should be carefully supervised as factors sometimes associated with aging, such as poor diet or impaired renal function may indirectly affect the dosage or tolerability.

Method of administration: Oral.

Contra-indications: Untreated cardiac failure, sick sinus syndrome (include sino-atrial block), second and third degree heart block, Prinzmetal's angina, history of bronchospasm and bronchial asthma (a warning stating 'do not take this medicine if you have a history of wheezing or asthma' will appear on the label), untreated phaeochromocytoma, metabolic acidosis, pronounced bradycardia, obstructive pulmonary disease, cor pulmonale, prolonged fasting hypokalaemia, refractory hypokalaemia, hyponatraemia, hypercalcaemia, Addison's disease, severe renal or hepatic impairment and symptomatic hyperuricaemia. Viskaldix should not be used with agents which inhibit calcium transport e.g. verapamil.

Special warnings and precautions for use: Especially in patients with ischaemic heart disease, treatment should not be discontinued suddenly. The dosage should be gradually reduced, i.e. over 1–2 weeks, if necessary at the same time initiating replacement therapy, to prevent exacerbation of angina pectoris.

Patients with a poor cardiac reserve should be stabilised with digitalis before treatment with Viskaldix to prevent impairment of myocardial contractility.

As with all beta-blockers, Viskaldix should be used with caution in patients with a history of non-asthmatic chronic obstructive lung disease or recent myocardial infarction.

Patients with spontaneous hypoglycaemia or diabetes should be monitored closely as concomitant use of beta-blockers may intensify the blood sugar lowering effect of insulin and other antidiabetic drugs and also as thiazide diuretics can lower insulin tolerance. Use of beta-blockers may mask the symptoms of hypoglycaemia (tachycardia, tremor). Beta-blockers may also mask the symptoms of thyrotoxicosis.

During treatment with Viskaldix, patients should not undergo anaesthesia with agents causing myocardial depression (e.g. Halothane, cyclopropane, trichlorethylene, ether, chloroform). Viskaldix should be gradually withdrawn before elective surgery. In emergency surgery or cases where withdrawal of Viskaldix would cause deterioration in cardiac condition, atropine sulphate 1 to 2 mg intravenously should be given to prevent severe bradycardia.

If a beta-blocker is indicated in a patient with phaeochromocytoma it must always be given in conjunction with an alpha-blocker, Pre-existing peripheral vascular disorders may be aggravated by beta-blockers. Patients with known psoriasis should take beta-blockers only after careful consideration.

Beta-blockers may increase both the sensitivity towards allergens and the seriousness of anaphylactic reactions.

There have been reports of skin rashes and/or dry eyes associated with the use of beta-adrenoceptor blocking drugs. The reported incidence is small and in most cases the symptoms have cleared when treatment was withdrawn. Discontinuance of the drug should be considered if any such reaction is not otherwise explicable. Cessation of therapy with a beta-blocker should be gradual.

In severe renal failure a further impairment of renal function following beta blockade has been reported in a few cases. Potassium levels should be checked in patients with renal or hepatic failure and urate levels should be checked in patients with gout.

Dilutional hyponatraemia may occur in hot weather in oedematous patients on Viskaldix. The appropriate therapy is water restriction rather than the administration of salt, except in rare instances when the hyponatraemia is life-threatening. In true salt depletion, appropriate replacement is the treatment of choice.

Interaction with other medicaments and other forms

of interaction: Viskaldix should not be used during concomitant administration of lithium, or by patients with known hypersensitivity to sulphonamides.

Calcium-channel blocking agents: Viskaldix should not be used with calcium-channel blockers with negative ionotropic effects e.g. verapamil and to a lesser extent diltiazem. The concomitant use of oral beta-blockers and calcium antagonists of the dihydropyridine type can be useful in hypertension or angina pectoris. However, because of their potential effect on the cardiac conduction system and contractility, the I.V. route must be avoided. The concomitant use with dihydropyridines e.g. nifedipine may increase the risk of hypotension. In patients with cardiac insufficiency, treatment with beta-blocking agents may lead to cardiac failure.

Use of digitalis glycosides in association with beta-blockers may increase atrio-ventricular conduction time.

Clonidine: when therapy is discontinued in patients receiving a beta-blocker and clonidine concurrently, the beta-blockers should be gradually discontinued several days before clonidine is discontinued, in order to reduce the potential risk of a clonidine withdrawal hypertensive crisis.

MAO inhibitors: concurrent use with beta-blockers is not recommended. Possibly significant hypertension may theoretically occur up to 14 days following discontinuation of the MAO inhibitor.

Caution should be exercised in the concurrent use of beta-blocking agents with class 1 antiarrhythmics (e.g. disopyramide, quinidine) and amiodarone.

Concomitant use of beta-blockers may intensify the blood sugar lowering effect of insulin and other antidiabetic drugs.

Cimetidine, hydralazine and alcohol may induce increased plasma level of beta-blockers.

Prostaglandin synthetase inhibiting drugs may decrease the hypotensive effects of beta-blockers.

Sympathomimetics with beta-adrenergic stimulant activity and xanthines: concurrent use with beta-blockers may result in mutual inhibition of therapeutic effects; in addition, beta-blockers may decrease theophylline clearance.

Concomitant use of beta-blockers with tricyclic antidepressants, barbiturates and phenothiazines as well as other anti-hypertensive agents may increase the blood pressure lowering effect.

Reserpine: concurrent use may result in an additive and possibly excessive beta-adrenergic blockade.

Pregnancy and lactation: Viskaldix should not be given to pregnant or lactating women.

Effects on ability to drive and to use machines: Because dizziness or fatigue may occur during initiation of treatment with antihypertensive drugs, patients driving vehicles or operating machinery should exercise caution until their individual reaction to treatment has been determined.

Undesirable effects: Side-effects associated with beta-blockade: bradycardia, a slowed av-conduction or increase of an existing av-block, hypotension, heart failure, cold and cyanotic extremities, Raynaud's phenomenon, paraesthesia of the extremities, increase of an existing intermittent claudication. Fatigue, headaches, impaired vision, hallucinations, psychoses, confusion, impotence, dizziness, sleep disturbances, depression, nightmares. Gastro-intestinal problems, nausea, vomiting, diarrhoea. Bronchospasm in patients with bronchial asthma or a history of asthmatic complaints. Disorder of the skin, especially rash. Dry eyes. Beta-blockers may mask the symptoms of thyrotoxicosis or hypoglycaemia. An increase in ANA (anti nuclear antibodies) has been seen; its clinical relevance is not clear.

Thiazide diuretics may cause postural hypotension and mild gastrointestinal effects; impotence (reversible on withdrawal of treatment); hypokalaemia, hypomagnesaemia, hyponatraemia, hypercalcaemia, hypochloraemic alkalosis, hyperuricaemia, gout, hyperglycaemia, and increases in plasma cholesterol. Less commonly rashes, photosensitivity; blood disorders (including neutropenia and thrombocytopenia), pancreatitis; intrahepatic cholestatis and hypersensitivity reactions (including pneumonitis, pulmonary oedema, severe skin reactions) have also been reported.

Overdose: Overdosage may cause alterations in heart rate, nausea, vomiting, orthostatic disturbances, collapse, hypokalaemia and its accompanying disorders. Treatment by elimination of any unabsorbed drug and general supportive measures.

Plasma electrolytes should be closely monitored. Marked bradycardia, as a result of overdosage (or idiosyncrasy) should be treated with atropine sulphate 1–2 mg iv.

If necessary isoprenaline hydrochloride can be administered by slow iv under constant supervision beginning with 25 mcg (5 mcg/min) until desired effect is achieved. A cardiac pacemaker may be required. Glucagon (5 to 10 mg) iv has been reported to overcome some of the features of serious overdosage.

Pharmacological properties

Pharmacodynamic properties: Viskaldix is a combination of pindolol and clopamide, both acting to lower blood pressure, although by two separate mechanisms.

Pindolol is a non-selective Beta-adrenergic antagonist which blocks both B1 and B2 adrenoceptors for more than 24 hours following administration. It has negligible membrane stabilising activity. The intrinsic sympathomimetic activity (ISA) provides the heart with basal stimulation similar to that elicited by normal resting sympathetic activity. Thus resting cardiac output and heart rate are not unduly depressed, subsequently reducing the risk of bradycardia.

Clopamide enhances the elimination of sodium and chloride by inhibiting their reabsorption in the renal tubules which in turn leads to increased water excretion. The mechanistic relationship to the diuretic action and reduced blood pressure is not fully understood, however the diuretic effect is proportional to the dosage. Diuresis is initiated after about 2 hours and can last for up to 24 hours with maximal effect after 3 to 6 hours.

This combination can produce a clear antihypertensive effect after a few days, but in some cases, to achieve the full effect, two to three weeks treatment may be necessary.

Pharmacokinetic properties: The pharmacokinetics of the two active ingredients are very similar and are not influenced by their combination or by being taken with food. Both components are rapidly and almost completely absorbed. They show negligible hepatic first-pass metabolism. Thus the bioavailability of both is at least 85%. The maximum plasma concentration of pindolol is reached within one hour after ingestion, and that of clopamide, one or two hours after ingestion. Plasma protein binding is 40% for pindolol, and 46% for clopamide. The volume of distribution is about 2 L/kg for pindolol, and 1.5 L/kg for clopamide. The total body clearance of pindolol is 400 ml/min, that of clopamide is 165 ml/min. The elimination half-life is 3–4 hours for pindolol, and 6 hours for clopamide. Approximately one third of the dose of both drugs is excreted unchanged in the urine. The excretion of clopamide occurs mainly via the kidneys, whereas pindolol shows a balanced excretion between the renal and hepatic routes.

Preclinical safety data: There are no pre-clinical data of relevance to the prescriber which are additional to that already included in other sections of the SPC.

Pharmaceutical particulars

List of excipients: Magnesium stearate , maize starch and lactose.

Incompatibilities: None.

Shelf life: 5 years from date of manufacture.

Special precautions for storage: None.

Nature and contents of container: PVDC opaque blister pack containing 28 tablets.

Instructions for use/handling: None.

Marketing authorisation holder: Novartis Pharmaceuticals UK Limited, trading as Sandoz Pharmaceuticals, Frimley Business Park, Frimley, Camberley, Surrey, GU16 5SG.

Marketing authorisation number 00101/0113

Date of approval/revision of SPC 23 April 1997.

Legal category POM.

VISKEN*

Presentation *5 mg Tablets:* Visken 5 mg is available as white, round, flat, bevel-edged tablets of 7 mm diameter, and weighing 120 mg. The tablets are marked VISKEN 5 on one side with a single break line on the reverse. Each tablet contains 5 mg Pindolol PhEur.

Uses *Principal action:* Visken is a specific beta-adrenoceptor blocking agent with low cardiodepressant activity at therapeutic dose. Its beta-blocking activity prevents excessive sympathetic drive to the heart, resulting in a fall in heart rate, and a decrease in cardiac work and myocardial oxygen consumption. Visken possesses some intrinsic sympathomimetic activity even at low dosage which may prevent reduction of resting sympathetic tone to an undesirably low level and minimise myocardial depression.

Indications: Hypertension: For reduction of blood pressure in essential hypertension. Onset of action of Visken is usually rapid, most patients showing a response within the first one to two weeks of treatment. However, maximum response may take several weeks to develop.

Angina pectoris: Prophylactic treatment with Visken reduces the frequency and severity of anginal attacks and increases work capacity.

Dosage and administration *Hypertension:* Initially one 5 mg tablet two or three times daily. Most patients respond to a once-daily dose of from 15 mg to 30 mg.

If necessary, dosage may be increased at weekly intervals up to a maximum of 45 mg daily in single or divided doses. Patients not responding after three to four weeks at this dosage level rarely benefit from further elevations in dosage. Addition of Visken to existing diuretic therapy increases the hypotensive effect and combination with other antihypertensives enables reduction in dosage of these agents.

Angina pectoris: Usually half to one 5 mg tablet up to three times a day according to response.

Use in the elderly: No evidence exists that elderly patients require different dosages or show different side-effects from younger patients.

Use in children: Experience with Visken in children is still limited. Its use in children cannot, therefore, be recommended.

Contra-indications, warnings, etc

Contra-indications: Cardiac failure unless satisfactorily controlled by digitalis (see also 'Precautions'). Atrio-ventricular block, pronounced bradycardia, obstructive pulmonary disease, bronchial asthma, cor pulmonale, metabolic acidosis, prolonged fasting, severe renal failure.

Visken should not be taken in conjunction with agents which inhibit calcium transport, e.g. verapamil.

Use in pregnancy and lactation: Visken is contra-indicated in pregnancy and passes in small quantities into breast milk.

Precautions: Patients with a poor cardiac reserve should be stabilised with digitalis before treatment with Visken to prevent impairment of myocardial contractility.

As with all beta-blockers, Visken should be used with caution in patients with a history of non-asthmatic chronic obstructive lung disease or recent myocardial infarction. Caution must be exercised when beta-blocking agents are administered to patients with spontaneous hypoglycaemia or diabetics under treatment with insulin or oral hypoglycaemic agents, since hypoglycaemia may occur during prolonged fasting and some of its symptoms (tachycardia, tremor) may be masked.

During treatment with Visken, patients should not undergo anaesthesia with agents causing myocardial depression (e.g. halothane, cyclopropane, trichlorethylene, ether, chloroform). Visken should be gradually withdrawn before elective surgery. In emergency surgery or cases where withdrawal of Visken would cause deterioration in cardiac condition, atropine sulphate 1 to 2 mg intravenously should be given to prevent severe bradycardia.

If a beta-blocker is indicated in a patient with a phaeochromocytoma it must always be given in conjunction with an alpha-blocker. Pre-existing peripheral vascular disorders may be aggravated by beta-blockers.

In severe renal failure a further impairment of renal function following beta blockade has been reported in a few cases.

There have been reports of skin rashes and/or dry eyes associated with the use of beta-adrenoceptor blocking drugs. The reported incidence is small and in most cases the symptoms have cleared when treatment was withdrawn. Discontinuance of the drug should be considered if any such reaction is not otherwise explicable. Cessation of therapy with a beta-blocker should be gradual.

Because dizziness or fatigue may occur during the initial phase of treatment with antihypertensive drugs, patients driving vehicles or operating machinery should exercise caution until their individual response to treatment has been determined.

Drug interactions:

Calcium-channel blocking agents: experience has shown that the concomitant use of oral beta-blockers and calcium antagonists of the dihydropyridine type can be useful in hypertension or angina pectoris. However, because of their potential effect on the cardiac conduction system and contractility, the i.v. route must be avoided.

Cimetidine may increase the plasma level of beta-blockers, possibly by interference with hepatic metabolism.

Clonidine: when therapy is discontinued in patients receiving a beta-blocker and clonidine concurrently, the beta-blockers should be gradually discontinued several days before clonidine is discontinued, in order to reduce the potential risk of a clonidine withdrawal hypertensive crisis.

MAO inhibitors: concurrent use with beta-blockers is not recommended. Possibly significant hypertension may theoretically occur up to 14 days following discontinuation of the MAO inhibitor.

Non-steroidal anti-inflammatory drugs (NSAIDs): the effect of many antihypertensive agents, including beta-blockers, may be reduced when they are used concurrently with these drugs, possibly as a result of the inhibition of renal prostaglandin synthesis and sodium and fluid retention caused by NSAIDs.

Phenothiazines: concurrent use with beta-blockers may result in an increased plasma concentration of either drug.

Reserpine: concurrent use may result in an additive and possibly excessive beta-adrenergic blockade.

Sympathomimetics with beta-adrenergic stimulant activity and xanthines: concurrent use with beta-blockers may result in mutual inhibition of therapeutic effects; in addition, beta-blockers may decrease theophylline clearance.

Side-effects: Few serious side-effects have been reported. Depression, gastrointestinal distubances (including diarrhoea, nausea and epigastric pain), muscle cramps, tremors, insomnia, headaches, sleep disturbance, fatigue, dizziness and hypotension have occurred but are usually transient and disappear if dosage is reduced. Allergic skin reactions have occasionally been reported.

Overdosage: Treat by elimination of any unabsorbed drug and general supportive measures. Marked bradycardia as a result of overdosage or idiosyncrasy should be treated with atropine sulphate 1 to 2 mg intravenously. If necessary, isoprenaline hydrochloride can be administered by a slow intravenous injection, under constant supervision, beginning with 25 micrograms (5 micrograms/min) until the desired effect is achieved. A cardiac pacemaker may be required; i.v. glucagon (5 to 10 mg) has been reported to overcome some of the features of serious overdosage and may be useful.

Pharmaceutical precautions Nil.

Legal category POM.

Package quantities Blister pack of 56 (OP).

Further information Nil.

Product licence number 0101/0065

Product licence holder: Novartis Pharmaceuticals UK Limited, trading as Sandoz Pharmaceuticals, Frimley Business Park, Camberley, Surrey, GU16 5SG.

Date of last revision April 1998.

VISKEN TABLETS 15 mg

Qualitative and quantitative composition Each tablet contains 15 mg pindolol.

Pharmaceutical form Tablet.

Clinical particulars

Therapeutic indications: For the treatment of hypertension and the prophylaxis of angina pectoris.

Posology and method of administration

Adults: Hypertension: initially one 15 mg tablet daily, with breakfast, or 5 mg two or three times daily. Most patients respond to a once daily dose of from 15–30 mg. If necessary, dosages may be increased at weekly intervals up to a maximum of 45 mg daily in single or divided doses. Patients not responding after 3–4 weeks at this dosage level rarely benefit from further elevation in dosage. Addition of VISKEN to existing diuretic therapy increases the hypotensive effect and combination with other antihypertensives enables reduction in dosage of these other agents.

Children: Experience with VISKEN in children is limited.

Use in the elderly: No data are available to show that elderly patients require different dosages or show different side effects from younger patients.

Method of administration: Oral.

Contra-indications: Untreated cardiac failure, cardiogenic shock, sick sinus syndrome, second and third degree heart block, Prinzmetals angina, history of bronchospasm and bronchial asthma (a warning stating 'do not take this medicine if you have a history of wheezing or asthma' will appear on the label), untreated phaeochromocytoma, peripheral circulatory disease, pronounced bradycardia, obstructive pulmonary disease, history of cor pulmonale, metabolic acidosis, prolonged fasting, severe renal failure. VISKEN should not be taken in conjunction with agents which inhibit calcium transport, e.g. verapamil.

Special warnings and special precautions for use: Patients with a poor cardiac reserve should be stabilised before treatment with VISKEN to prevent impairment of myocardial contractility.

As for other beta-blockers, and especially in patients with ischaemic heart disease, treatment should not be discontinued suddenly. The dosage should gradually be reduced, i.e. over 1–2 weeks, if necessary at the same time initiating replacement therapy, to prevent exacerbation of angina pectoris.

As with all beta-blockers, VISKEN should be used with caution in patients with a history of non-asthmatic chronic obstructive lung disease or recent myocardial infarction. Caution must be exercised when beta-blocking agents are administered to patients with spontaneous hypoglycaemia or diabetes under treatment with insulin or oral hypoglycaemic agents, since hypoglycaemia may occur during prolonged fasting and some of its symptoms (tachycardia, tremor) may be masked. Beta blockers may also mask the symptoms of thyrotoxicosis. During treatment with VISKEN, patients should not undergo anaesthesia with agents causing myocardial depression (e.g. Halothane, cyclopropane, trichlorethylene, ether, chloroform). VISKEN should be gradually withdrawn before elective surgery. In emergency surgery or cases where withdrawal of VISKEN would cause deterioration in cardiac condition, atropine sulphate 1 to 2 mg intravenously should be given to prevent severe bradycardia.

If a beta-blocker is indicated in a patient with phaeochromocytoma it must always be given in conjunction with an alpha-blocker. Pre-existing peripheral vascular disorders may be aggravated by beta-blockers.

In severe renal failure a further impairment of renal function following beta blockage has been reported in a few cases.

There have been reports of skin rashes and/or dry eyes associated with the use of beta-adrenoceptor blocking drugs. The reported incidence is small and in most cases the symptoms have cleared when treatment is withdrawn. Discontinuance of the drug should be considered if any such reaction is not otherwise explicable.

Patients with known psoriasis should take beta-blockers only after careful consideration.

Beta blockers may increase both the sensitivity towards allergens and the seriousness of anaphylactic reactions.

Interaction with other medicaments and other forms of interaction: Calcium-channel blocking agents: VISKEN should not be used with calcium-channel blockers with negative ionotropic effects e.g. verapamil and to a lesser extent diltiazem. The concomitant use of oral beta-blockers and calcium antagonists of the dihydropyridine type can be useful in hypertention or angina pectoris. However, because of their potential effect on the cardiac conduction system and contractility, the i.v. route must be avoided. The concomitant use with dihydropyridines, e.g. Nifedapine, may increase the risk of hypotension. In patients with cardiac insufficiency, treatment with beta-blocking agents may lead to cardiac failure.

Use of digitalis glycosides, in association with beta-adrenoceptor blocking drugs, may increase atrio-ventricular conduction time.

Clonidine: when therapy is discontinued in patients receiving a beta-blocker and clonidine concurrently, the beta-blockers should be gradually discontinued several days before clonidine is discontinued, in order to reduce the potential risk of a clonidine withdrawal hypertensive crisis.

MAO inhibitors: concurrent use with beta-blockers is not recommended. Possibly significant hypertension may theoretically occur up to 14 days following discontinuation of the MAO inhibitor.

Caution should be exercised in the concurrent use of beta-blocking agents with class 1 antiarrhythmics (e.g. disopyramide, quinidine) and amiodarone.

Concomitant use of beta-blockers may intensify the blood sugar lowering effect of insulin and other antidiabetic drugs. Use of beta-blockers may prevent appearance of the signs of hypocalcaemia (tachycardia).

Cimetidine, hydralazine and alcohol may increase the plasma levels of hepatically metabolised beta-blockers.

Prostaglandin synthetase inhibiting drugs may decrease the hypotensive effects of beta-blockers.

Sympathomimetics with beta-adrenergic stimulant activity and xanthines: concurrent use with beta-blockers may result in mutual inhibition of therapeutic effects; in addition, beta-blockers may decrease theophylline clearance.

Concomitant use of beta-blockers with tricyclic antidepressants, barbiturates and phenothiazines as well as other anti-hypertensive agents may increase the blood pressure lowering effect.

Reserpine: concurrent use may result in an additive and possibly excessive beta-adrenergic blockade.

Pregnancy and lactation: VISKEN is contraindicated in pregnancy and passes in small quantities into breast milk. Breastfeeding is therefore not recommended following administration.

Effects on ability to drive and to use machines: Because dizziness or fatigue may occur during initiation of treatment with antihypertensive drugs, patients driving vehicles or operating machinery should exercise caution until their individual reaction to treatment has been determined.

Undesirable effects: Bradycardia, a slowed AV-conduction or increase of an existing AV-block, hypotension, heart failure, cold and cyanotic extremities, Raynaud's phenomenon, paraesthesia of the extremities, increase of an existing intermittent claudication. Fatigue, headaches, impaired vision, hallucinations, psychoses, confusion, impotence, dizziness, sleep disturbances, depression, nightmares. Gastro-intestinal problems, nausea, vomiting, diarrhoea. Bronchospasm in patients with bronchial asthma or a history of asthmatic complaints. Disorder of the skin, especially rash. Dry eyes. Beta-blockers may mask the symptoms of thyreotoxicosis or hypoglycaemia. An increase in ANA (anti nuclear antibodies) has been seen; its clinical relevance is not clear.

Overdose: Treat by elimination of any unabsorbed drug and general supportive measures. Marked bradycardia as a result of overdosage or idiosyncrasy should be treated with atropine sulphate 1 or 2 mg intravenously. If necessary, isoprenaline hydrochloride can be administered by a slow intravenous injection, under constant supervision, beginning with 25 mcg (5 mcg/min) until the desired effect is achieved. A cardiac pacemaker may be required, i.v. glucagon (5–10 mg) has been reported to overcome some of the features of serious overdosage and may be useful.

Pharmacological properties

Pharmacodynamic properties: VISKEN is a specific beta-adrenoceptor blocking agent with low cardio-depressant activity at therapeutic doses. Its beta-blocking activity prevents excessive sympathetic drive to the heart, resulting in a fall in heart rate and a decrease in cardiac work and myocardial oxygen consumption. VISKEN possesses some intrinsic sympathomimetic activity even at low dosage, which may prevent reduction of resting sympathetic tone to an undesirably low level and minimise myocardial depression.

Pharmacokinetic properties: The rapid nearly complete absorption (>95%) and the negligible hepatic first-pass effect (13%) of VISKEN result in a high bioavailability (87%). Maximum plasma concentration is reached within one hour after oral administration. VISKEN has a plasma protein binding of 40%, a volume of distribution of 2–3 L/kg and a total clearance of 500 ml/min. The elimination half-life of VISKEN is 3–4 hours. 30–40% is excreted unchanged in the urine, while 60–70% is excreted via kidney and liver as inactive metabolites. VISKEN crosses the placental barrier and passes in small quantities into breast milk.

Preclinical safety data: There are no pre-clinical data of relevance to the prescriber which are additional to that already included in other sections of the SmPC.

Pharmaceutical particulars

List of excipients: Microcrystalline cellulose, starch, colloidal anhydrous silica, magnesium stearate.

Incompatibilities: None.

Shelf life: 5 years from date of manufacture.

Special precautions for storage: None.

Nature and contents of container: PVDC opaque blister packs in a cardboard carton containing 28 tablets.

Instructions for use/handling: None.

Marketing authorisation holder: Novartis Pharmaceuticals UK Limited, trading as Sandoz Pharmaceuticals, Frimley Business Park, Frimley, Camberley, Surrey GU16 5SG.

Marketing authorisation number PL0101/0110.

Date of first authorisation/renewal of the authorisation 30 April 1997.

Date of (partial) revision of the text 23rd April 1997.

Legal category POM.

VOLTAROL* AMPOULES

Qualitative and quantitative composition The active ingredient is sodium-[o-[(2,6-dichlorophenyl)-amino]-phenyl]-acetate) (diclofenac sodium).

Each 3 ml ampoule contains 75 mg diclofenac sodium.

Pharmaceutical form Solution for injection in ampoules.

Clinical particulars

Therapeutic indications:

Ampoules for intramuscular use: The ampoules are effective in acute forms of pain, including renal colic, exacerbations of osteo- and rheumatoid arthritis, acute back pain, acute gout, acute trauma and fractures, and post-operative pain.

Ampoules used in intravenous infusion: For treatment or prevention of post-operative pain in the hospital setting.

Posology and method of administration:

Adults: Voltarol Ampoules (given i.m. or i.v.) should not be given for more than two days; if necessary, treatment can be continued with Voltarol Tablets or Suppositories.

Intramuscular injection: The following directions for

intramuscular injection must be adhered to in order to avoid damage to a nerve or other tissue at the injection site.

One ampoule once (or in severe cases twice) daily intramuscularly by deep intragluteal injection into the upper outer quadrant. If two injections daily are required it is advised that the alternative buttock be used for the second injection. Alternatively, one ampoule of 75 mg can be combined with other dosage forms of Voltarol (Tablets or Suppositories) up to the maximum daily dosage of 150 mg.

Renal colic: One 75 mg ampoule intramuscularly. A further ampoule may be administered after 30 minutes if necessary. The recommended maximum daily dose of Voltarol is 150 mg.

Intravenous infusion: Immediately before initiating an intravenous infusion, Voltarol must be diluted with 100–500 ml of either sodium chloride solution (0.9%) or glucose solution (5%). Both solutions should be buffered with sodium bicarbonate solution (0.5 ml 8.4% or 1 ml 4.2%). Only clear solutions should be used.

Voltarol must not be given as an intravenous bolus injection.

Two alternative regimens are recommended:

For the *treatment* of moderate to severe post-operative pain, 75 mg should be infused continuously over a period of 30 minutes to 2 hours. If necessary, treatment may be repeated after 4–6 hours, not exceeding 150 mg within any period of 24 hours.

For the *prevention* of post-operative pain, a loading dose of 25 mg–50 mg should be infused after surgery over 15 minutes to 1 hour, followed by a continuous infusion of approx. 5 mg per hour up to a maximum daily dosage of 150 mg.

Children: Voltarol Ampoules are not recommended for use in children.

Elderly: Although the pharmacokinetics of Voltarol are not impaired to any clinically relevant extent in elderly patients, non-steroidal anti-inflammatory drugs should be used with particular caution in such patients who, generally, are more prone to adverse reactions. In particular, it is recommended that the lowest effective dosage be used in frail elderly patients or those with a low body weight (see also *Precautions*).

The recommended maximum daily dose of Voltarol is 150 mg.

Contra-indications: Active or suspected gastro-intestinal ulcers or bleeding.

Previous sensitivity to diclofenac.

Patients in whom attacks of asthma, urticaria or acute rhinitis are precipitated by aspirin or other non-steroidal anti-inflammatory agents.

Hypersensitivity to the excipients sodium metabisulphite, benzyl alcohol, propylene glycol, mannitol.

Specifically for iv use: Concomitant NSAID or anti-coagulant use (including low dose heparin).

History of haemorrhagic diathesis, a history of confirmed or suspected cerebrovascular bleeding.

Operations associated with a high risk of haemorrhage.

A history of asthma.

Moderate or severe renal impairment (serum creatinine >160 μmol/l).

Hypovolaemia or dehydration from any cause.

Special warnings and special precautions for use

Warnings: Gastro-intestinal: Close medical surveillance is imperative in patients with symptoms indicative of gastro-intestinal disorders, with a history suggestive of gasto-intestinal ulceration, with ulcerative colitis or with Crohn's disease.

Gastro-intestinal bleeding or ulcerative/perforation, haematemesis and melaena have, in general, more serious consequences in the elderly. They can occur at any time during treatment, with or without warning symptoms or a previous history. In the rare instances, where gastro-intestinal bleeding or ulceration occurs in patients receiving Voltarol, the drug should be withdrawn.

Hepatic: Close medical surveillance is also imperative in patients suffering from severe impairment of hepatic function.

Hypersensitivity reactions: As with other non-steroidal anti-inflammatory drugs, allergic reactions, including anaphylactic/anaphylactoid reactions, can also occur without earlier exposure to the drug.

Like other NSAIDs, Voltarol may mask the signs and symptoms of infection due to its pharmacodynamic properties.

Precautions: Renal: Patients with renal, cardiac or hepatic impairment and the elderly should be kept under surveillance, since the use of NSAIDs may result in deterioration of renal function. The lowest effective dose should be used and renal function monitored.

The importance of prostaglandins in maintaining renal blood flow should be taken into account in patients with impaired cardiac or renal function, those being treated with diuretics or recovering from major surgery. Effects on renal function are usually reversible on withdrawal of Voltarol.

Hepatic: If abnormal liver function tests persist or worsen, clinical signs or symptoms consistent with liver disease develop or if other manifestations occur (eosinophilia, rash), Voltarol should be discontinued. Hepatitis may occur without prodromal symptoms.

Use of Voltarol in patients with hepatic porphyria may trigger an attack.

Haematological: Voltarol may reversibly inhibit platelet aggregation (see *Anticoagulants* in *Drug interactions*). Patients with defects of haemostasis, bleeding diathesis or haematological abnormalities should be carefully monitored.

Long-term treatment: All patients who are receiving non-steroidal anti-inflammatory agents should be monitored as a precautionary measure e.g. renal function, hepatic function (elevation of liver enzymes may occur) and blood counts. This is particularly important in the elderly.

Interaction with other medicaments and other forms of interaction:

Lithium and digoxin: Voltarol may increase plasma concentrations of lithium and digoxin.

Anticoagulants: Although clinical investigations do not appear to indicate that Voltarol has an influence on the effect of anticoagulants, there are isolated reports of an increased risk of haemorrhage with the combined use of diclofenac and anticoagulant therapy. Therefore, to be certain that no change in anticoagulant dosage is required, close monitoring of such patients is required. As with other non-steroidal anti-inflammatory agents, diclofenac in a high dose can reversibly inhibit platelet aggregation.

Antidiabetic agents: Clinical studies have shown that Voltarol can be given together with oral antidiabetic agents without influencing their clinical effect. However, there have been isolated reports of hypoglycaemic and hyperglycaemic effects which have required adjustment to the dosage of hypoglycaemic agents.

Cyclosporin: Cases of nephrotoxicity have been reported in patients receiving concomitant cyclosporin and NSAIDs, including Voltarol. This might be mediated through combined renal antiprostaglandin effects of both the NSAID and cyclosporin.

Methotrexate: Cases of serious toxicity have been reported when methotrexate and NSAIDs are given within 24 hours of each other. This interaction is mediated through accumulation of methotrexate resulting from impairment of renal excretion in the presence of the NSAID.

Quinolone antimicrobials: Convulsions may occur due to an interaction between quinolones and NSAIDs. This may occur in patients with or without a previous history of epilepsy or convulsions. Therefore, caution should be exercised when considering the use of a quinolone in patients who are already receiving an NSAID.

Other NSAIDs and steroids: Co-administration of Voltarol with other systemic NSAIDs and steroids may increase the frequency of side-effects. Concomitant therapy with aspirin lowers the plasma levels of each, although no clinical significance is known.

Diuretics: Various NSAIDs are liable to inhibit the activity of diuretics. Concomitant treatment with potassium-sparing diuretics may be associated with increased serum potassium levels, hence serum potassium should be monitored.

Pregnancy and lactation: Although animal studies have not demonstrated teratogenic effects, Voltarol should not be prescribed during pregnancy, unless there are compelling reasons for doing so. The lowest effective dosage should be used.

Use of prostaglandin synthetase inhibitors may result in premature closure of the ductus arteriosus or uterine inertia; such drugs are, therefore, not recommended during the last trimester of pregnancy.

Following doses of 50 mg enteric coated tablets every 8 hours, traces of active substance have been detected in breast milk, but in quantities so small that no undesirable effects on the infant are to be expected.

Effects on ability to drive and use machines: Patients who experience dizziness or other central nervous disturbances, while taking NSAIDs should refrain from driving or operating machinery.

Undesirable effects: If serious side-effects occur, Voltarol should be withdrawn.

Frequency estimate: *frequent:* >10%, *occasional:* >1–10%, *rare:* >0.001–1%, *isolated cases:* <0.001%.

Gastro-intestinal tract: Occasional: Epigastric pain, other gastro-intestinal disorders (e.g. nausea, vomiting, diarrhoea, abdominal cramps, dyspepsia, flatulence, anorexia). *Rare:* Gastro-intestinal bleeding (haematemesis, melaena, bloody diarrhoea), gastro-intestinal ulcers with or without bleeding or perforation. *Isolated cases:* Aphthous stomatitis, glossitis, oesophageal lesions, lower gut disorders (e.g. non-specific haemorrhagic colitis and exacerbations of ulcerative colitis or Crohn's proctocolitis, colonic damage and stricture formation), pancreatitis, constipation.

Central nervous system: Occasional: Headache, dizziness, or vertigo. *Rare:* drowsiness, tiredness. *Isolated cases:* Disturbances of sensation, paraesthesia, memory disturbance, disorientation, insomnia, irritability, convulsions, depression, anxiety, nightmares, tremor, psychotic reactions, aseptic meningitis.

Special senses: Isolated cases: Disturbances of vision (blurred vision, diplopia), impaired hearing, tinnitus, taste disturbances.

Skin: Occasional: Rashes or skin eruptions. *Rare:* Urticaria. *Isolated cases:* Bullous eruptions, eczema, erythema multiforme, Stevens-Johnson syndrome, Lyell's syndrome (acute toxic epidermolysis), erythroderma (exfoliative dermatitis), loss of hair, photosensitivity reactions, purpura including allergic purpura.

Kidney: Rare: Oedema. *Isolated cases:* Acute renal insufficiency, urinary abnormalities (e.g. haematuria, proteinuria), interstitial nephritis, nephrotic syndrome, papillary necrosis.

Liver: Occasional: Elevation of serum aminotransferase enzymes (ALT, AST). *Rare:* Liver function disorders including hepatitis (in isolated cases fulminant) with or without jaundice.

Blood: Isolated cases: Thrombocytopenia, leucopenia, agranulocytosis, haemolytic anaemia, aplastic anaemia.

Hypersensitivity: Rare: Hypersensitivity reactions (e.g. bronchospasm, anaphylactic/anaphylactoid systemic reactions including hypotension). *Isolated cases:* Vasculitis, pneumonitis.

Cardiovascular system: Isolated cases: palpitations, chest pain, hypertension, congestive heart failure.

Reactions to the intramuscular injection: Occasional: Reactions such as local pain and induration. *Isolated cases:* Abscesses and local necrosis at the intramuscular injection site.

Overdose: Management of acute poisoning with NSAIDs essentially consists of supportive and symptomatic measures. There is no typical clinical picture resulting from Voltarol overdosage. Supportive and symptomatic treatment should be given for complications such as hypotension, renal failure, convulsions, gastro-intestinal irritation, and respiratory depression; specific therapies such as forced diuresis, dialysis or haemoperfusion are probably of no help in eliminating NSAIDs due to their high rate of protein binding and extensive metabolism.

Pharmacological properties

Pharmacodynamic properties:

Pharmacotherapeutic group: Non-steroidal anti-inflammatory drugs (NSAIDs).

Mechanism of action: Voltarol is a non-steroidal agent with marked analgesic/anti-inflammatory properties. It is an inhibitor of prostaglandin synthetase (cyclo-oxygenase). Diclofenac sodium *in vitro* does not suppress proteoglycan biosynthesis in cartilage at concentrations equivalent to the concentrations reached in human beings. When used concomitantly with opioids for the management of post-operative pain, Voltarol often reduces the need for opioids.

Pharmacokinetic properties:

Absorption: After administration of 75 mg diclofenac by intramuscular injection, absorption sets in immediately, and mean peak plasma concentrations of about 2.558±0.968 mcg/ml (2.5 mcg/ml≡8 μmol/l) are reached after about 20 minutes. The amount absorbed is in linear proportion to the size of the dose.

Intravenous infusion: When 75 mg diclofenac is administered as an intravenous infusion over 2 hours, mean peak plasma concentrations are about 1.875±0.436 mcg/ml (1.9 mcg/ml≡5.9 μmol/l). Shorter infusions result in higher peak plasma concentrations, while longer infusions give plateau concentrations proportional to the infusion rate after 3 to 4 hours. This is in contrast to the rapid decline in plasma concentrations seen after peak levels have been achieved with oral, rectal or intramuscular administration.

Bioavailability: The area under the concentration curve (AUC) after intramuscular or intravenous administration is about twice as large as it is following oral or rectal administration as this route avoids 'first-pass' metabolism.

Distribution: The active substance is 99.7% protein bound, mainly to albumin (99.4%).

Diclofenac enters the synovial fluid, where maximum concentrations are measured 2–4 hours after the peak plasma values have been attained. The apparent half-life for elimination from the synovial fluid is 3–6 hours. Two hours after reaching the peak plasma values, concentrations of the active substance are already higher in the synovial fluid than they are in the plasma and remain higher for up to 12 hours.

Metabolism: Biotransformation of diclofenac takes place partly by glucuronidation of the intact molecule, but mainly by single and multiple hydroxylation and methoxylation, resulting in several phenolic metabolites, most of which are converted to glucuronide conjugates. Two phenolic metabolites are biologically active, but to a much lesser extent than diclofenac.

Elimination: Total systemic clearance of diclofenac in plasma is 263±56 ml/min (mean value±SD). The terminal half-life in plasma is 1–2 hours. Four of the metabolites, including the two active ones, also have short plasma half-lives of 1–3 hours.

About 60% of the administered dose is excreted in the urine in the form of the glucuronide conjugate of the intact molecule and as metabolites, most of which are also converted to glucuronide conjugates. Less than 1% is excreted as unchanged substance. The rest of the dose is eliminated as metabolites through the bile in the faeces.

Characteristics in patients: Elderly: No relevant age-dependent differences in the drug's absorption, metabolism or excretion have been observed, other than the finding that in five elderly patients, a 15 minute iv infusion resulted in 50% higher plasma concentrations than expected with young healthy subjects.

Patients with renal impairment: In patients suffering from renal impairment, no accumulation of the unchanged active substance can be inferred from the single-dose kinetics when applying the usual dosage schedule. At a creatinine clearance of <10 ml/min, the calculated steady-state plasma levels of the hydroxy metabolites are about 4 times higher than in normal subjects. However, the metabolites are ultimately cleared through the bile.

Patients with hepatic disease: In patients with chronic hepatitis or non-decompensated cirrhosis, the kinetics and metabolism of diclofenac are the same as in patients without liver disease.

Preclinical safety data: None stated.

Pharmaceutical particulars

List of excipients: Voltarol Ampoules also contain mannitol, sodium metabisulphite (E.223), benzyl alcohol, propylene glycol, sodium hydroxide and water.

Incompatibilities: The ampoules used im or iv as an infusion should not be mixed with other injection solutions.

Shelf life: Two years.

Special precautions for storage: Protect from light and heat (store below 30°C).

Medicines should be kept out of the reach of children.

The infusion solution should not be used if crystals or precipitates are observed.

Nature and contents of container: The glass ampoules (PhEur Type I) contain colourless to faintly yellow liquid and come in packs of 2 and 10.

Instructions for use/handling: Intravenous infusions should be freshly made up and used immediately. Once prepared, the infusion should not be stored.

Marketing authorisation holder: Novartis Pharmaceuticals UK Limited, trading as Geigy Pharmaceuticals.

Marketing authorisation number 00101/0466.

Date of approval/revision of SPC September 1997.

Legal category POM.

VOLTAROL* DISPERSIBLE TABLETS

Qualitative and quantitative composition The active ingredient is o-[(2,6-dichlorophenyl)amino]phenyl-acetic acid (diclofenac). Each tablet contains 46.5 mg diclofenac free acid, which is equivalent to 50 mg of diclofenac sodium.

Pharmaceutical form Tablet.

Clinical particulars

Therapeutic indications:

Adults and elderly: The rapid onset of absorption of diclofenac from Voltarol Dispersible makes this preparation more suitable for *short-term* use in acute conditions for which treatment is required for no more than 3 months including: acute episodes of arthritic conditions, acute musculo-skeletal disorders and acute pain resulting from trauma.

There is no information on the use of Voltarol Dispersible for more than 3 months.

Posology and method of administration:

Adults: 100–150 mg daily in two or three divided doses. The Voltarol Dispersible tablet should be dropped into a glass of water, and the liquid stirred to aid dispersion, before swallowing.

The recommended maximum daily dose of Voltarol is 150 mg.

Children: Not recommended.

Elderly: Although the pharmacokinetics of Voltarol are not impaired to any clinically relevant extent in elderly patients, non-steroidal anti-inflammatory drugs should be used with particular caution in such patients who, generally, are more prone to adverse reactions. In particular, it is recommended that the lowest effective dosage be used in frail elderly patients or those with a low body weight (see also *Precautions*).

Contra-indications: Active or suspected gastro-intestinal ulcers or bleeding. Previous sensitivity to diclofenac. Patients in whom attacks of asthma, urticaria or acute rhinitis are precipitated by aspirin or other non-steroidal anti-inflammatory agents.

Special warnings and special precautions for use

Warnings: Gastro-intestinal: Close medical surveillance is imperative in patients with symptoms indicative of gastro-intestinal disorders, with a history suggestive of gastro-intestinal ulceration, with ulcerative colitis, or with Crohn's disease.

Gastro-intestinal bleeding or ulcerative/perforation, haematemesis and melaena have, in general, more serious consequences in the elderly. They can occur at any time during treatment, with or without warning symptoms or a previous history. In the rare instances when gastro-intestinal bleeding or ulceration occurs in patients receiving Voltarol, the drug should be withdrawn.

In choosing to prescribe Voltarol Dispersible it should be remembered that any liquid NSAID preparation does not have the advantages of an enteric-coated tablet in relation to gastric tolerability. In clinical trials of three months duration, a slight increase in the frequency and reported severity of G.I. side-effects and higher rates of withdrawal because of these have been noted in patients receiving dispersible tablets compared with those receiving enteric-coated tablets.

An endoscopy study also revealed Voltarol Dispersible to have a slightly higher mucosal injury score than enteric-coated tablets, although no ulcers occurred with either treatment. These observations must be taken into account and weighed against the advantages of the dispersible formulation.

Hepatic: Close medical surveillance is also imperative in patients suffering from severe impairment of hepatic function.

Hypersensitivity reactions: As with other non-steroidal anti-inflammatory drugs, allergic reactions, including anaphylactic/anaphylactoid reactions, can also occur without earlier exposure to the drug.

Like other NSAIDs, Voltarol may mask the signs and symptoms of infection due to its pharmacodynamic properties.

Precautions:

Renal: Patients with renal, cardiac or hepatic impairment and the elderly should be kept under surveillance, since the use of NSAIDs may result in deterioration of renal function. The lowest effective dose should be used and renal function monitored.

The importance of prostaglandins in maintaining renal blood flow should be taken into account in patients with impaired cardiac or renal function, those being treated with diuretics or recovering from major surgery. Effects on renal function are usually reversible on withdrawal of Voltarol.

Hepatic: If abnormal liver function tests persist or worsen, clinical signs or symptoms consistent with liver disease develop or if other manifestations occur (eosinophilia, rash), Voltarol should be discontinued. Hepatitis may occur without prodromal symptoms.

Use of Voltarol in patients with hepatic porphyria may trigger an attack.

Haematological: Voltarol may reversibly inhibit platelet aggregation (see *Anticoagulants* in *Drug interactions*). Patients with defects of haemostasis, bleeding diathesis or haematological abnormalities should be carefully monitored.

Long-term treatment: All patients who are receiving non-steroidal anti-inflammatory agents should be monitored as a precautionary measure e.g. renal function, hepatic function (elevation of liver enzymes may occur) and blood counts. This is particularly important in the elderly.

Interaction with other medicaments and other forms of interaction:

Lithium and digoxin: Voltarol may increase plasma concentrations of lithium and digoxin.

Anticoagulants: Although clinical investigations do not appear to indicate that Voltarol has an influence on the effect of anticoagulants, there are isolated reports of an increased risk of haemorrhage with the combined use of diclofenac and anticoagulant therapy. Therefore, to be certain that no change in anticoagulant dosage is required, close monitoring of such patients is required. As with other non-steroidal anti-inflammatory agents, diclofenac in high dose can reversibly inhibit platelet aggregation.

Antidiabetic agents: Clinical studies have shown that Voltarol can be given together with oral antidiabetic agents without influencing their clinical effect. However, there have been isolated reports of hypoglycaemic and hyperglycaemic effects which have required adjustment to the dosage of hypoglycaemic agents.

Cyclosporin: Cases of nephrotoxicity have been reported in patients receiving concomitant cyclosporin and NSAIDs, including Voltarol. This might be mediated through combined renal antiprostaglandin effects of both the NSAID and cyclosporin.

Methotrexate: Cases of serious toxicity have been reported when methotrexate and NSAIDs are given within 24 hours of each other. This interaction is mediated through accumulation of methotrexate resulting from impairment of renal excretion in the presence of the NSAID.

Quinolone antimicrobials: Convulsions may occur due to an interaction between quinolones and NSAIDs. This may occur in patients with or without a previous history of epilepsy or convulsions. Therefore, caution should be exercised when considering the use of a quinolone in patients who are already receiving an NSAID.

Other NSAIDs and steroids: Co-administration of Voltarol with other systemic NSAIDs and steroids may increase the frequency of unwanted effects. Concomitant therapy with aspirin lowers the plasma levels of each, although no clinical significance is known.

Diuretics: Various NSAIDs are liable to inhibit the activity of diuretics. Concomitant treatment with potassium-sparing diuretics may be associated with increased serum potassium levels, hence serum potassium should be monitored.

Pregnancy and lactation: Although animal studies have not demonstrated teratogenic effects, Voltarol should not be prescribed during pregnancy, unless there are compelling reasons for doing so. The lowest effective dosage should be used.

Use of prostaglandin synthetase inhibitors may result in premature closure of the ductus arteriosus or uterine inertia; such drugs are, therefore, not recommended during the last trimester of pregnancy.

Following doses of 50 mg enteric coated tablets every 8 hours, traces of active substance have been detected in breast milk, but in quantities so small that no undesirable effects on the infant are to be expected.

Effects on ability to drive and use machines: Patients who experience dizziness or other central nervous disturbances while taking NSAIDs should refrain from driving or operating machinery.

Undesirable effects: If serious side-effects occur, Voltarol should be withdrawn.

Frequency estimate: *frequent:* >10%, *occasional:* >1–10%, *rare:* >0.001–1%, *isolated cases:* <0.001%.

Gastro-intestinal tract: Occasional: Epigastric pain, other gastro-intestinal disorders (e.g. nausea, vomiting, diarrhoea, abdominal cramps, dyspepsia, flatulence, anorexia). *Rare:* Gastro-intestinal bleeding (haematemesis, melaena, bloody diarrhoea), gastro-intestinal ulcers with or without bleeding or perforation. *Isolated cases:* Aphthous stomatitis, glossitis, oesophageal lesions, lower gut disorders (e.g. non-specific haemorrhagic colitis and exacerbations of ulcerative colitis or Crohn's proctocolitis, colonic damage and stricture formation), pancreatitis, constipation.

Central nervous system: Occasional: Headache, dizziness, or vertigo. *Rare:* drowsiness, tiredness. *Isolated cases:* Disturbances of sensation, paraesthesia, memory disturbance, disorientation, insomnia, irritability, convulsions, depression, anxiety, nightmares, tremor, psychotic reactions, aseptic meningitis.

Special senses: Isolated cases: Disturbances of vision (blurred vision, diplopia), impaired hearing, tinnitus, taste disturbances.

Skin: Occasional: Rashes or skin eruptions. *Rare:* Urticaria. *Isolated cases:* Bullous eruptions, eczema, erythema multiforme, Stevens-Johnson syndrome, Lyell's syndrome (acute toxic epidermolysis), erythroderma (exfoliative dermatitis), loss of hair, photosensitivity reactions, purpura including allergic purpura.

Kidney: Rare: Oedema. *Isolated cases:* Acute renal insufficiency, urinary abnormalities (e.g. haematuria, proteinuria), interstitial nephritis, nephrotic syndrome, papillary necrosis.

Liver: Occasional: Elevation of serum aminotransferase enzymes (ALT, AST). *Rare:* Liver function disorders including hepatitis (in isolated cases fulminant) with or without jaundice.

Blood: In isolated cases: Thrombocytopenia, leucopenia, agranulocytosis, haemolytic anaemia, aplastic anaemia.

Hypersensitivity: Rare: Hypersensitivity reactions (e.g. bronchospasm, anaphylactic/anaphylactoid systemic reactions including hypotension). *Isolated cases:* Vasculitis, pneumonitis.

Cardiovascular system: Isolated cases: Palpitations, chest pain, hypertension, congestive heart failure.

Overdose: Management of acute poisoning with NSAIDs essentially consists of supportive and symptomatic measures. There is no typical clinical picture resulting from Voltarol overdosage. The therapeutic measures to be taken are: supportive and symptomatic treatment should be given for complications such as hypotension, renal failure, convulsions, gastro-intestinal irritation, and respiratory depression; specific therapies such as forced diuresis, dialysis or haemoperfusion are probably of no help in eliminating NSAIDs due to their high rate of protein binding and extensive metabolism.

Pharmacological properties

Pharmacodynamic properties:

Pharmacotherapeutic group: Non-steroidal anti-inflammatory drugs (NSAIDs).

Mechanism of action: Voltarol is a non-steroidal agent with marked analgesic/anti-inflammatory properties. It is an inhibitor of prostaglandin synthetase (cyclo-oxygenase).

Diclofenac sodium *in vitro* does not suppress proteoglycan biosynthesis in cartilage at concentrations equivalent to the concentrations reached in human beings.

Pharmacokinetic properties:

Absorption: Absorption begins immediately upon administration. Mean peak plasma concentrations of diclofenac are reached at about 1 hour 0.9±0.0.4 mcg/ml (1 mcg/ml≡3 μmol/l). Ingestion of dispersible tablets together with or immediately after a meal does not delay the onset of absorption but reduces the amount absorbed by an average of about 16% and the maximum concentrations by about 50%.

Bioavailability: The bioavailability is 82% of that of enteric-coated tablets. Ingestion with food affects the bioavailability (see above).

Pharmacokinetic behaviour does not change on repeated administration. Accumulation does not occur, provided the recommended dosage intervals are observed.

Distribution: The active substance is 99.7% protein bound, mainly to albumin (99.4%).

Diclofenac enters the synovial fluid, where maximum concentrations are measured 2–4 hours after the peak plasma values have been attained. The apparent half-life for elimination from the synovial fluid is 3–6 hours. Two hours after reaching the peak plasma values, concentrations of the active substance are already higher in the synovial fluid than they are in the plasma and they remain higher for up to 12 hours.

Metabolism: Biotransformation of diclofenac takes place partly by glucuronidation of the intact molecule, but mainly by single and multiple hydroxylation and methoxylation, resulting in several phenolic metabolites, most of which are converted to glucuronide conjugates. Two phenolic metabolites are biologically active, but to a much lesser extent than diclofenac.

Elimination: The total systemic clearance of diclofenac in plasma is 263±56 ml/min (mean value±SD). The terminal half-life in plasma is 1–2 hours. Four of the metabolites, including the two active ones, also have short plasma half-lives of 1–3 hours.

About 60% of the administered dose is excreted in the urine in the form of the glucuronide conjugate of the intact molecule and as metabolites, most of which are also converted to glucuronide conjugates. Less than 1% is excreted as unchanged substance. The rest of the dose is eliminated as metabolites through the bile in the faeces.

Characteristics in patients: Elderly: No relevant age-dependent differences in the drug's absorption, metabolism, or excretion have been observed, other than the finding that in five elderly patients, a 15 minute iv infusion resulted in 50% higher plasma concentrations than expected with young healthy subjects.

Patients with renal impairmment: In patients suffering from renal impairment, no accumulation of the unchanged active substance can be inferred from the single-dose kinetics when applying the usual dosage schedule. At a creatinine clearance of <10 ml/min, the calculated steady-state plasma levels of the hydroxy metabolites are about 4 times higher than in normal subjects. However, the metabolites are ultimately cleared through the bile.

Patients with hepatic disease: In patients with chronic hepatitis or non-decompensated cirrhosis, the kinetics and metabolism of diclofenac are the same as in patients without liver disease.

Preclinical safety data: None stated.

Pharmaceutical particulars

List of excipients: The dispersible tablets also contain microcrystalline cellulose, croscarmellose sodium type A, sodium starch glycollate, sodium saccharin, hydrogenated caster oil, purified talc special, colloidal anhydrous silica, blackcurrant and F.D. and C. red No. 3.

Incompatibilities: None known.

Shelf life: Five years.

Special precautions for storage: Protect from heat (store below 30°C) and moisture. Medicines should be kept out of the reach of children.

Nature and contents of container: The tablets are pink speckled with white, triangular shaped, uncoated tablets, impressed GEIGY on one side with an embossed 'V' on the other, with a blackcurrant odour and come in aluminium blister packs of 21.

Instructions for use/handling: The dispersible tablets should be dissolved in water.

Market authorisation holder: Novartis Pharmaceuticals UK Limited, trading as Geigy Pharmaceuticals.

Marketing authorisation number 00101/0467.

Date of approval/revision of SPC September 1997.

Legal category POM.

VOLTAROL* EMULGEL

Qualitative and quantitative composition Diethylammonium-{-o-[2,6-dichlorophenyl)-amino]-phenyl}-acetate. 100 g of Voltarol Emulgel contains 1.16 g of the active substance diclofenac diethylammonium, which corresponds to 1 g diclofenac sodium.

Pharmaceutical form Gel for topical administration.

Clinical particulars

Therapeutic indications:

For the local symptomatic relief of pain and inflammation in:

- trauma of the tendons, ligaments, muscles and joints, e.g. due to sprains, strains and bruises
- localised forms of soft tissue rheumatism

It is recommended that treatment be reviewed after 14 days in these indications.

For the treatment of osteoarthritis of superficial joints such as the knee.

In the treatment of osteoarthritis, therapy should be reviewed after 4 weeks.

Posology and method of administration:

Adults: Voltarol Emulgel should be rubbed gently into the skin. Depending on the size of the affected site to be treated 2–4 g (a circular shaped mass approximately 2.0–2.5 cm in diameter) should be applied 3–4 times a day. After application, the hands should be washed unless they are the site being treated.

Use in the elderly: The usual adult dosage may be used.

Children: Voltarol Emulgel is not recommended for use in children as dosage recommendations and indications for use in this group of patients have not been established.

Voltarol Emulgel is suitable for the transmission of ultrasound and may be used as a couplant in combination with ultrasound therapy. If large areas of the body are covered with gel, systemic absorption will be greater and the risk of side-effects increased, especially if the therapy is used frequently.

Contra-indications: Patients with or without chronic asthma in whom attacks of asthma, urticaria or acute rhinitis are precipitated by aspirin or other non-steroidal anti-inflammatory agents. Hypersensitivity to diclofenac, acetylsalicylic acid or other non-steroidal anti-inflammatory drugs. Hypersensitivity to propylene glycol, isopropanol or other components of the gel base.

Special warnings and special precautions for use:

Warnings: None stated.

Precautions: Concomitant use of oral NSAIDs should be cautioned as the incidence of untoward effects, particularly systemic side effects, may increase (see also *Interactions*).

Voltarol Emulgel should not be co-administered with other products containing diclofenac.

Voltarol Emulgel should be applied only to intact, non-diseased skin and not to skin wounds or open injuries. It should not be used with occlusion. It should not be allowed to come into contact with the eyes or mucous membranes, and should never be taken by mouth.

Some possibility of gastro-intestinal bleeding in those with a significant history of this condition has been reported in isolated cases.

Interactions with other medicaments and other forms of interaction: Systemic absorption of Voltarol Emulgel is low and hence the risk of an interaction is small. There are no known interactions with Volterol Emulgel but for a list of interactions known with oral diclofenac the SPC for oral dosage forms should be consulted.

Pregnancy and lactation: Since no experience has been acquired with Voltarol Emulgel in pregnancy or lactation, it is not recommended for use in these circumstances.

During the last trimester of pregnancy the use of prostaglandin synthetase inhibitors may result in premature closure of the ductus arteriosus, or in uterine inertia.

Animal data have shown an increased incidence of dystonia and delayed parturition when drug administration is continued into late pregnancy.

Effects on ability to drive and use machines: None known.

Undesirable effects: Local reactions: Voltarol Emulgel is usually well tolerated. *Occasional:* allergic or non-allergic contact dermatitis (with symptoms and signs such as itching, reddening, oedema, papules, vesicles, bullae or scaling of skin).

Systemic reactions: Isolated cases: generalised skin rash, hypersensitivity reactions (e.g. asthmatic attacks, angio-oedema), photosensitivity reactions.

Patients should be warned against excessive exposure to sunlight in order to reduce the incidence of photosensitivity.

General: Systemic absorption of Voltarol Emulgel is low compared with plasma levels obtained following administration of oral forms of Voltarol and the likelihood of systemic side-effects occurring with topical diclofenac is small compared with the frequency of side-effects associated with oral diclofenac. However, where Voltarol Emulgel is applied to a relatively large area of skin and over a prolonged period, the possibility of systemic side-effects cannot be completely excluded. If such usage is envisaged, the SPC on Voltarol oral dosage forms should be consulted.

Asthma has been rarely reported in patients using topical NSAID preparations.

Overdose:

Signs and symptoms: The low systemic absorption of Voltarol Emulgel renders overdosage extremely unlikely. In the event of accidental ingestion, resulting in significant systemic side-effects, general therapeutic measures normally adopted to treat poisoning with non-steroidal anti-inflammatory drugs should be used.

Treatment: Management of overdosage with NSAIDs essentially consists of supportive and symptomatic measures. There is no typical clinical picture resulting from Voltarol overdosage. Supportive and symptomatic treatment should be given for complications such as hypotension, renal failure, convulsions, gastro-intestinal irritation, and respiratory depression; specific therapies such as forced diuresis, dialysis or haemoperfusion are probably of no help in eliminating NSAIDs due to their high rate of protein binding and extensive metabolism.

Pharmacological properties

Pharmacodynamic properties: Voltarol Emulgel is a non-steroidal anti-inflammatory (NSAID) and analgesic preparation designed for external application. Due to an aqueous-alcoholic base the gel exerts a soothing and cooling effect.

Pharmacokinetic properties: When Voltarol Emulgel is applied locally, the active substance is absorbed through the skin. In healthy volunteers approximately 6% of the dose applied is absorbed, as determined by urinary excretion of diclofenac and its hydroxylated metabolites. Findings in patients confirm that diclofenac penetrates inflamed areas following local application of Voltarol Emulgel.

After topical administration of Voltarol Emulgel to hand and knee joints diclofenac can be measured in plasma, synovial tissue and synovial fluid. Maximum plasma concentrations of diclofenac are about 100 times lower than after oral administration of Voltarol.

Preclinical safety data: None known.

Pharmaceutical particulars

List of excipients: Diethylamine, carbopol 934P, cetomacrogol 1000, cetiol LC, isopropyl alcohol, liquid paraffin heavy, perfume creme 45, propylene glycol dist., and water.

Incompatibilities: None known.

Shelf life: Three years.

Special precautions for storage: Protect from heat (store below 30°C). Voltarol Emulgel should be kept out of the reach of children.

Nature and contents of container: Aluminium tubes with protective inner coating, available in packs of 10 g, 20 g and 100 g.

Instructions for use/handling: None.

Marketing authorisation holder: Novartis Pharmaceuticals UK Limited, trading as Geigy Pharmaceuticals.

Marketing authorisation number 00101/0468.

Date of approval/revision of SPC 29/04/98.

Legal category POM.

VOLTAROL* TABLETS

Qualitative and quantitative composition The active substance is sodium-[o-[(2,6-dichlorophenyl)-amino]-phenyl]-acetate (diclofenac sodium).

Each enteric-coated tablet contains either 25 mg or 50 mg diclofenac sodium PhEur.

Pharmaceutical form Enteric coated tablet.

Clinical particulars

Therapeutic indications:

Adults and elderly: Relief of all grades of pain and inflammation in a wide range of conditions, including:

(i) arthritic conditions: rheumatoid arthritis, osteoarthritis, ankylosing spondylitis, acute gout,
(ii) acute musculo-skeletal disorders such as periarthritis (for example, frozen shoulder), tendinitis, tenosynovitis, bursitis,
(iii) other painful conditions resulting from trauma, including fracture, low back pain, sprains, strains, dislocations, orthopaedic, dental and other minor surgery.

Children (aged 1–12 years): Juvenile chronic arthritis (25 mg enteric-coated tablets only).

Posology and method of administration

Adults: 75–150 mg daily in two or three divided doses.

The recommended maximum daily dose of Voltarol is 150 mg.

Children (aged 1–12 years) 25 mg enteric-coated tablets only: 1–3 mg/kg per day individed doses.

Elderly: Although the pharmacokinetics of Voltarol are not impaired to any clinically relevant extent in elderly patients, non-steroidal anti-inflammatory drugs should be used with particular caution in such patients who, generally, are more prone to adverse reactions. In particular, it is recommended that the lowest effective dosage be used in frail, elderly patients or those with a low body weight (see also *Precautions*).

Contra-indications: Active or suspected gastro-intestinal ulcers or bleeding.

Previous sensitivity to diclofenac.

Patients in whom attacks of asthma, urticaria or acute rhinitis are precipitated by aspirin or other non-steroidal anti-inflammatory agents.

Special warnings and special precautions for use:

Warnings: Close medical surveillance is imperative in patients with symptoms indicative of gastro-intestinal disorders, with a history suggestive of gastric or intestinal ulceration, with ulcerative colitis, or with Crohn's disease.

Gastro-intestinal bleeding or ulceration/perforation, haematemesis and melaena have, in general, more serious consequences in the elderly. They can occur at any time during treatment, with or without warning symptoms or a previous history. In the rare instances when gastro-intestinal bleeding or ulceration occurs in patients receiving Voltarol, the drug should be withdrawn.

Hepatic: Close medical surveillance is also imperative in patients suffering from severe impairment of hepatic function.

Hypersensitivity reactions: As with other non-steroidal anti-inflammatory drugs, allergic reactions, including anaphylactic/anaphylactoid reactions, can also occur without earlier exposure to the drug.

Like other NSAIDs, Voltarol may mask the signs and symptoms of infection due to its pharmacodynamic properties.

Precautions:

Renal: Patients with renal, cardiac or hepatic impairment and the elderly should be kept under surveillance, since the use of NSAIDs may result in deterioration of renal function. The lowest effective dose should be used and renal function monitored.

The importance of prostaglandins in maintaining renal blood flow should be taken into account in patients with impaired cardiac or renal function, those being treated with diuretics or recovering from major surgery. Effects on renal function are usually reversible on withdrawal of Voltarol.

Hepatic: If abnormal liver function tests persist or worsen, clinical signs or symptoms consistent with liver disease develop or if other manifestations occur (eosinophilia, rash), Voltarol should be discontinued. Hepatitis may occur without prodromal symptoms.

Use of Voltarol in patients with hepatic porphyria may trigger an attack.

Haematological: Voltarol may reversibly inhibit platelet aggregation (see *Anticoagulants* in *Drug interactions*). Patients with defects of haemostasis, bleeding diathesis or haematological abnormalities should be carefully monitored.

Long-term treatment: All patients who are receiving non-steroidal anti-inflammatory agents should be monitored as a precautionary measure e.g. renal function, hepatic function (elevation of liver enzymes may occur) and blood counts. This is particularly important in the elderly.

Interaction with other medicaments and other forms of interaction:

Lithium and digoxin: Voltarol may increase plasma concentrations of lithium and digoxin.

Anticoagulants: Although clinical investigations do not appear to indicate that Voltarol has an influence on the effect of anticoagulants, there are isolated reports of an increased risk of haemorrhage with the combined use of diclofenac and anticoagulant therapy. Therefore, to be certain that no change in anticoagulant dosage is required, close monitoring of such patients is required. As with other non-steroidal anti-inflammatory agents, diclofenac in high dose can reversibly inhibit platelet aggregation.

Antidiabetic agents: Clinical studies have shown that Voltarol can be given together with oral antidiabetic agents without influencing their clinical effect. However there have been isolated reports of hypoglycaemic and hyperglycaemic effects which have required adjustment to the dosage of hypoglycaemic agents.

Cyclosporin: Cases of nephrotoxicity have been reported in patients receiving concomitant cyclosporin and NSAIDs, including Voltarol. This might be mediated through combined renal antiprostaglandin effects of both the NSAID and cyclosporin.

Methotrexate: Cases of serious toxicity have been reported when methotrexate and NSAIDs are given within 24 hours of each other. This interaction is mediated through accumulation of methotrexate resulting from impairment of renal excretion in the presence of the NSAID.

Quinolone antimicrobials: Convulsions may occur due to an interaction between quinolones and NSAIDs. This may occur in patients with or without a previous history of epilepsy or convulsions. Therefore, caution should be exercised when considering the use of a quinolone in patients who are already receiving an NSAID.

Other NSAIDs and steroids: Co-administration of Voltarol with other systemic NSAIDs and steroids may increase the frequency of unwanted effects. Concomitant therapy with aspirin lowers the plasma levels of each, although no clinical significance is known.

Diuretics: Various NSAIDs are liable to inhibit the activity of diuretics. Concomitant treatment with potassium-sparing diuretics may be associated with increased serum potassium levels, hence serum potassium should be monitored.

Pregnancy and lactation: Although animal studies have not demonstrated teratogenic effects, Voltarol should not be prescribed during pregnancy, unless there are compelling reasons for doing so. The lowest effective dosage should be used.

Use of prostaglandin synthetase inhibitors may result in premature closure of the ductus arteriosus or uterine inertia; such drugs are, therefore, not recommended during the last trimester of pregnancy.

Following doses of 50 mg enteric coated tablets every 8 hours, traces of active substance have been detected in breast milk, but in quantities so small that no undesirable effects on the infant are to be expected.

Effects on ability to drive and use machines: Patients who experience dizziness or other central nervous disturbances, while taking NSAIDs should refrain from driving or operating machinery.

Undesirable effects: If serious side-effects occur, Voltarol should be withdrawn.

Frequency estimate: *frequent:* >10%, *occasional:* >1–10%, *rare:* >0.001–1%, *isolated cases:* <0.001%.

Gastro-intestinal tract: Occasional: Epigastric pain, other gastro-intestinal disorders (e.g. nausea, vomiting, diarrhoea, abdominal cramps, dyspepsia, flatulence, anorexia). *Rare:* Gastro-intestinal bleeding (haematemesis, melaena, bloody diarrhoea), gastro-intestinal ulcers with or without bleeding or perforation. *Isolated cases:* Aphthous stomatitis, glossitis, oesophageal lesions, lower gut disorders (e.g. non-specific haemorrhagic colitis and exacerbations of ulcerative colitis or Crohn's proctocolitis, colonic damage and stricture formation), pancreatitis, constipation.

Central nervous system: Occasional: Headache, dizziness, or vertigo. *Rare:* drowsiness, tiredness. *Isolated cases:* Disturbances of sensation, paraesthesia, memory disturbance, disorientation, insomnia, irritability, convulsions, depression, anxiety, nightmares, tremor, psychotic reactions, aseptic meningitis.

Special senses: Isolated cases: Disturbances of vision (blurred vision, diplopia), impaired hearing, tinnitus, taste disturbances.

Skin: Occasional: Rashes or skin eruptions. *Rare:* Urticaria. *Isolated cases:* Bullous eruptions, eczema, erythema multiforme, Stevens-Johnson syndrome, Lyell's syndrome (acute toxic epidermolysis), erythroderma (exfoliative dermatitis), loss of hair, photosensitivity reactions, purpura including allergic purpura.

Kidney: Rare: Oedema. *Isolated cases:* Acute renal insufficiency, urinary abnormalities (e.g. haematuria, proteinuria), interstitial nephritis, nephrotic syndrome, papillary necrosis.

Liver: Occasional: Elevation of serum aminotransferase enzymes (ALT, AST). *Rare:* Liver function disorders including hepatitis (in isolated cases fulminant) with or without jaundice.

Blood: Isolated cases: Thrombocytopenia, leucopenia, agranulocytosis, haemolytic anaemia, aplastic anaemia.

Hypersensitivity: Rare: Hypersensitivity reactions (e.g. bronchospasm, anaphylactic/anaphylactoid systemic reactions including hypotension). *Isolated cases:* Vasculitis, pneumonitis.

Cardiovascular system: Isolated cases: Palpitations, chest pain, hypertension, congestive heart failure.

Overdose: Management of acute poisoning with NSAIDs essentially consists of supportive and symptomatic measures. There is no typical clinical picture resulting from Voltarol overdosage. The therapeutic measures to be taken are: Supportive and symptomatic treatment should be given for complications such as hypotension, renal failure, convulsions, gastro-intestinal irritation, and respiratory depression; special therapies such as forced diuresis, dialysis or haemoperfusion are probably of no help in eliminating NSAIDs due to their high rate of protein binding and extensive metabolism.

Pharmacological properties

Pharmacodynamic properties

Pharmacotherapeutic group: Non-steroidal anti-inflammatory drugs (NSAIDs).

Mechanism of action: Voltarol is a non-steroidal agent with marked analgesic/anti-inflammatory properties. It is an inhibitor of prostaglandin synthetase (cyclo-oxygenase).

Diclofenac sodium *in vitro* does not suppress proteoglycan biosynthesis in cartilage at concentrations equivalent to the concentrations reached in human beings.

Pharmacokinetic properties:

Absorption: Absorption is complete but onset is delayed until passage through the stomach, which may be affected by food, which delays stomach emptying. The mean peak plasma diclofenac concentration reached at about 2 hours (50 mg dose produces 1.48±0.65 mcg/ml (1.5 mcg/ml≡5 μmol/l)).

Bioavailability: About half of the administered diclofenac is metabolised during its first passage through the liver ('first-pass' effect), the area under the concentrations curve (AUC) following oral administration is about half that following an equivalent parenteral dose.

Pharmacokinetic behaviour does not change on repeated administration. Accumulation does not occur, provided the recommended dosage intervals are observed.

25 mg enteric-coated tablet only: The plasma concentrations attained in children given equivalent doses (mg/kg, b.w.) are similar to those obtained in adults.

Distribution: The active substance is 99.7% protein bound, mainly to albumin (99.4%).

Diclofenac enters the synovial fluid, where maximum concentrations are measured 2–4 hours after the peak plasma values have been attained. The apparent half-life for elimination from the synovial fluid is 3–6 hours. Two hours after reaching the peak plasma values, concentrations of the active substance are already higher in the synovial fluid than they are in the plasma and remain higher for up to 12 hours.

Metabolism: Biotransformation of diclofenac takes place partly by glucuronidation of the intact molecule, but mainly by single and multiple hydroxylation and methoxylation, resulting in several phenolic metabolites, most of which are converted to glucuronide conjugates. Two phenolic metabolites are biologically active, but to a much lesser extent than diclofenac.

Elimination: Total systemic clearance of diclofenac in plasma is 263±56 ml/min (mean value±SD). The terminal half-life in plasma is 1–2 hours. Four of the metabolites, including the two active ones, also have short plasma half-lives of 1–3 hours.

About 60% of the administered dose is excreted in the urine in the form of the glucuronide conjugate of the intact molecule and as metabolites, most of which are also converted to glucuronide conjugates. Less than 1% is excreted as unchanged substance. The rest of the dose is eliminated as metabolites through the bile in the faeces.

Characteristics in patients: Elderly: No relevant age-dependent differences in the drug's absorption, metabolism or excretion have been observed, other than the finding that in five elderly patients, a 15 minute iv infusion resulted in 50% higher plasma concentrations than expected with young healthy subjects.

Patients with renal impairment: In patients suffering from renal impairment, no accumulation of the unchanged active substance can be inferred from the single-dose kinetics when applying the usual dosage schedule. At a creatinine clearance of <10 ml/min, the calculated steady-state plasma levels of the hydroxy metabolites are about 4 times higher than in normal subjects. However, the metabolites are ultimately cleared through the bile.

Patients with hepatic disease: In patients with chronic hepatitis or non-decompensated cirrhosis, the kinetics and metabolism of diclofenac are the same as in patients without liver disease.

Preclinical safety data: None stated.

Pharmaceutical particulars

List of excipients: The enteric-coated tablets also contain colloidal anhydrous silica, lactose, maize starch, sodium starch glycollate, povidone (K30), microcrystalline cellulose, magnesium stearate, hydroxypropylmethylcellulose, Cremophor RH40, yellow iron oxide (E.172), red iron oxide (E.172) (*50 mg tablet only*) purified talc special, titanium dioxide (E.171), eudragit L30D-55, polyethylene glycol 8000 flakes, silicone antifoam emulsion SE2, ammonia 25% and purified water.

Incompatibilities: None known.

Shelf life: 5 years.

Special precautions for storage: Protect from moisture. Store below 30°C. Medicines should be kept out of the reach of children.

Nature and contents of container: The 25 mg tablets are yellow, round, biconvex, film coated tablets, impressed GEIGY on one face and VOLTAROL 25 on the other, and come in PVC/PVdC blister packs of 84.

The 50 mg tablets are light brown, round, biconvex, film coated tablets, impressed GEIGY on one face and VOLTAROL 50 on the other, and come in PVC/PVdC blister packs of 14 and 84.

Instructions for use/handling: The enteric-coated tablets should be swallowed whole, preferably before meals.

Market authorisation holder: Novartis Pharmaceuticals UK Limited, trading as Geigy Pharmaceuticals.

Marketing authorisation numbers

25 mg	00101/0476
50 mg	00101/0477

Date of approval/revision of SPC September 1997.

Legal category POM.

VOLTAROL* SR and RETARD TABLETS

Qualitative and quantitative composition The active substance is sodium-[o-[(2,6-dichlorophenyl)-amino]-phenyl]-acetate (diclofenac sodium).

Each slow release/retard tablet contains 75 mg or 100 mg diclofenac sodium PhEur.

Pharmaceutical forms Slow/sustained release, film-coated tablet.

Clinical particulars

Therapeutic indications:

Adults and elderly: Relief of all grades of pain and inflammation in a wide range of conditions, including:

(i) arthritic conditions: rheumatoid arthritis, osteoarthritis, ankylosing spondylitis, acute gout,

(ii) acute musculo-skeletal disorders such as periarthritis (for example, frozen shoulder), tendonitis, tenosynovitis, bursitis,

(iii) other painful conditions resulting from trauma, including fracture, low back pain, sprains, strains, dislocations, orthopaedic, dental and other minor surgery.

Children: Voltarol 75 mg SR tablets and Retard tablets 100 mg are not suitable for children.

Posology and method of administration:

Adults: One tablet once or twice daily, taken whole with liquid, preferably at meal times.

The recommended maximum daily dose of Voltarol is 150 mg.

Children: Voltarol 75 mg SR tablets and Retard tablets 100 mg are not suitable for children.

Elderly: Although the pharmacokinetics of Voltarol are not impaired to any clinically relevant extent in elderly patients, non-steroidal anti-inflammatory drugs should be used with particular caution in such patients who, generally, are more prone to adverse reactions. In particular, it is recommended that the lowest effective dosage be used in frail, elderly patients or those with a low body weight (see also *Precautions*).

Contra-indications: Active or suspected gastro-intestinal ulcers or bleeding.

Previous sensitivity to diclofenac.

Patients in whom attacks of asthma, urticaria or acute rhinitis are precipitated by aspirin or other non-steroidal anti-inflammatory agents.

Special warnings and special precautions for use:

Warnings: Close medical surveillance is imperative in patients with symptoms indicative of gastro-intestinal disorders, with a history suggestive of gastric or intestinal ulceration, with ulcerative colitis, or with Crohn's disease.

Gastro-intestinal bleeding or ulceration/perforation, haematemesis and melaena have, in general, more serious consequences in the elderly. They can occur at any time during treatment, with or without warning symptoms or a previous history. In the rare instances when gastro-intestinal bleeding or ulceration occur in patients receiving Voltarol, the drug should be withdrawn.

Hepatic: Close medical surveillance is also imperative in patients suffering from severe impairment of hepatic function.

Hypersensitivity reactions: As with other non-steroidal anti-inflammatory drugs, allergic reactions, including anaphylactic/anaphylactoid reactions, can also occur without earlier exposure to the drug.

Like other NSAIDs, Voltarol may mask the signs and symptoms of infection due to its pharmacodynamic properties.

Precautions: Renal: Patients with renal, cardiac or hepatic impairment and the elderly should be kept under surveillance, since the use of NSAIDs may result in deterioration of renal function. The lowest effective dose should be used and renal function monitored.

The importance of prostaglandins in maintaining renal blood flow should be taken into account in patients with impaired cardiac or renal function, those being treated with diuretics or recovering from major surgery. Effects on renal function are usually reversible on withdrawal of Voltarol.

Hepatic: If abnormal liver function tests persist or worsen, clinical signs or symptoms consistent with liver disease develop or if other manifestations occur (eosinophilia, rash), Voltarol should be discontinued. Hepatitis may occur without prodromal symptoms.

Use of Voltarol in patients with hepatic porphyria may trigger an attack.

Haematological: Voltarol may reversibly inhibit platelet aggregation (see *Anticoagulants* in *Drug interactions*). Patients with defects of haemostasis, bleeding diathesis or haematological abnormalities should be carefully monitored.

Long-term treatment: All patients who are receiving non-steroidal anti-inflammatory agents should be monitored as a precautionary measure e.g. renal function, hepatic function (elevation of liver enzymes may occur) and blood counts. This is particularly important in the elderly.

Interaction with other medicaments and other forms of interaction:

Lithium and digoxin: Voltarol may increase plasma concentrations of lithium and digoxin.

Anticoagulants: Although clinical investigations do not appear to indicate that Voltarol has an influence on the effect of anticoagulants, there are isolated reports of an increased risk of haemorrhage with the combined use of diclofenac and anticoagulant therapy. Therefore, to be certain that no change in anticoagulant dosage is required, close monitoring of such patients is required. As with other non-steroidal anti-inflammatory agents, diclofenac in high dose can reversibly inhibit platelet aggregation.

Antidiabetic agents: Clinical studies have shown that Voltarol can be given together with oral antidiabetic agents without influencing their clinical effect. However, there have been isolated reports of hypoglycaemic and hyperglycaemic effects which have required adjustment to the dosage of hypoglycaemic agents.

Cyclosporin: Cases of nephrotoxicity have been reported in patients receiving concomitant cyclosporin and NSAIDs, including Voltarol. This might be mediated through combined renal antiprostaglandin effects of both the NSAID and cyclosporin.

Methotrexate: Cases of serious toxicity have been reported when methotrexate and NSAIDs are given within 24 hours of each other. This interaction is mediated through accumulation of methotrexate resulting from impairment of renal excretion in the presence of the NSAID.

Quinolone antimicrobials: Convulsions may occur due to an interaction between quinolones and NSAIDs. This may occur in patients with or without a previous history of epilepsy or convulsions. Therefore, caution should be exercised when considering the use of a quinolone in patients who are already receiving an NSAID.

Other NSAIDs and steroids: Co-administration of Voltarol with other systemic NSAIDs and steroids may increase the frequency of unwanted effects. Concomitant therapy with aspirin lowers the plasma levels of each, although no clinical significance is known.

Diuretics: Various NSAIDs are liable to inhibit the activity of diuretics. Concomitant treatment with potassium-sparing diuretics may be associated with increased serum potassium levels, hence serum potassium should be monitored.

Pregnancy and lactation: Although animal studies have not demonstrated teratogenic effects, Voltarol should not be prescribed during pregnancy, unless there are compelling reasons for doing so. The lowest effective dosage should be used.

Use of prostaglandin synthetase inhibitors may result in premature closure of the ductus arteriosus or uterine inertia; such drugs are therefore not recommended during the last trimester of pregnancy.

Following doses of 50 mg enteric coated tablets every 8 hours, traces of active substance have been detected in breast milk, but in quantities so small that no undesirable effects on the infant are to be expected.

Effects on ability to drive and use machines: Patients who experience dizziness or other central nervous disturbances, while taking NSAIDs should refrain from driving or operating machinery.

Undesirable effects: If serious side-effects occur, Voltarol should be withdrawn.

Frequency estimate: *frequent:* >10%, *occasional:* >1–10%, rare: >0.001–1%, *isolated cases:* <0.001%.

Gastro-intestinal tract: Occasional: Epigastric pain, other gastro-intestinal disorders (e.g. nausea, vomiting, diarrhoea, abdominal cramps, dyspepsia, flatulence, anorexia). *Rare:* Gastro-intestinal bleeding (haematemesis, melaena, bloody diarrhoea), gastro-intestinal ulcers with or without bleeding or perforation. *Isolated cases:* Aphthous stomatitis, glossitis, oesophageal lesions, lower gut disorders (e.g. non-specific haemorrhagic colitis and exacerbations of ulcerative colitis or Crohn's proctocolitis, colonic damage and stricture formation), pancreatitis, constipation.

Central nervous system: Occasional: Headache, dizziness, or vertigo. *Rare:* drowsiness, tiredness. *Isolated cases:* Disturbances of sensation, paraesthesia, memory disturbance, disorientation, insomnia, irritability, convulsions, depression, anxiety, nightmares, tremor, psychotic reactions, aseptic meningitis.

Special senses: Isolated cases: Disturbances of vision (blurred vision, diplopia), impaired hearing, tinnitus, taste disturbances.

Skin: Occasional: Rashes or skin eruptions. *Rare:* Urticaria. *Isolated cases:* Bullous eruptions, eczema, erythema multiforme, Steven's-Johnson syndrome, Lyell's syndrome (acute toxic epidermolysis), erythroderma (exfoliative dermatitis), loss of hair, photosensitivity reactions, purpura including allergic purpura.

Kidney: Rare: Oedema. *Isolated cases:* Acute renal insufficiency, urinary abnormalities (e.g. haematuria, proteinuria), interstitial nephritis, nephrotic syndrome, papillary necrosis.

Liver: Occasional: Elevation of serum aminotransferase enzymes (ALT, AST). *Rare:* Liver function disorders including hepatitis (in isolated cases fulminant) with or without jaundice.

Blood: Isolated cases: Thrombocytopenia, leucopenia, agranulocytosis, haemolytic anaemia, aplastic anaemia.

Hypersensitivity: Rare: Hypersensitivity reactions (e.g. bronchospasm, anaphylactic/anaphylactoid systemic reactions including hypotension). *Isolated cases:* Vasculitis, pneumonitis.

Cardiovascular system: Isolated cases: Palpitations, chest pain, hypertension, congestive heart failure.

Overdose: Management of acute poisoning with NSAIDs essentially consists of supportive and symptomatic measures. There is no typical clinical picture resulting from Voltarol overdosage. The therapeutic measures to be taken are: supportive and symptomatic treatment should be given for complications such as hypotension, renal failure, convulsions, gastro-intestinal irritation, and respiratory depression; special therapies such as forced diuresis, dialysis or haemoperfusion are probably of no help in eliminating NSAIDs due to their high rate of protein binding and extensive metabolism.

Pharmacological properties

Pharmacodynamic properties:

Pharmacotherapeutic group: Non-steroidal anti-inflammatory drugs (NSAIDs).

Mechanism of action: Voltarol is a non-steroidal agent with marked analgesic/anti-inflammatory properties. It is an inhibitor of prostaglandin synthetase (cyclo-oxygenase).

Diclofenac sodium *in vitro* does not suppress proteoglycan biosynthesis in cartilage at concentrations equivalent to the concentrations reached in human beings.

Pharmacokinetic properties:

Absorption: The same amount of active substance is released and absorbed from SR and Retard tablets as from enteric-coated tablets. Mean peak plasma concentrations of diclofenac are reached at 4 hours, 0.508±0.185 mcg/ml (0.5 mcg/mL≡1.6 μmol/l) or 0.4±0.184 mcg/ml (0.4 mcg/mL≡1.25 μmol/l) after Retard 100 mg or 75 mg SR, respectively. 75 mg SR and Retard 100 mg are modified release preparations and plasma concentrations of diclofenac of 13 ng/ml (40 μmol/l) can be recorded at 24 hours (Retard 100 mg) and 16 hours (75 mg SR) after administration. Absorption is unaffected by food.

Bioavailability: The systemic availability of diclofenac from the SR formulations is on average 82% of that achieved with the same dose of enteric-coated tablets (possibly due to release rate dependent first-pass metabolism). As a result of the slower release of active substance, peak plasma concentrations are lower than for the equivalent enteric-coated tablets.

Pharmacokinetic behaviour does not change on repeated administration. Accumulation does not occur, provided the recommended dosage intervals are observed. Trough levels of diclofenac in the plasma after Retard 100 mg daily or 75 mg SR twice daily are around 22 ng/ml or 25 ng/ml (70 nmol/l or 80 nmol/l), respectively.

Distribution: The active substance is 99.7% protein bound, mainly to albumin (99.4%).

Diclofenac enters the synovial fluid, where maximum concentrations are measured 2–4 hours after the peak plasma values have been attained. The apparent half-life for elimination from the synovial fluid is 3–6 hours. Two hours after reaching the peak plasma values, concentrations of the active substance are already higher in the synovial fluid than they are in the plasma and remain higher for up to 12 hours.

Metabolism: Biotransformation of diclofenac takes place partly by glucuronidation of the intact molecule, but mainly by single and multiple hydroxylation and methoxylation, resulting in several phenolic metabolites, most of which are converted to glucuronide conjugates. Two phenolic metabolites are biologically active, but to a much lesser extent than diclofenac.

Elimination: The total systemic clearance of diclofenac in plasma is 263±56 ml/min (mean value±SD). The terminal half-life in plasma is 1–2 hours. Four of the metabolites, including the two active ones, also have short plasma half-lives of 1–3 hours.

About 60% of the administered dose is excreted in the urine in the form of the glucuronide conjugate of the intact molecule and as metabolites, most of which are also converted to glucuronide conjugates. Less than 1% is excreted as unchanged substance. The rest of the dose is eliminated as metabolites through the bile in the faeces.

Characteristics in patients: Elderly: No relevant age-dependent differences in the drug's absorption, metabolism or excretion have been observed, other than the finding that in five elderly patients, a 15 minute iv infusion resulted in 50% higher plasma concentrations than expected with young healthy subjects.

Patients with renal impairment: In patients suffering from renal impairment, no accumulation of the unchanged active substance can be inferred from the single-dose kinetics when applying the usual dosage schedule. At a creatinine clearance of <10 ml/min, the calculated steady-state plasma levels of the hydroxy metabolites are about 4 times higher than in normal subjects. However, the metabolites are ultimately cleared through the bile.

Patients with hepatic disease: In patients with chronic hepatitis or non-decompensated cirrhosis, the kinetics and metabolism of diclofenac are the same as in patients without liver disease.

Preclinical safety data: None stated.

Pharmaceutical particulars

List of excipients: 75 mg SR and Retard 100 mg tablets also contain colloidal anhydrous silica, cetyl alcohol, sucrose (powder), povidone, magnesium stearate, hydroxypropylmethylcellulose, polysorbate 80, purified talc, titanium dioxide (E.171), red iron oxide (E.172) and purified water.

Incompatibilities: None known.

Shelf life: 75 mg SR tablets: Three years. Retard 100 mg tablets: Five years.

Special precautions for storage: 75 mg SR tablets: Protect from moisture and heat (store below 30°C).

Retard 100 mg tablets: No special precautions for storage.

Medicines should be kept out of the reach of children.

Nature and contents of container: 75 mg SR tablets are pale pink, triangular film coated tablets embossed GEIGY on one face, V 75 SR on the other, and come in PVC/PVdC blister packs of 2, 7, 28, 56 and 70.

The Retard 100 mg tablets are pale red, round, slightly convex, film coated tablets, impressed GEIGY on one side and VOLTAROL R on the other, and come in PVC/PVdC blister packs of 7, 28 and 70.

Instructions for use/handling: The tablets should be swallowed whole with liquid, preferably with meals.

Marketing authorisation holder: Novartis Pharmaceuticals UK Limited, trading as Geigy Pharmaceuticals.

Marketing authorisation numbers

75 mg SR tablets	00101/0471
Retard 100 mg tablets	00101/0470

Date of approval/revision of SPC September 1997.

Legal category POM.

VOLTAROL* SUPPOSITORIES

Qualitative and quantitative composition The active substance is sodium-[o-[(2,6-dichlorophenyl)-amino]-phenyl]-acetate (diclofenac sodium).

Each suppository contains 12.5 mg, 25 mg, 50 mg and 100 mg diclofenac sodium.

Pharmaceutical form Suppositories.

Clinical particulars

Therapeutic indications:

Adults and elderly: Relief of all grades of pain and inflammation in a wide range of conditions, including:

(i) arthritic conditions: rheumatoid arthritis, osteoarthritis, ankylosing spondylitis, acute gout,
(ii) acute musculo-skeletal disorders such as periarthritis (for example, frozen shoulder), tendinitis, tenosynovitis, bursitis,
(iii) other painful conditions resulting from trauma, including fracture, low back pain, sprains, strains, dislocations, orthopaedic, dental and other minor surgery.

Children (aged 1–12 years): Juvenile chronic arthritis (12.5 mg and 25 mg suppositories only).

Posology and method of administration:

Adults: 25 mg, 50 mg and 100 mg: 75–150 mg daily, in divided doses.

The recommended maximum daily dose of Voltarol is 150 mg. This may be administered using a combination of dosage forms, e.g. tablets and suppositories.

Children (aged 1–12 years) 12.5 mg and 25 mg suppositories only: 1–3 mg/kg per day in divided doses.

Elderly: Although the pharmacokinetics of Voltarol are not impaired to any clinically relevant extent in elderly patients, non-steroidal anti-inflammatory drugs should be used with particular caution in such patients who, generally, are more prone to adverse reactions. In particular it is recommended that the lowest effective dosage be used in frail, elderly patients or those with a low body weight (see also *Precautions*).

Contra-indications: Active or suspected gastro-intestinal ulcers or bleeding.

Previous sensitivity to diclofenac.

Patients in whom attacks of asthma, urticaria or acute rhinitis are precipitated by aspirin or other non-steroidal anti-inflammatory agents.

In ulcerative or acute inflammatory conditions of the anus, rectum (proctitis) and sigmoid colon.

Special warnings and special precautions for use:

Warnings: Close medical surveillance is imperative in patients with symptoms indicative of gastro-intestinal disorders, with a history suggestive of gastric or intestinal ulceration, with ulcerative colitis, or with Crohn's disease.

Gastro-intestinal bleeding or ulceration/perforation, haematemesis and melaena have, in general, more serious consequences in the elderly. They can occur at any time during treatment, with or without warning symptoms or a previous history. In the rare instances when gastro-intestinal bleeding or ulceration occur in patients receiving Voltarol, the drug should be withdrawn.

Hepatic: Close medical surveillance is also imperative in patients suffering from severe impairment of hepatic function.

Hypersensitivity reactions: As with other non-steroidal anti-inflammatory drugs, allergic reactions, including anaphylactic/anaphylactoid reactions, can also occur without earlier exposure to the drug.

Like other NSAIDs, Voltarol may mask the signs and symptoms of infection due to its pharmacodynamic properties.

Precautions: Renal: Patients with renal, cardiac or hepatic impairment and the elderly should be kept under surveillance, since the use of NSAIDs may result in deterioration of renal function. The lowest effective dose should be used and renal function monitored.

The importance of prostaglandins in maintaining renal blood flow should be taken into account in patients with impaired cardiac or renal function, those being treated with diuretics or recovering from major surgery. Effects on renal function are usually reversible on withdrawal of Voltarol.

Hepatic: If abnormal liver function tests persist or worsen, clinical signs or symptoms consistent with liver disease develop or if other manifestations occur (eosinophilia, rash), Voltarol should be discontinued. Hepatitis may occur without prodromal symptoms.

Use of Voltarol in patients with hepatic porphyria may trigger an attack.

Haematological: Voltarol may reversibly inhibit platelet aggregation (see *Anticoagulants* in *Drug interactions*). Patients with defects of haemostasis, bleeding diathesis or haematological abnormalities should be carefully monitored.

Long-term treatment: All patients who are receiving non-steroidal anti-inflammatory agents should be monitored as a precautionary measure e.g. renal function, hepatic function (elevation of liver enzymes may occur) and blood counts. This is particularly important in the elderly.

Interaction with other medicaments and other forms of interaction:

Lithium and digoxin: Voltarol may increase plasma concentrations of lithium and digoxin.

Anticoagulants: Although clinical investigations do not appear to indicate that Voltarol has an influence on the effect of anticoagulants, there are isolated reports of an increased risk of haemorrhage with the combined use of diclofenac and anticoagulant therapy. Therefore, to be certain that no change in anticoagulant dosage is required, close monitoring of such patients is required. As with other non-steroidal anti-inflammatory agents, diclofenac in high dose can reversibly inhibit platelet aggregation.

Antidiabetic agents: Clinical studies have shown that Voltarol can be given together with oral antidiabetic agents without influencing their clinical effect. However, there have been isolated reports of hypoglycaemic and hyperglycaemic effects which have required adjustment to the dosage of hypoglycaemic agents.

Cyclosporin: Cases of nephrotoxicity have been reported in patients receiving concomitant cyclosporin and NSAIDs, including Voltarol. This might be mediated through combined renal antiprostaglandin effects of both the NSAID and cyclosporin.

Methotrexate: Cases of serious toxicity have been reported when methotrexate and NSAIDs are given within 24 hours of each other. This interaction is mediated through accumulation of methotrexate resulting from impairment of renal excretion in the presence of the NSAID.

Quinolone antimicrobials: Convulsions may occur due to an interaction between quinolones and NSAIDs. This may occur in patients with or without a previous history of epilepsy or convulsions. Therefore, caution should be exercised when considering the use of a quinolone in patients who are already receiving an NSAID.

Other NSAIDs and steroids: Co-administration of Voltarol with other systemic NSAIDs and steroids may increase the frequency of unwanted effects. Concomitant therapy with aspirin lowers the plasma levels of each, although no clinical significance is known.

Diuretics: Various NSAIDs are liable to inhibit the activity of diuretics. Concomitant treatment with potassium-sparing diuretics may be associated with increased serum potassium levels, hence serum potassium should be monitored.

Pregnancy and lactation: Although animal studies have not demonstrated teratogenic effects, Voltarol should not be prescribed during pregnancy, unless there are compelling reasons for doing so. The lowest effective dosage should be used.

Use of prostaglandin synthetase inhibitors may result in premature closure of the ductus arteriosus or uterine inertia; such drugs are, therefore, not recommended during the last trimester of pregnancy.

Following doses of 50 mg enteric coated tablets every 8 hours, traces of active substance have been detected in breast milk, but in quantities so small that no undesirable effects on the infant are to be expected.

Effects on ability to drive and use machines: Patients who experience dizziness or other central nervous disturbances, while taking NSAIDs should refrain from driving or operating machinery.

Undesirable effects: If serious side-effects occur, Voltarol should be withdrawn.

Frequency estimate: *frequent:* >10%, *occasional:* >1–10%, *rare:* >0.001–1%, *isolated cases:* <0.001%.

Gastro-intestinal tract: Occasional: Epigastric pain, other gastro-intestinal disorders (e.g. nausea, vomiting, diarrhoea, abdominal cramps, dyspepsia, flatulence, anorexia). *Rare:* Gastro-intestinal bleeding (haematemesis, melaena, bloody diarrhoea), gastro-intestinal ulcers with or without bleeding or perforation. *Isolated cases:* Aphthous stomatitis, glossitis, oesophageal lesions, lower gut disorders (e.g. non-specific haemorrhagic colitis and exacerbations of ulcerative colitis or Crohn's proctocolitis, colonic damage and stricture formation), pancreatitis, constipation.

Suppositories only: Occasional: Local reactions (e.g. itching, burning and increased bowel movement). *Isolated cases:* exacerbation of haemorrhoids.

Central nervous system: Occasional: Headache, dizziness, or vertigo. *Rare:* drowsiness, tiredness. *Isolated cases:* Disturbances of sensation, paraesthesia, memory disturbance, disorientation, insomnia, irritability, convulsions, depression, anxiety, nightmares, tremor, psychotic reactions, aseptic meningitis.

Special senses: Isolated cases: Disturbances of vision (blurred vision, diplopia), impaired hearing, tinnitus, taste disturbances.

Skin: Occasional: Rashes or skin eruptions. *Rare:* Urticaria. *Isolated cases:* Bullous eruptions, eczema, erythema multiforme, Steven's-Johnson syndrome, Lyell's syndrome (acute toxic epidermolysis), erythroderma (exfoliative dermatitis), loss of hair, photosensitivity reactions, purpura including allergic purpura.

Kidney: Rare: Oedema. In isolated cases: Acute renal insufficiency, urinary abnormalities (e.g. haematuria, proteinuria), interstitial nephritis, nephrotic syndrome, papillary necrosis.

Liver: Occasional: Elevation of serum aminotransferase enzymes (ALT, AST). *Rare:* Liver function disorders including hepatitis (in isolated cases fulminant) with or without jaundice.

Blood: Isolated cases: Thrombocytopenia, leucopenia, agranulocytosis, haemolytic anaemia, aplastic anaemia.

Hypersensitivity: Rare: Hypersensitivity reactions (e.g. bronchospasm, anaphylactic/anaphylactoid systemic reactions including hypotension). *Isolated cases:* Vasculitis, pneumonitis.

Cardiovascular system: Isolated cases: Palpitations, chest pain, hypertension, congestive heart failure.

Overdose: Management of acute poisoning with NSAIDs essentially consists of supportive and symptomatic measures. There is no typical clinical picture resulting from Voltarol overdosage. The therapeutic measures to be taken are: Supportive and symptomatic treatment should be given for complications such as hypotension, renal failure, convulsions, gastro-intestinal irritation, and respiratory depression; specific therapies such as forced diuresis, dialysis or haemoperfusion are probably of no help in eliminating NSAIDs due to the high rate of protein binding and extensive metabolism.

Pharmacological properties

Pharmacodynamic properties:

Pharmacotherapeutic group: Non-steroidal anti-inflammatory drugs (NSAIDs).

Mechanism of action: Voltarol is a non-steroidal agent with marked analgesic/anti-inflammatory properties. It is an inhibitor of prostaglandin synthetase (cyclo-oxygenase).

Diclofenac sodium *in vitro* does not suppress proteoglycan biosynthesis in cartilage at concentrations equivalent to the concentrations reached in human beings.

Pharmacokinetic properties:

Absorption: Absorption is rapid; although the rate of absorption is slower than from enteric-coated tablets administered orally. After the administration of 50 mg suppositories, peak plasma concentrations are attained on average within 1 hour, but maximum concentrations per dose unit are about two thirds of those reached after administration of enteric-coated tablets (1.95±0.8 mcg/ml (1.9 mcg/ml≡5.9 μmol/l)).

Bioavailability: As with oral preparations, the AUC is approximately a half of the value obtained from a parenteral dose.

Pharmacokinetic behaviour does not change on repeated administration. Accumulation does not occur, provided the recommended dosage intervals are observed. The plasma concentrations attained in children given equivalent doses (mg/kb, b.w.) are similar to those obtained in adults.

Distribution: The active substance is 99.7% protein bound, mainly to albumin (99.4%).

Diclofenac enters the synovial fluid, where maximum concentrations are measured 2–4 hours after the peak plasma values have been attained. The apparent half-life for elimination from the synovial fluid is 3–6 hours. Two hours after reaching the peak plasma values, concentrations of the active substance are already higher in the synovial fluid than they are in the plasma and remain higher for up to 12 hours.

Metabolism: Biotransformation of diclofenac takes place partly by glucuronidation of the intact molecule, but mainly by single and multiple hydroxylation and methoxylation, resulting in several phenolic metabolites, most of which are converted to glucuronide conjugates. Two phenolic metabolites are biologically active, but to a much lesser extent than diclofenac.

Elimination: The total systemic clearance of diclofenac in plasma is 263±56 ml/min (mean value±SD). The terminal half-life in plasma is 1–2 hours. Four of the metabolites, including the two active ones, also have short plasma half-lives of 1–3 hours.

About 60% of the administered dose is excreted in the urine in the form of the glucuronide conjugate of the intact molecule and as metabolites, most of which are also converted to glucuronide conjugates. Less than 1% is excreted as unchanged substance. The rest of the dose is eliminated as metabolites through the bile in the faeces.

Characteristics in patients: No relevant age-dependent differences in the drug's absorption, metabolism or excretion have been observed, other than the finding that in five elderly patients, a 15 minute iv infusion resulted in 50% higher plasma concentrations than expected with young healthy subjects.

Patients with renal impairment: In patients suffering from renal impairment, no accumulation of the unchanged active substance can be inferred from the single-dose kinetics when applying the usual dosage schedule. At a creatinine clearance of <10 ml/min, the calculated steady-state plasma levels of the hydroxy metabolites are about 4 times higher than in normal subjects. However, the metabolites are ultimately cleared through the bile.

Patients with hepatic disease: In patients with chronic hepatitis or non-decompensated cirrhosis, the kinetics and metabolism of diclofenac are the same as in patients without liver disease.

Preclinical safety data: None stated.

Pharmaceutical particulars

List of excipients: Voltarol Suppositories also contain suppository mass 5 (a waxy base composed of hard fat).

Incompatibilities: None known.

Shelf life: Three years.

Special precautions for storage: Protect from heat (store below 30°C). Medicines should be kept out of the reach of children.

Nature and contents of container: The suppositories are white to yellowish, torpedo-shaped, with smooth surfaces and a slightly fatty odour and are sealed in white laminated, plastic film of polyamide and peel-off seal of polyethylene. They come in packs of 10.

Instructions for use/handling: For rectal use only.

Marketing authorisation numbers

12.5 mg	00101/0472
25 mg	00101/0473
50 mg	00101/0474
100 mg	00101/0475

Marketing authorisation holder: Novartis Pharmaceuticals UK Limited, trading as Geigy Pharmaceuticals.

Date of approval/revision of SPC September 1997.

Legal category POM.

ZADITEN*

Presentation *1 mg capsules:* White, opaque, oblong, gelatin capsules, size 4, weighing 182 mg. Each capsule contains 1.38 mg ketotifen hydrogen fumarate (equivalent to 1 mg ketotifen base). Coded CS in red.

1 mg tablets: White, uncoated, round, flat, bevel-edged tablets weighing 130 mg, 7 mm diameter. The tablets are marked ZADITEN 1 on one side and scored on the other. Each tablet contains 1.38 mg ketotifen hydrogen fumarate (equivalent to 1 mg ketotifen base).

Elixir: Clear, colourless, strawberry flavoured elixir. Each 5 ml spoonful contains 1.38 mg ketotifen hydrogen fumarate (equivalent to 1 mg ketotifen base).

For information on excipients, refer to *Further information.*

Uses *Principal action:* Ketotifen is a non-bronchodilator anti-asthmatic drug which inhibits the effect of certain endogenous substances known to be inflammatory mediators, and thereby exerts anti-allergic activity.

Laboratory experiments indicate that this anti-asthmatic activity may be due to the inhibition of release of allergic mediators such as histamine and leukotrienes and the inhibition of the development of airway hyperactivity associated with activation of platelets by PAF (platelet activating factor) or caused by neural activation following the use of sympathomimetic drugs or the exposure to allergen. In addition, ketotifen exerts a non-competitive blocking effect on histamine (H1) receptors.

Experimental investigations in asthmatic subjects have shown that Zaditen is as effective orally as a selective mast cell stabiliser administered by inhalation: antihistamines are ineffective in these tests.

The effectiveness of Zaditen in the prevention of bronchial asthma has been studied in long term clinical trials. Asthma attacks were reduced in number, severity and duration and in some cases the patients were completely freed from attacks. Progressive reduction of corticosteroids and/or bronchodilators was also possible.

The prophylactic activity of Zaditen may take several weeks to become fully established.

Zaditen will not abort established attacks of asthma.

Indications: Prophylactic treatment of bronchial asthma. Symptomatic treatment of allergic conditions including rhinitis and conjunctivitis.

Dosage and administration *Adults:* 1 mg twice daily with food. If necessary the dose may be increased to 2 mg twice daily.

Patients known to be easily sedated should begin treatment with 0.5 to 1 mg at night for the first few days.

Children from two years: 1 mg twice daily with food.

Use in the elderly: No evidence exists that elderly patients require different dosages or show different side effects from younger patients.

Contra-indications, warnings, etc

Contra-indications: Hypersensitivity to ketotifen or any of the excipients (see *Further information*). A reversible fall in the thrombocyte count in patients receiving Zaditen concomitantly with oral antidiabetic agents has been observed in a few cases. This combination of drugs should therefore be avoided until this phenomenon has been satisfactorily explained.

Use in pregnancy and lactation: Although there is no evidence of any teratogenic effect, recommendations for Zaditen in pregnancy cannot be given. Ketotifen is excreted in breast milk, therefore mothers receiving Zaditen should not breast feed.

Precautions: Post-marketing surveillance has shown exacerbation of asthma in approximately 2 per 1000 patients. Since some of these asthmatic attacks might have been related to stopping existing treatment, it is important to continue such treatment for a minimum of two weeks after starting Zaditen. Symptomatic and prophylactic anti-asthmatic drugs already in use should never be withdrawn abruptly when long-term treatment with Zaditen is begun. This applies especially to systemic corticosteroids and ACTH because of the possible existence of adrenocortical insufficiency in steroid-dependent patients; in such cases recovery of a normal pituitary-adrenal response to stress may take up to one year. If it is necessary to withdraw Zaditen, this should be done progressively over a period of 2 to 4 weeks. Symptoms of asthma may recur.

If intercurrent infection occurs Zaditen treatment must be supplemented by specific antimicrobial therapy.

During the first days of treatment with Zaditen reactions may be impaired. Patients should be warned not to take charge of vehicles or machinery until the effect of Zaditen treatment on the individual is known. Patients should be advised to avoid alcoholic drinks.

Zaditen may potentiate the effects of sedatives, hypnotics, antihistamines and alcohol.

Side-effects: Drowsiness and, in isolated cases, dry mouth and slight dizziness may occur at the beginning of treatment, but usually disappear spontaneously after a few days. Occasionally symptoms of CNS stimulation have been observed. Weight gain has also been reported. Cystitis has been rarely described in association with Zaditen. Isolated cases of severe skin reactions (erythema multiforme, Stephen's-Johnson Syndrome) have been reported.

Overdosage: The reported features of overdosage include confusion, drowsiness, nystagmus, headache, disorientation, tachycardia, hypotension, reversible coma; especially in children, hyperexcitability or convulsions. Bradycardia and respiratory depression should be watched for. Elimination of the drug with gastric lavage or emesis is recommended. Otherwise general supportive treatment is all that is required.

Pharmaceutical precautions Nil.

Legal category POM.

Package quantities *1 mg capsules:* Blister pack of 60 capsules (OP).

1 mg tablets: Blister pack of 60 tablets (OP).

Elixir 1 mg/5 ml: Bottles of 150 ml. Bottles of 300 ml.

Further information Zaditen capsules: the excipients are colloidal anhydrous silica, magnesium stearate, maize starch and mannitol. The capsule shell is made of gelatin and contains titanium dioxide.

Zaditen tablets: the excipients are magnesium stearate, maize starch, lactose and pre-gel corn starch.

Zaditen elixir: the excipients are propyl hydroxybenzoate, methyl hydroxybenzoate, strawberry flavour, citric acid, disodium phosphate, ethyl alcohol, Lycasin* 80/55 (hydrogenated glucose syrup) and purified water.

Zaditen elixir is sugar free. It contains the sweetening agent Lycasin* 80/55 (hydrogenated glucose syrup) at a concentration of 4 g in 5 ml. Lycasin* 80/55 contains 45% readily absorbable carbohydrate. This should be considered if prescribing the drug for diabetic patients.

The bioavailability of Zaditen is not influenced by food. After oral administration, the absorption of Zaditen is almost complete. Bioavailability amounts to approximately 50% owing to a first-pass effect of about 50% in the liver. Maximal plasma concentrations are reached within 2 to 4 hours. Protein binding is 75%. Ketotifen is eliminated biphasically, with a short half-life of 3 to 5 hours and a longer one of 21 hours. About 1% of the substance is excreted unchanged in the urine within 48 hours and 60 to 70% is excreted as metabolites. The main metabolite is ketotifen-N-glucuronide. This is practically inactive.

Product licence numbers

1 mg capsules	0101/0105
1 mg tablets	0101/0125
Elixir 1 mg/5 ml	0101/0137

Product licence holder: Novartis Pharmaceuticals, trading as Sandoz Pharmaceuticals.

**Trade Mark*

Novex Pharma Ltd

Innovex House
Marlow Park
Marlow
Bucks., SL7 1TB

☎ 01628 491500 🗋 01628 487799

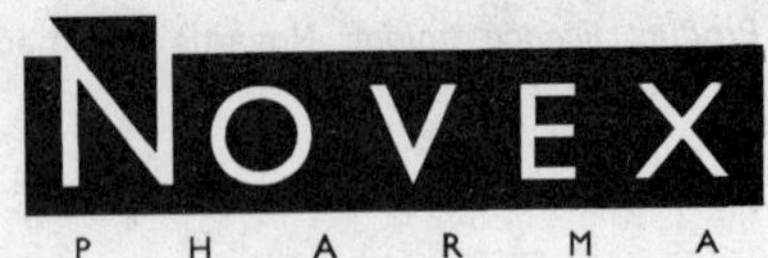

ALVEDON* SUPPOSITORIES 60 mg

Qualitative and quantitative composition Each suppository contains Paracetamol PhEur 60 mg in a hard fat base.

Pharmaceutical form Suppositories.

Clinical particulars
Therapeutic indications: For the treatment of mild to moderate pain and pyrexia in children. Alvedon Suppositories may be especially useful in patients unable to take oral forms of paracetamol, e.g. post-operatively or with nausea or vomiting.

Posology and method of administration:
Children: 3 months to 1 year, 1–2 suppositories.
The dosage should be based on age and weight, i.e.

3 months (5 kg)–60 mg (1 suppository)
1 year (10 kg)–120 mg (2 suppositories).

These doses may be repeated up to 4 times daily.

Infants under 3 months: One suppository (60 mg) is suitable for babies who develop a fever following immunisation at 2 months. Otherwise only use in babies aged less than 3 months on a doctor's advice.

Contra-indications: Hypersensitivity to paracetamol.

Special warnings and special precautions for use: Paracetamol should be given with care to patients with impaired kidney or liver function.

Interaction with other medicaments and other forms of interaction: Drugs which induce hepatic microsomal enzymes such as alcohol, barbiturates and other anticonvulsants, may increase the hepatotoxicity of paracetamol particularly after overdosage.

Pregnancy and lactation: Not applicable.

Effects on ability to drive and use machines: None known.

Undesirable effects: Side-effects at therapeutic doses are rare. Isolated cases of liver damage and allergic reactions such as skin rash have been reported.

Redness of the mucous membrane of the rectum and minor local vascular changes have been reported after the use of Alvedon Suppositories. Hepatic necrosis may occur after overdosage (see below).

Overdosage: Clinical symptoms of liver damage are manifested usually after 48 hours. Overdosage results in saturation of the conjugation capacity of the liver and irreversible binding of a reactive intermediate metabolite in the hepatocytes. N-acetylcysteine intravenously or L-methionine orally protects the liver if administered within 10–12 hours of ingesting an overdose.

Pharmacological properties
Pharmacodynamic properties: Paracetamol is an aniline derivative with analgesic and antipyretic actions similar to those of aspirin but with no demonstrable anti-inflammatory activity. Paracetamol is less irritant to the stomach than aspirin. It does not affect thrombocyte aggregation or bleeding time. Paracetamol is generally well tolerated by patients hypersensitive to acetylsalicylic acid.

Pharmacokinetic properties: Paracetamol is well absorbed by both oral and rectal routes. Peak plasma concentrations occur about 2 to 3 hours after rectal administration. The plasma half life is about 2 hours.

Paracetamol is primarily metabolised in the liver by conjugation to glucuronide and sulphate. A small amount (about 3–10% of a therapeutic dose) is metabolised by oxidation and the reactive intermediate metabolite thus formed is bound preferentially to the liver glutathione and excreted as cystein and mercapturic acid conjugates. Excretion occurs via the kidneys. 2–3% of a therapeutic dose is excreted unchanged; 80–90% as glucuronide and sulphate and a smaller amount as cystein and mercapturic acid derivatives.

Preclinical safety data: None.

Pharmaceutical particulars
List of excipients: Hard fat (Witepsol H12).

Incompatibilities: None known.

Shelf-life: 3 years.

Special precautions for storage: Store below 25°C.

Nature and contents of container: Alvedon Suppositories are packed in cartons of 10, each containing two PVC/polyethylene blister strips of 5 suppositories.

Instructions for use/handling: Peel the wrapper apart to remove the suppository, gently push into the rectum pointed end first.

Marketing authorisation holder: Astra Pharmaceuticals Ltd, Home Park, Kings Langley, Hertfordshire WD4 8DH.

Marketing authorisation number PL 0017/0339.

Date of first authorisation 17 June 1997.

Date of (partial) revision of the text May 1997.

ALVEDON* SUPPOSITORIES 125 mg

Qualitative and quantitive composition Paracetamol 125 mg

Pharmaceutical form Suppositories

Clinical particulars
Therapeutic indications: For treatment of mild to moderate pain and pyrexia in children. Alvedon suppositories may be especially useful in patients unable to take oral forms of paracetamol eg post-operatively or with nausea or vomiting.

Posology and method of administration:
Children: 1-5 years, 1-2 suppositories. The dosage should be based on age and weight i.e.
1 year (10 kg) 1 suppository
5 years (20 kg) 2 suppositories.
These doses may be repeated up to 4 times daily.

Contra-indications: Hypersensivity to paracetamol

Special warnings and special precautions for use: Paracetamol should be given with care to patients with impaired kidney or liver function

Interaction with other medicaments and other forms of interaction: Drugs which induce hepatic microsomal enzymes such as alcohol, barbiturates and other anticonvulsants may increase the hepatotoxicity of paracetamol particularly after overdosage

Using during pregnancy. Not applicable

Effects on ability to drive and use machines: None known.

Undesirable effects: Side-effects at therapeutic doses are rare. Isolated cases of liver damage and allergic reactions such as skin rash have been reported.

Redness of the mucous membrane of the rectum and minor local vascular changes have been reported after the use of Alvedon Suppositories. Hepatic necrosis may occur after overdosage.

Overdosage: Clinical symptoms of liver damage are manifested usually after 48 hours.

Overdosage results in saturation of the conjugation capacity of the liver and irreversible binding of a reactive intermediate metabolite in the hepatocytes. N-acetylcysteine intravenously or L-methionine orally protects the liver if administered within 10-12 hours of ingesting an overdose.

Pharmacological properties
Pharmacodynamic properties: Paracetamol is an aniline derivative with analgesic and antipyretic actions similar to those of aspirin but with no demonstrable anti-inflammatory activity.

Paracetamol is less irritant to the stomach than aspirin. It does not affect thrombocyte aggregation or bleeding time. Paracetamol is generally well tolerated by patients hypersensitive to acetylsalicyclic acid.

Pharmacokinetic properties: Paracetamol is well absorbed by both oral and rectal routes.

Peak plasma concentrations occur about 2 to 3 hours after rectal administration. The plasma half life is about 2 hours.

Paracetamol is primarily metabolised in the liver by conjugation to glucuronide and sulphate. A small amount (about 3-10% of a therapeutic dose) is metabolised by oxidation and the reactive intermediate metabolite thus formed is bound preferentially to the liver glutathione and excreted as cystein and mercapturic acid conjugates. Excretion occurs via the kidneys. 2-3% of a therapeutic dose is excreted unchanged: 80-90% as glucuronide and sulphate and a smaller amount as cystein and mercapturic acid derivatives.

Pharmaceutical particulars
List of excipients: Hard fat (Witepsol H12).

Incompatibilities: None.

Shelf-life: 3 years.

Special precautions for storage: Store below 25°C.

Nature and contents of container: PVC/Polyethylene strips each containing 5 suppositories. Packs of 5, 10 or 50 suppositories.

PVC/Polyethylene strips each containing 1 suppository. Packs of 10 suppositories.

Instructions for use/handling: Not applicable.

Marketing authorisation holder: Astra Pharmaceuticals Ltd, Home Park, Kings Langley, Hertfordshire WD4 8DH.

Marketing authorisation number 0017/0250

Date of approval/revision of SPC October 1995

Legal category P

ALVEDON* SUPPOSITORIES 250 mg

Qualitative and quantitative composition Each suppository contains Paracetamol PhEur 250 mg in a hard fat base.

Pharmaceutical form Suppositories.

Clinical particulars
Therapeutic indications: For treatment of mild to moderate pain and pyrexia in children. Alvedon Suppositories may be especially useful in patients unable to take oral forms of paracetamol, e.g. post-operatively or with nausea or vomiting.

Posology and method of administration:
Children: 6–12 years, 1–2 suppositories.
The dosage should be based on age and weight, i.e.

6 years (20 kg)–250 mg (1 suppository)
12 years (40 kg)–500 mg (2 suppositories).

These doses may be repeated up to 4 times daily.

Contra-indications: Hypersensitivity to paracetamol.

Special warnings and special precautions for use: Paracetamol should be given with care to patients with impaired kidney or liver function.

Interaction with other medicaments and other forms of interaction: Drugs which induce hepatic microsomal enzymes such as alcohol, barbiturates and other anticonvulsants, may increase the hepatotoxicity of paracetamol particularly after overdosage.

Pregnancy and lactation: Not applicable.

Effects on ability to drive and use machines: None known.

Undesirable effects: Side-effects at therapeutic doses are rare. Isolated cases of liver damage and allergic reactions such as skin rash have been reported.

Redness of the mucous membrane of the rectum and minor local vascular changes have been reported after the use of Alvedon Suppositories. Hepatic necrosis may occur after overdosage (see below).

Overdosage: Clinical symptoms of liver damage are manifested usually after 48 hours. Overdosage results in saturation of the conjugation capacity of the liver and irreversible binding of a reactive intermediate metabolite in the hepatocytes. N-acetylcysteine intravenously or L-methionine orally protects the liver if administered within 10–12 hours of ingesting an overdose.

Pharmacological properties
Pharmacodynamic properties: Paracetamol is an aniline derivative with analgesic and antipyretic actions similar to those of aspirin but with no demonstrable anti-inflammatory activity. Paracetamol is less irritant to the stomach than aspirin. It does not affect thrombocyte aggregation or bleeding time. Paracetamol is generally well tolerated by patients hypersensitive to acetylsalicylic acid.

Pharmacokinetic properties: Paracetamol is well absorbed by both oral and rectal routes. Peak plasma concentrations occur about 2 to 3 hours after rectal administration. The plasma half life is about 2 hours.

Paracetamol is primarily metabolised in the liver by conjugation to glucuronide and sulphate. A small amount (about 3–10% of a therapeutic dose) is metabolised by oxidation and the reactive intermediate metabolite thus formed is bound preferentially to the liver glutathione and excreted as cystein and mercapturic acid conjugates. Excretion occurs via the kidneys. 2–3% of a therapeutic dose is excreted unchanged; 80–90% as glucuronide and sulphate and a smaller amount as cystein and mercapturic acid derivatives.

Preclinical safety data: None.

Pharmaceutical particulars

List of excipients: Hard fat (Witepsol H12).

Incompatibilities: None known.

Shelf-life: 3 years.

Special precautions for storage: Store below 25°C.

Nature and contents of container: Alvedon Suppositories are packed in cartons of 10, each containing two PVC/polyethylene blister strips of 5 suppositories.

Instructions for use/handling: Peel the wrapper apart to remove the suppository, gently push into the rectum pointed end first.

Marketing authorisation holder: Astra Pharmaceuticals Ltd, Home Park, Kings Langley, Hertfordshire WD4 8DH.

Marketing authorisation number PL 0017/0340.

Date of first authorisation 17 June 1997.

Date of (partial) revision of the text May 1997.

FENOPRON* 300

Qualitative and quantitative composition Each tablet contains as active ingredient, fenoprofen calcium equivalent to 300 mg of fenoprofen.

Pharmaceutical form Tablet

Clinical particulars

Therapeutic indications: For the treatment of osteoarthritis, rheumatoid arthritis and ankylosing spondylitis. For the relief of mild/moderate pain.

Posology and method of administration: For oral administration to adults only and not recommended for administration to children.

Dosage: 300-600 mg three or four times a day.

Fenopron 300: Recommended initial dosage is 2 tablets three times per day, then adjusted to the needs of the patient.

Fenopron 600: Recommended initial dosage is one tablet three times per day plus one at night if necessitated by a more severe condition. The dosage may then be adjusted to the needs of the patient.

The maximum daily dose should not exceed 3 g.

If fenoprofen is administered with meals the total amount absorbed is not affected, although peak blood levels are delayed and diminished.

The elderly: There is no difference in the metabolism or pharmacokinetics of fenoprofen in the elderly. However, it may be advisable to start therapy with a low dose, as side-effects of non-steroidal anti-inflammatory drugs are more pronounced in this patient population.

Contra-indications: Hypersensitivity to the drug. Active or a history of, peptic or intestinal ulceration. Fenoprofen should not be given to patients in whom aspirin and other non-steroidal anti-inflammatory drugs induce the symptoms of asthma, rhinitis or urticaria because cross-sensitivity to these drugs occurs in a high proportion of patients. Patients with a history of significantly impaired renal function.

Special warnings and special precautions:

Gastro-intestinal: Serious toxicity, such as bleeding, ulceration and perforation, can occur at any time, without warning symptoms, in patients treated chronically. Elderly or debilitated patients tolerate ulceration or bleeding less well than other individuals and most spontaneous reports of fatal gastro-intestinal events are in this population. Minor upper gastro-intestinal problems, such as dyspepsia are common, usually developing early in therapy.

Fenoprofen should only be given under close supervision to patients with a history of upper gastro-intestinal disease or peptic ulcer risk factors.

Genito-urinary: The most frequently reported problems have been episodes of dysuria, cystitis, haematuria, interstitial nephritis and nephrotic syndrome. This syndrome may be preceded by the appearance of fever, rash, arthralgia, oliguria and uraemia, and may progress to anuria. Early recognition of the syndrome and withdrawal of the drug have been followed by rapid recovery. Patients who have had similar reactions with other non-steroidal anti-inflammatory drugs should not be given fenoprofen. Patients likely to have compromised renal function should be monitored periodically.

Bronchospasm may be precipitated in patients suffering from, or with a previous history of, bronchial asthma or allergic disease.

In patients with conditions leading to reduction in renal blood flow or blood volume, administration of non-steroidal anti-inflammatory drugs may precipitate overt renal decompensation. Patients at greatest risk of this reaction are those with impaired renal function, heart failure, liver dysfunction, those taking diuretics and the elderly. Discontinuation of therapy is typically followed by recovery to the pre-treatment state.

Since fenoprofen is eliminated primarily by the kidneys, patients with possibly compromised renal function (such as the elderly) should be closely monitored, especially during long term therapy: a lower daily dosage should be anticipated to avoid excessive drug accumulation.

Some patients have developed elevation of serum transaminase, LDH and alkaline phosphatase and it is recommended that fenoprofen be discontinued if any significant liver abnormalities occur. Borderline elevations of one or more liver function tests may occur in up to 15% of patients. Severe hepatic reactions, including jaundice and cases of fatal hepatitis, have been reported. Patients in whom an abnormal liver test has occurred should be evaluated for evidence of more severe hepatic reactions. During long-term therapy, liver function tests should be monitored periodically. If fenoprofen is used in the presence of impaired liver function, it must be done under strict observation.

Patients with initial low haemoglobin values who are receiving long-term therapy with fenoprofen should have a haemoglobin determination at reasonable intervals.

Peripheral oedema has been observed in some patients taking fenoprofen, therefore, it should be used with caution in patients with compromised cardiac function or hypertension. The possibility of renal involvement should be considered.

Studies to date have not shown changes in the eyes attributable to the administration of fenoprofen. However, adverse ocular effects have been observed with other anti-inflammatory drugs, so eye examinations should be performed if visual disturbances occur in patients taking fenoprofen.

Since the safety of fenoprofen has not been established in patients with impaired hearing, these patients should have periodic tests of auditory function during chronic therapy

Fenoprofen decreases platelet aggregation and may prolong bleeding time.

Interaction with other medicaments and other forms of interaction:

Laboratory test interactions: Values of total and free triiodothyronine in patients receiving fenoprofen have been reported as falsely elevated. Thyroid stimulating hormones, total thyroxine and thyrotropin releasing hormone response are not affected.

Drug interactions: The concurrent use of fenoprofen and salicylates is not recommended.

Chronic administration of phenobarbitone may be associated with a decrease in the plasma half life of fenoprofen. Dosage adjustment of fenoprofen may be required

Patients treated with fenoprofen may be resistant to the effects of loop diuretics.

In-vitro studies have shown that fenoprofen may displace other drugs, for example hydantoins, sulphonamides, or sulphonylureas, from their binding sites and this may lead to drug interaction. Theoretically, fenoprofen could likewise be displaced. In patients receiving coumarin-type anti-coagulants, the addition of fenoprofen could prolong the prothrombin time.

Pregnancy and lactation: Usage in pregnancy: The safety of fenoprofen for use during pregnancy has not be established; therefore it should not be used during pregnancy unless considered essential by the physician. Animal studies showed prolongation of parturition, but no evidence of teratogenicity.

Usage in nursing mothers: Safety has not been established, therefore, administration to nursing mothers is not recommended.

Effects on the ability to drive and use machines: Caution should be exercised by patients whose activities require alertness if they experience central nervous system side-effects.

Undesirable effects:

Gastro-intestinal: These are the most commonly observed side-effects and include dyspepsia, constipation, diarrhoea, nausea, vomiting, anorexia, ulceration of the buccal mucosa, abdominal pain, flatulence, dry mouth, gastritis, metallic taste, pancreatitis and occult blood in the stool. Cases of peptic ulceration, including some complicated by bleeding or perforation have occurred.

Renal: Cases of acute renal insufficiency, in association with interstitial nephritis, nephrotic syndrome or papillary necrosis, have been reported. Episodes of dysuria, cystitis and haematuria, oliguria, azotaemia and anuria have occurred.

Hepatic: Severe hepatic reactions, including jaundice and fatal hepatitis, have been reported rarely. Increases in alkaline phosphatase, LDH and AST have been observed.

Haematological: Various syndromes involving the bone marrow have been reported rarely: thrombocytopenia, pancytopenia and aplastic anaemia have occurred. Purpura, bruising, haemorrhage, haemolytic anaemia and agranulocytosis have also been reported.

Allergic skin: Pruritus, rash, urticaria, anaphylaxis, Stevens-Johnson syndrome, angioneurotic oedema, increased sweating, exfoliative dermatitis, toxic epidermal necrolysis and alopecia have been reported

Neurological: Reactions reported include headache, somnolence, dizziness, tremor, confusion and insomnia, depression, disorientation, seizures and trigeminal neuralgia.

Cardiovascular: Palpitations, tachycardia, atrial fibrillation, pulmonary oedema, ECG changes and supraventricular tachycardia have been reported.

Miscellaneous: Tinnitus, hearing decrease, amblyopia, blurred vision, diplopia, optic neuritis, nervousness, peripheral oedema, asthenia, dyspnoea, fatigue, malaise, burning tongue, personality change, lymphadenopathy, mastodynia, fever, upper respiratory infection and nasopharyngitis have been reported.

Overdose: Symptoms of overdose appear within several hours and generally involve the gastro-intestinal and central nervous systems. They include dyspepsia, nausea, vomiting, abdominal pain, dizziness, headache, ataxia, tinnitus, tremor, drowsiness and confusion. Hyperpyrexia, tachycardia, hypotension and acute renal failure may occur rarely following overdose. Respiratory depression and metabolic acidosis have also been reported following overdose with certain non-steroidal anti-inflammatory drugs.

Treatment: Standard therapy to evacuate gastric contents and to support vital functions should be employed. Alkalinisation of the urine, forced diuresis, peritoneal dialysis, haemodialysis and charcoal haemoperfusion do not enhance systemic drug elimination.

Pharmacological properties

Pharmacodynamic properties: Fenoprofen calcium is a nonsteroidal, anti-inflammatory, antiarthritic drug that also possess analgesic and antipyretic activities. Its exact mode of action is unknown, but it is thought that prostaglandin synthetase inhibition is involved.

Pharmacokinetic properties: Under fasting conditions, fenoprofen is rapidly absorbed, and peak plasma levels of 50 mgc/L are achieved within 2 hours after oral administration of 600 mg doses. Good dose proportionality was observed between 200 mg and 600 mg doses in fasting male volunteers. The plasma half-life is approximately 3 hours. About 90% of a single oral dose is eliminated within 24 hours as fenoprofen glucuronide and 4-hydroxyfenoprofen glucuronide, the major urinary metabolites of fenoprofen. Fenoprofen is highly bound (99%) to albumin. The concomitant administration of antacid (containing both aluminium and magnesium hydroxide) does not interfere with absorption of fenoprofen.

Preclinical safety data: Reproduction studies in rats have shown fenoprofen calcium to be associated with prolonged labour and difficult parturition when given during late pregnancy, but no evidence of teratogenicity has been seen.

Fenoprofen shows anti-inflammatory effects in rodents by inhibiting the development of redness and oedema in acute inflammatory conditions by reducing soft tissue swelling and bone damage associated with chronic inflammation. It exhibits analgesic activity in rodents by inhibiting the writhing response caused by the introduction of an irritant into the peritoneal cavities of mice and by elevating pain thresholds that are related to pressure in edematous hindpaws of rats. In rats made febrile by the subcutaneous administration of brewer's yeast, fenoprofen produces antipyretic action.

In chronic studies in rats, high doses of fenoprofen calcium caused elevation of serum transaminase and hepatocellular hypertrophy.

Pharmaceutical particulars

List of excipients: Calcium hydrogen phosphate; maize starch; polacrilin potassium; magnesium stearate; stearic acid powder; methylhydroxypropylcellulose; polyethylene glycol 8000; propylene glycol; titanium dioxide; sunset yellow (E110).

Incompatibilities: Not applicable

Shelf life: Two years, when stored appropriately

Special precautions for storage: Store at room temperature (15°-25°C)

Nature and contents of container: Screw capped, high density polyethylene bottles of 100 tablets

Instruction for use/handling: No special instructions

Marketing authorisation number 11157/0005

Date of approval/ revision of SPC October 1996

Legal category POM

FENOPRON* 600

Presentation Fenoprofen Calcium Tablets BP, each containing fenoprofen calcium equivalent to 600 mg fenoprofen.

Fenopron 600 tablets are orange, para-capsule, 20 mm long and marked 4021.

Uses For the treatment of osteoarthritis, rheumatoid arthritis and ankylosing spondylitis.

For the relief of mild/moderate pain.

Dosage and administration For oral administration to adults only, and not recommended for administration to children.

Dosage: 300 to 600 mg three or four times per day.

Fenopron 600: Recommended initial dosage is 1 tablet three times per day, plus one at night if necessitated by a more severe condition. The dosage may then be adjusted to the needs of the patient.

The maximum daily dose should not exceed 3 g.

If fenoprofen is administered with meals the total amount absorbed is not affected, although peak blood levels are delayed and diminished.

The elderly: There is no difference in the metabolism or pharmacokinetics of fenoprofen in the elderly. However, it may be advisable to start therapy with a low dose, as side-effects of non-steroidal anti-inflammatory drugs are more pronounced in this patient population.

Contra-indications, warnings, etc

Contra-indications: Hypersensitivity to the drug. Active, or a history of, peptic or intestinal ulceration.

Fenoprofen should not be given to patients in whom aspirin and other non-steroidal anti-inflammatory drugs induce the symptoms of asthma, rhinitis, or urticaria, because cross-sensitivity to these drugs occurs in a high proportion of patients.

Patients with a history of significantly impaired renal function.

Warnings

Gastro-intestinal: Serious toxicity, such as bleeding, ulceration and perforation, can occur at any time, without warning symptoms, in patients treated chronically. Elderly or debilitated patients tolerate ulceration or bleeding less well than other individuals and most spontaneous reports of fatal gastro-intestinal events are in this population. Minor upper gastro-intestinal problems, such as dyspepsia, are common, usually developing early in therapy.

Fenoprofen should only be given under close supervision to patients with a history of upper gastro-intestinal disease or peptic ulcer risk factors.

Genito-urinary: The most frequently reported problems have been episodes of dysuria, cystitis, haematuria, interstitial nephritis and nephrotic syndrome. This syndrome may be preceded by the appearance of fever, rash, arthralgia, oliguria and uraemia, and may progress to anuria. Early recognition of the syndrome and withdrawal of the drug have been followed by rapid recovery. Patients who have had similar reactions with other non-steroidal anti-inflammatory drugs should not be given fenoprofen. Patients likely to have compromised renal function should be monitored periodically.

Bronchospasm may be precipitated in patients suffering from, or with a previous history of, bronchial asthma or allergic disease.

Usage in pregnancy: The safety of fenoprofen for use during pregnancy has not been established; therefore it should not be used during pregnancy unless considered essential by the physician. Animal studies showed prolongation of parturition, but no evidence of teratogenicity.

Usage in nursing mothers: Safety has not been established, therefore administration to nursing mothers is not recommended.

Precautions: In patients with conditions leading to reduction in renal blood flow or blood volume, administration of non-steroidal anti-inflammatory drugs may precipitate overt renal decompensation. Patients at greatest risk of this reaction are those with impaired renal function, heart failure, liver dysfunction, those taking diuretics, and the elderly. Discontinuation of therapy is typically followed by recovery to the pre-treatment state.

Since fenoprofen is eliminated primarily by the kidneys, patients with possibly compromised renal function (such as the elderly) should be closely monitored, especially during long-term therapy; a lower daily dosage should be anticipated to avoid excessive drug accumulation.

Some patients have developed elevation of serum transaminase, LDH and alkaline phosphatase and it is recommended that fenoprofen be discontinued if any significant liver abnormalities occur. Borderline elevations of one or more liver function tests may occur in up to 15% of patients. Severe hepatic reactions, including jaundice and cases of fatal hepatitis, have been reported. Patients in whom an abnormal liver test has occurred should be evaluated for evidence of more severe hepatic reactions. During long-term therapy, liver function tests should be monitored periodically. If fenoprofen is used in the presence of impaired liver function, it must be done under strict observation.

Patients with initial low haemoglobin values who are receiving long-term therapy with fenoprofen should have a haemoglobin determination at reasonable intervals.

Peripheral oedema has been observed in some patients taking fenoprofen, therefore it should be used with caution in patients with compromised cardiac function or hypertension. The possibility of renal involvement should be considered.

Studies to date have not shown changes in the eyes attributable to the administration of fenoprofen. However, adverse ocular effects have been observed with other anti-inflammatory drugs, so eye examinations should be performed if visual disturbances occur in patients taking fenoprofen.

Caution should be exercised by patients whose activities require alertness if they experience central nervous system side-effects.

Since the safety of fenoprofen has not been established in patients with impaired hearing, these patients should have periodic tests of auditory function during chronic therapy.

Fenoprofen decreases platelet aggregation and may prolong bleeding time.

Laboratory test interactions: Values of total and free triiodothyronine in patients receiving fenoprofen have been reported as falsely elevated. Thyroid stimulating hormones, total thyroxine and thyrotropin releasing hormone response are not affected.

Drug interactions: The concurrent use of fenoprofen and salicylates is not recommended.

Chronic administration of phenobarbitone may be associated with a decrease in the plasma half-life of fenoprofen. Dosage adjustment of fenoprofen may be required.

Patients treated with fenoprofen may be resistant to the effects of loop diuretics.

In vitro studies have shown that fenoprofen may displace other drugs, for example hydantoins, sulphonamides, or sulphonylureas, from their binding sites and this may lead to drug interaction. Theoretically, fenoprofen could likewise be displaced. In patients receiving coumarin-type anti-coagulants, the addition of fenoprofen could prolong the prothrombin time.

Side-effects

Gastro-intestinal: These are the most commonly observed side-effects and include dyspepsia, constipation, diarrhoea, nausea, vomiting, anorexia, ulceration of the buccal mucosa, abdominal pain, flatulence, dry mouth, gastritis, metallic taste, pancreatitis and occult blood in the stool. Cases of peptic ulceration, including some complicated by bleeding or perforation have occurred.

Renal: Cases of acute renal insufficiency, in association with interstitial nephritis, nephrotic syndrome or papillary necrosis, have been reported. Episodes of dysuria, cystitis and haematuria, oliguria, azotaemia and anuria have occurred.

Hepatic: Severe hepatic reactions, including jaundice and fatal hepatitis, have been reported rarely. Increases in alkaline phosphatase, LDH and AST have been observed.

Haematological: Various syndromes involving the bone marrow have been reported rarely; thrombocytopenia, pancytopenia and aplastic anaemia have occurred. Purpura, bruising, haemorrhage, haemolytic anaemia and agranulocytosis have also been reported.

Allergic/skin: Pruritus, rash, urticaria, anaphylaxis, Stevens-Johnson syndrome, angioneurotic oedema, increased sweating, exfoliative dermatitis, toxic epidermal necrolysis and alopecia have been reported.

Neurological: Reactions reported include headache, somnolence, dizziness, tremor, confusion and insomnia, depression, disorientation, seizures and trigeminal neuralgia.

Cardiovascular: Palpitations, tachycardia, atrial fibrillation, pulmonary oedema, ECG changes and supraventricular tachycardia have been reported.

Miscellaneous: Tinnitus, hearing decrease, amblyopia, blurred vision, diplopia, optic neuritis, nervousness, peripheral oedema, asthenia, dyspnoea, fatigue, malaise, burning tongue, personality change, lymphadenopathy, mastodynia, fever, upper respiratory infection and nasopharyngitis have been reported.

Overdosage: Symptoms of overdose appear within several hours and generally involve the gastro-intestinal and central nervous systems. They include dyspepsia, nausea, vomiting, abdominal pain, dizziness, headache, ataxia, tinnitus, tremor, drowsiness and confusion. Hyperpyrexia, tachycardia, hypotension and acute renal failure may occur rarely following overdose. Respiratory depression and metabolic acidosis have also been reported following overdose with certain non-steroidal anti-inflammatory drugs.

Treatment: Standard therapy to evacuate gastric contents and to support vital functions should be employed. Alkalinisation of the urine, forced diuresis, peritoneal dialysis, haemodialysis and charcoal haemoperfusion do not enhance systemic drug elimination.

Pharmaceutical precautions Nil.

Legal category POM.

Package quantities
Bottles of 100 tablets

Further information Nil.

Product licence number 11157/0006

HAELAN CREAM

Qualitative and quantitative composition Flurandrenolone (Fludroxycortide) 0.0125% w/w.

Pharmaceutical form Cream for topical administration.

Clinical particulars

Therapeutic indications: Adults and children: Eczema and dermatitis of all types including childhood and adult atopic eczema, photodermatitis, primary irritant and allergic dermatitis, lichen planus, lichen simplex, prurigo nodularis, discoid lupus erythematosus, necrobiosis lipoidica, pretibial myxoedema and erythroderma.

Posology and method of administration: For moist, weeping lesions, the cream should be applied gently to the affected area two or three times daily.

The elderly: As the skin is likely to be thin, apply sparingly to avoid development of atrophy.

Dilution is not recommended, but if considered necessary, aqueous cream BP may be used.

Contra-indications: Tuberculosis of the skin, facial rosacea, acne vulgaris, perioral dermatitis, perianal and genital pruritus, dermatoses in infancy including eczema, dermatitic napkin eruption, bacterial (impetigo), viral (herpes simplex) and fungal (candida or dermatophyte) infections. Use in patients with a history of hypersensitivity to any of the components in the preparation.

Special warnings and special precautions for use: Preparations of Haelan are not intended for ophthalmic use.

Local and systemic toxicity is common especially following long-term continuous use, continued use on large areas of damaged skin, flexures and with polythene occlusion.

Systemic absorption of topical corticosteroids has produced reversible hypothalamic-pituitary-adrenal (HPA) axis suppression (see *Undesirable effects*). Therefore, patients receiving a large dose of a potent topical steroid applied to a large surface area or under an occlusive dressing should be evaluated periodically for evidence of HPA axis suppression by using urinary-free cortisol and ACTH stimulation tests. If HPA axis suppression is noted, an attempt should be made to withdraw the drug, to reduce the frequency of application or to substitute a less potent steroid. Recovery of HPA axis function is generally prompt and complete on discontinuation of the drug. Infrequently, signs and symptoms of steroid withdrawal may occur, so that supplemental systemic corticosteroids are required.

Long-term continuous therapy should be avoided in all patients irrespective of age.

Application under occlusion should be restricted to dermatoses in very limited areas.

If used on the face, courses should be limited to five days and occlusion should not be used.

In the presence of skin infections, the use of an appropriate antifungal or antibacterial agent should be instituted. If a favourable response does not occur promptly, flurandrenolone should be discontinued until the infection has been adequately controlled.

Usage in children: If used in childhood courses should be limited to five days and occlusion should not be used.

Children may absorb proportionally larger amounts of topical corticosteroids and thus may be more susceptible to systemic toxicity. Children may also demonstrate greater susceptibility to topical corticosteroid induced HPA axis suppression and Cushing's Syndrome than do mature patients because of a large skin surface to body weight ratio. Administration of topical corticosteriods to children should be limited to the least amount compatible with an effective therapeutic regimen. Chronic corticosteroid therapy may interfere with the growth and development of children.

As with all topical steroids, the activity can be enhanced by the use of occlusive dressings. Preparations of Haelan are recommended only as a supplement to, and not as a substitute for, preparations (lotions, wet dressings, etc.) used in the conventional management of skin lesions. Haelan Cream does not contain parahydroxybenzoates or lanolin.

Interaction with other medicaments and other forms of interaction: Not known.

Pregnancy and lactation: Usage in pregnancy: There is inadequate evidence of safety in human pregnancy. There may be a very small risk of cleft palate and intra-uterine growth retardation as well as suppression of the neonatal HPA axis. There is evidence of harmful effects in animals.

Use in pregnancy only when there is no safer alternative and when the disease itself carries risks for mother and child.

Usage in nursing mothers: It is not known whether topical administration of corticosteroids could result in sufficient systemic absorption to produce detectable quantities in the breast milk of nursing mothers. Systemically administered corticosteroids are secreted into breast milk in quantities not likely to have a deleterious effect on the infant. Nevertheless, caution should be exercised when topical corticosteroids are administered to nursing mothers.

Effects on ability to drive and to use machines: Not applicable.

Undesirable effects: The following local adverse reactions are reported infrequently with topical corticosteroids but may occur more frequently with the use of occlusive dressings. These reactions are listed in approximate decreasing order of occurrence; burning, itching, irritation, dryness, folliculitis, hypertrichosis, acneform eruptions, hypopigmentation, perioral dermatitis, allergic contact dermatitis, maceration of the skin, secondary infection, skin atrophy, miliaria, striae and thinning and dilatations of the superficial blood vessels producing telangiectasia.

Prolonged use of large doses to extensive areas can result in sufficient systemic absorption to produce generalised manifestations of steroid toxicity and may result in depression of HPA function on discontinuing treatment.

Manifestations of Cushing's syndrome, hyperglycaemia and glycosuria have occurred in some patients.

Manifestations of adrenal suppression in children include linear growth retardation, delayed weight gain, low plasma cortisol levels and absence of response to ACTH stimulation. Intracranial hypertension including bulging fontanelles, headaches and bilateral papilloedema have also been reported in children receiving topical corticosteroids.

Infected skin lesions, viral, bacterial or fungal may be substantially exacerbated by topical steroid therapy. Wound healing is significantly retarded.

Hypersensitivity reactions may occur.

Overdose: Topically applied corticosteroids can be absorbed in sufficient amounts to produce systemic effects (see *Special warnings and special precautions for use*).

Pharmacological properties

Pharmacodynamic properties: Flurandrenolone is a fluorinated, synthetic, moderately potent corticosteroid.

As with other topical steroids, the therapeutic effect is primarily the result of its anti-inflammatory, antimitotic and anti-synthetic activities.

Pharmacokinetic properties: Flurandrenolone applied under occlusive dressing has shown therapeutic improvement without disturbance of electrolyte, liver or renal function or suppression of adrenal function.

Preclinical safety data: There are no preclinical data of relevance to the prescriber in addition to that summarised in other sections of the Summary of Product Characteristics.

Pharmaceutical particulars

List of excipients: Stearic acid, cetyl alcohol, polyoxyl 40 stearate, liquid paraffin, propylene glycol, sodium citrate, citric acid anhydrous, water purified

Incompatibilities: None known.

Shelf life: 24 months.

Special precautions for storage: None.

Nature and contents of container: 60 g aluminium tubes with screw cap.

Instructions for use/handling: No special instructions for handling.

Marketing authorisation number 11157/0008.

Date of approval/revision of SPC December 1996

Legal category POM

HAELAN* OINTMENT

Presentation Collapsible tubes containing 0.0125% flurandrenolone in an ointment base. The ointment is translucent in colour.

Uses *Adults and children:* Eczema and dermatitis of all types including childhood and adult atopic eczema, photodermatitis, primary irritant and allergic dermatitis, lichen planus, lichen simplex, prurigo nodularis, discoid lupus erythematosus, necrobiosis lipoidica, pretibial myxoedema and erythroderma.

Dosage and administration For topical administration.

For dry, scaly lesions, the ointment should be applied as a thin film to the affected area two or three times daily.

The elderly: As the skin is likely to be thin, apply sparingly to avoid development of atrophy.

Dilution is not recommended, but if considered necessary White Soft Paraffin BP may be used.

Contra-indications, warnings, etc

Contra-indications: Tuberculosis of the skin. Facial rosacea. Acne vulgaris. Perioral dermatitis. Perianal and genital pruritus. Dermatoses in infancy including eczema, dermatitic napkin eruption, bacterial (impetigo), viral (herpes simplex) and fungal (candida or dermatophyte) infections. Use in patients with a history of hypersensitivity to any of the components in the preparation.

Warnings and precautions: Preparations of Haelan are not intended for ophthalmic use.

Local and systemic toxicity is common especially following long-term continuous use, continued use on large areas of damaged skin, flexures and with polythene occlusion.

Systemic absorption of topical corticosteroids has produced reversible hypothalamic-pituitary-adrenal (HPA) axis suppression (see 'Side-effects'). Therefore, patients receiving a large dose of a potent topical steroid applied to a large surface area or under an occlusive dressing should be evaluated periodically for evidence of HPA axis suppression by using urinary-free cortisol and ACTH stimulation tests. If HPA axis suppression is noted, an attempt should be made to withdraw the drug, to reduce the frequency of application or to substitute a less potent steroid. Recovery of HPA axis function is generally prompt and complete on discontinuation of the drug. Infrequently, signs and symptoms of steroid withdrawal may occur, so that supplemental systemic corticosteroids are required.

Long-term continuous therapy should be avoided in all patients irrespective of age.

Application under occlusion should be restricted to dermatoses in very limited areas.

If used on the face, courses should be limited to five days and occlusion should not be used.

In the presence of skin infections, the use of an appropriate antifungal or antibacterial agent should be instituted. If a favourable response does not occur promptly, flurandrenolone should be discontinued until the infection has been adequately controlled.

Usage in children: If used in childhood, courses should be limited to five days and occlusion should not be used.

Children may absorb proportionally larger amounts of topical corticosteroids and thus may be more susceptible to systemic toxicity. Children may also demonstrate greater susceptibility to topical corticosteroid induced HPA axis suppression and Cushing's syndrome than do mature patients because of a larger skin surface to body weight ratio. Administration of topical corticosteroids to children should be limited to the least amount compatible with an effective therapeutic regimen. Chronic corticosteroid therapy may interfere with the growth and development of children.

Usage in pregnancy: There is inadequate evidence of safety in human pregnancy. There may be a very small risk of cleft palate and intra-uterine growth retardation as well as suppression of the neonatal HPA axis. There is evidence of harmful effects in animals.

Use in pregnancy only when there is no safer alternative and when the disease itself carries risks for mother and child.

Usage in nursing mothers: It is not known whether topical administration of corticosteroids could result in sufficient systemic absorption to produce detectable quantities in the breast milk of nursing mothers. Systemically administered corticosteroids are secreted into breast milk in quantities not likely to have a deleterious effect on the infant. Nevertheless, caution should be exercised when topical corticosteroids are administered to nursing mothers.

Side-effects: The following local adverse reactions are reported infrequently with topical corticosteroids but may occur more frequently with the use of occlusive dressings. These reactions are listed in an approximate decreasing order of occurrence: burning, itching, irritation, dryness, folliculitis, hypertrichosis, acneform eruptions, hypopigmentation, perioral dermatitis, allergic contact dermatitis, maceration of the skin, secondary infection, skin atrophy, miliaria, striae and thinning and dilatations of superficial blood vessels producing telangiectasia.

Prolonged use of large doses to extensive areas can result in sufficient systemic absorption to produce generalised manifestations of steroid toxicity and may result in depression of HPA function on discontinuing treatment.

Manifestations of Cushing's syndrome, hyperglycaemia and glycosuria have occurred in some patients.

Manifestations of adrenal suppression in children include linear growth retardation, delayed weight gain, low plasma cortisol levels and absence of response to ACTH stimulation. Intracranial hypertension including bulging fontanelles, headaches and bilateral papilloedema have also been reported in children receiving topical corticosteroids.

Infected skin lesions, viral, bacterial or fungal may be substantially exacerbated by topical steroid therapy. Wound healing is significantly retarded.

Hypersensitivity reactions may occur.

Overdosage: Topically applied corticosteroids can be absorbed in sufficient amounts to produce systemic effects (see 'Warnings and precautions').

Pharmaceutical precautions Do not store above 25°C.

See *Administration* for diluents.

Legal category POM.

Package quantities

Haelan Ointment (0.0125% flurandrenolone): Tubes of 60 g

Further information As with all topical steroids, the activity can be enhanced by the use of occlusive dressings. Preparations of Haelan are recommended only as a supplement to, and not as a substitute for, preparations (lotions, wet dressings, etc.) used in the conventional management of skin lesions. Haelan preparations do not contain parahydroxybenzoates or lanolin.

Product licence number 11157/009

HAELAN* TAPE

Qualitative and quantitative composition The tape is impregnated with 4 micrograms flurandrenolone per square centimetre.

Pharmaceutical form Occlusive tape

Clinical particulars

Therapeutic indications: Occlusive topical steroid. Adjunctive therapy for chronic, localised, recalcitrant dermatoses that may respond to topical corticosteroids and particularly dry, scaling lesions.

Posology and method of administration:

Adults and the elderly: For application to the skin, which should be clean, dry and shorn of hair. In most instances the tape need only remain in place for 12 out of 24 hours. Cosmetics may be applied over the tape.

Application: The tape is cut so as to cover the lesion and a quarter inch margin of normal skin. Corners should be rounded off. After removing the lining paper, the tape is applied to the centre of the lesion with gentle pressure and worked to the edges, avoiding excessive tension of the skin. If longer strips of tape are to be applied, the lining paper should be removed progressively.

If irritation or infection develops, remove tape and consult a physician.

Children: If used in childhood, courses should be limited to five days and occlusion should not be used (see *Special warnings and special precautions for use*).

Contra-indications: Chicken pox. Vaccinia. Tuberculosis of the skin. Hypersensitivity to any of the components. Facial rosacea. Acne vulgaris. Perioral dermatitis. Perianal and genital pruritus. Dermatoses in infancy including eczema, dermatitic napkin eruption, bacterial (impetigo), viral (herpes simplex) and fungal (candida or dermatophyte) infections.

Special warnings and special precautions for use: Not advocated for acute and weeping dermatoses.

Local and systemic toxicity of medium and high potency topical corticosteroids is common, especially following long-term continuous use, continued use on large areas of damaged skin, flexures and with polythene occlusion.

Systemic absorption of topical corticosteroids has produced reversible hypothalamic-pituitary-adrenal (HPA) axis suppression (see *Undesirable effects*). Therefore, patients receiving a large dose of a potent topical steroid applied to a large surface area or under an occlusive dressing should be evaluated periodically for evidence of HPA axis suppression by using urinary-free cortisol and ACTH stimulation tests. If HPA axis suppression is noted, an attempt should be made to withdraw the drug, to reduce the frequency of application or to substitute a less potent steroid. Recovery of HPA axis function is generally prompt and complete on discontinuation of the drug. Infrequently, signs and symptoms of steroid withdrawal may occur, so that supplemental systemic corticosteroids are required.

Long-term continuous therapy should be avoided in all patients irrespective of age.

Application under occlusion should be restricted to dermatoses in very limited areas.

If used on the face, courses should be limited to five days and occlusion should not be used.

In the presence of skin infections, the use of an appropriate antifungal or antibacterial agent should be instituted. If a favourable response does not occur promptly, flurandrenolone should be discontinued until the infection has been adequately controlled.

Children may absorb proportionally larger amounts of topical corticosteroids and thus may be more susceptible to systemic toxicity. Children may also demonstrate greater susceptibility to topical corticosteroid induced HPA axis suppression and Cushing's syndrome than do mature patients because of a larger skin surface to bodyweight ratio. Administration of topical corticosteroids to children should be limited to the least amount compatible with an effective therapeutic regimen. Chronic corticosteroid therapy may interfere with the growth and development of children.

Interaction with other medicaments and other forms of interaction: None known.

Pregnancy and lactation: Usage in pregnancy: There is inadequate evidence of safety in human pregnancy. There may be a very small risk of cleft palate and intra-uterine growth retardation as well as suppression of the neonatal HPA axis. There is evidence of harmful effects in animals.

Use in pregnancy only when there is no safer alternative and when the disease itself carries risks for mother and child.

Usage in nursing mothers: It is not known whether topical administration of corticosteroids could result in sufficient systemic absorption to produce detectable quantities in the breast milk of nursing mothers. Systemically administered corticosteroids are secreted into breast milk in quantities not likely to have a deleterious effect on the infant. Nevertheless, caution should be exercised when topical corticosteroids are administered to nursing mothers.

Effects on the ability to drive and use machines: Not applicable.

Undesirable effects: The following local adverse reactions are reported infrequently with topical corticosteroids but may occur more frequently with the use of occlusive dressings. These reactions are listed in an approximate decreasing order of occurrence: burning, itching, irritation, dryness, folliculitis, hypertrichosis, acneform eruptions, hypopigmentation, perioral dermatitis, allergic contact dermatitis, maceration of the skin, secondary infection, skin atrophy, miliaria, striae and thinning and dilatations of superficial blood vessels producing telangiectasia.

Prolonged use of large doses to extensive areas can result in sufficient systemic absorption to produce generalised manifestations of steroid toxicity and may result in depression of HPA function on discontinuing treatment.

Manifestations of Cushing's syndrome, hyperglycaemia and glycosuria have occurred in some patients.

Manifestations of adrenal suppression in children include linear growth retardation, delayed weight gain, low plasma cortisol levels and absence of response to ACTH stimulation. Intracranial hypertension including bulging fontanelles, headaches and bilateral papilloedema have also been reported in children receiving topical corticosteroids. Infected skin lesions, viral, bacterial or fungal, may be substantially exacerbated by topical steroid therapy. Wound healing is significantly retarded.

Hypersensitivity reactions may occur.

Overdose: Topically applied corticosteroids can be absorbed in sufficient amounts to produce systemic affects (see *Special warnings and special precautions for use*).

Pharmacological properties

Pharmacodynamic properties: Flurandrenolone is a fluorinated, synthetic, moderately potent, topical corticosteroid. As with other topical steroids, the therapeutic effect is primarily the result of its anti-inflammatory, antimitotic and antisynthetic activities.

Pharmacokinetic properties: When applied topically, particularly to large areas, when skin is broken, or under occlusive dressings, corticosteroids may be absorbed in sufficient amounts to cause systemic effects.

Preclinical safety data: There are no preclinical data of relevance to the prescriber in addition to that summarised in other sections of the Summary of Product Characteristics.

Pharmaceutical particulars

List of excipients: Blenderm brand surgical tape.

Incompatibilities: None known.

Shelf life: 3 years.

Special precautions for storage: Store in a dry place, below 25°C.

Nature and contents of container: Polypropylene dispenser, in a cardboard box, containing 50cm or 200cm of translucent, polythene adhesive film, 7.5cm wide, protected by a removable paper liner.

Instructions for use/handling: Not applicable.

Marketing authorisation number 11157/0007

Date of approval/revision of SPC January 1997

Legal category POM

**Trade Mark*

Novo Nordisk Pharmaceuticals Limited

Novo Nordisk House, Broadfield Park
Brighton Road, Pease Pottage
Crawley, West Sussex, RH11 9RT

☎ 01293 613555   🗋 01293 613535

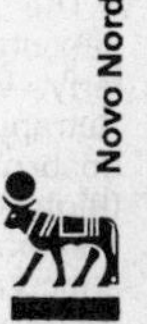

ACTRAPID* PENFILL* 3 ml
INSULATARD* PENFILL* 3 ml
MIXTARD* 10 PENFILL* 3 ml
MIXTARD* 20 PENFILL* 3 ml
MIXTARD* 30 PENFILL* 3 ml
MIXTARD* 40 PENFILL* 3 ml
MIXTARD* 50 PENFILL* 3 ml

Qualitative and quantitative composition

Actrapid Penfill 3 ml: Insulin Injection.
Insulatard Penfill 3 ml: Isophane Insulin Injection.
Mixtard 10 Penfill 3 ml: Biphasic Isophane Insulin Injection 10/90.
Mixtard 20 Penfill 3 ml: Biphasic Isophane Insulin Injection 20/80.
Mixtard 30 Penfill 3 ml: Biphasic Isophane Insulin Injection 30/70.
Mixtard 40 Penfill 3 ml: Biphasic Isophane Insulin Injection 40/60.
Mixtard 50 Penfill 3 ml: Biphasic Isophane Insulin Injection 50/50.

Active ingredient: Human insulin (pyr) 100 iu/ml.

Pharmaceutical form

Actrapid Penfill 3 ml: Sterile solution for injection.
Insulatard Penfill 3 ml and Mixtard Penfill 3 ml range: Sterile suspension for injection.

Clinical particulars

Therapeutic indications: The treatment of insulin-requiring diabetics.

Posology and method of administration: The dosage is determined by the physician according to the needs of the patient.

The Penfill preparations are usually administered subcutaneously but may also be given intramuscularly. When injected subcutaneously, injection of Actrapid Penfill 3 ml into the abdominal wall ensures a faster absorption than from other regions of the body. The thigh is the recommended site for injection of Insulatard Penfill 3 ml, the abdominal wall or thigh for subcutaneous injection of Mixtard Penfill 3 ml preparations. Injection into a lifted skin fold minimises the risk of intramuscular injection.

When used alone Actrapid Penfill 3 ml is usually given three or more times daily; it is more commonly used in regimens where an intermediate or long-acting insulin is given in addition.

Insulatard Penfill 3 ml and the Mixtard Penfill 3 ml preparations may be given once or, more commonly, twice daily. Insulatard Penfill 3 ml may also be supplemented with shorter-acting insulin.

Penfill insulin cartridges are designed to be used with NovoPen insulin pens and NovoFine needles. The Penfill preparations are intended for use by one person only. The Penfill cartridges must not be used with conventional syringes or refilled.

Use in the elderly: There are no precautions concerning the use of insulin which are specific to the elderly diabetic. However, injection procedures may be difficult for the infirm or the confused patient, and the simplest regimen consistent with keeping the patient symptom-free should be considered.

Contra-indications: Insulin is contra-indicated in hypoglycaemia.

Special warnings and special precautions for use: Injection of Actrapid Penfill 3 ml or the Mixtard Penfill 3 ml preparations should be followed by a meal within approximately 30 minutes of administration.

The use of dosages which are inadequate, or discontinuation of treatment, especially in insulin-dependent diabetics, may lead to hyperglycaemia and diabetic ketoacidosis; conditions which are potentially lethal.

When patients are transferred from other insulins to highly purified human insulin the change should be made according to the following general guidelines:

For patients currently controlled on highly purified human or porcine insulin preparations no dosage change is anticipated other than the routine adjustments made in order to maintain stable diabetic control. Patients currently stabilised on mixed species or bovine insulin may require a dosage adjustment dependent upon dosage, purity, species and formulation of the insulin preparation(s) currently administered. Variations in glycaemic control may occur and adjustments in therapy should be made under the guidance of a physician. A few patients have reported that after being transferred to human insulin the early warning symptoms for hypoglycaemia were less pronounced than they were with animal-source insulin.

Patients whose blood glucose is greatly improved, e.g. by intensified insulin therapy, may experience a change in their usual warning symptoms of hypoglycaemia and possibly lose some or all of the symptoms, and should be advised accordingly.

Interaction with other medicaments and other forms of interaction: Concomitant use of other drugs may influence insulin requirements. The following substances may enhance the hypoglycaemic effect of insulin: alcohol, non-selective beta adrenergic blocking agents, monoamine oxidase inhibitors (MAOI), ACE inhibitors, salicylate, anabolic steroids.

Other drugs may increase insulin requirements: oral contraceptives, thyroid hormones, corticosteroids, thiazides and sympathomimetics. Beta adrenergic blocking agents may blur the symptoms of hypoglycaemia. Alcohol may intensify and prolong the hypoglycaemic effect of insulin.

Diabetic patients treated with drugs other than insulin should discuss possible interactions with the prescribing physician.

Pregnancy and lactation: Intensified control in the treatment of pregnant insulin-dependent diabetics is recommended. Insulin requirements usually fall in the first trimester and increase during the second and third trimester. Insulin does not pass the placental barrier.

Effects on ability to drive and use machines: The ability to drive or use machinery may be impaired during hypoglycaemia or severe hyperglycaemia.

Undesirable effects: At initiation of insulin therapy, oedema and refraction anomalies may occur; these are usually transitory. The same applies to local hypersensitivity reactions (swelling and itching at the injection site) which usually disappear during continued treatment.

Persistent allergies to human insulin are very rare and are mostly due to cross-reacting antibodies to animal insulins. Lipodystrophy at injection sites is also rare and should be prevented by constantly changing injection sites.

Overdose: Overdosage causes hypoglycaemia; symptoms are variable but may include confusion, palpitations, sweating, malaise and loss of consciousness. In the event of an overdose, glucose should be given if the patient is conscious. Where the patient is unconscious an intramuscular, subcutaneous or intravenous injection of glucagon should be given and oral carbohydrate administered when the patient responds. Alternatively intravenous glucose may be administered; it must be given if there is no response to glucagon. If severe hypoglycaemia is not treated it can cause temporary or permanent brain damage and death.

Pharmacological properties

Pharmacodynamic properties: Human insulin (pyr) is identical to pancreatic human insulin. It has hypoglycaemic actions in man, promotes uptake of glucose into liver, muscle and adipose tissue, inhibits gluconeogenesis and promotes lipogenesis.

Pharmacokinetic properties: Actrapid Penfill 3 ml is a neutral solution of human insulin (pyr). When injected subcutaneously it has a duration of action of some ½ to 8 hours and its maximum effect is exerted between 1 and 3 hours after injection. Insulatard Penfill 3 ml is an isophane insulin preparation. When injected subcutaneously it has a duration of action of some 1½ up to 24 hours and its maximum effect is exerted between 4 and 12 hours after injection.

The Mixtard Penfill 3 ml preparations consist of soluble human insulin and isophane human insulin in the ratios:

Mixtard 10 Penfill 3 ml – 10/90
Mixtard 20 Penfill 3 ml – 20/80
Mixtard 30 Penfill 3 ml – 30/70
Mixtard 40 Penfill 3 ml – 40/60
Mixtard 50 Penfill 3 ml – 50/50

They are intermediate acting insulins with a pronounced initial effect. When injected subcutaneously they have a duration of action of some ½ up to 24 hours and their maximum effect is exerted between 2 and 8 hours after injection.

Pharmaceutical particulars

List of excipients: Glycerol (E422), m-cresol, zinc oxide, sodium hydroxide, hydrochloric acid, water for injections.

Plus, Insulatard Penfill 3 ml and Mixtard Penfill 3 ml preparations: sodium phosphate dihydrate, phenol, protamine sulphate.

Incompatibilities: Not applicable.

Shelf life: 30 months. Cartridges in use or carried as a spare may be kept at ambient temperature (e.g. in the pocket or handbag) for up to one month but should not be exposed to excessive heat or sunlight.

Special precautions for storage: Store between 2 and 8°C. Avoid freezing. Cartridges in use must not be stored in a refrigerator.

Nature and contents of container: 3 ml glass cartridges closed at one end with an aluminium cap and natural rubber/bromobutyl rubber laminate disc, and at the other end with a bromobutyl piston. A threaded colour-coded plastic cap is placed over the aluminium cap. Pack size: 5×3 ml cartridges.

Instructions for use/handling: Each carton contains a patient information leaflet with instructions for use; the leaflet includes a reference to the instruction manual accompanying the NovoPen 3 device.

Marketing authorisation numbers

Actrapid Penfill 3 ml	03132/0105
Insulatard Penfill 3 ml	03132/0091
Mixtard 10 Penfill 3 ml	03132/0092
Mixtard 20 Penfill 3 ml	03132/0093
Mixtard 30 Penfill 3 ml	03132/0094
Mixtard 40 Penfill 3 ml	03132/0095
Mixtard 50 Penfill 3 ml	03132/0096

Date of approval/revision of SPC July 1996, 18 March 1998.

Legal category POM.

ACTRAPID* PEN
HUMAN INSULATARD* PEN
HUMAN MIXTARD* 10 PEN
HUMAN MIXTARD* 20 PEN
HUMAN MIXTARD* 30 PEN
HUMAN MIXTARD* 40 PEN
HUMAN MIXTARD* 50 PEN

Human Mixtard 10 Pen, Human Mixtard 20 Pen, Human Mixtard 30 Pen, Human Mixtard 40 Pen and Human Mixtard 50 Pen were formerly named PenMix 10/90, PenMix 20/80, PenMix 30/70, PenMix 40/60 and PenMix 50/50 respectively.

Qualitative and quantitative composition

Actrapid Pen: Insulin Injection
Human Insulatard Pen: Isophane Insulin Injection
Human Mixtard 10 Pen: Biphasic Isophane Insulin Injection 10/90
Human Mixtard 20 Pen: Biphasic Isophane Insulin Injection 20/80
Human Mixtard 30 Pen: Biphasic Isophane Insulin Injection 30/70
Human Mixtard 40 Pen: Biphasic Isophane Insulin Injection 40/60
Human Mixtard 50 Pen: Biphasic Isophane Insulin Injection 50/50

Active ingredient: Human insulin (pyr) 100 iu/ml.

Pharmaceutical form

Actrapid Pen: Sterile solution for injection.
Human Insulatard Pen and Human Mixtard Pen range: Sterile suspension for injection.

Clinical particulars

Therapeutic indications: The treatment of insulin-requiring diabetics.

Posology and method of administration: The dosage is determined by the physician according to the needs of the patient.

The Pen preparations are usually administered subcutaneously but may also be given intramuscularly. When injected subcutaneously, injection of Actrapid Pen into the abdominal wall ensures a faster absorption than from other regions of the body. The thigh is the recommended site for injection of Human Insulatard Pen, the abdominal wall or thigh for subcutaneous injection of Human Mixtard Pen preparations. Injection into a lifted skin fold minimises the risk of intramuscular injection.

When used alone Actrapid Pen is usually given three or more times daily; it is more commonly used in regimens where an intermediate or long-acting insulin is given in addition.

Human Insulatard Pen and the Human Mixtard Pen preparations may be given once or, more commonly, twice daily. Human Insulatard Pen may also be supplemented with shorter-acting insulin.

NovaFine needles are designed to be used with the Pen prefilled insulin syringes. The Pen preparations are for single-patient use only.

Use in the elderly: There are no precautions concerning the use of insulin which are specific to the elderly diabetic. However, injection procedures may be difficult for the infirm or the confused patient, and the simplest regimen consistent with keeping the patient symptom-free should be considered.

Contra-indications: Insulin is contra-indicated in hypoglycaemia.

Special warnings and special precautions for use: Injection of Actrapid Pen or the Human Mixtard Pen preparations should be followed by a meal within approximately 30 minutes of administration.

The use of dosages which are inadequate, or discontinuation of treatment, especially in insulin-dependent diabetics, may lead to hyperglycaemia and diabetic ketoacidosis; conditions which are potentially lethal.

When patients are transferred from other insulins to highly purified human insulin the change should be made according to the following general guidelines:

For patients currently controlled on highly purified human or porcine insulin preparations no dosage change is anticipated other than the routine adjustments made in order to maintain stable diabetic control. Patients currently stabilised on mixed species or bovine insulin may require a dosage adjustment dependent upon dosage, purity, species and formulation of the insulin preparation(s) currently administered. Variations in glycaemic control may occur and adjustments in therapy should be made under the guidance of a physician. A few patients have reported that after being transferred to human insulin the early warning symptoms for hypoglycaemia were less pronounced than they were with animal-source insulin.

Patients whose blood glucose is greatly improved, e.g. by intensified insulin therapy, may experience a change in their usual warning symptoms of hypoglycaemia and possibly lose some or all of the symptoms, and should be advised accordingly.

Interaction with other medicaments and other forms of interaction: Concomitant use of other drugs may influence insulin requirements. The following substances may enhance the hypoglycaemic effect of insulin: alcohol, non-selective beta adrenergic blocking agents, monoamine oxidase inhibitors (MAOI), ACE inhibitors, salicylate, anabolic steroids.

Other drugs may increase insulin requirements: oral contraceptives, thyroid hormones, corticosteroids, thiazides and sympathomimetics. Beta adrenergic blocking agents may blur the symptoms of hypoglycaemia. Alcohol may intensify and prolong the hypoglycaemic effect of insulin.

Diabetic patients treated with drugs other than insulin should discuss possible interactions with the prescribing physician.

Pregnancy and lactation: Instensified control in the treatment of pregnant insulin-dependent diabetics is recommended. Insulin requirements usually fall in the first trimester and increase during the second and third trimester. Insulin does not pass the placental barrier.

Effects on ability to drive and use machines: The ability to drive or use machinery may be impaired during hypoglycaemia or severe hyperglycaemia.

Undesirable effects: At initiation of insulin therapy, oedema and refraction anomalies may occur; these are usually transitory. The same applies to local hypersensitivity reactions (swelling and itching at the injection site) which usually disappear during continued treatment.

Persistent allergies to human insulin are very rare and are mostly due to cross-reacting antibodies to animal insulins. Lipodystrophy at injection sites is also rare and should be prevented by constantly changing injection sites.

Overdose: Overdosage causes hypoglycaemia; symptoms are variable but may include confusion, palpitations, sweating, malaise and loss of consciousness. In the event of an overdose, glucose should be given if the patient is conscious. Where the patient is unconscious an intramuscular, subcutaneous or intravenous injection of glucagon should be given and oral carbohydrate administered when the patient responds. Alternatively intravenous glucose may be administered; it must be given if there is no response to glucagon. If severe hypoglycaemia is not treated it can cause temporary or permanent brain damage and death.

Pharmacological properties

Pharmacodynamic properties: Human insulin (pyr) is identical to pancreatic human insulin. It has hypoglycaemic actions in man, promotes uptake of glucose into liver, muscle and adipose tissue, inhibits gluconeogenesis and promotes lipogenesis.

Pharmacokinetic properties: Actrapid Pen is a neutral solution of human insulin (pyr). When injected subcutaneously it has a duration of action of some ½ to 8 hours and its maximum effect is exerted between 1 and 3 hours after injection. Human Insulatard Pen is an isophane insulin preparation. When injected subcutaneously it has a duration of action of some 1½ up to 24 hours and its maximum effect is exerted between 4 and 12 hours after injection.

The Human Mixtard Pen preparations consist of soluble human insulin and isophane human insulin in the ratios:

Human Mixtard 10 Pen – 10/90
Human Mixtard 20 Pen – 20/80
Human Mixtard 30 Pen – 30/70
Human Mixtard 40 Pen – 40/60
Human Mixtard 50 Pen – 50/50

They are intermediate acting insulins with a pronounced initial effect. When injected subcutaneously they have a duration of action of some ½ up to 24 hours and their maximum effect is exerted between 2 and 8 hours after injection.

Pharmaceutical particulars

List of excipients: Glycerol (E422), m-cresol, zinc oxide, sodium hydroxide, hydrochloric acid, water for injections.

Plus, Human Insulatard Pen and Human Mixtard Pen preparations: sodium phosphate dihydrate, phenol, protamine sulphate.

Incompatibilities: Not applicable.

Shelf life: 30 months.

Special precautions for storage: Store between 2 and 8°C. Avoid freezing. Pens in use or carried as a spare may be kept at ambient temperature (maximum 25°C) for up to one month but should not be exposed to excessive heat or sunlight. Pens in use must not be refrigerated.

Nature and contents of container: 3 ml glass cartridges closed at one end with an aluminium cap and natural rubber/bromobutyl rubber laminate disc, and at the other end with a bromobutyl piston, and which is contained within a disposable injection device.

Pack size: 5×3 ml prefilled, disposable injection device.

Instructions for use/handling: Each carton contains a patient information leaflet with instructions for use.

Marketing authorisation numbers

Actrapid Pen	03132/0104
Human Insulatard Pen	03132/0067
Human Mixtard 10 Pen	03132/0068
Human Mixtard 20 Pen	03132/0069
Human Mixtard 30 Pen	03132/0070
Human Mixtard 40 Pen	03132/0071
Human Mixtard 50 Pen	03132/0072

Date of approval/revision of SPC 21 April 1997, 18 March 1998.

Legal category POM.

HUMAN ACTRAPID* PENFILL*
HUMAN INSULATARD* PENFILL*
HUMAN MIXTARD* 10 PENFILL*
HUMAN MIXTARD* 20 PENFILL*
HUMAN MIXTARD* 30 PENFILL*
HUMAN MIXTARD* 40 PENFILL*
HUMAN MIXTARD* 50 PENFILL*

Human Insulatard Penfill was formerly named Human Protaphane Penfill. Human Mixtard 10 Penfill, Human Mixtard 20 Penfill, Human Mixtard 30 Penfill, Human Mixtard 40 Penfill and Human Mixtard 50 Penfill were formerly named PenMix 10/90 Penfill, PenMix 20/80 Penfill, PenMix 30/70 Penfill, PenMix 40/60 Penfill and PenMix 50/50 Penfill respectively.

Presentation *Human Actrapid Penfill* (Insulin Injection) is a clear neutral solution of human insulin (pyr), containing glycerol and m-cresol as added preservative.

Human Insulatard Penfill (Isophane Insulin Injection) is a neutral suspension of isophane human insulin (pyr).

The Human Mixtard Penfill preparations are neutral suspensions of human insulin (pyr) consisting of soluble human insulin and isophane human insulin in the ratios:

Human Mixtard 10 Penfill – 10/90
Human Mixtard 20 Penfill – 20/80
Human Mixtard 30 Penfill – 30/70
Human Mixtard 40 Penfill – 40/60
Human Mixtard 50 Penfill – 50/50

Human Insulatard Penfill and the Human Mixtard Penfill preparations also contain glycerol, sodium phosphate, protamine sulphate as retarding agent, and m-cresol and phenol as added preservatives.

The Penfill preparations are contained in 1.5 ml cartridges; when agitated up and down the suspensions appear white and cloudy. Each preparation is available in a strength of 100 iu/ml.

Uses The treatment of insulin-requiring diabetics.

Dosage and administration

Adults and children: The dosage is determined by the physician according to the needs of the patient.

Penfill insulin cartridges are designed to be used with the NovoPen insulin pens and NovoFine needles. When used in these devices they are given by subcutaneous injection. Instructions for use of these preparations in NovoPen insulin pens are included with the devices and must be carefully followed. Prior to injection the suspensions should be agitated up and down until the insulin is white and cloudy; a glass ball is included in the cartridge to facilitate resuspension.

When injected subcutaneously, Human Actrapid Penfill has a duration of action of some ½ to 8 hours and its maximum effect is exerted between 1 and 3 hours after injection. When used alone it is usually given three or more times daily; it is most commonly used in regimens where an intermediate or long acting insulin is given in addition.

When injected subcutaneously, Human Insulatard Penfill has a duration of action of some 1½ up to 24 hours and its maximum effect is exerted between 4 and 12 hours after injection, and the Human Mixtard Penfill preparations have a duration of action of some ½ to 24 hours and their maximum effect is exerted between 2 and 8 hours after injection. Human Insulatard Penfill and the Human Mixtard Penfill preparations may be given once, or more commonly, twice daily. The Human Mixtard Penfill preparations are used especially when a strong initial effect is desired. Human Insulatard Penfill may also be supplemented with shorter-acting insulin.

When injected subcutaneously, injection of Human Actrapid Penfill into the abdominal wall ensures a faster absorption than from other regions of the body. The thigh is the recommended site for subcutaneous injection of Human Insulatard Penfill, the abdominal wall or thigh for subcutaneous injection of Human Mixtard Penfill preparations. Injection into a lifted skin fold minimises the risk of intramuscular injection.

The Penfill preparations must not be used with conventional syringes, or refilled.

Use in the elderly: There are no precautions concerning the use of insulin which are specific to the elderly diabetic. However, injection procedures may be difficult for the infirm, the poorly sighted, or the confused patient, and the simplest regimen consistent with keeping the patient symptom-free should be considered.

Contra-indications, warnings, etc

Contra-indications: Insulin is contra-indicated in hypoglycaemia.

Precautions: Owing to their strong early effect, injections of Human Actrapid Penfill or the Human Mixtard Penfill preparations should be followed by a meal within 30 minutes of administration.

The use of dosages which are inadequate or discontinuation of treatment, especially in insulin-dependent diabetics, may lead to hyperglycaemia and diabetic ketacidosis; conditions which are potentially lethal.

When patients are transferred from other insulins to Human Monocomponent insulin the change should be made according to the following general guidelines:

For patients currently controlled on Human Monocomponent, porcine monocomponent or other highly purified human or porcine insulin preparations, no dosage change is anticipated other than the routine adjustments made in order to maintain stable diabetic control.

Patients currently stabilised on mixed species or bovine insulin may require a dosage adjustment dependent upon dosage, purity, species and formulation of the insulin preparation(s) currently administered. Variations in glycaemic control may occur and adjustments in therapy should be made under the guidance of a physician.

A few patients have reported that after being transferred to human insulin, the early warning symptoms for hypoglycaemia were less pronounced than they were with animal source insulin.

Patients whose blood glucose control is greatly improved, e.g. by intensified insulin therapy, may experience a change in their usual warning symptoms of hypoglycaemia, and possibly lose some or all of the symptoms, and should be advised accordingly.

Use in pregnancy: Intensified control in the treatment of pregnant insulin-dependent diabetics is recommended. Insulin requirements usually fall in the first trimester and increase during the second and third trimester. Insulin does not pass the placental barrier.

Concomitant use of other drugs may influence insulin requirements. The following substances may enhance the hypoglycaemic effect of insulin: alcohol, non-selective beta-adrenergic blocking agents, monoamine oxidase inhibitors (MAOI), ACE inhibitors, salicylate, anabolic steroids. Other drugs may increase insulin requirements: oral contraceptives, thyroid hormones, corticosteroids, thiazides and sympathomimetics. Beta-adrenergic blocking agents may blur the symptoms of hypoglycaemia. Alcohol may intensify and prolong the hypoglycaemic effect of insulin. Diabetic patients treated with other drugs than insulin should discuss possible interactions with the prescribing physician.

Side-effects: At initiation of insulin therapy, oedema and refraction anomalies may occur; these are usually transitory. The same applies to local hypersensitivity reactions (swelling and itching at the injection site) which usually disappear during continued treatment.

Persistent allergies to human insulin are very rare and are mostly due to cross-reacting antibodies to animal insulins. Lipo-dystrophy at injection sites is also rare and should be prevented by constantly changing injection sites.

Overdosage: Overdosage causes hypoglycaemia, symptoms are variable but may include confusion, palpitations, sweating, malaise, and loss of consciousness.

In the event of an overdose, glucose should be given orally if the patient is conscious. Where the patient is unconscious an intra-muscular, subcutaneous or intravenous injection of glucagon should be given and oral carbohydrate administered when the patient responds. Alternatively intravenous glucose may be administered; it must be given if there is no response to glucagon.

If severe hypoglycaemia is not treated it can cause temporary or permanent brain damage and death.

Pharmaceutical precautions The Penfill cartridge preparations should be stored between 2 and 8°C, and should not be allowed to freeze. Cartridges in use or carried as a spare may be kept at ambient temperature (e.g. in the pocket or handbag) for up to one month, but should not be exposed to excessive heat or sunlight. Cartridges in use must not be stored in a refrigerator.

Legal category POM.

Package quantities Pack of 5×1.5 ml cartridges.

Further information Nil.

Product licence numbers

Human Actrapid Penfill	4668/0024
Human Insulatard Penfill	4668/0019
Human Mixtard 10 Penfill	4668/0032
Human Mixtard 20 Penfill	4668/0033
Human Mixtard 30 Penfill	4668/0020
Human Mixtard 40 Penfill	4668/0034
Human Mixtard 50 Penfill	4668/0035

Product licence holder: Novo Nordisk A/S.

HUMAN ACTRAPID*
HUMAN MONOTARD*
HUMAN INSULATARD* GE
HUMAN MIXTARD* 30 GE
HUMAN ULTRATARD*

Human Insulatard ge and Human Mixtard 30 ge were formerly named Human Protaphane and Human Actraphane 30/70; they are not identical to the products Human Insulatard and Human Mixtard 30/70 which contained human insulin (emp) and which were discontinued in April 1995.

Presentation Human Actrapid (Insulin Injection) is a clear neutral solution of human insulin (pyr), containing glycerol, and m-cresol as added preservative.

Human Monotard (Insulin Zinc Suspension) is a neutral suspension of amorphous (30%) and crystalline (70%) human insulin (pyr).

Human Insulatard ge (Isophane Insulin Injection) is a neutral suspension of isophane human insulin (pyr).

Human Mixtard 30 ge (Biphasic Isophane Insulin Injection) is a neutral suspension of human insulin (pyr), consisting of soluble human insulin and isophane human insulin in the ratio 3:7.

Human Ultratard (Insulin Zinc Suspension Crystalline) is a neutral suspension of crystalline human insulin (pyr).

Human Monotard and Human Ultratard contain sodium chloride, sodium acetate, zinc as retarding agent and methyl parahydroxybenzoate as added preservative. Human Insulatard ge and Human Mixtard 30 ge contain glycerol, sodium phosphate, protamine sulphate as retarding agent, and m-cresol and phenol as added preservative. When shaken, the suspensions appear white and cloudy.

Each preparation is available in a strength of 100 iu/ml.

Uses The treatment of insulin-requiring diabetics.

Dosage and administration

Adults and children: The dosage is determined by the physician according to the needs of the patient.

Human Actrapid may be given by subcutaneous, intramuscular or intravenous injection. When injected subcutaneously it has a duration of action of some ½ to 8 hours and its maximum effect is exerted between 1 and 3 hours after injection.

The suspensions may be given by subcutaneous or intramuscular injection. The vial should be gently shaken before use to ensure that the insulin is uniformly distributed throughout the liquid. The dose should then be immediately drawn into the syringe and injected.

Human Monotard and Human Insulatard ge may be used in once, or more commonly, twice daily injection regimens. When injected subcutaneously, Human Monotard has a duration of action of some 2½ to 24 hours and its maximum effect is exerted between 7 and 15 hours after injection, and Human Insulatard ge has a duration of action of some 1½ to 24 hours and its maximum effect is exerted between 4 and 12 hours after injection.

Human Mixtard 30 ge may be given once, or more commonly, twice daily, especially when a strong initial effect is desired. When injected subcutaneously it has a duration of action of some ½ to 24 hours and its maximum effect is exerted between 2 and 8 hours after injection.

Human Ultratard is usually given as a once daily insulin but may also be given twice daily if required. It is often used as a basal insulin in multiple injection regimens. Human Ultratard may be used as a once daily injection (if necessary with the addition of rapid acting insulin) in maturity onset diabetes when diet or oral hypoglycaemic drugs fail to produce good control. When injected subcutaneously Human Ultratard has a duration of action of some 4 to 28 hours and its maximum effect is exerted between 8 and 24 hours after injection.

The suspensions may be mixed in the syringe with Human Actrapid to intensify the initial effect. The Human Actrapid should be drawn into the syringe first and the injection given immediately after mixing. When injected subcutaneously, injection of Human Actrapid into the abdominal wall ensures a faster absorption than from other regions of the body. The thigh is the recommended site for subcutaneous injection of Human Insulatard ge, Human Monotard, or Human Ultratard, the abdominal wall or thigh for subcutaneous injection of Human Mixtard 30 ge. Injection into a lifted skin fold minimises the risk of intramuscular injection.

Infusion pumps: Due to the risk of precipitation in some pump catheters, Human Actrapid is not recommended for use in ambulatory insulin infusion pumps.

The suspensions must not be used in insulin infusion pumps.

Use in the elderly: There are no precautions concerning the use of insulin which are specific to the elderly diabetic. However the injection procedure may be difficult for the infirm, the poorly sighted, or the confused patient, and the simplest regimen consistent with keeping the patient symptom-free should be considered.

Contra-indications, warnings, etc

Contra-indications: Insulin is contra-indicated in hypoglycaemia.

Precautions: Owing to their strong early effect, injections of Human Actrapid or Human Mixtard 30 ge should be followed by a meal within 30 minutes of administration.

The use of dosages which are inadequate or discontinuation of treatment, especially in insulin-dependent diabetics, may lead to hyperglycaemia and diabetic ketoacidosis; conditions which are potentially lethal.

When patients are transferred from other insulins to Human Monocomponent insulin the change should be made according to the following general guidelines:

For patients currently controlled on Human Monocomponent, porcine monocomponent, or other highly purified human or porcine insulin preparation, no dosage change is anticipated other than the routine adjustments made in order to maintain stable diabetic control.

Patients currently stabilised on mixed species or bovine insulin may require a dosage adjustment dependent upon dosage, purity, species, and formulation of the insulin preparation(s) currently administered. Variations in glycaemic control may occur and adjustment in therapy should be made under the guidance of a physician.

A few patients have reported that after being transferred to human insulin, the early warning symptoms for hypoglycaemia were less pronounced than they were with animal source insulin.

Patients whose blood glucose control is greatly improved, e.g. by intensified insulin therapy, may experience a change in their usual warning symptoms of hypoglycaemia, and possibly lose some or all of the symptoms, and should be advised accordingly.

Use in pregnancy: Intensified control in the treatment of pregnant insulin dependent diabetics is recommended. Insulin requirements usually fall in the first trimester and increase during the second and third trimester. Insulin does not pass the placental barrier.

Concomitant use of other drugs may influence insulin requirements. The following substances may enhance the hypoglycaemic effect of insulin: alcohol, non-selective beta-adrenergic blocking agents, monoamine oxidase inhibitors (MAOI), ACE inhibitors, salicylate, anabolic steroids. Other drugs may increase insulin requirements: oral contraceptives, thyroid hormones, corticosteroids, thiazides and sympathomimetics. Beta-adrenergic blocking agents may blur the symptoms of hypoglycaemia. Alcohol may intensify and prolong the hypoglycaemic effect of insulin. Diabetic patients treated with other drugs than insulin should discuss possible interactions with the prescribing physician.

Side-effects: At initiation of insulin therapy, oedema and refraction anomalies may occur; these are usually transitory. The same applies to local hypersensitivity reactions (swelling and itching at the injection site) which usually disappear during continued treatment.

Persistent allergies to human insulin are very rare and are mostly due to cross-reacting antibodies to animal insulins. Lipo-dystrophy at injection sites is also rare and should be prevented by constantly changing injection sites.

Overdosage: Overdosage causes hypoglycaemia, symptoms are variable but may include confusion, palpitations, sweating, malaise, and loss of consciousness.

In the event of an overdose, glucose should be given orally if the patient is conscious. Where the patient is unconscious an intra-muscular, subcutaneous or intravenous injection of glucagon should be given and oral carbohydrate administered when the patient responds. Alternatively intravenous glucose may be administered; it must be given if there is no response to glucagon.

If severe hypoglycaemia is not treated it can cause temporary or permanent brain damage and death.

Pharmaceutical precautions The human insulin preparations should be stored between 2° and 8°C. They should not be exposed to excessive heat or sunlight and should not be allowed to freeze. The vial in use may be kept at room temperature (max. 25°C) for up to four weeks.

Legal category POM.

Package quantities 10 ml glass vials.

Further information Nil.

Product licence numbers

Human Actrapid	4668/0025
Human Monotard	4668/0021
Human Insulatard ge	4668/0018
Human Mixtard 30 ge	4668/0023
Human Ultratard	4668/0022

Product licence holder: Novo Nordisk A/S.

HUMAN MIXTARD* 50

Qualitative and quantitative composition Biphasic Isophane Insulin Injection 50/50. *Active ingredient:* Insulin Human, Biosynthetic (pyr); 50% as soluble insulin, 50% as isophane insulin, 100 iu/ml.

Pharmaceutical form Sterile suspension for injection (subcutaneously).

Clinical particulars
Therapeutic indications: Treatment of diabetes mellitus.

Posology and method of administration: Dosage is individual and determined by the physician in accordance with the needs of the patient. Concomitant disease, especially if the patient is febrile, usually increases insulin requirements. Blood glucose monitoring is recommended.

The preparation is administered subcutaneously into the abdominal wall or the thigh. Each injection should be followed within 30 minutes by a meal containing carbohydrate. The physician determines whether one or several daily injections are necessary. Injection into a lifted skin fold minimises the risk of intramuscular injection.

Contra-indications: Insulin should never be given to patients with hypoglycaemia. Hypersensitivity to human insulin or to one of the excipients. Insulin suspensions must not be administered intravenously.

Special warnings and special precautions for use: The use of too low doses or discontinuation of treatment may lead to hyperglycaemia and diabetic ketoacidosis. These conditions are potentially lethal. For diabetic ketoacidosis treatment soluble insulin should be used. Transfer of patients to this human insulin may lead to change in glycaemic control; adjustments in therapy should be made under the guidance of a physician. The following general guidelines apply:

For patients currently controlled on human or porcine highly purified insulin, no dosage change is anticipated other than routine adjustments to maintain stable diabetic control.

Patients currently controlled on mixed species or bovine insulin may require adjustment of their insulin dosage dependent upon purity, species and formulation of their current insulin preparation(s).

A few patients have reported that after being transferred to human insulin the early warning symptoms for hypoglycaemia were less pronounced than experienced with animal source insulin.

Patients whose blood glucose control is greatly improved, e.g. by intensified insulin therapy, may experience a change in their usual warning symptoms of hypoglycaemia, and should be advised accordingly.

Interaction with other medicaments and other forms of interaction: Omission of a meal or unplanned, vigorous physical exercise may lead to hypoglycaemia, see *Overdose*.

Concomitant use of other drugs may influence insulin requirements.

The following substances may enhance the hypoglycaemic effect of insulin: monoamine oxidase inhibitors (MAOI), non-selective beta-blocking agents, ACE inhibitors, salicylate, alcohol, anabolic steroids.

Other drugs may decrease the effect: oral contraceptives, thiazides, corticosteroids, thyroid hormones and sympathomimetics.

Beta-blocking agents may mask the symptoms of hypoglycaemia. Alcohol may intensify and prolong the hypoglycaemic effect of insulin.

Diabetic patients treated with other drugs than insulin should discuss possible interactions with their prescribing physician.

Pregnancy and lactation: Insulin does not pass the placental barrier. Breast-feeding involves no risk for the baby.

Intensified control of pregnant insulin-dependent diabetic patients is recommended. Insulin requirements usually fall in the first trimester and increase during the second and third trimester.

Effects on ability to drive and use machines: The ability to drive or use machines can be impaired depending on the tendency to experience hypoglycaemia.

Undesirable effects: Oedema and refraction anomalies may occur at initiation of insulin therapy. These conditions are usually of transitory nature. The same applies to local hypersensitivity reactions (redness, swelling and itching at the injection site), which usually disappear during continued treatment. Persistent allergic reactions and lipoatrophy rarely occur when using this human insulin. Lipohypertrophy may occur as a consequence of too frequent injections into the same small area.

Overdose: Hypoglycaemia, accompanied by a variety of symptoms, is a common phenomenon with insulin treatment. Hypoglycaemia is potentially lethal. In the event of an overdose causing hypoglycaemia, sugar or food rich in carbohydrate should be given immediately if the patient is conscious. If the patient is unconscious, a subcutaneous, intramuscular or intravenous injection of glucagon (0.5–1 mg) may be given, followed by oral carbohydrate when the patient regains consciousness. An alternative to glucagon is intravenous glucose; it must be given if there is no response to glucagon within 10–15 minutes.

Pharmacological properties
Pharmacodynamic properties: The blood glucose lowering effect of insulin occurs when the molecules facilitate the uptake of glucose by binding to insulin receptors on muscle and fat cells – and simultaneously inhibit the output of glucose from the liver.

Pharmacokinetic properties: Insulin in the blood stream has a half-life of only a few minutes. Consequently, the time-action profile of an insulin preparation is determined solely by its absorption characteristics. This process is influenced by several factors, which is why considerable intra- and inter-patient variations are seen. An approximate action profile following s.c. administration indicates:

Onset:	½ hour
Maximum:	2–8 hours
Duration:	up to 24 hours

Preclinical safety data: Not applicable.

Pharmaceutical particulars
List of excipients: Zinc chloride; protamine sulphate; glycerol; disodium phosphate dihydrate; m-cresol; phenol; water for injection; stabilising agent; protracting principle; isotonic agent; buffering agent; preservative; preservative.

Incompatibilities: Insulin is compatible with simple infusion fluids, however, other drugs added to the fluid together with insulin may cause degradation of the insulin, e.g. if the drugs contain substances such as thiols or sulphites.

It is therefore recommended not to mix insulin with other drugs. Only soluble insulin (i.e. not insulin suspensions) should be added to infusion fluids. An unpredictable amount of insulin will be absorbed to the infusion material. Monitoring of the patient's blood glucose during infusion is therefore recommended.

Shelf life: 30 months at 2°C to 8°C

Special precautions for storage: Insulin preparations should be stored between 2°C and 8°C, not near a freezing compartment. Insulin which has been frozen must not be used. Insulin should be protected from excessive heat or sunlight. Insulin vials can be kept at room temperature for up to 6 weeks (max. 25°C).

Nature and contents of container: 10 ml vial made of glass, closed with a rubber disc. Packed in a carton.

Instructions for use/handling: Immediately before use, the vial should be turned upside down several times in order to resuspend the insulin crystals. The liquid should appear uniformly white and cloudy. Each carton contains a patient insert with instructions for use.

Marketing authorisation number 3132/0120.

Date of approval/revision of SPC August 1996, 18 March 1998.

Legal category POM.

HUMAN VELOSULIN*

Qualitative and quantitative composition Insulin Injection.

Active ingredient: Insulin human (emp) 100 iu/ml.

Pharmaceutical form Sterile solution for injection.

Clinical particulars
Therapeutic indications: The treatment of insulin-requiring diabetics.

Posology and method of administration
Adults and children: The dosage is determined by the physician according to the needs of the patient.

Human Velosulin has a rapid onset and a short duration of action, making it particularly suitable for the treatment of diabetic coma and precoma.

Human Velosulin is usually administered subcutaneously, but may also be given by intramuscular or intravenous injection or by infusion. When injected subcutaneously, injection into the abdominal wall ensures a faster absorption than from other regions of the body; injection into a lifted skin fold minimises the risk of intra-muscular injection.

Human Velosulin is most commonly used in regimens where an intermediate or long-acting insulin is given in addition.

Use in the elderly: Clearance rates may be reduced in the elderly due to declining renal function. Insulin may, therefore, have a more prolonged action. Dose requirements should be regularly reviewed.

Contra-indications: Insulin is contra-indicated in hypoglycaemia.

Hypersensitivity to human insulin or any of the excipients.

Special warnings and special precautions for use: Injection of Human Velosulin should be followed by a meal within approximately 30 minutes of administration.

Variations in lifestyle and other factors, e.g. infection and pregnancy, can affect insulin requirements.

The use of dosages which are inadequate, or discontinuation of treatment, especially in insulin-dependent diabetics, may lead to hyperglycaemia and diabetic ketoacidosis; conditions which are potentially lethal.

Some patients previously treated with insulin of beef or pork origin may require a dosage adjustment on transfer to highly purified human insulin (emp). This is more likely in patients previously treated with beef or mixed beef/pork insulin.

A few patients have reported that after being transferred to human insulin, their early warning symptoms for hypoglycaemia were less pronounced than they had been with beef or porcine insulin. Patients should be alerted to this possibility on being transferred to human insulin.

Patients whose blood glucose is greatly improved, e.g. by intensified insulin therapy, may experience a change in their usual warning symptoms of hypoglycaemia and possibly lose some or all of the symptoms and should be advised accordingly.

Interaction with other medicaments and other forms of interaction: Concomitant use of other drugs may influence insulin requirements. The following substances may enhance the hypoglycaemic effect of insulin: alcohol, non-selective beta adrenergic blocking agents, monoamine oxidase inhibitors (MAOI), ACE inhibitors, salicylate, anabolic steroids.

Other drugs may increase insulin requirements: oral contraceptives, thyroid hormones, corticosteroids, thiazides and sympathomimetics. Beta adrenergic blocking agents may blur the symptoms of hypoglycaemia. Alcohol may intensify and prolong the hypoglycaemic effect of insulin.

Diabetic patients treated with drugs other than insulin should discuss possible interactions with the prescribing physician.

Pregnancy and lactation: Intensified control in the treatment of pregnant insulin-dependent diabetics is recommended. Insulin requirements usually fall in the first trimester and increase during the second and third trimester.

Breast feeding is not contra-indicated.

Effects on ability to drive and use machinery: The patient's ability to concentrate and react may be impaired as a result of hypoglycaemia. This may constitute a risk in situations where these abilities are of special importance (e.g. driving a car or operating machinery).

Patients should be advised to take precautions to avoid hypoglycaemia whilst driving, this is particularly important in those who have reduced or absent awareness of the warning signs of hypoglycaemia or have frequent episodes of hypoglycaemia. The advisability of driving should be considered in these circumstances.

Undesirable effects: At initiation of insulin therapy, oedema and refraction anomalies may occur; these are usually transitory. The same applies to local hypersensitivity reactions (swelling and itching at the injection site) which usually disappear during continued treatment.

Persistent allergies to human insulin are very rare and are mostly due to cross-reacting antibodies to animal insulins. Lipodystrophy at injection sites is also rare and should be prevented by constantly changing injection sites.

Overdose: Overdosage causes hypoglycaemia; symptoms are variable but may include confusion, palpitations, sweating, malaise and loss of consciousness.

In the event of an overdose, glucose should be given if the patient is conscious. Where the patient is unconscious an intramuscular, subcutaneous or intravenous injection of glucagon should be given and oral carbohydrate administered when the patient responds. Alternatively intravenous glucose may be administered; it must be given if there is no response to glucagon.

If severe hypoglycaemia is not treated it can cause temporary or permanent brain damage and death.

Pharmacological properties
Pharmacodynamic properties: Insulin has a blood glucose lowering effect.

Pharmacokinetic properties: Human Velosulin has an onset of action of approximately half an hour after subcutaneous injection with a duration of about 8 hours, the maximum effect being exerted between 1 and 3 hours after injection. Following intramuscular injection, the onset of action is more rapid, while the overall duration of action is shorter, provided the injection site is well perfused muscle.

Preclinical safety data: None stated.

Pharmaceutical particulars
List of Excipients: Glycerol (E422); m-Cresol; Disodium Phosphate Dihydrate; Sodium Hydroxide; Hydrochloric Acid; Water for injections

Incompatibilities: Human Velosulin should not be mixed with insulin zinc suspensions, since the phosphate buffer can interact with the zinc in the suspensions and may alter the timing of action of the mixture in an unpredictable way.

Shelf life: 36 months.

Special precautions for storage: Store at 2° and 8°C. Avoid freezing and direct sunlight.

Nature and cotents of container: 10 ml glass vial closed with a rubber disc and aluminium cap.

The rubber disc/aluminium cap is covered with a plastic, tamper-evident cap which must be removed before use of the vial. The plastic cap cannot be replaced once removed from the vial.

Instructions for use/handling: Each carton contains a patient information leaflet with instructions for use.

Marketing authorisation number PL 3132/0031.

Date of first authorisation/renewal
First authorised: 4 January 1988.
Last renewal: 17 June 1997.

Date of (partial) revision of the text June 1997, 19 March 1998, 24 March 1998, 15 April 1998.

Legal category POM.

PORK ACTRAPID*
PORK INSULATARD*
PORK MIXTARD* 30

Qualitative and quantitative composition
Pork Actrapid: Insulin Injection.
Pork Insulatard: Isophane Insulin Injection.
Pork Mixtard 30: Biphasic Isophane Insulin Injection 30/70.
Active ingredient: Porcine insulin 100 iu/ml.

Pharmaceutical form
Pork Actrapid: Sterile solution for injection.
Pork Insulatard and Pork Mixtard 30: Sterile suspension for injection.

Clinical particulars
Therapeutic indications: Treatment of diabetes mellitus.

Posology and method of administration
Adults and children: The dosage is determined by the physician according to the needs of the patient.

Pork Actrapid is usually administered subcutaneously, but may also be given by intramuscular or intravenous injection. When injected subcutaneously, injection into the abdominal wall ensures a faster absorption than from other regions of the body; injection into a lifted skin fold minimises the risk of intramuscular injection.

When used alone Pork Actrapid is usually given three or four times daily; it is most commonly used in regimens where an intermediate or long-acting insulin is given in addition. Pork Actrapid may be mixed in the syringe with insulin suspensions to intensify their initial effect. The Pork Actrapid should be drawn into the syringe first and the injection given immediately after mixing.

Pork Actrapid does not contain a buffer; for this reason it should not be used in ambulatory insulin infusion pumps because of the risk of needle or catheter blockage.

Pork Insulatard and Pork Mixtard are usually administered subcutaneously, but may also be given intramuscularly. The thigh is the recommended site for subcutaneous injection of Pork Insulatard; the abdominal wall or thigh for subcutaneous injection of Pork Mixtard 30. Injection into a lifted skin fold minimises the risk of intramuscular injection.

Use in the elderly: There are no precautions concerning the use of insulin which are specific to the elderly diabetic. However, injection procedures may be difficult for the infirm or the confused patient and the simplest regimen consistent with keeping the patient symptom-free should be considered.

Contra-indications: Insulin is contra-indicated in hypoglycaemia.

Hypersensitivity to porcine insulin or any of the excipients.

Special warnings and special precautions for use: Injection of Pork Actrapid or Pork Mixtard 30 should be followed by a meal within approximately 30 minutes of administration.

The use of dosages which are inadequate, or discontinuation of treatment, especially in insulin-dependent diabetics, may lead to hyperglycaemia and diabetic ketoacidosis; conditions which are potentially lethal.

Transfer of patients to this highly purified porcine insulin may lead to changes in glycaemic control; adjustments in therapy should be made under the guidance of a physician. The following general guidelines apply:

For patients currently controlled on highly purified porcine insulin no dosage change is expected other than routine adjustments made in order to maintain stable diabetic control. Patients currently controlled on mixed species or bovine insulin may require a dosage adjustment dependent upon dosage, purity, species and formulation of the insulin preparation(s) currently administered.

Patients whose blood glucose control is greatly improved, e.g. by intensified insulin therapy, may experience a change in their usual warning symptoms of hypoglycaemia and possibly lose some or all of the symptoms and should be advised accordingly.

Interaction with other medicaments and other forms of interaction: Concomitant use of other drugs may influence insulin requirements. The following substances may enhance the hypoglycaemic effect of insulin: alcohol, non-selective beta adrenergic blocking agents, monoamine oxidase inhibitors (MAOI), ACE inhibitors, salicylate, anabolic steroids.

Other drugs may increase insulin requirements: oral contraceptives, thyroid hormones, corticosteroids, thiazides and sympathomimetics. Beta adrenergic blocking agents may blur the symptoms of hypoglycaemia. Alcohol may intensify and prolong the hypoglycaemic effect of insulin.

Diabetic patients treated with drugs other than insulin should discuss possible interactions with the prescribing physician.

Pregnancy and lactation: Intensified control in the treatment of pregnant insulin-dependent diabetics is recommended. Insulin requirements usually fall in the first trimester and increase during the second and third trimester. Insulin does not pass the placental barrier. Breast feeding is not contra-indicated.

Effects on ability to drive and use machinery: The patient's ability to concentrate and react may be impaired as a result of hypoglycaemia. This may constitute a risk in situations where these abilities are of special importance (e.g. driving a car or operating machinery).

Patients should be advised to take precautions to avoid hypoglycaemia whilst driving, this is particularly important in those who have reduced or absent awareness of the warning signs of hypoglycaemia or have frequent episodes of hypoglycaemia. The advisability of driving should be considered in these circumstances.

Undesirable effects: At initiation of insulin therapy, oedema and refraction anomalies may occur; these are usually transitory. The same applies to local hypersensitivity reactions (swelling and itching at the injection site) which usually disappear during continued treatment.

Persistent allergies to this insulin are very rare. Lipodystrophy at injection sites is also rare and should be prevented by constantly changing injection sites.

Overdose: Overdosage causes hypoglycaemia; symptoms are variable but may include confusion, palpitations, sweating, malaise and loss of consciousness.

In the event of an overdose, glucose should be given if the patient is conscious. Where the patient is unconscious an intramuscular, subcutaneous or intravenous injection of glucagon should be given and oral carbohydrate administered when the patient responds. Alternatively intravenous glucose may be administered; it must be given if there is no response to glucagon.

If severe hypoglycaemia is not treated it can cause temporary or permanent brain damage and death.

Pharmacological properties
Pharmacodynamic properties: Porcine insulin is a hypoglycaemic agent in man; promotes uptake of glucose into liver, muscle and adipose tissue, inhibits gluconeogenesis and promotes lipogenesis.

Pharmacokinetic properties: Pork Actrapid is a neutral solution of porcine insulin. When injected subcutaneously it has a duration of action of some ½ to 8 hours and its maximum effect is exerted between 1 and 3 hours after injection.

Pork Insulatard is an isophane porcine insulin preparation. When injected subcutaneously it has a duration of action of some 1½ to 24 hours and its maximum effect is exerted between 4 and 12 hours after injection.

Pork Mixtard 30 consists of soluble and isophane porcine insulin in the ratio 3:7. When injected subcutaneously it has a duration of action of some ½ up to 24 hours and its maximum effect is exerted between 4 and about 8 hours after injection.

When Pork Insulatard and Pork Mixtard 30 are injected intramuscularly, the onset of action is more rapid, while the overall duration of action is shorter, provided the injection site is well perfused muscle.

Preclinical safety data: Not applicable.

Pharmaceutical particulars
List of Excipients: Glycerol (E422); m-Cresol; Phenol (Pork Insulatard and Pork Mixtard 30); Disodium phosphate dihydrate (Pork Insulatard and Pork Mixtard 30); Sodium Hydroxide; Hydrochloric Acid; Zinc Oxide (Pork Insulatard and Pork Mixtard 30); Protamine Sulphate (Pork Insulatard and Pork Mixtard 30); Water for injections.

Incompatibilities: Due to the high risk of precipitation in some pump catheters, Pork Actrapid is not recommended for use in ambulatory insulin infusion pumps.

Shelf life: 30 months.

Special precautions for storage: Store between 2°C and 8°C. Avoid freezing and direct sunlight.

Nature and contents of container: 10 ml glass vial, closed with rubber disc and aluminium cap. The rubber disc/aluminium cap is covered with a plastic, tamper-evident cap which must be removed before use of the vial. The plastic cap cannot be replaced once removed from the vial.

Instructions for use/handling: Each carton contains a patient information leaflet with instructions for use.

Marketing authorisation number
Pork Actrapid: PL 3132/0121.
Pork Insulatard: PL 3132/0018.
Pork Mixtard 30: PL 3132/0021.

Date of first authorisation/renewal

Pork Actrapid	Date of first grant: 10.7.98
Pork Insulatard	Date of first grant: 8.2.82
	Date of last renewal: 20.5.97
Pork Mixtard 30	Date of first grant: 8.2.82
	Date of last renewal: 19.5.98

Date of (partial) revision of the text
Pork Actrapid: March 1997.
Pork Insulatard, Pork Mixtard 30: December 1997, 19 March 1998, 24 March 1998.

Legal category POM.

LENTARD* MC

Qualitative and quantitative composition Insulin Zinc Suspension.
Active ingredient: Porcine insulin 34 iu/ml
Bovine insulin 66 iu/ml.

Pharmaceutical form Sterile suspension for injection.

Clinical particulars
Therapeutic indications: The treatment of insulin-requiring diabetics.

Posology and method of administration
Adults and children: The dosage is determined by the physician according to the needs of the patient.

Lentard MC is usually administered subcutaneously, but may also be given intramuscularly. The thigh is the recommended site for subcutaneous injection; injection into a lifted skin fold minimises the risk of intramuscular injection.

Lentard MC may be given once or twice a day. It may be mixed in the syringe with Human Actrapid to intensify the initial effect. The soluble insulin should be drawn into the syringe first and the injection given immediately after mixing.

Use in the elderly: There are no precautions concerning the use of insulin which are specific to the elderly diabetic. However, injection procedures may be difficult for the infirm, the poorly sighted or the confused patient and the simplest regimen consistent with keeping the patient symptom-free should be considered.

Contra-indications: Insulin is contra-indicated in hypoglycaemia.

Special warnings and special precautions for use: The use of dosages which are inadequate, or discontinuation of treatment, especially in insulin-dependent diabetics, may lead to hyperglycaemia and diabetic ketoacidosis; conditions which are potentially lethal.

Patients transferred from conventional insulins may require a smaller dosage. The dosage reduction may occur immediately after transfer or gradually over a period of weeks or months. In order to reduce the risk of hypoglycaemia, the patient and the physician should be aware of the possibility that the insulin requirement may be reduced.

If the daily dosage is below 40 iu the risk is considered minimal. However, when higher dosages are required, stricter supervision of the patient is necessary. Insulin resistant patients receiving over 100 units daily should be referred to hospital for transfer.

Patients whose blood glucose control is greatly improved, e.g. by intensified insulin therapy, may experience a change in their usual warning symptoms of hypoglycaemia and possibly lose some or all of the symptoms and should be advised accordingly.

Interaction with other medicaments and other forms of interaction: Concomitant use of other drugs may influence insulin requirements. The following substances may enhance the hypoglycaemic effect of insulin: alcohol, non-selective beta adrenergic blocking agents, monoamine oxidase inhibitors (MAOI), ACE inhibitors, salicylate, anabolic steroids.

Other drugs may increase insulin requirements: oral contraceptives, thyroid hormones, corticosteroids, thiazides and sympathomimetics. Beta adrenergic blocking agents may blur the symptoms of hypoglycaemia. Alcohol may intensify and prolong the hypoglycaemic effect of insulin.

Diabetic patients treated with drugs other than insulin should discuss possible interactions with the prescribing physician.

Pregnancy and lactation: Intensified control in the treatment of pregnant insulin-dependent diabetics is recommended. Insulin requirements usually fall in the first trimester and increase during the second and third trimester.

Breast feeding is not contra-indicated.

Effects on ability to drive and use machinery: The patient's ability to concentrate and react may be impaired as a result of hypoglycaemia. This may constitute a risk in situations where these abilities are of special importance (e.g. driving a car or operating machinery).

Patients should be advised to take precautions to avoid hypoglycaemia whilst driving, this is particularly important in those who have reduced or absent awareness of the warning signs of hypoglycaemia or have frequent episodes of hypoglycaemia. The advisability of driving should be considered in these circumstances.

Undesirable effects: At initiation of insulin therapy, oedema and refraction anomalies may occur; these are usually transitory. The same applies to local hypersensitivity reactions (swelling and itching at the injection site) which usually disappear during continued treatment.

Persistent allergies to purified insulin are rare. Lipodystrophy at injection sites is also rare and should be prevented by constantly changing injection sites.

Overdose: Overdosage causes hypoglycaemia; symptoms are variable but may include confusion, palpitations, sweating, malaise and loss of consciousness.

In the event of an overdose, glucose should be given if the patient is conscious. Where the patient is unconscious an intramuscular, subcutaneous or intravenous injection of glucagon should be given and oral carbohydrate administered when the patient responds. Alternatively intravenous glucose may be administered; it must be given if there is no response to glucagon.

If severe hypoglycaemia is not treated it can cause temporary or permanent brain damage and death.

Pharmacological properties

Pharmacodynamic properties: Porcine/bovine insulins are hypoglycaemic agents in man; promotes uptake of glucose into liver, muscle and adipose tissue, inhibits gluconeogenesis and promotes lipogenesis.

Pharmacokinetic properties: Lentard MC is a zinc suspension comprising of 30% procine insulin and 70% bovine insulin. When injected subcutaneously it has a duration of action of some 2½ to 24 hours and its maximum effect is exerted between 7 and 15 hours after injection.

Preclinical safety data: —

Pharmaceutical particulars

List of excipients: Zinc Acetate; Zinc Oxide; Sodium Chloride; Sodium Acetate; Methyl Parahydroxybenzoate; Sodium Hydroxide; Hydrochloric Acid; Water for injections

Incompatibilities: Lentard MC must not be used in insulin infusion pumps.

Shelf life: 36 months.

Special precautions for storage: Store between 2°C and 8°C. Avoid freezing.

The vial in use may be kept at room temperature (max 25°C) for up to one month.

Nature and contents of container: 10 ml glass vial, closed with a rubber disc and aluminium cap. The rubber disc/aluminium cap is covered with a plastic, tamper-evident cap which must be removed before use of the vial. The plastic cap cannot be replaced once removed from the vial.

Instructions for use/handling: Each carton contains a patient information leaflet with instructions for use.

Marketing authorisation number PL 3132/0090.

Date of first authorisation/renewal

Date of first grant: 30 July 1992.
Date of last renewal: 22 August 1997.

Date of (partial) revision of the text December 1997, 19 March 1998, 24 March 1998.

Legal category POM.

GLUCAGEN* KIT 1 mg
GLUCAGEN* 1 mg

Qualitative and quantitative composition GlucaGen Kit 1 mg consists of a vial containing 1 mg (1 iu) glucagon (rys) and a pre-filled syringe containing 1.1 ml Water for Injections.

GlucaGen 1 mg consists of a vial containing 1 mg (1 iu) glucagon (rys) and a vial containing 1.1 ml Water for Injections.

Active substance: Glucagon biosynthetic (rys), structurally identical to human glucagon.

Glucagon hydrochloride equivalent to 1 mg (1 iu) glucagon.

Pharmaceutical form Powder for injection with accompanying diluent for preparation of a solution for injection.

Clinical particulars

Indications

Therapeutic indications: Treatment of severe hypoglycaemic reactions which may occur in the management of diabetic patients receiving insulin.

Diagnostic indications

Inhibition of motility:

(i) As a motility inhibitor in examinations of the gastrointestinal tract, e.g. double contrast radiography and endoscopy.

(ii) As a motility inhibitor in computerised tomography (CT), nuclear magnetic resonance scanning (NMR) and digital subtraction angiography (DSA).

Posology and method of administration: Dissolve the freeze-dried product in the accompanying solvent, as described under *Instructions for use/handling*. The reconstituted solution may be administered by intravenous, intramuscular or subcutaneous injection.

Severe hypoglycaemia

(a) *Administration by medical personnel:* Administer 1.0 mg (adults and children above 25 kg or 6–8 years) or 0.5 mg (children below 25 kg or 6–8 years) by subcutaneous, intramuscular or intravenous injection. The patient will normally respond within 10 minutes. When the patient has responded to the treatment, give oral carbohydrate to restore the liver glycogen and prevent relapse of hypoglycaemia. If the patient does not respond within 10 minutes, intravenous glucose should be given.

(b) *Administration to the patient by a relative:* Inject GlucaGen as indicated below.

Administer 1.0 mg (adults and children above 25 kg or 6–8 years) or 0.5 mg (children below 25 kg or 6–8 years) by subcutaneous or intramuscular injection. The patient will normally respond whithin 10 minutes. When the patient has responded to the treatment, give oral carbohydrate to restore the liver glycogen and prevent relapse of hypoglycaemia.

Medical assistance is required for all patients with severe hypoglycaemia.

Diagnostic indications

Inhibition of motility: Onset of action after an intravenous injection of 0.2–0.5 mg occurs within one minute and the duration of effect is between 5 and 20 minutes depending on the organ under examination. The onset of action after an intramuscular injection of 1–2 mg occurs after 5–15 minutes and lasts approximately 10–40 minutes depending on the organ.

(i) Dose ranges from 0.2–2 mg depending on the diagnostic technique used and the route of administration. The usual diagnostic dose for relaxation of the stomach, duodenal bulb, duodenum and small bowel is 0.2–0.5 mg given intravenously or 1 mg given intramuscularly; the usual dose to relax the colon is 0.5–0.75 mg intravenously or 1–2 mg intramuscularly.

(ii) In CT-scanning, NMR and DSA intravenous doses of up to 1 mg are used.

Contra-indications: Hypersensitivity to glucagon or any of the excipients. GlucaGen is contra-indicated in phaeochromocytoma.

Special warnings and special precautions for use: It should be borne in mind that glucagon reacts antagonistically towards insulin. Caution should be observed if GlucaGen is used in patients with insulinoma or glucagonoma. Caution should also be observed when GlucaGen is used in diabetic patients or in elderly patients with known cardiac disease, as an adjunct in endoscopy or radiography. The presence of fibril formation (viscous appearance) or solid particles in the solution is a contra-indication to its use at any time.

Interaction with other medicaments and other forms of interaction: Insulin: Reacts antagonistically towards glucagon.

Indomethacin: Glucagon may lose its ability to raise blood glucose or, paradoxically, may even produce hypoglycaemia.

Warfarin: Glucagon may increase the anticoagulant effect of warfarin.

Interactions of clinical significance between GlucaGen and other drugs are not known when GlucaGen is used in the approved indications.

Pregnancy and lactation: Glucagon does not cross the human placental barrier. The use of glucagon has been reported in pregnant women with diabetes and no harmful effects are known with respect to the course of pregnancy and the health of the unborn and the neonate.

Glucagon is cleared from the bloodstream very fast (mainly by the liver) (T/2=3–6 min.), thus the amount excreted in the milk of nursing mothers following treatment of severe hypoglycaemic reactions will be extremely small. As glucagon is degraded in the digestive tract and cannot be absorbed in its intact form, it will not exert any metabolic effect in the child.

Effects on ability to drive and use machines: GlucaGen is not known to produce any effect on the ability to drive and to operate machines.

It is not recommended to drive or operate machines following severe hypoglycaemia, due to the clinical features of hypoglycaemia and its possible recurrence.

Undesirable effects: Severe side effects are rare, although nausea and vomiting may occur occasionally, especially with dosages higher than 1 mg or with rapid injection (less than 1 minute).

Glucagon exerts positive inotropic and chronotropic effects (tachycardia).

Hypersensitivity reactions may occur in rare cases. Side effects indicating toxicity of glucagon have not been reported.

Overdose: Adverse effects of overdose have not been reported. See *Undesirable effects.*

In case of suspected overdosing (i.e. above therapeutic dosages) the serum potassium may decrease and should be monitored and corrected, if needed.

Pharmacological properties

Pharmacodynamic properties: Pharmacotherapeutic Group: H 04 AA 01.

Glucagon is a hyperglycaemic agent that mobilises hepatic glycogen which is released into the blood as glucose. Glucagon will not be effective in patients whose liver glycogen is depleted. For that reason, glucagon has little or no effect when the patient is fasting or is suffering from adrenal insufficiency, chronic hypoglycaemia or alcohol-induced hypoglycaemia.

Glucagon, unlike adrenaline, has no effect upon muscle phosphorylase and therefore cannot assist in the transference of carbohydrate from the much larger stores of glycogen that are present in the skeletal muscle.

Glucagon stimulates the release of catecholamines. In the presence of phaeochromocytoma, glucagon can cause the tumour to release large amounts of catecholamines which will cause an acute hypertensive reaction.

Glucagon inhibits the tone and motility of the smooth muscle in the gastrointestinal tract.

Pharmacokinetic properties: Metabolic clearance rate of glucagon in humans is approximately 10 ml/kg/min. It is degraded enzymatically in the blood plasma and in the organs to which it is distributed. The liver and kidney are major sites of glucagon clearance, each organ contributing about 30% to the overall metabolic clearance rate.

Glucagon has a short half-life in the blood of about 3–6 minutes.

Onset of effect occurs within 1 min. after an intravenous injection. Duration of action is in the range of 5–20 min. depending upon dose and the organ under examination. The onset of effect occurs within 5–15 minutes after an intramuscular injection, with a duration of 10–40 min. depending upon dose and organ.

When used in treatment of severe hypoglycaemia, an effect on blood glucose is usually seen within 10 minutes.

Preclinical safety data: No relevant preclinical data exist that provide information useful to the prescriber.

Pharmaceutical particulars

List of excipients: Lactose Monohydrate, Hydrochloric Acid (pH adjuster), Sodium Hydroxide (pH adjuster), Water for Injections.

After reconstitution with the solvent provided (Sterilised Water for Injections), the solution contains glucagon 1 mg/ml and lactose monohydrate 107 mg/ml.

Incompatibilities: Not applicable.

Shelf life: Prior to reconstitution, the shelf life of the product is 36 months when stored between 2°C and 8°C.

The reconstituted GlucaGen should be used immediately after preparation.

Special precautions for storage: The sealed container

should be protected from light and stored between 2°C and 8°C. Freezing should be avoided. Packs carried for use may be kept at room temperature (maximum 25°C) for up to 18 months provided that the expiry date is not exceeded.

The reconstituted GlucaGen should be used immediately after preparation. If in rare cases it shows any signs of fibril formation (viscous appearance) or insoluble matter it should be discarded. Any portion of the solution remaining after use should be discarded.

Nature and contents of container: Container for GlucaGen (both packs): Vial made of glass type 1, PhEur, closed with a bromobutyl rubber stopper and covered with an aluminium cap.

Container for diluent (GlucaGen Kit): 1.5 ml glass syringe with a stainless steel needle, natural rubber needle shield and a bromobutyl rubber piston.

Container for diluent (GlucaGen 1 mg): Vial made of glass type I, PhEur closed with a bromobutyl rubber stopper and teflon disc and covered with an aluminium cap.

The vials are provided with tamper-evident plastic caps which must be removed before use.

Instructions for use/handling

Reconstitution: GlucaGen Kit: Inject the Sterilised Water for Injections (1.1 ml) into the vial containing the freeze-dried glucagon. Shake the vial gently until the glucagon is completely dissolved and the solution is clear. Withdraw the solution back into the syringe.

GlucaGen 1 mg: Draw up the Sterilised Water for Injections (1.1 ml) in a disposable syringe. Inject the Sterilised Water for Injections into the vial containing the freeze-dried glucagon. Shake the vial gently until the glucagon is completely dissolved and the solution is clear. Withdraw the solution back into the syringe.

The reconstituted solution forms an injection of 1 mg (1 IU) per ml to be administered subcutaneously, intramuscularly or intravenously.

Marketing authorisation holder: Novo Nordisk A/S (GlucaGen, Diluent in syringe).

Marketing Authorisation number

PL 4668/0027	GlucaGen 1 mg
PL 4668/0028	Diluent for GlucaGen 1 mg
PL 3132/0082	Water for Injection, PhEur

Date of first authorisation/renewal of authorisation
First authorised: 30 September 1991.
Date of renewal of authorisation: 15 October 1996.

Date of revision of the text 1 August 1997.

Legal category POM.

KLIOFEM*

Qualitative and quantitative composition
Active ingredients: Estradiol 2 mg and Norethisterone acetate 1 mg.

The tablets also contain lactose and maize starch, but do not contain clinically significant amounts of gluten.

Pharmaceutical form Film-coated tablet for oral administration.

Clinical particulars
Therapeutic indications:

1. The treatment of symptoms due to oestrogen deficiency.
2. The prophylaxis of postmenopausal osteoporosis in women at risk of developing fractures.

At present there is no established screening programme for determining women at risk of developing osteoporotic fractures. Epidemiological studies suggest a number of individual risk factors which contribute to the development of postmenopausal osteoporosis. These include: early menopause, family history of osteoporosis, thin, small frame; cigarette use; recent prolonged systemic cortico-steroid use.

If several of these risk factors are present in a patient, consideration should be given to oestrogen replacement therapy.

Kliofem is for use in postmenopausal women with an intact uterus. In perimenopausal women treated with Kliofem the incidence of vaginal bleeding is unacceptably high and therefore therapy should not be initiated earlier than one year after the last natural menstrual period.

Posology and method of administration

Dosage: Adults: Menopausal symptoms and prophylaxis of osteoporosis.

Kliofem is administered orally, without chewing, one tablet daily without interruption, preferably at the same time each day.

Prophylaxis of osteoporosis: Hormone replacement therapy (HRT) has been found to be effective in the prevention of osteoporosis especially when started soon after the menopause and used for 5 years and probably up to 10 years or more. Treatment should ideally start as soon as possible after the onset of the menopause and certainly within 2 to 3 years, but benefit may also be obtained even if treatment is started at a later date. Protection appears to be effective for as long as treatment is continued. However, data beyond 10 years are limited. A careful re-appraisal of the risk-benefit ratio should be undertaken before treating for longer than 5 to 10 years.

Not intended for children or males.

Use in the elderly: There are no special dosage requirements.

Administration: In women not previously treated with HRT, treatment may be started on any convenient day. In women transferred from sequential HRT, treatment should probably be started at the end of the scheduled bleed.

During the first few months of Kliofem therapy, a high proportion of patients will experience bleeding or spotting. About half of women will become amenorrhoeic after 3–4 months' treatment with Kliofem. In a further group, bleeding or spotting may still occur infrequently but will remain acceptable. This means that after 3 months treatment the majority of women will derive benefit from Kliofem in terms of either having no bleeding at all or only light spotting. Some women may experience continued unacceptable bleeding and in these cases Kliofem should be discontinued. All patients on Kliofem require the routine follow up examinations which are recommended every 6 to 12 months (see below).

If, at any time, bleeding or spotting is unacceptable, Kliofem should be discontinued; if all bleeding subsides completely within 3 weeks of stopping Kliofem, then no further investigation is needed.

Bleeding after a period of amenorrhoea or heavy bleeding after a period of light bleeding may indicate poor compliance or concurrent antibiotics use. However, any doubt as to the cause of the bleeding is a reason for endometrial evaluation including some form of endometrial biopsy.

Before initiation of therapy it is recommended that the patient is fully informed of all likely benefits and potential risks. She should have a full physical and gynaecological examination, with special emphasis on blood pressure, breasts, abdominal and pelvic organs. Endometrial assessment should be carried out if indicated; this may be particularly relevant in patients who are, or who have been, previously treated with oestrogens unopposed by a progestogen. The patient should be asked to keep a diary of any spotting or bleeding that occurs during treatment with Kliofem. After the first 6 months, follow-up examinations are recommended every 6 to 12 months and should include examination of the diary.

Since progestogens are only administered to protect against hyperplastic changes of the endometrium patients without a uterus should be treated with an oestrogen-only preparation.

Contra-indications:

1. Known, suspected, or past history of cancer of the breast.
2. Known or suspected oestrogen-dependent neoplasia. Vaginal bleeding of unknown aetiology.
3. Known or suspected pregnancy.
4. Active deep venous thrombosis, thromboembolic disorders or a history of confirmed venous thromboembolism. See also *Special warnings and special precautions,* number 4.
5. Acute or chronic liver disease or history of liver disease where the liver function tests have failed to return to normal.
6. Rotor's syndrome or Dubin-Johnson syndrome.
7. Severe cardiac or renal disease.
8. Allergy to one or more of the constituents.

Special warnings and special precautions for use:

1. In the female there is an increased risk of endometrial hyperplasia and carcinoma associated with unopposed oestrogen administered long term (for more than one year). However, the appropriate addition of a progestogen to an oestrogen regimen lowers this additional risk.

2. There has been concern about the possible risk of breast cancer in oestrogen-treated women. Although many studies have failed to disclose an increased incidence of breast cancer, some have shown a small increase upon prolonged therapy (e.g. 5 years or longer). It is not known whether concurrent progestogen use influences the risk of breast cancer in post-menopausal women taking HRT. Women on long-term therapy should have regular breast examinations, and should be instructed in self breast examination. Regular mammographic investigations should be conducted where considered appropriate.

There is a need for caution when prescribing oestrogens in women who have a history of, or known breast nodules or fibrocystic disease. Breast status should be closely monitored, supported by regular mammography.

3. Certain diseases may be made worse by hormone replacement therapy and patients with these conditions should be closely monitored. These include otosclerosis, multiple sclerosis, systemic lupus erythematosus, porphyria, melanoma, epilepsy, migraine and asthma. In addition, pre-existing uterine fibroids may increase in size during oestrogen therapy and symptoms associated with endometriosis may be exacerbated.

4. Epidemiological studies have suggested that hormone replacement therapy (HRT) is associated with a higher relative risk of developing venous thromboembolism (VTE), i.e. deep vein thrombosis or pulmonary embolism. The studies find a 2–3 fold higher risk for users compared with non-users which for healthy women amounts to one extra case of VTE each year for every 5000 patients taking HRT.

Generally recognised risk factors for VTE include a personal or family history and severe obesity (Body Mass Index >30 kg/m^2). In women with these factors the benefits of treatment with HRT need to be carefully weighed against risks. There is no consensus about the possible role of varicose veins in VTE.

The risk of VTE may be temporarily increased with prolonged immobilisation, major trauma or major surgery. In women on HRT scrupulous attention should be given to prophylactic measures to prevent VTE following surgery. Where prolonged immobilisation is liable to follow elective surgery, particularly abdominal or orthopaedic surgery to the lower limbs, consideration should be given to temporarily stopping HRT four weeks earlier, if possible.

If venous thromboembolism develops after initiating therapy the drug should be discontinued.

5. Oestrogens may cause fluid retention and, therefore, patients with cardiac or renal dysfunction should be carefully observed.

6. If jaundice, migraine-like headaches, visual disturbance, or a significant increase in blood pressure develop after initiating therapy, the medication should be discontinued while the cause is investigated.

7. Kliofem is not a contraceptive, neither will it restore fertility.

8. Most studies indicate that oestrogen replacement therapy has little effect on blood pressure and some indicate that oestrogen use may be associated with a small decrease in B.P. In addition, most studies on combined therapy, including Kliofem, indicate that the addition of a progestogen also has little effect on blood pressure. Rarely, idiosyncratic hypertension may occur.

However, when oestrogens are administered to hypertensive women, supervision is necessary and blood pressure should be monitored at regular intervals.

9. Diabetic patients should be carefully observed when initiating hormone replacement therapy, as worsening glucose tolerance may occur.

10. Changed oestrogen levels may affect certain endocrine and liver function tests.

11. It has been reported that there is an increase in the risk of surgically confirmed gall bladder disease in women receiving postmenopausal oestrogens.

Interactions with other medicaments and other forms of interaction: Drugs such as barbiturates, phenytoin, rifampicin and carbamazepine which induce the activity of microsomal drug metabolising enzymes may decrease the effectiveness of Kliofem.

Pregnancy and lactation: Kliofem is contra-indicated during pregnancy and lactation.

Effects on ability to drive and use machinery: No effects known.

Undesirable effects: The following side-effects have been reported with oestrogen/progestogen therapy:

1. Genitourinary system – breakthrough bleeding, spotting, change in menstrual flow, dysmenorrhoea, premenstrual-like syndrome, increase in size of uterine fibromyomata, vaginal candidiasis, change in cervical erosion and in degree of cervical secretion, cystitis-like syndrome.
2. Breasts – tenderness, enlargement, secretion.
3. Gastrointestinal – nausea, vomiting, abdominal cramps, bloating, cholestatic jaundice.
4. Skin – chloasma or melasma which may persist when drug is discontinued, erythema multiforme, erythema nodosum, haemorrhagic eruption, loss of scalp hair, hirsutism.
5. Eyes – steepening of corneal curvature, intolerance to contact lenses.
6. CNS – headaches, migraine, dizziness, mental depression, chorea.
7. Miscellaneous – increase or decrease in weight, reduced carbohydrate tolerance, aggravation of porphyria, oedema, change in libido, leg cramps.

Overdose: Overdosage may be manifested by nausea and vomiting. There is no specific antidote and treatment should be symptomatic.

Pharmacological properties
Pharmacodynamic properties: The oestrogen component of Kliofem substitutes for the loss of endogenous oestrogen production in postmenopausal women, whilst the progestogen component counter-

acts hyperstimulation of the endometrium. A regular shedding of the endometrium is not induced by Kliofem. Studies based on measurement of bone mineral content have shown that Kliofem is effective in the prevention of progressive bone loss following the menopause.

Pharmacokinetic properties: The micronised oestradiol in Kliofem is rapidly and efficiently absorbed from the gastrointestinal tract, maximum plasma concentration being reached after 2–4 hours. Oestrogens are partly bound to plasma proteins. Oestradiol is oxidised to oestrone which, in turn, is hydrated to oestriol; both transformations take place mainly in the liver. Oestrogens are excreted into the bile and then undergo reabsorption from the intestine. During this entero-hepatic circulation, degradation of the oestrogens occur. They are excreted in the urine (90–95%) as biologically inactive glucuronide and sulphate conjugates or in the faeces (5–10%) most conjugated.

Norethisterone acetate is rapidly absorbed and transformed to norethisterone, then metabolised and excreted as glucuronide and sulphate conjugates. About half the dose is recovered in the urine within 24 hours, the remainder being reduced to less than 1% of the dose within 5–6 days. Mean plasma half-life is 3–6 hours.

Pharmaceutical particulars

List of excipients: Lactose; maize starch; gelatin; talc; magnesium stearate; methyl hydroxypropyl cellulose (E464); titanium dioxide (E171); iron oxide (E172); propylene glycol; purified water.

Incompatibilities: None known.

Shelf life: 48 months.

Special precautions for storage: Store at room temperature; protect from light and moisture.

Nature and contents of container: Polypropylene/polystyrene calendar dial pack containing 28 tablets. Calendar dial packs (3×28 tablets) are contained within outer carton.

Instructions for use/handling: Each carton contains a patient information leaflet with instructions for use of the calendar dial pack.

Marketing authorisation number 3132/0080.

Date of revision/approval of SPC February 1998.

Legal category POM.

KLIOVANCE*

Qualitative and quantitative composition

Each tablet contains: Estradiol hemihydrate 1.03 mg equivalent to anhydrous estradiol 1 mg and norethisterone acetate 0.5 mg.

Pharmaceutical form Film coated tablet.

Clinical particulars

Therapeutic indications: Hormone Replacement Therapy (HRT) for estrogen deficiency symptoms in women who are more than one year past the menopause.

Experience of treating women older than 65 years is limited.

Posology and method of administration: Kliovance is a continuous-combined hormone replacement product intended for use in women with an intact uterus. One tablet should be taken orally once a day without interruption, preferably at the same time of the day.

A switch to a higher dose combination product could be indicated if the response after three months is insufficient for satisfactory symptom relief.

In women with amenorrhea and not taking HRT or women transferring from another continuous combined HRT product, treatment with Kliovance may be started on any convenient day. In women transferring from sequential HRT regimens, treatment should start as soon as their withdrawal bleeding has ended.

Contra-indications: Pregnancy or suspected pregnancy.

Lactation.

Known, suspected or past history of breast cancer.

Known or suspected estrogen-dependent tumours.

Undiagnosed vaginal bleeding.

Active or recent thromboembolic processes.

Acute or chronic liver disease or a history of liver disease as long as liver function tests have failed to return to normal.

Known hypersensitivity to any of the ingredients.

Special warnings and special precautions for use: Before initiating or reinstituting HRT, a complete personal and family medical history should be taken, together with a thorough general and gynaecological examination guided by the contraindications and warnings for use. During treatment periodic check-ups are recommended of a frequency and nature adapted to the individual woman.

A careful appraisal of the risk/benefit ratio should be undertaken over time in women treated with estrogen/progestogen therapy.

If any of the following conditions are present, have occurred previously and/or have aggravated during pregnancy or previous hormone treatment, the benefits of treatment should be weighed against the possible risks. In these cases the patient should be closely supervised.

It should be taken into account that these conditions may, in rare cases, recur or be aggravated during treatment with Kliovance:

A history of estrogen-dependent tumours.

Leiomyoma, endometriosis, hyperplasia of the endometrium.

Fibrocystic disease of the breast.

A history of thromboembolic disorders or the presence of risk factors (see below).

Hypertension.

Diabetes mellitus with vascular involvement.

Liver disorders (e.g. porphyria, liver adenoma).

Cholelithiasis.

Otosclerosis.

Migraine or (severe) headache.

Estrogens may cause fluid retention and, therefore, patients with cardiac or renal dysfunction should be carefully observed. Patients with end-stage renal disease should be closely monitored as it would be expected that the circulating levels of the active components of Kliovance would be increased. In case of aggravation of asthma, epilepsy or diabetes mellitus HRT should be reconsidered.

Epidemiological studies have suggested that hormone replacement therapy (HRT) is associated with a higher relative risk of developing venous thromboembolism (VTE), i.e. deep vein thrombosis or pulmonary embolism. The studies find a 2–3 fold higher risk for users compared with non-users, which for healthy women amounts to one extra case of VTE for every 5000 patients taking HRT.

Generally recognised risk factors for VTE include a personal history or family history, severe obesity (Body Mass Index >30 kg/m²) and systemic lupus erythematosus (SLE). In women with risk factors, the benefits of treatment with HRT need to be carefully weighed against risks. There is no consensus about the possible role of varicose veins in VTE.

The risk of VTE may be temporarily increased with prolonged immobilisation, major trauma or major surgery. As in all post-operative patients, scrupulous attention should be given to prophylactic measures to prevent VTE following surgery. Where prolonged immobilisation is liable to follow elective surgery, particularly abdominal or orthopaedic surgery to the lower limbs, consideration should be given to temporarily stopping HRT four to six weeks earlier, if possible.

If VTE develops after initiating therapy, the drug should be discontinued.

Use of HRT for more than five years is associated with an increase in the risk of breast cancer. The risk increases with the time of the treatment and decreases after the treatment has been stopped, so that the risk of breast cancer is at the same level as for untreated women five years after withdrawal. Breast cancers found in women on HRT tend to be more limited than those not associated with HRT. The findings may be due to an earlier diagnosis, the biological effects of HRT, or a combination of both. The absolute increase in risk is small to moderate. During the period between 50 and 70 years of age, about 45 in every 1000 will have breast cancer diagnosed. Among those who use HRT for 5 years, 2 extra cases of breast cancer in every 1000 will be detected during the same period of age. For those who use HRT for 10 to 15 years, there will be 6 and 12 extra cases of breast cancer respectively in every 1000 women.

Regular breast examination and, where appropriate, mammography should be carried out in women on HRT. Breast status should also be closely monitored in women with a history of or known breast nodules, fibrocystic disease, or with a family history of breast cancer.

It has been confirmed that there is an increase in the risk of surgically confirmed gall bladder disease in postmenopausal women receiving estrogens.

An increased risk of developing systemic lupus erythematosus during HRT treatment has been reported.

The use of estrogen may influence the results of certain endocrine and liver function tests.

Breakthrough bleeding and spotting often occur during the initial months of treatment. If at any time bleeding or spotting is unacceptable Kliovance should be discontinued. If bleeding occurs after a period of amenorrhea or persists after treatment has been discontinued, the aetiology of the bleeding should be investigated. This may include an endometrial biopsy.

Interaction with other medicaments and other forms of interaction: Drugs that induce the activity of hepatic microsomal drug metabolising enzymes e.g. barbiturates, phenytoin, rifampicin and carbamazepine may accelerate the metabolism of the active substances in Kliovance. Drugs that inhibit the activity of hepatic microsomal drug metabolising enzymes e.g. ketoconazole, may increase circulating levels of the active substances in Kliovance.

Food delays the absorption of norethisterone and decreases C_{max}, however, the extent of absorption is not decreased. There is no clinical relevance to this finding.

Pregnancy and lactation: Kliovance is contraindicated during pregnancy and lactation.

Effects on ability to drive and use machines: No effects known.

Undesirable effects: The most frequently reported adverse event during treatment in clinical trials was breast tenderness, which was mainly reported during the initial months of treatment.

Other adverse events associated with estrogen-progestogen treatment have been reported with Kliovance in clinical trials: headache, vaginal bleeding, abdominal pain, nausea, flatulence, breast enlargement, increase in size of uterine fibroids, skin rash and pruritus, insomnia, depression, venous thromboembolism and oedema.

Additional adverse events associated with estrogen-progestogen treatment:

Gastrointestinal: dyspepsia, vomiting, bloating, gallbladder disease, gallstones.

Skin: loss of scalp hair, hirsuitism.

CNS: migraine, dizziness.

Urogenital: vaginal candidiasis.

Cardiovascular: increase in blood pressure.

Miscellaneous: increase or decrease in weight, changes in libido, leg cramps.

Exceptional cases of chloasma, erythema multiforme, erythema nodosum and haemorrhagic eruption have been reported in women using HRT.

Overdose: Overdose may be manifested by nausea and vomiting. Treatment should be symptomatic.

Pharmacological properties

Pharmacodynamic properties: ATC code G03F A01.

The oestrogen component of Kliovance is 17β-estradiol, identical to the endogenous human 17β-estradiol and classified as a natural oestrogen. The component norethisterone acetate is a synthetic progestogen.

The oestrogen component of Kliovance substitutes for the loss of oestrogen production in menopausal women, and alleviates menopausal symptoms. The progestogen component of Kliovance provides protection for the oestrogen-induced increased risk of endometrial hyperplasia and carcinoma, and against the oestrogen-induced proliferative changes in the endometrium, as shown in one-year studies with Kliovance. In clinical trials with Kliovance, the addition of the norethisterone acetate component enhanced the vasomotor symptom relieving effect of 17β-estradiol.

The biological activity of Kliovance on the hypothalamic-pituitary axis can be observed by the reduction of menopausal serum FSH levels. In addition, an effect has been found on vaginal cytology, as shown by an increase in vaginal superficial epithelial cells during Kliovance treatment.

Relief of menopausal symptoms is achieved during the first few weeks of treatment.

Kliovance is a continuous combined HRT given with the intent of avoiding the regular withdrawal bleeding associated with cyclic or sequential HRT. During the first months of treatment breakthrough bleeding and spotting are quite common but tend to decrease with time. After 9–12 months of treatment about 80% of women have become amenorrheic.

Kliovance has influence on metabolic processes. In placebo-controlled clinical trials, Kliovance reduced total cholesterol, LDL-cholesterol, and lipoprotein (a). A decrease in HDL-cholesterol over time was observed without any change in the LDL/HDL ratio. Kliovance did not increase triglycerides levels. In addition, Kliovance did not alter glucose tolerance or insulin sensitivity.

Pharmacokinetic: Following oral administration of 17β-estradiol in micronised form, rapid absorption from the gastrointestinal tract occurs. It undergoes extensive first-pass metabolism in the liver and other enteric organs and reaches a peak plasma concentration of approximately 35 pg/ml (range 21–52 pg/ml) within 5–8 hours. The half-life of 17β-estradiol is about 12–14 hours. It circulates bound to SHBG (37%) and to albumin (61%), while only approximately 1–2% is unbound. Metabolism of 17β-estradiol, occurs mainly in the liver and gut but also in target organs, and involves the formation of less active or inactive metabolites, including estrone, catecholestrogens and several estrogen sulphates and glucuronides. Estrogens are excreted with the bile, where they are hydrolysed and reabsorbed (enterohepatic circulation), and are excreted mainly in urine in biologically inactive form.

After oral administration norethisterone acetate is

rapidly absorbed and transformed to norethisterone (NET). It undergoes first-pass metabolism in the liver and other enteric organs and reaches a peak plasma concentration of approximately 3.9 ng/ml (range 1.4–6.8 ng/ml) within 0.5–1.5 hour. The terminal half-life of NET is about 8–11 hours. NET binds to SHBG (36%) and to albumin (61%). The most important metabolites are isomers of 5α-dihydro-NET and of tetrahydro-NET, which are excreted mainly in the urine as sulphate or glucuronide conjugates.

The pharmacokinetics in the elderly have not been studied.

Preclinical safety data: The toxicity profiles of estradiol and norethisterone acetate are well known. There are no preclinical data of relevance to the prescriber which are additional to that already included in other sections of the SPC.

Pharmaceutical particulars

List of excipients: Lactose monohydrate PhEur/NF; Maize starch PhEur/NF; Copovidone PhEur; Talc PhEur/USP; Magnesium stearate PhEur/NF; Hypromellose PhEur/USP; Glycerol triacetate PhEur/USP.

Incompatibilities: None.

Shelf life: 2 years.

Special precautions for storage: Store in a dry place, protected from light. Store below 25°C. Do not refrigerate.

Keep out of reach of children.

Nature and contents of container: The tablets are contained in calendar dial packs; each calendar dial pack contains 28 tablets.

Packs containing 3 calendar dial packs are available (3×28 tablets).

The calendar dial pack with 28 tablets consists of the following 3 parts:

- The base made of coloured non-transparent polypropylene.
- The ring-shaped lid made of transparent polystyrene.
- The centre-dial made of coloured non-transparent polystyrene.

Instructions for use/handling

1. *Set the day reminder:* Use a coin to turn the inner disc to set the selected day of the week opposite the little plastic tab.
2. *How to take the first tablet:* Break the plastic tab and tip out the first tablet.
3. *Every day:* Simply move the transparent dial clockwise one space as indicated by the arrow. Tip out the next tablet.

The transparent dial can only be turned after the tablet in the opening has been removed.

Marketing authorisation number PL 03132/0125.

Date of first authorisation/renewal of authorisation 20 August 1998.

Date of (partial revision) of the text 2 July 1998.

Legal category POM.

NORDITROPIN* 12 IU
NORDITROPIN PENSET 12
NORDITROPIN PENSET 24

Qualitative and quantitative composition

Norditropin Vials and PenSet: Active ingredient Somatropin 12 IU (4 mg) and 24 IU (8 mg) (biosynthetic human growth hormone).

Solvent contains 0.9% benzyl alcohol.

Inactive ingredients: Mannitol, glycine, sodium hydrogen carbonate.

Pharmaceutical form Powder for injection supplied with diluent.

Route of administration: Subcutaneous injection.

Clinical particulars

Therapeutic indications

Children: Growth failure due to growth hormone insufficiency. Turner syndrome. Growth retardation in prepubertal children due to chronic renal disease.

Adults: Growth hormone insufficiency with known hypothalamic-pituitary disease where there is evidence of deficiency in at least one other axis (prolactin excepted) or pronounced growth hormone deficiency demonstrated by two different dynamic growth hormone stimulation tests. Tests for growth hormone deficiency should be undertaken only after adequate replacement therapy has been instituted for deficiencies in any other axis. Patients with childhood onset growth hormone deficiency should be retested as adults and the deficiency should be confirmed by two dynamic tests.

Posology and method of administration: The dosage is individual, based on body weight or body surface area and must always be adjusted in accordance with the individual's response to therapy. Generally, daily subcutaneous administration in the evening is recommended. The injection site should be varied to prevent lipoatrophy.

Generally recommended dosages:
Children
Growth hormone insufficiency:
0.07–0.1 IU/kg (2–3 IU/m²/day)
Equal to: 0.02–0.03 mg/kg/day or 0.7–1.0 mg/m²/day
Turner syndrome:
0.14 IU/kg/day (4.3 IU/m²/day)
Equal to: 0.05 mg/kg/day or 1.4 mg/m²/day
Chronic renal disease:
0.14 IU/kg/day (4.3 IU/m²/day)
Equal to: 0.05 mg/kg/day or 1.4 mg/m²/day

Replacement therapy in adults: The dosage must be adjusted to the need of the individual patient. It is recommended to start treatment with a very low dose like 0.5 IU (0.17 mg) per day or not more than 0.02 IU/kg/day, equal to 0.007 mg/kg/day. The starting dosage may be increased step-wise up to 0.04 IU/kg/day, equal to 0.013/mg/kg/day over a period of one or two months, depending on the obtained treatment results. Insulin-like Growth Factor 1 (IGF-1) in serum should be used as guidance. Dose requirements decline with age.

Daily dosage	*IU/kg*	*mg/kg*
Starting dose 0.5 IU (0.17 mg) not more than	0.02	0.007
Maximum maintenance dosage	0.04	0.013

Administration: Patients should be reminded to wash their hands thoroughly with soap and water and/or disinfectant prior to mixing the dry powder and solvent. The solution should not be shaken vigorously at any time.

Norditropin PenSet: Norditropin PenSet 12 and 24 should be prescribed only for use with Nordiject 12 and Nordiject 24 pen injection devices respectively. Instructions for preparing the cartridge for use and for using Nordiject are provided within the respective packs. Patients should be advised to read these instructions very carefully.

Norditropin 12 IU: Norditropin 12 IU is reconstituted by adding 3 ml solvent to the dry powder for injection. Prior to administration the rubber seals of the vials should be wiped with antiseptic solution. The solvent is then drawn into a syringe and injected into the vial containing the dry powder whilst directing the stream against the glass wall of the vial. The powder is dissolved by inverting the vial several times, avoiding vigorous shaking.

Contra-indications: Norditropin should not be used where there is evidence of active tumour. Anti-tumour therapy should be completed prior to the institution of therapy. Norditropin should be discontinued if there is any evidence of recurrent tumour growth.

In children with chronic renal disease treatment with Norditropin should be discontinued at renal transplantation.

Treatment during pregnancy and lactation is not recommended (see *Pregnancy and lactation* section).

Hypersensitivity to Norditropin preparations.

Special warnings and special precautions for use: Patients treated with Norditropin should be regularly assessed by a specialist in child growth. Norditropin treatment should always be instigated by a physician with special knowledge of growth hormone insufficiency and its treatment. This is also true for the management of Turner syndrome and chronic renal disease.

The stimulation of skeletal growth in children can only be expected until the epiphysial discs are closed.

Data on final adult height following the use of Norditropin in children with Turner syndrome and chronic renal disease are not available.

The dosage in children with chronic renal disease is individual and must be adjusted according to the individual response to therapy. The growth disturbance should be clearly established before treatment by following the growth on optimal conservative treatment for a minimum of 1 year. Conservative management of uraemia should be maintained during therapy. Patients with chronic renal disease normally experience a decline in renal function. During Norditropin treatment renal function should be observed for an excessive decline or an increase in the glomerular filtration rate (which could be attributed to hyper filtration).

Somatropin has been found to influence carbohydrate metabolism and, therefore, patients should be observed for evidence of glucose intolerance.

A state of hypothyroidism may develop during growth hormone treatment. Since untreated hypothyroidism may interfere with the response to Norditropin, patients should have a periodic thyroid function test and should be treated with thyroid hormone when indicated.

Patients with growth hormone deficiency secondary to an intracranial lesion should be examined frequently for progression or recurrence of the underlying disease process.

Leukaemia has been reported in a small number of growth hormone deficient patients, some of whom have been treated with somatropin. Based on current evidence, it is unlikely that somatropin is associated with this risk.

Slipped capital femoral epiphysis may occur more frequently in patients with endocrine disorders. This may result in the development of a limp or complaints of hip or knee pain in patients treated with somatropin and parents should be alerted to this possibility.

In the event of severe or recurrent headache, visual problems, nausea and/or vomiting, a funduscopy for papilloedema is recommended. If papilloedema is confirmed, a diagnosis of benign intracranial hypertension should be considered and if appropriate the growth hormone treatment should be discontinued. At present there is insufficient evidence to guide clinical decision making in patients with resolved intracranial hypertension. If growth hormone treatment is restarted, careful monitoring for symptoms of intracranial hypertension is necessary.

Experience in patients above 60 years of age is lacking. Experience with prolonged treatment in adults is limited.

Interaction with other medicaments and other forms of interaction: Concomitant glucocorticoid therapy may inhibit the growth promoting effect of Norditropin.

Pregnancy and lactation: There is currently insufficient evidence of safety of human growth hormone therapy during pregnancy. Norditropin is, therefore, contra-indicated during pregnancy. In the event of pregnancy occurring during treatment, Norditropin therapy should be discontinued.

The possibility that human growth hormone is secreted in breast milk cannot be discounted.

Effect of ability to drive and use machines: No effects.

Undesirable effects: Fluid retention with peripheral oedema may occur. It is normally transient and dependent on the dosage.

Formation of antibodies directed against somatropin has rarely been observed during Norditropin therapy. The titres and binding capacities of these antibodies have been very low and have not interfered with the growth response to Norditropin.

During treatment with Norditropin a few children developed transient local skin reactions. General reactions are very rarely seen.

Some rare cases of benign intracranial hypertension have been reported.

Rare cases of hypersensitivity to the preservative benzyl alcohol may occur.

Overdose: Acute overdosage could lead initially to hypoglycaemia and subsequently to hyperglycaemia. Long-term overdosage could result in signs and symptoms consistent with the known effects of human growth hormone excess.

Pharmacological properties

Pharmacodynamic properties: Norditropin contains somatropin, which is human growth hormone produced by recombinant DNA-technology. It is an anabolic peptide of 191 amino acids stabilised by two disulphide bridges with a molecular weight of approximately 22.000 Daltons. The major effect is stimulation of skeletal and somatic growth and in addition to Norditropin's growth promoting effect, it has also other metabolic effects. When growth hormone deficiency is treated a normalisation of body composition takes place resulting in an increase in lean body mass and a decrease in fat mass.

The lipolytic and protein sparing effects become particularly important during stress. Somatropin exerts most of its actions through insulin-like growth factors (IGF). IGF is produced in tissues throughout the body, the most important contribution coming from hepatic synthesis. More than 90% of IGF is bound to binding proteins (IGF-BP) of which IGF-BP-3 is the most important.

Pharmacokinetic properties: Following i.v. infusion of Norditropin (33 ng/kg/min for 3 hours) in nine growth hormone deficient patients, the following results were found. Serum half-life was 21.1±1.7 min, metabolic clearance rate was 2.33±0.58 ml/kg/min and the distribution space was 67.6±14.6 ml/kg.

Preclinical safety data: The toxicity of Norditropin has been tested in mice, rats and monkeys and no findings of toxicological relevance were revealed. Norditropin has also been tested for mutagenic potential and none of the tests showed any mutagenic properties of the product.

Pharmaceutical particulars

List of excipients: Lyophilised powder contains Glycine BP, Sodium Hydrogen Carbonate PhEur and Mannitol PhEur. Solvent contains Benzyl Alcohol PhEur 9 mg/ml as preservative in Water for Injections PhEur.

Incompatibilities: None.

Shelf life:

Norditropin 12 IU in vials: Powder for injection: 2 years (2–8°C). Reconstituted powder for injection: 14 days (2–8°C).

Norditropin PenSet 12 IU and 24 IU: Powder for injection: 3 years (2–8°C). Reconstituted powder for injection: 14 days (2–8°C).

Special precautions for storage: Avoid freezing. Protect from light. Storage between 2°C and 8°C.

Nature and contents of container

Norditropin vials and PenSet:

(a) Powder for injection: Colourless vials of glass.

(b) Solvent: Colourless vials or cartridge vials of glass.

Vials with powder for injection and its respective solvent are packed together in a light cardboard carton.

The PenSet package contains mixing devices packed in a carton.

Marketing authorisation numbers

Norditropin PenSet 12	3132/0060
Norditropin PenSet 24	3132/0061
Norditropin 12 IU	3132/0046
Diluent for Norditropin PenSet	3132/0062
Norditropin Diluent	3132/0065

Dat of approval/revision of SPC July 1997.

Legal category CD (Sch 4), POM.

NOVONORM* 0.5 MG TABLETS ▼
NOVONORM* 1 MG TABLETS 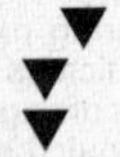
NOVONORM* 2 MG TABLETS ▼

Qualitative and quantitative composition Each tablet contains: Repaglinide 0.5 mg or Repaglinide 1 mg or Repaglinide 2 mg, respectively.

Pharmaceutical form Tablet.

Repaglinide tablets are white (0.5 mg), yellow (1 mg), or red (2 mg), round and convex and engraved with Novo Nordisk logo (Apis bull).

Clinical particulars

Therapeutic indications: Repaglinide is indicated in patients with Type 2 diabetes (non insulin-dependent diabetes mellitus (NIDDM)) whose hyperglycaemia can no longer be controlled satisfactorily by diet, weight reduction and exercise. Repaglinide is also indicated in combination with metforminin Type 2 diabetes patients who are not satisfactorily controlled on metformin alone.

Treatment should be initiated as an adjunct to diet and exercise to lower the blood glucose in relation to meals.

Posology and method of administration: Repaglinide is given preprandially and is titrated individually to optimise the glycaemic control. In addition to the usual self-monitoring by the patient of blood and/or urinary glucose, the patient's blood glucose must be monitored periodically by the physician to determine the minimum effective dose for the patient. Glycosylated haemoglobin levels are also of value in monitoring the patient's response to therapy. Periodic monitoring is necessary to detect inadequate lowering of blood glucose at the recommended maximum dose level (i.e. primary failure) and to detect loss of adequate blood-glucose-lowering response after an initial period of effectiveness (i.e. secondary failure).

Short-term administration of repaglinide may be sufficient during periods of transient loss of control in Type 2 diabetic patients usually controlled well on diet.

Repaglinide should be taken before main meals (i.e. preprandially).

Initial dose: The dosage should be determined by the physician, according to the patient's requirements.

The recommended starting dose is 0.5 mg. One to two weeks should elapse between titration steps (as determined by blood glucose response). If patients are transferred from another oral hypoglycaemic agent the recommended starting dose is 1 mg.

Maintenance: The recommended maximum single dose is 4 mg taken with main meals. The total maximum daily dose should not exceed 16 mg.

Specific patient groups: Repaglinide is primarily excreted via the bile and excretion is therefore not affected by renal disorders.

Only 8% of one dose of repaglinide is excreted through the kidneys and total plasma clearance of the product is decreased in patients with renal impairment. As insulin sensitivity is increased in diabetic patients with renal impairment, caution is advised when titrating these patients.

No clinical studies have been conducted in patients >75 years of age or in patients with hepatic insufficiency. See *Special warnings and special precautions for use.*

In debilitated or malnourished patients the initial and maintenance dosage should be conservative and careful dose titration is required to avoid hypoglycaemic reactions.

Patients receiving other oral hypoglycaemic agents (OHAs): Patients can be transferred directly from other oral hypoglycaemic agents to repaglinide. However, no exact dosage relationship exists between repaglinide and the other oral hypoglycaemic agents. The recommended maximum starting dose of patients transferred to repaglinide is 1 mg given before main meals.

Repaglinide can be given in combination with metformin, when the blood glucose is insufficiently controlled with metformin alone. In this case, the dosage of metformin should be maintained and repaglinide administered concomitantly. The starting dose of repaglinide is 0.5 mg, taken before main meals; titration is according to blood glucose response as for monotherapy.

Contra-indications: Known hypersensitivity to repaglinide or any of the excipients in NovoNorm.

Type 1 diabetes (Insulin-Dependent Diabetes Mellitus: IDDM), C-peptide negative.

Diabetic ketoacidosis, with or without coma.

Pregnancy and lactation (See *Pregnancy and lactation*).

Children < 12 years of age.

Severe renal or hepatic function disorders.

Concomittant therapy with medicinal products, inhibiting or inducing CYP3A4 (See *Interaction with other medicaments and other forms of interaction*).

Special warnings and special precautions for use

General: Repaglinide should only be prescribed if poor blood glucose control and symptoms of diabetes persist despite adequate attempts at dieting, exercise and weight reduction.

Repaglinide like other insulin secretagogues, is capable of producing hypoglycaemia.

The blood glucose lowering effect of oral hypoglycaemic agents decreases in many patients over time. This may be due to progression of the severity of the diabetes or to diminished responsiveness to the product. This phenomenon is known as secondary failure, to distinguish it from primary failure, where the drug is ineffective in an individual patient when first given. Adjustment of dose and adherence to diet and exercise should be assessed before classifying a patient as a secondary failure.

Repaglinide acts through a distinct binding site with a short action on the β-cells. Use of repaglinide in case of secondary failure to *insulin* secretagogues has not been investigated in clinical trials.

Trials investigating the combination with other insulin secretagogues and acarbose have not been performed.

No trials of combination therapy with insulin or thiazolidenediones have been performed.

Combination treatment with metformin is associated with an increased risk of hypoglycaemia.

When a patient stabilised on any oral hypoglycaemic agent is exposed to stress such as fever, trauma, infection or surgery, a loss of glycaemic control may occur. At such times, it may be necessary to discontinue repaglinide and treat with insulin on a temporary basis.

Specific patient groups: No clinical studies have been conducted in patients with impaired hepatic function. No clinical studies have been performed in children and adolescents <18 years of age or in patients >75 years of age. Therefore, treatment is not recommended in these patient groups.

Interaction with other medicaments and other forms of interaction: A number of drugs are known to influence glucose metabolism, possible interactions should therefore be taken into account by the physician.

The following substances may enhance the hypoglycaemic effect of repaglinide: Monoamine oxidase inhibitors (MAOI), non selective beta blocking agents, angiotensin converting enzyme (ACE)-inhibitors, salicylates, NSAIDS, octreotide, alcohol, and anabolic steroids.

The following substances may reduce the hypoglycaemic effect of repaglinide: Oral contraceptives, thiazides, corticosteriods, danazol, thyroid hormones and sympathomimetics.

When these medications are administered to or withdrawn from a patient receiving repaglinide, the patient should be observed closely for changes in glycaemic control.

Repaglinide had no clinically relevant effect on the pharmacokinetic properties of digoxin, theophylline or warfarin at steady state, when administered to healthy volunteers. Dosage adjustment of these compounds when co-administered with repaglinide is therefore not necessary.

Co-administration of cimetidine with multiple dosing of repaglinide did not significantly alter the absorption and disposition of repaglinide and no change in hypoglycaemic symptomatology of repaglinide was seen.

β-blocking agents may mask the symptoms of hypoglycaemia. Alcohol may intensify and prolong the hypoglycaemic effect of repaglinide.

In vitro studies indicate that repaglinide is primarily metabolised by CYP3A4. Although no *in vivo* studies have been performed, it is expected that CYP3A4 inhibitors, like ketoconazole, itraconazole, erythromycin, fluconazole and mibefradil, increase the plasma levels of repaglinide. Compounds that induce CYP3A4, like rifampicin or phenytoin, may decrease the plasma levels of repaglinide. Since the magnitude of an inducing or inhibiting effect is not known, these drug combinations are contra-indicated.

When repaglinide is used together with other drugs that are mainly secreted by the bile like repaglinide any potential interaction should be considered.

Pregnancy and lactation: There are no studies of repaglinide in pregnant or lactating women. Therefore the safety of repaglinide in pregnant women cannot be assessed. Up to now repaglinide showed not to be teratogenic in animal studies. Embryotoxicity, abnormal limb development in foetuses and new born pups, was observed in rats exposed to high doses in the last stage of pregnancy and during the lactation period. Repaglinide is detected in the milk of experimental animals. For that reason repaglinide should be avoided during pregnancy and should not be used in lactating women.

Effects on ability to drive and use machines: Patients should be advised to take precautions to avoid hypoglycaemia whilst driving. This is particularly important in those who have reduced or absent awareness of the warning signs of hypoglycaemia or have frequent episodes of hypoglycaemia. The advisability of driving should be considered in these circumstances.

Undesirable effects: Based on the experience with repaglinide and with other hypoglycaemic agents the following side effects have been seen:

Hypoglycaemia: As with other hypoglycaemic agents, hypoglycaemic reactions have been observed after administration of repaglinide. These reactions are mostly mild and easily handled through intake of carbohydrates. If severe, infusion of glucose may be necessary. The occurrence of such reactions depends, as for every diabetes therapy, on individual factors, such as dietary habits, dosage, exercise and stress (see also *Special warnings and special precautions for use*).

Visual disturbances: Changes in blood glucose levels have been known to result in transient visual disturbances, especially at the commencement of treatment. Such disturbances have only been reported in very few cases after initiation of repaglinide treatment. No such cases have led to discontinuation of repaglinide treatment in clinical trials.

Gastro-intestinal: Complaints such as abdominal pain, diarrhoea, nausea, vomiting and constipation have been reported in clinical trials. The rate and severity of these symptoms did not differ from that seen with other oral insulin secretagogues.

Liver enzymes: Isolated cases of increase in liver enzymes have been reported during treatment with repaglinide. Most cases were mild and transient, and very few patients discontinued treatment due to increase in liver enzymes.

Allergy: Hypersensitivity reactions of the skin may occur as itching, rashes and urticaria. There is no reason to suspect cross-allergenicity with sulphonylurea drugs due to the difference of the chemical structure.

Overdose: Repaglinide has been given with weekly escalating doses from 4–20 mg four times daily in a 6 week period. No safety concerns were raised. As hypoglycaemia in this study was avoided through increased calorie intake, a relative overdose may result in an exaggerated glucose lowering effect with development of hypoglycaemic symptoms (dizziness, sweating, tremor, headache etc.). Should these symptoms occur, adequate action should be taken to correct the low blood glucose (oral carbohydrates). More severe hypoglycaemia with seizure, loss of consciousness or coma should be treated with i.v. glucose.

Pharmacological properties

Pharmacodynamic properties: Pharmaco-therapeutic group: Carbamoylmethyl benzoic acid derivative (ATC code: A 10 B H01).

Repaglinide is a novel short-acting oral secretagogue. Repaglinide lowers the blood glucose levels acutely by stimulating the release of insulin from the pancreas, an effect dependent upon functioning β-cells in the pancreatic islets.

Repaglinide closes ATP-dependent potassium channels in the β-cell membrane via a target protein different from other secretagogues. This depolarises the β-cell and leads to an opening of the calcium channels. The resulting increased calcium influx induces insulin secretion from the β-cell.

In Type 2 diabetic patients, the insulinotropic

response to a meal occurred within 30 minutes after an oral dose of repaglinide. This resulted in a blood glucose-lowering effect throughout the meal period. The elevated insulin levels did not persist beyond the time of the meal challenge. Plasma repaglinide levels decreased rapidly, and low drug concentrations were seen in the plasma of Type 2 diabetic patients 4 hours post-administration.

A dose-dependent decrease in blood glucose was demonstrated in Type 2 diabetic patients when administered in doses from 0.5 to 4 mg repaglinide. Clinical study results have shown that repaglinide is optimally dosed in relation to main meals (preprandial dosing). Doses are usually taken within 15 minutes of the meal, but time may vary from immediately preceding the meal to as long as 30 minutes before the meal.

Pharmacokinetic properties: Repaglinide is rapidly absorbed from the gastrointestinal tract, which leads to a rapid increase in the plasma concentration of the drug. The peak plasma level occurs within one hour post administration. After reaching a maximum, the plasma level decreases rapidly, and repaglinide is eliminated within 4–6 hours. The plasma elimination half-life is approximately one hour.

Repaglinide pharmacokinetics is characterised by a mean absolute bioavailability of 63% (CV 11%), low volume of distribution, 30 L (consistent with distribution into intracellular fluid), and rapid elimination from the blood.

A high interindividual variability (60%) in repaglinide plasma concentrations has been detected in the clinical trials. Intraindividual variability is low to moderate (35%) and as repaglinide should be titrated against the clinical response, efficacy is not affected by interindividual variability.

Repaglinide exposure is increased in patients with hepatic and renal insufficiency and in the elderly Type 2 diabetic patients. The AUC (SD) after 2 mg single dose exposure (4 mg in patients with hepatic insufficiency) was 31.4 ng/ml×hr (28.3) in healthy volunteers, 75.2 ng/ml×hr (67.7) in patients with renal insufficiency, 304.9 ng/ml×hr (228.0) in patients with hepatic insufficiency, and 117.9 ng/ml×hr (13.8) in the elderly Type 2 diabetic patients.

Repaglinide is highly bound to plasma proteins in humans (greater than 98%).

No clinically relevant differences were seen in the pharmacokinetics of repaglinide, when repaglinide was administered 0, 15 or 30 minutes before a meal or in fasting state.

Repaglinide is almost completely metabolised, and no metabolites with clinically relevant hypoglycaemic effect have been identified. Repaglinide and its metabolites are excreted primarily via the bile. A small fraction (less than 8%) of the administered dose appears in the urine, preliminary as metabolites. Less than 1% of the parent drug is recovered in faeces.

Preclinical safety data: Preclinical data revealed no special hazard for humans based on conventional studies of safety pharmacology, repeated dose toxicity, genotoxicity and carcinogenic potential.

Pharmaceutical particulars

List of excipients: Microcrystalline cellulose (E460); calcium hydrogen phosphate, anhydrous; maize starch; amberlite (Polacrilin potassium); povidone (Polyvidone); glycerol 85%; magnesium stearate; meglumine; poloxamer; iron oxide, yellow (1 mg tablets only) (E172); iron oxide, red (2 mg tablets only) (E172).

Incompatibilities: Not applicable.

Shelf-life: 2 years.

Special precautions for storage: Store in the original package and keep the container tightly closed.

Nature and content of container: Blister packs (aluminium/aluminium) containing 30 tablets (0.5 mg, 1 mg tablets) or 90 tablets (0.5 mg, 1 mg, 2 mg tablets) are available.

Instructions for use and handling: Not applicable.

Marketing authorisation holder

Novo Nordisk A/S, DK-2880 Bagsværd, Denmark.

Marketing authorisation mumber

NovoNorm 0.5 mg×30 tablets	EU/1/98/076/004
NovoNorm 0.5 mg×90 tablets	EU/1/98/076/005
NovoNorm 1 mg×30 tablets	EU/1/98/076/011
NovoNorm 1 mg×90 tablets	EU/1/98/076/012
NovoNorm 2 mg×90 tablets	EU/1/98/076/019

Date of first authorisation/renewal of the authorisation 17 August 1998.

Legal category POM.

NOVOSEVEN* ▼

Qualitative and quantitative composition Recombinant Coagulation Factor VIIa. Human Factor VII was cloned and expressed in baby hamster kidney cells (BHK cells). Recombinant Factor VII is secreted from the BHK cells and is activated during the purification procedure. NovoSeven Recombinant Coagulation Factor VIIa is structurally very similar to plasma-derived activated Factor VII (Human).

INN: eptacog alfa (activated).

Solvent: Water for injections PhEur.

Quantitative composition: Recombinant Coagulation Factor VIIa (rFVIIa) 60 KIU/vial (corresponds to 1.2 mg/vial). Water for injections PhEur 2.2 ml.

Recombinant Coagulation Factor VIIa 120 KIU/vial (corresponds to 2.4 mg/vial). Water for injections PhEur 4.3 ml.

Recombinant Coagulation Factor VIIa 240 KIU/vial (corresponds to 4.8 mg/vial). Water for injections PhEur 8.5 ml.

Please note that the above units are international units, measured with reference to the first international standard of FVIIa 89/688. Thus, these units should not be mistaken for units of other coagulation factors including FVII. 1 KIU equals 1000 IU (International Units). After reconstitution with the appropriate volume of diluent each vial contains 30 KIU/ml (0.6 mg/ml).

Pharmaceutical form Recombinant Coagulation Factor VIIa is supplied as a powder for injections. After reconstitution with the supplied diluent (Water for injections PhEur 2.2 ml, 4.3 ml or 8.5 ml) NovoSeven is administered intravenously as a bolus injection.

Clinical particulars

Therapeutic indications: Bleeding episodes and surgery in patients with inherited or acquired haemophilia with inhibitors to coagulation factors (FVIII or FIX) >10 BU or in patients with antibody titre <10 BU who are expected to have a high anamnestic response to Factor VIII or Factor IX.

Posology and method of administration

Dosage:

Serious bleeding episodes and surgery: From 3–6 KIU (60–120 μg) per kg body weight per single dose given by intravenous bolus injection. Administration time is 2–5 minutes.

Dose intervals: 2–3 hours initially, then 4–12 hours.

Serious bleeding episodes: The dosage varies according to the type and severity of the haemorrhages. As a guideline, an initial dosage of 4.5 KIU (90 μg) per kg body weight is recommended and could be administered on the way to the hospital where the patient is usually treated. Dosing frequency should initially be every second hour until clinical improvement is observed. If continued therapy is indicated the dosage interval can then be increased to 3 hours for 1–2 days. Thereafter, the dosage interval can be increased successively to every 4, 6, 8 or 12 hours for the period of time treatment is judged as being indicated. A major bleeding episode may be treated for 2–3 weeks but can be extended beyond this if clinically warranted.

Surgery: An initial dose of 4.5 KIU (90 μg) per kg body weight should be given immediately before the procedure. The dose should be repeated after 2 hours and then at 2–3 hour intervals for the first 24–48 hours depending on the surgery performed and the clinical status of the patient. In major surgery the dosage should be continued at 2–4 hour intervals for 6–7 days. The dosage interval may then be increased to 6–8 hours for another 2 weeks of treatment. Patients undergoing major surgery may be treated for up to 2–3 weeks until healing has occurred.

For patients with Factor IX inhibitors or acquired antibodies to Factor VIII, only experience of the use of NovoSeven in minor surgery exists.

Mild to moderate bleeding episodes: In the home-treatment setting early intervention doses of 4.5 KIU/kg b.w. (90 μg/kg b.w.) have been efficacious to treat mild to moderate joint, muscle and mucocutaneous bleeds. Treatment with 1 to 3 doses was administered at 3-hour intervals to achieve haemostasis and 1 additional dose was given to maintain haemostasis. The duration of the home treatment should not exceed 24 hours.

Administration: Dissolve the preparation as described under Instructions for use/handling and administer as an intravenous bolus injection.

NovoSeven should not be mixed with infusion solutions or be given in a drip.

Contra-indications: Known hypersensitivity to mouse, hamster or bovine protein may be a contra-indication to the use of NovoSeven.

Special warnings and special precautions for use: In pathological conditions in which tissue factor can be expected in circulating blood there is a possibility of a thrombogenic potential or induction of DIC in association with NovoSeven treatment. Such situations may include patients with advanced atherosclerotic disease, crush injury, septicaemia or DIC and surgery with major tissue destruction.

As Recombinant Coagulation Factor VIIa NovoSeven contains trace amounts of mouse IgG (maximum of 1.2 ng/mg rFVIIa), bovine IgG (maximum of 45 ng/ml rFVIIa) and hamster and other bovine proteins (maximum of 23 ng BHK protein/mg rFVIIa) the remote possibility exists that patients treated with this product may develop hypersensitivity to these proteins.

In case of severe bleeds the product should be administered in hospitals preferably specialised in treatment of haemophilia patients with coagulation Factor VIII or IX inhibitors or, if not possible, in close collaboration with a physician specialised in haemophilia treatment.

In case of mild or moderate bleeding episodes the product may be administered at home, however this should only be done in close collaboration with a haemophilia centre where the patient is regularly followed up.

All usages of NovoSeven and the results of it should be reported immediately (e.g. by telephone) to the supervising hospital.

The duration of home-treatment should not exceed 24 hours. If bleeding is not kept under control hospital care is mandatory.

Interaction with other medicaments and other forms of interaction: The risk of a potential interaction between NovoSeven and coagulation factor concentrates is unknown. Simultaneous use of prothrombin complex concentrates, activated or not, should be avoided.

Anti-fibrinolytics have been reported to reduce blood loss in association with surgery in haemophilia patients, especially in regions rich in fibrinolytic activity, such as the oral cavity. Preliminary experience indicates that concomitant use of anti-fibrinolytic therapy in minor and major surgery is clinically safe.

Laboratory tests: The relationship between the prothrombin time (PT), activated partial thromboplastin time (aPTT) and levels of the plasma FVII clotting activity FVII:C has been investigated in one core laboratory.

The therapeutic range has not been identified for any of the assays.

FVII:C was measured in a one step coagulation system containing FVII-deficient plasma (immunodepleted, Novo Nordisk A/S) and rabbit brain thromboplastin (type C, Manchester Comparative Reagents Ltd., UK). Coagulation was started by adding thromboplastin and Ca^{++}. Pooled citrated plasma from healthy normal subjects was used as calibrator and was assigned an arbitrary potency of 1 U/ml.

PT shortens to 7 seconds and seems to reach a plateau at plasma FVII:C levels of approximately 5 U/ml. Preliminary data indicate that a clinical improvement is associated with a shortening of the PT to 3–4 seconds from baseline and that this shortening is maintained throughout the treatment with therapeutic doses. The PT cannot be used to differentiate plasma FVII:C levels >5 U/ml. The PT assay is performed according to the instructions given in the kit 'IL TEST (TM) PT-Fibrinogen: Calcium thromboplastin for the simultaneous *in vitro* determination of Prothrombin Time (PT) and Fibrinogen in plasma' from Instrumentation Laboratory. CAVE: Penicillins cause a reduction in prothrombin time.

Although administration of NovoSeven shortens the aPTT, normalisation is usually not observed in doses shown to induce clinical improvement. Experience so far indicates that a shortening of 15–20 seconds was associated with clinical improvement. It is not known if aPTT is helpful in the monitoring of treatment. The aPTT assay is performed according to the instructions given in the kit 'IL TEST (TM) APTT-Micronised Silica: Cephalin with Micronised silica for the *in vitro* determination of activated partial thromboplastin time (APTT) in plasma' from Instrumentation Laboratory.

For all the assay different thromboplastins may give different results.

Pregnancy and lactation: From an animal reproduction study it was concluded that intravenous administration of NovoSeven to male and female rats at dose levels up to 3.0 mg/kg b.w./day (150 KIU/kg b.w./day had no effect upon mating performance, fertility and litter responses. It is not known whether NovoSeven can cause foetal harm when administered to a pregnant woman or can affect reproduction capacity. NovoSeven should only be given to a pregnant woman if clearly needed.

Use during lactation: It is not known whether this drug is excreted in human milk but, since many drugs are, caution should be exercised when NovoSeven is administered to lactating women.

Effects on ability to drive and use machines: None known.

Undesirable effects: During the clinical studies conducted, a total of 1940 treatment episodes were evaluated for adverse events. Eight % of treatment episodes resulted in one or more possibly related adverse events. When analysed by body system, the majority of the adverse events possibly related to NovoSeven treatment occurred with an incidence of

1% or less, except for the following body systems: platelet, bleeding and clotting (4%), cardiovascular (3%) and body as a whole (2%). The serious adverse events possibly related to treatment included renal failure, ataxia, liver dysfunction, cerebrovascular disorder, angina pectoris, supraventricular tachycardia, circulatory shock, thrombophlebitis, pulmonary embolism and disseminated intravascular coagulation. The most frequent possibly related, non-serious adverse events reported were hypertension, fever, headache, epistaxis and skin related reactions (e.g. rash, itching).

One FVII deficient patient has developed antibodies against FVII after treatment with NovoSeven.

Overdose: From human use no thrombotic complications to overdose have been reported, even after accidental administration of 800 µg/kg b.w. (40 KIU/kg b.w.).

Pharmacological properties

Pharmacodynamic properties: Pharmacotherapeutic Group: Coagulation factors, ATC code B02B D08.

NovoSeven contains activated Recombinant Coagulation Factor VII. The working mechanism of FVIIa in the induction of haemostasis includes a direct activation of FX into FXa which then initiates the conversion of prothrombin into thrombin leading to the formation of the haemostatic plug by converting fibrinogen into fibrin. In addition, FVIIa activates FIX into FIXa. Accordingly, a pharmacodynamic effect of FVIa should give rise to an increased formation of FIXa and FXa as well as thrombin. However, the activity of FVIIa increases tremendously when it forms a complex with tissue factor/phospholipid which are exposed locally following an injury to the vessel wall. Therefore, the activity of rFVIIa will induce local haemostatsis only.

Systemic activation of the coagulation system may occur in patients suffering from underlying diseases predisposing for DIC.

Pharmacokinetic properties: Using a FVII clot assay, the pharmacokinetic properties of NovoSeven were investigated in 25 non-bleeding and in 5 bleeding study episodes. NovoSeven was given as a single dose of 17.5 mcg (0.875 KIU), 35 mcg (1.75 KIU) and 70 mcg (3.5 KIU) per kilo b.w.

Single dose pharmacokinetics of NovoSeven, 17.5, 35 and 70 mcg/kg (0.875, 1.75 and 3.5 KIU/kg) exhibited linear behaviour. FVII clotting activities measured in plasma drawn prior to and during a 24-hour period after NovoSeven administration were analysed. In non-bleeding episodes the median apparent volume of distribution at steady state and at elimination were 106 and 122 ml/kg and in bleeding episodes the figures were 107 and 121 ml/kg respectively. Median clearance was 31.0 ml/h×kg non-bleeding episodes and 32.6 ml/h×kg in bleeding episodes. The elimination of the drug was described also by mean residence time and half-time. In non-bleeding episodes mean residence time was 3.44 h and half-time was 2.89 h (median values). In bleeding episodes the elimination seemed faster, mean residence time being 2.97 h and half-time being 2.30 h (median values).

The median *in vivo* plasma recovery was 45.6% in non-bleeding episodes and 43.5% in bleeding episodes. A significantly lower plasma recovery was found in bleeding episodes than in non-bleeding episodes, indicating a consumption of rFVIIa in connection with tissue damage.

Preclinical safety data: All findings in the pre-clinical safety programme were related to the pharmacological effect of Recombinant Coagulation Factor VIIa.

Pharmaceutical particulars

List of excipients: Sodium chloride; calcium chloride; glyclyglycine; polysorbate 80; mannitol.

After reconstitution with the appropriate volume of diluent (water for injections, PhEur) each bottle contains NovoSeven 30 KIU/ml (0.6 mg/ml). Sodium chloride 3 mg/ml, calcium chloride dihydrate 1.5 mg/ml, glycylglycine 1.3 mg/ml, polysorbate 80 0.1 mg/ml and mannitol 30 mg/ml are present in the preparation.

Incompatibilities: NovoSeven should not be mixed with infusion solutions or be given in a drip.

Shelf life: The shelf life for the product packed for sale is 2 years. The reconstituted product should be administered within 3 hours.

Special precautions for storage: NovoSeven should be stored under refrigeration (2°–8°C). Do not use after the expiry date.

Freezing should be avoided to prevent damage to the diluent bottle.

Avoid exposure to direct sunlight.

Nature and contents of container

Vials for NovoSeven: Glass type 1 PhEur, closed with a bromobutyl rubber plug, covered with an aluminium cap. The closed vials are equipped with a snap-off cap made of polypropylene for sealing.

Vials for diluent: Glass type 1 PhEur, closed with a bromobutyl rubber disc with teflon, covered with an aluminium cap. The closed vials are equipped with a snap-off cap made of polypropylene for sealing.

Syringe for reconstitution and administration: The disposable syringe is made of polypropylene and the size is 3 ml, 6 ml and 12 ml for 60 KIU/vial, 120 KIU/vial and 240 KIU/vial respectively.

Instructions for use/handling

Reconstitution – Always use aseptic technique:

1. Bring NovoSeven (powder) and water for injections, PhEur (diluent) to room temperature (but not above 37°C).
2. Remove caps from powder and diluent bottles to expose central portion of rubber stoppers.
3. Cleanse stoppers with alcohol swab and allow to dry prior to use.
4. To take the needle out of the package, press the needle end. Remove protective covering from the needle and attach the disposable syringe supplied in the package.
5. Draw back the plunger to admit air into the syringe.
6. Insert needle through the diluent bottle stopper at its centre and inject air into the bottle. Hold the bottle upside down, then withdraw the total content of the bottle into the syringe.
7. Inject the diluent from the syringe into the bottle containing the powder through the centre of the stopper (the powder bottle does not contain vacuum).
8. Gently swirl until all material is dissolved.

The enclosed disposable syringe should be used for reconstitution and administration of the preparation.

NovoSeven is for intravenous bolus injection only and should not be mixed with infusion solutions or be given in a drip.

Administration should preferably take place immediately or at least within 3 hours after reconstitution.

The enclosed disposable syringe is compatible with the reconstituted preparation, but **do not** store reconstituted NovoSeven in plastic syringes.

Parental drug products should be inspected visually for particulate matter and discolouration prior to administration whenever solution and container permit.

Marketing authorisation holder: Novo Nordisk A/S, Novo Alle, DK-2880 Bagsvaerd, Denmark.

Marketing authorisation numbers

NovoSeven 60 KIU	EU/1/96/006/001
NovoSeven 120 KIU	EU/1/96/006/002
NovoSeven 240 KIU	EU/1/96/006/003

Date of approval/revision of SPC December 1997.

Legal category POM.

TRISEQUENS* TRISEQUENS* FORTE

Qualitative and quantitative composition

Trisequens: 28 sequential tablets: 12 blue, 10 white, 6 red.

Active ingredients:

Blue tablets: Estradiol hemihydrate EP corresponding to estradiol 2 mg.

White tablets: Estradiol hemihydrate EP corresponding to estradiol 2 mg, Norethisterone acetate EP 1 mg.

Red tablets: Estradiol hemihydrate EP corresponding to estradiol 1 mg.

Trisequens Forte: 28 sequential tablets: 12 yellow, 10 white, 6 red.

Active ingredients:

Yellow tablets: Estradiol hemihydrate EP corresponding to estradiol 4 mg.

White tablets: Estradiol hemihydrate EP corresponding to estradiol 4 mg, Norethisterone acetate EP 1 mg.

Red tablets: Estradiol hemihydrate EP corresponding to estradiol 1 mg.

Pharmaceutical form Film-coated tablets for oral administration.

Clinical particulars

Therapeutic indications:

(a) The treatment of symptoms due to oestrogen deficiency.
(b) The prophylaxis of postmenopausal osteoporosis in women at risk of developing fractures (Trisequens only).

At present there is no established diagnostic test for determining women at risk of developing osteoporotic fractures. Epidemiological studies suggest a number of individual risk factors which contribute to the development of postmenopausal osteoporosis. These include: early menopause, family history of osteoporosis, thin, small frame, cigarette use, recent prolonged systemic cortico-steroid use.

If several of these risk factors are present in a patient, consideration should be given to oestrogen replacement therapy.

Posology and method of administration

Dosage: Adults: Menopausal symptoms and prophylaxis of osteoporosis. Trisequens and Trisequens Forte are administered orally, without chewing, one tablet daily without interruption, starting with the blue or yellow tablets respectively.

For menopausal symptoms treatment should be instituted with Trisequens. If the clinical response is unsatisfactory, Trisequens Forte may be tried. Treatment with Trisequens Forte should be replaced by Trisequens as soon as symptoms can be relieved with the lower dose.

Prophylaxis of osteoporosis: Hormone replacement therapy (HRT) has been found to be effective in the prevention of osteoporosis, especially when started soon after the menopause and used for 5 years and probably up to 10 years or more. Treatment should ideally start as soon as possible after the onset of the menopause and certainly within 2 to 3 years. Protection appears to be effective for as long as treatment is continued. However, data beyond 10 years are limited. A careful re-appraisal of the risk-benefit ratio should be undertaken before treating for longer than 5 to 10 years.

Use in the elderly: There are no special dosage requirements.

Not intended for children or males.

Administration: In menstruating women the first tablet should be taken on the fifth day of menstrual bleeding. If menstruation has stopped altogether or is infrequent and sporadic (2–4 monthly intervals) the first tablet can be taken at any time.

A regular shedding of the endometrium is usually induced during the red tablet phase or at the end of the white tablet phase.

Before initiation of therapy it is recommended that the patient is fully informed of all likely benefits and potential risks. She should have a full physical and gynaecological examination with special emphasis on blood pressure, breasts, abdominal and pelvic organs. Endometrial assessment should be carried out if indicated; this may be particularly relevant in patients who are, or who have been, treated with oestrogen unopposed by a progestogen. During long-term treatment with Trisequens or Trisequens Forte, follow-up examinations are recommended every 6–12 months.

Since progestogens are only administered to protect against hyperplastic changes of the endometrium, patients without a uterus should be treated with an oestrogen-only preparation.

Contra-indications:

1. Known, suspected or past history of cancer of the breast.
2. Known or suspected oestrogen-dependent neoplasia.
3. Undiagnosed irregular vaginal bleeding.
4. Known or suspected pregnancy.
5. Active deep venous thrombosis, thromboembolic disorders or a history of confirmed venous thromboembolism.
6. Active or chronic liver disease or history of liver disease where the liver function tests have failed to return to normal.
7. Rotor's syndrome or Dubin-Johnson syndrome.
8. Severe cardiac or renal disease.
9. Hypersensitivity to one or more of the constituents.

Special warnings and special precautions for use:

1. In the female there is an increased risk of endometrial hyperplasia and carcinoma associated with unopposed oestrogen administered long term (for more than one year). However, the appropriate addition of a progestogen to an oestrogen regimen lowers this additional risk.

2. There has been concern about the possible risk of breast cancer in oestrogen-treated women. Although many studies have failed to disclose an increased incidence of breast cancer, some have shown a small increase upon prolonged therapy (e.g. 5 years or longer). It is not known whether concurrent progestogen use influences the risk of breast cancer in post-menopausal women taking HRT. Women on long-term therapy should have regular breast examinations and should be instructed in self breast examination. Regular mammographic investigations should be conducted where considered appropriate.

There is a need for caution when prescribing oestrogens in women who have a history of, or known, breast nodules or fibrocystic disease. Breast status should be closely monitored, supported by regular mammography.

3. Certain diseases may be made worse by hormone replacement therapy and patients with these conditions should be closely monitored. These include otosclerosis, multiple sclerosis, systemic lupus erythematosus, porphyria, melanoma, epilepsy, migraine and asthma. In addition, pre-existing uterine fibroids may increase in size during oestrogen therapy and symptoms associated with endometriosis may be exacerbated.

4. Epidemiological studies have suggested that hormone replacement therapy (HRT) is associated with a higher relative risk of developing venous thromboembolism (VTE) i.e. deep vein thrombosis or pulmonary embolism. The studies find a 2–3 fold higher risk for users compared with non-users which for healthy women amounts to one extra case of VTE each year for every 5000 patients taking HRT.

Generally recognised risk factors for VTE include a personal history or family history and severe obesity (Body Mass Index >30 kg/m^2). In women with these factors the benefits of treatment with HRT need to be carefully weighed against the risks. There is no consensus about the possible role of varicose veins in VTE.

The risk of VTE may be temporarily increased with prolonged immobilisation, major trauma or major surgery. In women on HRT scrupulous attention should be given to prophylactic measures to prevent VTE following surgery. Where prolonged immobilisation is likely to follow elective surgery, particularly abdominal or orthopaedic surgery to the lower limbs, consideration should be given to temporarily stopping HRT 4 weeks earlier, if possible.

If venous thromboembolism develops after initiating therapy the drug should be discontinued.

5. Oestrogens may cause fluid retention and, therefore, patients with cardiac or renal dysfunction should be carefully observed.

6. If jaundice, migraine-like headaches, visual disturbance or a significant increase in blood pressure develop after initiating therapy, the medication should be discontinued while the cause is investigated.

7. Trisequens and Trisequens Forte are not contraceptives, neither will they restore fertility.

8. Most studies indicate that oestrogen replacement therapy has little effect on blood pressure and some indicate that oestrogen use may be associated with a small decrease in B.P. In addition, most studies on combined therapy, including Trisequens, indicate that the addition of a progestogen also has little effect on blood pressure. Rarely, idiosyncratic hypertension may occur.

However, when oestrogens are administered to hypertensive women, supervision is necessary and blood pressure should be monitored at regular intervals.

9. Diabetic patients should be carefully observed when initiating hormone replacement therapy, as worsening glucose tolerance may occur.

10. Changed oestrogen levels may affect certain endocrine and liver function tests.

11. It has been reported that there is an increase in the risk of surgically confirmed gall bladder disease in women receiving postmenopausal oestrogens.

12. If abnormal or irregular vaginal bleeding occurs during or shortly after therapy, diagnostic measures, including endometrial sampling when indicated, should be undertaken to rule out the possibility of uterine malignancy.

Interaction with other medicaments and other forms of interaction: May potentiate side effects of phenothiazines. Drugs such as barbiturates, phenytoin and rifampicin, which induce the activity of hepatic microsomal drug metabolising enzymes, may decrease the effectiveness of Trisequens and Trisequens Forte. Mineral oil may decrease the intestinal absorption of Trisequens and Trisequens Forte.

Pregnancy and Lactation: Trisequens and Trisequens Forte are contra-indicated during pregnancy and lactation.

Effects on ability to drive and use machines: No effects known.

Undesirable effects: The following side effects have been reported with oestrogen/progestogen therapy:

1. Genitourinary system: irregular vaginal bleeding, pre-menstrual-like syndrome, increase in size of uterine fibromyomata.
2. Breasts - tenderness, enlargement, secretion.
3. Gastrointestinal - nausea, vomiting, abdominal cramps, bloating, cholestatic jaundice.
4. Skin - chloasma or melasma which may persist when drug is discontinued, erythema multiforme, erythema nodosum, haemorrhagic eruption, loss of scalp hair, hirsutism.
5. Eyes - steepening of corneal curvature, intolerance to contact lenses.
6. CNS - headaches, migraine, dizziness, mental depression, chorea.
7. Miscellaneous - increase or decrease in weight, reduced carbohydrate tolerance, aggravation of porphyria, oedema, change in libido, leg cramps.

Overdose: Overdosage may be manifested by nausea and vomiting. There is no specific antidote and treatment should be symptomatic.

Pharmacological properties
Pharmacodynamic properties: The oestrogen component of Trisequens and Trisequens Forte substitutes for the loss of endogenous oestrogen production which occurs in women around the time of the menopause, whilst the progestogen component counteracts hyperstimulation of the endometrium. A regular shedding of the endometrium is usually induced during the red tablet phase or at the end of the white tablet phase.

Studies based on measurement of bone mineral content have shown that Trisequens is effective in the prevention of progressive bone loss following the menopause.

During treatment with Trisequens total cholesterol and LDL-C are lowered significantly whereas HDL-C and triglycerides are unchanged.

Pharmacokinetic properties: The micronised 17β-estradiol in Trisequens and Trisequens Forte is absorbed rapidly and efficiently from the gastrointestinal tract, reaching a peak plasma concentration in 2–4 hours. Following administration of Trisequens, the steady state plasma level of estradiol ranges from between 70–100 pg/ml. Estradiol has a half life of approximately 14–16 hours. In the blood stream more than 90% of estradiol is bound to plasma proteins. Estradiol is oxidized to oestrone, which is coverted to oestriol. Both transformations take place mainly in the liver. Oestrogens are excreted into the bile and then undergo reabsorption from the intestine. During this enterohepatic circulation, degradation occurs. Estradiol and its metabolites are excreted either in the urine (90–95%) as biologically inactive glucuronide and sulphate conjugates or in the faeces (5–10%) mostly unconjugated.

Norethisterone acetate is rapidly absorbed and transformed to norethisterone, then metabolised and excreted as glucuronide and sulphate conjugates. About half the dose is recovered in the urine within 24 hours, the remainder being reduced to less than 1% of the dose within 5–6 days. The mean plasma half life is 3–6 hours.

Pharmaceutical particulars
List of excipients: Lactose monohydrate; maize starch; gelatin; talc; magnesium stearate; methyl hydroxypropyl cellulose; purified water.

Blue tablets: Indigo carmine (E132); titanium dioxide (E171); polyethylene glycol

Yellow tablets: Iron oxide (E172); titanium dioxide (E171); propylene glycol.

White tablets: Triacetin.

Red tablets: Iron oxide (E172); titanium dioxide (E171); propylene glycol.

Incompatibilities: None known.

Shelf life: 48 months.

Special precautions for storage: Store in a dry place, protected from light. Store below 25°C. Do not refrigerate.

Nature and contents of container: Polypropylene/polystyrene calendar dial pack containing 28 tablets. Calendar dial packs (3×28 tablets) are contained within outer carton.

Instructions for use/handling: Each carton contains a patient information leaflet with instructions for use of the calendar dial pack.

Marketing authorisation number
Trisequens: PL3132/0122.
Trisequens Forte: PL3132/0123.

Date of first authorisation/renewal 29 January 1998.

Date of (partial) revision of the text February 1998.

Legal category POM.

VAGIFEM*

Qualitative and quantitative composition Active ingredient, Oestradiol 25 micrograms.

Pharmaceutical form Film-coated vaginal tablet inset in disposable applicator.

Clinical particulars
Therapeutic indications: The treatment of atrophic vaginitis due to oestrogen deficiency.

Posology and method of administration
Dosage: Vagifem is administered intravaginally using the applicator. An initial dose of 1 tablet daily for two weeks will usually improve vaginal atrophy and associated symptoms; a maintenance dose of 2 tablets per week may then be instituted. Treatment should be discontinued after about 3 months to assess whether further therapy is necessary.

Not intended for children or males.

Use in the elderly: there are no special dosage requirements.

Administration: The applicator is inserted into the vagina up to the end of the smooth part of the applicator (approximately 9 cms). The tablet is released by pressing the plunger. The applicator is then withdrawn and disposed of.

Contra-indications:
1. Known, suspected, or past history of carcinoma of the breast.
2. Known or suspected oestrogen-dependent neoplasia, e.g. endometrial carcinoma or other hormone-dependent tumours.
3. Abnormal genital bleeding of unknown aetiology.
4. Acute thrombophlebitis or thromboembolic disorders, or a past history of these conditions associated with previous oestrogen use.

Special warnings and special precautions for use: Although the dose of oestradiol is low and the treatment is local, a minor degree of systemic absorption may occur. Because of this, the increased risk of endometrial cancer after treatment with unopposed oestrogens should be kept in mind. Endometrial hyperplasia (atypical or adenomatous) often precedes endometrial cancer.

Patients with the following conditions who are treated with Vagifem should be monitored more frequently and if any of the conditions worsen Vagifem treatment should be withdrawn:

- Acute or chronic liver disease or history of liver disease where the liver function tests have failed to return to normal.
- Thrombophlebitis, thromboembolic disorders or cerebro vascular accident, or a past history of these disorders.
- Haemoglobinopathies or sickle cell anaemia.
- Porphyria.
- Epilepsy.
- Migraine.
- Diabetes.
- Asthma.
- Cardiac dysfunction.
- Hypertension requiring treatment.

Before initiation of therapy with Vagifem, it is advisable to undertake a thorough examination to exclude any possibility of genital or mammary tumours. Vaginal infections should be treated before initiation of Vagifem therapy.

Persistent or recurring vaginal bleeding should be investigated.

The present bulk of evidence shows that oestrogens given to post-menopausal women do not increase the risk of breast cancer.

Interactions with other medicaments and other forms of interaction: Not applicable due to the low systemic absorption.

Pregnancy and lactation: Vagifem is contra-indicated in pregnant women.

Effects on ability to drive and to use machines: No effects known.

Undesirable effects: Few side-effects have been observed. Slight vaginal bleeding, vaginal discharge and skin rash have rarely been reported.

Overdose: Vagifem is intended for intravaginal use. The dose of oestradiol is so low that a considerable number of tablets would have to be ingested to approach a significant dose.

Pharmacological properties
Pharmacodynamic properties: 17-β oestradiol is the principal and most active of the naturally occurring human oestrogens. It has pharmacological actions in common with all oestrogenic compounds. The action on the vagina is to increase maturation of vaginal epithelial cells and increase cervical secretory activity.

Pharmacokinetic properties: Oestrogens are well absorbed from the vagina. After treatment with Vagifem, marginal elevations of plasma oestradiol and conjugated oestrogens as well as suppression of pituitary gonadotrophins have been observed. This indicates that there is an absorption of the oestradiol. This absorption is, however, low and no other systemic oestrogen effect could be determined.

Pharmaceutical particulars
List of excipients: Methyl hydroxypropyl cellulose (E464), lactose, maize starch, magnesium stearate, polyethylene glycol 6000, purified water.

Incompatibilities: None known.

Shelf life: 36 months.

Special precautions for storage: Store in a dry place, protect from light. Store below 25°C. Do not refrigerate.

Nature and contents of container: Laminated bubble strips containing 5 applicators with inset tablet. Packed in cartons containing 3 strips (15 tablets and applicators).

Instructions for use/handling: Each carton contains a patient information leaflet with instructions for use.

Marketing authorisation holder: Novo Nordisk A/S, Novo Alle, DK-2880 Bagsvaerd, Denmark.

Marketing authorisation number 4668/0026.

Date of approval/revision of SPC August 1995.

Legal category POM.

**Trade Mark*

Nycomed Amersham Plc

Amersham Place
Little Chalfont
Buckinghamshire
HP7 9NA

☎ 01494 544000 Fax 01494 543588

ABDOSCAN*

Qualitative and quantitative composition Granules for Oral Suspension 23.4 mg Fe/sachet.

One sachet contains: Ferristene (USAN) 100 mg, equivalent to 23.4 mg Fe.

Ferristene (USAN) = Iron ferrite with carrier particles.

The carrier particles are monosized spheres of polystyrenesulphonate.

The product is a superparamagnetic MRI-contrast medium for oral use.

Pharmaceutical form Granules for Oral Suspension.

The product is dark brown to grey granules, delivered in sachets (containing 6 grams). The contents of each sachet should be mixed with 200 ml water before use.

Clinical particulars

Indications: Oral contrast medium for diagnostic magnetic resonance imaging (MRI) in adults with suspected or known abdominal pathology.

For labelling of the bowel during MRI-assessment of masses in abdomen, pelvis and retroperitoneum, e.g. in pancreatic disease, enlarged lymph nodes and tumours.

Posology and method of administration: The patient should be fasting from approximately 4 hours prior to contrast medium intake.

The contents of each sachet should be mixed with 200 ml of drinking water. Scanning should be started immediately after the contents of the last sachet have been ingested.

Dosage for adults:

Complete abdomen: 4 sachets are needed for each investigation.

The contents of one sachet should be ingested every 30-40 minutes, starting 2 hours prior to imaging.

Upper abdomen: 2 sachets are needed for each investigation.

The contents of each sachet should be ingested with an interval of 30 minutes prior to imaging.

Children: Safety and efficacy in patients below the age of 18 have not been established.

Contra-indications: ABDOSCAN should not be used in patients with:

- Phenylketonuria (because of the aspartame content)
- Suspected or known perforation of the GI-tract or intestinal obstruction

Special warnings and special precautions for use: The administration of ABDOSCAN to patients below the age of 18 has not yet been investigated.

Care should be exercised in patients with:

- severe nausea and vomiting
- colitis, Crohn's disease, fistula in the GI-tract
- known or suspected GI-damage due to radiation therapy.

Interaction with other medicaments and other forms of interaction: None known.

Pregnancy and lactation: The safety of ABDOSCAN during pregnancy and lactation has not been demonstrated clinically. However, due to the fact that essentially no absorption of ABDOSCAN from the gastrointestinal tract has been found, it is unlikely therefore that there would be any foetal transfer. However, the product should only be used during pregnancy if an MR-investigation is essential.

Similarly, during lactation, transfer of ABDOSCAN to the breast fed infant is unlikely.

No specific precautions during lactation apply.

Effects on ability to drive and use machines: None known.

Undesirable effects: The reported adverse events are mainly gastrointestinal disturbances such as nausea, vomiting, constipation or loose stools. The events have predominantly been of mild or moderate intensity.

No serious adverse events have been reported from the clinical trials.

Overdose: Overdosage is unlikely to occur as there is essentially no absorption of the product and also due to the consistency of the suspension and the relatively large volume of the normal dose. Oral intake of the dry powder is disagreeable, and accidental ingestion of significant amounts by children is not likely to occur. Should intake of product at doses higher than the recommended actually take place, treatment is symptomatic.

Pharmacological properties

Pharmacodynamic properties: The product is a superparamagnetic contrast agent for oral use in MRI of the abdomen. ABDOSCAN consists of small crystals of magnetic iron oxide deposited on the surfaces of monosized polymer particles. The use of ABDOSCAN is based on the ability of the magnetic material to disturb or create inhomogeneities in the magnetic field and thereby reduce the relaxation time T_2* of the water protons. Signals from the gastrointestinal tract filled with ABDOSCAN will be reduced and the gut will turn black in the MR-image (negative contrast). The differentiation of the bowel and other organs in the abdomen will be improved, thus facilitating the identification of abdominal pathology.

Pharmacokinetic properties: Essentially no absorption of the product has been found in the preclinical animal studies or in the pharmacokinetic study in human volunteers.

The product is excreted in the faeces.

Preclinical safety data: None of the animals died after the acute toxicity studies/administration of the maximal possible dose (9.6 g/kg, mouse).

There are no findings in the preclinical studies which identify any requirement regarding warnings for safe use of the product in humans.

Pharmaceutical particulars

List of excipients: The excipients of ABDOSCAN are: Microcrystalline cellulose and carboxymethyl-cellulose sodium (Avicel), Maize starch, Xanthan gum, Polyvidone, Methylhydroxypropylcellulose, Talc, Aspartame.

The excipients give an increased viscosity and ensure that the particles of the active ingredient in the suspension are well dispersed in the GI-tract.

Incompatibilities: None known.

Shelf life: The shelf life is 24 months.[1]

[1] Text in the package leaflet: The expiry date is stated on the label.

Special precautions for storage: No special storage temperature required. The reconstituted product may be stored for up to 6 hours at +2–+8°C.

Nature and content of container: The product is supplied in sachets made from an aluminium-plastic laminate. Each sachet contains 6 grams of granules corresponding to 23.4 mg Fe.

The product is supplied as: Cardboard boxes with 20 sachets of 6 grams.

Instructions for use/handling: The contents of each sachet should be mixed with 200 ml of drinking water immediately before ingestion.

Reconstitution of granules in the sachet: Use a graduated mixing beaker with some shaking volume.

Add the content of one sachet by sprinkling it into 200 ml of water. Put on the lid and shake well until the granules are evenly suspended (a few seconds). If the suspension is not used immediately, shake again before administration.

Marketing authorisation holder: NYCOMED IMAGING AS, Nycoveien 1-2, P.O. Box 4220 Torshov, N-0401 OSLO, NORWAY.

Marketing authorisation number
UK: PL 0637/0022

Legal Category POM

Date of first authorisation 26 January 1994 in UK

CERETEC*

Kit for the preparation of Technetium [^{99m}Tc] Exametazime Injection

Qualitative and quantitative composition Exametazime 0.5 mg.

Pharmaceutical form Powder for injection.

Clinical particulars

Indications:

(i) Technetium [^{99m}Tc] Exametazime Injection is indicated for brain scintigraphy. The product is to be used for the diagnosis of abnormalities of regional cerebral blood flow, such as those occurring following stroke and other cerebrovascular disease, epilepsy, Alzheimer's Disease and other forms of dementia, transient ischaemic attack, migraine and tumours of the brain.

(ii) Technetium [^{99m}Tc] Exametazime Injection is also indicated for *in vitro* technetium-99 m leucocyte labelling, the labelled leucocytes subsequently being re-injected and scintigraphy carried out to image the sites of localisation. This procedure may be used in the detection of sites of focal infection (e.g. abdominal abscess), in the investigation of pyrexia of unknown origin and in the evaluation of inflammatory conditions not associated with infection such as inflammatory bowel disease.

Posology and method of administration: The route of administration is direct intravenous injection for brain scintigraphy studies and intravenous injection of labelled leucocytes post labelling *in vitro*.

Dose for adults and the elderly:

(i) for brain scintigraphy, 350–500 MBq

(ii) for *in vivo* localisation of technetium-99 m-labelled leucocytes, 200 MBq

Normally a once-only diagnostic procedure

Technetium [^{99m}Tc]-Exametazime and Technetium-99 m-labelled leucocytes are not recommended for administration to children.

Contra-indications: There are no specific contra-indications.

Special warnings and precautions for use: Radiopharmaceutical agents should only be used by qualified personnel with the appropriate government authorisation for the use and manipulation of radionuclides. They may be received, used and administered only by authorised persons in designated clinical settings. Their receipt, storage, use, transfer and disposal are subject to the regulations and/or appropriate licences of the local competent official organisations.

Radiopharmaceuticals should be prepared by the user in a manner which satisfies both radiation safety and pharmaceutical quality requirements. Appropriate aseptic precautions should be taken, complying with the requirements of Good Manufacturing Practice for pharmaceuticals. Normal safety precautions for the handling of blood products should be observed in the preparation and administration of labelled leucocytes.

When preparing technetium-99 m-labelled leucocytes it is essential that cells are washed free of sedimentation agents before they are re-injected into the patient as materials used in cell separation may cause hypersensitivity reactions.

Interaction with other medicaments and other forms of interaction: No drug interactions have been reported to date.

Pregnancy and lactation: No data are available on the use of this product in human pregnancy. Animal reproduction studies have not been performed.

When it is necessary to administer radioactive medicinal products to women of childbearing potential, information should always be sought about pregnancy. Any woman who has missed a period should be assumed to be pregnant until proven otherwise. Where uncertainty exists it is important that radiation exposure should be the minimum consistent with achieving the desired clinical information. Alternative techniques which do not involve ionising radiation should be considered. Radionuclide procedures carried out on pregnant women also involve radiation doses to the foetus. Only imperative investigations should be carried out during pregnancy, when the likely benefit exceeds the risk incurred by the mother and the foetus.

Before administering a radioactive medicinal product to a mother who is breast feeding consideration should be given as to whether the investigation could be reasonably delayed until after the mother has ceased breast feeding and as to whether the most appropriate choice of radiopharmaceutical has been made, bearing in mind the secretion of activity in breast milk. If the administration is considered necessary, breast feeding should be interrupted for 12 hours and the expressed feeds discarded. Breast feeding can be restarted when the level in the milk will not result in a radiation dose to the child greater than 1 mSv.

Effects on ability to drive and use machines: No effects on the ability to drive or to operate machines have been reported to date.

Undesirable effects: A very few cases of mild hypersensitivity evidenced by the development of an urticarial erythematous rash have been reported following direct intravenous injection of the reconstituted product. A very few reports have also been received of hypersensitivity reactions, possibly anaphylactic in nature, following administration of technetium-99 m-labelled leucocytes prepared using Technetium [^{99m}Tc]-exametazime.

For each patient, exposure to ionising radiation must be justifiable on the basis of likely benefit. The activity administered must be such that the resulting radiation dose is as low as reasonably achievable bearing in mind the need to obtain the intended diagnostic result.

Exposure to ionising radiation is linked with cancer induction and a potential for development of hereditary defects. For diagnostic nuclear medicine investigations the current evidence suggests that these adverse effects will occur with low frequency because of the low radiation doses incurred.

For most diagnostic investigations using a nuclear medicine procedure the radiation dose (EDE) is less than 20 mSv. Higher doses may be justified in some clinical circumstances.

Overdose: In the event of the administration of a radiation overdose frequent micturition and defecation should be encouraged in order to minimise the absorbed dose to patient.

Pharmacological properties

Pharmacodynamic properties: At the chemical concentrations and activities used for diagnostic procedures technetium [^{99m}Tc]-exametazime and technetium-99 m-labelled leucocytes do not appear to exert any pharmacodynamic effects.

Pharmacokinetic properties:

(i) Direct intravenous injection

The technetium-99 m complex of the active ingredient is uncharged, lipophilic and of sufficiently low molecular weight to cross the blood-brain barrier. It is rapidly cleared from the blood after intravenous injection. Uptake in the brain reaches a maximum of 3.5-7.0% of the injected dose within one minute of injection. Up to 15% of the cerebral activity washes out of the brain 2 minutes post injection after which there is little loss of activity for the following 24 hours except by physical decay of technetium-99 m. The activity not associated with the brain is widely distributed throughout the body particularly in muscle and soft tissue. About 20% of the injected dose is removed by the liver immediately after injection and excreted through the hepatobiliary system. About 40% of the injected dose is excreted through the kidneys and urine over the 48 hours after injection resulting in a reduction in general muscle and soft tissue background.

(ii) Injection of labelled leucocytes

Technetium-99 m-labelled leucocytes distribute between the marginating pools of the liver (within 5 minutes) and spleen (within about 40 minutes), and the circulating pool, (the latter represents approximately 50% of the leucocyte pool). Approximately 37% of the cell associated technetium-99 m is recoverable from the circulating pool 40 minutes after injection. Technetium-99 m activity is slowly eluted from the cells and is excreted partly by the kidneys and partly via the liver into the gall bladder. This results in increasing amounts of activity being seen in the intestines.

Preclinical Safety Data There are no additional preclinical safety data of relevance for the prescriber in recognising the safety profile of the product used for the authorised indications.

Radiation dosimetry data: Technetium-99 m disintegrates with the emission of gamma radiation with an energy of 140 keV and a half-life of 6 hours to technetium-99 which can be regarded as quasi-stable.

(i) Brain scintigraphy

According to ICRP 62 (International Commission on Radiological Protection) the estimated absorbed radiation doses to various organs following administration of technetium [^{99m}Tc]-exametazime to adults are in the table below:

Organ	*Absorbed dose per unit activity administered (mGy/MBq[1]) Adult*
Adrenals	5.3E–03
Bladder	2.3E–02
Bone surfaces	5.1E–03
Brain	6.8E–03
Breast	2.0E–03
Gall bladder	1.8E–02
GI tract	
Stomach	6.4E–03
SI	1.2E–02
ULI	1.8E–02
LLI	1.5E–02
Heart	3.7E–03
Kidneys	3.4E–02
Liver	8.6E–03
Lungs	1.1E–02
Muscles	2.8E–03
Oesophagus	2.6E–03
Ovaries	6.6E–03
Pancreas	5.1E–03
Red marrow	3.4E–03
Skin	1.6E–03
Spleen	4.3E–03
Testes	2.4E–03
Thymus	2.6E–03
Thyroid	2.6E–02
Uterus	6.6E–03
Remaining organs	3.2E–03
Effective dose equivalent (mSv/MBq)	1.1E–02

[1] Effective Dose (E) is 4.7 mSv/500 MBq (70 kg individual).

(ii) *In vivo* localisation of technetium-99 m-labelled leucocytes

The estimated absorbed radiation doses to various organs following the intravenous administration of technetium-99 m-labelled leucocytes to adults given by ICRP 53 are in the table below:

Organ	*Absorbed dose per unit activity administered (mGy/MBq[2]) Adult*
Adrenals	8.9E–03
Bladder wall	2.6E–03
Bone surfaces	1.3E–02
Breast	3.1E–03
GI tract	
Stomach wall	8.0E–03
Small intestine	4.9E–03
ULI wall	4.9E–03
LLI wall	3.9E–03
Heart	9.0E–03
Kidneys	9.9E–03
Liver	2.0E–02
Lungs	6.9E–03
Ovaries	4.2E–03
Pancreas	1.4E–02
Red marrow	2.2E–02
Spleen	1.5E–01
Testes	1.7E–03
Thyroid	2.4E–03
Uterus	3.8E–03
Other tissue	3.4E–03
Effective dose equivalent (mSv/MBq)	1.7E–02

[2] Effective Dose (E) is 2.2 mSv/200 MBq (70 kg individual).

Pharmaceutical particulars

List of excipients: The finished product contains the following excipients: Sodium chloride BP, Stannous chloride dihydrate DAB, Nitrogen gas USP

Incompatibilities: There are no known incompatibilities.

Shelf-life: The shelf-life of the product is 26 weeks from the day of manufacture. The labelled product must be injected within 30 minutes of reconstitution.

Special precautions for storage: Store the unopened product at any temperature in the range 2-25°C. Store the reconstituted product at 15-25°C. Storage should be in accordance with national regulations for radioactive materials.

Nature and contents of the container: The product is supplied in a glass vial sealed with a chlorobutyl rubber closure and metal overseal.

Instructions for use/handling: Procedure for preparation of technetium [^{99m}Tc]exametazime for intravenous injection or *in vitro* leucocyte labelling:

Use aseptic technique throughout

(i) Place the vial in a shielding container and swab the closure with the sanitising swab provided.

(ii) Using a 10 ml syringe, inject into the shielded vial 5 ml of sterile eluate from a ^{99m}Tc generator (see notes 1–6). Before withdrawing the syringe from the vial withdraw 5 ml of gas from the space above the solution to normalise the pressure in the vial. Shake the shielded vial for 10 seconds to ensure complete dissolution of the powder.

(iii) Assay the total activity and calculate the volume to be injected or used for *in vitro* technetium-99 m-leucocyte labelling.

(iv) Complete the label provided and attach to the vial.

(v) Use within a maximum of 30 minutes after reconstitution. Discard any unused material.

Note:

1. For the highest radiochemical purity reconstitute with freshly eluted ^{99m}Tc generator eluate.

2. Use only eluate which was eluted less than 2 hours previously from a generator which was eluted within 24 hours.

3. 0.37–1.11GBq (10–30 mCi) technetium-99 m may be added to the vial.

4. Before reconstitution the generator eluate may be adjusted to the correct radioactive concentration (0.37–1.11GBq in 5 ml) by dilution with saline for injection.

5. Pertechnetate complying with the specifications prescribed by the USP and BP/PhEur monographs on Sodium Pertechnetate [^{99m}Tc] Injection should be used.

6. The pH of the prepared injection/labelling agent is in the range 9.0–9.8.

Procedure for separation of leucocytes and subsequent in vitro labelling with techentium [^{99m}Tc] exametazime.

Use aseptic technique throughout.

(i) Draw 9 ml of acid-citrate-dextrose[a] into each of two 60 ml plastic non-heparinized syringes.

(ii) Withdraw 51 ml of patient's blood into each syringe, using a 19G Butterfly needle infusion set. Close the syringes with sterile hubs.

(iii) Dispense 2 ml sedimentation agent[b] into each of 5 Universal containers or tubes.

(iv) Without attaching a needle to the syringes dispense 20 ml of blood into each of the 5 Universal tubes containing sedimentation agent. Dispense the remaining 20 ml of blood into a tube without sedimentation agent.

TIP To avoid bubbles and frothing run the blood gently down the sides of the tubes.

(v) Mix the blood and sedimentation agent with one gentle inversion. Remove the cap of the Universal tube and burst the bubble formed at the top using a sterile needle. Replace the cap and allow the tubes to stand for 30–60 minutes for erythrocyte sedimentation to take place.

TIP The period of time for erythrocyte sedimentation depends on the patient's condition. As a guideline it should be stopped when the blood has sedimented to give approximately half the volume as sedimented red cells.

(vi) Meanwhile centrifuge the tube containing 20 ml of blood and no sedimentation agent at 2000 g for 10 minutes. This will yield supernatant cell-free plasma (CFP) containing ACD which is retained, at room temperature, for use as a cell labelling and re-injection medium.

(vii) When sufficient red cell sedimentation has taken place [see (v)] carefully transfer 15 ml aliquots of the cloudy straw-coloured supernatant into clean Universal tubes. Take care to avoid withdrawing any sedimented erythrocytes. The supernatant is leucocyte-rich, platelet-rich plasma [LRPRP].

TIP Do not use needles on sampling syringes to avoid unnecessary cell damage.

(viii) Centrifuge the LRPRP at 150 g for 5 minutes to give supernatant, platelet-rich plasma (PRP) and a pellet of 'mixed' leucocytes.

(ix) Remove as much of the PRP as possible into clean Universal tubes and further centrifuge at 2000 g for 10 minutes to give more supernatant, cell-free plasma (CFP) containing sedimentation agent. This will be used to wash the cells after labelling.

(x) Meanwhile loosen the pellets of 'mixed' leucocytes by *very* gently tapping and swirling the Universal tubes. Using a syringe, without an attached needle, pool all the cells into one tube then, using the same syringe, add 1 ml of cell-free plasma containing ACD (from vi) and *gently* swirl to resuspend.

(xi) Reconstitute a vial of Ceretec with 5 ml of ^{99m}Tc generator eluate containing approximately 500MBq (13.5 mCi) of $^{99m}TcO_4^-$ (using the procedure described above).

(xii) *Immediately* following reconstitution add 4 ml of the resulting technetium [^{99m}Tc] exametazime solution to the 'mixed' leucocytes in CFP (from x).

(xiii) *Gently* swirl to mix and incubate for 10 minutes at room temperature.

(xiv) If required, immediately spot the chromatography strips for assessment of radiochemical purity of the technetium [^{99m}Tc] exametazime, as instructed overleaf.

(xv) On completion of incubation *carefully* add 10 ml of CFP containing sedimentation agent (from ix) to the cells, in order to stop labelling. Gently invert the cells to mix.

(xvi) Centrifuge at 150 g for 5 minutes.

(xvii) Remove and retain all of the supernatant.

TIP It is critical that all the supernatant which contains unbound technetium [^{99m}Tc] exametazime is removed at this stage. This can be best achieved using a syringe with a wide-bore [19G] needle.

(xviii) Gently resuspend the technetium-99 m labelled mixed leucocyte preparation in 5-10 ml of CFP containing ACD from (vi). Gently swirl to mix.

(xix) Measure the radioactivity in the cells and in the supernatant from (xvii). Calculate the labelling efficiency [LE] which is defined as the activity in the cells as a percentage of the sum of the activity in the cells and the activity in the supernatant.

TIP Labelling efficiency depends on the patient's leucocyte count and will vary according to the volume of the initial blood sample. Using the volumes in (ii), a LE of about 55% might be expected.

(xx) Without attaching a needle, carefully draw up the labelled cells into a plastic, non-heparinised syringe and close it with a sterile hub. Measure the radioactivity.

(xxi) Labelled cells are now ready for re-injection. This should be performed without delay.

Note:

(a) Acid-citrate-dextrose (ACD) should be made up as follows:

NIH Formula A. For 1 litre add 22 g trisodium citrate, 8 g citric acid, 22.4 g dextrose and make up to 1 litre with Water for Injections PhEur. The product should be manufactured under aseptic condition. Commercial preparations of the product are also available. The product should be stored under the conditions recommended by the manufacturer and should be used only up to the expiry date given by the manufacturer.

(b) 6% hydroxyethyl starch should be manufactured under aseptic conditions. Commercial preparations of the product are available. The product should be stored under the conditions recommended by the manufacturer and should be used only up to the expiry date given by the manufacturer.

Radiochemical purity measurement: Three potential radiochemical impurities may be present in the prepared exametazime injection. These are a secondary technetium [^{99m}Tc]-exametazime complex, free pertechnetate and reduced-hydrolysed-technetium-99 m. A combination of two chromatographic systems is necessary for the determination of the radiochemical purity of the injection.

Test samples are applied by needle approximately 2.5 cm from the bottom of two Gelman ITLC/SG strips (2.5 cm x 20 cm). The strips are then immediately placed in prepared ascending chromatography development tanks, one containing butan-2-one and the other 0.9% aq. sodium chloride (1 cm depth fresh solvent). After a 15 cm elution the strips are removed, solvent fronts marked, the strips dried and the distribution of activity determined using suitable equipment.

Interpretation of chromatograms.

System 1 (ITLC:butan-2-one(MEK))

Secondary technetium [^{99m}Tc] exametazime complex and reduced-hydrolysed-technetium remain at the origin.

Lipophilic technetium [^{99m}Tc] exametazime complex and pertechnetate migrate at Rf 0.8-1.0.

System 2 (ITLC:0.9% sodium chloride)

Lipophilic technetium [^{99m}Tc] exametazime complex, secondary technetium [^{99m}Tc] exametazime complex and reduced-hydrolysed-Tc remain at the origin.

Pertechnetate migrates at Rf 0.8-1.0.

(i) Calculate the percentage of activity due to both secondary technetium [^{99m}Tc] exametazime complex and reduced-hydrolysed-technetium[^{99m}Tc] from System 1 (A%). Calculate the percentage of activity due to pertechnetate from System 2 (B%).

(ii) The radiochemical purity (as percentage lipophilic technetium [^{99m}Tc] exametazime complex) is given by: 100-(A%+B%) where:

A% represents the level of secondary technetium [^{99m}Tc] exametazime complex plus reduced-hydrolysed technetium-99 m

B% represents the level of pertechnetate.

A radiochemical purity of at least 80% may be expected provided the test samples have been taken and analysed within 30 minutes of reconstitution.

Marketing authorisation number PL 0221/0126

Date of approval/revision of SPC October 1997

Legal category POM

METASTRON*

Qualitative and quantitative composition A solution of the active ingredient strontium-89 chloride, (150 MBq) in 4 ml water.

Physical characteristics: Strontium-89 is a pure beta emitter with an energy of 1.463 MeV and a half-life of 50.5 days.

Pharmaceutical form Sterile aqueous solution for intravenous injection.

Clinical particulars

Therapeutic Indications: Metastron is indicated as an adjunct to and as an alternative to external beam radiotherapy for the palliation of pain from bone metastases secondary to prostatic carcinoma at the stage of hormone therapy failure.

Posology and method of administration: Metastron is an aqueous solution for intravenous injection and should be used without dilution. The recommended dose is 150 MBq (4 mCi) per injection. Alternatively in particularly heavy or light framed patients a dose of 2 MBq (55 TCi)/kg 'fat-free' body weight may be used. This dosage is suitable for the elderly. Repeat administrations should not be performed within 3 months of the previous Metastron injection. Further administrations are not indicated in patients who have not responded to a previous administration of Metastron. The product is not for administration to children.

Contra-indications: Use of the product in patients with evidence of seriously compromised bone marrow, particularly low neutrophil and platelet counts, is not recommended unless the potential benefit of the treatment is considered to outweigh the risk.

Metastron should not be used as a primary treatment for cord compression secondary to spinal metastases where more rapid treatment may be necessary.

Special warnings and precautions for use: Special precautions, such as urinary catheterisation, should be taken following administration of Metastron to patients who are significantly incontinent to minimise risks of radioactive contamination. International guidelines for disposal of radioactive waste must be followed.

It is recommended that the haematology of patients should be monitored. In considering repeat administration of Metastron the patient's haematological response to his initial dose, his current platelet levels and any other evidence of marrow depletion should all be carefully considered.

A cytotoxic agent may be administered to a patient who has previously received Metastron provided that his haematological parameters are stable and within the normal range. An interval of 12 weeks is recommended between administration of the two therapies.

The expected time of onset of pain relief (10 to 20 days following Metastron administration) should be taken into account in patient management. It is not recommended that Metastron is administered to patients with very short life expectancies.

Care should be exercised in the pre-treatment assessment of the haematological status of patients who, for the same cause, have previously received extensive bone radiation and/or another injectable bone-seeking isotope.

It is important that written information concerning this treatment and the associated safety precautions are given to the patient, relatives and hospital staff. Users should refer to the accompanying Patient Information.

Interaction with other medicaments and other forms of interaction: Calcium therapy should be discontinued at least two weeks before Metastron administration.

Pregnancy and lactation: Not relevant due to indication.

Effects on ability to drive and use machines: None known.

Undesirable effects: Adverse effects may include an exacerbation of pain within the first few days of administration. In clinical trials this effect was temporary and controlled with analgesics. Some degree of haematological toxicity, including thrombocytopenia and leucopenia, is to be expected following administration of Metastron. Typically platelets will be depressed by about 30% (95% confidence limits 10–55%) compared to pre-administration levels. Because of the natural progress of their disease more severe depression of platelet levels may be observed in some patients.

Overdose: Not applicable.

Pharmacological properties

Pharmacodynamic properties: The chemical properties of strontium enable it to imitate calcium *in vivo*, rapidly localising in proliferating bone. Strontium-89 is a beta emitter (100%), with a physical half-life of 50.5 days. The range of ϑ-particles in tissue is 0.8cm.

Pharmacokinetic properties: The extent of uptake and retention of strontium-89 will depend on the metastatic involvement of the skeleton. Strontium is retained in lesions with a long biological half life compared to the physical half-life of strontium-89, whilst strontium taken up into normal bone exhibits a half life of about 14 days. The longer retention of strontium-89 in metastatic lesions enables the isotope to deliver a larger radiation dose to metastases whilst delivering a relatively small dose to bone marrow.

Strontium which is not localised in the skeleton is excreted mainly via the urine with a small amount via the faeces.

Preclinical safety data: The chemical toxicity of non-radioactive strontium chloride is well-documented and of little consequence, particularly in terms of the risk/benefit to the patient for whom this product is intended.

Radiation dosimetry: The estimated radiation doses that would be received by normal healthy adults from the intravenous administration of 1 MBq of strontium-89 are given in the table below. Data are taken from the ICRP publication 'Radiation Dose to Patients from Radiopharmaceuticals' ICRP 53.

Radiation doses to normal adults from the intravenous injection of strontium-89.

Organ	*Absorbed radiation dose mGy/MBq*
Bone surfaces	17.0
Red bone marrow	11.0
Lower large intestine wall	4.7
Bladder wall	1.3
Testes	0.78

When osseous metastases are present significantly enhanced localisation of the radiopharmaceutical will occur with correspondingly higher doses to the metastases relative to other organs.

The absorbed dose to vertebral metastases has been measured in a group of 10 patients with widely varying extends of disease*. The minimum, maximum and mean doses in this group are listed below.

* Blake, G M *et al* Strontium-89 therapy: Measurement of absorbed dose to skeletal metastases. J Nucl Med 1988; 29(4), 549-557. The effective dose equivalent (EDE) for strontium-89 is 435 mSv per 150 MBq.

Radiation dose to vertebral metastases from intravenous injection of strontium-89.

	Absorbed radiation dose mGy/MBq
Minimum	60
Maximum	610
Mean	230

Pharmaceutical particulars

List of excipients: Strontium chloride and Water for Injections PhEur.

Incompatibilities: None

Shelf Life: The shelf life of the product is 28 days post the radioactivity reference date.

Special precautions for storage: The product should be stored at room temperature.

Nature and contents of container: The product is supplied in a neutral glass vial as an aqueous solution. The vial is sealed with a PTFE coated rubber closure and metal overseal.

Instructions for use/handling: The normal precautions for handling radioactive materials should be observed.

After use, all materials associated with the preparation and administration of radiopharmaceuticals, including any unused product and its container, should be decontaminated or treated as radioactive waste and disposed of in accordance with the conditions specified by the local competent authority. Contaminated materials must be disposed of as radioactive waste via an authorised route.

Marketing authorisation number PL 0221/0127

Date of approval/revision of SPC February 1993

Legal category POM

MYOVIEW*

Kit for the preparation of Technetium [^{99m}Tc]Tetrofosmin Injection

Qualitative and quantitative composition Tetrofosmin 0.23 mg/vial.

Pharmaceutical form Lyophilisate for injection, intended for reconstitution with 4-8 ml of sterile Sodium Pertechnetate [^{99m}Tc] Injection PhEur at a radioactive concentration not exceeding 1.1 GBq/ml.

Clinical particulars

Indication: Myoview is a myocardial perfusion agent indicated as an adjunct in the diagnosis and localisation of myocardial ischaemia and/or infarction.

Posology and method of administration: For the diagnosis and localisation of myocardial ischaemia the recommended procedure involves two intravenous injections of ^{99m}Tc-tetrofosmin. For adults and the elderly 185–250 MBq is given at peak exercise, followed by 500–750 MBq given at rest approximately 4 hours later. The activity administered should be restricted to 1000 MBq in any one day.

As an adjunct in the diagnosis and localisation of myocardial infarction, one injection of ^{99m}Tc-tetrofosmin (185–250 MBq) at rest is sufficient.

Myoview is not recommended for use in children or adolescents as data are not available for these age groups.

Patients should be requested to fast overnight or to have only a light breakfast on the morning of the procedure.

Planar or preferably SPECT imaging should begin no earlier than 15 minutes post-injection. There is no evidence for significant changes in myocardial concentration or redistribution of ^{99m}Tc-tetrofosmin, therefore, images may be acquired up to at least four hours post-injection. For planar imaging the standard views (anterior, LAO 40°–45°, LAO 65°–70° and/or left lateral) should be acquired.

Contra-indications: Myoview is contraindicated in pregnancy and in patients with known hypersensitivity to tetrofosmin.

Special warnings and precautions for use: Radiopharmaceutical agents should only be used by qualified personnel with the appropriate government authorisation for the use and manipulation of radionuclides. They may be received, used and administered only by authorised persons in designated clinical settings. Their receipt, storage, use, transfer and disposal are subject to the regulations and/or appropriate licences of the local competent official organisations.

Radiopharmaceuticals should be prepared by the user in a manner which satisfies both radiation safety and pharmaceutical quality requirements. Appropriate aseptic precautions should be taken, complying with the requirements of Good Manufacturing Practice for pharmaceuticals.

Interaction with other medicaments and other forms of interaction: The interaction of Myoview with other drugs has not been systematically investigated, however no interactions were reported in clinical studies in which Myoview was administered to patients receiving comedication. Drugs which influence myocardial function and/or blood flow, e.g. beta blockers, calcium antagonists or nitrates, can lead to false negative results in diagnosis of coronary artery disease. The results of imaging studies should always, therefore, be considered in the light of current medication.

Pregnancy and lactation: Myoview is contraindicated in pregnancy. Animal reproductive toxicity studies have not been performed with this product. Radionuclide procedures carried out on pregnant women also involve radiation doses to the foetus. Administration of ^{99m}Tc-tetrofosmin at doses of 250 MBq at exercise, followed by 750 MBq at rest results in an absorbed dose to the uterus of 8.1 mGy. A radiation dose above 0.5 mGy (equivalent to that exposure from annual background radiation) would be regarded as a potential risk to the foetus.

When it is necessary to administer radioactive medicinal products to women of childbearing potential, information should always be sought about pregnancy. Any woman who has missed a period should be assumed to be pregnant until proven otherwise. Where uncertainty exists it is important that radiation exposure should be the minimum consistent with achieving the desired clinical information. Alternative techniques which do not involve ionising radiation should be considered.

Before administering a radioactive medicinal product to a mother who is breast feeding consideration should be given as to whether the investigation could be reasonably delayed until the mother has ceased breast feeding and as to whether the most appropriate choice of radiopharmaceutical has been made, bearing in mind the secretion of activity in breast milk. It is not known whether ^{99m}Tc-tetrofosmin is secreted in human milk, therefore if administration is considered necessary, formula feeding should be substituted for breast feeding for at least 12 hours.

Effects on ability to drive and use machines: None known.

Undesirable effects: No serious adverse effects have been reported following ^{99m}Tc-tetrofosmin injection. A few patients experienced a feeling of bodily warmth, vomiting (12–24 hours post-injection), a transient metallic taste, disturbance of smell or a mild burning sensation in the mouth after injection. Transient rises in white blood cell counts have been reported in a small number of patients.

For each patient, exposure to ionising radiation must be justifiable on the basis of likely benefit. The activity administered must be such that the resulting radiation dose is as low as reasonably achievable bearing in mind the need to obtain the intended diagnostic result. Exposure to ionising radiation are linked with cancer induction and a potential for development of hereditary defects. For diagnostic nuclear medicine investigations the current evidence suggests that these adverse events will occur with negligible frequency because of the low radiation dose incurred.

For most diagnostic investigations using a nuclear medicine procedure the radiation dose (EDE) delivered is less than 20 mSv. Higher doses may be justified in some clinical circumstances.

Overdose: In cases of overdosage of radioactivity frequent micturition and defaecation should be encouraged in order to minimize radiation dosage to the patient.

Pharmacological properties

Pharmacodynamic properties: Pharmacological effects are not expected following intravenous administration of reconstituted Myoview at the recommended dosage. Studies in animals have shown that myocardial uptake of ^{99m}Tc-tetrofosmin is linearly related to coronary blood flow, confirming the effectiveness of the complex as a myocardial perfusion imaging agent.

Pharmacokinetic properties: ^{99m}Tc-tetrofosmin is rapidly cleared from the blood after intravenous injection; less than 5% of the administered activity remains in whole blood at 10 minutes post-injection. Uptake in the myocardium is rapid, reaching a maximum of about 1.2% of injected dose with sufficient retention to allow imaging of the myocardium by planar or SPECT techniques from 5 minutes up to 4 hours post-administration. Background tissue clearance is rapid from lung and liver and activity is reduced in these organs following exercise, with enhanced sequestration in skeletal muscle. Approximately 66% of the injected activity is excreted within 48 hours post-injection, with approximately 40% excreted in the urine and 26% in the faeces.

Preclinical safety data: Acute toxicity studies employing Myoview at dosage levels of approximately 1050 times the maximum human single dose failed to reveal mortality or any significant signs of toxicity in rats or rabbits. In repeated dose studies some evidence of toxicity was observed in rabbits, but only at cumulative doses exceeding 10,000 times the maximum human single dose. In rats receiving these doses there was no significant evidence of toxicity. Studies on reproductive toxicity have not been conducted. Tetrofosmin showed no evidence of mutagenic potential in *in vitro* or *in vivo* mutagenicity studies. Studies to assess the carcinogenic potential of Myoview have not been performed.

Radiation dosimetry data: The estimated absorbed radiation dose to an average adult patient (70 kg) from intravenous injections of ^{99m}Tc-tetrofosmin are listed in the table below. The values are calculated assuming urinary bladder emptying at 3.5 hour intervals.

Frequent bladder emptying should be encouraged after dosing to minimise radiation exposure.

Organ	*Absorbed radiation dose (μGy/MBq)* Exercise	Rest
Gallbladder wall	33.2	48.6
Upper large intestine	20.1	30.4
Lower large intestine	15.3	22.2
Urinary bladder wall	15.6	19.3
Small intestine	12.1	17.0
Kidney	10.4	12.5
Salivary glands	8.0	11.6
Ovaries	7.9	9.6
Uterus	7.3	8.4
Bone surface	6.2	5.6
Thyroid	4.3	5.8
Pancreas	5.0	5.0
Stomach	4.6	4.6
Adrenals	4.3	4.1
Red Marrow	4.1	4.0
Heart wall	4.1	4.0
Spleen	4.1	3.8
Muscle	3.5	3.3
Testes	3.4	3.1
Liver	3.2	4.2
Thymus	3.1	2.5
Brain	2.7	2.2
Lungs	2.3	2.1
Skin	2.2	1.9
Breasts	2.2	1.8
Total body	3.8	3.7

The effective dose equivalent (EDE) resulting from the administration of doses of reconstituted Myoview of 250 MBq after exercise and 750 MBq at rest is 2.15 mSv after exercise and 8.38 mSv at rest (per 70 kg individual).

Sodium Pertechnetate [^{99m}Tc] Injection is produced by a [^{99}Mo/^{99m}Tc] generator. [^{99m}Tc] Technetium disintegrates with the emission of gamma radiation (energy 141 keV) and a half-life of 6.02 hours.

Pharmaceutical particulars

List of excipients: Stannous chloride dihydrate DAB, disodium sulphosalicylate, sodium D-gluconate, sodium hydrogen carbonate, Nitrogen gas USP.

Incompatibilities: None known, however ^{99m}Tc-tetrofosmin should not be mixed or diluted with any substance other than those recommended for reconstitution.

Shelf-life: The shelf-life of the packaged product is 26 weeks and that of the prepared injection 8 hours after reconstitution with Sodium Pertechnetate [^{99m}Tc] Injection PhEur.

Special precautions for storage: Store the product at 2–8°C before and after reconstitution.

Nature and contents of the container: The product is supplied in a clear glass vial sealed with a chlorobutyl rubber closure and metal overseal.

Instructions for use/handling: Normal safety precautions for the handling of radioactive materials should be observed in addition to the use of aseptic technique to maintain sterility of the vial contents.

Procedure for the preparation of ^{99m}Tc-tetrofosmin:

1. Place the vial in a suitable shielding container and sanitize the rubber septum with the swab provided.
2. Using a shielded, 10 ml sterile syringe, inject the required activity of Sodium Pertechnetate [^{99m}Tc] Injection PhEur (appropriately diluted with 0.9% Sodium Chloride Injection BP) into the shielded vial (see Notes 1 and 2). Before removing the syringe from the vial, withdraw a volume of gas from above the solution equal to the volume of eluate added, to normalise the pressure inside the vial. Shake the vial to ensure complete dissolution of the powder.
3. Incubate at room temperature for 15 minutes.
4. During this time assay the total activity, complete the user label provided and attach it to the vial.
5. Store the reconstituted injection at 2–8°C and use within 8 hours of preparation. Dispose of any unused material and its container via an authorised route.

Notes:

1. The Sodium Pertechnetate [^{99m}Tc] Injection PhEur used for reconstitution should contain less than 5ppm aluminium.
2. The volume of diluted Sodium Pertechnetate [^{99m}Tc] Injection PhEur added to the vial must be in the range 4–8 ml.
3. The radioactive concentration of the diluted Sodium Pertechnetate [^{99m}Tc] Injection PhEur must not exceed 1.1 GBq/ml when it is added to the vial.
4. The pH of the prepared injection is in the range 7.5–9.0.

Radiochemical purity measurement: Radiochemical purity may be checked according to the following procedure:

Equipment and eluent:

1. Gelman ITLC/SG strip (2 cm x 20 cm)
2. Ascending chromatography tank and cover
3. 35:65 v/v mixture of acetone and dichloromethane
4. 1 ml syringe with 22–25G needle
5. Suitable counting equipment

Method:

1. Pour the 35:65 acetone:dichloromethane mixture into the chromatography tank to a depth of 1cm and cover the tank to allow the solvent vapour to equilibrate.
2. Mark an ITLC/SG strip with a pencil line at 3 cm from the bottom and, using an ink marker pen, at 15 cm from the pencil line. The pencil line indicates the origin where the sample is to be applied and movement of colour from the ink line will indicate the position of the solvent front when upward elution should be stopped.
3. Cutting positions at 3 cm and 12 cm above the origin (Rf's 0.2 and 0.8 respectively) should also be marked in pencil.
4. Using a 1 ml syringe and needle, apply a 10–20 μl sample of the prepared injection at the origin of the strip. Do not allow the spot to dry. Place the strip in the chromatography tank immediately and replace the cover. Ensure that the strip is not adhering to the walls of the tank.

Note: A 10–20 μl sample will produce a spot with a diameter of 7–10 mm. Smaller sample volumes have been shown to give unreliable radiochemical purity values.

5. When the solvent reaches the ink line, remove the strip from the tank and allow it to dry.
6. Cut the strip into 3 pieces at the marked cutting positions and measure the activity on each using suitable counting equipment. Try to ensure similar counting geometry for each piece and minimize equipment dead time losses.
7. Calculate the radiochemical purity from:-

% ^{99m}Tc-tetrofosmin

$$= \frac{\text{Activity of centre piece}}{\text{Total activity of all 3 pieces}} \times 100$$

Note: Free [^{99m}Tc] pertechnetate runs to the top piece of the strip. ^{99m}Tc-tetrofosmin runs to the centre piece of the strip. Reduced hydrolysed-^{99m}Tc and any hydrophilic complex impurities remain at the origin in the bottom piece of the strip.

Do not use material if the radiochemical purity is less than 90%.

Marketing authorisation number PL 00221/0128

Date of approval/revision of SPC October 1997

Legal category POM

OMNIPAQUE*

Qualitative and quantitative composition

Active ingredient: Iohexol (INN)[1]

Strength	Content per. ml.
140 mg I/ml	302 mg equiv. 140 mg I
180 mg I/ml	388 mg equiv. 180 mg I
240 mg I/ml	518 mg equiv. 240 mg I
300 mg I/ml	647 mg equiv. 300 mg I
350 mg I/ml	755 mg equiv. 350 mg I

[1] Iohexol is a non-ionic, monomeric, triiodinated, water-soluble X-ray contrast medium. Omnipaque in the concentration of 140 mg I/ml is isotonic with blood and tissue fluid.

The osmolality and viscosity values of Omnipaque are as follows:

Concentration	Osmolality[2] Osm/kg H_2O	Viscosity (mPa·s)	
	37°C	20°C	37°C
140 mg I/ml	0.29	2.3	1.5
180 mg I/ml	0.36	3.2	2.0
240 mg I/ml	0.51	5.6	3.3
300 mg I/ml	0.64	11.6	6.1
350 mg I/ml	0.78	23.3	10.6

[2] In aqueous solutions of iohexol.

Pharmaceutical form Solution for injection.

Clinical particulars

Indications: X-ray contrast medium for use in adults and children for urography, phlebography, i.v. DSA, CT, arteriography, cardioangiography and i.a. DSA. Myelography. For use in body cavities: Arthrography, ERP/ERCP, herniography, hysterosalpingography, sialography and use in the G-I tract.

Posology and method of administration: The dosage depends on the type of investigation and the technique used. Usually the same iodine concentration and volume is used as for other iodinated X-ray contrast media in current use.

Adequate hydration should be assured before and after administration as for other contrast media.

The product is for intravenous, intra-arterial and intrathecal use, and use in body cavities.

The following dosages may serve as a guide:

Guidelines for Intravenous use.

Indication	Concentration	Volume	Comments
Urography			
adults:	300 mg I/ml or 350 mg I/ml	40–80 ml 40–80 ml	
children <7 kg:	240 mg I/ml or 300 mg I/ml	4 ml/kg 3 ml/kg	
children >7 kg:	240 mg I/ml or 300 mg I/ml	3 ml/kg 2 ml/kg	
Phlebography (leg)	240 mg I/ml or 300 mg I/ml	20–100 ml/leg	
Digital subtraction angiography, intravenous.			
adults:	140 mg I/ml	up to 3 ml per kg body weight	
	300 mg I/ml or 350 mg I/ml	20–60 ml/inj. 20–60 ml/inj.	
children:	140 mg I/ml	dependent upon age, weight and pathology	
CT-enhancement			
adults:	140 mg I/ml or 240 mg I/ml or 300 mg I/ml or 350 mg I/ml	100–400 ml 100–250 ml 100–200 ml 100–150 ml	

Guidelines for Intra-arterial use

Indication	Concentration	Volume	Comments
Arteriographies			
arch aortography	300 mg I/ml	30–40 ml/inj.	
selective cerebral	300 mg I/ml	5–10 ml/inj.	
aortography	350 mg I/ml	40–60 ml/inj.	
femoral	300 mg I/ml or 350 mg I/ml	30–50 ml/inj.	
other	300 mg I/ml	depending on type of examination	
Cardioangiography			
adults:			
left ventricle and aortic root inj.	350 mg I/ml	30–60 ml/inj.	
selective coronary arteriography	350 mg I/ml	4–8 ml/inj.	
children:	300 mg I/ml or 350 mg I/ml	depending on age, weight and pathology (max 8 ml/kg)	
Digital subtraction angiography, intra-arterial			
adults:	140 mg I/ml or 240 mg I/ml or 300 mg I/ml	4–10 ml/inj. 1–15 ml/inj. 1–15 ml/inj.	
children:	140 mg I/ml	dependent on age, weight and pathology	

Contra-indications: Manifest thyrotoxicosis. History of serious reaction to Omnipaque.

Special warnings and special precautions for use: Special precautions for use of non-ionic monomeric contrast media in general: A positive history of allergy, asthma, or untoward reactions to iodinated contrast media indicates a need for special caution. Premedication with corticosteroids or histamine H_1 and H_2 antagonists might be considered in these cases.

The risk of serious reactions in connection with use of Omnipaque is regarded as minor. However, iodinated contrast media may provoke anaphylactoid reactions or other manifestations of hypersensitivity. A course of action should therefore be planned in advance, with necessary drugs and equipment available for immediate treatment, should a serious reaction occur. It is advisable always to use an indwelling cannula or catheter for quick intravenous access throughout the entire X-ray procedure.

When performing vascular catheterisation procedures one should pay meticulous attention to the angiographic technique and flush the catheter frequently (e.g.: with heparinised saline) so as to minimize the risk of procedure-related thrombosis and embolism.

Adequate hydration should be assured before and after contrast media administration. This applies especially to patients with multiple myeloma, diabetes mellitus, renal dysfunction, as well as to infants, small children and elderly patients. Young infants (age < 1 year) and especially neonates are susceptible to electrolyte disturbance and haemodynamic alterations.

Care should also be taken in patients with serious cardiac disease and pulmonary hypertension as they may develop haemodynamic changes or arrhythmias.

Patients with acute cerebral pathology, tumours or a history of epilepsy are predisposed for seizures and merit particular care. Also alcoholics and drug addicts have an increased risk for seizures and neurological reactions. A few patients have experienced a temporary hearing loss or even deafness after myelography, which is believed to be due to a drop in spinal fluid pressure by the lumbar puncture per se.

To prevent acute renal failure following contrast media administration, special care should be exercised in patients with preexisting renal impairment and diabetes mellitus as they are at risk. Patients with paraproteinemias (myelomatosis and Waldenström's macroglobulinemia) are also at risk.

Preventive measures include:

- Identification of high risk patients
- Ensuring adequate hydration. If necessary by maintaining an i.v. infusion from before the procedure until the contrast medium has been cleared by the kidneys.
- Avoiding additional strain on the kidneys in the form of nephrotoxic drugs, oral cholecystographic agents, arterial clamping, renal arterial angioplasty, or major surgery, until the contrast medium has been cleared.
- Postponing a repeat contrast medium examination until renal function returns to pre-examination levels.

Particular care is required in patients with severe disturbance of both renal and hepatic function as they may have significantly delayed contrast medium clearance. Patients on haemodialysis may receive contrast media for radiological procedures provided dialysis is performed immediately afterwards.

The administration of iodinated contrast media may aggravate the symptoms of myasthenia gravis. In patients with phaeochromocytoma undergoing interventional procedures, alpha blockers should be given as prophylaxis to avoid a hypertensive crisis. Special care should be exercised in patients with hyperthyroidism. Patients with multinodular goiter may be at risk of developing hyperthyroidism following injection of iodinated contrast media. One should also be aware of the possibility of inducing transient hypothyroidism in premature infants receiving contrast media.

Extravasation of contrast media occurs rarely and gives local pain and oedema, which usually recedes without sequela.However, inflammation and even tissue necrosis have been seen. Elevating and cooling the affected site is recommended as routine measures. Surgical decompression may be necessary in cases of compartment syndrome.

Observation time: After contrast medium administration the patient should be observed for at least 30 minutes, since the majority of serious side effects occurs within this time. However, delayed reactions may occur.

Intrathecal use: Following myelography the patient should rest with the head and thorax elevated by 20° for one hour. Thereafter he/she may ambulate carefully but bending down must be avoided. The head and thorax should be kept elevated for the first 6 hours if remaining in bed. Patients suspected of having a low seizure threshold should be observed during this period. Outpatients should not be completely alone for the first 24 hours.

Interaction with other medicaments and other forms of interaction: Use of contrast media may result in a transient impairment of renal function and this may precipitate lactic acidosis in diabetics who are taking biguanides (metformine). As a precaution, biguanides should be stopped 48 hours prior to the contrast medium examination and reinstated only after renal function has stabilized.

Patients treated with interleukin-2 less than two weeks previously have been associated with an increased risk for delayed reactions (flu-like symptoms or skin reactions).

All iodinated contrast media may interfere with tests on thyroid function, thus the iodine binding capacity of the thyroid may be reduced for up to several weeks.

High concentrations of contrast media in serum and urine can interfere with laboratory tests for bilirubin, proteins or inorganic substances (e.g. iron, copper, calcium and phosphate). These substances should therefore not be assayed on the day of examination.

Guidelines for Intrathecal use.

Indication	*Concentration*	*Volume*	*Comments*
Lumbar and thoracic myelography	180 mg I/ml or 240 mg I/ml	10–15 ml 8–12 ml	
Cervical myelography (lumbar injection)	240 mg I/ml or 300 mg I/ml	10–12 ml 7–10 ml	
Cervical myelography (cervical injection)	240 mg I/ml or 300 mg I/ml	6–10 ml 6–8 ml	
CT cisternography	180 mg I/ml or 240 mg I/ml	5–15 ml 4–12 ml	
Paediatric myelography			
<2 years	180 mg I/ml	2–6 ml	
2–6 years	180 mg I/ml	4–8 ml	
>6 years	180 mg I/ml	6–12 ml	

To minimise possible adverse reactions a total dose of 3 g iodine should not be exceeded.

Guidelines for Body cavities

Indication	*Concentration*	*Volume*	*Comments*
Arthrography	240 mg I/ml or 300 mg I/ml or 350 mg I/ml	5–20 ml 5–15 ml 5–10 ml	
ERP/ERCP	240 mg I/ml	20–50 ml	
Herniography	240 mg I/ml	50 ml	
Hysterosalpingography	240 mg I/ml or 300 mg I/ml	15–50 ml 15–25 ml	
Sialography	240 mg I/ml or 300 mg I/ml	0.5–2 ml 0.5–2 ml	
Gastrointestinal studies	180 mg I/ml or 350 mg I/ml	10–200 ml 10–20 ml	

Pregnancy and lactation: The safety of Omnipaque for use in human pregnancy has not been established. An evaluation of experimental animal studies does not indicate direct or indirect harmful effects with respect to reproduction, development of the embryo or fetus, the course of gestation and peri- and postnatal development.

Since whenever possible, radiation exposure should be avoided during pregnancy, the benefits of an X-ray examination, with or without contrast media, should be carefully weighed against the possible risk. Omnipaque should not be used in pregnancy unless the benefit outweighs risk and it is considered essential by the physician.

Contrast media are poorly excreted in human breast milk and minimal amounts are absorbed by the intestine. Harm to the nursing infant is therefore unlikely. The amount of iohexol in breast milk excreted in 24 hours after injection was 0.5% of the weight adjusted dose in a trial. The amount of iohexol ingested by the baby in the first 24 hours after injection corresponds to only 0.2% of the paediatric dose.

Effects on ability to drive and use machines: It is not advisable to drive a car or use machines during the first 24 hours following myelography. However, individual judgement must be performed if persistent post myelography symptoms.

Undesirable effects: General (applies to all uses of iodinated contrast media):

Below are listed possible general side effects in relation with radiographic procedures which include the use of non-ionic monomeric contrast media. For side effects specific to mode of administration, please refer to these specific sections.

Undesirable effects associated with the use of iodinated contrast media are usually mild to moderate and transient in nature, and less frequent with non-ionic than with ionic contrast media. Serious reactions as well as fatalities are only seen on very rare occasions.

The most frequent adverse event is a mild, general sensation such as a feeling of warmth or a transient metallic taste.

Abdominal discomfort/pain is very rare (incidence <1:1000) and gastrointestinal reactions like nausea or vomiting are rare (incidence <1:100, but >1:1000).

Hypersensitivity reactions are rare and usually present as mild respiratory or cutaneous symptoms like dyspnoea, rash, erythema, urticaria, pruritus and angioedema. They may appear either immediately after the injection or up to a few days later. Severe manifestations such as laryngeal oedema, bronchospasm or pulmonary oedema are very rare.

Anaphylactoid reactions may occur irrespectively of the dose and mode of administration and mild symptoms of hypersensitivity may represent the first signs of a serious reaction. Administration of the contrast medium must be discontinued immediately and, if necessary, specific therapy instituted via the vascular access. In patients using beta blockers the bradycardia may not respond to shock and thereby these patients present with atypical symptoms of anaphylaxis which may be misinterpreted as a vagal reaction.

Vagal reactions giving hypotension and bradycardia are seen on very rare occasions.

Severe skin reactions such as Stevens-Johnsons or toxic epidermal necrolysis are seen very rarely. Pyrexia with rigors are seen on rare occasions.

Iodism or 'iodide mumps' is a very rare complication of iodinated contrast media resulting in swelling and tenderness of the salivary glands for up to approximately 10 days after the examination.

Intra-arterial use: Please first read the section labelled 'General'. Below, only undesireable events with frequency during intraarterial use of non-ionic monomeric contrast media are described.

The nature of the undesirable effects specifically seen during intraarterial use depend on the site of injection and dose given. Selective arteriographies and other procedures in which the contrast medium reaches a particular organ in high concentrations may be accompanied by complications in that particular organ.

Distal pain or heat sensation in peripheral angiography is common (incidence >1:10).

A transient increase in S-creatinine is common, but usually of no clinical relevance. Renal failure is very rare. However, fatalities have been reported.

Arterial spasm may follow injection into coronary, cerebral or renal arteries and result in transient ischaemia.

Neurological reactions are very rare. They may include seizures or transient motor or sensory disturbances. On very rare occasions the contrast medium may cross the blood-brain barrier resulting in uptake of contrast medium in the cerebral cortex being visible on CT-scanning until the day following examination, sometimes associated with transient confusion or cortical blindness.

Serious cardiac complications which include arrhythmias cardiac depression or signs of ischaemia are very rare.

Intravenous use: Please first read the section labelled 'General'. Below, only undesireable events with frequency during intravenous use of non-ionic monomeric contrast media are described.

Post phlebographic thrombophlebitis or thrombosis is very rare. A very few cases of arthralgia has been reported.

Intrathecal use: Please first read the section labelled 'General'. Below, only undesireable events with frequency during intrathecal use of non-ionic monomer contrast media are described.

Undesirable effects following intrathecal use may be delayed and present some hours or even days after the procedure. The frequency is similar to lumbar puncture alone.

Headache, nausea, vomiting or dizziness are common and may largely be attributed to pressure loss in the subarachnoid space resulting from leakage at the puncture site. Some of these patients may experience a severe headache lasting for several days. Excessive removal of cerebrospinal fluid should be avoided in order to minimize pressure loss.

Mild local pain, paraesthesia and radicular pain occasionally (incidence <1:10, but >1:100) occur at the site of injection. Cramping and pain in the lower limbs are seen on very rare occasions.

Meningeal irritation giving photophobia and meningism happens occasionally. Frank chemical meningitis appears on very rare occasions. The possibility of an infective meningitis should also be considered.

On very rare occasions, manifestations of transient cerebral dysfunction are seen. These include seizures, transient confusion or transient motor or sensory dysfunction. Changes in the EEG may be noted in a few of these patients.

Use in Body Cavities: Please first read the section labelled 'General'. Below, *only* undesireable events with frequency during use of non-ionic monomeric contrast media in body cavities are described.

Systemic hypersensitivity reactions are rare.

Endoscopic Retrograde Choleangio Pancreatography (ERCP): Some elevation of amylase levels is common. Post ERCP renal opacification is seen on rare occasions and is associated with an increased risk of post ERCP pancreatitis. Rare cases of necrotizing pancreatitis have also been described.

Oral use: Gastrointestinal upset occasionally occur.

Hysterosalpingography (HSG): Transient and mild pain in the lower abdomen is common.

Arthrography: Post procedural pain is common. Frank arthritis is rare. The possibility of infective arthritis should be considered in such cases.

Herniography: Mild postprocedural pain is common.

Overdose: Preclinical data indicate a high safety margin for Omnipaque and no fixed upper dose level has been established for routine intravascular use. Symptomatic overdosing is unlikely unless the patient has received an excess of 2000 mg I/kg body-weight over a limited period of time. The duration of the procedure is important for the renal tolerability of high doses of contrast media ($t_{1/2}$~2 hours). Accidental overdosing is most likely following complex angiographic procedures in children, particularly when multiple injections of contrast medium with high-concentration are given.

In cases of overdose, any resulting water- or electrolyte imbalance must be corrected. Renal function should be monitored for the next 3 days. If needed, haemodialysis may be used for clearance of excessive contrast medium. There is no specific antidote.

Pharmacological properties

Pharmacodynamic properties: For most of the haemodynamic, clinical-chemical and coagulation parameters examined following intravenous injection of iohexol in healthy volunteers, no significant deviation from preinjection values has been found. The few changes observed in the laboratory parameters were minor and considered to be of no clinical importance.

Pharmacokinetic properties: Close to 100 per cent of the intravenously injected iohexol is excreted unchanged through the kidneys within 24 hours. The maximum urinary concentration of iohexol appears approximately 1 hour after injection. No metabolites have been detected. The protein binding of Omnipaque is very low (less than 2%).

Preclinical safety data: Iohexol has a very low acute intravenous and intrathecal toxicity in mice and rats. Animal studies have shown that iohexol has a very low protein binding and is well tolerated by the kidneys.

Pharmaceutical particulars

List of excipients: The following excipients are included:

Trometamol, sodium calcium edetate, hydrochloric acid (pH adjustment) and water for injections.

The pH of the product is 6.8–7.6.

Incompatibilities: Omnipaque should not be directly mixed with other drugs. A separate syringe should be used.

Shelf life: The shelf life is 3 years for glass vials and – bottles and for polypropylene bottles.

The expiry date is indicated on the label.

Special precautions for storage: Omnipaque should be stored at or below 30°C protected from light and secondary X-rays. The product in glass vials and bottles may be stored at 37°C for up to 3 months prior to use.

The product in polypropylene bottles may be stored at 37°C for up to 1 month prior to use.

Nature and content of container:

Glass vials and bottles: The product is filled in injection vials (10, 15, 20 and 40 ml) and infusion bottles (50, 75, 100 and 200 ml). Both containers are made of colourless highly resistant borosilicate glass (PhEur Type I), closed with chlorobutyl rubber stoppers (PhEur Type I), and sealed with combined 'flip off seal/tear off seal–flat plast disc'.

Polypropylene bottles: The product is filled in

polypropylene bottles (40 and 50 ml). The bottle is a rigid stand-up bottle with a twist-off top.

The product is supplied as:

140 mg I/ml:	10 bottles of 50 ml:
	6 bottles of 200 ml
180 mg I/ml:	10 vials of 10 ml
	10 vials of 15 ml
240 mg I/ml:	10 vials of 10 ml
	10 vials of 15 ml
300 mg I/ml:	10 vials of 10 ml
	6 vials of 20 ml
	25 vials of 20 ml
	10 bottles of 50 ml
	10 bottles of 75 ml
	10 bottles of 100 ml
	6 bottles of 200 ml
	10 polypropylene bottles of 40 ml
	10 polypropylene bottles of 50 ml
350 mg I/ml:	10 vials of 10 ml
	6 vials of 20 ml
	25 vials of 20 ml
	10 vials of 40 ml
	10 bottles of 50 ml
	10 bottles of 75 ml
	10 bottles of 100 ml
	6 bottles of 200 ml
	10 polypropylene bottles of 40 ml
	10 polypropylene bottles of 50 ml

Instructions for use/handling: Like all parenteral products, Omnipaque should be inspected visually for particulate matter, discolouration and the integrity of the container prior to use.

The product should be drawn into the syringe immediately before use. Vials are intended for single use only, any unused portions must be discarded.

Marketing authorisation holder: Nycomed Imaging AS, Nycoveien 1-2, P.O.Box 4220, Torshov, N-0401 OSLO, NORWAY

Marketing authorisation numbers

Omnipaque 140 mg I/ml	PL 4517/0006
Omnipaque 180 mg I/ml	PL 4517/0005
Omnipaque 240 mg I/ml	PL 4517/0002
Omnipaque 300 mg I/ml	PL 4517/0003
Omnipaque 350 mg I/ml	PL 4517/0004

Date of first authorisation/renewal of authorisation
20 April 1983

OMNISCAN*

Qualitative and quantitative composition

Active ingredient: GADODIAMIDE (GdDTPA-BMA) equiv. 0.5 mmol/ml.

Content per ml	*Function*
287 mg	MRI-contrast agent

OMNISCAN injection is a non-ionic paramagnetic contrast medium with the following physicochemical properties:

Osmolality (mOsm/kg H_2O) at 37°C	780
Viscosity (mPa·s) at 20°C	2.8
Viscosity (mPa·s) at 37°C	1.9
Density at 20°C (kg/l)	1.15
Molar relaxivity	
r_1 ($mM^{-1} \cdot s^{-1}$) at 20 MHz and 37°C	3.9
r_1 ($mM^{-1} \cdot s^{-1}$) at 10 MHz and 37°C	4.6
r_2 ($mM^{-1} \cdot s^{-1}$) at 10 MHz and 37°C	5.1
pH 6.0–7.0	

Gadodiamide is freely soluble in water.

Pharmaceutical form Injection, for intravenous use. The product is a clear, colourless to slightly yellow aqueous solution.

Clinical particulars

Indications: Contrast medium for cranial and spinal magnetic resonance imaging (MRI) and for general MRI of the body after intravenous administration.

The product provides contrast enhancement and facilitates visualisation of abnormal structures or lesions in various parts of the body including the CNS

Posology and method of administration: No special preparation of the patient is required. OMNISCAN should be drawn into the syringe immediately before use. Both the vial and the bottle are intended for one patient only. Contrast medium not used in one examination must be discarded.

CNS and Whole Body:

Dosage for adults and children from 2 years of age: The recommended dosage is 0.1 mmol/kg body weight (equivalent to 0.2 ml/kg b.w.) up to 100 kg. Above 100 kg body weight 20 ml is usually sufficient to provide diagnostically adequate contrast.

OMNISCAN has also been used in a limited number of children below 2 years of age.

The required dose should be administered as a single intravenous injection. To ensure complete injection of the contrast medium, the intravenous line may be flushed with sodium chloride injection 0.9%.

Contrast-enhanced MRI should start shortly after administration of the contrast medium, depending on the pulse sequences used and the protocol for the examination. Optimal enhancement is observed within the first minutes after injection (time depending on type of lesion/tissue). Enhancement is generally lasting up to 45 minutes after contrast medium injection. T_1-weighted scanning sequences are particularly suitable for contrast-enhanced examinations with OMNISCAN. In the investigated range of field strengths, from 0.15 Tesla up to 1.5 Tesla, the relative image contrast was found to be independent of the applied field strength.

Contra-indications: OMNISCAN should not be used in patients known to have hypersensitivity to OMNISCAN or its constituents.

There is no experience of the use of Omniscan in patients with impaired renal function (GFR <30 ml/min). OMNISCAN should therefore not be used in these patients.

Special warnings and special precautions for use: The possibility of a reaction, including serious, life-threatening, fatal, anaphylactoid or cardiovascular reactions or other idiosyncratic reactions should always be considered, especially in those patients with a known clinical hypersensitivity or a history of asthma or other allergic respiratory disorders. A course of action should therefore be planned in advance, with necessary drugs and equipment available for immediate treatment should a serious reaction occur.

Transitory changes in serum iron (within the normal range in the majority of cases) have been observed in some patients after administration of OMNISCAN. The clinical significance of this, if any, is not known, but all patients in whom this effect was observed remained asymptomatic.

OMNISCAN interferes with serum calcium measurements with some colorimetric (complexometric) methods commonly used in hospitals. It may also interfere with determinations of other electrolytes (e.g. iron). Thus it is recommended not to use such methods for 12–24 hours after administration of OMNISCAN. If such measurements are necessary, the use of other methods is recommended.

Interaction with other medicaments and other forms of interaction: None known.

Pregnancy and lactation: There is no experience of the use of OMNISCAN during human pregnancy. The product should not be used during pregnancy, unless an enhanced MR investigation is essential, and no suitable alternative is available.

OMNISCAN had no effects on fertility or reproductive performance in rats or in teratology studies in rats and rabbits at doses that did not cause maternal toxicity.

The degree of excretion into human milk is not known, although expected to be low. Breast feeding should be discontinued prior to administration and should not be re-commenced until at least 24 hours after the administration of OMNISCAN.

Effects on ability to drive and use machines: No effects are known.

Undesirable effects: All events have been transient and the majority of mild intensity. Discomfort with general sensation of warmth, coolness or a sensation of local pressure or pain at the injection site are occasionally seen. Less frequently reported are dizziness, nausea, headache and a perverted sensation of taste or smell. Rare reactions are vomiting, somnolence, paraesthesia or allergy-like symptoms such as urticaria, itching or an irritation in the throat. Anaphylactoid reactions may occur.

In very rare cases convulsions have been observed after the administration of OMNISCAN as is the case for other paramagnetic MR contrast media. However, a causal relationship seems to be questionable.

Transient renal failure was observed in one patient included in the clinical trials. The patient had received an X-ray contrast medium for myelography 22 hours prior to the injection of OMNISCAN. The causality for the reaction has not been established.

Overdose: Clinical consequences of overdose have not been reported and acute symptoms of toxicity are unlikely in patients with a normal renal function. Treatment is symptomatic. There is no antidote for this contrast medium. In patients with delayed elimination due to renal insufficiency and in patients who have received excessive doses, the contrast medium may theoretically be eliminated by haemodialysis.

Pharmacological properties

Pharmacodynamic properties: The paramagnetic properties of OMNISCAN provides contrast enhancement during MRI.

There were no clinically significant deviations from preinjection values in haemodynamic and blood and urine laboratory parameters following intravenous injection of gadodiamide in healthy volunteers. However, a minor transient change in serum iron levels 8 to 48 hours after gadodiamide injection was observed.

OMNISCAN does not cross the intact blood-brain barrier. Administration of OMNISCAN causes signal enhancement from areas where blood-brain barrier dysfunction has been induced by pathological processes, and may provide greater diagnostic yield than unenhanced MRI. Lack of enhancement need not indicate absence of pathology since some types of low grade malignancies or inactive MS-plaques fail to enhance; it can be used for differential diagnosis between different pathologies.

Pharmacokinetic properties: Gadodiamide is rapidly distributed in the extracellular fluid. The volume of distribution is equivalent to that of extracellular water. The distribution half-life is approximately 4 minutes and the elimination half-life is approximately 70 minutes.

Gadodiamide is excreted through the kidneys by glomerular filtration. Approximately 85% of the administered dose is recovered in the urine by 4 hours and 95–98% by 24 hours after intravenous injection. The renal and total clearance rates of gadodiamide are nearly identical, and are similar to that of substances excreted primarily by glomerular filtration.

No dose dependent kinetics have been observed after injection of 0.l and 0.3 mmol/kg.

No metabolites have been detected. No protein binding has been observed.

Preclinical safety data: The efficacy of OMNISCAN as a contrast enhancing agent during MRI has been demonstrated in a series of animal studies.

Safety pharmacology studies in dogs and rats have demonstrated that OMNISCAN has no significant effects on the cardiovascular system. *In vitro* studies have demonstrated no or insignificant effects on mast cell histamine release, human serum complement activation factors, human erythrocyte cholinesterase activity, lysozyme activity, human erythrocyte fragility and morphology, and on tension in isolated bovine blood vessels. No evidence of antigenicity was seen in a dermal test in Guinea pigs.

Pharmacokinetic studies in several animal species have demonstrated OMNISCAN to be rapidly distributed in the extracellular volume, and quantitatively excreted via the kidneys by glomerular filtration. The elimination half-lives in man and monkey are similar. The calculated distribution volume is approximately 25% of body size.

Toxicological studies have demonstrated a high acute tolerance of OMNISCAN, the approximate LD_{50} in mice was >30 mmol/kg. The common finding after high single doses or repeated dosing was proximal tubular vacuolation, which was reversible, and was not associated with altered renal function. OMNISCAN was found to be non-irritating after intravenous, intra-arterial, paravenous, intramuscular and subcutaneous administration, or when applied to the skin or the eye.

OMNISCAN had no effects on fertility or reproductive performance in rats or in teratology studies in rats and rabbits at doses that did not cause maternal toxicity.

Pharmaceutical particulars

List of excipients: The following excipients are included:

Caldiamide sodium, sodium hydroxide 1 M or hydrochloric acid 1 M, water for injections.

Incompatibilities: OMNISCAN should not be directly mixed with other drugs. A separate syringe and needle should be used.

Shelf life: The shelf life of the glass vials and the polypropylene bottles is 3 years when stored below 30°C and protected from light and freezing.

Special precautions for storage: OMNISCAN in glass and polypropylene bottles should be stored below 30°C and protected from light and freezing. Both the vial and the bottle are intended for one patient only. Any unused portions must be discarded.

Nature and content of container: The product is filled in injection vials with a fill volume of 5 ml, 10 ml, 15 and 20 ml and in polypropylene bottles with a fill volume of 10, 15, 20, 40 ml and 50 ml. The vials are made of colourless highly resistant borosilicate glass (PhEur Type I) and are closed with grey halo-butyl isoprene blend rubber stoppers (PhEur Type I) size 20 mm, sealed with complete tear off capsules of aluminium with coloured plastic 'flip-off' tops.

The product is supplied as:

1 vial of 5 ml	10 polypropylene bottles of 10 ml
10 vials of 5 ml	10 polypropylene bottles of 15 ml
10 vials of 10 ml	10 polypropylene bottles of 20 ml
10 vials of 15 ml	10 polypropylene bottles of 40 ml
10 vials of 20 ml	10 polypropylene bottles of 50 ml

Marketing authorisation holder: NYCOMED IMAGING AS, Nycoveien 1-2, P.O. Box 4220 Torshov, N-0401 OSLO, NORWAY.

Marketing authorisation numbers
PL 0637/0015 in UK (Glass vials)
PL 0637/0025 in UK (Polypropylene bottles)

Date of first authorisation 25 September 1992 in UK

TESLASCAN*

Qualitative and quantitative composition

Active Ingredient	*Content per ml*
Mangafodipir trisodium (anhydrous)	7.57 mg equiv. 0.01 mmol (10 μmol)
corresp. mangafodipir	6.91 mg

Pharmaceutical form 0.01 mmol/ml solution for infusion (a clear bright to dark yellow solution).

Clinical particulars
Therapeutic indications: Contrast medium for diagnostic Magnetic Resonance Imaging (MRI) for the detection of lesions of the liver suspected to be due to metastatic disease or hepatocellular carcinomas.

Posology and method of administration: The product is for single intravenous use only as repeated dosing has not been studied. It should be administered as an intravenous infusion at the rate of 2–3 ml/min.

Near maximal enhancement of the normal liver parenchyma is generally observed 15–20 minutes from start of administration and lasts for approximately 4 hours.

At the clinical dose the contrast agent has no T_2-effect, and pre- and post-T_2-weighted images are equivalent. The clinical use of TESLASCAN has been investigated at field strengths from 0.5 to 2.0 Tesla.

Dosage for adults: The recommended dosage is 0.5 ml/kg b.w. (5 μmol/kg b.w.). This corresponds to a dose of 35 ml for a 70 kg person. Above 100 kg body weight, 50 ml is usually sufficient to provide a diagnostically adequate contrast effect.

Dosage for elderly: Pharmacokinetics in the elderly have not been investigated. However, clinical studies to date do not suggest that a dose adjustment is required.

Children: Safety and efficacy in patients below the age of 18 have not been documented.

Contra-indications: Pregnancy and lactation.

Hypersensitivity to the product or its constituents. Phaeochromocytoma. Severely reduced liver function (Child-Pugh class C), especially severe obstructive hepatobiliary disease. Severely reduced renal function.

Special warnings and special precautions for use: Rarely, hypersensitivity reactions (urticaria and other possible allergic phenomena) may occur. As anaphylactic reactions have been observed with other contrast media, such reactions cannot be excluded after TESLASCAN.

Familiarity with the practice and technique of resuscitation and treatment of anaphylaxis is essential. Appropriate drugs and instruments should be readily available.

Care should be exercised in patients with severe cardiac disease and in patients with injuries of the blood brain barrier and severe cerebral disease.

The fact that long term parenteral nutrition with manganese supplementation can cause manganese accumulation in the basal ganglia should be considered when administering TESLASCAN to patients on such treatment

Interaction with other medicaments and other forms of interaction: No specific interaction studies have been performed with TESLASCAN.

Pregnancy and lactation: The safety of TESLASCAN in human pregnancy has not been established. TESLASCAN must not be used during pregnancy (see below). Prior to administration of TESLASCAN to women of child bearing potential pregnancy should be excluded.

Experimental studies in rats have established teratogenic effects when TESLASCAN was given repeatedly during major organogenesis. TESLASCAN causes foetotoxicity and embryotoxicity in rabbits. TESLASCAN is not teratogenic in rabbits. TESLASCAN has no effect on male or female fertility in rats.

The degree of excretion into human breast milk is not known. Breast-feeding should be discontinued from administration and should not be recommenced until 14 days after administration of TESLASCAN.

Effects on ability to drive and use machines: No effects are known.

Undesirable effects: Most of the adverse reactions reported were transient and of mild intensity. Those most commonly reported were: feeling of warmth/flushing, headache, nausea, vomiting, other gastrointestinal symptoms (like abdominal pain, diarrhoea, flatulence) and taste sensations. Less frequent reactions are hypersensitivity reactions (such as skin reactions, rhinitis, pharyngitis), dizziness, palpitation, chest pain, hypertension and injection associated discomfort. Rarely, visual disturbances, fever and paraesthesia have been reported.

Mangafodipir can cause transient increases of bilirubin and liver transaminases and transient decreases in plasma zinc.

The frequency of mild and moderate, non-serious adverse reactions, mainly transient warmth and flushing is likely to increase if TESLASCAN is administered at a faster rate than that advised.

Overdose: Serious adverse events have not been reported in healthy subjects with dosages up to 5 times the normal clinical dose (maximum dose investigated).

High doses of manganese can have negative inotropic and vasodilatory effects as well as effects on heart rhythm and conduction because of calcium antagonism.

Treatment of an overdose should be symptomatic and directed towards the support of vital functions. There is no antidote to this contrast medium.

Mangafodipir and its metabolites pass membranes with cut-off thresholds of 10–30 kDa and are, therefore, most probably dialysable with conventional membranes.

Pharmacological properties
Pharmacodynamic properties: Pharmaco-therapeutic group: Paramagnetic MRI contrast medium ATC Code: V08C A05.

Mangafodipir is a chelate containing the metal manganese – which has paramagnetic properties and is responsible for the contrast enhancement effect in MRI – and the ligand fodipir (dipyridoxyl diphosphate). Manganese is preferentially taken up by normal liver parenchyma so that contrast enhancement between abnormal tissue and normal liver tissue can be expected.

The effect of the product is to shorten the longitudinal relaxation time (T_1) of targeted tissues during MRI, leading to an increase in signal intensity (brightness) of, for example, liver parenchyma. Liver enhancement is near maximal for up to approx. 4 hours after the end of administration, and lesion related enhancement of certain types of lesions, such as metastases and hepatocellular carcinomas, may be detectable for up to 24 hours. Clinical studies have demonstrated that TESLASCAN facilitates the detection of liver lesions in patients with such lesions.

TESLASCAN is isotonic with blood and normal body fluids.

Pharmacokinetic properties: Mangafodipir trisodium is metabolised (dephosphorylated) and manganese ions are released from the mangafodipir by exchange with plasma zinc (mainly) after intravenous administration. Manganese and the ligand (fodipir), which have different pharmacokinetics, are eliminated by different routes.

The mean initial plasma half-life of manganese is 20 minutes or less, with significant uptake into the liver, pancreas, kidneys and spleen. The initial plasma half-life of ligand is about 50 minutes. The volume of distribution for manganese is between 0.5 and 1.5 l/kg, and for fodipir 0.17 to 0.45 l/kg. Following its metabolism, nearly all the ligand (fodipir) is excreted in urine within 24 hours, with negligible amounts being eliminated via the faeces. About 15–20% of the manganese is eliminated in the urine within the first 24 hours, most of the remainder is excreted in the faeces over the following 4 days.

In whole human blood *in vitro*, the protein binding of manganese is approximately 27% but binding of fodipir to protein is negligible.

Preclinical safety data: Preclinical studies reveal no special hazard for humans based on conventional studies of genotoxicity, safety pharmacology and validating kinetics and metabolism. Relevant adverse effects from repeated dose toxicity studies were as follows:

Liver toxicity (cholangiohepatitis) was observed at relatively low dosages in dogs, while sufficient margins of safety were determined in rats and monkeys.

Mangafodipir is teratogenic in rats; it causes increased foetal skeletal abnormalities when given daily by intravenous injection to female rats at dosages slightly greater than clinical dosages. Embryo- and foetotoxicity has been observed in rabbits.

Pharmaceutical particulars
List of excipients: The following excipients are included:

Ascorbic acid, sodium chloride, sodium hydroxide and/or hydrochloric acid (pH adjustment), water for injections.

TESLASCAN has the following physicochemical properties:

Osmolality (mosmol/kg H_2O) at 37°C	290
Viscosity (mP·s) at 20°C	1.0
Viscosity (mP·s) at 37°C	0.7
Density (g/ml) at 20°C	1.01

Incompatibilities: TESLASCAN should not be directly mixed with other drugs.

A separate cannula should be used.

Shelf life: The shelf life is 24 months when stored protected from light.

Special precautions for storage: TESLASCAN should be stored protected from light.

Nature and content of container: The product is filled in 50 ml narrow-necked vials (PhEur Type 1, sulphur treated) made of uncoloured highly resistant borosilicate glass. The containers are closed with 20 mm Carbonblack rubber stoppers and sealed with aluminium caps with coloured polypropylene lids. TESLASCAN is supplied in packs of 1 x 50 ml and 10 x 50 ml vials.

Instructions for use/handling: As for all parenteral products, vials of TESLASCAN should be visually inspected for particulate matter and the integrity of the container prior to use. Vials are intended for single use only, any unused portions must be discarded.

The required volume to be given to the patient should be determined and administered appropriately (intravenous infusion). Any excess volume should be withdrawn from the vial before infusion.

Connective tubing may be flushed with physiological saline (0.9% sodium chloride), to ensure complete administration of the contrast medium.

Marketing authorisation holder: NYCOMED IMAGING AS, Nycoveien 1-2, P.O. Box 4220 Torshov, N-0401 OSLO, NORWAY.

Number in the community register of medicinal products
EU/1/97/040/001 (single pack)
EU/1/94/040/002 (multiple pack)

Date of first authorisation/renewal of authorisation
22 May 1997

VISIPAQUE*

Qualitative and quantitative composition
Active ingredient: Iodixanol (INN)[1]

Strength	*Content pr. ml.*
150 mg I/ml	305 mg equiv. 150 mg I
270 mg I/ml	550 mg equiv. 270 mg I
320 mg I/ml	652 mg equiv. 320 mg I

[1] Iodixanol is a non-ionic, dimeric, hexaiodinated, water-soluble X-ray contrast medium.

Pure aqueous solutions of iodixanol in all clinical relevant concentrations have a lower osmolality than whole blood and the corresponding strengths of the non-ionic monomeric contrast media. VISIPAQUE is made isotonic with normal body fluids by addition of electrolytes.

The osmolality and viscosity values of VISIPAQUE are as follows:

Concentration	*Osmolality*[2] *mOsm/kg H_2O*	*Viscosity (mPa·s)*	
	37°C	20°C	37°C
150 mg I/ml	290	2.7	1.7
270 mg I/ml	290	11.3	5.8
320 mg I/ml	290	25.4	11.4

[2] Method: Vapour-pressure osmometry.

Pharmaceutical form Solution for injection. VISIPAQUE injections are supplied ready to use as clear, colourless to pale yellow aqueous solutions.

Clinical particulars
Indications: X-ray contrast medium for use in adults for cardioangiography, cerebral angiography (conventional and i.a. DSA), peripheral arteriography (conventional and i.a. DSA), abdominal angiography (i.a. DSA), urography, venography and CT-enhancement, and for children in cardioangiography, urography and CT-enchancement.

Posology and method of administration: The dosage may vary depending on the type of examination, the age, weight, cardiac output and general condition of the patient and the technique used. Usually approximately the same iodine concentration and volume is used as with other iodinated X-ray contrast media in current use, but adequate diagnostic information has also been obtained in some studies with iodixanol injection with somewhat lower iodine concentration. Adequate hydration should be assured before and after administration as for other contrast media.

The product is for intravenous and intra-arterial use.

The following dosages may serve as a guide. The doses given for intra-arterial use are for single injections that may be repeated.

Elderly: As for other adults.
Contra-indications: Manifest thyrotoxicosis. History of serious hypersensitivity reaction to VISIPAQUE.

Intra-arterial use:

Indication/Investigation	*Concentration*	*Volume*
Arteriographies; adults only		
Selective cerebral	270/320[1] mg I/ml	5–10 ml per inj.
Selective cerebral i.a. DSA	150 mg I/ml	5–10 ml per inj.
Aortography	270/320 mg I/ml	40–60 ml per inj.
Peripheral	270/320 mg I/ml	30–60 ml per inj.
Peripheral i.a. DSA	150 mg I/ml	30–60 ml per inj.
Selective visceral i.a. DSA	270 mg I/ml	10–40 ml per inj.
Cardioangiography, adults		
Left ventricle and aortic root inj.	320 mg I/ml	30–60 ml per inj.
Selective coronary arteriography	320 mg I/ml	4–8 ml per inj.
Children	270/320 mg I/ml	Depending on age, weight and pathology (recommended max total dose 10 ml/kg).

[1] Both strengths are documented, but 270 mg I/ml is recommended in most cases.

Intravenous Use:

Indication/Investigation	*Concentration*	*Volume*
Urography		
Adults	270/320 mg I/ml	40–80 ml[2]
Children <7 kg	270/320 mg I/ml	2–4 ml/kg
Children >7 kg	270/320 mg I/ml	2–3 ml/kg All doses depending on age, weight and pathology (max. 50 ml)
Venography; adults only	270 mg I/ml	50–150 ml/leg
CT-enhancement		
CT of the head, adults	270/320 mg I/ml	50–150 ml
CT of the body, adults	270/320 mg I/ml	75–150 ml
Children, CT of the head and body	270/320 mg I/ml	2–3 ml/kg up to 50 ml (in a few cases up to 150 ml may be given)

[2] In high-dose urography higher doses can be used.

Special warnings and special precautions for use:
Special precautions for use of non-ionic contrast media in general: A positive history of allergy, asthma, or untoward reactions to iodinated contrast media indicates a need for special caution. Premedication with corticosteroids or histamine H_1 and H_2 antagonists might be considered in these cases.

The risk of serious reactions in connection with use of VISIPAQUE is regarded as minor. However, iodinated contrast media may provoke anaphylactoid reactions or other manifestations of hypersensitivity. A course of action should therefore be planned in advance with necessary drugs and equipment available for immediate treatment, should a serious reaction occur. It is advisable always to use an indwelling cannula or catheter for quick intravenous access throughout the entire X-ray procedure.

Non-ionic contrast media have less effect on the coagulation system *in vitro*, compared to ionic contrast media. When performing vascular catheterisation procedures one should pay meticulous attention to the angiographic technique and flush the catheter frequently (e.g.: with heparinised saline) so as to minimize the risk of procedure-related thrombosis and embolism.

Adequate hydration should be assured before and after contrast media administration. This applies especially to patients with multiple myeloma, diabetes mellitus, renal dysfunction, as well as to infants, small children and elderly patients. Young infants (age <1 year) and especially neonates are susceptible to electrolyte disturbance and haemodynamic alterations.

Care should also be taken in patients with serious cardiac disease and pulmonary hypertension as they may develop haemodynamic changes or arrhythmias.

Patients with acute cerebral pathology, tumours or a history of epilepsy are predisposed for seizures and merit particular care. Also alcoholics and drug addicts have an increased risk for seizures and neurological reactions.

To prevent acute renal failure following contrast media administration, special care should be exercised in patients with preexisting renal impairment and diabetes mellitus as they are at risk. Patients with paraproteinemias (myelomatosis and Waldenström's macroglobulinemia) are also at risk.

Preventive measures include:

- Identification of high risk patients.
- Ensuring adequate hydration. If necessary by maintaining an i.v. infusion from before the procedure until the contrast medium has been cleared by the kidneys.
- Avoiding additional strain on the kidneys in the form of nephrotoxic drugs, oral cholecystographic agents, arterial clamping, renal arterial angioplasty, or major surgery, until the contrast medium has been cleared.
- Postponing a repeat contrast medium examination until renal function returns to pre-examination levels.

Particular care is required in patients with severe disturbance of both renal and hepatic function as they may have significantly delayed contrast medium clearance. Patients on haemodialysis may receive contrast media for radiological procedures provided dialysis is performed immediately afterwards.

The administration of iodinated contrast media may aggravate the symptoms of myasthenia gravis. In patients with phaeochromocytoma undergoing interventional procedures, alpha blockers should be given as prophylaxis to avoid a hypertensive crisis. Special care should be exercised in patients with hyperthyroidism. Patients with multinodular goiter may be at risk of developing hyperthyroidism following injection of iodinated contrast media. One should also be aware of the possibility of inducing transient hypothyroidism in premature infants receiving contrast media.

Extravasation of VISIPAQUE has not been reported, but it is likely that VISIPAQUE due to its isotonicity gives rise to less local pain and extravascular oedema than hyperosmolar contrast media. In case of extravasation, elevating and cooling the affected site is recommended as routine measures. Surgical decompression may be necessary in cases of compartment syndrome.

Observation time: After contrast medium administration the patient should be observed for at least 30 minutes, since the majority of serious side effects occur within this time. However, delayed reactions may occur.

Interaction with other medicaments and other forms of interaction: All iodinated contrast media may interfere with tests on thyroid function, thus the iodine binding capacity of the thyroid may be reduced for up to several weeks. High concentrations of contrast medium in serum and urine can interfere with laboratory tests for bilirubin, proteins or inorganic substances (e.g. iron, copper, calcium and phosphate). These substances should therefore not be assayed on the day of examination.

Use of iodinated contrast media may result in a transient impairment of renal function and this may precipitate lactic acidosis in diabetics who are taking biguanides (metformine). As precaution, biguanides should be stopped 48 hours prior to the contrast medium examination and reinstated only after renal function has stabilised.

Patients treated with interleukin-2 less than two weeks previous to an iodinated contrast medium injection have been associated with an increased risk for delayed reactions (flu-like symptoms or skin reactions).

Pregnancy and lactation: The safety of VISIPAQUE for use in human pregnancy has not been established. An evaluation of experimental animal studies does not indicate direct or indirect harmful effects with respect to reproduction, development of the embryo or fetus, the course of gestation and peri- and postnatal development.

Since, wherever possible, radiation exposure should be avoided during pregnancy, the benefits of any X-ray examination, with or without contrast media, should be carefully weighed against the possible risk. The product should not be used in pregnancy unless benefit outweighs risk and it is considered essential by the physician.

The degree of excretion into human milk is not known, although expected to be low. Breast feeding should be discontinued prior to administration and should not be recommenced until at least 24 hours after the administration of VISIPAQUE.

Effects on ability to drive and use machines: No effects are known.

Undesirable effects: Below are listed possible side effects in relation with radiographic procedures which include the use of VISIPAQUE.

Intravascular use: Undesirable effects associated with the use of iodinated contrast media are usually mild to moderate and transient in nature, and less frequent with non-ionic than with ionic contrast media. Serious reactions as well as fatalities are only seen on very rare occasions.

The most frequent adverse event is a mild, general feeling of warmth or cold. Heat sensation in peripheral angiography is common (Incidence: >1:10), while distal pain occurs occasionally (Incidence <1:10, but >1:100).

Abdominal discomfort/pain is very rare (Incidence <1:1000) and gastrointestinal reactions like nausea or vomiting are rare (Incidence <1:100, but >1:1000). Some patients have experienced taste and smell alterations.

Hypersensitivity reactions occur occasionally and usually present as mild respiratory or cutaneous symptoms like dyspnoea, rash, erythema, urticaria, pruritus and angioedema. They may appear either immediately after the injection or up to a few days later. Hypotension or fever may occur. Severe and even toxic skin reactions have been reported. Severe manifestations such as laryngeal oedema, bronchospasm, pulmonary oedema and anaphylactic shock are very rare.

Anaphylactoid reactions may occur irrespectively of the dose and mode of administration and mild symptoms of hypersensitivity may represent the first signs of a serious reaction. Administration of the contrast medium must be discontinued immediately and, if necessary, specific therapy instituted via the vascular access. Patients using beta blockers may present with atypical symptoms of anaphylaxis which may be misinterpreted as a vagal reaction.

Vagal reactions giving hypotension and bradycardia are seen on very rare occasions.

Iodism or 'iodide mumps' is a very rare complication of iodinated contrast media resulting in swelling and tenderness of the salivary glands for up to approximately 10 days after the examination.

A minor transient increase in S-creatinine is common after iodinated contrast media, but usually of no clinical relevance. Renal failure is very rare. However, fatalities have been reported in high risk patient groups.

Arterial spasm may follow injection into coronary, cerebral or renal arteries and result in transient ischaemia.

Neurological reactions are very rare. They may include headache, dizziness, seizures or transient motor or sensory disturbances. On very rare occasions the contrast medium may cross the blood-brain barrier resulting in uptake of contrast medium in the cerebral cortex being visible on CT-scanning until the day following examination, sometimes associated with transient confusion or cortical blindness.

Cardiac complications are very rare, including arrhythmias, depression or signs of ischaemia. Hypertension may occur.

Post phlebographic thrombophlebitis or thrombosis is very rare. A very few cases of arthralgia have been reported.

Overdose: Overdosage is unlikely in patients with a normal renal function. The duration of the procedure is important for the renal tolerability of high doses of contrast media (t~2 hours). In the event of accidental overdosing, the water and electrolyte losses must be compensated by infusion. Renal function should be monitored for at least the next 3 days. If needed, haemodialysis may be used to remove iodixanol from the patient's system. There is no specific antidote.

Pharmacological properties
Pharmacodynamic properties: The organically bound iodine absorbs radiation in the blood vessels/tissues when it is injected.

For most of the haemodynamic, clinical-chemical and coagulation parameters examined following intravenous injection of iodixanol in healthy volunteers, no significant deviation from preinjection values has been found. The few changes observed in the laboratory parameters were minor and considered to be of no clinical importance.

VISIPAQUE induces only minor effects on renal function in patients. The release of enzymes (alkaline phosphatase and N-acetyl-β-glucosaminidase) from the proximal tubular cells is less than after injections of non-ionic monomeric contrast media and the same trend is seen compared to ionic dimeric contrast media. VISIPAQUE is also well tolerated by the glomerulus.

Cardiovascular parameters such as LVEDP, LVSP, heart rate and QT-time as well as femoral blood flow were less influenced after VISIPAQUE than after other contrast media, where measured.

Pharmacokinetic properties: Iodixanol is rapidly distributed in the body with a mean distribution half-life of approximately 21 minutes. The apparent volume of distribution is of the same magnitude as the extracellular fluid (0.26 l/kg b.w.), indicating that iodixanol is distributed in the extra-cellular volume only.

No metabolites have been detected. The protein binding is less than 2%.

The mean elimination half-life is approximately 2 hours in normal adults. In infants the elimination of iodixanol is prolonged ($t_{1/2}$ approx. 4 hours in newborns). Iodixanol is excreted mainly through the kidneys by glomerular filtration. Approximately 80% of the administered dose is recovered unmetabolised in the urine within 4 hours and 97% within 24 hours after intravenous injection in healthy volunteers. Only about 1.2% of the injected dose is excreted in faeces within 72 hours. The maximum urinary concentration appears within approximately 1 hour after injection.

No dose dependent kinetics have been observed in the recommended dose range.

Preclinical safety data: Reproduction studies in rats and rabbits have revealed no evidence of impaired fertility or teratogenicity due to iodixanol.

Pharmaceutical particulars

List of excipients: The following excipients are included: Trometamol, sodium chloride, calcium chloride, sodium calcium edetate, hydrochloric acid (pH adjustment) and water for injections.

The pH of the product is 6.8–7.6.

Incompatibilities: No incompatibility has been found. However, VISIPAQUE should not be directly mixed with other drugs. A separate syringe should be used.

Shelf life: The shelf life is 3 years when stored at or below 30°C, protected from light.

Special precautions for storage: VISIPAQUE should be stored at or below 30°C, protected from light and secondary X-rays. The product in glass containers and 40 and 50 ml in polypropylene bottles can be stored for up to 1 month at 37°C, protected from light. The product in 10 and 20 ml polypropylene bottles can be stored for up to 1 week at 37°C, protected from light, prior to use.

Nature and content of container: The product is filled in injection vials (20 ml), infusion bottles (50, 75, 100 and 200 ml) and polypropylene bottles (10, 20, 40 and 50 ml). The glass vials/bottles are made of colourless highly resistant borosilicate glass (PhEur Type I), closed with black chlorobutyl rubber stoppers (PhEur Type I), and sealed with complete tear off caps with coloured plastic 'flip-off' tops.

The product is supplied as:

150 mg I/ml:	10 bottles of 50 ml
	1 bottle of 200 ml
	6 bottles of 200 ml
	10 polypropylene bottles of 50 ml
270 mg I/ml:	10 vials of 20 ml
	10 bottles of 50 ml
	10 bottles of 75 ml
	1 bottle of 100 ml
	10 bottles of 100 ml
	1 bottle of 200 ml
270 mg I/ml:	6 bottles of 200 ml
	10 polypropylene bottles of 10 ml
	10 polypropylene bottles of 20 ml
	10 polypropylene bottles of 40 ml
	10 polypropylene bottles of 50 ml
320 mg I/ml:	10 vials of 20 ml
	10 bottles of 50 ml
	1 bottle of 100 ml
	10 bottles of 100 ml
	1 bottle of 200 ml
	6 bottles of 200 ml
	10 polypropylene bottles of 10 ml
	10 polypropylene bottles of 20 ml
	10 polypropylene bottles of 40 ml
	10 polypropylene bottles of 50 ml

Instructions for use/handling: Like all parenteral products, VISIPAQUE should be inspected visually for particulate matter, discolouration and the integrity of the container prior to use.

The product should be drawn into the syringe immediately before use. Vials are intended for single use only, any unused portions must be discarded.

VISIPAQUE may be warmed to body temperature before administration.

Marketing authorisation holder: NYCOMED IMAGING AS, Nycoveien 1-2, P.O. Box 4220 Torshov, N-0401 OSLO, NORWAY.

Marketing authorisation numbers

PL 0637/0017-19 (Glass vials/bottles)
PL 0637/0026-28 (Polypropylene bottles)

Date of first authorisation UK: 31 March 1993

Text in the package leaflet: The expiry date is stated on the label.

**Trade Mark*

Organon Laboratories Limited
Cambridge Science Park
Milton Road
Cambridge CB4 0FL

☎ 01223 423445   🗋 01223 424368

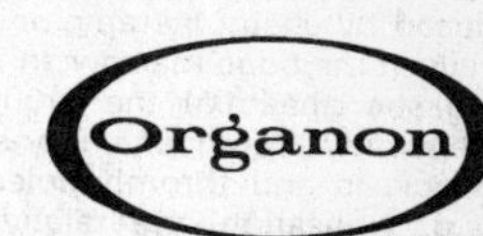

DECA-DURABOLIN*

Presentation Deca Durabolin is a clear, sterile, oily, solution for injection containing Nandrolone Decanoate PhEur, 25 mg or 50 mg per ml.

Other constituents: Benzyl Alcohol PhEur, 0.1 ml and Arachis Oil PhEur, to 1.0 ml.

Uses For use in osteoporosis in post-menopausal women.

Established osteoporosis should have been diagnosed by the following parameters:

i) crush or wedge fractures of the vertebrae
ii) other osteoporotic fractures
iii) established reduction in bone mineral content as measured by accepted BMC measurements.

Dosage and administration

Dosage: Post-menopausal women–50 mg every three weeks.

Children: There are no recommendations for use in children.

Administration: The duration of treatment depends on the clinical response and the possible occurrence of side-effects.

We would recommend that the effectiveness of therapy be monitored with the appropriate methods for osteoporosis on a 6-12 monthly basis.

Deca-Durabolin should be administered by deep intramuscular injection.

Contra-indications, warnings, etc.

Contra-indications: Pregnancy. Known or suspected carcinoma of prostate or mammary carcinoma in the male.

Use in pregnancy and lactation: This medicine is contraindicated during pregnancy because of possible masculinization of the foetus. There are insufficient data on the use of this medicine during breast-feeding to assess potential harm to the infant or a possible influence on milk production.

Warnings and precautions: If signs of virilisation develop, discontinuation of the treatment should be considered.

Patients, especially the elderly, with the following conditions should be monitored: Latent or overt cardiac failure, renal dysfunction, hypertension, epilepsy or migraine (or a history of these conditions), since anabolic steroids may occasionally induce sodium and water retention;

Incomplete statural growth, since anabolic steroids in high dosages may accelerate epiphyseal closure;

Skeletal metastases, since anabolic steroids may induce hypercalcaemia and hypercalciuria in these patients;

Liver dysfunction.

Effects on ability drive and use machines: None known

Interactions: Anabolic steroids may improve the glucose tolerance and decrease the need for insulin or other antidiabetic drugs in diabetics.

Overdosage: The acute toxicity of nandrolone decanoate in animals is very low. There are no reports of acute overdosage with Deca-Durabolin in the human.

Adverse reactions: Deca-Durabolin at the *recommended* dosages is unlikely to produce virilising effects.

High dosages, prolonged treatment and/or too frequent administration may cause:

Virilisation which appears in sensitive women as hoarseness, acne, hirsutism and increase of libido; in prepubertal boys as an increased frequency of erections and phallic enlargement, and in girls as an increase of pubic hair and clitoral hypertrophy. Hoarseness may be the first symptom of vocal change which may end in long-lasting, sometimes irreversible deepening of the voice;

Amenorrhoea and inhibition of spermatogenesis; Premature epiphyseal closure;

Sodium and water retention.

Abnormal liver function tests have been reported in patients treated with (high doses) of Deca-Durabolin. Liver tumours have been reported.

Liver tumours have been reported occasionally on prolonged treatment with orally active C17-alpha alkylated anabolic steroids. A relationship between liver tumours and non-C17-alkylated injectable steroids, such as nandrolone esters, appears to be highly unlikely, but cannot be absolutely excluded.

Pharmaceutical precautions Protect from light. Store below 25°C.

Legal category POM.

Package quantities *25 mg per ml:* 1 ml ampoules in carton of 1 and 1 ml ampoules in cartons of 3.

50 mg per ml: 1 ml ampoules in carton of 1 and 1 ml ampoules in cartons of 3

Further information Nandrolone is chemically related to testosterone and shows enhanced anabolic and a reduced androgenic activity.

In humans Deca-Durabolin has been shown to positively influence calcium metabolism and to increase bone mass in osteoporosis.

Androgenic effects (e.g. virilisation) are relatively uncommon at the recommended dosages. Nandrolone lacks the C17 alpha-alkyl group which is associated with the occurrence of liver dysfunction and cholestasis.

Nandrolone decanoate is slowly released from the injection site into the blood with a half-life of 6 days. The ester is rapidly hydrolysed to nandrolone in the blood with a half-life of one hour or less. The half-life for the combined process of hydrolysis of nandrolone decanoate and of distribution and elimination of nandrolone is 4.3 hours.

Nandrolone is metabolised by the liver. 19-norandrosterone, 19-noretiocholanolone and 19-norepiandrosterone have been identified as metabolites in the urine. It is not known whether these metabolites display a pharmacological action.

Product licence numbers
25 mg/ml 0065/5005R
50 mg/ml 0065/5063R.

DECA-DURABOLIN 100*

Qualitative and quantitative composition Each ml of Deca Durabolin 100 contains 100 mg nandrolone decanoate BP.

Pharmaceutical form 1 ml clear PhEur type ampoules containing a sterile pale yellow oily liquid intended for intramuscular injection in human beings.

Clinical particulars

Therapeutic indications: Anaemia of chronic renal failure. Aplastic anaemia. Anaemia due to cytotoxic therapy

Posology and method of administration

Dosage: Adults: Anaemia of chronic renal failure. Males: 200 mg weekly. Females: 100 mg weekly.

Aplastic anaemia. The usual dose is 50 to 150 mg weekly.

Anaemia due to cytotoxic therapy.

The usual dose is 200 mg weekly commencing 2 weeks prior to the course of cytotoxic therapy. This treatment should be continued throughout cytotoxic therapy and thereafter during the recovery period until the blood count has returned to normal.

NB: Treatment with DECA-DURABOLIN "100' does not substitute for other therapeutic measures.

The onset of a therapeutic effect may vary widely among patients. If no satisfactory response occurs after 3-6 months of treatment, administration should be discontinued.

After a satisfactory improvement or a normalisation of the red blood picture has been obtained, treatment should be withdrawn gradually on the basis of regular monitoring of the haematological parameters. Should a relapse occur at any time whilst the dose is being reduced or after stopping the treatment, re-institution of therapy should be considered.

Children: There is insufficient clinical experience to permit specific recommendations

Administration: Deep Intramuscular injection

Contra-indications: Pregnancy. Known or suspected carcinoma of prostate or mammary carcinoma in males.

Special warnings and special precautions for use: The recommended doses should not be exceeded. If signs of virilisation develop, discontinuation of the treatment should be considered, preferably in consultation with the patient.

It is recommended that patients with any of the following conditions should be monitored:

- latent or overt cardiac failure, renal dysfunction, hypertension or migraine (or a history of these conditions), since anabolic steroids may occasionally induce fluid retention;
- incomplete statural growth, since anabolic steroids in high dosages may accelerate epiphyseal closure;
- skeletal metastases of breast carcinoma. In these patients hypercalcaemia may develop both spontaneously and as a result of anabolic steroid therapy. The latter can be indicative of a positive tumour response to the treatment. Nevertheless, the hypercalcaemia should first be treated appropriately and after restoration of normal calcium levels the therapy can be resumed;
- liver dysfunction.

The use of anabolic steroids to enhance athletic ability may carry severe risks to the user's health and should be discouraged.

Interaction with other medicaments and other forms of interaction: Anabolic steroids may improve glucose tolerance and decrease the need for insulin or other antidiabetic medicines in diabetes.

Although only one possible case of interaction with an oral anticoagulant has been observed, it is advisable to check the prothrombin time regularly when Deca Durabolin 100 is used in conjunction with such an agent.

Pregnancy and lactation: This medicine is contraindicated during pregnancy because of possible masculinisation of the foetus. There are insufficient data on the use of this medicine during breast-feeding to assess potential harm to the infant or a possible influence on milk production.

Effects on ability to drive and use of machines: As far as is known Deca Durabolin 100 has no effect on alertness and concentration.

Undesirable effects: The high dosages which are required to obtain a therapeutic effect in the indications mentioned may cause:

- Virilisation which appears in sensitive women as hoarseness, acne, hirsutism and increase of libido; in prepubertal boys as an increased frequency of erections and phallic enlargement, and in girls as an increase of pubic hair and clitoral hypertrophy. Hoarseness may be the first symptom of vocal change which may end in a long-lasting, sometimes irreversible deepening of the voice
- Amenorrhoea
- Inhibition of spermatogenesis
- Premature epiphyseal closure
- Fluid retention
- Occasionally, abnormal values in some liver function tests. These changes appear to be reversible after completion of the treatment course.

Overdosage: The acute toxicity of nandrolone decanoate in animals is very low. There are no reports of acute overdosage with Deca-Durabolin '100' in man.

Pharmacological properties

Pharmacodynamic properties: DECA-DURABOLIN '100' is a high dosage form of nandrolone decanoate designed especially for adjuvant therapy in the treatment of certain blood disorders. Nandrolone, the pharmacologically active substance of the preparation, is chemically related to testosterone. Compared to testosterone, it has an enhanced anabolic and a reduced androgenic activity. This has been demonstrated in animal bioassays and explained by receptor binding studies. The low androgenicity of nandrolone is confirmed in clinical use.

In animals, nandrolone decanoate possesses an erythropoiesis-stimulating effect probably by directly stimulating the haematopoietic stem cells in the bone marrow and by increasing the release of erythropoietin. It also affords protection against the bone marrow depression caused by cytotoxic agents.

In the human, DECA-DURABOLIN '100' stimulates erythropoiesis as demonstrated by rises in the red blood cell mass, and in the haemoglobin and haematocrit values. This effect is utilised therapeutically in the treatment of anaemia due to a decreased production of erythropoietin, bone marrow depression induced by chemotherapy, or hypoplasia of the stem cells in the bone marrow. In the latter condition (e.g. aplastic anaemia) the erythropoiesis response is frequently accompanied by a positive effect on leucopoiesis and thrombopoiesis. Androgenic effects (e.g. virilisation) are relatively uncommon at the recommended dosages. Nandrolone lacks the C17alpha-alkyl group which is associated with the occurrence of liver dysfunction and cholestasis.

Pharmacokinetic properties: Nandrolone decanoate is slowly released from the injection site into the blood with a half-life of 6 days. In the blood, the ester is rapidly hydrolysed to nandrolone with a half-life of one hour or less. The half-life for the combined process of hydrolysis of nandrolone decanoate and of distribution and elimination of nandrolone is 4.3 hours. Nandrolone is metabolised by the liver. 19-Norandrosterone, 19-noretiocholanolone and 19-norepiandrosterone have been identified as metabolites in the urine. It is not known whether these metabolites display a pharmacological action

Preclinical safety data: Not applicable

Pharmaceutical particulars
List of excipients: Benzyl alcohol EP; Arachis oil EP

Incompatibilities: None known

Shelf-life: 5 years

Special precautions for storage: Protect from light. Store at room temperature 15-25°C.

Nature and contents of containers: 1 ml clear glass ampoule with ring snap neck.

Instructions for use/handling: Not applicable.

Marketing authorisation number 0065/0036

Date of approval/revision June 1995

Legal category POM

DEXAMETHASONE INJECTION 5 mg/ml

Qualitative and quantitative composition Dexamethasone sodium phosphate BP 5.0 mg/ml(vials)

Dexamethasone sodium phosphate BP 5.0 mg/ml (ampoules)

Pharmaceutical form Solution for injection.

Clinical particulars
Therapeutic indications: Dexamethasone injection can be used for all forms of general and local glucocorticoid injection therapy and all acute conditions in which intravenous glucocorticoids may be life-saving.

Posology and method of administration:
Dosage: **N.B.** All doses are expressed as mg dexamethasone sodium phosphate.

In general, glucocorticoid dosage depends on the severity of the condition and response of the patient. Under certain circumstances, for instance in stress, extra dosage adjustments may be necessary. If no favourable response is noted within a couple of days, glucocorticoid therapy should be discontinued.

Adults and elderly: Once the disease is under control the dosage should be reduced or tapered off to the lowest suitable level under continuous monitoring and observation of the patient. (See *Special warnings and special precautions for use*).

For acute life-threatening situations (e.g. anaphylaxis, acute severe asthma) substantially higher dosages may be needed. Cerebral oedema (adults): initial dose 10-20 mg iv followed by 6 mg iv or im every 6 hours, until a satisfactory result has been obtained. In brain surgery these dosages may be necessary until several days after the operation. Thereafter, the dosage has to be tapered off gradually. Increase of intracranial pressure associated with brain tumours can be counteracted by continuous treatment.

For local treatment, the following dosages can be recommended:

- intra-articulary: 2–4 mg large joints; 0.8-1 mg small joints
- intrabursally: 2- 4 mg;
- in tendon sheaths: 0.4–1 mg

The frequency of these injections may vary from every 3-5 days to every 2 -3 weeks.

For rectal drip in cases of ulcerative colitis: 5 mg diluted in 120 ml saline.

Suggested doses for children: Dosage requirements are variable and may have to be changed according to individual needs. Usually 0.25 mg/kg to 0.5 mg/kg of body weight daily.

Administration: Dexamethasone Injection may be administered intravenously, subcutaneously, intramuscularly, by local injection or as a rectal drip. For administration by intravenous infusion: (See section on 'compatibility with infusion fluids'). With intravenous administration high plasma levels can be obtained rapidly.

Rapid intravenous injection of massive doses of glucocorticoids may sometimes cause cardiovascular collapse; the injection should therefore be given slowly over a period of several minutes.

Intra-articular injections should be given under strictly aseptic conditions.

Contra-indications: Systemic infection unless specific anti-infective therapy is employed.

Hypersensitivity to any ingredient.

Local injection of a glucocorticoid is contraindicated in bacteraemia and systemic fungal infections, unstable joints, infection at the injection site e.g. septic arthritis resulting from gonorrhoea or tuberculosis.

Special warnings and special precautions for use: **A patient information leaflet should be supplied with this product.**

Undesirable effects may be minimised by using the lowest effective dose for the minimum period, and by administering the daily requirement as a single morning dose or whenever possible as a single morning dose on alternative days. Frequent patient review is required to appropriately titrate the dose against disease activity.

After parenteral administration of glucocorticoids serious anaphylactoid reactions, such as glottis oedema, urticaria and bronchospasm, have occasionally occurred, particularly in patients with a history of allergy. If such an anaphylactoid reaction occurs, the following measures are recommended: immediate slow intravenous injection of 0.1–0.5 ml of adrenaline (solution of 1:1000: 0.1–0.5 mg adrenaline dependent on body weight), intravenous administration of aminophylline and artificial respiration if necessary.

Dexamethasone withdrawal: Adrenal cortical atrophy develops during prolonged therapy and may persist for years after stopping treatment. Withdrawal of corticosteroids after prolonged therapy must therefore always be gradual to avoid acute adrenal insufficiency, being tapered off over weeks or months according to the dose and duration of treatment.

In patients who have received more than physiological doses of systemic corticosteroids (approximately 1 mg dexamethasone) for greater than 3 weeks, withdrawal should not be abrupt. How dose reduction should be carried out depends largely on whether the disease is likely to relapse as the dose of systemic corticosteroids is reduced. Clinical assessment of disease activity may be needed during withdrawal. If the disease is unlikely to relapse on withdrawal of systemic corticosteroids but there is uncertainty about HPA suppression, the dose of systemic corticosteroid *may* be reduced rapidly to physiological doses. Once a daily dose of 1 mg dexamethasone is reached, dose reduction should be slower to allow the HPA-axis to recover.

Abrupt withdrawal of systemic corticosteroid treatment, which has continued up to 3 weeks is appropriate if it is considered that the disease is unlikely to relapse. Abrupt withdrawal of doses of up to 6 mg daily of dexamethasone for 3 weeks is unlikely to lead to clinically relevant HPA-axis suppression in the majority of patients. In the following patient groups, gradual withdrawal of systemic corticosteroid therapy should be *considered* even after courses lasting 3 weeks or less:

Patients who have had repeated courses of systemic corticosteroids, particularly if taken for greater than 3 weeks.

When a short course has been prescribed within one year of cessation of long-term therapy (months or years).

Patients who may have reasons for adrenocortical insufficiency other than exogenous corticosteroid therapy.

Patients receiving doses of systemic corticosteroid greater than 6 mg daily of dexamethasone.

Patients repeatedly taking doses in the evening.

During prolonged therapy any intercurrent illness, trauma or surgical procedure will require a temporary increase in dosage; if corticosteroids have been stopped following prolonged therapy they may need to be temporarily re-introduced.

Patients should carry 'Steroid treatment' cards which give clear guidance on the precautions to be taken to minimise risk and which provide details of prescriber, drug, dosage and the duration of treatment.

Anti-inflammatory/immunosuppressive effects and infection: Suppression of the inflammatory response and immune function increases the susceptibility to infections and their severity. The clinical presentation may often be atypical, and serious infections such as septicaemia and tuberculosis may be masked and may reach an advanced stage before being recognised.

Appropriate antimicrobial therapy should accompany glucocorticoid therapy when necessary e.g. in tuberculosis and viral and fungal infections of the eye.

Chickenpox is of particular concern since this normally minor illness may be fatal in immunosuppressed patients. Patients (or parents of children) without a definite history of chickenpox should be advised to avoid close personal contact with chickenpox or herpes zoster and if exposed they should seek urgent medical attention. Passive immunisation with varicella zoster immunoglobulin (VZIG) is needed by exposed non-immune patients who are receiving systemic corticosteroids or who have used them within the previous 3 months; this should be given within 10 days of exposure to chickenpox. If a diagnosis of chickenpox is confirmed, the illness warrants specialist care and urgent treatment. Corticosteroids should not be stopped and the dose may need to be increased.

Live vaccines should not be given to individuals with impaired immune responsiveness. The antibody response to other vaccines may be diminished.

Special precautions: Particular care is required when considering the use of systemic corticosteroids in patients with the following conditions and frequent patient monitoring is necessary.

a. Osteoporosis (post-menopausal females are particularly at risk).
b. Hypertension or congestive heart failure.
c. Existing or previous history of severe affective disorders (especially previous steroid psychosis).
d. Diabetes mellitus (or a family history of diabetes).
e. History of tuberculosis, since glucocorticoids may induce reactivation.
f. Glaucoma (or a family history of glaucoma).
g. Previous corticosteroid-induced myopathy.
h. Liver failure.
i. Renal insufficiency.
j. Epilepsy.
k. Gastro-intestinal ulceration.
l. Migraine.
m. Certain parasitic infestations in particular amoebiasis.
n. Incomplete statural growth since glucocorticoids on prolonged administration may accelerate epiphyseal closure.
o. Patients with Cushing's syndrome.

In the treatment of conditions such as tendinitis or tenosynovitis care should be taken to inject into the space between the tendon sheath and the tendon as cases of ruptured tendon have been reported.

Use in children: Corticosteroids cause dose-related growth retardation in infancy, childhood and adolescence, which may be irreversible.

Use in the elderly: The common adverse effects of systemic corticosteroids may be associated with more serious consequences in old age, especially osteoporosis, hypertension, hypokalaemia, diabetes, susceptibility to infection and thinning of the skin. Close clinical supervision is required to avoid life-threatening reactions.

Interactions with other medicaments and other forms of interaction: Rifampicin, rifabutin, ephedrine, carbamazepine, phenylbutazone, phenobarbitone, phenytoin, primidone, and aminoglutethimide enhance the metabolism of corticosteroids and its therapeutic effects may be reduced.

The desired effects of hypoglycaemic agents (including insulin), anti-hypertensives, cardiac glycosides and diuretics are antagonised by corticosteroids, and the hypokalaemic effects of acetazolamide, loop diuretics, thiazide diuretics and carbenoxolone are enhanced.

The efficacy of coumarin anticoagulants may be enhanced by concurrent corticosteroid therapy and close monitoring of the INR or prothrombin time is required to avoid spontaneous bleeding.

The renal clearance of salicylates is increased by corticosteroids and steroid withdrawal may result in salicylate intoxication. There may be interaction with salicylates in patients with hypoprothrombinaemia.

Pregnancy and lactation: The ability of corticosteroids to cross the placenta varies between individual drugs, however, dexamethasone readily crosses the placenta.

Administration of corticosteroids to pregnant animals can cause abnormalities of foetal development including cleft palate, intra-uterine growth retardation and affects on brain growth and development. There is no evidence that corticosteroids result in an increased incidence of congenital abnormalities, such as cleft palate/lip in man. However, when administered for prolonged periods or repeatedly during pregnancy, corticosteroids may increase the risk of intra-uterine growth retardation. Hypoadrenalism may, in theory, occur in the neonate following prenatal exposure to corticosteroids but usually resolves spontaneously following birth and is rarely clinically important. As with all drugs, corticosteroids should only be prescribed when the benefits to the mother and child outweigh the risks. When corticosteroids are essential however, patients with normal pregnancies may be treated as though they were in the non-gravid state.

Lactation: Corticosteroids may pass into breast milk, although no data are available for dexamethasone. Infants of mothers taking high doses of systemic corticosteroids for prolonged periods may have a degree of adrenal suppression.

Effects on ability to drive and use of machines: None known

Undesirable effects: Side-effects: Local adverse reactions include post-injection flare, and a painless destruction of the joint reminiscent of Charcots arthropathy especially with repeated intra-articular injection.

The incidence of predictable undesirable effects, including hypothalamic-pituitary-adrenal suppression correlates with the relative potency of the drug, dosage, timing of administration and the duration of treatment. Cases of ruptured tendon have been reported. (See *Special warnings and special precautions for use*).

Local injection of glucocorticoid may produce systemic effects.

Endocrine/metabolic: Suppression of the hypothalamic-pituitary-adrenal axis, premature epiphyseal closure, growth suppression in infancy, childhood and adolescence, menstrual irregularity and amenorrhoea. Cushiongoid faces, hirsutism, weight gain, impaired carbohydrate tolerance with increased requirement for anti-diabetic therapy. Negative protein and calcium balance. Increased appetite.

Anti-inflammatory and immunosuppressive effects: Increased susceptibility and severity of infections with suppression of clinical symptoms and signs. Diminished lymphoid tissue and immune response. Opportunistic infections, recurrence of dormant tuberculosis and decreased responsiveness to vaccination and skin tests. (See *Special warnings and special precautions for use*).

Musculoskeletal: Osteoporosis, vertebral and long bone fractures, avascular osteonecrosis, tendon rupture. Proximal myopathy.

Fluid and electrolyte disturbance: Sodium and water retention, hypertension, potassium loss, hypokalaemic alkalosis.

Neuropsychiatric: Psychological dependence, depression, insomnia, and aggravation of schizophrenia. Increased intra-cranial pressure with papilloedema in children (pseudotumour cerebri), usually after treatment withdrawal. Aggravation of epilepsy. Psychic disturbances ranging from euphoria to frank psychotic manifestations.

Ophthalmic: Increased intra-ocular pressure, glaucoma, papilloedema, posterior subcapsular cataracts, corneal or scleral thinning, exacerbation of opthalmic viral or fungal diseases.

Gastrointestinal: Dyspepsia, peptic ulceration with perforation and haemorrhage, acute pancreatitis, candidiasis.

Dermatological: Impaired healing, skin atrophy, bruising, telangiectasia, striae, increased sweating and acne.

General: Hypersensitivity including anaphylaxis, has been reported. Leucocytosis. Thromboembolism.

A transient burning or tingling sensation mainly in the perineal area following intravenous injection of large doses of corticosteroid phosphates.

Withdrawal symptoms and signs: Too rapid a reduction of corticosteroid dosage following prolonged treatment can lead to acute adrenal insufficiency, hypotension and death. (See *Special warnings and special precautions for use*).

A 'withdrawal syndrome' may also occur including, fever, myalgia, arthralgia, rhinitis, conjunctivitis, painful itchy skin nodules and loss of weight.

Overdosage: It is difficult to define an excessive dose of a corticosteroid as the therapeutic dose will vary according to the indication and patient requirements. Massive i.v. corticosteroid doses given as a pulse in emergencies are relatively free from hazardous effects.

Exaggeration of corticosteroid related adverse effects may occur. Treatment should be asymptomatic and supportive as necessary.

Pharmacological properties

Pharmacodynamic properties: Dexamethasone is a synthetic adrenocorticoid with approximately a 7 times higher anti-inflammatory potency than prednisolone and 30 times that of hydrocortisone. Adrenocorticoids act on the HPA at specific receptors on the plasma membrane. On other tissues the adrenocorticoids diffuse across cell membranes and complex with specific cytoplasmic receptors which enter the cell nucleus and stimulate protein synthesis. Adrenocorticoids have anti-allergic, antitoxic, antishock, antipyretic and immunosuppressive properties. Dexamethasone has only minor mineralocorticoid activities and does therefore, not induce water and sodium retention.

Pharmacokinetic properties: After administration of dexamethasone injection, dexamethasone sodium phosphate is rapidly hydrolysed to dexamethasone. After an iv dose of 20 mg dexamethasone plasma levels peak within 5 minutes. Dexamethasone is bound (up to 77%) by plasma proteins, mainly albumin. There is a high uptake of dexamethasone by the liver, kidney and adrenal glands. Metabolism in the liver is slow and excretion is mainly in the urine, largely as unconjugated steroids. The plasma half life is 3.5-4.5 hours but as the effects outlast the significant plasma concentrations of steroids the plasma half-life is of little relevance and the use of biological half life is more applicable. The biological half life of dexamethasone is 36-54 hours, therefore dexamethasone is especially suitable in conditions where continuous glucocorticoid action is desirable.

Preclinical safety data: Not applicable

Pharmaceutical particulars

List of excipients:

Amps	*Vials*
Glycerol PhEur	Glycerol PhEur
Disodium edetate PhEur	Disodium edetate PhEur
Water for injections PhEur	Methyl paraben PhEur
Sodium hydroxide PhEur or	Propyl paraben PhEur
Phosphoric acid PhEur	Water for injections PhEur
	Sodium hydroxide PhEur or
	Phosphoric acid PhEur

Incompatibilities: None known

Shelf-life: 2 years

Special precautions for storage: Store below 25°C. Protect from light. Do not freeze the ampoules.

Nature and contents of containers:

1 ml glass ampoules in cartons of 5, 10 or 25, 2 ml glass vials cartons of 1 or 10.

Instructions for use/handling

Use with infusion fluids: Dexamethasone Injection has been shown to retain its potency for at least 24 hours at room temperature, and in daylight conditions, when diluted with one of the following infusion fluids:

sodium chloride 0.9%
anhydrous glucose 5%
invert sugar 10%
sorbitol 5%
Ringer's solution
Hartmann's solution (ringer-lactate)
Rheomacrodex
Haemaccel

Using these infusion fluids, Dexamethasone Injection can also be injected into the infusion line without causing precipitation of the ingredients. Direct injection into the infusion line is also possible with the following infusion fluids:

mannitol 10%
Vamin N (See *Special warnings and special precautions for use*).

Marketing authorisation numbers

2 ml vial	PL 0065/5013R
1 ml ampoule	PL 0065/0106R

Date of partial revision of the text April 1998.

Legal category POM.

DEXAMETHASONE TABLETS

Qualitative and quantitative composition 500 microgram tablet contains 500 mg dexamethasone PhEur. 2.0 mg tablet contains 2.0 mg dexamethasone PhEur.

Pharmaceutical form Tablet

Clinical particulars

Therapeutic indications: Indicated in a wide variety of disorders amenable to glucocorticoid therapy, as well as an adjunct in the control of cerebral oedema.

Posology and method of administration: In general, glucocorticoid dosage depends on the severity of the condition and response of the patient. Under certain circumstances, for instance in stress, and changed clinical picture, extra dosage adjustments may be necessary. If no favourable response is noted within a couple of days, glucocorticoid therapy should be discontinued.

Adults: Usually, daily oral dosages of 0.5–10 mg are sufficient. In some patients higher dosages may be temporarily required to control the disease. Once the disease is under control the dosage should be reduced or tapered off to the lowest suitable level under continuous monitoring and observation of the patient. (See *Special warnings and special precautions for use*).

For a short dexamethasone suppression test, 1 mg dexamethasone is given at 11 p.m. and plasma cortisol measured the next morning. Patients who do not show a decrease in cortisol can be exposed to a longer test: 500 micrograms dexamethasone is given at 6 hourly intervals for 48 hours followed by 2 mg every 6 hours for a further 48 hours. 24 hour-urine collections are made before, during and at the end of the test for determination of 17-hydroxycorticosteroids.

Children: 0.01-0.1 mg/kg of body weight daily. Dosage of glucocorticoids should be adjusted on the basis of the individual patient's response.

Contra-indications: Systemic infection unless specific anti-infective therapy is employed. Hypersensitivity to any ingredient. In general no contra-indications apply in conditions where the use of glucocorticoids may be life saving.

Special warnings and special precautions for use: **A patient information leaflet should be supplied with this product**. Undesirable effects may be minimised by using the lowest effective dose for the minimum period, and by administering the daily requirement as a single morning dose or whenever possible as a single morning dose on alternative days. Frequent patient review is required to appropriately titrate the dose against disease activity. (See *Posology and method of administration*).

Dexamethasone withdrawal: Adrenal cortical atrophy develops during prolonged therapy and may persist for years after stopping treatment. Withdrawal of corticosteroids after prolonged therapy must therefore always be gradual to avoid acute adrenal insufficiency, being tapered off over weeks or months according to the dose and duration of treatment.

In patients who have received more than physiological doses of systemic corticosteroids (approximately 1 mg dexamethasone) for greater than 3 weeks, withdrawal should not be abrupt. How dose reduction should be carried out depends largely on whether the disease is likely to relapse as the dose of systemic corticosteroids is reduced. Clinical assessment of disease activity may be needed during withdrawal. If the disease is unlikely to relapse on withdrawal of systemic corticosteroids but there is uncertainty about HPA suppression, the dose of systemic corticosteroid *may* be reduced rapidly to physiological doses. Once a daily dose of 1 mg dexamethasone is reached, dose reduction should be slower to allow the HPA-axis to recover.

Abrupt withdrawal of systemic corticosteroid treatment, which has continued up to 3 weeks is appropriate if it is considered that the disease is unlikely to relapse. Abrupt withdrawal of doses of up to 6 mg daily of dexamethasone for 3 weeks is unlikely to lead to clinically relevant HPA-axis suppression in the majority of patients. In the following patient groups, gradual withdrawal of systemic corticosteroid therapy should be *considered* even after courses lasting 3 weeks or less:

Patients who have had repeated courses of systemic corticosteroids, particularly if taken for greater than 3 weeks.

When a short course has been prescribed within one year of cessation of long-term therapy (months or years).

Patients who may have reasons for adrenocortical insufficiency other than exogenous corticosteroid therapy.

Patients receiving doses of systemic corticosteroid greater than 6 mg daily of dexamethasone.

Patients repeatedly taking doses in the evening.

During prolonged therapy any intercurrent illness, trauma or surgical procedure will require a temporary increase in dosage; if corticosteroids have been stopped following prolonged therapy they may need to be temporarily re-introduced.

Patients should carry 'Steroid treatment' cards which give clear guidance on the precautions to be taken to minimise risk and which provide details of prescriber, drug, dosage and the duration of treatment.

Anti-inflammatory/immunosuppressive effects and infection: Suppression of the inflammatory response and immune function increases the susceptibility to infections and their severity. The clinical presentation may often be atypical, and serious infections such as septicaemia and tuberculosis may be masked and may reach an advanced stage before being recognised.

Appropriate anti-microbial therapy should accompany glucocorticoid therapy when necessary e.g. in tuberculosis and viral and fungal infections of the eye.

Chickenpox is of particular concern since this normally minor illness may be fatal in immunosuppressed patients. Patients (or parents of children) without a definite history of chickenpox should be advised to avoid close personal contact with chickenpox or herpes zoster and if exposed they should seek urgent medical attention. Passive immunisation with varicella zoster immunoglobulin (VZIG) is needed by exposed non-immune patients who are receiving systemic corticosteroids or who have used them within the previous 3 months; this should be given within 10 days of exposure to chickenpox. *If a diagnosis of chickenpox is confirmed, the illness warrants specialist care and urgent treatment. Corticosteroids should not be stopped and the dose may need to be increased.*

Live vaccines should not be given to individuals with impaired immune responsiveness. The antibody response to other vaccines may be diminished.

Particular care is required when considering the use of systemic corticosteroids in patients with the following conditions and frequent patient monitoring is necessary.

a. Osteoporosis (post-menopausal females are particularly at risk).
b. Hypertension or congestive heart failure.
c. Existing or previous history of severe affective disorders (especially previous steroid psychosis).
d. Diabetes mellitus (or a family history of diabetes).
e. History of tuberculosis.
f. Glaucoma (or a family history of glaucoma).
g. Previous corticosteroid-induced myopathy.
h. Liver failure.
i. Renal insufficiency.
j. Epilepsy.
k. Peptic ulceration.
l. Migraine
m. Certain parasitic infestations in particular amoebiasis
n. Incomplete natural growth since glucocorticoids on prolonged administration may accelerate epiphyseal closure.

After administration of glucocorticoids serious anaphylactoid reactions such as glottis oedema, urticaria and bronchospasm have occasionally occurred particularly in patients with a history of allergy.

If such an anaphylactoid reaction occurs, the following measures are recommended: immediate slow intravenous injection of 0.1-0.5 ml of adrenaline (solution of 1:1000: 0.1-0.5 mg adrenaline dependent on body weight), intravenous administration of aminophylline and artificial respiration if necessary.

Use in children: Corticosteroids cause dose-related growth retardation in infancy, childhood and adolescence, which may be irreversible.

Use in the elderly: The common adverse effects of systemic corticosteroids may be associated with more serious consequences in old age, especially osteoporosis, hypertension, hypokalaemia, diabetes, susceptibility to infection and thinning of the skin. Close clinical supervision is required to avoid life-threatening reactions.

Interaction with other medicaments and other forms of interaction: Rifampicin, rifabutin, carbamazepine, phenobarbitone, phenytoin, primidone, and aminoglutethimide enhance the metabolism of corticosteroids and its therapeutic effects may be reduced.

The desired effects of hypoglycaemic agents (including insulin), anti-hypertensives and diuretics are antagonised by corticosteroids, and the hypokalaemic effects of acetazolamide, loop diuretics, thiazide diuretics and carbenoxolone are enhanced.

The efficacy of coumarin anticoagulants may be enhanced by concurrent corticosteroid therapy and close monitoring of the INR or prothrombin time is required to avoid spontaneous bleeding.

The renal clearance of salicylates is increased by corticosteroids and steroid withdrawal may result in salicylate intoxication.

Patients taking NSAIDs should be monitored since the incidence and/or severity of gastro-intestinal ulceration may increase.

Antacids, especially those containing magnesium trisilicate have been reported to impair the gastrointestinal absorption of glucocorticoid steroids. Therefore, doses of one agent should be spaced as far as possible from the other.

Pregnancy and lactation: The ability of corticosteroids to cross the placenta varies between individual drugs, however, dexamethasone readily crosses the placenta.

Administration of corticosteroids to pregnant animals can cause abnormalities of foetal development including cleft palate, intra-uterine growth retardation and affects on brain growth and development. There is no evidence that corticosteroids result in an increased incidence of congenital abnormalities, such as cleft palate/lip in man. However, when administered for prolonged periods or repeatedly during pregnancy, corticosteroids may increase the risk of intrauterine growth retardation. Hypoadrenalism may, in theory, occur in the neonate following prenatal exposure to corticosteroids but usually resolves spontaneously following birth and is rarely clinically important. As with all drugs, corticosteroids should only be prescribed when the benefits to the mother and child outweigh the risks. When corticosteroids are essential however, patients with normal pregnancies may be treated as though they were in the non-gravid state.

Lactation: Corticosteroids may pass into breast milk, although no data are available for dexamethasone. Infants of mothers taking high doses of systemic corticosteroids for prolonged periods may have a degree of adrenal suppression.

Effects on ability to drive and use machines: None known

Undesirable effects: The incidence of predictable undesirable effects, including hypothalamic-pituitary-adrenal suppression correlates with the relative potency of the drug, dosage, timing of administration and the duration of treatment. (See *Special warnings and precautions for use*).

Endocrine/metabolic: Suppression of the hypothalamic-pituitary-adrenal axis, growth suppression in infancy, childhood and adolescence, menstrual irregularity and amenorrhoea. Cushingoid faces, hirsutism, weight gain, premature epiphyseal closure, impaired carbohydrate tolerance with increased requirement for anti-diabetic therapy. Negative protein and calcium balance. Increased appetite.

Anti-inflammatory and immunosuppressive effects: Increased susceptibility and severity of infections with suppression of clinical symptoms and signs, opportunistic infections, recurrence of dormant tuberculosis. (See *Special warnings and precautions for use*). Decreased responsiveness to vaccination and skin tests.

Musculoskeletal: Osteoporosis, vertebral and long bone fractures, avascular osteonecrosis, tendon rupture. Proximal myopathy.

Fluid and electrolyte disturbance: Sodium and water retention, hypertension, potassium loss, hypokalaemic alkalosis.

Neuropsychiatric: Psychological dependence, depression, insomnia, and aggravation of schizophrenia. Increased intra-cranial pressure with papilloedema in children (pseudotumour cerebri), usually after treatment withdrawal. Aggravation of epilepsy. Psychic disturbances ranging from euphoria to frank psychotic manifestations.

Ophthalmic: Increased intra-ocular pressure, glaucoma, papilloedema, posterior subcapsular cataracts, corneal or scleral thinning, exacerbation of opthalmic viral or fungal diseases.

Gastrointestinal: Dyspepsia, peptic ulceration with perforation and haemorrhage, acute pancreatitis, candidiasis. Abdominal distension and vomiting.

Dermatological: Impaired healing, skin atrophy, bruising, telangiectasia, striae, acne.

General: Hypersensitivity including anaphylaxis, has been reported. Leucocytosis. Thromboembolism.

Withdrawal symptoms and signs: Too rapid a reduction of corticosteroid dosage following prolonged treatment can lead to acute adrenal insufficiency, hypotension and death. (See *Special warnings and precautions for use*).

A 'withdrawal syndrome' may also occur including, fever, myalgia, arthralgia, rhinitis, conjunctivitis, painful itchy skin nodules and loss of weight.

Overdosage: It is difficult to define an excessive dose of a corticosteroid as the therapeutic dose will vary according to indication and patient requirements. Exaggeration of corticosteroid related adverse effects may occur. Treatment should be asymptomatic and supportive as necessary.

Pharmacological properties

Pharmacodynamic properties: Dexamethasone is a synthetic glucocorticoid whose anti-inflammatory potency is 7 times greater than prednisolone. Like other glucocorticoids, dexamethasone also has anti-allergic, antipyretic and immunosuppressive properties.

Dexamethasone has practically no water and salt-retaining properties and is, therefore, particularly suitable for the use in patients with cardiac failure or hypertension. Because of its long biological half-life (36-54 hours), dexamethasone is especially suitable in conditions where continuous glucocorticoid action is desired.

Pharmacokinetic properties: Corticosteroids, are, in general, readily absorbed from the gastro-intestinal tract. They are also well absorbed from sites of local application. Water-soluble forms of corticosteroids are given by intravenous injection for a rapid response; more prolonged effects are achieved using lipid-soluble forms of corticosteroids by intramuscular injection.

Corticosteroids are rapidly distributed to all body tissues. They cross the placenta and may be excreted in small amounts in breast milk.

Most corticosteroids in the circulation are extensively bound to plasma proteins, mainly to globulin and less so to albumin. The corticosteroid-binding globulin has high affinity but low binding capacity, while the albumin has low affinity but large binding capacity. The synthetic corticosteroids are less extensively protein bound than hydrocortisone (cortisol). They also tend to have longer half-lives.

Corticosteroids are metabolised mainly in the liver but also in the kidney, and are excreted in the urine. The slower metabolism of the synthetic corticosteroids with their lower protein-binding affinity may account for their increased potency compared with the natural corticosteroids.

Preclinical safety data: Not applicable

Pharmaceutical particulars

List of excipients:

0.5 mg tablet: Glycerol PhEur; potato starch PhEur; magnesium stearate PhEur; talc PhEur and lactose PhEur.

2 mg tablets: Potato starch PhEur; propylene glycol PhEur; magnesium stearate PhEur; and lactose PhEur.

Incompatibilities: None known.

Shelf-life: 5 years – when stored in polyethylene tampertainers. 3 years – when stored in polystyrene bottle.

Special precautions for storage: Store below 25°C protected from light.

Nature and contents of containers: Polyethylene tampertainers with child resistant closures Polystyrene bottles containing 50, 100 or 500 tablets.

Instructions for use/handling: Not applicable.

Marketing authorisation numbers
0065/5044R & 0065/0045R

Date of preparation of the text April 1998

Legal category: POM

LIVIAL*

Qualitative and quantitative composition Each Livial tablet contains as active substance 2.5 mg of the steroid tibolone.

Pharmaceutical form Tablets for oral use.

Clinical Particulars

Therapeutic indications: In oestrogen deficiency states for the treatment of vasomotor symptoms (such as hot flushes and sweating), depressed mood, decreased libido and prevention of osteoporosis in women at risk of developing fractures.

However at present there is no established screening programme for determining women at risk of developing osteoporosis and osteoporotic fractures. Epidemiological studies suggest a number of individual risk factors which contribute to the development of postmenopausal osteoporosis. These include early menopause, family history of osteoporosis, thinness, small frame, cigarette use and recent prolonged systemic corticosteroid use. If several of these risk factors are present in a patient, consideration should be given to hormone replacement therapy.

Posology and method of administration: Adults and the elderly: Livial tablets should be swallowed without chewing, preferably at the same time of day.

The dosage is one tablet per day. Improvement of symptoms generally occurs within a few weeks, but optimal results are obtained when therapy is continued for at least 3 months. At the recommended dosage, Livial may be used uninterrupted for longer periods. For prevention of osteoporosis in postmenopausal women long term therapy (5-10 years) is required.

Starting Livial: For the treatment of vasomotor symptoms and the prevention of osteoporosis.

- Women experiencing a natural menopause should commence treatment with Livial 12 months after their last natural bleed. If Livial is taken sooner than this irregular menstrual bleeding may occur.
- Women experiencing a surgical menopause may commence treatment with Livial immediately
- Women being treated with gonadotrophin releasing hormone (GnRH) analogues, for example, for endometriosis, may commence treatment with Livial immediately.

Switching from another HRT preparation: If changing from another HRT preparation the endometrium may already be stimulated, so induction of a withdrawal bleed with a progestogen is advisable.

Missed pills: A missed dose should be taken as soon as remembered, unless it is more than 12 hours overdue. In the latter case, the missed dose should be skipped and the next dose should be taken at the normal time.

Children: Not applicable.

Contra-indications:

- Hypersensitivity to the active ingredient or any of the constituents of the product.
- Pregnancy or lactation.
- Known or suspected hormone-dependent tumours.
- Cardiovascular or cerebrovascular disorders e.g. thrombophlebitis, thrombo-embolic processes, or a history of these conditions.
- Undiagnosed vaginal bleeding
- Severe liver disorders.

Special warnings and precautions for use:

- Livial is not intended for contraceptive use.
- Risk-benefit should be considered when any of the following medical conditions exist:
- liver disease or a history of this condition;
- hypercholesterolaemia
- Treatment should be discontinued if results of liver function tests become abnormal, or if cholestatic jaundice appears.
- During prolonged treatment with steroids with hormonal activity, periodic medical examination is advisable.
- In women experiencing a natural menopause Livial should not be prescribed in the premenopause

because, in view of the ovulation inhibition, cycle regularity may be disturbed.

- In postmenopausal women Livial does not stimulate the endometrium; the incidence of vaginal bleeding is no higher than that with placebo use. In women in whom some endogenous oestrogen is still produced, vaginal bleeding may occur during Livial therapy because of an apparently stimulated endometrium. Normally such a bleeding is of short duration. Bleeding commencing after three months of treatment or recurrent or persistent bleeding should be appropriately investigated, however in most cases no apparent cause of the bleeding is found.
- In women changing from another form of hormonal substitution therapy to Livial therapy, it is always advisable to induce a withdrawal bleed with a progestogen, because also in these women the endometrium may be stimulated.

Epidemiological studies have suggested that hormone replacement therapy (HRT) is associated with an increased relative risk of developing venous thromboembolism (VTE) i.e. deep vein thrombosis or pulmonary embolism. It is unclear whether tibolone carries the same risk as other types of HRT in this regard.

Generally recognised risk factors for VTE include a personal or family history and severe obesity (Body Mass Index >30 kg/m²). In women with these factors the benefits of treatment with tibolone need to be carefully weighed against possible risks. There is no consensus about the possible role of varicose veins in VTE.

The risk of VTE may be temporarily increased with prolonged immobilisation, major trauma or major surgery. In women on tibolone scrupulous attention should be given to prophylactic measures to prevent VTE following surgery. Where prolonged immobilisation is liable to follow elective surgery, particularly abdominal or orthopaedic surgery to the lower limbs, consideration should be given to temporarily stopping tibolone 4 weeks earlier.

- If venous thromboembolism develops after initiating therapy the drug should be discontinued.
- Patients with any of the following conditions should be monitored:
  - renal dysfunction, liver disease, epilepsy or migraine or a history of these conditions, since the use of steroids with hormonal activity may occasionally induce fluid retention;
  - hypercholesterolaemia, since during Livial treatment changes in the serum lipid profile have been observed.
  - impaired carbohydrate metabolism, since Livial may diminish glucose tolerance and increase the need for insulin or other antidiabetic drugs.

Interaction with other medicaments and other forms of interaction: No examples of interactions between Livial and other medicines have been reported in clinical practice. However, the following potential interactions should be considered on a theoretical basis:

Enzyme inducing compounds such as barbiturates, carbamazepine, hydantoins and rifampicin may enhance the metabolism of tibolone and thus decrease its therapeutic effect.

Since tibolone may increase blood fibrinolytic activity (lower fibrinogen levels, higher antithrombin III, plasminogen and fibrinolytic activity values) it may enhance the effect of anticoagulants.

Pregnancy and lactation: There is no clinical experience with Livial in pregnancy but animal studies have indicated that tibolone is fetotoxic. Livial is contraindicated in pregnancy and lactation.

Effects on ability to drive and use machines: Livial is not known to have any effects on alertness and concentration.

Undesirable effects: Occasionally, vaginal bleeding or spotting may occur, mainly during the first months of treatment. Other adverse events that have been observed occasionally include: change of body weight, dizziness, rash, pruritus, seborrhoeic dermatosis, increased facial hair growth, headache, migraine, visual disturbances (including blurred vision), gastrointestinal upset, abdominal pain, depression, oedema, effects on the musculoskeletal system such as arthralgia or myalgia and changes in liver function parameters. There have been reports of endometrial hyperplasia and endometrial cancer in patients treated with tibolone although a causal relationship has not been established.

Overdosage: The acute toxicity of tibolone in animals is very low. Therefore toxic symptoms are not expected to occur even when several tablets are taken simultaneously. In cases of acute overdose, nausea, vomiting and withdrawal bleeding in females may develop. No specific antidote is known. Symptomatic treatment can be given if necessary.

Pharmacological properties

Pharmacodynamic properties: After oral administration tibolone is rapidly metabolised into three compounds which contribute to the pharmacological effects of Livial. Two of these metabolites have predominantly oestrogenic activity, a third metabolite and the parent compound have predominantly progestagenic activity.

Livial has an oestrogen-like effect on hot flushes and other climacteric complaints. In addition, oestrogen-like effects are exerted on the vagina and bone. Due to its progestagenic effects Livial does not stimulate the endometrium. Therefore, if bleeding occurs, this usually results from an atrophic endometrium. Finally, Livial has effects on certain metabolic and haematological parameters such as a decrease in plasma high density lipoprotein cholesterol, triglycerides, lipoprotein (a) and an increase in blood fibrinolytic activity.

Pharmacokinetic properties: After oral administration tibolone is rapidly and extensively absorbed. Due to rapid metabolism the plasma levels of tibolone are very low. Pharmacokinetic data indicate linear kinetics. Peak plasma levels are reached after 1–4 hours and accumulation does not occur.

Excretion of tibolone is mainly in the form of polar and very polar metabolites. A small amount of the administered compound is excreted in the urine, but most is eliminated via the bile and the faeces.

Preclinical safety data: Livial is not genotoxic. Although a carcinogenic effect was seen in certain strains of rat (hepatic tumours) and mouse (bladder tumours), the relevance of this evidence to man is uncertain.

Pharmaceutical particulars

List of excipients: Potato starch; magnesium stearate; ascorbyl palmitate and lactose.

Incompatibilities: None known.

Shelf-life: When stored as indicated the tablets can be stored for up to two years.

Special precautions for storage: Livial tablets should be stored at room temperature (below 25°C), protected from moisture and light.

Nature and contents of container: Press-through strips of 28 or 30 tablets each containing 2.5 mg of tibolone. Cartons containing 1 strip or 3 strips.

Instructions for use/handling: Not applicable.

Marketing authorisation number 0065/0086.

Date of (partial) revison the text March 1998.

Legal Category POM.

MARVELON*

Presentation White, round, biconvex tablets, diameter 6 mm, coded TR5 on one side and ORGANON* on the reverse side.

Each pack of Marvelon contains 21 tablets.

Each tablet contains: desogestrel B.P. (a progestogen) 150 micrograms; ethinylestradiol EP (an estrogen) 30 micrograms.

Other ingredients: dl-alpha-tocopherol, potato starch, povidone, stearic acid, aerosil and lactose.

Uses Oral contraception.

Dosage and Administration It is preferable that tablet intake from the first pack is started on the first day of menstruation in which case no extra contraceptive precautions are necessary.

If menstruation has already begun,(that is 2, 3, or 4 days previously), tablet taking should commence on day 5 of the menstrual period. In this case additional contraceptive precautions must be taken for the first 7 days of tablet taking.

If menstruation began more than 5 days previously then the patient should be advised to wait until her next menstrual period before starting to take Marvelon.

How to take Marvelon: One tablet is taken daily at the same time,(preferably in the evening) without interruption for 21 days, followed by a break of 7 tablet-free days. Each subsequent pack is started after the 7 tablet-free days have elapsed.

Additional contraceptive precautions are not then required.

Use during pregnancy and breast feeding: Marvelon is contraindicated for use during pregnancy or suspected pregnancy and in mothers who are breast-feeding.

Post-partum administration: Following childbirth oral contraceptive administration to non-breast feeding mothers should be started 21 days post-partum in which case no additional contraceptive precautions are required.

If intercourse has taken place post-partum, oral contraceptive use should be delayed until the first day of the first menstrual period.

If post-partum administration of Marvelon begins more than 21 days after delivery then additional contraceptive precautions are required for the first 7 days.

N.B. Mothers who are breast feeding should be advised not to use the combined pill since this may reduce the amount of breast-milk, but may be advised instead to use a progestogen-only pill (POP).

After miscarriage or abortion administration should start immediately in which case no additional contraceptive precautions are required.

Changing from a 21 day pill or a 22 day pill to Marvelon: All tablets in the old pack should be finished. The first Marvelon tablet is taken the next day i.e. no gap is left between taking tablets nor does the patient need to wait for her period to begin. Tablets should be taken as instructed in 'How to take Marvelon'. Additional contraceptive precautions are not required. The patient will not have a period until the end of the first Marvelon pack, but this is not harmful, nor does it matter if she experiences some bleeding on tablet-taking days.

Changing from a combined Every Day Pill (28 day tablets) to Marvelon: Marvelon should be started after taking the last **active** tablet from the 'Every Day Pill' pack (i.e. after taking 21 or 22 tablets). The first Marvelon tablet is taken the next day i.e. no gap is left between taking tablets nor does the patient need to wait for her period to begin. Tablets should be taken as instructed in 'How to take Marvelon'. Remaining tablets from the Every Day (ED) pack should be discarded. The patient will not have a period until the end of the first Marvelon pack, but this is not harmful, nor does it matter if she experiences some bleeding on tablet-taking days.

Changing from a progestogen-only pill (POP or mini pill) to Marvelon: The first Marvelon tablet should be taken on the first day of the period, even if the patient has already taken a mini pill on that day. Tablets should be taken as instructed in 'How to take Marvelon'. All the remaining progestogen-only pills in the mini pill pack should be discarded.

If the patient is taking a (mini) pill, then she may not always have a period, especially when she is breast feeding. The first Marvelon tablet should be taken on the day *after* stopping the mini pill. All remaining pills in the mini pill packet must be discarded. Additional contraceptive precautions must be taken for the first 7 days.

Additional contraceptive precautions: When additional contraceptive precautions are required the patient should be advised either not to have sex, or to use a cap plus spermicide, or for her partner to use a condom. Rhythm methods should not be advised as the pill disrupts the usual cyclical changes associated with the natural menstrual cycle e.g. changes in temperature and cervical mucus.

To skip a period: To skip a period, a new pack of Marvelon should be started on the day after finishing the current pack (the patient skips the tablet-free days). Tablet-taking should be continued in the usual way. During the use of the second pack she may experience slight spotting or break-through bleeding but contraceptive protection will not be diminished provided there are no tablet omissions. The next pack of Marvelon is started after the usual 7 tablet-free days, regardless of whether the period has completely finished or not.

REDUCED RELIABILITY: The reliability of Marvelon may be reduced under the following circumstances:

Forgotten tablets: If the forgotten tablet is taken *within 12 hours*, no further precautions are necessary, further tablets should be taken at the usual time.

If one or more tablets are forgotten for *more than 12 hours*, contraceptive protection will be reduced. The patient should take the last forgotten tablet, even if this means taking two tablets in one day, and then continue to take tablets at the normal time. Additional contraceptive precautions should be taken for the next seven days, and the patient should follow the 'seven day rule'. (See *Precautions and Warnings* for further advice).

Vomiting or diarrhoea: If symptoms persist for more than 12 hours the patient should follow the '7-day rule'. (See *Precautions and Warnings* for further advice)

Interactions: The doctor should consider the possibility of interactions between oral contraceptives and other drugs commonly prescribed such as antibiotics, anticonvulsants and barbiturates. (See *Interactions* for further advice).

Surgery, varicose veins or immobilisation: It is advisable to discontinue oral contraceptive use at least 4 to 6 weeks prior to these procedures, and to (re)start not less than 2 weeks after full ambulation. (See *Precautions and Warnings* for further advice).

Contra-indications, warnings etc.
Absolute contra-indications:

- Pregnancy or suspected pregnancy (that cannot yet be excluded) or breast feeding.
- Circulatory disorders (cardiovascular or cerebrovascular) such as thrombophlebitis and thromboembolic processes (or a history of these conditions), moderate to severe hypertension, hyperlipoproteinaemia.
- In addition the presence of more than one of the risk factors for arterial disease which are discussed under 'Serious Adverse Reactions'.
- Severe liver disease, cholestatic jaundice or hepatitis (viral or non-viral), or a history of these conditions if the results of liver function tests have failed to return to normal, and for 3 months after liver function tests have been found to be normal; a history of jaundice of pregnancy or jaundice due to the use of steroids, Rotor syndrome and Dubin-Johnson syndrome, hepatic cell tumours and porphyria.
- Cholelithiasis
- Known or suspected estrogen-dependent tumours, (see *Serious adverse reactions*); endometrial hyperplasia; undiagnosed vaginal bleeding.
- Systemic lupus erythematosus or a history of this condition.
- A history during pregnancy or previous use of steroids of: severe pruritis; pemphigoid gestationis; a manifestation or deterioration of otosclerosis

Relative Contra-indications: If any of the relative contraindications listed below is present, the benefits of estrogen/progestogen-containing preparations must be weighed against the possible risks for each individual case and the patient kept under close supervision. In case of aggravation or appearance of any of these conditions whilst the patient is taking the pill, its use should be discontinued.

- Conditions implicating an increasing risk of developing venous thrombo-embolic complications, e.g. severe varicose veins or prolonged immobilisation or major surgery (see 'Precautions and Warnings'). Disorders of coagulation.
- Presence of any risk factor for arterial disease e.g. smoking, hyperlipidaemia or hypertension (see 'Serious Adverse Reactions').
- Other conditions associated with an increased risk of circulatory disease such as latent or overt cardiac failure, renal dysfunction, or a history of these conditions.
- Epilepsy or a history of this condition.
- Migraine or a history of this condition.
- A history of cholelithiasis.
- Presence of any risk factor for estrogen-dependent tumours; estrogen-sensitive gynaecological disorders such as uterine fibromyomata and endometriosis (see also under *Serious adverse reactions*).
- Diabetes mellitus.
- Severe depression or a history of this condition. If this is accompanied by a disturbance in tryptophan metabolism, administration of vitamin B_6 might be of therapeutic value.
- Sickle cell haemoglobinopathy, since under certain circumstances, e.g. during infections or anoxia, estrogen-containing preparations may induce thromboembolic processes in patients with this condition.
- If the results of liver function tests become abnormal, use should be discontinued.

Precautions and warnings:
Reduced reliability: When Marvelon is taken according to the directions for use the occurrence of pregnancy is highly unlikely. However, the reliability of oral contraceptives may be reduced under the following circumstances:

Forgotten tablets: Provided she is *less than 12 hours* late in taking her tablet the patient should take it as soon as she remembers, further tablets should be taken at the usual time. Marvelon will still give contraceptive protection during this cycle.

If she is *more than 12 hours late* in taking one or more tablets then she will *not* be protected for the next 7 days.

If one or more tablets are forgotten for *more than 12 hours*, contraceptive protection will be reduced. The patient should take the last forgotten tablet, even if this means taking two tablets in one day, and then continue to take tablets at the normal time. Additional contraceptive precautions should be taken for the next 7 days, and the patient should follow the '7-day rule'.

Vomiting or diarrhoea: If after tablet intake vomiting or diarrhoea occurs, a tablet may not be absorbed properly by the body. If the symptoms disappear within 12 hours of tablet-taking, the patient should take an extra tablet from a spare pack and continue with the rest of the pack as usual. However, if the symptoms continue beyond those 12 hours, additional contraceptive precautions are necessary for any sexual intercourse during the stomach or bowel upset and for the following 7 days (the patient must be advised to follow '7-day rule').

If the patient is taking certain other medicines: If the patient is taking any of the medicines given in the *Interactions* section she should be advised to follow the '7-day rule':

THE 7-DAY RULE

If any one tablet is forgotten for more than 12 hours:

If the patient has vomiting or diarrhoea for more than 12 hours:

If the patient is taking any of the drugs listed under 'Interactions':

The patient should continue to take her tablets as usual and:

• Additional contraceptive precautions must be taken for the next 7 days

• BUT–if these 7 days run beyond the end of the current pack, the next pack must be started as soon as the current one is finished, i.e. no gap should be left between packs. (This prevents an extended break in tablet taking which may increase the risk of the ovaries releasing an egg and thus reducing contraceptive protection). The patient will not have a period until the end of 2 packs but this is not harmful nor does it matter if she experiences some bleeding on tablet taking days.

If after taking Marvelon for several months there is a sudden occurrence of spotting or breakthrough bleeding (not observed in previous cycles) or the absence of withdrawal bleeding, contraceptive effectiveness may be reduced. If withdrawal bleeding fails to occur and none of the above mentioned events has taken place, pregnancy is highly unlikely and oral contraceptive use can be continued until the end of the next pack.(If withdrawal bleeding fails to occur at the end of the second cycle, tablet intake should be discontinued and pregnancy excluded before oral contraceptive use can be resumed.) However, if withdrawal bleeding is absent and any of the above mentioned events has occurred, tablet intake should be discontinued and pregnancy excluded before oral contraceptive use can be resumed.

Examination/consultation: A complete medical history and physical examination should be taken prior to the initiation or reinstitution of oral contraceptives and should be repeated periodically.

These physical examinations should include special reference to blood pressure, breasts, abdomen and pelvic organs, including cervical cytology and, where indicated by the medical or family history, relevant laboratory tests.

Caution should be observed when prescribing oral contraceptives to young women whose cycles are not yet stabilised.

Surgery, varicose veins or immobilisation: In patients using estrogen-containing preparations, the risk of deep-vein thrombosis may be temporarily increased when undergoing a major operation (e.g. abdominal, orthopaedic), any surgery to the legs, medical treatment for varicose veins or prolonged immobilisation. Therefore, it is advisable to discontinue oral contraceptive use at least 4 to 6 weeks prior to these procedures if performed electively and to (re)start not less than 2 weeks after full ambulation. The latter is also valid with regard to immobilisation after an accident or emergency surgery. In case of emergency surgery, thrombotic prophylaxis is usually indicated e.g. with subcutaneous heparin.

Chloasma: Chloasma may occasionally occur, especially in women with a history of chloasma gravidarum. Women with a tendency to chloasma should avoid exposure to the sun or ultraviolet radiation whilst taking this preparation.

Laboratory tests: The use of steroids may influence the results of certain laboratory tests. In the literature, at least a hundred different parameters have been reported to possibly be influenced by oral contraceptive use, predominantly by the estrogenic component. Among these are: biochemical parameters of the liver, thyroid, adrenal and renal function, plasma levels of (carrier) proteins and lipid/lipoprotein fractions and parameters of coagulation and fibrinolysis.

Adverse reactions: Various adverse reactions have been associated with oral contraceptive use. The serious reactions are dealt with in more detail. The first appearance of symptoms indicative of any one of these reactions necessitates immediate cessation of oral contraceptive use while appropriate diagnostic and therapeutic measures are undertaken.

Serious adverse reactions:

Various reports have associated oral contraceptive use with the occurrence of deep venous thrombosis, pulmonary embolism and other embolisms.

Other investigations involving oral contraceptives have suggested an increased risk of estrogen and/or progestogen dose-dependent coronary and cerebrovascular accidents, predominantly in heavy smokers. Thrombosis has very rarely been reported to occur in other veins or arteries, e.g. hepatic, mesenteric, renal or retinal. It should be noted that there is no consensus about the often contradictory findings obtained in early studies. The physician should bear in mind, the possibility of vascular events occurring and take into account the presence of risk factors for arterial disease and deep venous thrombosis when prescribing oral contraceptives. Risk factors for arterial disease include smoking, the presence of hyperlipidaemia, hypertension, or diabetes. Signs and symptoms of a thromboembolic event may include: sudden severe pain in the chest, whether or not reaching to the left arm; sudden breathlessness; any unusual severe, prolonged headache, especially if it occurs for the first time or gets progressively worse, or is associated with any of the following symptoms: sudden partial or complete loss of vision or diplopia, aphasia, vertigo, a bad fainting attack or collapse with or without focal epilepsy, weakness or very marked numbness suddenly affecting one side or one part of the body, motor disturbances; severe pain in the calf of one leg; acute abdomen.

Cigarette smoking increases the risk of serious cardiovascular adverse reactions to oral contraceptive use. This risk increases with age and with heavy smoking and is more marked in women over 35 years of age. Women who use oral contraceptives should be strongly advised not to smoke.

The use of estrogen-containing oral contraceptives may promote growth of existing sex steroid dependent tumours. For this reason, the use of these oral contraceptives in patients with such tumours is contraindicated.

Numerous epidemiological studies have been reported on the risks of ovarian, endometrial, cervical and breast cancer in women using combined oral contraceptives. The evidence is clear that combined oral contraceptives offer substantial protection against both ovarian and endometrial cancer.

An increased risk of cervical cancer in long term users of combined oral contraceptives has been reported in some studies, but there continues to be controversy about the extent to which this is attributable to the confounding effects of sexual behaviour and other factors.

A meta-analysis from 54 epidemiological studies reported that there is a slightly increased relative risk (RR = 1.24) of having breast cancer diagnosed in women who are currently using combined oral contraceptives (COCs). The observed pattern of increased risk may be due to an earlier diagnosis of breast cancer in COC users, the biological effects of COCs or a combination of both. The additional breast cancers diagnosed in current users of COCs or in women who have used COCs in the last ten years are more likely to be localised to the breast than those in women who never used COCs.

Breast cancer is rare among women under 40 years of age whether or not they take COCs. Whilst this background risk increases with age, the excess number of breast cancer diagnoses in current and recent COC users is small in relation to the overall risk of breast cancer (see bar chart).

The most important risk factor for breast cancer in COC users is the age women discontinue the COC; the older the age at stopping, the more breast cancers are diagnosed. Duration of use is less important and the excess risk gradually disappears during the course of the 10 years after stopping COC use such that by 10 years there appears to be no excess.

The possible increase in risk of breast cancer should be discussed with the user and weighed against the benefits of COCs taking into account the evidence that they offer substantial protection against the risk of developing certain other cancers (e.g. ovarian and endometrial cancer).

Malignant hepatic tumours have been reported on rare occasions in long-term users of oral contraceptives. Benign hepatic tumours have also been associated with oral contraceptive usage. A hepatic tumour should be considered in the differential diagnosis when upper abdominal pain, enlarged liver or signs of intra-abdominal haemorrhage occur.

The use of oral contraceptives may sometimes lead to the development of cholestatic jaundice or cholelithiasis.

On rare occasions the use of oral contraceptives may trigger or reactivate systemic lupus erythematosus.

A further rare complication of oral contraceptive use is the occurrence of Sydenhams' chorea which can be reversed by discontinuing the pill. The majority of cases of oral-contraceptive-induced chorea show a pre-existing predisposition which may relate to previous rheumatic fever.

Other Adverse Reactions:

Cardiovascular system: rise of blood pressure. If hypertension develops, treatment should be discontinued.

Genital tract: intermenstrual bleeding, post-medication amenorrhoea, changes in cervical secretion,

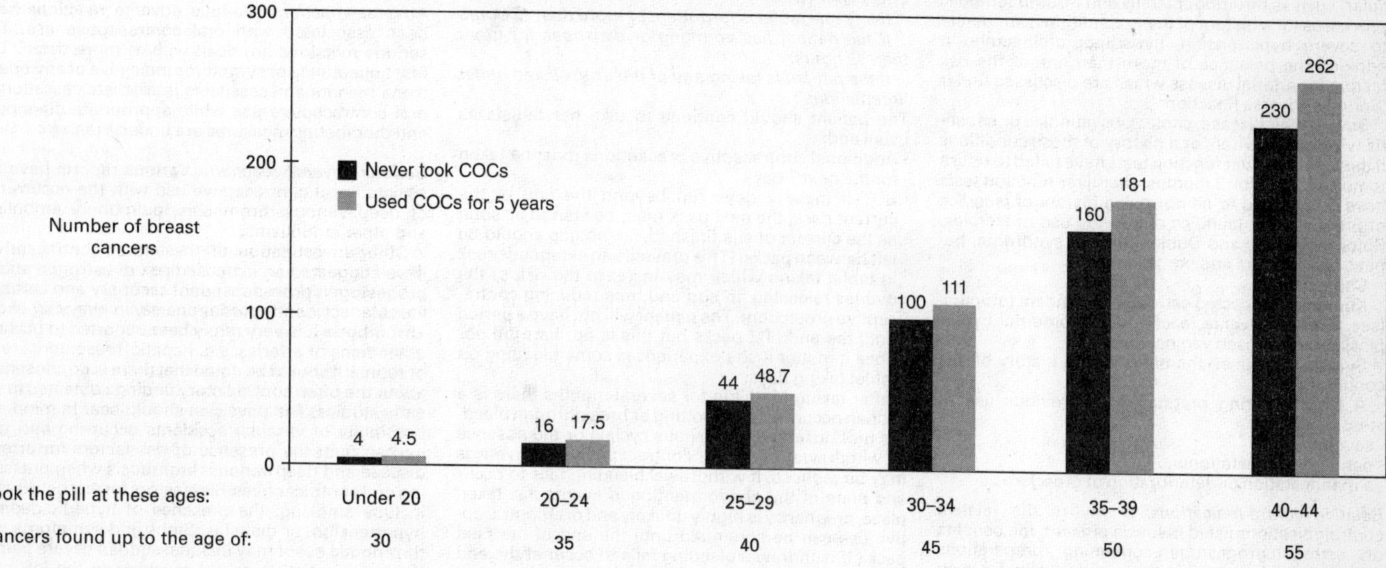

increase in size of uterine fibromyomata, aggravation of endometriosis and certain vaginal infections, e.g. candidiasis

Breast: tenderness, pain, enlargement, secretion.

Gastro-intestinal tract: nausea, vomiting, cholelithiasis, cholestatic jaundice.

Skin: erythema nodosum, rash, chloasma.

Eyes: discomfort of the cornea if contact lenses are used.

CNS: headache, migraine, mood changes, depression.

Metabolic: fluid retention, change in body weight, reduced glucose tolerance.

Interactions: Irregular cycles and reduced reliability of oral contraceptives may occur when these preparations are used concomitantly with drugs such as anticonvulsants, barbiturates, antibiotics, (e.g. tetracyclines, ampicillin, rifampicin, etc.), griseofulvin, activated charcoal and certain laxatives.

Special consideration should be given to patients being treated with antibiotics for acne.

They should be advised to use a non-hormonal method of contraception, or to use an oral contraceptive containing a progestogen showing minimal androgenicity, which have been reported as helping to improve acne without using an antibiotic.

Oral contraceptives may diminish glucose tolerance and increase the need for insulin or other antidiabetic drugs in diabetics.

Overdosage: There have been no reports of serious ill-effects from overdosage even when a considerable number of tablets have been taken by a small child. In general, it is therefore unnecessary to treat overdosage. However, if overdosage is discovered within two or three hours and is large, then gastric lavage can be safely used. There are no antidotes and further treatment should be symptomatic.

Pharmaceutical Precautions Store below 25° in a dry place and protect from light.

Legal category POM.

Package quantities Plastic/aluminium foil blister strips containing 21 tablets, overwrapped with a sealed aluminium laminated sachet. Pack of 3 strips.

Product licence number 0065/0071.

MERCILON*

Qualitative and quantitative composition
Desogestrel B.P. 150 micrograms.
Ethinylestradiol PhEur 20 micrograms.

Pharmaceutical form Tablets.

Clinical particulars
Therapeutic indications: Oral contraception.

Posology and method of administration:

How to take Mercilon: One tablet is taken daily at the same time,(preferably in the evening) without interruption for 21 days, followed by a break of 7 tablet-free days. Each subsequent pack is started after the 7 tablet-free days have elapsed. Additional contraceptive precautions are not then required.

How to start Mercilon: It is preferable that tablet intake from the first pack is started on the first day of menstruation in which case no extra contraceptive precautions are necessary.

If menstruation has already begun, (that is 2, 3, or 4 days previously), tablet taking should commence on day 5 of the menstrual period. In this case additional contraceptive precautions must be taken for the first 7 days of tablet taking.

If menstruation began more than 5 days previously then the patient should be advised to wait until her next menstrual period before starting to take Mercilon.

Post-partum administration: Following childbirth oral contraceptive administration to non-breast feeding mothers should be started 21 days post-partum in which case no additional contraceptive precautions are required.

If intercourse has taken place post-partum, oral contraceptive use should be delayed until the first day of the first menstrual period.

If post-partum administration of Mercilon begins more than 21 days after delivery then additional contraceptive precautions are required for the first 7 days.

N.B. Mothers who are breast feeding should be advised not to use the combined pill since this may reduce the amount of breast-milk, but may be advised instead to use a progestogen-only pill (POP).

After miscarriage or abortion administration should start immediately in which case no additional contraceptive precautions are required.

Changing from a 21 day pill or another 22 day pill to Mercilon: All tablets in the old pack should be finished. The first Mercilon tablet is taken the next day i.e. no gap is left between taking tablets nor does the patient need to wait for her period to begin. Tablets should be taken as instructed in 'How to take Mercilon'. Additional contraceptive precautions are not required. The patient will not have a period until the end of the first Mercilon pack, but this is not harmful, nor does it matter if she experiences some bleeding on tablet-taking days.

Changing from a combined Every Day Pill (28 day tablets) to Mercilon: Mercilon should be started after taking the last active tablet from the 'Every Day Pill' pack (i.e. after taking 21 or 22 tablets). The first Mercilon tablet is taken the next day i.e. no gap is left between taking tablets nor does the patient need to wait for her period to begin. One tablet is taken daily at the same time, without interruption for 21 days, followed by a 7 day tablet-free period. Each subsequent pack is started after the 7 day tablet-free period has elapsed. Additional contraceptive precautions are not required. Remaining tablets from the Every Day (ED) pack should be discarded. The patient will not have a period until the end of the first Mercilon pack, but this is not harmful, nor does it matter if she experiences some bleeding on tablet-taking days.

Changing from a progestogen-only pill (POP or mini pill) to Mercilon: The first Mercilon tablet should be taken on the first day of the period, even if the patient has already taken a mini pill on that day. One tablet is taken daily at the same time, without interruption for 21 days, followed by a 7 day tablet-free period. Each subsequent pack is started after the 7 day tablet-free period has elapsed. Additional contraceptive precautions are not then required. All the remaining progestogen-only pills in the mini pill pack should be discarded.

If the patient is taking a (mini) pill, then she may not always have a period, especially when she is breast feeding. The first Mercilon tablet should be taken on the day *after* stopping the mini pill. All remaining pills in the mini pill packet must be discarded. Additional contraceptive precautions must be taken for the first seven days.

Additional contraceptive precautions: When additional contraceptive precautions are required the patient should be advised either not to have sex, or to use a cap plus spermicide, or for her partner to use a condom. Rhythm methods should not be advised as the pill disrupts the usual cyclical changes associated with the natural menstrual cycle e.g. changes in temperature and cervical mucus.

How to skip a period: To skip a period, a new pack of Mercilon should be started on the day after finishing the current pack (the patient skips the tablet-free days). Tablet-taking should be continued in the usual way. During the use of the second pack she may experience slight spotting or break-through bleeding but contraceptive protection will not be diminished provided there are no tablet omissions. The next pack of Mercilon is started after the usual 7 tablet-free days, regardless of whether the period has completely finished or not.

Advice in case of missed pill: The reliability of Mercilon may be reduced under the following circumstances:

Forgotten tablets

If the forgotten tablet is taken **within 12 hours,** no further precautions are necessary, further tablets should be taken at the usual time.

If one or more tablets are forgotten for **more than 12 hours,** contraceptive protection will be reduced. The patient should take the last forgotten tablet, even if this means taking two tablets in one day, and then continue to take tablets at the normal time. Additional contraceptive precautions should be taken for the next seven days, and the patient should follow the 'seven day rule'. (See *Special warnings and special precautions for use*).

Advice in case of vomiting: If after tablet intake vomiting or diarrhoea occurs, a tablet may not be absorbed properly by the body. If the symptoms disappear within 12 hours of tablet-taking, the patient should take an extra tablet from a spare pack and continue with the rest of the pack as usual. However, if the symptoms continue beyond those 12 hours, additional contraceptive precautions are necessary for any sexual intercourse during the stomach or bowel upset and for the following 7 days (the patient must be advised to follow '7-day rule').

Surgery, varicose veins or immobilisation: It is advisable to discontinue oral contraceptive use at least 4 to 6 weeks prior to these procedures, and to (re)start not less than 2 weeks after full ambulation. (See *Special warnings and special precautions for use* for further advice).

Contra-indications: Pregnancy or suspected pregnancy (that cannot yet be excluded) or breast feeding.

Circulatory disorders (cardiovascular or cerebrovascular) such as thrombophlebitis and thromboembolic processes (or a history of these conditions), moderate to severe hypertension, hyperlipoproteinaemia. In addition the presence of more than one of the risk factors for arterial disease which are discussed under 'Serious Adverse Reactions'.

Severe liver disease, cholestatic jaundice or hepatitis (viral or non-viral), or a history of these conditions if the results of liver function tests have failed to return to normal, and for 3 months after liver function tests have been found to be normal; a history of jaundice of pregnancy or jaundice due to the use of steroids, Rotor syndrome and Dubin-Johnson syndrome, hepatic cell tumours and porphyria.

Cholelithiasis

Known or suspected estrogen-dependent tumours, (see *Serious adverse reactions*); endometrial hyperplasia; undiagnosed vaginal bleeding.

Systemic lupus erythematosus or a history of this condition.

A history during pregnancy or previous use of steroids of:
- severe pruritis
- pemphigoid gestationis
- a manifestation or deterioration of otosclerosis

Relative contra-indications: If any of the relative contraindications listed below is present, the benefits of estrogen/progestogen-containing preparations must be weighed against the possible risks for each individual case and the patient kept under close supervision. In case of aggravation or appearance of any of these conditions whilst the patient is taking the pill, its use should be discontinued.

Conditions implicating an increasing risk of developing venous thrombo-embolic complications, e.g. severe varicose veins or prolonged immobilisation or major surgery (*Special precautions and special warnings*). Disorders of coagulation.

Presence of any risk factor for arterial disease e.g. smoking, hyperlipidaemia or hypertension (see *Serious adverse reactions*).

Other conditions associated with an increased risk of circulatory disease such as latent or overt cardiac failure, renal dysfunction, or a history of these conditions.

Epilepsy or a history of this condition.

Migraine or a history of this condition.

A history of cholelithiasis.

Presence of any risk factor for estrogen-dependent tumours; estrogen-sensitive gynaecological disorders such as uterine fibromyomata and endometriosis. (See also under *Serious adverse reactions*).

Diabetes mellitus.

Severe depression or a history of this condition. If this is accompanied by a disturbance in tryptophan metabolism, administration of vitamin B_6 might be of therapeutic value.

Sickle cell haemoglobinopathy, since under certain circumstances, e.g. during infections or anoxia, estrogen-containing preparations may induce thromboembolic process in patients with this condition.

If the results of liver function tests become abnormal, use should be discontinued.

Special warnings and special precautions for use: Reduced reliability: When Mercilon is taken according to the directions for use the occurrence of pregnancy is highly unlikely. However, the reliability of oral contraceptives may be reduced under the following circumstances:

Forgotten tablets: Provided she is **less than 12 hours late** in taking her tablet the patient should take it as soon as she remembers. Further tablets should be taken at the usual time. Mercilon will still give contraceptive protection during this cycle.

If she is **more than 12 hours late** in taking one or more tablets then she will *not* be protected for the next 7 days.

If one or more tablets are forgotten for **more than 12 hours**, contraceptive protection will be reduced. The patient should take the last forgotten tablet, even if this means taking two tablets in one day, and then continue to take tablets at the normal time. Additional contraceptive precautions should be taken for the next 7 days, and the patient should follow the '7-day rule'.

Vomiting or diarrhoea: If after tablet intake vomiting or diarrhoea occurs, a tablet may not be absorbed properly by the body. If the symptoms disappear within 12 hours of tablet-taking, the patient should take an extra tablet from a spare pack and continue with the rest of the pack as usual. However, if the symptoms continue beyond those 12 hours, additional contraceptive precautions are necessary for any sexual intercourse during the stomach or bowel upset and for the following 7 days (the patient must be advised to follow '7-day rule').

If the patient is taking certain other medicines: If the patient is taking any of the medicines given in the 'Interactions' section she should be advised to follow the '7-day rule':

THE 7-DAY RULE

If any one tablet is forgotten for more than 12 hours

If the patient has vomiting or diarrhoea for more than 12 hours:

If the patient is taking any of the drugs listed under 'Interactions':

The patient should continue to take her tablets as usual and:
- Additional contraceptive precautions must be taken for the next 7 days
- BUT–if these 7 days run beyond the end of the current pack, the next pack must be started as soon as the current one is finished, i.e. no gap should be left between packs. (This prevents an extended break in tablet taking which may increase the risk of the ovaries releasing an egg and thus reducing contraceptive protection). The patient will not have a period until the end of 2 packs but this is not harmful nor does it matter if she experiences some bleeding on tablet taking days.

If after taking Mercilon for several months there is a sudden occurrence of spotting or breakthrough bleeding (not observed in previous cycles) or the absence of withdrawal bleeding, contraceptive effectiveness may be reduced. If withdrawal bleeding fails to occur and none of the above mentioned events has taken place, pregnancy is highly unlikely and oral contraceptive use can be continued until the end of the next pack.(If withdrawal bleeding fails to occur at the end of the second cycle, tablet intake should be discontinued and pregnancy excluded before oral contraceptive use can be resumed.) However, if withdrawal bleeding is absent and any of the above mentioned events has occurred, tablet intake should be discontinued and pregnancy excluded before oral contraceptive use can be resumed.

*Examination/consultation:*A complete medical history and physical examination should be taken prior to the initiation or reinstitution of oral contraceptives and should be repeated periodically.

These physical examinations should include special reference to blood pressure, breasts, abdomen and pelvic organs, including cervical cytology and, where indicated by the medical or family history, relevant laboratory tests.

Caution should be observed when prescribing oral contraceptives to young women whose cycles are not yet stabilised.

Surgery, varicose veins or immobilisation: In patients using estrogen-containing preparations, the risk of deep-vein thrombosis may be temporarily increased when undergoing a major operation (e.g. abdominal, orthopaedic), any surgery to the legs, medical treatment for varicose veins or prolonged immobilisation. Therefore, it is advisable to discontinue oral contraceptive use at least 4 to 6 weeks prior to these procedures if performed electively and to (re)start not less than 2 weeks after full ambulation. The latter is also valid with regard to immobilisation after an accident or emergency surgery. In case of emergency surgery, thrombotic prophylaxis is usually indicated e.g. with subcutaneous heparin.

Chloasma: Chloasma may occasionally occur, especially in women with a history of chloasma gravidarum. Women with a tendency to chloasma should avoid exposure to the sun or ultraviolet radiation whilst taking this preparation.

Laboratory tests: The use of steroids may influence the results of certain laboratory tests. In the literature, at least a hundred different parameters have been reported to possibly be influenced by oral contraceptive use, predominantly by the estrogenic component. Among these are: biochemical parameters of the liver, thyroid, adrenal and renal function, plasma levels of (carrier) proteins and lipid/lipoprotein fractions and parameters of coagulation and fibrinolysis.

Interaction with other medicaments and other forms of interaction: Irregular cycles and reduced reliability of oral contraceptives may occur when these preparations are used concomitantly with drugs such as anti-convulsants, barbiturates, antibiotics, (e.g. tetracyclines, ampicillin, rifampicin, etc.), griseofulvin, activated charcoal and certain laxatives.

Special consideration should be given to patients being treated with antibiotics for acne. They should be advised to use a non-hormonal method of contraception, or to use an oral contraceptive containing a progestogen showing minimal androgenicity, which have been reported as helping to improve acne without using an antibiotic.

Oral contraceptives may diminish glucose tolerance and increase the need for insulin or other antidiabetic drugs in diabetics.

Pregnancy and lactation: Mercilon is contraindicated for use during pregnancy or suspected pregnancy and in mothers who are breast-feeding.

Effects on ability to drive and use of machines: None stated

Undesirable effects:

Adverse reactions: Various adverse reactions have been associated with oral contraceptive use. The serious reactions are dealt with in more detail. The first appearance of symptoms indicative of any one of these reactions necessitates immediate cessation of oral contraceptive use while appropriate diagnostic and therapeutic measures are undertaken.

Serious adverse reactions: Various reports have associated oral contraceptive use with the occurrence of deep venous thrombosis, pulmonary embolism and other embolisms.

Other investigation of these oral contraceptives have suggested an increased risk of estrogen and/or progestogen dose-dependent coronary and cerebrovascular accidents, predominantly in heavy smokers. Thrombosis has very rarely been reported to occur in other veins or arteries, e.g. hepatic, mesenteric, renal or retinal. It should be noted that there is no consensus about the often contradictory findings obtained in the early studies. The physician should bear in mind, the possibility of vascular accidents occurring and take into account the presence of risk factors for arterial disease and deep venous thrombosis when prescribing oral contraceptives. Risk factors for arterial disease include smoking, the presence of hyperlipidaemia, hypertension, or diabetes. Signs and symptoms of a thrombotic event may include: sudden severe pain in the chest, whether or not reaching to the left arm; sudden breathlessness; any unusual severe, prolonged headache, especially if it occurs for the first time or gets progressively worse, or is associated with any of the following symptoms: sudden partial or complete loss of vision or diplopia, aphasia, vertigo, a bad fainting attack or collapse with or without focal epilepsy, weakness or very marked numbness suddenly affecting one side or one part of the body, motor disburbances; severe pain in the calf of one leg; acute abdomen.

Cigarette smoking increases the risk of serious cardiovascular adverse reactions to oral contraceptive use. This risk increases with age and with heavy smoking and is more marked in women over 35 years of age. Women who use oral contraceptives should be strongly advised not to smoke.

The use of estrogen-containing oral contraceptives may promote growth of existing sex steroid dependent tumours. For this reason, the use of these oral contraceptives in patients with such tumours is contraindicated.

Numerous epidemiological studies have been reported on the risks of ovarian, endometrial, cervical and breast cancer in women using combined oral contraceptives. The evidence is clear that combined oral contraceptives offer substantial protection against both ovarian and endometrial cancer.

An increased risk of cervical cancer in long term users of combined oral contraceptives has been reported in some studies, but there continues to be controversy about the extent to which this is attributable to the confounding effects of sexual behaviour and other factors.

A meta-analysis from 54 epidemiological studies reported that there is a slightly increased relative risk (RR=1.24) of having breast cancer diagnosed in women who are currently using combined oral contraceptives (COCs). The observed pattern of increased risk may be due to an earlier diagnosis of breast cancer in COC users, the biological effects of COCs or a combination of both. The additional breast cancers diagnosed in current users of COCs or in women who have used COCs in the last ten years are more likely to be localised to the breast than those in women who never used COCs.

Breast cancer is rare among women under 40 years of age whether or not they take COCs. Whilst this background risk increases with age, the excess number of breast cancer diagnoses in current and recent COC users is small in relation to the overall risk of breast cancer (see bar chart).

The most important risk factor for breast cancer in COC users is the age women discontinue the COC; the older the age at stopping, the more breast cancers are diagnosed. Duration of use is less important and the excess risk gradually disappears during the course of the 10 years after stopping COC use such that by 10 years there appears to be no excess.

The possible increase in risk of breast cancer should be discussed with the user and weighed against the benefits of COCs taking into account the evidence that they offer substantial protection against the risk of developing certain other cancers (e.g. ovarian and endometrial cancer).

Malignant hepatic tumours have been reported on rare occasions in long-term users of oral contraceptives. Benign hepatic tumours have also been associated with oral contraceptive usage. A hepatic tumour should be considered in the differential diagnosis

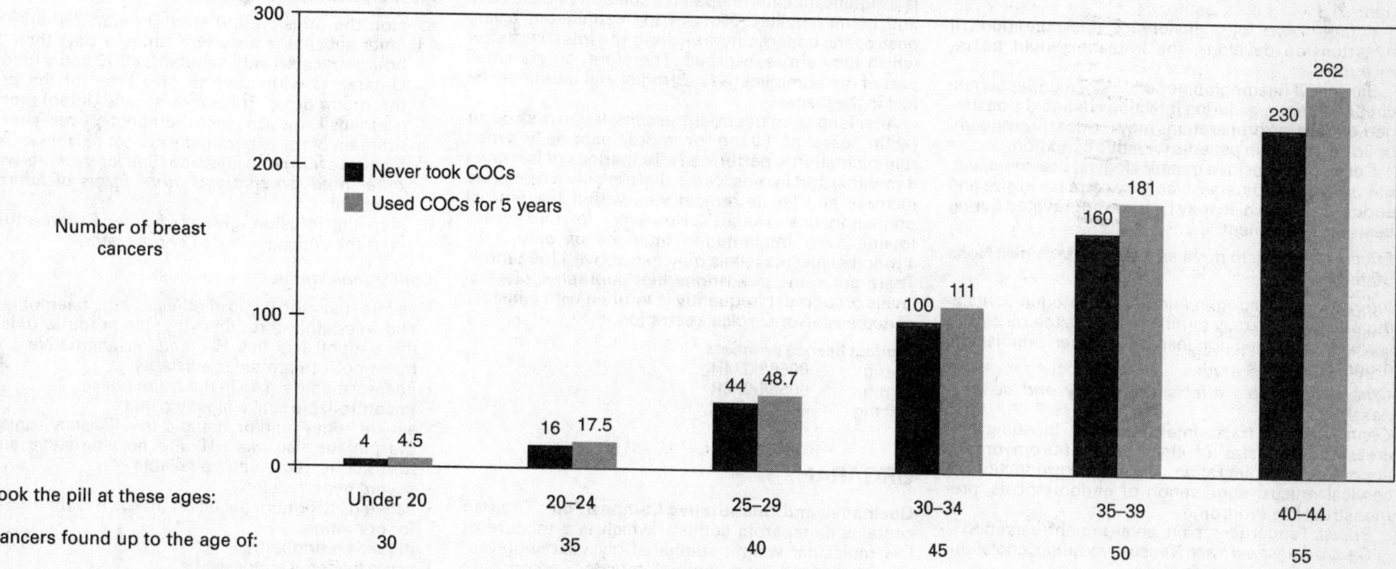

when upper abdominal pain, enlarged liver or signs of intra-abdominal haemorrhage occur.

The use of oral contraceptives may sometimes lead to the development of cholestatic jaundice or cholelithiasis.

On rare occasions the use of oral contraceptives may trigger or reactivate systemic lupus erythematosus.

A further rare complication of oral contraceptive use is the occurrence of Sydenhams' chorea which can be reversed by discontinuing the pill. The majority of cases of oral-contraceptive-induced chorea show a pre-existing predisposition which often relates to acute rheumatism.

Other adverse reactions:

- *Cardiovascular system:* rise of blood pressure. If hypertension develops, treatment should be discontinued.
- *Genital tract:* intermenstrual bleeding, post-medication amenorrhoea, changes in cervical secretion, increase in size of uterine fibromyomata, aggravation of endometriosis and certain vaginal infections, e.g. candidiasis
- *Breast:* tenderness, pain, enlargement, secretion.
- *Gastro-intestinal tract:* nausea, vomiting, cholelithiasis, cholestatic jaundice.
- *Skin:* erythema nodosum, rash, chloasma
- *Eyes:* discomfort of the cornea if contact lenses are used.
- *CNS:* headache, migraine, mood changes, depression.
- *Metabolic:* fluid retention, change in body weight, reduced glucose tolerance.

Overdosage: There have been no reports of serious ill-effects from overdosage even when a considerable number of tablets have been taken by a small child. In general, it is therefore unnecessary to treat overdosage. However, if overdosage is discovered within two or three hours and is large, then gastric lavage can be safely used. There are no antidotes and further treatment should be symptomatic.

Pharmacological properties

Pharmacodynamic properties: Mercilon is an oral contraceptive combination containing 150 micrograms desogestrel and 20 micrograms ethinylestradiol.

Ethinylestradiol is a well known synthetic estrogen.

Desogestrel is a synthetic progestogen. After oral administration it has a strong ovulation-inhibiting activity, a strong progestational and anti-estrogenic activity, no estrogenic activity, very weak androgenic/anabolic activity.

Pharmacokinetic properties: After oral administration, desogestrel shows rapid absorption, followed by distribution throughout the body, and subsequent excretion, not resulting in retention of the drug and/or its metabolites. The freely extractable fraction in serum of volunteers contains desogestrel 3-keto-desogestrel and polar metabolites. The level of the unchanged drug decreases rapidly and the level of the biologically active 3-keto-metabolite is still measurable 24 hours after dosing.

Preclinical safety data: The results of pre-clinical studies do not add to the information included in the other sections of the SmPC.

Pharmaceutical particulars

List of excipients: dl-alpha-tocopherol USP; Potato starch PhEur; Povidone USP; Stearic acid NF; Aerosil NF; Lactose PhEur.

Incompatibilities: None

Shelf-life: 3 years

Special precautions for storage: Store below 25°C protected from light and moisture.

Nature and contents of containers: Plastic/aluminium foil blister strips containing 21 tablets, overwrapped with a sealed aluminium laminated sachet.

Packs of 1, 3, 6 or 50 sachets.

Instructions for use/handling: See *Posology and method of administration.*

Marketing authorisation number 0065/0085

Date of preparation of the text JANUARY 1998

OESTRADIOL IMPLANTS

Presentation Pellets of fused, crystalline oestradiol for implantation. Each pellet contains either 25 mg, 50 mg, or 100 mg of Oestradiol.

The 25 mg weight has a diameter of 2.2 mm and the 50 mg and 100 mg weights have a diameter of 4.5 mm.

Uses *Indicated in females for:* Major post-menopausal symptoms due to oestrogen deficiency, including prevention of post-menopausal osteoporosis in hysterectomised patients.

Should women with an intact uterus be prescribed Oestradiol implants then the lowest effective dose should be used and it must be co-administered with a progestogen for 10-13 days in each cycle.

Dosage and Administration 25-100 mg. Frequency of replacement depends on the duration of activity of the implants administered and the severity of the symptoms. Patients require a further implant when symptoms return, usually every 4 to 8 months.

Because of the sustained absorption of oestradiol, the endometrium of post-menopausal or ovariectomised women is liable to progressive hypertrophy. Therefore, in women with an intact uterus, additional administration of a progestogen is essential, for 10-13 days in each cycle, to prevent endometrial hyperplasia.

When the patient no longer requires or seeks re-implantation with oestradiol pellets, it is recommended that, in those women with an intact uterus, cyclical administration of an oral progestogen should be continued until there is a cessation of withdrawal bleeding, in order to prevent the possibility of continued endometrial stimulation.

Oestradiol Implants should be inserted subcutaneously, (either by means of a trocar and cannula or in the wound at the time of laparotomy), into an area where there is relatively little movement or blood supply, such as the lower abdominal wall or the buttock. Insertion is made under local anaesthesia and the wound is closed either with an adhesive dressing or a fine suture. Full aseptic 'no touch' technique should be adopted.

Contra-indications, warnings, etc.

Contra-indications: Pregnancy. Cardiovascular or cerebrovascular disorders,

Active deep venous thrombosis, thromboembolic disorders, or a history of confirmed venous thromboembolism. Moderate to severe hypertension. Severe liver disease or history of this condition if results of liver function tests have failed to return to normal; cholestatic jaundice, a history of jaundice in pregnancy or jaundice due to the use of steroids; Rotor syndrome and Dubin-Johnson syndrome. Known or suspected oestrogen-dependent tumours: Endometrial hyperplasia. Undiagnosed vaginal bleeding. Porphyria. Hyperlipoproteinaemia, especially in the presence of other risk factors predisposing to cardiovascular disorders. A history during pregnancy or previous steroid use of severe pruritus or pemphigoid gestationis.

Use in pregnancy and lactation: Oestradiol implants are contraindicated during pregnancy. This is based on epidemiological evidence that use during pregnancy is harmful to the foetus.

Oestradiol implants are not recommended in lactating women.

Warnings and precautions: Epidemiological studies have suggested that hormone replacement therapy (HRT) is associated with an increased relative risk of developing venous thromboembolism (VTE) i.e. deep vein thrombosis or pulmonary embolism. The studies find a 2-3 fold increase for users compared with non-users which for healthy women amounts to a low risk of one extra case of VTE each year for every 5000 patients taking HRT.

Generally recognised risk factors for VTE include a personal or family history and severe obesity (Body Mass Index >30 kg/m²). In women with these factors the benefits of treatment with HRT need to be carefully weighed against risks. There is no consensus about the possible role of varicose veins in VTE

The risk of VTE may be temporarily increased with prolonged immobilisation, major trauma or major surgery. In women on HRT scrupulous attention should be given to prophylactic measures to prevent VTE following surgery. Removal of implants prior to surgery is not necessary in general.

If venous thromboembolism develops after initiating therapy the drug should be discontinued.

Chloasma is occasionally seen during the use of oestrogen and/or progestogen-containing preparations, especially in women with a history of chloasma gravidarum. Women with a tendency to chloasma should avoid exposure to the sun while taking this preparation.

Pain in the breasts or excessive production of cervical mucus may be indicative of too high a dosage.

The use of steroids may influence the results of certain laboratory tests e.g. thyroid function tests.

During prolonged treatment with oestrogen-containing preparations periodical medical examinations are advisable. Patients, especially the elderly, with the following conditions should be monitored: latent or overt cardiac failure, renal dysfunction, epilepsy or migraine (or a history of these conditions), since the use of steroids may occasionally induce fluid retention.

Hypertension (or a history of this condition); if hypertension develops, the implant should be removed.

Sickle cell haemoglobinopathy, since under certain circumstance, e.g. during infections or anoxia, oestrogen-containing preparations may induce thromboembolic processes in patients with this condition.

Oestrogen-sensitive gynaecological disorders, e.g. uterine fibromyomata which may increase in size and endometriosis which may become aggravated during oestrogen treatment.

Effects on ability to drive and to use machines: None Stated

Interactions: Oestrogen and/or progestogen-containing preparations may diminish glucose tolerance and increase the need for insulin or other antidiabetic drugs in diabetics.

Other undesirable effects (frequency and seriousness):
Genito-urinary tract: Intermenstrual bleeding, increase in the size of the uterine fibromyomata, endometrial proliferation, excessive production of cervical mucus, aggravation of endometriosis, premenstrual like syndrome.

Breast: Tenderness, pain, enlargement, secretion.

Gastro-intestinal tract: Nausea, vomiting, cholelithiasis, cholestatic jaundice.

Cardiovascular system: Thrombosis, rise of blood pressure.

Skin: Chloasma, erythema nodosum, rash.

Eyes: Discomfort of the cornea if contact lenses are used.

CNS: Headache, migraine, mood changes.

Metabolic: Sodium and water retention, reduced glucose tolerance, and change in body weight.

Changes in liver function.

High dosages and/or prolonged use of oestrogens may cause psychotic disturbances.

Prolonged exposure to unopposed oestrogens may increase risk of development of cardiac and renal disease, melanoma, otosclerosis, multiple sclerosis and systemic lupus erythematosus. If there is a history of breast nodules or fibrocystic disease then closely monitor breast status.

Overdosage: Acute overdose with oestradiol implants is not known to occur. With chronic use supraphysiological levels of oestradiol can be found, however these do not generally result in adverse symptoms, signs or metabolic effects. None the less it would seem prudent in the circumstances to withhold further implantation or other administration of exogenous oestrogens until oestradiol levels have fallen to within the pre-menopausal physiological range.

Pharmaceutical Precautions Store below 25°C. Protect from light

Legal Category POM

Package Quantities Each sterile implant is supplied singly, in a sealed glass tube, available in the following weights: 25 mg, 50 mg, and 100 mg.

Further Information

Pharmacodynamic: 17β Oestradiol is the main, naturally occurring female sex hormone. Among numerous effects Oestradiol is largely responsible for the development and maintenance of the reproductive system and secondary sexual characteristics in women.

Oestradiol implants are effective in relieving the major symptoms of the menopause due to oestrogen deficiency, whether naturally occurring or due to oophorectomy.

Oestradiol implants have also been shown to be effective in reducing the bone loss associated with oestrogen deficiency after the menopause.

Pharmacokinetic: After insertion of an implant into the subcutaneous fat the oestradiol plasma levels gradually increase and generally reach their maximum within approximately two months. Thereafter the concentrations remain nearly stationary until the 4th-6th month after insertion. As with other progestogens and oestrogens, there are large interindividual differences in oestradiol levels, but intraindividual variability appears to be small. Unlike oral oestrogen therapy, subcutaneous administration bypasses the gastrointestinal tract, where oestradiol is converted to oestrone and avoids the first-pass effect of the liver. Therefore more unconjugated oestradiol is observed and the liver is less burdened.

The transport, metabolism, and excretion of oestradiol released from the implants are comparable to those of endogenous oestradiol. Thus, about 38 per cent of circulatory oestradiol will be bound to SHBG, 60 per cent is bound to albumin, and only 2-3 per cent is free. The main metabolic end products are oestriol and 2-hydroxyestrone, which are synthesized after conversion of oestradiol to oestrone. Most of the oestradiol is excreted by the kidneys, mainly after conjugation with glucuronic and sulphuric acid. There is a significant enterohepatic circulation of oestradiol and its metabolites. Most of the conjugated biliary oestrogens undergo hydrolysis in the intestines after which they are reabsorbed. Therefore, only a small part of the administered oestradiol will ultimately be lost in the faeces.

After long-term treatment, accumulation may occur (with doses of 50 mg or more, especially when reimplantation is performed after periods of less than 6 months), but in most cases there is only a moderate increase and levels remain well within the normal premenopausal range. However, in rare cases (mainly with implantation intervals of only 3 or 4 months) plasma levels may rise above 1750 pmol/l. There are some indications that supraphysiological levels occur most frequently in women with a history of depression or surgical castration.

Product licence numbers

25 mg	0065/5074R
50 mg	0065/5075R
100 mg	0065/5076R

ORGARAN*

Qualitative and Quantitative Composition Orgaran contains danaparoid sodium, which is a mixture of low molecular weight sulphated glycosaminoglycuronans derived from animal mucosa, comprising heparan sulphate, dermatan sulphate and a minor amount of chondroitin sulphate. One ml contains 1250 amidolytic anti-factor Xa units danaparoid sodium and 0.15% (w/v) sodium sulphite. The anti-Xa unit is derived from the international heparin standard in an antithrombin-III containing buffer system.

Pharmaceutical form Orgaran is supplied in ampoules containing 750 anti-Xa units (0.6 ml), as a sterile, isotonic solution of pH7 in water for injections. Orgaran is administered by subcutaneous injection.

Clinical Particulars

Therapeutic indications: Prevention of deep vein thrombosis and its possible consequences in patients undergoing general or orthopaedic surgery.

Treatment of thrombo-embolic disorders in patients who require urgent parenteral anti-coagulation because of the development or history of heparin-induced thrombocytopenia (HIT)

Posology and method of administration:

a) *Non-HIT patients (DVT prophylaxis):* In general Orgaran should be administered by subcutaneous injection at a dose of 750 anti-factor Xa units, twice daily for 7 to 10 days or until the risk of thromboembolism has diminished. In surgical patients it is recommended to start this dosing pre-operatively and to give the last pre-operative dose 1-4 hours before surgery.

Plasma anti-Xa activity is linearly related to the dose of Orgaran given. If it is necessary to monitor anticoagulant activity, and for individual dose setting, a functional anti-factor Xa test using a chromogenic peptide substrate should be used. In this test Orgaran should be used as standard for constructing the reference curve.

b) *HIT patients:* The diagnosis of HIT should as a minimum be based on:

1) thrombocytopenia (platelet count $<100\times10^9$/L) occurring during heparin administration and

2) exclusion of all other causes of thrombocytopenia

In general monitoring of plasma anti-Xa activity is not necessary. However, in patients suffering from renal insufficiency and/or patients weighing over 90 kg, monitoring (using an amidolytic assay) is recommended.

Orgaran should be administered intravenously as a bolus of 2500 anti-Xa units (for patients less than 55 kg, 1250 units, if over 90 kg, 3750 units) followed by an intravenous infusion of 400units/h for 2 hours, then 300 units/h for 2 hours, then a maintenance infusion of 200 units/h for 5 days. The expected plasma anti-Xa levels are 0.5-0.7 units/ml 5-10 minutes after the bolus, not higher than 1.0units/ml during the adjustment phase of maintenance infusion and 0.5-0.8 units/ml during the maintenance infusion.

Dosage in the elderly: Clearance of anti-factor Xa activity has not been shown to be markedly reduced in the elderly and the usual dosage is recommended.

Children: There is insufficient experience with the use of Orgaran in children to suggest a dosage regimen for this group of patients.

Dosage in patients with moderately impaired renal and/or liver function: Orgaran should be used with caution in patients with moderately impaired renal and/or liver function with impaired haemostasis.

Conversion to anticoagulants is possible, however it is advisable only to start such a therapy once there is adequate antithrombotic control with Orgaran.

Oral anticoagulants can be given with the infusion (maximum rate 300 units/h) which can then be stopped when the international normalised ratio is ≥1.5. If the bleeding risk is high then either:

a. stop the infusion and start Orgaran 750 anti-Xa units subcutaneously two times a day, then 24 hours later start anticoagulants 48-72 hours before Orgaran is withdrawn to give time for the prothrombin time, Thrombotest and international normalised ratio to reach therapeutic levels (measurement of these parameters is not reliable within 5 hours of Orgaran injection (See *Interactions with other medicaments and other forms of interactions*)) or
b. stop the infusion, give no further Orgaran then start the anticoagulants 12 hours later.

Contra-indications:

- severe haemorrhagic diathesis, e.g. haemophilia and idiopathic thrombocytopenic purpura, unless the patient also has HIT and no alternative anti-thrombotic treatment is available
- haemorrhagic stroke in the acute phase
- uncontrollable active bleeding state
- severe renal- and/or hepatic insufficiency, unless the patient also has HIT and no alternative anti-thrombotic treatment is available
- severe hypertension
- active gastroduodenal ulcer, unless it is the reason for operation
- diabetic retinopathy
- acute bacterial endocarditis
- hypersensitivity to Orgaran
- a positive *in vitro* aggregation test for the heparin-induced antibody in the presence of Orgaran in patients with a history of thrombocytopenia induced by heparin or heparin-like anticoagulants
- hypersensitivity to sulphite.

Special warnings and special precautions for use: Orgaran should be used with caution in patients with moderately impaired renal, and/or liver function with impaired haemostasis, ulcerative lesions of the gastro-intestinal tract or other diseases which may lead to an increased danger of haemorrhage into a vital organ or site.

- Orgaran contains sodium sulphite. In asthma patients hypersensitive to sulphite the latter can result in bronchospasm and/or anaphylactic shock.
- Since Orgaran has been shown to have a low incidence (<10%) of (platelet) cross-reactivity with plasma from patients sensitised by heparin, Orgaran can be used for these patients but it is advisable to rule out cross-reactivity by an *in vitro* test. Although the risk of antibody-induced thrombocytopenia is very small, it is advisable to check the number of platelets regularly. If antibody-induced thrombocytopenia occurs, one should stop the use of Orgaran and consider alternative treatment
- Orgaran should not be given by the intramuscular route.
- The safety and efficacy of Orgaran in patients with non-haemorrhagic stroke remains to be confirmed
- No incidences of osteoporosis have been reported in patients treated with the recommended dose of Orgaran. However, as for heparin, treatment with glycosaminoglycuronan may result in osteoporosis if the dosage is inappropriate.
- It should be noted that the anti-Xa units of Orgaran have a different relationship to clinical efficacy than those of heparin and low molecular weight heparins.

Interactions with other medicaments and other forms of interaction: In clinical studies no clinically significant interactions with other medications have been found. Orgaran may be used together with oral anticoagulants, drugs which interfere with platelet function (such as aspirin and non-steroidal anti-inflammatory drugs) or potentially ulcerogenic drugs (such as corticosteroids), but caution remains necessary. Monitoring of anticoagulant activity of oral anticoagulants by prothrombin time and thrombotest is unreliable within 5 hours after Orgaran administration. There are no data available on the effect of Orgaran on thyroid function tests

Use during pregnancy and lactation: Animal studies have not demonstrated any teratogenic effect or placental transfer. There is no data available about Orgaran secretion into breast milk. In the few cases in which human umbilical cord blood was tested for the presence of anti-Xa activity, no activity was found.

Although Orgaran has been used with success in a small number of pregnancies, the available information is still considered to be insufficient to assess whether deleterious effects may occur in pregnancy during the use of Orgaran. Therefore Orgaran cannot be recommended during pregnancy and lactation.

Effects on ability to drive and use machines: Orgaran is not known to have any effect on the ability to drive and use machines.

Undesirable effects: Enhanced bleeding or haematoma may occur at the operation site.

Bruising and/or pain may occur at injection sites.

Skin rashes and other local or generalised hypersensitivity reactions have occasionally been observed.

Antibody induced thrombocytopenia, as can be caused by (low molecular weight) heparin, was observed in rare cases during the use of Orgaran, but only in patients who were already sensitised to either heparin or low molecular weight heparin. (see *Special warnings and specail precautions for use*).

Liver abnormalities such as changes in transaminase and alkaline phosphatase have been observed, but no clinical significance has been demonstrated.

Overdosage: In the event of serious bleeding other than caused by a surgical error, Orgaran should be stopped and a blood transfusion should be considered. Although protamine partially neutralises the anticoagulant activity of Orgaran the relevance for the reversal of the bleeding is not clear and therefore cannot be recommended.

Pharmacological properties

Pharmacodynamic properties: Danaparoid sodium has been shown both in animal models and in human studies to be an effective antithrombotic substance. At therapeutic doses danaparoid sodium has no or only a minor effect on haemostatic plug formation, platelet function and platelet aggregability with no significant effect on bleeding time at the recommended doses. Occasionally, after high intravenous or subcutaneous doses, a prolonged bleeding time has been observed.

The anticoagulant activity of danaparoid sodium in clotting assays such as prothrombin time, activated partial thromboplastin time, kaolin cephalin clotting time and prothrombin time is small, and characterised by a very flat dose-response curve up to relatively high doses.

The ultimate step in blood coagulation, the fibrinogen-fibrin conversion, is critically dependent on prothrombin generation to which Factor Xa and thrombin contribute substantially. The anticoagulant profile of danaparoid sodium is characterised by a high ratio of anti-factor Xa/antithrombin activities, resulting in an effective inhibition of thrombin generation and thrombus formation. The anti-Xa activity is mediated by antithrombin-III and is not inactivated by endogenous heparin-neutralising factors. The small antithrombin activity is mediated by heparin co-factor II and antithrombin-III. The heparan sulphate fraction with low affinity for antithrombin-III, lacking significant effects on coagulation factors Xa and IIa *in vitro*, has been shown in animal studies to contribute substantially to the antithrombotic activity by an as yet unexplained mechanism.

Organan shows low cross-reactivity (<10%) with the heparin induced antibody. This can be explained by the absence of heparin in Orgaran and its low degree of sulphation. (See 'Special warnings and special precautions for use').

Pharmacokinetic particulars: Pharmacokinetic studies have primarily been based on the kinetics of relevant anticoagulant activities of danaparoid sodium, because no specific chemical assay methods are available. In animal models the time courses of the long-lasting anti-Xa and antithrombotic activities of danaparoid sodium were strongly related.

The absolute bioavailability of danaparoid sodium after subcutaneous administration approaches 100%. In humans the time to reach peak plasma anti-Xa activity levels is approximately 4-5 hours.

The half-lives of elimination of anti-Xa and thrombin generation inhibiting activities of approximately 25 hours and 7 hours respectively, after both subcutaneous and intravenous administration are independent of the dose. Steady-state levels of plasma anti-Xa activity are usually reached within 4-5 days of dosing. Measured by thrombin generation inhibiting activity steady-state levels are reached earlier, i.e. within 1-2 days.

Danaparoid sodium is mainly eliminated by renal excretion and animal experiments indicate that the liver is not involved in its metabolism. In patients with severely impaired renal function the half-life of elimination of plasma anti-factor Xa activity may be prolonged.

Preclinical safety data: The results of pre-clinical studies do not add to the information included in the other sections of the SmPC.

Pharmaceutical particulars

List of excipients: Sodium sulphite BP; Sodium chloride PhEur; Hydrochloric acid PhEur; Water PhEur.

Incompatabilities: When administered as an intravenous bolus or infusion, Orgaran should be given separately and not mixed with other drugs. However, Orgaran is compatible with, and therefore can be added to, infusions of saline, dextrose or dextrose-saline.

Shelf-life: At least three years when stored at a temperature below 30°C and protected from light.

Special precautions for storage: Store protected from light at 2-30°C.

Nature and contents of container: 1-ml glass ampoules containing 750 anti-factor Xa units (0.6 ml) danaparoid sodium per ampoule (1250 anti-factor Xa units/ml) in packs of 10 or 20 ampoules.

Instructions for use/handling: See *Posology and method of administration.*

Product licence number 0065/0125

Date of revision of the text August 1997

Legal Category POM

OVESTIN* CREAM

Presentation An intravaginal cream containing 1 mg oestriol in 1 g of cream.

Other ingredients: 2 octyl-dodecanol (eutanol G); cetyl palmitate; glycerin; cetyl alcohol; stearyl alcohol; Polysorbate 60; sorbitan monostearate; chlorhexidine hydrochloride; lactic acid; sodium hydroxide to pH 4, purified water.

Uses Vulvo-vaginal complaints due to oestrogen deficiency associated with the climacteric and the post-menopause or after oophorectomy: atrophic vaginitis, kraurosis vulvae, pruritus vulvae, dyspareunia due to an atrophic vaginal mucosa and as pre-surgery therapy for vaginal operations and during subsequent convalescence.

Dosage and Administration Ovestin Cream should be given at the lowest dose to control the symptoms and for as short a time as is found necessary. Ovestin Cream is administered intravaginally by means of a calibrated applicator.

One applicator-dose (applicator filled to the ring mark) is 0.5 grams Ovestin Cream containing 0.5 mg oestriol.

Usual dose for vulvo-vaginal complaints associated with the menopause: One application per day for 2 to 3 weeks.

As maintenance dosage, one application twice a week is recommended.

Medication should be discontinued every 2 to 3 months for a period of 4 weeks to assess the necessity for further treatment.

Pre-surgery therapy (one application per day) should begin 2 weeks before the operation. Following surgery a period of at least 2 weeks should be allowed before resuming therapy.

Children: There are no clinical trials to support use in children.

The following 'Instructions for Use' should be given to the patient and are included in the package interior leaflet:

How to Apply the Cream

Use the applicator to apply the cream in the vagina. It is a good idea to do this before going to bed. 1 application (applicator filled to the ring mark) contains 0.5 grams Ovestin cream, which has 0.5 mg of oestriol in it.

1. Remove cap from the tube, invert it, and use the sharp point to open the tube.
2. Screw the end of the applicator onto the tube.
3. Squeeze tube to fill the applicator with the cream until the plunger stops (at the ring mark).
4. Unscrew applicator from tube and replace cap on tube.
5. To apply the cream, lie down, insert the end of the applicator deep into the vagina and slowly push plunger all the way in.

After use, pull plunger out of barrel and wash both in warm, soapy water. Do not use detergents. Rinse well afterwards.

DO NOT PUT THE APPLICATOR IN HOT OR BOILING WATER.

Contra-indications, warnings etc.

Contra-indications: Pregnancy or suspected pregnancy and during lactation.

Active deep venous thrombosis, thromboembolic disorders, or a history of confirmed venous thromboembolism. Known or suspected oestrogen-dependent tumours, e.g. mammary, genital carcinoma. Undiagnosed vaginal bleeding. Acute or chronic liver disease or history of liver disease where the liver function tests have failed to return to normal. Jaundice or history of jaundice in pregnancy. Rotor syndrome or Dubin-Johnson syndrome. Porphyria. Cerebrovascular or cardiovascular disease.

Hyperlipoproteinaemia, especially in the presence of other risk factors which may indicate a predisposition to cerebrovascular or cardiovascular disorders.

A history during pregnancy or previous use of steroids of severe pruritus, pemphigoid gestationis or a deterioration of otosclerosis.

Precautions and warnings: Medication should be discontinued every 2-3 months for a period of 4 weeks to assess the necessity for further treatment.

In the event of persistent or recurring vaginal bleeding, appropriate diagnostic measures should be taken to rule out malignancy. In case of vaginal infections these should be treated before therapy with Ovestin Cream is started.

Prolonged exposure to unopposed oestrogens may increase the risk of the development of endometrial carcinoma.

Pain in the breasts or excessive production of cervical mucus may be indicative of too high a dosage.

During prolonged treatment with oestrogens, periodic medical examinations are advisable.

A cervical smear should be taken at regular intervals.

Epidemiological studies have suggested that hormone replacement therapy (HRT) is associated with an increased relative risk of developing venous thromboembolism (VTE) i.e. deep vein thrombosis or pulmonary embolism. The studies find a 2-3 fold increase for users compared with non-users which for healthy women amounts to a low risk of one extra case of VTE each year for every 5000 patients taking HRT.

Generally recognised risk factors for VTE include a personal or family history and severe obesity (Body Mass Index >30 kg/m²). In women with these factors the benefits of treatment with HRT need to be carefully weighed against risks. There is no consensus about the possible role of varicose veins in VTE

The risk of VTE may be temporarily increased with prolonged immobilisation, major trauma or major surgery. In women on HRT scrupulous attention should be given to prophylactic measures to prevent VTE following surgery. Where prolonged immobilisation is liable to follow elective surgery, particularly abdominal or orthopaedic surgery to the lower limbs, consideration should be given to temporarily stopping HRT 4 weeks earlier, if this is possible.

If venous thromboembolism develops after initiating therapy the drug should be discontinued.

Patients, especially the elderly, with any of the following conditions should be monitored:

latent or overt cardiac failure
renal or hepatic dysfunction
hypertension
epilepsy or migraine or a history of these conditions
endometriosis
fibrocystic mastopathy
diabetes mellitus

Adverse reactions: As with any preparation that is to be applied to mucosal surfaces, Ovestin Cream may cause local irritation or itching at the beginning of treatment. During the first weeks of therapy, occasional mastodynia may occur. In general, these complaints are transient in nature.

Interactions: There is insufficient evidence to support the occurrence of clinically relevant interactions.

Overdosage: The acute toxicity of oestriol in animals is very low. Symptoms that may occur in the case of an acute oral overdosage are nausea, vomiting and possibly withdrawal bleeding in females. No specific antidote is known. If necessary a symptomatic treatment should be instituted.

Pharmaceutical Precautions The preparation should be stored at room temperature (15-25° C)

Legal Category POM

Package Quantities Tube (+applicator) containing 15 g cream.

Further Information

Pharmacological particulars: Oestriol, along with oestradiol and oestrone, is one of the three most important oestrogens found in the body.

Morphological and clinical investigations have shown that oestriol has a specific effect upon the cervix and upon the epithelium of the vagina and vulva, with only a mild proliferative effect upon the endometrium.

The local application of oestriol makes therapeutic use of its stimulating effect upon the epithelium of the vulva and vagina.

The vaginal mucosa reacts with a loosening up and hyperaemia of the sub epithelial tissue, and an increase in the desquamation of superficial and intermediate cells containing glycogen. Histological examination shows the vaginal smear exhibiting regular layering once again, which corresponds to the picture of oestrogen-stimulated tissue.

Oestriol is absorbed from the vagina into the general circulation as evidenced by a rise in plasma oestriol. There is no effect on plasma levels of oestradiol, oestrone and prolactin, nor on sex hormone binding globulin and corticosteroid binding globulin synthesis in the liver.

There is no clinically significant suppression of the

FSH/LH release. Oestriol administered at therapeutically effective dosages as Ovestin Cream, does not induce a general oestrogenic effect in the body.

In particular no effect on the endometrium is found.

No other pharmacological effects are observed.

Pharmacokinetic particulars: Intravaginal application of oestriol ensures optimal availability of the product at the site of action. After administration of Ovestin Cream, oestriol is also absorbed from the vagina into the general circulation, shown by a sharp rise in plasma oestriol, followed by a gradual decline.

After 3 weeks of administration of a single daily dose, a similar absorption pattern to that seen for a single application was observed.

Daily treatment with 0.5 mg of oestriol (in 0.5 g of cream) leads to a sharp rise in unconjugated plasma oestriol levels to 110 pg/ml at one hour from previously undetectable levels (<12 pg/ml). This was followed by a gradual decline during the next 5 hours to around 60 pg/ml.

On day 21 of treatment mean baseline oestriol levels of about 26 pg/ml rose to a mean peak value of 95 pg/ml at 1 hour. A decline similar to that seen on day 1 was observed during the next 5 hours.

Vaginal administration permits the absorption of the active (unconjugated, or free) form of oestriol into the blood for transport to the target tissues, prior to its inactivation via conjugation by enterohepatic enzymes.

Product Licence Number 0065/0074

OVESTIN TABLETS (1MG)

Qualitative and quantitative composition Estriol 1 mg.

Pharmaceutical form White, round, flat tablets, marked with Organon on one side and the code DG7 on the other side.

Clinical particulars

Therapeutic indications: In genito-urinary complaints due to estrogen deficiency such as vaginal atrophy, atrophic vaginitis and recurrent urogenital infections.

Infertility due to poor cervical penetration.

Posology and method of administration

Adults and the elderly: The tablets should be swallowed without chewing.

It is important that the total daily dose is taken at one time.

Genito-urinary complaints: 0.5–3 mg daily for up to 1 month. Maintenance dose 0.5-1 mg daily until restoration of the epithelial integrity and normal balance of vaginal flora is established.

Infertility due to poor cervix penetration:

0.25–1 mg per day on days 6–15 of cycle.

NB. Estrogen therapy should be reviewed according to the individual patient's requirements and clinical picture. Long-term therapy requires regular monitoring procedures.

Children: There is no recommended dose for children.

Contra-indications: Pregnancy, active deep venous thrombosis, thromboembolic disorders, or a history of confirmed venous thromboembolism, known or suspected estrogen-dependent tumours, undiagnosed vaginal bleeding, porphyria, severe hypertension, hepatic diseases.

Special warnings and special precautions for use: Prolonged exposure to unopposed estrogens may increase the risk of the development of endometrial carcinoma. Pain in the breasts or excessive production of cervical mucus may be indicative of too high a dosage.

During prolonged treatment with estrogens, periodical medical examinations are advisable.

With vaginal infections, a concomitant specific treatment is recommended.

Epidemiological studies have suggested that hormone replacement therapy (HRT) is associated with an increased relative risk of developing venous thromboembolism (VTE) i.e. deep vein thrombosis or pulmonary embolism. The studies find a 2-3 fold increase for users compared with non-users which for healthy women amounts to a low risk of one extra case of VTE each year for every 5000 patients taking HRT.

Generally recognised risk factors for VTE include a personal or family history and severe obesity (Body Mass Index >30 kg/m²). In women with these factors the benefits of treatment with HRT need to be carefully weighed against risks. There is no consensus about the possible role of varicose veins in VTE.

The risk of VTE may be temporarily increased with prolonged immobilisation, major trauma or major surgery. In women on HRT scrupulous attention should be given to prophylactic measures to prevent VTE following surgery. Where prolonged immobilisation is liable to follow elective surgery, particularly abdominal or orthopaedic surgery to the lower limbs, consideration should be given to temporarily stopping HRT 4 weeks earlier, if this is possible.

If venous thromboembolism develops after initiating therapy the drug should be discontinued.

Patients, with the following conditions should be monitored: latent or overt cardiac failure; fluid retention due to renal dysfunction; hypertension; epilepsy or migraine (or a history of these conditions); endometriosis; fibrocystic mastopathy; hyperlipoproteinaemia; diabetes mellitus; a history during pregnancy or previous use of steroids of severe pruritus or pemphigoid gestationis.

Interaction with other medicaments and other forms of interaction: There is insufficient evidence to support the potential occurrence of clinically relevant interactions.

Pregnancy and lactation: Ovestin tablets are contra-indicated during pregnancy. This is based on observations in the human which have indicated that the use of estrogens may be harmful in pregnancy.

There is insufficient data on the use of Ovestin tablets at recommended dosages during breast-feeding to assess potential harm to the child. It is known, however, that estriol is excreted in breast milk and may inhibit lactation.

Effects on ability to drive and use of machines: None stated.

Undesirable effects: The following adverse reactions, associated with estrogen treatment may occur during estriol therapy: Nausea and vomiting, breast tenderness or pain in the breasts, spotting during or on withdrawal of therapy, excessive production of cervical mucus, headache.

Overdosage: The acute toxicity of the natural hormone estriol is very low. Symptoms that may possibly occur in the case of an acute overdosage are nausea and vomiting. No specific antidote is known. If necessary a symptomatic treatment will probably be sufficient.

Pharmacological properties

Pharmacodynamic properties: Ovestin tablets contain the natural hormone estriol. In the years just before and after the menopause (whether naturally or surgically induced) estriol can be used in the treatment of symptoms and complaints related to estrogen deficiency. In cases of vaginal atrophy estriol induces normalisation of the vaginal epithelium and thus helps to restore the normal microflora and a physiological pH in the vagina. As a result it increases the resistance of the vaginal epithelial cells to infection and inflammation. Estriol also has a beneficial effect on the quality of cervical mucus allowing cervical penetration by spermatozoa, increasing the chances of conception in those less fertile women who have 'cervical hostility'.

Estriol is relatively short-acting estrogen due to its short nuclear retention time in endometrial cells, its low affinity for plasma proteins and partly as a result of this, its rapid metabolic clearance. Endometrial proliferation is not expected when estriol is given in a single daily dose, since this requires sustained, occupancy of the nuclear estrogen receptor. As a consequence, undesired vaginal bleeding rarely occurs during treatment with estriol and an increased risk of endometrial carcinoma is unlikely.

Pharmacokinetic properties: Estriol is rapidly absorbed into the general circulation with peak plasma levels occurring 1-2 hours after administration. Nearly all (90%) estriol is weakly bound to albumin in the plasma and in contrast with other estrogen's, hardly any estriol is bound to sex hormone-binding globulin (SHBG). The metabolism of estriol consists principally of conjugation and deconjugation during the enterohepatic circulation. Estriol, being a metabolic end product is mainly excreted via the urine in the conjugated form. Only a small part (±2%) is excreted via the faeces, mainly as unconjugated estriol.

Preclinical safety data: Not applicable.

Pharmaceutical particulars

List of excipients: Amylopectin; potato starch; magnesium stearate; lactose.

Incompatibilities: Not applicable.

Shelf-life: 36 months.

Special precautions for storage: Store between 2°C and 30°C. Protect from light.

Nature and contents of containers: Push through strips of 30 tablets.

Instructions for use/handling: Not applicable.

Marketing authorisation number 0065/0130

Date of (partial) revision of the text August 1998

Legal Category POM

PREGNYL*

Qualitative and quantitative composition Injection containing human chorionic gonadotrophin 5000IU.

Pharmaceutical form Freeze dried powder for injection

Clinical particulars

Therapeutic indications: In the male: Hypogonadotrophic hypogonadism. Delayed puberty associated with insufficient gonadotrophic pituitary function. Sterility in selected cases of deficient spermatogenesis.

In the female: Sterility due to the absence of follicle-ripening or ovulation.

In conjunction with HMG, in the promotion of controlled superovulation in medically assisted reproduction programmes.

Posology and method of administration

Dosage: In the male: *Hypogonadotrophic hypogonadism.* 500-1,000 Units 2-3 times weekly. *Delayed puberty associated with insufficient gonadotrophic pituitary function.*

1,500 Units twice weekly for at least 6 months.

Sterility in selected cases of deficient spermatogenesis.

Usually, 3,000 Units per week in combination with an HMG preparation.

In the female: Sterility due to the absence of follicle-ripening or ovulation.

5000-10 000 Units hCG to induce ovulation, following treatment with an HMG (human menopausal gonadotrophins) preparation. Up to 3 repeat injections of up to 5000 Units hCG each, may be given within the following 9 days to prevent insufficiency of the corpus luteum.

In conjunction with HMG, in the promotion of controlled superovulation in medically assisted reproduction programmes.

5000-10 000 Units hCG 30-40 hours after the last HMG injection. Pregnyl should not be administered if the following criteria have not been met: It is recommended that at least 3 follicles greater than 17 mm in diameter are present with 17β oestradiol levels of at least 3500 pmol/L (920 picogram/ml).

Oocyte collection is carried out 32-36 hours after the hCG injection.

Method of administration: After addition of the solvent to the freeze-dried substance, the solution should be given immediately by intramuscular or subcutaneous injection. Any unused solution should be discarded. Subcutaneous injection may be carried out by patient or partner, provided that proper instruction are given by the physician. Self administration of Pregnyl should only be performed by patients who are well-motivated, adequately trained and with access to expert advice.

Contra-indications: Known or suspected androgen-dependent tumours, carcinoma of the prostate or mammary carcinoma in males.

Special warnings and special precautions for use: Treatment of male patients with Pregnyl leads to increased androgen production. Therefore:

Pregnyl should be used cautiously in prepubertal boys to avoid premature epiphyseal closure or precocious sexual development.

Patients with latent or overt cardiac failure, renal dysfunction, hypertension, epilepsy or migraine (or a history of these conditions) should be monitored, since sodium and fluid retention have been observed after administration of high dosages of hCG.

Prior to treating patients for inadequate endogenous stimulation of the gonads, an examination should be performed to exclude anatomical abnormalities of the genital organs or nongonadal endocrinopathies (e.g. thyroid or adrenal disorders, diabetes). Primary ovarian failure should be excluded by the determination of gonadotrophin levels.

In the pregnancies occurring after induction of ovulation with gonadotrophic preparations, there is an increased risk of abortion and multiplets.

Unwanted hyperstimulation: During treatment of female patients, determinations of oestrogen levels and assessment of ovarian size and if possible, ultrasonography should be performed prior to treatment and at regular intervals during treatment. High dosages may cause oestrogen levels to rise excessively rapidly, e.g. more than doubling on 2 or 3 consecutive days, and possibly reaching excessively high pre-ovulatory values.

If unwanted hyperstimulation occurs (i.e. not as part of a treatment preparing for IVF/ET or GIFT or other assisted reproduction techniques), the administration of HMG should be discontinued immediately. hCG must not be given, because the administration of an hLH–active gonadotrophin at this stage may induce, in addition to multiple ovulations, the ovarian hyperstimulation syndrome. This warning is particularly important with respect to patients with polycystic ovarian disease.

The severe form of ovarian hyperstimulation syndrome may be life-threatening and is characterised by large ovarian cysts (prone to rupture), acute abdominal pain, ascites, very often hydrothrax and occasionally thrombo-embolic phenomena.

Interaction with other medicaments and other forms of interaction: None known

Pregnancy and lactation: Not applicable.

Effects on ability to drive and use machines: Not applicable.

Undesirable effects: Skin rashes have occasionally been reported.

Sodium and water retention is occasionally seen in males after administration of high dosages; this is regarded as a result of excessive androgen production.

Overdose: The toxicity of human chorionic gonadotrophic hormone is very low. However, too high a dose may lead to hyperstimulation of the ovaries. (See *Unwanted hyperstimulation*).

Pharmacological properties

Pharmacodynamic properties: Pregnyl is a preparation of human chorionic gonadotrophin obtained from the urine of pregnant women. It stimulates the steroidogenesis in the gonads by virtue of a biological effect similar to that of LH (Luteinizing hormone, which is the same as interstitial cell stimulating hormone). In the male it promotes the production of testosterone and in the female the production of estrogens and particularly of progesterone after ovulation. In certain cases, this preparation is used in combination with human menopausal gonadotrophin (HMG e.g. Humegon). Because HCG is of human origin, no antibody formation is to be expected.

Pharmacokinetic properties: Pregnyl has a half life of about 9h in its first phase and of about 30h in its second phase.

Preclinical safety data: There are no preclinical data of relevance to the prescriber which are additional to that already included in other sections of the SPC.

Pharmaceutical particulars

List of excipients:

Sodium carboxymethylcelluose USP 0.05MG

Mannitol USP 5.0MG

Disodium hydrogen phosphate, calculated as anhydrous EP 0.25MG

Sodium dihydrogen phosphate, calculated as anhydrous EP 0.25MG

Incompatibilities: None stated

Shelf life: 36 months

Special precautions for storage: Store between 2 and 15°C and protect from light.

Nature and contents of container: 2 ml ampoule containing freeze-dried powder with 1 ml ampoule of solvent sodium chloride 9 mg/ml.

Instructions for use/handling: Pregnyl should be reconstituted with the solvent provided. Do not use if the solution contains particles or if the solution is not clear. Since an opened ampoule cannot be resealed in such a way to further guarantee the sterility of the contents, the solution should be used immediately after reconstitution. Discard any remaining solution after single use.

Marketing Authorisation number 0065/5079R

Date of (partial) revision of the text 8/7/97

Legal category POM

PUREGON* ▼

Qualitative and quantitative composition Puregon consists of a freeze-dried powder and a solvent for reconstitution. The powder for injection contains the active ingredient recombinant follicle-stimulating hormone (FSH) (INN Follitropin beta).

One container of Puregon contains 50, 100 or 150 I.U. FSH activity corresponding to 5, 10 or 15 microgram of protein (specific in vivo bioactivity equal to approximately 10 000 I.U. FSH/ mg protein[1]). Puregon is in the form of a lyophilised sphere or lyosphere.(50 I.U., 100 I.U. or 150 I.U.).

[1] as determined by the PhEur. test for FSH in vivo bioactivity and on the basis of the molar extinction coefficient at 277 nm (εs ; $mg^{-1}cm^{-1}$) = 1.066.

Pharmaceutical form Powder for injection. Prior to use, Puregon is reconstituted with the solvent for parenteral use provided.

Clinical particulars

Therapeutic indications: Puregon is indicated for the treatment of female infertility in the following clinical situations:

Anovulation (including polycystic ovarian disease, PCOD) in women who have been unresponsive to treatment with clomiphene citrate.

Controlled ovarian hyperstimulation to induce the development of multiple follicles in medically assisted reproduction programmes [e.g. in vitro fertilisation/embryo transfer (IVF/ET), gamete intra-fallopian transfer (GIFT) and intracytoplasmic sperm injection (ICSI)].

Posology and method of administration

General: The dosage recommendations given below are in line with those usually applied for urinary FSH. These dosages were also applied in comparative clinical studies with Puregon and urinary FSH. In these studies it was shown that Puregon is more effective than urinary FSH in terms of a lower total dose and a shorter treatment period needed to achieve pre-ovulatory conditions. Therefore, it may be appropriate to give a lower dosage of Puregon than for urinary FSH. This advice is not only relevant in order to optimise follicular development but also to minimise the risk of unwanted ovarian hyperstimulation. For this purpose the dosage range of Puregon includes the strengths of 50 I.U. and 100 I.U.

Posology: There are great inter- and intra-individual variations in the response of the ovaries to exogenous gonadotropins. This makes it impossible to set a uniform dosage scheme. The dosage should, therefore, be adjusted individually depending on the ovarian response. This requires ultrasonography and monitoring of oestradiol levels.

After pituitary desensitisation induced by a GnRH agonist a higher dose of Puregon may be necessary to achieve an adequate follicular response.

Clinical experience with Puregon is based on up to three treatment cycles in both indications. Overall experience with IVF indicates that in general the treatment success rate remains stable during the first four attempts and gradually declines thereafter.

Anovulation: In general, a sequential treatment scheme is recommended. This usually starts with daily administration of 75 I.U. FSH activity. The starting dose is maintained for at least seven days. If there is no ovarian response, the daily dose is then gradually increased until follicle growth and/or plasma oestradiol levels indicate an adequate pharmacodynamic response. A daily increase of oestradiol levels of 40-100 per cent is considered to be optimal. The daily dose is then maintained until pre-ovulatory conditions are reached.

Pre-ovulatory conditions are reached when there is ultrasonographic evidence of a dominant follicle of at least 18 mm in diameter and/or when plasma oestradiol levels of 300-900 picograms/ml (1000-3000 pmol/L) are attained. Usually, 7 to 14 days of treatment is sufficient to reach this state. The administration of Puregon is then discontinued and ovulation can be induced by administering human chorionic gonadotropin (hCG).

If the number of responding follicles is too high or oestradiol levels increase too rapidly, i.e. more than a daily doubling for oestradiol for two or three consecutive days, the daily dose should be decreased.

Since follicles of over 14 mm may lead to pregnancies, multiple pre-ovulatory follicles exceeding 14 mm carry the risk of multiple gestations. In that case hCG should be withheld and pregnancy should be avoided in order to prevent multiple gestations.

Controlled ovarian hyperstimulation in medically assisted reproduction programmes: Various stimulation protocols are applied. A starting dose of 150-225 I.U. is recommended for at least the first four days. Thereafter, the dose may be adjusted individually, based upon ovarian response. In clinical studies it was shown that maintenance dosages ranging from 75-375 I.U. for six to twelve days are sufficient, although longer treatment may be necessary.

Puregon can be given either alone, or in combination with a GnRH agonist to prevent premature luteinisation. In the latter case a higher total treatment dose of Puregon may be required.

Ovarian response is monitored by ultrasonography and measurement of plasma oestradiol levels. When ultrasonographic evaluation indicates the presence of at least three follicles of 16-20 mm, and there is evidence of a good oestradiol response (plasma levels of about 300-400 picogram/ml (1000-1300 pmol/l) for each follicle with a diameter greater than 18 mm), the final phase of maturation of the follicles is induced by administration of hCG. Oocyte retrieval is performed 34-35 hours later.

Method of administration: Puregon should be reconstituted with the solvent provided. The reconstituted solution should be administered immediately.

To prevent painful injections and minimise leakage from the injection site the Puregon solution should be slowly administered intramuscularly or subcutaneously. The subcutaneous injection site should be alternated to prevent lipoatrophy. Any unused solution should be discarded.

Subcutaneous injection of Puregon may be carried out by patient or partner, provided that proper instructions are given by the physician. Self administration of Puregon should only be performed by patients who are well-motivated, adequately trained and with access to expert advice.

Contra-indications: Tumours of the ovary, breast, uterus, pituitary or hypothalamus. Pregnancy or lactation. Undiagnosed vaginal bleeding. Hypersensitivity to any of the substances in Puregon. Primary ovarian failure. Ovarian cysts or enlarged ovaries, not related to polycystic ovarian disease (PCOD). Malformations of the sexual organs incompatible with pregnancy. Fibroid tumours of the uterus incompatible with pregnancy.

Special warnings and special precautions for use: The presence of uncontrolled non-gonadal endocrinopathies (e.g. thyroid, adrenal or pituitary disorders) should be excluded.

In pregnancies occurring after induction of ovulation with gonadotropic preparations, there is an increased risk of multiple gestations.

There have been no reports of hypersensitivity to Puregon, but there remains the possibility of anaphylactic responses. The first injection of Puregon should only be performed under direct medical supervision.

Since infertile women undergoing assisted reproduction, and particularly IVF, often have tubal abnormalities the incidence of ectopic pregnancies might be increased. Early ultrasound confirmation that a pregnancy is intrauterine is therefore important.

Rates of pregnancy loss in women undergoing ART are higher than in the normal population.

Unwanted ovarian hyperstimulation: In the treatment of female patients, ultrasonographic assessment of follicular development, and determination of oestradiol levels should be performed prior to treatment and at regular intervals during treatment. Apart from the development of a high number of follicles, oestradiol levels may rise very rapidly, e.g. more than a daily doubling for two or three consecutive days, and possibly reaching excessively high values. The diagnosis of ovarian hyperstimulation may be confirmed by ultrasound examination. If this unwanted ovarian hyperstimulation occurs (i.e. not as part of controlled ovarian hyperstimulation in medically assisted reproduction programmes), the administration of Puregon should be discontinued. In that case pregnancy should be avoided and hCG must be withheld, because it may induce, in addition to multiple ovulation, the ovarian hyperstimulation syndrome. Clinical symptoms and signs of mild ovarian hyperstimulation syndrome are abdominal pain, nausea, diarrhoea, and mild to moderate enlargement of ovaries and ovarian cysts. In rare cases severe ovarian hyperstimulation syndrome occurs, which may be life-threatening. This is characterised by large ovarian cysts (prone to rupture), ascites, often hydrothorax and weight gain. In rare instances, arterio-thromboembolic processes have been associated with other gonadotropin therapy. This may also occur with Puregon/hCG.

Interaction with other medicaments and other forms of interaction: Concomitant use of Puregon and clomiphene citrate may enhance the follicular response. After pituitary desensitisation induced by a GnRH agonist, a higher dose of Puregon may be necessary to achieve an adequate follicular response.

Pregnancy and lactation: Puregon must not be used during pregnancy and lactation.

Effects on ability to drive and use machines: As far as known this medicine has no influence on alertness and concentration.

Undesirable effects: Unwanted ovarian hyperstimulation has been observed in 5% of subjects treated with Puregon. Characteristic symptoms of these conditions have been described. (See *Special warnings and special precautions for use*).

Clinical use of Puregon by the i.m. or s.c. routes may lead to reactions at the site of injection such as bruising, pain, redness, swelling and itching, the majority of which are mild. Generalised reactions have not been observed.

Formation of antibodies against follitropin beta or host cell-derived proteins have not been observed during therapy.

A slightly increased risk of ectopic pregnancy and multiple pregnancies has been seen.

In rare instances, arterio-thromboembolisms have been associated with menotrophin/human chorionic gonadotrophin therapy. This may also occur with Puregon/hCG therapy.

Overdosage: No data on acute toxicity of Puregon in humans is available, but the acute toxicity of Puregon and of urinary gonadotropin preparations in animal studies has been shown to be very low. Too high a dosage of FSH may lead to hyperstimulation of the ovaries. (See 'Unwanted ovarian hyperstimulation').

Pharmacological properties

Pharmacodynamic properties: (ATC classification: gonadotrophins, GO3G)

Puregon contains a recombinant FSH. This is

produced by recombinant DNA technology, using a Chinese hamster ovary cell line transfected with the human FSH subunit genes. The primary amino acid sequence is identical to that of natural human FSH. Small differences in the carbohydrate chain structure are known to exist. FSH is indispensable in normal follicular growth and maturation, and gonadal steroid production. In the female the level of FSH is critical for the onset and duration of follicular development, and consequently for the timing and number of follicles reaching maturity. Puregon can thus be used to stimulate follicular development and steroid production in selected cases of disturbed gonadal function. Furthermore Puregon can be used to promote multiple follicular development in medically assisted reproduction programmes [e.g. in vitro fertilisation/ embryo transfer (IVF/ET), gamete intra-fallopian transfer (GIFT) and intracytoplasmic sperm injection (ICSI)]. Treatment with Puregon is generally followed by administration of hCG to induce the final phase of follicle maturation, resumption of meiosis and rupture of the follicle.

Pharmacokinetic properties: After intramuscular or subcutaneous administration of Puregon, maximum concentrations of FSH are reached within about 12 hours. Due to the sustained release from the injection site and the elimination half-life of about 40 hours (ranging from 12 to 70 hours), FSH levels remain increased for 24-48 hours. Due to the relatively long elimination half-life, repeated administration of the same dose will lead to plasma concentrations of FSH that are approximately 1.5-2.5 times higher than after single dose administration. This increase enables therapeutic FSH concentrations to be reached.

There are no significant pharmacokinetic differences between intramuscular and subcutaneous administration of Puregon. Both have an absolute bioavailability of approximately 77 per cent. Recombinant FSH is biochemically very similar to urinary human FSH and is distributed, metabolised, and excreted in the same way.

Preclinical safety data: Single-dose administration of Puregon to rats induced no toxicologically significant effects. In repeated-dose studies in rats (two weeks) and dogs (13 weeks) up to 100-fold the maximal human dose, Puregon induced no toxicologically significant effects. Puregon showed no mutagenic potential in the Ames test or in the in vitro chromosome aberration test with human lymphocytes.

Pharmaceutical particulars

List of excipients: The powder for injection contains sucrose, sodium citrate, and polysorbate 20. The pH may have been adjusted with sodium hydroxide and/ or hydrochloric acid. The ampoule of solvent contains sodium chloride (4.5 mg) and water for injections (1.0 ml). The quality of all excipients is in accordance with the specifications of the European Pharmacopoeia (PhEur.)

Incompatibilities: Incompatibilities with other medication have not been investigated and mixing with other medication should therefore be avoided.

Shelf-life: The shelf-life of Puregon is two years under the conditions specified below in "special precautions for storage" Puregon may be used until the expiration date indicated on the package.

Special precautions for storage: Store below 30°C. Protect from light. Do not freeze. Store Puregon out of reach of children

Nature and contents of containers: Boxes of Puregon contain:

1 ampoule of follitropin beta plus 1 ampoule solvent or

5 ampoules of follitropin beta plus 5 ampoules solvent or

Ampoules of Puregon contain a sterile lyophilised sphere (called lyosphere) corresponding to 50, 100 or 150 I.U. FSH activity. Ampoules solvent contain 1 ml saline 0.45%.

Instructions for use/handling: Puregon should be reconstituted with the solvent provided using a gentle, swirling motion. Vigorous shaking should be avoided. Do not use if the solution contains particles or if the solution is not clear.

Since an opened ampoule cannot be resealed in such a way to further guarantee the sterility of the contents, the solution should be used immediately after reconstitution. The content of a vial should also be used immediately after reconstitution. Discard any remaining solution after single use.

Marketing authorisation holder N.V. Organon, P O Box 20, 5340 BH Oss, The Netherlands

Marketing authorisation numbers

50 IU	1 ampoule	EU/1/96/008/001
	5 ampoules	EU/1/96/008/003
100 IU	1 ampoule	EU/1/96/008/009
	5 ampoules	EU/1/96/008/011
150 IU	1 ampoule	EU/1/96/008/013
	5 ampoules	EU/1/96/008/015

Date of (partial) revision of the text 9 August 1996

Legal category POM

RESTANDOL*

Qualitative and quantitative composition Each capsule contains Testosterone Undecanoate 40.0 mg.

Pharmaceutical form Brown soft gelatin capsule printed Org D_3V.

Clinical particulars

Therapeutic indications: Testosterone replacement therapy in male hypogonadal disorders, for example: after castration; eunuchoidism; hypopituitarism; endocrine impotence; male climacteric symptoms like decreased libido and decreased mental and physical activity; certain types of infertility due to disorders of spermatogenesis

Testosterone therapy may also be indicated in osteoporosis due to androgenic deficiency.

Posology and method of administration

Dosage:

Adults: The initial dosage required will usually be 120-160 mg daily for 2-3 weeks. Subsequent dosage (40-120 mg daily) should be based on the clinical effect obtained during the first weeks of therapy.

Elderly patients: It should be noted that smaller and less frequent doses may achieve the same response.

Children: Not applicable.

Administration: Oral. The capsules should be taken after meals, if necessary with a little water, and be swallowed whole without chewing. It is preferable that half of the daily dose be taken in the morning and the other half in the evening. If an uneven number of capsules is taken daily, the greater part should be taken in the morning.

Contra-indications: Known or suspected prostatic or mammary carcinoma; hypercalciuria, hypercalcaemia, nephrotic syndrome, ischaemic heart disease or untreated congestive heart failure.

Special warnings and special precautions for use: Patients, especially the elderly, with the following conditions should be monitored: latent or overt cardiac failure, renal or hepatic dysfunction, hypertension, epilepsy or migraine (or a history of these conditions), since androgens may occasionally induce sodium and water retention. Mammary carcinoma, hypernephroma, bronchial carcinoma, and skeletal metastases, since these conditions may produce hypercalcaemia or hypercalciuria which may in turn be exacerbated by androgen therapy. If hypercalcaemia or hypercalciuria develops treatment should be discontinued.

A decrease in protein-bound iodine (PBI) may occur, but this has no clinical significance.

Androgens should be used cautiously in prepubertal boys to avoid premature epiphyseal closure or precocious sexual development.

Androgen therapy should only be used in male hypogonadism in which testosterone levels have been demonstrated to be low.

In treating males, stimulation to the point of increasing nervous, mental and physical activities beyond the patient's cardiovascular capacity should be avoided.

Tumours and other histological abnormalities and disturbances of liver function have been reported in patients subjected to prolonged treatment with some testosterone derivatives. Most of these compounds were 17-alpha alkyl derivatives but a smaller number of cases has occurred with certain 17-beta esters of testosterone. The possibility that such changes result from the use of Restandol has not been excluded.

Interaction with other medicaments and other forms of interaction: Concurrent administration of liver enzyme inducing drugs such as rifampicin, barbiturates, carbamazepine, dichloralphenazone, phenylbutazone, phenytoin or primidone may decrease the effect of Restandol.

Pregnancy and lactation: Not applicable (only male indications).

Effects on ability to drive and use of machines: Restandol will not effect ability to drive or use machines.

Undesirable effects: Restandol, like any other androgen therapy, may give rise to the following adverse reactions: priapism and other signs of excessive sexual stimulation. Precocious sexual development, an increased frequency of erections, phallic enlargement and premature epiphyseal closure in pre-pubertal males. Sodium and water retention. Oligospermia and a decreased ejaculatory volume.

Treatment should be interrupted until these symptoms have disappeared, after which it should be continued at a lower dosage.

Hoarseness of the voice may be the first symptom of vocal change which may lead to irreversible lowering of the voice. If signs of virilisation, particularly lowering of the voice, develop, treatment should be discontinued.

Overdosage: Treatment of overdosage is by gastric lavage with appropriate supportive therapy. Standard resuscitative measures should be given as required.

Pharmacological properties

Pharmacodynamic properties: The pharmacological action of testosterone undecanoate can be attributed to the testosterone content, an androgenic hormone which controls the development and maintenance of the male sex organs and male secondary sex characteristics

Pharmacokinetic properties: Testosterone undecanoate, a fatty acid ester of the natural androgen testosterone, is an orally effective testosterone preparation. Testosterone is inactive on oral administration because it is prematurely inactivated by the liver. Testosterone undecanoate is able to by-pass the liver via the lymphatic system and is therefore orally active.

Preclinical safety data: Not applicable.

Pharmaceutical particulars

List of excipients: Oleic Acid PhEur; Capsule shell: Glycerol (85%) PhEur; sorbitol concentrate (Karion 83) HSE; sodium ethylhydroxybenzoate FRP; sodium propylhydroxybenzoate BP; titanium dioxide PhEur; iron oxide (Red) NF; gelatin PhEur.

Incompatibilities: None stated.

Shelf-life: 3 years

Special precautions for storage: Wholesaler/pharmacy: Store in the refrigerator (2-8°C). Protect from light and moisture. *Patient:* Store at room temperature (up to 30°C). Protect from light and moisture.

Nature and contents of containers: Polyethylene tampertainers 28. Polyethylene tampertainers 56

Instructions for use/handling: Not applicable

Marketing authorisation number 0065/0059

Date of first authorisation 14/1/81

Date of preparation of the text October 1995

Legal Category: POM

SANDRENA

Qualitative and quantitative composition

Oestradiol hemihydrate corresponding to: 0.5 mg oestradiol/dose (in single dose units containing 0.5 g gel).

Oestradiol hemihydrate corresponding to: 1.0 mg oestradiol/dose (in single dose units containing 1.0 g gel).

Pharmaceutical form Gel

Clinical particulars

Therapeutic indications: Treatment of the climacteric syndrome associated with natural or artificial menopause (oestrogenic deficiency, e.g. hot flushes, night sweats, urogenital atrophy).

Posology and method of administration: Sandrena can be used for continuous or cyclical treatment.

The dose can be adjusted individually from 0.5 g to 1.5 g per day, corresponding to 0.5 to 1.5 mg oestradiol per day. The usual starting dose is 1.0 mg oestradiol (1.0 g gel) daily and can be readjusted after 2-3 cycles.

In patients with an intact uterus, it is recommended to combine Sandrena treatment with an adequate dose of progestogen, for adequate duration e.g. for 10-12 consecutive days per month.

The Sandrena dose is applied once daily on the skin of the lower trunk of the right or left thigh, on alternate days. The application surface should be 1-2 times the size of the hand. Sandrena should not be applied on the breasts, on the face or on irritated skin. After application the gel should be allowed to dry for a few minutes and the application site should not be washed within 1 hour. Accidental contact of the gel with the eyes should be avoided. Hands should be washed after application.

If the patient forgets to apply a dose, it should be applied as soon as possible, unless the dose is more than 12 hours late. If the dose is more than 12 hours late, it should be skipped. Missed doses may induce breakthrough bleeding.

Contra-indications:

- Undiagnosed vaginal bleeding,
- Active or recent thromboembolic disease or thrombophlebitis,
- Severe hepatic disease (including Dubin-Johnson and Rotor's syndrome),
- Oestrogen dependent cancer (e.g. of the breast or endometrium),
- Hypersensitivity to the constituents of the preparation.

Special warnings and special precautions for use: Before therapy is initiated, a thorough medical history should be taken. A complete gynaecological examination should be performed and repeated at least once a year during therapy.

Prolonged use without addition of a progestogen may cause endometrial hyperplasia. Therefore, in women with an intact uterus, Sandrena treatment should be combined with cyclic progestogen administration. Withdrawal bleeding resembling normal menstruation will usually occur after each course of progestogen. The cause of unexpected or prolonged uterine bleeding during therapy should be clarified. Atypical adenomatous hyperplasia of the endometrium must be treated before commencing oestrogen therapy.

Consider discontinuation prior to surgery or prolonged immobilisation. Development of de novo frequent severe headaches or migraine should be investigated and possible prodromal symptoms of vascular occlusion should be clarified.

The risks and benefits of treatment should be evaluated and close monitoring performed for patients with:

- endometriosis
- uterine leiomyoma
- endometrial hyperplasia (simple glandular hyperplasia or hyperplasia glandularis cystica)
- diseases of the cardiovascular system including cerebrovascular disorders,
- a history of thromboembolic disease,
- severe hypertension,
- history of (or close family history of) breast cancer,
- severe disturbances of lipid metabolism,
- renal dysfunction
- systemic lupus erythematosus
- porphyria

At present there is suggestive evidence of a slight increase in the relative risk of carcinoma of the breast with long-term hormone replacement therapy, however, the results are contradictory. Regular breast examinations and mammography, where appropriate, should be carried out in women on hormone replacement therapy.

Some conditions may be aggravated during oestrogen therapy or pregnancy. Women on Sandrena treatment with one of the following conditions (or with a history thereof during previous pregnancy or hormone use) should therefore be closely monitored.

These conditions include:

- mild hypertension,
- migraine or severe headache,
- benign breast disease,
- liver function disturbances,
- cholestasis,
- cholelithiasis,
- diabetes mellitus,
- asthma,
- otosclerosis,
- multiple sclerosis,
- galactorrhea, elevated prolactin levels,
- history of herpes gestationis,
- epilepsy.

Interaction with other medicaments and other forms of interaction: No interactions between Sandrena and other medicines have been reported. There are some indications that oestrogens may reduce the effects of antihypertensive, anticoagulant and antidiabetic drugs. Concomitant treatment with potent inducers of liver enzymes (e.g. barbiturates, carbamazepine, griseofulvin and rifampicin) may reduce the plasma levels of oestradiol. The significance of these interactions in transdermal application has not been elucidated.

Pregnancy and lactation: Sandrena is not indicated in women of child-bearing capacity. It has no contraceptive efficacy. Sandrena should not be used during pregnancy or lactation.

Effects on ability to drive and use machines: Oestrogens such as Sandrena do not affect the ability to drive or use machines.

Undesirable effects: Adverse drug reactions are usually mild and only seldom lead to discontinuation of treatment. If they do occur, it will usually be during the first months of treatment.

Occasionally for oestrogens in general: Breast tenderness, headache, oedema, weight increase, unscheduled vaginal bleeding or spotting.

Rarely for oestrogens in general: Migraine, changes in libido and mood, gastrointestinal discomfort (e.g. nausea, vomiting, stomach cramps), hypertension, alterations in liver function and biliary flow.

In clinical trials dermal irritation has been very infrequent with Sandrena.

Overdosage: Generally, oestrogens are well tolerated even in massive doses. Possible symptoms of overdose include those listed under undesirable effects. Treatment is symptomatic.

Pharmacological properties Therapeutic classification: G03 CA 03, Oestrogen preparation for hormone replacement therapy.

Pharmacodynamic properties: The pharmacodynamics of Sandrena are similar to those of oral oestrogens, but the major difference to oral administration lies in the pharmacokinetic profile.

The clinical efficacy of Sandrena in the treatment of menopausal symptoms is comparable to that of peroral oestrogen. Combined with medroxyprogesterone acetate, percutaneous oestradiol lowers total cholesterol without reducing the HDL cholesterol level.

Pharmacokinetic properties: Sandrena is an alcohol-based oestradiol gel. When applied to the skin the alcohol evaporates rapidly and oestradiol is absorbed through the skin into the circulation. To some extent, however, the oestradiol is stored in the subcutaneous tissue from where it is released gradually into circulation. Percutaneous administration circumvents the hepatic first-pass metabolism. For these reasons, the fluctuations in the plasma oestrogen concentrations with Sandrena are less pronounced than peroral oestrogen.

A 1.5 mg percutaneous dose of oestradiol (1.5 g Sandrena) results in a plasma concentration of about 340 pmol/l, which corresponds to the level of early follicular stage in premenopausal women. During Sandrena treatment the oestradiol/oestrone ratio remains at 0.7, while during peroral oestrogen treatment it usually drops to less than 0.2.

The mean oestradiol exposure at steady state of Sandrena is 82 per cent compared with an equivalent oral dose of oestradiol valerate. Otherwise the metabolism and excretion of transdermal oestradiol follow the fate of natural oestrogens.

Preclinical safety data: Oestradiol is a natural female hormone with an established clinical use, therefore no toxicological studies have been performed with Sandrena. The necessary studies on the irritant effects of the gel have been studied in rabbits and skin sensitisation in guinea pig. Based on the results from these studies it can be concluded that Sandrena could very infrequently cause mild skin irritation. The frequency of the occurrence of dermal irritation can be reduced by daily change of the application site.

Pharmaceutical particulars

List of excipients: Carbomer 934 BP; Sodium hydroxide; Propylene glycol PhEur; Spir. fort.–Ethanol 96% BP. Aq. purif.–Purified water PhEur.

Incompatibilities: No incompatibilities have been found.

Shelf life: 3 years.

Special precautions for storage: At room temperature (below 25°C).

Nature and contents of container: Single dose aluminium foil sachets supplied in packages containing 28 of either dose or 91 sachets of 1 mg dose.

Instructions for use/handling: None

Marketing authorisation holder

Orion Corporation, Orioninite 1, P.O. Box 65, FIN-02101, ESPOO, FINLAND

Distributed by Organon Laboratories Limited, Cambridge Science Park, Milton Road, Cambridge, CB4 0FL.

Marketing authorisation number 13911/0004-0005

Date of (partial) revision of the text October 1996

Legal Category POM

SUSTANON* 100

Qualitative and quantitative composition

Testosterone propionate PhEur 20 mg
Testosterone phenylpriopionate BP 40 mg
Testosterone isocaproate BP 40 mg
(Equivalent to a total of 74 mg of testosterone)

Pharmaceutical form Sustanon 100 is a clear, sterile, oily solution for deep intramuscular injection.

Clinical particulars

Therapeutic indications: Testosterone replacement therapy in male hypogonadal disorders, for example: after castration; eunuchoidism; hypopituitarism; endocrine impotence; male climacteric symptoms like decreased libido; certain types of infertility due to disorders of spermatogenesis.

Testosterone therapy may also be indicated for the prevention and treatment of osteoporosis in hypogonadal males

Posology and method of administration:

Dosage: In general, dosage should be adjusted to the individual response of the patient.

Adults: Usually, one injection of 1 ml per two weeks is adequate.

Elderly: It should be noted that smaller and less frequent doses may achieve the same response.

Children: It should be noted that smaller and less frequent doses may achieve the same response.

Administration: Deep intramuscular injection

Contra-indications: Known or suspected prostatic or mammary carcinoma. Pregnancy. Breast-feeding. Hypersensitivity to one of the excipients.

Special warnings and special precautions for use: Patients, especially the elderly, with the following conditions should be monitored: ischaemic heart disease, since androgens may produce hypercholesterolaemia; latent or overt cardiac failure, renal dysfunction, hypertension, epilepsy or migraine (or a history of these conditions), since androgens may occasionally induce fluid and sodium retention; skeletal metastases, since androgens may induce hypercalcaemia or hypercalciuria in these patients.

The use of steroids may influence the results of certain laboratory tests.

Androgens should be used cautiously in prepubertal boys to avoid premature epiphyseal closure or precocious sexual development.

If androgen-associated adverse reactions occur, Sustanon 100 treatment should be interrupted and, after disappearance of the symptoms, be resumed at a lower dosage.

Interaction with other medicaments and other forms of interaction: Enzyme-inducing agents may exert increasing or decreasing effects on testosterone levels. Therefore adjustment of the dose, and/or intervals between injections may be required.

Pregnancy and lactation: On the basis of its pharmacological effect, Sustanon 100 is suspected to cause birth defects and/or other irreversible adverse effects on pregnancy outcome. Therefore, Sustanon 100 is contraindicated during pregnancy and lactation.

Effects on ability to drive and use of machines: As far as is known Sustanon 100 has no influence on alertness and concentration

Undesirable effects: The following adverse reactions have been associated with androgen therapy in general: In prepubertal boys, precocious sexual development, an increased frequency of erections, phallic enlargement and premature epiphyseal closure; priapism and other signs of excessive sexual stimulation; water and sodium retention; oligospermia and a decreased ejaculatory volume.

Treatment should be interrupted until these symptoms have disappeared, after which it should be continued at a lower dosage.

Hoarseness of the voice may be the first symptom of vocal change which may lead to irreversible lowering of the voice. If signs of virilisation, particularly lowering of the voice, develop, treatment should be discontinued.

Overdosage: The acute intramuscular toxicity of Sustanon 100 is very low. Therefore toxic symptoms are not expected to occur.

Pharmacological properties

Pharmacodynamic properties: Testosterone is the principal endogenous hormone essential for normal growth and development of the male sex organs and male secondary sex characteristics. During adult life testosterone is essential for the functioning of the testes and accessory structures, and for the maintenance of libido, sense of well-being, erectile potency, prostate and seminal vesicle function.

Treatment of hypogonadal males with Sustanon 100 results in a clinically significant rise of plasma concentrations of testosterone, dihydrotestosterone and androstenedione, as well as a decrease of SHBG (sex hormone binding globulin). In the males with primary (hypergonadotropic) hypogonadism treatment with Sustanon results in a normalisation of pituitary function.

Pharmacokinetic properties: Sustanon 100 contains a number of esters of testosterone with different durations of action. The esters are hydrolysed into the natural hormone testosterone, as soon as they enter the general circulation.

A single dose of Sustanon 100 leads to an increase of total plasma testosterone, with peak level reached approximately 24-48hrs (t_{max}) after administration. Plasma testosterone levels return to the lower limit of the normal range in males after approximately 21 days.

Testosterone is metabolised via the normal pathways. Excretion mainly takes place via the urine as conjugates of etiocholanolone and androsterone.

Preclinical safety data: Not applicable.

Pharmaceutical particulars

List of excipients:

Benzyl Alcohol PhEur 0.1 ml
Arachis Oil PhEur to 1.0 ml

Incompatibilities: No relevant incompatibilities are known.

Shelf-life: 5 years.

Special precautions for storage: Store between 15-25°C, protect from light.

Nature and contents of containers: 1 ml ampoules in boxes of 3.

Instructions for use/handling: not applicable.

Marketing authorisation number 0065/5019

Date of first authorisation 28 February 1973

Date of preparation of the text March 1995

Legal category POM

SUSTANON* 250

Qualitative and quantitative composition
Testosterone propionate PhEur 30 mg
Testosterone phenylpriopionate BP 60 mg
Testosterone isocaproate BP 60 mg
Testosterone decanoate BP 100 mg
(equivalent to a total of 176 mg of Testosterone)

Pharmaceutical form Sustanon 250 is a clear, sterile, oily solution for deep intramuscular injection.

Clinical particulars
Therapeutic indications: Testosterone replacement therapy in male hypogonadal disorders, for example: after castration; eunuchoidism; hypopituitarism; endocrine impotence; male climacteric symptoms like decreased libido; certain types of infertility due to disorders of spermatogenesis.

Testosterone therapy may also be indicated for the prevention and treatment of osteoporosis in hypogonadal males

Posology and method of administration:
Dosage: In general, dosage should be adjusted to the individual response of the patient.

Adults: Usually, one injection of 1 ml per three weeks is adequate.

Elderly: It should be noted that smaller and less frequent doses may achieve the same response.

Children: It should be noted that smaller and less frequent doses may achieve the same response.

Administration: Deep intramuscular injection

Contra-indications: Known or suspected prostatic or mammary carcinoma. Pregnancy. Breast-feeding. Hypersensitivity to one of the excipients.

Special warnings and special precautions for use: Patients, especially the elderly, with the following conditions should be monitored: ischaemic heart disease, since androgens may produce hypercholesterolaemia. Latent or overt cardiac failure, renal dysfunction, hypertension, epilepsy or migraine (or a history of these conditions), since androgens may occasionally induce fluid and sodium retention. Skeletal metastases, since androgens may induce hypercalcaemia or hypercalciuria in these patients.

The use of steroids may influence the results of certain laboratory tests.

Androgens should be used cautiously in prepubertal boys to avoid premature epiphyseal closure or precocious sexual development.

If androgen-associated adverse reactions occur, Sustanon 250 treatment should be interrupted and, after disappearance of the symptoms, be resumed at a lower dosage.

Interaction with other medicaments and other forms of interaction: Enzyme-inducing agents may exert increasing or decreasing effects on testosterone levels. Therefore adjustment of the dose, and/or intervals between injections may be required.

Pregnancy and lactation: On the basis of its pharmacological effect, Sustanon 250 is suspected to cause birth defects and/or other irreversible adverse effects on pregnancy outcome. Therefore, Sustanon 250 is contraindicated during pregnancy and lactation.

Effects on ability to drive and use of machines: As far as is known Sustanon 250 has no influence on alertness and concentration.

Undesirable effects: The following adverse reactions have been associated with androgen therapy in general:

In prepubertal boys, precocious sexual development, an increased frequency of erections, phallic enlargement and premature epiphyseal closure; priapism and other signs of excessive sexual stimulation; water and sodium retention; oligospermia and a decreased ejaculatory volume.

Treatment should be interrupted until these symptoms have disappeared, after which it should be continued at a lower dosage.

Hoarseness of the voice may be the first symptom of vocal change which may lead to irreversible lowering of the voice. If signs of virilisation, particularly lowering of the voice, develop, treatment should be discontinued.

Overdosage: The acute intramuscular toxicity of Sustanon 250 is very low. Therefore toxic symptoms are not expected to occur.

Pharmacological properties
Pharmacodynamic properties: Testosterone is the principal endogenous hormone essential for normal growth and development of the male sex organs and male secondary sex characteristics. During adult life testosterone is essential for the functioning of the testes and accessory structures, and for the maintenance of libido, sense of well-being, erectile potency, prostate and seminal vesicle function.

Treatment of hypogonadal males with Sustanon 250 results in a clinically significant rise of plasma concentrations of testosterone, dihydrotestosterone and androstenedione, as well as a decrease of SHBG (sex hormone binding globulin). In the males with primary (hypergonadotropic) hypogonadism treatment with Sustanon results in a normalisation of pituitary function.

Pharmacokinetic properties: Sustanon 250 contains a number of esters of testosterone with different durations of action. The esters are hydrolysed into the natural hormone testosterone as soon as they enter the general circulation.

A single dose of Sustanon 250 leads to an increase of total plasma testosterone with peak-levels of approximately 70 nmol\1 (C_{max}), which are reached approximately 24-48h (t_{max}) after administration. Plasma testosterone levels return to the lower limit of the normal range in males in approximately 21 days.

Testosterone is metabolised via the normal pathways. Excretion mainly takes place via the urine as conjugates of etiocholanolone and androsterone.

Preclinical safety data: Not applicable.

Pharmaceutical particulars
List of excipients:
Benzyl Alcohol PhEur 0.1 ml
Arachis Oil PhEur to 1.0 ml

Incompatibilities: No relevant incompatibilities are known.

Shelf-life: 5 years

Special precautions for storage: Store between 15-25°C, protect from light

Nature and contents of containers: 1 ml ampoules in boxes of 3

Instructions for use/handling: not applicable.

Marketing authorisation number 0065/5086

Date of first authorisation 28 February 1973

Date of preparation of the text March 1995

Legal category POM

TESTOSTERONE IMPLANT

Presentation Testosterone implants are pellets containing 50, 100 or 200 mg testosterone in glass ampoules.

Uses In the male: testosterone replacement therapy in primary or secondary hypogonadal disorders, for example:

- after castration,
- eunuchoidism,
- hypopituitarism,
- endocrine impotence,
- infertility due to spermatogenic disorders,
- male climacteric symptoms such as decreased libido and decreased mental and physical activity.

Moreover, testosterone therapy may be indicated in osteoporosis in the male due to androgen deficiency.

In the female as an adjunct to oestrogen replacement therapy in postmenopausal women to alleviate symptoms, such as decreased libido and/or loss of energy.

Dosage and administration
In males: 100-600 mg depending on individual requirements. A dosage of 600 mg (6 x 100 mg) usually maintains plasma testosterone levels within the normal physiological range for 4-5 months.

In females: 50-100 mg as an adjunct to oestradiol implants.

Method of implantation: Testosterone implants should be inserted subcutaneously into an area where there is relatively little movement or blood supply, such as the lower abdominal wall or the buttock. Insertion is made under local anaesthesia using a trocar and a cannula. The wound is closed either with an adhesive dressing or a fine suture. The implants must be placed subcutaneously to facilitate removal if necessary. Full aseptic 'no touch' technique should be adopted.

Contra-indications, warnings, etc.
Contra-indications: Known or suspected prostatic carcinoma or breast carcinoma in the male. Pregnancy. Breast-feeding.

Use in pregnancy and lactation: Testosterone implants are contra-indicated during pregnancy and lactation.

Warnings and precautions:

- Androgens should be used with caution in women to avoid unacceptable and irreversible virilization. Female patients should therefore be counselled to report any deepening or hoarsening of the voice without delay.
- Androgens should be used with caution in prepubertal boys to avoid premature epiphyseal closure or precocious sexual development. Skeletal maturation should be monitored regularly.
- Due to the long-lasting action and the difficulty of removal, Testosterone implants should be used with extra caution. Therefore, it may be advisable to establish the beneficial effect and tolerance for androgen therapy by prior treatment with a shorter-acting testosterone preparation. This applies in particular to (pre)pubertal boys, women and elderly men.
- Patients with latent or overt cardiac failure, renal or hepatic dysfunction, hypertension, epilepsy or migraine (or a history of these conditions) should be kept under close medical supervision, since aggravation of recurrence may occasionally be induced.
- If androgen-associated adverse reactions occur the implant should be removed if possible.
- The use of steroids may influence the results of certain laboratory tests.

Effects on ability to drive and to use machines: As far as is known Testosterone implants have no effects on alertness and concentration.

Interactions: Enzyme-inducing drugs may influence plasma testosterone levels.

Other undesirable effects (frequency and seriousness): The following adverse reactions have been associated with androgen therapy:

- *in general:* water and sodium retention, hypercalcaemia;
- *in women:* symptoms of virilization, such as voice changes (deepening, hoarsening) and hirsutism;
- *in prepubertal boys:* precocious sexual development, increased frequency of erections, phallic enlargement and premature epiphyseal closure;
- *in men:* priapism and other signs of excessive sexual stimulation, oligospermia and decreased ejaculatory volume

Overdosage: The acute toxicity of testosterone is low. Priapism in men and undesired deepening of the voice in women are symptoms of chronic overdosage. In this case the implant(s) should be removed.

Pharmaceutical precautions Store below 25°C and protect from light

Incompatibilities: None.

Legal category POM.

Package quantities Each sterile implant is supplied singly, in a sealed glass tube.

Further information Testosterone is a naturally-occurring hormone formed in the interstitial cells of the testes under the control of the anterior lobe of the pituitary gland which controls the development and maintenance of the male sex organs and male secondary sex characteristics. Testosterone also produces systemic effects, such as increasing the retention of nitrogen, calcium, sodium, potassium, chloride and phosphate leading to an increase in skeletal weight, water retention and an increase in the growth of bone.

Testosterone implants, when inserted subcutaneously release testosterone into the bloodstream at a relatively even rate supplying near physiological plasma testosterone levels.

Surface area of the implants is the most important factor influencing the rate of absorption. In general the absorption rate estimated by removal of implants at intervals and weighing appears to be appreciably more rapid than when the rate is assessed upon the clinical requirement. In addition to clinical evidence individual variation in the rate of absorption of implants must be taken into account.

The average daily absorption of testosterone has been estimated at 0.5 mg for a 100 mg implant with an approximate duration of 30 weeks.

Product licence numbers
50 mg 0065/5082R
100 mg 0065/5083R
200 mg 0065/5084R

ZISPIN ▼

Qualitative and quantitative composition Each tablet contains 30 mg of mirtazapine.

Pharmaceutical form Tablet

Clinical particulars

Therapeutic Indications: Treatment of depressive illness.

Posology and method of administration: The tablets should be taken orally, if necessary with fluid, and swallowed without chewing.

Adults: Treatment should begin with 15 mg daily. The dosage generally needs to be increased to obtain an optimal clinical response. The effective daily dose is usually between 15 and 45 mg.

Elderly: The recommended dose is the same as that for adults. In elderly patients an increase in dosing should be done under close supervision to elicit a satisfactory and safe response.

Children: Since safety and efficacy of Zispin has not been established in children, it is not recommended to treat children with Zispin.

The clearance of mirtazapine may be decreased in patients with renal or hepatic insufficiency. This should be taken into account when prescribing Zispin to this category of patients.

Mirtazapine has a half-life of 20-40 hours and therefore Zispin is suitable for once-a-day administration. It should be taken preferably as a single night-time dose before going to bed. Zispin may also be given in subdoses equally divided over the day (once in the morning and once at night-time).

Treatment should preferably be continued until the patient has been completely symptom-free for 4-6 months. After this, treatment can be gradually discontinued. Treatment with an adequate dose should result in a positive response within 2-4 weeks. With an insufficient response, the dose can be increased up to the maximum dose. If there is no response within a further 2-4 weeks, then treatment should be stopped.

Contra-indications: Hypersensitivity to mirtazapine or any of the other ingredients of Zispin.

Special warnings and special precautions for use: Reversible white blood cell disorders including agranulocytosis, leukopenia and granulocytopenia have been reported with Zispin. With respect to agranulocytosis the physician should be alert to symptoms such as fever, sore throat, stomatitis or other signs of infection; when such symptoms occur, treatment should be stopped and blood counts taken. Patients should also be advised of the importance of these symptoms.

Careful dosing as well as regular and close monitoring is necessary in patients with:

- epilepsy and organic brain syndrome; from clinical experience it appears that insults occur rarely in patients treated with Zispin
- hepatic or renal insufficiency
- cardiac diseases like conduction disturbances, angina pectoris and recent myocardial infarct, where normal precautions should be taken and concomitant medicines carefully administered
- low blood pressure.

As with other antidepressants care should be taken in patients with:

- micturation disturbances like prostate hypertrophy (although problems are not to be expected because Zispin possesses only very weak anticholinergic activity)
- acute narrow-angle glaucoma and increased intra-ocular pressure (also here little chance of problems with Zispin because of its very weak anticholinergic activity)
- diabetes mellitus.

Treatment should be discontinued if jaundice occurs.

Moreover, as with other antidepressants, the following should be taken into account:

- worsening of psychotic symptoms can occur when antidepressants are administered to patients with schizophrenia or other psychotic disturbances; paranoid thoughts can be intensified
- when the depressive phase of manic-depressive psychosis is being treated, it can transform into the manic phase
- with regard to the chance of suicide, in particular at the beginning of treatment, only a limited number of Zispin tablets should be given to the patient
- although antidepressants are not addictive, the abrupt termination of treatment after long-term administration may result in nausea, headache and malaise
- elderly patients are often more sensitive, especially with regard to the side-effects of antidepressants.

During clinical research with Zispin, side-effects have not been reported more often in elderly patients than in other age groups; however experience until now is limited.

Interaction with other medicaments and other forms of interaction:

- Mirtazapine may potentiate the central nervous dampening action of alcohol; patients should therefore be advised to avoid alcohol during treatment with Zispin.
- Zispin should not be administered concomitantly with MAO inhibitors or within two weeks of cessation of therapy with these agents.
- Mirtazapine may potentiate the sedative effects of benzodiazepines; caution should be taken when these drugs are prescribed together with Zispin.
- No data are available from formal clinical studies on interactions with neuroleptics.
- In vitro data suggest that mirtazapine is a very weak competitive inhibitor of the cytochrome P450 enzymes CYP1A2, CYP2D6 and CYP3A and clinically significant interactions are unlikely with mirtazapine.

Pregnancy and lactation: The safety of Zispin in human pregnancy has not been established.

Reproduction studies in pregnant rats and rabbits at doses up to 100 mg/kg and 40 mg/kg (approx. 3 and 5 times respectively the maximum recommended human dose on the basis of exposure) have revealed no evidence of teratogenic effects. There was, however, in rats an increase in post-implantation loss; there was also an increase in pup deaths during the first three days of lactation (cause of death unknown) and a decrease in pup birth weights. These findings are common with CNS-active drugs at high dose levels in animals.

As the relevance of these findings to humans is not certain the use of Zispin during pregnancy is not recommended. Women of child bearing potential should employ an adequate method of contraception if taking Zispin.

Although animal experiments show that mirtazapine is excreted only in very small amounts in the milk, the use of Zispin in nursing mothers is not recommended since no human data in breast milk are available.

Effects on ability to drive and use machines: Zispin has sedative properties and may impair concentration and alertness. Patients treated with Zispin should avoid the performance of potentially dangerous tasks, which require alertness and good concentration, such as driving a motor vehicle or operating machinery.

Undesirable effects: Depressed patients display a number of symptoms that are associated with the illness itself. It is therefore sometimes difficult to ascertain which symptoms are a result of the illness itself and which are a result of treatment with Zispin.

The following adverse effects have been reported:

Common: (>1/100) Increase in appetite and weight gain. Drowsiness/sedation, generally occurring during the first few weeks of treatment. (N.B. dose reduction generally does not lead to less sedation but can jeopardize antidepressant efficacy).

Less common: Increases in liver enzyme levels.

Rare: (<1/1000) Oedema and accompanying weight gain.

Reversible agranulocytosis has been reported as a rare occurrence with Zispin. (See also 'Special warnings and special precautions for use'). (Orthostatic) hypotension. Exanthema. Mania, convulsions (insults), tremor, myoclonus.

Overdose: Toxicity studies in animals suggest that clinically relevant cardiotoxic effects will not occur after overdosing with Zispin. Experience in clinical trials and from the market has shown that no serious adverse effects have been associated with Zispin in overdose. Symptoms of acute overdosage are confined to prolonged sedation.

Cases of overdose should be treated by gastric lavage with appropriate symptomatic and supportive therapy for vital functions.

Pharmacological properties

Zispin (mirtazapine) is an antidepressant, which can be given as treatment for episodes of major depression. The presence of symptoms such as anhedonia, psychomotor inhibition, sleep disturbances (early wakening) and weight loss, increase the chance of a positive response. Other symptoms are: loss of interest, suicidal thoughts and changes in mood (better in the evening than in the morning). Zispin begins to exert its effect in general after 1-2 weeks of treatment.

Pharmacodynamic properties: Mirtazapine is a centrally active presynaptic α_2-antagonist, which increases central noradrenergic and serotonergic neurotransmission. The enhancement of serotonergic neurotransmission is specifically mediated via 5-HT_1 receptors, because 5-HT_2 and 5-HT_3 receptors are blocked by mirtazapine. Both enantiomers of mirtazapine are presumed to contribute to the antidepressant activity, the S(+) enantiomer by blocking α_2 and 5-HT_2 receptors and the R(-) enantiomer by blocking 5-HT_3 receptors.

The histamine H_1-antagonistic activity of mirtazapine is responsible for its sedative properties. Mirtazapine is generally well tolerated. It has practically no anticholinergic activity and, at therapeutic doses, has practically no effect on the cardiovascular system.

Pharmacokinetic properties: After oral administration of Zispin tablets, the active constituent mirtazapine is rapidly and well absorbed (bioavailability ≈ 50%), reaching peak plasma levels after about 2 hours. Binding of mirtazapine to plasma proteins is approx. 85%. The mean half-life of elimination is 20-40 hours; longer half-lives, up to 65 hours, have occasionally been recorded and shorter half-lives have been seen in young men. The half-life of elimination is sufficient to justify once-a-day dosing. Steady state is reached after 3-4 days, after which there is no further accumulation. Mirtazapine displays linear pharmacokinetics within the recommended dose range. Food intake has no influence on the pharmacokinetics of mirtazapine. Mirtazapine is extensively metabolized and eliminated via the urine and faeces within a few days. Major pathways of biotransformation are demethylation and oxidation, followed by conjugation. In vitro data from human liver microsomes indicate that cytochrome P450 enzymes CYP2D6 and CYP1A2 are involved in the formation of the 8-hydroxy metabolite of mirtazapine, whereas CYP3A4 is considered to be responsible for the formation of the N-demethyl and N-oxide metabolites. The demethyl metabolite is pharmacologically active and appears to have the same pharmacokinetic profile as the parent compound. There are no differences in the pharmacokinetic parameters of racemic mirtazapine or its demethyl metabolite in extensive and poor metabolisers. Plasma metabolite profiles for the individual enantiomers are qualitatively similar in extensive and poor metabolisers.

The clearance of mirtazapine may be decreased as a result of renal or hepatic insufficiency.

Preclinical safety data: No special particulars.

Pharmaceutical particulars

List of excipients:

Core: maize starch; hydroxypropyl cellulose; magnesium stearate; colloidal silicon dioxide; lactose.

Coating layer: hydroxypropyl methylcellulose; polyethylene glycol 8000; titanium dioxide (E171) yellow iron oxide (E172) and red iron oxide (E172).

Incompatibilities: Not applicable.

Shelf life: The shelf life for Zispin tablets is 3 years, if stored in the dark and dry at 2-30 °C. Zispin tablets should not be used after the expiry date on the package.

Special precautions for storage: Zispin should be stored in the dark and dry.

Nature and contents of containers:

Zispin tablets are oval, biconvex, scored and marked with 'Organon' on one side and a code on the other side.

Zispin tablets are packed in child-safe, push-through strips made of opaque white polyvinyl chloride film and aluminium foil containing a heat-seal coating on the side in contact with the tablets.

The following packages are available: 4 push-through strips with 7 red-brown tablets each containing 30 mg mirtazapine (code TZ/5).

Instructions for use/handling: Not applicable

Marketing authorisation number 0065/0145

Date of first authorisation/renewal of authorisation
May 1997

Legal Category POM

**Trade Mark*

Organon Teknika Limited
Science Park
Milton Road
Cambridge CB4 0FL

☎ 01223 423650 ⎙ 01223 420264

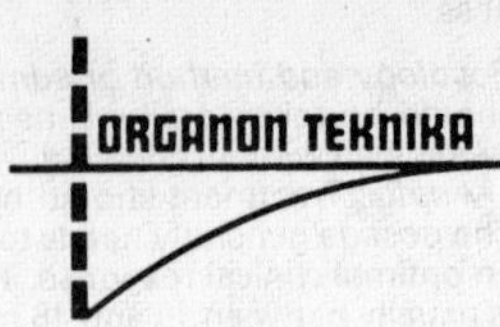

ESMERON

Qualitative and quantitative composition Each ml Esmeron contains 10 mg rocuronium bromide.

Pharmaceutical form Esmeron is supplied as a solution for intravenous injection.

Clinical particulars

Therapeutic indications: Esmeron is indicated as an adjunct to general anaesthesia to facilitate endotracheal intubation during routine and rapid sequence induction, to provide skeletal muscle relaxation, during surgery. Esmeron is also indicated as an adjunct in the intensive care unit (ICU) to facilitate intubation and mechanical ventilation.

Posology and method of administration:

Dosage: As with other neuromuscular blocking agents, the dosage of Esmeron should be individualized in each patient. The anaesthetic method used, the expected duration of surgery, the possible interaction with other drugs that are administered before and/or during anaesthesia and the condition of the patient should be taken into account when determining the dose. The routine use of an appropriate neuromuscular monitoring technique is recommended for the evaluation of neuromuscular block and recovery.

Inhalational anaesthetics do potentiate the neuromuscular blocking effects of Esmeron. This potentiation, however, only becomes clinically relevant in the course of anaesthesia when the volatile agents have reached the tissue concentrations required for this interaction. Consequently, adjustments with Esmeron should be made by administering smaller maintenance doses at less frequent intervals or by using lower infusion rates of Esmeron during long lasting procedures (longer than 1 hour) under inhalational anaesthesia (see Interaction with other medicaments and other forms of interaction).

In adult patients the following dosage recommendations may serve as a general guideline for endotracheal intubation and muscle relaxation for short to long lasting surgical procedures and for use in the intensive care unit.

Surgical Procedures: Endotracheal intubation: The intubating dose is 0.6 mg Esmeron per kg body weight. This dose can also be used for facilitating intubation during rapid sequence induction of anaesthesia. However as part of a rapid sequence induction technique a dose of 1.0 mg of rocuronium bromide per kg of body weight is recommended.

Maintenance dosing: The recommended maintenance dose is 0.15 mg Esmeron per kg body weight; in case of long-term inhalational anaesthesia this should be reduced to 0.075-0.1 mg of rocuronium bromide per kg body weight. The maintenance doses should best be given when twitch height has recovered to 25% of control twitch height.

Continuous infusion: If Esmeron is administered by continuous infusion, it is recommended to give a loading dose of 0.6 mg Esmeron per kg body weight and, when neuromuscular block starts to recover, to start administration by infusion. The infusion rate should be adjusted to maintain twitch response at 10% of control twitch height. In adults, the infusion rate required to maintain neuromuscular block at this level ranges from 0.3-0.6 $mg.kg^{-1}.hour^{-1}$ (300-600 $micrograms.kg^{-1}.hour^{-1}$) and under inhalational anaesthesia the infusion ranges from 0.3-0.4 $mg.kg^{-1}.h^{-1}$. Continuous monitoring of neuromuscular block is essential since infusion rate requirements vary from patient to patient and with the anaesthetic method used.

Dosing in paediatric patients: Children (1-14 years) and infants (1-12 months) under halothane anaesthesia manifest similar sensitivity to Esmeron as adults. Onset of action is faster in infants and children than in adults. Clinical duration is shorter in children than in adults. There are no data to support recommendations for the use of Esmeron in neonates (0-1 month).

Dosing in geriatric patients and patients with hepatic and/or biliary tract disease and/or renal failure: The intubation dose for geriatric patients and patients with hepatic and/or biliary tract disease and/or renal failure is 0.6 mg rocuronium bromide per kg body weight. Regardless of the anaesthetic technique used, the recommended maintenance dose for these patients is 0.075-0.1 mg rocuronium bromide per kg body weight, and the recommended infusion rate is 0.3-0.4 $mg.kg^{-1}.h^{-1}$. (see also *Continuous infusion*).

Dosing in overweight and obese patients: When used in overweight or obese patients (defined as patients with a body weight of 30% or more above ideal body weight) doses should be reduced taking into account a lean body mass.

Intensive care procedures: Endotracheal intubation: For endotracheal intubation, the same doses should be used as described above under surgical procedures.

Dosing to facilitate mechanical ventilation: The use of an initial loading dose of 0.6 mg rocuronium bromide per kg body weight is recommended, followed by a continuous infusion as soon as twitch height recovers to 10% or upon reappearance of 1 to 2 twitches to train of four stimulation. Dosage should always be titrated to effect in the individual patient. The recommended initial infusion rate for the maintenance of a neuromuscular block of 80–90% (1 to 2 twitches to TOF stimulation) in adult patients is 0.3–0.6 $mg.kg^{-1}.h^{-1}$ during the first hour of administration, which will need to be decreased during the following 6–12 hours, according to the individual response. Thereafter, individual dose requirements remain relatively constant. A large between patient variability in hourly infusion rates has been found in controlled clinical studies, with mean hourly infusion rates ranging from 0.06–0.50 $mg.kg^{-1}.h^{-1}$ depending on nature and extent of organ failure(s), concomitant medication and individual patient characteristics. To provide optimal individual patient control, monitoring of neuromuscular transmission is strongly recommended. Administration up to 7 days has been investigated. There are no data to support dose recommendations for the facilitation of mechanical ventilation in paediatric and geriatric patients.

Administration: Esmeron is administered intravenously either as a bolus injection or as a continuous infusion (see also *Instructions for use/handling*).

Contraindications: Former anaphylactic reactions to rocuronium or to the bromide ion.

Special warnings and special precautions for use: Since Esmeron causes paralysis of the respiratory muscles, ventilatory support is mandatory for patients treated with this drug until adequate spontaneous respiration is restored. As with all neuromuscular blocking agents it is important to anticipate intubation difficulties particularly when used as part of a rapid sequence induction technique. Anaphylactic reactions to neuromuscular blocking agents in general have been reported. Although these are very rarely seen with Esmeron, precautions for treating such reactions if they would occur should always be taken (see also *Undesirable effects*).

Dose levels greater than 0.9 mg Esmeron per kg body weight may increase the heart rate; this effect could counteract the bradycardia produced by other anaesthetic agents or by vagal stimulation. In general, following long term use of muscle relaxants in the ICU, prolonged paralysis and/or skeletal muscle weakness has been noted. In order to help preclude possible prolongation of neuromuscular block and/or overdosage it is strongly recommended that neuromuscular transmission is monitored throughout the use of muscle relaxants. Furthermore, muscle relaxants should be titrated to effect in the individual patients by or under supervision of experienced clinicians who are familiar with their actions and with appropriate neuromuscular monitoring techniques. Because Esmeron is always used with other agents and because the occurrence of malignant hyperthermia during anaesthesia is possible, even in the absence of known triggering agents, clinicians should be familiar with early signs, confirmatory diagnosis and treatment of malignant hyperthermia prior to the start of any anaesthesia. In animal studies Esmeron was shown not to be a triggering factor for malignant hyperthermia. The following conditions may influence the pharmacokinetics and/or pharmacodynamics of Esmeron:

Hepatic and/or biliary tract disease and renal failure: Because rocuronium is excreted in urine and bile, Esmeron should be used with caution in patients with clinically significant hepatic and/or biliary diseases and/or renal failure. In these patient groups prolongation of action has been observed with doses of 0.6 mg rocuronium bromide per kg body weight.

Prolonged circulation time: Conditions associated with prolonged circulation time such as cardiovascular disease, old age and oedematous state resulting in an increased volume of distribution, may contribute to a slower onset of action.

Neuromuscular disease: Like other neuromuscular blocking agents, Esmeron should be used with extreme caution in patients with a neuromuscular disease or after poliomyelitis since the response to neuromuscular blocking agents may be considerably altered in these cases. The magnitude and direction of this alteration may vary widely. In patients with myasthenia gravis or with the myasthenic (Eaton-Lambert) syndrome, small doses of Esmeron may have profound effects and Esmeron should be titrated to the response.

Hypothermia: In surgery under hypothermic conditions, the neuromuscular blocking effect of Esmeron is increased and the duration prolonged.

Obesity: Like other neuromuscular blocking agents, Esmeron may exhibit a prolonged duration and a prolonged spontaneous recovery in obese patients when the administered doses are calculated on actual body weight.

Burns: Patients with burns are known to develop resistance to non-depolarizing neuromuscular blocking agents. It is recommended that the dose is titrated to response.

Conditions which may increase the effects of Esmeron:

Hypokalaemia (e.g. after severe vomiting, diarrhoea and diuretic therapy), hypermagnesaemia, hypocalcaemia (after massive transfusions), hypoproteinaemia, dehydration, acidosis, hypercapnia, cachexia.

Severe electrolyte disturbances, altered blood pH or dehydration should therefore be corrected when possible.

Interaction with other medicaments and other forms of interaction: The following drugs have been shown to influence the magnitude and/or duration of action of non-depolarizing neuromuscular blocking agents.

Increased effect:

Anaesthetics:
- halothane, ether, enflurane, isoflurane, methoxyflurane, cyclopropane.
- high doses of thiopentone, methohexitone, ketamine, fentanyl, gammahydroxybutyrate, etomidate and propofol.

Other non-depolarising neuromuscular blocking agents.

- Prior administration of suxamethonium.

Other drugs:
- antibiotics: aminoglycoside and polypeptide antibiotics, acylamino-penicillin antibiotics, high doses of metronidazole.
- diuretics, β-adrenergic blocking agents, thiamine, MAO inhibiting agents, quinidine, protamine, α-adrenergic blocking agents, magnesium salts.

Decreased effect:
- neostigmine, edrophonium, pyridostigmine, aminopyridine derivatives.
- prior chronic administration of corticosteroids, phenytoin or carbamazepine.
- noradrenaline, azathioprine (only transient and limited effect), theophylline, calcium chloride.

Note: Single doses of the antibiotics netilmicin, cefuroxime, metronidazole and the combination of cefuroxime and metronidazole do not potentiate the effect of Esmeron.

Pregnancy and lactation: In animal studies neither embryotoxicity nor teratogenicity was observed that could be attributed to treatment with rocuronium bromide.

There are no data on the use of Esmeron during human pregnancy to assess potential harm to the foetus. Esmeron should be given to pregnant women only when the attending physician decides that the benefits outweigh the risks. In patients undergoing Caesarean section, Esmeron can be used as part of a rapid sequence induction technique, provided no intubation difficulties are anticipated and a sufficient dose of anaesthetic agent is administered or following succinylcholine facilitated intubation. Esmeron, administered in doses of 0.6 mg per kg body weight, has been shown to be safe in parturients undergoing Caesarean section. Esmeron does not affect Apgar score, foetal muscle tone or cardiorespiratory adaptation. From umbilical cord blood sampling it is apparent that only limited placental transfer of rocuronium bromide occurs which does not lead to the observation of clinical adverse effects in the newborn.

Note: doses of 1.0 $mg.kg^{-1}$ have been investigated during rapid sequence induction of anaesthesia, but not in Caesarean section patients. In patients receiving magnesium sulphate, the dose of Esmeron should be reduced and be carefully titrated to twitch response.

Insignificant levels of rocuronium bromide were found in the milk of lactating rats. There are no human data on the use of Esmeron during lactation. Esmeron should be given to lactating women only when the attending physician decides that the benefits outweigh the risks.

Effects on ability to drive and use of machines: It is not recommended to use potentially dangerous machinery or drive a car within 24 hours after the full recovery from the neuromuscular blocking action of Esmeron.

Undesirable effects: Anaphylactic reactions: Anaphylactic reactions to neuromuscular blocking agents in general have been reported. Although these are very rarely seen with Esmeron, precautions for treating such reactions if they would occur should always be taken. Particularly in the case of former anaphylactic reactions to neuromuscular blocking agents, special caution should be taken since allergic cross-reactivity between neuromuscular blocking agents has been reported.

Histamine release and histaminoid reactions: Since neuromuscular blocking agents are known to be capable of inducing histamine release both locally and systemically, the possible occurrence of itching and erythematous reaction at the site of injection and/or generalised histaminoid (anaphylactoid) reactions such as bronchospasm and cardiovascular changes should always be taken into consideration when administering these drugs.

Although slight increases in mean plasma histamine levels have been observed following rapid bolus administration of 0.3-0.9 mg Esmeron per kg body weight, no clinically significant tachycardia, hypotension or other clinical signs of histamine release associated with the administration of Esmeron, have been reported.

Local injection site reactions: During rapid sequence induction of anaesthesia, pain on injection has been reported, especially when the patient has not yet completely lost consciousness and particularly when propofol is used as the induction agent. In clinical studies, pain on injection has been noted in 16% of the patients who underwent rapid sequence induction of anaesthesia with propofol and in less than 0.5% of the patients who underwent rapid sequence induction of anaesthesia with fentanyl and thiopental.

Overdosage: In the event of overdosage and prolonged neuromuscular block, the patient should continue to receive ventilatory support and upon start of spontaneous recovery an acetylcholinesterase inhibitor (e.g. neostigmine, edrophonium, pyridostigmine) should be administered in adequate doses. When administration of an acetylcholinesterase inhibiting agent fails to reverse the neuromuscular effects of Esmeron, ventilation must be continued until spontaneous breathing is restored. Repeated dosage of an acetylcholinesterase inhibitor can be dangerous. In animal studies, severe depression of cardiovascular function, ultimately leading to cardiac collapse did not occur until a cumulative dose of 750 x ED_{90} (135 mg per kg body weight) was administered.

Pharmacological properties

Pharmacodynamic properties: Esmeron is a fast onset, intermediate acting non-depolarizing neuromuscular blocking agent, possessing all of the characteristic pharmacological actions of this class of drugs (curariform). It acts by competing for nicotinic cholinoceptors at the motor end-plate. This action is antagonised by acetylcholinesterase inhibitors such as neostigmine, edrophonium and pyridostigmine. The ED_{90} (dose required to produce 90% depression of the twitch response of the thumb to stimulation of the ulnar nerve) during balanced anaesthesia is approximately 0.3 mg per kg body weight. Within 60 seconds following intravenous administration of a dose of 0.6 mg Esmeron per kg body weight (2 x ED_{90} under balanced anaesthesia), adequate intubation conditions can be achieved in nearly all patients of which in 80% intubation conditions are rated excellent; within 2 minutes general muscle paralysis adequate for any type of surgery is established. The clinical duration (the duration until spontaneous recovery to 25% of control twitch height) with this dose is 30-40 minutes. The total duration (time until spontaneous recovery to 90% of control twitch height) is 50 minutes. The mean time of spontaneous recovery of twitch response from 25 to 75% (recovery index) after a bolus dose of 0.6 mg Esmeron per kg body weight is 14 minutes. With lower dosages of 0.3-0.45 mg Esmeron per kg body weight (1-1½ x ED_{90}), onset of action is slower and duration of action is shorter (13-26 mins). After administration of 0.45 mg Esmeron per kg body weight, acceptable intubation conditions are present after 90 seconds. During rapid sequence induction of anaesthesia under propofol or fentanyl/thiopental anaesthesia, adequate intubation conditions are achieved within 60 seconds in 93% and 96% of the patients respectively, following a dose of 1.0 mg rocuronium bromide per kg body weight. Of these, 70% are rated excellent. The clinical duration with this dose approaches 1 hour, at which time the neuromuscular block can be safely reversed. Following a dose of 0.6 mg rocuronium bromide per kg body weight, adequate intubation conditions are achieved within 60 seconds in 81% and 75% of the patients during a rapid sequence induction technique with propofol or fentanyl/thiopental, respectively. With doses higher than 3 x ED_{90} the intubation conditions will not improve appreciably; the duration of action, however, will be prolonged. Doses higher than 4 x ED_{90} have not been studied. The duration of action of maintenance doses of 0.15 mg Esmeron per kg body weight might be somewhat longer under enflurane and isoflurane anaesthesia in geriatric patients and in patients with hepatic or renal disease (approximately 20 minutes) than in patients without impairment of excretory organ functions under intravenous anaesthesia (approximately 13 minutes). No cumulation of effect (progressive increase in duration of action) with repetitive maintenance dosing at the recommended level has been observed. Following continuous infusion in the Intensive Care Unit, the time to recovery of the train of four ratio to 0.7 depends on the level of block at the end of the infusion. After a continuous infusion for 20 hours or more the mean (± SD) time between return of T_2 to train of four stimulation and recovery of the train of four ratio to 0.7 approximates 2 (± 1) hours in patients without multiple organ failure and 4 (± 2.5) hours in patients with multiple organ failure. In patients scheduled for cardiovascular surgery the most common cardiovascular changes during the onset of maximum block following 0.6-0.9 mg Esmeron per kg body weight are a slight and clinically insignificant increase in heart rate up to 9% and an increase in mean arterial blood pressure up to 16% from the control values. Administration of acetylcholinesterase inhibitors, such as neostigmine, pyridostigmine or edrophonium, antagonises the action of Esmeron.

Pharmacokinetic properties: After intravenous administration of a single bolus dose of rocuronium bromide the plasma concentration time course runs in three exponential phases. In normal adults, the mean (95%CI) elimination half-life is 73 (66-80) minutes, the (apparent) volume of distribution at steady state conditions is 203 (193-214) $ml.kg^{-1}$ and plasma clearance is 3.7 (3.5-3.9) $ml.kg^{-1}.min^{-1}$. In controlled studies the plasma clearance in geriatric patients and in patients with renal dysfunction was reduced, in most studies however without reaching the level of statistical significance. In patients with hepatic disease, the mean elimination half-life is prolonged by 30 minutes and the mean plasma clearance is reduced by 1 $ml.kg^{-1}.min^{-1}$. (See also Posology and method of administration). When administered as a continuous infusion to facilitate mechanical ventilation for 20 hours or more, the mean elimination half-life and the mean (apparent) volume of distribution at steady state are increased. A large between patient variability is found in controlled clinical studies, related to nature and extent of (multiple) organ failure and individual patient characteristics. In patients with multiple organ failure a mean (± SD) elimination half-life of 21.5 (± 3.3) hours, a (apparent) volume of distribution at steady state of 1.5 (± 0.8) $l.kg^{-1}$ and a plasma clearance of 2.1 (± 0.8) $ml.kg^{-1}.min^{-1}$ were found. See also Posology and method of administration. Rocuronium is excreted in urine and bile. Excretion in urine approaches 40% within 12-24 hours. After injection of a radiolabeled dose of rocuronium bromide, excretion of the radiolabel is on average 47% in urine and 43% in faeces after 9 days. Approximately 55% is recovered as the parent compound. No metabolites are detected in plasma.

Preclinical safety data: Acute toxicity: In acute toxicity studies rocuronium bromide was intravenously administered to cats and dogs up to a dose of 350 x ED_{90} and 750 x ED_{90} respectively. This last dose was administered in 4 consecutive doses at intervals of 30 minutes (9, 18, 36 and 72 mg per kg body weight) and resulted in death due to cardiac collapse.

Subacute toxicity: In subacute toxicity studies rocuronium bromide was intravenously administered to cats and dogs up to a dose of 37 x ED_{90} and 60 x ED_{90} respectively two times per week for a period of 4 weeks. Unforeseen mortalities occurred in three out of seven dogs at the dose of 60 x ED_{90} (10.8 mg per kg body weight). The cause of death could not be established, but was considered to be related to interactions between rocuronium treatment and experimental procedures and/or instrumentation and anaesthesia.

Chronic toxicity: Chronic toxicity studies have not been performed with rocuronium bromide.

Mutagenicity and carcinogenicity: In vivo and in vitro mutagenicity studies revealed no mutagenic potential of rocuronium bromide. Carcinogenicity studies have not been performed with rocuronium bromide.

Reproductive toxicity: Studies in rats with administration of rocuronium bromide during organogenesis using subpharmacological intravenous doses revealed no evidence of embryolethality, teratological changes or suppression of growth of the foetuses.

Pharmacceutical particulars

List of excipients: Esmeron contains the following excipients: sodium acetate; sodium chloride; acetic acid and water for injections.

Incompatibilities: Physical incompatibility has been documented for Esmeron when added to solutions containing the following drugs: amphotericin, amoxycillin, azathioprine, cefazolin, cloxacillin, dexamethasone, diazepam, enoximone, erythromycin, famotidine, frusemide, hydrocortisone sodium succinate, insulin, intralipid, methohexitone, methylprednisolone, prednisolone sodium succinate, thiopentone, trimethoprim and vancomycin.

Shelf-life: Esmeron can be stored for three years provided it is stored under the prescribed conditions (see Special precautions for storage). The date mentioned behind 'exp.:' on the label of the vial is the expiry date; this is the date up to which Esmeron may be used. Since Esmeron does not contain a preservative, it is recommended to discard any unused solution.

Special precautions for storage: Storage in the Refrigerator: Esmeron should be stored at 2–8°C in the dark and used within the expiry date given on the pack.

Storage out of the refrigerator: Esmeron may also be stored between 8–30°C for up to 3 months, after which it should be discarded. Once stored at 8–30°C Esmeron should not be returned to the refrigerator.

Nature and contents of containers:

Esmeron 50 mg in 5 ml (10 mg/ml)

Packaging of 12 vials each containing 50 mg rocuronium bromide.

Esmeron 100 mg in 10 ml (10 mg/ml)

Packaging of 10 vials each containing 100 mg rocuronium bromide.

Esmeron 250 mg in 25 ml (10 mg/ml)

Packaging of 4 vials each containing 250 mg rocuronium bromide.

Instructions for use/handling: Compatibility studies with the following infusion fluids have been performed. Esmeron has been shown to be compatible with: 0.9% NaCl, 5% dextrose, 5% dextrose in saline, sterile water for injections, Lactated Ringers and Haemaccel 35. Solutions should be used within 24 hours after mixing. Unused solutions should be discarded.

Esmeron can be injected into the intravenous line of a running infusion containing most of the commonly used intravenous drugs, except those mentioned under Incompatibilities.

Marketing authorisation number 3524/0025

Date of (partial) revision of the text May 1998.

Legal category POM

NORCURON*

Trade Name of the medicinal product Norcuron 10 mg

Qualitative and quantitative composition Norcuron 10 mg, 1 vial contains: Vecuronium bromide 10 mg

Pharmaceutical form Powder for injection.

Clinical particulars

Therapeutic indications: Norcuron is indicated as an adjunct to general anaesthesia to facilitate endotracheal intubation and to provide skeletal muscle relaxation during surgery.

Posology and method of administration:

Dosage: As with all other neuromuscular blocking agents, the dosage of Norcuron should be individualised in each patient. The anaesthetic method used, the expected duration of surgery, the possible interaction with other drugs that are administered before or during anaesthesia and the condition of the patient should be taken into account when determining the dose. The use of a peripheral nerve stimulator is recommended to monitor neuromuscular blockade and recovery.

The following dosages may serve as general guidelines for initial and maintenance intravenous bolus dose requirements of Norcuron to assure appropriate muscle relaxation throughout short, medium and long lasting surgical procedures under balanced anaesthesia, with and without the use of Norcuron for facilitation of endotracheal intubation.

Adults and children (see also use in paediatrics): Intubating dose: 80 to 100 micrograms vecuronium bromide per kg body weight.

Dosages of Norcuron for surgical procedures after intubation with succinylcholine: 30 to 50 micrograms vecuronium bromide per kg body weight.

If succinylcholine is used for intubation, the administration of Norcuron should be delayed until the patient has clinically recovered from the neuromuscular block induced by succinylcholine.

Maintenance dose: 20 to 30 micrograms vecuronium bromide per kg body weight.

These maintenance doses should best be given when twitch height has recovered to 25% of control twitch height.

Notes: In obese patients, these doses should be reduced taking into account a lean body mass.

Since inhalational anaesthetics potentiate the action of Norcuron (see interactions), doses of Norcuron in general should be reduced during surgical procedures where these anaesthetics are used.

Should there be reason for selection of larger doses in individual patients, initial doses ranging from 150 micrograms up to 300 micrograms vecuronium bromide per kg body weight have been administered during surgery both under halothane and neurolept anaesthesia without adverse cardiovascular effects being noted as long as ventilation is properly maintained. The use of these high dosages of Norcuron pharmacodynamically decreases the onset time and increases the duration of action.

In caesarean section and neonatal surgery the dose should not exceed 100 micrograms/kg.

Neonates and infants up to one year of age: Because of the possible variations of the sensitivity of the neuromuscular junction, especially in neonates (up to 4 weeks) and probably in infants (up to 4 months of age), it is recommended that an initial test dose of 10 to 20 micrograms vecuronium bromide per kg body weight followed by incremental doses until 90 to 95% depression of twitch response is achieved is recommended. Dose requirements in infants of 5 months to 1 year of age are the same as in adults. However, since the onset time of Norcuron in these patients is considerably shorter than in adults and children, the use of high intubating doses in general is not required for early development of good intubating conditions. Since the duration of action and recovery time with Norcuron is longer in neonates and infants than in children and adults, maintenance doses could be lower and are required less frequently. (see also Use in Paediatrics in the section 'Special Warnings and Precautions for Use'.)

Dose requirements for administration of Norcuron by continuous infusion: If Norcuron is administered by continuous infusion, it is recommended that a bolus dose of ED_{90} or $2xED_{90}$ (40-100 micrograms per kg) is administered first and, when neuromuscular block starts to recover, administration of Norcuron by infusion is commenced. The infusion rate should be adjusted to maintain twitch response at 10% of control twitch height. In adults, the infusion rate required to maintain neuromuscular block at this level, ranges from 0.8 to 1.4 micrograms vecuronium bromide/kg/min. For neonates and infants see above. Repeated monitoring of neuromuscular block is essential since infusion rate requirements vary from patient to patient and with the anaesthetic method used.

Administration: Norcuron should be administered intravenously.

Contra-indications: Former anaphylactic reactions to vecuronium or the bromide ion.

Special warnings and precautions for use: As with other neuromuscular blocking agents, Norcuron should only be administered by, or under supervision of experienced clinicians who are familiar with the action and use of these drugs. Since Norcuron causes relaxation of the respiratory muscles, mechanical ventilation until spontaneous respiration is restored, is necessary for patients treated with this drug. Anaphylactic reactions to neuromuscular blocking agents in general have been reported. Although these are very rarely seen with Norcuron, precautions for treating such reactions if they would occur should always be taken (see also Undesirable effects). Since Norcuron has no cardiovascular effects within the clinical dosage range, it does not attenuate bradycardia that may occur due to the use of some types of anaesthetics and opiates or due to vagal reflexes during surgery. Therefore, reassessment of the use and/or dosage of vagolytic drugs such as atropine for premedication or at induction of anaesthesia, may be of value for surgical procedures during which vagal reactions are more likely to occur (e.g. surgical procedures where anaesthetic drugs with known vagal stimulatory effects are used, opthalmic abdominal or anorectal surgery, etc.). Presently there are insufficient data to give recommendations for the use of Norcuron in the Intensive Care Unit. As with other muscle relaxants prolonged neuromuscular block following long term use of Norcuron in seriously ill patients in the Intensive Care Unit has been reported. It is essential that during continuous neuromuscular block patients receive adequate analgesia and sedation and that neuromuscular transmission is monitored throughout; furthermore, muscle relaxants should be administered in carefully adjusted doses, sufficient for the maintenance of less than complete block by or under the supervision of experienced clinicians who are familiar with its actions with appropriate neuromuscular monitoring techniques.

The following disease states may influence the pharmacokinetics and/or pharmacodynamics of Norcuron: *Hepatic and/or biliary tract disease:* Despite the fact that Norcuron is excreted mainly via the bile, in general only moderate changes of the course of neuromuscular block induced by Norcuron are found in patients with hepatic and/or biliary tract diseases. In addition, these changes are dose dependent. With a dose of 100 micrograms vecuronium bromide per kg body weight, a slight, statistically not significant prolongation of the onset time and decrease of the duration of action were found as compared to normal patients. At doses of 150 and 200 micrograms vecuronium bromide per kg body weight, the prolongation of the onset time was even less pronounced (150 micrograms/kg) or absent (200 micrograms/kg), and no alterations of the duration of action were found in the 150 micrograms/kg group, while significant increases in the duration of action and in the recovery time were observed in the 200 micrograms/kg group.

Renal failure: Only limited changes of pharmacodynamic parameters were reported with Norcuron when administered to patients with renal failure. As with other non-depolarising neuromuscular blocking agents, a limited degree of resistance to the action of Norcuron may occur in patients with renal failure. A slight, clinically not relevant, prolongation of onset time and recovery time may occur when Norcuron is administered to patients with renal failure.

Prolonged circulation time: Conditions associated with prolonged circulation time such as cardiovascular disease, old age, oedematous state resulting in an increased volume of distribution, may contribute to an increase in the onset time of neuromuscular block.

Neuromuscular disease: As with other neuromuscular blocking agents, Norcuron should be used with extreme caution in cases of neuromuscular disease or after poliomyelitis since the response to neuromuscular blocking agents may be considerably altered in these patients. The magnitude and direction of this alteration may vary widely. In patients with myasthenia gravis or the myasthenic (Eaton Lambert) syndrome, small doses of Norcuron may have profound effects and Norcuron should be titrated to the response.

Hypothermia: In operations under hypothermia, the neuromuscular blocking effect of Norcuron is prolonged.

Other conditions which may increase the effects of Norcuron are: hypokalaemia (e.g. after severe vomiting, diarrhoea, and diuretic therapy), hypermagnesaemia, hypocalcaemia (after massive transfusions), hypoproteinaemia, dehydration, acidosis, hypercapnoea, cachexia.

Severe electrolyte disturbances, altered blood pH or dehydration should therefore be corrected when possible. Like pancuronium bromide, d-tubocurarine or other non-depolarising neuromuscular blocking agents, Norcuron may cause a reduction in the partial thromboplastin time and the prothrombin time.

Interaction with other medicaments and other forms of interaction: The following drugs have shown to influence the magnitude and/or duration of action of non-depolarising neuromuscular blocking agents:

Increased effect:
Anaesthetics:
- halothane, ether, enflurane, isoflurane, methoxyflurane, cyclopropane, propofol
- High doses of thiopentone, methohexitone, ketamine, fentanyl, gammahydroxybutyrate, etomidate

Other non-depolarising neuromuscular blocking agents:
- Prior administration of succinylcholine (1 mg/kg).

Other drugs:
- antibiotics: aminoglycoside and polypeptide antibiotics, acylaminopenicillin antibiotics, high doses of metronidazole
- diuretics, β-adrenergic blocking agents, thiamine, MAO inhibiting agents, quinidine, protamine, α-adrenergic blocking agents, magnesium salts.

Decreased effect:
- neostigmine, edrophonium, pyridostigmine, aminopyridine derivatives.
- prior chronic administration of corticosteroids, phenytoin or carbamazepine
- noradrenaline, azathioprine (only transient and limited effect), theophylline, $CaCl_2$

Variable effect:
- depolarising muscle relaxants, e.g. succinylcholine, given after the administration of Norcuron may produce potentiation or attenuation of the neuromuscular blocking effect of Norcuron.

Pregnancy and lactation: There are insufficient data on the use of Norcuron during animal or human pregnancy to assess potential harm to the foetus. Norcuron should be given to a pregnant woman only when the attending physician decides that the benefits outweigh the risks.

Caesarean section: Studies with Norcuron, administered in doses up to 100 micrograms/kg, have shown its safety for use in Caesarean section. Norcuron does not affect Apgar score, foetal muscle tonus nor cardiorespiratory adaptation. From umbilical cord blood sampling it is apparent that only very little placental transfer of Norcuron does occur which did not lead to the observation of any clinical adverse effect in the newborn.

Remark: Reversal of Norcuron-induced neuromuscular block may be unsatisfactory in patients receiving magnesium sulphate for toxaemia of pregnancy because magnesium salts enhance neuromuscular blockade.

Therefore, in patients receiving magnesium sulphate, the dosage of Norcuron should be reduced and be carefully titrated to twitch response.

Effects on ability to drive and use machines: It is not recommended to use potentially dangerous machinery or drive a car within 24 hours after the full recovery from the neuromuscular blocking action of Norcuron.

Undesirable effects
Anaphylactic and histaminoid reactions:
Anaphylactic reactions: Anaphylactic reactions to neuromuscular blocking agents in general have been reported. Although these are very rarely seen with Norcuron, precautions for treating such reactions if they would occur should always be taken. Particularly in the case of former anaphylactic reactions to neuromuscular blocking agents, special caution should be taken since allergic cross-reactivity between neuromuscular blocking agents has been reported.

Histamine release and histaminoid reactions: Since neuromuscular blocking agents are known to be capable of inducing histamine release both locally and systematically, the possible occurrence of itching and erythematous reactions at the site of injection and/or generalised histaminoid (anaphylactoid) reactions such as bronchospasm and cardiovascular changes should always be taken into consideration when administering these drugs.

Experimental studies with intradermal injection of Norcuron have demonstrated that this drug has only a weak capacity for inducing local histamine release. Controlled studies in man failed to demonstrate any significant rise in plasma histamine levels after intravenous administration of Norcuron. Nevertheless, such cases have rarely been reported during large scale use of Norcuron.

Overdose: In the event of overdosage and prolonged neuromuscular block, the patient should remain under mechanical ventilation and a cholinesterase inhibitor (e.g. neostigmine, pyridostigmine, edrophonium) in adequate doses should be administered as an antidote. When administration of a cholinesterase inhibiting agent fails to reverse the neuromuscular effects of Norcuron, ventilation must be continued until spontaneous breathing is restored. Repeated dosage of a cholinesterase inhibitor can be dangerous.

Pharmacological properties

Pharmacodynamic properties: Norcuron (vecuronium bromide) is a non-depolarising neuromuscular blocking agent, chemically designated as the aminosteroid 1-(3α, 17β-diacetoxy-2β piperidino-5α-androstan-16β-yl)-1 methylpiperidinium bromide. Norcuron blocks the transmission process between the motor nerve-ending and striated muscle by binding competitively with acetylcholine to the nicotinic receptors located in the motor end-plate region of striated muscle.

Unlike depolarising neuromuscular blocking agents, such as succinylcholine, Norcuron does not cause muscle fasciculations. Within 90 to 120 seconds following intravenous administration of a dose of 80 to 100 micrograms vecuronium bromide per kg body weight (approximately $2xED_{90}$ under neurolept anaesthesia), good to excellent conditions for endotracheal intubation occur and within 3 to 4 minutes following administration of these dosages, general muscle paralysis adequate for any type of surgery is established.

The duration of action to 25% recovery of control twitch height (clinical duration) with this dose is 20 to 30 minutes. The time to 95% recovery of control twitch height following this dose is approximately 40 to 50 minutes. With higher dosages of Norcuron, onset time to maximal block is shortened and duration of action is prolonged. At dosages of 150, 200, 250 and 300 micrograms vecuronium bromide per kg body weight, the mean onset time under neurolept anaesthesia amounts to 146, 110, 92 and 77 seconds respectively. The mean clinical duration of action with these is 41, 55, 70 and 86 minutes respectively. With these high dosages, also a gradual, but relatively slight increase of the recovery rate from neuromuscular block occurs. When Norcuron is administered by continuous intravenous infusion, a steady state neuromuscular blockade of 90% can be maintained at a constant rate of drug delivery and without clinically significant prolongation of the recovery time from neuromuscular block at termination of the infusion. Norcuron has no cumulative effects if maintenance doses are administered at 25% recovery of control twitch height. Several maintenance doses can therefore be give in succession. These properties allow the use of Norcuron in short, medium and long lasting surgical procedures. Within the clinical dosage range, Norcuron exerts no vagolytic no ganglion blocking activity. Administration of acetylcholinesterase inhibitors, such as neostigmine, pyridostigmine or edrophonium, antagonises the action of Norcuron.

Pharmacokinetic properties: After intravenous administration of Norcuron, the distribution half-life of vecuronium amounts to approx. 2.2 (± 1.4) minutes. Vecuronium is mainly distributed in the extracellular fluid compartment. At steady state, the volume of distribution averages 0.27 l.kg^{-1} and its plasma elimination half-life averages 71 (±20) minutes. The extent of metabolism of vecuronium is relatively low. In humans, a 3-hydroxy derivative having approximately 50% less neuromuscular blocking potency than vecuronium could be demonstrated in the urine and bile as metabolite of Norcuron. In patients not suffering from renal or hepatic failure, the plasma concentration of this derivative is below detection limit, and does not contribute to the neuromuscular block occurring after administration of Norcuron.

Biliary excretion is the main elimination route. It is estimated that within 24 hours after intravenous administration of Norcuron, 40 to 80% of the dose administered is excreted into the bile as monoquaternary compounds. Approximately 95% of these monoquaternary compounds is unchanged vecuronium and 5% is 3-hydroxy vecuronium. Renal elimination is relatively low. The amount of monoquaternary compounds excreted in the urine collected by intravesical catheter for 24 hours following Norcuron administration averages 30% of the dose administered.

Use in paediatrics: Neonates and infants: In neonates and infants the ED_{90} dose of vecuronium bromide under halothane anaesthesia was found to be approximately the same (approx. 28 micrograms/kg body weight) as in adults. The onset time of Norcuron in neonates and infants is considerably shorter as compared to children and adults, probably due to the shorter circulation time and larger cardiac output. Also, a greater sensitivity of the neuromuscular junction to the action of neuromuscular blocking agents in these patients may account for a more rapid onset of action. The duration of action and recovery time with Norcuron is longer in neonates and infants than in adults. Maintenance doses of Norcuron should therefore be less frequently administered.

Children: In children the ED_{90} dose of vecuronium bromide under halothane anaesthesia was found to be somewhat higher (approx. 32 micrograms/kg body weight), although statistically not significant, than in adults. In comparison to adults, the duration of action and recovery time with Norcuron in children are in general approximately 30% and 20-30% shorter respectively. Similar to adults, cumulative effects with repeat maintenance doses of approximately one quarter of the initial dose and administered at 25% recovery of control twitch height are not observed in paediatric patients. The longer recovery time of Norcuron in neonates and infants is not of a magnitude which would require routine use of reversal agents. If used, these reversal agents are as efficacious for antagonising the neuromuscular block in neonates and infants as they are in children and adults.

Preclinical safety data: In animal studies, at high doses, a toxicity related to the pharmacological activity of vecuronium bromide was seen.

Pharmaceutical particulars

List of Excipients: Norcuron is supplied as a freeze dried powder containing citric acid monohydrate, disodium hydrogen phosphate dihydrate, mannitol, sodium hydroxide (for pH correction) and phosphoric acid (for pH correction). No preservative has been added.

Incompatibilities: As is the case for many other drugs, incompatibility has been documented for Norcuron when added to thiopentone or thiopentone containing solutions. Except for those solutions with which Norcuron has been shown to be compatible, it is not recommended that Norcuron should be mixed with other solutions or drugs in the same syringe or bag (see Instructions for use/handling–compatibility).

Shelf life: Norcuron can be kept until the expiry date indicated on the packaging, provided it is stored under the prescribed conditions.

The shelf life is as follows: Norcuron 10 mg–2 years.

When reconstituted as indicated under 'Reconstitution' or diluted as described under 'Compatibility', the solution obtained can be kept for 24 hours at room temperature and in daylight. However, in order to avoid microbiological contamination it is recommended to discard any unused solution.

Special precautions for storage: Norcuron should be stored at a temperature below 25°C, protected from light.

Nature and contents of container: Packaging of 20 vials each containing 10 mg vecuronium bromide, and 20 ampoules each containing 5 ml water for injections (solvent). It is possible that one or more of the above mentioned presentations is not available in this country.

Instructions for use/handling: Reconstitution: Norcuron 10 mg.

Addition of 5 ml water for injections results in an isotonic solution of pH 4 containing 2 mg vecuronium bromide per ml. (2 mg/ml).

Alternatively, in order to obtain a solution with a lower concentration Norcuron 10 mg may be reconstituted with a volume up to 10 ml respectively of the following infusion fluids:

5% glucose injection fluid
0.9% sodium chloride injection fluid
Lactated Ringer's solution
Lactated Ringer's injection and 5% glucose
Glucose 5% and 0.9% sodium chloride injection
Water for injections

Compatibilities: Norcuron can be injected into the line of a running infusion containing the following drugs: fentanyl, droperidol, nicomorphinehydrochloride and pancuronium bromide.

Compatibility studies with other drugs have not been performed.

When Norcuron is reconstituted with water for injections, the resultant solution can be mixed with the following infusion fluids, packed in PVC or glass, to a dilution up to 40 mg/litre:

0.9% NaCl solution
5% glucose solution
Ringer's solution
Ringer's glucose

The above-mentioned reconstituted solution can also be injected in to the line of a running infusion of the following fluids:

Lactated Ringer's solution
Lactated Ringer's solution and 5% glucose
Glucose 5% and 0.9% NaCl solution
Haemaccel
Dextran-40 5% in 0.9% NaCl solution
Water for injections

Compatibility studies with other infusion fluids have not been performed.

Marketing authorisation number 3524/0019

Date of partial revision of the text June 1996

Legal Category POM

OncoTICE* ▼

Qualitative and quantitative composition Tice BCG 12.5 mg equivalent to 2-8 x 10^8 cfu

Pharmaceutical form Freeze dried powder for intravesical instillation fluid

Clinical particulars

Therapeutic indications: OncoTICE is indicated for treatment of primary or concurrent carcinoma-in-situ of the urinary bladder and for the prevention of recurrence of high grade and/or relapsing superficial papillary transitional cell carcinoma of the urinary bladder (Stage Ta or T1) after transurethral resection.

Posology and method of administration: Reconstitution: Add 1 ml of a sterile physiological saline solution to the freeze dried powder by means of a sterile syringe and allow to stand for a few minutes. Then gently swirl the ampoule/vial until a homogenous suspension is obtained, forceful agitation should be avoided.

Intravesical instillation: Insert a catheter via the urethra into the bladder and drain the bladder completely. Connect the 50 ml syringe containing the prepared OncoTICE suspension to the catheter, and instil the suspension into the bladder. After instillation, remove the catheter. The instilled OncoTICE suspension must remain in the bladder for a period of 2 hours. During this period care should be taken that the instilled OncoTICE suspension has sufficient contact with the whole mucosal surface of the bladder. Therefore the patient should not be immobilised or, in case of a bed-ridden patient, should be turned over from back to prone and vice versa every 15 minutes. After two hours, have the patient void the instilled suspension in a sitting position.

NOTE: The patient is not allowed any fluid for a period of 4 hours prior to instillation, nor during the time that the OncoTICE suspension remains in the bladder (2 hours).

Dosage:

Adults and the elderly: The contents of one ampoule/vial of OncoTICE, reconstituted and diluted as indicated, are instilled into the urinary bladder.

Initiation of Treatment: OncoTICE should be administered ten to fourteen days after TUR, biopsy or traumatic catheterisation. Treatment should be delayed in cases of gross haematuria or major bladder irritability.

Carcinoma in situ with or without papillary carcinoma of the bladder: A standard treatment schedule consists of one intravesical instillation of OncoTICE per week for six consecutive weeks. This schedule may be repeated if tumour remission has not been achieved and if the clinical circumstances warrant. After a treatment-free interval of 2 weeks intravesical OncoTICE administration should continue at monthly intervals for at least 6 months. Maintenance treatment for up to 24 months may be required in some patients. The duration of treatment should be determined by clinical response.

Prophylaxis of papillary tumour after transurethral resection: A weekly instillation for six consecutive weeks, followed by a treatment free period of 2 weeks. Subsequent treatments to be given monthly for the next 11 months.

Children: Not recommended.

Contra-indications: Impaired immune response irrespective of whether this impairment is congenital or caused by disease, drugs or other therapy. Positive HIV serology. Pregnancy and lactation. In patients with a positive Mantoux test, OncoTICE instillations are contra-indicated only if there is supplementary medical evidence for an active tuberculous infection. Urinary tract infections. Therapy with OncoTICE should be interrupted until the bacterial culture from urine becomes negative and therapy with antibiotics and/or urinary antiseptics is stopped.

Special warnings and special precautions for use: Before the first intravesical instillation of OncoTICE, a Mantoux test (PPD) should be performed. If the test is positive, OncoTICE instillations are contraindicated only if there is supplementary medical evidence for an active tuberculous infection. OncoTICE should not be administered intravenously, subcutaneously or intramuscularly. Reconstitution and preparation of the OncoTICE suspension for instillation and administration should be performed under aseptic conditions.

Spillage of OncoTICE solution should be treated with a disinfectant such as strong hypochlorite. Spillage on the skin should be treated with dilute hypochlorite. Traumatic catheterization can promote systemic BCG infection. Administration of OncoTICE should be delayed in such patients until mucosal damage has healed. In patients with known risk factors for HIV infection, it is recommended that adequate HIV assays are performed prior to therapy.

Interactions with other medicaments and other forms of interaction: Tice BCG is sensitive to the routinely used tuberculostatic chemotherapeutic agents such as streptomycin, para-amino salicylic acid (PAS), isoniazid (INH), rifampicin and ethambutol. Studies on interactions with other drugs have not been performed.

Pregnancy and lactation: OncoTICE instillation for carcinoma of the bladder is contraindicated during pregnancy and lactation.

Effects on ability to drive and use machines: Not applicable.

Undesirable effects: Common side effects: The intravesical administration of BCG frequently produces symptoms of cystitis or bladder irritation such as dysuria, urinary frequency and haematuria. The cystitis and inflammatory reaction (granulomata) may be an essential part of the antitumour activity. In most cases the symptoms disappear within two days after instillation and the cystitis does not require treatment. Where necessary the irritative bladder effects can be managed symptomatically. Severe or prolonged (greater than 48 hours) frequency and dysuria may be treated with isoniazid (300 mg daily) and analgesics until the symptoms resolve. BCG treatment should be withheld until symptoms have resolved completely. Malaise, low grade fever and/or a flu-like syndrome.

These symptoms usually appear within 4 hours of administration and last for 24–48 hours and should be managed by standard symptomatic treatment.

Less frequent complications: BCG infection. Systemic BCG infection is a serious side effect of OncoTICE administration, and fatalities have occurred. BCG infection may be more common after traumatic bladder catheterisation or bladder perforation. BCG treatment should be delayed in such patients until mucosal damage has healed. Treatment should be delayed for 10-14 days after TUR or biopsy of bladder lesions. All patients receiving the product should be carefullly monitored and advised to report all incidences of fever and other events outside the urinary tract. Fever lasting over 24 hours and any unusual event should be investigated to exclude another cause and to try and isolate organisms. Blood cultures and samples from affected sites should be cultured for BCG. The infection may manifest as pneumonitis, hepatitis and/or cytopenia after a period of fever and malaise. Fever lasting more than 48 hours for which there is no other explanation and any other unexplained reactions should be treated with antituberculous therapy, following the regular treatment schedules for tuberculosis. OncoTICE is sensitive to Isoniazid, Rifampicin and Ethambutol. No further treatment with BCG should be given.

In rare cases, arthritis/arthralgias, major haematuria, skin rash, transient urethral obstruction, orchitis or bladder contracture may occur. If these rare complications of OncoTICE instillation occur, it is almost exclusively during the maintenance treatment regimen. In most cases of arthritis, arthralgias and skin rash, these can be attributed to hypersensitivity reactions of the patient to BCG.

Overdose: Patients with manifest symptoms of therapy-induced BCG infections should be adequately treated with antituberculosis chemotherapeutics, following the normal treatment schedules used for tuberculosis infections.

Pharmacological properties

Pharmacodynamic properties: The precise mode of action of intravesical BCG instillation in the treatment and/or recurrence prophylaxis of superficial bladder cancer is still largely unknown. The primary mode of action is thought to involve local and systemic immunological mechanisms.

Pharmacokinetic properties: For the treatment and recurrence prophylaxis of bladder cancer, the attachment of BCG to the bladder wall after voiding has been shown to be important. This allows a targeted pharmacological effect at the site of application.

Preclinical safety data: As a result of the wide clinical application of BCG vaccination in the preceding decades the risks of BCG in human subjects are well-characterised. Intra-vesical administration to dogs has been found to be safe and without significant toxicity. No evidence of birth defects, genetic damage or carcinogenecity in humans are available from the extensive adverse reaction literature of BCG used as a vaccine.

Pharmaceutical particulars

List of excipients: Lactose PhEur; Asparagine USP; Citric Acid PhEur; Dibasic potassium phosphate USP; Magnesium sulphate PhEur; Ferric Ammonium Citrate USP; Glycerol PhEur; Zinc Formate HSE and Ammonium Hydroxide PhEur.

Incompatibilities: OncoTICE is incompatible with hypo and hypertonic solutions.

Shelf-life: 12 months.

Once reconstituted: The solution in ampoules should be used within 1 hour.

The solution in vials should be used within 2 hours.

Special precautions for storage: Store at 2-8°C, protect from light.

Nature and contents of containers: 2 ml glass ampoules in packs of 1, 3 & 6. 2 ml glass vials in packs of 1 & 3

Instructions for use/handling: See *Posology and method of administration.*

Marketing authorisation number

Ampoules, 03524/0016.

Vials 03524/0027.

Date of partial revision of text October 1997.

Legal category POM

PAVULON*

Presentation Pancuronium bromide BP 2 ml ampoules. A clear, aqueous solution. Active ingredient: Each 2 ml ampoule contains pancuronium bromide BP 4 mg. Other ingredients: sodium chloride, sodium acetate acetic acid to pH 4 and water for injection.

Uses Pavulon is a non-depolarising neuromuscular blocking agent with a medium duration of action. It is used in adjunct to surgical anaesthesia to obtain relaxation of the skeletal muscles in a wide range of surgical procedures. Pavulon is also used for neuromuscular blockade during intensive care therapy for a variety of pathologies, including intractable status asthmaticus and tetanus.

Dosage and Administration Pavulon is administered intravenously. When determining the dose, the method of anaesthesia, expected duration of surgery, potential interaction with other drugs that are administered before or during anaesthesia and the condition of the patient should be taken into account. The use of a peripheral nerve stimulator is recommended for monitoring neuromuscular block and recovery. The following may be used as a general guide to dosage:

Adult surgery:

Initial dose: 50–80 micrograms/kg (intubation accomplished within 150–120 seconds)

or 80–100 micrograms/kg (intubation accomplished within 120–90 seconds).

Incremental doses: 10–20 micrograms/kg.

Child surgery:

Initial dose: 60–100 micrograms/kg Incremental doses: 10–20 micrograms/kg.

Neonatal surgery: 30–40 micrograms/kg.

Incremental doses: As neonates are sensitive this dose should be adjusted according to the initial response but generally incremental doses lie in the range 10–20 micrograms/kg body weight. If succinylcholine is used for intubation the administration of Pavulon should be delayed until the patient has clinically recovered from the neuromuscular block induced by succinylcholine. Following the administration of suxamethonium the dosage of Pavulon may be considerably reduced:

Adults: Initial dose 20–60 micrograms/kg. Incremental doses 10–20 micrograms/kg

Children: Initial dose: 20–60 micrograms/kg. Incremental doses 10–20 micrograms/kg

In obese patients all of these doses should be reduced. The duration of action depends upon the clinical condition of the patient and the dose administered, but in normal subjects receiving perioperative muscle relaxant doses the duration of action is usually 45–60 minutes.

Pavulon is longer-acting in the intensive-care patient, and an intravenous dose of 60 micrograms/kg every one to one and a half hours, or even less frequently, is usually adequate.

The neuromuscular blocking activity of Pavulon is prolonged in the elderly. In the control of tetanus, duration of Pavulon relaxation probably depends on the severity of the spasm: duration of effect can therefore be variable. Pavulon should not be mixed with other agents in the same syringe, or with solutions for intravenous infusion, as a change in pH may induce precipitation. Any unused solution should be discarded.

Contra-indications, warnings, etc.

Contra-indications: Patients with a known hypersensitivity to Pavulon injection.

Use in Pregnancy and lactation: There are insufficient data on the use of Pavulon during animal or human pregnancy to assess potential harm to the foetus. The drug should only be administered to a pregnant woman when the attending physician decides that the benefits outweigh the risks.

Lactation: There is no available evidence that breast-feeding, after a mother has been given Pavulon, has any adverse effects on the baby.

Caesarean section: Studies with Pavulon have shown its safety for use in Caesarean section. Pavulon does not affect Apgar score, foetal muscle tonus nor cardiorespiratory adaptation of the new-born. From assays of the Pavulon concentration in umbilical blood samples it is apparent that only very limited placental transfer of Pavulon occurs.

Warning: Reversal of neuromuscular block induced by Pavulon may be unsatisfactory in patients receiving magnesium sulphate for toxaemia of pregnancy because magnesium salts enhance neuromuscular blockade. Dosages should be reduced in such cases.

Precautions and warnings: Pavulon should be administered only by anaesthetists familiar with its use, and only when facilities for controlled ventilation insufflation with oxygen and endotracheal intubation are available for immediate use. Since Pavulon causes relaxation of the respiratory muscles, respiration must be assisted in all patients. It is essential to ensure that the patient is breathing spontaneously, deeply and regularly before leaving the theatre after anaesthesia. The neuromuscular blockade achieved with Pavulon can be reversed with a cholinesterase inhibiting agent (e.g. neostigmine) in an adequate dose, together with atropine as an anticholinergic agent. Care should be exercised if there is a danger of regurgitation when intubating the patient, for example during crash induction. Pavulon (like d-tubocurarine) causes a reduction in the partial thromboplastin time and the prothrombin time. The following disease states may influence the pharmacokinetics and/or pharmacodynamics of Pavulon:

Renal failure: Since renal excretion is the major elimination route of Pavulon, the elimination half-life is prolonged and the plasma clearance is reduced in patients with renal failure. Pavulon should be used with caution in patients with severe renal impairment as the duration of action can be prolonged. The prolongation of half-life in patients with renal failure is often but not always associated with an extended duration of neuromuscular blockade. In these patients the recovery from neuromuscular block may also be prolonged.

Hyperdiuresis may result in a decreased neuromuscular blocking effect.

Hepatic and/or biliary tract disease: Despite the modest role of the liver in the elimination of Pavulon, major pharmacokinetic changes have been observed in patients with liver disease.

Resistance to the neuromuscular blocking activity of Pavulon may occur, because these conditions are characterised by a considerable increase (up to 50%) in the volume of distribution of the drug. At the same time hepatic and/or biliary tract disease can prolong the elimination half-life of Pavulon and prolong the recovery from neuromuscular block. The possibility of slower onset, higher total dosage requirements and prolongation of neuromuscular blockade and recovery time must be taken into consideration when Pavulon is used in these patients.

Altered circulation time: Conditions associated with slower circulation time, such as cardiovascular disease, old age, oedematous states resulting in an increased volume of distribution, may contribute to an increase of onset time.

Neuromuscular disease: As is the case with other curariform agents, in cases of neuromuscular disease or after poliomyelitis, Pavulon should be used with extreme caution since the response to neuromuscular blocking agents may be considerably altered in these patients. The magnitude and direction of this alteration may vary widely. In patients with myasthenia gravis or the myasthenic (Eaton Lambert) syndrome, small doses of Pavulon may have profound effects and only very small doses of Pavulon should be used initially.

Hypothermia: In operations requiring hypothermia the neuromuscular blockade of non-depolarising drugs is decreased and increases when re-warming the patient. Hypothermia in neonates therefore, requires a reduced dosage of Pavulon.

Other conditions which may increase the effect of Pavulon are: hypokalaemia (e.g. after severe vomiting, diarrhoea, digitalisation and diuretic therapy), hypermagnesaemia, hypocalcaemia (after massive transfusions), hypoproteinaemia, dehydration, acidosis, hypercapnoea, cachexia. Severe electrolyte disturbances, altered blood pH or dehydration should therefore be corrected when possible. Patients with carcinomatosis especially when associated with bronchial carcinoma, may exhibit a marked sensitivity to this agent, and the neuromuscular block produced may respond poorly to neostigmine.

Effects on ability to drive and to use machines: It is not recommended to use potentially dangerous machinery or drive a car within 24 hours after full recovery from the neuromuscular blocking action of Pavulon.

Interactions: The following drugs have been shown to influence the magnitude and/or duration of action of non-depolarising neuromuscular blocking agents:

Increased effect: Anaesthetics: halothane, ether, enflurane, isoflurane, methoxyflurane, cyclopropane, thiopentone, methohexital, ketamine, fentanyl, gammahydroxybutyrate, etomidate.

Other drugs: other non-depolarising muscle relaxants, prior administration of succinylcholine, aminoglycoside and polypeptide antibiotics, diuretics, beta-adrenergic blocking agents, thiamine, M.A.O. inhibiting agents, quinidine, protamine, phenytoin, alpha-adrenergic blocking agents, imidazoles, metronidazole, nitroglycerin, diazepam, magnesium sulphate, narcotic analgesics.

Decreased effect: Anaesthetics: Neurolept analgesia, propanidid. Other drugs: neostigmine, edrophonium, pyridostigmine, prior chronic administration of corticosteroids, noradrenaline, adrenaline, azathioprine, theophylline, KCl, $CaCl_2$, heparin (temporary decrease).

Variable effect: depolarising muscle relaxants given after the administration of Pavulon may produce potentiation or attenuation of the neuromuscular blocking effect. The non-depolarising drug increases resistance towards the neuromuscular blocking effect of the depolarising drug. Therefore high doses of a depolarising drug are necessary before muscular relaxation can be obtained. These high doses of a depolarising drug may cause endplate desensitisation and prolong post-operative apnoea. Unlike a non-depolarising block, a depolarising block cannot be overcome by, and may even be worsened by an anticholinesterase agent.

Influence on the cardiovascular system: Pavulon does not intensify the hypotension induced by halothane; in addition the cardiac depression is partly restored. The excessive bradycardia induced by neurolept analgesia and some of the cholinergic effects of morphine derivatives are counteracted by Pavulon.

Pavulon should be given with caution to a patient receiving chronic tricyclic antidepressant therapy who is anaesthetised with halothane or any inhalation anaesthetic, since this enhances the predisposition to the development of cardiac arrhythmias associated with tricyclic antidepressants. Recent evidence suggests that alkylating drugs (nitrogen mustards) should be considered a possible hazard when given to patients during anaesthesia involving the use of muscle relaxants.

Side effects: After Pavulon a slight to moderate rise in arterial pressure may occur. Increased pulse rate and cardiac output are frequently reported, showing Pavulon to have weak vagolytic activity. In general this is considered to be a favourable effect. Pavulon decreases intra-ocular pressure and induces miosis, both effects being favourable in ophthalmic surgery. A few cases of localised reactions at the site of injection have been reported. Although rare instances of bronchospasm have been reported, Pavulon has in general a lack of associated bronchospasm.

Overdosage: In the event of an overdosage i.e. a failure of neostigmine to reverse the neuromuscular block, the patient must continue to be ventilated. When administration of a cholinesterase inhibiting agent fails to reverse the neuromuscular blocking effects of Pavulon, ventilation must be continued until spontaneous breathing is restored. Repeated dosage of a cholinesterase inhibitor can be dangerous.

Pharmaceutical Precautions Pavulon should be stored at 2–8°C and protected from light. Any unused solution should be discarded.

Legal Category POM

Package Quantities Boxes of 25 x 2 ml ampoules.

Further Information *Pharmacological particulars:* Pavulon (pancuronium bromide) is a non-depolarising neuromuscular blocking agent chemically designated as the amino-steroid 1,1'-(3α, 17β-diacetoxy-5α-androstan-2β, 16β-ylene) bis (1-methylpiperidinium) dibromide. Pavulon blocks the transmission process between the motor nerve-ending and the striated muscle by binding competitively with acetylcholine to the nicotinic receptors located in the motor end-plate region of striated muscle. Unlike depolarising neuromuscular blocking agents such as succinylcholine, Pavulon does not cause muscle fasciculations. Pavulon has no hormonal activity. Pavulon exerts a slight and dose dependent vagolytic action. Within the clinical dose range it has no ganglion blocking action. Acetylcholinesterase inhibitors such as neostigmine, pyridostigmine or edrophonium antagonise the action of Pavulon. The ED_{95} (dose required to produce 95% suppression of twitch height) is approximately 0.06 mg pancuronium bromide per kilogram of bodyweight under neurolept anaesthesia. The time from administration to occurrence of the maximal effect (onset time) and the duration of action largely depend on the dose administered. With a dose of 0.06 mg pancuronium bromide per kg body-weight (ED_{95} under neurolept anaesthesia), the onset time is approximately 5 minutes and the time from administration to 25% recovery of control twitch height (duration of action) is approximately 35 minutes. The time from administration to 90% recovery of control twitch height with this dose averages 73 minutes . Higher doses up to 0.1 mg pancuronium bromide per kg bodyweight as used to facilitate endotracheal intubation, will reduce the onset time and prolong the duration of action.

Pharmacokinetic particulars: Following intravenous injection, the plasma half-life of the drug during the distribution phase ($T_{1/2}\alpha$) is less than 5 minutes. This rapid initial disappearance from the plasma is compatible with the assumption that a stable distribution of pancuronium between plasma and extracellular fluid is attained within 5 minutes of drug administration in man. The plasma elimination half-life ($T_{1/2}\beta$) of pancuronium bromide averages 110 to 120 minutes. Renal excretion is the major route of elimination. Approximately 40 to 50% of the initial dose of pancuronium is excreted unchanged in the urine. 11% is excreted in the bile as unchanged pancuronium or its metabolites. The metabolites of pancuronium are 3-OH, 17-OH 3,17 di-OH derivatives. These derivatives do not significantly contribute to the neuromuscular block occurring after the administration of Pavulon.

Product licence number 0065/5014R.

**Trade Mark*

Orion Pharma (UK) Limited

1st Floor, Leat House
Overbridge Square
Hambridge Lane
Newbury Berkshire RG14 5UX

☎ 01635 520300 🖷 01635 520319

COMTESS*

Qualitative and quantitative composition Active substance: entacapone. Each film-coated tablet contains 200 mg entacapone.

Pharmaceutical form Film-coated tablet. Brownish-orange, oval, biconvex film-coated tablet with Comtess engraved on one side.

Clinical particulars Entacapone should only be used in combination with levodopa/benserazide or levodopa/carbidopa. The prescribing information for these levodopa preparations is applicable to their concomitant use with entacapone.

Therapeutic indications: Entacapone is indicated as an adjunct to standard preparations of levodopa/benserazide or levodopa/carbidopa for use in patients with Parkinson's disease and end-of-dose motor fluctuations, who cannot be stabilised on those combinations.

Posology and method of administration:

Method of administration: Entacapone is administered orally and simultaneously with each levodopa/carbidopa or levodopa/benserazide dose. Entacapone can be used with standard preparations of levodopa. Efficacy of entacapone as an adjunct to controlled-release levodopa/dopa decarboxylase inhibitor preparations has not been proven.

Entacapone can be taken with or without food (see *Pharmacokinetic properties*).

Posology: One 200 mg tablet is taken with each levodopa/dopa decarboxylase inhibitor dose. The maximum recommended dose is 200 mg ten times daily, i.e. 2,000 mg of entacapone.

Entacapone enhances the effects of levodopa. Hence, to reduce levodopa-related dopaminergic adverse effects, e.g. dyskinesias, nausea, vomiting and hallucinations, it is often necessary to adjust levodopa dosage within the first days to first weeks after initiating entacapone treatment. The daily dose of levodopa should be reduced by about 10–30% by extending the dosing intervals and/or by reducing the amount of levodopa per dose, according to the clinical condition of the patient.

If entacapone treatment is discontinued, it is necessary to adjust the dosing of other antiparkinsonian treatments, especially levodopa, to achieve a sufficient level of control of the parkinsonian symptoms.

Entacapone increases the bioavailability of levodopa from standard levodopa/benserazide preparations slightly (5–10%) more than from standard levodopa/carbidopa preparations. Hence, patients who are taking standard levodopa/benserazide preparations may need a larger reduction of levodopa dose when entacapone is initiated.

Renal insufficiency does not affect the pharmacokinetics of entacapone and there is no need for dose adjustment. However, for patients who are receiving dialysis therapy, a longer dosing interval may be considered (see *Pharmacokinetic properties*).

Elderly: No dosage adjustment of entacapone is required for elderly patients.

Children: As entacapone has not been studied in patients under 18 years of age, the use of the medicinal product in patients under this age cannot be recommended.

Contra-indications: Known hypersensitivity to entacapone or any of the excipients of the medicinal product (see *List of excipients*).

Pregnancy and breast-feeding (see *Pregnancy and lactation*).

Liver impairment.

Entacapone is contra-indicated in patients with pheochromocytoma due to the increased risk of hypertensive crisis.

Concomitant use of entacapone and non-selective monoamine oxidase (MAO-A and MAO-B) inhibitors (e.g. phenelzine, tranylcypromine) is contra-indicated. Similarly, concomitant use of a selective MAO-A inhibitor plus a selective MAO-B inhibitor and entacapone is contra-indicated. Entacapone may be used with selegiline (a selective MAO-B inhibitor), but the daily dose of selegiline should not exceed 10 mg (see *Interaction with other medicinal products and other forms of interaction*).

A previous history of Neuroleptic Malignant Syndrome (NMS) and/or non-traumatic rhabdomyolysis.

Special warnings and special precautions for use: Rhabdomyolysis secondary to severe dyskinesias or Neuroleptic Malignant Syndrome (NMS) has been observed rarely in patients with Parkinson's disease, although it has not been reported during entacapone treatment.

NMS, including rhabdomyolysis and hyperthermia, is characterised by motor symptoms (rigidity, myoclonus, tremor), mental status changes (e.g. agitation, confusion, coma), hyperthermia, autonomic dysfunction (tachycardia, labile blood pressure) and elevated serum creatine phosphokinase (CPK) which may be a consequence of rhabdomyolysis. In individual cases, only some of these symptoms and/or findings may be evident.

Neither NMS nor rhabdomyolysis have been reported in association with entacapone treatment from controlled trials in which entacapone was discontinued abruptly. Nevertheless, because NMS has been reported rarely in Parkinson's disease patients when other dopaminergic medications were withdrawn abruptly, prescribers should exercise caution when discontinuing entacapone treatment. When considered necessary, withdrawal should proceed slowly, and if signs and/or symptoms occur despite a slow withdrawal of entacapone, an increase in levodopa dosage may be necessary.

Because of its mechanism of action, entacapone may interfere with the metabolism of medicinal products containing a catechol group and potentiate their action. Thus, entacapone should be administered cautiously to patients being treated with medicinal products metabolised by catechol-O-methyl transferase (COMT), e.g. rimiterole, isoprenaline, adrenaline, noradrenaline, dopamine, dobutamine, alpha-methyldopa, and apomorphine (see also *Interaction with other medicinal products and other forms of interaction*).

Entacapone is always given as an adjunct to levodopa treatment. Hence, the precautions valid for levodopa treatment should also be taken into account for entacapone treatment. Entacapone increases the bioavailability of levodopa from standard levodopa/benserazide preparations 5–10% more than from standard levodopa/carbidopa preparations. Consequently, undesirable dopaminergic effects may be more frequent when entacapone is added to levodopa/benserazide treatment (see also *Undesirable effects*). To reduce levodopa-related dopaminergic adverse effects, it is often necessary to adjust levodopa dosage within the first days to first weeks after initiating entacapone treatment, according to the clinical condition of the patient (see *Posology and method of administration* and *Undesirable effects*).

Entacapone may aggravate levodopa-induced orthostatic hypotension. Entacapone should be given cautiously to patients who are taking other medicinal products which may cause orthostatic hypotension.

In clinical studies, undesirable dopaminergic effects, e.g. dyskinesia, were more common in patients who received entacapone and dopamine agonists (such as bromocriptine), selegiline or amantadine compared to those who received placebo with this combination. The doses of other antiparkinsonian medications may need to be adjusted when entacapone treatment is initiated.

Interaction with other medicinal products and other forms of interaction: No interaction of entacapone with carbidopa has been observed with the recommended treatment schedule. Pharmacokinetic interaction with benserazide has not been studied.

In single-dose studies in healthy volunteers, no interactions were observed between entacapone and imipramine or between entacapone and moclobemide. Similarly, no interactions between entacapone and selegiline were observed in repeated-dose studies in parkinsonian patients. However, the experience of the clinical use of entacapone with several drugs, including MAO-A inhibitors, tricyclic antidepressants, noradrenaline reuptake inhibitors such as desipramine, maprotiline and venlafaxine, and catechol-structured medicinal products that are metabolised by COMT is still limited. Concomitant use of entacapone with these medicinal products is not recommended (see also *Contra-indications* and *Special warnings and special precautions for use*).

Entacapone may form chelates with iron in the gastrointestinal tract. Entacapone and iron preparations should be taken at least 2–3 hours apart (see *Undesirable effects*).

Entacapone binds to human albumin binding site II which also binds several other medicinal products, including diazepam and ibuprofen. Clinical interaction studies with diazepam and non-steroidal anti-inflammatory drugs have not been carried out. According to *in vitro* studies, significant displacement is not anticipated at therapeutic concentrations of the medicinal products.

Pregnancy and lactation: Pregnancy: No overt teratogenic or primary foetotoxic effects were observed in animal studies in which the exposure levels of entacapone were markedly higher than the therapeutic exposure levels. As there is no experience in pregnant women, entacapone should not be used during pregnancy (see *Contra-indications*).

Lactation: In animal studies entacapone was excreted in milk. The safety of entacapone in infants is unknown. Women should not breast-feed during treatment with entacapone (see *Contra-indications*).

Effects on ability to drive and use machines: Comtess together with levodopa may cause dizziness and symptomatic orthostatism. Therefore, caution should be exercised when driving or using machines.

Undesirable effects: The most frequent undesirable effects caused by entacapone relate to the increased dopaminergic activity and occur most commonly at the beginning of treatment. Reduction of levodopa dosage decreases the severity and frequency of these effects. The other major class of undesirable effects are gastointestinal symptoms, including e.g. nausea, vomiting, abdominal pains, constipation and diarrhoea. Urine may be discoloured reddish-brown by entacapone, but this is a harmless phenomenon.

Usually undesirable effects caused by entacapone are mild to moderate. Most commonly undesirable effects leading to discontinuation of entacapone treatment have been gastrointestinal symptoms (e.g. diarrhoea, 2.5%) and increased dopaminergic undesirable effects of levodopa (e.g. dyskinesias, 1.7%).

Dyskinesias (27%), nausea (11%), diarrhoea (8%), abdominal pain (7%) and dry mouth (4.2%) were reported significantly more often with entacapone than with placebo.

Some of the adverse events, such as dyskinesia, nausea, and abdominal pain, may be more common with the higher doses (1400 to 2000 mg per day) than with the lower doses of entacapone.

Undesirable effects occurring in at least 2% of patients treated for 6 months with entacapone or placebo with levodopa/DDCI (dopa decarboxylase inhibitors) in double-blind phase III studies are presented in the following table:

SYSTEM ORGAN CLASS Preferred term	*Entacapone (n=406) % of patients*	*Placebo (n=296) % of patients*
AUTONOMIC NERVOUS SYSTEM DISORDERS		
Hypertension postural	2.0	2.0
BODY AS A WHOLE – GENERAL DISORDERS		
Fatigue	4.2	2.4
Sweating increased	2.7	1.7
Headache	2.5	2.7
CENTRAL & PERIPHERAL SYSTEM DISORDERS		
Dyskinesia	27.3	13.9
Parkinsonism aggravated	8.1	7.1
Dizziness	7.4	5.4
Dystonia	2.7	2.4
Hyperkinesia	2.5	1.0
Leg cramps	2.0	2.4
Vertigo	1.5	2.0
Tremor	1.2	2.7
Gait abnormal	0.7	2.0

SYSTEM ORGAN CLASS Preferred term	*Entacapone (n=406) % of patients*	*Placebo (n=296) % of patients*
GASTRO-INTESTINAL SYSTEM DISORDERS		
Nausea	11.1	6.4
Diarrhoea	8.4	3.0
Abdominal pain	7.1	2.7
Mouth dry	4.2	0.0
Constipation	3.0	2.0
PSYCHIATRIC DISORDERS		
Insomnia	4.4	3.7
Hallucinations	3.4	2.4
Confusion	2.0	1.0
Paroniria	2.0	1.4
SECONDARY TERMS-EVENTS		
Fall	2.0	0.7
URINARY SYSTEM DISORDERS		
Urine abnormal	12.6	0.0

Slight decreases in haemoglobin, erythrocyte count and hematocrit have been reported during entacapone treatment. The underlying mechanism may involve decreased absorption of iron from the gastrointestinal tract. During long-term treatment (6 months) with entacapone a clinically significant decrease in haemoglobin have been observed in 1.5% of patients.

Rare reports of clinically significant increases in liver enzymes have been received.

Overdose: No cases of overdose have been reported with entacapone. The highest dose of entacapone given to man is 2400 mg daily. Management of acute overdosing is symptomatic.

Pharmacological properties

Pharmacodynamic properties: Pharmacotherapeutic group: catechol-O-methyl transferase inhibitor, ATC code: NO4BX02.

Entacapone belongs to a new therapeutic class, catechol-O-methyl transferase (COMT) inhibitors. It is a reversible, specific, and mainly peripherally acting COMT inhibitor designed for concomitant administration with levodopa preparations. Entacapone decreases the metabolic loss of levodopa to 3-O-methyldopa (3-OMD) by inhibiting the COMT enzyme. This leads to a higher levodopa AUC. The amount of levodopa available to the brain is increased. Entacapone thus prolongs the clinical response to levodopa.

Entacapone inhibits the COMT enzyme mainly in peripheral tissues. COMT inhibition in red blood cells closely follows the plasma concentrations of entacapone, thus clearly indicating the reversible nature of COMT inhibition.

Clinical studies: In two phase III double-blind studies in altogether 376 patients with Parkinson's disease and end-of-dose motor fluctuations, entacapone or placebo was given with each levodopa/dopa decarboxylase inhibitor dose. The results are given in the following table. In study I, daily ON time (hours) was measured from home diaries. In study II, the proportion of daily ON time was measured.

Study I

	Entacapone (n=85) Mean (±S.D.)	*Placebo (n=86) Mean (±S.D.)*	*Difference*
Baseline*	9.3±2.2	9.2±2.5	
Week 8–24*	10.7±2.2	9.4±2.6	1 h 20 min (8.3%) $CI_{95\%}$ 45 min, 1 h 56

Study II

	Entacapone (n=103)	*Placebo (n=102)*	*Difference*
Baseline**	60.0±15.2	60.8±14.0	
Week 8–24**	66.8±14.5	62.8±16.80	4.5% (0 h 35 min) $CI_{95\%}$ 0.93%, 7.97%

* daily ON time (h)
** proportion ON time%

There were corresponding decreases in OFF time.

The % change from baseline in OFF time was –24% in the entacapone group and 0% in the placebo group in study I. The corresponding figures in study II were –18% and –5%.

Pharmacokinetic properties:

a) General characteristics of the active substance:

Absorption: There are large intra- and interindividual variations in the absorption of entacapone.

The peak concentration (C_{max}) in plasma is usually reached about one hour after a 200 mg entacapone tablet. The drug is subject to extensive first-pass metabolism. The bioavailability of entacapone is about 35% after an oral dose. Food does not affect the absorption of entacapone to any significant extent.

Distribution: After absorption from the gastrointestinal tract, entacapone is rapidly distributed to the peripheral tissues with a distribution volume of 181 litres. Approximately 92% of the dose is eliminated during β-phase with a short elimination half-life of 30 minutes. The total clearance of entacapone is about 800 ml/min.

Entacapone is extensively bound to plasma proteins, mainly to albumin. In human plasma the unbound fraction is about 2.0% in the therapeutic concentration range. At therapeutic concentrations, entacapone does not displace other extensively bound drugs (e.g. warfarin, salicylic acid, phenylbutazone, or diazepam), nor is it displaced to any significant extent by any of these drugs at therapeutic or higher concentrations.

Metabolism: A small amount of entacapone, the (E)-isomer, is converted to its (Z)-isomer. The (E)-isomer accounts for 95% of the AUC of entacapone. The (Z)-isomer and traces of other metabolites account for the remaining 5%.

Elimination: The elimination of entacapone occurs mainly by non-renal metabolic routes. It is estimated that 80–90% of the dose is excreted in faeces, although this has not been confirmed in man. Approximately 10–20% is excreted in urine. Only traces of entacapone are found unchanged in urine. The major part (95%) of the product excreted in urine is conjugated with glucuronic acid. Of the metabolites found in urine only about 1% have been formed through oxidation.

b) Characteristics in patients: The pharmacokinetic properties of entacapone are similar in both young and elderly adults. The metabolism of the medicinal product is slowed in patients with mild to moderate liver insufficiency (Child-Pugh Class A and B), which leads to an increased plasma concentration of entacapone both in the absorption and elimination phases (see *Contra-indications*). Renal impairment does not affect the pharmacokinetics of entacapone. However, a longer dosing interval may be considered for patients who are receiving dialysis therapy.

Preclinical safety data: Preclinical data revealed no special hazard for humans based on conventional studies of safety pharmacology, repeated dose toxicity, genotoxicity, and carcinogenic potential. In repeated dose toxicity studies, anaemia most likely due to iron chelating properties of entacapone was observed. Regarding reproduction toxicity, decreased foetal weight and a slightly delayed bone development were noticed in rabbits at systemic exposure levels in the therapeutic range.

Pharmaceutical particulars

List of excipients: Microcrystalline cellulose, mannitol, croscarmellose sodium, hydrogenated vegetable oil, hypromellose, polysorbate 80, glycerol 85%, sucrose, magnesium stearate, yellow iron oxide, red iron oxide, titanium dioxide.

Incompatibilities: Not applicable.

Shelf life: 3 years.

Special precautions for storage: None.

Nature and contents of container: White high-density polyethylene (HPDE) bottles with white tamper proof HD-polyethylene closures containing 30, 60, 100 or 350 tablets.

Instructions for use/handling and disposal (if appropriate): No special requirements.

Marketing authorisation holder: Orion Corporation, Orionintie 1, FIN-02200 Espoo, Finland.

Number in the community register of medicinal products EU/1/98/082/001-004

Date of first authorisation/renewal of the authorisation 16 September 1998

Date of revision of the text 19 November 1998

ELDEPRYL*

Qualitative and quantitative composition

Tablets: Eldepryl tablets 5 mg—selegiline hydrochloride 5 mg, Constit. q.s.

Eldepryl tablets 10 mg—selegiline hydrochloride 10 mg, Constit. q.s.

Eldepryl tablets 10 mg/5 ml—selegiline hydrochloride 2 mg/ml, Constit. q.s.

Pharmaceutical form: Tablets for peroral administration.

Syrup for peroral administration.

Clinical particulars

Therapeutic indications: Selegiline is indicated for the treatment of Parkinson's disease, or symptomatic parkinsonism. It may be used alone to delay the need for levadopa (with or without decarboxylase inhibitor) or as an adjunct to levodopa (with or without decarboxylase inhibitor).

Posology and method of administration: 10 mg daily either alone or as an adjunct to levodopa or levodopa/peripheral decarboxylase inhibitor. Selegiline may be administered either as a single dose in the morning or in two divided doses of 5 mg, taken at breakfast and lunch. When selegiline is added to a levodopa regimen it is possible to reduce the levodopa dosage by an average of 30%.

Contra-indications: Known hypersensitivity to selegiline or other components of the formulation.

Special warnings and precautions for use: Selegiline should be administered cautiously to patients with peptic or duodenal ulcer, labile hypertension, cardiac arrhythmias, severe angina pectoris or psychosis.

In higher doses (more than 30 mg daily) the selectivity of selegiline begins to diminish resulting in increased inhibition of MAO-A. Thus in higher doses there is a risk of hypertension after ingestion of food rich in tyramine.

Interactions with other medicinal products and other forms of interaction: Foods containing tyramine have not been reported to induce hypertensive reactions during selegiline treatment at doses used in the treatment of Parkinson's disease. Concomitant use of non-selective MAO-inhibitors may cause severe hypotension.

No tolerability problems have been reported when a combination of selegiline and moclobemide, an inhibitor of MAO-A, has been used. However, when they are used together, the tyramine sensitivity factor may increase up to 8-9 (being 1 for selegiline alone and 2-3 for moclobemide alone). Although tyramine induced hypersensitive reactions are unlikely when selegiline and moclobemide are used together, dietary restrictions (excluding foods with large amounts of tyramine such as aged cheese and yeast products) are recommended when prescribing this combination.

Interactions between nonselective MAO-inhibitors and pethidine, as well as selegiline and pethidine have been described. The mechanism of this interaction is not fully understood and therefore, use of pethidine concomitantly with selegiline should be avoided.

Serious reactions with signs and symptoms that may include diaphoresis, flushing, ataxia, tremor, hyperthermia, hyper/hypotension, seizures, palpitation, dizziness and mental changes that include agitation, confusion and hallucinations progressing to delirium and coma have been reported in some patients receiving a combination of selegiline and fluoxetine. Similar experiences have been reported in patients receiving selegiline and either of two other serotonin re-uptake inhibitors, sertraline and paroxetine. Since the mechanisms of these reactions are not fully understood, it is recommended to avoid the combinations of selegiline and fluoxetine, sertraline or paroxetine. A minimum period of five weeks should be allowed between discontinuation of fluoxetine and initiation of selegiline treatment, due to the long half-lives of fluoxetine and its active metabolite. As the half-lives of selegiline and its metabolites are short, a wash-out period of 14 days after selegiline treatment would be sufficient before starting fluoxetine.

Severe CNS toxicity has been reported in patients with the combination of tricyclic antidepressants and selegiline. In one patient receiving amitriptyline and selegiline this included hyperpyrexia and death, and another patient receiving protriptyline and selegiline experienced tremor, agitation, and restlessness followed by unresponsiveness and death two weeks after selegiline was added.

Other adverse reactions occasionally reported in patients receiving a combination of selegiline with various tricyclic antidepressants include hyper/hypotension, dizziness, diaphoresis, tremor, seizures, and changes in behavioural and mental status. Since the mechanisms of these reactions are not fully understood, it is recommended to be cautious when using selegiline together with tricyclic antidepressants.

Pregnancy and lactation: The available safety data concerning the use during pregnancy and lactation is insufficient to justify the use in these patient groups.

Effects on ability to drive and use machines: No effects on ability to drive or operate machines.

Undesirable effects: In monotherapy, selegiline has been found to be well tolerated. Dry mouth, transient rise of serum alanine aminotransferase (ALAT) values and sleeping disorders have been reported more frequently than in patients receiving placebo.

Because selegiline potentiates the effects of levodopa, the adverse reactions of levodopa, e.g. abnormal movements, nausea, agitation, confusion, hallucinations, headache, postural hypotension, cardiac arrhythmias and vertigo, may be emphasised, particularly if the dose of levodopa is too high. Such adverse reactions usually disappear when the levodopa dosage is decreased. Levodopa dosage can be reduced by an average of 30% when selegiline is added to the treatment.

Micturition difficulties and skin reactions have also been reported during selegiline treatment.

Follow-up of these possible adverse reactions is important.

Overdose: No overdosage cases are known. However,

experience gained during selegiline's development reveals that some individuals exposed to doses of 600 mg/day selegiline suffered severe hypotension and psychomotor agitation.

Theoretically, overdosage causes significant inhibition of both MAO-A and MAO-B and thus, symptoms of overdosage may resemble those observed with non-selective MAO-inhibitors, such as different central nervous and cardiovascular system disorders (e.g. drowsiness, dizziness, faintness, irritability, hyperactivity, agitation, severe headache, hallucination, hypertension, hypotension, vascular collapse, rapid and irregular pulse, precordial pain, respiratory depression and failure, hyperpyrexia and diaphoresis).

There is no specific antidote and treatment is symptomatic.

Pharmacological properties

Pharmacodynamic properties: Selegiline is a selective MAO-B-inhibitor which prevents dopamine breakdown in the brain. It also inhibits the re-uptake of dopamine at the pre-synaptic dopamine receptor. These effects potentiate dopaminergic function in the brain and help to even out and prolong the effect of exogenous and endogenous dopamine. Thus, selegiline potentiates and prolongs the effect of levodopa in the treatment of parkinsonism.

Double-blind studies on early phase Parkinsonian patients showed that patients receiving selegiline monotherapy manage significantly longer without levodopa therapy than controls receiving placebo. These patients could also maintain their ability to work longer.

The addition of selegiline to levodopa (with or without decarboxylase inhibitor) therapy helps to alleviate dose related fluctuations and end of dose deterioration. When selegiline is added to such a regimen it is possible to reduce the levodopa dosage by an average of 30%. Unlike conventional MOA-inhibitors, which inhibit both the MAO-A and MAO-B enzyme, selegiline is a specific MAO-B inhibitor and can be given safely with levodopa.

Selegiline HCl does not cause the so called 'cheese effect' either when used alone as monotherapy, or when used with other drugs, except for moclobemide or nonselective MAO-inhibitors.

Pharmacokinetic properties: Selegiline HCl is readily absorbed from the gastrointestinal tract. The maximal concentrations are reached in half an hour after oral administration. The bioavailability is low; 10% (on the average; interindividual variation is large) of unchanged selegiline can reach the systemic circulation.

Selegiline is lipophilic, slightly basic compound which quickly penetrates into tissues, also into brain. Selegiline HCl inhibits MAO irreversibly and enzyme activity only increases again after new enzyme is synthesised. The inhibitory effect of a single 10 mg dose lasts for 24 hours. Selegiline is rapidly distributed throughout the body, the apparent volume of distribution being 500 litres after an intravenous 10 mg dose. 75–85% of selegiline is bound to plasma proteins at therapeutic concentrations.

Selegiline is rapidly metabolised, mainly in the liver, into desmethylselegiline, l-methamphetamine and to l-amphetamine. In humans, the three metabolites have been identified in plasma and urine after single and multiple does of selegiline. The mean elimination half-life is 1.6 hours for selegiline. The total body clearance of selegiline is about 240 L/hour. Metabolites of selegiline are excreted mainly via the urine with about 15% occurring in the faeces.

Preclinical safety data: No mutagenicity or carcinogenicity due to selegiline have emerged in routine studies.

Pharmaceutical particulars

List of excipients:

Tablets: mannitol, maize starch, microcrystalline cellulose, povidone, ethanol and magnesium stearate.

Syrup: methyl parahydroxybenzoate, propyl parahydroxybenzoate, butyl parahydroxybenzoate, sucrose, xanthan gum T, saccharin sodium, flavour mango, purified water.

Incompatibilities: No other incompatibilities noted.

Shelf life:

Tablets: 60 months bottle.
36 months blister.

Syrup: 36 months

Special precautions for storage:

Tablets: Protect from heat, moisture and light. Keep tablets in the original container.

Syrup: Store your medicine at room temperature. Do not store in a fridge. Keep container closed.

Nature and contents of container:

Tablets 5 mg: White polyethylene bottle with polyethylene closure; 100 tablets

Al/Al blister: 30, 50, 60, 100 tablets.

Tablets 10 mg: White polyethylene bottle with polyethylene closure; 50, 100 tablets.

Al/Al blister: 30, 50, 60, 100 tablets.

Syrup: Amber glass bottle (200 ml) sealed with a pilfer-proof type EPE/Aluminium Melinex screw cap. The container is packed in a cardboard box with a graduated dose dispenser.

Instructions for use/handling: None.

Marketing authorisation holder: Orion Corporation, Orionintie 1, FIN-02200 Espoo, Finland.

Marketing numbers/authorisation number

Tablets 5 mg: PL 06043/0011.
Tablets 10 mg: PL 06043/0012.
Syrup: PL 06043/0013.

Date of first authorisation/renewal of authorisation 1.7.1993/28.6.1997 (Tablets).
27.7.1997 (Syrup).

Date of (partial) revision of the text November 1996

Legal category POM.

FRUSENE* TABLETS

Qualitative and quantitative composition Frusemide PhEur 40.0 mg, Triamterene PhEur 50.0 mg.

Pharmaceutical form Frusene is presented as pale yellowish, scored TABLETS of 9 mm diameter. Each tablet contains 40 mg frusemide and 50 mg triamterene.

Clinical particulars

Therapeutic indications: Frusene is indicated when a prompt diuresis is required and where potassium conservation is important: congestive heart failure, cardiac oedema, hepatic oedema and ascites.

Posology and method of administration: The dosage will depend on individual requirements. The usual adult dose is ½–2 tablets, taken in the morning. Maximum daily dose: 6 tablets.

Contra-indications: Frusene is contra-indicated in severe renal or hepatic failure or if the serum potassium level is elevated. Known sensitivity to frusemide, triamterene or any of the other ingredients.

Special warnings and precautions for use: In patients with mild renal failure, serum creatinine and electrolytes should be monitored regularly.

Frusemide may affect metabolic control in diabetes. Insulin requirements could increase, or latent diabetes become manifest. Triamterene may cause a blue fluorescence of the urine under certain light conditions.

Interactions with other medicinal products and other forms of interaction: Hyperkalaemia may occur if Frusene is used in combination with other drugs which raise plasma potassium levels, including ACE-inhibitors, potassium sparing diuretics or potassium supplements. Concomitant administration of potent diuretics may increase the toxic effects of antibiotics known to exhibit nephrotoxicity. Plasma lithium levels may rise when frusemide is given with lithium. The effects of curariform muscle relaxants may be increased by frusemide. The dosage of concurrently administered cardiac glycosides or antihypertensive agents may require adjustment. The effects of theophylline may be potentiated.

Salicylates and certain other non-steroidal anti-inflammatory agents may antagonise the action of diuretics such as frusemide and may cause renal failure in pre-existing hypovolaemia. Rare cases of renal failure have been reported due to an interaction between triamterene and indomethacin.

Pregnancy and lactation: Frusene should be used with caution during the first trimester of pregnancy. Frusemide and triamterene are known to pass into breast milk. Therefore, Frusene should be used with caution in breast-feeding women.

Effects on ability to drive and use machines: None known.

Undesirable effects: Frusene is a combination of frusemide and triamterene and side effects due to either component are possible. Reported side effects are as follows:

Frusemide: Frusemide is generally well tolerated. Side effects of a minor nature such as nausea, malaise or gastric upset may occur, but are not usually severe enough to cause withdrawal of treatment. The incidence of allergic reactions such as skin rashes is very low, but when these occur, treatment should be withdrawn. In common with other sulphonamide-based diuretics, hyperuricaemia may occur and in rare cases, clinical gout may be precipitated. Bone marrow depression has been reported as a rare complication and necessitates withdrawal of treatment. As with other diuretics, electrolytes and water balance may be disturbed as a result of diuresis after prolonged therapy. This may cause symptoms such as headache, hypotension and muscle cramps. Ototoxicity has been rarely reported with high doses.

Triamterene: Nausea, diarrhoea, fatigue, headache, dry mouth or rash have been reported. If renal function is impaired, triamterene has been reported to cause elevation of BUN and the uric acid level. Leucopenia or photosensitivity have been rarely reported in association with the use of triamterene. Hyperkalaemia or hypokalaemia have been observed in some patients. Megaloblastic anaemia may rarely be induced by triamterene in patients with depleted folic acid stores.

Triamterene may rarely result in adverse effects on renal function.

Overdose: Treatment of overdose consists of fluid replacement and correction of the electrolyte imbalance.

Pharmacological properties

Pharmacodynamic properties:

Frusemide: Frusemide is a potent diuretic with a rapid action. Its effects are evident within 1 hour after a dose by mouth and lasts for about 4 to 6 hours. It has been reported to exert inhibiting effects on electrolyte reabsorption in the proximal and distal renal tubules and in the ascending Loop of Henle.

Excretion of sodium, potassium and chloride ions is increased and water excretion enhanced.

Unlike thiazide diuretics where, owing to their flat dose response curve, very little is gained by increasing the dose, frusemide has a steep dose-response curve, which gives it a wide therapeutic range.

Triamterene: Triamterene is a mild diuretic which appears mainly to act on the distal renal tubules. It produces a diuresis in about 2 to 4 hours, reaching a maximum effect in about 6 hours. Triamterene adds to the natriuretic but diminishes the kaliuretic effects of other diuretics and is used as an adjunct to frusemide to conserve potassium, in the treatment of refractory oedema associated with hepatic cirrhosis, congestive heart failure and the nephrotic syndrome.

Pharmacokinetic properties:

Frusemide: Frusemide is incompletely but fairly rapidly absorbed from the gastro-intestinal tract. It has a biphasic half-life in the plasma with a terminal elimination phase that has been estimated to range up to about 1½ hours. It is up to 99% bound to plasma proteins and is mainly excreted in the urine, largely unchanged, but also in the form of the glucuronide and free amine metabolites. Variable amounts are also excreted in the bile, non renal elimination being considerably increased in renal failure. Frusemide crosses the placental barrier and is excreted in the breast milk.

Triamterene: Triamterene is incompletely but fairly rapidly absorbed from the gastro-intestinal tract. It has been estimated to have a plasma half-life of about 2 hours. It is extensively metabolised and is excreted in the urine in the form of metabolites with some unchanged triamterene. Variable amounts are also excreted in the bile. Animal studies have indicated that triamterene crosses the placental barrier and is excreted in the breast milk.

Preclinical safety data: None stated.

Pharmaceutical particulars

List of excipients: Lactose, maize starch, STa-Rx 1500 = pre-gelatinised starch, sodium starch glycolate = Explotab, Prejel PA5, polysorbate 80, gelatin, magnesium stearate.

Incompatibilities: None known.

Shelf life: 60 months.

Special precautions for storage: Store below 30°C, in a dry place protected from sunlight.

Nature and contents of container: Either a white PVC/aluminium foil blister strip containing 56 tablets or a white polyethylene bottle with snap cap containing 100 tablets.

Instructions for use/handling: None stated.

Marketing authorisation holder: Orion Corporation, PO Box 65, FIN-02101 Espoo, Finland.

Marketing authorisation number PL 6043/0020.

Date of first authorisation/renewal of authorisation 20 December 1996.

Date of (partial) revision of text November 1996.

Legal category POM.

FARESTON* TABLETS 60 mg

Qualitative and quantitative composition

Active ingredient: Toremifene 60 mg (as toremifene citrate).

Inactive ingredients: Maize starch, lactose, povidone, sodium starch glycolate, microcrystalline cellulose, colloidal anhydrous silica, magnesium stearate.

Pharmaceutical form Tablet for oral administration.

Clinical particulars

Therapeutic indications: First line hormone treatment of hormone-dependent metastatic breast cancer in postmenopausal patients. Fareston is not recommended for patients with oestrogen receptor negative tumours.

Posology and method of administration: The recommended dose is 60 mg, one tablet, daily.

No dose adjustment is needed in renal insufficiency. Toremifene should be used cautiously in patients with hepatic impairment (see also *Pharmacokinetic properties,* (b) *Characteristics in patients*).

Contra-indications: Pre-existing endometrial hyperplasia and severe hepatic failure are contra-indications in long-term use of toremifene.

Special warnings and special precautions for use: Experience of the long-term use (more than one year) of toremifene is limited.

Patients with non-compensated cardiac insufficiency or severe angina pectoris should be closely monitored.

Because hypercalcaemia may occur at the beginning of the treatment patients with bone metastases should also be closely monitored.

There is no data on the bone effect of toremifene.

Patients with history of severe thromboembolic disease should generally not be treated.

There is no clinical data available in patients with labile or poorly controlled diabetes, in patients with severely altered performance status or in patients with non-compensated cardiac insufficiency or serious angina pectoris.

Interaction with other medicinal products and other forms of interaction: No specific interaction studies have been performed.

Drugs which decrease renal calcium excretion e.g. thiazide diuretics, may increase the risk of hypercalcaemia. Enzyme inducers, like phenobarbital, phenytoin and carbamazepine, may increase the rate of toremifene metabolism thus lowering the steady-state concentration in serum. In such cases doubling of the daily dose may be necessary.

There is a known interaction between anti-oestrogens and warfarin-type anticoagulants leading to a seriously increased bleeding time. Therefore, the concomitant use of toremifene with such drugs should be avoided.

Theoretically the metabolism of toremifene is inhibited by drugs known to inhibit the CYP 3A4-6 enzyme system which is reported to be responsible for its main metabolic pathways. Examples of such drugs are ketoconazole and similar antimycotics, erythromycin and troleandomycin. Concomitant use of those drugs with toremifene should be carefully considered.

Pregnancy and lactation: Toremifene is recommended for postmenopausal patents.

Owing to the lack of specific data in humans toremifene should not be used during pregnancy and lactation.

In the animal reproduction studies toremifene has shown to prevent implantation, to induce parturition failures, and to reduce perinatal survival. In addition, treatment during organogenesis induces changes in ossification, rib abnormalities, and oedematous foetuses.

In rats, decreased body weight gain of the offspring during lactation was observed.

Effects on ability to drive and use machines: None.

Undesirable effects: Adverse drug reactions are usually mild. They are mostly due to the hormonal action of toremifene.

In clinical studies, the most frequent adverse reaction is hot flushes (up to 20%). Other common adverse reactions include sweating (14%), nausea (8%), leucorrhea (8%), dizziness (4%), oedema (3%), pain (2%) and vomiting (2%). Less frequent adverse reactions (frequency <1%) include vaginal bleeding, chest pain, fatigue, back pain, headache, skin discoloration, weight increase, insomnia, constipation, dyspnea, paresis, tremor, vertigo, pruritus, anorexia, reversible cornea verticillata (reversible corneal opacity) and asthenia. Thromboembolic events have been reported, although the causal relationship to toremifene treatment remains conjectural.

Rare adverse reactions with unclear causal relationship to toremifene include dermatitis, alopecia, emotional lability, depression, jaundice and stiffness.

Treatment was discontinued due to adverse reactions in about 3% of patients. Most of the cases were due to nausea, vomiting, vertigo, hypercalcaemia and vaginal bleeding. Development of hypercalcaemia in the beginning of the treatment is possible especially in patients with bone metastases.

Endometrial hypertrophy may develop during the treatment due to the hormonal (partial oestrogenic) effect of toremifene. There is a risk of increased endometrial changes including hyperplasia, polyps and cancer. This may be due to the underlying mechanism/oestrogenic stimulation.

Overdose: No overdose cases are known.

Vertigo, headache and dizziness were observed in healthy volunteer studies at daily dose of 680 mg. There is no specific antidote and the treatment is symptomatic.

Pharmacological properties

Pharmacodynamic properties: Toremifene is a non-steroidal triphenylethylene derivative. As other members of this class, e.g. tamoxifen and clomifene, toremifene binds to oestrogen receptors and may produce oestrogenic or anti-oestrogenic, or both, effects, depending upon the duration of treatment, animal species, gender, target organ and variable selected. In general, however, nonsteroidal triphenylethylene derivatives are predominantly anti-oestrogenic in rats and man and oestrogenic in mice.

In female rats the lowest dose of toremifene that produces an intrinsic oestrogenic effect on the uterus is about 40 times higher than that of tamoxifen. In the same model the minimum anti-oestrogenically effective dose is 10 times higher than that of tamoxifen suggesting a lower oestrogenic to anti-oestrogenic ratio for toremifene than for tamoxifen. No data is available on this ratio in humans. In post-menopausal volunteers receiving oestrogen by oral or transdermal routes, toremifene was shown to exert an anti-oestrogenic effect on vaginal mucous, by reducing the cornification index. The latter effect was reproducibly found for toremifene doses ranging from 20 to 200 mg daily and could not be distinguished from that of 20 mg tamoxifen. Lower doses of toremifene did not oppose the oestrogenic stimulation of vaginal epithelium.

Toremifene binds specifically to oestrogen receptors, competitively with oestradiol, and inhibits oestrogen-induced stimulation of DNA synthesis and cell replication. In some experimental cancers and/or using high-dose, toremifene displays anti-tumour effects which are not oestrogen-dependent.

The anti-tumour effect of toremifene in breast cancer is mainly due to the anti-oestrogenic effect, although other mechanisms (changes in oncogene expression, growth factor secretion, induction of apoptosis and influence on cell cycle kinetics) may also be involved in the anti-tumour effect.

Pharmacokinetic properties:

(a) General characteristics: Toremifene is readily absorbed after oral administration. Peak concentrations in serum are obtained within 3 (range 2-5) hours. Food intake has no effect on the extent of absorption but may delay the peak concentrations by 1.5–2 hours. The changes due to food intake are not clinically significant.

The serum concentration curve can be described by a biexponential equation.

The half-life of the first (distribution) phase is 4 (range 2-12) hours, and of the second (elimination) phase 5 (range 2-10) days. The basal disposition parameters (CL and V) could not be estimated due to the lack of intravenous study. Toremifene binds extensively (>99.5%) to serum proteins, mainly to albumin. Toremifene obeys linear serum kinetics at oral daily doses between 11 and 680 mg. The mean concentration of toremifene at steady-state is 0.9 (range 0.6–1.3) μ g/ml at the recommended dose of 60 mg per day.

Toremifene is extensively metabolised. In human serum the main metabolite is N-demethyltoremifene with mean half-life of 11 (range 4-20) days. Its steady-state concentrations are about twice compared to those of the parent compound. It has similar anti-oestrogenic, albeit weaker anti-tumour activity than the parent compound. It is bound to plasma proteins even more extensively than toremifene, the protein bound fraction being > 99.9%. Three minor metabolites have been detected in human serum: (deaminohydroxy) toremifene, 4-hydroxytoremifene, and N,N-didemethyltoremifene. Although they have theoretically interesting hormonal effects, their concentrations during toremifene treatment are too low to have any major biological importance.

Toremifene is eliminated mainly as metabolites to the faeces. Enterohepatic circulation can be expected. About 10% of the administered dose is eliminated via urine as metabolites. Owing to the slow elimination, steady-state concentrations in serum are reached in 4 to 6 weeks.

(b) Characteristics in patients: Clinical anti-tumour efficacy and serum concentrations have no positive correlation at the recommended daily dose of 60 mg.

No information is available concerning polymorphic metabolism. Enzyme complex, known to be responsible for the metabolism of toremifene in humans, is cytochrome P450-dependent hepatic mixed function oxidase. The main metabolic pathway, N-demethylation, is mediated mainly by CYP 3A4/3A5.

Pharmacokinetics of toremifene were investigated in an open study with four parallel groups of ten subjects: normal subjects, patients with impaired (mean AST 57 U/L–mean ALT 76 U/L–mean gamma GT 329 U/L) or activated liver function (mean AST 25 U/L–mean ALT 30 U/L–mean gamma GT 91 U/L), patients treated with antiepileptics and patients with impaired renal function (creatinine: 176 μ mol/L). In this study the kinetics of toremifene in patients with impaired renal function were not significantly altered as compared to normal subjects. The elimination of toremifene and its metabolites was significantly increased in patients with activated liver function and decreased in patients with impaired liver function.

Preclinical safety data: The acute toxicity of toremifene is low with LD-50 in rats and mice of more than 2000 mg/kg. In repeated toxicity studies the cause of death in rats is gastric dilatation. In the acute and chronic toxicity studies most of the findings are related to the hormonal effects of toremifene. The other findings are not toxicologically significant. Toremifene has not shown any genotoxicity and has not been found to be carcinogenic in rats. In mice, oestrogens induce ovarian and testicular tumours as well as hyperostosis and osteosarcomas. Toremifene has a species-specific oestrogen-like effect in mice and causes similar tumours. These findings are postulated to be of little relevance for the safety in man, where toremifene acts mainly as an anti-oestrogen.

Pharmaceutical particulars

List of excipients: Maize starch; lactose; povidone; purified water; sodium starch glycolate; magnesium stearate; microcrystalline cellulose; colloidal anhydrous silica.

Incompatibilities: None.

Shelf life: 5 years between +15°C and +30°C.

Special precautions for storage: None.

Nature and contents of container: Green PVC foil and aluminium foil blister in a cardboard box. Package sizes: 30 and 100 tablets.

Instructions for use/handling: None.

Marketing authorisation holder: Orion Corporation, Orionintie 1, PO Box 65, FIN-02101 Espoo, Finland.

Marketing authorisation numbers

Fareston 60 mg, 30 tablets EU/1/96/004/001
Fareston 60 mg, 100 tablets EU/1/96/004/002

Date of first authorisation 14 February 1996.

Date of latest revision of text 21 March 1996.

Legal category POM.

TRIDESTRA TABLETS

Qualitative and quantitative composition

Tridestra tablet (white): Oestradiol valerate 2 mg
Tridestra tablet (blue): Oestradiol valerate 2 mg, Medroxyprogesterone acetate 20 mg
Tridestra tablet (yellow): Placebo

Pharmaceutical form Tablet for oral administration.

Clinical particulars

Therapeutic indications:

(i) The treatment of climacteric symptoms associated with the menopause.

(ii) The prevention of postmenopausal osteoporosis in women considered at risk of developing fractures. Epidemiological studies suggest a number of risk factors may contribute to postmenopausal osteoporosis, including:

- early menopause (either natural or surgically induced),
- family history of osteoporosis,
- recent corticosteroid therapy,
- a small frame,
- thinness, and
- cigarette smoking.

Posology and method of administration: Dosage is according to the calendar pack, one tablet daily, continuously, in cycles of 91 days.

Tridestra is an oestrogen-progestogen combination product consisting of 91 tablets in a blister pack bearing calendar markings. The dosage during days 1 to 70 (inclusive) of the cycle is 2 mg oestradiol valerate (white tablets). From day 71 to day 84 (inclusive) it is 2 mg of oestradiol valerate and 20 mg of medroxyprogesterone acetate (blue tablets). From day 85 to day 91 (inclusive) a placebo preparation (yellow tablets) is taken.

Contra-indications: Tridestra is contraindicated in pregnancy (known or suspected); severe cardiac or renal disease, severe disturbances of liver function; previous or existing liver tumours; jaundice or pruritus during a previous pregnancy; Dubin-Johnson syndrome; Rotor syndrome; active deep venous thrombosis, thromboembolic disorders, or a history of confirmed venous thromboembolism, sickle cell anaemia; suspected or existing hormone-dependent disorders or tumours of the uterus and breast or other organs: undiagnosed abnormal vaginal bleeding; endometriosis: a history of herpes gestationis: otosclerosis with deterioration in previous pregnancies: severe diabetes with vascular changes.

Special warnings and special precautions for use: Before starting Tridestra, patients should have a thorough general medical and gynaecological examination with special emphasis on body weight, skin, legs, blood pressure, heart, breast, pelvic organs with endometrial assessment if indicated. Regular follow-up examinations are recommended during treatment, at least annually.

Before starting treatment, pregnancy must be excluded. If expected withdrawal bleeding fails to occur at about 91 days intervals, treatment should be stopped until pregnancy has been ruled out. In women of childbearing potential, hormonal contraception should be stopped when treatment is started for the first time, and the patient advised to use non-hormonal contraception.

If used perimenopausally, breakthrough bleeding may occur due to endogenous sex hormone production. Persistent breakthrough bleeding during treatment is an indication for endometrial assessment which may include biopsy. Pre-existing fibroids may increase in size under the influence of oestrogens. If this is observed, treatment should be discontinued.

Epidemiological studies have suggested that hormone replacement therapy (HRT) is associated with increased relative risk of developing venous thromboembolism (VTE) i.e. deep vein thrombosis or pulmonary embolism. The studies find a 2–3 fold increase for users compared with non-users which for healthy women amounts to a low risk of one extra case of VTE each year for every 5000 patients taking HRT.

Generally recognised risk factors for VTE include a personal or family history and severe obesity (Body Mass Index>30 kg/m^2). In women with these factors the benefits of treatment with HRT need to be carefully weighed against risks.

The risk of VTE may be temporarily increased with prolonged immobilisation, major trauma or major surgery. In women on HRT scrupulous attention should be given to prophylactic measures to prevent VTE following surgery. Where prolonged immobilisation is liable to follow elective surgery, particularly abdominal or orthopaedic surgery to the lower limbs, consideration should be given to temporarily stopping HRT 4 weeks earlier, if this is possible.

If venous thromboembolism develops after initiating therapy the drug should be discontinued.

In patients with mild chronic liver disease, liver function should be checked every 8 to 12 weeks. Some women are predisposed to cholestasis during steroid therapy. Patients with gallstones should be closely monitored.

Treatment should be stopped at once and investigations undertaken if jaundice or pregnancy occurs, or if there is a significant rise in blood pressure, the occurrence of thromboembolic disease or epileptic seizures.

Diseases that are known to be subject to deterioration during pregnancy (e.g. multiple sclerosis, epilepsy, diabetes, benign breast disease, hypertension, cardiac or renal dysfunction, asthma, porphyria, tetany and otosclerosis) and women with a strong family history of breast cancer should be carefully observed during treatment.

At the present time there is evidence which suggests a slight increase in the relative risk of breast cancer in postmenopausal women receiving long-term hormone replacement therapy.

A careful appraisal of the risk/benefit ratio should be undertaken before treating for longer than 5 to 10 years.

In rare cases, benign and in even rarer cases, malignant liver tumours leading in isolated cases to life-threatening intra-abdominal haemorrhage have been observed after the use of hormonal substances such as those contained in Tridestra. A hepatic tumour should be considered in the differential diagnosis if abdominal pain, enlarged liver, or signs of intra-abdominal haemorrhage occur.

Interaction with other medicinal products and other forms of interaction: Drugs which induce hepatic microsomal enzymes, for example barbiturates, phenytoin, and rifampicin accelerate the metabolism of oestrogen-progestogen combinations such as Tridestra, and may reduce their efficacy.

Pregnancy and lactation: Tridestra is contraindicated during pregnancy and lactation. Milk/plasma ratio for both E_2V and MPA is about 0.5. Use of Tridestra during lactation may induce gynaecomastia and vaginal bleeding in the child, and may also prolong postnatal jaundice.

Effects on ability to drive and use machines: None recorded.

Undesirable effects: Side effects are most common in the first months of the treatment. They are usually mild, improving with the continuation of the treatment. Side effects include: nausea, oedema, breast tenderness or enlargement, headache, migraine, visual disturbances, tiredness, increase in body weight, and changes in mood and libido. Breakthrough bleeding may also occur, particularly during the first year of treatment, but the incidence reduces by the second year of treatment.

The use of oestrogen-progestogen combinations may affect clinical laboratory results: there may be an increase in serum transaminases, alkaline phosphatase, gamma-glutamyltransferase and bilirubin. Thyroid-binding globulin may rise leading to erroneous results in thyroid function tests.

Overdose: Overdosage of oestrogen may cause nausea, headache and withdrawal bleeding. Serious ill effects have not been reported following acute ingestion of large doses of oestrogens and progestogens in contraceptive formulations by young children. When needed, therapy is symptomatic.

Pharmacological properties

Pharmacodynamic properties: Oestradiol valerate (E_2V), an ester, is absorbed after oral intake and metabolised to free oestradiol, a potent natural oestrogen. At a dose of 2 mg/day, E_2V is effective in the treatment of postmenopausal symptoms.

Oestradiol valerate exerts its effects through iteraction with specific receptors in the cytoplasm or oestrogen sensitive tissues. It is involved in the development and maintenance of the female sex organs, secondary sexual characteristics, control of mammary glands, proliferation of endometrium, development of decidua and cyclic changes in the cervix and vagina.

Medroxyprogesterone acetate (MPA) is a derivative of natural progesterone, a 17-α-hydroxy-6-methylprogesterone acetate. It has a similar effect to progesterone with slight androgenic activity. MPA acts on the endometrium to convert the proliferative phase to secretory phase, and acts by binding to progestogen-specific receptors. MPA is established as a contraceptive, in the treatment of malignant disease (endometrial, ovarian and breast cancer), and in the treatment of dysfunctional uterine bleeding, secondary amenorrhoea and mild to moderate endometriosis.

The progestogen component of Tridestra is added to reduce the risk of endometrial hyperplasia which may occur with unopposed long-term oestrogen therapy. Fixed combinations of oestrogen and progestogens developed to date have been based on a 28-day cycle of use. A major reason for discontinuation of such therapy is the unacceptability of monthly menstruation to some women. Tridestra, which only causes menstruation at the end of a 3-month cycle, is likely to be more acceptable to this group of women, particularly those who are postmenopausal.

In addition of its effect on climacteric symptoms, Tridestra prevents postmenopausal osteoporosis by reducing bone loss.

Pharmacokinetic properties: Maximum plasma levels of oestradiol (about 0.2 nmol/l) are reached in about 8 hours. In circulation, natural oestrogens are bound to sex hormone binding globulin and albumin. Free oestradiol is metabolised in the liver and partly converted to less active oestrogens like oestrone. Maximum plasma levels of oestrone (about 2 nmol/l) are reached in 6–7 hours after intake of the tablet. Oestrone is subjected to an enterohepatic cycle and its half life is 15–20 hours. The majority of oestrogens are excreted via kidneys as conjugates (sulphates or glucuronides).

MPA is well absorbed from the gastrointestinal tract and rapidly distributed from the circulation to extravascular tissues. After the intake of Tridestra combination tablet, the maximum plasma level of MPA (about 5 μg/l) is reached in 2 hours. The elimination half-life is 40–50 hours. MPA is metabolised in the liver and excreted as glucoronides both in urine and bile. The extent of absorption from the combination tablet is comparable to MPA given alone.

Pharmaceutical particulars

List of excipients: Tridestra tablet (white): Lactose, maize starch, gelatine, purified water, magnesium stearate, talc.

Tridestra tablet (blue): Lactose, maize starch, gelatine, purified water, magnesium stearate, indigo carmine (E132).

Tridestra tablet (yellow): Lactose, maize starch, gelatine, purified water, magnesium stearate, yellow iron oxide (E172).

Incompatibilities: None.

Shelf life: 3 years.

Special precautions for storage: At a temperature not exceeding 25°C in a dry place.

Nature and contents of container: A PVC/PVDC/AL thromofoiled blister pack. Quantity; 91.

Market authorisation holder: Orion Pharma A/S, Bøgeskovvej 9, DK-3590, Kvistgard, Denmark.

Market authorisation numbers 13910/0003.

Date of first authorisation/renewal or authorisation: 13.10.95.

Date of (partial) revision of the text 26.05.97.

Legal category POM.

ZOLEPTIL*

Qualitative and quantitative composition

Zoleptil 25 tablets contain zotepine 25 mg
Zoleptil 50 tablets contain zotepine 50 mg
Zoleptil 100 tablets contain zotepine 100 mg

Pharmaceutical form

Zoleptil 25 are white sugar-coated tablets for oral administration printed with Z 25

Zoleptil 50 are yellow sugar-coated tablets for oral administration printed with Z 50

Zoleptil 100 are pink sugar-coated tablets for oral administration printed with Z 100

Clinical particulars

Therapeutic indications: Zoleptil is indicated for the treatment of schizophrenia.

Posology and method of administration: Zoleptil is given orally in divided doses with or without food.

Children: Zoleptil is not recommended for use in children (under 18 years of age).

Adults: The effective adult dose is 75 to 300 mg daily. The recommended starting dose for Zoleptil is 25 mg taken three times daily. The dose may be adjusted according to clinical response up to a recommended maximum of 100 mg three times daily. It is recommended that dosage adjustments be made at intervals of four days.

Doses above 100 mg three times daily are not recommended because they may increase the risk of seizure.

Elderly patients and patients with established hepatic and/or renal impairment: The starting dose of Zoleptil should be reduced to 25 mg twice daily in the elderly and patients with established renal and/or hepatic impairment. Titration should be gradual, based on tolerability and efficacy up to a maximum of 75 mg twice daily.

Contra-indications: Zoleptil should not be used in patients with a known hypersensitivity to zotepine or any of its excipients.

Zoleptil should not be used in patients suffering from acute intoxication with CNS depressants including alcohol.

As with other uricosuric agents, due to the increased risk of renal stone formation, Zoleptil should not be used in patients with acute gout or a history of nephrolithiasis.

Nursing mothers taking Zoleptil should not breast-feed.

Special warnings and precautions for use: Zoleptil is known to lower the seizure threshold and PMS data have shown a clear dose-related proconvulsive effect. Zoleptil should not be used to treat patients with a personal or close family history of epilepsy unless the individual benefit outweighs the risk. Data from controlled clinical trials indicate that the seizure rate associated with Zoleptil treatment when used up to a maximum total daily dose of 300 mg is about 1%. At total daily doses above the recommended maximum of 300 mg there is an appreciable increase in the incidence of seizures. It is therefore recommended that total daily doses above 300 mg are not used. High doses of other antipsychotics should not be co-prescribed with zotepine as this may further lower the seizure threshold. Caution should be exercised when withdrawing concomitantly prescribed CNS depressants.

Clinical trials showed a dose related QTc interval prolongation. Caution is therefore advised in relation to the use of Zoleptil in patients at risk of arrhythmias such as patients with coronary heart disease, patients taking other drugs known to cause QTc prolongation or those at risk of hypokalaemia. When treating patients from these groups, it is recommended that an ECG is performed prior to initiation of treatment, to enable the exclusion of those patients with a pre-existing QTc prolongation. Zoleptil is associated with an increase in heart rate and should be used with caution in patients who suffer from angina pectoris due to coronary artery disease.

In common with other antipsychotics isolated reports of Neuroleptic Malignant Syndrome (NMS) have occurred during treatment with Zoleptil. This potentially fatal syndrome includes muscle rigidity, stupor, hyperpyrexia, labile pulse or blood pressure, elevation of plasma creatinine kinase, myoglobinaemia and acute renal failure. If NMS occurs all antipsychotic drugs including Zoleptil should be discontinued immediately and expert advice sought.

As with all compounds that possess α_1-adrenergic blocking properties, Zoleptil may cause orthostatic hypotension, especially during initiation of therapy and increase in dosage. Patients should be advised to rise slowly from the recumbent position and blood pressure should be measured periodically as with other antipsychotics. A dose reduction or more gradual titration should be considered if orthostatic hypotension occurs. Anaesthesia may increase the risk of hypotension. Zoleptil should be used with caution in patients with known severe cardiovascular disease including severe hypertension or severely restricted cardiac output.

As with other antipsychotic drugs a reduction in white cell count can occur. Extensive clinical usage of Zoleptil suggests that this poses minimal risk to patient safety. If a reduction in white cell count is suspected (e.g. infection) then a white cell count should be performed and specialist advice sought if appropriate.

Caution should be exercised when prescribing Zoleptil to patients with established hepatic impairment. Weekly monitoring of Liver Function Tests is recommended for at least for first 3 months of therapy in patients with hepatic impairment.

A lower starting dose, gradual titration and a reduced maximum daily dose should be used in the elderly, renally or hepatically impaired patients (see *Posology and method of administration*).

As with other antipsychotics, patients should be advised of the possibility for weight gain and given dietary advice.

Isolated reports of tardive dyskinesia have occurred during clinical trials and marketing experience but no causality has been established. If tardive dyskinesia does occur the discontinuation or reduction in dose of all antipsychotic drugs should be considered.

Zoleptil possesses anticholinergic properties and should be used with caution in patients with prostatic hypertrophy, retention of urine, narrow angle glaucoma and paralytic ileus.

Zoleptil has uricosuric properties and thus, in the unlikely event of treating a patient with a history of gout or hyperuricaemia, Zoleptil should be started with care, maintaining a good urine output until serum uric acid returns to normal levels. As with all uricosurics, Zoleptil should not be started within three weeks of the resolution of an episode of acute gout. There is a theoretical risk of increased urate renal stone formation and Zoleptil should not be used in patients with a history of nephrolithiasis. In practice this risk appears to be low.

As with other antipsychotics, thermoregulation of the body may be adversely affected by treatment with Zoleptil giving rise to hyperpyrexia or hypothermia.

Theoretically Zoleptil may cause a deterioration in patients with Parkinson's disease.

Caution should be exercised in treating patients with tumours of the adrenal medulla, e.g. phaeochromocytoma or neuroblastoma.

Interaction with other medicinal products and other forms of interaction: Zoleptil is a CNS depressant, therefore it should be used with caution in combination with other CNS depressant drugs. Antipsychotics are known to lower the seizure threshold and PMS data for Zoleptil have shown a clear dose-related proconvulsive effect. If co-prescription of high doses of other antipsychotics is considered necessary, the prescriber should be aware that this may further lower the seizure threshold.

As Zoleptil possesses significant α_1-blocking properties, caution should be exercised when it is co-prescribed with hypotensive agents, including some anaesthetic agents. Through its effect on α-adrenoceptors, the simultaneous administration of adrenaline may lead to a fall in blood pressure. Theoretically the effects of α-methyldopa, guanethidine and clonidine may be reduced.

In a desipramine co-administration study no clinical interaction was found with respect to the CYP 2D6 isoenzyme suggesting that antidepressants and other drugs dependent on this isoenzyme are unlikely to interact with Zoleptil.

Co-administration with fluoxetine or diazepam leads to increased plasma concentrations of zotepine and norzotepine, and caution is advised when these drugs are co-prescribed.

No specific clinical interaction studies have been conducted with anticonvulsants or lithium.

Food taken with a single oral dose of Zoleptil delayed by 30% the appearance of Zoleptil in plasma but had no effect on the extent of absorption of Zoleptil; the effect of food is unlikely to be significant on chronic administration.

Pregnancy and lactation: Use in pregnancy: The drug plasma concentrations (AUC) in the animal reproduction studies were generally lower than those seen in patients. Whilst animal studies have shown no teratogenic effects in rats and rabbits, some indirect prolactin- and CNS-mediated effects were observed in rats including reduced fertility in females and increased neonatal mortality. The use of Zoleptil during human pregnancy has not been investigated, therefore, Zoleptil should not be used during pregnancy unless the benefits to the mother outweigh the potential risk to the baby. Women of child-bearing potential should employ adequate contraception whilst taking Zoleptil.

Lactation: There is evidence that Zoleptil and its metabolites may be secreted in the milk of lactating rats, and a case report indicates similar secretion may occur in humans. Therefore, women taking Zoleptil should not breast-feed.

Effects on ability to drive and use machines: Zoleptil may cause sedation and/or impair mental alertness. Patients should be advised not to drive or operate machinery, during treatment, until their susceptibility has been established.

Undesirable effects: The following adverse events have been reported on at least four occasions in association with Zoleptil therapy in clinical trials and spontaneously during extensive clinical usage (approximately 1.98 million patients treated).

The adverse events occurring in each body system are classified according to the following frequency estimates: frequent >10%, occasional 1–10%, rare 0.001–1%, isolated cases <0.001%.

Body as a whole: Frequent: asthenia, chills, headache, infection, pain. *Occasional:* abdominal pain, chest pain, fever, flu syndrome, malaise. *Rare:* abdominal enlargement, allergic reaction, facial oedema, hypothermia, neuroleptic malignant syndrome. *Isolated cases:* shock.

Cardiovascular: Frequent: hypotension, tachycardia. *Occasional:* arrhythmia, ECG abnormality, hypertension, postural hypotension, syncope. *Rare:* bradycardia, palpitations.

Digestive: Frequent: constipation, dyspepsia, elevated liver function tests. *Occasional:* anorexia, appetite increased, diarrhoea, nausea, vomiting. *Rare:* ileus.

Endocrine: Occasional: prolactin increased. *Rare:* inappropriate lactation.

Haemic and lymphatic: Frequent: changes in ESR, leucocytosis, leucopenia. *Occasional:* abnormal blood cells, anaemia, thrombocythaemia. *Rare:* thrombocytopenia.

Metabolic and nutritional: Frequent: weight increase. *Occasional:* creatinine increased, hyperglycaemia, hypoglycaemia, hyperlipidaemia, hypouricaemia, oedema, thirst, weight loss.

Musculo-skeletal: Occasional: arthralgia, joint disease, myalgia. *Rare:* myasthenia.

Nervous: Frequent: agitation, anxiety, depression, dizziness, dry mouth, EEG abnormal, extrapyramidal syndrome (akathisia, dyskinesia, dystonias, Parkinsonism), insomnia, salivation increased, somnolence. *Occasional:* confusion, convulsions, dysautonomia, hostility, libido decreased, nervousness, speech disorder, vertigo. *Rare:* amnesia, ataxia, CNS stimulation, coma, delirium, hypaesthesia, myoclonus.

Respiratory: Frequent: rhinitis. *Occasional:* cough increase, dyspnoea. *Rare:* epistaxis.

Skin and appendages: Frequent: sweating. *Occasional:* acne, dry skin, rash. *Rare:* alopecia, photosensitivity.

Special senses: Frequent: blurred vision. *Occasional:* conjunctivitis.

Urogenital: Occasional: impotence, urinary incontinence. *Rare:* abnormal ejaculation, menstrual disorder, retention of urine.

Overdose: Symptoms of overdose: Overdose may result in exaggerated pharmacological effects which include hypotension, tachycardia, arrhythmias, agitation, pronounced extrapyramidal motor effects, hypothermia, hyperthermia, seizures, respiratory depression, stupor or even coma.

In the event of overdosage, the posibility of multiple drug involvement should be considered.

Management of overdose: There is no specific antidote to Zoleptil, therefore appropriate supportive measures should be instituted. A clear airway should be established and maintained, and adequate oxygenation and ventilation ensured. Gastric lavage (after endotracheal intubation if the patient is unconscious) and administration of activated charcoal together with a laxative should be considered. Cardiovascular monitoring should commence immediately and should include continuous ECG monitoring to detect possible arrhythmias. Hypotension and circulatory collapse should be treated by plasma volume expansion and other appropriate measures. If sympathomimetic agents are used for vascular support, adrenaline and dopamine should not be used, since beta-stimulation combined with α_1 antagonism associated with Zoleptil may worsen hypertension. Cardiac arrhythmias may respond to correction of circulatory and metabolic disturbance, however, if persistent or life-threatening, appropriate antiarrhythmic treatment may be considered. In the case of severe extrapyramidal symptoms, anticholinergic medication should be administered. Seizures may be treated with intravenous diazepam, preferably in emulsion form (artificial respiration equipment and expertise should be available in the event of respiratory depression). Close medical supervision and monitoring should continue until the patient recovers.

Pharmacological properties

Pharmacodynamic properties: Zoleptil is an antipsychotic drug.

Zoleptil's antipsychotic effects are almost certainly mediated by reducing CNS dopamine function via antagonism of both D_1-like and D_2-like receptors. Zoleptil also binds to four 5-hydroxytryptamine (5-HT) subtypes, namely 5-HT_{2A}, 5-HT_{2C}, and the more recently discovered 5-HT_6 and 5-HT_7 receptors. Zoleptil binds to α_1-adrenoceptors and histamine H_1 receptors; it also inhibits noradrenaline reuptake which may compensate in part, for Zoleptil's α_1-adrenergic antagonist effects.

Pharmacokinetic properties: Zotepine is well absorbed and undergoes extensive first-pass metabolism. Peak plasma levels were achieved after 2 to 3 hours, followed by a multiphasic decline with an elimination half-life of about 14 hours. Linear kinetics have been demonstrated over the dose range 25 to 100 mg with no dose-related change in elimination of half-lives and a dose proportionate increase in plasma concentrations. Zotepine concentrations tended to be around three times higher than those of the generally equipotent metabolite norzotepine, which followed a similar time course.

Zotepine is not excreted unchanged in any significant amounts but is converted into inactive polar metabolites which have been identified as conjugates of hydroxylated, demethylated and S-oxide derivatives. Metabolites are excreted in both urine and faeces (urine:faeces ratio 4:6).

Elderly subjects, subjects with hepatic impairment and subjects with renal dysfunction had 2 or 3 fold higher plasma levels of zotepine compared to young, healthy volunteers for a given dose. With regard to gender, data pooled from a number of studies revealed a tendency to higher plasma concentrations in healthy females after a single dose but no gender differences were reported for patients at steady-state.

On administration of Zoleptil three times a day to schizophrenic patients, steady-state was achieved within approximately four days. Cmax and AUC were three-to-four-fold higher at steady-state, reflecting the accumulation expected from the observed elimination rates. At steady-state, Cmax was less than two-fold higher than Cmin and the pharmacokinetics of zotepine were generally consistent with linear kinetics. Plasma concentrations of norzotepine were approximately 30% of zotepine concentrations.

Standard *in vitro* metabolism studies have indicated no specific mechanism likely to lead to significant drug interactions with Zoleptil. *In vitro* hepatic microsome studies indicated that CYP 1A2 and CYP 3A4 are the major cytochrome P450 isoenzymes responsible for zotepine metabolism.

There was no pharmacokinetic interaction when zotepine was co-administered with desipramine, confirming that CYP 2D6 (debrisoquine oxidase) was not affected by or involved in zotepine metabolism.

In a clinical interaction study, co-administration with fluoxetine increased plasma AUC of zotepine by approximately 10% and doubled that of norzotepine. A study in Japanese patients reported that zotepine steady state plasma concentrations increased by approximately one quarter when diazepam was added to the medication.

Plasma protein binding of zotepine and norzotepine (a pharmacologically active metabolite of zotepine) is 97%; the relatively low plasma concentrations indicate that protein-displacement based drug-drug interactions will not occur.

Preclinical safety data: Single dose studies have been conducted with zotepine in mice, rats, dogs and rabbits and repeated-dose studies up to one year's duration in dogs and two years' duration in rats have been performed. The two-year study in rats was a combined toxicity and carcinogenicity study; a separate carcinogenicity study has been completed in mice. In addition, a full battery of *in vivo* and *in vitro* genotoxicity studies has been performed. Reproduction studies have been conducted in rats and rabbits. The toxicological reactions elicited by zotepine in this preclinical programme were consistent with the class effects of antipsychotic drugs, though the drug plasma AUC levels were generally lower than those seen in patients. There was no evidence of eye toxicity or of blood dyscrasias. Zotepine was not teratogenic. Dietary carcinogenicity studies, at doses giving drug plasma AUC levels lower than those following therapeutic doses in patients, showed minimal toxicity but no indication of carcinogenicity; zotepine is not mutagenic and there is no pharmacological or chemical structural association with carcinogenic compounds.

Pharmaceutical particulars

List of excipients: Zoleptil Tablets 25 mg: Sucrose, lactose, microcrystalline cellulose, calcium carbonate, maize starch, polyethylene glycol, hydroxypropylcellulose, titanium dioxide (E171), liquid glucose, povidone, magnesium stearate, carnauba wax, potassium dihydrogen orthophosphate, either shellac, iron oxide black (E172) or shellac, iron oxide black (E172), soya lecithin, dimethylpolysiloxane.

Zoleptil Tablets 50 mg: Sucrose, lactose, microcrystalline cellulose, calcium carbonate, maize starch, polyethylene glycol, hydroxypropylcellulose, liquid glucose, povidone, talc, magnesium stearate, titanium dioxide (E171), carnauba wax, potassium dihydrogen orthophosphate, iron oxide yellow (E172), methyl-4-hydroxybenzoate sodium salt, propyl-4-hydroxybenzoate sodium salt, either shellac, iron oxide black (E172) or shellac, iron oxide black (E172), soya lecithin, dimethylpolysiloxane.

Zoleptil Tablets 100 mg: Sucrose, lactose, microcrystalline cellulose, calcium carbonate, maize starch, polyethylene glycol, hydroxypropylcellulose, titanium dioxide (E171), liquid glucose, povidone, magnesium stearate, carnauba wax, potassium dihydrogen orthophosphate, iron oxide red (E172), methyl-4-hydroxybenzoate sodium salt, propyl-4-hydroxybenzoate sodium salt, either shellac, iron oxide black (E172) or shellac, iron oxide black (E172), soya lecithin, dimethylpolysiloxane.

Incompatibilities: None.

Shelf life: 3 years 6 months.

Special precautions for storage: For tablets in PVC/PVDC blister packs: Do not store above 25°C. Store in original packaging.

For tablets in HDPE bottles: Do not store above 25°C. Keep the container tightly closed.

Nature and contents of container: Zoleptil tablets 25 mg, 50 mg and 100 mg provided in: PVC/PVDC blister strip packs of 10, 20, 21, 28, 30, 50, 60, 84, 90, 100, 500 or 1000 tablets and HDPE bottles with screw caps containing 10, 20, 30, 50, 60, 90, 500 or 1000 tablets.

Instructions for use/handling: None.

Marketing authorisation holder: Knoll Ltd, 9 Castle Quay, Castle Boulevard, Nottingham NG7 1FW, England.

Marketing authorisation numbers
PL 00169/0110 (25 mg)
PL 00169/0111 (50 mg)
PL 00169/0112 (100 mg)

Date of first authorisation 21 September 1998

Legal category POM

**Trade Mark*

Paines & Byrne Limited
Yamanouchi House
Pyrford Road
West Byfleet
Surrey KT14 6RA

☎ 01932 355405 🗋 01932 353458

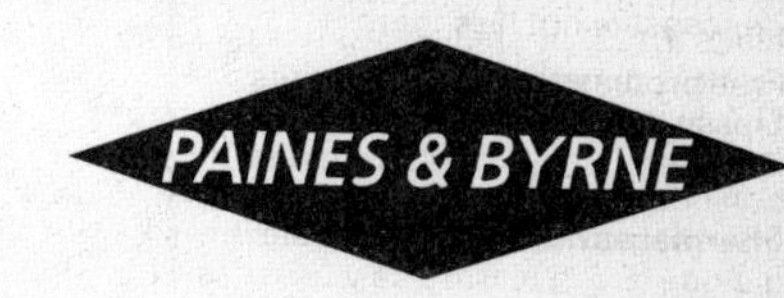

KETOVITE* LIQUID

Qualitative and quantitative composition

Vitamin A as palmitate (1.7×10⁶ units/g)	HSE 2.5 kU
Vitamin D_2 (ergocalciferol)	BP 400.0 U
Cyanocobalamin	BP 12.5 µg
Choline chloride	HSE 150.0 mg

Pharmaceutical form Oral emulsion.

Clinical particulars

Therapeutic indications: As a sugar-free therapeutic supplement for the prevention of vitamin deficiency in conditions such as galactosaemia, disaccharide intolerance, phenylketonuria and other disorders or carbohydrate or amino acid metabolism, as well as in patients who are on restricted, specialised or synthetic diets.

Posology and method of administration
For adults, children and the elderly: 5 ml daily, by oral administration.

Contra-indications: Hypersensitivity to the product. Hypercalcaemia.

Special warnings and special precautions for use: The recommended dose should not be exceeded without medical advice. No other vitamin supplement containing Vitamins A and D should be taken with Ketovite Liquid except under medical supervision.

Warning: do not exceed the stated dose.

Interaction with other medicaments and other forms of interaction: Absorption of some vitamins in this preparation may be reduced in conditions of fat malabsorption or with the concurrent use of neomycin, cholestyramine, liquid paraffin, aminoglycosides, aminosalicylic acid, anticonvulsants, biguanides, chloramphenicol, cimetidine, colchicine, potassium salts and methyl-dopa. Serum B_{12} concentrations may be decreased by concurrent administration of oral contraceptives.

Pregnancy and lactation: Caution should be used in pregnancy as excessive doses of Vitamin A may be teratogenic, especially when taken in the first trimester.

Large doses of Vitamin D in lactating mothers may cause hypercalcaemia in infants.

Effects on ability to drive and to use machines: None known.

Undesirable effects: None, in the absence of overdosage.

Overdose: Symptoms of overdosage may include anorexia, nausea, vomiting, rough dry skin, polyuria, thirst, loss of hair, painful bones and joints as well as raised plasma and urine calcium and phosphate concentration.

No emergency procedure or antidote is applicable and symptoms are rapidly reduced upon withdrawal of the preparation.

Pharmacological properties

Pharmacodynamic properties: The product is a multivitamin supplemental product.

Pharmacokinetic properties: The pharmacokinetics of the active substances would not differ from that of the same substance when derived naturally from oral foodstuffs.

Preclinical safety data: No relevant pre-clinical data has been generated.

Pharmaceutical particulars

List of excipients

Methyl cellulose (methocel E4M)	HSE
Saccharin	BP
Methyl hydroxybenzoate	BP
Polysorbate 80	BP
Ascorbic acid	BP
DL-α tocopherol	HSE
Terpeneless orange oil	BP
Ammonia solution 0.88 m	HSE
Deionised water	HSE

Incompatibilities: None known.

Shelf life: 24 months.

Special precautions for storage: Store between 5°C–15°C.

Nature and contents of container: Amber glass bottle with plastic screw cap.

Instruction for use/handling: Not applicable.

Marketing authoristion number 0051/5080R.

Date of first authorisation/renewal of authorisation
First authorisation granted 30 January 1990. Renewal granted 23 February 1995.

Date of (partial) revision of the text 7 February 1995.

KETOVITE* TABLETS

Presentation Yellow biconvex tablets. Each tablet contains the following vitamins in a formulation which does not contain sucrose, glucose, fructose, lactose, starch, sodium, artificial colouring or preservatives:

Thiamine Hydrochloride BP	1.0 mg
Riboflavine BP	1.0 mg
Pyridoxine Hydrochloride BP	330 micrograms
Nicotinamide BP	3.3 mg
Calcium Pantothenate PhEur	1.16 mg
Ascorbic Acid BP	16.6 mg
Alpha Tocopheryl Acetate BP	5.0 mg
Inositol	50.0 mg
Biotin	170 micrograms
Folic Acid BP	250 micrograms
Acetomenaphthone 1973 BP	500 micrograms

Uses As a therapeutic supplement for the prevention of vitamin deficiency in conditions such as galactosaemia, disaccharide intolerance, phenylketonuria and other disorders of carbohydrate or amino acid metabolism, as well as in patients who are on restricted, specialised or synthetic diets.

Dosage and administration Ketovite Tablets should be administered orally. The dose for adults, children and the elderly is one tablet three times a day.

Contra-indications, warnings, etc

Contra-indications: Hypersensitivity to the product.

Interactions: Pyridoxine may increase the peripheral metabolism of levodopa reducing therapeutic efficacy in patients with Parkinson's disease.

Effects on ability to drive and to use machines: None known.

Other undesirable effects: None known.

Use in pregnancy and lactation: The recommended dose should not be exceeded without medical advice.

Overdose: Large overdosages of water-soluble vitamins are readily excreted in the urine.

No emergency procedure or antidote is applicable and any symptoms are rapidly reduced upon withdrawal of the preparation.

Incompatibilities (major): None known.

Pharmaceutical precautions Store in a cool dry place.

Legal category POM.

Package quantities 100.

Further information For complete vitamin supplementation, Ketovite Tablets should be used in conjunction with Ketovite Liquid. Ketovite Tablets are available on NHS prescription.

Product licence number 0051/5079R.

PANCREX* GRANULES

Qualitative and quantitative composition Pancreatin BP (Pancreas powder EP) to provide enzymic activity per gram not less than:

Free protease	300 BP units
Lipase	5000 BP units
Amylase	4000 BP units

Pharmaceutical form Granules.

Clinical particulars

Therapeutic indications: Pancrex is used to compensate for reduced intestinal enzyme activity in pancreatic deficiency states.

It is indicated for the treatment of fibrocystic disease of the pancreas (cystic fibrosis), chronic pancreatitis and pancreatic steatorrhoea following pancreatectomy. It may also be indicated following gastrectomy as an aid to digestion.

Posology and method of administration: Dosage should be adjusted according to the needs of the individual patient and the amount and type of food consumed.

The following dosage ranges provide a suitable basis for adjustment.

Adults, the elderly and children: 5–10 g swallowed dry or mixed with a little water or milk just before meals.

Contra-indications: None known.

Special warnings and special precautions for use: It is possible that some irritation of the skin of the mouth may occur if the granules are chewed or retained in the mouth. Irritation of the anus may also occur. A barrier cream may prevent this local irritation.

If the granules are mixed with liquids the resulting mixture should not be allowed to stand for more than one hour prior to use.

Interaction with other medicaments and other forms of interaction: None known.

Pregnancy and lactation: Safety in pregnancy has not been established. However, no teratogenic effects have been observed in clinical use.

Effects on ability to drive and use machines: None.

Undesirable effects: Rare cases of hyperuricosuria and hyperuricaemia have been reported when extremely high doses of pancreatin have been taken.

Strictures of the ileo-caecum and large bowel, and colitis, have been reported in children with cystic fibrosis taking high doses of pancreatic enzyme supplements. To date Pancrex and Pancrex V presentations have not been implicated in the development of colonic damage. However unusual abdominal symptoms or changes in abdominal symptoms should be reviewed to exclude the possibility of colonic damage especially if the patient is taking in excess of 10,000 units/kg/day of lipase.

Overdose: None stated.

Pharmacological properties

Pharmacodynamic properties: Pancreatin is derived from mammalian pancreas and contains the enzymes, amylase, protease and lipase. The enzymes have the same actions as pancreatic juice and when administered to patients with pancreatic insufficiency improve the ability to metabolise starches, proteins and fats.

Pharmacokinetic properties: Pancreatin hydrolyses fats to glycerol and fatty acids, changes proteins into proteoses and derived substances, and converts starch into dextrins and sugars.

Preclinical safety data: No relevant pre-clinical safety data has been generated.

Pharmaceutical particulars

List of excipients: Lactose, acacia, polyvinyl acetate phthalate.

Incompatibilities: None known.

Shelf life: 2 years.

Special precautions for storage: Store at a temperature not exceeding 15°C.

Nature and contents of container: Securitainer; 100, 300 and 500 g.

Instructions for use/handling: Not applicable.

Marketing authorisation number 0051/5003R.

Date of first authorisation/renewal of authorisation
First authorisation granted 1 May 1987. Renewed Feb 1998.

Date of (partial) revision of the text 21 July 1997.

PANCREX* V CAPSULES 125 mg

Qualitative and quantitative composition Pancreatin BP (Pancreas powder EP) to provide enzymic activity per capsule not less than:

Free protease	160 BP units
Lipase	2950 BP units
Amylase	3300 BP units

Pharmaceutical form Capsule.

Clinical particulars
Therapeutic indications: Pancrex is used to compensate for reduced intestinal enzyme activity in pancreatic deficiency states.

It is indicated for the treatment of fibrocystic disease of the pancreas (cystic fibrosis), chronic pancreatitis and pancreatic steatorrhoea following pancreatectomy. It may also be indicated following gastrectomy as an aid to digestion.

Posology and method of administration: These low dose capsules may be used when small amounts of Pancrex are required, for example for neonates.

Dosage should be adjusted according to the needs of the individual patient and the amount of food consumed.

The following dosage scale provides a suitable basis for adjustment.

Neonates: the contents of 1–2 capsules mixed with feeds.

Contra-indications: None known.

Special warnings and special precautions for use: It is possible that some irritation of the skin of the mouth may occur if capsules 125 mg are chewed or the contents retained in the mouth. Irritation of the anus may also occur. A barrier cream may prevent this local irritation.

Allergic/asthmatic reactions have occasionally occurred on handling the capsule contents.

If the capsule contents are mixed with liquids or feeds the resulting mixture should not be allowed to stand for more than one hour prior to use.

Interaction with other medicaments and other forms of interaction: None known.

Pregnancy and lactation: Safety in pregnancy has not been established. However, no teratogenic effects have been observed in clinical use.

Effects on ability to drive and use machines: None.

Undesirable effects: Rare cases of hyperuricosuria and hyperuricaemia have been reported when extremely high doses of pancreatin have been taken.

Strictures of the ileo-caecum and large bowel, and colitis, have been reported in children with cystic fibrosis taking high doses of pancreatic enzyme supplements. To date Pancrex and Pancrex V presentations have not been implicated in the development of colonic damage. However unusual abdominal symptoms or changes in abdominal symptoms should be reviewed to exclude the possibility of colonic damage especially if the patient is taking in excess of 10,000 units/kg/day of lipase.

Overdose: None stated.

Pharmacological properties
Pharmacodynamic properties: Pancreatin is derived from mammalian pancreas and contains the enzymes, amylase, protease and lipase. The enzymes have the same actions as pancreatic juice and when administered to patients with pancreatic insufficiency improve the ability to metabolise starches, proteins and fats.

Pharmacokinetic properties: Pancreatin hydrolyses fats to glycerol and fatty acids, changes proteins into proteoses and derived substances, and converts starch into dextrins and sugars.

Preclinical safety data: No relevant pre-clinical safety data has been generated.

Pharmaceutical particulars
List of excipients: Aluminium oxide, magnesium stearate, microcrystalline cellulose.

Incompatibilities: None known.

Shelf life: 2 years.

Special precautions for storage: Store at a temperature not exceeding 15°C.

Nature and contents of container: Securitainer; 300 and 500 capsules.

Instructions for use/handling: Not applicable.

Marketing authorisation number 0051/5104R.

Date of first authorisation/renewal of authorisation First authorisation granted 13 November 1985. Renewed August 1997.

Date of (partial) revision of the text 18 July 1997.

PANCREX* V CAPSULES

Qualitative and quantitative composition Pancreatin BP (Pancreas powder EP) to provide enzymic activity per capsule not less than:

Free protease	430 BP units
Lipase	8000 BP units
Amylase	9000 BP units

Pharmaceutical form Capsule.

Clinical particulars
Therapeutic indications: Pancrex is used to compensate for reduced intestinal enzyme activity in pancreatic deficiency states.

It is indicated for the treatment of fibrocystic disease of the pancreas (cystic fibrosis), chronic pancreatitis and pancreatic steatorrhoea following pancreatectomy. It may also be indicated following gastrectomy as an aid to digestion.

Posology and method of administration: Dosage should be adjusted according to the needs of the individual patient and the amount and type of food consumed.

The following dosage ranges provide a suitable basis for adjustment.

Infants: the contents of 1–2 capsules mixed with feeds.

Older children and adults: the contents of 2–6 capsules with each snack or meal.

The capsules may provide a suitable alternative to the enteric coated presentations in cases where the pH of the duodenum is not sufficiently alkaline to dissolve the enteric coat.

Capsules provide a simple and convenient method of dose measurement of pancreatin for administration to younger children requiring a low dose.

Contra-indications: None known.

Special warnings and special precautions for use: It is possible that some irritation of the skin of the mouth may occur if capsules are chewed or the contents retained in the mouth. Irritation of the anus may also occur. A barrier cream may prevent this local irritation.

Allergic/asthmatic reactions have occasionally occurred on handling the capsule contents.

If the capsule contents are mixed with liquids or feeds the resulting mixture should not be allowed to stand for more than one hour prior to use.

Interaction with other medicaments and other forms of interaction: None known.

Pregnancy and lactation: Safety in pregnancy has not been established. However, no teratogenic effects have been observed in clinical use.

Effects on ability to drive and use machines: None.

Undesirable effects: Rare cases of hyperuricosuria and hyperuricaemia have been reported when extremely high doses of pancreatin have been taken.

Strictures of the ileo-caecum and large bowel, and colitis, have been reported in children with cystic fibrosis taking high doses of pancreatic enzyme supplements. To date Pancrex and Pancrex V presentations have not been implicated in the development of colonic damage. However unusual abdominal symptoms or changes in abdominal symptoms should be reviewed to exclude the possibility of colonic damage especially if the patient is taking in excess of 10,000 units/kg/day of lipase.

Overdose: None stated.

Pharmacological properties
Pharmacodynamic properties: Pancreatin is derived from mammalian pancreas and contains the enzymes, amylase, protease and lipase. The enzymes have the same actions as pancreatic juice and when administered to patients with pancreatic insufficiency improve the ability to metabolise starches, proteins and fats.

Pharmacokinetic properties: Pancreatin hydrolyses fats to glycerol and fatty acids, changes proteins into proteoses and derived substances, and converts starch into dextrins and sugars.

Preclinical safety data: No relevant pre-clinical safety data has been generated.

Pharmaceutical particulars
List of excipients: Aluminium oxide, magnesium stearate, microcrystalline cellulose.

Incompatibilities: None known.

Shelf life: 2 years.

Special precautions for storage: Store at a temperature not exceeding 15°C.

Nature and contents of container: Securitainer; 100, 300 and 500 capsules.

Instructions for use/handling: Not applicable.

Marketing authorisation number 0051/5043R.

Date of first authorisation/renewal of authorisation First authorisation granted 13 November 1985. Renewed March 1996.

Date of (partial) revision of the text 18 July 1997.

PANCREX* V POWDER

Qualitative and quantitative composition Pancreatin BP (Pancreas powder EP) to provide enzymic activity per gram not less than:

Free protease	1,400 BP units
Lipase	25,000 BP units
Amylase	30,000 BP units

Pharmaceutical form Powder.

Clinical particulars
Therapeutic indications: Pancrex is used to compensate for reduced intestinal enzyme activity in pancreatic deficiency states.

It is indicated for the treatment of fibrocystic disease of the pancreas (cystic fibrosis), chronic pancreatitis and pancreatic steatorrhoea following pancreatectomy. It may also be indicated following gastrectomy as an aid to digestion.

Posology and method of administration: Dosage should be adjusted according to the needs of the individual patient and the amount and type of food consumed.

The following dosage ranges provide a suitable basis for adjustment.

Adults, the elderly and children: 0.5 g–2 g swallowed dry or mixed with a little water or milk before each snack or meal.

New-born infants: 0.25 g–0.5 g with each feed.

Contra-indications: None known.

Special warnings and special precautions for use: It is possible that some irritation of the skin of the mouth may occur if the powder is retained in the mouth. Irritation of the anus may also occur. A barrier cream may prevent this local irritation.

Allergic/asthmatic reactions have occasionally occurred on handling the powder.

If the powder is mixed with liquids or feeds the resulting mixture should not be allowed to stand for more than one hour prior to use.

Interaction with other medicaments and other forms of interaction: None known.

Pregnancy and lactation: Safety in pregnancy has not been established. However, no teratogenic effects have been observed in clinical use.

Effects on ability to drive and use machines: None.

Undesirable effects: Rare cases of hyperuricosuria and hyperuricaemia have been reported when extremely high doses of pancreatin have been taken.

Strictures of the ileo-caecum and large bowel, and colitis, have been reported in children with cystic fibrosis taking high doses of pancreatic enzyme supplements. To date Pancrex and Pancrex V presentations have not been implicated in the development of colonic damage. However unusual abdominal symptoms or changes in abdominal symptoms should be reviewed to exclude the possibility of colonic damage especially if the patient is taking in excess of 10,000 units/kg/day of lipase.

Overdose: None stated.

Pharmacological properties
Pharmacodynamic properties: Pancreatin is derived from mammalian pancreas and contains the enzymes, amylase, protease and lipase. The enzymes have the same actions as pancreatic juice and when administered to patients with pancreatic insufficiency improve the ability to metabolise starches, proteins and fats.

Pharmacokinetic properties: Pancreatin hydrolyses fats to glycerol and fatty acids, changes proteins into proteoses and derived substances, and converts starch into dextrins and sugars.

Preclinical safety data: No relevant pre-clinical safety data has been generated.

Pharmaceutical particulars
List of excipients: None.

Incompatibilities: None known.

Shelf life: 2 years.

Special precautions for storage: Store at a temperature not exceeding 15°C.

Nature and contents of container: Securitainer; 100 g, 300 g and 500 g.

Instructions for use/handling: Not applicable.

Marketing authorisation number 0051/5004R.

Date of first authorisation/renewal of authorisation First authorisation granted 13 November 1985. Renewed March 1998.

Date of (partial) revision of the text 18 July 1997.

PANCREX* V TABLETS

Qualitative and quantitative composition Pancreatin BP (Pancreas powder EP) to provide enzymic activity per capsule not less than:

Free protease	110 BP units
Lipase	1900 BP units
Amylase	1700 BP units

Pharmaceutical form Tablet.

Clinical particulars

Therapeutic indications: Pancrex is used to compensate for reduced intestinal enzyme activity in pancreatic deficiency states.

It is indicated for the treatment of fibrocystic disease of the pancreas (cystic fibrosis), chronic pancreatitis and pancreatic steatorrhoea following pancreatectomy. It may also be indicated following gastrectomy as an aid to digestion.

Posology and method of administration: Dosage should be adjusted according to the needs of the individual patient and the amount and type of food consumed.

The following dosage ranges provide a suitable basis for adjustment.

Adults, the elderly and children: 5–15 tablets before each snack or meal, swallowed whole.

Contra-indications: None known.

Special warnings and special precautions for use: Variations in response to treatment may be due to enteric coating. It is possible that some irritation of the skin of the mouth may occur if tablets are chewed or preparations retained in the mouth. Irritation of the anus may also occur. A barrier cream may prevent this local irritation.

Interaction with other medicaments and other forms of interaction: None known.

Pregnancy and lactation: Safety in pregnancy has not been established. However, no teratogenic effects have been observed in clinical use.

Effects on ability to drive and use machines: None.

Undesirable effects: Rare cases of hyperuricosuria and hyperuricaemia have been reported when extremely high doses of pancreatin have been taken.

Strictures of the ileo-caecum and large bowel, and colitis, have been reported in children with cystic fibrosis taking high doses of pancreatic enzyme supplements. To date Pancrex and Pancrex V presentations have not been implicated in the development of colonic damage. However unusual abdominal symptoms or changes in abdominal symptoms should be reviewed to exclude the possibility of colonic damage especially if the patient is taking in excess of 10,000 units/kg/day of lipase.

Overdose: None stated.

Pharmacological properties

Pharmacodynamic properties: Pancreatin is derived from mammalian pancreas and contains the enzymes, amylase, protease and lipase. The enzymes have the same actions as pancreatic juice and when administered to patients with pancreatic insufficiency improve the ability to metabolise starches, proteins and fats.

Pharmacokinetic properties: Pancreatin hydrolyses fats to glycerol and fatty acids, changes proteins into proteoses and derived substances, and converts starch into dextrins and sugars.

Preclinical safety data: No relevant pre-clinical safety data has been generated.

Pharmaceutical particulars

List of excipients: Lactose, povidine, stearic acid, Opaseal P28-7117, talc, sucrose, acacia, calcium carbonate, titanium dioxide, Opalux AS 7000B, syrup, Opagloss 6000P.

Incompatibilities: None known.

Shelf life: 2 years.

Special precautions for storage: Store at a temperature not exceeding 15°C.

Nature and contents of container: Securitainer; 100, 300 and 500 tablets.

Instructions for use/handling: Not applicable.

Marketing authorisation number 0051/5002R.

Date of first authorisation/renewal of authorisation First authorisation granted 30 October 1985. Renewed March 1998.

Date of (partial) revision of the text 21 July 1997.

PANCREX* V FORTE TABLETS

Qualitative and quantitative composition Pancreatin BP (Pancreas powder EP) to provide enzymic activity per capsule not less than:

Free protease	330 BP units
Lipase	5600 BP units
Amylase	5000 BP units

Pharmaceutical form Tablet.

Clinical particulars

Therapeutic indications: Pancrex is used to compensate for reduced intestinal enzyme activity in pancreatic deficiency states.

It is indicated for the treatment of fibrocystic disease of the pancreas (cystic fibrosis), chronic pancreatitis and pancreatic steatorrhoea following pancreatectomy. It may also be indicated following gastrectomy as an aid to digestion.

Posology and method of administration: Dosage should be adjusted according to the needs of the individual patient and the amount and type of food consumed.

The following dosage ranges provide a suitable basis for adjustment.

Adults, the elderly and children: 6–10 tablets before each snack or meal, swallowed whole.

Contra-indications: None known.

Special warnings and special precautions for use: Variations in response to treatment may be due to enteric coating. It is possible that some irritation of the skin of the mouth may occur if capsules are chewed or the contents retained in the mouth. Irritation of the anus may also occur. A barrier cream may prevent this local irritation.

Allergic/asthmatic reactions have occasionally occurred on handling the capsule contents.

If the capsule contents are mixed with liquids or feeds the resulting mixture should not be allowed to stand for more than one hour prior to use.

Interaction with other medicaments and other forms of interaction: None known.

Pregnancy and lactation: Safety in pregnancy has not been established. However, no teratogenic effects have been observed in clinical use.

Effects on ability to drive and use machines: None.

Undesirable effects: Rare cases of hyperuricosuria and hyperuricaemia have been reported when extremely high doses of pancreatin have been taken.

Strictures of the ileo-caecum and large bowel, and colitis, have been reported in children with cystic fibrosis taking high doses of pancreatic enzyme supplements. To date Pancrex and Pancrex V presentations have not been implicated in the development of colonic damage. However unusual abdominal symptoms or changes in abdominal symptoms should be reviewed to exclude the possibility of colonic damage especially if the patient is taking in excess of 10,000 units/kg/day of lipase.

Overdose: None stated.

Pharmacological properties

Pharmacodynamic properties: Pancreatin is derived from mammalian pancreas and contains the enzymes, amylase, protease and lipase. The enzymes have the same actions as pancreatic juice and when administered to patients with pancreatic insufficiency improve the ability to metabolise starches, proteins and fats.

Pharmacokinetic properties: Pancreatin hydrolyses fats to glycerol and fatty acids, changes proteins into proteoses and derived substances, and converts starch into dextrins and sugars.

Preclinical safety data: No relevant pre-clinical safety data has been generated.

Pharmaceutical particulars

List of excipients: Lactose, povidone, stearic acid, Opaseal P28-7117, talc, sucrose, acacia, calcium carbonate, titanium dioxide, Opalux AS 7000B, syrup, Opagloss 6000P.

Incompatibilities: None known.

Shelf life: 2 years.

Special precautions for storage: Store at a temperature not exceeding 15°C.

Nature and contents of container: Securitainer; 100, 250, 300 and 500 tablets.

Instructions for use/handling: Not applicable.

Marketing authorisation number 0051/5000R.

Date of first authorisation/renewal of authorisation First authorisation granted 22 November 1985. Renewed March 1998.

Date of (partial) revision of the text 18 July 1997.

*Trade Mark

Parke Davis
Lambert Court
Chestnut Avenue
Eastleigh
Hampshire SO53 3ZQ

☎ 01703 620500 🗋 01703 629819

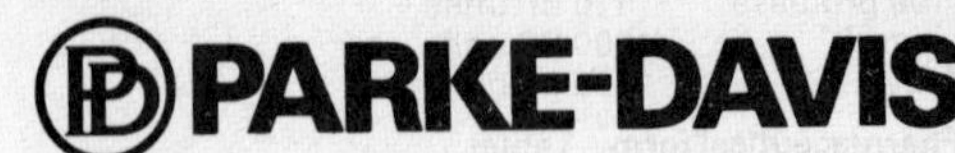

ACCUPRO*

Qualitative and quantitative composition Each Accupro 5 mg tablet contains: Quinapril hydrochloride 5.416 mg (equivalent to 5 mg quinapril base).

Each Accupro 10 mg tablet contains Quinapril hydrochloride 10.832 mg (equivalent to 10 mg quinapril base).

Each Accupro 20 mg tablet contains Quinapril hydrochloride 21.664 mg (equivalent to 20 mg quinapril base).

Each Accupro 40 mg tablet contains Quinapril hydrochloride 43.328 mg (equivalent to 40 mg quinapril base).

Pharmaceutical form Accupro is supplied as brown film coated tablets imprinted with the dosage strength. The 5 mg tablet is elliptical. The 10 mg tablet is triangular. The 20 mg tablet is round. The 40 mg tablet is elliptical.

Clinical particulars

Therapeutic indications: (1) For the treatment of all grades of essential hypertension. Accupro is effective as monotherapy or concomitantly with diuretics in patients with hypertension. (2) For the treatment of congestive heart failure when given concomitantly with a diuretic and/or cardiac glycoside. Treatment of congestive heart failure with Accupro should always be initiated under close medical supervision.

Posology and method of administration: For oral use *Adults: Hypertension: Monotherapy:* The recommended initial dosage is 10 mg once daily in uncomplicated hypertension. Depending upon clinical response, patient's dosage may be titrated (by doubling the dose allowing adequate time for dosage adjustment) to a maintenance dosage of 20 to 40 mg/day given as a single dose or divided into 2 doses. Long-term control is maintained in most patients with a single daily dosage regimen. Patients have been treated with dosages up to 80 mg/day.

Concomitant diuretics: In order to determine if excess hypotension will occur, an initial dosage of 2.5 mg of Accupro is recommended in patients who are also being treated with a diuretic. After this the dosage of Accupro should be titrated (as described above) to the optimal response.

Congestive heart failure: In order to closely monitor patients for symptomatic hypotension, a single 2.5 mg initial dose is recommended. After this, patients should be titrated to an effective dose (up to 40 mg/day) given in 1 or 2 doses with concomitant diuretic and/or cardiac glycoside therapy. Patients are usually maintained effectively on doses of 10-20 mg/day given with concomitant therapy.

In the treatment of severe or unstable congestive heart failure, Accupro should always be initiated in hospital under close medical supervision.

Other patients who may also be considered to be at higher risk and should have treatment initiated in hospital include: patients who are on high dose loop diuretics (e.g. > 80 mg frusemide) or on multiple diuretic therapy, have hypovolaemia, hyponatraemia (serum sodium < 130 mgeq/l) or systolic blood pressure < 90 mm Hg, are on high dose vasodilator therapy, have a serum creatinine > 150 micromol/l or are aged 70 years or over.

Elderly/Renal impairment: In elderly patients and in patients with a creatinine clearance of less than 40 ml/min, an initial dosage in essential hypertension of 2.5 mg is recommended followed by titration to the optimal response.

Children (6-12 years): Not recommended. Safety and efficacy in children has not been established.

Contra-indications: Hypersensitivity to any of the ingredients. Pregnancy: Accupro is contraindicated throughout pregnancy. Accupro has been shown to be foetotoxic in rabbits. When ACE inhibitors have been used during the second and third trimesters of pregnancy, there have been reports of hypotension, renal failure, skull hypoplasia, and/or death in the newborn. Oligohydramnios has also been reported, presumably representing decreased renal function in the foetus; limb contractures, craniofacial deformities, hypoplastic lung development, and intrauterine growth retardation have been reported in association with oligohydramnios. Should a woman become pregnant while receiving ACE inhibitors, the drug should be discontinued as soon as possible. Infants exposed *in utero* to ACE inhibitors should be closely observed for hypotension, oliguria, and hyperkalaemia. If oliguria occurs, attention should be directed toward support of blood pressure and renal perfusion.

Special warnings and special precautions for use: Accupro should not be used in patients with aortic stenosis or outflow obstruction.

In patients with renal insufficiency, monitoring of renal function during therapy should be performed as deemed appropriate, although in the majority renal function will not alter or may improve.

As a consequence of inhibiting the renin-angiotensin-aldosterone system, changes in renal function may be anticipated in susceptible individuals. In patients with severe heart failure whose renal function may depend on the activity of the renin-angiotensin-aldosterone system, treatment with ACE inhibitors including quinapril, may be associated with oliguria and/or progressive azotemia and rarely acute renal failure and/or death.

Patients haemodialysed using high-flux polyacrylonitrile ('AN69') membranes are highly likely to experience anaphylactoid reactions if they are treated with ACE inhibitors. This combination should therefore be avoided, either by use of alternative antihypertensive drugs or alternative membranes for haemodialysis.

The half-life of quinaprilat is prolonged as creatinine clearance falls. Patients with a creatinine clearance of <40 ml/min require a lower initial dosage of quinapril. These patients' dosage should be titrated upwards based upon therapeutic response, and renal function should be closely monitored although initial studies do not indicate that quinapril produces further deterioration in renal function.

In clinical studies in hypertensive patients with unilateral or bilateral renal artery stenosis, increases in blood urea nitrogen and serum creatinine have been observed in some patients following ACE inhibitor therapy. These increases were almost always reversible upon discontinuation of the ACE inhibitor and/or diuretic therapy. In such patients, renal function should be monitored during the first few weeks of therapy.

Some patients with hypertension or heart failure with no apparent pre-existing renal vascular disease have developed increases (>1.25 times the upper limit of normal) in blood urea and serum creatinine, usually minor and transient, especially when quinapril has been given concomitantly with a diuretic and has been observed in 4% and 3% respectively of patients on monotherapy. This is more likely to occur in patients with pre-existing renal impairment. Dosage reduction and/or discontinuation of a diuretic and/or quinapril may be required.

Angioedema: Angioedema has been reported in patients treated with angiotensin- converting enzyme inhibitors. If laryngeal stridor or angioedema of the face, tongue, or glottis occur, treatment should be discontinued immediately, the patient treated appropriately in accordance with accepted medical care, and carefully observed until the swelling disappears. In instances where swelling is confined to the face and lips, the condition generally resolves without treatment; antihistamines may be useful in relieving symptoms. Angioedema associated with laryngeal involvement may be fatal. Where there is involvement of the tongue, glottis, or larynx likely to cause airway obstruction, appropriate therapy eg, subcutaneous adrenaline solution 1:1000 (0.3 to 0.5 ml) should be promptly administered.

Hypotension: Symptomatic hypotension was rarely seen in hypertensive patients treated with Accupro but is a possible consequence of ACE inhibition therapy particularly in salt/volume depleted patients such as those previously treated with diuretics, who have a dietary salt reduction, or who are on dialysis. If symptomatic hypotension occurs, the patient should be placed in the supine position and, if necessary, receive an intravenous infusion of normal saline. A transient hypotensive response is not a contraindication to further doses; however, lower doses of quinapril or any concomitant diuretic therapy should be considered if this event occurs.

Neutropenia/agranulocytosis: ACE inhibitors have been rarely associated with agranulocytosis and bone marrow depression in patients with uncomplicated hypertension but more frequently in patients with renal impairment, especially if they also have collagen vascular disease. As with other ACE inhibitors, monitoring of white blood cell counts in patients with collagen vascular disease and/or renal diseases should be considered.

Interaction with other medicaments and other forms of interaction: Tetracycline: Because of the presence of magnesium carbonate in the formulation Accupro has been shown in healthy volunteers to reduce the absorption of tetracycline in concomitant administration by 28-37%. It is recommended that concomitant administration with tetracycline be avoided.

Concomitant diuretic therapy: Patients treated with diuretics may occasionally experience an excessive reduction of blood pressure after initiation of therapy with Accupro. This hypotensive effect may be effectively minimised by either discontinuing the diuretic or increasing the salt intake prior to the initial dose of Accupro. If discontinuation of the diuretic is not possible, medical supervision should be provided for up to two hours following administration of the initial dose.

Surgery/anaesthesia: Although no data are available to indicate there is an interaction between Accupro and anaesthetic agents that produces hypotension, caution should be exercised when patients undergo major surgery or anaesthesia since ACE inhibitors have been shown to block angiotensin II formation secondary to compensatory renin release. This may lead to hypotension which can be corrected by volume expansion.

Agents increasing serum potassium: Concomitant treatments with potassium sparing diuretics, potassium supplements or potassium containing salts should be used with caution and with appropriate monitoring of serum potassium. As with other ACE inhibitors, patients on quinapril alone may have increased serum potassium levels. When administered concomitantly, quinapril may reduce the hypokalaemia induced by thiazide diuretics.

Lithium: Increased serum lithium levels and symptoms of lithium toxicity have been reported in patients receiving concomitant lithium and ACE inhibitor therapy due to the sodium-losing effect of these agents. These drugs should be co-administered with caution and frequent monitoring of serum lithium levels is recommended. If a diuretic is also used, it may increase the risk of lithium toxicity.

Pregnancy and lactation:
Pregnancy: See under *Contra-indications.*

Lactation: Since it is not known if this drug is secreted in human milk caution should be exercised when the product is given to a nursing mother.

Effects on ability to drive or use machines: None known.

Undesirable effects: The most frequent clinical adverse reactions in hypertension and congestive heart failure are headache, dizziness, rhinitis, coughing, upper respiratory tract infection, fatigue, and nausea and vomiting. Other less frequent side effects are dyspepsia, myalgia, chest pain, abdominal pain, diarrhoea, back pain, sinusitis, insomnia, paraesthesia, nervousness, asthenia, pharyngitis, hypotension, palpitations, flatulence, depression, pruritus, rash, impotence, oedema, arthralgia, amblyopia.

Renal dysfunction, angioedema, hypotension, hyperkalaemia, neutropenia, agranulocytosis (see *Special warnings and special precautions of use*).

Pancreatitis has been reported rarely in patients treated with ACE inhibitors; in some cases this has proved fatal.

Overdose: No data are available with respect to overdosage in humans. The most likely clinical manifestation would be symptoms attributable to severe hypotension, which should normally be treated by intravenous volume expansion.

Haemodialysis and peritoneal dialysis have little effect on the elimination of quinapril and quinaprilat.

Pharmacological properties
Pharmacodynamic properties: Quinapril is rapidly de-esterified to quinaprilat (quinapril diacid, the principal metabolite), which is a potent angiotensin-converting enzyme (ACE) inhibitor. ACE is a peptidyl dipeptidase that catalyzes the conversion of angiotensin I to the vasoconstrictor angiotensin II which is involved in vascular control and function through many different mechanisms, including stimulation of aldosterone secretion by the adrenal cortex. The mode of action of quinapril in humans and animals is to inhibit circulating and tissue ACE activity, thereby decreasing vasopressor activity and aldosterone secretion. In animal studies, the antihypertensive effect of quinapril outlasts its inhibitory effect on circulating ACE, whereas, tissue ACE inhibition more closely correlates with the duration of antihypertensive effects. Administration of 10-40 mg of quinapril to patients with mild to severe hypertension results in a reduction of both sitting and standing blood pressure with minimal effect on heart rate. Antihypertensive activity commences within one hour with peak effects usually achieved by two to four hours after dosing. Achievement of maximum blood pressure lowering effects may require two weeks of therapy in some patients. At the recommended doses, antihypertensive effects are maintained in most patients throughout the 24-hour dosing interval and continue during long-term therapy.

Pharmacokinetic properties: Peak plasma Accupro concentrations are observed within 1 hour of oral administration. The extent of absorption is approximately 60% and is not influenced by food. Following absorption, Accupro is deesterified to its major active metabolite, quinaprilat and to minor inactive metabolites. Accupro has an apparent half-life of approximately one hour. Peak plasma quinaprilat concentrations are observed approximately 2 hours following an oral dose of quinapril. Quinaprilat is eliminated primarily by renal excretion and has an effective accumulation half-life of 3 hours. In patients with renal insufficiency and creatinine clearance of ≤ 40 ml/min, peak and trough quinaprilat concentrations increase, time to peak concentration increases, apparent half-life increases and time to steady state may be delayed. The elimination of quinaprilat is also reduced in elderly patients (>65 years) and correlates well with the impaired renal function which frequently occurs in the elderly. Quinaprilat concentrations are reduced in patients with alcoholic cirrhosis due to impaired deesterification of Accupro. Studies in rats indicate that Accupro and its metabolites do not cross the blood-brain barrier.

Preclinical safety data: The results of the pre-clinical tests do not add anything of further significance to the prescriber.

Pharmaceutical particulars
List of excipients: Accupro tablets contain the following excipients: Magnesium carbonate, lactose, gelatin, crospovidone, magnesium stearate, candelilla wax, colourings: red iron oxide (E172) and titanium dioxide (E171).

Incompatibilities: None known.

Shelf life: Not less than 3 years when stored in the original packaging.

Special precautions for storage: Store below 25°C

Nature and contents of container: Polyamide/aluminium/PVC blister containing 28 tablets.

Instructions for use/handling: No special requirements.

Marketing authorisation numbers

Accupro 5 mg	PL 0019/0123
Accupro 10 mg	PL 0019/0124
Accupro 20 mg	PL 0019/0125
Accurpo 40 mg	PL 0019/0126

Date of last revision October 1997

Legal category POM

ACCURETIC*

Presentation Pink, scored, elliptical, biconvex film coated tablets.

Composition: Tablets containing 10 mg quinapril and 12.5 mg of hydrochlorothiazide.

Uses
Indications: Hydrochlorothiazide: For the treatment of essential hypertension.

Quinapril: For the treatment of all grades of essential hypertension where the standard therapy is ineffective or inappropriate because of adverse events.

Accuretic: For the treatment of hypertensive patients who have been stabilised on their individual components given in the same proportions.

Dosage and administration Oral.
Adults: Effective blood pressure control is usually achieved with a daily dosage of 10/12.5 mg to a maximum of 20/25 mg.

Renal impairment: Accuretic is not recommended for use in patients with creatinine clearance of less than 40 ml/min.

Elderly: The dose should be kept as low as possible commensurate with achievement of adequate blood pressure control.

Children: Not recommended. Safety and efficacy in children has not been established.

Contra-indications, warnings, etc
Contra-indications: Accuretic is contra-indicated in patients with anuria or hypersensitivity to quinapril, thiazides or any sulfonamide derived drug.

Pregnancy: Accuretic is contra-indicated throughout pregnancy. Quinapril has been shown to be foetoxic in rabbits. Use of ACE inhibitors in the second and third trimesters have been associated with oligohydramnios. Hypotension and renal failure have occurred in the newborn.

Accuretic should not be used in nursing mothers.

Precautions: Sensitivity reactions may occur in patients with or without a history of allergy or bronchial asthma, e.g. purpura, photosensitivity, urticaria, necrotising angiitis, respiratory distress including pneumonitis and pulmonary oedema.

Stevens-Johnson syndrome and exacerbations or activation of systemic lupus erythematosus have been reported with thiazides.

In patients with renal insufficiency, monitoring of renal function during therapy should be performed as deemed appropriate.

Renal failure has been reported in association with ACE inhibitors and has occurred mainly in patients with severe congestive heart failure or underlying renal disease, including renal artery stenosis. If recognised promptly and treated appropriately, renal failure is usually reversible.

Accuretic should be used cautiously in patients with impaired hepatic function or progressive liver disease because of the known risks associated with alterations in fluid and electrolyte balance resulting from thiazide treatment.

Patients receiving Accuretic should be observed for clinical signs of thiazide–induced fluid or electrolyte imbalance. In such patients, periodic determination of serum electrolytes should be performed. Because quinapril reduces the production of aldosterone, its combination with hydrochlorothiazide may minimise diuretic induced hypokalaemia. However, some patients may still require potassium supplements.

Patients haemodialysed using high-flux polyacrylonitrile ('AN69') membranes are highly likely to experience anaphylactoid reactions if they are treated with ACE inhibitors. This combination should therefore be avoided, either by use of alternative antihypertensive drugs or alternative membranes for haemodialysis.

Drug interactions: Tetracycline: Because of the presence of magnesium carbonate in the formulation it is recommended that concomitant administration of Accuretic with tetracycline be avoided.

Agents increasing serum potassium: Accuretic contains a diuretic. The addition of a potassium sparing diuretic is not recommended since these may cause a significant increase in serum potassium.

Surgery/anaesthesia: Although no data are available to indicate there is an interaction between Accuretic and anaesthetic agents that produce hypotension, caution should be exercised when patients undergo major surgery or anaesthesia since ACE inhibitors have been shown to block angiotensin II formation secondary to compensatory renin release. This may lead to hypotension which can be corrected by volume expansion.

Thiazides may decrease the arterial response to noradrenaline. In emergency surgery pre-anaesthetic and anaesthetic agents should be administered in reduced doses. Thiazides may increase the response to tubocurarine.

Lithium: Increased serum lithium levels and symptoms of lithium toxicity have been reported in patients receiving concomitant lithium and ACE inhibitor therapy or lithium and thiazide therapy. Lithium should not generally be given with Accuretic since the risk of lithium toxicity may be increased.

Corticosteroids, ACTH: Intensified electrolyte depletion, particularly hypokalaemia has been observed.

Non-steroidal anti-inflammatory drugs: In some patients, the administration of a non-steroidal anti-inflammatory agent can reduce the diuretic, natriuretic, and antihypertensive effects of loop, potassium-sparing, and thiazide diuretics. Therefore, when Accuretic and non-steroidal anti-inflammatory agents are used concomitantly the patients should be observed closely to determine if the desired effect of Accuretic is obtained.

Side effects: The most frequent clinical adverse reactions in hypertension are headache, dizziness, rhinitis, coughing and fatigue. Other adverse experiences include myalgia, viral infection, nausea and vomiting, abdominal pains, back pain and upper respiratory infection. Less frequent side effects are dyspepsia, chest pain, diarrhoea, insomnia, bronchitis, somnolence, asthenia, pharyngitis, vasodilatation and vertigo.

Increases (>1.25 times the upper limit of normal) in serum creatinine and blood urea nitrogen were observed in 3% and 4% respectively of the patients treated with Accuretic. These increases were almost always reversible upon discontinuation of ACE inhibitor therapy. In such patients renal function should be monitored during the first few weeks of therapy.

Increases in cholesterol and triglyceride levels may be associated with thiazide diuretic therapy.

Angioedema: Angioedema has been reported in patients treated with ACE inhibitors. If laryngeal stridor or angioedema of the face, tongue, or glottis occur, treatment should be discontinued immediately, the patient treated appropriately in accordance with accepted medical care, and carefully observed until the swelling disappears. In instances where swelling is confined to the face and lips, the condition generally resolves without treatment; antihistamines may be useful in relieving symptoms. Angioedema associated with laryngeal involvement may be fatal. Where there is involvement of the tongue, glottis, or larynx likely to cause airway obstruction, appropriate therapy eg subcutaneous adrenaline solution 1:1000 (0.3 to 0.5 ml) should be promptly administered.

Hypotension: Symptomatic hypotension is a possible consequence of ACE inhibition therapy in volume depleted patients such as those previously treated with thiazides.

Neutropenia/agranulocytosis: ACE inhibitors have been rarely associated with agranulocytosis and bone marrow depression in patients with uncomplicated hypertension but more frequently in patients with renal impairment, especially if they also have collagen vascular disease. As with other ACE inhibitors, monitoring of white blood cell counts in patients with collagen vascular disease and/or renal diseases should be considered. With thiazides leucopenia, agranulocytosis thrombocytopenia and aplastic anaemia have been reported.

Metabolic disorders: Hyperuricaemia may occur or frank gout be precipitated by thiazides in certain patients. Insulin requirements in diabetic patients may be altered by thiazides and latent diabetes mellitus may occur.

Pancreatitis has been reported rarely in patients treated with ACE inhibitors; in some cases this has proved fatal.

Overdosage: No data are available with respect to overdosage in humans. The most likely clinical manifestation would be symptoms attributed to severe hypotension. Treatment is symptomatic and supportive. Therapy with Accuretic should be discontinued and the patient observed closely.

Haemodialysis and peritoneal dialysis have little effect on the elimination of quinapril and quinaprilat.

Pharmaceutical precautions Store at a temperature not exceeding 25°C.

Legal category POM.

Package quantities Blister strips of 7 tablets, 4 strips in a carton (28 tablets).

Further information *Clinical chemistry:* Accuretic may cause a false positive urine test for Acetone.

Accuretic is designed to aid compliance by providing a convenient once daily preparation of quinapril combined with hydrochlorothiazide for the treatment of all grades of essential hypertension.

Significant antihypertensive activity is detectable throughout a 24 hour period following oral therapy. Quinaprilat is highly potent at binding to arterial and cardiac ACE.

By combining lower doses than might be required with each component used alone, side effects, especially the hypokalaemia associated with diuretics can be minimised.

Product licence number 0019/0127

Revised October 1997

ANUGESIC* HC CREAM

Qualitative and quantitative composition
Each 100 g of cream contains:

Zinc oxide PhEur	12.35 g
Balsam peru PhEur	1.85 g
Benzyl benzoate PhEur	1.2 g
Pramoxine hydrochloride USP	1.0 g
Bismuth oxide	0.875 g
Hydrocortisone acetate PhEur	0.5 g

Pharmaceutical form Buff coloured cream.

Clinical particulars
Therapeutic indications: Anugesic HC Cream provides antiseptic, astringent, emollient and decongestant properties. In addition hydrocortisone exerts an anti-inflammatory effect. Pramoxine is a rapidly acting local anaesthetic. The cream may be used to provide lubrication for suppositories.

Anugesic HC Cream is indicated for the comprehensive symptomatic treatment of severe and acute discomfort or pain associated with internal and external haemorrhoids, and pruritus ani.

Posology and method of administration: For topical use only.

Adults: Apply cream to the affected area at night, in the morning and after each evacuation. Thoroughly cleanse the affected area, dry and apply cream by gently smoothing onto the affected area. For internal conditions use rectal nozzle provided and clean it after each use.

Not to be taken orally.

Elderly (over 65 years): As for adults.

Children: Not recommended.

Contra-indications Tubercular, fungal and most viral lesions including herpes simplex, vaccinia and varicella.

History of sensitivity to any of the constituents.

Special warnings and special precautions for use: As with all products containing topical steroids the possibility of systemic absorption should be borne in mind.

Prolonged or excessive use may produce systemic corticosteroid effects, and use for periods longer than seven days is not recommended.

Following symptomatic relief definite diagnosis should be established.

Interaction with other medicaments and other forms of interaction: None known.

Pregnancy and lactation: There is inadequate evidence of safety in human pregnancy and there may be a very small risk of cleft palate and intrauterine growth retardation as well as suppression of the neonatal HPA axis. There is evidence of harmful effects in animals. Use in pregnancy only when there is no safer alternative and when the disease itself carries risks for the mother or child.

Effects on ability to drive and use machines: None known.

Undesirable effects: Rarely, sensitivity reactions. Patients may occasionally experience transient burning on application, especially if the anoderm is not intact.

Overdose: If swallowed, fever, nausea, vomiting, stomach cramps and diarrhoea may develop 3-12 hours after ingestion.

Pramoxine is relatively non-toxic and less sensitising than other local anaesthetics.

Hydrocortisone does not normally produce toxic effects in an acute single overdose.

Treatment of a large acute overdosage should include gastric lavage, purgation with magnesium sulphate and complete bed rest. If necessary, give oxygen and general supportive measures. Methaemoglobinaemia should be treated by intravenous methylene blue.

Pharmacological properties
Pharmacodynamic properties: Pramoxine hydrochloride is a surface anaesthetic used on the skin and mucous membranes to relieve surface pain and pruritus. Hydrocortisone acetate has the general properties of hydrocortisone and the anti-inflammatory action is of primary interest in this product. Benzyl benzoate is used as a solubilizing agent and has mild antiseptic and preservative properties, bismuth oxide exerts a protective action on mucous membranes and raw surfaces. It is weakly astringent and is reported to have antiseptic properties. Balsam peru has protective properties and a very mild antiseptic action by virtue of its content of cinnamic and benzoic acids. It is believed to promote the growth of epithelial cells, zinc oxide acts as astringent and mild antiseptic.

Pharmacokinetic properties: It is well known that topically applied corticosteroids can be absorbed percutaneously. This appears to be more likely upon repeated or prolonged use. The remaining active ingredients in Anugesic HC Cream exert their therapeutic effect without being absorbed into the systemic circulation. These observations are supported by evidence from various studies and reviews.

Preclinical safety data: Preclinical data does not add anything of further significance to the prescriber.

Pharmaceutical particulars
List of excipients: Liquid paraffin, Glyceryl monostarate, Propylene glycol, Polysorbate 60, Sorbitan monostearate, Titanium dioxide, Methyl hydroxybenzoate, Propyl hydroxybenzoate, Purified water.

Incompatibilities: None known.

Shelf life: Thirty six months.

Special precautions for storage: Store at a temperature not exceeding 25°C.

Nature and contents of container: Externally printed and internally lacquered aluminium tube with plastic cap containing 30 g.

Instructions for use/handling: Not applicable.

Marketing authorisation number PL 0019/0151

Date of first authorisation 22/01/90

Date of revision 07/02/95

Legal category POM

ANUGESIC* HC SUPPOSITORIES

Presentation Buff coloured suppositories.

Each 2.8 g suppository contains:

Pramoxine hydrochloride USP	27 mg
Hydrocortisone acetate Ph Eur	5 mg
Benzyl benzoate Ph Eur	33 mg
Bismuth oxide	24 mg
Bismuth subgallate BP	59 mg
Balsam peru Ph Eur	49 mg
Zinc oxide Ph Eur	296 mg

Uses Anugesic H.C. suppositories provide antiseptic, astringent, emollient and decongestant properties. In addition hydrocortisone exerts an anti-inflammatory effect. Pramoxine is a rapidly acting local anaesthetic.

Anugesic-HC Suppositories are indicated for the comprehensive symptomatic treatment of severe and acute discomfort or pain associated with internal haemorrhoids and pruritus ani.

Dosage and administration
Adults: Remove plastic cover and insert one suppository into the anus at night, in the morning and after each evacuation.

Not to be taken orally.

Elderly (over 65 years): As for adults.

Children: Not recommended.

Contra-indications, warnings, etc
Contra-indications: Tubercular, fungal and most viral lesions including herpes simplex, vaccinia and varicella. History of sensitivity to any of the constituents.

Warnings: As with all products containing topical steroids the possibility of systemic absorption should be borne in mind.

Prolonged or excessive use may produce systemic corticosteroid effects, and use for periods longer than seven days is not recommended.

Use in pregnancy: There is inadequate evidence of safety in human pregnancy and there may be a very small risk of cleft palate and intrauterine growth retardation as well as suppression of the neonatal HPA axis. There is evidence of harmful effects in animals. Use in pregnancy only when there is no safer alternative and when the disease itself carries risks for the mother or child.

Precautions: Following symptomatic relief definitive diagnosis should be established.

Side effects: Rarely, sensitivity reactions.

Patients may occasionally experience transient burning on application, especially if the anoderm is not intact.

Overdosage: If swallowed, fever, nausea, vomiting, stomach cramps and diarrhoea may develop 3-12 hours after ingestion.

Pramoxine is relatively non-toxic and less sensitising than other local anaesthetics.

Hydrocortisone normally does not produce toxic effects in an acute single overdose.

Treatment of a large acute overdosage should include gastric lavage, purgation with magnesium sulphate and complete bed rest. If necessary, give oxygen and general supportive measures. Methaemoglobinaemia should be treated by intravenous methylene blue.

Pharmaceutical precautions Store in a dry place, at a temperature not exceeding 25°C.

Legal category POM.

Package quantities Box of 12 suppositories.

Further information Nil

Product licence number PL 0019/0152

DICLOMAX RETARD* AND SR*

Qualitative and quantitative composition *Diclomax Retard* is supplied in opaque white capsules containing 100 mg Diclofenac Sodium in a modified release formulation.

Diclomax SR is supplied in opaque yellow capsules containing 75 mg Diclofenac Sodium in a modified release formulation.

Pharmaceutical form Modified release capsule for oral use.

Clinical particulars
Therapeutic indications: Diclomax SR and Diclomax Retard are indicated for rheumatoid arthritis; osteoarthritis; low back pain; acute musculo-skeletal disorders and trauma such as periarthritis (especially frozen shoulder), tendinitis, tenosynovitis, bursitis, sprains, strains and dislocations; relief of pain in fractures; ankylosing spondylitis; acute gout; control in pain and inflammation in orthopaedic, dental and other minor surgery.

Posology and method of administration: For oral administration.

Adults: Diclomax Retard: One 100 mg capsule taken whole daily, preferably with food or after food.

Diclomax SR: One or two 75 mg capsules daily taken whole in single or divided doses preferably with or after food.

Elderly: Studies indicate the pharmacokinetics of diclofenac sodium are not impaired to any clinical extent in the elderly, however, as with all non-steroidal anti-inflammatory drugs, Diclomax should be used with caution in elderly patients and the lowest effective dose used. (See also *Precautions*).

Children: Not recommended.

Contra-indications: Diclomax is contra-indicated in patients with a known sensitivity to diclofenac sodium, patients with active peptic ulcer or gastrointestinal bleeding, asthmatic patients in whom attacks of asthma, urticaria or acute rhinitis are precipitated by aspirin or other non-steroidal anti-inflammatory agents.

Special warnings and special precautions for use: As with all non-steroidal anti-inflammatory drugs (NSAIDs) Diclomax should only be given to the elderly and to patients with a history of peptic ulcer after other forms of treatment have been carefully considered.

NSAIDs in general, have been reported to cause nephrotoxicity, interstitial nephritis, nephrotic syndrome and renal failure. In patients with renal, cardiac or hepatic impairment caution is required since the use of NSAIDs may result in deterioration of renal function. The dose should be kept as low as possible and renal function should be monitored in these patients.

Diclomax should be used with caution in patients with gastro-intestinal ulceration, haematemesis or melaena, ulcerative colitis, Crohn's disease, bleeding diathesis or haematological abnormalities.

Patients with severe hepatic, cardiac or renal insufficiency or the elderly should be kept under close surveillance.

All patients who are receiving long-term treatment with non-steroidal anti-inflammatory agents should be monitored as a precautionary measure, eg. renal, hepatic function (elevation of liver enzymes may occur) and blood counts.

If abnormal liver function tests persist or worsen, clinical signs or symptoms consistent with liver disease develop or if other manisfestations occur (eosinophilia, rash), Diclomax should be discontinued.

Use of Diclomax in patients with hepatic porpyhria may trigger an attack.

The importance of prostaglandins in maintaining renal blood flow should be taken into account in patients with impaired cardiac or renal function, those being treated with diuretics or recovering from major surgery. Effects on renal function are usually reversible on withdrawal of Diclomax.

Diclomax in common with other NSAIDs, can reversibly inhibit platelet aggregation.

Interaction with other medicaments and other forms of interaction: Drug interactions: Diclomax may increase plasma concentrations of lithium and digoxin.

Clinical investigations do not appear to indicate that Diclomax affects the activity of anticoagulants but there have been isolated reports of an increased risk of haemorrhage with the combined use of these agents. Close monitoring is therefore recommended. Clinical studies have shown that Diclomax can be given together with oral antidiabetic agents without influencing their clinical effect. However there have been isolated reports of hyperglycaemic effects which have required adjustments to the dosage of hypoglycaemic agents.

Cyclosporin nephrotoxicity may be increased by the effect of non-steroidal anti-inflammatory drugs on renal prostaglandins.

Caution should be exercised if NSAIDs and methotrexate are administered within 24 hours of each other, since NSAIDs may increase methotrexate plasma levels, resulting in increased toxicity.

Concomitant therapy with other systemic NSAIDs may increase the frequency of side effects.

Various NSAIDs are liable to inhibit the activity of

diuretics. Concomitant treatment with potassium-sparing diuretics may be associated with increased serum potassium levels hence serum potassium should be monitored.

Pregnancy and lactation: Diclofenac sodium should not be prescribed during pregnancy unless the benefits outweigh the risk. Use of Diclomax in the last trimester of pregnancy is not recommended as regular use of NSAIDs may result in closure of the fetal ductus arteriosus in utero and possibly persistant pulmonary hypertension of the newborn, delay onset and increase duration of labour.

Traces of diclofenac sodium have been found in breast milk following oral doses of 50 mg every 8 hours.

Effects on ability to drive and use machines: None reported.

Undesirable effects: There have been occasional reports of epigastric pain, other gastrointestinal disorders, headache, dizziness, vertigo, rashes or skin eruptions and elevation of serum aminotransferase enzymes (SGOT, SGPT). Rare reports of gastrointestinal bleeding, peptic ulcer, bloody diarrhoea, drowsiness, tiredness, urticaria, liver function disorders including hepatitis with or without jaundice, oedema and hypersensitivity reactions have been reported.

Overdose: Symptomatology of overdose with diclofenac sodium is not well documented. The management of NSAID overdose should be supportive and the treatment symptomatic.

Should a patient ingest a large amount of Diclomax the stomach may be emptied, treatment with charcoal may reduce absorption. Haemodialysis is unlikely to decrease plasma protein concentration due to the high degree of protein binding.

Pharmacological properties

Pharmacodynamic properties: Diclofenac Sodium is a non-steroidal agent with marked analgesic/anti-inflammatory and anti-pyretic properties. It is an inhibitor of prostaglandin synthetase (cyclo-oxygenase).

Pharmacokinetic properties: Diclofenac Sodium is rapidly absorbed from the gut and is subject to first-pass metabolism. Capsules give peak plasma concentrations after approximately 2.5 hours. The active substance is 99.7% protein bound and plasma half-life for the terminal elimination phase is 1-2 hours. Approximately 60% of the administered dose is excreted via the kidneys in the form of metabolites and less than 1% in unchanged form. About 30% of the dose is excreted via the bile in metabolised form.

The Diclomax modified release preparations:

(i) increase the duration of action of the drug
(ii) maintain a relatively constant rate of absorption in the gastointestinal tract over a longer period of time
(iii) increase the fraction of the ingested dose absorbed in the G.I. tract
(iv) regulate the rate at which the drug is made available for absorption, thereby reducing the possibility of malabsorption and occurrence of side-effects.

Pharmaceutical particulars

List of excipients: Diclomax Retard capsules contain the following excipients: Sucrose EP, Maize Starch EP, purified stearic acid NF, polyethylene glycol 6000 NF, Ammonio methacrylate copolymer type A NF, Talc EP, Lactose EP and polysorbate 80 EP.

Diclomax SR capsules contain the following excipients: Sucrose EP, maize starch EP, purified stearic acid NF, polyethylene glycol 6000 NF, ammonio methacrylate copolymer type A NF, talc EP, lactose EP, polysorbate 80 EP, gelatin EP, titanium dioxide (E171) EP, iron oxide yellow (E172), opacode S-1-8100HV Black 1007 HSE.

Incompatibilities: None known.

Shelf life: Diclomax Retard capsules: Two years. *Diclomax SR* capsules: 18 months.

Special precautions for storage: Store between 10°C and 25°C. Protect from moisture. Do not refrigerate

Nature and contents of container: Diclomax Retard: White opaque PVC/Al blister strips or white opaque PVC/PE/PVDC/Al blister strips in packs of 28 capsules

Diclomax SR: White opaque PVC/hard tempered aluminium foil or white opaque PVC/PE/PVDC hard tempered aluminium foil blister strips in packs of 56 capsules

Instructions for use/handling: None.

Marketing authorisation numbers

Diclomax Retard	PL0019/0155
Diclomax SR	PL0019/0156

Date of revision *Diclomax Retard:* February 1998. *Diclomax SR:* September 1997.

Legal category POM.

EPANUTIN* CAPSULES 25 mg, 50 mg, 100 mg, 300 mg EPANUTIN* SUSPENSION and EPANUTIN INFATABS

Qualitative and quantitative composition Epanutin Capsules containing 25 mg, 50 mg, 100 mg or 300 mg phenytoin sodium Ph Eur. Epanutin Suspension containing phenytoin BP 30 mg/5 ml. Epanutin Infatabs containing phenytoin BP 50 mg.

Pharmaceutical form

Epanutin Capsules 25 mg: A white powder in a No 4 hard gelatin capsule with a white opaque body and purple cap, radially printed 'EPANUTIN 25'.

Epanutin Capsules 50 mg: A white powder in a No 4 hard gelatin capsule with a white opaque body and a pale pink opaque cap, radially printed 'EPANUTIN 50'.

Epanutin Capsules 100 mg: A white powder in a No 3 hard gelatin capsule with a white opaque body and orange cap, radially printed 'EPANUTIN 100'.

Epanutin Capsules 300 mg: A white powder in a No 1 hard gelatin capsule with a white opaque body and dark green cap, radially imprinted 'EPANUTIN 300'.

Epanutin Suspension: Cherry red suspension

Epanutin Infatabs: A yellow triangular tablet with a breaking line on one side.

Clinical particulars

Therapeutic indications: Control of tonic-clonic seizures (grand mal epilepsy), partial seizures (focal including temporal lobe) or a combination of these and the prevention and treatment of seizures occurring during or following neurosurgery and/or severe head injury. Epanutin has also been employed in the treatment of trigeminal neuralgia but it should only be used as second line therapy if carbamazepine is ineffective or patients are intolerant to carbamazepine.

Posology and method of administration: For oral administration only.

Dosage should be individualised, as there may be wide interpatient variability in phenytoin serum levels with equivalent dosage. Epanutin should be introduced in small dosages with gradual increments until control is achieved or until toxic effects appear. In some cases serum level determinations may be necessary for optimal dosage adjustments–the clinically effective level is usually 10–20 mg/l (40–80 micromoles/l) although some cases of tonic-clonic seizures may be controlled with lower serum levels of phenytoin. With recommended dosage a period of seven to ten days may be required to achieve steady state serum levels with Epanutin and changes in dosage should not be carried out at intervals shorter than seven to ten days. Maintenance of treatment should be the lowest dose of anticonvulsant consistent with control of seizures.

Epanutin Capsules, Suspension and Infatabs: Epanutin Capsules contain phenytoin sodium whereas Epanutin Suspension and Epanutin Infatabs contain phenytoin. Although 100 mg of phenytoin sodium is equivalent to 92 mg of phenytoin on a molecular weight basis, these molecular equivalents are not necessarily biologically equivalent. Physicians should therefore exercise care in those situations where it is necessary to change the dosage form and serum level monitoring is advised.

Adults: Initially 3 to 4 mg/kg/day with subsequent dosage adjustment if necessary. For most adults a satisfactory maintenance dose will be 200 to 500 mg daily in single or divided doses. Exceptionally, a daily dose outside this range may be indicated. Dosage should normally be adjusted according to serum levels where assay facilities exist.

Elderly (over 65 years): As with adults the dosage of Epanutin should be titrated to the patient's individual requirements using the same guidelines.

As elderly patients tend to receive multiple drug therapies, the possibility of drug interactions should be borne in mind.

Infants and children: Initially, 5 mg/kg/day in two divided doses, with subsequent dosage individualised to a maximum of 300 mg daily. A recommended daily maintenance dosage is usually 4-8 mg/kg.

Epanutin Infatabs may be chewed.

Neonates: The absorption of phenytoin following oral administration in neonates is unpredictable. Furthermore, the metabolism of phenytoin may be depressed. It is therefore especially important to monitor serum levels in the neonate.

Contra-indications: Hypersensitivity to hydantoins.

Special warnings and special precautions for use: Abrupt withdrawal of phenytoin in epileptic patients may precipitate status epilepticus. When, in the judgement of the clinician, the need for dosage reduction, discontinuation, or substitution of alternative anti-epileptic medication arises, this should be done gradually. However, in the event of an allergic or hypersensitivity reaction, rapid substitution of alternative therapy may be necessary. In this case, alternative therapy should be an anti-epileptic drug not belonging to the hydantoin chemical class.

Phenytoin is highly protein bound and extensively metabolised by the liver. Reduced dosage to prevent accumulation and toxicity may therefore be required in patients with impaired liver function. Where protein binding is reduced, as in uraemia, total serum phenytoin levels will be reduced accordingly. However, the pharmacologically active free drug concentration is unlikely to be altered. Therefore, under these circumstances therapeutic control may be achieved with total phenytoin levels below the normal range of 10–20 mg/l (40–80 micromoles/l). Patients with impaired liver function, elderly patients or those who are gravely ill may show early signs of toxicity.

Phenytoin should be discontinued if a skin rash appears. If the rash is exfoliative, purpuric, or bullous or if lupus erythematosus or Stevens-Johnson syndrome or toxic epidermal necrolysis is suspected, use of the drug should not be resumed (see Adverse Reactions). If the rash is of a milder type (measles-like or scarlatiniform), therapy may be resumed after the rash has completely disappeared. If the rash recurs upon reinstitution of therapy, further phenytoin medication is contraindicated.

Phenytoin is not effective for absence (petit mal) seizures. If tonic-clonic (grand mal) and absence seizures are present together, combined drug therapy is needed.

Phenytoin may affect glucose metabolism and inhibit insulin release. Hyperglycaemia has been reported in association with toxic levels. Phenytoin is not indicated for seizures due to hypoglycaemia or other metabolic causes.

Serum levels of phenytoin sustained above the optimal range may produce confusional states referred to as 'delirium,' 'psychosis,' 'encephalopathy,' or rarely irreversible cerebellar dysfunction. Accordingly, at the first sign of acute toxicity, serum drug level determinations are recommended. Dose reduction of phenytoin therapy is indicated if serum levels are excessive; if symptoms persist, termination of therapy with phenytoin is recommended.

Phenytoin therapy may interfere with Vitamin D metabolism. In the absence of an adequate dietary intake of Vitamin D or exposure to sunlight, osteomalacia, hypocalcemia or rickets may develop.

In view of isolated reports associating phenytoin with exacerbation of porphyria, caution should be exercised in using the medication in patients suffering from this disease.

Interaction with other medicaments and other forms of interaction:

1. Drugs which may *increase* phenytoin serum levels include: Amiodarone, antifungal agents, (such as, but not limited to, amphotericin B, fluconazole, ketoconazole, miconazole and itraconazole), chloramphenicol, chlordiazepoxide, diazepam, dicoumarol, disulfiram, H2-antagonists, halothane, isoniazid, methylphenidate, omeprazole, oestrogens, phenothiazines, phenylbutazone, salicylates, succinimides, sulphonamides, tolbutamide, trazodone and viloxazine.
2. Drugs which may *decrease* phenytoin serum levels include: carbamazepine, folic acid, reserpine, sucralfate and vigabatrin.
3. Drugs which may either *increase* or *decrease* phenytoin serum levels include: Phenobarbitone, valproic acid, sodium valproate antineoplastic agents, certain antacids and ciprofloxacin. Similarly, the effect of phenytoin on phenobarbitone and valproic acid and sodium valproate serum levels is unpredictable.

   Acute alcohol intake may increase phenytoin serum levels while chronic alcoholism may decrease serum levels.
4. Although not a true pharmacokinetic interaction, tricylic antidepressants and phenothiazines may precipitate seizures in susceptible patients and phenytoin dosage may need to be adjusted.
5. Drugs whose effect is *impaired* by phenytoin include: antifungal agents, antineoplastic agents, clozapine, corticosteroids, dicoumarol, digitoxin, doxycycline, frusemide, oestrogens, oral contraceptives, quinidine, rifampicin, theophylline and vitamin D.
6. Drugs whose effect is *altered* by phenytoin include: warfarin. The effect of phenytoin on warfarin is variable and prothrombin times should be determined when these agents are combined.

Serum level determinations are especially helpful when possible drug interactions are suspected.

Drug/laboratory test interactions: Phenytoin may cause a slight decrease in serum levels of total and free thyroxine, possibly as a result of enhanced peripheral metabolism. These changes do not lead to clinical hypothyroidism and do not affect the levels of circulating TSH. The latter can therefore be used for diagnosing hypothyroidism in the patient on phenytoin. Phenytoin does not interfere with uptake and suppression tests used in the diagnosis of hypothyroidism. It may, however, produce lower than normal values for dexamethasone or metapyrone tests. Phenytoin may cause raised serum levels of glucose, alkaline phosphatase, gamma glutamyl transpeptidase and lowered serum levels of calcium and folic acid. It is recommended that serum folate concentrations be measured at least once every 6 months and folic acid supplements given if necessary. Phenytoin may affect blood sugar metabolism tests.

Pregnancy and lactation: There are intrinsic methodologic problems in obtaining adequate data on drug teratogenicity in humans. Genetic factors or the epileptic condition itself may be more important than drug therapy in leading to birth defects. The great majority of mothers on anticonvulsant medication deliver normal infants. It is important to note that anticonvulsant drugs should not be discontinued in patients in whom the drug is administered to prevent major seizures because of the strong possibility of precipitating status epilepticus with attendant hypoxia and threat to life. In individual cases where the severity and frequency of the seizure disorder are such that the removal of medication does not pose a serious threat to the patient, discontinuation of the drug may be considered prior to and during pregnancy although it cannot be said with any confidence that even minor seizures do not pose some hazard to the developing embryo or foetus.

Anticonvulsants including phenytoin may produce congenital abnormalities in the offspring of a small number of epileptic patients. The exact role of drug therapy in these abnormalities is unclear and genetic factors, in some studies, have also been shown to be important. Epanutin should only be used during pregnancy, especially early pregnancy, if in the judgement of the physician the potential benefits clearly outweigh the risk.

In addition to the reports of increased incidence of congenital malformations, such as cleft lip/palate and heart malformations in children of women receiving phenytoin and other antiepileptic drugs, there have more recently been reports of a foetal hydantoin syndrome. This consists of prenatal growth deficiency, micro-encephaly and mental deficiency in children born to mothers who have received phenytoin, barbiturates, alcohol or trimethadione. However, these features are all interrelated and are frequently associated with intrauterine growth retardation from other causes.

There have been isolated reports of malignancies, including neuroblastoma, in children whose mothers received phenytoin during pregnancy.

An increase in seizure frequency during pregnancy occurs in a proportion of patients and this may be due to altered phenytoin absorption or metabolism. Periodic measurement of serum phenytoin levels is particularly valuable in the management of a pregnant epileptic patient as a guide to an appropriate adjustment of dosage. However, postpartum restoration of the original dosage will probably be indicated.

Neonatal coagulation defects have been reported within the first 24 hours in babies born to epileptic mothers receiving phenytoin. Vitamin K1 has been shown to prevent or correct this defect and may be given to the mother before delivery and to the neonate after birth.

Infant breast-feeding is not recommended for women taking phenytoin because phenytoin appears to be secreted in low concentrations in human milk.

Effects on ability to drive and use machines: None known.

Undesirable effects: Central nervous system: The most common manifestations encountered with phenytoin therapy are referable to this system and are usually dose-related. These include nystagmus, ataxia, slurred speech, decreased coordination, mental confusion, paraesthesia, drowsiness and vertigo. Dizziness, insomnia, transient nervousness, motor twitchings and headaches have also been observed. There have also been rare reports of phenytoin induced dyskinesias, including chorea, dystonia, tremor and asterixis, similar to those induced by phenothiazine and other neuroleptic drugs. There are occasional reports of irreversible cerebellar dysfunction associated with severe phenytoin overdosage. Peripheral neuropathy has been reported on rare occasions.

Gastrointestinal: Nausea, vomiting and constipation, toxic hepatitis and liver damage.

Dermatological: Dermatological manifestations sometimes accompanied by fever have included scarlatiniform or morbilliform rashes. A morbilliform rash is the most common; dermatitis is seen more rarely. Other more serious and rare forms have included bullous, exfoliative or purpuric dermatitis, lupus erythematosus, Stevens- Johnson syndrome and toxic epidermal necrolysis (see *Special precautions and special warnings for use*).

Connective tissue: Coarsening of the facial features, enlargement of the lips, gingival hyperplasia, hirsutism, hypertrichosis, Peyronie's Disease and Dupuytren's contracture may occur rarely.

Haemopoietic: Haemopoietic complications, some fatal, have occasionally been reported in association with administration of phenytoin. These have included thrombocytopenia, leucopenia, granulocytopenia, agranulocytosis, pancytopenia with or without bone marrow suppression and aplastic anaemia. While macrocytosis and megaloblastic anaemia have occurred, these conditions usually respond to folic acid therapy.

There have been a number of reports suggesting a relationship between phenytoin and the development of lymphadenopathy (local and generalised) including benign lymph node hyperplasia, pseudolymphoma, lymphoma and Hodgkin's Disease. Although a cause and effect relationship has not been established, the occurrence of lymphadenopathy indicates the need to differentiate such a condition from other types of lymph node pathology. Lymph node involvement may occur with or without symptoms and signs resembling serum sickness, e.g. fever, rash and liver involvement. In all cases of lymphadenopathy, follow-up observation for an extended period is indicated and every effort should be made to achieve seizure control using alternative antiepileptic drugs.

Frequent blood counts should be carried out during treatment with phenytoin.

Immune system: Hypersensitivity syndrome has been reported and may in rare cases be fatal (the syndrome may include, but is not limited to, symptoms such as arthralgias, eosinophilia, fever, liver dysfunction, lymphadenopathy or rash), systemic lupus erythematosus, polyarteritis nodosa and immunoglobulin abnormalities may occur. Several individual case reports have suggested that there may be an increased, although still rare, incidence of hypersensitivity reactions, including skin rash and hepatotoxicity, in black patients.

Other: Polyarthropathy, interstitial nephritis, pneumonitis.

Overdose: The lethal dose in children is not known. The mean lethal dose for adults is estimated to be 2 to 5 g. The initial symptoms are nystagmus, ataxia and dysarthria. The patient then becomes comatose, the pupils are unresponsive and hypotension occurs followed by respiratory depression and apnoea. Death is due to respiratory and circulatory depression.

There are marked variations among individuals with respect to phenytoin serum levels where toxicity may occur. Nystagmus on lateral gaze usually appears at 20 mg/l, ataxia at 30 mg/l, dysarthria and lethargy appear when the serum concentration is greater than 40 mg/l, but a concentration as high as 50 mg/l has been reported without evidence of toxicity.

As much as 25 times therapeutic dose has been taken to result in serum concentration over 100 mg/l (400 micromoles/l) with complete recovery.

Treatment: Treatment is non-specific since there is no known antidote. If ingested within the previous 4 hours the stomach should be emptied. If the gag reflex is absent, the airway should be supported. Oxygen and assisted ventilation may be necessary for central nervous system, respiratory and cardiovascular depression. Haemodialysis can be considered since phenytoin is not completely bound to plasma proteins. Total exchange transfusion has been utilised in the treatment of severe intoxication in children.

Pharmacological properties
Pharmacodynamic properties: Phenytoin is effective in various animal models of generalised convulsive disorders, reasonably effective in models of partial seizures but relatively ineffective in models of myoclonic seizures. It appears to stabilise rather than raise the seizure threshold and prevents spread of seizure activity rather than abolish the primary focus of seizure discharge. The mechanism by which phenytoin exerts its anticonvulsant action has not been fully elucidated however, possible contributory effects include: 1. Non-synaptic effects to reduce sodium conductance, enhance active sodium extrusion, block repetitive firing and reduce post-titanic potentiation. 2. Post-synaptic action to enhance gaba-mediated inhibition and reduce excitatory synaptic transmission. 3. Pre-synaptic actions to reduce calcium entry and block release of neurotransmitter.

Pharmacokinetic properties: Phenytoin is absorbed from the small intestine after oral administration. Various formulation factors may affect the bioavailability of phenytoin, however, non-linear techniques have estimated absorption to be essentially complete. After absorption it is distributed into body fluids, including CSF. Its volume of distribution has been estimated to be between 0.52 and 1.19 litres/kg, and it is highly protein bound (usually 90% in adults). The plasma half-life of phenytoin in man averages 22 hours with a range of 7 to 42 hours. Steady state therapeutic drug levels are achieved at least 7 to 10 days after initiation of therapy. Phenytoin is hydroxylated in the liver by an enzyme system which is saturable. Small incremental doses may produce very substantial increases in serum levels when these are in the upper range of therapeutic concentrations. The parameters controlling elimination are also subject to wide interpatient variation. The serum level is achieved by a given dose is therefore also subject to wide variation.

Preclinical safety data: Pre-clinical safety data does not add anything of further significance to the prescriber.

Pharmaceutical particulars
List of excipients:

Epanutin Capsules 25 mg: Each capsule contains lactose and magnesium stearate. The gelatin capsule shell also contains E127 (erythrosine), E131 (patent blue V) and E171 (titanium dioxide).

Epanutin Capsules 50 mg: Each capsule contains lactose and magnesium stearate. The gelatin capsule shell also contains E127 (erythrosine), E104 (quinoline yellow) and E171 (titanium dioxide).

Epanutin Capsules 100 mg: Each capsule contains lactose and magnesium stearate. The gelatin capsule shell also contains E127 (erythrosine), E104 (quinoline yellow) and E171 (titanium dioxide).

Epanutin Capsules 300 mg: Each capsule contains lactose, magnesium stearate and silica. The gelatin capsule shell also contains E104 (quinoline yellow), E131 (patent blue V) and E171 (titanium dioxide).

Epanutin Infatabs: Sugar (icing sugar), maize starch, saccharin sodium, spearmint flavour, sugar solution (66.6%w/w), magnesium stearate, purified talc and E104 (quinoline yellow).

Epanutin Suspension: Aluminium magnesium silicate, sodium benzoate, citric acid, sodium carboxymethylcellulose, glycerol, polysorbate 40, sugar mineral water, ethanol, vanillin, banana flavour, orange oil, carmoisine (E122), sunset yellow (E110) and water.

Incompatibilities: None known.

Shelf life: Epanutin Capsules 25 mg, 50 mg, 100 mg, Epanutin Infatabs and Epanutin Suspension: 36 months.

Epanutin Capsules 300 mg: 24 months.

Special precautions for storage: Epanutin Capsules and Infatabs: Store at a temperature not exceeding 30°C.

Epanutin Suspension: Store at a temperature not exceeding 25°C.

Nature and contents of container:

Epanutin Capsules 25 mg, and 50 mg: White HDPE container with white LDPE cap, containing 500 capsules.

Epanutin Capsules 100 mg: White HDPE container with white LDPE cap, containing 100, 500 or 1000 capsules.

Epanutin Capsules 300 mg: PVC/PVdC blister pack containing 100 capsules.

Epanutin Infatabs: White HDPE container with white LDPE cap, containing 100 tablets.

Epanutin Suspension: Amber glass bottle with aluminium cap containing 500 ml.

Instructions for use/handling: No special requirements.

Marketing authorisation numbers

Epanutin Capsules 25 mg	PL0019/0130
Epanutin Capsules 50 mg	PL0019/0131
Epanutin Capsules 100 mg	PL0019/0132
Epanutin Capsules 300 mg	PL0019/0133
Epanutin Infatabs	PL0019/0134
Epanutin Suspension	PL0019/0136

Date of renewal of authorisation
Epanutin Capsules 25 mg, 50 mg, 100 mg: 9/8/96.
Epanutin Capsules 300 mg, Epanutin Suspension, Epanutin Infatabs: 31/10/97.

Date of revision
Epanutin Capsules 25 mg, 50 mg, 100 mg: January 1998. Epanutin Capsules 300 mg, Epanutin Suspension, Epanutin Infatabs: July 1998.

Legal category POM

EPANUTIN* READY-MIXED PARENTERAL

Qualitative and quantitative composition Each 5 ml ampoule contains Phenytoin sodium PhEur 250 mg.

Pharmaceutical form Clear, sterile solution for injection

Clinical particulars
Therapeutic indications: Parenteral Epanutin is indicated for the control of status epilepticus of the tonic-clonic (grand mal) type and prevention and treatment of seizures occurring during or following neurosurgery and/or severe head injury.

It is of use in the treatment of cardiac arrhythmias

where first line therapy is not effective. It is of particular value when these are digitalis induced.

Posology and method of administration:
For parenteral administration:

Parenteral drug products should be inspected visually for particulate matter and discolouration prior to administration, whenever solution and container permit. Parenteral Epanutin is suitable for use as long as it remains free of haziness and precipitate. Upon refrigeration or freezing a precipitate might form; this will dissolve again after the solution is allowed to stand at room temperature. The product is still suitable for use. Only a clear solution should be used. A faint yellow colouration may develop, however, this has no effect on the potency of this solution.

There is a relatively small margin between full therapeutic effect and minimally toxic doses of this drug. Optimum control without clinical signs of toxicity occurs most often with serum levels between 10 and 20 mg/l (40–80 micromoles/l).

Parenteral Epanutin should be injected **slowly** directly into a large vein through a large-gauge needle or intravenous catheter.

Each injection or infusion of intravenous Epanutin should be preceded and followed by an injection of sterile saline through the same needle or catheter to avoid local venous irritation due to alkalinity of the solution (see warning section).

For infusion administration the parenteral phenytoin should be diluted in 50–100 ml of normal saline, with the final concentration of phenytoin in the solution not exceeding 10 mg/ml. Administration should commence immediately after the mixture has been prepared and must be completed within one hour (the infusion mixture should not be refrigerated). An in-line filter (0.22–0.50 microns) should be used. The diluted form is suitable for use as long as it remains free of haziness and precipitate.

Continuous monitoring of the electrocardiogram and blood pressure is essential. Cardiac resuscitative equipment should be available. The patient should be observed for signs of respiratory depression. If administration of intravenous Epanutin does not terminate seizures, the use of other measures, including general anaesthesia, should be considered.

Epanutin Ready Mixed Parenteral contains phenytoin sodium whereas Epanutin Suspension and Epanutin Infatabs contain phenytoin. Although 100 mg of phenytoin sodium is equivalent to 92 mg of phenytoin on a molecular weight basis, these molecular equivalents are not necessarily biologically equivalent. Physicians should therefore exercise care in those situations where it is necessary to change the dosage form and serum level monitoring is advised.

Status epilepticus: In a patient having continuous seizure activity, as compared to the more common rapidly recurring seizures, i.e. serial epilepsy, injection of intravenous diazepam or a short acting barbiturate is recommended because of their rapid onset of action, prior to administration of Epanutin.

Following the use of diazepam in patients having continuous seizures and in the initial management of serial epilepsy a loading dose of Epanutin 10–15 mg/kg should be injected **slowly** intravenously, at a rate not exceeding 50 mg per minute in adults (this will require approximately 20 minutes in a 70 kg patient). The loading dose should be followed by maintenance doses of 100 mg orally or intravenously every 6 to 8 hours.

Recent work in neonates has shown that absorption of phenytoin is unreliable after oral administration, but a loading dose of 15–20 mg/kg of Epanutin intravenously will usually produce serum concentrations of phenytoin within the generally accepted therapeutic range (10–20 mg/l). The drug should be injected slowly intravenously at a rate of 1–3 mg/kg/min.

Determination of phenytoin serum levels is advised when using Epanutin in the management of status epilepticus and in the subsequent establishing of maintenance dosage. The clinically effective level is usually 10–20 mg/l although some cases of tonic-clonic seizures may be controlled with lower serum levels of phenytoin.

Intramuscular administration should not be used in the treatment of status epilepticus because the attainment of peak plasma levels may require up to 24 hours.

Use in cardiac arrhythmias: 3.5–5 mg per kg of bodyweight intravenously initially, repeated once if necessary. The solution should be injected slowly, intravenously and at a uniform rate which should not exceed 1 ml (50 mg) per minute.

Other clinical conditions: It is not possible to set forth a universally applicable dosage schedule. **The intravenous route of administration is preferred**. Dosage and dosing interval will, of necessity, be determined by the needs of the individual patient. Factors such as previous antiepileptic therapy, seizure control, age and general medical condition must be considered. Notwithstanding the slow absorption of Epanutin when given intra-muscularly its use in certain conditions may be appropriate.

When short term intramuscular administration is necessary for a patient previously stabilised orally, compensating dosage adjustments are essential to maintain therapeutic serum levels. An intramuscular dose 50% greater than the oral dose is necessary to maintain these levels. When returned to oral administration, the dose should be reduced by 50% of the original oral dose, for the same period of time the patient received Epanutin intra-muscularly, to prevent excessive serum levels due to continued release from intramuscular tissue sites.

Neurosurgery: In a patient who has not previously received the drug, Parenteral Epanutin 100–200 mg (2–4 ml) may be given intramuscularly at approximately 4-hour intervals prophylactically during neurosurgery and continued during the postoperative period for 48–72 hrs. The dosage should then be reduced to a maintenance dose of 300 mg and adjusted according to serum level estimations.

If the patient requires more than a week of intramuscular Epanutin alternative routes should be explored such as gastric intubation. For time periods less than one week, the patient switched from intramuscular administration should receive one half the original oral dose for the same period of time the patient received Epanutin intra-muscularly. Measurement of serum levels is of value as a guide to an appropriate adjustment of dosage.

Elderly (over 65 years): As for adults. However, complications may occur more readily in elderly patients.

Neonates: Recent work in neonates has shown that absorption of phenytoin is unreliable after oral administration, but a loading dose of 15–20 mg/kg of Epanutin intravenously will usually produce serum concentrations of phenytoin within the generally accepted therapeutic range (10–20 mg/l). The drug should be injected slowly intravenously at a rate of 1–3 mg/kg/min.

Infants and children: As for adults. However, it has been shown that children tend to metabolise phenytoin more rapidly than adults. This should be borne in mind when determining dosage regimens. The use of serum level monitoring being particularly beneficial in such cases.

Contra-indications: Phenytoin is contraindicated in patients who are hypersensitive to phenytoin or other hydantoins.

Intra arterial administration must be avoided in view of the high pH of the preparation.

Because of its effect on ventricular automaticity, phenytoin is contraindicated in sinus bradycardia, sino-atrial block, and second and third degree A-V block and patients with Adams-Stokes syndrome.

Special warnings and special precautions for use: In adults, intravenous administration should not exceed 50 mg per minute. In neonates, the drug should be administered at a rate of 1–3 mg/kg/min.

The most notable signs of toxicity associated with the intravenous use of this drug are cardiovascular collapse and/or central nervous system depression. Severe cardiotoxic reactions and fatalities due to depression of atrial and ventricular conduction and ventricular fibrillation, respiratory arrest and tonic seizures have been reported particularly in elderly or gravely ill patients, if the preparation is given too rapidly or in excess.

Hypotension usually occurs when the drug is administered rapidly by the intravenous route.

Soft tissue irritation and inflammation has occurred at the site of injection with and without extravasation of intravenous phenytoin. Soft tissue irritation may vary from slight tenderness to extensive necrosis, sloughing and in rare instances has led to amputation. Subcutaneous or perivascular injection should be avoided because of the highly alkaline nature of the solution.

The intramuscular route is not recommended for the treatment of status epilepticus because of slow absorption. Serum levels of phenytoin in the therapeutic range cannot be rapidly achieved by this method.

General: Intravenous Epanutin should be used with caution in patients with hypotension and severe myocardial insufficiency.

Phenytoin should be discontinued if a skin rash appears. If the rash is exfoliative, purpuric, or bullous or if lupus erythematosus, Stevens- Johnson syndrome, or toxic epidermal necrolysis is suspected, use of this drug should not be resumed and alternative therapy should be considered. If the rash is of a milder type (measles-like or scarlatiniform), therapy may be resumed after the rash has completely disappeared. If the rash recurs upon reinstitution of therapy, further phenytoin medication is contraindicated.

Phenytoin is not effective for absence (petit mal) seizures. If tonic-clonic (grand mal) and absence (petit mal) seizures are present together, combined drug therapy is needed.

Serum levels of phenytoin sustained above the optimal range may produce confusional states referred to as 'delirium,' 'psychosis,' or 'encephalopathy,' or rarely irreversible cerebellar dysfunction. Accordingly, at the first sign of acute toxicity, serum drug level determinations are recommended. Dose reduction of phenytoin therapy is indicated if serum levels are excessive; if symptoms persist, termination of therapy with phenytoin is recommended.

Phenytoin is highly protein bound and extensively metabolised by the liver.

Reduced maintenance dosage to prevent accumulation and toxicity may therefore be required in patients with impaired liver function. Where protein binding is reduced, as in uraemia, total serum phenytoin levels will be reduced accordingly. However, the pharmacologically active free drug concentration is unlikely to be altered. Therefore, under these circumstances therapeutic control may be achieved with total phenytoin levels below the normal range of 10–20 mg/l. Dosage should not exceed the minimum necessary to control convulsions.

The liver is the chief site of biotransformation of phenytoin. Patients with impaired liver function, elderly patients, or those who are gravely ill may show early signs of toxicity.

Phenytoin may affect glucose metabolism and inhibit insulin release. Hyperglycaemia has been reported. Phenytoin is not indicated for seizures due to hypoglycaemia or other metabolic causes. Caution is advised when treating diabetic patients.

In view of isolated reports associating phenytoin with exacerbation of porphyria, caution should be exercised in using this medication in patients suffering from this disease.

Laboratory tests: Phenytoin serum level determinations may be necessary to achieve optimal dosage adjustments.

Interaction with other medicaments and other forms of interaction:

1. Drugs which may *increase* phenytoin serum levels include: Amiodarone, antifungal agents, (such as, but not limited to, amphotericin B, fluconazole, ketoconazole, miconazole and itraconazole), chloramphenicol, chlordiazepoxide, diazepam, dicoumarol, disulfiram, H2-antagonists, halothane, isoniazid, methylphenidate, omeprazole, oestrogens, phenothiazines, phenylbutazone, salicylates, succinimides, sulphonamides, tolbutamide, trazodone and viloxazine.
2. Drugs which may *decrease* phenytoin serum levels include: carbamazepine, folic acid, reserpine, sucralfate and vigabatrin.
3. Drugs which may either *increase* or *decrease* phenytoin serum levels include: Phenobarbitone, valproic acid, sodium valproate, antineoplastic agents, certain antacids and ciprofloxacin. Similarly, the effect of phenytoin on phenobarbitone and valproic acid and sodium valproate serum levels is unpredictable.

   Acute alcohol intake may increase phenytoin serum levels while chronic alcoholism may decrease serum levels.
4. Although not a true pharmacokinetic interaction, tricylic antidepressants and phenothiazines may precipitate seizures in susceptible patients and phenytoin dosage may need to be adjusted.
5. Drugs whose effect is *impaired* by phenytoin include: antifungal agents, antineoplastic agents, clozapine, corticosteroids, dicoumarol, digitoxin, doxycycline, frusemide, oestrogens, oral contraceptives, quinidine, rifampicin, theophylline and vitamin D.
6. Drugs whose effect is *enhanced* by phenytoin include: warfarin.

Serum level determinations are especially helpful when possible drug interactions are suspected.

Drug/laboratory test interactions: Phenytoin may cause decreased serum levels of protein-bound iodine (PBI). It may also produce lower than normal values for dexamethasone or metyrapone tests. Phenytoin may cause raised serum levels of glucose, alkaline phosphatase, gamma glutamyl transpeptidase and lowered serum levels of calcium and folic acid. Phenytoin may affect blood sugar metabolism tests.

Pregnancy and lactation: In considering the use of Epanutin intravenously in the management of status epilepticus in pregnancy, the following information should be weighed in assessing the risks and the benefits. The potential adverse effects upon the foetus of status epilepticus, specifically hypoxia, make it imperative to control the condition in the shortest possible time.

There are intrinsic methodologic problems in obtaining adequate data on drug teratogenicity in humans. Genetic factors or the epileptic condition itself may be more important than drug therapy in leading to birth defects.

The great majority of mothers on anticonvulsant medication deliver normal infants. It is important to note that anticonvulsant drugs should not be discontinued in patients in whom the drug is administered to prevent major seizures because of the strong possibility of precipitating status epilepticus and attendant hypoxia and threat to life. In individual cases where the severity and frequency of the seizure disorder are such that the removal of medication does not pose a serious threat to the patient, discontinuation of the drug may be considered prior to and during pregnancy although it cannot be said with any confidence that even minor seizures do not pose some hazard to the developing embryo or foetus.

There is some evidence that phenytoin may produce congenital abnormalities in the offspring of a small number of epileptic patients, therefore it should not be used as first drug during pregnancy, especially early pregnancy, unless in the judgement of the physician the potential benefits outweigh the risk.

In addition to the reports of increased incidence of congenital malformations, such as cleft lip/palate and heart malformations in children of women receiving phenytoin and other anti-epileptic drugs, there have more recently been reports of a foetal hydantoin syndrome. This consists of prenatal growth deficiency, microencephaly and mental deficiency in children born to mothers who have received phenytoin, barbiturates, alcohol or trimethadione. However, these features are all interrelated and are frequently associated with intrauterine growth retardation from other causes.

There have been isolated reports of malignancies, including neuroblastoma, in children whose mothers received phenytoin during pregnancy.

An increase in seizure frequency during pregnancy occurs in a proportion of patients, because of altered phenytoin absorption or metabolism. Periodic measurement of serum phenytoin levels is particularly valuable in the management of a pregnant epileptic patient as a guide to an appropriate adjustment of dosage. However, post partum restoration of the original dosage will probably be indicated. Neonatal coagulation defects have been reported within the first 24 hours in babies born to epileptic mothers receiving phenytoin. Vitamin K has been shown to prevent or correct this defect and may be given to the mother before delivery and to the neonate after birth.

Infant breast-feeding is not recommended for women taking this drug because phenytoin appears to be secreted in low concentrations in human milk.

Effects on ability to drive and use machines: None known.

Undesirable effects: Signs of toxicity are associated with cardiovascular and central nervous system depression.

Central nervous system: The most common manifestations encountered with phenytoin therapy are referable to this system and are usually dose-related. These include nystagmus, ataxia, slurred speech, decreased coordination, mental confusion, paraesthesia, drowsiness and vertigo. Dizziness, insomnia, transient nervousness, motor twitching, and headache have also been observed. There have also been rare reports of phenytoin-induced dyskinesia, including chorea, dystonia, tremor and asterixis, similar to those induced by phenothiazine and other neuroleptic drugs. A predominantly sensory peripheral polyneuropathy has been observed in patients receiving long-term phenytoin therapy. Tonic seizures have also been reported.

Cardiovascular: Severe cardiotoxic reactions and fatalities have been reported with atrial and ventricular conduction depression and ventricular fibrillation. Severe complications are most commonly encountered in elderly or gravely ill patients.

Respiratory: Alterations in respiratory function including respiratory arrest may occur.

Injection site: Local irritation, inflammation and tenderness. Necrosis and sloughing have been reported after subcutaneous or perivascular injection. Subcutaneous or perivascular injection should be avoided. Soft tissue irritation and inflammation have occurred at the site of injection with and without extravasation of intravenous phenytoin.

Dermatological system: Dermatological manifestations sometimes accompanied by fever have included scarlatiniform or morbilliform rashes. A morbilliform rash (measles-like) is the most common. Other types of dermatitis are seen more rarely. Other more serious forms which may be fatal have included bullous, exfoliative or purpuric dermatitis, lupus erythematosus, Stevens-Johnson syndrome and toxic epidermal necrolysis.

Haemopoietic system: Haemopoietic complications, some fatal, have occasionally been reported in association with administration of phenytoin. These have included thrombocytopenia, leucopenia, granulocytopenia, agranulocytosis and pancytopenia with or without bone marrow suppression and aplastic anaemia. While macrocytosis and megaloblastic anaemia have occurred, these conditions usually respond to folic acid therapy. There have been a number of reports suggesting a relationship between phenytoin and the development of lymphadenopathy (local or generalised) including benign lymph node hyperplasia, pseudolymphoma, lymphoma and Hodgkin's Disease. Although a cause and effect relationship has not been established, the occurrence of lymphadenopathy indicates the need to differentiate such a condition from other types of lymph node pathology. Lymph node involvement may occur with or without symptoms and signs resembling serum sickness, eg fever, rash and liver involvement.

In all cases of lymphadenopathy, follow-up observation for an extended period is indicated and every effort should be made to achieve seizure control using alternative antiepileptic drugs.

Gastrointestinal system: Nausea, vomiting, constipation, toxic hepatitis and liver damage.

Connective tissue system: Coarsening of the facial features, enlargement of the lips, gingival hyperplasia, hirsutism, hypertrichosis, Peyronie's disease and Dupuytren's contracture may occur rarely.

Immune system: Hypersensitivity syndrome has been reported and may in rare cases be fatal (the syndrome may include, but is not limited to, symptoms such as arthralgias, eosinophilia, fever, liver dysfunction, lymphadenopathy or rash), systemic lupus erythematosus, periarteritis nodosa and immunoglobulin abnormalities may occur. Several individual case reports have suggested that there may be an increased, although still rare, incidence of hypersensitivity reactions, including skin rash and hepatotoxicity, in black patients.

Other: Polyarthropathy, interstitial nephritis, pneumonitis.

Overdose: The lethal dose in children is not known. The mean lethal dose in adults is estimated to be 2 to 5 grams. The initial symptoms are nystagmus, ataxia and dysarthria. Other signs are tremor, hyperflexia, lethargy, nausea, vomiting. The patient may become comatose and hypotensive. Death is due to respiratory and circulatory depression.

Attempts to relate serum levels of the drug to toxic effects have shown wide interpatient variation. Nystagmus on lateral gaze usually appears at 20 mg/l and ataxia at 30 mg/l, dysarthria and lethargy appear when the serum concentration is >40 mg/l, but a concentration as high as 50 mg/l has been reported without evidence of toxicity.

As much as 25 times the therapeutic dose, which resulted in a serum concentration of 100 mg/l was taken with complete recovery.

Treatment: Treatment is non-specific since there is no known antidote. The adequacy of the respiratory and circulatory systems should be carefully observed and appropriate supportive measures employed. Haemodialysis can be considered since phenytoin is not completely bound to plasma proteins. Total exchange transfusion has been used in the treatment of severe intoxication in children.

In acute overdosage the possibility of other CNS depressants, including alcohol, should be borne in mind.

Pharmacological properties

Pharmacodynamic properties: Phenytoin is effective in various animal models of generalised convulsive disorders, reasonably effective in models of partial seizures but relatively ineffective in models of myoclonic seizures. It appears to stabilise rather than raise the seizure threshold and prevents spread of seizure activity rather than abolish the primary focus of seizure discharge. The mechanism by which phenytoin exerts its anticonvulsant action has not been fully elucidated however, possible contributory effects include: 1. Non-synaptic effects to reduce sodium conductance, enhance active sodium extrusion, block repetitive firing and reduce post-titanic potentiation. 2. Post-synaptic action to enhance gaba-mediated inhibition and reduce excitatory synaptic transmission. 3. Pre-synaptic actions to reduce calcium entry and block release of neurotransmitter.

Pharmacokinetic properties: After injection phenytoin is distributed into body fluids including CSF. Its volume of distribution has been estimated to be between 0.52 and 1.19 litres/kg and it is highly protein bound (usually 90% in adults). In serum, phenytoin binds rapidly and reversibly to proteins. About 90% of phenytoin in plasma is bound to albumin. The plasma half-life of phenytoin in man averages 22 hours with a range of 7 to 42 hours. Phenytoin is hydroxylated in the liver by an enzyme system which is saturable. Small incremental doses may produce very substantial increases in serum levels when these are in the upper range of therapeutic concentrations. The parameters controlling elimination are also subject to wide interpatient variation. The serum level is achieved by a given dose is therefore also subject to wide variation.

Preclinical safety data: Pre-clinical safety data does not add anything of further significance to the prescriber.

Pharmaceutical particulars

List of excipients: Each 5 ml contains: propylene glycol, ethanol 96%, water for injection, sodium hydroxide.

Incompatibilities: None stated.

Shelf life: 36 months.

Special precautions for storage: Store at room temperature not exceeding 25°C. Protect from light. The product should not be used if a precipitate or haziness develops in the solution in the ampoule. Epanutin Ready Mixed Parenteral should not be mixed with other drugs because of precipitation of phenytoin acid.

Nature and contents of container: Colourless neutral glass, Type 1, PH Eur, white colour break band. Each pack contains 10 ampoules.

Instructions for use/handling: See *Posology and method of administration* for further information.

Marketing authorisation number PL 00019/0135

Date of renewal of authorisation 31/07/1997.

Date of revision January 1998.

Legal category POM.

KETALAR*

Qualitative and quantitative composition Each 1 ml of solution contains: Ketamine Hydrochloride Ph.Eur equivalent to 10 mg, 50 mg and 100 mg Ketamine base per ml.

Pharmaceutical form A clear solution for injection

Clinical particulars

Therapeutic indications: Ketalar is recommended:

1. as the sole anaesthetic agent for diagnostic and surgical procedures. When used by intravenous or intramuscular injection, Ketalar is best suited for short procedures. With additional doses, or by intravenous infusion, Ketalar can be used for longer procedures. If skeletal muscle relaxation is desired, a muscle relaxant should be used and respiration should be supported.
2. for the induction of anaesthesia prior to the administration of other general anaesthetic agents.
3. to supplement other anaesthetic agents.

Specific areas of application or types of procedures:

1. when the intramuscular route of administration is preferred.
2. debridement, painful dressings, and skin grafting in burned patients, as well as other superficial surgical procedures.
3. neurodiagnostic procedures such as pneumoencephalograms, ventriculograms, myelograms, and lumbar punctures.
4. diagnostic and operative procedures of the eye, ear, nose, and mouth, including dental extractions. *Note:* Eye movements may persist during ophthalmological procedures.
5. anaesthesia in poor-risk patients with depression of vital functions or where depression of vital functions must be avoided, if at all possible.
6. orthopaedic procedures such as closed reductions, manipulations, femoral pinning, amputations, and biopsies.
7. sigmoidoscopy and minor surgery of the anus and rectum, circumcision and pilonidal sinus.
8. cardiac catheterisation procedures.
9. Caesarian section; as an induction agent in the absence of elevated blood pressure.
10. anaesthesia in the asthmatic patient, either to minimise the risks of an attack of bronchospasm developing, or in the presence of bronchospasm where anaesthesia cannot be delayed.

Posology and method of administration: For intravenous infusion, intravenous injection or intramuscular injection. **Note**: All doses are given in terms of ketamine base

Adults, elderly (over 65 years) and children: For surgery in elderly patients ketamine has been shown to be suitable either alone or supplemented with other anaesthetic agents.

Preoperative preparations:

1. Ketalar has been safely used alone when the stomach was not empty. However, since the need for supplemental agents and muscle relaxants cannot be predicted, when preparing for elective surgery it is advisable that nothing be given by mouth for at least six hours prior to anaesthesia.
2. Atropine, hyoscine, or another drying agent should be given at an appropriate interval prior to induction.
3. Midazolam, diazepam, lorazepam, or flunitrazepam used as a premedicant or as an adjunct to ketamine, have been effective in reducing the incidence of emergence reactions.

Onset and duration: As with other general anaesthetic agents, the individual response to Ketalar is somewhat varied depending on the dose, route of administration, age of patient, and concomitant use of other agents, so that dosage recommendation cannot be absolutely fixed. The dose should be titrated against the patient's requirements.

Because of rapid induction following intravenous injection, the patient should be in a supported position during administration.

An intravenous dose of 2 mg/kg (1 mg/lb) of bodyweight usually produces surgical anaesthesia within 30 seconds after injection and the anaesthetic effect usually lasts 5 to 10 minutes. An intramuscular dose of 10 mg/kg (5 mg/lb) of body-weight usually produces surgical anaesthesia within 3 to 4 minutes following injection and the anaesthetic effect usually lasts 12 to 25 minutes. Return to consciousness is gradual.

A. Ketalar as the sole anaesthetic agent:

Intravenous infusion: The use of Ketalar by continuous infusion enables the dose to be titrated more closely, thereby reducing the amount of drug administered compared with intermittent administration. This results in a shorter recovery time and better stability of vital signs.

A solution containing 1 mg/ml of ketamine in dextrose 5% or sodium chloride 0.9% is suitable for administration by infusion.

Induction: An infusion corresponding to 0.5–2 mg/kg as total induction dose.

Maintenance of anaesthesia: Anaesthesia may be maintained using a microdrip infusion of 10–45 microgram/kg/min (approximately 1–3 mg/min)

The rate of infusion will depend on the patient's reaction and response to anaesthesia. The dosage required may be reduced when a long acting neuromuscular blocking agent is used.

Intermittent injection:

Induction:

Intravenous route: The initial dose of Ketalar administered intravenously may range from 1 mg/kg to 4.5 mg/kg (0.5 to 2 mg/lb)*. The average amount required to produce 5 to 10 minutes of surgical anaesthesia has been 2.0 mg/kg (1 mg/lb). It is recommended that intravenous administration be accomplished slowly (over a period of 60 seconds). More rapid administration may result in respiratory depression.

Intramuscular route: The initial dose of Ketalar administered intramuscularly may range from 6.5 to 13 mg/kg (3 to 6 mg/lb)*. A low initial intramuscular dose of 4 mg/kg (2 mg/lb) has been used in diagnostic manoeuvres and procedures not involving intensely painful stimuli. A dose of 10 mg/kg (5 mg/lb) will usually produce 12 to 25 minutes of surgical anaesthesia.

Maintenance of anaesthesia: Lightening of anaesthesia may be indicated by nystagmus, movements in response to stimulation, and vocalization. Anaesthesia is maintained by the administration of additional doses of Ketalar by either the intravenous or intramuscular route.

Each additional dose is from ½ to the full induction dose recommended above for the route selected for maintenance, regardless of the route used for induction.

The larger the total amount of Ketalar administered, the longer will be the time to complete recovery.

Purposeless and tonic-clonic movements of extremities may occur during the course of anaesthesia. These movements do not imply a light plane and are not indicative of the need for additional doses of the anaesthetic.

*In terms of ketamine base.

B. Ketalar as induction agent prior to the use of other general anaesthetics: Induction is accomplished by a full intravenous or intramuscular dose of Ketalar as defined above. If Ketalar has been administered intravenously and the principal anaesthetic is slow-acting, a second dose of Ketalar may be required 5 to 8 minutes following the initial dose. If Ketalar has been administered intramuscularly and the principal anaesthetic is rapid-acting, administration of the principal anaesthetic may be delayed up to 15 minutes following the injection of Ketalar.

C. Ketalar as supplement to anaesthetic agents: Ketalar is clinically compatible with the commonly used general and local anaesthetic agents when an adequate respiratory exchange is maintained. The dose of Ketalar for use in conjunction with other anaesthetic agents is usually in the same range as the dosage stated above; however, the use of another anaesthetic agent may allow a reduction in the dose of Ketalar.

D. Management of patients in recovery: Following the procedure the patient should be observed but left undisturbed. This does not preclude the monitoring of vital signs. If, during the recovery, the patient shows any indication of emergence delirium, consideration may be given to the use of diazepam (5 to 10 mg I.V in an adult). A hypnotic dose of a thiobarbiturate (50 to 100 mg I.V) may be used to terminate severe emergence reactions. If any one of these agents is employed, the patient may experience a longer recovery period.

Contra-indications: Ketalar is contra-indicated in persons in whom an elevation of blood pressure would constitute a serious hazard (see Undesirable effects) and in those who have shown hypersensitivity to the drug. Ketalar should not be used in patients with eclampsia or pre-eclampsia.

Special warnings and special precautions for use:

1. To be used only in hospitals by or under the supervision of experienced medically qualified anaesthetists except under emergency conditions.
2. As with any general anaesthetic agent, resuscitative equipment should be available and ready for use.
3. Emergence delirium phenomena may occur during the recovery period. The incidence of these reactions may be reduced if verbal and tactile stimulation of the patient is minimised during the recovery period. This does not preclude the monitoring of vital signs.
4. Because pharyngeal and laryngeal reflexes usually remain active, mechanical stimulation of the pharynx should be avoided unless muscle relaxants, with proper attention to respiration, are used.
5. Although aspiration of contrast medium has been reported during Ketalar anaesthesia under experimental conditions (Taylor, P A and Towey, R M, Brit. Med. J. 1971, 2: 688) in clinical practice aspiration is seldom a problem.
6. Cardiac function should be continually monitored during the procedure in patients found to have hypertension or cardiac decompensation.
7. Since an increase in cerebrospinal fluid pressure has been reported during Ketalar anaesthesia, Ketalar should be used with special caution in patients with preanaesthetic elevated cerebrospinal fluid pressure.
8. Respiratory depression may occur with overdosage of Ketalar, in which case supportive ventilation should be employed. Mechanical support of respiration is preferred to the administration of analeptics.
9. The intravenous dose should be administered over a period of 60 seconds. More rapid administration may result in transient respiratory depression or apnoea.
10. In surgical procedures involving visceral pain pathways, Ketalar should be supplemented with an agent which obtunds visceral pain.
11. Use with caution in the chronic alcoholic and the acutely alcohol- intoxicated patient.
14. When Ketalar is used on an outpatient basis, the patient should not be released until recovery from anaesthesia is complete and then should be accompanied by a responsible adult.

Interaction with other medicaments and other forms of interaction: Prolonged recovery time may occur if barbiturates and/or narcotics are used concurrently with Ketalar.

Ketalar is chemically incompatible with barbiturates because of precipitate formation. Therefore, these should not be mixed in the same syringe or infusion fluid.

Pregnancy and lactation: Ketalar crosses the placenta. This should be borne in mind during operative obstetric procedures in pregnancy.

With the exception of administration during surgery for abdominal delivery or vaginal delivery, no controlled studies in pregnancy have been conducted. The safe use in pregnancy has not been established and such use is not recommended.

Effects on ability to drive and use machines: Patients should be cautioned that driving a car, operating hazardous machinery or engaging in hazardous activities should not be undertaken for 24 hours or more after anaesthesia.

Undesirable effects:

Cardiovascular: Temporary elevation of blood pressure and pulse rate is frequently observed following administration of ketamine hydrochloride. However, hypotension and bradycardia have been reported. Arrhythmia has also occurred. The medium peak rise of blood pressure has ranged from 20 to 25 per cent of preanaesthetic values. Depending on the condition of the patient, this elevation of blood pressure may be considered an adverse reaction or a beneficial effect.

Respiratory: Depression of respiration or apnoea may occur following over rapid intravenous administration or high doses of ketamine hydrochloride. Laryngospasm and other forms of airway obstruction have occurred during ketamine hydrochloride anaesthesia.

Ocular: Diplopia and nystagmus may occur following ketamine hydrochloride administration. A slight elevation in intraocular pressure may also occur.

Psychological: During recovery from anaesthesia the patient may experience emergence delirium, characterised by vivid dreams (pleasant or unpleasant), with or without psychomotor activity, manifested by confusion and irrational behaviour. The fact that these reactions are observed less often in the young (15 years of age or less) makes Ketalar especially useful in paediatric anaesthesia. These reactions are also less frequent in the elderly (over 65 years of age) patient. The incidence of emergence reactions is reduced as experience with the drug is gained. No residual psychological effects are known to have resulted from the use of Ketalar.

Neurological: In some patients, enhanced skeletal muscle tone may be manifested by tonic and clonic movements sometimes resembling seizures. These movements do not imply a light plane of anaesthesia and are not indicative of a need for additional doses of the anaesthetic.

Gastrointestinal: Anorexia, nausea, and vomiting have been observed; however, these are minimal and are not usually severe. The great majority of patients are able to take liquids by mouth shortly after regaining consciousness.

Other: Local pain and exanthema at the injection site have infrequently been reported. Transient erythema and/or morbilliform rash have also been reported. Increased salivation leading to respiratory difficulties may occur unless an antisialogogue is used.

Overdose: Respiratory depression can result from an overdosage of ketamine hydrochloride. Supportive ventilation should be employed. Mechanical support of respiration that will maintain adequate blood oxygen saturation and carbon dioxide elimination is preferred to administration of analeptics.

Ketalar has a wide margin of safety; several instances of unintentional administration of overdoses of Ketalar (up to 10 times that usually required) have been followed by prolonged but complete recovery.

Pharmacological properties

Pharmacodynamic properties: Ketamine is a rapidly acting general anaesthetic for intravenous or intramuscular use with a distinct pharmacological action. Ketamine hydrochloride produces dissociative anaesthesia characterised by catalepsy, amnesia and marked analgesia, which may persist into the recovery period.

Pharmacokinetic properties: Ketamine is rapidly distributed into perfused tissues including brain and placenta. Animal studies have shown ketamine to be highly concentrated in body fat, liver and lung. Biotransformation takes place in liver. Termination of anaesthetic is partly by redistribution from brain to other tissues and partly by metabolism. Elimination half-life is approximately 2-3 hours, and excretion renal, mostly as conjugated metabolites.

Preclinical safety data: Preclinical safety data does not add anything of further significance to the prescriber.

Pharmaceutical particulars

List of excipients: All strengths contain: Benzethonium chloride and water for injection Ketalar 10 mg/ml vials also contain Sodium chloride.

Incompatibilities: Ketalar is chemically incompatible with barbiturates because of precipitate formation. Therefore, these should not be mixed in the same syringe or infusion fluid.

Shelf life: 3 years

Special precautions for storage: Store at a temperature not exceeding 25°C. Protect from light. Do not freeze. Discard any unused product at the end of each operating session.

Nature and contents of container: 20 ml white neutral glass vial with rubber closure and aluminium flip-off cap containing 10 mg Ketamine base per ml. 12 ml vials containing 10 ml of solution as 50 mg Ketamine base per ml. 12 ml vials containing 10 ml of solution as 100 mg Ketamine base per ml.

Instructions for use/handling: See *Incompatibilities.*

Marketing authorisation numbers

Ketalar 10 mg per ml	PL 0019/0118
Ketalar 50 mg per ml	PL 0019/0119
Ketalar 100 mg per ml	PL 0019/0120

Date of renewal of authorisation 31st October 1997.

Date of revision 14 July 1998.

Legal category POM.

LENTIZOL*

Qualitative and quantitative composition Lentizol 50 mg is supplied in white pellets in a size 2 capsule with a pink body and a red cap radially marked LENTIZOL 50, each capsule contains Amitriptyline Hydrochloride BP 50 mg.

Lentizol 25 mg is supplied in white pellets in a size 3 all-pink capsule radially marked LENTIZOL 25, each capsule contains Amitriptyline Hydrochloride BP 25 mg.

Pharmaceutical form Oral capsules.

Clinical particulars

Therapeutic indications: Symptoms of depressive illness especially where sedation is required.

Posology and method of administration: Oral administration.

Adults and adolescents over 16 years old: Initially 50-100 mg as a single dose at night, increasing to 200 mg/day according to clinical response. Once a satisfactory response has been obtained, the dosage should be reduced to the lowest dose that will maintain the symptomatic benefit. The usual maintenance dose is 50 -100 mg as a single dose at night.

Elderly (over 65 years): Initially 25-75 mg a day. Since the elderly are particularly prone to experience adverse effects such as agitation, confusion and postural hypotension; the initial dose should only be increased with caution under close medical supervision. Half the normal maintenance dose may be sufficient to produce a satisfactory clinical response.

Children (under 16 years): Not recommended.

Contra-indications: Recent cardiac infarction and patients with any degree of heart block or disorders of cardiac rhythm and those suffering from coronary artery insufficiency. Patients with mania, severe liver disease, or known hypersensitivity to dibenzazepines. Co-administration with monoamine oxidase inhibitors. Lactation. Porphyria.

Special warnings and special precautions for use: As improvement may not occur during the first 2-4 weeks of treatment, patients should be closely monitored during this period especially those posing a high suicidal risk.

Cardiac arrhythmias and severe hypotension are likely to occur with high dosage or in deliberate overdosage. They may also occur in patients with pre-existing heart disease taking normal dosage.

Unless essential it is inadvisable to combine Lentizol with ECT.

When Lentizol is used for the depressive component of schizophrenia, psychotic symptoms may be aggravated. In manic-depressives, a shift towards the manic phase may occur; paranoid delusions, with or without associated hostility, may be aggravated.

Avoid if possible in patients with a history of urinary retention, narrow angle glaucoma, impaired liver function, or increased ocular pressure, symptoms suggestive of prostatic hypertrophy and a history of epilepsy. Lentizol should be used with caution in hyperthyroid patients.

Anaesthetics given during tri/tetracyclic antidepressant therapy may increase the risk of arrhythmias and hypotension.

If possible, discontinue Lentizol several days before surgery; if emergency surgery is unavoidable, the anaesthetist should be informed that the patient is being so treated.

Hyperpyrexia has been reported with tricyclic antidepressants when administered with anticholinergic or with neuroleptic medications.

Abrupt withdrawal of Lentizol should be avoided.

Interaction with other medicaments and other forms of interaction: Lentizol should not be administered concurrently, or within 14 days of termination of treatment with MAO inhibitors. It should not be given with sympathomimetic agents such as adrenaline, ephedrine, isoprenaline, noradrenaline, phenylephrine, and phenylpropanolamine, and should be used with caution when administered concurrently with anticholinergic drugs, or thyroid medications.

Lentizol may counteract the effect of adrenergic neurone blocking agents, and possibly clonidine, and therefore it would be advisable to review all antihypertensive therapy during treatment.

The action of Lentizol may be decreased by barbiturates, and potentiated by methylphenidate. Lentizol may enhance the response to alcohol, barbiturates and other CNS depressants.

Cimetidine is reported to reduce hepatic metabolism of certain tricyclic antidepressants.

Delirium has been reported in patients taking amitriptyline with disulfiram.

Pregnancy and lactation: Do not use during pregnancy, especially during the first and last trimesters, unless there are compelling reasons. There is no, or inadequate, evidence of safety of the drug in human pregnancy. There is evidence of harmful effects in pregnancy in animals, when given in exceptionally high doses.

Adverse effects such as withdrawal symptoms, respiratory depression and agitation have been reported in neonates whose mothers had taken amitriptyline during the last trimester of pregnancy.

Amitriptyline is detectable in breast milk. Because of the potential for serious adverse reactions in infants from amitriptyline, Lentizol should not be given to mothers during breast-feeding. A decision should be made whether to discontinue breast-feeding or discontinue the drug.

Effects on ability to drive and use machines: Amitriptyline may initially impair alertness and also potentiate the CNS depressant effects of alcohol. Patients should be warned of the possible hazard when driving or operating machinery. This can usually be controlled by reducing the dose. If necessary the dose can be subsequently increased gradually.

Undesirable effects: The following adverse effects, although not necessarily all reported with amitriptyline, have occurred with tricyclic antidepressants.

Anticholinergic: Excessive perspiration, dryness of mouth, blurred vision, mydriasis, disturbed accommodation, increased intraocular pressure, hyperpyrexia, urinary retention, and urinary tract dilatation. These symptoms are common but usually lessen on continuing therapy.

Cardiovascular reactions: Hypotension, syncope, postural hypotension, hypertension, tachycardia, palpitations, myocardial infarction, arrhythmias, heart block, stroke, non-specific ECG and AV conduction changes.

CNS and neuromuscular: Confusional states, disturbed concentration, disorientation, delusions, hallucinations, hypomania, excitement, anxiety, restlessness, drowsiness, insomnia, nightmares, numbness, tingling, and paraesthesiae of the extremities, peripheral neuropathy, incoordination, ataxia, tremors, coma, convulsions, alteration of EEG, extrapyramidal symptoms, including abnormal involuntary movements and tardive dyskinesia, dysarthria, tinnitus, dizziness, weakness, fatigue, headache.

Allergic: Skin rash, urticaria, photosensitisation, oedema of face and tongue.

Haematological: Bone-marrow depression including agranulocytosis, leucopenia, eosinophilia, purpura, thrombocytopenia.

Gastrointestinal: Nausea, epigastric distress, vomiting, anorexia, stomatitis, unpleasant taste, diarrhoea, weight loss, increased appetite and weight gain (may be a drug reaction or due to relief of the depression), parotid swelling, black tongue, rarely hepatitis (including altered liver function and cholestatic jaundice) constipation, paralytic ileus.

Endocrine: Testicular swelling, gynaecomastia, breast enlargement, galactorrhoea, increased or decreased libido, impotence, interference with sexual function, elevation or lowering of blood sugar levels, inappropriate ADH (antidiuretic hormone) secretion.

Other: Oedema, urinary frequency, alopecia

Withdrawal symptoms may occur on abrupt cessation of therapy and include insomnia, irritability, nausea, headache and excessive perspiration.

Mania or hypomania has been reported rarely within 2–7 days of stopping chronic therapy with tricyclic antidepressants.

Overdose: Amitriptyline exerts an anticholinergic effect as well as antihistamine and adrenaline blocking actions. Large doses produce temporary confusion, disturbed concentration, transient visual hallucinations, drowsiness, hypothermia, convulsions, coma, apnoea, tachycardia and other rhythm dysfunctions such as bundle branch block, ECG evidence of impaired conduction, congestive heart failure, dilated pupils, disorders of ocular motility, severe hypotension, stupor, polyradiculoneuropathy, and intestinal stasis.

Other symptoms may be agitation, hyperactive reflexes, muscle rigidity, vomiting, hyperpyrexia, or any of those listed as adverse effects.

Treatment: Gastric lavage and emesis if appropriate. Following lavage, activated charcoal may be given during the first 24–48 hours at a dosage of 20–30 g every four to six hours. Vital signs should be continuously monitored and patients should be treated in hospital wherever possible. General supportive measures should be initiated with careful attention to electrolyte balance. An ECG should be taken and close monitoring of cardiac function instituted if there is any sign of abnormality. Cardiac irregularities may need controlling with antiarrhythmic drugs and physostigmine salicylate may be indicated. If convulsions occur, paraldelyde, diazepam or inhalation anaesthetics, but not barbiturates, may be indicated. Forced diuresis and haemodialysis have no place in treatment. An open airway and an adequate fluid intake should be maintained, and body temperature regulated.

Pharmacological properties

Pharmacodynamic properties: Amitriptyline is a tricyclic antidepressant. It prevents re-uptake and hence inactivation of noradrenaline and serotonin at nerve terminals. The precise mechanism by which an antidepressant effect is achieved remains unclear.

Pharmacokinetic properties: After release from Lentizol capsules, amitriptyline is readily absorbed from the gastro-intestinal tract. Peak serum levels are reached between 6 and 12 hours after administration of Lentizol.

Amitriptyline is extensively demethylated in the liver to its primary active metabolite, nortriptyline. Paths of metabolism of both amitriptyline and nortriptyline include hydroxylation (possibly to active metabolites), n-oxidation, and conjugation with glucuronic acid. Amitriptyline is excreted in the urine, mainly in the form of its metabolites, either free or in conjugated form. Amitriptyline and nortriptyline are widely distributed throughout the body and are extensively bound to plasma and tissue protein. Amitriptyline has been estimated to have a half-life ranging from 9 to 25 hours, which may be considerably extended in overdosage. Plasma concentrations of amitriptyline and nortriptyline vary very widely between individuals and simple correlation with therapeutic reponse has been established. Amitriptyline and nortriptyline cross the placental barrier and are excreted in breast milk.

Preclinical safety data: Pre-clinical safety data does not add anything of further significance to the prescriber.

Pharmaceutical particulars

List of excipients: Lentizol 50 mg capsules contain the following excipients–Active pellets: Sucrose, maize starch, stearic acid, diffulac (shellac), povidone and talc. Neutral pellets: Sucrose, maize starch, stearic acid, talc and diffulac (shellac). Gelatin capsule shell: E127, E132, E122.

Lentizol 25 mg capsules contain the following excipients - Active pellets: Sucrose, maize starch, stearic acid, diffulac (shellac), povidone and talc. Neutral pellets: Sucrose, maize starch, stearic acid, talc and diffulac (shellac). Gelatin capsule shell: E127, E132.

Incompatibilities: Not applicable.

Shelf life: Two years.

Special precautions for storage: Store in a dry place, at a temperature not exceeding 30°C.

Nature and contents of container: PVC/PVdC blister pack, containing 56 capsules.

Instructions for use/handling: No special requirements.

Marketing authorisation numbers

Lentizol 50 mg PL 0019/0140
Lentizol 25 mg PL 0019/0139

Date of revision October 1997

Legal category POM

LIPITOR* 

Qualitative and quantitative composition Lipitor Tablets contain atorvastatin calcium (trihydrate) equivalent to 10, 20 and 40 mg atorvastatin per tablet.

Pharmaceutical form Lipitor is supplied as 10, 20, and 40 mg film-coated tablets for oral administration.

Clinical particulars

Therapeutic indications: Lipitor is indicated as an adjunct to diet for reduction of elevated total cholesterol, LDL-cholesterol, apolipoprotein B and triglycerides in patients with primary hypercholesterolaemia, heterozygous familial hypercholesterolaemia or combined (mixed) hyperlipidaemia when response to diet and other nonpharmacological measures is inadequate.

Lipitor is also indicated as an adjunct to diet and other non-dietary measures in reducing elevated total cholesterol, LDL-cholesterol and apolipoprotein B in patients with homozygous familial hypercholesterolaemia when response to these measures is inadequate.

Posology and method of administration: The patient should be placed on a standard cholesterol-lowering diet before receiving Lipitor and should continue on this diet during treatment with Lipitor. The usual starting dose is 10 mg once a day. Doses should be individualised according to baseline LDL-C levels, the goal of therapy and patient response. Adjustment of dosage should be made at intervals of 4 weeks or more. The maximum dose is 80 mg once a day. Doses may be given at any time of day with or without food.

Primary hypercholesterolaemia and combined (mixed) hyperlipidaemia: The majority of patients are controlled with 10 mg Lipitor once a day. A therapeutic response is evident within 2 weeks and the maximum response is usually achieved within 4 weeks. The response is maintained during chronic therapy.

The following treatment guidelines may be used to establish treatment goals (Table 1).

TABLE 1. European Atherosclerosis Society Treatment Goals for Lipid Management

Patient Population		*Treatment Goal mg/dL*	*mmol/L*
No risk factors and no CHD	LDL-C	155-175	4-4.5
One risk factor and no CHD	LDL-C	135-155	3.5-4
Two or more risk factors, CHD, PVD, or famililal hypercholesterolaemia	LDL-C	115-135	3-3.5

CHD = Coronary heart disease; PVD = Peripheral vascular disease.

Heterozygous familial hypercholesterolaemia: Patients should be started with Lipitor 10 mg daily. Doses should be individualised and adjusted every 4 weeks to 40 mg daily. Thereafter, either the dose may be increased to a maximum of 80 mg daily or a bile acid sequestrant (eg, colestipol) may be combined with 40 mg Lipitor.

Homozygous familial hypercholesterolaemia: Adults: In a compassionate-use study of patients with homozygous familial hypercholesterolaemia, most patients responded to a dose of 80 mg of Lipitor (see *Pharmacodynamic properties*).

Children: Treatment experience in a paediatric population with doses of Lipitor up to 80 mg/day is limited.

Dosage in patients with renal insufficiency: Renal disease has no influence on the plasma concentrations nor lipid effects of Lipitor; thus, no adjustment of dose is required.

Dosage in patients with hepatic dysfunction: In patients with moderate to severe hepatic dysfunction, the therapeutic response to Lipitor is unaffected but exposure to the drug is greatly increased. Cmax increases by approximately 16 fold and AUC (0-24) by approximately 11 fold. Therefore, caution should be exercised in patients who consume substantial quantities of alcohol and/or have a history of liver disease.

Geriatric use: Adequate treatment experience in adults age 70 or older with doses of Lipitor up to 80 mg/day has been obtained. Efficacy and safety in older patients using recommended doses is similar to that seen in the general population.

Contra-indications: Lipitor is contra-indicated in patients with hypersensitivity to any component of this medication, active liver disease or unexplained persistent elevations of serum transaminases exceeding 3 times the upper limit of normal, during pregnancy, while breast-feeding, and in women of child-bearing potential not using appropriate contraceptive measures.

Special warnings and special precautions for use: Liver effects: Liver function tests should be performed before the initiation of treatment and periodically thereafter. Patients who develop any signs or symptoms suggestive of liver injury should have liver function tests performed. Patients who develop increased transaminase levels should be monitored until the abnormality(ies) resolve. Should an increase in ALT or AST of greater than 3 times the upper limit of normal persist, reduction of dose or withdrawal of Lipitor is recommended.

Lipitor should be used with caution in patients who consume substantial quantities of alcohol and/or have a history of liver disease.

Skeletal muscle effects: Uncomplicated myalgia has been reported in Lipitor-treated patients. Lipitor therapy should be discontinued if markedly elevated CPK levels occur or myopathy is diagnosed or suspected. Patients who develop any signs or symptoms suggestive of myopathy should have CPK levels measured. Should significant increases in CPK persist, reduction of dose or withdrawal of Lipitor is recommended.

These CPK elevations should be considered when evaluating the possibility of myocardial infarction in the differential diagnosis of chest pain.

Rhabdomyolysis with renal dysfunction secondary to myoglobinuria has been reported with other drugs in this class.

Interaction with other medicaments and other forms of interaction: The risk of myopathy during treatment with other drugs in this class is increased with concurrent administration of cyclosporin, fibric acid derivatives, erythromycin, azole antifungals, or niacin. This increase in risk may also occur when combining these drugs with Lipitor.

Phenazone (antipyrine) is a non-specific model for evaluation of drug metabolism by the hepatic microsomal enzyme system. Administration of multiple doses of Lipitor with phenazone showed little or no detectable effect on the pharmacokinetics of phenazone in healthy subjects (no change in the clearance of phenazone but the formation clearance of 4-hydroxyphenazone increased by 20% and that of norphenazone by 8%).

More specific *in vitro* studies using human hepatic microsomes and cells expressing human cytochrome P450 isozymes show that atorvastatin, like other HMG-CoA reductase inhibitors, is metabolised by cytochrome P450 3A4 indicating the possibility of an interaction with drugs also metabolised by this isozyme. When combining Lipitor with other drugs which are the substrate of this isozyme (eg, immunomodulators, many antiarrhythmic agents, some calcium channel antagonists and some benzodiazepines) the possibility of a change in the plasma drug levels of either drug should be considered. In clinical studies in which Lipitor was administered with antihypertensives (including ACE inhibitors, beta-blockers, calcium channel antagonists, and diuretics) or hypoglycaemic agents no clinically significant interactions were seen.

Based on experience with other HMG-CoA reductase inhibitors caution should also be exercised when Lipitor is administered with inhibitors of cytochrome P450 3A4 (eg, macrolide antibiotics and azole antifungals). The effect of inducers of cytochrome P450 3A4 (eg, rifampicin or phenytoin) on Lipitor is unknown.

Digoxin: Administration of multiple doses of Lipitor with digoxin increased steady-state plasma digoxin concentrations by approximately 20%. Patients taking digoxin should be monitored appropriately.

Erythromycin: In healthy individuals, administration of Lipitor with erythromycin (500 mg QID), a known inhibitor of cytochrome P450 3A4, was associated with higher plasma concentrations of atorvastatin.

Oral contraceptives: Administration of Lipitor with an oral contraceptive containing norethisterone and ethinyl oestradiol produced increases in plasma concentrations of norethisterone and ethinyl oestradiol. These increased concentrations should be considered when selecting oral contraceptive doses.

Colestipol: Plasma concentrations of atorvastatin were lower (approximately 25%) when colestipol was administered with Lipitor. However, lipid effects were greater when Lipitor and colestipol were administered together than when either drug was given alone.

Antacid: Administration of Lipitor with an oral antacid suspension containing magnesium and aluminium hydroxides decreased atorvastatin plasma concentrations approximately 35%; however, LDL-C reduction was not altered.

Warfarin: Administration of Lipitor with warfarin caused a minimal decrease in prothrombin time (mean ± SE of 1.7±0.4 seconds) during the first 4 days of dosing with 80 mg Lipitor. Dosing continued for 15 days and prothrombin time returned to normal by the end of Lipitor treatment. Nevertheless, patients receiving warfarin should be closely monitored when Lipitor is added to their therapy.

Cimetidine: An interaction study with cimetidine and Lipitor was conducted, and no interaction was seen.

Pregnancy and lactation: Lipitor is contraindicated in pregnancy and while breast-feeding. Women of child-bearing potential should use appropriate contraceptive measures. An interval of 1 month should be allowed from stopping Lipitor treatment to conception in the event of planning a pregnancy.

In animal studies atorvastatin had no effect on fertility and was not teratogenic, however, at maternally toxic doses foetal toxicity was observed in rats and rabbits. The development of the rat offspring was delayed and post-natal survival reduced during exposure of the dams to atorvastatin equivalent to 6 and 21 times that expected in man, respectively.

In rats, plasma concentrations of atorvastatin are similar to those in milk. It is not known whether this drug or its metabolites is excreted in human milk.

Effects on ability to drive and use machines: There is no pattern of reported adverse events suggesting that patients taking Lipitor will have any impairment of ability to drive and use hazardous machinery.

Undesirable effects: Lipitor is generally well tolerated. Adverse reactions have usually been mild and transient. Less than 2% of patients were discontinued from clinical trials due to side effects attributed to Lipitor.

The most frequent (1% or more) adverse effects associated with Lipitor therapy, in patients participating in controlled clinical studies are constipation, flatulence, dyspepsia, abdominal pain, headache, nausea, myalgia, asthenia, diarrhoea and insomnia.

Elevated serum ALT levels have been reported in 1.3% of patients receiving Lipitor. Clinically important (>3 times upper normal limit) elevations in serum ALT levels occurred in 19 of the 2483 (0.8%) patients on Lipitor. It was dose related and was reversible in all 19 patients. In 10 cases, the increase was first observed within 12 weeks of starting the treatment. Only 1 case occurred after 36 weeks and only 1 patient had symptoms suggestive of hepatitis. Treatment was discontinued in only 9 of these 19 cases.

Elevated serum CPK levels (>3 times upper normal limit) occurred in 62 of the 2452 (2.5%) patients on Lipitor compared with 3.1% with other HMG-CoA reductase inhibitors in clinical trials. Levels above 10 times the normal upper range occurred in only 11 (0.4%) Lipitor-treated patients. Only 3 (0.1%) of these 11 patients had concurrent muscle pain, tenderness or weakness.

The following additional adverse effects have been reported in clinical trials. Not all effects listed have necessarily been associated with Lipitor therapy: angioneurotic oedema, muscle cramps, myositis, myopathy, paraesthesia, peripheral neuropathy, pancreatitis, hepatitis, cholestatic jaundice, anorexia, vomiting, alopecia, pruritus, rash, impotence, hyperglycaemia and hypoglycaemia. Chest pain, dizziness, angina, and allergic reactions have also been reported in isolated cases.

Overdose: Specific treatment is not available for Lipitor overdosage. Should an overdose occur, the patient should be treated symptomatically and supportive measures instituted as required. Liver function tests and serum CPK levels should be monitored. Due to extensive drug binding to plasma proteins, haemodialysis is not expected to significantly enhance atorvastatin clearance.

Pharmacological properties

Pharmacodynamic properties: Atorvastatin is a selective, competitive inhibitor of HMG-CoA reductase, the rate-limiting enzyme responsible for the conversion of 3-hydroxy-3-methyl-glutaryl-coenzyme A to mevalonate, a precursor of sterols, including cholesterol. Triglycerides and cholesterol in the liver are incorporated into VLDL and released into the plasma for delivery to peripheral tissues. Low-density lipoprotein (LDL) is formed from VLDL and is catabolised primarily through the high affinity LDL receptor.

Atorvastatin lowers plasma cholesterol and lipoprotein levels by inhibiting HMG-CoA reductase and cholesterol synthesis in the liver and increases the number of hepatic LDL receptors on the cell surface for enhanced uptake and catabolism of LDL.

Atorvastatin reduces LDL production and the number of LDL particles. Atorvastatin produces a profound and sustained increase in LDL receptor activity coupled with a beneficial change in the quality of circulating LDL particles.

Approximately 70% of circulating inhibitory activity for HMG-CoA reductase is attributed to active metabolites (see Pharmacokinetic Properties).

Atorvastatin has been shown to reduce total-C, LDL-C, apolipoprotein B and triglycerides while producing variable increases in HDL-C in a dose-response study as shown in Table 2 below.

TABLE 2. Dose Response in Patients With Primary Hypercholesterolaemia

Lipitor Dose (mg)	*N*	*Total-C*	*LDL-C*	*Apo B*	*TG*	*HDL-C*
Placebo	12	5	8	6	-1	-2
10	11	-30	-41	-34	-14	4
20	10	-35	-44	-36	-33	12
40	11	-38	-50	-41	-25	-3
80	11	-46	-61	-50	-27	3

Adjusted mean % change from baseline

These results are consistent in patients with heterozygous familial hypercholesterolaemia, nonfamilial forms of hypercholesterolaemia and mixed hyperlipidaemia, including patients with noninsulin-dependent diabetes mellitus.

Atorvastatin produced a variable but small increase in apolipoprotein AI. However, there was no clear dose response effect.

Lipitor is effective in reducing LDL-C in patients with homozygous familial hypercholesterolaemia, a population that has not usually responded to lipid-lowering medication. In a compassionate use study, 41 patients aged 6 to 51 years with homozygous familial hypercholesterolaemia or with severe hypercholesterolaemia, who had ≤15% reduction in LDL-C in response to previous maximum dose combination drug therapy, received daily doses of 40 to 80 mg of Lipitor. Twenty four patients with homozygous familial hypercholesterolaemia received 80 mg Lipitor. Nineteen of these 24 patients responded with a greater than 15% reduction of LDL-C (mean 26%, range 18% to 42%).

Pharmacokinetic properties:

Absorption: Atorvastatin is rapidly absorbed after oral administration; maximum plasma concentrations occur within 1 to 2 hours. Extent of absorption increases in proportion to atorvastatin dose. Lipitor tablets are bioequivalent to atorvastatin solutions. The absolute bioavailability of atorvastatin is approximately 12% and the systemic availability of HMG-CoA reductase inhibitory activity is approximately 30%. The low systemic availability is attributed to presystemic clearance in gastrointestinal mucosa and/or hepatic first-pass metabolism.

Distribution: Mean volume of distribution of atorvastatin is approximately 565 L. Atorvastatin is ≥98% bound to plasma proteins.

Metabolism: Atorvastatin is metabolised by cytochrome P450 3A4 to ortho- and parahydroxylated derivatives and various beta-oxidation products. In-vitro, inhibition of HMG-CoA reductase by ortho- and parahydroxylated metabolites is equivalent to that of atorvastatin. Approximately 70% of circulating inhibitory activity for HMG-CoA reductase is attributed to active metabolites.

Excretion: Atorvastatin is eliminated primarily in bile following hepatic and/or extrahepatic metabolism. However, the drug does not appear to undergo significant enterohepatic recirculation. Mean plasma elimination half-life of atorvastatin in humans is approximately 14 hours. The half-life of inhibitory activity for HMG-CoA reductase is approximately 20 to 30 hours due to the contribution of active metabolites.

Special populations:

Geriatric: Plasma concentrations of atorvastatin are higher in healthy elderly subjects than in young adults while the lipid effects were comparable to those seen in younger patient populations.

Paediatric: Pharmacokinetic data in the paediatric population are not available.

Gender: Concentrations of atorvastatin in women differ (approximately 20% higher for Cmax and 10% lower for AUC) from those in men. These differences were of no clinical significance, resulting in no clinically significant differences in lipid effects among men and women.

Renal insufficiency: Renal disease has no influence on the plasma concentrations or lipid effects of atorvastatin.

Hepatic insufficiency: Plasma concentrations of atorvastatin are markedly increased (approximately 16-fold in Cmax and 11-fold in AUC) in patients with chronic alcoholic liver disease (Childs-Pugh B).

Preclinical safety data: Atorvastatin was not carcinogenic in rats. The maximum dose used was 63-fold higher than the highest human dose (80 mg/day) on a mg/kg body-weight basis and 8 to 16-fold higher based on AUC (0-24) values as determined by total inhibitory activity. In a 2-year study in mice, incidences of hepatocellular adenoma in males and hepatocellular carcinomas in females were increased at the maximum dose used, and the maximum dose used was 250-fold higher than the highest human dose on a mg/kg body-weight basis. Systemic exposure was 6 to 11-fold higher based on AUC (0-24). Atorvastatin did not demonstrate mutagenic or clastogenic potential in 4 in-vitro tests with and without metabolic activation and in 1 in-vivo assay.

Pharmaceutical particulars

List of excipients: The 10, 20, and 40 mg dosage forms each contain the following excipients: Calcium Carbonate, Microcrystalline Cellulose, Lactose (Hydrous), Croscarmellose Sodium, Polysorbate 80, Hydroxypropyl Cellulose, Magnesium Stearate, Opadry White YS-1-7040 (Hydroxypropyl methylcellulose, Polyethylene glycol, Titanium dioxide, Talc), Simethicone Emulsion (Simethicone, Stearate emulsifiers, Sorbic acid, Water), Candelilla Wax

Incompatibilities: None.

Shelf life: Two years.

Special precautions for storage: None.

Nature and contents of container: Foil/foil blisters consisting of a polyamide/aluminium foil/polyvinyl chloride unit-dose blister and a paper/polyester/aluminium foil/vinyl heat-seal coated backing or an aluminium foil/vinyl heat-seal coated backing.

Lipitor is supplied in packs of 28 tablets.

Instructions for use/handling: No special requirements needed.

Marketing authorisation numbers

Lipitor Tablets 10 mg	PL16051/0001
Lipitor Tablets 20 mg	PL16051/0002
Lipitor Tablets 40 mg	PL16051/0003

Date of first authorisation August 1997.

Date of revision August 1997.

Legal category POM.

LOESTRIN*

Qualitative and quantitative composition Each Loestrin 20 tablet contains: Norethisterone Acetate Ph Eur 1 mg and Ethinyloestradiol Ph Eur 20 microgrammes.

Each Loestrin 30 tablet contains Norethisterone Acetate BP 1.5 mg and Ethinyloestradiol Ph Eur 30 microgrammes.

Pharmaceutical form Loestrin 20: Blue convex film coated tablet. Loestrin 30: Pale green convex film coated tablet.

Clinical particulars

Therapeutic indications: For the prevention of pregnancy in women who elect to use oral contraceptives. The efficacy of any contraceptive method, except sterilisation, depends on the reliability with which it is used. Correct and consistent use of methods can result in lower failure rates.

Posology and method of administration: For Oral administration.

One Loestrin tablet should be taken daily at approximately the same time of day for three weeks, starting on the first day of menstrual bleeding, and then an interval of one week allowed before commencing the second course of tablets. If starting on the fourth day of the cycle or later, additional contraceptive precautions should be used for the first seven days. Second and subsequent courses should be taken for three weeks with one week without tablets between courses. Thus each new course of tablets is always started on the same day of the week. It is important that the tablets are taken as directed and should be taken without regard to menstrual bleeding except in the initial cycle.

Missed pills: If a tablet is not taken at the usual time, it must be taken as soon as possible and the next tablet taken at the normal time. If the delay exceeds twelve hours, additional contraception (barriers and spermicides) should be used for the next 7 days whilst continuing to take Loestrin. Additionally, if pills have been missed during the last 7 days of a pack, there should be no break before the next pack is started.

Gastrointestinal upset: Vomiting or diarrhoea may reduce efficacy by preventing full absorption. Barriers and spermicides should therefore be used during and for 7 days after recovery and if these 7 days overrun the end of a pack, the next pack should be started without a break. In this case, a withdrawal bleed should not be expected until the end of the second pack. If the patient does not have a withdrawal bleed at the end of the second pack, she must return to the doctor to exclude the possibility of pregnancy.

Changing from another 21 day combined oral contraceptive to Loestrin: The first Loestrin tablet should be taken on the first day immediately after the end of the previous oral contraceptive course. Additional contraception is not required. A withdrawal bleed should not be expected until the end of the first Loestrin pack.

Changing from an every day (ED) 28 day combined oral contraceptive to Loestrin: The first tablet of Loestrin should be taken on the day immediately after the day on which the last active pill in the ED pack has been taken. The remaining (inactive) tablets in the ED pack should be discarded. Additional contraception is not required. A withdrawal bleed should not be expected until the end of the first pack of Loestrin.

Changing from a progestogen-only-pill (POP) to Loestrin: The first tablet of Loestrin should be taken on the first day of menstruation, even if the POP for that day has already been taken. The remaining tablets in the POP pack should be discarded. Additional contraception is not required.

Post-partum and post-abortum use: After pregnancy combined oral contraception can be started in non-lactating women 21 days after a vaginal delivery, provided that the patient is fully ambulant and there are no puerperal complications.

If the pill is started later than 21 days after delivery, then barriers and spermicides should be used until oral contraception is started and for the first 7 days of pill-taking. If unprotected intercourse has taken place after 21 days post partum, then oral contraception should not be started until the first menstrual bleed after childbirth.

After a miscarriage or abortion, oral contraceptives may be started immediately.

Contra-indications:

1. Known or suspected pregnancy and lactation.
2. Thrombo-embolic disorders, or a past history of these conditions, ischaemic heart disease, severe hypertension or coagulation abnormalities.
3. Liver disease including disorders of hepatic excretion e.g. Dublin Johnson or Rotor syndromes, infective hepatitis (until liver function returns to normal), known or suspected disorders of lipid metabolism, porphyria, liver adenoma or carcinoma, gall stones or jaundice with prior pill use.
4. Sickle cell anaemia.
5. Known or suspected carcinoma of the breast or oestrogen dependent neoplasms.
6. Undiagnosed abnormal vaginal bleeding
7. History during pregnancy of idiopathic jaundice, severe pruritus, chorea, herpes or deterioration of otosclerosis.
8. Focal, severe or crescendo migraine or transient cerebral ischaemic attacks without headaches.

Special warnings and special precautions for use: The following information is principally based on studies in patients who used oral contraceptives with higher concentrations of oestrogens and progestogens than those in common use today. The effect of long-term use of the oral contraceptives with lower concentrations of both oestrogens and progestogens remains to be determined. The efficacy of any contraceptive method, except sterilisation, depends upon the reliability with which it is used. Correct and consistent use of methods can result in lower failure rates.

Thrombo-embolism: The use of oral contraceptives has been shown to be associated with an increased risk of thrombo-embolic disorders. The physician should be alert to the earliest manifestations of these disorders (thrombophlebitis, cerebrovascular disorders, pulmonary embolism, and retinal thrombosis). Should any of these occur or be suspected, Loestrin should be discontinued immediately.

Certain factors may predispose to the development of thrombosis e.g. smoking, obesity, age, the presence of varicose veins, cardiovascular disease, diabetes and migraine. The suitability of combined oral contraceptives for patients with any of these conditions should be discussed with the patient before a final decision is taken.

Cigarette smoking increases the risk of serious cardiovascular side effects from oral contraceptive use. This risk increases with age and with heavy smoking (15 or more cigarettes a day) and is quite marked in women over 35 years of age. Women who use oral contraceptives should be strongly advised not to smoke.

Hepatic tumours: Benign hepatic tumours have been associated with oral contraceptive usage. Malignant hepatic tumours have also been reported on rare occasions in long term users of oral contraceptives. A hepatic tumour should be considered in the differential diagnosis when upper abdominal pain, enlarged liver or signs of intra-abdominal haemorrhage occur.

Ovarian, endometrial, cervical and breast cancer: Numerous epidemiological studies have been reported on the risks of ovarian, endometrial, cervical and breast cancer in women using combined oral contraceptives. The evidence is clear that combined oral contraceptives offer substantial protection against both ovarian and endometrial cancer.

An increased risk of cervical cancer in long term users of combined oral contraceptives has been reported in some studies, but there continues to be controversy about the extent to which this is attributable to the confounding effects of sexual behaviour and other factors.

A meta-analysis from 54 epidemiological studies reported that there is a slightly increased relative risk (RR=1.24) of having breast cancer diagnosed in women who are currently using combined oral contraceptives (COCs). The observed pattern of increased risk may be due to an earlier diagnosis of breast cancer in COC users, the biological effects of COCs, or a combination of both. The additional breast cancers diagnosed in current users of COCs, or in women who have used COCs in the last ten years, are more likely to be localised to the breast than in those women who have never used COCs.

Breast cancer is rare among women under 40 years of age, whether or not they take COCs, Whilst this background risk increases with age, the excess number of breast cancer diagnoses in current and recent COC users is small in relation to the overall risk of breast cancer.

The most important risk factor for breast cancer in COC users is the age women discontinue the COC; the older the age at stopping, the more breast cancers are diagnosed. Duration of use is less important and the excess risk gradually disappears during the course of the ten years after stopping COC use such that by 10 years there appears to be no excess (see graph).

The possible increase in risk of breast cancer should be discussed with the user and weighed against the benefits of COCs taking into account the evidence that they offer substantial protection against the risk of developing certain other cancers (e.g. ovarian and endometrial cancer).

Reasons for stopping Loestrin immediately:

1. Occurrence of migraine in patients who have never previously suffered from it. Any unusually frequent or severe headaches.
2. Any kind of visual disturbance eg. proptosis or diplopia and migraine.
3. Suspicion of thrombosis or infarction.
4. Combined oral contraceptives should be stopped at least six weeks before elective surgery and during and following prolonged immobilisation eg. after accidents etc.
5. Loestrin should be discontinued if the patient becomes jaundiced or has a significant rise in blood pressure.
6. Patients with a history of depression should be carefully observed and the drug discontinued if the depression recurs to a serious degree.
7. Since the safety of Loestrin in pregnancy has not been demonstrated, it is recommended that for any patient who has missed a period, the absence of pregnancy should be established before continuing the contraceptive regimen.
8. Clear exacerbation of conditions known to be capable of deteriorating during oral contraception or pregnancy.

A complete medical history and physical examination should be undertaken prior to the initiation or reinstitution of oral contraceptives and periodically thereafter. The physical examination may be deferred until after initiation of the oral contraceptive if requested by the patient and judged appropriate by the clinician.

The pre-treatment and periodic physical examination should include special reference to blood pressure, breast, abdomen and pelvic organs, including relevant laboratory tests and Papanicolaou smear since oestrogens have been known to produce tumours, some of them malignant in five species of subprimate animals.

In case of undiagnosed, persistent or recurrent abnormal vaginal bleeding, appropriate diagnostic

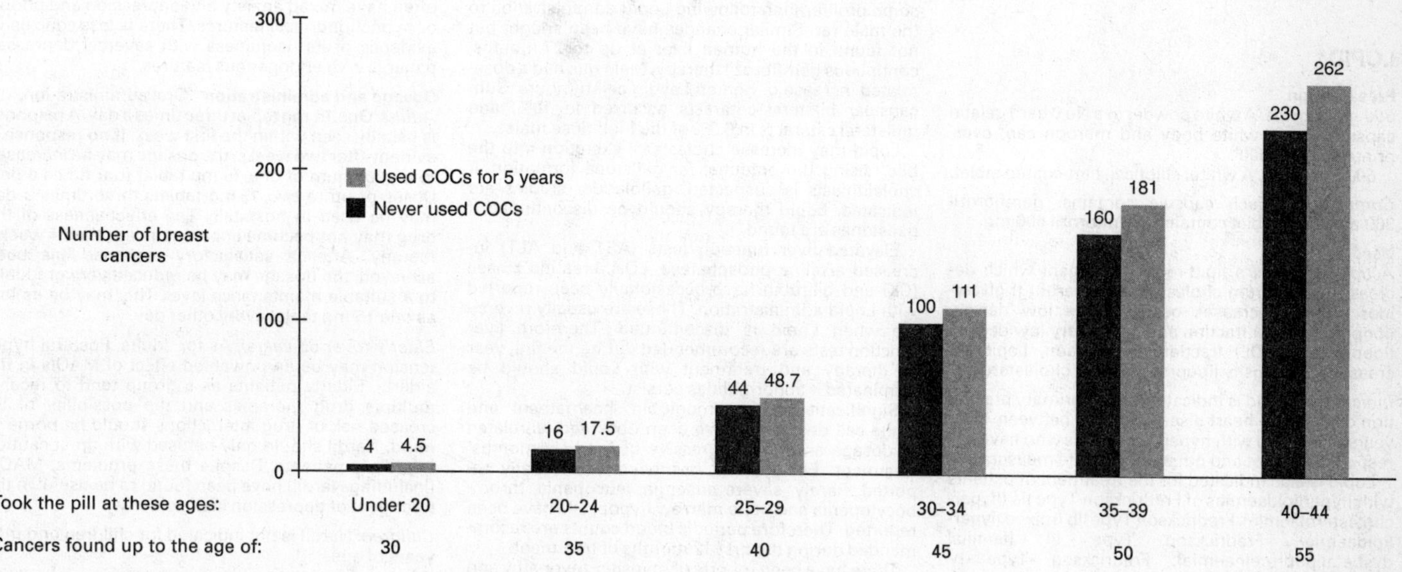

measures should be conducted to rule out malignancy. Women with a strong family history of breast cancer or who have breast nodules should be monitored with particular care.

Oestrogen-progestogen preparations should be used with caution in patients with a history of hypertension and some women experience an increase in blood pressure following the administration of contraceptive steroids. Pregnancy should be excluded before starting treatment. Because these agents may cause some degree of fluid retention, patients with conditions which might be influenced by this such as epilepsy, migraine, asthma and cardiac or renal dysfunction should be carefully monitored.

A decrease in glucose tolerance has been observed in a significant percentage of patients on oral contraceptives. The mechanism of this decrease is obscure. For this reason, prediabetic and diabetic patients should be carefully observed whilst receiving Loestrin.

Under the influence of oestrogen-progestogen preparations, pre-existing uterine fibroleiomyomata may increase in size. Loestrin may mask the onset of the climacteric.

The following conditions also require careful consideration: multiple sclerosis, porphyria, tetany, disturbed liver function, gall stones, cardiovascular disease, renal disease, chloasma or any disease that is prone to worsen during pregnancy. The deterioration or first appearance of any of these conditions may indicate that the oral contraceptive should be stopped. Contact lens wearers who develop visual changes or changes to lens tolerance should be assessed by an optometrist.

Interference with laboratory tests: The following laboratory results may be altered by the use of oral contraceptives: hepatic function (increased sulphobromophthalein retention and other tests); thyroid function (increased thyroid binding globulin (TBG) leading to increased circulating total thyroid hormone as measured by protein-bound iodine (PBI), T4 by column, or by radioimmunoassay. Free T3 resin uptake is decreased, reflecting the elevated TBG. Free T4 concentration is unaltered.); haematological tests (increased prothrombin and factors VII, VIII, IX and X, decreased antithrombin 3 and increased adrenaline induced platelet aggregation); measurement of pregnanediol excretion (reduced). Other binding proteins may be elevated in the serum, sex-binding globulins are increased, triglycerides may be increased and serum folate levels may be depressed. Therefore, if such tests are abnormal in a patient taking Loestrin, it is recommended that they be repeated after Loestrin has been withdrawn for two months. The pathologist should be advised of the administration of Loestrin when relevant specimens are submitted. Any influence of prolonged administration of Loestrin on pituitary, ovarian, adrenal, hepatic and uterine functions is unknown at present.

Interaction with other medicaments and other forms of interaction: The effectiveness of combined oral contraceptives may be considerably reduced by interaction with drugs that induce hepatic enzyme activity eg. carbamazepine, griseofulvin, phenytoin, phenobarbitone, primidone and rifampicin. Other drugs suspected of having the capacity to reduce the efficacy of oral contraceptives include ampicillin and other broad-spectrum antibiotics.

Additional contraceptive precautions should be taken whilst taking enzyme inducing drugs and some antibiotics and for at least seven days after stopping them. If these seven days run beyond the end of the packet the new packet should be started immediately without a break. Rifampicin is such a potent inducer that even if a course lasts for less than 7 days, the additional contraceptive precautions should be continued for at least 4 weeks after stopping it.

Pregnancy and lactation: Loestrin is not recommended for use during pregnancy, suspected pregnancy and in lactating mothers. Studies do not suggest a teratogenic effect, paticularly in so far as cardiac anomalies and limb reduction defects are concerned, when oral contraceptives are taken inadvertently during early pregnancy. The administration of oral contraceptives to induce withdrawal bleeding should not be used as a test for pregnancy. Oral contraceptives should not be used during pregnancy to treat threatened or habitual abortion.

Effects on ability to drive and use machines: None known.

Undesirable effects: The following adverse effects which have been reported in patients receiving oral contraceptives are believed to be drug-related.

Nausea, vomiting, gastro-intestinal symptoms (such as abdominal cramps and bloating), breakthrough bleeding, spotting, change in menstrual flow, amenorrhoea during and after treatment, oedema, chloasma, or melasma, breast changes (tenderness, enlargement and secretion), change in weight, cervical erosion and changes in cervical secretion, suppression of lactation when given immediately post-partum, cholestastic jaundice, migraine, rash (allergic), rise in blood pressure, depression, and thromboembolic disorders, temporary infertility after discontinuation of treatment, reduced tolerance to carbohydrates, vaginal candidiasis, change in corneal curvature (steepening) and intolerance to contact lenses.

Although the following adverse effects have been reported in women taking oral contraceptives, an association has been neither confirmed nor refuted: prolonged amenorrhoea after discontinuing oral contraceptives, pre-menstrual like syndrome, headache, nervousness, dizziness, fatigue, cataract, backache, hirsutism, loss of scalp hair, erythema multiforme, erythema nodusum, haemorrhagic eruption, itching, changes in appetite, cystitis-like syndrome, vaginitis, porphyria, impaired renal function, haemolytic uraemic syndrome, Budd-Chiari syndrome, acne, changes in libido and colitis.

Menstrual changes: Breakthrough bleeding and spotting are sometimes encountered, especially during the first three months of use. Non-hormonal causes should be considered and adequate diagnostic measures taken to rule out malignancy or pregnancy in the event of breakthrough bleeding, as in the case of any abnormal vaginal bleeding. If pathology has been excluded, time or a change to another formulation may solve the problem.

Overdose: The usual effects in children are nausea and drowsiness. Slight vaginal bleeding occasionally occurs in girls. In view of the low toxicity following overdosage with oral contraceptives, it is suggested that treatment should be conservative.

Pharmacological properties

Pharmacodynamic properties: Loestrin achieves contraceptive effect primarily by inhibition of ovulation through gonadotrophin suppression. It is thought that other sites of action such as changes in cervical mucus and in the endometrium may contribute to the efficacy of combined oral contraceptives.

Pharmacokinetic properties: Ethinyloestradiol is rapidly and almost completely absorbed and peak serum levels are usually attained within an hour of oral administration. At this time, the majority of drug is already conjugated, largely as the sulphate. These conjugates have a primary serum half-life of approximately 7 hours and a terminal half-life of 48 hours, and are excreted in urine and faeces.

Norethisterone aceate undergoes rapid absorption with peak serum concentrations ocurring at one hour after oral administration. Less than 5% is cleared as unchanged norethisterone; glucuronide and sulphate conjugates are excreted in urine and faeces. the terminal half-life for norethisterone conjugates has been estimated at 70 hours (range: 42–84 hours).

Preclinical safety data: The results of the preclinical tests do not add anything of further significance to the prescriber.

Pharmaceutical particulars

List of excipients: Each Loestrin 20 tablet contains the following excipients: Lactose, sucrose, maize starch, talc, powdered acacia, magnesium stearate, industrial methylated spirit*, purified water*, dichloromethane*, propylene glycol*, hypromellose 15, carnauba wax, E104, E127, E132, E171 and hydroxypropylcellulose.

Each Loestrin 30 tablet contains the following excipients: Lactose, sucrose, maize starch, talc, powdered acacia, magnesium stearate, industrial methylated spirit*, purified water*, dichloromethane*, propylene glycol*, hypromellose 15, carnauba wax, E104, E110, E131, E171 and hydroxypropylcellulose.

* not present in final product

Incompatibilities: Not known.

Shelf life: 3 years.

Special precautions for storage: Store below 30°C.

Nature and contents of container: Printed aluminium foil blister strip contained in a cardboard carton together with a product leaflet. Supplied in packs of 21 and 63 tablets.

Instructions for use/handling: No special instructions needed.

Marketing authorisation numbers
Loestrin 20 PL/0019/0137
Loestrin 30 PL/0019/0138

Date of renewal of authorisation 17th October 1997.

Legal category POM.

LOPID*

Presentation
300 mg capsule: A white powder in a No 0 hard gelatin capsule with a white body and maroon cap, overprinted 'LOPID 300'.
600 mg tablet: A white, elliptical, film-coated tablet.

Composition: Each capsule contains: gemfibrozil 300 mg. Each tablet contains: gemfibrozil 600 mg

Uses
Action: LOPID is a lipid-regulating agent which decreases total serum cholesterol and serum triglycerides. These decreases occur in the low density lipoprotein (LDL) fraction and in the very low density lipoprotein (VLDL) fraction. In addition, Lopid increases high density lipoprotein (HDL) cholesterol.

Indications: Lopid is indicated for the primary prevention of coronary heart disease in men between 40-55 years of age and with hyperlipidaemias who have not responded to diet and other appropriate measures.

Lopid is also indicated for the treatment of patients with hyperlipidaemias of Fredrickson Type IIa (hypercholesterolaemia), Fredrickson Type IIb (mixed hyperlipidaemia), Fredrickson Type III (familial dysbetalipoproteinaemia), Fredrickson Type IV (hypertriglyceridaemia) and Type V (hypertriglyceridaemia). Lopid should be prescribed only for patients with lipid or lipoprotein abnormalities demonstrated by laboratory tests and where diet alone is insufficient to correct the condition.

Dosage and administration
Adult: 1200 mg daily in divided doses usually twice daily. 900 mg as a total daily dose may be given in cases of intolerance at normal dosage. When maximum triglyceride reduction is desired as in Type V patients, up to 1500 mg daily may be needed.

Elderly: As for adults. Patients 60 years or older with lipid levels consistent with increased risk of coronary heart disease should be treated with diet for at least three months. If diet therapy is not effective, treatment with gemfibrozil in this age group should be considered. The incidence of side effects associated with treatment with Lopid has not been shown to be different in elderly subjects compared with younger ones.

Children: Not recommended.

Contra-indications, warnings etc
Contra-indications: Hypersensitivity to gemfibrozil, alcoholism, hepatic dysfunction, pre-existing gall stones.

Use in pregnancy and lactation: Safe use in human pregnancy has not been established. It is not known whether gemfibrozil is secreted in human milk. Like most drugs, gemfibrozil should normally be avoided during pregnancy and lactation.

Warnings and precautions: Before instituting treatment with Lopid, attempts should be made to control serum lipids with appropriate diet, exercise, cessation of smoking, limitation of alcohol intake, weight loss in obese patients, and treatment of the causes of secondary hyperlipidaemias such as hypothyroidism and diabetes mellitus.

Since long-term administration of Lopid is recommended, all baseline values including lipid profile, blood count and liver function tests, should be measured before treatment and periodic determinations of serum lipids should be obtained. The drug should be withdrawn or additional therapy instituted if the lipid response is inadequate after 3 months. In addition, Lopid should be withdrawn if after 3 months the response is paradoxical. Paradoxical response has been occasionally observed, usually in patients with alcoholic hepatic disease. The blood level of LDL cholesterol occasionally rises on treatment with Lopid. A further estimation of LDL cholesterol should therefore be made during treatment to confirm that the desired therapeutic effect has been achieved.

Adverse effects have not been reported in patients with renal disease, but such patients should start treatment at 900 mg daily, which may be increased after careful assessment of response and renal function.

Long-term toxicity studies in rats and mice were carried out at one and ten times the human dose on a weight for weight basis. In male rats receiving ten times the human dose, there was a significant increase in incidence of benign liver nodules and liver carcinomas. Male rats receiving a dose equivalent to the human dose had no statistically significant increase in the incidence of liver carcinomas. In high dose female rats there was a significant increase in the combined incidence of benign and malignant liver neoplasms. In mice (both male and female), there were no statistically significant differences from controls in the incidence of liver tumours. Electron microscopy demonstrated a marked hepatic peroxisome proliferation following Lopid administration to the male rat. Similar changes have been sought but not found in the human liver at up to 27 months' continuous gemfibrozil therapy. Male rats had a dose-related increase of benign Leydig cell tumours. Subcapsular bilateral cataracts occurred in 10%, and unilateral cataracts in 6.3% of the high dose males.

Lopid may increase cholesterol excretion into the bile raising the potential for gallstone formation. If cholelithiasis is suspected, gallbladder studies are indicated. Lopid therapy should be discontinued if gallstones are found.

Elevated liver function tests (AST and ALT) increased alkaline phosphatase, LDH, creatine kinase (CK) and bilirubin have occasionally been reported with Lopid administration. These are usually reversible when Lopid is discontinued. Therefore liver function tests are recommended during the first year of therapy and treatment with Lopid should be terminated if abnormalities persist.

Significant mild haemoglobin, haematocrit and white cell decreases have been observed, unrelated to dosage and not progressive beyond six months' treatment. Eosinophilia has been occasionally reported. Rarely, severe anaemia, leucopenia, thrombocytopenia and bone marrow hypoplasia have been reported. Therefore periodic blood counts are recommended during the first 12 months of treatment.

There have been reports of myositis, myopathy and marked elevations of creatine phosphokinase associated with Lopid. Rhabdomyolysis has also been reported rarely. Patients who develop signs of muscle toxicity should be monitored closely and CPK levels checked. Treatment with Lopid should be stopped if myopathy is suspected or if CPK rises to >10 times the upper limit of normal. The risk of serious muscle toxicity is increased if Lopid is used concomitantly with HMG-CoA reductase inhibitors or other fibrates. Combination therapy should be used with caution and patients monitored closely for signs of muscle toxicity.

Drug interactions: Concomitant anticoagulant dosage may need to be reduced and frequent determinations of prothrombin carried out to confirm that the desired prothrombin level has been re-established.

Reduced bioavailability of gemfibrozil may result when given simultaneously with resin-granule drugs such as colestipol. Administration of the drugs two hours or more apart is recommended.

Adverse effects: Significant side effects in decreasing order of frequency were abdominal pain, diarrhoea, nausea, epigastric pain, vomiting and flatulence. Occasionally and possibly attributable to Lopid are rash, dermatitis, pruritus, urticaria, impotence, headache, dizziness, blurred vision, cholestatic jaundice, angioedema, laryngeal oedema, atrial fibrillation, pancreatitis, myaesthenia, myopathy, rhabdomyolysis, painful extremities and myalgia accompanied by increases in creatine kinase.

Other reactions where a causal relationship is difficult to establish to which the physician should be alert: dry mouth, constipation, anorexia, dyspepsia, back pain, arthralgia, muscle cramps, swollen joints, vertigo, insomnia, paraesthesia, tinnitus, leucopenia, hypokalaemia, fatigue, malaise, syncope, peripheral neuritis, and acute appendicitis. Viral and bacterial infections (common cold, cough and urinary tract infections) were more common in Lopid than in placebo-treated patients.

Overdose: Overdosage has been reported with gemfibrozil. In one case of accidental overdosage, where a child ingested nine grams of gemfibrozil, non specific symptoms of nausea and vomiting were reported. The patient fully recovered.

Symptomatic supportive measures should be taken should overdose occur.

Pharmaceutical precautions Lopid 300 and Lopid 600: Store at a temperature not exceeding 30°C.

Legal category POM

Package quantities Lopid 300 mg – Blister packs containing 112 capsules.
Lopid 600 mg – Blister packs containing 56 tablets.

Product licence numbers
Lopid 300 mg 0019/0153
Lopid 600 mg 0019/0154

Date of preparation January 1998.

NARDIL*

Presentation Orange film-coated tablets, each containing 15 mg phenelzine (as the sulphate BP).

Uses
Indications: Phenelzine is a monoamine oxidase inhibitor (MAOI). It has been found to be effective in depressed patients clinically characterised as 'atypical', 'nonendogenous', 'neurotic' or where treatment with other antidepressants has failed. These patients often have mixed anxiety and depression and phobic or hypochondriacal features. There is less conclusive evidence of its usefulness with severely depressed patients with endogenous features.

Dosage and administration Oral administration.
Adults: One 15 mg tablet three times a day. A response is usually seen within the first week. If no response is evident after two weeks, the dosage may be increased to a maximum of one 15 mg tablet four times a day. Doses of up to two 15 mg tablets three times a day may be used in hospitals. The effectiveness of the drug may not become apparent in less than 4 weeks' therapy. After a satisfactory response has been achieved, the dosage may be reduced very gradually to a suitable maintenance level. This may be as low as one 15 mg tablet every other day.

Elderly (over 65 years): As for adults. Postural hypotension may be an unwanted effect of MAOIs in the elderly. Elderly patients as a group tend to receive multiple drug therapies and the possibility of increased risk of drug interactions should be borne in mind. Nardil should only be used with great caution in elderly patients. Despite these problems, MAOIs (including Nardil) have been found to be useful in the treatment of depression in the elderly.

Children: Nardil is not indicated for children under 16 years of age.

Contra-indications, warnings, etc
Contra-indications: Nardil should not be used in patients who are hypersensitive to phenelzine or with phaeochromocytoma, cerebrovascular disease, congestive heart failure, a history of liver disease or with abnormal liver function tests.

Phenelzine sulphate should not be administered at the same time as, or within 14 days of treatment with other MAOIs, buspirone, or dibenzazaepine derivative drugs (including tricyclic antidepressant agents, perphenazine or carbamazepine). It is recognised that there is some division of consultant opinion with respect to concomitant use of MAOIs and tricyclic antidepressants. There have been reports of serious reactions (including hyperthermia, rigidity, myoclonic movements and death) when serotonin reuptake inhibitors or serotonin/noradrenaline inhibitors (e.g. venlafaxine) have been combined with MAOIs. Therefore, Nardil should not be used in combination with these drugs and before initiating Nardil, a sufficent amount of time must be allowed for clearance of the drugs and its metabolites. For example, five weeks in the case of fluoxetine and two weeks with paroxetine. Conversely, these drugs should not be started within 14 days of discontinuing phenelzine.

Phenelzine sulphate should not be used in combination with guanethidine, dextromethorphan, or with CNS depressants such as alcohol and narcotic analgesics. Death has been reported in patients receiving a single dose of pethidine.

Use in pregnancy and lactation: Do not use during pregnancy, especially during the first and last trimesters, unless there are compelling reasons. There is no evidence as to drug safety in human pregnancy nor is there evidence from animal work that it is free from hazard.

It is not known if phenelzine is excreted in breast milk. Because of the potential for serious adverse effects to the infant, a decision should be made whether to discontinue the drug or not to breast-feed.

Precautions: Nardil should be withdrawn two weeks before elective surgery/dentistry. Nardil should not be given with cocaine or local anaesthesia containing sympathomimetic vasoconstrictors and the possible combined hypotensive effects of Nardil and spinal anaesthesia should be kept in mind.

Potentially suicidal patients should be carefully observed until control of depresssion is attained.

Patients should be warned against self-medication, particularly cold cures, and about potential food interactions.

Patients under treatment with Nardil should avoid high protein food that has undergone breakdown by ageing, fermentation, pickling, smoking or bacterial contamination. Patients should avoid cooked or plain cheese, Oxo, Bovril, Marmite, brewer's yeast etc. during treatment and up to 14 days after ceasing treatment. Flavoured textured vegetable protein, hung game, pickled herrings, dry sausage (salami, pepperoni etc), liver, yoghurt and broad bean pods may also present a hazard patients should not consume alcoholic drinks or non-alcoholic beers, lagers or wines and excessive amounts of tea and coffee should be avoided.

Where a reaction between Nardil and certain foodstuffs occurs the intensity of the reaction is usually related to the tyramine content of the food. The reaction is now well-recognised and serious hypertensive episodes are extremely rare. Should such a reaction occur, the hypertension should be controlled promptly by slow administration of phentolamine 5-10 mg I.V repeated if necessary. Care should be taken to administer this drug slowly to avoid an excessive hypotensive effect.

Nardil should only be used with great caution in agitated patients or those who have cardiovascular disease, epilepsy, blood dyscrasias, porphyria, or diabetes; and in patients taking diuretics.

Blood pressure should be observed frequently to detect any pressor response and therapy discontinued if palpitations or frequent headaches occur.

Patients should also be closely followed for symptoms of postural hypotension. Hypotensive side effects have occured in hypertensive as well as normotensive and hypotensive patients.

Nardil may also potentiate the effects of alcohol.

Drug interactions: See *Contra-indications.* Nardil may potentiate the action of pethidine, morphine, adrenaline, amphetamines and other sympathomimetic amines such as fenfluramine, ephedrine, phenylpropanolamine, dopamine and levodopa.

Nardil may also potentiate the effects of antihypertensives, hypoglycaemic agents, sympathomimetics, anti-Parkinson drugs, local anaesthetics and CNS depressants, including barbiturates.

The combination of MAOIs and tryptophan has been reported to cause behavioural and neurological symptoms.

Side effects: Side effects tend to be mild or moderate in severity, often subside as treatment continues, and can be minimised by adjusting dosage; rarely is it necessary to discontinue Nardil.

The most important reaction associated with Nardil is the occurrence of hypertensive crises, which have been associated with intracranial bleeding and have sometimes been fatal.

Common side-effects include: dizziness, drowsiness, weakness and fatigue, oedema and gastro-intestinal disturbances (nausea, vomiting, dryness of the mouth, constipation), insomnia, blurred vision, adverse effects on driving ability, postural hypotension, twitching, myoclonic movement, hyperreflexia, elevated serum transaminases and anorgasmia.

Less common side-effects are headache, nervousness, euphoria, paraesthesia, sweating, increased appetite and weight, rash, pruritus, difficulty in micturition, muscle tremor, peripheral neuritis, behavioural changes, arrhythmias, convulsions, impotence and delayed ejaculation, purpura, blood dyscrasias, jitteriness, palilalia, nystagmus, hypernatraemia and glaucoma.

Although reported less frequently, sometimes only once, additional severe side effects include: ataxia, shock-like coma, toxic delirium, manic reaction, acute anxiety reaction, precipitation of schizophrenia, transient respiratory and cardiovascular depression following ECT, fatal progressive necrotising hepatocellular damage, reversible jaundice, hypermetabolic syndrome, oedema of the glottis and fever associated with increased muscle tone.

Withdrawal may be associated with nausea, vomiting and malaise.

An uncommon withdrawal syndrome following abrupt withdrawal of Nardil has been infrequently reported. Signs and symptoms of this syndrome generally commence 24 to 72 hours after drug discontinuation and may vary from vivid nightmares with agitition to frank psychosis and convulsions. This syndrome generally responds to reinstitution of low-dose Nardil therapy followed by cautious downward titration and discontinuation.

Overdosage: Signs and symptoms may be absent or minimal during the initial 12 hour period following ingestion and may develop slowly thereafter, reaching a maximum in 24-48 hours. Death has been reported following overdosage. Therefore immediate hospitalisation with continuous patient observation and monitoring throughout this period is essential.

Large doses may produce hypomania, euphoria, followed by coma with hypotension, or acute hypertension sometimes with sub-arachnoid haemorrhage. In a few cases extra-pyramidal symptoms have been recorded.

Other symptoms may be: drowsiness, dizziness, faintness, irritability, hyperactivity, agitation, severe headache, hallucinations, trismus, opisthotonos, rigidity, convulsions, rapid and irregular pulse, precordial pain, respiratory depression and failure, hyperpyrexia, diaphoresis and cool, clammy skin.

Treatment: Gastric lavage with instillation of charcoal slurry may be helpful in early poisoning (tablets dissolve slowly in stomach).

Absolute bed rest, raise feet in hypotension. Vasopressors are best avoided. Hypertension should be urgently controlled with phentolamine IV. Avoid hypnotics, such as morphine, pethidine, barbiturates. Body temperature should be monitored, and fever managed by cooling.

Use intravenous therapy to maintain fluid and electrolyte balance and use a slow IV injection of diazepam for any CNS stimulation. In deep coma and severe hypotension, hydrocortisone by injection may be tried.

There is no specific antidote for Nardil.

Haemodialysis, peritoneal dialysis and charcoal haemoperfusion may be of value in massive overdosage, but sufficent data is not available to recommend their routine use in these cases.

Pharmaceutical precautions Store between 2–8°C in a refrigerator, unless unavoidable for short periods.

Legal category POM.

Package quantities Bottles of 100 tablets.

Further information Nil

Product licence number 0019/0141

NEURONTIN* ▼

Qualitative and quantitative composition Neurontin Capsules 100 mg contain 100 mg gabapentin per capsule. Neurontin Capsules 300 mg contain 300 mg gabapentin per capsule. Neurontin Capsules 400 mg contain 400 mg gabapentin per capsule.

Pharmaceutical form Neurontin is supplied in capsules containing 100 mg, 300 mg, and 400 mg of active drug substance for oral administration.

Clinical particulars

Therapeutic indications: Neurontin is an antiepileptic drug indicated as add-on therapy for partial seizures and partial seizures with secondary generalisation in patients who have not achieved satisfactory control with or who are intolerant to standard anticonvulsants used alone or in combination.

Posology and method of administration: For oral administration only.

Adults: The anti-epileptic effect of Neurontin generally occurs at 900-1200 mg/day. It is not necessary to monitor Neurontin plasma concentrations to optimise Neurontin therapy.

Titration to an effective dose can progress rapidly and can be accomplished over a few days by administering 300 mg once a day on day 1, 300 mg twice a day on day 2, and 300 mg three times a day on day 3.

Thereafter, the dose can be increased to 1200 mg per day given in three equally divided doses, and if necessary, further titration can occur using increments of 300 mg per day given in three equally divided doses up to a maximum of 2400 mg per day.

The maximum time between doses in a three times daily schedule should not exceed 12 hours.

If Neurontin is discontinued and/or an alternate anticonvulsant medication is added to the therapy, this should be done gradually over a minimum of one week.

Elderly: Elderly patients may require dosage adjustment because of declining renal function with age (see Ttable 1 below).

Dosage in patients with compromised renal function or those undergoing haemodialysis: Dosage adjustment is recommended in patients with compromised renal function or those undergoing haemodialysis (see Table 1 below).

Table 1. Maintenance dosage of Neurontin in adults with reduced renal function

Renal Function Creatinine Clearance (ml/min)	*Total Daily Dose (mg/day)*	*Dose Regimen (mg)*
60-90	1200 mg	400 mg three times a day
30-60	600 mg	300 mg twice daily
15-30	300 mg	300 mg once daily
<15	150 mg	300 mg once daily every other day
Haemodialysis[a]	–	200-300[b]

[a] Loading dose of 300 to 400 mg
[b] Maintenance dose of 200 to 300 mg gabapentin following each 4 hours of haemodialysis.

Children under 12 years of age: Not recommended.

Contra-indications: Neurontin is contra-indicated in patients who are hypersensitive to Neurontin or to the product's components.

Special warnings and special precautions for use: Although there is no evidence of rebound seizures with Neurontin, abrupt withdrawal of anticonvulsant agents in epileptic patients may precipitate status epilepticus. When in the judgement of the clinician there is a need for dose reduction, discontinuation or substitution of alternative anticonvulsant medication, this should be done gradually over a minimum of one week.

Neurontin is not generally considered effective in the treatment of absence seizures.

Patients with epilepsy can be the subject of mood and behavioural disturbances. Such reports have been noted in patients on Neurontin although a causal link has not been established.

Interaction with other medicaments and other forms of interaction: Neurontin may be used in combination with other anti-epileptic drugs without concern for alteration of the plasma concentrations of Neurontin or serum concentrations of other anti-epileptic drugs.

There is no interaction between Neurontin and phenytoin, valproic acid, carbamazepine or phenobarbital. Neurontin steady-state pharmacokinetics are similar for healthy subjects and patients with epilepsy receiving antiepileptic agents.

Co-administration of Neurontin with oral contraceptives including norethisterone and/or ethinyl estradiol does not influence the steady-state pharmacokinetics of either component.

In a clinical study where Neurontin and an aluminium and magnesium containing antacid were given at the same time, Neurontin's bioavailability was reduced by up to 24%. It is recommended that Neurontin is taken about two hours following any such antacid administration.

Renal excretion of Neurontin is unaltered by probenecid. The slight decrease in renal excretion of Neurontin observed when co-administered with cimetidine is not expected to be of clinical importance.

Food has no effect on Neurontin pharmacokinetics.

Because false positive readings were reported with the Ames N-Multistix SG;® dipstick test when Neurontin or placebo was added to other anticonvulsant drugs, the more specific sulphosalicylic acid precipitation procedure is recommended to determine urine protein.

Pregnancy and lactation: Safe use in human pregnancy has not been established.

Reproduction studies in mice at doses up to 80 times the human dose and in rats and rabbits at doses up to 40 times the human dose revealed no evidence of impaired fertility or harm to the foetus due to Neurontin administration. However, because animal reproduction studies are not always predictive of human response, this drug should be used during pregnancy only if clearly needed.

It is not known if Neurontin is excreted in human milk. Because many drugs are excreted in human milk and because of the potential for serious adverse reactions in nursing infants from Neurontin, a decision should be made whether to discontinue nursing or to discontinue the drug, taking into account the importance of the drug to the mother.

Effects on ability to drive and use machines: As with all anticonvulsants, Neurontin acts on the central nervous system and may produce drowsiness, dizziness or other related symptoms. These otherwise mild or moderate adverse events could be potentially dangerous in patients driving or operating machinery, particularly until such time as the individual patient's experience with the drug is established.

Undesirable effects: Neurontin has been evaluated for safety in more than 2000 subjects and patients and was well tolerated.

Since Neurontin was most often administered in combination with other antiepileptic agents, it is not possible to determine which agents, if any, are associated with adverse events. However, based on placebo-controlled, double blind studies, possible side effects are: somnolence, dizziness, ataxia, fatigue, nystagmus, headache, tremor, diplopia, nausea and/or vomiting, rhinitis and amblyopia. Less common side effects are: pharyngitis, dysarthria, weight increase, dyspepsia, amnesia, nervousness and myalgia.

Post-marketing surveillance: As with the other AEDs there have been rare reports of pancreatitis, elevated liver function tests, erythema multiforme, Stevens Johnson Syndrome and sudden unexplained deaths where a causal relationship to treatment has not been established.

Overdose: In limited experience with overdoses, dizziness, double vision and slurred speech have been noted. Overdoses of Neurontin, up to 30 g ingested at one time, have been reported. Symptoms were drowsiness and mild diarrhoea with a full recovery. Therefore, acute, life-threatening toxicity has not been observed with Neurontin overdoses of up to 30 g per day. Reduced absorption of Neurontin at higher doses may limit drug absorption at the time of overdosing and, hence, toxicity from overdoses.

Although Neurontin can be removed by hemodialysis, it is not usually required. However, in patients with renal impairment, hemodialysis may be indicated.

Pharmacological properties

Pharmacodynamic properties: Neurontin is an anticonvulsant structurally related to the neurotransmitter gamma-aminobutyric acid (GABA) but its mechanism of action is different from that of several drugs that interact with GABA synapses. The identification and function of the gabapentin binding site remains to be elucidated and the relevance of its various actions to the anticonvulsant effect remains to be established.

Pharmacokinetic properties: Mean plasma gabapentin concentrations C_{max} occurred approximately 3 hours (T_{max}) following single oral doses of Neurontin regardless of dose size of formulation. Mean T_{max} values following multiple dose administration were approximately 1 hour shorter than the values following single-dose administration.

Mean C_{max} and AUC values increased with increasing dose; however, the increase was less than dose proportional. Deviation from linearity was very slight up to 600 mg for both parameters and thus should be minimal at doses of 300 mg to 400 mg three times daily where the antiepileptic effect generally occurs.

Following repeated Neurontin administration, steady-state was achieved within 1 to 2 days after the start of the multiple dosing and was maintained throughout the dosing regime.

Plasma gabapentin concentration-time profiles were similar between gabapentin solution and capsule formulations following single doses of 300 and 400 mg. Absolute bioavailability of a 300 mg oral dose of Neurontin was approximately 60%. At doses of 300 mg and 400 mg, Neurontin bioavailability was unchanged following multiple-dose administration.

The presence of food did not influence the bioavailabilty of Neurontin.

Gabapentin is not metabolised in humans and does not induce hepatic mixed function oxidase enzymes.

Gabapentin elimination from plasma following IV administration was best described by linear pharmacokinetics. Elimination half-life ($T_{\frac{1}{2}}$) of gabapentin ranged from 5 to 7 hours. Gabapentin elimination parameters, apparent plasma $T_{\frac{1}{2}}$ and renal clearance (CL_R) were independent of dose and remained unchanged following repeated administration. Renal clearance was the sole elimination pathway for gabapentin. Since gabapentin is not metabolised in humans, the amount of drug recovered in urine is indicative of gabapentin bioavailability. Following a single 200 mg oral dose of [C_{14}] gabapentin recovery of radioactivity was essentially complete with approximately 80% and 20% of the dose recovered in urine and faeces, respectively.

As renal function (as determined by creatinine clearance) decreases with increasing age, gabapentin oral clearance, renal clearance and elimination-rate constant decrease proportionally.

Preclinical safety data: Gabapentin was given in the diet to mice at 200, 600 and 2000 mg/kg/day and to rats at 250, 1000 and 2000 mg/kg/day for two years. A statistically significant increase in the incidence of pancreatic acinar cell tumours was found only in male rats at the highest dose. Peak plasma drug concentrations and areas under the concentration time curve in rats at 2000 mg/kg is 20 times higher than the therapeutic concentrations in humans given the recommended maximum therapeutic dose and is 14 times higher than the therapeutic concentrations in humans given the recommended maximum tolerated dose (2400 mg/day).

The pancreatic acinar cell tumours in male rats are low grade malignancies, did not affect survival, did not metastasise or invade surrounding tissue and were similar to those seen in concurrent controls. The relevance of these pancreatic acinar cell tumours in male rats to carcinogenic risk in humans is therefore of uncertain significance.

Gabapentin has no genotoxic potential. It was not mutagenic in the Ames bacterial plate incorporation assay or at the HGPRT locus in mammalian cells in the presence or absence of metabolic activation. Gabapentin did not induce structural chromosome aberrations in mammalian cells in vitro or in vivo, and did not induce micronucleus formation in the bone marrow of hamsters.

Pharmaceutical particulars

List of excipients: The 100 mg, 300 mg and 400 mg capsules contain the following excipients: lactose (hydrous), corn starch and talc. The capsule shells for Neurontin 100 mg, 300 mg and 400 mg consist of Gelatin. The capsule shell for Neurontin 100 mg also contain E171 (Titanium Dioxide). The capsule shell for Neurontin 300 mg also contains E171 (Titanium Dioxide) and E172 (Yellow Iron Oxide). The capsule shell for Neurontin 400 mg also contains E171 (Titanium Dioxide), E172 (Yellow Iron oxide) and E172 (Red Iron Oxide).

Incompatibilities: None.

Shelf life: 3 years

Special precautions for storage: Store in a dry place at a temperature between 15–30°C.

Nature and contents of container: Neurontin Capsules 100 mg, 300 mg and 400 mg are packed in PVC/PVDC blister packs with vinyl heat seal/aluminium coating backing containing 100 capsules.

Instructions for use/handling: None.

Marketing authorisation numbers

Neurontin Capsules 100 mg	PL0019/0172
Neurontin Capsules 300 mg	PL0019/0173
Neurontin Capsules 400 mg	PL0019/0174

Date of revision 31 December 1997.

Legal category POM.

OPILON*

Qualitative and quantitative composition Each tablet contains Thymoxamine hydrochloride BP 45.22 mg (equivalent to thymoxamine base 40 mg).

Pharmaceutical form A pale yellow film-coated tablet.

Clinical particulars

Therapeutic indications: Thymoxamine is an alpha-adrenergic blocking agent. Opilon is indicated in the short term control of the symptoms of primary Raynaud's Phenomenon.

Posology and method of administration: Oral administration

Adults: Initially one tablet to be taken four times a day. This may be increased to two tablets four times a day if initial response is poor. For patients exposed to the cold during the daytime, one tablet should be administered every three hours during the period when symptoms are most likely to occur. In the event that a response is not evident within 2 weeks, the drug should be discontinued.

Elderly (over 65 years): As for adults. No clinical or pharmacokinetic data specific to this age group is available. Whilst at normal dosage no problems have been reported, caution nevertheless is advised when Opilon is prescribed in the elderly.

Children: Opilon tablets are not indicated for use in children.

Contra-indications: Opilon Tablets are contraindicated in those with hypersensitivity to any of the ingredients, or have active liver disease.

Special warnings and special precautions for use: The alpha-adrenergic blocking action of Opilon will produce a vasodilating effect which may theoretically potentiate the effect of a number of drugs used in the management of hypertension. In practice, with the recommended dosage of Opilon, this has not been reported.

Opilon should be used with caution in diabetes as, theoretically, insulin requirements may be reduced. Tricyclic antidepressants may increase any hypotensive effect produced by alpha blockade.

Interaction with other medicaments and other forms of interaction: See *Special warnings and special precautions for use.*

Pregnancy and lactation: The safety of Opilon for use during pregnancy and lactation has not been established. It should not therefore be used by women who are pregnant or breast-feeding.

Effects on ability to drive and use machines: None known.

Undesirable effects: Occasionally, mild nausea, diarrhoea, vertigo, headache, facial flushing and rash may be encountered. These are, however, rare and transient. There have also been rare reports of hepatotoxicity, including cases of hepatitis and cholestatic jaundice, which are reversible on stopping treatment. Opilon should be withdrawn promptly if hepatic dysfunction develops.

Overdose: In excessive overdosage, a fall in blood pressure is the main symptom. The patient should be nursed in the supine position until the blood pressure has been restored to normal.

Pharmacological properties

Pharmacodynamic properties: Thymoxamine is an alpha-adrenergic blocking agent which is used for the treatment of the symptoms of Raynaud's phenomenon.

Pharmacokinetic properties: Thymoxamine is rapidly absorbed after oral administration. In plasma, the drug is rapidly converted to desacetylthymoxamine (metabolite I) and desmethyldesacetylthymoxamine (metabolite II) which are pharmacologically active. Other circulatory species are the sulphate and glucuronide conjugates of metabolites i and ii. Excretion is almost exclusively via the kidneys. The half life of total radioacitivity, after radiolabelled thymoxamine was administered to man, was 1-2 hours.

Preclinical safety data: Preclinical safety data does not add anything of further significance to the prescriber.

Pharmaceutical particulars

List of excipients: Lactose, Colloidal silicon dioxide, Microcrystalline cellulose, Magnesium stearate, Maize starch. The film coating contains: Methylhydroxypropylcellulose, Propylene glycol, Opaspray M-1-22900 (E464, E171, E104, E124 and E132).

Incompatibilities: None known.

Shelf life: 36 months.

Special precautions for storage: Store at a temperature not exceeding 30°C.

Nature and contents of container: Blister pack comprising white PVC and aluminium foil backing containing 112 tablets.

Instructions for use/handling: Not applicable.

Marketing authorisation number PL 0019/0121

Date of renewal of authorisation 17th October 1997

Date of revision 19 August 1998

Legal category POM

PRO-EPANUTIN* CONCENTRATE FOR INJECTION ▼

Qualitative and quantitative composition One ml of Pro-Epanutin contains 75 mg of fosphenytoin sodium (equivalent to 50 mg of phenytoin sodium) referred to as 50 mg PE.

Each 10 ml vial contains 750 mg of fosphenytoin sodium (equivalent to 500 mg of phenytoin sodium) and referred to as 500 mg PE.

Pharmaceutical form Solution for injection or infusion

Clinical particulars

Therapeutic indications: Pro-Epanutin is indicated: for the control of status epilepticus of the tonic-clonic (grand mal) type (see posology and method of administration); for prevention and treatment of seizures occurring in connection with neurosurgery and/or head trauma; as a substitute for oral phenytoin if oral administration is not possible and/or contra-indicated.

Posology and method of administration:

Phenytoin sodium equivalents (PE): 1.5 mg of fosphenytoin sodium is equivalent to 1 mg PE (phenytoin sodium equivalent).

To avoid the need to perform molecular weight-based adjustments when initiating therapy with Pro-Epanutin or substituting Epanutin and fosphenytoin sodium for each other, Pro-Epanutin should always be prescribed and dispensed in PE units. The concentration and rate of administration of solutions for the parenteral administration of Pro-Epanutin are expressed as phenytoin sodium equivalents (PE).

Administration: Pro-Epanutin may be administered by IV infusion or by IM injection. Pro-Epanutin should not be administered by IM route in emergency situations such as status epilepticus. Products with particulate matter or discoloration should not be used.

Intravenous infusion: For IV infusion, Pro-Epanutin should be diluted in 5% dextrose or 0.9% sodium chloride solution. The concentration should range from 1.5 to 25 mg PE/ml. Because of the risk hypotension, the recommended rate of administration by IV infusion in routine clinical settings is 50–100 mg PE/minute. Even in an emergency, it should not exceed 150 mg PE/minute. The use of a device controlling the rate of infusion is recommended.

Continuous monitoring of electrocardiogram, blood pressure and respiratory function for the duration of the infusion is essential. The patient should also be observed throughout the period where maximal plasma phenytoin concentrations occur. This is approximately 10 to 20 minutes after the end of the Pro-Epanutin infusions.

Cardiac resuscitative equipment should be available.

Dosage in adults: status epilepticus: loading dose: In order to obtain rapid seizure control in patients with continuous seizure activity IV diazepam or lorazepam should be administered prior to administration of Pro-Epanutin. The loading dose of Pro-Epanutin is 15 mg PE/kg administered by IV infusion at a rate of 100 to 150 mg PE/min. The rate of IV infusion, even in this emergency use, should not exceed 150 mg PE/minute.

Intramuscular administration of Pro-Epanutin is contraindicated in the treatment of status epilepticus. If administration of Pro-Epanutin does not terminate seizures, the use of alternative anticonvulsants should be considered.

Maintenance dose: Initial maintenance doses of Pro-Epanutin of 4 to 5 mg PE/kg/day may be given by IV infusion or by IM injection. The recommended rate of IV infusion for maintenance dosing up 50 to 100 mg PE/minute.

Maintenance doses should be adjusted according

to patient response and trough plasma phenytoin concentrations (See *Therapeutic drug monitoring*).

Transfer to maintenance therapy with oral phenytoin should be made when appropriate.

Treatment or prophylaxis of seizures: loading dose: The loading dose of Pro-Epanutin is 10 to 15 mg PE/kg given by IV infusion or by IM injection. The recommended rate of IV infusion for treatment of prophylaxis of seizures is 50 to 100 mg PE/minute.

Maintenance dose: Initial maintenance doses of Pro-Epanutin of 4 to 5 mg PE/kg/day may be given by IV infusion or by IM injection. The recommended rate of IV infusion for maintenance dosing is 50 to 100 mg PE/minute.

Maintenance doses should be adjusted according to patient response and trough plasma phenytoin concentrations (see *Therapeutic drug monitoring*).

Transfer to maintenance therapy with oral phenytoin should be made when appropriate.

Temporary substitution of oral phenytoin therapy with Pro-Epanutin: The same dose and dosing frequency as for oral phenytoin therapy should be used.

Fosphenytoin has not been evaluated systemically for more than 5 days.

Dosage in children: Pro-Epanutin may be administered to children (ages 5 and above) by IV infusion, at the same mg PE/kg dose used for adults. The doses of Pro-Epanutin for children have been predicted from the known pharmacokinetics of Pro-Epanutin in adults and children aged 5 to 10 years and of parenteral phenytoin in adults and children.

As for adults, the recommend rate of IV infusion in routine clinical settings is 50 to 100 mg PE/minute (1 to 2 mg PE/kg/minute). In an emergency for the treatment of status epilepticus, the rate of IV infusion is 100 to 150 mg PE/minute (2 to 3 mg PE/kg/minute) and should not exceed 3 mg PE/kg/minute (150 mg PE/minute). In order to obtain rapid seizure control in patients with continuous seizure activity IV diazepam or lorazepam should be administered prior to administration of Pro-Epanutin.

The following table represents the dosing schedules for Pro-Epanutin for children (see below).

Elderly patients: A lower loading dose and / or infusion rate and lower or less frequent maintenance dosing of Pro-Epanutin may be required. Phenytoin metabolism is slightly decreased in elderly patients. A 10% to 25% reduction is dose or rate may be considered.

Patients with renal or hepatic disease: Except in the treatment of status epilepticus, a lower loading dose and/or infusion rate, and lower or less frequent maintenance dosing may be required in patients with renal and/or hepatic disease or in those with hypoalbuminaemia. A 10% to 25% reduction in dose or rate may be considered.

The rate of conversion of IV Pro-Epanutin to phenytoin but not the clearance of phenytoin may be increased in these patients. Plasma unbound phenytoin concentrations may also be elevated. It may therefore, be more appropriate to measure plasma unbound phenytoin concentrations rather than plasma total phenytoin concentrations in these patients.

Therapeutic drug monitoring: Prior to complete conversion, immunoanalytical techniques may significantly overestimate plasma phenytoin concentrations due to cross-reactivity with fosphenytoin. Chromatographic assay methods (e.g. HPLC) accurately quantitate phenytoin concentrations in biological fluids in the presence of fosphenytion. It is advised that blood samples to assess phenytoin concentration *should not* be obtained for at least 2 hours after IV Pro-Epanutin infusion or 4 hours after IM Pro-Epanutin injection.

Optimal seizure control without clinical signs of toxicity occurs most often with plasma total phenytoin concentrations of between 10 and 20 mg/l (40 and 80 micromoles/l) or plasma unbound phenytoin concentration of between 1 and 2 mg/l (4 and 8 micromoles/l).

Plasma phenytoin concentrations sustained above the optimal range may produce signs of acute toxicity (see *Special warnings and special precautions for use*).

Phenytoin capsules are approximately 90% bioavailable by the oral route. Phenytoin, supplied as Pro-Epanutin, is 100% bioavailable by both the IM and IV routes. For this reason, plasma phenytoin concentrations may increase when IM or IV Pro-Epanutin is substituted for oral phenytoin sodium therapy. However, it is not necessary to adjust the initial doses when substituting oral phenytoin with Pro-Epanutin or vice versa.

Therapeutic drug monitoring may be useful whenever switching between products and/or routes of administration.

Contra-indications: Hypersensitivity to fosphenytoin sodium or the excipients of Pro-Epanutin, or to phenytoin or other hydantoins.

Parenteral phenytoin affects ventricular automaticity. Pro-Epanutin is therefore contraindicated in patients with sinus bradycardia, sino-atrial block, second and third degree A-V block and Adams-Stokes syndrome.

Acute intermittent porphyria.

Special warnings and special precautions for use: Doses of Pro-Epanutin are expressed as their phenytoin equivalents in this labelling (PE = phenytoin sodium equivalent). When Pro-Epanutin is dosed as PE it is therefore not necessary to make any adjustment in the recommended doses when substituting Pro-Epanutin for phenytoin sodium or vice versa.

Phenytoin is not effective in absence seizures. If tonic-clonic seizures are present simultaneously with absence seizures, combined drug therapy is recommended.

Withdrawal precipitated seizure/status epilepticus: Abrupt withdrawal of antiepileptic drugs may increase seizure frequency and may lead to status epilepticus.

Rash: Pro-Epanutin should be discontinued if a skin rash or signs of an allergic or hypersensitivity reaction or syndrome appear. Rapid substitution with an alternative antiepileptic drug not belonging to the hydantoin chemical class may be necessary.

Hypersensitivity syndrome and hepatoxicity: A hypersensitivity reaction or syndrome has been associated with phenytoin administration. Fever, skin eruptions and lymphadenopathy may occur within the first two months of treatment. Hepatotoxicity is often associated with this hypersensitivity syndrome. Acute hepatotoxicities, including acute hepatic failure, jaundice, hepatomegaly and elevated serum transaminase levels have also been reported. Recovery from acute hepatotoxicity may be prompt, however fatal outcomes have also occurred. Pro-Epanutin should be discontinued immediately following signs of acute hepatotoxicity and not readministered. Leucocytosis, eosinophilia and arthralgias may also occur. Although still rare, there may be an increased incidence of hypersensitivity reactions in black patients.

Lymphadenopathy: Lymphadenopathy (local or generalised) including benigh lymph node hyperplasia, pseudolymphoma, lymphoma and Hodgkins Disease have been associated with administration of phenytoin, although a cause and effect relationship has not been established. It is therefore, important to eliminate other types of lymph node pathology before discontinuing therapy with Pro-Epanutin. Lymph node involvement may occur with or without symptoms and signs resembling serum sickness, e.g. fever, rash and liver involvement, as part of the hypersensitivity syndrome described above. In all cases of lymphadenopathy, long term follow-up observations are indicated and every effort should be made to achieve seizure control using alternative antiepileptic drugs.

Acute toxicity: Confessional states referred to as "delirium", "psychosis" or "encephalopathy" or rarely irreversible cerebellar dysfunction may occur if plasma phenytoin concentrations are sustained above the optimal therapeutic range. Plasma phenytoin concentrations should be determined at the first sign of acute toxicity (see Posology and Method of Administration: Therapeutic Drug Monitoring). If plasma phenytoin concentrations are excessive, the dose of Pro-Epanutin should be reduced. If symptoms persist, administration of Pro-Epanutin should be discontinued.

Cardiovascular disease: Pro-Epanutin should be used with caution in patients with hypotension and severe myocardial insufficiency. Severe cardiovascular reactions including atria and ventricular conduction depression and ventricular fibrillation, and sometimes fatalities have been reported following phenytoin administration. Hypotension may also occur following IV administration of high doses and/or high infusion rates of Pro-Epanutin. A reduction in the rate of administration or discontinuation of dosing may be necessary (see *Posology and method of administration*).

Renal or hepatic disease: Pro-Epanutin should be used with caution in patients with renal and/or hepatic disease, or in those with hypoalbuminaemia. Alterations in dosing may be necessary in patients with impaired kidney or liver function, elderly patients or those who are gravely ill (see *Posology and method of administration*). These patients may show early signs of phenytoin toxicity or an increase in the severity of adverse events due to alterations in Pro-Epanutin and phenytoin pharmacokinetics.

The phosphate load provided by Pro-Epanutin is 0.0037 mmol phosphate/mg fosphenytoin sodium. Caution is advised when administering Pro-Epanutin in patients requiring phosphate restriction, such as those with severe renal impairment.

Sensory disturbances: Overall these occur in 13% of the patients exposed to Pro-Epanutin. Transient itching, burning, warmth or tingling in the groin during and shortly after intravenous infusion of Pro-Epanutin may occur. The sensations are not consistent with the signs of an allergic reaction and may be avoided or minimised, by using a slower rate of IV infusion or by temporarily stopping the infusion.

Diabetes: Phenytoin may raise blood glucose in diabetic patients.

Alcohol use: Acute alcohol intake may increase plasma phenytoin concentrations while chronic alcohol use may decrease plasma phenytoin concentrations.

Interaction with other medicaments and other forms of interaction: Drug interactions which may occur following the administration of Pro-Epanutin are those that are expected to occur with drugs known to interact with phenytoin. Phenytoin metabolism is saturable and other drugs that utilise the same metabolic pathways may alter plasma phenytoin concentrations. There are many drugs which may increase or decrease plasma phenytoin concentrations. Equally phenytoin may affect the metabolism of a number of other drugs because of its potent enzyme-inducing potential. Determination of plasma phenytoin concentrations is especially helpful when possible drug interactions are suspected (see *Posology and method of administration: Therapeutic drug monitoring*).

No drugs are known to interfere with the conversion of fosphenytoin to phenytoin.

Phenytoin is extensively bound to plasma proteins and is prone to competitive displacements. Drugs highly bound to albumin could also increase the fosphenytoin unbound fraction with the potential to increase the rate of conversion of fosphenytoin to phenytoin. Phenytoin is metabolised by hepatic cyto-

Recommended doses and rates of Pro-Epanutin administration for adults

Indication	*Route*	*Pro-Epanutin[a] dose*	*IV Infusion rate*	*Dose frequency*
Loading dose administration				
Status epilepticus	IV	15 mg PE/kg	100 to 150 mg PE/min	Single-dose
Treatment or prophylaxis of seizures	IM/IV	10 to 15 mg PE/kg	50 to 100 mg PE/min	Single-dose
Maintenance dose administration				
Maintenance following loading dose	IM/IV	4 to 5 mg PE/kg[b]	50 to 100 mg PE/min	Once or twice daily
Temporary substitution for oral phenytoin	IM/IV	Current daily oral phenytoin dose	50 to 100 mg PE/min	Same frequency as oral phenytoin

[a] Dose expressed as Phenytoin sodium equivalents (PE).
1 mg PE = 1.5 mg fosphenytoin sodium.
[b] Initial dose; subsequent doses are dependent on patient response and trough plasma phenytoin concentrations.

Recommended doses and rates of Pro-Epanutin administration for children

Indication	*Route*	*Pro-Epanutin[a] dose*	*IV Infusion rate*	*Dose frequency*
Loading dose administration				
Status epilepticus	IV	15 mg PE/kg	2 to 3 mg PE/kg/min	Single-dose
Treatment or prophylaxis of seizures	IV	10 to 15 mg PE/kg	1 to 2 mg PE/kg/min	Single-dose
Maintenance dose administration				
Maintenance following loading dose	IV	4 to 5 mg PE/kg[b]	1 to 2 mg PE/kg/min	Up to four times daily
Temporary substitution for oral phenytoin	IV	Current daily oral phenytoin dose	1 to 2 mg PE/kg/min	Same frequency as oral phenytoin

[a] Dose expressed as Phenytoin sodium equivalents (PE).
1 mg PE = 1.5 mg fosphenytoin sodium
[b] Initial dose; subsequent doses are dependent on patient response and trough plasma phenytoin concentrations.

chrome P450 enzymes. Inhibition of phenytoin metabolism may produce significant increases in plasma phenytoin concentrations and increase the risk of phenytoin toxicity. Phenytoin is also a potent inducer of hepatic drug-metabolising enzymes.

The following drug interactions are the most commonly occurring drug interactions with phenytoin: Drugs that may *increase* plasma phenytoin concentrations include: acute alcohol intake, amiodarone, chloramphenicol, chlordiazepoxide, diazepam, dicoumarol, disulfiram, oestrogens, fluoxetine, H_2-antagonists (e.g. cimetidine), halothane, isoniazid, methylphenidate, phenothiazines, phenylbutazone, salicylates, succinimides (e.g. ethosuximide), sulphonamides, tolbutamide, trazodone, viloxazine, antifungal agents (e.g. amphotericin B, fluconazole, ketoconazole, miconazole, and itraconazole) and omeprazole.

Drugs that may *decrease* plasma phenytoin concentrations include carbamazepine, chronic alcohol abuse, reserpine, folic acid, sucralfate and vigabatrin.

Drugs that may either *increase* or *decrease* plasma phenytoin concentrations include: phenobarbitone, valproic acid, sodium valproate, antineoplastic agents, ciprofloxacin and certain antacids. Similarly, the effects of phenytoin on plasma phenobarbitone, valproic acid and sodium valproate concentrations are unpredictable.

Although not a true pharmacokinetic interaction, tricyclic antidepressants and phenothiazines may precipitate seizures in susceptible patients and Pro-Epanutin dosage may need to be adjusted.

Drugs whose efficacy is impaired by phenytoin include: anticoagulants, corticosteroids, dicoumarol, digitoxin, doxycycline, oestrogens, frusemide, oral contraceptives, rifampicin, quinidine, theophylline, vitamin D, antifungal agents, antineoplastic agents and clozapine.

Drugs whose effect is enhanced by phenytoin include: warfarin.

Drug/laboratory test interactions: Phenytoin may decrease serum concentrations of T_4. It may also produce low results in dexamethasone or metyrapone tests. This may be an artefact. Phenytoin may cause increased blood glucose or serum concentrations of alkaline phosphatase and gamma glutamyl transpeptidase (GGT).

Phenytoin may affect blood calcium and blood sugar metabolism tests.

Phenytoin has the potential to lower serum folate levels.

Pregnancy and lactation: An increase in seizure frequency may occur during pregnancy because of altered phenytoin pharmacokinetics. Periodic measurement of plasma phenytoin concentrations may be valuable in the management of pregnant women as a guide to appropriate adjustment of dosage (see *Posology and method of administration: Therapeutic drug monitoring*). However, postpartum restoration of the original dosage will probably be indicated.

If this drug is used during pregnancy, or if the patient becomes pregnant while taking the drug, the patient should be informed of the potential harm to the foetus. Prenatal exposure to phenytoin may increase the risks for congenital malformations and other adverse developmental outcomes. Increased frequencies of major malformations (such as orofacial clefts and cardiac defects), minor anomalies (dysmorphic facial features, nail and digit hypoplasia), growth abnormalities (including microcephaly) and mental deficiency have been reported among children born to epileptic women who took phenytoin alone or in combination with other antiepileptic drugs during pregnancy. There have also been several reported cases of malignancies, including neuroblastoma, in children whose mothers received phenytoin during pregnancy. The overall incidence of malformations for children of epileptic women treated with antiepileptic drugs (phenytoin and/or others) during pregnancy is about 10% or two- to three-fold that in the general population. However, the relative contribution of antiepileptic drugs and other factors associated with epilepsy to this increased risk are uncertain and in most cases it has not been possible to attribute specific developmental abnormalities to particular antiepileptic drugs.

It might be necessary to give vitamin K to the mother during the last gestational month. Neonates of the mother receiving Pro-Epanutin should be monitored for haemorrhagic diathesis and if necessary additional vitamin K should be administered.

Foetal toxicity, developmental toxicity, and teratogenicity were observed in offspring of rats given fosphenytoin during pregnancy, similar to those reported with phenytoin. No developmental effects were observed in offspring of pregnant rabbits given fosphenytoin; malformations have been reported in offspring of pregnant rabbits with phenytoin at ≥75 mg/kg.

It is not known whether Pro-Epanutin is excreted in human milk.

Following administration of oral phenytoin, phenytoin appears to be excreted in low concentrations in human milk. Therefore, breast-feeding is not recommended for women receiving Pro-Epanutin.

Effects on ability to drive and use machines: Caution is recommended in patients performing skilled tasks (eg, driving or operating machinery) as treatment with fosphenytoin may cause central nervous system adverse effects such as dizziness and drowsiness.

Undesirable effects: The following adverse events have been reported in clinical trials in adults receiving Pro-Epanutin. The list also includes adverse effects that have been reported following both the acute and chronic use of phenytoin.

Central nervous system: Central nervous system effects are the most common side effects seen following administration of Pro-Epanutin or phenytoin and are usually dose-related, nystagmus, dizziness, paraesthesia, ataxia, tremor, incoordination, stupor, vertigo, euphoria, drowsiness, motor twitching, transient nervousness, slurred speech, mental confusion, insomnia.

There have also been rare reports of phenytoin-induced dyskinesias, including chorea, dystonia, and asterixis, similar to those induced by phenothiazines or other neuroleptic drugs. A predominantly sensory peripheral polyneuropathy has been observed in patients receiving long-term phenytoin therapy. Tonic seizures have also been reported.

The incidence and severity of adverse events related to the CNS and sensory disturbances were greater at higher doses and rates.

Cardiovascular and respiratory systems: Hypotension, vasodilation, atria and ventricular conduction depression, ventricular fibrillation, and cardiovascular collapse (see *Special warnings and special precautions for use),* alterations in respiratory function (including respiratory arrest), pneumonitis.

Haemopoietic system: Ecchymosis, thrombocytopenia, leucopenia, granulocytopenia, agranulocytosis, pancytopenia with or without bone marrow suppression, and aplastic anaemia have been occasionally reported with phenytoin administration. Some of these reports have been fatal.

Liver or kidney: Toxic hepatitis, liver damage, interstitial nephritis.

Gastrointestinal system: Nausea, vomiting, dry mouth, taste perversion, constipation.

Skin and connective tissue: Pruritus, rash (see *Special warnings and special precautions for use*), coarsening of the facial features, enlargement of the lips, gingival hyperplasia, hirsutism, hypertrichosis, Peyronie's disease and Dupuytren's contracture may occur rarely.

Special senses: Tinnitus, ear disorder, taste perversion, abnormal vision.

Immune system: Hypersensitivity syndrome (see *Special warnings and special precautions for use*), systemic lupus erythematosus, periarteritis nodosa, immunoglobulin abnormalities.

Body as a whole: Headache, pain, asthenia, chills, injection site reaction, injection site pain, polyarthropathy, hyperglycaemia.

No trends in laboratory changes were observed in Pro-Epanutin treated patients.

Overdose: There is no experience with Pro-Epanutin overdosage in humans. Initial symptoms of Pro-Epanutin toxicity are those associated with acute phenytoin toxicity. These are nystagmus, ataxia, and dysarthria. Other signs include tremor, hyperreflexia, lethargy, slurred speech, nausea, vomiting, coma, and hypotension. There is a risk of potentially fatal respiratory or circulatory depression. There are marked variations among individuals with respect to plasma phenytoin concentrations where toxicity occurs. Lateral gaze nystagmus usually appears at 20 mg/l, ataxia at 30 mg/l, and dysarthria and lethargy appear when the plasma concentration is over 40 mg/l. However, phenytoin concentrations as high as 50 mg/l have been reported without evidence of toxicity. As much as 25 times the therapeutic phenytoin dose has been taken, resulting in plasma phenytoin concentrations over 100 mg/l, with complete recovery.

Treatment is non-specific since there is no known antidote to Pro-Epanutin or phenytoin overdosage. The adequacy of the respiratory and circulatory systems should be carefully observed and appropriate supportive measures employed. Haemodialysis can be considered since phenytoin is not completely bound to plasma proteins. Total exchange transfusion has been used in the treatment of severe intoxication in children. In acute overdosage the possibility of the use of other CNS depressants, including alcohol, should be borne in mind.

Formate and phosphate are metabolites of fosphenytoin and, therefore, may contribute to signs of toxicity following overdosage. Signs of formate toxicity are similar to those of methanol toxicity and are associated with severe anion-gap metabolic acidosis. Large amounts of phosphate, delivered rapidly, could potentially cause hypocalcaemia with paraesthesia, muscle spasms and seizures. Ionised free calcium levels can be measured and, if low, used to guide treatment.

Pharmacological properties

Pharmacodynamic properties: N03AB. Pro-Epanutin is a prodrug of phenytoin and accordingly, its anticonvulsant effects are attributable to phenytoin. The pharmacological and toxicological effects of fosphenytoin sodium include those of phenytoin.

The cellular mechanisms of phenytoin thought to be responsible for its anticonvulsant actions include modulation of voltage-dependent sodium channels of neurones, inhibition of calcium flux across neuronal membranes, modulation of voltage-dependent calcium channels of neurones and enhancement of the sodium-potassium ATPase activity of neurones and glial cells. The modulation of sodium channels may be a primary anticonvulsant mechanism because this property is shared with several other anticonvulsants in addition to phenytoin.

Pharmacokinetic properties: Fosphenytoin is a prodrug of phenytoin and it is rapidly converted into phenytoin mole for mole.

Fosphenytoin pharmacokinetics: Absorption/Bioavailability: When Pro-Epanutin is administered by IV infusion, maximum plasma fosphenytoin concentrations are achieved at the end of the infusion. Fosphenytoin is completely bioavailable following IM administration of Pro-Epanutin. Peak concentrations occur at approximately 30 minutes postdose. Plasma fosphenytoin concentrations following IM administration are lower but more sustained than those following IV administration due to the time required for absorption of fosphenytoin from the injection site.

Distribution: Fosphenytoin is extensively bound (95% to 99%) to human plasma proteins, primarily albumin. Binding to plasma proteins is saturable with the result that the fraction unbound increases as total fosphenytoin concentrations increase. Fosphenytoin displaces phenytoin from protein binding sites. The volume of distribution of fosphenytoin increases with fosphenytoin sodium dose and rate, and ranges from 4.3 to 10.8 L.

Metabolism and excretion: The hydrolysis of fosphenytoin to phenytoin yields 2 metabolites, phosphate and formaldehyde. Formaldehyde is subsequently converted to formate, which is in turn metabolised via a folate dependent mechanism. Although phosphate and formaldehyde (formate) have potentially important biological effects, these effects typically occur at concentrations considerably in excess of those obtained when Pro-Epanutin is administered under conditions of use recommended in this labelling.

The conversion half-life of fosphenytoin to phenytoin is approximately 15 minutes. The mechanism of fosphenytoin conversion has not been determined, but phosphatases probably play a major role. Each mmol of fosphenytoin is metabolised to 1 mmol of phenytoin, phosphate and formate.

Fosphenytoin is not excreted in urine.

Phenytoin pharmacokinetics (after Pro-Epanutin administration): The pharmacokinetics of phenytoin following IV administration of Pro-Epanutin, are complex and when used in an emergency setting (e.g., status epilepticus), differences in rate of availability of phenytoin could be critical. Studies have, therefore, empirically determined an infusion rate for Pro-Epanutin that gives a rate and extent of phenytoin systemic availability similar to that of a 50 mg/min phenytoin sodium infusion. Because Pro-Epanutin is completely absorbed and converted to phenytoin following IM administration, systemic phenytoin concentrations are generated that are similar enough to oral phenytoin to allow essentially interchangeable use and to allow reliable IM loading dose administration.

Absorption/bioavailability: Fosphenytoin sodium is rapidly and completely converted to phenytoin following IV or IM Pro-Epanutin administration. Therefore, the bioavailability of phenytoin following administration of Pro-Epanutin is the same as that following parenteral administration of phenytoin.

Distribution: Phenytoin is highly bound to plasma proteins, primarily albumin, although to a lesser extent than fosphenytoin. In the absence of fosphenytoin, approximately 12% of total plasma phenytoin is unbound over the clinically relevant concentration range. However, fosphenytoin displaces phenytoin from plasma protein binding sites. This increases the fraction of phenytoin unbound (up to 30% unbound) during the period required for conversion of fosphenytoin to phenytoin (approximately 0.5 to 1 hour postinfusion). The volume of distribution for phenytoin ranges from 24.9 to 36.8 L.

Metabolism and excretion: Phenytoin derived from administration of Pro-Epanutin is extensively metabolised in the liver and excreted in urine primarily as 5-(p-hydroxy-phenyl)-5-phenylhydantoin and its glucuronide; little unchanged phenytoin (1%-5% of the

The following table displays pharmacokinetic parameters of fosphenytoin and phenytoin following IV and IM Pro-Epanutin administration.

Route	Dose (mg PE)	Dose (mg PE/kg)	Infusion rate (mg PE/min)	Fosphenytoin			Total phenytoin		Free (unbound) phenytoin	
				Cmax (mcg/ml)	tmax (hr)	$t_{\frac{1}{2}}$ (min)	Cmax (mcg/ml)	Tmax (hr)	Cmax (mcg/ml)	tmax (hr)
Intramuscular	855	12.4	–	18.5	0.61	41.2	14.3	3.23	2.02	4.16
Intravenous	1200	15.6	100	139	0.19	18.9	26.9	1.18	2.78	0.52
Intravenous	1200	15.6	150	156	0.13	20.5	28.2	0.98	3.18	0.58

Dose = Fosphenytoin dose (phenytoin sodium equivalents [mgPE] or phenytoin sodium equivalents/kg [mg PE/kg]).
Infusion rate = Fosphenytoin infusion rate (mg phenytoin sodium equivalents/min [mg PE/min]).
Cmax = Maximum plasma analyte concentration (mcg/ml).
Tmax = Time of Cmax (hr).
$t_{\frac{1}{2}}$ = Terminal elimination half-life (min).

Pro-Epanutin dose) is recovered in urine. Phenytoin hepatic metabolism is saturable, and following administration of single IV Pro-Epanutin doses of 400 to 1200 mg PE, total and unbound phenytoin AUC values increase disproportionately with dose. Mean total phenytoin half-life values (12.0 to 28.9 hr) following Pro-Epanutin administration at these doses are similar to those after equal doses of parenteral phenytoin and tend to be longer at higher plasma phenytoin concentrations.

Characteristics in patients: patients with renal or hepatic disease: Fosphenytoin conversion to phenytoin is more rapid in patients with renal or hepatic disease than with other patients because of decreased plasma protein binding secondary to hypoalbuminaemia occurring in these disease states. The extent of conversion to phenytoin is not affected. Phenytoin metabolism may be reduced in patients with hepatic impairment resulting in increased plasma phenytoin concentrations (see *Posology and method of administration*).

Elderly patients: Patient age had no significant impact on fosphenytoin pharmacokinetics. Phenytoin clearance tends to decrease with increasing age (20% less in patients over 70 years of age relative to that in patients 20-30 years of age) (see *Posology and method of administration*).

Gender: Gender had no significant impact on fosphenytoin or phenytoin pharmacokinetics.

Children: Limited studies in children (age 5 to 10) receiving Pro-Epanutin have shown similar concentration-time profiles of fosphenytoin and phenytoin to those observed in adult patients receiving comparable mg PE/kg doses.

Preclinical safety data: The systemic toxicity of fosphenytoin is qualitatively and quantitatively similar to that of phenytoin at comparable exposures.

Carcinogenicity studies with fosphenytoin are not available. Since fosphenytoin is a prodrug of phenytoin, the carcinogenicity results with phenytoin can be extrapolated. An increased incidence of hepatocellular tumors was observed after administration of phenytoin in 1 of 3 studies in rats and 2 of 3 studies in mice. Lymphomas were also observed in susceptible strains of mice. These rodent tumors are of uncertain clinical significance.

Genetic toxicity studies showed that fosphenytoin was not mutagenic in bacteria or in mammalian cells in vitro. It was clastogenic in cultured V79 Chinese hamster lung cells in the presence of metabolic activation, but not in an in vivo mouse bone marrow micronucleus test. Phenytoin is not genotoxic in vivo.

Local irritation following IV or IM dosing or inadvertent perivenous administration was less severe with fosphenytoin than with phenytoin, and was generally comparable to that observed with vehicle injections. The potential of fosphenytoin to induce intra-arterial irritation was not assessed.

Pharmaceutical particulars

List of excipients: Water for injection, trometanol buffer adjusted to pH 8.6 to 9.0 with hydrochloric acid.

Incompatibilities: None known

Shelf life: 24 months.

When Pro-Epanutin injection is diluted with 5% dextrose or 0.9% saline, it is suitable only for immediate and single use.

Special precautions for storage: Store under refrigeration at 2°C to 8°C. The undiluted product should not be stored at room temperature (below 25°C) for more than 24 hours. Vials that develop particulate matter should not be used.

Nature and contents of container: Ten-ml glass vials (containing 10-ml solution) with a Teflon coated stopper, an aluminium seal and flip-off cap.

Boxes of 10 vials with 10 ml solution for injection.

Instructions for use/handling: Pro-Epanutin must be diluted to a concentration ranging from 1.5 to 25 mgPE/ml prior to infusion, with 5% dextrose or 0.9% saline solution for injection.

Marketing authorisation number PL 00019/0157

Date of first authorisation 4th February 1998

Date of Revision 10th June 1998

Legal category POM.

ZARONTIN*

Presentation *Elixir:* A clear, red, raspberry flavoured, syrup.

Capsules: Clear pale yellow, dye free oblong soft gelatin capsules containing a clear solution.

Composition: Each 5 ml Zarontin Syrup contains: Ethosuximide B.P. 250 mg in a pleasantly flavoured syrup.

Each soft gelatin capsule contains: Ethosuximide Ph Eur 250 mg.

Uses

Action: Ethosuximide suppresses the paroxysmal spike and wave pattern common to absence (petit mal) seizures. The frequency of epileptiform attacks is reduced, apparently by depression of the motor cortex and elevation of the threshold of the central nervous system to convulsive stimuli. Compared with other succinimide anticonvulsants, ethosuximide is more specific for pure absence seizures.

Indications: Primarily useful in absence seizures. When generalised tonic clonic seizures (grand mal) and other forms of epilepsy co-exist with absence seizures, Zarontin may be administered in combination with other antiepileptic drugs.

Dosage and administration Oral.

Adults and children over six years: Initially two capsules or two 5 ml spoonfuls daily and adjusted thereafter to the patient's needs; daily dosage should be increased by small increments, for example, by one capsule or 5 ml every 4 to 7 days until control is achieved with minimal side effects. Although four to six capsules or 20-30 ml daily in divided doses often produces control of seizures, higher doses up to 8 capsules or 40 ml daily may occasionally be required.

Children and infants under 6 years: The initial dose is 5 ml daily which is adjusted by small increments until control is achieved with minimal side effects. The optimal dose for most children is 20 mg/kg/day. This dose has given average plasma levels within the accepted therapeutic range of 40 to 100 mg/l.

Contra-indications, warnings, etc

Contra-indications: Hypersensitivity to succinimides.

Use in pregnancy and lactation: There is some evidence that the succinimides may produce congenital abnormality in the offspring of a small number of epileptic patients and therefore they should only be used in pregnancy if in the judgement of the physician the potential benefits outweigh the risk.

Ethosuximide may be excreted in breast milk therefore breast-feeding is best avoided.

Precautions and warnings: Ethosuximide is capable of producing morphological and funtional changes in the animal liver. In humans, abnormal liver and renal function studies have been reported. Zarontin should be used with caution in patients with impaired hepatic or renal function. Periodic urinalysis and liver function studies are advised for all patients receiving the drug.

Psychotic states thought to be induced or exacerbated by anticonvulsant therapy have been reported.

Ethosuximide may impair the mental and/or physical abilities required for the performance of potentially hazardous tasks such as driving or other such activities requiring alertness; therefore the patient should be cautioned accordingly.

Blood dyscrasias including some with fatal outcome have been reported to be associated with the use of ethosuximide. Should symptoms or signs of infection (e.g.sore throat, fever) develop, blood count determinations should be performed.

In most cases of leucopenia, the blood picture has been restored to normal on reduction of the dosage or discontinuation of the drug. Where leucopenia has occurred with other drugs, the polymorph count has in some cases increased steadily after starting treatment with ethosuximide and discontinuing the previous medication.

Ethosuximide when used alone in mixed types of epilepsy, may increase the frequency of generalised tonic-clonic (grand mal) seizures in some patients.

If the patient has been receiving other antiepileptic medications the sudden withdrawal of these drugs may precipitate a series of attacks before Zarontin has been given in sufficient amounts to exercise control. This may be avoided by gradually replacing the antiepileptic medication previously used with Zarontin.

Sudden withdrawal of Zarontin should be avoided.

Drug Interactions: Since ethosuximide may interact with concurrently administered antiepileptic drugs, periodic serum level determinations of these drugs may be necessary (e.g., ethosuximide may elevate phenytoin serum levels and valproic acid has been reported to both increase and decrease ethosuximide levels).

Adverse reactions: Mild side effects, which are usually transient, may occur initially. These include apathy, drowsiness, depression, mild euphoria, extrapyramidal side effects, headache, ataxia, dizziness, anorexia, gastric upset, nausea and vomiting.

Skin rashes have been seen in a few patients. Systemic lupus erythematosus has occasionally been associated with the use of ethosuximide. Additionally, lupus-like reactions have been reported in children given ethosuximide. They vary in severity from systemic immunological disorders, which include the nephrotic syndrome, to the asymptomatic presence of antinuclear antibodies. The nephrotic syndrome is rare and a complete recovery has usually been reported on drug withdrawal. Stevens-Johnson syndrome has also occurred during administration.

Cases of leucopenia, agranulocytosis, pancytopenia and aplastic anaemia have been reported. Monocytosis, leucocytosis and transitory mild eosinophilia have also been noted.

Other adverse reactions reported include: weight loss, diarrhoea, abdominal pain, gum hypertrophy, swelling of the tongue, hiccoughs, irritability, hyperactivity, lethargy, fatigue, sleep disturbances, night terrors, inability to concentrate, aggressiveness, paranoid psychosis, increased libido, myopia, and vaginal bleeding.

Overdosage: Acute overdoses may produce nausea, vomiting and CNS depression including coma with respiratory depression. A relationship between ethosuximide toxicity and its plasma levels has not been established.

If less than 2 g have been taken, fluids should be given by mouth. If a larger dose has been taken the stomach should be emptied, respiration maintained and any other symptoms treated accordingly. Activated charcoal and purgatives are known to be used in the treatment of overdosage. Haemodialysis may be useful. Forced diuresis and exchange transfusions are ineffective.

Pharmaceutical precautions *Capsules:* Store at a temperature not exceeding 30°C.

Syrup: Store at a temperature not exceeding 25°C.

Recommended diluent–Syrup B.P. When diluted use within 14 days of preparation.

Legal category POM.

Package quantities Capsules 250 mg: 56. Syrup: 300 ml.

Further information Nil

Product licence numbers
Zarontin Capsules 0019/0169
Zarontin Syrup 0019/0170

**Trade Mark*

Pasteur Mérieux MSD Ltd
Mallards Reach
Bridge Avenue
Maidenhead
Berkshire
SL6 1QP

☎ 01628 785291   01628 671722

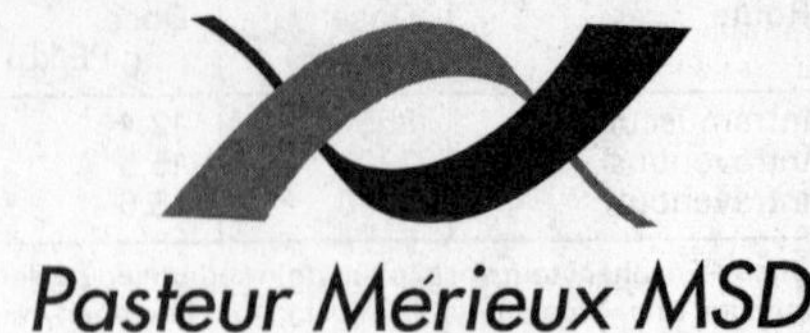

ACT-HIB*

Haemophilus type b conjugate vaccine Pasteur Merieux

Presentation Act-HIB is a sterile solution of inactivated conjugate polysaccharide vaccine against *Haemophilus influenzae* type b invasive disease.

Each 0.5 ml dose contains not less than 10 mcg of lyophilised Haemophilus type b polysaccharide conjugated to tetanus protein, with TRIS and sucrose added as stabilisers. Sodium chloride (0.4%) diluent is supplied with each dose. The product does not contain thiomersal or aluminium hydroxide.

Uses Active immunisation against invasive diseases caused by *Haemophilus influenzae* type b.

Dosage and administration By deep subcutaneous or intramuscular injection.

Primary immunisation: The vaccine is indicated for children from 2 months of age. The immunisation schedule is three injections each of 0.5 ml with an interval of 4 weeks between the first and second doses and not less than 4 weeks between the second and third doses.

In cases where both adsorbed diphtheria, tetanus and pertussis vaccine and haemophilus type b conjugate vaccine are indicated, Adsorbed Diphtheria, Tetanus and Pertussis Vaccine BP, Pasteur Mérieux may be used to reconstitute ACT-HIB. The combined vaccine can then be administered as a single injection. No other adsorbed diphtheria, tetanus and pertussis vaccine should be used.

Haemophilus influenzae type b conjugate vaccine from the same manufacturer should be used for the whole primary immunisation course.

Children over 13 months should receive a single dose of 0.5 ml of Act-HIB, which may be administered simultaneously with measles, mumps and rubella vaccine, at a different site.

Children of any age may receive Act-HIB but the vaccine would not normally be required in those over 4 years of age.

The vaccine should be reconstituted using the diluent provided.

Record the dose, batch number and date of administration.

Instructions for mixing adsorbed Diphtheria, Tetanus and Pertussis Vaccine BP, Pasteur Mérieux (DTP Pasteur Mérieux) with ACT-HIB: Inject the entire contents of an ampoule or pre-filled syringe of DTP Pasteur Mérieux into a vial of ACT-HIB. Shake gently for 30 seconds. Allow the vial to stand, shaking it occasionally. Examine the base of the vial for any remaining undissolved particles of ACT-HIB. Administer the combined vaccine immediately after reconstitution.

Contra-indications, warnings, etc

Contra-indications: Acute infectious illness. Hypersensitivity to the vaccine or any component. Severe reaction to a previous dose of Act-HIB.

Warnings: Act-HIB confers protection specific to *Haemophilus influenzae* type b. Immunisation does not protect against other serogroups of *Haemophilus influenzae* or against meningitis caused by meningococci or other organisms.

Side-effects: These are normally mild and short lasting with no serious sequelae. Local reactions including erythema, swelling, tenderness or pain may occur at the injection site. Less commonly systemic reactions may occur; reactions reported include fever, headache, malaise, irritability, inconsolable and high pitched crying.

Rarely seizures have been reported. One case of transient cyanosis of the lower limbs, and one case of erythema multiforme have been reported.

Precautions: Although anaphylaxis is extremely rare, facilities for its management should always be available during vaccination.

Use in pregnancy: No reproductive studies have been conducted in animals. There is no data on the use of this vaccine in pregnancy or lactation. The vaccine should not normally be used in pregnancy or during lactation.

Pharmaceutical precautions Store at +2°C to +8°C, do not freeze the diluent.

After reconstitution, use within one hour. Any vaccine remaining after this time should be discarded.

Shake before use.

Legal category POM.

Package quantities Box of 1 single vial of lyophilised vaccine + 1 syringe of diluent (0.5 ml).

Box of 10 vials of lyophilised vaccine + 10 syringes of diluent (0.5 ml).

Box of 10 vials of lyophilised vaccine + 10 ampoules of diluent (0.5 ml).

Further information The tetanus protein in the vaccine does not replace the need for routine tetanus immunisation.

Product licence numbers

Vaccine	6745/0041
Diluent syringe	6745/0042
Diluent ampoule	6745/0054

Date of preparation 07/95

ACT-HIB* DTP d.c. ▼

Haemophilus type b conjugate vaccine in a dual chamber syringe with Adsorbed Diphtheria, Tetanus and Pertussis Vaccine BP (DTP Pasteur Merieux)

Qualitative and quantitative composition

Purified diphtheria toxoid ≥ 30 IU (≤ 30 Lf)
Purified tetanus toxoid ≥ 60 IU (≤ 12 Lf)
Bordetella pertussis ≥ 4 IU (≤ 16 opacity units)
Haemophilus type b polysaccharide conjugated to tetanus protein equivalent to 10 mcg of polysaccharide
Aluminium (as aluminium hydroxide) ≤ 1.25 mg

The DTP Pasteur Mérieux is a sterile aqueous suspension containing a mixture of the diphtheria, tetanus and pertussis antigens adsorbed onto aluminium hydroxide with thiomersal added as preservative. The ACT-HIB is in lyophilised form to optimise its stability.

Pharmaceutical form The DTP Pasteur Mérieux vaccine is in the form of a sterile liquid suspension; the ACT-HIB is lyophilised. When reconstituted, ACT-HIB DTP d.c. comprises a 0.5 ml dose suspension for intramuscular or deep subcutaneous injection only.

Clinical particulars

Therapeutic indications: Active immunisation against diphtheria, tetanus, pertussis and against invasive diseases caused by Haemophilus influenzae type b (e.g. meningitis, septicaemia, cellulitis, arthritis, epiglottitis).

Posology and method of administration: Administer by intramuscular or deep subcutaneous injection only.

Primary immunisation: Three injections each of 0.5 ml with an interval of at least 4 weeks between the first and second doses and at least 4 weeks between the second and the third doses. The vaccine may be administered to infants from 2 months of age.

If a primary course is interrupted it should be resumed allowing appropriate intervals between the remaining doses of ACT-HIB DTP d.c.

Reinforcing doses: In some children it may have been decided initially not to immunise against pertussis and they may have received one or more doses of adsorbed diphtheria and tetanus vaccine and Haemophilus type b conjugate vaccine. If in such cases, subsequently it is decided to immunise against pertussis, ACT-HIB DTP d.c. may be administered to complete the 3 dose immunisation course of adsorbed diphtheria and tetanus vaccine and Haemophilus type b conjugate vaccine. Monovalent pertussis vaccine may be given thereafter at monthly intervals to complete the 3 dose course of pertussis immunisation.

ACT-HIB DTP d.c. is not recommended for children presenting for their pre-school diphtheria and tetanus booster. Such children will not normally need Haemophilus type b conjugate vaccine.

Children aged 4 years and over adults and elderly: ACT-HIB DTP d.c. vaccine is not recommended for persons aged 4 years or over.

Other information: Oral poliomyelitis vaccine BP may be given simultaneously.

Record the dose, batch number and date of administration.

Contra-indications: The following recommendations are in line with those of the Department of Health as issued in its 1992 guidelines 'Immunisation against Infectious Diseases' (HMSO).

Hypersensitivity to any vaccine component is a contra-indication to ACT-HIB DTP d.c.

Specialist advice: No child should either be immunised or denied immunisation without serious thought as to the consequences, both for the individual and the community. Where there is any doubt, advice should be sought from a Consultant Paediatrician, Consultant in Public Health Medicine or District (Health Board) Immunisation Co-ordinator.

Alternative vaccination: If pertussis vaccine is contra-indicated or refused by parents, then DT/Vac/Ads (Child) should be offered.

Acute illness: If the child is suffering from any acute illness, immunisation should be postponed until the child has recovered. Minor infections without fever or systemic upset are not reasons to postpone immunisation.

General reactions: The following are regarded as severe general reactions: fever equal to or more than 39.5°C within 48 hours of vaccine; anaphylaxis; bronchospasm; laryngeal oedema; generalised collapse. Prolonged unresponsiveness; prolonged inconsolable or high-pitched screaming for more than 4 hours; convulsions or encephalopathy occurring within 72 hours. General reactions to ACT-HIB DTP d.c. are considered most likely to be due to the pertussis component. Children who have a history of severe general reaction to a preceding dose of a pertussis-containing vaccine (including ACT-HIB DTP d.c.) should not receive the whole cell pertussis again. They should receive DT vaccine in one limb and Haemophilus influenzae type b conjugate vaccine in another limb. If another severe general reaction occurs, primary immunisation should be discontinued and expert advice should be sought.

Local reactions: The following are regarded as severe local reactions: an extensive area of redness and swelling which becomes indurated and involves most of the antero-lateral surface of the thigh or a major part of the circumference of the upper arm. Since local reactions to ACT-HIB DTP d.c. may be due to one or more of its components, it is recommended that children who have a history of a severe local reaction to a preceding dose of ACT-HIB DTP d.c. be given DTP in one limb and Haemophilus influenzae type b conjugate vaccine in another limb. Despite the previous severe local reaction with ACT-HIB DTP d.c., the need to adequately immunise the child outweighs the risk of a further severe local reaction. If another severe local reaction occurs to one or both of these vaccines, the vaccine(s) concerned should not be re-administered.

Personal history of epilepsy: Specialist advice (see above) should be sought prior to performing immunisation on children with a personal history of epilepsy.

Family history of epilepsy: In a recent British study, children with a family history of epilepsy were immunised with pertussis vaccine without any significant adverse events. These children's developmental progress has been normal. In children with a close family history (first degree relative) of idiopathic epilepsy, there may be a risk of developing a similar condition, irrespective of vaccine. Immunisation is recommended for these children.

Febrile convulsions: When there is a personal or family history of febrile convulsions, there is an increased risk of these occurring after pertussis immunisation. In such children, immunisation is recommended but advice on the prevention of fever should be given at the time of immunisation.

Evolving neurological disease: Where there is an ongoing evolving neurological problem, immunisation should be deferred until the condition is stable.

Stable neurological disease: Stable neurological conditions such as occur in certain patients with cerebral palsy or spina bifida are not a contra-indication to immunisation.

Cerebral damage in the neonatal period: When there has been a documented history of cerebral damage in the neonatal period, immunisation should be carried out unless there is evidence of an evolving neurological abnormality. If pertussis immunisation is to be deferred, then this should be stated on the neonatal discharge summary and DT and Haemophilus type b conjugate vaccines given at the appropriate chronological age.

Allergy: A personal or family history of allergy is not a contra-indication to immunisation.

Special warnings and precautions for use: HIV positive individuals may receive ACT-HIB DTP d.c. but efficacy may be reduced.

Not for intradermal injection.

Although anaphylaxis is rare, facilities for its management should always be available during vaccination.

ACT-HIB DTP d.c. is not recommended for use in individuals aged 4 years or over. Use in individuals aged 10 years or over may be associated with severe hypersensitivity reactions (due to the adsorbed diphtheria, tetanus and pertussis vaccine component).

ACT-HIB DTP d.c. confers protection specific to Haemophilus influenzae type b. It does not protect against other serotypes of Haemophilus influenzae or against meningitis caused by meningococci or other organisms.

Interaction with other medicaments and other forms of interaction: ACT-HIB DTP d.c. should not be mixed with other vaccines or drugs prior to administration.

Pregnancy or lactation: No reproductive studies have been conducted in animals. There is no data on the use of this vaccine in pregnancy or lactation. The vaccine is not recommended for use in pregnancy or during lactation.

Effects on ability to drive and use machines: Not applicable.

Undesirable effects: Pain tenderness, swelling or redness may occur at the injection site. Generalised reactions may include headache, fever, malaise, irritability, pallor, crying. Attacks of inconsolable and high pitched screaming, limpness and convulsions may occur.

Rarely seizures, erythema multiforme and transient cyanosis of the lower limbs have been reported.

More severe neurological conditions including encephalopathy and prolonged convulsions have been reported after pertussis vaccine.

Acute allergic reactions may occur, including anaphylaxis, dyspnoea and bronchospasm, urticaria and laryngeal oedema. Peripheral neuropathy has been reported.

A persistent nodule may occur at the site of injection particularly if the vaccine is administered into superficial layers of the subcutaneous tissue.

Overdose: Not applicable.

Pharmacological properties
Pharmacodynamic properties: The Adsorbed Diphtheria, Tetanus and Pertussis vaccine component is a pharmacopoieal product used for active immunisation.

The ACT-HIB component contains the purified capsular polysaccharide (polyribosylribitol phosphate, PRP) of Haemophilus influenzae type b conjugated covalently to tetanus toxin protein.

When administered alone PRP induces a serological response but it is weakly immunogenic in infants. The covalent binding of PRP to tetanus protein renders it a T-cell dependent immunogen which induce a specific IgG anti-PRP response in infants and which can instil an immunological memory.

Immunogenicity studies in infants vaccinated with ACT-HIB DTP d.c. at 2, 3, 4 months of age have shown that a PRP antibody titre of ≥ 0.15 mcg/ml was reached in 97.9–100% of subjects after 3 doses. An anti-PRP titre of ≥ 1.00 mcg/ml was achieved in 82.5–92% after 3 doses. A marked anamnestic response was seen to a single test dose of plain PRP vaccine given at 14 months of age after a primary course using a vial of ACT-HIB reconstituted with a syringe of DTP vaccine at 3, 4, 5 months of age. The geometric mean titre of serum PRP antibody rose 20 fold after the single test dose of plain PRP vaccine given at 14 months.

Pharmacokinetic properties: Not applicable.

Preclinical safety data: Not applicable.

Pharmaceutical particulars
List of excipients: Thiomersal, TRIS (hydroxymethylaminomethane), sucrose, water for injections, sodium chloride, disodium phosphate, monopotassium phosphate.

Incompatibilities: None known.

Shelf life: 24 months at +2°C to +8°C.

Special precautions for storage: Store at +2°C to +8°C. Do not freeze.

Nature and contents of container: ACT-HIB DTP d.c. is supplied in a dual chamber syringe with lyophilised ACT-HIB in the first chamber and DTP Pasteur Mérieux suspension in the second chamber.

The containers are a type I glass dual chamber syringe with a disposable stainless steel needle and a plastic plunger rod. Closures are Elastomer tip-cap and plunger stoppers.

Instructions for use/handling: The dual chamber syringe should be shaken well prior to use to achieve a homogenous DTP Pasteur Mérieux suspension. Remove the rubber tip-cap and mount the needle. Whilst holding the syringe upright, depress the plunger carefully and expel the DTP Pasteur Mérieux suspension from the second chamber into the first chamber where it reconstitutes the lyophilised ACT-HIB.

Shake the syringe until a homogeneous suspension is achieved (the suspension is whitish/cloudy) and examine the syringe for any remaining undissolved particles of ACT-HIB. Continue shaking if necessary. Administer ACT-HIB DTP d.c. immediately after reconstitution.

Marketing authorisation number 6745/0079.

Date of approval/revision of SPC February 1997.

Legal category POM.

Date of preparation 02/97

ADSORBED DIPHTHERIA AND TETANUS VACCINE BP PASTEUR MÉRIEUX

Presentation Adsorbed diphtheria and tetanus vaccine is a sterile aqueous suspension containing a mixture of purified tetanus and diphtheria toxoids. The toxoids are adsorbed onto aluminium hydroxide with thiomersal added as preservative. Each 0.5 ml dose contains not less than 40 IU of tetanus toxoid and not less than 30 IU of diphtheria toxoid.

Uses For active immunisation against diphtheria and tetanus. Reinforcement of immunity to diphtheria and tetanus.

Dosage and administration By deep subcutaneous or intramuscular injection. Shake before use.

(a) Primary immunisation: 3 injections each of 0.5 ml with an interval of 4 weeks between the first and second doses and 4 weeks between the second and third doses.

(b) Reinforcing doses: A single reinforcing dose of adsorbed diphtheria and tetanus vaccine may be administered preferably after at least 3 years from the last dose of the primary immunisation course.

Children aged 10 years and over, adults, elderly: Adsorbed diphtheria and tetanus vaccine is *not* normally administered to persons aged 10 years or over. In this age group, if immunisation against diphtheria is indicated, an adult (low dose) diphtheria preparation should be used without the need for prior Schick testing.

Contra-indications, warnings, etc
Contra-indications: Aged 10 years or over. Acute infectious illness. Severe reaction to a previous dose. Hypersensitivity to any component of the vaccine.

Warnings: Not for intradermal injection.

Side-effects: Local reactions such as transient erythema, swelling, tenderness or pain at the injection site or rarely systemic effects such as fever, headache, malaise and pallor may occur. Acute allergic reactions have been reported after administration of adsorbed diphtheria and tetanus vaccines, including dyspnoea, urticaria, angioneurotic oedema, peripheral neuropathy and rarely, anaphylaxis. A persistent nodule at the site of vaccination may occur with all adsorbed vaccines, particularly if administered into the superficial layers of the subcutaneous tissue.

Precautions: Although anaphylaxis is extremely rare, facilities for its management should always be available during vaccination.

Use in pregnancy: Not recommended as there is insufficient data on the use of this type of vaccine in pregnancy.

Overdosage: Not applicable.

Pharmaceutical precautions Store in a refrigerator between +2°C and +8°C. Do not freeze. Shake well immediately before use.

Legal category POM.

Package quantities 0.5 ml single dose prefilled syringe (unit pack). 0.5 ml single dose ampoule (pack of 5).

Further information Use of Adsorbed Diphtheria and Tetanus Vaccine BP in individuals aged 10 years or over may be associated with severe hypersensitivity reactions.

Product licence number 6745/0046.

Date of preparation 05/97

ADSORBED DIPHTHERIA TETANUS AND PERTUSSIS VACCINE, BP PASTEUR MERIEUX

Presentation Adsorbed diphtheria, tetanus and pertussis vaccine is a sterile aqueous suspension containing a mixture of purified diphtheria and tetanus toxoids and killed *Bordetella pertussis* organisms adsorbed onto aluminium hydroxide with thiomersal added as preservative. Each 0.5 ml dose has a potency of not less than 30 IU of diphtheria toxoid, not less than 60 IU of tetanus toxoid and not less than 4 IU of *Bordetella pertussis* cells.

Uses For active immunisation against diphtheria, tetanus and pertussis.

Dosage and administration Administer by intramuscular or deep subcutaneous injection.

Primary immunisation: Three injections each of 0.5 ml with an interval of at least 4 weeks between the first and second doses and at least 4 weeks between the second and the third doses. The vaccine may be administered to infants from 2 months of age.

In cases where both adsorbed diphtheria, tetanus and pertussis vaccine and haemophilus type b conjugate vaccine are indicated, Adsorbed Diphtheria, Tetanus and Pertussis Vaccine BP, Pasteur Mérieux may be used to reconstitute ACT-HIB. The combined vaccine can then be administered as a single injection. No other adsorbed diphtheria, tetanus and pertussis vaccine should be used.

If a primary course is interrupted it should be resumed allowing appropriate intervals between the remaining doses.

Reinforcing doses: Once primary immunisation is completed, a single reinforcing dose of adsorbed diphtheria and tetanus vaccine may be administered preferably at least 3 years after the last dose of the primary course.

Where adsorbed diphtheria and tetanus vaccine (DT/Vac/Ads (child)) has been administered at the start of a primary course, adsorbed diphtheria, tetanus and pertussis vaccine may be administered for subsequent doses. Once three doses of adsorbed diphtheria and tetanus have been administered, monovalent pertussis vaccine may be given at monthly intervals to complete the course.

Children presenting for their pre-school diphtheria and tetanus booster who have not previously been immunised against pertussis may be given a single dose of adsorbed diphtheria, tetanus and pertussis vaccine with 2 subsequent doses of monovalent pertussis vaccine given at monthly intervals.

Children aged 10 years and over, adults and elderly: Adsorbed diphtheria, tetanus and pertussis vaccine is not recommended for persons aged 10 years or over.

Instructions for mixing adsorbed Diphtheria, Tetanus and Pertussis Vaccine BP, Pasteur Mérieux (DTP Pasteur Mérieux) with ACT-HIB: Inject the entire contents of an ampoule or pre-filled syringe of DTP Pasteur Mérieux into a vial of ACT-HIB. Shake gently for 30 seconds. Allows the vial to stand, shaking it occasionally. Examine the base of the vial for any remaining undissolved particles of ACT-HIB. Administer the combined vaccine immediately after reconstitution.

Contra-indications, warnings, etc
Department of Health recommendations: These recommendations are from the 1992 guidelines "immunisation against Infectious Diseases" (HMSO).

Specialist advice: No child should be either immunised or denied immunisation without serious thought as to the consequences, both for the individual child and the community. Where there is any doubt, advice should be sought from a Consultant Paediatrician, Consultant in Public Health Medicine or District (Health Board) Immunisation Co-ordinator.

Alternative vaccination: If pertussis vaccine is contra-indicated or refused by parents, then DT/Vac/Ads should be offered.

Acute illness: If the child is suffering from any acute illness, immunisation should be postponed until the child has recovered. Minor infections without fever or systemic upset are not reasons to postpone immunisation.

Local or general reactions: Immunisation should not be carried out in children who have a history of severe local or general reaction to a preceding dose. Immunisation should be completed with DT vaccine. The following reactions should be regarded as severe:

Local: An extensive area of redness and swelling which becomes indurated and involves most of the antero-lateral surface of the thigh or a major part of the circumference of the upper arm.

General: Fever equal to or more than 39.5°C within 48 hours of vaccine; anaphylaxis; bronchospasm; laryngeal oedema; generalised collapse. Prolonged unresponsiveness; prolonged inconsolable or high-pitched screaming for more than 4 hours; convulsions or encephalopathy occurring within 72 hours.

Personal history of epilepsy: Specialist advice should be sought prior to performing immunisation on children with a personal history of epilepsy (see above).

Family history of epilepsy: In a recent British study, children with a family history of epilepsy were immunised with pertussis vaccine without any significant adverse events. These children's developmental progress has been normal. In children with a close family history (first degree relative) of idiopathic epilepsy, there may be a risk of developing a similar condition, irrespective of vaccine. Immunisation is recommended for these children.

Febrile conclusions: When there is a personal or family history of febrile convulsions, there is an increased risk of these occurring after pertussis immunisation. In such children, immunisation is recommended but advice on the prevention of fever should be given at the time of immunisation.

Evolving neurological disease: Where there is an ongoing evolving neurological problem, immunisation should be deferred until the condition is stable.

Stable neurological disease: Stable neurological conditions such as occur in certain patients with cerebral palsy or spina bifida are not a contraindication to immunisation.

Cerebral damage in the neonatal period: When there has been a documented history of cerebral damage in the neonatal period, immunisation should be carried out unless there is evidence of an evolving neurological abnormality. If immunisation is to be deferred, then this should be stated on the neonatal discharge summary.

Allergy: A personal or family history or allergy is not a contraindication to immunisation.

HIV: HIV positive individuals may receive DTP vaccine but pertussis efficacy may be reduced.

Warnings: Not for intradermal injection.

Side-effects: Pain, tenderness, swelling or redness may occur at the injection site. Generalised reactions may include headache, malaise, pallor, crying, screaming and fever. Attacks of high pitched screaming, limpness and convulsions may occur.

More severe neurological conditions including encephalopathy and prolonged convulsions have been reported after pertussis vaccine.

Acute allergic reactions may occur, including anaphylaxis, dyspnoea and bronchospasm, urticaria and laryngeal oedema. Peripheral neuropathy has been reported.

A persistent nodule may occur at the site of injection particularly if the vaccine is administered into superficial layers of the subcutaneous tissue.

Precautions: Although anaphylaxis is rare, facilities for its management should always be available during vaccination.

Use in pregnancy and lactation: No reproductive studies have been conducted in animals. There are no data on the use of this vaccine in pregnancy or lactation. The vaccine should not normally be used in pregnancy or during lactation.

Treatment of overdose: Not applicable.

Pharmaceutical precautions Store at +2°C to +8°C. Do not freeze. Shake before use.

Legal category POM.

Package quantities 0.5 ml single dose pre-filled syringe (unit pack). 0.5 ml single dose ampoule (pack of 5).

Further information Use of adsorbed diphtheria, tetanus and pertussis vaccine in individuals aged 10 years or over may be associated with severe hypersensitivity reactions.

Oral poliomyelitis vaccine may be given simultaneously.

Product licence number 6745/0043.

Date of preparation 07/95

ADSORBED TETANUS VACCINE BP PASTEUR MERIEUX (TET/VAC/ADS)

Presentation A sterile aqueous suspension of purified tetanus toxoid. The toxoid is adsorbed onto aluminium hydroxide with thiomersal added as preservative.

Each 0.5 ml dose contains not less than 40 International Units (IU) of tetanus toxoid.

Uses Active immunisation against tetanus. Reinforcement of immunity to tetanus.

Dosage and administration By deep subcutaneous or intramuscular injection. Shake before use.

Primary immunisation: 3 injections each of 0.5 ml with an interval of 4 weeks between the first and second doses and 4 weeks between the second and third doses.

Reinforcing doses: Following primary immunisation, a reinforcing dose of 0.5 ml is recommended after 10 years and a further 0.5 ml dose 10 years later.

Management of tetanus prone wounds: Following a tetanus prone injury, a single dose of the vaccine should be administered to persons who have not received a booster dose nor completed a primary course during the preceding 10 years. Persons who have never received a primary course or in whom the immunisation history is not known, should commence or complete a primary course in addition to tetanus immunoglobulin, as appropriate.

Adsorbed tetanus vaccine may be administered simultaneously with tetanus immunoglobulin but must be given at a separate site.

Contra-indications, warnings, etc
Contra-indications: Acute infectious illness except when used in the management of tetanus prone injuries. The vaccine should not be given to persons who have had a severe reaction to a previous dose.

Warnings: Not for intradermal injection.

In immunised adults, booster doses at less than 10 year intervals are unnecessary and may cause excess reactions.

Side effects: General reactions are uncommon but may include transient pyrexia, headache, malaise, local swelling, redness and tenderness (especially in adults), acute allergic reactions, pallor, dyspnoea, urticaria, angioneurotic oedema, acute anaphylactic reactions and rarely, peripheral neuropathy. A small painless nodule may form at the injection site especially if administered into the superficial layers of subcutaneous tissue.

Precautions: Although anaphylaxis is extremely rare, facilities for its management should always be available during vaccination.

Pharmaceutical precautions Store in a refrigerator between +2° and +8°C. Do not freeze. Shake well immediately before use.

Multidose containers which are partly used should be discarded at the end of the vaccination session.

Legal category POM.

Package quantities Single dose pre-filled syringe (unit pack and pack of 10); single dose ampoule (pack of 5).

Further information Active immunisation against tetanus is recommended for everybody. Adsorbed tetanus vaccine may be administered to persons of any age.

Product licence number 6745/0045

Date of preparation 04/98

AVAXIM* ▼

Inactivated Hepatitis A vaccine

Qualitative and quantitative composition Each 0.5 millilitre dose contains:
Active ingredient:
Inactivated hepatitis A virus* 160 antigen units**

Other components:
Aluminium hydroxide (expressed as aluminium) 0.3 milligram
2-phenoxyethanol 2.5 microlitres
Formaldehyde 12.5 micrograms
Medium 199***, Water for Injections up to 0.5 millilitre

This vaccine contains polysorbate 80 and undetectable traces of neomycin.

* GBM strain cultured on MRC-5 human diploid cells.
** In the absence of an international standardised reference, the antigen content is expressed using an in-house reference.
*** Medium 199 is a mixture of aminoacids, mineral salts, vitamins and other components.

Pharmaceutical form Suspension for injection.

Clinical particulars
Therapeutic indications: AVAXIM is indicated for active immunisation against infection caused by hepatitis A virus in susceptible adults and adolescents (of 16 years and over).

Individuals having grown up in areas of high endemicity and/or with a history of jaundice may be immune to hepatitis A, in which case the vaccine is unnecessary. Testing for antibodies to hepatitis A prior to a decision on immunisation should be considered in such situations. If not, seropositivity against hepatitis A is not a contra-indication. AVAXIM is as well tolerated in seropositive as in seronegative subjects (see section 4.8).

Posology and method of administration: Recommended dosage is 0.5 millilitre for each injection.

Primary immunisation is achieved with one single dose of vaccine. In order to provide long term protection, a booster should be given 6 to 12 months later. The long term duration of serum antibodies to hepatitis A virus is unknown. AVAXIM may be used as a booster in subjects previously vaccinated with another inactivated hepatitis A vaccine.

Long term antibody persistence data following vaccination with AVAXIM are not currently available. It is predicted that HAV antibodies persist for many years (at least 10 years) after the booster. In case of doubt the serum hepatitis antibody titre should be determined.

As AVAXIM is adsorbed, the vaccine must be injected by the intramuscular route (i.m.) in order to minimise local reactions.

AVAXIM should be administered by intramuscular injection in the deltoid region. AVAXIM must not be administered intradermally or intravenously.

Before using AVAXIM*, shake the syringe well.

In exceptional circumstances (e.g. in patients with thrombocytopenia or in patients at risk of haemorrhage), the vaccine may be injected by the subcutaneous route.

In the event of case contact, AVAXIM may be given simultaneously with human immunoglobulin at different sites, after consideration of whether or not the subject is likely to be at long term risk of exposure.

Contra-indications: Usual contra-indications to any immunisation: vaccination should be delayed in subjects with current severe febrile infections.

True hypersensitivity to any AVAXIM component.

Special warnings and special precautions for use: Injection of AVAXIM should only be performed by a physician or health care worker trained in the administration of vaccines.

As AVAXIM has not been extensively studied in subjects less than or equal to 15 years of age, it is not indicated in this age group.

Do not administer AVAXIM by intradermal or intravenous injection. Ensure that the needle does not penetrate a blood vessel.

As with all vaccines, appropriate facilities and medication such as epinephrine (adrenaline) should be readily available for immediate use in case of anaphylaxis or hypersensitivity following injection.

Individuals who develop symptoms suggestive of hypersensitivity after an injection of AVAXIM should not receive further injections of the vaccine (see contra-indications).

The vaccine should not be administered into the buttocks, due to the varying amount of fatty tissue in this region, contributing to variability in effectiveness of the vaccine.

Following vaccination with AVAXIM*, protection develops against infection caused by hepatitis A virus. This protection does not occur immediately but over 90% of individuals will have protective levels of antibodies after 2 weeks. As with any vaccine, vaccination may not result in a protective response in all susceptible vaccinees.

AVAXIM does not provide protection against infection caused by hepatitis B virus, hepatitis C virus, hepatitis E virus or by other liver pathogens.

In the event that the booster vaccination has been delayed, there may be a decreased anti-hepatitis A antibody response. If long term protection is required, the serum anti-hepatitis A antibody titre may be determined after AVAXIM administration.

AVAXIM has not been studied in patients with impaired immunity. Immunogenicity of AVAXIM could be impaired by immunosuppressive treatment or in immunodeficiency. In such cases, it is recommended to measure the antibody response to be sure of protection and, if necessary, to wait for the end of any suppressive treatment before vaccination. Nevertheless, vaccination of subjects with chronic immunodeficiency such as HIV infection is recommended if the underlying pathology allows the induction of an antibody response, even if limited.

Because of the incubation period of hepatitis A, infection may be present but not clinically apparent at the time of vaccination. The effect of AVAXIM on individuals late in the incubation period of hepatitis A has not been documented.

As no studies have been performed with AVAXIM in subjects with liver disease, the use of this vaccine in such subjects should be considered with care.

Interaction with other medicaments and other forms of interaction: Concomitant administration of immunoglobulin and AVAXIM at two separate sites may be performed. Seroconversion rates are not modified, but antibody titres could be lower than after vaccination with AVAXIM alone.

As AVAXIM is inactivated, association with other inactivated vaccine(s) given at another injection site is unlikely to interfere with immune responses. Seroconversion rates and acute tolerance were not modified when AVAXIM was given concurrently at different sites with a Vi polysaccharide typhoid vaccine or with a yellow fever vaccine reconstituted with a Vi polysaccharide typhoid vaccine. When concurrent administration is considered necessary, AVAXIM must not be mixed with other vaccines in the same syringe, and other vaccines should be administered at different sites with different syringes and needles. Studies on the current administration of AVAXIM with concurrent recombinant hepatitis B virus vaccine have not been performed.

There is no change to safety or immunogenicity when AVAXIM* is used as a booster in subjects previously vaccinated with another inactivated hepatitis A vaccine.

No interaction with other medicinal products is currently known.

Pregnancy and lactation: The effect of AVAXIM on embryofoetal development has not been assessed. AVAXIM is not recommended in pregnancy unless there is a high risk of hepatitis A infection. The vaccine should be given to a pregnant woman only if clearly needed.

There is no data on the effect of administration of AVAXIM during lactation. AVAXIM is therefore not recommended during lactation.

Effects on ability to drive and use machines: None known.

Undesirable effects: In clinical trials, adverse reactions were usually mild and confined to the first few days after vaccination with spontaneous recovery. As with all pharmaceuticals however, it is possible that expanded commercial use of the vaccine could reveal rare adverse effects.

The most common reactions with an incidence of 1% to 10% were mild local pain (10% of injections), asthenia (10%), myalgia/arthralgia (7.9%), headache (7.2%), gastro-intestinal tract disorders (nausea, vomiting, decreased appetite, diarrhoea, abdominal pain) (4.3%) and mild fever (3.7%).

Those with an incidence less than 1% included redness at the injection site (0.5%). On rare occasions a nodule was observed at the injection site (less than 0.1%).

Mild reversible elevation of serum transaminases has been observed on rare occasions.

Reactions were less frequently reported after the booster dose than after the first dose. In subjects seropositive against hepatitis A virus, AVAXIM was as well tolerated as in seronegative subjects.

Although there have been no observations of allergic reactions or neurological manifestations following administration of AVAXIM*, such events have occurred with related vaccines.

Overdosage effects: None known.

Pharmacological properties

Pharmacodynamic properties: AVAXIM is prepared from hepatitis A virus cultured, purified and then inactivated by formaldehyde. AVAXIM confers immunity against hepatitis A virus by inducing antibody titres greater than those obtained after passive immunisation with immunoglobulin. Immunity appears shortly after the first injection and 14 days after vaccination more than 90% of immunocompetent subjects are protected (titre above 20 mIU/millilitre).

One month after first injection virtually 100% of subjects are protected. Immunity persists for at least 12 months and is reinforced after a first booster dose.

Long term protection of serum antibodies to hepatitis A virus after booster dose of AVAXIM is under evaluation. Nevertheless, antibody titres obtained two years after the first booster are consistent with a projected 10 year protection.

Pharmacokinetic properties: Not relevant.

Preclinical safety data: Preclinical safety data reveal no special hazard to humans based on conventional studies of acute toxicity, repeated dose toxicity, local tolerance and hypersensitivity.

Pharmaceutical particulars

List of excipients: Aluminium hydroxide, 2-phenoxyethanol, Formaldehyde, Medium 199

Incompatibilities: None known.

Shelf life: 2 years.

Special precautions for storage: Store between + 2°C and + 8°C (in a refrigerator).

The vaccine must not be frozen. If frozen, the vaccine should be discarded.

Nature and contents of container: Glass type I container: One dose (0.5 millilitre) prefilled syringe

Closure: Elastomer plunger-stopper

Instructions for use/handling: Shake before injection to obtain a homogeneous suspension.

Marketing authorisation number
UNITED KINGDOM: PL 6745/0070

Date of first authorisation/renewal of authorisation
30 April 1996

Date of (partial) revison of the text June 1998

Legal category POM

DIFTAVAX*

Adsorbed Diphtheria and Tetanus Vaccine for Adults and Adolescents BP

Presentation Sterile aqueous suspension containing purified tetanus and low dose diphtheria toxoids. Each 0.5 ml dose contains not less than 40 IU of tetanus toxoid and not less than 4 IU of diphtheria toxoid. The toxoids are adsorbed onto aluminium hydroxide; thiomersal is added as preservative.

Uses Active immunisation against tetanus and diphtheria for persons over ten years.

Dosage and administration By deep subcutaneous or intramuscular injection.

Primary immunisation: Three injections each of 0.5 ml, with an interval of at least 4 weeks between the first and the second doses, and at least 4 weeks between the second and third doses. If a course is interrupted it may be resumed; there is no need to recommence a primary course.

Reinforcing doses: A reinforcing dose of 0.5 ml is recommended after 10 years.

Use in children: Adsorbed Diphtheria and Tetanus Vaccine for Adults and Adolescents BP would not normally be administered to children under 10 years. Children under this age may receive Adsorbed Diphtheria and Tetanus Vaccine BP (DT/Vac/Ads (child)) which contains a higher amount of diphtheria toxoid.

Use in elderly: No special comment.

Contra-indications, warnings, etc

Contra-indications: Acute infectious illness. Severe reaction to a previous dose, or known hypersensitivity to any component of the vaccine. Immunisation with either diphtheria or tetanus toxoid within the preceding month.

Precautions: Adults and adolescents over 10 years requiring combined diphtheria and tetanus immunisation must always receive vaccine containing low dose diphtheria (not less than 4 IU).

Although anaphylaxis is extremely rare, facilities for its management should always be available during vaccination.

Warnings: Not for intradermal injection.

Schick testing is not necessary prior to immunisation.

Primary immunisation should only be considered for adults and adolescents who have not received a primary DTP or DT immunisation series in childhood.

Routine reinforcing doses at intervals of less than 10 years are not normally indicated and may be associated with an increased incidence and severity of reactions.

When diphtheria immunisation is indicated for subjects immunised against tetanus within the previous 10 years, the benefits of immunisation should be assessed against the possible risk of reactions.

Adsorbed Diphtheria and Tetanus Vaccine for Adults and Adolescents BP may normally be given to subjects requiring tetanus toxoid for wound management, to help ensure continuing diphtheria immunity, unless they have received a diphtheria toxoid containing vaccine in the last 10 years.

Adverse reactions: Local reactions such as transient erythema, swelling, tenderness or pain at the injection site or rarely systemic effects such as fever, headache, malaise and pallor may occur. Acute allergic reactions have been reported after administration of adsorbed diphtheria and tetanus vaccines, including dyspnoea, urticaria, angioneurotic oedema, peripheral neuropathy and rarely, anaphylaxis. A persistent nodule at the site of vaccination may occur with all adsorbed vaccines, particularly if administered into the superficial layers of the subcutaneous tissue.

Use in pregnancy and lactation: No reproductive studies have been conducted in animals. There are no data on the use of this vaccine in pregnancy or lactation. The vaccine should not normally be used in pregnancy or during lactation unless the benefit outweighs the risk.

Pharmaceutical precautions Store in a refrigerator between +2°C and +8°C. Do not freeze. Shake well immediately before use.

Legal category POM.

Package quantities 0.5 ml single dose pre-filled syringe unit pack.

Further information Nil.

Product licence number 6745/0055

Date of preparation 04/98

FLUZONE*

Inactivated Influenza Vaccine (Split Virion) BP

Qualitative and quantitative composition Influenza virus propagated on eggs, split by Triton* X-100, inactivated by formaldehyde, purified, containing antigens equivalent to †:

†A/Sydney/5/97 (H_3N_2)-like strain
(A/Sydney/5/97/IVR-108) .... 15 mcg haemagglutinin
†A/Beijing/262/95 (H_1N_1)-like strain
(A/Beijing/262/95/X-127) .... 15 mcg haemagglutinin
†B/Beijing/184/93-like strain
(B-Harbin/7/94) .... 15 mcg haemagglutinin

Prefilled syringe containing one 0.5 millilitre vaccination dose

† The vaccine complies with the WHO recommendation (northern hemisphere) and EU decision for the 98/99 season

Pharmaceutical form Suspension for injection.

Clinical particulars

Therapeutic indications: Prophylaxis of influenza, especially in those who run an increased risk of associated complications.

Posology and method of administration: Adults and children from 36 months: 0.5 millilitre.

Children from 6 months to 35 months: Clinical data are limited. Dosages of 0.25 millilitre or 0.5 millilitre have been used.

For children who have not previously been infected or vaccinated, a second dose should be given after an interval of at least 4 weeks.

Immunisation should be carried out by intramuscular or deep subcutaneous injection.

Contra-indications: Hypersensitivity to eggs, chicken protein or any constituents of the vaccine. Immunisation should be postponed in patients with febrile illness or acute infection.

Special warnings and precautions for use: As with all injectable vaccines, appropriate medical treatment and supervision should always be readily available in case of a rare anaphylactic event following the administration of the vaccine.

FLUZONE* should under no circumstances be administered intravascularly.

Antibody response in patients with endogenous or iatrogenic immunosuppression may be insufficient.

Interaction with other medicaments and other forms of interaction: FLUZONE* may be given at the same time as other vaccines. Immunisation should be carried out on separate limbs. It should be noted that the adverse reactions may be intensified.

The immunological response may be diminished if the patient is undergoing immunosuppressant treatment.

Following influenza vaccination, false positive results in serology tests using the ELISA method to detect antibodies against HIV1, Hepatitis C and especially HTLV1 have been observed. The Western Blot technique disproves the results. The transient false positive reactions could be due to IgM response by the vaccine.

Pregnancy and lactation: No relevant animal data are available. In humans, up to now, the data are inadequate to assess teratogenic or foetotoxic risk during pregnancy. In pregnant high risk patients the possible risks of clinical infection should be weighed against the possible risks of vaccination.

FLUZONE* may be used during lactation.

Effects on ability to drive and use machines: The vaccine is unlikely to produce an effect on the ability to drive and use machinery.

Undesirable effects: The following reactions are most common:

- Local reactions: redness, swelling, pain, ecchymosis, induration

- Systemic reactions: fever, malaise, shivering, fatigue, headache, sweating, myalgia, arthralgia.

These reactions usually disappear within 1–2 days without treatment.

The following events are observed rarely: neuralgia, paraesthesia, convulsions, transient thrombocytopenia.

Allergic reactions, in rare cases leading to shock, have been reported.

Vasculitis with transient renal involvement has been reported in very rare cases.

Rarely neurological disorders, such as encephalomyelitis, neuritis and Guillain Barré syndrome have been reported. An increased risk of Guillain Barré syndrome has not been demonstrated with currently used influenza vaccines.

Overdose: Overdosage is unlikely to have any untoward effect.

Pharmacological properties
Pharmacodynamic properties: Seroprotection is generally obtained within 2 to 3 weeks. The duration of post vaccinal immunity varies but is usually 6–12 months.

Pharmacokinetic properties: Not applicable.

Preclinical safety data: Not applicable.

Pharmaceutical particulars
List of excipients:
- Thiomersal
- Gelatin
- Phosphate Buffered Saline
- Sodium chloride
- Monobasic sodium phosphate
- Dibasic sodium phosphate
- Water for Injections
- Formaldehyde
- Sucrose
- Triton* X-100

Incompatibilities: FLUZONE* should not be mixed with other injection fluids.

Shelf life: The expiry date is indicated on the label and packaging. The shelf-life is 12 months.

Special precautions for storage: This product should be stored between +2°C and +8°C (in a refrigerator). Do not freeze. Protect from light.

Nature and contents of container: 0.5 millilitre of suspension in a prefilled syringe (glass) – packs of 1 syringe or 10 syringes.

Instructions for use/handling: The vaccine should be allowed to reach room temperature before use.

Shake before use.

For children, when one dose of 0.25 millilitre is indicated, push the plunger exactly to the edge of the mark so that half of the volume is eliminated. The remaining volume should be injected.

Marketing authorisation number PL 6745/0099

Date of first authorisation/renewal of authorisation 9th September 1997

Date of (partial) revision of the text May 1998

Legal category POM

HB-VAX* II 40

Recombinant Hepatitis B Vaccine 40 micrograms/ 1 millilitre, suspension for injection (IM), for dialysis and predialysis patients

Qualitative and quantitative composition
HBsAg†
Hepatitis B surface antigen,
recombinant ....40 micrograms
Thiomersal (sodium
mercurothiolate) ....50 micrograms
Aluminium hydroxide†† ......0.5×10^3 microgram
Sodium chloride ....9.00×10^3 microgram
Sodium borate ....70.0 micrograms
Water for Injections ....q.s. 1 millilitre
For a vial.
† Surface antigen of hepatitis B virus produced from recombinant strain of the yeast *Saccharomyces cerevisiae* (strain 2150-2-3).
†† Expressed as Al^{3+}.

Pharmaceutical form Suspension for intramuscular administration.

Clinical particulars
Therapeutic indications: This vaccine is indicated for dialysis and predialysis patients, for the active immunisation against hepatitis B virus infection caused by all known subtypes in subjects of all ages considered at risk of exposure to hepatitis B virus (HBV).

Posology and method of administration:
Posology: Dialysis and predialysis patients.

The volume and dose of vaccine recommended for each injection is 40 micrograms in 1 millilitre.

A course of vaccination should include at least three doses as follows:

1st injection: at elected date
2nd injection: ≥ 1 month after the first immunisation
3rd injection: ≥ 1 month after the second immunisation

The most commonly used schedule in Europe is:

0, 1, 6 months: Two injections with an interval of one month; a third injection 6 months after the first administration.

Booster: A booster dose may be required if the anti-HBs level is less than 10 international units per litre (IU/L).

In dialysis patients and persons with an impaired immune system, administration of additional doses of vaccine may be needed to obtain a protective anti-HBs titre.

Method of administration: This vaccine is for intramuscular injection. The deltoid muscle is the preferred site for injection.

Exceptionally, the vaccine may be administered subcutaneously in patients with thrombocytopenia or to persons at risk of haemorrhage.

Contra-indications:
- Severe febrile illness
- Known hypersensitivity to any component of the vaccine or allergic reaction after previous vaccine administration.

Special warnings and special precautions for use: Because of the long incubation period of hepatitis B, it is possible for unrecognised hepatitis B infection to be present at the time of immunisation. The vaccine may not prevent hepatitis B infection in such cases.

The vaccine will not prevent infection caused by other agents such as hepatitis A, hepatitis C and hepatitis E and other pathogens known to infect the liver.

As with all injectable vaccines, appropriate medical treatment should always be readily available in case of rare anaphylactic reactions following the administration of the vaccine.

Exceptionally, the vaccine may be administered subcutaneously in patients with thrombocytopenia or to persons at risk of haemorrhage.

This vaccine contains Thiomersal (Sodium Mercurthiolate) as a preservative.

This vaccine may contain traces of formaldehyde and potassium thiocyanate which are used during the manufacturing process.

Interaction with other medicaments and other forms of interaction: This vaccine can be administered with hepatitis B immunoglobulin (HBIG), at a separate injection site.

This vaccine can be used to complete a primary immunisation course or as a booster dose in subjects who have previously received another HBV vaccine.

Pregnancy and lactation: The effect of the HBsAg on foetal development has not been assessed. However, as with all inactivated viral vaccines, one does not expect harm for the foetus. Utilisation during pregnancy requires that the potential benefit justifies the potential risk to the foetus.

The effect on breast fed infants of the administration of this vaccine has not been assessed; nevertheless, this situation is not a contra-indication.

Effects on ability to drive and use machines: There are no specific data. Some of the rare effects mentioned under *Undesirable effects,* such as dizziness, headache, may affect the ability to drive or operate machinery.

Undesirable effects: The following undesirable effects have been reported following the widespread use of the vaccine. As with other hepatitis B vaccines, in many instances, the causal relationship to the vaccine has not been established.

Common reactions: Local reactions in injection site: transient soreness, erythema, induration.

Rare:
- elevation of liver enzymes, fatigue, fever, malaise, influenza-like symptoms, bronchospasm-like symptoms, serum sickness, thrombocytopenia
- dizziness, headache, paresthesia
- nausea, vomiting, diarrhoea, abdominal pain
- arthralgia, myalgia
- rash, pruritis, urticaria, anaphylaxis
- hypotension, syncope
- paralysis (Bell's palsy), neuropathy, neuritis (including Guillain-Barré Syndrome), myelitis (including transverse myelitis), encephalitis, optic neuritis
- angioedema, erythema multiforme
- lymphadenopathy

Overdose: There are no data with regard to overdosage.

Pharmacological properties
J: Anti-infectious. Vaccines/hepatitis B

Pharmacodynamic properties: The vaccine induces specific humoral antibodies against HBsAg (anti-HBs). Development of an anti-HBs titre above 10 international units per litre (IU/L) measured 1–2 months after the last injection correlates with protection to HBV infection.

Pharmacokinetic properties: Not applicable.

Preclinical safety data: Each lot of vaccine must pass the Abnormal Toxicity Test of the European Pharmacopoeia in mice and guinea pigs; a single dose acute toxicity test has been conducted in mice. Animal reproduction studies have not been conducted.

Relevant information for vaccinees: Although the duration of the protective effect of HB-VAX* II 40 in healthy vaccinees is unknown, follow-up over 5–9 years of approximately 3000 high-risk subjects given a similar plasma-derived vaccine has revealed no cases of clinical apparent hepatitis B infection.

In addition, persistence of vaccine-induced immunologic memory for HBsAg has been demonstrated through an anamnestic antibody response to a booster dose of HB-VAX* II 40 in healthy adults given plasma-derived vaccine 5 to 7 years earlier.

Pharmaceutical particulars
List of excipients: See *Qualitative and quantitative composition* above.

Incompatibilities: The vaccine should not be mixed in the same syringe with other vaccines or parenterally administered drugs.

Shelf life: 36 months.

Special precautions for storage: The vaccine should be stored between +2°C and +8°C. DO NOT FREEZE.

Nature and contents of container: Type I USP glass 2 millilitre vial with West n° 888 butyl rubber stopper and aluminium seal. Flip-off plastic cap.

Vial of 1 millilitre.

Instructions for use/handling: Immediately before use, the vaccine should be well shaken to obtain a slightly opaque white suspension.

Marketing authorisation number PL 6745/0098

Date of first authorisation/renewal of the authorisation 23 October 1997.

Date of (partial) revision of the text December 1998.

Legal category POM.

HB-VAX* II

Recombinant Hepatitis B Vaccine 10 micrograms/ 1 millilitre, suspension for injection (IM), adults and adolescents

Qualitative and quantitative composition
HBsAg†
Hepatitis B surface antigen,
recombinant ....10 micrograms
Thiomersal (sodium
mercurothiolate) ....50 micrograms
Aluminium hydroxide†† ......0.50×10^3 microgram
Sodium chloride ....9.00×10^3 microgram
Sodium borate ....70 micrograms
Water for Injections ....q.s. 1 millilitre
For a vial and prefilled syringe.
† Surface antigen of hepatitis B virus produced from recombinant strain of the yeast *Saccharomyces cerevisiae* (strain 2150-2-3).
†† Expressed as Al^{3+}.

Pharmaceutical form Suspension for intramuscular administration.

Clinical particulars
Therapeutic indications: This vaccine is indicated for active immunisation against hepatitis B virus infection caused by all known subtypes in subjects of all ages considered at risk of exposure to hepatitis B virus (HBV).

Groups identified at increased risk of infection:

Health care personnel: Oral surgeons, dentists, physicians and surgeons, nurses, dental hygienists, paramedical personnel in close contact with patients, staff in haemodialysis, haematology and oncology units, laboratory personnel handling blood and other clinical specimens, emergency and first aid workers, ambulance staff, blood bank and plasma fractionation workers, cleaning staff in hospitals handling waste, chiropodists, morticians and embalmers.

Patients frequently receiving blood products: Patients in haemodialysis and oncology units, patients suffering from thalassaemia, sickle cell anaemia, liver cirrhosis, haemophilia, and patients receiving frequent blood transfusion or clotting factor concentrates, patients receiving organ transplants.

Personnel collecting, sorting out, handling the specific waste and household rubbish.

Personnel and residents of institutions: Persons with frequent and/or close contacts with high risk groups, prisoners and prison staff, residents and staff of institutions for mentally handicapped.

Personnel at increased risk due to their sexual behaviour: Persons with multiple sexual partners, patients with a Sexually Transmitted Disease (STD), persons seeking treatment for an STD, prostitutes and male homosexuals.

Illicit users of addictive injectable drugs.

Travellers to areas with a high endemicity of HBV.

Persons originating from areas with a high endemicity of HBV: Adoptees, immigrants and refugees.

Others: Police personnel, fire brigade personnel, armed forces personnel and anybody who through their work or personal lifestyle may be exposed to HBV.

Household contacts of any of the above groups and contacts with acute or chronic HBV infection.

Nevertheless, the recommendations should be adjusted in line with national vaccination policies since in some countries generalisation of vaccination is highly recommended.

Posology and method of administration:

Posology: Adolescents and adults (16 years of age and older).

The volume and dose of vaccine recommended for each injection is 10 micrograms in 1 millilitre.

A course of vaccination should include at least three doses as follows:

1st injection: at elected date

2nd injection: ≥1 month after the first immunisation

3rd injection: ≥31 month after the second immunisation

This schedule allows the incorporation of several schemes in national vaccination recommendations.

The most commonly used schedules in Europe are:

0, 1, 6 months: two injections with an interval of one month; a third injection 6 months after the first administration

0, 1, 2, 12 months: three injections with an interval of one month; a fourth dose should be administered at 12 months

The accelerated schedule (0, 1, 2, 12 months) may induce protective antibody levels earlier in a slightly larger proportion of vaccinees.

The timing of successive injections in a vaccination series may need to be adjusted to local programmes, especially where hepatitis B vaccine is integrated with the administration of other paediatric vaccines.

Booster:

Immunocompetent vaccinees: The duration of the protective effect of HB-VAX* II in healthy vaccinees is unknown at present and the need for booster doses is not yet defined. However, some national vaccination schedules currently include recommendations for periodic booster doses.

Immunoincompetent vaccinees (e.g. dialysis patients): A booster dose may be considered in these vaccinees if the anti-HBs level is less than 10 international units per litre (IU/L).

Special dosage recommendations:

- *Recommendations for known or presumed exposure to HBV (dosage 10 micrograms / 1.0 millilitre) (e.g. needlestick with contaminated needle):*

Hepatitis B immunoglobulin (HBIG) should be given as soon as possible after exposure (within 24 hours). The first dose of the vaccine should be given within 7 days of exposure and can be given simultaneously with hepatitis B immunoglobulin, however it must be administered at a separate injection site.

Subsequent doses of vaccine, if necessary, (i.e. according to the serologic status of the patient) should be given as the recommended schedule for this vaccine.

Method of administration: This vaccine is for intramuscular injection. The deltoid muscle is the preferred site for injection.

Exceptionally, the vaccine may be administered subcutaneously in patients with thrombocytopenia or to persons at risk of haemorrhage.

Contra-indications

- Severe febrile illness.
- Known hypersensitivity to any component of the vaccine or allergic reaction after previous vaccine administration.

Special warnings and special precautions for use: Because of the long incubation period of hepatitis B, it is possible for unrecognised hepatitis B infection to be present at the time of immunisation. The vaccine may not prevent hepatitis B infection in such cases.

The vaccine will not prevent infection caused by other agents such as hepatitis A, hepatitis C and hepatitis E and other pathogens known to infect the liver.

In dialysis patients and persons with an impaired immune system, administration of additional doses of vaccine may be needed to obtain a protective anti-HBs titre.

As with all injectable vaccines, appropriate medical treatment should always be readily available in case of rare anaphylactic reactions following the administration of the vaccine.

Exceptionally, the vaccine may be administered subcutaneously in patients with thrombocytopenia or to persons at risk of haemorrhage.

This vaccine contains thiomersal (sodium mercurothiolate) as a preservative.

This vaccine may contain traces of formaldehyde and potassium thiocyanate which are used during the manufacturing process.

Interaction with other medicaments and other forms of interaction: This vaccine can be administered with hepatitis B immunoglobulin, at a separate injection site.

This vaccine can be used to complete a primary immunisation course or as a booster dose in subjects who have previously received another HBV vaccine.

Pregnancy and lactation: The effect of the HBsAg on foetal development has not been assessed. However, as with all inactivated viral vaccines, one does not expect harm for the foetus. Utilisation during pregnancy requires that the potential benefit justifies the potential risk to the foetus.

The effect on breast fed infants of the administration of this vaccine has not been assessed; nevertheless, this situation is not a contra-indication.

Effects on ability to drive and use machines: There are no specific data. Some of the rare effects mentioned under *Undesirable effects*, such as dizziness, headache, may affect the ability to drive or operate machinery.

Undesirable effects: The following undesirable effects have been reported following the widespread use of the vaccine. As with other hepatitis B vaccines, in many instances, the causal relationship to the vaccine has not been established.

Common reactions: Local reactions at injection site: transient soreness, erythema, induration.

Rare:

- elevation of liver enzymes, fatigue, fever, malaise, influenza-like symptoms, bronchospasm-like symptoms, serum sickness, thrombocytopenia
- dizziness, headache, paraesthesia
- nausea, vomiting, diarrhoea, abdominal pain
- arthralgia, myalgia
- rash, pruritus, urticaria, anaphylaxis
- hypotension, syncope
- paralysis (Bell's palsy), neuropathy, neuritis (including Guillain-Barré Syndrome), myelitis (including transverse myelitis), encephalitis, optic neuritis
- angioedema, erythema multiforme
- lymphadenopathy

Overdose: There are no data with regard to overdosage.

Pharmacological properties

J: Anti-infectious. Vaccines/hepatitis B.

Pharmacodynamic properties: The vaccine induces specific humoral antibodies against HBsAg (anti-HBs). Development of an anti-HBs titre above 10 international units per litre (IU/L) measured 1-2 months after the last injection correlates with protection to HBV infection.

Pharmacokinetic properties: Not applicable.

Preclinical safety data: Each lot of vaccine must pass the Abnormal Toxicity Test of the European Pharmacopoeia in mice and guinea pigs; a single dose acute toxicity test has been conducted in mice. Animal reproduction studies have not been conducted.

Relevant information for vaccinees: In clinical trials, 96% of 1497 healthy infants, children, adolescents and adults given a 3 dose course of HB-VAX* II developed a protective level of anti-HBs (≥10 international units per litre–IU/L).

The protective efficacy of a dose of HBIG at birth followed by 3 doses of HB-VAX* II has been demonstrated for neonates born to mothers positive for both HBsAg and HBeAg. Among 130 vaccinated infants, the estimated efficacy in prevention of chronic hepatitis B infection was 95% as compared to the infection rate in untreated historical controls.

Although the duration of the protective effect of HB-VAX* II in healthy vaccinees is unknown, follow-up over 5-9 years of approximately 3000 high-risk subjects given a similar plasma-derived vaccine has revealed no cases of clinical apparent hepatitis B infection.

In addition, persistence of vaccine-induced immunologic memory for HBsAg has been demonstrated through an anamnestic antibody response to a booster dose of HB-VAX* II in healthy adults given plasma-derived vaccine 5 to 7 years earlier.

Pharmaceutical particulars

List of excipients: See *Qualitative and quantitative composition* above.

Incompatibilities: The vaccine should not be mixed in the same syringe with other vaccines or parenterally administered drugs.

Shelf life: 36 months.

Special precautions for storage: The vaccine should be stored between +2°C and +8°C.

DO NOT FREEZE.

Nature and contents of container: Vial of 1 millilitre of suspension. Type I USP glass 2 millilitre vial with West n° 888 butyl rubber stopper and aluminium seal. Flip-off plastic cap.

Prefilled syringe (glass) 1 millilitre of suspension.

Instructions for use/handling: Before use, the vaccine should be well shaken to obtain a slightly opaque white suspension.

Marketing authorisation number

UNITED KINGDOM: PL 6745/0096

Date of first authorisation/renewal of the authorisation 14 December 1993.

Date of (partial) revision of the text December 1998.

Legal category POM.

HB VAX* II PAEDIATRIC

Recombinant Hepatitis B Vaccine 5 micrograms/0.5 millilitre, suspension for injection (IM), paediatric

Qualitative and quantitative composition

HBsAg†

Hepatitis B surface antigen, recombinant ....5 micrograms

Thiomersal (sodium mercurothiolate) ....25 micrograms

Aluminium hydroxide†† ......0.25×10^3 microgram

Sodium chloride ....4.50×10^3 microgram

Sodium borate ....35 micrograms

Water for Injections ....q.s. 0.5 millilitre

For a prefilled syringe.

† Surface antigen of hepatitis B virus produced from recombinant strain of the yeast *Saccharomyces cerevisiae* (strain 2150-2-3).

†† Expressed as Al^{3+}

Pharmaceutical form Suspension for intramuscular administration.

Clinical particulars

Therapeutic indications: This vaccine is indicated for active immunisation against hepatitis B virus infection caused by all known subtypes in subjects up to and including 15 years of age, considered at risk of exposure to hepatitis B virus (HBV).

Groups identified at increased risk of infection:

Children frequently receiving blood products: Children in haemodialysis and oncology units, children suffering from thalassaemia, sickle cell anaemia, haemophilia, and children receiving frequent blood transfusions or clotting factor concentrates, organ transplants.

Infants born of mothers who are HBV carriers.

Children residents of institutions: Children residents of institutions for mentally handicapped.

Children travelling to areas with a high endemicity of HBV.

Children originating from areas with a high endemicity of HBV: Adoptees, immigrants and refugees.

Others: Children through their personal lifestyle may be exposed to HBV.

Household contacts of anyone at increased risk of HBV infection and contacts with acute or chronic HBV infection.

Nevertheless, the recommendations should be adjusted in line with national vaccination policies since in some countries generalisation of vaccination is highly recommended.

Posology and method of administration:

Posology: Neonates and children (birth through 15 years of age).

The volume and dose of vaccine recommended for each injection is 5 micrograms in 0.5 millilitre.

A course of vaccination should include at least three doses as follows:

1st injection: at elected date

2nd injection: ≥ 1 month after the first immunisation

3rd injection: ≥ 1 month after the second immunisation

This schedule allows the incorporation of several schemes in national vaccination recommendations.

The most commonly used schedules in Europe are:

0, 1, 6 months: two injections with an interval of one month; a third injection 6 months after the first administration.

0, 1, 2, 12 months: three injections with an interval of one month; a fourth dose should be administered at 12 months.

The accelerated schedule (0,1,2,12 months) may induce protective antibody levels earlier in a slightly larger proportion of vaccinees.

The timing of successive injections in a vaccination series may need to be adjusted to local programmes, especially where hepatitis B vaccine is integrated with the administration of other paediatric vaccines.

Booster:

Immunocompetent vaccinees: The duration of the protective effect of HB-VAX* II in healthy vaccinees is unknown at present and the need for booster doses is not yet defined. However, some national vaccination schedules currently include recommendations for periodic booster doses.

Immunoincompetent vaccinees (e.g. dialysis patients): A booster dose may be considered in these vaccinees if the anti-HBs level is less than 10 international units per litre (IU/L).

Special dosage recommendations:

Neonates born of mothers who are HBV carriers (dosage 5 micrograms/0.5 millilitre): At birth, one dose of hepatitis B immunoglobulin (within 24 hours). The first dose of the vaccine should be given within 7 days of birth and can be given simultaneously with HB immunoglobulin at birth, but administered at a separate injection site.

Subsequent doses of vaccine should be given to complete a 0-1-6 months (or possibly at 0-1-2-12 months) schedule.

Known or presumed exposure to HBV (e.g. needle-stick with contaminated needle): Hepatitis B immunoglobulin (HBIG) should be given as soon as possible after exposure (within 24 hours). The first dose of the vaccine should be given within 7 days of exposure and can be given simultaneously with hepatitis B immunoglobulin, however it must be administered at a separate injection site.

Subsequent doses of vaccine, if necessary, (i.e. according to the serologic status of the patient) should be given as the recommended schedule for this vaccine.

Method of administration: This vaccine is for intramuscular injection. The anterolateral thigh is the preferred site for injection in neonates, infants and young children.

Exceptionally, the vaccine may be administered subcutaneously in patients with thrombocytopenia or to persons at risk of haemorrhage.

Contra-indications:

- Severe febrile illness.
- Known hypersensitivity to any component of the vaccine or allergic reaction after previous vaccine administration.

Special warnings and special precautions for use: Because of the long incubation period of hepatitis B, it is possible for unrecognised hepatitis B infection to be present at the time of immunisation. The vaccine may not prevent hepatitis B infection in such cases.

The vaccine will not prevent infection caused by other agents such as hepatitis A, hepatitis C and hepatitis E and other pathogens known to infect the liver.

In dialysis patients and persons with an impaired immune system, administration of additional doses of vaccine may be needed to obtain a protective anti-HBs titre.

As with all injectable vaccines, appropriate medical treatment should always be readily available in case of rare anaphylactic reactions following the administration of the vaccine.

Exceptionally, the vaccine may be administered subcutaneously in patients with thrombocytopenia or to persons at risk of haemorrhage.

This vaccine contains thiomersal as a preservative.

This vaccine may contain traces of formaldehyde and potassium thiocyanate which are used during the manufacturing process.

Interaction with other medicaments and other forms of interaction: This vaccine can be administered with hepatitis B immunoglobulin, at a separate injection site.

This vaccine can be used to complete a primary immunisation course or as a booster dose in subjects who have previously received another HBV vaccine.

Pregnancy and lactation: Not relevant.

Effects on ability to drive and use machines: Not relevant.

Undesirable effects: The following undesirable effects have been reported following the widespread use of the vaccine. As with other hepatitis B vaccines, in many instances, the causal relationship to the vaccine has not been established.

Common reactions: Local reactions at injection site: transient soreness, erythema, induration.

Rare:

- elevation of liver enzymes, fatigue, fever, malaise, influenza-like symptoms, bronchospasm-like symptoms, serum sickness, thrombocytopenia
- dizziness, headache, paraesthesia
- nausea, vomiting, diarrhoea, abdominal pain
- arthralgia, myalgia
- rash, pruritus, urticaria, anaphylaxis
- hypotension, syncope
- paralysis (Bell's palsy), neuropathy, neuritis (including Guillain-Barré Syndrome), myelitis (including transverse myelitis), encephalitis, optic neuritis
- angioedema, erythema multiforme
- lymphadenopathy

Overdose: There are no data with regard to overdosage.

Pharmacological properties

J: Anti-infectious. Vaccines/hepatitis B

Pharmacodynamic properties: The vaccine induces specific humoral antibodies against HBsAg (anti-HBs). Development of an anti-HBs titre above 10 international units per litre (IU/L) measured 1-2 months after the last injection correlates with protection to HBV infection.

Pharmacokinetic properties: Not applicable.

Preclinical safety data: Each lot of vaccine must pass the Abnormal Toxicity Test of the European Pharmacopoeia in mice and guinea pigs. A single dose acute toxicity test has been conducted in mice. Animal reproduction studies have not been conducted.

Relevant information for vaccinees: In clinical trials, 96% of 1497 healthy infants, children, adolescents and adults given a 3 dose course of HB-VAX* II developed a protective level of anti-HBs (10 international units per litre–IU/L).

The protective efficacy of a dose of HBIG at birth followed by 3 doses of HB-VAX* II has been demonstrated for neonates born to mothers positive for both HBsAg and HBeAg. Among 130 vaccinated infants, the estimated efficacy in prevention of chronic hepatitis B infection was 95% as compared to the infection rate in untreated historical controls.

Although the duration of the protective effect of HB-VAX* II in healthy vaccinees is unknown, follow-up over 5-9 years of approximately 3000 high-risk subjects given a similar plasma-derived vaccine has revealed no cases of clinically apparent hepatitis B infection.

In addition, persistence of vaccine-induced immunologic memory for HBsAg has been demonstrated through an anamnestic antibody response to a booster dose of HB-VAX* II in healthy adults given plasma-derived vaccine 5 to 7 years earlier.

Pharmaceutical particulars

List of excipients: See *Quantitative and qualitative composition* above.

Incompatibilities: The vaccine should not be mixed in the same syringe with other vaccines or parenterally administered drugs.

Shelf life: 36 months.

Special precautions for storage: The vaccine should be stored between +2°C and +8°C.

DO NOT FREEZE.

Nature and contents of container: 0.5 millilitre of suspension in prefilled syringes (glass).

Instructions for use/handling: Before use, the vaccine should be well shaken to obtain a slightly opaque white suspension.

Marketing authorisation number
UNITED KINGDOM: PL 6745/0097

Date of first authorisation/renewal of the authorisation 14 December 1993.

Date of (partial) revision of the text December 1998

Legal category POM.

INACTIVATED INFLUENZA VACCINE (SPLIT VIRION) BP PASTEUR MÉRIEUX

Qualitative and quantitative composition Influenza virus propagated on eggs, split by Octoxynol-9, inactivated by formaldehyde, purified, containing antigens equivalent to *:

A/Sydney/5/97 (H_3N_2) - like strain (A/Sydney/5/97-IVR108) 15 micrograms haemagglutinin

A/Beijing/262/95 (H_1N_1) - like strain (A/Beijing/262/95-X127) 15 micrograms haemagglutinin

B/Beijing/184/93 - like strain (B/Harbin/7/94) 15 micrograms haemagglutinin

Prefilled syringe containing one 0.5 millilitre vaccination dose

* The vaccine complies with the WHO recommendation (northern hemisphere) and EU decision for the 98/99 season

Pharmaceutical form Suspension for injection.

Clinical particulars

Therapeutic indications: Prophylaxis of influenza, especially in those who run an increased risk of associated complications.

Posology and method of administration: Adults and children from 36 months: 0.5 millilitre.

Children from 6 months to 35 months: Clinical data are limited. Dosages of 0.25 millilitre or 0.5 millilitre have been used.

For children who have not previously been infected or vaccinated, a second dose should be given after an interval of at least 4 weeks.

Immunisation should be carried out by intramuscular or deep subcutaneous injection.

Contra-indications: Hypersensitivity to eggs, chicken protein or any constituents of the vaccine. Immunisation should be postponed in patients with febrile illness or acute infection.

Special warnings and special precautions for use: As with all injectable vaccines, appropriate medical treatment and supervision should always be readily available in case of a rare anaphylactic event following the administration of the vaccine.

Inactivated Influenza Vaccine (Split Virion) BP Pasteur Mérieux should under no circumstances be administered intravascularly.

Antibody response in patients with endogenous or iatrogenic immunosuppression may be insufficient.

Since this vaccine contains traces of neomycin due to the use of this substance during production, it should be used with caution in subjects with a hypersensitivity to this substance.

Interaction with other medicaments and other forms of interaction: Inactivated Influenza Vaccine (Split Virion) BP Pasteur Mérieux may be given at the same time as other vaccines. Immunisation should be carried out on separate limbs. It should be noted that the adverse reactions may be intensified.

The immunological response may be diminished if the patient is undergoing immunosuppressant treatment.

Following influenza vaccination, false positive results in serology tests using the ELISA method to detect antibodies against HIV1, Hepatitis C and especially HTLV1 have been observed. The Western Blot technique disproves the results. The transient false positive reactions could be due to IgM response by the vaccine.

Pregnancy and lactation: No relevant animal data are available. In humans, up to now, the data are inadequate to assess teratogenic or foetotoxic risk during pregnancy. In pregnant high risk patients the possible risks of clinical infection should be weighed against the possible risks of vaccination.

Inactivated Influenza Vaccine (Split Virion) BP Pasteur Mérieux may be used during lactation.

Effects on ability to drive and use machines: The vaccine is unlikely to produce an effect on the ability to drive and use machinery.

Undesirable effects: The following reactions are most common:

- Local reactions: redness, swelling, pain, ecchymosis, induration;
- Systemic reactions: fever, malaise, shivering, fatigue, headache, sweating, myalgia, arthralgia.

These reactions usually disappear within 1-2 days without treatment.

The following events are observed rarely: neuralgia, paraesthesia, convulsions, transient thrombocytopenia.

Allergic reactions, in rare cases leading to shock, have been reported.

Vasculitis with transient renal involvement has been reported in very rare cases.

Rarely neurological disorders, such as encephalomyelitis, neuritis and Guillain Barré syndrome have been reported. An increased risk of Guillain Barré syndrome has not been demonstrated with currently used influenza vaccines.

Overdose: Overdosage is unlikely to have any untoward effect.

Pharmacological properties

Pharmacodynamic properties: Seroprotection is generally obtained within 2 to 3 weeks. The duration of post vaccinal immunity varies but is usually 6-12 months.

Pharmacokinetic properties: Not applicable.

Preclinical safety data: Not applicable.

Pharmaceutical particulars

List of excipients:

- Thiomersal
- Buffer solution (pH 7.2)
- Sodium chloride
- Potassium chloride
- Disodium phosphate dihydrate
- Potassium dihydrogen phosphate
- Water for Injections
- Formaldehyde
- Octoxynol-9
- Residue of the manufacturing process: neomycin

Incompatibilities: Inactivated Influenza Vaccine (Split Virion) BP Pasteur Mérieux should not be mixed with other injection fluids.

Shelf life: The expiry date is indicated on the label and packaging. The shelf-life is 12 months.

Special precautions for storage: This product should be stored between +2°C and +8°C (in a refrigerator). Do not freeze. Protect from light.

Nature and contents of container: 0.5 0. millilitre of suspension in a prefilled syringe (glass) equipped with an elastomer plunger stopper - packs of 1 syringe or 10 syringes.

Instructions for use/handling: The vaccine should be allowed to reach room temperature before use.

Shake before use.

For children, when one dose of 0.25 millilitre is indicated, push the plunger exactly to the edge of the mark so that half of the volume is eliminated. The remaining volume should be injected.

Marketing authorisation number
UK: PL 6745/0095

Date of first authorisation/renewal of authorisation
23 March 1998

Date of (partial) revision of the text March 1998

Legal category POM

MENGIVAC A+C*

Meningococcal Polysaccharide Vaccine BP

Presentation An inactivated polysaccharide vaccine against *Neisseria meningitidis* Serogroups A and C.

Each 0.5 ml dose contains not less than 50 µg each of lyophilised, Group A and Group C polysaccharides and 2 mg of lactose as stabiliser. Isotonic buffered diluent is supplied with each dose.

Indications Active immunisation against meningococcal meningitis caused by N. meningitidis Serogroups A and C.

(a) Travel: Vaccination should be offered to travellers visiting parts of the world where the risk of meningococcal meningitis is high. These regions include countries within the African Meningitis Belt (countries whose borders are between the Equator and latitude 15° North), parts of the Middle East and parts of the Indian Sub-Continent.

(b) Contacts of cases: Family members and close contacts of disease cases of Group A and Group C meningococcal meningitis should be immunised. The vaccine does not protect against Group B disease.

(c) Local outbreaks: To help control local outbreaks of meningococcal Group A and Group C disease, vaccination may be recommended by appropriate Public Health Authorities.

Post vaccination immunity lasts at least 3 years.

Dosage and administration 0.5 ml reconstituted vaccine by deep subcutaneous or intramuscular injection. The vaccine should be reconstituted using the diluent provided.

Shake before use.

Record the dose, batch number and date of administration.

Contra-indications, warnings, etc
Contra-indications: Acute infectious illness. Hypersensitivity to the vaccine or any component.

Precautions: Mengivac A+C confers protection specific to meningococci of Groups A and C. Immunisation does not protect against meningococci of other serogroups or against meningitis caused by other organisms.

Warnings: Facilities for the management of anaphylaxis should always be available during vaccination.

Adverse reactions: These are normally mild and short lasting. Local reactions may occur at the injection site and less commonly, systemic reactions may occur. Pyrexial reactions may occur more frequently in young children.

Use in pregnancy and lactation is not routinely recommended.

Pharmaceutical precautions Store at +2°C to +8°C. Do not freeze the diluent. After reconstitution, use within 1 hour. Shake well immediately before use.

Legal category POM.

Package quantities Carton of 1 single dose vial of lyophilised vaccine + 1 syringe of diluent (0.5 ml).

Further information Young children and infants respond less well to the vaccine than older children and adults, with little response to the Group C polysaccharide under 18 months of age and a poor response to Group A polysaccharide under 3 months of age.

Additionally, protection in infants under 18 months of age is of shorter duration.

Product licence numbers
Diluent 6745/0029
Lyophilised vaccine 6745/0048.

Date of preparation 04/98

MMR* II

Measles, Mumps and Rubella vaccine, Live, Attenuated

Qualitative and quantitative composition Each 0.5 ml dose when reconstituted contains not less than equivalent of:

1,000 $TCID_{50}$† of Measles Vaccine Live (the more attenuated Enders Line of the Edmonston strain).
20,000 $TCID_{50}$ of Mumps Vaccine Live (Jeryl Lynn* Level B strain).
1,000 $TCID_{50}$ of Rubella Vaccine Live (Wistar, RA 27/Strain).
† Tissue Culture Infectious Dose.

Pharmaceutical form A lyophilised powder for subcutaneous or intramuscular injection, after reconstitution with sterile water.

Clinical particulars *Therapeutic indications:* For simultaneous immunisation against measles, mumps and rubella in the following groups:

Children: Recommended for both primary and booster immunisation of both boys and girls 12 months of age or older.

Non-pregnant adolescent and adult females: Immunisation of susceptible non-pregnant adolescent and adult females of childbearing age is indicated when the potential vaccinee agrees not to become pregnant for the next 3 months after vaccination and is informed of the reason, and is told of the frequent occurrence of generally self-limiting arthralgia and/or arthritis beginning 2–4 weeks after vaccination.

International travellers: Individuals planning travel abroad who are known to be susceptible to one or more of these diseases can receive either a single antigen vaccine (measles, mumps or rubella) or a combined antigen vaccine as appropriate. MMR II is preferred for persons likely to be susceptible to mumps and rubella as well as measles.

Posology and method of administration: The vaccine is administered by subcutaneous or intramuscular injection preferably into the outer aspect of the arm.

Adults and children: After suitably cleansing the injection site, 0.5 ml of reconstituted vaccine should be injected. MMR II must not be given intravenously.

Do not give immunoglobulin with MMR II.

Warning: A sterile syringe and epinephrine (adrenaline) injection should be available for immediate use should an anaphylactic reaction occur.

Elderly: No special comment.

Revaccination: A second dose of MMR vaccine is recommended in the national immunisation schedule.

Children receiving their first dose of MMR vaccine younger than 12 months of age should be revaccinated at 15 months of age. They may still receive a further dose at the time indicated in the national immunisation schedule (MMR II is not recommended for infants under 12 months of age).

Use with other vaccines: Vaccines containing diphtheria, tetanus and pertussis antigens and/or oral poliomyelitis vaccine can be administered at the same time as MMR II. For concurrent parenteral vaccination, separate syringes and separate sites for injection should be used. MMR II should not be given less than one month before or after immunisation with other vaccines.

Contra-indications: Do not give MMR II to pregnant females; the possible effects of the vaccine on foetal development are unknown at this time. Pregnancy must be avoided for three months following vaccination of post-pubertal females.

Anaphylactic or anaphylactoid reactions to a previous dose of vaccine or to neomycin or any other vaccine constituent. (Each dose of reconstituted vaccine contains approximately 25 mcg neomycin.)

History of anaphylactic or anaphylactoid reactions to eggs (see *Hypersensitivity to eggs, chicken, or chicken feathers*).

Any febrile respiratory illness, or other active or suspected infection.

Those with impaired immune responsiveness, whether occurring naturally or as a result of therapy with steroids, radiotherapy, cytotoxic or other agents. This contra-indication does not apply to patients receiving corticosteroids as replacement therapy, e.g. for Addison's disease.

Patients with active untreated tuberculosis, blood dyscrasias such as thrombocytopenia, leukaemia, malignant disease including lymphomas of any type or other malignant neoplasms affecting the bone marrow or lymphatic systems.

Primary and acquired immunodeficiency states, including patients who are immunosuppressed in association with AIDS or other clinical manifestations with human immunodeficiency viruses; cellular immune deficiencies; and hypogammaglobulinaemic and dysgammaglobulinaemic states.

Those patients with a family history of congenital hereditary immunodeficiency until their immune competence has been demonstrated.

Children below 12 months of age: Children below 12 months of age should not normally be given MMR II unless they are at special risk, since the presence of maternal antibody may interfere with their ability to respond. They may be given human normal immunoglobulin. However, where immunisation below the age of 12 months is deemed necessary, a second dose of vaccine should be given at 15 months of age and a further dose may still be given at the usual time.

Special warnings and special precautions for use: Epinephrine (adrenaline) should be available for immediate use should an anaphylactic or anaphylactoid reaction occur.

Hypersensitivity to eggs: There is increasing evidence that MMR* II vaccine can be given safely to children even if they have previously had an anaphylactic reaction (generalised urticaria, swelling of the mouth and throat, difficulty in breathing, hypotension or shock) following food containing egg. Nevertheless, caution should be observed and if there is concern, paediatric advice should be sought with a view to immunisation under controlled conditions such as admission to hospital as a day case.

MMR II should be given with caution to those with an individual or family history of cerebral injury or any other condition in which stress due to fever should be avoided. The physician should be alert to the rise in temperature that may follow vaccination.

Children and young adults who are known to be infected with, or have a history of immunodeficiency viruses, but without overt clinical manifestations of immunosuppression, may be vaccinated; however, the vaccinees should be closely monitored for exposure to vaccine-preventable diseases because immunisation may be less effective than for uninfected persons. In selected cases, confirmation of circulating antibody levels may be indicated to help guide appropriate protective measures, including immunoprophylaxis if immunity has waned to non-protective levels.

Excretion of small amounts of live attenuated rubella virus from the nose and throat has occurred in the majority of susceptible individuals 7–28 days after vaccination. There is no definite evidence to indicate that such a virus is transmitted to susceptible persons who are in contact with vaccinated individuals. Consequently transmission, while accepted as a theoretical possibility, has not been regarded as a significant risk. However, transmission of the vaccine virus via breast milk has been documented.

There are no reports of transmission of live attenuated measles or mumps viruses from vaccinees to susceptible contacts.

Children under treatment for tuberculosis have not experienced exacerbation of the disease when immunised with live measles virus vaccine; no studies have been reported to date of the effect of measles virus vaccines on untreated tuberculous children.

Parents of children with a personal or family history of convulsions or idiopathic epilepsy should be advised that such children have a small increased risk of seizures following vaccination and be informed in advance of procedures for their management.

Interaction with other medicaments and other forms of interaction: Vaccination should be deferred for at least three months following blood or plasma transfusions or administration of any human immune serum globulin. If any of these substances has been used near to the time of vaccination with MMR II, a test should subsequently be made to confirm successful seroconversions.

Where anti-Rho (D) globulin (human) and rubella vaccine are required in the immediate post-partum period, rubella vaccine alone and not MMR II should be used.

It has been reported that live attenuated measles, mumps and rubella vaccine may temporarily depress tuberculin skin sensitivity. If a tuberculin test is to be done, it should be administered before or simultaneously with MMR II.

Pregnancy and lactation: Pregnant females must NOT be given MMR II. Furthermore, pregnancy should be avoided for three months following vaccination (see *Contra-indications*).

Animal reproduction studies have not been conducted with MMR II. It is also not known whether MMR II can cause foetal harm when given to pregnant women or affect reproductive capacity.

If a woman is inadvertently vaccinated or if she becomes pregnant within three months of vaccination, she should be counselled by her physician. It has been established that: (1) in a ten-year study involving 700 pregnant women who received rubella vaccination within three months of conception, none of their new-born infants had abnormalities compatible with a congenital rubella syndrome; (2) although mumps virus is capable of infecting the placenta and foetus, there is no good evidence that it causes congenital malformations in humans.

Mumps vaccine virus has also been shown to affect the placenta, but the virus has not been isolated from foetal tissues taken from susceptible women who were vaccinated and underwent elective abortions; and (3) reports indicate that contracting natural measles during pregnancy increases the rates of spontaneous abortion, stillbirth, congenital defects and prematurity. Although there are no adequate studies on the attenuated (vaccine) strain in pregnancy, it would be prudent to assume that the strain of the virus in the vaccine is also capable of inducing adverse foetal effects.

Breast-feeding mothers: Caution should be exercised when MMR II is given to a breast-feeding mother. Although it is not known whether measles or mumps vaccine virus is secreted in human milk, studies have shown that breast-feeding mothers immunised with live attenuated RA 27/3 strain rubella vaccine transmit the virus via breast milk. In those babies with serological evidence of rubella, none showed clinical disease.

Effects on ability to drive and use machines: None reported.

Undesirable effects: Adverse reactions: Adverse reactions associated with MMR II are similar to those to be expected from the administration of monovalent vaccines given separately.

The following adverse reactions occur commonly: Burning and/or stinging at the injection site for a short period.

The following adverse reactions occur occasionally: Body as a whole: Fever (101°F [38.3°C] or higher).

Skin: Rash, usually minimal but may be generalised.

Generally, fever, rash or both appear between the 5th and the 12th days.

Mild, local reactions such as erythema; induration and tenderness.

The following adverse reactions occur rarely: Body as a whole: Sore throat, malaise.

Digestive: Parotitis, nausea, vomiting, diarrhoea.

Haematologic/lymphatic: Regional lymphadenopathy, thrombocytopenia, purpura.

Hypersensitivity: Allergic reactions such as wheal and flare at injection site, anaphylaxis and anaphylactoid reactions, urticaria.

Musculoskeletal: Arthralgia and/or arthritis (usually transient and rarely chronic), myalgia.

Nervous/psychiatric: Febrile convulsions in children, afebrile convulsion or seizures, headache, dizziness, paraesthesia, polyneuritis, Guillain-Barré syndrome, ataxia. Encephalitis/encephalopathy have been reported approximately once for every 3 million doses. In no cases has it been shown that reactions were actually caused by vaccine. The risk of such serious neurological disorders following live measles virus vaccine administered remains for less than that for encephalitis and encephalopathy with natural measles (1 per 2000 reported cases).

Skin: Erythema multiforme.

Special senses: Forms of optic neuritis, including retrobulbar neuritis, papillitis, and retinitis; ocular palsies, otitis media, nerve deafness, conjunctivitis.

Urogenital: Orchitis.

There have been reports of subacute sclerosing panencephalitis (SSPE) in children who did not have a history of natural measles but did receive measles vaccine. Some of these cases may have resulted from unrecognised measles in the first year of life or possibly from the measles vaccination. Based on the estimated nationwide measles vaccine distribution in the USA, the association of SSPE cases to measles vaccination is about one case per million vaccine doses distributed. This is far less than the association with natural measles: 6–22 cases of SSPE per million cases of measles.

A study suggests that the overall effect of measles vaccine has been to protect against SSPE by preventing measles with its inherent higher risk of SSPE.

Local reactions characterised by marked swelling, redness and vesiculation at the injection site of attenuated live measles virus vaccines and systemic reactions including atypical measles have occurred in vaccinees who had previously received killed measles vaccine. Rarely, there have been reports of more severe reactions, including prolonged high fevers and extensive local reactions requiring hospitalisation. Panniculitis has also been reported rarely following vaccination with measles vaccine.

Arthralgia or arthritis or both are usually transient and rarely chronic features of natural infection, their frequency and severity vary with age and sex, begin greatest in adult females and least in prepubertal children.

The chronic arthritis associated with natural rubella has been related to virus and/or viral antigen found in body tissues. Only rarely have vaccinees developed chronic joint symptoms and causal relationship is unknown.

Following vaccination in children, reactions in joints are uncommon and generally of brief duration. In women, incidence rates for arthritis are generally higher than those seen in children (children 0–3%; women 12–20%) and the reactions tend to be more marked and of longer duration. Symptoms may persist for a matter of months or, on rare occasions, for years. In adolescent girls, the rections appear to be intermediate in incidence between those seen in children and in adult women. Even in older women (35–45 years) these reactions are generally well tolerated and rarely interfere with normal activities. Such reactions occur much less frequently after revaccination than primary vaccination.

Overdose: Poisoning is unlikely. Swallowing MMR II would render the live attenuated vaccine benign, and the content of the neomycin (25 mcg/ml) is not likely to cause toxicity. No case of overdosage has been reported.

Pharmacological properties

Pharmacodynamic properties: MMR II Vaccine is a mixture of live attenuated measles, mumps and rubella viruses to provide active immunisation against these diseases.

Clinical studies in 279 triple seronegative children aged 11 months to 7 years, showed that MMR II is highly immunogenic and generally well-tolerated. In these studies, a single injection of the vaccine induced measles haemogglutination-inhibition (HI) antibodies in 95%, mumps neutralising antibodies in 96% and rubella HI antibodies in 99% of susceptible persons.

Based on available evidence a second dose of MMR vaccine in the national immunisation schedule has the potential to prevent epidemics of measles and overall is as well-tolerated as primary immunisation.

Vaccine induced antibody levels following administration of MMR II have been shown to persist for over 11 years.

Pharmacokinetic properties: Not applicable.

Preclinical safety data: No further information available.

Pharmaceutical particulars

List of excipients: Before lyophilisation each unit of vaccine comprises the component virus in 0.5 ml of a medium with the following composition:

The quantities shown are of initial amounts of materials. Nutrients used for viral growth will be depleted in the final vehicle of the viruses.

Albumin, Human USP	300.0 mcg
Dipotassium Hydrogen Phosphate USP	30.0 mcg
Disodium Hydrogen Phosphate PhEur	30.0 mcg
Gelatine, Hydrolysed HSE	14.5 mg
Medium 199 HSE	3.4 mg
Minimum Essential Medium, Eagle HSE	140.0 mcg
Monosodium L-Glutamate USP	20.0 mcg
Neomycin Sulphate USP	25.0 mcg
Phenol Red HSE	3.4 mcg
Potassium Dihydrogen Phosphate USP	100.0 mcg
Sodium Bicarbonate PhEur	400.0 mcg
Sodium Dihydrogen Phosphate PhEur	100.0 mg
Sorbitol	14.5 mg
Sucrose	1.9 mg

Incompatibilities: None known.

Shelf life: 18 months

Special precautions for storage: Store between +2°C to +8°C.

Nature and contents of container: 3 ml type 1 glass tubing vials with 13 mm (West Co gray butyl 1816) lyophilisation stoppers and 13 mm 1 piece flip-off aluminium seal with plastic cap.

Instructions for use/handling: To reconstitute the vaccine, all the diluent provided should be injected into a vial of lyophilised vaccine, and this agitated to ensure thorough mixing. All the reconstituted vaccine is then drawn into the syringe and injected subcutaneously or intramuscularly.

Only the diluent supplied should be used for reconstitution, since it is free of preservatives and other antiviral substances that may inactivate the vaccine.

A separate sterile disposable needle and syringe should be used for each vaccinee.

It is good practice to record title, dose and batch number of all vaccines and dates of administration.

Pharmaceutic particulars During shipment, the vaccine must be maintained at a temperature of 10°C (50°F) or less to ensure no loss of potency.

Before reconstitution, MMR II should be stored between +2°C to +8°C (35.6°F to 46.4°F) and protected from light. Do not freeze.

MMR II retains at least 8 times the minimum immunising dose even after 6 weeks at 22°C or 1 week at 37°C. Storage at tempeatures above +2°C to +8°C cannot be recommended due to the difficulty in monitoring the exact temperature and monitoring repeated exposures to time out of refrigeration.

When reconstituted, the vaccine is yellow. It is acceptable for use only when clear and free from particulate matter.

The vaccine should be used as soon as possible and not later than one hour after reconstitution. Protect from light at all times, since exposure may inactivate the virus.

Marketing authorisation number 6745/0076.

Date of first authorisation/renewal of authorisation 1 March 1995.

Date of (partial) revision of the text December 1998

Legal category POM.

PNEUMOVAX II*

Pneumococcal Vaccine, Polyvalent

Presentation Single-dose vial containing, in 0.5 ml, 25 mcg of each polysaccharide type derived from capsules of the 23 most prevalent pneumococci dissolved in isotonic saline containing 0.25% phenol.

Uses A pneumococcal vaccine.

Pneumovax II is a sterile liquid vaccine consisting of a mixture of highly purified capsular polysaccharides from the 23 most prevalent or invasive pneumococcal types accounting for at least 90% of pneumococcal blood isolates and at least 85% of all pneumococcal isolates from usually sterile sites determined by ongoing surveillance (see chart).

23 pneumococcal capsular types included in Pneumovax II

Nomenclature	*Pneumococcal types*									
Danish	1	2	3	4	5	6B	7F	8	9N	9V
U.S.	1	2	3	4	5	26	51	8	9	68
Danish	10A	11A	12F	14	15B	17F	18C	19F	19A	20
U.S.	34	43	12	14	54	17	56	19	57	20
Danish	22F	23F	33F							
U.S.	22	23	70							

Protective capsular type-specific antibody levels usually develop by the third week following vaccination.

Pneumovax II is indicated for immunisation against pneumococcal disease caused by those pneumococcal types included in the vaccine. Pneumovax II will not immunise against capsular types of pneumococcus other than those contained in the vaccine. It should be considered for all persons 2 years of age or older in whom there is an increased risk of morbidity and mortality from pneumococcal pneumonia.

Pneumovax II may not be effective in preventing infection resulting from basilar skull fracture or from external communication with cerebrospinal fluid.

Dosage and administration *Do not inject intravenously; avoid intradermal administration.*

Administer a single 0.5 ml dose of Pneumovax II subcutaneously or intramuscularly (preferably in the deltoid muscle or lateral mid-thigh) with appropriate precautions to avoid intravascular administration.

Revaccination

Adults: Routine vaccination of adults with Pneumovax II is not recommended because of an increased incidence and severity of adverse reactions among healthy adults revaccinated with pneumococcal vaccines at intervals under three years. This was probably due to sustained high antibody levels. Also, persons who received the 14-valent vaccine should not be routinely revaccinated with the 23-valent vaccine, as increased coverage is modest and duration of protection is not well defined.

Although routine revaccination is not recommended, revaccination is recommended for adults with chronic conditions which increase the risk of fatal pneumococcal infection and for those shown to have a rapid decline in pneumococcal antibody levels (e.g. patients with nephrotic syndrome, renal failure, or transplant recipients).

Based on clinical study results, revaccination with Pneumovax II is recommended for adults at highest risk of fatal pneumococcal infection who were initially vaccinated with Pneumovax (Pneumococcal Vaccine, Polyvalent, MSD) four or more years previously without a serious or severe reaction.

In addition, it is recommended that revaccination should be considered for adults at highest risk who received the 23-valent vaccine six or more years previously.

Children: It is recommended that revaccination after three to five years should be considered for children at highest risk for pneumococcal infection (e.g. children with asplenia, sickle cell disease, or nephrotic syndrome) who would be 10 years old or younger at revaccination. Such children should not, however, be revaccinated within three years.

Children at highest risk for pneumococcal infection may have lower peak antibody levels and/or more rapid antibody decline than do healthy adults. There is evidence that some of these high-risk children (e.g. asplenic children) benefit from revaccination with vaccine containing antigen 7F, 8, 19F.

Contra-indications, warnings, etc
Contra-indications: Hypersensitivity to any component of the vaccine. Adrenaline injection BP (1:1,000) must be immediately available should an acute anaphylactoid reaction occur.

Revaccination with Pneumovax II is contra-indicated, except as described under '*Revaccination*'.

Do not use Pneumovax II less than ten days prior to or during immuno-suppressive therapy.

Patients with Hodgkin's disease who have received extensive chemotherapy and/or nodal irradiation.

Pneumovax II should not be given to pregnant women, since it is not known whether the vaccine can cause fetal harm, or affect the outcome of pregnancy.

Breast-feeding mothers should not be given Pneumovax II.

Warnings: The expected serum antibody response may not be obtained in patients receiving immuno-suppressive therapy.

Intradermal administration may cause severe local reactions.

Precautions: Caution and appropriate care should be exercised in administering Pneumovax II to individuals with severely compromised cardiac and/or pulmonary function in whom a systemic reaction would pose a significant risk.

Delay the use of Pneumovax II in any febrile respiratory illness or other active infection, except when this delay may involve even greater risk.

Required prophylactic antibiotic therapy against pneumococcal infection should not be stopped after immunisation with Pneumovax II.

It is recommended that a clear note of vaccination with Pneumovax II be kept in the patient's hospital and general practitioner records.

Children under 2 years of age: Pneumovax II is not recommended because antibody response to capsular types that most often cause pneumococcal disease in this age group may be poor. Safety and efficacy in children under 2 years have not been established.

Adverse reactions: Adverse reactions occurring commonly are:

Local injection site soreness, erythema, and induration.

Adverse reactions occurring occasionally are: *Body as a whole*—Low-grade fever (<100.9°F/38.3°C).

Adverse reactions occurring rarely are: *Body as a whole*—Headache, fever (>102°F/38.9°C), malaise, asthenia; *Haematologic/Lymphatic*—Adenitis; *Hypersensitivity*—Anaphylactoid reactions, serum sickness; *Musculoskeletal*—Arthralgia, myalgia, arthritis; *Skin*—Rash, urticaria.

On rare occasions, patients with otherwise stabilised idiopathic thrombocytopenic purpura have relapsed with a thrombocytopenia that has recurred 2–14 days after vaccination, and lasted for up to two weeks.

Reactions of greater severity, duration, or extent are unusual. Neurological disorders such as paraesthesiae and acute radiculoneuropathy, including the Guillain-Barré syndrome, have rarely been reported at the time of vaccination, but with no established cause-and-effect relationship.

Pharmaceutical precautions Store in a refrigerator between +2°C and +8°C. The vaccine is used directly as supplied. No dilution or reconstitution is necessary. Phenol 0.25% is present as preservative. All vaccine must be discarded after the expiration date.

Pneumovax II should be inspected before injection to see that it is a clear, colourless liquid without suspended particles.

Legal category POM.

Package quantities A single-dose vial.

Further information Invasive pneumococcal disease causes high morbidity and mortality in spite of effective antimicrobial control by antibiotics. These effects of pneumococcal disease appear to be due to irreversible pathological damage caused by bacteria during the first five days following onset of illness, irrespective of antimicrobial therapy.

Although the duration of the protective effect of Pneumovax II is presently unknown, previous studies with other pneumococcal vaccines suggest that induced antibodies may persist for five years. Type-specific antibody levels induced by 14-valent Pneumovax decline over a 42-month period of observation, but remain significantly higher than prevaccination levels in almost all recipients who responded initially.

Product licence number 0025/0293.

Product licence holder: Merck Sharp & Dohme Limited, Hertford Road, Hoddesdon, Hertfordshire, EN11 9BU.

Distributed by: Pasteur Mérieux MSD Ltd, Clivemont House, Clivemont Road, Maidenhead, Berkshire, SL6 7BU.

Date of preparation 04/97

RABIES VACCINE BP PASTEUR MERIEUX

Human Diploid Cell Rabies Vaccine

Presentation The vaccine is a lyophilised, stabilised suspension of inactivated Wistar rabies virus strain PM/WI38 1503–3M, cultured on human diploid cells (MRC_5) and inactivated by beta-propiolactone. The dry vaccine is coloured off-white but, after reconstitution with the diluent supplied, it turns a pinkish colour due to the presence of phenol red. The potency of the reconstituted vaccine is not less than 2.5 International Units per dose (1 ml).

Uses
(a) Prophylactic immunisation against rabies.
(b) Treatment of patients following suspected rabies contact.

Dosage and administration The dose of reconstituted vaccine in all cases is 1 ml given by deep subcutaneous or intramuscular injection. The vaccine should be administered into the deltoid region but not the gluteal region. Reconstitution: Inject the diluent from the syringe into the vial, agitate to ensure complete reconstitution and withdraw the contents back into the syringe.

(a) Prophylaxis: Three injections each of 1 ml given on days 0, 7 and 28. A single reinforcing dose should be given at two or three year intervals to those at continued risk. If, for whatever reason, it has not been possible to give a full course of three injections, it is probable that, in the majority of subjects, two doses may be adequate to confer protection, provided these were given four weeks apart. Subjects receiving only two injections who remain at continued risk should receive a reinforcing dose 6–12 months later, with further reinforcing doses given at two to three year intervals.

(b) Treatment:

(i) *In persons known to have adequate prophylaxis.* In the event of contact with a suspected rabid animal, two further boosters should be given on day 0 and on day 3 to 7.

(ii) *In persons with no, or possibly inadequate, prophylaxis.* The first injection of rabies vaccine should be given as soon as possible after the suspected contact (day 0) and followed by five further doses on days 3, 7, 14, 30 and 90. The use of Human Rabies Immunoglobulin on day 0 should be considered but only in persons with no adequate prophylaxis. The treatment schedule may be stopped if the animal concerned is found conclusively to be free of rabies.

Contra-indications, warnings, etc There are no absolute contra-indications to HDCV, although if there were evidence of severe hypersensitivity, subsequent doses should not be given except for treatment. Redness, swelling or tenderness at the site of injection may occur during the first 48 hours. A mild fever, malaise and influenza-like symptoms have been reported.

Although anaphylaxis is extremely rare remedial facilities such as adrenaline should always be available during vaccination.

The vaccine contains traces of neomycin.

Use in pregnancy: Because of the potential consequences of inadequately treated rabies exposure and because there is no indication that foetal abnormalities have been associated with rabies vaccination, pregnancy is not considered a contra-indication to post-exposure prophylaxis. If there is substantial risk of exposure to rabies, pre-exposure prophylaxis may also be indicated during pregnancy.

Pharmaceutical precautions Store at +2°C to +8°C. Do not freeze. Use immediately after reconstituting the vaccine. Discard any vaccine unused one hour after reconstitution.

Legal category POM.

Package quantities A vial of lyophilised vaccine containing one dose together with a disposable syringe containing 1 ml of diluent. The diluent is Water for Injections with no added preservatives.

Further information The British National Formulary and DoH Immunisation against Infectious Disease (HMSO) both contain reference to rabies.

Product licence numbers 6745/0053 (vaccine)
6745/0024 (diluent)

Date of preparation 04/98

TYPHIM Vi*

Vi Capsular Polysaccharide Typhoid Vaccine

Qualitative and quantitative composition Each dose of 0.5 millilitre contains:
Purified Vi capsular polysaccharide of *Salmonella typhi* - 25 micrograms

Pharmaceutical form Sterile solution.

Clinical particulars
Therapeutic indications: Active immunisation against typhoid fever.

Posology and method of administration: Adults and Children over 18 months of age:

A single dose of 0.5 millilitre administered by deep subcutaneous or intramuscular injection.

Children under 18 months of age:

Since the response to the vaccine may be sub-optimal, the use of the product should be based upon the risk of exposure to the disease.

Elderly:

As for adults and children over 18 months of age.

Revaccination: A single dose at 3 yearly intervals in subjects who remain at risk from typhoid fever.

Contra-indications: Acute infectious illness.

Hypersensitivity to the vaccine or its components.

Special warnings and special precautions for use: The vaccine does not protect against paratyphoid fever. As with all vaccines, facilities for the management of anaphylaxis should always be available during vaccination.

Interaction with other medicaments and other forms of interaction: None known

Pregnancy and lactation: No reproductive studies have been conducted in animals. There are no data on the use of this vaccine in pregnancy and lactation. The vaccine should not normally be used in pregnancy or during lactation unless the benefit outweighs the risk.

Effects on ability to drive and use machines: Not applicable

Undesirable effects: Local reactions including pain, swelling and erythema at the injection site may occur in two thirds of vaccinees. Systemic reactions including fever, headache, malaise and nausea occur infrequently (in less than 8% of recipients).

Overdose: Not applicable

Pharmaceutical properties
Pharmacodynamic properties: Not applicable

Pharmacokinetic properties: Not applicable

Preclinical safety data: Not applicable

Pharmaceutical particulars
List of excipients:

Phenol (preservative)	<1.250 milligrams
Isotonic buffer solution†	q.s. 0.5 millilitre

†Composition of the isotonic buffer solution:

Sodium Chloride	4.150 milligrams
Disodium phosphate	0.065 milligram
Monosodium phosphate	0.023 milligram
Water for Injections	q.s. 0.5 millilitre

Incompatibilities: Not applicable

Shelf life: 36 months

Special precautions for storage: Store between +2°C and +8°C. Do not freeze.

Nature and contents of container: The vaccine is supplied in single dose prefilled syringes (0.5 millilitre); in single syringe packs and packs of 10 syringes

Instructions for use/handling: Shake well immediately before use.

Marketing authorisation number
UK: PL 6745/0039

Date of first authorisation/renewal of authorisation
5 May 1992 / 30 May 1997

Date of (partial) revision of the text October 1997

Legal category POM

VAQTA* PAEDIATRIC 

Hepatitis A Vaccine, Purified Inactivated, for Children and Adolescents

Qualitative and quantitative composition Each 0.5 millilitre dose contains approximately 25U of hepatitis A virus antigen adsorbed onto approximately 0.225 milligram of aluminium provided as aluminium hydroxide, and 35 microgram of sodium borate as a pH stabiliser, in 0.9% sodium chloride. Neomycin and formaldehyde are used in the manufacturing process.

Pharmaceutical form VAQTA Paediatric is a sterile suspension for intramuscular use.

Clinical particulars
Therapeutic indications: VAQTA Paediatric is indicated for active pre-exposure prophylaxis against disease caused by hepatitis A virus. Vaccination is recommended in healthy children and adolescents 2 years of age up to and including 17 years of age, who

are at risk of contracting or spreading infection or who are at risk of life-threatening disease if infected.

Subjects at high risk of hepatitis A infection include those travelling to, or living in, medium or high endemicity areas. Other high risk groups include recent close contacts of infected individuals and potential contacts of cases such as childcare or health workers. In event of a case contact, human normal immunoglobulin should be given simultaneously with VAQTA Paediatric at different sites. Individuals who potentially play a key role in transmitting infection, e.g. food-handlers, might also be considered for vaccination.

VAQTA Paediatric will not prevent hepatitis caused by infectious agents other than hepatitis A virus.

Posology and method of administration: VAQTA Paediatric should be injected INTRAMUSCULARLY in the deltoid region. The vaccine should not be administered subcutaneously or intradermally since administration by these routes may result in a less than optimal antibody response.

VAQTA Paediatric should never be administered intravenously.

The vaccination series consists of one primary dose and one booster dose given according to the following schedule:

Individuals 2 to 17 years of age should receive a single 0.5 millilitre (~25U) dose of vaccine at elected date and a booster dose of 0.5 millilitre (~25U) 6 to 18 months later.

Known or Presumed Exposure to HAV/Travel to Endemic Areas /Use with Immunoglobulin

VAQTA* Paediatric may be administered concomitantly with immunoglobulin using separate sites and syringes. The vaccination regimen for VAQTA Paediatric should be followed as stated above. Consult the appropriate Summary of Product Characteristics/Data Sheet for the dosage of immunoglobulin. A booster dose of VAQTA Paediatric should be administered at the appropriate time as outlined above (see Interaction with Other Medicaments and Other Forms of Interaction).

Contra-indications: Hypersensitivity to any component of the vaccine.

Vaccination should be delayed in subjects with current severe febrile infections.

VAQTA Paediatric is not to be used in children under 2 years of age.

Special warnings and special precautions for use: Individuals who develop symptoms suggestive of hypersensitivity after an injection of VAQTA Paediatric should not receive further injections of the vaccine (see Contra-Indications).

Duration of antibodies: The long-term duration of serum antibodies to hepatitis A virus is unknown. In cases of doubt, the serum anti-hepatitis A antibody titre should be determined.

However, immune memory persists in seroconverted vaccinees even if antibody titres wane to undetectable levels, and such individuals generally respond anamnestically to a booster

Testing for antibodies to hepatitis A prior to a decision on immunisation should be performed in patients born in areas of high endemicity and/or with a history of jaundice.

VAQTA Paediatric does not cause immediate protection against hepatitis A, and there may be a period of 2 to 4 weeks before antibody induction occurs.

VAQTA Paediatric will not prevent hepatitis caused by infectious agents other than hepatitis A virus. Because of the long incubation period (approximately 20 to 50 days) for hepatitis A, it is possible for unrecognised hepatitis A infection to be present at the time the vaccine is given. The vaccine may not prevent hepatitis A in such individuals.

As with any vaccine, adequate treatment provisions, including epinephrine (adrenaline), should be available for immediate use should an anaphylactic or anaphylactoid reaction occur.

As with any vaccine, vaccination with VAQTA Paediatric may not result in a protective response in all susceptible vaccinees.

As no studies have been performed with VAQTA Paediatric in subjects with liver disease the use of this vaccine in such subjects should be considered with care.

Interaction with other medicaments and other forms of interaction: If VAQTA Paediatric is used in individuals with malignancies or those receiving immunosuppressive therapy or who are otherwise immunocompromised, the expected immune response may not be obtained.

Use with immunoglobulin: For individuals requiring either post exposure prophylaxis or combined immediate and longer term protection (e.g. travellers departing on short notice to endemic areas), VAQTA Paediatric may be administered concomitantly with immunoglobulin using separate sites and syringes (see Posology and Method of Administration)

Use with other vaccines: When concurrent administration is necessary, VAQTA Paediatric must not be mixed with other vaccines in the same syringe, and other vaccines should be administered at different sites.

Pregnancy and lactation: Animal reproduction studies have not been conducted with VAQTA Paediatric.

It is not known whether VAQTA Paediatric can cause foetal harm when administered to a pregnant woman or can affect reproduction capacity. VAQTA Paediatric is not recommended in pregnancy unless there is a high risk of hepatitis A infection, and the attending physician judges that the possible benefits of vaccination outweigh the risks to the foetus.

It is not known whether VAQTA Paediatric is excreted in human milk, and the effect on breast fed infants following administration of VAQTA Paediatric to mothers has not been studied. Hence, VAQTA Paediatric should be used with caution in women who are breast feeding.

Effects on ability to drive and use machines: There are no specific data. However, asthenia/fatigue and headache have been reported following administration of VAQTA Paediatric.

Undesirable effects: No serious vaccine related adverse experiences were observed during clinical trials.

In combined clinical trials involving 2,595 healthy children and adolescents who received one or more ~25U doses of hepatitis A vaccine, fever and local complaints were observed during a 5 day period following vaccination and systemic complaints during a 14 day period following vaccination. Injection site complaints, generally mild and transient, were the most frequently reported complaints. Listed below are the complaints (^{3} 1%) reported, without regard to causality, in decreasing order of frequency, within each body system.

Localised injection-site reactions: (generally mild and transient) pain (18.7%); tenderness (16.8%); warmth (8.6%); swelling (7.3%); erythema (7.5%); ecchymosis (1.3%).

Body as a whole: fever (^{3} 38.9°C, oral) (3.1%); abdominal pain (1.6%).

Digestive system: diarrhoea (1.0%); vomiting (1.0%).

Nervous system/psychiatric: headache (2.3%).

Respiratory system: pharyngitis (1.5%); upper respiratory infection (1.1%); cough (1.0%).

As with any vaccine, there is a possibility that use of VAQTA Paediatric in very large populations might reveal adverse experiences not observed in clinical trials.

Overdose: There are no data with regard to overdose.

Pharmacological properties

Pharmacodynamic properties: VAQTA Paediatric is derived from hepatitis A virus grown in cell culture in human MRC-5 diploid fibroblasts. It contains inactivated virus of a strain which was originally derived by further serial passage of a proven attenuated strain. The virus is grown, harvested, highly purified, formalin inactivated and then adsorbed onto aluminium hydroxide.

Pharmacokinetic properties: The onset of seroconversion following a single dose of VAQTA Paediatric was shown to parallel the onset of protection against clinical hepatitis A disease. A very high degree of protection has been demonstrated after a single dose of VAQTA Paediatric in 1037 children and adolescents 2 to 16 years of age in a US community with recurrent outbreaks of hepatitis A (The Monroe Efficacy Study). Seroconversion was achieved in more than 99% of vaccine recipients within 4 weeks of the vaccination. The protective efficacy of a single dose of VAQTA Paediatric was observed to be 100%. A booster dose was administered to most vaccinees 6, 12 or 18 months after the primary dose. The effectiveness of VAQTA Paediatric for use in this community has been demonstrated by the fact that after 3 years, no cases of hepatitis A disease ^{3}16 days after vaccination have occurred in the vaccinees.

Clinical studies showed seroconversion rates of 97% in children and adolescents within 4 weeks after the recommended primary dose.

Seropositivity was shown to persist up to 18 months in children and adolescents from the Monroe Efficacy Study and up to 6 months in adults (studies ongoing). Persistence of immunologic memory was demonstrated with an anamnestic antibody response to a booster dose given 6 to 18 months after the primary dose in children and adolescents.

A mathematical model predicts duration of protection lasting for many years after the booster.

Preclinical safety data: None Stated.

Pharmaceutical particulars

List of excipients: VAQTA Paediatric contains aluminium hydroxide, sodium borate, and sodium chloride.

Incompatibilities: Do not mix in the same syringe with other vaccines/drugs.

Booster vaccine following primary immunisation with VAQTA Paediatric should be performed with VAQTA Paediatric.

Shelf life: 24 months when stored between +2°C and +8°C.

Expiry date has been printed on the package (month followed by year) and is applicable only if the vaccine has been stored between +2°C and +8°C. Potency of this vaccine is not significantly affected after exposure to temperatures up to 28°C for up to 3 months. However this is NOT a storage recommendation and if kept longer than three months at this temperature it should not be used.

Special precautions for storage: Store vaccine between +2°C and +8°C (+36°F and +46°F).

DO NOT FREEZE since freezing destroys potency.

Nature and contents of container: Single dose prefilled syringe is available as a single unit pack and a pack of 10.

Instructions for use/handling: The vaccine should be used as supplied; no reconstitution is necessary.

Shake well immediately before withdrawal and use. Thorough agitation is necessary to maintain suspension of the vaccine.

Parenteral drug products should be inspected visually for extraneous particulate matter and discoloration prior to administration. After thorough agitation, VAQTA Paediatric is a slightly opaque white suspension.

Marketing authorisation number PL 6745/0064

Date of first authorisation/renewal of authorisation 15 August 1996

Date of (partial) revision of the text May 1998

Legal category POM

**Trade Mark*

Penn Pharmaceuticals Ltd
Tafarnaubach Industrial Estate
Tredegar
Gwent NP2 3AA

☎ 01495 711222 🗋 01495 711225/718285

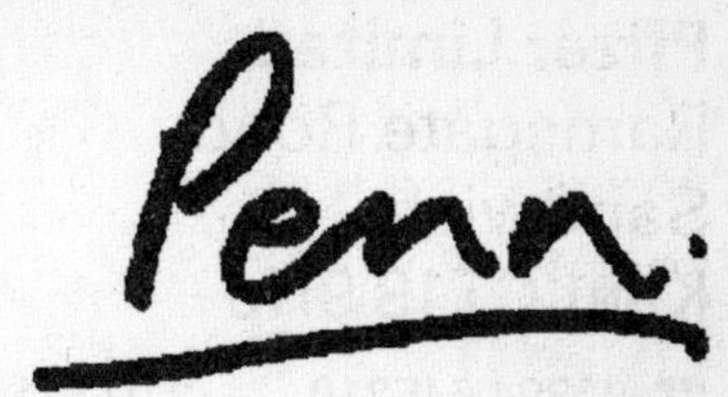

CARBOMIX*

Presentation Black, odourless, tasteless granules for mixing with water before administration.

Carbomix is available in bottles containing activated charcoal 25 g and 50 g.

Carbomix granules also contain citric acid, acacia and glycerol.

Uses Emergency treatment of acute oral poisoning or drug overdose. Carbomix absorbs toxic substances and reduces or prevents systemic absorption. The shorter the time interval between ingestion of the toxicant and the administration of Carbomix, the greater is the benefit to the patient. However, as the absorption of massive drug overdoses is often retarded in acute conditions of intoxication, even the delayed administration of Carbomix may be beneficial.

In severe intoxications, repeated administration of Carbomix is recommended to prevent absorbed drug being released (in an unbound state) in the lower intestinal tract or to expedite the elimination and prevent the re-absorption of any drug undergoing entero-hepatic circulation.

Dosage and administration
Adults (including the elderly): 50 g activated charcoal (one standard treatment pack), repeated if necessary.

Children under 12 years: 25 g activated charcoal (one small treatment pack or half the contents of the standard pack), repeated if necessary. If a large quantity of toxicant has been ingested, and where there is a risk to life, a dose of 50 g is recommended.

Carbomix should be given as soon as possible after the ingestion of the potential poison.

The contents of the bottle are made up to the red band with water and shaken thoroughly. The suspension is then taken orally or given by intragastric tube using the applicator provided. Carbomix may be administered after emesis or gastric lavage and may be used concurrently with parenteral antidotes such as acetylcysteine.

Contra-indications, warnings, etc
Contra-indications: There are no contra-indications to the use of Carbomix but see under *Precautions* for inappropriate concomitant use.

Precautions: The value of Carbomix in the treatment of poisoning by strong acids, alkalis and other corrosive substances is limited. It should also be borne in mind that the presence of charcoal will render difficult any immediate endoscopy that may be required. Carbomix is poor in binding cyanide, iron salts and some solvents including methanol, ethanol and ethylene glycol.

In cases where the toxicant has diuretic properties or has been ingested with alcohol, plenty of fluid should be given after the administration of Carbomix.

Carbomix should not be used concurrently with systemically active oral emetics or oral antidotes such as methionine since such agents would be absorbed by the charcoal.

Pregnancy and lactation: There is no evidence to suggest that Carbomix should not be used during pregnancy or lactation. The product is not systemically absorbed.

Side-effects: In general, Carbomix is well tolerated. Some patients may however experience constipation or diarrhoea. Faecal impaction has been reported in a patient treated for an overdose of a diuretic with alcohol.

Interactions: The purpose of the product is to interact with other medicaments and toxicants taken in overdosage. There are no systemic interactions because the product is not absorbed from the gut.

Overdose: Not applicable. In theory, severe constipation would result from excessive use and this could be treated with laxatives.

Pharmaceutical precautions Store below 25°C. Dispose of any unused suspension after 24 hours.

Legal category P.

Package quantities Treatment packs containing 50 g activated charcoal in 61.5 g granules (standard pack) and 25 g activated charcoal in 30.75 g granules.

Further information Activated charcoal has well-documented adsorptive properties and is effective in reducing the absorption of a wide variety of toxicants, including drugs taken in overdose, from the gut. In addition, there is evidence that the administration of activated charcoal can enhance the elimination of some compounds by creating an effective concentration gradient from the circulation to the gut. Activated charcoal is not systemically absorbed.

Product licence number 4351/0002.

Date of preparation: September 1994.

PARADOTE*

Qualitative and quantitative composition Paracetamol 500 mg and DL-Methionine 100 mg (co-methiamol 100/500).

Pharmaceutical form White, capsuloid, film-coated tablets, marked 'CM'.

Clinical particulars
Therapeutic indications: Paradote tablets are indicated for use in most painful and febrile conditions such as headache, toothache, colds, influenza, rheumatic pain and dysmenorrhoea. Methionine is added to this preparation as it may prevent liver damage occurring if an overdose is taken.

Posology and method of administration: Paradote tablets are for oral administration only.

Adults (including the elderly): Two tablets to be taken every four hours as required. No more than eight tablets should be taken in 24 hours.

Children aged 12 and under: Not recommended.

Contra-indications: Hypersensitivity to paracetamol, methionine or any of the other constituents. The product should not be used by patients taking mono-amine-oxidase inhibitors (MAOIs) or in the presence of hepatic diseases as there is an increased risk of psychosis or encephalopathy.

Special warnings and special precautions for use: Care is advised in the administration of paracetamol to patients with severe renal or hepatic impairment. The hazard of overdose is greater in those with non-cirrhotic alcoholic liver disease.

Patients should be advised not to exceed the recommended dose and not to take other paracetamol-containing products concurrently.

Interactions with other medicaments and other forms of medication: The speed of absorption of paracetamol may be increased by metoclopramide or domperidone and absorption reduced by cholestyramine. The anticoagulant effect of warfarin and other coumarins may be enhanced by prolonged regular daily use of paracetamol with increased risk of bleeding; occasional doses have no significant effect. Concurrent administration of methionine may inhibit the effect of levodopa.

Use in pregnancy and lactation: Epidemiological studies in human pregnancy have shown no ill effects due to paracetamol used in the recommended dosage and methionine is an essential amino acid. Paracetamol is excreted in breast milk but not in a clinically significant amount. Available data do not contraindicate breast feeding. However, the product should be used with caution during pregnancy and lactation.

Effects on ability to drive and to use machines: None.

Undesirable effects: Adverse effects of paracetamol are rare but hypersensitivity, including skin rash, may occur. There have been a few reports of blood dyscrasias, including thrombocytopenia and agranulocytosis, but these were not necessarily related to paracetamol.

Overdose: Symptoms of paracetamol overdosage in the first 24 hours are pallor, nausea, vomiting, anorexia and abdominal pain. Liver damage may become apparent 12 to 48 hours after ingestion. Abnormalities of glucose metabolism and metabolic acidosis may occur. Acute renal failure with acute tubular necrosis may develop even in the absence of severe liver damage. Cardiac arrhythmias and pancreatitis have been reported.

Liver damage is possible in adults who have taken 10 g or more of paracetamol. It is considered that excess quantities of a toxic metabolite, usually adequately detoxified by glutathione when normal doses of paracetamol are ingested, become irreversibly bound to liver tissue. Death may result from paracetamol overdosage when liver glutathione stores are exhausted so that hepatic necrosis results. Concurrent ingestion of methionine (which enables the liver cells to manufacture more glutathione) in Paradote tablets is designed to help protect the liver against the hepatotoxic effects of excessive amounts of paracetamol.

Immediate treatment is essential in the management of paracetamol overdose and this should still be followed in the case of Paradote tablets. Despite lack of early symptoms, patients should be referred to hospital urgently for immediate medical attention and any patient who has ingested around 7.5 g or more of paracetamol in the preceding 4 hours should undergo gastric lavage or be given activated charcoal. Administration of additional oral methionine or intravenous acetylcysteine, which may have a beneficial effect up to at least 48 hours after the overdose, may be required, taking into account the amount of methionine already ingested. General supportive measures must be available.

Pharmacological properties
Pharmacodynamic properties: Paracetamol possesses analgesic and antipyretic properties but has no useful anti-inflammatory activity. DL-methionine is a racemic mixture of the essential amino acid L-methionine and its D-isomer. Methionine enhances hepatic synthesis of glutathione which is used to inactivate the toxic quinone metabolite of paracetamol by conjugation.

Pharmacokinetic properties: Paracetamol is rapidly absorbed from the small intestine, the rate of absorption being dependent on the rate of gastric emptying. Peak plasma levels occur between 30 minutes and 2 hours after ingestion. It has been shown for this preparation that the presence of DL-methionine does not significantly alter the bioavailability of paracetamol. The plasma half-life of paracetamol varies between 1.5 and 2.5 hours; it is extensively metabolised in the liver and excreted in the urine, mainly as the sulphate and glucuronide conjugates. A small proportion (5–10%) is converted to a highly reactive quinone metabolite which is normally inactivated by conjugation with liver glutathione.

Methionine is rapidly and completely absorbed. The plasma half-life of methionine is about 2 hours which is similar to that of paracetamol. Utilisation of L-methionine is 100%. About 50% of the D-methionine is excreted in the urine and, although the remaining 50% is not directly available for synthesis of glutathione, its sulphur moiety is transferred to serine to form L-cysteine which can be used for glutathione synthesis. In the event of overdose, all the L-methionine and about half the D-methionine can provide a source of glutathione.

Preclinical safety data: No findings have been reported from pre-clinical safety studies which add to the prescribing information given in other sections.

Pharmaceutical particulars
List of excipients: Sodium Starch Glycollate BP; Colloidal Silicon Dioxide NF (Aerosil 200); Magnesium Stearate PhEur; Povidone PhEur (Kollidon 90); stearic acid; acrylic polymer coating (Eudragit E); Talc BP; Titanium Dioxide BP; Polyethylene Glycol 300 BP.

Incompatibilities: None.

Shelf life: 24 months, unopened.

Special precautions for storage: Store below 25°C in a dry place.

Nature and contents of container: The product is blister-packed in strips of 12 and presented in cartons of 12, 24 and 96 tablets.

Instructions for use/handling: None.

Marketing authorisation number 04351/0017.

Date of approval/revision of SPC November 1995.

Legal category P.

**Trade Mark*

Pfizer Limited
Ramsgate Road
Sandwich
Kent CT13 9NJ

☎ 01304 645210 📠 01304 656221

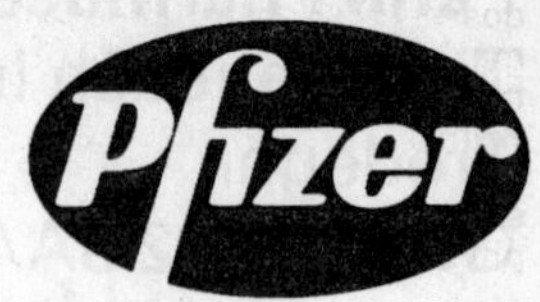

ATARAX* TABLETS

Qualitative and quantitative composition
Hydroxyzine hydrochloride 10 mg
Hydroxyzine hydrochloride 25 mg

Pharmaceutical form 10 mg sugar coated tablets, coloured orange and coded on one side with 'Pfizer'.

25 mg sugar coated tablets, coloured green and coded on one side with 'Pfizer'.

Clinical particulars
Therapeutic indications: Atarax is indicated to assist in the management of anxiety in adults.

Atarax is indicated for the management of pruritus associated with acute and chronic urticaria, including cholinergic and physical types, and atopic and contact dermatitis in adults and children.

Posology and method of administration: Method of administration: oral.
Dosage:
Anxiety
Adults: 50-100 mg four times daily.
Pruritus
Adults: Starting dose of 25 mg at night increasing as necessary to 25 mg three or four times daily.

Use in the elderly: Atarax may be used in elderly patients with no special precautions other than the care always necessary in this age group. The lowest effective maintenance dose and careful observation for side-effects are important.

Use in children: From 6 months to 6 years 5-15 mg rising to 50 mg daily in divided doses and for children over 6 years, 15-25 mg rising to 50-100 mg daily in divided doses.

As with all medications, the dosage should be adjusted to according to the patient's response to therapy.

Renal impairment: The total daily dosage should be reduced by half (see *Special warnings and special precautions for use*).

Contra-indications: Atarax is contra-indicated in patients who have shown previous hypersensitivity to it.

Special warnings and special precautions for use: Atarax should be used caution in patients with impaired renal function (see *Posology and method of administration*). It is uncertain whether the drug may accumulate or have other adverse effects in such patients. Atarax is completely metabolised and one of the metabolites is the active metabolite cetirizine. Cetirizine is renally excreted and clearance is reduced in patients with moderate renal impairment and on dialysis compared to normal volunteers.

Interactions with other medicaments and other forms of interaction: Patients should be warned that Atarax may enhance their response to alcohol, barbituates and other CNS depressants.

Pregnancy and lactation: Atarax is contra-indicated in early pregnancy. Hydroxyzine, when administered to the pregnant mouse, rat and rabbit, induced foetal abnormalities at doses substantially above the human therapeutic range. Clinical data in humans are inadequate to establish safety in early pregnancy. There is inadequate evidence of safety in the later stages of pregnancy. Use in pregnancy only when there is no safe alternative or when the disease itself carries risks for the mother or child.

Use in nursing mothers: It is not known whether Atarax is excreted in human milk. Since many drugs are so excreted, Atarax should not be given to nursing mothers.

Effects on ability to drive and use machines: Patients should be warned that Atarax may impair their ability to perform activities requiring mental alertness or physical coordination such as operating machinery or driving a vehicle.

Undesirable effects: Therapeutic doses of Atarax seldom produce marked impairment of mental alertness. Drowsiness may occur; if so, it is usually transitory and may disappear after a few days of continued therapy or upon reduction of the dose. Dryness of the mouth may be encountered at higher doses. Dizziness, weakness, headache and confusion have been reported.

Extensive clinical use has substantiated the absence of toxic effects on the liver or bone marrow when administered for over four years of uninterrupted therapy. The absence of side-effects has been further demonstrated in experimental studies in which excessively high doses were administered.

Involuntary motor activity, including rare instances of tremor and convulsions, have been reported, usually with doses considerably higher than those recommended. Continuous therapy with over 1 g/day has been employed in some patients without these effects having been encountered.

Overdose: The most common manifestation of Atarax overdosage is hypersedation. As in the management of overdosage with any drug, it should be borne in mind that multiple agents may have been taken. If vomiting has not occurred spontaneously in conscious patients it should be induced. Immediate gastric lavage is also recommended. General supportive care, including frequent monitoring of the vital signs and close observation of the patient is indicated. Hypotension, though unlikely, may be controlled with intravenous fluids and noradrenaline, or metaraminol. Adrenaline should not be used in this situation as Atarax counteracts its pressor action.

There is no specific antidote. It is doubtful whether haemodialysis has any value in the treatment of overdosage with Atarax. However, if other agents such as barbiturates have been ingested concomitantly, haemodialysis may be indicated.

Pharmacological properties
Pharmacodynamic properties: Atarax is unrelated chemically to phenothiazine, reserpine and meprobamate.

Atarax has been shown clinically to be a rapid-acting anxiolytic with a wide margin of safety. It induces a calming effect in anxious tense adults. It is not a cortical depressant, but its action may be due to a suppression of activity in certain key regions of the subcortical area of the central nervous system.

Antihistamine effects have been demonstrated experimentally and confirmed clinically; it is highly effective in alleviating pruritus.

Pharmacokinetic properties: Atarax is rapidly absorbed from the gastro-intestinal tract and effects are usually noted within 15 to 30 minutes after oral administration.

Preclinical safety data: None stated.

Pharmaceutical particulars
List of excipients: Tablet core: Lactose anhydrous Ph.Eur., Calcium Phosphate Dibasic Anhydrous USP, Pregelatinised Starch NF, Magnesium Stearate Ph.Eur., Sodium Lauryl Sulphate Ph.Eur.

Tablet coating: Sucrose Ph.Eur., Gum Acacia Ph.Eur., Calcium Sulphate Dihydrate NF, Talc Ph.Eur., Butyl Parahydroxybenzoate Ph.Eur., Beeswax Ph.Eur., Carnuba Wax NF, Dewaxed Orange Shellac, Opalux AS.3563 Dye (10 mg only) and Opalux AS.5994 Dye (25 mg only).

Incompatibilities: None stated.

Shelf life: 24 months.

Special precautions for storage: Store below 30°C

Nature and contents of container: White opaque 250 micron PVC/PVdC–20 micron aluminium foil blister strips containing 84×10 mg tablets, (6 blister strips per carton) or 28×25 mg tablets (2 blister strips per carton).

Instruction for use/handling: No special requirements.

Marketing authorisation numbers
Atarax 10 mg Tablets PL 0057/5003R
Atarax 25 mg Tablets PL 0057/5004R

Date of first authorisation/renewal of authorisation
Atarax 10 mg Tablets 27 April 1987/30 July 1997
Atarax 25 mg Tablets 24 July 1985/24 July 1997

Date of (partial) revision of the text November 1998

Legal category POM

CARDURA*

Qualitative and quantitative composition Doxazosin mesylate:
1.213 mg equivalent to 1 mg doxazosin,
2.43 mg equivalent to 2 mg doxazosin,
4.86 mg equivalent to 4 mg doxazosin.

Pharmaceutical form Tablets for oral administration.

1 mg pentagonal tablets: marked DXP1 on one side and 'PFIZER' on the other.

2 mg ovoid tablets: marked DXP2 on one side and 'PFIZER' on the other.

4 mg square tablets: marked DXP4 on one side and 'PFIZER' on the other.

Clinical particulars
Therapeutic indications:
Hypertension: Cardura is indicated for the treatment of hypertension and can be used as the sole agent to control blood pressure in the majority of patients. In patients inadequately controlled on single antihypertensive therapy, Cardura may be used in combination with a thiazide diuretic, beta-adrenoceptor blocking agent, calcium antagonist or an angiotensin-converting enzyme inhibitor.

Benign prostatic hyperplasia: Cardura is indicated for the treatment of urinary outflow obstruction and symptoms associated with benign prostatic hyperplasia (BPH).

Posology and method of administration:
Hypertension: Cardura is used in a once daily regimen: the initial dose is 1 mg. Dosage may then be increased after one or two weeks of therapy to 2 mg and thereafter, if necessary to 4 mg. The majority of patients who respond to Cardura will do so at a dose of 4 mg or less. Dosage can be further increased if necessary to 8 mg or the maximum recommended dose of 16 mg.

Benign prostatic hyperplasia: The initial dosage of Cardura is 1 mg given once daily. Depending on the individual patient's response dosage may then be increased to 2 mg and thereafter to 4 mg and up to the maximum recommended dose of 8 mg. The recommended titration interval is 1–2 weeks. The usual recommended dose is 2–4 mg daily.

Children: There is insufficient exprience to recommend the use of Cardura in children.

Elderly: Normal adult dosage.

Patients with renal impairment: Since there is no change in pharmacokinetics in patients with impaired renal function the usual adult dose of Cardura is recommended. Cardura is not dialysable.

Patients with hepatic impairment: There have been no pharmacokinetic studies in patients with liver impairment, nor in patients taking drugs known to influence hepatic metabolism (e.g. cimetidine). Cardura should be used with care in such patients.

Contra-indications: Cardura is contra-indicated in patients with a known hypersensitivity to quinazolines.

Use during lactation: Animal studies have shown that doxazosin accumulates in breast milk. The clinical safety of Cardura during lactation has not been established, consequently Cardura is contra-indicated in nursing mothers.

Special warnings and precautions for use:
Impaired liver function: As with any drug wholly metabolised by the liver, Cardura should be administered with caution to patients with evidence of impaired hepatic function (see *Pharmacokinetic properties*).

Interactions with other medicaments and other forms of interaction: Doxazosin is highly bound to plasma proteins (98%). *In vitro* data in human plasma indicates that doxazosin has no effect on protein binding of the drugs tested (digoxin, phenytoin, warfarin or indomethacin). No adverse drug interactions have been observed with thiazide diuretics, frusemide, beta-blocking agents, non-steroidal anti-inflammatory drugs, antibiotics, oral hypoglycaemic drugs, uricosuric agents, or anticoagulants.

Pregnancy and lactation:
Use during pregnancy: Although no teratogenic ef-

fects were seen in animal testing, reduced fetal survival was observed in animals at extremely high doses. These doses were approximately 300 times the maximum recommended human dose. As there are no adequate and well controlled studies in pregnant women, the safety of Cardura's use during pregnancy has not yet been established. Accordingly, Cardura should be used only when, in the opinion of the physician, potential benefit outweighs potential risk.

Use during lactation: Contra-indicated (see *Contra-indications*).

Effects on ability to drive and use machines: The ability to drive or use machinery may be impaired, especially when initiating therapy.

Undesirable effects:
Hypertension: In clinical trials involving patients with hypertension, the most common reactions associated with Cardura therapy were of a postural type (rarely associated with fainting) or non-specific and included: dizziness, headache, fatigue/malaise, postural dizziness, vertigo, oedema, asthenia, somnolence, nausea and rhinitis.

In post-marketing experience, the following additional adverse events have been reported: rare cases of non-specific gastric complaints such as abdominal pain, diarrhoea and vomiting; rare cases of agitation and tremor.

Rare cases of urinary incontinence were reported; this may be related to Cardura's pharmacological action.

Isolated reports of priapism and impotence have been reported to be associated with alpha-1-antagonists, including Cardura.

Rare cases of skin rash, pruritis, thrombocytopenia, purpura, epistaxis, leucopenia, haematuria, cholestasis, hepatitis, jaundice, abnormal liver function tests and blurred vision have also been reported.

The following additional adverse events have been reported in marketing experience among patients treated for hypertension. In general, these are not distinguishable from symptoms that might have occurred in the absence of exposure to Cardura: tachycardia, palpitations, chest pain, angina pectoris, myocardial infarction, cerebrovascular accidents and cardiac arrhythmias.

Benign prostatic hyperplasia: Experience in controlled clinical trials in BPH indicates a similar adverse event profile to that seen in hypertension.

Overdose: Should overdosage lead to hypotension, the patient should be immediately placed in a supine, head down position. Other supportive measures may be appropriate in individual cases. Since Cardura is highly protein bound, dialysis is not indicated.

Pharmacological properties
Pharmacodynamic properties: Doxazosin is a potent and selective post-junctional alpha-1-adrenoceptor antagonist. This action results in a decrease in systemic blood pressure. Cardura is appropriate for oral administration in a once daily regimen in patients with essential hypertension.

Cardura has been shown to be free of adverse metabolic effects and is suitable for use in patients with co-existent diabetes mellitus, gout and insulin resistance.

Cardura is suitable for use in patients with co-existent asthma, left ventricular hypertrophy and in elderly patients. Treatment with Cardura has been shown to result in regression of left ventricular hypertrophy, inhibition of platelet aggregation and enhanced activity of tissue plasminogen activator. Additionally, Cardura improves insulin sensitivity in patients with impairment.

Cardura, in addition to its antihypertensive effect, has in long term studies produced a modest reduction in plasma total cholesterol, LDL-cholesterol and triglyceride concentrations and therefore may be of particular benefit to hypertensive patients with concomitant hyperlipidaemia.

Administration of Cardura to patients with symptomatic BPH results in a significant improvement in urodynamics and symptoms. The effect in BPH is thought to result from selective blockade of the alpha-adrenoceptors located in the prostatic muscular stroma, capsule and bladder neck.

Pharmacokinetic properties: Following oral administration in humans (young male adults or the elderly of either sex), doxazosin is well absorbed and approximately two thirds of the dose is bioavailable. The mean plasma elimination half-life is 22 hours thus making the drug suitable for once daily administration.

Doxazosin is extensively metabolised in man and in the animal species tested, with the faeces being the predominant route of excretion.

After oral administration of Cardura the plasma concentrations of the metabolites are low. The most active (6' hydroxy) metabolite is present in man at one fortieth of the plasma concentration of the parent compound which suggests that the antihypertensive activity is in the main due to doxazosin.

Preclinical safety data: None stated.

Pharmaceutical particulars
List of excipients: Lactose, magnesium stearate, microcrystalline cellulose, sodium lauryl sulphate and sodium starch glycolate.

Incompatibilities: None stated.

Shelf life: 5 years.

Special precautions for storage: Store below 30°C.

Nature and contents of container: Cardura 1 mg, 2 mg and 4 mg Tablets are available as calendar packs of 28 tablets. Aluminium/PVC/PVdC blister strips, 14 tablets/strip, 2 strips in a carton box.

Instruction for use/handling: No special requirements.

Marketing authorisation numbers
Cardura 1 mg PL 0057/0276
Cardura 2 mg PL 0057/0277
Cardura 4 mg PL 0057/0278

Date of first authorisation/renewal of authorisation 20 October 1993.

Date of (partial) revision of the text August 1998.

Legal category POM.

DELTACORTRIL* ENTERIC

Qualitative and quantitative composition Prednisolone 2.5 mg or 5 mg.

Pharmaceutical form Tablets 2.5 mg, uniformly brown in colour and coded 'Pfizer'.

Tablets 5 mg, uniformly red in colour and coded 'Pfizer'.

Clinical particulars
Therapeutic indications:
Allergy and anaphylaxis: Bronchial asthma, drug hypersensitivity reactions, serum sickness, angioneurotic oedema, anaphylaxis.

Arteritis/collagenosis: Giant cell arteritis/polymyalgia rheumatica, mixed connective tissue disease, polyarteritis nodosa, polymyositis.

Blood disorders: Haemolytic anaemia (autoimmune), leukaemia (acute and chronic lymphocytic), lymphoma, multiple myeloma, idiopathic thrombocytopenic purpura.

Cardiovascular disorders: Post myocardial infarction syndrome, rheumatic fever with severe carditis.

Endocrine disorders: Primary and secondary adrenal insufficiency, congenital adrenal hyperplasia.

Gastro-intestinal disorders: Crohn's disease, ulcerative colitis, persistent coeliac syndrome (coeliac disease unresponsive to gluten withdrawal), autoimmune chronic active hepatitis, multisystem disease affecting liver, biliary peritonitis.

Hypercalcaemia: Sarcoidosis, vitamin D excess.

Infections (with appropriate chemotherapy): Helminthic infestations, Herxheimer reaction, infectious mononucleosis, miliary tuberculosis, mumps orchitis (adult), tuberculous meningitis, rickettsial disease.

Muscular disorders: Polymyositis, dermatomyositis.

Neurological disorders: Infantile spasms, Shy-Drager syndrome, sub-acute demyelinating polyneuropathy.

Ocular disease: Scleritis, posterior uveitis, retinal vasculitis, pseudo tumours of the orbit, giant cell arteritis, malignant ophthalmic Graves disease.

Renal disorders: Lupus nephritis, acute interstitial nephritis, minimal change glomerulonephritis.

Respiratory disease: Allergic pneumonitis, asthma, occupational asthma, pulmonary aspergillosis, pulmonary fibrosis, pulmonary alveolitis, aspiration of foreign body, aspiration of stomach contents, pulmonary sarcoid, drug induced lung disease, adult respiratory distress syndrome, spasmodic croup.

Rheumatic disorders: Rheumatoid arthritis, polymyalgia rheumatica, juvenile chronic arthritis, systemic lupus erythematosus, dermatomyositis, mixed connective tissue disease.

Skin disorders: Pemphigus vulgaris, bullous pemphigoid, systemic lupus erythematosus, pyoderma gangrenosum.

Miscellaneous: Sarcoidosis, hyperpyrexia, Behçets disease, immunosuppression in organ transplantation.

Posology and method of administration: The initial dosage of Deltacortril Enteric may vary from 5 mg to 60 mg daily depending on the disorder being treated. Divided daily dosage is usually used.

The following therapeutic guidelines should be kept in mind for all therapy with corticosteroids:

Corticosteroids are palliative symptomatic treatment by virtue of their anti-inflammatory effects; they are never curative.

The appropriate individual dose must be determined by trial and error and must be re-evaluated regularly according to activity of the disease.

As corticosteroid therapy becomes prolonged and as the dose is increased, the incidence of disabling side-effects increases.

In general, initial dosage shall be maintained or adjusted until the anticipated response is observed. The dose should be gradually reduced until the lowest dose which will maintain an adequate clinical response is reached. Use of the lowest effective dose may also minimise side-effects – see *Special warnings and special precautions for use.*

In patients who have received more than the physiological dose for systemic corticosteroids (approximately 7.5 mg prednisolone or equivalent) for greater than 3 weeks, withdrawal should not be abrupt. How dose reduction should be carried out depends largely on whether the disease is likely to relapse as the dose of systemic corticosteroids is reduced. Clinical assessment of disease activity may be needed during withdrawal. If the disease is unlikely to relapse on withdrawal of systemic corticosteroids but there is uncertainty about hypothalamic-pituitary-adrenal (HPA) suppression, the dose of corticosteroid may be reduced rapidly to physiological doses. Once a daily dose equivalent to 7.5 mg of prednisolone is reached, dose reduction should be slower to allow the HPA-axis to recover.

Abrupt withdrawal of systemic corticosteroid treatment, which has continued up to 3 weeks is appropriate if it is considered that the disease is unlikely to relapse. Abrupt withdrawal of doses of up to 40 mg daily of prednisolone, or equivalent for 3 weeks is unlikely to lead to clinically relevant HPA-axis suppression, in the majority of patients. In the following patient groups, gradual withdrawal of systemic corticosteroid therapy should be considered even after courses lasing 3 weeks or less:

- Patients who have had repeated courses of systemic corticosteroids, particularly if taken for greater than 3 weeks.
- When a short course has been prescribed within one year of cessation of long-term therapy (months or years).
- Patients who may have reasons for adrenocortical insufficiency other than exogenous corticosteroid therapy.
- Patients receiving doses of systemic corticosteroid greater than 40 mg daily of prednisolone (or equivalent).
- Patients repeatedly taking doses in the evening.

(See *Special warnings and special precautions for use* and *Undesirable effects.*)

During prolonged therapy, dosage may need to be temporarily increased during periods of stress or during exacerbations of the disease. (See *Special warnings and special precautions for use.*)

If there is lack of a satisfactory clinical response to Deltacortril Enteric, the drug should be gradually discontinued and the patient transferred to alternative therapy.

Intermittent dosage regimen: A single dose of Deltacortril Enteric in the morning on alternate days or at longer intervals is acceptable therapy for some patients. When this regimen is practical, the degree of pituitary-adrenal suppression can be minimised.

Specific dosage guidelines: The following recommendations for some corticosteroid-responsive disorders are for guidance only. Acute or severe disease may require initial high dose therapy with reduction to the lowest effective maintenance dose as soon as possible. Dosage reductions should not exceed 5–7.5 mg daily during chronic treatment.

Allergic and skin disorders: Initial doses of 5–15 mg daily are commonly adequate.

Collagenosis: Initial doses of 20–30 mg daily are frequently effective. Those with more severe symptoms may require higher doses.

Rheumatoid arthritis: The usual initial dose is 10–15 mg daily. The lowest daily maintenance dose compatible with tolerable symptomatic relief is recommended.

Blood disorders and lymphoma: An initial daily dose of 15–60 mg is often necessary with reduction after an adequate clinical or haematological response. Higher doses may be necessary to induce remission in acute leukaemia.

Use in children: Although appropriate fractions of the actual dose may be used, dosage will usually be determined by clinical response as in adults (see also *Precautions*). Alternate day dosage is preferable where possible.

Use in elderly: Treatment of elderly patients, particularly if long-term, should be planned bearing in mind the more serious consequences of the common side-effects of corticosteroids in old age (see also *Special warnings and special precautions for use*).

Contra-indications: Systemic infections unless specific anti-infective therapy is employed. Hypersensitivity to any ingredient. Ocular herpes simplex because of possible perforation.

Special warnings and special precautions for use: Caution is necessary when oral corticosteroids, including Deltacortril Enteric, are prescribed in patients with the following conditions, and frequent patient monitoring is necessary.

- Tuberculosis: Those with a previous history of, or X-ray changes characteristic of, tuberculosis. The emergence of active tuberculosis can, however, be prevented by the prophylactic use of antituberculosis therapy.
- Hypertension.
- Congestive heart failure.
- Liver failure.
- Renal insufficiency.
- Diabetes mellitus or in those with a family history of diabetes.
- Osteoporosis: This is of special importance in post-menopausal females who are at particular risk.
- Glaucoma or in those with a family history of glaucoma.
- Patients with a history of severe affective disorders and particularly those with a previous history of steroid-induced psychoses.
- Epilepsy.
- Peptic ulceration.
- Previous Steroid Myopathy.

A Patient Information Leaflet is supplied with this product.

Undesirable effects may be minimised by using the lowest effective dose for the minimum period and by administering the daily requirement as a single morning dose on alternate days. Frequent patient review is required to titrate the dose appropriately against disease activity (see *Dosage* section).

Adrenal suppression: Adrenal cortical atrophy develops during prolonged therapy and may persist for years after stopping treatment. Withdrawal of corticosteroids after prolonged therapy must therefore always be gradual to avoid acute adrenal insufficiency, being tapered off over weeks or months according to the dose and duration of treatment. (See *Posology and method of administration.*) During prolonged therapy any intercurrent illness, trauma, or surgical procedure will require a temporary increase in dosage; if corticosteroids have been stopped following prolonged therapy they may need to be temporarily re-introduced.

Patients should carry 'Steroid treatment' cards which give clear guidance on the precautions to be taken to minimise risk and which provide details of prescriber, drug, dosage and the duration of treatment.

Anti-inflammatory/immunosuppressive effects and infection: Suppression of the inflammatory response and immune function increases the susceptibility to infections and their severity. The clinical presentation may often be atypical and serious infections such as septicaemia and tuberculosis may be masked and may reach an advanced stage before being recognised.

Chickenpox: Chickenpox is of particular concern since this normally minor illness may be fatal in immunosuppressed patients. Patients (or parents of children) without a definite history of chickenpox should be advised to avoid close personal contact with chickenpox or herpes zoster and if exposed they should seek urgent medical attention. Passive immunisation with varicella-zoster immunoglobulin (VZIG) is needed by exposed non-immune patients who are receiving systemic corticosteroids or who have used them within the previous 3 months; this should be given within 10 days of exposure to chickenpox. If a diagnosis of chickenpox is confirmed, the illness warrants specialist care and urgent treatment. Corticosteroids should not be stopped and the dose may need to be increased.

The effect of corticosteroids may be enhanced in patients with hypothyroidism and in those with chronic liver disease with impaired hepatic function.

Use in children: Corticosteroids cause growth retardation in infancy, childhood and adolescence, which may be irreversible. Treatment should be limited to the minimum suppression of the hypothalamo-pituitary adrenal axis and growth retardation. Treatment should be administered where possible as a single dose on alternate days.

Use in the elderly: Treatment of elderly patients, particularly if long term, should be planned bearing in mind the more serious consequences of the common side-effects of corticosteroids in old age, especially osteoporosis, diabetes, hypertension, hypokalaemia, susceptibility to infection and thinning of the skin. Close clinical supervision is required to avoid life threatening reactions.

Interactions with other medicaments and other forms of interaction:

Hepatic microsomal enzyme inducers: Drugs which can cause liver enzyme induction such as phenobarbitone, phenytoin, rifampicin, rifabutin, carbamazepine, primidone and aminoglutethimide may reduce the therapeutic efficacy of corticosteroids by increasing the rate of metabolism. Lack of expected response may be observed and dosage of Deltacortril Enteric may need to be increased.

Non-steroidal anti-inflammatory drugs: Concomitant administration of ulcerogenic drugs such as indomethacin during corticosteroid therapy may increase the risk of GI ulceration. Aspirin should be used cautiously in conjunction with glucocorticoids in patients with hypoprothrombinaemia. Although concomitant therapy with salicylate and corticosteroids does not appear to increase the incidence or severity of GI ulceration, the possibility of this effect should be considered.

Serum salicylate concentrations may decrease when corticosteroids are administered concomitantly. The renal clearance of salicylates is increased by corticosteroids and steroid withdrawal may result in salicylate intoxication. Salicylates and corticosteroids should be used concurrently with caution. Patients receiving both drugs should be observed closely for adverse effects of either drug.

Anticoagulants: Response to anticoagulants may be reduced or, less often, enhanced by corticosteroids. Close monitoring of the INR or prothrombin time is required to avoid spontaneous bleeding.

Vaccines: Live vaccines should not be given to individuals with impaired immune responsiveness. The antibody response to other vaccines may be diminished.

Oestrogens: Oestrogens may potentiate the effects of glucocorticoids and dosage adjustment may be required if oestrogens are added to or withdrawn from a stable dosage regimen.

Other: The desired effects of hypoglycaemic agents (including insulin), anti-hypertensives and diuretics are antagonised by corticosteroids and the hypokalaemic effect of acetazolamide, loop diuretics, thiazide diuretics and carbenoxolone are enhanced.

Pregnancy and lactation:

Use in pregnancy: The ability of corticosteroids to cross the placenta varies between individual drugs, however, 88% of prednisolone is inactivated as it crosses the placenta. Administration of corticosteroids to pregnant animals can cause abnormalities of foetal development including cleft palate, intra-uterine growth retardation and affects on brain growth and development. There is no evidence that corticosteroids result in an increased incidence of congenital abnormalities, such as cleft palate/lip in man. However, when administered for prolonged periods or repeatedly during pregnancy, corticosteroids may increase the risk of intra-uterine growth retardation. Hypoadrenalism may, in theory, occur in the neonate following prenatal exposure to corticosteroids but usually resolves spontaneously following birth and is rarely clinically important. As with all drugs, corticosteroids should only be prescribed when the benefits to the mother and child outweigh the risks. When corticosteroids are essential however, patients with normal pregnancies may be treated as though they were in the non-gravid state. Patients with pre-eclampsia or fluid retention require close monitoring.

Use in lactation: Corticosteroids are excreted in small amounts in breast milk. However doses of up to 40 mg daily of prednisolone are unlikely to cause systemic effects in the infant. Infants of mothers taking higher doses than this may have a degree of adrenal suppression but the benefits of breast feeding are likely to outweigh any theoretical risk.

Effects of ability to drive and use machines: Deltacortril Enteric is unlikely to affect ability to drive and use machines.

Undesirable effects: The incidence of predictable undesirable effects, including hypothalmic-pituitary adrenal suppression correlates with the relative potency of the drug, dosage, timing of administration and the duration of treatment. (See *Special warnings and special precautions for use*).

Gastro-intestinal: Dyspepsia, peptic ulceration with perforation and haemorrhage, abdominal distension, oesophageal ulceration, oesophageal candidiasis, acute pancreatitis.

Musculo-skeletal: Proximal myopathy, osteoporosis, vertebral and long bone fractures, avascular osteonecrosis, tendon rupture.

Fluid and electrolyte disturbance: Sodium and water retention, hypertension, hypokalaemic alkalosis.

Dermatological: Impaired healing, skin atrophy, bruising, striae, telangiectasia, acne.

Endocrine/metabolic: Suppression of the hypothalamo-pituitary adrenal axis, growth suppression in infancy, childhood and adolescence, menstrual irregularity and amenorrhoea. Cushingoid facies, hirsutism, weight gain, impaired carbohydrate tolerance with increased requirement for antidiabetic therapy, negative nitrogen and calcium balance. Increased appetite.

Neuropsychiatric: Euphoria, psychological dependence, depression, insomnia. Raised intracranial pressure with papilloedema (pseudotumor cerebri) in children, usually after treatment withdrawal . Aggravation of schizophrenia. Aggravation of epilepsy.

Ophthalmic: Increased intra-ocular pressure, glaucoma, papilloedema, posterior subcapsular cataracts, corneal or scleral thinning, exacerbation of ophthalmic viral or fungal disease.

Anti-inflammatory and immunosuppressive effects: Increased susceptibility to, and severity of infections with suppression of clinical symptoms and signs, opportunistic infections, recurrence of dormant tuberculosis (see Other special warnings and precautions).

General: Leucocytosis, hypersensitivity including anaphylaxis, thromboembolism, nausea, malaise.

Withdrawal symptoms: Too rapid a reduction of corticosteroid dosage following prolonged treatment can lead to acute adrenal insufficiency, hypotension and death (see *Special warnings and special precautions for use* and *Posology and method of administration*). A 'withdrawal syndrome' may also occur including: fever, myalgia, arthralgia, rhinitis, conjunctivitis, painful itchy skin nodules and loss of weight.

Overdose: Reports of acute toxicity and/or death following overdosage of glucocorticoids are rare. No specific antidote is available; treatment is supportive and symptomatic. Serum electrolytes should be monitored.

Pharmacological properties

Pharmacodynamic properties: Naturally occurring glucocorticoids (hydrocortisone and cortisone), which also have salt-retaining properties, are used as replacement therapy in adrenocortical deficiency states. Their synthetic analogs are primarily used for their potent anti-inflammatory effect in disorders of many organ systems.

Glucocorticoids cause profound and varied metabolic effects. In addition, they modify the body's immune responses to diverse stimuli.

Pharmacokinetic properties: Prednisolone is rapidly and apparently almost completely absorbed after oral administration; it reaches peak plasma concentrations after 1–3 hours. There is however wide inter-subject variation suggesting impaired absorption in some individuals. Plasma half-life is about 3 hours in adults and somewhat less in children.

Although peak plasma prednisolone levels are somewhat lower after administration of Deltacortril Enteric and absorption is delayed, total absorption and bioavailability are the same as after plain prednisolone.

Prednisolone shows dose dependent pharmacokinetics, with an increase in dose leading to an increase in volume of distribution and plasma clearance. The degree of plasma protein binding determines the distribution and clearance of free, pharmacologically active drug. Reduced doses are necessary in patients with hypoalbuminaemia. Liver disease prolongs the half-life of prednisolone and, if the patient has hypoalbuminaemia, also increases the proportion of unbound drug and may thereby increase adverse effects.

Pharmaceutical particulars

List of excipients: 5 mg tablets: acacia, azo-dye (E124), beeswax, calcium carbonate, carnauba wax, cellulose acetate phthalate, citroflex A-2, kaolin, lactose, magnesium stearate, maize starch, shellac, sucrose and talc.

2.5 mg tablets: acacia, red/brown iron oxide (E172), beeswax, calcium carbonate, carnauba wax, cellulose acetate phthalate, citroflex A-2, kaolin, lactose, magnesium stearate, maize starch, shellac, sucrose and talc.

Incompatibilities: None.

Shelf life: 24 months.

Storage conditions: Store below 25°C.

Nature and contents of container: Polypropylene tablet container with HDPE Child-Resistant screw cap.

30 or 100 tablets per container in a carton box containing a Patient Information Leaflet.

Instructions for use/handling: None.

Marketing authorisation numbers
2.5 mg 0057/5012R
5 mg 0057/0128

Date of renewal of the authorisation 23 December 1996

Date of (partial) revision of the text May 1998

Legal category POM.

DIFLUCAN* 150 CAPSULE

Qualitative and quantitative composition Diflucan 150 capsule contains as its active ingredient fluconazole 150 mg.

Pharmaceutical form Diflucan 150 capsules are light turquoise blue, coded 'FLU 150' and 'PFIZER'.

Clinical particulars

Therapeutic indications: Diflucan 150 is indicated for the treatment of the following conditions:

Genital candidiasis. Vaginal candidiasis, acute or recurrent. Candidal balanitis. The treatment of partners who present with symptomatic genital candidiasis should be considered.

Posology and method of administration
In adults: Vaginal candidiasis or candidal balanitis – 150 mg single oral dose.

In children: Despite extensive data supporting the use of Diflucan in children there are limited data available on the use of Diflucan for genital candidiasis in children below 16 years. Use at present is not recommended unless antifungal treatment is imperative and no suitable alternative agent exists.

Use in elderly: The normal adult dose should be used.

Use in renal impairment: Fluconazole is excreted predominantly in the urine as unchanged drug. No adjustments in single dose therapy are required.

Contra-indications: Diflucan 150 should not be used in patients with known hypersensitivity to fluconazole or to related azole compounds or any other ingredient in the formulation.

Coadministration of terfenadine or cisapride is contraindicated in patients receiving Diflucan. (See *Interactions with other medicaments and other forms of interaction*).

Special warnings and special precautions for use: In some patients, particularly those with serious underlying diseases such as AIDS and cancer, abnormalities in haematological, hepatic, renal and other biochemical function test results have been observed during treatment with Diflucan but the clinical significance and relationship to treatment is uncertain.

Very rarely, patients who died with severe underlying disease and who have received multiple dose Diflucan, had post-mortem findings which included hepatic necrosis. These patients were receiving multiple concomitant medications, some known to be potentially hepatotoxic, and/or had underlying diseases which could have caused the hepatic necrosis. Consequently, because a causal relationship with Diflucan cannot be excluded, the risk-benefit ratio of continued Diflucan treatment should be assessed in those patients in whom a significant rise of liver enzymes occurs.

Patients have rarely developed exfoliative cutaneous reactions, such as Stevens-Johnson Syndrome and toxic epidermal necrolysis, during treatment with fluconazole. AIDS patients are more prone to the development of severe cutaneous reactions to many drugs.

If a rash develops in a patient which is considered attributable to Diflucan 150, further therapy with this agent is not recommended.

In rare cases, as with other azoles, anaphylaxis has been reported.

Interactions with other medicaments and other forms of interaction: The following drug interactions relate to the use of multiple-dose Diflucan, and the relevance to single-dose Diflucan 150 has not yet been established:

Anticoagulants: In an interaction study, Diflucan increased the prothrombin time after warfarin administration in healthy males. Though the magnitude of change was small (12%), careful monitoring of prothrombin time in patients receiving coumarin-type anticoagulants is recommended.

Sulphonylureas: Diflucan has been shown to prolong the serum half-life of concomitantly administered oral sulphonylureas (chlorpropamide, glibenclamide, glipizide and tolbutamide) in healthy volunteers. Diflucan and oral sulphonylureas may be co-administered to diabetic patients, but the possibility of a hypoglycaemic episode should be borne in mind.

Hydrochlorothiazide: In a kinetic interaction study, co-administration of multiple-dose hydrochlorothiazide to healthy volunteers receiving Diflucan increased plasma concentrations of fluconazole by 40%. An effect of this magnitude should not necessitate a change in the Diflucan dose regimen in subjects receiving concomitant diuretics, although the prescriber should bear it in mind.

Phenytoin: Concomitant administration of Diflucan and phenytoin may increase the levels of phenytoin to a clinically significant degree. If it is necessary to administer both drugs concomitantly, phenytoin levels should be monitored and the phenytoin dose adjusted to maintain therapeutic levels.

Oral contraceptives: Two kinetic studies with combined oral contraceptives have been performed using multiple doses of Diflucan. There were no relevant effects on either hormone level in the 50 mg Diflucan study, while at 200 mg daily the AUCs of ethinyloestradiol and levonorgestrel were increased 40% and 24% respectively. Thus multiple dose use of Diflucan at these doses is unlikely to have an effect on the efficacy of the combined oral contraceptive.

Rifampicin: Concomitant administration of Diflucan and rifampicin resulted in a 25% decrease in the AUC and 20% shorter half-life of fluconazole. In patients receiving concomitant rifampicin, an increase in the Diflucan dose should be considered.

Endogenous steroid: Diflucan 50 mg daily does not affect endogenous steroid levels in females: 200-400 mg daily has no clinically significant effect on endogenous steroid levels or on ACTH stimulated response in healthy male volunteers.

Cyclosporin: A kinetic study in renal transplant patients found Diflucan 200 mg daily to slowly increase cyclosporin concentrations. However, in another multiple dose study with 100 mg daily, Diflucan did not affect cyclosporin levels in patients with bone marrow transplants. Cyclosporin plasma concentration monitoring in patients receiving Diflucan is recommended.

Theophylline: In a placebo controlled interaction study, the administration of Diflucan 200 mg for 14 days resulted in an 18% decrease in the mean plasma clearance of theophylline. Patients who are receiving high doses of theophylline or who are otherwise at increased risk for theophylline toxicity should be observed for signs of theophylline toxicity while receiving Diflucan, and the therapy modified appropriately if signs of toxicity develop.

Terfenadine: Because of the occurrence of serious dysrhythmias secondary to prolongation of the QTc interval in patients receiving other azole antifungals in conjunction with terfenadine, interactions studies have been performed. One study at a 200 mg daily dose of Diflucan failed to demonstrate a prolongation in QTc interval. Another study at a 400 mg and 800 mg daily dose of Diflucan demonstrated that Diflucan taken in multiple doses of 400 mg per day or greater significantly increased plasma levels of terfenadine when taken concomitantly. There have been spontaneously reported cases of palpitations, tachycardia, dizziness, and chest pain in patients taking concomitant Diflucan and terfenadine where the relationship of the reported adverse events to drug therapy or underlying medical conditions was not clear. Because of the potential seriousness of such an interaction, it is recommended that terfenadine not be taken in combination with Diflucan. (See *Contra-indications*).

Cisapride: There have been reports of cardiac events including torsades de pointes in patients to whom Diflucan and cisapride were coadministered. In most of these cases, the patients appear to have been predisposed to arrhythmias or had serious underlying illnesses, and the relationship of the reported events to a possible Diflucan-cisapride drug interaction is unclear. There have been no formal drug interaction studies with Diflucan and cisapride. Because of the potential seriousness of such an interaction, it is recommended that cisapride not be taken in combination with Diflucan. (See *Contra-indications*).

Zidovudine: Two kinetic studies resulted in increased levels of zidovudine most likely caused by the decreased conversion of zidovudine to its major metabolite. One study determined zidovudine levels in AIDS or ARC patients before and following Diflucan 200 mg daily for 15 days. There was a significant increase in zidovudine AUC (20%). A second randomised, two-period, two-treatment cross-over study examined zidovudine levels in HIV infected patients. On two occasions, 21 days apart, patients received zidovudine 200 mg every eight hours either with or without Diflucan 400 mg daily for seven days. The AUC of zidovudine significantly increased (74%) during coadministration with Diflucan. Patients receiving this combination should be monitored for the development of zidovudine-related adverse reactions.

Rifabutin: There have been reports that an interaction exists when Diflucan is administered concomitantly with rifabutin, leading to increased serum levels of rifabutin. There have been reports of uveitis in patients to whom Diflucan and rifabutin were coadministered. Patients receiving rifabutin and Diflucan concomitantly should be carefully monitored.

Tacrolimus: There have been reports that an interaction exists when Diflucan is administered concomitantly with tacrolimus, leading to increased serum levels of tacrolimus. There have been reports of nephrotoxicity in patients to whom Diflucan and tacrolimus were coadministered. Patients receiving tacrolimus and Diflucan concomitantly should be carefully monitored.

The use of Diflucan in patients concurrently taking astemizole, rifabutin, tacrolimus, or other drugs metabolised by the cytochrome P450 system may be associated with elevations in serum levels of these drugs. In the absence of definitive information, caution should be used when coadministering Diflucan. Patients should be carefully monitored.

Interaction studies have shown that when oral Diflucan is co-administered with food, cimetidine, antacids or following total body irradiation for bone marrow transplantation, no clinically significant impairment of fluconazole absorption occurs.

Physicians should be aware that drug-drug interaction studies with other medications have not been conducted, but that such interactions may occur.

Pregnancy and lactation: Use during pregnancy:
There has been little use during human pregnancy. Accordingly, Diflucan 150 should not be used in pregnancy, or in women of childbearing potential unless adequate contraception is employed.

Use during lactation:
Fluconazole is found in human breast milk at concentrations similar to plasma, hence its use in nursing mothers is not recommended.

Effects on ability to drive and use machines: Experience with Diflucan indicates that therapy is unlikely to impair a patient's ability to drive or use machinery.

Undesirable effects: Diflucan 150 is generally well tolerated. The commonest side effects associated with Diflucan are symptoms related to the gastrointestinal tract. These include nausea, abdominal discomfort, diarrhoea and flatulence. Other adverse events such as rash are rarely encountered (incidences less than 1%). Headache has been associated with Diflucan.

Exfoliative skin disorders (see *Special warnings and special precautions for use*), seizures, leukopenia, thrombocytopenia and alopecia have occurred under conditions where a causal association is uncertain.

In rare cases, as with other azoles, anaphylaxis has been reported.

Overdose: There has been a reported case of overdosage with Diflucan. A 42 year-old patient infected with human immunodeficiency virus developed hallucinations and exhibited paranoid behaviour after reportedly ingesting 8200 mg of Diflucan, unverified by his physician. The patient was admitted to the hospital and his condition resolved within 48 hours.

In the event of overdosage, supportive measures and symptomatic treatment, with gastric lavage if necessary, may be adequate.

As fluconazole is largely excreted in the urine, forced volume diuresis would probably increase the elimination rate. A three hour haemodialysis session decreases plasma levels by approximately 50%.

Pharmacological properties
Pharmacodynamic properties: Fluconazole, a member of the triazole class of antifungal agents, is a potent and selective inhibitor of fungal enzymes necessary for the synthesis of ergosterol.

Fluconazole shows little pharmacological activity in a wide range of animal studies. Some prolongation of pentobarbitone sleeping times in mice (p.o.), increased mean arterial and left ventricular blood pressure and increased heart rate in anaesthetised cats (i.v.) occurred. Inhibition of rat ovarian aromatase was observed at high concentrations.

Pharmacokinetic properties: Fluconazole has high systemic oral bioavailability (greater than 90%) and absorption is unaffected by food. Peak plasma concentrations in the fasting state occur at 0.5-1.5 hours post dose with a plasma elimination half-life of approximately 30 hours. 90% steady state levels occur by day 4-5 after multiple once daily dosing. Plasma concentrations are proportional to dose and apparent volume of distribution approximates to total body water. Plasma protein binding is low (12%).

The major route of excretion is renal with approximately 80% of drug appearing unchanged in urine. Fluconazole clearance is proportional to creatinine clearance. There is no evidence of circulating metabolites.

The long plasma elimination half-life provides the basis for single dose therapy for genital candidiasis.

Preclinical safety data: Reproductive Toxicity:
Increases in foetal anatomical variants (supernumerary ribs, renal pelvis dilation) and delays in ossification were observed at 25 and 50 mg/kg and higher doses. At doses ranging from 80 mg/kg to 320 mg/kg embryolethality in rats was increased and foetal abnormalities included wavy ribs, cleft palate and abnormal cranio-facial ossification.

Carcinogenesis: Fluconazole showed no evidence of carcinogenic potential in mice and rats treated orally for 24 months at doses of 2.5, 5 or 10 mg/kg/day. Male rats treated with 5 and 10 mg/ kg/day had an increased incidence of hepatocellular adenomas.

Mutagenesis: Fluconazole, with or without metabolic activation, was negative in tests for mutagenicity in 4 strains of *S. typhimurium* and in the mouse lymphoma L5178Y system. Cytogenetic studies *in vivo* (murine bone marrow cells, following oral administration of fluconazole) and *in vitro* (human lymphocytes exposed to fluconazole at 1000 μg/ml) showed no evidence of chromosomal mutations.

Impairment of fertility: Fluconazole did not affect the fertility of male or female rats treated orally with daily doses of 5, 10 or 20 mg/kg or with parenteral doses of 5, 25 or 75 mg/kg, although the onset of parturition was slightly delayed at 20 mg/kg p.o. In an intravenous perinatal study in rats at 5, 20 and 40 mg/kg, dystocia and prolongation of parturition were observed in a few dams at 20 mg/kg and 40 mg/kg, but not at 5 mg/kg. The disturbances in parturition were reflected by a slight increase in the number of still-born pups and decrease of neonatal survival at these dose levels. The effects on parturition in rats are consistent with the species specific oestrogen-lowering property produced by high doses of fluconazole. Such a hormone change has not been observed in women treated with Diflucan.

Pharmaceutical particulars

List of excipients: Diflucan 150 capsules contain lactose, maize starch, colloidal silicon dioxide, magnesium stearate and sodium lauryl sulphate as excipients.

In addition, capsule shells contain: patent blue V (E131), titanium dioxide (E171) and gelatin.

Incompatibilities: No specific incompatibilities have been noted.

Shelf life: Current stability data support a shelf life of 5 years.

Special precautions for storage: Store below 30°C.

Nature and contents of container: Diflucan 150 capsules will be supplied as a pack containing one capsule in clear or opaque PVC blister packs with aluminium foil backing.

Instruction for use/handling: Diflucan 150 capsules should be swallowed whole.

Marketing authorisation number PL 00057/0290

Date of first authorisation/renewal of authorisation 24 August 1994

Date of (partial) revision of the text 15 May 1998

Legal category POM

DIFLUCAN CAPSULES 50 MG AND 200 MG
DIFLUCAN POWDER FOR ORAL SUSPENSION 50 MG/5 ML AND 200 MG/5 ML
DIFLUCAN INTRAVENOUS INFUSION 2 MG/ML

Qualitative and quantitative composition Diflucan contains as its active ingredient fluconazole 50 mg and 200 mg as capsules, 50 mg or 200 mg per 5 ml as powder for oral suspension on reconstitution with water, and as 2 mg/ml in a saline solution for intravenous infusion.

Pharmaceutical form Diflucan 50 mg capsules are light turquoise blue and white, coded 'FLU 50' and 'PFIZER'.

Diflucan 200 mg capsules are purple and white, coded 'FLU 200' and 'PFIZER'.

Diflucan Powder for Oral Suspension is a dry white to off-white powder which yields, on reconstitution with water (24 ml), an orange flavoured suspension containing the equivalent of 50 mg or 200 mg fluconazole per 5 ml.

Diflucan Intravenous Infusion 2 mg/ml is available in a 0.9% aqueous sodium chloride solution presented in glass infusion vials (25 or 100 ml).

Clinical particulars

Therapeutic indications: Therapy may be instituted before the results of the cultures and other laboratory studies are known; however, once these results become available, anti-infective therapy should be adjusted accordingly.

Diflucan is indicated for the treatment of the following conditions:

1. Genital candidiasis. Vaginal candidiasis, acute or recurrent. Candidal balanitis. The treatment of partners who present with symptomatic genital candidiasis should be considered.
2. Mucosal candidiasis. These include oropharyngeal, oesophageal, non-invasive bronchopulmonary infections, candiduria, mucocutaneous and chronic oral atrophic candidiasis (denture sore mouth). Normal hosts and patients with compromised immune function may be treated.
3. Tinea pedis, tinea corporis, tinea cruris, tinea versicolor and dermal *Candida* infections. Diflucan is not indicated for nail infections.
4. Systemic candidiasis including candidaemia, disseminated candidiasis and other forms of invasive candidal infection. These include infections of the peritoneum, endocardium and pulmonary and urinary tracts. Candidal infections in patients with malignancy, in intensive care units or those receiving cytotoxic or immunosuppressive therapy, may be treated.
5. Cryptococcosis, including cryptococcal meningitis and infections of other sites (e.g. pulmonary, cutaneous). Normal hosts and patients with acquired immune deficiency syndrome (AIDS), organ transplants or other causes of immunosuppression may be treated. Diflucan can be used as maintenance therapy to prevent relapse of cryptococcal disease in patients with AIDS.
6. For the prevention of fungal infections in immunocompromised patients considered at risk as a consequence of neutropenia following cytotoxic chemotherapy or radiotherapy, including bone marrow transplant patients.

Posology and method of administration: Diflucan may be administered either orally, or by intravenous infusion at a rate of approximately 5-10 ml/min, the route being dependent on the clinical state of the patient. On transferring from the intravenous route to the oral route or vice versa, there is no need to change the daily dose. Diflucan intravenous infusion is formulated in 0.9% sodium chloride solution, each 200 mg (100 ml bottle) containing 15 mmol each of Na^+ and Cl^-.

The daily dose of Diflucan should be based on the nature and severity of the fungal infection. Most cases of vaginal candidiasis respond to single dose therapy. Therapy for those types of infections requiring multiple dose treatment should be continued until clinical parameters or laboratory tests indicate that active fungal infection has subsided. An inadequate period of treatment may lead to recurrence of active infection. Patients with AIDS and cryptococcal meningitis usually require maintenance therapy to prevent relapse.

Adults:

1. Candidal vaginitis or balanitis: 150 mg single oral dose.
2. Mucosal Candidiasis

   Oropharyngeal candidiasis: the usual dose is 50 mg once daily for 7 to 14 days. Treatment should not normally exceed 14 days except in severely immunocompromised patients.

   Atrophic oral candidiasis associated with dentures: the usual dose is 50 mg once daily for 14 days administered concurrently with local antiseptic measures to the denture.

   For other candidal infections of the mucosa, (except genital candidiasis see above), e.g. oesophagitis, non-invasive bronchopulmonary infections, candiduria, mucocutaneous candidiasis etc.: the usual effective dose is 50 mg daily, given for 14 to 30 days.

   In unusually difficult cases of mucosal candidal infections the dose may be increased to 100 mg daily.
3. For tinea pedis, corporis, cruris, versicolor and dermal *Candida* infections the recommended dosage is 50 mg once daily. Duration of treatment is normally 2 to 4 weeks but tinea pedis may require treatment for up to 6 weeks. Duration of treatment should not exceed 6 weeks.
4. For candidaemia, disseminated candidiasis and other invasive candidal infections: the usual dose is 400 mg on the first day followed by 200 mg daily. Depending on the clinical response the dose may be increased to 400 mg daily. Duration of treatment is based upon the clinical response.

5a. For cryptococcal meningitis and cryptococcal infections at other sites: the usual dose is 400 mg on the first day followed by 200 mg–400 mg once daily. Duration of treatment for cryptococcal infections will depend on the clinical and mycological response, but is usually at least 6 to 8 weeks for cryptococcal meningitis.

5b. For the prevention of relapse of cryptococcal meningitis in patients with AIDS, after the patient receives a full course of primary therapy, Diflucan may be administered indefinitely at a daily dose of 100–200 mg.

6. For the prevention of fungal infections in immunocompromised patients considered at risk as a consequence of neutropenia following cytotoxic chemotherapy or radiotherapy, the dose should be 50–400 mg once daily, based on the patient's risk for developing fungal infection. For patients at high risk of systemic infection, e.g. patients who are anticipated to have profound or prolonged neutropenia such as during bone marrow transplantation, the recommended dose is 400 mg once daily. Diflucan administration should start several days before the anticipated onset of neutropenia and continue for seven days after the neutrophil count rises above 1000 cells per mm³.

Use in children: As with similar infections in adults, the duration of treatment is based on the clinical and mycological response. Diflucan is administered as a single dose each day.

Children over four weeks of age: The recommended dose of Diflucan for mucosal candidiasis is 3 mg/kg daily. A loading dose of 6 mg/kg may be used on the first day to achieve steady state levels more rapidly.

For the treatment of systemic candidiasis and cryptococcal infection, the recommended dosage is 6–12 mg/kg daily, depending on the severity of disease.

For the prevention of fungal infections in immunocompromised patients considered at risk as a consequence of neutropenia following cytotoxic chemotherapy or radiotherapy, the dose should be 3-12 mg/kg daily depending on the extent and duration of the induced neutropenia (see adult dosing).

A maximum dosage of 400 mg daily should not be exceeded in children.

Children below four weeks of age: Neonates excrete fluconazole slowly. In the first two weeks of life the same mg/kg dosing as in older children should be used but administered every 72 hours. During weeks 2–4 of life the same dose should be given every 48 hours.

A maximum dosage of 12 mg/kg every 72 hours should not be exceeded in children below two weeks of life. For children between 2–4 weeks of life 12 mg/kg every 48 hours should not be exceeded.

For children with impaired renal function the daily dose should be reduced in accordance with the guidelines given for adults.

To facilitate accurate measurement of doses less than 10 mg, Diflucan should only be administered to children in hospital using the 50 mg/5 ml suspension orally or the intravenous infusion, depending on the clinical condition of the child. A suitable measuring device should be used for administration of the suspension. Once reconstituted, the suspension should not be further diluted.

Use in the elderly: The normal dose should be used if there is no evidence of renal impairment. In patients with renal impairment (creatinine clearance less than 50 ml/min) the dosage schedule should be adjusted as described below.

Use in renal impairment: Fluconazole is excreted predominantly in the urine as unchanged drug. No adjustments in single dose therapy are required. In patients with impaired renal function who will receive multiple doses of Diflucan, the normal recommended dose (according to indication) should be given on day 1, followed by a daily dose based on the following table:

Creatinine clearance (ml/min)	*Percent of recommended dose*
>50	100%
11–50	50%
Patients receiving regular dialysis	One dose after every dialysis session

Compatibility of intravenous infusion: Although further dilution is unnecessary Diflucan Intravenous Infusion is compatible with the following administration fluids:

a) Dextrose 20%
b) Ringer's solution
c) Hartmann's solution
d) Potassium chloride in dextrose
e) Sodium bicarbonate 4.2%
f) Normal saline (0.9%)

Diflucan may be infused through an existing line with one of the above listed fluids. No specific incompatibilities have been noted, although mixing with any other drug prior to infusion is not recommended.

Contra-indications: Diflucan should not be used in patients with known hypersensitivity to fluconazole or to related azole compounds.

Co-administration of terfenadine or cisapride is contra-indicated in patients receiving Diflucan. (See *Interactions of other medicaments and other forms of interactions.*)

Special warnings and precautions for use: In some patients, particularly those with serious underlying diseases such as AIDS and cancer, abnormalities in haematological, hepatic, renal, and other biochemical function tests have been observed during treatment with Diflucan but the clinical significance and relationship to treatment is uncertain.

Very rarely, patients who died with severe underlying disease and who had received multiple dose Diflucan, had post-mortem findings which included hepatic necrosis. These patients were receiving multiple concomitant medications, some known to be potentially hepatotoxic, and/or had underlying diseases which could have caused the hepatic necrosis. Consequently, because a causal relationship with Diflucan cannot be excluded, the risk-benefit ratio of continued Diflucan treatment should be assessed in those patients in whom a significant rise of liver enzymes occurs.

Patients have rarely developed exfoliative cutaneous reactions, such as Stevens-Johnson Syndrome and toxic epidermal necrolysis, during treatment with fluconazole. AIDS patients are more prone to the development of severe cutaneous reactions to many drugs.

If a rash develops in a patient treated for a superficial fungal infection which is considered attributable to Diflucan, further therapy with this agent should be discontinued. If patients with invasive/systemic fungal infections develop rashes, they should be monitored closely and Diflucan discontinued if bullous lesions or erythema multiforme develop.

In rare cases, as with other azoles, anaphylaxis has been reported

Interactions with other medicaments and other forms of interaction: The following drug interactions relate to the use of multiple-dose Diflucan, and the relevance to single-dose Diflucan 150 mg has not yet been established:

Anticoagulants: In an interaction study, Diflucan increased the prothrombin time after warfarin administration in healthy males. Though the magnitude of change was small (12%), careful monitoring of prothrombin time in patients receiving coumarin-type anticoagulants is recommended.

Sulphonylureas: Diflucan has been shown to prolong the serum half-life of concomitantly administered oral sulphonylureas (chlorpropamide, glibenclamide, glipizide and tolbutamide) in healthy volunteers. Diflucan and oral sulphonylureas may be co-administered to diabetic patients, but the possibility of a hypoglycaemic episode should be borne in mind.

Hydrochlorothiazide: In a kinetic interaction study, co-administration of multiple-dose hydrochlorothiazide to healthy volunteers receiving Diflucan increased plasma concentrations of fluconazole by 40%. An effect of this magnitude should not necessitate a change in the Diflucan dose regimen in subjects receiving concomitant diuretics, although the prescriber should bear it in mind.

Phenytoin: Concomitant administration of Diflucan and phenytoin may increase the levels of phenytoin to a clinically significant degree. If it is necessary to administer both drugs concomitantly, phenytoin levels should be monitored and the phenytoin dose adjusted to maintain therapeutic levels.

Oral contraceptives: Two kinetic studies with combined oral contraceptives have been performed using multiple doses of Diflucan. There were no relevant effects on either hormone level in the 50 mg Diflucan study, while at 200 mg daily the AUCs of ethinyloestradiol and levonorgestrel were increased 40% and 24% respectively. Thus multiple dose use of Diflucan at these doses is unlikely to have an effect on the efficacy of the combined oral contraceptive.

Rifampicin: Concomitant administration of Diflucan and rifampicin resulted in a 25% decrease in the AUC and 20% shorter half-life of fluconazole. In patients receiving concomitant rifampicin, an increase in the Diflucan dose should be considered.

Endogenous steroid: Diflucan 50 mg daily does not affect endogenous steroid levels in females. 200-400 mg daily has no clinically significant effect on endogenous steroid levels or on ACTH stimulated response in healthy male volunteers.

Cyclosporin: A kinetic study in renal transplant patients found Diflucan 200 mg daily to slowly increase cyclosporin concentrations. However, in another multiple dose study with 100 mg daily, Diflucan did not affect cyclosporin levels in patients with bone marrow transplants. Cyclosporin plasma concentration monitoring in patients receiving Diflucan is recommended.

Theophylline: In a placebo-controlled interaction study, the administration of Diflucan 200 mg for 14 days resulted in an 18% decrease in the mean plasma clearance of theophylline. Patients who are receiving high doses of theophylline or who are otherwise at increased risk for theophylline toxicity should be observed for signs of theophylline toxicity while receiving Diflucan, and the therapy modified appropriately if signs of toxicity develop.

Terfenadine: Because of the occurrence of serious dysrhythmias secondary to prolongation of the QTc interval in patients receiving other azole antifungals in conjunction with terfenadine, interactions studies have been performed. One study at a 200 mg daily dose of Diflucan failed to demonstrate a prolongation in QTc interval. Another study at a 400 mg and 800 mg daily dose of Diflucan demonstrated that Diflucan taken in multiple doses of 400 mg per day or greater significantly increased plasma levels of terfenadine when taken concomitantly. There have been spontaneously reported cases of palpitations, tachycardia, dizziness, and chest pain in patients taking concomitant Diflucan and terfenadine where the relationship of the reported adverse events to drug therapy or underlying medical conditions was not clear. Because of the potential seriousness of such an interaction, it is recommended that terfenadine not be taken in combination with Diflucan. (See *Contra-indications*.)

Cisapride: There have been reports of cardiac events including torsades de pointes in patients to whom Diflucan and cisapride were co-administered. In most of these cases, the patients appear to have been predisposed to arrhythmias or had serious underlying illnesses, and the relationship of the reported events to a possible Diflucan-cisapride drug interaction is unclear. There have been no formal drug interaction studies with Diflucan and cisapride. Because of the potential seriousness of such an interaction, it is recommended that cisapride not be taken in combination with Diflucan. (See *Contra-indications*.)

Zidovudine: Two kinetic studies resulted in increased levels of zidovudine most likely caused by the decreased conversion of zidovudine to its major metabolite. One study determined zidovudine levels in AIDS or ARC patients before and following Diflucan 200 mg daily for 15 days. There was a significant increase in zidovudine AUC (20%). A second randomised, two-period, two-treatment cross-over study examined zidovudine levels in HIV infected patients. On two occasions, 21 days apart, patients received zidovudine 200 mg every eight hours either with or without Diflucan 400 mg daily for seven days. The AUC of zidovudine significantly increased (74%) during co-administration with Diflucan. Patients receiving this combination should be monitored for the development of zidovudine-related adverse reactions.

Rifabutin: There have been reports that an interaction exists when Diflucan is administered concomitantly with rifabutin, leading to increased serum levels of rifabutin. There have been reports of uveitis in patients to whom Diflucan and rifabutin were co-administered. Patients receiving rifabutin and Diflucan concomitantly should be carefully monitored.

Tacrolimus: There have been reports that an interaction exists when Diflucan is administered concomitantly with tacrolimus, leading to increased serum levels of tacrolimus. There have been reports of nephrotoxicity in patients to whom Diflucan and tacrolimus were co-administered. Patients receiving tacrolimus and Diflucan concomitantly should be carefully monitored.

The use of Diflucan in patients concurrently taking astemizole, rifabutin, tacrolimus, or other drugs metabolised by the cytochrome P450 system may be associated with elevations in serum levels of these drugs. In the absence of definitive information, caution should be used when co-administering Diflucan. Patients should be carefully monitored.

Interaction studies have shown that when oral Diflucan is co-administered with food, cimetidine, antacids or following total body irradiation for bone marrow transplantation, no clinically significant impairment of fluconazole absorption occurs.

Physicians should be aware that drug-drug interaction studies with other medications have not been conducted, but that such interactions may occur.

Pregnancy and lactation:
Use in pregnancy: There has been little use during human pregnancy. Accordingly, Diflucan should not be used in pregnancy, or in women of child-bearing potential unless adequate contraception is employed.

Use during lactation: Fluconazole is found in human breast milk at concentrations similar to plasma, hence its use in nursing mothers is not recommended.

Effects on ability to drive and use machines: Experience with Diflucan indicates that therapy is unlikely to impair a patient's ability to drive or use machinery.

Undesirable effects: Diflucan is generally well tolerated. The commonest side-effects associated with Diflucan are symptoms associated with the gastrointestinal tract. These include nausea, abdominal discomfort, diarrhoea and flatulence. Other adverse events such as rash are rarely encountered (incidences less than 1%). Headache has been associated with Diflucan.

Exfoliative skin disorders (see *Warnings and special precautions for use*), seizures, leukopenia, thrombocytopenia and alopecia have occurred under conditions where a causal association is uncertain.

In rare cases, as with other azoles, anaphylaxis has been reported.

Overdose: There has been a reported case of overdosage with Diflucan. A 42 year-old patient infected with human immunodeficiency virus developed hallucinations and exhibited paranoid behaviour after reportedly ingesting 8200 mg of Diflucan, unverified by his physician. The patient was admitted to the hospital and his condition resolved within 48 hours.

In the event of overdosage, supportive measures and symptomatic treatment, with gastric lavage if necessary, may be adequate.

As fluconazole is largely excreted in the urine, forced volume diuresis would probably increase the elimination rate. A three hour haemodialysis session decreases plasma levels by approximately 50%.

Pharmacological properties
Pharmacodynamic properties: Fluconazole, a member of the triazole class of antifungal agents, is a potent and selective inhibitor of fungal enzymes necessary for the synthesis of ergosterol.

Fluconazole shows little pharmacological activity in a wide range of animal studies. Some prolongation of pentobarbitone sleeping times in mice (p.o.), increased mean arterial and left ventricular blood pressure and increased heart rate in anaesthetised cats (i.v.) occurred. Inhibition of rat ovarian aromatase was observed at high concentrations.

Pharmacokinetic properties: Fluconazole has high systemic oral bioavailability (greater than 90%) and absorption is unaffected by food. Peak plasma concentrations in the fasting state occur at 0.5–1.5 hours post dose with a plasma elimination half-life of approximately 30 hours. 90% steady state levels occur by day 4–5 after multiple once daily dosing. Plasma concentrations are proportional to dose and apparent volume of distribution approximates to total body water. Plasma protein binding is low (12%).

The major route of excretion is renal with approximately 80% of drug appearing unchanged in urine. Fluconazole clearance is proportional to creatinine clearance. There is no evidence of circulating metabolites.

The long plasma elimination half-life provides the basis for single dose therapy for genital candidiasis and once daily dosing for other indications.

Preclinical safety data: Reproductive Toxicity:
Increases in foetal anatomical variants (supernumerary ribs, renal pelvis dilation) and delays in ossification were observed at 25 and 50 mg/kg and higher doses. At doses ranging from 80 mg/kg to 320 mg/kg embryolethality in rats was increased and foetal abnormalities included wavy ribs, cleft palate and abnormal cranio-facial ossification.

Carcinogenesis: Fluconazole showed no evidence of carcinogenic potential in mice and rats treated orally for 24 months at doses of 2.5, 5 or 10 mg/kg/day. Male rats treated with 5 and 10 mg/kg/day had an increased incidence of hepatocellular adenomas.

Mutagenesis: Fluconazole, with or without metabolic activation, was negative in tests for mutagenicity in 4 strains of *S. typhimurium* and in the mouse lymphoma L5178Y system. Cytogenetic studies *in vivo* (murine bone marrow cells, following oral administration of fluconazole) and *in vitro* (human lymphocytes exposed to fluconazole at 1000 µg/ml) showed no evidence of chromosomal mutations.

Impairment of fertility: Fluconazole did not affect the fertility of male or female rats treated orally with daily doses of 5, 10 or 20 mg/kg or with parenteral doses of 5, 25 or 75 mg/kg, although the onset of parturition was slightly delayed at 20 mg/kg p.o. In an intravenous perinatal study in rats at 5, 20 and 40 mg/kg, dystocia and prolongation of parturition were observed in a few dams at 20 mg/kg and 40 mg/kg, but not at 5 mg/kg. The disturbances in parturition were reflected by a slight increase in the number of still-born pups and decrease of neonatal survival at these dose levels. The effects on parturition in rats are consistent with the species specific oestrogen-lowering property produced by high doses of fluconazole. Such a hormone change has not been observed in women treated with Diflucan.

Pharmaceutical particulars
List of excipients:
Diflucan Capsules (all strengths) contain lactose, maize starch, colloidal silicon dioxide, magnesium stearate and sodium lauryl sulphate as excipients.

In addition, capsule shells contain:

50 mg–patent blue V (E131), titanium dioxide (E171) and gelatin.

200 mg–titanium dioxide (E171), erythrosine (E127), indigotine (E132) and gelatin.

Diflucan Intravenous Infusion: is a sterile aqueous solution which is made iso-osmotic with sodium chloride.

Diflucan Powder for Oral Suspension: contains sucrose (2.88 g per 50 mg dose; 2.73 g per 200 mg dose), colloidal silicon dioxide, titanium dioxide, xanthan gum, sodium citrate dihydrate, citric acid anhydrous, sodium benzoate and natural orange flavour.

Incompatibilities: No specific incompatibilities have been noted.

Shelf life: Current stability data support a shelf life of 5 years for the capsules, 5 years for the intravenous infusion and 2 years for the dry powder for oral suspension. There is a use period of 14 days for the reconstituted suspension.

Special precautions for storage: Store below 30°C.

Reconstituted suspension should be stored at 5°C–30°C.

Do not freeze reconstituted suspension or intravenous infusion.

Nature and contents of container:
Diflucan Capsules: will be supplied in clear or opaque PVC blister packs with aluminium foil backing, as follows:

7×50 mg or 200 mg Diflucan capsules for multiple dose therapy.

Diflucan Intravenous Infusion: will be supplied in clear Type I glass infusion vials (25 or 100 ml) sealed with rubber bungs on crimping with aluminium overcaps.

Diflucan Powder for Oral Suspension: will be supplied in high density polyethylene bottles with child resistant closures, containing 35 ml of suspension

(50 mg/5 ml or 200 mg/5 ml) on reconstitution with 24 ml of water.

Instruction for use/handling: Diflucan Capsules should be swallowed whole.

Diflucan Intravenous Infusion: do not freeze. The infusion does not contain any preservative. It is for single use only. Discard any remaining solution.

To reconstitute the Diflucan Powder for Oral Suspension: Tap the bottle to loosen powder. Add 24 ml of water. Shake well. Shake immediately prior to use. Where doses of less than 5 ml are required, a suitable measuring device should be used. Dilution is not appropriate.

Marketing authorisation numbers

Diflucan Capsules 50 mg	PL 00057/0289
Diflucan Capsules 200 mg	PL 00057/0317
Diflucan Intravenous Infusion 2 mg/ml	PL 00057/0315
Diflucan Powder for Oral Suspension 50 mg/5 ml	PL 00057/0343
Diflucan Powder for Oral Suspension 200 mg/5 ml	PL 00057/0344

Date of first authorisation/renewal of authorisation

Diflucan Capsules 50 mg	24 August 1994
Diflucan Capsules 200 mg	30 May 1996
Diflucan IV Infusion	24 November 1994
Diflucan POS	18 December 1996

Date of (partial) revision of the text December 1997.

Legal category POM

FASIGYN*

Presentation Fasigyn (tinidazole) is available as 500 mg film coated white tablets.

Inactive excipients: alginic acid, hydroxypropylmethyl cellulose, magnesium stearate, maize starch, microcrystalline cellulose, propylene glycol, sodium lauryl sulphate and titanium dioxide.

Uses

Actions: Fasigyn is rapidly and completely absorbed following oral administration. In studies with healthy volunteers receiving 2 g tinidazole orally, peak serum levels of 40–51 micrograms/ml were achieved within two hours and decreased to between 11–19 micrograms/ml at 24 hours. Plasma levels decline slowly and tinidazole can be detected in plasma at concentrations of up to 1 microgram/ml at 72 hours after oral administration. The plasma elimination half-life for tinidazole is between 12–14 hours.

Tinidazole is widely distributed in all body tissues and also crosses the blood brain barrier, obtaining clinically effective concentrations in all tissues. The apparent volume of distribution is about 50 litres. About 12% of plasma tinidazole is bound to plasma protein.

Tinidazole is excreted by the liver and kidneys. Studies in healthy patients have shown that over 5 days, 60–65% of an administered dose is excreted by the kidneys with 20–25% of the administered dose excreted as unchanged tinidazole. Approximately 12% of the administered dose is excreted in the faeces.

Studies in patients with renal failure (creatinine clearance <22 ml/min) indicate that there is no statistically significant change in tinidazole pharmacokinetic parameters in these patients. Thus no adjustments in dosing are required in these patients.

Fasigyn is active against both protozoa and obligate anaerobic bacteria. The activity against protozoa involves *Trichomonas vaginalis, Entamoeba histolytica* and *Giardia lamblia.*

Fasigyn is active against *Gardnerella vaginalis* and most anaerobic bacteria including *Bacteroides fragilis, Bacteroides melaninogenicus,* Bacteroides spp., Clostridium spp., Eubacterium spp., Fusobacterium spp., Peptococcus spp., Peptostreptococcus spp., and Veillonella spp.

The mode of action of Fasigyn against anaerobic bacteria and protozoa involves penetration of the drug into the cell of the micro-organism and subsequent damage of DNA strands or inhibition of their synthesis.

Indications:

1. Prophylaxis: The prevention of post-operative infections caused by anaerobic bacteria, especially those associated with colonic, gastro-intestinal and gynaecological surgery.

2. Treatment of anaerobic infections such as:
Intraperitoneal infections: peritonitis, abscess.
Gynaecological infections: endometritis, endomyometritis, tubo-ovarian abscess.
Bacterial septicaemia.
Post-operative wound infections.
Skin and soft tissue infections.
Upper and lower respiratory tract infections: pneumonia, empyema, lung abscess.

3. Non-specific vaginitis.
4. Acute ulcerative gingivitis.
5. Urogenital trichomoniasis in both male and female patients.
6. Giardiasis.
7. Intestinal amoebiasis.
8. Amoebic involvement of the liver.

Dosage and administration

1. *Prevention of post-operative infections: Adults:* A single oral dose of 2 g approximately 12 hours before surgery.

Children less than 12 years: Data are not available to allow dosage recommendations for children below the age of 12 years in the prophylaxis of post-operative infections.

2. *Treatment of anaerobic infections: Adults:* An initial dose of 2 g the first day followed by 1 g daily given as a single dose or as 500 mg twice daily.

Treatment for 5 to 6 days will generally be adequate but clinical judgement must determine the duration of therapy, particularly when eradication of infection from certain sites may be difficult.

Regular clinical and laboratory observation is advised if it is considered necessary to continue therapy for more than 7 days.

Children less than 12 years: Data are not available to allow dosage recommendations for children below the age of 12 years in the treatment of anaerobic infections.

3. *Non-specific vaginitis: Adults:* Non-specific vaginitis is treated with a single oral dose of 2 g. Higher cure rates have been achieved with 2 g single daily doses for two consecutive days (total dosage 4 g).

4. *Acute ulcerative gingivitis: Adults:* A single oral dose of 2 g.

5. *Urogenital trichomoniasis:* When infection with *Trichomonas vaginalis* is confirmed, simultaneous treatment of the consort is recommended.

Adult preferred regimen: A single dose of 2 g.

Children: A single dose of 50 to 75 mg/kg of body weight. It may be necessary to repeat this dose once in some cases.

6. *Giardiasis: Adults:* A single dose of 2 g.

Children: A single dose of 50 to 75 mg/kg of body weight. It may be necessary to repeat this dose once in some cases.

7. *Intestinal amoebiasis: Adults:* A single daily dose of 2 g for two or three days. Occasionally when a three day single daily dose is ineffective, treatment may be continued up to six days.

Children: A single dose of 50 to 60 mg/kg of body weight per day for three successive days.

8. *Amoebic involvement of the liver: Adults:* Total dosage varies from 4.5 to 12g, depending on the virulence of the *Entamoeba histolytica.*

For amoebic involvement of the liver, the evacuation of pus may be required in addition to therapy with Fasigyn.

Initiate treatment with 1.5 to 2 g as a single oral daily dose for three days. Occasionally when a three-day course is ineffective, treatment may be continued for up to six days.

Children: A single daily dose of 50 to 60 mg/kg of body weight per day for five successive days.

It is recommended that Fasigyn be taken during or after a meal.

Use in the elderly: There are no special recommendations for this age group.

Contra-indications, warnings, etc

Contra-indications: Use of Fasigyn is contra-indicated during the first trimester of pregnancy, in nursing mothers, in patients with organic neurologic disorders and in patients with known hypersensitivity to any of the components of Fasigyn. As with other drugs of similar structure, Fasigyn is also contra-indicated in patients having a history of or with blood dyscrasias, although no persistent haematologic abnormalities have been noted in clinical or animal studies with tinidazole.

Use in pregnancy: Fertility studies in rats receiving 100 mg or 300 mg tinidazole/kg had no effect on fertility, adult and pup weights, gestation, viability or lactation. There was a slight, not significant, increase in resorption rate at the 300 mg/kg dose.

Tinidazole crosses the placental barrier. Since the effects of compounds of this class on foetal development are unknown, the use of tinidazole during the first trimester is contra-indicated. There is no evidence that Fasigyn is harmful during the latter stages of pregnancy, but its use during the second and third trimesters requires that the potential benefits be weighed against possible hazards to mother or foetus.

Use in nursing mothers: Tinidazole is excreted in breast milk. Tinidazole may continue to appear in breast milk for more than 72 hours after administration. Women should not nurse until at least 3 days after having discontinued taking Fasigyn.

Precautions: As with related compounds, alcoholic beverages should be avoided during Fasigyn therapy because of the possibility of a disulfiram-like reaction (flushing, abdominal cramps, vomiting, tachycardia). Alcohol should be avoided until 72 hours after discontinuing Fasigyn.

Driving/use of machinery: No special precautions should be necessary. However, drugs of similar chemical structure, including Fasigyn, have been associated with various neurological disturbances such as dizziness, vertigo, ataxia, peripheral neuropathy (paraesthesia, sensory disturbances, hypoaesthesia) and rarely convulsions. If any abnormal neurological signs develop during Fasigyn therapy, the drug should be discontinued.

Side-effects: Reported side-effects have generally been infrequent, mild and self-limiting. Gastro-intestinal side-effects include nausea, vomiting, anorexia, diarrhoea, metallic taste and abdominal pain.

Hypersensitivity reactions, occasionally severe, may occur in rare cases in the form of skin rash, pruritus, urticaria and angioneurotic oedema.

Neurological disturbances associated with Fasigyn include dizziness, vertigo, ataxia, peripheral neuropathy (paraesthesia, sensory disturbances, hypoaesthesia) and rarely convulsions.

As with related compounds, Fasigyn may produce transient leucopenia. Other rarely reported side-effects are headache, tiredness, furry tongue and dark urine.

Overdosage: In acute animal studies with mice and rats, the LD_{50} for mice was >3600 mg/kg and >2300 mg/kg for oral and intraperitoneal administration, respectively. For rats, the LD_{50} was >2000 mg/kg for both oral and intraperitoneal administration.

There are no reported overdoses in humans with Fasigyn.

There is no specific antidote for treatment of overdosage with tinidazole. Treatment is symptomatic and supportive. Gastric lavage may be useful. Tinidazole is easily dialysable.

Pharmaceutical precautions Store below 25°C in a dry place, away from light.

Legal category POM.

Package quantities 20×500 mg tablets.

Further information Nil.

Product licence number 0057/0150.

FELDENE* CAPSULES
FELDENE* 20 CAPSULES
FELDENE* DISPERSIBLE TABLETS
FELDENE* SUPPOSITORIES
FELDENE* I.M. INTRAMUSCULAR INJECTION
FELDENE MELT*

Presentation Feldene capsules are available in two strengths: 10 mg maroon and blue capsules, coded 'Pfizer' and 'FEL 10' containing 10 mg piroxicam. Feldene 20 capsules are maroon capsules coded 'Pfizer' and 'FEL 20' containing 20 mg piroxicam.

Feldene dispersible tablets are available in two strengths: 10 mg – white to off-white flat round tablets coded 'FEL' and '10' on one side, with an incised line between and 'Pfizer' on the other. 20 mg – white to off-white capsular tablets coded 'FEL 20' on one side and lettered 'PFIZER' on the other.

Feldene Melt tablets: Off-white, round, freeze-dried, fast dissolving tablets containing 20 mg piroxicam.

Feldene suppositories (white to off-white) containing 20 mg piroxicam.

Feldene I.M.: Sterile, pyrogen-free, clear solution in ampoule containing 1 ml of piroxicam solution (20 mg/ml) for intramuscular injection.

Inactive excipients: Feldene capsules (both strengths): lactose, maize starch, magnesium stearate, sodium lauryl sulphate. In addition, capsule shells contain erythrosine, gelatin, indigotine and titanium dioxide.

Feldene dispersible tablets (both strengths); lactose, microcrystalline cellulose, hydroxypropyl cellulose, sodium stearyl fumarate.

Feldene Melt tablets: aspartame, citric acid anhydrous, gelatin, mannitol.

Feldene suppositories: Lunacera M, propyl gallate, suppocire AM.

Feldene IM: benzyl alcohol, ethanol, nicotinamide, propylene glycol and other ingredients.

Uses Feldene is a non-steroidal anti-inflammatory drug indicated for a variety of conditions requiring anti-inflammatory and/or analgesic activity.

Capsules; dispersible tablets; suppositories; Melt tablets: Rheumatoid arthritis, osteoarthritis (arthrosis, degenerative joint disease), ankylosing spondylitis, acute musculoskeletal disorders and acute gout. Pain following orthopaedic, dental and other minor surgery.

Dispersible tablets: Children with definitely diagnosed juvenile chronic arthritis (Still's disease).

Intramuscular injection: Initial treatment of acute conditions (acute gout, acute musculoskeletal disorders) and acute exacerbations of chronic conditions (rheumatoid arthritis, osteoarthritis, ankylosing spondylitis).

Dosage and administration

Adults:

Rheumatoid arthritis, osteoarthritis, ankylosing spondylitis: The recommended starting dose is 20 mg given as a single daily dose. The majority of patients will be maintained on 20 mg daily. A relatively small group of patients may be maintained on 10 mg daily. Some patients may require up to 30 mg daily given in single or divided doses. Administration of doses exceeding 20 mg daily (of more than several days duration) carries an increased risk of gastro-intestinal side-effects.

Acute gout: Therapy should be initiated by a single dose of 40 mg, followed on the next four to six days with 40 mg daily, given in single or divided doses. Feldene is not indicated for the long-term management of gout.

Acute musculoskeletal disorders: Therapy should be initiated with 40 mg daily for the first two days, given in single or divided doses. For the remainder of the seven to fourteen day treatment period, the dose should be reduced to 20 mg daily.

Post-operative pain:

Dental and other minor surgery: The recommended starting and maintenance dose is 20 mg once daily. Doses of 40 mg daily, in single or divided doses, for the first two days of treatment may provide faster onset of action.

Orthopaedic surgery: Therapy should be initiated with 40 mg daily for the first two days, given in single or divided doses. For the remainder of the treatment period, the dose should be reduced to 20 mg daily.

Children:

Juvenile chronic arthritis (Still's disease): As little data are available in very young children, it is recommended that only children aged 6 years and older are treated with Feldene dispersible tablets according to the following dosage schedule:

Body weight (kg)	*Once-daily dose*
less than 15	5 mg
16–25	10 mg
26–45	15 mg
46 and above	20 mg

Dosage recommendations and indications for use in children other than in juvenile chronic arthritis have not been established.

Feldene dispersible tablets: These can be swallowed whole with a fluid, or may be dispersed in a minimum of 50 ml of water and then swallowed.

Feldene Melt tablets: These should be placed on the tongue to disperse and then swallowed with the saliva. Feldene Melt dissolves almost instantly in the mouth in the presence of saliva.

Feldene Suppositories: For each indication (excluding juvenile chronic arthritis), the dosage of Feldene suppositories when used alone, is identical with the dosage of Feldene capsules or dispersible tablets.

Feldene I.M. intramuscular injection: The dosage of Feldene I.M. intramuscular injection is identical to the dosage of oral Feldene. For continuation of treatment oral or suppository dose forms should be used. Feldene I.M. intramuscular injection should be administered by deep intramuscular injection into the upper, outer quadrant of the buttock. Feldene I.M. intramuscular injection should not be administered intravenously.

Combined administration: The total daily dosage of Feldene administered as capsules, dispersible tablets, Melt tablets, suppositories and intramuscular injection should not exceed the maximum recommended daily dosage as indicated above.

Use in the elderly: Elderly, frail or debilitated patients may tolerate side-effects less well and such patients should be carefully supervised.

As with other non-steroidal anti-inflammatory drugs, caution should be used in the treatment of elderly patients who are more likely to be suffering from impaired renal, hepatic or cardiac function.

Contra-indications, warnings, etc

Contra-indications:

1. Active peptic ulceration or a history of recurrent ulceration.

2. Feldene should not be used in those patients who have previously shown a hypersensitivity to the drug. The potential exists for cross sensitivity to aspirin and other non-steroidal anti-inflammatory drugs. Feldene should not be given to patients in whom aspirin and other non-steroidal anti-inflammatory drugs induce the symptoms of asthma, nasal polyps, angioneurotic oedema or urticaria.

3. Feldene suppositories should not be used in patients with any inflammatory lesions of the rectum or anus, or in patients with a recent history of rectal or anal bleeding.

Warnings:

Use in pregnancy: Although no teratogenic effects were seen in animal testing, the use of Feldene during pregnancy is not recommended. Feldene inhibits prostaglandin synthesis and release through a reversible inhibition of the cyclo-oxygenase enzyme. This effect, as with other non-steroidal anti-inflammatory drugs has been associated with an increased incidence of dystocia and delayed parturition in pregnant animals when drug administration was continued into late pregnancy. Non-steroidal anti-inflammatory drugs are also known to induce closure of the ductus arteriosus in infants.

Nursing mothers: A study indicates that piroxicam appears in breast milk at about 1% to 3% of the maternal plasma concentrations. No accumulation of piroxicam occurred in milk relative to that in plasma during treatment for up to 52 days. Feldene is not recommended for use in nursing mothers as clinical safety in neonates has not been established.

Precautions: Drug administration should be closely supervised in patients with a history of upper gastro-intestinal disease. Feldene should be withdrawn if peptic ulceration or gastro-intestinal bleeding occurs.

In rare cases, non-steroidal anti-inflammatory drugs may cause interstitial nephritis, glomerulonephritis, papillary necrosis and the nephrotic syndrome. Such agents inhibit the synthesis of renal prostaglandin which plays a supportive role in the maintenance of renal perfusion in patients whose renal blood flow and blood volume are decreased. In these patients, administration of a non-steroidal anti-inflammatory drug may precipitate overt renal decompensation which is typically followed by recovery to pretreatment state upon discontinuation of non-steroidal anti-inflammatory therapy. Patients at greatest risk of such a reaction are those with congestive heart failure, liver cirrhosis, nephrotic syndrome and overt renal disease. Such patients should be carefully monitored whilst receiving therapy with a non-steroidal anti-inflammatory drug.

Patients with phenylketonuria: Due to aspartame content of Feldene Melt each tablet contains 0.14 mg phenylalanine.

Because of reports of adverse eye findings with non-steroidal anti-inflammatory drugs, it is recommended that patients who develop visual complaints during treatment with Feldene have ophthalmic evaluation.

Drug interactions: Non-steroidal anti-inflammatory drugs may cause sodium, potassium and fluid retention and may interfere with the natriuretic action of diuretic agents. These properties should be kept in mind when treating patients with compromised cardiac function or hypertension since they may be responsible for a worsening of those conditions.

As with other non-steroidal anti-inflammatory drugs, bleeding has been reported rarely when Feldene has been administered to patients on coumarin-type anticoagulants. Patients should be monitored closely if Feldene and oral anticoagulants are administered together.

Feldene, like other non-steroidal anti-inflammatory drugs, decreases platelet aggregation and prolongs bleeding time. This effect should be kept in mind when bleeding times are determined.

As with other non-steroidal anti-inflammatory drugs, the use of Feldene in conjunction with aspirin or the concomitant use of two non-steroidal anti-inflammatory drugs is not recommended because data are inadequate to demonstrate that the combination produces greater improvement than that achieved with the drug alone and the potential for adverse reactions is increased.

Studies in man have shown that the concomitant administration of Feldene and aspirin resulted in a reduction of plasma levels of piroxicam to about 80% of the normal values. Concomitant administration of antacids had no effect on piroxicam plasma levels. Neither did concurrent therapy with Feldene and digoxin, or Feldene and digitoxin, affect the plasma levels of either drug.

Feldene is highly protein-bound and therefore might be expected to displace other protein-bound drugs. The physician should closely monitor patients for change in dosage requirements when administering Feldene to patients on highly protein-bound drugs.

Non-steroidal anti-inflammatory drugs, including Feldene, have been reported to increase steady state plasma lithium levels. It is recommended that these levels are monitored when initiating, adjusting and discontinuing Feldene.

Results of two separate studies indicate a slight but significant increase in absorption of piroxicam following cimetidine administration but no significant changes in elimination rate constants or half-life. The small increase in absorption is unlikely to be clinically significant.

Side-effects: Gastro-intestinal: These are the most commonly encountered side-effects but in most instances do not interfere with the course of therapy. They include stomatitis, anorexia, epigastric distress, nausea, constipation, abdominal discomfort, flatulence, diarrhoea, abdominal pain and indigestion, rare cases of pancreatitis have been reported. Objective evaluations of gastric mucosal appearances and intestinal blood loss show that 20 mg/day of Feldene administered either in single or divided daily doses is significantly less irritating to the gastro-intestinal tract than aspirin. Peptic ulceration, perforation and gastro-intestinal bleeding, in rare cases fatal, have been reported with Feldene.

Some epidemiological studies have suggested that piroxicam is associated with a higher risk of gastro-intestinal adverse reactions compared with some other NSAIDS, but this has not been confirmed in all studies. Administration of doses exceeding 20 mg daily (of more than several days duration) carries an increased risk of gastro-intestinal side-effects, but they may also occur with lower doses. See Dosage and Administration.

Ano-rectal reactions to suppositories have presented as local pain, burning, pruritus and tenesmus. Rare instances of rectal bleeding have occurred.

Oedema: As with other non-steroidal anti-inflammatory drugs, oedema, mainly of the ankle, has been reported in a small percentage of patients and the possibility of precipitating congestive cardiac failure in elderly patients or those with compromised cardiac function should therefore be borne in mind.

CNS: Dizziness, headache, somnolence, insomnia, depression, nervousness, hallucinations, mood alterations, dream abnormalities, mental confusion, paraesthesias and vertigo have been reported rarely.

Dermal hypersensitivity: Rash and pruritus. Onycholysis and alopecia have rarely been reported. Photosensitivity reactions occur infrequently. As with other non-steroidal anti-inflammatory drugs, toxic epidermal necrolysis (Lyell's disease) and Stevens-Johnson syndrome may develop in rare cases. Vesiculo-bullous reactions have been reported rarely.

Hypersensitivity reactions: Hypersensitivity reactions such as anaphylaxis, bronchospasm, urticaria/angioneurotic oedema, vasculitis and serum sickness have been reported rarely.

Renal function: Interstitial nephritis, nephrotic syndrome, renal failure and renal papillary necrosis have been reported rarely. (See Precautions).

Haematological: Decreases in haemoglobin and haematocrit, unassociated with obvious gastro-intestinal bleeding, have occurred. Anaemia, thrombocytopenia, non-thrombocytopenic purpura (Henoch-Schoenlein), leucopenia and eosinophilia have been reported. Cases of aplastic anaemia, haemolytic anaemia and epistaxis have rarely been reported.

Liver function: Changes in various liver function parameters have been observed. As with most other non-steroidal anti-inflammatory drugs, some patients may develop increased serum transaminase levels during treatment with Feldene. Severe hepatic reactions, including jaundice and cases of fatal hepatitis have been reported. Although such reactions are rare, if abnormal liver function tests persist or worsen, if clinical signs and symptoms consistent with liver disease develop, or if systemic manifestations occur (e.g. eosinophilia, rash), Feldene should be discontinued.

Other: The following have been reported rarely: palpitations and dyspnoea, anecdotal cases of positive ANA, anecdotal cases of hearing impairment, metabolic abnormalities such as hypoglycaemia, hyperglycaemia, weight increase or decrease.

Swollen eyes, blurred vision and eye irritations have been reported. Routine ophthalmoscopy and slit-lamp examination have revealed no evidence of ocular changes. Malaise and tinnitus may occur.

Intramuscular: Transient pain upon injection has occasionally been reported. Local adverse reactions (burning sensations) or tissue damage (sterile abscess formation, fatty tissue necrosis) may occasionally occur at the site of injection.

Overdosage: In the event of overdosage with Feldene, supportive and symptomatic therapy is indicated. Studies indicate that administration of activated charcoal may result in reduced absorption and re-absorption of piroxicam thus reducing the total amount of active drug available.

Pharmaceutical precautions

Capsules: Store below 30°C.
Dispersible Tablets: Store below 30°C.
Suppositories: Store below 25°C. Do not refrigerate.
Intramuscular injection: Store below 25°C.
Melt Tablets: Store below 25°C.

Legal category POM.

Package quantities
Feldene Capsules 10 mg: Containers of 56 (Original pack).
Feldene 20 Capsules 20 mg: Containers of 28 (Original pack).
Feldene Dispersible Tablets 10 mg: Containers of 56 (Original pack).
Feldene Dispersible Tablets 20 mg: Containers of 28 (Original pack).
Feldene Suppositories 20 mg: Foil strip of 10 (Original pack).
Feldene I.M. Intramuscular injection 20 mg/ml: Pack of 1×1 ml ampoule.
Feldene Melt Tablets 20 mg: Containers of 28 (Original pack).

Further information Feldene pharmacokinetics are similar following oral or rectal administration. Following oral administration with food there is a slight delay in the rate but not the extent of absorption. The plasma half-life is approximately 50 hours in man and stable plasma concentrations are maintained throughout the day on once-daily dosage. Continuous treatment with 20 mg/day for periods of one year produces similar blood levels to those seen once steady state is first achieved.

Feldene Melt and Feldene capsules are bioequivalent. A multiple dose study of the pharmacokinetics and the bioavailability of Feldene Melt compared to oral capsules for 14 days has shown that after once daily administration the piroxicam concentration time profiles were nearly superimposable. Single dose studies demonstrated bioequivalent with capsules when Feldene Melt is taken with or without water.

Feldene I.M. intramuscular injection and Feldene capsules are bioequivalent. However, Feldene intramuscular injection provides significantly higher plasma levels of piroxicam during the first 45 minutes on the first day and 30 minutes on the second day.

Feldene is extensively metabolised and less than 5% of the daily dose is excreted unchanged in urine and faeces. One important metabolic pathway is hydroxylation of the pyridyl ring of the piroxicam side chain, followed by conjugation with glucuronic acid and urinary elimination.

Product licence numbers

Feldene Capsules 10 mg	0057/0145
Feldene 20 Capsules 20 mg	0057/0146
Feldene Dispersible Tablets 10 mg	0057/0240
Feldene Dispersible Tablets 20 mg	0057/0242
Feldene Suppositories 20 mg	0057/0219
Feldene I.M. Intramuscular injection 20 mg/ml	0057/0320
Feldene Melt Tablets 20 mg	0057/0352

FELDENE* GEL

Presentation Topical Feldene is available as a clear pale yellow gel containing 5 mg piroxicam in each gram. Topical Feldene is available in two tube sizes: 60 g Feldene Gel and 112 g Feldene Gel.

Inactive excipients: These are benzyl alcohol, carbopol 940, di-isopropanolamine, ethyl alcohol, hydroxyethyl cellulose, propylene glycol and water.

Uses Feldene Gel contains piroxicam, a non-steroidal anti-inflammatory agent indicated for a variety of conditions characterised by pain and inflammation, or stiffness.

Feldene Gel is effective in the treatment of osteoarthritis of superficial joints such as the knee, acute musculoskeletal injuries, periarthritis, epicondylitis, tendinitis and tenosynovitis.

Feldene Gel is for topical use only.

Dosage and administration Feldene Gel is for external use only. No occlusive dressings should be employed. Apply 1 g of the Gel, corresponding to 3 cms, (approximately 1¼ inches) and rub into the affected site three to four times daily leaving no residual material on the skin. Therapy should be reviewed after four weeks.

Use in children: Dosage recommendations and indications for the use of Feldene Gel in children have not been established.

Use in the elderly: No special precautions are required.

Contra-indications, warnings, etc
Contra-indications: Feldene Gel should not be used in those patients who have previously shown a hypersensitivity to the Gel or piroxicam in any of its forms. The potential exists for cross sensitivity to aspirin and other non-steroidal anti-inflammatory agents.

Feldene Gel should not be given to patients in whom aspirin and other non-steroidal anti-inflammatory agents induce the symptoms of asthma, nasal polyps, angioneurotic oedema or urticaria.

Precautions: If local irritation develops, the use of the Gel should be discontinued and appropriate therapy instituted as necessary.

Keep away from the eyes and mucosal surfaces. Do not apply to any sites affected by open skin lesions, dermatoses or infection.

Use in Pregnancy: Although no teratogenic effects were seen when Feldene was orally administered in animal testing, the use of Feldene Gel during pregnancy or during lactation is not recommended.

Nursing mothers: Feldene Gel is not recommended for use in nursing mothers as clinical safety has not been established.

Side-effects: Feldene Gel is well tolerated. Mild to moderate local irritation, erythema, pruritus and dermatitis may occur at the application site. The systemic absorption of Feldene Gel is very low. In common with other topical NSAIDs, systemic reactions occur infrequently and have included minor gastro-intestinal side-effects such as nausea and dyspepsia. Cases of abdominal pain and gastritis have been reported rarely. There have been isolated reports of bronchospasm and dyspnoea (see also *Contra-indications*).

Overdosage: Overdosage is unlikely to occur with this topical preparation.

Pharmaceutical precautions None.

Legal category POM.

Package quantities
Feldene Gel: 112 g tube.
Feldene Gel: 60 g tube.

Further information On the basis of various pharmacokinetic and tissue distribution studies in animals, with the Gel, the highest concentrations of piroxicam were achieved in the tissues below the site of application with low concentrations being reached in the plasma. The Gel was continuously and gradually released from the skin to underlying tissues, equilibrium between skin and muscle or synovial fluid appeared to be reached rapidly, within a few hours of application.

From a pharmacokinetic study in man, 2 g of the Gel was applied to the shoulders of normal volunteers twice daily (corresponding to 20 mg piroxicam/day) for 14 days, plasma levels of piroxicam rose slowly, reaching steady state after about 11 days. The plasma levels at this time were between 300–400 ng/ml, or one-twentieth of those observed in subjects receiving 20 mg orally.

The Gel was well tolerated in volunteers with a history of contact allergy.

Product licence number
Feldene Gel (60 g and 112 g) 0057/0284

GASTROMAX*

Qualitative and quantitative composition Active ingredient: Metoclopramide Hydrochloride PhEur 30 mg.

Pharmaceutical form Opaque orange/yellow capsules for oral administration. Controlled release formulation.

Clinical particulars
Therapeutic indications: For the relief of upper gastro-intestinal symptoms in patients aged over 20 years, including heartburn, dyspepsia and flatulence associated with such conditions as peptic ulcer, reflux oesophagitis, gastric reflux, gastritis, duodenitis and hiatus hernia.

For the relief of nausea and vomiting due to gastro-intestinal disorders. Also for use as an anti-emetic for nausea and vomiting associated with cytotoxic drugs.

Posology and method of administration:
Adults over 20 years of age: Gastromax should be swallowed whole with liquid, preferably before a meal. Dosage is one capsule, once daily, either morning or evening dependent upon timing of symptoms.

For example, in cases of nocturnal reflux and heartburn, the capsule should be taken in the evening. If symptoms are mainly associated with daytime activity e.g. after meals, bending, stooping, etc., the capsule should be taken in the morning.

One capsule (30 mg) is the maximum recommended dose and should not be exceeded.

Children and young adults under 20 years of age: Not recommended.

Elderly: The usual adult dose is recommended. Since tardive dyskinesia is more likely to occur in the elderly, especially during long term therapy, treatment should be regularly reviewed.

Use in hepatic or renal impairment: In patients with clinically significant hepatic or renal impairment, the clearance of Gastromax may be impaired. Such patients should be observed carefully, and treatment discontinued if side-effects occur.

Contra-indications: Gastromax is contra-indicated in patients under 20 years of age, in nursing mothers and during the first trimester of pregnancy (see *Pregnancy and lactation*).

Gastromax is contra-indicated in patients with phaeochromocytoma.

Gastromax is also contra-indicated in patients who have shown hypersensitivity to metoclopramide or any component of the product.

Special warnings and special precautions for use: If vomiting persists, the patient should be assessed to exclude the possibility of underlying disease.

Patients with hepatic or renal insufficiency should be observed carefully. Treatment should be discontinued if side-effects occur.

Cases of neuroleptic malignant syndrome, an idiosyncratic response characterised by hyperthermia, muscle rigidity, altered consciousness including coma and elevated CPK have been reported with metoclopramide. Tardive dyskinesia may occur principally in the elderly, after prolonged treatment. The dose in the elderly should be strictly adhered to and treatment should be regularly reviewed.

Gastromax should not be administered to patients undergoing gastrointestinal surgery, e.g. gut anastomosis, until a sufficient period for healing has elapsed.

Metoclopramide has been classified as porphyrinogenic and is potentially unsafe in patients with acute porphyria.

Interaction with other medicaments and other forms of interaction: The absorption of any orally co-administered medication may be affected by the effects of Gastromax on gastro-intestinal motility. Drugs known to be affected in this way include: asprin, paracetamol, digoxin and alcohol.

The effects of Gatromax on the gastro-intestinal tract are antagonised by anti-muscarinics and by opioid analgesics.

Since extrapyramidal symptoms may occur with both Gastromax and other centrally acting medication (e.g. lithium, phenothiazines, anticonvulsants), particular care should be exercised in the event of co-administration of these drugs.

Gastromax should be used with care in association with other drugs acting at central dopamine receptors, such as levodopa and bromocriptine.

Gastromax should be used with care in association with drugs that enhance sympathomimetic activity such as MAOIs.

Pregnancy and lactation: Gastromax is contra-indicated during the first trimester of pregnancy. In later stages of pregnancy, Gastromax should only be used where there are compelling reasons to do so.

Since metoclopramide is found in breast milk, Gastromax is contra-indicated in nursing mothers.

Effects of ability to drive and use machines: Rarely, Gastromax may cause drowsiness and affect reaction times. Patients should be warned of the possibility and cautioned against driving a car or operating machinery if so affected.

Undesirable effects: Fatigue, dizziness, drowsiness, restlessness and diarrhoea have been reported.

Raised prolactin levels manifesting as mammary engorgement or galactorrhoea may occur. These symptoms are usually associated with long-term therapy and disappear on discontinuation of therapy. Depression has been reported very rarely.

Various extrapyramidal reactions, usually of the dystonic type, have been reported. Symptoms which can occur include: spasm of facial, extra-ocular or cervical muscles which may be constant or rhythmic. There may also be a generalised increase in muscle tone. Should treatment of a dystonic reaction be required, an anticholinergic anti-Parkinsonian drug may be used.

Tardive dyskinesia may occur, principally in the elderly after prolonged treatment (see under *Special warnings and special precautions for use*).

Overdose: Gastric lavage and intensive supportive therapy should be initiated. Dystonic symptoms should be treated with atropine, benztropine or other anticholinergic agents.

Pharmacological properties
Pharmacodynamic properties: Metoclopramide increases lower oesophageal sphincter pressure, accelerates gastric emptying and increases the amplitude of gastric contractions. As well as a central effect on the 'vomit centre' metoclopramide exerts an increase in gastric motor activity and encourages normal peristaltic action. This anti-emetic effect is useful in post-operative nausea and vomiting, drug-induced vomiting, radiation sickness and non-specific vomiting.

Pharmacokinetic properties: Following administration, the Gastromax capsule disintegrates to release pellets into the gastrointestinal tract. Metoclopramide is released from these pellets by a controlled delivery system.

One 30 mg Gastromax capsule, once daily, can replace 10 mg metoclopramide three times daily, minimising peaks and troughs in plasma metoclopramide concentration.

Pharmaceutical particulars
List of excipients: The capsules contain the following inert ingredients: Colloidal silicon dioxide, sucrose PhEur, maize starch PhEur, talc PhEur, shellac, ethyl cellulose, titanium dioxide (E171), iron (II) oxide yellow (E172), erythrosine (E127), Gelatin BP.

Incompatibilities: None known.

Shelf life: 36 months.

Special precautions for storage: None.

Nature and contents of container: Packs of 28 capsules. Aluminium/PVC blister strips, 14 capsules/strip, 2 strips in a carton box.

Instructions for use/handling: None.

Marketing authorisation number 0057/0395.

Date of renewal of the authorisation 11 November 1996.

Date of (partial) revision of the text March 1996.

Legal category POM.

GLIBENESE*

Presentation Glibenese (glipizide) is available as white capsular scored tablets engraved Y2 on one side and bisected. Each tablet contains 5 mg glipizide.

Uses *Actions:* Glibenese is an orally active sulphonylurea which effectively reduces blood glucose to the normal range in properly selected patients with non-insulin-dependent diabetes mellitus (NIDDM). It eliminates or diminishes glycosuria and ameliorates symptoms such as polyuria, polydipsia and pruritus.

The primary mode of action of Glibenese in experimental animals is the stimulation of insulin secretion from the beta-cells of pancreatic islet tissue. In man, stimulation of insulin secretion by Glibenese in response to a meal is undoubtedly of major importance. Fasting insulin levels are not elevated even on long-term Glibenese administration, but the post-prandial insulin response continues to be enhanced after at least 6 months of treatment. The insulinotropic response to a meal occurs within 30 minutes after an oral dose of Glibenese in diabetic patients, but elevated insulin levels do not persist beyond the time of the meal challenge. There is also increasing evidence that extrapancreatic effects involving potentiation of insulin action form a significant component of the activity of Glibenese.

Blood sugar control persists for up to 24 hours after a single dose of Glibenese even though plasma levels have declined to a small fraction of peak levels by that time. Once-daily administration of doses up to 15 mg has been shown to be safe and effective maintenance therapy in selected patients.

Some patients fail to respond initially, or gradually lose their responsiveness to sulphonylurea drugs, including Glibenese. Alternatively, Glibenese, may be effective in some patients who have not responded or have ceased to respond to other sulphonylureas.

Gastrointestinal absorption of Glibenese in man is uniform, rapid and essentially complete. Peak plasma concentrations occur 1–3 hours after a single oral dose. The half-life of elimination ranges from 2–4 hours in normal subjects, whether given intravenously or orally. The metabolic and excretory patterns are similar with the two routes of administration, indicating that first-pass metabolism is not significant. Glibenese does not accumulate in plasma on repeated oral administration. Total absorption and disposition of an oral dose was unaffected by food in normal volunteers, but absorption was delayed by about 40 minutes. Thus, Glibenese was more effective when administered about 30 minutes before, rather than with a test meal in diabetic patients. Protein binding was studied in serum from volunteers who received either oral or intravenous Glibenese and found to be 98–99% one hour after either route of administration. The apparent volume of distribution of Glibenese after intravenous administration was 11 litres, indicative of localisation within the extracellular fluid compartment.

The metabolism of Glibenese is extensive and occurs mainly in the liver. The primary metabolites are inactive hydroxylation products and polar conjugates and are excreted mainly in the urine. Less than 10% unchanged Glibenese is found in the urine.

In a placebo-controlled, crossover study in normal volunteers, Glibenese showed no anti-diuretic activity, and, in fact, led to a slight increase in free water clearance.

Indications: Glibenese is indicated as an adjunct to diet to lower the blood glucose in patients with non-insulin-dependent diabetes mellitus (type II, NIDDM), formerly known as maturity onset diabetes, whose hyperglycaemia cannot be controlled by diet alone.

In initiating treatment for non-insulin dependent diabetes, diet should be emphasised as the primary form of treatment. Caloric restriction and weight loss are essential in the obese diabetic patient. Proper dietary management alone may be effective in controlling the blood glucose and symptoms of hyperglycaemia. The importance of regular physical activity should also be stressed, cardiovascular risk factors should be identified and corrective measures taken where possible.

Use of Glibenese must be viewed by both the physician and patient as a treatment in addition to diet, and not as a substitute for diet or as a convenient mechanism for avoiding dietary restraint. Furthermore, loss of blood glucose control on diet alone also may be transient, thus requiring only short-term administration of Glibenese.

Patient selection: The most likely patient for therapy is one in whom diabetes is of the NIDDM type, stable, and not controlled by dietary regulation alone. A past history of diabetic coma does not necessarily preclude successful therapeutic control with Glibenese. A trial period may be indicated in certain patients who might be expected to respond to this type of medication, but who failed in initial trials with, or after having been on other oral sulphonylurea agents, or in patients whose diabetic control on such agents has not been satisfactory. Glibenese may prove effective and provide improved control of the diabetes. The final evaluation of response in patients who qualify as candidates for Glibenese is a therapeutic trial for a period of at least seven days. During the trial period, the absence of ketonuria together with a satisfactory control, indicates that the patient is responsive and amenable to control with the drug. However, the development of ketonuria within 24 hours after withdrawal of insulin usually will be indicative of a poor response. The patient is considered unresponsive if he fails to achieve satisfactory lowering of blood sugar levels or fails to obtain objective or subjective clinical improvement and if he develops ketonuria or glycosuria. Insulin is indicated for the therapy of such patients.

Dosage and administration There is no fixed dosage regimen for the management of diabetes mellitus with Glibenese or any other hypoglycaemic agent. In addition to the usual monitoring of urinary glucose, the patient's blood glucose must also be monitored periodically to determine the minimum effective dose for the patient, to detect primary failure: i.e., inadequate lowering of blood glucose at the maximum recommended dose of medication, and to detect secondary failure; i.e., loss of adequate blood-glucose-lowering response after an initial period of effectiveness. Glycosylated haemoglobin levels may also be of value in monitoring the patient's response to therapy.

Short term administration of Glibenese may be sufficient during periods of transient loss of control in patients usually controlled well on diet.

In general, Glibenese should be given approximately 30 minutes before a meal to achieve the greatest reduction in post-prandial hyperglycaemia.

Initial dose: The recommended starting dose is 5 mg, given before breakfast or the midday meal. Mild diabetics, elderly patients or those with liver disease may be started on 2.5 mg.

Titration: Dosage adjustments should ordinarily be in increments of 2.5 to 5 mg, as determined by blood glucose response. At least several days should elapse between titration steps. The maximum recommended single dose is 15 mg. Doses above 15 mg should ordinarily be divided.

Maintenance: Some patients may be effectively controlled on a once-a-day regimen. Total daily dosage above 15 mg should ordinarily be divided. Total daily dosage above 30 mg has been safely given on a twice daily basis to long term patients. Patients can usually be stabilised on a dosage ranging from 2.5 to 30 mg daily. The maximum recommended daily dosage is 40 mg.

Use in the elderly: Elderly diabetics are more sensitive to the hypoglycaemic effect of sulphonylurea drugs and should therefore be prescribed a low starting dose of 2.5 mg daily. The elderly are also particularly susceptible to the effects of hypoglycaemia. Hypoglycaemia may be difficult to recognise in the elderly.

In elderly, debilitated or malnourished patients, and patients with an impaired renal or hepatic function, the initial and maintenance dosing should be conservative to avoid hypoglycaemic reactions (see Precautions section).

Use in children: Safety and effectiveness in children have not been established.

Patients receiving insulin: As with other sulphonylurea class hypoglycaemics, many stable non-insulin-dependent diabetic patients receiving insulin may be safely placed on Glibenese. When transferring patients from insulin to Glibenese, the following general guidelines should be considered.

For patients whose daily insulin requirement is 20 units or less, insulin may be discontinued and Glibenese therapy begun at usual dosages. Several days should elapse between Glibenese titration steps.

For patients whose daily insulin requirement is greater than 20 units, the insulin dose should be reduced by 50% and Glibenese therapy initiated at usual dosages. Subsequent reductions in insulin dosage should depend on individual patient response. Several days should elapse between Glibenese steps.

During the insulin withdrawal period, the patient should test urine samples for sugar and ketone bodies at least three times daily. Patients should be instructed to contact the prescriber immediately if these tests are abnormal. In some cases, especially when the patient has been receiving greater than 40 units of insulin daily, it may be advisable to consider hospitalisation during the transition period.

Patients receiving other oral hypoglycaemic agents: As with other sulphonylurea class hypoglycaemics, no transition period is necessary when transferring patients to Glibenese. Patients should be observed carefully (1–2 weeks) for hypoglycaemia when being transferred from longer half-life sulphonylureas (e.g. chlorpropamide) to Glibenese due to potential overlapping of drug effect.

Concurrent biguanide therapy: As with other sulphonylureas, a proportion of patients who do not achieve optimal control with Glibenese alone, or who experience secondary failure, may be expected to have their control improved or restored by the addition of a biguanide.

For such patients, it is suggested that the dosage of Glibenese should be maintained and the biguanide chosen should be added using low doses initially and increasing the dosage of the biguanide progressively until adequate control is achieved or restored. Should gastrointestinal side-effects appear, an attempt should be made to reduce the dosage of the biguanide.

Contra-indications, warnings, etc
Contra-indications: Glibenese is contra-indicated in the following conditions:

1. Known hypersensitivity to Glibenese.
2. Diabetic ketoacidosis, with or without coma. This condition should be treated with insulin.
3. Insulin dependent (juvenile-onset) diabetes.
4. Severe renal, hepatic or thyroid impairment; coexistent renal and hepatic disease.

Warnings: The metabolism and excretion of Glibenese may be slowed in patients with impaired renal and/or hepatic function. If hypoglycaemia should occur in such patients, it may be prolonged.

Precautions
General: Hypoglycaemia: All sulphonylurea drugs are capable of producing severe hypoglycaemia. Proper patient selection, dosage, and instructions are important to avoid hypoglycaemic episodes. Renal or hepatic insufficiency may cause elevated blood levels of Glibenese and the latter may also diminish gluconeogenic capacity, both of which increase the risk of serious hypoglycaemic reactions. Elderly, debilitated or malnourished patients, and those with adrenal or pituitary insufficiency are particularly susceptible to the hypoglycaemic action of glucose-lowering drugs. Hypoglycaemia may be difficult to recognise in the elderly, and in people who are taking beta-adrenergic blocking drugs. Hypoglycaemia is more likely to occur when caloric intake is deficient, after severe or prolonged exercise, when alcohol is ingested, or when more than one glucose-lowering drug is used.

Loss of control of blood glucose: When a patient stabilised on any diabetic regimen is exposed to stress such as fever, trauma, infection, or surgery, a loss of control may occur. At such times, it may be necessary to discontinue Glibenese and administer insulin.

The effectiveness of any oral hypoglycaemic drug, including Glibenese, in lowering blood glucose to a desired level decreases in many patients over a period of time, which may be due to progression of the severity of the diabetes or to diminished responsiveness to the drug. This phenomenon is known as secondary failure, to distinguish it from primary failure in which the drug is ineffective in an individual patient when first given.

Information for patients: Patients should be informed of the potential risks and advantages of Glibenese and of alternative modes of therapy. They should also be informed about the importance of adherence to dietary instructions, of a regular exercise programme, and of regular testing of urine and/or blood glucose.

The risk of hypoglycaemia, its symptoms and treatment, and conditions that predispose to its development should be explained to patients and responsible family members. Primary and secondary failure should also be explained.

Laboratory tests: Blood and urine glucose should be monitored periodically. Measurement of glycosylated haemoglobin may be useful.

Driving/use of machinery: Clinical experience with

Glibenese indicates that it is unlikely to impair a patient's ability to drive or use machinery.

Use in pregnancy: Glibenese is contra-indicated during pregnancy. Diabetes in pregnancy should be treated with insulin and not sulphonylureas. Recent evidence suggests that hyperglycaemia in pregnancy is associated with a higher incidence of congenital abnormalities.

Nursing mothers: Although it is not known whether Glibenese is excreted in human milk, some sulphonylurea drugs are known to be excreted in human milk. Caution is therefore necessary if a sulphonylurea drug is prescribed because of the possibility of hypoglycaemia in the infant.

Use in renal insufficiency: Glibenese is not recommended in patients with renal insufficiency.

Drug interactions: The hypoglycaemic action of sulphonylureas may be potentiated by certain drugs including nonsteroidal anti-inflammatory agents and other drugs that are highly protein bound, salicylates, sulphonamides, chloramphenicol, probenecid, coumarins, monoamine oxidase inhibitors and beta-adrenergic blocking agents. When such drugs are administered to a patient receiving Glibenese, the patient should be observed closely for hypoglycaemia. When such drugs are withdrawn from a patient receiving Glibenese, the patient should be observed closely for loss of control.

Certain drugs tend to produce hyperglycaemia and may lead to loss of control. These drugs include the thiazides and other diuretics, corticosteroids, phenothiazines, thyroid products, oestrogens, oral contraceptives, phenytoin, nicotinic acid, sympathomimetics, calcium antagonists and isoniazid. When such drugs are administered to or withdrawn from a patient receiving Glibenese, the patient should be closely observed for loss of control.

In the mouse, Glibenese pre-treatment did not cause an accumulation of acetaldehyde after ethanol administration. Clinical experience has confirmed the virtual absence of an alcohol interaction in man.

Side-effects: The majority of side-effects have been dose related, transient, and have responded to dose reduction or withdrawal of the medication. However, clinical experience thus far has shown that, as with other sulphonylureas some side-effects associated with hypersensitivity may be severe and deaths have been reported in some instances.

Hypoglycaemia: See *Precautions* and *Overdosage* sections.

Gastrointestinal: Gastrointestinal complaints include nausea, diarrhoea, constipation and gastralgia. They appear to be dose related and usually disappear on division or reduction of dosage.

Dermatological: Allergic skin reactions including erythema, morbilliform or maculopapular reactions, urticaria, pruritus and eczema have been reported. They frequently disappear with continued therapy. However, if they persist, the drug should be discontinued.

Miscellaneous: Dizziness, drowsiness and headache have each been reported in patients treated with Glibenese. They are usually transient and seldom require discontinuance of therapy.

Laboratory tests: The pattern of laboratory test abnormalities observed with Glibenese is similar to that for other sulphonylureas. Occasional mild to moderate elevations of AST (SGOT), LDH, alkaline phosphatase, BUN and creatinine were noted. One case of jaundice was reported. The relationship of these abnormalities to Glibenese is uncertain, and they have rarely been associated with clinical symptoms.

Overdosage: There is no well documented experience with Glibenese overdosage. The acute oral toxicity was extremely low in all species tested (LD_{50} greater than 4g/kg).

Overdosage of sulphonylureas including Glibenese can produce hypoglycaemia. Mild hypoglycaemic symptoms without loss of consciousness or neurological findings should be treated aggressively with oral glucose and adjustments in drug dosage and/or meal patterns. Close monitoring should continue until the physician is assured that the patient is out of danger. Severe hypoglycaemic reactions with coma, seizure, or other neurological impairment occur infrequently, but constitute medical emergencies requiring immediate hospitalisation. If hypoglycaemic coma is diagnosed or suspected, the patient should be given a rapid intravenous injection of concentrated (50%) glucose solution. This should be followed by continuous infusion of a more dilute (10%) glucose solution at a rate that will maintain the blood glucose at a level above 5.6 mmol/l (100 mg/dl). Patients should be closely monitored for a minimum of 24 to 48 hours since hypoglycaemia may recur after apparent clinical recovery. Clearance of Glibenese from plasma would be prolonged in persons with liver disease. Because of the extensive protein binding of Glibenese, dialysis is unlikely to be of benefit.

Pharmaceutical precautions Store below 25°C.

Legal category POM.

Package quantities Glibenese tablets 5 mg: Original packs of 56 tablets.

Further information Nil.

Product licence number 0057/0113R.

Date of revision January 1997.

HYPOVASE*

Presentation Hypovase is available in tablets containing prazosin hydrochloride BP equivalent to the following quantities of prazosin:

500 microgram white tablets, unscored: marked 'Pfizer' on one side.
1 mg scored orange tablets: marked HYP/1 on one side.
2 mg scored white tablets: marked HYP/2 on one side and 'Pfizer' on the other.

Inactive excipients: Tablets (all strengths): avicel pH 101, calcium phosphate dibasic anhydrous, magnesium stearate, maize starch, sodium lauryl sulphate. In addition, the 1 mg tablet contains the azo-dye, sunset yellow E110.

Uses
Actions: Hypovase causes a decrease in total peripheral vascular resistance thought to be mediated by selective inhibition of post-synaptic alpha-1-adrenoceptors in vascular smooth muscle. The results of forearm plethysmographic studies in humans demonstrate that the resultant peripheral vasodilatation is a balanced effect on both resistance vessels (arterioles) and capacitance vessels (veins).

In hypertensive patients, blood pressure is lowered in both the supine and standing positions; this effect is more pronounced on the diastolic blood pressure. Tolerance to the antihypertensive effect has not been observed in long-term clinical use; relatively little tachycardia or change in renin levels has been noted. Rebound elevation of blood pressure does not occur following abrupt cessation of Hypovase therapy.

The therapeutic efficacy of Hypovase in patients with congestive heart failure is ascribed to a reduction in left ventricular filling pressure, reduction in cardiac impedance and an augmentation of cardiac output. The use of Hypovase in congestive heart failure does not provoke a reflex tachycardia and blood pressure reduction is minimal in normotensive patients.

Hypovase has been found to successfully reduce the severity of the signs, symptoms, frequency and duration of attacks, in patients with Raynaud's disease.

In low dosage, antagonism of alpha-1-receptors on prostatic and urethral smooth muscle has been shown to improve the urinary pressure profile in men and to improve symptoms of benign prostatic hypertrophy.

Clinical studies have shown that Hypovase therapy is not associated with adverse changes in the serum lipid profile.

Following oral administration in normal volunteers and hypertensive patients, plasma concentrations reach a peak in one to two hours, with a plasma half-life of two to three hours. Pharmacokinetic data in a limited number of patients with congestive heart failure, most of whom showed evidence of hepatic congestion, indicates that peak plasma concentrations are reached in 2.5 hours and plasma half-life is approximately 7 hours. Hypovase is highly bound to plasma protein. Studies indicate that Hypovase is extensively metabolised, primarily by demethylation and conjugation, and excreted mainly via bile and faeces.

Renal blood flow and glomerular filtration rate are not impaired by long term oral administration and thus Hypovase can be used with safety in patients with impaired renal function.

Indications: Hypertension: Hypovase is indicated in the treatment of all grades of essential (primary) hypertension and of all grades of secondary hypertension of varied aetiology. It can be used as the initial and sole agent or it may be employed in a treatment regimen in conjunction with a diuretic and/or other antihypertensive drug as needed for proper patient response.

Congestive heart failure: Hypovase may be used alone or added to the therapeutic regimen in those patients with congestive heart failure who are resistent or refractory to conventional therapy with diuretics, and/or cardiac glycosides.

Raynaud's phenomenon and Raynaud's disease: Hypovase is indicated for the symptomatic treatment of patients with Raynaud's phenomenon and Raynaud's disease.

Benign prostatic hyperplasia: Hypovase is indicated as an adjunct in the symptomatic treatment of urinary obstruction caused by benign prostatic hyperplasia, and may therefore be of value in patients awaiting prostatic surgery.

Dosage and administration
Hypertension: The dosage range is from 500 micrograms – 20 mg daily. It is recommended that therapy be initiated at the lowest dose, 500 micrograms, twice or three times daily for three to seven days, with the starting dose administered in the evening. This dose should be increased to 1 mg twice or three times daily for a further three to seven days. Thereafter, the daily dose should be increased gradually as determined by the patient's response to the blood pressure lowering effect. Most patients are likely to be maintained on a dosage regimen of Hypovase alone of up to 15 mg daily in divided doses. Maximum recommended daily dosage: 20 mg in divided doses.

The b.d. starter pack is available for the convenience of prescribers to initiate treatment up to 2 mg twice daily.

Patients receiving other antihypertensive therapy but with inadequate control: The dosage of the other drug should be reduced to a maintenance level and Hypovase initiated at 500 micrograms in the evening, then continuing with 500 micrograms twice or three times daily. Subsequent dosage increase, should be made gradually depending upon the patient's response.

There is evidence that adding Hypovase to angiotensin converting enzyme inhibitor, beta-adrenergic antagonist or calcium antagonist therapy may bring about a substantial reduction in blood pressure. Therefore, the low initial dosage regimen is recommended.

Congestive cardiac failure: The recommended starting dose is 500 micrograms two, three or four times daily, increasing to 4 mg in divided doses. Dosage should be adjusted according to the patient's clinical response, based on careful monitoring of cardiopulmonary signs and symptoms, and when indicated, haemodynamic studies. Dosage may be adjusted as often as every two to three days in patients under close medical supervision. In severely ill, decompensated patients, rapid dosage adjustment over one to two days may be indicated and is best done when haemodynamic monitoring is available. In clinical studies, the therapeutic dosages ranged from 4 mg to 20 mg daily in divided doses. Adjustment of dosage may be required in the course of Hypovase therapy in some patients to maintain optimal clinical improvement.

Usual daily maintenance dosage: 4 mg to 20 mg in divided doses.

Raynaud's phenomenon and Raynaud's disease: The recommended starting dosage is 500 micrograms twice daily given for a period of three to seven days and should be adjusted according to the patient's clinical repsonse. Usual maintenance dosage 1 mg or 2 mg twice daily.

Benign prostatic hyperplasia: The recommended dosage is 500 micrograms twice daily for a period of 3 to 7 days, with the initial dose administered in the evening. The dosage should then be adjusted according to clinical response. The usual maintenance dosage is 2 mg twice daily. This dose should not be exceeded, unless the patient requires Hypovase as antihypertensive therapy.

Patients with BPH receiving antihypertensive therapy: It is recommended that patients receiving antihypertensive therapy are administered Hypovase for BPH only under supervision of the practitioner responsible for treating the patient's hypertension.

Patients with moderate to severe grades of renal impairment: Evidence to date shows that Hypovase does not further compromise renal function when used in patients with renal impairment. As some patients in this category have responded to small doses of Hypovase, it is recommended that therapy be initiated at 500 micrograms daily and that dosage increases be instituted cautiously.

Patients with hepatic dysfunction: No information is available on the use of Hypovase in this patient group, however, since Hypovase normally undergoes substantial first pass metabolism and subsequent metabolism and excretion by the liver, it is recommended that therapy be initiated at 500 micrograms daily and that dosage increases be instituted cautiously.

Use in the elderly: Since the elderly may be more susceptible to hypotension, therapy should be initiated with the lowest possible dose.

Use in children: Hypovase is not recommended for the treatment of children under the age of 12 years since safe conditions for its use have not been established.

Contra-indications, warnings, etc
Contra-indications: Sensitivity to Hypovase or related quinazolines.
Warnings:
Use in pregnancy or lactation: Although no teratogenic effects were seen in animal testing, the safety of Hypovase during pregnancy has not yet been estab-

lished. The use of prazosin and a beta-blocker for the control of severe hypertension in 44 pregnant women revealed no drug-related foetal abnormalities or adverse effects. Therapy with prazosin was continued for as long as 14 weeks.

Prazosin has also been used alone or in combination with other hypotensive agents in severe hypertension of pregnancy. No foetal or neonatal abnormalities have been reported with the use of prazosin.

Studies to date are inadequate to establish the safety of Hypovase in pregnancy, accordingly, it should be used only when, in the opinion of the physician, potential benefit outweighs potential risk. Hypovase has been shown to be excreted in small amounts in human milk. Caution should be exercised when Hypovase is administered to nursing mothers.

In patients with congestive cardiac failure: Hypovase is not recommended in the treatment of congestive cardiac failure due to mechanical obstruction such as aortic valve stenosis, mitral valve stenosis, pulmonary embolism and restrictive pericardial disease. Adequate data are not yet available to establish efficacy in patients with heart failure due to recent myocardial infarction.

Benign prostatic hyperplasia: Hypovase is not recommended for patients with a history of micturition syncope.

Precautions:

In patients with hypertension: A very small percentage of patients may respond in an abrupt and exaggerated manner to the initial dose of Hypovase. Postural hypotension evidenced by dizziness and weakness, or rarely loss of consciousness, has been reported, particularly with the commencement of therapy, but this effect is readily avoided by initiating treatment with a low dose of Hypovase and with small increases in dosage during the first one to two weeks of therapy. The effect when observed, is not related to the severity of hypertension, is self-limiting and in most patients does not recur after the initial period of therapy or during subsequent dosage increments.

When instituting therapy with any effective antihypertensive agent, the patient should be advised how to avoid symptoms resulting from postural hypotension and what measures to take should they develop.

In patients with congestive cardiac failure: When Hypovase is initially administered to patients with congestive cardiac failure who have undergone vigorous diuretic or other vasodilator treatment, particularly in higher than the recommended starting dose, the resultant decrease in left ventricular filling pressure may be associated with a significant fall in cardiac output and systemic blood pressure. In such patients, observance of the recommended starting dose of Hypovase followed by gradual dosage increase is particularly important. (See *Dosage and administration*).

The clinical efficacy of Hypovase in congestive cardiac failure has been reported to diminish after several months of treatment, in a proportion of patients. In these patients there is usually evidence of weight gain or peripheral oedema indicating fluid retention. Since spontaneous deterioration may occur in such severely ill patients a causal relationship to prazosin therapy has not been established. Thus, as with all patients with congestive cardiac failure, careful adjustment of diuretic dosage according to the patient's clinical condition is required to prevent excessive fluid retention and consequent relief of symptoms.

In those patients without evidence of fluid retention, when clinical improvement has diminished, an increase in the dosage of Hypovase will usually restore clinical efficacy.

Raynaud's phenomenon and Raynaud's disease: Because Hypovase decreases peripheral vascular resistance, careful monitoring of blood pressure during initial administration and during subsequent dosage increments of Hypovase is suggested. Close observation is especially recommended for patients already taking medications that are known to lower blood pressure.

Benign prostatic hyperplasia: Hypovase decreases peripheral vascular resistance and since many patients with this disorder are elderly, careful monitoring of blood pressure during initial administration and during adjustment of dosage is recommended. The possibility of postural hypotension, or rarely, loss of consciousness, as reported in other patient groups should be borne in mind. Hypovase may augment the efficacy of antihypertensive therapy, consequently, close observation is especially recommended for patients taking medications that are known to lower blood pressure. Hypovase should not normally be administered to patients already receiving another alpha-1-antagonist.

Driving/use of machinery: The patient should be advised that the ability to drive or use machinery may be impaired should dizziness or weakness occur during the initiation of Hypovase therapy.

Drug interactions: Hypovase has been administered without any adverse drug interaction in clinical experience to date with the following:

(1) cardiac glycosides – digitalis and digoxin;
(2) hypoglycaemic agents – insulin, chlorpropamide, phenformin, tolazamide and tolbutamide;
(3) tranquillizers and sedatives – chlordiazepoxide, diazepam and phenobarbitone;
(4) agents for treatment of gout – allopurinol, colchicine and probenecid;
(5) anti-arrhythmic agents – procainamide and quinidine;
(6) analgesic, antipyretic, and anti-inflammatory agents – dextropropoxyphene, aspirin, indomethacin and phenylbutazone;

There is evidence that adding Hypovase to beta-adrenergic antagonist or calcium antagonist therapy may produce a substantial reduction in blood pressure. Therefore, the low initial dosage regimen is recommended.

Drug/laboratory test interactions: False positive results may occur in screening tests for phaeochromocytoma (urinary vanillylmandelic acid (VMA) and methoxyhydroxyphenyl glycol (MHPG) metabolites of noradrenaline) in patients who are being treated with Hypovase.

Side-effects: In patients with hypertension: The most common side-effects associated with Hypovase therapy are: dizziness, headache, drowsiness, lack of energy, weakness, nausea, and palpitations. In most instances side-effects will disappear with continued therapy or may be tolerated with no decrease in dosage of the drug.

In addition, the following reactions have been associated with Hypovase therapy: vomiting, diarrhoea, constipation, abdominal discomfort and/or pain, liver function abnormalities, pancreatitis, oedema, dyspnoea, faintness, transient temporary loss of consciousness, tachycardia, nervousness, vertigo, hallucinations, depression, paraesthesia, rash, pruritus, alopecia, lichen planus, urinary frequency, impotence, incontinence, priapism, blurred vision, reddened sclera, epistaxis, tinnitus, dry mouth, nasal congestion, diaphoresis, fever, positive ANA titre and arthralgia.

Some of these reactions have occurred rarely, and in many instances the exact causal relationships have not been established.

Literature reports exist associating Hypovase therapy with a worsening of pre-existing narcolepsy. A causal relationship is uncertain in these cases.

In patients with congestive cardiac failure: The following side-effects have been observed when Hypovase is used in conjunction with cardiac glycosides and diuretics: drowsiness, dizziness, postural hypotension, blurred vision, oedema, dry mouth, palpitations, nausea, diarrhoea, impotence, headache, and nasal congestion. In most instances these occurrences have been mild to moderate in severity and have resolved with continued therapy or have been tolerated with no decrease in drug dosage.

Raynaud's phenomenon and Raynaud's disease: The most common, although infrequently reported side-effect, is mild dizziness.

Benign prostatic hyperplasia: The most common, although infrequently reported side-effect, is dizziness.

Overdosage: Should overdosage lead to hypotension, support of the cardiovascular system is of first importance. Restoration of blood pressure and normalisation of heart rate may be accomplished by keeping the patient in the supine position. If this measure is inadequate, shock should first be treated with volume expanders. If necessary, vasopressors including angiotensin should then be used. Renal function should be monitored and supported as needed. Laboratory data indicate Hypovase is not dialysable because it is protein bound.

Pharmaceutical precautions Store below 30°C.

Legal category POM.

Package quantities b.d. starter pack, for the convenience of patients initiating Hypovase therapy, containing 8×500 microgram Hypovase tablets and 32×1 mg Hypovase tablets (see 'Further information').

Hypovase 500 microgram: Original packs of 56 tablets (in blister strips of 4×14 tablets).
Hypovase 1 mg: Original packs of 56 tablets (in blister strips of 4×14 tablets).
Hypovase 2 mg: Original packs of 56 tablets (in blister strips of 4×14 tablets).

Further information The two week b.d. starter pack has the following instructions to the patient:

'Step 1 (500 microgram tablets) – evening day 1 to morning day 5
Step 2 (1 mg tablets) – evening day 5 to morning day 9
Step 3 (2×1 mg tablets) – evening day 9 to morning day 15
Your doctor will wish you to follow further dosage instructions beyond Step 3 and you should follow those instructions or see your doctor before the end of Step 3.'

The tablets (500 microgram and 1 mg) are carefully packed in sequence, in blister strips to ensure correct usage.

Product licence numbers

500 microgram tablet	0057/0149R
1 mg tablet	0057/0106R
2 mg tablet	0057/0107R

Date of issue of this document January 1997

ISTIN*

Qualitative and quantitative composition Active ingredient: amlodipine. The tablets contain amlodipine besylate (equivalent to 5 mg and 10 mg amlodipine).

Pharmaceutical form Tablet for oral administration.
5 mg tablets coded 'ITN5' on one side and 'PFIZER' on the other.

10 mg tablets coded 'ITN10' on one side and 'PFIZER' on the other.

Clinical particulars

Therapeutic indications: Hypertension.

Prophylaxis of chronic stable angina pectoris.

Prinzmetal's (variant) angina when diagnosed by a cardiologist.

In hypertensive patients, Istin has been used in combination with a thiazide diuretic, alpha blocker, beta-adrenoceptor blocking agent, or an angiotensin converting enzyme inhibitor. For angina, Istin may be used as monotherapy or in combination with other antianginal drugs in patients with angina that is refractory to nitrates and/or adequate doses of beta blockers.

Istin is well tolerated in patients with heart failure and a history of hypertension or ischaemic heart disease.

Posology and method of administration:

In adults: For both hypertension and angina the usual initial dose is 5 mg Istin once daily which may be increased to a maximum dose of 10 mg depending on the individual patient's response.

No dose adjustment of Istin is required upon concomitant administration of thiazide diuretics, beta blockers, and angiotensin-converting enzyme inhibitors.

Use in children: Not recommended.

Use in the elderly: The time to reach peak plasma concentrations of amlodipine is similar in elderly and younger subjects. Amlodipine clearance tends to be decreased with resulting increases in AUC and elimination half-life in elderly patients. Increases in AUC and elimination half-life in patients with congestive heart failure were as expected for the patient age group studied. Istin, used at similar doses in elderly or younger patients, is equally well tolerated. Therefore normal dosage regimens are recommended.

Patients with hepatic impairment: As with all calcium antagonists, amlodipine's half-life is prolonged in patients with impaired liver function and dosage recommendations have not been established. The drug should therefore be administered with caution in these patients.

Patients with renal impairment: Amlodipine is extensively metabolised to inactive metabolites with 10% excreted as unchanged drug in the urine. Changes in amlodipine plasma concentrations are not correlated with degree of renal impairment, therefore the normal dosage is recommended. Amlodipine is not dialysable.

Contra-indications: Istin is contra-indicated in patients with a known sensitivity to dihydropyridines.

Istin should not be used in cardiogenic shock, clinically significant aortic stenosis, unstable angina (excluding Prinzmetal's angina).

Pregnancy and lactation (see also under *Pregnancy and lactation* section).

Special warnings and precautions for use: There are no data to support the use of Istin alone, during or within one month of a myocardial infarction.

The safety and efficacy of Istin in hypertensive crisis has not been established.

Interactions with other medicaments and other forms of interaction: Istin has been safely administered with thiazide diuretics, alpha blockers, beta blockers, angiotensin-converting enzyme inhibitors, long-acting nitrates, sublingual glyceryl trinitrate, non-steroidal anti-inflammatory drugs, antibiotics, and oral hypoglycaemic drugs.

Pharmacokinetic studies with cyclosporin have demonstrated that amlodipine does not significantly alter the pharmacokinetics of cyclosporin.

Special studies have indicated that the co-administration of Istin with digoxin did not change serum digoxin levels or digoxin renal clearance in normal volunteers, and that co-administration of cimetidine did not alter the pharmacokinetics of amlodipine.

In healthy male volunteers, the co-administration of Istin does not significantly alter the effect of warfarin on prothrombin response time.

In vitro data from studies with human plasma, indicate that amlodipine has no effect on protein binding of digoxin, phenytoin, warfarin or indomethacin.

Grapefruit juice may interact with Istin to increase the plasma concentration. However this increase is too small to significantly alter blood pressure or heart rate.

Pregnancy and lactation: Although some dihydropyridine compounds have been found to be teratogenic in animals, data in the rat and rabbit for amlodipine provide no evidence for a teratogenic effect. There is, however, no clinical experience with the preparation in pregnancy or lactation. Accordingly, Istin should not be administered during pregnancy, or lactation, or to women of childbearing potential unless effective contraception is used (see under *Contra-indications*).

Effects on ability to drive and use machines: Clinical experience with Istin indicates that therapy is unlikely to impair a patient's ability to drive or use machinery.

Undesirable effects: The most commonly reported side-effects of Istin are headache, oedema, rash, fatigue, nausea, flushing and dizziness. Gingival hyperplasia has been reported after Istin. The following adverse reactions have been reported rarely: pruritus, palpitations, dyspnoea, abdominal pain, dyspepsia, muscle cramps, asthenia, somnolence, altered bowel habit, myalgia, arthralgia, mood changes, increased urinary frequency, impotence and visual disturbances. The following adverse reactions have been reported very rarely: abnormal liver function tests, jaundice, erythema multiforme and gynaecomastia.

As with other calcium channel blockers the following adverse events have been rarely reported and cannot be distinguished from the natural history of the underlying disease: myocardial infarction, arrhythmia (including ventricular tachycardia and atrial fibrillation) and chest pain.

Overdose: In humans, experience with intentional overdose is limited. Gastric lavage may be worthwhile in some cases. Available data suggest that gross overdosage could result in excessive peripheral vasodilatation with subsequent marked and probably prolonged systemic hypotension. Clinically significant hypotension due to Istin overdosage calls for active cardiovascular support including frequent monitoring of cardiac and respiratory function, elevation of extremities, and attention to circulating fluid volume and urine output. A vasoconstrictor may be helpful in restoring vascular tone and blood pressure, provided that there is no contra-indication to its use. Intravenous calcium gluconate may be beneficial in reversing the effects of calcium channel blockade. Since Istin is highly protein-bound, dialysis is not likely to be of benefit.

Pharmacological properties

Pharmacodynamic properties: Istin is a calcium ion influx inhibitor of the dihydropyridine group (slow channel blocker or calcium ion antagonist) and inhibits the transmembrane influx of calcium ions into cardiac and vascular smooth muscle.

The mechanism of the antihypertensive action of Istin is due to a direct relaxant effect on vascular smooth muscle. The precise mechanism by which Istin relieves angina has not been fully determined but Istin reduces total ischaemic burden by the following two actions:

(1) Istin dilates peripheral arterioles and thus, reduces the total peripheral resistance (afterload) against which the heart works. Since the heart rate remains stable, this unloading of the heart reduces myocardial energy consumption and oxygen requirements.

(2) The mechanism of action of Istin also probably involves dilatation of the main coronary arteries and coronary arterioles, both in normal and ischaemic regions. This dilatation increases myocardial oxygen delivery in patients with coronary artery spasm (Prinzmetal's or variant angina).

In patients with hypertension, once daily dosing provides clinically significant reductions of blood pressure in both the supine and standing positions throughout the 24 hour interval. Due to the slow onset of action, acute hypotension is not a feature of Istin administration.

In patients with angina, once daily administration of Istin increases total exercise time, time to angina onset, and time to 1 mm ST segment depression, and decreases both angina attack frequency and glyceryl trinitrate tablet consumption.

Istin has not been associated with any adverse metabolic effects or changes in plasma lipids and is suitable for use in patients with asthma, diabetes and gout.

Haemodynamic studies and exercise based controlled clinical trials in NYHA Class II–IV heart failure patients have shown that Istin did not lead to clinical deterioration as measured by exercise tolerance, left ventricular ejection fraction and clinical symptomatology.

A placebo controlled study (PRAISE) designed to evaluate patients in NYHA Class III-IV heart failure receiving digoxin, diuretics and ACE inhibitors has shown that Istin did not lead to an increase in risk of mortality or combined mortality and morbidity with heart failure.

Pharmacokinetic properties

Absorption, distribution, plasma protein binding: After oral administration of therapeutic doses, amlodipine is well absorbed with peak blood levels between 6–12 hours post dose. Absolute bioavailability has been estimated to be between 64 and 80%. The volume of distribution is approximately 21 l/kg. *In vitro* studies have shown that approximately 97.5% of circulating amlodipine is bound to plasma proteins.

Biotransformation/elimination: The terminal plasma elimination half-life is about 35–50 hours and is consistent with once daily dosing. Amlodipine is extensively metabolised by the liver to inactive metabolites with 10% of the parent compound and 60% of metabolites excreted in the urine.

Preclinical safety data: None.

Pharmaceutical particulars

List of excipients: Microcrystalline Cellulose PhEur, dibasic calcium phosphate anhydrous NF, Sodium Starch Glycollate BP and Magnesium Stearate PhEur.

Incompatibilities: None stated.

Shelf life: 60 months.

Special precautions for storage: None specified.

Nature and contents of container: Istin is available as: Calendar packs of 28 tablets. Aluminium/PVC blister strips, 14 tablets/strip, 2 strips in a carton box.

Instructions for use/handling: No special requirements.

Marketing authorisation numbers

Istin Tablets 5 mg	0057/0297
Istin Tablets 10 mg	0057/0298

Date of first authorisation/renewal of authorisation 30 January 1995.

Date of (partial) revision of text April 1997.

Legal category POM.

LUSTRAL*

Qualitative and quantitative composition Sertraline hydrochloride equivalent to 50 mg or 100 mg sertraline.

Pharmaceutical form 50 mg white, capsular shaped, film-coated tablets coded 'LTL-50' on one side and 'PFIZER' on the other.

100 mg white, capsular shaped, film-coated tablets coded 'LTL-100' on one side and 'PFIZER' on the other.

Clinical particulars

Therapeutic indications: Lustral is indicated for the treatment of symptoms of depressive illness, including accompanying symptoms of anxiety. Following satisfactory response, continuation with Lustral therapy is effective in preventing relapse of the initial episode of depression or recurrence of further depressive episodes, including accompanying symptoms of anxiety.

Posology and method of administration:

Adults: Lustral should be given as a single daily dose. Lustral tablets can be administered with or without food. The starting dose is 50 mg daily and the usual therapeutic dose is 50 mg daily.

In some patients doses higher than 50 mg daily may be required. In patients with incomplete response but good toleration at lower doses, dosage adjustments should be made in 50 mg increments over a period of weeks to a maximum of 200 mg daily.

Once optimal therapeutic response is achieved the dose should be reduced, depending on therapeutic response, to the lowest effective level. Doses of 150 mg or more should not be used for periods exceeding 8 weeks. Dosage during prolonged maintenance therapy should be kept at the lowest effective level, with subsequent adjustments depending on therapeutic response. The onset of therapeutic effect may be seen within 7 days, although 2–4 weeks are usually necessary for full antidepressant activity.

Lustral tablets are for oral administration only.

Use in patients with renal or hepatic impairment: As with many other medications, sertraline should be used with caution in patients with renal and hepatic impairment (see *Contra-indications, precautions*).

Use in children: The use of Lustral in children is not recommended as safety and efficacy have not been established.

Use in the elderly: No special precautions are required. The usual adult dose is recommended. Several hundred elderly patients have participated in clinical studies with Lustral. The pattern and incidence of adverse reactions in the elderly is similar to that in younger patients.

Contra-indications: Lustral is contra-indicated in patients with a known hypersensitivity to sertraline.

Concomitant use in patients taking monoamine oxidase inhibitors (MAOIs) is contra-indicated (see *Special warnings and special precautions for use*).

Use in hepatic impairment: Sertraline is extensively metabolised by the liver. A single dose pharmacokinetic study in subjects with mild, stable cirrhosis demonstrated a prolonged elimination half-life and increased AUC in comparison to normal subjects.

There is insufficient clinical experience in patients with significant hepatic dysfunction and accordingly Lustral should not be used in such patients.

Special warnings and special precautions for use:

Monoamine oxidase inhibitors: Cases of serious reactions have been reported in patients receiving Lustral in combination with a monoamine oxidase inhibitor (MAOI), including the selective MAOI selegiline and the reversible MAOI (reversible inhibitor of monoamine oxidase RIMA), moclobemide. Some cases presented with features resembling the serotonin syndrome. Similar cases, sometimes fatal, have been reported with other antidepressants during combined treatment with a MAOI and in patients who have recently discontinued an antidepressant drug and have been started on a MAOI. Symptoms of a drug interaction between an SSRI and a MAOI include: hyperthermia, rigidity, myoclonus, autonomic instability with possible rapid fluctuations of vital signs, mental status changes that include confusion, irritability and extreme agitation progressing to delirium and coma. Therefore, Lustral should not be used in combination with a MAOI or within 14 days of discontinuing treatment with a MAOI. Similarly, at least 14 days should elapse after discontinuing Lustral treatment before starting a MAOI.

Electroconvulsive therapy (ECT): There are no clinical studies establishing the risks or benefits of the combined use of ECT and Lustral.

Activation of mania/hypomania: As with other antidepressants, activation of mania/hypomania has been reported in a small proportion of patients.

Seizures: Seizures are a potential risk with antidepressant drugs. Lustral should be avoided in patients with unstable epilepsy and patients with controlled epilepsy should be carefully monitored. The drug should be discontinued in any patient who develops seizures.

Suicide: Since the possibility of a suicide attempt is inherent in depression and may persist until significant remission occurs, patients should be closely supervised during the early course of therapy.

Haemorrhage: There have been reports of cutaneous bleeding abnormalities such as ecchymoses and purpura with SSRIs.

Caution is advised in patients taking SSRIs, particularly in concomitant use with drugs known to affect platelet function (*e.g.* atypical antipsychotics and phenothiazines, most tricyclic antidepressants, aspirin and non-steroidal anti-inflammatory drugs (NSAIDs)) as well as in patients with a history of bleeding disorders.

Use in renal insufficiency: Since sertraline is extensively metabolised, excretion of unchanged drug in urine is a minor route of elimination. In patients with mild to moderate renal impairment (creatinine clearance 20–50 ml/min) or severe renal impairment (creatinine clearance <20 ml/min), single dose pharmacokinetic parameters were not significantly different compared with controls. However, steady state pharmacokinetics of sertraline have not been adequately studied in this patient population and caution is advised when treating patients with renal impairment.

Use in the elderly: Several hundred elderly patients have participated in clinical studies with Lustral. The pattern and incidence of adverse reactions in the elderly is similar to that in younger patients.

Interactions with other medicaments and other forms of interaction:

Monoamine oxidase inhibitors: (see *Special warnings and special precautions for use*).

Centrally active medication: Caution is advised if Lustral is administered with other centrally active medication.

Alcohol: In 11 healthy subjects administered Lustral

(200 mg daily) for 9 days, there was no adverse effect on cognitive or psychomotor performance relative to placebo, following a single dose of 500 mg/kg alcohol. However, the concomitant use of Lustral and alcohol in depressed patients is not recommended.

Lithium: In placebo-controlled trials in normal volunteers, the co-administration of Lustral and lithium did not significantly alter lithium pharmacokinetics, however it is recommended that plasma lithium levels be monitored following initiation of lithium therapy.

Co-administration of Lustral with lithium did result in an increase in tremor relative to placebo, indicating a possible pharmacodynamic interaction. As with other SSRIs, caution is recommended when co-administering sertraline with medications, such as lithium, which may act via serotonergic mechanisms.

Serotonergic drugs: There is limited controlled experience regarding the optimal timing of switching from other antidepressant drugs to Lustral. Care and prudent medical judgment should be exercised when switching, particularly from long-acting agents. The duration of the washout period which should intervene before switching from one selective serotonin reuptake inhibitor (SSRI) to another has not been established.

Until further data are available, serotonergic drugs, such as tryptophan, sumatriptan or fenfluramine, should not be used concomitantly with Lustral.

Other drug interactions: Since Lustral is bound to plasma proteins, the potential of Lustral to interact with other plasma protein bound drugs should be borne in mind.

Formal drug interaction studies have been performed with Lustral. Co-administration of Lustral (200 mg daily) with diazepam or tolbutamide resulted in small, statistically significant changes in some pharmacokinetic parameters. Co-administration with cimetidine caused a substantial decrease in sertraline clearance. The clinical significance of these changes is unknown. Lustral had no effect on the beta-adrenergic blocking ability of atenolol. No interaction with Lustral (200 mg daily) was observed with glibenclamide or digoxin.

Co-administration of Lustral (200 mg daily) with warfarin resulted in a small but statistically significant increase in prothrombin time, the clinical significance of which is unknown. Accordingly, prothrombin time should be carefully monitored when Lustral therapy is initiated or stopped.

Lustral (200 mg daily), did not potentiate the effects of carbamazepine, haloperidol or phenytoin on cognitive and psychomotor performance in healthy subjects.

Pregnancy and lactation:
Use in pregnancy: Reproduction studies have been performed in rats and rabbits at doses up to approximately 20 times and 10 times the maximum daily human dose, respectively. There was no evidence of teratogenicity or embryotoxicity at any dose level. At the dose level corresponding to approximately 2.5 to 10 times the maximum daily human dose, however, sertraline was associated with delayed ossification in foetuses, probably secondary to effects on the dams.

There was decreased neonatal survival following maternal administration of sertraline at doses approximately 5 times the maximum human dose. Similar effects on neonatal survival have been described for other antidepressant drugs. The clinical significance of these effects is unknown.

There are no adequate and well-controlled studies in pregnant women. Since animal reproduction studies are not always predictive of human response, Lustral should be used during pregnancy only if the perceived benefits outweigh the risks. Women of childbearing potential should employ an adequate method of contraception if taking Lustral.

Use during lactation: Limited data concerning sertraline levels in breast milk are available, hence use in nursing mothers is not recommended.

Effects of ability to drive and use machines: Since antidepressant drugs may impair the abilities required to perform potentially hazardous tasks such as driving a car or operating machinery, the patient should be cautioned accordingly. Lustral should not be administered with benzodiazepines or other tranquillisers in patients who drive or operate machinery.

Undesirable effects: Side-effects which occurred significantly more frequently with Lustral than placebo in multiple dose studies were: nausea, diarrhoea/loose stools, anorexia, dyspepsia, tremor, dizziness, insomnia, somnolence, increased sweating, dry mouth and sexual dysfunction (principally ejaculatory delay in males).

Post-marketing spontaneous reports include the following:

Gastrointestinal: vomiting, abdominal pain.

Nervous system: amnesia, confusion, paraesthesia, hypoaesthesia, depressive symptoms, hallucinations, aggressive reaction, agitation, anxiety and psychosis.

Convulsions (Seizures). Lustral should be discontinued in any patient who develops seizures. See *Special warnings and special precautions for use.*

Movement disorders (such as extrapyramidal symptoms and gait abnormalities); most of these have occurred in patients on concomitant neuroleptic medication or with pre-existing movement disorder.

Hepatic/pancreatic: Rarely, pancreatitis and serious liver events (including hepatitis, jaundice and liver failure). Asymptomatic elevations in serum transaminases (SGOT and SGPT) have been reported infrequently (approximately 0.8%) in association with sertraline administration. The abnormalities usually occurred within the first 1 to 9 weeks of drug treatment and promptly diminished upon drug discontinuation.

Reproductive: hyperprolactinemia, galactorrhoea, menstrual irregularities.

Skin: Rash (including rare reports of erythema multiforme, photosensitivity), angioedema.

Cardiovascular: tachycardia.

Metabolic: Rare cases of hyponatremia have been reported and appeared to be reversible when sertraline was discontinued. Some cases were possibly due to the syndrome of inappropriate antidiuretic hormone secretion. The majority of reports were associated with older patients, and patients taking diuretics or other medications.

Haematologic: There have been rare reports of altered platelet function and/or abnormal clinical laboratory results in patients taking sertraline. While there have been reports of thrombocytopenia, abnormal bleeding or purpura in several patients taking sertraline, it is unclear whether sertraline had a causative role. See also *Special warnings and special precautions for use.*

Musculo-skeletal: arthralgia, myalgia.

General: malaise.

Other: Withdrawal reactions have been reported with Lustral. Common symptoms include dizziness, paraesthesia, headache, anxiety and nausea. Abrupt discontinuation of treatment with Lustral should be avoided. The majority of symptoms experienced on withdrawal of Lustral are non-serious and self-limiting.

Overdose: On the evidence available, Lustral has a wide margin of safety in overdose. Overdoses of Lustral alone of up to 8 g have been reported. Deaths involving overdoses of Lustral in combination with other drugs and/or alcohol have been reported. Therefore, any overdosage should be treated aggressively.

No specific therapy is recommended and there are no specific antidotes to Lustral. Establish and maintain an airway, ensure adequate oxygenation and ventilation. Activated charcoal, which may be used with sorbitol, may be as or more effective than emesis or lavage, and should be considered in treating overdose. Cardiac and vital signs monitoring is recommended along with general symptomatic and supportive measures. Due to the large volume of distribution of sertraline, forced diuresis, dialysis, haemoperfusion and exchange transfusion are unlikely to be of benefit.

Pharmacological properties
Pharmacodynamic properties: Sertraline is a potent and specific inhibitor of neuronal serotonin (5-HT) uptake *in vitro* and *in vivo*, but is without affinity for muscarinic, serotonergic, dopaminergic, adrenergic, histaminergic, GABA or benzodiazepine receptors.

Sertraline is devoid of stimulant, sedative or anticholinergic activity or cardiotoxicity in animals.

Unlike tricyclic antidepressants, no weight gain is observed with treatment for depression.

Lustral has not been observed to produce physical or psychological dependence.

Pharmacokinetic properties: Sertraline exhibits dose proportional pharmacokinetics over a range of 50–200 mg. After oral administration of sertraline in man, peak blood levels occur at about 4.5–8.4 hours. Daily doses of sertraline achieve steady-state after one week. Sertraline has a plasma half-life of approximately 26 hours with a mean half-life for young and elderly adults ranging from 22–36 hours. Sertraline is approximately 98% bound to plasma proteins. The principal metabolite, N-desmethylsertraline, is inactive in *in vivo* models of depression and has a half-life of approximately 62–104 hours. Sertraline and N-desmethylsertraline are both extensively metabolised in man and the resultant metabolites excreted in faeces and urine in equal amounts. Only a small amount (<0.2%) of unchanged sertraline is excreted in the urine.

The pharmacokinetics of sertraline in elderly patients are similar to younger adults.

Food does not significantly change the bioavailability of Lustral tablets.

Preclinical safety data: Extensive chronic safety evaluation studies in animals show that sertraline is generally well tolerated at doses that are appreciable multiples of those that are clinically effective.

Pharmaceutical particulars
List of excipients: Sertraline tablets include the following inert ingredients: calcium hydrogen phosphate, microcrystalline cellulose, hydroxypropylcellulose, sodium starch glycollate, magnesium stearate, hydroxypropylmethylcellulose, polyethylene glycol, polysorbate-80, titanium dioxide (E171).

Incompatibilities: None.

Shelf life: Current stability data for tablets supports a shelf life of 5 years.

Special precautions for storage: None.

Nature and contents of container: Lustral is available as: Calendar packs of 28 tablets. Aluminium/PVC blister strips, 14 tablets/strip, 2 strips in a carton box.

Instructions for use/handling: No special requirements.

Marketing authorisation numbers
Lustral Tablets 50 mg 0057/0308
Lustral Tablets 100 mg 0057/0309

Date of renewal of the authorisation 30 September 1997

Date of (partial) revision of the text 26 August 1998

Legal category POM.

NEPHRIL* TABLETS

Qualitative and quantitative composition Active ingredient: Polythiazide equivalent to 1 mg.

Pharmaceutical form Tablets. White round tablets scored and marked NEP/1 on one side and 'Pfizer' on the reverse.

Clinical particulars
Therapeutic indications: Nephril is indicated as adjunctive therapy in oedema associated with congestive heart failure, hepatic cirrhosis and corticosteroid and oestrogen therapy.

Nephril has also been found useful in oedema due to various forms of renal dysfunction such as nephrotic syndrome, acute glomerulonephritis and chronic renal failure.

Nephril is indicated in the management of hypertension either as the sole therapeutic agent or to enhance the effectiveness of other antihypertensive drugs in the more severe forms of hypertension.

Posology and method of administration: Nephril is administered by the oral route.

The usual dosage of Nephril for diuretic therapy is 1 to 4 mg daily.

For antihypertensive therapy the usual maintenance dose is between 2 mg and 4 mg daily although some patients may be optimally controlled on 500 micrograms or 1 mg daily.

Use in children: Nephril is not recommended for children.

Use in the elderly: Elderly patients are especially liable to the adverse effects of diuretic agents. It is therefore particularly important that the dose should be the lowest possible consistent with adequate effect (see dosage above). The possibility of drug interactions should also be considered in view of the frequency of multiple drug therapy in this age group.

Use in renal insufficiency: Thiazides should be used with caution in severe renal disease. In patients with renal disease, thiazides may precipitate azotaemia. Cumulative effects of the drug may develop in patients with impaired renal function. If progressive renal impairment becomes evident, as indicated by a rising non-protein nitrogen or blood urea nitrogen, a careful reappraisal of therapy is necessary with probably cessation of treatment.

Use in hepatic disease: Thiazides should be used with caution in patients with impaired hepatic function or progressive liver disease, since minor alterations of fluid and electrolyte balance may precipitate hepatic coma.

Contra-indications: Anuria, hypersensitivity to polythiazide and other thiazide diuretics and other sulphonamide derived drugs.

Special warnings and precautions for use: All patients receiving thiazide therapy should have periodic determinations of serum electrolytes at appropriate intervals to detect possible electrolyte imbalance. Such patients should also be observed for clinical signs of fluid or electrolyte imbalance, namely hyponatraemia, hypochloraemic alkalosis and hypokalaemia. Serum and urine electrolyte determinations are particularly important when the patient is vomiting or receiving parenteral fluids. Warning signs of possible electrolyte imbalance, irrespective of cause, are: dryness of mouth, thirst, weakness, lethargy, drowsiness, restlessness, muscle pains or cramps, muscular fatigue, hypotension, oliguria, tachycardia and gastro-intestinal disturbances such as nausea and vomiting.

Hypokalaemia may develop with thiazides as with any other potent diuretics, especially with brisk diuresis, when severe cirrhosis is present, or during concomitant use of corticosteroids or ACTH.

Interference with adequate oral electrolyte intake will also contribute to hypokalaemia.

Hypokalaemia may exaggerate metabolic effects of digitalis therapy especially with reference to myocardial activity.

Any chloride deficit is generally mild and usually does not require specific treatment except under extraordinary circumstances (as in liver disease or renal disease). Dilutional hyponatraemia may occur in oedematous patients in hot weather; appropriate therapy is water restriction, rather than administration of salt except in those rare instances when the hyponatraemia is life threatening. In actual salt depletion, appropriate replacement is the therapy of choice.

Hyperuricaemia may occur or frank gout may be precipitated in certain patients receiving thiazide therapy.

Insulin requirements in diabetic patients may be increased, decreased or unchanged. Latent diabetes mellitus may become manifest during thiazide administration.

Thiazide drugs may increase the responsiveness to tubocurarine.

The antihypertensive effects of thiazides may be enhanced in the post-sympathectomy patient. Thiazides may decrease arterial responsiveness to noradrenaline. This diminution is not sufficient to preclude effectiveness of the pressor agent for therapeutic use.

If progressive renal impairment becomes evident, as indicated by a rising non-protein nitrogen or blood urea nitrogen a careful reappraisal of therapy is necessary with probable discontinuation of therapy with Nephril.

Thiazides may decrease serum protein-bound iodine levels without signs of thyroid disturbance.

Interactions with other medicaments and other forms of interaction:

Corticosteroids or ACTH: When co-prescribed with polythiazide, corticosteroids or ACTH may enhance total potassium loss. It is recommended that electrolyte balance is carefully monitored.

Cardiac glycosides/antiarrhythmics: The possibility that the toxicity of cardiac glycosides, e.g. digitoxin or antiarrhythmics may be enhanced by polythiazide induced hypokalaemia should be borne in mind. Additional care should be taken in prescribing quinidine since plasma levels may be raised due to the urine alkalizing effect of thiazides.

Antihypertensive drugs: Thiazides may add to or potentiate the action of other antihypertensive drugs. Potentiation occurs with ganglionic or peripheral adrenergic blocking drugs.

Antidiabetic drugs: Requirement for antidiabetic therapy may be increased, decreased or unchanged. Diabetic patients should be monitored for possible decreased diabetic control.

Tubocurarine: Thiazide drugs may increase responsiveness to tubocurarine.

Pregnancy and lactation:

Use in pregnancy: The routine use of diuretics in healthy pregnant women is inappropriate and may expose mother and foetus to unnecessary hazard. Diuretics do not prevent development of toxaemia of pregnancy and there is no satisfactory evidence that they are useful in the treatment of established toxaemia.

Oedema during pregnancy may arise from pathological cause or from physiological and mechanical consequences of pregnancy. Physiological hypervolaemia during pregnancy may be associated with generalised oedema including dependent oedema. This oedema is properly treated by recumbency and support hose. Thiazides may be indicated in pregnancy when oedema is due to pathological causes other than toxaemia. Rarely, short courses of thiazides are indicated when physiological oedema is unrelieved by rest and where the oedema causes extreme discomfort.

Thiazides cross the placental barrier and appear in cord blood. The use of thiazides in pregnant women requires that the anticipated benefit be weighed against possible hazards to the foetus. These hazards include foetal or neonatal jaundice, thrombocytopenia and other side-effects which have occurred in the adult.

Use in lactation: Thiazides appear in breast milk. If use of Nephril is deemed essential, breast feeding should be discontinued.

Effects on ability to drive and use machines: None stated.

Undesirable effects:

Gastrointestinal: Anorexia, gastric irritation, nausea, vomiting, cramping, diarrhoea, constipation, jaundice (intrahepatic cholestatic jaundice), pancreatitis.

Central nervous system: Dizziness, vertigo, paraesthesia, headache, xanthopsia.

Haematological: Leucopenia, agranulocytosis, thrombocytopenia, aplastic anaemia.

Dermatological: Purpura, photosensitivity, rash, urticaria, necrotising angiitis (vasculitis) (cutaneous vasculitis).

Cardiovascular: Orthostatic hypotension may occur and be aggravated by alcohol, barbiturates or narcotics.

Other: Hyperglycaemia, glycosuria, hyperuricaemia, muscle spasm, weakness, restlessness.

Whenever adverse reactions are moderate or severe, thiazide dosage should be reduced or therapy withdrawn.

Thiazides may add to or potentiate the action of other hypertensive drugs. Potentiation occurs with ganglionic or peripheral adrenergic blocking drugs.

Sensitivity reactions may occur in patients with a history of allergy or bronchial asthma. The possibility of exacerbation or activation of systemic lupus erythematosus has been reported.

Overdose: Gastric lavage and supportive therapy. Treatment of acute renal failure if present. Potassium supplements.

Pharmacological properties

Pharmacodynamic properties: Nephril (polythiazide) is one of the thiazide diuretics, all of which have an identical mode of action as diuretic agents. The chief mechanism of action is interference with the distal renal tubular mechanism of electrolyte reabsorption and, in particular, at the cortical diluting site. Thiazides are also antihypertensive agents although their mode of action is uncertain. Their use as antihypertensive agents is initially associated with a fall in plasma volume and, in the longer term, with a modest reduction in total peripheral resistance.

The therapeutic effects, mode of action and adverse effects of the thiazide diuretics are identical. Such differences as exist between the various compounds are related to milligram potency and duration of action.

Pharmacokinetic properties: Nephril has a long duration of action in man (24–48 hours) and an elimination half-life of approximately 26 hours. It is rapidly absorbed from the gastrointestinal tract and usually shows an effect within 1 hour of administration.

Increased lipid solubility, compared with other thiazides, is associated with larger apparent volume of distribution, lower renal clearance and binding to tissue elements.

Preclinical safety data: None.

Pharmaceutical particulars

List of excipients: Calcium phosphate dibasic, lactose, maize starch, vanillin, magnesium stearate, sodium lauryl sulphate, purified water for starch paste (not present in final product).

Incompatibilities: None stated.

Shelf life: 5 years.

Special precautions for storage: Store below 25°C.

Nature and contents of container: White opaque HDPE bottle with child resistant cap, containing 28 tablets.

Instructions for use/handling: None.

Date of renewal of the authorisation 6 March 1992.

Marketing authorisation number 0057/5024R.

Date of (partial) revision of the text 7 October 1996.

Legal category POM.

SINEQUAN*

Qualitative and quantitative composition Active Ingredient: Doxepin Hydrochloride BP

The capsules contain Doxepin Hydrochloride BP equivalent to 10, 25, 50 or 75 mg doxepin.

Pharmaceutical form Capsules for oral administration.

Clinical particulars

Therapeutic indications: Symptoms of depressive illness, especially where sedation is required.

Posology and method of administration:

Dosage: The optimum oral dose depends on the severity of the condition and the individual patient's response. The dose varies from 30-300 mg daily. Doses up to 100 mg daily may be given on a divided or once daily schedule. Should doses over 100 mg daily be required, they should be administered in three divided doses daily. 100 mg is the maximum dose recommended at any one time. This dose may be given at bedtime.

For the majority of patients with moderate or severe symptoms, it is recommended that treatment commences with an initial dose of 75 mg daily. Many of these patients will respond satisfactorily at this dose level. For patients who do not, the dosage may be adjusted according to individual response. In more severely ill patients, it may be necessary to administer a dose of up to 300 mg in divided doses daily, to obtain a clinical response.

In patients where insomnia is a troublesome symptom, it is recommended that the total daily dose be divided so that a higher proportion is given for the evening dose; similarly, if drowsiness is experienced as a side effect of treatment, Sinequan may be administered by this regimen or the dosage may be reduced. It is often possible, having once obtained a satisfactory therapeutic response, to reduce the dose for maintenance therapy.

The optimal antidepressant effect may not be evident for two to three weeks.

Use in children: The use of Sinequan in children under 12 years is not recommended because safe conditions for its use have not been established.

Use in the elderly: In general, lower doses are recommended. Where the presenting symptoms are mild in nature, it is advisable to initiate treatment at a dose of 10–50 mg daily. A satisfactory clinical response is obtained in many of these patients at a daily dose of 30–50 mg. The dosage may be adjusted according to the individual response.

Use in hepatic impairment: Dosage reduction may be required in patients with hepatic impairment. (See under *Special warnings and special precautions for use*).

Use in renal impairment: (See under *Special warnings and special precautions for use*).

Contra-indications: Hypersensitivity, mania, severe liver disease, lactation, glaucoma, tendency to urinary retention.

Special warnings and special precautions for use: The once-a-day dosage regimen of Sinequan in patients with intercurrent illness or patients taking other medications should be carefully adjusted. This is especially important in patients receiving other medications with anticholinergic effects.

The use of Sinequan on a once-a-day dosage regimen in geriatric patients should be adjusted carefully on the basis of the patient's condition. The elderly are particularly liable to experience toxic effects, especially agitation, confusion and postural hypotension. The initial dose should be increased with caution under close supervision. Half the normal maintenance dose may be sufficient to produce a satisfactory clinical response.

Patients should be warned that drowsiness may occur with the use of Sinequan. Patients should also be cautioned that their response to alcohol may be potentiated.

Use with caution in patients with severe cardiovascular disease, including patients with heart block, cardiac arrhythmia and those who have experienced a recent myocardial infarction.

Use in hepatic/renal impairment: Use with caution in patients with hepatic and/or renal impairment.

Use in patients with epilepsy: Use with caution in patients with a history of epilepsy.

Since suicide is an inherent risk in any depressed patient until significant improvement has occurred, patients should be closely supervised during early therapy.

Interactions with other medicaments and other forms of treatment: Combined use with other antidepressants, alcohol or anti-anxiety agents should be undertaken with due recognition of the possibility of potentiation. It is known, for example, that monoamine oxidase inhibitors may potentiate other drug effects, therefore Sinequan should not be given concurrently, or within two weeks of cessation of therapy, with monoamine oxidase inhibitors.

Cimetidine has been reported to produce clinically significant fluctuations in steady-state serum concentrations of various tricyclic antidepressants.

Sinequan should not be given with sympathomimetic agents such as ephedrine, isoprenaline, noradrenaline, phenylephrine and phenylpropanolamine.

General anaesthetics and local anaesthetics (containing sympathomimetics) given during tricyclic or tetracyclic antidepressant therapy may increase the risk of arrhythmias and hypotension, or hypertension. If surgery is necessary, the anaesthetist should be informed that a patient is being so treated.

Sinequan may decrease the antihypertensive effect of agents such as debrisoquine, bethanidine, guanethidine and possibly clonidine. It usually requires daily doses of Sinequan in excess of 150 mg before any effect on the action of guanethidine is seen. It would be advisable to review all antihypertensive therapy during treatment with tricyclic antidepressants.

Barbiturates may increase the rate of metabolism of Sinequan.

The dose of thyroid hormone medication may need reducing if Sinequan is being given concurrently.

Tolazamide: a case of severe hypoglycaemia, 11 days after the addition of doxepin (75 mg/day) has been reported in a non-insulin dependent diabetic patient maintained on tolazamide (1 g/day).

Pregnancy and lactation: Doxepin crosses the placenta. Reproduction studies have been performed in rats, rabbits and monkeys and there was no evidence

of harm to the animal foetus. The relevance to humans is not known. Since there is insufficient experience in pregnant women who have received this drug, its safety in pregnancy has not been established.
Doxepin and its active metabolite desmethyldoxepin are excreted in breast milk. There has been a report of apnoea and drowsiness occurring in a nursing infant whose mother was taking doxepin . The use of Sinequan is contraindicated during lactation.

Effects on ability to drive and use machines: Since drowsiness may occur with the use of Sinequan, patients should be warned of the possibility and cautioned against driving a car or operating machinery while taking this drug.

Undesirable effects: Sinequan is well tolerated. Most side-effects are mild and generally disappear with continued treatment, or if necessary a reduction in dose.

Note: Some of the side-effects noted below have not been specifically reported with Sinequan. However, due to the close pharmacological similarities amongst the tricyclics, the reactions should be considered when prescribing Sinequan.

The most common side-effects to Sinequan are drowsiness, dry mouth and constipation. For further details see below under central nervous system and anticholinergic effects.

Anticholinergic effects: Anticholinergic effects are relatively common and may occur immediately following the first dose of a tricyclic antidepressant. Dry mouth and constipation are the most common anticholinergic effects. Blurred vision and sweating occur occasionally. Urinary retention is rare except in predisposed males who have an enlarged prostate gland. Tolerance is often achieved if treatment is continued. If these undesirable effects do not subside with continued therapy, or if they become severe, it may be necessary to reduce the dosage.

Central nervous system effects: Drowsiness is the most commonly noticed side effect. This tends to disappear as therapy is continued. Other infrequently reported CNS side effects are confusion, disorientation, agitation, numbness or paraesthesiae, tremor (which is usually mild). But at high doses, in susceptible individuals (particularly the elderly) other extrapyramidal symptoms may occur including tardive dyskinesia. Rarely reported are hallucinations, ataxia (generally where mixtures of CNS drugs have been given), and convulsions. Convulsions are unlikely except in people predisposed to seizure activity by brain damage or alcohol and drug abuse.

Psychotic manifestations, including mania and paranoid delusions may be exacerbated during treatment with tricyclic antidepressants.

Cardiovascular: Although Sinequan carries less risk than other tricyclic antidepressants, caution should be observed in the treatment of patients with heart block or cardiac arrhythmias. Cardiovascular effects including postural hypotension, and tachycardia have been reported occasionally.

Allergic: Allergic reactions to tricyclic antidepressants are uncommon . They include skin rash, facial oedema, photosensitisation and pruritus.

Haematological: Rare cases of eosinophilia and bone marrow depression manifesting as agranulocytosis, leucopenia, thrombocytopenia and purpura.

Gastro-intestinal: Nausea, vomiting, indigestion, taste disturbances, diarrhoea, anorexia and aphthous stomatitis have been reported. (See *Anticholinergic effects*).

Endocrine: Occasional reports of raised or lowered libido, testicular swelling, raised or lowered blood sugar levels. Rarely the syndrome of inappropriate antidiuretic hormone secretion, gynaecomastia, enlargement of breasts and galactorrhoea in the female.

Other: Dizziness, weight gain, chills, fatigue, weakness, flushing, alopecia, headache, exacerbation of asthma and hyperpyrexia (in association with chlorpromazine) have been occasionally observed. Rare reports of jaundice and of tinnitus.

Withdrawal: Withdrawal symptoms may occur on abrupt cessation of tricyclic antidepressant therapy and include insomnia, irritability and excessive perspiration. Withdrawal symptoms in neonates whose mothers received tricyclic antidepressants during the third trimester have also been reported and include respiratory depression, convulsions and "jitteriness" (hyper-reflexia).

Overdose: Signs and symptoms:

1. Mild: drowsiness, stupor, blurred vision, excessive dryness of mouth.

2. Severe: respiratory depression, hypotension, coma, convulsions, cardiac arrhythmias and tachycardias.

Also: urinary retention (bladder atony), decreased gastrointestinal motility (paralytic ileus), hyperthermia (or hypothermia), hypertension, dilated pupils, hyperactive reflexes.

Management and treatment:

1. Mild: observation and supportive therapy is all that is usually necessary.

2. Severe: medical management of severe Sinequan overdosage consists of aggressive supportive therapy. If the patient is conscious, gastric lavage with appropriate precautions to prevent pulmonary aspiration should be performed even though Sinequan is rapidly absorbed. The use of activated charcoal has been recommended, as has been continuous gastric lavage with saline for 24 hours or more. An adequate airway should be established in comatose patients and assisted ventilation used if necessary. ECG monitoring may be required for several days, since relapse after apparent recovery has been reported. Arrhythmias should be treated with the appropriate anti-arrhythmic agent. It has been reported that many of the cardiovascular and CNS symptoms of tricyclic antidepressant poisoning in adults may be reversed by the slow intravenous administration of 1 mg to 3 mg of physostigmine salicylate.

Because physostigmine is rapidly metabolised, the dosage should be repeated as required. Convulsions may respond to standard anticonvulsant therapy. However, barbiturates may potentiate any respiratory depression. Dialysis and forced diuresis generally are not of value in the management of overdosage due to high tissue and protein binding of Sinequan.

Pharmacological properties

Pharmacodynamic poperties: The mechanism of action of Sinequan is not definitely known. It is not a central nervous system stimulant nor a monoamine oxidase inhibitor. The current hypothesis is that the clinical effects are due, at least in part, to influences on the adrenergic activity at the synapses so that deactivation of noradrenaline by reuptake into the nerve terminals is prevented. In animal studies anticholinergic, antiserotonergic and antihistaminergic effects on smooth muscle have been demonstrated. At higher than usual clinical doses, adrenaline response was potentiated in animals. This effect was not demonstrated in humans.

Pharmacokinetic Properties: Doxepin is well absorbed from the gastrointestinal tract. Approximately 55%–87% of orally administered doxepin undergoes first pass metabolism in the liver, forming the primary active metabolite desmethyldoxepin.

In healthy volunteers, a single oral dose of 75 mg resulted in peak plasma concentrations for doxepin ranging from 8.8–45.8 ng/ml (mean 26.1 ng/ml). Peak levels were reached between 2 and 4 hours (mean 2.9 hours) after administration. Peak levels for the primary metabolite desmethyldoxepin ranged from 4.8–14.5 ng/ml (mean 9.7 ng/ml) and were achieved between 2 and 10 hours after administration. The mean apparent volume of distribution for doxepin is approximately 20 l/kg. The protein binding for doxepin is approximately 76%. In healthy volunteers the plasma elimination half-life of doxepin ranged from 8 to 24 hours (mean 17 hours). The half-life of desmethyldoxepin ranged from 33–80 hours (mean 51 hours). Mean plasma clearance for doxepin is approximately 0.84 l/kg.hr. Paths of metabolism of doxepin include demethylation, N-oxidation, hydroxylation and glucuronide formation. Doxepin is excreted primarily in the urine, mainly as its metabolites, either free or in conjugate form.

Pharmaceutical particulars

List of excipients: Sinequan 10 mg capsule: lactose, magnesium stearate, maize starch dried, sodium lauryl sulphate; capsule shell constituents: amaranth (E123), erythrosine (E127), gelatin, sunset yellow (E110) and titanium dioxide (E171).

Sinequan 25 mg capsule: lactose, magnesium stearate, maize starch dried, sodium lauryl sulphate; capsule shell constituents: amaranth (E123), erythrosine (E127), gelatin, patent blue V(E131), sunset yellow (E110) and titanium dioxide (E171).

Sinequan 50 mg capsule: lactose, magnesium stearate, maize starch dried, sodium lauryl sulphate; capsule shell constituents: erythrosine (E127), gelatin, patent blue V (E131) and titanium dioxide (E171).

Sinequan 75 mg capsule: magnesium stearate, maize starch dried, sodium lauryl sulphate; capsule shell constituents: erythrosine (E127), gelatin, patent blue V (E131) , quinoline yellow (E104), and titanium dioxide (E171).

Sinequan capsules are free of gluten and sucrose.

Incompatibilities: None known.

Shelf life: 3 years.

Storage conditions: Store below 25°C.

Nature and contents of container: Sinequan 10 mg capsules are available as:

Packs of 56 capsules. Aluminium/PVC blister strips; 2 rows of 7 capsules per strip, 4 strips in a carton box.

Packs of 560 capsules in a capsule container (not manufactured).

Sinequan 25 mg capsules are available as:

Packs of 28 capsules. Aluminium/PVC blister strips; 2 rows of 7 capsules per strip, 2 strips in a carton box.

Packs of 560 capsules in a capsule container (not manufactured).

Sinequan 50 mg capsules are available as:

Packs of 28 capsules. Aluminium/PVC blister strips; 2 rows of 7 capsules per strip, 2 strips in a carton box.

Packs of 280 capsules in a capsule container (not manufactured).

Sinequan 75 mg capsules are available as:

Packs of 28 capsules. Aluminium/PVC blister strips; 2 rows of 7 capsules per strip, 2 strips in a carton box.

Packs of 280 capsules in a capsule container (not manufactured).

Instructions for use/handling: No special requirements.

Marketing authorisation numbers

Sinequan capsules 10 mg	PL 0057/5032R
Sinequan capsules 25 mg	PL 0057/5033R
Sinequan capsules 50 mg	PL 0057/5034R
Sinequan capsules 75 mg	PL 0057/0133

Date of renewal of the authorisation

Sinequan capsules 10 mg	30/09/96
Sinequan capsules 25 mg	30/09/96
Sinequan capsules 50 mg	30/09/96
Sinequan capsules 75 mg	12/09/96

Date of (partial) revision of the text September 1996

Legal category POM

TERRAMYCIN*

Presentation Terramycin (oxytetracycline) is available as:

Tablets 250 mg: Sugar-coated yellow tablets, containing 250 mg Oxytetracycline Dihydrate PhEur and coded 'Pfizer'.

Capsules 250 mg: Hard gelatin capsules, opaque yellow cap and body printed TER250 and 'Pfizer', each containing 250 mg Oxytetracycline as the Hydrochloride PhEur.

Inactive excipients: Terramycin capsules: magnesium stearate, maize starch and sodium lauryl sulphate. In addition the capsule shell contains: erythrosine, gelatin, quinoline yellow and titanium dioxide.

Terramycin tablets: alginic acid, magnesium stearate and maize starch. In addition, the tablet coating contains: beeswax white, carnauba wax, gelatin, gum acacia, kaolin, methyl hydroxybenzoate, quinoline yellow, shellac orange, sucrose, sunset yellow, talc and titanium dioxide.

Uses *Actions:* Oxytetracycline is primarily bacteriostatic and is thought to exert its antimicrobial effect by the inhibition of protein synthesis. Terramycin is active against a wide range of Gram-negative and Gram-positive organisms.

The drugs in the tetracycline class have closely similar antimicrobial spectra, and cross resistance among them is common.

Oxytetracycline and its salts are readily absorbed orally and are 10–40% bound to plasma proteins. Between 40 and 70% is excreted unchanged in the urine via glomerular filtration. A serum half-life of 6–10 hours has been reported for Terramycin in patients with normal renal function.

Oxytetracycline diffuses readily through the placenta into the foetal circulation, into the pleural fluid and, under some circumstances, into the cerebrospinal fluid. It appears to be well concentrated in the hepatic system and excreted in the bile, so that it appears in the faeces, as well as in the urine, in a biologically active form.

Indications: Respiratory tract infections: Pneumonia and other lower respiratory tract infections due to susceptible strains of *Streptococcus pneumoniae, Haemophilus influenzae, Klebsiella pneumoniae* and other organisms. *Mycoplasma pneumoniae* pneumonia. Treatment of chronic bronchitis.

Urinary tract infections: caused by susceptible strains of the Klebsiella species. Enterobacter species, *Escherichia coli, Streptococcus faecalis* and other organisms.

Sexually transmitted diseases: Infections due to *Chlamydia trachomatis* including uncomplicated urethral, endocervical or rectal infections. Non-gonococcal urethritis caused by *Ureaplasma urealyticum.* Terramycin is also indicated in chancroid, granuloma inguinale and lymphogranuloma venereum.

Terramycin is an alternative drug in the treatment of gonorrhoea and syphilis.

Skin infections: Acne vulgaris when antibiotic therapy is considered necessary and severe rosacea.

Ophthalmic infections: Trachoma, although the infectious agent, as judged by immunofluorescence, is not always eliminated. Inclusion conjunctivitis may be treated with oral Terramycin alone or in combination with topical agents.

Rickettsial infections: Rocky Mountain spotted fever, typhus group, Q fever and Coxiella endocarditis and tick fevers.

Other infections: Stagnant loop syndrome. Psittacosis, brucellosis (in combination with streptomycin), cholera, bubonic plague, louse and tick-borne relapsing fever, tularaemia, glanders, melioidosis and acute intestinal amoebiasis (as an adjunct to amoebicides).

Terramycin is an alternative drug in the treatment of leptospirosis, gas-gangrene and tetanus.

Dosage and administration The usual daily dose of Terramycin is 1–2 g, given in four equal doses, depending on the severity of the infection.

Therapy should be continued for at least 24–48 hours after symptoms and fever have subsided.

Food, milk and some dairy products interfere with absorption. Tetracyclines should be given one hour before or two hours after meals.

Administration of adequate amounts of fluid along with capsules and tablet forms of drugs in the tetracycline class is recommended to reduce the risk of oesophageal irritation and ulceration.

Dosage recommendation in specific infections:

Acne vulgaris and severe rosacea: Terramycin 250–500 mg daily in single or divided doses.

Brucellosis: Terramycin 500 mg, four times daily in combination with streptomycin.

Sexually Transmitted Diseases: Terramycin 500 mg four times daily for 7 days is recommended in the following infections: uncomplicated gonococcal infections (except anorectal infections in man); uncomplicated urethral, endocervical or rectal infection caused by *Chlamydia trachomatis*; non-gonococcal urethritis caused by *Ureaplasma urealyticum*.

Acute epididymo-orchitis caused by *Chlamydia trachomatis*, or *Neisseria gonorrhoeae*, Terramycin 500 mg, four times daily for 10 days.

Primary and secondary syphilis: Terramycin 500 mg, four times daily for 15 days. Syphilis of more than 1 year's duration, (latent syphilis of uncertain or more than 1 year's duration, cardiovascular or late benign syphilis) except neurosyphilis, should be treated with Terramycin 500 mg, four times daily for 30 days. Patient compliance with this regimen may be difficult so care should be taken to encourage optimal compliance. Close follow-up, including laboratory tests, is recommended.

Use in the elderly: See 'Precautions' section.

Use in children: Terramycin is contra-indicated in children under the age of 12 years. See 'Contra-indications' section.

Contra-indications, warnings, etc

Contra-indications: Terramycin is contra-indicated in persons who have shown hypersensitivity to any of the tetracyclines.

Pregnancy: Terramycin is contra-indicated in pregnancy. If this drug is used during pregnancy, or if the patient becomes pregnant while taking this drug, the patient should be apprised of the potential hazard to the foetus.

Results of animal studies with the tetracycline family of antimicrobials indicate that tetracyclines cross the placenta, are found in foetal tissues and can have toxic effects on the developing foetus. Evidence of embryo-toxicity has also been noted in animals treated early in pregnancy.

It appears that the risks associated with the use of tetracyclines during pregnancy are predominantly due to effects on teeth and skeletal development. (See below about use during tooth development).

Nursing mothers: Tetracyclines are excreted into milk and are therefore contra-indicated in nursing mothers.

Children: Terramycin is contra-indicated in children under the age of 12 years. As with other tetracyclines, Terramycin forms a stable calcium complex in any bone-forming tissue. A decrease in the fibula growth rate has been observed in premature infants given oral tetracyclines in doses of 25 mg/kg every six hours. This reaction was shown to be reversible when the drug was discontinued.

The use of drugs of the tetracycline class during tooth development (pregnancy, infancy and childhood up to the age of 12 years) may cause permanent discolouration of the teeth (yellow-grey-brown) and enamel hypoplasia. This adverse reaction is more common during long-term use of the drug but has been observed following repeated short-term courses.

Renal impairment: Administration of usual doses may lead to excessive systemic accumulation of the drug and liver toxicity.

The anti-anabolic action of the tetracyclines may cause an increase in blood urea; while this is not a problem in those with normal renal function, in patients with significantly impaired renal function, higher levels of tetracycline may lead to azotaemia, hyperphosphataemia and acidosis.

Precautions: Terramycin should be administered with caution to patients with hepatic impairment or those receiving potentially hepatotoxic drugs.

The use of antibiotics may occasionally result in the overgrowth of nonsusceptible organisms including *Candida*. Constant observation of the patient is essential. If a resistant organism appears, the antibiotic should be discontinued and appropriate therapy instituted.

When treating venereal disease, where co-existent syphilis is suspected, proper diagnostic procedures should be utilized. In all such cases monthly serological tests should be made for at least four months.

Terramycin should not be given concurrently with bactericidal drugs such as penicillins.

In long term therapy, periodic laboratory evaluation of organ systems, including haematopoietic, renal and hepatic studies should be performed.

All infections due to Group A beta-haemolytic streptococci should be treated for at least 10 days.

Use in the elderly: Terramycin may be given in the usual adult dosage. The possibility of sub-clinical renal insufficiency should be kept in mind, as it may lead to drug accumulation (see *Contra-indications*).

Drug interactions: Antacids containing aluminium, calcium, magnesium, zinc or iron salts, may impair absorption of oxytetracycline.

In long term therapy, tetracyclines depress plasma prothrombin activity and reduced doses of concomitant anticoagulants may be necessary.

A few cases of pregnancy or breakthrough bleeding have been attributed to the concurrent use of tetracycline or oxytetracycline with oral contraceptives.

The concurrent use of tetracyclines and methoxyflurane has been reported to result in fatal renal toxicity.

Side-effects: Gastro-intestinal: Anorexia, nausea, vomiting, diarrhoea, glossitis, dysphagia, enterocolitis, and inflammatory lesions (with candidial overgrowth) in the anogenital regions. Rare instances of oesophagitis and oesophageal ulceration have been reported in patients receiving capsule and tablet forms of drugs in the tetracycline class. Most of these patients took medication immediately before going to bed.

Skin: Maculopapular and erythematous rashes. Exfoliative dermatitis has been reported but is uncommon. Photosensitivity manifested by an exaggerated sunburn reaction has been observed in some individuals taking tetracyclines. Patients likely to be exposed to direct sunlight or ultraviolet light should be advised that this reaction can occur with tetracyclines and treatment should be discontinued at the first evidence of skin erythema.

Hypersensitivity reactions: Urticaria, angioneurotic oedema, anaphylaxis, anaphylactoid purpura, pericarditis, and exacerbation of systemic lupus erythematosus.

Bulging fontanelles in infants and benign intracranial hypertension in adults have been reported in individuals receiving full therapeutic dosages of tetracyclines. These conditions disappeared rapidly when the drug was discontinued.

Blood: Haemolytic anaemia, thrombocytopenia, neutropenia and eosinophilia have been reported with tetracyclines.

When given over prolonged periods, tetracyclines have been reported to produce brown-black microscopic discolouration of thyroid tissue. No abnormalities of thyroid function are known to occur.

Overdosage: Acute overdosage with antibiotics is rare. In the event of overdosage, gastric lavage plus appropriate supportive treatment is indicated.

Pharmaceutical precautions Store below 25°C. Protect from light.

Legal category POM.

Package quantities Tablets 250 mg: Original packs of 28 tablets. Capsules 250 mg: Original packs of 28 capsules.

Further information Nil.

Product licence numbers

Tablets 250 mg	0057/5080R
Capsules 250 mg	0057/5036R

TERRA-CORTRIL* TOPICAL OINTMENT

Presentation Terra-Cortril Topical Ointment contains 30 mg Oxytetracycline as the Hydrochloride PhEur and 10 mg Hydrocortisone PhEur in each gram of paraffin base, comprising white soft and liquid paraffin.

Uses

Actions: Terra-Cortril Topical Ointment possesses both the anti-inflammatory activity of hydrocortisone and the broad-spectrum antibacterial activity of oxytetracycline, which is active against a wide variety of Gram-positive and Gram-negative organisms.

Where topical therapy with hydrocortisone is of value the concurrent use of oxytetracycline may help eradicate secondary bacterial infection.

Indications: Terra-Cortril Topical Ointment is indicated in the following disorders: exudative and secondarily infected eczema including atopic eczema, primary irritant dermatitis, allergic and seborrhoeic dermatitis. Secondarily infected insect bite reactions.

In exudative flexural intertrigo Terra-Cortril Topical Ointment can be used for up to seven days.

Like other tetracyclines, oxytetracycline is generally ineffective against Pseudomonas and Proteus species. Because these are recognised secondary infecting organisms in exudative dermatoses, preliminary identification of the organism and determination of antibiotic sensitivity is important.

Terra-Cortril Topical Ointment is for topical administration only.

Dosage and administration

Adults: After thorough cleansing of the affected skin areas, a small amount of the ointment should be applied gently two to four times daily.

Use in the elderly: No special precautions.

Use in children: Not recommended. See 'Contra-indications'.

Contra-indications, warnings, etc

Contra-indications:

1. Hypersensitivity to any of the components of the preparation.
2. Primary bacterial infections, e.g. impetigo, pyoderma, furunculosis.
3. Acute herpes simplex, vaccinia and varicella.
4. Tuberculosis of the skin.
5. Fungal diseases of the skin.
6. Pregnancy, and in infants and small children because of the theoretical risk of damage to permanent dentition.

Precautions: If irritation develops, the product should be discontinued.

Terra-Cortril Topical Ointment should not be continued for more than seven days in the absence of any clinical improvement, since in this situation occult extension of infection may occur due to the masking effect of the steroid.

Extended or recurrent application may increase the risk of contact sensitization and should be avoided.

The use of oxytetracycline and other antibiotics may result in an overgrowth of resistant organisms – particularly *Candida* and Staphylococci. Careful observation of the patient for this possibility is essential. If new infections due to nonsusceptible bacteria or fungi appear during therapy, Terra-Cortril Topical Ointment should be discontinued.

If extensive areas are treated or if the occlusive technique is used, there may be increased systemic absorption of the corticosteroid and suitable precautions should be taken.

Terra-Cortril Topical Ointment is not recommended for ophthalmic use.

Side-effects: Hydrocortisone and oxytetracycline are well tolerated by the epithelial tissues and may be used topically with minimal untoward effects. Allergic reactions may occur occasionally, but are rare.

The following local side-effects have been reported with topical corticosteroids, especially under occlusive dressings: burning, itching, irritation, dryness, folliculitis, hypertrichosis, acneiform eruptions, hypopigmentation, perioral dermatitis, allergic contact dermatitis, maceration of the skin, secondary infection, skin atrophy, striae, miliaria.

The use of Terra-Cortril Topical Ointment should be discontinued if such reactions occur.

Overdosage: No cases of overdosage with Terra-Cortril Topical Ointment have been reported. No special antidotes are required following accidental ingestion.

Pharmaceutical precautions Store below 25°C.

Legal category POM.

Package quantities 15 g tube; 30 g tube.

Further information Nil.

Product licence number 0057/5076R.

TERRA-CORTRIL* NYSTATIN CREAM

Presentation Terra-Cortril Nystatin Cream contains 30 mg Oxytetracycline as Oxytetracycline Calcium BP., 10 mg Hydrocortisone PhEur and 100,000 units Nystatin BP in each gram of perfumed homogeneous yellow cream.

Inactive excipients: These are sodium metabisulphite, polysorbate 80, soft white paraffin, liquid paraffin, stearyl alcohol, stearic acid, cetomacrogol 1000, di-sodium hydrogen ortho-phosphate anhydrous, sodium dihydrogen orthophosphate dihydrate, sodium hydroxide, propyl and methyl hydroxybenzoates, propylene glycol, fragrance lavender-citrus.

Uses *Actions:* Terra-Cortril Nystatin Cream is ideal for use in conditions where topical, non-systemic action is desired. The oxytetracycline present will prevent or overcome superficial infections caused by organisms susceptible to it. Concomitantly, the concentration of hydrocortisone supplied is ample for inflammatory reactions resulting from allergy, infection or trauma. Nystatin is an antifungal antibiotic which is both fungistatic and fungicidal *in vitro* against a wide variety of yeasts and yeast-like fungi. It is effective for the treatment of cutaneous infections caused by *Candida albicans* and other *Candida* as well as other yeasts.

Thus this product provides the combined broad-spectrum activity of oxytetracycline against the primarily causative or secondarily infecting organisms, and the effectiveness of hydrocortisone, an anti-allergic, anti-inflammatory hormone, which controls excessive tissue reaction to infections, allergens and trauma along with nystatin which prevents or eradicates secondary fungal infections.

Indications: The use of Terra-Cortril Nystatin Cream is indicated in the treatment of steroid-responsive dermatoses. The added presence of oxytetracycline and nystatin will serve to prevent or eradicate secondary bacterial and fungal complications. Since varying degrees of bacterial and/or fungal infection frequently complicate those skin conditions for which hydrocortisone topical therapy is indicated, this combined preparation may offer therapeutic advantages over the use of hydrocortisone alone.

Among these conditions are: Atopic dermatitis: including allergic eczema, both disseminated and circumscribed neurodermatitis, pruritus with lichenification, eczematoid dermatitis and food eczema.

Cutaneous infections: including superficial pyogenic infections, pyoderma, pustular dermatitis, and infections associated with minor burns or wounds.

Contact dermatitis: due to plants, drugs, cosmetics, clothing material and miscellaneous substances.

Non-specific pruritus: of the anus, vulva or scrotum.

Dosage and administration

Adults: After thorough cleansing of the affected skin areas, a small amount of the cream should be applied gently. Applications should be made two to four times daily. When actual infection is present, the cream may be applied on sterile gauze and, by this means, kept in contiguous contact with the affected area. Care should be taken not to discontinue therapy too soon after the initial response has been obtained.

Supplementary therapy with oral antibiotics is advisable in the treatment of severe infections or those which may become systemic.

Use in the elderly: No special precautions.

Use in children: Not recommended. See *Contra-indications.*

Contra-indications, warnings, etc

Contra-indications:

1. Acute herpes simplex, vaccinia and varicella.
2. Tuberculosis of the skin.
3. Hypersensitivity to any of the components of the cream.
4. Acute purulent infections.
5. Pregnancy, and in infants and small children because of the theoretical risk of damage to permanent dentition.

Precautions: The use of oxytetracycline and other antibiotics may result in an overgrowth of resistant organisms. Observation of the patient for this possibility is required.

If irritation develops, the product should be discontinued and appropriate therapy instituted.

If a favourable response does not occur promptly, the corticosteroid should be discontinued until the infection has been adequately controlled.

If extensive areas are treated or if the occlusive technique is used there will be increased systemic absorption of the corticosteroid and suitable precautions should be taken.

Terra-Cortril Nystatin Cream is not for ophthalmic use.

Side-effects: Oxytetracycline, hydrocortisone and nystatin are well tolerated by the epithelial tissues and may be used topically with minimal untoward effects. Allergic reactions may occur occasionally, but are rare.

The following local side-effects have been reported with topical corticosteroids, especially under occlusive dressings: burning, itching, irritation, dryness, folliculitis, hypertrichosis, acneiform eruptions, hypopigmentation, perioral dermatitis, allergic contact dermatitis, maceration of the skin, secondary infection, skin atrophy, striae, miliaria.

The use of Terra-Cortril Nystatin Cream should be discontinued if such reactions occur.

Overdosage: No cases of overdosage with Terra-Cortril Nystatin Cream have been reported. No special antidotes are required following accidental ingestion.

Pharmaceutical precautions Store below 25°C.

Legal category POM.

Package quantities 30 g tube.

Further information Nil.

Product licence number 0057/0099.

TROSYL* NAIL SOLUTION

Qualitative and quantitative composition

Active ingredient	*mg/ml*
Tioconazole	283

Pharmaceutical form Clear pale yellow solution for topical application.

Clinical particulars

Therapeutic indications: Tioconazole is a broad spectrum imidazole antifungal agent. Trosyl Nail Solution is indicated for the topical treatment of nail infections due to susceptible fungi (dermatophytes and yeasts) and bacteria.

Posology and method of administration:

Adults: The solution should be applied to the affected nails and immediately surrounding skin every twelve hours using the applicator brush supplied.

The duration of treatment is up to six months but may be extended to twelve months.

Use in the elderly: No special precautions are required. Use the adult dose.

Use in children: No special precautions are required. Use the adult dose.

Contra-indications: Trosyl Nail Solution is contra-indicated in individuals who have been shown to be hypersensitive to imidazole antifungal agents, or to any of the components of the solution.

Use is contra-indicated during pregnancy.

Special warnings and precautions for use: Trosyl Nail Solution is not for ophthalmic use.

Interactions with other medicaments and other forms of interaction: None known.

Pregnancy and lactation

Use in pregnancy: In animal studies tioconazole was not teratogenic. At high doses it increased the incidence of renal abnormalities in rat embryos, but this effect was minor and transient and was not evident in weaned animals. There is insufficient evidence as to the drug's safety in human pregnancy although absorption after topical administration is negligible. Because of the extensive duration of treatment required for nail infections, the use of Trosyl Nail Solution is contra-indicated throughout pregnancy.

Effects on ability to drive and use machines: None known.

Undesirable effects: Trosyl Nail Solution is well tolerated following local application. Symptoms of local irritation have been reported by some patients, but are usually seen during the first week of treatment and are transient and mild.

However, if a sensitivity reaction develops with the use of Trosyl Nail Solution, treatment should be discontinued and appropriate therapy instituted.

Overdose: No cases of overdosage with Trosyl Nail Solution have been reported. In the event of excessive oral ingestion, gastrointestinal symptoms may occur. Appropriate means of gastric lavage should be considered.

Pharmacological properties

Pharmacodynamic properties: Tioconazole is an imidazole which is active against commonly occurring dermatophyte and yeast-like fungal species. It is fungicidal in murine models vs. Candida spp., *T. rubrum* and *T. mentacrophytes. In vitro* it is fungicidal to pathenogenic dermatophytes, yeasts and other fungi. All dermatophytes and Candida spp. were inhibited by 6.25 or 12.5 mg/l respectively. It is also inhibitory vs. Staph. spp. and Strep. spp. at 100 mg/l or less.

Oral doses (200 mg/kg) did not affect behaviour in rats but 25 mg/kg i.v. produced dose-related respiratory distress, gasping, tremors and prostration. Slight but dose-related impairment of performance of mice on the rotating rod occurred from 25 mg/kg. Slight anti-cholinergic and anti-histamine (H_1) activity was recorded *in vitro* but no effect on mice pupil size *in vivo.* Oral tioconazole prolonged alcohol and pentobarbitone sleeping time at 150 and 37.5 mg/kg respectively.

In the anaesthetised cat i.v. tioconazole 2.5–10 mg/kg produced brief falls in blood pressure and increased heart rate, haematuria, tremors and twitches.

Pharmacokinetic Properties: Absorption is rapid and extensive on oral administration to rats, monkeys and man, the major metabolite being a glucuronide conjugate of tioconazole. Tissue uptake in rat and monkey was highest in liver, kidney and intestinal tract with excretion in all species mainly in faeces.

Rat studies using oral, dermal and vaginal administration of C^{14} labelled tioconazole confirm significantly lower absorption via the topical route.

In man, oral formulations of tioconazole (500 mg) gave plasma concentrations of 1300 ng/ml. Topical administration of dermal cream 1% (20 mg/day) for 28 days, or vaginal cream 2% (100 mg/day) for 30 days gave negligible mean peak plasma levels, i.e. 10.1 and 11.5 ng/ml respectively.

After single dose administration of tioconazole vaginal ointment 6.5% w/w (tioconazole 300 mg) the mean peak plasma concentration was 18 ng/ml in humans, achieved approximately 8 hours post dose.

Preclinical safety data: None relevant to the prescriber.

Pharmaceutical particulars

List of excipients: Undecylenic acid, ethyl acetate.

Incompatibilities: None known.

Shelf life: 24 months when stored between 4°C and 30°C.

Special precautions for storage: Avoid flame and heat.

Nature and contents of container: Trosyl Nail Solution is contained in an amber glass bottle with a screw cap fitted with an applicator containing 12 ml.

Instruction for use/handling: No special instructions are required.

Marketing authorisation number PL 00057/0236

Date of first authorisation/renewal of authorisation 14 July 1994

Date of (partial) revision of the text August 1998

VIAGRA* 25 mg film-coated tablets ▼
VIAGRA* 50 mg film-coated tablets
VIAGRA* 100 mg film-coated tablets

Qualitative and quantitative composition Each tablet contains 25 mg , 50 mg or 100 mg sildenafil as citrate.

Pharmaceutical form Film-coated tablet.

The 25 mg tablets are blue film-coated, rounded diamond-shaped tablets, marked 'PFIZER' on one side and 'VGR 25' on the other.

The 50 mg tablets are blue film-coated, rounded diamond-shaped tablets, marked 'PFIZER' on one side and 'VGR 50' on the other.

The 100 mg tablets are blue film-coated, rounded diamond-shaped tablets, marked 'PFIZER' on one side and 'VGR 100' on the other.

Clinical particulars

Therapeutic indications: Treatment of erectile dysfunction, which is the inability to achieve or maintain a penile erection sufficient for satisfactory sexual performance.

In order for Viagra to be effective, sexual stimulation is required.

Viagra is not indicated for use by women.

Posology and method of administration: For oral use.

Use in adults: The recommended dose is 50 mg taken as needed approximately one hour before sexual activity. Based on efficacy and toleration, the dose may be increased to 100 mg or decreased to 25 mg. The maximum recommended dose is 100 mg. The maximum recommended dosing frequency is once per day. If Viagra is taken with food, the onset of activity may be delayed compared to the fasted state (see *Pharmacokinetic properties – Absorption*).

Use in the elderly: Since sildenafil clearance is reduced in elderly patients (see *Pharmacokinetic properties*), a first dose of 25 mg should be used. Based on efficacy and toleration, the dose may be increased to 50 mg and 100 mg.

Use in patients with impaired renal function: The dosing recommendations described in *Use in adults* apply to patients with mild to moderate renal impairment (creatinine clearance = 30–80 ml/min).

Since sildenafil clearance is reduced in patients with severe renal impairment (creatinine clearance < 30 ml/min) a 25 mg dose should be considered. Based on efficacy and toleration, the dose may be increased to 50 mg and 100 mg.

Use in patients with impaired hepatic function: Since sildenafil clearance is reduced in patients with hepatic impairment (e.g. cirrhosis) a 25 mg dose should be considered. Based on efficacy and toleration, the dose may be increased to 50 mg and 100 mg.

Use in children: Viagra is not indicated for individuals below 18 years of age.

Contra-indications: Consistent with its known effects on the nitric oxide/cyclic guanosine monophosphate (cGMP) pathway (see *Pharmacodynamic properties*), sildenafil was shown to potentiate the hypotensive effects of nitrates, and its co-administration with nitric oxide donors (such as amyl nitrite) or nitrates in any form is therefore contra-indicated.

Agents for the treatment of erectile dysfunction, including sildenafil, should not be used in men for whom sexual activity is inadvisable (e.g. patients with severe cardiovascular disorders such as unstable angina or severe cardiac failure).

The safety of sildenafil has not been studied in the following sub-groups of patients and its use is therefore contra-indicated until further information is available: severe hepatic impairment, hypotension (blood pressure <90/50 mmHg), recent history of stroke or myocardial infarction and known hereditary degenerative retinal disorders such as retinitis pigmentosa (a minority of these patients have genetic disorders of retinal phosphodiesterases).

Hypersensitivity to the active substance or to any of the excipients.

Special warnings and special precautions for use: A medical history and physical examination should be undertaken to diagnose erectile dysfunction and determine potential underlying causes, before pharmacological treatment is considered.

Prior to initiating any treatment for erectile dysfunction, physicians should consider the cardiovascular status of their patients, since there is a degree of cardiac risk associated with sexual activity. Sildenafil has vasodilator properties, resulting in mild and transient decreases in blood pressure (see *Pharmacodynamic properties*) and as such potentiates the hypotensive effect of nitrates (see *Contra-indications*).

Agents for the treatment of erectile dysfunction, including sildenafil, should be used with caution in patients with anatomical deformation of the penis (such as angulation, cavernosal fibrosis or Peyronie's disease), or in patients who have conditions which may predispose them to priapism (such as sickle cell anaemia, multiple myeloma or leukaemia).

The safety and efficacy of combinations of sildenafil with other treatments for erectile dysfunction have not been studied. Therefore the use of such combinations is not recommended.

Studies with human platelets indicate that sildenafil potentiates the antiaggregatory effect of sodium nitroprusside *in vitro*. There is no safety information on the administration of sildenafil to patients with bleeding disorders or active peptic ulceration. Therefore sildenafil should be administered to these patients only after careful benefit-risk assessment.

Interaction with other medicinal products and other forms of interaction

Effects of other medicinal products on sildenafil: ***In vitro* studies**: Sildenafil metabolism is principally mediated by the cytochrome P450 (CYP) isoforms 3A4 (major route) and 2C9 (minor route). Therefore, inhibitors of these isoenzymes may reduce sildenafil clearance.

***In vivo* studies**: Cimetidine (800 mg), a cytochrome P450 inhibitor and non-specific CYP3A4 inhibitor, caused a 56% increase in plasma sildenafil concentrations when co-administered with sildenafil (50 mg) to healthy volunteers. When a single 100 mg dose of sildenafil was administered with erythromycin, a specific CYP3A4 inhibitor, at steady state (500 mg b.i.d. for 5 days), there was a 182% increase in sildenafil systemic exposure (AUC).

Population pharmacokinetic analysis of clinical trial data indicated a reduction in sildenafil clearance when co-administered with CYP3A4 inhibitors (such as ketoconazole, erythromycin, cimetidine). Although no increased incidence of adverse events was observed in these patients, when sildenafil is administered concomitantly with CYP3A4 inhibitors, a starting dose of 25 mg should be considered.

Single doses of antacid (magnesium hydroxide/aluminium hydroxide) did not affect the bioavailability of sildenafil.

Although specific interaction studies were not conducted for all medicinal products, population pharmacokinetic analysis showed no effect of concomitant medication on sildenafil pharmacokinetics when grouped as CYP2C9 inhibitors (such as tolbutamide, warfarin, phenytoin), CYP2D6 inhibitors (such as selective serotonin reuptake inhibitors, tricyclic antidepressants), thiazide and related diuretics, loop and potassium sparing diuretics, angiotensin converting enzyme inhibitors, calcium channel blockers, beta-adrenoreceptor antagonists or inducers of CYP450 metabolism (such as rifampicin, barbiturates).

Effects of sildenafil on other medicinal products: ***In vitro* studies:**

Sildenafil is a weak inhibitor of the cytochrome P450 isoforms 1A2, 2C9, 2C19, 2D6, 2E1 and 3A4 (IC_{50} >150 microM). Given sildenafil peak plasma concentrations of approximately 1 microM after recommended doses, it is unlikely that Viagra will alter the clearance of substrates of these isoenzymes.

There are no data on the interaction of sildenafil and non-specific phosphodiesterase inhibitors such as theophylline or dipyridamole.

***In vivo* studies:**

No significant interactions were shown when sildenafil (50 mg) was coadministered with tolbutamide (250 mg) or warfarin (40 mg), both of which are metabolised by CYP2C9.

Sildenafil (50 mg) did not potentiate the increase in bleeding time caused by acetyl salicylic acid (150 mg).

Sildenafil (50 mg) did not potentiate the hypotensive effects of alcohol in healthy volunteers with mean maximum blood alcohol levels of 80 mg/dl.

Pooling of the following classes of antihypertensive medication; diuretics, beta-blockers, ACE inhibitors, angiotensin II antagonists, antihypertensive medicinal products (vasodilator and centrally-acting), adrenergic neurone blockers, calcium channel blockers and alpha-adrenoceptor blockers, showed no difference in the side effect profile in patients taking sildenafil compared to placebo treatment. In a specific interaction study, where sildenafil (100 mg) was co-administered with amlodipine in hypertensive patients, there was an additional reduction on supine systolic blood pressure of 8 mmHg. The corresponding additional reduction in supine diastolic blood pressure was 7 mmHg. These additional blood pressure reductions were of a similar magnitude to those seen when sildenafil was administered alone to healthy volunteers (see *Pharmacodynamic properties*).

Consistent with its known effects on the nitric oxide/cGMP pathway (see *Pharmacodynamic properties*), sildenafil was shown to potentiate the hypotensive effects of nitrates, and its co-administration with nitric oxide donors or nitrates in any form is therefore contra-indicated (see *Contra-indications*).

Use during pregnancy and lactation: Viagra is not indicated for use by women.

No relevant adverse effects were found in reproduction studies in rats and rabbits following oral administration of sildenafil.

Effects on ability to drive and use machines: As dizziness and altered vision were reported in clinical trials with sildenafil, patients should be aware of how they react to Viagra, before driving or operating machinery.

Undesirable effects: The following adverse reactions (with incidence > 1%) were reported in patients treated with the recommended dosing regimen in clinical trials:

Cardiovascular: Headache (12.8%), Flushing (10.4%), Dizziness (1.2%)

Digestive: Dyspepsia (4.6%)

Respiratory: Nasal congestion (1.1%)

Special senses: Altered vision (1.9%; mild and transient, predominantly colour tinge to vision, but also increased perception of light or blurred vision).

In fixed dose studies, dyspepsia (12%), and altered vision (11%) were more common at 100 mg than at lower doses.

In addition, there were reports of muscle aches when sildenafil was administered more frequently than the recommended dosing regimen. In post marketing surveillance, priapism has been reported.

Adverse reactions were mild to moderate in nature and the incidence and severity increased with dose.

Overdose: In single dose volunteer studies of doses up to 800 mg, adverse reactions were similar to those seen at lower doses, but the incidence rates and severities were increased. Doses of 200 mg did not result in increased efficacy but the incidence of adverse reactions (headache, flushing, dizziness, dyspepsia, nasal congestion, altered vision) was increased.

In cases of overdose, standard supportive measures should be adopted as required. Renal dialysis is not expected to accelerate clearance as sildenafil is highly bound to plasma proteins and not eliminated in the urine.

Pharmacological properties

Pharmacodynamic properties: Pharmacotherapeutic group: Drugs used in erectile dysfunction. ATC Code: G04B E (proposed).

Sildenafil is an oral therapy for erectile dysfunction. In the natural setting, i.e. with sexual stimulation, it restores impaired erectile function by increasing blood flow to the penis.

The physiological mechanism responsible for erection of the penis involves the release of nitric oxide (NO) in the corpus cavernosum during sexual stimulation. Nitric oxide then activates the enzyme guanylate cyclase, which results in increased levels of cyclic guanosine monophosphate (cGMP), producing smooth muscle relaxation in the corpus cavernosum and allowing inflow of blood.

Sildenafil is a potent and selective inhibitor of cGMP specific phosphodiesterase type 5 (PDE5) in the corpus cavernosum, where PDE5 is responsible for degradation of cGMP. Sildenafil has a peripheral site of action on erections. Sildenafil has no direct relaxant effect on isolated human corpus cavernosum but potently enhances the relaxant effect of NO on this tissue. When the NO/cGMP pathway is activated, as occurs with sexual stimulation, inhibition of PDE5 by sildenafil results in increased corpus cavernosum levels of cGMP. Therefore sexual stimulation is required in order for sildenafil to produce its intended beneficial pharmacological effects.

Studies *in vitro* have shown that sildenafil has between 80 and 10,000-fold greater selectivity for PDE5 than for other phosphodiesterase isoforms (PDE's 1,2,3 and 4). In particular, sildenafil has greater than 4,000-fold selectivity for PDE5 over PDE3, the cAMP-specific phosphodiesterase isoform involved in the control of cardiac contractility. There is a 10-fold selectivity over PDE6 which is involved in the phototransduction pathway in the retina.

Two clinical studies were specifically designed to assess the time window after dosing during which sildenafil could produce an erection in response to sexual stimulation. In a penile plesthysmography (RigiScan) study of fasted patients, the median time to onset for those who obtained erections of 60% rigidity (sufficient for sexual intercourse) was 25 minutes (range 12-37 minutes) on sildenafil. In a separate RigiScan study, sildenafil was still able to produce an erection in response to sexual stimulation 4-5 hours post-dose.

Sildenafil causes mild and transient decreases in blood pressure which, in the majority of cases, do not translate into clinical effects. The mean maximum decreases in supine systolic blood pressure following 100 mg oral dosing of sildenafil was 8.4 mmHg. The corresponding change in supine diastolic blood pressure was 5.5 mmHg. These decreases in blood pressure are consistent with the vasodilatory effects of sildenafil, probably due to increased cGMP levels in vascular smooth muscle. Single oral doses of sildenafil up to 100 mg in healthy volunteers produced no clinically relevant effects on ECG.

Mild and transient differences in colour discrimination (blue/green) were detected in some subjects using the Farnsworth-Munsell 100 hue test at 1 hour following a 100 mg dose, with no effects evident after 2 hours post-dose. The postulated mechanism for this change in colour discrimination is related to inhibition of PDE6, which is involved in the phototransduction cascade of the retina. Sildenafil has no effect on visual acuity or contrast sensitivity.

There was no effect on sperm motility or morphology after single 100 mg oral doses of sildenafil in healthy volunteers.

Further information on clinical trials: In clinical trials sildenafil was administered to more than 3000 patients aged 19-87. The following patient groups were represented: elderly (21%), patients with hypertension (24%), diabetes mellitus (16%), ischaemic heart disease and other cardiovascular diseases (14%), hyperlipidaemia (14%), spinal cord injury (6%), depression (5%), transurethral resection of the prostate (5%), radical prostatectomy (4%). The following groups were not well represented or excluded from clinical trials: patients with pelvic surgery, patients post-radiotherapy, patients with severe renal or hepatic impairment and patients with certain cardiovascular conditions (see *Contra-indications*).

In fixed dose studies, the proportions of patients reporting that treatment improved their erections were 62% (25 mg), 74% (50 mg) and 82% (100 mg) compared to 25% on placebo. In controlled clinical trials, the discontinuation rate due to sildenafil was low and similar to placebo.

Across all trials, the proportion of patients reporting improvement on sildenafil were as follows: psychogenic erectile dysfunction (84%), mixed erectile dysfunction (77%), organic erectile dysfunction (68%), elderly (67%), diabetes mellitus (59%), ischaemic heart disease (69%), hypertension (68%), TURP (61%), radical prostatectomy (43%), spinal cord injury (83%), depression (75%). The safety and efficacy of sildenafil was maintained in long term studies.

Pharmacokinetic properties: Absorption: Sildenafil is rapidly absorbed. Maximum observed plasma concentrations are reached within 30 to 120 minutes (median 60 minutes) of oral dosing in the fasted state. The mean absolute oral bioavailability is 41% (range 25–63%). After oral dosing of sildenafil AUC and C_{max} increase in proportion with dose over the recommended dose range (25–100 mg).

When sildenafil is taken with food, the rate of absorption is reduced with a mean delay in T_{max} of 60 minutes and a mean reduction in C_{max} of 29%.

Distribution: The mean steady state volume of distribution (V_{ss}) for sildenafil is 105 l, indicating distribution into the tissues. Sildenafil and its major circulating N-desmethyl metabolite are both approximately 96% bound to plasma proteins. Protein binding is independent of total drug concentrations.

In healthy volunteers receiving sildenafil (100 mg single dose), less than 0.0002% (average 188 ng) of the administered dose was present in ejaculate 90 minutes after dosing.

Metabolism: Sildenafil is cleared predominantly by the CYP3A4 (major route) and CYP2C9 (minor route) hepatic microsomal isoenzymes. The major circulating metabolite results from N-demethylation of sildenafil. This metabolite has a phosphodiesterase selectivity profile similar to sildenafil and an *in vitro* potency for PDE5 approximately 50% that of the parent drug. Plasma concentrations of this metabolite are approximately 40% of those seen for sildenafil.

The N-desmethyl metabolite is further metabolised, with a terminal half life of approximately 4 h.

Elimination: The total body clearance of sildenafil is 41 l/h with a resultant terminal phase half life of 3–5 h. After either oral or intravenous administration, sildenafil is excreted as metabolites predominantly in the faeces (approximately 80% of administered oral dose) and to a lesser extent in the urine (approximately 13% of administered oral dose).

Pharmacokinetics in special patient groups:

Elderly: Healthy elderly volunteers (65 years or over) had a reduced clearance of sildenafil, resulting in approximately 90% higher plasma concentrations of sildenafil and the active N-desmethyl metabolite compared to those seen in healthy younger volunteers (18–45 years). Due to age-differences in plasma protein binding, the corresponding increase in free sildenafil plasma concentration was approximately 40%.

Renal insufficiency: In volunteers with mild to moderate renal impairment (creatinine clearance = 30–80 ml/min), the pharmacokinetics of sildenafil were not altered after receiving a 50 mg single oral dose. The mean AUC and C_{max} of the N-desmethyl metabolite increased 126% and 73% respectively, compared to age-matched volunteers with no renal impairment. However, due to high inter-subject variability, these differences were not statistically significant. In volunteers with severe renal impairment (creatinine clearance <30 ml/min), sildenafil clearance was reduced, resulting in mean increases in AUC and C_{max} of 100% and 88% respectively compared to age-matched volunteers with no renal impairment. In addition, N-desmethyl metabolite AUC and C_{max} values were significantly increased 79% and 200% respectively.

Hepatic insufficiency: In volunteers with mild to moderate hepatic cirrhosis (Child-Pugh A and B) sildenafil clearance was reduced, resulting in increases in AUC (84%) and C_{max} (47%) compared to age-matched volunteers with no hepatic impairment. The pharmacokinetics of sildenafil in patients with severely impaired hepatic function have not been studied.

Preclinical safety data: Preclinical data revealed no special hazard for humans based on conventional studies of safety pharmacology, repeated dose toxicity, genotoxicity, carcinogenicity, and toxicity to reproduction.

Pharmaceutical particulars

List of excipients: Tablet core: microcrystalline cellulose, calcium hydrogen phosphate (anhydrous), croscarmellose sodium, magnesium stearate.

Film coat: hypromellose, titanium dioxide (E171), lactose, triacetin, indigo carmine aluminium lake (E132).

Incompatibilities: Not applicable.

Shelf-life: 2 years.

Special precautions for storage: Do not store above 30°C. Keep tablets in the original package, protected from moisture.

Nature and content of container: Aclar/Aluminium foil blisters in cartons of 1, 4, 8 or 12 tablets.

Instructions for use and handling: Not applicable.

Number(s) in the community register of medicinal products

EU/1/98/077/001 – Viagra tablets 25 mg; pack size 1 tablet
EU/1/98/077/002 – Viagra tablets 25 mg; pack size 4 tablets
EU/1/98/077/003 – Viagra tablets 25 mg; pack size 8 tablets
EU/1/98/077/004 – Viagra tablets 25 mg; pack size 12 tablets
EU/1/98/077/005 – Viagra tablets 50 mg; pack size 1 tablet
EU/1/98/077/006 – Viagra tablets 50 mg; pack size 4 tablets
EU/1/98/077/007 – Viagra tablets 50 mg; pack size 8 tablets
EU/1/98/077/008 – Viagra tablets 50 mg pack size 12 tablets
EU/1/98/077/009 – Viagra tablets 100 mg; pack size 1 tablet
EU/1/98/077/010 – Viagra tablets 100 mg; pack size 4 tablets
EU/1/98/077/011 – Viagra tablets 100 mg; pack size 8 tablets
EU/1/98/077/012 – Viagra tablets 100 mg; pack size 12 tablets

Date of first authorisation/renewal of the authorisation September 1998

Date of revision of the text August 1998

Legal category POM

VIBRAMYCIN*
VIBRAMYCIN 50*
VIBRAMYCIN*-D

Qualitative and quantitative composition Active Ingredient: doxycycline.

Vibramycin 50 Capsules contain 50 mg doxycycline as doxycycline hyclate PhEur.

Vibramycin Capsules contain 100 mg doxycycline as doxycycline hyclate PhEur.

Vibramycin-D Dispersible Tablets contain l00 mg doxycycline PhEur.

Pharmaceutical form Vibramycin 50 capsules are green and ivory, coded 'Pfizer' and 'VBM 50'.

Vibramycin capsules 100 mg are green, coded 'Pfizer' and 'VBM 100'.

Vibramycin-D Dispersible Tablets are off-white buff tablets coded 'D 9' on one side and 'Pfizer' on the other.

Clinical particulars

Therapeutic indications: Vibramycin has been found clinically effective in the treatment of a variety of infections caused by susceptible strains of Gram-positive and Gram-negative bacteria and certain other micro-organisms.

Respiratory tract infections: Pneumonia and other lower respiratory tract infections due to susceptible strains of *Streptococcus pneumoniae, Haemophilus influenzae, Klebsiella pneumoniae* and other organisms. *Mycoplasma pneumoniae* pneumonia. Treatment of chronic bronchitis, sinusitis.

Urinary tract infections caused by susceptible strains of Klebsiella species, Enterobacter species, *Escherichia coli, Streptococcus faecalis* and other organisms.

Sexually transmitted diseases: Infections due to *Chlamydia trachomatis* including uncomplicated urethral, endocervical or rectal infections. Non-gonococcal urethritis caused by *Ureaplasma urealyticum* (T-mycoplasma). Vibramycin is also indicated in chancroid, granuloma inguinale and lymphogranuloma venereum. Vibramycin is an alternative drug in the treatment of gonorrhoea and syphilis.

Skin infections: Acne vulgaris, when antibiotic therapy is considered necessary.

Since Vibramycin is a member of the tetracycline series of antibiotics, it may be expected to be useful in the treatment of infections which respond to other tetracyclines, such as:

Ophthalmic infections: Due to susceptible strains of gonococci, staphylococci and Haemophilus influenzae. Trachoma, although the infectious agent, as judged by immunofluorescence, is not always eliminated. Inclusion conjunctivitis may be treated with oral Vibramycin alone or in combination with topical agents.

Rickettsial infections: Rocky Mountain spotted fever, typhus group, Q fever, Coxiella endocarditis and tick fevers.

Other infections: Psittacosis, brucellosis (in combination with streptomycin), cholera, bubonic plague, louse and tick-borne relapsing fever, tularaemia, glanders, melioidosis, chloroquine-resistant falciparum malaria and acute intestinal amoebiasis (as an adjunct to amoebicides).

Vibramycin is an alternative drug in the treatment of leptospirosis, gas gangrene and tetanus.

Vibramycin is indicated for prophylaxis in the following conditions: Scrub typhus, travellers' diarrhoea (enterotoxigenic *Escherichia coli)*, leptospirosis.

Posology and method of administration: Dosage:

Adults: The usual dosage of Vibramycin for the treatment of acute infections in adults is 200 mg on the first day (as a single dose or in divided doses) followed by a maintenance dose of 100 mg/day. In the management of more severe infections, 200 mg daily should be given throughout treatment.

Capsules and Dispersible Tablets are for oral administration only.

Vibramycin-D tablets are administered by drinking a suspension of the tablets in a small amount of water.

Vibramycin capsules should be administered with adequate amounts of fluid. This should be done in the sitting or standing position and well before retiring at night to reduce the risk of oesophageal irritation and ulceration. If gastric irritation occurs, it is recommended that Vibramycin be given with food or milk. Studies indicate that the absorption of Vibramycin is not notably influenced by simultaneous ingestion of food or milk.

Exceeding the recommended dosage may result in an increased incidence of side effects. Therapy should be continued for at least 24 to 48 hours after symptoms and fever have subsided.

When used in streptococcal infections, therapy should be continued for 10 days to prevent the development of rheumatic fever or glomerulonephritis.

Dosage recommendations in specific infections:

Acne vulgaris: 50 mg daily with food or fluid for 6 to 12 weeks.

Sexually transmitted diseases: 100 mg twice daily for 7 days is recommended in the following infections: uncomplicated gonococcal infections (except anorectal infections in men); uncomplicated urethral, endocervical or rectal infection caused by *Chlamydia trachomatis;* non-gonococcal urethritis caused by *Ureaplasma urealyticum.* Acute epididymo-orchitis caused by *Chlamydia trachomatis* or *Neisseria gonorrhoea* 100 mg twice daily for 10 days. Primary and secondary syphilis: 300 mg a day in divided doses for at least 10 days.

Louse and tick-borne relapsing fevers: A single dose of 100 or 200 mg according to severity.

Chloroquine-resistant falciparum malaria: 200 mg daily for at least 7 days. Due to the potential severity of the infection, a rapid-acting schizonticide such as quinine should always be given in conjunction with Vibramycin; quinine dosage recommendations vary in different areas.

For the prevention of scrub typhus: 200 mg as a single dose.

For the prevention of travellers' diarrhoea in adults: 200 mg on the first day of travel (administered as a single dose or as 100 mg every 12 hours) followed by 100 mg daily throughout the stay in the area. Data on the use of the drug prophylactically are not available beyond 21 days.

For the prevention of leptospirosis: 200 mg once each week throughout the stay in the area and 200 mg at the completion of the trip. Data on the use of the drug prophylactically are not available beyond 21 days.

Use for children: See under *Contra-indications.*

Use in the elderly: Vibramycin may be prescribed in the elderly in the usual dosages with no special precautions. No dosage adjustment is necessary in the presence of renal impairment. The Vibramycin-D dispersible tablet may be preferred for the elderly since it is less likely to be associated with oesophageal irritation and ulceration.

Use in patients with impaired hepatic function: see under *Special warnings/precautions.*

Use in patients with renal impairment: Studies to date have indicated that administration of Vibramycin at the usual recommended doses does not lead to accumulation of the antibiotic in patients with renal impairment see under *Special warnings/precautions.*

Contra-indications: Persons who have shown hypersensitivity to any of the tetracyclines. The use of drugs of the tetracycline class during tooth development (pregnancy, infancy and childhood to the age of 12 years) may cause permanent discolouration of the teeth (yellow-grey-brown). This adverse reaction is more common during long-term use of the drugs but has been observed following repeated short-term courses. Enamel hypoplasia has also been reported. Vibramycin is therefore contraindicated in these groups of patients.

Pregnancy: Vibramycin is contraindicated in pregnancy. It appears that the risks associated with the use of tetracyclines during pregnancy are predominantly due to effects on teeth and skeletal development. (See above about use during tooth development).

Nursing mothers: Tetracyclines are excreted into milk and are therefore contraindicated in nursing mothers. (See above about use during tooth development).

Children: Vibramycin is contraindicated in children under the age of 12 years. As with other tetracyclines, Vibramycin forms a stable calcium complex in any bone-forming tissue. A decrease in the fibula growth rate has been observed in prematures given oral tetracyclines in doses of 25 mg/kg every 6 hours. This reaction was shown to be reversible when the drug was discontinued. (See above about use during tooth development).

Special warnings and special precautions for use: Use in patients with impaired hepatic function: Vibramycin should be administered with caution to patients with hepatic impairment or those receiving potentially hepatotoxic drugs.

Use in patients with renal impairment: Excretion of doxycycline by the kidney is about 40%/72 hours in individuals with normal renal function. This percentage excretion may fall to a range as low as 1–5%/72 hours in individuals with severe renal insufficiency (creatinine clearance below 10 ml/min). Studies have shown no significant difference in the serum half-life of doxycycline in individuals with normal and severely impaired renal function. Haemodialysis does not alter the serum half-life of doxycycline. The anti-anabolic action of the tetracyclines may cause an increase in blood urea. Studies to date indicate that this does not occur with the use of Vibramycin in patients with impaired renal function.

Photosensitivity: Photosensitivity manifested by an exaggerated sunburn reaction has been observed in some individuals taking tetracyclines. Patients likely to be exposed to direct sunlight or ultraviolet light should be advised that this reaction can occur with tetracycline drugs and treatment should be discontinued at the first evidence of skin erythema.

Microbiological overgrowth: The use of antibiotics may occasionally result in the overgrowth of nonsusceptible organisms including Candida. If a resistant organism appears, the antibiotic should be discontinued and appropriate therapy instituted.

Venereal disease: When treating venereal disease, where co-existent syphilis is suspected, proper diagnostic procedures including dark-field examinations should be utilised. In all such cases monthly serological tests should be made for at least four months.

Beta-haemolytic streptococci Infections: Infections due to group A beta-haemolytic streptococci should be treated for at least 10 days.

Interaction with other medicaments and other forms of treatment: The absorption of doxycycline may be impaired by concurrently administered antacids containing aluminium, calcium or magnesium; oral zinc, iron salts or bismuth preparations.

Since bacteriostatic drugs may interfere with the bactericidal action of penicillin, it is advisable to avoid giving Vibramycin in conjunction with penicillin.

Tetracyclines depress plasma prothrombin activity and reduced doses of concomitant anticoagulants may be necessary.

The serum half-life of doxycycline may be shortened when patients are concurrently receiving barbiturates, carbamazepine or phenytoin. An increase in the daily dosage of Vibramycin should be considered.

Alcohol may decrease the half-life of doxycycline.

A few cases of pregnancy or breakthrough bleeding have been attributed to the concurrent use of tetracycline antibiotics with oral contraceptives.

Pregnancy and lactation: See under *Contra-indications.*

Effects on ability to drive and use machines: Vibramycin has to date not been associated with effects on the ability to drive and to use machinery.

Undesirable effects: Due to virtually complete absorption of Vibramycin gastro-intestinal side-effects are infrequent. The following adverse reactions have been observed in patients receiving tetracyclines.

Gastro-intestinal: Gastrointestinal symptoms are usually mild and seldom necessitate discontinuation of treatment. Anorexia, nausea, vomiting, diarrhoea, glossitis, dysphagia, enterocolitis and inflammatory lesions (with candidal overgrowth) in the anogenital region. Rare instances of oesophagitis and oesophageal ulceration have been reported in patients receiving Vibramycin. A significant proportion of these occurred with the hyclate salt in the capsule form. Most of the patients took medication immediately before going to bed.

Hepatic toxicity: Abnormal hepatic function has been reported.

Skin: Maculopapular and erythematous rashes occur, but were uncommon in clinical trials. Exfoliative dermatitis has been reported but is uncommon. Photosensitivity is discussed in the 'Special warnings and special precautions for use' section.

Hypersensitivity reactions: Urticaria, angioneurotic oedema, anaphylaxis, anaphylactoid purpura, serum sickness, pericarditis, and exacerbation of systemic lupus erythematosus.

Bulging fontanelles in infants and benign intracranial hypertension in adults have been reported in individuals receiving full therapeutic dosages of tetracyclines. These conditions disappeared rapidly when the drug was discontinued.

Blood: Haemolytic anaemia, thrombocytopenia, neutropenia and eosinophilia have been reported with tetracyclines.

When given over prolonged periods, tetracyclines have been reported to produce brown-black microscopic discolouration of thyroid tissue. No abnormalities of thyroid function are known to occur.

Overdose: Acute overdosage with antibiotics is rare. In the event of overdosage discontinue medication. Gastric lavage plus appropriate supportive treatment is indicated.

Dialysis does not alter serum half-life and thus would not be of benefit in treating cases of overdosage.

Pharmacological properties

Pharmacodynamic properties: Vibramycin is primarily bacteriostatic and is believed to exert its antimicrobial effect by the inhibition of protein synthesis. Vibramycin is active against a wide range of Gram-positive and Gram-negative bacteria and certain other microorganisms.

Pharmacokinetic properties: Tetracyclines are readily absorbed and are bound to plasma proteins in varying degrees. They are concentrated by the liver in the bile and excreted in the urine and faeces at high concentrations and in a biologically active form. Doxycycline is virtually completely absorbed after oral administration. Studies reported to date indicate that the absorption of doxycycline, unlike certain other tetracyclines, is not notably influenced by the ingestion of food or milk. Following a 200 mg dose, normal adult volunteers averaged peak serum levels of 2.6 micrograms/ml of doxycycline at 2 hours decreasing to 1.45 micrograms/ml at 24 hours. Doxycycline has a high degree of lipid solubility and a low affinity for calcium. It is highly stable in normal human serum. Doxycycline will not degrade into an epianhydro form.

Pharmaceutical particulars

List of excipients: Vibramycin 100 mg capsules: Maize Starch PhEur, Lactose PhEur, alginic acid, magnesium stearate NF, Sodium Lauryl Sulphate PhEur. The capsule shell contains: gelatin BP, titanium dioxide (E171), patent blue V (E131) and quinoline yellow (E104).

Vibramycin 50 mg capsules: Maize Starch PhEur, Lactose PhEur, alginic acid, magnesium stearate NF, Sodium Lauryl Sulphate PhEur. In addition the capsule shell cap contains: gelatin BP, titanium dioxide (E171), patent blue V (E131) and quinoline yellow (E104) and the body contains yellow iron oxide (E172), indigotine (E132) and titanium dioxide (E171).

Vibramycin D Dispersible tablets: Colloidal silicon dioxide PhEur, microcrystalline cellulose PhEur and Magnesium Stearate PhEur.

Incompatibilities: None stated.

Shelf life: Vibramycin 50 and 100 mg capsules 48 months

Vibramycin-D Dispersible tablets 48 months

Storage conditions: Store below 25°C

Nature and contents of container: Vibramycin Capsules 100 mg are available as:

Packs of 8 Capsules. Aluminium/PVC blister strips, a single strip of 8 capsules in a carton box.

Vibramycin 50 Capsules 50 mg are available as: Calendar Packs of 28 Capsules. Aluminium/PVC blister strips, 14 capsules per strip, 2 strips in a carton box.

Vibramycin-D Dispersible Tablets 100 mg are available as:

Packs of 8 Tablets. Aluminium/PVC blister strips, a single strip of 8 tablets in a carton box.

Instructions for use/handling: No special requirements.

Marketing authorisation numbers

Vibramycin Capsules 100 mg	0057/5059R
Vibramycin Capsules 50 mg	0057/0238
Vibramycin-D Dispersible Tablets I00 mg	0057/0188

Date of renewal of the authorisation

Vibramycin Capsules 100 mg	25/10/95
Vibramycin Capsules 50 mg	25/10/95
Vibramycin-D Dispersible Tablets I00 mg	25/10/95

Date of (partial) revision of the text 16 April 1998

Legal category POM

VIBRAMYCIN* ACNE PACK

Qualitative and quantitative composition Doxycycline base (as doxycycline hyclate PhEur) 50 mg.

Pharmaceutical form Capsules.

Hard gelatin capsules coloured pale green and white and marked 'VBM C50', containing spherical yellow to yellowish coated microgranules, intended for oral administration to human beings.

Clinical particulars

Therapeutic indications: As a bacteriostatic antibiotic, doxycycline is clinically effective in the treatment of a variety of infections caused by a wide range of gram-negative and gram-positive bacteria, as well as certain other micro-organisms.

Dermatological infections: *acne vulgaris.*

Posology and method of administration: Use in adults.

Acne vulgaris: In the treatment of *acne vulgaris* the recommended dose is 50 mg daily with food or fluid. Duration of treatment will vary from 6 to 12 weeks.

Conventional capsule forms of the tetracycline class of drugs are liable to cause oesophageal irritation and ulceration. Administration of adequate amounts of fluid is therefore recommended to combat this problem. If, however, gastric irritation does occur, doxycycline capsules can be given with food or milk. The absorption of doxycycline is not markedly influenced by simultaneous ingestion of food or milk.

Use in children: Vibramycin is contra-indicated in children under 12 years of age.

For children over 12 years of age, the usual adult dose should be used.

Use in Patients with renal/hepatic impairment: See *Special warnings and special precautions for use.*

Contra-indications: Persons who have shown hypersensitivity to any of the tetracyclines.

The use of drugs of the tetracycline class during tooth development (pregnancy, infancy and childhood to the age of 12 years) may cause permanent discolouration of the teeth (yellow-grey-brown). This adverse reaction is more common during long-term use of the drugs but has been observed following repeated short-term courses. Enamel hypoplasia has also been reported. Vibramycin is therefore contra-indicated in these groups of patients.

Pregnancy: Vibramycin is contraindicated in pregnancy. It appears that the risks associated with the use of tetracyclines during pregnancy are predominantly due to effects on teeth and skeletal development. (See above about use during tooth development).

Nursing mothers: Tetracyclines are excreted into milk and are therefore contra-indicated in nursing mothers. (See above about use during tooth development).

Children: Vibramycin is contra-indicated in children under the age of 12 years. As with other tetracyclines, Vibramycin forms a stable calcium complex in any bone-forming tissue. A decrease in the fibula growth rate has been observed in prematures given oral tetracyclines in doses of 25 mg/kg every 6 hours. This reaction was shown to be reversible when the drug was discontinued. (See above about use during tooth development).

Special warnings and special precautions for use:

Photosensitivity: Photosensitivity manifested by an exaggerated sunburn reaction has been observed in some individuals taking tetracyclines. Patients likely to be exposed to direct sunlight or ultraviolet light should be advised that this reaction can occur with tetracycline drugs and treatment should be discontinued at the first evidence of skin erythema.

Microbiological overgrowth: The use of antibiotics may occasionally result in the overgrowth of nonsusceptible organisms including *Candida.* If a resistant organism appears, the antibiotic should be discontinued and appropriate therapy instituted.

Patients known to have, or suspected to have, achlorhydria should not be prescribed Vibramycin Acne Pack.

Use in patients with renal impairment: No dosage adjustment is necessary in the presence of renal impairment.

Excretion of doxycycline by the kidney is about 40%/72 hours in individuals with normal renal function. This percentage excretion may fall to a range as low as 1–5%/72 hours in individuals with severe renal insufficiency (creatinine clearance below 10 ml/min). Studies have shown no significant difference in the serum half-life of doxycycline in individuals with normal and severely impaired renal function. Haemodialysis does not alter the serum half-life of doxycycline. The anti-anabolic action of the tetracyclines may cause an increase in blood urea. Studies to date indicate that this does not occur with the use of Vibramycin in patients with impaired renal function.

Use in patients with impaired hepatic function: Vibramycin should be administered with caution to patients with hepatic impairment or those receiving potentially hepatotoxic drugs.

Interactions with other medicaments and other forms of interaction: The absorption of doxycycline may be impaired by concurrently administered antacids containing aluminium, calcium or magnesium; oral zinc, iron salts or bismuth preparations.

Tetracyclines depress plasma prothrombin activity and reduced doses of concomitant anticoagulants may be necessary.

The serum half-life of doxycycline may be shortened when patients are concurrently receiving barbiturates, carbamazepine or phenytoin.

A few cases of pregnancy or breakthrough bleeding have been attributed to the concurrent use of tetracycline antibiotics with oral contraceptives.

Since bacteriostatic drugs may interfere with the bactericidal action of penicillin, it is advisable to avoid giving Vibramycin in conjunction with penicillin.

Alcohol may decrease the half-life of doxycycline.

Pregnancy and lactation: See under *Contra-indications.*

Effects on ability to drive and use machinery: There is no evidence to suggest that doxycycline may have an effect on the ability to drive or operate machinery.

Undesirable effects: Due to virtually complete absorption of Vibramycin, gastro-intestinal side-effects are infrequent.

The following adverse reactions have been observed in patients receiving tetracyclines:

Gastro-intestinal: Gastro-intestinal symptoms are usually mild and seldom necessitate discontinuation of treatment. Anorexia, nausea, vomiting, diarrhoea, glossitis, dysphagia, enterocolitis and inflammatory lesions (with candidal overgrowth) in the anogenital region.

Hepatic toxicity: Abnormal hepatic function has been reported.

Skin: Maculopapular and erythematous rashes occur, but were uncommon in clinical trials. Exfoliative dermatitis has been reported but is uncommon. Photosensitivity is discussed in the *Special warnings and special precautions for use.*

Hypersensitivity reactions: Urticaria, angioneurotic oedema, anaphylaxis, anaphylactoid purpura, serum sickness, pericarditis, and exacerbation of systemic lupus erythematosus.

Bulging fontanelles in infants and benign intracranial hypertension in adults have been reported. Treatment should be withdrawn if evidence of raised intracranial pressure develops. These conditions disappeared rapidly when the drug was discontinued.

Blood: Haemolytic anaemia, thrombocytopenia, neutropenia and eosinophilia have been reported with tetracyclines.

When given over prolonged periods, tetracyclines have been reported to produce brown-black microscopic discolouration of thyroid tissue. No abnormalities of thyroid function are known to occur.

Overdose: Acute overdosage with antibiotics is rare. In the event of overdosage discontinue medication. Gastric lavage plus appropriate supportive treatment is indicated.

Dialysis does not alter the serum half-life and thus would not be of benefit in treating cases of overdosage.

Pharmacological properties

Pharmacodynamic properties: As an antibiotic, doxycycline exerts its antimicrobial effect by the inhibition of protein synthesis and is considered to be primarily bacteriostatic.

Doxycycline is clinically effective in the treatment of a variety of infections caused by a wide range of gram-negative and gram-positive bacteria, as well as certain other micro-organisms.

Pharmacokinetic properties: Absorption:

- absorption is rapid (effective concentrations are attained as from the first hour), and the peak serum concentration occurs after 2 to 4 hours.
- almost all of the product is absorbed in the upper part of digestive tract.
- absorption is not notably modified by administration with meals, milk has little effect.

Distribution: In adults, an oral dose of 200 mg results in:

- a peak serum concentration of more than 3 µg/ml
- a residual concentration of more than 1 µg/ml after 24 hours
- a serum half-life of 16–22 hours
- protein binding varying between 82 and 93% (labile binding).

Intra- and extracellular diffusion is good.

With usual doses, effective concentrations are found in the skin, ovaries, uterine tubes, uterus, placenta, testicles, prostate, bladder, kidneys, lung tissue, muscles, lymph glands, sinus secretions, maxillary sinus, nasal polyps, tonsils, liver, hepatic and gallbladder bile, gall bladder, stomach, intestine, appendix, omentum, saliva and gingival fluid. Only small amounts are diffused into the cerebrospinal fluid.

Excretion: The antibiotic is concentrated in the bile. About 40% of the administered dose is eliminated in 3 days in active form in the urine and about 32% in the faeces. Urinary concentrations are roughly 10 times higher than plasma concentrations at the same time. In the presence of impaired renal function, urinary elimination decreases, faecal elimination increases and the half-life remains unchanged. The half-life is not affected by haemodialysis.

Preclinical safety data: Not applicable.

Pharmaceutical particulars

List of excipients: Sucrose and maize starch microgranules, Crospovidone, Polymethacrylate, Talc.

Gelatin (capsule shell)

Colourants–capsule shell: Titanium dioxide (E 171), Indigo Carmine (E 132), Quinoline Yellow (E 104), Iron Oxide (E 172).

Incompatibilities: Nil.

Shelf life: 4 years.

Special precautions for storage: Store below 25°C.

Nature and contents of container: Doxycycline capsules are packed in blister packs (200 micron rigid, opaque white polyvinylchloride and 20 micron aluminium).

Doxycycline capsules 50 mg are supplied in packs of 2 and 56 capsules.

Instructions for handling: See *Posology and method and administration.*

Marketing authorisation number PL 0057/0410

Date of first authorisation/renewal of authorisation 29 May 1997.

Date of (partial) revision of the text 16 July 1997.

ZITHROMAX* CAPSULES
ZITHROMAX* SUSPENSION
ZITHROMAX* TABLETS

Qualitative and quantitative composition Active ingredient: azithromycin.

Zithromax Capsules contain azithromycin dihydrate equivalent to 250 mg azithromycin.

Zithromax Powder for Oral Suspension is a dry blend of azithromycin dihydrate containing the equivalent of 200 mg azithromycin per 5 ml on reconstitution with water.

Zithromax Tablets contain azithromycin dihydrate equivalent to 500 mg azithromycin.

Pharmaceutical form Zithromax Capsules are white, hard gelatin capsules marked Pfizer and ZTM 250.

Zithromax Powder for Oral Suspension is a dry powder which reconstitutes with water to give a cherry/banana flavoured suspension with a slight vanilla odour.

Zithromax Tablets are white, film-coated tablets, marked ZTM 500.

Clinical particulars

Therapeutic indications: Zithromax is indicated for infections caused by susceptible organisms; in lower respiratory tract infections including bronchitis and pneumonia, skin and soft tissue infections, otitis media and in upper respiratory tract infections including sinusitis and pharyngitis/tonsillitis.

In sexually transmitted diseases in men and women, Zithromax is indicated in the treatment of uncomplicated genital infections due to *Chlamydia trachomatis.*

Posology and method of administration: Zithromax should be given as a single daily dose. In common with many other antibiotics Zithromax Capsules should be taken at least 1 hour before or 2 hours after food.

Zithromax Suspension and Zithromax Tablets can be taken with food.

Adults: For the treatment of sexually transmitted diseases caused by *Chlamydia trachomatis,* the dose is 1 g given as a single dose.

For all other indications, the dose is 1.5g, which should be given 500 mg daily for 3 days.

In the elderly: The same dose range as in younger patients may be used in the elderly.

In children: Zithromax Suspension should be used for children under 45 kg. There is no information on children under 6 months of age. The dose in children is 10 mg/kg as a single daily dose for 3 days:

Up to 15 kg (less than 3 years): Measure the dose as closely as possible using the 10 ml oral dosing syringe provided. The syringe is graduated in 0.25 ml divisions, providing 10 mg of azithromycin in every graduation.

For children weighing more than 15 kg: Zithromax Suspension should be administered using the spoon provided according to the following guidance:

15–25 kg (3–7 years): 5 ml (200 mg) given as 1 x 5 ml spoonful, once daily for 3 days.

26–35 kg (8–11 years): 7.5 ml (300 mg) given as 1 x 7.5 ml spoonful, once daily for 3 days.

36–45 kg (12–14 years): 10 ml (400 mg) given as 1 x 10 ml spoonful, once daily for 3 days.

Over 45 kg: Dose as per adults.

See *Nature and contents of container,* for appropriate pack size to use depending on age/body weight of child.

The specially supplied measure should be used to administer Zithromax suspension to children.

In patients with renal impairment: No dosage adjustment is needed in patients with mild renal impairment (creatinine clearance >40 ml/min). For patients with more severe renal impairment, see *Special warnings and special precautions for use.*

In patients with hepatic impairment: See *Special warnings and special precautions for use.*

Zithromax Capsules, Tablets and Zithromax Suspension are for oral administration only.

Contra-indications: Zithromax is contra-indicated in patients with a known hypersensitivity to azithromycin or any of the macrolide antibiotics.

Because of the theoretical possibility of ergotism, Zithromax and ergot derivatives should not be co-administered.

Special warnings and special precautions for use: As with erythromycin and other macrolides, rare serious allergic reactions including angioneurotic oedema and anaphylaxis (rarely fatal), have been reported. Some of these reactions with Zithromax have resulted in recurrent symptoms and required a long period of observation and treatment.

As with any antibiotic preparation, observation for signs of superinfection with non-susceptible organisms, including fungi is recommended.

Use in renal impairment: No dose adjustment is needed in patients with mild renal impairment (creatinine clearance >40 ml/min), but there are no data regarding Zithromax in patients with more severe renal impairment, thus caution should be exercised in using Zithromax in these patients.

Use in hepatic impairment: As the liver is the principal route of excretion of azithromycin, it should not be used in patients with hepatic disease.

Interaction with other medicaments and other forms of interaction

Antacids: In patients receiving Zithromax and antacids, Zithromax should be taken at least 1 hour before or 2 hours after the antacid.

Carbamazepine: In a pharmacokinetic interaction study in healthy volunteers, no significant effect was observed on the plasma levels of carbamazepine or its active metabolite.

Cimetidine: A single dose of cimetidine administered 2 hours before Zithromax had no effect on the pharmacokinetics of azithromycin.

Cyclosporin: Some of the related macrolide antibiotics interfere with the metabolism of cyclosporin. In the absence of conclusive data from pharmacokinetic studies or clinical data investigating potential interaction between Zithromax and cyclosporin, caution should be exercised before co-administration of these two drugs. If co-administration is necessary, cyclosporin levels should be monitored and the dose adjusted accordingly.

Digoxin: Some of the macrolide antibiotics have been reported to impair the metabolism of digoxin (in the gut) in some patients. Therefore, in patients receiving concomitant Zithromax and digoxin the possibility of raised digoxin levels should be borne in mind, and digoxin levels monitored.

Ergot derivatives: Because of the theoretical possibility of ergotism, Zithromax and ergot derivatives should not be co-administered.

Methylprednisolone: In a pharmacokinetic interaction study in healthy volunteers, Zithromax had no significant effect on the pharmacokinetics of methylprednisolone.

Theophylline: There is no evidence of any pharmacokinetic interaction when Zithromax and theophylline are co-administered to healthy volunteers. In general, however, theophylline levels should be monitored.

Terfenadine: Because of the occurrence of serious dysrhythmias secondary to prolongation of the QTc interval in patients receiving other anti-infectives in conjunction with terfenadine, interaction studies have been performed. Pharmacokinetic studies have reported no evidence of an interaction between azithromycin and terfenadine. There have been rare cases reported where the possibility of such an interaction could not be entirely excluded; however there was no specific evidence that such an interaction had occurred. As with other macrolides, Zithromax should be administered with caution in combination with terfenadine.

Warfarin: In a pharmacodynamic interaction study, Zithromax did not alter the anticoagulant effect of a single 15 mg dose of warfarin administered to healthy volunteers. Zithromax and warfarin may be co-administered, but monitoring of the prothrombin time should be continued as routinely performed.

Pregnancy and lactation

Use in pregnancy: Animal reproduction studies have demonstrated that azithromycin crosses the placenta, but have revealed no evidence of harm to the foetus. There are no adequate and well controlled studies in pregnant women. Since animal studies are not always predictive of human response, Zithromax should be used during pregnancy only if adequate alternatives are not available.

Use in lactation: No data on secretion of azithromycin in breast milk are available, so that Zithromax should only be used in lactating women where adequate alternatives are not available.

Effects on ability to drive and use machines: There is no evidence to suggest that Zithromax may have an effect on a patient's ability to drive or operate machinery.

Undesirable effects: Zithromax is well tolerated with a low incidence of side effects.

The majority of side effects were gastrointestinal in origin with anorexia, nausea, vomiting/diarrhoea (rarely resulting in dehydration) and loose stools, dyspepsia, abdominal discomfort (pain/cramps), constipation and flatulence being occasionally observed.

Allergic reactions such as rash, photosensitivity, arthralgia, oedema or urticaria have occurred and there have also been rare reports of serious hypersensitivity reactions – See *Special warnings/precautions.*

Abnormal liver function, including hepatitis and cholestatic jaundice, as well as rare cases of hepatic necrosis and hepatic failure, which have rarely resulted in death.

Dizziness/vertigo, convulsions (as seen with other macrolides), headache and somnolence have been reported.

Transient mild reductions in neutrophil counts have occasionally been observed in clinical trials.

Hearing impairment has been reported with macrolide antibiotics. There have been rare reports of hearing impairment, including hearing loss, deafness and/or tinnitus in some patients receiving azithromycin. Many of these have been associated with prolonged use of high doses in investigational studies. In those cases where follow-up information was available the majority of these events were reversible.

There have been rare reports of taste disturbances.

Interstitial nephritis and acute renal failure have been reported.

Palpitations and arrythmias including ventricular tachycardia (as seen with macrolides) have been reported.

Rarely, serious skin reactions including erythema multiforme, Stevens Johnson Syndrome and toxic epidermal necrolysis have occurred.

Asthenia and paraesthesia have been reported.

Overdose: There are no data on overdosage with Zithromax. Typical symptoms of overdosage with macrolide antibiotics include hearing loss, severe nausea, vomiting and diarrhoea. Gastric lavage and general supportive measures are indicated.

Pharmacological properties

Pharmacodynamic properties: Zithromax is an azalide, derived from the macrolide class of antibiotics. The mode of action of azithromycin is inhibition of protein synthesis in bacteria by binding to the 50s ribosomal subunit and preventing translocation of peptides.

Azithromycin demonstrates activity *in vitro* against a wide variety of Gram-positive and Gram-negative bacteria including: *Staphylococcus aureus, Streptococcus pneumoniae, Streptococcus pyogenes* (Group A) and other Streptococcal species; *Haemophilus influenzae* and *parainfluenzae; Branhamella catarrhalis;* anaerobes including *Bacteroides fragilis; Escherichia coli; Bordetella pertussis; Bordetella parapertussis; Borrelia burgdorferi; Haemophilus ducreyi; Neisseria gonorrhoeae* and *Chlamydia trachomatis.* Azithromycin also demonstrates *in vitro* activity against *Legionella pneumophila, Mycoplasma pneumoniae* and *hominis,* Campylobacter sp., *Toxoplasma gondii* and *Treponema pallidum.*

Pharmacokinetic properties: Following oral administration in humans, azithromycin is widely distributed throughout the body; bioavailability is approximately 37%. The time taken to peak plasma levels is 2–3 hours. The plasma terminal elimination half-life closely reflects the tissue depletion half-life of 2 to 4 days.

Kinetic studies have shown markedly higher azithromycin levels in tissue than in plasma (up to 50 times the maximum observed concentration in plasma) indicating that the drug is heavily tissue bound. Concentrations in target tissues such as lung, tonsil, and prostate exceed the MIC90 for likely pathogens after a single dose of 500 mg.

Pharmaceutical particulars

List of excipients

Zithromax Capsules contain: Lactose, magnesium stearate, maize starch, and sodium lauryl sulphate. The capsule shells contain: Gelatin, iron oxide-black (E172), shellac, sulphur dioxide and titanium dioxide.

Zithromax Powder for Oral Suspension contains: Hydroxypropylcellulose, sodium phosphate tribasic anhydrous, sucrose, xanthan gum. Flavours: artificial banana, artificial cherry, artificial creme de vanilla.

Zithromax Tablets contain: calcium phosphate dibasic anhydrous, croscarmellose sodium, hydroxypropylmethylcellulose, lactose, magnesium stearate, sodium lauryl sulphate, starch, titanium dioxide (E171) and triacetin.

Incompatibilities: None known

Shelf life: Zithromax Capsules 4 years.

Powder for Oral Suspension 3 years.

Once reconstituted with water, Zithromax Suspension has a shelf-life of 5 days.

Zithromax Tablets 2 years.

Special precautions for storage: No special storage conditions required.

Nature and contents of container: Zithromax Capsules are available as:

Packs of 4 capsules. Aluminium/PVC blister strips, 4 capsules per strip, 1 strip in a carton box.

Pack of 6 capsules. Aluminium/PVC blister strips, 6 capsules per strip, 1 strip in a carton box.

Zithromax Powder for Oral Suspension is available as:

600 mg (15 ml) Pack: (Recommended for use in children up to 7 years (25 kg)).

Packs of powder equivalent to 600 mg azithromycin in a polypropylene container with child resistant screw cap, in a carton box. Pack contains a multi-dosing spoon and 10 ml oral dosing syringe with detachable adaptor. A sticker for the syringe is appended to the bottle label. Reconstitute with 8 ml of water to give 15 ml suspension.

900 mg (22.5 ml) Pack: (Recommended for use in children aged from 8–11 years (26–35 kg)). Packs of powder equivalent to 900 mg azithromycin in a polypropylene container with child resistant screw cap, in a carton box. Pack contains a multi-dosing spoon. Reconstitute with 11 ml of water to give 22.5 ml suspension.

1200 mg (30 ml) Pack: (Recommended for use in children aged from 12–14 years (36–45 kg)). Packs of powder equivalent to 1200 mg azithromycin in a polypropylene container with child resistant screw cap, in a carton box. Pack contains a multi-dosing spoon. Reconstitute with 14 ml of water to give 30 ml suspension.

Multi-dosing spoon delivers doses as follows:

Small end to graduation	2.5 ml	(100 mg)
brimful	5 ml	(200 mg)
Large end to graduation	7.5 ml	(300 mg)
brimful	10 ml	(400 mg)

Zithromax 500 mg Tablets are available as:

Pack of 3 tablets. Aluminium/PVC blister strip, 3 tablets per strip, 1 strip in a carton box.

Each Pack contains a Patient information/instruction leaflet.

Instructions for use/handling: When dispensing the 15 ml pack, advice should be given as to whether the dose should be measured using the oral dosing syringe or the spoon provided and on correct usage.

If the dose is to be given using the oral dosing syringe, before dispensing, the syringe adaptor should be detached from the syringe and inserted into the bottle neck and the cap replaced.

The sticker provided should be used to mark the syringe at the appropriate level once the correct daily dosage has been calculated.

When dispensing 22.5 ml and 30 ml packs, advice should be given as to the correct usage of the multi-dosing spoon.

Zithromax Tablets and Capsules should be swallowed whole.

Marketing authorisation numbers

Zithromax Capsules 250 mg	0057/0335
Zithromax Powder for Oral Suspension 200 mg/5 ml	0057/0336
Zithromax Tablets 500 mg	0057/0391

Date of renewal of the authorisation

Zithromax Capsules 250 mg:	4 April 1996.
Zithromax Powder for Oral Suspension 200 mg/5 ml:	4 April 1996.
Zithromax Tablets 500 mg:	17 September 1996

Date of (partial) revision of the text 22 July 1998

Legal category POM

**Trade Mark*

Pfizer Consumer Healthcare
Wilsom Road
Alton, Hampshire GU34 2TJ

☎ 01420 84801 🗋 01420 89376

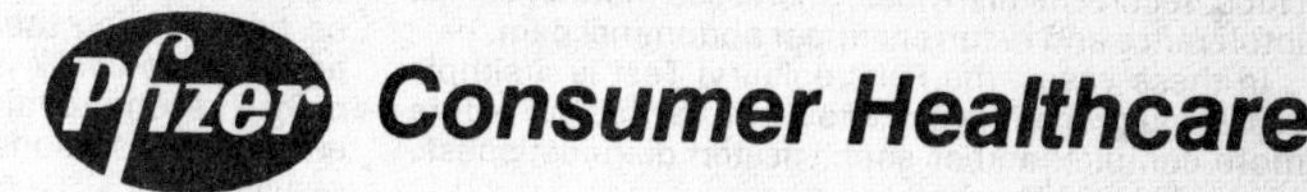

ISOGEL*

Presentation Isogel is a preparation of Ispaghula Husk BP, which consists of the epidermis and collapsed adjacent layers removed from the dried ripe seeds of Plantago ovata Forssk.

Isogel is supplied as small, reddish-brown granules in containers of 200 g.

Uses Isogel is not absorbed from the gastrointestinal tract, but it absorbs water to form a mucilaginous mass. This results in a purely mechanical stimulus to mass peristalsis without any purgative effect. It is for this reason that Isogel is not only an effective remedy for constipation but is also of value in the treatment of diarrhoea, irritable bowel syndrome and the management of patients with a colostomy. Isogel is indicated in habitual constipation, including cases due to spastic colon, dietary insufficiencies and in patients with haemorrhoids or diabetes. It can be used to normalise bowel movement in patients with mucous or ulcerative colitis.

Isogel is of help to patients with a colostomy as the formation of a well-formed, easily passed stool assists in the maintenance of cleanliness and the establishment of control.

Dosage and administration The required quantity of Isogel should be stirred briskly into half a glass of water and swallowed at once. Carbonated water is frequently preferred and may make swallowing easier.

Adults and the elderly: Two teaspoonfuls once or twice daily, preferably at mealtimes. Elderly or debilitated patients should be supervised whilst taking Isogel.

Children: One teaspoonful once or twice daily, preferably at mealtimes.

The above dosage is only a general guide and it should be adjusted to suit the needs of each individual patient.

In diarrhoea the dose, usually one teaspoonful, is taken three times daily until symptoms abate.

Contra-indications, warnings, etc
Contra-indications: Nil.

Precautions: A few cases of inhalation of the mucilaginous mass which forms on allowing an Isogel/water mixture to stand have been reported. In consequence, it is important that Isogel should be swallowed immediately after mixing, and elderly or debilitated patients should be supervised whilst taking it.

Use in pregnancy: No known adverse effects in pregnancy. However, as with all medicines, care should be taken during pregnancy, particularly during the first trimester. No adverse effects in lactation.

Side-effects: Nil.

Overdosage: As Isogel is not absorbed and it has no purgative action the problem of overdosage does not arise.

Pharmaceutical precautions Store below 25 deg C in a dry place.

Legal category GSL.

Package quantities Isogel is supplied in containers of 200 g.

Further information Nil.

Product licence number 01906/0008.

MIGRALEVE*

Qualitative and quantitative composition
Migraleve combines two dosage forms, Migraleve Pink and Migraleve Yellow tablets.

Each Migraleve Pink tablet contains:

Paracetamol DC 96% (equivalent to Paracetamol PhEur 500 mg)	520 mg
Codeine Phosphate PhEur	8 mg
Buclizine Hydrochloride BP	6.25 mg

Each Migraleve Yellow tablet contains:

Paracetamol DC 96% (equivalent to Paracetamol PhEur 500 mg)	520 mg
Codeine Phosphate PhEur	8 mg

Pharmaceutical form Pink (Migraleve Pink) or yellow (Migraleve Yellow) aqueous film-coated tablets.

Clinical particulars
Therapeutic indications: For the treatment of migraine attacks which can include the symptoms of migraine headache, nausea and vomiting. Route of administration - oral.

Posology and method of administration:
Adults and the elderly: Two Migraleve Pink tablets to be swallowed immediately it is known that a migraine attack has started or is imminent. If further treatment is required, two Migraleve Yellow tablets every four hours.

Maximum dose: eight tablets (two Migraleve Pink and six Migraleve Yellow) in 24 hours.

Children 10–14 years: One Migraleve Pink tablet to be swallowed immediately it is known that a migraine attack has started or is imminent. If further treatment is required, one Migraleve Yellow tablet every four hours.

Maximum dose: four tablets (one Migraleve Pink and three Migraleve Yellow) in 24 hours.

Do not give to children under 10 years of age except under medical supervision.

Contra-indications: Do not give to children under 10 years of age except under medical supervision. Hypersensitivity to any of the ingredients.

Special warnings and precautions for use: Migraine should be medically diagnosed. Because some medicines do not combine, if you are already taking prescribed medicines please consult your doctor. If symptoms persist, consult your doctor. Migraleve tablets contain potent medicaments and should not be taken continuously for extended periods without the advice of a doctor. Do not exceed the stated dose. Migraleve Pink tablets only: May cause drowsiness. If affected, do not drive or operate machinery. Avoid alcoholic drink. Should be used with caution in patients with severe renal disease or liver dysfunction.

Interaction with other medicaments and other forms of interaction: None known.

Pregnancy and lactation: Although experiments in some animal species gave rise to adverse effects following the administration of buclizine to pregnant animals e.g. foetal abnormalities and maternal deaths, these occurred at doses in excess of 120 times the human daily dose. Whilst there are no specific reasons for contra-indicating Migraleve during pregnancy, as with all drugs it is recommended that Migraleve be used in pregnancy only when the physician has considered the need in respect of the patients' welfare. Migraleve is not contra-indicated in breast-feeding mothers.

Effects on ability to drive and use machinery: Migraleve Pink tablets only: May cause drowsiness. If affected do not drive or operate machinery. Avoid alcoholic drink.

Undesirable effects: Rare allergic reactions to paracetamol, such as skin rashes, hives or itching. Codeine may cause constipation. Buclizine hydrochloride may cause drowsiness.

Overdose: Symptoms of paracetamol overdosage are often delayed for at least 24 hours, but to prevent damage, treatment should be given as soon as possible and within 10 hours of ingestion. Treatment is by the administration of i.v. acetylcysteine. Oral methionine may be used, but is less certain in its effect because of its need for G.I. absorption. Once hepatic failure has developed, standard measures of management should be employed.

Patients on enzyme-inducing agents (such as barbiturates) and chronic non-cirrhotic alcoholics may be more susceptible to the toxicity of paracetamol overdosage.

Symptoms of codeine overdosage include nausea and vomiting, and circulatory and respiratory depression. Initial treatment includes gastric lavage. If CNS depression is severe, artificial respiration, oxygen and parenteral naloxone may be required.

Pharmacological particulars
Pharmacodynamics: Paracetamol has analgesic, antipyretic and mild, acute anti-inflammatory properties. Paracetamol inhibits prostaglandin synthesis, especially in the CNS. Paracetamol does not inhibit chronic inflammatory reactions.

Codeine is an opioid analgesic. Codeine also has anti-tussive properties.

The combination of paracetamol and codeine has been shown to have hyperadditive analgesic effects in animals.

Buclizine is a piperazine derivative with the actions and uses of H_1-receptor antagonists. It has antimuscarinic and central sedative properties. It is used mainly for its anti-emetic properties.

Pharmacokinetics: Paracetamol is rapidly absorbed from the upper G.I. tract after oral administration, with the small intestine being an important site of absorption. Peak blood levels of 15–20 µg/ml after normal 1 g oral doses of paracetamol occur within 30–90 minutes. Depending upon dosage form, it is rapidly distributed throughout the body and is primarily metabolised in the liver with excretion via the kidney. Elimination half-life is about 2 hours after reaching a peak following a 1 g oral dose. Paracetamol crosses the placental barrier and is present in breast milk.

Codeine is absorbed from the gastro-intestinal tract and peak plasma concentrations occur after one hour. Codeine is metabolised by O- and N-demethylation in the liver to morphine, norcodeine and other metabolites. Codeine and its metabolites are excreted almost entirely by the kidney, mainly as conjugates with glucuronic acid. Codeine is not extensively bound to plasma proteins. The plasma half-life has been reported to be between 3 and 4 hours.

Buclizine hydrochloride is more slowly absorbed from the G.I. tract (T_{max} 3 hours). The elimination half-life is approximately 15 hours.

Preclinical safety data: No data presented.

Pharmaceutical particulars
List of excipients:
Migraleve Pink Tablets
Magnesium Stearate PhEur; Colloidal Silicon Dioxide NF; Stearic Acid BP; Starch Pregelatinised NF; Colour Dispersed Pink 11150 (E127); Opadry OY-1367 Pink*

*Opadry OY-1367 Pink contains: Hypromellose PhEur; Titanium Dioxide BP (E171); Macrogol 400; Erythrosine Lake (E127)**

**consists of Erythrosine (E127) and Aluminium Oxide

Migraleve Yellow Tablets
Magnesium Stearate PhEur; Colloidal Silicon Dioxide NF; Stearic Acid BP; Starch Pregelatinised NF; Opadry OY-6126 Yellow*

*Opadry OY-6126 Yellow contains: Hypromellose PhEur; Titanium Dioxide BP (E171); Macrogol 400; Quinoline Yellow Aluminium Lake (E104)**; Iron Oxide Yellow (E172)

**consists of Quinoline Yellow (E104) and Aluminium Oxide

Incompatibilities: None known.

Shelf-life: 36 months.

Special precautions for storage: None.

Nature and contents of container: Clear amber PVC/Aluminium foil blister strips.

Packs of 48 tablets (32 Migraleve Pink and 16 Migraleve Yellow). Also continuation packs of 48 Migraleve Pink and 48 Migraleve Yellow.

Instructions for use/handling: None.

Marketing authorisation holder
Unicliffe Ltd T/A Pfizer Consumer Healthcare, Wilsom Road, Alton, Hampshire GU34 2TJ.

Marketing authorisation numbers

PL 01906/0026	Migraleve Pink
PL 01906/0027	Migraleve Yellow
PL 01906/0028	Migraleve

Date of approval/revision of SPC June 1998.

Legal category POM.

PANCREOLAURYL* TEST

Qualitative and quantitative composition
Each blue capsule contains: 174.25 mg (=0.25 mmol) Fluorescein dilaurate.
Each red capsule contains: 94.07 mg (=0.25 mmol) Fluorescein Sodium BP.

Pharmaceutical form Capsules.

Clinical particulars
Therapeutic indications: Pancreolauryl Test is used to detect abnormally low pancreatic exocrine function in

patients who have symptoms associated with disturbances of pancreatic function. These symptoms include recurrent diarrhoea, increased flatulence, fat intolerance and recurrent upper abdominal pain.

In these cases, the Pancreolauryl Test is a simple screening procedure and should be carried out before more complex and/or sophisticated diagnostic tests are performed.

Route of administration – oral.

Posology and method of administration:

Adults and the elderly: The patient can eat and drink as usual on the evening prior to the test, but no medicines containing vitamins should be taken. It is recommended that Pfizer Consumer Healthcare are consulted prior to the concomitant administration of pancreatic enzyme preparations and Pancreolauryl Test.

Test Day No 1: For 10 hours after the start of the test, i.e. administration of 2 blue capsules with the standard meal, all urine is collected including a final emptying of the bladder at exactly 10 hours after the start of the test. The total quantity of urine collected can be tested by the laboratory immediately. If there is any delay the contained should be stored in a refrigerator; preservatives need not be added.

Test Day No 2: Two red control capsules can be taken the following day ensuring that the same procedure is followed.

Children: Although satisfactory results have been obtained in children, the test is not currently recommended for children.

Contra-indications: Acute necrotising pancreatitis. Pregnancy.

Special warnings and special precautions for use: Although satisfactory results have been obtained in children, the test is not currently recommended for children.

Interactions with other medicaments and other forms of interaction: No drug interactions known. However, test results may be affected by concomitant use of vitamins. Sulphasalazine can interfere with photometric measurements. Pancreatic enzyme preparations sold in the U.K. as of June 1992 may continue to be taken during the test. However, if in doubt, it is advisable to check with Pfizer Consumer Healthcare before recommending continued use of pancreatic enzyme preparations to prevent interference with test results.

Pregnancy and lactation: Contra-indicated in pregnancy. No information in lactation.

Effects on ability to drive and use machines: No known effects.

Undesirable effects: No side-effects have been reported.

Overdosage: General supportive measures. Administration of activated charcoal.

Pharmacological particulars

Pharmacodynamic properties: Cholesterol ester hydrolase, secreted by the pancreas, is able to break down fluorescein dilaurate into free, water-soluble fluorescein and lauric acid. Absence of this enzyme, as in cases of pancreatic insufficiency, will result in a T/K ratio 20 or below, when the urinary fluorescein concentration after fluorescein dilaurate capsules is compared to urinary fluorescein concentration after water-soluble fluorescein sodium capsules.

Pharmacokinetic properties: The blue capsules contain fluorescein dilaurate which has low water solubility and is not absorbed systemically. When administered with a standard meal, pancreatic exocrine function is stimulated and enzymes secreted. The pancreatic enzymes lyse the fluorescein dilaurate releasing fluorescein which is absorbed and excreted in the urine.

The urine is collected for a period of ten hours following administration of the test capsule and the total quantity of fluorescein dye excreted is determined by direct measurement of fluorescein concentration.

The amount of fluorescein excreted in the urine depends on pancreatic function and on individual variations in gastro-intestinal absorption and renal excretion.

To assess the absorption and excretion characteristics for individual patients; a repeat test using the control capsules is carried out the next day. The control capsule is red and contain unesterified fluorescein (Fluorescein Sodium).

The quantity of fluorescein excreted from the test capsule is expressed as a percentage of the quantity of fluorescein excreted from the control capsule. This value is termed the T/K ratio, and is used as a parameter of pancreatic function.

Pre-clinical safety data: No further data presented.

Pharmaceutical particulars

List of excipients:

Fluorescein dilaurate capsules: Povidone BP; Microcrystalline cellulose DAB; Gelatin DAB; Titanium Dioxide (E171); Indigotin (E132).

Fluorescein sodium capsules: Povidone BP; Lactose PhEur; Zinc Stearate DAC '79; Gelatin DAB; Indigotin (E132); Titanium Dioxide (E171); Erythrosine (E127).

Incompatibilities: None known.

Shelf-life: 36 months.

Special precautions for storage: Store in a cool, dry place.

Nature of contents and container: 20 um aluminium foil strips, yellow, heat sealable, lacquered.

Packs of 4 capsules (2 Test plus 2 Control); and 10×4 capsules (10×2 Test plus 2 Control); and 6×4 capsules (6×2 Test plus 2 Control).

Instructions for use/handling: None.

Marketing authorisation holder Unicliffe Ltd T/A Pfizer Consumer Healthcare, Wilsom Road, Alton, Hampshire GU34 2TJ.

Marketing authorisation number PL 01906/0020.

Date of approval/revision of SPC March 1996.

Legal category POM.

**Trade Mark*

Pharmacia & Upjohn
Davy Avenue
Knowlhill
Milton Keynes
Bucks MK5 8PH

☎ 01908 661101 🖷 01908 690091

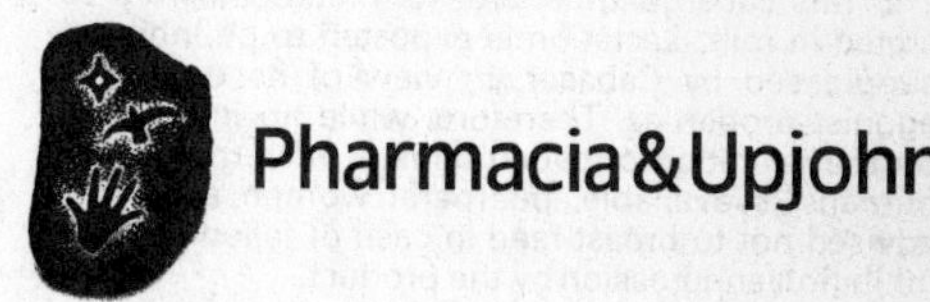

AMINOGLUTETHIMIDE

Presentation Practically white, round, scored tablets, containing 250 mg aminoglutethimide.

Uses Aminoglutethimide is indicated for treatment of metastatic carcinoma of the breast in post-menopausal or oophorectomised women.

Aminoglutethimide is also indicated in Cushing's syndrome due to malignant disease, where surgical treatment is inappropriate or as an adjunct to surgery, either pre-operatively in the management of metabolic disturbances or post-operatively for the treatment of relapse.

Dosage and administration
Adults: Metastatic carcinoma of the breast: administration should start at 250 mg twice daily for two weeks. In the absence of severe side-effects the dose may be increased to 250 mg four times daily.

Cushing's syndrome due to malignant disease: treatment should be started at 250 mg daily, increasing gradually up to 1 g daily. In some cases, especially ectopic ACTH syndrome, higher doses may be necessary to achieve adequate suppression.

Elderly: The adult dosage schedules may be given without modification.

Children: Not recommended.

Contra-indications, warnings, etc
Contra-indications: Use during pregnancy and lactation is contra-indicated as foetal abnormalities have been seen in animal studies and cases of pseudohermaphroditism have been reported in neonates of women treated with aminoglutethimide.

Warnings: Aminoglutethimide suppresses production of glucocorticoids and in patients with breast carcinoma supplementary glucocorticoids will be needed.

During initial treatment of Cushing's syndrome due to malignant disease, no corticosteroids should be necessary. Plasma cortisol levels should be monitored regularly and if adrenocortical insufficiency occurs supplementary glucocorticoids may be given.

The suppression of aldosterone synthesis may lead to hyponatraemia, hyperkalaemia, hypotension and dizziness, in which case a mineralocorticoid should be given.

Blood count and plasma electrolytes should be checked regularly. Aminoglutethimide has been found occasionally to diminish thyroid function. If, during treatment of breast carcinoma signs of Cushing's syndrome appear which are due to concomitant glucocorticoid medication, the dosage of the glucocorticoid should be reduced.

Aminoglutethimide may increase the rate of metabolism of some drugs such as coumarin anticoagulants, oral hypoglycaemic agents and dexamethasone and dosage of these may need adjustment.

Side-effects: Aminoglutethimide tolerability varies greatly and CNS side-effects such as dizziness, somnolence and lethargy are relatively common and dose dependent; unsteadiness occurs only in the highest dosage range. Gastrointestinal effects are less frequent but usually dose-dependent. A drug rash, sometimes accompanied by fever, may develop after 7–14 days. This usually subsides within 7–10 days even though treatment is continued: if it should not subside, treatment should be stopped temporarily. Alternatively the dose of concomitant glucocorticoid may be increased. Rarely pancytopenia, leucopenia and agranulocytosis have been reported.

Overdosage: Following overdosage of aminoglutethimide, no serious outcome has been reported. However, gastric lavage should be performed as soon as possible and full supportive measures should be employed. In severe cases, haemodialysis or charcoal haemoperfusion may be useful. Steroid replacement should be maintained or initiated, as necessary.

Pharmaceutical precautions Protect from heat, light and moisture.

Legal category POM.

Package quantities Cartons of 100 tablets.

Further information Aminoglutethimide inhibits steroid biosynthesis in the adrenal cortex causing a chemical adrenalectomy. This inhibition occurs at an early stage in the biosynthesis. Suppression of oestrogen production in peripheral tissue may also occur.

Product licence number 3433/0104.

CABASER* 

Qualitative and quantitative composition Cabergoline INN 1, 2 and 4 mg

Pharmaceutical form
1 mg tablets: oval, 4.58 x 7.12 mm, scored, white tablets

2 mg tablets: convex, capsule-shaped, 5 x 10 mm, scored, white tablets

4 mg tablets: oval, biconvex 7.14 x 12.7 mm, scored white tablets.

Container: Type I amber glass bottles with aluminium tamper resistant screw caps, containing silica gel desiccant.

Each bottle contains 20 tablets of either 1 mg or 2 mg strength, or 16 tablets of 4 mg strength, and is enclosed in an outer cardboard carton.

The tablets are for oral administration.

Clinical particulars
Therapeutic indications: Treatment of Parkinson's disease.

Cabaser is indicated for the treatment of symptoms of Parkinson's disease, as adjuvant therapy to levodopa plus dopa-decarboxylase inhibitor, in patients affected by "on-off" mobility problems with daily fluctuations in motor performance.

Controlled clinical studies have demonstrated that cabergoline administered once daily at an average dose of 4 mg/day following titration (up to 5–6 mg/day in the different studies) is effective in decreasing daily fluctuations in motor performance in Parkinsonian patients receiving levodopa/carbidopa therapy. Improvement of motor deficit has been demonstrated, while substantially decreasing the levodopa/carbidopa dose.

Posology and method of administration: Cabaser is for oral administration. Since the tolerability of dopaminergic agents is improved when administered with food, it is recommended that Cabaser be taken with meals.

Cabaser is intended for chronic, long term treatment.

Adults and elderly patients: As expected for dopamine agonists, dose response for both efficacy and side effects appears to be linked to individual sensitivity. Optimization of dose should be obtained through slow initial dose titration, from starting doses of 1 mg daily. The dosage of concurrent levodopa may be gradually decreased, while the dosage of Cabaser is increased, until the optimum balance is determined. In view of the long half-life of the compound, increments of the daily dose of 0.5–1 mg should be done at weekly (initial weeks) or bi-weekly intervals, up to optimal doses.

The recommended therapeutic dosage is 2 to 6 mg/day as adjuvant therapy to levodopa/carbidopa. Cabaser should be given as a single daily dose. Maximum doses higher than 6 mg/day and up to 20 mg/day have been administered in a small proportion of patients during clinical studies.

Use in children: The safety and efficacy of Cabaser have not been investigated in children as Parkinson's disease does not affect this population.

Contra-indications: Hypersensitivity to any ergot alkaloid.

Special warnings and special precautions for use: While renal insufficiency has been shown not to modify cabergoline kinetics, hepatic insufficiency of severe degree (> 10 Child-Pugh score, maximum score 12) has been shown to be associated with an increase of AUC, thus indicating that dose regimens in Parkinsonian patients with severe hepatic insufficiency should be modified accordingly.

Pleural effusion/fibrosis has been infrequently reported following long term administration of Cabaser, and usually when given to patients previously treated with ergolinic DA agonists. Therefore Cabaser should be given with caution to patients with a history or clinical symptoms of respiratory disorders linked to fibrotic tissue degeneration. A chest x-ray examination is recommended if clinical symptoms of respiratory disorders are observed. Where x-ray examination indicates pleural effusion/fibrosis, discontinuation of Cabaser is expected to lead to immediate improvement of symptoms.

Erythrocyte sedimentation rate has been found to be abnormally increased in association with pleural effusion/fibrosis. Chest x-ray examination is recommended in cases of unexplained ESR increases to abnormal values.

In addition, by analogy with other ergot derivatives, Cabaser should be given with caution to patients suffering from severe cardiovascular disease, Raynaud's syndrome, peptic ulcer, gastrointestinal bleeding or a history of serious, particularly psychotic mental disease. Symptomatic hypotension can occur following adminstration of Cabaser: particular attention should be paid when administering Cabaser concomitantly with other drugs known to lower blood pressure.

The effects of alcohol on overall tolerability of Cabaser are currently unknown.

Interaction with other medicaments and other forms of interaction: No pharmacokinetic interaction with L-Dopa or selegiline was observed in the studies carried out in parkinsonian patients. The concomitant use of other drugs, particularly other antiparkinsonian non-dopamine-agonist agents, was not associated with detectable interactions modifying the efficacy and safety of Cabaser.

No other information is available about possible interaction between Cabaser and other ergot alkaloids: therefore the concomitant use of these medications during long term treatment with Cabaser is not recommended.

Since Cabaser exerts its therapeutic effect by direct stimulation of dopamine receptors, it should not be concurrently administered with drugs which have dopamine antagonist activity (such as phenothiazines, butyrophenones, thioxanthenes, metoclopramide) since these might reduce the therapeutic effect of Cabaser.

By analogy with other ergot derivatives, Cabaser should not be used in association with macrolide antibiotics (e.g erythromycin) since the systemic bioavailability of Cabaser and adverse effects could increase.

Pregnancy and lactation: Cabaser has been shown to cross the placenta in rats: it is unknown whether this occurs also in humans.

Animal studies in rats and mice have not demonstrated any teratogenic effect or any effect of the compound on global reproductive performance. In clinical studies there have been over 100 pregnancies in women treated with cabergoline for hyperprolactinemic disorders. The compound was generally taken during the first 8 weeks after conception. Among the pregnancies evaluable so far, there were approximately 85% live births and about 10% spontaneous abortions. Three cases of congenital abnormalities (Down's syndrome, hydrocephalus, malformation of lower limbs) which led to therapeutic abortion and three cases of minor abnormalities in live births were observed.

These incidence rates are comparable with those quoted for normal populations and for women exposed to other ovulation-inducing drugs. Based on the above data, the use of the product does not appear to be associated with an increased risk of abortion, premature delivery, multiple pregnancy or congenital abnormalities.

Because clinical experience is still limited and the drug has a long half-life, as a precautionary measure it is recommended that women seeking pregnancy discontinue Cabaser one month before intended conception, in order to prevent possible foetal exposure to the drug. If conception occurs during therapy, treatment is to be discontinued as soon as pregnancy is confirmed, to limit foetal exposure to the drug.

In rats cabergoline and/or its metabolites are excreted in milk. Lactation is expected to be inhibited/suppressed by Cabaser, in view of its dopamine-agonist properties. Therefore, while no information on the excretion of cabergoline in maternal milk in humans is available, puerperal women should be advised not to breast-feed in case of failed lactation inhibition/suppression by the product.

Effects on ability to drive and use machines: During treatment with Cabaser, patients should be cautioned about engaging in activities requiring rapid and precise responses, such as driving or operating machinery.

Undesirable effects: About 1070 parkinsonian patients have received Cabaser as adjuvant therapy to L-dopa in clinical studies; of these 74% had at least one adverse event, mainly of mild to moderate severity and transient in nature, and requiring discontinuation in a small proportion of cases.

In the majority of cases (51%), events were related to the nervous system: most frequently reported events were dyskinesia, hyperkinesia, hallucinations or confusion. The gastrointestinal system was involved in 33% of cases: events most frequently reported were nausea, vomiting, dyspepsia and gastritis. The cardiovascular system was involved in 27% of cases, most frequently reported events being dizziness and hypotension. The respiratory system was involved in 13% of cases, symptomatic pleural effusion/fibrosis being reported with a frequency <2%.

Other adverse events expected for the pharmacological class, in view of the vasoconstrictive properties, include angina (reported in about 1% of the patients on cabergoline) and erythromelalgia (observed in 0.4% of the patients). Similarly expected for the pharmacological class, peripheral oedema occurred in 6% of patients.

Gastric upset was more frequent in female than in male patients, while CNS events were more frequent in the elderly.

A blood pressure decrease of clinical relevance was observed mainly on standing in a minority of patients. The effect was mainly evident in the first weeks of therapy. Neither modification of heart rate nor consistent changes of ECG tracing were observed during Cabaser treatment.

Alterations in standard laboratory tests are uncommon during long term therapy with Cabaser.

Overdose: The acute toxicity studies carried out in animals indicate very low toxicity, with a wide safety margin with respect to pharmacologically active doses. Clinical signs and cause of death, if any, were related to CNS stimulation.

There is no experience in humans of overdosage with Cabaser in the proposed indication: it is likely to lead to symptoms due to over-stimulation of dopamine receptors. These might include nausea, vomiting, gastric complaints, hypotension, confusion/psychosis or hallucinations. The vomiting stimulating properties of dopamine agonists are expected to favour removal of unabsorbed drug. Supportive measures should be directed to maintain blood pressure, if necessary. In addition, in case of pronounced central nervous system effects (hallucinations) the administration of dopamine antagonist drugs may be advisable.

Pharmacological properties

Pharmacodynamic properties: Cabaser is a dopaminergic ergoline derivative endowed with potent and long-lasting dopamine D2 receptor agonist properties. In rats the compound, acting at D2 dopamine receptors on pituitary lactotrophic cells, decreases PRL secretion at oral doses of 3-25 mcg/kg, and *in vitro* at a concentration of 45 pg/ml. In addition, Cabaser exerts a central dopaminergic effect via D2 receptor stimulation at doses higher than those effective in lowering serum PRL levels. Improvement of motor deficit in animal models of parkinson's disease was present at oral daily doses of 1–2.5 mg/kg in rats and at s.c. doses of 0.5–1 mg/kg in monkeys.

In healthy volunteers the administration of Cabaser at single oral doses of 0.3–2.5 mg was associated with a significant decrease in serum PRL levels. The effect is prompt (within 3 hours of administration) and persistent (up to 7–28 days). The PRL-lowering effect is dose-related both in terms of degree of effect and duration of action.

The pharmacodynamic actions of Cabaser not linked to the therapeutic effect relate only to blood pressure decrease. The maximal hypotensive effect of Cabaser as a single dose usually occurs during the first 6 hours after drug intake and is dose-dependent both in terms of maximal decrease and frequency.

Pharmacokinetic properties: The pharmacokinetic and metabolic profiles of Cabaser have been studied in healthy volunteers of both sexes, in female hyperprolactinemic patients and in parkinsonian patients. After oral administration of the labelled compound, radioactivity was rapidly absorbed from the gastrointestinal tract as the peak of radioactivity in plasma was between 0.5 and 4 hours. Ten days after administration about 18/20% and 55/72% of the radioactive dose (^{3}H-cabergoline/^{14}C-cabergoline) was recovered in urine and faeces, respectively. Unchanged drug in urine accounted for 2–3% of the dose.

In urine, the main metabolite identified was 6-allyl-8b-carboxy-ergoline, which accounted for 4–6% of the dose. Three additional metabolites were identified in urine, which accounted overall for less than 3% of the dose. The metabolites have been found to be much less potent than Cabaser as D_2 dopamine receptor agonists '*in vitro*'.

The low urinary excretion of unchanged Cabaser has been confirmed also in studies with non-radioactive product. The elimination half-life of Cabaser, estimated from urinary excretion rates, is long (63–68 hours in healthy volunteers, 79–115 hours in hyperprolactinemic patients).

The pharmacokinetics of Cabaser seem to be dose-independent both in healthy volunteers (doses of 0.5–1.5 mg) and parkinsonian patients (steady state of daily doses up to 7 mg/day).

On the basis of the elimination half-life, steady state conditions should be achieved after 4 weeks, as confirmed by the mean peak plasma levels of Cabaser obtained after a single dose (37±8 pg/ml) and after a 4 week multiple-regimen (101±43 pg/ml). '*In vitro*' experiments showed that the drug at concentrations of 0.1–10 ng/ml is 41–42% bound to plasma proteins.

Food does not appear to affect absorption and disposition of Cabaser.

While renal insufficiency has been shown not to modify cabergoline kinetics, hepatic insufficiency of severe degree (> 10 Child-Pugh score, maximum score 12) has been shown to be associated with an increase of AUC.

Preclinical safety data: Almost all the findings noted throughout the series of preclinical safety studies are a consequence of the central dopaminergic effects or the long-lasting inhibition of PRL in rodents with a specific hormonal physiology different to man.

Preclinical safety studies of Cabaser indicate a consistent safety margin for this compound in rodents and in monkeys, as well as a lack of teratogenic, genotoxic or carcinogenic potential.

Pharmaceutical particulars

List of excipients:

Lactose anhydrous	NF USP
Leucine	PhEur

Incompatibilities: Not applicable

Shelf life: 24 months at room temperature (25°C).

Special precautions for storage: There are no special precautions for storage.

Nature and contents of container: The tablets are contained in Type I amber glass bottles with tamper resistant screw caps which contain silica gel desiccant.

Each bottle contains 20 tablets of either 1 mg or 2 mg strength or 16 tablets of 4 mg strength and is enclosed in an outer cardboard carton.

Instructions for use/handling: Bottles of Cabaser are supplied with desiccant in the caps. This desiccant must not be removed.

Marketing authorisation numbers

1 mg tablets	0022/0169
2 mg tablets	0022/0170
4 mg tablets	0022/0171

Legal category POM.

Date of first authorisation/renewal of authorisation
14 February 1996

Date of (partial) revision of the text January 1997.

CAVERJECT* POWDER FOR INJECTION 5 MICROGRAMS
CAVERJECT POWDER FOR INJECTION 10 MICROGRAMS
CAVERJECT POWDER FOR INJECTION 20 MICROGRAMS
CAVERJECT POWDER FOR INJECTION 40 MICROGRAMS

Qualitative and quantitative composition Alprostadil USP 5, 10, 20 or 40 micrograms

Pharmaceutical form Powder for Injection

Clinical particulars

Therapeutic indications: Caverject is indicated for the treatment of erectile dysfunction in adult males due to neurogenic, vasculogenic, psychogenic or mixed aetiology.

Caverject may be a useful adjunct to other diagnostic tests in the diagnosis of erectile dysfunction.

Posology and method of administration: Caverject is administered by direct intracavernous injection. A 1/2-inch, 27- to 30-gauge needle is generally recommended. The dose of Caverject should be individualised for each patient by careful titration under supervision by a physician.

The intracavernosal injection must be done under sterile conditions. The site of injection is usually along the dorsolateral aspect of the proximal third of the penis. Visible veins should be avoided. Both the side of the penis that is injected and the site of injection must be alternated; prior to the injection, the injection site must be cleansed with an alcohol swab.

To reconstitute Caverject using the prefilled diluent syringe: flip off the plastic cap from the vial, and use one of the swabs to wipe the rubber cap. Fit the 22 gauge needle to the syringe.

Inject the 1 ml of diluent into the vial, and shake to dissolve the powder entirely. Withdraw slightly more than the required dose of Caverject solution, remove the 22 gauge needle, and fit the 30 gauge needle. Adjust volume to the required dose for injection. Following administration, any unused contents of the vial or syringe should be discarded.

As an aid to aetiologic diagnosis: Subjects without evidence of neurological dysfunction; 20 micrograms alprostadil to be injected into the corpus cavernosum and massaged through the penis. Should an ensuing erection persist for more than one hour detumescent therapy (please refer to *Overdose*) should be employed prior to the subject leaving the clinic to prevent a risk of priapism.

Over 80% of subjects may be expected to respond to a single 20 micrograms dose of alprostadil. At the time of discharge from the clinic, the erection should have subsided entirely and the penis must be in a completely flaccid state.

Subjects with evidence of neurological dysfunction: these patients can be expected to respond to lower doses of alprostadil. In subjects with erectile dysfunction caused by neurologic disease/trauma the dose for diagnostic testing must not exceed 10 micrograms and an initial dose of 5 micrograms is likely to be appropriate. Should an ensuing erection persist for more than one hour detumescent therapy (please refer to *Overdose*) should be employed prior to the subject leaving the clinic to prevent a risk of priapism. At the time of discharge from the clinic, the erection should have subsided entirely and the penis must be in a completely flaccid state.

Treatment: The initial dose of alprostadil in patients with erectile dysfunction of neurogenic origin secondary to spinal cord injury is 1.25 micrograms, with a second dose of 2.5 micrograms, a third of 5 micrograms, and subsequent incremental increases of 5 micrograms until an optimal dose is achieved. For erectile dysfunction of vasculogenic, psychogenic, or mixed aetiology, the initial dose is 2.5 micrograms. The second dose should be 5 micrograms if there is a partial response, and 7.5 micrograms if there is no response. Subsequent incremental increases of 5–10 micrograms should be given until an optimal dose is achieved. If there is no response to the administered dose, then the next higher dose may be given within 1 hour. If there is a response, there should be at least a 1-day interval before the next dose is given. The usual maximum recommended frequency of injection is no more than once daily and no more than three times weekly.

The first injections of alprostadil must be done by medically trained personnel. After proper training and instruction, alprostadil may be injected at home. If self-administration is planned, the physician should make an assessment of the patient's skill and competence with the procedure. It is recommended that patients are regularly monitored (e.g. every 3 months) particularly in the initial stages of self injection therapy when dose adjustments may be needed.

The dose that is selected for self-injection treatment should provide the patient with an erection that is satisfactory for sexual intercourse. It is recommended that the dose administered produces a duration of the erection not exceeding one hour. If the duration is longer, the dose should be reduced. The majority of patients achieve a satisfactory response with doses in the range of 5 to 20 micrograms. Doses of greater than 60 micrograms of alprostadil are not recommended. The lowest effective dose should be used.

Contra-indications: Caverject should not be used in patients who have a known hypersensitivity to any of the constituents of the product; in patients who have conditions that might predispose them to priapism, such as sickle cell anaemia or trait, multiple myeloma, or leukaemia; or in patients with anatomical deformation of the penis, such as angulation, cavernosal fibrosis, or Peyronie's disease. Patients with penile implants should not be treated with Caverject.

Caverject should not be used in men for whom sexual activity is inadvisable or contra-indicated.

Special warnings and precautions for use: Prolonged

erection and/or priapism may occur. Patients should be instructed to report to a physician any erection lasting for a prolonged time period, such as 4 hours or longer. Treatment of priapism should not be delayed more than 6 hours (please refer to *Overdose*).

Painful erection is more likely to occur in patients with anatomical deformations of the penis, such as angulation, phimosis, cavernosal fibrosis, Peyronie's disease or plaques. Penile fibrosis, including angulation, fibrotic nodules and Peyronie's disease may occur following the intracavernosal administration of Caverject. The occurrence of fibrosis may increase with increased duration of use. Regular follow-up of patients, with careful examination of the penis, is strongly recommended to detect signs of penile fibrosis or Peyronie's disease. Treatment with Caverject should be discontinued in patients who develop penile angulation, cavernosal fibrosis, or Peyronie's disease.

Patients on anticoagulants such as warfarin or heparin may have increased propensity for bleeding after the intracavernous injection.

Underlying treatable medical causes of erectile dysfunction should be diagnosed and treated prior to initiation of therapy with Caverject.

Use of intracavernosal alprostadil offers no protection from the transmission of sexually transmitted diseases. Individuals who use alprostadil should be counselled about the protective measures that are necessary to guard against the spread of sexually transmitted diseases, including the human immunodeficiency virus (HIV). In some patients, injection of Caverject can induce a small amount of bleeding at the site of injection. In patients infected with blood-born diseases, this could increase the transmission of such diseases to their partner.

Reconstituted solutions of Caverject are intended for single use only, they should be used immediately and not stored.

Interaction with other medicaments and other forms of interaction: No known interactions. Caverject is not intended for co-administration with any other agent for the treatment of erectile dysfunction.

Pregnancy and lactation: Not applicable. (High doses of alprostadil (0.5 to 2.0 mg/kg subcutaneously) had an adverse effect on the reproductive potential of male rats, although this was not seen with lower doses (0.05 to 0.2 mg/kg). Alprostadil did not affect rat spermatogenesis at doses 200 times greater than the proposed human intrapenile dose.

Effects on ability to drive and use machines: Not applicable.

Undesirable effects: The most frequent adverse reaction after intracavernosal injection of Caverject is penile pain. In studies, 37% of the patients reported penile pain at least once; however, this event was associated with only 11% of the administered injections. In the majority of the cases, penile pain was rated mild or moderate in intensity. 3% of patients discontinued treatment because of penile pain.

Prolonged erection (defined as an erection that lasts for 4 to 6 hours) after intracavernosal administration of Caverject was reported in 4% of patients. The frequency of priapism (defined as an erection that lasts 6 hours or longer) was 0.4%. (Please refer to *Special warnings and precautions for use*). In the majority of cases, spontaneous detumescence occurred.

Penile fibrosis, including angulation, fibrotic nodules and Peyronie's disease was reported in 3% of clinical trial patients overall, however, in one self-injection study in which the duration of use was up to 18 months, the incidence of penile fibrosis was 7.8% (please refer to Section 4.4).

Haematoma and ecchymosis at the site of injection, which is related to the injection technique rather than to the effects of alprostadil, occurred in 3% and 2% of patients, respectively. Penile oedema or rash was reported by 1% of alprostadil treated patients.

The following local adverse reactions were reported by fewer than 1% of patients in clinical studies following intracavernosal injection of Caverject: balanitis, injection site haemorrhage, injection site inflammation, injection site itching, injection site swelling, injection site oedema, urethral bleeding and penile warmth, numbness, yeast infection, irritation, sensitivity, phimosis, pruritus, erythema, venous leak, painful erection and abnormal ejaculation.

In terms of systemic events, 2 to 4% of alprostadil-treated patients reported headache, hypertension, upper respiratory infection, flu-like syndrome, prostatic disorder, localised pain (buttocks pain, leg pain, genital pain, abdominal pain), trauma, and sinusitis. One percent of patients reported each of the following: dizziness, back pain, nasal congestion and cough. The following were reported for less than 1% of patients in clinical trials and were judged to be possibly related to Caverject use: testicular pain, scrotal disorder (redness, pain, spermatocele), scrotal oedema, haematuria, testicular disorder (warmth, swelling, mass, thickening), impaired urination, urinary frequency, urinary urgency, pelvic pain, hypotension, vasodilatation, peripheral vascular disorder, supraventricular extrasystoles, vasovagal reactions, hypaesthesia, non-generalised weakness, diaphoresis, rash, non-application site pruritus, skin neoplasm, nausea, dry mouth, increased serum creatinine, leg cramps and mydriasis.

Haemodynamic changes, manifested as decreases in blood pressure and increases in pulse rate, were observed during clinical studies, principally at doses above 20 micrograms and above 30 micrograms of Caverject, respectively and appeared to be dose-dependent. However, these changes were usually clinically unimportant; only three patients (0.2%) discontinued the treatment because of symptomatic hypotension.

Caverject had no clinically important effect on serum or urine laboratory tests.

Overdose: The pharmacotoxic signs of alprostadil are similar in all animal species and include depression, soft stools or diarrhoea and rapid breathing. In animals, the lowest acute LD_{50} was 12 mg/kg which is 12,000 times greater than the maximum recommended human dose of 60 micrograms.

In man, prolonged erection and/or priapism are known to occur following intracavernous administration of vasoactive substances, including alprostadil. Patients should be instructed to report to a physician any erection lasting for a prolonged time period, such as 4 hours or longer.

The treatment of priapism (prolonged erection) should not be delayed more than 6 hours. Initial therapy should be by penile aspiration. Using aseptic technique, insert a 19–21 gauge butterfly needle into the corpus cavernosum and aspirate 20–50 ml of blood. This may detumesce the penis. If necessary, the procedure may be repeated on the opposite side of the penis until a total of up to 100 ml blood has been aspirated. If still unsuccessful, intracavernous injection of alpha-adrenergic medication is recommended. Although the usual contra-indication to intrapenile administration of a vasoconstrictor does not apply in the treatment of priapism, caution is advised when this option is exercised. Blood pressure and pulse should be continuously monitored during the procedure. Extreme caution is required in patients with coronary heart disease, uncontrolled hypertension, cerebral ischaemia, and in subjects taking monoamine oxidase inhibitors. In the latter case, facilities should be available to manage a hypertensive crisis. A 200 microgram/ml solution of phenylephrine should be prepared, and 0.5 to 1.0 ml of the solution injected every 5 to 10 minutes. Alternatively, a 20 microgram/ml solution of adrenaline should be used. If necessary, this may be followed by further aspiration of blood through the same butterfly needle. The maximum dose of phenylephrine should be 1 mg, or adrenaline 100 micrograms (5 ml of the solution). As an alternative metaraminol may be used, but it should be noted that fatal hypertensive crises have been reported. If this still fails to resolve the priapism, urgent surgical referral for further management, which may include a shunt procedure, is required.

Pharmacological properties

Pharmacodynamic properties: Alprostadil is present in various mammalian tissues and fluids. It has a diverse pharmacologic profile, among which some of its more important effects are vasodilation, inhibition of platelet aggregation, inhibition of gastric secretion, and stimulation of intestinal and uterine smooth muscle. The pharmacologic effect of alprostadil in the treatment of erectile dysfunction is presumed to be mediated by inhibition of $alpha_1$-adrenergic activity in penile tissue and by its relaxing effect on cavernosal smooth muscle.

Pharmacokinetic properties: Following intracavernous injection of 20 micrograms of alprostadil, mean peripheral levels of alprostadil at 30 and 60 minutes after injection are not significantly greater than baseline levels of endogenous PGE_1. Peripheral levels of the major circulating metabolite, 15-oxo-13,14-dihydro-PGE_1, increase to reach a peak 30 minutes after injection and return to pre-dose levels by 60 minutes after injection. Any alprostadil entering the systemic circulation from the corpus cavernosum will be rapidly metabolized. Following intravenous administration, approximately 80% of the circulating alprostadil is metabolized in one pass through the lungs, primarily by beta- and omega-oxidation. The metabolites are excreted primarily by the kidney and excretion is essentially complete within 24 hours. There is no evidence of tissue retention of alprostadil or its metabolites following intravenous administration.

Pre-clinical safety data: No relevant information additional to that already contained in this SPC.

Pharmaceutical particulars

List of excipients: Lactose, sodium citrate, hydrochloric acid, sodium hydroxide.

Incompatibilities: Caverject is not intended to be mixed or coadministered with any other products.

The presence of benzyl alcohol in the reconstitution vehicle decreases the degree of binding to package surfaces. Therefore, a more consistent product delivery is produced when Bacteriostatic Water for Injection containing benzyl alcohol is used.

Shelf life: Caverject 5, 10 and 20 micrograms: 24 months. Reconstituted solutions should be used immediately and not stored.

Caverject 40 micrograms: 24 months under refrigerated conditions (2–8°C). After dispensing, 3 months at room temperature (at or below 25°C), included in 24 months shelf life. The reconstituted solution can be kept at or below 25°C for up to 6 hours.

Special precautions for storage: Caverject 5, 10 and 20 micrograms: Store at room temperature (at or below 25°C). Reconstituted solutions are intended for single use only, they should be used immediately and not stored.

Caverject 40 micrograms: Store at 2–8°C until dispensed. After dispensing, may be stored at or below 25°C for up to 3 months. Reconstituted solutions can be kept for 6 hours at or below 25°C; do not refrigerate or freeze.

Nature and contents of container: Single packs containing a vial of Caverject 5, 10, 20 or 40 microgram powder and a syringe of diluent.

Packs also each contain a sterile 22 G and a 30 G needle plus pre-injection swab.

For hospital use only, a dose titration pack containing 8 individual boxes of Caverject 10 micrograms.

Instructions for use/handling: None stated.

Marketing authorisation numbers

Caverject Powder for Injection 5 micrograms	0032/0214
Caverject Powder for Injection 10 micrograms	0032/0203
Caverject Powder for Injection 20 micrograms	0032/0188
Caverject Powder for Injection 40 micrograms	0032/0227
Bacteriostatic Water for Injections diluent	0032/0193

Date of first authorisation/renewal of authorisation

Caverject Powder for Injection 5 micrograms - Granted: 25 March 1997

Caverject Powder for Injection 10 micrograms - Granted: 8 February 1996

Caverject Powder for Injection 20 micrograms - Granted: 15 March 1994

Caverject Powder for Injection 40 micrograms - Granted: 23 June 1998

Bacteriostatic Water for Injections diluent - Granted: 15 March 1994.

Date of (partial) revision of the text 22 May 1998

Legal category POM.

CEDOCARD RETARD*-20

Presentation Round yellow sustained-release tablets, embossed CCSR and scored on reverse side, each containing 20 mg isosorbide dinitrate.

Uses For the prophylaxis of angina pectoris.

The active principle of Cedocard Retard-20 is isosorbide dinitrate which relaxes vascular smooth muscle and produces coronary vasodilation, reduction in peripheral resistance and venous return, alteration of myocardial metabolism, and reduction of the myocardial oxygen demand.

Dosage and administration For oral administration.

Adult dose: One tablet in the morning and 1 tablet before retiring to sleep. Onset of action 20–30 minutes and the duration of action is 10–12 hours.

Dosage for the elderly: The dosage of nitrates in cardiovascular disease is usually determined by patient response and stabilisation. Clinical experience has not necessitated alternative advice for use in elderly patients. The pharmacokinetics of isosorbide dinitrate in patients with severe renal failure and liver cirrhosis are similar to those in normal subjects.

There is no recommended dose for children.

Contra-indications, warnings, etc

Contra-indication: A history of sensitivity to the drug.

Precautions: Tolerance and cross-tolerance to other nitrates may occur.

Adverse reactions: Cutaneous vasodilation with flushing, transient episodes of dizziness and weakness, and other signs of cerebral ischaemia, may occur with postural hypotension.

Use in pregnancy: No data have been reported which would indicate the possibility of adverse effects resulting from the use of isosorbide dinitrate in pregnancy. Safety in pregnancy, however, has not been established. Isosorbide dinitrate should only be used in pregnancy if, in the opinion of the physician, the possible benefits of treatment outweigh the possible hazards.

Treatment of overdosage: In rare cases of overdosage, gastric lavage is indicated. Passive exercise of the extremities of the recumbent patient will promote venous return.

Pharmaceutical precautions *Storage:* Protect from heat and moisture.

Legal category P.

Package quantities Blister strips of 60 (OP) tablets.

Further information Nil.

Product licence number 0424/0007.

CEDOCARD* RETARD-40

Qualitative and quantitative composition Isosorbide Dinitrate BP 40.0 mg

Pharmaceutical form Uncoated sustained release tablets for oral administration.

Clinical particulars
Therapeutic indications: Cedocard Retard is indicated for prophylactic treatment of angina pectoris.

Posology and method of administration:
Children: There is no recommended dose for children.
Adults: One or two tablets to be taken twice daily.
Elderly: Dosage as for other adults.

Contra-indications: Isosorbide dinitrate is contra-indicated in patients with a history of sensitivity to the drug.

Special warnings and special precautions for use: Tolerance and cross-tolerance to other nitrates and nitrites may occur.

Interaction with other medicaments and other forms of interaction: Alcohol may potentiate the effect of isosorbide dinitrate.

Use in pregnancy and lactation: No data have been reported which would indicate the possibility of adverse effects resulting from the use of isosorbide dinitrate in pregnancy. Safety in pregnancy however, has not been established. Isosorbide dinitrate should only be used in pregnancy if, in the opinion of the physician, the possible benefits of treatment outweigh the possible hazards. Lactation–there are no data available on the transfer of isosorbide dinitrate in breast milk or its effect on breast fed children.

Effects on ability to drive and use machines: Side effects include throbbing headache and dizziness. Patients are advised not to drive or operate machinery if so affected.

Undesirable effects: A headache may occur at the start of treatment, but this usually disappears after a few days. Rarely, occasional episodes of dizziness and weakness may occur.

Overdose: No available data.

Pharmacological properties
Pharmacodynamic properties: Isosorbide dinitrate is a vasodilator. It relaxes vascular smooth muscle and produces coronary vasodilation, reduction in peripheral resistance and venous return, alteration of myocardial metabolism and reduction of the myocardial oxygen demand.

Pharmacokinetic properties: The mean plasma concentrations of ISDN at the end of each 12 hour dosage interval (Cmin) during the period of administration of 40 mg as the sustained release tablets were 0.6 ng/ml, 0.6 ng/ml, 0.9 ng/ml and 0.6 ng/ml after the first, second, third and fourth doses respectively and was 0.9 ng/ml at 12 hours after the last dose. At 1, 4 and 8 hours after the first dose the mean plasma levels of ISDN were 1.3 ng/ml, 4.0 ng/ml and 2.2 ng/ml respectively. At 1, 4 and 8 hours after the 3rd dose the mean plasma levels of ISDN were 2.1 ng/ml, 4.0 ng/ml and 2.0 ng/ml respectively and after the last dose, the peak plasma concentrations of ISDN of 12.7 ng/ml occurred at 5 hours and thereafter mean concentrations of ISDN declined to 0.4 ng/ml at 14 hours after the last dose.

Preclinical safety data: Due to the age and well established safety nature of this product, preclinical data has not been included.

Pharmaceutical particulars
List of excipients

Lactose	PhEur
Talc	PhEur
Magnesium stearate	PhEur
Polyvinyl acetate	
Red (E124)	
Yellow-orange S (E110)	
Potato starch	PhEur
Methylene chloride	USP
Water	
Sodium chloride	
Sodium sulphate	

Incompatibilities: None known.

Shelf life: 60 months.

Special precautions for storage: Protect from heat and moisture.

Nature and contents of container: PVC/Aluminium blisters in packs of 60 or 1000 tablets.

Instructions for use/handling: There are no special instructions for handling.

Marketing authorisation holder:
Tillotts Laboratories
Davy Avenue
Milton Keynes
MK5 8PH

Marketing authorisation number 0424/0050

Date of first authorisation/renewal of authorisation 18 November 1986/18 November 1991

Date of (partial) revision of the text 6 March 1997.

Legal category POM.

CISPLATIN

Presentation Cisplatin powder for injection: Yellowish-white freeze-dried cake in vials containing 10 mg or 50 mg cisplatin (cis-diamminedichloroplatinum). The formulation also contains sodium chloride and mannitol.

Uses Cisplatin has antitumour activity either as a single agent or in combination chemotherapy particularly in the treatment of testicular and metastatic ovarian tumours, also cervical tumours, lung carcinoma and bladder cancer.

Dosage and administration Cisplatin powder should be dissolved in Water for Injections such that the reconstituted solution contains 1 mg/ml of cisplatin. Cisplatin reconstituted powder should be diluted in 2 litres of 0.9% saline or a dextrose/saline solution (to which 37.5 g of mannitol may be added) and administration should be over a 6–8 hour period.

Single agent therapy: Adults and children: The usual dose regimen given as a single agent is 50–120 mg/m^2 by infusion once every 3 to 4 weeks or 15–20 mg/m^2 by infusion daily for five consecutive days, every 3 to 4 weeks.

Combination chemotherapy: Dosage may be adjusted if the drug is used in combination with other antitumour chemotherapy.

With multiple drug treatment schedules cisplatin is usually given in doses from 20 mg/m^2 upward every 3 to 4 weeks. Dosage should be reduced for patients with renal impairment or depressed bone marrow function (see *Contra-indications, Warnings etc*).

Pre-treatment hydration with 1 to 2 litres of fluid infused for 8 to 12 hours prior to the cisplatin will initiate diuresis. Adequate subsequent hydration should maintain diuresis during the 24 hours following administration.

Contra-indications, warnings, etc
Contra-indications: Cisplatin is contra-indicated in patients who have had previous allergic reactions to cisplatin or other platinum compounds as anaphylactic-like reactions have been reported. Relative contra-indications are pre-existing renal impairment, hearing disorders and depressed bone marrow function which may increase toxicity (see *Warnings*).

Warnings: This agent should only be administered under the direction of physicians experienced in cancer chemotherapy.

Nephrotoxicity of cisplatin is cumulative and serum creatinine, BUN and creatinine clearance should be measured before starting each course of therapy. Repeat courses of cisplatin should not be given unless levels of serum creatinine are below 1.5 mg/100 ml (100 mcmol/l) or blood urea below 55 mg/100 ml (9 mmol/l) and circulating blood elements are at an acceptable level.

Diuresis should be controlled and serum electrolyte levels monitored regularly. Adequate pre-treatment and 'during treatment' hydration should be ensured and such agents as mannitol given to minimise hazards of renal toxicity. In addition, adequate post-treatment hydration and urinary output should be monitored. Concomitant use of nephrotoxic drugs may seriously impair kidney function.

Ototoxicity is cumulative and occurs with high dose regimens. Hearing function should be evaluated before, and regularly during therapy (see Adverse Reactions).

Haematologic toxicity is dose-related and may be cumulative; RBC, WBC and platelet counts should be monitored.

The nephrotoxicity, ototoxicity and myelosuppression induced by cisplatin will be additive to existing impairment or to the similar toxicity of agents such as cephaloridine, frusemide, aminoglycosides, etc. administered concurrently.

Anaphylactic-like reactions to cisplatin have been observed. These reactions can be controlled by administration of antihistamines, adrenaline and/or glucocorticoids.

Neurotoxicity secondary to cisplatin administration has been reported and therefore neurological examinations are recommended (see *Adverse reactions*). Cisplatin has been shown to be mutagenic. It may also have an anti-fertility effect. Other antineoplastic substances have been shown to be carcinogenic and this possibility should be borne in mind in long term use of cisplatin.

Cisplatin has been shown to be teratogenic and embryotoxic in animals. The use of the drug should be avoided in pregnant or nursing women if possible.

Adverse reactions:
Nephrotoxicity: Immediate renal toxicity is greatly reduced when extensive saline hydration is used but cumulative toxicity may remain a problem and requires careful monitoring when repeat courses of cisplatin are administered.

Renal function impairment is evidenced by an increase in blood urea nitrogen, creatinine and serum uric acid levels and by a decreased creatinine clearance.

Cisplatin induces pathological lesions in the distal renal tubules and the collecting ducts.

Gastrointestinal toxicity: Nausea and vomiting occur in the majority of patients, usually starting within 1 hour of treatment and lasting up to 24 hours. Anorexia, nausea and occasional vomiting may persist for up to a week.

Myelosuppression: Cisplatin can cause suppression of all three blood elements.

Leucopenia is dose-related, possibly cumulative, usually reversible. The onset of leucopenia occurs usually between days 6 and 26 and the time of recovery ranges from 21 to 45 days. Thrombocytopenia is also a dose-limiting effect of cisplatin but is usually reversible. The onset of thrombocytopenia is usually from days 10 to 26 and the time of recovery ranges from about 28 to 45 days.

The incidence of cisplatin-induced anaemia (haemoglobin drop of 2 g/100 ml) ranges from 9% to 40%, although this is a difficult toxic effect to assess because it may have a complex aetiology in cancer patients.

Ototoxicity: Unilateral or bilateral tinnitus, which is usually reversible, and/or hearing loss in the high frequency range may occur.

The overall incidence of audiogram abnormalities is 24%, but large variations exist. These abnormalities usually appear within 4 days after drug administration and consist of at least a 15 decibel loss in pure tone threshold. The damage seems to be cumulative and is not reversible. The audiogram abnormalities are most common in the 4000–8000 Hz frequencies.

Neurotoxicity: Peripheral neuropathies with paraesthesia in both upper and lower extremities, tremor and loss of taste have been observed in some patients, generally those treated with repeated courses.

Anaphylactic-like reactions: Anaphylactic-like reactions such as flushing, facial oedema, wheezing, tachycardia and hypotension may occur within a few minutes after intravenous administration. Antihistamines, adrenaline and/or glucocorticoids control all these reactions.

Hyperuricaemia: Hyperuricaemia occurring with cisplatin is more pronounced with doses greater than 50 mg/m^2. Allopurinol effectively reduces uric acid levels.

Hypomagnesaemia: Asymptomatic hypomagnesaemia has been documented in a certain number of patients treated with cisplatin. Symptomatic hypomagnesaemia has been observed in a limited number of cases.

Pharmaceutical precautions The unopened vials of the freeze-dried powder should be stored at room temperature protected from light. Solutions of cisplatin must not be cooled or refrigerated as cooling may result in precipitation; they should be stored at room temperature protected from light and used within 20 hours. It is recommended that diluted infusion solutions of cisplatin be protected from light during administration.

Any unused solution should be discarded.

Cisplatin is degraded on contact with aluminium. Aluminium containing equipment should not be used for administration of cisplatin.

It is recommended that personnel handling cisplatin wear protective gloves. Spillage or leakage should be mopped up wearing protective gloves and all cleaning materials should be placed in high-risk, waste-disposal bags and then incinerated. Contaminated surfaces should be washed with copious amounts of water.

Legal category POM.

Package quantities Cisplatin 10, 50: Individual vials.

Further information Nil.

Product licence numbers
Cisplatin 10 3433/0061
Cisplatin 50 3433/0063

COLESTID* ORANGE

Qualitative and quantitative composition Colestipol Hydrochloride USP 5.0 gram

Pharmaceutical form Granules for oral administration.

Clinical particulars
Therapeutic indications: Colestid is indicated as adjunctive therapy to diet in the management of patients with elevated cholesterol levels who have not responded adequately to diet. It may be used alone or in combination with additional lipid lowering agents.

Dietary therapy specific for the type of hypercholesterolaemia should be the initial treatment of choice. Excess body weight may be an important factor and weight reduction should be attempted prior to drug therapy in the overweight. The use of drugs should be considered only when reasonable attempts have been made to obtain satisfactory results with non-drug methods. When drug therapy is begun, the patient should be instructed of the importance of adhering to the correct diet.

Although Colestid is effective in all types of hypercholesterolaemia, it is medically most appropriate in patients with Fredrickson's type II hyperlipoproteinaemia.

Posology and method of administration:
Route of administration: Oral, mixed with water or other fluids.

Adults: The recommended initial daily adult dosage of colestipol hydrochloride is 5 grams either once or twice daily.

For adults colestipol hydrochloride is recommended in doses of 5–30 grams taken as one dose or two divided doses. Initiation of therapy is recommended at 5 grams either once or twice daily with 5 gram increments at one month intervals. Appropriate use of lipid profiles including LDL-cholesterol and triglycerides is advised so that optimal, but not excessive doses are used to obtain the desired therapeutic effect on LDL-cholesterol level. If the desired therapeutic effect is not obtained at a dose of 5–30 grams/day with good compliance and acceptable side-effects, combined therapy or alternate treatment should be considered.

Patients should take other drugs at least one hour before or four hours after Colestid to minimise possible interference with their absorption. However, Colestid and gemfibrozil may be used in the same patient when administered 2 hours apart. (See *Interactions*).

Preparation: Colestid should always be taken mixed in a liquid such as orange or tomato juice, water, skimmed milk or non-carbonated beverage. The contents of the sachet or level scoopful should be added to 100 ml or more of the preferred aqueous vehicle and mixed thoroughly until dispersed. Colestid may also be taken in soups or with cereals, pulpy fruits with a high water content or yoghurt.

Elderly patients: At present there are no extensive clinical studies with colestipol in patients over the age of 65. Review of available data does not suggest that the elderly are more predisposed to side-effects attributable to colestipol than the general population; however, therapy should be individualised and based on each patient's clinical characteristics and tolerance to the medication.

Children: Dosage in children has not been established.

Contra-indications: Colestipol is contra-indicated in individuals who have previously demonstrated hypersensitivity to its use.

Special warnings and special precautions for use:
Warnings: Before instituting therapy with Colestid, diseases contributing to increased blood cholesterol such as hypothyroidism, diabetes mellitus, nephrotic syndrome, dysproteinaemias and obstructive liver diseases should be looked for and specifically treated.

To avoid accidental inhalation or oesophageal distress, Colestid should not be taken in its dry form.

Colestid Orange contains 0.0325 g aspartame per sachet or level scoopful. This should be taken into consideration in patients suffering from phenylketonuria since excessive amounts of aspartame may interfere with the control of this condition.

Colestid may elevate serum triglyceride levels when used as sole therapy. This elevation is generally transient but may persist in some individuals. A significant rise in triglyceride level should be considered as an indication for dose reduction, drug discontinuation, or combined or alternate therapy.

The use of Colestid in children has been limited; however, it does appear to be effective in lowering serum cholesterol in older children and young adults. Because bile acid sequestrants may interfere with the absorption of fat-soluble vitamins, appropriate monitoring of growth and development is essential. Dosage and long term safety in children have not been established.

Precautions: Because it sequesters bile acids, Colestid may interfere with normal fat absorption and thus may alter absorption of fat soluble vitamins such as A, D, E and K. A study in humans found only one patient in whom a prolonged prothombin time was noted. Most studies did not show a decrease in vitamin A, D or E levels during the administration of Colestid; however, if Colestid is to be given for a long period these vitamin levels should be monitored and supplements given if necessary.

Interaction with other medicaments and other forms of interaction: In man, Colestid may delay or reduce the absorption of certain concomitant oral drugs (digitalis and its glycosides, propranolol, chlorothiazide and hydrochlorothiazide, tetracycline hydrochloride, penicillin G and gemfibrozil). Particular caution should be taken with digitalis preparations since conflicting results have been obtained for the effect of Colestid on the availability of digoxin and digitoxin. Colestid has been shown not to interfere with the absorption of clindamycin, clofibrate, aspirin, tolbutamide, warfarin, methyldopa and phenytoin. The clinical response to concomitant medication should be closely monitored and appropriate adjustments made.

Repeated doses of Colestid given prior to a single dose of propranolol in human trials have been reported to decrease propranolol absorption. However, in a follow-up study in normal subjects, single dose administration of Colestid and propranolol or multiple dose administration of both agents did not affect the extent of propranolol absorption. Effects on the absorption of other beta-blockers have not been determined. Patients on propranolol should be observed when Colestid is either added or deleted from a therapeutic regimen.

Pregnancy and lactation: Safety for use in pregnant women has not been established. The use of Colestid in pregnancy or lactation or by women of childbearing age requires that the potential benefits of treatment be weighed against the possible hazards to the mother and child.

Effects on ability to drive and use machines: No adverse effect has been reported.

Undesirable effects:
Side-effects: The most common adverse reactions reported with Colestid have been of a functional gastro-intestinal nature. The most frequent is constipation which is usually mild, transient and responsive to the usual adjunctive measures. At times, constipation can be severe and may be accompanied by impaction. As such, haemorrhoids can be aggravated, and infrequent blood in the stools has been reported. Less frequent gastro-intestinal complaints are abdominal discomfort, belching, flatulence, indigestion, nausea, vomiting and diarrhoea. Rarely, peptic ulceration and bleeding, cholelithiasis and cholecystitis have been reported, although these are not necessarily drug related.

Transient and modest elevation of SGOT and alkaline phosphatase have been observed. No medical significance is attached to these observed changes.

Although not necessarily drug-related, the following non-gastro-intestinal medical events have been reported during clinical trials at a similar incidence to placebo.

Cardiovascular: Chest pain, angina, and tachycardia have been infrequently reported.

Hypersensitivity: Rash has been infrequently reported. Urticaria and dermatitis have been rarely noted.

Musculoskeletal: Musculoskeletal pain, aches and pains in the extremities, joint pain and arthritis, and backache have been reported.

Neurological: Headache, migraine headache and sinus headache have been reported. Other infrequently reported complaints include dizziness, light-headedness, and insomnia.

Miscellaneous: Anorexia, fatigue, weakness, shortness of breath, and swelling of the hands or feet, have been infrequently reported.

Overdose: No toxic effects due to overdosage have been reported. Should overdosage occur, obstruction of the gastro-intestinal tract would be expected to occur. Treatment should be determined by the location and degree of obstruction.

Pharmacological properties
Pharmacodynamic properties: Ion exchange resin which lowers plasma cholesterol through binding with bile acids in the intestinal lumen.

Pharmacokinetics: Colestid is not absorbed; its action is limited to the lumen of the gastro-intestinal tract, and it is passed in the faeces. It binds bile acids in the intestinal lumen and causes them to be excreted in the faeces together with the polymer. When the enterohepatic circulation of bile acids is interrupted, cholesterol conversion to bile acids is enhanced and plasma cholesterol levels are thereby lowered.

Preclinical safety data: Both clinical usage and animal studies with Colestid have provided no evidence of drug related intestinal neoplasms. Colestid is not mutagenic in the ames test.

Pharmaceutical particulars
List of excipients:

Mannitol	PhEur
Methylcellulose (15CPS)	PhEur
Citric Acid	PhEur
Orange Durarome Wonf	HSE
Aspartame Powder	NF
Maltol	HSE
Ethyl Vanillin	NF
Beta Carotene 1%	HSE
Glycerol	PhEur
Purified Water	PhEur

Incompatibilities: None.

Shelf life: 24 months.

Special precautions for storage: Store at controlled room temperature (15–30°C).

Nature and contents of container: HDPE bottle with plastic caps or tinplate screwcaps containing 450 grams or foil sachets in packs of 8, 28, 30, 56, 60 and 250 sachets.

Instructions for use/handling: None.

Marketing authorisation number 0032/0172

Date of first authorisation/renewal of authorisation
Date of Grant: 25 February 1992
Date of Renewal: 18 April 1997.

Date of (partial) revision of the text 20 November 1996.

Legal category POM.

COLESTID* SACHETS 5 g

Qualitative and quantitative composition Colestipol hydrochloride USP 5.0 grams

Pharmaceutical form Granules for oral administration.

Clinical Particulars
Therapeutic indications: Colestid is indicated as adjunctive therapy to diet in the management of patients with elevated cholesterol levels who have not responded adequately to diet. It may be used alone or in combination with additional lipid lowering agents.

Dietary therapy specific for the type of hypercholesterolaemia should be the initial treatment of choice. Excess body weight may be an important factor and weight reduction should be attempted prior to drug therapy in the overweight. The use of drugs should be considered only when reasonable attempts have been made to obtain satisfactory results with non-drug method. When drug therapy is begun, the patient should be instructed of the importance of adhering to the correct diet.

Although Colestid is effective in all types of hypercholesterolaemia, it is medically most appropriate in patients with Fredrickson's type II hyperlipoproteinaemia.

Posology and method of administration:
Route of administration: Oral, mixed with water or other fluids.

Adults: The recommended initial daily adult dosage of colestipol hydrochloride is 5 grams either once or twice daily.

For adults colestipol hydrochloride is recommended in doses of 5–30 grams taken as one dose or two divided doses. Initiation of therapy is recommended at 5 grams either once or twice daily with 5 gram increments at one month intervals. Appropriate use of lipid profiles including LDL-cholesterol and triglycerides is advised so that optimal, but not excessive doses are used to obtain the desired therapeutic effect on LDL-cholesterol level. If the desired therapeutic effect is not obtained at a dose of 5–30 grams/day with good compliance and acceptable side-effects, combined therapy or alternate treatment should be considered.

Patients should take other drugs at least one hour before or four hours after Colestid to minimise possible interference with their absorption. However, Colestid and Gemfibrozil may be used in the same patient when administered 2 hours apart (see Interactions).

Preparation: Colestid Granules should always be taken mixed in a liquid such as orange or tomato juice, water, skimmed milk or non-carbonated beverage. The contents of the sachet or level scoopful should be added to 100 ml or more of the preferred aqueous vehicle and mixed thoroughly until dispersed. Colestid may also be taken in soups or with cereals, pulpy fruits with a higher water content or yoghurt.

Elderly patients: At present there are no extensive clinical studies with colestipol in patients over the age of 65. Review of available data does not suggest that the elderly are more predisposed to side effects attributable to colestipol than the general population; however, therapy should be individualised and based on each patient's clinical characteristics and tolerance to the medication.

Children: Dosage in children has not been established.

Contra-indications: Colestipol is contra-indicated in individuals who have previously demonstrated hypersensitivity to its use.

Special warnings and precautions for use:
Warnings: Before instituting therapy with Colestid, diseases contributing to increased blood cholesterol such as hypothyroidism, diabetes mellitus, nephrotic syndrome, dysproteinaemias and obstructive liver disease should be looked for and specifically treated.

To avoid accidental inhalation or oesophageal distress, Colestid should not be taken in its dry form.

Colestid may elevate serum triglyceride levels when used as sole therapy. This elevation is generally transient but may persist in some individuals. A significant rise in triglyceride level should be considered as an indication for dose reduction, drug discontinuation, or combined or alternate therapy.

The use of Colestid in children has been limited; however, it does appear to be effective in lowering serum cholesterol in older children and young adults. Because bile acid sequestrants may interfere with the absorption of fat soluble vitamins, appropriate monitoring of growth and development is essential. Dosage and long term safety in children has not been established.

Precautions: Because it sequesters bile acids, Colestid may interfere with normal fat absorption and thus may alter absorption of fat soluble vitamins such as A, D, E and K. A study in humans found only one patient in whom a prolonged prothombin time was noted. Most studies did not show a decrease in vitamin A, D or E levels during the administration of Colestid; however, if Colestid is to be given for a long period these vitamin levels should be monitored and supplements given if necessary.

Both clinical usage and animal studies with Colestid have provided no evidence of drug related intestinal neoplasms. Colestid is not mutagenic in the Ames test.

Interaction with other medicaments and other forms of interaction: In man, Colestid may delay or reduce the absorption of certain concomitant oral drugs (digitalis and its glycosides, propranolol, chlorothiazide and hydrochlorothiazide, tetracycline hydrochloride, penicillin G, gemfibrozil). Particular caution should be taken with digitalis preparations since conflicting results have been obtained for the effect of Colestid on the availability of digoxin and digitoxin. Colestid has been shown not to interfere with the absorption of clindamycin, clofibrate, aspirin, tolbutamide, warfarin, methyldopa and phenytoin. The clinical response to concomitant medication should be closely monitored and appropriate adjustments made.

Repeated doses of Colestid given prior to a single dose of propranolol in human trials have been reported to decrease propranolol absorption. However, in a follow-up study in normal subjects, single dose administration of Colestid and propranolol or multiple dose administration of both agents did not affect the extent of propranolol absorption. Effects on the absorption of other beta-blockers have not been determined. Patients on propranolol should be observed when Colestid is either added or deleted from a therapeutic regimen.

Pregnancy and lactation: Safety for use in pregnant women has not been established. The use of Colestid in pregnancy or lactation or by women of childbearing age requires that the potential benefits of treatment be weighed against the possible hazards to the mother and child.

Effects on ability to drive and use machines: No adverse effect has been reported.

Undesirable effects: Side-effects:

The most common adverse reactions reported with Colestid have been of a functional gastro-intestinal nature. The most frequent is constipation which is usually mild, transient and responsive to the usual adjunctive measures. At times, constipation can be severe and may be accompanied by impaction. As such, haemorrhoids can be aggravated, and infrequent blood in the stools has been reported. Less frequent gastro-intestinal complaints are abdominal discomfort, belching, flatulence, indigestion, nausea, vomiting and diarrhoea. Rarely, peptic ulceration and bleeding, cholelithiasis and cholecystitis have been reported, although these are not necessarily drug related.

Transient and modest elevation of SGOT and alkaline phosphatase have been observed. No medical significance is attached to these observed changes.

Although not necessarily drug-related, the following non gastro-intestinal medical events have been reported during clinical trials at a similar incidence to placebo.

Cardiovascular: Chest pain, angina and tachycardia have been infrequently reported.

Hypersensitivity: Rash has been infrequently reported. Urticaria and dermatitis have been rarely noted.

Musculoskeletal: Musculoskeletal pain, aches and pains in the extremities, joint pain and arthritis, and backache have been reported.

Neurological: Headache, migraine headache and sinus headache have been reported. Other infrequently reported complaints include dizziness, lightheadedness, and insomnia.

Miscellaneous: Anorexia, fatigue, weakness, shortness of breath, and swelling of the hands or feet, have been infrequently reported.

Overdose: No toxic effects due to overdosage have been reported. Should overdosage occur, obstruction of the gastro-intestinal tract would be expected to occur. Treatment would be determined by the location and degree of obstruction.

Pharmacological properties
Pharmacodynamic properties: Ion exchange resin which lowers plasma cholesterol through binding with bile acids in the intestinal lumen.

Pharmacokinetic properties: Colestid is not absorbed; its action is limited to the lumen of the gastro-intestinal tract, and it is passed in the faeces. It binds bile acids in the intestinal lumen and causes them to be excreted in the faeces together with the polymer. When the enterohepatic circulation of bile acids is interrupted, cholesterol conversion to bile acids is enhanced and plasma cholesterol levels are thereby lowered.

Preclinical safety data: Both clinical and animal studies with Colestid have provided no evidence of drug related intestinal neoplasms. Colestid is not mutagenic in the Ames test.

Pharmaceutical particulars
List of excipients: Colloidal Silicon Dioxide NF.

Incompatibilities: None.

Shelf life: 48 months.

Special precautions for storage: None.

Nature and contents of container: Paper/Aluminium foil/vinyl sachets of 5 gm (in packs of 10 or 30 sachets).
Pack sizes: 5 gm
Amber glass bottle with screw cap or HDPE bottle with screw cap or tamper-evident cap.
Pack size: 250 gm

Instructions for use/handling: None

Marketing authorisation number 0032/0055

Date of first authorisation/renewal of authorisation 26 October 1992.

Date of (partial) revision of the text July 1997.

Legal category POM.

COLPERMIN*

Qualitative and quantitative composition Peppermint Oil BP 0.2 ml

Pharmaceutical form Prolonged release capsule, hard, size 1. Body opaque light blue, cap opaque blue, with a blue band between body and cap.

Clinical particulars
Therapeutic indications: For the relief of the symptoms of Irritable Bowel Syndrome.

Posology and method of administration: For oral use.

Adults: One capsule three times a day. This dosage may be increased to two capsules three times a day if discomfort is severe.

The capsules should be taken until symptoms resolve which would normally be within one or two weeks. The treatment can be continued for longer periods of between 2 to 3 months, when symptoms are more persistent.

Elderly: As adult dose.

Children: There is no experience in the use of these capsules in children under the age of 15.

Contra-indications: None.

Special warnings and special precautions for use: The capsules should be swallowed whole, ie not broken or chewed. Patients who already suffer from heartburn sometimes have an exacerbation of this symptom after taking Colpermin. Treatment should be discontinued in these patients.

The patient should be advised to consult a doctor before use in the following circumstances:

First presentation of these symptoms for confirmation of IBS; aged 40 years or over and it is some time since the last attack, or the symptoms have changed; blood has been passed from the bowel; there is a feeling of sickness or there is vomiting; loss of appetite or loss of weight; paleness and tiredness; severe constipation; fever; recent foreign travel; pregnancy or planning a pregnancy or possibly pregnant; abnormal vaginal bleeding or discharge; difficulty or pain in passing urine

If there are new symptoms or worsening of the condition or failure to improve over two weeks, the patient should consult their doctor.

Interaction with other medicaments and other forms of interaction: The capsules should not be taken immediately after food. Indigestion remedies should not be taken at the same time as Colpermin.

Pregnancy and lactation: There are no data available to establish the safety of Colpermin in pregnancy, therefore it should be used only if, in the opinion of the physician, the possible benefits of treatment outweighs the possible hazards. Levels of menthol were not detectable in plasma or saliva following administration of Colpermin indicating rapid first pass metabolism. Significant levels of menthol in breast milk are thought to be unlikely.

Effects on ability to drive and use machines: None.

Undesirable effects: Occasional heartburn, perianal irritation; allergic reactions to menthol, which are rare, include erythematous rash, headache, bradycardia, muscle tremor and ataxia, which may occur in conjunction with alcohol.

Overdose: In the event of overdosage, the stomach should be emptied by gastric lavage. Observations should be carried out with symptomatic treatment if necessary.

Pharmacological properties
Pharmacodynamic properties: Antispasmodic and carminative.

The mode of action is local rather than systemic. The enteric coating delays opening of the capsule until it reaches the distal small bowel. Peppermint oil is then slowly released as the matrix passes along the gut. The oil exerts a local effect of colonic relaxation and a fall of intra-colonic pressure.

Pharmacological studies have demonstrated that peppermint oil exerts its inhibitory effect on gastrointestinal smooth muscle by interference with the mobilisation of calcium ions.

Pharmacokinetic properties: Not relevant.

Preclinical safety data: Not relevant.

Pharmaceutical particulars
List of excipients: White beeswax, Arachis oil, Colloidal Silica, Gelatin, Titanium dioxide, Indigotine (E132), Eudragit S100, Eudragit L30 D55, Triethyl citrate, Ammonia solution 10%, Monostearin, Polyethyleneglycol 4000, Talc, Purified Water.

Incompatibilities: None.

Shelf life: 36 months.

Special precautions for storage: Store below 25°C; avoid direct sunlight.

Nature and contents of container: Aluminium foil/PVC blister pack containing 10 capsules (250 μm PVC, 20 μm Al).
Marketed packs 20 and 100.

Instructions for use/handling: Not applicable.

Marketing authorisation number 0032/0218.

Date of first authorisation/renewal of authorisation 2 August 1996.

Date of (partial) revision of the text October 1997.

Legal category GSL.

CONVULEX*

Presentation Enteric-coated soft gelatin capsules containing 150, 300 and 500 mg Valproic Acid USP.

Uses For the treatment of epilepsy, both generalised and partial seizures, by oral medication.

Dosage and administration Convulex capsules should be swallowed whole.

Adults: Starting with a daily dose of 15 mg/kg body weight the dosage should be slowly increased by

5–10 mg/kg body weight up to 30 mg/kg body weight or until the patient no longer suffers from seizures.

Children: Starting with a daily dose of 15 mg/kg body weight the dosage should be slowly increased by 5–10 mg/kg body weight up to 30 mg/kg body weight or until the patient no longer suffers from seizures.

Elderly: Dosage should be determined by seizure control.

It is recommended that Convulex be given as a divided dose i.e. half the daily dose b.d. In some circumstances the daily dose can be split into 3 or 4 administrations.

Substitution: A one to one dose relationship of Convulex and products containing sodium valproate has been demonstrated in pharmacokinetic trials. In patients previously receiving sodium valproate therapy, Convulex should be initiated at the same total daily dose.

Combination therapy: During therapy with concurrently administered anticonvulsant drugs, Convulex dosages may have to be increased or decreased to maintain seizure control.

Contra-indications, warnings, etc
Contra-indications: Disturbances of hepatic function, known hypersensitivity to valproic acid and sodium valproate.

Warnings and precautions: The following laboratory tests should be determined before the start of therapy, subsequently at two-monthly intervals and before dosage increase; liver function tests, blood coagulation time, thrombocyte aggregation and fibrinogen levels.

Valproic acid should be discontinued or not started if the following abnormalities occur; hypofibrinogenaemia and/or coagulation disturbances, a threefold increase of transaminase values, an increase of alkaline phosphatase and bilirubin in serum in connection with clinical symptoms of toxic hepatitis. If only a slight increase in transaminase values is discovered the dosage should be reduced and liver function and coagulation tests should be monitored. If severe abdominal pain and vomiting occurs serum amylase values should be determined. If the results show pathological values, valproic acid should be discontinued. During treatment with valproic acid urine analysis for ketones may be false-positive. The platelet counts and bleeding time should be measured prior to surgical interventions.

Convulex may enhance the sedating effect of other preparations, especially that of the barbiturates. It may potentiate the CNS depressant action of alcohol, neuroleptics and antidepressants and may interact with concurrently administered anti-epileptic drugs. The effect of drugs affecting coagulation may be enhanced.

Adverse effects:
Hepatic: Liver function disturbances may occur during Convulex therapy. Rarely non-dose related severe hepatic damage has been reported within the first six months of treatment.

Minor abnormalities of liver function tests may occur during therapy but usually normalise after dosage adaption.

Valproic acid should be discontinued after the occurrence of clinical symptoms of hepatic damage eg recurrent epigastric complaints, anorexia etc. The patient should be instructed to report immediately any such symptoms to the treating physician.

Pancreatic: Pancreatic effects (acute pancreatitis) have been observed in rare cases. The treatment should be stopped immediately if symptoms and laboratory tests suggest pancreatitis. Patients should be instructed to report acute abdominal pain to the treating physician.

Haematological: Thrombocytopenia and inhibition of platelet aggregation have been observed. Monitoring of platelet function is therefore recommended especially prior to surgical intervention. The treatment should be stopped immediately after the manifestation of any coagulation disturbances.

Neurological: Sedation, aggression, hyperactivity, ataxia and tremor may occur rarely. In isolated cases states of confusion, stupor and coma have been observed some days after reaching therapeutic plasma levels.

Effects on ability to drive and use machines: Patients should be advised not to drive or use machinery if fatigue occurs.

Gastro-intestinal: Gastro-intestinal disturbances are among the most frequent side effects. Minor gastric irritation and nausea occur mostly at the onset of therapy and disappear with dose adjustment and/or taking the capsules during meals. Increased appetite and weight gain have been observed.

Dermatological: Allergic skin reactions occur very rarely. Transient loss of hair has been observed in isolated cases.

Use during pregnancy and lactation: In pregnancy, the possible benefits should be weighed against possible risks. Up to the 40th day, dosage should be as low as possible (15–20 mg/kg of body weight). Combination with other drugs is to be avoided as much as possible. There is no contra-indication to its use in lactating mothers.

Treatment of overdosage: At plasma concentrations of up to 5–6 times the maximum therapeutic levels there are unlikely to be any symptoms other than nausea, vomiting and dizziness.

In massive overdose, ie with plasma concentrations 10–20 times maximum therapeutic levels, there may be serious CNS depression and respiration may be impaired. Full recovery is usual following treatment including induced vomiting, gastric lavage, assisted ventilation and other supportive measures. Naloxone 0.01 mg/kg i.v. has been reported to reverse the CNS depressant effect of Valproic acid.

Pharmaceutical precautions Do not store above 25°C. Protect from light.

Legal category POM.

Package quantities Blister packs of 100 capsules.

Further information Nil.

Product licence numbers
150 mg 8298/0004
300 mg 8298/0002
500 mg 8298/0003

Product licence holder: Gerot Pharmaceuticals, Austria.

CYCLOPHOSPHAMIDE

Presentation Pink, biconvex, sugar coated tablets containing 53.5 mg Cyclophosphamide BP (equivalent to 50 mg anhydrous cyclophosphamide).

Cyclophosphamide for injection is a sterile white powder in clear glass vials, with rubber caps and aluminium seals, containing 107 mg, 214 mg, 535 mg or 1070 mg Cyclophosphamide BP (equivalent to 100 mg, 200 mg, 500 mg or 1000 mg anhydrous cyclophosphamide) with sodium chloride.

Uses Alkylating, antineoplastic agent. Cyclophosphamide has been used successfully to induce and maintain regressions in a wide range of neoplastic conditions, including leukaemias, lymphomas, soft tissue and osteogenic sarcomas, paediatric malignancies and adult solid tumours; in particular, breast and lung carcinomas.

Cyclophosphamide is frequently used in combination chemotherapy regimens involving other cytotoxic drugs.

Dosage and administration The dosage regimen should be tailored to the individual requirements of the patient, depending on his general condition, concurrent therapy, the type and state of tumour, and the patient's response. Three samples regimens may serve as guides:

Low dose: 80 to 240 mg/m^2 (2 to 6 mg/kg) as a single dose weekly i.v., or in divided doses orally.

Medium dose: 400 to 600 mg/m^2 (10 to 15 mg/kg) as a single dose weekly i.v.

High dose: 800 to 1,600 mg/m^2 (20 to 40 mg/kg) as a single dose i.v. at 10–20 day intervals.

Higher doses should be used only at the discretion of a physician experienced in cytotoxic chemotherapy.

It is recommended that the calculated dose of cyclophosphamide be reduced when it is given in combination with other anti-neoplastic agents or radiotherapy, and in patients with bone marrow depression.

Cyclophosphamide tablets should be swallowed whole, preferably on an empty stomach, but if gastric irritation is severe, they may be taken with meals.

Cyclophosphamide injection should be reconstituted with Water for Injections, 5 ml for each 100 mg of anhydrous cyclophosphamide. After reconstitution the solution should remain stable at room temperature for 2–3 hours. It should be given by slow intravenous injection over a period of 2–3 minutes or into the tubing of a freely running intravenous infusion over a period of 2–3 minutes.

A minimum output of 100 ml/hour should be maintained during therapy with conventional doses to avoid cystitis. If the larger doses are used, an output of at least this level should be maintained for 24 hours following administration, if necessary by forced diuresis. Alkalinisation of the urine is not recommended. Cyclophosphamide should be given early in the day and the bladder voided frequently. The patient should be well hydrated and maintained in fluid balance.

Mesna (Uromitexan) can be used concurrently with Cyclophosphamide to reduce urotoxic effects (for dosage see Uromitexan data sheet). If mesna (Uromitexan) is used to reduce uroethelial toxicity, frequent emptying of the bladder should be avoided.

If the leucocyte count is below 4,000/mm^3 or the platelet count is below 100,000/mm^3, treatment with Cyclophosphamide should be temporarily withheld until the blood count returns to normal levels.

Contra-indications, warnings, etc Cyclophosphamide should be used only under the direction of physicians experienced in cytotoxic or immunosuppressant therapy.

Contra-indications: Hypersensitivity and haemorrhagic cystitis.

Warnings: Cyclophosphamide should be withheld in the presence of severe bone marrow depression and reduced doses should be used in the presence of lesser degrees of bone marrow depression. Single doses will produce a leucopenia which may be severe but usually returns to normal within 21 days. Regular blood counts should be performed in patients who are pregnant or to mothers who are breastfeeding. It should not normally be given to patients with severe infections and should be withdrawn if such infections become life-threatening.

Cyclophosphamide should be used with caution in debilitated patients and those with renal and/or hepatic failure. Cyclophosphamide is not recommended in patients with a plasma creatinine greater than 120 μmol/l (1.5 mg/100 ml) bilirubin greater than 17 μmol (1 mg/100 ml); or serum transaminases or alkaline phosphatase more than 2–3 times the upper limit of normal. In all such cases, dosage should be reduced. Oral hypoglycaemic agents may be potentiated by cyclophosphamide.

Amenorrhoea and azoospermia often occur during treatment with cyclophosphamide but in most cases are reversible. Alkylating agents, including cyclophosphamide, have been shown to possess mutagenic, teratogenic and carcinogenic potential. Pregnancy should therefore be avoided during cyclophosphamide therapy and three months thereafter.

Cyclophosphamide is excreted mainly in the urine, largely in the form of active metabolites. These may give rise to a chemical cystitis which may be haemorrhagic. Because of this, a high fluid intake should be maintained with frequent emptying of the bladder. However, cyclophosphamide may give rise to fluid retention with subsequent water intoxication. Should this arise, a diuretic may be given. Cyclophosphamide may cause myocardial toxicity, especially at high dosage.

Cyclophosphamide may induce permanent sterility in children.

Adverse reactions: In addition to those noted above, the following may accompany cyclophosphamide therapy: hair loss, which may be total, although generally reversible; mucosal ulceration, anorexia, nausea and vomiting, pigmentation typically affecting the palms and nails of the hands and the soles of the feet, and interstitial pulmonary fibrosis.

Haematuria may occur during or after therapy with Cyclophosphamide. Acute sterile haemorrhagic cystitis may occur in up to 10% of patients not given mesna (Uromitexan) in conjunction with Cyclophosphamide. Late sequelae of this cystitis are bladder contracture and fibrosis.

Cyclophosphamide therapy may lead to inappropriate secretion of anti-diuretic hormone, fluid retention and hyponatremia, with subsequent water intoxication. Should this occur, diuretic therapy should be instigated.

Overdosage: Myelosuppression (particularly granulocytopenia) and haemorrhagic cystitis are the most serious consequences of overdosage. Recovery from myelosuppression will occur by the 21st day after the overdose in the great majority of patients (at doses up to 200 mg/kg i.v.) while granulocytopenia is usually seen by day 6 and lasts for a mean period of 12 days up to 18 days. A broad spectrum antibiotic may be administered until recovery occurs. Transfusion of whole-blood, platelets or white cells and reverse barrier nursing may be necessary.

If the drug has been taken in the form of tablets, early gastric lavage may reduce the amount of drug absorbed. During the first 24 hours and possibly up to 48 hours after overdosage, i.v. mesna may be beneficial in ameliorating damage to the urinary system. Normal supportive measures such as analgesics and maintenance of fluid balance should be instituted. If the cystitis does not resolve, more intensive treatment may be necessary. No further courses should be given until the patient has fully recovered.

Pharmaceutical precautions *Tablets:* Store in a cool dry place and protect from light.

Injection: Store in a cool place and protect from light. If heated above 32°C, cyclophosphamide may decompose to a damp-looking gel. It is, therefore, recommended that this product is never stored where heat build-up may occur such as near radiators, etc.

Legal category POM.

Package quantities
Tablets: Containers of 100 tablets of 50 mg.
Injection:
Vials of 100 mg in packs of 10.
Vials of 200 mg in packs of 10.
Vials of 500 mg in packs of 10.
Vials of 1000 mg in packs of 5.
Each vial contains dry powder for reconstitution.

Further information The dosage regimen for mesna (Uromitexan) varies according to the dose of Cyclophosphamide administered. In general i.v. Uromitexan is given as 60% w/w of the dose of i.v. Cyclophosphamide in three equal doses of 20% at 0, 4 and 8 hours. With the higher doses of Cyclophosphamide, the dose and frequency of administration may need to be increased. Uromitexan Tablets are also available; full prescribing information for both presentations is available on the appropriate data sheet.

Product licence numbers
Cyclophosphamide tablets 50 mg 3433/0036
Cyclophosphamide Injection 100 mg 3433/0037
Cyclophosphamide Injection 200 mg 3433/0038
Cyclophosphamide Injection 500 mg 3433/0039
Cyclophosphamide Injection 1000 mg 3433/0040

CYKLOKAPRON* INJECTION

Qualitative and quantitative composition
Active ingredient: Tranexamic Acid BP/EP 500 mg

Pharmaceutical form Ampoules containing 5 ml colourless solution

Clinical particulars
Therapeutic indications:
Local fibrinolysis: For short term use in prophylaxis and treatment in patients at high risk of per- and post-operative haemorrhage following:
prostatectomy
conisation of the cervix
surgical procedures and dental extractions in haemophiliacs

General fibrinolysis: haemorrhagic complications in association with thrombolytic therapy.

Haemorrhage associated with disseminated intravascular coagulation with predominant activation of the fibrinolytic system.

Posology and method of administration: Route of administration: by slow intravenous injection.

Local fibrinolysis: the recommended standard dose is 5–10 ml (500–1000 mg) by slow intravenous injection (1 ml/min), three times daily. If treatment continues for more than three days, consideration should be given to the use of Cyklokapron tablets or syrup. Alternatively, following an initial intravenous injection, subsequent treatment may proceed by intravenous infusion. Following addition to a suitable diluent (see *Interaction with other medicaments and other forms of interaction* section), Cyklokapron may be administered at a rate of 25–50 mg/kg body wt/day.

Children: According to body weight (10 mg/kg body wt/ 2–3 times daily)

Elderly patients: No reduction in dosage is necessary unless there is evidence of renal failure.

General fibrinolysis: In disseminated intravascular coagulation with predominant activation of the fibrinolytic system, usually a single dose of 10 ml (1 g) is sufficient to control bleeding.

Neutralisation of thrombolytic therapy; 10 mg/kg body wt by slow intravenous injection.

Contra-indications: Cyklokapron is contra-indicated in patients with a history of thromboembolic disease.

Special warnings and precautions for use: In patients with renal insufficiency, because of the risk of accumulation. The dose should be reduced according to the following table:

Serum creatinine	*Dose iv*	*Dose Frequency*
120–250 mcmol/l	10 mg/kg	Twice daily
250–500 mcmol/l	10 mg/kg	Every 24 hours
> 500 mcmol/l	5 mg/kg	Every 24 hours

In massive haematuria from the upper urinary tract (especially in haemophilia) since, in a few cases, ureteric obstruction has been reported.

In patients with disseminated intravascular coagulation (DIC) treatment must be restricted to those in whom there is predominant activation of the fibrinolytic system with acute severe bleeding. Characteristically, the haematological profile approximates to the following: reduced euglobulin clot lysis time; prolonged prothrombin time; reduced plasma levels of fibrinogen, factors V and VIII, plasminogen and alpha-2 macroglobulin; normal plasma levels of P and P complex; ie factors II (prothrombin), VIII and X; increased plasma levels of fibrinogen degradation products; a normal platelet count. The foregoing presumes that the underlying disease state does not modify the various elements in this profile. In such acute cases a single dose of 1 g tranexamic acid is frequently sufficient to control bleeding. The fibrinolytic activity in the blood will be reduced for about 4 hours if renal function is normal. Anticoagulation with heparin should be instigated in order to prevent further fibrin deposition. Administration of Cyklokapron in DIC should be considered only when appropriate haematological laboratory facilities and expertise are available. Cyklokapron must not be administered in DIC with predominant activation of the coagulation system.

Interaction with other medicaments and other forms of interaction: The solution for injection may be mixed with the following solutions: isotonic sodium chloride; isotonic glucose; 20% fructose; 10% invertose; dextran 40; dextran 70; ringer's solution.

Cyklokapron solution for injection may be mixed with Heparin.

Pregnancy and lactation: Although there is no evidence from animal studies of a teratogenic effect, the usual caution with the use of drugs in pregnancy should be observed.

Tranexamic acid passes into breast milk to a concentration of approximately one hundreth of the concentration in the maternal blood. An antifibrinolytic effect in the infant is unlikely.

Effects on ability to drive and use machines: None known.

Undesirable effects: Gastro-intestinal disorders (nausea, vomiting, diarrhoea) may occur but disappear when the dosage is reduced. Rapid intravenous injection may cause dizziness and/or hypotension.

Overdose: No cases of overdosage have been reported. Symptoms may be nausea, vomiting, orthostatic symptoms and/or hypotension. Maintain a high fluid intake to promote renal excretion.

Pharmacological properties
Pharmacodynamic properties: Tranexamic acid is an antifibrinolytic agent which competitively inhibits the activation of plasminogen to plasmin.

Pharmacokinetic properties: Approximately 90% of an intravenously administered tranexamic acid dose is excreted, largely unchanged, in the urine within 24 hours. The plasma half-life is approximately 2 hours.

Preclinical safety data: There are no preclinical data of relevance to the prescriber which are additional to that already included in other sections of the Summary of Product Characteristics.

Pharmaceutical particulars
List of excipients: Water for injections.

Incompatibilities: Cyklokapron solution for injection should not be added to blood for transfusion, or to injections containing penicillin.

Shelf life: 3 years.

Special precautions for storage: None.

Nature and contents of container: Type I glass 5 ml ampoules packed in outer cardboard carton.

Instructions for use/handling: See Posology and Method of Administration Section.

Marketing authorisation number 0022/0004R.

Date of first authorisation/renewal of authorisation
Granted: 9 February 1987
Renewed: 9 February 1992

Date of (partial) revision of the text N/A

Legal category POM.

CYKLOKAPRON* SYRUP

Qualitative and quantitative composition
Active ingredient: Tranexamic acid EP 500 mg/5 ml

Pharmaceutical form A colourless or slightly yellow syrup with an orange taste.

Clinical particulars
Therapeutic indications: Short-term use for haemorrhage or risk of haemorrhage in increased fibrinolysis or fibrinogenolysis. Local fibrinolysis as occurs in the following conditions:
- Prostatectomy and bladder surgery
- Menorrhagia
- Epistaxis
- Conisation of the cervix
- Traumatic hyphaema
- Hereditary angioneurotic oedema
- Management of dental extraction in haemophiliacs

Posology and method of administration: Route of administration: Oral.

Local fibrinolysis: The recommended standard dosage is 15–25 mg/kg bodyweight (10–15 ml syrup) 2–3 times daily. For the indications listed below the following doses may be used:

Prostatectomy: Prophylaxis and treatment of haemorrhage in high risk patients should commence per- or post-operatively with Cyklokapron

Injection; thereafter 10 ml syrup 3–4 times daily until macroscopic haematuria is no longer present.

Menorrhagia: 10–15 ml syrup 3–4 times daily for 3–4 days. Cyklokapron therapy should be initiated only after heavy bleeding has started.

Epistaxis: Where recurrent bleeding is anticipated oral therapy (10 ml syrup 3 times daily) should be administered for 7 days.

Conisation of the cervix: 15 ml syrup 3 times daily.

Traumatic hyphaema: 10-15 ml syrup 3 times a day. The dose is based on 25 mg/kg 3 times a day.

Hereditary angioneurotic oedema: Some patients are aware of the onset of the illness; suitable treatment for these patients is intermittently 10–15 ml syrup 2–3 times daily for some days. Other patients are treated continuously at this dosage.

Haemophilia: In the management of dental extractions 10–15 ml syrup every eight hours. The dose is based on 25 mg/kg.

Children: Dosage should be calculated according to body weight at 25 mg/kg/dose.

Elderly patients: No reduction in dosage is necessary unless there is evidence of renal failure (please refer to section *Special warnings and precautions for use*).

Contra-indications: Patients with a history of thromboembolic disease.

Special warnings and precautions for use: In patients with renal insufficiency, because of the risk of accumulation. By extrapolation from clearance data relating to the intravenous dosage form, the following reduction in the oral dosage is recommended:

Serum creatinine	*Oral dose*	*Dose frequency*
120–250 mmol/l	25 mg/kg	Twice daily
250–500 mmol/l	25 mg/kg	Every 24 hours
> 500 mmol/l	12.5 mg/kg	Every 24 hours

In massive haematuria from the upper urinary tract (especially in haemophilia) since, in a few cases, ureteric obstruction has been reported.

In the long-term treatment of patients with hereditary angioneurotic oedema, regular eye examinations (e.g. visual acuity, slit lamp, intraocular pressure, visual fields) and liver function tests should be performed.

Interaction with other medicaments and other forms of interaction: Cyklokapron will counteract the thrombolytic effect of fibrinolytic preparations.

Pregnancy and lactation
Pregnancy: Although there is no evidence from animal studies of a teratogenic effect, the usual caution with the use of drugs in pregnancy should be observed.

Lactation: Tranexamic acid passes into breast milk to a concentration of approximately one hundredth of the concentration in the maternal blood. An antifibrinolytic effect in the infant is unlikely.

Effects on ability to drive and use machines: None known.

Undesirable effects: Gastrointestinal disorders (nausea, vomiting, diarrhoea) may occur but disappear when the dosage is reduced. Rare instances of colour vision disturbances have been reported. Patients who experience disturbance of colour vision should be withdrawn from treatment.

Overdose: No cases of overdosage have been reported. Symptoms may be nausea, vomiting, orthostatic symptoms and/or hypotension. Initiate vomiting, then stomach lavage, and charcoal therapy. Maintain a high fluid intake to promote renal excretion.

Pharmacological properties
Pharmacodynamic properties: Tranexamic acid is an antifibrinolytic compound which is a potent competitive inhibitor of the activation of plasminogen to plasmin. At much higher concentrations it is a non-competitive inhibitor of plasmin. The inhibitory effect of tranexamic acid in plasminogen activation by urokinase has been reported to be 6–100 times and by streptokinase 6-40 times greater than that of aminocaproic acid. The antifibrinolytic activity of tranexamic acid is approximately ten times greater than that of aminocaproic acid.

Pharmacokinetic properties: Following oral administration, 1.13% and 39% of the administered dose were recovered after 3 and 24 hours respectively. Tranexamic acid administered parenterally is distributed in a two compartment model. Tranexamic acid crosses the placenta, and may reach one hundredth of the serum peak concentration in the milk of lactating women. Tranexamic acid crosses the blood brain barrier.

Following intravenous administration, the biological half-life of tranexamic acid has been determined to be 1.9 hours and 2.7 hours.

Preclinical safety data: There are no preclinical data of

relevance to the prescriber which are additional to that already included in other sections of the Summary of Product Characteristics.

Pharmaceutical particulars
List of excipients: Xylitol; Citric Acid anhydrous; Methyl parahydroxybenzoate; Propyl parahydroxybenzoate; Orange Aroma 3174; Purified Water

Incompatibilities: None known.

Shelf life: Unopened: 24 months; Opened: 3 months.

Special precautions for storage: Store below 25°C.

Nature and contents of container: 300 ml, brown soda-lime glass bottles (Type III, PhEur) with white polypropylene tamper-proof closure consisting of lip and pour part or 300 ml, amber PET bottles with polypropylene screw caps.

Instructions for use/handling: Cyklokapron Syrup may be diluted with syrup BP and the resulting mixture stored for up to 14 days.

Marketing authorisation number 0022/0044.

Date of first authorisation/renewal of authorisation
Granted: 17 March 1981
Renewed: 12 June 1991.

Date of (partial) revision of the text March 1996.

Legal category POM.

CYKLOKAPRON* TABLETS

Presentation White, film-coated oblong tablets, 8×18 mm, engraved CY with an arc above and below the lettering. Each tablet contains Tranexamic Acid 500 mg.

Uses
Action: Tranexamic acid is an antifibrinolytic agent which competitively inhibits the activation of plasminogen to plasmin.

Indications: Short-term use for haemorrhage or risk of haemorrhage in increased fibrinolysis or fibrinogenolysis.

1. Local fibrinolysis as occurs in the following conditions:
a. Prostatectomy
b. Menorrhagia
c. Epistaxis
d. Conisation of the cervix
e. Traumatic hyphaema

2. Management of dental extraction in haemophiliacs.

3. Hereditary angioneurotic oedema.

Dosage and administration
Local fibrinolysis: The recommended standard dose is 15–25 mg/kg body wt, i.e. 2–3 tablets two to three times daily. For the indications listed below the following doses may be used:

1a. *Prostatectomy:* Prophylaxis and treatment of haemorrhage in high risk patients should commence per- or post-operatively with Cyklokapron Injection; thereafter 2 tablets, three to four times daily until macroscopic haematuria is no longer present.

1b. *Menorrhagia:* 2–3 tablets three to four times daily for three to four days. Cyklokapron therapy is initiated only after heavy bleeding has started.

1c. *Epistaxis:* Where recurrent bleeding is anticipated, oral therapy (2 tablets three times daily) should be administered for seven days.

1d. *Conisation of the cervix:* 3 tablets three times daily.

1e. *Traumatic hyphaema:* 2–3 tablets three times daily. The dose is based on 25 mg/kg three times a day.

2. *Haemophilia:* In the management of dental extractions 2–3 tablets every eight hours. The dose is based on 25 mg/kg.

3. *Hereditary angioneurotic oedema:* Some patients are aware of the onset of the illness; suitable treatment for these patients is intermittently 2–3 tablets two to three times daily for some days. Other patients are treated continuously at this dosage.

Children's dosage: This should be calculated according to body weight, at 25 mg/kg per dose.

Elderly patients: No reduction in dosage is necessary unless there is evidence of renal failure (see guidelines below).

Contra-indications, warnings, etc Cyklokapron is contra-indicated in patients with a history of thromboembolic disease.

Precautions:

1. In patients with renal insufficiency, because of the risk of accumulation. By extrapolation from clearance data relating to the intravenous dosage form, the following reduction in the oral dosage is recommended.

Serum creatinine	*Oral dose*	*Dose frequency*
120–250 micromol/l	25 mg/kg	twice daily
250–500 micromol/l	25 mg/kg	every 24th hour
>500 micromol/l	12.5 mg/kg	every 24th hour

2. In massive haematuria from the upper urinary tract (especially in haemophilia) since, in a few cases, ureteric obstruction has been reported.

3. When disseminated intravascular coagulation is in progress.

4. In the long-term treatment of patients with hereditary angioneurotic oedema regular eye examination (e.g. visual acuity, slit lamp, intra-ocular pressure, visual fields) and liver function tests should be performed.

Pregnancy: Although there is no evidence from animal studies of a teratogenic effect, the usual caution with use of drugs in pregnancy should be observed.

Lactation: Tranexamic acid passes into breast milk to a concentration of approximately one hundredth of the concentration in the maternal blood. An antifibrinolytic effect in the infant is unlikely.

Side-effects: Gastro-intestinal disorders (nausea, vomiting, diarrhoea) may occur but disappear when the dosage is reduced. Rare instances of transient colour vision disturbance have been reported. Patients who experience disturbance of colour vision should be withdrawn from treatment.

Overdosage: No cases of overdosage have been reported. Symptoms may be nausea, vomiting, orthostatic symptoms and/or hypotension. Initiate vomiting, then stomach lavage and charcoal therapy. Maintain a high fluid intake to promote renal excretion.

Legal category POM.

Package quantities Carton containing 5 blister strips of 12 tablets each.

Further information Absorption of tranexamic acid from the gastro-intestinal tract is 30–40%. The plasma half-life is approximately 2 hours.

Product licence number 0022/0003R.

CYTOSAR* 100 mg and 500 mg

Qualitative and quantitative composition Cytarabine EP 100 mg or 500 mg.

Pharmaceutical form Powder for injection.

Clinical particulars
Therapeutic indications: Cytotoxic for induction of remission in acute myeloid leukaemia in adults and for other acute leukaemias of adults and children.

Posology and method of administration: By intravenous infusion or injection, or subcutaneous injection. Water for Injections, 0.9% saline or 5% dextrose should be used for preparing a solution of cytarabine in the vial. When the accompanying diluent (Water for Injections) is used, such solution contains 20 mg/ml (100 mg vial) or 50 mg/ml (500 mg vial) cytarabine.

The physician is reminded that in practice Cytosar has been administered in combination with a variety of other cytotoxic agents using a number of different dosage schedules, and reference to the current literature before commencing treatment is recommended.

Dosage recommendations may be converted from those in terms of bodyweight to those related to surface area by means of nomograms such as are presented in Documenta Geigy.

1) Remission induction:
a) Continuous treatment:
i) Rapid injection - 2 mg/kg/day is a judicious starting dose. Administer for 10 days. Obtain daily blood counts. If no antileukaemic effect is noted and there is no apparent toxicity, increase to 4 mg/kg/day and maintain until therapeutic response or toxicity is evident. Almost all patients can be carried to toxicity with these doses.

ii) 0.5–1.0 mg/kg/day may be given in an infusion of up to 24 hours duration. Results from one-hour infusions have been satisfactory in the majority of patients. After 10 days this initial daily dose may be increased to 2 mg/kg/day subject to toxicity. Continue to toxicity or until remission occurs.

b) Intermittent treatment:
3–5 mg/kg/day are administered intravenously on each of five consecutive days. After a two to nine-day rest period, a further course is given. Continue until response or toxicity occurs.

The first evidence of marrow improvement has been reported to occur 7–64 days (mean 28 days) after the beginning of therapy.

In general, if a patient shows neither toxicity nor remission after a fair trial, the cautious administration of higher doses is warranted. As a rule, patients have been seen to tolerate higher doses when given by rapid intravenous injection as compared with slow infusion. This difference is due to the rapid metabolism of Cytosar and the consequent short duration of action of the high dose.

2) Maintenance therapy: Remissions which have been induced by cytarabine, or by other drugs, may be maintained by intravenous or subcutaneous injection of 1 mg/kg once or twice weekly.

Children: Children appear to tolerate higher doses than adults and, where dose ranges are quoted, the children should receive the higher dose and the adults the lower.

Elderly patients: There is no information to suggest that a change in dosage is warranted in the elderly. Nevertheless, the elderly patient does not tolerate drug toxicity as well as the younger patient, and particular attention should thus be given to drug induced leucopenia, thrombocytopenia, and anaemia, with appropriate initiation of supportive therapy when indicated.

Contra-indications: Therapy with Cytosar should not be considered in patients with pre-existing drug-induced bone marrow suppression, unless the clinician feels that such management offers the most hopeful alternative for the patient. Cytosar should not be used in the management of non-malignant disease, except for immunosuppression.

Special warnings and special precautions for use: Cytosar is a potent bone marrow suppressant. Therapy should be started cautiously in patients with pre-existing drug-induced bone marrow suppression. Patients receiving this drug must be under close medical supervision and, during induction therapy, should have leucocyte and platelet counts performed daily. Bone marrow examinations should be performed frequently after blasts have disappeared from the peripheral blood. Facilities should be available for management of complications, possibly fatal, of bone marrow suppression (infection resulting from granulocytopenia and other impaired body defences, and haemorrhage secondary to thrombocytopenia). One case of anaphylaxis that resulted in acute cardiopulmonary arrest and required resuscitation has been reported. This occurred immediately after the intravenous administration of Cytosar.

Severe and at times fatal CNS, GI and pulmonary toxicity (different from that seen with conventional therapy regimens of Cytosar) has been reported following some experimental Cytosar dose schedules. These reactions include reversible corneal toxicity; cerebral and cerebellar dysfunction, usually reversible; severe gastro-intestinal ulceration, including pneumatosis cystoides intestinalis, leading to peritonitis; sepsis and liver abscess; and pulmonary oedema.

Cytosar has been shown to be carcinogenic in animals. The possibility of a similar effect should be borne in mind when designing the long-term management of the patient.

Patients receiving Cytosar must be monitored closely. Frequent platelet and leucocyte counts are mandatory. Suspend or modify therapy when drug-induced marrow depression has resulted in a platelet count under 50,000 or a polymorphonuclear count under 1,000 per cubic mm. Counts of formed elements in the peripheral blood may continue to fall after the drug is stopped, and reach lowest values after drug-free intervals of five to seven days. If indicated, restart therapy when definite signs of marrow recovery appear (on successive bone marrow studies). Patients whose drug is withheld until 'normal' peripheral blood values are attained may escape from control.

When intravenous doses are given quickly, patients are frequently nauseated and may vomit for several hours afterwards. This problem tends to be less severe when the drug is infused.

The human liver apparently detoxifies a substantial fraction of an administered dose. Use the drug with caution and at reduced dose in patients whose liver function is poor.

Periodical checks of bone marrow, liver and kidney functions should be performed in patients receiving Cytosar.

The safety of this drug for use in infants is not established.

Like other cytotoxic drugs, Cytosar may induce hyperuricaemia secondary to rapid lysis of neoplastic cells. The clinician should monitor the patient's blood uric acid level and be prepared to use such supportive and pharmacological measures as may be necessary to control this problem.

Interaction with other medicaments and other forms of interaction: None have been reported.

Pregnancy and lactation: Cytosar is known to be teratogenic in some animal species. The use of Cytosar in women who are, or who may become, pregnant should be undertaken only after due consideration of the potential benefits and hazards.

This product should not normally be administered to patients who are pregnant or to mothers who are breast-feeding.

Effects on ability to drive and use machines: No adverse effect has been reported.

Undesirable effects: Adverse reactions seen with cytarabine treatment have included those seen with cytotoxic agents having an effect on bone marrow, such as: leucopenia, thrombocytopenia, anaemia, bone marrow suppression and megaloblastosis. Other side-effects have included: nausea, vomiting, diarrhoea, oral ulceration, hepatic dysfunction. Occasional adverse experiences have been reported as follows: renal dysfunction, anorexia, sepsis, gastro-intestinal haemorrhage, irritation or sepsis at site of injection, neuritis or neurotoxicity, rash, freckling, oesophagitis, skin and mucosal bleeding, chest pain, joint pain and reduction in reticulocytes.

A Cytosar syndrome has been described. It is characterised by fever, myalgia, bone pain, occasionally chest pain, maculopapular rash, conjunctivitis and malaise. It usually occurs 6–12 hours following drug administration. Corticosteroids have been shown to be beneficial in treating or preventing this syndrome. If the symptoms of the syndrome are serious enough to warrant treatment, corticosteroids should be contemplated as well as continuation of therapy with Cytosar.

Cytosar is not recommended for intrathecal use; however, the following side-effects have been reported with such use. Expected systemic reactions: bone marrow depression, nausea, vomiting. Occasionally, severe spinal cord toxicity even leading to quadriplegia and paralysis, necrotising encephalopathy, blindness and other isolated neurotoxicities have been reported.

Overdose: Cessation of therapy, followed by management of ensuing bone marrow depression including whole blood or platelet transfusion and antibiotics as required.

Pharmacological properties

Pharmacodynamic properties: Cytarabine, a pyrimidine nucleoside analogue, is an antineoplastic agent which inhibits the synthesis of deoxyribonucleic acid. It also has antiviral and immunosuppressant properties. Detailed studies on the mechanism of cytotoxicity in vitro suggests that the primary action of cytarabine is inhibition of deoxycytidine synthesis, although inhibition of cytidylic kinases and incorporation of the compound into nucleic acids may also play a role in its cytostatic and cytocidal actions.

Pharmacokinetic properties: Cytarabine is deaminated to arabinofuranosyl uracil in the liver and kidneys. After intravenous administration to humans, only 5.8% of the administered dose is excreted unaltered in the urine within 12–24 hours, 90% of the dose is excreted as the deaminated product. Cytosar appears to be metabolised rapidly, primarily by the liver and perhaps by the kidney. After single high intravenous doses, blood levels fall to unmeasurable levels within 15 minutes in most patients. Some patients have in demonstrable circulating drug as early as 5 minutes after injection.

Pharmaceutical particulars

List of excipients: None.

Incompatibilities: None.

Shelf-life: Shelf-life of the medicinal product as packaged for sale: 60 months.

Solutions reconstituted with Water for Injections, 0.9% saline, or 5% dextrose must be used immediately and not stored. When reconstituted with the accompanying diluent, solutions should be stored at room temperature and used within 48 hours.

Discard any solution in which a slight haze develops.

Special precautions for storage: Store at room temperature.

Nature and contents of container: Type I flint glass vial with butyl rubber plug and aluminium flip off seal.

Each vial contains 100 mg or 500 mg of cytarabine.

Instructions for use/handling: No special requirements.

Marketing authorisation numbers
0032/5037 100 mg
0032/0109 500 mg

Date of renewal of authorisation
0032/5037 date of renewal:
0032/0109 date of renewal: 7 August 1989

Date of revision of the text August 1996.

Legal category POM.

DALACIN* C CAPSULES 75 MG, 150 MG

Presentation

Hard-filled, gelatin capsules (lavender/lavender) containing clindamycin hydrochloride equivalent to 75 mg clindamycin. Also contains: lactose, maize starch, talc, magnesium stearate, gelatin, E132 and E127.

Hard-filled, gelatin capsules (maroon/lavender) containing clindamycin hydrochloride equivalent to 150 mg clindamycin. Also contains: lactose, maize starch, talc, magnesium stearate, gelatin, E132, E127 and E171.

Uses

Indications: Antibacterial. Serious infections caused by susceptible Gram-positive organisms, staphylococci (both penicillinase- and non-penicillinase-producing), streptococci (except *Streptococcus faecalis*) and pneumococci. It is also indicated in serious infections caused by susceptible anaerobic pathogens.

Clindamycin does not penetrate the blood/brain barrier in therapeutically effective quantities.

Mechanism of action: Lincosamides such as clindamycin bind to the 50S subunit of the bacterial ribosome similarly to macrolides such as erythromycin and inhibit the early stages of protein synthesis. The action of clindamycin is predominantly bacteriostatic although high concentrations may be slowly bactericidal against sensitive strains.

Pharmacology: Clindamycin is a lincosamide antibiotic with a primarily bacteriostatic action against Gram-positive aerobes and a wide range of anaerobic bacteria. Most Gram-negative aerobic bacteria, including the Enterobacteriaceae, are resistant to clindamycin. Clindamycin demonstrates cross-resistance with lincomycin. When tested by *in vitro* methods, some staphylococcal strains originally resistant to erythromycin rapidly developed resistance to clindamycin. The mechanisms for resistance are the same as for erythromycin, namely methylation of the ribosomal binding site, chromosomal mutation of the ribosomal protein and in a few staphylococcal isolates enzymic inactivation by a plasmid-mediated adenyltransferase.

Pharmacokinetics: About 90% of a dose of clindamycin hydrochloride is absorbed from the gastro-intestinal tract; concentrations of 2 to 3 micrograms per ml occur within one hour after a 150 mg dose of clindamycin, with average concentrations of about 0.7 micrograms per ml after 6 hours. After doses of 300 and 600 mg peak plasma concentrations of 4 and 8 micrograms per ml, respectively, have been reported. Absorption is not significantly diminished by food in the stomach, but the rate of absorption may be reduced.

Clindamycin is widely distributed in body fluids and tissues including bone, but it does not reach the cerebrospinal fluid in significant concentrations. It diffuses across the placenta into the fetal circulation and appears in breast milk. High concentrations occur in bile. It accumulates in leucocytes and macrophages. Over 90% of clindamycin in the circulation is bound to plasma proteins. The half-life is 2 to 3 hours, although this may be prolonged in pre-term neonates and patients with severe renal impairment.

Clindamycin undergoes metabolism, presumably in the liver, to the active *N*-demethyl and sulphoxide metabolites and also some inactive metabolites. About 10% of the drug is excreted in the urine as active drug or metabolites and about 4% in the faeces; the remainder is excreted as inactive metabolites. Excretion is slow and takes place over several days. It is not effectively removed from the blood by dialysis.

Dosage and administration

Oral. Absorption of Dalacin C is not appreciably modified by the presence of food.

Dalacin C Capsules should always be taken with a glass of water

Adults: Moderately severe infection, 150–300 mg every six hours; severe infection, 300 -- 450 mg every six hours.

Elderly patients: The half-life, volume of distribution and clearance, and extent of absorption after administration of clindamycin hydrochloride are not altered by increased age. Analysis of data from clinical studies has not revealed any age-related increase in toxicity. Dosage requirements in elderly patients, therefore, should not be influenced by age alone. See *Precautions* for other factors which should be taken into consideration.

Children: Dalacin C Paediatric is recommended for use in children, however, where capsules are preferred, the recommended dosage is 3–6 mg/kg every six hours depending on the severity of the infection. In children under one year or weighing 10 kg or less the minimum recommended dose is 2.5 ml (37.5 mg) every eight hours.

Note: In cases of beta-haemolytic streptococcal infection, treatment with Dalacin C should continue for at least 10 days to diminish the likelihood of subsequent rheumatic fever or glomerulonephritis.

Contra-indications, warnings, etc

Contra-indications: Dalacin C is contra-indicated in patients previously found to be sensitive to clindamycin or lincomycin.

Interaction with other medicaments and other forms of interaction: Clindamycin has been shown to have neuromuscular blocking properties that may enhance the action of other neuromuscular blocking agents. It should be used with caution, therefore, in patients receiving such agents.

Antagonism has been demonstrated between clindamycin and erythromycin *in vitro*. Because of possible clinical significance the two drugs should not be administered concurrently.

Effects on ability to drive and to use machines: Not applicable.

Other undesirable effects: Gastro-intestinal tract: Nausea, vomiting, abdominal pain and diarrhoea (see *Warnings*).

Haematopoietic: Transient neutropenia (leucopenia), eosinophilia, agranulocytosis and thrombocytopenia have been reported. No direct aetiologic relationship to concurrent clindamycin therapy could be made in any of the foregoing.

Skin and mucous membranes: Pruritus, vaginitis and rare instances of exfoliative and vesiculobullous dermatitis have been reported.

Hypersensitivity reactions: Maculopapular rash and urticaria have been observed during drug therapy. Generalised mild to moderate morbilliform-like skin rashes are the most frequently reported reactions. Rare instances of erythema multiforme, some resembling Stevens-Johnson syndrome, have been associated with clindamycin. A few cases of anaphylactoid reactions have been reported.

Liver: Jaundice and abnormalities in liver function tests have been observed during clindamycin therapy.

Use in pregnancy and lactation: Safety for use in pregnancy has not yet been established.

Clindamycin is excreted in human milk. Caution should be exercised when Dalacin C is administered to a nursing mother. It is unlikely that a nursing infant can absorb a significant amount of clindamycin from its gastro-intestinal tract.

Other special warnings and precautions:

Warnings: Dalacin C should only be used in the treatment of serious infections. In considering the use of the product, the practitioner should bear in mind the type of infection and the potential hazard of the diarrhoea which may develop, since cases of colitis have been reported during, or even two or three weeks following, the administration of clindamycin.

Studies indicate a toxin(s) produced by clostridia (especially *Clostridium difficile*) is the principal direct cause of antibiotic-associated colitis. These studies also indicate that this toxigenic clostridium is usually sensitive *in vitro* to vancomycin. When 125 mg to 500 mg of vancomycin are administered orally four times a day for 7–10 days, there is a rapid observed disappearance of the toxin from faecal samples and a coincident clinical recovery from the diarrhoea. (Where the patient is receiving cholestyramine in addition to vancomycin, consideration should be given to separating the times of administration).

Colitis is a disease which has a clinical spectrum from mild, watery diarrhoea to severe, persistent diarrhoea, leucocytosis, fever, severe abdominal cramps, which may be associated with the passage of blood and mucus. If allowed to progress, it may produce peritonitis, shock and toxic megacolon. This may be fatal.

The appearance of marked diarrhoea should be regarded as an indication that the product should be discontinued immediately. The disease is likely to follow a more severe course in older patients or patients who are debilitated. Diagnosis is usually made by the recognition of the clinical symptoms, but can be substantiated by endoscopic demonstration of pseudomembranous colitis. The presence of the disease may be further confirmed by culture of the stool for *Clostridium difficile* on selective media and assay of the stool specimen for the toxin(s) of *C. difficile*.

Precautions: Caution should be used when prescribing Dalacin C to individuals with a history of gastro-intestinal disease, especially colitis.

Periodic liver and kidney function tests should be carried out during prolonged therapy. Such monitoring is also recommended in neonates and infants.

The dosage of Dalacin C may require reduction in patients with renal or hepatic impairment due to prolongation of the serum half-life.

Prolonged administration of Dalacin C, as with any anti-infective, may result in super-infection due to organisms resistant to clindamycin.

Care should be observed in the use of Dalacin C in atopic individuals.

Overdosage: In cases of overdosage no specific treatment is indicated.

The serum biological half-life of clindamycin is 2.4

hours. Clindamycin cannot readily be removed from the blood by dialysis or peritoneal dialysis.

If an allergic adverse reaction occurs, therapy should be with the usual emergency treatments, including corticosteroids, adrenaline and antihistamines.

Incompatibilities: None known.

Pharmaceutical precautions Store below 25°C.

Legal category POM.

Package quantities 75 mg capsules in packs of 24. 150 mg capsules in packs of 24 and 100.

Product licence numbers
0032/5006 Dalacin C Capsules 75 mg
0032/5007 Dalacin C Capsules 150 mg

Date of preparation or last review August 1998

DALACIN* C PAEDIATRIC

Qualitative and quantitative composition Each 2 g granules or 5 ml reconstituted suspension contains clindamycin palmitate hydrochloride equivalent to 75 mg clindamycin.

Pharmaceutical form Off-white, sucrose-based granules for paediatric suspension.

Clinical particulars
Therapeutic indications: Antibacterial. Serious infections caused by susceptible Gram-positive organisms, staphylococci (both penicillinase- and non-penicillinase-producing), streptococci (except *Streptococcus faecalis*) and pneumococci. It is also indicated in serious infections caused by susceptible anaerobic pathogens.

Clindamycin does not penetrate the blood/brain barrier in therapeutically effective quantities.

Posology and method of administration: Oral. Absorption of Dalacin C is not appreciably modified by the presence of food.

To each 100 ml bottle of granules add 74 ml purified water and shake.

Children: 3–6 mg/kg every six hours depending on the severity of the infection.

In children under one year or weighing 10 kg or less the minimum recommended dose is 2.5 ml (37.5 mg) every eight hours.

The following paediatric dose regime is recommended as a guide:

Moderately severe infection: 0–11 months: 3.5–9.0 kg: 2.5 ml every eight hours.
1–3 years: 10–15 kg: 2.5 ml every six hours.
4–7 years: 16–25 kg: 5 ml every six hours.
8–12 years: 26–38 kg: 7.5 ml every six hours.

Severe infection: 0 - 11 months: 3.5–9.0 kg: 2.5 ml every six hours.
1–3 years: 10–15 kg: 5 ml every six hours.
4–7 years: 16–25 kg: 7.5 ml every six hours.
8–12 years: 26–38 kg: 10 ml every six hours.

Adults: moderately severe infection: 10 ml every six hours; severe infection: 20 ml every six hours.

Treatment for infections caused by beta-haemolytic streptococci should be continued for at least 10 days to guard against subsequent rheumatic fever or glomerulonephritis.

Elderly patients: The half-life, volume of distribution and clearance, and extent of absorption after administration of clindamycin hydrochloride are not altered by increased age. Analysis of data from clinical studies has not revealed any age-related increase in toxicity. Dosage requirements in elderly patients, therefore, should not be influenced by age alone. See *Precautions* for other factors which should be taken into consideration.

Contra-indications: Dalacin C Paediatric is contra-indicated in patients previously found to be sensitive to clindamycin or lincomycin.

Special warnings and special precautions for use: Warnings: Dalacin C Paediatric should only be used in the treatment of serious infections. In considering the use of the product, the practitioner should bear in mind the type of infection and the potential hazard of the diarrhoea which may develop, since cases of colitis have been reported during, or even two or three weeks following, the administration of clindamycin.

Studies indicate a toxin(s) produced by clostridia (especially *Clostridium difficile*) is the principal direct cause of antibiotic-associated colitis. These studies also indicate that this toxigenic clostridium is usually sensitive *in vitro* to vancomycin. When 125 mg to 500 mg of vancomycin are administered orally four times a day for 7–10 days, there is a rapid observed disappearance of the toxin from faecal samples and a coincident clinical recovery from the diarrhoea. (Where the patient is receiving cholestyramine in addition to vancomycin, consideration should be given to separating the times of administration).

Colitis is a disease which has a clinical spectrum from mild, watery diarrhoea to severe, persistent diarrhoea, leucocytosis, fever, severe abdominal cramps, which may be associated with the passage of blood and mucus. If allowed to progress, it may produce peritonitis, shock and toxic megacolon. This may be fatal. The appearance of marked diarrhoea should be regarded as an indication that the product should be discontinued immediately. The disease is likely to follow a more severe course in older patients or patients who are debilitated. Diagnosis is usually made by the recognition of the clinical symptoms, but can be substantiated by endoscopic demonstration of pseudomembranous colitis. The presence of the disease may be further confirmed by culture of the stool for *C. difficile* on selective media and assay of the stool specimen for the toxin(s) of *C. difficile.*

Precautions: Caution should be used when prescribing Dalacin C Paediatric to individuals with a history of gastro-intestinal disease, especially colitis.

Periodic liver and kidney function tests should be carried out during prolonged therapy. Such monitoring is also recommended in neonates and infants.

The dosage of Dalacin C Paediatric may require reduction in patients with renal or hepatic impairment due to prolongation of the serum half-life.

Prolonged administration of Dalacin C Paediatric, as with any anti-infective, may result in super-infection due to organisms resistant to clindamycin.

Care should be observed in the use of Dalacin C Paediatric in atopic individuals.

Interaction with other medicaments and other forms of interaction: Clindamycin has been shown to have neuromuscular blocking properties that may enhance the action of other neuromuscular blocking agents. It should be used with caution, therefore, in patients receiving such agents.

Antagonism has been demonstrated between clindamycin and erythromycin *in vitro.* Because of possible clinical significance, the two drugs should not be administered concurrently.

Pregnancy and lactation: Pregnancy Code B1: Safety for use in pregnancy has not been established.

Clindamycin is excreted in human milk. Caution should be exercised when Dalacin C Paediatric is administered to a nursing mother. It is unlikely that a nursing infant can absorb a significant amount of clindamycin from its gastro-intestinal tract.

Effects on ability to drive and use machines: None known.

Undesirable effects: Gastro-intestinal tract: Nausea, vomiting, abdominal pain and diarrhoea (see *Warnings*).

Haematopoietic: Transient neutropenia (leucopenia), eosinophilia, agranulocytosis and thrombocytopenia have been reported. No direct aetiologic relationship to concurrent clindamycin therapy could be made in any of the foregoing.

Skin and mucous membranes: Pruritus, vaginitis and rare instances of exfoliative and vesiculobullous dermatitis have been reported.

Hypersensitivity reactions: Maculopapular rash and urticaria have been observed during drug therapy. Generalised mild to moderate morbilliform-like skin rashes are the most frequently reported reactions. Rare instances of erythema multiforme, some resembling Stevens-Johnson syndrome, have been associated with clindamycin. A few cases of anaphylactoid reactions have been reported.

Liver: Jaundice and abnormalities in liver function tests have been observed during clindamycin therapy.

Overdose: In cases of overdosage no specific treatment is indicated.

The serum biological half-life of clindamycin is 2.4 hours. Clindamycin cannot readily be removed from the blood by dialysis or peritoneal dialysis.

If an allergic adverse reaction occurs, therapy should be with the usual emergency treatments, including corticosteroids, adrenaline and antihistamines.

Pharmacological properties
Pharmacodynamic properties: Clindamycin is a lincosamide antibiotic with a primarily bacteriostatic action against Gram-positive aerobes and a wide range of anaerobic bacteria. Lincosamides such as clindamycin bind to the 50S subunit of the bacterial ribosome similarly to macrolides such as erythromycin and inhibit the early stages of protein synthesis. The action of clindamycin is predominantly bacteriostatic although high concentrations may be slowly bactericidal against sensitive strains.

Most Gram-negative aerobic bacteria, including the Enterobacteriaceae, are resistant to clindamycin. Clindamycin demonstrates cross-resistance with lincomycin. When tested by *in vitro* methods, some staphylococcal strains originally resistant to erythromycin rapidly developed resistance to clindamycin. The mechanisms for resistance are the same as for erythromycin, namely methylation of the ribosomal binding site, chromosomal mutation of the ribosomal protein and in a few staphylococcal isolates enzymic inactivation by a plasmid-mediated adenyltransferase.

Pharmacokinetic properties:
General characteristics of active substance: Clindamycin palmitate hydrochloride is rapidly hydrolysed to clindamycin following oral administration. Clindamycin is widely distributed in body fluids and tissues including bone, but it does not reach the cerebrospinal fluid in significant concentrations. It diffuses across the placenta into the fetal circulation and appears in breast milk. High concentrations occur in bile. It accumulates in leucocytes and macrophages. Over 90% of clindamycin in the circulation is bound to plasma proteins.

The half-life is 2 to 3 hours, although this may be prolonged in pre-term neonates and patients with severe renal impairment.

Clindamycin undergoes metabolism, presumably in the liver, to the active *N*-demethyl and sulphoxide metabolites and also some inactive metabolites. About 10% of the drug is excreted in the urine as active drug or metabolites and about 4% in the faeces; the remainder is excreted as inactive metabolites. Excretion is slow and takes place over several days, It is not effectively removed from the blood by dialysis.

Characteristics in patients: No special characteristics. See section 4.4 'Special warnings and special precautions for use' for further information.

Pharmaceutical particulars
List of excipients: Sucrose, Pluronic F-68, Sorbic acid, Dimethicone, Pineapple flavour Pharmaceutical flavour IFF CO 654).

Incompatibilities: None known.

Shelf-life: 48 months.

Special precautions for storage for product and admixture storage: Store at room temperature (18–25°C). Following reconstitution, the paediatric suspension is stable for up to two weeks at room temperature.

Nature and contents of container: Amber glass bottle containing paediatric granules to make 100 ml suspension.

Sachet containing paediatric granules to make 5 ml suspension (single dose sachet).

Instructions for use/handling: Do not dispense in its current dry state.

To each 100 ml bottle of granules add 74 ml purified water and shake. Where further dilution is required use purified water.

Marketing authorisation number 0032/0023R.

Date of grant of authorisation 16 July 1991.

Date of revision of the text 3 August 1998.

Legal category POM.

DALACIN* C PHOSPHATE

Qualitative and quantitative composition Each ml of solution contains clindamycin phosphate BP equivalent to 150 mg clindamycin.

Pharmaceutical form Clear, colourless, sterile solution for intramuscular or intravenous use.

Clinical particulars
Therapeutic indications: Antibacterial. Serious infections caused by susceptible Gram-positive organisms, staphylococci (both penicillinase- and non-penicillinase-producing), streptococci (except *Streptococcus faecalis*) and pneumococci. It is also indicated in serious infections caused by susceptible anaerobic pathogens such as *Bacteroides spp, Fusobacterium spp, Propionibacterium spp, Peptostreptococcus spp.* and microaerophilic streptococci.

Clindamycin does not penetrate the blood/brain barrier in therapeutically effective quantities.

Posology and method of administration: Parenteral (i.m. or iv administration). Dalacin C Phosphate must be diluted prior to iv administration and should be infused over at least 10--60 minutes.

Adults: Serious infections: 600 mg -- 1.2 g/day in two, three or four equal doses.

More severe infections: l.2--2.7 g/day in two, three or four equal doses.

Single i.m. injections of greater than 600 mg are not recommended nor is administration of more than 1.2 g in a single one-hour infusion.

For more serious infections, these doses may have to be increased. In life-threatening situations, doses as high as 4.8 g daily have been given intravenously to adults.

Alternatively, the drug may be administered in the form of a single rapid infusion of the first dose followed by continuous iv infusion.

Children (over 1 month of age): Serious infections: 15–25 mg/kg/day in three or four equal doses.

More severe infections: 25–40 mg/kg/day in three or

four equal doses. In severe infections it is recommended that children be given no less than 300 mg/day regardless of body weight.

Elderly patients: The half-life, volume of distribution and clearance and extent of absorption after administration of clindamycin phosphate are not altered by increased age. Analysis of data from clinical studies has not revealed any age-related increase in toxicity. Dosage requirements in elderly patients should not be influenced, therefore, by age alone. See 'Precautions' for other factors which should be taken into consideration.

Treatment for infections caused by beta-haemolytic streptococci should be continued for at least 10 days to guard against subsequent rheumatic fever or glomerulonephritis.

Contra-indications: Dalacin C Phosphate is contra-indicated in patients previously found to be sensitive to clindamycin or lincomycin.

Special warnings and special precautions for use
Warnings: This product contains benzyl alcohol. Benzyl alcohol has been reported to be associated with a fatal 'Gasping syndrome' in premature infants.

Dalacin C Phosphate should only be used in the treatment of serious infections. In considering the use of the product, the practitioner should bear in mind the type of infection and the potential hazard of the diarrhoea which may develop, since cases of colitis have been reported during, or even two or three weeks following, the administration of clindamycin.

Studies indicate a toxin(s) produced by clostridia (especially *Clostridium difficile*) is the principal direct cause of antibiotic-associated colitis. These studies also indicate that this toxigenic clostridium is usually sensitive *in vitro* to vancomycin. When 125 mg to 500 mg of vancomycin are administered orally four times a day for 7–10 days, there is a rapid observed disappearance of the toxin from faecal samples and a coincident clinical recovery from the diarrhoea. (Where the patient is receiving cholestyramine in addition to vancomycin, consideration should be given to separating the times of administration).

Colitis is a disease which has a clinical spectrum from mild, watery diarrhoea to severe, persistent diarrhoea, leucocytosis, fever, severe abdominal cramps, which may be associated with the passage of blood and mucus. If allowed to progress, it may produce peritonitis, shock and toxic megacolon. This may be fatal. The appearance of marked diarrhoea should be regarded as an indication that the product should be discontinued immediately. The disease is likely to follow a more severe course in older patients or patients who are debilitated. Diagnosis is usually made by the recognition of the clinical symptoms, but can be substantiated by endoscopic demonstration of pseudomembranous colitis. The presence of the disease may be further confirmed by culture of the stool for *C. difficile* on selective media and assay of the stool specimen for the toxin(s) of *C. difficile*.

Precautions: Caution should be used when prescribing Dalacin C Phosphate to individuals with a history of gastro-intestinal disease, especially colitis.

Periodic liver and kidney function tests should be carried out during prolonged therapy. Such monitoring is also recommended in neonates and infants. Safety and appropriate dosage in infants less than one month old have not been established.

The dosage of Dalacin C Phosphate may require reduction in patients with renal or hepatic impairment due to prolongation of the serum half-life.

Prolonged administration of Dalacin C Phosphate, as with any anti-infective, may result in super-infection due to organisms resistant to clindamycin.

Care should be observed in the use of Dalacin C Phosphate in atopic individuals.

Interaction with other medicaments and other forms of interaction: Clindamycin has been shown to have neuromuscular blocking properties that may enhance the action of other neuromuscular blocking agents. It should be used with caution, therefore, in patients receiving such agents.

Antagonism has been demonstrated between clindamycin and erythromycin *in vitro*. Because of possible clinical significance, the two drugs should not be administered concurrently.

Pregnancy and lactation: Pregnancy Code B1: Safety for use in pregnancy has not been established.

Clindamycin is excreted in human milk. Caution should be exercised when Dalacin C Phosphate is administered to a nursing mother. It is unlikely that a nursing infant can absorb a significant amount of clindamycin from its gastro-intestinal tract.

Effects on ability to drive and use machines: None known

Undesirable effects: Gastro-intestinal tract: Nausea, vomiting, abdominal pain and diarrhoea (see *Warnings*).

Haematopoietic: Transient neutropenia (leucopenia), eosinophilia, agranulocytosis and thrombocytopenia have been reported. No direct aetiologic relationship to concurrent clindamycin therapy could be made in any of the foregoing.

Skin and mucous membranes: Pruritus, vaginitis and rare instances of exfoliative and vesiculobullous dermatitis have been reported.

Hypersensitivity reactions: Maculopapular rash and urticaria have been observed during drug therapy. Generalised mild to moderate morbilliform-like skin rashes are the most frequently reported reactions. Rare instances of erythema multiforme, some resembling Stevens-Johnson syndrome, have been associated with clindamycin. A few cases of anaphylactoid reactions have been reported.

Liver: Jaundice and abnormalities in liver function tests have been observed during clindamycin therapy.

Cardiovascular: Rare instances of cardiopulmonary arrest and hypotension have been reported following too rapid intravenous administration. (See Dosage and administration section)

Local reactions: Local irritation, pain, abscess formation have been seen with i.m. injection. Thrombophlebitis has been reported with iv injection. These reactions can be minimized by deep i.m. injection and avoiding the use of an indwelling catheter.

Overdose: In cases of overdosage no specific treatment is indicated.

The serum biological half-life of clindamycin is 2.4 hours. Clindamycin cannot readily be removed from the blood by dialysis or peritoneal dialysis.

If an allergic adverse reaction occurs, therapy should be with the usual emergency treatments, including corticosteroids, adrenaline and antihistamines.

Pharmacological properties
Pharmacodynamic properties: Clindamycin is a lincosamide antibiotic with a primarily bacteriostatic action against Gram-positive aerobes and a wide range of anaerobic bacteria. Lincosamides such as clindamycin bind to the 50S subunit of the bacterial ribosome similarly to macrolides such as erythromycin and inhibit the early stages of protein synthesis. The action of clindamycin is predominantly bacteriostatic although high concentrations may be slowly bactericidal against sensitive strains.

Most Gram-negative aerobic bacteria, including the Enterobacteriaceae, are resistant to clindamycin. Clindamycin demonstrates cross-resistance with lincomycin. When tested by *in vitro* methods, some staphylococcal strains originally resistant to erythromycin rapidly developed resistance to clindamycin. The mechanisms for resistance are the same as for erythromycin, namely methylation of the ribosomal binding site, chromosomal mutation of the ribosomal protein and in a few staphylococcal isolates, enzymic inactivation by a plasmid-mediated adenyltransferase.

Pharmacokinetic properties: General characteristics of active substance.

Following parenteral administration, the biologically inactive clindamycin phosphate is hydrolysed to clindamycin. When the equivalent of 300 mg of clindamycin is injected intramuscularly, a mean peak plasma concentration of 6 microgram/ml is achieved within three hours; 600 mg gives a peak concentration of 9 microgram/ml. In children, peak concentration may be reached within one hour. When the same doses are infused intravenously, peak concentrations of 7 and 10 micrograms per ml respectively are achieved by the end of infusion.

Clindamycin is widely distributed in body fluids and tissues including bone, but it does not reach the cerebrospinal fluid in significant concentrations. It diffuses across the placenta into the fetal circulation and appears in breast milk. High concentrations occur in bile. It accumulates in leucocytes and macrophages. Over 90% of clindamycin in the circulation is bound to plasma proteins. The half-life is 2 to 3 hours, although this may be prolonged in pre-term neonates and patients with severe renal impairment.

Clindamycin undergoes metabolism, to the active *N*-demethyl and sulphoxide metabolites and also some inactive metabolites. About 10% of the drug is excreted in the urine as active drug or metabolites and about 4% in the faeces; the remainder is excreted as inactive metabolites. Excretion is slow and takes place over several days, It is not effectively removed from the blood by dialysis.

Characteristics in patients: No special characteristics. See *Special warnings and special precautions for use* for further information.

Pharmaceutical particulars
List of excipients: Benzyl alcohol, disodium edetate, sterilised Water for Injections

Incompatibilities: Solutions of clindamycin salts have a low pH and incompatibilities may reasonably be expected with alkaline preparations or drugs unstable at low pH. Incompatibility has been reported with: ampicillin sodium, aminophylline, barbiturates, calcium gluconate, ceftriaxone sodium, idarubicin hydrochloride, magnesium sulphate, phenytoin sodium and ranitidine hydrochloride.

Shelf-life: Dalacin C Phosphate has a shelf-life of 24 months when stored below 25°C, avoiding refrigeration.

Special precautions for storage for product and admixture storage: Store below 25°C.

Nature and contents of container: Type 1 flint glass ampoule containing 2 ml or 4 ml sterile, aqueous solution, packed in cardboard carton, together with a leaflet.

Instructions for use/handling: Dalacin C Phosphate has been known to be physically and chemically compatible for at least 24 hours in dextrose 5% water and sodium chloride injection solutions containing the following antibiotics in usually administered concentrations: Amikacin sulphate, aztreonam, cefamandole nafate, cephazolin sodium, cefotaxime sodium, cefoxitin sodium, ceftazidime sodium, ceftizoxime sodium, gentamicin sulphate, netilmicin sulphate, piperacillin and tobramycin.

The compatibility and duration of stability of drug admixtures will vary depending upon concentration and other conditions.

Marketing authorisation number 0032/0042R

Date of renewal of authorisation 17 January 1996

Date of revision of the text February 1996.

Legal category POM.

DALACIN* T TOPICAL LOTION

Qualitative and quantitative composition White to off-white emulsion containing clindamycin phosphate (equivalent to clindamycin 10 mg/ml) in an aqueous base.

Pharmaceutical form Topical Emulsion

Clinical particulars
Therapeutic indication: Dalacin T Topical is indicated for the treatment of acne vulgaris.

Posology and method of administration: Apply a thin film of Dalacin T Topical Lotion twice daily to the affected area.

Contra-indications: Dalacin T is contra-indicated in patients previously found to be hypersensitive to this antibiotic. Although cross-sensitisation to lincomycin has not been demonstrated, it is recommended that Dalacin T is not used in patients who have demonstrated lincomycin sensitivity.

Special warnings and special precautions for use: Oral and parenteral clindamycin, as well as most other antibiotics, have been associated with severe pseudomembranous colitis. However, post-marketing studies have indicated a very low incidence of colitis with Dalacin T Solution. The physician should, nonetheless, be alert to the development of antibiotic-associated diarrhoea or colitis. If diarrhoea occurs, the product should be discontinued immediately.

Studies indicate a toxin(s) produced by *Clostridium difficile* is the major cause of antibiotic-associated colitis. Colitis is usually characterized by persistent, severe diarrhoea and abdominal cramps. Endoscopic examination may reveal pseudomembranous colitis. Stool culture for *C. difficile* and/or assay for *C. difficile* toxin may be helpful to diagnosis.

Vancomycin is effective in the treatment of antibiotic-associated colitis produced by *C. difficile*. The usual dose is 125–500 mg orally every 6 hours for 7–10 days. Additional supportive medical care may be necessary.

Mild cases of colitis may respond to discontinuance of clindamycin alone. Cholestyramine and colestipol resins have been shown to bind *C. difficile* toxin *in vitro*, and cholestyramine has been effective in the treatment of some mild cases of antibiotic-associated colitis. Cholestyramine resins have been shown to bind vancomycin; therefore, when both cholestyramine and vancomycin are used concurrently, their administration should be separated by at least two hours.

The lotion has an unpleasant taste and caution should be exercised when applying medication around the mouth.

Interaction with other medicaments and other forms of interaction: None.

Pregnancy and lactation: Safety for use in pregnancy has not been established.

Reproduction studies have been performed in rats and mice using subcutaneous and oral doses of clindamycin ranging from 100 to 600 mg/kg/day and have revealed no evidence of impaired fertility or harm to the foetus due to clindamycin. There are, however, no adequate and well-controlled studies in pregnant women. Because animal reproduction studies are not always predictive of human response, this drug should be used during pregnancy only if clearly needed.

It is not known whether clindamycin is excreted in human milk following use of Dalacin T Topical Lotion. However, orally and parenterally administered clindamycin has been reported to appear in breast milk. As a general rule, breastfeeding should not be undertaken while a patient is on a drug since many drugs are excreted in human milk.

Effects on ability to drive and use machines: None.

Undesirable effects
Side-effects: Adverse reactions reported in clinical trials have been minor and of a similar incidence to placebo.

Overdose: Improbable given route of application.

Pharmacological properties
Pharmacodynamic properties: The active constituent, clindamycin, is a known antibiotic. When applied topically it is found in comedone samples at sufficient levels to be active against most strains of *P. acnes*.

Pharmacokinetic properties: When applied topically in an alcoholic solution, clindamycin has been shown to be absorbed from the skin in small amounts. Very low levels, more than 1,000 times lower than those from normal systemic doses of clindamycin, have been found in the plasma. Using a sensitive RIA method, clindamycin has been detected in the urine at levels of < 1 to 53 ng/ml, 0.15-0.25% of the cumulative dose being recovered from the urine. No clindamycin has been detected in the serum following topical application.

Pharmaceutical particulars
List of excipients: Glycerol, sodium lauroyl sarcosinate, stearic acid, tegin, cetostearyl alcohol, isostearyl alcohol, methylparaben, purified water.

Incompatibilities: None.

Shelf-life: 36 months.

Special precautions for storage: Store below 25°C.

Nature and contents of container: HDPE bottle, polypropylene roller-ball and cap containing 30 ml and 50 ml of Dalacin Topical Lotion.

Instructions for use/handling: None.

Marketing authorisation number 0032/0156

Date of first authorisation/renewal of authorisation
Date of first authorisation: 18th September 1990
Renewal date: 23 February 1996.

Date of revision of the text February 1996.

Legal category POM.

DALACIN* T TOPICAL SOLUTION

Qualitative and quantitative composition Clindamycin phosphate BP equivalent to clindamycin 10 mg/ml.

Pharmaceutical form Topical solution.

Clinical particulars
Therapeutic indications: Dalacin T Topical Solution is indicated in the treatment of acne vulgaris.

Posology and method of administration: Apply a thin film of Dalacin T Topical Solution twice daily to the affected area.

Contra-indications: Dalacin T is contra-indicated in patients previously found to be hypersensitive to this antibiotic. Although cross-sensitisation to lincomycin has not been demonstrated, it is recommended that Dalacin T is not used in patients who have demonstrated lincomycin sensitivity.

Special warnings and precautions for use: Products containing benzoyl peroxide should not be used concurrently with Dalacin T Topical Solution.

Oral and parenteral clindamycin, as well as most other antibiotics, have been associated with severe pseudomembranous colitis. Post-marketing studies, however, have indicated a very low incidence of colitis with Dalacin T Topical Solution. The physician should, nonetheless, be alert to the development of antibiotic associated diarrhoea or colitis. If significant or prolonged diarrhoea occurs, the product should be discontinued immediately.

Studies indicate a toxin(s) produced by *Clostridium difficile* is the major cause of antibiotic associated colitis. Colitis is usually characterised by persistent, severe diarrhoea and abdominal cramps. Endoscopic examination may reveal pseudomembranous colitis. Stool culture for *C. difficile* and/or assay for *C. difficile* toxin may be helpful to diagnosis.

Vancomycin is effective in the treatment of antibiotic-associated colitis produced by *C. difficile*. The usual dose is 125–500 mg orally every 6 hours for 7–10 days. Additional supportive medical care may be necessary.

Mild cases of colitis may respond to discontinuance of clindamycin alone. Cholestyramine and colestipol resins have been shown to bind *C. difficile* toxin *in vitro*, and cholestyramine has been effective in the treatment of some mild cases of antibiotic-associated colitis. Cholestyramine resins have been shown to bind vancomycin; therefore, when both cholestyramine and vancomycin are used concurrently, their administration should be separated by at least two hours.

Dalacin T Topical Solution contains an alcohol base which can cause burning and irritation of the eye. In the event of accidental contact with sensitive surfaces (eye, abraded skin, mucous membranes), bathe with copious amounts of cool tap water. The solution has an unpleasant taste and caution should be exercised when applying medication around the mouth.

Interaction with other medicaments and other forms of interaction: Not known.

Pregnancy and lactation: Safety for use in pregnancy has not been established.

It is not known if clindamycin is excreted in breast milk following the use of Dalacin T Topical Solution.

Effects on ability to drive and use machines: Not applicable.

Undesirable effects: Skin dryness is the most common side-effect reported. Other side-effects include skin irritation, contact dermatitis, oily skin, stinging of the eye, Gram-negative folliculitis, gastro-intestinal disturbances and abdominal pain.

Overdose: Not applicable.

Pharmacological properties
Pharmacodynamic properties: The active constituent, clindamycin, is a known antibiotic. When applied topically it is found in comedone samples at sufficient levels to be active against most strains of *Propionibacterium acnes*.

Pharmacokinetic properties: When applied topically, clindamycin has been shown to be absorbed from the skin in small amounts.

Very low levels, more than 1000 times lower than those from normal systemic doses of clindamycin, have been found in the plasma. Using a sensitive RIA method clindamycin has been detected in the urine at levels of < 1 to 53 nanograms/ml, 0.15–0.25% of the cumulative dose being recovered from the urine. No clindamycin has been detected in the serum following topical applications.

Preclinical safety data: No further pre-clinical safety data are available.

Pharmaceutical particulars
List of excipients:
Isopropyl alcohol BP
Propylene glycol BP
Purified water BP
Hydrochloric acid (10%) BP
Sodium hydroxide (10%)

Incompatibilities: Not applicable.

Shelf life: 24 months.

Special precautions for storage: None.

Nature and contents of container: Dab-O-Matic bottle containing 30 ml, 50 ml or 60 ml.
Novonette wipe (1 g)
Webril wipe (2 g)

Instructions for use/handling: None.

Marketing authorisation number 0032/0135.

Date of first authorisation/renewal of authorisation
Date of first authorisation: 18 January 1988
Date of renewal of authorisation: 18 January 1998.

Date of (partial) revision of the text December 1997.

Legal category POM.

DALACIN* CREAM 2%

Qualitative and quantitative composition Each gram of cream contains clindamycin phosphate BP equivalent to 20 mg clindamycin.

Pharmaceutical form White, semi-solid cream.

Clinical particulars
Therapeutic indications: Antibiotic for the treatment of bacterial vaginosis.

Posology and method of administration: One applicator full (approximately 5 grams) intravaginally at bedtime for 7 consecutive days.

In patients in whom a shorter treatment course is desirable, a 3 day regimen has been shown to be effective.

Children and the elderly: No clinical studies have been conducted in populations younger than 15 or older than 60. Dalacin Cream is not recommended in children under 12 years of age.

Contra-indications: Dalacin Cream is contra-indicated in patients previously found to be hypersensitive to preparations containing clindamycin or any of the components of the cream base (see *Qualitative and quantitative composition, List of excipients*). Although cross-sensitisation to lincomycin has not been demonstrated, it is recommended that Dalacin Cream should not be used in patients who have demonstrated lincomycin sensitivity.

Special warnings and special precautions for use: As there are no data available on the use of Dalacin Cream in patients younger than 12 years of age, it should not be used in this population. The use of clindamycin may result in the overgrowth of non-susceptible organisms, particularly yeasts.

Virtually all antibiotics have been associated with diarrhoea and in some cases pseudomembranous colitis. Therefore, even though only a minimal amount of drug is absorbed, if significant diarrhoea occurs, the drug should be discontinued and appropriate diagnostic procedures and treatment provided as necessary.

Dalacin Cream contains oil-based components. Some of these have been shown to weaken the rubber of condoms and diaphragms and make them less effective as a barrier method of contraception or as protection from sexually transmitted disease, including AIDS. Do not rely on condoms and diaphragms when using Dalacin Cream.

Interaction with other medicaments and other forms of interaction: Cross resistance has been demonstrated between clindamycin and lincomycin, and erythromycin and clindamycin. Antagonism has been demonstrated between clindamycin and erythromycin *in vitro*.

No information is available on concomitant use with other intravaginal products, which is not recommended.

Pregnancy and lactation: Pregnancy: Reproduction studies have been performed in rats and mice using subcutaneous and oral doses of clindamycin ranging from 20 to 600 mg/kg/day and have revealed no evidence of impaired fertility or harm to the foetus due to clindamycin. In one mouse strain, cleft palates were observed in treated foetuses; this response was not produced in other mouse strains or in other species, and is therefore considered to be a strain specific effect.

There are no adequate and well-controlled studies in pregnant women during their first trimester, and because animal reproduction studies are not always predictive of human response, this drug should be used during the first trimester of pregnancy only if clearly needed. In a clinical trial in pregnant women during the second trimester, Dalacin Cream was effective in treating bacterial vaginosis, and no drug-related medical events were reported in the neonates. However, as with any drug used during pregnancy, a careful risk-benefit assessment should take place beforehand.

Lactation: It is not known if clindamycin is excreted in breast milk following the use of vaginally administered clindamycin phosphate. However, orally and parenterally administered clindamycin has been reported to appear in breast milk. Therefore, a full assessment of benefit-risk should be made when consideration is given to using vaginal clindamycin phosphate in a nursing mother.

Effects on ability to drive and use machines: Not applicable.

Undesirable effects: In clinical trials medical events judged to be related, probably related, or possibly related to vaginally administered clindamycin phosphate cream were reported for (24%) of patients as indicated below:

Genital tract:	cervicitis/vaginitis (14%); vulvo-vaginal irritation (6%).
Central nervous system:	dizziness, headache, vertigo.
Gastro-intestinal:	heartburn, nausea, vomiting, diarrhoea, constipation, abdominal pain.
Dermatological:	rash, exanthema.
Hypersensitivity:	urticaria.

(Events without percentages were reported by less than 1% of the patients.)

Overdose: Intravaginal overdose is not possible. Accidental ingestion of the product could be accompanied by effects related to therapeutic levels of oral clindamycin.

Pharmacological properties
Pharmacodynamic properties: Clindamycin is an antimicrobial agent which has been shown to be effective in the treatment of infection caused by susceptible anaerobic bacteria or susceptible strains of Gram positive aerobic bacteria. It has been shown to have *in-vitro* activity against the following organisms which are associated with bacterial vaginosis.: Gardnerella vaginalis; Mobiluncus spp; Bacteroides spp; Mycoplasma hominis; Peptostreptococcus spp.

Pharmacokinetic properties: Following once a day dosing of 100 mg of vaginally administered clindamycin phosphate, at a concentration equivalent to 20 mg of clindamycin per gram of cream, peak serum clindamycin levels average 20 nanograms/ml (range 3–93 nanograms/ml in normal volunteers. Approximately 3% (range 0.1–7%) of the administered dose is absorbed systematically.

In women with bacterial vaginosis, the amount of clindamycin absorbed following vaginal administration of 100 mg of Dalacin Cream (20 mg/g) is 4% (range 0.8-8%), which is approximately the same as in normal women.

Characteristics in patients: No special characteristics. See *Special warnings and special precautions for use* for further information.

Pharmaceutical particulars
List of excipients: Sorbitan monostearate, polysorbate 60, propylene glycol, stearic acid, cetostearyl alcohol, cetyl palmitate, liquid paraffin, benzyl alcohol and water.

Incompatibilities: None known

Shelf-life: Dalacin Cream has a shelf-life of 18 months.

Special precautions for storage for product and admixture storage: None.

Nature and contents of container: Laminate tube with polypropylene cap containing 7.8 g*, 20 g* or 40 g cream, packed in cardboard carton, together with a leaflet.
(* Not currently marketed.)

Instructions for use/handling: None.

Marketing authorisation number 0032/0176

Date of first authorisation/renewal of authorisation Date of first authorisation: 27 April 1993

Date of (partial) revision of the text 8 September 1998

Legal category POM

DEBRISAN*

Presentation Sterile, straw-coloured spherical beads of dextranomer of 0.1–0.3 mm diameter, packed in plastic castors.

Uses A dressing for moist wounds and indolent ulcers, whether clean or infected and small area burns.

Dosage and administration A 3 mm layer of Debrisan should be sprinkled onto the wound and kept in place by a pad of lint or a perforated plastic sheet. Debrisan is hydrophilic and the tissue exudate is drawn up into the layer. The Debrisan should be renewed before saturation occurs. Depending on the rate of exudation this may be necessary from one to five times a day. Once or twice daily is usually adequate. When Debrisan is changed the old material is readily rinsed off with water or saline and new material may then be sprinkled onto the wound.

Shallow wounds, or those in awkward positions, may be dressed more easily by using Debrisan Paste, or by mixing four parts of Debrisan with one part of sterile glycerol to form a stiff paste. This should be spread into the wound with a spatula to a depth of 3 mm or more. Dressing continues as above. The paste should be prepared freshly at each application. Once the wound is clean and poorly secreting, change therapy to an antiseptic dressing, e.g. chlorhexidine tulle, or a sterile pad.

Full instructions for use are enclosed with each pack. Treated in this manner the wound will remain soft and pliable during healing.

Elderly: No special instructions.

Contra-indications, warnings, etc
1. Do not leave Debrisan for more than 24 hours on wounds with a very low exudation rate as it may dry and form a crust which may be difficult to wash off.
2. Occlusive dressings may lead to maceration of skin round the wound under treatment.
3. When deep infected wounds are treated, care must be taken to wash Debrisan from the depths of the wound.
4. No side-effects have been reported.

Warning: Debrisan spillage can render surfaces very slippery. Clear spillages promptly.

Precautions:
1. Not to be used on dry wounds.
2. When exudate has been markedly removed by Debrisan alternative treatment should be substituted.
3. In order to avoid cross-infection it is recommended that the contents of a castor be confined to the treatment of a single patient for one day.

Pharmaceutical precautions Keep in a dry place in well-closed containers.

Package quantities Castors of 60 g.

Legal category P.

Further information Each gram of Debrisan absorbs 4 grams of exudate. Capillary action carries debris and bacteria away from the wound surface. Local oedema is reduced so that the wound may look larger initially. Debrisan is non sensitising and controls malodour.

DEBRISAN* PASTE

Presentation Foil-plastic laminate pouches containing 10 g of a sterile soft, white, granular paste consisting of: Dextranomer 6.4 g, polyethylene glycol 600 and water to 10 g.

Uses Treatment of exudative and infected wounds such as surgical or post-traumatic wounds, decubital ulcers and leg ulcers. As the paste is adherent it may be preferred to Debrisan beads on shallow wounds, or those where retention of the beads is a problem.

Dosage and administration After cleaning the wound with sterile water or saline the Paste is applied firmly with a spatula to a depth of not less than 3 mm. The wound is covered and the Paste changed at intervals governed by the exudation rate of the wound, the Paste being renewed before it is entirely discoloured and saturated with secretion and debris. Debrisan Paste should be changed from twice daily to every two days according to the rate of exudation. Stop Debrisan Paste once the wound is granulating and free of exudate, changing to sterile or antiseptic dressings.

Elderly: No special instructions.

Contra-indications, warnings, etc Use with caution: When applied near the eyes; in deep fistulae etc. with a narrow opening where paste removal might be difficult.

Occasionally pain may be experienced in the wound after application. This can be avoided by wetting the wound before applying the Paste.

Pharmaceutical precautions Stored at room temperature the shelf life is 3 years.

Legal category P.

Package quantities 6×10 g.

Further information Nil.

DEPO-MEDRONE*

Qualitative and quantitative composition Methylprednisolone Acetate BP 40 mg/ml.

Pharmaceutical form Sterile, aqueous suspension.

Clinical particulars
Therapeutic indications: Depo-Medrone may be used locally or systemically, particularly where oral therapy is not feasible.

Depo-Medrone may be used by any of the following routes: intramuscular, intra-articular, periarticular, intrabursal, intralesional or into the tendon sheath. It *must not* be used by the intrathecal or intravenous routes (see Contra-indications and Undesirable effects).

Intramuscular administration:
Rheumatic disorders: Rheumatoid arthritis
Collagen diseases/arteritis: Systemic lupus erythematosus
Dermatological diseases: Severe erythema multiforme (Stevens-Johnson syndrome).
Allergic states: Bronchial asthma; Severe seasonal and perennial allergic rhinitis; Drug hypersensitivity reactions; Angioneurotic oedema.
Gastro-intestinal diseases: Ulcerative colitis; Crohn's disease.
Respiratory diseases: Fulminating or disseminated tuberculosis (with appropriate antituberculous chemotherapy); Aspiration of gastric contents.
Miscellaneous: TB meningitis (with appropriate antituberculous chemotherapy).

Intra-articular administration: Rheumatoid arthritis; Osteo-arthritis with an inflammatory component.

Soft tissue administration (intrabursal, periarticular, into tendon sheath): Synovitis not associated with infection; Epicondylitis; Tenosynovitis; Plantar fasciitis; Bursitis.

Intralesional: Keloids; Localized lichen planus; Localized lichen simplex; Granuloma annulare; Discoid lupus erythematosus; Alopecia areata.

Posology and method of administration: Depo-Medrone should not be mixed with any other suspending agent or solution. Parenteral drug products should be inspected visually for particulate matter and discoloration prior to administration, whenever suspension and container permit. Depo-Medrone may be used by any of the following routes: intramuscular, intra-articular, periarticular, intrabursal, intralesional and into the tendon sheath. It must not be used by the intrathecal or intravenous routes (see *Contra-indications* and *Undesirable effects*).

Undesirable effects may be minimised by using the lowest effective dose for the minimum period (see *Special warnings and special precautions for use*).

Depo-Medrone vials are intended for single dose use only.

Intramuscular – for sustained systemic effect: Allergic conditions (severe seasonal and perennial allergic rhinitis, asthma, drug reactions), 80–120 mg (2–3 ml).

Dermatological conditions, 40–120 mg (1–3 ml).

Rheumatic disorders and collagen diseases (rheumatoid arthritis, SLE), 40–120 mg (1–3 ml) per week.

Dosage must be individualized and depends on the condition being treated and its severity.

Note: Depo-Medrone is not intended for the prophylaxis of severe seasonal and perennial allergic rhinitis or other seasonal allergies and should be administered only when symptoms are present.

The frequency of intramuscular injections should be determined by the duration of clinical response.

In the case of seasonal allergic rhinitis a single injection is frequently sufficient. If necessary, however, a second injection may be given after two to three weeks.

On average the effect of a single 2 ml (80 mg) injection may be expected to last approximately two weeks.

Intra-articular: Rheumatoid arthritis, osteo-arthritis. The dose of Depo-Medrone depends upon the size of the joint and the severity of the condition. Repeated injections, if needed, may be given at intervals of one to five or more weeks depending upon the degree of relief obtained from the initial injection. A suggested dosage guide is: large joint (knee, ankle, shoulder), 20–80 mg (0.5–2 ml); medium joint (elbow, wrist), 10–40 mg (0.25–1 ml); small joint (metacarpophalangeal, interphalangeal, sternoclavicular, acromioclavicular), 4–10 mg (0.1–0.25 ml).

Intrabursal: Subdeltoid bursitis, prepatellar bursitis, olecranon bursitis. For administration directly into bursae, 4–30 mg (0.1–0.75 ml). In most cases, repeat injections are not needed.

Intralesional: Keloids, localised lichen planus, localized lichen simplex, granuloma annulare, alopecia areata, and discoid lupus erythematosus. For administration directly into the lesion for local effect in dermatological conditions, 20–60 mg (0.5–1.5 ml). For large lesions, the dose may be distributed by repeated local injections of 20–40 mg (0.5–1 ml). One to four injections are usually employed. Care should be taken to avoid injection of sufficient material to cause blanching, since this may be followed by a small slough.

Peri-articular: Epicondylitis. Infiltrate 4–30 mg (0.1–0.75 ml) into the affected area.

Into the tendon sheath: Tenosynovitis, epicondylitis. For administration directly into the tendon sheath, 4–30 mg (0.1–0.75 ml). In recurrent or chronic conditions, repeat injections may be necessary.

Special precautions should be observed when administering Depo-Medrone. Intramuscular injections should be made deeply into the gluteal muscles. The usual technique of aspirating prior to injection should be employed to avoid intravascular administration. Doses recommended for intramuscular injection must not be administered superficially or subcutaneously.

Intra-articular injections should be made using precise, anatomical localisation into the synovial space of the joint involved. The injection site for each joint is determined by that location where the synovial cavity is most superficial and most free of large vessels and nerves. Suitable sites for intra-articular injection are the knee, ankle, wrist, elbow, shoulder, phalangeal and hip joints. The spinal joints, unstable joints and those devoid of synovial space are not suitable. Treatment failures are most frequently the result of failure to enter the joint space. Intra-articular injections should be made with care as follows: ensure correct positioning of the needle into the synovial space and aspirate a few drops of joint fluid. The aspirating syringe should then be replaced by another containing Depo-Medrone. To ensure position of the needle, synovial fluid should be aspirated and the injection made. After injection the joint is moved slightly to aid mixing of the synovial fluid and the suspension. Subsequent to therapy care should be taken for the patient not to overuse the joint in which benefit has been obtained. Negligence in this matter may permit an increase in joint deterioration that will more than offset the beneficial effects of the steroid.

Intrabursal injections should be made as follows: the area around the injection site is prepared in a sterile way and a wheal at the site made with 1 per cent procaine hydrochloride solution. A 20 to 24 gauge needle attached to a dry syringe is inserted into the bursa and the fluid aspirated. The needle is left in place and the aspirating syringe changed for a small syringe containing the desired dose. After injection, the needle is withdrawn and a small dressing applied. In the treatment of tenosynovitis care should be taken to inject Depo-Medrone into the tendon sheath rather than into the substance of the tendon. Due to the absence of a true tendon sheath, the Achilles tendon should not be injected with Depo-Medrone.

Children: Dosage may be reduced for infants and children but should be governed more by the severity of the condition and response of the patient, than by age or size.

Elderly patients: When used according to instructions, there is no information to suggest that a change in dosage is warranted in the elderly. However, treatment of elderly patients, particularly if long-term, should be planned bearing in mind the more serious consequences of the common side-effects of corticosteroids in old age and close clinical supervision is required (see Special warnings and special precautions for use).

Contra-indications: Depo-medrone is contra-indicated where there is known hypersensitivity to components and in systemic infection unless specific anti-infective therapy is employed.

Due to its potential for neurotoxicity, Depo-Medrone *must not* be given by the intrathecal route. In addition, as the product is a suspension it *must not* be given by the intravenous route (see *Undesirable effects*).

Special warnings and special precautions for use
Warnings and precautions: A Patient Information Leaflet is provided in the pack by the manufacturer.

Undesirable effects may be minimised by using the lowest effective dose for the minimum period. Frequent patient review is required to appropriately titrate the dose against disease activity (see *Posology and method of administration*).

Patients should carry 'Steroid Treatment' cards which give clear guidance on the precautions to be taken to minimise risk and which provide details of prescriber, drug, dosage and the duration of treatment.

Depo-Medrone vials are intended for single dose use only. Any multidose use of the product may lead to contamination.

Depo-Medrone is not recommended for epidural, intranasal, intra-ocular, or any other unapproved route of administration. See Undesirable effects section for details of side-effects reported from some non-recommended routes of administration.

Due to the absence of a true tendon sheath, the Achilles tendon should not be injected with Depo-Medrone.

While crystals of adrenal steroids in the dermis suppress inflammatory reactions, their presence may cause disintegration of the cellular elements and physiochemical changes in the ground substance of the connective tissue. The resultant infrequently occurring dermal and/or subdermal changes may form depressions in the skin at the injection site. The degree to which this reaction occurs will vary with the amount of adrenal steroid injected. Regeneration is usually complete within a few months or after all crystals of the adrenal steroid have been absorbed. In order to minimize the incidence of dermal and subdermal atrophy, care must be exercised not to exceed recommended doses in injections. Multiple small injections into the area of the lesion should be made whenever possible. The technique of intra-articular and intramuscular injection should include precautions against injection or leakage into the dermis. Injection into the deltoid muscle should be avoided because of a high incidence of subcutaneous atrophy.

Intralesional doses should not be placed too superficially, particularly in easily visible sites in patients with deeply pigmented skins, since there have been rare reports of subcutaneous atrophy and depigmentation.

Systemic absorption of methylprednisolone occurs following intra-articular injection of Depo-Medrone. Systemic as well as local effects can therefore be expected.

Intra-articular corticosteroids are associated with a substantially increased risk of inflammatory response in the joint, particularly bacterial infection introduced with the injection. Charcot-like arthropathies have been reported particularly after repeated injections. Appropriate examination of any joint fluid present is necessary to exclude any bacterial infection, prior to injection.

Following a single dose of Depo-Medrone, plasma cortisol levels are reduced and there is evidence of hypothalamic-pituitary-adrenal (HPA) axis suppression. This suppression lasts for a variable period of up to 4 weeks. The usual dynamic tests of HPA axis function can be used to diagnose evidence of impaired activity (e.g. Synacthen test).

Adrenal cortical atrophy develops during prolonged therapy and may persist for months after stopping treatment. In patients who have received more than physiological doses of systemic corticosteroids (approximately 6 mg methylprednisolone) for greater than 3 weeks, withdrawal should not be abrupt. How dose reduction should be carried out depends largely on whether the disease is likely to relapse as the dose of systemic corticosteroids is reduced. Clinical assessment of disease activity may be needed during withdrawal. If the disease is unlikely to relapse on withdrawal of systemic corticosteroids, but there is uncertainty about HPA suppression, the dose of systemic corticosteroid *may* be reduced rapidly to physiological doses. Once a daily dose of 6 mg methylprednisolone is reached, dose reduction should be slower to allow the HPA-axis to recover.

Abrupt withdrawal of systemic corticosteroid treatment, which has continued up to 3 weeks is appropriate if it is considered that the disease is unlikely to relapse. Abrupt withdrawal of doses up to 32 mg daily of methylprednisolone for 3 weeks is unlikely to lead to clinically relevant HPA-axis suppression, in the majority of patients. In the following patient groups, gradual withdrawal of systemic corticosteroid therapy should be *considered* even after courses lasting 3 weeks or less:

Patients who have had repeated courses of systemic corticosteroids, particularly if taken for greater than 3 weeks; When a short course has been prescribed within one year of cessation of long-term therapy (months or years); Patients who may have reasons for adrenocortical insufficiency other than exogenous corticosteroid therapy; Patients receiving doses of systemic corticosteroid greater than 32 mg daily of methylprednisolone; Patients repeatedly taking doses in the evening.

Since mineralocorticoid secretion may be impaired, salt and/or a mineralocorticoid should be administered concurrently.

Because rare instances of anaphylactic reactions have occurred in patients receiving parenteral corticosteroid therapy, appropriate precautionary measures should be taken prior to administration, especially when the patient has a history of drug allergy.

Corticosteroids may mask some signs of infection, and new infections may appear during their use. Suppression of the inflammatory response and immune function increases the susceptibility to fungal, viral and bacterial infections and their severity. The clinical presentation may often be atypical and may reach an advanced stage before being recognised.

Chickenpox is of serious concern since this normally minor illness may be fatal in immunosuppressed patients. Patients (or parents of children) without a definite history of chickenpox should be advised to avoid close personal contact with chickenpox or herpes zoster and if exposed they should seek urgent medical attention. Passive immunization with varicella/zoster immunoglobin (VZIG) is needed by exposed non-immune patients who are receiving systemic corticosteroids or who have used them within the previous 3 months; this should be given within 10 days of exposure to chickenpox. If a diagnosis of chickenpox is confirmed, the illness warrants specialist care and urgent treatment. Corticosteroids should not be stopped and the dose may need to be increased.

Live vaccines should not be given to individuals with impaired immune responsiveness. The antibody response to other vaccines may be diminished.

The use of Depo-Medrone in active tuberculosis should be restricted to those cases of fulminating or disseminated tuberculosis in which the corticosteroid is used for the management of the disease in conjunction with an appropriate antituberculous regimen. If corticosteroids are indicated in patients with latent tuberculosis or tuberculin reactivity, close observation is necessary as reactivation of the disease may occur. During prolonged corticosteroid therapy, these patients should receive chemoprophylaxis.

Care should be taken for patients receiving cardioactive drugs such as digoxin because of steroid induced electrolyte disturbance/potassium loss (see *Undesirable effects*).

The following precautions apply for parenteral corticosteroids: Following intra-articular injection, the occurrence of a marked increase in pain accompanied by local swelling, further restriction of joint motion, fever, and malaise are suggestive of septic arthritis. If this complication occurs and the diagnosis of sepsis is confirmed, appropriate antimicrobial therapy should be instituted.

Local injection of a steroid into a previously infected joint is to be avoided.

Corticosteroids should not be injected into unstable joints.

Sterile technique is necessary to prevent infections or contamination.

The slower rate of absorption by intramuscular administration should be recognised.

Special precautions: Particular care is required when considering the use of systemic corticosteroids in patients with the following conditions and frequent patient monitoring is necessary.

Osteoporosis (post-menopausal females are particularly at risk).
Hypertension or congestive heart failure.
Existing or previous history of severe affective disorders (especially previous steroid psychosis).
Diabetes mellitus (or a family history of diabetes).
History of tuberculosis.
Glaucoma (or a family history of glaucoma).
Previous corticosteroid-induced myopathy.
Liver failure or cirrhosis.
Renal insufficiency.
Epilepsy.
Peptic ulceration.
Fresh intestinal anastomoses.
Predisposition to thrombophlebitis.
Abscess or other pyogenic infections.
Ulcerative colitis.
Diverticulitis.
Myasthenia gravis.
Ocular herpes simplex, for fear of corneal perforation.
Hypothyroidism.

Use in children: Corticosteroids cause growth retardation in infancy, childhood and adolescence which may be irreversible. Treatment should be limited to the minimum dosage for the shortest possible time.

Use in the elderly: The common adverse effects of systemic corticosteroids may be associated with more serious consequences in old age, especially osteoporosis, hypertension, hypokalaemia, diabetes, susceptibility to infection and thinning of the skin. Close clinical supervision is required to avoid life-threatening reactions.

Interaction with other medicaments and other forms of interaction: Convulsions have been reported with concurrent use of methylprednisolone and cyclosporin. Since concurrent administration of these agents results in a mutual inhibition of metabolism, it is possible that convulsions and other adverse effects associated with the individual use of either drug may be more apt to occur.

Drugs that induce hepatic enzymes, such as rifampicin, rifabutin, carbamazepine, phenobarbitone, phenytoin, primidone, and aminoglutethimide enhance the metabolism of corticosteroids and its therapeutic effects may be reduced.

Drugs such as erythromycin and ketoconazole may inhibit the metabolism of corticosteroids and thus decrease their clearance.

Steroids may reduce the effects of anticholinesterases in myasthenia gravis. The desired effects of hypoglycaemic agents (including insulin), anti-hypertensives and diuretics are antagonised by corticosteroids, and the hypokalaemic effects of acetazolamide, loop diuretics, thiazide diuretics and carbenoxolone are enhanced.

The efficacy of coumarin anticoagulants may be enhanced by concurrent corticosteroid therapy and close monitoring of the INR or prothrombin time is required to avoid spontaneous bleeding.

The renal clearance of salicylates is increased by corticosteroids and steroid withdrawal may result in salicylate intoxication. Salicylates and non-steroidal anti-inflammatory agents should be used cautiously in conjunction with corticosteroids in hypothrombinaemia.

Steroids have been reported to interact with neuromuscular blocking agents such as pancuronium with partial reversal of the neuromuscular block.

Pregnancy and lactation
Pregnancy: The ability of corticosteroids to cross the placenta varies between individual drugs, however, methylprednisolone does cross the placenta.

Administration of corticosteroids to pregnant animals can cause abnormalities of foetal development including cleft palate, intra-uterine growth retardation and affects on brain growth and development. There is no evidence that corticosteroids result in an increased incidence of congenital abnormalities, such as cleft palate in man, however, when administered for long periods or repeatedly during pregnancy, corticosteroids may increase the risk of intra-uterine growth retardation. Hypoadrenalism may, in theory, occur in the neonate following prenatal exposure to corticosteroids but usually resolves spontaneously following birth and is rarely clinically important. As with all drugs, corticosteroids should only be prescribed when the benefits to the mother and child outweigh the risks. When corticosteroids are essential, however, patients with normal pregnancies may be treated as though they were in the non-gravid state.

Lactation: Corticosteroids are excreted in small amounts in breast milk, however, doses of up to 40 mg daily of methylprednisolone are unlikely to cause systemic effects in the infant. Infants of mothers taking higher doses than this may have a degree of adrenal suppression, but the benefits of breastfeeding are likely to outweigh any theoretical risk.

Effects on ability to drive and use machines: None stated.

Undesirable effects: The incidence of predictable undesirable side-effects associated with the use of corticosteroids, including hypothalamic-pituitary-adrenal suppression correlates with the relative potency of the drug, dosage, timing of administration and duration of treatment (see Special warnings and special precautions for use).

Parenteral corticosteroid therapy: Anaphylactic reaction or allergic reactions, hypopigmentation or hyperpigmentation, subcutaneous and cutaneous atrophy, sterile abscess, post injection flare (following intra-articular use), Charcot-like arthropathy, rare instances of blindness associated with intralesional therapy around the face and head.

Gastro-intestinal: Dyspepsia, peptic ulceration with perforation and haemorrhage, abdominal distension, oesophageal ulceration, oesophageal candidiasis, acute pancreatitis, perforation of bowel.

Increases in alanine transaminase (ALT, SGPT) aspartate transaminase (AST, SGOT) and alkaline phosphatase have been observed following corticosteroid treatment. These changes are usually small, not associated with any clinical syndrome and are reversible upon discontinuation.

Anti-inflammatory and immunosuppressive effects: Increased susceptibility and severity of infections with suppression of clinical symptoms and signs, opportunistic infections, may suppress reactions to skin tests, recurrence of dormant tuberculosis (see *Special warnings and special precautions for use*).

Musculoskeletal: Proximal myopathy, osteoporosis, vertebral and long bone fractures, avascular osteonecrosis, tendon rupture, aseptic necrosis, muscle weakness.

Fluid and electrolyte disturbance: Sodium and water retention, potassium loss, hypertension, hypokalaemic alkalosis, congestive heart failure in susceptible patients.

Dermatological: Impaired healing, petechiae and ecchymosis, thin fragile skin, skin atrophy, bruising, striae, telangiectasia, acne.

Endocrine/metabolic: Suppression of the hypothalamo-pituitary-adrenal axis, growth suppression in infancy, childhood and adolescence, menstrual irregularity and amenorrhoea. Cushingoid facies, hirsutism, weight gain, impaired carbohydrate tolerance with increased requirement for antidiabetic therapy, negative nitrogen and calcium balance. Increased appetite.

Neuropsychiatric: Euphoria, psychological dependence, mood swings, depression, personality changes, insomnia. Increased intra-cranial pressure with papilloedema in children (pseudotumour cerebri), usually after treatment withdrawal. Psychosis, aggravation of schizophrenia, seizures.

Ophthalmic: Increased intra-ocular pressure, glaucoma, papilloedema, cataracts with possible damage to the optic nerve, corneal or scleral thinning, exacerbation of ophthalmic viral or fungal disease, exophthalmos.

General: Leucocytosis, hypersensitivity including anaphylaxis, thrombo-embolism, nausea, vertigo.

Withdrawal symptoms: Too rapid a reduction of corticosteroid dosage following prolonged treatment can lead to acute adrenal insufficiency, hypotension and death. However, this is more applicable to corticosteroids with an indication where continuous therapy is given (see Special warnings and special precautions for use).

A 'withdrawal syndrome' may also occur including, fever, myalgia, arthralgia, rhinitis, conjunctivitis, painful itchy skin nodules and loss of weight.

Certain side-effects reported with some non-recommended routes of administration

Intrathecal: Usual systemic corticoid adverse reactions, headache, meningismus, meningitis, paraplegia, spinal fluid abnormalities, nausea, vomiting, sweating, arachnoiditis, convulsions.

Extradural: Wound dehiscence, loss of sphincter control.

Intranasal: Permanent/temporary blindness, rhinitis.

Ophthalmic: (Subconjunctival)–Redness and itching, abscess, slough at injection site, residue at injection site, increased intra-ocular pressure, decreased vision–blindness, infection.

Miscellaneous injection sites: Scalp, tonsillar fauces, sphenopalatine ganglion: blindness.

Overdose: There is no clinical syndrome of acute overdosage with Depo-Medrone. Following overdosage the possibility of adrenal suppression should be guarded against by gradual diminution of dose levels over a period of time. In such event the patient may require to be supported during any further traumatic episode.

Pharmacological properties

Pharmacodynamic properties: Methylprednisolone acetate is a synthetic glucocorticoid. An aqueous suspension may be injected directly into joints and soft tissues in the treatment of rheumatoid arthritis, osteoarthritis, bursitis and similar inflammatory conditions. For prolonged systemic effect it may be administered intramuscularly.

Pharmacokinetic properties: Methylprednisolone acetate is absorbed from joints in a few days, with peak serum levels being reached 2–12 hours after injection.

It is more slowly absorbed following deep intramuscular injection with plasma levels detected up to 17 days afterwards.

Methylprednisolone acetate is less soluble than methylprednisolone.

Pharmaceutical particulars

List of excipients: Polyethylene glycol, sodium chloride, myristyl-gamma-picolinium chloride and sterile water for injections.

Incompatibilities: None stated.

Shelf-life: Shelf-life of the medicinal product as packaged for sale: 60 months. Depo-Medrone should not be mixed with any other fluid. Discard any remaining suspension after use.

Special precautions for storage: Depo-Medrone should be protected from freezing.

Nature and contents of container: Type I flint glass vial with a butyl rubber plug and metal seal. Each vial contains 1 ml, 2 ml, or 3 ml of Depo-Medrone 40 mg/ml.

Instructions for use/handling: No special requirements.

Marketing authorisation number 0032/5038.

Date of first authorisation/renewal of authorisation

Date of first authorisation: 7 March 1989.

Last renewal date: 5 September 1996.

Date of revision of the text July 1998.

Legal category POM.

DEPO-MEDRONE* WITH LIDOCAINE

Qualitative and quantitative composition Methyprednisolone BP 4%, Lidocaine Hydrochloride BP 1%

Pharmaceutical form White, sterile aqueous suspension for injection.

Clinical particulars

Therapeutic indications: Corticosteroid (glucocorticoid). Depo-Medrone with Lidocaine is indicated in conditions requiring a glucocorticoid effect: e.g. anti-inflammatory or anti-rheumatic. It is recommended for local use where the added anaesthetic effect would be considered advantageous.

Depo-Medrone with Lidocaine may be used as follows:

Intra-articular administration: Rheumatoid arthritis; Osteo-arthritis with an inflammatory component.

Periarticular administration: Epicondylitis.

Intrabursal administration: Subacromial bursitis; Prepatellar bursitis; Olecranon bursitis

Tendon sheath administration: Tendinitis; Tenosynovitis; Epicondylitis

Therapy with Depo-Medrone with Lidocaine does not obviate the need for the conventional measures usually employed. Although this method of treatment will ameliorate symptoms, it is in no sense a cure and the hormone has no effect on the cause of the inflammation.

Posology and method of administration: Depo-Medrone with Lidocaine should not be mixed with any other preparation as flocculation of the product may occur. Parenteral drug products should be inspected visually for particulate matter and discoloration prior to administration whenever suspension and container permit. Depo-Medrone with Lidocaine may be used by any of the following routes: intra-articular, periarticular, intrabursal, and into the tendon sheath. It *must not* be used by the intrathecal or intravenous routes (see *Contra-indications* and *Side-effects*).

Adults:

Intra-articular: Rheumatoid arthritis, osteo-arthritis. The dose of Depo-Medrone with Lidocaine depends on the size of the joint and the severity of the condition. Repeated injections, if needed, may be given at intervals of one to five or more weeks depending upon the degree of relief obtained from the initial injection. A suggested dosage guide is: large joint (knee, ankle, shoulder), 0.5–2 ml (20–80 mg of steroid); medium joint (elbow, wrist), 0.25–1 ml (10–40 mg of steroid); small joint (metacarpophalangeal, interphalangeal, sternoclavicular, acromioclavicular), 0.1–0.25 ml (4–10 mg of steroid).

Periarticular: Epicondylitis. Infiltrate 0.1–0.75 ml (4–30 mg of steroid) into the affected area.

Intrabursal: Subdeltoid bursitis, prepatellar bursitis, olecranon bursitis. For administration directly into bursae, 0.1–0.75 ml (4–30 mg of steroid). In most acute cases, repeat injections are not needed.

Into the tendon sheath: Tendinitis, tenosynovitis, epicondylitis. For administration directly into the tendon sheath, 0.1–0.75 ml (4–30 mg of steroid). In recurrent or chronic conditions, repeat injections may be necessary.

Children: For infants and children, the recommended dosage should be reduced, but dosage should be governed by the severity of the condition rather than by strict adherence to the ratio indicated by age or body weight.

Elderly: When used according to instructions, there is no information to suggest that a change in dosage is warranted in the elderly. However, treatment of elderly patients, particularly if long-term, should be planned bearing in mind the more serious consequences of the common side-effects of corticosteroids in old age and close clinical supervision is required (see *Other special warnings and precautions*).

Special precautions should be observed when administering Depo-Medrone with Lidocaine:

Intra-articular injections should be made using precise, anatomical localisation into the synovial space of the joint involved. The injection site for each joint is determined by that location where the synovial cavity is most superficial and most free of large vessels and nerves. Suitable sites for intra-articular injection are the knee, ankle, wrist, elbow, shoulder, phalangeal and hip joints. The spinal joints, unstable joints and those devoid of synovial space are not suitable. Treatment failures are most frequently the result of failure to enter the joint space. Intra-articular injections should be made with care as follows: ensure correct positioning of the needle into the synovial space and aspirate a few drops of joint fluid. The aspirating syringe should then be replaced by another containing Depo-Medrone with Lidocaine. To ensure position of the needle synovial fluid should be aspirated and the injection made.

After injection the joint is moved slightly to aid mixing of the synovial fluid and the suspension. Subsequent to therapy care should be taken for the patient not to overuse the joint in which benefit has been obtained. Negligence in this matter may permit an increase in joint deterioration that will more than offset the beneficial effects of the steroid.

Intrabursal injections should be made as follows: the area around the injection site is prepared in a sterile way and a wheal at the site made with 1 percent procaine hydrochloride solution. A 20 to 24 gauge needle attached to a dry syringe is inserted into the bursa and the fluid aspirated. The needle is left in place and the aspirating syringe changed for a small syringe containing the desired dose. After injection, the needle is withdrawn and a small dressing applied. In the treatment of tenosynovitis and tendinitis, care should be taken to inject Depo-Medrone with Lidocaine into the tendon sheath rather than into the substance of the tendon. Due to the absence of a true tendon sheath, the Achilles tendon should not be injected with Depo-Medrone with Lidocaine.

Contra-indications: Depo-Medrone with Lidocaine is contra-indicated where there is known hypersensitivity to components or to any local anaesthetics of the amide type and in systemic infection unless anti-infective therapy is employed.

Due to its potential for neurotoxicity, Depo-Medrone with Lidocaine *must not* be given by the intrathecal route. In addition, as the product is a suspension it *must not* be given by the intravenous route (see *Side-effects*).

Special warnings and special precautions for use: Undesirable effects may be minimised by using the lowest effective dose for the minimum period. Frequent patient review is required to appropriately titrate the dose against disease activity (see *Dosage and administration*).

Patients should carry 'Steroid Treatment' cards which give clear guidance on the precautions to be taken to minimise risk and which provide details of prescriber, drug, dosage and the duration of treatment.

Depo-Medrone with Lidocaine vials are intended for single dose use only. Any multidose use of the product may lead to contamination.

Depo-Medrone with Lidocaine is not recommended for epidural, intranasal, intra-ocular, or any other unapproved route of administration. See *Side-effects* section for details of side-effects reported from some non-recommended routes of administration.

Due to the absence of a true tendon sheath, the Achilles tendon should not be injected with Depo-Medrone with Lidocaine.

While crystals of adrenal steroids in the dermis suppress inflammatory reactions, their presence may cause disintegration of the cellular elements and physiochemical changes in the ground substance of the connective tissue. The resultant infrequently occurring dermal and/or subdermal changes may form depressions in the skin at the injection site and the possibility of depigmentation. The degree to which this reaction occurs will vary with the amount of adrenal steroid injected. Regeneration is usually complete within a few months or after all crystals of the adrenal steroid have been absorbed. In order to minimize the incidence of dermal and subdermal atrophy, care must be exercised not to exceed recommended doses in injections. Multiple small injections into the area of the lesion should be made whenever possible. The technique of intra-articular injection should include precautions against injection or leakage into the dermis.

Systemic absorption of methylprednisolone occurs following intra-articular injection of Depo-Medrone with Lidocaine. Systemic as well as local effects can therefore be expected.

Intra-articular corticosteroids are associated with a substantially increased risk of inflammatory response in the joint, particularly bacterial infection introduced with the injection. Charcot-like arthropathies have been reported particularly after repeated injections. Appropriate examination of any joint fluid present is necessary to exclude any bacterial infection, prior to injection.

Following a single dose of Depo-Medrone with Lidocaine, plasma cortisol levels are reduced and there is evidence of hypothalamic-pituitary-adrenal axis (HPA) suppression. This suppression lasts for a variable period of up to 4 weeks. The usual dynamic tests of HPA axis function can be used to diagnose evidence of impaired activity (e.g. Synacthen test).

Adrenal cortical atrophy develops during prolonged therapy and may persist for months after stopping treatment. In patients who have received more than physiological doses of systemic corticosteroids (approximately 6 mg methylprednisolone) for greater than 3 weeks, withdrawal should not be abrupt. How dose reduction should be carried out depends largely on whether the disease is likely to relapse as the dose of systemic corticosteroids is reduced. Clinical assessment of disease activity may be needed during withdrawal. If the disease is unlikely to relapse on withdrawal of systemic corticosteroids, but there is uncertainty about HPA suppression, the dose of systemic corticosteroid *may* be reduced rapidly to physiological doses. Once a daily dose of 6 mg methylprednisolone is reached, dose reduction should be slower to allow the HPA-axis to recover.

Abrupt withdrawal of systemic corticosteroid treatment, which has continued up to 3 weeks is appropriate if it is considered that the disease is unlikely to relapse. Abrupt withdrawal of doses up to 32 mg daily of methylprednisolone for 3 weeks is unlikely to lead to clinically relevant HPA-axis suppression, in the majority of patients. In the following patient groups, gradual withdrawal of systemic corticosteroid therapy should be *considered* even after courses lasting 3 weeks or less:

Patients who have had repeated courses of systemic corticosteroids, particularly if taken for greater than 3 weeks.

When a short course has been prescribed within one year of cessation of long-term therapy (months or years).

Patients who may have reasons for adrenocortical insufficiency other than exogenous corticosteroid therapy.

Patients receiving doses of systemic corticosteroid greater than 32 mg daily of methylprednisolone.

Patients repeatedly taking doses in the evening.

Since mineralocorticoid secretion may be impaired, salt and/or a mineralocorticoid should be administered concurrently.

Because rare instances of anaphylactic reactions have occurred in patients receiving parenteral corticosteroid therapy, appropriate precautionary measures should be taken prior to administration, especially when the patient has a history of drug allergy.

Corticosteroids may mask some signs of infection, and new infections may appear during their use. Suppression of the inflammatory response and immune function increases the susceptibility to fungal, viral and bacterial infections and their severity. The clinical presentation may often be atypical and may reach an advanced stage before being recognised.

Chickenpox is of serious concern since this normally minor illness may be fatal in immunosuppressed patients. Patients (or parents of children) without a definite history of chickenpox should be advised to avoid close personal contact with chickenpox or herpes zoster and if exposed they should seek urgent medical attention. Passive immunization with varicella/zoster immunoglobin (VZIG) is needed by exposed non-immune patients who are receiving systemic corticosteroids or who have used them within the previous 3 months; this should be given within 10 days of exposure to chickenpox. If a diagnosis of chickenpox is confirmed, the illness warrants specialist care and urgent treatment. Corticosteroids should not be stopped and the dose may need to be increased.

Live vaccines should not be given to individuals with impaired immune responsiveness. The antibody response to other vaccines may be diminished.

If corticosteroids are indicated in patients with latent tuberculosis or tuberculin reactivity, close observation is necessary as reactivation of the disease may occur. During prolonged corticosteroid therapy, these patients should receive chemoprophylaxis.

This product contains benzyl alcohol. Benzyl alcohol has been reported to be associated with a fatal 'Gasping Syndrome' in premature infants.

Care should be taken for patients receiving cardioactive drugs such as digoxin because of steroid induced electrolyte disturbance/potassium loss (see *Side-effects*).

The following precautions apply for parenteral corticosteroids: Following intra-articular injection, a marked increase in pain accompanied by local swelling, further restriction of joint motion, fever, and malaise are suggestive of septic arthritis. If this complication occurs and the diagnosis of sepsis is confirmed, appropriate antimicrobial therapy should be instituted.

No additional benefit derives from the intramuscular administration of Depo-Medrone with Lidocaine. Where parenteral corticosteroid therapy for sustained systemic effect is desired, plain Depo-Medrone should be used.

Local injection of a steroid into a previously infected joint is to be avoided.

Corticosteroids should not be injected into unstable joints.

Sterile technique is necessary to prevent infections or contamination.

Special precautions: Particular care is required when considering the use of systemic corticosteroids in patients with the following conditions and frequent patient monitoring is necessary.

Osteoporosis (post-menopausal females are particularly at risk).
Hypertension or congestive heart failure.
Existing or previous history of severe affective disorders (especially previous steroid psychosis).
Diabetes mellitus (or a family history of diabetes).
History of tuberculosis.
Glaucoma (or a family history of glaucoma).
Previous corticosteroid-induced myopathy.
Liver failure or cirrhosis.
Renal insufficiency.
Epilepsy.
Peptic ulceration.
Fresh intestinal anastomoses.
Predisposition to thrombophlebitis.
Abscess or other pyogenic infections.
Ulcerative colitis.
Diverticulitis.
Myasthenia gravis.
Ocular herpes simplex, for fear of corneal perforation.
Hypothyroidism.

Use in children: Corticosteroids cause growth retardation in infancy, childhood and adolescence which may be irreversible. Treatment should be limited to the minimum dosage for the shortest possible time.

Use in the elderly: The common adverse effects of systemic corticosteroids may be associated with more serious consequences in old age, especially osteoporosis, hypertension, hypokalaemia, diabetes, susceptibility to infection and thinning of the skin. Close clinical supervision is required to avoid life-threatening reactions.

Interaction with other medicaments and other forms of interaction: Convulsions have been reported with concurrent use of methylprednisolone and cyclosporin. Since concurrent administration of these agents results in a mutual inhibition of metabolism, it is possible that convulsions and other adverse effects associated with the individual use of either drug may be more apt to occur.

Drugs that induce hepatic enzymes, such as rifampicin, rifabutin, carbamazepine, phenobarbitone, phenytoin, primidone, and aminoglutethimide enhance the metabolism of corticosteroids and its therapeutic effects may be reduced.

Drugs such as erythromycin and ketoconazole may inhibit the metabolism of corticosteroids and thus decrease their clearance.

Steroids may reduce the effects of anticholinesterases in myasthenia gravis. The desired effects of hypoglycaemic agents (including insulin), anti-hypertensives and diuretics are antagonised by corticosteroids, and the hypokalaemic effects of acetazolamide, loop diuretics, thiazide diuretics and carbenoxolone are enhanced.

The efficacy of coumarin anticoagulants may be enhanced by concurrent corticosteroid therapy and close monitoring of the INR or prothrombin time is required to avoid spontaneous bleeding.

The renal clearance of salicylates is increased by corticosteroids and steroid withdrawal may result in salicylate intoxication. Salicylates and non-steroidal anti-inflammatory agents should be used cautiously in conjunction with corticosteroids in hypothrombinaemia.

Steroids have been reported to interact with neuromuscular blocking agents such as pancuronium with partial reversal of the neuromuscular block.

Pregnancy and lactation:
Pregnancy: The ability of corticosteroids to cross the placenta varies between individual drugs, however, methylprednisolone does cross the placenta.

Administration of corticosteroids to pregnant animals can cause abnormalities of foetal development including cleft palate, intra-uterine growth retardation and affects on brain growth and development. There is no evidence that corticosteroids result in an increased incidence of congenital abnormalities, such as cleft palate in man, however, when administered for long periods or repeatedly during pregnancy, corticosteroids may increase the risk of intra-uterine growth retardation. Hypoadrenalism may, in theory, occur in the neonate following prenatal exposure to corticosteroids but usually resolves spontaneously following birth and is rarely clinically important. As with all drugs, corticosteroids should only be prescribed when the benefits to the mother and child outweigh the risks. When corticosteroids are essential, however, patients with normal pregnancies may be treated as though they were in the non-gravid state.

The use of local anaesthetics such as lidocaine during labour and delivery may be associated with adverse effects on mother and foetus. Lidocaine readily crosses the placenta.

Lactation: Corticosteroids are excreted in small amounts in breast milk, however, doses of up to 40 mg daily of methylprednisolone are unlikely to cause systemic effects in the infant. Infants of mothers taking higher doses than this may have a degree of adrenal suppression, but the benefits of breastfeeding are likely to outweigh any theoretical risk.

It is not known whether lidocaine is excreted in human breast milk.

Effects on ability to drive and use machines: None stated.

Undesirable effects: The incidence of predictable undesirable side-effects associated with the use of corticosteroids, including hypothalamic-pituitary-adrenal suppression correlates with the relative potency of the drug, dosage, timing of administration and duration of treatment (See other special warnings and precautions).

Side-effects for the Depo-Medrone component may be observed including:

Parenteral corticosteroid therapy : Anaphylactic reaction or allergic reactions, hypopigmentation or hyperpigmentation, subcutaneous and cutaneous atrophy, sterile abscess, post injection flare (following intra-articular use), charcot-like arthropathy.

Gastro-intestinal: Dyspepsia, peptic ulceration with perforation and haemorrhage, abdominal distension, oesophageal ulceration, oesophageal candidiasis, acute pancreatitis, perforation of bowel.

Increases in alanine transaminase (ALT, SGPT) aspartate transaminase (AST, SGOT) and alkaline phosphatase have been observed following corticosteroid treatment. These changes are usually small, not associated with any clinical syndrome and are reversible upon discontinuation.

Anti-inflammatory and immunosuppressive effects: Increased susceptibility and severity of infections with suppression of clinical symptoms and signs, opportunistic infections, may suppress reactions to skin tests, recurrence of dormant tuberculosis (see *Other special warnings and precautions*).

Musculoskeletal: Proximal myopathy, osteoporosis, vertebral and long bone fractures, avascular osteonecrosis, tendon rupture, aseptic necrosis, muscle weakness.

Fluid and electrolyte disturbance: Sodium and water retention, potassium loss, hypertension, hypokalaemic alkalosis, congestive heart failure in susceptible patients.

Dermatological: Impaired healing, petechiae and ecchymosis, thin fragile skin, skin atrophy, bruising, striae, telangiectasia, acne.

Endocrine/metabolic: Suppression of the hypothalamo-pituitary-adrenal axis; growth suppression in infancy, childhood and adolescence; menstrual irregularity and amenorrhoea. Cushingoid facies, hirsutism, weight gain, impaired carbohydrate tolerance with increased requirement for antidiabetic therapy, negative nitrogen and calcium balance. Increased appetite.

Neuropsychiatric: Euphoria, psychological dependence, mood swings, depression, personality changes, insomnia. Increased intra-cranial pressure with papilloedema in children (pseudotumour cerebri), usually after treatment withdrawal. Psychosis, aggravation of schizophrenia, seizures.

Ophthalmic: Increased intra-ocular pressure, glaucoma, papilloedema, cataracts with possible damage to the optic nerve, corneal or scleral thinning, exacerbation of ophthalmic viral or fungal disease, exophthalmos.

General: Leucocytosis, hypersensitivity including anaphylaxis, thrombo-embolism, nausea, vertigo.

Withdrawal symptoms: Too rapid a reduction of corticosteroid dosage following prolonged treatment can lead to acute adrenal insufficiency, hypotension and death. However, this is more applicable to corticosteroids with an indication where continuous therapy is given (see *Other special warnings and precautions*).

A 'withdrawal syndrome' may also occur including, fever, myalgia, arthralgia, rhinitis, conjunctivitis, painful itchy skin nodules and loss of weight.

Side-effects for the Lidocaine component include:
Central nervous system: Lightheadedness, nervousness, apprehension, euphoria, confusion, dizziness, drowsiness, tinnitus, blurred or double vision, vomiting, sensation of heat, cold, numbness, twitching, tremors, convulsions, loss of consciousness, respiratory depression, respiratory arrest.

Cardiovascular system: Bradycardia, hypotension, cardiovascular collapse, cardiac arrest.

Allergic reactions: Cutaneous lesions, urticaria, oedema, anaphylactic reactions.

Certain side-effects reported with some non recommended routes of administration:
Intrathecal: Usual systemic corticoid adverse reactions, headache, meningismus, meningitis, paraplegia, spinal fluid abnormalities, nausea, vomiting, sweating, arachnoiditis, convulsions.

Extradural: Wound dehiscence, loss of sphincter control.

Intranasal: Permanent/temporary blindness, allergic reactions, rhinitis.

Ophthalmic (Subconjunctival): Redness and itching, abscess, slough at injection site, residue at injection site, increased intra-ocular pressure, decreased vision–blindness, infection.

Miscellaneous: Scalp, tonsillar fauces, sphenopalatine ganglion: blindness.

Overdose: There is no clinical syndrome of acute overdosage with Depo-Medrone with Lidocaine. Following overdosage the possibility of adrenal suppression should be guarded against by gradual diminution of dose levels over a period of time. In such event the patient may require to be supported during any further traumatic episode.

Pharmacological properties
Pharmacodynamic properties: Methylprednisolone acetate is a synthetic glucocorticoid with the actions and use of natural corticosteroids. However the slower metabolism of the synthetic corticosteroid with their lower protein-binding affinity may account for their increased potency compared with the natural corticosteroids.

Lidocaine has the actions of a local anaesthetic.

Pharmacokinetic properties: Administration of methylprednisolone acetate 40 mg intramuscularly produced measurable plasma concentrations of methylprednisolone for 11–17 days. The average peak plasma concentration was 14.8 ng per ml and occurred after 6–8 hours.

Plasma concentrations of lidocaine decline rapidly after an intravenous dose with an initial half life of less than 30 minutes; the elimination half life is 1–2 hours.

Preclinical safety data: Due to the age and well established safety nature of this product, preclinical data has not been included.

Pharmaceutical particulars
List of excipients: Sodium chloride, myristyl-gamma-picolinium chloride, benzyl alcohol, polyethylene glycol, sodium hydroxide, hydrochloric acid and water for injection.

Incompatibilities: None.

Shelf life: 24 months.

Special precautions for storage: Store at room temperature. Protect from freezing.

Nature and contents of container: Glass vials with rubber cap containing 1 or 2 ml of suspension.

Instructions for use/handling: None.

Marketing authorisation number 0032/0076

Date of first authorisation/renewal of authorisation
MA granted: 3 March 1981.
MA renewed: 25 November 1991.

Date of (partial) revision of the text July 1998.

Legal category POM.

DEPO-PROVERA* 150 mg/ml

Qualitative and quantitative composition Each ml of suspension contains 150 mg medroxyprogesterone acetate PhEur.

Pharmaceutical form Sterile suspension for injection.

Clinical particulars
Therapeutic indications: Progestogen: for contraception.

Depo-Provera is a long-term contraceptive agent suitable for use in women who have been appropriately counselled concerning the likelihood of menstrual disturbance and the potential for a delay in return to full fertility.

Depo-Provera may also be used for short-term contraception in the following circumstances:

(i) For partners of men undergoing vasectomy, for protection until the vasectomy becomes effective.

(ii) In women who are being immunised against rubella, to prevent pregnancy during the period of activity of the virus.

(iii) In women awaiting sterilisation.

It is of the greatest importance that adequate explanations of the long-term nature of the product, of its possible side-effects and of the impossibility of immediately reversing the effects of each injection are given to potential users and that every effort is made to ensure that each patient receives such counselling as to enable her to fully understand these explanations. Patient information leaflets are supplied by the manufacturer. It is recommended that the doctor uses these leaflets to aid counselling of the patient.

Consistent with good clinical practice a general medical as well as gynaecological examination should be undertaken before administration of Depo-Provera and at appropriate intervals thereafter.

Posology and method of administration: The sterile aqueous suspension of Depo-Provera should be vigorously shaken just before use to ensure that the dose being given represents a uniform suspension of Depo-Provera.

Doses should be given by deep intramuscular injection.

Adults:
First injection: To provide contraceptive cover in the first cycle of use, an injection of 150 mg i.m. should be given during the first five days of a normal menstrual cycle. If the injection is carried out according to these instructions, no additional contraceptive cover is required.

Post partum: To increase assurance that the patient is not pregnant at the time of first administration, this injection should be given within 5 days post partum if not breast-feeding.

There is evidence that women prescribed Depo-Provera in the immediate puerperium can experience prolonged and heavy bleeding. Because of this, the drug should be used with caution in the puerperium. Women who are considering use of the product immediately following delivery or termination should be advised that the risk of heavy or prolonged bleeding may be increased. Doctors are reminded that in the non breast-feeding, post partum patient, ovulation may occur as early as week 4.

If the puerperal woman will be breast-feeding, the initial injection should be delayed until six weeks post partum, when the infant's enzyme system is more fully developed. Further injections should be given at 12 week intervals.

Further doses: These should be given at 12 week intervals, however, as long as the injection is given no later than five days after this time, no additional contraceptive measures (e.g. barrier) are required. (N.B. For partners of men undergoing vasectomy a second injection of 150 mg i.m. 12 weeks after the first may be necessary in a small proportion of patients where the partner's sperm count has not fallen to zero.) If the interval from the preceding injection is greater than 89 days (12 weeks and five days) for any reason, then pregnancy should be excluded before the next injection is given and the patient should use additional contraceptive measures (e.g. barrier) for fourteen days after this subsequent injection.

Elderly: Not appropriate.

Children: Not appropriate.

Contra-indications: Depo-Provera is contra-indicated in patients with a known sensitivity to medroxyprogesterone acetate or any ingredient of the vehicle.

Depo-Provera should not be used during pregnancy, either for diagnosis or therapy.

Depo-Provera is contra-indicated as a contraceptive at the above dosage in known or suspected hormone-dependent malignancy of breast or genital organs.

Whether administered alone or in combination with oestrogen, Depo-Provera should not be employed in patients with abnormal uterine bleeding until a definite diagnosis has been established and the possibility of genital tract malignancy eliminated.

Special warnings and special precautions for use:
Warnings:
Menstrual irregularity: The administration of Depo-Provera usually causes disruption of the normal menstrual cycle. Bleeding patterns include amenorrhoea (present in up to 30% of women during the first 3 months and increasing to 55% by month 12 and 68% by month 24); irregular bleeding and spotting; prolonged (>10 days) episodes of bleeding (up to 33% of women in the first 3 months of use decreasing to 12% by month 12). Rarely, heavy prolonged bleeding may occur. Evidence suggests that prolonged or heavy bleeding requiring treatment may occur in 0.5–4 occasions per 100 women years of use. If abnormal bleeding persists or is severe, appropriate investigation should take place to rule out the possibility of organic pathology and appropriate treatment should be instituted when necessary. Excessive or prolonged bleeding can be controlled by the co-administration of oestrogen. This may be delivered either in the form of a low dose (30 micrograms oestrogen) combined oral contraceptive pill or in the form of oestrogen replacement therapy such as conjugated equine oestrogen (0.625–1.25 mg daily). Oestrogen therapy may need to be repeated for 1–2 cycles. Long-term co-administration of oestrogen is not recommended.

Return to fertility: There is no evidence that Depo-Provera causes permanent infertility. Pregnancies have occurred as early as 14 weeks after a preceding injection, however, in clinical trials, the mean time to return of ovulation was 5.3 months following the preceding injection. Women should be counselled that there is a potential for delay in return to full fertility following use of the method, regardless of the duration of use, however, 83% of women may be expected to conceive within 12 months of the first 'missed' injection (i.e. 15 months after the last injection administered). The median time to conception was 10 months (range 4–31) after the last injection.

Cancer risks: Long-term case-controlled surveillance of Depo-Provera users found no overall increased risk of ovarian, liver, or cervical cancer and a prolonged, protective effect of reducing the risk of endometrial cancer in the population of users. A meta-analysis in 1996 from 54 epidemiological studies reported that there is a slight increased relative risk of having breast cancer diagnosed in women who are currently using hormonal contraceptives. The observed pattern of increased risk may be due to an earlier diagnosis of breast cancer in hormonal contraceptive users, biological effects or a combination of both. The additional breast cancers diagnosed in current users of hormonal contraceptives or in women who have used them in the last ten years are more likely to be localised to the breast than those in women who never used hormonal contraceptives.

Breast cancer is rare among women under 40 years of age whether or not they use hormonal contraceptives. In the meta-analysis the results for injectable progestogens (1.5% of the data) and progestogen only pills (0.8% of the data) did not reach significance although there was no evidence that they differed from other hormonal contraceptives. Whilst the background risk of breast cancer increases with age, the excess number of breast cancer diagnoses in current and recent injectable progestogen (IP) users is small in relation to the overall risk of breast cancer, possibly of similar magnitude to that associated with combined oral contraceptives. However, for IPs, the evidence is based on much smaller populations of users (less than 1.5% of the data) and is less conclusive than for combined oral contraceptives. It is not possible to infer from these data whether it is due to an earlier diagnosis of breast cancer in ever-users, the biological effects of hormonal contraceptives, or a combination of reasons.

The most important risk factor for breast cancer in IP users is the age women discontinue the IP; the older the age at stopping, the more breast cancers are diagnosed. Duration of use is less important and the excess risk gradually disappears during the course of the 10 years after stopping IP use, such that by 10 years there appears to be no excess.

The evidence suggests that compared with never-users, among 10,000 women who use IPs for up to 5 years but stop by age 20, there would be much less than 1 extra case of breast cancer diagnosed up to 10 years afterwards. For those stopping by age 30 after 5 years use of the IP, there would be an estimated 2–3 extra cases (additional to the 44 cases of breast cancer per 10,000 women in this age group never exposed to oral contraceptives). For those stopping by age 40 after 5 years use, there would be an estimated 10 extra cases diagnosed up to 10 years afterwards (additional to the 160 cases of breast cancer per 10,000 never-exposed women in this age group).

It is important to inform patients that users of all hormonal contraceptives appear to have a small increase in the risk of being diagnosed with breast cancer, compared with non-users of hormonal contraceptives, but that this has to be weighed against the known benefits.

Bone mineral density changes: Data from a small cross-sectional study has given rise to a concern that Depo-Provera may be considered among the risk factors for osteoporosis. There is evidence that bone loss is reversible in premenopausal women and that structure and bone mass is restored after Depo-Provera usage ends. Pending the result of larger well controlled studies, women who reach the menopause and have a history of prolonged usage of Depo-Provera could be considered candidates for hormone replacement therapy.

Weight gain: There is a tendency for women to gain weight while on Depo-Provera therapy. Studies indicate that over the first 1–2 years of use, average weight gain was 5–8 lbs. Women completing 4–6 years of therapy gained an average of 14–16.5 lbs. There is evidence that weight is gained as a result of increased fat and is not secondary to an anabolic effect or fluid retention.

Anaphylaxis: Very few reports of anaphylactoid reactions have been received.

Thrombo-embolic disorders: Should the patient experience pulmonary embolism, cerebrovascular disease or retinal thrombosis while receiving Depo-Provera, the drug should not be readministered.

Psychiatric disorders: Patients with a history of endogenous depression should be carefully monitored. Some patients may complain of premenstrual-type depression while on Depo-Provera therapy.

Precautions: History or emergence of the following conditions require careful consideration and appropriate investigation: migraine or unusually severe headaches, acute visual disturbances of any kind, pathological changes in liver function and hormone levels. Patients with thromboembolic or coronary vascular disease should be carefully evaluated before using Depo-Provera.

A decrease in glucose tolerance has been observed in some patients treated with progestogens. The mechanism for this decrease is obscure. For this reason, diabetic patients should be carefully monitored while receiving progestogen therapy.

Rare cases of thrombo-embolism have been reported with use of Depo-Provera, but causality has not been established.

The effects of medroxyprogesterone acetate on lipid metabolism have been studied with no clear impact demonstrated. Both increases and decreases in total cholesterol, triglycerides and low-density lipoprotein (LDL) cholesterol have been observed in studies. The use of Depo-Provera appears to be associated with a 15–20% reduction in serum high density lipoprotein (HDL) cholesterol levels which may protect women from cardiovascular disease. The clinical consequences of this observation are unknown. The potential for an increased risk of coronary disease should be considered prior to use.

Doctors should carefully consider the use of Depo-Provera in patients with recent trophoblastic disease before levels of human chorionic gonadotrophin have returned to normal.

Physicians should be aware that pathologists should be informed of the patient's use of Depo-Provera if endometrial or endocervical tissue is submitted for examination.

The results of certain laboratory tests may be affected by the use of Depo-Provera. These include gonadotrophin levels (decreased), plasma progesterone levels (decreased), urinary pregnanediol levels (decreased), plasma oestrogen levels (decreased), plasma cortisol levels (decreased), glucose tolerance test, metyrapone test, liver function tests (may increase), thyroid function tests (protein bound iodine levels may increase and T3 uptake levels may decrease). Coagulation test values for prothrombin (Factor II), and Factors VII, VIII, IX and X may increase.

Interaction with other medicaments and other forms of interaction: Aminoglutethimide administered concurrently with Depo-Provera may significantly depress the bioavailability of Depo-Provera.

Interactions with other medicinal treatments (including oral anticoagulants) have rarely been reported, but causality has not been determined. The possibility of interaction should be borne in mind in patients receiving concurrent treatment with other drugs.

The clearance of medroxyprogesterone acetate is approximately equal to the rate of hepatic blood flow. Because of this fact, it is unlikely that drugs which induce hepatic enzymes will significantly affect the kinetics of medroxyprogesterone acetate. Therefore, no dose adjustment is recommended in patients receiving drugs known to affect hepatic metabolising enzymes.

Pregnancy and lactation: Doctors should check that patients are not pregnant before initial injection of Depo-Provera, and also if administration of any subsequent injection is delayed beyond 89 days (12 weeks and five days).

Infants from accidental pregnancies that occur 1–2 months after injection of Depo-Provera may be at an increased risk of low birth weight, which in turn is associated with an increased risk of neonatal death. The attributable risk is low because such pregnancies are uncommon.

Children exposed to medroxyprogesterone acetate *in utero* and followed to adolescence, showed no evidence of any adverse effects on their health including their physical, intellectual, sexual or social development.

Medroxyprogesterone acetate and/or its metabolites are secreted in breast milk, but there is no evidence to suggest that this presents any hazard to the child. Infants exposed to medroxyprogesterone via breast milk have been studied for developmental and behavioural effects to puberty. No adverse effects have been noted.

Effects on ability to drive and use machines: None.

Undesirable effects: In a large clinical trial of over 3900 women, who were treated with Depo-Provera for up to 7 years, the following adverse events were reported.

The following adverse events were commonly (by more than 5% of subjects) reported: menstrual irregularities (bleeding and/or amenorrhoea), weight changes, headache, nervousness, abdominal pain or discomfort, dizziness, asthenia (weakness or fatigue).

Adverse events reported by 1% to 5% of subjects using Depo-Provera were: decreased libido or anorgasmia, backache, leg cramps, depression, nausea, insomnia, leucorrhoea, acne, vaginitis, pelvic pain, breast pain, no hair growth or alopecia, bloating, rash, oedema, hot flushes.

Other events were reported infrequently (by fewer than 1% of subjects), and included: galactorrhoea, melasma, chloasma, convulsions, changes in appetite, gastrointestinal disturbances, jaundice, genitourinary infections, vaginal cysts, dyspareunia, paraesthesia, chest pain, pulmonary embolus, allergic reactions, anaemia, syncope, dyspnoea, thirst, hoarseness, pain at injection site, blood dyscrasia, rectal bleeding, changes in breast size, breast lumps or nipple bleeding, axillary swelling, prevention of lactation, sensation of pregnancy, lack of return to fertility, paralysis, facial palsy, scleroderma, osteoporosis, uterine hyperplasia, varicose veins, dysmenorrhoea, thrombophlebitis, deep vein thrombosis.

Overdose: No positive action is required other than cessation of therapy.

Pharmacological properties

Pharmacodynamic properties: Medroxyprogesterone acetate exerts anti-oestrogenic, anti-androgenic and antigonadotrophic effects.

Pharmacokinetic properties: Parenteral medroxyprogesterone acetate (MPA) is a long acting progestational steroid. The long duration of action results from its slow absorption from the injection site. Immediately after injection of 150 mg/ml MPA, plasma levels were 1.7±0.3 nmol/l. Two weeks later, levels were 6.8±0.8 nmol/l. Concentrations fell to the initial levels by the end of 12 weeks. At lower doses, plasma levels of MPA appear directly related to the dose administered. Serum accumulation over time was not demonstrated. MPA is eliminated via faecal and urinary excretion. Plasma half-life is about six weeks after a single intramuscular injection. At least 11 metabolites have been reported. All are excreted in the urine, some, but not all, conjugated.

Pharmaceutical particulars

List of excipients: Excipients are methylparaben, polyethylene glycol, polysorbate 80, propylparaben, sodium chloride, hydrochloric acid, sodium hydroxide and water for injections.

Incompatibilities: None known.

Shelf-life: 36 months.

Special precautions for storage: Store below 25°C. Protect from freezing.

Nature and contents of container: 1 ml disposable syringe with plunger stopper and tip cap.

Instructions for use/handling: No special instructions are applicable.

Marketing authorisation number 0032/0082.

Date of first authorisation/renewal of authorisation
Date of Grant: 27 August 1991
Date of Renewal: 6 February 1997.

Date of revision of the text July 1998.

Legal category POM.

DEPO-PROVERA ONCOLOGY* 150 mg/ml

Qualitative and quantitative composition Each ml of suspension contains 150 mg medroxyprogesterone acetate PhEur.

Pharmaceutical form Sterile suspension for injection.

Clinical particulars

Therapeutic indications: Progestogen. As adjunctive therapy in certain classes of malignant tumours exhibiting a degree of hormone sensitivity.

Posology and method of administration: The sterile aqueous suspension should be vigorously shaken just before use to ensure that the dose being given represents a uniform suspension of Depo-Provera Oncology.

Doses should be given by deep intramuscular injection.

Adults: Endometrial or renal carcinoma: the normal initial dose lies in the range 400-1000 mg per week, but doses in excess of 1000 mg per day have been used without serious adverse effects. If improvement is noted within a few weeks or months and the disease appears stabilised, it may be possible to maintain the improvement with as little as 400 mg per month. Depo-Provera Oncology is not recommended as primary therapy, but as adjunctive and palliative treatment in advanced inoperable cases including those with recurrent or metastatic disease.

Breast carcinoma: the recommended schedule is 500 mg/day for 28 days. The patient should then be placed on a maintenance schedule of 500 mg twice weekly as long as the patient is responding to treatment.

Progression of disease at any time during therapy indicates treatment with Depo-Provera should be terminated, although response to hormonal therapy may not be evident until after at least 8--10 weeks of therapy.

Where large doses are being administered, consideration should be given to dividing the dose between two separate sites.

Elderly patients: Medroxyprogesterone acetate has been extensively used in both the young (ages 20--35) and older age groups (ages 50--75). Its use in the young has been primarily for contraception while its use in the older age group has been for the treatment of malignancies. There appears to be no evidence to suggest that the older aged patient is less well prepared to handle the drug metabolically than is the younger aged patient, therefore, in the treatment of carcinoma of the breast, kidney and endometrium, the same dosage, contra-indications and precautions would apply to either age group.

Children: Not appropriate

Contra-indications: Depo-Provera Oncology is contra-indicated in patients with a known sensitivity to medroxyprogesterone acetate or any ingredient of the vehicle.

Depo-Provera Oncology should not be used during pregnancy, either for diagnosis or therapy.

Depo-Provera Oncology is contra-indicated in cancer patients with liver dysfunction or disease.

Depo-Provera Oncology is contra-indicated as a contraceptive at the above dosage in known or suspected hormone-dependent malignancy of breast or genital organs.

Special warnings and special precautions for use:
Warnings: This form of therapy should only be administered under the direction of specialist units having facilities for appropriate surveillance of the patients.

Patients with thromboembolic or coronary vascular disease should be carefully evaluated before using Depo-Provera Oncology.

Any patient who develops an acute impairment of vision, proptosis, diplopia or migraine headache should be carefully evaluated ophthalmologically to exclude the presence of papilloedema or retinal vascular lesions before continuing medication.

Following repeated injections in women, amenorrhoea and anovulation may persist for periods up to 18 months and, in rare instances, for longer periods.

Anaphylactic and anaphylactoid reactions have occasionally been reported.

Animal studies show that medroxyprogesterone acetate possesses adrenocorticoid activity. This has also been reported in man, therefore patients receiving large doses continuously and for long periods of time should be observed closely.

Precautions: Discard any remaining contents after use.

Because progestogens may cause some degree of fluid retention, conditions which might be influenced by this factor, such as epilepsy, migraine, asthma, cardiac or renal dysfunction, require careful observation.

For patients with a history of endogenous depression, the physician should bear in mind the prolonged action of the product when considering the use of Depo-Provera Oncology.

A decrease in glucose tolerance has been observed in some patients on progestogens. The mechanism for this decrease is obscure. For this reason diabetic patients should be carefully observed while receiving progestogen therapy.

Physicians should be aware that pathologists should be informed of the patient's use of Depo-Provera Oncology if endometrial or endocervical tissue is submitted for examination.

The results of certain laboratory tests may be affected by the use of Depo-Provera Oncology. These include gonadotrophin levels (decreased), plasma progesterone levels (decreased), urinary pregnanediol levels (decreased), plasma testosterone levels (in the male), plasma oestrogen levels (in the female) (decreased), plasma cortisol levels (decreased), glucose tolerance test, metyrapone test, liver function tests (may increase), thyroid function tests (protein bound iodine levels may increase and T3 uptake levels may decrease). Coagulation test values for prothrombin (Factor II), and Factors VII, VIII, IX and X may increase.

In the treatment of carcinoma of the breast occasional cases of hypercalcaemia have been reported.

The high doses of medroxyprogesterone used may, in some cases, produce Cushingoid symptoms, e.g. moon facies, fluid retention, glucose intolerance, and blood pressure elevation.

Gynaecomastia, hirsutism and other evidence of virilisation may develop after prolonged courses of Depo-Provera Oncology.

Rare cases of thrombo-embolism have been reported with use of medroxyprogesterone acetate, but causality has not been established.

History or emergence of the following conditions require careful consideration and appropriate investigation: migraine or unusually severe headaches, acute visual disturbances of any kind, pathological changes in liver function and hormone levels.

The effects of medroxyprogesterone acetate on lipid metabolism have been studied with no clear impact demonstrated. Both increases and decreases in total cholesterol, triglycerides and low-density lipoprotein (LDL) cholesterol have been observed in studies. The use of Depo-Provera appears to be associated with a 15–20% reduction in serum high density lipoprotein (HDL) cholesterol levels which may protect women from cardiovascular disease. The clinical consequences of this observation are unknown. The potential for an increased risk of coronary disease should be considered prior to use.

Doctors should carefully consider the use of Depo-Provera Oncology in patients with recent trophoblastic disease before levels of human chorionic gonadotrophin have returned to normal.

Interaction with other medicaments and other forms of interaction: Aminoglutethimide administered concurrently with Depo-Provera Oncology may significantly depress the bioavailability of medroxyprogesterone acetate.

Interactions with other medicinal treatments (including oral anticoagulants) have rarely been reported, but causality has not been determined. The possibility of interaction should be borne in mind in patients receiving concurrent treatment with other drugs.

The clearance of medroxyprogesterone acetate is approximately equal to the rate of hepatic blood flow. Because of this fact, it is unlikely that drugs which induce hepatic enzymes will significantly affect the kinetics of medroxyprogesterone acetate. Therefore, no dose adjustment is recommended in patients receiving drugs known to affect hepatic metabolising enzymes.

Pregnancy and lactation: Depo-Provera Oncology should not be used in pregnancy, either for diagnosis or therapy. Doctors should therefore check that patients are not pregnant before initial injection of Depo-Provera Oncology and also if administration of any subsequent injection is overdue. Congenital anomalies, including female foetal masculinisation and clitoral hypertrophy have been observed following larger doses of progestogens.

Effects on ability to drive and use machines: None.

Undesirable effects: Depending on the volume injected, some patients may be expected to show undesirable sequelae at the site of injection such as residual lump, change in colour of skin or sterile abscess. Other adverse reactions noted, particularly with large doses have been:

Breast: in a few instances breast tenderness or galactorrhoea has occurred.

Psychic: an occasional patient has experienced nervousness, insomnia, somnolence, fatigue or dizziness.

Skin and mucous membranes: sensitivity reactions ranging from pruritus, urticaria, angioneurotic oedema, to generalised rash and anaphylaxis have occasionally been reported. Acne, alopecia or hirsutism have been reported in a few cases.

Gastro-intestinal: rarely nausea has been reported. Jaundice has been noted in a few instances.

Miscellaneous: hyperpyrexia, weight gain and moon facies.

Overdose: No action required other than cessation of therapy.

Pharmacological properties

Pharmacodynamic properties: Medroxyprogesterone acetate exerts anti-oestrogenic, anti-androgenic and antigonadotrophic effects.

Pharmacokinetic properties: Parenteral medroxyprogesterone acetate (MPA) is a long acting progestational steroid. The long duration of action results from its slow absorption from the injection site. Immediately after injection of 150 mg/ml MPA, plasma levels were 1.7 ± 0.3 nmol/l. Two weeks later, levels were 6.8 ± 0.8 nmol/l. Concentrations fell to the initial levels by the end of 12 weeks. At lower doses, plasma levels of MPA appear directly related to the dose administered. Serum accumulation over time was not demonstrated. MPA is eliminated via faecal and urinary excretion. Plasma half-life is about six weeks after a single intramuscular injection. At least 11 metabolites have been reported. All are excreted in the urine, some, but not all, conjugated.

Preclinical safety data: None stated.

Pharmaceutical particulars

List of excipients: Methylparaben, polyethylene glycol, polysorbate 80, propylparaben, sodium chloride, hydrochloric acid, sodium hydroxide and water for injection.

Incompatibilities: None known.

Shelf life: 36 months.

Special precautions for storage: Store below 25° C. Protect from freezing.

Nature and contents of container: Vial with stopper closure.

Instructions for use/handling: Do not mix the suspension with any other agents prior to injection. Discard any remaining contents after use.

Marketing authorisation number 0032/0225.

Date of first authorisation/renewal of authorisation 25 November 1997.

Date of (partial) revision of the text 3 November 1997.

Legal category POM.

DETRUSITOL* 1 mg and 2 mg

Qualitative and quantitative composition Each film-coated tablet contains tolterodine L-tartrate 1 mg or 2 mg corresponding to 0.68 mg or 1.37 mg tolterodine respectively.

Pharmaceutical form Filmcoated tablet.

Clinical particulars

Therapeutic indications: For the treatment of unstable bladder with symptoms of urgency, frequency or urge incontinence.

Posology and method of administration: The recommended dose is 2 mg b.i.d. except in patients with impaired liver function for whom the recommended dose is 1 mg b.i.d. In case of troublesome side-effects the dose may be reduced from 2 mg to 1 mg b.i.d.

After 6 months the need for further treatment should be considered.

Safety and effectiveness in children have not yet been established. Therefore Detrusitol is not recommended for children, until more information is available.

Contra-indications: Tolterodine is contra-indicated in patients with: urinary retention; uncontrolled narrow angle glaucoma; myasthenia gravis; known hypersensitivity to tolterodine or excipients; severe ulcerative colitis; toxic megacolon.

Special warnings and precautions for use: Tolterodine should be used with caution in patients with : significant bladder outlet obstruction at risk of urinary retention; gastrointestinal obstructive disorders e.g. pyloric stenosis; renal disease; hepatic disease. The dosage should not exceed 1 mg b.i.d.; autonomic neuropathy; hiatus hernia

Warning: Organic reasons for urge and frequency should be considered before treatment.

Concomitant treatment with potent CYP3A4 inhibitors, such as macrolide antibiotics (erythromycin and clarithromycin) or antifungal agents (ketoconazole, itraconazole and miconazole) should be avoided until further data are available.

Interaction with other medicaments and other forms of interaction: Concomitant medication with other drugs that possess anticholinergic properties may result in more pronounced therapeutic effect and side-effects. Conversely, the therapeutic effect of tolterodine may be reduced by concomitant administration of muscarinic cholinergic receptor agonists. The effects of prokinetics like metoclopramide and cisapride may be decreased by tolterodine.

Pharmacokinetic interactions are possible with other drugs metabolised by or inhibiting cytochrome P450 2D6 (CYP2D6), or CYP3A4. However, concomitant treatment with fluoxetine, a potent CYP2D6 inhibitor which is metabolised to norfluoxetine, (a CYP3A4 inhibitor), results in only minor increase in the combined exposure of unbound tolterodine and the equipotent 5-hydroxymethyl metabolite. This does not result in a clinically significant interaction.

Patients on concomitant medication with more potent CYP3A4 inhibitors, such as macrolide antibiotics (erythromycin and clarithromycin) or antifungal agents (ketoconazole, itraconazole and miconazole) should be treated with caution until further data are available.

Clinical studies have shown no interactions with warfarin or combined oral contraceptives (ethinyl estradiol/levonorgestrol).

A clinical study with metabolic probe drugs has not given any evidence that the activity of CYP2D6, 2C19, 3A4 or 1A2 will be inhibited by tolterodine.

Pregnancy and lactation: No pregnant women have been included in the clinical studies. Studies in pregnant mice have shown that high doses cause reduced foetal weight, embryolethality and increased incidence of foetal malformations. Until more information is available pregnant women should not be treated with tolterodine.

Women of fertile age should be considered for treatment only if using adequate contraception.

Use of tolterodine during lactation should be avoided since no data in humans are available.

Effects on ability to drive and use machines: Since this drug may cause accommodation disturbances and influence reaction time, the ability to drive and use machines may be negatively affected.

Undesirable effects: Tolterodine may cause mild to moderate anticholinergic effects like dryness of the mouth, dyspepsia and reduced lacrimation.

Common (> 1/100)	*Autonomic Nervous System:* Dry mouth
	GI: Dyspepsia, constipation, abdominal pain, flatulence, vomiting
	General: Headache
	Vision: Xerophthalmia
	Skin: Dry skin
	Psychiatric: Somnolence, nervousness
	CNS: Paraesthesia
Less common (<1/100)	*Autonomic nervous system:* Accommodation disturbance
	General: Chest pain
Uncommon(1/1000):	*General:* Allergic reactions
	Urinary: Urinary retention
	CNS: Confusion

Overdose: The highest dose given to human volunteers of tolterodine L-tartrate is 12.8 mg as a single dose. The most severe adverse events observed were accommodation disturbances and micturition difficulties.

In the event of tolterodine overdose, treat with gastric lavage and give activated charcoal. Treat symptoms as follows:

Severe central anticholinergic effects (e.g. hallucinations, severe excitation):	treat with physostigmine
Convulsions or pronounced excitation:	treat with benzodiazepines
Respiratory insufficiency:	treat with artificial respiration
Tachycardia:	treat with beta-blockers
Urinary retention:	treated with catheterization
Mydriasis:	treat with pilocarpine eye drops and/or place patient in dark room

Pharmacological properties

Pharmacodynamic properties: Tolterodine is a competitive, specific cholinergic receptor antagonist with a selectivity for the urinary bladder rather than salivary glands in-vivo. One of the tolterodine metabolites (5-hydroxymethyl derivative) exhibits a pharmacological profile similar to that of the parent compound. In extensive metabolisers this metabolite contributes significantly to the therapeutic effect.

Effect of the treatment can be expected within 4 weeks.

Effect of treatment with Detrusitol 2 mg twice daily after 4 and 12 weeks, respectively, compared with placebo (pooled data). Absolute change and percentage change relative to baseline (see table).

Pharmacokinetic properties: Tolterodine is rapidly absorbed. Both tolterodine and the 5-hydroxymethyl metabolite reach maximal serum concentrations 1-3 hours after dose. The average peak serum concentrations of tolterodine and the metabolite increase

Variable	4-week studies			12-week studies		
	Detrusitol 2 mg b.i.d.	*Placebo*	*Statistical significance vs. placebo*	*Detrusitol 2 mg b.i.d.*	*Placebo*	*Statistical significance vs. placebo*
Number of micturitions per 24 hours	−1.6 (−14%) n=392	−0.9 (−8%) n=189	*	−2.3 (−20%) n=354	−1.4 (−12%) n=176	**
Number of incontinence episodes per 24 hours	−1.3 (−38%) n=288	−1.0 (−26%) n=151	n.s.	−1.6 (−47%) n=299	−1.1 (−32%) n=145	*
Mean volume voided per micturition (ml)	+25 (+17%) n=385	+12 (+8%) n=185	***	+35 (+22%) n=354	+10 (+6%) n=176	***
Number of patients with no or minimal bladder problems after treatment (%)	16% n=394	7% n=190	**	19% n=356	15% n=177	n.s.

n.s.= not significant; *= p≤0.05; **= p≤0.01; ***= p≤0.001

proportionally in the dose interval 1 to 4 mg. Tolterodine is mainly metabolised by the polymorphic enzyme CYP2D6 leading to the formation of a pharmacologically active 5-hydroxymethyl metabolite. The systemic serum clearance of tolterodine in extensive metabolisers is about 30 L/h and the terminal half-life is 2 – 3 hours. The half-life of the 5-hydroxymethyl metabolite is 3 – 4 hours. In poor metabolisers (deficient of CYP2D6) tolterodine is dealkylated via CYP34A isoenzymes whereby N-dealkylated tolterodine is formed. This metabolite does not contribute to the clinical effect. The reduced clearance and prolonged half-life (about 10 hours) of the parent compound in poor metabolisers lead to increased concentrations of tolterodine (about 7-fold) associated with undetectable concentrations of the 5-hydroxymethyl metabolite. As a result, the exposure (AUC) of unbound tolterodine in poor metabolisers is similar to the combined exposure of unbound tolterodine and the 5-hydroxymethyl metabolite in patients with CYP2D6 activity given the same dosage regimen. The safety, tolerability and clinical response are similar irrespective of phenotype. Steady state concentrations are reached within 2 days.

The absolute bioavailability of tolterodine is 65% in poor metabolisers (devoid of CYP2D6) and 17% in extensive metabolisers (the majority of the patients).

Food does not influence the exposure to the unbound tolterodine and the active 5-hydroxymethyl metabolite in extensive metabolisers, although the tolterodine levels increase when taken with food. Clinically relevant changes are likewise not expected in poor metabolisers.

Tolterodine and the 5-hydroxymethyl metabolite bind primarily to orosomucoid. The unbound fractions are 3.7 and 36%, respectively. The volume of distribution of tolterodine is 113 L. The excretion of radioactivity after [^{14}C]-tolterodine is approximately 77% in urine and 17% in faeces. Less than 1% of the dose is excreted as unchanged drug and about 4% of the 5-hydroxymethyl metabolite. The carboxylated metabolite and the corresponding dealkylated metabolite account for about 51% and 29% of the urinary recovery, respectively.

About 2-fold higher exposure of unbound tolterodine and the 5-hydroxymethyl metabolite is found in liver cirrhosis subjects.

Preclinical safety data: In toxicity, genotoxicity, carcinogenicity and safety pharmacology studies no clinically relevant effects have been observed, except those related to the pharmacological effect of the drug.

Reduced foetal weight, embryolethality and increased incidence of foetal malformations have been observed in pregnant mice treated with high doses. No effects were observed at a systemic exposure (measured as C_{max} or AUC for unbound tolterodine and its active metabolite) 9–50 times higher than in humans after the highest recommended dose.

In dogs a slight prolongation of the QT interval has been observed at high concentrations of tolterodine or its main metabolite (50–100 times therapeutic levels). In clinical trials, no QT interval prolongation has been found in a large and representative patient sample, on recommended doses of Detrusitol.

Pharmaceutical particulars

List of excipients

Core: Cellulose, microcrystalline
Calcium hydrogen phosphate dihydrate
Sodium starch glycollate (type B)
Magnesium stearate
Colloidal anhydrous silica

Film coating: Coating granules containing:
hypromellose
cellulose, microcrystalline
stearic acid
titanium dioxide

Incompatibilities: No incompatibilities are known.

Shelf life: 24 months

Special precautions for storage: No.

Nature and contents of container: Tablets are packed in blister packages made of PVC/PVDC and aluminium foil with a heat seal coating of PVDC.

Tablet description:

1 mg tablet: White, round, biconvex, filmcoated tablet. Engraved with arcs above and below the letters TO.

2 mg tablet: White, round, biconvex, filmcoated tablet. Engraved with arcs above and below the letters DT.

Package sizes: Detrusitol 1 mg and 2 mg in cartons of 56 containing 4 blister strips of 14 tablets each.

Instructions for use/handling: N/A.

Marketing authorisation numbers

Detrusitol 1 mg tablets 0032/0222
Detrusitol 2 mg tablets 0032/0223

Date of first authorisation/renewal of authorisation Not applicable.

Date of (partial) revision of the text 19 December 1997.

Legal category POM.

DIPENTUM*

Presentation Caramel coloured capsules containing 250 mg olsalazine sodium.

Yellow capsule shaped tablets containing 500 mg olsalazine sodium with 'KPh' on one side and code '110' and score line on the other.

Uses Oral treatment of acute mild ulcerative colitis and the maintenance of remission. Olsalazine consists of two molecules of 5-amino-salicylic acid (5-ASA) joined through an azo-bond. The systemic absorption of olsalazine is minimal. 99% of an oral dose will reach the colon. Olsalazine is activated in the colon where it is converted into 5-ASA. The release of 5-ASA is neither pH nor time dependent. 5-ASA acts topically on the colonic mucosa and local colonic concentrations of 5-ASA are more than 1000 time that found in the serum.

Dosage and administration

General: Olsalazine taken on an empty stomach may sometimes lead to loose stools or diarrhoea. By taking the drug at the end of a meal, this may be avoided.

Acute mild disease

Adults including the elderly: Commence on 1 g daily in divided doses taken at the end of meals. Depending on the patient's response, the dose may be titrated upwards over a period of 1 week to a maximum of 3 g daily.

A single dose should not exceed 1 g.

Remission

Adults including the elderly: A dose of 0.5 g should be taken twice daily, at the end of meals.

Olsalazine has been used concomitantly with glucocorticosteroids.

Contra-indications, warnings, etc

Contra-indications: Hypersensitivity to salicylates.

There is no experience of the use of olsalazine in patients with significant renal impairment. Olsalazine is contra-indicated in patients with significant renal impairment.

Precautions: Serious blood dyscrasias have been reported very rarely with olsalazine. Haematological investigations should be performed if the patient develops unexplained bleeding, bruising, purpura, anaemia, fever or sore throat. Treatment should be stopped if there is a suspicion or evidence of a blood dyscrasia.

Pregnancy and lactation: Reproduction studies performed in mice, rats and rabbits have revealed no evidence of impaired fertility, harm to the foetus or teratogenic effects due to olsalazine administration. However, the experience of use in pregnant women is limited.

Dipentum should not be used during pregnancy unless the clinician considers that the potential benefit outweighs the possible risk to the foetus.

Adverse reactions: As with sulphasalazine and mesalazine gastrointestinal side-effects are the most common. The most frequently reported adverse reactions are diarrhoea, arthralgia and rash.

A watery diarrhoea occurs in some patients. This is usually controlled by taking the drug at the end of a meal, as directed. Dose reduction or titration may also help.

Blood dyscrasias have been reported in a few patients: leucopenia, neutropenia, aplastic anaemia, pancytopenia, thrombocytopenia, anaemia and haemolytic anaemia.

Treatment of overdosage: There is no specific antidote to olsalazine. Treatment should be supportive.

Pharmaceutical precautions Store in a dry place.

Legal category POM.

Package quantities Containers of 60 tablets Containers of 112 capsules.

Further information Olsalazine has been used concomitantly with gluco-corticosteroids.

Product licence numbers

Capsules: 0022/0134
Tablets: 0022/0135

DOSTINEX* ▼

Presentation Flat, capsule-shaped, 4×8 mm, scored, white tablets, each containing 0.5 mg cabergoline, in type I amber glass bottles with tamper resistant screw caps and containing silica gel dessicant. Each bottle contains 8 tablets and is enclosed in an outer cardboard carton. The tablets are for oral administration.

Uses

Inhibition/suppression of physiological lactation: Dostinex is indicated for the inhibition of physiological lactation soon after delivery and for suppression of already established lactation: 1. After parturition, when the mother elects not to breast feed the infant or when breast feeding is contraindicated due to medical reasons related to the mother or the newborn.

2. After stillbirth or abortion.

Treatment of hyperprolactinemic disorder: Dostinex is indicated for the treatment of dysfunctions associated with hyperprolactinemia, including amenorrhea, oligomenorrhea, anovulation and galactorrhea. Dostinex is indicated in patients with prolactin-secreting pituitary adenomas (micro- and macroprolactinomas), idiopathic hyperprolactinemia, or empty sella syndrome with associated hyperprolactinemia, which represent the basic underlying pathologies contributing to the above clinical manifestations.

Dosage and administration Dostinex is to be administered by the oral route. Since in clinical studies Dostinex has been mainly administered with food and since the tolerability of this class of compounds is improved with food, it is recommended that Dostinex be preferably taken with meals for all the therapeutic indications.

Inhibition/suppression of physiological lactation: For INHIBITION of lactation Dostinex should be administered during the first day post-partum. The recommended therapeutic dosage is 1 mg (two 0.5 mg tablets) given as a single dose.

For SUPPRESSION of established lactation the recommended therapeutic dosage regimen is 0.25 mg (one-half 0.5 mg tablet) every 12 hours for two days (1 mg total dose). This dosage regimen has been demonstrated to be better tolerated than the single dose regimen in women electing to suppress lactation having a lower incidence of adverse events, in particular of hypotensive symptoms.

Treatment of hyperprolactinemia disorders: The recommended initial dosage of Dostinex is 0.5 mg per week given in one or two (one-half of one 0.5 mg tablet) doses (e.g. on Monday and Thursday) per week. The weekly dose should be increased gradually, preferably by adding 0.5 mg per week at monthly intervals until an optimal therapeutic response is achieved. The therapeutic dosage is usually 1 mg per week and ranges from 0.25 mg to 2 mg per week. Doses of Dostinex up to 4.5 mg per week have been used in hyperprolactinemic patients. The weekly dose may be given as a single administration or divided into two or more doses per week according to patient tolerability. Division of the weekly dose into multiple administrations is advised when doses higher than 1 mg per week are to be given since the tolerability of doses greater than 1 mg taken as a single weekly dose has been evaluated only in a few patients. Patients should be evaluated during dose escalation to determine the lowest dosage that produces the therapeutic response. Monitoring of serum prolactin levels at monthly intervals is advised since, once the effective therapeutic dosage regimen has been reached, serum prolactin normalisation is usually observed within two to four weeks. After Dostinex withdrawal, recurrence of hyperprolactinemia is usually observed. However, persistent suppression of prolactin levels has been observed for several months in some patients. Of the group of women followed-up 23–29 had ovulatory cycles which continued for greater than 6 months.

Use in children: The safety and efficacy of Dostinex has not been established in subjects less than 16 years of age.

Use in the elderly: As a consequence of the indications for which Dostinex is presently proposed, the experience in elderly is very limited. Available data do not indicate a special risk.

Contra-indications, warnings, etc

Contra-indications: Hypersensitivity to any ergot alkaloid. Dostinex is contra-indicated in patients with hepatic insufficiency and with toxaemia of pregnancy. Dostinex should not be co-administered with anti-psychotic medications or administered to women with a history of puerperal psychosis.

Precautions: The safety and efficacy of Dostinex have not yet been established in patients with renal and hepatic disease. Dostinex should be given with caution to subjects with cardiovascular disease, Raynaud's syndrome, renal insufficiency, peptic ulcer, gastrointestinal bleeding or a history of serious, particularly psychotic, mental disease. Particular care should be taken when patients are taking concomitant psychoactive medication. Symptomatic hypotension can occur with Dostinex administration for any indication. Care should be exercised when administering Dostinex concomitantly with other drugs known to lower blood pressure. The effects of alcohol on overall tolerability of Dostinex are currently unknown. Before Dostinex administration, pregnancy should be excluded and after treatment pregnancy should be prevented for at least one month.

Inhibition/suppression of physiological lactation: By analogy with other ergot derivatives, Dostinex should not be used in women with pre-eclampsia and should be used with caution in patients with post-partum hypertension. In post-partum studies with Dostinex, blood pressure decreases were mostly symptomatic and were frequently observed on a single occasion 2 to 4 days after treatment. Since decreases in blood pressure are frequently noted during the puerperium, independently of drug therapy, it is likely that many of the observed decreases in blood pressure after Dostinex administration were not drug-induced. However, periodic monitoring of blood pressure, particularly during the first days after Dostinex administration, is advised. Dostinex should not be administered as a single dose greater than 0.25 mg in nursing women treated for suppression of established lactation since a clinical study exploring the efficacy and tolerability of 0.5 mg of Dostinex given as a single dose for suppression of lactation has shown that the risk of side effects is approximately doubled in this indication if the drug is administered as a single dose of 0.5 mg. In rats Dostinex and/or its metabolites are excreted in milk. Therefore, while no information on the excretion of Dostinex in maternal milk in humans is available, puerperal women should be advised not to breast-feed in case of failed lactation inhibition/suppression by Dostinex.

Treatment of hyperprolactinemic disorders: Since hyperprolactinemia with amenorrhea/galactorrhea and infertility may be associated with pituitary tumours, a complete evaluation of the pituitary is indicated before treatment with Dostinex is initiated. Dostinex restores ovulation and fertility in women with hyperprolactinemic hypogonadism: since pregnancy might occur prior to reinitiation of menses, a pregnancy test is recommended at least every four weeks during the amenorrheic period and, once menses are reinitiated, every time a menstrual period is delayed by more than three days. Women not seeking pregnancy should be advised to use mechanical contraception during treatment and after Dostinex withdrawal until recurrence of anovulation. Because of the still limited experience on the safety of fetal exposure to Dostinex, until further data become available it is advisable that women seeking pregnancy conceive at least one month after Dostinex discontinuation given that ovulatory cycles persist in some patients for 6 months after drug withdrawal. Should pregnancy occur during treatment, Dostinex is to be discontinued. As a precautionary measure, women who become pregnant should be monitored to detect signs of pituitary enlargement since expansion of pre-existing pituitary tumours may occur during gestation. Regular gynaecological assessment, including cervical and endometrial cytology, is recommended for patients taking Dostinex for extensive periods.

Interactions: The concomitant use of other drugs during early puerperium, particularly of ergot alkaloids, was not associated with detectable interactions modifying the efficacy and safety of Dostinex. Although there is no conclusive evidence of an interaction between Dostinex and other ergot alkaloids the concomitant use of these medications during long term treatment with Dostinex is not recommended. Since Dostinex exerts its therapeutic effect by direct stimulation of dopamine receptors, it should not be concurrently administered with drugs which have dopamine antagonist activity (such as phenothiazines, butyrophenones, thioxanthenes, metoclopramide) since these might reduce the prolactin-lowering effect of Dostinex. By analogy with other ergot derivatives, Dostinex should not be used in association with macrolide antibiotics (e.g. erythromycin) since the systemic bioavailability and also adverse effects could increase.

Pregnancy and lactation: Dostinex crosses the placenta in rats: it is unknown whether this occurs also in humans. Studies in animal models have not demonstrated any teratogenic effect. In clinical studies there have been over 100 pregnancies in women treated for hyperprolactinemic disorders. Dostinex was generally taken during the first 8 weeks after conception. Among the pregnancies evaluable so far, there were approximately 85% live births and about 10% spontaneous abortions. Three cases of congenital abnormalities (Down's syndrome, hydrocephalus, malformation of lower limbs) which led to therapeutic abortion and three cases of minor abnormalities in live births were observed. These incidence rates are comparable with those quoted for normal populations and for women exposed to other ovulation-inducing drugs. Based on the above data, the use of Dostinex does not appear to be associated with an increased risk of abortion, premature delivery, multiple pregnancy, or congenital abnormalities. Because clinical experience is still limited and the drug has a long half life, as a precautionary measure it is recommended that once regular ovulatory cycles have been achieved women seeking pregnancy discontinue Dostinex one month before intended conception. This will prevent possible fetal exposure to the drug and will not interfere with the possibility of conception since ovulatory cycles persist in some cases for six months after withdrawal. If conception occurs during therapy, treatment is to be discontinued as soon as pregnancy is confirmed to limit fetal exposure to the drug. Before Dostinex administration, pregnancy should be excluded and after treatment pregnancy should be prevented for at least one month. Dostinex should not be administered to mothers who elect to breast-feed their infants since it prevents lactation and no information is available on excretion of the drug in maternal milk.

Effects on ability to drive and use machines: During the first days of Dostinex administration, patients should be cautioned about re-engaging in activities requiring rapid and precise responses such as driving an automobile or operating machinery.

Undesirable effects:

Inhibition suppression of lactation: Approximately 14% of women treated with a single 1 mg Dostinex for inhibition of physiological lactation complained of at least one side effect. All side effects were mild to moderate in severity and of a transient nature. The most frequently occurring adverse events were dizziness/vertigo, headache, nausea and abdominal pain. In addition, rarely palpitations, epigastric pain, somnolence, epistaxis and transient hemianopsia were reported. Asymptomatic decreases in blood pressure (≥20 mm Hg systolic and ≥10 mm Hg diastolic) may occur usually once during the first 3–4 days post-partum. Adverse effects have been observed in approximately 14% of nursing women treated with 0.25 mg of Dostinex every 12 hours for two days for *suppression of lactation.* The most frequent symptoms were dizziness/vertigo, headache, nausea, somnolence, abdominal pain. In addition, rarely, vomiting, syncope, asthenia, and hot flushes were reported. Most side effects were transient and mild to moderate in severity.

Hyperprolactinemic disorders: Data obtained in a controlled clinical trial of 6 months therapy with doses ranging between 1 and 2 mg per week given in two weekly administrations, indicate a 68% incidence of adverse events during Dostinex therapy; this was significantly lower than the incidence observed for the reference standard compound. Moreover, the symptoms were generally mild to moderate in degree, mainly appearing during the first two weeks of therapy, and mostly disappearing despite continued therapy. Severe adverse events were reported at least once during therapy by 14% of patients but therapy was discontinued because of adverse events in only approximately 3% of patients. Dostinex withdrawal results in reversal of side effects, usually within a few days after discontinuation. The most common symptoms in decreasing rank of frequency were nausea, headache, dizziness/vertigo, abdominal pain/dyspepsia/gastritis, asthenia/fatigue, constipation, vomiting, breast pain, hot flushes, depression and paraesthesia. Dostinex generally exerts a hypotensive effect in patients treated chronically: however, symptomatic hypotension or fainting have been rarely reported. Being an ergot derivative, Dostinex may also act in some patients as a vasoconstrictor: digital vasospasm and leg cramps have been occasionally reported. Side effects are generally dose-related. In patients known to be intolerant of dopaminergic drugs, side effects may be lessened by starting Dostinex therapy with reduced doses (e.g. 0.25 mg once a week) with subsequent gradual increase until the therapeutic range is reached. In case of persistent or severe adverse events, temporary reduction of dosage followed by a more gradual increase (e.g. in steps of 0.25 mg per week fortnightly) may result in reversal of side effects once they have occurred. Alterations in standard laboratory tests are uncommon during long term therapy with Dostinex: a decrease in haemoglobin values have been observed in amenorrheic women during the first few months after menses resumption.

Overdose: There is no experience in humans of overdosage of Dostinex in the proposed indications: it is likely to lead to symptoms due to over-stimulation of dopamine receptors. These might include nausea, vomiting, gastric complaints, hypotension, confusion/psychosis or hallucinations. General supportive measures should be undertaken to remove any unabsorbed drug and maintain blood pressure if necessary. In addition, the administration of dopamine antagonist drugs may be advisable.

Pharmaceutical precautions Bottles of Dostinex are supplied with dessicant in caps. This dessicant must not be removed.

Legal category POM.

Package quantities Bottles of 8 tablets.

Further information Nil.

Product licence number 3433/0169.

DOXORUBICIN RAPID DISSOLUTION

Qualitative and quantitative composition
Doxorubicin Hydrochloride HSE 10.0 mg
Doxorubicin Hydrochloride HSE 50.0 mg

Pharmaceutical form Freeze-dried powder for injection.

Clinical particulars

Therapeutic indications: The treatment of a wide range of neoplastic diseases including acute leukaemia, lymphoma, paediatric malignancies and adult solid tumours, in particular, breast and lung carcinomas.

Posology and method of administration

Route of administration: The proposed routes of administration are intravenous and intra-arterial injection and intravesical instillation. Doxorubicin cannot be used as an antibacterial agent.

The vial contents must be reconstituted before use with water for injections or normal saline.

Adults and children: Intravenous administration: The reconstituted solution is given via the tubing of a freely-running intravenous infusion, taking 2–3 minutes over the injection. Commonly used acceptable solutions are sodium chloride injection, dextrose injection 5% or sodium chloride and dextrose injection.

Dosage is usually calculated on the basis of body surface area. On this basis, 60–70 mg/m² may be given every three weeks when doxorubicin is used alone. If it is used in combination with other antitumour agents having overlapping toxicity, the dosage for doxorubicin may need to be reduced to 30–40 mg/m² every three weeks. If dosage is to be calculated on the basis of body weight, 1.2–2.4 mg/kg should be given as a single dose every three weeks.

It has been shown that giving doxorubicin as a single dose every three weeks greatly reduces the distressing toxic effect, mucositis; however there are still some who believe that dividing the dose over three successive days (0.4–0.8 mg/kg or 20–25 mg/m² on each day) gives greater effectiveness even though at the cost of high toxicity.

Administration of doxorubicin in a weekly regimen has been shown to be as effective as the 3-weekly regimen. The recommended dosage is 20 mg/m² weekly although objective responses have been seen at 6-12 mg/m². Weekly administration leads to a reduction in cardiotoxicity.

Dosage may need to be reduced for patients who have had prior treatment with other cytotoxic agents.

Dosage may also need to be reduced in children and the elderly.

If hepatic function is impaired, doxorubicin should be reduced according to the following table:

Serum bilirubin levels	*BSP retention*	*Recommended dose*
1.2–3.0 mg/100 ml	9–15%	50% normal dose
>3.0 mg/100 ml	>15%	25% normal dose

Intra-arterial administration: Intra-arterial injection has been used in attempts to produce intense local activity while keeping the total dose low and therefore reducing general toxicity. It should be emphasised that this technique is potentially extremely hazardous and can lead to widespread necrosis of the perfuse tissue unless due precautions are taken.

Intra-arterial injection should only be attempted by those fully conversant with this technique.

Intravesical administration: Doxorubicin is being increasingly used by intravesical administration for the treatment of transitional cell carcinoma, papillary bladder tumours and carcinoma-in-situ. It should not be employed in this way for the treatment of invasive tumours which have penetrated the bladder wall. It has also been found useful to instil doxorubicin into the bladder at intervals after transurethral resection of a tumour in order to reduce the probability of recurrence.

While at present many regimens are in use, making interpretation difficult, the following may be helpful guides:

The concentration of doxorubicin in the bladder should be 50 mg per 50 ml.

To avoid undue dilution with urine, the patient should be instructed not to drink any fluid in the 12 hours prior to instillation.

This should limit urine production to approximately 50 ml per hour. The patient should be rotated a quarter turn every 15 minutes while the drug is in situ.

Exposure to the drug solution for one hour is generally adequate and the patient should be instructed to void at the end of this time.

Contra-indications: Hypersensitivity to hydroxybenzoates is a contra-indication. Dosage should not be repeated in the presence of bone-marrow depression or buccal ulceration. The latter may be preceded by premonitory buccal burning sensations and repetition in the presence of this symptom is not advised.

Special warnings and precautions for use: A cumulative dose of 450–550 mg/m² should only be exceeded with extreme caution. Above this level, the risk of irreversible congestive cardiac failure increases greatly. The total dose of doxorubicin administered to the individual patient should also take account of any previous of concomitant therapy with other potentially cardiotoxic agents such as high-dose i.v. cyclophosphamide, mediastinal irradiation or related anthracycline compounds such as daunorubicin. Administration of doxorubicin weekly has been shown to be associated with reduced cardiotoxicity compared with a 3-weekly schedule allowing patients to be treated to a higher cumulative dose. It should be noted that cardiac failure may also occur several weeks after administration and may not respond to treatment.

Baseline and follow-up ECGs during and immediately after drug administration are advisable. Transient ECG changes, such as T-wave flattening, S-T segment depression and arrhythmias, are not considered indications for the suspension of doxorubicin therapy. A reduction of the QRS wave is considered more indicative of cardiac toxicity. If this change occurs, the benefit of continued therapy must be carefully evaluated against the risk of producing irreversible cardiac damage.

Accidental contact with the skin or eyes should be treated immediately by copious lavage with water or soap and water or if available sodium bicarbonate solution.

Interaction with other medicaments and other forms of interaction: None stated.

Pregnancy and lactation: There is no conclusive evidence as to whether doxorubicin may adversely affect human fertility or cause teratogenesis. Experimental data, however, suggest that doxorubicin may harm the foetus and should, therefore, not be administered to pregnant women or to mothers who are breast-feeding.

Effects on ability to drive and use machines: None stated.

Undesirable effects: Haematological monitoring should be undertaken regularly in both haematological and non-haematological conditions, because of the possibility of bone-marrow depression which may become evident around ten days from the time of administration.

The occurrence of secondary acute myeloid leukaemia with or without a pre-leukaemic phase has been reported rarely in patients concurrently treated with doxorubicin in association with DNA-damaging antineoplastic agents. Such cases could have a short (1–3 year) latency period.

Cardiotoxicity may be manifested in tachycardia including supraventricular tachycardia and ECG changes. Routine ECG monitoring is recommended and caution should be exercised in patients with impaired cardiac function.

Severe cardiac failure may occur suddenly, without premonitory ECG changes.

Doxorubicin Rapid Dissolution may impart a red colour to the urine, particularly to the first specimen passed after the injection, and patients should be advised that this is no cause for alarm.

Alopecia occurs frequently, including the interruption of beard growth, but all hair growth normally resumes after treatment is stopped. Nausea, vomiting and diarrhoea may also occur.

The risk of thrombophlebitis at the injection site may be minimised by following the procedure for administration recommended above. A stinging or burning sensation at the site of administration signifies a small degree of extravasation and the infusion should be stopped and re-started in another vein.

Overdose: Single doses of 250 mg and 500 mg of doxorubicin have proved fatal. Such doses may cause acute myocardial degeneration within 24 hours and severe myelosuppression, the effects of which are greatest between 10 and 15 days after administration. Treatment should aim to support the patient during this period and should utilise such measures as blood transfusions and reverse barrier nursing.

Delayed cardiac failure may occur up to six months after the overdose. Patients should be observed carefully and should signs of cardiac failure arise, be treated along conventional lines.

Pharmacological properties

Pharmacodynamic properties: Doxorubicin is an antitumour agent. Tumour cells are probably killed through drug-induced alterations of nucleic acid synthesis although the exact mechanism of action have not yet been clearly elucidated.

Proposed mechanism of action include:

DNA intercalation (leading to an inhibition of synthesis of DNA, RNA and proteins), formation of highly reactive free-radicals and superoxides, chelation of divalent cations, the inhibition of Na-K ATPase and the binding of doxorubicin to certain constituents of cell membranes (particularly to the membrane lipids, spectrin and cardiolipin). Highest drug concentrations are attained in the lung, liver, spleen, kidney, heart, small intestine and bone-marrow. Doxorubicin does not cross the blood-brain barrier.

Pharmacokinetic properties: After i.v. administration, the plasma disappearance curve of doxorubicin is triphasic with half-lives of 12 minutes, 3.3 hours and 30 hours. The relatively long terminal elimination half-life reflects doxorubicin's distribution into a deep tissue compartment. Only about 33 to 50% of fluorescent or tritiated drug (or degradation products), respectively, can be accounted for in urine, bile and faeces for up to 5 days after i.v. administration. The remainder of the doxorubicin and degradation products appear to be retained for long periods of time in body tissues.

In cancer patients, doxorubicin is reduced to adriamycinol, which is an active cytotoxic agent. This reduction appears to be catalysed by cytoplasmic nadph-dependent aldo-keto reductases that are found in all tissues and play an important role in determining the overall pharmacokinetics of doxorubicin.

Microsomal glycosidases present in most tissues split doxorubicin and adriamycinol into inactive aglycones. The aglycones may then undergo 0-demethylation, followed by conjugation to sulphate or glucuronide esters, and excretion in the bile.

Preclinical safety data: No further preclinical safety data available.

Pharmaceutical particulars

List of excipients:

Lactose	PhEur.
Methyl hydroxybenzoate	PhEur.
Water for Injections	PhEur.

Incompatibilities: Doxorubicin Rapid Dissolution should not be mixed with heparin as a precipitate may form and it is not recommended that Doxorubicin Rapid Dissolution be mixed with other drugs.

Shelf life: The shelf-life for Doxorubicin Rapid Dissolution is 48 months. Once reconstituted, the solution should be used straight away. If not it may be stored for up to 24 hours.

Special precautions for storage: None.

Nature and contents of container: Glass vial, type III, with white or grey rubber stopper, aluminium seal and snap cap (10 and 50 mg vials).

Instructions for use/handling: The vial contents are under a negative pressure to minimise aerosol formation during reconstitution, particular care should be taken when the needle is inserted. Inhalation of any aerosol produced during reconstitution must be avoided.

The following protective recommendations are given due to the toxic nature of this substance:

Personnel should be trained in good technique for reconstitution and handling.

Pregnant staff should be excluded from working with this drug.

Personnel handling Doxorubicin should wear protective clothing: goggles, gowns and disposable gloves and masks.

A designated area should be defined for reconstitution (preferably under a laminar flow system). The work surface should be protected by disposable plastic-backed absorbent paper.

All items used for reconstitution, administration or cleaning, including gloves, should be placed in high-risk waste-disposal bags for high temperature incineration.

The reconstituted solution contains 0.02% methylhydroxybenzoate. This is not a preservative solution. Discard any unused solution.

Accidental contact with the skin or eyes should be treated immediately by copious lavage with water, or soap and water, or sodium bicarbonate solution: medical attention should be sought.

Spillage or leakage should be treated with dilute sodium hypochlorite (1% available chlorine) solution, preferably soaking overnight and then water. All cleaning materials should be disposed of as indicated previously.

Marketing authorisation number 3433/0110.

Date of first authorisation/renewal of authorisation 25 June 1987/25 June 1992.

Date of (partial) revision of the text 4 April 1998.

Legal category POM.

DOXORUBICIN SOLUTION FOR INJECTION

Qualitative and quantitative composition Doxorubicin Hydrochloride 2 mg/ml

Pharmaceutical form Solution for intravenous use.

Clinical particulars

Therapeutic indications: Antimitotic and cytotoxic. Doxorubicin has been used successfully to produce regression in a wide range of neoplastic conditions including acute leukaemia, lymphomas, soft-tissue and osteogenic sarcomas, paediatric malignancies and adult solid tumours; in particular breast and lung carcinomas.

Doxorubicin is frequently used in combination chemotherapy regimens with other cytotoxic drugs. Doxorubicin cannot be used as an antibacterial agent.

Posology and method of administration: The solution is given via the tubing of a freely running intravenous infusion, taking 2 to 3 minutes over the injection. This technique minimises the risk of thrombosis or perivenous extravasation which can lead to severe cellulitis and vesication.

Dosage is usually calculated on the basis of body surface area. On this basis, 60–75 mg/m² may be given every three weeks when doxorubicin is used alone. If it used in combination with other antitumour agents having overlapping toxicity, the dosage of doxorubicin may need to be reduced to 30–40 mg/m² every three weeks.

If dosage is calculated on the basis of body weight, it has been shown that giving doxorubicin as a single dose every three weeks greatly reduces the distressing toxic effect, mucositis; however, there are still some who believe that dividing the dose over three successive days (0.4–0.8 mg/kg or 20–25 mg/m² on each day) gives greater effectiveness though at the cost of higher toxicity.

Administration of doxorubicin in a weekly regimen has been shown to be as effective as the 3-weekly regimen. The recommended dosage is 20 mg/m² weekly, although, objective responses have been seen at 16 mg/m² . Weekly administration leads to a reduction in cardiotoxicity.

Dosage may also need to be reduced in children and the elderly.

If hepatic function is impaired, doxorubicin dosage should be reduced according to the following table:

Serum bilirubin levels	*BSP retention*	*Recommended dose*
1.2–3.0 mg/100 ml	9–15%	50% Normal dose
>3.0 mg/100 ml	>15%	25% Normal Dose

Contra-indications: Dosage should not be repeated in the presence of bone marrow depression or buccal ulceration. The latter may be preceded by premonitory buccal burning sensations and repetition in the presence of this symptom is not advised.

Special warnings and precautions for use: A cumulative dose of 450–500 mg/m² should only be exceeded with extreme caution. Above this level, the risk of irreversible congestive cardiac failure increases greatly. The total dose of doxorubicin administered to the individual patient should also take into account any previous or concomitant therapy with other potentially cardiotoxic agents such as high-dose i.v. cyclophosphamide, mediastinal irradiation or related anthracycline compounds such as daunorubicin.

Administration weekly has been shown to be associated with reduced cardiotoxicity compared with a 3-weekly schedule, allowing patients to be treated with a higher cumulative dose.

It should be noted that cardiac failure may also occur several weeks after administration and may not respond to treatment. Baseline and follow-up ECGs during and immediately after drug administration are advisable. Transient ECG changes, such as T-wave flattening, S-T segment depression and arrhythmias are not considered indications for suspension of doxorubicin therapy. A reduction of the QRS wave is considered more indicative of cardiac toxicity. If this change occurs, the benefit of continued therapy must be carefully evaluated against the risk of producing irreversible cardiac damage.

Interaction with other medicaments and other forms of interaction: None stated.

Pregnancy and lactation: There is no conclusive evidence as to whether doxorubicin may adversely affect human fertility or cause teratogenesis. Experimental data however suggest that doxorubicin may harm the foetus and should not therefore be administered to pregnant women or those who are breast feeding.

Effects on ability to drive and use machines: None stated.

Undesirable effects: Haematological monitoring should be undertaken regularly in both haematological and non haematological conditions, because of the possibility of bone-marrow depression which may become evident around ten days from the time of administration.

The occurrence of secondary acute myeloid leukaemia with or without a pre-leukaemic phase has been reported rarely in patients concurrently treated with doxorubicin in association with DNA damaging antineoplastic agents. Such cases could have a short (1–3 year) latency period.

Cardiotoxicity may be manifested in tachycardia including supraventricular tachycardia and ECG changes. Routine ECG monitoring is recommended and caution should be exercised in patients with impaired cardiac function. Severe cardiac failure may occur suddenly, without premonitory ECG changes.

Doxorubicin solution for injection may impart a red colour to the urine particularly to the first specimen passed after the injection, and patients should be advised that there is no cause for alarm.

Alopecia occurs frequently, including the interruption of beard growth, but all hair growth normally returns after treatment is stopped. Nausea, vomiting and diarrhoea may also occur.

The risk of thrombophlebitis at the injection site may be minimised by following the procedure for administration recommended above. A stinging or burning sensation signifies a small degree of extravasation and the infusion should be stopped and restarted in another vein.

Overdose: Single doses of 250 mg and 500 mg of doxorubicin have proved fatal. Such doses may cause acute myocardial degeneration within 24 hours and severe myelosupression, the effects of which are greatest between 10 and 15 days after administration. Treatment should aim to support the patient during this period and should utilise such measures as blood transfusions and reverse barrier nursing.

Delayed cardiac failure may occur up to six months after the overdosage. Patients should be observed carefully and should signs of cardiac failure arise, be treated along conventional lines.

Pharmacological properties

Pharmacodynamic properties: Doxorubicin is an antitumour agent which forms a strong complex with DNA which is associated with various physical changes in the DNA molecule. The DNA and RNA polymerase reactions are inhibited and consequently nucleic acid synthesis is reduced. Free radicals generated by interactions with phospholipids may provide the mechanisms for cellular damage leading to cell death.

Pharmacokinetic properties: After IV injection, doxorubicin is rapidly cleared form the blood and taken up by the tissues. Drug retention is pronounced and persistent in the spleen, lymph nodes and bone marrow. Relatively low but persistent levels are found in tumour tissue.

Doxorubicin does not cross the blood-brain barrier.

Drug elimination takes place mainly through the bile with a t_{50} of about 7 days

Doxorubicin is metabolised initially to adriamycinol and subsequently to minor metabolites.

Preclinical safety data: No information in addition to that presented elsewhere in this Summary of Product Characteristics is available.

Pharmaceutical particulars

List of excipients: Water for Injections PhEur, Sodium chloride PhEur, Hydrochloric acid PhEur.

Incompatibilities: Doxorubicin should not be mixed with heparin as a precipitate may form and it is not recommended that doxorubicin be mixed with other drugs.

Shelf life: 2 years.

Special precautions for storage: Store refrigerated between 2–8°C.

Nature and contents of container: Single glass vials of 5 ml (10 mg), 10 ml (20 mg), 25 ml (50 mg) and 100 ml (200 mg).

Single Cytosafe™ polypropylene vials of 5 ml (10 mg), 10 ml (20 mg), 25 ml (50 mg) and 100 ml (200 mg).

Instructions for use/handling: For use only under the direction of those experienced in cytotoxic therapy.

Unused solution should be discarded after use

Marketing authorisation number 3433/0127.

Date of first authorisation/renewal of authorisation Renewed 25 January 1995.

Date of (partial) revision of the text 24 October 1997.

Legal category POM.

EDRONAX* 

Qualitative and quantitative composition Reboxetine 4.0 mg (equivalent to 5.224 mg reboxetine methanesulphonate).

Pharmaceutical form 4.0 mg strength: white, round, convex, 8 mm diameter tablet with a breakline on one side. A "P" will be marked on the left side of the breakline. A "U" will be marked on the right side of the breakline. The side opposite the breakline will be marked "7671".

Clinical particulars

Therapeutic indications: Reboxetine is indicated for the acute treatment of depressive illness/major depression and for maintaining the clinical improvement in patients initially responding to treatment.

Posology and method of administration: Edronax tablets are for oral administration.

Use in adults: The recommended therapeutic dose is 4 mg b.i.d. (8 mg/day) administered orally. The full therapeutic dose can be given upon starting treatment. After 3–4 weeks, this dose can be increased to 10 mg/day in case of incomplete clinical response. The maximum daily dose should not exceed 12 mg. The minimum effective dose has not yet been established.

Use in the elderly: Elderly patients have been studied in clinical trials at doses of 2 mg b.i.d. However, safety and efficacy have not been evaluated in placebo-controlled conditions. Therefore, as for other antidepressants that have not been studied in placebo-controlled conditions, reboxetine cannot be recommended.

Use in children: The use of reboxetine in children is not recommended since safety and efficacy have not been evaluated in this population.

Use in patients with renal or hepatic insufficiency: The starting dose in patients with renal or hepatic insufficiency should be 2 mg b.i.d which can be increased based on patient tolerance.

Contra-indications: Hypersensitivity to one of the constituents of the formulation.

Reboxetine is contra-indicated in pregnancy and lactation.

Special warnings and precautions for use: As reboxetine has not been tested in patients with convulsive disorders in clinical studies and since rare cases of seizures have been reported in clinical studies, it should be given under close supervision to subjects with a history of convulsive disorders and it must be discontinued if the patient develops seizures.

Concomitant use of MAO-inhibitors and reboxetine should be avoided in view of the potential risk (tyramine effect) based on their mechanisms of action.

Concomitant use of reboxetine with other antidepressants (tricyclics, MAO inhibitors, SSRIs and lithium) has not been evaluated during clinical trials.

As with all antidepressants, switches to mania/hypomania have occurred during the clinical studies. Close supervision of bipolar patients is, therefore, recommended.

The risk of a suicidal attempt is inherent in depression and may persist until significant remission occurs: close patient supervision during initial drug therapy is, therefore, recommended.

Clinical experience with reboxetine in patients affected by serious concomitant systemic illnesses is limited. Close supervision should be applied in patients with current evidence of urinary retention, prostatic hypertrophy, glaucoma and history of cardiac disease.

At doses higher than the maximum recommended, orthostatic hypotension has been observed with greater frequency. Particular attention should be paid when administering reboxetine with other drugs known to lower blood pressure.

Clinical experience with reboxetine in the long-term treatment of elderly patients is, at present, limited. In this population, lowering of mean potassium levels was found starting from week 14; the magnitude of this reduction did not exceed 0.8 mmol/litre and potassium levels never dropped below normal limits.

Interaction with other medicaments and other forms of interaction: The route of metabolism of reboxetine is unknown and it is therefore difficult to predict interactions between reboxetine and other drugs. The cytochrome P450 enzyme CYP2D6 does not seem to be involved in reboxetine metabolism. Because of reboxetine's narrow therapeutic margin, inhibition of its elimination is a major concern. The potential for co-prescribed drugs to inhibit reboxetine elimination has not been tested. Edronax, therefore, should not be given together with drugs known to inhibit other major drug metabolising enzymes other than CYP2D6, such as the azole antifungal agents, macrolide antibiotics such as erythromycin or fluvoxamine.

Information regarding reboxetine's potential to influence the pharmacokinetics of other drugs is limited. In vivo data indicate that glucuronidation is not influenced, nor is CYP3A4 induced, by reboxetine. In vitro data show that reboxetine in high concentrations inhibits CYP3A4 and CYP2D6. Until further in vivo data are available, reboxetine should be used with caution when prescribed with drugs metabolised by CYP3A4 or CYP2D6 that have a narrow therapeutic margin such as the antiarrhythmic drugs, antipsychotic drugs, tricyclic antidepressant drugs or cyclosporin.

No significant reciprocal pharmacokinetic interaction has been found between reboxetine and lorazepam. During their co-administration in healthy volunteers, mild to moderate drowsiness and short lasting orthostatic acceleration of heart rate have been observed.

Reboxetine does not appear to potentiate the effect of alcohol on cognitive functions in healthy volunteers.

Concomitant use of MAO-inhibitors and reboxetine should be avoided in view of the potential risk (tyramine effect) based on their mechanisms of action.

Concomitant use of reboxetine with other antidepressants (tricyclics, MAO inhibitors, SSRIs and lithium) has not been evaluated during clinical trials.

Concomitant use of ergot derivatives and reboxetine might result in increased blood pressure.

Food intake delayed the absorption of reboxetine, but did not significantly influence the extent of absorption.

Although data are not available from clinical studies, the possibility of hypokalaemia with concomitant use of potassium losing diuretics should be considered.

Pregnancy and lactation: Studies in animals have not demonstrated any teratogenic effect or any effect of the compound on global reproductive performance. Dosages that produced plasma concentrations within the therapeutic range for humans induced an impairment of growth and development and long term behavioural changes in offspring of rats.

In humans experience is very limited. Therefore, administration during pregnancy should be avoided. If conception occurs during therapy, treatment is to be discontinued as soon as pregnancy is confirmed to limit foetal exposure to the drug.

In rats reboxetine is excreted in milk. Therefore, while no information on the excretion of reboxetine in maternal milk in humans is available, reboxetine administration is not recommended in breast feeding women.

Effects on ability to drive and use machines: Reboxetine is not sedative per se. No cognitive or psychomotor impairment has been observed with reboxetine in clinical studies, also when the compound was co-administered with alcohol. However, as with all psychoactive drugs, patients should be cautioned about operating machinery and driving.

Undesirable effects: About 1500 patients received reboxetine in clinical studies, 200 of which received reboxetine for at least 1 year.

Information reported in the tables below refers to placebo-controlled trials.

Short-term studies		
	Reboxetine	Placebo
Patient nos.	373	373
Total adverse events	69%	57%
Withdrawal due to AEs	8%	7.5%
AEs causing withdrawal at least twice as much on reboxetine		
Insomnia	1.3%	0.5%
Increased sweating	1.1%	0.3%
Dizziness or hypotension	0.8%	0%
Paraesthesia	0.8%	0.3%
Impotence, UTI, dysuria	0.5%	0%
AEs significantly higher on reboxetine than placebo		
Dry mouth	27%	16%
Constipation	17%	8%
Insomnia	14%	5%
Increased sweating	14%	7%
Symptomatic tachycardia	5%	2%
Vertigo	2%	0%
Urinary hesitancy/retention	5%	2%
(retention)	(2%)	(1%)
Impotence	5%	0%

As for long-term tolerability, 143 reboxetine-treated and 140 placebo-treated adult patients participated in a long term placebo controlled study. Adverse events newly emerged on long term treatment in 28% of the reboxetine treated patients and 23% of the placebo-treated patients and caused discontinuation in 4% and 1% of the cases respectively. There was a similar risk of the development of individual events with reboxetine and placebo. In the long term studies, no individual events were seen which have not been seen on short term treatment.

The most relevant between gender difference in adverse event rate was related to the frequency of urinary hesitancy/retention complained of mainly by male patients (10% vs. 2% in females on short term treatment; 14% vs. 1% in females on long term treatment).

In the elderly population, frequency of total adverse events, as well as of individual events, was no higher than that reported above.

Signs and symptoms newly reported on abrupt discontinuation were infrequent and less frequent in patients treated with reboxetine (4%) than in those treated with placebo (6%).

During medical examination an increase in heart rate *vs.* baseline (either >20% or, to values ≥ 100 beats/min) was observed, mainly in adult patients (20% of the patients on short-term treatment compared with 6% on placebo and 23% of the patients on long-term treatment compared with 17% on placebo).

Overdose: The acute toxicity studies carried out in animals indicate a very low toxicity, with a wide safety margin with respect to the pharmacologically active doses. Clinical signs and cause of death were related to CNS stimulation (mainly convulsive symptoms).

In a few cases doses higher than those recommended were administered to patients (12 mg to 20 mg/day) for a period ranging from a few days to some weeks during clinical studies: newly reported complaints include postural hypotension, anxiety and hypertension. Elderly might be particularly vulnerable to overdose.

Two cases of self-overdosing with reboxetine were reported by the patients during the clinical studies. No major adverse events were observed.

In case of overdose, monitoring of cardiac function and vital signs is recommended. General symptomatic supportive and/or emetic measures might be required.

Pharmacological properties
Pharmacodynamic properties: Reboxetine is a highly selective and potent inhibitor of norepinephrine reuptake. It has only a weak effect on the 5-HT reuptake and does not affect the uptake of dopamine.

Norepinephrine reuptake inhibition and the consequent increase of norepinephrine availability in the synaptic cleft and modification of noradrenergic transmission, reportedly is among the most relevant mechanisms of action of known antidepressant drugs.

In vitro, studies have shown that reboxetine has no significant affinity for adrenergic (α_1, α_2, β) and muscarinic receptors; antagonism of such receptors has been described to be associated with cardiovascular, anticholinergic and sedative side effects of other antidepressant drugs.

Reboxetine is devoid of in-vitro binding affinity for either α_1 or α_2 adrenoceptors, however, a functional interference with α-adrenoceptors at high doses in-vivo cannot be excluded.

Pharmacokinetic properties: After oral administration of a single 4 mg reboxetine dose to healthy volunteers, peak levels of about 130 ng/ml are achieved within 2 h post-dosing. Data indicate that absolute bioavailability is at least 60%.

Reboxetine plasma levels decreased monoexponentially with a half-life of about 13 h. Steady-state conditions are observed within 5 days. Linearity of the pharmacokinetics was shown in the range of single oral doses in the clinically recommended dose-ranges.

The drug appears to be distributed into total body water. Reboxetine is 97 % bound to human plasma proteins in young and 92% in elderly (with affinity markedly higher for α_1 acid glycoprotein than albumin), with no significant dependence of the concentration of drug.

The metabolic routes for reboxetine are insufficiently characterised and in vivo interaction studies are limited, hence predictions of potential interactions are difficult and reboxetine should only with caution be coprescribed with drugs known to influence CYP450 enzymes other than CYP2D6 or drugs with a narrow therapeutic margin which are metabolised by CYP2D6 or CYP3A4.

The amount of radioactivity excreted in urine accounts for 78 % of the dose. Even though unchanged drug is predominant in the systemic circulation (70% of total radioactivity, in terms of AUC), only 10% of the dose is excreted as unchanged drug in urine. These findings suggest that biotransformation rules the overall elimination of reboxetine and that metabolites excretion is limited by their formation. The main metabolic pathways identified are 2-O-dealkylation, hydroxylation of the ethoxyphenoxy ring and oxidation of the morpholine ring, followed by partial or complete glucuro- or sulpho-conjugation.

The drug is available as a racemic mixture (with both enantiomers being active in the experimental models): no chiral inversion, nor reciprocal pharmacokinetic interferences between enantiomers have been observed. Plasma levels of the more potent SS enantiomer are about two times lower and urinary excretion two times higher than those of the enantiomeric counterpart. No significant differences were observed in the terminal half-lives of the two enantiomers.

Increases in systemic exposure and half-life of approximately two-fold are observed in patients with renal insufficiency and hepatic insufficiency . Similar or somewhat greater (3-fold) increases in systemic exposure also occur in elderly patients relative to young healthy volunteers.

Preclinical safety data: The preclinical safety studies indicated no evidence of teratogenic, genotoxic or carcinogenic potential of reboxetine. Haemosiderosis was reported in toxicity studies in rats only.

Pharmaceutical particulars
List of excipients: Cellulose microcrystalline; Calcium hydrogen phosphate dihydrate; Crospovidone; Silica, colloidal hydrated; Magnesium stearate.

Incompatibilities: None known.

Shelf life: 36 months.

Special precautions for storage: Storage at or below 25°C.

Nature and contents of container: The tablets are contained in aluminium-PVDC/PVC-PVDC opaque blisters.

Each pack contains: 60 tablets in blisters.

Instructions for use/handling: There are no special instructions for handling.

Marketing authorisation number
Edronax 4 mg tablets 0032/0216.

Date of first authorisation/renewal of authorisation 10 April 1997.

Date of (partial) revision of the text 4 December 1997.

Legal category POM.

ESTRACYT* CAPSULES

Qualitative and quantitative composition Estramustine phosphate 140 mg as estramustine sodium phosphate.

Pharmaceutical form Gelatin capsules.

Clinical particulars
Therapeutic indications: Carcinoma of the prostate, especially in cases unresponsive to, or relapsing after, treatment by conventional oestrogens (stilboestrol, polyoestradiol phosphate etc.) or by orchidectomy.

Posology and method of administration
Adult and the elderly: Dosage range may be from 1 to 10 capsules a day by mouth. The capsules should be taken not less than 1 hour before or 2 hours after meals. The capsules should not be taken with milk or milk products. Standard starting dosage is 4–6 capsules a day in divided doses with later adjustment according to response and gastrointestinal tolerance.

Children: Estracyt should not be administered to children.

Contra-indications: Use in patients with peptic ulceration, or those with severe liver dysfunction or myocardial insufficiency. Use in children. Use in patients hypersensitive to oestradiol or nitrogen mustard.

Special warnings and precautions for use: Use with caution in patients with moderate to severe bone marrow depression, thrombophlebitis, thrombosis, thromboembolic disorders, cardiovascular disease, coronary artery disease and congestive heart failure.

Caution should also be exercised in patients with diabetes, hypertension, epilepsy, hepatic and renal impairment and diseases associated with hypercalcaemia. Blood counts, liver function tests and serum calcium in hypercalcaemia should be performed at regular intervals.

Interaction with other medicaments and other forms of interaction: Milk, milk products or drugs containing calcium may impair the absorption of Estracyt and should not be taken simultaneously with Estracyt.

Pregnancy and lactation: Not applicable.

Effects on ability to drive and use machines: No adverse effects on a patient's ability to drive or operate heavy machinery have been reported.

Undesirable effects: Gastro-intestinal disturbances (most commonly transient nausea, but occasionally vomiting and rarely diarrhoea) sometimes occur at the beginning of therapy. In a few cases thrombocytopenia, leukopenia and elevated transaminases/bilirubin have been noted. Cardiovascular effects including oedema, worsening angina, congestive cardiac failure. Myocardial infarction has rarely been reported. Thromboembolic disorders, gynaecomastia, reduced libido and potency may occur as with other oestrogenic drugs. Occasionally allergy (manifested as rash and/or fever) is encountered.

Overdose: There is no specific antidote. Treatment is symptomatic and supportive and in the event of dangerously low red cell, white cell or platelet count, whole blood should be given as necessary. Liver function should be monitored.

Pharmacological properties
Pharmacodynamic properties: Estracyt is a chemical compound of oestradiol and nitrogen mustard. It is effective in the treatment of advanced prostatic carcinoma.

Estracyt has a dual mode of action. The intact molecule acts as an anti-miotic agent; after hydrolysis of the carbamate ester, the metabolites act to bridge the released oestrogens and exert an anti-gonadotrophic effect. The low level of clinical side effects may be due to the fact that estramustine binds to a protein present in the tumour tissue, so resulting in accumulation of the drug at the target site. Estracyt also has weak oestrogenic and anti-gonadotrophic properties.

Estracyt causes little or no bone marrow depression at usual therapeutic dosage. Estracyt is effective in patients who have not previously received drug therapy, as well as in those who have shown no response to conventional hormone treatment.

Pharmacokinetic properties: Estramustine phosphate sodium is rapidly dephosphorylated in the intestine and prostate to estramustine and estromustine, which accumulate in the prostatic tissue. The plasma half-lives of these metabolites are 10 – 20 hours. Estramustine and estromustine are further metabolised before excretion.

Preclinical safety data: No particular information is presented given the experience gained with the use of estramustine phosphate sodium in humans over the past several years.

Pharmaceutical particulars
List of excipients: Talcum, sodium lauryl sulphate, colloidal silicon dioxide, magnesium stearate, titanium dioxide (E171), hard gelatin capsule, black ink.

Incompatibilities: None that are relevant.

Shelf life: Three years.

Special precautions for storage: Store out of the sight and reach of children.

Nature and contents of container: Brown glass bottle containing 100 capsules.

Instructions for use/handling: No special instructions.

Marketing authorisation number 0022/0106.

Date of first authorisation/renewal of authorisation 7 July 1992.

Date of (partial) revision of the text August 1997.

Legal category POM.

ESTRING*

Qualitative and quantitative composition Each vaginal ring contains:

Active constituent: Estradiol (INN) 2.0 mg.

Pharmaceutical form Estradiol vaginal ring is a slightly opaque ring, made of a silicone elastomer, with a whitish core, containing a drug reservoir of 2 mg Estradiol Hemihydrate PhEur. The product has the following dimensions: outer diameter–55 mm; cross sectional diameter–9 mm; core diameter–2 mm.

Clinical particulars

Therapeutic indications: Treatment of postmenopausal atrophic vaginitis. Estring is only suitable for the treatment of urogenital complaints due to oestrogen deficiency. Its pharmacokinetic profile shows that there is no significant systemic effect and therefore it is not suitable for postmenopausal complaints which require a systemically active dose of oestrogen (e.g vasomotor symptoms), neither is it suitable for osteoporosis prophylaxis.

Posology and method of administration: Estring releases small amounts of oestradiol 7.5 µg/24 hours, in a consistent stable manner for at least 90 days.

Adults including the elderly: One ring to be inserted into the upper third of the vagina, to be worn continuously for 3 months, then replaced by a new ring as appropriate. The maximum recommended duration of continuous therapy is two years.

Instructions for use are available in a Patient Information Leaflet enclosed in each pack.

Estring is only intended for treatment of postmenopausal women.

Children: Estring is not recommended for use in children.

Contra-indications: Known or suspected oestrogen-dependent malignancy, e.g endometrial carcinoma or other oestrogen-dependent tumours.

Undiagnosed abnormal genital bleeding.

Known or suspected pregnancy.

Special warnings and special precautions for use: Some women may be unsuitable for treatment with Estring, in particular those with short narrow vaginas due to previous surgery or the effect of atrophy, or those with a degree of uterovaginal prolapse severe enough to prevent retention of the ring.

During long-term treatment with oestrogens, periodic medical examinations are advisable. In addition, any woman with symptoms/signs of abnormal vaginal discharge, vaginal discomfort, or any vaginal bleeding should be examined fully to exclude ulceration, infection, or unresponsive atrophic vaginitis. Minor signs of irritation are often transient. Any woman experiencing persistent or severe discomfort due to the presence of the ring or excessive movement of the ring should be withdrawn from treatment. Patients with signs of ulceration or severe inflammation due to unresponsive atrophic vaginitis should also be withdrawn from treatment. Patients with vaginal infection should be treated appropriately. In the case of systemic therapy, Estring treatment may continue without interruption.

However, removal of Estring should be considered while using vaginal preparations.

Treatment with Estring will result in very low plasma levels of oestradiol, similar to those seen in untreated postmenopausal women. It has been estimated that approximately 4 µg of 17β-oestradiol are absorbed systemically per 24 hours. It is unlikely that this level of oestradiol would be associated with any of the known risks of systemic oestrogen treatment. However, it is advisable that patients with endometrial hyperplasia; thromboembolic disease; acute or chronic liver disease (including Dubin Johnson Syndrome and Rotor Syndrome) or acute intermittent porphyria should be treated with caution. Accordingly, these patients should be carefully assessed prior to treatment and monitored during therapy including measurement of appropriate parameters.

Patients on long-term corticosteroid treatment or those with conditions causing poor skin integrity, e.g Cushing's Disease, may be unsuitable for treatment as they may have vaginal atrophy unresponsive to oestrogen therapy.

There have been incidences of both the ring falling out and movement of the ring, generally at defaecation. Therefore, if the woman is constipated she should remove the ring before defaecation. There may also be other instances when some women wish to remove the ring, e.g prior to sexual intercourse. Comprehensive advice for removal and reinsertion of the ring are provided in the Patient Information Leaflet which is included in every pack.

Interaction with other medicaments and other forms of interaction: As the oestrogen is administered vaginally and due to the low levels released, it is unlikely that any clinically relevant drug interactions will occur with Estring.

Removal of Estring should be considered when using other vaginal preparations.

Pregnancy and lactation: Estring is indicated for postmenopausal treatment. Women of child bearing potential and lactating women should, therefore, not be prescribed Estring.

Effects on ability to drive and use machines: Estring is unlikely to have any effect on alertness or coordination.

Undesirable effects: Adverse reactions with Estring are rare. Adverse reactions reported with a frequency of 1% or more in clinical trials, in order of decreasing frequency, were vaginal irritation, abdominal pain/lower abdominal pain/abdominal discomfort, vulvovaginal infection, urogenital pruritus, pressure symptoms in vagina/on bladder/on rectum, generalised pruritus, urinary tract infection and increased sweating. However, some of these symptoms occur more frequently in untreated post-menopausal women, e.g vaginal irritation, urinary tract infection, urogenital pruritus, vulvovaginal infection and increased sweating.

A few cases of vaginal ulceration were reported in clinical trials. While these were minor and transient it is recommended that any patient who develops an ulcer should be withdrawn from treatment.

In the Patient Information Leaflet, patients are advised that if they experience any undesirable effects they should consult their doctor. Furthermore, if these effects are severe the leaflet gives instructions on how to remove the ring themselves, if they wish, before seeing their doctor.

Overdosage: This is not relevant due to the mode of administration.

Pharmacological properties

Pharmacodynamic properties: Estring is a vaginal ring which delivers approximately 7.5 µg/24 hours of 17β-oestradiol for 3 months. The active ingredient, Estradiol is well known as it is an endogenously occurring hormone produced primarily by the ovaries and to some extent by the adrenal glands. The circulating oestradiol is transported into cells and bound to oestrogen receptors in the nucleus, where it initiates protein synthesis resulting in, for example, cell growth.

Important target organs for oestrogens are the uterus, vagina and urethra. The surface linings, as well as the musculature of these organs, are affected to varying degrees by the hormone.

Oestradiol and other oestrogens are also known to increase the α-adrenoreceptor content and the noradrenaline-induced contractility of the urethra, and to increase the α- and β-adrenoreceptor content of the uterus. It has also been reported that even low doses of oestradiol are able to considerably increase the blood flow in urogenital organs.

The oestradiol from the ring acts locally to eliminate or reduce symptoms and signs of post-menopausal urogenital oestrogen deficiency. Estring therapy restores vaginal pH to premenopausal values and returns the histology and physiology of the vaginal and urethral epithelia to premenopausal states. The very low, constant release of oestradiol from Estring does not exert adverse systemic effects, ie induces no increase in SHBG (Sex Hormone Binding Globulin) or α_2-PAG (Pregnancy Zone Protein). Therefore, theoretically, it should not cause endometrial proliferation. Estring can, therefore, be used continuously without the addition of progestogens and consequently, no uterine bleeding will result from treatment.

Pharmacokinetic properties: Oestradiol is mainly metabolized in the liver. Its main metabolites are oestriol, oestrone, and their conjugates. The plasma half life of oestradiol is 1-2 hours. Metabolic plasma clearance varies between 450-625 ml/min/m². The metabolites are mainly excreted via the kidneys as glucuronides and sulphates. Oestrogens also undergo enterohepatic circulation.

After a brief initial peak, the release of oestradiol from Estring is constant (7.5 µg/24 h), according to Fick's law, for at least 90 days. As a consequence of the initial release peak, plasma levels of oestradiol reach about 200 pmol/l within 3 hours.

After this initial peak, plasma oestradiol concentrations decline rapidly and constant levels are achieved after 2-3 days. These levels are maintained at, or near, the quantification limit (20-30 pmol/l) throughout the rest of the treatment period.

The levels are considerably lower than the lowest levels commonly detected in pre-menopausal women, i.e during the early follicular phase.

Estring presumably increases local oestradiol target concentrations, while maintaining very low and stable systemic plasma concentrations. The maximum duration of use during clinical trials was 2 years and, therefore, the maximum recommended duration of continuous therapy is 2 years.

Preclinical safety data: One of the well-documented adverse effects of oestrogen replacement therapy is its stimulation of cell growth with resultant endometrial proliferation. However, the very low, stable plasma oestradiol concentrations resulting from treatment with Estring should not be sufficient to yield this effect. Likewise, the risk of adverse systemic effects on other organs and tissues is considered minimal.

Silicone elastomer in Estring: The biological safety of the silicone elastomer has been studied in various in-vitro and in-vivo test models.

The results show that the silicone elastomer was non-toxic in in-vitro studies, and non-pyrogenic, non-irritant, and non-sensitizing in short term in-vivo tests. Long-term implantation induced encapsulation equal to or less than the negative control (polyethylene) used in the prescribed USP test. No toxic reaction or further formation was observed with the silicone elastomer.

Pharmaceutical particulars

List of excipients:

Silicone elastomer	Q7-4735 A	Filler	4992 mg
Silicone elastomer	Q7-4735 B	Filler	4992 mg
Silicone Fluid	SFD 119	Dispersing agent	8.7 mg
Barium sulphate	PhEur	Marker	5.9 mg

Incompatibilities: No incompatibilities are known.

Shelf-life: Results from stability studies indicate that Estring is stable for at least 24 months when stored at room temperature (below 30°C).

Special precautions for storage: Store at room temperature (below 30°C)

Nature and contents of container: One ring is individually packed in a heat-sealed rectangular pouch consisting of, from outside to inside: Polyester/Aluminium foil/Low density Poly-ethylene. Each pouch is provided with a tear-off notch on one side and is packed into a cardboard carton. Each carton contains a Patient Information Leaflet.

Instructions for use/handling: Comprehensive details are provided in the Patient Information Leaflet.

Marketing authorisation number 0022/0115

Date of approval/revision of SPC 12 July 1996

Legal category POM

FARLUTAL*

Qualitative and quantitative composition Medroxyprogesterone Acetate BP, 20.0 w/v.

Pharmaceutical form White sterile suspension for injection which settles on standing but readily disperses on shaking.

Clinical particulars

Therapeutic indications: Palliative treatment of hormone-sensitive malignancies. Farlutal has been successfully used to produce regressions in breast, endometrial, prostatic and renal cell carcinoma. High dose Farlutal therapy has proved especially useful in breast carcinoma and in achieving subjective improvements in terminally ill patients, notably pain relief and improved performance status.

Posology and method of administration: Route of administration: Intramuscular injection

Suggested dosage schemes are as follows:

Breast carcinoma: Initial dose: 500 – 1000 mg/day i.m. for 4 weeks. Maintenance: 500 mg i.m. twice a week

Endometrial carcinoma: Initial dose: 500 mg i.m. twice weekly for 3 months. Maintenance: 500 mg i.m. weekly

Renal adenocarcinoma: Initial dose: 500 mg i.m. on alternate days for 30 days. Maintenance: 500 mg i.m. twice weekly until 60th day, then 250 mg i.m. weekly

Prostatic Adenocarcinoma: Initial dose: 500 mg i.m. twice weekly. Maintenance: 500 mg i.m. weekly.

Children and elderly: None stated.

Contra-indications: Thrombophlebitis, thrombo-embolic disorders, severe hepatic insufficiency and hypercalcaemia as may occur in patients with osseous metastases; also, suspected or early breast carcinoma, missed abortion, metrorrhagia, pregnancy and known hypersensitivity to medroxyprogesterone acetate, or, for the injectable formulation, hydroxybenzoates (excipients).

Special warnings and precautions for use: Farlutal should be used under the direction of those experienced in cancer chemotherapy.

Since medroxyprogesterone acetate appears to enhance blood clotting potential, treatment should be discontinued upon the appearance of thrombo-embolic episodes, migraine or associated ocular problems such as sudden partial or total loss of vision, diplopia or vascular lesions of the retina.

In the event of vaginal bleeding occurring, an accurate diagnosis should be made. If a histological examination is indicated, the laboratory should be informed that the patient has been receiving a progestogen.

Animal studies have shown that medroxyprogesterone acetate possesses adrenocorticoid activity and this effect has also been observed in humans. Patients treated with high doses continuously over long periods should be carefully observed for signs normally associated with adrenocorticoid therapy, such as hypertension, sodium retention, oedema, etc. and care is needed in treating patients with diabetes and/or arterial hypertension.

Farlutal may raise plasma calcium levels; some cases of hypercalcaemia have been reported in the treatment of breast carcinoma.

Interactions with other medicaments and other forms of interaction: None known.

Pregnancy and lactation: Administration of progesterone during the first months of pregnancy may possibly be associated with the occurrence of congenital cardiac malformations in the neonate. In addition, instances of masculinisation of female foetuses have been reported following high dose therapy during pregnancy. For these reasons, Farlutal is contra-indicated during pregnancy.

It should be noted that long term administration of medroxyprogesterone acetate to beagle dogs has resulted in the development of mammary nodules which were occasionally found to be malignant. The relevance of these findings to humans has, however, not been established.

Effects on ability to drive and use machines: Not applicable.

Undesirable effects: As is generally found after intramuscular administration of large volumes of suspension, the i.m. preparation may cause local lesions at the injection site, such as sterile abscesses or inflammatory infiltrates. Therefore, the suspension should be well shaken before use and injected deeply into healthy gluteal muscle.

In common with other progestogens, Farlutal may cause mastodynia, galactorrhoea, vaginal bleeding, changes in menstrual flow, amenorrhoea, cervical erosions and modifications of cervical secretions. Farlutal also exerts a corticoid-like effect which may lead to facies lunaris, cushingoid syndrome and weight changes; and an adrenergic-like action which may result in fine hand tremors, sweating and cramps in the calves at night. Cholestatic jaundice has occasionally been reported.

Overdose: No positive action is required.

Pharmacological properties

Pharmacodynamic properties: MPA has an antigonadotrophic effect, it blocks the pre-ovulatory intermenstrual oestrogen peak by direct action on the ovary. Its effects at low doses include contraceptive action, secretion by the endometrium, delay in the menstrual flow, a decrease in the viscosity of cervical mucus and a reduction in the vaginal karyopycnotic index.

At higher doses, oncological actions are evident. There is a direct cytotoxic action on tumour cells manifested by a decrease in DNA and RNA synthesis.

Pharmacokinetic properties: The absorption and metabolism of the MPA are affected by both the administration route used and the type of pharmaceutical preparation.

After i.m. administration of MPA in an aqueous solution, absorption is slow. The highest blood levels are found during the first 2 days, measurable amounts being found up to 100 days after treatment. Variations in plasma concentrations are interpreted as being due to irregular release from the injection site.

Only 3–6% of the administered dose is recovered in urine after 24 hours. After 6 days approximately 11% is found in the urine and 3% in the faeces, hence elimination is slow after i.m. administration. Traces of metabolites have been found in the urine up to 6 months after high doses of MPA. Only a slight increase in porter-silber steroids is found in the urine of patients treated by the i.m. route.

Preclinical safety data: No further preclinical safety data available.

Pharmaceutical particulars

List of excipients:

Polysorbate 80	BP
Sodium Chloride	PhEur
Carbowax 400	BP
Methyl Hydroxybenzoate	BP
Propyl Hydroxybenzoate	BP
Water for Injections	BP

Incompatibilities: None known.

Shelf life: 48 months

Special precautions for storage: The vials should be stored between 15°–30°C and should not be frozen.

Nature and contents of container: Colourless siliconised glass vial (Type I) with grey chlorobutyl rubber stopper and aluminium seal containing 2.5 or 5 ml of suspension.

Instruction for use/handling: None stated.

Marketing authorisation holder:
Farmitalia Carlo Erba Limited, Davy Avenue, Milton Keynes, MK5 8PH, UK

Marketing authorisation number 3433/0045

Date of first authorisation/renewal of authorisation
Date of First Authorisation: 14 August 1981
Date of Renewal of Authorisation: 15 January 1993

Date of (partial) revision of the text 4 September 1997

Legal category POM

FLEXOTARD MR

Qualitative and quantitative composition Diclofenac sodium 100 mg.

Pharmaceutical form Biconvex, pink coloured, film-coated tablets marked DICL on one face, in a sustained-release preparation.

Clinical partiulcars

Therapeutic indications: For the treatment of acute gout, pain and inflammation in rheumatic disease and in other musculoskeletal disorders. These include rheumatoid arthritis, juvenile rheumatoid arthritis, osteoarthritis, periarthritis (especially frozen shoulder), low back pain, tendinitis, tenosynovitis, bursitis, sprains, strains and dislocations, relief of pain in fractures; ankylosing spondylitis. It may be used in the control of pain and inflammation in orthopaedic, dental and other minor surgery.

Posology and method of administration: By oral administration:

Adults: One 100 mg diclofenac sodium sustained release tablet (Flexotard MR) daily. If necessary the daily dosage can be increased to 150 mg by supplementation with conventional dosage forms of diclofenac sodium 25 mg or 50 mg.

Elderly adults: The pharmacokinetics of diclofenac sodium do not indicate impairment of any clinical significance in the elderly and therefore, there is no requirement for reduction of the usual adult dosage. However, close surveillance of elderly patients is advisable.

Contra-indications: Active or suspected peptic ulceration or gastro-intestinal bleeding. Hypersensitivity to diclofenac sodium, asthma, urticaria or rhinitis, where these are precipitated by non-steroidal, anti-inflammatory agents.

Special warnings and precautions for use: Side effects are generally more serious in the elderly and if serious diclofenac sodium should be withdrawn. Patients on long term treatment should be monitored and patients with severe hepatic, cardiac or renal insufficiency should be kept under close surveillance.

If there is a persistency in abnormal liver function tests or there are symptoms consistent with liver disease or if there are other manifestations such as rash or eosinophilia, diclofenac sodium treatment should be discontinued. Attacks of hepatic porphyria may be triggered in susceptible patients. Patients with impaired cardiac or renal function or recovering from major surgery or being treated with diuretics should be considered because of the importance of prostaglandins in maintaining blood flow. Diclofenac sodium in common with other non-steroidal anti-inflammatory drugs (NSAIDs) can reversibly inhibit platelet aggregation.

Interaction with other medicaments and other forms of interaction: The plasma concentrations of digoxin and lithium may be increased by diclofenac sodium. Increased risk of haemorrhage when used in conjunction with anti-coagulants has been reported, as too have hypoglycaemic effects when used in conjunction with non-steroidal anti-inflammatory agents.

The effect on renal prostaglandins may increase cyclosporin nephrotoxicity.

Methotrexate plasma levels may be increased and result in increased toxicity, therefore, caution should be exercised if diclofenac sodium and methotrexate are administered within 24 hours of each other. Serum potassium levels may be raised and should be monitored where there is concomitant treatment with potassium sparing diuretics.

Pregnancy and lactation: Diclofenac sodium should be used in pregnancy only if the benefits outweigh the risk, when the lowest effective dose should be employed. Use of prostaglandin synthetase inhibitors may result in premature closure of the ductus arteriosus or uterine inertia and therefore are not recommended during the last trimester of pregnancy.

Traces have been detected in breast milk but the level is so low as to be thought not to affect the infant.

Effects on ability to drive and use machines: It is advisable not to drive or operate machinery if headaches, dizziness or drowsiness occur whilst taking diclofenac sodium.

Undesirable effects: Gastro-intestinal disorders (rarely with bleeding) and lower intestinal disorders, in some cases with exacerbation of exisiting conditions such as ulcerative colitis may occur. Pancreatitis, apthous stomatitis, glossitis and constipation may occur and occasionally there are effects on the CNS such as headache, dizziness, vertigo, drowsiness, disturbance of taste, vision, hearing and sensation. There may be insomnia, anxiety or depression, tremor or psychotic reactions. Skin reactions, including loss of hair and photosensitivity reactions occur occasionally. Kidney and urinary abnormalities occur on rare occasions, as do liver function disorders.

Isolated cases of thrombocytopenia, leucopenia, agranulocytosis, haemolytic anaemia and aplastic anaemia have been reported. Hypersensitivity reactions, anaphylactoid systemic reactions and hypertension have been reported.

Overdose: Treatment should be symptomatic and supportive. Gastric lavage and treatment with active charcoal, as soon as possible, to prevent absorption together with symptomatic measures to treat gastro-intestinal irritation and other complications such as hypotension, convulsions, respiratory disorders and renal failure are indicated. The extensive metabolism and high rate of protein binding of NSAIDs obviate the use of specific therapies such as forced diuresis, haemoperfusion or dialysis.

Pharmacological properties

Pharmacodynamic properties: Diclofenac sodium is a non-steroidal anti-inflammatory agent which has analgesic and antipyretic properties. It is a prostaglandin synthetase (cyclo-oxygenase) inhibitor.

Pharmacokinetic properties: Following ingestion, diclofenac sodium is completely absorbed from the intestinal tract but undergoes first pass metabolism and peak plasma concentrations occur in about 2 to 4 hours; at therapeutic concentrations it is more than 99% bound to plasma proteins. Diclofenac is almost entirely metabolised in the liver and the terminal plasma half-life is about 1 – 2 hours, with metabolic excretion mainly via the kidneys and also in the bile.

Preclinical safety data: Diclofenac sodium is a well established drug for which there are adequate published safety data. This application is an abridged authorisation application submitted under Article 4.8.1(iii) of Directive 65/65/EEC and therefore, preclinical data have not been submitted.

Pharmaceutical particulars

List of excipients:

Granulating fluid:	BP
Cetostearyl alcohol	
Core:	
Colloidal silicon dioxide	USP
Compressible sugar	USP
Talc	BP
Povidone	BP
Magnesium stearate	BP
Subcoat:	DAB
Copolyvidon	BP
Sucrose	
Pigmented film-coat:	HSE
Opadry OY-S-1387	
Polish:	BP
Carnauba wax	

Incompatibilities: None known.

Shelf life: 60 months when stored at 25°C.

Special precautions for storage: To be stored at 25°C

Nature and contents of container: The tablets are presented in aluminium/PVC blisters, strips of which are contained within a printed cardboard carton. Each carton contains 28 tablets.

Instructions for use/handling: No specific statement.

Marketing authorisation number
Flexotard 100 mg: 14017/0008

Date of first authorisation/renewal of authorisation
3 December 1996.

Date of (partial) revision of the text 1 May 1997.

FRAGMIN* AMPOULES

Qualitative and quantitative composition

Active ingredient: Dalteparin sodium (INN); Quality according to PhEur and in-house specification.

Potency is described in International anti-Factor Xa units (IU) of the 1st International Standard for Low Molecular Weight Heparin.

Content of active ingredient: Fragmin 10,000 IU/4 ml: Ampoules containing dalteparin sodium corresponding to 2,500 IU (anti-Factor Xa)/ml.

Fragmin 10,000 IU/1 ml: Ampoules containing dalteparin sodium, 10,000 IU (anti-Factor Xa) in 1 ml.

Pharmaceutical form Solution for injection for intravenous or subcutaneous administration.

Clinical particulars
Therapeutic indications: Prevention of clotting in the extracorporeal circulation during haemodialysis or haemofiltration, in patients with chronic renal insufficiency or acute renal failure.

Treatment of acute deep venous thrombosis.

Unstable coronary artery disease, defined as newly developed or increased angina or ongoing chest pain, with the electrocardiogram changes of non Q-wave myocardial infarction.

Posology and method of administration
Recommended dosage for adults:
Prevention of clotting during haemodialysis and haemofiltration: In chronic renal insufficiency for patients with no known additional bleeding risk, the dosage is:

Long-term haemodialysis or haemofiltration – duration of haemodialysis/haemofiltration more than 4 hours: An i.v bolus injection of Fragmin 30–40 IU (anti-Factor Xa)/kg bodyweight, followed by an infusion of 10–15 IU (anti-Factor Xa)/kg bodyweight/hour.

Short-term haemodialysis or haemofiltration – duration of haemodialysis/haemofiltration less than 4 hours: Either as above, or, a single i.v bolus injection of Fragmin 5000 IU (anti-Factor Xa).

Both for long and short-term haemodialysis and haemofiltration, the plasma anti-Factor Xa levels should be within the range 0.5–1.0 IU (anti-Factor Xa)/ml.

In acute renal failure, or chronic renal failure in patients with a high risk of bleeding, the dosage is:

An i.v bolus injection of Fragmin 5–10 IU (anti-Factor Xa)/kg bodyweight, followed by an infusion of 4–5 IU (anti-Factor Xa)/kg bodyweight/hour.

The plasma anti-Factor Xa levels should be within the range 0.2–0.4 IU (anti-Factor Xa)/ml.

When considered necessary, it is recommended that the antithrombotic effect of Fragmin be monitored by analysing anti-Factor Xa activity using a suitable chromogenic substrate assay. This is because Fragmin has only a moderate prolonging effect on clotting time assays such as APTT or thrombin time.

Treatment of deep venous thrombosis (10,000 IU/1 ml presentation): Fragmin can be administered subcutaneously either as a single daily injection or as twice daily injections.

Once daily administration: 200 IU/kg body weight is administered s.c once daily. Monitoring of the anticoagulant effect is not necessary. The single daily dose should not exceed 18,000 IU.

Twice daily administration: A dose of 100 IU/kg body weight administered s.c twice daily can be used for patients with increased risk of bleeding. Monitoring of the treatment is generally not necessary but can be performed with a functional anti-Factor Xa assay. Maximum plasma levels are obtained 3–4 hours after s.c injection, when samples should be taken. Recommended plasma levels are between 0.5–1.0 IU (anti-Factor Xa)/ml.

Simultaneous anticoagulation with oral vitamin K antagonists can be started immediately. Treatment with Fragmin is continued until the prothrombin complex levels (factor II, VII, IX and X) have decreased to a therapeutic level. At least five days of combined treatment is normally required.

Unstable coronary artery disease (10,000 IU/1 ml presentation): 120 IU/kg body weight subcutaneously twelve hourly. The maximum dose is 10,000 IU/12 hours.

The recommended treatment period is 5 – 8 days. Concomitant therapy with low dose aspirin is recommended.

Children: Not recommended for children.

Elderly: Fragmin has been used safely in elderly patients without the need for dosage adjustment.

Contra-indications: Known hypersensitivity to Fragmin or other low molecular weight heparins and/or heparins e.g. history of confirmed or suspected immunologically mediated heparin induced thrombocytopenia, acute gastroduodenal ulcer; cerebral haemorrhage; known haemorrhagic diathesis; subacute endocarditis; injuries to and operations on the central nervous system, eyes and ears. In patients being treated with Fragmin for acute deep venous thrombosis, regional anaesthesia is contraindicated due to an increased risk of bleeding.

Special warnings and special precautions for use: Do not administer by the intramuscular route.

Caution should be exercised in patients in whom there is an increased risk of bleeding complications, e.g. following surgery or trauma, haemorrhagic stroke, severe liver or renal failure, thrombocytopenia or defective platelet function, uncontrolled hypertension, hypertensive or diabetic retinopathy, patients receiving concurrent anticoagulant/antiplatelet agents (see *Interactions*).

It is recommended that platelets be counted before starting treatment with Fragmin and monitored regularly. Special caution is necessary in rapidly developing thrombocytopenia and severe thrombocytopenia (<100,000/µl) associated with positive or unknown results of in-vitro tests for anti-platelet antibody in the presence of Fragmin or other low molecular weight (mass) heparins and/or heparin.

Fragmin induces only a moderate prolongation of the APTT and thrombin time. Accordingly, dosage increments based upon prolongation of the APTT may cause overdosage and bleeding. Therefore, prolongation of the APTT should only be used as a test of overdosage.

Anti-Factor Xa levels should be regularly monitored in new patients on chronic haemodialysis during the first weeks, later less frequent monitoring is generally required. Patients undergoing acute haemodialysis have a narrower therapeutic dose range and should be monitored frequently in accordance with the individual course of the disease.

Patients with severely disturbed hepatic function may need a reduction in dosage and should be monitored accordingly.

If a transmural myocardial infarction occurs in patients with unstable coronary artery disease, thrombolytic treatment might be appropriate. This does not necessitate discontinuation of treatment with Fragmin, but might increase the risk of bleeding.

As individual low molecular weight (mass) heparins have differing characteristics, switching to an alternative low molecular weight heparin should be avoided. The directions for use relating to each specific product must be observed as different dosages may be required.

Interaction with other medicaments and other forms of interaction: The possibility of the following interactions with Fragmin should be considered:

An enhancement of the anticoagulant effect by anticoagulant/antiplatelet agents e.g. aspirin/ dipyridamole, vitamin K antagonists, NSAIDs e.g. indomethacin, cytostatics, dextran, sulphinpyrazone, probenecid, and ethacrynic acid. However, unless specifically contraindicated, patients with unstable coronary artery disease should receive oral low dose aspirin.

A reduction of the anticoagulant effect may occur with concomitant administration of antihistamines, cardiac glycosides, tetracycline and ascorbic acid.

Pregnancy and lactation: This medicinal product has been assessed in pregnant women and no harmful effects are known with respect to the course of pregnancy and the health of the unborn and neonate.

No information is available as to whether Fragmin passes into breast milk.

Effects on ability to drive and use machines: Fragmin does not affect the ability to drive or operate machinery.

Undesirable effects: Bleeding may be provoked, especially at high dosages corresponding with anti-Factor Xa levels greater than 1.5 IU/ml. However, at recommended dosages bleeding rarely occurs.

Transient, slight to moderate, elevation of liver transaminases (ASAT, ALAT) has been observed, but no clinical significance has been demonstrated.

Commonly reported side-effects include: Subcutaneous haematomas at the injection site, mild thrombocytopenia (type I) which is usually reversible during treatment.

Allergic reactions (urticaria, pruritus, hair loss and skin necrosis) occur rarely.

A few cases of anaphylactoid reactions and of severe immunologically mediated thrombocytopenia (type II) with arterial and/or venous thrombosis or thromboembolism have been observed.

Osteoporosis has been associated with long-term heparin treatment and therefore cannot be excluded with Fragmin.

Overdose: The anticoagulant effect (i.e. prolongation of the APTT) induced by Fragmin is inhibited by protamine. Since protamine itself has an inhibiting effect on primary haemostasis it should be used only in an emergency.

The prolongation of the clotting time induced by Fragmin may be fully neutralised by protamine, but the anti-Factor Xa activity is only neutralised to about 25–50%. 1 mg of protamine inhibits the effect of 100 IU (anti-Factor Xa) of Fragmin.

Pharmacological properties
Pharmacodynamic properties: Dalteparin sodium is a low molecular weight heparin fraction (average molecular weight 4000-6000 Daltons) produced from porcine-derived sodium heparin.

Dalteparin sodium is an antithrombotic agent, which acts mainly through its ability to potentiate the inhibition of Factor Xa and thrombin by antithrombin. It has a relatively higher ability to potentiate Factor Xa inhibition than to prolong plasma clotting time (APTT).

Compared with standard, unfractionated heparin, dalteparin sodium has a reduced adverse effect on platelet function and platelet adhesion, and thus has only a minimal effect on primary haemostasis. Some of the antithrombotic properties of dalteparin sodium are thought to be mediated through the effects on vessel walls or the fibrinolytic system.

Pharmacokinetic properties: The half life following i.v and s.c administration is 2 hours and 3.5–4 hours respectively, twice that of unfractionated heparin.

The bioavailability following s.c injection is approximately 87 per cent and the pharmacokinetics are not dose dependent. The half life is prolonged in uraemic patients as dalteparin sodium is eliminated primarily through the kidneys.

Preclinical safety data: The acute toxicity of dalteparin sodium is considerably lower than that of heparin. The only significant finding, which occurred consistently throughout the toxicity studies after subcutaneous administration of the higher dose levels was local haemorrhage at the injection sites, dose-related in incidence and severity. There was no cumulative effect on injection site haemorrhages.

The haemorrhagic reaction was reflected in dose related changes in the anticoagulant effects as measured by APTT and anti-Factor Xa activities.

It was concluded that dalteparin sodium did not have a greater osteopenic effect than heparin since at equivalent doses the osteopenic effect was comparable.

The results revealed no organ toxicity irrespective of the route of administration, doses or the duration of treatment. No mutagenic effect was found. No embryotoxic or teratogenic effects and no effect on fertility reproductive capacity or peri- and postnatal development was shown.

Pharmceutical particulars
List of excipients: Sodium chloride (PhEur); Water for injections (PhEur)

Incompatibilities: The compatibility of Fragmin with products other than those mentioned under 6.6 has not been investigated.

Shelf life: 36 months.

Special precautions for storage: Store at room temperature (below 30°C).

Nature and contents of container: Clear glass ampoules (PhEur Type 1) containing dalteparin sodium, 10,000 IU (anti-factor Xa) in 1 ml or 10,000 IU (anti-factor Xa) in 4 ml.

Instructions for use/handling: Fragmin solution for injection is compatible with isotonic sodium chloride (9 mg/ml) or isotonic glucose (50 mg/ml) infusion solutions in glass bottles and plastic containers for up to 24 hours. Compatibility between Fragmin and other products has not been studied.

Marketing authorisation number
Fragmin 10,000 IU/4 ml – 0022/0074
Fragmin 10,000 IU/1 ml – 0022/0075

Date of first authorisation/renewal of authorisation
Fragmin 10,000 IU/4 ml – Product Licence granted 26/04/90, renewed 12/05/95
Fragmin 10,000 IU/1 ml – Product Licence granted 26/04/90, renewed 12/05/95

Date of (partial) revision of the text September 19 1997.

Legal category POM.

FRAGMIN* GRADUATED SYRINGE

Qualitative and quantitative composition
Active ingredient: Dalteparin sodium (INN); Quality according to PhEur and in-house specification.

Potency is described in International anti-Factor Xa units (IU) of the 1st International Standard for Low Molecular Weight Heparin.

Single dose syringe containing dalteparin sodium 10,000 IU (anti-Factor Xa) in 1.0 ml solution.

Fragmin Graduated Syringes do not contain preservatives.

Pharmaceutical form Solution for injection for subcutaneous administration.

Clinical particulars
Therapeutic indications: Unstable coronary artery disease, defined as newly developed or increased angina or ongoing chest pain, with the electrocardiogram changes of non Q-wave myocardial infarction.

Posology and method of administration:
Adults: 120 IU/kg body weight subcutaneously twelve hourly. The maximum dose is 10,000 IU/12 hours.

The recommended treatment period is 5–8 days. Concomitant therapy with low dose aspirin is recommended.

Children: Not recommended for children.

Elderly: Fragmin has been used safely in elderly patients without the need for dosage adjustment.

Method of administration: Following the determination of the required dose, excess solution should be ejected from the syringe.

Administration is by subcutaneous injection, preferably into the abdominal subcutaneous tissue anterolaterally or posterolaterally, or into the lateral part of the thigh. Patients should be supine and the total length of the needle should be introduced vertically, not at an angle, into the thick part of a skin fold, produced by squeezing the skin between thumb and forefinger; the skin fold should be held throughout the injection.

Syringes should be discarded after use

Contra-indications: Known hypersensitivity to Fragmin or other low molecular weight heparins and/or heparins e.g. history of confirmed or suspected immunologically mediated heparin induced thrombocytopenia; acute gastroduodenal ulcer; cerebral haemorrhage; known haemorrhagic diathesis; subacute endocarditis; injuries to and operations on the central nervous system, eyes and ears.

Special warnings and precautions for use: Do not administer by the intramuscular route.

Caution should be exercised in patients in whom there is an increased risk of bleeding complications, e.g. following surgery or trauma, haemorrhagic stroke, severe liver or renal failure, thrombocytopenia or defective platelet function, uncontrolled hypertension, hypertensive or diabetic retinopathy, patients receiving concurrent anticoagulant/antiplateletagents (see Interactions Section).

It is recommended that platelets be counted before starting treatment with Fragmin and monitored regularly. Special caution is necessary in rapidly developing thrombocytopenia and severe thrombocytopenia (<100,000/µl) associated with positive or unknown results of *in-vitro* tests for anti-platelet antibody in the presence of Fragmin or other low molecular weight (mass) heparins and/or heparin.

Patients with severely disturbed hepatic function may need a reduction in dosage and should be monitored accordingly.

If a transmural myocardial infarction occurs, thrombolytic treatment might be appropriate. This does not necessitate discontinuation of treatment with Fragmin, but might increase the risk of bleeding.

As individual low molecular weight (mass) heparins have differing characteristics, switching to an alternative low molecular weight heparin should be avoided. The directions for use relating to each specific product must be observed as different dosages may be required.

Interaction with other medicaments and other forms of interaction: The possibility of the following interactions with Fragmin should be considered:

i) An enhancement of the anticoagulant effect by anticoagulant/antiplatelet agents e.g. aspirin/dipyridamole, vitamin K antagonists, NSAIDs e.g. indomethacin, cytostatics, dextran, sulphinpyrazone, probenecid, and ethacrynic acid. However, unless specifically contra-indicated, patients should receive oral low-dose aspirin.

ii) A reduction of the anticoagulant effect may occur with concomitant administration of antihistamines, cardiac glycosides, tetracycline and ascorbic acid.

Pregnancy and lactation: This medicinal product has been assessed in pregnant women and no harmful effects are known with respect to the course of pregnancy and the health of the unborn and neonate.

No information is available as to whether Fragmin passes into breast milk.

Effects on ability to drive and use machines: Fragmin does not affect the ability to drive or operate machinery.

Undesirable effects: Bleeding may be provoked, especially at high dosages corresponding with anti-Factor Xa levels greater than 1.5 IU/ml. However, at recommended dosages bleedings rarely occur.

Transient, slight to moderate, elevation of liver transaminases (ASAT, ALAT) has been observed, but no clinical significance has been demonstrated.

Commonly reported side-effects include subcutaneous haematomas at the injection site and mild thrombocytopenia (type I) which is usually reversible during treatment.

Allergic reactions (urticaria, pruritus, hair loss and skin necrosis) occur rarely.

A few cases of anaphylactoid reactions and of severe immunologically mediated thrombocytopenia (type II) with arterial and/or venous thrombosis or thromboembolism have been observed.

Osteoporosis has been associated with long-term heparin treatment and therefore cannot be excluded with Fragmin.

Overdose: The anticoagulant effect (i.e. prolongation of the APTT) induced by Fragmin is inhibited by protamine. Since protamine itself has an inhibiting effect on primary haemostasis it should be used only in an emergency. The prolongation of the clotting time induced by Fragmin may be fully neutralised by protamine, but the anti-Factor Xa activity is only neutralised to about 25–50%. 1 mg of protamine inhibits the effect of 100 IU (anti-Factor Xa) of Fragmin.

Pharmacological properties

Pharmacodynamic properties: Dalteparin sodium is a low molecular weight heparin fraction (average molecular weight 4000-6000 Daltons) produced from porcine-derived sodium heparin.

Dalteparin sodium is an antithrombotic agent, which acts mainly through its ability to potentiate the inhibition of Factor Xa and thrombin by antithrombin. It has a relatively higher ability to potentiate Factor Xa inhibition than to prolong plasma clotting time (APTT).

Compared with standard, unfractioned heparin, dalteparin sodium has a reduced adverse effect on platelet function and platelet adhesion, and thus has only a minimal effect on primary haemostasis. Some of the antithrombotic properties of dalteparin sodium are thought to be mediated through the effects on vessel walls or the fibrinolytic system.

Pharmacokinetic properties: The half life following s.c. administration is 3.5–4 hours, twice that of unfractioned heparin.

The bioavailability following s.c. injection is approximately 87 per cent and the pharmacokinetics are not dose dependent. The half life is prolonged in uraemic patients as dalteparin sodium is eliminated primarily thought the kidneys.

Preclinical safety data: The acute toxicity of dalteparin sodium is considerably lower than that of heparin. The only significant finding, which occurred consistently throughout the toxicity studies after subcutaneous administration of the higher dose levels was local haemorrhage at the injection sites, dose-related in incidence and severity. There was no cumulative effect on injection site haemorrhages.

The haemorrhagic reaction was reflected in dose related changes in the anticoagulant effects as measured by APTT and anti-Factor Xa activities.

It was concluded that dalteparin sodium did not have a greater osteopenic effect than heparin since at equivalent doses the osteopenic effect was comparable.

The results revealed no organ toxicity irrespective of the route of administration, doses or duration of treatment. No mutagenic effect was found. No embryotoxic or teratogenic effects and no effect on fertility reproductive capacity or peri- and postnatal development was shown.

Pharmaceutical particulars

List of excipients

Sodium Chloride PhEur
Water for Injections PhEur
Sodium hydroxide or hydrochloric acid for pH adjustment

Incompatibilities: Not applicable.

Shelf life: 36 months.

Special precautions for storage: Store at room temperature (below 25°C).

Nature and contents of container: 1 ml single dose syringe (glass PhEur Type I) with chlorobutyl rubber stopper containing dalteparin sodium 10,000 IU (anti-Factor Xa) in 1 ml.

Instructions for use/handling: Fragmin Graduated Syringes are for single dose use only.

Marketing authorisation number

Fragmin Graduated Syringe 0022/0202

Date of first authorisation/renewal of authorisation

Pending.

Date of (partial) revision of the text April 16, 1998.

Legal category POM.

FRAGMIN* MULTIDOSE VIAL

Qualitative and quantitative composition Fragmin 100,000 IU/4 ml Multidose Vial.

Active ingredient: Dalteparin sodium (INN); Quality according to PhEur and in-house specification.

Potency is described in International anti-Factor Xa units (IU) of the 1st International Standard for Low Molecular Weight Heparin.

Content of active ingredient: Fragmin 100,000 IU/4 ml: Multidose vial containing dalteparin sodium corresponding to 25,000 IU (anti-Factor Xa)/ml.

Pharmaceutical form Solution for injection for subcutaneous administration.

Clinical particulars

Therapeutic indications: Treatment of acute deep venous thrombosis.

Posology and method of administration

Recommended dosage for adults:

Treatment of deep venous thrombosis: Fragmin can be administered subcutaneously either as a single daily injection or as twice daily injections.

Once daily administration: 200 IU/kg body weight is administered s.c once daily. Monitoring of the anticoagulant effect is not necessary. The single daily dose should not exceed 18,000 IU.

Twice daily administration: A dose of 100 IU/kg body weight administered s.c twice daily can be used for patients with increased risk of bleeding. Monitoring of the treatment is generally not necessary but can be performed with a functional anti-Factor Xa assay. Maximum plasma levels are obtained 3–4 hours after s.c injection, when samples should be taken. Recommended plasma levels are between 0.5–1.0 IU (anti-Factor Xa)/ml.

Simultaneous anticoagulation with oral vitamin K antagonists can be started immediately. Treatment with Fragmin is continued until the prothrombin complex levels (factor II, VII, IX and X) have decreased to a therapeutic level. At least five days of combined treatment is normally required.

Children: Not recommended for children.

Elderly: Fragmin has been used safely in elderly patients without the need for dosage adjustment.

Contra-indications: Known hypersensitivity to Fragmin, other low molecular weight heparins and/or heparins e.g. history of confirmed or suspected immunologically mediated heparin induced thrombocytopenia, or benzyl alcohol; acute gastroduodenal ulcer; cerebral haemorrhage; known haemorrhagic diathesis; subacute endocarditis; injuries to and operations on the central nervous system, eyes and ears. In patients treated with Fragmin for acute deep venous thrombosis, regional anaesthesia is contraindicated due to an increased risk of bleeding.

Special warnings and special precautions for use: Do not administer by the intramuscular route.

Caution should be exercised in patients in whom there is an increased risk of bleeding complications, e.g. following surgery or trauma, haemorrhagic stroke, severe liver or renal failure, thrombocytopenia or defective platelet function, uncontrolled hypertension, hypertensive or diabetic retinopathy, patients receiving concurrent anticoagulant/antiplateletagents (see interactions section).

It is recommended that platelets be counted before starting treatment with Fragmin and monitored regularly. Special caution is necessary in rapidly developing thrombocytopenia and severe thrombocytopenia (<100,000/µl) associated with positive or unknown results of in-vitro tests for anti-platelet antibody in the presence of Fragmin or other low molecular weight (mass) heparins and/or heparin.

Fragmin induces only a moderate prolongation of the APTT and thrombin time. Accordingly, dosage increments based upon prolongation of the APTT may cause overdosage and bleeding. Therefore, prolongation of the APTT should only be used as a test of overdosage.

Patients with severely disturbed hepatic function may need a reduction in dosage and should be monitored accordingly.

As individual low molecular weight (mass) heparins have differing characteristics, switching to an alternative low molecular weight heparin should be avoided. The directions for use relating to each specific product must be observed as different dosages may be required.

Interaction with other medicaments and other forms of interaction: The possibility of the following interactions with Fragmin should be considered:

An enhancement of the anticoagulant effect by anticoagulant/antiplatelet agents e.g. aspirin/ dipyridamole, vitamin K antagonists, NSAIDs e.g. indomethacin, cytostatics, dextran, sulphinpyrazone, probenecid, and ethacrynic acid.

A reduction of the anticoagulant effect may occur with concomitant administration of antihistamines, cardiac glycosides, tetracycline and ascorbic acid.

Pregnancy and lactation: Fragmin multidose vial contains benzyl alcohol as a preservative and is not recommended for use during pregnancy. Benzyl alcohol may cross the placenta. One should bear in mind the potential toxicity for premature infants.

No information is available as to whether Fragmin passes into breast milk.

Effects on ability to drive and use machines: Fragmin does not affect the ability to drive or operate machinery.

Undesirable effects: Bleeding may be provoked, especially at high dosages corresponding with anti-Factor Xa levels greater than 1.5 IU/ml. However, at recommended dosages bleeding rarely occurs.

Transient, slight to moderate, elevation of liver

transaminases (ASAT, ALAT) has been observed, but no clinical significance has been demonstrated.

Commonly reported side-effects include: Subcutaneous haematomas at the injection site. Mild thrombocytopenia (type I) which is usually reversible during treatment.

Allergic reactions (urticaria, pruritus, hair loss and skin necrosis) occur rarely.

Few cases of anaphylactoid reactions and of severe immunologically mediated thrombocytopenia (type II) with arterial and/or venous thrombosis or thromboembolism have been observed.

Osteoporosis has been associated with long-term heparin treatment and therefore cannot be excluded with Fragmin.

Overdose: The anticoagulant effect (i.e. prolongation of the APTT) induced by Fragmin is inhibited by protamine. Since protamine itself has an inhibiting effect on primary haemostasis it should be used only in an emergency. The prolongation of the clotting time induced by Fragmin may be fully neutralised by protamine, but the anti-Factor Xa activity is only neutralised to about 25–50%. 1 mg of protamine inhibits the effect of 100 IU (anti-Factor Xa) of Fragmin.

Pharmacological properties
Pharmacodynamic properties: Dalteparin sodium is a low molecular weight heparin fraction (average molecular weight 4000–6000 Daltons) produced from porcine-derived sodium heparin.

Dalteparin sodium is an antithrombotic agent, which acts mainly through its ability to potentiate the inhibition of Factor Xa and thrombin by antithrombin. It has a relatively higher ability to potentiate Factor Xa inhibition than to prolong plasma clotting time (APTT).

Compared with standard, unfractionated heparin, dalteparin sodium has a reduced adverse effect on platelet function and platelet adhesion, and thus has only a minimal effect on primary haemostasis. Still some of the antithrombotic properties of dalteparin sodium are thought to be mediated through the effects on vessel walls or the fibrinolytic system.

Pharmacokinetic properties: The half life following i.v and s.c administration is 2 hours and 3.5–4 hours respectively, twice that of unfractionated heparin.

The bioavailability following s.c injection is approximately 87 per cent and the pharmacokinetics are not dose dependent. The half life is prolonged in uraemic patients as dalteparin sodium is eliminated primarily through the kidneys.

Preclinical safety data: The acute toxicity of dalteparin sodium is considerably lower than that of heparin. The only significant finding, which occurred consistently throughout the toxicity studies after subcutaneous administration of the higher dose levels was local haemorrhage at the injection sites, dose-related in incidence and severity. There was no cumulative effect on injection site haemorrhages.

The haemorrhagic reaction was reflected in dose related changes in the anticoagulant effects as measured by APTT and anti-Factor Xa activities.

It was concluded that dalteparin sodium did not have a greater osteopenic effect than heparin since at equivalent doses the osteopenic effect was comparable.

The results revealed no organ toxicity irrespective of the route of administration, doses or the duration of treatment. No mutagenic effect was found. No embryotoxic or teratogenic effects and no effect on fertility reproductive capacity or peri- and postnatal development was shown.

Pharmaceutical particulars
List of excipients: Benzyl alcohol (PhEur) Water for injections (PhEur)

Incompatibilities: Not applicable.

Shelf life: 24 months. Once opened, the solution should be used within 14 days.

Special precautions for storage: Store at room temperature (below 30°C).

Nature and contents of container: Multidose vial (Ph Eur Type 1) with bromobutyl rubber stopper, secured with aluminium overseal with flip off cap, containing dalteparin sodium 100,000 IU (anti-Factor Xa) in 4 ml.

Instructions for use/handling: As with other multidose preparations, care should be taken to avoid any risk of cross-contamination during use.

Marketing authorisation number 0022/0177

Date of first authorisation/renewal of authorisation Product Licence granted 31st July 1996.

Date of (partial) revision of the text September 16 1997.

Legal category POM.

FRAGMIN* 10,000 IU, 12,500 IU, 15,000 IU AND 18,000 IU SYRINGES

Qualitative and quantitative composition
Active ingredient: Dalteparin sodium (INN). Quality according to PhEur and in-house specification.

Potency is described in International anti-Factor Xa units (IU) of the 1st International Standard for Low Molecular Weight Heparin.

Fragmin 10,000 IU: single dose syringe containing dalteparin sodium 10,000 IU (anti-Factor Xa) in 0.4 ml solution.

Fragmin 12,500 IU: single dose syringe containing dalteparin sodium 12,500 IU (anti-Factor Xa) in 0.5 ml solution.

Fragmin 15,000 IU: single dose syringe containing dalteparin sodium 15,000 IU (anti-Factor Xa) in 0.6 ml solution.

Fragmin 18,000 IU: single dose syringe containing dalteparin sodium 18,000 IU (anti-Factor Xa) in 0.72 ml solution.

Fragmin does not contain preservatives.

Pharmaceutical form Solution for injection for subcutaneous administration.

Clinical particulars
Therapeutic indications: Treatment of acute deep venous thrombosis (DVT).

Posology and method of administration
Adult: A single dose of Fragmin is administered subcutaneously, once daily according to the following weight ranges. Monitoring of the anticoagulant effect is not usually necessary.

Weight (kg)	*Dose*
46–56	10,000 IU
57–68	12,500 IU
69–82	15,000 IU
83 and over	18,000 IU

Simultaneous anti-coagulation with vitamin K antagonists can be started immediately. Treatment with Fragmin is continued until the prothrombin complex levels (Factor II, VII, IX and X) have decreased to a therapeutic level. At least five days of combined treatment is normally required.

For patients with an increased risk of bleeding, it is recommended that Fragmin be administered according to the twice daily regimen detailed in the Summary of Product Characteristics for Fragmin 10,000 IU/1 ml ampoules or Fragmin Multidose Vial.

Children: Not recommended for children.

Elderly: Fragmin has been used safely in elderly patients without the need for dosage adjustment.

Method of administration: By subcutaneous injection, preferably into the abdominal subcutaneous tissue anterolaterally or posterolaterally, or into the lateral part of the thigh. Patients should be supine and the total length of the needle should be introduced vertically, not at an angle, into the thick part of a skin fold, produced by squeezing the skin between thumb and forefinger; the skin fold should be held throughout the injection.

Contra-indications: Known hypersensitivity to Fragmin or other low molecular weight heparins and/or heparins e.g. history of confirmed or suspected immunologically mediated heparin induced thrombocytopenia; acute gastroduodenal ulcer; cerebral haemorrhage; known haemorrhagic diathesis; subacute endocarditis; injuries to and operations on the central nervous system, eyes and ears.

In patients being treated with Fragmin for acute deep venous thrombosis, regional anaesthesia is contra-indicated due to an increased risk of bleeding.

Special warnings and precautions for use: Caution should be exercised in patients in whom there is an increased risk of bleeding complications, e.g. following trauma, haemorrhagic stroke, severe liver or renal failure, thrombocytopenia or defective platelet function, uncontrolled hypertension, hypertensive or diabetic retinopathy, patients receiving concurrent anticoagulant/antiplatelet agents (see *Interactions*).

It is recommended that platelets be counted before starting treatment with Fragmin and monitored regularly. Special caution is necessary in rapidly developing thrombocytopenia and severe thrombocytopenia ($<100{,}000/\mu l$) associated with positive or unknown results of in-vitro tests for anti-platelet antibody in the presence of Fragmin or other low molecular weight (mass) heparins and/or heparin.

Fragmin induces only a moderate prolongation of the APTT and thrombin time. Accordingly, dosage increments based upon prolongation of the APTT may cause overdosage and bleeding. Therefore, prolongation of the APTT should only be used as a test of overdosage.

As individual low molecular weight (mass) heparins have differing characteristics, switching to an alternative low molecular weight heparin should be avoided. The directions for use relating to each specific product must be observed as different dosages may be required.

Do not administer by the intramuscular route.

Interaction with other medicaments and other forms of interaction: The possibility of the following interactions with Fragmin should be considered:

i) An enhancement of the anticoagulant effect by anticoagulant/antiplatelet agents e.g. aspirin/dipyridamole, Vitamin K antagonists, NSAIDs e.g. indomethacin, cytostatics, dextran, sulphinpyrazone, probenecid, and ethacrynic acid.

ii) A reduction of the anticoagulant effect may occur with concomitant administration of antihistamines, cardiac glycosides, tetracycline and ascorbic acid.

Pregnancy and lactation: This medicinal product has been assessed in pregnant women and no harmful effects are known with respect to the course of pregnancy and the health of the unborn and neonate.

No information is available as to whether Fragmin passes into breast milk.

Effects on ability to drive and use machines: Fragmin does not affect the ability to drive or operate machinery.

Undesirable effects: Bleeding may be provoked, especially at high dosages corresponding with anti-Factor Xa levels greater than 1.5 IU/ml. However, at recommended dosages bleedings rarely occur.

Transient, slight to moderate, elevation of liver transaminases (ASAT, ALAT) has been observed, but no clinical significance has been demonstrated.

Commonly reported side-effects include subcutaneous haematomas at the injection site and mild thrombocytopenia (type I) which is usually reversible during treatment.

Allergic reactions (urticaria, pruritus, hair loss and skin necrosis) occur rarely.

A few cases of anaphylactoid reactions and of severe immunologically mediated thrombocytopenia (type II) with arterial and/or venous thrombosis or thromboembolism have been observed.

Osteoporosis has been associated with long-term heparin treatment and therefore cannot be excluded with Fragmin.

Overdose: The anticoagulant effect (i.e. prolongation of the APTT) induced by Fragmin is inhibited by protamine. Since protamine itself has an inhibiting effect on primary haemostasis it should be used only in an emergency. The prolongation of the clotting time induced by Fragmin may be fully neutralised by protamine, but the anti-Factor Xa activity is only neutralised to about 25–50%. 1 mg of protamine inhibits the effect of 100 IU (anti-Factor Xa) of Fragmin.

Pharmacological properties
Pharmacodynamic properties: Dalteparin sodium is a low molecular weight heparin fraction (average molecular weight 4000–6000 daltons) produced from porcine-derived sodium heparin.

Dalteparin sodium is an antithrombotic agent, which acts mainly through its ability to potentiate the inhibition of Factor Xa and thrombin by antithrombin. It has a relatively higher ability to potentiate Factor Xa inhibition than to prolong plasma clotting time (APTT).

Compared with standard, unfractioned heparin, dalteparin sodium has a reduced adverse effect on platelet function and platelet adhesion, and thus has only a minimal effect on primary haemostasis. Still some of the antithrombotic properties of dalteparin sodium are thought to be mediated through the effects on vessel walls or the fibrinolytic system.

Pharmacokinetic properties: The half life following i.v. and s.c. administration is 2 hours and 3.5–4 hours respectively, twice that of unfractioned heparin.

The bioavailability following s.c. injection is approximately 87 per cent and the pharmacokinetics are not dose dependent. The half life is prolonged in uraemic patients as dalteparin sodium is eliminated primarily though the kidneys.

Preclinical safety data: The acute toxicity of dalteparin sodium is considerably lower than that of heparin. The only significant finding, which occurred consistently throughout the toxicity studies after subcutaneous administration of the higher dose levels was local haemorrhage at the injection sites, dose-related in incidence and severity. There was no cumulative effect on injection site haemorrhages.

The haemorrhagic reaction was reflected in dose related changes in the anticoagulant effects as measured by APTT and anti-Factor Xa activities.

It was concluded that dalteparin sodium did not have a greater osteopenic effect than heparin since at equivalent doses the osteopenic effect was comparable.

The results revealed no organ toxicity irrespective of the route of administration, doses or duration of treatment. No mutagenic effect was found. No embryotoxic or teratogenic effects and no effect on fertility reproductive capacity or peri- and postnatal development was shown.

Pharmaceutical particulars
List of excipients: Water for Injections (PhEur); Sodium chloride (PhEur); Sodium hydroxide or hydrochloric acid for pH adjustment.

Incompatibilities: Not applicable.

Shelf life: 24 months.

Special precautions for storage: Store at room temperature (below 25°C).

Nature and contents of container: 1 ml single dose syringe (glass PhEur Type I) with chlorobutyl rubber stopper containing dalteparin sodium 10,000 IU (anti-Factor Xa) in 0.4 ml or 12,500 IU (anti-Factor Xa) in 0.5 ml or 15,000 IU (anti-Factor Xa) in 0.6 ml or 18,000 IU (anti-Factor Xa) in 0.72 ml.

Instructions for use/handling: Not applicable.

Marketing authorisation numbers
Fragmin 10,000 IU 0022/0197
Fragmin 12,500 IU 0022/0198
Fragmin 15,000 IU 0022/0199
Fragmin 18,000 IU 0022/0200

Date of first authorisation/renewal of authorisation 11 February 1998.

Date of (partial) revision of the text 30 January 1998.

Legal category POM.

FRAGMIN* 2500 IU AND 5000 IU SYRINGES

Qualitative and quantitative composition
Active ingredient: Dalteparin sodium (INN); Quality according to PhEur and in-house specification.

Potency is described in International anti-Factor Xa units (IU) of the 1st International Standard for Low Molecular Weight Heparin.

Content of active ingredient: Fragmin 2500 IU: single dose syringe containing dalteparin sodium 2,500 IU (anti-Factor Xa) in 0.2 ml solution.

Fragmin 5000 IU: single dose syringe containing dalteparin sodium 5000 IU (anti-Factor Xa) in 0.2 ml solution.

Fragmin syringes do not contain preservatives.

Pharmaceutical form Solution for injection for subcutaneous administration.

Clinical particulars
Therapeutic indications: Peri- and post-operative surgical thromboprophylaxis.

Posology and method of administration:
Adults:

Surgical thromboprophylaxis in patients at moderate risk of thrombosis: 2,500 IU is administered subcutaneously 1–2 hours before the surgical procedure and thereafter 2,500 IU subcutaneously each morning until the patient is mobilised, in general 5-7 days or longer.

Surgical thromboprophylaxis in patients at high risk of thrombosis: 2,500 IU is administered subcutaneously 1–2 hours before the surgical procedure and 2,500 IU subcutaneously 8-12 hours later. On the following days, 5,000 IU subcutaneously each morning.

As an alternative, 5,000 IU is administered subcutaneously the evening before the surgical procedure and 5,000 IU subcutaneously the following evenings.

Treatment is continued until the patient is mobilised, in general 5–7 days or longer.

Prolonged thromboprophylaxis in hip replacement surgery: 5,000IU is given subcutaneously the evening before the operation and 5,000IU subcutaneously the following evenings. Treatment is continued for five post-operative weeks.

Children: Not recommended for children.

Elderly: Fragmin has been used safely in elderly patients without the need for dosage adjustment.

Method of administration: By subcutaneous injection, preferably into the abdominal subcutaneous tissue anterolaterally or posterolaterally, or into the lateral part of the thigh. Patients should be supine and the total length of the needle should be introduced vertically, not at an angle, into the thick part of a skin fold, produced by squeezing the skin between the thumb and forefinger; the skin fold should be held throughout the injection.

Contra-indications: Known hypersensitivity to Fragmin or other low molecular weight heparins and/or heparins e.g. history of confirmed or suspected immunologically mediated heparin induced thrombocytopenia; acute gastroduodenal ulcer; cerebral haemorrhage; known haemorrhagic diathesis; subacute endocarditis; injuries to and operations on the central nervous system, eyes and ears.

Special warnings and special precautions for use: Caution should be exercised in patients in whom there is an increased risk of bleeding complications, e.g. following trauma, haemorrhagic stroke, severe liver or renal failure, thrombocytopenia or defective platelet function, uncontrolled hypertension, hypertensive or diabetic retinopathy, patients receiving concurrent anticoagulant/anitplatelet agents (see Interactions Section).

It is recommended that platelets be counted before starting treatment with Fragmin and monitored regularly.Special caution is necessary in rapidly developing thrombocytopenia and severe thrombocytopenia (<100,000/μl) associated with positive or unknown results of in-vitro tests for anti-platelet antibody in the presence of Fragmin or other low molecular weight (mass) heparins and/or heparin.

Fragmin when administered in a dose of 2,500–5,000 IU (anti-Factor Xa)/day does not generally accumulate, and therefore monitoring of the effect is not usually required. However, if considered necessary, chromogenic substrate assays can be used to measure anti-Factor Xa activity (Fragmin has only a moderate prolonging effect on clotting time assays such as APTT or thrombin time).

As individual low molecular weight (mass) heparins have differing characteristics, switching to an alternative low molecular weight heparin should be avoided. The directions for use relating to each specific product must be observed as different dosages may be required.

Do not administer by the intramuscular route.

Interaction with other medicaments and other forms of interaction: The possibility of the following interactions with Fragmin should be considered:

An enhancement of the anticoagulant effect by anticoagulant/antiplatelet agents e.g. aspirin/dipyridamole, Vitamin K antagonists, NSAIDS e.g. indomethacin, cytostatics, dextran, sulphinpyrazone, probenecid, and ethacrynic acid.

A reduction of the anticoagulant effect may occur with concomitant administration of antihistamines, cardiac glycosides, tetracycline and ascorbic acid.

Pregnancy and lactation: This medicinal product has been assessed in pregnant women and no harmful effects are known with respect to the course of pregnancy and the health of the unborn and neonate.

No information is available as to whether Fragmin passes into breast milk.

Effects on ability to drive and use machines: Fragmin does not affect the ability to drive or operate machinery.

Undesirable effects: Bleeding may be provoked, especially at high dosages corresponding with anti-Factor Xa levels greater than 1.5 IU/ml. However, at recommended dosages bleeding rarely occurs.

Transient, slight to moderate, elevation of liver transaminases (ASAT, ALAT) has been observed, but no clinical significance has been demonstrated.

Commonly reported side-effects include: Subcutaneous haematomas at the injection site. Mild thrombocytopenia (type I) which is usually reversible during treatment.

Allergic reactions (urticaria, pruritus, hair loss and skin necrosis) occur rarely.

A few cases of anaphylactoid reactions and of severe immunologically mediated thrombocytopenia (type II) with arterial and/or venous thrombosis or thromboembolism have been observed.

Osteoporosis has been associated with long-term heparin treatment and therefore cannot be excluded with Fragmin.

Overdose: The anticoagulant effect (i.e. prolongation of the APTT) induced by Fragmin is inhibited by protamine. Since protamine itself has an inhibiting effect on primary haemostasis it should be used only in an emergency. The prolongation of the clotting time induced by Fragmin may be fully neutralised by protamine, but the anti-Factor Xa activity is only neutralised to about 25–50%. 1 mg of protamine inhibits the effect of 100 IU (anti-Factor Xa) of Fragmin.

Pharmacological properties
Pharmacodynamic properties: Dalteparin sodium is a low molecular weight heparin fraction (average molecular weight 4000–6000 daltons) produced from porcine-derived sodium heparin.

Dalteparin sodium is an antithrombotic agent, which acts mainly through its ability to potentiate the inhibition of Factor Xa and thrombin by antithrombin. It has a relatively higher ability to potentiate Factor Xa inhibition than to prolong plasma clotting time (APTT).

Compared with standard, unfractionated heparin, dalteparin sodium has a reduced adverse effect on platelet function and platelet adhesion, and thus has only a minimal effect on primary haemostasis. Still some of the antithrombotic properties of dalteparin sodium are thought to be mediated through the effects on vessel walls or the fibrinolytic system.

Pharmacokinetic properties: The half-life following i.v. and s.c. administration is 2 hours and 3.5–4 hours respectively, twice that of unfractionated heparin.

The bioavailability following s.c. injection is approximately 87 per cent and the pharmacokinetics are not dose dependent. The half life is prolonged in uraemic patients as dalteparin sodium is eliminated primarily through the kidneys.

Preclinical safety data: The acute toxicity of dalteparin sodium is considerably lower than that of heparin. The only significant finding, which occurred consistently throughout the toxicity studies after subcutaneous administration of the higher dose levels was local haemorrhage at the injection sites, dose-related in incidence and severity. There was no cumulative effect on injection site haemorrhages.

The haemorrhagic reaction was reflected in dose related changes in the anticoagulant effects as measured by APTT and anti-Factor Xa activities.

It was concluded that dalteparin sodium did not have a greater osteopenic effect than heparin since at equivalent doses the osteopenic effect was comparable.

The results revealed no organ toxicity irrespective of the route of administration, doses or duration of treatment. No mutagenic effect was found. No embryotoxic or teratogenic effects and no effect on fertility, reproductive capacity or peri- and post natal development was shown.

Pharmaceutical particulars
List of excipients: Sodium chloride (PhEur) (2,500 IU presentation only) Water for Injections (PhEur) (2,500 IU and 5,000 IU presentations).

Incompatibilities: Not applicable.

Shelf life: 36 months

Special precautions for storage: Store at room temperature (below 30°C).

Nature and contents of container: Single dose syringe (glass PhEur Type I) with chlorobutyl rubber stopper containing dalteparin sodium 2500 IU (anti-Factor Xa) in 0.2 ml or 5000 IU (anti-Factor Xa) in 0.2 ml.

Instructions for use/handling: Not applicable.

Marketing authorisation numbers
Fragmin 2,500 IU 0022/0076
Fragmin 5,000 IU 0022/0077

Date of first authorisation/renewal of authorisation
Fragmin 2,500 IU–Product Licence granted 15 April 1991

Fragmin 5,000 IU–Product Licence granted 15 April 1991

Date of (partial) revision of the text September 19 1997.

Legal category POM.

GENOTROPIN* 2IU (0.7 mg), 3IU (1 mg), 4 IU (1.3 mg) KABIQUICK, GENOTROPIN* 4 IU (1.3 mg), GENOTROPIN* 4 IU (1.3 mg) KABIVIAL MULTIDOSE, GENOTROPIN* 16 IU (5.3 mg), GENOTROPIN* 16 IU (5.3 mg) KABIVIAL MULTIDOSE, GENOTROPIN* 36 IU (12 mg)

Qualitative and quantitative composition Active constituent: Somatropin (rbe) 2IU (0.7 mg), 3IU (1 mg), 4IU (1.3 mg), 16IU (5.3 mg) or 36IU (12 mg)

Pharmaceutical form Powder and solvent for solution for injection (with or without preservative) for subcutaneous (sc) administration.

Clinical particulars
Therapeutic indications: Growth disturbance due to insufficient secretion of growth hormone or associated with gonadal dysgenesis (Turner syndrome).

Growth disturbance in prepubertal children with chronic renal insufficiency.

Replacement therapy in adults with pronounced growth hormone deficiency as diagnosed in two different dynamic tests for growth hormone deficiency. Patients must also fulfil the following criteria:

Childhood onset: Patients, who were diagnosed as growth hormone deficient during childhood, must be retested and their growth hormone deficiency confirmed before replacement therapy with Genotropin is started.

Adult onset: Patients must have growth hormone deficiency as a result of hypothalamic or pituitary disease and at least one other hormone deficiency diagnosed (except for prolactin) and adequate replacement therapy instituted, before replacement therapy using growth hormone may begin.

Posology and method of administration: The dosage and administration schedule should be personalised for each individual.

The injection site should be varied to prevent lipoatrophy.

Growth disturbance due to insufficient secretion of growth hormone in children: Generally a dose of 0.07–0.10IU/kg (0.025–0.035 mg/kg) body weight per day or 2.1–3.0IU/m² (0.7–1.0 mg/m²) body surface area per day is recommended. Even higher doses have been used.

Growth disturbance due to gonadal dysgenesis (Turner syndrome): A dose of 0.14IU/kg (0.045–0.050 mg/kg) body weight per day or 4.3IU/m² (1.4 mg/m²) body surface area per day is recommended.

Growth disturbance in chronic renal insufficiency: A dose of 4.3IU/m² (1.4 mg/m²) body surface area per day (approximately 0.14IU/kg (0.045–0.050 mg/kg) body weight per day) is recommended. Higher doses can be needed if growth velocity is too low. A dose correction can be needed after six months of treatment.

Growth hormone deficient adult patients: The recommended dosage at the start of therapy is 0.018 IU/kg (0.006 mg/kg) per day. The dose should be gradually increased according to individual patient requirements to a maximum of 0.036 IU/kg (0.012 mg/kg) per day. Side effects of the patients as well as determination of insulin-like growth factor-I (IGF-I) in serum should be used as guidance for dose titration. The minimum effective dose should be used and dose requirements may decline with increasing age.

(See Table.)

Contra-indications: Genotropin should not be used when there is any evidence of activity of a tumour. Intracranial lesions must be inactive and antitumour therapy completed prior to starting therapy.

Genotropin should not be used for growth promotion in children with closed epiphyses.

Special warnings and special precautions for use: Diagnosis and therapy with Genotropin should be initiated and monitored by physicians who are appropriately qualified and experienced in the diagnosis and management of patients with growth hormone deficiency.

In diabetes mellitus, the dose of insulin might require adjustment when Genotropin is instituted.

A state of hypothyroidism may develop during somatropin treatment. Since untreated hypothyroidism may interfere with the response to somatropin, patients should have a periodic thyroid function test and should be treated with thyroid hormone when indicated.

In growth hormone deficiency secondary to treatment of malignant disease, it is recommended to pay attention to signs of relapse of the malignancy.

In patients with endocrine disorders, including growth hormone deficiency, slipped epiphyses of the hip may occur more frequently. Each child with limping during treatment with growth hormone should be examined clinically.

In patients with (pan) hypopituitarism, standard replacement therapy has to be monitored closely.

In case of severe or recurrent headache, visual problems, nausea and/or vomiting, a funduscopy for papilloedema is recommended. If papilloedema is confirmed, a diagnosis of benign intracranial hypertension should be considered and, if appropriate, the growth hormone treatment should be discontinued.

At present there is insufficient evidence to guide clinical decision making in patients with resolved intracranial hypertension. If growth hormone treatment is restarted, careful monitoring for symptoms of intracranial hypertension is necessary.

No information on the final height in Turner syndrome is available yet.

In chronic renal insufficiency, the renal function should have decreased below 50 per cent of normal before institution of therapy. To verify the growth disturbance, the growth should have been followed for a year preceding institution of therapy. Conservative treatment for the renal insufficiency should have been established and should be maintained during treatment. The treatment should be discontinued after renal transplantation.

Experience in patients above 60 years is lacking.

Experience with prolonged treatment in adults is limited.

Interaction with other medicaments and other forms of interaction: Patients with diabetes mellitus may require adjustment of their antidiabetic therapy (see under *Special warnings and special precautions for use*).

Pregnancy and lactation:
Pregnancy: No clinical experience of the use in pregnant women is available. Animal experimental data are incomplete. Treatment with Genotropin should be interrupted if pregnancy occurs.

Lactation: No information is available as to whether peptide hormones pass into breast milk, but absorption of intact protein from the gastrointestinal tract of the infant is extremely unlikely.

Effects on ability to drive and use machines: The ability to react is not influenced by somatropin.

Undesirable effects: Side effects have been noted in approximately 10% of the patients participating in clinical trials in children with short stature.

In clinical trials in adults, side effects have been noted in approximately 30–40% of the patients primarily related to symptoms of fluid retention. These events have an early onset after initiation of therapy with a reduction in incidence and prevalence over time and rarely influencing daily activities.

Common (> 1/100) side effects are: Transient local skin reactions at the injection site. Symptoms of fluid retention (peripheral oedema, arthralgia/myalgia).

Genotropin has given rise to the formation of antibodies in a few patients. The binding capacity of these antibodies has been low.

It has been reported that patients may develop hypothyroidism during treatment with Genotropin which should be considered.

In vitro chromosome aberrations have been reported during growth hormone therapy; the clinical significance is unknown.

Some cases of leukaemia have been reported in growth hormone deficient children, untreated as well as treated with growth hormone, and might possibly represent a slightly increased incidence compared with non growth hormone deficient children. A causal relationship to growth hormone therapy has not been established.

Some rare cases of benign intracranial hypertension have been reported.

Overdose: No overdose or intoxication is known.

Acute overdosage could lead initially to hypoglycaemia and subsequently to hyperglycaemia. Long-term overdosage could result in signs and symptoms consistent with the known effects of human growth hormone excess.

Pharmacological properties
Pharmacodynamic properties: Genotropin stimulates linear growth and increases growth rate in children who lack adequate endogenous growth hormone. In adults with growth hormone deficiency, Genotropin reduces fat mass, increases muscle mass and improves energy, vitality and subjective well-being.

Treatment of growth hormone deficient patients with Genotropin normalises serum IGF-I (Insulin-like Growth Factor-I/Somatomedin C) levels.

Genotropin has been studied with regard to its primary and secondary pharmacological effects and the effects of Genotropin are equal to those of pituitary growth hormone.

In addition, the following actions have been demonstrated for Genotropin and/or somatropin.

Tissue growth: Stimulation of skeletal muscle growth in patients with growth hormone deficiency (GHD) as well as increasing the number and size of muscle cells.

Protein metabolism: Nitrogen retention demonstrated by decreased urinary nitrogen excretion and decreased serum urea nitrogen.

Carbohydrate metabolism: Children with hypopituitarism sometimes experience fasting hypoglycaemia that is improved by treatment with Genotropin. Large doses of human growth hormone may impair glucose tolerance.

Lipid metabolism: In GHD patients, administration of somatropin has resulted in lipid mobilisation, reduction in body fat stores and increased plasma fatty acids.

Mineral metabolism: Retention of sodium, potassium and phosphorus is induced by somatropin. Serum concentrations of inorganic phosphate are increased in patients with GHD after therapy with Genotropin or somatropin. Serum calcium is not significantly altered by either Genotropin or somatropin.

Pharmacokinetic properties: Approximately 80% of Genotropin is absorbed following sc injection and maximum serum concentrations are achieved after 3–4 hours.

Preclinical safety data: Genotropin has been studied regarding general toxicity, local tolerance and genotoxicity using pituitary growth hormone as a reference. Genotropin has shown an equivalent toxicological profile to pituitary growth hormone. Based on the experimental studies, a large safety margin is provided for the treatment of growth failure. Preclinical studies on point mutations and inductions of chromosome aberrations have been negative.

Pharmaceutical particulars
List of excipients:
Genotropin 2IU (0.7 mg), 3IU (1 mg), 4IU (1.3 mg) KabiQuick, respectively:

Glycine PhEur 12.0 mg, 18.0 mg, 24.0 mg; Sodium dihydrogen phosphate anhydrous PhEur 0.13 mg, 0.20 mg, 0.26 mg; Disodium phosphate anhydrous PhEur 0.13 mg, 0.19 mg, 0.26 mg; Water for injections PhEur to 0.5 ml, 0.75 ml, 1.0 ml

Genotropin 4IU (1.3 mg): Glycine PhEur 24.0 mg, Sodium dihydrogen phosphate anhydrous PhEur 0.26 mg, Disodium phosphate anhydrous PhEur 0.26 mg

Genotropin 4IU (1.3 mg) KabiVial Multidose: Glycine PhEur 24.0 mg, Sodium dihydrogen phosphate anhydrous PhEur 0.26 mg, Disodium phosphate anhydrous Ph Eur 0.26 mg, m-Cresol 3.0 mg, Water for injections PhEur to 1.0 ml

Genotropin 16IU (5.3 mg)/Genotropin 16IU (5.3 mg) KabiVial Multidose: Glycine PhEur 2.0 mg, Mannitol PhEur 41.0 mg, Sodium dihydrogen phosphate anhydrous PhEur 0.29 mg, Disodium phosphate anhydrous PhEur 0.28 mg, m-cresol 3.0 mg, Water for injections PhEur to 1.0 ml

Genotropin 36IU (12 mg): Glycine PhEur 2.0 mg, Mannitol PhEur 40.0 mg, Sodium dihydrogen phosphate anhydrous PhEur 0.41 mg, Disodium phosphate anhydrous PhEur 0.40 mg, m-cresol 3.0 mg, Water for injections PhEur to 1.0 ml

Incompatibilities: Should only be reconstituted in the supplied solvent.

Shelf life: The powder for injection is assigned a shelf life of 24 months (Genotropin 36IU (12 mg) – 18 months) when stored cold at 2–8°C. Storage for one month can take place at room temperature.

Genotropin 2IU (0.7 mg), 3IU (1 mg), 4IU (1.3 mg) KabiQuick, Genotropin 4IU (1.3 mg): The reconstituted product may be stored cold at 2–8°C for 24 hours protected from light.

Genotropin 4IU (1.3 mg) KabiVial Multidose: The reconstituted product may be stored cold at 2–8°C for 2 weeks protected from light.

Genotropin 16IU (5.3 mg)/Genotropin 16IU (5.3 mg) KabiVial Multidose, Genotropin 36IU (12 mg): The reconstituted product may be stored cold at 2–8°C for 3 weeks protected from light.

Special precautions for storage: Powder which has been frozen should not be used. Store cold at 2–8°C protected from light.

Nature and contents of container:
Genotropin 2IU (0.7 mg), 3IU (1 mg), 4IU (1.3 mg) KabiQuick: Two compartment glass cartridge with separating rubber stoppers in a plastic injection device, KabiQuick.

Genotropin 4IU (1.3 mg): Glass vial containing lyophilised powder together with glass ampoule containing 1 ml water for injection for reconstitution.

Genotropin 4IU (1.3 mg) KabiVial Multidose: Two compartment glass cartridge with separating rubber stoppers in a plastic reconstitution device, KabiVial.

Genotropin 16IU (5.3 mg)/Genotropin 16IU (5.3 mg) KabiVial Multidose: Two compartment glass cartridge with separating rubber stoppers intended to be used in either an injection device or a plastic, multiuse reconstitution device, Genotropin Mixer. The cartridge is also supplied intact in a plastic reconstitution device, KabiVial.

Genotropin 36IU (12 mg): Two compartment glass cartridge with separating rubber stoppers intended to be used in either an injection device or a plastic, multiuse reconstitution device, Genotropin Mixer.

Instructions for use/handling:
Genotropin 4IU (1.3 mg): Add solvent to vial containing powder for injection. Gently dissolve the drug with a slow, swirling motion. Do not shake vigorously; this might denature the active ingredient.

Genotropin 2IU (0.7 mg), 3IU (1 mg), 4IU (1.3 mg) KabiQuick, Genotropin 4IU (1.3 mg) KabiVial Multidose, Genotropin 16IU (5.3 mg)/Genotropin 16IU (5.3 mg) KabiVial Multidose, Genotropin 36IU (12 mg): The solution is prepared by screwing the reconstitution or injection device together so that the solvent

	IU/kg body weight dose per day	*mg/kg body weight dose per day*	*IU/m² body surface area dose per day*	*mg/m² body surface area dose per day*
Growth hormone deficiency in children	0.07–0.10	0.025–0.035	2.1–3.0	0.7–1.0
Turner syndrome	0.14	0.045–0.050	4.3	1.4
Chronic renal insufficiency	0.14	0.045–0.050	4.3	1.4
Growth hormone deficiency in adults	0.018–0.036	0.006–0.012	—	—

will be mixed with the powder in the two compartment cartridge. Gently dissolve the drug with a slow, swirling motion. Do not shake vigorously; this might denature the active ingredient.

When using an injection device, the injection needle should be screwed on before reconstitution.

Marketing authorisation numbers
Genotropin 2IU (0.7 mg), 3IU (1 mg), 4IU (1.3 mg) KabiQuick 0022/0089-91
Genotropin 4IU (1.3 mg) 0022/0071
Genotropin 4IU (1.3 mg) KabiVial Multidose 0022/0088
Genotropin 16IU (5.3 mg)/16IU (5.3 mg) KabiVial Multidose 0022/0085
Genotropin 36IU (12 mg) 0022/0098

Date of first authorisation/renewal of authorisation 1 February 1995.

Date of (partial) revision of the text May 1998.

Legal category CD (Sch 4, Part I), POM.

HARMOGEN* 1.5 MG TABLETS

Qualitative and quantitative composition Each tablet contains Estropipate USP (piperazine oestrone sulphate) equivalent to 0.93 mg oestrone.

Pharmaceutical form Tablets for oral administration

Clinical particulars

Therapeutic indications: For oral use. Menopausal and post-menopausal oestrogen replacement therapy for vasomotor symptoms, senile atrophic vaginitis, vulvitis. Harmogen is also indicated in the prophylaxis of postmenopausal osteoporosis in women identified to be at risk of this condition. These women include those suffering from an early menopause, receiving recent prolonged corticosteroid therapy, having a family history of osteoporosis, of small frame, who are thin, smokers and those with an excess alcohol intake.

In women with an intact uterus the addition of a progestogen is essential.

Posology and method of administration: Oral.

Adults: Postmenopausal osteoporosis: 1.5 mg daily.

Other indications: 1.5 mg -- 3.0 mg daily taken as a single or divided dose.

Harmogen should be given continuously and, in women with an intact uterus, a progestogen should be added for 10–13 days at the end of each 28-day cycle. If the patient has undergone hysterectomy, the addition of a progestogen is not necessary.

Elderly: As for adults

Children: Not recommended

Contra-indications:
1. Known or suspected pregnancy;
2. Cardiovascular or cerebrovascular disorders, e.g. thrombophlebitis, thrombosis, or thromboembolic disorders, moderate to severe hypertension, hyperlipoproteinaemia or a history of these conditions;
3. Known or suspected oestrogen dependent tumours;
4. Endometrial hyperplasia, uterine fibromyomata, undiagnosed vaginal bleeding;
5. Severe liver disease including Rotor syndrome and Dubin-Johnson syndrome;
6. Porphyria.

Special warnings and special precautions for use:
Warnings:
1. Prolonged exposure to unopposed oestrogens increases the risk of endometrial neoplasia, however, the addition of a progestogen to the oestrogen regimen reduces the incidence of endometrial hyperplasia and cancer.
2. Severe varicose veins–the benefits of oestrogen-containing preparations must be weighed against the possible risks.
3. Cardiac failure, latent or overt.
4. Epilepsy or migraine, or a history of these conditions.
5. Sickle cell haemoglobinopathy, since under certain circumstances, e.g. infections or anoxia, oestrogen-containing preparations may induce thromboembolic processes in patients with this condition.
6. Untreated polycythaemia or pulmonary hypertension.
7. Epidemiological studies have suggested that hormone replacement therapy (HRT) is associated with an increased relative risk of developing venous thromboembolism (VTE) i.e. deep vein thrombosis or pulmonary embolism. The studies find a 2–3 fold increase for users compared with non-users which for healthy women amounts to a low risk of one extra case of VTE each year for every 5000 patients taking HRT.

Generally recognised risk factors for VTE include a personal or family history and severe obesity (Body Mass Index > 30 kg/m^2). In women with these factors the benefits of treatment with HRT need to be carefully weighed against risks.

The risk of VTE may be temporarily increased with prolonged immobilisation, major trauma or major surgery. In women on HRT scrupulous attention should be given to prophylactic measures to prevent VTE following surgery. Where prolonged immobilisation is liable to follow elective surgery, particularly abdominal or orthopaedic surgery to the lower limbs, consideration should be given to temporarily stopping HRT 4 weeks earlier, if this is possible.

If venous thromboembolism develops after initiating therapy the drug should be discontinued.

Precautions:
1. Before initiation of therapy, a complete medical and family history should be taken. The pretreatment and periodic physical examination should include special emphasis on blood pressure, breasts, abdomen and pelvic organs including cervical cytology and endometrial assessment where possible. Regular follow-up examinations are recommended every 6–12 months. The benefit of continued treatment should be reviewed periodically.
2. Caution should be exercised when administering Harmogen to women with a family history of breast cancer or who have breast nodules, fibrocystic disease or abnormal mammograms. There is suggestive evidence of a small increased risk of breast cancer with oestrogen replacement therapy used for long-term (greater than 5 years). Some studies have reported an increased risk of breast cancer in long-term users. Others, however, have not shown this relationship. It is not known whether concurrent progestogen use influences the risk of breast cancer in post-menopausal women taking hormone replacement therapy. Women on long-term therapy should have regular breast examinations.
3. Mild hypertension or a history of it. If hypertension develops in patients receiving Harmogen, treatment should be stopped.
4. Pre-existing uterine fibromyomata may increase in size during oestrogen therapy. The pathologist should be advised of the patient's use of Harmogen when submitting relevant samples.
5. Glucose tolerance may be lowered and may, therefore, increase the need for insulin of other antidiabetic drugs in diabetics.
6. Thyroid hormone binding globulin may be increased leading to increased circulating total thyroid hormone, therefore care must be taken in interpreting thyroid function tests.
7. History of gall stones, cholestatic jaundice in pregnancy or jaundice due to oral contraceptives. If jaundice develops or liver function tests become abnormal in any patient receiving Harmogen, the medication should be stopped while the cause is investigated.
8. Renal dysfunction.
9. Major depression
10. Contact lens wearers.

Interaction with other medicaments and other forms of interaction: Glucose tolerance may be lowered and may, therefore, increase the need for insulin or other anti-diabetic drugs in diabetics.

Thyroid hormone binding globulin may be increased leading to increased circulating total thyroid hormone, therefore care must be taken in interpreting thyroid function test.

Pregnancy and lactation: Pregnancy code: D

The indications for Harmogen are such that it is not likely to be used in pregnant or lactating women. Harmogen is contra-indicated in known or suspected pregnancy. In the unlikely event of the use of Harmogen in breast-feeding women, it should be remembered that oestrogens are excreted in breast milk and inhibit lactation.

Effects on ability to drive and use machines: None known.

Undesirable effects: The incidence of side-effects with Harmogen is low. The following adverse reactions have been reported with oestrogen therapy:
1. *Genito-urinary tract:* Endometrial neoplasia, intermenstrual bleeding, increase in the size of uterine fibromyomata, endometrial proliferation or aggravation of endometriosis, changes in cervical eversion and excessive production of cervical mucus;
2. *Breast:* Tenderness, pain, enlargement or secretion;
3. *Gastro-intestinal tract:* Nausea, vomiting, cholelithiasis, cholestatic jaundice, abdominal cramp, bloating;
4. *Cardiovascular system:* Hypertension, thrombosis, thrombophlebitis, thrombo-embolism;
5. *Skin:* Chloasma which may persist when the drug is discontinued, erythema multiforme, erythema nodosum, rash, loss of scalp hair, hirsutism;
6. *Eyes:* Steepening of corneal curvature, intolerance to contact lenses;
7. *CNS:* Headache, migraine, dizziness, mood changes (elation or depression), chorea;
8. *Miscellaneous:* Sodium and water retention, reduced glucose tolerance, change in body weight, aggravation of porphyria, changes in libido.

Overdose: Overdosage is unlikely to cause serious problems, although the following symptoms may be present, i.e. nausea and withdrawal bleeding in women. However gastric lavage or emesis may be used when considered appropriate.

Pharmacological properties

Pharmacodynamic properties: Estropipate is a semi-synthetic oestrogen conjugate. Its action is due to oestrone, to which it is hydrolysed in the body. Oestrogens are important in the development and maintenance of the female reproductive system and secondary sex characteristics. They promote growth and development of the vagina, uterus and fallopian tubes and enlargement of the breasts. Indirectly, they contribute to the shaping of the skeleton, maintenance of tone and allow for the pubertal growth spurt and its termination, growth of axillary and pubic hair and pigmentation of the nipples and genitals. Along with other hormones such as progesterone, oestrogens are intricately involved in the process of menstruation. Oestrogens also affect the release of pituitary gonadotrophins.

A depletion of endogenous oestrogens occurs postmenopausally as a result of a decline in ovarian function and may cause symptomatic vulvovaginal epithelial atrophy.

Pharmacokinetic properties:

General characteristics of active substance: Oestradiol is rapidly hydrolysed in the body to oestrone, which in turn may be hydrated to the less active oestriol. These transformations occur readily, mainly in the liver where there is also free interconversion between oestrone and oestradiol.

Gastro-intestinal absorption of orally administered (tablets) oestrogens is usually prompt and complete, inactivation of oestrogens in the body occurs mainly in the liver. During cyclic passage through the liver, oestrogens in the body are degraded to less active oestrogenic compounds and conjugated with sulphuric and glucuronic acids. Oestrone is 50–80% bound as it circulates in the blood, primarily as a conjugate with sulphate.

Characteristics in patients: Estropipate is metabolised in the liver, so any form of liver impairment will result in reduced metabolism. See 'Special warnings and special precautions for use' for further information.

Preclinical safety data: No special information. See *Special warnings and special precautions for use* for further information.

Pharmaceutical particulars

List of excipients:
Ingredient:
Lactose (monohydrate) NF
Lactose (anhydrous) NF
Dibasic potassium phosphate USP
Tromethamine USP
Hydroxypropyl cellulose NF
Sodium starch glycollate NF
Microcrystalline cellulose NF
Colloidal silicon dioxide NF
Magnesium stearate NF
Hydrogenated vegetable oil wax
Dye E110
Purified water USP
Alcohol 200 proof

Incompatibilities: None known.

Shelf life: Two years.

Special precautions for storage: None.

Nature and contents of container: The containers comprise an HDPE container with tamper-evident cap or securitainer holding 100 estropipate tablets or a PVC/Aluminium foil blister pack, holding 28 tablets, which, together with a Patient Information Leaflet are packed in a carton.

Instructions for use/handling: No special instructions

Marketing authorisation holder:
Abbott Laboratories Limited
Queenborough
Kent
ME11 5EL

Marketing authorisation number 0037/5064R

Date of first authorisation/renewal of authorisation 13 April 1992

Date of (partial) revision of the text January 1998.

HEALONID*

Presentation Disposable single use cartridge/syringe assemblies containing a sterile isotonic buffered solution of sodium hyaluronate:

Sodium hyaluronate (5000)	10 mg
Sodium chloride	8.5 mg
Disodium hydrogen phosphate dihydrate	0.28 mg
Sodium dihydrogen phosphate hydrate	0.04 mg
Water for injection	to 1 ml

Uses
Properties: Sodium hyaluronate is a polysaccharide normally found in the aqueous humour. Presented as Healonid, the solution has viscoelastic properties, being a clear viscous solution at rest yet under pressure able to pass easily through a fine needle or cannula. The average molecular weight of sodium hyaluronate in Healonid is approximately 4 million.

Indications: Introduction into the eye during anterior segment surgery helps maintain the shape of the anterior chamber and the space in which to work. The solution can be used as a soft tool to move tissues and objects. During surgery Healonid protects tissues from trauma and dehydration and reduces endothelial cell loss. Healonid may also be used in posterior segment surgery.

At close of surgery Healonid should be removed by aspiration or irrigation. Excess residues left in the eye may cause a rise in intraocular pressure a few hours after closure.

Dosage and administration The volume of Healonid will vary according to the procedure and technique employed.

The volume will be increased if the viscoelastic is used to coat the intraocular lens or tips of instruments, or where bleeding necessitates replacement on one or more occasions. At close of surgery Healonid should be aspirated or irrigated out. Excessive residues in the eye may lead to raised intraocular pressure postoperatively.

As a guide to volumes used, the anterior chamber has a volume of 0.2–0.3 ml.

No special directions are given for use in the elderly or children.

Prior to use, Healonid should be allowed to warm to room temperature over 30–60 minutes.

Contra-indications, warnings, etc
Warnings:

(i) Rarely inflammatory reactions have been reported; their connection with Healonid has not been established.

(ii) With traces of avian protein being present in Healonid there is the remote possibility of an idiosyncratic reaction.

Precautions: Healonid is viscous and thus residues left in the eye may impair drainage of aqueous humour through the trabecular meshwork. Consequently at close of surgery Healonid should be irrigated or aspirated out and intraocular pressure monitored over the first 24 hours, rises being most likely after 4–8 hours. In keratoplasty and trabeculectomy it is permissible to leave some Healonid *in situ* to prevent 'shallowing' of the anterior chamber due to leakage or excessive drainage. Again, intraocular pressure should be monitored. Excessive rises in pressure may be treated with appropriate therapy such as beta blockers or carbonic anhydrase inhibitors.

Pregnancy and lactation: There is no adverse animal evidence and Healonid has been widely used for many years without apparent ill consequence. Considering also the small amounts entering the body from what may be an isolated procedure, safety in pregnancy and lactation is likely.

Interactions and incompatibilities: Do not use with hyaluronidase. Healonid may become turbid due to precipitation in the presence of cationic agents such as benzalkonium chloride or detergents residual in some recycled cannulae. Avoid recycled cannulae.

Pharmaceutical precautions: Healonid has a shelf life of three years when stored at 2–8°C, protected from light and freezing. These conditions should be adhered to routinely. Healonid should be allowed to warm to room temperature over 30–60 minutes before use.

Legal category POM.

Package quantities Disposable cartridge/syringe assemblies containing 0.55 or 0.85 ml. A sterile cannula (27 G) is supplied.

Further information Healonid may be used in anterior segment surgery in situations such as trauma; intra- and extra-capsular lens extraction; corneal graft; glaucoma surgery; intraocular lens insertion; to facilitate manipulation within the eye; to protect the corneal endothelium and other sensitive tissues; to manoeuvre and separate tissues and bodies within the eye; to control vitreous bulge; to maintain a deep anterior chamber; to provide a support for corneal graft at suturing. Posterior segment surgery may include procedures for vitreal replacement and retinal detachment repair.

Evidence from animals suggests that Healonid is no longer present in the anterior chamber six days after introduction.

Product licence number 0022/0131.

HEALONID* GV INJECTION

Qualitative and quantitative composition Sodium hyaluronate 7000 14 mg/ml

Pharmaceutical form Injection for intra-ocular use.

Clinical particulars
Therapeutic indications: Healonid GV (Greater Viscosity) is used intra-ocularly in anterior segment surgical procedures such as cataract extraction, intra-ocular lens insertion and corneal transplant surgery where the surgeon requires greater visco-elastic properties than Healonid offers.

Posology and method of administration: Prior to use , Healonid GV should be allowed to warm to room temperature over 30–60 minutes.

The volume of Healonid GV will vary according to the procedure and technique employed. The volume will be increased if the visco-elastic is used to coat the intra-ocular lens or tips of the instruments, or when bleeding necessitates replacement on one or more occasions. At close of surgery, Healonid GV should be aspirated or irrigated out, the texture facilitating the procedure (see Special Warnings and Precautions for Use).

As a guide to volumes used, the anterior chamber has a volume of 0.2 ml to 0.3 ml.

No special directions are given for use in the elderly or children.

Contra-indications: No known contra-indications

Special warnings and precautions for use: At close of surgery, Healonid GV should be aspirated or irrigated from the anterior chamber. Healonid GV is very viscous and residues left in the eye may impair the drainage of aqueous humour thought the trabecular meshwork. In turn, this may give rise to an increase in intra-ocular pressure.

Intra-ocular pressure should be monitored for 24 hours, any rises usually becoming apparent between 4–8 hours post-operatively. Treatment with beta-blockers or carbonic anhydrase inhibitors may be indicated. Healonid GV may be more prone to cause such rises than Healonid.

Interactions with other medicaments and other forms of interaction: No known interactions with drugs used in ocular surgery.

Pregnancy and lactation: There has been limited use of Healonid GV in humans but there is no adverse animal evidence and Healonid has been in wide use for many years without apparent ill consequence. Considering the small amounts entering the body, safety in pregnancy and lactation is likely.

Effects on ability to drive and use machines: Not applicable

Undesirable effects: With traces of avian protein being present, there is the remote possibility of an idiosyncratic reaction.

Rarely, inflammatory reactions have been reported. Their connection with Healonid GV has not been established.

If excessive levels of Healonid GV are left in the eye at close of surgery, a rise in intra-ocular pressure may occur within 24 hours of surgery. (See Special Warnings and Precautions)

Overdose: Any excess Healonid GV may be aspirated or irrigated from the anterior chamber, the texture of the product aiding identification and removal. If excess is left in the eye at close of surgery, intra-ocular pressure should be monitored for 24 hours and any increases treated with beta-blockers or carbonic anhydrase inhibitors as necessary.

Pharmacological properties
Pharmacodynamic properties: Sodium hyaluronate is a natural constituent of the aqueous humour. In the eyes there is evidence for a monolayer held on the surface of the corneal endothelium and for specific binding sites. During surgery, sodium hyaluronate protects surfaces from trauma, contact with other surfaces and from dehydration.

Sodium hyaluronate's gel properties allow use as a soft tool for supporting and manoeuvring tissues and objects with minimal trauma. Endothelial cell loss is reduced. Although extremely viscous at rest, its visco-elasticity allows it under pressure to pass readily through a fine needle or cannula.

In certain surgical situations, the high viscosity of Healonid GV allows the surgeon to control and manoeuvre tissues or bodies within the eye to a degree not possible with less viscous preparations.

Pharmacokinetic properties: Experiments in animals suggest that injected sodium hyaluronate is no longer in the anterior chamber six days after introduction. Sodium hyaluronate is removed from the eye largely unchanged through the Canal of Schlemm to join the body pool. Receptor mediated uptake in the liver is the major route of destruction, a rate of 5 mg/kg/day being the upper limit, normal being about 10% of this. Catabolism to lactate and water is rapid. It is estimated that a maximum of 2.8 mg of hyaluronate as Healonid GV could be left in the eye, which would represent less than 1% of the body's maximal daily metabolic capacity.

Experimental studies suggest that initial loss from the eye is decreased by the volume and viscosity of the hyaluronate and estimates of half life range up to 13 hours. The more viscous the solution, the more slowly it passed through the trabecular meshwork, viscosity being reduced through mixing into the aqueous humour and drainage.

Preclinical safety data: No information relevant to the use of the product, other than that presented in other sections of the Summary of Product Characteristics is available.

Pharmaceutical particulars
List of excipients: Sodium Chloride PhEur; Disodium hydrogen phosphate dihydrate; Sodium Dihydrogen phosphate hydrate; Water for Injections PhEur.

Incompatibilities: Incompatible with hyaluronidase. Sodium hyaluronate may become turbid due to precipitation in the presence of cationic agents such as benzalkonium chloride or detergent residue present in recycled cannulae.

Shelf life: 36 months.

Special precautions for storage: Store at 2–8°C routinely. May be stored for up to 3 weeks at room temperature by the user. Protect from light.

Nature and contents of container: Single-use glass cartridges of 0.55 ml or 0.85 ml contained within a sterile syringe assembly. Syringe/cartridge assemblies are enclosed in individual sterile blister-packs.

Instruction for use/handling: Not applicable.

Date of first authorisation/renewal of authorisation 17 October 1997

Date of (partial) revision of the text 4 August 1997

Legal status POM

HEMABATE* STERILE SOLUTION

Presentation Colourless, sterile, aqueous solution containing carboprost tromethamine equivalent to carboprost 250 micrograms/ml.

The product also contains benzyl alcohol, sodium chloride, tromethamine and water.

Uses Treatment of post-partum haemorrhage due to uterine atony and refractory to conventional methods of treatment with oxytocic agents and ergometrine used either alone or in combination.

Conventional therapy should usually consist of 0.5–1 mg ergometrine with up to 50 units of oxytocin infused intravenously over periods of time from 20 minutes to 12 hours. The dosage and duration of administration should reflect the seriousness of the clinical situation.

Dosage and administration Parenteral drug products should be inspected visually for particulate matter and discolouration prior to administration whenever solution and container permit.

An initial dose of 250 micrograms (1.0 ml) of Hemabate should be administered as a deep intramuscular injection.

If necessary, further doses of 250 micrograms may be administered at intervals of approximately 1.5 hours. In severe cases the interval between doses may be reduced at the discretion of the attending physician, but it should not be less than 15 minutes. The total dose of Hemabate should not exceed 2 mg (8 doses).

Elderly: Not applicable.

Children: Not applicable.

Contra-indications, warnings, etc
Contra-indications: There are no absolute contra-indications to the use of Hemabate, however, its use is not recommended in the following circumstances:

1. Hypersensitivity to any of the components of the preparation.
2. Acute pelvic inflammatory disease.
3. Patients with known cardiac, pulmonary, renal or hepatic disease.

Interaction with other medicaments and other forms of interaction: Since prostaglandins may potentiate the effect of oxytocin, it is recommended that the use of these drugs simultaneously or in sequence should be carefully monitored.

Effects on ability to drive and to use machines: None.

Other undesirable effects: The adverse effects of

Hemabate are generally transient and reversible when therapy ends.

The most frequent side-effects observed with the use of Hemabate are related to its contractile effect on smooth muscle. Thus nausea, vomiting and diarrhoea have been reported as commonly encountered. The incidence of vomiting and diarrhoea may be decreased by pre-treatment and concomitant use during treatment of anti-emetic and antidiarrhoeal agents.

Hyperthermia and flushing have been observed after intramuscular Hemabate, but if not complicated by endometritis, the temperature will usually return to normal within several hours of the last injection.

Asthma and wheezing have been noted with Hemabate treatment.

Less frequent, but potentially more serious adverse effects are elevated blood pressure, dyspnoea and pulmonary oedema. Other less serious adverse effects noted include chills, headache, diaphoresis, dizziness and injection site erythema and pain.

Use in pregnancy and lactation: Not applicable.

Other special warnings and precautions
Warnings: This preparation should not be used for induction of labour.

Hemabate, as with other potent oxytocic agents, should be used only with strict adherence to recommended dosages. Hemabate should be used by medically trained personnel and is available only to hospitals and clinics with specialised obstetric units where 24 hour resident medical cover is provided.

Hemabate must not be given intravenously.

Very rare cases of cardiovascular collapse have been reported following the use of prostaglandins. This should always be considered when using Hemabate.

Precautions: Hemabate should be used with caution in patients with a history of glaucoma or raised intra-ocular pressure, asthma, hypertension or hypotension, cardiovascular disease, renal disease, hepatic disease, anaemia, jaundice, diabetes or epilepsy.

As with other oxytocic agents, Hemabate should be used with care in patients with compromised (scarred) uteri. The possibility of uterine rupture should be borne in mind where high tone myometrial contractions are sustained.

Animal studies lasting several weeks at high doses have shown that prostaglandins of the E and F series can induce proliferation of bone. Such effects have also been noted in newborn infants who have received prostaglandin E1 during prolonged treatment. There is no evidence that short-term administration of Hemabate can cause similar bone effects.

Decreases in maternal arterial oxygen content have been observed in patients treated with carboprost tromethamine. A causal relationship to carboprost tromethamine has not been established, however, it is recommended that patients with pre-existing cardio-pulmonary problems receiving Hemabate are monitored during treatment and given additional oxygen if necessary.

Overdosage: Treatment of overdosage must be, at this time, symptomatic, as clinical studies with prostaglandin antagonists have not progressed to the point where recommendations may be made.

If evidence of excessive uterine activity or side-effects appear, the rate of infusion or frequency of administration should be decreased or discontinued.

In cases of massive overdosage resulting in extreme uterine hypertonus, appropriate obstetric procedures are indicated.

Incompatibilities: None.

Pharmaceutical precautions Hemabate must be stored in a refrigerator between 2 and 8°C. At 4°C it has a shelf-life of 48 months.

Legal category POM.

Package quantities Pack containing 10 x 1 ml ampoules of Hemabate Sterile Solution 250 micrograms/ml.

Further information Carboprost tromethamine stimulates the myometrium of the gravid uterus to contract in a manner that is similar to that observed in the term uterus during labour. Whether or not this action results from a direct effect of carboprost tromethamine on the myometrium has not been determined with certainty at this time.

When Hemabate is given post-partum, the resulting myometrial contractions provide haemostasis at the site of placentation and hence prevent further blood loss.

Product licence number 0032/0152.

INDOMOD*

Presentation
Indomod 25 mg: Hard gelatin orange capsules with the imprint '27' in light type, containing 25 mg indomethacin, in modified release form (Repro-Dose).

Indomod 75 mg: Hard gelatin brown capsules with imprint '26' in light type, containing 75 mg indomethacin, in modified release form (Repro-Dose).

Uses Inflammatory rheumatic diseases such as rheumatoid arthritis, ankylosing spondylitis and gout. Inflammatory phases in osteoarthrosis. Inflammatory conditions such as bursitis, tendinitis, and tenosynovitis.

Dosage and administration
Dosage: Use as directed by physician. The dose should be adjusted individually. In chronic rheumatoid disease the initial daily dose is normally 50–75 mg, which is increased by 25 mg or 50 mg at weekly intervals until a satisfactory effect is achieved. The daily dose should never exceed 200 mg.

In acute conditions, e.g. gouty arthritis, a dose of 100 mg is given initially, followed by 75 mg b.i.d. for controlling the pain. Then the dose is rapidly reduced and medication is discontinued. (See 'Further information').

Paediatric usage not established.

Contra-indications, warnings, etc
Contra-indications: Active peptic ulcer or a history of recurrent gastrointestinal lesions; ulcerative colitis.

Haemophilia and other bleeding disorders. Allergy to non-steroidal anti-inflammatory drugs (salicylates, etc.).

Warnings and precautions: To be used with caution in patients with psychiatric disturbances, parkinsonism, or epilepsy. NSAIDs have been reported to cause nephrotoxicity in various forms and their use can lead to interstitial nephritis, nephrotic syndrome and renal failure. The symptoms of infection may be masked by indomethacin. The use of indomethacin is not recommended during pregnancy or lactation. Serum levels of indomethacin are raised by the concurrent administration of probenicid. Indomethacin reduces the natriuretic effect of frusemide.

Side-effects: Headache, dizziness, light-headedness, confusion and other reactions from the central nervous system are correlated to plasma concentrations and less likely to occur when high peak levels are avoided, as in the case with Indomod. Dyspepsia is another frequent side-effect of indomethacin likely to be modified by Indomod, due to the bypass of the stomach. Gastrointestinal bleeding and ulceration, fluid retention, disturbed renal or hepatic function, fatigue, tinnitus, drowsiness or insomnia may occur.

In patients with renal, cardiac or hepatic impairment caution is required since the use of NSAIDs may result in deterioration of renal function. The dose should be kept as low as possible and renal function should be monitored.

Anaphylactic reactions in hypersensitive patients.

Pharmaceutical precautions No special requirements or precautions.

Legal category POM.

Package quantities
Indomod 25 mg: Blister packs of 120 modified release capsules.

Indomod 75 mg: Blister packs of 30 modified release capsules.

Further information Due to the special indomethacin plasma profile obtained with Indomod, doses may be taken at intervals of 8–12 hours, and a capsule of 75 mg taken at bedtime can be expected to relieve the next day's morning stiffness.

Product licence numbers
Indomod 25 mg 4338/0006
Indomod 75 mg 4338/0007

Product licence holder: Benzon Pharma A/S, 29 Halmtorvet, DK-1700 Copenhagen, Denmark.

KABIGLOBULIN*

Presentation Ampoules containing Human Normal Immunoglobulin solution 16%, a clear pale straw colour. The active constituent is gamma globulin.

Uses *Main pharmacological action:* The immunoglobulins present in Kabiglobulin may be used prophylactically and therapeutically to provide passive immunity against infectious diseases.

Indications: Prophylaxis against infectious hepatitis (Hepatitis A). Prophylaxis against Rubella following exposure during pregnancy. Prevention, or modification of symptoms, following measles exposure in susceptible individuals. Antibody deficiency syndromes; to reduce the incidence and severity of infections in agammaglobulinaemia, hypogammaglobulinaemia and dysgammaglobulinaemia. Following burns injury.

Dosage and administration *Route of administration:* By intramuscular injection only.

Recommended dosage: Infectious hepatitis (Hepatitis A): for prophylaxis against infectious hepatitis for up to 3 months, in adults and children, 0.02–0.04 ml per kg body weight is recommended by WHO. In massive exposure, e.g. to people visiting highly endemic areas, 0.06–0.12 ml per kg body weight is recommended. The effect of the larger injection lasts for a period of at least four months.

Rubella in pregnancy: 20 ml is administered as soon as possible following exposure. The effect of an injection lasts about 3 weeks and therefore the dosage should be repeated after this time in the case of renewed exposure to the disease.

Measles prevention: 0.2 ml per kg body weight is injected within five days of exposure. The preventive effect of an injection normally lasts three weeks. The dosage should therefore be repeated after that period of time in the case of renewed exposure to the disease.

Measles modification: 0.04 ml per kg body weight is injected within five days of exposure.

Antibody deficiency syndromes: agammaglobulinaemia, hypogammaglobulinaemia, dysgammaglobulinaemia. As an initial dosage, 1.3 ml per kg body weight (maximum 60 ml) injected in divided doses over 48 hours. Half this dosage, 0.65 ml per kg (maximum 30 ml), is then given every three to four weeks.

Burns injury: during the first week following the trauma a total of about 50 g gamma globulin in the form of Kabiglobulin should be given in addition to plasma and blood. From the third up to the tenth day, 15–30 ml (2.5–5.0 g gamma globulin) per day is administered.

Contra-indications, warnings, etc Kabiglobulin should not be given at the same time as live vaccines, such as measles, mumps, rubella and oral polio vaccines (Sabin). If Kabiglobulin (2 ml) has been administered these vaccines should not be given for 3 months. This period should be increased to 4 months for the 5 ml injection. Following administration of live vaccines a period of 2–3 weeks should elapse before giving Kabiglobulin. Kabiglobulin may be given at the same time as tetanus, typhoid, diphtheria, cholera, polio [the inactivated form (Salk)] and yellow fever; although a live vaccine, Kabiglobulin donors are unlikely to possess the antibody to yellow fever.

Pregnancy and lactation: There is no evidence of safety nor of toxicity of Kabiglobulin in human pregnancy or lactation, but it has been commonly used for many years without apparent ill consequence. If such therapy is needed in pregnancy or lactation, Kabiglobulin can be used if there is no alternative course of action.

Side-effects: In exceptional cases, intramuscular injections of gamma globulin may give rise to adverse reactions of the following types:

Local reactions: at the site of injection such as erythema, swelling, tenderness and induration, which generally subside within a few days after the injection.

General reactions: such as fever (38–40°C), chills and general malaise. These symptoms have appeared 6–8 hours after the injection and have generally subsided by the following day.

Hypersensitivity reactions: such as exanthema and pruritus. Flush, tachycardia and shock are rare. The reactions are more frequent in patients with hypogammaglobulinaemia or dysgammaglobulinaemia and may be delayed for some hours following administration.

Overdosage: There have been no reports of overdosage with Kabiglobulin. There is no specific antidote and in the unlikely event of any reactions occurring following overdosage, they should be treated symptomatically.

Pharmaceutical precautions Store between 2°C and 8°C.

Legal category POM.

Package quantities Ampoules of 2.0 and 5.0 ml.

Further information The IgA content of Kabiglobulin does not exceed 0.01% of the total protein content. Kabiglobulin contains no preservative agents. Based on results from model experiments and from clinical follow-up, several organisations such as the Food and Drug Administration, Centers for Disease Control and World Health Organisation have drawn the conclusion that immunoglobulin preparations, manufactured according to standard methods are safe with respect to transmission of HIV infectivity.

Product licence number 0022/5009.

KABIKINASE*

Presentation Vial containing a straw coloured lyophilised powder, containing 250,000 iu of streptokinase. Human albumin and buffering agents are present as stabilisers.

Uses
Action: By activating the fibrinolytic system streptokinase induces dissolution of intravascular thrombi and emboli.

Indications: Thrombolytic therapy by intravenous Kabikinase infusion is indicated in the treatment of deep vein thrombosis, acute major pulmonary embolism, acute arterial thromboembolism.

Additionally, thrombolytic therapy by local streptokinase administration is indicated in the treatment of myocardial infarction (see b, below) and in the clearance of clotted haemodialysis shunts (see c, below).

Dosage and administration *Routes of administration:* By intravascular infusion; intracoronary infusion.

Recommended dosage for adults:
a. Standard intravenous infusion regimen: The standard intravenous dosage scheme includes a loading dose sufficient to neutralise circulating streptococcal antibody, followed by a maintenance dose to maintain an appropriate degree of fibrinolysis.

Loading dose: Streptokinase 600,000 iu is infused via a peripheral vein over a period of 30–60 minutes.

Maintenance dose: Streptokinase 100,000 iu/hour is infused for 72 hr. If further treatment is considered necessary it should be continued for not more than a further 3 days.

b. Intracoronary administration in myocardial infarction: Intracoronary thrombolysis is performed using standard techniques for selective coronary angiography by either the brachial or femoral approach. Early intervention is recommended, ideally within 6 hours following onset of chest pain.

Using a standard 7 or 8 French catheter, angiography is used to identify the presence and location of the thrombus. Nitroglycerin (100–400 micrograms) is administered into the involved vessel, to relieve coronary artery spasm. Initially a bolus dose of streptokinase 10,000–25,000 iu is administered followed by a continuous infusion of 4,000 iu/minute, which is continued until vessel patency is restored, or for 60–75 minutes (total dose 240,000–300,000 iu). If reperfusion is achieved prior to this time then the infusion rate may be reduced when patency is restored, and infusion should continue for an additional 30–60 minutes (80,000–100,000 iu streptokinase) in order to lyse any remaining residual thrombus.

Subsequent anticoagulant treatment with heparin is necessary in order to prevent rethrombosis in the infarct-related coronary artery. However, in the majority of patients intracoronary streptokinase administration produces significant fibrinogen (and plasminogen) depletion. Additionally, circulating fibrin/fibrinogen degradation products exert an anticoagulant effect. Accordingly heparin should be administered incrementally and judiciously during the first 24 hr following treatment. The partial thromboplastin time should be monitored at regular intervals, and the heparin dosage adjusted to maintain the former within the range 2–2.5 times normal.

c. Local application in occluded haemodialysis shunts: Kabikinase 100,000 iu is dissolved in normal saline 100 ml. 10,000–25,000 iu (10–25 ml) is deposited in the clotted portion of the shunt, which is then sealed on the venous side with forceps. A sterile single-dose syringe is attached on the arterial side to form an air cushion against which the artery can pulsate. If required, the treatment may be repeated after 30–45 minutes.

Recommended dosage for infants: Although the standard dosage scheme may be reduced proportionally to circulating volume, it may be preferable to titrate the initial dose followed by a maintenance dose of 1300–1400 iu/kg body weight/hr for 3 days. Response normally occurs within this period but if further therapy is considered it should not be for more than an additional 3 days.

Preparation of solution: The contents of a vial of Kabikinase are dissolved at room temperature in 5 ml water for injections carefully avoiding the formation of a foam. The concentrated solution thus obtained is transferred aseptically into an infusion bottle of glucose or saline of suitable volume, according to the needs of the patient. The rate of infusion is then adjusted to give the required dosage rate.

Standard intravenous infusion regimen: For the loading dose; 600,000 iu Kabikinase is made up in 100 ml 5% glucose or physiological saline and is administered over 30 minutes.

For the maintenance dose; 600,000 iu is made up in 500 ml 5% glucose or physiological saline, and is administered at a rate of 80 ml per hr (100,000 iu hourly). If desired, smaller volumes can be employed, to enable the use of a syringe pump.

Intracoronary administration: The contents of a reconstituted vial are added to a volume of 5% glucose or physiological saline in order to achieve a final streptokinase concentration of not less than 1,000 iu/ml.

Control of therapy (standard intravenous infusion regimen): Therapy is controlled by the thrombin clotting time performed at intervals and should be within the limits of two to four times the normal value.

Contra-indications, warnings, etc
Contra-indications: Kabikinase should not be administered intramuscularly. Since thrombolytic therapy increases the risk of bleeding, Kabikinase is contra-indicated in the following:
1. Surgery within the last 10 days.
2. Invasive procedures during the last 10 days.
3. Gastrointestinal bleeding within the last six months.
4. Thrombocytopenia or other evidence of defective haemostasis.
5. Liver or kidney disease.
6. Cerebrovascular accident.
7. Severe hypertension treated and untreated.
8. Parturition (within the last 10 days).
9. Ulcerative colitis.
10. Visceral carcinoma.
11. Menstrual bleeding.
12. During the first 18 weeks of pregnancy (see note below).
13. Sub-acute bacterial endocarditis.

Precautions and warnings: Following 7–10 days' treatment with streptokinase, the patient's anti-streptokinase antibody titre increases considerably, and returns to normal only after up to 6 months. Normally, a second treatment with streptokinase should not be considered within 6 months of the first. If a second treatment is considered necessary within 6 months then the initial loading dose should be individually determined. The titrated initial dose may be calculated following determination of the smallest quantity of Kabikinase required to lyse a clot, formed from 1.0 ml of the patient's blood within 10 minutes.

If heparin or oral anticoagulants have been given before commencing Kabikinase thrombolytic therapy, further administration should cease (it is not advisable to give Kabikinase and heparin simultaneously). The Kabikinase infusion can then be started after 4 hours. If immediate Kabikinase therapy is required the heparin in the blood should be neutralised with protamine sulphate.

On termination of Kabikinase treatment, the patient should be given anticoagulants in an attempt to prevent rethrombosis. Preferably heparin should be used, starting four hours after the end of thrombolysis, and then oral anticoagulants may be introduced in the usual manner. Drugs which affect blood platelet function, such as salicylic acid preparations, pyrazolone, or indole derivatives, should not be administered concurrently with Kabikinase since the risk of bleeding will be increased.

Streptokinase should be used with caution in patients with haemorrhagic retinopathy.

Pregnancy: Thrombolytic therapy with Kabikinase during the first 18 weeks of pregnancy should be avoided, since there may be a risk of placental separation.

Negligible amounts of streptokinase cross the placenta. The foetal blood concentration reaches about one thousandth of the maternal blood concentration. Fibrinolytic effects in the foetus are unlikely.

Elderly patients: The incidence of cerebral haemorrhage resulting from thrombolytic therapy is increased in elderly patients. Therapy should be restricted to those patients in whom the benefit of treatment outweighs this additional hazard.

Side-effects: Kabikinase therapy may be accompanied by a slight to moderate elevation in body temperature. Mild allergic reactions such as urticaria occur uncommonly. Anaphylaxis occurs extremely rarely. These reactions may be controlled by the prior administration of corticosteroids (25 mg prednisolone or a corresponding amount of another glucocorticoid).

Streptokinase administration has been associated with low back pain. This may indicate an allergic response and it may be appropriate to discontinue the infusion. In some cases, without other features of allergy, infusion has been continued with analgesic cover, without adverse consequence.

A few allergic reactions such as polyneuropathy and uveitis have been temporally related to the administration of streptokinase. Guillain-Barre Syndrome has been reported after streptokinase treatment.

Haemorrhage can occur in any tissue and organ in the body and can present with symptoms affecting any body system, including the abdomen, cardiovascular system, joints and CNS. Haemorrhage should be considered as a potential cause of unusual symptoms occurring after administration.

Minor oozing or bleeding occurring at injection sites may be controlled by applying local pressure.

Exceptionally there may be severe haemorrhage, in which case administration of Kabikinase must be discontinued. If necessary, the antifibrinolytic agent Cyklokapron (tranexamic acid-10 mg/kg body weight) should be given immediately by slow intravenous injection. Cryoprecipitate may be used to correct haemostatic deficiency.

Antidote: Tranexamic acid 10 mg/kg body weight by slow intravenous injection.

Pharmaceutical precautions Vials of Kabikinase should be stored below 25°C before reconstitution. Reconstituted vials may be stored for up to 24 hr when kept in a refrigerator. Kabikinase solutions diluted for infusion should be used within 12 hours of preparation.

Legal category POM.

Package quantities Vial of 250,000 iu.

Further information Kabikinase is a highly purified streptokinase preparation. It is prepared from beta-haemolytic streptococci culture filtrates. Subsequent purification ensures that Kabikinase is virtually free from streptodornase, streptolysin, hyaluronidase and other enzymes. Kabikinase is soluble in water, is non-toxic and is non-pyrogenic, but is weakly antigenic. Kabikinase is stabilised with sterile human albumin and this imparts a faint straw colour to the preparation.

Product licence number 0022/5012R.

KABIKINASE* 750,000 IU

Presentation Vial of straw coloured lyophilised powder containing 750,000 iu of streptokinase. Human albumin and buffering agents are present as stabilisers.

Uses
Action: By activating the fibrinolytic system, streptokinase induces dissolution of intravascular thrombi and emboli.

Indication: Acute myocardial infarction.

Dosage and administration
Recommended dosage for adults: Streptokinase 1.5 million iu in physiological saline or dextrose 5% is administered as an intravenous infusion, at a constant rate, over 60 minutes.

Preparation of solution: Dissolve the contents of 2 vials of Kabikinase 750,000 iu by adding 5 ml Water for Injections, to each vial.

The solution should be prepared at room temperature. Care should be taken to avoid the formation of foam. The concentrated solution thus obtained is transferred aseptically into an infusion bottle or PVC bag, containing 100 ml of physiological saline, or dextrose 5%.

Contra-indications, warnings, etc
Contra-indications: Kabikinase should not be administered intramuscularly. Since thrombolytic therapy increases the risk of bleeding, Kabikinase is contra-indicated in the following:

1. Invasive or traumatic procedures within the previous 10 days including the following: surgery; central venous cannulation, or puncture of a non-compressible vessel; external cardiac compression; endotracheal intubation; biopsy.

2. Defective haemostasis including: thrombocytopenia or any other platelet disorder; coagulation disorder (including those caused by hepatic or renal impairment); acute systemic infection, bacteraemia or septicaemia; oral or intravenous anticoagulant therapy (see under Precautions, paragraph 2).

3. Potential for gastrointestinal haemorrhage including: oesophageal varices; history of peptic ulceration; visceral carcinoma; ulcerative colitis; diverticulitis.

4. Increased risk of cerebral haemorrhage/infarction as evidenced by any of the following: stroke; cerebral tumour; hypertension (treated or untreated); hypertensive or diabetic retinopathy; transient ischaemic attacks.

5. Obstetric or gynaecological conditions likely to predispose to haemorrhage, including: menstruation; pregnancy – see also Pregnancy section; parturition within the previous 18 weeks.

6. Potential for cardiac thromboemboli, including: active or recent infective endocarditis; atrial valve disease with atrial fibrillation.

7. Increased risk of pulmonary haemorrhage, including: active tuberculosis; pneumothorax.

8. Previous streptokinase therapy, more than 5 days and up to 6 months previously, or recent streptococcal infection, since an elevated titre of anti-streptokinase antibody may render the treatment ineffective.

9. Coma.

Precautions: Patients should not receive streptokinase unless they will be managed within a hospital setting, under expert medical supervision. It is recommended that patients should be treated in a coronary care (or intensive care) unit.

1. The *diagnosis* of acute myocardial infarction should initially be based upon both clinical signs and ECG evidence. Specific ECG changes diagnostic of recent myocardial infarction should be present. The following diagnoses, which can be associated with ECG changes, and in which administration of thrombolytic therapy might result in life-threatening haemorrhage **MUST** be excluded;

aortic dissection; acute pericarditis, oesophageal rupture; acute abdominal emergencies, including pancreatitis and perforation of the duodenum; intracranial haemorrhage; (see also 2., below).

A chest X-ray should be performed in order to assist in eliminating ruptured oesophagus (pneumomediastinum) or duodenum (air under the diaphragm) and aortic dissection (wide mediastinum). Aortic dissection should be suspected particularly when pain radiates into the back, aortic regurgitation is evident on auscultation or there are absent pulses. Pericarditis should be suspected when ST-segment elevation occurs in all ECG leads. Raised blood amylase is an indication of pancreatitis.

2. Thrombolytic therapy should be considered only in the case of patients for whom a well documented *medical history* is available. It is essential that thrombolytic therapy is not instituted in patients with co-existing medical conditions likely to exacerbate the risk of haemorrhage (e.g. peptic ulceration, history of cerebro-vascular accident, cerebral tumour, visceral carcinoma, see also 'Contraindications'). Additionally, caution should be exercised in patients who are receiving other drug therapies which are likely to predispose to increased risk of haemorrhagic complications.

3. In most patients, infarction probably is complete within 4–6 hrs and, accordingly, only patients in whom therapy can be initiated within this time interval should be considered for treatment. (But see statement on Q waves below). *Myocardial salvage* is possible only when recanalisation of the infarct-related artery is effected within a critical time interval following coronary occlusion. The rate of progression of myocardial necrosis is inversely related to the extent of residual perfusion of the ischaemic myocardium. When infarction is due to sub-total coronary occlusion (ca 10–25% of patients) and there is some residual antegrade perfusion, the rate of necrosis is less than when infarction results from complete coronary occlusion. Similarly, in some patients (ca 5–10%) a well developed collateral circulation may retard the progress and reduce the severity of ischaemia. The maximum time delay commensurate with myocardial salvage and reduction in mortality is not known. In patients treated within one hour following symptomatic onset, the risk of death is halved. Generally, the presence of marked pathological Q waves in the ECG should be considered as evidence that transmural infarction is complete and that appreciable myocardial salvage is not possible.

Conversely, benefit may be derived up to 18 hours following symptom onset, in patients in whom pathological Q waves are absent, or symptoms are intermittent.

4. *Hypokalaemia* predisposes to ventricular arrhythmias and, if present should be corrected.

5. If *venous access* is considered necessary (e.g. for cardiac pacing) the risk of haemorrhage from central venous cannulation must be considered, and preference should be given to the antecubital route.

6. Thrombolytic therapy with Kabikinase induces a *systemic fibrinolytic state.* The presence of circulating free plasmin results in consumption of fibrinogen and of coagulation factors (predominantly Factors V, VIII and XII). Additionally, circulating degradation products of fibrinogen and fibrin exert an anticoagulant effect. Accordingly thrombolytic therapy increases the risk of haemorrhage both throughout the period of streptokinase infusion, and for approximately 12–24 hours thereafter, i.e. until the serum fibrinogen exceeds 100 mg%.

7. Care should be exercised when moving the patient to avoid trauma-induced haematomas. Unnecessary venepunctures should be avoided.

8. Streptokinase should be used with caution in patients with haemorrhagic retinopathy.

9. *Reperfusion* is usually accompanied by relief of chest pain. Occasionally, reperfusion is preceded by a period of fluctuation in the severity of chest pain. Reperfusion is followed by resolution of the ischaemic ST segment changes. An ECG lead with distinct ST segment elevation should be selected for continuous monitoring, and the initial positions of the ST segment and the peak of the T waves marked. The time of reperfusion may then be recorded. In patients who have sustained minimal necrosis there may be no development of Q waves. However, development of Q waves may not imply complete necrosis, since myocardium subjected to prolonged ischaemia ('stunned myocardium') may take several days to recover.

10. In some patients with inferior wall infarction reperfusion is associated with *vagal reactions* of nausea, vomiting, sinus bradycardia and hypotension. It has been proposed that these result from the triggering of the Bezold-Jarisch reflex by the restoration of perfusion to the inferior and posterior wall of the left ventricle. These vagal reactions usually respond to intravenous atropine.

11. Accelerated idioventricular rhythm occurs at the time of reperfusion or shortly thereafter in approximately 50–60% of patients. Reperfusion is also associated with ventricular ectopic beats occurring late in diastole. These may be single or may give rise to ventricular bigeminy or trigeminy, or may form fusion beats. These ventricular arrhythmias (frequently referred to as '*reperfusion arrhythmias*') are probably related to increased automaticity. Sustained ventricular tachycardia and ventricular fibrillation are rare, occurring no more commonly than in patients receiving standard management, and should be managed in the normal way.

12. The titre of circulating antistreptokinase antibody rises abruptly at 5–7 days following Kabikinase administration, and may reach levels sufficient to neutralise subsequent Kabikinase dosages administered within the following 3–6 months.

Accordingly,

a. Information relating to the administration of Kabikinase therapy should be recorded clearly in the patient's notes.
b. Kabikinase therapy should not be repeated within the period of 5 days to 6 months following the initial treatment.
c. Patients with on-going, or recent, streptococcal infections may be resistant to Kabikinase therapy.

13. Subsequent *anticoagulant treatment* with heparin is generally considered necessary in order to prevent rethrombosis in the infarct-related coronary artery, since following thrombolysis, the thrombogenic segment is again exposed to circulating blood, and may again induce thrombosis in the affected artery. Reocclusion occurs in approximately 10–20% of successfully reperfused patients. If anticoagulant treatment is considered appropriate, then heparin should be administered incrementally and judiciously during the first 24 hr following treatment. The partial thromboplastin time should be monitored at regular intervals, and the heparin dosage adjusted to maintain the former within the range 2–2.5 times normal. The optimal duration of anticoagulant therapy is not known. The use of thrombolytic therapy should not necessarily lead to any change in the normal patient management of acute myocardial infarction.

14. Successful thrombolytic therapy will not obviate the requirement for further expert cardiological assessment and patient management.

Side-effects: Kabikinase therapy may be accompanied by a slight to moderate pyrexia. Mild allergic reactions such as urticaria are uncommon, particularly when the total duration of infusion is less than 2 hours. Anaphylaxis occurs extremely rarely (ca 0.1%). These reactions may be controlled by the prior intravenous administration of corticosteroids (e.g. hydrocortisone 100 mg, or prednisolone 25 mg). If streptokinase infusion is to be administered for more than 2 hours, or is to be repeated within 6 months, the prior administration of intravenous corticosteroid and/or an antihistamine should be considered, in order to reduce the incidence of allergic reactions.

Streptokinase administration has been associated with low back pain. This may indicate an allergic response and it may be appropriate to discontinue the infusion. In some cases, without other features of allergy, infusion has been continued with analgesic cover, without adverse consequences.

A few allergic reactions such as polyneuropathy and uveitis have been temporally related to the administration of streptokinase. Guillain-Barre Syndrome has been reported after streptokinase treatment.

Haemorrhagic complications largely result from inappropriate anticoagulant therapy, rather than from fibrinolysis *per se.*

Haemorrhage can occur in any tissue and organ in the body and can present with symptoms affecting any body system, including the abdomen, cardiovascular system, joints and CNS. Haemorrhage should be considered as a potential cause of unusual symptoms occurring after administration. Minor bleeding, predominantly at puncture sites, occurs with an incidence of approximately 3–4%. Major haemorrhagic episodes requiring transfusion of 2 or more units of blood (gastrointestinal and retroperitoneal haemorrhage) occur with an incidence of approximately 0.3%. Cerebral haemorrhage and stroke occurs with a frequency of approximately 0.1%. Though there is a theoretical risk of haemorrhagic infarction and haemorrhage into the pericardium, these are extremely rarely encountered. In cases of severe haemorrhage administration of Kabikinase must be discontinued. If necessary, the antifibrinolytic agent Cyklokapron (tranexamic acid – 10 mg/kg body weight), should be given immediately by slow intravenous injection. Fresh frozen plasma, or preferably cryoprecipitate, should be administered, to correct haemostatic deficiencies.

Antidote: Tranexamic acid 10 mg/kg body weight by slow intravenous injection.

Pregnancy: Thrombolytic therapy with Kabikinase is contraindicated during pregnancy, since there may be increased risk of placental separation.

Elderly patients: The incidence of cerebral haemorrhage may be increased in elderly compared with young patients.

Children: Not recommended.

Pharmaceutical precautions Vials of Kabikinase should be stored below 25°C before reconstitution. The overall reconstituted shelf life is 12 hours. The concentrate should be stored at 2–8°C. Diluted material should be used as soon as possible and not longer than 12 hours after initial reconstitution.

Legal category POM.

Package quantities Vials containing 750,000 iu streptokinase.

Further information Kabikinase is a highly purified streptokinase preparation. It is prepared from beta-haemolytic streptococci culture filtrates. Subsequent purification ensures that Kabikinase is virtually free from streptodornase, streptolysin, hyaluronidase and other enzymes. Kabikinase is soluble in water, is non-toxic and is non-pyrogenic but is weakly antigenic.

Kabikinase is stabilised with sterile human albumin and this imparts a faint straw colour to the preparation.

Product licence number 0022/0069.

KABIKINASE* 1.5 Million IU

Presentation Vial of straw coloured lyophilised powder containing 1.5 million iu of streptokinase. Human albumin and buffering agents are present as stabilisers.

Uses
Action: By activating the fibrinolytic system, streptokinase induces dissolution of intravascular thrombi and emboli.

Indication: Acute myocardial infarction.

Dosage and administration
Recommended dosage for adults: Streptokinase 1.5 million iu in physiological saline or dextrose 5% is administered as an intravenous infusion, at a constant rate, over 60 minutes.

Preparation of solution: Dissolve the contents of the vial by adding 10 ml Water for Injections.

The solution should be prepared at room temperature. Care should be taken to avoid the formation of foam. The concentrated solution thus obtained is transferred aseptically into an infusion bottle or PVC bag, containing 100 ml of physiological saline, or dextrose 5%.

Contra-indications, warnings, etc
Contra-indications: Kabikinase should not be administered intramuscularly. Since thrombolytic therapy increases the risk of bleeding, Kabikinase is contra-indicated in the following:

Invasive or traumatic procedures within the previous 10 days including the following: Surgery; central venous cannulation, or puncture of a non-compressible vessel; external cardiac compression; endotracheal intubation biopsy.

Defective haemostasis including: Thrombocytopenia or any other platelet disorder; coagulation disorders (including those caused by hepatic or renal impairment); acute systemic infection, bacteraemia or septicaemia; oral or intravenous anticoagulant therapy (see under 'Precautions', paragraph 2).

Potential for gastro-intestinal haemorrhage including: Oesophageal varices; history of peptic ulceration; visceral carcinoma; ulcerative colitis; diverticulitis.

Increased risk of cerebral haemorrhage/infarction as evidenced by any of the following: Stroke; cerebral tumour; hypertension (treated or untreated); hypertensive or diabetic retinopathy; transient ischaemic attacks.

Obstetric or gynaecological conditions likely to predispose to haemorrhage, including: Menstruation; pregnancy – see also 'Pregnancy' section; parturition within the previous 18 weeks.

Potential for cardiac thromboemboli, including: Active or recent infective endocarditis; atrial valve disease with atrial fibrillation.

Increased risk of pulmonary haemorrhage, including: Active tuberculosis; pneumothorax.

Previous streptokinase therapy, more than 5 days and up to 6 months previously, or recent streptococcal infection, since an elevated titre of anti-streptokinase antibody may render the treatment ineffective.

Coma.

Precautions: Patients should not receive streptokinase unless they will be managed within a hospital setting, under expert medical supervision. It is recommended that patients should be treated in a coronary care (or intensive care) unit.

1. The *diagnosis* of acute myocardial infarction should initially be based upon both clinical signs and ECG evidence. Specific ECG changes diagnostic of recent myocardial infarction should be present. The following diagnoses, which can be associated with ECG changes, and in which administration of thrombolytic therapy might result in life-threatening haemorrhage **MUST** be excluded:

aortic dissection; acute pericarditis; oesophageal rupture; acute abdominal emergencies, including pancreatitis and perforation of the duodenum; intracranial haemorrhage; (see also 2. below).

A chest X-ray should be performed in order to assist in eliminating ruptured oesophagus (pneumomediastinum) or duodenum (air under the diaphragm) and aortic dissection (wide mediastinum). Aortic dissection should be suspected particularly when pain radiates into the back, aortic regurgitation is evident on auscultation or there are absent pulses. Pericarditis should be suspected when ST-segment elevation occurs in all ECG leads. Raised blood amylase is an indication of pancreatitis.

2. Thrombolytic therapy should be considered only in the case of patients for whom a well documented *medical history* is available. It is essential that thrombolytic therapy is not instituted in patients with co-existing medical conditions likely to exacerbate the risk of haemorrhage (e.g. peptic ulceration, history of cerebro-vascular accident, cerebral tumour, visceral carcinoma, see also 'Contra-indications'). Additionally, caution should be exercised in patients who are receiving other drug therapies which are likely to predispose to increased risk of haemorrhagic complications.

3. In most patients, infarction probably is complete within 4–6 hrs and, accordingly, only patients in whom therapy can be iniated within this time interval should be considered for treatment. (But see statement on Q waves below.) *Myocardial salvage* is possible only when recanalisation of the infarct-related artery is effected within a critical time interval following coronary occlusion. The rate of progression of myocardial necrosis is inversely related to the extent of residual perfusion of the ischaemic myocardium. When infarction is due to sub-total coronary occlusion (ca 10–25% of patients) and there is some residual antegrade perfusion, the rate of necrosis is less than when infarction results from complete coronary occlusion. Similarly, in some patients (ca 5–10%) a well developed collateral circulation may retard the progress and reduce the severity of ischaemia. The maximum time delay commensurate with myocardial salvage and reduction in mortality is not known. In patients treated within one hour following symptomatic onset, the risk of death is halved. Generally, the presence of marked pathological Q waves in the ECG should be considered as evidence that transmural infarction is complete and that appreciable myocardial salvage is not possible.

Conversely, benefit may be derived up to 18 hours following symptoms onset, in patients in whom pathological Q waves are absent, or symptoms are intermittent.

4. *Hypokalaemia* predisposes to ventricular arrhythmias and, if present should be corrected.

5. If *venous access* is considered necessary (e.g. for cardiac pacing) the risk of haemorrhage from central venous cannulation must be considered, and preference should be given to the antecubital route.

6. Thrombolytic therapy with Kabikinase induces a *systemic fibrinolytic state.* The presence of circulating free plasmin results in consumption of fibrinogen and of coagulation factors (predominantly Factors V, VIII and XII). Additionally, circulating degradation products of fibrinogen and fibrin exert an anticoagulant effect. Accordingly thrombolytic therapy increases the risk of haemorrhage both throughout the period of streptokinase infusion, and for approximately 12–24 hours thereafter, i.e. until the serum fibrinogen exceeds 100 mg%.

7. Care should be exercised when moving the patient to avoid trauma-induced haematomas. Unnecessary venepunctures should be avoided.

8. Streptokinase should be used with caution in patients with haemorrhagic retinopathy.

9. *Reperfusion* is usually accompanied by relief of chest pain. Occasionally, reperfusion is preceded by a period of fluctuation in the severity of chest pain. Reperfusion is followed by resolution of the ischaemic ST segment changes. An ECG lead with distinct ST segment elevation should be selected for continuous monitoring, and the initial positions of the ST segment and the peak of the T waves marked. The time of reperfusion may then be recorded. In patients who have sustained minimal necrosis there may be no development of Q waves. However, development of Q waves may not imply complete necrosis, since myocardium subjected to prolonged ischaemia ('stunned myocardium') may take several days to recover.

10. In some patients with inferior wall infarction reperfusion is associated with *vagal reactions,* of nausea, vomiting, sinus bradycardia and hypotension. It has been proposed that these result from the triggering of the Bezold-Jarisch reflex by the restoration of perfusion to the inferior and posterior wall of the left ventricle. These vagal reactions usually respond to intravenous atropine.

11. Accelerated idioventricular rhythm occurs at the time of reperfusion or shortly thereafter in approximately 50–60% of patients. Reperfusion is also associated with ventricular ectopic beats occurring late in diastole. These may be single or may give rise to ventricular bigeminy or trigeminy, or may form fusion beats. These ventricular arrhythmias (frequently referred to as '*reperfusion arrhythmias*') are probably related to increased automaticity. Sustained ventricular tachycardia and ventricular fibrillation are rare, occurring no more commonly than in patients receiving standard management, and should be managed in the normal way.

12. The titre of circulating antistreptokinase antibody rises abruptly at 5–7 days following Kabikinase administration, and may reach levels sufficient to neutralise subsequent Kabikinase dosages administered within the following 6 months.

Accordingly,

a. Information relating to the administration of Kabikinase therapy should be recorded clearly in the patient's notes.
b. Kabikinase therapy should not be repeated within the period of 5 days to 6 months following the initial treatment.
c. Patients with on-going, or recent, streptococcal infections may be resistant to Kabikinase therapy.

13. Subsequent *anticoagulant treatment* with heparin is generally considered necessary in order to prevent rethrombosis in the infarct-related coronary artery, since following thrombolysis, the thrombogenic segment is again exposed to circulating blood, and may again induce thrombosis in the affected artery. Reocclusion occurs in approximately 10–20% of successfully reperfused patients. If anticoagulant treatment is considered appropriate, then heparin should be administered incrementally and judiciously during the first 24 hr following treatment. The partial thromboplastin time should be monitored at regular intervals, and the heparin dosage adjusted to maintain the former within the range 2–2.5 times normal. The optimal duration of anticoagulant therapy is not known. The use of thrombolytic therapy should not necessarily lead to any change in the normal patient management of acute myocardial infarction.

14. Successful thrombolytic therapy will not obviate the requirement for further expert cardiological assessment and patient management.

Side-effects: Kabikinase therapy may be accompanied by a slight to moderate pyrexia. Mild allergic reactions such as urticaria are uncommon, particularly when the total duration of infusion is less than 2 hours. Anaphylaxis occurs extremely rarely (ca 0.1%). These reactions may be controlled by the prior intravenous administration of corticosteroids (e.g. hydrocortisone 100 mg, or prednisolone 25 mg). If streptokinase infusion is to be administered for more than 2 hours, or is to be repeated within 6 months, the prior administration of intravenous corticosteroid and/or an antihistamine should be considered, in order to reduce the incidence of allergic reactions.

Streptokinase administration has been associated with low back pain. This may indicate an allergic response and it may be appropriate to discontinue the infusion. In some cases, without other features of allergy, infusion has been continued with analgesic cover, without adverse consequences.

A few allergic reactions such as polyneuropathy and uveitis have been temporally related to the administration of streptokinase. Guillain-Barre Syndrome has been reported after streptokinase treatment.

Haemorrhagic complications largely result from inappropriate anticoagulant therapy, rather than from fibrinolysis *per se.* Haemorrhage can occur in any tissue and organ in the body and can present with symptoms affecting any body system, including the abdomen, cardiovascular system, joints and CNS. Haemorrhage should be considered as a potential cause of unusual symptoms occurring after administration. Minor bleeding, predominantly at puncture sites, occurs with an incidence of approximately 3–4%. Major haemorrhagic episodes requiring transfusion of 2 or more units of blood (gastro-intestinal and retroperitoneal haemorrhage) occur with an incidence of approximately 0.3%. Cerebral haemorrhage and stroke occurs with a frequency of approximately 0.1%. Though there is a theoretical risk of haemorrhagic infarction and haemorrhage into the pericardium, these are extremely rarely encountered. In cases of severe haemorrhage administration of Kabikinase must be discontinued. If necessary, the antifibrinolytic agent Cyklokapron, (tranexamic acid – 10 mg/kg body weight) should be given immediately by slow intravenous injection. Fresh frozen plasma, or preferably cryoprecipitate, should be administered, to correct haemostatic deficiencies.

Antidote: Tranexamic acid 10 mg/kg body weight by slow intravenous injection.

Pregnancy: Thrombolytic therapy with Kabikinase is contra-indicated during pregnancy, since there may be an increased risk of placental separation.

Elderly patients: The incidence of cerebral haemorrhage may be increased in elderly compared with young patients.

Children: Not recommended.

Pharmaceutical precautions Vials of Kabikinase should be stored below 25°C before reconstitution. The overall reconstituted shelf life is 12 hours. The concentrate should be stored at 2–8°C. Diluted material should be used as soon as possible and not longer than 12 hours after initial reconstitution.

Legal category POM.

Package quantities Vials containing 1.5 million iu streptokinase.

Further information Kabikinase is a highly purified streptokinase preparation. It is prepared from beta-haemolytic streptococci culture filtrates. Subsequent purification ensures that Kabikinase is virtually free from streptodornase, streptolysin, hyaluronidase and other enzymes. Kabikinase is soluble in water, is non-toxic and is non-pyrogenic, but is weakly antigenic.

Kabikinase is stabilised with sterile human albumin and this imparts a faint straw colour to the preparation.

Product licence number 0022/0070.

KELFIZINE W*

Presentation White, uncoated tablets each containing sulfametopyrazine 2 g stamped white flat, uncoated tablets, marked 'LONGUM' on one side.

Uses The treatment of infections due to sulphonamide-sensitive organisms. Kelfizine W is recommended in the management of chronic bronchitis (including prophylaxis), it is also indicated for use in urinary tract infections.

Dosage and administration

Adults: 2 g once weekly by mouth.

Children: Not recommended.

Elderly: As hepatic conjugation and renal clearance occur at a reduced rate in the elderly, caution is advised when prescribing the drug for long periods of time, to avoid accumulation.

The tablet should be stirred into half a tumblerful of water or orange squash.

Contra-indications, warnings, etc

Contra-indications: Not to be taken by persons sensitive to sulphonamides.

Warnings: Occasionally severe reactions such as erythema multiforme and the Stevens–Johnson syndrome, epidermal necrolysis, eosinophilia, agranulocytosis, granulocytopenia, purpura and leucopenia have been reported in patients treated with sulphonamides.

Sulphonamides, and thus sulfametopyrazine, may potentiate the effects of coumarin derivatives, some oral antidiabetic agents (sulphonylureas) and some diaminopyrimidine derivatives (trimethoprim, pyrimethamine). Paraminobenzoic acid can antagonize the antibacterial activity of sulfametopyrazine.

Adverse reactions: Other side-effects reported with the use of sulphonamides include nausea, vomiting and rashes: these are usually mild and transient with Kelfizine W.

Precautions: Sulfametopyrazine should be used with caution in patients with renal or hepatic dysfunction, dehydration, or blood dyscrasias.

Use in pregnancy and lactation: There is no evidence of the drug's safety in human pregnancy nor is there evidence from animal work that it is free from hazard. Kelfizine W is contra-indicated during the third trimester of pregnancy and during breast-feeding.

Overdosage: Doses up to 8 g have been taken over 36 hours without evidence of ill effects. To increase excretion a high fluid intake should be maintained for seven days and the urine rendered alkaline with Potassium Citrate mixture BP or sodium bicarbonate. The sulphonamide will then be retained in the urine in higher concentrations in the form of the alkali metal salt.

Legal category POM.

Package quantities Pack of 5 tablets individually foil wrapped.

Further information Sulfametopyrazine has a long half-life. This is due not to a high degree of serum protein binding (which is only 60%) but to a high degree of renal tubular re-absorption coupled with a low rate of hepatic metabolism of the drug.

Product licence number 3433/5916R.

KEMICETINE* SUCCINATE

Presentation Individual glass vials of chloramphenicol sodium succinate for injection containing the equivalent of 1 g of chloramphenicol.

Uses Kemicetine (chloramphenicol) is a broad-spectrum antibiotic and is active against many gram-positive and gram-negative organisms, spirillae and rickettsia. Kemicetine should not be used for trivial infections due to the possibility of severe blood dyscrasias, which may prove fatal.

Kemicetine succinate is indicated for typhoid, meningitis caused by *H. influenzae* infections and other serious infections. It is also indicated wherever chloramphenicol is deemed the antibiotic of choice and oral administration is not possible, or higher than usual blood concentrations are required.

Dosage and administration

In order to ensure rapid attainment of high blood levels, Kemicetine succinate is best administered by i.v. injection. Where this is not possible, however, intramuscular administration may be used, although it should be borne in mind that absorption may be slow and unpredictable.

The injection should be reconstituted with Water for Injections, Sodium Chloride Injection, or Dextrose Injection 5%. The following dilution table may be useful for the administration of a proportion of the contents of a vial:

Concentration	*Solution strength*	*Volume of diluent to be added*	*Total volume after dilution*
40%	400 mg/ml	1.7 ml	2.5 ml
25%	250 mg/ml	3.2 ml	4.0 ml
20%	200 mg/ml	4.2 ml	5.0 ml
10%	100 mg/ml	9.2 ml	10.0 ml

The dose administered and the concentration used is dependent on the severity of the infection. The recommended standard dosage is as follows:

Adults: The equivalent of 1 g chloramphenicol every 6–8 hours.

Children: The equivalent of 50 mg/kg chloramphenicol, according to body weight, daily in divided doses every 6 hours (this dose should not be exceeded). The patient should be carefully observed for signs of toxicity.

Elderly: The usual adult dosage should be given subject to normal hepatic and renal function.

Neonates and premature infants: 25 mg/kg in divided doses.

Certain infections, such as meningitis or septicaemia, may require substantially higher doses.

The 10% solution should be given by intravenous injection over a period of about a minute, or in a larger volume of fluid, by slow intravenous infusion.

The concurrent administration of i.v. Kemicetine succinate with topical treatment has been found to be very effective in the treatment of osteomyelitic foci, abscesses, empyema and skin and urinary infections.

Contra-indications, warnings, etc Kemicetine succinate is contra-indicated in patients with a previous history of sensitivity and/or toxic reaction to chloramphenicol. It is also contra-indicated in pregnancy and whilst breast feeding. Kemicetine is to be administered only under the direction of a medical practitioner. Chloramphenicol may cause severe bone marrow depression which may lead to agranulocytosis, thrombocytopenic purpura or aplastic anaemia. These effects on the haemopoietic system are usually associated with a high dose, prolonged administration, or repeated courses, but they may occur at relatively low doses. Chloramphenicol should not be used in the treatment of any infection for which a less toxic antibiotic is available. It is also advisable to perform blood tests in the case of prolonged or repeated administration. Evidence of any detrimental effect on blood elements is an indication to discontinue therapy immediately.

Other adverse reactions which may become apparent after chloramphenicol treatment are: dryness of the mouth, nausea and vomiting, diarrhoea, urticaria, optic neuritis with blurring or temporary loss of vision, peripheral neuritis, headache and depression. Superinfection by fungi, e.g. *C. albicans* in the gastrointestinal tract, or vagina, may also occur due to the disturbance of normal bacterial flora.

Chloramphenicol has been shown to interact with, and enhance the effects of, coumarin anticoagulants, some hypoglycaemic agents (e.g. tolbutamide) and phenytoin. When given concurrently, a dose reduction of these agents may, therefore, be necessary. Plasma concentrations of chloramphenicol may be reduced with concomitant usage of phenobarbitone and rifampicin. Chloramphenicol may also impede the development of immunity and should therefore not be given during active immunisation.

The drug should be used with great caution in patients with impairment of hepatic or renal function. The dosage should be reduced in these patients. 'The Grey Syndrome' may occur after administration, in patients with immature hepatic metabolic capacity, i.e. infants and neonates, usually in those treated with doses substantially in excess of those recommended.

Because of its toxic nature, it is important to monitor serum levels of this antibiotic particularly in newborn and premature infants, in the elderly, in patients with renal or hepatic disease and in those receiving other drugs with which chloramphenicol may interact.

Overdosage: General supportive therapy should be given.

Pharmaceutical precautions Any Kemicetine succinate solution remaining in the vial after use should be discarded, as chloramphenicol sodium succinate is not bactericidal or bacteriostatic.

Legal category POM.

Package quantities Cartons containing 25 individual vials.

Further information Nil.

Product licence number 3433/5903R.

LONITEN* TABLETS 2.5 mg, 5 mg, and 10 mg

Qualitative and quantitative composition Each Loniten Tablet contains 2.5 mg, 5 mg or 10 mg minoxidil USP.

Pharmaceutical form Tablet.

Clinical particulars

Therapeutic indications: Loniten is indicated for the treatment of severe hypertension.

It should not be used as the sole agent to initiate therapy. It is a peripheral vasodilator and should be given in conjunction with a diuretic, to control salt and water retention and a beta-adrenergic blocking agent or appropriate substitute, to control reflex tachycardia.

Posology and method of administration: Oral administration

Adults and patients over 12 years of age: An initial daily dose of 5 mg, which may be given as a single or divided dosage, is recommended. This dose may first be increased to 10 mg daily and subsequent increases should be by increments of 10 mg in the daily dose. Dosage adjustments should be made at intervals of not less than three days, until optimum control of blood pressure is achieved. It is seldom necessary to exceed 50 mg per day although, in exceptional circumstances, doses up to 100 mg per day have been used. Twice-daily dosage is satisfactory. Where diastolic pressure reduction of less than 30 mm Hg is required, once daily dosing has been reported as effective.

Dosage requirements may be lower in dialysis patients. Minoxidil is removed from the blood by dialysis, but its pharmacological action, once established is not reversed. Therefore, haemodialysis patients should take Loniten either after or at least two hours before dialysis.

Children: For patients of 12 years of age or under, the initial dose should be 200 micrograms per kilogram (0.2 mg/kg) given as a single or divided daily dosage. Incremental increases of 100 -- 200 micrograms per kilogram (0.1--0.2 mg/kg) in the daily dose are recommended at intervals of not less than three days until optimum blood pressure control has been achieved, or the maximum daily dose of 1.0 mg/kg has been reached.

Rapid reduction of blood pressure: Under hospital monitoring conditions, rapid reduction of blood pressure can be achieved using continuous blood pressure monitoring and incremental doses of 5 mg every six hours.

Concomitant antihypertensive therapy: It is recommended that, where possible, antihypertensive therapy, other than a beta-adrenergic blocking agent and a diuretic be discontinued before Loniten treatment is started. It is recognised that some antihypertensive agents should not be abruptly discontinued. These drugs should be gradually discontinued during the first week of Loniten treatment.

Loniten causes sodium retention and, if used alone, can result in several hundred milli-equivalents of salt being retained together with a corresponding volume of water.

Therefore, in all patients who are not on dialysis, Loniten must be given in conjunction with a diuretic in sufficient dosage to maintain salt and water balance. Examples of the daily dosages of diuretics commonly used when starting therapy with Loniten include: hydrochlorothiazide (100 mg) or other thiazides at equi-effective dosage; chlorthalidone (100 mg); frusemide (80 mg).

If excessive water retention results in a weight gain of more than 3 pounds when a thiazide or chlorthalidone is being used, diuretic therapy should be changed to frusemide, the dose of which may be increased in accordance with the patient's requirements. Diuretic dosage in children should be proportionally less in relation to weight.

Patients will require a sympathetic nervous system suppressant to limit a Loniten-induced rise in heart rate. The preferred agent is a beta-blocker equivalent to an adult propranolol dosage of 80--160 mg/day. Higher doses may be required when pre-treated patients have an increase in heart rate exceeding 20 beats per minute or when simultaneous introduction causes an increase exceeding 10 beats per minute. When beta-blockers are contra-indicated, alternatives such as methyldopa may be used instead and should be started 24 hours prior to Loniten.

Elderly patients: At present there are no extensive clinical studies with minoxidil in patients over age 65. There is data indicating that elevated systolic and diastolic pressures are important risk factors for cardiovascular disease in individuals over age 65. However, elderly patients may be sensitive to the blood pressure lowering effect of minoxidil and thus caution is urged in initiating therapy as orthostatic hypotension may occur. It is suggested that 2.5 mg per day be used as the initial starting dose in patients over 65 years of age.

Contra-indications: Loniten is contra-indicated in patients with a phaeochromocytoma.

Special warnings and special precautions for use: If used alone, Loniten can cause a significant retention of salt and water leading to positive physical signs such as oedema and to clinical deterioration of some patients with heart failure. Diuretic treatment alone or in combination with restricted salt intake is, therefore, necessary for all patients taking Loniten.

Patients who have had myocardial infarction should only be treated with Loniten after a stable post-infarction state has been established.

The physician should bear in mind that if not controlled by sympathetic suppressants, the rise in cardiac rate and output that follows the use of potent vasodilators may induce anginal symptoms in patients with undiagnosed coronary artery disease or may aggravate pre-existing angina pectoris.

The effect of Loniten may be additive to concurrent antihypertensive agents. The interaction of Loniten with sympathetic-blocking agents such as guanethidine or bethanidine may produce excessive blood pressure reduction and/or orthostasis.

Hypertrichosis occurs in most patients treated with Loniten and all patients should be warned of this possibility before starting therapy. Spontaneous reversal to the pre-treatment state can be expected one to three months after cessation of therapy.

Soon after starting Loniten therapy approximately 60% of patients exhibit ECG alterations in the direction and magnitude of their T waves. Large changes may encroach on the ST segment, unaccompanied by evidence of ischaemia. These asymptomatic changes usually disappear with continuing Loniten treatment. The ECG reverts to the pre-treatment state if Loniten is discontinued.

Pericardial effusion has been detected in patients treated with a Loniten-containing regime. A cause and effect relationship has not been established. Most effusions have either been present before Loniten was given or occurred among uraemic patients. However, it is suggested that Loniten-treated patients should be periodically monitored for signs or symptoms of pericardial effusion and appropriate therapy instituted if necessary.

Salt and water retention in excess of 2 to 3 pounds may diminish the effectiveness of Loniten. Patients should, therefore, be carefully instructed about compliance with diuretic therapy and a detailed record of body weight should be maintained.

Interaction with other medicaments and other forms of interaction: The effect of Loniten may be additive to concurrent antihypertensive agents. The interaction of Loniten with sympathetic-blocking agents such as guanethidine or bethanidine may produce excessive blood pressure reduction and/or orthostasis.

Pregnancy and lactation: The safety of Loniten in pregnancy remains to be established. Minoxidil has been shown to reduce the conception rate in rats and to show evidence of increased fetal absorption in rabbits. There was no evidence of teratogenic effects in rats and rabbits. Minoxidil has been reported to be secreted in breast milk. Therefore, breast-feeding should not be undertaken while a patient is on Loniten Tablets.

Effects on ability to drive and use machines: No adverse effects reported.

Undesirable effects: Most patients receiving Loniten experience a diminution of pre-existing side-effects attributable to their disease or previous therapy. New events or side-effects likely to increase include peripheral oedema, associated with or independent of weight gain; increases in heart rate; hypertrichosis; and a temporary rise in creatinine and blood urea nitrogen. Gastro-intestinal intolerance, rash and breast tenderness are infrequently reported side-effects of Loniten therapy.

Overdose: If exaggerated hypotension is encountered, it is most likely to occur in association with residual sympathetic nervous system blockade (guanethidine-like effects or alpha-adrenergic blockade). Recommended treatment is intravenous administration of normal saline. Sympathomimetic drugs, such as noradrenaline or adrenaline, should be avoided because of their excessive cardiac-stimulating action. Phenylephrine, angiotensin II and vasopressin, which reverse the effect of Loniten, should be used only if inadequate perfusion of a vital organ is evident.

Pharmacological properties
Pharmacodynamic properties: Minoxidil is an anti-hypertensive agent which acts predominantly by causing direct peripheral vasodilation of the arterioles.

Pharmacokinetic properties: About 90% of an oral dose of minoxidil has been reported to be absorbed from the GI tract.

Following oral administration the maximum hypotensive effect usually occurs after 2–3 hours. The action may persist for up to 75 hours. The plasma half life is about 4.2 hours.

Minoxidil is not bound to plasma proteins. It is extensively metabolised in the liver primarily by conjugation with glucuronic acid and is excreted in the urine mainly in the form of metabolites.

Pharmaceutical particulars
List of excipients: Lactose hydrous, microcrystalline cellulose, starch, colloidal silicon dioxide and magnesium stearate.

Incompatibilities: None

Shelf-life: Shelf-life of the medicinal product as packaged for sale: 36 months.

Special precautions for storage: Store below 25°C.

Nature and contents of container: High density polyethylene (HDPE) bottles with LDPE caps. Each bottle contains 100 tablets.

20–25 micron aluminium foil/250 micron opaque pvc blister. Pack contains 60 tablets.

Instructions for use/handling: No special requirements.

Marketing authorisation numbers
2.5 mg 0032/0064
5 mg 0032/0065
10 mg 0032/0066

Date of first authorisation/renewal of authorisation
0032/0064–0066 date of first authorisation: 14 November 1979

Renewal dates 14 November 1984, 11 January 1990, 24 May 1995.

Date of revision of the text March 1995.

Legal category POM.

MAXTREX*

Presentation *Maxtrex Tablets:* Round, uncoated, convex tablets diameter 6 mm, containing 2.5 mg (pale yellow tablets marked 'M2.5' on one side) and 10 mg (deep yellow tablets marked 'M10' on one side and scored on the other) methotrexate.

Uses Methotrexate is a folic acid antagonist and is classified as an antimetabolite cytotoxic agent.

Methotrexate has been used to produce regression in a wide range of neoplastic conditions including acute leukaemias, non-Hodgkin's lymphoma, soft-tissue and osteogenic sarcomas, and solid tumours particularly breast, lung, head and neck, bladder, cervical ovarian, and testicular carcinoma.

Methotrexate has also been used in the treatment of severe, uncontrolled psoriasis which is non-responsive to other therapy.

Dosage and administration Single doses, not exceeding 30 mg/m², on not more than 5 consecutive days. A rest period of at least two weeks is recommended between treatments, in order to allow the bone marrow to return to normal.

Methotrexate has been used both alone and in combination chemotherapy with radiotherapy and surgery. Dosage regimens may therefore vary considerably. Leucovorin rescue regimens are discussed briefly under 'Further information'.

If methotrexate is administered in combination chemotherapy regimens, the dosage should be reduced, taking into consideration any overlapping toxicity of the other drug components.

Dosage for psoriasis: A test dose of 5–10 mg parentally is recommended, one week prior to therapy to detect idiosyncratic adverse reactions For the treatment of severe psoriasis 10 – 25 mg orally, once weekly, is recommended. Dosage should be adjusted according to the patient's response and the haematological toxicity.

Contra-indications, warnings, etc Maxtrex is usually intended for use under the direction of those experienced in cytotoxic therapy.

Contra-indications: Methotrexate is contra-indicated in the presence of severe renal or hepatic impairment and serious anaemia, leucopenia or thrombocytopenia. Maxtrex should not be used concomitantly with drugs with antifolate properties (eg co-trimoxazole)

Warnings: Methotrexate should be used with caution in patients with haematological depression, renal impairment, diarrhoea, ulcerative disorders of the G.I. tract and psychiatric disorders and in the elderly and very young. Hepatic toxicity has been observed. Renal lesions may develop if the urinary flow is impeded and urinary pH is low, especially if large doses have been administered.

The administration of low doses of methotrexate for prolonged periods may give rise, in particular, to hepatic toxicity. Liver function tests should be periodically carried out and abnormalities are indication for discontinuing treatment for at least a period of 2 weeks. Particular care and possible cessation of treatment are indicated if stomatitis or G.I. toxicity occurs as haemorrhagic enteritis and intestinal perforation may result. After intrathecal administration, leucoencephalopathies have been observed, especially with concomitant cerebral radiotherapy.

Reversible eosinophilic pulmonary reactions and treatment-resistant, interstitial fibrosis may occur, particularly after long-term treatment.

Methotrexate is teratogenic and should not ordinarily be administered to patients who are pregnant or to mothers who are breast-feeding. The drug affects spermatogenesis and oogenesis and may therefore decrease fertility. The effect appears to be reversible after discontinuation of therapy. Conception should be prevented for at least 6 months after administration has ceased.

There are isolated reports in the literature of tumours occurring in patients following treatment with methotrexate, and in some studies in animals. However, controlled animal studies and human epidemiological surveys have not demonstrated carcinogenicity. Nevertheless, the possibility of such an effect should be borne in mind when designing long-term management.

Methotrexate is immunosuppressive and may therefore reduce immunological response to concurrent vaccination. Severe antigenic reactions may occur if a live vaccine is given concurrently.

Precautions: Complete haematological analysis, together with urinalysis and renal and hepatic function tests should be carried out every 2–3 months. Haemopoietic depression may occur suddenly even with low doses. A severe reduction of any blood element requires immediate cessation of treatment and suitable supportive measures such as blood transfusion and reverse barrier nursing. During therapy urine should be kept alkaline, if necessary, by giving oral or i.v. sodium bicarbonate, to prevent crystal deposition.

The disappearance of methotrexate from plasma should be monitored, if possible. This is recommended in particular when high, or very high doses are administered, in order to permit calculation of an adequate dose of leucovorin rescue. (See under 'Further Information').

Radiotherapy to the CNS should not be given concomitantly with intrathecally administered methotrexate.

After intrathecal administration the drug is transported into the general circulation and may therefore still give rise to systemic toxicity, particularly myelosuppression.

Drug interactions: Methotrexate is extensively protein bound and may displace, or be displaced by, other acidic drugs. The concurrent administration of agents such as aminobenzoic acid, chloramphenicol, phenytoin, propionic acid anti-inflammatory agents, salicylates, sulphonamides, tetracyclines, thiazide diuretics, probenecid or sulpinpyrazone will decrease the methotrexate transport function of renal tubules, thereby reducing excretion and almost certainly increasing methotrexate toxicity. Methotrexate dosage should be monitored if concomitant treatment with NSAIDs is commenced.

Side-effects: Common side-effects are leucopenia and thrombocytopenia (which are usually reversible), nausea and vomiting, diarrhoea and stomatitis. Other side-effects include G.I. ulceration, alopecia, erythematous skin reactions and suppression of ovarian and testicular function.

Megaloblastic anaemia has been reported. Renal and hepatic damage may occur, particularly after high doses or prolonged administration, respectively. Reversible, eosinophilic pulmonary reactions and treatment-resistant interstitial fibrosis have been recorded.

CNS side-effects that may follow intrathecal or intraventricular use are headache, drowsiness, blurred vision, ataxia and, rarely, dementia and convulsions.

Overdose: Leucovorin is a specific antidote for methotrexate and, following accidental overdosage, should be administered within one hour at a dosage equal to, or greater than, the methotrexate dose. It may be administered by i.v. bolus or infusion. Further doses may be required. The patient should be observed carefully and blood transfusions, renal dialysis and reverse barrier nursing may be necessary.

Pharmaceutical precautions Maxtrex should be stored at room temperature protected from light.

Legal category POM

Package quantities:
Maxtrex 2.5 tablets: Bottles of 100 tablets
Maxtrex 10 tablets: Bottles of 100 tablets

Further information Methotrexate is a folic acid antagonist and its major site of action is the enzyme dihydrofolate reductase. Its main effect is inhibition of DNA synthesis, but it also acts directly both on RNA and protein synthesis. Methotrexate is a phase specific substance, the main effect being directed during the S-phase of cell division.

The inhibition of dihydrofolate reductase can be circumvented by the use of leucovorin (folinic acid; citrovorum factor) and protection of normal tissues can be carried out by properly timed administration of leucovorin calcium. Dosage regimens for leucovorin rescue vary, depending on the dose of methotrexate administered. Up to 120 mg are generally given (as the calcium salt), usually in divided doses over 12 – 24 hours, by i.m. or i.v. bolus, or intravenous infusion in normal saline. This is followed by 12 – 15 mg i.m. or 15 mg orally every 6 hours for 48 hours.

Product licence numbers
Maxtrex 2.5 tablets: 3433/0071
Maxtrex 10 tablets: 3433/0072

MEDRONE* TABLETS 2 mg AND 4 mg

Presentation Oval single-scored pink tablet containing 2 mg methylprednisolone.

Oval single-scored white tablet containing 4 mg methylprednisolone.

Tablets also contain lactose, sucrose, maize starch and calcium stearate. Medrone Tablets 2 mg also contain E123 and E127.

Uses Medrone is indicated for conditions requiring glucocorticoid activity such as:
Endocrine disorders: Primary and secondary adrenal insufficiency; Congenital adrenal hyperplasia

Rheumatic disorders: Rheumatoid arthritis; Juvenile chronic arthritis; Ankylosing spondylitis

Collagen diseases/arteritis: Systemic lupus erythematosus; Systemic dermatomyositis (polymyositis); Rheumatic fever with severe carditis: Giant cell arteritis/polymyalgia rheumatica

Dermatological diseases: Pemphigus vulgaris

Allergic states: Severe seasonal and perennial allergic rhinitis; Drug hypersensitivity reactions; Serum sickness; Allergic contact dermatitis; Bronchial asthma

Ophthalmic diseases; Anterior uveitis (iritis, iridocyclitis); Posterior uveitis; Optic neuritis

Respiratory diseases; Pulmonary sarcoid; Fulminating or disseminated tuberculosis (with appropriate anti-tuberculous chemotherapy); Aspiration of gastric contents

Haematological disorders: Idiopathic thrombocytopenic purpura; Haemolytic anaemia (autoimmune)

Neoplastic diseases: Leukaemia (acute and lymphatic); Malignant lymphoma

Gastro-intestinal diseases: Ulcerative colitis; Crohn's disease

Miscellaneous: Tuberculous meningitis (with appropriate antituberculous chemotherapy); Transplantation

Dosage and administration The dosage recommendations shown in the table below are suggested initial daily doses and are intended as guides. The average total daily dose recommended may be given either as a single dose or in divided doses (excepting in alternate day therapy when the minimum effective daily dose is doubled and given every other day at 8.00 am).

The initial suppressive dose level may vary depending on the condition being treated. This is continued until a satisfactory clinical response is obtained, a period usually of three to seven days in the case of rheumatic diseases (except for acute rheumatic carditis), allergic conditions affecting the skin or respiratory tract and ophthalmic diseases. If a satisfactory response is not obtained in seven days, re-evaluation of the case to confirm the original diagnosis should be made. As soon as a satisfactory clinical response is obtained, the daily dose should be reduced gradually, either to termination of treatment in the case of acute conditions (e.g. seasonal asthma, exfoliative dermatitis, acute ocular inflammations) or to the minimal effective maintenance dose level in the case of chronic conditions (e.g. rheumatoid arthritis, systemic lupus erythematosus, bronchial asthma, atopic dermatitis). In chronic conditions, and in rheumatoid arthritis especially, it is important that the reduction in dosage from initial to maintenance dose levels be accomplished as clinically appropriate. Decrements of not more than 2 mg at intervals of 7–10 days are suggested. In rheumatoid arthritis, maintenance steroid therapy should be at the lowest possible level.

In alternate-day therapy, the minimum daily corticoid requirement is doubled and administered as a single dose every other day at 8.00 am. Dosage requirements depend on the condition being treated and response of the patient.

Elderly patients: Treatment of elderly patients, particularly if long-term, should be planned bearing in mind the more serious consequences of the common side-effects of corticosteroids in old age, particularly osteoporosis, diabetes, hypertension, susceptibility to infection and thinning of skin.

Children: In general, dosage for children should be based upon clinical response and is at the discretion of the physician. Treatment should be limited to the minimum dosage for the shortest period of time. If possible, treatment should be administered as a single dose on alternate days.

Dosage recommendations:

Indications	*Recommended initial daily dosage*
Rheumatoid arthritis	
severe	12–16 mg
moderately severe	8–12 mg
moderate	4–8 mg
children	4–8 mg
Systemic dermatomyositis	48 mg
Systemic lupus erythematosus	20–100 mg
Acute rheumatic fever	48 mg until ESR normal for one week
Allergic diseases	12–40 mg
Bronchial asthma	up to 64 mg single dose/alternate day up to 100 mg maximum
Ophthalmic diseases	12–40 mg
Haematological disorders and leukaemias	16–100 mg
Malignant lymphoma	16–100 mg
Ulcerative colitis	16–60 mg
Crohn's disease	up to 48 mg per day in acute episodes
Organ transplantation	up to 3.6 mg/kg/day
Pulmonary sarcoid	32–48 mg on alternate days
Giant cell arteritis/ polymyalgia rheumatica	64 mg
Pemphigus vulgaris	80–360 mg

Contra-indications, warnings, etc

Contra-indications: Medrone is contra-indicated in known hypersensitivity to components and in systemic fungal infections. Immunization procedures should not be undertaken in patients who are on corticosteroids, especially on high doses, due to the possibility of neurological complications and lack of antibody response.

Interactions: Convulsions have been reported with concurrent use of methylprednisolone and cyclosporin. Since concurrent administration of these agents results in a mutual inhibition of metabolism, it is possible that convulsions and other adverse effects associated with the individual use of either drug may be more apt to occur.

Drugs that induce hepatic enzymes, such as rifampicin, rifabutin, carbamazepine, phenobarbitone, phenytoin, primidone, and aminoglutethimide enhance the metabolism of corticosteroids and its therapeutic effects may be reduced.

Drugs such as erythromycin and ketoconazole may inhibit the metabolism of corticosteroids and thus decrease their clearance.

Steroids may reduce the effects of anticholinesterases in myasthenia gravis. The desired effects of hypoglycaemic agents (including insulin), anti-hypertensives and diuretics are antagonised by corticosteroids, and the hypokalaemic effects of acetazolamide, loop diuretics, thiazide diuretics and carbenoxolone are enhanced.

The efficacy of coumarin anticoagulants may be enhanced by concurrent corticosteroid therapy and close monitoring of the INR or prothrombin time is required to avoid spontaneous bleeding.

The renal clearance of salicylates is increased by corticosteroids and steroid withdrawal may result in salicylate intoxication. Salicylates and non-steroidal anti-inflammatory agents should be used cautiously in conjunction with corticosteroids in hypothrombinaemia.

Steroids have been reported to interact with neuromuscular blocking agents such as pancuronium with partial reversal of the neuromuscular block.

Effects on ability to drive and use machines: None stated.

Other undesirable effects (frequency and seriousness): The incidence of predictable undesirable side-effects associated with the use of corticosteroids, including hypothalamic-pituitary-adrenal suppression correlates with the relative potency of the drug, dosage, timing of administration and duration of treatment (see Other special warnings and precautions).

Gastro-intestinal: Dyspepsia, peptic ulceration with perforation and haemorrhage, abdominal distension, oesophageal ulceration, oesophageal candidiasis, acute pancreatitis, perforation of bowel.

Increases in alanine transaminase (ALT, SGPT) aspartate transaminase (AST, SGOT) and alkaline phosphatase have been observed following corticosteroid treatment. These changes are usually small, not associated with any clinical syndrome and are reversible upon discontinuation.

Anti-inflammatory and immunosuppressive effects: Increased susceptibility and severity of infections with suppression of clinical symptoms and signs, opportunistic infections, may suppress reactions to skin tests, recurrence of dormant tuberculosis (see *Other special warnings and precautions*).

Musculoskeletal: Proximal myopathy, osteoporosis, vertebral and long bone fractures, avascular osteonecrosis, tendon rupture, muscle weakness.

Fluid and electrolyte disturbance: Sodium and water retention, hypertension, hypokalaemic alkalosis, potassium loss, congestive heart failure in susceptible patients.

Dermatological: Impaired healing, skin atrophy, bruising, striae, telangiectasia, acne, petechiae and ecchymosis.

Endocrine/metabolic: Suppression of the hypothalamo-pituitary-adrenal axis; growth suppression in infancy, childhood and adolescence; menstrual irregularity and amenorrhoea. Cushingoid facies, hirsutism, weight gain, impaired carbohydrate tolerance with increased requirement for antidiabetic therapy, negative nitrogen and calcium balance. Increased appetite.

Neuropsychiatric: Euphoria, psychological dependence, mood swings, depression, personality changes, insomnia. Increased intra-cranial pressure with papilloedema in children (pseudotumour cerebri), usually after treatment withdrawal. Psychosis, aggravation of schizophrenia, seizures.

Ophthalmic: Increased intra-ocular pressure, glaucoma, papilloedema, cataracts with possible damage to the optic nerve, corneal or scleral thinning, exacerbation of ophthalmic viral or fungal disease, exophthalmos.

General: Leucocytosis, hypersensitivity reactions including anaphylaxis, thrombo-embolism, nausea, malaise.

Withdrawal symptoms: Too rapid a reduction of corticosteroid dosage following prolonged treatment can lead to acute adrenal insufficiency, hypotension and death (see *Other special warnings and precautions*).

A 'withdrawal syndrome' may also occur including, fever, myalgia, arthralgia, rhinitis, conjunctivitis, painful itchy skin nodules and loss of weight.

Use in pregnancy and lactation:
Pregnancy: The ability of corticosteroids to cross the placenta varies between individual drugs, however, methylprednisolone does cross the placenta.

Administration of corticosteroids to pregnant animals can cause abnormalities of foetal development including cleft palate, intra-uterine growth retardation and affects on brain growth and development. There is no evidence that corticosteroids result in an increased incidence of congenital abnormalities, such as cleft palate in man, however, when administered for long periods or repeatedly during pregnancy, corticosteroids may increase the risk of intra-uterine growth retardation. Hypoadrenalism may, in theory, occur in the neonate following prenatal exposure to corticosteroids but usually resolves spontaneously following birth and is rarely clinically important. As with all drugs, corticosteroids should only be prescribed when the benefits to the mother and child outweigh the risks. When corticosteroids are essential, however, patients with normal pregnancies may be treated as though they were in the non-gravid state.

Lactation: Corticosteroids are excreted in small amounts in breast milk, however, doses of up to 40 mg daily of methylprednisolone are unlikely to cause systemic effects in the infant. Infants of mothers taking higher doses than this may have a degree of adrenal suppression, but the benefits of breastfeeding are likely to outweigh any theoretical risk.

Other special warnings and precautions: Warnings : A Patient Information Leaflet is provided in the pack by the manufacturer.

Undesirable effects may be minimised by using the lowest effective dose for the minimum period, and by administering the daily requirement as a single morning dose or whenever possible as a single morning dose on alternative days. Frequent patient review is required to appropriately titrate the dose against disease activity (see Dosage and administration).

Adrenal cortical atrophy develops during prolonged therapy and may persist for months after stopping treatment. In patients who have received more than physiological doses of systemic corticosteroids (approximately 6 mg methylprednisolone) for greater than 3 weeks, withdrawal should not be abrupt. How dose reduction should be carried out depends largely on whether the disease is likely to relapse as the dose of systemic corticosteroids is reduced. Clinical assessment of disease activity may be needed during withdrawal. If the disease is unlikely to relapse on withdrawal of systemic corticosteroids, but there is uncertainty about HPA suppression, the dose of systemic corticosteroid *may* be reduced rapidly to physiological doses. Once a daily dose of 6 mg methylprednisolone is reached, dose reduction should be slower to allow the HPA-axis to recover.

Abrupt withdrawal of systemic corticosteroid treatment, which has continued up to 3 weeks is appropriate if it is considered that the disease is unlikely to relapse. Abrupt withdrawal of doses up to 32 mg daily of methylprednisolone for 3 weeks is unlikely to lead to clinically relevant HPA-axis suppression, in the majority of patients. In the following patient groups, gradual withdrawal of systemic corticosteroid therapy should be ***considered*** even after courses lasting 3 weeks or less:

Patients who have had repeated courses of systemic corticosteroids, particularly if taken for greater than 3 weeks.

When a short course has been prescribed within one year of cessation of long-term therapy (months or years).

Patients who may have reasons for adrenocortical insufficiency other than exogenous corticosteroid therapy.

Patients receiving doses of systemic corticosteroid greater than 32 mg daily of methylprednisolone.

Patients repeatedly taking doses in the evening.

Since mineralocorticoid secretion may be impaired, salt and/or a mineralocorticoid should be administered concurrently.

Patients should carry 'Steroid Treatment' cards which give clear guidance on the precautions to be taken to minimise risk and which provide details of prescriber, drug, dosage and the duration of treatment.

Corticosteroids may mask some signs of infection, and new infections may appear during their use. Suppression of the inflammatory response and immune function increases the susceptibility to infections and their severity.

Chickenpox is of serious concern since this normally minor illness may be fatal in immunosuppressed patients. Patients (or parents of children) without a definite history of chickenpox should be advised to avoid close personal contact with chickenpox or herpes zoster and if exposed they should seek urgent medical attention. Passive immunization with varicella/zoster immunoglobin (VZIG) is needed by exposed non-immune patients who are receiving systemic corticosteroids or who have used them within the previous 3 months; this should be given within 10 days of exposure to chickenpox. If a diagnosis of chickenpox is confirmed, the illness warrants specialist care and urgent treatment. Corticosteroids should not be stopped and the dose may need to be increased.

Live vaccines should not be given to individuals with impaired immune responsiveness. The antibody response to other vaccines may be diminished.

The use of Medrone in active tuberculosis should be restricted to those cases of fulminating or disseminated tuberculosis in which the corticosteroid is used for the management of the disease in conjunction with an appropriate antituberculous regimen. If corticosteroids are indicated in patients with latent tuberculosis or tuberculin reactivity, close observation is necessary as reactivation of the disease may occur. During prolonged corticosteroid therapy, these patients should receive chemoprophylaxis.

Care should be taken for patients receiving cardioactive drugs such as digoxin because of steroid induced electrolyte disturbance/potassium loss (see *Side-effects*).

Special precautions: Particular care is required when considering the use of systemic corticosteroids in patients with the following conditions and frequent patient monitoring is necessary.

Osteoporosis (post-menopausal females are particularly at risk).
Hypertension or congestive heart failure.
Existing or previous history of severe affective disorders (especially previous steroid psychosis).
Diabetes mellitus (or a family history of diabetes).
History of tuberculosis.
Glaucoma (or a family history of glaucoma).
Previous corticosteroid-induced myopathy.
Liver failure or cirrhosis.
Renal insufficiency.
Epilepsy.
Peptic ulceration.
Fresh intestinal anastomoses.
Predisposition to thrombophlebitis.
Abscess or other pyogenic infections.
Ulcerative colitis.
Diverticulitis.
Myasthenia gravis.
Ocular herpes simplex, for fear of corneal perforation.
Hypothyroidism.

Use in children: Corticosteroids cause growth retardation in infancy, childhood and adolescence. Treatment should be limited to the minimum dosage for the shortest possible time. In order to minimise suppression of the hypothalamo-pituitary-adrenal axis and growth retardation, treatment should be administered where possible as a single dose on alternate days.

Use in the elderly: The common adverse effects of systemic corticosteroids may be associated with more serious consequences in old age, especially osteoporosis, hypertension, hypokalaemia, diabetes, susceptibility to infection and thinning of the skin. Close clinical supervision is required to avoid life-threatening reactions.

Overdosage: Administration of Medrone should not be discontinued abruptly but tailed off over a period of time. Appropriate action should be taken to alleviate the symptoms produced by any side-effect that may become apparent. It may be necessary to support the patient with corticosteroids during any further period of trauma occurring within two years of overdosage.

There is no clinical syndrome of acute overdose with Medrone. Methylprednisolone is dialysable.

Incompatibilities (major): None stated.

Pharmaceutical precautions Store below 25°C.

Legal category POM.

Package quantities 2 and 4 mg tablets in packs of 30.

Further information Medrone has achieved a clinically acceptable split between glucocorticoid effect and undesired mineralocorticoid effect. Weight for weight, methylprednisolone has five times the anti-inflammatory activity of hydrocortisone but has little tendency to cause salt and water retention.

Information on Medrone Tablets 16 mg and 100 mg is available separately and this details those indications for which high dose oral steroid therapy is appropriate.

Product licence numbers
Medrone Tablets 2 mg 0032/5017
Medrone Tablets 4 mg 0032/5018

Date of preparation or last review August 1998.

MEDRONE* TABLETS 16 MG

Presentation Oval single-scored white tablet marked 'UPJOHN 73' containing 16 mg methylprednisolone. Medrone Tablets 16 mg also contain lactose, sucrose, maize starch, mineral oil and calcium stearate.

Uses Medrone is a potent corticosteroid with an anti-inflammatory activity at least five times that of hydrocortisone. An enhanced separation of glucocorticoid and mineralocorticoid effect results in a reduced incidence of sodium and water retention.

These products are indicated for conditions requiring glucocorticoid activity such as :-

Collagen diseases/arteritis: Systemic lupus erythematosus; Systemic dermatomyositis (polymyositis); Rheumatic fever with severe carditis ; Giant cell arteritis/polymyalgia rheumatica.

Dermatological diseases: Pemphigus vulgaris

Allergic states: Bronchial asthma

Respiratory diseases: Pulmonary sarcoid

Haematological disorders: Idiopathic thrombocytopenic purpura ; Haemolytic anaemia (autoimmune)

Neoplastic diseases: Leukaemia (acute and lymphatic) ; Malignant lymphoma

Gastro-intestinal diseases: Crohn's disease

Miscellaneous: Tuberculous meningitis (with appropriate antituberculous chemotherapy) ; Transplantation

Dosage and administration The dosage recommendations shown in the table below are suggested initial daily doses and are intended as guides. The average total daily dose recommended may be given either as a single dose or in divided doses (excepting in alternate day therapy when the minimum effective daily dose is doubled and given every other day at 8.00 a.m.). It is envisaged that the 100 mg tablet will be used for high initial daily or alternate day doses in acute situations, with tapering of dosage achieved by using the 16 mg tablet.

Undesirable effects may be minimised by using the lowest effective dose for the minimum period (see Other special warnings and precautions).

The initial suppressive dose level may vary depending on the condition being treated. As soon as a satisfactory clinical response is obtained, the daily dose should be reduced gradually, either to termination of treatment in the case of acute conditions or to the minimal effective maintenance dose level in the case of chronic conditions. In chronic conditions it is important that the reduction in dosage from initial to maintenance dose levels be accomplished as clinically appropriate.

In alternate-day therapy, the minimum daily corticoid requirement is doubled and administered as a single dose every other day at 8.00 a.m. Dosage requirements depend on the condition being treated and response of the patient.

Elderly patients: Treatment of elderly patients, particularly if long-term, should be planned bearing in mind the more serious consequences of the common side-effects of corticosteroids in old age and close clinical supervision is required (see *Other special warnings and precautions*).

Children: In general, dosage for children should be based upon clinical response and is at the discretion of the clinician. Treatment should be limited to the minimum dosage for the shortest period of time. If possible, treatment should be administered as a single dose on alternate days (see *Other special warnings and precautions*).

Dosage recommendations:

Indications	*Recommended initial daily dosage*
Systemic lupus erythematosus	20–100 mg
Systemic dermatomyositis	48 mg
Acute rheumatic fever	48 mg until ESR normal for one week.
Giant cell arteritis/polymyalgia rheumatica	64 mg
Pemphigus vulgaris	80–360 mg
Bronchial asthma	up to 64 mg single dose/alternate day up to 100 mg maximum.
Pulmonary sarcoid	32–48 mg on alternate days.
Haematological disorders and leukaemias	16–100 mg
Malignant lymphoma	16–100 mg
Crohn's disease	up to 48 mg per day in acute episodes.
Organ transplantation	up to 3.6 mg/kg/day

Contra-indications, warnings, etc

Contra-indications: Medrone is contra-indicated where there is known hypersensitivity to components and in systemic fungal infection unless specific anti-infective therapy is employed.

Interactions: Convulsions have been reported with concurrent use of methylprednisolone and cyclosporin. Since concurrent administration of these agents results in a mutual inhibition of metabolism, it is possible that convulsions and other adverse effects associated with the individual use of either drug may be more apt to occur.

Drugs that induce hepatic enzymes, such as rifampicin, rifabutin, carbamazepine, phenobarbitone, phenytoin, primidone, and aminoglutethimide enhance the metabolism of corticosteroids and its therapeutic effects may be reduced.

Drugs such as erythromycin and ketoconazole may inhibit the metabolism of corticosteroids and thus decrease their clearance.

Steroids may reduce the effects of anticholinesterases in myasthenia gravis. The desired effects of hypoglycaemic agents (including insulin), anti-hypertensives and diuretics are antagonised by corticosteroids, and the hypokalaemic effects of acetazolamide, loop diuretics, thiazide diuretics and carbenoxolone are enhanced.

The efficacy of coumarin anticoagulants may be enhanced by concurrent corticosteroid therapy and close monitoring of the INR or prothrombin time is required to avoid spontaneous bleeding.

The renal clearance of salicylates is increased by corticosteroids and steroid withdrawal may result in salicylate intoxication. Salicylates and non-steroidal anti-inflammatory agents should be used cautiously in conjunction with corticosteroids in hypothrombinaemia.

Steroids have been reported to interact with neuromuscular blocking agents such as pancuronium with partial reversal of the neuromuscular block.

Effects on ability to drive and use machines: None stated.

Other undesirable effects (frequency and seriousness):

Side-effects: The incidence of predictable undesirable side-effects associated with the use of corticosteroids, including hypothalamic-pituitary-adrenal suppression correlates with the relative potency of the drug, dosage, timing of administration and duration of treatment (see *Other special warnings and precautions*).

Gastro-intestinal: Dyspepsia, peptic ulceration with perforation and haemorrhage, abdominal distension, oesophageal ulceration, oesophageal candidiasis, acute pancreatitis, perforation of bowel.

Increases in alanine transaminase (ALT, SGPT) aspartate transaminase (AST, SGOT) and alkaline phosphatase have been observed following corticosteroid treatment. These changes are usually small, not associated with any clinical syndrome and are reversible upon discontinuation.

Anti-inflammatory and immunosuppressive effects: Increased susceptibility and severity of infections with suppression of clinical symptoms and signs, opportunistic infections, may suppress reactions to skin tests, recurrence of dormant tuberculosis (see *Other special warnings and precautions*).

Musculoskeletal: Proximal myopathy, osteoporosis, vertebral and long bone fractures, avascular osteonecrosis, tendon rupture, muscle weakness.

Fluid and electrolyte disturbance: Sodium and water retention, hypertension, hypokalaemic alkalosis, potassium loss, congestive heart failure in susceptible patients.

Dermatological: Impaired healing, skin atrophy, bruising, striae, telangiectasia, acne, petechiae and ecchymosis.

Endocrine/metabolic: Suppression of the hypothalamo-pituitary-adrenal axis; growth suppression in infancy, childhood and adolescence; menstrual irregularity and amenorrhoea. Cushingoid facies, hirsutism, weight gain, impaired carbohydrate tolerance with increased requirement for antidiabetic therapy, negative nitrogen and calcium balance. Increased appetite.

Neuropsychiatric: Euphoria, psychological dependence, mood swings, depression, personality changes, insomnia. Increased intra-cranial pressure with papilloedema in children (pseudotumour cerebri), usually after treatment withdrawal. Psychosis, aggravation of schizophrenia, seizures.

Ophthalmic: Increased intra-ocular pressure, glaucoma, papilloedema, cataracts with possible damage to the optic nerve, corneal or scleral thinning, exacerbation of ophthalmic viral or fungal disease, exophthalmos.

General: Leucocytosis, hypersensitivity reactions including anaphylaxis, thrombo-embolism, nausea, malaise.

Withdrawal symptoms: Too rapid a reduction of corticosteroid dosage following prolonged treatment can lead to acute adrenal insufficiency, hypotension and death (see *Other special warnings and precautions*).

A 'withdrawal syndrome' may also occur including, fever, myalgia, arthralgia, rhinitis, conjunctivitis, painful itchy skin nodules and loss of weight.

Use in pregnancy and lactation:

Pregnancy: The ability of corticosteroids to cross the placenta varies between individual drugs, however, methylprednisolone does cross the placenta.

Administration of corticosteroids to pregnant animals can cause abnormalities of foetal development including cleft palate, intra-uterine growth retardation and affects on brain growth and development. There is no evidence that corticosteroids result in an increased incidence of congenital abnormalities, such as cleft palate in man, however, when administered for long periods or repeatedly during pregnancy, corticosteroids may increase the risk of intra-uterine growth retardation. Hypoadrenalism may, in theory , occur in the neonate following prenatal exposure to corticosteroids but usually resolves spontaneously following birth and is rarely clinically important. As with all drugs, corticosteroids should only be prescribed when the benefits to the mother and child outweigh the risks. When corticosteroids are essential, however, patients with normal pregnancies may be treated as though they were in the non-gravid state.

Lactation: Corticosteroids are excreted in small amounts in breast milk, however, doses of up to 40 mg daily of methylprednisolone are unlikely to cause systemic effects in the infant. Infants of mothers taking higher doses than this may have a degree of adrenal suppression, but the benefits of breastfeeding are likely to outweigh any theoretical risk.

Other special warnings and precautions:
Warnings: A Patient Information Leaflet is provided in the pack by the manufacturer.

Undesirable effects may be minimised by using the lowest effective dose for the minimum period, and by administering the daily requirement as a single morning dose or whenever possible as a single morning dose on alternative days. Frequent patient review is required to appropriately titrate the dose against disease activity (see *Dosage and administration*).

Adrenal cortical atrophy develops during prolonged therapy and may persist for months after stopping treatment. In patients who have received more than physiological doses of systemic corticosteroids (approximately 6 mg methylprednisolone) for greater than 3 weeks, withdrawal should not be abrupt. How dose reduction should be carried out depends largely on whether the disease is likely to relapse as the dose of systemic corticosteroids is reduced. Clinical assessment of disease activity may be needed during withdrawal. If the disease is unlikely to relapse on withdrawal of systemic corticosteroids, but there is uncertainty about HPA suppression, the dose of systemic corticosteroid *may* be reduced rapidly to physiological doses. Once a daily dose of 6 mg methylprednisolone is reached, dose reduction should be slower to allow the HPA-axis to recover.

Abrupt withdrawal of systemic corticosteroid treatment, which has continued up to 3 weeks is appropriate if it is considered that the disease is unlikely to relapse. Abrupt withdrawal of doses up to 32 mg daily of methylprednisolone for 3 weeks is unlikely to lead to clinically relevant HPA-axis suppression, in the majority of patients. In the following patient groups, gradual withdrawal of systemic corticosteroid therapy should be ***considered*** even after courses lasting 3 weeks or less:

Patients who have had repeated courses of systemic corticosteroids, particularly if taken for greater than 3 weeks.

When a short course has been prescribed within one year of cessation of long-term therapy (months or years).

Patients who may have reasons for adrenocortical insufficiency other than exogenous corticosteroid therapy.

Patients receiving doses of systemic corticosteroid greater than 32 mg daily of methylprednisolone.

Patients repeatedly taking doses in the evening.

Since mineralocorticoid secretion may be impaired, salt and/or a mineralocorticoid should be administered concurrently.

Patients should carry 'Steroid Treatment' cards which give clear guidance on the precautions to be taken to minimise risk and which provide details of prescriber, drug, dosage and the duration of treatment.

Corticosteroids may mask some signs of infection, and new infections may appear during their use. Suppression of the inflammatory response and immune function increases the susceptibility to infections and their severity.

Chickenpox is of serious concern since this normally minor illness may be fatal in immunosuppressed patients. Patients (or parents of children) without a definite history of chickenpox should be advised to avoid close personal contact with chickenpox or herpes zoster and if exposed they should seek urgent medical attention. Passive immunization with varicella/zoster immunoglobin (VZIG) is needed by exposed non-immune patients who are receiving systemic corticosteroids or who have used them within the previous 3 months; this should be given within 10 days of exposure to chickenpox. If a diagnosis of chickenpox is confirmed, the illness warrants specialist care and urgent treatment. Corticosteroids should not be stopped and the dose may need to be increased.

Live vaccines should not be given to individuals with impaired immune responsiveness. The antibody response to other vaccines may be diminished.

The use of Medrone in active tuberculosis should be restricted to those cases of fulminating or disseminated tuberculosis in which the corticosteroid is used for the management of the disease in conjunction with an appropriate antituberculous regimen. If corticosteroids are indicated in patients with latent tuberculosis or tuberculin reactivity, close observation is necessary as reactivation of the disease may occur. During prolonged corticosteroid therapy, these patients should receive chemoprophylaxis.

Care should be taken for patients receiving cardioactive drugs such as digoxin because of steroid induced electrolyte disturbance/potassium loss (see *Side-effects*).

Special precautions: Particular care is required when considering the use of systemic corticosteroids in patients with the following conditions and frequent patient monitoring is necessary.

Osteoporosis (post-menopausal females are particularly at risk).
Hypertension or congestive heart failure.
Existing or previous history of severe affective disorders (especially previous steroid psychosis).
Diabetes mellitus (or a family history of diabetes).
History of tuberculosis.
Glaucoma (or a family history of glaucoma).
Previous corticosteroid-induced myopathy.
Liver failure or cirrhosis.
Renal insufficiency.
Epilepsy.
Peptic ulceration.
Fresh intestinal anastomoses.
Predisposition to thrombophlebitis.
Abscess or other pyogenic infections.
Ulcerative colitis.
Diverticulitis.
Myasthenia gravis.
Ocular herpes simplex, for fear of corneal perforation.
Hypothyroidism.

Use in children: Corticosteroids cause growth retardation in infancy, childhood and adolescence. Treatment should be limited to the minimum dosage for the shortest possible time. In order to minimise suppression of the hypothalamo-pituitary-adrenal axis and growth retardation, treatment should be administered where possible as a single dose on alternate days.

Use in the elderly: The common adverse effects of systemic corticosteroids may be associated with more serious consequences in old age, especially osteoporosis, hypertension, hypokalaemia, diabetes, susceptibility to infection and thinning of the skin. Close clinical supervision is required to avoid life-threatening reactions.

Overdosage: Administration of Medrone should not be discontinued abruptly but tailed off over a period of time. Appropriate action should be taken to alleviate the symptoms produced by any side-effect that may become apparent. It may be necessary to support the patient with corticosteroids during any further period of trauma occurring within two years of overdosage.

There is no clinical syndrome of acute overdose with Medrone. Methylprednisolone is dialysable.

Incompatibilities (major): None stated.

Pharmaceutical precautions Store below 25°C.

Legal category POM.

Package quantities Packs of 30 tablets

Further information Medrone has achieved a clinically acceptable split between glucocorticoid effect and undesired mineralocorticoid effect. Weight for weight, methylprednisolone has five times the anti-inflammatory activity of hydrocortisone but has little tendency to cause salt and water retention. The 16 mg tablet gives opportunity for use of alternate day therapy in long term use in chronic conditions.

A separate data sheet is available for Medrone Tablets 2 mg and 4 mg and includes additional indications in which low dose therapy is appropriate.

Product licence numbers 0032/0024

Date of preparation or last review August 1998.

MEDRONE* TABLETS 100 MG

Qualitative and quantitative composition Each Medrone Tablet contains 100 mg methylprednisolone PhEur.

Pharmaceutical form Tablet.

Clinical particulars

Therapeutic indications: Medrone is a potent corticosteroid with an anti-inflammatory activity at least five times that of hydrocortisone. An enhanced separation of glucocorticoid and mineralocorticoid effect results in a reduced incidence of sodium and water retention.

Medrone is indicated for conditions requiring glucocorticoid activity such as:

Collagen diseases/arteritis: Systemic lupus erythematosus ; Systemic dermatomyositis (polymyositis) ; Rheumatic fever with severe carditis ; Giant cell arteritis/polymyalgia rheumatica
Dermatological diseases: Pemphigus vulgaris
Allergic states: Bronchial asthma
Respiratory diseases: Pulmonary sarcoid
Haematological disorders: Idiopathic thrombocytopenic purpura;
Haemolytic anaemia (autoimmune)
Neoplastic diseases: Leukaemia (acute and lymphatic); Malignant lymphoma
Gastro-intestinal diseases: Crohn's disease
Miscellaneous: Tuberculous meningitis (with appropriate antituberculous chemotherapy); Transplantation

Posology and method of administration: The dosage recommendations shown in the table below are suggested initial daily doses and are intended as guides. The average total daily dose recommended may be given either as a single dose or in divided doses (excepting in alternate day therapy when the minimum effective daily dose is doubled and given every other day at 8.00 a.m.). It is envisaged that the 100 mg tablet will be used for high initial daily or alternate day doses in acute situations, with tapering of dosage achieved by using the 16 mg tablet.

Undesirable effects may be minimised by using the lowest effective dose for the minimum period (see *Special warnings and special precautions for use*).

The initial suppressive dose level may vary depending on the condition being treated. As soon as a satisfactory clinical response is obtained, the daily dose should be reduced gradually, either to termination of treatment in the case of acute conditions or to the minimal effective maintenance dose level in the case of chronic conditions. In chronic conditions it is important that the reduction in dosage from initial to maintenance dose levels be accomplished as clinically appropriate.

In alternate-day therapy, the minimum daily corticoid requirement is doubled and administered as a single dose every other day at 8.00 a.m. Dosage requirements depend on the condition being treated and response of the patient.

Elderly patients: Treatment of elderly patients, particularly if long-term, should be planned bearing in mind the more serious consequences of the common side-effects of corticosteroids in old age and close clinical supervision is required (see *Special warnings and special precautions for use*).

Children: In general, dosage for children should be based upon clinical response and is at the discretion of the clinician. Treatment should be limited to the minimum dosage for the shortest period of time. If possible, treatment should be administered as a single dose on alternate days (see *Special warnings and special precautions for use*).

Dosage recommendations:

Indications	*Recommended initial daily dosage*
Systemic lupus erythematosus	20–100 mg
Systemic dermatomyositis	48 mg
Acute rheumatic fever	48 mg until ESR normal for one week.
Giant cell arteritis/polymyalgia rheumatica	64 mg
Pemphigus vulgaris	80–360 mg
Bronchial asthma	up to 64 mg single dose/alternate day up to 100 mg maximum.
Pulmonary sarcoid	32–48 mg on alternate days.
Haematological disorders and leukaemias	16–100 mg
Malignant lymphoma	16–100 mg
Crohn's disease	up to 48 mg per day in acute episodes.
Organ transplantation	up to 3.6 mg/kg/day

Contra-indications: Medrone is contra-indicated where there is known hypersensitivity to components and in systemic fungal infection unless specific anti-infective therapy is employed.

Special warnings and special precautions for use:
Warnings and precautions: A Patient Information Leaflet is provided in the pack by the manufacturer.

Undesirable effects may be minimised by using the lowest effective dose for the minimum period, and by administering the daily requirement as a single morning dose or whenever possible as a single morning dose on alternative days. Frequent patient review is required to appropriately titrate the dose against disease activity (see *Posology and method of administration*).

Adrenal cortical atrophy develops during prolonged therapy and may persist for months after stopping treatment. In patients who have received more than physiological doses of systemic corticosteroids (approximately 6 mg methylprednisolone) for greater than 3 weeks, withdrawal should not be abrupt. How dose reduction should be carried out depends largely on whether the disease is likely to relapse as the dose of systemic corticosteroids is reduced. Clinical assessment of disease activity may be needed during withdrawal. If the disease is unlikely to relapse on withdrawal of systemic corticosteroids, but there is uncertainty about HPA suppression, the dose of systemic corticosteroid *may* be reduced rapidly to physiological doses. Once a daily dose of 6 mg methylprednisolone is reached, dose reduction should be slower to allow the HPA-axis to recover.

Abrupt withdrawal of systemic corticosteroid treatment, which has continued up to 3 weeks is appropriate if it is considered that the disease is unlikely to relapse. Abrupt withdrawal of doses up to 32 mg daily of methylprednisolone for 3 weeks is unlikely to lead to clinically relevant HPA-axis suppression, in the majority of patients. In the following patient groups, gradual withdrawal of systemic corticosteroid therapy should be *considered* even after courses lasting 3 weeks or less:

Patients who have had repeated courses of systemic corticosteroids, particularly if taken for greater than 3 weeks.

When a short course has been prescribed within one year of cessation of long-term therapy (months or years).

Patients who may have reasons for adrenocortical insufficiency other than exogenous corticosteroid therapy.

Patients receiving doses of systemic corticosteroid greater than 32 mg daily of methylprednisolone.

Patients repeatedly taking doses in the evening.

Since mineralocorticoid secretion may be impaired, salt and/or a mineralocorticoid should be administered concurrently.

Patients should carry 'Steroid Treatment' cards which give clear guidance on the precautions to be taken to minimise risk and which provide details of prescriber, drug, dosage and the duration of treatment.

Corticosteroids may mask some signs of infection, and new infections may appear during their use. Suppression of the inflammatory response and immune function increases the susceptibility to infections and their severity.

Chickenpox is of serious concern since this normally minor illness may be fatal in immunosuppressed patients. Patients (or parents of children) without a definite history of chickenpox should be advised to avoid close personal contact with chickenpox or herpes zoster and if exposed they should seek urgent medical attention. Passive immunization with varicella/zoster immunoglobin (VZIG) is needed by exposed non-immune patients who are receiving systemic corticosteroids or who have used them within the previous 3 months; this should be given within 10 days of exposure to chickenpox. If a diagnosis of chickenpox is confirmed, the illness warrants specialist care and urgent treatment. Corticosteroids should not be stopped and the dose may need to be increased.

Live vaccines should not be given to individuals with impaired immune responsiveness. The antibody response to other vaccines may be diminished.

The use of Medrone in active tuberculosis should be restricted to those cases of fulminating or disseminated tuberculosis in which the corticosteroid is used for the management of the disease in conjunction with an appropriate antituberculous regimen. If corticosteroids are indicated in patients with latent tuberculosis or tuberculin reactivity, close observation is necessary as reactivation of the disease may occur. During prolonged corticosteroid therapy, these patients should receive chemoprophylaxis.

Care should be taken for patients receiving cardioactive drugs such as digoxin because of steroid induced electrolyte disturbance/potassium loss (see *Undesirable effects*).

Special precautions: Particular care is required when considering the use of systemic corticosteroids in patients with the following conditions and frequent patient monitoring is necessary.

Osteoporosis (post-menopausal females are particularly at risk).
Hypertension or congestive heart failure.
Existing or previous history of severe affective disorders (especially previous steroid psychosis).
Diabetes mellitus (or a family history of diabetes).
History of tuberculosis.
Glaucoma (or a family history of glaucoma).
Previous corticosteroid-induced myopathy.
Liver failure or cirrhosis.
Renal insufficiency.
Epilepsy.
Peptic ulceration.
Fresh intestinal anastomoses.
Predisposition to thrombophlebitis.
Abscess or other pyogenic infections.
Ulcerative colitis.
Diverticulitis.
Myasthenia gravis.
Ocular herpes simplex, for fear of corneal perforation.
Hypothyroidism.

Use in children: Corticosteroids cause growth retardation in infancy, childhood and adolescence. Treatment should be limited to the minimum dosage for the shortest possible time. In order to minimise suppression of the hypothalamo-pituitary-adrenal axis and growth retardation, treatment should be administered where possible as a single dose on alternate days.

Use in the elderly: The common adverse effects of systemic corticosteroids may be associated with more serious consequences in old age, especially osteoporosis, hypertension, hypokalaemia, diabetes, susceptibility to infection and thinning of the skin. Close clinical supervision is required to avoid life-threatening reactions.

Interaction with other medicaments and other forms of interaction: Convulsions have been reported with concurrent use of methylprednisolone and cyclosporin. Since concurrent administration of these agents results in a mutual inhibition of metabolism, it is possible that convulsions and other adverse effects associated with the individual use of either drug may be more apt to occur.

Drugs that induce hepatic enzymes, such as rifampicin, rifabutin, carbamazepine, phenobarbitone, phenytoin, primidone, and aminoglutethimide enhance the metabolism of corticosteroids and its therapeutic effects may be reduced.

Drugs such as erythromycin and ketoconazole may inhibit the metabolism of corticosteroids and thus decrease their clearance.

Steroids may reduce the effects of anticholinesterases in myasthenia gravis. The desired effects of hypoglycaemic agents (including insulin), anti-hypertensives and diuretics are antagonised by corticosteroids, and the hypokalaemic effects of acetazolamide, loop diuretics, thiazide diuretics and carbenoxolone are enhanced.

The efficacy of coumarin anticoagulants may be enhanced by concurrent corticosteroid therapy and close monitoring of the INR or prothrombin time is required to avoid spontaneous bleeding.

The renal clearance of salicylates is increased by corticosteroids and steroid withdrawal may result in salicylate intoxication. Salicylates and non-steroidal anti-inflammatory agents should be used cautiously in conjunction with corticosteroids in hypothrombinaemia.

Steroids have been reported to interact with neuromuscular blocking agents such as pancuronium with partial reversal of the neuromuscular block.

Pregnancy and lactation:
Pregnancy: The ability of corticosteroids to cross the placenta varies between individual drugs, however, methylprednisolone does cross the placenta.

Administration of corticosteroids to pregnant animals can cause abnormalities of foetal development including cleft palate, intra-uterine growth retardation and affects on brain growth and development. There is no evidence that corticosteroids result in an increased incidence of congenital abnormalities, such as cleft palate in man, however, when administered for long periods or repeatedly during pregnancy, corticosteroids may increase the risk of intra-uterine growth retardation. Hypoadrenalism may, in theory, occur in the neonate following prenatal exposure to corticosteroids but usually resolves spontaneously following birth and is rarely clinically important. As with all drugs, corticosteroids should only be prescribed when the benefits to the mother and child outweigh the risks. When corticosteroids are essential, however, patients with normal pregnancies may be treated as though they were in the non-gravid state.

Lactation: Corticosteroids are excreted in small amounts in breast milk, however, doses of up to 40 mg daily of methylprednisolone are unlikely to cause systemic effects in the infant. Infants of mothers taking higher doses than this may have a degree of adrenal suppression, but the benefits of breastfeeding are likely to outweigh any theoretical risk.

Effects on ability to drive and use machines: None stated.

Undesirable effects: The incidence of predictable undesirable side-effects associated with the use of corticosteroids, including hypothalamic-pituitary-adrenal suppression correlates with the relative potency of the drug, dosage, timing of administration and duration of treatment (see *Special warnings and special precautions for use*).

Gastro-intestinal: Dyspepsia, peptic ulceration with perforation and haemorrhage, abdominal distension, oesophageal ulceration, oesophageal candidiasis, acute pancreatitis, perforation of bowel.

Increases in alanine transaminase (ALT, SGPT) aspartate transaminase (AST, SGOT) and alkaline phosphatase have been observed following corticosteroid treatment. These changes are usually small, not associated with any clinical syndrome and are reversible upon discontinuation.

Anti-inflammatory and immunosuppressive effects: Increased susceptibility and severity of infections with suppression of clinical symptoms and signs, opportunistic infections, may suppress reactions to skin tests, recurrence of dormant tuberculosis (see *Special warnings and special precautions for use*).

Musculoskeletal: Proximal myopathy, osteoporosis, vertebral and long bone fractures, avascular osteonecrosis, tendon rupture, muscle weakness.

Fluid and electrolyte disturbance: Sodium and water retention, hypertension, hypokalaemic alkalosis, potassium loss, congestive heart failure in susceptible patients.

Dermatological: Impaired healing, skin atrophy, bruising, striae, telangiectasia, acne, petechiae and ecchymosis.

Endocrine/metabolic: Suppression of the hypothalamo-pituitary-adrenal axis, growth suppression in infancy, childhood and adolescence, menstrual irregularity and amenorrhoea. Cushingoid facies, hirsutism, weight gain, impaired carbohydrate tolerance with increased requirement for antidiabetic therapy, negative nitrogen and calcium balance. Increased appetite.

Neuropsychiatric: Euphoria, psychological dependence, mood swings, depression, personality changes, insomnia. Increased intra-cranial pressure with papilloedema in children (pseudotumour cerebri), usually after treatment withdrawal. Psychosis, aggravation of schizophrenia, seizures.

Ophthalmic: Increased intra-ocular pressure, glaucoma, papilloedema, cataracts with possible damage to the optic nerve, corneal or scleral thinning, exacerbation of ophthalmic viral or fungal disease, exophthalmos.

General: Leucocytosis, hypersensitivity reactions including anaphylaxis, thrombo-embolism, nausea, malaise.

Withdrawal symptoms: Too rapid a reduction of corticosteroid dosage following prolonged treatment can lead to acute adrenal insufficiency, hypotension and death (see *Special warnings and special precautions for use*).

A 'withdrawal syndrome' may also occur including, fever, myalgia, arthralgia, rhinitis, conjunctivitis, painful itchy skin nodules and loss of weight.

Overdose: Administration of Medrone should not be discontinued abruptly but tailed off over a period of time. Appropriate action should be taken to alleviate the symptoms produced by any side-effect that may become apparent. It may be necessary to support the patient with corticosteroids during any further period of trauma occurring within two years of overdosage.

There is no clinical syndrome of acute overdose with Medrone. Methylprednisolone is dialysable.

Pharmacological properties
Pharmacodynamic properties: Methylprednisolone is a potent anti-inflammatory steroid. It has greater anti-inflammatory potency than prednisolone and less tendency than prednisolone to induce sodium and water retention. The relative potency of methylprednisolone to hydrocortisone is at least four to one.

Pharmacokinetic properties: The mean elimination half-life ranges from 2.4 to 3.5 hours in normal, healthy adults and appears to be independent of the route of administration.

Methylprednisolone is metabolised in the liver to inactive metabolites, the major ones being 20 b-hydroxymethylprednisolone and 20 b-hydroxy-a-methylprednisolone.

Methylprednisolone clearance is altered by concurrent administration of troleandomycin, erythromycin, rifampicin, anticonvulsants and theophylline. No dosing adjustments are necessary in renal failure. Methylprednisolone is haemodialyzable.

Pharmaceutical particulars
List of excipients: Methylcellulose, sodium starch glycolate, microcrystalline cellulose, magnesium stearate and E132.

Incompatibilities: None stated.

Shelf-life: 48 months.

Special precautions for storage: Store below 25°C.

Nature and contents of container: Amber glass bottle with LDPE cap and bulb–each bottle contains 20 tablets.

Instructions for use/handling: No special requirements.

Marketing authorisation number 0032/0145

Date of first authorisation/renewal of authorisation Date of first authorisation: 3 May 1991.
Last renewal dates: 25 March 1997.

Date of revision of the text July 1998.

Legal category POM.

MINODIAB* 2.5 mg

Qualitative and quantitative composition Glipizide 2.5 mg.

Pharmaceutical form White biconvex tablets.

Clinical particulars

Therapeutic indications: As an adjunct to diet, in non-insulin-dependent diabetics (NIDDM), when proper dietary management alone has failed.

Posology and method of administration:

Route of administration: Oral.

As for any hypoglycaemic agent, dosage must be adapted for each individual case.

Short term administration of glipizide may be sufficient during periods of transient loss of control in patients usually controlled well on diet.

In general, glipizide should be given shortly before a meal to achieve the greatest reduction in post-prandial hyperglycaemia.

Initial dose: The recommended starting dose is 5 mg, given before breakfast or the midday meal. Mild diabetics, geriatric patients or those with liver disease may be started on 2.5 mg.

Titration: Dosage adjustments should ordinarily be in increments of 2.5 to 5 mg, as determined by blood glucose response. At least several days should elapse between titration steps. The maximum recommended single dose is 15 mg. If this is not sufficient, splitting the daily dosage may prove effective. Doses above 15 mg should ordinarily be divided.

Maintenance: Some patients may be effectively controlled on a once-a-day regimen. Total daily dosage above 15 mg should ordinarily be divided.

The maximum recommended daily dosage is 20 mg.

Use in children: Safety and effectiveness in children have not been established.

Use in elderly and in high risk patients: In elderly patients, debilitated or malnourished patients and patients with an impaired renal or hepatic function, the initial and maintenance dosing should be conservative to avoid hypoglycaemic reactions (see initial dose and special warnings and special precautions for use sections).

Patients receiving other oral hypoglycaemic agents: As with other sulfonylurea class hypoglycaemics, no transient period is necessary when transferring patients to glipizide. Patients should be observed carefully (1–2 weeks) for hypoglycaemia when being transferred from longer half-life sulfonylureas (e.g. chlorpropamide) to glipizide due to potential overlapping of drug effect.

Contra-indications: Glipizide is contraindicated in patients with:

Hypersensitivity to glipizide, other sulfonylureas or sulphonamides, or any excipients in the tablets;

Insulin-dependent diabetes, diabetic ketoacidosis, diabetic coma;

Severe renal or hepatic insufficiency;

Patients treated with miconazole (see section Interactions with other Medicaments and other forms of Interaction);

Pregnancy and lactation

Special warnings and precautions for use:

Hypoglycaemia: All sulfonylurea drugs are capable of producing severe hypoglycaemia. Proper patient selection, dosage, and instructions are important to avoid hypoglycaemic episodes. Regular, timely carbohydrate intake is important to avoid hypoglycaemic events occurring when a meal is delayed or insufficient food is eaten or carbohydrate intake is unbalanced. Renal or hepatic insufficiency may cause elevated blood levels of glipizide and the latter may also diminish gluconeogenic capacity, both of which increase the risk of serious hypoglycaemic reactions. Elderly, debilitated or malnourished patients and those with adrenal or pituitary insufficiency are particularly susceptible to the hypoglycaemic action of glucose-lowering drugs.

Hypoglycaemia may be difficult to recognise in the elderly, and in people who are taking beta-adrenergic blocking drugs (see interactions). Hypoglycaemia is more likely to occur when caloric- intake is deficient, after severe or prolonged exercise, when alcohol is ingested, or when more than one glucose-lowering drug is used.

Loss of control of blood glucose: When a patient stabilised on a diabetic regimen is exposed to stress such as fever, trauma, infection, or surgery, a loss of control may occur. At such times, it may be necessary to discontinue glipizide and administer insulin.

The effectiveness of any oral hypoglycaemic drug, including glipizide, in lowering blood glucose to a desired level decreases in many patients over a period of time, which may be due to progression of the severity of diabetes or to diminished responsiveness to the drug. This phenomenon is known as secondary failure, to distinguish it from primary failure in which the drug is ineffective in an individual patient when first given. Adequate adjustment of dose and adherence to diet should be assessed before classifying a patient as a secondary failure.

Renal and hepatic disease: The pharmacokinetics and/or pharmacodynamics of glipizide may be affected in patients with impaired renal or hepatic function. If hypoglycaemia should occur in such patients, it may be prolonged and appropriate management should be instituted.

Information for patients: Patients should be informed of the potential risks and advantages of glipizide and of alternative modes of therapy. They should also be informed about the importance of adherence to dietary instructions, of a regular exercise program, and of regular testing of urine and/or blood glucose.

The risks of hypoglycaemia, its symptoms and treatment, and conditions that predispose to its development should be explained to patients and responsible family members. Primary and secondary failure should also be explained.

Laboratory tests: Blood and urine glucose should be monitored periodically. Measurement of glycosylated haemoglobin may be useful.

Interaction with other medicaments and other forms of interaction: The following products are likely to increase the hypoglycaemic effect:

Contra-indicated combinations: Miconazole: increase in hypoglycaemic effect, possibly leading to symptoms of hypoglycaemia or even coma.

Inadvisable combinations: Nonsteroidal anti-inflammatory agents (NSAIDS) e.g. phenylbutazone: increase in hypoglycaemic effect of sulfonylureas (displacement of sulfonylurea binding to plasma proteins and/or decrease in sulfonylurea elimination).

Alcohol: increase in hypoglycaemic reaction which can lead to hypoglycaemic coma.

Combinations requiring precaution: Fluconazole: increase in the half-life of the sulfonylurea, possibly giving rise to symptoms of hypoglycaemia.

Salicylates (acetylsalicylic acid): increase in hypoglycaemic effect by high doses of acetylsalicylic acid (hypoglycaemic action of the acetylsalicylic acid).

Beta-blockers: all beta-blockers mask some of the symptoms of hypoglycaemia, i.e. palpitations and tachycardia. Most non cardioselective beta-blockers increase the incidence and severity of hypoglycaemia.

Angiotensin converting enzyme inhibitors: the use of angiotensin converting enzyme inhibitors may lead to an increased hypoglycaemic effect in diabetic patients treated with sulfonylureas.

Cimetidine: the use of cimetidine may be associated with a reduction in post prandial blood glucose in patients treated with glipizide.

The hypoglycaemic action of sulfonylureas in general may also be potentiated by monoamine oxidase inhibitors and drugs that are highly protein bound, such as sulfonamides, chloramphenicol, probenecid, coumarins and fibrates.

When such drugs are administered to (or withdrawn from) a patient receiving glipizide, the patient should be observed closely for hypoglycaemia (or loss of control).

The following products could lead to hyperglycaemia:

Inadvisable combinations:

Danazol: diabetogenic effect of danazol. If it cannot be avoided, warn the patient and step up self monitoring of blood glucose and urine. Possibly adjust the dosage of antidiabetic agent during treatment with danazol and after its discontinuation.

Combinations requiring precaution: Phenothiazines (e.g. chlorpromazine) at high doses (> 100 mg per day of chlorpromazine): elevation in blood glucose (reduction in insulin release).

Corticosteroids: elevation in blood glucose.

Sympathomimetics (e.g. ritodrine, salbutamol, terbutaline): elevation in blood glucose due to beta-2-adrenoceptor stimulation.

Progestogens: diabetogenic effects of high-dose progestogens. Warn the patient and step up self-monitoring of blood glucose and urine. Possibly adjust the dosage of antidiabetic agent during treatment with the neuroleptics, corticoids or progestogen and after discontinuation.

Other drugs that may produce hyperglycaemia and lead to a loss of control include the thiazides and other diuretics, thyroid products, oestrogens, oral contraceptives, phenytoin, nicotinic acid, calcium channel blocking drugs, and isoniazid.

When such drugs are withdrawn from a patient receiving glipizide, the patient should be observed closely for hypoglycaemia.

Pregnancy and lactation:

Pregnancy: Glipizide is contraindicated in pregnancy.

Glipizide was found to be mildly fetotoxic in rat reproductive studies. No teratogenic effects were found in rat or rabbit studies.

Prolonged severe hypoglycaemia (4 to 10 days) has been reported in neonates born to mothers who were receiving a sulfonylurea drug at the time of delivery.

Because recent information suggests that abnormal blood glucose levels during pregnancy are associated with a higher incidence of congenital abnormalities, many experts recommend that insulin be used during pregnancy to maintain blood glucose levels as close to normal as possible.

Lactation: No data are available on secretion into breast milk. Therefore glipizide is contraindicated in lactation.

Effects on ability to drive and use machines: The effect of glipizide on the ability to drive or operate machinery has not been studied. However, there is no evidence to suggest that glipizide may affect these abilities. Patients should be aware of the symptoms of hypoglycaemia and be careful about driving and the use of machinery, especially when optimum stabilisation has not been achieved, for example during the change-over from other medications or during irregular use.

Undesirable effects: The majority of side effects have been dose related, transient, and have responded to dose reduction or withdrawal of the medication. However, clinical experience thus far has shown that, as with other sulfonylureas, some side effects associated with hypersensitivity may be severe and deaths have been reported in some instances.

Hypoglycaemia: See Special Warnings and Special Precautions for Use and Overdose sections.

Gastrointestinal: Gastrointestinal complaints include nausea, diarrhoea, constipation and gastralgia. They appear to be dose related and usually disappear on division or reduction of dosage.

Dermatologic: Allergic skin reactions including erythema, morbilliform or maculopapular reactions, urticaria, pruritus and eczema have been reported. They frequently disappear with continued therapy. However, if they persist, the drug should be discontinued. As with other sulfonylureas, photosensitivity reactions have been reported.

Miscellaneous: Confusion, dizziness, drowsiness, headache, tremor, and visual disturbances have each been reported in patients treated with glipizide. They are usually transient and do not require discontinuance of therapy; however, they may also be symptoms of hypoglycaemia.

Laboratory test: The pattern of laboratory test abnormalities observed with glipizide is similar to that for other sulfonylureas. Occasional mild to moderate elevations of SGOT, LDH, alkaline phosphatase, BUN and creatinine were noted. The relationship of these abnormalities to glipizide is uncertain, and they have rarely been associated with clinical symptoms.

Hepatic disorder: Cholestatic jaundice, impaired hepatic function, and hepatitis have been reported. Discontinue treatment if cholestatic jaundice occurs.

Haematologic reactions: Leucopenia, agranulocytosis, thrombocytopenia, haemolytic anaemia, aplastic anaemia and pancytopenia have been reported.

Metabolic reactions: Hepatic porphyria and porphyria cutanea tarda have been reported. Disulfiram-like reactions have been reported with other sulfonylureas.

Endocrine reactions: Hyponatraemia has been reported.

Overdose: There is no well documented experience with glipizide overdosage.

Overdosage of sulfonylureas including glipizide can produce glycaemia. Mild hypoglycaemic symptoms without loss of consciousness or neurologic findings should be treated actively with oral glucose and adjustments in drug dosage and/or meal patterns. Close monitoring should continue until the physician is assured that the patient is out of danger. Severe hypoglycaemic reactions with coma, seizure, or other neurological impairment occur infrequently, but constitute medical emergencies requiring immediate hospitalisation. If hypoglycaemic coma is diagnosed or suspected, the patient should be given a rapid intravenous injection of concentrated (50%) glucose solution. This should be followed by a continuous infusion of a more dilute (10%) glucose solution at a rate that will maintain the blood glucose at a level above 100 mg/dL (5.55 mmol/L). Patients should be closely monitored for a minimum of 48 hours and depending on the status of the patient at this time the physician should decide whether further monitoring is required. Clearance of glipizide from plasma may be prolonged in persons with liver disease. Because of the extensive protein binding of glipizide, dialysis is unlikely to be of benefit.

Pharmacological properties

Pharmacodynamic properties: Glipizide is an oral blood glucose lowering drug of the sulfonylurea class. The primary mode of action of glipizide is the stimulation of insulin secretion from the beta-cells of pancreatic islet tissue. Stimulation of insulin secretion by glipizide in response to a meal is of major importance. Fasting insulin levels are not elevated even on long-term glipizide administration, but the post-prandial insulin response continues to be enhanced after at least 6 months of treatment. The insulinotropic response to a meal occurs within 30 minutes after oral dose of glipizide in diabetic patients, but elevated insulin levels do not persist beyond the time of the meal challenge. There is also increasing evidence that extrapancreatic effects involving potentiation of insulin action form a significant component of the activity of glipizide.

Blood sugar control persists for up to 24 hours after a single dose of glipizide, even though plasma levels have declined to a small fraction of peak levels by that time (see "Pharmacokinetics" below).

Pharmacokinetic properties: Gastrointestinal absorption of glipizide in man is uniform, rapid and essentially complete. Peak plasma concentrations occur 1–3 hours after a single oral dose. The half-life of elimination ranges from 2–4 hours in normal subjects, whether given intravenously or orally. The metabolic and excretory patterns are similar with the two routes of administration, indicating that first-pass metabolism is not significant. Glipizide does not accumulate in plasma on repeated oral administration. Total absorption and disposition of an oral dose was unaffected by food in normal volunteers, but absorption was delayed by about 40 minutes. Thus, glipizide was more effective when administered about 30 minutes before, rather than with, a test meal in diabetic patients. Protein binding was studies in serum from volunteers who received either oral or intravenous glipizide and found to be 98–99% one hour after either route of administration. The apparent volume of distribution of glipizide after intravenous administration was 11 litres, indicative of localisation within the extracellular fluid compartment. In mice, no glipizide or metabolites were detectable autoradiographically in the brain or spinal cord of males or females, nor in the foetuses of pregnant females. In another study, however, very small amounts of radioactivity were detected in the foetuses of rats given labelled drug.

The metabolism of glipizide is extensive and occurs mainly in the liver. The primary metabolites are inactive hydroxylation products and polar conjugates and are excreted mainly in the urine. Less than 10% unchanged glipizide is found in urine.

Preclinical safety data: Acute toxicity studies showed no specific susceptibility. The acute oral toxicity of glipizide was extremely low in all species tested (LD50 greater than 4 g/kg). Chronic toxicity tests in rats and dogs at doses up to 8.0 mg/kg did not show any evidence of toxic effects.

A 20-month study in rats and an 18-month study in mice at doses up to 75 times the maximum human dose revealed no evidence of drug related carcinogenicity. Bacterial and in vivo mutagenicity tests were uniformly negative. Studies in rats of both sexes at doses up to 75 times the human dose showed no effects on fertility.

Pharmaceutical particulars

List of excipients:

Microcrystalline cellulose	PhEur
Starch	PhEur
Stearic acid	HSE
Lactose	PhEur

Incompatibilities: None stated.

Shelf life: 60 months.

Special precautions for storage: None.

Nature and contents of container:
Blister strips containing 28 tablets
Blister strips containing 60 tablets

Instructions for use/handling: None.

Marketing authorisation number 3433/0022

Date of first authorisation/renewal of authorisation 23 July 1976/31 September 1997.

Date of (partial) revision of the text 30 September 1997.

Legal category POM.

MINODIAB* 5 mg

Qualitative and quantitative composition Glipizide 5.0 mg

Pharmaceutical form White biconvex scored tablets.

Clinical particulars

Therapeutic indications: As an adjunct to diet, in non-insulin-dependent diabetics (NIDDM), when proper dietary management alone has failed.

Posology and method of administration:
Route of administration: Oral.

As for any hypoglycaemic agent, dosage must be adapted for each individual case.

Short term administration of glipizide may be sufficient during periods of transient loss of control in patients usually controlled well on diet.

In general, glipizide should be given shortly before a meal to achieve the greatest reduction in post-prandial hyperglycaemia.

Initial dose: The recommended starting dose is 5 mg, given before breakfast or the midday meal. Mild diabetics, geriatric patients or those with liver disease may be started on 2.5 mg.

Titration: Dosage adjustments should ordinarily be in increments of 2.5 to 5 mg, as determined by blood glucose response. At least several days should elapse between titration steps. The maximum recommended single dose is 15 mg. If this is not sufficient, splitting the daily dosage may prove effective. Doses above 15 mg should ordinarily be divided.

Maintenance: Some patients may be effectively controlled on a once-a-day regimen. Total daily dosage above 15 mg should ordinarily be divided.

The maximum recommended daily dosage is 20 mg.

Use in children: Safety and effectiveness in children have not been established.

Use in elderly and in high risk patients: In elderly patients, debilitated or malnourished patients and patients with an impaired renal or hepatic function, the initial and maintenance dosing should be conservative to avoid hypoglycaemic reactions (see Initial Dose and Special Warnings and Special Precautions for Use sections).

Patients receiving other oral hypoglycaemic agents: As with other sulfonylurea class hypoglycaemics, no transient period is necessary when transferring patients to glipizide. Patients should be observed carefully (1–2 weeks) for hypoglycaemia when being transferred from longer half-life sulfonylureas (e.g. chlorpropamide) to glipizide due to potential overlapping of drug effect.

Contra-indications: Glipizide is contraindicated in patients with:

Hypersensitivity to glipizide, other sulfonylureas or sulphonamides, or any excipients in the tablets;
Insulin-dependent diabetes, diabetic ketoacidosis, diabetic coma;
Severe renal or hepatic insufficiency;
Patients treated with miconazole (see section Interactions with other Medicaments and other forms of Interaction);
Pregnancy and lactation

Special warnings and precautions for use:
Hypoglycaemia: All sulfonylurea drugs are capable of producing severe hypoglycaemia. Proper patient selection, dosage, and instructions are important to avoid hypoglycaemic episodes. Regular, timely carbohydrate intake is important to avoid hypoglycaemic events occurring when a meal is delayed or insufficient food is eaten or carbohydrate intake is unbalanced. Renal or hepatic insufficiency may cause elevated blood levels of glipizide and the latter may also diminish gluconeogenic capacity, both of which increase the risk of serious hypoglycaemic reactions. Elderly, debilitated or malnourished patients and those with adrenal or pituitary insufficiency are particularly susceptible to the hypoglycaemic action of glucose-lowering drugs.

Hypoglycaemia may be difficult to recognise in the elderly, and in people who are taking beta-adrenergic blocking drugs (see interactions). Hypoglycaemia is more likely to occur when caloric- intake is deficient, after severe or prolonged exercise, when alcohol is ingested, or when more than one glucose-lowering drug is used.

Loss of control of blood glucose: When a patient stabilised on a diabetic regimen is exposed to stress such as fever, trauma, infection, or surgery, a loss of control may occur. At such times, it may be necessary to discontinue glipizide and administer insulin.

The effectiveness of any oral hypoglycaemic drug, including glipizide, in lowering blood glucose to a desired level decreases in many patients over a period of time, which may be due to progression of the severity of diabetes or to diminished responsiveness to the drug. This phenomenon is known as secondary failure, to distinguish it from primary failure in which the drug is ineffective in an individual patient when first given. Adequate adjustment of dose and adherence to diet should be assessed before classifying a patient as a secondary failure.

Renal and hepatic disease: The pharmacokinetics and/or pharmacodynamics of glipizide may be affected in patients with impaired renal or hepatic function. If hypoglycaemia should occur in such patients, it may be prolonged and appropriate management should be instituted.

Information for patients: Patients should be informed of the potential risks and advantages of glipizide and of alternative modes of therapy. They should also be informed about the importance of adherence to dietary instructions, of a regular exercise program, and of regular testing of urine and/or blood glucose.

The risks of hypoglycaemia, its symptoms and treatment, and conditions that predispose to its development should be explained to patients and responsible family members. Primary and secondary failure should also be explained.

Laboratory tests: Blood and urine glucose should be monitored periodically. Measurement of glycosylated haemoglobin may be useful.

Interaction with other medicaments and other forms of interaction: The following products are likely to increase the hypoglycaemic effect:

Contra-indicated combinations: Miconazole: increase in hypoglycaemic effect, possibly leading to symptoms of hypoglycaemia or even coma.

Inadvisable combinations: Nonsteroidal anti-inflammatory agents (NSAIDS) e.g. phenylbutazone): increase in hypoglycaemic effect of sulfonylureas (displacement of sulfonylurea binding to plasma proteins and/or decrease in sulfonylurea elimination).

Alcohol: increase in hypoglycaemic reaction which can lead to hypoglycaemic coma.

Combinations requiring precaution: Fluconazole: increase in the half-life of the sulfonylurea, possibly giving rise to symptoms of hypoglycaemia.

Salicylates (acetylsalicylic acid): increase in hypoglycaemic effect by high doses of acetylsalicylic acid (hypoglycaemic action of the acetylsalicylic acid).

Beta-blockers: all beta-blockers mask some of the symptoms of hypoglycaemia, i.e. palpitations and tachycardia. Most non cardioselective beta-blockers increase the incidence and severity of hypoglycaemia.

Angiotensin converting enzyme inhibitors: the use of angiotensin converting enzyme inhibitors may lead to an increased hypoglycaemic effect in diabetic patients treated with sulfonylureas.

Cimetidine: the use of cimetidine may be associated with a reduction in post prandial blood glucose in patients treated with glipizide.

The hypoglycaemic action of sulfonylureas in general may also be potentiated by monoamine oxidase inhibitors and drugs that are highly protein bound, such as sulfonamides, chloramphenicol, probenecid, coumarins and fibrates.

When such drugs are administered to (or withdrawn from) a patient receiving glipizide, the patient should be observed closely for hypoglycaemia (or loss of control).

The following products could lead to hyperglycaemia:
Inadvisable combinations:
Danazol: diabetogenic effect of danazol. If it cannot be avoided, warn the patient and step up self monitoring of blood glucose and urine. Possibly adjust the dosage of antidiabetic agent during treatment with danazol and after its discontinuation.

Combinations requiring precaution: Phenothiazines (e.g. chlorpromazine) at high doses (>100 mg per day of chlorpromazine): elevation in blood glucose (reduction in insulin release).

Corticosteroids: elevation in blood glucose.

Sympathomimetics (e.g. ritodrine, salbutamol, terbutaline): elevation in blood glucose due to beta-2-adrenoceptor stimulation.

Progestogens: diabetogenic effects of high-dose progestogens. Warn the patient and step up self-monitoring of blood glucose and urine. Possibly adjust the dosage of antidiabetic agent during treatment with the neuroleptics, corticoids or progestogen and after discontinuation.

Other drugs that may produce hyperglycaemia and lead to a loss of control include the thiazides and other diuretics, thyroid products, oestrogens, oral contraceptives, phenytoin, nicotinic acid, calcium channel blocking drugs, and isoniazid.

When such drugs are withdrawn from a patient receiving glipizide, the patient should be observed closely for hypoglycaemia.

Pregnancy and lactation:
Pregnancy: Glipizide is contraindicated in pregnancy.

Glipizide was found to be mildly fetotoxic in rat reproductive studies. No teratogenic effects were found in rat or rabbit studies.

Prolonged severe hypoglycaemia (4 to 10 days) has been reported in neonates born to mothers who were receiving a sulfonylurea drug at the time of delivery.

Because recent information suggests that abnormal blood glucose levels during pregnancy are associated with a higher incidence of congenital abnormalities, many experts recommend that insulin be used during pregnancy to maintain blood glucose levels as close to normal as possible.

Lactation: No data are available on secretion into breast milk. Therefore glipizide is contraindicated in lactation.

Effects on ability to drive and use machines: The effect of glipizide on the ability to drive or operate machinery has not been studied. However, there is no evidence to suggest that glipizide may affect these abilities. Patients should be aware of the symptoms of hypoglycaemia and be careful about driving and the use of machinery, especially when optimum stabilisation has not been achieved, for example during the change-over from other medications or during irregular use.

Undesirable effects: The majority of side effects have been dose related, transient, and have responded to dose reduction or withdrawal of the medication. However, clinical experience thus far has shown that, as with other sulfonylureas, some side effects associated with hypersensitivity may be severe and deaths have been reported in some instances.

Hypoglycaemia: See Special Warnings and Special Precautions for Use and Overdose sections.

Gastrointestinal: Gastrointestinal complaints include nausea, diarrhoea, constipation and gastralgia. They appear to be dose related and usually disappear on division or reduction of dosage.

Dermatologic: Allergic skin reactions including erythema, morbilliform or maculopapular reactions, urticaria, pruritus and eczema have been reported. They frequently disappear with continued therapy. However, if they persist, the drug should be discontinued. As with other sulfonylureas, photosensitivity reactions have been reported.

Miscellaneous: Confusion, dizziness, drowsiness, headache, tremor, and visual disturbances have each been reported in patients treated with glipizide. They are usually transient and do not require discontinuance of therapy; however, they may also be symptoms of hypoglycaemia.

Laboratory test: The pattern of laboratory test abnormalities observed with glipizide is similar to that for other sulfonylureas. Occasional mild to moderate elevations of SGOT, LDH, alkaline phosphatase, BUN and creatinine were noted. The relationship of these abnormalities to glipizide is uncertain, and they have rarely been associated with clinical symptoms.

Hepatic disorder: Cholestatic jaundice, impaired hepatic function, and hepatitis have been reported. Discontinue treatment if cholestatic jaundice occurs.

Haematologic reactions: Leucopenia, agranulocytosis, thrombocytopenia, haemolytic anaemia, aplastic anaemia and pancytopenia have been reported.

Metabolic reactions: Hepatic porphyria and porphyria cutanea tarda have been reported. Disulfiram-like reactions have been reported with other sulfonylureas.

Endocrine reactions: Hyponatraemia has been reported.

Overdose: There is no well documented experience with glipizide overdosage.

Overdosage of sulfonylureas including glipizide can produce glycaemia. Mild hypoglycaemic symptoms without loss of consciousness or neurologic findings should be treated actively with oral glucose and adjustments in drug dosage and/or meal patterns. Close monitoring should continue until the physician is assured that the patient is out of danger. Severe hypoglycaemic reactions with coma, seizure, or other neurological impairment occur infrequently, but constitute medical emergencies requiring immediate hospitalisation. If hypoglycaemic coma is diagnosed or suspected, the patient should be given a rapid intravenous injection of concentrated (50%) glucose solution. This should be followed by a continuous infusion of a more dilute (10%) glucose solution at a rate that will maintain the blood glucose at a level above 100 mg/dL (5.55 mmol/L). Patients should be closely monitored for a minimum of 48 hours and depending on the status of the patient at this time the physician should decide whether further monitoring is required. Clearance of glipizide from plasma may be prolonged in persons with liver disease. Because of the extensive protein binding of glipizide, dialysis is unlikely to be of benefit.

Pharmacological properties

Pharmacodynamic properties: Glipizide is an oral blood glucose lowering drug of the sulfonylurea class. The primary mode of action of glipizide is the stimulation of insulin secretion from the beta-cells of pancreatic islet tissue. Stimulation of insulin secretion by glipizide in response to a meal is of major importance. Fasting insulin levels are not elevated even on long-term glipizide administration, but the post-prandial insulin response continues to be enhanced after at least 6 months of treatment. The insulinotropic response to a meal occurs within 30 minutes after oral dose of glipizide in diabetic patients, but elevated insulin levels do not persist beyond the time of the meal challenge. There is also increasing evidence that extrapancreatic effects involving potentiation of insulin action form a significant component of the activity of glipizide.

Blood sugar control persists for up to 24 hours after a single dose of glipizide, even though plasma levels have declined to a small fraction of peak levels by that time (see "Pharmacokinetics" below).

Pharmacokinetic properties: Gastrointestinal absorption of glipizide in man is uniform, rapid and essentially complete. Peak plasma concentrations occur 1–3 hours after a single oral dose. The half-life of elimination ranges from 2–4 hours in normal subjects, whether given intravenously or orally. The metabolic and excretory patterns are similar with the two routes of administration, indicating that first-pass metabolism is not significant. Glipizide does not accumulate in plasma on repeated oral administration. Total absorption and disposition of an oral dose was unaffected by food in normal volunteers, but absorption was delayed by about 40 minutes. Thus, glipizide was more effective when administered about 30 minutes before, rather than with, a test meal in diabetic patients. Protein binding was studies in serum from volunteers who received either oral or intravenous glipizide and found to be 98–99% one hour after either route of administration. The apparent volume of distribution of glipizide after intravenous administration was 11 litres, indicative of localisation within the extracellular fluid compartment. In mice, no glipizide or metabolites were detectable autoradiographically in the brain or spinal cord of males or females, nor in the foetuses of pregnant females. In another study, however, very small amounts of radioactivity were detected in the foetuses of rats given labelled drug.

The metabolism of glipizide is extensive and occurs mainly in the liver. The primary metabolites are inactive hydroxylation products and polar conjugates and are excreted mainly in the urine. Less than 10% unchanged glipizide is found in urine.

Preclinical safety data: Acute toxicity studies showed no specific susceptibility. The acute oral toxicity of glipizide was extremely low in all species tested (LD50 greater than 4 g/kg). Chronic toxicity tests in rats and dogs at doses up to 8.0 mg/kg did not show any evidence of toxic effects.

A 20-month study in rats and an 18-month study in mice at doses up to 75 times the maximum human dose revealed no evidence of drug related carcinogenicity. Bacterial and in vivo mutagenicity tests were uniformly negative. Studies in rats of both sexes at doses up to 75 times the human dose showed no effects on fertility.

Pharmaceutical particulars

List of excipients:

Microcrystalline cellulose	PhEur
Starch	PhEur
Stearic acid	HSE
Lactose	PhEur

Incompatibilities: None stated.

Shelf life: 60 months.

Special precautions for storage: None.

Nature and contents of container:
Blister strips containing 28 tablets.
Blister strips containing 60 tablets.

Instructions for use/handling: None.

Marketing authorisation number 3433/0023

Date of first authorisation/renewal of authorisation 23 July 1976/31 September 1997.

Date of (partial) revision of the text 30 September 1997.

Legal category POM.

MONO-CEDOCARD*-10

Qualitative and quantitative composition Isosorbide 5-mononitrate 10 mg

Pharmaceutical form Round, flat, bevel edged, orange tablet, scored on one side and imprinted with C MONO C on the other side.

Clinical particulars

Therapeutic indications: For the prophylaxis and maintenance of angina pectoris. Isosorbide mononitrate is the active constituent of isosorbide dinitrate. It has significant vasodilator activity, the strongest effect being exerted on the venous system, and a lesser effect on the arterial circulation. As a consequence the heart has less work to perform against diminished resistance and therefore oxygen requirement is reduced.

Posology and method of administration:
Route of Administration: Oral.

Children: There is no dose recommendation for children.

Adult dose: One tablet, two-three times daily. The tablets should be swallowed (without chewing) with a little water. Where therapeutic efficacy with the usual dosage proves insufficient, the daily dosage may be increased to 120 mg according to individual need.

Elderly adults: The dosage of nitrates in cardiovascular disease is usually determined by patient response and stabilisation. Clinical experience has not necessitated alternative advice for use in elderly patients.

Contra-indications: Hypotension. Acute myocardial infarction with low filling pressures. Acute circulatory failure (shock, vascular collapse). When the blood pressure is very low. During the first three months of pregnancy.

Special warnings and precautions for use: Consumption of alcohol should be avoided during treatment, as reaction capacity may be reduced and the vasodilator activity of isosorbide mononitrate may be enhanced.

Protect from heat and moisture.

Interaction with other medicaments and other forms of interaction: Some of the effects of alcohol and the action of hypotensive agents may be potentiated by this product.

Pregnancy and lactation: Mono-Cedocard 10 should not be used during the first three months of pregnancy.

Effects on ability to drive and use machines: Side effects include throbbing headache and dizziness. Patients are advised not to drive or operate machinery if so affected.

Undesirable effects: Generally, no serious adverse effects are to be expected. Headache, dizziness, fatigue, palpitations, orthostatic hypotension and flushing may occur, especially at the beginning of the treatment. These reactions can usually be controlled by a temporary dosage reduction.

Overdose: Passive exercise of the extremities of the encumbent patient will promote venous return.

Pharmacological properties

Pharmacodynamic properties: Isosorbide-5-mononitrate is the major pharmacologically active metabolite of isosorbide dinitrate. It has significant vasodilator activity, the strongest effect being exerted on the venous system and to a lesser extent on the arterial circulation. As a consequence the heart has less work to perform against diminished resistance, thus reducing oxygen requirement.

Pharmacokinetic properties: After oral administration isosorbide-5-mononitrate is very rapidly and completely absorbed from the gastro-intestinal tract without any first pass metabolism. The absorption half-life is 15 minutes and drug is detected in plasma at 3.5±0.6 minutes after an oral dose of 20 mg. A maximum concentration of 480.6±23.1 mg/l is reached within 1.2±0.1 h after administration.

Haemodynamic effects are demonstrable at 20 minutes after oral administration of drug.

The anti-anginal effect of a 20 mg dose persists for more than 4 hours after oral administration.

Preclinical safety data: Isosorbide mononitrate is a well established drug for which there are adequate published safety data.

Pharmaceutical particulars

List of excipients

Lactose	PhEur
Talc	PhEur
Colloidal silicon dioxide	PhEur
Microcrystalline cellulose	PhEur
Potato Starch	PhEur
Aluminium stearate	HSE
Anstead No. 11348 (dispersed orange lake)	HSE

Incompatibilities: None stated.

Shelf life: 60 months.

Special precautions for storage: Protect from heat and moisture.

Nature and contents of container: The tablets are presented in aluminium/PVC blisters, strips of which are contained within a printed cardboard carton.

Pack size: 60 tablets.

Instructions for use/handling: No specific statement.

Marketing authorisation holder:
JB Tillotts Limited
Davy Avenue
Milton Keynes
MK5 8PH
UK

Marketing authorisation number 0424/0072

Date of first authorisation/renewal of authorisation
Date of First Authorisation: 25 March 1988
Renewal of Authorisation: 25 March 1993

Date of (partial) revision of the text 18 March 1998.

Legal category P

MONO-CEDOCARD*-20

Presentation Round white tablets, embossed 'MONO CC', reverse side scored, containing 20 mg isosorbide 5-mononitrate.

Uses For the prophylaxis of angina pectoris.

Isosorbide mononitrate, the active constituent of Mono-Cedocard-20, is the major active metabolite of isosorbide dinitrate. It has significant vasodilator activity, the strongest effect being exerted on the venous system and a lesser effect on the arterial circulation. As a consequence, the heart has less work to perform against diminished resistance and therefore oxygen requirement is reduced.

Dosage and administration For oral administration.

Adult dose: One tablet two or three times a day taken after meals. The tablet should be swallowed (without chewing) with a little water. The dosage may be increased to two tablets three times a day.

Dosage for the elderly: The dosage of nitrates in cardiovascular disease is usually determined by patient response and stabilisation. Clinical experience has not necessitated alternative advice for use in elderly patients.

There is no dose recommendation for children.

Contra-indications, warnings, etc
Contra-indications: In acute myocardial infarction with low filling pressures. Acute circulatory failure (shock, vascular collapse). When blood pressure is very low. During the first three months of pregnancy.

Warnings/precautions: Consumption of alcohol should be avoided during treatment, as reaction capacity may be reduced, and the vasodilator activity of isosorbide mononitrate may be enhanced. Symptoms of circulatory collapse can arise in patients already taking ACE inhibitors.

Adverse effects: Generally, no serious adverse effects are to be expected. Headache, dizziness, fatigue, palpitations, orthostatic hypotension and flushing may occur, especially at the beginning of treatment. These reactions can usually be controlled by a temporary dosage reduction.

Treatment of overdosage: Gastric lavage; passive exercise of the extremities of the recumbent patient will promote venous return.

Pharmaceutical precautions
Storage: Protect from heat and moisture.

Legal category P.

Package quantities Packs of 100 tablets (OP).

Further information The plasma half-life of isosorbide mononitrate is 4.2 hours.

After oral administration, isosorbide mononitrate is well absorbed, a haemodynamic effect being measurable within 15–20 minutes. In contrast to isosorbide dinitrate, the mononitrate is not subject to first-pass metabolism.

Product licence number 0424/0040.

MONO-CEDOCARD*-40

Qualitative and quantitative composition Isosorbide-5-mononitrate-lactose 40 mg.

Pharmaceutical form Round, flat, bevel edged, white tablet, scored on one side and imprinted 40 MONO 40 on the other side.

Clinical particulars
Therapeutic indications: For the prophylaxis and maintenance of angina pectoris.

Posology and method of administration: By oral administration:

Children: There is no recommended dose for children.

Adults: One tablet to be taken twice daily after meals.

Elderly adults: As for adult dose.

Contra-indications: Acute myocardial infarction with low filling pressures; acute circulatory failure (shock and vascular collapse). Severe hypotension. During the first trimester of pregnancy.

Special warnings: Consumption of alcohol should be avoided during treatment, as reaction capacity may be reduced and the vasodilator activity of isosorbide mononitrate may be enhanced.

Interaction with other medicaments and other forms of interaction: Nitrates may potentiate the effects of anti-hypertensive agents. The vasodilator activity of isosorbide mononitrate may be enhanced by alcohol.

Use during pregnancy and lactation: No data have been reported which would indicate the possibility of adverse effects resulting from the use of nitrates in pregnancy. However, safety in pregnancy has not been established. Isosorbide mononitrate should only be used in pregnancy if, in the opinion of the practitioner, the possible benefits of treatment outweigh the possible hazards.

Effects on ability to drive and use machines: Side effects include throbbing headache and dizziness. Patients are advised not to drive or operate machinery if so affected.

Undesirable effects: Most commonly transient headaches which can usually be controlled by temporary dosage reduction. Less frequently, cutaneous vasodilation with flushing, transient episodes of dizziness and weakness and other signs of cerebral ischaemia can occur with postural hypotension.

Overdosage: Symptoms and signs of overdosage include vomiting, hypotension, restlessness, syncope, cyanosis, headache, flushing, dizziness, collapse, convulsions and methaemoglobinaemia. Treatment should include emesis or gastric lavage, if appropriate. Symptomatic and supportive measures should be provided. Syncope should be treated by keeping the patient in recumbent position. Fluid replacement with or without vasopressors may be indicated. Methaemoglobinaemia should be treated with intravenous injection of 1 mg to 4 mg/kg of methylene blue.

Pharmacological properties
Pharmacodynamic properties: Isosorbide-5-mononitrate is a vasodilator.

Pharmacokinetic properties: Isosorbide-5-mononitrate is readily absorbed from the gastrointestinal tract following oral administration; it does not undergo first-pass hepatic metabolism and it is eliminated more slowly than is isosorbide dinitrate.

Preclinical safety data: Isosorbide mononitrate is a well established drug for which there are adequate published safety data.

Pharmaceutical particulars
Excipients:

Lactose	PhEur
Talc	PhEur
Colloidal Silicon Dioxide (Aerosil 200)	DAB
Microcrystalline Cellulose	DAB
Potato starch	PhEur
Aluminium stearate	HSE

Incompatibilities: None stated.

Shelf life: 5 years when stored at room temperature

Special precautions for storage: To be protected from heat and moisture.

Nature and contents of container: The tablets are presented in aluminium/PVC blisters, strips of which are contained within a printed cardboard carton.

Instructions for use/handling: No specific statement

Marketing authorisation number 0424/0054

Date of approval/revision of SPC 8 July 1996.

Legal Category POM.

MCR-50* (MONO CEDOCARD RETARD-50)

Presentation Hard gelatin slow release capsules (size 3) containing 50 mg isosorbide mononitrate. Each capsule contains white micro pellets which are specially formulated to release 30% of the dose initially and the remaining 70% as a maintenance dose.

Uses For the prophylaxis of angina pectoris.

Dosage and administration The capsules are for oral administration and should be swallowed whole.

Adults: One capsule to be taken in the morning.

Elderly patients: The dosage of nitrates in cardiovascular disease is usually determined by patient response and stabilisation. Clinical experience has not necessitated alternative advice for use in elderly patients.

Children: The safety and efficacy of MCR-50 in children has yet to be established.

For patients with higher nitrate requirements the dose may be increased to two capsules daily.

Contra-indications, warnings, etc
Contra-indications: MCR-50 should not be used in cases of acute myocardial infarction with low filling pressures, acute circulatory failure (shock, vascular collapse) or very low blood pressure.

This product should not be given to patients with a known sensitivity to nitrates.

MCR-50 should not be used in patients with marked anaemia, head trauma, cerebral haemorrhage, severe hypotension or hypovolaemia.

Precautions and warnings: This preparation may give rise to postural hypotension and syncope at higher doses. This may be avoided if treatment is started with the lowest dose possible.

Some of the effects of alcohol and the action of hypotensive agents may be potentiated by this product. MCR-50 should be used with caution in patients who are pre-disposed to closed angle glaucoma.

A headache may occur at the start of the treatment but this usually disappears after a few days.

This product should not be used during pregnancy or lactation unless considered essential by the physician. MCR-50 should be used with caution in patients suffering from hypothyroidism, hypothermia, malnutrition, severe liver or renal disease.

Symptoms of circulatory collapse may arise after the first dose, particularly in patients with labile circulation.

Pharmaceutical precautions None.

Legal category P.

Package quantities MCR-50 is calendar packed in cartons of 28 capsules (OP).

Further information MCR-50 is a long-acting nitrate which is effective for twenty four hours. The total amount of drug is divided into micro pellets which distribute themselves throughout the gastro-intestinal tract, thus giving a controlled and predictable release of isosorbide 5-mononitrate.

Each micro pellet releases 30% of the dose initially and the remaining 70% as a maintenance dose.

Isosorbide mononitrate is the British Approved Name for isosorbide 5-mononitrate.

MCR-50 lacks any significant first pass metabolism providing consistently uniform plasma levels of isosorbide mononitrate thereby laying the foundation for improved clinical response.

Product licence number 0424/0081.

MOTRIN*

Presentation Film-coated tablets containing Ibuprofen BP:

400 mg -round, biconvex, orange tablet marked U on one side;

600 mg -elliptical, peach tablet marked U on one side;

800 mg -elliptical, capsule shaped, white tablet marked MOTRIN 800 on one side.

Motrin Tablets 400 mg, 600 mg also contain maize starch, colloidal silicon dioxide, pregelatinised starch, stearic acid and carnauba wax. In addition, Motrin Tablets 400 mg and 600 mg contain hydroxypropyl methylcellulose, propylene glycol and E110.

Motrin Tablets 800 mg contain silicon dioxide, croscarmellose sodium, magnesium stearate, microcrystalline cellulose, talc, E464, E171, propylene glycol and carnauba wax.

Uses Non-steroidal, anti-inflammatory agent with analgesic and antipyretic properties. Motrin is indicated for the relief of the signs and symptoms of rheumatoid arthritis (including Still's Disease), osteoarthritis, ankylosing spondylitis and seronegative (non-rheumatoid) arthropathies. It may also be used in non-articular rheumatic conditions and soft tissue injuries; these include low back pain, capsulitis, bursitis, tenosynovitis, sprains and strains.

Dosage and administration
Adults: 1200 -- 1800 mg daily in three divided doses; up to 2400 mg daily may be given in severe conditions.

Children: 20 mg/kg daily in divided doses. In juvenile rheumatoid arthritis, up to 40 mg/kg daily in divided doses may be taken. In those children weighing less than 30 kg, the total dose in 24 hours should not exceed 500 mg.

If gastro-intestinal complaints occur, administer Motrin with food or milk.

Elderly patients: It appears that advanced age has a minimal influence on the pharmacokinetics of ibuprofen. However, the following should be considered:

Ibuprofen may increase levels of digoxin concentration, presumably from reduced renal excretion of digoxin.

Ibuprofen has been reported to have an antagonistic effect on frusemide-induced diuresis in cardiac failure.

Ibuprofen has been reported to be associated with cognitive dysfunction in the elderly.

Ibuprofen should be used with caution in association with anti-coagulants (warfarin).

Contra-indications, warnings etc
Contra-indications: Active peptic ulceration. Motrin Tablets should not be given to patients who have previously shown hypersensitivity to the drug, or to those patients in whom aspirin, Motrin or other non-steroidal anti-inflammatory drugs induce the syndrome of nasal polyps, bronchospastic reactivity or angioedema. Fatal asthmatic and anaphylactoid reactions have occurred in such patients.

Warnings: Use with extreme caution in those patients with asthma. Fatal asthmatic and anaphylactic reactions have been reported.

Serious gastro-intestinal toxicity such as bleeding, ulceration and perforation of the stomach, small intestine or large intestine, have been reported in patients receiving ibuprofen. Motrin should be given under close supervision to patients with a history of upper gastro-intestinal tract disease.

Treatment should be discontinued in patients reporting blurred or diminished vision, scotomata and/or changes in colour vision.

Precautions: Administration of Motrin is not recommended during pregnancy. Reproductive studies conducted in rats and rabbits at doses somewhat less than the clinical maximum dose did not demonstrate any evidence of developmental abnormalities. As there are no adequate and well-controlled studies in pregnant women, this drug should be used during pregnancy only if clearly needed. Because of the known effects of non-steroidal anti-inflammatory drugs on the foetal cardiovascular system (closure of ductus arteriosus), use during late pregnancy should be avoided. As with other drugs known to inhibit prostaglandin synthesis, an increased incidence of dystocia and delayed parturition occurred in rats.

In limited studies, an assay capable of detecting 1 microgram/ml did not demonstrate ibuprofen in the milk of lactating women. However, due to the limited nature of the studies and the possible adverse effects of prostaglandin-inhibiting drugs on neonates, Motrin is not recommended for use in nursing mothers.

Pre-existing asthma: About 10% of patients with asthma may have aspirin-sensitive asthma. The use of aspirin in patients with aspirin-sensitive asthma has been associated with severe bronchospasm which can be fatal. Since cross-reactivity, including bronchospasm, between aspirin and other non-steroidal anti-inflammatory drugs has been reported in such aspirin-sensitive patients, Motrin Tablets should not be administered to patients with this form of aspirin-sensitivity and should be used with caution in all patients with pre-existing asthma.

Fluid retention and oedema have been reported in association with Motrin; therefore, the drug should be used with caution in patients with a history of cardiac decompensation or hypertension.

As with other non-steroidal anti-inflammatory drugs, long-term administration of ibuprofen to animals has resulted in renal papillary necrosis and other abnormal renal pathology. In humans, there have been reports of acute interstitial nephritis with haematuria, proteinuria and occasionally nephrotic syndrome.

A second form of renal toxicity has been seen in patients with prerenal conditions leading to a reduction in renal blood flow or blood volume, where the renal prostaglandins have a supportive role in the maintenance of renal perfusion. In these patients, administration of a non-steroidal anti-inflammatory drug may cause a dose dependent reduction in prostaglandin formation and may precipitate overt renal decompensation. Patients at greatest risk of this reaction are those with impaired renal function, heart failure, liver dysfunction, those taking diuretics and the elderly. Discontinuation of non-steroidal anti-inflammatory drug therapy is typically followed by recovery to the pre-treatment state.

Since ibuprofen is eliminated primarily by the kidneys, patients with significantly impaired renal function should be closely monitored and a reduction in dosage should be anticipated to avoid drug accumulation.

Those patients at high risk of developing renal dysfunction during long-term treatment should have renal function monitored periodically.

Ibuprofen, like other non-steroidal anti-inflammatory drugs, can inhibit platelet aggregation, but the effect is quantitatively less and of shorter duration than that seen with aspirin. Motrin has been shown to prolong bleeding time (but within the normal range) in normal subjects. Because this prolonged bleeding effect may be exaggerated in patients with underlying haemostatic defects, Motrin should be used with caution in persons with intrinsic coagulation defects and those on anticoagulant therapy.

Patients on Motrin should report to their physicians signs or symptoms of gastro-intestinal ulceration or bleeding, blurred vision or other eye symptoms, skin rash, weight gain or oedema.

The antipyretic and anti-inflammatory activity of ibuprofen may reduce fever and inflammation, thus diminishing their utility as diagnostic signs in detecting complications of presumed non-infectious, non-inflammatory painful conditions.

Drug interactions:

Coumarin-type anticoagulants: Several short-term controlled studies failed to show that Motrin significantly affected prothrombin times, or a variety of other clotting factors, when administered to individuals on coumarin-type anticoagulants.

Aspirin: Animal studies show that aspirin given with non-steroidal anti-inflammatory drugs, including Motrin, causes a net decrease in anti-inflammatory activity with lowered blood levels of the non-aspirin drug.

Methotrexate: Motrin and other non-steroidal anti-inflammatory drugs have been reported to reduce renal tubular secretion of methotrexate *in vitro*. This may lead to enhanced toxicity of methotrexate. Caution should be used if Motrin is administered concomitantly with methotrexate.

Diuretics: Motrin has been shown to reduce the natriuretic effect of frusemide, thiazide or other diuretics in some patients, probably due to inhibition of renal prostaglandin synthesis by Motrin and other non-steroidal anti-inflammatory drugs. Patients being treated concomitantly with Motrin and frusemide, thiazide or other diuretics should therefore be observed closely.

Anti-hypertensive agents: Antagonism of the anti-hypertensive effect of beta-adrenergic blocking agents by non-steroidal anti-inflammatory drugs including Motrin has been reported. During the co-administration of these drugs, as well as other anti-hypertensive medications, care should be taken to monitor blood pressure.

Lithium: Motrin has been shown to produce a clinically relevant elevation of plasma lithium levels and a reduction in renal lithium clearance in a volunteer study. This effect has been attributed to inhibition of renal prostaglandin synthesis. Thus, when Motrin and lithium are administered concurrently, subjects should be carefully observed for signs of lithium toxicity.

Cardiac glycosides: Increased plasma levels of cardiac glycosides may occur during concomitant administration with ibuprofen.

Quinolones: The CNS excitatory effects of 4-quinolones may be increase by concomitant administration of non-steroidal anti-inflammatory drugs.

Adverse reactions: A decrease in haemoglobin content of 1 gram or more has been observed in 20% of patients.

Gastro-intestinal effects are a frequent adverse reaction to Motrin Tablets.

The following adverse reactions may occur in 3–9% of patients taking Motrin Tablets: nausea, epigastric pain, dizziness, non-specific rash, elevated serum creatinine levels and anaemia.

The following rarely occurring adverse reactions have been reported in patients taking Motrin Tablets: renal failure, lupus erythematosus syndrome with aseptic meningitis, jaundice, abnormal liver function tests, blood dyscrasias including thrombocytopenia, colitis, exacerbation of inflammatory bowel disease, perforation of the colon, inflammation of the small intestine with loss of blood and protein, collagenous colitis, small bowel perforation, ulcer or stricture, complications of colonic diverticula (perforation, fistula). Aseptic meningitis is probably more common in patients with systemic lupus erythematosus and related connective tissue diseases.

Treatment of overdosage: Gastric lavage. No specific antidote. It is theoretically advantageous to administer alkali and induce diuresis as the drug is acidic and excreted in the urine.

Pharmaceutical precautions Motrin Tablets 400 mg and 600 mg should be stored below 25°C in a well-closed container. Motrin Tablets 800 mg should be stored below 25°C.

Legal category POM.

Package quantities 400 mg, 600 mg and 800 mg strengths–packs of 90 tablets.

Further information The absorption profile shows Motrin to be of particular value in relieving morning stiffness.

Product licence numbers
400 mg 0032/0105
600 mg 0032/0106
800 mg 0032/0134

Date of preparation or last review January 1997.

MYCIFRADIN* SULPHATE TABLETS 0.5 g

Qualitative and quantitative composition Each tablet contains 500 mg neomycin sulphate.

Pharmaceutical form An off-white, biconvex oval tablet for oral use.

Clinical particulars

Therapeutic indications: Antibacterial.

For pre-operative suppression of bacterial bowel flora. Also for reduction of ammonia-forming bacteria in the intestine in hepatic coma.

Posology and method of administration: Oral.

Adults: Bowel surgery: One gram every 4 hours. Dosage should not continue longer than 72 hours.

Hepatic coma: 4–12 grams per day in divided doses for up to 6 days.

Elderly patients: It should be borne in mind that elderly patients may have some degree of renal impairment and thus not excrete neomycin normally. See '*Special warnings and special precautions for use*' section for other factors which should be taken into consideration.

Children: Safety and efficacy in patients under 18 years of age have not been established.

Contra-indications: The product is contra-indicated in patients who are receiving or have received, other ototoxic medications such as aminoglycosides or potent diuretics, in patients with ulcerative colitis, malabsorption syndrome or intestinal obstruction, in patients with renal insufficiency and in patients hypersensitive to neomycin.

Special warnings and special precautions for use:
Warnings: Systemic absorption of neomycin occurs following oral administration and toxic reactions may occur.

Neurotoxicity (including ototoxicity) and nephrotoxicity have been reported following oral administration of neomycin even when used in recommended doses. Higher doses of neomycin or administration for longer periods than recommended may give rise to ototoxicity and nephrotoxicity even in patients with normal renal function. The risk of hearing loss continues after drug withdrawal. The risk of ototoxicity and nephrotoxicity is greater in patients with impaired renal function. Use in such patients should be considered only when alternative therapy is clearly contra-indicated.

Neuromuscular blockade and respiratory paralysis have been reported following the oral use of neomycin. Concurrent administration of neomycin with a neuromuscular blocking agent may enhance neuromuscular blockade and lead to respiratory paralysis. Thus, the use of neomycin in patients receiving such agents or in patients with myasthenia gravis, should be avoided.

Concurrent and/or sequential systemic, oral or topical use of other aminoglycoside antibiotics and other potentially nephrotoxic or neurotoxic drugs should be avoided because the toxicity may be additive.

The concurrent use of neomycin with potent diuretics such as ethacrynic acid or frusemide should be avoided since certain diuretics by themselves may cause ototoxicity. In addition, when administered intravenously, diuretics may enhance neomycin toxicity by altering the antibiotic concentration in serum and tissue.

Precautions: As with other antibiotics, use of neomycin may result in the overgrowth of nonsusceptible organisms, particularly fungi.

Cross allergenicity among aminoglycosides has been demonstrated.

Laboratory Tests: Patients with renal insufficiency may develop toxic neomycin blood levels unless doses are properly regulated. If renal insufficiency develops during treatment, the dosage should be reduced or the antibiotic discontinued. To avoid nephrotoxicity and eighth nerve damage associated with high doses and prolonged treatment, the following should be performed prior to and periodically during therapy: urinalysis for increased excretion of protein, decreased specific gravity, casts and cells; renal function tests such as serum creatinine, BUN or creatinine clearance; tests of the vestibulocochlearis nerve (eighth cranial nerve) function. During prolonged treatment, neomycin serum concentrations should be monitored to detect the presence of systemic absorption. Ototoxicity has been reported in cases with neomycin blood levels as low as 0.4 – 1.2 microgram/ml.

Serial vestibular and audiometric tests should be performed (especially in high risk patients). Since elderly patients may have reduced renal function which may not be evident in the results of routine screening tests such as BUN or serum creatinine, a creatinine clearance determination may be more useful.

Interaction with other medicaments and other forms of interaction: Oral neomycin at high doses may produce a malabsorption syndrome for a variety of substances including fat, nitrogen, cholesterol, carotene, glucose, xylose, lactose, sodium, calcium, cyanocobalamin and iron.

Although the clinical significance has not been established clearly, neomycin has been reported to decrease the gastro-intestinal absorption of penicillin, methotrexate and 5-fluorouracil and digoxin. Oral neomycin may enhance the effect of coumarin in anticoagulation by decreasing vitamin K availability.

Pregnancy and lactation: Some aminoglycosides cross the placenta and although serious side-effects to the foetus or newborn have not been reported in the treatment of the pregnant woman with neomycin, the potential for harm exists. Because of this risk, use in pregnancy is not recommended unless clearly indicated based on an assessment of benefit-risk

Aminoglycosides are excreted in human milk. Administration to nursing mothers is not recommended unless it is clearly indicated based on an assessment of benefit-risk.

Effects on ability to drive and use machines: None.

Undesirable effects: The most common adverse reactions to oral neomycin are nausea, vomiting and diarrhoea.

Overdose: In the event of signs or symptoms of

ototoxicity or nephrotoxicity occurring, discontinue treatment immediately.

Pharmacological properties

Pharmacodynamic properties: Neomycin is a broad spectrum bactericidal aminoglycoside antibiotic, with activity against both Gram-positive and Gram-negative organisms.

Pharmacokinetic properties: About 97% of an oral dose is excreted unchanged with faeces and a daily intake of 10 g for 3 days yields a blood level below that associated with systemic toxicity. Approximately 0.7% of the total oral dose is excreted in the urine within 24 hours. Gastro-intestinal ulceration does not seem to affect absorption, although gastroenteritis in children may augment it.

Pharmaceutical particulars

List of excipients: Povidone, calcium stearate.

Incompatibilities: None.

Shelf-life: 60 months.

Special precautions for storage: Keep container tightly closed. Store below 25°C.

Nature and contents of container: Amber glass tablet bottle with screw cap containing 100 tablets. High density polyethylene bottle with white LDPE tamper evident cap containing 100 or 500 tablets.

Instructions for use/handling: None.

Marketing authorisation number 0032/5012R

Date of first authorisation 25th January 1991.

Date of revision of the text October 1995.

Legal category POM.

MYCOBUTIN*

Qualitative and quantitative composition Rifabutin INN 150.0 mg

Pharmaceutical form Opaque, red-brown, hard gelatin capsules Size No.0 containing 150 mg rifabutin in transparent PVC/Al blisters or in amber glass bottles.

The capsules are for oral administration.

Clinical particulars

Therapeutic indications: Mycobutin is indicated for:
- the prophylaxis of *M. avium intracellulare complex* (MAC) infections in patients with HIV disease with CD4 counts lower than 75 cells/mcl.
- the treatment of non-tuberculous mycobacterial disease (such as that caused by MAC and M. xenopi).
- pulmonary tuberculosis.

Posology and method of administration: Mycobutin can be administered as a single, daily, oral dose at any time independently of meals.

Adults:
- prophylaxis of *M. avium intracellulare complex* (MAC) infections in patients with HIV disease with CD4 counts lower than 75 cells/mcl.: 300 mg (2 capsules) as a single agent.
- treatment of non-tuberculous mycobacterial disease:

450–600 mg (3–4 capsules) in combination regimens for up to 6 months after negative cultures are obtained.

When Mycobutin is given in association with clarithromycin (or other macrolides) and/or fluconazole (or related compounds) the Mycobutin dosage may need to be reduced to 300 mg (see Interactions with other Medicaments and other forms of Interaction Section).

- treatment of pulmonary tuberculosis:

150 – 450 mg (1 – 3 capsules) in combination regimens for at least 6 months.

In accordance with the commonly accepted criteria for the treatment of mycobacterial infections, Mycobutin should always be given in combination with other anti-mycobacterial drugs not belonging to the family of rifamycins.

Children: There are inadequate data to support the use of Mycobutin in children at the present time.

Elderly: No specific recommendations for dosage alterations in the elderly are suggested.

Contra-indications: Mycobutin is contra-indicated in patients with a history of hypersensitivity to rifabutin or other rifamycins (eg rifampicin).

Due to insufficient clinical experience in pregnant and breast-feeding women and in children, Mycobutin should not be used in these patients.

Special warnings and precautions for use: Before starting Mycobutin prophylaxis, patients should be assessed to ensure that they do not have active disease caused by pulmonary tuberculosis or other mycobacteria.

Prophylaxis against MAC infection may need to be continued throughout the patient's lifetime.

Mycobutin may impart a red-orange colour to the urine and possibly to skin and body secretions. Contact lenses, especially soft, may be permanently stained.

Mild hepatic impairment does not require a dose modification. Mycobutin should be used with caution in cases of severe liver insufficiency. Mild to moderate renal impairment does not require any dosage adjustment.

Severe renal impairment (creatinine clearance below 30 ml/min) requires a dosage reduction of 50%.

It is recommended that white blood cell and platelet counts and liver enzymes be monitored periodically during treatment.

Because of the possibility of occurrence of uveitis, patients should be carefully monitored when rifabutin is given in combination with clarithromycin (or other macrolides) and/or fluconazole (and related compounds). If such an event occurs, the patient should be referred to an ophthalmologist and, if considered necessary, Mycobutin treatment should be suspended.

Uveitis associated with Mycobutin must be distinguished from other ocular complications of HIV.

Interaction with other medicaments and other forms of interaction: Rifabutin has been shown to induce the enzymes of the cytochrome P450 3A subfamily and therefore may affect the pharmacokinetic behaviour of drugs metabolised by the enzymes belonging to this subfamily. Upward adjustment of the dosage of such drugs may be required when administered with Mycobutin.

For this reason, during Mycobutin therapy oral contraception may not be adequate and patients should be advised to use other forms of contraception.

Similarly, Mycobutin might reduce the activity of analgesics, anticoagulants, corticosteroids, cyclosporin, digitalis (although not digoxin), dapsone, oral hypoglycaemics, narcotics, phenytoin and quinidine.

Although pharmacokinetic data have shown that Mycobutin when given in combination with zidovudine reduces the plasma levels of the latter, a large controlled clinical study has shown that these changes are of no clinical relevance. Clinical studies have shown that Mycobutin does not affect the pharmacokinetics of didanosine (DDI), isoniazid (for the latter refer also to Undesirable Effects). On the basis of the above metabolic considerations no significant reaction may be expectes with ethambutol, theophylline, sulphonamides, pyrazinamide and zalcitabine (DDC).

An interaction, leading to an increase in rifabutin plasma levels, occurs when Mycobutin is administered together with clarithromycin and/or fluconazole. This may apply to drugs of the same classes (refer to Undesirable Effects and Special Precautions). However, Mycobutin does not affect the pharmacokinetics of fluconazole.

As p-aminosalicylic acid has been shown to impede GI absorption of rifamycins it is recommended that when it and Mycobutin are both to be administered they be given with an interval of 8 – 12 hours.

Pregnancy and lactation: Due to lack of data in pregnant women, as a precautionary measure, Mycobutin should not be administered to pregnant women or those breast-feeding children even though in experimental animal studies the drug was not teratogenic.

Mycobutin may interact with oral contraceptives (see Interactions and other Medicaments and other forms of Interaction Section).

Effects on ability to drive and use machines: There have been no reports of adverse effects on ability to drive and use machines.

Undesirable effects: The tolerability of Mycobutin in multiple drug regimens, was assessed in both immunocompetent and immunocompromised patients, suffering from tuberculosis and non-tuberculous mycobacteriosis in long term studies with daily dosages up to 600 mg.

Bearing in mind that Mycobutin was often given in these studies as part of a multidrug regimen it is not possible to define with certainty a drug-event relationship. Treatment discontinuation was necessary only in a very few cases. The most commonly reported adverse events, were primarily related to:

- the gastro-intestinal system, such as nausea, vomiting, increase of liver enzymes, jaundice;
- the blood and lymphatic system, such as leucopenia, neutropenia, thrombocytopenia and anemia, where the frequency and severity of haematologic reactions could be increased by combined administration of isoniazid;
- the musculo-skeletal system: arthralgia and myalgia.

Also, fever, rash and rarely other hypersensitivity reactions such as eosinophilia, bronchospasm and shock might occur as has been seen with other antibiotics.

In addition, mild to severe, reversible uveitis has been reported. The risk appears to be low, when Mycobutin is used at 300 mg as monotherapy in MAC prophylaxis, but increases when Mycobutin is administered at higher doses in combination with clarithromycin (or other macrolides) for MAC treatment (see Special Warnings and Precautions for use Section). The possible role of fluconazole (and related compounds) has not been established yet. Asymptomatic corneal opacities have been reported after long term therapy. Pseudojaundice (yellow skin discolouration with normal plasma bilirubin) has been reported with high doses of rifabutin. Flu-like syndrome, chest pressure or pain with dyspnoea and rarely hepatitis and haemolysis. Clostridium difficile diarrhoea has been reported rarely.

Overdose: Gastric lavage and diuretic treatment should be carried out. Supportive care and symptomatic treatment should be administered.

Pharmacological properties

Pharmacodynamic properties: In vitro activity of rifabutin against laboratory strains and clinical isolates of *M. tuberculosis* has been shown to be very high. *In vitro* studies carried out so far have shown that from one-third to half of *M.tuberculosis* strains resistant to rifampicin are susceptible to rifabutin, indicating that cross-resistance between the two antibiotics is incomplete.

The *in vivo* activity of rifabutin on experimental infections caused by *M. tuberculosis* was about 10 times greater than that of rifampicin in agreement with the *in vitro* findings.

Rifabutin was seen to be active against non-tuberculous (atypical) mycobacteria including *M. avium-intracellulare* (MAC), *in vitro* as well as in experimental infections caused by these pathogens in mice with induced immuno-deficiency.

Pharmacokinetic properties: In man, rifabutin is rapidly absorbed and maximum plasma concentrations are reached around 2–4 hours after oral administration. The pharmacokinetics of rifabutin is linear after single administration of 300, 450, and 600 mg to healthy volunteers. With these doses, C max is in the range of 0.4–0.7 μg/ml. Plasma concentrations are maintained above the MIC values for *M. tuberculosis* up to about 30 hours from administration.

Rifabutin is widely distributed in various animal organs with the exception of the brain. In particular, in human lung tissue the concentrations measured up to 24 hours after dosing were about 5–10 times higher than the plasma levels.

The intracellular penetration of rifabutin is very high as demonstrated by intracellular/extracellular concentration ratios which ranged from 9 in neutrophils to 15 in monocytes, both obtained from human sources.

The high intracellular concentration is likely to play a crucial role in sustaining the efficacy of rifabutin against intracellular pathogens such as mycobacteria.

Rifabutin and its metabolites are eliminated mainly by the urinary route. The $t_{½}\beta$ of rifabutin in man is approximately 35–40 hours.

Preclinical safety data: Preclinical safety studies of rifabutin indicate a good safety margin in rodents and in monkeys.

In repeated dose studies, target organs were identified at doses producing blood levels higher than those achieved with recommended doses for human therapy. The main target organs are liver and, to a lesser degree, erythrocytes.

Rifabutin did not show any teratogenic, mutagenic or carcinogenic potential.

Pharmaceutical particulars

List of excipients: Microcrystalline cellulose; Sodium lauryl sulphate; Magnesium stearate; Silica gel

Incompatibilities: None known.

Shelf life: 24 months at room temperature.

Special precautions for storage: None.

Nature and contents of container: Transparent PVC/Al blisters in cardboard cartons containing 30 capsules or amber glass bottles containing 30 or 100 capsules.

Instructions for use/handling: There are no special instructions for handling.

Marketing authorisation number 3433/0168

Date of first authorisation/renewal of authorisation 15 October 1993.

Date of (partial) revision of the text 30 July 1997.

Legal category POM.

NICORETTE*

Presentation Square pieces of chewing gum containing 2 mg nicotine in a chewing gum base.

Uses

Pharmacology: When Nicorette is chewed, nicotine is slowly released into the mouth and is absorbed through the buccal mucosa, the desired action is relief of unpleasant symptoms associated with smoking cessation. A proportion, by the swallowing of nicotine-containing saliva, reaches the stomach and intestine where it is inactivated.

Indications: Nicorette is intended to help smokers who want to give up smoking, but experience great difficulty in doing so because of their nicotine dependence.

Dosage and administration
Adults (including the elderly): The rate of gum use should depend upon the previous smoking habits of the individual.

Nicorette should be chewed slowly when there is an urge to smoke, up to a maximum of 15 pieces per day; however the patient's individual need may be considerably less than this. If more than 15 pieces of Nicorette per day are required, treatment with 4 mg nicotine gum (Nicorette Plus) may be considered. Most patients require about 10 pieces of gum per day initially. All available nicotine is released from a piece of gum after about 30 minutes chewing. Since effective absorption is through the buccal mucosa, the rate of chewing should be adjusted to minimise the swallowing and inactivation of nicotine contained in saliva.

After 3 months ad libitum dosage, Nicorette should be gradually withdrawn.

Children: Not to be administered to children.

Contra-indications, warnings, etc
Contra-indications: Nicotine in any form is contra-indicated in pregnancy.

Precautions: Swallowed nicotine may exacerbate symptoms in patients suffering from gastritis or peptic ulcers.

Nicotine's cardiovascular effects may be deleterious to patients with angina or a history of coronary artery disease. Nicorette presents a lesser hazard, however, than smoking, which introduces carbon monoxide as an additional toxic factor.

Warnings and adverse effects: Nicorette in the recommended dose has not been found to cause any serious adverse effects. Nicotine from the gum may sometimes cause a slight irritation of the throat at the start of treatment, and may also cause increased salivation. Allergic reactions such as angiodema and urticaria, and ulcerative stomatitis have been reported.

Excessive swallowing of dissolved nicotine may, at first, cause hiccuping. Those with a tendency of indigestion may suffer initially from minor degrees of indigestion or heartburn, slower chewing will usually overcome this problem.

Dependence is a rare side-effect and is both less harmful and easier to break than smoking dependence.

Excessive consumption of Nicorette by patients who have not been in the habit of inhaling tobacco smoke could possibly lead to nausea, faintness or headaches (as may be experienced by such a patient if tobacco smoke is inhaled).

Smokers who wear dentures may experience difficulty in chewing Nicorette.

Overdosage: Overdosage of Nicorette can occur only if many pieces are chewed simultaneously. The fatal acute dose of nicotine in man is probably about 60 mg. Risk of overdosage with Nicorette is, however, small since nausea or vomiting usually occurs at an early stage.

Risk of poisoning by swallowing the gum is also small, since the release of nicotine from the gum is slow. Therefore very little nicotine is absorbed from the stomach and intestine and any that is will be inactivated in the liver. Nicotine is excreted in acid urine four times as rapidly as in alkaline urine.

Treatment of overdosage: In the event of overdosage vomiting should be induced with syrup of ipecacuanha or gastric lavage carried out (wide bore tube). A suspension of activated charcoal should then be passed through the tube and left in the stomach. Artificial respiration with oxygen should be instituted if needed and continued for as long as necessary. Other therapy, including treatment of shock, is purely symptomatic.

Pharmaceutical precautions No special storage conditions are necessary. The preparation has a shelf-life at room temperature of 30 months from the date of manufacture.

Legal category P.

Package quantities Packages of 30 or 105 pieces, in the form of blister-packed strips each containing 15 pieces.

Further information Nicorette should be chewed slowly. Sufficient nicotine may be released from the gum by chewing intermittently and leaving the gum under the lip or in the corner of the mouth between chews. Nicorette is sugar-free.

Product licence number 0022/0101

NICORETTE PLUS*

Presentation Square pieces of chewing gum containing 4 mg nicotine in a chewing gum base.

Uses
Pharmacology: When Nicorette Plus is chewed, nicotine is slowly released into the mouth and is absorbed through the buccal mucosa, the desired action is relief of unpleasant symptoms associated with smoking cessation. A proportion, by the swallowing of nicotine-containing saliva, reaches the stomach and intestine where it is inactivated.

Indications: Nicorette Plus is intended to help smokers who want to give up smoking, but experience great difficulty in doing so because of their nicotine dependence, particularly those patients who are heavy smokers or who require more than 15 pieces of 2 mg nicotine gum (Nicorette) per day.

Dosage and administration
Adults (including the elderly): The rate of gum use should depend upon the previous smoking habits of the individual.

Nicorette Plus should be chewed slowly when there is an urge to smoke, up to a maximum of 15×4 mg pieces per day; however the patient's individual need may be considerably less than this. All available nicotine is released from a piece of gum after about 30 minutes chewing. Since effective absorption is through the buccal mucosa, the rate of chewing should be adjusted to minimise the swallowing and inactivation of nicotine contained in saliva.

After 3 months ad libitum dosage, Nicorette Plus should be gradually withdrawn.

Children: Not to be administered to children.

Contra-indications, warnings, etc
Contra-indications: Nicotine in any form is contra-indicated in pregnancy.

Precautions:

1. Swallowed nicotine may exacerbate symptoms in patients suffering from gastritis or peptic ulcers.
2. Nicotine's cardiovascular effects may be deleterious to patients with angina or a history of coronary artery disease. Nicorette Plus presents a lesser hazard, however, than smoking, which introduces carbon monoxide as an additional toxic factor.

Warnings and adverse effects: Nicorette Plus in the recommended dose has not been found to cause any serious adverse effects. Nicotine from the gum may sometimes cause a slight irritation of the throat at the start of treatment, and may also cause increased salivation. Allergic reactions such as angiodema and urticaria, and ulcerative stomatitis have been reported.

Excessive swallowing of dissolved nicotine may, at first, cause hiccuping. Those with a tendency of indigestion may suffer initially from minor degrees of indigestion or heartburn if Nicorette Plus is used; slower chewing and the use of 2 mg nicotine gum (Nicorette) (if necessary more frequently) will usually overcome this problem.

Dependence is a rare side-effect and is both less harmful and easier to break than smoking dependence.

Excessive consumption of Nicorette Plus by patients who have not been in the habit of inhaling tobacco smoke could possibly lead to nausea, faintness or headaches (as may be experienced by such a patient if tobacco smoke is inhaled).

Smokers who wear dentures may experience difficulty in chewing Nicorette Plus.

Overdosage: Overdosage of Nicorette Plus can occur only if many pieces are chewed simultaneously. The fatal acute dose of nicotine in man is probably about 60 mg. Risk of overdosage with Nicorette Plus is, however, small since nausea or vomiting usually occurs at an early stage.

Risk of poisoning by swallowing the gum is also small, since the release of nicotine from the gum is slow. Therefore very little nicotine is absorbed from the stomach and intestine and any that is will be inactivated in the liver. Nicotine is excreted in acid urine four times as rapidly as in alkaline urine.

Treatment of overdosage: In the event of overdosage vomiting should be induced with syrup of ipecacuanha or gastric lavage carried out (wide bore tube). A suspension of activated charcoal should then be passed through the tube and left in the stomach. Artificial respiration with oxygen should be instituted if needed and continued for as long as necessary. Other therapy, including treatment of shock, is purely symptomatic.

Pharmaceutical precautions No special storage conditions are necessary. The preparation has a shelf-life at room temperature of 30 months from the date of manufacture.

Legal category P.

Package quantities Blister packed strips each containing 15 pieces supplied in packs of 105 pieces.

Further information Nicorette Plus should be chewed slowly. Sufficient nicotine may be released from the gum by chewing intermittently and leaving the gum under the lip or in the corner of the mouth between chews. Nicorette Plus is sugar-free.

Product licence number 0022/0102

NICORETTE* MINT

Presentation Square pieces of chewing gum containing 2 mg nicotine in a mint flavoured chewing gum base.

Uses
Pharmacology: When Nicorette Mint is chewed, nicotine is slowly released into the mouth and is absorbed through the buccal mucosa, the desired action is relief of unpleasant symptoms associated with smoking cessation. A proportion, by the swallowing of nicotine-containing saliva, reaches the stomach and intestine where it is inactivated.

Indications: Nicorette Mint is intended to help smokers who want to give up smoking, but experience great difficulty in doing so because of their nicotine dependence.

Dosage and administration
Adults (including the elderly): The rate of gum use should depend upon the previous smoking habits of the individual.

Nicorette Mint should be chewed slowly when there is an urge to smoke, up to a maximum of 15 pieces per day; however the patient's individual need may be considerably less than this. If more than 15 pieces of Nicorette Mint per day are required, treatment with 4 mg nicotine gum (Nicorette Mint Plus) may be considered. Most patients require about 10 pieces of gum per day initially. All available nicotine is released from a piece of gum after about 30 minutes chewing. Since effective absorption is through the buccal mucosa, the rate of chewing should be adjusted to minimise the swallowing and inactivation of nicotine contained in saliva.

After 3 months ad libitum dosage, Nicorette Mint should be gradually withdrawn.

Children: Not to be administered to children.

Contra-indications, warnings, etc
Contra-indications: Nicotine in any form is contra-indicated in pregnancy.

Precautions: Swallowed nicotine may exacerbate symptoms in patients suffering from gastritis or peptic ulcers.

Nicotine's cardiovascular effects may be deleterious to patients with angina or a history of coronary artery disease. Nicorette Mint presents a lesser hazard, however, than smoking, which introduces carbon monoxide as an additional toxic factor.

Warnings and adverse effects: Nicorette Mint in the recommended dose has not been found to cause any serious adverse effects. Nicotine from the gum may sometimes cause a slight irritation of the throat at the start of treatment, and may also cause increased salivation. Allergic reactions such as angiodema and urticaria, and ulcerative stomatitis have been reported.

Excessive swallowing of dissolved nicotine may, at first, cause hiccuping. Those with a tendency of indigestion may suffer initially from minor degrees of indigestion or heartburn, slower chewing will usually overcome this problem.

Dependence is a rare side-effect and is both less harmful and easier to break than smoking dependence.

Excessive consumption of Nicorette Mint by patients who have not been in the habit of inhaling tobacco smoke could possibly lead to nausea, faintness or headaches (as may be experienced by such a patient if tobacco smoke is inhaled).

Smokers who wear dentures may experience difficulty in chewing Nicorette Mint.

Overdosage: Overdosage of Nicorette Mint can occur only if many pieces are chewed simultaneously. The fatal acute dose of nicotine in man is probably about 60 mg. Risk of overdosage with Nicorette Mint is, however, small since nausea or vomiting usually occurs at an early stage.

Risk of poisoning by swallowing the gum is also small, since the release of nicotine from the gum is slow. Therefore very little nicotine is absorbed from the stomach and intestine and any that is will be inactivated in the liver. Nicotine is excreted in acid urine four times as rapidly as in alkaline urine.

Treatment of overdosage: In the event of overdosage vomiting should be induced with syrup of ipecacuanha or gastric lavage carried out (wide bore tube). A suspension of activated charcoal should then be passed through the tube and left in the stomach. Artificial respiration with oxygen should be instituted if needed and continued for as long as necessary.

Other therapy, including treatment of shock, is purely symptomatic.

Pharmaceutical precautions No special storage conditions are necessary. The preparation has a shelf-life at room temperature of 30 months from the date of manufacture.

Legal category P.

Package quantities Packages of 15, 30 or 105 pieces, in the form of blister-packed strips each containing 15 pieces.

Further information Nicorette Mint should be chewed slowly. Sufficient nicotine may be released from the gum by chewing intermittently and leaving the gum under the lip or in the corner of the mouth between chews. Nicorette Mint is sugar-free.

Product licence number 0022/0112

NICORETTE MINT PLUS*

Presentation Square pieces of chewing gum containing 4 mg nicotine in a mint flavoured chewing gum base.

Uses

Pharmacology: When Nicorette Mint Plus is chewed, nicotine is slowly released into the mouth and is absorbed through the buccal mucosa, the desired action is relief of unpleasant symptoms associated with smoking cessation. A proportion, by the swallowing of nicotine-containing saliva, reaches the stomach and intestine where it is inactivated.

Indications: Nicorette Mint Plus is intended to help smokers who want to give up smoking, but experience great difficulty in doing so because of their nicotine dependence, particularly those patients who are heavy smokers or who require more than 15 pieces of 2 mg nicotine gum (Nicorette Mint) per day.

Dosage and administration

Adults (including the elderly): The rate of gum use should depend upon the previous smoking habits of the individual.

Nicorette Mint Plus should be chewed slowly when there is an urge to smoke, up to a maximum of 15×4 mg pieces per day; however the patient's individual need may be considerably less than this. All available nicotine is released from a piece of gum after about 30 minutes chewing. Since effective absorption is through the buccal mucosa, the rate of chewing should be adjusted to minimise the swallowing and inactivation of nicotine contained in saliva.

After 3 months ad libitum dosage, Nicorette Mint Plus should be gradually withdrawn.

Children: Not to be administered to children.

Contra-indications, warnings, etc

Contra-indications: Nicotine in any form is contra-indicated in pregnancy.

Precautions:

1. Swallowed nicotine may exacerbate symptoms in patients suffering from gastritis or peptic ulcers.

2. Nicotine's cardiovascular effects may be deleterious to patients with angina or a history of coronary artery disease. Nicorette Mint Plus presents a lesser hazard, however, than smoking, which introduces carbon monoxide as an additional toxic factor.

Warnings and adverse effects: Nicorette Mint Plus in the recommended dose has not been found to cause any serious adverse effects. Nicotine from the gum may sometimes cause a slight irritation of the throat at the start of treatment, and may also cause increased salivation. Allergic reactions such as angiodema and urticaria, and ulcerative stomatitis have been reported.

Excessive swallowing of dissolved nicotine may, at first, cause hiccuping. Those with a tendency of indigestion may suffer initially from minor degrees of indigestion or heartburn if Nicorette Mint Plus is used; slower chewing and the use of 2 mg nicotine gum (Nicorette Mint) (if necessary more frequently) will usually overcome this problem.

Dependence is a rare side-effect and is both less harmful and easier to break than smoking dependence.

Excessive consumption of Nicorette Mint Plus by patients who have not been in the habit of inhaling tobacco smoke could possibly lead to nausea, faintness or headaches (as may be experienced by such a patient if tobacco smoke is inhaled).

Smokers who wear dentures may experience difficulty in chewing Nicorette Mint Plus.

Overdosage: Overdosage of Nicorette Mint Plus can occur only if many pieces are chewed simultaneously. The fatal acute dose of nicotine in man is probably about 60 mg. Risk of overdosage with Nicorette Mint Plus is, however, small since nausea or vomiting usually occurs at an early stage.

Risk of poisoning by swallowing the gum is also small, since the release of nicotine from the gum is slow. Therefore very little nicotine is absorbed from the stomach and intestine and any that is will be inactivated in the liver. Nicotine is excreted in acid urine four times as rapidly as in alkaline urine.

Treatment of overdosage: In the event of overdosage vomiting should be induced with syrup of ipecacuanha or gastric lavage carried out (wide bore tube). A suspension of activated charcoal should then be passed through the tube and left in the stomach. Artificial respiration with oxygen should be instituted if needed and continued for as long as necessary. Other therapy, including treatment of shock, is purely symptomatic.

Pharmaceutical precautions No special storage conditions are necessary. The preparation has a shelf-life at room temperature of 30 months from the date of manufacture.

Legal category P.

Package quantities Packages of 15, 30 or 105 pieces, in the form of blister-packed strips each containing 15 pieces.

Further information Nicorette Mint Plus should be chewed slowly. Sufficient nicotine may be released from the gum by chewing intermittently and leaving the gum under the lip or in the corner of the mouth between chews. Nicorette Mint Plus is sugar-free.

Product licence number 0022/0113.

NICORETTE* INHALATOR

Qualitative and quantitative composition Nicotine 10 mg per cartridge.

Pharmaceutical form Inhalation cartridge for oromucosal use.

Clinical particulars

Therapeutic indications: The treatment of nicotine dependence and for the relief of withdrawal symptoms associated with smoking cessation.

Posology and method of administration: Adults (Including elderly).

Dosage: The frequency of use should depend on the previous smoking habit of the individual. Nicorette Inhalator should be used whenever the urge to smoke is felt, up to a maximum usage of 12 cartridges per day.

In the treatment of nicotine dependence, a course not exceeding three months is suggested, the patient stopping smoking completely at the start of the course.

a) For up to 8 weeks the patient uses not less than six and not more than 12 cartridges each day, to relieve craving.

b) Over the following two weeks the aim is to reduce the number of cartridges used by half, and over the next two weeks to reduce the number to zero by the last day.

c) Counselling and support from family, friends and health professionals can improve the chances of abstinence.

d) Patients who revert to smoking during or upon completion of the course should see a doctor before attempting a new course. Similarly, where a course extends into chronic use because of inability to cut down use of the Inhalator, medical advice should be sought.

Method of administration: The cartridge is inserted into the mouthpiece according to the instructions. The patient draws air into the mouth through the mouthpiece: there is a greater effort needed than with a cigarette. The patient may find deep drawing or short sucks on the mouthpiece most effective–patients soon find a favoured technique. Nicotine vapour passing through the mouth is absorbed by the buccal mucosa: little reaches the lungs. After about 20 minutes of intense use the maximal dose is achieved and it is about then that the nicotine amounts released from the cartridge begin to fall away, such that the cartridge is rejected by the user.

The actual time that the cartridge is active depends on the intensity of use.

Children: Nicorette Inhalator should not be administered to individuals under 18 years of age.

Concomitant disease: Only severe renal impairment would be expected to affect the clearance of nicotine or its metabolites from the circulation. In patients smoking and undergoing haemodialysis, elevated nicotine levels have been seen.

Patients with obstructive lung disease may find use of the Inhalator difficult. Nicotine Gum, Patch or Nasal Spray may be preferred in such cases.

Contra-indications:

(i) The product should not be administered to non tobacco users or to patients known to be intolerant of nicotine or menthol.

(ii) Nicotine in any form should be avoided during pregnancy and lactation.

(iii) Nicorette Inhalator is contraindicated in persons up to 18 years of age.

Special warnings and special precautions for use: The patient should stop smoking or using other sources of nicotine completely when initiating therapy with the product. Patients who continue smoking or use other sources of nicotine when using the Nicorette Inhalator may experience adverse effects due to peak nicotine levels being higher than those experienced from smoking alone.

Nicorette Inhalator is best used at room temperature. Low temperature (below 15°C) may depress the release of nicotine, whilst high temperature (above 30°C) may increase release. Patients should avoid use in high temperatures or make fewer inhalations.

The cardiovascular effects of nicotine may be deleterious to patients with a history of angina pectoris. Nicorette Inhalator should be used with caution in patients with a history of peptic ulcer, recent myocardial infarction, serious cardiac arrhythmias, systemic hypertension, peripheral vascular disease, gastritis or renal or hepatic impairment.

Nicotine can stimulate production of adrenaline. Nicorette Inhalator should be used with caution in patients with diabetes mellitus, hyperthyroidism or phaeochromocytoma.

Interaction with other medicaments and other forms of interaction: Smoking cessation, with or without nicotine replacement, may alter the pharmacokinetics of certain concomitant medications.

May require a decrease in dose at cessation of smoking	*Possible mechanism of action*
Paracetamol, caffeine, pentazocine, imipramine, oxazepam, propranolol, theophylline	Deinduction of hepatic enzymes on smoking cessation
Insulin	Increase of subcutaneous insulin absorption with smoking cessation
Adrenergic antagonists (eg: prazosin, labetalol)	Decrease in circulating catecholamines with smoking cessation
May require an increase in dose at cessation of smoking	*Possible mechanism of action*
Adrenergic agonists (eg isoprenaline, phenylephrine)	Decrease in circulating catecholamines with smoking cessation

Pregnancy and lactation: Nicotine in any form is contra-indicated in pregnancy. As nicotine passes freely into breast milk it should also be avoided by nursing mothers.

Effects on ability to drive and use machines: None.

Undesirable effects: The most frequently reported adverse events are local, ie: cough and irritation in mouth and throat. During controlled clinical trials the following events were reported at an incidence of greater by 1% in the active than with placebo treatment:

cough	27%
headache	26%
throat irritation	24%
rhinitis	18%
pharyngitis	15%
stomatitis	15%
dyspepsia	14%
anxiety	13%
nausea	10%
sinusitis	8%
dry mouth	7%
chest pain	5%
skeletal pain	5%
diarrhoea	4%
flatulence	4%
local paraesthesia	4%
allergy	3%
depression	3%
vomiting	2%
dyspnoea	2%
thirst	2%
gingival irritation	2%
hiccup	2%

Some symptoms, such as dizziness, headache and sleeplessness, may be related to withdrawal symptoms associated with smoking cessation. Increased frequency of aphthous ulcer may occur after smoking cessation. The causality is unclear. Maintained nicotine dependence may occur.

Overdose: Overdosage with nicotine can occur if the patient has very low nicotine dependence or uses other forms of nicotine concomitantly. During non-clinical forced inhalation techniques, maximum plasma levels produced were in the range found when smoking.

Symptoms of overdosage are those of acute nicotine poisoning and include nausea, salivation, abdominal pain, diarrhoea, sweating, headache, dizziness, disturbed hearing and marked weakness. In extreme cases, these symptoms may be followed by hypotension, rapid, weak, irregular pulse, breathing difficulties, prostration, circulatory collapse and terminal convulsions.

The minimum acute lethal dose of nicotine in man is believed to be 40–60 mg.

Management of overdosage: All nicotine intake should cease immediately and the patient should be treated symptomatically. Artificial respiration with oxygen should be instituted if necessary.

Pharmacological properties

Pharmacodynamic properties: Nicorette Inhalator facilitates uptake of nicotine through the buccal mucosa into the venous circulation. The amount taken up alleviates the craving symptoms caused by the absence of nicotine from smoking.

Pharmacokinetic properties: Nicotine given iv has a volume of distribution of 2 or 3 L/kg with a half life of 1–2 hours. Average plasma clearance is about 1–2 L/min mainly in the liver. More than 20 metabolites are known, all less active than nicotine: cotinine, with a half life of 15–20 hours and concentrations ten times that of nicotine is the main one.

Plasma binding of nicotine below 5% means significant displacement of drugs or nicotine are unlikely. Nicotine is excreted in the urine principally as cotinine (15%), 3-hydroxycotinine (45%), nicotine (10%).

Most inhaled nicotine is absorbed via the buccal mucosa. Forced rapid inhalation over 20 minutes will remove 40% of the nicotine from the cartridge. Uptake is slow and free of the peaks resultant from cigarette smoking. In normal use, plasma levels of 6–8 ng/ml nicotine are obtained–about one third that from smoking, and equivalent to an hourly 2 mg nicotine chewing gum.

Peak plasma levels occur within 15 minutes after the end of inhalation. Forced rapid inhalation for 20 minutes per hour for 12 hours achieved steady state plasma levels of 20–25 ng/ml.

Ambient temperature affects volatilisation of nicotine, the biologically available dose rising by 35% for each 10°C above 20°C. Use below 15°C is not recommended.

Because the pattern of use is decided by the patient up to a limit of 12 cartridges per day to relieve craving, therapeutic levels of nicotine are individual, dictated by the level of dependence.

Preclinical safety data: None stated.

Pharmaceutical particulars

List of excipients: Levomenthol and porous plug.

Incompatibilities: None relevant.

Shelf-life: Two years.

Special precautions for storage: Store below 30°C.

Nature and contents of container: Aluminium foil sealed plastic cartridge.

Instructions for use/handling:

1. Remove the Aluminium foil sealed tray and the mouthpiece from the carton box.
2. Peel back the foil from the tray.
3. Pull the mouthpiece apart and insert a cartridge, whereby the seal of the inserted end of the cartridge is perforated.
4. Push the other part of the mouthpiece back into place over the cartridge: the product is ready for use.
5. Grip the mouthpiece with the lips.

As air is inhaled, the nicotine is vaporised and absorbed in the mouth.

Disposal instructions: Because of residual nicotine, used cartridges may be a hazard to children, animals and fish and so should never be thrown away or left lying around. They should be kept in the case and disposed of with household rubbish.

Cleaning of mouthpiece: The empty mouthpiece should be rinsed in water several times a week.

Nicorette Inhalator should be used when the patient has the urge for a cigarette or feels the onset of other withdrawal symptoms, up to a maximum of twelve cartridges per day.

The number, frequency, puffing/inhalation time and technique vary individually. Studies show that different inhalation techniques give similar effects: deep inhalation (the cigarette smoker's way) or shallow puffing (the pipe smoker's way). The amount of nicotine from a puff is less than that from a cigarette.

To compensate for less nicotine delivery from a puff it is necessary to inhale more often than when smoking a cigarette, ie use the Nicorette Inhalator for longer periods at a time. After using a few cartridges the patient will have found a method that suits him/her and gives the best effect.

This product works best at room temperature. In cold conditions (below 15°C) the nicotine evaporates less rapidly and it will be necessary to inhale more frequently, whilst in warm conditions (above 30°C) nicotine will evaporate more readily and inhalation should be less frequent to avoid overdose.

Marketing authorisation number 0022/0163

Date of first authorisation/renewal of authorisation 15 July 1997.

Date of approval/revision of SPC 1 July 1997.

Legal category P.

NICORETTE* MICROTAB

Qualitative and quantitative composition Nicotine β-cyclodextrin complex 17.4 mg, equivalent to 2 mg nicotine.

Pharmaceutical form Sublingual tablet.

Clinical particulars

Therapeutic indications: Nicorette Microtab is intended to help smokers who want to give up smoking, but who experience difficulty in doing so owing to their dependence on nicotine.

Posology and method of administration: Adults and the elderly: The patient should be urged to stop smoking completely when initiating therapy with Nicorette Microtab.

The initial dose is based on the individual's nicotine dependence. The tablet is used sublingually with a recommended dose of one tablet per hour or, for heavy smokers (smoking more than 20 cigarettes per day), two tablets per hour. Increasing to two tablets per hour may be considered for patients who fail to stop smoking with the one tablet-per-hour regimen or for those whose nicotine withdrawal symptoms remain so strong as to foresee a relapse.

Most smokers require 8 to 12 or 16 to 24 tablets per day, not to exceed 40 tablets. The duration of treatment is individual, but at least three months of treatment is recommended. The nicotine dose should then be gradually reduced, by decreasing the total number of tablets used per day. The treatment should be stopped when the daily consumption is down to one or two tablets. Nicotine dosage beyond six months is not generally recommended.

Children: The safety of Nicorette Microtab has not been established in individuals below eighteen years of age. The product should not be used in these subjects.

Concomitant disease: Only severe renal impairment would be expected to affect the clearance of nicotine or its metabolites from the circulation. Elevated nicotine levels have been seen in patients smoking and undergoing renal haemodialysis.

Contra-indications: Nicotine in any form is contraindicated in pregnancy.

Special warnings and precautions for use: It is important that the treatment is supported with other activities in order to facilitate the smoking cessation. Individuals who continue smoking when using Nicorette Microtab may experience adverse effects due to peak nicotine levels higher than those from smoking alone.

The cardiovascular effects of nicotine may be deleterious to patients with a history of angina pectoris. Nicorette Microtab should be used with caution in patients with a history of peptic ulcer, recent myocardial infarction, serious cardiac arrhythmia, systemic hypertension, peripheral vascular disease or hepatic, renal or gastric disease.

Nicotine can stimulate production of epinephrine (adrenaline). Nicorette Microtab should be used with caution in patients with diabetes mellitus, hyperthyroidism or phaeochromocytoma.

Interactions with other medicaments and other forms of interaction: Smoking cessation with or without nicotine replacement may alter the pharmacokinetics of certain concomitant medicines.

May require a decrease in dose at cessation of smoking	*Possible mechanism of action*
Caffeine, imipramine, oxazepam, paracetamol, pentazocine, propanolol, theophylline	Deinduction of hepatic enzymes with smoking cessation
Insulin	Increase of subcutaneous insulin absorption with smoking cessation
Adrenergic antagonists (e.g. prazosin, labetalol)	Decrease in circulating catecholamines with smoking cessation
May require an increase in dose at cessation of smoking	*Possible mechanism of action*
Adrenergic agonists (e.g. isoprenaline, phenylephrine)	Decrease in circulating catacholamines with smoking cessation

Pregnancy and lactation: Pregnancy: Nicotine passes over to the foetus and influences the breathing pattern and circulation of the foetus. The effect on the foetal circulation is dose dependent. Nicorette sublingual tablets should therefore be avoided during pregnancy except by women who are unable to give up smoking without nicotine substitution.

Breast feeding: Nicotine passes over into breast milk in such amounts that it may affect the infant even with therapeutic doses.

Effects on ability to drive and use machines: Not applicable.

Undesirable effects: Nicorette Microtab may give rise to the adverse events noted for nicotine replacement therapy in general. Adverse events, at a frequency of over one percent compared to placebo, include headache, dyspepsia, nausea, vomiting, diarrhoea, dyspnoea and thirst.

In clinical studies of Nicorette Microtab, the following adverse events were reported: heartburn, mouth irritation, hiccups, nausea, dizziness, unpleasant taste, headache and sensation of a lump in the throat. The pattern is similar to that reported for nicotine chewing gum.

The adverse events occur mainly during the first weeks following initiation of treatment, and are due to the dose-dependent local or systemic pharmacological effects of nicotine.

Symptoms such as dizziness, headache and sleeplessness, may be related to withdrawal symptoms associated with smoking cessation. Increased incidence of aphthous ulcer may occur after smoking cessation. The causality is unclear. Maintained nicotine dependence may occur.

Overdose: Overdosage can occur if many tablets are taken simultaneously or in rapid succession. The consequences of an overdose are most likely to be minimised by the early nausea and vomiting known to occur with excessive nicotine intake. Nicotine is also subject to a significant first-pass metabolism.

Symptoms of overdosage are those of acute nicotine poisoning and include nausea, salivation, abdominal pain, diarrhoea, sweating, headache, dizziness, disturbed hearing and marked weakness. In extreme cases, these symptoms may be followed by hypotension, rapid or weak or irregular pulse, breathing difficulties, prostration, circulatory collapse and terminal convulsions.

The minimum lethal dose of nicotine in a non-tolerant man has been estimated to be 40 to 60 mg.

Management of overdosage: All nicotine intake should cease immediately and the patient should be treated symptomatically. Artificial respiration with oxygen should be instituted if necessary.

Pharmacological Properties

Pharmacodynamic properties: The pharmacological effects of nicotine are well documented. Those resulting from using Nicorette Microtab are comparatively small. The response at any one time represents a summation of stimulant and depression actions from direct, reflex and chemical mediator influences on several organs. The principal pharmacological actions are central stimulation and/or depression; transient hyperpnoea; peripheral vasoconstriction (usually associated with a rise in systolic pressure); suppression of appetite and stimulation of peristalsis.

Pharmacokinetic properties: Most of the absorption of nicotine from Nicorette Microtab occurs directly through the buccal mucosa. The absolute bioavailability, after sublingual administration of the tablet, is approximately 50%. The systemic bioavailability of orally administered nicotine is lower due to the amount removed initially by the liver (the first-pass effect). Hence, the high and rapidly rising nicotine concentrations seen after smoking are rarely produced by treatment with Nicorette Microtab.

Nicotine from smoking is rapidly absorbed from the lungs into arterial plasma whereas nicotine from sublingual tablets passes more slowly into the venous system.

Steady-state trough nicotine plasma concentrations, achieved after ten hourly doses of one tablet, are in the order of magnitude of 10 ng/mL, which is about 50% of normal smoking levels.

There is a slight deviation from dose-linearity of AUC_{inf} and C_{max} when single doses of one, two and three tablets are given. This deviation may be explained by a larger fraction of the higher doses being swallowed and subject to first-pass elimination.

The therapeutic blood concentrations of nicotine, i.e. the blood levels which relieve craving, are based on the individual's nicotine dependence.

Preclinical safety data: Preclinical data indicate that nicotine is neither mutagenic nor genotoxic.

Pharmaceutical Particulars

List of excipients: Crospovidone, β-cyclodextrin, colloidal anhydrous silica, magnesium stearate.

Incompatibilities: Not applicable.

Shelf-life: Three (3) years.

Special precautions for storage: Do not store above 30°C.

Nature and contents of container: Aluminium foil/PVC-PVDC circular-shaped blister strips (discs) of fifteen (15) tablets assembled in cartons, together with a dispenser. The dispenser is used to remove the tablets from the disc.

Package sizes:
Starter pack: Two discs (30 tablets), together with the dispenser.
Refill: Seven discs (105 tablets).

Instructions for use/handling:

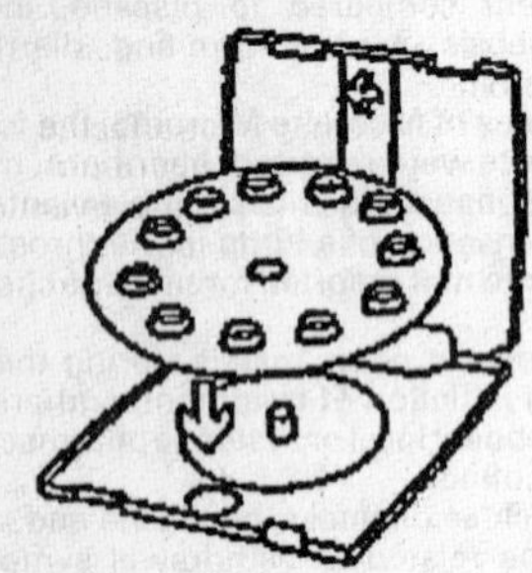

Figure 1

1. Place the disc on the peg in the tablet dispenser with the flat side facing downwards (**Figure 1**).

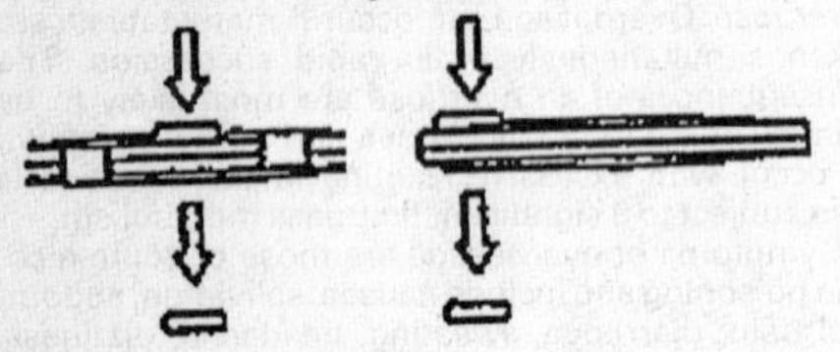

Figure 2

2. Close the dispenser and press on the punch to push the tablet out of the strip (**Figure 2**).

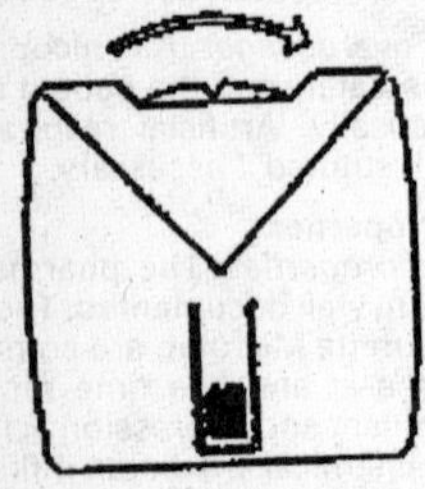

Figure 3

3. Turn the disc in the direction of the arrow to place the next tablet into position (**Figure 3**). The disc should **not** be turned in the opposite direction to the arrow.

Marketing authorisation number 0032/0239.

Date of first authorisation/renewal of authorisation 23 October 1998

Date of (partial) revision of the text July 1998.

Legal Category P

NICORETTE* NASAL SPRAY

Presentation A metered spray bottle containing 10 ml of a 10 mg/ml solution of nicotine for intranasal use. Each 50 microlitre spray contains 0.5 mg nicotine.

Uses
Pharmacology: Nicotine solution applied to the nasal passages is rapidly absorbed into the circulation, reaching a maximum in 10–15 minutes. About 50% is absorbed.

Indications: Nicorette Nasal Spray is for the rapid relief of nicotine withdrawal symptoms in the treatment of nicotine dependent persons as a part of a supervised smoking cessation programme. It may be of particular use in the most heavily dependent smokers.

Dosage and administration
Children and young adults: The product is not for use by any person under the age of 16 years.

Adults and elderly: Use of Nicorette Nasal Spray should be restricted to 3 months. The spray is to be used as part of a supervised smoking cessation programme for nicotine dependency. Counselling should be part of this procedure.

The method of use of the spray is illustrated in the package insert.

A 50 μl dose of solution is sprayed into the nostril when the unit is activated. This is described as a 'spray' and dosage is described using this term. Each spray delivers 0.5 mg of nicotine, about half of which is absorbed.

On commencing treatment the patient uses the spray to treat craving as required, subject to a limit of one spray to each nostril twice an hour. The daily limit of use is 32 mg of nicotine (64 sprays) which is the equivalent of two sprays to each nostril every hour for 16 hours.

The 3 month course should take the following pattern:

a. For 8 weeks the patient uses the spray as required, subject to the maxima described above, to relieve craving.
b. After this period the patient reduces usage until after 4 more weeks treatment has ended. It is suggested that after 2 weeks into this period usage will have been reduced by a half and usage be zero by the last day.
c. In order to avoid substituted dependence, treatment should be limited to 3 months within the rehabilitation programme. No other nicotine containing drugs, or tobacco products should be used during the treatment. The patient should understand the aim of decreasing the use of the spray to make a final break with nicotine at the end of the course.

Contra-indications, warnings, etc
Contra-indications:

(i) The product should not be administered to non tobacco users or to patients known to be allergic to components of the spray.

(ii) Nicotine in any form should be avoided during pregnancy and lactation.

(iii) Nicorette Nasal Spray is contra-indicated in persons up to 16 years of age.

(iv) Other nicotine-containing preparations or tobacco products must not be used during the Nicorette Nasal Spray course.

Interaction with other medicaments and other forms of interactions:

May require a decrease in dose at cessation of smoking	*Possible mechanism of action*
Paracetamol, caffeine, imipramine, oxazepam, pentazocine, propranolol, theophylline.	Deinduction of hepatic enzymes on smoking cessation.
Insulin.	Increase of subcutaneous insulin absorption with smoking cessation.
Adrenergic antagonists (e.g. prazosin, labetalol).	Decrease in circulating catecholamines with smoking cessation.

May require an increase in dose at cessation of smoking	Possible mechanism of action
Adrenergic agonists (e.g. isoprenaline, phenylephrine).	Decrease in circulating catecholamines with smoking cessation.

Effects on ability to drive and use machines: The nasal spray should not be used whilst the user is driving or operating machinery as sneezing and watering eyes can contribute to accidents which may result in serious injury.

Other undesirable effects: Nicorette Nasal Spray may cause adverse reactions similar to those produced by nicotine given by other means, including smoking.

Principal adverse effects: These occur commonly at start of therapy but usually decline within the first couple of weeks or treatment.
Local: Nasal irritation (sneezing, running nose), watering eyes and throat irritation.
Systemic: Headache and dizziness.
Other: Additionally an incidence greater than 1% compared with placebo was noted in clinical studies for the following: Sore nose, ear sensations, increased urination, tingling or burning sensation in the head, nose bleed, dyspepsia.

Pregnancy and lactation: Nicotine in any form is contra-indicated in pregnancy. As nicotine passes freely into breast milk, it should also be avoided by nursing mothers.

Other special warnings and special precautions for use: The patient should be urged to stop smoking completely when initiating therapy with the product. Patients who continue smoking when using the spray may experience adverse effects due to peak nicotine levels higher than those experienced from smoking alone. Similarly adverse effects may occur if nicotine products are used at the same time as nasal spray.

The cardiovascular effects of nicotine may be deleterious to patients with a history of angina pectoris. Nicorette Nasal Spray should be used with caution in patients with a history of peptic ulcer and chronic nasal disorders (polyposis, vasomotor rhinitis, perennial rhinitis), recent myocardial infarction, serious cardiac arrhythmias, systemic hypertension or peripheral vascular disease.

Nicotine can stimulate production of adrenaline; Nicorette Nasal Spray should be used with caution in patients with diabetes mellitus, hyperthyroidism or phaeochromocytoma.

Substituted dependence: The practitioner should be aware of the possibility of substituted dependence and accordingly limit treatment to 3 months.

Concomitant disease: Only severe renal impairment would be expected to affect the clearance of nicotine or its metabolites from the circulation. In patients smoking and undergoing haemodialysis elevated nicotine levels have been seen.

Overdosage: Overdosage with nicotine can only occur, if the patient has very low nicotine dependence or uses other forms of nicotine concomitantly. Should Nicorette Nasal Spray be used orally, the risk of poisoning is small due to high first pass metabolism. Due to the nature of the container it will not be possible to take the product without using the spraying device.

Symptoms of overdosage are those of acute nicotine poisoning and include nausea, salvation, abdominal pain, diarrhoea, sweating, headache, dizziness, disturbed hearing and marked weakness. In extreme cases, these symptoms may be followed by hypotension, rapid, weak, irregular pulse, breathing difficulties, prostration, circulatory collapse and terminal convulsions.

The acute minimum lethal oral dose of nicotine in man is believed to be 40–60 mg.

Management of overdosage: All nicotine intake should cease immediately and the patient should be treated symptomatically. Artificial respiration with oxygen should be instituted if necessary.

Pharmaceutical precautions Protect from light. Shelf life is 2 years at room temperature.

Legal category POM.

Package quantities Metered spray bottle, 10 ml in packs of one.

Further information Contains methyl and propyl parabens as preservatives.

Product licence number 0022/0141

NICORETTE* PATCH

Presentation Nicorette Patch is a transdermal delivery system for topical application, available in sizes of 30, 20 and 10 cm² each containing 0.83 mg/cm² of nicotine, releasing 15 mg, 10 mg and 5 mg respectively over 16 hours. Each patch is rectangular in shape and comprises 3 distinct layers; an outer beige matt finish backing layer, a patterned silvery middle layer and an inner clear release liner, which is removed prior to use. Each patch is packaged in a heat sealed multilaminate sachet.

Uses
Pharmacology: When the patch is applied, nicotine is slowly released and absorbed through the skin. Blood levels of nicotine are lower than the peaks associated with smoking but sufficient to relieve smoking withdrawal symptoms. The patch is designed to be applied during waking hours only (16 hours).

Pharmacokinetics: Taking into account the residual concentration of nicotine in the transdermal system, the nicotine released from the system is efficiently absorbed: a bioavailability of between 80–108% has been reported. There is no clinically significant difference in bioavailability when the patch is applied to the hip, upper arm or chest.

Steady state concentrations of plasma nicotine in volunteers were examined during a study period of six days. Although nicotine was detectable 24 hours after the first dose, the data did not indicate any accumulation.

Tmax of nicotine after application of a 30 cm² nicotine transdermal system has been shown to vary between 6±2 and 9±3 hours; Cmax has been shown to vary between 13±3 and 16±5 ng/ml. No differences in these pharmacokinetic parameters have been observed between males and females.

All Nicorette Patches are labelled by the average amount of nicotine absorbed by the patient over 16 hours.

Indications: The treatment of nicotine dependence, and the relief of withdrawal symptoms associated with smoking cessation.

Dosage and administration
Adults (including elderly): The recommended treatment programme for Nicorette Patch should occupy 3 months. Nicorette Patch should not be used concurrently with any other nicotine products and patients must stop smoking completely when starting treatment.

The daily dose is one patch delivering 15 mg, 10 mg or 5 mg nicotine as appropriate, with application limited to 16 hours in a 24 hour period in each case.

Daily treatment commences with one 15 mg (30 cm^2) patch, applied on waking (usually in the morning) and removed 16 hours later (usually at bedtime). Treatment should continue at this dose for an initial period of 8 weeks. Patients who have successfully abstained from smoking during this 8 week period should be supported through a further 4 week weaning period, using the lower strength patches. Downward titration of dose is achieved by applying one 10 mg (20 cm^2) patch daily for 2 weeks followed by one 5 mg (10 cm^2) patch daily for a further 2 weeks. Patients should be reviewed at 3 months. Following this review, if abstinence has not been achieved, further courses of treatment may be recommended if it is considered that the patient would benefit.

Nicorette Patch should be applied to clean, dry intact areas of hairless skin, for example on the hip, upper arm, or chest. These areas should be varied each day and the same site should not be used on consecutive days.

There is no clinically significant difference in bioavailability of nicotine when the patch is applied to the hip, upper arm or chest.

After removal, used patches should be disposed of carefully (see below).

Experience with treatment of nicotine dependence shows that success rates are improved if patients also receive supportive therapy and counselling.

Children: Nicorette Patches should not be administered to individuals under 18 years of age.

Contra-indications, warnings, etc
Contra-indications: Not to be administered to non-tobacco users. Nicorette Patch should not be administered to patients with known hypersensitivity to nicotine or any component of the patch.

Pregnancy and lactation: Nicotine in any form, is contra-indicated during pregnancy or whilst breast feeding. Nicotine has been shown in animal studies to cause harm to the foetus including non-specific retardation of growth and skeletal abnormalities. It is therefore presumed nicotine could cause harm to the human foetus if administered to pregnant women. The effect of nicotine delivered by Nicorette Patch has not been examined in pregnancy, although the harmful effects of smoking on maternal and foetal health are clearly established.

Precautions: Due to the cardiovascular effects of nicotine, Nicorette Patch should be used with caution in patients with a history of angina, recent myocardial infarction or cerebrovascular accident, serious cardiac arrythmias, systemic hypertension or peripheral vascular disease. Nicorette Patch should be used with caution in patients with a history of peptic ulcer.

Nicotine can stimulate production of adrenaline; Nicorette Patch should be used with caution in patients with diabetes mellitus, hyperthyroidism or phaeochromocytoma.

Patients with chronic generalised dermatological disorders such as psoriasis, chronic dermatitis or urticaria should not use Nicorette Patch.

After removal, the patch should be folded in half, adhesive side innermost, and placed inside the opened sachet, or in a piece of aluminium foil. The used patch should then be disposed of carefully, away from the reach of children or animals.

Warnings: Erythema may occur. If it is severe or persistent, treatment should be discontinued.

Drug interactions: Smoking cessation, with or without nicotine replacement, may alter the pharmacokinetics of certain concomitant medications.

May require a decrease in dose at cessation of smoking	*Possible mechanism*
Paracetamol, caffeine, imipramine, oxazepam, pentazocine, propranolol, theophylline, warfarin, oestrogens, lignocaine, phenacetin.	Deinduction of hepatic enzymes on smoking cessation.
Insulin.	Increase of subcutaneous insulin absorption with smoking cessation.
Adrenergic antagonists (e.g. prazosin, labetalol).	Decrease in circulating catecholamines with smoking cessation.

May require an increase in dose at cessation of smoking	*Possible mechanism*
Adrenergic agonists (e.g. isoprenaline, phenylephrine).	Decrease in circulating catecholamines with smoking cessation.

Other effects, associated with smoking, include reduced analgesic efficacy with propoxyphene, reduced diuretic response to frusemide and reduced rates of ulcer healing with H_2 antagonists.

Side-effects: Nicorette patch may cause adverse reactions similar to those associated with nicotine administered by other means.

During controlled clinical studies, the following adverse events were reported at an incidence of greater than 1% and more frequently with active than with placebo treatment: application site reactions (e.g. erythema and itching), headache, dizziness, nausea, palpitations, dyspepsia and myalgia.

Other subjective sensations associated with smoking cessation may occur, such as impaired concentration, fatigue, anxiety, irritability and increased appetite.

Concurrent smoking may be associated with symptoms of nicotine overdose.

Overdosage: Overdosage with nicotine can occur if many patches are used simultaneously, or if the patient has very low nicotine dependence or uses other forms of nicotine concomitantly. Should Nicorette Patch be swallowed, the risk of poisoning is small due to slow release of nicotine and high first pass metabolism.

Symptoms of overdosage are those of acute nicotine poisoning and include, nausea, salivation, abdominal pain, diarrhoea, sweating, headache, dizziness, disturbed hearing and marked weakness. In extreme cases, these symptoms may be followed by hypotension, rapid weak irregular pulse, breathing difficulties, prostration, circulatory collapse and terminal convulsions.

The acute minimum lethal oral dose of nicotine in man is believed to be 40–60 mg.

Treatment of overdosage: All nicotine patches should be removed and the patient should be treated symptomatically. Artificial respiration with oxygen should be instituted if necessary.

Pharmaceutical precautions No special storage conditions are necessary. The storage sachet should remain unopened until Nicorette Patch is administered.

Legal category P.

Package quantities Cartons containing Nicorette Patches in single sachets in the following quantities:
Nicorette Patch 15 mg boxes of 7
Nicorette Patch 10 mg boxes of 7
Nicorette Patch 5 mg boxes of 7

Further information Nil.

Product licence numbers

Nicorette Patch 15 mg	0022/0105
Nicorette Patch 10 mg	0022/0104
Nicorette Patch 5 mg	0022/0103

OLBETAM*

Qualitative and quantitative composition Acipimox INN 250 mg

Pharmaceutical form -brown/dark pink hard gelatin capsules, size no. 1, containing a white to cream powder.

Clinical particulars
Therapeutic indications: Olbetam is indicated for the treatment of lipid disorders characterised, according to Fredrickson, by elevated plasma levels of triglycerides (type IV hyperlipo-proteinaemia), or cholesterol (type IIA hyperlipoproteinaemia) and triglycerides and cholesterol (type IIB hyperlipoproteinaemia).

Posology and method of administration: To be given orally.

The daily dosage should be adjusted individually depending on plasma triglyceride and cholesterol levels.

The recommended dosage is one 250 mg capsule 2 or 3 times daily to be taken with or after meals. The lower dose is advised in type IV and the higher dose in types IIA and IIB hyperlipoproteinaemias.

Daily dosages of up to 1200 mg have been safely administered for long periods. Improvement in the plasma lipid's picture is usually seen within the first month of therapy.

In patients with slight renal impairment (creatinine clearance values > 60 ml/min) no dose reduction is required. For patients with moderate to severe renal impairment creatinine clearance values between 60 and 30 ml/min) the dose needs to be reduced accordingly. Acipimox is eliminated entirely through the kidneys, therefore, accumulation can be expected and is related to the degree of renal impairment. It is advised that longer intervals are left between doses of the drug in patients with renal impairment.

Contra-indications: Olbetam is contra-indicated in patients who are hypersensitive to the drug and those with peptic ulceration.

Olbetam should not be given to patients with severe renal impairment (creatinine clearance < 30 ml/min)

Special warnings and precautions for use: Modification of hyperlipidaemia is recommended only for patients with hyperlipoproteinaemia of a degree and type considered appropriate for treatment.

Low cholesterol and low-fat diets, together with cessation of alcohol consumption, are preferable therapeutic approaches to be tried before starting treatment with Olbetam.

The absorption of Olbetam is not affected by the concomitant administration of cholestyramine.

Evidence of clinical efficacy in the prevention of heart disease has not been established.

The possible beneficial and adverse, long-term consequences of some drugs used in the hyperlipidaemias are still the subject of scientific discussion.

Interaction with other medicaments and other forms of interaction: None stated.

Pregnancy and lactation: There is no evidence from the animal studies that acipimox is teratogenic. However, a higher incidence of immature and underweight foetuses was seen in pregnant animals given higher doses of acipimox. This effect may be due to maternal toxicity.

There is only limited experience to date of administration of acipimox to humans therefore epidemiological data is not available. Taking into account the present experience of administration to humans of acipimox and that the safety of acipimox in human pregnancy has not yet been ascertained, it is recommended, therefore, that acipimox not be administered to women who are, or may be pregnant.

In the absence of animal data on the levels of acipimox excreted in milk, Olbetam should not be administered to women who are breast-feeding.

Effects on ability to drive and use machines: None stated.

Undesirable effects: The drug may induce skin vasodilatation giving rise to a sensation of heat, flushing or itching, especially at the beginning of therapy and also rash and erythema. These reactions usually disappear rapidly during the first day of treatment. Moderate gastric disturbances (heartburn, epigastric pain, nausea and diarrhoea) have been reported occasionally, as well as headache, malaise, eye symptoms (dry or gritty eye) and urticaria. On rare occasions patients have developed angioedema and bronchospasm; and anaphylactoid reactions have also been reported.

Overdose: If toxic effects are observed, supportive care and symptomatic treatment should be administered.

Pharmacological properties
Pharmacodynamic properties: Acipimox inhibits the release of fatty acids from adipose tissue and reduces the blood concentrations of very low density lipoproteins (VLDL or Pre-beta) and low density lipoproteins (LDL or beta) with a subsequent overall reduction in triglyceride and cholesterol levels.

Acipimox also has a favourable effect on high density lipoproteins (HDL or alpha) which increase during treatment.

Pharmacokinetic properties: Acipimox is rapidly and completely absorbed orally, reaching peak plasma levels within two hours. The half-life is about two hours. It does not bind to plasma proteins; it is not significantly metabolised and is eliminated almost completely intact by the urinary route.

Preclinical safety data: There is no evidence from the animal studies that acipimox is teratogenic. However, a higher incidence of immature and underweight foetuses was seen in pregnant animals given higher doses of acipimox. This effect may be due to maternal toxicity.

Pharmaceutical particulars
List of excipients: Physically modified corn starch (STA-RX 1500), Silica gel (Syloid 244) USP, Magnesium stearate PhEur, Sodium lauryl sulphate PhEur.

Hard gelatin capsules shell: Gelatin USP, Titanium dioxide (E171), Iron oxide red (E172), Iron oxide yellow (E172).

Incompatibilities: None stated.

Shelf life: 48 months

Special precautions for storage: Store at a temperature below 30°C in a dry place.

Nature and contents of container: Packed in blisters of 10 capsules per strip, inside cartons. Each carton contains 90 capsules.

Instructions for use/handling: None given.

Marketing authorisation number 3433/0097

Date of first authorisation/renewal of authorisation 18 September 1987/18 September 1997.

Date of (partial) revision of the text 19 September 1997.

Legal category POM.

PHARMORUBICIN* RAPID DISSOLUTION

Presentation Sterile, pyrogen-free, red, freeze-dried powder in vials containing 10 mg, 20 mg and 50 mg of epirubicin hydrochloride with lactose and hydroxybenzoate.

Uses Pharmorubicin has produced responses in a wide range of neoplastic conditions, including breast, ovarian, gastric, lung and colorectal carcinomas, malignant lymphomas, leukaemias and multiple myeloma.

Intravesical administration of Pharmorubicin has been found to be beneficial in the treatment of papillary transitional cell carcinoma of the bladder, carcinoma-in-situ and in the prophylaxis of recurrences after transurethral resection.

Dosage and administration For reconstitution the contents of the 10 mg vial should be dissolved in 5 ml of Water for Injections or Sodium Chloride Injection, the 20 mg vial in 10 ml of Water for Injections or Sodium Chloride Injection and the 50 mg vial in 25 ml of Water for Injections or Sodium Chloride Injection.

After adding the diluent the vial contents will dissolve with gentle shaking, without inversion, within 30 seconds. The approximate displacement value of the contents of a 50 mg vial after 25 ml of solvent have been added is 0.15 ml.

Intravenous administration: Pharmorubicin is not active when given orally and should not be injected intramuscularly or intrathecally.

It is advisable to give the drug via the tubing of a freely-running i.v. saline infusion after checking that the needle is well placed in the vein. This method minimises the risk of drug extravasation and makes sure that the vein is flushed with saline after the administration of the drug. Extravasation of Pharmorubicin from the vein during injection may give rise to severe tissue lesions, even necrosis. Venous sclerosis may result from injection into small vessels or repeated injections into the same vein.

Conventional doses: When Pharmorubicin is used as a single agent, the recommended dosage in adults is 60–90 mg/m² body area; the drug should be injected i.v. over 3–5 minutes and, depending on the patient's haematomedullary status, the dose should be repeated at 21 day intervals.

High doses: Pharmorubicin as a single agent for the treatment of lung cancer at high doses should be administered according to the following regimens:

Small cell lung cancer (previously untreated): 120 mg/m² day 1, every 3 weeks.

Non-small cell lung cancer (squamous, large cell, and adenocarcinoma previously untreated): 135 mg/m² day 1 or 45 mg/m² day 1, 2, 3, every 3 weeks.

The drug should be given as an i.v. bolus over 3–5 minutes or as an infusion up to 30 minutes. Lower doses (60–75 mg/m² for conventional treatment and 105–120 mg/m² for high dose schedules) are recommended for patients whose bone marrow function has already been impaired by previous chemotherapy or radiotherapy, by age, or neoplastic bone-marrow infiltration. The total dose per cycle may be divided over 2–3 successive days. When the drug is used in combination with other antitumour agents, the doses need to be adequately reduced. Since the major route of elimination of Pharmorubicin is the hepatobiliary system, the dosage should be reduced in patients with impaired liver function, in order to avoid an increase of overall toxicity.

Moderate liver impairment (bilirubin: 1.4–3 mg/100 ml) requires a 50% reduction of dose, while severe impairment (bilirubin>3 mg/100 ml) necessitates a dose reduction of 75%.

Moderate renal impairment does not appear to require a dose reduction in view of the limited amount of Pharmorubicin excreted by this route.

Intravesical administration: Pharmorubicin may be given by intravesical administration for the treatment of *superficial bladder cancer* and carcinoma-in-situ. It should not be used in this way for the treatment of invasive tumours which have penetrated the bladder wall where systemic therapy or surgery is more appropriate. Epirubicin has also been successfully used intravesically as a prophylactic agent after transurethral resection of superficial tumours in order to prevent recurrences.

While many regimens have been used, the following may be helpful as a guide: for therapy 8 x weekly instillations of 50 mg/50 ml (diluted with saline or distilled sterile water). In the case of local toxicity (chemical cystitis), a dose reduction to 30 mg per 50 ml is advised. For carcinoma-in-situ, depending upon the individual tolerability of the patient, the dose may be increased up to 80 mg per 50 ml. For prophylaxis, 4 x weekly administrations of 50 mg per 50 ml followed by 11 x monthly instillations at the same dosage, is the schedule most commonly used.

The solution should be retained intravesically for 1 hour. To avoid undue dilution with urine, the patient should be instructed not to drink any fluid in the 12 hours prior to instillation. During the instillation, the patient should be rotated occasionally and should be instructed to void at the end of the instillation time.

Contra-indications, warnings, etc

Contra-indications: Pharmorubicin Rapid Dissolution is contra-indicated in patients with marked myelosuppression induced by previous treatment with other antitumour agents or by radiotherapy and in patients already treated with maximal cumulative doses of other anthracyclines such as doxorubicin or daunorubicin. The drug is contra-indicated in patients with a current or previous history of cardiac impairment.

Warnings: Pharmorubicin Rapid Dissolution should be administered only under the supervision of a qualified physician experienced in antiblastic and cytotoxic therapy.

Treatment with high dose Pharmorubicin in particular requires the availability of facilities for the care of patients with possible clinical complications due to myelosuppression.

Initial treatment calls for careful baseline monitoring of various laboratory parameters and cardiac function.

Precautions: During each cycle of treatment with Pharmorubicin Rapid Dissolution, patients must be carefully and frequently monitored. Red and white blood cells, neutrophils and platelet counts should be carefully assessed both before and during each cycle of therapy. Leukopenia and neutropenia are usually transient both with conventional and high doses, reaching a nadir between the 10th and 14th day and returning to normal values by the 21st day: they are more severe with high dose schedules. Very few patients, even receiving high doses, experience thrombocytopenia (<100,000 platelets/mm³).

Before starting therapy and if possible during treatment, liver function should be evaluated (SGOT, SGPT, alkaline phosphatase, bilirubin). A cumulative dose of 900–1000 mg/m² should only be exceeded with extreme caution with both conventional and high doses. Above this level the risk of irreversible congestive cardiac failure increases greatly. There is objective evidence that cardiac toxicity may rarely occur below this range. However, cardiac function must be carefully monitored during treatment to minimize the risk of heart failure of the type described for other anthracyclines.

Heart failure can appear even several weeks after discontinuing treatment and may prove unresponsive to specific medical treatment. The potential risk of cardiotoxicity may increase in patients who have received concomitant, or prior, radiotherapy to the mediastinal pericardial area.

In establishing the maximal cumulative doses of Pharmorubicin, any concomitant therapy with potentially cardiotoxic drugs should be taken into account.

It is recommended that an ECG before and after treatment cycle should be carried out. Alterations in the ECG tracing, such as flattening or inversion of the T wave, depression of the S-T segment, or the onset of arrhythmias, generally transient and reversible, need not necessarily be taken as indications to discontinue treatment.

Cardiomyopathy induced by anthracyclines is associated with a persistent reduction of the QRS voltage, prolongation beyond normal limits of the systolic interval (PEP/LVET) and a reduction of the ejection fraction. Cardiac monitoring of patients receiving Pharmorubicin treatment is highly important and it is advisable to assess cardiac function by non-invasive techniques such as ECG, echocardiography and, if necessary, measurement of ejection fraction by radionuclide angiography.

Like other cytotoxic agents, Pharmorubicin may induce hyperuricemia as a result of rapid lysis of neoplastic cells. Blood uric acid levels should therefore be carefully checked so that this phenomenon may be controlled pharmacologically.

Pharmorubicin Rapid Dissolution may impart a red colour to the urine for 1–2 days after administration.

Adverse reactions: Apart from myelosuppression and cardiotoxicity (described under Precautions) the following adverse reactions have been described:

- alopecia, normally reversible, appears in 60–90% of treated cases; it is accompanied by lack of beard growth in males.
- mucositis may appear 5–10 days after the start of treatment and usually involves stomatitis with areas of painful erosions, mainly along the side of the tongue and on the sublingual mucosa.
- gastro-intestinal disturbances, such as nausea, vomiting and diarrhoea.
- hyperpyrexia.

Fever, chills and urticaria have been rarely reported; anaphylaxis may occur.

High doses of Pharmorubicin have been safely administered in a large number of untreated patients having various solid tumours and has caused adverse events which are no different from those seen at conventional doses with the exception of reversible severe neutropenia (<500 neutrophils/mm³ for <7 days) which occurred in the majority of patients. Only a few patients have required hospitalization and supportive therapy for severe infectious complications at high doses.

During intravesical administration, as drug absorption is minimal, systemic side effects are rare; more frequently chemical cystitis, sometimes haemorrhagic, has been observed.

The occurrence of secondary acute myeloid leukaemia with or without a pre-leukaemic phase has been reported rarely in patients concurrently treated with epirubicin in association with DNA-damaging antineoplastic agents. Such cases should have a short (1–3 year) latency period.

Use during pregnancy and lactation: There is no conclusive information as to whether epirubicin may adversely affect human fertility or cause teratogenesis. Experimental data, however, suggest that epirubicin may harm the foetus. This product should not normally be administered to patients who are pregnant or to mothers who are breast-feeding. Like most other anticancer agents, epirubicin has shown mutagenic and carcinogenic properties in animals.

Overdosage: Very high single doses of Pharmorubicin may be expected to cause acute myocardial degeneration within 24 hours and severe myelosuppression within 10–14 days. Treatment should aim to support the patient during this period and should utilise such measures as blood transfusions and reverse barrier nursing. Delayed cardiac failure has been seen with the anthracyclines up to 6 months after the overdose. Patients should be observed carefully and should, if signs of cardiac failure arise, be treated along conventional lines.

Pharmaceutical precautions The following protective recommendations are given due to the toxic nature of this substance:

- personnel should be trained in good technique for reconstitution and handling.
- pregnant staff should be excluded from working with this drug.
- personnel handling Pharmorubicin Rapid Dissolution should wear protective clothing: goggles, gowns and disposable gloves and masks.
- a designated area should be defined for reconstitution (preferably under a laminar flow system). The work surface should be protected by disposable, plastic-backed, absorbent paper.
- all items used for reconstitution, administration or cleaning, including gloves, should be placed in high-risk, waste-disposal bags for high temperature incineration.

The reconstituted solution is chemically stable when stored for up to 48 hours at 2°C to 8°C or 24 hours at room temperature; however, it is recommended that, in line with good pharmaceutical practice, the solution should not normally be stored for longer than 24 hours at 2°C to 8°C. Avoid exposure of the product to sunlight or direct light. Discard any unused solution.

Prolonged contact with any solution of an alkaline pH should be avoided as it will result in hydrolysis of the drug. Pharmorubicin should not be mixed with heparin due to chemical incompatibility which may lead to precipitation when the drugs are in certain proportions.

Pharmorubicin can be used in combination with other antitumour agents, but it is not recommended that it be mixed with these drugs in the same syringe.

Accidental contact with the skin or eyes should be treated immediately by copious lavage with water, or soap and water, or sodium bicarbonate solution; medical attention should be sought.

Spillage or leakage should be treated with dilute sodium hypochlorite (1% available chlorine) solution, preferably by soaking, and then water.

All cleaning materials should be disposed of as indicated previously.

Legal category POM.

Package quantities 10 mg, 20 mg, 50 mg and 200 mg vials for injection.

Further information In patients with normal hepatic and renal function, plasma levels, after i.v. injection of 60–150 mg/m² of the drug, follow a tri-exponential decrease with a very fast first phase and a slow terminal phase corresponding to a half-life of about 40 hours. These doses are within the limits of pharmacokinetic linearity both in terms of plasma clearance values and metabolic pathway. Plasma levels of the main metabolite, the 13-OH derivative, are constantly lower and virtually parallel those of the unchanged drug. Pharmorubicin is eliminated mainly through the liver; high plasma clearance values (0.9 l/min) indicate that the slow elimination is due to extensive tissue distribution. The drug does not cross the blood–brain barrier.

When Pharmorubicin is administered intravesically, the systemic absorption is minimal.

Product licence number 3433/0082.

PHARMORUBICIN* SOLUTION FOR INJECTION

Qualitative and quantitative composition Epirubicin hydrochloride HSE 0.2% w/v

Pharmaceutical form Sterile red mobile solution in vials containing 10 mg, 20 mg, 50 mg or 200 mg of epirubicin hydrochloride as a 2 mg/ml solution in 0.9% sodium chloride.

Clinical particulars

Therapeutic indications: Pharmorubicin has produced responses in a wide range of neoplastic conditions, including breast, ovarian, gastric, lung, and colorectal carcinomas, malignant lymphomas, leukaemias and multiple myeloma.

Intravesical administration of epirubicin has been found to be beneficial in the treatment of superficial bladder cancer, carcinoma-in-situ and in the prophylaxis of recurrences after transurethral resection.

Posology and method of administration: Pharmorubicin is not active when given orally and should not be injected intramuscularly or intrathecally.

It is advisable to give the drug via the tubing of a freely-running i.v. saline infusion after checking that the needle is well placed in the vein. This method minimises the risk of drug extravasation and makes sure that the vein is flushed with saline after the administration of the drug. Extravasation of Pharmorubicin from the vein during injection may give rise to severe tissue lesions, even necrosis. Venous sclerosis may result from injection into small vessels or repeated injections into the same vein.

Conventional doses: When Pharmorubicin is used as a single agent, the recommended dosage in adults is 60–90 mg/m² body area; the drug should be injected i.v. over 3–5 minutes and depending on the patient's haematomedullary status, the dose should be repeated at 21-day intervals.

High doses: Pharmorubicin as a single agent for the treatment of lung cancer at high doses should be administered according to the following regimens : *Small cell lung cancer (previously untreated):* 120 mg/m² day 1, every 3 weeks. *Non small cell lung cancer (squamous, large cell, and adenocarcinoma previously untreated):* 135 mg/m² day 1, 2, 3, every 3 weeks.

The drug should be given as an i.v. bolus over 3–5 minutes or as an infusion up to 30 minutes. Lower doses (60–75 mg/m² for conventional treatment and 105–120 mg/m² for high dose schedules) are recommended for patients whose bone marrow function has already been impaired by previous chemotherapy or radiotherapy, by age, or neoplastic bone-marrow infiltration. The total dose per cycle may be divided over 2–3 succesive days.

When the drug is used in combination with other anti-tumour agents, the doses need to be adequately reduced. Since the major route of elimination of Pharmorubicin is the hepatobiliary system, the dosage should be reduced in patients with impaired liver function, in order to avoid an increase of overall toxicity. Moderate liver impairment (bilirubin: 1.4–3 mg/100 ml) requires a 50% reduction of dose, while sever impairment (>3 mg/100 ml) necessitates a dose reduction of 75%.

Moderate renal impairment does not appear to require a dose reduction in view of the limited amount of Pharmorubicin excreted by this route.

Intravesical administration: Pharmorubicin can be given by intravesical administration for the treatment of superficial bladder cancer and carcinoma-in-situ. It should not be used in this way for the treatment of invasive tumours which have penetrated the bladder wall where systemic therapy or surgery is more appropriate. Epirubicin has also been successfully used intravesicularly as a prophylactic agent after transurethral resection of superficial tumours in order to prevent recurrences.

While many regimens have been used, the following may be helpful as a guide: for therapy, 8 x weekly instillations of 50 mg/50 ml (diluted with saline or distilled sterile water). In the case of local toxicity (chemical cystitis), a dose reduction to 30 mg/50 ml is advised. For carcinoma-in-situ, depending on the individual tolerability of the patient, the dose may be increased up to 80 mg/50 ml. For prophylaxis, 4 x weekly administrations of 50 mg/ 50 ml followed by 11 x monthly instillations at the same dosage, is the schedule most commonly used.

The solution should be retained intravesically for 1 hour. To avoid undue dilution with urine, the patient should be instructed not to drink any fluid in the 12 hours prior to instillation. During the instillation, the patient should be rotated occasionally and should be instructed to void at the end of the instillation time.

Contra-indications: Pharmorubicin Solution for Injection is contraindicated in patients with marked myelosuppression induced by previous treatments with other anti-tumour agents or by radiotherapy and in patients already treated with maximal cumulative doses of other anthracyclines such as doxorubicin or daunorubicin. The drug is contraindicated in patients with a current or previous history of cardiac impairment.

Special warnings and precautions for use: Pharmorubicin Solution for Injection should be administered only under the supervision of qualified physicians experienced in antiblastic and cytotoxic therapy. Treatment with high dose Pharmorubicin in particular requires the availability of facilities for the care of possible clinical complications due to myelosuppression.

Initial treatment calls for a careful baseline monitoring of various laboratory parameters and cardiac function.

During each cycle of treatment with Pharmorubicin Solution for Injection, patients must be carefully and frequently monitored. Red and white blood cells, neutrophils and platelet counts should be carefuilly assessed both before and during each cycle of therapy. Leukopenia and neutropenia are usually transient with conventional and high-dose schedules, reaching a nadir between the 10th and 14th day and returning to normal values by the 21st day; they are more severe with high dose schedules. Very few patients, even receiving high doses, experience thrombocytopenia (< 100,000 platelets/mm³).

Before starting therapy and if possible during treatment, liver function should be evaluated (SGOT, SGPT, alkaline phosphatase, bilirubin). A cumulative dose of 900–1000 mg/m² should only be exceeded with extreme caution with both conventional and high doses.

Above this level the risk of irreversible congestive cardiac failure increases greatly. There is objective evidence that the cardiac toxicity may occur rarely below this range. However, cardiac function must be carefully monitored during treatment to minimise the risk of heart failure of the type described for other anthracyclines.

Heart failure can appear even several weeks after discontinuing treatment, and may prove unresponsive to specific medical treatment. The potential risk of cardiotoxicity may increase in patients who have received concomitant, or prior, radiotherapy to the mediastinal pericardial area.

In establishing the maximal cumulative doses of Pharmorubicin, any concomitant therapy with potentially cardiotoxic drugs should be taken into account. It is recommended that an ECG before and after each treatment cycle should be carried out. Alterations in the ECG tracing, such as flattening or inversion of the T-wave, depression of the S-T segment, or the onset of arrhythmias, generally transient and reversible, need not necessarily be taken as indications to discontinue treatment.

Cardiomyopathy induced by anthracyclines, is associated with a persitent reduction of the QRS voltage, prolongation beyond normal limits of the systolic interval (PEP/LVET) and a reduction of the ejection fraction. Cardiac monitoring of patients receiving Pharmorubicin treatment is highly important and it is advisable to assess cardiac function by non-invasive techniques such as ECG, echocardiography and, if necessary, measurement of ejection fraction by radionuclide angiography.

Like other cytotoxic agents, Pharmorubicin may induce hyperuricaemia as a result of rapid lysis of neoplastic cells. Blood uric acid levels should therefore be carefully checked so that this phenomenon may be controlled pharmacologically.

Pharmorubicin Solution for Injection may impart a red colour to the urine for 1–2 days after administration.

Interaction with other medicaments and other forms of interaction: It is not recommended that Pharmorubicin Solution for Injection be mixed with other drugs. But Pharmorubicin can be used in combination with other anticancer drugs.

Pregnancy and lactation: There is no conclusive information as to whether epirubicin may adversely affect human fertility or cause teratogenesis. Experimental data, however, suggest that epirubicin may harm the foetus. This product should not normally be administered to patients who are pregnant or to mothers who are breast-feeding. Like most other anti-cancer agents, epirubicin has shown mutagenic and carcinogenic properties in animals.

Effects on ability to drive and use machines: There have been no reports of particular adverse events relating to effects on ability to drive and to use machines.

Undesirable effects: Apart from myelosuppression and cardiotoxicity, the following adverse reactions have been described: Alopecia, normally reversible, appears in 60–90% of treated cases; it is accompanied by lack of beard growth in males. Mucositis may appear 5–10 days after the start of treatment, and usually involves stomatitis with areas of painful erosions, mainly along the side of the tongue and on the sublingual mucosa. Gastro-intestinal disturbances, such as nausea, vomiting and diarrhoea. Hyperpyrexia.

Fever, chills and urticaria have been rarely reported; anaphylaxis may occur.

High doses of Pharmorubicin have been safely administered in a large number of untreated patients having various solid tumours and has caused adverse events which are no different from those seen at conventional doses with the exception of reversible severe neutropenia (<500 neutrophils/mm³ for <7 days) which occurred in the majority of patients. Only a few patients have required hospitalisation and supportive therapy for severe infectious complications at high doses.

During intravesical administration, as drug absorption is minimal, systemic side effects are rare; more frequently chemical cystitis, sometimes haemorrhagic, has been observed.

Haematologic: The occurrence of secondary acute myeloid leukaemia with or without a pre-leukaemic phase has been reported rarely in patients concurrently treated with epirubicin in association with DNA-damaging antineoplastic agents, such cases could have a short (1–3 year) latency period.

Overdose: Very high single doses of epirubicn may be expected to cause acute myocardial degeneration within 24 hours and severe myelosuppression within 10–14 days. Treatment should aim to support the patient during this period and should utilise such measures as blood transfusion and reverse barrier nursing. Delayed cardiac failure has been seen with the anthracyclines up to 6 months after the overdose. Patients should be obserbved carefully and should, if signs of cardiac failure arise, be treated along conventional lines.

Pharmacological properties

Pharmacodynamic properties: The mechanism of action of Pharmorubicin is related to its ability to bind to DNA. Cell culture studies have shown rapid cell penetration, localisation in the nucleus and inhibition of nucleic acid synthesis and mitosis. Pharmorubicin has proved to be active on a wide spectrum of experimental tumours including L1210 and P388 leukaemias, sarcomas SA180 (solid and ascitic forms), B16 melanoma, mammary carcinoma, Lewis lung carcinoma and colon carcinoma 38. It has also shown activity against human tumours transplanted into athymic nude mice (melanoma, mammary, lung, prostatic and ovarian carcinomas).

Pharmacokinetic properties: In patients with normal hepatic and renal function, plasma levels after i.v. injection of 60–150 mg/m² of the drug follow a tri-exponential decreasing pattern with a very fast first phase and a slow terminal phase with a mean half-life of about 40 hours. These doses are within the limits of pharmacokinetic linearity both in terms of plasma clearance values and metabolic pathway. The major metabolites that have been identified are epirubicinol (13-OH epirubicin) and glucuronides of epirubicin and eprirubicinol.

The 4'-O-glucuronidation distinguishes epirubicin from doxorubicin and may account for the faster elimination of epirubicin and its reduced toxicity. Plasma levels of the main metabolite, the 13-OH derivative (epirubicinol) are consistently lower and virtually parallel those of the unchanged drug.

Pharmorubicin is eliminated mainly through the liver; high plasma clearance values (0.9 l/min) indicate that this slow elimination is due to extensive tissue distribution. Urinary excretion accounts for approximately 9–10% of the administered dose in 48 hours.

Biliary excretion represents the major route of elimination, about 40% of the administered dose being recovered in the bile in 72 hours. The drug does not cross the blood brain-barrier.

Preclinical safety data: No further information is given.

Pharmaceutical particulars

List of excipients: Hydrochloric acid PhEur, Sodium chloride PhEur, Water for Injections PhEur

Incompatibilities: Prolonged contact with any solution of an alkaline pH should be avoided as it will result in hydrolysis of the drug.

Pharmorubicin should not be mixed with heparin

due to chemical incompatibility which may lead to precipitation when the drugs are in certain proportions.

Pharmorubicin can be used in combination with other antitumour agents, but it is not recommended that it be mixed with other drugs.

Shelf life:
Glass vials: 36 months.
Polypropylene Cytosafe™ vials: 24 months.

Special precautions for storage: Store at 2°C – 8°C.

Nature and contents of container: Colourless glass 5 ml, 10 ml, 25 ml, or 100 ml vial (type I), with teflon-faced chlorobutyl rubber bung and aluminium cap with inset grey polypropylene disk.

Colourless polypropylene 5 ml, 10 ml, 25 ml or 100 ml vial with Teflon faced halobutyl-rubber stopper and aluminium cap with plastic flip-off top.

Instructions for use/handling: The following protective recommendations are given due to the toxic nature of this substance:

Personnel should be trained in good technique for handling.

Pregnant staff should be excluded from working with this drug.

Personnel handling Pharmorubicin Solution for Injection should wear protective clothing: goggles, gowns and disposable gloves and masks.

All items used for administration or cleaning, including gloves, should be placed in high-risk, waste disposal bags for high temperature incineration.

Spillage or leakage should be treated with dilute sodium hypochlorite (1% available chlorine) solution, preferably by soaking, and then water. All cleaning materials should be disposed of as indicated previously. Accidental contact with the skin or eyes should be treated immediately by copious lavage with water, or soap and water, or sodium bicarbonate solution; medical attention should be sought.

The drug should be used within 24 hours of first penetration of the rubber stopper. Pharmorubicin Solution for Injection should be stored at 2–8°C. Discard any unused solution.

Marketing authorisation number 3433/0135

Date of first authorisation/renewal of authorisation 18 January 1991.

Date of (partial) revision of the text 14 July 1997.

Legal category POM.

PREPIDIL* GEL 500 MICROGRAMS

Presentation Translucent, thixotropic, sterile gel containing 500 micrograms dinoprostone per 3 g (2.5 ml). Also contains silicon dioxide and triacetin.

Uses Pre-induction cervical softening and dilation in pregnant women with at term or near term, gestation and unfavourable induction features, when there are no fetal or maternal contra-indications.

Dosage and administration The entire contents of the syringe are administered into the cervical canal just below the level of the internal cervical os using the accompanying catheter. The patient should be instructed to remain recumbent for 10–15 minutes.

Contra-indications, warnings, etc
Contra-indications: Prepidil Gel 0.5 mg should not be used where the patient is sensitive to prostaglandins or other constituents of the gel.

Prepidil Gel 0.5 mg is not recommended in the following circumstances: For patients in whom oxytocic drugs are generally contra-indicated or where prolonged contractions of the uterus are considered inappropriate such as: cases with a history of Caesarean section or major uterine surgery; cases where there is cephalopelvic disproportion; cases in which fetal malpresentation is present; cases where there is clinical suspicion or definite evidence of pre-existing fetal distress; cases in which there is a history of difficult labour and/or traumatic delivery; grand multiparae with over five previous term pregnancies.

Patients with ruptured membranes.

In patients with a past history of, or existing, pelvic inflammatory disease, unless adequate prior treatment has been instituted.

In patients where there is clinical suspicion or definite evidence of placenta praevia or unexplained vaginal bleeding during this pregnancy.

Patients with active cardiac, pulmonary, renal or hepatic disease.

Special warnings and special precautions for use:
This product is only available to hospitals and clinics with specialised obstetric units and should only be used where 24-hour resident medical cover is provided.

Use the total contents of the syringe for one patient only. Discard after use. Use caution in handling this product to prevent contact with skin. Wash hands thoroughly with soap and water after administration.

Care should be taken not to administer Prepidil Gel 0.5 mg above the level of the internal os, as placement of the gel into the extra-amniotic space has been associated with uterine hyperstimulation.

Caution should be exercised in the administration of Prepidil Gel 0.5 mg in patients with: asthma or a history of asthma; epilepsy or a history of epilepsy; glaucoma or raised intra-ocular pressure; compromised cardiovascular, hepatic or renal function; hypertension.

As with any oxytocic agent, Prepidil Gel 0.5 mg should be used with caution in patients with compromised (scarred) uteri.

Cephalopelvic relationships should be carefully evaluated before use of Prepidil Gel 0.5 mg. During use, uterine activity, fetal status and the cervical dilation and effacement should be carefully monitored to detect possible evidence of undesired responses, e.g. hypertonus, sustained uterine contractions or fetal distress.

In cases where there is a known history of hypertonic uterine contractility or tetanic uterine contractions, it is recommended that uterine activity and the state of the fetus (where applicable) should be continuously monitored throughout labour. The possibility of uterine rupture should be borne in mind where high-tone uterine contractions are sustained.

Animal studies lasting several weeks at high doses have shown that prostaglandins of the E and F series can induce proliferation of bone. Such effects have also been noted in newborn infants who received prostaglandin E_1 during prolonged treatment. There is no evidence that short-term administration of prostaglandin E_2 can cause similar bone effects.

Interaction with other medicaments and other forms of interaction: Since it has been found that prostaglandins potentiate the effect of oxytocin, it is recommended that if these drugs are used in sequence, the patient's uterine activity should be carefully monitored.

Pregnancy and lactation: Prepidil Gel 0.5 mg is only used during pregnancy, for pre-induction of labour.

Prostaglandins are excreted in breast milk. This is not expected to be a hazard given the circumstances in which the product is used.

Effects on ability to drive and use machines: Not applicable

Undesirable effects: The most commonly reported events are vomiting, nausea and diarrhoea. Certain rare events that should be especially noted are: hypersensitivity to the drug; uterine rupture and cardiac arrest. Other adverse events, in decreasing order of severity, reported with use of dinoprostone are: pulmonary/amniotic fluid embolism; abruptio placenta; stillbirth, neonatal death; uterine hypercontractility or hypertonus; fetal distress; hypertension – systemic (maternal); bronchospasm/asthma; rapid cervical dilation; fever; backache; rash; vaginal symptoms – warmth, irritation, pain.

In addition, other adverse reactions that have been seen with the use of prostaglandin E_2 for term labour induction have included: uterine hypercontractility with fetal bradycardia; uterine hypercontractility without fetal bradycardia and low Apgar scores in the newborn.

Overdose: Uterine hypertonus or unduly severe uterine contractions have rarely been encountered, but might be anticipated to result from overdosage. Where there is evidence of fetal distress or uterine hypertonus, then prompt delivery is indicated. Treatment of overdosage must be, at this time, symptomatic, since clinical studies with prostaglandin antagonists have not progressed to the point where recommendations may be made.

Incompatibilities: None known

Pharmaceutical precautions Store in a refrigerator at 2°C–8°C. Use the total contents of the syringe for one patient only. Discard after use.

Legal category POM.

Package quantities Prepidil Gel is supplied as a 2.5 ml pre-filled disposable syringe containing 500 micrograms dinoprostone.

Further information Prepidil Gel exhibits the capacity of other prostaglandins to influence uterine activity at any stage of gestation. Other forms of dinoprostone (Prostin E2) are available for induction of labour (oral, vaginal and i.v. routes), fetal death in utero (i.v. route), therapeutic termination of pregnancy (i.v. and extra-amniotic routes), missed abortion and hydatidiform mole (i.v. route).

Product licence number 0032/0138

PROSTIN* E2 ORAL TABLETS 0.5 mg

Qualitative and quantitative composition Each tablet contains 500 micrograms (0.5 mg) dinoprostone (plus 5% overage).

Pharmaceutical form White, roughly rectangular tablets embossed on one side to resemble the letter 'U' and marked '76' on the other side.

Clinical particulars
Therapeutic indications: Oxytocic. Prostin E2 Oral Tablets 0.5 mg are indicated for the induction of labour when there are no fetal or maternal contra-indications.

Posology and method of administration: Adults: The dosage of Prostin E2 Oral Tablets 0.5 mg must be adapted to the patient's response and should always be maintained at the lowest level which will produce satisfactory uterine response. All doses should be taken with a small glass of water.

An initial dose of 500 micrograms (1 tablet) should be given. Thereafter, doses should be given hourly. The usual dose will be 500 micrograms (1 tablet), but if uterine activity is inadequate, 1 mg (2 tablets) may be given hourly until such time as adequate uterine activity is established. Thereafter, it may be possible to reduce the dosage to 500 micrograms (1 tablet) hourly. It is recommended that a total single dose of 1.5 mg (3 tablets) is not exceeded.

Elderly: Not applicable

Children: Not applicable

Contra-indications: Prostin E2 Oral Tablets 0.5 mg should not be used where the patient is sensitive to prostaglandins or any other constituents of the tablet.

Prostin E2 Oral Tablets 0.5 mg are not recommended in the following circumstances:

For patients in whom oxytocic drugs are generally contra-indicated or where prolonged contractions of the uterus are considered inappropriate such as: cases with a history of Caesarean section or major uterine surgery; cases where there is cephalopelvic disproportion; cases in which fetal malpresentation is present; cases where there is clinical suspicion or definite evidence of pre-existing fetal distress; cases in which there is a history of difficult labour and/or traumatic delivery; grand multiparae with over five previous term pregnancies.

In patients with a past history of, or existing, pelvic inflammatory disease, unless adequate prior treatment has been instituted.

In patients where there is clinical suspicion or definite evidence of placenta praevia or unexplained vaginal bleeding during this pregnancy.

Patients with active cardiac, pulmonary, renal or hepatic disease.

Special warnings and special precautions for use: This product is only available to hospitals and clinics with specialised obstetric units and should only be used where 24-hour resident medical cover is provided.

Use caution in handling this product to prevent contact with skin. Wash hands thoroughly with soap and water after administration.

Caution should be exercised in the administration of Prostin E2 Oral Tablets 0.5 mg for the induction of labour in patients with: asthma or a history of asthma; epilepsy or a history of epilepsy; glaucoma or raised intra-ocular pressure; compromised cardiovascular, hepatic, or renal function; hypertension

As with any oxytocic agent, Prostin E2 Oral Tablets 0.5 mg should be used with caution in patients with compromised (scarred) uteri.

In labour induction, cephalopelvic relationships should be carefully evaluated before use of Prostin E2 Oral Tablets 0.5 mg. During use, uterine activity, fetal status and the progression of cervical dilation should be carefully monitored to detect possible evidence of undesired responses, e.g. hypertonus, sustained uterine contractions or fetal distress. In cases where there is a known history of hypertonic uterine contractility or tetanic uterine contractions, it is recommended that uterine activity and the state of the fetus (where applicable) should be continuously monitored throughout labour. The possibility of uterine rupture should be borne in mind where high-tone uterine contractions are sustained.

Animal studies lasting several weeks at high doses have shown that prostaglandins of the E and F series can induce proliferation of bone. Such effects have also been noted in newborn infants who received prostaglandin E_1 during prolonged treatment. There is no evidence that short-term administration of prostaglandin E_2 can cause similar bone effects.

Interaction with other medicaments and other forms of interaction: Since it has been found that prostaglandins potentiate the effect of oxytocin, it is not recommended that these drugs are used together. If used in sequence, the patient's uterine activity should be carefully monitored.

Pregnancy and lactation: Pregnancy Code A

Prostin E2 Oral Tablets 0.5 mg are only used during pregnancy, to induce labour.

Prostaglandins are excreted in breast milk. This is not expected to be a hazard given the circumstances in which the product is used.

Effects on ability to drive and use machines: Not applicable

Undesirable effects: The most commonly reported events are vomiting, nausea and diarrhoea. Certain rare events that should be especially noted are: hypersensitivity to the drug; uterine rupture and cardiac arrest. Other adverse events, in decreasing order of severity, reported with use of dinoprostone are: pulmonary/amniotic fluid embolism; abruptio placenta; stillbirth, neonatal death; uterine hypercontractility or hypertonus; fetal distress; hypertension – systemic (maternal); bronchospasm/asthma; rapid cervical dilation; fever; backache; rash.

In addition, other adverse reactions that have been seen with the use of prostaglandin E_2 for term labour induction have included: altered fetal heart rate patterns; uterine hypercontractility with fetal bradycardia; uterine hypercontractility without fetal bradycardia and low Apgar scores in the newborn.

Overdose: Uterine hypertonus or unduly severe uterine contractions have rarely been encountered, but might be anticipated to result from overdosage. Where there is evidence of fetal distress or uterine hypertonus, then prompt delivery is indicated. Treatment of overdosage must be, at this time, symptomatic, since clinical studies with prostaglandin antagonists have not progressed to the point where recommendations may be made. It is currently believed that vomiting produced by overdosage may act as a self-limiting factor in protecting the patient.

Pharmacological properties

Pharmacodynamic properties: Dinoprostone is a prostaglandin of the E series with actions on smooth muscle; the endogenous substance is termed prostaglandin E2 (PGE_2). It induces contraction of uterine muscle at any stage of pregnancy and is reported to act predominantly as a vasodilator on blood vessels and as a bronchodilator on bronchial muscle.

Pharmacokinetic properties: General characteristics of active substance

Following ingestion of the tablet, PGE_2 absorption (as measured by the presence of PGE_2 metabolites) was detectable at 15 minutes, with a peak level occurring at about 45 minutes after the first oral dose. There was little evidence of accumulative effects when a second dose was administered after one hour.

There is a possibility that oral prostaglandin E_2 is converted in the stomach into prostaglandin A_2 and subsequently into its metabolites, which may contribute to uterine action.

There has been found to be considerable inter-patient variability in the time courses and in the absolute levels of PGE_2 metabolites in plasma following the administration of oral PGE_2 tablets. This seems likely to reflect differences in the rates of absorption of PGE_2 and in its metabolic transformations, but it may also incorporate varying contributions from endogenous prostaglandin production–although this is unlikely to be significant.

Characteristics in patients: No special characteristics. See 'Special warnings and special precautions for use' for further information.

Preclinical safety data: In mice and rats, the oral LD_{50} values were >500 mg/kg and 141–513 mg/kg respectively.

Three month oral administration to rats resulted in significantly heavier stomach weights for treated compared with untreated rats, which effect was reversible on treatment cessation. Treated rats had a dose related acanthotic squamous glandular junction and thickened glandular gastric mucosal epithelium. No significant alterations were recognized in routine evaluation of the sternebrae and the femur.

A fourteen day oral toxicity study in dogs showed a maximum tolerated dose of 6–20 mg/kg/day. All treated dogs had microscopic evidence of increased fundic and pyloric mucus. The fundic and pyloric mucosa were thickened, having a cobblestone appearance and had an increased gastric mucus in both 20 mg/kg/day treated dogs and the 60 mg/kg/day male dog. These were the only gross and microscopic drug related changes observed.

Satisfactory results were obtained in intravenous and intramuscular tolerability tests performed in dog and monkey.

Teratogenic effects were observed in rats injected subcutaneously with 0.5 mg/animal. No teratogenic effects were seen in the rabbit at dosage levels of up to 1.5 mg/kg day.

No evidence of mutagenicity was obtained using the Ames Assay, the DNA Damage/Alkaline Elution Assay and the micronucleus test.

Pharmaceutical particulars

List of excipients: Lactose, microcrystalline cellulose, maize starch, magnesium stearate and colloidal silicon dioxide.

Incompatibilities: None known.

Shelf life: Prostin E2 Oral Tablets 0.5 mg have a shelf-life of 24 months when stored at 4°C.

Special precautions for product and admixture storage: Store in a refrigerator. The tablets should be used within three months of opening the bottle.

Nature and contents of container: Amber glass bottle with screw cap and tac seal. Each bottle contains a desiccant capsule.

Instructions for use/handling: Use caution in handling this product to prevent contact with skin. Wash hands thoroughly with soap and water after administration.

Marketing authorisation number 0032/0040R

Date of renewal of authorisation 21 February 1996.

Date of revision of the text September 1995.

Legal category POM

PROSTIN* E2 STERILE SOLUTION 1 mg/ml

Presentation Colourless, sterile solution containing 1 mg/ml dinoprostone (prostaglandin E2). Also contains ethanol.

Uses

Indications: Oxytocic agent. Prostin E2 Sterile Solution 1 mg/ml is indicated for the induction of labour.

Mechanism of action: Dinoprostone induces contraction of uterine muscle.

Pharmacology: Dinoprostone is a prostaglandin of the E series with actions on smooth muscle. It induces contraction of uterine muscle at any stage of labour.

Pharmacokinetics: Dinoprostone is rapidly metabolised in the body. Intravenous administration results in very rapid distribution and metabolism, with only 3% of unchanged drug remaining in the blood after 15 minutes. At least nine prostaglandin E2 metabolites have been identified in human blood and urine.

Dosage and administration Prostin E2 Sterile Solution 1 mg/ml is administered by the intravenous route.

The ampoule contents must be diluted before use and full instructions on method of dilution and dosage are given on the package insert which should be consulted prior to initiation of therapy. The dose of Prostin E2 used, normally depends not only upon the indication, but also on patient response.

The following is a guide to dosage:

Dilute with normal saline or 5% dextrose according to the package insert to produce a 1.5 micrograms/ml solution. The 1.5 micrograms/ml solution is infused at 0.25 micrograms/minute for 30 minutes and then maintained or increased. Cases of fetal death *in utero* may require higher doses. An initial rate of 0.5 micrograms/minute may be used with stepwise increases, at intervals of not less than one hour.

The appearance of fetal distress or uterine hypertonus requires cessation of therapy until the state returns to normal. The situation should be re-assessed and, if necessary, the infusion can be recommenced but at lower dosage rates, 50% of the last dose level used.

If no response is seen within the first 12–24 hours of treatment, the medication should be discontinued.

Children and elderly patients: Not applicable

Contra-indications, warnings etc

Contra-indications: Prostin E2 Sterile Solution 1 mg/ml should not be used where the patient is sensitive to prostaglandins.

Prostin E2 Sterile Solution 1 mg/ml is not recommended in the following circumstances:

For patients in whom oxytocic drugs are generally contra-indicated or where prolonged contractions of the uterus are considered inappropriate, such as: cases with a history of Caesarean section or major uterine surgery; cases in which there is cephalopelvic disproportion; cases in which fetal malpresentation is present; cases in which there is clinical suspicion or definite evidence of pre-existing fetal distress; cases in which there is a history of difficult labour and/or traumatic delivery; grand multiparae with six or more previous term pregnancies.

In patients with a past history of, or existing, pelvic inflammatory disease, unless adequate prior treatment has been instituted.

In patients where there is clinical suspicion or definite evidence of placenta praevia or unexplained vaginal bleeding during this pregnancy.

Patients with active cardiac, pulmonary, renal or hepatic disease.

Interaction with other medicaments and other forms of interaction: Since it has been found that prostaglandins potentiate the effect of oxytocin, it is not recommended that these drugs are used together. If used in sequence, the patient's uterine activity should be carefully monitored.

Effects on ability to drive and use machines: Not applicable.

Other undesirable effects: The most commonly reported events are vomiting, nausea and diarrhoea. Certain rare events that should be especially noted are: hypersensitivity to the drug; uterine rupture and cardiac arrest. Other adverse events,in decreasing order of severity, reported with use of dinoprostone are: Pulmonary/amniotic fluid embolism; abruptio placenta; stillbirth, neonatal death; uterine hypercontractility or hypertonus; fetal distress; hypertension – systemic (maternal); bronchospasm/asthma; rapid cervical dilation; fever; back ache; rash.

Transient vasovagal symptoms , including flushing, shivering, headache and dizziness, have been recorded with intravenous use of Prostin E2. Local tissue irritation and erythema have occurred. No evidence of thrombophlebitis has been recorded and local tissue erythema at the infusion site has disappeared within two to five hours after infusion. A temporary pyrexia and elevated WBC are not unusual, but both have reverted after termination of infusion.

In addition, other adverse reactions that have been seen with the use of prostaglandin E_2 for term labour induction have included: altered fetal heart rate patterns; uterine hypercontractility with fetal bradycardia; uterine hypercontractility without fetal bradycardia and low Apgar scores in the newborn.

Use in pregnancy and lactation: Prostin E2 Sterile Solution 1 mg/ml is only used during pregnancy, to induce labour.

Prostaglandins are excreted in breast milk. This is not expected to be a hazard given the circumstances in which the product is used.

Other special warnings and precautions:

Warnings: This product is available only to hospitals and clinics with specialised obstetric units and should only be used where 24-hour resident medical cover is provided.

It is advised that Prostin E2 Sterile Solution 1 mg/ml should not be administered by the intramyometrial route since there have been reports of a possible association between this route of administration and cardiac arrest in severely ill patients.

Precautions: Use caution in handling this product to prevent contact with skin. Wash hands thoroughly with soap and water after administration. Caution should be exercised in the administration of Prostin E2 Sterile Solution 1 mg/ml for the induction of labour in patients with: asthma or a history of asthma; epilepsy or a history of epilepsy; glaucoma or raised intra-ocular pressure; compromised cardiovascular, hepatic or renal function; hypertension.

As with any oxytocic agent, Prostin E2 Sterile Solution should be used with caution in patients with compromised (scarred) uteri.

In labour induction, cephalopelvic relationships should be carefully evaluated before use of Prostin E2 Sterile Solution 1 mg/ml. During use, uterine activity, fetal status and the progression of cervical dilation should be carefully monitored to detect possible evidence of undesired responses, e.g. hypertonus, sustained uterine contractions or fetal distress.

In cases where there is a known history of hypertonic uterine contractility or tetanic uterine contractions, it is recommended that uterine activity and the state of the fetus (where applicable) should be continuously monitored throughout labour. The possibility of uterine rupture should be borne in mind where high-tone uterine contractions are sustained.

Animal studies lasting several weeks at high doses have shown that prostaglandins of the E and F series can induce proliferation of bone. Such effects have also been noted in newborn infants who received prostaglandin E_1 during prolonged treatment. There is no evidence that short-term administration of prostaglandin E_2 can cause similar bone effects.

Overdose: Uterine hypertonus or unduly severe uterine contractions have rarely been encountered, but might be anticipated to result from overdosage. In the rare instance where temporary discontinuation of therapy is not effective in reversing fetal distress or uterine hypertonus, then prompt delivery is indicated. Treatment of overdosage must be, at this time, symptomatic, since clinical studies with prostaglandin antagonists have not progressed to the point where recommendations may be made.

Incompatibilities: None known.

Pharmaceutical precautions Prostin E2 Sterile Solution 1 mg/ml must be refrigerated at 4°C. It should be diluted before use only with the diluents stated. Diluted solutions should be used within 24 hours (48 hours for extra-amniotic).

Legal category POM.

Package quantities Pack containing 1 x 0.75 ml ampoule of Prostin E2 Sterile Solution 1 mg/ml.

Further information Oral Prostin E2 Tablets, Prostin

E2 Vaginal Tablets and Prostin E2 Vaginal Gel are also available for the induction of labour.

Product licence number 0032/0020R.

PROSTIN* E2 STERILE SOLUTION 10 mg/ml

Presentation Colourless sterile solution containing 10 mg/ml dinoprostone (prostaglandin E2). Also contains ethanol.

Uses

Indications: Oxytocic agent. Prostin E2 Sterile Solution 10 mg/ml is indicated for the therapeutic termination of pregnancy, missed abortion and hydatidiform mole.

Mechanism of action: Dinoprostone induces contraction of uterine muscle

Pharmacology: Dinoprostone is a prostaglandin of the E series with actions on smooth muscle. It induces contraction of uterine muscle at any stage of labour.

Pharmacokinetics: Dinoprostone is rapidly metabolised in the body. Intravenous administration results in very rapid distribution and metabolism, with only 3% of unchanged drug remaining in the blood after 15 minutes. At least nine prostaglandin E2 metabolites have been identified in human blood and urine.

Dosage and administration Prostin E2 Sterile Solution 10 mg/ml is administered by the intravenous route.

The ampoule contents must be diluted before use and full instructions on method of dilution and dosage are given in the package insert which should be consulted prior to initiation of therapy. The dose of Prostin E2 Sterile Solution 10 mg/ml used, normally depends not only upon the indication, but also on patient response. Increase in dosage above that recommended is possible, but may produce excessive uterine activity and be governed by the unacceptable appearance of dose-related side-effects, such as nausea and vomiting.

The following is a guide to dosage:

Dilute with normal saline or 5% dextrose according to package insert to produce a 5 micrograms/ml solution. The 5 micrograms/ml solution is infused at 2.5 micrograms/minute for 30 minutes and then maintained or increased to 5 micrograms/minute. The rate should be maintained for at least four hours before increasing further.

Continuous administration of the drug for more than 2 days is not recommended.

Children and elderly patients: Not applicable.

Contra-indications, warnings etc

Contra-indications: Prostin E2 Sterile Solution 10 mg/ml should not be used where the patient is sensitive to prostaglandins.

Prostin E2 Sterile Solution 10 mg/ml is not recommended in the following circumstances:

For patients in whom oxytocic drugs are generally contra-indicated or where prolonged contractions of the uterus are considered inappropriate such as: cases with a history of Caesarean section or major uterine surgery; cases where there is evidence of a potential for obstructed labour;

In therapeutic termination of pregnancy where known pelvic infection exists, unless adequate prior treatment has been instituted.

Patients with active cardiac, pulmonary, renal or hepatic disease.

Interaction with other medicaments and other forms of interaction: Since it has been found that prostaglandins potentiate the effect of oxytocin, it is not recommended that these drugs are used together. If used in sequence, the patient's uterine activity should be carefully monitored.

Effects on ability to drive and use machines: Not applicable.

Other undesirable effects: The most commonly reported events are vomiting, nausea and diarrhoea. Certain rare events that should be especially noted are: hypersensitivity to the drug; uterine rupture; and cardiac arrest. Other adverse events, in decreasing order of severity, reported with use of dinoprostone are: pulmonary/amniotic fluid embolism; uterine hypercontractility or hypertonus; hypertension – systemic (maternal); bronchospasm/asthma; rapid cervical dilation; fever; back ache; rash.

In addition, with intravenous use, transient vasovagal symptoms, including flushing, shivering, headache and dizziness, have been recorded. Local tissue irritation and erythema have occurred. No evidence of thrombophlebitis has been recorded and local tissue erythema at the infusion site has disappeared within two to five hours after infusion. A temporary pyrexia and elevated WBC are not unusual, but both have reverted after termination of infusion.

Use in pregnancy and lactation: Prostin E2 Sterile Solution 10 mg/ml is only used during pregnancy for therapeutic termination of pregnancy, missed abortion and hydatidiform mole. There has been some evidence in animals of a low order of teratogenic activity, Therefore, if abortion does not occur or is suspected to be incomplete as a result of prostaglandin therapy, (as in spontaneous abortion, where the process is sometimes incomplete), the appropriate treatment for complete evacuation of the pregnant uterus should be instituted in all instances.

Prostaglandins are excreted in breast milk. This is not expected to be a hazard given the circumstances in which the product is used.

Other special warnings and precautions:
Warnings: This product is only available to hospitals and clinics with specialised obstetric units and should only be used where 24-hour resident medical cover is provided.

It is advised that Prostin E2 Sterile Solution should not be administered by the intramyometrial route since there have been reports of a possible association between this route of administration and cardiac arrest in severely ill patients.

Precautions: Use caution in handling this product to prevent contact with skin. Wash hands thoroughly with soap and water after administration.

Caution should be exercised in the administration of Prostin E2 Sterile Solution 10 mg/ml to patients with asthma or a history of asthma; epilepsy or a history of epilepsy; glaucoma or raised intra-ocular pressure; compromised cardiovascular, hepatic or renal function; hypertension.

As with any oxytocic agent, Prostin E2 should be used with caution in patients with compromised (scarred) uteri.

Animal studies lasting several weeks at high doses have shown that prostaglandins of the E and F series can induce proliferation of bone. Such effects have also been noted in newborn infants who received prostaglandin E_1 during prolonged treatment. There is no evidence that short-term administration of prostaglandin E_2 can cause similar bone effects.

Overdosage: Uterine hypertonus or unduly severe uterine contractions have rarely been encountered, but might be anticipated to result from overdosage. Treatment of overdosage must be, at this time, symptomatic, as clinical studies with prostaglandin antagonists have not progressed to the point where recommendations may be made. If evidence of excessive uterine activity or side-effects appears, the rate of infusion should be decreased or discontinued. In cases of massive overdosage resulting in extreme uterine hypertonus, appropriate obstetric procedures are indicated.

Pharmaceutical precautions Prostin E2 Sterile Solution 10 mg/ml must be refrigerated at 4°C. It should be diluted before use only with the diluents stated. Diluted solutions should be used within 24 hours.

Legal category POM.

Package quantities Pack containing 1×0.5 ml ampoule of Prostin E2 Sterile Solution 10 mg/ml.

Product licence numbers 0032/0021R.

PROSTIN* E2 STERILE SOLUTION 10 mg/ml (EXTRA-AMNIOTIC PACK)

Qualitative and quantitative composition Each ml contains 10 mg dinoprostone.

Pharmaceutical form Colourless, sterile solution, which after appropriate dilution is intended for extra-amniotic administration to human beings.

Clinical particulars

Therapeutic indications: Oxytocic agent. The therapeutic termination of pregnancy by the extra-amniotic route.

Posology and method of administration:
Adults: Ampoule contents must be diluted before use and full instructions on method of dilution and dosage are given on the package insert which should be consulted prior to initiation of therapy. The following is a guide to dosage:

Dilute with the 50 ml of diluent provided according to the package insert to produce a 100 micrograms/ml solution. The 100 micrograms/ml solution is instilled via a 12–14 french gauge foley catheter. Initial instillation is 1 ml, then dependent on uterine response, 1 or 2 ml usually at two hour intervals.

Elderly: Not applicable. *Children:* Not applicable.

Contra-indications: Prostin E2 Sterile Solution should not be used where the patient is sensitive to prostaglandins.

Prostin E2 Sterile Solution 10 mg/ml is not recommended in the following circumstances:

For patients in whom oxytocic drugs are generally contra-indicated or where prolonged contractions of the uterus are considered inappropriate such as: Cases with a history of Caesarean section or major uterine surgery; Cases where there is evidence of a potential for obstructed labour;

In patients with a past history of, or existing, pelvic inflammatory disease, unless adequate prior treatment has been instituted.

In patients with cervicitis or vaginal infections.

Patients with active cardiac, pulmonary, renal or hepatic disease.

Special warnings and special precautions for use
This product is only available to hospitals and clinics with specialised obstetric units and should only be used where 24-hour resident medical cover is provided

Use caution in handling this product to prevent contact with skin. Wash hands thoroughly with soap and water after administration.

It is advised that Prostin E2 Sterile Solution should not be administered by the intramyometrial route since there have been reports of a possible association between this route of administration and cardiac arrest in severely ill patients.

Caution should be exercised in the administration of Prostin E2 Sterile Solution to patients with:
(i) asthma or a history of asthma;
(ii) epilepsy or a history of epilepsy;
(iii) glaucoma or raised intra-ocular pressure;
(iv) compromised cardiovascular, hepatic, or renal function;
(v) hypertension.

As with any oxytocic agent, Prostin E2 Sterile Solution should be used with caution in patients with compromised (scarred) uteri.

Animal studies lasting several weeks at high doses have shown that prostaglandins of E and F series can induce proliferation of bone. Such effects have also been noted in newborn infants who received prostaglandin E_1 during prolonged treatment. There is no evidence that short-term administration of prostaglandin E_2 can cause similar bone effects.

Interaction with other medicaments and other forms of interaction : Since it has been found that prostaglandins potentiate the effect of oxytocin, it is not recommended that these drugs are used together. If used in sequence, the patient's uterine activity should be carefully monitored.

Pregnancy and lactation: Pregnancy Code D: Prostin E2 Sterile Solution 10 mg/ml is only used during pregnancy for therapeutic termination of pregnancy. There has been some evidence in animals of a low order of teratogenic activity, therefore, if abortion does not occur or is suspected to be incomplete as a result of prostaglandin therapy, (as in spontaneous abortion, where the process is sometimes incomplete), the appropriate treatment for complete evacuation of the pregnant uterus should be instituted in all instances.

Prostaglandins are excreted in breast milk. This is not expected to be a hazard given the circumstances in which the product is used.

Effects on ability to drive and use machines: Not applicable.

Undesirable effects: The most commonly reported events are vomiting, nausea and diarrhoea. Certain rare events that should be especially noted are: hypersensitivity to the drug; uterine rupture; and cardiac arrest. Other adverse events, in decreasing order of severity, reported with use of dinoprostone are: Pulmonary/amniotic fluid embolism; Uterine hypercontractility or hypertonus; Hypertension–systemic maternal); Bronchospasm/asthma; Rapid cervical dilation; Fever; Back ache; Rash.

A temporary pyrexia and elevated WBC are not unusual, but both have reverted after termination of therapy. In extra-amniotic therapy, the possibility of local infection must be considered and appropriate therapy initiated if necessary.

Overdose: Uterine hypertonus or unduly severe uterine contractions have rarely been encountered, but might be anticipated to result from overdosage. Treatment of overdosage must be, at this time, symptomatic, as clinical studies with prostaglandin antagonists have not progressed to the point where recommendations may be made. If evidence of excessive uterine activity or side-effects appears, the rate of infusion should be decreased or discontinued. In cases of massive overdosage resulting in extreme uterine hypertonus, appropriate obstetric procedures are indicated.

Pharmacological properties

Pharmacodynamic properties: Dinoprostone is a prostaglandin of the E series with actions on smooth muscle. It induces contraction of uterine muscle at any stage of pregnancy.

Pharmacokinetic properties:
General characteristics of active substance: Dinopro-

stone is rapidly metabolised in the body. Intravenous administration results in very rapid distribution and metabolism, with only 3% of unchanged drug remaining in the blood after 15 minutes. At least nine prostaglandin E_2 metabolites have been identified in human blood and urine.

Characteristics in patients: No special characteristics. See 'Special warnings and special precautions for use' for further information.

Preclinical safety data: In mice and rats, the oral LD_{50} values were >500 mg/kg and 141–513 mg/kg respectively.

Three month oral administration to rats resulted in significantly heavier stomach weights for treated compared with untreated rats, which effect was reversible on treatment cessation. Treated rats had a dose related acanthotic squamous glandular junction and thickened glandular gastric mucosal epithelium. No significant alterations were recognized in routine evaluation of the sternebrae and the femur.

A fourteen day oral toxicity study in dogs showed a maximum tolerated dose of 6–20 mg/kg/day. All treated dogs had microscopic evidence of increased fundic and pyloric mucus. The fundic and pyloric mucosa were thickened, having a cobblestone appearance and had an increased gastric mucus in both 20 mg/kg/day treated dogs and the 60 mg/kg/day male dog. These were the only gross and microscopic drug related changes observed.

Satisfactory results were obtained in intravenous and intramuscular tolerability tests performed in dog and monkey.

Teratogenic effects were observed in rats injected subcutaneously with 0.5 mg/animal. No teratogenic effects were seen in the rabbit at dosage levels of up to 1.5 mg/kg day.

No evidence of mutagenicity was obtained using the Ames Assay, the DNA Damage/Alkaline Elution Assay and the micronucleus test.

Pharmaceutical particulars
List of excipients: Dehydrated alcohol BP.

Incompatibilities: None known.

Shelf life: 24 months.

Special precautions for product and admixture storage: Store in a refrigerator at 4°C. Once diluted, the diluted solution should be stored in a refrigerator and used within 48 hours.

Nature and contents of container: PhEur. Type I glass ampoule, containing 0.5 ml sterile solution, packed in a carton, together with a vial containing diluent.

Instructions for use/handling: Use caution in handling this product to prevent contact with skin. Wash hands thoroughly with soap and water after administration.

Marketing authorisation number 0032/0026R

Date of first authorisation/renewal of authorisation
Date of Grant: 1 July 1986
Date of Renewal: 18 March 1997

Date of revision of the text March 1997.

Legal category POM.

PROSTIN* E2 VAGINAL GEL 1 mg AND 2 mg

Presentation Translucent thixotropic gel containing 1 or 2 mg dinoprostone per 3 g (2.5 ml). Also contains silicon dioxide and triacetin.

Uses Oxytocic. Prostin E2 Vaginal Gel is indicated for the induction of labour, when there are no fetal or maternal contra-indications.

Dosage and administration
In primigravida patients with unfavourable induction features (Bishop score of 4 or less), an initial dose of 2 mg should be administered vaginally. In other patients an initial dose of 1 mg should be administered vaginally.

In both groups of patients, a second dose of 1 mg or 2 mg may be administered after 6 hours as follows:

1 mg should be used where uterine activity is insufficient for satisfactory progress of labour.

2 mg may be used where response to the initial dose has been minimal.

Maximum dose 4 mg in unfavourable primigravida patients or 3 mg in other patients (see 'Precautions').

The gel should be inserted high into the posterior fornix avoiding administration into the cervical canal. The patient should be instructed to remain recumbent for at least 30 minutes.

Contra-indications, warnings, etc
Contra-indications: Prostin E2 Vaginal Gel should not be used where the patient is sensitive to prostaglandins or other constituents of the gel.

Prostin E2 Vaginal Gel is not recommended in the following circumstances: For patients in whom oxytocic drugs are generally contra-indicated or where prolonged contractions of the uterus are considered inappropriate such as: cases with a history of caesarean section or major uterine surgery; cases where there is cephalopelvic disproportion; cases in which fetal malpresentation is present; cases where there is clinical suspicion or definite evidence of pre-existing fetal distress; cases in which there is a history of difficult labour and/or traumatic delivery; grand multiparae with over five previous term pregnancies.

Patients with ruptured membranes.

In patients with a past history of, or existing, pelvic inflammatory disease, unless adequate prior treatment has been instituted.

In patients where there is clinical suspicion or definite evidence of placenta praevia or unexplained vaginal bleeding during this pregnancy.

Patients with active cardiac, pulmonary, renal or hepatic disease.

Interaction with other medicaments and other forms of interaction: Since it has been found that prostaglandins potentiate the effect of oxytocin, it is not recommended that these drugs are used together. If used in sequence, the patient's uterine activity should be carefully monitored.

Effects on ability to drive and use machines: Not applicable.

Other undesirable effects (frequency and seriousness): The most commonly reported events are vomiting, nausea and diarrhoea. Certain rare events that should be especially noted are: hypersensitivity to the drug; uterine rupture and cardiac arrest. Other adverse events, in decreasing order of severity, reported with use of dinoprostone, are: pulmonary/amniotic fluid embolism; abruptio placenta; stillbirth, neonatal death; uterine hypercontractility or hypertonus; fetal distress; hypertension – systemic (maternal); bronchospasm/asthma; rapid cervical dilation; fever; back ache; rash; vaginal symptoms – warmth, irritation, pain.

In addition, other adverse reactions that have been seen with the use of prostaglandin E_2 for term labour induction have included: altered fetal heart rate patterns; uterine hypercontractility with fetal bradycardia; uterine hypercontractility without fetal bradycardia and low Apgar scores in the newborn.

Use in pregnancy and lactation: Prostin E2 Vaginal Gel is only used during pregnancy, to induce labour.

Prostaglandins are excreted in breast milk. This is not expected to be a hazard given the circumstances in which the product is used.

Other special warnings and precautions: This product is only available to hospitals and clinics with specialised obstetric units and should only be used where 24- hour resident medical cover is provided.

Use the total contents of the syringe for one patient only. Discard after use. Use caution in handling this product to prevent contact with skin. Wash hands thoroughly with soap and water after administration.

Prostin E2 Vaginal Gel and Prostin E2 Vaginal Tablets are not bioequivalent.

Caution should be exercised in the administration of Prostin E2 Vaginal Gel for the induction of labour in patients with: asthma or a history of asthma; epilepsy or a history of epilepsy; glaucoma or raised intra-ocular pressure; compromised cardiovascular, hepatic, or renal function; hypertension.

As with any oxytocic agent, Prostin E2 Vaginal Gel should be used with caution in patients with compromised (scarred) uteri.

In labour induction, cephalopelvic relationships should be carefully evaluated before use of Prostin E2 Vaginal Gel. During use, uterine activity, fetal status and the progression of cervical dilation should be carefully monitored to detect possible evidence of undesired responses, e.g. hypertonus, sustained uterine contractions or fetal distress.

In cases where there is a known history of hypertonic uterine contractility or tetanic uterine contractions, it is recommended that uterine activity and the state of the fetus (where applicable) should be continuously monitored throughout labour. The possibility of uterine rupture should be borne in mind where high-tone uterine contractions are sustained.

Animal studies lasting several weeks at high doses have shown that prostaglandins of the E and F series can induce proliferation of bone. Such effects have also been noted in newborn infants who received prostaglandin E_1 during prolonged treatment. There is no evidence that short-term administration of prostaglandin E_2 can cause similar bone effects.

Overdose: Uterine hypertonus or unduly severe uterine contractions have rarely been encountered, but might be anticipated to result from overdosage. Where there is evidence of fetal distress or uterine hypertonus, then prompt delivery is indicated. Treatment of overdosage must be, at this time, symptomatic, since clinical studies with prostaglandin antagonists have not progressed to the point where recommendations may be made.

Incompatibilities: None known.

Pharmaceutical precautions Store in a refrigerator at 2–8°C. The contents of one syringe to be used for one patient. Discard after use.

Legal category POM.

Package quantities Prostin E2 Vaginal Gel is available in single packs of 1 mg or 2 mg.

Further information Unlike other oxytocics, Prostin E2 exhibits the capacity of the prostaglandins to influence uterine activity at any stage of gestation. Other Prostin E2 dosage forms are available for induction of labour (oral, vaginal and i.v. routes), foetal death in utero (i.v. route), therapeutic termination of pregnancy (i.v. and extra-amniotic routes), missed abortion and hydatidiform mole (i.v. route).

Product licence numbers
Prostin E2 Vaginal Gel 1 mg 0032/0123
Prostin E2 Vaginal Gel 2 mg 0032/0124

PROSTIN* E2 VAGINAL TABLETS

Presentation Prostin E2 Vaginal Tablets are presented as white, biconvex, oblong tablets with radiused corners marked 'UPJOHN' and '715' on one side. Each tablet contains 3 mg dinoprostone. Also contains: lactose, microcrystalline cellulose, silicon dioxide, maize starch and magnesium stearate.

Uses Oxytocic. Prostin E2 Vaginal Tablets are indicated for the induction of labour, especially in patients with favourable induction features, when there are no fetal or maternal contra-indications.

Dosage and administration One tablet (3 mg) to be inserted high into the posterior fornix. A second tablet may be inserted after six to eight hours if labour is not established. Maximum dose 6 mg.

Contra-indications, warnings, etc
Contra-indications: Prostin E2 Vaginal Tablets should not be used where the patient is sensitive to prostaglandins or other constituents of the tablet.

Prostin E2 Vaginal Tablets are not recommended in the following circumstances: For patients in whom oxytocic drugs are generally contra-indicated or where prolonged contractions of the uterus are considered inappropriate such as: cases with a history of caesarean section or major uterine surgery; cases where there is cephalopelvic disproportion; cases in which fetal malpresentation is present; cases where there is clinical suspicion or definite evidence of pre-existing fetal distress; cases in which there is a history of difficult labour and/or traumatic delivery; grand multiparae with over five previous term pregnancies.

Patients with ruptured membranes.

In patients with a past history of, or existing, pelvic inflammatory disease, unless adequate prior treatment has been instituted.

In patients where there is clinical suspicion or definite evidence of placenta praevia or unexplained vaginal bleeding during this pregnancy.

Patients with active cardiac, pulmonary, renal or hepatic disease.

Interaction with other medicaments and other forms of interaction: Since it has been found that prostaglandins potentiate the effect of oxytocin, it is not recommended that these drugs are used together. If used in sequence, the patient's uterine activity should be carefully monitored.

Effects on ability to drive and use machines: Not applicable.

Other undesirable effects (frequency and seriousness): The most commonly reported events are vomiting, nausea and diarrhoea. Certain rare events that should be especially noted are: hypersensitivity to the drug; uterine rupture and cardiac arrest. Other adverse events, in decreasing order of severity, reported with use of dinoprostone, are: pulmonary/amniotic fluid embolism; abruptio placenta; stillbirth, neonatal death; uterine hypercontractility or hypertonus; fetal distress; hypertension– systemic (maternal); bronchospasm/asthma; rapid cervical dilation; fever; back ache; rash; vaginal symptoms – warmth, irritation, pain.

In addition, other adverse reactions that have been seen with the use of prostaglandin E_2 for term labour induction have included: altered fetal heart rate patterns; uterine hypercontractility with fetal bradycardia; uterine hypercontractility without fetal bradycardia and low Apgar scores in the newborn.

Use in pregnancy and lactation: Prostin E2 Vaginal Tablets are only used during pregnancy, to induce labour.

Prostaglandins are excreted in breast milk. This is not expected to be a hazard given the circumstances in which the product is used.

Other special warnings and precautions: This product is only available to hospitals and clinics with specialised obstetric units and should only be used where 24- hour resident medical cover is provided.

Use caution in handling the product to prevent contact with skin. Wash hands thoroughly with soap and water after administration.

Caution should be exercised in the administration of Prostin E2 Vaginal Tablets for the induction of labour in patients with: asthma or a history of asthma; epilepsy or a history of epilepsy; glaucoma or raised intra-ocular pressure; compromised cardiovascular, hepatic or renal function; hypertension

As with any oxytocic agent, Prostin E2 Vaginal Tablets should be used with caution in patients with compromised (scarred) uteri.

In labour induction, cephalopelvic relationships should be carefully evaluated before use of Prostin E2 Vaginal Tablets. During use, uterine activity, fetal status and the progression of cervical dilation should be carefully monitored to detect possible evidence of undesired responses, e.g. hypertonus, sustained uterine contractions or fetal distress.

In cases where there is a known history of hypertonic uterine contractility or tetanic uterine contractions, it is recommended that uterine activity and the state of the fetus (where applicable) should be continuously monitored throughout labour. The possibility of uterine rupture should be borne in mind where high-tone uterine contractions are sustained.

Animal studies lasting several weeks at high doses have shown that prostaglandins of the E and F series can induce proliferation of bone. Such effects have also been noted in newborn infants who received prostaglandin E_1 during prolonged treatment. There is no evidence that short-term administration of prostaglandin E_2 can cause similar bone effects.

Overdose: Uterine hypertonus or unduly severe uterine contractions have rarely been encountered, but might be anticipated to result from overdosage. Where there is evidence of fetal distress or uterine hypertonus, then prompt delivery is indicated. Treatment of overdosage must be, at this time, symptomatic, since clinical studies with prostaglandin antagonists have not progressed to the point where recommendations may be made.

Incompatibilities: None known.

Pharmaceutical precautions Prostin E2 Vaginal Tablets have a shelf-life of 24 months when stored at 4°C. Store in a refrigerator.

Legal category POM.

Package quantities Prostin E2 Vaginal Tablets are supplied in packs of 8 tablets.

Further information Tablet disintegration and release of prostaglandin is moisture dependent. In a small proportion of women, tablet remains may be seen in the vagina a few hours after insertion and may contain some prostaglandin. However, this is rarely of clinical significance.

Unlike other oxytocics, Prostin E2 exhibits the capacity of the prostaglandins to influence uterine activity at any stage of gestation. Other Prostin E2 dosage forms are available for a number of indications, including induction of labour.

Product licence number 0032/0074.

PROSTIN* VR STERILE SOLUTION

Qualitative and quantitative composition Each 1 ml contains 500 micrograms (0.5 mg) alprostadil.

Pharmaceutical form Sterile solution for injection.

Clinical particulars
Therapeutic indications: Prostin VR is indicated to temporarily maintain the patency of the ductus arteriosus until corrective or palliative surgery can be performed in infants who have congenital defects and who depend upon the patent ductus for survival. Such congenital heart defects include pulmonary atresia, pulmonary stenosis, tricuspid atresia, tetralogy of Fallot, interruption of the aortic arch, co-arctation of the aorta, aortic stenosis, aortic atresia, mitral atresia, or transposition of the great vessels with or without other defects.

Posology and method of administration: For administration by intravenous drip or constant rate infusion pump.

In infants with lesions restricting pulmonary blood flow (blood is flowing through the ductus arteriosus from the aorta to the pulmonary artery), Prostin VR may be administered by continuous infusion through an umbilical artery catheter placed at or just above the junction of the descending aorta and the ductus arteriosus, or intravenously. Adverse effects have occurred with both routes of administration, but the types of reactions are different. A higher incidence of flushing has been associated with intra-arterial than with intravenous administration.

The infusion is generally initiated at a rate of 0.05 to 0.1 micrograms alprostadil per kilogram of body weight per minute. The most experience has been with 0.1 micrograms/kg/min. After a therapeutic response (an increase in pO_2 in neonates with restricted pulmonary blood flow or an increase in systemic blood pressure and blood pH in neonates with restricted systemic blood flow) has been obtained, the infusion rate should be reduced to the lowest possible dosage that will maintain the desired response.

Dilution instructions: To prepare infusion solutions, dilute 1 ml of Prostin VR Sterile Solution with sterile 0.9% Sodium Chloride Intravenous Infusion or sterile 5% Dextrose Intravenous Infusion. If undiluted Prostin VR Sterile Solution comes in direct contact with a plastic container, plasticisers are leached from the sidewalls. The solution may turn hazy and the appearance of the container may change. Should this occur, the solution should be discarded and the plastic container should be replaced. This appears to be a concentration-dependent phenomenon. To minimise the possibility of haze formation, Prostin VR Sterile Solution should be added directly to the intravenous infusion solution, avoiding contact with the walls of plastic containers. Dilute to volumes appropriate for the delivery system available. Prepare fresh infusion solutions every 24 hours. Discard any solution more than 24 hours old.

PARTICULAR CARE SHOULD BE TAKEN IN CALCULATING AND PREPARING DILUTIONS OF PROSTIN VR

Contra-indications: None.

Special warnings and special precautions for use:
Warnings: Only the recommended Prostin VR dosages should be administered and only by medically trained personnel in hospitals or other facilities with immediately available intensive care.

Approximately 10--12% of neonates with congenital heart defects treated with Prostin VR Sterile Solution experienced apnoea. Apnoea is most often seen in neonates weighing less than 2 kg at birth and usually appears during the first hour of drug infusion. Therefore, Prostin VR Sterile Solution should be used where ventilatory assistance is immediately available.

Precautions: Prostin VR Sterile Solution (alprostadil) should be infused for the shortest time and at the lowest dose which will produce the desired effects. The risk of long-term infusion of Prostin VR should be weighed against the possible benefits that critically ill infants may derive from its administration.

Cortical proliferation of the long bones has followed long-term infusions of alprostadil in infants and dogs. The proliferation in infants regressed after withdrawal of the drug.

Use Prostin VR Sterile Solution cautiously in neonates with histories of bleeding tendencies.

Care should be taken to avoid the use of Prostin VR Sterile Solution in neonates with respiratory distress syndrome (hyaline membrane disease), which sometimes can be confused with cyanotic heart disease. If full diagnostic facilities are not immediately available, cyanosis (pO_2 less than 40 mm Hg) and restricted pulmonary blood flow apparent on an X-ray are good indicators of congenital heart defects.

In all infants, commencing when infusion starts, intermittently monitor arterial pressure by umbilical artery catheter, auscultation, or with a Doppler transducer. Should arterial pressure fall significantly, decrease the rate of infusion immediately.

A weakening of the wall of the ductus arteriosus and pulmonary artery has been reported, particularly during prolonged administration.

The administration of alprostadil to neonates may result in gastric outlet obstruction secondary to antral hyperplasia. This effect appears to be related to duration of therapy and cumulative dose of the drug. Neonates receiving alprostadil at recommended doses for more than 120 hours should be closely monitored for evidence of antral hyperplasia and gastric outlet obstruction.

Long-term carcinogenicity and fertility studies have not been done. The Ames and Alkaline Elution assays reveal no potential for mutagenesis.

Interaction with other medicaments and other forms of interaction: No drug interactions have been reported to occur between Prostin VR and the standard therapy employed in neonates with congenital heart defects. Standard therapy includes antibiotics, such as penicillin or gentamicin; vasopressors, such as dopamine or isoproterenol; cardiac glycosides; and diuretics, such as frusemide.

Pregnancy and lactation: This product is for use in children only.

Effects on ability to drive and use machines: Not applicable.

Undesirable effects: The most frequent adverse reactions observed with Prostin VR infusion in neonates with ductal-dependent congenital heart defects are related to the drug's known pharmacological effects. These include, in decreasing frequency, transient pyrexia, apnoea, bradycardia, seizures, hypotension, tachycardia, and diarrhoea. The relationship of the following adverse events, in decreasing frequency, to the drug is unknown: sepsis, cardiac arrest, disseminated intravascular coagulation, hypokalaemia, and oedema. Cutaneous vasodilation (flushing) is the only event related to the route of administration, occurring more frequently during intra-arterial administration.

Overdose: Apnoea, bradycardia, pyrexia, hypotension and flushing may be signs of drug overdose. If apnoea or bradycardia occur, the infusion should be discontinued and the appropriate medical treatment initiated. Caution should be used if the infusion is restarted. If pyrexia or hypotension occur, the infusion rate should be reduced until these symptoms subside. Flushing is usually attributed to incorrect intra-arterial catheter placement and is usually alleviated by repositioning the tip of the catheter.

Pharmacological particulars
Pharmacodynamic properties: Prostaglandins are potent vasoactive derivatives of arachadonic acid that exert vasomotor, metabolic and cellular effects on the pulmonary and coronary circulation. The E series of prostaglandins produces vasodilation of the systemic and coronary circulation in most species: these prostaglandins have been used for maintaining the patency of the ductus arteriosus in children.

Pharmacokinetic properties: Based on studies in several animal species, intravenous or arterially administered prostaglandin E_1 is very rapidly metabolised and distributed throughout the entire body, with the exception of the CNS, where distribution, though detectable, is markedly reduced. The primary organisms for metabolism and inactivation of prostaglandin E_1 are probably the lung, liver and kidney which remove and metabolise 40–95% of the prostaglandin E_1 in a single pass through the organ. A number of other tissues possess lesser, but significant, capacity to metabolise prostaglandin E_1. The predominant metabolites found in plasma, 15-oxo-prostaglandin E_1 and 13,14-dihydro-15 oxo-prostaglandin E_1 are extensively metabolised by β and ω-oxidation prior to excretion, primarily by the kidney. Few urinary metabolites of prostaglandin E_1 have been characterised, but are widely believed to be analogous to those reported in detail for prostaglandin E_2 and prostaglandin $F_{2\alpha}$. Excretion is essentially complete within 24 hours after dosing, with no intact prostaglandin E_1 being found in urine and no evidence of tissue retention of prostaglandin E_1 or metabolites. In three species, rat, rabbit and lamb, the prostaglandin metabolising activity of lung from near-term fetal animals has been shown to be at least as effective as that of adults.

Preclinical safety data: See section "Undesirable effects".

Pharmaceutical particulars
List of excipients: Dehydrated ethanol.

Incompatibilities: Diluted solutions of Prostin VR should be infused from glass or hard plastic containers, or PVC infusion bags. If undiluted Prostin VR Sterile Solution comes in direct contact with a plastic container, plasticisers are leached from the sidewalls. This appears to be a concentration-dependent phenomenon.

Shelf life: Three years.

Special precautions for product storage: Store in a refrigerator.

Nature and contents of container: Glass ampoule, containing 1 ml solution.

Instructions for use/handling: Diluted solutions should be used within 24 hours.

Marketing authorisation number 0032/0083

Date of first authorisation/renewal of authorisation
Date of Grant: 23 July 1981
Date of Renewal: 17 April 1997

Date of (partial) revision of the text 1 April 1997.

Legal category POM.

PROVERA TABLETS 2.5 mg AND 5 mg

Presentation 2.5 mg: Orange, compressed tablets scored on one face and marked U64 on the other face, containing 2.5 mg medroxyprogesterone acetate.

Also contains: lactose, sucrose, maize starch, liquid paraffin, talc, calcium stearate and E110.

5 mg: Blue, compressed tablets scored on one face, marked 286 on either side of the score and marked 'U' on the other face, containing 5 mg medroxyprogesterone acetate.

Also contains: lactose, sucrose, maize starch, liquid paraffin, talc, calcium stearate and E132.

Uses Progestogen.

Indicated for dysfunctional (anovulatory) uterine

bleeding, secondary amenorrhoea and for mild to moderate endometriosis.

Dosage and administration Oral.

Dysfunctional (anovulatory) uterine bleeding: 2.5 – 10 mg daily for 5 – 10 days commencing on the assumed or calculated 16th – 21st day of the cycle. Treatment should be given for two consecutive cycles. When bleeding occurs from a poorly developed proliferative endometrium, conventional oestrogen therapy may be employed in conjunction with medroxyprogesterone acetate in doses of 5 – 10 mg for 10 days.

Secondary amenorrhoea: 2.5 – 10 mg daily for 5 – 10 days beginning on the assumed or calculated 16th to 21st day of the cycle. Repeat the treatment for three consecutive cycles. In amenorrhoea associated with a poorly developed proliferative endometrium, conventional oestrogen therapy may be employed in conjunction with medroxyprogesterone acetate in doses of 5 – 10 mg for 10 days.

Mild to moderate endometriosis: Beginning on the first day of the menstrual cycle, 10 mg three times a day for 90 consecutive days. Breakthrough bleeding, which is self-limiting, may occur. No additional hormonal therapy is recommended for the management of this bleeding.

Contra-indications, warnings, etc

Contra-indications: Use in patients with a known sensitivity to medroxyprogesterone acetate.

Use in patients with impaired liver function or with active liver disease.

Before using Provera, the general medical condition of the patient should be carefully evaluated. This evaluation should exclude the presence of genital or breast neoplasia before considering the use of Provera.

Warnings: Doses of up to 30 mg a day may not suppress ovulation and patients should be advised to take adequate contraceptive measures, where appropriate.

Precautions: A negative pregnancy test should be demonstrated before starting therapy with Provera.

Whether administered alone or in conjunction with oestrogens, Provera should not be employed in patients with abnormal uterine bleeding until a definite diagnosis has been established and the possibility of genital malignancy eliminated.

Provera, especially in high doses, may cause weight gain and fluid retention. With this in mind, caution should be exercised in treating any patient with a pre-existing medical condition, such as epilepsy, migraine, asthma, cardiac or renal dysfunction, that may be adversely affected by weight gain or fluid retention.

Some patients receiving Provera may exhibit a decreased glucose tolerance. The mechanism for this is not known. This fact should be borne in mind when treating all patients, especially known diabetics.

Rare cases of thrombo-embolism have been reported with use of Provera, especially at higher doses. Causality has not been established.

Patients with a history of treatment for mental depression should be carefully monitored while receiving Provera therapy. Some patients may complain of premenstrual-like depression while on Provera therapy.

Medroxyprogesterone acetate and its metabolites are secreted in breast milk, however, there is no evidence to suggest that this presents any hazard to the child.

Interactions: Aminoglutethimide administered concurrently with Provera may significantly depress the bioavailability of Provera.

Interactions with other medicinal treatments (including oral anti-coagulants) have rarely been reported, but causality has not been determined. The possibility of interaction should be borne in mind in patients receiving concurrent treatment with other drugs.

Side-effects: The following medical events, listed in order of seriousness rather than frequency of occurrence, have been associated occasionally to rarely with the use of progestogens:

Rare anaphylactoid-like reactions.

Psychic: nervousness, insomnia, somnolence, fatigue, depression, dizziness and headache.

Skin and mucous membranes: urticaria, pruritus, rash, acne, hirsutism and alopecia.

Gastro-intestinal: nausea.

Breast tenderness and galactorrhoea.

Miscellaneous: change in weight.

Overdosage: In animals, Provera has been shown to be capable of exerting an adreno-corticoid effect: this has not been reported in the human, following usual dosages. The oral administration of Provera at a rate of 100 mg per day has been shown to have no effect on adrenal function.

Pharmaceutical precautions None.

Legal category POM.

Package quantities 2.5 mg: Packs of 30. 5 mg: Packs of 10 and 100.

Further information Pathologists should be informed of the patient's ingestion of Provera if endometrial or endocervical tissue is submitted for examination.

The results of certain laboratory tests may be affected by the use of Provera; these include gonadotrophin levels, plasma progesterone levels, urinary pregnanediol levels, plasma testosterone levels (in the male), plasma oestrogen levels (in the female), plasma cortisol levels, glucose tolerance test and metyrapone tests.

Product licence numbers

2.5 mg 0032/0168

5 mg 0032/5035R

Date of preparation or last review May 1994.

PROVERA TABLETS 10 mg

Qualitative and quantitative composition Each tablet contains 10 mg medroxyprogesterone acetate PhEur.

Pharmaceutical form Tablets for oral use.

Clinical particulars

Therapeutic indications: Progestogen. Indicated for dysfunctional (anovulatory) uterine bleeding, secondary amenorrhoea and for mild to moderate endometriosis.

Posology and method of administration: Oral.

Adults: Dysfunctional (anovulatory) uterine bleeding: 2.5 – 10 mg daily for 5 – 10 days commencing on the assumed or calculated 16th – 21st day of the cycle. Treatment should be given for two consecutive cycles. When bleeding occurs from a poorly developed proliferative endometrium, conventional oestrogen therapy may be employed in conjunction with medroxyprogesterone acetate in doses of 5 – 10 mg for 10 days.

Secondary amenorrhoea: 2.5 – 10 mg daily for 5 – 10 days beginning on the assumed or calculated 16th to 21st day of the cycle. Repeat the treatment for three consecutive cycles. In amenorrhoea associated with a poorly developed proliferative endometrium, conventional oestrogen therapy may be employed in conjunction with medroxyprogesterone acetate in doses of 5 – 10 mg for 10 days.

Mild to moderate endometriosis: Beginning on the first day of the menstrual cycle, 10 mg three times a day for 90 consecutive days. Breakthrough bleeding, which is self-limiting, may occur. No additional hormonal therapy is recommended for the management of this bleeding.

Elderly: Not applicable.

Children: Not applicable.

Contra-indications: Use in patients with a known sensitivity to medroxyprogesterone acetate.

Use in patients with impaired liver function or with active liver disease.

Before using Provera, the general medical condition of the patient should be carefully evaluated. This evaluation should exclude the presence of genital or breast neoplasia before considering the use of Provera.

Special warnings and special precautions for use: Whether administered alone or in conjunction with oestrogens, Provera should not be employed in patients with abnormal uterine bleeding until a definite diagnosis has been established and the possibility of genital malignancy eliminated.

Rare cases of thrombo-embolism have been reported with use of Provera, especially at higher doses. Causality has not been established.

Doses of up to 30 mg a day may not suppress ovulation and patients should be advised to take adequate contraceptive measures, where appropriate.

Provera, especially in high doses, may cause weight gain and fluid retention. With this in mind, caution should be exercised in treating any patient with a pre-existing medical condition, such as epilepsy, migraine, asthma, cardiac or renal dysfunction, that might be adversely affected by weight gain or fluid retention.

Some patients receiving Provera may exhibit a decreased glucose tolerance. The mechanism for this is not known. This fact should be borne in mind when treating all patients and especially known diabetics.

Patients with a history of treatment for mental depression should be carefully monitored while receiving Provera therapy. Some patients may complain of premenstrual like depression while on Provera therapy.

Interaction with other medicaments and other forms of interaction: Aminoglutethimide administered concurrently with Provera may significantly depress the bioavailability of Provera.

Interactions with other medicinal treatments (including oral anti-coagulants) have rarely been reported, but causality has not been determined. The possibility of interaction should be borne in mind in patients receiving concurrent treatment with other drugs.

Pregnancy and lactation: A negative pregnancy test should be demonstrated before starting therapy. Medroxyprogesterone acetate and its metabolites are secreted in breast milk, but there is no evidence to suggest that this presents any hazard to the child.

Effects on ability to drive and use machines: No adverse effect has been reported.

Undesirable effects: The following medical events, listed in order of seriousness rather than frequency of occurrence, have been occasionally to rarely associated with the use of progestogens:

Rare anaphylactoid-like reactions.

Psychic: nervousness, insomnia, somnolence, fatigue, depression, dizziness and headache.

Skin and mucous membranes: urticaria, pruritus, rash, acne, hirsutism and alopecia.

Gastro-intestinal: nausea.

Breast: tenderness and galactorrhoea.

Miscellaneous: change in weight.

Overdose: In animals Provera has been shown to be capable of exerting an adreno-corticoid effect, but this has not been reported in the human, following usual dosages. The oral administration of Provera at a rate of 100 mg per day has been shown to have no effect on adrenal function.

Pharmacological properties

Pharmacodynamic properties: Medroxyprogesterone acetate has actions and uses similar to those of progesterone.

MPA has minimal androgenic activity compared to progesterone and virtually no oestrogenic activity.

Progestogens are used in the treatment of dysfunctional uterine bleeding, secondary amenorrhoea and endometriosis.

Pharmacokinetic properties: MPA is rapidly absorbed from the GI tract with a single oral dose of 10–250 mg. The time taken to reach the peak serum concentration (T_{max}) was 2 – 6 hours and the average peak serum concentration (C_{max}) was 13 – 46.89 mg/ml.

Unmetabolised MPA is highly plasma protein bound. MPA is metabolised in the liver.

Pharmaceutical particulars

List of excipients: Lactose, Sucrose, Maize starch, Liquid paraffin, Talc, Calcium stearate.

Incompatibilities: None known.

Shelf-life: Five years.

Special precautions for storage: None.

Nature and contents of container: HDPE tamper-evident bottles with LDPE push-fit tamper evident caps, containing 50 tablets.

Aluminium foil/PVC blisters, containing 10, 90 and 100 tablets.

Instructions for use/handling: None.

Marketing authorisation number 0032/0151.

Date of approval/revision of SPC 8 January 1996.

Legal category POM.

PROVERA* TABLETS 100 mg, 200 mg AND 400 mg

Presentation 100 mg: White, circular, flat bevelled tablets marked 'U 467' on one side and scored on the reverse, containing 100 mg medroxyprogesterone acetate.

200 mg: White, circular, biconvex tablets marked 'U 320' on one side and scored on the reverse, containing 200 mg medroxyprogesterone acetate.

400 mg: White, capsule shaped, compressed tablets marked 'Upjohn 421' on one side only, containing 400 mg medroxyprogesterone acetate.

Provera Tablets (all strengths) also contain microcrystalline cellulose, maize starch, byco C, polyethylene glycol, sodium starch glycollate, docusate sodium, sodium benzoate and magnesium stearate.

Uses Progestogen.

Indicated for the treatment of certain hormone dependent neoplasms, such as endometrial carcinoma, renal cell carcinoma and carcinoma of breast in post-menopausal women.

Dosage and administration Oral.

For endometrial and renal cell carcinoma: 200 – 400 mg daily.

For breast carcinoma: 400 – 800 mg per day. Doses of 1000 mg daily have been given although the incidence of minor side-effects, such as indigestion and weight gain, increase with the increase in dose. Response to hormonal therapy may not be evident until after at least 8 – 10 weeks of therapy.

Elderly patients: These products have been used primarily in the older age group for the treatment of malignancies. There is no evidence to suggest that the older aged group is any less prepared to handle the drug metabolically than is the younger aged patient. Therefore, the same dosage, contra-indications and precautions would apply to either age group.

Contra-indications, warnings, etc

Contra-indications: Use in patients with a known sensitivity to medroxyprogesterone acetate.

Use in patients with impaired liver function or active liver disease.

Warnings: In the treatment of carcinoma of breast, occasional cases of hypercalcaemia have been reported.

Any patient who develops an acute impairment of vision, proptosis, diplopia or migraine headache should be carefully evaluated ophthalmologically to exclude the presence of papilloedema or retinal vascular lesions before continuing medication.

Medroxyprogesterone acetate and/or its metabolites are secreted in breast milk but there is no evidence to suggest that this presents any hazard to the child.

Precautions: Animal studies show that Provera possesses adrenocorticoid activity. This has also been reported in man, therefore, patients receiving large doses continuously and for long periods should be observed closely.

The administration of large doses to pregnant women has resulted in the observation of some instances of female foetal masculinization. Doctors should, therefore, check that patients are not pregnant before commencing treatment.

Because progestogens may cause some degree of fluid retention, conditions which might be influenced by this factor, such as epilepsy, migraine, asthma, cardiac or renal dysfunction, require careful observation.

Rare cases of thrombo-embolism have been reported with use of Provera, but causality has not been established.

Patients who have a history of mental depression should be carefully observed and the drug discontinued if the depression recurs to a serious degree.

A decrease in glucose tolerance has been observed in some patients on progestogens. The mechanism of this decrease is obscure. For this reason, diabetic patients should be carefully observed while receiving progestogen therapy.

Before using Provera, the general medical condition of the patient should be carefully evaluated.

This product should be used under the supervision of a specialist and the patients kept under regular surveillance.

Interactions: Aminoglutethimide administered concomitantly with Provera may significantly depress the bioavailability of Provera.

Interactions with other medicinal treatments (including oral anti-coagulants) have rarely been reported, but causality has not been determined. The possibility of interaction should be borne in mind in patients receiving concurrent treatment with other drugs.

Side-effects: Reactions occasionally associated with the use of progestogens, particularly in high doses, are:

Breast: tenderness or galactorrhoea.

Psychic: nervousness, insomnia, somnolence, fatigue, dizziness, depression and headache.

Skin and mucous membranes: sensitivity reactions ranging from pruritus, urticaria, angioneurotic oedema to generalised rash and anaphylaxis have occasionally been reported. Acne, alopecia or hirsutism have been reported in a few cases.

Gastro-intestinal: nausea and indigestion have been noted particularly with the higher doses.

Miscellaneous: hyperpyrexia, weight gain, moon facies, increased blood pressure.

Overdosage: No action required other than cessation of therapy.

Pharmaceutical precautions Keep containers tightly closed.

Provera Tablets should be stored at controlled room temperature (15 – 30°C).

Legal category POM.

Package quantities Provera Tablets 100 mg in packs of 60 and 100 tablets.
Provera Tablets 200 mg in packs of 30 (OP) and 100 tablets.
Provera Tablets 400 mg in packs of 30 tablets (OP).

Further information The results of certain laboratory tests may be affected by the use of Provera; these include gonadotrophin levels, plasma progesterone levels, urinary pregnanediol levels, plasma testosterone levels (in the male), plasma oestrogen levels (in the female), plasma cortisol levels, glucose tolerance and metyrapone tests.

Pathologists should be informed of the patient's ingestion of Provera if endometrial or endocervical tissue is submitted for examination.

Product licence numbers
100 mg Tablet 0032/0111
200 mg Tablet 0032/0112
400 mg Tablet 0032/0131

REFOLINON*

Presentation Clear, pale yellow liquid for injection containing leucovorin 3 mg/ml (as the calcium salt) in ampoules of 10 ml.

Pale yellow, round, convex, uncoated tablet marked with an 'F' on one side and 'CF' on the other; diameter 9 mm containing 15 mg leucovorin (as the calcium salt).

Uses Leucovorin (folinic acid) is the formyl derivative of tetrahydrofolic acid and is an intermediate product of the metabolism of folic acid. Leucovorin is used in cytotoxic therapy as an antidote to folic acid antagonists such as methotrexate. Leucovorin is effective in the treatment of megaloblastic anaemia due to folate deficiency.

Dosage and administration (Adults and children)

Leucovorin rescue: Depending upon the dose of methotrexate administered, dosage regimens of leucovorin calcium vary. Up to 120 mg leucovorin calcium are generally given, usually in divided doses over 12–24 hours by intramuscular injection, bolus intravenous injection or intravenous infusion in normal saline. This is followed by 12–15 mg intramuscularly or 15 mg orally every 6 hours for 48 hours. Rescue therapy is usually started 24 hours after the commencement of methotrexate administration.

If overdosage of methotrexate is suspected, the dose of leucovorin calcium should be equal to or greater than the dose of methotrexate and should be administered within one hour of the methotrexate administration.

Megaloblastic anaemia (folate deficiency): 15 mg (one tablet) leucovorin per day.

Contra-indications, warnings, etc Calcium folinate should not be used for the treatment of pernicious anaemia or other megaloblastic anaemia where vitamin B12 is deficient.

Leucovorin should not be given simultaneously with a folic acid antagonist, for the purpose of reducing or preventing clinical toxicity, as the therapeutic effect of the antagonist may be nullified.

High-dose methotrexate therapy together with leucovorin rescue should only be carried out under the direction of physicians experienced in antitumour chemotherapy.

Adverse reactions to leucovorin calcium are rare, but following parenteral administration occasional pyrexial reactions have been reported.

Pharmaceutical precautions Protect from light.

Refolinon for injection has been shown to be compatible with 0.9% sodium chloride solution. Under normal light conditions and at room temperature solutions of calcium folinate in 0.9% sodium chloride have been shown to be stable for 24 hours.

Legal category POM.

Package quantities
Refolinon for Injection 5×10 ml ampoules
Refolinon Tablets Containers of 30 tablets

Further information Nil.

Product licence numbers
Refolinon for Injection 3433/0079
Refolinon Tablets 3433/0078

REGAINE* REGULAR STRENGTH

Presentation Clear, colourless to light yellow liquid containing minoxidil 20 mg per ml in a solution of ethanol, propylene glycol and water.

Uses Regaine Regular Strength is indicated for the treatment of alopecia androgenetica. There is also evidence that Regaine slows hair loss in patients with diagnosed male pattern baldness.

After only four months of treatment, little regrowth of terminal hair should be expected (the average length of the scalp hair cycle is three years). Physicians observed 8% of subjects to have moderate or dense terminal hair regrowth after four months, increasing to 39% of the subjects after treatment for 12 months. Twenty-six percent of patients assessed themselves as having moderate to dense hair regrowth after four months, increasing to 48% of subjects treated for 12 months. At 12 months, 36% of patients had minimal regrowth as assessed by both the patients themselves as well as the treating physicians. In these, patients loss of hair from affected areas was considered to be reduced. Onset and degree of hair regrowth may be variable among patients and it may take at least four months of continuous twice daily use before evidence of hair regrowth can be expected. Although trends in the data suggest that those patients who are younger, who have been balding for a shorter period of time or who have a smaller area of baldness on the vertex are more likely to respond to Regaine, individual response cannot be predicted. If hair regrowth occurs, twice daily applications of Regaine are necessary for continued hair growth. Anecdotal reports indicate that regrown hair may disappear three to four months after stopping Regaine application and the balding process will continue. Patients should discontinue treatment if there is no improvement after one year.

Dosage and administration Hair and scalp should be thoroughly dry prior to topical application of Regaine. A dose of 1 ml Regaine Regular Strength should be applied to the total affected areas of the scalp twice daily. The total dosage should not exceed 2 ml. If fingertips are used to facilitate drug application, hands should be washed afterwards.

The method of application varies according to the disposable applicator used:

Pump spray applicator: This is useful for large areas. Aim the pump at the centre of the bald area, press once and spread with fingertips over the entire bald area. Repeat for a total of 6 times to apply a dose of 1 ml. Avoid breathing spray mist.

Extended spray tip applicator: This is useful for small areas or under hair. The pump spray applicator must be in place in order to use this additional applicator. Use in the same way as the pump spray.

Rub-on applicator: Squeeze the upright bottle once to fill the 1 ml chamber to the black line. Invert bottle, dab on scalp and spread Regaine over the entire bald area until chamber is empty.

Contra-indications, warnings, etc

Contra-indications: Regaine is contra-indicated in patients with a history of sensitivity to minoxidil, ethanol or propylene glycol.

Warnings: Use of Regaine Regular Strength results in slight absorption (an average of 1.4% of the applied topical dose) of minoxidil from the skin surface. Although not causally related to the use of Regaine in clinical trials, the following potential systemic effects should be considered: sodium and water retention, tachycardia, aggravation of pre-existing angina pectoris or the induction of anginal symptoms in patients with undiagnosed coronary artery disease. Patients should be instructed to discontinue use of Regaine and contact their physician if any of the above systemic effects occur.

Precautions: Patients with hypertension, including those under treatment with antihypertensive agents, should be monitored closely when treated with Regaine Regular Strength.

Regaine contains an alcohol base which will cause burning and irritation of the eye. In the event of accidental contact with sensitive surfaces (eye, abraded skin and mucous membranes), the area should be bathed with large amounts of cool tap water.

Inhalation of the spray mist should be avoided. Regaine should not be used in conjunction with other topical agents including corticosteroids, retinoids and petrolatum or agents that are known to enhance cutaneous drug absorption.

As is the case with other topically applied drugs, decreased integrity of the epidermal barrier caused by inflammation or disease processes in the skin (e.g. excoriations of the scalp, scalp psoriasis or severe sunburn) may increase percutaneous absorption of minoxidil.

Regaine is for external use only. Do not apply to areas of the body other than the scalp.

The safety and effectiveness of Regaine in patients under 18 or over 65 years of age has not been established.

There is no evidence as to drug safety in human pregnancy nor is there evidence from animal work that it is free from hazard. Regaine should not be used during pregnancy or lactation.

Side-effects: When incidences of medical events in placebo-controlled trials of topical minoxidil were compared, they revealed that only reports involving the dermatological system were present at a significantly greater level in the minoxidil group than in the placebo group. In both groups in all body systems, the overall incidence of medical events reported by females was approximately five times that of males.

Details of percentage occurrences after 4–8 months treatment with minoxidil (n=3857) or placebo (n=2717) were as follows:

Body system	Minoxidil % occurrence	Placebo % occurrence
Respiratory (bronchitis, URTI, sinusitis)	7.16	8.58
Dermatological (irritant dermatitis, allergic contact dermatitis)	7.36	5.41
Gastro-intestinal (diarrhoea, nausea, vomiting)	4.33	6.55
Neurology (headache, dizziness, faintness, lightheadedness)	3.42	3.46
Musculoskeletal (fractures, back pain, tendinitis, aches and pains)	2.59	2.21
Cardiovascular (oedema, chest pain, blood pressure increases/decreases, palpitations, pulse rate increases/decreases)	1.53	1.55

In other systems monitored (allergy, special senses, metabolic-nutritional, urinary tract, genital tract, psychiatric, haematology, endocrine) occurrences were all below 1.5% (range 0.31– 1.29).

Interactions: There are currently no known drug interactions associated with the use of Regaine Topical Solution. Although it has not been clinically demonstrated, there exists the theoretical possibility of absorbed minoxidil potentiating orthostatic hypotension caused by guanethidine.

Overdosage: Increased systemic absorption of minoxidil may potentially occur if higher than recommended doses of Regaine are applied to larger surface areas of the body or areas other than the scalp. There are no known cases of minoxidil overdosage resulting from topical administration of Regaine.

Because of the concentration of minoxidil in Regaine, accidental ingestion has the potential of producing systemic effects related to the pharmacological action of the drug (5 ml of Regaine contains 100 mg minoxidil, the maximum recommended adult dose for oral minoxidil administration in the treatment of hypertension). Signs and symptoms of minoxidil overdosage would most likely be cardiovascular effects associated with sodium and water retention and tachycardia. Fluid retention can be managed with appropriate diuretic therapy. Clinically significant tachycardia can be controlled by administration of a beta adrenergic blocking agent.

If encountered, hypotension should be treated by intravenous administration of normal saline. Sympathomimetic drugs, such as noradrenaline and adrenaline, should be avoided because of their excessive cardiac stimulating activity.

Pharmaceutical precautions Regaine Regular Strength should be stored at room temperature. The solution is flammable.

Legal category P.

Package quantities Regaine Regular Strength is supplied in bottles of 60 ml with one or more of the following disposable applicators: pump spray, extended tip or rub-on assemblies.

Further information The mechanism of action of minoxidil in the treatment of male pattern baldness is currently not known.

Following application of Regaine, minoxidil is poorly absorbed from normal intact skin with an average of 1.4% (range 0.3–4.5%) of the total applied dose reaching the systemic circulation. Therefore, a 1 ml dose of Regaine Regular Strength, delivering 20 mg of minoxidil solution to the skin, would result in absorption of approximately 0.28 mg minoxidil. This compares with greater than 95% absorption from the gastro-intestinal tract of orally administered minoxidil as tablets. Serum levels resulting from administration of Regaine are governed by the drug's percutaneous absorption rate. Following cessation of topical dosing of Regaine, approximately 95% of systemically absorbed minoxidil is eliminated within four days.

Product licence number 0032/0136.

REGAINE* EXTRA STRENGTH

Qualitative and quantitative composition Minoxidil 50 mg/ml (5%w/v).

Pharmaceutical form Topical Solution

Clinical particulars

Therapeutic indications: Regaine Extra Strength is indicated for the treatment of alopecia androgenetica in men

Onset and degree of hair regrowth may be variable among users. Although trends in the data suggest that those users who are younger, who have been balding for a shorter period of time or who have a smaller area of baldness on the vertex are more likely to respond to Regaine Extra Strength, individual responses cannot be predicted.

Posology and method of administration: Men aged 18-65: Hair and scalp should be thoroughly dry prior to topical application of Regaine Extra Strength. A dose of 1 ml Regaine Extra Strength topical solution should be applied to the total affected areas of the scalp twice daily. The total dosage should not exceed 2 ml. If fingertips are used to facilitate drug application, hands should be washed afterwards.

It may take twice daily applications for 2 months or more before evidence of hair growth can be expected.

If hair regrowth occurs, twice daily applications of Regaine Extra Strength are necessary for continued hair growth. Anecdotal reports indicate that regrown hair may disappear three to four months after stopping Regaine Extra Strength application and the balding process will continue.

Users should discontinue treatment if there is no improvement after one year.

The method of application varies according to the disposable applicator used:

Pump spray applicator: this is useful for large areas. Aim the pump at the centre of the bald area, press once and spread with fingertips over the entire bald area. Repeat for a total of 6 times to apply a dose of 1 ml. Avoid breathing spray mist.

Extended spray tip applicator: this is useful for small areas, or under hair. The pump spray applicator must be in place in order to use this additional applicator. Use in the same way as the pump spray.

Rub-on applicator: squeeze the upright bottle once to fill the 1 ml chamber to the black line. Invert bottle, dab on scalp, and spread Regaine Extra Strength over the entire bald area until chamber is empty.

Children and the elderly: Not recommended. The safety and effectiveness of Regaine Extra Strength in users aged under 18 or over 65 has not been established.

Contra-indications: Regaine Extra Strength is contra-indicated:

in women;
in users with a history of sensitivity to minoxidil, ethanol, or propylene glycol;
in users with treated or untreated hypertension;
in users with any scalp abnormality (including psoriasis and sunburn);
in users with a shaved scalp;
if occlusive dressings or other topical medical preparations are being used.

Special warnings and special precautions for use: Before using Regaine Extra Strength, the user should determine that the scalp is normal and healthy.

Regaine Extra Strength is for external use only. Do not apply to areas of the body other than the scalp

Hands should be washed thoroughly after applying the solution. Inhalation of the spray mist should be avoided.

Regaine Extra Strength Topical Solution contains alcohol, which will cause burning and irritation of the eye. In the event of accidental contact with sensitive surfaces (eye, abraded skin and mucous membranes) the area should be bathed with large amounts of cool tap water.

Users should be aware that, whilst extensive use of Regaine Extra Strength has not revealed evidence that sufficient minoxidil is absorbed to have systemic effects, greater absorption because of misuse, individual variability, unusual sensitivity or decreased integrity of the epidermal barrier caused by inflammation or disease processes in the skin (eg. excoriations of the scalp, or scalp psoriasis) could lead, at least theoretically, to systemic effects.

Interaction with other medicaments and other forms of interaction: Topical drugs, such as tretinoin or dithranol, which alter the stratum corneum barrier, could result in increased absorption of minoxidil if applied concurrently. Although it has not been demonstrated clinically, there exists the theoretical possibility of absorbed minoxidil potentiating orthostatic hypotension caused by peripheral vasodilators.

Pregnancy and lactation: There is no evidence as to drug safety in human pregnancy nor is there evidence from animal work that it is free from hazard. Regaine should not be used during pregnancy or lactation.

Effects on ability to drive and use machines: Based on the pharmacodynamic and overall safety profile of minoxidil, it is not expected that Regaine Extra Strength would interfere with the ability to drive or operate machinery.

Undesirable effects: Several thousand patients have used topical minoxidil in clinical trials where a comparison with an inactive solution was made. Dermatological reactions (e.g. irritation, itching) occurred in patients using both solutions. This has been explained by the presence of propylene glycol in both the active and inactive solution.

Reactions reported in commercial marketing experience include: hypertrichosis (unwanted non-scalp hair including facial hair growth in women), local erythema, itching, dry skin/scalp flaking, and exacerbation of hair loss.

Some consumers reported increased hair shedding upon initiation of therapy with Regaine Extra Strength. This is most likely due to minoxidil's action of shifting hairs from the resting telogen phase to the growing anagen phase (old hairs fall out as new hairs grow in their place). This temporary increase in hair shedding generally occurs two to six weeks after beginning treatment and subsides within a couple of weeks. If shedding persists (>2 weeks), users should stop using Regaine Extra Strength and consult their doctor.

Particular attention was paid to body systems, such as cardiovascular and metabolic, which might have some relevance based on the pharmacology of minoxidil. There was no increased risk to users due to drug related medical reactions in these, or other, body system categories.

Users should stop using Regaine Extra Strength if they experience, chest-pain, tachycardia, faintness, dizziness, sudden unexplained weight gain, swollen hands or feet or persistent redness or irritation of the scalp.

Overdose: Increased systemic absorption of minoxidil may potentially occur if higher-than-recommended doses of Regaine Extra Strength are applied to larger surface areas of the body or areas other than the scalp. There are no known cases of minoxidil overdosage resulting from topical administration of Regaine Extra Strength.

Because of the concentration of minoxidil in Regaine Extra Strength, accidental ingestion has the potential of producing systemic effects related to the pharmacological action of the drug (2 ml of Regaine Extra Strength contains 100 mg; the maximum recommended adult dose for oral minoxidil administration in the treatment of hypertension),. Signs and symptoms of minoxidil overdosage would primarily be cardiovascular effects associated with sodium and water retention, and tachycardia. Fluid retention can be managed with appropriate diuretic therapy. Clinically significant tachycardia can be controlled by administration of a beta-adrenergic blocking agent.

Pharmacological properties

Pharmacodynamic properties: Regaine Extra Strength stimulates hair growth in men with androgenetic alopecia (expressed as baldness of the vertex of the scalp). There is also evidence that topical minoxidil slows hair loss due to androgenetic alopecia.

The mechanism by which minoxidil stimulates hair growth is not fully understood, but minoxidil can reverse the hair loss process of androgenetic alopecia.

In trials comparing Regaine Extra Strength with Regaine Regular Strength, users of Regaine Extra Strength who responded to treatment experienced the same degree of hair regrowth associated with 4 months of treatment with Regaine Regular Strength after 2 months. After 12 months, Regaine Extra Strength produced 43% more regrowth than Regaine Regular Strength.

Regaine Extra Strength may therefore be considered by men who wish to achieve earlier hair regrowth and/or a greater degree of hair regrowth than would be expected through the use of Regaine Regular Strength.

Pharmacokinetic properties: The failure to detect evidence of systemic effects during treatment with Regaine Extra Strength reflects the poor absorption of topical minoxidil, which averages about 1.7% (range 0.3–4.5%) of the total applied dose from normal intact skin. Absorption is about 2% when applied topically to shaved scalps of hypertensive users. Increasing the amount of drug applied or increasing the frequency of application of Regaine Extra Strength also results in increased absorption.

The use of Regaine Extra Strength in conjunction with occlusion (plastic dressings), application to sunburn areas, and increasing the surface area of application has minimal to no effect on the absorption of topical minoxidil. Results of extensive pharmacokinetic studies indicate that the three major factors by which topical minoxidil absorption are increased by are: Increasing the dose applied, increasing the frequency of dosing and decreasing the barrier function of the stratum corneum.

Serum minoxidil levels and systemic effects resulting from administration of Regaine Extra Strength are governed by the drug's absorption rate through the skin. Following cessation of topical dosing of Regaine Extra Strength, approximately 95% of the systemically absorbed drug is eliminated within 4 days. Minoxidil and its metabolites are excreted principally in the urine.

Pharmaceutical particulars
List of excipients: Propylene glycol, ethanol, water.

Incompatibilities: None known.

Shelf-life: 24 months.

Special precautions for storage: Regaine Extra Strength solution is flammable. Store below 25°C

Nature and contents of container: HDPE bottle with spray-pump/dabbing applicator containing 60 ml of solution. Packs contain either one or three bottles.

Instructions for use/handling: The solution is flammable and exposure of the container and contents to naked flames should be avoided during use, storage and disposal.

Marketing authorisation number 0032/0183.

Date of first authorisation/renewal of authorisation
Date of first authorisation: 30 November 1995
Renewal dates:

Dates of revision of the text November 2, 1998.

Legal category P.

SALAZOPYRIN* TABLETS, ENEMAS, SUPPOSITORIES AND SUSPENSION

Presentation Tablets: Yellow, 13.5 mm diameter tablets, tasteless, scored deeply on one side, with KPh on one side and 101 on the other, containing Sulphasalazine PhEur 0.5 g. Excipients: Maize starch, PVP, magnesium stearate, colloidal silicon dioxide.

Enema: Round, soft, polyethylene 135 ml enema bottle with screw-on cap/spout (elastomer valve in spout) containing sulphasalazine 3 g, vehicle to 100 mls. Excipients: Normal saline, methyl and propyl parabens.

Suppositories: Yellow, odourless, torpedo-shaped containing sulphasalazine 0.5 g. Excipients: PVP, hard fat.

Suspension: Yellow suspension, orange-lemon flavour 250 mg/5 ml in polythene bottle with tamper evident cap. Excipients: Xanthan gum, microcrystalline cellulose, sucrose, orange/lemon flavouring, polysorbate 80, sodium benzoate, water.

Uses Treatment of ulcerative colitis and Crohn's disease.

Dosage and administration
Adults and elderly: The dose is adjusted according to the severity of the disease and the patient's tolerance to the drug, as detailed below.

1. Tablets: Induction and maintenance of remission of ulcerative colitis; treatment of active Crohn's disease.

   Severe attack: Salazopyrin 2–4 tablets four times a day may be given in conjunction with steroids as part of an intensive management regime. Rapid passage of the tablets may reduce effect of the drug. Night-time interval between doses should not exceed eight hours.

   Mild-moderate attack: 2–4 tablets four times a day may be given in conjunction with steroids.

   Maintenance therapy: With induction of remission reduce the dose gradually to 4 tablets per day. This dosage should be continued indefinitely, since discontinuance even several years after an acute attack is associated with a four fold increase in risk of relapse.
2. Enemas: Treatment of ulcerative colitis and Crohn's colitis.

   One enema should be given daily, preferably at bedtime.
3. Suppositories: Treatment of ulcerative colitis and Crohn's colitis affecting the rectum.

   Two suppositories to be inserted in the morning and two at bedtime after defaecation. After three weeks it may be possible to gradually reduce the dosage as the patient improves.

   Adjunct to oral therapy: In severe generalised disease affecting the rectum or rectosigmoid, and in cases slow to respond to oral therapy, one or two suppositories may be given morning and evening in addition.
4. Suspension: Dosage as for tablets, 10 ml being taken instead of each 0.5 g tablet.

Children
1. Tablets: The dose is reduced in proportion to body weight.

Severe attack:	40–60 mg/kg per day
Mild–moderate attack:	40–60 mg/kg per day
Maintenance:	20–30 mg/kg per day

2. Enema: The enema presentation contains an adult dose and is not recommended for children.
3. Suppositories: Reduce the adult dosage on the basis of body weight.
4. Suspension: 5 ml contains 250 mg sulphasalazine. Reduce adult dosage on the basis of body weight.

Severe attack:	0.8–1.2 ml/kg per day
Mild–moderate attack:	0.8–1.2 ml/kg per day
Maintenance therapy:	0.4–0.6 ml/kg per day

Contra-indications, warnings, etc
Contra-indications:
a. History of sensitivity to sulphonamides or salicylates.
b. Infants under 2 years of age.
c. In the case of the Enema, subjects sensitive to methyl or propyl parabens.
d. In the case of Suspension, subjects sensitive to sodium benzoate.

Precautions: Haematological and hepatic side effects may occur. Differential white cell, red cell and platelet counts should be performed initially and at least monthly for a minimum of the first three months of treatment. The patient should also be counselled to report immediately with any sore throat, fever, malaise or unexpected non specific illness. The treatment should be stopped immediately if there is suspicion or laboratory evidence of a potentially serious blood dyscrasia.

A patient information leaflet should be supplied specifically advising patients on blood dyscrasias.

Liver function tests should be carried out at monthly intervals for the first three months of treatment. Kidney function should be checked initially and at regular intervals during treatment.

Patients with allergy, or renal or hepatic disease should be treated with caution. Patients with glucose-6-phosphate dehydrogenase deficiency should be closely observed for signs of haemolytic anaemia (Heinz body anaemia).

The uptake of digoxin and folate may be reduced. An acute attack may be precipitated in patients with porphyria.

Adverse effects: Overall, about 75% of ADRs occur within 3 months of starting therapy, and over 90% by 6 months. Some undesirable effects are dose dependent and symptoms can often be alleviated by reduction of the dose.

Since sulphasalazine is metabolised to sulphapyridine and 5-amino salicylic acid, side-effects of sulphonamides or salicylates may occur. Patients with slow acetylator status are more likely to experience adverse effects due to sulphapyridine. The most commonly encountered reactions are nausea, headache, rash, loss of appetite and raised temperature.

The following adverse reactions have been reported:

Haematological: Potentially fatal leucopenia, neutropenia, agranulocytosis, aplastic anaemia and thrombocytopenia. Leucopenia, which is normally mild and transient, may occur in up to 1.5% of patients and agranulocytosis in up to 1 in 700 patients during the second month of therapy.

Heinz body anaemia, methaemoglobinaemia, hypoprothrombinaemia, haemolytic anaemia, megaloblastic anaemia.

Hypersensitivity reactions: Generalised skin eruptions, Stevens–Johnson syndrome, exfoliative dermatitis, epidermal necrolysis, pruritus, urticaria, photosensitisation, anaphylaxis, serum sickness, drug fever, periorbital oedema, conjunctival and scleral injection, arthralgia, allergic myocarditis, polyarteritis nodosa, LE-phenomenon and lung complications with dyspnoea, fever, cough, eosinophilia, fibrosing alveolitis.

Gastro-intestinal reactions: Stomatitis, parotitis, pancreatitis, hepatitis.

CNS reactions: Vertigo, tinnitus, peripheral neuropathy, ataxia, convulsions, insomnia, mental depression, aseptic meningitis and hallucinations.

Fertility: Oligospermia, reversible on discontinuance of drug.

Renal reactions: Crystalluria, haematuria, proteinuria and nephrotic syndrome. An acute attack may be precipitated in patients with porphyria.

Overdosage: There is no specific antidote to Salazopyrin.

Pregnancy and lactation: Long term clinical usage and experimental studies have failed to reveal any teratogenic or icteric hazards. The amounts of drug present in the milk should not present a risk to a healthy infant.

Pharmaceutical precautions Store suppositories in a cool place.

Legal category POM.

Package quantities

Tablets:	Bottles of 112
Suppositories:	Boxes of 10
Enemas:	Boxes of 7×100 mls.
Suspension:	Bottles of 500 ml.

Further information The drug may colour the urine orange-yellow.

Extended-wear soft contact lenses (Bausch and Lomb 70) have been reported as being permanently stained during sulphasalazine treatment. Daily-wear soft contact and gas-permeable types should respond to standard cleansing.

When gastro-intestinal intolerance to Salazopyrin tablets occurs, Salazopyrin EN-tabs may be used instead. These film-coated enteric tablets are subject to a separate Data Sheet.

The suspension contains 33 g/100 ml sucrose.

Product licence numbers

Tablets:	0022/0158
Suppositories:	0022/0156
Enemas:	0022/0154
Suspension:	0022/0157

SALAZOPYRIN* EN-TABS

Presentation Yellow elliptical convex film coated enteric tablets, containing 0.5 g of sulphasalazine. One side of the tablet has KPh with 102 on the reverse. Excipients: maize starch, P.V.P., magnesium stearate, enteric coating, colloidal silicon dioxide.

Uses
1. The treatment of Rheumatoid Arthritis which has failed to respond to non-steroidal anti-inflammatory drugs (NSAIDs).
2. Induction and maintenance of remission of Ulcerative Colitis.
3. The treatment of active Crohn's disease.

Dosage and administration
Rheumatoid arthritis

Adults including the elderly: Commence treatment with 0.5 g daily (one tablet) for one week, thereafter increasing the dose by one tablet each week, to a maximum of 3 g/day (six tablets) as in the following table.

	1st Week	*2nd Week*	*3rd Week*	*4th Week*
Morning	—	1 tablet	1 tablet	2 tablets
Evening	1 tablet	1 tablet	2 tablets	2 tablets†

† etc to 3 g/day maximum.

Should a patient experience nausea, the dose should be reduced to a previously tolerated dose for one week and then increased. EN-tabs should not be broken or crushed. Alternatively, the total daily dose may be divided and taken three times or four times daily.

In rheumatoid arthritis Salazopyrin EN-tabs have a 'disease-modifying' action: clinical and haematological response is often seen after one month but may be delayed for up to 12 weeks following the commencement of treatment.

Salazopyrin EN-tabs do not possess analgesic activity, therefore NSAIDs or analgesic treatment should not be reduced or stopped abruptly until clinical response has been achieved.

Patients have been maintained on Salazopyrin EN-tabs for several years.

No recommendations are made for the treatment of children with rheumatoid arthritis.

Ulcerative colitis
Adults:
Severe: 2–4 tablets four times a day may be given in conjunction with steroids as part of an intensive management regime. The night-time interval between doses should not exceed eight hours. In severe disease rapid passage of the tablets may reduce the effect of the drug.

Mild–moderate: 2–4 tablets four times a day may be given in conjunction with steroids.

Maintenance: With induction of remission reduce the dose gradually to four tablets per day in divided doses. This dosage should be continued indefinitely, since discontinuance even several years after an acute attack has been shown to be associated with a four fold increase in the risk of relapse.

Salazopyrin EN-tabs should not be broken or crushed.

Children: The dose is reduced in proportion to body weight.

Severe:	40–60 mg/kg per day
Mild–Moderate:	40–60 mg/kg per day
Maintenance:	20–30 mg/kg per day

Crohn's disease
In active Crohn's disease, Salazopyrin EN-tabs should be administered as for severe ulcerative colitis.

Contra-indications, warnings, etc
Contra-indications:
a. History of sensitivity to sulphonamides or salicylates.
b. Infants under 2 years of age.

Precautions: Haematological and hepatic side effects may occur. Differential white cell, red cell and platelet counts should be performed initially and at least monthly for a minimum of the first three months of treatment. The patient should also be counselled to report immediately with any sore throat, fever, malaise or unexpected non specific illness. Treatment should be stopped immediately if there is suspicion or laboratory evidence of a potentially serious blood dyscrasia.

A patient information leaflet should be supplied specifically advising patients on blood dyscrasias.

Liver function tests should be carried out at monthly intervals for the first three months of treatment. Kidney function should be checked initially and at intervals during treatment.

Patients with allergy, or renal or hepatic disease should be treated with caution. Patients with glucose-6-phosphate dehydrogenase deficiency should be closely observed for signs of haemolytic anaemia (Heinz body anaemia).

The uptake of digoxin and folate may be reduced. An acute attack may be precipitated in patients with porphyria.

Adverse effects: Overall, about 75% of ADRs occur within 3 months of starting therapy, and over 90% by 6 months. Some undesirable effects are dose dependent and symptoms can often be alleviated by reduction of the dose.

Since sulphasalazine is metabolised to sulphapyridine and 5-amino salicylic acid, effects of sulphonamides or salicylates may occur. Patients with slow acetylator status are more likely to experience adverse effects due to sulphapyridine. The most commonly encountered reactions are nausea, headache, rash, loss of appetite and raised temperature.

The following adverse reactions have been reported:

Haematological: Potentially fatal leucopenia, neutropenia, agranulocytosis, aplastic anaemia and thrombocytopenia. Leucopenia, which is normally mild and transient, may occur in up to 1.5% of patients and agranulocytosis in up to 1 in 700 patients during the second month of therapy.

The risk of sulphasalazine associated blood disorders is substantially higher in patients treated for rheumatoid arthritis than it is for patients treated for inflammatory bowel disease.

Heinz body anaemia, methaemoglobinaemia, hypoprothrombinaemia, haemolytic anaemia, megaloblastic anaemia.

Hypersensitivity reactions: Generalised skin eruptions, Stevens–Johnson syndrome, exfoliative dermatitis, epidermal necrolysis, pruritis, urticaria, photosensitisation, anaphylaxis, serum sickness, drug fever, periorbital oedema, conjunctival and scleral injection, arthralgia, allergic myocarditis, polyarteritis nodosa, LE-phenomenon and lung complications with dyspnoea, fever, cough, eosinophilia, fibrosing alveolitis.

Gastro-intestinal reactions: Stomatitis, parotitis, pancreatitis, hepatitis.

CNS reactions: Vertigo, tinnitus, peripheral neuropathy, ataxia, convulsions, insomnia, mental depression, aseptic meningitis and hallucinations.

Fertility: Oligospermia, reversible on discontinuance of drug.

Renal reactions: Crystalluria, haematuria, proteinuria and nephrotic syndrome.

Overdosage: There is no specific antidote to Salazopyrin EN-tabs.

Pregnancy and lactation: Long term clinical usage and experimental studies have failed to reveal any teratogenic or icteric hazards. The amounts of drug present in the milk should not present a risk to a healthy infant.

Legal category POM.

Package quantities EN-tabs: Containers of 112 (special easily-opened pack for the disabled).

Further information The drug may colour the urine orange-yellow.

Extended-wear soft contact lenses (Bausch and Lomb 70) have been reported as being permanently stained during sulphasalazine treatment. Daily-wear soft contact and gas-permeable types should respond to standard cleansing.

Product licence number 0022/0155.

SOLU-CORTEF*

Qualitative and quantitative composition Hydrocortisone sodium succinate 133.7 mg equivalent to hydrocortisone 100.0 mg.

Pharmaceutical form White, freeze dried powder for parenteral use.

Clinical particulars

Therapeutic indications: Anti-inflammatory agent.

Solu-Cortef is indicated for any condition in which rapid and intense corticosteroid effect is required such as:

Endocrine disorders: Primary or secondary adrenocortical insufficiency

Collagen diseases: Systemic lupus erythematosus

Dermatological diseases: Severe erythema multiforme (Stevens-Johnson syndrome)

Allergic states: Bronchial asthma, anaphylactic reactions

Gastro-intestinal diseases: Ulcerative colitis, Crohn's disease

Respiratory diseases: Aspiration of gastric contents

Medical emergencies: Solu-Cortef is indicated in the treatment of shock secondary to adrenocortical insufficiency or shock unresponsive to conventional therapy when adrenocortical insufficiency may be present.

Posology and method of administration: Solu-Cortef may be administered by intravenous injection, by intravenous infusion, or by intramuscular injection, the preferred method for initial emergency use being intravenous injection. Following the initial emergency period, consideration should be given to employing a longer-acting injectable preparation or an oral preparation.

Dosage usually ranges from 100 mg to 500 mg depending on the severity of the condition, administered by intravenous injection over a period of one to ten minutes. This dose may be repeated at intervals of 2, 4 or 6 hours as indicated by the patient's response and clinical condition.

In general high-dose corticosteroid therapy should be continued only until the patient's condition has stabilised - usually not beyond 48 to 72 hours. If hydrocortisone therapy must be continued beyond 48 to 72 hours hypernatraemia may occur, therefore it may be preferable to replace Solu-Cortef with a corticosteroid such as methylprednisolone sodium succinate as little or no sodium retention occurs. Although adverse effects associated with high dose, short-term corticoid therapy are uncommon, peptic ulceration may occur. Prophylactic antacid therapy may be indicated.

Patients subjected to severe stress following corticoid therapy should be observed closely for signs and symptoms of adrenocortical insufficiency.

Corticosteroid therapy is an adjunct to, and not a replacement for, conventional therapy.

Elderly patients: Solu-Cortef is primarily used in acute short-term conditions. There is no information to suggest that a change in dosage is warranted in the elderly. However, treatment of elderly patients should be planned bearing in mind the more serious consequences of the common side-effects of corticosteroids in old age and close clinical supervision is required (see Special warnings and special precautions for use).

Children: While the dose may be reduced for infants and children, it is governed more by the severity of the condition and response of the patient than by age or body weight but should not be less than 25 mg daily (see Special warnings and special precautions for use).

Preparation of solutions: For intravenous or intramuscular injection prepare the solution aseptically by adding not more than 2 ml of Sterile Water for Injections to the contents of one vial of Solu-Cortef 100 mg, shake and withdraw for use.

For intravenous infusion, first prepare the solution by adding not more than 2 ml of Sterile Water for Injections to the vial; this solution may then be added to 100 ml – 1000 ml (but not less than 100 ml) of 5% dextrose in water (or isotonic saline solution or 5% dextrose in isotonic saline solution if patient is not on sodium restriction).

When reconstituted as directed the pH of the solution will range from 7.0 to 8.0.

Contra-indications: Solu-Cortef is contra-indicated where there is known hypersensitivity to components and in systemic fungal infection unless specific anti-infective therapy is employed.

Special warnings and special precautions for use: Warnings and precautions: A Patient Information Leaflet is provided in the pack by the manufacturer.

Undesirable effects may be minimised by using the lowest effective dose for the minimum period. Frequent patient review is required to appropriately titrate the dose against disease activity (see Posology and method of administration).

Adrenal cortical atrophy develops during prolonged therapy and may persist for months after stopping treatment. In patients who have received more than physiological doses of systemic corticosteroids (approximately 30 mg hydrocortisone) for greater than 3 weeks, withdrawal should not be abrupt. How dose reduction should be carried out depends largely on whether the disease is likely to relapse as the dose of systemic corticosteroids is reduced. Clinical assessment of disease activity may be needed during withdrawal. If the disease is unlikely to relapse on withdrawal of systemic corticosteroids, but there is uncertainty about HPA suppression, the dose of systemic corticosteroid *may* be reduced rapidly to physiological doses. Once a daily dose of 30 mg hydrocortisone is reached, dose reduction should be slower to allow the HPA-axis to recover.

Abrupt withdrawal of systemic corticosteroid treatment, which has continued up to 3 weeks is appropriate if it is considered that the disease is unlikely to relapse. Abrupt withdrawal of doses up to 160 mg hydrocortisone for 3 weeks is unlikely to lead to clinically relevant HPA-axis suppression, in the majority of patients. In the following patient groups, gradual withdrawal of systemic corticosteroid therapy should be ***considered*** even after courses lasting 3 weeks or less:

Patients who have had repeated courses of systemic corticosteroids, particularly if taken for greater than 3 weeks; When a short course has been prescribed within one year of cessation of long-term therapy (months or years); Patients who may have reasons for adrenocortical insufficiency other than exogenous corticosteroid therapy; Patients receiving doses of systemic corticosteroid greater than 160 mg of hydrocortisone.

Patients repeatedly taking doses in the evening: Patients should carry 'Steroid Treatment' cards which give clear guidance on the precautions to be taken to minimise risk and which provide details of prescriber, drug, dosage and the duration of treatment.

Corticosteroids may mask some signs of infection, and new infections may appear during their use. Suppression of the inflammatory response and immune function increases the susceptibility to fungal, viral and bacterial infections and their severity. The clinical presentation may often be atypical and may reach an advanced stage before being recognised.

Chickenpox is of serious concern since this normally minor illness may be fatal in immunosuppressed patients. Patients (or parents of children) without a definite history of chickenpox should be advised to avoid close personal contact with chickenpox or herpes zoster and if exposed they should seek urgent medical attention. Passive immunization with varicella/zoster immunoglobin (VZIG) is needed by exposed non-immune patients who are receiving systemic corticosteroids or who have used them within the previous 3 months; this should be given within 10 days of exposure to chickenpox. If a diagnosis of chickenpox is confirmed, the illness warrants specialist care and urgent treatment. Corticosteroids should not be stopped and the dose may need to be increased.

Live vaccines should not be given to individuals with impaired immune responsiveness. The antibody response to other vaccines may be diminished.

The use of Solu-Cortef in active tuberculosis should be restricted to those cases of fulminating or disseminated tuberculosis in which the corticosteroid is used for the management of the disease in conjunction with appropriate antituberculosis regimen. If corticosteroids are indicated in patients with latent tuberculosis or tuberculin reactivity, close observation is necessary as reactivation of the disease may occur. During prolonged corticosteroid therapy, these patients should receive chemoprophylaxis.

Rarely anaphylactoid reactions have been reported following parenteral Solu-Cortef therapy. Physicians using the drug should be prepared to deal with such a possibility. Appropriate precautionary measures should be taken prior to administration, especially when the patient has a history of drug allergy.

Care should be taken for patients receiving cardioactive drugs such as digoxin because of steroid induced electrolyte disturbance/potassium loss (see Undesirable effects).

Special precautions: Particular care is required when considering the use of systemic corticosteroids in patients with the following conditions and frequent patient monitoring is necessary.

Osteoporosis (post-menopausal females are particularly at risk) ; Hypertension or congestive heart failure ; Existing or previous history of severe affective disorders (especially previous steroid psychosis) ; Diabetes mellitus (or a family history of diabetes) ; History of tuberculosis ; Glaucoma (or a family history of glaucoma) ; Previous corticosteroid-induced myopathy ; Liver failure or cirrhosis ; Renal insufficiency ; Epilepsy ; Peptic ulceration ; Fresh intestinal anastomoses ; Predisposition to thrombophlebitis ; Abscess or other pyogenic infections ; Ulcerative colitis ; Diverticulitis ; Myasthenia gravis ; Ocular herpes simplex, for fear of corneal perforation ; Hypothyroidism.

Use in children: Corticosteroids cause growth retardation in infancy, childhood and adolescence, which may be irreversible. Treatment should be limited to the minimum dosage for the shortest possible time. The use of steroids should be restricted to the most serious indications.

Use in the elderly: The common adverse effects of systemic corticosteroids may be associated with more serious consequences in old age, especially osteoporosis, hypertension, hypokalaemia, diabetes, susceptibility to infection and thinning of the skin. Close clinical supervision is required to avoid life-threatening reactions.

Interaction with other medicaments and other forms of interaction: Convulsions have been reported with concurrent use of corticosteroids and cyclosporin. Since concurrent administration of these agents results in a mutual inhibition of metabolism, it is possible that convulsions and other adverse effects associated with the individual use of either drug may be more apt to occur.

Drugs that induce hepatic enzymes, such as rifampicin, rifabutin, carbamazepine, phenobarbitone, phenytoin, primidone, and aminoglutethimide enhance the metabolism of corticosteroids and its therapeutic effects may be reduced.

Drugs such as erythromycin and ketoconazole may inhibit the metabolism of corticosteroids and thus decrease their clearance.

Steroids may reduce the effects of anticholinesterases in myasthenia gravis. The desired effects of hypoglycaemic agents (including insulin), anti-hypertensives and diuretics are antagonised by corticosteroids, and the hypokalaemic effects of acetazolamide, loop diuretics, thiazide diuretics and carbenoxolone are enhanced.

The efficacy of coumarin anticoagulants may be enhanced by concurrent corticosteroid therapy and close monitoring of the INR or prothrombin time is required to avoid spontaneous bleeding.

The renal clearance of salicylates is increased by corticosteroids and steroid withdrawal may result in salicylate intoxication. Salicylates and non-steroidal anti-inflammatory agents should be used cautiously in conjunction with corticosteroids in hypothrombinaemia.

Steroids have been reported to interact with neuromuscular blocking agents such as pancuronium with partial reversal of the neuromuscular block.

Pregnancy and lactation:

Pregnancy: The ability of corticosteroids to cross the placenta varies between individual drugs, however, hydrocortisone readily crosses the placenta.

Administration of corticosteroids to pregnant animals can cause abnormalities of foetal development including cleft palate, intra-uterine growth retardation and affects on brain growth and development. There is no evidence that corticosteroids result in an increased incidence of congenital abnormalities, such as cleft palate in man, however, when administered for long periods or repeatedly during pregnancy, corticosteroids may increase the risk of intra-uterine growth retardation. Hypoadrenalism may, in theory , occur in the neonate following prenatal exposure to corticosteroids but usually resolves spontaneously following birth and is rarely clinically important. As with all drugs, corticosteroids should only be prescribed when the benefits to the mother and child outweigh the risks. When corticosteroids are essential, however, patients with normal pregnancies may be treated as though they were in the non-gravid state.

Lactation: Corticosteroids are excreted in breast milk, although no data are available for hydrocortisone. Doses up to 160 mg daily of hydrocortisone are unlikely to cause systemic effects in the infant. Infants of mothers taking higher doses than this may have a degree of adrenal suppression, but the benefits of breastfeeding are likely to outweigh any theoretical risk.

Effects on ability to drive and use machines: None stated.

Undesirable effects: Since Solu-Cortef is normally employed on a short-term basis it is unlikely that side-effects will occur; however, the possibility of side-effects attributable to corticosteroid therapy should be recognised (see Special warnings and special precautions for use). Such side-effects include:

Parenteral corticosteroid therapy: Anaphylactoid reaction e.g. bronchospasm, hypopigmentation or hyperpigmentation, subcutaneous and cutaneous atrophy, sterile abscess, laryngeal oedema and urticaria.

Gastro-intestinal: Dyspepsia, peptic ulceration with perforation and haemorrhage, abdominal distension, oesophageal ulceration, oesophageal candidiasis, acute pancreatitis, perforation of bowel.

Increases in alanine transaminase (ALT, SGPT) aspartate transaminase (AST, SGOT) and alkaline phosphatase have been observed following corticosteroid treatment. These changes are usually small, not associated with any clinical syndrome and are reversible upon discontinuation.

Anti-inflammatory and immunosuppressive effects: Increased susceptibility and severity of infections with suppression of clinical symptoms and signs, opportunistic infections, may suppress reactions to skin tests, recurrence of dormant tuberculosis (see Special warnings and special precautions for use).

Musculoskeletal: Proximal myopathy, osteoporosis, vertebral and long bone fractures, avascular osteonecrosis, tendon rupture, aseptic necrosis, muscle weakness.

Fluid and electrolyte disturbance: Sodium and water retention, potassium loss, hypertension, hypokalaemic alkalosis, congestive heart failure in susceptible patients.

Dermatological: Impaired healing, petechiae and ecchymosis, skin atrophy, bruising, striae, increased sweating, telangiectasia, acne.

Endocrine/metabolic: Suppression of the hypothalamo-pituitary-adrenal axis; growth suppression in infancy, childhood and adolescence; menstrual irregularity and amenorrhoea, Cushingoid facies, hirsutism, weight gain, impaired carbohydrate tolerance with increased requirement for antidiabetic therapy, negative nitrogen and calcium balance. Increased appetite.

Neuropsychiatric: Euphoria, psychological dependence, mood swings, depression, personality changes, insomnia, convulsions. Increased intra-cranial pressure with papilloedema in children (pseudotumour cerebri), usually after treatment withdrawal. Psychosis, aggravation of schizophrenia, seizures.

Ophthalmic: Increased intra-ocular pressure, glaucoma, papilloedema, cataracts with possible damage to the optic nerve, corneal or scleral thinning, exacerbation of ophthalmic viral or fungal disease, exophthalmos.

General: Leucocytosis, hypersensitivity reactions including anaphylaxis, thrombo-embolism, nausea, malaise.

Withdrawal symptoms: Too rapid a reduction of corticosteroid dosage following prolonged treatment can lead to acute adrenal insufficiency, hypotension and death. However, this is more applicable to corticosteroids with an indication where continuous therapy is given (see Special warnings and special precautions for use).

A 'withdrawal syndrome' may also occur including, fever, myalgia, arthralgia, rhinitis, conjunctivitis, painful itchy skin nodules and loss of weight.

Overdose: There is no clinical syndrome of acute overdosage with Solu-Cortef. Hydrocortisone is dialysable.

Pharmacological properties

Pharmacodynamic properties: Hydrocortisone sodium succinate has the same metabolic and anti-inflammatory actions as hydrocortisone. It is a glucocorticosteroid. Used in pharmacological doses, its actions supress the clinical manifestations of disease in a wide range of disorders.

Pharmacokinetic properties: Twelve normal subjects received 100, 200 or 400 mg Solu-Cortef intravenously. Radio-immunoassay results were as follows:-

DOSE (mg)	*CMAX (µg/100 ml)*	*TMAX (hr)*	*12-HR AUC (µg/100 ml×hr)*
100	132.3	0.35	418.0
200	231.8	0.25	680.0
400	629.8	0.37	1024.0

In another study, a 1 mg/kg i.m. dose of Solu-Cortef peaked in 30–60 minutes, with a plasma C_{max} of 80 µg/100 ml.

In analysing hydrocortisone metabolism, a 25 mg IV dose resulted in higher plasma concentrations in females than in males.

Pharmaceutical particulars

List of excipients: Sodium biphosphate, sodium phosphate.

Incompatibilities: None stated.

Shelf-life: Shelf-life of the medicinal product as packaged for sale: 60 months.

After reconstitution with Sterile Water for Injections, use immediately, discard any remainder.

Special precautions for storage: Store below 25°C. Refer to Section 4.2 Dosage and Administration. No diluents other than those referred to are recommended. Parenteral drug products should be inspected visually for particulate matter and discoloration prior to administration.

Nature and contents of container: Type I flint glass vials with a butyl rubber plug and metal seal. Each vial of Solu-Cortef 100 mg contains the equivalent of 100 mg hydrocortisone as the sodium succinate for reconstitution with 2 ml of Sterile Water for Injections.

Instructions for use/handling: No special requirements.

Marketing authorisation number 0032/5019.

Date of first authorisation/renewal of authorisation 0032/5019 date of first authorisation: 18 May 1990. Last renewal date: 7 December 1995

Date of revision of the text July 1998.

Legal category POM.

SOLU-MEDRONE*

Qualitative and quantitative composition

Solu-Medrone 40 mg : Methylprednisolone sodium succinate 53.0 mg equivalent to 40 mg of methylprednisolone.

Solu-Medrone 125 mg : Methylprednisolone sodium succinate 165.8 mg equivalent to 125 mg of methylprednisolone.

Solu-Medrone 500 mg : Methylprednisolone sodium succinate 663.0 mg equivalent to 500 mg of methylprednisolone.

Solu-Medrone 1 gram : Methylprednisolone sodium succinate 1.326 gm equivalent to 1.0 g of methylprednisolone.

Pharmaceutical form Powder for injection.

Clinical particulars

Therapeutic indications: Solu-Medrone is indicated to treat any condition in which rapid and intense corticosteroid effect is required such as:

Dermatological disease: Severe erythema multiforme (Stevens-Johnson syndrome)

Allergic states: Bronchial asthma; Severe seasonal and perennial allergic rhinitis; Angioneurotic oedema; Anaphylaxis

Gastro-intestinal diseases: Ulcerative colitis; Crohn's disease

Respiratory diseases: Aspiration of gastric contents; Fulminating or disseminated tuberculosis (with appropriate antituberculous chemotherapy)

Neurological disorders: Cerebral oedema secondary to cerebral tumour ; Acute exacerbations of multiple sclerosis superimposed on a relapsing-remitting background.

Miscellaneous: T.B. meningitis (with appropriate antituberculous chemotherapy); Transplantation

Posology and method of administration: Solu-Medrone may be administered intravenously or intramuscularly, the preferred method for emergency use being intravenous injection given over a suitable time interval. When administering Solu-Medrone in high doses intravenously it should be given over a period of at least 30 minutes. Doses up to 250 mg should be given intravenously over a period of at least five minutes.

For intravenous infusion the initially prepared solution may be diluted with 5% dextrose in water, isotonic saline solution, or 5% dextrose in isotonic saline solution. To avoid compatibility problems with other drugs Solu-Medrone should be administered separately, only in the solutions mentioned.

Undesirable effects may be minimised by using the lowest effective dose for the minimum period (see Other special warnings and precautions).

Parenteral drug products should wherever possible be visually inspected for particulate matter and discoloration prior to administration.

Adults: Dosage should be varied according to the severity of the condition, initial dosage will vary from 10 to 500 mg. In the treatment of graft rejection reactions following transplantation, a dose of up to 1 g/day may be required. Although doses and protocols have varied in studies using methylprednisolone sodium succinate in the treatment of graft rejection reactions, the published literature supports the use of doses of this level, with 500 mg to 1 g most commonly used for acute rejection. Treatment at these doses should be limited to a 48--72 hour period until the patient's condition has stabilised, as prolonged high dose corticosteroid therapy can cause serious corticosteroid induced side-effects (see Undesirable effects and Special warnings and special precautions for use).

Children: In the treatment of high dose indications, such as haematological, rheumatic, renal and dermatological conditions, a dosage of 30 mg/kg/day to a maximum of 1 g/day is recommended. This dosage may be repeated for three pulses either daily or on alternate days. In the treatment of graft rejection reactions following transplantation, a dosage of 10 to 20 mg/kg/day for up to 3 days, to a maximum of 1 g/day, is recommended. In the treatment of status asthmaticus, a dosage of 1 to 4 mg/kg/day for 1--3 days is recommended.

Elderly patients: Solu-Medrone is primarily used in acute short-term conditions. There is no information to suggest that a change in dosage is warranted in the elderly. However, treatment of elderly patients should be planned bearing in mind the more serious consequences of the common side-effects of corticosteroids in old age and close clinical supervision is required (see Special warnings and special precautions for use).

Detailed recommendations for adult dosage are as follows: In anaphylactic reactions: adrenaline or noradrenaline should be administered first for an immediate haemodynamic effect, followed by intravenous injection of Solu-Medrone (methylprednisolone sodium succinate) with other accepted procedures. There is evidence that corticosteroids through their prolonged haemodynamic effect are of value in preventing recurrent attacks of acute anaphylactic reactions.

In sensitivity reactions: Solu-Medrone is capable of providing relief within one half to two hours. In patients with status asthmaticus Solu-Medrone may be given at a dose of 40 mg intravenously, repeated as dictated by patient response. In some asthmatic patients it may be advantageous to administer by slow intravenous drip over a period of hours.

In graft rejection reactions following transplantation: doses of up to 1 g per day have been used to suppress rejection crises, with doses of 500 mg to 1 g most commonly used for acute rejection. Treatment should be continued only until the patient's condition has stabilised; usually not beyond 48--72 hours.

In cerebral oedema: corticosteroids are used to reduce or prevent the cerebral oedema associated with brain tumours (primary or metastatic).

In patients with oedema due to tumour, tapering the dose of corticosteroid appears to be important in order to avoid a rebound increase in intracranial pressure. If brain swelling does occur as the dose is reduced (intracranial bleeding having been ruled out), restart larger and more frequent doses parenterally. Patients with certain malignancies may need to remain on oral corticosteroid therapy for months or even life. Similar or higher doses may be helpful to control oedema during radiation therapy.

The following are suggested dosage schedules for oedemas due to brain tumour.

Schedule A (1)	*Dose (mg)*	*Route*	*Interval in hours*	*Duration*
Pre-operative:	20	IM	3-6	
During Surgery:	20 to 40	IV	hourly	
Post operative:	20	IM	3	24 hours
	16	IM	3	24 hours
	12	IM	3	24 hours
	8	IM	3	24 hours
	4	IM	3	24 hours
	4	IM	6	24 hours
	4	IM	12	24 hours

Schedule B (2)	*Dose (mg)*	*Route*	*Interval in hours*	*Days Duration*
Pre-operative:	40	IM	6	2-3
Post-operative:	40	IM	6	3-5
	20	Oral	6	1
	12	Oral	6	1
	8	Oral	8	1
	4	Oral	12	1
	4	Oral		1

Aim to discontinue therapy after a total of 10 days.

References: Fox JL, MD. 'Use of Methylprednisolone in Intracranial Surgery' Medical Annals of the District of Columbia, 34:261-265,1965.

Cantu RC, MD Harvard Neurological Service, Boston, Massachusetts. Letter on file, The Upjohn Company (February 1970).

In the treatment of *acute exacerbations of multiple sclerosis* in adults, the recommended dose is 1 g daily for 3 days. Solu-Medrone should be given as an intravenous infusion over at least 30 minutes.

In other indications, initial dosage will vary from 10 to 500 mg depending on the clinical problem being treated. Larger doses may be required for short-term management of severe, acute conditions. The initial dose, up to 250 mg, should be given intravenously over a period of at least 5 minutes, doses exceeding 250 mg should be given intravenously over a period of at least 30 minutes. Subsequent doses may be given intravenously or intramuscularly at intervals dictated by the patient's response and clinical condition. Corticosteroid therapy is an adjunct to, and not replacement for, conventional therapy.

Contra-indications: Solu-Medrone is contra-indicated where there is known hypersensitivity to components, in systemic infection unless specific anti-infective therapy is employed and in cerebral oedema in malaria.

Special warnings and special precautions for use: Warnings and precautions: A Patient Information Leaflet is provided in the pack by the manufacturer.

Undesirable effects may be minimised by using the lowest effective dose for the minimum period. Frequent patient review is required to appropriately titrate the dose against disease activity (see Posology and method of administration).

Adrenal cortical atrophy develops during prolonged therapy and may persist for months after stopping treatment. In patients who have received more than physiological doses of systemic corticosteroids (approximately 6 mg methylprednisolone) for greater than 3 weeks, withdrawal should not be abrupt. How dose reduction should be carried out depends largely on whether the disease is likely to relapse as the dose of systemic corticosteroids is reduced. Clinical assessment of disease activity may be needed during withdrawal. If the disease is unlikely to relapse on withdrawal of systemic corticosteroids, but there is uncertainty about HPA suppression, the dose of systemic corticosteroid *may* be reduced rapidly to physiological doses. Once a daily dose of 6 mg methylprednisolone is reached, dose reduction should be slower to allow the HPA-axis to recover.

Abrupt withdrawal of systemic corticosteroid treatment, which has continued up to 3 weeks is appropriate if it is considered that the disease is unlikely to relapse. Abrupt withdrawal of doses up to 32 mg daily of methylprednisolone for 3 weeks is unlikely to lead to clinically relevant HPA-axis suppression, in the majority of patients. In the following patient groups, gradual withdrawal of systemic corticosteroid therapy should be *considered* even after courses lasting 3 weeks or less:

Patients who have had repeated courses of systemic corticosteroids, particularly if taken for greater than 3 weeks.

When a short course has been prescribed within one year of cessation of long-term therapy (months or years).

Patients who may have reasons for adrenocortical insufficiency other than exogenous corticosteroid therapy.

Patients receiving doses of systemic corticosteroid greater than 32 mg daily of methylprednisolone.

Patients repeatedly taking doses in the evening.

Patients should carry 'Steroid Treatment' cards which give clear guidance on the precautions to be taken to minimise risk and which provide details of prescriber, drug, dosage and the duration of treatment.

Although Solu-Medrone is not approved in the UK for use in any shock indication, the following warning statement should be adhered to. Data from a clinical study conducted to establish the efficacy of Solu-Medrone in septic shock, suggest that a higher mortality occurred in subsets of patients who entered the study with elevated serum creatinine levels or who developed a secondary infection after therapy began. Therefore this product should not be used in the treatment of septic syndrome or septic shock.

There have been a few reports of cardiac arrhythmias and/or circulatory collapse and/or cardiac arrest associated with the rapid intravenous administration of large doses of Solu-Medrone (greater than 500 mg administered over a period of less than 10 minutes). Bradycardia has been reported during or after the administration of large doses of methylprednisolone sodium succinate, and may be unrelated to the speed and duration of infusion.

Corticosteroids may mask some signs of infection, and new infections may appear during their use. Suppression of the inflammatory response and immune function increases the susceptibility to fungal, viral and bacterial infections and their severity. The clinical presentation may often be atypical and may reach an advanced stage before being recognised.

Chickenpox is of serious concern since this normally minor illness may be fatal in immunosuppressed patients. Patients (or parents of children) without a definite history of chickenpox should be advised to avoid close personal contact with chickenpox or herpes zoster and if exposed they should seek urgent medical attention. Passive immunization with varicella/zoster immunoglobin (VZIG) is needed by exposed non-immune patients who are receiving systemic corticosteroids or who have used them within the previous 3 months; this should be given within 10 days of exposure to chickenpox. If a diagnosis of chickenpox is confirmed, the illness warrants specialist care and urgent treatment. Corticosteroids should not be stopped and the dose may need to be increased.

Live vaccines should not be given to individuals with impaired immune responsiveness. The antibody response to other vaccines may be diminished.

The use of Solu-Medrone in active tuberculosis should be restricted to those cases of fulminating or disseminated tuberculosis in which the corticosteroid is used for the management of the disease in conjunction with an appropriate anti-tuberculous regimen. If corticosteroids are indicated in patients with latent tuberculosis or tuberculin reactivity, close observation is necessary as reactivation of the disease may occur. During prolonged corticosteroid therapy, these patients should receive chemoprophylaxis.

Rarely anaphylactoid reactions have been reported following parenteral Solu-Medrone therapy. Physicians using the drug should be prepared to deal with such a possibility. Appropriate precautionary measures should be taken prior to administration, especially when the patient has a history of drug allergy.

Care should be taken for patients receiving cardioactive drugs such as digoxin because of steroid induced electrolyte disturbance/potassium loss (see Undesirable effects).

Special precautions: Particular care is required when considering the use of systemic corticosteroids in patients with the following conditions and frequent patient monitoring is necessary.

Osteoporosis (post-menopausal females are particularly at risk).
Hypertension or congestive heart failure.
Existing or previous history of severe affective disorders (especially previous steroid psychosis).
Diabetes mellitus (or a family history of diabetes).
History of tuberculosis.
Glaucoma (or a family history of glaucoma).
Previous corticosteroid-induced myopathy.
Liver failure or cirrhosis.
Renal insufficiency.
Epilepsy.
Peptic ulceration.
Fresh intestinal anastomoses.
Predisposition to thrombophlebitis.
Abscess or other pyogenic infections.
Ulcerative colitis.
Diverticulitis.
Myasthenia gravis.
Ocular herpes simplex, for fear of corneal perforation.
Hypothyroidism.

Use in children: Corticosteroids cause growth retardation in infancy, childhood and adolescence, which may be irreversible. Treatment should be limited to the minimum dosage for the shortest possible time. In order to minimise suppression of the hypothalamo-pituitary-adrenal axis and growth retardation, treatment should be administered where possible as a single dose on alternate days.

Use in the elderly: The common adverse effects of systemic corticosteroids may be associated with more serious consequences in old age, especially osteoporosis, hypertension, hypokalaemia, diabetes, susceptibility to infection and thinning of the skin. Close clinical supervision is required to avoid life-threatening reactions.

Interaction with other medicaments and other forms of interaction: Convulsions have been reported with concurrent use of methylprednisolone and cyclosporin. Since concurrent administration of these agents results in a mutual inhibition of metabolism, it is possible that convulsions and other adverse events associated with the individual use of either drug may be more apt to occur.

Drugs that induce hepatic enzymes, such as rifampicin, rifabutin, carbamazepine, phenobarbitone, phenytoin, primidone, and aminoglutethimide enhance the metabolism of corticosteroids and its therapeutic effects may be reduced.

Drugs such as erythromycin and ketoconazole may inhibit the metabolism of corticosteroids and thus decrease their clearance.

Steroids may reduce the effects of anticholinesterases in myasthenia gravis. The desired effects of hypoglycaemic agents (including insulin), anti-hypertensives and diuretics are antagonised by corticosteroids, and the hypokalaemic effects of acetazolamide, loop diuretics, thiazide diuretics and carbenoxolone are enhanced.

The efficacy of coumarin anticoagulants may be enhanced by concurrent corticosteroid therapy and close monitoring of the INR or prothrombin time is required to avoid spontaneous bleeding.

The renal clearance of salicylates is increased by corticosteroids and steroid withdrawal may result in salicylate intoxication. Salicylates and non-steroidal anti-inflammatory agents should be used cautiously in conjunction with corticosteroids in hypothrombinaemia.

Steroids have been reported to interact with neuromuscular blocking agents such as pancuronium with partial reversal of the neuromuscular block.

Pregnancy and lactation:
Pregnancy: The ability of corticosteroids to cross the placenta varies between individual drugs, however, methylprednisolone does cross the placenta.

Administration of corticosteroids to pregnant animals can cause abnormalities of foetal development including cleft palate, intra-uterine growth retardation and affects on brain growth and development. There is no evidence that corticosteroids result in an increased incidence of congenital abnormalities, such as cleft palate in man, however, when administered for long periods or repeatedly during pregnancy, corticosteroids may increase the risk of intra-uterine growth retardation. Hypoadrenalism may, in theory , occur in the neonate following prenatal exposure to corticosteroids but usually resolves spontaneously following birth and is rarely clinically important. As with all drugs, corticosteroids should only be prescribed when the benefits to the mother and child outweigh the risks. When corticosteroids are essential, however, patients with normal pregnancies may be treated as though they were in the non-gravid state.

Lactation: Corticosteroids are excreted in small amounts in breast milk, however, doses of up to 40 mg daily of methylprednisolone are unlikely to cause systemic effects in the infant. Infants of mothers taking higher doses than this may have a degree of adrenal suppression, but the benefits of breastfeeding are likely to outweigh any theoretical risk.

Effects on ability to drive and use machines: None stated.

Undesirable effects: Under normal circumstances Solu-Medrone therapy would be considered as short-term. However, the possibility of side-effects attributable to corticosteroid therapy should be recognised, particularly when high-dose therapy is being used (see *Special warnings and special precautions for use*). Such side-effects include:

Parenteral corticosteroid therapy: Anaphylactic reaction with or without circulatory collapse, cardiac arrest, bronchospasm, cardiac arrhythmias, hypotension or hypertension.

Gastro-intestinal: Dyspepsia, peptic ulceration with perforation and haemorrhage, abdominal distension, oesophageal ulceration, oesophageal candidiasis, acute pancreatitis. Nausea, vomiting and bad taste in mouth may occur especially with rapid administration.

Increases in alanine transaminase (ALT, SGPT) aspartate transaminase (AST, SGOT) and alkaline phosphatase have been observed following corticosteroid treatment. These changes are usually small, not associated with any clinical syndrome and are reversible upon discontinuation.

Anti-inflammatory and immunosuppressive effects: Increased susceptibility and severity of infections with suppression of clinical symptoms and signs, opportunistic infections, may suppress reactions to skin tests, recurrence of dormant tuberculosis (see *Special warnings and special precautions for use*).

Musculoskeletal: Proximal myopathy, osteoporosis, vertebral and long bone fractures, avascular osteonecrosis, tendon rupture.

Fluid and electrolyte disturbance: Sodium and water retention, potassium loss, hypertension, hypokalaemic alkalosis, congestive heart failure in susceptible patients.

Dermatological: Impaired healing, petechiae and ecchymosis, skin atrophy, bruising, striae, telangiectasia, acne.

Endocrine/metabolic: Suppression of the hypothalamo-pituitary-adrenal axis, growth suppression in infancy, childhood and adolescence, menstrual irregularity and amenorrhoea. Cushingoid facies, hirsutism, weight gain, impaired carbohydrate tolerance with increased requirement for antidiabetic therapy, negative nitrogen and calcium balance. Increased appetite.

Neuropsychiatric: Euphoria, psychological dependence, mood swings, depression, personality changes, insomnia. Increased intra-cranial pressure with papilloedema in children (pseudotumour cerebri), usually after treatment withdrawal. Psychosis, aggravation of schizophrenia, seizures.

Ophthalmic: Increased intra-ocular pressure, glaucoma, papilloedema, cataracts with possible damage to the optic nerve, corneal or scleral thinning, exacerbation of ophthalmic viral or fungal disease.

General: Leucocytosis, hypersensitivity including anaphylaxis, thrombo-embolism, malaise.

Withdrawal symptoms: Too rapid a reduction of corticosteroid dosage following prolonged treatment can lead to acute adrenal insufficiency, hypotension and death. However, this is more applicable to corticosteroids with an indication where continuous therapy is given (see *Special warnings and special precautions for use*).

A 'withdrawal syndrome' may also occur including, fever, myalgia, arthralgia, rhinitis, conjunctivitis, painful itchy skin nodules and loss of weight.

Overdose: There is no clinical syndrome of acute overdosage with Solu-Medrone. Methylprednisolone is dialysable. Following chronic overdosage the possibility of adrenal suppression should be guarded against by gradual diminution of dose levels over a period of time. In such event the patient may require to be supported during any further stressful episode.

Pharmacological properties
Pharmacodynamic properties: Medrone is a corticosteroid with an anti-inflammatory activity at least five times that of hydrocortisone. An enhanced separation of glucocorticoid and mineralocorticoid effect results in a reduced incidence of sodium and water retention.

Pharmacokinetic properties: Methylprednisolone is extensively bound to plasma proteins, mainly to globulin and less so to albumin. Only unbound corticosteroid has pharmacological effects or is metabolised. Metabolism occurs in the liver and to a lesser extent in the kidney. Metabolites are excreted in the urine.

Mean elimination half-life ranges from 2.4 to 3.5 hours in normal healthy adults and appears to be independent of the route of administration.

Total body clearance following intravenous or intramuscular injection of methylprednisolone to healthy adult volunteers is approximately 15–6l/hour. Peak methylprednisolone plasma levels of 33.67 mcg/100 ml were achieved in 2 hours after a single 40 mg i.m. injection to 22 adult male volunteers.

Pharmaceutical particulars
List of excipients: Sodium biphosphate and sodium phosphate. The 40 mg vial also contains lactose.

Incompatibilities: None stated.

Shelf-life: Shelf-life of the medicinal product as packaged for sale: 60 months. After reconstitution with Sterile Water for injections, use immediately, discard any remainder.

Special precautions for storage: Store below 25°C. Refer to Section 4.2 Dosage and Administration. No diluents other than those referred to are recommended. Parenteral drug products should be inspected visually for particulate matter and discoloration prior to administration.

Nature and contents of container: Type I clear glass vial with butyl rubber plug and flip top seal.

Each vial of Solu-Medrone 40 mg contains the equivalent of 40 mg of methylprednisolone as the sodium succinate for reconstitution with 1 ml of Sterile Water for Injections.

Each vial of Solu-Medrone 125 mg contains the equivalent of 125 mg of methylprednisolone as the sodium succinate for reconstitution with 2 ml of Sterile Water for Injections.

Each vial of Solu-Medrone 500 mg contains the equivalent of 500 mg of methylprednisolone as the sodium succinate for reconstitution with 7.8 ml of Sterile Water for Injections.

Each vial of Solu-Medrone 1 g contains the equivalent of 1 g of methylprednisolone as the sodium succinate for reconstitution with 15.6 ml of Sterile Water for Injections.

Instructions for use/handling: No special requirements.

Marketing authorisation numbers
Solu-Medrone 40 mg 0032/0033
Solu-Medrone 125 mg 032/0034
Solu-Medrone 500 mg 0032/0035
Solu-Medrone 1 g 0032/0039

Date of first authorisation/renewal of authorisation
0032/0033, 0034, 0035, date of first authorisation: 21 February 1990
0032/0039, date of first authorisation: 30 July 1990
Last renewal date: 20 August 1996.

Date of revision of the text July 1998.

Legal category POM.

SOLU-MEDRONE* 2 GRAM

Qualitative and quantitative composition Methylprednisolone sodium succinate 2.652 grams equivalent to 2 grams of methylprednisolone.

Pharmaceutical form Powder for injection.

Clinical particulars
Therapeutic indications: Solu-Medrone is indicated to treat any condition in which rapid and intense corticosteroid effect is required such as:
Dermatological disease: Severe erythema multiforme (Stevens-Johnson syndrome)

Allergic states: Bronchial asthma, Severe seasonal and perennial allergic rhinitis, Angioneurotic oedema, Anaphylaxis

Gastro-intestinal diseases: Ulcerative colitis, Crohn's disease

Respiratory diseases: Aspiration of gastric contents, Fulminating or disseminated tuberculosis (with appropriate antituberculous chemotherapy)

Neurological disorders: Cerebral oedema secondary to cerebral tumour

Miscellaneous: TB meningitis (with appropriate antituberculous chemotherapy), Transplantation

Acute spinal cord injury. The treatment should begin within eight hours of injury.

Posology and method of administration: Solu-Medrone may be administered intravenously or intramuscularly, the preferred method for emergency use being intravenous injection given over a suitable time interval. When administering Solu-Medrone in high doses intravenously it should be given over a period of at least 30 minutes. Doses up to 250 mg should be given intravenously over a period of at least five minutes.

For intravenous infusion the initially prepared solution may be diluted with 5% dextrose in water, isotonic saline solution, or 5% dextrose in isotonic saline solution. To avoid compatibility problems with other drugs Solu-Medrone should be administered separately, only in the solutions mentioned.

Undesirable effects may be minimised by using the lowest effective dose for the minimum period (see *Special warnings and special precautions for use*).

Parenteral drug products should wherever possible be visually inspected for particulate matter and discoloration prior to administration.

Adults: Dosage should be varied according to the severity of the condition, initial dosage will vary from 10 to 500 mg. In the treatment of graft rejection reactions following transplantation, a dose of up to 1 g/day may be required. Although doses and protocols have varied in studies using methylprednisolone sodium succinate in the treatment of graft rejection reactions, the published literature supports the use of doses of this level, with 500 mg to 1 g most commonly used for acute rejection. Treatment at these doses should be limited to a 48–72 hour period until the patient's condition has stabilised, as prolonged high dose corticosteroid therapy can cause serious corticosteroid induced side-effects (see *Undesirable effects* and *Special warnings and special precautions for use*).

Children: In the treatment of high dose indications, such as haematological, rheumatic, renal and dermatological conditions, a dosage of 30 mg/kg/day to a maximum of 1 g/day is recommended. This dosage may be repeated for three pulses either daily or on alternate days. In the treatment of graft rejection reactions following transplantation, a dosage of 10 to 20 mg/kg/day for up to 3 days, to a maximum of 1 g/day, is recommended. In the treatment of status asthmaticus, a dosage of 1 to 4 mg/kg/day for 1–3 days is recommended.

Solu-Medrone is not recommended for use in spinal cord injury in children.

Elderly patients: Solu-Medrone is primarily used in acute short-term conditions. There is no information to suggest that a change in dosage is warranted in the elderly. However, treatment of elderly patients should be planned bearing in mind the more serious consequences of the common side-effects of corticosteroids in old age and close clinical supervision is required (see *Special warnings and special precautions for use*).

Detailed recommendations for adult dosage are as follows:

In anaphylactic reactions: adrenaline or noradrenaline should be administered first for an immediate haemodynamic effect, followed by intravenous injection of Solu-Medrone (methylprednisolone sodium succinate) with other accepted procedures. There is evidence that corticosteroids through their prolonged haemodynamic effect are of value in preventing recurrent attacks of acute anaphylactic reactions.

In sensitivity reactions: Solu-Medrone is capable of providing relief within one half to two hours. In patients with status asthmaticus Solu-Medrone may be given at a dose of 40 mg intravenously, repeated as dictated by patient response. In some asthmatic patients it may be advantageous to administer by slow intravenous drip over a period of hours.

In graft rejection reactions following transplantation: doses of up to 1 g per day have been used to suppress rejection crises, with doses of 500 mg to 1 g most commonly used for acute rejection. Treatment should be continued only until the patient's condition has stabilised; usually not beyond 48–72 hours.

In cerebral oedema: corticosteroids are used to reduce or prevent the cerebral oedema associated with brain tumours (primary or metastatic).

In patients with oedema due to tumour, tapering the dose of corticosteroid appears to be important in order to avoid a rebound increase in intracranial pressure. If brain swelling does occur as the dose is reduced (intracranial bleeding having been ruled out), restart larger and more frequent doses parenterally. Patients with certain malignancies may need to remain on oral corticosteroid therapy for months or even life. Similar or higher doses may be helpful to control oedema during radiation therapy.

The following are suggested dosage schedules for oedemas due to brain tumour.

Schedule A (1)	*Dose (mg)*	*Route*	*Interval in hours*	*Duration*
Pre-operative:	20	IM	3-6	
During Surgery:	20 to 40	IV	hourly	
Post operative:	20	IM	3	24 hours
	16	IM	3	24 hours
	12	IM	3	24 hours
	8	IM	3	24 hours
	4	IM	3	24 hours
	4	IM	6	24 hours
	4	IM	12	24 hours

Schedule B (2)	*Dose (mg)*	*Route*	*Interval in hours*	*Days Duration*
Pre-operative:	40	IM	6	2-3
Post-operative:	40	IM	6	3-5
	20	Oral	6	1
	12	Oral	6	1
	8	Oral	8	1
	4	Oral	12	1
	4	Oral		1

Aim to discontinue therapy after a total of 10 days.

References: Fox JL, MD. 'Use of Methylprednisolone in Intracranial Surgery' Medical Annals of the District of Columbia, 34:261-265,1965.

Cantu RC, MD Harvard Neurological Service, Boston, Massachusetts. Letter on file, The Upjohn Company (February 1970).

For treatment of acute spinal cord injury: administer intravenously 30 mg methylprednisolone per kilogram of body weight in a bolus dose over a 15 minute period, followed by a 45 minute pause, and then a continuous infusion of 5.4 mg/kg per hour for 23 hours. There should be a separate intravenous site for the infusion pump. The treatment should begin within eight hours of injury.

In other indications: initial dosage will vary from 10 to 500 mg depending on the clinical problem being treated. Larger doses may be required for short-term management of severe, acute conditions. The initial dose, up to 250 mg, should be given intravenously over a period of at least 5 minutes, doses exceeding 250 mg should be given intravenously over a period of at least 30 minutes. Subsequent doses may be given intravenously or intramuscularly at intervals dictated by the patient's response and clinical condition. Corticosteroid therapy is an adjunct to, and not replacement for, conventional therapy.

Contra-indications: Solu-Medrone is contra-indicated where there is known hypersensitivity to components, in systemic fungal infections unless specific anti-infective therapy is employed and in cerebral oedema in malaria.

Special warnings and special precautions for use:
Warnings and precautions: A Patient Information Leaflet is provided in the pack by the manufacturer.

Undesirable effects may be minimised by using the lowest effective dose for the minimum period. Frequent patient review is required to appropriately titrate the dose against disease activity (see *Posology and method of administration*).

Adrenal cortical atrophy develops during prolonged therapy and may persist for months after stopping treatment. In patients who have received more than physiological doses of systemic corticosteroids (approximately 6 mg methylprednisolone) for greater than 3 weeks, withdrawal should not be abrupt. How dose reduction should be carried out depends largely on whether the disease is likely to relapse as the dose of systemic corticosteroids is reduced. Clinical assessment of disease activity may be needed during withdrawal. If the disease is unlikely to relapse on withdrawal of systemic corticosteroids, but there is uncertainty about HPA suppression, the dose of systemic corticosteroid *may* be reduced rapidly to physiological doses. Once a daily dose of 6 mg methylprednisolone is reached, dose reduction should be slower to allow the HPA-axis to recover.

Abrupt withdrawal of systemic corticosteroid treatment, which has continued up to 3 weeks is appropriate if it is considered that the disease is unlikely to relapse. Abrupt withdrawal of doses up to 32 mg daily of methylprednisolone for 3 weeks is unlikely to lead to clinically relevant HPA-axis suppression, in the majority of patients. In the following patient groups, gradual withdrawal of systemic corticosteroid therapy should be *considered* even after courses lasting 3 weeks or less:

Patients who have had repeated courses of systemic corticosteroids, particularly if taken for greater than 3 weeks; When a short course has been prescribed within one year of cessation of long-term therapy (months or years); Patients who may have reasons for adrenocortical insufficiency other than exogenous corticosteroid therapy; Patients receiving doses of systemic corticosteroid greater than 32 mg daily of methylprednisolone; Patients repeatedly taking doses in the evening.

Patients should carry 'Steroid Treatment' cards which give clear guidance on the precautions to be taken to minimise risk and which provide details of prescriber, drug, dosage and the duration of treatment.

Although Solu-Medrone is not approved in the UK for use in any shock indication, the following warning statement should be adhered to. Data from a clinical study conducted to establish the efficacy of Solu-Medrone in septic shock, suggest that a higher mortality occurred in subsets of patients who entered the study with elevated serum creatinine levels or who developed a secondary infection after therapy began. Therefore this product should not be used in the treatment of septic syndrome or septic shock.

There have been a few reports of cardiac arrhythmias and/or circulatory collapse and/or cardiac arrest associated with the rapid intravenous administration of large doses of Solu-Medrone (greater than 500 mg administered over a period of less than 10 minutes). Bradycardia has been reported during or after the administration of large doses of methylprednisolone sodium succinate, and may be unrelated to the speed and duration of infusion.

Corticosteroids may mask some signs of infection, and new infections may appear during their use. Suppression of the inflammatory response and immune function increases the susceptibility to fungal, viral and bacterial infections and their severity. The clinical presentation may often be atypical and may reach an advanced stage before being recognised.

Chickenpox is of serious concern since this normally minor illness may be fatal in immunosuppressed patients. Patients (or parents of children) without a definite history of chickenpox should be advised to avoid close personal contact with chickenpox or herpes zoster and if exposed they should seek urgent medical attention. Passive immunisation with varicella/zoster immunoglobin (VZIG) is needed by exposed non-immune patients who are receiving systemic corticosteroids or who have used them within the previous 3 months; this should be given within 10 days of exposure to chickenpox. If a diagnosis of chickenpox is confirmed, the illness warrants specialist care and urgent treatment. Corticosteroids should not be stopped and the dose may need to be increased.

Live vaccines should not be given to individuals with impaired immune responsiveness. The antibody response to other vaccines may be diminished.

The use of Solu-Medrone in active tuberculosis should be restricted to those cases of fulminating or disseminated tuberculosis in which the corticosteroid is used for the management of the disease in conjunction with an appropriate anti-tuberculous regimen. If corticosteroids are indicated in patients with latent tuberculosis or tuberculin reactivity, close observation is necessary as reactivation of the disease may occur. During prolonged corticosteroid therapy, these patients should receive chemoprophylaxis.

Rarely anaphylactoid reactions have been reported following parenteral Solu-Medrone therapy. Physicians using the drug should be prepared to deal with such a possibility. Appropriate precautionary measures should be taken prior to administration, especially when the patient has a history of drug allergy.

Care should be taken for patients receiving cardioactive drugs such as digoxin because of steroid induced electrolyte disturbance/potassium loss (see *Undesirable effects*).

Special precautions: Particular care is required when considering the use of systemic corticosteroids in patients with the following conditions and frequent patient monitoring is necessary.

Osteoporosis (post-menopausal females are particularly at risk); Hypertension or congestive heart failure; Existing or previous history of severe affective disorders (especially previous steroid psychosis); Diabetes mellitus (or a family history of diabetes); History of tuberculosis; Glaucoma (or a family history of glaucoma); Previous corticosteroid-induced myopathy; Liver failure or cirrhosis; Renal insufficiency; Epilepsy; Peptic ulceration; Fresh intestinal anastomoses; Predisposition to thrombophlebitis; Abscess or other pyogenic infections; Ulcerative colitis; Diverticulitis; Myasthenia gravis; Ocular herpes simplex, for fear of corneal perforation; Hypothyroidism.

Use in children: Corticosteroids cause growth retardation in infancy, childhood and adolescence, which may be irreversible. Treatment should be limited to the minimum dosage for the shortest possible time. In order to minimise suppression of the hypothalamo-pituitary-adrenal axis and growth retardation, treatment should be administered where possible as a single dose on alternate days.

Use in the elderly: The common adverse effects of systemic corticosteroids may be associated with more serious consequences in old age, especially osteoporosis, hypertension, hypokalaemia, diabetes, susceptibility to infection and thinning of the skin. Close clinical supervision is required to avoid life-threatening reactions.

Interaction with other medicaments and other forms of interaction: Convulsions have been reported with concurrent use of methylprednisolone and cyclosporin. Since concurrent administration of these agents results in a mutual inhibition of metabolism, it is possible that convulsions and other adverse events associated with the individual use of either drug may be more apt to occur.

Drugs that induce hepatic enzymes, such as rifampicin, rifabutin, carbamazepine, phenobarbitone, phenytoin, primidone, and aminoglutethimide enhance the metabolism of corticosteroids and its therapeutic effects may be reduced.

Drugs such as erythromycin and ketoconazole may inhibit the metabolism of corticosteroids and thus decrease their clearance.

Steroids may reduce the effects of anticholinesterases in myasthenia gravis. The desired effects of hypoglycaemic agents (including insulin), anti-hypertensives and diuretics are antagonised by corticosteroids, and the hypokalaemic effects of acetazolamide, loop diuretics, thiazide diuretics and carbenoxolone are enhanced.

The efficacy of coumarin anticoagulants may be enhanced by concurrent corticosteroid therapy and close monitoring of the INR or prothrombin time is required to avoid spontaneous bleeding.

The renal clearance of salicylates is increased by corticosteroids and steroid withdrawal may result in salicylate intoxication. Salicylates and non-steroidal anti-inflammatory agents should be used cautiously in conjunction with corticosteroids in hypothrombinaemia.

Steroids have been reported to interact with neuromuscular blocking agents such as pancuronium with partial reversal of the neuromuscular block.

Pregnancy and lactation:
Pregnancy: The ability of corticosteroids to cross the placenta varies between individual drugs, however, methylprednisolone does cross the placenta.

Administration of corticosteroids to pregnant animals can cause abnormalities of foetal development including cleft palate, intra-uterine growth retardation and affects on brain growth and development. There is no evidence that corticosteroids result in an increased incidence of congenital abnormalities, such as cleft palate in man, however, when administered for long periods or repeatedly during pregnancy, corticosteroids may increase the risk of intra-uterine growth retardation. Hypoadrenalism may, in theory, occur in the neonate following prenatal exposure to corticosteroids but usually resolves spontaneously following birth and is rarely clinically important. As with all drugs, corticosteroids should only be prescribed when the benefits to the mother and child outweigh the risks. When corticosteroids are essential, however, patients with normal pregnancies may be treated as though they were in the non-gravid state.

Lactation: Corticosteroids are excreted in small amounts in breast milk, however, doses of up to 40 mg daily of methylprednisolone are unlikely to cause systemic effects in the infant. Infants of mothers taking higher doses than this may have a degree of adrenal suppression, but the benefits of breastfeeding are likely to outweigh any theoretical risk.

Effects on ability to drive and use machines: None stated.

Undesirable effects: Under normal circumstances Solu-Medrone therapy would be considered as short-term. However, the possibility of side-effects attributable to corticosteroid therapy should be recognised, particularly when high-dose therapy is being used (see *Special warnings and special precautions for use*). Such side-effects include:

Parenteral corticosteroid therapy: Anaphylactic reaction with or without circulatory collapse, cardiac arrest, bronchospasm, cardiac arrhythmias, hypotension or hypertension.

Gastro-intestinal: Dyspepsia, peptic ulceration with perforation and haemorrhage, abdominal distension, oesophageal ulceration, oesophageal candidiasis, acute pancreatitis. Nausea, vomiting and bad taste in mouth may occur especially with rapid administration.

Increases in alanine transaminase (ALT, SGPT) aspartate transaminase (AST, SGOT) and alkaline phosphatase have been observed following corticosteroid treatment. These changes are usually small, not associated with any clinical syndrome and are reversible upon discontinuation.

Anti-inflammatory and immunosuppressive effects: Increased susceptibility and severity of infections with suppression of clinical symptoms and signs, opportunistic infections, may suppress reactions to skin tests, recurrence of dormant tuberculosis (see *Special warnings and special precautions for use*).

Musculoskeletal: Proximal myopathy, osteoporosis, vertebral and long bone fractures, avascular osteonecrosis, tendon rupture.

Fluid and electrolyte disturbance: Sodium and water retention, potassium loss, hypertension, hypokalaemic alkalosis, congestive heart failure in susceptible patients.

Dermatological: Impaired healing, petechiae and ecchymosis, skin atrophy, bruising, striae, telangiectasia, acne.

Endocrine/metabolic: Suppression of the hypothalamo-pituitary-adrenal axis; growth suppression in infancy, childhood and adolescence; menstrual irregularity and amenorrhoea. Cushingoid facies, hirsutism, weight gain, impaired carbohydrate tolerance with increased requirement for antidiabetic therapy, negative nitrogen and calcium balance. Increased appetite.

Neuropsychiatric: Euphoria, psychological dependence, mood swings, depression, personality changes, insomnia. Increased intra-cranial pressure with papilloedema in children (pseudotumour cerebri), usually after treatment withdrawal. Psychosis, aggravation of schizophrenia, seizures.

Ophthalmic: Increased intra-ocular pressure, glaucoma, papilloedema, cataracts with possible damage to the optic nerve, corneal or scleral thinning, exacerbation of ophthalmic viral or fungal disease.

General: Leucocytosis, hypersensitivity including anaphylaxis, thrombo-embolism, malaise.

Withdrawal symptoms: Too rapid a reduction of corticosteroid dosage following prolonged treatment can lead to acute adrenal insufficiency, hypotension and death. However, this is more applicable to corticosteroids with an indication where continuous therapy is given (see *Special warnings and special precautions for use*).

A 'withdrawal syndrome' may also occur including, fever, myalgia, arthralgia, rhinitis, conjunctivitis, painful itchy skin nodules and loss of weight.

Overdose: There is no clinical syndrome of acute overdosage with Solu-Medrone. Methylprednisolone is dialysable. Following chronic overdosage the possibility of adrenal suppression should be guarded against by gradual diminution of dose levels over a period of time. In such event the patient may require to be supported during any further stressful episode.

Pharmacological properties

Pharmacodynamic properties: Medrone is a corticosteroid with an anti-inflammatory activity at least five times that of hydrocortisone. An enhanced separation of glucocorticoid and mineralocorticoid effect results in a reduced incidence of sodium and water retention.

Pharmacokinetic properties: Methylprednisolone is extensively bound to plasma proteins, mainly to globulin and less so to albumin. Only unbound corticosteroid has pharmacological effects or is metabolised. Metabolism occurs in the liver and to a lesser extent in the kidney. Metabolites are excreted in the urine.

Mean elimination half-life ranges from 2.4 to 3.5 hours in normal healthy adults and appears to be independent of the route of administration.

Total body clearance following intravenous or intramuscular injection of methylprednisolone to healthy adult volunteers is approximately 15–16l/hour. Peak methylprednisolone plasma levels of 33.67 micrograms/100 ml were achieved in 2 hours after a single 40 mg i.m. injection to 22 adult male volunteers.

Pharmaceutical particulars

List of excipients: Sodium biphosphate and sodium phosphate.

Incompatibilities: None stated.

Shelf-life: Shelf-life of the medicinal product as packaged for sale: 60 months.

After reconstitution with Sterile Water for Injections, use immediately, discard any remainder.

Special precautions for storage: Store below 25°C. Refer to Section 4.2 Dosage and Administration. No diluents other than those referred to are recommended. Parenteral drug products should be inspected visually for particulate matter and discoloration prior to administration.

Nature and contents of container: Type I clear glass vial with butyl rubber plug and flip top seal. Each vial contains 2 grams of methylprednisolone as the sodium succinate for reconstitution with 31.2 ml of Sterile Water for Injections.

Instructions for use/handling: No special requirements.

Marketing authorisation number 0032/0073.

Date of first authorisation/renewal of authorisation

0032/0073 date of first authorisation: 20 February 1980

Last renewal dated: 17 October 1995

Date of revision of the text July 1998.

Legal category POM.

SULPITIL

Qualitative and quantitative composition Each tablet contains 200 mg sulpiride

Pharmaceutical form Round, white tablet with bevelled edge, marked 'L113' on one side and scored on the reverse.

Clinical particulars

Therapeutic indications: For the treatment of acute and chronic schizophrenia.

Posology and method of administration: For oral administration.

Adult dose: In mild cases, 400 mg to 800 mg daily given as one or two tablets twice daily. In severe cases, a maximum dosage of 1200 mg to 1800 mg per day may be given. A maintenance dose of 400 mg to 800 mg is recommended.

Children: 3 –5 mg/kg body weight daily is recommended. Clinical experience in children under the age of 14 years is insufficient to permit specific recommendations.

Dosage in the elderly: Elderly patients are usually more sensitive to all centrally-acting drugs, therefore an initial dose of 50 mg to 100 mg is recommended, increasing gradually to the normal adult dose. Reduced dosage should be used in patients with renal impairment.

Contra-indications: Phaeochromocytoma. Severe hepatic, renal or blood disease. Alcoholic intoxication and other disorders which depress CNS function.

Special warnings and special precautions for use: Sulpiride should be given with caution to patients suffering from extrapyramidal disturbances, hypertension, and to patients with tumours.

As with all drugs, of which the kidney is a major elimination pathway, the usual precautions should be taken in cases of renal failure.

Patients should be warned against taking alcohol with sulpiride as reaction capacity may be impaired.

Increased motor agitation has been reported at high doses in a small number of patients, i.e. in excessively agitated or excited phases of the disease process, this drug may aggravate symptoms. Care should be exercised when hypomania is present. If warranted, reduction in dosage or anti-parkinsonian medication is sufficient.

Interaction with other medicaments and other forms of interaction: Although no drug interactions are known, unnecessary polypharmacy should be avoided. Patients should be warned against taking alcohol with sulpiride, as reaction capacity may be impaired. Sulpiride has no anticholinergic or significant cardiovascular activity.

Pregnancy and lactation: Despite the negative results of teratogenicity studies in animals sensitive to the effects of thalidomide and the lack of teratogenic effect during widespread clinical use in other countries, this drug should not be considered an exception to the general principle of avoiding drug treatment during pregnancy, particularly during the first sixteen weeks, with potential benefits being weighed against probable hazards.

Effects on ability to drive and use machines: Patients should be advised not to drive or operate machinery if they experience symptoms of slowing of reaction time or loss of concentration.

Undesirable effects: Extrapyramidal symptoms can occur: tremor, tardive dyskinesia (rare), and akathisia. Insomnia and other sleep disturbances have been reported.

As is usual with neuroleptic and psychotropic drugs, sulpiride increases serum prolactin levels, sometimes causing gynaecomastia and galactorrhoea.

Sulpiride has a low toxicity and, unlike other neuroleptics, does not produce serious adverse effects on the autonomic nervous system.

Cases of convulsions, sometimes in patients with no previous history, have been reported.

Hepatic reactions have been reported.

Overdose: Overdosage may be treated with alkaline osmotic diuresis and anti-parkinsonian drugs to treat any extrapyramidal symptoms. An overdose of more than 7 g may cause coma which has been observed to last for up to four days and which should receive suitable treatment.

Pharmacological properties

Pharmacodynamic properties: Sulpiride belongs to a new class of neuroleptics, the benzamides, and has both antidepressant and neuroleptic properties. In high doses it controls florrid positive symptoms but in lower doses it has an alerting effect on apathetic withdrawn schizophrenics; further reductions in dosage increase this alerting effect.

Pharmacokinetic properties: The plasma half-life of sulpiride is 8 – 9 hours.

Preclinical safety data: In long-term animal studies with neuroleptic drugs, including sulpiride, an increased incidence of various endocrine tumours, some of which have been malignant, has been found in some, but not all, strains of rats and mice studied. The significance of these findings to man is not known. There is no current evidence of an association between neuroleptic use and tumour risk in man.

Pharmaceutical particulars

List of excipients:

Microcrystalline cellulose	PhEur
Maize starch	PhEur
Lactose	PhEur
Gelatin	BP
Talc	PhEur
Sodium stearyl fumarate (PRUV)	HSE

Incompatibilities: None stated.

Shelf life: 60 months.

Special precautions for storage: Store in a dry place below 25°C.

Nature and contents of container: Polyethylene containers each fitted with a tamper-evident strip closure and enclosed within a printed cardboard carton, containing either 28 or 112 tablets.

Instructions for use/handling: None stated.

Marketing authorisation number 0424/0066.

Date of first authorisation/renewal of authorisation 19 June 1996.

Date of (partial) revision of the text 29 April 1997.

Legal category POM

SUPRANE* ▼

Qualitative and quantitative composition Desflurane, supplied as pure drug substance.

Pharmaceutical form Volatile liquid for administration by inhalation.

Clinical particulars

Therapeutic indications: Desflurane is indicated as an inhalation agent for induction and/or maintenance of anaesthesia for inpatient and outpatient surgery in adults and maintenance of anaesthesia for inpatient and outpatient paediatric surgery.

Posology and method of administration: Method of administration: Desflurane is administered by inhalation. The concentration of desflurane should be delivered from a vaporizer specifically designed and designated for use with desflurane.

Premedication: Premedication should be selected according to the needs of the individual patient taking into account that salivary secretions are stimulated. The use of anticholinergic drugs is a matter of choice for the anaesthetist.

Dosage: The minimum alveolar concentration (MAC) of desflurane is age-specific and has been determined as listed below:

MAC

Age	*100% Oxygen*	*60% Nitrous Oxide*
0–1 year	8.95–10.65%	5.75–7.75%*
1–12 years	7.20–9.40%	5.75–7.00%**
18–30 years	6.35–7.25%	3.75–4.25%
30–65 years	5.75–6.25%	1.75–3.25%
over 65 years	NA***	NA***

* 3-12 months
** 1-5 years
*** NA = data not available

Induction: Inspired concentrations of 4–11% of desflurane usually produce surgical anaesthesia in 2–4 minutes. However, concentrations of up to 15% have been used in clinical trials. Suprane is not recommended for paediatric induction.

Maintenance: Surgical levels of anaesthesia may be sustained with 2–6% concentration of desflurane when nitrous oxide is used concomitantly. Desflurane at 2.5–8.5% may be required when administered using oxygen or oxygen enriched air. Although concentrations of up to 18% desflurane have been administered for short periods of time, if high concentrations are used with nitrous oxide it is important to ensure that the inspired mixture contains a minimum of 25% oxygen. Desflurane concentrations of greater than 17% are therefore not recommended.

If added relaxation is required, supplemental doses of muscle relaxants may be used.

Dosage in renal and hepatic impairment: Concentrations of 1–4% desflurane in nitrous oxide/ oxygen have been used successfully in patients with chronic renal or hepatic impairment and during renal transplantation surgery.

Contra-indications: Desflurane should not be used for patients in whom general anaesthesia is contraindicated. Desflurane is also contraindicated in patients with known sensitivity to halogenated agents and in patients with known or genetic susceptibility to malignant hyperthermia.

In patients with coronary artery disease, maintenance of normal haemodynamics is important to avoid myocardial ischaemia. Desflurane should not be used for anaesthetic induction in patients at risk of coronary artery disease or in patients where increases in heart rate or blood pressure are undesirable.

Special warnings and special precautions for use: Desflurane should only be administered by persons trained in the administration of general anaesthesia using a vaporizer specifically designed and designated for use with desflurane. Facilities for maintenance of a patent airway, artificial ventilation, oxygen enrichment and circulatory resuscitation must be immediately available. Hypotension and respiratory depression increase as anaesthesia is deepened.

Desflurane is not recommended for use as an inhalation induction agent in paediatric patients because of the frequent occurrence of cough, breath holding, apnoea, laryngospasm and increased secretions in children under 12 years.

Due to limited experience in neurosurgical patients, desflurane cannot be recommended in this group.

Desflurane, as other volatile anaesthetics, may increase CSF or intracranial pressure in patients with space occupying lesions.

Use of desflurane in hypovolaemic, hypotensive and debilitated patients has not been extensively investigated. As with other potent inhaled anaesthetics, a lower concentration is recommended for use in these patients.

Desflurane was shown to be a potential trigger of malignant hyperthermia. If malignant hyperthermia occurs, the use of dantrolene sodium will be indicated to reverse this hyperthermia. Desflurane should not be used in subjects known to be susceptible to MH.

Desflurane has been reported to interact with dry carbon dioxide absorbents to form carbon monoxide. In order to minimise the risk of formation of carbon monoxide in rebreathing circuits and the possibility of elevated carboxyhaemoglobin levels, carbon dioxide absorbents should not be allowed to dry out.

As with other halogenated anaesthetic agents, desflurane may cause sensitivity hepatitis in patients who have been sensitized by previous exposure to halogenated anaesthetics.

Interaction with other medicaments and other forms of interaction: Commonly used muscle relaxants are potentiated by desflurane. Lower doses of desflurane are required in patients receiving opioids, benzodiazepines or other sedatives. These interactions are illustrated below. In addition, concomitant nitrous oxide reduces desflurane MAC, as illustrated under dosage, above.

Non-depolarizing and depolarizing muscle relaxants: The doses of pancuronium, atracurium and suxamethonium needed to produce 95% (ED_{95}) depression in neuromuscular transmission at different concentrations of desflurane are given in Table 1. (These doses are similar to isoflurane.)

Opioids and benzodiazepines: Patients anaesthetized with different concentrations of desflurane who received increasing doses of fentanyl showed a marked reduction in the anaesthetic requirements or MAC. The administration of increasing doses of intravenous midazolam showed a small reduction in MAC. Results are reported in Table 2. These MAC reductions are similar to those observed with isoflurane. It is anticipated that there will be a similar influence on MAC with other opioid and sedative drugs.

Table 2–Desflurane 0.6–0.8 MAC/O_2

	**MAC (%)*	*% MAC Reduction*
No Fentanyl	*6.33–6.35*	*—*
Fentanyl (3 mg/kg)	*3.12–3.46*	*46–51*
Fentanyl (6 mg/kg)	*2.25–2.97*	*53–64*
No Midazolam	*5.85–6.86*	*—*
Midazolam (25 mg/kg)	*4.93*	*15.7*
Midazolam (50 mg/kg)	*4.88*	*16.6*

* Includes values for ages 18 – 65 years

Pregnancy and lactation: Developmental toxicity studies with desflurane, administered at 1 MAC to rats and rabbits have shown a possible anaesthetic-related fetotoxic effect at approximately 40 cumulative MAC-hours of exposure. No adverse effects were observed following 10 cumulative MAC-hours of exposure.

Increased post-implantation loss and reduced offspring weight gain during lactation were observed in rats following maternal desflurane exposure of 4 MAC-hours per day throughout gestation and lactation (approximately 37 days). No adverse effects on these parameters were observed following maternal exposure of 1 MAC-hour per day over this time course. All fetal or offspring effects observed were restricted to groups where maternal toxicity (mortalities and reduced weight gain) was noted, and therefore offspring effects may reflect the pharmacological effect of desflurane on the dams.

There are no adequate and well-controlled studies in pregnant women, therefore desflurane is not indicated for use during pregnancy.

Desflurane is not indicated for use in nursing mothers because it is not known whether it is excreted in human milk.

Effects on ability to drive and use machines: There is no information on the effects of desflurane on the ability to drive or operate machinery. However, patients should be advised that the ability to perform tasks such as driving or operation of machinery may be impaired after general anaesthesia, and it is advisable to avoid such tasks for a period of 24 hours.

Undesirable effects: As with all potent inhaled anaesthetics desflurane may cause dose-dependent cardio-respiratory depression. Most other adverse events are mild and transient. Nausea and vomiting have been observed in the postoperative period, common sequelae of surgery and general anaesthesia, which may be due to inhalational anaesthetic, other agents administered intraoperatively or post-operatively and to the patient's response to the surgical procedure.

Desflurane should not be used for anaesthetic induction in patients at risk of coronary artery disease or in patients where increase in heart rate or blood pressure are undesirable. In patients with coronary artery disease, maintenance of normal haemodynamics is important to avoid myocardial ischaemia.

Hepatitis may occur in patients sensitized by prior exposure to halogenated anaesthetics.

In adults, adverse reactions associated with desflurane during its use for inhaled induction of anaesthesia include cough, breath holding, salivation, apnoea and laryngospasm.

Desflurane is not recommended for use as an inhalation induction agent in paediatric patients because of the frequent occurrence of cough, breath holding, apnoea, laryngospasm and increased secretions in children under 12 years.

As with all other general anaesthetics, transient elevations in white blood count have been observed even in the absence of surgical stress.

As with other agents of this type, desflurane anaesthesia has been shown to trigger a skeletal muscle hypermetabolic state leading to high oxygen demand and the clinical syndrome known as malignant hyperthermia (MH). The syndrome includes nonspecific features such as hypercapnia, muscle rigidity, tachycardia, tachypnoea, cyanosis, arrhythmias and unstable blood pressure and an increase in overall metabolism may be reflected in an elevated temperature. Treatment includes discontinuation of triggering agents, administration of intravenous dantrolene sodium and application of supportive therapy. This effect has been observed in man with desflurane anaesthesia, in very rare cases, therefore, desflurane should not be used in subjects known to be susceptible to MH.

Overdose: Acute experience in animals: Preclinical toxicology data for desflurane suggest that it produces concentration related respiratory and cardiovascular depression which is predictable and controllable. It does not produce target organ toxicity or pathology.

Human experience: There is no experience of overdosage in humans.

Symptoms and treatment of overdosage: The symptoms of overdosage of desflurane are anticipated to be similar to those of other volatile agents with a deepening of anaesthesia, cardiac and/or respiratory depression in spontaneous breathing patients, and hypotension in ventilated patients in whom hypercarbia and hypoxia may occur only at a late stage.

In the event of overdosage or what may appear to be overdosage, the following actions should be taken: stop desflurane, establish a clear airway and initiate assisted or controlled ventilation with pure oxygen. Support and maintain adequate haemodynamics.

Pharmacological properties

Pharmacodynamic properties: Desflurane is one of a family of halogenated methylethylethers which are administered by inhalation producing a dose-related, reversible loss of consciousness and of pain sensations, suppression of voluntary motor activity, reduction of autonomic reflexes and sedation of respiration and the cardiovascular system. Other members of the series include enflurane and its structural isomer isoflurane which are halogenated with chlorine as well as fluorine. Desflurane is halogenated exclusively with fluorine. As suggested by its structure, the low blood/ gas partition coefficient of desflurane (0.42) is lower than that of other potent inhaled anaesthetics such as isoflurane (1.4) and even lower than that of nitrous oxide (0.46). These data indicate that desflurane would meet the need for an agent characterized by rapid recovery and that it is particularly suited for use in outpatient anaesthesia where this is an important property. Animal studies showed a more rapid induction and recovery from anaesthesia than for isoflurane, with a similar cardiorespiratory profile.

There were no signs of epileptogenic or other untoward effects on EEG, and adjuvant drugs produced no unanticipated or toxic EEG responses during anaesthesia with desflurane.

Studies in pigs bred to be susceptible to malignant hyperthermia (MH) indicated that desflurane is a potential trigger for MH.

Pharmacokinetic properties: General characteristics: As predicted from its physicochemical profile, pharmacokinetic studies in animals as in man indicate that desflurane washes into the body more rapidly than other volatile anaesthetic agents, suggesting a more rapid induction of anaesthesia. It also washes out of the body more rapidly, allowing quick recovery and flexibility in adjustment of the depth of anaesthesia. Desflurane is eliminated via the lungs, undergoing only minimal metabolism (0.02%).

Characteristics in patients: The pharmacological effect is proportional to the inspired concentration of desflurane. The main adverse effects are extensions of the pharmacological action.

MAC decreases with increasing age. A reduction of dosage is recommended in hypovolaemic, hypotensive and debilitated patients, as discussed under Warnings above.

Preclinical safety data: In swine, desflurane does not sensitize the myocardium to exogenously administered epinephrine (adrenaline). Desflurane appears to produce coronary vasodilation at arteriolar level in selected animal models, in a similar fashion to that of isoflurane. In an animal model simulating coronary artery disease with conscious, chronically instrumented dogs, desflurane does not appear to divert blood from collateral dependent myocardium to normally perfused areas ("coronary steal"). Clinical studies to date evaluating myocardial ischaemia, infarction and death as outcome parameters have not established that the coronary arteriolar property of Suprane is associated with coronary steal or myocardial ischaemia in patients with coronary artery disease.

Pharmaceutical particulars

List of excipients: Not applicable.

Incompatibilities: None.

Shelf-life: Two years.

Special precautions for storage: The product should be stored in an upright position at room temperature (25°C).

Nature and contents of container: Suprane is presented in amber glass bottles, containing 240 ml of desflurane. The closure is constructed of black, moulded phenol resin, fitted with a conical insert of polypropylene. Alternatively the glass bottle may be closed with a crimped-on valve directly compatible with the filling port of the desflurane vaporizer.

Instructions for use/handling: Desflurane should only be administered by persons trained in the administration of anaesthesia, using a vaporizer specifically designed and designated for use with desflurane.

Marketing authorisation number 0022/0120

Date of first authorisation/renewal of authorisation 19 July 1993

Date of (partial) revision of the text October 1998

Legal Category POM

TAMOFEN-10*

Qualitative and quantitative composition

Active ingredient: Tamoxifen Citrate BP 15.2 mg, equivalent to Tamoxifen 10.0 mg.

Pharmaceutical form Tablets

Clinical particulars

Therapeutic indications: To be used for the treatment of breast cancer and anovulatory infertility.

Posology and method of administration:
Route of administration: Oral.

Children: There is no recommended dose for children.

Adult dose:
Breast cancer: The recommended daily dose for tamoxifen is normally 20 mg. No additional benefit, in terms of delayed recurrence or improved survival in patients, has been demonstrated with higher doses. Substantive evidence supporting the use of treatment

Table 1–Dosage (mg/kg) of muscle relaxant causing 95% depression in neuromuscular transmission

Desflurane Concentration	*Pancuronium*	*Atracurium*	*Suxamethonium*
0.65 MAC/60%N_2O/O_2	*0.026*	*0.133*	**NA*
1.25 MAC/60%N_2O/O_2	*0.018*	*0.119*	**NA*
1.25 MAC/O_2	*0.022*	*0.120*	*0.360*

*NA = not available

with 30–40 mg per day is not available, although these doses have been used in some patients with advanced disease.

Anovulatory infertility: The possibility of pregnancy must be excluded before the commencement of treatment. In women with regular menstruation but anovular cycles, treatment should commence with 20 mg daily in either one or two doses administered on the 2nd, 3rd, 4th and 5th days of the menstrual cycle. If treatment is unsuccessful, further courses may be given during subsequent menstrual periods, increasing the dosage to 20 mg twice daily and then to 40 mg twice daily.

In women with irregular menstruation, the commencement of treatment may take place on any day. If this initial course is not successful then a further course may be initiated after an interval of 45 days with the higher dosage level (30 mg to 40 mg twice daily). If a patient responds with menstruation then the next course of treatment is started on the second day of the cycle.

Elderly patients: The adult dosage range has been used in elderly patients with breast cancer.

Contra-indications: Pregnancy.

Special warnings and special precautions for use:
Precautions: Tamoxifen may be given to pre-menopausal women only after thorough examination has excluded the possibility of pregnancy.

Interaction with other medicaments and other forms of interaction: Tamoxifen increases the dopaminergic effect of bromocriptine. Tamoxifen may potentiate the anti-coagulant action of warfarin if these drugs are used concomitantly. Patients taking coumarin-type anti-coagulants will require close monitoring on the introduction or withdrawal of tamoxifen.

Pregnancy and lactation: Tamoxifen is known to be associated with a serious risk of termination if administered during pregnancy. Tamoxifen causes a suppression of lactation. Tamoxifen is not recommended for use during lactation; it is not known whether it is excreted in human milk.

Effects on ability to drive and use machines: None stated.

Undesirable effects: Side effects are generally associated with long-term use. They can occasionally be controlled by reducing the dosage without loss of therapeutic effect. Persistent adverse effects may necessitate the discontinuation of treatment.

The following side-effects have been reported: hot flushes, rashes, dry skin, pruritus vulvae, vaginal discharge or bleeding, dizziness, confusion, headache, depression, muscle cramps, fatigue, fluid retention, alopecia, and gastrointestinal disturbances including nausea, vomiting and anorexia.

Occasional tumour flare and pain have been reported. In some patients with bony metastases, hypercalcaemia has been observed at the start of treatment.

The tendency towards thromboembolic phenomenon may increase. Changes in blood lipids have been reported and pulmonary embolism has occurred. Transient leucopenia and thrombocytopenia may occur. Decreased platelet counts–usually between 80,000–90,000–which have been reported in breast cancer patients, revert to normal without stopping treatment.

Rarely blurred vision, loss of visual acuity, retinopathy, corneal opacities and cataracts have been reported.

Menstruation is suppressed in a number of premenopausal women receiving tamoxifen.

Reversible cystic ovarian swellings have occasionally been observed when such women have been treated with 40 mg twice daily for short periods.

Endometrial hyperplasia, endometrial polyps and an increased incidence of endometrial carcinoma has been reported in association with tamoxifen treatment, abnormal vaginal bleeding including menstrual irregularities, vaginal discharge, and symptoms such as pelvic pain or pressure in patients receiving tamoxifen should be promptly investigated.

Tamoxifen has been associated with changes in liver enzyme levels and rarely with more severe liver abnormalities including fatty liver, cholestasis, and hepatitis.

Overdose: Overdosage causes anti-oestrogenic effects. In animals, extremely high doses (over 100 times the recommended daily dose) have caused oestrogenic effects. There is no special antidote to overdosage and treatment should therefore be symptomatic.

Pharmacological properties
Pharmacodynamic properties: Tamoxifen is a non-steroidal anti-oestrogen. It binds to oestrogen receptors preventing the stimulating effects of oestrogen on nucleic acid synthesis. The metabolites of tamoxifen are also anti-oestogens.

Pharmacokinetic properties: Maximum plasma levels of tamoxifen occur at 4–7 hours after administration. The elimination half-life is about 7 days. Considerable enterohepatic circulation is a probable reason for the slow elimination.

Preclinical safety data: In animals, extremely high doses (over 100 times the recommended daily dose) have caused oestrogenic effects

Pharmaceutical particulars
List of excipients

Lactose	PhEur
Maize starch	PhEur
Povidone 25 000	USP
Silicon Dioxide	USP
Talc	PhEur
Magnesium Stearate	PhEur
Purified Water	PhEur

Incompatibilities: None known.

Shelf life: 60 months.

Special precautions for storage: Store in a dry place, below 25°C.

Nature and contents of container: Aluminium/Aluminium foil strips containing 30 tablets or aluminium/aluminium foil blisters containing 250 tablets. Both strips and blisters are contained within a printed cardboard carton.

Instructions for use/handling: None stated.

Marketing authorisation holder: J B Tillott Limited, Davy Avenue, Milton Keynes MK5 8PH, UK

Marketing authorisation number 0424/0031.

Date of first authorisation/renewal of authorisation 18 October 1983/22 December 1994.

Date of (partial) revision of the text 10 July 1997.

Date of preparation 10 July 1997.

Legal category POM

TAMOFEN-20*

Qualitative and quantitative composition
Active ingredient: Tamoxifen Citrate BP 30.4 mg, equivalent to Tamoxifen 20.0 mg.

Pharmaceuticla form Tablets.

Clinical particulars
Therapeutic indications: To be used for the treatment of breast cancer and anovulatory infertility.

Posology and method of administration:
Route of administration: Oral.

Children: There is no recommended dose for children.

Adult dose: Breast cancer: The recommended daily dose for tamoxifen is normally 20 mg. No additional benefit, in terms of delayed recurrence or improved survival in patients, has been demonstrated with higher doses. Substantive evidence supporting the use of treatment with 30–40 mg per day is not available, although these doses have been used in some patients with advanced disease.

Anovulatory infertility: The possibility of pregnancy must be excluded before the commencement of treatment. In women with regular menstruation but anovular cycles, treatment should commence with 20 mg daily in either one or two doses administered on the 2nd, 3rd, 4th and 5th days of the menstrual cycle. If treatment is unsuccessful, further courses may be given during subsequent menstrual periods, increasing the dosage to 20 mg twice daily and then to 40 mg twice daily.

In women with irregular menstruation, the commencement of treatment may take place on any day. If this initial course is not successful then a further course may be initiated after an interval of 45 days with the higher dosage level (30 mg to 40 mg twice daily). If a patient responds with menstruation then the next course of treatment is started on the second day of the cycle.

Elderly patients: The adult dosage range has been used in elderly patients with breast cancer.

Contra-indications: Pregnancy.

Special warnings and special precautions for use:
Precautions: Tamoxifen may be given to pre-menopausal women only after thorough examination has excluded the possibility of pregnancy.

Interaction with other medicaments and other forms of interaction: Tamoxifen increases the dopaminergic effect of bromocriptine. Tamoxifen may potentiate the anti-coagulant action of warfarin if these drugs are used concomitantly. Patients taking coumarin-type anti-coagulants will require close monitoring on the introduction or withdrawal of tamoxifen.

Pregnancy and lactation: Tamoxifen is known to be associated with a serious risk of termination if administered during pregnancy. Tamoxifen causes a suppression of lactation. Tamoxifen is not recommended for use during lactation; it is not known whether it is excreted in human milk.

Effects on ability to drive and use machines: None stated.

Undesirable effects: Side effects are generally associated with long-term use. They can occasionally be controlled by reducing the dosage without loss of therapeutic effect. Persistent adverse effects may necessitate the discontinuation of treatment.

The following side-effects have been reported: hot flushes, rashes, dry skin, pruritus vulvae, vaginal discharge or bleeding, dizziness, confusion, headache, depression, muscle cramps, fatigue, fluid retention, alopecia, and gastrointestinal disturbances including nausea, vomiting and anorexia.

Occasional tumour flare and pain have been reported. In some patients with bony metastases, hypercalcaemia has been observed at the start of treatment.

The tendency towards thromboembolic phenomenon may increase. Changes in blood lipids have been reported and pulmonary embolism has occurred. Transient leucopenia and thrombocytopenia may occur. Decreased platelet counts–usually between 80,000–90,000–which have been reported in breast cancer patients, revert to normal without stopping treatment.

Rarely blurred vision, loss of visual acuity, retinopathy, corneal opacities and cataracts have been reported.

Menstruation is suppressed in a number of premenopausal women receiving tamoxifen.

Reversible cystic ovarian swellings have occasionally been observed when such women have been treated with 40 mg twice daily for short periods.

Endometrial hyperplasia, endometrial polyps and an increased incidence of endometrial carcinoma has been reported in association with tamoxifen treatment, abnormal vaginal bleeding including menstrual irregularities, vaginal discharge, and symptoms such as pelvic pain or pressure in patients receiving tamoxifen should be promptly investigated.

Tamoxifen has been associated with changes in liver enzyme levels and rarely with more severe liver abnormalities including fatty liver, cholestasis, and hepatitis.

Overdose: Overdosage causes anti-oestrogenic effects. In animals, extremely high doses (over 100 times the recommended daily dose) have caused oestrogenic effects. There is no special antidote to overdosage and treatment should therefore be symptomatic.

Pharmacological properties
Pharmacodynamic properties: Tamoxifen is a non-steroidal anti-oestrogen. It binds to oestrogen receptors preventing the stimulating effects of oestrogen on nucleic acid synthesis. The metabolites of tamoxifen are also anti-oestogens.

Pharmacokinetic properties: Maximum plasma levels of tamoxifen occur at 4–7 hours after administration. The elimination half-life is about 7 days. Considerable enterohepatic circulation is a probable reason for the slow elimination.

Preclinical safety data: In animals, extremely high doses (over 100 times the recommended daily dose) have caused oestrogenic effects

Pharmaceutical particulars
List of excipients

Lactose	PhEur
Maize starch	PhEur
Povidone 25 000	USP
Silicon Dioxide	USP
Talc	PhEur
Magnesium Stearate	PhEur
Purified Water	PhEur

Incompatibilities: None known.

Shelf life: 60 months.

Special precautions for storage: Store in a dry place, below 25°C.

Nature and contents of container: Aluminium/Aluminium foil strips containing 30 tablets or aluminium/aluminium foil blisters containing 250 tablets. Both strips and blisters are contained within a printed cardboard carton.

Instructions for use/handling: None stated.

Marketing authorisation holder: J B Tillott Limited, Davy Avenue, Milton Keynes MK5 8PH, UK.

Marketing authorisation number 0424/0043.

Date of first authorisation/renewal of authorisation 16 March 1984/17 January 1995.

Date of (partial) revision of the text 10 July 1997.

Date of preparation 10 July 1997.

Legal category POM

TAMOFEN-40*

Qualitative and quantitative composition
Active ingredient: Tamoxifen Citrate BP 60.8 mg, equivalent to Tamoxifen 40.0 mg.

Pharmaceutical form Tablets.

Clinical particulars
Therapeutic indications: To be used for the treatment of breast cancer and anovulatory infertility.

Posology and method of administration:
Route of administration: Oral.

Children: There is no recommended dose for children.

Adult dose:
Breast cancer: The recommended daily dose for tamoxifen is normally 20 mg. No additional benefit, in terms of delayed recurrence or improved survival in patients, has been demonstrated with higher doses. Substantive evidence supporting the use of treatment with 30–40 mg per day is not available, although these doses have been used in some patients with advanced disease.

Anovulatory infertility: The possibility of pregnancy must be excluded before the commencement of treatment. In women with regular menstruation but anovular cycles, treatment should commence with 20 mg daily in either one or two doses administered on the 2nd, 3rd, 4th and 5th days of the menstrual cycle. If treatment is unsuccessful, further courses may be given during subsequent menstrual periods, increasing the dosage to 20 mg twice daily and then to 40 mg twice daily.

In women with irregular menstruation, the commencement of treatment may take place on any day. If this initial course is not successful then a further course may be initiated after an interval of 45 days with the higher dosage level (30 mg to 40 mg twice daily). If a patient responds with menstruation then the next course of treatment is started on the second day of the cycle.

Elderly patients: The adult dosage range has been used in elderly patients with breast cancer.

Contra-indications: Pregnancy.

Special warnings and special precautions for use: Precautions: Tamoxifen may be given to pre-menopausal women only after thorough examination has excluded the possibility of pregnancy.

Interaction with other medicaments and other forms of interaction: Tamoxifen increases the dopaminergic effect of bromocriptine. Tamoxifen may potentiate the anti-coagulant action of warfarin if these drugs are used concomitantly. Patients taking coumarin-type anti-coagulants will require close monitoring on the introduction or withdrawal of tamoxifen.

Pregnancy and lactation: Tamoxifen is known to be associated with a serious risk of termination if administered during pregnancy. Tamoxifen causes a suppression of lactation. Tamoxifen is not recommended for use during lactation; it is not known whether it is excreted in human milk.

Effects on ability to drive and use machines: None stated.

Undesirable effects: Side effects are generally associated with long-term use. They can occasionally be controlled by reducing the dosage without loss of therapeutic effect. Persistent adverse effects may necessitate the discontinuation of treatment.

The following side-effects have been reported: hot flushes, rashes, dry skin, pruritus vulvae, vaginal discharge or bleeding, dizziness, confusion, headache, depression, muscle cramps, fatigue, fluid retention, alopecia, and gastrointestinal disturbances including nausea, vomiting and anorexia.

Occasional tumour flare and pain have been reported. In some patients with bony metastases, hypercalcaemia has been observed at the start of treatment.

The tendency towards thromboembolic phenomenon may increase. Changes in blood lipids have been reported and pulmonary embolism has occurred. Transient leucopenia and thrombocytopenia may occur. Decreased platelet counts–usually between 80,000–90,000–which have been reported in breast cancer patients, revert to normal without stopping treatment.

Rarely blurred vision, loss of visual acuity, retinopathy, corneal opacities and cataracts have been reported.

Menstruation is suppressed in a number of premenopausal women receiving tamoxifen.

Reversible cystic ovarian swellings have occasionally been observed when such women have been treated with 40 mg twice daily for short periods.

Endometrial hyperplasia, endometrial polyps and an increased incidence of endometrial carcinoma has been reported in association with tamoxifen treatment, abnormal vaginal bleeding including menstrual irregularities, vaginal discharge, and symptoms such as pelvic pain or pressure in patients receiving tamoxifen should be promptly investigated.

Tamoxifen has been associated with changes in liver enzyme levels and rarely with more severe liver abnormalities including fatty liver, cholestasis, and hepatitis.

Overdose: Overdosage causes anti-oestrogenic effects. In animals, extremely high doses (over 100 times the recommended daily dose) have caused oestrogenic effects. There is no special antidote to overdosage and treatment should therefore be symptomatic.

Pharmacological properties
Pharmacodynamic properties: Tamoxifen is a non-steroidal anti-oestrogen. It binds to oestrogen receptors preventing the stimulating effects of oestrogen on nucleic acid synthesis. The metabolites of tamoxifen are also anti-oestogens.

Pharmacokinetic properties: Maximum plasma levels of tamoxifen occur at 4–7 hours after administration. The elimination half-life is about 7 days. Considerable enterohepatic circulation is a probable reason for the slow elimination.

Preclinical safety data: In animals, extremely high doses (over 100 times the recommended daily dose) have caused oestrogenic effects

Pharmaceutical particulars
List of excipients

Lactose	PhEur
Maize starch	PhEur
Povidone 25 000	USP
Silicon Dioxide	USP
Talc	PhEur
Magnesium Stearate	PhEur
Purified Water	PhEur

Incompatibilities: None known.

Shelf life: 60 months.

Special precautions for storage: Store in a dry place, below 25°C.

Nature and contents of container: Aluminium/Aluminium foil strips containing 30 tablets or aluminium/aluminium foil blisters containing 250 tablets. Both strips and blisters are contained within a printed cardboard carton.

Instructions for use/handling: None stated.

Marketing authorisation holder: J B Tillott Limited, Davy Avenue, Milton Keynes MK5 8PH, UK.

Marketing authorisation number 0424/0055.

Date of first authorisation/renewal of authorisation 24 January 1985/25 January 1996.

Date of (partial) revision of the text 10 July 1997.

Date of preparation 10 July 1997.

Legal category POM

TEMAZEPAM ELIXIR

Presentation A clear, green, lemon-mint flavoured elixir containing 10 mg temazepam per 5 ml in a sugar free base.

Uses Temazepam Elixir is indicated for the short-term treatment of sleep disturbances considered severe or disabling or where insomnia is subjecting the individual to extreme distress. This product is especially useful in those patients for whom the persistence of hypnotic effect after rising would be undesirable.

Dosage and administration
Insomnia: Treatment should be as short as possible. Generally the duration of treatment should vary from a few days to two weeks with a maximum, including the tapering off process, of four weeks. In certain cases extension beyond the maximum treatment period may be necessary; if so, it should not take place without re-evaluation of the patient's status. The product should be taken on retiring or up to 30 minutes before going to bed.

Adults: 10–20 mg. In exceptional circumstances the dose may be increased to 30–40 mg.

Elderly: 10 mg. In exceptional circumstances the dose may be increased to 20 mg.

Treatment should be started with the lowest recommended dose. The maximum dose should not be exceeded. Patients with impaired liver function should have a reduced dose.

Contra-indications, warnings, etc
Contra-indications: Hypersensitivity to benzodiazepines, severe respiratory insufficiency, myasthenia gravis, sleep apnoea syndrome, children, severe hepatic insufficiency.

Warnings: Temazepam Elixir should not be taken in concomitant intake of alcohol. The sedative effect may be enhanced when the product is used in combination with alcohol. This affects the ability to drive or use machines.

Take into account combination with CNS depressants. Enhancement of the central depressive effect may occur during concomitant use with antipsychotics (neuroleptics), hypnotics, anxiolytics/sedatives, antidepressant agents, narcotic analgesics, antiepileptic drugs, anaesthetics and sedative antihistamines. In the case of narcotic analgesics enhancement of the euphoria may also occur leading to an increase in psychic dependence.

Sedation, amnesia, impaired concentration and impaired muscular function may adversely affect the ability to drive or to use machines. If insufficient sleep duration occurs, the likelihood of impaired alertness may be increased.

Use in pregnancy: Insufficient data are available on temazepam to assess its safety during pregnancy and lactation. If the product is prescribed to a woman of child-bearing age, she should be warned to contact her physician about stopping the product if she intends to become, or suspects that she is, pregnant. If for compelling medical reasons, temazepam is administered during the late phase of pregnancy, or during labour, effects on the neonate, such as hypothermia, hypotonia and moderate respiratory depression, can be expected due to the pharmacological action of the product. Moreover, infants born to mothers who took benzodiazepines chronically during the later stages of pregnancy may have developed physical dependence and may be at some risk of developing withdrawal symptoms in the postnatal period.

Since benzodiazepines are found in breast milk, temazepam should not be administered to breast-feeding mothers.

Adverse effects: Drowsiness during the day, numbed emotions, reduced alertness, confusion, fatigue, headaches, muscle weakness, ataxia, or double vision. These phenomena occur predominantly at the start of therapy and usually disappear thereafter. Other side effects like gastrointestinal disturbances, changes in libido or skin reactions have been reported occasionally. Anterograde amnesia may occur using therapeutic dosages, the risk increasing at higher dosages. Amnesia may be associated with inappropriate behaviour. (See also precautions). Pre-existing depression may be unmasked during benzodiazepine use. Reactions like restlessness, agitation, irritability, aggressiveness, delusion, rages, nightmares, hallucinations, psychoses, inappropriate behaviour and other adverse behavioral effects are known to occur when using benzodiazepines. Should this occur, use of the product should be discontinued. These reactions are more likely to occur in children and the elderly.

Use (even at therapeutic doses) may lead to the development of physical dependence: discontinuation of therapy may result in withdrawal or rebound phenomena (see also precautions). Psychic dependence may occur. Abuse has been reported in polydrug users.

Precautions: Tolerance – some loss of efficacy to the hypnotic effects of short acting benzodiazepines may develop after repeated use for a few weeks.

Dependence – use of benzodiazepines may lead to the development of physical and psychic dependence upon the products. The risk of dependence increases with dose and duration of treatment; it is also greater in patients with a history of alcohol and drug abuse. Once physical dependence has developed, abrupt termination of treatment will be accompanied by withdrawal symptoms. These may consist of headaches, muscle pain, extreme anxiety, tension, restlessness, confusion and irritability. In severe cases the following symptoms may occur: derealisation, depersonalisation, hyperacusis and tingling of the extremities, hypersensitivity to light, noise and physical contact, hallucinations or epileptic seizures.

Rebound insomnia – a transient syndrome whereby the symptoms that led to treatment with a benzodiazepine recur in an enhanced form, may occur on withdrawal of hypnotic treatment. It may be accompanied by other reactions including mood changes, anxiety and restlessness. Since the risk of withdrawal phenomena/rebound phenomena is greater after abrupt discontinuation of treatment it is recommended that the dosage is decreased gradually.

Duration of treatment – the duration of treatment should be as short as possible (see dosage), but should not exceed 4 weeks, including the tapering off process. Extension beyond this period should not take place without re-evaluation of the situation. It may be useful to inform the patient at the start of treatment that it will be of limited duration and to explain precisely how the dosage will be progressively decreased. Moreover, it is important that the patient should be made aware of the possibility of rebound phenomena to minimise anxiety over such symptoms should they occur while the medicinal product is being discontinued. There is some evidence to suggest that for benzodiazepines with a short duration of action, withdrawal phenomena can occur within the dosage interval, especially when the dosage is high.

Amnesia – benzodiazepines may induce anterograde amnesia. The condition occurs most often several hours after ingesting the product and therefore to reduce the risk, patients should ensure that they will be able to have an uninterrupted sleep of 7 – 8 hours (see also adverse effects).

Psychiatric and 'paradoxical reactions' – reactions like restlessness, agitation, irritability, aggressiveness, delusion, rages, nightmares, hallucinations, psychoses, inappropriate behaviour and other adverse behavioral effects are known to occur when using benzodiazepines. Should this occur, use of the product should be discontinued. These reactions are more likely to occur in children and in the elderly.

Specific patient groups – for the elderly see the dosage recommendation. A lower dose is also recommended for patients with a chronic respiratory insufficiency due to risk of respiratory depression. Benzodiazepines are contraindicated in patients with severe hepatic insufficiency as their use may precipitate encephalopathy. Benzodiazepines are not recommended for the primary treatment of psychotic illness. Benzodiazepines should not be used alone to treat depression or anxiety associated with depression (suicide may be precipitated in such patients). Benzodiazepines should be used with extreme caution in patients with a history of alcohol or drug abuse.

Overdosage: As with other benzodiazepines, overdose should not present a threat to life unless combined with other CNS depressants (including alcohol). In the management of overdose with any medicinal product, it should be borne in mind that multiple agents may have been taken.

Following overdose with oral benzodiazepines, vomiting should be induced (within one hour) if the patient is conscious or gastric lavage undertaken with the airway protected if the patient is unconscious. If there is no advantage in emptying the stomach, activated charcoal should be given to reduce absorption. The value of dialysis has not been determined for temazepam. 3-OH benzodiazepines are, as a rule not dialysable and their metabolites (glucuronides) only dialysable with difficulty. Special attention should be paid to respiratory and cardiovascular function in intensive care.

Overdose of benzodiazepines is usually manifested by degrees of central nervous system depression ranging from drowsiness to coma. In mild cases, symptoms include drowsiness, mental confusion and lethargy; in more serious cases, symptoms may include ataxia, hypotonia, hypotension, respiratory depression, rarely coma and very rarely death. Flumazenil may be used as an antidote.

Pharmaceutical precautions Store below 25°C and protect from light. Temazepam Elixir is sugar-free being based on a glycerol vehicle. If dilution of the elixir is required, glycerol BP is a suitable diluent.

Legal category CD(Sch.4) POM.

Package quantities Single dose containers of 5 ml (10 mg) and 10 ml (20 mg). Bottles of 300 ml.

Further information The formulation of temazepam as an elixir ensures rapid and complete absorption which, with its short half-life and lack of active metabolites, results in prompt induction of sleep and a low incidence of hangover effects.

Temazepam is a short-acting benzodiazepine. As accumulation tends not to occur, patients are less likely to experience excessive drowsiness or impairment in the performance of skilled tasks. The short half-life of this drug may offer advantages in the treatment of the elderly, in patients with impaired renal or liver function, and in situations where daytime alertness is desirable.

Product licence number 3433/0054.

TOLANASE* TABLETS 100 mg

Qualitative and quantitative composition Each tablet contains 100 mg tolazamide.

Pharmaceutical form Tablet for oral use.

Clinical particulars
Therapeutic indications: Sulphonylurea. Indicated in maturity-onset diabetes of mild to moderate severity.

Posology and method of administration: Oral.

Adults: 100--250 mg daily, or up to 1 g daily in divided doses if necessary. It is doubtful whether doses greater than 1 g daily will result in improved control. (For dose conversion from other oral hypoglycaemic agents see literature).

Depending on the results of urinary glucose tests and blood sugar determinations, the daily dose should be either raised or lowered by amounts of one tablet (100 mg or 250 mg) at weekly intervals.

Elderly patients: These agents have had their primary use in the older aged group. The contra-indications and precautions that appear below in this Summary of Product Characteristics should be carefully observed for all aged patients and any patient with significantly compromised liver or renal function should be very carefully followed if it is the election of the physician to use oral agents.

Contra-indications: Tolanase is not indicated in juvenile or labile (brittle) diabetes, or in patients with infections or those undergoing surgery or trauma. It is contra-indicated in patients with ketosis, acidosis or in coma, or who have a history of such.

Since Tolanase has not been studied extensively in diabetes complicated by pregnancy nor in diabetics with liver, kidney or endocrine disease, it is not recommended in these instances.

Special warnings and special precautions for use: The appearance of significant acetonuria in a patient transferred from insulin to tolazamide makes return to insulin therapy mandatory.

Interaction with other medicaments and other forms of interaction: The hypoglycaemic action of sulphonylureas may be potentiated by certain drugs including phenylbutazone, oxyphenbutazone, salicylates, sulphonamides, chloramphenicol, probenecid, coumarins, monoamine oxidase inhibitors and beta adrenergic blocking agents. When such drugs are administered to a patient receiving Tolanase, the patient should be closely observed for hypoglycaemia. When such drugs are withdrawn from a patient receiving Tolanase, the patient should be observed closely for loss of control.

Certain drugs tend to produce hyperglycaemia and may lead to loss of control. These drugs include the thiazides and other diuretics, corticosteroids, phenothiazines, thyroid products, oestrogens, oral contraceptives, phenytoin, nicotinic acid, sympathomimetics and isoniazid. When such drugs are administered to a patient receiving Tolanase, the patient should be observed for loss of control. When such drugs are withdrawn from a patient receiving Tolanase, the patients should be observed closely for hypoglycaemia.

Pregnancy and lactation: See Contra-indications section, above.

Effects on ability to drive and use machines: No information

Undesirable effects: The most commonly encountered symptoms are gastro-intestinal (1.8%), including nausea, anorexia, diarrhoea. Other minor occurrences, such as dizziness, weakness, insomnia, lethargy, have been reported. A disulfiram-like action after taking alcohol has been reported.

Overdose: Action should be taken to counteract the ensuing hypoglycaemic period. No known antidote.

Pharmacological properties
Pharmacodynamic properties: Tolazamide is a sulphonylurea which stimulates the islet tissue to secrete insulin. It is approximately 7 times as potent as tolbutamide in normal subjects, and 5 times in diabetics, on a milligram, single dose, basis. Hypoglycaemic effects begin 20 minutes after administration and peak at 2–4 hours. Hypoglycaemia is still apparent after 20 hours in fasted non-diabetics. With fasting diabetics, the peak effect occurs at 4–6 hours, with a duration of maximal effect of about 10 hours. Blood glucose levels begin to rise at 14–16 hours.

Pharmacokinetic properties: Peak serum concentrations occur 3–4 hours after a single oral dose. The average half-life is 7 hours. Accumulation stops after the first 4–6 doses, and peak and nadir values do not change after this time.

Tolazamide is metabolised to 5 major metabolites, with hypoglycaemic activity from 0–70%. They are excreted principally in the urine.

Pharmaceutical particulars
List of excipients: Calcium sulphate; Docusate sodium; Methyl cellulose; Sodium alginate; Magnesium stearate.

Incompatibilities: None known.

Shelf-life: 60 months (36 months in blisters).

Special precautions for storage: Store at room temperature (at or below 25°C).

Nature and contents of container: Amber glass bottle or HDPE bottle with tamper-evident LDPE cap containing 100 or 500 tablets.

PVC blister/aluminium foil strip of 15 tablets with two or six strips in a carton.

Instructions for use/handling: None.

Marketing authorisation number 0032/5043R.

Date of first authorisation/renewal of authorisation
Date of first authorisation: 2 May 1986
Renewal date: 24 June 2001

Date of (partial) revision of the text October 1996.

Legal status POM.

TOLANASE* TABLETS 250 mg

Qualitative and quantitative composition Each tablet contains 250 mg tolazamide

Pharmaceutical form Tablet for oral use.

Clinical particulars
Therapeutic indications: Sulphonylurea. Indicated in maturity-onset diabetes of mild to moderate severity.

Posology and method of administration: Oral.

Adults: 100--250 mg daily, or up to 1 g daily in divided doses if necessary. It is doubtful whether doses greater than 1 g daily will result in improved control. (For dose conversion from other oral hypoglycaemic agents see literature).

Depending on the results of urinary glucose tests and blood sugar determinations, the daily dose should be either raised or lowered by amounts of one tablet (100 mg or 250 mg) at weekly intervals.

Elderly patients: These agents have had their primary use in the older aged group. The contra-indications and precautions that appear below in this Summary of Product Characteristics should be carefully observed for all aged patients and any patient with significantly compromised liver or renal function should be very carefully followed if it is the election of the physician to use oral agents.

Contra-indications: Tolanase is not indicated in juvenile or labile (brittle) diabetes, or in patients with infections or those undergoing surgery or trauma. It is contra-indicated in patients with ketosis, acidosis or in coma, or who have a history of such.

Since Tolanase has not been studied extensively in diabetes complicated by pregnancy nor in diabetics with liver, kidney or endocrine disease, it is not recommended in these instances.

Special warnings and special precautions for use: The appearance of significant acetonuria in a patient transferred from insulin to tolazamide makes return to insulin therapy mandatory.

Interaction with other medicaments and other forms of interaction: The hypoglycaemic action of sulphonylureas may be potentiated by certain drugs including phenylbutazone, oxyphenbutazone, salicylates, sulphonamides, chloramphenicol, probenecid, coumarins, monoamine oxidase inhibitors and beta adrenergic blocking agents. When such drugs are administered to a patient receiving Tolanase, the patient should be closely observed for hypoglycaemia. When such drugs are withdrawn from a patient receiving Tolanase, the patient should be observed closely for loss of control.

Certain drugs tend to produce hyperglycaemia and may lead to loss of control. These drugs include the thiazides and other diuretics, corticosteroids, phenothiazines, thyroid products, oestrogens, oral contraceptives, phenytoin, nicotinic acid, sympathomimetics and isoniazid. When such drugs are administered to a patient receiving Tolanase, the patient should be observed for loss of control. When such drugs are withdrawn from a patient receiving Tolanase, the patients should be observed closely for hypoglycaemia.

Pregnancy and lactation: See *Contra-indications* section, above.

Effects on ability to drive and use machines: No information.

Undesirable effects: The most commonly encountered symptoms are gastro-intestinal (1.8%), including nausea, anorexia, diarrhoea. Other minor occurrences, such as dizziness, weakness, insomnia, lethargy, have been reported. A disulfiram-like action after taking alcohol has been reported.

Overdose: Action should be taken to counteract the ensuing hypoglycaemic period. No known antidote.

Pharmacological properties
Pharmacodynamic properties: Tolazamide is a sulphonylurea which stimulates the islet tissue to secrete insulin. It is approximately 7 times as potent as tolbutamide in normal subjects, and 5 times in diabetics, on a milligram, single dose, basis. Hypoglycaemic effects begin 20 minutes after administration and peak at 2–4 hours. Hypoglycaemia is still apparent after 20 hours in fasted non-diabetics. With fasting diabetics, the peak effect occurs at 4–6 hours, with a duration of maximal effect of about 10 hours. Blood glucose levels begin to rise at 14–16 hours.

Pharmacokinetic properties: Peak serum concentrations occur 3–4 hours after a single oral dose. The average half-life is 7 hours. Accumulation stops after the first 4–6 doses, and peak and nadir values do not change after this time.

Tolazamide is metabolised to 5 major metabolites,

with hypoglycaemic activity from 0–70%. They are excreted principally in the urine.

Pharmaceutical particulars
List of excipients: Calcium sulphate; Docusate sodium; Methyl cellulose; Sodium alginate; Magnesium stearate.

Incompatibilities: None known.

Shelf-life: 60 months (36 months in blisters).

Special precautions for storage: Store at room temperature (at or below 25°C).

Nature and contents of container: Amber glass bottle or HDPE bottle with tamper-evident LDPE cap containing 100 or 500 tablets.

PVC blister/aluminium foil strip of 10 tablets with three or nine strips in a carton.

Instructions for use/handling: None.

Marketing authorisation number 0032/5044R.

Date of first authorisation/renewal of authorisation
Date of first authorisation: 2 May 1986
Renewal date: 24 June 2001

Date of (partial) revision of the text March 1997.

Legal status POM.

TROBICIN*

Presentation Vial containing spectinomycin hydrochloride BP, equivalent to spectinomycin 2 g, as a sterile powder. Also ampoule containing Water for Injections PhEur, for use as diluent.

Uses Antibiotic for intramuscular injection in the treatment of ano-genital gonorrhoea.

Dosage and administration Add 3.2 ml water for injections to the vial containing Trobicin as the sterile powder. Shake the vial vigorously immediately after adding diluent and before withdrawing dose. When reconstituted according to direction, each vial yields 5 ml of a suspension containing 400 mg spectinomycin per millilitre.

Adults: A single dose of 2 grams (5 ml) by deep intramuscular injection. Up to 4 grams (10 ml) have been administered in difficult-to-treat cases and in areas where antibiotic resistance is known to occur. Intramuscular injections should be made deep into the upper outer quadrant of the gluteal muscle. The dose may be divided between two injection sites.

Elderly: There is no evidence to suggest that Trobicin is less well tolerated by patients of advanced age. The normal adult dose should be given.

Children: There are insufficient data to recommend the use of Trobicin in children. Doses of 40 mg/kg are reported to be effective in children of over 2 years of age and may be used where no alternative therapy exists. There are no data to support the use of Trobicin in infants.

Contra-indications, warnings, etc
Contra-indications: Trobicin is contra-indicated for patients previously found to be hypersensitive to it. Trobicin is not indicated for the treatment of syphilis.

Interaction with other medicaments and other forms of interaction: Spectinomycin increases lithium effect and toxicity due to decreased lithium clearance. This interaction is clinically significant.

Effects on ability to drive and use machines: None

Other undesirable effects: The following reactions have been observed during single dose clinical trials: soreness at the injection site; urticaria; dizziness; nausea; chills; fever and a reduction in urine output (without renal function changes indicative of renal toxicity).

The following reactions have been observed during multiple-dose tolerance studies in healthy volunteers: a decrease in haemoglobin, haematocrit and creatinine clearance and an elevation of alkaline phosphatase, blood urea nitrogen and serum glutamic pyruvic transaminase.

Anaphylaxis and anaphylactoid reactions have been reported on rare occasions.

Use in pregnancy and lactation: There are no adequate or well-controlled studies in pregnant women. Trobicin has been used successfully, at the standard adult dose level, to treat gonorrhoea in pregnant women either where the strain of *Neisseria gonorrhoeae* was resistant to penicillin or in whom penicillin had produced an allergic reaction. Reproductive studies conducted in rats, mice and rabbits, at doses above the clinical dose level, did not demonstrate any evidence of developmental abnormalities. Nevertheless, Trobicin should only be used during pregnancy if clearly needed.

Animal studies have demonstrated that only minute quantities of Trobicin are excreted in breast milk. There are, however, insufficient data to support the use of Trobicin in nursing mothers.

Other special warnings and precautions: Spectinomycin is excreted renally and where renal impairment exists, there has been shown to be a significant prolonging of the excretion time. As Trobicin is given as single-dose therapy, the increased excretion time is not considered to be a contra-indication to its use in renally impaired patients, nevertheless, Trobicin should be used only where alternative therapies are inappropriate. The standard adult dosage should be used.

The safety of use in patients with hepatic dysfunction has not been established.

Antibiotics used in high doses for short periods of time to treat gonorrhoea may mask or delay the symptoms of incubating syphilis. Since the treatment of acute syphilis demands prolonged therapy with an effective antibiotic, patients being treated for gonorrhoea should be closely observed clinically for a period of four to six weeks. Appropriate serological follow-up for at least four months should be instituted if a diagnosis of syphilis is suspected.

Development of resistance to antibiotics has been observed with *N. gonorrhoeae*. This appears, so far, to occur only rarely with Trobicin, however, the clinical effectiveness of Trobicin should be monitored to detect evidence of resistance development.

Overdosage: Overdosage is unlikely to be a problem in practice.

Incompatibilities: None known.

Pharmaceutical precautions Shake vial vigorously immediately after adding diluent and before withdrawing dose. Dilution of the reconstituted suspension should not be necessary. Prepare suspension immediately before use. Discard any unused suspension.

Legal category POM.

Package quantities 1×2 g vial plus diluent.

Further information Trobicin bears no structural or antigenic relationship to the penicillins. It is an inhibitor of protein synthesis in the bacterial cell, the site of action being the 30 S ribosomal subunit. Trobicin is rapidly absorbed after intramuscular injection, a single 2 g dose producing peak serum concentrations averaging 103 microgram/ml at one hour. Serum concentrations inhibitory to most gonococcal strains persist for up to eight hours. Up to 100% of the administered dose is excreted in the urine within 48 hours in a biologically active form.

Product licence number 0032/0032.

VISTIDE*

Qualitative and quantitative composition Each vial contains cidofovir equivalent to 375 mg/5 ml (75 mg/ml) cidofovir anhydrous. The formulation is adjusted to pH 7.4.

Pharmaceutical form Concentrate for solution for infusion.

Clinical particulars
Therapeutic indications: Cidofovir is indicated for the treatment of CMV retinitis in patients with acquired immunodeficiency syndrome (AIDS) and without renal dysfunction. Until further experience is gained, cidofovir should be used only when other agents are considered unsuitable.

Posology and method of administration: Before each administration of cidofovir, serum creatinine and urine protein levels should be investigated.

The recommended dosage, frequency, or infusion rate must not be exceeded. Cidofovir must be diluted in 100 millilitres 0.9% (normal) saline prior to administration. To minimise potential nephrotoxicity, oral probenecid and intravenous saline prehydration must be administered with each cidofovir infusion.

Dosage in adults:
Induction treatment: The recommended dose of cidofovir is 5 mg/kg body weight (given as an intravenous infusion at a constant rate over 1 hour) administered once weekly for two consecutive weeks.

Maintenance treatment: Beginning two weeks after the completion of induction treatment, the recommended maintenance dose of cidofovir is 5 mg/kg body weight (given as an intravenous infusion at a constant rate over 1 hour) administered once every two weeks.

Cidofovir therapy should be discontinued and intravenous hydration is advised if serum creatinine increases by ≥ 44 µmol/l (≥ 0.5 mg/dl), or if persistent proteinuria ≥ 2+ develops.

Probenecid: A course of probenecid, administered orally with each cidofovir dose may reduce the potential for nephrotoxicity. All clinical trials relevant to clinical efficacy evaluation were performed using probenecid concomitantly with cidofovir. Therefore to minimise the potential for nephrotoxicity, a course of probenecid should be administered orally with each cidofovir dose. Two grams should be administered 3 hours prior to the cidofovir dose and one gram administered at 2 and again at 8 hours after completion of the 1 hour cidofovir infusion (for a total of 4 grams). In order to reduce the potential for nausea and/or vomiting associated with administration of probenecid, patients should be encouraged to eat food prior to each dose of probenecid. The use of an anti-emetic may be necessary. In patients who develop allergic or hypersensitivity symptoms to probenecid (e.g., rash, fever, chills and anaphylaxis), prophylactic or therapeutic use of an appropriate antihistamine and/or paracetamol should be considered (see *Contra-indications*).

Hydration: To minimise the potential for nephrotoxicity, patients should receive a total of one litre of 0.9 % (normal) saline solution intravenously immediately prior to each infusion of cidofovir. Patients who can tolerate the additional fluid load may receive up to a total of 2 litres of 0.9% saline intravenously with each dose of cidofovir. The first litre of saline solution should be infused over a 1 hour period immediately before the cidofovir infusion, and the second litre, if given, infused over a 1-3 hour period beginning simultaneously with the cidofovir infusion or starting immediately after the infusion of cidofovir.

Dosage in elderly: The safety and efficacy of cidofovir have not been established for the treatment of CMV disease in patients over 60 years of age. Since elderly individuals frequently have reduced glomerular function, particular attention should be paid to assessing renal function before and during administration of cidofovir.

Dosage in children and neonates: The safety and efficacy of cidofovir have not been established for the treatment of CMV disease in patients under 18 years of age. Therefore, cidofovir is not recommended for use in children and neonates.

Dosage in renal insufficiency: Renal insufficiency is a contraindication for the use of cidofovir (See *Contra-indications*). Treatment with cidofovir should not be initiated in patients with serum creatinine > 133 µmol/l (> 1.5 mg/dl), creatinine clearance ≤ 0.92 ml/s (≤ 55 ml/min), or ≥ 2+ proteinuria (≥ 100 mg/dl), as the optimum induction and maintenance doses for patients with moderate to severe renal impairment are not known.

Dosage in hepatic insufficiency: The safety and efficacy of cidofovir have not been established in patients with hepatic disease.

Monitoring advice: Proteinuria appears to be an early and sensitive indicator of cidofovir-induced nephrotoxicity. Patients receiving cidofovir must have their serum creatinine and urine protein levels determined on specimens obtained within 24 hours prior to the administration of each dose of cidofovir. In patients exhibiting ≥ 2+ proteinuria, intravenous hydration should be performed and the test repeated. If following hydration, a ≥ 2+ proteinuria is still observed, cidofovir therapy should be discontinued. Continued administration of cidofovir to patients with persistent ≥ 2+ proteinuria following intravenous hydration may result in further evidence of proximal tubular injury, including glycosuria, decreases in serum phosphate, uric acid and bicarbonate, and elevations in serum creatinine.

During treatment, these parameters should be investigated prior to the administration of each infusion, and the treatment should be stopped in case of abnormality. In case of complete recovery, the reintroduction of cidofovir has not yet been evaluated.

White blood cell counts, including the differential neutrophil count, should also be performed prior to each dose of cidofovir.

Patients receiving cidofovir should be advised to have regular follow-up ophthalmologic examinations.

Contra-indications: Cidofovir is contra-indicated in patients with renal impairment [serum creatinine > 133 µmol/l (> 1.5 mg/dl) or creatinine clearance ≤ 0.92 ml/s (≤ 55 ml/min) or proteinuria ≥ 100 mg/dl (≥ 2+ proteinuria)]. The safety of cidofovir has not been evaluated in patients receiving other known potentially nephrotoxic agents such as aminoglycosides, amphotericin B, foscarnet, intravenous pentamidine and vancomycin. Concomitant administration of cidofovir and these agents is contra-indicated. Cidofovir is also contra-indicated in patients with hypersensitivity to the drug.

Direct intraocular injection of cidofovir is contraindicated; direct injection may be associated with significant decreases in intraocular pressure and impairment of vision.

Special warnings and special precautions for use: Cidofovir is formulated for intravenous infusion only and should not be administered by intraocular injection. Cidofovir should be infused only into veins with adequate blood flow to permit rapid dilution and distribution. Therapy should be accompanied by administration of oral probenecid and adequate intravenous saline prehydration. In patients unable to receive probenecid because of a clinically significant hypersensitivity to the drug or to other sulpha-containing medications, cidofovir administration should only be considered if the potential benefits of therapy outweigh the potential risks. Such use of cidofovir without concomitant probenecid has not been clinically investigated. A probenecid desensitization program is not recommended for use.

Renal function (serum creatinine and urine protein) must be monitored prior to each dose of cidofovir. Interruption, and possibly discontinuation, is required for changes in renal function (see *Posology and method of administration*).

Renal impairment: Dose-dependent nephrotoxicity is the major dose-limiting toxicity related to administration of cidofovir. Proteinuria, as measured by urinalysis in a clinical laboratory, may be an early indicator of nephrotoxicity. Patients receiving weekly intravenous cidofovir at a dose of 0.5 mg/kg or 1.0 mg/kg, without concomitant probenecid, with or without intravenous saline prehydration, did not show evidence of significant drug-related nephrotoxicity (as defined by serum creatinine ≥177 μmol/l (≥2.0 mg/dl), while patients treated at 3.0 mg/kg, 5.0 mg/kg or 10.0 mg/kg without concomitant probenecid developed evidence of proximal tubular cell injury, including glycosuria, and decreases in serum phosphate, uric acid and bicarbonate, and elevations in serum creatinine. The signs of nephrotoxicity were partially reversible in some patients.

Haematology: Reversible neutropenia has been observed in patients receiving cidofovir. This has not been associated with clinical sequelae and does not appear to be dose-dependent. Resolution has occurred in some cases while on continued cidofovir therapy and in others following discontinuation of the drug.

Laboratory tests: Renal function tests (routine urinalysis and serum creatinine) must be measured, and the results reviewed, prior to administration of each cidofovir dose. Neutrophil counts also should be monitored regularly.

Other: Cidofovir should be considered a potential carcinogen in humans (see *Preclinical safety data*).

Caution should be applied when considering cidofovir treatment of patients with diabetes mellitus due to the potential increased risk of developing ocular hypotony.

Male patients should be advised that cidofovir caused reduced testes weight and hypospermia in animals. Although not observed in clinical studies of cidofovir, such changes may occur in humans and cause infertility. Men should be advised to practice barrier contraceptive methods during and for 3 months after treatment with cidofovir.

Interaction with other medicaments and other forms of interaction: Probenecid is known to interact with the metabolism or renal tubular secretion of many drugs (e.g., paracetamol, acyclovir, angiotensin-converting enzyme inhibitors, aminosalicyclic acid, barbiturates, benzodiazepines, bumetanide, clofibrate, methotrexate, famotidine, furosemide, nonsteroidal anti-inflammatory agents, theophylline, and zidovudine).

Patients who are being treated with zidovudine should temporarily discontinue zidovudine administration or decrease their zidovudine dose by 50% on days when cidofovir is administered, because probenecid reduces the clearance of zidovudine.

Interactions of cidofovir, probenecid, and anti-HIV drugs, including anti-HIV protease inhibitors, have not been investigated in clinical trials.

Use during pregnancy and lactation: Cidofovir is embryotoxic in rats and rabbits at subtherapeutic dose levels. A significantly increased foetal incidence of external, soft tissue and skeletal anomalies occurred in rabbits at 1.0 mg/kg/day, which was also maternally toxic.

There are no studies of cidofovir in pregnant women. The drug should not be used during pregnancy.

Women of childbearing potential should be advised to use effective contraception during and after treatment with cidofovir.

It is not known whether cidofovir is excreted in human milk. Because many drugs are excreted in human milk, nursing mothers should be instructed to discontinue cidofovir or discontinue nursing if they continue to receive cidofovir. Passage of the placenta barrier of drug-related compound was observed in pregnant rats. Excretion of drug-related material into milk of lactating animals was not examined.

Refer to *Special warnings and special precautions for use* for further information.

Effects on ability to drive and use machines: Adverse effects such as asthenia may occur during cidofovir therapy. The physician is advised to discuss this issue with the patient, and based upon the condition of the disease and the tolerance of medication, give his recommendation in the individual case.

Undesirable effects: In controlled clinical trials with cidofovir in patients with AIDS and CMV retinitis, the most frequently reported adverse events were: proteinuria 51%, fever 43%, asthenia 32%, nausea with vomiting 26%, and rash 19%. These incidence figures were calculated independent of relationship to study drugs (cidofovir or probenecid) or severity. The adverse events reported as serious and which occurred in at least 5% of patients were: proteinuria 13%, neutropenia 10%, fever 9%, death 8%, infection 8%, creatinine increase 8%, dyspnea 7%, pneumonia 7%, asthenia 6%, and nausea with vomiting 5%. All deaths occurring during study were attributed to complications of AIDS and not to cidofovir.

The adverse events which occurred in at least 10% of the patients and were possibly or probably related to cidofovir were: proteinuria 41%, neutropenia 18%, asthenia 15%, creatinine increase 14%, fever 13%, alopecia 12%, and nausea without vomiting 10%.

The serious adverse events which occurred in at least 5% of patients and were possibly or probably related to cidofovir were: proteinuria 11%, neutropenia 9%, and creatinine increase 7%.

The adverse events which occurred in at least 10% of the patients and were possibly or probably related to probenecid were: fever 18%, rash 13%, nausea with vomiting 12%, and nausea without vomiting 10%.

The incidence of decreased intraocular pressure (≥50% decrease from pretreatment baseline) was 9%.

Overdose: Two cases of cidofovir overdose have been reported. In both cases, the overdose occurred during the first induction dose and no additional cidofovir therapy was administered. One patient received a single dose of 16.4 mg/kg and the other patient received a single dose of 17.3 mg/kg. Both patients were hospitalised and received prophylactic oral probenecid and vigorous hydration for 3 to 7 days. One of these patients experienced a minor transient change in renal function, while the other patient had no change in renal function.

Pharmacological properties

Pharmacodynamic properties: Antiviral for Systemic Use (ATC Code J05)

General: Cidofovir is a cytidine analogue with in vitro and in vivo activity against human cytomegalovirus (HCMV). HCMV strains resistant to ganciclovir may still be susceptible to cidofovir.

Mechanism of action: Cidofovir suppresses CMV replication by selective inhibition of viral DNA synthesis. Biochemical data support selective inhibition of HSV-1, HSV-2 and CMV DNA polymerases by cidofovir diphosphate, the active intracellular metabolite of cidofovir.

Cidofovir diphosphate inhibits these viral polymerases at concentrations that are 8- to 600-fold lower than those needed to inhibit human cellular DNA polymerases alpha, beta, and gamma. Incorporation of cidofovir into viral DNA results in reductions in the rate of viral DNA synthesis.

Cidofovir enters cells by fluid-phase endocytosis and is phosphorylated to cidofovir monophosphate and subsequently to cidofovir diphosphate. In addition, a cidofovir phosphate-choline adduct is formed. In contrast to ganciclovir, the metabolism of cidofovir is neither dependent on, nor facilitated by, viral infections. Prolonged antiviral effects of cidofovir are related to the half-lives of metabolites; cidofovir diphosphate persists inside cells with a half-life of 17-65 hours. Additionally, the phosphate-choline species has a half-life of 87 hours.

Antiviral activity: Cidofovir is active in vitro against CMV, a member of the herpesviridae family. Antiviral activity is seen at concentrations significantly below those which cause death in cell monolayers. The in vitro sensitivity to cidofovir is shown in the following table.

Cidofovir Inhibition of Virus Multiplication in Cell Culture

Virus	*IC_{50} (μM)*
wild-type CMV isolates	0.7 (±0.6)
ganciclovir-resistant CMV isolates	7.5 (± 4.3)
foscarnet-resistant CMV isolates	0.59 (±0.07)

In vivo activity against human CMV was confirmed with controlled clinical studies of cidofovir for the treatment of CMV retinitis in patients with AIDS, which demonstrated statistically significant delays in time to CMV retinitis progression for patients on cidofovir when compared to control patients. The median times to retinitis progression in the two studies relevant for efficacy assessment (studies GS-93-106 and GS-93-105, both conducted in patients previously untreated for CMV retinitis) were 120 days and not reached for the treatment arms vs. 22 days and 21 days for the untreated (deferred treatment) arms, respectively.

In study GS-93-107 conducted in patients who had relapsed after treatment with other agents, the median time to retinitis progression was 115 days.

Viral resistance: Following in vitro selection of ganciclovir-resistant human CMV isolates, cross-resistance between ganciclovir and cidofovir was seen with ganciclovir-selected mutations in the CMV DNA polymerase gene but not with mutations in the UL97 gene. No cross-resistance between foscarnet and cidofovir was seen with foscarnet-selected mutants. Cidofovir-selected mutants had a mutation in the DNA polymerase gene and were cross-resistant to ganciclovir, but susceptible to foscarnet.

Pharmacokinetic properties: The major route of elimination of cidofovir was by renal excretion of unchanged drug by a combination of glomerular filtration and tubular secretion. In patients with normal renal function, 80 to 100% of the intravenous dose was recovered in the urine over 24 hours as unchanged cidofovir. No metabolites of cidofovir have been detected in serum or urine of patients.

At the end of a one-hour infusion of cidofovir 5 mg/kg administered with concomitant oral probenecid, the mean (±SD) serum concentration of cidofovir was 19.6 (±7.18) mg/ml. The mean values of total serum clearance, volume of distribution at steady-state and terminal elimination half-life were 138 (±36) ml/hr/kg, 388 (±125) ml/kg and 2.2 (±0.5) hour, respectively.

Dose-independent kinetics were demonstrated with single doses of cidofovir given over the dose range 3 to 7.5 mg/kg.

In vitro protein binding: In vitro protein binding of cidofovir to plasma or serum protein was 10% or less over the cidofovir concentration range 0.25 to 25 mg/ml.

Preclinical safety data: Preclinical animal studies demonstrated that nephrotoxicity was the major dose-limiting toxicity of cidofovir. Evidence for a nephroprotective effect for probenecid was shown in a 52-week study conducted in cynomolgus monkeys administered cidofovir 2.5 mg/kg once weekly intravenously with 1 gram of probenecid given orally.

Carcinogenesis: In a 26-week intravenous toxicity study, a significant increase in incidence of mammary adenocarcinomas was seen in female rats and of Zymbal's gland carcinomas in male and female rats at subtherapeutic plasma levels of cidofovir. In a separate study, once weekly subcutaneous injections of cidofovir for 19 consecutive weeks resulted in mammary adenocarcinomas in female rats at doses as low as 0.6 mg/kg/week. In both studies, tumors were observed within 3 months of dosing. No tumours were observed in cynomolgus monkeys administered cidofovir intravenously once weekly for 52 weeks at doses up to 2.5 mg/kg/week.

Mutagenicity and reproductive toxicology: Studies have shown that cidofovir is clastogenic in vitro at 100 μg/ml and is embryotoxic in rats and rabbits.

No mutagenic response was elicited by cidofovir at dose levels up to 5 mg/plate, in the presence and absence of metabolic activation by rat liver S-9 fraction, in microbial assays involving Salmonella typhimurium for base pair substitutions or frameshift mutations (Ames) and Escherichia coli for reverse mutations.

An increase in formation of micronucleated polychromatic erythrocytes was observed in vivo in mice receiving a high, toxic intraperitoneal dose of cidofovir (≥2000 mg/kg).

Cidofovir induced chromosomal aberrations in human peripheral blood lymphocytes in vitro without metabolic activation (S-9 fraction). At the 4 cidofovir levels (12.5 to 100 μg/ml) tested, the percentage of damaged metaphases and number of aberrations per cell increased in a concentration-dependent manner.

No adverse effects on fertility or general reproduction were seen following once weekly intravenous injections of cidofovir in male rats for 13 consecutive weeks at doses up to 15 mg/kg/week. Female rats dosed intravenously once weekly at 1.2 mg/kg/week or higher for up to 6 weeks prior to mating and for 2 weeks post mating had decreased litter sizes and live births per litter and increased early resorptions per litter. Peri- and post-natal development studies in which female rats received subcutaneous injections of cidofovir once daily at doses up to 1.0 mg/kg/day from day 7 of gestation through day 21 postpartum (approximately 5 weeks) resulted in no adverse effects on viability, growth, behavior, sexual maturation or reproductive capacity in the offspring. Daily intravenous administration of cidofovir during the period of organogenesis led to reduced fetal body weights when administered to pregnant rats at 1.5 mg/kg/day and to pregnant rabbits at 1.0 mg/kg/day. The no-observable-effect dosages for embryotoxicity was 0.5 mg/kg/day in rats and 0.25 mg/kg/day in rabbits.

Pharmaceutical particulars
List of excipients: Sodium Hydroxide; Hydrochloric Acid; Water for Injection

Incompatibilities: The chemical and physical stability of VISTIDE admixed with saline has been demonstrated in glass bottles, in infusion bags composed of either polyvinyl chloride (PVC) or ethylene/propylene copolymer, and in PVC based vented I.V. administration sets. Other types of I.V. set tubing and infusion bags have not been studied.

No data are available to support the addition of other drugs or supplements to the recommended admixture for intravenous infusion. Compatibility with Ringer's Solution, Lactated Ringer's Solution or bacteriostatic infusion fluids has not been evaluated.

Shelf life: VISTIDE vials are stable for 36 months when stored between 15°C and 30°C.

Special precautions for storage: Store at a temperature between 15°C and 30°C.

If not intended for use immediately after preparation, VISTIDE infusion admixtures may be stored temporarily for up to 24 hours in a refrigerator (2–8°C) when reconstitution is performed under aseptic conditions. Storage beyond 24 hours or freezing is not recommended. Refrigerated solutions should be allowed to warm to room temperature prior to use.

VISTIDE is supplied in single-use vials. Partially used vials should be discarded.

Nature and contents of container: Sterile cidofovir solution is supplied in single use 5 ml clear glass vials with a 5 ml nominal fill volume. The container/closure components include: Type I clear borosilicate glass vials, Teflon™ faced grey butyl plug stoppers, and aluminum crimp seals with a flip off plastic tab. Each pack contains one 5 ml vial together with the package leaflet.

Instructions for use/handling:
Method of preparation and administration: As with all parenteral products, VISTIDE vials should be visually inspected for particulate matter and discolouration prior to administration.

With a syringe, transfer under aseptic conditions the appropriate dose of VISTIDE from the vial to an infusion bag containing 100 ml 0.9% (normal) saline solution, and mix thoroughly. The entire volume should be infused intravenously into the patient at a constant rate over a period of 1 hour by use of a standard infusion pump. VISTIDE should be administered by health care professionals adequately experienced in the care of AIDS patients.

Handling and disposal: Adequate precautions including the use of appropriate safety equipment are recommended for the preparation, administration and disposal of VISTIDE. The preparation of VISTIDE should be done in a laminar flow biological safety cabinet. Personnel preparing the drug should wear surgical gloves, safety glasses and a closed front surgical-type gown with knit cuffs. If VISTIDE contacts the skin, wash membranes and flush thoroughly with water. Excess VISTIDE and all other materials used in the admixture preparation and administration should be placed in a leak-proof, puncture-proof container for disposal.

Marketing authorisation holder: Pharmacia & Upjohn S.A., Route d'Esch 52, 1470 Luxembourg, G.D. Luxembourg.

Number in the community register of medicincal products EU/1/97/037/001

Date of first authorisation/renewal of authorisation 23rd April 1997.

Date of (partial) revision of text May 1998.

Legal category POM.

For further information, please contact the local representative of the Marketing Authorisation Holder.,
UK: Pharmacia & Upjohn Ltd, Davy Avenue, Milton Keynes, MK5 8PH.
Ireland: Pharmacia & Upjohn Ltd, PO Box 1752, Airways Industrial Estate, Boeing Road, Dublin 17.

XALATAN* ▼

Qualitative and quantitative composition

	1 ml eye drops contains:	One Bottle with 2.5 ml eye drops contains:
Latanoprost	50 micrograms	125 micrograms

One drop contains approximately 1.5 micrograms latanoprost.

Pharmaceutical form Eye drops, solution.

Clinical particulars
Therapeutic indications: Reduction of elevated intraocular pressure in patients with open angle glaucoma and ocular hypertension who are intolerant or insufficiently responsive to another intraocular pressure lowering medication.

Posology and method of administration:
Recommended dosage for adults (including the elderly):
Recommended therapy is one eye drop in the affected eye(s) once daily.

Optimal effect is obtained if Xalatan is administered in the evening.

The dosage of Xalatan should not exceed once daily since it has been shown that more frequent administration decreases the intraocular pressure lowering effect.

If one dose is missed treatment should continue with the next dose as normal.

If more than one topical ophthalmic drug is being used, the drugs should be administered at least five minutes apart.

Reduction of the intraocular pressure in man starts about three to four hours after administration and maximum effect is reached after eight to twelve hours. Pressure reduction is maintained for at least 24 hours.

Children: Safety and effectiveness in children has not been established. Therefore, Xalatan is not recommended for use in children.

Contra-indications: Known hypersensitivity to any component in Xalatan. Use of all contact lenses.

Special warnings and special precautions for use: Xalatan may gradually change the eye colour by increasing the amount of brown pigment in the iris. Before treatment is instituted patients should be informed of the possibility of a change in eye colour. Unilateral treatment can result in permanent heterochromia.

This change in eye colour has predominantly been seen in patients with mixed coloured irides, i.e, blue-brown, grey-brown, yellow-brown and green-brown. The colour change is due to increased melanin content in the stromal melanocytes of the iris. Typically the brown pigmentation around the pupil spreads concentrically towards the periphery in affected eyes, but the entire iris or parts of it may become more brownish. The effect, based on evidence from consecutive photographs, has been seen in 16% of all patients during 12 months of treatment in clinical trials. The highest incidence, about 50%, was found in patients with green-brown and yellow-brown irides. In patients with homogenously blue, grey, green or brown eyes, the change has only rarely been seen during two years of treatment in clinical trials.
The change in iris colour occurs slowly and may not be noticeable for several months to years. It has not been associated with any symptom or pathological changes in clinical trials to date.

No further increase in brown iris pigment has been observed after discontinuation of treatment, but the resultant colour change may be permanent. Neither naevi nor freckles of the iris have been affected by treatment.

To date, there are no clinical data on Xalatan treatment beyond two years. Accumulation of pigment in the trabecular meshwork or elsewhere in the anterior chamber has not been observed in clinical trials, but until further long term experience regarding increased iris pigmentation is available, patients should be examined regularly and, depending on the clinical situation, treatment may be stopped if increased iris pigmentation ensues. The effects of continuous treatment with Xalatan after the appearance of iris pigmentation are currently not known. There is no experience of Xalatan in inflammatory ocular conditions, inflammatory, neovascular, angle closure or congenital glaucoma and only limited experience in open angle glaucoma of pseudophakic patients and in pigmentary glaucoma. Xalatan has no or little effect on the pupil but there is no experience in acute attacks of closed angle glaucoma. Therefore, it is recommended that Xalatan should be used with caution in these conditions until more experience is obtained. Latanoprost has not been found to affect pulmonary function when studied in a small number of patients suffering from moderate asthma but there is no experience from patients with severe or brittle asthma. Such patients should therefore be treated with caution until there is sufficient experience.

Interaction with other medicaments and other forms of interaction: Definitive drug interaction data are not available.

Pregnancy and lactation:
Pregnancy: The safety of this medicinal product for use in human pregnancy has not been established. It has potential hazardous pharmacological effects with respect to the course of pregnancy, to the unborn or the neonate. Therefore Xalatan should not be used during pregnancy.

Lactation: Latanoprost and its metabolites may pass into breast milk and Xalatan should therefore not be used in nursing women or breast feeding should be stopped.

Effects on ability to drive and use machines: In common with other eye preparations, instillation of eye drops may cause transient blurring of vision.

Undesirable effects: Xalatan has caused an increase in brown pigmentation of the iris, predominantly in patients with mixed coloured irides, (i.e blue-brown, grey-brown, green-brown, yellow-brown) and is due to increased melanin content in the stromal melanocytes of the iris. The effect, based on evidence from consecutive photographs, has been seen in 16% of all patients during 12 months of treatment in clinical trials. The highest incidence, about 50%, was found in patients with green-brown and yellow-brown irides. The change in iris colour occurs slowly and may not be noticeable for several months to years. It has not been associated with any symptom or pathological changes in clinical trials. No further increase in brown iris pigment has been seen after discontinuation of treatment, but the resultant colour change may be permanent. The change has been seen only rarely in patients with homogenously blue, grey, green or brown eyes during two years of clinical trials, see also *Special warnings and special precautions for use.*

A slight foreign body sensation has been noted in about 13% of patients. Mild conjunctival hyperaemia has been noted in about 10% and moderate hyperaemia in about 1% of patients undergoing chronic treatment. Transient punctate epithelial erosions, mostly without symptoms, have been noted in about 8% of patients. Xalatan may cause darkening, thickening and lengthening of eye lashes. Macular oedema has been reported rarely during Xalatan treatment. These reports have mainly occurred in aphakic patients, in pseudophakic patients with anterior chamber lenses, or in patients with known risk factors for macular oedema (such as diabetic retinopathy and retinal vein occlusion). An association between the use of Xalatan and unexplained macular oedema cannot be excluded. Rare cases of iritis/uveitis have been reported. Darkening of the palpebral skin has very rarely been reported. Skin rash of unknown etiology has been reported rarely during Xalatan treatment.

Overdose: Apart from ocular irritation and conjunctival hyperaemia no other ocular side effects are known if Xalatan is overdosed.

If Xalatan is accidentally ingested the following information may be useful: One bottle contains 125 micrograms latanoprost. More than 90% is metabolised during the first pass through the liver. Intravenous infusion of 3 micrograms/kg in healthy volunteers induced no symptoms but a dose of 5.5–10 micrograms/kg caused nausea, abdominal pain, dizziness, fatigue, hot flushes and sweating. In monkeys latanoprost has been infused intravenously in doses of up to 500 micrograms/kg without major effects on the cardiovascular system.

Intravenous administration of latanoprost in monkeys has been associated with transient bronchoconstriction. However, in patients with moderate bronchial asthma, bronchoconstriction was not induced by latanoprost when applied topically on the eyes in a dose of seven times the clinical dose of Xalatan.

If overdosage with Xalatan occurs, treatment should be symptomatic.

Pharmacological properties
Pharmacodynamic properties: Pharmacotherapeutic group (ATC code): S 01 E X 03

The active substance latanoprost, a prostaglandin $F_{2\alpha}$ analogue, is a selective prostanoid FP receptor agonist which reduces the intraocular pressure by increasing the outflow of aqueous humour. Reduction of the intraocular pressure in man starts about three to four hours after administration and maximum effect is reached after eight to twelve hours. Pressure reduction is maintained for at least 24 hours.

Studies in animals and man indicate that the main mechanism of action is increased uveoscleral outflow, although some increase in outflow facility (decrease in outflow resistance) has been reported in man.

Pivotal studies have demonstrated that Xalatan is effective as a single drug therapy. Although definitive clinical trials of combination use have not been done, a three month study shows that latanoprost is effective in combination with beta-adrenergic antagonists (timolol). Short term (1 or 2 weeks) studies suggest that the effect of latanoprost is additive in combination with adrenergic agonists (dipivalyl epinephrine), oral carbonic anhydrase inhibitors (acetazolamide) and at least partly additive with cholinergic agonists (pilocarpine).

Clinical trials have shown that latanoprost has no significant effect on the production of aqueous humour. Latanoprost has not been found to have any effect on the blood-aqueous barrier.

Latanoprost has no or negligible effects on the intraocular blood circulation when used at the clinical dose and studied in monkeys. However, mild to moderate conjunctival or episcleral hyperaemia may occur during topical treatment.

Chronic treatment with latanoprost in monkey eyes which had undergone extracapsular lens extraction did not affect the retinal blood vessels as determined by fluorescein angiography.

Latanoprost has not induced fluorescein leakage in the posterior segment of pseudophakic human eyes during short term treatment.

Latanoprost in clinical doses has not been found to have any significant pharmacological effects on the cardiovascular or respiratory system.

Pharmacokinetic properties: Latanoprost (mw 432.58) is an isopropyl ester prodrug which per se is inactive, but after hydrolysis to the acid of latanoprost becomes biologically active.

The prodrug is well absorbed through the cornea and all drug that enters the aqueous humour is hydrolysed during the passage through the cornea.

Studies in man indicate that the peak concentration in the aqueous humour is reached about two hours after topical administration. After topical application in monkeys latanoprost is distributed primarily in the anterior segment, the conjunctivae and the eye lids. Only minute quantities of the drug reach the posterior segment.

There is practically no metabolism of the acid of latanoprost in the eye. The main metabolism occurs in the liver. The half life in plasma is 17 minutes in man. The main metabolites, the 1, 2-dinor and 1, 2, 3, 4-tetranor metabolites, exert no or only weak biological activity in animal studies and are excreted primarily in the urine.

Preclinical safety data: The ocular as well as systemic toxicity of latanoprost has been investigated in several animal species. Generally latanoprost is well tolerated with a safety margin between clinical ocular dose and systemic toxicity of at least 1000 times. High doses of latanoprost, approximately 100 times the clinical dose/kg body weight, administered intravenously to unanaesthetised monkeys have been shown to increase the respiration rate probably reflecting bronchoconstriction of short duration. In animal studies, latanoprost has not been found to have sensitising properties.

In the eye, no toxic effects have been detected with doses of up to 100 micrograms/eye/day in rabbits or monkeys (clinical dose is approximately 1.5 micrograms/eye/day). In monkeys, however, latanoprost has been shown to induce increased pigmentation of the iris.

The mechanism of increased pigmentation seems to be stimulation of melanin production in melanocytes of the iris with no proliferative changes observed. The change in iris colour may be permanent.

In chronic ocular toxicity studies, administration of latanoprost 6 micrograms/ eye/day has also been shown to induce increased palpebral fissure. This effect is reversible and occurs at doses above the clinical dose level. The effect has not been seen in humans.

Latanoprost was found negative in reverse mutation tests in bacteria, gene mutation in mouse lymphoma and mouse micronucleus test. Chromosome aberrations were observed in vitro with human lymphocytes. Similar effects were observed with prostaglandin $F_{2\alpha}$, a naturally occurring prostaglandin, and indicates that this is a class effect.

Additional mutagenicity studies on in vitro/in vivo unscheduled DNA synthesis in rats were negative and indicate that latanoprost does not have mutagenic potency. Carcinogenicity studies in mice and rats were negative.

Latanoprost has not been found to have any effect on male or female fertility in animal studies. In the embryotoxicity study in rats, no embryotoxicity was observed at intravenous doses (5, 50 and 250 micrograms/kg/day) of latanoprost. However, latanoprost induced embryolethal effects in rabbits in doses of 5 micrograms/kg/day and above.

The dose of 5 micrograms/kg/day (approximately 100 times the clinical dose) caused significant embryofoetal toxicity characterised by increased incidence of late resorption and abortion and by reduced foetal weight. No teratogenic potential has been detected.

Pharmaceutical particulars

List of excipients: Sodium chloride; Benzalkonium chloride (0.2 mg/ml); Sodium dihydrogen phosphate monohydrate; Disodium phosphate anhydrous; Water for injections.

Incompatibilities: In vitro studies have shown that precipitation occurs when eye drops containing thiomersal are mixed with Xalatan.

If such drugs are used the eye drops should be administered with an interval of at least five minutes.

Shelf life: 2 years: *Shelf life after opening of container:* 4 weeks.

Special precautions for storage: Store in a cold place (+2° to 8°C).

Protect from light. Once opened the container should be used within four weeks and may be stored at room temperature up to 25°C.

Nature and contents of container: Bottle (5 ml), dropper applicator (dropper tip), screw cap, tamper evident overcap of polyethylene.

Each bottle contains 2.5 ml eye drop solution corresponding to approximately 80 drops of solution.

Instructions for use/handling: The tamper evident overcap should be removed before use.

Marketing authorisation numbers

United Kingdom: 0032/0220 *Ireland:* 16/57/1

Date of first authorisation/renewal of authorisation

United Kingdom: 16 December 1996 *Ireland:* 25 July 1997

Date of (partial) revision of the text 14 May 1997.

Legal category POM.

XANAX* TABLETS 250 MICROGRAMS, 500 MICROGRAMS

Presentation White, oval, biconvex tablets with bevelled edges containing 250 micrograms (0.25 mg) alprazolam, scored on one side and marked 'Upjohn 29' on the other. Also contains lactose, microcrystalline cellulose, maize starch, magnesium stearate, docusate sodium, colloidal silicon dioxide and sodium benzoate.

Pink, oval, biconvex tablets with bevelled edges containing 500 micrograms (0.5 mg) alprazolam, scored on one side and marked 'Upjohn 55' on the other. Also contains lactose, microcrystalline cellulose, maize starch, magnesium stearate, docusate sodium, colloidal silicon dioxide, sodium benzoate and E127.

Uses Xanax is indicated for the short-term treatment of moderate or severe anxiety states and anxiety associated with depression. Xanax should not be used to treat short-term mild anxiety, such as anxiety or tension associated with the stress of everyday life. As the efficacy of Xanax in depression and in phobic or obsessional states has yet to be established, specific treatment may have to be considered.

Xanax tablets are recommended for short-term use. It is recommended that the patient be reassessed at the end of no longer than 4 weeks' treatment and the need for continued treatment be established. As with all benzodiazepines, physicians should be aware that long-term use may lead to dependence in certain patients.

Dosage and administration

Adults: The optimum dosage of Xanax should be based upon the severity of the symptoms and individual patient response. The lowest dose which can control symptoms should be used. Dosage should be reassessed at intervals of no more than 4 weeks. Xanax should not be used for long-term chronic treatment. The usual dosage is stated below; in the few patients who require higher doses, the dosage should be increased cautiously to avoid adverse effects. When higher dosage is required, the evening dose should be increased before the daytime doses. In general, patients who have not previously received psychotropic medications will require lower doses than those so treated, or those with a history of chronic alcoholism. Treatment should always be tapered off gradually. Patients who have taken benzodiazepines for a long time may require a longer period during which doses are reduced.

There is a reduced clearance of the drug and, as with other benzodiazepines, an increased sensitivity to the drug in elderly patients.

Anxiety: 250 micrograms (0.25 mg) to 500 micrograms (0.5 mg) three times daily increasing, if required, to a total of 3 mg daily.

Geriatric patients or in the presence of debilitating disease: 250 micrograms (0.25 mg) two to three times daily to be gradually increased if needed and tolerated.

If side-effects occur, the dose should be lowered. It is advisable to review treatment regularly and to discontinue use as soon as possible. Should longer term treatment be necessary, then intermittent treatment may be considered to minimize the risk of dependence.

Children: Not recommended.

Contra-indications, warnings etc

Contra-indications: Xanax should not be used in patients with a known sensitivity to benzodiazepines or in patients with acute pulmonary insufficiency.

Interaction with other medicaments and other forms of interaction: Potentiation of the sedative effect may be seen when the product is used in combination with alcohol. The concurrent use of other CNS depressant drugs should be avoided.

Effects on ability to drive and use machines: Performance at skilled tasks and alertness may be impaired. Patients should be warned of this hazard and advised not to drive or operate machinery during treatment. These effects are potentiated by alcohol.

Other undesirable effects (frequency and seriousness): Products should be used with caution in chronic pulmonary insufficiency and chronic renal or hepatic disease.

The safety and efficacy of Xanax in patients less than 18 years of age has not been established.

Administration to severely depressed or suicidal patients should be done with appropriate precautions and appropriate size of prescriptions.

In cases of loss or bereavement, psychological adjustment may be inhibited by benzodiazepines.

Common adverse effects include drowsiness, sedation, blurring of vision, unsteadiness and ataxia. These effects occur following single as well as repeated dosage and may persist well into the following day. Performance at skilled tasks and alertness may be impaired. The elderly are particularly liable to experience these symptoms together with confusion, especially if organic brain symptoms are present. Amnesia may occur.

As with other benzodiazepines, reactions such as concentration difficulties, confusion, hallucinations, stimulation and adverse behavioural effects such as irritability, agitation, rage and aggressive or hostile behaviour have been reported rarely. In many of the spontaneous case reports of adverse behavioural effects, patients were receiving other CNS drugs concomitantly and/or were described as having underlying psychiatric conditions. Isolated published reports involving small numbers of patients have suggested that patients who have borderline personality disorder, a prior history of violent or aggressive behaviour, or alcohol or substance abuse may be at risk for such events.

As with other benzodiazepines disinhibiting effects and aggressive behaviour towards self and others may be manifested in various ways. Extreme caution should be used, therefore, in prescribing benzodiazepines in patients with personality disorders.

Other rare adverse effects including hypotension, gastro-intestinal and visual disturbances, skin rashes, urinary retention, headache, vertigo, changes in libido, blood dyscrasias and jaundice have been reported also.

Use in pregnancy and lactation: If the product is prescribed to a woman of childbearing potential, she should be warned to contact her physician regarding discontinuance of the product if she intends to become or suspects that she is pregnant. If, for compelling medical reasons, the product is administered during the late phase of pregnancy, or during labour, effects on the neonate, such as hypothermia, hypotonia, and moderate respiratory depression, can be expected, due to the pharmacological action of the compound.

Infants born to mothers who took benzodiazepines chronically during the latter stages of pregnancy, may have developed physical dependence and may be at some risk of developing withdrawal symptoms in the postnatal period.

Since benzodiazepines are found in breast milk, benzodiazepines should not be given to breastfeeding mothers.

Other special warnings and precautions: Xanax is not recommended as the primary treatment for psychotic patients and should not be used in lieu of appropriate treatment for psychosis.

In general the dependence potential of benzodiazepines is low, but this increases when high dosage is attained, especially when given over long periods. This is particularly so in patients with a history of alcoholism, drug abuse or in patients with marked personality disorders. Regular monitoring of treatment in such patients is essential and routine repeat prescriptions should be avoided.

Treatment in all patients should be withdrawn gradually as symptoms such as depression, nervousness, rebound insomnia, irritability, sweating and diarrhoea have been reported following abrupt cessation of treatment, even in patients receiving normal therapeutic doses for short periods of time.

Abrupt withdrawal following excessive dosage may produce confusion, toxic psychosis, convulsions or a condition resembling delirium tremens.

Overdose: Manifestations of Xanax overdosage include extensions of its pharmacological activity, namely ataxia and somnolence. Induced vomiting and/or gastric lavage are indicated. As in all cases of drug overdosage, respiration, pulse and blood pressure should be monitored and supported by general measures when necessary. Intravenous fluids may be administered and an adequate airway maintained.

Animal experiments have suggested that forced diuresis or haemodialysis are probably of little value in treating overdosage.

As with the management of any overdosage, the

physician should bear in mind that multiple agents may have been ingested.

Incompatibilities: None known.

Pharmaceutical precautions Bottle packs should be kept tightly closed and protected from light.

Legal category CD (Sch 4) POM.

Package quantities Packs of 60 tablets.

Further information Alprazolam is readily absorbed. Following oral administration, peak concentrations in the plasma occur after 1-2 hours. The mean half-life is 12-15 hours. Repeated dosage may lead to accumulation and this should be borne in mind in elderly patients and those with impaired renal or hepatic function. Alprazolam and its metabolites are excreted primarily in the urine. Xanax did not affect the prothrombin times or plasma warfarin levels in male volunteers administered sodium warfarin orally.

Product licence numbers
0032/0092 250 micrograms (0.25 mg) tablet
0032/0093 500 micrograms (0.5 mg) tablet

Date of preparation or last review August 1997.

ZAVEDOS*

Presentation Sterile, pyrogen-free, orange-red, freeze-dried powder in vials containing 5 and 10 mg of idarubicin hydrochloride with 50 mg and 100 mg of lactose, respectively.

Uses Antimitotic and cytotoxic agent. Acute non-lymphocytic leukaemia (ANLL) in adults for remission induction in untreated patients or for remission induction in relapsed or refractory patients.

Acute lymphocytic leukaemia (ALL) as second line treatment in adults and children.

Zavedos may be used in combination chemotherapy regimens involving other cytotoxic agents.

Dosage and administration For reconstitution, the contents of the 5 mg vial should be dissolved in 5 ml of Water for Injections (PhEur) and the 10 mg vial in 10 ml of Water for Injections. Zavedos must be administered only by the intravenous route and the reconstituted solution should be given via the tubing of a freely running intravenous infusion of 0.9% Sodium Chloride Injection taking 5 to 10 minutes over the injection. This technique minimises the risk of thrombosis or perivenous extravasation which can lead to severe cellulitis and necrosis. Venous sclerosis may result from injection into small veins or repeated injections into the same vein.

Dosage is usually calculated on the basis of body surface area.

Acute non-lymphocytic leukaemia (ANLL): In adult ANLL the dose schedule suggested is 12 mg/m^2 i.v. daily for 3 days in combination with cytarabine.

Another dose-schedule which has been used in ANLL as a single agent and in combination is 8 mg/m^2 i.v. daily for 5 days.

Acute lymphocytic leukaemia (ALL): As single agent in ALL the suggested dose in adults is 12 mg/m^2 i.v. daily for 3 days and in children is 10 mg/m^2 i.v. daily for 3 days.

All of these dosage schedules should, however, take into account the haematological status of the patient and the dosages of other cytotoxic drugs when used in combination.

Contra-indications, warnings, etc
Contra-indications: Zavedos therapy should not be started in patients with severe renal and liver impairment or patients with uncontrolled infections. See also *Use during pregnancy and lactation.*

Warnings: Zavedos is intended for use under the direction of those experienced in leukaemia chemotherapy. The drug should not be given to patients with pre-existing bone marrow suppression induced by previous drug therapy or radiotherapy unless the benefit warrants the risk. Pre-existing heart disease and previous therapy with anthracyclines at high cumulative doses or other potentially cardiotoxic agents are co-factors for increased risk of idarubicin-induced cardiac toxicity and the benefit to risk ratio of Zavedos therapy in such patients should be weighed before starting treatment with Zavedos.

Like most other cytotoxic agents, idarubicin has mutagenic properties and it is carcinogenic in rats.

Bone marrow: Zavedos is a potent bone marrow suppressant. Myelosuppression, primarily of leukocytes, will therefore occur in all patients given a therapeutic dose of this agent and careful haematologic monitoring including granulocytes, red cells and platelets is required. Facilities with laboratory and supportive resources adequate to monitor drug tolerability and protect and maintain a patient compromised by drug toxicity should be available. It must be possible to treat rapidly and effectively a severe haemorrhagic condition and/or a severe infection.

Cardiac effects: Myocardial toxicity as manifested by potentially fatal congestive heart failure, acute life-threatening arrhythmias or other cardiomyopathies may occur during therapy or several weeks after termination of therapy. Treatment with digitalis, diuretics, sodium restriction and bed-rest is indicated.

Cardiac function should be carefully monitored during treatment in order to minimise the risk of cardiac toxicity of the type described for other anthracycline compounds. The risk of such myocardial toxicity may be higher following concomitant or previous radiation to the mediastinal-pericardial area or treatment with other potentially cardiotoxic agents or in patients with a particular clinical situation due to their disease (anaemia, bone marrow depression, infections, leukaemic pericarditis and/or myocarditis).

On the basis of the recommended dosage schedules the total cumulative dose administered over two courses can be expected to reach 60–80 mg/m^2. Although a cumulative dose limit cannot yet be defined, a specific cardiological evaluation in cancer patients showed no significant modifications of cardiac function in patients treated with Zavedos at a mean cumulative dose of 93 mg/m^2.

While there is no reliable method for predicting acute congestive heart failure, cardiomyopathy induced by anthracyclines is usually associated with persistent QRS voltage reduction, increase beyond normal limits of the systolic time interval (PEP/LVET) and decrease of the left ventricular ejection fraction (LVET) from pre-treatment baseline values. An electrocardiogram or echocardiogram and a determination of left ventricular ejection fraction should be performed prior to starting therapy and during treatment with Zavedos. Early clinical diagnosis of drug-induced myocardial damage appears to be important for pharmacological treatment to be useful.

Evaluation of hepatic and renal function: Since hepatic and/or renal function impairment can affect the disposition of idarubicin, liver and kidney function should be evaluated with conventional clinical laboratory tests (using serum bilirubin and serum creatinine as indicators) prior to, and during, treatment. In a number of Phase III clinical trials, treatment was not given if bilirubin and/or creatinine serum levels exceeded 2 mg%. With other anthracyclines, a 50% dose reduction is generally employed if bilirubin and creatinine levels are in the range 1.2–2.0 mg%.

Precautions: Therapy with Zavedos requires close observation of the patient and laboratory monitoring. Patients aged over 55 years should be given vigorous supportive treatment during the aplastic period.

Hyperuricemia secondary to rapid lysis of leukaemic cells may be induced: blood uric acid levels should be monitored and appropriate therapy initiated if hyperuricemia develops. Appropriate measures must be taken to control any systemic infection before beginning therapy.

Extravasation of Zavedos at the site of i.v. injection can cause severe local tissue necrosis. The risk of thrombophlebitis at the injection site may be minimised by following the recommended procedure for administration. A stinging or burning sensation at the site of administration signifies a small degree of extravasation and the infusion should be stopped and re-started in another vein.

Adverse reactions: Severe myelosuppression and cardiac toxicity are the two major adverse effects. Other adverse reactions include: reversible alopecia in most patients; acute nausea and vomiting; mucositis, usually involving the oral mucosa and appearing 3–10 days after starting treatment; oesophagitis and diarrhoea; fever, chills, skin rash; elevation of liver enzymes and bilirubin in about 20–30% of cases. Severe and sometimes fatal infections have been associated with Zavedos alone or in combination with cytarabine.

Zavedos may impart a red colour to the urine for 1–2 days after administration and patients should be advised that this is no cause for alarm.

Use in pregnancy and lactation: There is no information as to whether idarubicin may adversely affect human fertility, or cause teratogenesis. However, in rats (but not rabbits) it is teratogenic and embryotoxic. Women of child bearing potential should be advised to avoid pregnancy.

If Zavedos is to be used during pregnancy, or if the patient becomes pregnant during therapy, the patient should be informed of the potential hazard to the foetus. Mothers should be advised not to breast-feed while undergoing chemotherapy with this drug.

Interactions: Zavedos is a potent myelosuppressant and combination chemotherapy regimens which contain other agents having a similar action may be expected to lead to additive myelosuppressive effects.

Overdose: Very high doses of Zavedos may be expected to cause acute myocardial toxicity within 24 hours and severe myelosuppression within one or two weeks. Treatment should aim to support the patient during this period and should utilise such measures as blood transfusions and reverse-barrier nursing. Delayed cardiac failure has been seen with the anthracyclines up to several months after the overdose. Patients should be observed carefully and if signs of cardiac failure arise, should be treated along conventional lines.

Pharmaceutical precautions The vial contents are under a negative pressure to minimise aerosol formation during reconstitution: particular care should be taken when the needle is inserted. Inhalation of any aerosol produced during reconstitution must be avoided.

The following protective recommendations which are valid for all cytotoxic agents are given:

- Personnel should be trained in good technique for reconstitution and handling.
- Pregnant staff should be excluded from working with this drug.
- Personnel handling the drug should wear protective clothing: goggles, gowns and disposable gloves and masks.
- A designated area should be defined for reconstitution (preferably under a vertical laminar flow system). The work surface should be protected by disposable, plastic-backed, absorbent paper.
- All items used for reconstitution, administration or cleaning, including gloves, should be placed in high-risk, waste disposal bags for high temperature incineration.

Accidental contact with the skin or eyes should be treated immediately by copious lavage with water: medical attention should be sought.

Spillage or leakage should be treated with dilute sodium hypochlorite (1% available chlorine) solution, preferably by soaking, and then water. All cleaning materials should subsequently be disposed of as indicated previously.

The reconstituted solution is chemically stable when stored for at least 48 hours at 2°C–8°C and 24 hours at room temperature; however, it is recommended that, in line with good pharmaceutical practice, the solution should not normally be stored for longer than 24 hours at 2°C–8°C.

Discard any unused solution.

Prolonged contact with any solution of an alkaline pH should be avoided as it will result in degradation of the drug. Zavedos should not be mixed with heparin as a precipitate may form and it is not recommended that it be mixed with other drugs.

Legal category POM.

Package quantities 5 mg and 10 mg vials for injection.

Further information Nil.

Product licence numbers
Zavedos 5 mg 3433/0133
Zavedos 10 mg 3433/0134

ZAVEDOS* CAPSULES

Presentation *5 mg dosage:* opaque, red cap and red body, self-locking, hard gelatin capsule, marked with the trademark Zavedos, size No 4, containing idarubicin hydrochloride as an orange powder.

10 mg dosage: opaque, red cap and white body, self-locking, hard gelatin capsule, marked with the trademark Zavedos, size No 4, containing idarubicin hydrochloride as an orange powder.

25 mg dosage: opaque, white cap and white body, self-locking, hard gelatin capsule, marked with the trademark Zavedos, size No 2, containing idarubicin hydrochloride as an orange powder.

Uses Whenever intravenous idarubicin cannot be employed e.g. for medical, psychological or social reasons, oral idarubicin can be used for remission induction in patients with previously untreated, relapsed or refractory acute non-lymphocytic leukaemia (ANLL).

Zavedos capsules may be used in combination chemotherapy regimens involving other cytotoxic agents.

Zavedos can also be used as a single agent to treat advanced breast cancer after failure of frontline chemotherapy not including anthracyclines.

Dosage and administration Dosage is usually calculated on the basis of body surface area.

In adult ANLL the recommended dose schedule is 30 mg/m^2 orally given daily for 3 days as a single agent, or between 15 and 30 mg/m^2 orally daily for 3 days in combination with other anti-leukaemic agents.

In advanced breast cancer the recommended dose schedule as single agent is 45 mg/m^2 orally given either on a single day or divided over 3 consecutive days, to be repeated every 3 or 4 weeks based on the haematological recovery.

A maximum cumulative dose of 400 mg/m² is recommended.

These dosage schedules should, however, take into account the haematological status of the patient and the dosages of other cytotoxic drugs when used in combination.

In patients with hepatic impairment a dose reduction of Zavedos should be considered (see *Special warnings*).

The capsules should be swallowed whole with some water and should not be sucked, bitten or chewed.

Zavedos Capsules may also be taken with a light meal.

Contra-indications, warnings, etc

Contra-indications: Zavedos should not be administered to individuals with hypersensitivity to idarubicin and/or other anthracyclines.

Zavedos therapy should not be started in patients with severe renal and liver impairment or patients with uncontrolled infections. See also *Use during pregnancy and lactation.*

Warnings: Zavedos is intended for use under the direction of those experienced in leukaemia chemotherapy. The drug should not be given to patients with pre-existing bone marrow suppression induced by previous drug therapy or radiotherapy unless the benefit warrants the risk. Pre-existing heart disease and previous therapy with anthracyclines at high cumulative doses or other potentially cardiotoxic agents are co-factors for increased risk of idarubicin-induced cardiac toxicity and the benefit to risk ratio of Zavedos therapy in such patients should be weighed before starting treatment with Zavedos. In absence of sufficient data, the use of oral idarubicin is not recommended in patients with prior total body irradiation or bone marrow transplantation.

Like most other cytotoxic agents, idarubicin has mutagenic properties and it is carcinogenic in rats.

Bone marrow: Zavedos is a potent bone marrow suppressant. Myelosuppression, primarily of leukocytes, will therefore occur in all patients given a therapeutic dose of this agent and careful haematologic monitoring including granulocytes, red cells and platelets is required. Facilities with laboratory and supportive resources adequate to monitor drug tolerability and protect and maintain a patient compromised by drug toxicity should be available. It must be possible to treat rapidly and effectively a severe haemorrhagic condition and/or a severe infection.

Cardiac effects: Myocardial toxicity as manifested by potentially fatal congestive heart failure (CHF), acute life-threatening arrhythmias or other cardiomyopathies may occur during therapy or several weeks after termination of therapy. Although a cumulative dose limit cannot yet be defined, available data on patients treated with Zavedos capsules indicate that total cumulative doses up to at least 400 mg/m² have a low probability of cardiotoxicity.

Should CHF occur, treatment with digitalis, diuretics, sodium restriction and bed-rest is indicated.

Cardiac function should be carefully monitored during treatment in order to minimise the risk of cardiac toxicity of the type described for other anthracycline compounds. The risk of such myocardial toxicity may be higher following concomitant or previous radiation to the mediastinal-pericardial area or treatment with other potentially cardiotoxic agents or in patients with a particular clinical situation due to their disease (anemia, bone marrow depression, infections, leukaemic pericarditis and/or myocarditis).

While there is no reliable method of predicting acute congestive heart failure, cardiomyopathy induced by anthracyclines is usually associated with persistent QRS voltage reduction, increase beyond normal limits of the systolic time interval (PEP/LVET) and a significant decrease of the left ventricular ejection fraction (LVET) from pretreatment baseline values.

An electrocardiogram or echocardiogram and a determination of left ventricular ejection fraction should be performed prior to starting therapy and during treatment with Zavedos. Early clinical dignosis of drug-induced myocardial damage appears to be important for pharmacological treatment to be useful.

Evaluation of hepatic function: Since hepatic function impairment can affect the disposition of idarubicin, liver function should be evaluated with conventional clinical laboratory tests (using serum bilirubin as indicator) prior to, and during, treatment.

In a number of clinical trials, treatment was not given if bilirubin serum levels exceeded 2 mg/100 ml. With other anthracyclines a 50% dose reduction has been employed if bilirubin levels are in the range 1.2–2.0 mg/100 ml in acute leukaemias. In some studies in breast cancer the oral idarubicin dose was reduced by 50% if bilirubin rose to 2–3 mg/100 ml during treatment or withdrawn with a bilirubin level >3 mg/100 ml.

Occasionally episodes of serious gastro-intestinal events (such as perforation or bleeding) have been observed in patients receiving oral idarubicin who had either acute leukaemia or a history of other pathologies/medications that might have led to GI complications. Therefore in the case of patients with active GI disease with increased risk of bleeding and/or perforation the physician must balance the benefit of Zavedos therapy against the risk.

Precautions: Therapy with Zavedos requires close observation of the patient and laboratory monitoring. Patients over 55 years of age should be given vigorous supportive treatment during the aplastic period. Hyperuricemia secondary to rapid lysis of leukemic cells may be induced: blood uric acid levels should be monitored and appropriate therapy initiated if hyperuricemia develops. Appropriate measures must be taken to control any systemic infections before beginning therapy.

Adverse reactions: Severe myelosuppression and cardiac toxicity are the two major adverse effects. Other adverse reactions include: reversible alopecia in most patients treated at the dosage recommended in leukaemia and in about half of the patients treated at the doses recommended for breast cancer; acute nausea and vomiting; mucositis, usually involving the oral mucosa and appearing 3–10 days after starting treatment; oesophagitis; diarrhoea; fever and chills; skin rash; elevation of liver enzymes and bilirubin in about 10–20% of cases. Severe and sometimes fatal infections have been associated with idarubicin alone or in combination. Severe enterocolitis with perforation has been reported very rarely.

Idarubicin may impart a red colour to the urine for 1–2 days after administration and patients should be advised that this is no cause for alarm.

Use in pregnancy and lactation: There is no information as to whether idarubicin may adversely affect human fertility, or cause teratogenesis. However, in rats (but not in rabbits) it is teratogenic and embryotoxic. Women of child bearing potential should be advised to avoid pregnancy. If Zavedos is to be used during pregnancy, or if the patient becomes pregnant during therapy, the patient should be informed of the potential hazard to the foetus.

Mothers should be advised not to breast-feed while undergoing chemotherapy with this drug.

Interactions: Zavedos is a potent myelosuppressant and combination chemotherapy regimens which contain other agents having a similar action may be expected to lead to additive myelosuppressive effects.

An additive myelosuppressant effect is to be expected also with radiotherapy to metastases given concomitantly or within 2–3 weeks prior to treatment with Zavedos.

Food does not appear to reduce idarubicin absorption and Zavedos may therefore be given with a light meal.

Overdosage: Although the single-dose packaging is designed to minimise the risk of overdosage and no data on overdosage exists, should this occur gastric lavage should be carried out as soon as possible. The patient should be observed for possible gastrointestinal hemorrhage and severe mucosal damage.

Very high doses of idarubicin may be expected to cause acute myocardial toxicity within 24 hours and severe myelosuppression within one or two weeks. Treatment should further aim to support the patient during this period and should utilise such measures as blood transfusions and reverse-barrier nursing. Delayed cardiac failure has been seen with the anthracyclines up to several months after an overdose. Patients should be observed carefully and if signs of cardiac failure arise, should be treated along conventional lines.

Pharmaceutical precautions Before administration it should be ensured that the capsules are intact. They should be swallowed whole with some water and should not be sucked, bitten or chewed.

In case of accidental contact of the powder from the capsule with eye, skin or mucosa, the area should be immediately and thoroughly rinsed with water: medical attention should be sought.

Store in a dry place.

Legal category POM.

Package quantities 5 mg, 10 mg and 25 mg Capsules placed singly in bottles.

Further information Nil.

Product licence numbers

Zavedos 5 mg	3433/0158
Zavedos 10 mg	3433/0159
Zavedos 25 mg	3433/0160

**Trade Mark*

Pharmax Limited
(A Division of Forest Laboratories Europe)
Bourne Road
Bexley
Kent DA5 1NX
☎ 01322 550550   01322 558776

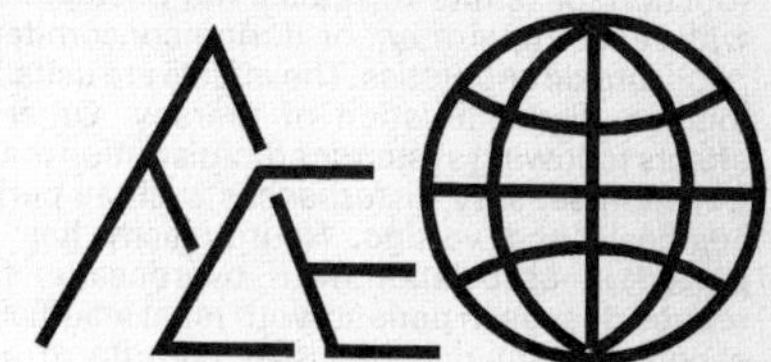

COLOMYCIN* INJECTION

Qualitative and quantitative composition Each vial contains either 1.0 or 0.5 mega units (MU) of Colistin Sulphomethate Sodium BP. 1 mg of colistin sulphomethate sodium is approximately 12,500 units.

Pharmaceutical form Sterile creamy-white crystalline powder for reconstitution.

Clinical particulars
Therapeutic indications: Colomycin Injection should only be used to treat severe systemic or localised infections caused by sensitive Gram-negative organisms, e.g. respiratory infection and septicaemia.

By aerosol inhalation, as adjunct therapy in patients already receiving standard antibiotic therapy. Parenterally or via other routes where routine antibiotic therapy has been unsuccessful.

Posology and method of administration: Colomycin Injection is administered by aerosol, intramuscularly or intravenously following reconstitution with sterile water or saline, but when indicated can be introduced via other routes such as subconjunctivally (used with 0.5% lidocaine) and by local instillation. Normal recommendations for systemic treatment are:

Children (up to 60 kg): 50,000 units/kg/body weight in 24 hours, divided into three eight-hourly doses. Serum levels should be measured if used in the newborn.

Adults (including elderly) (over 60 kg): 6,000,000 units in 24 hours (i.e. 2 x 1MU vials every eight hours)

Infusion therapy: Daily dosage as above. Infusion should preferably be completed within six hours.

Aerosol therapy: Daily dosage as above, concomitant with parenteral administration. For the aerosol, colistin is dissolved in water or saline for use in a suitable nebuliser attached to an air/oxygen supply.

Bladder irrigation: 1,000,000 units are dissolved in 50 ml water or saline and instilled during catheterisation. In the presence of infection administration is carried out twice daily.

The above are expressed as average doses. Should clinical or bacteriological response be slow, dosage may be increased as indicated by the patient's condition. Minimum of five days treatment is recommended.

Where there is moderate or severe renal impairment excretion of the antibiotic is delayed. Therefore, size of dose and dosage interval should be adjusted in relation to renal function. The table below is a guide to dosage modifications in order to prevent accumulation of Colomycin. It is stressed that adjustments may still have to be made on evaluation of the individual patient.

Blood level estimations are recommended : 10–15 micrograms/ml should be adequate.

Contra-indications: Colomycin Injection is contra-indicated in patients with known sensitivity to colistin.

Special warnings and precautions for use: None stated

Interaction with other medicaments and other forms of interaction: Curariform muscle relaxants should be used with extreme caution in patients receiving Colomycin Injection.

Pregnancy and lactation: Safety in human pregnancy has not been established. Animal studies do not indicate teratogenic properties; however, single dose studies in human pregnancy show that Colomycin crosses the placental barrier and there is a risk of foetal toxicity if repeated doses are given to pregnant patients.
Colomycin is secreted in breast milk and patients to whom the drug is administered should not breast-feed an infant.

Effects on ability to drive and use machines: None stated.

Undesirable effects: Adverse effects on renal function have been reported, usually following use of higher than recommended doses in patients with normal renal function, or failure to reduce the dosage in patients with renal impairment or during concomitant use of other nephrotoxic antibiotics. The effects are usually reversible on discontinuation of therapy. Other reversible adverse effects may include transient sensory disturbances such as facial paraesthesia and vertigo, and rarely, vasomotor instability, slurred speech, visual disturbances, confusion or psychosis. Neurotoxicity has been reported in association with overdosage, failure to reduce dosage in patients with renal insufficiency and concomitant use of either curariform agents or antibiotics with similar neurotoxic effects. Therapy need not be discontinued and reduction of dosage may alleviate symptoms.

Bronchospasm may occur on antibiotic inhalation; this may be treated with $beta_2$-agonists.

Permanent nerve damage such as deafness or vestibular damage has not been reported. Local irritation at the site of injection is minimal.

Overdose: Overdosage can result in renal insufficiency, muscle weakness and apnoea. There is no specific antidote. Management is by supportive treatment and measures to increase the rate of elimination of colistin e.g. mannitol diuresis, prolonged haemodialysis or peritoneal dialysis.

Pharmacological properties
Pharmacodynamic properties: Colistin is a polypeptide antibiotic derived from *Bacillus polymyxa var. colistinus*. It possesses a rapid bactericidal activity against a number of Gram-negative organisms including *Pseudomonas aeruginosa* and is largely free from the development or transference of resistance.

Pharmacokinetic properties: Colomycin Injection is a sterile powder for reconstitution using sterile water or saline prior to administration primarily via intravenous or intramuscular injection, or aerosol inhalation. Peak serum levels are usually attained within 2–3 hours following intramuscular injection and demonstrable amounts of Colomycin persist for at least 8 hours. Transpulmonary absorption has been reported following administration of Colomycin via aerosol inhalation and appears to be influenced by aerosol particle size. Clinical studies have, however, demonstrated the effectiveness of Colomycin in the lungs even in the absence of detectable serum levels of the antibiotic. Distribution of injected Colomycin occurs throughout the body fluids with excretion taking place via the kidneys thus producing high urine levels of Colomycin. Peak urine levels are obtained after 2–3 hours and up to 80% of the administered dose is recovered within approximately 8 hours.

Preclinical safety data: There are no preclinical data of relevance to the prescriber which are additional to those already included in other sections of the SPC.

Pharmaceutical particulars
List of excipients: None

Incompatibilities: None stated.

Shelf life: 36 months.

Special precautions for storage: Store below 25°C protected from light.

Nature and contents of container: Neutral glass vials in packs of 10.

Instructions for use/handling: Solutions of Colomycin Injection for parenteral administration should preferably be freshly prepared. Compatible infusion solutions are: normal saline, 5% dextrose, 5% fructose, Ringer's solution. Infusions should be completed within 6 hours. Mixed infusions or injections involving Colomycin should be avoided.

Marketing authorisation numbers
0.5 MU 0108/5005
1.0 MU 0108/5006

Date of approval/revision of SPC January 1996

Legal category POM

Creatinine clearance (ml/min)	*B.U.N. (mg/100 ml)*	*(mmol/l)*	*Adult Dosage*	*Childrens' Dosage*
20–72	> 6	>10	1–2 million units every 8 hr	12,500–16,000 units/kg every 8 hr
10–20	> 100	> 16.5	1 million units every 12–18 hr	12,500 units/kg every 12–18 hr
< 10	> 200	> 33	1 million units every 18–24 hr	8,000 units/kg every 18–24 hr

COLOMYCIN* STERILE POWDER

Qualitative and quantitative composition Vial containing 1 g Colistin Sulphate BP. 1 mg of colistin sulphate is approximately 19,500 units.

Pharmaceutical form A white to cream coloured powder.

Clinical particulars
Therapeutic indications: For the treatment of topical infections caused by sensitive Gram-negative organisms.

Posology and method of administration: *For adults, children and the elderly*: Colomycin Sterile Powder is applied topically as a 1% solution, dispersed powder or ointment according to the site of infection, as follows:

1% solution in water or saline for use as eye and ear drops, in wound irrigation, and for application to dressings.

1% dispersed powder in lactose or biosorb for application for infected leg ulcers and in other skin infections. Undiluted powder should not be applied topically.

1% ointment in Simple Cream BP, simple cream plus hydrous lanolin (90:10), Hydrous Ointment BP, Macrogel Ointment BPC, for use in skin infections.

Colomycin Sterile Powder must not be used for the preparation of injectable solutions.

Contra-indications: The preparation is contra-indicated in patients with known sensitivity to colistin. Colomycin Sterile Powder should not be used for the treatment of otitis externa if the tympanic membrane is perforated.

Special warnings and special precautions for use: Colistin absorption has not been detected following limited topical application. Absorption may, however, increase with prolonged use and absorption may be enhanced if colistin is applied to large areas of broken skin. Caution should be employed in the use of the preparation in patients with renal failure and in patients receiving curariform muscle relaxants.

Interaction with other medicaments and other forms of interaction: Neurotoxicity has been reported with concomitant use of either curariform agents or antibiotics with similar neurotoxic effects and systemic administration of colistin. Therapy need not be discontinued and reduction of dosage may alleviate symptoms.

Pregnancy and lactation: Safety in human pregnancy has not been established. Animal studies do not indicate teratogenic properties; however, parenteral single dose studies in human pregnancy show that colomycin crosses the placental barrier and there is a risk of foetal toxicity if repeated doses are given to pregnant patients. Colomycin is secreted in breast milk and patients to whom the drug is administered should not breast-feed an infant.

Effects on ability to drive and use machines: None stated.

Undesirable effects: Topical therapy is well tolerated. Transient irritation at the site of application has been reported infrequently. Allergic sensitisation has not been reported.

Systemic side effects have not been reported following topical administration. Following systemic therapy with colistin, adverse effects on renal function have been reported, usually following use of higher than recommended dose in patients with normal renal function, or failure to reduce the dosage in patients with renal impairment or during concomitant use of nephrotoxic antibiotics. The effects are usually reversible on discontinuation of therapy. Other adverse effects following systemic administration may include transient sensory disturbances such as perioral paraesthesia and vertigo. Neurotoxicity has been reported in association with overdosage, failure to reduce dosage in patients with renal insufficiency and a concomitant use of either curariform agents or antibiotics with similar neurotoxic effects. Therapy need not be discontinued and reduction of dosage may alleviate symptoms. Permanent nerve damage such as deafness or vestibular damage has not been reported.

Overdose: No symptoms of overdosage have been reported following topical use of colistin. However, use of the undiluted powder causes stinging and is not recommended. Following systemic administration overdosage can result in renal insufficiency, muscle weakness and apnoea. There is no specific antidote. Manage by supportive treatment and measures to increase the rate of elimination of colistin, e.g. mannitol diuresis, prolonged haemodialysis or peritoneal dialysis.

Pharmacological properties
Pharmacodynamic properties: Colistin is a polmyxin antibiotic derived from *Bacillus polymyxa var. colistinus.* It has a bactericidal action on most Gram-negative bacilli, including *Pseudomonas aeruginosa,* and use is largely free from the development or transference of resistance. It is not recommended for Proteus spp.

Pharmacokinetic properties: There is almost complete lack of absorption when colistin is applied to intact or denuded skin; it is poorly absorbed from mucus membranes and the surface of large burns.

Preclinical safety data: There are no preclinical data of relevance to the prescriber that might add to the safety data provided in other sections of this SPC.

Pharmaceutical particulars
List of excipients: None

Incompatibilities: None stated.

Shelf-life: Unopened product as packaged for sale: 60 months. Colomycin Sterile Powder solutions should be used within 24 hours of preparation and stored at 2°-8°C. Ointments or dispersed powders may be stored for up to 1 month at room temp. (25°C), as may preserved solutions.

Special precautions for storage: Unopened product should be stored below 25°C, protected from light.

Nature and contents of container: Neutral glass vial closed with an aluminium crimp ring. Each vial is individually packed in a cardboard carton.

Instructions for use/handling: Colomycin Sterile Powder should be formulated as a 1% solution, 1% dispersed powder or 1% ointment, according to the site of infection. Suitable formulations include: 1% solution prepared by dissolving 1 g of powder in 100 ml water or saline; 1% dispersed powder in lactose or Biosorb; a 1% ointment prepared by the addition of 1 g of powder to 100 ml of either Simple Cream BP, simple cream plus hydrous lanolin (90:10), Hydrous Ointment BP or Macrogel Ointment BPC. Colomycin Sterile Powder may be given orally as an alternative to Colomycin Tablets or Syrup by dissolving in a suitable vehicle.

Marketing authorisation number 0108/5010

Date of approval/revision of SPC November 1995

Legal category POM

COLOMYCIN* SYRUP COLOMYCIN* TABLETS

Qualitative and quantitative composition
Colomycin Syrup: Each bottle contains 4 MU of Colistin Sulphate BP, equivalent to 250,000 units/5 ml when dispensed.

Colomycin Tablets: Each tablet contains 1.5 MU Colistin Sulphate BP.

Pharmaceutical form White powder for reconstitution into syrup and a white bevelled edge tablet with 'P' in a hexagon on one face and two crossed score marks on the reverse.

Clinical particulars
Therapeutic indications: For the treatment of gastro-intestinal infections caused by sensitive Gram-negative organisms. Also for bowel preparation.

Colistin sulphate is not absorbed from the gastro-intestinal tract, except in infants under the age of 6 months, and must not be given orally for the treatment of systemic infection in any age group.

Posology and method of administration:
Adults over 30 kg (including the elderly): 1,500,000 to 3,000,000 units taken every 8 hours.

Children (15-30 kg): 750,000 to 1,500,000 units every 8 hours.

Children (up to 15 kg): 250,000 to 500,000 units every 8 hours.

A minimum of 5 days treatment is recommended. Dosage may be increased when clinical or bacteriological response is slow. For bowel preparation, a 24 hour course at the normal dosage above is given. Treatment should preferably finish 12 hours before surgery.

Contra-indications: Patients with known sensitivity to colistin.

Special warnings and special precautions for use: Colistin is subject to limited and unpredictable absorption from the G.I. tract in infants under 6 months. Studies in older children and adults have demonstrated no systemic absorption of colistin following oral administration. Nevertheless, caution should be employed in the use of these preparations in patients with renal failure and in patients receiving curariform muscle relaxants

Interaction with other medicaments and other forms of interaction: Neurotoxicity has been reported in association with the concomitant use of either curariform agents or antibiotics with similar neurotoxic effects. Therapy need not be discontinued and reduction of dosage may alleviate symptoms.

Pregnancy and lactation: Safety in human pregnancy has not been established. Animal studies do not indicate teratogenic properties however, parenteral single dose studies in human pregnancy show that Colomycin crosses the placental barrier and there is a risk of foetal toxicity if repeated doses are given to pregnant patients.

Colomycin is secreted in breast milk and patients to whom the drug is administered should not breast-feed an infant.

Effects on ability to drive and use machines: None stated.

Undesirable effects: No significant systemic absorption has been found to occur in older children and adults following oral administration nor have any systemic side effects been reported.

However, since the use of colistin may be associated with unpredictable, albeit limited, absorption in infants under 6 months, the potential adverse effects of systemic administration should be noted for this patient population. These adverse effects may include transient sensory disturbances such as perioral paraesthesia and vertigo.

Neurotoxicity and adverse effects on renal function have been reported in association with systemic overdosage, failure to reduce dosage in patients with renal insufficiency and the concomitant use of either curariform agents or antibiotics with similar neurotoxic effects.

Therapy need not be discontinued and reduction of dosage may alleviate symptoms. Permanent nerve damage such as deafness or vestibular damage has not been reported.

Overdose: No symptoms of overdosage have been reported following oral use of colistin. However, following systemic administration overdosage can result in renal insufficiency, muscle weakness and apnoea and this should be borne in mind in the oral therapy of infants under 6 months old.

There is no specific antidote. Manage by supportive treatment and measures to increase the rate of elimination of colistin, e.g. mannitol diuresis, prolonged haemodialysis or peritoneal dialysis.

Pharmacological properties
Pharmacodynamic properties: Colistin is a polymyxin antibiotic derived from *Bacillus polymyxa var. colistinus.* It has a bactericidal action on most Gram-negative bacilli, including *Pseudomonas aeruginosa,* and use is largely free from the development or transference of resistance. It is not recommended for Proteus spp.

Pharmacokinetic properties: In adults and older children, colistin sulphate taken orally is not absorbed from the G.I. tract. However, in small infants less than 6 months old, some very limited and unpredictable absorption may occur.

Preclinical safety data: There are no preclinical data of relevance to the prescriber that might add to the safety data provided in other sections of this SPC.

Pharmaceutical particulars
List of excipients: Syrup: Sucrose PhEur, Sodium Citrate PhEur, Cherry flavour, Benzoic Acid BP, Sodium Methyl Hydroxybenzoate BP.

Tablets: Microcrystalline Cellulose BPC, Maize Starch PhEur, Colloidal Silicon Dioxide NF, Cutina HR.

Incompatibilities: None stated.

Shelf life: Syrup: 36 months. Tablets: 60 months

Special precautions *for storage:* Store below 25°C in a dry place, protected from light.

Nature and contents of container: Syrup: Amber glass bottle for preparation of 80 ml of syrup. *Tablets:* Plastic containers of 50 tablets.

Instructions for use/handling: Colomycin Syrup Powder is reconstituted by adding 58 ml of water, and shaking the bottle until the powder is dissolved.

Marketing authorisation numbers
Colomycin Syrup 0108/5009
Colomycin Tablets 0108/5008

Date of approval/revision of SPC
Colomycin Syrup: November 1995
Colomycin Tablets: July 1996

Legal category POM

FLETCHERS' ARACHIS OIL RETENTION ENEMA*

Presentation Ready-to-use, self-contained, single-dose, disposable enema containing Arachis Oil BP 130 ml.

Uses To soften impacted faeces.

Dosage and administration For rectal administration only.
Adults and elderly patients: 1 enema as required.

Children: Reduce adult dose in proportion to body-weight.

Children under 3 years: Not recommended.

The enema should be warmed before use by placing in warm water.

Contra-indications, warnings, etc
Contra-indications: Hypersensitivity to arachis oil or peanuts. Inflammatory bowel disease except under the instruction of a medical practitioner.

Precautions and warnings: Not for use in children unless under medical supervision. Use with caution in patients with intestinal obstruction.

Care should be taken not to use undue force in administration of the enema especially in elderly or debilitated patients or those with neurological disorders.

Use in pregnancy and lactation: The use of enemas is not recommended during pregnancy except under medical advice.

Side-effects: Like other rectally applied substances arachis oil may produce local irritation.

Pharmaceutical precautions Store at room temperature.

Legal category P

Package quantities Box of 10 enemas.

Further information Contains peanut oil.

Product licence number 0108/5016

FLETCHERS' ENEMETTE*

Presentation Ready-to-use, self-contained, single-dose, disposable microenema of 5 ml liquid containing: Docusate Sodium BP 90 mg, Glycerol PhEur 3780 mg.

This product also contains sorbic acid and polyethylene glycol.

Uses Routine treatment of constipation. Pre- and post-operative cleansing of the bowel, in obstetrics and prior to proctoscopy, sigmoidoscopy or X-ray examination.

Dosage and administration For rectal administration only.
Adults, elderly and children over 3 years: 1 enema as required.

Children under 3 years: Not recommended.

Contra-indications, warnings, etc
Contra-indications: Nil

Precautions: Use with caution in patients with intestinal obstruction.

Care should be taken not to use undue force in administration of the enema especially in elderly or debilitated patients or those with neurological disorders.

Pharmaceutical precautions Store below 25°C. Protect from heat.

Legal category P

Package quantities Box of 12 microenemas.

Further information The formulation of docusate sodium, a faecal softening agent, in glycerol (which when administered rectally promotes peristalsis and evacuation of the lower bowel) and polyethylene glycol, provides an easy-to-use, efficacious, low-volume enema.

Product licence number 0108/0078

FLETCHERS' PHOSPHATE ENEMA*

Qualitative and quantitative composition Each 128 ml enema contains: Sodium Acid Phosphate BP 10.0% w/v and Sodium Phosphate PhEur 8.0% w/v. The formulation is equivalent to Phosphates Enema BP Formula B.

Pharmaceutical form Single dose enema

Clinical particulars
Therapeutic indications: Routine treatment of constipation. Pre- and post-operative cleansing of the bowel, in obstetrics and prior to proctoscopy, sigmoidoscopy or X-ray examination.

Posology and method of administration:
Adults including the elderly: One enema as required.

Children over 3 years of age: Reduce adult dosage in proportion to body weight.

Children under 3 years of age: Not recommended.

For rectal administration only. The enema may be administered at room temperature or warmed in water before use.

Contra-indications: Use in patients with inflammatory or ulcerative conditions of the bowel, in those with increased colonic absorptive capacity e.g. Hirschsprung's disease and in those with acute gastrointestinal conditions.

Special warnings and precautions for use: Prolonged use may lead to irritation of the anal canal. Use with caution in patients requiring a reduced sodium intake and electrolyte balance should be maintained during extended use. Use with caution in patients with intestinal obstruction. Care should be taken not to use undue force in administration of the enema, especially in elderly or debilitated patients or those with neurological disorders.

Interaction with other medicaments and other forms of interaction: None known.

Pregnancy and lactation: No special warnings.

Effects on ability to drive and use machines: Not applicable.

Undesirable effects: There have been occasional reports of apparent vasovagal attacks occurring in elderly patients following administration of phosphate enemata.

Overdose: There have been no reports of overdose. In the event of overdosage electrolyte levels should be monitored and balance restored where appropriate.

Pharmacological properties
Pharmacodynamic properties: Fletchers' Phosphate Enema is a solution of sodium acid phosphate and sodium phosphate. The formulation is equivalent to Phosphates Enema BP Formula B. Following rectal administration the active ingredients exert their laxative effect via their osmotic properties. The resulting fluid retention in the bowel encourages evacuation.

Pharmacokinetic properties: Saline laxatives are poorly and slowly absorbed following rectal administration. Under normal usage only minimal absorption is likely to occur.

Pharmaceutical particulars
List of excipients: Benzalkonium Chloride BP, Disodium Edetate BP, Purified Water PhEur.

Shelf life: Bag presentation: 12 months. Bottle presentation: 36 months

Special precautions for storage: Store below 25°C.

Nature and contents of container:
(a) Translucent LDPE bottle with rubber non-return valve, plastic nozzle and nozzle plug containing 128 ml solution packed singly in a cardboard carton.
(b) Translucent PVC bag containing 128 ml solution with a plastic extension tube with nozzle and plug (long-tube enema) in packs of 50.

Marketing authorisation number 0108/5015R

Date of approval/revision of SPC May 1995

Legal category P

INFACOL*

Qualitative and quantitative composition Simethicone USP 40 mg/ml.

Pharmaceutical form An orange-flavoured, colourless, translucent suspension for oral administration.

Clinical particulars
Therapeutic indications: An antiflatulent for the relief of griping pain, colic or wind due to swallowed air.

Posology and method of administration: Infants: 20 mg (0.5 ml) administered before each feed. If necessary this may be increased to 40 mg (1 ml). Treatment with Infacol may provide a progressive improvement in symptoms over several days.

Adults and the elderly: Not applicable.

Contra-indications: None stated.

Special warnings and precautions for use: If symptoms persist, seek medical advice.

Interactions with other medicaments and other forms of interaction: None stated.

Pregnancy and lactation: Not applicable.

Effects on ability to drive and use machines: Not applicable.

Undesirable effects: None stated.

Overdose: In the event of deliberate or accidental overdosage, treat symptoms on appearance.

Pharmacological properties
Pharmacodynamic properties: Physiologically the active ingredient is a chemically inert, non-systemic, gastric defoaming agent that works by altering the elasticity of interfaces of mucus-embedded bubbles in the gastro-intestinal tract.

The gas bubbles are thus broken down or coalesced and in this form gas is more easily eliminated through eructation or passing flatus.

Pharmacokinetic properties: Simethicone is not absorbed from the gastro-intestinal tract.

Preclinical safety data: There are no pre clinical data of relevance to the prescriber which are additional to that already included in other sections of the SPC.

Pharmaceutical particulars
List of excipients: Saccharin Sodium BP, Hydroxypropyl Methylcellulose USP, Orange flavour, Methyl Paraben PhEur, Propyl Paraben PhEur, Purified Water PhEur.

Incompatibilities: None stated.

Shelf life: 24 months.

Special precautions for storage: Store at room temperature (below 25°C).

Nature and contents of container: High density polyethylene bottle containing 50 ml of liquid fitted with a low density polyethylene dropper and evoprene teat.

Instruction for use/handling: None.

Marketing authorisation number 0108/0100

Date of approval/revision of SPC July 1996

Legal category GSL

LASMA*

Qualitative and quantitative composition Each tablet contains 300 mg Theophylline PhEur.

Pharmaceutical form Sustained release tablets for oral administration.

Clinical particulars
Therapeutic indications: Treatment and prophylaxis of bronchospasm associated with asthma, (including nocturnal asthma) and bronchitis.

Posology and method of administration: Tablets should be swallowed and not sucked or chewed.

Adults (including the elderly): Therapy should commence with 2 tablets (600 mg). In patients of 70 kg body weight or over the dosage should be increased after 1 week to 3 tablets (900 mg) daily.

The daily dosage is administered as 1 or 1½ tablets every 12 hours, preferably after food. The dosage may be increased, as necessary, by half-tablet increments.

Children: Not recommended.

Nocturnal asthma: In patients where nocturnal symptoms predominate therapeutic benefit of up to 12 hours duration may be achieved by administration of Lasma Tablets as a single dose in the late evening. This will prevent the characteristic 'early-morning dip' in peak expiratory flow rate, thus allowing patients an uninterrupted night's sleep. Any day-time symptoms may then be controlled by inhaled bronchodilators.

Contra-indications: There are no absolute contraindications to theophylline, however caution should be exercised in the treatment of patients with cardiac arrhythmias, peptic ulcers or severe hypertension. Cardiac failure or hepatic dysfunction decreases theophylline clearance and patients with such conditions should be carefully monitored.

Special warnings and precautions for use: It is recommended, as with all xanthine preparations, that patients are individually titrated to their correct daily dosage by blood level estimations. Once a patient is stabilised on an effective dosage regime of Lasma Tablets this should not be changed, nor should an alternative product be substituted without re-titration of the dosage by clinical assessment and blood-level estimations.

Theophylline is not recommended for patients with a history of seizure activity as seizures have been reported in children whose theophylline levels are within the therapeutic range.

Interaction with other medicaments and other forms of interaction: Lasma should not be used concurrently with other preparations containing xanthine derivatives. Theophylline has been reported to interact with a number of drugs.

The following increase clearance and it may therefore be necessary to increase dosage to ensure a therapeutic effect: phenytoin, carbamazepine, rifampicin, sulphinpyrazone and barbiturates. Smoking and alcohol consumption can also increase clearance of theophylline. The following reduce clearance and a reduced dosage may therefore be necessary to avoid side-effects: the calcium-channel blockers verapamil and diltiazem, allopurinol, cimetidine, erythromycin, thiabendazole, ciprofloxacin, isoprenaline and oral contraceptives. Factors such as viral infections, liver disease and heart failure also reduce theophylline clearance. There are conflicting reports concerning the potentiation of theophylline by influenza vaccine and physicians should be aware that interaction may occur. A reduction of dosage may also be necessary in the elderly patient.

The concomitant use of theophylline and fluvoxamine should usually be avoided. Where this is not possible, patients should have their theophylline dose halved and plasma theophylline should be monitored closely.

The following should also be used with caution in patients taking theophylline preparations: halothane, lomustine and lithium.

Xanthines can potentiate hypokalaemia resulting from $beta_2$ agonist therapy, steroids, diuretics and hypoxia. Particular caution is advised in severe asthma. It is recommended that serum potassium levels are monitored in such situations.

Pregnancy and lactation: Safety in human pregnancy has not been established. Theophylline crosses the placental barrier and is secreted in breast milk. Theophylline should be used with caution in pregnancy and lactation.

Effects on ability to drive and use machines: None known.

Undesirable effects: Reported side-effects include gastro-intestinal disturbances, headache, CNS stimulation and tremor. Side-effects (particularly tremor) are rare at plasma concentrations of less than 20 mg/litre.

Overdose: Symptoms may include nausea, vomiting, gastro-intestinal irritation, cramps, convulsions, tachycardia and hypotension.

The stomach contents should be emptied and supportive measures employed to maintain circulation, respiration and fluid and electrolyte balance. Electrocardiographic monitoring should be carried out and in severe poisoning charcoal haemoperfusion should be used.

Pharmacological properties
Pharmacodynamic properties: Theophylline is a xanthine bronchodilator effecting dilatation of bronchial smooth muscle through as yet unknown mechanisms. Efficacy has been established at blood levels of 3–5 mg/litre with a log-blood level response relationship. The benefit of efficacy at higher levels is curtailed by side-effects which occur above 15 mg/litre and become increasingly serious as blood levels are increased especially above 20 mg/litre.

Pharmacokinetic properties: The reported elimination half-life for theophylline is 3½ hrs in children and 6–9 hrs in adults. The apparent volume of distribution is 400–500 ml/kg and plasma protein binding is approx. 50%. Lasma is a sustained release tablet and in a multiple dose kinetic study one tablet given 12 hourly produced a Cmin of 4.54 mg/litre and a Cmax of 8.41 mg/litre, the Tmax was 4.06 hrs. The relative bioavailability of the tablet is 88% of an oral liquid. When given as a 900 mg single daily dose the peak to trough difference was 9 mg/litre and the Cmax 14.9 mg/litre.

Preclinical safety data: Theophylline has been in use for many years and there are no preclinical safety data that are of additional value to the prescriber.

Pharmaceutical particulars
List of excipients: Hydroxypropyl Methylcellulose USP, Stearic Acid NF, Magnesium Stearate NF, Colloidal Silicon Dioxide NF.

Incompatibilities: None known.

Shelf life: 36 months.

Special precautions for storage: None.

Nature and contents of container: Amber glass bottle containing 60 tablets.

Instructions for use/handling: Not applicable.

Marketing authorisation number 0108/0075

Date of approval/revision of SPC February 1997

Legal category P

MUCOGEL* SUSPENSION

Presentation A white mint flavoured suspension. Each 5 ml contains: Aluminium Hydroxide equivalent to Dried Gel BP 220 mg and Magnesium Hydroxide BP 195 mg. This product also contains methyl and propyl parabens.

Uses Antacid therapy in gastric and duodenal ulcer, gastritis, heartburn, gastric hyperacidity. Treatment of indigestion.

Relief of symptoms of heartburn and dyspepsia associated with gastric reflux in hiatus hernia, reflux oesophagitis and similar conditions.

Dosage and administration
Adults, elderly and children over 12 years old: 10–20 ml three times daily 20 minutes to one hour after meals and at bedtime, or as required.

Children under 12 years: Not recommended.

Contra-indications, warnings, etc
Contra-indications: Mucogel should not be used in patients who are severely debilitated or suffering from kidney failure. Antacids inhibit the absorption of tetracyclines and vitamins and should not be taken concomitantly.

Adverse effects: Gastrointestinal side-effects are uncommon. This formulation minimises the problems of diarrhoea and constipation.

Use in pregnancy and lactation: Unnecessary drug therapy should be avoided in the first trimester of pregnancy.

Overdosage: Serious symptoms are unlikely to follow overdosage.

Pharmaceutical precautions Store below 25°C. Do not freeze. Use within 28 days of opening.

Legal category GSL

Package quantities Bottles of 500 ml

Further information Mucogel is a pleasant-tasting, well tolerated antacid containing balanced quantities of aluminium and magnesium.

Product licence number 0108/0074

PREDENEMA*

Qualitative and quantitative composition Each 100 ml enema contains 35 mg prednisolone metasulphobenzoate sodium equivalent to prednisolone 20 mg.

Pharmaceutical form Single dose enema.

Clinical particulars
Therapeutic indications: Local treatment of ulcerative colitis.

Posology and method of administration:
Adults (including the elderly): One enema nightly for 2-4 weeks, the course may be extended when a good response is obtained.
Children: Not recommended.
Predenema is to be used for rectal administration only.

Contra-indications: In local conditions where the use of Predenema might mask infection or impair healing, such as peritonitis, sinus infection, fistulae, intestinal obstruction, perforation of the bowel.

Special warnings and special precautions for use: Symptoms of adrenal insufficiency have not been reported, but prolonged therapy should be carefully monitored. Use with caution in patients with intestinal obstruction.

Interaction with other medicaments and other forms of interaction: None stated.

Pregnancy and lactation: Topical administration of corticosteroids to pregnant animals can cause abnormalities of foetal development. The relevance of this finding to human beings has not been established. However, physicians should be aware of the possibility of teratogenic effects, and also of potential suppression of the HPA axis, and should weigh up the risk/benefit ratio before using Predenema in pregnancy.

If treatment is instituted with Predenema, the minimum dosage and frequency of administration required for clinical control should be employed and prolonged usage should be avoided.

Effects on ability to drive and use machines: None stated.

Undesirable effects: Administration of prednisolone via this route, for this indication is seldom associated with adverse effects.

Overdosage: Overdose is not likely with this route of administration.

Pharmacological properties
Pharmacodynamic properties: Prednisolone 21-sodium metasulphobenzoate has the general properties of prednisolone as a potent anti-inflammatory agent with immuno-suppressant glucocorticoid properties. Esterification of prednisolone at the 21 position increases the topical activity of the drug.

Pharmacokinetic properties: Following rectal administration of prednisolone 21-sodium metasulphobenzoate in the form of an enema, the action of the drug is predominantly local. The peak plasma levels obtained following this treatment are significantly lower than those obtained following treatment with prednisolone 21-phosphate.

Following absorption, the drug is hydrolysed to *m*-sulphobenzoic acid (and salts) and free prednisolone.

At the low plasma levels obtained, following rectal administration of prednisolone 21-sodium metasulphobenzoate the precautions generally applied to the use of prednisolone are considered to be unnecessary.

Preclinical safety data: There are no pre-clinical data of relevance to the prescriber which are additional to those already included in other sections of the SPC.

Pharmaceutical particulars
List of excipients: Disodium Edetate PhEur, Nipastat and Purified Water PhEur.

Incompatibilities: None stated.

Shelf life: 12 months

Special precautions for storage: Store below 25°C, protected from light.

Nature and contents of container: Predenema is presented as a ready to use, single dose, disposable plastic enema bag containing 100 ml of solution. It is available with a standard tube in packs of 10 or with an extension tube (long tube) in packs of 7.

Instructions for use/handling: Predenema may be administered at room temperature or warmed in warm water before use. Hold the bag with tube upwards and squeeze base of tube where it joins the bag. Remove cap and lubricate tube before inserting into rectum. The patient should lie in bed with knees drawn up. Squeeze bag gently until fluid is expelled and discard container hygienically. The patient should lie face down for a few minutes to retain the fluid before going to sleep in the usual position. The long tube presentation facilitates self-administration.

Marketing authorisation number 0108/5018R

Date of approval/revision of SPC September 1995.

Legal category POM

PREDFOAM*

Presentation A white, mucoadherent aerosol foam containing prednisolone metasulphobenzoate sodium equivalent to 20 mg prednisolone per metered dose.

This product also contains disodium edetate, phenoxyethanol and sorbic acid.

Uses Treatment of proctitis and distal ulcerative colitis.

Dosage and administration
Adults and elderly patients: One metered dose inserted rectally once or twice daily for two weeks, extending treatment for a further two weeks when a good response is obtained. Use should be discontinued at the discretion of the physician once the disease is stable and under control.

Children: Not recommended.

Contra-indications, warnings, etc
Contra-indications: Local conditions where infection might be masked or healing impaired e.g. peritonitis, fistulae, intestinal obstruction, perforation of the bowel.

Precautions: This product should be used with extreme caution in the presence of severe ulcerative colitis. The possible occurrence of masking of local or systemic infection should be borne in mind when using this product. For rectal use only.

Side-effects: The consequences of systemic absorption should be considered with extensive use over prolonged periods. As with all rectal corticosteroids, prolonged continuous use is undesirable.

Use in pregnancy and lactation: There is inadequate evidence of safety in human pregnancy. Topical administration of corticosteroids to pregnant animals can cause abnormalities of foetal development including cleft palate and intra-uterine growth retardation. There may therefore be a very small risk of such effects in the human foetus.

Overdosage: Overdosage by this route is unlikely.

Pharmaceutical precautions Pressurised container containing a flammable propellant. Store below 25°C. Protect from sunlight and do not expose to temperatures above 50°C. Do not pierce or burn even after use. Do not spray on naked flame or any incandescent material. Shake before use.

Legal category POM

Package quantities Carton containing an aerosol canister containing sufficient for 14 applications plus 14 disposable applicators.

Further information Nil

Product licence number 0108/0101

SAVENTRINE i.v.*

Qualitative and quantitative composition Ampoule containing 2 ml of a 1 mg/ml solution of Isoprenaline Hydrochloride BP.

Pharmaceutical form Glass ampoules containing a sterile stabilised solution of Isoprenaline Hydrochloride BP for injection.

Clinical particulars
Therapeutic indications:
1. Cardiogenic or endotoxic shock.
2. Acute Stokes-Adams attacks and other cardiac emergencies.
3. Severe bradycardia precipitated by beta-adrenergic antagonists and disopyramide.
4. Evaluation of congenital heart defects.

Posology and method of administration: The usual route is by intravenous infusion in 5% dextrose solution or Water for Injections. Widely varying doses have been used with success.

Adults and elderly patients:
1. Shock states: 0.5–10 micrograms/min or alternatively injection of 0.1 mg in 10 ml water.
2. Acute Stokes-Adams attack: 4–8 micrograms/min or alternatively intracardiac injection of 0.1 mg in 10 ml water.
3. Severe bradycardia: 1–4 micrograms/min.
4. Evaluation of congenital cardiac defects: 1.5–4 micrograms/min.

Children: Adjust above dosage in proportion to body weight.

Contra-indications: Saventrine i.v. is contraindicated in acute coronary disease and in patients prone to episodes of ventricular fibrillation or tachycardia secondary to their slow rate.

Isoprenaline may precipitate ventricular extrasystoles and arrhythmias especially in patients who may be hypersensitive to the drug. In such cases the infusion rate should be reduced or possibly discontinued.

Special warnings and precautions for use: Use with caution in patients with hyperthyroidism, diabetes, left ventricular failure, ischaemic heart disease, angina, cardiac arrhythmia or hypertension. This product is not suitable for oral administration.

Interaction with other medicaments and other forms of interaction: Do not use in patients who are receiving monoamine oxidase inhibitors or within 14 days of stopping such treatment.

Isoprenaline may induce arrhythmias when administered with halothane, cyclopropane and trichlorethylene. Use with caution if isoprenaline is given concomitantly with digoxin, digitoxin, guanethidine, methyldopa or tricyclic antidepressants.

Pregnancy and lactation: Safety during pregnancy and lactation has not been established. The risk to benefit ratio should be assessed in individual circumstances.

Effects on ability to drive and use machines: None stated.

Undesirable effects: These may include palpitations, tremor, precordial pain, sweats, facial flushing and headache.

Overdose: Symptoms of overdosage are listed in the 'Undesirable effects' section above. Fatality may also occur in cases of serious overdosage. A beta-adrenergic blocking drug may diminish toxic effects and should be accompanied by monitoring of heart rhythm.

Pharmacological properties
Pharmacodynamic properties: Isoprenaline hydrochloride is a beta-adrenergic agonist, which has a powerful stimulant action on the heart, increasing cardiac output and cardiac rate.

It also produces peripheral vasodilation, a reduction in diastolic blood pressure and maintains or slightly increases systolic blood pressure.

Pharmacokinetic properties: Saventrine i.v. administered by intravenous injection allows isoprenaline to become immediately available within the bloodstream, and has a plasma half-life of one to several minutes dependent on injection rate.

Isoprenaline is excreted mainly in the urine as unchanged isoprenaline and metabolites.

Preclinical safety data: There are no preclinical data of relevance to the prescriber which are additional to those already included in other sections of the SPC.

Pharmaceutical particulars

List of excipients: Ascorbic Acid PhEur, Disodium Edetate BP, Hydrochloric Acid, Water for Injections PhEur.

Incompatibilities: None stated.

Shelf life: 2 years from the date of manufacture.

Special precautions for storage: Store below 25°C, protected from light.

Nature and contents of container: 2 ml glass ampoules, packed into cartons of 10.

Instructions for use/handling: None stated.

Marketing authorisation number 0108/5030R

Date of approval/revision of SPC June 1996

Legal category POM

SUSCARD* BUCCAL TABLETS

Qualitative and quantitative composition Tablets containing 1 mg, 2 mg, 3 mg or 5 mg of glyceryl trinitrate as Diluted Nitroglycerin USP.

Pharmaceutical form Circular biconvex off-white controlled release tablets for buccal administration.

Clinical particulars

Therapeutic indications: Management and treatment of angina pectoris. This product may also be of benefit in the in-patient management of unstable angina.

Acute and congestive cardiac failure.

Posology and method of administration: For buccal administration.

Dosage:

Adults and elderly patients:

Angina: Administration of Suscard Tablets should start with the 2 mg strength. If angina occurs while the tablet is in place, the dosage strength used should be increased to 3 mg where necessary. The 5 mg strength should be reserved for patients with severe angina pectoris refractory to treatment with the lower dosage strengths.

A 1 mg dosage strength is also available and may be considered for the small number of patients who may initially show intolerance to the 2 mg strength as a starting dose.

Suggested dosage frequency in angina:

For patients suffering only occasional angina pectoris – the tablets may be administered on a p.r.n. basis to relieve the acute attack.

For patients suffering angina pectoris in response to known stimuli – the tablet may be administered a few minutes prior to encountering the angina precipitating stimulus.

For patients in whom chronic therapy is indicated, the tablet should be administered on a thrice daily basis or as dictated by the dissolution rate of the tablet in an individual patient. If angina occurs during the period between the disappearance of one tablet and the time the next tablet is due to be put in place, dosage frequency should be increased.

Note that if an acute attack of angina pectoris is suffered while a tablet is in place, an additional tablet may be positioned on the opposite side of the mouth.

Unstable angina: Dosage should be rapidly titrated upwards in order to relieve and prevent symptoms. Suscard Tablets may be used in addition to pre-existing anti-anginal therapy, where considered appropriate.

As indicated in the above section the higher 5 mg dosage strength may be required to achieve a satisfactory therapeutic response in patients exhibiting severe symptoms. Unstable angina is a serious condition managed under hospitalised conditions and involving continuous monitoring of ECG changes with frequent monitoring of appropriate haemodynamic variables. In common with other nitrate therapy a fall in systolic blood pressure of 10-15 mm Hg may occur.

Acute heart failure: Administer 5 mg, repeated as indicated by the patient response, until the symptoms abate.

Congestive cardiac failure: Dosage should commence with the 5 mg strength, administered three times daily. In moderately severe or severe cases, particularly where patients have not responded to standard therapy (digitalis/diuretics), the dosage may need to be increased to 10 mg (2 x 5 mg tablets) t.i.d. over a period of three or four days. In such instances one tablet should be placed between the upper lip and the gum, on each side of the front teeth.

Method of administration: Suscard is for buccal administration. The Suscard tablet is placed high up between the upper lip and gum to either side of the front teeth. (see diagrams).

The onset of action of Suscard is extremely rapid and the tablets may be substituted for sublingual glyceryl trinitrate tablets in the treatment of acute angina pectoris. The duration of action of the Suscard Tablet, once in place correlates with the dissolution time of the tablet. This is normally 3-5 hours. However, the first few doses may dissolve more rapidly until the patient is used to the presence of the tablet.

During the dissolution period the tablet will soften and adhere to the gum; in practice the presence of the tablet is not noticeable to the patient after a short time.

Patients should be instructed as to the correct placement of the tablet and should note the following points

A) The tablet should not be moved about the mouth with the tongue, as this will cause it to dissolve more rapidly.

B) A slight stinging sensation (as for sublingual glyceryl trinitrate) may be felt for a few minutes after placement of the tablet.

C) If a tablet is accidentally swallowed it may be replaced by a further tablet.

D) In patients who wear dentures, the tablet may be placed in any comfortable position between the lip and the gum.

E) The patient may alternate the placement of successive tablets on the right and left sides of the front teeth.

The tablets should not be placed under the tongue, chewed or intentionally swallowed.

Contra-indications: As for glyceryl trinitrate. Suscard Tablets should not be used in patients with marked anaemia, head trauma, cerebral haemorrhage or closed angle glaucoma.

Special warnings and precautions for use: Rarely prolonged use in susceptible individuals with poor dental hygiene and associated plaque may lead to an increased risk of dental caries. Patients should therefore be instructed to alternate the site of application and careful attention should be paid to dental hygiene, particularly in those areas where the tablet is applied. In conditions where xerostomia (dry mouth) may occur, e.g. during concomitant medication with drugs having anticholinergic effects, patients should be instructed to moisten the buccal mucosa with the tongue, or with a little water, prior to insertion of Suscard.

Interactions with other medicaments and other forms of interaction: None known.

Pregnancy and lactation: There is no information on the safety of nitrates in pregnancy and lactation. Nitrates should not be administered to pregnant women and nursing mothers unless considered essential by the physician.

Effects on ability to drive and use machines: None known.

Undesirable effects: Side effects are predominantly headache, dizziness, facial flushing and postural hypotension. In the unlikely event of severe side effects, the tablet may simply be removed from the mouth.

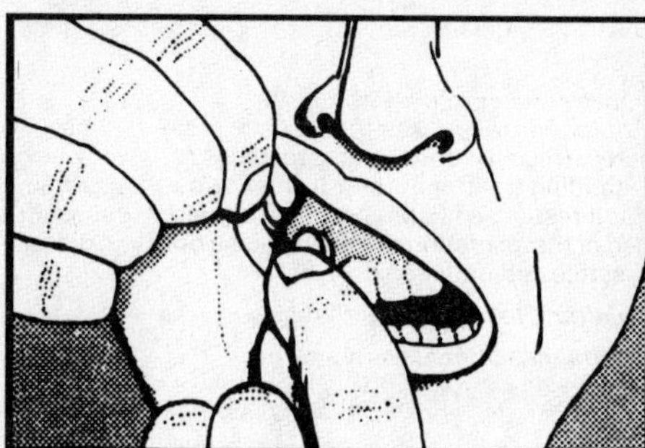

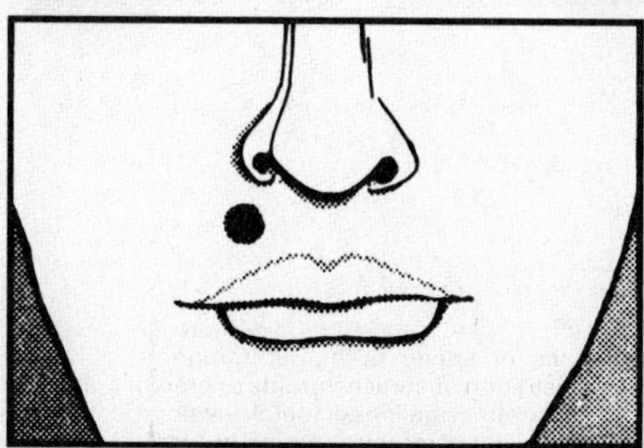

Overdose: Toxic effects of glyceryl trinitrate include vomiting, restlessness, cyanosis, methaemoglobinaemia and syncope. Overdosage (i.e. if large numbers of tablets have been swallowed) should be treated with gastric aspiration and lavage plus attention to the respiratory and circulatory systems.

Pharmacological properties

Pharmacodynamic properties: The principal action of glyceryl trinitrate is relaxation of vascular smooth muscle producing a vasodilator effect on both peripheral arteries and veins. Dilation of the post-capillary vessels, including large veins, promotes peripheral pooling of blood pressure and decreases venous return to the heart, thereby reducing left ventricular end-diastolic pressure (preload). Arteriolar relaxation reduces systemic vascular resistance and arterial pressure (afterload). Myocardial oxygen consumption or demand for a given level of exercise is decreased by both the arterial and venous effects of nitroglycerin. Dilatation of the large epicardial coronary arteries by nitroglycerin contributes to the relief of exertional angina.

Pharmacokinetic properties: Bioavailability relative to sublingual GTN: 107%.

Mean plasma levels of 0.7ng/ml obtained with 5 mg Buccal Tablet over 5 hours compared with 0.4ng/ml over 30 minutes with 0.4 mg sublingual GTN.

Maximum plasma concentration: 1.7ng/ml following 5 mg Buccal compared with 0.9ng/ml following 0.4 mg sublingual GTN.

Time to maximum plasma concentration: 1.52 hours following Buccal GTN compared with 6 minutes following sublingual GTN.

Apparent elimination half-life: 1.30 hours for Buccal GTN compared with an elimination half-life of 5 minutes following sublingual GTN.

Pharmacodynamic studies have shown a dose-related response with a rapid onset equivalent to sublingual GTN, together with a prolonged duration of activity of 4-5 hours.

Preclinical safety data: There are no pre clinical data of relevance to the prescriber which are additional to that already included in other sections of the SPC.

Pharmaceutical particulars

List of excipients: Lactose hydrous, hydroxypropyl methylcellulose, purified water, peppermint flavour, spearmint flavour, stearic acid, silica gel.

Incompatibilities: None stated.

Shelf life: 36 months.

Special precautions for storage: None.

Nature and contents of container: Aluminium foil blister strips in packs of 100 tablets.

Instruction for use/handling: None stated.

Marketing authorisation number
1 mg tablet: 0108/0067
2 mg tablet: 0108/0069
3 mg tablet: 0108/0073
5 mg tablet: 0108/0071

Date of approval/revision of SPC Suscard 1 mg, 2 mg and 5 mg tablets: June 1997
Suscard 3 mg tablets: November 1997

Legal category P

SUSTAC*

Qualitative and quantitative composition Tablets containing glyceryl trinitrate 2.6 mg, 6.4 mg and 10 mg (as Diluted Nitroglycerin USP)

Pharmaceutical form Slow release tablets for oral administration

Clinical particulars

Therapeutic indications: The prophylaxis of angina pectoris

Posology and method of administration: Oral. Sustac tablets must be swallowed whole and not chewed. They are not for sublingual administration. Tablets should be taken between meals.

Adults and elderly patients: Dosage should be tailored to the requirements of the individual patient but will usually be 1 or 2 tablets of the 2.6 mg or 6.4 mg strength taken three times daily or 1 tablet of the 10 mg strength taken two or three times daily.

Children: Not recommended.

Contra-indications: As for glyceryl trinitrate. Sustac should not be used in patients with marked anaemia, head trauma, cerebral haemorrhage or close angle glaucoma.

Special warnings and precautions for use: As with other drugs for the treatment of angina pectoris, abrupt discontinuation of therapy may lead to exacerbation of symptoms. When discontinuing long term treatment, the dosage should be reduced gradually over several days, and the patient carefully monitored.

Interactions with other medicaments and other forms of interaction: May enhance the effects of peripheral vasodilators.

Pregnancy and lactation: There is no evidence relating

to the safety of nitrates in pregnancy and lactation. Nitrates should not be administered to pregnant women and nursing mothers unless considered essential by the physician.

Effects on ability to drive and use machines: None stated.

Undesirable effects: Side effects include facial flushing and headache. Toxic effects of glyceryl trinitrate include vomiting, restlessness, cyanosis, methaemoglobinaemia and syncope.

Overdose: In the event of accidental or deliberate overdosage toxic effects of glyceryl trinitrate include vomiting, restlessness, cyanosis, methaemoglobinaemia, tachycardia and syncope. Patients should receive gastric aspiration and lavage and be given respiratory and circulatory support. The physician should be aware that tablets in the intestine will release their content over several hours.

Pharmacological properties

Pharmacodynamic properties: Glyceryl trinitrate is a potent coronary vasodilator. It also reduces venous return and thus left ventricular work.

Pharmacokinetic properties: Following oral administration glyceryl trinitrate is rapidly metabolised to glyceryl 1,2 dinitrate and glyceryl 1,3 dinitrate. Although less potent the metabolites probably provide the predominant pharmacological effect. Studies with Sustac 2.6 mg and 6.4 mg demonstrate a t_{max} for both metabolites of approx. 1 hr and an apparent $t_{\frac{1}{2}}$ of approx. 2 hrs. There is evidence of activity extending over 6 hours or more.

Preclinical safety data: There are no preclinical data of relevance to the prescriber which are additional to safety data already included in other sections of the SPC.

Pharmaceutical particulars

List of excipients: Compressible sugar, E127, magnesium stearate, ethyl cellulose, castor oil, shellac, lactose, sucrose, corn starch, talc.

Incompatibilities: None stated.

Shelf life: 3 years

Special precautions for storage: Store at room temperature.

Nature and contents of container: Sustac 2.6 mg and 6.4 mg: Plastic containers of 90
Sustac 10 mg: Plastic containers of 60

Instruction for use/handling: None stated.

Marketing authorisation number

Sustac 2.6 mg 0108/5031
Sustac 6.4 mg 0108/5032
Sustac 10 mg 0108/0064

Date of approval/revision of SPC

Sustac 2.6 mg: and 6.4 mg tablets: November 1997
Sustac 10 mg tablets: December 1996

Legal category P

**Trade Mark*

Pierre Fabre Limited
Hyde Abbey House
23 Hyde Street
Winchester
Hampshire
SO23 7DR

☎ 01962 856956 ⎙ 01962 844014

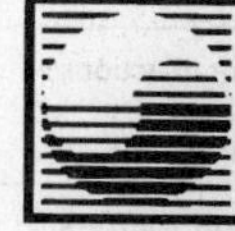

Pierre Fabre Ltd

NAVELBINE*

Qualitative and quantitative composition

Active ingredient	*Formulation* 10 mg/1 ml	40 mg/4 ml	50 mg/5 ml
vinorelbine tartrate (mg)	13.85	55.40	69.25
equivalent to vinorelbine (INN) base (mg)	10.00	40.00	50.00

Pharmaceutical form Injectable solution for intravenous infusion.

Clinical particulars

Therapeutic indications:

– As a single agent or in combination for the first line treatment of stage 3 or 4 non-small cell lung cancer.
– Treatment of advanced breast cancer stage 3 and 4 relapsing after or refractory to an anthracycline containing regimen.

Posology and method of administration:

Strictly by intravenous injection through an infusion line.

The use of intra-thecal route is contra-indicated.

In adults:

- Navelbine is usually given at 25–30 mg/m² weekly.
- Navelbine may be administered by slow bolus (5–10 minutes) after dilution in 20–50 ml of normal saline solution or by a short infusion (20–30 minutes) after dilution in 125 ml of normal saline solution. Administration should always be followed by a normal saline infusion to flush the vein.

Dose modifications: Vinorelbine metabolism and clearance are mostly hepatic: only 18.5% is excreted unchanged in the urine. No prospective study relating altered metabolism of the drug to its pharmacodynamic effects is available in order to establish guidelines for Vinorelbine dose reduction in patients with impaired liver or kidney function.

However, in breast cancer patients, Vinorelbine clearance is not altered in presence of moderate liver metastases (i.e. ≤75% of liver volume replaced by the tumour). In these patients, there is no pharmacokinetic rationale for reducing Vinorelbine doses.

In patients with massive liver metastases (i.e. >75% of liver volume replaced by the tumour), it is empirically suggested that the dose be reduced by ⅓ and the haematological toxicity closely followed-up.

There is no pharmacokinetic rationale for reducing Vinorelbine dose in patients with impaired kidney function.

The dose limiting toxicity of Vinorelbine is mainly neutropenia. This usually occurs between day 8 and day 12 after drug administration, is short-lived, and is not cumulative. If the neutrophil count is <2000/mm³ and/or platelet number is <75000/mm³, then the treatment should be delayed until recovery. Drug administration is expected to be delayed by 1 week in about 35% of treatment courses.

The maximum tolerated dose per administration: 35.4 mg/m².

The maximum total dose per administration: 60 mg.

Contra-indications:

Pregnancy and lactation: Severe hepatic insufficiency not related to the tumoural process.

Special warnings and special precautions for use:

- Navelbine must only be administered by the intravenous route. **The use of intra-thecal route is contra-indicated.** Administration should always be followed by a normal saline infusion to flush the vein.
- Treatment should be undertaken with close haematological monitoring (determination of haemoglobin level and number of leucocytes, granulocytes and platelets before each new injection); if the neutrophil count is <2000/mm³, treatment should be delayed until recovery and the patient should be observed.
- If the patient presents signs or symptoms suggestive of infection, a prompt investigation should be carried out.
- If there is significant hepatic impairment the dose should be reduced.
- In case of renal impairment, because of the low level of renal excretion, no dose modification is necessary.
- Navelbine should not be given concomitantly with radiotherapy if the treatment field includes the liver.
- All contact with the eye should be strictly avoided: risk of severe irritation and even corneal ulceration if the drug is sprayed under pressure. Immediate liberal washing of the eye with normal saline solution should be undertaken if any contact occurs.

Interaction with other medicaments and other forms of interaction: The combination Vinorelbine-Cisplatin shows no interaction on the pharmacokinetic parameters.

Pregnancy and lactation: In animal reproductive studies Navelbine was embryo- and feto-lethal and teratogenic.

Women should not become pregnant during treatment with Navelbine.

This product should not be used during pregnancy.

If pregnancy should occur during treatment, the possibility of genetic counselling should be used.

It is not known whether Navelbine passes into the breast milk. Lactation must therefore be discontinued before treatment with this medicine.

Effects on ability to drive and use machines: Not applicable.

Undesirable effects:

- **Haematological tolerance**
  – The limiting toxicity is neutropenia (G1: 9.7%; G2: 15.2%; G3: 24.3%; G4: 27.8%) which is rapidly reversible (5 to 7 days) and non-cumulative; it is maximal between 5 and 7 days after administration. Further treatment may be given after recovery of the granulocyte count.
  – Anaemia (G1–2: 61.2%; G3–4: 7.4%) and thrombocytopenia (G1–2: 5.1%; G3–4: 2.5%) are seldom severe.
- **Neurological tolerance**
  – Peripheral
  This is generally limited to loss of deep tendon reflexes; severe paraesthesiae are uncommon (G1: 17.2%; G2: 3.6%; G3: 2.6%; G4: 0.1%). The effects are dose dependent but reversible when treatment is discontinued.
  – Autonomic neuropathy
  The main symptom is intestinal paresis causing constipation (G1: 16.9%; G2: 4.9%) which rarely progresses to paralytic ileus (G3: 2%; G4: 0.7%). Treatment may be resumed after recovery of normal bowel mobility.
- **Gastrointestinal tolerance**
  – Constipation (see Autonomic neuropathy)
  – Diarrhoea (G1: 7.6%; G2: 3.6%; G3: 0.7%; G4: 0.1%): severe diarrhoea is uncommon.
  – Nausea-vomiting (G1: 19.9%; G2: 8.3%; G3: 1.9%; G4: 0.3%): severe nausea and vomiting may occasionally occur. Conventional anti-emetic therapy reduces these undesirable effects.
- **Allergic reactions**

As with other vinca alkaloids, Navelbine may occasionally produce dyspnoea and bronchospasm and more rarely local or generalised cutaneous reactions.

- **Venous tolerance**

Burning pain at the injection site and local phlebitis (G1: 12.3%; G2: 8.2%; G3: 3.6%; G4: 0.1%) may be observed with repeated injections of Navelbine.

Bolus injection followed by liberal flushing of the vein can limit this effect. Insertion of a central venous line may be necessary.

- **Other undesirable effects**
  - Alopecia is mild and may appear progressively with extended courses of treatment (G1–2: 21%; G3–4: 4.1%)
  - Jaw pain has occasionally been reported.
  - Any extravasation may induce local reactions which rarely progress to necrosis (see *Posology and method of administration*).

Overdose:

- Studies of acute toxicity in animals:
  The symptoms of overdose are pilo erection, behaviour abnormalities (lethargy, prostration), pulmonary lesions, weight loss and bone marrow hypoplasia more or less severe in animals sacrificed during the course of the study.
- Accidental overdosages have been reported in humans: they may produce a period of bone marrow aplasia sometimes associated with fever, infection and possibly paralytic ileus. Management of the infectious complications is by broad-spectrum antibiotic therapy and the paralytic ileus is managed by naso-gastric aspiration.

Pharmacological properties

Pharmacodynamic properties: Navelbine is a cytostatic antineoplastic drug of the vinca alkaloid family with a molecular action on the dynamic equilibrium of tubulin in the microtubular apparatus of the cell. It inhibits tubulin polymerisation and binds preferentially to mitotic microtubules, only affecting axonal microtubules at high concentration. The induction of tubulin spiralisation is less than that produced by vincristine. Navelbine blocks mitosis at G2-M, causing cell death in interphase or at the following mitosis.

Pharmacokinetic properties: After intravenous administration of Navelbine 30 mg/m² in patients, the plasma concentration of the active ingredient is characterised by a three exponential elimination curve. The end-elimination phase reflects a long half-life greater than 40 hours. Total clearance of vinorelbine is high (1.3 l/h/kg) with excretion occurring mainly by the biliary route; renal excretion is minimal (18.5% of label is recovered in urine).

The active ingredient is widely distributed in the body with a volume of distribution greater than 40 l/kg. There is moderate binding to plasma proteins (13.5%), but strong binding to platelets (78%). Penetration of vinorelbine into pulmonary tissue is significant with tissue/plasma concentration ratios of greater than 300 in a study involving surgical biopsy.

Small concentrations of deacetyl vinorelbine have been recovered in humans, but vinorelbine is principally detected as the parent compound in urine.

Preclinical safety data:

- **Mutagenic and carcinogenic potential**
  The interaction of Navelbine with the spindle apparatus during mitosis can cause an incorrect distribution of chromosomes. In animal studies Navelbine induced aneuploidy and polyploidy. It is therefore to be assumed that Navelbine can also cause mutagenic effects (induction of aneuploidy) in man.
  The carcinogenicity studies, in which Navelbine was administered only once every two weeks in order to avoid the toxic effects of the drug, are negative.
- **Reproductive toxicity**
  In animal reproductive studies Navelbine was embryo- and feto-lethal and teratogenic.
  The NOEL in the rat was 0.26 mg/kg every 3 days.
  Following peri/postnatal administration in the rat at doses of 1.0 mg/kg every 3 days i.v., retarded weight gain was found in the offspring up to the 7th week of life.
- **Safety pharmacology**
  Bibliographic review concerning the tolerance of vinca alkaloids on the cardiovascular system shows the occurence of some cardiac events (such as angina, myocardial infarction), but the incidence of these is low.
  Haemodynamic and electrocardiographic studies on animals have been carried out by Pierre Fabre Médicament Laboratories; no haemodynamic effects have been found using a maximal tolerated dose in dogs, however only some non significant disturbances of repolarisation were found for all vinca alkaloids tested. No effect on the cardiovascular system has been detected using repeated doses (study 39 weeks) of Navelbine on primates.

Pharmaceutical particulars
List of excipients:

Excipients	*Formulation* 10 mg/1 ml	40 mg/4 ml	50 mg/5 ml
Water for injections (ml) qs	1.00	4.00	5.00
nitrogen qs	inert filling	inert filling	inert filling

Incompatibilities
- Navelbine solution (10 mg/ml) may be diluted in a solution for infusion of normal saline or 5% dextrose.
- The volume of dilution depends on the mode of administration:
  bolus=20–50 ml
  infusion=125 ml
- Navelbine should not be diluted in alkaline solutions (risk of precipitate)
- In case of polychemotherapy, Navelbine should not be mixed with other agents.
- Navelbine is not absorbed to or affected by either PVC or clear neutral glass.

Shelf life:
- The product is stable for 3 years.
- After diluting Navelbine in normal saline solution or dextrose solution, the product should be used either immediately or it can be stored in the clear glass vials or in the PVC perfusion bags during 24 hours in a refrigerator (+2°C to +8°C).

Special precautions for storage: Navelbine should be stored in a refrigerator (+2°C to +8°C) and shielded from light.

Nature and contents of container: The drug is distributed in glass vials (type I) of appropriated volume closed by a butyl or chlorobutyl stopper. The stopper is covered with a crimped-on aluminium cap equipped with a polypropylene seal.

Vials of 1, 4 and 5 ml.

Instructions for use/handling: Navelbine has a more or less yellow colouration which does not affect the quality of the product.

Handling guidelines: the preparation and administration of Navelbine should be carried out only by trained staff and as with all cytotoxic agents, precautions should be taken to avoid exposing staff during pregnancy.

Preparation of solution for administration should be carried out in a designated handling area and working over a washable tray or disposable plastic-backed absorbent paper.

Suitable eye protection, disposable gloves, face mask and disposable apron should be worn.

Syringes and infusion sets should be assembled carefully to avoid leakage (use of Luer lock fittings is recommended).

Actual spillage or leakage should be mopped up wearing protective gloves.

All contact with the eye should be strictly avoided: risk of severe irritation and even corneal ulceration if the drug is sprayed under pressure. Immediate liberal washing of the eye with normal saline solution should be undertaken if any contact occurs.

On completion, any exposed surface should be thoroughly cleaned and hands and face washed.

Navelbine may be administered by slow bolus (5–10 minutes) after dilution in 20–50 ml of normal saline solution or by a short infusion (20–30 minutes) after dilution in 125 ml of normal saline solution. Administration should always be followed by a normal saline infusion to flush the vein.

Navelbine must be given strictly intravenously: it is very important to make sure that the cannula is accurately placed in the vein before starting to infuse Navelbine.

If the drug extravasates during intravenous administration, a substantial local reaction may occur. In this case, the injection should be stopped and the rest of the dose should be administered in another vein.

Disposal guidelines: all sharps should be placed in an appropriate container and all other disposable items and cleaning materials in a sealed plastic bag which should be incinerated with other clinical waste.

Waste material may be disposed of by incineration.

Marketing authorisation number PL 00603/0028

Date of the first authorisation/renewal of the authorisation 10 May 1996

Date of last revision of the text 18 September 1998

**Trade Mark*

Procter & Gamble Pharmaceuticals UK Limited

Lovett House
Lovett Road
Staines
Middlesex TW18 3AZ

☎ 01784 495000 🗋 01784 495297

ALPHADERM* CREAM

Qualitative and quantitative composition Alphaderm cream contains the active ingredients Hydrocortisone, PhEur 1% w/w and Urea, BP 10% w/w.

Pharmaceutical form Alphaderm is a translucent white cream containing Hydrocortisone and Urea in a specially formulated base which assists the percutaneous transportation of the active ingredients to the site of action. Due to this formulation Alphaderm acts as a moderately potent topical corticosteroid. The base is self-occlusive and fulfils the functions of both an ointment and a cream.

Clinical particulars

Therapeutic indications: For the treatment of all dry ichthyotic, eczematous conditions of the skin, including atopic, infantile, chronic allergic and irritant eczema, asteatotic, hyperkeratotic and lichenified eczema, neurodermatitis and prurigo.

Posology and method of administration: Adults, children and the elderly. A small amount should be applied topically to the preferably dry affected areas twice daily. In resistant lesions occlusive dressings may be used but this is usually unnecessary because of the self occlusive nature of the special base.

Contra-indications: Primary bacterial, viral and fungal diseases of the skin and secondarily infected eczemas or intertrigo and, in general, should not be used on weeping surfaces.

Known hypersensitivity to the cream or any of its excipients.

Special warnings and special precautions for use: Caution should be exercised when using in children. In infants and children, long term continuous therapy should be avoided, as adrenal suppression can occur even without occlusion. Excessive absorption may occur when applied under napkins.

Application to moist or fissured skin may cause temporary irritation.

As with corticosteroids in general, prolonged application to the face and eyelids is undesirable.

Interaction with other medicaments and other forms of interaction: Urea may enhance the absorption of the corticosteroid and this should be borne in mind, especially when long term treatment is contemplated.

Pregnancy and lactation: There is inadequate evidence for safety in human pregnancy. Topical administration of corticosteroids to pregnant animals can cause abnormalities of foetal development including cleft palate and intra-uterine growth retardation. There may, therefore, be a very small risk of such effects in the human foetus.

Effects on ability to drive and use machines: Alphaderm does not interfere with the ability to drive or use machines.

Undesirable effects: If used correctly Alphaderm is unlikely to cause side effects.

Overdose: Chronically, grossly excessive over-use on large areas of skin in, for example, children could result in adrenal suppression of the hypothalamic-pituitary axis (HPA) as well as topical and systemic signs and symptoms of high corticosteroid dosage. In such cases, treatment should not stop abruptly. Adrenal insufficiency may require treatment with systemic hydrocortisone. Ingestion of a large amount of Alphaderm would be expected to result in gastro-intestinal irritation, nausea, and possibly vomiting. Symptomatic and supportive care should be given. Liberal oral administration of milk or water may be helpful.

Pharmacological properties

Pharmacodynamic properties: Hydrocortisone is a naturally occurring glucocorticoid with proven anti-inflammatory and vasoconstrictive properties. Urea has been demonstrated to have hydrating, keratolytic and anti-pruritic properties. As such, urea has additional therapeutic effect in dry hyperkeratotic skin conditions.

Pharmacokinetic properties: Therapeutic activity of hydrocortisone depends upon the adequate penetration through the horny layer of the skin. The urea in the formulation solubilises part of the hydrocortisone and has a keratolytic effect. Both these factors increase penetration of the hydrocortisone.

Pharmaceutical particulars

List of excipients: White soft paraffin, maize starch, isopropyl myristate, sycrowax HR-C, palmitic acid, sorbitan monolaurate and Arlatone G.

Incompatibilities: See (*Interactions with other medicaments and other forms of interaction*).

Shelf life: Two years.

Special precautions for storage: Store below 25°C.

Nature and contents of container: Supplied in tubes of 30 g and 100 g.

Instructions for use/handling: A patient leaflet is provided with details of use and handling of the product.

Marketing authorisation number PL 0364/0019R.

Date of first authorisation/renewal of authorisation 13 February 1990

Legal status POM

AQUADRATE* CREAM

Qualitative and quantitative composition Aquadrate cream contains urea BP 10% w/w.

Pharmaceutical form A smooth, unperfumed, non greasy, off white cream for topical administration.

Clinical particulars

Therapeutic indications: For the treatment of ichthyosis and hyperkeratotic skin conditions associated with atopic eczema, xeroderma, iasteatosis and other chronic dry skin conditions.

Posology and method of administration: Aquadrate is applied topically. Wash affected areas well, rinse off all traces of soap, dry, and apply sparingly twice daily. Occlusive dressings may be used but are usually unnecessary because of the self-occlusive nature of the cream.

Contra-indications: Known hypersensitivity to the product.

Special warnings and special precautions for use: Avoid application to moist or broken skin.

Interaction with other medicaments and other forms of interaction: Aquadrate may increase the penetration through the skin barrier of other topically applied medicaments.

Pregnancy and lactation: Animal reproduction studies have not been conducted with Aquadrate. Aquadrate should only be used if the anticipated benefits outweigh the risks.

Effects on ability to drive and use machines: Aquadrate does not interfere with the ability to drive or use machines.

Undesirable effects: May produce stinging if applied to sensitive, moist or fissured skin.

Overdose: Topical applications of excessive amounts of Aquadrate might cause skin irritation but no other effects would be expected. Ingestion of a large amount of Aquadrate would be expected to result in gastro-intestinal irritation (nausea and vomiting). Symptomatic and supportive care should be given. Liberal oral administration of milk or water may be helpful.

Pharmacological properties

Pharmacodynamic properties: Urea has a therapeutic effect in chronic dry skin conditions through its hydrating, keratolytic and anti-pruritic properties.

Pharmacokinetic properties: There is no information available on the pharmacokinetics of urea.

Pharmaceutical particulars

List of excipients: The cream also contains white soft paraffin, maize starch, isopropyl myristate, syncrowax HR-C, palmitic acid, sorbitan monolaurate and arlatone G.

Incompatibilities: None known.

Shelf life: Two years.

Special precautions for storage: Store below 30°C.

Nature and contents of container: Aquadrate is available in tubes of 30 g and 100 g.

Instructions for use/handling: A patient leaflet is provided with details of use and handling of the product.

Marketing authorisation number PL 0364/0018R

Date of first authorisation/renewal of authorisation 10 September 1991

Date of (partial) revision of the text July 1997

CACIT* D3 effervescent granules, 500 mg/440 IU

Qualitative and quantitative composition Cacit D3 500 mg/440 IU contains 1250 mg of calcium carbonate (equivalent to 500 mg of elemental calcium) and 440 IU of cholecalciferol (vitamin D3) per sachet of 4 g.

Pharmaceutical form Effervescent granules for oral solution.

Clinical particulars

Therapeutic indications: For correction of vitamin D and calcium combined deficiency in elderly people. Cacit D3 may be used as an adjunct to specific therapy for osteoporosis, in patients with either established vitamin D and calcium combined deficiencies or in those patients at high risk of needing such therapeutic supplements.

Posology and method of administration:

Dosage: One or two sachets of Cacit D3 effervescent granules, 500 mg/440 IU per day.

Method of administration: Oral, after reconstitution.

Pour the contents of the sachet into a glass, add a large quantity of water, stir, then drink immediately the solution is obtained.

Contra-indications:

- hypercalcaemia, hypercalciuria.
- long-term immobilisation accompanied by hypercalciuria and/or hypercalcaemia.
- calci-lithiasis.
- hypersensitivity to one of the ingredients.

Special warnings and special precautions for use: With long-term treatment it is advisable to monitor serum and urinary calcium levels and kidney function, and reduce or interrupt treatment temporarily if urinary calcium exceeds 7.5 mmol/24 hours (300 mg/24 hours).

The product should be used with caution in patients with renal insufficiency and the effects on calcium and phosphate homeostasis should be monitored.

In the case of combined treatment with digitalis, bisphosphonate, sodium fluoride, thiazide diuretics, tetracyclines (see *Interaction with other medicaments and other forms of interaction*).

Allowances should be made for vitamin D/calcium supplements from other sources. Additional administration of vitamin D or calcium should be carried out under strict medical supervision, with weekly monitoring of serum and urinary calcium.

The product should be prescribed with caution in patients with sarcoidosis because of possible increased metabolism of vitamin D to its active form. These patients should be monitored for serum and urinary calcium.

Interaction with other medicaments and other forms of interaction: The effects of digitalis and other cardiac glycosides may be accentuated with the oral administration of calcium combined with vitamin D (increases the toxicity of digitalis and therefore the risk of dysrhythmia). Strict medical supervision, and if necessary, monitoring ECG and calcaemia are necessary.

In case of concomitant treatment with a bisphosphonate or with sodium fluoride, it is advisable to allow a minimum period of two hours before taking the calcium (risk of reduction of the gastrointestinal absorption of bisphosphonate and sodium fluoride).

Thiazide diuretics increase the renal absorption of calcium, so the risk of hypercalcaemia should be considered. Strict medical supervision of calcaemia is recommended.

Concomitant treatment with phenytoin or barbiturates can decrease the effect of vitamin D because of metabolic inactivation.

Concomitant use of a glucocorticosteroid can decrease the effect of vitamin D.

Calcium salts reduce the absorption of tetracyclines. It is advisable to delay taking Cacit D3 by at least three hours.

Possible interactions with food (e.g. containing oxalic acid, phosphate or phytinic acid).

Pregnancy and lactation
The product may be used during pregnancy and lactation. However, the daily intake should not exceed 1500 mg calcium and 600 IU vitamin D.

Overdoses of vitamin D have shown teratogenic effects in pregnant animals. In humans overdoses of vitamin D must be avoided, as permanent hypercalcaemia can lead to physical and mental retardation, supravalvular aortic stenosis and retinopathy in the child. There are several case reports of administration of very high doses in hypoparathyroidism in the mother, where normal children were born.

Vitamin D and its metabolites pass into the breast milk.

Effects on ability to drive and use machines: No data are known about the effect of this product on driving capacity. However, an effect is unlikely.

Undesirable effects: Constipation, flatulence, nausea, gastric pain, diarrhoea.

Hypercalciuria and in rare cases hypercalcaemia with long-term treatment in high doses.

Overdose: The most serious consequence of acute or chronic overdose would be hypercalciuria and hypercalcaemia due to vitamin D toxicity. Symptoms include nausea, vomiting, thirst, polydipsia, polyuria and constipation. Chronic overdoses can lead to vascular and organ calcifications as a result of hypercalcaemia. Treatment would consist of stopping all intake of calcium and vitamin D and rehydration.

Pharmacological properties
Pharmacodynamic properties: Vitamin D corrects an insufficient intake of vitamin D and increases intestinal absorption of calcium. The optimal amount of vitamin D in the elderly is 500–1000 IU/day. Calcium corrects an insufficient intake of calcium in the diet. The commonly accepted requirement of calcium in the elderly is 1500 mg/day.

Vitamin D and calcium correct secondary senile hyperparathyroidism.

Pharmacokinetic properties: During dissolution the calcium salt contained in Cacit D3 is transformed into calcium citrate. Calcium citrate is well absorbed (approximately 30% to 40% of the ingested dose). Calcium is eliminated in the urine and faeces and secreted in the sweat.

Vitamin D is absorbed in the intestine and transported by protein binding in the blood to the liver (first hydroxylation) then to the kidney (second hydroxylation).

The non-hydroxylated vitamin D is stored in reserve compartments such as adipose and muscle tissue. Its plasma half-life is several days; it is eliminated in the faeces and the urine.

Pre-clinical safety data: No remarkable findings.

Pharmaceutical particulars
List of excipients: Citric acid, malic acid, gluconolactone, maltodextrin, sodium cyclamate, saccharin sodium, lemon flavouring (containing: sorbitol, mannitol, D-gluconolactone, dextrin, gum arabic, lemon oil), rice starch, corn starch, potassium carbonate, α-tocopherol, vegetable oils, gelatin, and sucrose.

One sachet of Cacit D3 500 mg/440 IU contains a total of 0.22 mmol of sodium (5 mg).

Incompatibilities: None known.

Shelf life: 3 years.

Special precautions for storage: Store below 25°C.

Nature and contents of container: Paper/aluminium/polyethylene sachets packed in boxes of 30.

Instructions for use: Pour the contents of the sachet into a glass, add a large quantity of water, stir, then drink immediately the solution is obtained.

Marketing authorisation numbers PL 0364/0060 and PA 170/18/1 Cacit D3 500 mg/440 IU

Date of approval/renewal of authorisation March 1996

Date of last revision of SmPC January 1997

Legal category P

CACIT* TABLETS

Presentation Cacit tablets are round, flat, white tablets with pink speckles and a distinctive orange odour and flavour. Each tablet contains 1.25 g of Calcium Carbonate, PhEur, which when dispersed in water provides 500 mg of calcium as calcium citrate.

Uses
1. Treatment of calcium deficiency states including osteomalacia, rickets and malabsorption syndromes affecting the upper gastrointestinal tract.
2. An adjunct to conventional therapy in the arrest or slowing down of bone demineralisation in osteoporosis.
3. In the arrest or slowing down of bone demineralisation in osteoporosis, where other effective treatment is contra-indicated.
4. As a therapeutic supplement during times when intake may be inadequate, particularly those associated with the increased demand of childhood, old age, pregnancy and lactation.

Dosage and administration The tablets must be dissolved in a glass of water and the solution should then be drunk immediately after complete dissolution of the tablets.

Adults and the elderly: For simple calcium deficiency states and malabsorption, the dosage should be tailored to the individual patient's needs. In osteomalacia 1–3 g per day is recommended.

For the treatment of osteoporosis a dose of up to 1.5 g per day is normally required. In women with adequate dietary calcium intake (at least 1 g/day), 500 mg daily may be sufficient.

Up to 1.5 g of calcium per day is the recommended dosage for therapeutic supplementation.

Children: For calcium deficiency states, malabsorption and rickets the recommendation given under adult dosage should be followed.

For therapeutic supplementation a dose of up to 1 g per day is recommended.

Contra-indications, warnings, etc
Contra-indications: Hypercalcaemia (e.g. due to hyperparathyroidism, hypervitaminosis D, decalcifying tumours, severe renal failure, bone metastases), severe hypercalciuria and renal calculi.

Precautions and warnings: In mild hypercalciuria (exceeding 7.5 mmol/24 hours in adults or 0.12–0.15 mmol/kg/24 hours in children) or renal failure, or where there is evidence of stone formation in the urinary tract; adequate checks must be kept on urinary calcium excretion. If necessary the dosage should be reduced or calcium therapy discontinued.

Interactions with other drugs: Concomitant administration with vitamin D causes an increase in calcium absorption and plasma levels may continue to rise after stopping vitamin D therapy.

The effects of digoxin and other cardiac glycosides may be accentuated by calcium and toxicity may be produced, especially in combination with vitamin D.

Calcium salts reduce the absorption of some drugs, in particular tetracyclines. It is therefore recommended that administration of Cacit tablets be separated from these products by at least 3 hours.

Thiazide diuretics increase renal absorption of calcium, so the risk of hypercalcaemia should be considered.

Side effects: Mild gastrointestinal disturbances have occurred rarely (e.g. nausea, abdominal pain, constipation, flatulence and eructation).

Use in pregnancy and lactation: Calcium supplements have been in wide use for many years without apparent ill consequence.

Overdosage: The amount of calcium absorbed will depend on the individuals calcium status. Deliberate overdosage is unlikely with effervescent preparations and acute overdosage has not been reported. It might cause gastrointestinal disturbance but would not be expected to cause hypercalcaemia, except in patients treated with excessive doses of vitamin D. Treatment should be aimed at lowering serum calcium levels, e.g. administration of oral phosphates.

Pharmaceutical precautions Cacit tablets are hygroscopic and should be dispensed in the original container. Store in a dry place.

Legal category P

Packaging quantities Cacit tablets, 500 mg, are supplied in boxes of 76 (4 tubes each containing 19 tablets).

Further information Cacit tablets, 500 mg contain no sugar and have a low sodium content.

Product licence number PL 0364/0045

Date of preparation September 1995

DANTRIUM* INTRAVENOUS

Qualitative and quantitative composition Each vial contains 20 mg dantrolene sodium, 3 g mannitol and sufficient sodium hydroxide to yield a pH of approximately 9.5 when reconstituted with 60 ml of water for injection.

Pharmaceutical form A sterile lyophilised substance for reconstitution with sterile water for injection.

Clinical particulars
Therapeutic indications: For the treatment of malignant hyperthermia.

Posology and method of administration: As soon as the malignant hyperthermia syndrome is recognised all anaesthetic agents should be discontinued. An initial Dantrium intravenous dose of 1 mg/kg should be given rapidly into the vein. If the physiological and metabolic abnormalities persist or reappear, this dose may be repeated up to a cumulative dose of 10 mg/kg. Clinical experience to date has shown that the average dose of Dantrium intravenous required to reverse the manifestations of malignant hyperthermia has been 2.5 mg/kg. If a relapse or recurrence occurs, Dantrium intravenous should be readministered at the last effect dose.

Contra-indications: None stated.

Special warnings and special precautions for use: In some subjects as much as 10 mg/kg of Dantrium intravenous has been needed to reverse the crisis. In a 70 kg man this dose would require approximately 36 vials. Such a volume has been administered in approximately one and a half hours.

Because of the high pH of the intravenous formulation of Dantrium, care must be taken to prevent extravasation of the intravenous solution into the surrounding tissues.

The use of Dantrium intravenous in the management of malignant hyperthermia is not a substitute for previously known supportive measures. It will be necessary to discontinue the suspect triggering agents, attend to increased oxygen requirements and manage the metabolic acidosis. When necessary institute cooling, attend to urinary output and monitor for electrolyte imbalance.

Interaction with other medicaments and other forms of interaction: The combination of therapeutic doses of intravenous dantrolene sodium and verapamil in halothane/alpha-chloralose anaesthetised swine has resulted in ventricular fibrillation and cardiovascular collapse in association with marked hyperkalaemia. It is recommended that the combination of intravenous dantrolene sodium and calcium channel blockers, such as verapamil, is not used during the reversal of a malignant hyperthermia crisis until the relevance of these findings to humans is established.

Pregnancy and lactation: The safety of Dantrium intravenous in pregnant women has not been established; it should be given only when the potential benefits have been weighed against the possible risk to mother and child.

Effects on ability to drive and use machines: None stated.

Undesirable effects: No side-effects have been attributed to Dantrium intravenous in patients treated with short-term therapy for malignant hyperthermia. The nature of the emergency and the complexity of concomitant therapy will make it extremely difficult to isolate cause and effect relationships for any of the drugs used. Hepatotoxic reactions have been noted in a small number of subjects given long-term oral dantrolene therapy.

Overdose: None stated.

Pharmacological properties
Pharmacodynamic properties:
Molecular pharmacology: The receptor molecule for dantrolene has not been identified. Radiolabelled dantrolene sodium binds to specific components of the striated muscle cell, namely the t-tubules and the sarcoplasmic reticulum. However, the kinetics of binding vary between these two organelles. The binding of ryanodine is thought to compete with the binding of calcium in these organelles; further evidence for the specificity of binding is that dantrolene inhibits the binding of ryanodine to heavy sarcoplasmic reticulum vesicles from rabbit skeletal muscle. Under some conditions, dantrolene will lower intrasarcoplasmic calcium concentrations in the resting state. This may be more important in diseased muscle [e.g. in malignant hyperthermia in humans and swine stress syndrome] than in muscle with normal function.

Dantrolene does not bind to the same sites as calcium channel blocking drugs such as nitrendipine or calmodulin. There is no electrophysiological evidence that dantrolene interferes with the influx of calcium from outside the cell. This may be one reason why paralysis by dantrolene has never been reported in animals or man; the muscle cell has alternative sources of calcium which are not influenced by dantrolene.

Biochemical pharmacology: Whatever the molecular mechanism, the cardinal property of dantrolene sodium is that it lowers intracellular calcium concentration in skeletal muscle. Calcium concentrations may be lower in both the quiescent state, and as a result of a reduction in the release of calcium from the sarcoplasmic reticulum in response to a standard stimulus. This effect has been observed in striated muscle fibres from several species, and is not seen in myocardium. Fast fibres may be more sensitive than slow fibres to the action of dantrolene sodium.

Diverse other properties of dantrolene sodium have been observed *in vitro*, and in animal studies. Dantrolene sodium may inhibit the release of calcium from the smooth endoplasmic reticulum of smooth muscle, but the significance of this observation is questionable; for example, dantrolene sodium has no effect on isolated human urinary bladder smooth muscle. Calcium dependent, pre-synaptic neurotransmitter release may also be inhibited by dantrolene sodium. Again, the clinical significance of this has not been demonstrated.

Studies on isolated, functional muscle: Elevation of intracellular, free calcium ion concentration is an obligatory step in excitation-contraction coupling of skeletal muscle. Dantrolene sodium, therefore, acts as a muscle relaxant by a peripheral mechanism which is quite different, and easily distinguishable from neuromuscular junction blocking drugs. In contrast with compounds that relax skeletal muscle by acting principally on the central nervous system, dantrolene sodium acts directly on skeletal muscle cells. In rabbit atria, dantrolene sodium has no effect alone, but it may antagonise inotropic agents which act by increasing intramyocardial cell calcium e.g. anthopleurin-a.

Pharmacokinetic properties:

Distribution: Dantrolene sodium is a highly lipophobic drug. In addition, it lacks hydrophilicity. Dantrolene sodium binds to human serum albumin (HSA) with a molar ratio of 0.95 to 1.68 *in vitro*. The association constant *in vitro* is 2.3 to 5.4×10^{-5} per mol. *In vitro* dantrolene sodium can be displaced from HSA by warfarin, clofibrate and tolbutamide but these interactions have not been confirmed in humans (re manufacturer's database). Single intravenous dose studies suggest that the primary volume of distribution is about 15 litres.

Metabolism and excretion: The biological half life in plasma in most human subjects is between 5 and 9 hours, although half-lives as long as 12.1±1.9 hours have been reported after a single intravenous dose. Inactivation is by hepatic metabolism in the first instance. There are two alternative pathways. Most of the drug is hydroxylated to 5-hydroxy-dantrolene. The minor pathway involves nitro-reduction to aminodantrolene which is then acetylated (compound F-490). The 5-hydroxy metabolite is a muscle relaxant with nearly the same potency as the parent molecule, and may have a longer half life than the parent compound. Compound F-490 is much less potent and is probably inactive at the concentrations achieved in clinical samples. Metabolites are subsequently excreted in the urine in the ratio of 79 5-hydroxy dantrolene: 17 compound F-490: 4 unaltered dantrolene (salt or free acid). The proportion of drug excreted in the faeces depends upon dose size.

Preclinical safety data: Whilst there is no clinical evidence of carcinogenicity in humans, this possibility cannot be absolutely excluded. Dantrolene sodium has shown some evidence of tumourgenicity at high dose levels in Sprague-Dawley female rats, but these effects have not been seen in other studies in Fischer 344 rats or HaM/ICR mice.

Pharmaceutical particulars

List of excipients: Mannitol and sodium hydroxide.

Incompatibilities: Dantrium intravenous should not be mixed with other intravenous infusions.

Shelf life: Three years.

Special precautions for storage: Each vial of Dantrium intravenous should be reconstituted by adding 60 ml of water for injection PhEur, and shaking until the solution is clear. The contents of the vial must be protected from direct light and used within six hours of reconstitution. Protect the reconstituted solution from temperatures above 30°C and below 15°C. Store the unreconstituted product below 30°C.

Because of the nature of the freeze-drying process used in the manufacture of Dantrium intravenous, the freeze-dried cake of Dantrium intravenous may have a mottled orange/white appearance or be in the form of loose aggregates. This is an entirely normal artefact and in no way compromises the stability of the product.

Nature and contents of container: Dantrium intravenous is available in packs of twelve 70 ml vials, each containing 20 mg dantrolene sodium.

Instruction for use/handling: A leaflet is provided for details of use and handling the product.

Marketing authorisation number PL 0364/0030

Date of first authorisation/renewal of authorisation 14 February 1980

Date of (partial) revision of the text August 1997

DANTRIUM* 100 mg CAPSULES

Qualitative and quantitative composition Dantrium 100 mg capsules contain 100 mg dantrolene sodium per capsule.

Pharmaceutical form Dantrium capsules are presented in orange/light brown capsules. The 100 mg capsule carries the monogram Dantrium 100 mg on the cap and 0149, 0033 and triple coding bars on the body.

Clinical particulars

Therapeutic indications: For the treatment of chronic, severe spasticity of skeletal muscle in adults.

Posology and method of administration:

Adults: For the individual patient, the lowest dose compatible with optimal response is recommended.

A recommended dosage increment scale is shown below:

Week	*Recommended dosage*
First	One 25 mg capsule daily
Second	One 25 mg capsule twice daily
Third	Two 25 mg capsules twice daily
Fourth	Two 25 mg capsules three times daily
Fifth	Three 25 mg capsules three times daily
Sixth	Three 25 mg capsules four times daily
Seventh	One 100 mg capsule four times daily

Each dosage level should be maintained for seven days in order to determine the patient's response. Therapy with a dose four times daily may offer maximum benefit to some patients. The maximum daily dose should not exceed 400 mg. In view of the potential for hepatoxicity in long term use, if no observable benefit is derived from the administration of Dantrium after a total of 45 days, therapy should be discontinued.

Elderly: A similar dosage scheme should be used with the elderly.

Children: Dantrium is not recommended for use in children.

Contra-indications: Dantrium is contra-indicated where spasticity is utilised to sustain upright posture and balance in locomotion or whenever spasticity is utilised to obtain or maintain increased function. Dantrium is contra-indicated in patients with evidence of hepatic dysfunction. Dantrium is not indicated for the treatment of acute skeletal muscle spasm. Dantrium should not be administered to children.

Special warnings and special precautions for use: Fatal and non-fatal liver disorders of an idiosyncratic or hypersensitivity type may occur with Dantrium therapy.

At the start of Dantrium therapy, it is desirable to do liver function studies (SGOT/ALT, SGPT/AST, alkaline phosphatase, total bilirubin) for a baseline or to establish whether there is pre-existing liver disease. If baseline liver abnormalities exist and are confirmed, there is a clear possibility that the potential for Dantrium hepatoxicity could be enhanced, although such a possibility has not yet been established.

Liver function studies (e.g. serum, SGOT/AST, SGPT/ALT) should be performed at appropriate intervals during Dantrium therapy. If such studies reveal abnormal values, therapy should generally be discontinued. Only where benefits of the drug have been of major importance to the patient, should re-introduction or continuation of therapy be considered. Some patients have revealed a return to normal laboratory values in the face of continued therapy while others have not.

If symptoms compatible with hepatitis, accompanied by abnormalities in liver function tests or jaundice appear, Dantrium should be discontinued. If caused by Dantrium and detected early, the abnormalities in liver function have reverted to normal when the drug was discontinued.

Dantrium has been re-introduced in a few patients who have developed clinical signs, or elevated serum enzymes, of hepatocellular injury.

Re-introduction of Dantrium therapy should only be contemplated in patients who clearly need the drug, and only after complete reversal of the signs of hepatotoxicity and liver function tests. Patients being re-challenged with Dantrium should be hospital in-patients, and small, gradually increasing doses should be used. Laboratory test monitoring should be frequent, and the drug should be withdrawn immediately if there is any indication of recurrent liver abnormality. Some patients have reacted with unmistakable signs of liver abnormality upon administration of a challenge dose, whilst others have not.

The use of Dantrium with other potentially hepatotoxic drugs should be avoided.

There are isolated cases of possibly significant effects of Dantrium on the cardiovascular and respiratory systems. These cases also have other features suggesting a pre-disposition to cardiovascular disease, and impaired respiratory function, particularly obstructive pulmonary disease. Dantrium should be used with caution in such patients.

Dantrolene sodium showed some evidence of tumourgenicity at high dose levels in Sprague-Dawley female rats. However, these effects were not seen in other studies in Fischer 344 rats or HaM/ICR mice. There is no clinical evidence of carcinogenicity in humans, however, this possibility cannot be absolutely excluded.

Caution should be exercised in the simultaneous administration of tranquillising agents and alcohol.

Interaction with other medicaments and other forms of interaction: An idiosyncratic interaction between verapamil and intravenous Dantrium, involving hypotension, hyperkalaemia, and myocardial depression, has been reported as a single case. This interaction has been replicated in dogs and pigs.

Pregnancy and lactation: Although teratological studies in animals have proved satisfactory, the use of Dantrium is not advised in pregnant or nursing mothers.

Effects on ability to drive and use machines: Patients should be advised not to drive a motor vehicle or to undertake potentially dangerous work until Dantrium therapy has been stabilised, because some patients experience drowsiness and dizziness.

Undesirable effects: The most frequently reported unwanted effects associated with the use of Dantrium have been drowsiness, dizziness, weakness, general malaise, fatigue and diarrhoea. These effects are generally transient, occur early in treatment, and can often be obviated by careful determination and regulation of the dosage. Diarrhoea may be severe, and may necessitate temporary withdrawal of Dantrium. If diarrhoea recurs upon re-introduction of Dantrium, then Dantrium therapy should probably be withdrawn permanently. Other frequent side effects include anorexia, nausea, headache and skin rash. Less frequent side effects include constipation, dysphagia, speech disturbance, visual disturbance, confusion, nervousness, depression, seizures, increased urinary frequency, and insomnia. Rare reports include tachycardia, erratic blood pressure, dyspnoea, haematuria, crystalluria (unconfirmed reports), urinary incontinence, and urinary retention. Pleural effusion and/or pericarditis in patients using Dantrium have been rarely reported. Chills and fever have occasionally been reported.

Dantrium has a potential for hepatotoxicity. Symptomatic hepatitis (fatal and non-fatal) has been reported at various dose levels although the incidence is greater in patients taking more than 400 mg/day. Liver dysfunction as evidenced by blood chemical abnormalities alone (liver enzyme elevation) has been observed in patients exposed to Dantrium for varying periods of time.

Overt hepatitis has occurred at varying intervals after initiation of therapy, but has most frequently been observed between the second and twelfth month of treatment. The risk of hepatic injury appears to be greater in females, in patients over 30 years old and in patients taking concomitant medication. There is some evidence that hepatic injury is more likely in patients using concomitant oral oestrogen.

Overdose: For acute overdosage, general supportive measures and gastric lavage should be employed as well as measures to reduce the absorption of Dantrium. The theoretical possibility of crystalluria in overdose has not been reported for Dantrium, but would be treated according to general principles, including administration of fluids.

Pharmacological properties

Pharmacodynamic properties:

Molecular pharmacology: The receptor molecule for dantrolene has not been identified. Radiolabelled dantrolene sodium binds to specific components of the striated muscle cell, namely the t-tubules and the sarcoplasmic reticulum; however, the kinetics of binding varies between these two organelles. The binding of ryanodine is thought to compete with the binding of calcium in these organelles; further evidence for the specificity of binding is that dantrolene inhibits the binding of the insecticide ryanodine to heavy sarcoplasmic reticulum vesicles from rabbit skeletal muscle. Under some conditions, dantrolene will lower intra-sarcoplasmic calcium concentrations in the resting state. This may be more important in diseased muscle (e.g. in malignant hyperthermia in humans and swine stress syndrome) than in muscle with normal function.

Dantrolene does not bind to the same sites as calcium channel blocking drugs such as nitrendipine or calmodulin. There is no electrophysiological evidence that dantrolene interferes with the influx of calcium from outside the cell. This may be one reason why paralysis by dantrolene has never been reported in animals or man; the muscle cell has alternative sources of calcium which are not influenced by dantrolene.

Biochemical pharmacology: Whatever the molecular mechanism, the cardinal property of dantrolene sodium is that it lowers intracellular calcium concentration in skeletal muscle. Calcium concentrations may be lower in both the quiescent state, and as a result of a reduction in the release of calcium from the sarcoplasmic reticulum in response to a standard stimulus. This effect has been observed in striated muscle fibres from several species, and is not seen in myocardium. Fast fibres may be more sensitive than slow fibres to the action of dantrolene sodium.

Diverse other properties of dantrolene sodium have been observed *in vitro*, and in animal studies. Dantrolene sodium may inhibit the release of calcium from the smooth endoplasmic reticulum of smooth muscle, but the significance of this observation is questionable; for example, dantrolene sodium has no effect on isolated human urinary bladder smooth muscle. Calcium dependent, pre-synaptic neurotransmitter release may also be inhibited by dantrolene sodium. Again, the clinical significance of this has not been demonstrated.

Studies on isolated, functional muscle: Elevation of intracellular, free calcium ion concentration is an obligatory step in excitation-contraction coupling of skeletal muscle. Dantrolene sodium, therefore, acts as a muscle relaxant by a peripheral mechanism which is quite different, and easily distinguishable from neuromuscular junction blocking drugs. In contrast with compounds that relax skeletal muscle by acting principally on the central nervous system, dantrolene sodium acts directly on skeletal muscle cells. In rabbit atria, dantrolene sodium has no effect alone, but it may antagonise inotropic agents which act by increasing intramyocardial cell calcium e.g. the experimental drug anthopleurin-A.

Pharmacokinetic properties:
Absorption: Dantrium is easily and almost completely absorbed from the gastrointestinal tract. After dosing on an empty stomach, plasma dantrolene levels peak within three hours in most subjects.

Distribution: Dantrolene sodium is a highly lipophobic drug. In addition it lacks hydrophilicity. Dantrolene sodium binds to human serum albumin (HSA) with a molar ratio of 0.95 to 1.68 *in vitro*. The association constant *in vitro* is higher (2.3 to 5.4×10^{-5} per mol). *In vitro* dantrolene sodium can be displaced from HSA by warfarin, clofibrate and tolbutamide but these interactions have not been confirmed in humans (re manufacturer's database). Single intravenous dose studies suggest that the primary volume of distribution is about 15 litres. Single oral doses achieve peak plasma concentration of about a quarter of that for similarly sized intravenous dose.

Metabolism and excretion: The biological half life in plasma in most human subjects is between 5 and 9 hours, although half-lives as long as 12.1 ± 1.9 hours have been reported after a single intravenous dose. Inactivation is by hepatic metabolism in the first instance. There are two alternative pathways. Most of the drug is hydroxylated to 5-hydroxy-dantrolene. The minor pathway involves nitro-reduction to amino-dantrolene which is then acetylated (compound F-490). The 5-hydroxy metabolite is a muscle relaxant with nearly the same potency as the parent molecule, and may have a longer half life than the parent compound. Compound F-490 is much less potent and is probably inactive at the concentrations achieved in clinical samples. Metabolites are subsequently excreted in the urine in the ratio of 79 5-hydroxy-dantrolene: 17 compound F-490: 4 unaltered dantrolene (salt or free acid). The proportion of drug excreted in the faeces depends upon dose size.

Preclinical safety data: Sprague-Dawley female rats fed dantrolene sodium for 18 months at dosage levels of 15, 30 and 60 mg/kg/day showed an increased incidence of benign and malignant mammary tumours compared with concurrent controls. At the highest dose level, there was an increase in the incidence of benign hepatic lymphatic neoplasms. In a 30-month study at the same dose levels also in Sprague-Dawley rats, dantrolene sodium produced a decrease in the time of onset of mammary neoplasms. Female rats at the highest dose level showed an increased incidence of hepatic lymphangiomas and hepatic angiosarcomas.

The only drug-related effect seen in a 30-month study in Fischer-344 rats was a dose-related reduction in the time of onset of mammary and testicular tumours. A 24-month study in HaM/ICR mice revealed no evidence of carcinogenic activity.

The significance of carcinogenicity data relative to use of dantrolene sodium in humans is unknown.

Dantrolene sodium has produced positive results in the Ames S. Typhimurium bacterial mutagenesis assay in the presence and absence of a liver activating system.

Dantrolene sodium administered to male and female rats at dose levels up to 45 mg/kg/day showed no adverse effects on fertility or general reproductive performance.

Pharmaceutical particulars
List of excipients: Gelatin, starch, talc, magnesium stearate, lactose, E110, E171 and E172.

Incompatibilities: None.

Shelf life: Three years.

Special precautions for storage: Store below 30°C.

Nature and contents of container: Dantrium 100 mg capsules are supplied in polypropylene containers of 100 capsules.

Instructions for use/handling: A patient leaflet is provided for details of use and handling of the product.

Marketing authorisation number PL 0364/0016R

Date of first authorisation/renewal of authorisation 25 October 1989

Date of (partial) revision of the text June 1997

DANTRIUM* 25 mg CAPSULES

Qualitative and quantitative composition Dantrium 25 mg capsules contain 25 mg dantrolene sodium per capsule.

Pharmaceutical form Dantrium capsules are presented in orange/light brown capsules. The 25 mg capsule carries the monogram Dantrium 25 mg on the cap and 0149, 0030 and a single coding bar on the body.

Clinical particulars
Therapeutic indications: For the treatment of chronic, severe spasticity of skeletal muscle in adults.

Posology and method of administration:
Adults: For the individual patient, the lowest dose compatible with optimal response is recommended.

A recommended dosage increment scale is shown below:

Week	*Recommended dosage*
First	One 25 mg capsule daily
Second	One 25 mg capsule twice daily
Third	Two 25 mg capsules twice daily
Fourth	Two 25 mg capsules three times daily
Fifth	Three 25 mg capsules three times daily
Sixth	Three 25 mg capsules four times daily
Seventh	One 100 mg capsule four times daily

Each dosage level should be maintained for seven days in order to determine the patient's response. Therapy with a dose four times daily may offer maximum benefit to some patients. The maximum daily dose should not exceed 400 mg. In view of the potential for hepatoxicity in long term use, if no observable benefit is derived from the administration of Dantrium after a total of 45 days, therapy should be discontinued.

Elderly: A similar dosage scheme should be used with the elderly.

Children: Dantrium is not recommended for use in children.

Contra-indications: Dantrium is contra-indicated where spasticity is utilised to sustain upright posture and balance in locomotion or whenever spasticity is utilised to obtain or maintain increased function. Dantrium is contra-indicated in patients with evidence of hepatic dysfunction. Dantrium is not indicated for the treatment of acute skeletal muscle spasm. Dantrium should not be administered to children.

Special warnings and special precautions for use: Fatal and non-fatal liver disorders of an idiosyncratic or hypersensitivity type may occur with Dantrium therapy.

At the start of Dantrium therapy, it is desirable to do liver function studies (SGOT/ALT, SGPT/AST, alkaline phosphatase, total bilirubin) for a baseline or to establish whether there is pre-existing liver disease. If baseline liver abnormalities exist and are confirmed, there is a clear possibility that the potential for Dantrium hepatoxicity could be enhanced, although such a possibility has not yet been established.

Liver function studies (e.g. serum, SGOT/AST, SGPT/ALT) should be performed at appropriate intervals during Dantrium therapy. If such studies reveal abnormal values, therapy should generally be discontinued. Only where benefits of the drug have been of major importance to the patient, should re-introduction or continuation of therapy be considered. Some patients have revealed a return to normal laboratory values in the face of continued therapy while others have not.

If symptoms compatible with hepatitis, accompanied by abnormalities in liver function tests or jaundice appear, Dantrium should be discontinued. If caused by Dantrium and detected early, the abnormalities in liver function have reverted to normal when the drug was discontinued.

Dantrium has been re-introduced in a few patients who have developed clinical signs, or elevated serum enzymes, of hepatocellular injury.

Re-introduction of Dantrium therapy should only be contemplated in patients who clearly need the drug, and only after complete reversal of the signs of hepatotoxicity and liver function tests. Patients being re-challenged with Dantrium should be hospital in-patients, and small, gradually increasing doses should be used. Laboratory test monitoring should be frequent, and the drug should be withdrawn immediately if there is any indication of recurrent liver abnormality. Some patients have reacted with unmistakable signs of liver abnormality upon administration of a challenge dose, whilst others have not.

The use of Dantrium with other potentially hepatotoxic drugs should be avoided.

There are isolated cases of possibly significant effects of Dantrium on the cardiovascular and respiratory systems. These cases also have other features suggesting a pre-disposition to cardiovascular disease, and impaired respiratory function, particularly obstructive pulmonary disease. Dantrium should be used with caution in such patients.

Dantrolene sodium showed some evidence of tumourgenicity at high dose levels in Sprague-Dawley female rats. However, these effects were not seen in other studies in Fischer 344 rats or HaM/ICR mice. There is no clinical evidence of carcinogenicity in humans, however, this possibility cannot be absolutely excluded.

Caution should be exercised in the simultaneous administration of tranquillising agents and alcohol.

Interaction with other medicaments and other forms of interaction: An idiosyncratic interaction between verapamil and intravenous Dantrium, involving hypotension, hyperkalaemia, and myocardial depression, has been reported as a single case. This interaction has been replicated in dogs and pigs.

Pregnancy and lactation: Although teratological studies in animals have proved satisfactory, the use of Dantrium is not advised in pregnant or nursing mothers.

Effects on ability to drive and use machines: Patients should be advised not to drive a motor vehicle or to undertake potentially dangerous work until Dantrium therapy has been stabilised, because some patients experience drowsiness and dizziness.

Undesirable effects: The most frequently reported unwanted effects associated with the use of Dantrium have been drowsiness, dizziness, weakness, general malaise, fatigue and diarrhoea. These effects are generally transient, occur early in treatment, and can often be obviated by careful determination and regulation of the dosage. Diarrhoea may be severe, and may necessitate temporary withdrawal of Dantrium. If diarrhoea recurs upon re-introduction of Dantrium, then Dantrium therapy should probably be withdrawn permanently. Other frequent side effects include anorexia, nausea, headache and skin rash. Less frequent side effects include constipation, dysphagia, speech disturbance, visual disturbance, confusion, nervousness, depression, seizures, increased urinary frequency, and insomnia. Rare reports include tachycardia, erratic blood pressure, dyspnoea, haematuria, crystalluria (unconfirmed reports), urinary incontinence, and urinary retention. Pleural effusion and/or pericarditis in patients using Dantrium have been rarely reported. Chills and fever have occasionally been reported.

Dantrium has a potential for hepatoxicity. Symptomatic hepatitis (fatal and non-fatal) has been reported at various dose levels although the incidence is greater in patients taking more than 400 mg/day. Liver dysfunction as evidenced by blood chemical abnormalities alone (liver enzyme elevation) has been observed in patients exposed to Dantrium for varying periods of time.

Overt hepatitis has occurred at varying intervals after initiation of therapy, but has most frequently been observed between the second and twelfth month of treatment. The risk of hepatic injury appears to be greater in females, in patients over 30 years old and in patients taking concomitant medication. There is some evidence that hepatic injury is more likely in patients using concomitant oral oestrogen.

Overdose: For acute overdosage, general supportive measures and gastric lavage should be employed as well as measures to reduce the absorption of Dantrium. The theoretical possibility of crystalluria in overdose has not been reported for Dantrium, but would be treated according to general principles, including administration of fluids.

Pharmacological properties
Pharmacodynamic properties:
Molecular pharmacology: The receptor molecule for dantrolene has not been identified. Radiolabelled dantrolene sodium binds to specific components of the striated muscle cell, namely the t-tubules and the sarcoplasmic reticulum; however, the kinetics of binding varies between these two organelles. The binding of ryanodine is thought to compete with the binding of calcium in these organelles; further evidence for the specificity of binding is that dantrolene inhibits the binding of the insecticide ryanodine to heavy sarcoplasmic reticulum vesicles from rabbit skeletal muscle. Under some conditions, dantrolene will lower intra-sarcoplasmic calcium concentrations

in the resting state. This may be more important in diseased muscle (e.g. in malignant hyperthermia in humans and swine stress syndrome) than in muscle with normal function.

Dantrolene does not bind to the same sites as calcium channel blocking drugs such as nitrendipine or calmodulin. There is no electrophysiological evidence that dantrolene interferes with the influx of calcium from outside the cell. This may be one reason why paralysis by dantrolene has never been reported in animals or man; the muscle cell has alternative sources of calcium which are not influenced by dantrolene.

Biochemical pharmacology: Whatever the molecular mechanism, the cardinal property of dantrolene sodium is that it lowers intracellular calcium concentration in skeletal muscle. Calcium concentrations may be lower in both the quiescent state, and as a result of a reduction in the release of calcium from the sarcoplasmic reticulum in response to a standard stimulus. This effect has been observed in striated muscle fibres from several species, and is not seen in myocardium. Fast fibres may be more sensitive than slow fibres to the action of dantrolene sodium.

Diverse other properties of dantrolene sodium have been observed *in vitro*, and in animal studies. Dantrolene sodium may inhibit the release of calcium from the smooth endoplasmic reticulum of smooth muscle, but the significance of this observation is questionable; for example, dantrolene sodium has no effect on isolated human urinary bladder smooth muscle. Calcium dependent, pre-synaptic neurotransmitter release may also be inhibited by dantrolene sodium. Again, the clinical significance of this has not been demonstrated.

Studies on isolated, functional muscle: Elevation of intracellular, free calcium ion concentration is an obligatory step in excitation-contraction coupling of skeletal muscle. Dantrolene sodium, therefore, acts as a muscle relaxant by a peripheral mechanism which is quite different, and easily distinguishable from neuromuscular junction blocking drugs. In contrast with compounds that relax skeletal muscle by acting principally on the central nervous system, dantrolene sodium acts directly on skeletal muscle cells. In rabbit atria, dantrolene sodium has no effect alone, but it may antagonise inotropic agents which act by increasing intramyocardial cell calcium e.g. the experimental drug anthopleurin-A.

Pharmacokinetic properties:

Absorption: Dantrium is easily and almost completely absorbed from the gastrointestinal tract. After dosing on an empty stomach, plasma dantrolene levels peak within three hours in most subjects.

Distribution: Dantrolene sodium is a highly lipophobic drug. In addition it lacks hydrophilicity. Dantrolene sodium binds to human serum albumin (HSA) with a molar ratio of 0.95 to 1.68 *in vitro*. The association constant *in vitro* is higher (2.3 to 5.4×10^{-5} per mol). *In vitro* dantrolene sodium can be displaced from HSA by warfarin, clofibrate and tolbutamide but these interactions have not been confirmed in humans (re manufacturer's database). Single intravenous dose studies suggest that the primary volume of distribution is about 15 litres. Single oral doses achieve peak plasma concentration of about a quarter of that for similarly sized intravenous dose.

Metabolism and excretion: The biological half life in plasma in most human subjects is between 5 and 9 hours, although half-lives as long as 12.1 ± 1.9 hours have been reported after a single intravenous dose. Inactivation is by hepatic metabolism in the first instance. There are two alternative pathways. Most of the drug is hydroxylated to 5-hydroxy-dantrolene. The minor pathway involves nitro-reduction to aminodantrolene which is then acetylated (compound F-490). The 5-hydroxy metabolite is a muscle relaxant with nearly the same potency as the parent molecule, and may have a longer half life than the parent compound. Compound F-490 is much less potent and is probably inactive at the concentrations achieved in clinical samples. Metabolites are subsequently excreted in the urine in the ratio of 79 5-hydroxydantrolene: 17 compound F-490: 4 unaltered dantrolene (salt or free acid). The proportion of drug excreted in the faeces depends upon dose size.

Preclinical safety data: Sprague-Dawley female rats fed dantrolene sodium for 18 months at dosage levels of 15, 30 and 60 mg/kg/day showed an increased incidence of benign and malignant mammary tumours compared with concurrent controls. At the highest dose level, there was an increase in the incidence of benign hepatic lymphatic neoplasms. In a 30-month study at the same dose levels also in Sprague-Dawley rats, dantrolene sodium produced a decrease in the time of onset of mammary neoplasms. Female rats at the highest dose level showed an increased incidence of hepatic lymphangiomas and hepatic angiosarcomas.

The only drug-related effect seen in a 30-month study in Fischer-344 rats was a dose-related reduction in the time of onset of mammary and testicular tumours. A 24-month study in HaM/ICR mice revealed no evidence of carcinogenic activity.

The significance of carcinogenicity data relative to use of dantrolene sodium in humans is unknown.

Dantrolene sodium has produced positive results in the Ames S. Typhimurium bacterial mutagenesis assay in the presence and absence of a liver activating system.

Dantrolene sodium administered to male and female rats at dose levels up to 45 mg/kg/day showed no adverse effects on fertility or general reproductive performance.

Pharmaceutical particulars

List of excipients: Gelatin, starch, talc, magnesium stearate, lactose, E110, E171 and E172.

Incompatibilities: None.

Shelf life: Three years.

Special precautions for storage: Store below 30°C.

Nature and contents of container: Dantrium 25 mg capsules are supplied in polypropylene containers of 100 capsules.

Instructions for use/handling: A patient leaflet is provided for details of use and handling of the product.

Marketing authorisation number PL 0364/0015R

Date of first authorisation/renewal of authorisation 25 October 1989

Date of (partial) revision of the text June 1997

DIDRONEL* 200 mg TABLETS

Qualitative and quantitative composition Each tablet contains 200 mg of Etidronate Disodium, USP.

Pharmaceutical form White rectangular tablets marked with 'P&G' on one face and '402' on the other.

Clinical particulars

Therapeutic indications:

Paget's disease of bone: Effectiveness has been demonstrated primarily in patients with polyostotic Paget's disease with symptoms of pain and with clinically significant elevations of urinary hydroxyproline and serum alkaline phosphatase. In other circumstances in which there is extensive involvement of the skull or the spine with the prospect of irreversible neurological damage, or when a weight-bearing bone may be involved, the use of Didronel may also be considered.

Posology and method of administration: 5 mg/kg/day to 20 mg/kg/day as detailed below.

Didronel should be given on an empty stomach. It is recommended that patients take the therapy with water, at the mid point of a four hour fast (i.e. two hours before and two after food).

Adults and elderly: The recommended initial dose of Didronel for most patients is 5 mg/kg body weight/day, for a period not exceeding six months. Doses above 10 mg/kg should be reserved for use when there is an overriding requirement for suppression of increased bone turnover associated with Paget's disease or when the patient requires more prompt reduction of elevated cardiac output. Treatment with doses above 10 mg/kg/day should be approached cautiously and should not exceed three months duration. Doses in excess of 20 mg/kg/day are not recommended.

Re-treatment should be undertaken only after a drug-free period of at least three months and after it is evident that reactivation of the disease has occurred and biochemical indices of the disease have become substantially re-elevated or approach pretreatment values (approximately twice the upper limit of normal or 75% of pre-treatment value). In no case should duration of treatment exceed the maximum duration of the initial treatment. Premature re-treatment should be avoided. In clinical trials the biochemical improvements obtained during drug therapy have generally persisted for a period of three months to 2 years after drug withdrawal.

Daily dosage guide

Body weight		Required daily regimen of 200 mg tablets		
Kilograms	Stones	5 mg/kg*	10 mg/kg*	20 mg/kg†
50	8	1	3	5
60	9.5	2	3	6
70	11	2	4	7
80	12.5	2	4	8
90	14	2	5	9

* Course of therapy – 6 months
† Course of therapy – 3 months

Children: Disorders of bone in children, referred to as juvenile Paget's disease, have been reported rarely. The relationship to adult Paget's disease has not been established. Didronel has not been studied in children for Paget's disease.

Contra-indications: None.

Special warnings and special precautions for use: In Pagetic patients the physician should adhere to the recommended dose regimen in order to avoid overtreatment with Didronel. The response to therapy may be of slow onset and may continue even for months after treatment with the drug has been discontinued. Dosage should not be increased prematurely nor should treatment be resumed before there is clear evidence of reactivation of the disease process. Retreatment should not be initiated until the patient has had at least a three-month drug-free interval.

Didronel is not metabolised but excreted unchanged via the kidney; therefore, a reduced dose should be used in patients with mild renal impairment and treatment of patients with moderate to severe renal impairment should be avoided.

It is recommended that serum phosphate, serum alkaline phosphatase and if possible urinary hydroxyproline be measured before commencing medication and at three month intervals during treatment. If after three months of medication the pre-treatment levels have not been reduced by at least 25%, the patient may be relatively resistant to therapy. If the serum phosphate level is unchanged in the 'resistant' patient, consideration should be given to increasing the dose since the absorption of pharmacologically active amounts of Didronel is typically accompanied by a rise in serum phosphate. This rise usually correlates with reductions in the biochemical indices of disease activity. If after three or more months of medication elevations of serum phosphate above the upper limit of normal are not accompanied by clinical or biochemical evidence of reduced activity, resistance of the disease to the action of Didronel is probable and termination of Didronel medication should be considered. Patients in whom serum phosphate elevations are high and reductions of disease activity are low may be particularly prone to retarded mineralisation of new osteoid. In those cases where 200 mg per day (a single tablet) may be excessive, doses may be administered less frequently.

Patients with Paget's disease of bone should maintain an adequate intake of calcium and vitamin D. Patients with low vitamin D and calcium intake may be particularly sensitive to drugs that affect calcium homeostasis and should be closely monitored during Didronel therapy.

Etidronate disodium does not adversely affect serum levels of parathyroid hormone or calcium.

Hyperphosphataemia has been observed in patients receiving etidronate disodium, usually in association with doses of 10–20 mg/kg/day. No adverse effects have been traced to this, and it does not constitute grounds for discontinuing therapy. It is apparently due to a drug-related increase in renal tubular reabsorption of phosphate. Serum phosphate levels generally return to normal 2–4 weeks post therapy.

Didronel therapy has been withheld from patients with enterocolitis because of increased frequency of bowel movements.

Increased or recurrent bone pain at existing Pagetic sites and/or the appearance of pain at sites previously asymptomatic have been reported at a dose of 5 mg/kg/day.

Fractures are recognised as a common feature in patients with Paget's disease. There has been no evidence of increased risk of fractures at the recommended dose at 5 mg/kg/day for six months. At doses of 20 mg/kg/day in excess of three months' duration, mineralisation of newly formed osteoid may be impaired and the risk of fracture may be increased. The risk of fracture may also be greater in patients with extensive and severe disease, a history of multiple fractures, and/or rapidly advancing osteolytic lesions. It is therefore recommended that the drug is discontinued when fractures occur and therapy not reinstated until the fracture healing is complete.

The incidence of osteogenic sarcoma is known to be increased in Paget's disease. Pagetic lesions, with or without therapy, may appear by X-ray to progress markedly, possibly with some loss of definition of periosteal margins. Such lesions should be evaluated carefully to differentiate these from osteogenic sarcoma.

Interaction with other medicaments and other forms of interaction: Food in the stomach or upper portions of the small intestine, particularly materials with a high calcium content such as milk, may reduce absorption of etidronate disodium. Vitamins with mineral supplements such as iron, calcium supplements, laxatives containing magnesium, or antacids containing calcium or aluminium should not be taken within two hours of dosing etidronate disodium.

Pregnancy and lactation: The safety of this medicinal product for use in human pregnancy has not been established. Reproductive studies have shown skeletal abnormalities in rats. It is therefore recommended that Didronel should not be used in women of childbearing potential unless adequate contraceptive measures are taken.

It is not known whether this drug is excreted in human milk, and therefore caution should be exercised when Didronel is administered to a nursing woman.

Effects on ability to drive and use machines: Etidronate disodium does not interfere with the ability to drive or use machines.

Undesirable effects:

Gastro-intestinal: The most common effects reported are diarrhoea and nausea.

Dermatological/hypersensitivity: Hypersensitivity reactions, including angio-oedema/urticaria, rash and/or pruritus, have been reported rarely.

Haematological: In patients receiving etidronate disodium, there have been rare reports of leucopenia, agranulocytosis and pancytopenia; however a causal relationship has not been established.

Overdose: Overdose would manifest as the signs and symptoms of hypocalcaemia. Treatment should involve cessation of therapy and correction of hypocalcaemia with administration of Ca^{2+} intravenously.

Pharmacological properties

Pharmacodynamic properties: Etidronate acts primarily on bone. It can inhibit the formation, growth and dissolution of hydroxyapatite crystals and amorphous precursors by chemisorption to calcium phosphate surfaces. Inhibition of crystal resorption occurs at lower doses than are required for the inhibition of crystal growth. Both effects increase as dose increases.

Pharmacokinetic properties: Etidronate is not metabolised. Absorption averages about 1% of an oral dose of 5 mg/kg body weight/day. This increases to about 1.5% at 10 mg/kg/day and 6% at 20% mg/kg/day. Most of the drug is cleared from the blood within 6 hours. Within 24 hours about half of the absorbed dose is excreted in the urine. The remainder is chemically absorbed to bone, especially to areas of elevated osteogenesis, and is slowly eliminated. Unabsorbed drug is excreted in the faeces.

Preclinical safety data: In long term studies in mice and rats, there was no evidence of carcinogenicity with etidronate disodium. All *in vitro* and *in vivo* assays conducted to assess the mutagenic potential of etidronate disodium have been negative.

Pharmaceutical particulars

List of excipients: Starch, magnesium stearate and microcrystalline cellulose.

Incompatibilities: See *Interaction with other medicaments and other forms of interaction.*

Shelf life: Four years.

Special precautions for storage: None.

Nature and contents of container: Supplied in high density polypropylene bottles or amber glass bottles of 60 tablets.

Instructions for use/handling: None.

Marketing authorisation number PL 0364/0039

Date of first authorisation/renewal of authorisation 26th November 1987

Date of (partial) revision of the text October 1998

DIDRONEL* PMO

Qualitative and quantitative composition A two component therapy consisting of 14 Didronel 400 mg tablets and 76 Cacit 500 mg effervescent tablets (equivalent to 500 mg elemental calcium). Each Didronel tablet contains 400 mg of etidronate disodium, USP. Each Cacit 500 mg effervescent tablet contains 1250 mg of calcium carbonate, PhEur, which when dispersed in water provides 500 mg of elemental calcium as calcium citrate.

Pharmaceutical form Each Didronel 400 mg tablet is white, capsule-shaped and marked with 'NE' on one face and '406' on the other. The Cacit 500 mg effervescent tablet is round, flat, white with pink speckles and has a distinctive orange flavour.

Clinical particulars

Therapeutic indications: Treatment of osteoporosis, and prevention of bone loss in postmenopausal women considered at risk of developing osteoporosis. Didronel PMO is particularly indicated in patients who are unable or unwilling to take oestrogen replacement therapy. Didronel PMO is also indicated for the prevention and treatment of corticosteroid-induced osteoporosis.

Posology and method of administration: Didronel PMO therapy is a long-term cyclical regimen administered in 90-day cycles. Each cycle consists of Didronel 400 mg tablets for the first 14 days, followed by Cacit 500 mg tablets for the remaining 76 days.

The majority of patients have been treated for 3 years, with a small number of patients treated for up to 7 years, with no clinical safety concerns. The optimum duration of treatment has not been established.

**Didronel 400 mg component:* One tablet should be taken each day for 14 consecutive days on an empty stomach. It is recommended that patients take the tablet with water at the midpoint of a four hour fast (i.e. two hours before and two hours after food).

**Cacit 500 mg component:* Following 14 days treatment with Didronel 400 mg tablets, one Cacit tablet should be taken on a daily basis. The Cacit tablet should be dissolved in water and drunk immediately after complete dissolution.

Adult and elderly: The patient should adhere to the prescribed regimen above. Modification of the dosage for the elderly is not required.

Children: No data exists in the use of this therapy in juvenile osteoporosis.

Contra-indications: Known hypersensitivity to etidronate disodium. Treatment of patients with severe renal impairment. Patients with hypercalcaemia or hypercalciuria. Not recommended in patients with clinically overt osteomalacia. Use in pregnancy and lactation.

Special warnings and special precautions for use: Clinicians should advise patients to adhere to the recommended treatment regimen, and compliance pack.

In long-term trials no clinical osteomalacia was observed in patients receiving cyclical etidronate. Following long-term therapy in excess of 4 years, analysis of bone biopsies showed an increased prevalence of peritrabecular fibrosis and histologically defined atypical and focal osteomalacia (not to be confused with the syndrome associated with 'clinical osteomalacia' due to vitamin D deficiency). In addition, these laboratory findings were not associated with any clinical consequences. Osteoid, which may accumulate at high doses of continuous etidronate therapy (10–20 mg/kg/day) mineralises normally after discontinuation of therapy.

Therapy should be withheld from patients with enterocolitis because of increased frequency of bowel movements.

Caution should be taken in patients with impaired renal function, or a history of renal stone formation.

Etidronate disodium does not adversely effect serum levels of parathyroid hormone or calcium.

Hyperphosphataemia has been observed in patients receiving etidronate disodium, usually in association with doses of 10–20 mg/kg/day. No adverse effects have been traced to this, and it does not constitute grounds for discontinuing therapy. It is apparently due to a drug-related increase in renal tubular reabsorption of phosphate. Serum phosphate levels generally return to normal 2–4 weeks post therapy.

Interaction with other medicaments and other forms of interaction: Food in the stomach or upper gastro-intestinal tract, particularly materials with a high calcium content such as milk, may reduce absorption of etidronate disodium. Vitamins with mineral supplements such as iron, calcium supplements, laxatives containing magnesium, or antacids containing calcium or aluminium should not be taken within two hours of dosing etidronate disodium.

A small number of patients in clinical trials (involving more than 600 patients) received either thiazide diuretics or intravaginal oestrogen while on this treatment. The concomitant use of either of these agents did no interfere with the positive effects of the therapy on vertebral bone mass or fracture rates.

Calcium salts may reduce the absorption of some drugs, e.g. tetracyclines. It is therefore suggested that administration of Cacit tablets be separated from these products by at least three hours.

Vitamin D causes an increase in calcium absorption and plasma calcium levels may continue to rise after stopping vitamin D therapy. Concomitant administration of Cacit tablets and vitamin D should therefore be carried out with caution.

The effects of digoxin and other cardiac glycosides may be accentuated by calcium and toxicity may be produced, especially in combination with vitamin D therapy.

Pregnancy and lactation: Contra-indicated.

Effects on ability to drive and use machines: Etidronate disodium does not interfere with the ability to drive or use machines.

Undesirable effects:

Gastro-intestinal: In clinical studies of 2–3 years duration, the incidence of these events were comparable to placebo. The most common effects reported in order of incidence were diarrhoea, nausea, flatulence, dyspepsia, abdominal pain, constipation and vomiting.

Dermatological/hypersensitivity: Hypersensitivity reactions including angio-oedema, urticaria, rash and/or pruritus have been reported rarely.

Nervous system: Headache, paraesthesia, peripheral neuropathy.

Haematological: There have been rare reports of leucopaenia, agranulocytosis and pancytopaenia; however a causal relationship has not been established.

Other: Occasional mild leg cramps have been reported in less than 5% of patients on the Didronel PMO regimen. These cramps were transient, often nocturnal and generally associated with other underlying conditions.

Overdose: Clinical experience of acute overdosage with etidronate is limited and unlikely with this compliance kit. Theoretically it would be manifested as the signs and symptoms of hypocalcaemia and possibly paraesthesia of the fingers. Treatment would consist of gastric lavage to remove unabsorbed drug along with correction of hypocalcaemia with administration of Ca^{2+} intravenously.

Prolonged continuous treatment (chronic overdose) has been reported to cause nephrotic syndrome and fractures.

Pharmacological properties

Pharmacodynamic properties: Etidronate in an intermittent cyclical regimen, works indirectly to increase bone mass. By timing delivery and withdrawal, the etidronate disodium component acts to modulate osteoclasts and reduce the mean resorption depth of the affected basic multicellular units (BMU). Calcium is an essential element which has been shown to help prevent bone loss.

Epidemiological studies have suggested that there are a number of risk factors associated with post-menopausal osteoporosis, such as early menopause, a family history of osteoporosis, prolonged exposure to corticosteroid therapy, small and thin skeletal frame and excessive cigarette smoking.

Pharmacokinetic properties: Within 24 hours, about one half of the absorbed dose of etidronate is excreted in the urine. The remainder is chemically absorbed on bone and is slowly eliminated. Unabsorbed drug is excreted in the faeces. Etidronate disodium is not metabolised. After oral doses of up to 1600 mg of the disodium salt, the amount of drug absorbed is approximately 3–4%. In normal subjects, plasma half life ($t_{\frac{1}{2}}$) of etidronate, based on non-compartmental pharmacokinetics is 1–6 hours.

Calcium carbonate is converted into soluble calcium salts in the stomach under the influence of hydrochloric acid. 30–80% of orally ingested calcium is absorbed both by active transport (primarily in the upper small intestine) and by passive diffusion. The distribution of calcium in the body is subject to the mechanism of physiological regulation controlled by parathyroid hormone, calcitonin, calciferol and other hormones.

When calcium effervescent tablets are added to water, insoluble calcium carbonate is converted into calcium citrate.

Preclinical safety data: In long-term studies in mice and rats, there was no evidence of carcinogenicity with etidronate disodium. All *in vitro* and *in vivo* assays conducted to assess the mutagenic potential of etidronate disodium have been negative.

Pharmaceutical particulars

List of excipients: Etidronate disodium tablets contain microcrystalline cellulose, pregelatinised starch and magnesium stearate. Cacit tablets contain citric acid, sodium saccharin, sodium cyclamate, sunset yellow (E110) and orange flavouring.

Incompatibilities: None.

Shelf life: The expiry date for the compliance pack should not exceed 3 years from the date of its manufacture.

Special precautions for storage: Store in a dry place below 30°C. Since Cacit 500 mg tablets are hygroscopic, the stopper should be carefully replaced after use.

Nature and contents of container: 14 Didronel 400 mg tablets in a blister plus four polypropylene tubes, each containing 19 Cacit 500 mg tablets, all packaged in a compliance kit.

Instructions for use/handling: None.

Marketing authorisation number PL 0364/0051

Date of first authorisation/renewal of authorisation 1 November 1991

Date of (partial) revision of the text May 1997

FURADANTIN* TABLETS

Qualitative and quantitative composition Furadantin tablets contain 50 mg or 100 mg Nitrofurantoin PhEur.

Pharmaceutical form Furadantin tablets are yellow and pentagonal. Each tablet has a break line on one face and the tablet strength on the opposite face.

Clinical particulars
Therapeutic indications: For the treatment of and prophylaxis against acute or recurrent, uncomplicated lower urinary tract infections or pyelitis either spontaneous or following surgical procedures.

Nitrofurantoin is specifically indicated for the treatment of infections due to susceptible strains of *Escherichia coli, Enterococci, Staphylococci, Citrobacter, Klebsiella* and *Enterobacter.*

Most strains of *Proteus* and *Serratia* are resistant. All *Pseudomonas* strains are resistant.

Furadantin is not indicated for the treatment of associated renal cortical or peri-nephric abscesses.

Posology and method of administration:
Adults and children over ten years of age: The dose should be taken with food or milk (e.g. at meal times).

Acute uncomplicated urinary tract infections: 50 mg four times daily for seven days.

Severe chronic recurrent infections: 100 mg four times daily for seven days. In the event of severe nausea the dose may be reduced, but not below the adult equivalent of 200 mg/day. Should nausea persist the drug should be withdrawn.

Long term suppressive therapy: 50–100 mg once a day at bedtime is suggested.

Surgical prophylaxis: 50 mg four times daily on the day of the procedure and for the three days after.

Elderly: Provided there is no significant renal impairment, the dosage should be that for any normal adult.

Children over the age of three months:
Acute urinary tract infections: 3 mg/kg/day in four divided doses for seven days.

Suppressive therapy: 1 mg/kg/day once a day.

Contra-indications: Patients suffering from renal dysfunction with a creatinine clearance of less than 60 ml/minute or elevated serum creatinine.

In infants under three months of age as well as pregnant patients at term (during labour and delivery) because of the theoretical possibility of haemolytic anaemia in the foetus or in the newborn infant due to immature erythrocyte enzyme systems.

Patients with known hypersensitivity to nitrofurantoin or other nitrofurans.

Special warnings and special precautions for use: Gastrointestinal reactions may be minimised by taking the drug with food or milk or by adjustment of dosage.

Nitrofurantoin is not effective for the treatment of parenchymal infections of a unilaterally non-functioning kidney.

Nitrofurantoin should be used with caution in patients with pulmonary disease, hepatic dysfunction, neurological disorders, allergic diathesis, anaemia, diabetes mellitus, electrolyte imbalance, and vitamin B (particularly folate) deficiency.

Nitrofurantoin may cause haemolysis in patients with glucose-6-phosphate dehydrogenase deficiency (ten percent of black patients and a variable percentage of ethnic groups of Mediterranean, Near Eastern and Asian origin). Haemolysis ceases when the drug is discontinued.

Discontinue treatment with nitrofurantoin if otherwise unexplained pulmonary, hepatotoxic, haematological or neurologic syndromes occur. For long term treatment monitor patient closely for appearance of hepatic, pulmonary or neurological symptoms and other evidence of toxicity.

Interaction with other medicaments and other forms of interaction: Concomitant administration of magnesium trisilicate with nitrofurantoin reduces absorption.

Uricosuric drugs such as probenecid and sulphinpyrazone may inhibit renal tubular secretion of nitrofurantoin. The resulting increase in serum levels may increase toxicity. Decreased urinary levels could reduce its efficacy as a urinary tract antibacterial.

Concurrent use with quinolones is not recommended.

There may be decreased antibacterial activity for nitrofurantoin in the presence of carbonic anhydrase inhibitors and urine alkalinising agents.

Pregnancy and lactation: Animal studies with nitrofurantoin have shown no teratogenic effects. Nitrofurantoin has been in extensive clinical use since 1952 and its suitability in human pregnancy has been well documented.

Nitrofurantoin is however contra-indicated in infants under three months of age and in pregnant women during *labour and delivery,* because of the possible risk of haemolysis of the infants immature red cells.

Effects on ability to drive and use machines: Furadantin does not interfere with the ability to drive or use machines.

Undesirable effects:
Respiratory: If any of the following respiratory reactions occur the drug should be discontinued.

Acute pulmonary reactions usually occur within the first week of treatment and are reversible with cessation of therapy.

Subacute reactions may take several months to resolve once the drug has been stopped.

Chronic pulmonary reactions rarely occur in patients who have received continuous therapy for six months or longer and are more common in elderly patients. Changes in ECG have occurred, associated with pulmonary reactions. Symptoms such as fever, chills, cough and dyspnoea may be significant. Collapse and cyanosis have seldom been reported. The severity of chronic pulmonary reactions and their degree of resolution appear to be related to the duration of therapy after the first clinical signs appear. It is important to recognise symptoms as early as possible. Pulmonary function may be impaired permanently, even after cessation of therapy.

Hepatic: Hepatic reactions including cholestatic jaundice and chronic active hepatitis, both of which occur rarely. Fatalities have been reported. Cholestatic jaundice is generally associated with short-term therapy (usually up to two weeks). Chronic active hepatitis, occasionally leading to hepatic necrosis is generally associated with long-term therapy (usually after six months). The onset may be insidious. Treatment should be stopped at the first sign of hepatotoxicity.

Neurological: Peripheral neuropathy (including optical neuritis) with symptoms of sensory as well as motor involvement, which may become severe or irreversible, has been reported infrequently. Less frequent reactions of unknown causal relationship are depression, euphoria, confusion, psychotic reactions, nystagmus, vertigo, dizziness, asthenia, headache and drowsiness. Treatment should be stopped at the first sign of neurological involvement.

Gastrointestinal: Nausea and anorexia have been reported. Emesis, abdominal pain and diarrhoea are less common gastrointestinal reactions.

Hypersensitivity: Exfoliative dermatitis and erythema multiforme (including Stevens-Johnson syndrome) have been reported rarely.

Allergic skin reactions manifesting as angioneurotic oedema, maculopapular, erythematous or eczematous eruptions, urticaria, rash, and pruritus have occurred. Lupus-like syndrome associated with pulmonary reaction to nitrofurantoin has been reported.

Other hypersensitivity reactions include anaphylaxis, sialadenitis, pancreatitis, drug fever, and arthralgia.

Haematological: Agranulocytosis, leucopenia, granulocytopaenia, haemolytic anaemia, thrombocytopaenia, glucose-6-phosphate dehydrogenase deficiency, anaemia, megaloblastic anaemia and eosinophilia have occurred. Cessation of therapy has generally returned the blood picture to normal. Aplastic anaemia has been reported rarely.

Other: Transient alopecia and benign intercranial hypertension.

Superinfections by fungi or resistant organisms such as Pseudomonas may occur. However, these are limited to the genito-urinary tract.

Overdose: Symptoms and signs of overdosage include gastric irritation, nausea and vomiting. There is no known specific antidote. Nitrofurantoin can be haemodialysed. Standard treatment is by induction of emesis or by gastric lavage in cases of recent ingestion. Monitoring of full blood count, liver function tests and pulmonary function, are recommended. A high fluid intake should be maintained to promote urinary excretion of the drug.

Pharmacological properties
Pharmacodynamic properties: Nitrofurantoin is a broad spectrum antibacterial agent, active against the majority of urinary tract pathogens. The mechanism of action of nitrofurantoin is based on reduction to reactive intermediates. These inhibit enzymes involved in energy metabolism, such as in the Krebs cycle, interfering with the energy supply for normal growth and maintenance of bacteria. They also bind to bacterial ribosomal proteins at different sites, resulting in disruption of bacterial protein synthesis. Transferable resistance to nitrofurantoin is a rare phenomenon. There is no cross resistance to antibiotics and sulphonamides.

Pharmacokinetic properties: Nitrofurantoin is readily absorbed in the upper gastrointestinal tract. Intake with food or milk increases absorption. Nitrofurantoin is highly soluble in urine but plasma concentrations are low with peak levels usually less than 1 mg/ml.

Nitrofurantoin is loosely bound to plasma albumin (60–70%). The molecule is readily distributed into intra and extracellular compartments. However, substantial tissue concentrations are not expected since the drug is rapidly excreted and readily degraded by tissue enzymes. The drug crosses the placenta in small amounts.

The elimination half life in blood or plasma after IV injection is about 20 minutes; and after oral administrations of macrocrystals, less than 60 minutes. Following a single dose of nitrofurantoin about 25% is found unchanged in the urine over 24 hours.

Pharmaceutical particulars
List of excipients: Furadantin tablets also contain lactose, maize starch, talc, alginic acid and magnesium stearate.

Incompatibilities: None known.

Shelf life: The expiry date for the tablets should not exceed 3 years from the date of manufacture.

Special precautions for storage: The tablets should be packaged in light-proof and preferably moisture-resistant containers. Storage temperatures must not exceed 30°C.

Nature and contents of container: Furadantin tablets are supplied in packs of 30 and 100 tablets.

Instructions for use/handling: Used as directed by physician.

Marketing authorisation numbers
PL 0364/0008R (50 mg tablets)
PL 0364/0009R (100 mg tablets)

Date of first authorisation/renewal of authorisation
21 February 1990

Date of (partial) revision of the text May 1998

MACROBID* CAPSULES

Qualitative and quantitative composition Macrobid is a modified release, hard gelatin capsule containing the equivalent of 100 mg of Nitrofurantoin in the form of nitrofurantoin macrocrystals and nitrofurantoin monohydrate.

Pharmaceutical form The 100 mg capsule has an opaque blue cap and opaque yellow body and bears the monogram 'Eaton BID'.

Clinical particulars
Therapeutic indications: For the treatment of and prophylaxis against acute or recurrent, uncomplicated lower urinary tract infections or pyelitis either spontaneous or following surgical procedures.

Macrobid is specifically indicated for the treatment of infections when due to susceptible strains of *Escherichia coli, Enterococci, Staphylococci, Citrobacter, Klebsiella* and *Enterobacter.*

Most strains of *Proteus* and *Serratia* are resistant. All *Pseudomonas* strains are resistant.

Macrobid is not indicated for the treatment of associated renal cortical or peri-nephric abscesses.

Posology and method of administration:
Adults and children over 12 years old: The dose should be taken with food or milk (e.g. at meal times).

Acute or recurrent uncomplicated UTI and pyelitis: 100 mg twice daily for 7 days.

Surgical prophylaxis: 100 mg twice daily on the day of the procedure and three days thereafter.

Elderly patients: Provided there is no significant renal dysfunction, in which nitrofurantoin is contra-indicated, the dosage should be that for any normal adult.

See precautions and risks to elderly patients associated with long term therapy.

Children under 12 years old: Macrobid is a fixed dosage and is therefore not suitable for children under 12 years.

Contra-indications: Patients suffering from renal dysfunction with a creatinine clearance of less than 60 ml/minute or elevated serum creatinine.

In infants under three months of age as well as pregnant patients at term (during labour and delivery) because of the theoretical possibility of haemolytic anaemia in the foetus or in the newborn infant due to immature erythrocyte enzyme systems.

Patients with known hypersensitivity to nitrofurantoin or other nitrofurans.

Special warnings and special precautions for use: Nitrofurantoin is not effective for the treatment of parenchymal infections of a unilaterally functioning kidney. A surgical cause for infection should be excluded in recurrent or severe cases.

Peripheral neuropathy which may become severe or irreversible has occurred and may be life threatening. Nitrofurantoin should be used with caution in patients with anaemia, diabetes mellitus, electrolyte imbalance, debilitating conditions, and vitamin B (particularly folate) deficiency since these conditions may enhance the occurrence of peripheral neuropathy. Therefore, treatment should be stopped at the first signs of neural involvement (paraesthesiae).

Since pre-existing conditions may mask hepatic or pulmonary adverse reactions, nitrofurantoin should be used with caution in patients with pulmonary disease, hepatic dysfunction, neurological disorders and allergic diathesis.

Acute, subacute or chronic pulmonary reactions have been observed in patients treated with nitrofurantoin. If these reactions occur, Macrobid should be discontinued and appropriate measures taken. Reports have cited pulmonary reactions as a contributing cause of death.

Chronic pulmonary reactions (diffuse interstitial pneumonitis or pulmonary fibrosis or both) can develop insidiously. These reactions occur rarely and generally in patients receiving therapy for six months or longer. Chronic pulmonary reactions may occur more commonly in elderly patients. Close monitoring of the pulmonary condition of patients receiving long term therapy is warranted and requires that the benefits of therapy be weighed against potential risks.

Hepatic reactions, including cholestatic jaundice and chronic active hepatitis, occur rarely. Fatalities have been reported. Cholestatic jaundice is generally associated with short-term therapy (usually up to two weeks). Chronic active hepatitis is generally associated with long-term therapy (usually after six months); the onset may be insidious, and patients should be monitored periodically for changes in liver function. If hepatitis occurs, the drug should be withdrawn immediately and appropriate measures taken.

Ten percent of black patients and a variable percentage of ethnic groups of Mediterranean, Near Eastern and Asian origin, suffer from a deficiency of glucose-6-phosphate dehydrogenase in their blood cells. In such people nitrofurantoin, in common with many other therapeutic agents, may cause haemolysis. This enzyme deficiency is extremely rare in caucasians. Any sign of haemolysis is an indication to discontinue the drug. Haemolysis ceases when the drug is withdrawn.

Discontinue treatment with nitrofurantoin if otherwise unexplained pulmonary, hepatotoxic, haematological or neurologic syndromes occur. For long term treatment monitor the patient closely for appearance of hepatic or pulmonary symptoms and other evidence of toxicity.

Interaction with other medicaments and other forms of interaction: Concomitant administration of magnesium trisilicate with nitrofurantoin reduces absorption. Uricosuric drugs such as probenecid and sulphinpyrazone may inhibit renal tubular secretion of nitrofurantoin. The resulting increase in serum levels may increase toxicity. Decreased urinary levels could lessen its efficacy as a urinary tract antibacterial. Concurrent use with quinolones is not recommended. There may be decreased antibacterial activity for nitrofurantoin in the presence of carbonic anhydrase inhibitors and urine alkalinising agents.

Pregnancy and lactation: Animal studies with nitrofurantoin have shown no teratogenic effects. Nitrofurantoin has been in extensive clinical use since 1952 and its suitability in human pregnancy has been well documented.

Nitrofurantoin is however contra-indicated in infants under three months of age and in pregnant women during *labour and delivery* because of the possible risk of haemolysis of the infants immature red cells.

Effects on ability to drive and use machines: Macrobid does not interfere with the ability to drive or use machines.

Undesirable effects:

Respiratory: If any of the following respiratory reactions occur the drug should be discontinued.

Acute pulmonary reactions usually occur within the first week of treatment and are reversible with cessation of therapy.

Subacute reactions may take several months to resolve once the drug has been stopped.

Chronic pulmonary reactions occur rarely in patients who have received continuous therapy for six months or longer and are more common in elderly patients. Changes in ECG have occurred, associated with pulmonary reactions. Symptoms such as fever, chills, cough and dyspnoea may be significant. Collapse and cyanosis have seldom been reported. The severity of chronic pulmonary reactions and their degree of resolution appear to be related to the duration of therapy after the first clinical signs appear. It is important to recognise symptoms as early as possible. Pulmonary function may be impaired permanently, even after cessation of therapy.

Hepatic: Hepatic reactions including cholestatic jaundice and chronic active hepatitis occur rarely. Fatalities have been reported. Cholestatic jaundice is generally associated with short-term therapy (usually up to two weeks). Chronic active hepatitis, occasionally leading to hepatic necrosis is generally associated with long-term therapy (usually after six months). The onset may be insidious. Treatment should be stopped at the first sign of hepatotoxicity.

Neurological: Peripheral neuropathy (including optical neuritis) with symptoms of sensory as well as motor involvement, which may become severe or irreversible, has been reported infrequently. Less frequent reactions of unknown causal relationship are depression, euphoria, confusion, psychotic reactions, nystagmus, vertigo, dizziness, asthenia, headache and drowsiness. Treatment should be stopped at the first sign of neurological involvement.

Gastrointestinal: Nausea and anorexia have been reported. Emesis, abdominal pain and diarrhoea are less common gastrointestinal reactions.

Hypersensitivity: Exfoliative dermatitis and erythema multiforme (including Stevens-Johnson syndrome) have been reported rarely.

Allergic skin reactions manifesting as angioneurotic oedema, maculopapular, erythematous or eczematous eruptions, urticaria, rash, and pruritus have occurred. Lupus-like syndrome associated with pulmonary reaction to nitrofurantoin has been reported.

Other hypersensitivity reactions include anaphylaxis, sialadenitis, pancreatitis, drug fever, and arthralgia.

Haematological: Agranulocytosis, leucopenia, granulocytopaenia, haemolytic anaemia, thrombocytopaenia, glucose-6-phosphate dehydrogenase deficiency, anaemia, megaloblastic anaemia and eosinophilia have occurred. Cessation of therapy has generally returned the blood picture to normal. Aplastic anaemia has been reported rarely.

Other: Transient alopecia and benign intercranial hypertension.

Superinfections by fungi or resistant organisms such as *Pseudomonas* may occur. However, these are limited to the genito-urinary tract.

Overdose: Symptoms and signs of overdosage include gastric irritation, nausea and vomiting. There is no known specific antidote. Nitrofurantoin can be haemodialysed. Standard treatment is by induction of emesis or by gastric lavage in cases of recent ingestion. Monitoring of full blood count, liver function tests and pulmonary function, are recommended. A high fluid intake should be maintained to promote urinary excretion of the drug.

Pharmacological properties

Pharmacodynamic properties: Nitrofurantoin is a broad spectrum antibacterial agent, active against the majority of urinary pathogens. It is bactericidal in renal tissue and throughout the urinary tract. The wide range of organisms sensitive to the bactericidal activity include *Escherichia coli, Enterococcus faecalis, Klebsiella* species, *Enterobacter* species, *Staphylococcus* species (e.g. *S. aureus, S. saprophyticus, S. epidermidis*).

Clinically, most common urinary pathogens are sensitive to nitrofurantoin. Some strains of *Enterobacter* and *Klebsiella* are resistant. Nitrofurantoin is not active against most strains of *Proteus* species or *Serratia* species. It has no activity against *Pseudomonas* species.

Pharmacokinetic properties:

Clinical pharmacology: Each Macrobid capsule contains two forms of nitrofurantoin. Twenty-five percent of the dose is macrocrystalline nitrofurantoin which has slower dissolution and absorption than nitrofurantoin microcrystals. The remaining 75% of the dose is microcrystalline nitrofurantoin contained in a powder blend which, upon exposure to gastric and intestinal fluids, forms a gel matrix resulting in a modified release of active ingredient over time. Combined, these systems provide a clinically effective bactericidal urine concentration at therapeutic doses. Approximately 20–25% of the total single dose of nitrofurantoin is recovered from the urine unchanged over 24 hours.

Plasma nitrofurantoin concentrations at therapeutic doses of the Macrobid capsule are low, with peak levels usually less than 1 mg/ml. Nitrofurantoin is highly soluble in urine, to which it may impart a brown colour. Unlike many drugs, the presence of food or agents delaying gastric emptying increases the bioavailability of the Macrobid capsule.

Pharmaceutical particulars

List of excipients: Macrobid capsules also contain talc, corn starch, lactose, carbopol, povidone, sugar, magnesium stearate, gelatin, sodium lauryl sulphate and colouring agents (E104, E132, E171).

Incompatibilities: None known.

Shelf life: The expiry date for the product should not exceed 2 years from the date of its manufacture.

Special precautions for storage: Capsules should be stored in light and moisture resistant containers. Storage temperature should not exceed 30°C.

Nature and contents of container: There are two pack sizes, one consists of 14 capsules and the other is a sample pack containing 2 capsules.

Instructions for use/handling: A patient information leaflet is provided with the product.

Marketing authorisation number PL 0364/0055.

Date of first authorisation/renewal of authorisation 5 February 1992.

Date of (partial) revision of the text March 1998.

MACRODANTIN* CAPSULES

Presentation Macrodantin is presented in hard gelatin capsules, containing 50 mg or 100 mg Nitrofurantoin PhEur in macrocrystalline form.

The 50 mg capsule has an opaque yellow cap and opaque white body marked 'Eaton 008'. The 100 mg capsule has an opaque yellow cap and body, marked 'Eaton 009'.

Uses For the treatment of and prophylaxis against acute or recurrent, uncomplicated lower urinary tract infections or pyelitis either spontaneous or following surgical procedures.

Nitrofurantoin is specifically indicated for the treatment of infections when due to susceptible strains of Escherichia coli, enterococci, staphylococci, Citrobacter, Klebsiella and Enterobacter.

Most strains of Proteus and Serratia are resistant. All Pseudomonas strains are resistant.

Macrodantin is not indicated for the treatment of associated renal cortical or perinephric abscesses.

Dosage and administration

Adults and children over ten years of age: The dose should be taken with food or milk (e.g. at meal times).

Acute uncomplicated urinary tract infections: 50 mg four times daily for seven days.

Severe chronic recurrent infections: 100 mg four times daily for seven days. In the event of severe nausea the dose may be reduced, but not below the adult equivalent of 200 mg/day. Should it persist the drug should be withdrawn.

Long term suppressive therapy: 50–100 mg once a day at bedtime is suggested.

Surgical prophylaxis: 50 mg four times daily on the day of the procedure and for the three days after.

Elderly: Provided there is no significant renal impairment, the dosage should be that for any normal adult.

Children over the age of three months:

Acute urinary tract infections: 3 mg/kg/day in four divided doses for seven days.

Suppressive therapy: 1 mg/kg/day once a day.

Contra-indications, warings, etc

Contra-indications: Patients suffering from renal dysfunction with a creatinine clearance of less than 60 ml/minute or elevated serum creatinine.

In infants under three months of age as well as pregnant patients at term (during labour and delivery) because of the theoretical possibility of haemolytic anaemia in the foetus or in the newborn infant due to immature erythrocyte enzyme systems.

Patients with known hypersensitivity to nitrofurantoin or other nitrofurans.

Precautions and warnings: Gastrointestinal reactions may be minimised by taking the drug with food or milk or by adjustment of dosage.

Nitrofuratoin is not effective for the treatment of parenchymal infections of unilaterally non-functioning kidney.

Nitrofurantoin should be used with caution in patients with pulmonary disease, hepatic dysfunction, neurological disorders, allergic diathesis, anaemia, diabetes mellitus, electrolyte imbalance, and vitamin B (particularly folate) deficiency.

Nitrofurantoin may cause haemolysis in patients with glucose-6-phosphate dehydrogenase deficiency (ten percent of black patients and a variable percentage of ethnic groups of Mediterranean, Near Eastern and Asian origin). Haemolysis ceases when the drug is discontinued.

Discontinue treatment with nitrofurantoin if otherwise unexplained pulmonary, hepatotoxic, haematological or neurologic syndromes occur. For long term treatment monitor patient closely for appearance of hepatic, pulmonary of neurological symptoms and other evidence of toxicity.

Interactions with other drugs: Concomitant administration of magnesium trisilicate with nitrofurantoin reduces absorption.

Uricosuric drugs such as probenecid and sulphinpyrazone may inhibit renal tubular secretion of nitrofurantoin. The resulting increase in serum levels may increase toxicity. Decreased urinary levels could reduce efficacy as a urinary tract antibacterial.

Concurrent use with quinolones is not recommended.

There may be decreased antibacterial activity for nitrofurantoin in the presence of carbonic anhydrase inhibitors and urine alkalinising agents.

Side effects:

Respiratory: If the following reactions occur the drug should be discontinued.

Acute pulmonary reactions usually occur within the first week of treatment and are reversible with cessation of therapy.

Subacute reactions may take several months to resolve once the drug has been stopped.

Chronic pulmonary reactions occur rarely in patients who have received continuous therapy for six months or longer and are more common in elderly patients. Changes in ECG have occurred, associated with pulmonary reactions. Minor symptoms such as fever, chills, cough and dyspnoea may be significant. Collapse and cyanosis have seldom been reported. The severity of chronic pulmonary reactions and their degree of resolution appear to be related to the duration of therapy after the first clinical signs appear. It is important to recognise symptoms as early as possible. Pulmonary function may be impaired permanently, even after cessation of therapy.

Hepatic: Hepatic reactions including cholestatic jaundice and chronic active hepatitis occur rarely. Fatalities have been reported. Cholestatic jaundice is generally associated with short-term therapy (usually up to two weeks). Chronic active hepatitis, occasionally leading to hepatic necrosis is generally associated with long-term therapy (usually after six months). The onset may be insidious. Treatment should be stopped at the first sign of hepatotoxicity.

Neurological: Peripheral neuropathy (including optical neuritis) with symptoms of sensory as well as motor involvement, which may become severe or irreversible, has been reported infrequently. Less frequent reactions of unknown causal relationship are depression, euphoria, confusion, psychotic reactions, nystagmus, vertigo, dizziness, asthenia, headache and drowsiness. Treatment should be stopped at the first sign of neurological involvement.

Gastrointestinal: Nausea and anorexia have been reported. Emesis, abdominal pain and diarrhoea are less common gastrointestinal reactions.

Hypersensitivity: Exfoliative dermatitis and erythema multiforme (including Stevens-Johnson syndrome) have been reported rarely.

Allergic skin reactions manifesting as angioneurotic oedema, maculopapular, erythematous or eczematous eruptions, urticaria, rash, and pruritus have occurred. Lupus-like syndrome associated with pulmonary reaction to nitrofurantoin has been reported.

Other hypersensitivity reactions include anaphylaxis, sialadenitis, pancreatitis, drug fever, and arthralgia.

Haematological: Agranulocytosis, leucopenia, granulocytopaenia, haemolytic anaemia, thrombocytopaenia, glucose-6-phosphate dehydrogenase deficiency, anaemia, megaloblastic anaemia and eosinophilia have occurred. Cessation of therapy has generally returned the blood picture to normal. Aplastic anaemia has been reported rarely.

Other: Transient alopecia and benign intercranial hypertension.

Superinfections by fungi or resistant organisms such as Pseudomonas may occur. However, these are limited to the genito-urinary tract.

Use in pregnancy and lactation: Animal studies with nitrofurantoin have shown no teratogenic effects. Nitrofurantoin has been in extensive clinical use since 1952 and its suitability in human pregnancy has been well documented.

Nitrofurantoin is however contra-indicated in infants under three months of age and in pregnant women during labour and delivery, because of the possible risk of haemolysis of the infants immature red cells.

Overdosage: Symptoms and signs of overdosage include gastric irritation, nausea and vomiting. There is no known specific antidote. Nitrofurantoin can be haemodialysed. Standard treatment is by induction of emesis or by gastric lavage in cases of recent ingestion. Monitoring of full blood count, liver function tests and pulmonary function, are recommended. A high fluid intake should be maintained to promote urinary excretion of the drug.

Pharmaceutical precautions Macrodantin capsules 100 mg should be dispensed in light-proof and preferably moisture-resistant containers. Storage temperatures for both 50 mg and 100 mg capsules must not exceed 30°C.

Legal category POM.

Packaging quantities Macrodantin capsules 100 mg are supplied in a blister pack of 30.

Macrodantin capsules 50 mg are supplied in a blister pack of 30.

Further information The nitrofurantoin macrocrystals of Macrodantin are specially formulated. The crystal size controls the rate of absorption and thus reduces the incidence of nausea. Clinical and animal studies indicate that Macrodantin therapy decreases the likelihood of nausea in patients who might experience these symptoms on nitrofurantoin therapy.

The urine of patients receiving Macrodantin may be coloured a dark yellow or brown. This results from the presence of drug and/or metabolite(s) and is quite harmless. Macrodantin can interfere with certain laboratory tests. False positive or spuriously high readings may be produced with urine glucose tests utilising the copper sulphate reduction method, e.g. Benedict's reagent, Clinitest (Ames). However, there is no interference with the Clinistix test.

Product licence numbers
PL 0364/0005R (50 mg)
PL 0364/0006R (100 mg)

Date of preparation July 1993

LEMON/LIME FLAVOUR REGULAN*

Qualitative and quantitative composition Lemon/Lime Flavour Regulan contains 3.4 g of Ispaghula Husk, BP.

Pharmaceutical form Premeasured, single-dose sachets containing a lemon/lime flavoured beige, fine ground powder, which when reconstituted with water is intended for oral administration.

Clinical particulars
Therapeutic indications: For the relief of constipation and for patients who need to increase their daily fibre intake.

Posology and method of administration: The measured dosage should be poured into a glass and 150 ml (¼ pint) of cool water, milk, fruit juice or other liquid added, stirred, and taken immediately. Additional liquid may be taken if required. Adequate fluid intake should be maintained.

Adults and children over 12 years: Usual dosage is the entire contents of one sachet taken one to three times daily.

Elderly: No alteration in dosage necessary.

Children 6–12 years: A reduced dosage based upon age of the child should be given. ½–1 level teaspoonful one to three times daily.

Contra-indications: Not to be given to patients with intestinal obstruction, faecal impaction, colonic atony or hypersensitivity to ispaghula.

Special warnings and special precautions for use: Lemon/Lime Flavour Regulan should always be taken as a liquid suspension and should be drunk immediately after mixing. The last dose should not be taken immediately before going to bed since impaired or reduced gastric motility may impair the intestinal passage and then cause sub-obstruction. The drug may cause allergic reactions in people sensitive to inhaled or ingested ispaghula powder.

It may be advisable to supervise treatment in the elderly or debilitated and patients with intestinal narrowing or decreased motility, as rare instances of gastrointestinal obstruction have been reported with mucilloid preparations when taken, contrary to the administration instructions, with insufficient liquid.

Each sachet contains 3 mg of phenylalanine and this should be considered in phenylketonuric patients.

Interaction with other medicaments and other forms of interaction: None known.

Pregnancy and lactation: Controlled studies in pregnant and lactating women are not available, but the product has been in wide use for many years without apparent ill consequence and animal studies have shown no hazard. Ispaghula is not thought to be absorbed nor is it thought to enter breast milk. Nevertheless the benefits of therapy should be weighed against the possible risks if used during pregnancy and lactation.

Effects on ability to drive and use machines: None known.

Undesirable effects: Allergy and gastrointestinal obstruction or impaction have been reported with hydrophilic mucilloid preparations.

Overdose: No instances of true overdosage have been reported. If overdosage should occur there is no specific treatment and symptomatic measures should be employed.

Pharmacological properties
Pharmacodynamic properties: The active constituent, ispaghula husk, is the epidermis and collapsed adjacent layers removed from the dried ripe seeds of plantago ovata, containing mucilage and hemicelluloses.

The ispaghula husk is not absorbed and produces its effect as a bulking agent by physical means alone.

Pharmacokinetic properties: Not applicable.

Pharmaceutical particulars
List of excipients: Contains maltodextrin, citric acid, citrus flavour, sodium saccharin, aspartame and E160a. Regulan is sugar free and gluten free. Each sachet contains 0.23 mmol of sodium.

Incompatibilities: None known.

Shelf life: Two years.

Special precautions for storage: Store in a dry place below 30°C.

Nature and contents of container: Paper/foil/polyethylene sachets. The product is available in pack sizes of 10 and 30 sachets.

Instructions for use/handling: A patient leaflet is provided with details of use and handling of the product.

Marketing authorisation holder: Procter & Gamble (Health & Beauty Care) Limited, The Heights, Brooklands, Weybridge, Surrey KT13 0XP.

Marketing authorisation number PL 0129/0113.

Date of first authorisation/renewal of authorisation 15 September 1992.

Date of (partial) revision of the text Feb 1998.

ORANGE FLAVOUR REGULAN*

Qualitative and quantitative composition Orange Flavour Regulan contains 3.4 g of Ispaghula Husk, BP.

Pharmaceutical form Premeasured, single-dose sachets containing an orange flavoured beige, fine ground powder, which when reconstituted with water is intended for oral administration.

Clinical particulars
Therapeutic indications: For the relief of constipation and for patients who need to increase their daily fibre intake.

Posology and method of administration: The measured dosage should be poured into a glass and 150 ml (¼ pint) of cool water, milk, fruit juice or other liquid added, stirred, and taken immediately. Additional liquid may be taken if required. Adequate fluid intake should be maintained.

Adults and children over 12 years: Usual dosage is the entire contents of one sachet taken one to three times daily.

Elderly: No alteration in dosage necessary.

Children 6–12 years: A reduced dosage based upon age of the child should be given. ½–1 level teaspoonful one to three times daily.

Contra-indications: Not to be given to patients with intestinal obstruction, faecal impaction, colonic atony or hypersensitivity to ispaghula.

Special warnings and special precautions for use: Orange Flavour Regulan should always be taken as a liquid suspension and should be drunk immediately after mixing. The last dose should not be taken immediately before going to bed since impaired or reduced gastric motility may impair the intestinal passage and then cause sub-obstruction. The drug may cause allergic reactions in people sensitive to inhaled or ingested ispaghula powder.

It may be advisable to supervise treatment in the elderly or debilitated and patients with intestinal narrowing or decreased motility, as rare instances of gastrointestinal obstruction have been reported with mucilloid preparations when taken, contrary to the administration instructions, with insufficient liquid.

Each sachet contains 3 mg of phenylalanine and this should be considered in phenylketonuric patients.

Interaction with other medicaments and other forms of interaction: None known.

Pregnancy and lactation: Controlled studies in pregnant and lactating women are not available, but the product has been in wide use for many years without apparent ill consequence and animal studies have shown no hazard. Ispaghula is not thought to be absorbed nor is it thought to enter breast milk. Nevertheless the benefits of therapy should be weighed against the possible risks if used during pregnancy and lactation.

Effects on ability to drive and use machines: None known.

Undesirable effects: Allergy and gastrointestinal obstruction or impaction have been reported with hydrophilic mucilloid preparations.

Overdose: No instances of true overdosage have been reported. If overdosage should occur there is no specific treatment and symptomatic measures should be employed.

Pharmacological properties
Pharmacodynamic properties: The active constituent, ispaghula husk, is the epidermis and collapsed adjacent layers removed from the dried ripe seeds of plantago ovata, containing mucilage and hemicelluloses.

The ispaghula husk is not absorbed and produces its effect as a bulking agent by physical means alone.

Pharmacokinetic properties: Not applicable.

Pharmaceutical particulars
List of excipients: Contains maltodextrin, citric acid, orange flavour, sodium saccharin, aspartame, E160a and E160e. Orange flavour Regulan is sugar free and gluten free. Each sachet contains 0.23 mmol of sodium.

Incompatibilities: None known.

Shelf life: Two years.

Special precautions for storage: Store in a dry place below 30°C.

Nature and contents of container: Paper/foil/polyethylene sachets. The product is available in pack sizes of 10 and 30 sachets.

Instructions for use/handling: A patient leaflet is provided with details of use and handling of the product.

Marketing authorisation holder: Procter & Gamble (Health & Beauty Care) Limited, The Heights, Brooklands, Weybridge, Surrey KT13 0XP.

Marketing authorisation number PL 0129/0114.

Date of first authorisation/renewal of authorisation 15 September 1992.

Date of (partial) revision of the text Feb 1998.

**Trade Mark*

Quinoderm Limited
Manchester Road
Oldham OL8 4PB

☎ 0161 624 9307 0161 627 0928

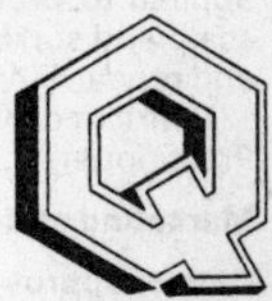

CEANEL* CONCENTRATE

Presentation
Active constituents:

Phenylethyl Alcohol USP	7.5%
Cetrimide BP	10%
Undecenoic Acid BP	1%

Other constituents: Lauric diethanolamide, diethanolamine, poly oxy propylene stearyl ether.

Appearance: Ceanel Concentrate is a clear, viscous, golden yellow coloured liquid.

Uses *Main pharmacological action:* Cetrimide is particularly active against Gram-positive organisms. This feature combined with the bactericidal action of phenylethyl alcohol and the fungicidal properties of undecenoic acid makes Ceanel Concentrate particularly effective in the treatment of dermatological conditions. Ceanel Concentrate is effective in removing debris and scale in seborrhoea capitis, and psoriasis of the scalp.

Indications: As an adjunct in the management of psoriasis of the scalp, seborrhoeic dermatitis, dandruff, psoriasis of the trunk and limbs.

Dosage and administration
Adults, children and the elderly: Scalp conditions: Wet the scalp and hair with warm water. Protect the eyes with a towel to avoid discomfort. Apply ½–1 teaspoonful of Ceanel to the wetted scalp. Then apply a small amount of water and work up into a lather. Rinse and repeat. Finally rinse the hair and scalp *thoroughly.* Use three times in the first week and twice weekly thereafter.

Other areas of the body: Wet the area to be treated with warm water; apply sufficient Ceanel Concentrate by gentle massage to cover the wetted area. Allow to remain in contact for two minutes. Remove the Ceanel by thorough rinsing with warm water. Use as required.

Contra-indications, warnings, etc *Precaution:* The eyes should be protected during treatment. A simple way to do this is with a towel.

Overdosage: Ceanel Concentrate is for external use only. Following accidental ingestion, nausea and vomiting may occur as well as respiratory problems and hypotension. Treatment is supportive and symptomatic avoiding gastric lavage.

Warning: There is inadequate evidence of safety in human pregnancy, but it has been in wide use for many years without apparent ill consequence. As with other medicaments it may be used during pregnancy if the anticipated benefits outweigh the risks. No problems are anticipated during lactation.

Pharmaceutical precautions *Storage:* No special precaution required.

Diluents: Ceanel Concentrate is easily removed by warm water.

Legal category P.

Package quantities Available in packs of 50 ml, 150 ml and 500 ml.

Further information Nil.

Product licence number 0291/5002R.

GELCOSAL*

Qualitative and quantitative composition

Strong Coal Tar Solution BPC	5.0%
Tar BP (Pine Tar)	5.0%
Salicylic Acid BP	2.0%

Pharmaceutical form Gelcosal is a light-brown thixotropic gel which spreads easily and cleanly on the skin. It is non-sticky, non-greasy and being water-miscible is easily removed and does not permanently stain the skin.

Clincial particulars
Therapeutic indications: Gelcosal is indicated in the treatment of psoriasis in the chronic scaling phase and the treatment of dermatitis in the chronic scaling phase.

Posology and method of administration:
Route of administration: For topical use only.
Adults, children and the elderly: By gentle massage over all the affected area twice daily. Unless hands are being treated, rinse hands following application.

Contra-indications: Patients with known sensitivity or intolerance to any of the ingredients should not use Gelcosal. If sensitivity occurs or infection appears discontinue use and institute appropriate therapy.

Special warnings and special precautions for use:
Precautions: For topical use only. Contact with eyes and other mucosal surfaces should be avoided.

Warning: Prolonged use over large areas of topical preparations containing salicylic acid may result in symptoms of salicylism e.g. tinnitus. In view of this, extra caution should be exercised when treating children.

Interaction with other medicaments and other forms of interaction: None known.

Pregnancy and lactation: Gelcosal is not contra-indicated in pregnancy or lactation.

Effects on ability to drive and use machines: Not applicable.

Undesirable effects: None known.

Overdose: Not applicable. Gelcosal is for topical use only.

Pharmacological properties The combination of two different tars in Gelcosal provides a preparation with antipruritic, keratolytic and antiseptic properites. The combination also provides the usual therapeutic activity of tars.

Salicylic acid provides a keratolytic action.

The salicylic acid constituent of Gelcosal allows removal of scale and thus access of the tar components to the underlying diseased areas.

The base has been developed with the objective of providing a cosmetically acceptable thixotropic formulation at the same time as retaining the therapeutic efficacy of crude tar.

Pharmaceutical particulars
List of excipients: Poly oxy propylene stearyl ether, Hypromellose BP, Purified Water BP.

Incompatibilities: Not applicable.

Shelf life: Three years.

Special precautions for storage: Gelcosal should be stored in a cool, dry place avoiding extremes of temperature i.e. not less than 5°C and not more than 30°C.

Nature and contents of container: Gelcosal is packed in low density polyethylene tubes with flush fitting ribbed cap containing 50 g of product. Each tube is cartoned and contains a patient information leaflet.

Instructions for use/handling: By gentle massage over all the affected area twice daily. Unless hands are being treated, rinse hands thoroughly following application.

Marketing authorisation number 0291/0019.

Date of approval/revision of SPC October 1995.

Legal category P.

GELCOTAR*

Presentation
Active constituents:

Strong Coal Tar Solution BPC	5%
Tar BP (Pine tar)	5%

Other constituents: Poly oxy propylene stearyl ether, Hypromellose BP.

Appearance: Gelcotar is a light-brown thixotropic gel which spreads easily and cleanly on the skin. It is non-sticky, non-greasy and being water-miscible is easily removed and does not permanently stain the skin.

Uses *Main pharmacological action:* The combination of two different tars in Gelcotar provides a preparation with antipruritic, keratolytic and antiseptic properties. The combination also provides the usual therapeutic activity of tars.

The base has been developed with the objective of providing a cosmetically acceptable thixotropic formulation at the same time as retaining the efficacy of crude tar.

Indications: Treatment of psoriasis.
Treatment of dermatitis in the chronic phase.

Dosage and administration *Adults and children:* By gentle massage over all the affected area twice daily.

Contra-indications, warnings, etc
Contra-indications: Known sensitivity or intolerance to any of the ingredients.

Precautions: For external use only. Keep away from the eyes and other mucosal surfaces.

Overdosage: Not applicable.

Main side-effects/adverse reactions: None reported.

Pharmaceutical precautions *Storage:* Store in a cool place.

Legal category P.

Package quantities 50 g and 500 g.

Further information If sensitivity occurs or infection appears discontinue use and institute appropriate therapy.

Gelcotar is water-miscible and does not permanently stain the skin.

Product licence number 0291/0011.

GELCOTAR* LIQUID

Qualitative and quantitative composition

Strong Coal Tar Solution BP	1.25%
Cade Oil BPC	0.5%

Pharmaceutical form Gelcotar Liquid is a completely clear deep red/brown viscous liquid.

Clinical particulars
Therapeutic indications: Psoriasis of the scalp, seborrhoeic dermatitis and dandruff.

Posology and method of administration:
Route of administration: For topical use only.
Adults, children and elderly: Wet the scalp and hair with warm water. Sufficient Gelcotar Liquid should be applied to produce a generous lather. Massage the scalp and surrounding area with the fingertips. Rinse and repeat. Finally rinse the hair and scalp thoroughly.
Use twice weekly or as directed by the medical practitioner.

Contra-indications: Patients with known sensitivity or intolerance to strong coal tar solution or cade oil should not use Gelcotar liquid.

Special warnings and special precautions in use: Contact with eyes and other mucosal surfaces should be avoided. All medicines should be kept out of the reach of children. Gelcotar Liquid can be easily removed by warm water.

Interaction with other medicaments and other forms of interaction: None known.

Pregnancy and lactation: Gelcotar Liquid is not contra-indicated in pregnancy or lactation.

Effects on ability to drive and use machines: Not applicable.

Undesirable effects: None known.

Overdose: Not applicable. Gelcotar Liquid is for topical use only.

Pharmacological properties The combination of strong coal tar solution and cade oil provides a preparation with antiseptic and keratolytic properties to be used as a medicated scalp cleanser.

Pharmaceutical particulars
List of excipients: Coconut diethanolamide, Chlorocresol BP, poly ethylene mono tallowate, disodium fatty acid monoethanolamide sulpho succinate, ricinoleic propyl amido trimethyl ammonium metho sulphate, triethanolamine lauryl sulphate, lecithin, Purified Water BP.

Incompatibilities: Not applicable. Gelcotar Liquid is for topical use only.

Shelf life: 2 years.

Special precautions for storage: Gelcotar Liquid should be stored in a dry place avoiding extremes of temperature i.e. not less than 5°C and not more than 30°C.

Nature and contents of container: Gelcotar Liquid is packed in printed polyethylene bottles of 150 ml and 350 ml.

Instructions for use/handling: Wet the scalp and hair

with warm water. Sufficient Gelcotar Liquid should be applied to produce a generous lather. Massage the scalp and surrounding area with the fingertips. Rinse and repeat. Finally rinse the hair and scalp thoroughly.

Use twice weekly or as directed by the Medical Practitioner.

Marketing authorisation number 0291/0018

Date of approval/revision of SPC October 1995.

Legal category GSL.

HIOXYL* CREAM

Qualitative and quantitative composition Hydrogen Peroxide 1.50%

Pharmaceutical form Hioxyl Cream is a smooth, white, non-greasy cream with virtually no odour.

Clinical particulars

Therapeutic indications: Hioxyl Cream is indicated in the treatment of leg ulcers, pressure sores, minor wounds and infections of the skin.

Posology and method of administration:

Route of administration: For topical use only.

Adults, children and the elderly: Hioxyl Cream is applied freely using a piece of lint or gauze. If necessary it may be covered with a dressing. The application is repeated as required.

Contra-indications: There are no known contra-indications except true hypersensitivity to the active ingredient.

Special warnings and special precautions for use: Care should be taken to avoid usage with other medicaments due to possible interaction negating the active ingredient. Care should be taken to avoid contact with dyed fabrics as this product may adversely affect dye fastness.

Interaction with other medicaments and other forms of interaction: Hydrogen peroxide is an oxidising agent and should not be used in conjunction with other topical agents which would react with an oxidising agent.

Pregnancy and lactation: Hioxyl Cream is not contra-indicated in pregnancy or lactation.

Effects on ability to drive and use machines: Not applicable. Hioxyl Cream is for topical use only.

Undesirable effects: Not applicable.

Overdose: Not applicable. Hioxyl Cream is for topical use only.

Pharmacological properties The antiseptic effect of hydrogen peroxide is a result of its ready release of oxygen when applied to tissues. The effect only lasts as long as oxygen is being released, and for solutions of hydrogen peroxide, this is of only short duration.

Hioxyl Cream is a unique formulation in which hydrogen peroxide has been stabilised in a soothing, easy to apply cream to give prolonged antiseptic action.

Pharmaceutical particulars

List of excipients: Lactic Acid BP, White Soft Paraffin BP, Sodium Acid Phosphate BP, Maize Starch BP, cetyl stearyl alcohol, sodium cetyl stearyl sulphate, PEG 40 castor oil, Purified Water BP.

Incompatibilities: Hioxyl Cream should not be used at the same time as other topical medicaments. It is an oxidising agent and other topical agents may negate the effect of the active ingredient.

Shelf life: 18 months.

Special precautions for storage: Hioxyl Cream should be stored in a cool, dry place avoiding extremes of temperature i.e. not less than 5°C and not more than 30°C.

Nature and contents of container: Hioxyl Cream is packed in low density polythene tubes of 25 g and 100 g with flush fitting cap.

Instructions for use/handling: For topical use only. *Adults, children and the elderly:* Hioxyl Cream is applied freely using a piece of lint or gauze. If necessary it may be covered with a dressing. The application is repeated as required.

Marketing authorisation number 0291/0008.

Date of approval/revision of SPC January 1997.

Legal Category P.

HYDROMOL* CREAM

Qualitative and quantitative composition

Arachis (Peanut) Oil BP	10.0%
Isopropyl Myristate BP	5.0%
Liquid Paraffin BP	10.0%
Sodium Pyrrolidone Carboxylate	2.5%
Sodium Lactate	1.0%

Pharmaceutical form Hydromol Cream is a soft, white, oil-in-water cream which can be massaged easily into the skin.

Clinical particulars

Therapeutic indications: Any condition in which 'dry skin' is a feature, including all forms of dermatitis/ eczema and all degrees of ichthyosis and senile pruritus.

Posology and method of administration

Route of administration: For topical use only.

Adults, children and the elderly: Apply liberally to the affected area and massage well into the skin. Hydromol Cream may be used as often as required.

Hydromol Cream is especially beneficial when used immediately after washing or bathing, when the resultant warmth of the skin enhances absorption.

Contra-indications: There are no contra-indications except true hypersensitivity to any of the ingredients.

Special warnings and precautions for use: The formulation is not designed for use as a diluent.

Interactions with other medicaments and other forms of interaction: None known.

Pregnancy and lactation: Hydromol Cream is not contra-indicated in pregnancy or lactation.

Effects on ability to drive and use machines: Not applicable.

Undesirable effects: None known.

Overdose: Not applicable. Hydromol Cream is for topical use only.

Pharmacological properties

Pharmacodynamic properties: The combination of oils used in Hydromol Cream helps to lubricate and hydrate the skin. Moisture loss from the stratum corneum is reduced by the formation of an occlusive film by arachis oil and liquid paraffin on the surface of the skin. Isopropyl myristate, a fatty acid ester, is easily absorbed into the skin and helps to improve skin softness.

Pharmacokinetic properties: The combination of sodium pyrrolidone carboxylate and sodium lactate positively aids the hydration of the skin.

Preclinical safety data: None stated.

Pharmaceutical particulars

List of excipients: Ceto Macrogol Emulsifying Wax BP, Myristyl Myristate, Ceto Macrogol 1000 BP, hydroxybenzoates (parabens), phenoxyethanol, Purified Water BP.

Incompatibilities: Not applicable, Hydromol Cream is for topical use only.

Shelf life: Two years.

Special precautions for storage: Hydromol Cream should be stored in a dry place avoiding extremes of temperature i.e. not less than 5°C and not more than 30°C.

Nature and contents of container: Hydromol Cream is packed in low density polythene tubes of 50 g and 100 g with a flush fitting cap. It is also available in polypropylene tubs containing 500 g with screw cap and dispenser.

Instruction for use/handling: No special instructions.

Marketing authorisation number PL 0291/0023

Date of approval/revision of SPC January 1998

Legal category GSL

HYDROMOL* EMOLLIENT

Qualitative and quantitative composition

Light Liquid Paraffin BP	37.8%
Isopropyl Myristate BP	13.0%

Pharmaceutical form Hydromol Emollient is a clear, colourless bath additive.

Clinical particulars

Therapeutic indications: For the treatment of dry skin conditions such as eczema, ichthyosis and senile pruritus.

Posology and method of administration

Route of administration: Hydromol Emollient should be used topically and is either added to water or applied to wet skin.

1. For use in the bath

(a) Adults, children and the elderly: Add 1–3 capfuls to an 8 inch bath of water. Soak for 10–15 minutes.

(b) Infants: Add ½–2 capfuls to a small bath of water.

2. For application to the skin as a sponge bath or in the shower

Adults, children and the elderly: Pour a small quantity on to a wet sponge or flannel and rub onto wet skin. Rinse and pat dry.

Contra-indications: Known sensitivity to any of the ingredients.

Special warnings and special precautions for use: Keep away from eyes. Take care to avoid slipping in the bath/shower. If there is aggravation of the condition consult the doctor.

Interaction with other medicaments and other forms of interaction: None known.

Pregnancy and lactation: Hydromol Emollient is not contra-indicated in pregnancy or lactation.

Effects on ability to drive and use machines: Not applicable.

Undesirable effects: Patients should be advised to take care to avoid slipping in the bath.

Overdose: Not applicable. Hydromol Emollient is for topical use only.

Pharmacological properties

Pharmacodynamic properties: The combination of oils used in Hydromol Emollient are deposited on the skin surface during bathing and thus reduce moisture loss, provide anti-pruritic action, lubricate and soften the skin.

Hydromol Emollient is particularly suitable for infant bathing. The preparation can also be used as a cleanser where soaps are best avoided.

Pharmacokinetic properties: Hydromol Emollient is a water-dispersible bath additive resulting in an emulsion of dispersed oils together with an homogenised film on the surface.

Preclinical safety data: None stated.

Pharmaceutical particulars

List of excipients: C12–C14 alcohol with 3 molecules of ethylene oxide, polyol fatty acid ester, iso-octyl stearate.

Incompatibilities: Not applicable, Hydromol Emollient is for topical use only.

Shelf life: Three years.

Special precautions for storage: Hydromol Emollient should be stored in a cool, dry place avoiding extremes of temperature i.e. not less than 5°C and not more than 30°C.

Nature and contents of containers: Hydromol Emollient is packed in printed polyethylene bottles of 150 ml, 350 ml, and 1 litre capacity.

Instructions for use/handling: Hydromol Emollient should be used topically and is either added to water or applied to wet skin.

1. For use in the bath

(a) Adults, children and the elderly: Add 1–3 capfuls to an 8 inch bath of water. Soak for 10–15 minutes.

(b) Infants: Add ½–2 capfuls to a small bath of water.

2. For application to the skin as a sponge bath or in the shower

Adults, children and the elderly: Pour a small quantity on to a wet sponge or flannel and rub onto wet skin. Rinse and pat dry.

Marketing authorisation number PL 0291/0022

Date of approval/revision of SPC May 1997

Legal category GSL

QUINOCORT* CREAM

Qualitative and quantitative composition

Potassium Hydroxyquinoline Sulphate BP	0.5%
Hydrocortisone BP	1.0%

Pharmaceutical form Quinocort Cream is a faintly yellow vanishing cream. It is intended for topical use only.

Clinical particulars

Therapeutic indications: The treatment of infected eczema, intertrigo and other steroid-responsive dermatoses where anti-infective cover is appropriate.

Posology and method of administration:

Route of administration: For topical use only.

Adults, children and the elderly: By gentle massage over all the affected area two to three times daily.

Contra-indications: Patients with known sensitivity or intolerance to any of the ingredients.

Special warnings and special precautions for use: Contact with eyes and other mucosal surfaces should be avoided. Caution should be exercised when using this preparation in infants. Long term continuous topical therapy should be avoided in infants – adrenal suppression can occur even without occlusion.

Interaction with other medicaments and other forms of interaction: Not applicable.

Pregnancy and lactation: In pregnant animals administration of corticosteroids can cause abnormalities of foetal development. The relevance of this finding in human beings has not been established. However, topical steroids should not be used extensively in pregnancy i.e. in large amounts for long periods.

Effects on ability to drive and use machines: Not applicable.

Undesirable effects: Not applicable.

Overdose: Not applicable.

Pharmacological properties Hydrocortisone provides anti-inflammatory action yet is the least potent topical corticosteroid available. Potassium hydroxyquinoline sulphate provides broad spectrum antibacterial and anticandidal activity. The combination facilitates treatment of steroid-responsive dermatoses where complication by infection with bacteria or yeasts is evident suspected, or a possibility.

Pharmaceutical particulars
List of excipients: Lactic Acid BP, White Soft Paraffin BP, Edetic Acid BP, Sodium Acid Phosphate BP, Maize Starch BP, cetyl stearyl alcohol, sodium cetyl stearyl sulphate, PEG 40 castor oil, Chlorocresol BP, Purified Water BP.

Incompatibilities: Not applicable.

Shelf life: Two years.

Special precautions for storage: Quinocort Cream should be stored in a cool, dry place avoiding extremes of temperature i.e. not less than 5°C and not more than 30°C.

Nature and contents of container: Quinocort Cream is available in heat sealed low density polyethylene tubes with flush fitting cap containing 30 g of product. Each tube is cartoned and contains a patient information leaflet.

Instructions for use/handling: For topical use only.

Marketing authorisation number 0291/0014.

Date of approval/revision of SPC May 1995.

Legal category POM.

QUINODERM* CREAM

Qualitative and quantitative composition

Benzoyl Peroxide BP	10.0%
Potassium Hydroxyquinoline Sulphate BP	0.5%

Pharmaceutical form Quinoderm Cream is a creamy white astringent vanishing cream. It is intended for topical use only.

Clinical particlars
Therapeutic indications: Acne vulgaris, acneform eruptions, folliculitis.

Posology and method of administration:
Route of administration: For topical use only.
Adults, children and the elderly: By gentle massage over all the affected area two or three times daily.

Contra-indications: Acne rosacea. Patients with known sensitivity to either of the active ingredients should not use Quinoderm Cream.

Special warnings and special precautions for use: Contact with mouth and eyes should be avoided. Care should be taken to avoid contact with dyed fabrics as this product may adversely affect dye fastness.

In a few isolated cases, overreaction to Quinoderm Cream may occur. To minimise this possibility, select a small area of skin behind the ear, apply the cream and leave for twelve hours. If severe irritation or pronounced redness occurs, do not proceed with treatment.

Interaction with other medicaments and other forms of interaction: Benzoyl peroxide is an oxidising agent. Hence, Quinoderm Cream should not be used at the same time as other topical agents which would react with an oxidising agent.

Pregnancy and lactation: Quinoderm Cream is not contra-indicated in pregnancy or lactation.

Effects on ability to drive and use machines: Not applicable.

Undesirable effects: Not applicable.

Overdose: Not applicable.

Pharmacological properties The combination of the mild keratolytic properties of benzoyl peroxide and the antibacterial and antifungal properties of potassium hydroxyquinoline sulphate in a specially formulated bland water-miscible base make this preparation valuable in the treatment of acne vulgaris, acneform eruptions and folliculitis.

Pharmaceutical particulars
List of excipients: Lactic Acid BP, White Soft Paraffin BP, Edetic Acid BP, Sodium Acid Phosphate BP, Maize Starch BP, cetyl stearyl alcohol, sodium cetyl stearyl sulphate, PEG 40 castor oil, Purified Water BP.

Incompatibilities: Not applicable.

Shelf life: Three years.

Special precautions for storage: Quinoderm Cream should be stored in a cool, dry place avoiding extremes of temperature i.e. not less than 5°C and not more than 30°C.

Nature and contents of container: Quinoderm Cream is available in heat sealed low density polythene tubes with flush fitting cap containing 25 g and 50 g of product. Each tube is cartoned and contains a patient information leaflet.

Instructions for use/handling: For topical use only.

Marketing authorisation number 0291/5000R.

Date of approval/revision of SPC May 1995.

Legal category P.

QUINODERM* CREAM 5

Presentation
Active constituents:

Benzoyl Peroxide BP	5.0%
Potassium Hydroxyquinoline Sulphate BP	0.5%

Other constituents: Lactic Acid BP, White Soft Paraffin BP, Edetic Acid BP, Sodium Acid Phosphate BP, Maize Starch BP, cetyl stearyl alcohol, sodium cetyl stearyl sulphate, PEG 40 castor oil.

Appearance: Quinoderm Cream 5 is a creamy white astringent vanishing cream.

Uses *Main pharmacological action:* The combination of the mild keratolytic properties of benzoyl peroxide and the antibacterial and antifungal properties of potassium hydroxyquinoline sulphate in a specially formulated bland water-miscible base make this preparation valuable in the treatment of pustular affections of the skin particularly when associated with staphylococcal infection.

Indications: Acne vulgaris, acneform eruptions, folliculitis.

Dosage and administration *Adults, children and the elderly:* By gentle massage over all the affected area, two or three times daily.

Contra-indications, warnings, etc
Contra-indications: Quinoderm Cream 5 is contra-indicated in acne rosacea. Patients with known sensitivity to either of the active ingredients should not use Quinoderm Cream 5. Quinoderm Cream 5 is used topically.

Precaution: In a few isolated cases overreaction to Quinoderm Cream 5 may occur. To minimise this possibility, select a small area of skin behind the ear, apply the cream and leave for 12 hours. If severe irritation or pronounced redness occurs do not proceed.

All medicines should be kept out of the reach of children.

Pharmaceutical precautions *Storage:* Quinoderm Cream 5 should be stored in a cool place, avoiding extremes of temperature.

Diluents, etc: Quinoderm Cream 5 can be easily removed by warm water and soap.

Legal category P.

Package quantities Quinoderm Cream 5 is supplied in tubes of 50 g.

Further information Contact with mouth and eyes should be avoided. Care should be taken to avoid contact with dyed fabrics as this preparation may adversely affect dye fastness.

Product licence number 0291/0012.

QUINODERM* LOTIO-GEL 5%

Qualitative and quantitative composition

Benzoyl Peroxide BP	5.0%
Potassium Hydroxyquinoline Sulphate BP	0.5%

Pharmaceutical form Quinoderm Lotio-gel 5% is a homogeneous astringent gel formulated to give the colour and consistency of a creamy white lotion. It is intended for topical use only.

Clinical particulars
Therapeutic indications: Acne.

Posology and method of administration:
Route of administration: For topical use only.
Adults, children and the elderly: By gentle massage over all the affected area one to three times daily.

Contra-indications: Patients with known sensitivity to either of the active constituents should not use Quinoderm Lotio-gel 5%.

Special warnings and special precautions for use: Contact with mouth and eyes should be avoided. Care should be taken to avoid contact with dyed fabrics as this product may adversely affect dye fastness.

In a few isolated cases, overreaction to Quinoderm Lotio-gel 5% may occur. To minimise this possibility, select a small area of skin behind the ear, apply the cream and leave for twelve hours. If severe irritation or pronounced redness occurs, do not proceed with treatment.

Interaction with other medicaments and other forms of interaction: Benzoyl peroxide is an oxidising agent. Hence, Quinoderm Lotio-gel 5% should not be used at the same time as other topical agents which would react with an oxidising agent.

Pregnancy and lactation: Quinoderm Lotio-gel 5% is not contra-indicated in pregnancy or lactation.

Effects on ability to drive and use machines: Not applicable.

Undesirable effects: If symptoms persist or if the condition worsens or if irritation, itch or rash occurs, treatment should be discontinued and the Physician or Pharmacist consulted for advice.

Overdose: If accidentally ingested symptomatic and supportive management is advised.

Pharmacological properties The main pharmacological action of benzoyl peroxide is considered to be keratolytic and comedolytic. Potassium hydroxyquinoline sulphate has broad spectrum antibacterial activity. This combination is formulated in a specifically researched and developed base and is designed to aid the resolution of the polymorphic lesions of acne.

The base has been developed with the objective of providing a stable pharmaceutical form which maximises the advantages of a gel and lotion in a system which does not employ organic solvents and therefore has a correspondingly lower irritancy, toxicity and abuse potential.

Pharmaceutical particulars
List of excipients: Light Liquid Paraffin BP, Edetic Acid BP, Sodium Acid Phosphate BP, Maize Starch BP, Lactic Acid BP, Cetomacrogol 1000 BP, cetyl stearyl alcohol, sodium cetyl stearyl sulphate, PEG 40 castor oil, Purified Water BP.

Incompatibilities: Any topical agent that would react with an oxidising agent.

Shelf life: 3 years.

Special precautions for storage: Quinoderm Lotio-gel 5% should be stored in a cool, dry place avoiding extremes of temperature, i.e. not less than 5°C and not more than 30°C.

Nature and contents of container: Quinoderm Lotio-gel 5% is available in polyethylene bottles with a flip-top cap containing 30 ml of product. Each bottles is cartoned and contains a package insert.

Instructions for use/handling: By gentle massage over all the affected area one to three times daily.

Marketing authorisation number 0291/0009

Date of approval/revision of SPC September 1995.

Legal category P.

QUINOPED* CREAM

Qualitative and quantitative composition

Benzoyl Peroxide BP	5.0%
Potassium Hydroxyquinoline Sulphate BP	0.5%

Pharmaceutical form Quinoped Cream is a cream-coloured astringent cream.

Clinical particulars
Therapeutic indications: Quinoped Cream is indicated in the treatment of tinea pedis (athlete's foot) and other related fungal infections.

Posology and method of administration
Route of administration: For topical use only.
Adults, children and the elderly: Spread thinly over all the affected area and gently massage until no trace of the cream can be seen on the skin surface. Apply morning and night.

Contra-indications: Known sensitivity to either of the active ingredients. Quinoped Cream is for topical use only.

Special warnings and precautions for use: Care should be taken to avoid contact with dyed fabrics as this preparation may adversely affect dye fastness. In a few isolated cases overreaction to Quinoped Cream may occur. To avoid this possibility select a small area of skin on the feet, apply the cream and leave for twelve hours. If severe irritation or pronounced redness occurs do not proceed.

Interactions with other medicaments and other forms of interaction: Benzoyl Peroxide is an oxidising agent. Hence Quinoped Cream should not be used at the same time as other topical agents which would react with an oxidising agent.

Pregnancy and lactation: Quinoped Cream is not contra-indicated in pregnancy or lactation.

Effects on ability to drive and use machines: Not applicable.

Undesirable effects: Not applicable.

Overdose: Not applicable.

Pharmacological properties

Pharmacodynamic properties: Benzoyl Peroxide functions as a keratolytic and facilitates the removal of macerated tissue and associated debris. Potassium Hydroxyquinoline Sulphate has anti-fungal and deodorant properties. In addition Quinoped Cream is formulated in an astringent cream base which helps dry the infected toe clefts.

Pharmacokinetic properties: Not applicable. Quinoped Cream is for topical use only.

Preclinical safety data: None stated.

Pharmaceutical particulars

List of excipients: Lactic Acid BP, White Soft Paraffin BP, Edetic Acid BP, Sodium Acid Phosphate BP, Maize Starch BP, cetyl stearyl alcohol, sodium cetyl stearyl sulphate, PEG 40 castor oil, Purified Water BP.

Incompatibilities: Not applicable.

Shelf life: Three years.

Special precautions for storage: Quinoped Cream should be stored in a cool dry place avoiding extremes of temperature i.e. not less than 5°C and not more than 30°C.

Nature and contents of container: Quinoped Cream is available in low density polyethylene tubes with flush fitting cap containing 25 g of product.

Instruction for use/handling: No special instructions.

Marketing authorisation number PL 0291/0002

Date of approval/revision of SPC January 1998

Legal category P

**Trade Mark*

Reckitt & Colman Products

Dansom Lane
Hull HU8 7DS

☎ 01482 326151 📠 01482 582532

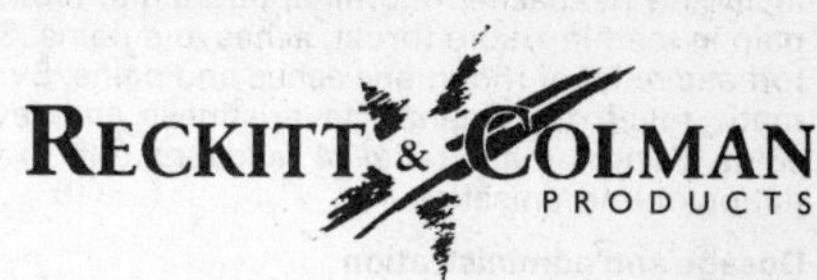

BONJELA* ORAL PAIN RELIEVING GEL

Presentation Bonjela is a clear, almost colourless gel containing choline salicylate 8.7% w/w and cetalkonium chloride 0.01% w/w, in a sugar free base containing ethanol, menthol, glycerol, hypromellose, aniseed oil and sodium cyclamate.

Uses For the relief of pain and discomfort of common mouth ulcers, cold sores, denture sore spots and infant teething.

Dosage and administration By topical application to the oral mucosa.

Adults: Using a clean finger, massage approximately half an inch of the gel onto the sore area, not more than once every three hours.

Children: (from 4 months): using a clean finger, massage approximately one quarter inch of gel onto the sore area, not more than once every three hours and not more than six doses in any twenty-four hour period.

Elderly: There is no evidence that dosage need be modified for the elderly.

Denture sore spots: Apply Bonjela to the gums and leave at least 30 minutes before reinsertion of the dentures. Do not apply this product directly to the dentures.

Contra-indications, warnings, etc Preparations containing aspirin should not be given to children under 12 during Bonjela treatment. Unwanted effects are those of salicylates. Bonjela should not be given to patients suffering from active peptic ulceration or known to be allergic to salicylates. Not to be used in infants under four months.

Salicylates may precipitate bronchospasm, and induce attacks of asthma in susceptible subjects.

Use in pregnancy: There is clinical evidence of the safety of salicylates in pregnancy but they may prolong bleeding and contribute to maternal and neonatal bleeding and are best avoided at term.

Use in lactation: Salicylates are excreted in low concentrations in breast milk but are unlikely to adversely affect the breast fed infant.

Drug interactions: Salicylates may enhance the effect of anticoagulants and inhibit the action of uricosurics.

Interferences with laboratory tests: Salicylates may produce falsely increased results for blood creatinine, urate (low dose aspirin) and urea. Falsely decreased results may be obtained for blood thyroxine and urate (>4 g/day aspirin) and for urinary 5-HIAA (with nitrosonaphthol method). Urinary VMA (HMMA) levels may be falsely increased or decreased depending on the method of analysis.

Treatment of overdosage: The usual procedure for salicylate overdosage should be followed, including general supportive measures and gastric lavage if necessary.

Pharmaceutical precautions None.

Legal category GSL.

Package quantities Tubes of 15 g.

Product licence number 0107/5002.

BUCCASTEM*

Presentation Buccastem tablets are circular, biconvex, pale yellow and uncoated with J1 engraved on the face; the reverse is plain. They contain 3 mg prochlorperazine maleate. This product contains sucrose.

Uses Buccastem is a potent phenothiazine neuroleptic. It is indicated in the symptomatic treatment of vertigo due to Meniere's disease, labyrinthitis and other causes; for nausea and vomiting from whatever cause and in the treatment of migraine.

Dosage and administration
Dosage: Adults and children aged 12 years and over: One or two 3 mg Buccastem tablets twice a day.

Elderly patients: For the indications shown above, there is no evidence that the dosage needs to be modified but the lower dosage is recommended for initial use.

Administration: The tablet should be placed high up between the upper lip and the gums to either side of the front teeth, where it will soften and adhere to the gum.

Patients should be instructed as to the correct placement of the tablet and should note the following points:

(a) The tablet should be left undisturbed.
(b) Slight numbness of the gum and tongue may be observed but this is transient.
(c) If a tablet is accidentally swallowed during insertion, it may be replaced by a further tablet.
(d) In patients who wear dentures, the tablet may be placed in any comfortable position between the lip and the gum.

Contra-indications, warnings, etc
Contra-indications: Buccastem is contra-indicated in patients with impaired renal or liver function, existing blood dyscrasias, known hypersensitivity to the active ingredient, epilepsy, Parkinson's disease, prostatic hypertrophy, and narrow angle glaucoma.

Use in pregnancy and lactation: There is inadequate evidence of safety in human pregnancy, although prochlorperazine has been used widely for many years without apparent ill effects. However, as with other drugs, use of Buccastem in the first trimester of pregnancy should be avoided unless absolutely necessary. Since data from animal studies show that prochlorperazine may be found in breast milk, Buccastem should not be used during lactation.

Warnings: Hypotension, usually postural, may occur, particularly in elderly or volume depleted subjects.

Parkinsonism or tardive dyskinesia may occur occasionally, although are normally associated with higher doses than are recommended for Buccastem.

Alcohol and other CNS depressants should be used with caution, as should α-adrenoreceptor blocking antihypertensives.

Patients who drive or operate machinery should be warned of the possibility of drowsiness.

Adverse reactions: Drowsiness, dizziness, dry mouth, insomnia, agitation and mild skin reactions may occur. Extrapyramidal reactions are very unlikely at the recommended dosage.

Other adverse effects which have occurred rarely with prochlorperazine and other phenothiazine neuroleptics include jaundice, blood dyscrasias and, very rarely, hyperprolactinaemic effects. Neuroleptic malignant syndrome (hyperthermia, rigidity, autonomic dysfunction and altered consciousness) may occur with any neuroleptic.

Overdosage: The signs and symptoms will be predominantly extrapyramidal and may be accompanied by either restlessness and agitation or central nervous depression. Hypotension may also occur. Treatment is essentially symptomatic and supportive. There is no specific antidote. Gastric lavage is helpful, particularly when carried out within 6 hours of ingestion. Do not induce vomiting. Particular attention must be directed to maintaining a clear airway, since this may be threatened by the extrapyramidal muscle dystonias. Severe dystonic reactions usually respond to procyclidine (5–10 mg) or orphenadrine (20–40 mg) given i.m. or i.v. If convulsions occur they should be treated using i.v. diazepam. If hypotension is present strict attention to ventilation and posturing of the patient will often secure the desired effect but failing this, consideration should be given to volume expansion by i.v. fluids. If this is insufficient, positive inotropic agents such as dopamine may be tried, but peripheral vasoconstrictor agents are not generally recommended. Adrenaline should *not* be used.

Pharmaceutical precautions Protect from light.

Legal category POM.

Package quantities Packs of 60 tablets, in blister foils of 15 tablets each.

Further information Pharmacokinetic studies have shown that prochlorperazine is absorbed via the buccal mucosa. One Buccastem tablet administered twice daily produces steady state plasma levels equivalent to those achieved after oral administration of 5 mg three times daily.

Product licence number 0063/0011

DISPRIN CV*

Presentation Modified release tablets in a 28 day calendar pack.

1. White capsule-shaped tablets containing 100 mg Aspirin PhEur impressed on one side with a heart shape and the other a scoreline.

2. White capsule-shaped tablets containing 300 mg Aspirin PhEur impressed on one side with a heart shape and the other with 3C.

Uses Disprin CV 100. For the prevention of graft occlusion following aortocoronary by-pass surgery.

Disprin CV 300. To reduce the risk of myocardial infarction in patients who have had a previous attack or in patients with unstable angina and to reduce the risk of occlusive stroke and recurrent transient cerebral ischaemic attacks in patients with a history of such thrombotic events.

Dosage and administration Disprin CV is a modified release tablet which should be swallowed whole with water.

Adults and children over 12: 1 tablet to be taken every day, preferably at the same time each day.

Not to be given to children under 12 years, unless the expected benefits outweigh the possible risks.

Elderly: Risk/benefit ratios in the elderly have not yet been fully evaluated.

Contra-indications, warnings, etc The patient should start treatment only after consulting a doctor and is advised to consult a doctor if symptoms which were there before starting treatment persist. Disprin CV should not be given to patients suffering from active peptic ulceration or haemophilia, or patients known to be allergic to aspirin.

Aspirin may induce gastric irritation and gastrointestinal haemorrhage, occasionally major. Disprin CV should not be given to patients with asthma.

Use in pregnancy and lactation: There is clinical and epidemiological evidence of the safety of aspirin in pregnancy but it may prolong labour and contribute to maternal and neonatal bleeding and is best avoided in the last trimester of pregnancy unless recommended by a doctor.

Aspirin is excreted in low concentrations in breast milk but it is unlikely to adversely affect the breast-fed infant.

Drug interactions: Aspirin may enhance the effects of anticoagulants, oral hypoglycaemics and methotrexate and decrease the action of uricosurics.

Interference with laboratory tests: Salicylates may produce falsely increased results for blood creatinine, urate (low dose aspirin) and urea. Falsely decreased results may be obtained for blood thyroxine and urate (>4 g/day aspirin) and for urinary 5-HIAAA (with nitrosonaphthol method). Urinary VMA (HMMA) levels may be falsely increased or decreased depending on the method of analysis.

Treatment of overdosage: The major toxic signs of aspirin overdose arise from stimulation and terminal depression of the central nervous system. Symptoms include tinnitus, difficulty in hearing, dizziness, sweating, mental confusion and hyperventilation.

Treat symptomatically. Gastric lavage may be required. Blood tests should be undertaken to determine treatment.

Pharmaceutical precautions Store below 25°C.

Legal category P.

Package quantities Calendar packs of 28 tablets in individual blisters.

Further information Nil.

Product licence numbers
Disprin CV100 4338/0019
Disprin CV300 4338/0020

DISPROL* PAEDIATRIC

Presentation Disprol Paediatric is a pale yellow suspension contained in an amber glass bottle fitted with an expanded polythene wad and an aluminium roll-on pilfer-proof cap. Each 5 ml dose contains paracetamol PhEur 120 mg in a base containing hydrogenated glucose syrup, glycerol, carbomer, sodium hydroxide, methyl hydroxybenzoate, citric acid, sodium saccharin, banana flavour and riboflavin.

Uses For the treatment of mild to moderate pain, including headache, migraine, neuralgia, toothache, pain in teething, sore throat, aches and pains. Symptomatic relief of rheumatic aches and pains. Symptomatic relief of influenza, feverishness and feverish colds. Symptomatic relief of reactions due to vaccination or immunisation.

Dosage and administration
Children 3–12 months: Half to one 5 ml spoonful every four hours.

1 year to under 6 years: One to two 5 ml spoonfuls every four hours.

6 to 12 years: Two to four 5 ml spoonfuls every four hours.

Dosage for children under 3 months is at a physician's discretion.

Disprol Paediatric may be diluted with an equal volume of boiled then cooled water to produce a 12 mg/ml solution (60 mg/5 ml spoonful) with a 14 day shelf life.

For babies who develop fever following vaccination at 2 months, a 2.5 ml dose is suitable. When prescribed for a baby weighing less than 4.4 kg dose at 0.5 ml/kg (12 mg/kg) using an oral measuring syringe. In all other cases, not to be given to children under 3 months without doctor's advice.

Not more than 4 doses should be administered in any 24-hour period.

Dosage should not be continued for more than 3 days without consulting a doctor.

Contra-indications, warnings, etc Disprol Paediatric should not be given to patients with a history of hypersensitivity to paracetamol. It should be used with caution in patients with hepatic or renal dysfunction.

Each 5 ml dose of suspension contains approximately 3.25 g of hydrogenated glucose syrup (up to 12 Kcal). This should be borne in mind when treating diabetic children.

Side-effects from paracetamol administered in normal doses are rare. There have been isolated reports of agranulocytosis, methaemoglobinaemia and thrombocytopenic purpura, and after overdosage or prolonged administration, isolated cases of chronic hepatic necrosis, acute pancreatitis and nephrotoxicity.

Drug interactions: Drugs which induce hepatic microsomal enzymes, such as alcohol, barbiturates and tricyclic antidepressants, may increase the hepatotoxicity of paracetamol particularly after overdosage.

Interferences with laboratory tests: In paracetamol overdosage, the following tests for blood glucose may be distorted:

Reduction methods and YSI analyser – falsely increased results.

Glucose oxidase method – falsely decreased results.

There is no interference with the hexokinase method.

There may be analytical interference with catecholamine estimations.

Treatment of overdosage: Overdosage should be treated promptly by gastric lavage followed by an infusion of N-acetylcysteine or oral methionine since liver damage following overdosage does not become apparent for 1–6 days after ingestion. Initial mild symptoms consist of nausea, vomiting and pallor. Measurement of the blood paracetamol level and the time elapsed since ingestion is important in order to determine whether further therapy with N-acetylcysteine is necessary.

Pharmaceutical precautions Store below 25°C and protect from light, avoid freezing.

Legal category P.

Package quantities 500 ml bottles.

Product licence number 0063/0021.

FYBOGEL*, FYBOGEL* ORANGE and FYBOGEL* LEMON

Presentation Fybogel, Fybogel Orange and Fybogel Lemon (hereafter referred to as Fybogel) are buff coloured granules, presented in sachets and enclosed in an outer cardboard carton. The granules form a suspension in water. Each sachet contains Ispaghula Husk BP 3500 mg in a base containing citric acid, potassium bicarbonate, sodium bicarbonate, povidone, aspartame.

The variants are coloured and flavoured as follows:

Fybogel – betacarotene, no flavouring
Fybogel Orange – betacarotene, orange flavouring
Fybogel Lemon – curcumin, lemon flavouring

Fybogel is gluten free and contains no mono or disaccharides. Fybogel is low in sodium and potassium, containing approximately 0.4 mmol sodium and 0.7 mmol potassium per sachet.

Uses Fybogel is recommended for the treatment of patients requiring a high-fibre regimen: for example, for the relief of constipation including constipation in pregnancy and the maintenance of regularity; for the management of bowel function in patients with colostomy, ileostomy, haemorrhoids, anal fissure, chronic diarrhoea associated with diverticular disease, irritable bowel syndrome and ulcerative colitis.

Dosage and administration Fybogel effervescent granules disperse readily to form a palatable drink in water. The contents of one sachet should be stirred into approximately ¼ pint (150 ml) water and taken as quickly as possible, preferably after meals.

Adults and children over 12 years: One sachet morning and evening.

Children 6–12 years: Half to one level 5 ml spoonful depending on age and size, morning and evening. If there has been no bowel movement after 3 days of treatment a doctor should be consulted.

Children under 6 years: To be taken only on medical advice: Dose half to one level 5 ml spoonful, depending on age and size, morning and evening.

Elderly: There is no indication that dosage needs to be modified for the elderly.

The unflavoured variant may be added to foods with a high liquid content, as an alternative method of administration.

Contra-indications, warnings, etc Fybogel is contra-indicated in cases of intestinal obstruction, faecal impaction and colonic atony such as senile megacolon.

Due to its aspartame content, Fybogel should not be given to patients with phenylketonuria.

Fybogel should not be taken in the dry form. Gastrointestinal obstruction or impaction have been reported with hydrophilic mucinoid preparations when taken with insufficient liquid, contrary to administration instructions.

Use in pregnancy and lactation: May be used during pregnancy and lactation since the ispaghula is not absorbed from the gastrointestinal tract.

Drug interactions: There have been no interactions reported when Fybogel granules have been used with other drugs.

Interference with laboratory tests: Fybogel has no known effects on diagnostic laboratory tests.

Treatment of overdosage: In the event of overdosage, conservative measures should be taken. The patient may notice abdominal discomfort and flatulence. Attention should be paid to maintaining an adequate fluid intake, particularly if the granules have been taken without water, contrary to the administration instructions.

Side-effects: Flatulence and bloating may be experienced during the first few days of treatment but diminish during continued treatment.

Further information Ispaghula husk is capable of absorbing up to forty times its own weight of water in vitro, and part of its activity can be attributed to its action as a simple bulking agent. In addition, colonic bacteria are believed to use the hydrated material as a metabolic substrate. This results in an increase in the bacterial cell mass which softens the faeces to allow easy evacuation and avoiding episodes of straining.

Pharmaceutical precautions Store below 30°C in a dry place.

Legal category GSL

Package quantities 30 sachets (prescription pack – all variants). 10 sachets (OTC pack – orange or lemon variants).

Product licence numbers

Fybogel	0063/0023
Fybogel Orange	0063/0026
Fybogel Lemon	0063/0024

FYBOGEL* MEBEVERINE

Presentation Buff coloured granules containing orange spheroids, presented in sachets and enclosed in an outer cardboard carton. The product forms an orange suspension in water. Each individual sachet contains Ispaghula Husk BP 3500 mg and Mebeverine Hydrochloride BP 135 mg, in a base containing microcrystalline cellulose, eudragit, sterilised talc, polyethylene glycol, apocarotenal, citric acid, potassium bicarbonate, povidone, orange flavour, sodium saccharin and beta-carotene. The potassium content is 7 mmol per sachet.

Uses Fybogel Mebeverine is indicated for the treatment of the symptoms of abdominal pain and bowel dysfunction associated with irritable bowel syndrome or other gastrointestinal diseases.

Dosage and administration
Adults and children over 12 years: One sachet morning and evening before meals. An additional sachet may be taken before the midday meal if necessary.

Children under 12 years: Not recommended.

Elderly: There is no indication that the dosage need be modified for the elderly.

The contents of one sachet should be stirred into a glass of cold water (approx. ¼ pint) and taken immediately.

Contra-indications, warnings, etc Fybogel Mebeverine is contraindicated in cases of intestinal obstruction, faecal impaction and colonic atony such as senile megacolon.

Use in pregnancy and lactation: In common with most drugs, care should be taken in prescribing during pregnancy and lactation.

Drug interactions: None known.

Treatment of overdosage: In the event of overdosage, conservative measures should be taken. The patient may notice abdominal discomfort and flatulence, and attention should be paid to maintaining an adequate fluid intake, particularly if the product has been taken without water contrary to the administration instructions.

Interference with laboratory tests: None known.

Pharmaceutical precautions Store below 30°C in a dry place.

Legal category POM.

Package quantities 10 sachet packs.

Further information Studies by Ritchie and Truelove (1979, 1980) have demonstrated that a combination of ispaghula and mebeverine gave better overall relief of the symptoms of irritable bowel syndrome when compared to bran or another antispasmodic agent. Fybogel Mebeverine is presented as effervescent granules which disperse readily in water. References: Ritchie, J. A. & Truelove, S. C. (1979) Br. Med. J. 1, 376, Ritchie. J. A. & Truelove, S. C. (1980) Br. Med J. 281, 1317.

Product licence number 0063/0025.

FYBOZEST* ORANGE

Qualitative and quantitative composition A standard does of Fybozest Orange contins 3.5 g Ispaghula Husk BP.

Pharmaceutical form Granules for the preparation of an oral suspension.

Clinical particulars
Therapeutic indications: Primary hypercholesterolaemia. Fybozest Orange is indicated for reduction of mild to moderately elevated total serum cholesterol levels (6.5–7.8 mmol/l) and for the maintenance of lowered levels thereafter.

To be used in conjunction with dietary modification.

Posology and method of administration: For oral administration. Fybozest Orange should be stirred into at least 150 ml water and taken as quickly as possible.

Adults: The standard dose is 3.5 g ispaghula husk morning and evening (one measure of Fybozest Orange).

Elderly: Dosage need not be modified for use in elderly patients.

Children: Not recommended.

For packs to be used to fill prescriptions only: A higher dose of 5.25 g ispaghula husk morning and evening (one and a half measures of Fybozest Orange) may be taken for the initial two to three months of treatment by patients for whom an earlier onset of maximum serum cholesterol reduction is desirable for either clinical or motivational reasons.

Contra-indications: In cases of intestinal obstruction, faecal impaction and colonic atony such as senile megacolon.

Hypersensitivity to any of the ingredients.

Owing to its aspartame content, Fybozest Orange should not be taken by patients with phenylketonuria.

Special warnings and special precautions for use: Ispaghula husk should not be taken in the dry form. Gastrointestinal obstruction or impaction have been reported with hydrophilic mucilloid preparations when taken with insufficient liquid contrary to administration instructions.

Patients with diabetes mellitus should only take Fybozest Orange under medical supervision. A reduction in insulin dose may be necessary.

Interactions with other medicaments and other forms of interaction:
Drug interactions: None known.
Interference with laboratory tests: None known.

Pregnancy and lactation: Ispaghula husk has no

systemic activity and consequently can be taken during pregnancy and lactation.

Effects on ability to drive and use machines: None.

Undesirable effects: Flatulence and abnominal bloating may be experienced during the first few days of treatment, but should diminish during continued treatment. If abdominal discomfort is noticed on commencing treatment, the dosage may be reduced to one level measure per day until the effects subside.

Overdose: In the event of overdose, symptomatic treatment should be given. The patient may notice abdominal discomfort and flatulence. Attention should be paid to maintaining an adequate fluid intake, especially if the product was taken without fluid, contrary to administration instructions.

Pharmacological properties
Pharmacodynamic particulars: Ispaghula husk consists of both soluble and insoluble dietary fibre. It exerts a bulking effect in the gut as a result of its ability to absorb and hold water, up to 40 times its own weight of water *in vitro*. The hydrated material is used by bacteria as a metabolic substrate resulting in an increase in bacterial cell mass and enhancement of the bulking effect. Several hypotheses have been proposed to explain the reduction in serum cholesterol levels caused by soluble dietary fibre. These include a reduction in the absorption of cholesterol and fatty acids from the gut due to the viscous nature of the hydrated fibre or as a result of binding between bile acids/lipids and fibre, increased faecal excretion of bile acids and, to a small extent, inhibitiion of cholesterol synthesis by short chain fatty acids produced during fermentation of dietary fibre by colonic bacteria.

Pharmacokinetic particulars: Although the majority of isphagula husk passes through the digestive system unchanged, gut fermentation by colonic bacteria may lead to the formation of short chain fatty acids, primarily acetate with some propionate and butyrate. These SCFAs are further metabolised in the colon (mainly butyrate) or passed to the portal vein and cleared by the liver. Acetate and butyrate are converted to acetyl-coenzyme A, whilst propionate is converted to succinyl-coenzyme A. Further metabolism occurs in the same way as that of endogenous acetyl-coenzyme A and succinyl-coenzyme A via the citric acid cycle.

Preclinical safety data: No preclinical findings relevant to the prescriber have been reported.

Pharmaceutical particulars
List of excipients: Povidone K90, citric acid, potassium bicarbonate, sodium bicarbonate, aspartame, beta-carotene (E160a), orange flavour.

Incompatibilities: None known.

Shelf life: Tubs – three years.

Special precautions for storage: Store below 30°C.

Nature and contents of container: Polyethylene container with a polypropylene flip top lid and containing 265 g Fybozest Orange.

A propylene dose measure sits inside the flip top lid.

Instructions for use/handling: No special instructions.

Marketing authorisation number 0063/0043

Date of approval/revision of SPC October 1996.

Legal category P.

GAVISCON* ADVANCE

Qualitative and quantitative composition Each 10 ml dose contains:

Sodium Alginate BP	1000.0 mg
Potassium Bicarbonate USP	200.0 mg

Pharmaceutical form Oral suspension.

Clinical particulars
Therapeutic indications: Gastric reflux, reflux oesophagitis, heartburn, hiatus hernia, flatulence associated with gastric reflux, heartburn of pregnancy. All cases of epigastric and retrosternal distress where the underlying cause is gastric reflux.

Posology and method of administration:
Adults and children 12 years and over: 5–10 ml after meals and at bedtime.

Children under 12 years: Should be given only on medical advice.

Elderly: No dose modification is required for this age group.

Contra-indications: Hypersensitivity to any of the ingredients.

Special warnings and special precautions for use: Each 10 ml dose has a sodium content of 106 mg (4.6 mmol) and a potassium content of 78 mg (2.0 mmol). This should be taken into account when a highly restricted salt diet is recommended as in some renal and cardiovascular conditions.

If symptoms do not improve after seven days, the doctor should be consulted.

Interactions with other medicaments and other forms of interaction: None known.

Use in pregnancy and lactation: Alginic acid has no systemic activity and consequently can be taken during pregnancy and lactation.

Effect on ability to drive and to use machines: None.

Undesirable effects: Very rarely patients sensitive to the ingredients may develop allergic manifestations such as urticaria or bronchospasm.

Overdose: In the event of overdosage symptomatic treatment should be given. The patient may notice abdominal distension.

Pharmacological properties
Pharmacodynamic properties: On ingestion the suspension reacts with gastric acid to form a raft of alginic acid gel having a near-neutral pH and which floats on the stomach contents effectively impeding gastro-oesophageal reflux. In severe cases the raft itself may be refluxed into the oesophagus in preference to the stomach contents and exert a demulcent effect.

Pharmacokinetic properties: The mode of action of Gaviscon Advance is physical and does not depend on absorption into the systemic circulation.

Preclinical safety data: No preclinical findings of relevance to the prescriber have been reported.

Pharmaceutical particulars *List of excipients:* Calcium carbonate, carbomer, ethyl hydroxybenzoate, sodium butyl hydroxybenzoate, saccachrin sodium, fennel flavour, sodium hydroxide, purified water.

Incompatibilities: None known.

Shelf life: Two years.

Special precautions for storage: Store below 30°C. Do not refrigerate.

Nature and contents of container: Amber glass bottles with moulded polypropylene cap with polyethylene tamper-evident strip, lined with an expanded polyethylene wad and containing 140 ml or 500 ml of suspension.

Instructions for use/handling: To be taken orally. Shake well before use. Check that the cap seal is unbroken before first taking the product.

Marketing authorisation number 0063/0097

Date of approval/revision of SPC November 1996.

Legal category GSL.

LIQUID GAVISCON* LIQUID GAVISCON* PEPPERMINT FLAVOUR

Presentation Liquid Gaviscon is a pink suspension with a flavour of fennel (similar to aniseed) and Liquid Gaviscon Peppermint Flavour is a white suspension with a flavour of peppermint. Each 10 ml of liquid contains Sodium Alginate BP 500 mg, Sodium Bicarbonate PhEur 267 mg, Calcium Carbonate PhEur 160 mg in a base containing carbomer, methyl hydroxybenzoate, propyl hydroxybenzoate, sodium saccharin, sodium hydroxide and water. The fennel – flavoured liquid also contains erythrosine and fennel flavour, and the peppermint – flavoured liquid contains peppermint oil.

Liquid Gaviscon is gluten free and sugar free.

Uses Liquid Gaviscon and Liquid Gaviscon Peppermint Flavour (hereafter referred to as Gaviscon) alleviate the painful conditions resulting from the reflux of gastric acid and bile into the oesophagus by suppressing the reflux itself.

On ingestion, Gaviscon reacts with gastric acid to produce in the stomach a floating viscous gel of near neutral pH which effectively impedes reflux. In severe cases the gel itself may be refluxed into the oesophagus, where it protects the inflamed mucosa, thus allowing healing to take place and preventing further inflammation. Gaviscon is indicated in heartburn including heartburn of pregnancy, dyspepsia associated with gastric reflux, hiatus hernia, reflux oesophagitis, regurgitation and all cases of epigastric and retrosternal distress where the underlying cause is gastric reflux.

Dosage and administration
Adults, children over 12 years: 10–20 ml after meals and at bedtime.

Children 6 years to under 12 years: 5–10 ml after meals and at bedtime.
Children 2–6 years: Should only be given on medical advice.
Infants: Not recommended, Infant Gaviscon is available for Infants.

Elderly: There is no indication that dosage need be modified for the elderly.

If desired, the standard dose of Liquid Gaviscon may be taken diluted with not more than an equal quantity of water, well stirred.

Contra-indications, warnings, etc There are no specific contra-indications.

The sodium content of a dose of 10 ml is 141 mg (6.2 mmol). This may be of importance when a highly restricted salt diet is required as in some renal and cardiovascular conditions.

Very rarely, patients sensitive to the ingredients may develop allergic manifestations such as urticaria or bronchospasm.

Use in pregnancy: Liquid Gaviscon is indicated for heartburn in pregnancy.

Use in lactation: May be used in lactation since alginate is not absorbed from the gastrointestinal tract.

Drug interactions: There have been no interactions reported when Liquid Gaviscon has been used with other drugs.

Treatment of overdosage: As Gaviscon's mode of action is physical, overdosage in terms of alginate presents virtually no hazard. The only likely consequence is abdominal distention which is best treated conservatively.

Pharmaceutical precautions Store below 30°C; do not refrigerate.

Legal category GSL.

Package quantities 500 ml bottles.

Product licence numbers
Liquid Gaviscon 0063/0031
Liquid Gaviscon Peppermint Flavour 0063/0032

GAVISCON TABLETS* GAVISCON TABLETS* LEMON FLAVOUR

Presentation Matt, white, flat and circular tablets with bevelled edges. "GAVISCON", and the sword and circle symbol are impressed on both surfaces. The tablets are presented in polypropylene tubes with snap on caps, inside a cardboard carton. Each tablet contains Alginic Acid BP 500 mg, Sodium Bicarbonate EP 170 mg, Aluminium Hydroxide Gel BP 100 mg and Magnesium Trisilicate EP 25 mg in a base containing mannitol, xylitol, povidone, magnesium stearate, calcium carbonate and sodium saccharin.

Gaviscon Tablets, which are peppermint flavoured, also contain vanillin and peppermint oil. Gaviscon Tablets Lemon Flavour also contain lemon flavouring. The tablets are free from gluten, lactose and sugar.

Uses Gaviscon Tablets and Gaviscon Tablets Lemon Flavour (hereafter referred to as Gaviscon) alleviate the painful conditions resulting from the reflux of gastric acid and bile into the oesophagus by suppressing the reflux itself.

On ingestion, Gaviscon reacts with gastric acid to produce in the stomach a floating viscous gel of near neutral pH which effectively impedes reflux. In severe cases the gel itself may be refluxed into the oesophagus, where it protects the inflamed mucosa, thus allowing healing to take place and preventing further inflammation. Gaviscon is indicated for heartburn including heartburn of pregnancy, dyspepsia associated with gastric reflux, hiatus hernia, reflux oesophagitis, regurgitation and all cases of epigastric and restrosternal distress where the underlying cause is gastric reflux.

Dosage and administration
Adults and children over 12 years: One or two tablets after meals and at bedtime.

Children 6–12 years: One tablet after meals and at bedtime.

Children 2–6 years: Should be given only on medical advice. Dose: One tablet after meals and at bedtime.

Infants: Not recommended. Infant Gaviscon is available for infants.

Elderly: There is no indication that dosage need be modified for the elderly. Tablets should be thoroughly chewed. It is recommended they be broken in half and chewed a little at a time. This may be followed by a drink of water.

Contra-indications, warnings, etc There are no specific contra-indications.

Aluminium hydroxide containing products should be used with caution in patients with renal dysfunction or hypophosphataemia. The sodium content of a tablet is 47 mg (2.04 mmol). This may be of importance when a highly restricted salt diet is required as in some renal and cardiovascular conditions.

Use in pregnancy: Gaviscon is indicated for heartburn, including heartburn of pregnancy.

Use in lactation: May be used during lactation since the alginate is not absorbed from the gastrointestinal tract.

Drug interactions: There have been no interactions reported when Gaviscon has been used with other drugs. Although large doses of antacids interfere with the absorption of some drugs, the amount of antacid in the recommended dose of Gaviscon is unlikely to interact with other drugs.

Interference with laboratory tests: Gaviscon has no known effects on diagnostic laboratory tests.

Treatment of overdosage: As Gaviscon's mode of action is physical, overdosage in terms of the alginate presents virtually no hazard. The only likely consequence is abdominal distension which is best treated conservatively.

Pharmaceutical precautions Store below 30°C in a dry place.

Legal category GSL.

Package quantities Carton containing 60 Tablets (3 tubes of 20 tablets).

Product licence numbers
Gaviscon Tablets 0063/0033
Gaviscon Tablets Lemon Flavour 0063/0029

GAVISCON INFANT*

Qualitative and quantitative composition Each unit dose sachet of 0.65 g powder contains 225 mg sodium alginate and 87.5 mg magnesium alginate.

Pharmaceutical form Sachet of powder.

Clinical particulars
Therapeutic indications: Gaviscon Infant helps to prevent gastric regurgitation in infants where competence of the cardiac sphincter has not been fully established.

The indications for use are gastric regurgitation, gastro-oesophageal reflux and reflux associated with hiatus hernia in infants and young children.

Posology and method of administration: For oral use after mixing with water or milk feed.

Mix immediately before use as directed below:

Breast-fed infants: Under 4.5 kg (10 lb) – one dose.
Over 4.5 kg (10 lb) – two doses.

Add 5 ml of cooled, boiled water to the powder in a glass, mix to a smooth paste, add another 10 mL of the water and mix. Give after each feed using a spoon or feeding bottle.

Bottle-fed infants: Under 4.5 kg (10 lb) – one dose to be mixed into not less than 115 mL of each feed in the bottle and shaken well.

Over 4.5 kg (10 lb) – two doses to be mixed into not less than 225 mL of each feed in the bottle and shaken well.

Young children: Two doses prepared as for breast-fed infants, to be taken after each meal.

Not appropriate for adults or elderly.

Treatment should not be administered more than six times per 24 hours.

Contra-indications: Contra-indicated in cases of intestinal obstruction and in cases of established diarrhoea. Not to be used except on a doctor or other health professional's recommendation.

Not to be used in premature infants or infants under one year except under medical supervision, or in situations where excessive water loss is likely, e.g. fever, diarrhoea, vomiting or high room temperature. Not to be used in gastroenteritis, where the appropriate treatment is rehydration with fluid replacement.

Not to be used when treating infants with known or suspected impairment of renal function as the sodium content (approximately 21 mg or 0.92 mmol per dose) may add to the risk of hypernatraemia.

Special warnings and special precautions for use: Follow dosage instructions exactly to avoid an excessive amount of product per feed and the possible risk of hypernatraemia.

Hypernatraemia should be treated with oral fluids and monitoring of the infant's electrolytes. Severe cases should be treated by the cautious use of hypo-osmotic solutions.

A medical review of the patient's condition should be undertaken seven days after initiating treatment or before if symptoms worsen.

Interaction with other medicaments and other forms of interaction: Not to be used with thickening agents or infant milk preparations containing a thickening agent as this could lead to over-thickening of the stomach contents.

Pregnancy and lactation: Not appropriate.

Effect on ability to drive and use machines: Not applicable.

Undesirable effects: Gaviscon Infant's mode of action is physical, resulting in a thickening of the gastric contents. An excessive concentration of Gaviscon Infant may lead to gastric distension.

Overdose: Rare instances have occurred in which an intragastric mass has developed, comprising Gaviscon Infant and milk proteins. Overdosage may have contributed to the development of such masses. The majority resolved spontaneously when the child was admitted to hospital, Gaviscon Infant was discontinued and a regime of adequate fluid intake and monitoring of fluid and electrolyte balance was installed. If spontaneous resolution of the mass does not occur, removal by surgical or endoscopic means may be required.

Pharmacological properties
Pharmacodynamic properties: The mode of action of Gaviscon Infant is physical. By reacting with acidic gastric contents to form a viscous gel it stabilises stomach activity so reducing the incidence of gastro-oesophageal reflux.

Pharmacokinetic properties: The mode of action of Gaviscon Infant is physical and does not depend on absorption into the systemic circulation.

Preclinical safety data: No preclinical findings of relevance to the prescriber have been reported.

Pharmaceutical particulars
List of excipients: Mannitol and colloidal silica.

Incompatibilities: None known.

Shelf life: Three years.

Special precautions for storage: None.

Nature and contents of container: A cardboard outer carton containing 30 unit dose sachets joined in pairs. The sachets are composed of paper (41 gsm), low density polyethylene (12 gsm), aluminium foil (21.6 gsm) with Surlyn 1652 laminate (18 gsm).

Instructions for use/handling: Gaviscon Infant should be mixed with milk or water before taking. As the powder is sterile the sachet should not be opened until immediately before mixing.

Marketing authorisation number PL 0063/0099

Date of renewal of authorisation 21 April 1997

Date of revision of the text
14 April 1998

SENOKOT*

Presentation *Tablets:* Small brown tablets engraved on one side only with the word Senokot and a sword symbol. One tablet contains standardised senna equivalent to 7.5 mg total sennosides calculated as sennoside B. Senokot tablets contain lactose and parabens.

Granules: Brown chocolate-flavoured granules. One 5 ml level spoonful (2.73 g) contains standardised senna equivalent to 15 mg total sennosides calculated as sennoside B. Senokot granules contain sucrose.

Syrup: Brown, fruit-flavoured syrup. One 5 ml spoonful contains standardised senna extract equivalent to 7.5 mg total sennosides calculated as sennoside B. Senokot syrup contains sucrose and ethanol.

Uses In the management of constipation, including:
Simple constipation, whether self-induced or environmental, e.g. neglect of the call to stool or poor sanitary conditions.
Constipation in old age, especially where maintenance treatment is required.
Constipation in pregnancy and the puerperium.
Idiopathic slow-transit constipation.
Constipation in the irritable bowel syndrome.
Conservative treatment of haemorrhoids.
Avoidance of straining after surgery and in cerebral and cardiovascular disease.

The physiological action of the anthrone glycoside in Senokot is virtually colon specific. The anthroquinones are protected by a natural sugar moiety which safeguards their transport to the large bowel, where bacterial action breaks the sugar-anthrone bond and releases the active fraction. Peristalsis is then stimulated via the submucosal and myenteric plexuses.

Being colon specific, Senokot does not affect the vital nutritional functions of the upper gastro-intestinal tract.

Dosage and administration The correct dose of Senokot is the smallest required to produce a comfortable soft-formed motion. It varies between individuals, but is generally found within the following ranges:

Adults: 2 tablets (up to 4 on medical advice) or one 5 ml spoonful of granules (up to 10 ml on medical advice) or 10 ml of syrup (up to 20 ml on medical advice) at bedtime.

Children over 6 years: Half the adult dosages, taken in the morning.

Children 2–6 years: Use Senokot syrup ½ to one 5 ml spoonful. Tablets and Granules are not recommended for children 6 and under.

There is no indication that dosage need be modified for the elderly.

New users should start with the lowest dose of the preferred formulation. These are available from a range of general sales packs advising only the lowest dose and available for self medication as described above. Alternatively the product may be dispensed to allow, if necessary, an increase by half the initial dose each day until a comfortable formed motion is produced. If no bowel action has occurred after three days' progressively increased dosage a medical examination should be considered.

Senokot is best taken as a single dose, at bedtime by adults and in the morning by children. The tablets can be taken with a drink, the granules can be stirred into hot milk, sprinkled on food, or eaten as they are.

Once regularity has been achieved, dosage should be reduced and can usually be stopped.

Contra-indications, warnings, etc Senokot like all laxatives, should not be given when any undiagnosed acute or persistent abdominal symptoms are present. Temporary mild griping may occur during adjustment of dosage.

Diabetic patients should use the tablets as these have a negligible sugar content.

Use in lactation: Clinical studies have shown that breast fed infants of mothers taking Senokot did not show any side effects of the drug.

Interference with laboratory tests: Senokot has no known effects on diagnostic laboratory tests.

Treatment of overdosage: In cases of accidental overdosage, where diarrhoea is severe, conservative measures are usually sufficient: generous amounts of fluid especially fruit drinks should be given.

Pharmaceutical precautions The tablets and granules should be kept in closed airtight containers, and the syrup in amber bottles as supplied. Store in a cool place.

Legal category GSL, sales restricted to pharmacies.

Package quantities
Tablets: 20, 60 and 100 in blisters; 500 in Securitainers.
Granules: 100 g in Securitainers.
Syrup: Bottles of 100 ml and 500 ml.

Further information Nil.

Product licence numbers
Tablets 0063/5000R
Granules 0063/5002
Syrup 0063/5003

TIMODINE*

Presentation A pale yellow cream presented in an internally laquered aluminium tube, in an outer cardboard carton. Each 30 g tube contains w/w Nystatin BP 100,000 i.u./g. Hydrocortisone Ph Eur 0.5 %, Benzalkonium Chloride solution BP 0.2% and Dimethicone 350 BP 10.0%, in a base containing: butylated hydroxyanisole, cetostearyl alcohol, cellulose nitrate, dibutyl phthalate, glyceryl monostearate, methyl and propyl hydroxybenzoate, sorbic acid, stearic acid and sodium metabisulphate.

Uses For the treatment of dermatoses, including intertrigo, eczema, seborrhoeic dermatitis, "housewive's eczema" and pruritus ani and vulvae, in which infection with Candida albicans is a factor. For the treatment of severe napkin rash in which Candida albicans is a factor.

Timodine is particularly indicated in the treament of dermatoses occurring in sites, such as the skin folds, in which the special environmental conditions present predispose to maceration and chafing, leading to secondary infection with Candida albicans and bacteria, and causing additional inflammation and persistent pruritis.

Dosage and administration *Dermatoses:* A thin layer of Timodine should be applied to cover the lesion. It should then be massaged into the skin until the cream disappears. The treatment should be repeated three times a day until the lesion has healed.

There is no indication that dosage need be modified for the elderly.

Napkin rash: After removal of the soiled napkin, the affected areas should be cleaned and dried and a thin layer of Timodine applied. The treatment should be repeated after every napkin change. In infants the long term continuous topical steroid therapy should be avoided and a course of treatment should not normally exceed seven days.

Contra-indications, warnings, etc Use only on the skin. Timodine should not be used by anyone who is allergic to the product or any of its ingredients.

Precautions: Keep away from eyes.

Use in pregnancy: Topical administration of corticosteroids to pregnant animals can cause abnormalities of foetal development. The relevance of this finding to human beings has not been established; however, topical steroids should not be used extensively in pregnancy, ie: in large amounts or for prolonged periods.

Use in lactation: There is no information about effects on lactation.

Side-effects: None have been reported.

Interference with laboratory tests: Timodine has no known effects on diagnostic laboratory tests.

Pharmaceutical precautions Store below 15°C.

Legal category POM.

Package quantities 30 g tubes.

Further information Nil.

Product licence number 1839/0001

Product licence holder: Lloyd-Hamol Limited.

**Trade Mark*

Rhône-Poulenc Rorer Limited

West Malling
Kent ME19 4AH

☎ 01732 584000 📠 01732 584080

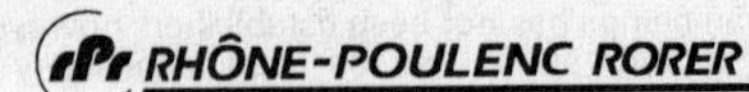

ALGICON* TABLETS AND SUSPENSION

Qualitative and quantitative composition
Ingredients
Tablets: Magnesium Alginate 500 mg, Aluminium Hydroxide/Magnesium Carbonate Co-gel 360 mg
Magnesium Carbonate Heavy BP 320 mg, Potassium Bicarbonate USP 100 mg
Suspension: Per 5 ml dose, Magnesium Alginate 250 mg
Aluminium Hydroxide/Magnesium Carbonate Co-gel 140 mg
Magnesium Carbonate BP 175 mg, Potassium Bicarbonate USP 50 mg

Pharmaceutical form Tablets or Suspension.

Clinical particulars
Therapeutic indications: Indications for which product may be sold as a GSL product:
Heartburn, Indigestion and excess stomach acid.
Indications for which product may be sold through registered Pharmacies:
Heartburn associated with gastric reflux, reflux oesophagitis, hiatus hernia, pregnancy and hyperacidity.

Posology and method of administration:
Tablets: Adults: Chew 1 or 2 tablets four times a day or as directed by a physician. Tablets should be taken after meals and at bedtime or as needed.

Children: Not recommended for children under 12 years.

Elderly: No special precautions required

Suspension: Adults: 10 to 20 ml four times a day or as directed by a Physician. The suspension should be taken after meals and at bedtime or as needed.

Children: Not recommended.

Elderly: No specific precautions are necessary in normal use.

Route of administration: Oral

Contra-indications: Algicon should not be administered to patients who have kidney disease or are severely debilitated or to patients who are taking an antibiotic containing tetracycline.

Special warnings and special precautions for use: Due to the high sugar content of the tablets care should be exercised in the treatment of diabetic patients with this dosage presentation. Do not freeze Suspension.

Interactions with other medicaments and other forms of interaction: None known.

Use during pregnancy and lactation: There is no information on the use of Algicon in pregnancy and lactation.

Effects on ability to drive and use machines: Algicon would not be expected to affect the ability to drive or to use machinery.

Undesirable effects: None stated.

Overdose: In overdose, abdominal distension is the most likely occurrence, and appropriate conservative measures should be taken.

Pharmacological properties
Pharmacodynamic properties: Algicon is an alginate antacid formulation. When taken by mouth the magnesium reacts with the gastric contents to form an insoluble gel-like foam which forms a layer above the gastric contents. The aluminium hydroxide/magnesium carbonate component gives the product antacid properties.

Pharmacokinetic properties: Algicon acts directly on the stomach contents; systemic absorption is not significant.

Preclinical safety data: Not applicable.

Pharmaceutical particulars
List of excipients: Tablets: Compressible sugar USP, Pregelatinised starch USP, Spray dried natural lemon flavour, Swiss creme powder, Peppermint flavour, Magnesium stearate.
Suspension: Precipitated calcium carbonate EP, Sorbitol Solution BP, Xanthan gum NF, Methylparaben EP, Propylparaben EP, Calcium saccharin USP, Natural lemon concentrate, Swiss creme flavour, Peppermint oil EP, Hydrogen peroxide 30% solution BP, Quinoline yellow (E 104), water.

Incompatibilities: None stated.

Shelf life: Tablets: 36 months, *Suspension:* 24 months

Special precautions for storage: Tablets: Store below 25°C in a dry place. *Suspension:* Keep from freezing.

Nature and contents of container: Tablets: PVC/ACLAR or PVC/PVDC blisters or amber glass bottles containing 2, 10, 50 or 60 tablets.
Suspension: White HDPE plastic bottles with polypropylene cap containing 500 ml or single dose paper/foil plastic sachets containing 10 ml.

Marketing authorisation number
Tablets PL 05272/0010
Suspension PL 05272/0009

Date of approval/revision of SPC Tablets: 28th April 1993
Suspension: 16th April 1993

Legal category GSL.

ASCABIOL* EMULSION 25% W/V

Qualitative and quantitative composition Benzyl benzoate B.P. 25% w/v.

Pharmaceutical form White emulsion.

Clinical particulars
Therapeutic indications: Ascabiol is an efficient acaricide and is indicated for the treatment of scabies and pediculosis.

Posology and method of administration: Topical.
Adults: Scabies – after a hot bath and drying, Ascabiol is applied to the whole body except the head and face. If the application is thorough, one treatment should suffice, but the possibility of failure is lessened if a second application is made within five days of the first.
Alternatively Ascabiol can be applied to the whole body, except the head and face, on three occasions at 12-hourly intervals. The patient has a hot bath 12 hours after the last application and changes to clean clothes and sheets.
Pediculosis–the affected region is coated with Ascabiol followed by a wash 24 hours later with soap and water. In severe cases this procedure may need to be repeated two or three times. An examination should always be made a week after the last treatment to confirm disinfestation.

Elderly patients: No specific recommendations.

Children: Ascabiol can be diluted with an equal quantity of water for older children and with three parts of water for babies.

Contra-indications: none.

Special warnings and special precautions for use: The emulsion may damage plastic or acrylic bathroom furniture, Care should be taken not to splash the emulsion on such surfaces.

Interaction with other medicaments and other forms of interaction: not applicable.

Pregnancy and lactation: There is inadequate evidence of the safety of Ascabiol in human pregnancy, but it has been in widespread use for many years without apparent ill consequence. Nevertheless Ascabiol should not be used during pregnancy unless considered essential.
Breast feeding should be suspended during treatment with Ascabiol. Feeding may be restarted after the emulsion has been washed off the body.

Effects on ability to drive and use machines: Not applicable.

Undesirable effects: Ascabiol causes little skin irritation, but may cause a transient burning sensation. This is usually mild but can occasionally be severe in sensitive individuals. In the event of a severe skin reaction the preparation should be washed off using soap and warm water. Ascabiol is also irritating to the eyes therefore these should be protected if it is applied to the scalp.

Overdose: If Ascabiol is accidentally taken by mouth, treatment should consist of gastric lavage or the administration of an emetic. An anticonvulsant should be given if necessary, otherwise treatment is symptomatic.
Urinary retention in adults and convulsions in infants, have been reported following excessive use of topical benzyl benzoate. The body should be washed to remove excess benzyl benzoate. Otherwise treatment is symptomatic.

Pharmacological properties
Pharmacodynamic properties: Benzyl benzoate is lethal to *Sarcoptes scabei* and to the larval and adult forms of head lice.

Pharmacokinetic properties: No data available by the topical route.

Preclinical safety data: There are no pre-clinical data of relevance to the prescriber which are additional to that already included in other sections of the SPC.

Pharmaceutical particulars
List of excipients: Stearic acid powder, Triethanolamine, Terpineol, Oil Cinnamon Leaf Ceylon, Silicone MS Antifoam A, Demineralised Water,

Incompatibilities: Not applicable.

Shelf life: 36 months.

Special precautions for storage: Store below 25°C.

Nature and contents of container: Amber glass bottles with a screw cap containing 100 ml and 200 ml sizes.

Instructions for use/handling: The emulsion may damage plastic or acrylic bathroom furniture. Care should be taken not to splash the emulsion on such surfaces.

Marketing authorisation number PL 0012/5104R.

Date of approval/revision of SPC January 1997.

Legal category: P.

CALCITARE*

Presentation For intramuscular or subcutaneous use only.
Each vial contains 160 international units Calcitonin (Pork) BP.

Uses For short term treatment in
i) Paget's disease of bone
ii) *Hypercalcaemia:* The calcium lowering effect of calcitonin is usually rapid. Treatment should be regarded as an adjunct to more specific long-term measures. The fall in serum calcium is more pronounced in hypercalcaemic patients with a raised bone turnover, e.g. Paget's disease and thyrotoxicosis. Treatment may also be beneficial in patients with hypercalcaemia due to immobilisation in Paget's disease, malignancy, vitamin D intoxication and hyperparathyroidism. Calcitonin is of particular value when such patients have concurrent renal or cardiac failure.

Dosage and administration Calcitare can be given subcutaneously or intramuscularly.
1. *Paget's disease of bone:* Clinical and biochemical improvement has been observed with dosage regimens ranging from 80 international units three times a week to 160 international units daily in single or divided doses.
Daily injections of 80 international units or 160 international units are recommended for three to six months in patients with bone pain or nerve compression syndromes.
Clinical improvement is usually seen within three months but may occasionally be delayed for as long as a year. When clinical improvement occurs, an attempt to reduce the dose and/or frequency of injection may be made, consistent with maintaining a remission. Alternatively, treatment can be stopped and restarted at a later date when necessary. Duration of dosage should be a maximum of two six month courses.
Biochemical improvement is shown by a reduction in serum alkaline phosphatase and urinary hydroxyproline excretion, the fall in urinary hydroxyproline often occurring in a matter of days. The fall in serum alkaline phosphatase occurs in a matter of weeks. Serum alkaline phosphatase and urinary hydroxyproline levels return slowly towards pre-treatment values (at different rates) on withdrawal of calcitonin therapy.
When changing from synthetic salmon calcitonin

(Calsynar) to porcine calcitonin (Calcitare), 80 international units of Calcitare may be conveniently substituted for 50 international units of Calsynar and 160 international units for 100 international units respectively.

2. *Hypercalcaemia:* The optimum dosage pattern must essentially be gauged by the magnitude of the hypocalcaemic response obtained in a particular patient. In general the greatest response will be observed in cases of rapid bone turnover. Four international units per kg per day of Calcitare may produce a fall in serum calcium. However, larger doses of calcitonin may be necessary, but are inconvenient to administer as Calcitare, in which case treatment with Calsynar is advised.

Elderly: No special precautions.

Children: Calcitare should not be given to children for more than a few weeks unless the physician considers that longer treatment is indicated on compelling medical grounds; careful surveillance of bone growth is recommended.

Contra-indications, warnings and side-effects A species and strain-specific dose-related increase of pituitary adenomas has been observed in long term toxicity studies in the rat. As the significance of these findings to man is uncertain, long term use is not recommended.

Calcitonin may cause nausea, vomiting, facial flushing and tingling of the hands. An unpleasant taste and inflammatory reactions at the injection site have been reported. The nausea and flushing are usually transient and rarely necessitate withdrawal of treatment. If necessary, the injections can be administered at night with an antiemetic. Administration of Calcitare has been reported in a few cases to cause serious allergic type reactions which should be differentiated from generalised flushing and hypotension.

In any patient with a history of allergy, a scratch (or intradermal) test should be conducted prior to administration of Calcitare using a 1:100 dilution in Sodium Chloride Injection BP. To detect gelatin sensitivity a similar test should be carried out using gelatin diluent in the same dilution.

Some patients will develop porcine calcitonin binding antibodies after several months of treatment. The antibodies are generally of low titre and are more likely to occur in patients on the higher doses. The development of these antibodies is not usually related to loss of clinical efficacy. It is possible that this may be analogous to treated diabetic patients in whom insulin binding antibodies frequently develop, but who rarely manifest clinical resistance to insulin. The presence of these antibodies appears to bear no relationship to allergic reactions which are very rare. Secondary hyperparathyroidism is not thought to occur following calcitonin therapy.

There are several reports of the value of calcitonin in the acute treatment of severe hypercalcaemia in patients with concurrent renal or cardiac failure; however, care should be exercised when treating such patients.

Trace amounts of T_3/T_4 are present in Calcitare. Experience over a number of years has not revealed any significant metabolic effects due to T_3 and T_4, when Calcitare has been given at the maximum recommended dose for Paget's disease of 160 international units daily. At higher doses (e.g. 4 international units/kg) used in the treatment of hypercalcaemia, the amounts of T_3/T_4 normally detected in the product are most unlikely to have any adverse effect, except in highly susceptible patients such as those with significant ischaemic heart disease.

Use in pregnancy and lactation: Studies have not been carried out in pregnant patients. Animal studies have suggested a possible relationship between calcitonin and retardation of foetal growth and inhibition of lactation. Unless considered essential, calcitonin should not be used in women of child bearing potential or nursing mothers.

Treatment of overdosage: No specific antidote. Following overdosage, e.g., 600 international units as a single injection one might experience flushing of the face and/or extremities or gastrointestinal disturbance. Acute hypocalcaemia is unlikely to occur.

Pharmaceutical precautions Calcitare is presented as a sterile, lyophilised powder providing 160 international units porcine calcitonin per vial. Calcitare should normally be used immediately after aseptic reconstitution. The reconstituted product will, however, maintain its potency for up to 24 hours at room temperature or 7 days in a refrigerator (2°–8°C). Typically, however, the reconstituted product should be stored at 2°–8°C and used within 48 hours.

The lyophilised powder when stored at less than 25°C will retain its potency for three years.

Legal category POM.

Package quantities *For intramuscular or subcutaneous use:* Boxes of 5 vials Calcitare 160 international units per vial sterile, lyophilised, with 5 ampoules gelatin diluent, sterile (2 ml).

Boxes of 10 vials Calcitare 160 international units per vial sterile, lyophilised, with 10 ampoules gelatin diluent, sterile (2 ml).

Further information The calcium lowering ability of the calcitonins is measured in international units. The international unit is based on a rat bioassay in which one fortieth of the weight of salmon calcitonin, as compared with weights of porcine and human calcitonin, produces the same fall in serum calcium. The weights of pure calcitonin equivalent to 100 international units in this assay are: human calcitonin, 1 mg, porcine calcitonin, 1 mg, and salmon calcitonin, 0.025 mg.

Product licence number 00012/0296

CALSYNAR*

Presentation

Multidose vials: An aqueous solution containing 400 international units of synthetic Salmon Calcitonin in 2 mls of solution. The injection also contains Sodium Chloride, Sodium Acetate, Acetic Acid and Phenol.

Ampoule: An aqueous solution containing 100 international units of Synthetic Salmon Calcitonin in 1 ml of solution. The injection also contains Sodium Chloride, Sodium Acetate and Acetic Acid.

Uses For the short term treatment of:

a. Paget's disease of bone.
b. Advancing osteolytic hypercalcaemia of malignancy.
c. Pain associated with advanced metastatic bone cancer: The use of Calsynar has been reported to be beneficial in the relief of pain in some patients with advanced metastatic bone cancer.
d. Postmenopausal osteoporosis: Studies based on total body calcium determinations have indicated that Calsynar may be effective in the prevention of progressive loss of bone mass in the treatment of postmenopausal osteoporosis.

Dosage and administration For subcutaneous or intramuscular use only.

(a) Paget's disease of bone: Clinical and biochemical improvement has been observed with dosage regimens ranging from 50 international units three times a week to 100 international units daily in single or divided doses.

When clinical improvement occurs, a dosage reduction may maintain a remission in some patients. Alternatively, treatment can be stopped and restarted at a later date when necessary.

Biochemical improvement is shown by a reduction in serum alkaline phosphatase and urinary hydroxyproline excretion, the fall in urinary hydroxyproline often occurring in a matter of days, the fall in serum alkaline phosphatase and urinary hydroxyproline levels return slowly towards pretreatment values (at different rates) on withdrawal of calcitonin therapy.

When changing from porcine calcitonin (Calcitare) to synthetic salmon calcitonin (Calsynar) 50 international units of Calsynar may be conveniently substituted for 80 international units of Calcitare and 100 international units for 160 international units of Calcitare.

(b) Advancing osteolytic hypercalcaemia of malignancy: Treatment should be adjusted to the patient's clinical and biochemical response.

Severe hypercalcaemia may require high doses of Calsynar and initially 400 international units may be given every 6 or 8 hours. Lower doses may be satisfactory in some patients and dosage may be adjusted according to the patient's clinical and biochemical response. There is no additional benefit to be gained from doses in excess of 8 international units per kg given every 6 hours.

(c) Pain associated with metastatic bone cancer: The usual dose is 200 international units, 6-hourly or 400 international units 12-hourly for 48 hours. Concomitant analgesic medication may be reduced as appropriate. The treatment course may be repeated at the discretion of the physician.

Many patients with advanced malignant disease already suffer from anorexia and nausea. In these cases, prior administration of anti-emetic therapy may reduce the incidence of nausea and vomiting sometimes associated with calcitonin therapy.

(d) Post menopausal osteoporosis: The recommended dose of Calsynar is 100 international units per day. Patients should also receive supplementary calcium (equivalent to 600 mg elemental calcium daily) and vitamin D (400 units daily). An adequate diet is also essential. (See also *Further information*).

Elderly: No special precautions.

Children: Calsynar should not be given to children for periods of more than a few weeks unless the physician considers that longer treatment is indicated on compelling medical grounds. Careful surveillance of bone growth is recommended.

Contra-indications, warnings, etc

Precautions: Rat carcinogenicity studies have shown a dose related excess of pituitary tumours. As the significance of this finding is uncertain, long term use is not recommended.

There are several reports of the value of Calcitonin in the acute treatment of severe hypercalcaemia in patients with concurrent renal or cardiac failure, however, care should be exercised when treating such patients.

Following injections of calcitonin serum calcium levels may be transiently lowered to below normal values. This effect is noted most frequently on initiation of therapy where bone turnover is abnormally high, but diminishes as osteoclastic activity is reduced with Calsynar. Whilst this phenomenon does not usually give rise to complications, care should be exercised in patients who are receiving concurrent cardiac glycosides as dosage adjustments of these drugs may be necessary in view of the fact that their effect may be modified by changes in cellular electrolyte concentrations.

Prior to treatment with Calsynar any patients with a history of allergy should undergo a scratch (or intradermal) test using a 1:100 dilution of Calsynar in Sodium Chloride injection BP.

Side-effects: Calcitonin may cause nausea, vomiting, facial flushing, tingling of the hands and an unpleasant taste. Inflammatory reactions at the injection site have been reported. The nausea and flushing are usually transient and rarely necessitate withdrawal of treatment. If necessary, the injections can be administered at night with an antiemetic.

Some patients will develop salmon calcitonin binding antibodies after several months of treatment. The antibodies are generally of low titre and are more likely to occur in patients on the higher doses. The development of these antibodies is not usually related to loss of clinical efficacy. It is possible that this may be analogous to treated diabetic patients in whom insulin binding antibodies frequently develop, but who rarely manifest clinical resistance to insulin. The presence of antibodies appears to bear no relationship to allergic reactions which are very rare. Secondary hyperparathyroidism is not thought to occur following calcitonin therapy.

Administration of salmon calcitonin has been reported in a few cases to cause serious allergic type reactions (e.g. bronchospasm, swelling of the tongue or throat and anaphylactic shock). Allergic reactions should be differentiated from generalised flushing and hypotension.

Use in pregnancy and lactation: Studies have not been carried out in pregnant women. Animal studies have suggested a possible relationship between Calcitonin and retardation of foetal growth and inhibition of lactation. Hence unless considered essential, Calcitonin should not be used in women of child bearing potential or nursing mothers.

Treatment of overdosage: Symptoms following overdosage, e.g. 400 international units administered as a single injection, may include flushing of the face and or extremities, and gastrointestinal disturbance. Acute hypocalcaemia is unlikely to occur. There is no specific antidote.

Pharmaceutical precautions

Calsynar multidose vials: Store between 2–8°C. Do not freeze.

Calsynar Ampoules: Store between 2–8°C. Do not freeze.

Legal category POM.

Package quantities Multidose vial: Box of 1 and cartons of 4 vials.

Ampoules: Cartons of 5.

Further information

Postmenopausal osteoporosis: There is evidence from published literature on postmenopausal osteoporosis that cyclical therapy may be useful in some patients.

Units and potency: The calcium lowering ability of the calcitonins is measured in international units. The international unit is based on a rat bioassay in which one fortieth of the weight of salmon calcitonin, as compared with weights of porcine and human calcitonin, produces the same fall in serum calcium. The weights of pure calcitonin equivalent to 100 international units in this assay are approximately: human calcitonin 1 mg; porcine calcitonin 1 mg and salmon calcitonin 0.025 mg.

Product licence numbers

Multidose vials: 00012/0297
Ampoules: 00012/0298

CAMPTO* ▼

Qualitative and quantitative composition Vials of Campto contain 40 mg or 100 mg of irinotecan hydrochloride, trihydrate.

Pharmaceutical form Concentrate for solution for infusion.

Clinical particulars

Therapeutic indications: Campto is indicated for the second-line treatment of adult patients with metastatic colorectal cancer who have failed an established 5-fluorouracil (5FU) containing treatment regimen.

Posology and method of administration: Recommended Dosage: The recommended dosage of Campto is 350 mg/m² administered as an intravenous infusion over a 30 to 90 minute period every three weeks (see *Instructions for use/handling*).

Dosage adjustments: In patients who experienced asymptomatic severe neutropenia (neutrophil count <500 cells/mm³), fever or infections associated with neutropenia (temperature ≥38°C and neutrophil count ≤1,000 cells/mm³) or severe diarrhoea (requiring an intravenous rehydration), dosage should be reduced from 350 mg/m² to 300 mg/m² in subsequent cycles. If at 300 mg/m², the patient again experiences severe neutropenia, fever or infections associated with neutropenia as defined above or severe diarrhoea, the dosage should be decreased from 300 mg/m² to 250 mg/m² at the next cycle.

Delayed dosing: Campto should not be administered until the neutrophil count returns to above 1,500 cells/mm³. In patients who experienced severe neutropenia or severe gastrointestinal adverse events such as diarrhoea, nausea and vomiting, (see *Special warnings and special precautions for use*), dosing of Campto should be delayed until there has been a full recovery of these symptoms, especially diarrhoea.

Treatment duration: Treatment with Campto should be continued until there is an objective progression of the disease or an unacceptable toxicity.

Special populations: Patients with impaired hepatic function: In patients with a bilirubin >1.0 and ≤1.5 times the upper limit of the normal range (ULN), the risk of severe neutropenia is increased. Thus frequent monitoring of complete blood counts should be conducted in this patient population. In patients with a bilirubin >1.5 times the ULN, patients should not be treated with Campto [see *Contra-indications* and *Special warnings and special precautions for use*]. *Patients with impaired renal function:* Campto is not recommended for use in patients with impaired renal function, as studies in this population have not been conducted. (see *Special warnings and special precautions for use* and *Pharmacokinetic properties*). *Elderly:* No specific pharmacokinetic studies have been performed in the elderly. However, the dose should be chosen carefully in this population due to their greater frequency of decreased biological functions, in particular hepatic function. (see *Special warnings and special precautions for use*).

Contra-indications: Campto is contraindicated in patients who have chronic inflammatory bowel disease and/or bowel obstruction (see *Special warnings and special precautions for use*). Campto is contraindicated in patients who have a history of severe hypersensitivity reactions to irinotecan hydrochloride trihydrate or to one of the excipients of Campto. Campto is contraindicated during pregnancy and lactation (see *Pregnancy and lactation* and *Special warnings and special precautions for use*). Campto is contraindicated in patients with a bilirubin >1.5 times the upper limit of the normal range (see *Special warnings and special precautions for use*). Campto is contraindicated in patients with severe bone marrow failure. Campto is contraindicated in patients with WHO performance status >2

Special warnings and special precautions for use: The use of Campto should be confined to units specialised in the administration of cytotoxic chemotherapy and it should only be administered under the supervision of a physician qualified in the use of anticancer chemotherapy.

Given the nature and incidence of adverse events, Campto will only be prescribed in the following cases after the expected benefits have been weighed against the possible therapeutic risks:

• in patients presenting a risk factor, particularly those with a WHO performance status = 2.

• in the few rare instances where patients are deemed unlikely to observe recommendations regarding management of side effects (need for immediate and prolonged antidiarrhoeal treatment combined with high fluid intake at onset of delayed diarrhoea). Strict hospital supervision is recommended for such patients.

Campto should not be administered as an intravenous bolus or an intravenous infusion shorter than 30 minutes and longer than 90 minutes (see *Posology and method of administration*).

Delayed diarrhoea: Patients should be made aware of the risk of delayed diarrhoea occurring more than 24 hours after the administration of Campto and at any time before the next cycle. The median time of onset of the first liquid stool was on day 5 after the infusion of Campto. They should quickly inform their physician of its occurrence and start appropriate therapy immediately. Patients with an increased risk of diarrhoea are those who had a previous abdominal/pelvic radiotherapy, those with baseline hyperleucocytosis and those with performance status ≥ 2. If not properly treated, diarrhoea can be life-threatening, especially if the patient is concomitantly neutropenic.

As soon as the first liquid stool occurs, the patient should start drinking large volumes of beverages containing electrolytes and an appropriate antidiarrhoeal therapy must be initiated immediately. This antidiarrhoeal treatment will be prescribed by the department where Campto has been administered. After discharge from the hospital, the patients should obtain the prescribed drugs so that they can treat the diarrhoea as soon as it occurs. In addition, they must inform their physician or the department administering Campto when/if diarrhoea is occurring.

The currently recommended antidiarrhoeal treatment consists of high doses of loperamide (2 mg every 2 hours). This therapy should continue for 12 hours after the last liquid stool and should not be modified. In no instance should loperamide be administered for more than 48 consecutive hours at these doses, because of the risk of paralytic ileus, nor for less than 12 hours.

In addition to the antidiarrhoeal treatment, a prophylactic broad spectrum antibiotic should be given, when the diarrhoea is associated with severe neutropenia (neutrophil count <500 cells/mm³).

In addition to the antibiotic treatment, hospitalisation is recommended for management of the diarrhoea, in the following cases:

–diarrhoea associated with fever,

–severe diarrhoea (requiring intravenous rehydration),

–diarrhoea persisting beyond 48 hours following the initiation of high dose loperamide therapy.

Loperamide should not be given prophylactically, even in patients who experienced delayed diarrhoea at previous cycles.

In patients who experienced severe diarrhoea, a reduction in dose is recommended for subsequent cycles. (see *Posology and method of administration*).

Haematology: Weekly monitoring of complete blood cell counts is recommended during Campto treatment. Patients should be aware of the risk of neutropenia and the significance of fever. Febrile neutropenia (temperature >38°C and neutrophil count ≤1,000 cells/mm³) should be urgently treated in the hospital with broad-spectrum intravenous antibiotics. Campto administration should be delayed until the neutrophil count is ≥1,500 cells/mm³. In patients who experienced severe asymptomatic neutropenia (<500 cells/mm³), fever (temperature >38°C) or infections associated with neutropenia (neutrophil count ≤1,000 cells/mm³), the dose of Campto should be reduced (see *Posology and method of administration*). There is an increased risk of infections and haematological toxicity in patients with severe diarrhoea. In patients with severe diarrhoea, complete blood cell counts should be performed.

Liver impairment: Liver function tests should be performed at baseline and before each cycle. Patients with impaired liver function (bilirubin >1 and ≤1.5 times the ULN and transaminases >5 times the ULN) are at greater risk of developing febrile neutropenia or severe neutropenia. Campto should not be used in patients with a bilirubin >1.5 times the ULN (see *Contra-indications*).

Nausea and vomiting: A prophylactic treatment with an antiemetic is recommended before each treatment with Campto. Nausea and vomiting have been frequently reported. Patients with vomiting associated with delayed diarrhoea should be hospitalised as soon as possible for treatment.

Acute cholinergic syndrome: If acute cholinergic syndrome appears (defined as early diarrhoea and various other symptoms such as sweating, abdominal cramping, lachrymation, myosis and salivation), atropine sulphate (0.25 mg subcutaneously) should be administered unless clinically contraindicated (see *Undesirable effects*). Caution should be exercised in patients with asthma. In patients who experienced an acute and severe cholinergic syndrome, the use of prophylactic atropine sulphate is recommended with subsequent doses of Campto.

Elderly: Due to the greater frequency of decreased biological functions, in particular hepatic function, in elderly patients, dose selection with Campto should be cautious in this population (see *Posology and method of administration*).

Patients with bowel obstruction: Patients must not be treated with Campto until resolution of the bowel obstruction (see *Contra-indications*).

Patients with impaired renal function: Studies in this population have not been conducted. (see *Posology and method of administration* and *Pharmacokinetic properties*).

Others: Contraceptive measures must be taken during and for at least three months after cessation of therapy.

Interaction with other medicaments and other forms of interaction: There have been no clinical studies to evaluate the drug interactions of irinotecan with other drugs. Interaction between irinotecan and neuromuscular blocking agents cannot be ruled out. Drugs with anticholinesterase activity may prolong the neuromuscular blocking effects of suxamethonium and the neuromuscular blockade of non-depolarising drugs may be antagonised.

Pregnancy and lactation:

Pregnancy: There is no information on the use of Campto in pregnant women. Campto has been shown to be embryotoxic, foetotoxic and teratogenic in rabbits and rats. Therefore, Campto must not be used during pregnancy. Women of childbearing age receiving Campto should be advised to avoid becoming pregnant, and to inform the treating physician immediately should this occur (see *Contra-indications* and *Special warnings and special precautions for use*).

Lactation: In lactating rats, ¹⁴C-irinotecan was detected in milk. It is not known whether irinotecan is excreted in human milk. Consequently, because of the potential for adverse reactions in nursing infants, breast-feeding must be discontinued for the duration of Campto therapy (see *Contra-indications*).

Effects on ability to drive and use machines: Patients should be warned about the potential for dizziness or visual disturbances which may occur within 24 hours following the administration of Campto, and advised not to drive or operate machinery if these symptoms occur.

Undesirable effects: The adverse reactions considered to be possibly or probably related to the administration of Campto at the recommended dose of 350 mg/m², have been reported from 765 patients.

Gastrointestinal: Delayed diarrhoea.

Diarrhoea (occurring more than 24 hours after administration) is a dose-limiting toxicity of Campto. Severe diarrhoea is observed in 20% of patients who follow recommendations for the management of diarrhoea.

The median time of onset of the first liquid stool was on day 5 after the infusion of Campto. Uncommon cases of pseudo-membranous colitis have been reported, one of which has been documented bacteriologically (Clostridium difficile).

Nausea and vomiting: Nausea and vomiting were severe in approximately 10% of patients treated with antiemetics.

Other gastrointestinal events: Episodes of dehydration commonly associated with diarrhoea and/or vomiting have been reported.

Constipation relative to Campto and/or loperamide has been observed in less than 10% of patients. Infrequent cases of intestinal obstruction or ileus were reported.

Other mild effects include anorexia, abdominal pain and mucositis.

Haematology: Neutropenia is a dose-limiting toxic effect. Neutropenia was observed in 78.7% of patients and was severe (neutrophil count <500 cells/mm³) in 22.6% of patients. Of the evaluable cycles, 18% had a neutrophil count below 1,000 cells/mm³ including 7.6% with a neutrophil count <500 cells/mm³. Neutropenia was reversible and not cumulative; the median day to nadir was 8 days and total recovery was usually reached by day 22.

Fever with severe neutropenia was reported in 6.2% of patients (1.7% of cycles). Infectious episodes occurred in about 10.3% of patients (2.5 % of cycles) and were associated with severe neutropenia in about 5.3% of patients (1.1% of cycles) and resulted in death in 2 cases.

Anaemia was reported in about 58.7% of patients (8% with haemoglobin <8 g/dl and 0.9% with haemoglobin <6.5 g/dl).

Thrombocytopenia (<100,000 cells/mm³) was observed in 7.4% of patients and 1.8% of cycles (0.9% with platelets count ≤50,000 cells/mm³ and 0.2% of cycles). Nearly all the patients showed a recovery by day 22.

One case of peripheral thrombocytopenia with antiplatelet antibodies has been reported in the post-marketing experience.

Acute cholinergic syndrome: Severe transient acute cholinergic syndrome was observed in 9% of patients. The main symptoms were defined as early diarrhoea and various other symptoms such as abdominal pain, conjunctivitis, rhinitis, hypotension, vasodilatation, sweating, chills, malaise, dizziness, visual disturbances, myosis, lacrimation and increased salivation occurring during or within the first 24 hours after the infusion of Campto. These symptoms disappear after atropine administration (see *Special warning and special precautions for use*)

Other effects: Early effects such as dyspnoea, muscular contraction or cramps and paraesthesia have been reported. Asthenia was severe in less than 10% of patients. The causal relationship to Campto has not been clearly established.

Alopecia was very common and reversible.

Fever in the absence of infection or severe neutropenia occurred in 12% of the patients.

Mild cutaneous reactions, allergy and infusion site reactions have been reported, although uncommonly.

Laboratory Tests: Transient and mild to moderate increases in serum levels of either transaminases, alkaline phosphatase or bilirubin were observed in 9.2%, 8.1% and 1.8% of the patients, respectively, in the absence of progressive liver metastasis.

Transient and mild to moderate increases of serum levels of creatinine have been observed in 7.3% of the patients.

Overdose: There have been no reports of overdosage. Doses as high as 750 mg/m² have been used in a phase I study under careful monitoring. The most significant adverse reactions reported were severe neutropenia and diarrhoea. Consequently, in case of overdosage, the patients should be kept in a specialised unit. There is no known antidote for Campto.

Pharmacological properties

Pharmacodynamic properties: Cytostatic topoisomerase I inhibitor.

Experimental data: Irinotecan is a semi-synthetic derivative of camptothecin. It is an antineoplastic agent which acts as a specific inhibitor of DNA topoisomerase I. It is metabolised by carboxylesterase in most tissues to SN-38, which was found to be more active than irinotecan in purified topoisomerase I and more cytotoxic than irinotecan against several murine and human tumour cell lines. The inhibition of DNA topoisomerase I by irinotecan or SN-38 induces single-strand DNA lesions which blocks the DNA replication fork and are responsible for the cytotoxicity. This cytotoxic activity was found time-dependent and was specific to the S-phase.

In vitro, irinotecan and SN-38 were not found to be significantly recognised by the P-glycoprotein^{MDR}, and display cytotoxic activities against doxorubicin- and vinblastine-resistant cell lines.

Furthermore, irinotecan has a broad antitumour activity in vivo against murine tumour models (PO3 pancreatic ductal adenocarcinoma, MA-16/C mammary adenocarcinoma, C38 and C51 colon adenocarcinomas) and against human xenografts (Co-4 colon adenocarcinoma, MX-1 mammary adenocarcinoma, St-15 and SC-6 gastric adenocarcinomas). Irinotecan is also active against tumours expressing the P-glycoprotein^{MDR} (vincristine- and doxorubicin-resistant P388 leukaemias).

Beside the antitumour activity of Campto, the most relevant pharmacological effect of irinotecan is the inhibition of acetylcholinesterase.

Clinical data: Clinical studies were performed in more than 980 patients with metastatic colorectal cancer who failed a previous 5-FU-based regimen. The efficacy of Campto was evaluated in 765 patients with documented progression on 5-FU at study entry.

Pharmacokinetic/pharmacodynamic data: The intensity of the major toxicities encountered with Campto (e.g., leuconeutropenia and diarrhoea) are related to the exposure (AUC) to parent drug and metabolite SN-38. Significant correlations were observed between haematological toxicity (decrease in white blood cells and neutrophils at nadir) or diarrhoea intensity and both irinotecan and metabolite SN-38 AUC values.

Pharmacokinetic properties: The pharmacokinetic properties of both irinotecan and SN-38 (its active metabolite) were evaluated in 60 patients during phase I studies using the recommended dosage regimen, i.e. 30-minute intravenous infusion of 100 to 750 mg/m². The kinetic profile of irinotecan is dose independent. The different irinotecan administration schedules investigated were pharmacokinetically similar in patients enrolled in the clinical trials.

The plasma decay was either biphasic or triphasic. The mean plasma half-life of the first phase of the triphasic model was 12 minutes, the second phase was 2.5 hours, and the terminal phase half-life was 14.2 hours. The mean irinotecan and SN-38 peak plasma concentrations, achieved at the end of the infusion at the recommended dose of 350 mg/m², were 7.7 μg/ml and 56 ng/ml, respectively, with corresponding area under the curve (AUC) values of 34 μg.h/ml and 451 ng.h/ml. The volume of distribution at steady state (Vdss) was large and remained relatively stable as a function of dose with a mean value of 157 l/m². The total body clearance had a mean value of 15 l/h/m², and did not vary between cycles in the same patient. A wide interindividual variability of pharmacokinetic parameters is observed mainly for SN-38. The mean 24 hour-urinary excretion of irinotecan and SN-38 was 19.9% and 0.25% of the administered dose, respectively. A pharmacokinetic phase II analysis has been performed with irinotecan in 72 cancer patients. Pharmacokinetic parameters estimated by a limited sampling model were very close to those estimated from phase I studies. *In vitro*, the plasma protein binding for irinotecan and SN-38 were approximately 65% and 95% respectively.

Preclinical safety data: Irinotecan and SN-38 have been shown to be mutagenic *in vitro* in the chromosomal aberration test on CHO-cells as well as in the *in vivo* micronucleus test in mice. However, they have been shown to be devoid of any mutagenic potential in the Ames test. In rats treated once a week during 13 weeks at the maximum dose of 150 mg/m² (which is less than half the human recommended dose), no treatment related tumours were reported 91 weeks after the end of treatment. Single- and repeated-dose toxicity studies with Campto have been carried out in mice, rats and dogs. The main toxic effects were seen in the haematopoietic and lymphatic systems. In dogs, delayed diarrhoea associated with atrophy and focal necrosis of the intestinal mucosa was reported. Alopecia was also observed in the dog. The severity of these effects was dose-related and reversible.

Pharmaceutical particulars:

List of excipients: Sorbitol, lactic acid and water for injections. The pH of the solution is adjusted to 3.5 with sodium hydroxide.

Incompatibilities: None known. Do not admix with other medications.

Shelf life: The shelf-life of unopened vials is 24 months. The Campto solution should be used immediately after reconstitution as it contains no antibacterial preservative. If reconstitution and dilution are performed under strict aseptic conditions (e.g. on laminar air flow bench) Campto solution should be used (infusion completed) within 12 hours at room temperature or 24 hours if stored 2°–8°C after the first breakage.

Special precautions for storage Vials of Campto concentrate for infusion should be protected from light.

Nature and contents of container:

Campto 40 mg 2-ml brown glass vial, with a halobutyl rubber closure coated with teflon on the inner side.

Campto 100 mg 5-ml brown glass vial, with a halobutyl rubber closure coated with teflon on the inner side.

Instructions for use/handling: As with other antineoplastic agents, Campto must be prepared and handled with caution. The use of glasses, mask and gloves is required. If Campto solution or infusion solution should come into contact with the skin, wash immediately and thoroughly with soap and water. If Campto solution or infusion solution should come into contact with the mucous membranes, wash immediately with water.

Preparation for the intravenous infusion administration: As with any other injectable drugs, Campto solution must be prepared aseptically (see *Shelf life*). Aseptically withdraw the required amount of Campto solution from the vial with a calibrated syringe and inject into a 250 ml infusion bag or bottle containing either 0.9% sodium chloride solution or 5% dextrose solution. The infusion should then be thoroughly mixed by manual rotation.

Campto infusion solution should be infused into a peripheral or central vein.

Campto should not be delivered as an intravenous bolus or an intravenous infusion shorter than 30 minutes or longer than 90 minutes.

Disposal: All materials used for dilution and administration should be disposed of according to hospital standard procedures applicable to cytotoxic agents.

Marketing authorisation numbers

Campto 40 mg/2 ml PL 0012/0302
Campto 100 mg/5 ml PL 0012/0303

Date of approval/revision of SPC November 1997

Legal classification POM

	Phase II	Phase III			
		Campto versus supportive care		Campto versus 5-FU	
		Campto	Supportive care	Campto	5-FU
	n = 455	n = 183	n = 90	n = 127	n = 129
Progression Free Survival at 6 months (%)	30	NA	NA	33.5* (p=0.03)	26.7
Survival at 12 months (%)	NA	36.2* (p=0.001)	13.8	44.8 (p=0.0351)	32.4
Median Survival (months)	9	9.2* (p=0.001)	6.5	10.8* (p=0.0351)	8.5

NA: Non Applicable
*: Statistically significant difference

CERUBIDIN*

Qualitative and quantitative composition The active ingredient in Cerubidin is daunorubicin hydrochloride Ph Eur Each vial contains 21.4 mg daunorubicin hydrochloride (equivalent to 20 mg as base).

Pharmaceutical form Vial containing a red lyophilised powder for intravenous administration following reconstitution in Water for Injections and dilution with saline.

Clinical particulars

Therapeutic indications: Cerubidin is indicated for the following: Inducing remissions of acute myelogenous and lymphocytic leukaemias.

Posology and method of administration: For intravenous administration. *Adults:* 40-60 mg/m² on alternate days for a course of up to three injections for the induction of remissions.

Acute myelogenous leukaemia: The recommended dose is 45 mg/m²/day

Acute lymphocytic leukaemia: The recommended dose is 45 mg/m²/day.

Children: Over 2 years - Same as for adults. *Under 2 years or if less than 0.5 m²2 surface area*: 1 mg/kg/day.

Elderly: Cerubidin should be used with care in patients with inadequate bone marrow reserves due to old age. A reduction of 50% in dosage is recommended.

The number of injections required varies widely from patient to patient and must be determined in each case according to response and tolerance.

The dosage should be reduced in patients with impaired hepatic or renal function. A 25% reduction is recommended in patients with serum bilirubin concentrations of 20–50 μmol/l or creatinine of 105–265 μmol/l. A 50% reduction is recommended in cases with serum bilirubin concentrations of above 50 μmol/l or creatinine of above 265 μmol/l.

Cerubidin is extremely irritating to tissues and may only be administered intravenously after dilution. Cerubidin should be administered through a large vein and the infusion should be kept free flowing. When second or subsequent injections are given, the doses and time intervals depend on the effect of the previous doses and must be the subject of careful deliberation, examination of the peripheral blood and, under some circumstances, of the bone marrow.

The effect of Cerubidin on the disease process and on normal blood precursors cannot be exactly predicted for any particular case. The difference between incomplete treatment, a satisfactory remission and overdosage with possible irreversible aplasia of the bone marrow depends on the correct choice of dosage, time intervals and total number of doses.

Contra-indications: Cerubidin should not be used in patients recently exposed to, or with existing chicken pox or herpes zoster.

Do not administer by the intramuscular or subcutaneous route.

Special warnings and special precautions for use: Cerubidin should be used under the direction of a clinician conversant with the management of acute leukaemia and cytotoxic chemotherapy. The haematological status of patients should be monitored regularly.

Cerubidin should be used with care in patients at risk of hyperuricaemia (eg in the presence of gout, urate and renal calculi), tumour cell infiltration of the bone marrow and in patients with inadequate bone marrow reserves due to previous cytotoxic drug or radiation therapy. The cumulative dose of Cerubidin should be limited to 400 mg/m² when radiation therapy to the mediastinum has been previously administered. The dose of Cerubidin should not be repeated in the presence of bone marrow depression or buccal ulceration.

Care should be taken to avoid extravasation during intravenous administration. All steps should be taken to avoid tissuing and bandages should be avoided.

Facial flushing or erythematous streaking along veins indicates too rapid injection. If tissue necrosis is suspected, the infusion should be stopped immediately and resumed in another vein. Where extravasation has occurred, an attempt should be made to aspirate the fluid back through the needle., The affected area may be injected with hydrocortisone. Sodium bicarbonate (5 ml of 8.4% w/v solution) may also be injected in the hope that through pH change the drug will hydrolyse. The opinion of a plastic surgeon should be sought as skin grafting may be required.

Application of ice packs may help decrease discomfort and also prevent extension. Liberal application of corticosteriod cream and dressing the area with sterile gauze should then be carried out.

Each patient should be given a clinical and bacteriological examination to determine whether infection is present; any infections should be adequately eliminated before treatment with Cerubidin which might depress the bone marrow to the point where anti-infective agents would no longer be effective. If facilities are available, patients should be treated in a germ-free environment or, where this is not possible, reverse barrier nursing and aseptic precautions should be employed.

Anti-infective therapy should be employed in the presence of suspected or confirmed infection and during a phase of aplasia. It should be continued for some time after the marrow has regenerated. Care should also be used in patients at risk of infection.

Interactions with other medicaments and other forms of interaction: None.

Pregnancy and lactation: Daunorubicin crosses the placenta and experiments in animals have shown it to be mutagenic, carcinogenic and teratogenic.

There is also the possibility that treatment during pregnancy may produce delayed effects in the offspring. If appropriate, the mother should be offered the opportunity of a therapeutic abortion.

Owing to potential toxic risk to the infant, breast-feeding should be discontinued during treatment.

Effects on ability to drive and use machines: Not applicable.

Undesirable effects: Bone marrow depression: In every patient bone marrow function will be depressed by treatment with Cerubidin and in a variable proportion of cases, severe aplasia will develop.

Leucopenia is usually more significant than thrombocytopenia. The nadir for leucopenia usually occurs between 10-14 days and recovery occurs gradually over the next 1-2 weeks. Bone marrow depression must be anticipated in every case by eliminating infection before treatment, by isolating the patient from infection during treatment and by means of supportive therapy. This includes the continuous administration of anti-infective agents, the administration of platelet-rich plasma or fresh whole blood transfusion and, under some circumstances, the transfusion of white cell concentrates.

Other less serious reactions have been reported (in order of frequency) are: stomatitis, alopecia, phlebitis, fever, anaemia, nausea, vomiting, mucositis, diarrhoea and rash. The urine may be temporarily coloured red after treatment.

Rapid destruction of a large number of leukaemia cells may cause a rise in blood uric acid or urea and so it is a wise precaution to check these concentrations three or four times a week during the first week of treatment. Fluids should be administered and allopurinol used in severe cases to prevent the development of hyperuricaemia.

Patients with heart disease should not be treated with this potentially cardiotoxic drug. Cardiotoxicity if it occurs is likely to be heralded by either a persistent tachycardia, shortness of breath, swelling of feet and lower limbs or by minor changes in the electrocardiogram and for this reason an electrocardiographic examination should be made at regular intervals during the treatment. Cardiotoxicity usually appears within 1 to 6 months after initiation of therapy. It may develop suddenly and not be detected by routine ECG. It may be irreversible and fatal but responds to treatment if detected early.

The risk of congestive heart failure increases significantly when the total cumulative dosage exceeds 600 mg/m^2 in adults, 300 mg/m^2 in children over 2 years or 10 mg/kg in children under 2 years. Cardiotoxicity may be more frequent in children and the elderly. The dosage should be modified if previous or concomitant cardiotoxic drug therapy is used.

Overdose: Although no cases of overdosage have been reported to our knowledge, overdosage may result in drastic myelosuppression and severe cardiotoxicity with or without transient reversible ECG changes leading to congestive heart failure. Treatment should be supportive and symptomatic.

Pharmacological properties

Pharmacodynamic properties: Cerubidin is an anthracycline glycoside antibiotic and is a potent antileukaemic agent. It also has immunosuppressant effects.

The exact mechanism of antineoplastic action is uncertain but may involve binding to DNA by intercalation between base pairs and inhibition of DNA and RNA synthesis by template disordering and steric obstruction. Daunorubicin is most active in the S-phase of cell division but is not cycle phase-specific. Tumour cell cross-resistance has been observed between daunorubicin and doxorubicin.

Pharmacokinetic properties: Daunorubicin is rapidly taken up by the tissues, especially by the kidneys, spleen, liver and heart. It does not cross the blood-brain barrier, subsequent release of drug and its metabolites from the tissues is slow ($T_{\frac{1}{2}}$=55 hours). Daunorubicin is rapidly metabolised in the liver. The major metabolite daunorubicinol is also active. Daunorubicin is excreted slowly in the urine, mainly as metabolites with 25% excreted in the first 5 days. Biliary excretion also makes a significant (40%) contribution to elimination.

Preclinical safety data: No further information available.

Pharmaceutical particulars

List of excipients: Mannitol.

Incompatibilities: The reconstituted solution is incompatible with heparin sodium injection and dexamethasone sodium phosphate injection.

Shelf life: The shelf-life of Cerubidin is 3 years. After reconstitution Cerubidin should be used within 24 hours.

Special precautions for storage: Cerubidin vials should be stored below 25°C, protected from light. After reconstitution Cerubidin should be stored at 2–8°C, protected from light.

Nature and content of container: Glass vial with rubber cap containing 21.4 mg of daunorubicin hydrochloride (equivalent to 20 mg as base).

Instructions for use/handling: The contents of a vial should be reconstituted with 4 ml of Water for Injection giving a concentration of 5 mg per ml. The calculated dose of Cerubidin should be further diluted with normal saline to give a final concentration of 1 mg per ml. The solution should be injected over a 20 minute period into the tubing or side arm, of a well placed, rapidly flowing i.v. infusion of normal saline (to minimise extravasation and possible tissue necrosis).

Alternatively, the Cerubidin may be added to a minibag of sodium chloride injection 0.9% and this solution infused into the side arm of a rapidly flowing infusion of normal saline.

Marketing authorisation number PL 0012/0220

Date of approval/revision of SPC February 1997

Legal category POM

CLEXANE* INJECTION

Qualitative and quantitative composition

20 mg Injection Enoxaparin 20 mg (equivalent to 2,000 IU anti-Xa activity) in 0.2 ml Water for Injections

40 mg Injection Enoxaparin 40 mg (equivalent to 4,000 IU anti-Xa activity) in 0.4 ml Water for Injections

60 mg Injection Enoxaparin 60 mg (equivalent to 6,000 IU anti-Xa activity) in 0.6 ml Water for Injections

80 mg Injection Enoxaparin 80 mg (equivalent to 8,000 IU anti-Xa activity) in 0.8 ml Water for Injections

100 mg Injection Enoxaparin 100 mg (equivalent to 10,000 IU anti-Xa activity) in 1.0 ml Water for Injections

Pharmaceutical form Sterile pyrogen-free solution for injection contained in ready-to-use prefilled syringes.

Clinical particulars

Therapeutic indications: The prophylaxis of thromboembolic disorders of venous origin, in particular those which may be associated with orthopaedic or general surgery.

The treatment of deep vein thrombosis with or without pulmonary embolism.

The treatment of unstable angina and non-Q-wave myocardial infarction, administered concurrently with aspirin.

The prevention of thrombus formation in the extra-corporeal circulation during haemodialysis.

Posology and method of administration: Adults: Prophylaxis of venous thromboembolism: In patients with a low to moderate risk of venous thromboembolism the recommended dosage is 20 mg (2000 IU) once daily for 7 to 10 days, or until the risk of thromboembolism has diminished. In patients undergoing surgery, the initial dose should be given approximately 2 hours pre-operatively. In patients with a higher risk, such as in orthopaedic surgery, the dosage should be 40 mg (4,000 IU) daily with the initial dose administered approximately 12 hours before surgery.

Treatment of deep vein thrombosis: Clexane should be administered as a single injection of 1.5 mg/kg (150 IU/kg). Clexane treatment is usually prescribed for at least 5 days and until adequate oral anticoagulation is established.

Treatment of unstable angina and non-Q-wave myocardial infarction: The recommended dose is 1 mg/kg Clexane every 12 hours by subcutaneous injection, administered concurrently with oral aspirin (100 to 325 mg once daily).

Treatment with Clexane in these patients should be prescribed for a minimum of 2 days and continued until clinical stabilisation. The usual duration of treatment is 2 to 8 days.

Prevention of extracorporeal thrombus formation during haemodialysis: A dose equivalent to 1 mg/kg (100 IU/kg) introduced into the arterial line at the beginning of a dialysis session is usually sufficient for a 4 hour session. If fibrin rings are found, such as after a longer than normal session, a further dose of 0.5 to 1 mg/kg (50 to 100 IU/kg) may be given. For patients at a high risk of haemorrhage the dose should be reduced to 0.5 mg/kg (50 IU/kg) for double vascular access or 0.75 mg/kg (75 IU/kg) for single vascular access.

Elderly: No dose adjustment necessary.

Children: Not recommended, as dosage not established.

Renal impairment: No adjustment of the prophylaxis dose is required. Patients with severe renal impairment should be closely monitored when receiving treatment doses.

Hepatic impairment: In the absence of clinical studies, caution should be exercised.

Clexane is administered by subcutaneous injection for the prevention of venous thromboembolic disease or treatment of deep vein thrombosis or for the treatment of unstable angina and non-Q-wave myocardial infarction; and through the arterial line of a dialysis circuit for the prevention of thrombus formation in the extra-corporeal circulation during haemodialysis. It must not be administered by the intramuscular route.

Subcutaneous injection technique: The prefilled disposable syringe is ready for immediate use. Clexane should be administered when the patient is lying down by deep subcutaneous injection. The administration should be alternated between the left and right anterolateral or posterolateral abdominal wall. The whole length of the needle should be introduced vertically into a skin fold held between the thumb and index finger. The skin fold should not be released until the injection is complete. Do not rub the injection site after administration.

Contra-indications: Contra-indicated in patients with acute bacterial endocarditis; major bleeding disorders; thrombocytopenia in patients with a positive *in-vitro* aggregation test in the presence of enoxaparin; active gastric or duodenal ulceration; hypersensitivity to enoxaparin; stroke (unless due to systemic emboli); other patients with an increased risk of haemorrhage.

Special warnings and special precautions for use: As different low molecular weight heparins may not be equivalent, alternative products should not be substituted during a course of treatment. Enoxaparin is to be used with extreme caution in patients with a history of heparin-induced thrombocytopenia with or without thrombosis. As there is a risk of antibody-mediated heparin-induced thrombocytopenia also occurring with low molecular weight heparins, regular platelet count monitoring should be considered prior to and during therapy with these agents. Thrombocytopenia, should it occur, usually appears between the 5th and the 21st day following the beginning of therapy. If platelet count is significantly reduced (30 to 50 % of the initial value), therapy must be discontinued immediately and an alternative therapy initiated. Enoxaparin injection, as with any other anticoagulant therapy, should be used with caution in conditions with increased potential for bleeding, such as: impaired haemostasis, history of peptic ulcer, recent ischaemic stroke, uncontrolled severe arterial hypertension, diabetic retinopathy, recent neuro- or ophthalmologic surgery. As with other anti-coagulants, there have been rare cases of intra-spinal haematomas reported with the concurrent use of enoxaparin and spinal/epidural anaesthesia resulting in long term or permanent paralysis. The risk of these rare events may be higher with the use of post-operative indwelling catheters.

Interaction with other medicaments and other forms of interaction: It is recommended that agents which affect haemostasis should be discontinued prior to enoxaparin therapy unless their use is essential, such as: systemic salicylates, acetylsalicylic acid, NSAIDs including ketorolac, dextran and ticlopidine, systemic glucocorticoids, thrombolytics and anticoagulants. If the combination cannot be avoided, enoxaparin should be used with careful clinical and laboratory monitoring.

Pregnancy and lactation: Pregnancy: Animal studies have not shown any evidence of foetotoxicity or teratogenicity. In the pregnant rat, the transfer of ^{35}S-enoxaparin across the maternal placenta to the foetus is minimal. In humans, there is no evidence that enoxaparin crosses the placental barrier during the second trimester of pregnancy. There is no information available concerning the first and the third trimesters. As there are no adequate and well-controlled studies in pregnant women and because animal studies are not always predictive of human response, this drug should not be used in pregnant patients unless no safer alternative is available.

Lactation: In lactating rats, the concentration of ^{35}S-enoxaparin or its labelled metabolites in milk is very low. It is not known whether unchanged enoxaparin is excreted in human breast milk. The oral absorption of enoxaparin is unlikely. However, as a precaution, lactating mothers receiving enoxaparin should be advised to avoid breast-feeding.

Effects on ability of drive and use machines: Enoxaparin has no effect on the ability to drive and operate machines

Undesirable effects: Bleeding may occur during enoxaparin therapy in the presence of associated risk factors such as: organic lesions liable to bleed or the use of medications affecting haemostasis (see *Interaction* section). Mild, transient, asymptomatic thrombocytopenia has been reported during the first days of therapy. Immuno-allergic thrombocytopenia, with or without thrombosis, has rarely been reported. Pain, haematoma and mild local irritation may follow the subcutaneous injection of enoxaparin. Rarely, hard inflammatory nodules which are not cystic enclosures of enoxaparin, have been observed at the injection site. They resolve after a few days and should not cause therapy discontinuation. Exceptional cases of skin necrosis at the injection site have been reported with heparins and low molecular weight heparins. These phenomena are usually preceded by purpura or erythematous plaques, infiltrated and painful. Enoxaparin must be discontinued. Although rare, cutaneous or systemic allergic reactions may occur. In some cases discontinuation of therapy may be necessary. Asymptomatic and reversible increases in platelet counts and liver enzyme levels have been reported. Long term therapy with heparin has been associated with a risk of osteoporosis. Although this has not been observed with enoxaparin the risk of osteoporosis cannot be excluded. There have been rare reports of intra-spinal haematomas with the concurrent use of enoxaparin and spinal/epidural anaesthesia and post-operative indwelling catheters. These events have resulted in varying degrees of neurological injuries including long term or permanent paralysis.

Overdose: Orally administered enoxaparin is poorly absorbed and even large oral doses should not lead to any serious consequences. This may be checked by plasma assays of anti-Xa and anti-IIa activities. Accidental overdose following parenteral administration may produce haemorrhagic complications. These may be largely neutralised by slow intravenous injection of protamine sulphate or hydrochloride. The dose of protamine should be equal to the dose of enoxaparin injected, that is, 100 anti-heparin units of protamine should neutralise the anti-IIa activity generated by 1 mg (100 IU) of enoxaparin. However, even with high doses of protamine, the anti-Xa activity of enoxaparin is never completely neutralised (maximum about 60%).

Pharmacological properties

Pharmacodynamic properties: Enoxaparin is a low molecular weight heparin which has antithrombotic activity. It is characterised by a higher ratio of antithrombotic activity to anticoagulant activity than unfractionated heparin. At recommended does, it does not significantly influence platelet aggregation, binding of fibrinogen to platelets or global clotting tests such as APTT and prothrombin time.

Pharmacokinetic properties: Enoxaparin is rapidly and completely absorbed following subcutaneous injection. The maximum plasma anti-Xa activity occurs 1 to 4 hours after injection with peak activities in the order of 0.16 IU/ml and 0.38 IU/ml after doses of 20 mg or 40 mg respectively. The anti-Xa activity generated is localised within the vascular compartments and elimination is characterised by a half life of 4 to 5 hours. Following a 40 mg dose, anti-Xa activity may persist in the plasma for 24 hours. The enoxaparin elimination rate remains unchanged in renal insufficiency. Hepatic metabolism by desulphation and depolymerisation also contributes to elimination. The elimination half life may be prolonged in elderly patients although no dosage adjustment is necessary. Enoxaparin, as detected by anti-Xa activity, does not cross the placental barrier during the second trimester of pregnancy.

Preclinical safety data: There are no pre-clinical data of relevance to the prescriber which are additional to that already included in other sections of the SPC

Pharmaceutical particulars

List of excipients: Water for Injections BP

Incompatibilities: Clexane should not be mixed with any other injections or infusions

Shelf life: 2 years

Special precautions for storage: Store at room temperature (22°C±4°C).

Nature and contents of container: Hypak SCF pre-filled syringes (Becton Dickinson) in packs of 10

Instructions for use/handling: See *Posology and method of administration.*

Marketing authorisation number PL 0012/0196

Date of approval/revision of SPC June 1998

Legal classification POM

DIORALYTE* SACHETS PLAIN, BLACKCURRANT AND CITRUS

Qualitative and quantitative composition

Sodium Chloride BP	0.47 g
Potassium Chloride BP	0.30 g
Glucose BP	3.56 g
Disodium Hydrogen Citrate BP	0.53 g

Pharmaceutical form Powder for reconstitution with 200 ml water.

Clinical particulars

Therapeutic indications: Oral correction of fluid and electrolyte loss in infants, children and adults. Treatment of watery diarrhoea of various aetiologies including gastro-enteritis in all age groups.

Posology and method of administration: Reconstitution: The contents of each sachet should be dissolved in 200 ml (approximately 7 fluid ounces) of drinking water. Use fresh drinking water for adults and children. For infants, and where drinking water is unavailable, the water should be freshly boiled and cooled. The solution should be made up immediately before use. If refrigerated, the solution may be stored for up to 24 hours, otherwise any solution remaining an hour after reconstitution should be discarded. The solution must not be boiled.

The actual volume of reconstituted Dioralyte to be taken should be decided by the clinician, taking into consideration the weight of the patient and the stage and severity of the condition. A basic principle of treatment of diarrhoea is to replace lost fluid and electrolytes and then to maintain sufficient fluid intake to replace fluid loss from stools. Severe dehydration may need to be corrected by parenteral fluids initially, followed by oral maintenance if indicated.

Dioralyte should not be administered to infants under 1 year of age except on medical advice.

Daily intake may be based on a volume of 150 ml/kg body weight for infants and 20–40 ml/kg body weight for adults and children. A reasonable approximation is:

Infants: One to one and a half times the usual 24 hour feed volume.

Children: One sachet after every loose motion.

Adults (including elderly): One or two sachets after every loose motion.

More may be required initially to ensure early and full volume repletion.

In the initial stage of treatment of diarrhoea all foods, including cow's or artificial milk should be stopped. However, breast milk need not be withheld. In breast fed infants it is suggested that the infant is given the same volume of Dioralyte as the bottle fed baby and then put to the breast until satisfied. Expression of residual milk from the breasts may be necessary during this period. After 24-48 hours, when symptoms are subsiding, the normal diet should be resumed but this should be gradual to avoid exacerbation of the condition.

When vomiting is present with the diarrhoea, it is advisable that small amounts of Dioralyte be taken frequently. However, it is important that the whole of the required volume of Dioralyte be taken. Where the kidneys are functioning normally, it is difficult to overhydrate by mouth and where there is doubt about the dosage, more rather than less should be taken. If no improvement is seen within 36 hours, it is recommended that the patient be reassessed.

Contra-indications: There are no known contra-indications to Dioralyte. However, there may be a number of conditions where treatment with Dioralyte will be inappropriate, e.g. intestinal obstruction requiring surgical intervention.

Special warnings and precautions for use: For oral administration only. Dioralyte should not be reconstituted in diluents other than water. Each sachet should always be dissolved in 200 ml water. A weaker solution than recommended will not contain the optimal glucose and electrolyte concentration and a stronger solution than recommended may give rise to electrolyte imbalance.

Dioralyte should not be administered to infants under 1 year of age except on medical advice.

If diarrhoea persists unremittingly for longer than 36 hours the patient should be reassessed by the physician.

No specific precautions are necessary in the elderly. However, care should be taken when administering glucose electrolyte solutions in cases of severe renal or hepatic impairment or other conditions where the normal electrolyte balance may be disturbed.

Interactions with other medicaments and other forms of interaction: None stated

Pregnancy and lactation: Dioralyte is not contra-indicated in pregnancy or during lactation.

Effects on ability to drive and use machines: Dioralyte could not be expected to affect the ability to drive or use machines

Undesirable effects: None stated

Overdose: In the event of significant overdose, serum electrolytes should be evaluated as soon as possible, appropriate steps taken to correct any abnormalities and levels monitored until return to normal levels is established. This is particularly important in the very young and in cases of severe hepatic or renal failure.

Pharmacological properties

Pharmacodynamic properties: Dioralyte is an oral rehydration therapy. The combination of electrolytes stimulates water and electrolyte absorption from the gastro-intestinal tract and therefore prevents or reverses dehydration in diarrhoea.

Pharmacokinetic properties: Sodium and glucose are actively transported via the membrane into the enterocytes. Sodium is then extruded into the intercellular spaces and the resulting osmotic gradient causes water and electrolytes to be drawn from the gut and then into the circulation.

Preclinical safety data: Not applicable

Pharmaceutical particulars

List of excipients: Silicon dioxide EP and Saccharin Sodium BP (PL 5272/0016)

Silicon dioxide EP, Saccharin sodium BP and Lemon/Lime flavour. (PL 5272/0023)

Silicon dioxide EP, Saccharin Sodium BP and Blackcurrant flavour (PL 5272/0022)

Incompatibilities: None

Shelf life: 24 months

Special precautions for storage: Store in a cool dry place.

Nature of and contents of container: Foil/Laminate sachets containing powder for reconstitution with 200 ml water.

Marketing authorisation numbers

Dioralyte Plain	5272/0016
Dioralyte Blackcurrant	5272/0022
Dioralyte Citrus	5272/0023

Date of approval/revision of SPC February 1997

Legal category P

DIORALYTE* EFFERVESCENT TABLETS BLACKCURRANT AND CITRUS

Qualitative and quantitative composition::

Glucose BP	1.62 g
Sodium Bicarbonate BP	0.336 g
Potassium Chloride BP	0.186 g
Citric Acid Anhydrous BP	0.384 g
Sodium Chloride BP	0.117 g

Pharmaceutical form Effervescent tablets

Clinical particulars Oral treatment of fluid and electrolyte loss and the management of conditions associated with mild to moderate dehydration in all age groups particularly acute diarrhoea of varying aetiologies.

Dosage and administration: Two tablets should be dissolved in 200 ml (approximately 7 fluid ounces) of drinking water. Use fresh drinking water for adults and children. For infants and where drinking water is unavailable, the water should be freshly boiled and cooled. The solution should be made up immediately before use. If refrigerated, the solution may be stored for up to 24 hours, otherwise any solution remaining an hour after reconstitution should be discarded. The solution must not be boiled.

The actual volume of reconstituted Dioralyte effervescent tablets to be taken should be decided by the clinician, taking into consideration the weight of the patient and the stage and severity of the condition.

A basic principle of treatment of diarrhoea is to replace lost fluid and the electrolytes and then to maintain sufficient fluid intake to replace fluid loss from stools.

Severe dehydration may need to be corrected by parenteral fluids initially followed by oral maintenance with Dioralyte if indicated.

Dioralyte should not be administered to infants under 1 year of age except on medical advice

Daily intake may be based on a volume of 150 ml/kg body weight for infants and 20–40 ml/kg body weight for adults and children. A reasonable approximation is:

Infants: One to one and a half times the usual 24 hour feed volume.

Children: Two tablets after every loose motion.

Adults (including elderly): Two or four tablets after every loose motion.

More may be required initially to ensure early and full volume repletion.

In the initial stages of treatment of diarrhoea all foods, including cow's or artificial milk should be stopped. However, breast milk need not be withheld. In breast fed infants it is suggested that the infant is given the same volume of Dioralyte as the bottle fed baby and then put to the breast until satisfied. Expression of residual milk from the breasts may be necessary during this period. After 24-48 hours, when symptoms have subsided, the normal diet should be resumed but this should be gradual to avoid exacerbation of the condition.

When vomiting is present with the diarrhoea it is advisable that small amounts of Dioralyte effervescent be taken frequently. However, it is important that the whole of the required volume of Dioralyte be taken. Where the kidneys are functioning normally, it is difficult to overhydrate by mouth and where there is doubt about the dosage, more rather than less should be taken. If no improvement is seen within 36 hours it is recommended that the patient be reassessed..

Contra-indications: There are no known absolute contra-indications to Dioralyte effervescent.

However, there may be a number of dehydrating conditions where treatment with Dioralyte Effervescent will be inappropriate, e.g., acute abdominal obstructive conditions. Treatment is also inappropriate in renal failure with oliguria or anuria, intractable vomiting and severe dehydration or severe infantile diarrhoea when parenteral therapy is required.

Special warnings and special precautions for use: Two tablets should always be dissolved in 200 ml of water. A weaker solution than recommended will not contain the optimal glucose and electrolyte concentration and a stronger solution than recommended may give rise to electrolyte imbalance.

Dioralyte should not be administered to infants under 1 year of age except on medical advice.

In administration to infants the effervescence should be allowed to subside before use.

If diarrhoea persists unremittingly for longer than 36 hours the patient should be reassessed by the physician.

No specific precautions are necessary in the elderly. However, care should be taken when administering glucose electrolyte solutions in cases of severe renal or hepatic impairment or other conditions where the normal electrolyte balance may be disturbed.

Interactions: None stated

Use in pregnancy and lactation: No special precautions in normal pregnancy and lactation.

Effects on ability to drive and use machines: Dioralyte effervescent could not be expected to affect the ability to drive or use machines.

Undesirable effects: None stated

Overdose: In the event of significant overdose serum electrolytes should be evaluated as soon as possible, appropriate steps taken to correct any abnormalities and levels monitored until return to normal levels is established. This is particularly important in the very young and in cases of severe hepatic or renal failure.

Pharmacological properties

Pharmacodynamic properties: Dioralyte effervescent tablet is an oral rehydration therapy. The combination of electrolytes stimulates water and electrolyte absorption from the GI tract and therefore prevents or reverses dehydration in diarrhoea.

Pharmacokinetic properties: Sodium and glucose are actively transported via the membrane into the enterocytes. Sodium is then extruded into the intercellular spaces and the resulting osmotic gradient causes water and electrolyte to be drawn from the gut and then into the circulation.

Preclinical safety data: Not applicable

Pharmaceutical particulars

List of excipients: Saccharin sodium and Blackcurrant flavour (PL 5272/0025).

Saccharin sodium and Lemon/Lime flavour (PL 5272/0042)

Incompatibilities: None.

Shelf life: 24 months.

Special precautions for storage: Store in original container in a cool (below 25°C) and dry place. Immediately after removal of a tablet replace the cap.

Nature and contents of container: Plastic tube with a push on/off cap containing a desiccant as a moisture proof seal. Each pack contains 10 tablets, available in packs containing one or four tubes.

Instructions for use/handling: Two tablets should be dissolved in 200 ml of drinking water. The tablets should not be reconstituted in other diluents other than water.

Marketing authorisations numbers

Dioralyte Blackcurrant Effervescent Tablets	5272/0025
Dioralyte Citrus Effervescent Tablets	5272/0042

Date of approval/revision of SPC February 1997

Legal category P

FLAGYL* INJECTION

Qualitative and quantitative composition Metronidazole BP 0.5% w/v.

Pharmaceutical form A clean, bright, pale yellow sterile isotonic solution for intravenous infusion.

Clinical particulars

Therapeutic indications: Flagyl is indicated in the prophylaxis and treatment of infections in which anaerobic bacteria have been identified or are suspected to be the cause. Flagyl is active against a wide range of pathogenic micro-organisms notably species of *Bacteroides, Fusobacteria, Clostridia, Eubacteria,* anaerobic cocci and *Gardnerella vaginalis.*

It is indicated in: 1. The prevention of postoperative infections due to anaerobic bacteria, particularly species of bacteroides and anaerobic streptococci. 2. The treatment of septicaemia, bacteraemia, peritonitis, brain abscess, necrotising pneumonia, osteomyelitis, puerperal sepsis, pelvic abscess, pelvic cellulitis, and post-operative wound infections from which pathogenic anaerobes have been isolated.

Posology and method of administration: Flagyl injection should be infused intravenously at an approximate rate of 5 ml/minute. Oral medication should be substituted as soon as feasible.

Anaerobic infections: Treatment for seven days should be satisfactory for most patients but, depending upon clinical and bacteriological assessments, the physician might decide to prolong treatment e.g. for the eradication of infection from sites which cannot be drained or are liable to endogenous recontamination by anaerobic pathogens from the gut, oropharynx or genital tract.

Prophylaxis against anaerobic infection: Chiefly in the context of abdominal (especially colorectal) and gynaecological surgery.

Adults: 500 mg shortly before operation, repeated 8 hourly. Oral doses of 200 mg or 400 mg 8 hourly to be started as soon as feasible.

Children: 7.5 mg/kg (1.5 ml/kg) 8 hourly.

Treatment of established anaerobic infection: Intravenous route is to be used initially if patient's symptoms preclude oral therapy.

Adults: 500 mg 8 hourly.

Children: 7.5 mg/kg 8 hourly.

Elderly: Caution is advised in the elderly. Particularly at high doses although there is limited information available on modification of dosage.

Contra-indications: Known hypersensitivity to metronidazole.

Special warnings and special precautions for use: Metronidazole has no direct activity against anaerobic or facultative anaerobic bacteria. Regular clinical and laboratory monitoring are advised if administration of Flagyl for more than 10 days is considered to be necessary. There is a possibility that after Trichomonas vaginalis has been eliminated a gonococcal infection might persist. The elimination half-life of metronidazole remains unchanged in the presence of renal failure. The dosage of metronidazole therefore needs no reduction. Such patients however retain the metabolites of metronidazole. The clinical significance of this is not known at present. In patients undergoing haemodialysis metronidazole and metabolites are efficiently removed during an eight hour period of dialysis. Metronidazole should therefore be re-administered immediately after haemodialysis. No routine adjustment in the dosage of Flagyl need be made in patients with renal failure undergoing intermittent peritoneal dialysis (IDP) or continuous ambulatory peritoneal dialysis (CAPD). Metronidazole is mainly metabolised by hepatic oxidation. Substantial impairment of metronidazole clearance may occur in the presence of advanced hepatic insufficiency. Significant cumulation may occur in patients with hepatic encephalopathy and the resulting high plasma concentrations of metronidazole may contribute to the symptoms of the encephalopathy. Flagyl should therefore, be administered with caution to patients with hepatic encephalopathy. The daily dosage should be reduced to one third and may be administered once daily. Aspartate amino transferase assays may give spuriously low values in patients being treated with Metronidazole depending on the method used. Flagyl should be used with caution in patients with active disease of the CNS.

Interaction with other medicaments and other forms of interaction: Patients should be advised not to take alcohol during metronidazole therapy and for at least 48 hours afterwards because of the possibility of a disulfiram-like (antabuse effect) reaction. Some potentiation of anticoagulant therapy has been reported when metronidazole has been used with the warfarin type oral anticoagulants. Dosage of the latter may require reducing. Prothrombin times should be monitored. There is no interaction with heparin. Lithium retention accompanied by evidence of possible renal damage has been reported in patients treated simultaneously with lithium and metronidazole. Lithium treatment should be tapered or withdrawn before administering metronidazole. Plasma concentrations of lithium, creatinine and electrolytes should be monitored in patients under treatment with lithium while they receive metronidazole. Patients receiving phenobarbitone metabolise metronidazole at a much greater rate than normally, reducing the half-life to approximately 3 hours.

Pregnancy and lactation: There is inadequate evidence of the safety of metronidazole in pregnancy. Flagyl should not therefore be given during pregnancy or during lactation unless the physician considers it essential; in these circumstances the short, high-dosage regimens are not recommended.

Effects on ability to drive and use machines: None stated.

Undesirable effects: During intensive and/or prolonged metronidazole therapy, a few instances of peripheral neuropathy or transient epileptiform seizures have been reported. In most cases neuropathy disappeared after treatment was stopped or when dosage was reduced. A moderate leucopenia has been reported in some patients but the white cell count has always returned to normal before or after treatment has been completed. Clinicians who contemplate continuous therapy for the relief of chronic conditions for periods longer than those recommended are advised to consider the possible therapeutic benefit against the risk of peripheral neuropathy. Serious adverse reactions occur rarely with standard recommended regimens. Unpleasant taste in the mouth, furred tongue, nausea, vomiting, gastro-intestinal disturbances, urticaria and angioedema occur occasionally. Anaphylaxis may occur rarely. Erythema multiforme may occur, which may be reversed on drug withdrawal. Abnormal liver function tests, cholestatic hepatitis and jaundice, reversible on drug withdrawal, have been reported very rarely. Agranulocytosis, neutropenia, thrombocytopenia and pancytopenia, often reversible on drug withdrawal, have very rarely been reported, although fatalities have occurred. Drowsiness, dizziness, headaches, ataxia, skin rashes, pruritus, inco-ordination of movement, darkening of urine (due to metronidazole metabolite) myalgia and arthralgia have been reported but very rarely.

Overdose: There is no specific treatment for gross overdosage of Flagyl

Pharmacological properties

Pharmacodynamic properties: Metronidazole has antiprotozoal and antibacterial actions and is effective against Trichomonas vaginalis and other protozoa including Entamoeba histolytica and Giardia lamblia and against anaerobic bacteria.

Pharmacokinetic properties: Metronidazole is widely distributed in body tissues after injection. At least half the dose is excreted in the urine as metronidazole and its metabolities, including an acid oxidation product, a hydroxy derivative and glucuronide. Metronidazole diffuses across the placenta, and is found in breast milk of nursing mothers in concentrations equivalent to the serum. 10% of the dose is bound in plasma.

Clearance: 1.3±0.3 ml/min/kg. *Volume of distribution:* 1.1±0.4 litres/kg.

Half-life: 8.5±2.9 hours. *Effective concentration:* 3-6 micrograms/ml.

Preclinical safety data: There are no pre-clinical data of relevance to the prescriber which are additional to that already included in other sections of the SPC.

Pharmaceutical particulars
List of excipients: Sodium phosphate, citric acid anhydrous, sodium chloride and water for injections.

Incompatibilities: Flagyl injection should not be mixed with cefamandole nafate, cefoxitin sodium, dextrose 10% w/v, compound sodium lactate injection, penicillin G potassium.

Shelf life: 24 months.

Special precautions for storage: store below 25°C, protect from light.

Nature and contents of container: Cartons containing 20 x 100 ml Viaflex minibags.

Instructions for use/handling: Cefotaxime sodium is physically and chemically compatible with Flagyl. The following drugs have been shown to be physically compatible in terms of pH and appearance with Flagyl injection over the normal period of administration, although there is no evidence of chemical stability: amikacin sulphate, ampicillin sodium, carbenicillin sodium, cephazolin sodium, cefotaxime sodium, cephalothin sodium, chloramphenicol sodium succinate, clindamycin phosphate, gentamicin sulphate, hydrocortisone sodium succinate, latamoxef disodium, netilmicin sulphate and tobramycin sulphate. In patients maintained on intravenous fluids, Flagyl injection may be diluted with appropriate volumes of normal saline, dextrose-saline, dextrose 5% w/v or potassium chloride infusions (20 and 40 mmol/litre). Apart from the above, Flagyl should on no account be mixed with any other substance.

Marketing authorisation number PL 0012/0107

Date of approval/revision of SPC February 1997

Legal classification POM

IKOREL* TABLETS ▼

Presentation Ikorel is presented as off-white, bevelled edge, circular tablets which are scored on one face. Ikorel 10 mg tablets contain nicorandil 10 mg and bear the identification code IK10. Ikorel 20 mg tablets contain nicorandil 20 mg and are coded IK20. The tablets are provided in blister packs with an integral silica gel desiccant.

Uses *Pharmacology:* Nicorandil provides a dual mode of action leading to relaxation of vascular smooth muscle. A potassium channel opening action provides arterial vasodilation, thus reducing afterload, while the nitrate component promotes venous relaxation and a reduction in preload. Nicorandil has a direct effect on coronary arteries without leading to a steal phenomenon. The overall action improves blood flow to post-stenotic regions and the oxygen balance in the myocardium

Kinetics: Nicorandil is well absorbed with no significant first-pass metabolism. Maximum plasma concentrations are achieved in 30 to 60 minutes and are dose related. Metabolism is mainly by denitration of the molecule into the nicotinamide pathway with approximately 20% of an administered dose being excreted in the urine mainly as metabolites. The main phase of elimination has a half-life of about 1 hour. Nicorandil is only slightly bound to plasma proteins. No clinically relevant modifications in the pharmacokinetic profile have been seen in the elderly or in patients with liver disease or chronic renal failure.

Indications: Ikorel tablets are indicated for the prevention and long-term treatment of chronic stable angina pectoris

Dosage and administration *Adults:* The recommended starting dose is 10 mg nicorandil twice daily although 5 mg twice daily may be employed in patients particularly susceptible to headache. Subsequently the dosage should be titrated upward depending on the clinical response. The usual therapeutic dosage is in the range 10 to 20 mg nicorandil twice daily, although up to 30 mg twice daily may be employed if necessary. *Elderly:* There is no special requirement for dosage adjustment in elderly patients. As with all medicines the lowest effective dosage should be used. *Children:* A paediatric dosage has not been established and use of nicorandil is not recommended.

Contra-indications Warnings etc:
Contra-indications: Ikorel is contra-indicated in patients with cardiogenic shock, left ventricular failure with low filling pressures and in hypotension. It is also contra-indicated in patients who have demonstrated an idiosyncratic response or hypersensitivity to nicorandil.

Warnings: The use of nicorandil should be avoided in patients with depleted blood volume, low systolic blood pressure, acute pulmonary oedema or acute myocardial infarction with acute left ventricular failure and low filling pressures. Therapeutic doses of nicorandil may lower the blood pressure of hypertensive patients and therefore nicorandil, as with other antianginal agents, should be used with care when prescribed with antihypertensive drugs. Alternative treatment should be considered if persistent aphtosis or severe mouth ulceration occurs.

Pregnancy: Animal studies have not revealed any harmful effect of nicorandil on the foetus although there is no experience in humans. It should not be used in pregnant patients unless there is no safer alternative.

Lactation: As it is not known whether nicorandil is excreted in human milk, breast feeding should be avoided by lactating patients who require therapy.

Precautions: Patients should be warned not to drive or operate machinery until it is established that their performance is unimpaired by nicorandil.

Interactions: No pharmacological or pharmacokinetic interactions have been observed in humans or animals with beta-blockers, digoxin, rifampicin, cimetidine, nicoumalone, a calcium antagonist or a combination of digoxin and frusemide. Nevertheless, there is the possibility that nicorandil may potentiate the blood pressure lowering effect of other vasodilators, tricyclic antidepressants or alcohol.

Adverse effects: The most frequent effect to be anticipated is headache, usually of a transitory nature, especially when treatment is initiated. Cutaneous vasodilation with flushing is less frequent. Nausea, vomiting, dizziness and a feeling of weakness have been reported occasionally. Myalgia and different types of rash have been reported rarely. Hypotension may occur at high therapeutic doses. An increase in heart rate may occur at high doses. Rare cases of persistent aphtosis or mouth ulcers which were occasionally severe have been reported. These resolved following treatment discontinuation.

Overdosage: Acute overdosage is likely to be associated with peripheral vasodilation, decreased blood pressure and reflex tachycardia. Cardiac function should be monitored and general supportive measures employed. If necessary, circulating plasma volume should be increased by infusion of suitable fluid. In life-threatening situations administration of vasopressors should be considered. There is no experience of massive overdosage in humans although the LD_{50} in dogs is in the range 62.5 to 125 mg/kg and in rodents it is in the order of 1200 mg/kg.'

Pharmaceutical precautions Ikorel tablets should be stored at a temperature not exceeding 25°C and in a dry place.

Legal category POM

Package quantities Blister packs of 60 tablets.

Further information Nil

Product licence numbers
10 mg tablet 0012/0229
20 mg tablet 0012/0230

Date of issue February 1997

INTAL* NEBULISER SOLUTION

Qualitative and quantitative composition Sodium Cromoglycate BP 1% w/v

Pharmaceutical form A clear, colourless or very pale yellow, sterile, aqueous solution for use in a nebuliser.

Clinical particulars
Therapeutic indications: Intal Nebuliser Solution is indicated for the preventative treatment of bronchial asthma which may be due to allergy, exercise, cold air, or chemical and occupational irritants.

Posology and method of administration: Intal Nebuliser Solution should be administered from a power-operated (air driven or ultrasonic) or foot-pump operated nebuliser machine, via a face-mask or mouthpiece.

Since Intal Nebuliser Solution therapy is essentially preventative, it is important that regular dosage is maintained, as distinct from intermittent use to relieve symptoms.

Adults (including the elderly) and children: The contents of one ampoule are administered by nebulisation four times a day, i.e. night and morning and at intervals of 3–6 hours. In severe cases, frequency of administration may be increased to 5–6 times daily.

Concomitant steroid therapy: In patients currently treated with steroids, the addition of Intal Nebuliser Solution to the regimen may make it possible to reduce the maintenance dose, or discontinue steroids completely. The patient must be carefully supervised while the steroid dose is reduced; a rate of reduction of 10% weekly is suggested. An increase in steroid dosage may be necessary if symptoms increase, and at times of infection, severe antigen challenge or stress.

If reduction of a steroid dosage has been possible, Intal Nebuliser Solution should not be withdrawn until steroid cover has been re-instituted.

Concomitant bronchodilator therapy: If bronchodilators are used concomitantly, patients may find that the frequency of bronchodilator usage can be reduced as their asthma is stabilised with Intal Nebuliser Solution.

Contra-indications: Intal Nebuliser Solution is contra-indicated in patients with a known sensitivity to sodium cromoglycate. Intal Nebuliser Solution must not be given by injection.

Special warnings and precautions for use: Withdrawal of Intal Nebuliser Solution: Since sodium cromoglycate acts prophylactically, it is important to continue treatment in those patients who benefit. If it is necessary to withdraw this treatment, it should be done progressively over a period of one week. Symptoms of asthma may recur.

Interactions with other medicaments and other forms of interaction: None known.

Pregnancy and lactation: As with all medication, caution should be exercised especially during the first trimester of pregnancy. Cumulative experience with sodium cromoglycate suggests that it has no adverse effects on foetal development. It should only be used in pregnancy where there is a clear need.

It is not known whether sodium cromoglycate is excreted in the breast milk but on the basis of its physico-chemical properties this is considered unlikely. There is no information to suggest that the use of sodium cromoglycate has any undesirable effects on the baby.

Effects on ability to drive and use machines: None known.

Undesirable effects: Mild throat irritation, coughing and transient bronchospasm may occur. Very rarely severe bronchospasm associated with a marked fall in pulmonary function has been reported. In such cases treatment should be stopped and should not be reintroduced.

Overdose: No action other than medical supervision should be necessary.

Pharmacological properties
Pharmacodynamic properties: Sodium cromoglycate has multiple actions in the lung. It inhibits the release from sensitised mast cells of mediators of the allergic reaction. In the lung, this inhibition of mediator release prevents both the immediate and late asthmatic response to immunological stimuli.

It is also known that sodium cromoglycate offers protection against many types of immunologic and non-immunologic challenge systems, some of which are thought to produce bronchoconstriction by mechanisms independent of mast cells.

It has also been shown that sodium cromoglycate inhibits reflex bronchoconstriction, probably by acting on sensory nerve endings in the lung.

Pharmacokinetic properties: Sodium cromoglycate is poorly absorbed from the gastro-intestinal tract. Following inhalation as a solution, about 8% of a dose is reported to be deposited in the lungs, from where it is rapidly absorbed and excreted unchanged in the urine and bile.

Preclinical safety data: Animal studies have shown that sodium cromoglycate has a very low order of local or systemic toxicity.

Pharmaceutical particulars
List of excipients: Purified Water EP

Incompatibilities: None known.

Shelf life: Glass ampoule: 60 months, Plastic ampoule: 36 months

Special precautions for storage: Glass ampoule: Store below 30°C–protect from direct sunlight.

Plastic ampoule: Store below 25°C – protect from direct sunlight.

Nature and contents of container: Glass ampoules, double ended (in boxes of 48 ampoules).

Natural low density polyethylene ampoules (strips of 12 ampoules) in cartons of 60 or 120 ampoules overwrapped with PVDC film.

Instructions for use/handling: Instructions for use are supplied with each pack.

Marketing authorisation number 0113/0068R

Date of approval/revision of SPC March 1998

Legal category POM

INTAL* SPINCAPS

Qualitative and quantitative composition Sodium Cromoglycate BP 20.0 mg

Pharmaceutical form Intal is presented as a hard gelatin capsule containing a micronised powder for inhalation through the Spinhaler device.

Clinical particulars
Therapeutic indications: Intal is indicated for the preventative treatment of bronchial asthma, in adults and children, which may be due to allergy, exercise, cold air or chemical and occupational irritants.

Posology and method of administration: Intal Spincaps must be administered via a Spinhaler inhalation device. The capsules are not effective if swallowed. Since Intal therapy is essentially preventative, it is important that the patient is instructed to maintain regular dosage, as distinct from inhaling the drug intermittently to relieve symptoms.

Adults (including the elderly) and children: The normal dose is one Spincap four times daily, i.e. one night and morning and at intervals of 3–6 hours in between. It may be necessary to increase this to 6–8 times daily in more severe cases or during periods of severe antigen challenge. Additional doses may be taken before exertion to prevent exercise induced asthma or before exposure to other trigger factors.

When the asthmatic condition is stabilised, it may be possible to reduce the dosage, provided that adequate control of the asthma is maintained.

Concomitant steroid therapy: In patients currently treated with steroids, the addition of Intal to the regime may make it possible to reduce the maintenance dose, or discontinue steroids completely. The patient must be carefully supervised while the steroid dose is reduced; a rate of reduction of 10% weekly is suggested.

An increase in steroid dosage may be necessary if symptoms increase and at times of infection, severe antigen challenge or stress.

If reduction of a steroid dosage has been possible, Intal should not be withdrawn until steroid cover has been re-instituted.

Concomitant bronchodilator therapy: If bronchodilators are used concomitantly, patients may find that the frequency of bronchodilator usage can be reduced as their asthma is stabilised with Intal.

Contra-indications: Intal are contraindicated in patients with a known sensitivity to sodium cromoglycate.

Special warnings and precautions for use: Intal must not be used for relief of an acute attack of bronchospasm.

Withdrawal of Intal therapy: Since sodium cromoglycate acts prophylactically, it is important to continue treatment in those patients who benefit. If it is necessary to withdraw Intal, this should be done progressively over a period of one week. Symptoms of asthma may recur.

Interactions with other medicaments and other forms of interaction: None known.

Pregnancy and lactation: As with all medication caution should be exercised especially during the first trimester of pregnancy. Cumulative experience with sodium cromoglycate suggests that it has no adverse effects on foetal development. Intal should only be used in pregnancy where there is a clear need.

It is not known whether sodium cromoglycate is excreted in the breast milk but on the basis of its physico-chemical properties this is considered unlikely. There is no information to suggest that the use of sodium cromoglycate has any undesirable effects on the baby.

Effects on ability to drive and use machines: None known.

Undesirable effects: Mild throat irritation, coughing and transient bronchospasm may occur. This may be overcome by changing to Intal Compound. Very rarely severe bronchospasm associated with a marked fall in pulmonary function has been reported. In such cases treatment should be stopped and should not be reintroduced.

Overdose: No action other than medical supervision should be necessary.

Pharmacological properties
Pharmacodynamic properties: Sodium cromoglycate has multiple actions in the lung. It inhibits the release from sensitised mast cells of mediators of the allergic reaction. In the lung inhibition of mediator release prevents both the immediate and late asthmatic response to immunological stimuli.

It is also known that sodium cromoglycate offers protection against many types of immunologic and non-immunologic challenge systems, some of which are thought to produce bronchoconstriction by mechanisms independent of mast cells.

It has also been shown that sodium cromoglycate inhibits reflex bronchoconstriction probably by acting on sensory nerve endings in the lung.

Pharmacokinetic properties: Sodium cromoglycate is poorly absorbed from the gastro-intestinal tract. Following inhalation as a fine powder only about 8% of a dose is reported to be deposited in the lungs from where it is rapidly absorbed and excreted unchanged in the urine and bile.

Preclinical safety data: Animal studies have shown that sodium cromoglycate has a very low order of local or systemic toxicity.

Pharmaceutical particulars
List of excipients: Gelatin capsule.

Incompatibilities: None known.

Shelf life: 60 months.

Special precautions for storage: Store in a cool, dry place, protect from light. Intal Spincaps can be adversely affected by moisture ingress. To prevent possible deterioration of this product, it is essential that the cartridges are kept in their containers at all times.

It is acceptable for up to four of the Spincaps to be stored in the spinhaler carrying case for up to 24 hours.

Nature and contents of container: An aluminium can with aluminium screw cap containing 50 or 56 Spincaps, a blister foil in laminated sachet containing 30, 50 or 100 Spincaps or a high density polypropylene (HDPE) bottle with Clicklok cap and induction seal membrane containing 50 or 56 Spincaps. The HDPE bottle may also be packed as 2 x 56.

Instructions for use/handling: Instructions for use are supplied with each pack.

Marketing authorisation number PL 0113/5022R
Date of approval/revision of SPC March 1998

Legal category POM

INTAL* INHALER

Qualitative and quantitative composition Sodium cromoglycate BP 5.0 mg

Pharmaceutical form Intal is presented as a metered dose pressurised aerosol containing sodium cromoglycate as a suspension in chlorofluorocarbon propellants, for inhalation.

Clinical particulars
Therapeutic indications: Intal is indicated for the preventative treatment of bronchial asthma, in adults and children.

Posology and method of administration: Adults and children: The initial dose is two inhalations of the aerosol four times daily. Once adequate control of symptoms has been achieved it may be possible to reduce to a maintenance dose of one inhalation four times daily. However, the dose may be increased to two inhalations six or eight times daily in more severe cases or during periods of severe antigen challenge. An additional dose before exercise may also be taken.

Elderly: No current evidence for alteration of the recommended adult dose.

Concomitant bronchodilator therapy: Where a concomitant aerosol bronchodilator is prescribed it is recommended that this be administered prior to Intal.

Concomitant steroid therapy: In patients currently treated with steroids, the addition of Intal to the regimen may make it possible to reduce the maintenance dose, or discontinue therapy completely. The patient must be carefully supervised while the steroid dose is reduced; a rate of 10% weekly is suggested. If reduction of a steroid dosage has been possible, Intal should not be withdrawn until steroid cover has been reinstituted.

Contra-indications: Intal is contra-indicated in patients with known hypersensitivity to sodium cromoglycate, sorbitan trioleate or aerosol propellants.

Special warnings and special precautions for use: Intal must not be used for relief of an acute attack of bronchospasm.

Withdrawal of Intal therapy: Since the therapy is prophylactic, it is important to continue therapy in those patients who benefit. If it is necessary to withdraw this treatment, it should be done progressively over a period of one week. Symptoms of asthma may recur.

Interactions with other medicaments and other forms of interaction: None

Pregnancy and lactation: As with all medication, caution should be exercised especially during the first trimester of pregnancy. Cumulative experience with sodium cromoglycate suggests that it has no adverse effects on foetal development. It should only be used in pregnancy where there is a clear need. It is not known whether sodium cromoglycate is excreted in the breast milk but on the basis of its physico-chemical properties this is considered unlikely. There is no evidence to suggest that the use of sodium cromoglycate has any undesirable effects on the baby.

Effects on ability to drive and use machines: None.

Undesirable effects: Mild throat irritation, coughing and transient bronchospasm may occur. Very rarely severe bronchospasm associated with a marked fall in pulmonary function has been reported. In such cases treatment should be stopped and should not be reintroduced.

Overdose: No action other than medical supervision should be necessary.

Pharmacological properties
Pharmacodynamic properties: Sodium cromoglycate has multiple actions in the lung. It inhibits the release from sensitised mast cells of mediators of the allergic reaction. In the lung, this inhibition of mediator release prevents both the immediate and late asthmatic response to immunological stimuli. It is also known that sodium cromoglycate offers protection against many types of immunologic and non-immunologic challenge systems, some of which are thought to produce bronchoconstriction by mechanisms independent of mast cells. It has also been shown that sodium cromoglycate inhibits reflex bronchoconstriction, probably by acting on sensory nerve endings in the lung.

Pharmacokinetic properties: Sodium cromoglycate is poorly absorbed from the gastro-intestinal tract. Following inhalation as a fine powder, about 8% of a dose is reported to be deposited in the lungs, from where it is rapidly absorbed and excreted unchanged in the urine and bile..

Preclinical safety data: Animal studies have shown that sodium cromoglycate has a very low order of local or systemic toxicity.

Pharmaceutical particulars
List of excipients: Sorbitan trioleate, propellant mixture of dichlorotetrafluoroethane (propellant 114) and dichlorodifluoromethane (propellant 12).

Incompatibilities: None known.

Shelf life: 36 months.

Special precautions for storage: Store below 30°C, not in a refrigerator. The aerosol canister is pressurised and should be protected from direct sunlight, heat and frost and must not be punctured or burnt, even when empty.

Nature and contents of container: The aluminium can is fitted with a metering valve which delivers 112 actuations each containing 5 mg of sodium cromoglycate.

Intal Inhaler: The cartoned pack consists of an aerosol canister and a plastic adapter with a dustcap.

Intal Fisonair: The cartoned pack consists of an aerosol canister and a plastic adapter with a dustcap and a holding chamber.

Intal Syncroner: The cartoned pack consists of two aerosol canisters, each with a spacer device and dustcap.

Instructions for use/handling: Instructions for use are supplied with each pack.

Marketing authorisation number PL 0113/0109

Date of approval/last revision of SPC March 1998

Legal category POM

MAALOX* TC SUSPENSION AND TABLETS

Presentation *Suspension:* White, peppermint flavoured suspension. Each 5 ml contains:

Dried Aluminium Hydroxide BP	600 mg
Magnesium Hydroxide BP	300 mg

Other ingredients include parabens.

Tablets: White, peppermint flavoured tablets marked 'Maalox TC' on one face and 'Rorer' on the other face. Each tablet contains:

Dried Aluminium Hydroxide BP	600 mg
Magnesium Hydroxide BP	300 mg

Other ingredients include sucrose.

Uses
Indications: The management of the symptoms of heartburn, gastric hyperacidity and gastritis.

The treatment of duodenal ulcer.

The management of the symptoms of peptic ulceration.

The prevention of duodenal ulcer recurrence.

Dosage and administration Maalox TC is administered orally and can be taken with milk or water if required.

Adult doses (including elderly):

Management of heartburn, gastric hyperacidity, gastritis and peptic ulceration:

Suspension: 5–10 ml four times daily taken 20 minutes to 1 hour after meals and at bedtime.

Tablets: 1–2 tablets four times daily taken 20 minutes to 1 hour after meals and at bedtime.

Treatment of duodenal ulcer:

Suspension: 15 ml four times daily taken 1 hour after meals and at bedtime.

Tablets: 3 tablets four times daily taken 1 hour after meals and at bedtime.

Prevention of duodenal ulcer recurrence:

Suspension: 15 ml in the morning, after food, and 15 ml at bedtime.

Tablets: 3 tablets in the morning, after food, and 3 tablets at bedtime.

Children: Not recommended.

Contra-indications, warnings, etc Contra-indicated in hypersensitivity to any of the active or inactive ingredients. Alkalosis, hypermagnesaemia or hypophosphataemia, where distension may be due to partial or complete intestinal obstruction. Not recommended for severely debilitated patients or those with impaired renal function.

Precautions: Magnesium salts, in the presence of renal insufficiency may cause CNS depression. Aluminium hydroxide, in the presence of low phosphorus diets, may cause phosphorus deficiency.

Maalox TC is a balanced formulation of antacids which will minimise bowel reaction, however, mild diarrhoea may be experienced at high doses.

Do not administer concomitantly with tetracycline antibiotics or iron preparations as antacids may interfere with the absorption of these drugs.

Use in pregnancy: The safety of Maalox TC in pregnancy has not been established.

Treatment of overdosage: Serious symptoms are unlikely following overdosage and specific therapy is rarely required.

Pharmaceutical precautions The suspension must be kept from freezing.

Legal category GSL.

Package quantities Suspension: Plastic bottle containing 500 ml.

Tablets: Carton containing 100 strip-packed tablets.

Further information Nil.

Product licence numbers

Suspension 5272/0021

Tablets 5272/0019.

MAALOX* SUSPENSION

Qualitative and quantitative composition Dried Aluminium Hydroxide Gel BP 220 mg, and Magnesium Hydroxide BP 195 mg per 5 ml.

Pharmaceutical form Suspension.

Clinical particulars

Therapeutic indications: Antacid therapy in gastric and duodenal ulcer, gastritis, heartburn and gastric hyperacidity.

Posology and method of administration: Oral.

Adult and elderly: 10–20 ml taken 20 minutes to one hour after meals and at bedtime, or as required. Maalox can be taken with water or milk if required.

Children: Not recommended for children under 14 years.

Contra-indications: Maalox should not be used in patients who are severely debilitated or suffering from renal insufficiency or if there is severe abdominal pain and/or the possibility of bowel obstruction.

Special warnings and special precautions for use: none stated.

Interactions with other medicaments and other forms of interaction: Antacids are known to interfere with the absorption of certain drugs including tetracyclines, vitamins, ciprofloxacin, ketoconazole, hydroxychlororquine, chloroquine, chlorpromazine and rifampicin.

Pregnancy and lactation: it is wise to avoid taking preparations containing antacids in the first trimester of pregnancy and during lactation.

Effects on ability to drive and use machines: none stated.

Undesirable effects: Gastro-intestinal side effects are uncommon. However, occasional diarrhoea or constipation may occur if use is excessive.

Overdose: serious symptoms are unlikely following overdose. Discontinue medication and correct fluid deficiency if necessary.

Pharmacological properties

Pharmacodynamic properties: Maalox is a balanced mixture of two antacids; aluminium hydroxide is a slow acting antacid and magnesium hydroxide is a quick-acting one. The two are frequently combined in antacid mixtures. Aluminium hydroxide on its own is astringent and may cause constipation. This effect is balanced by the effect of magnesium hydroxide, which, in common with other magnesium salts, may cause diarrhoea. Gastro-intestinal side-effects are thus rare with Maalox and makes it especially suitable when long-term therapy is necessary.

Pharmacokinetic properties: The absorption of aluminium and magnesium from antacids is small. Aluminium hydroxide is slowly converted to aluminium chloride in the stomach. Some absorption of soluble aluminium salts occurs in the gastro-intestinal tract with urinary excretion. Any absorbed magnesium is likewise excreted in the urine. Aluminium containing antacids should not be administered to patients with renal impairment where increased plasma concentration may occur.

Preclinical safety data: no relevant data.

Pharmaceutical particulars

List of excipients: Methylparaben NF, propylparaben NF, citric acid (anhydrous) USP, sodium saccharin (granular) USP, sorbitol solution 70% USP, mannitol powder USP, hydrogen peroxide solution 35%, hydrochloric acid BP, peppermint oil NF and purified water.

Incompatibilities: None stated.

Shelf life: Unopened: 24 months. After opening: 28 days.

Special precautions for storage: Protect from freezing. Store away from direct sunlight.

Nature and contents of container: White plastic bottles with polypropylene cap containing 300 or 500 ml.

Instructions for use/handling: Maalox can be taken with milk of water if required.

Marketing authorisation number 0050/5002.

Date of approval/revision of SPC February 1997

Legal category GSL.

MENOREST*

Qualitative and quantitative composition The active component of the Menorest patch is 17β-oestradiol (17β-estradiol-INN). The remaining components of the patch are pharmacologically inactive.

Three Menorest patches are available, see below:

The composition of the patch per unit area is identical.

	Nominal delivery (μg/day)	*17β-oestradiol content (mg)*	*Surface area (cm²)*	*Shape*
Menorest 37.5	37.5	3.29	11	Round
Menorest 50	50	4.33	14.5	Round
Menorest 75	75	6.57	22.0	Oval

Pharmaceutical form Transdermal patch.

Clinical particulars

Therapeutic indications: The Menorest patch is indicated for the following:

Symptoms of oestrogen deficiency due to natural or surgically induced menopause.

Prevention of postmenopausal osteoporosis in women at risk of developing fractures. Epidemiological studies suggest a number of individual risk factors which contribute to the development of postmenopausal osteoporosis. These include: early menopause; family history of osteoporosis; thin, small frame; cigarette use; prolonged corticosteroid use. If several of these risk factors are present in a patient consideration should be given to oestrogen replacement therapy.

Posology and method of administration: Adults and elderly: Menopausal symptoms: Therapy should be initiated with one Menorest 50 patch applied every 3 to 4 days (see *Instructions for use/handling*). The dose should be adjusted monthly depending on efficacy and signs of intolerance (e.g. breast tenderness). Dosage adjustment can be made using Menorest 37.5 and 75 patches. For maintenance therapy the lowest effective dose should be used.

Prevention of postmenopausal osteoporosis: Therapy should be initiated with one Menorest 50 patch applied every 3 to 4 days. The dosage may be adjusted monthly depending on signs of intolerance (e.g. breast tenderness) and yearly based upon bone mineral density assessment. Dosage adjustment can be made using Menorest 75 patch. Doses of less than 50 micrograms/day have not been shown to be effective in the prevention of osteoporosis.

Treatment with Menorest should commence as soon as possible after the onset of menopause and certainly within 2-3 years. Treatment should continue for at least 5 years and probably 10 years. Protection appears to be effective as long as the treatment is continued, however data beyond 10 years is limited. A careful reappraisal of the risk/benefit ratio should be undertaken before treating for longer than 5-10 years. For long term use see also *Special warnings and special precautions for use.*

Women undergoing a premature menopause, e.g. surgically induced menopause, may need to take Menorest for longer periods.

Therapeutic regimen: Menorest should be used as a continuous treatment. In patients with an intact uterus, progestogen therapy should be administered for at least 12 days per month normally during the second half of the month. Bleeding may occur after the progestogen treatment is completed.

Children: Menorest is not to be used by children.

Contra-indications: Oestrogens should not be used by women with any of the following conditions:

Known or suspected pregnancy.

Lactation.

History of, known or suspected cancer of the breast.

Known or suspected oestrogen-dependant neoplasia.

Undiagnosed abnormal vaginal bleeding.

Acute or chronic liver disease or history of liver disease where the liver function tests are still abnormal. Rotor syndrome or Dubin-Johnson syndrome.

Severe renal or cardiac disease.

Active deep venous thrombosis, thromboembolic disorders, or a past history of these conditions (see also *Special warnings and special precautions for use*).

Hypersensitivity to oestrogen or to components of this product.

Special warnings and special precautions for use: A complete medical and family history should be taken prior to the initiation of any oestrogen therapy. The pre-treatment and periodic physical examination should include special reference to blood pressure, breasts, abdomen, and pelvic organs and should include a Papanicolaou smear if not performed recently. Regular examination of the breasts is desirable in patients with a family history of breast cancer. As a general rule, oestrogen should not be prescribed for longer than 1 year without another physical examination being performed.

Some studies have suggested a possible increased incidence of breast cancer in postmenopausal women receiving long term (greater than 5 years) hormone replacement therapy. An assessment of the risk/benefit ratio should be undertaken before treating patients for longer than 5 years. Women on long-term therapy should have regular breast examinations and be instructed on self-breast examination. Regular mammographic investigation should be conducted where considered appropriate.

The long term administration (greater than 1 year) of unopposed oestrogen to women with an intact uterus increases the risk of endometrial hyperplasia and carcinoma. Women with an intact uterus should always receive a progestogen for at least 12 days of the menstrual cycle.

Patients with asthma, epilepsy, migraine, benign breast disease, otosclerosis, melanoma, multiple sclerosis, systemic lupus erythematosis, porphyria or hypophyseal tumours require careful observation as these conditions may be made worse by hormone replacement therapy.

Oestrogens may cause fluid retention and therefore patients with cardiac or renal dysfunction should be carefully observed.

Most studies indicate that oestrogen replacement therapy has little effect on blood pressure and some indicate that oestrogen use may be associated with a small decrease. In addition, most studies of combined therapy indicate that the addition of a progestogen also has little effect on blood pressure. Rarely, idiosyncratic hypertension may occur. When oestrogens are administered to hypertensive women, supervision is necessary and blood pressure should be monitored at regular intervals.

Epidemiological studies have suggested that hormone replacement therapy (HRT) is associated with an increased risk of developing venous thromboembolism (VTE) i.e. deep vein thrombosis or pulmonary embolism. The studies find a 2–3 fold increase for users compared with non-users which for healthy women amounts to a low risk of one extra case of VTE each year for every 5,000 patients taking HRT. Generally recognised risk factors for VTE include a personal or family history and severe obesity (Body Mass Index >30 kg/m2). In women with these factors the benefits of treatment with HRT need to be carefully weighed against risks. The risk of VTE may be temporarily increased with prolonged immobilisation, major trauma or major surgery. In women on HRT scrupulous attention should be given to prophylactic measures to prevent VTE following surgery. Where prolonged immobilisation is liable to follow elective surgery, particularly abdominal or orthopaedic surgery to the lower limbs, consideration should be given to temporarily stopping HRT 4 weeks earlier, if this is possible. If venous thromboembolism develops after initiating therapy the drug should be discontinued.

Oral oestrogen therapy may be associated with elevations of plasma triglycerides, leading to pancreatitis and other complications in patients with familial defects of lipoprotein metabolism.

Certain patients may develop undesirable manifestations of oestrogenic stimulation, such as irregular uterine bleeding, enlargement of fibroids, and mastodynia.

Changed oestrogen levels may affect certain endocrine and liver function tests.

Menorest is not a contraceptive neither will it restore fertility. If Menorest is administered to women of child bearing potential they should be advised to adhere to non-hormonal contraceptive methods.

Interactions with other medicaments and other forms of interaction: Preparations inducing microsomal liver enzymes, e.g. barbiturates, hydantoins, anticonvulsants (including carbamazepine), meprobamate, phenylbutazone, antibiotics (including rifampicin) and activated charcoal, may impair the activity of oestrogens (irregular bleeding and recurrence of symptoms may occur). The extent of interference with transdermally administered oestradiol is not known; these problems may be reduced by the transdermal route of administration which avoids any first pass hepatic metabolism.

Pregnancy and lactation: Oestrogens should not be used during pregnancy or while breast feeding.

Effects on ability to drive and use machines: On the basis of pharmacodynamic profile of Menorest, it is presumed to be safe or unlikely to produce an effect on driving performance or the operation of machines.

Undesirable effects: See *Special warnings and special precautions for use.*

Headache was the most commonly reported adverse reaction during clinical trials. Mild itching and rash were also reported around the application site and transient skin redness was observed after removing the patch.

The following adverse reactions have been reported with oral oestrogen therapy:

Urogenital system: Changes in vaginal bleeding pattern and abnormal withdrawal bleeding or flow; breakthrough bleeding; spotting; increase in size of uterine leoimyomata; vaginal candidiasis; change in amount of cervical secretion.

Breasts: Tenderness, enlargement.

Gastrointestinal: Nausea, vomiting; abdominal cramps, bloating; cholestatic jaundice.

Skin: Erythema and pruritus.

Eyes: Steepening of corneal curvature; intolerance to contact lenses.

Central nervous system: Headache, migraine, dizziness; mental depression, chorea.

Miscellaneous: Increase or decrease in weight; reduced carbohydrate tolerance, aggravation of porphyria, oedema; changes in libido.

As in the case with all oestrogens when administered without progestogen treatment, Menorest may induce hyperplasia of the endometrium.

Overdose: If signs of overdosage should appear the patch should be removed. The effects of overdosage with oral oestrogens are breast tenderness, nausea, vomiting and/or metrorrhagia.

Pharmacological properties

Pharmacodynamic properties: The Menorest patch is an efficient and systemic therapy for oestrogen replacement therapy which alleviates the symptoms of oestradiol deficiency in menopausal women as oestradiol is largely responsible for the development and maintenance of the female urogenital system and of secondary sexual characteristics.

Loss of ovarian secretion after menopause can result in instability of thermoregulation causing hot flushes and sweating associated with sleep disturbances.

Oestrogen therapy promotes growth and development of the urogenital epithelium providing an efficient therapy to avoid vaginal discomfort, dyspareunia, urinary urgency and frequency; in particular, vaginal cytology is converted to a pattern similar to that found in the premenopausal women, by increasing the proportion of superficial cells and concomitantly decreasing the number of basal and prebasal cells.

Oral oestrogen therapy changes the plasma lipid metabolism by a decrease in plasma levels of total and low density (LDL) cholesterol and by an increase in plasma high density lipoprotein (HDL) cholesterol. Although such alterations in the lipid profile are consistent with a reduction in the risk of coronary heart disease, plasma concentrations of triglycerides (a risk factor for coronary heart disease) may be elevated.

Oestrogen mainly exerts an anti-resorbitive and thus anti-activating effect on bone, leading to a reduction in bone turnover. Oestrogen therapy significantly reduces urinary calcium, hydroxyproline cross-links and serum alkaline phosphatase which are markers of bone turnover.

Oestrogen exerts a proliferative effect on endometrium which is prevented by concomitant progestogen administration.

Pharmacokinetic properties: The transdermal route achieves similar oestradiol plasma levels in the range of those observed in the pre-menopausal women at the early to mid-follicular phase. Following oral administration, oestradiol undergoes extensive first-pass metabolism to less active metabolites. The transdermal absorption of oestradiol avoids this first pass metabolism and thereby produces therapeutic plasma levels with a smaller total daily dose.

In pharmacokinetic studies it has been shown that following the application of Menorest patches delivering 25, 50 and 100 μg/day, the average plasma oestradiol concentrations and oestrone to oestradiol ratios were comparable with the physiological range reported for premenopausal women. Following the application of Menorest 50 patch twice-a-week for 3 weeks, the average oestradiol plasma concentration at steady-state was 57 pg/ml. At the end of the application period, the average plasma concentration of oestradiol was 29 pg/ml. Plasma oestradiol and oestrone concentrations with different dosages of Menorest increases linearly. Plasma concentrations of oestradiol and oestrone declined to baseline levels within 22 hours after removal of the patch.

Pre-clinical safety data: There are no pre-clinical data of relevance to the prescriber which are additional to that already included in other sections of the SPC.

Pharmaceutical particulars

List of excipients: Duro-Tak* adhesive; Morstik* adhesive; polyisobutylene (Vistanex LM-MS-LC*); 1,3 butylene glycol; oleic acid; mineral oil; bentonite; dipropylene glycol; vinyl acetate resin (Elvax 40W*); Alcolec 622/PG*.

Incompatibilities: Not applicable

Shelf life: The shelf life of the Menorest patch is 2 years when stored below 25°C.

Special precautions for storage: The Menorest patch should be stored below 25°C. Do not refrigerate.

Nature and contents of container: The Menorest patch is individually heat-sealed in foil laminate pouches of a paper/polyethylene/aluminium foil/polyethylene composite. They are available in packs of 8 patches.

Instructions for use/handling: The adhesive side of Menorest patch should be placed on a clean, dry area of the skin of the buttocks, abdomen, back or upper portion of the thighs. The Menorest patch should not be applied on or near to the breasts. The Menorest patch should be replaced every 3 to 4 days. The sites of application must be rotated, with an interval of at least 1 week allowed between applications to a particular site. The area selected should not be oily, abraded, or irritated. The waistline should be avoided, since tight clothing may rub the patch off. The patch should be applied immediately after opening the pouch and removing the protective liner. The patch should be pressed firmly in place with the palm of the hand for about 10 seconds, making sure there is good contact, especially around the edges. In the unlikely event that a patch should fall off, the same patch may be reapplied. If necessary, a new patch may be applied. In either case, the original treatment schedule should be continued. The patch may be worn during exercise or bathing. The patch should not be exposed to direct sunlight.

Menorest either new or used should always be kept out of the reach of children.

The Menorest patch should not be applied to any skin surface that is greasy, as this will affect the adhesive properties of the patch. Creams and lotions should not be used in the area of the patch for similar reasons.

The Menorest patch is used only once; after use the patch should be folded and disposed of with normal household waste.

Marketing authorisation numbers

Menorest 37.5	0012/0283
Menorest 50	0012/0268
Menorest 75	0012/0269

Date of approval/revision of SPC September 1997

Legal category POM

MUCODYNE* CAPSULES

Qualitative and quantitative composition In terms of the active ingredient Carbocisteine 375 mg.

Pharmaceutical form Size 1, yellow Lok-cap Capsules printed 'Mucodyne 375' in black.

Clinical particulars

Therapeutic indications: Carbocisteine is a mucolytic agent for the adjunctive therapy of respiratory tract dirorders characterised by excessive, viscous mucus, including suppurative otitis media (glue ear) and chronic obstructive airway disease.

Posology and method of administration: Adults including the elderly: Dosage is based upon an initial daily dosage of 2250 mg carbocisteine in divided doses, reducing to 1500 mg daily in divided doses when a satisfactory response is obtained e.g. two capsules three times a day reducing to one capsule four times a day.

Children: This formulation is not recommended for children. The normal daily dosage is 20 mg/kg bodyweight in divided doses. It is recommended that this is achieved with Mucodyne paediatric syrup.

Mucodyne capsules are for oral administration.

Contra-indications: Active peptic ulceration.

Special warnings and special precautions for use: None stated.

Interaction with other medicaments and other forms of interaction: None stated.

Pregnancy and lactation: Although tests in mammalian species have revealed no teratogenic efforts, Mucodyne is not recommended during the first trimester of pregnancy.

Use in lactation: Effects not known.

Effects on ability to drive and use machines: None stated.

Undesirable effects: There have been rare reports of skin rashes or gastronintestinal bleeding occurring during treatment with Mucodyne.

Overdose: Gastric lavage may be beneficial, followed by observation. Gastrointestinal disturbance is most likely symptom of Mucodyne overdosage.

Pharmacological properties

Pharmacodynamic properties: Carbocisteine (S-carboxymethyl L-cysteine) has been shown in normal and bronchitic animal models to affect the nature and amount of mucus glycoprotein which is secreted by the respiratory tract. An increase in the acid:neutral glycoprotein ratio of the mucus and a transformation of serous cells to mucus cells is known to be the intial response to irritation and will normally be followed by hypersecretion. The administration of carbocisteine to animals exposed to irritants indicates that the glycoprotein that is secreted remains normal; administration after exposure indicates that return to the normal state is accelerated. Studies in humans have demonstrated that carbocisteine reduces goblet cell hyperplasia.

Carbocisteine can therefore be demonstrated to have a role in the management of disorders characterised by abnormal mucus.

Pharmacokinetic properties: Carbocisteine is rapidly absorbed from the GI tract. In an 'in-house' study, at steady state (7 days) Mucodyne capsules 375 mg given as 2 capsules t.d.s. to healthy volunteers gave the following pharmacokinetic parameters:

Plasma Determinations	*Mean*	*Range*
T Max (Hr)	2.0	1.0-3.0
$T_{\frac{1}{2}}$(Hr)	1.87	1.4-2.5
K_{EL} (Hr^{-1})	0.387	0.28-0.50
AUC0-7.5(mcg.Hr.m1^{-1})	39.26	26.0-62.4
Derived Pharmacokinetic Parameters		
*CL_s(1}Hr^{-1})	20.2	—
CL_s (ml.min^{-1})	331	—
V_D(L)	105.2	—
V_D (L Kg^{-1})	1/75	—

*Calculated from dose for day 7 of study.

Preclinical safety data: No additional data of relevance to the prescriber.

Pharmaceutical particulars

List of excipients: Magnesium stearate (E572) BP, Aerosil 200 (E551), Lactose (spray dried) BP, Sodium lauryl sulphate BP, Size 1 yellow (Methuen 4A8-4A7) opaque gelatin lok-caps.

Incompatibilities: None stated.

Shelf life: 60 months.

Special precautions for storage: None stated.

Nature and contents of container: Grey HDPE tamper-tainer bottles with white LDPE cap or child resistant cap, or grey polypropylene securitainer bottles with white LDPE cap, containing 100 or 30 capsules. Blister packs of 18 or 6 capsules.

Instructions for use/handling: None stated.

Marketing authorisation number PL 0012/0238

Date of approval/revision of SPC December 1996

Legal category POM

MUCODYNE* PAEDIATRIC SYRUP

Qualitative and quantitative composition In terms of the active ingredient Carbocisteine 125 mg/5 ml.

Pharmaceutical form Clear, red syrup.

Clinical particulars:
Therapeutic indications: Carbocisteine is a mucolytic agent for the adjunctive therapy of respiratory tract dirorders characterised by excessive, viscous mucus.

Posology and method of administration: Children 5–12 years: 10 ml three times daily.
Children 2–5 years: 2.5–5 ml four times daily.
Mucodyne Paediatric Syrup is for oral administration.

Contra-indications: None.

Special warnings and precautions for use: None stated.

Interactions with other medicaments and other forms of interaction: None.

Pregnancy and lactation: Although tests in mammalian species have revealed no teratogenic efforts, Mucodyne is not recommended during the first trimester of pregnancy.

Use in lactation: Effects not known.

Effects on ability to drive and use machines: None.

Undesirable effects: None stated.

Overdose: Gastric lavage may be beneficial, followed by observation. Gastrointestinal disturbance is most likely symptom of Mucodyne overdosage.

Pharmacological properties
Pharmacodynamic properties: Carbocisteine (S-carboxymethyl L-cysteine) has been shown in normal and bronchitic animal models to affect the nature and amount of mucus glycoprotein which is secreted by the respiratory tract. An increase in the acid:neutral glycoprotein ratio of the mucus and a transformation of serous cells to mucus cells is known to be the intial response to irritation and will normally be followed by hypersecretion. The administration of carbocisteine to animals exposed to irritants indicates that the glycoprotein that is secreted remains normal; administration after exposure indicates that return to the normal state is accelerated. Studies in humans have demonstrated that carbocisteine reduces goblet cell hyperplasia.

Carbocisteine can therefore be demonstrated to have a role in the management of disorders characterised by abnormal mucus.

Pharmacokinetic properties: Carbocisteine is rapidly absorbed from the GI tract. In an 'in-house' study, at steady state (7 days) Mucodyne capsules 375 mg given as 2 capsules t.d.s to healthy volunteers gave the following pharmacokinetic parameters:

Plasma Determinations	*Mean*	*Range*
T Max (Hr)	2.0	1.0-3.0
$T\frac{1}{2}$(Hr)	1.87	1.4-2.5
K_{EL} (Hr^{-1})	0.387	0.28-0.50
AUC0-7.5(mcg.Hr.$m1^{-1}$)	39.26	26.0-62.4
*CL_s(1}Hr^{-1})	20.2	—
CL_s (ml.$min^{-1)}$	331	—
V_D(L)	105.2	—
V_D (L Kg^{-1})	1/75	—

*Calculated from dose for day 7 of study.

Preclinical safety data: No additional data of relevance to the prescriber.

Pharmaceutical particulars
List of excipients: Sucrose BP, Sodium methylhydroxybenzoate BP, Vanillin BP, Raspberry flavour, Cherry flavour, Red Ponceau 4R (E124), Sodium hydroxide solution 32% w/w (E524), Hydrochloric acid (E507), Distilled water BP.

Incompatibilities: None stated.

Shelf life: 36 months.

Special precautions for storage: Syrup should be stored in a cool place. Dilution may be effected with unpreserved syrup BP but diluted preparations should not be kept for more than 14 days.

Nature and contents of container: Clear PVC bottle with white plypropylene cap containing 200 or 300 ml (with measuring beaker).

Instructions for use/handling: None stated.

Marketing authorisation number PL 0012/0240

Date of approval/revision of SPC October 1996

Legal category POM

MUCODYNE* SYRUP

Qualitative and quantitative composition In terms of the active ingredient Carbocisteine 250 mg/5 ml.

Pharmaceutical form A clear amber syrup smelling of rum and slightly of cinnamon.

Clinical particulars:
Therapeutic indications: Carbocisteine is a mucolytic agent for the adjunctive therapy of respiratory tract dirorders characterised by excessive, viscous mucus, including suppurative otitis media (glue ear) and chronic obstructive airway disease.

Posology and method of administration: Adults including the elderly: Dosage is based upon an initial daily dosage of 2250 mg carbocisteine in divided doses, reducing to 1500 mg daily in divided doses when a satisfactory response is obtained e.g. for normal syrup 15 ml t.d.s reducing to 10 ml t.d.s.
Children: This formulation is not recommended for children. The normal daily dosage is 20 mg/kg bodyweight in divided doses. It is recommended that this is achieved with Mucodyne paediatric syrup.
Mucodyne syrup is for oral administration.

Contra-indications: Active peptic ulceration.

Special warnings and special precautions for use: None stated.

Interactions with other medicaments and other forms of interaction: None stated.

Pregnancy and lactation: Although tests in mammalian species have revealed no teratogenic efforts, Mucodyne is not recommended during the first trimester of pregnancy.

Use in lactation: Effects not known.

Effects on ability to drive and use machines: None stated.

Undesirable effects: There have been rare reports of skin rashes or gastrointestinal bleeding occurring during treatment with Mucodyne.

Overdose: Gastric lavage may be beneficial, followed by observation. Gastrointestinal disturbance is most likely symptom of Mucodyne overdosage.

Pharmacological properties
Pharmacodynamic properties: Carbocisteine (S-carboxymethyl L-cysteine) has been shown in normal and bronchitic animal models to affect the nature and amount of mucus glycoprotein which is secreted by the respiratory tract. An increase in the acid:neutral glycoprotein ratio of the mucus and a transformation of serous cells to mucus cells is known to be the intial response to irritation and will normally be followed by hypersecretion. The administration of carbocisteine to animals exposed to irritants indicates that the glycoprotein that is secreted remains normal; administration after exposure indicates that return to the normal state is accelerated. Studies in humans have demonstrated that carbocisteine reduces goblet cell hyperplasia.

Carbocisteine can therefore be demonstrated to have a role in the management of disorders characterised by abnormal mucus.

Pharmacokinetic properties: Carbocisteine is rapidly absorbed from the GI tract. In an 'in-house' study, at steady state (7 days) Mucodyne capsules 375 mg given as 2 capsules t.d.s to healthy volunteers gave the following pharmacokinetic parameters:

Plasma Determinations	*Mean*	*Range*
T Max (Hr)	2.0	1.0-3.0
$T\frac{1}{2}$(Hr)	1.87	1.4-2.5
K_{EL} (Hr^{-1})	0.387	0.28-0.50
AUC0-7.5(mcg.Hr.$m1^{-1}$)	39.26	26.0-62.4
Derived Pharmacokinetic Parameters		
*CL_s(1}Hr^{-1})	20.2	—
CL_s (ml.$min^{-1)}$	331	—
V_D(L)	105.2	—
V_D (L Kg^{-1})	1/75	—

*Calculated from dose for day 7 of study.

Preclinical safety data: No additional data of relevance to the prescriber.

Pharmaceutical particulars
List of excipients: Nipagin in sodium BP, Sucrose (granulated sugar) BP, Caramel liquid (E150), Rum flavour A662, Cinnamon flavour no. 1 NA, Sodium hydroxide solution 32% w/v (E524), Hydrochloric acid (E527) BP, Deionised water.

Incompatibilities: Mixture with linctus of pholcodine causes precipitation of carbocisteine from solution.

Shelf life: 36 months.

Special precautions for storage: Store below 25°C. Dilution may be effected with unpreserved syrup BP but diluted preparations should not be kept more than 14 days.

Nature and contents of container: Clear PVC bottle with white polypropylene cap containing 100 or 300 ml (with graduated dosage beaker).

Instructions for use/handling: None stated.

Marketing authorisation number PL 0012/0241

Date of approval/revision of SPC October 1996

Legal category POM

NIVAQUINE* TABLETS AND INJECTION

Presentation
Tablets: Yellowish buff film-coated tablets containing 200 mg chloroquine sulphate (equivalent to 150 mg chloroquine base) impressed 'Nivaquine 200' on one face, reverse plain. The tablets also contain glucose.
Injection: A colourless injection solution of chloroquine sulphate 5.45% w/v equivalent to 40 mg chloroquine base per ml in ampoules of 5 ml.

Uses Chloroquine is a 4-aminoquinoline derivative, which has a high degree of activity against the asexual erythrocytic forms of all species of malaria parasites. It is indicated for the suppression and clinical cure of all forms of malaria and, in addition, produces radical cure of falciparum malaria.

Nivaquine exerts a beneficial effect in certain collagen diseases and protects against the effects of solar radiation. It is also indicated in the treatment of rheumatoid arthritis, juvenile rheumatoid arthritis, discoid and systemic lupus erythematosus and skin conditions aggravated by sunlight.

Nivaquine is also active against Entamoeba histolytica and Giardia lamblia and when metronidazole is not available it may be used in hepatic amoebiasis and giardiasis.

Dosage and administration
Suppression of malaria: It is advisable to start taking Nivaquine 1 week before entering an endemic area and to continue for 4 weeks after leaving.

Age group	*Dose to be taken once a week on the same day each week*
Adults	Two Nivaquine tablets (300 mg chloroquine base)
Infants and children up to twelve years	5 mg chloroquine base per kg bodyweight

These dosages are those recommended by the World Health Organisation.

Treatment of malaria
(1) Non-immune subjects
(a) Oral route
Adults:

Day of treatment	*Dosage*
Day 1	Four Nivaquine tablets (600 mg chloroquine base) in one dose followed by a further two tablets (300 mg chloroquine base) six hours later.
Day 2	Two Nivaquine tablets (300 mg chloroquine base).
Day 3	Two Nivaquine tablets (300 mg chloroquine base).

The above dosage is intended as a guide in the treatment of Plasmodium falciparum malaria. However, due to variation in the strain sensitivity, it may sometimes be necessary to increase the duration of treatment by administering two Nivaquine tablets (300 mg chloroquine base) daily on days 4 to 7.

Infants and children: Nivaquine syrup can be conveniently used in this age group to permit flexibility of dosage.

(b) Injection
Adults and children: Slow intravenous infusion: 10 mg/kg bodyweight chloroquine base to be administered in sodium chloride 0.9% injection by slow intravenous infusion over eight hours followed by three further 8 hour infusions containing 5 mg base/kg (total dose 25 mg base/kg over 32 hours). The dose should not be modified in renal or hepatic disease.

Exceptionally, where intravenous administration is not possible, Nivaquine may be given by intramuscular or subcutaneous injection in small divided doses of 3.5 mg chloroquine base/kg bodyweight every 6 hours or 2.5 mg base/kg every 4 hours.

(2) Partially immune subjects
Adults: A single dose of four Nivaquine tablets (600 mg chloroquine base) will provide an effective course of treatment.
Infants and children: Repeated infection with many species and strains of malaria parasite prevalent in highly endemic malarial areas eventually produces a high degree of immune response frequently resulting in modification of the symptoms of clinical attack. This is particularly obvious in adults but less so in adolescents and children. Immunity is uncommon in very young age groups with the exception of infants up to the age of about 6 months who are partly

protected by trans-placentally derived maternal antibodies. It is therefore advisable to treat previously exposed children in the same way as non-immune children.

Other indications:

Indication	*Age group*	*Dose*
Rheumatoid arthritis	Adults	One Nivaquine tablet (150 mg chloroquine base) daily.
	Children	3 mg/kg bodyweight as base per day
Systemic lupus erythematosus	Adults	One Nivaquine tablet (150 mg chloroquine base) daily until maximum improvement is obtained followed by a smaller maintenance dosage.
	Children	3 mg/kg bodyweight as base per day.
Light-sensitive skin eruptions	Adults	One or two Nivaquine tablets (150 mg to 300 mg chloroquine base) daily during the period of maximum light exposure.
	Children	3 mg/kg bodyweight as base per day during the period of maximum light exposure.

Treatment should be discontinued if no improvement has occurred after 6 months.

Dosage in the elderly: No specific dosage recommendations.

Contra-indications, warnings, etc

Precautions: Caution is advised in cases of porphyria, severe gastrointestinal, neurological and blood disorders and in patients receiving anticolagulant therapy. Nivaquine should be used with care in patients with a history of epilepsy as it has been reported to provoke seizures. Caution should be exercised in patients with hepatic or renal disease. Retinopathy: Irreversible retinal damage may occur with prolonged treatment. Ophthalmological examination should always be carried out before and regularly (3–6 monthly intervals) during treatment. Retinal damage is particularly likely to occur if treatment has been given for longer than one year or if the total dosage has exceeded 1.6 g/kg bodyweight. These precautions also apply to patients receiving chloroquine continuously at weekly intervals as a prophylactic against malarial attack for more than three years.

Nivaquine has a temporary effect on visual accommodation and patients should be warned regarding driving or operating machinery.

Use in pregnancy: Nivaquine is generally contraindicated in pregnancy. However, clinicians may decide to administer Nivaquine to pregnant women for the prevention or treatment of malaria. Ocular or inner ear damage may occur in infants born of mothers who receive high doses of chloroquine throughout pregnancy.

Side-effects: The more common side-effects include gastro-intestinal disturbances, headache and skin eruptions. Psoriasis may be exacerbated. Depigmentation or loss of hair may also occur. These effects usually disappear on cessation of treatment. Convulsions have been reported rarely (these may result from cerebral malaria, such patients should receive an injection of phenobarbitone to prevent seizures in a dose of 3.5 mg/kg in addition to intravenous administration of Nivaquine). Bone marrow depression, including aplastic anaemia, occurs rarely. Full blood counts should therefore be carried out regularly during extended treatment. Allergic and anaphylactic reactions have occurred rarely. Changes in liver function, including hepatitis and abnormal liver function tests, have occurred rarely.

Treatment of overdosage: Chloroquine is highly toxic in overdose; children are particularly susceptible to toxic doses of chloroquine. The chief symptoms of overdosage include circulatory collapse due to a potent cardiotoxic effect, respiratory arrest and coma. Symptoms may progress rapidly after initial nausea and vomiting.

Death may result from circulatory or respiratory failure or cardiac dysrhythmia.

Gastric lavage should be carried out urgently, first protecting the airway and instituting artificial ventilation where necessary. There is a risk of cardiac arrest following aspiration of gastric contents in more serious cases. Activated charcoal left in the stomach may reduce the absorption of any remaining chloroquine from the gut. Circulatory status (with central venous pressure measurement), respiration, plasma electrolytes and blood gases should be monitored, with correction of hypokalaemia and acidosis if indicated. Cardiac arrhythmias should not be treated unless life threatening; drugs with quinidine-like effect should be avoided.

Early administration of the following has been shown to improve survival in cases of serious poisoning:

1. Adrenaline infusion 0.25 micrograms/kg/min initially with increments of 0.25 micrograms/kg/min until adequate systolic blood pressure (more than 100 mm Hg) is restored; adrenaline reduces the effects of chloroquine on the heart through its inotropic and vasoconstrictor effects.
2. Diazepam infusion (2 mg/kg over 30 minutes as a loading dose, followed by 1–2 mg/kg/day for up to 2–4 days). Diazepam may minimise cardiotoxicity.

Acidification of the urine, haemodialysis, peritoneal dialysis or exchange transfusion have not been shown to be of value in treating chloroquine poisoning. Chloroquine is excreted very slowly, therefore symptomatic cases merit observation for several days.

Pharmaceutical precautions

Tablets: Protect from light.
Injection: Protect from light.

Legal category Nivaquine Tablets POM, but when supplied for prevention of malaria in a container specifically labelled for that purpose, P.

Nivaquine Injection POM.

Package quantities 28×200 mg Tablets. Injection: 10 ampoules of 5 ml per carton.

Further information Nil.

Product licence numbers

Injection 0012/5048
Tablets 0012/5260

NIVAQUINE* SYRUP

Qualitative and quantitative composition Nivaquine Syrup contains Chloroquine Sulphate BP 68 mg/5 ml.

Pharmaceutical form Syrup.

Clinical particulars

Therapeutic indications: Nivaquine is a 4-aminoquinoline compound which has a high degree of activity against the asexual erythrocytic forms of all species of malaria parasites. It is indicated for the suppression and clinical cure of all forms of malaria and, in addition, produces radical cure of falciparum malaria.

Nivaquine also exerts a beneficial effect in certain collagen diseases and protects against the effects of solar radiation. It is employed in the treatment of rheumatoid arthritis, juvenile arthritis, discoid and systemic lupus erythematosus and skin conditions aggravated by sunlight.

Nivaquine is also active against entamoeba histolica and giardia lamblia and when flagyl (metronidazole) is not available it may be used in hepatic amoebiasis and giardiasis.

Packs for supply directly to the public: For the prevention of malaria.

Posology and method of administration: Route of administration oral.

Rheumatoid arthritis: Adults: 3×5 ml Nivaquine Syrup (150 mg chloroquine base) daily. *Children:* 3 mg/kg bodyweight daily. Treatment should be discontinued if no improvement has occurred after 6 months.

Systemic lupus erythematosus: Adults: 3×5 ml Nivaquine Syrup (150 mg chloroquine base) daily until maximum improvement is obtained followed by smaller maintenance dosage. *Children:* 3 mg/kg bodyweight daily. Treatment should be discontinued if no improvement has occurred after 6 months.

Light sensitive skin eruptions: Adults: 3 to 6×5 ml Nivaquine Syrup (150 mg to 300 mg chloroquine base) daily during the period of maximum light exposure. *Children:* 3 mg/kg body weight daily. Treatment should be discontinued if no improvement has occurred after 6 months.

Suppression of malaria: Adults: 6×5 ml Nivaquine Syrup (300 mg chloroquine base) to be taken once a week on the same day each week. *Infants and children up to 12 years:* 5 mg Chloroquine base per kg bodyweight to be taken once a week on the same day each week. It is advisable to start taking Nivaquine 1 week before entering an endemic area and to continue for 4 weeks after leaving.

Treatment of malaria: 1. *Partially immune adults:* A single dose of 12×5 ml Nivaquine Syrup (600 mg chloroquine base) will provide a safe and effective course of treatment. 2. *Non-immune adults:* Day 1: 12×5 ml Nivaquine syrup (600 mg chloroquine base) in one dose followed by a further 6×5 ml syrup (300 mg chloroquine base) six hours later. Day 2: 6×5 ml Nivaquine syrup (300 mg chloroquine base). Day 3: 6×5 ml Nivaquine Syrup (300 mg chloroquine base). The above dosage is intended as a guide in the treatment of plasmodium falciparum malaria. However, due to a variation in the strain sensitivity, it may sometimes be necessary to increase the duration of treatment by administering 6×5 ml Nivaquine Syrup (300 mg chloroquine base) daily on days 4 to 7. 3. *Non-immune or partially immune infants and children:* Nivaquine Syrup can be conveniently used in patients in this age group to permit flexibility of dosage. Day 1: 10 mg chloroquine base/kg bodyweight (maximum 600 mg base) followed by 5 mg chloroquine base/kg bodyweight (maximum 300 mg base) six hours later. Day 2: 5 mg chloroquine base/kg bodyweight (maximum 300 mg base). Day 3: 5 mg chloroquine base/kg bodyweight (maximum 300 mg base).

Contra-indications: Nivaquine is generally contraindicated in pregnancy. However, clinicians may decide to administer Nivaquine to pregnant women for the prevention or treatment of malaria. Ocular or inner ear damage may occur in infants born of mothers who receive high doses of chloroquine throughout pregnancy.

Special warnings and precautions for use: Nivaquine should be used with care in patients with a history of epilepsy as it has been reported to provoke seizures. Caution is advised in cases of porphyria, hepatic or renal disease, severe gastrointestinal, neurological and blood disorders and in patients receiving anticoagulant therapy.

Interactions with other medicaments and other forms of interaction: Caution is advised in patients receiving anticoagulant therapy.

Pregnancy and lactation: Nivaquine is generally contraindicated in pregnancy. However, clinicians may decide to administer Nivaquine to pregnant women for the prevention or treatment of malaria. Ocular or inner ear damage may occur in infants born of mothers who receive high doses of chloroquine throughout pregnancy.

Effects on ability to drive and use machines: Nivaquine has a temporary effect on visual accommodation and patients should be warned that they should not drive or operate machinery if they are affected.

Undesirable effects: The more common side effects include gastrointestinal disturbances, headache, skin eruptions, and disturbance of visual accommodation. Psoriasis may be exacerbated. Depigmentation or loss of hair may also occur. Bone marrow depression, including aplastic anaemia occurs rarely. Full blood counts should therefore be carried out regularly during extended treatment.

Irreversible retinal damage may occur with prolonged treatment. Ophthalmological examination should always be carried out before and regularly (3–6 monthly intervals) during treatment. Retinal damage is particularly likely to occur if treatment has been given for longer than one year, or if the total dosage has exceeded 1.6 g/kg bodyweight. These precautions also apply to patients receiving chloroquine continuously at weekly intervals as a prophylactic against malarial attack for more than three years. Convulsions have been reported rarely (these may result from cerebral malaria. Such patients should receive an injection of phenobarbitone to prevent seizures, in a dose of 3.5 mg/kg in addition to intravenous administration of Nivaquine). Allergic and anaphylactic reactions have occurred rarely.

Changes in liver function, including hepatitis and abnormal liver function tests, have been reported rarely.

Overdosage: Chloroquine is highly toxic in overdosage; children are particularly susceptible to toxic doses of chloroquine. The chief symptoms of overdose include circulatory collapse due to a potent cardiotoxic effect, respiratory arrest and coma. Symptoms may progress rapidly after initial nausea and vomiting. Death may result from circulatory or respiratory failure or cardiac dysrhythmia. Gastric lavage should be carried out urgently, first protecting the airways and instituting artificial ventilation where necessary. There is a risk of cardiac arrest following aspiration of gastric contents in more serious cases. Activated charcoal left in the stomach may reduce absorption of any remaining chloroquine from the gut. Circulatory status (with central venous pressure measurement) respiration, plasma electrolytes and blood gases should be monitored, with correction of hypokalaemia and acidosis if indicated. Cardiac arrhythmias should not be treated unless life threatening; drugs with quinidine-like effects should be avoided. Early administration of the following has been shown to improve survival in cases of serious poisoning.

1) Adrenaline infusion (0.25 micrograms/kg/min initially, with increments of 0.25 micrograms/kg/min until adequate systolic blood pressure (more than 100 mm mercury is restored; adrenaline reduces the effects of chloroquine on the heart through its inotropic and vasoconstrictor effects.

2) Diazepam infusion (2 mg/kg over 30 minutes as a loading dose, followed by 1–2 mg/kg/day for up to 2–4 days). Diazepam may minimise cardiotoxicity.

Acidification of the urine, haemodialysis, peritoneal dialysis or exchange transfusions have not been shown to be of value in treating chloroquine poisoning. Chloroquine is excreted very slowly, therefore symptomatic cases merit observation for several days.

Pharmacological properties
Pharmacodynamic properties: Chloroquine is used for the suppression and treatment of malaria. It has rapid schizonticidal effect and appears to affect cell growth by interfering with DNA; its activity also seems to depend on preferential accumulation in the infected erythrocyte. Chloroquine kills the erythrocytic forms of malaria parasites at all stages of development. In addition to its antimalarial properties, it possesses other pharmacological properties. Its anit-inflammatory properties enable Nivaquine to be used in certain collagen diseases and it protects against the effects of solar radiation. Nivaquine is also active against entamoeba histolytica and giardia lamblia. It may be used in hepatic amoebiasis and giardiasis.

Pharmacokinetic properties: Chloroquine is readily absorbed from the gastro-intestinal tract and about 55% in the circulation is bound to plasma proteins. It accumulates in high concentrations in some tissues, such as kidneys, liver, lungs and spleen and is strongly bound in melanin containing cells such as those in the eyes and the skin; it is also bound to double stranded DNA, present in red blood cells containing schizonts. Chloroquine in eliminated very slowly from the body and it may persist in tissues for a long period. Up to 70% of a dose may be excreted unchanged in urine and up to 25% may be excreted also in the urine as the desethyl metabolite. The rate of urinary excretion of chloroquine is increased at low pH values.

Pharmaceutical particulars
List of excipients: Liquid sugar gran. liquors, Sodium L glutamate, Saccharin sodium BP, Propylene glycol, Methyl hydroxybenzoate BP, Propyl hydroxybenzoate BP, Oil peppermint (Chinese), Witham pineapple flavour (F), Caramel HT, Demineralised water BP.

Incompatibilities: None known.

Shelf life: 36 months.

Special precautions for storage: Nivaquine should be stored below 25°C, protected from light.

Nature and contents of container: Amber glass bottle containing 100 ml.

Instructions for use/handling: None stated.

Marketing authorisation number PL 0012/5020

Date of approval/revision of SPC November 1997

Legal classification POM.
When used solely for the prevention of malaria: Pharmacy Medicine.

OPTICROM* AQUEOUS EYE DROPS

Presentation A clear colourless aqueous solution of Sodium Cromoglycate BP 2% w/v, with benzalkonium chloride 0.01% w/v.

Inactive ingredients: Benzalkonium Chloride USNF, Disodium Edetate BP.

Uses For the prophylaxis and symptomatic treatment of acute allergic conjunctivitis such as hay fever, chronic allergic conjunctivitis and vernal kerato conjunctivitis. Sodium cromoglycate inhibits the release from sensitised mast cells of mediators of the allergic reaction.

Dosage and administration *Adults (including the elderly) and children:* One or two drops into each eye four times daily.

Contra-indications, warnings, etc
Contra-indications: Opticrom is contra-indicated in patients with known sensitivity to any ingredient.

Warnings: As with other ophthalmic solutions containing benzalkonium chloride, soft contact lenses should not be worn during the treatment period.

Effects on ability to drive and use machinery: As with all eye drops, instillation of Opticrom may cause a transient blurring of vision.

Side-effects: Transient stinging and burning may occur after instillation. Other symptoms of local irritation have been recorded rarely.

Use in pregnancy and lactation: As with all medication caution should be exercised especially during the first trimester of pregnancy. Cumulative experience with sodium cromoglycate suggests it has no adverse effects on foetal development. It should only be used in pregnancy where there is a clear need.

It is not known whether sodium cromoglycate is excreted in the breast milk but on the basis of its physico-chemical properties this is considered unlikely. There is no information to suggest that the use of sodium cromoglycate has any undesirable effects on the baby.

Overdosage: No action other than medical observation should be necessary.

Pharmaceutical precautions Store below 30°C. Protect from direct sunlight.

Legal category POM.

Package quantities 13.5 ml.

Further information Discard any remaining contents four weeks after opening the bottle.

Product licence number 0113/0039R.

OPTICROM* EYE OINTMENT

Presentation Opticrom Eye Ointment is a cream coloured opaque sterile ointment containing 4% w/w Sodium Cromoglycate BP.

Inactive ingredients: Liquid Paraffin BP, Yellow Soft Paraffin BP, Modulan (acetylated lanolin)

Uses For the prophylactic relief and treatment of allergic conjunctivitis such as hay fever, chronic allergic conjunctivitis and vernal kerato conjunctivitis. Sodium cromoglycate inhibits the release from sensitised mast cells of mediators of the allergic reaction.

Dosage and administration *Adults (including the elderly) and children:* To be applied to the eye two to three times daily. Opticrom Ointment should be used regularly to ensure optimal control of symptoms. It is recommended that treatment is continued during the period of exposure to allergen even when free of symptoms.

Care should be taken to avoid direct contact between the eye and the tube nozzle.

Contra-indications, warnings, etc
Contra-indications: Known sensitivity to any ingredient.

Warnings: As with other ophthalmic ointments, transient blurring of vision may occur. The ointment should not be used if contact lenses are being worn.

Side-effects: Transient blurring of vision, stinging and burning may occur after application. Other symptoms of local irritation have been reported rarely.

Use in pregnancy and lactation: As with all medication caution should be exercised especially during the first trimester of pregnancy. Cumulative experience with sodium cromoglycate suggests that it has no adverse effects on foetal development. It should only be used in pregnancy where there is a clear need.

It is not known whether sodium cromoglycate is excreted in the breast milk but on the basis of its physico-chemical properties this is considered unlikely. There is no information to suggest that the use of sodium cromoglycate has any undesirable effects on the baby.

Pharmaceutical precautions Store below 25°C. Protect from direct sunlight. The contents should be discarded four weeks after opening.

Legal category POM.

Package quantities 5 g.

Further information Patients may prefer to use Opticrom Aqueous Eye Drops during the day and Opticrom Eye Ointment at night.

Product licence number 0113/0103.

PHENERGAN* TABLETS AND ELIXIR PHENERGAN* NIGHTIME

Qualitative and quantitative composition
Phenergan Elixir contains Promethazine Hydrochloride BP 5 mg / 5 ml

Phenergan 10 mg tablets contain Promethazine Hydrochloride BP 10 mg

Phenergan 25 mg tablets Phenergan Nightime contain Promethazine Hydrochloride BP 25 mg

Pharmaceutical form
Phenergan Elixir is a clear golden syrupy liquid

Phenergan tablets are pale blue and marked PN 10 (10 mg tablets) and PN 25 (25 mg tablets) on one side.

Clinical particulars
Therapeutic indications: As symptomatic treatment for allergic conditions of the upper respiratory tract and skin including allergic rhinitis, urticaria and anaphylactic reactions to drugs and foreign proteins. As an adjunct in preoperative sedation in surgery and obstetrics. As an antiemetic.

For short term use: Sedation and treatment of insomnia in adults. As a paediatric sedative.

Phenergan Nightime: For short term treatment of insomnia (sleeplessness) in adults.

Posology and method of administration: Route of administration: Oral

Not for use in children under the age of 2 years because the safety of such use has not been established.

Contra-indications: Phenergan should not be used in patients in coma or suffering from CNS depression of any cause. It must not be given to neonates, premature infants or patients hypersensitive to phenothiazines. Phenergan should be avoided in patients taking monoamine oxidase inhibitors up to 14 days previously. The Elixir contains hydrogenated glucose syrup and is not suitable for diabetics.

Special warnings and special precautions for use: Phenergan may thicken or dry lung secretions and impair expectoration. It should therefore be used with caution in patients with asthma, bronchitis or bronchiectasis. Use with care in patients with severe coronary artery disease, narrow angle glaucoma, epilepsy or hepatic and renal insufficiency. Caution should be exercised in patients with bladder neck or pyloro-duodenal obstruction. Promethazine may mask the warnings signs of ototoxicity caused by ototoxic drugs e.g. salicylates. It may also delay the early diagnosis of intestinal obstruction or raised intracranial pressure through the suppression of vomiting. Phenergan Elixir should not be used for longer than 7 days without seeking medical advice.

Interaction with other medicaments and other forms of interaction: Phenergan will enhance the action of any anticholinergic agent, tricyclic anti-depressant, sedative or hypnotic. Alcohol should be avoided during treatment. Phenergan may interfere with immunological urine pregnancy tests to produce false-positive or false-negative results. Phenergan should be discontinued at least 72 hours before the start of skin tests as it may inhibit the cutaneous histamine response thus producing false negative results.

Pregnancy and lactation: There is epidemiological evidence for the safety of promethazine in pregnancy and animal studies have shown no hazard. Nevertheless, it should not be used in pregnancy unless the physician considers it essential. The use of Phenergan is not recommended in the 2 weeks prior to delivery in view of the risk of irritability and excitement in the neonate. Available evidence suggests that the amount excreted in milk is insignificant. However, there are risks of neonatal irritability and excitement.

Effects on ability to drive and use machines: Because the duration of action may be up to 12 hours, patients should be advised that if they feel drowsy they should not drive or operate heavy machinery.

Undesirable effects: Side effects may be seen in a few patients: drowsiness, dizziness, restlessness, headaches, nightmares, tiredness, and disorientation. Anticholinergic side effects such as blurred vision, dry mouth and urinary retention occur occasionally. Infants are susceptible to the anticholinergic effects of promethazine, while other children may display paradoxical hyperexcitability. The elderly are particularly susceptible to the anticholinergic effects and confusion due to promethazine. Other side-effects include anorexia, gastric irritation, palpitations, hypotension, arrhythmias, extrapyramidal effects, muscle spasms and tic-like movements of the head and face. Anaphylaxis, jaundice and blood dyscrasias including haemolytic anaemia rarely occur. Photosensitive skin reactions have been reported. Strong sunlight should be avoided during treatment.

The preservatives used in Phenergan Elixir have been reported to cause hypersensitivity reactions, characterised by circulatory collapse with CNS de-

	Elixir	10 mg tablets	25 mg tablets
As an antihistamine in allergy			
Children 2-5 years	Either: 5-15 mg as a single dose Or 5 mg bd Maximum daily dose 15 mg	The use of the Elixir is recommended for this age group	The use of the Elixir is recommended for this age group
Children 5-10 years	Either 10-25 mg as a single dose Or: 5-10 mg bd Maximum daily dose 25 mg	Either 10 or 20 mg as a single dose† Or 10 mg bd Maximum daily dose 20 mg	25 mg as a single dose† Maximum daily dose 25 mg
Children over 10 years, adults (inc elderly)	Initially 10 mg bd Increasing to a maximum of 20 mg tds as required	Initially 10 mg bd Increasing to a maximum of 20 mg tds as required	25 mg as a single dose† Increasing to 25 mg bd as required
As an antiemetic			
Children 2-5 years	5 mg to be taken the night before the journey To be repeated after 6-8 hours as required	The use of the Elixir is recommended for this age group	The use of the Elixir is recommended for this age group
Children 5-10 years	10 mg to be taken the night before the journey To be repeated after 6-8 hours as required	10 mg to be taken the night before the journey. To be repeated after 6-8 hours as required	The use of the Elixir or 10 mg tablets is recommended for this age group
Children over 10 years and adults (including elderly)	25 mg to be taken the night before the journey To be repeated after 6-8 hours as required.	20 mg to be taken the night before the journey. To be repeated after 6-8 hours as required	25 mg to be taken the night before the journey. To be repeated after 6-8 hours as required
Short term sedation			
Children 2-5 years	15 or 20 mg as a single night time dose	The use of Phenergan Elixir is recommended for this age group	The use of Phenergan Elixir is recommended for this age group
Children 5-10 years	20 or 25 mg as a single night time dose	20 mg as a single night time dose	25 mg as a single night time dose
Children over 10 years and adults (including elderly)	25 or 50 mg as a single night time dose. The use of Phenergan tablets to provide these doses is recommended.	20 to 50 mg as a single night time dose	25 or 50 mg as a single night time dose Phenergan Nightime: 25 or 50 mg as a single night time dose.

pression in certain susceptible individuals with allergic tendencies.

Overdose: Symptoms of severe overdosage are variable. They are characterised in children by various combinations of excitation, ataxia, incoordination, athetosis and hallucinations, while adults may become drowsy and lapse into coma. Convulsions may occur in both adults and children. Coma may precede their occurrence. Tachycardia may develop. Cardiorespiratory depression is not uncommon. If the patient is seen soon enough after ingestion, it should be possible to induce vomiting with ipecacuanha despite the antiemetic effect of promethazine; alternatively, gastric lavage may be used.

Treatment is otherwise supportive with attention to maintenance of adequate respiratory and circulatory status. Convulsions should be treated with diazepam or other suitable anticonvulsant.

Pharmacological properties

Pharmacodynamic properties: Potent, long acting, antihistamine with additional anti-emetic central sedative and anticholinergic properties.

Pharmacokinetic properties: Promethazine is distributed widely in the body. It enters the brain and crosses the placenta. Promethazine is slowly excreted via urine and bile. Phenothiazines may pass into the milk at low concentrations.

Preclinical safety data: No additional pre-clinical data of relevance to the prescriber.

Pharmaceutical particulars

List of excipients:

Phenergan Elixir: Hydrogenated glucose syrup, citric acid anhydrous BP (E330), sodium citrate BP (E331), ascorbic acid BP (E300), sodium sulphite anhydrous BP (E221), sodium metabisulphite BP (E223), sodium benzoate BP (E211), Orange juice flavour, Caramel, acesulphame potassium (E950), demineralised water BP

Phenergan tablets Lactose BP, maize starch BP,Povidone K30 BP, magnesium stearate BP, polyethylene glycol 200, Opaspray M-1-4210A and (contains E132 and E171), Pharmacoat 606.

Incompatibilities: None stated.

Shelf life:

Phenergan Elixir: 24 months when unopened. 1 month when opened

Phenergan tablets: 60 months

Special Precautions for storage

Phenergan Elixir: Protect from light. Store below 25°C

Phenergan tablets: Protect from light. Store below 30°C

Nature and contents of container

Phenergan Elixir: Amber glass bottles containing 100 mg

Phenergan tablets: Blister packs of 56 tablets

Phenergan Nightime: Blister packs of 14 tablets

Instructions for use/handling: No special instructions

Marketing authorisation numbers

Phenergan Elixir PL 0012/5025R
Phenergan 10 mg tablets PL 0012/5285R
Phenergan 25 mg tablets PL 0012/5286R

Date of approval/revision of SPC June 1997

Legal classification P

PHENERGAN* INJECTION

Qualitative and quantitative composition Phenergan Injection contains Promethazine Hydrochloride BP 2.5%w/v

Pharmaceutical form Solution for injection

Clinical particulars

Therapeutic indications: A symptomatic treatment for allergic conditions of the upper respiratory tract and skin including allergic rhinitis, urticaria and anaphylactic reactions to drugs and foreign proteins.

Sedation and treatment of insomnia in adults.

As an adjunct in preoperative sedation in surgery and obstetrics.

As a paediatric sedative.

Not for use in children under 2 years of age because the safety of such use has not been established.

Posology and method of administration: For Intramuscular or intravenous use. The usual dose is 25–50 mg by deep intramuscular injection, or, in emergency, by slow intravenous injection after dilution of the 2.5% solution to 10 times its volume with water for injections immediately before use.

Maximum parenteral dose 100 mg.

Elderly: No specific dosage recommendations.

Children: 6.25–12.5 mg for children from 5–10 years by deep intramuscular injection.

Contra-indications: Phenergan should not be used in patients in coma or suffering from CNS depression of any cause. It must not be given to neonates, premature infants or patients hypersensitive to phenothiazines. Phenergan should be avoided in patients taking monoamine oxidase inhibitors up to 14 days previously.

Special warnings and precautions for use: Phenergan may thicken or dry lung secretions and impair expectoration. It should therefore be used with caution in patients with asthma, bronchitis or bronchiectasis. Use with care in patients with severe coronary artery disease, narrow angle glaucoma, epilepsy or hepatic and renal insufficiency. Caution should be exercised in patients with bladder neck or pyloro-duodenal obstruction. Promethazine may mask the warning signs of ototoxicity caused by ototoxic drugs e.g. Salicylates. It may also delay the early diagnosis of intestinal obstruction or raised intracranial pressure through the suppression of vomiting. Accidental intra-arterial injection may lead to peripheral gangrene and necrosis while subcutaneous injections may lead to local necrosis.

Interactions with other medicaments and other forms of interaction: Phenergan will enhance the action of any anticholinergic agent, tricyclic anti-depressant, sedative or hypnotic. Alcohol should be avoided during treatment. Phenergan may interfere with immunological urine pregnancy tests to produce false-positive or false-negative results. Phenergan should be discontinued at least 72 hours before the start of skin tests as it may inhibit the cutaneous histamine response thus producing false-negative results. Phenergan injection may increase glucose tolerance.

Pregnancy and lactation: There is epidemiological evidence for the safety of promethazine in pregnancy and animal studies have shown no hazard. Nevertheless it should not be used in pregnancy unless the physician considers it essential. The use of Phenergan is not recommended in the 2 weeks prior to delivery in view of the risk of irritability and excitement in the neonate.

Available evidence suggests that the amount excreted in milk is insignificant. However, there are risks of neonatal irritability and excitement.

Effects on ability to drive and use machines: Ambulant patients receiving Phenergan for the first time should not be in control of vehicles or machinery for the first few days until it is established that they are not hypersensitive to the central nervous effects of the drug and do not suffer from disorientation, confusion or dizziness.

Undesirable effects: Side effects may be seen in a few patients: drowsiness, dizziness, restlessness, headaches, nightmares, tiredness, and disorientation. Anticholinergic side effects such as blurred vision, dry mouth and urinary retention occur occasionally. Newborn and premature infants are susceptible to the anticholinergic effects of promethazine, while other children may display paradoxical hyperexcitability. The elderly are particularly susceptible to the anticholinergic effects and confusion due to promethazine. Other side-effects include anorexia, gastric irritation, palpitations, hypotension, arrhythmias, extrapyramidal effects, muscle spasms and tic-like movements of the head and face. Anaphylaxis, jaundice and blood dyscrasias including haemolytic anaemia rarely occur. Photosensitive skin reactions have been reported; strong sunlight should be avoided during treatment.

The preservatives used in Phenergan injection have been reported to cause hypersensitivity reactions, characterised by circulatory collapse with CNS depression in certain susceptible individuals with allergic tendencies.

Overdosage: Symptoms of severe overdosage are variable. They are characterised in children by various combinations of excitation, ataxia, incoordination, athetosis and hallucinations, while adults may become drowsy and lapse into coma. Convulsions may occur in both adults and children: coma or excitement may precede their occurrence. Cardiorespiratory depression is uncommon. If the patient is seen soon enough after ingestion, it should be possible to induce vomiting with ipecacuanha despite the antiemetic effect of promethazine; alternatively, gastric lavage may be used.

Treatment is otherwise supportive with attention to maintenance of adequate respiratory and circulatory status. Convulsions should be treated with diazepam or other suitable anticonvulsant.

Pharmacological properties

Pharmacodynamic properties: Potent, long acting, antihistamine with additional anti-emetic central sedative and anti-cholinergic properties.

Pharmacokinetic properties: Promethazine is slowly excreted via urine and bile. It is distributed widely in the body. It enters the brain and crosses the placenta. Phenothiazines pass into the milk at low concentrations.

Preclinical safety data: No additional data of relevance to the prescriber.

Pharmaceutical particulars

List of excipients: Sodium Sulphite anhydrous (E221), Sodium Metabisulphite (E223), Water for Injections

Incompatibilities: None stated.

Shelf life: 60 months.

Special precautions for storage: Protect from light.

Nature and contents of container: Cardboard carton containing 10×1 ml ampoules.

Instructions for use/handling: Discoloured solutions should not be used.

Marketing authorisation number PL 0012/5054R

Date of approval/revision of SPC February 1997

Legal classification POM

RAPITIL*

Qualitative and quantitative composition Nedocromil sodium 2.0% w/v

Pharmaceutical form Rapitil is presented as a 5 ml sterile, preserved, aqueous solution containing 2% nedocromil sodium in a dropper bottle for administration to the eye.

Clinical particulars

Therapeutic indications: Rapitil is recommended for the prevention, relief and treatment of allergic conjunctivitis, perennial allergic conjunctivitis and vernal kerato-conjunctivitis

Posology and method of administration: Adults (including the elderly) and children aged 6 years and over: In seasonal allergic conjunctivitis: one drop into each eye twice daily, increasing when necessary to four times daily. In seasonal allergic conjunctivitis: therapy should be restricted to 12 weeks. In vernal kerato-conjunctivitis: one drop into each eye four times daily.

Adults (including the elderly): In perennial allergic conjunctivitis: one drop into each eye twice daily, increasing when necessary to four times daily.

Rapitil should be used regularly to ensure optimum control of symptoms.

There is only limited trial evidence with Rapitil in children aged below 6 years, therefore use in this age range cannot be recommended.

Contra-indications: Rapitil is contra-indicated in patients with known hypersensitivity to any constituent of the formulation.

Special warnings and special precautions for use: Patients who use soft contact lenses should be advised not to wear them during the treatment period. In patients who continue to use hard or gas-permeable contact lenses during Rapitil treatment, the lenses should be taken out of the eye prior to instillation and not inserted again for at least 10 minutes.

Interactions with other medicaments and other forms of interaction: None have been reported.

Pregnancy and lactation: Studies in pregnant lactating animals have failed to reveal a hazard with nedocromil sodium. However, as with all medications caution should be exercised during pregnancy (especially during the first trimester) and whilst breast feeding.

On the basis of animal studies and its physiochemical properties it is considered that only negligible amounts of nedocromil sodium may pass into human breast milk. There is no information to suggest that the use of nedocromil sodium by nursing mothers has any undesirable effects on the baby.

Effects on ability to drive and use machines: No sedative effects have been reported with Rapitil.

Undesirable effects: Transient stinging and burning may occur after instillation. Other symptoms of local irritation have been reported rarely. Some patients have reported a distinctive taste.

Overdose: Animal studies have not shown evidence of toxic effects of nedocromil sodium even at high dosage, nor have extended human studies revealed any safety hazard with the drug. Overdosage is unlikely, therefore to cause problems. However, if suspected, treatment should be supportive and directed to the control of the relevant symptoms.

Pharmacological properties

Pharmacodynamic properties: Rapitil, the ophthalmic preparation of nedocromil sodium, displays specific anti-allergic and anti-inflammatory properties. Nedocromil sodium has been shown to prevent the release of inflammatory mediators from a range of inflammatory cell types

Pharmacokinetic properties: Following topical ophthalmic administration, less than 4% of the dose is absorbed following multiple dosing. Absorption occurs primarily through the nasal mucosa as approximately 80% of the ophthalmic dose drains into the nose via the naso-lachrymal duct, although 1-2% of the dose may be absorbed orally.

Nedocromil sodium is reversibly bound to plasma proteins and is not metabolised, but is excreted unchanged in bile and urine. The drug is rapidly cleared from the plasma (plasma clearance 10.2±1.3 ml/min/kg-elimination half-life 5.3±0.9 min) and accumulation does not occur.

Preclinical safety data: Animal studies have failed to reveal toxic effects with nedocromil sodium even at high doses.

Pharmaceutical particulars

List of excipients: Benzalkonium chloride, sodium chloride, disodium edetate.

Incompatibilities: None known.

Shelf life: 36 months.

Special precautions for storage: Store below 25°C, away from direct sunlight. Discard any remaining contents four weeks after opening the bottle.

Nature and contents of container: A plastic dropper bottle containing 5 ml of sterile, aqueous Rapitil solution for administration to the eye.

Instructions for use/handling: Please refer to enclosed package insert.

Marketing authorisation numbers PL 0113/0152

Date of approval/ revision of SPC February 1997

Legal category POM

REVASC

Qualitative and quantitative composition One vial of Revasc contains 15 mg desirudin (INN) corresponding to approximately 270 000 antithrombin units (ATU) or 18 000 ATU per mg of desirudin with reference to the WHO Second International Standard for α-thrombin. Desirudin is a recombinant DNA product derived from yeast cells.

Desirudin is a single chain polypeptide consisting of 65 amino acid residues and 3 disulphide bridges.

Vials of desirudin are supplied with solvent ampoules containing pyrogen-free Mannitol Ph. Eur. in Water for injections Ph. Eur.

Pharmaceutical form Powder and solvent for solution for injection.

Clinical particulars

Therapeutic indications: Prevention of deep venous thrombosis in patients undergoing elective hip and knee replacement surgery.

Posology and method of administration: Adult and elderly patients: The recommended dose is 15 mg twice daily. The first injection should be initiated 5 to 15 minutes before surgery but after induction of regional block anaesthesia, if used. Treatment with desirudin is then continued twice daily post-operatively for 9 to a maximum of 12 days or until the patient is fully ambulant, whichever occurs first. Currently, there is no clinical experience to support the use of desirudin beyond 12 days.

Administration is by subcutaneous injection, preferably at an abdominal site. Injections should be rotated between at least four different sites.

Children: There is no clinical experience with desirudin in children.

Patients with renal impairment: Desirudin is contra-indicated in patients with severe renal impairment (creatinine clearance of less than 30 ml/min corresponding to a serum creatinine >2.5 mg/dl or 221 μmol/l). In patients with moderate renal impairment (creatinine clearance between 31 and 60 ml/min; see Precautions) activated partial thromboplastin time (aPTT) should be monitored.

Patients with liver impairment: Desirudin is contraindicated in severe hepatic impairment. In patients with mild to moderate liver impairment (see *Precautions*) aPTT monitoring is recommended.

Contra-indications: Desirudin is contra-indicated in patients with known hypersensitivity to natural or recombinant hirudins, in patients with active bleeding and/or irreversible coagulation disorders, in severe renal and hepatic impairment and during pregnancy (see *Pregnancy and lactation*). Desirudin is also contra-indicated in patients with severe uncontrolled hypertension and subacute bacterial endocarditis.

Special warnings and special precautions for use: Warnings: Desirudin should not be administered by intramuscular injection owing to the risk of local haematoma.

Desirudin, like other anticoagulants, should be used with caution in conditions with increased risks of haemorrhage such as major surgery, biopsy or puncture of a non-compressible vessel within the last month; a history of haemorrhagic stroke, intracranial or intraocular bleeding including diabetic (haemorrhagic) retinopathy; a cerebral ischaemic attack within the last 6 months, a known haemostatic disorder (congenital or acquired, e.g. antithrombin III, protein C or protein S deficiencies, liver disease) or a history of gastrointestinal or pulmonary bleeding within the past 3 months.

Precautions: aPTT should be monitored in patients with increased risk of bleeding complications, hepatic dysfunction and/or moderate renal impairment and in combined therapy with oral anticoagulants. In these patients peak aPTT should not exceed 85 seconds or twice the upper limit of the normal aPTT range. If necessary, therapy with desirudin should be interrupted until aPTT falls within this therapeutic range at which time treatment with desirudin can be resumed at a reduced dose.

Desirudin should be used with care in patients receiving anticoagulants, and/or platelet inhibitors, and/or non-steroidal anti-inflammatory drugs. Monitoring for evidence of bleeding is advised (see Interactions). The concomitant use of desirudin with thrombolytics and ticlopidine has not been investigated in this patient population.

The anticoagulant effect of desirudin may be poorly reversible. aPTT levels can, however, be reduced by intravenous administration of DDAVP (desmopressin).

Interaction with other medicinal products and other forms of interaction: During prophylaxis, concomitant medication with heparins (unfractionated and low-molecular weight heparins) and dextrans is not recommended. The effects of desirudin and unfractionated heparins on prolongation of aPTT have been shown to be additive.

Desirudin prolongs prothrombin time (PT). When desirudin is given with oral anticoagulants, a period of at least 24 hours should elapse after the last dose of desirudin before blood is drawn to obtain a valid PT. Whilst desirudin and an oral anticoagulant are being administered concurrently, aPTT and PT should be monitored until the oral anticoagulant has entered its therapeutic range as measured by INR. Desirudin should then be discontinued.

As with other anticoagulants desirudin should be used with caution in conjunction with drugs which affect platelet function such as acetylsalicylic acid and other non-steroidal anti-inflammatory drugs.

Use during pregnancy and lactation: Desirudin is contraindicated during pregnancy; i.e. pregnancy must be excluded and a pregnancy test performed in women of childbearing age. Birth defects in animal experiments, characterized by spina bifida in rabbits and omphalocele in rats, were seen at doses comparable to or above the human therapeutic dose range and were causally related to the administration of desirudin.

It is not known whether desirudin is excreted in human milk. However, lactating mothers should be advised to avoid breast feeding or alternative drugs used.

Effects on ability to drive and use machines: Unknown.

Undesirable effects: The nature of the hip surgery operation and the mode of action of the two drugs studied account for most of the adverse experiences reported in controlled clinical trials investigating desirudin 15 mg twice daily and a standard dose of unfractionated heparin. As with other anticoagulants, bleeding is the most common adverse experience. All adverse experiences irrespective of trial drug relationship and reported with an incidence of more than 1.0% are by decreasing order of frequency the following:

Bleeding episodes, nausea, wound secretion, fever, injection site mass, haematomas, anaemia, hypotension, urinary retention, deep thrombophlebitis, hypokalaemia, insomnia, vomiting, hyperpyrexia, constipation, oedema in legs, urinary tract infection, cystitis, dizziness, haematuria, joint dislocation, pain in legs, pain, dyspnoea, impaired wound healing, hypertension and oliguria.

Other adverse experiences reported with a frequency equal or below 1% included:

epistaxis, abdominal and chest pain, confusion, haematemesis, increases in serum transaminases, rash and urticaria.

Allergic reactions have been reported in the same proportion (1.6 %) of patients treated with desirudin

(N=2367) or with unfractionated heparin (N=1134) in clinical trials, regardless of causality. Very rarely anti-hirudin antibodies have been detected upon reexposure to desirudin.

Overdose: There is no antidote for desirudin. Overdosage of desirudin could lead to bleeding complications. In such cases desirudin should be discontinued. If necessary, plasma expanders and/or blood transfusion may be used.

Pharmacological properties
Pharmacodynamic properties: Pharmacotherapeutic group: Anticoagulant, ATC code: B01 AX.

Mechanism of action: Desirudin is a highly potent and selective inhibitor of free circulating and clot-bound thrombin. A mean peak aPTT prolongation of around 1.4 times baseline value is observed following a subcutaneous (s.c.) b.i.d. injection of 15 mg desirudin. At therapeutic serum concentrations it has no effect on other enzymes of the haemostatic system such as factors IXa, Xa, kallikrein, plasmin, tPA, or activated protein C. In addition, it does not display any effect on other serine proteases, such as the digestive enzymes trypsin or chymotrypsin, or on complement activation by the classical or alternative pathways.

In two controlled double blind clinical trials, the overall rate of thromboembolic events in patients treated with desirudin 15 mg s.c. b.i.d. (N=370) was half that in patients treated with a standard dose of unfractionated heparin (N=396) (p<0.0001); the rate of proximal deep venous thrombosis was only one fifth that observed with the heparin (p<0.0001). To date clinical data are available on hip surgery only.

Pharmacodynamic effects: The anticoagulant properties of desirudin are demonstrated by its ability to prolong the clotting time of human or rat plasma whether induced directly (thrombin time) or via the intrinsic (aPTT) or extrinsic (PT) pathways. Desirudin has no profibrinolytic activity.

Pharmacokinetic properties: Absorption: Mean absorption time of s.c. desirudin is 4.1, 4.5 and 5.4 h for dose levels of 0.1, 0.3 and 0.5 mg/kg, respectively (overall mean = 4.6 h). Absorption is complete based on mean area under the curve (AUC) values.

Following administration of single s.c. doses of 0.1-0.75 mg/kg, plasma concentrations of desirudin increased rapidly to maximum levels (Cmax) between 1 and 3 h. Both Cmax and AUC values are dose proportional.

Distribution: Desirudin is distributed in the extracellular space with a distribution volume at steady state of 0.25 l/kg independently of the dose.

Metabolism and elimination: The disappearance of desirudin from plasma is rapid in the first phase with approximately 90 % of an intravenous (i.v.) bolus dose disappearing from the circulation within 2 hours of the injection. A slower terminal elimination phase follows with a dose-independent mean terminal elimination half-life of 2 to 3 h. The mean residence times are 1.7–2 h and 6–7 h after i.v. and s.c. administration, respectively.

The total urinary excretion of unchanged desirudin amounts to 40–50 % of the administered dose. Metabolites lacking one or two C-terminal amino acids constitutes a minor proportion of the material recovered from urine (<7%). In vitro and in vivo animal data indicate that desirudin is for the most part eliminated and metabolised by the kidney. Hepatic elimination of desirudin or the thrombin-desirudin complex does not appear to be significant.

Total clearance of desirudin has been found to be in the same range following either s.c. or i.v. administration (ca 1.95–2.20 ml/min/kg) and was dose-independent. The total and renal clearances of desirudin are slightly reduced in elderly subjects compared to young volunteers. This decrease can be considered unlikely to be of clinical significance, thus allowing no dose reduction.

Preclinical safety data: General toxicology studies with a variety of laboratory animal species have not displayed any evidence of target organ or systemic toxicity. Doses were limited by the pharmacological activity of desirudin, which was characterised by bleeding at the sites of injection and in some organs resulting from the inhibition of blood clotting activity. A low grade vasculitis and fibrinoid necrosis were only observed in the dog. These effects were associated with a low and inconsistent presence of antibodies specific to desirudin in the dog and as such they have been attributed to a dog specific immunological reaction. No such antibodies were found in rabbits or baboons.

Reproductive toxicology studies showed desirudin to be teratogenic with changes comprising spina bifida in rabbits and omphaloceles in rats. No mutagenic potential was demonstrated.

Pharmaceutical particulars
List of excipients: One vial contains, in addition to desirudin, magnesium chloride Ph. Eur. and sodium hydroxide for injections Ph. Eur. One solvent ampoule contains mannitol Ph. Eur. dissolved in water for injections Ph . Eur. No preservatives are included.

Incompatibilities: Desirudin should not be mixed/injected with other agents/solvents.

Shelf life: The shelf life of the packaged product is 18 months when stored under the recommended conditions.

Special precautions for storage: Protect from light and store below 25°C.

Nature and content of container: Powder for solution for injection: Colourless glass vial 2 ml, glass type I, according to Ph. Eur., with stoppers made from butyl rubber covered with a fluoropolymer film on the product side.

Solvent: Colourless glass ampoule 2 ml, hydrolytic glass type I, according to Ph. Eur.

Instructions for use and handling, and disposal (if appropriate): To prepare the reconstituted aqueous solution, 0.5 ml of the accompanying mannitol ampoule is added under aseptic conditions to the vial containing the dry substance. The drug is rapidly redispersed by shaking gently. The reconstituted solution should be used as soon as possible. It is, however, stable for 24 hours in the refrigerator (2–8°C); after this period, the reconstituted solution should be discarded.

Do not use reconstituted vials containing visible particles.

Market autorisation number EU/1//97/043/001-002

Date of approval/revision of SPC August 1998

Legal category POM

RILUTEK* ▼

Qualitative and quantitative composition riluzole 50 mg

Pharmaceutical form Capsule-shaped, white, film-coated tablets for oral use. The tablets are engraved with « RPR 202 » on one side of the tablet.

Clinical particulars
Therapeutic indications: Riluzole is indicated to extend life or the time to mechanical ventilation for patients with amyotrophic lateral sclerosis (ALS). (See *Pharmacodynamic properties*).

Clinical trials have demonstrated that RILUTEK extends survival for patients with ALS. Survival was defined as patients who were alive, not intubated for mechanical ventilation and tracheotomy-free. There is no evidence that riluzole exerts a therapeutic effect on motor function, lung function, fasciculations, muscle strength and motor symptoms. Riluzole has not been shown to be effective in the late stages of ALS. Safety and efficacy of riluzole has only been studied in ALS. Therefore, riluzole should not be used in any other form of motor neurone disease.

Posology and method of administration The recommended daily dose in adults or elderly is 100 mg (50 mg every 12 hours). No significant increased benefit can be expected from higher daily doses. Treatment with riluzole should only be initiated by specialist physicians with experience in the management of motor neurone diseases. Special populations: Children: Rilutek is not recommended for use in children, as the safety and effectiveness of riluzole in any neurodegenerative process occurring in children or adolescents have not been established. (see *Special warnings and special precautions for use*). Patients with Impaired Renal Function: Rilutek is not recommended for use in patients with impaired renal function, as studies at repeated doses have not been conducted in this population. (see *Special warnings and special precautions for use*). Elderly: Based on Pharmacokinetic data, there are no specific instructions for the use of Rilutek in this population. Patients with Impaired Hepatic Function: (see *Contra-indications* and *Special warnings and special precautions for use*).

Contra-indications: Patients who have a history of severe hypersensitivity reactions to riluzole or any of the tablet components. Patients who have hepatic disease or who have baseline transaminases greater than 3 times the upper limit of normal. Patients who are pregnant or lactating.

Special warnings and special precautions for use: Liver impairment: Riluzole should be prescribed with care in patients with a history of abnormal liver function, or in patients with slightly elevated serum transaminases (ALT/SGPT; AST/SGOT up to 3 times ULN), bilirubin and/or gamma-glutamyl transferase (GGT) levels. Baseline elevations of several liver function tests (especially elevated bilirubin) should preclude the use of riluzole (see *Undesirable effects*). It is recommended that serum transaminases, including ALT, be measured before and during therapy with riluzole. ALT should be measured every month during the first 3 months of treatment, every 3 months during the remainder of the first year, and periodically thereafter. ALT levels should be measured more frequently in patients who develop elevated ALT levels. Riluzole should be discontinued if the ALT levels increase to five times the ULN. There is no experience with dose reduction or rechallenge in patients who have developed an increase of ALT to 5 times ULN. Readministration of riluzole to patients in this situation cannot be recommended. *Neutropenia:* Patients should be warned to report any febrile illness to their physicians. The report of a febrile illness should prompt physicians to check white blood cell counts and to discontinue riluzole in case of neutropenia (see *Undesirable effects*). *Children:* The safety and effectiveness of riluzole in any neurodegenerative process occurring in children or adolescents have not been studied (see *Posology and method of administration*). *Patients with impaired renal function:* Studies at repeated doses have not been conducted in this population (see *Posology and method of administration*).

Interaction with other medicines and other forms of Interaction: There have been no clinical studies to evaluate the interactions of riluzole with other drugs.

In vitro studies using human liver microsomal preparations suggest that CYP 1A2 is the principal isozyme involved in the initial oxidative metabolism of riluzole. Inhibitors of CYP 1A2 (e.g. caffeine, diclofenac, diazepam, nicergoline, clomipramine, imipramine, fluvoxamine, phenacetin, theophylline, amitriptyline and quinolones) could potentially decrease the rate of riluzole elimination, while inducers of CYP 1A2 (e.g. cigarette smoke, charcoal-broiled food, rifampicin and omeprazole) could increase the rate of riluzole elimination.

Pregnancy and lactation:
Pregnancy: In the pregnant rat, the transfer of ^{14}C-riluzole across the placenta to the foetus has been detected. In rats, riluzole decreased the pregnancy rate and the number of implantations at exposure levels at least 2 times higher than the systemic exposure of humans given clinical therapy. No malformations were seen in animal reproductive studies.

Clinical experience with riluzole in pregnant women is lacking. Riluzole must not be used in pregnant women.

Lactation: In lactating rats, ^{14}C riluzole was detected in milk. It is not known whether riluzole is excreted in human milk. Riluzole must not be used in lactating women.

Effects on ability to drive and use machines: Patients should be warned about the potential for dizziness or vertigo, and advised not to drive or operate machinery if these symptoms occur.

Undesirable effects: Anaphylactoid reaction, angio dema and pancreatitis have been reported very rarely. In phase III studies conducted in Europe and North America the most frequent side-effects related to riluzole were asthenia, nausea and elevations in liver function tests. Elevations of alanine-aminotransferase (ALT) levels to more than 3 times the upper limit of the normal range (ULN) were observed in about 11% of the patients treated with riluzole compared to 4.2% in the placebo group; levels increased to more than 5 times the ULN in 3.8% of the patients treated with riluzole compared to 1.7% of the placebo treated patients. The increases in ALT usually appeared within 3 months after the start of therapy with riluzole; they were usually transient and levels returned to below 2 times the ULN after 2 to 6 months while treatment was continued. These increases were rarely associated with jaundice. In patients with increases in ALT to more than 5 times the ULN, treatment was discontinued and the levels returned to less than 2 times the ULN within 2 to 4 months. (see *Special warnings and special precautions for use*). The listing that follows describes all the adverse events that occurred at a frequency of 1% or more among ALS patients receiving riluzole 100 mg/day and were greater than placebo by 1%, or were serious adverse events with frequency greater than placebo.

*Adverse Events Occurring in Placebo-Controlled Clinical Trials—Percentage of patients reporting events**

*Adverse Event**	*Riluzole 100 mg/day (N=395)*	*Placebo (N=406)*
Asthenia	17.5	11.3
Nausea	14.2	9.1
Headache	6.8	5.7
Abdominal pain	5.1	3.7
Pain	4.8	2.0
Vomiting	3.8	1.5
Dizziness	3.3	2.2
Tachycardia	3.0	1.5
Somnolence	2.0	1.0
Circumoral paresthesia	1.3	0.0

* Where riluzole incidence is greater than placebo by 1%.

Among approximately 5000 patients given riluzole for ALS, there were three cases of marked neutropenia (absolute neutrophil count less than 500/mm³), all seen within the first 2 months of riluzole treatment. In one case, neutrophil counts rose on continued treatment. In a second case, counts rose after therapy was stopped. A third case was associated with marked anaemia (see *Special warnings and special precautions for use*).

Overdose: There have been no reports of overdose with riluzole; no specific treatment information or antidote are available. In case of overdosage, treatment is symptomatic and supportive.

Pharmacological properties Pharmaco-therapeutic Group: Other nervous system drugs, ATC code N07X.

Although the pathogenesis of ALS is not completely elucidated, it is suggested that glutamate (the primary excitatory neurotransmitter in the central nervous system) plays a role for cell death in the disease. Riluzole is proposed to act by inhibiting glutamate processes. The mode of action is unclear.

Clinical trial: Further information: In a trial, 155 patients were randomised to riluzole 100 mg/day (50 mg twice daily) or placebo and were followed-up for 12 to 21 months. Survival, as defined in the second paragraph of section 4.1. of the SPC, was significantly extended for patients who received riluzole as compared to patients who received placebo. The median survival time was 17.7 months versus 14.9 months for riluzole and placebo, respectively. In a dose-ranging trial, 959 patients with ALS were randomised to one of four treatment groups: riluzole 50, 100, 200 mg/day, or placebo and were followed-up for 18 months. In patients treated with riluzole 100 mg/day, survival was significantly higher compared to patients who received placebo. The effect of riluzole 50 mg/day was not statistically significant compared to placebo and the effect of 200 mg/day was essentially comparable to that of 100 mg/day. The median survival time approached 16.5 months versus 13.5 months for riluzole 100 mg/day and placebo, respectively. In a parallel group study designed to assess the efficacy and safety of riluzole in patients at a late stage of the disease, survival time and motor function under riluzole did not differ significantly from that of placebo. In this study, the majority of patients had a vital capacity ratio less than 60%.

In a double-blind placebo-controlled trial designed to assess the efficacy and safety of riluzole in Japanese patients, 204 patients were randomised to riluzole 100 mg/day (50 mg twice daily) or placebo and were followed-up for 18 months. In this study, the efficacy was assessed on inability to walk alone, loss of upper limb function, tracheostomy, need for artificial ventilation, gastric tube feeding or death. Tracheostomy-free survival in patients treated with riluzole did not differ significantly from placebo. However, the power of this study to detect differences between treatment groups was low. Meta-analysis including this study and those described above showed a less striking effect on survival for riluzole as compared to placebo although the differences remained statistically significant.

Pharmacokinetic properties: The pharmacokinetics of riluzole have been evaluated in healthy male volunteers after single oral administration of 25 to 300 mg and after multiple-dose oral administration of 25 to 100 mg bid. Plasma levels increase linearly with the dose and the pharmacokinetic profile is dose-independent. With multiple dose administration (10 day-treatment at 50 mg riluzole bid), unchanged riluzole accumulates in plasma by about 2 fold and steady-state is reached in less than 5 days.

Absorption: Riluzole is rapidly absorbed after oral administration with maximal plasma concentrations occurring within 60 to 90 minutes ($C_{max}=173\pm72$ (SD) ng/ml). About 90% of the dose is absorbed and the absolute bioavailability is $60\pm18\%$. The rate and extent of absorption is reduced when riluzole is administered with high-fat meals (decrease in Cmax of 44%, decrease in AUC of 17%). *Distribution:* Riluzole is extensively distributed throughout the body and has been shown to cross the blood brain barrier. The volume of distribution of riluzole is about 245 ± 69 l (3.4 l/kg). Riluzole is about 97% protein bound and it binds mainly to serum albumin and to lipoproteins. *Metabolism:* Unchanged riluzole is the main component in plasma and is extensively metabolised by cytochrome P450 and subsequent glucuronidation. In vitro studies using human liver preparations demonstrated that cytochrome P450 1A2 is the principal isoenzyme involved in the metabolism of riluzole. The metabolites identified in urine are 3 phenolic derivatives, one ureido-derivative and unchanged riluzole. The identified and non-conjugated metabolites do not contribute to the pharmacodynamic profile of riluzole in animals and therefore have not been investigated in humans. *Elimination:* The elimination half-life ranges from 9 to 15 hours. Riluzole is eliminated mainly in the urine. The overall urinary excretion accounts for about 90% of the dose. Glucuronides accounted for more than 85% of the metabolites in the urine. Only 2% of a riluzole dose was recovered in the urine as unchanged drug.

Special populations: Patients with impaired renal function: There is no significant difference in pharmacokinetic parameters between patients with moderate or severe chronic renal insufficiency (creatinine clearance between 10 and 50 ml/min⁻¹) and healthy volunteers after a single oral dose of 50 mg riluzole.

Elderly: The pharmacokinetic parameters of riluzole after multiple dose administration (4.5 days of treatment at 50 mg riluzole bid) are not affected in the elderly (>70 years).

Patients with impaired hepatic function: The AUC of riluzole after a single oral dose of 50 mg increases by about 1.7 fold in patients with mild chronic liver insufficiency and by about 3 fold in patients with moderate chronic liver insufficiency.

Preclinical safety data: Long-term studies to determine the carcinogenic potential of riluzole have not yet been completed.

Conventional genotoxicity assays in vitro, utilising rat liver S9 fraction to model metabolism, gave no evidence of genotoxic potential for riluzole. In vivo assays in rat and mouse also gave no indication of chromosomal damage. There remains the possibility that these models did not generate all metabolites relevant to humans, particularly since no metabolic characterisation of the S9 fraction was conducted. Reductions in red blood cell parameters and/or alterations in liver parameters were noted inconsistently in subacute and chronic toxicity studies in rats and monkeys. In dogs, haemolytic anaemia was observed. In a single toxicity study, the absence of corpora lutea was noted at a higher incidence in the ovary of treated compared to control female rats. This isolated finding was not noted in any other study or species. All these findings were noted at doses which were 2-10 times higher than the human dose of 100 mg/day. Fertility studies in rats revealed slight impairment of reproductive performance and fertility at doses of 15 mg/kg/day (which is higher than the therapeutic dose), probably due to sedation and lethargy.

Pharmaceutical particulars

List of excipients: core: dibasic calcium phosphate, anhydrous; micro crystalline cellulose; colloidal silica, anhydrous; magnesium stearate; cross linked carboxymethylcellulose sodium (croscarmellose sodium); **coating**: hydroxypropylmethyl cellulose; Macrogol 6000 and titanium dioxide (E171).

Incompatibilities: None known.

Shelf life: 24 months.

Special precautions for storage: Rilutek must be kept out of the reach of children.

Nature and contents of container: Rilutek® tablets are packaged in opaque PVC/Aluminium blister packs. Each package contains 4 blister cards of 14 tablets each.

Instructions for use/handling: Not applicable.

Marketing authorisation number EU/1/96/010/001

Date of approval/ revision of SPC 10 June 1996

Legal category POM

SUPRAX*

Qualitative and quantitative composition

Tablets 200 mg: Each tablet contains 200 mg cefixime (anhydrous).

Powder for Paediatric Oral Suspension: Each 5 ml of reconstituted suspension contains 100 mg cefixime (anhydrous).

Pharmaceutical form

Tablets 200 mg: Rectangular, white film-coated tablets with a break-line on each side engraved with 'SUPRAX' on one side and 'LL 200' on the other side.

Powder for Paediatric Oral Suspension: Bottles of powder for the preparation of suspension. When reconstituted each 5 ml volume contains 100 mg of cefixime. The suspension contains 2.5 mg of sucrose in 5 ml.

For oral administration.

Clinical particulars

Therapeutic indications: Suprax is an orally active cephalosporin antibiotic which has marked in-vitro bactericidal activity against a wide variety of Gram-positive and Gram-negative organisms.

It is indicated for the treatment of the following acute infections when caused by susceptible micro-organisms:

Upper respiratory tract infections (URTI): e.g. otitis media; and other URTI where the causative organism is known or suspected to be resistant to other commonly used antibiotics, or where treatment failure may carry significant risk.

Lower respiratory tract infection: e.g. bronchitis.

Urinary tract infections: e.g. cystitis, cystourethritis, uncomplicated pyeloneophritis.

Clinical efficacy has been demonstrated in infections caused by commonly occurring pathogens including *Streptococcus pneumoniae, Streptococcus pyogenes, Escherichia coli, Proteus mirabilis, Klebsiella* species, *Haemophilus influenzae* (beta-lactamase positive and negative), *Branhamella catarrhalis* (beta-lactamase positive and negative) and *Enterobacter* species. Suprax is highly stable in the presence of beta-lactamase enzymes.

Most strains of enterococci *(Streptococcus faecalis,* group D *Streptococci*) and *Staphylococci* (including coagulase positive and negative strains and methicillin-resistant strains) are resistant to Suprax. In addition, most strains of *Pseudomonas, Bacteriodes fragalis, Listeria monocytogenes* and *Clostridia* are resistant to Suprax.

Posology and method of administration: Absorption of Suprax is not significantly modified by the presence of food. The usual course of treatment is 7 days. This may be continued for up to 14 days if required.

Adult and children over 10 years: The recommended adult dosage is 200-400 mg daily according to the severity of infection, given either as a single dose or two divided doses.

The elderly: Elderly patients may be given the same dose as recommended for adults. Renal function should be assessed and dosage should be adjusted in severe renal impairment (See *Dosage in renal impairment*).

Children (use Paediatric Oral Suspension): The recommended dosage for children is 8 mg/kg/day administered as a single dose or in two divided doses. As a general guide for prescribing in children the following daily doses in terms of volume of Paediatric Oral Suspension are suggested:

6 months up to 1 year: 3.75 ml daily, children 1-4 years: 5 ml daily, Children 5-10 years: 10 ml daily.

Children weighing more than 50 kg or older than 10 years should be treated with the recommended adult dose (200–400 mg daily depending on the severity of infection). The safety and efficacy of cefixime has not been established in children less than 6 months.

Dosage in renal impairment: Suprax may be administered in the presence of impaired renal function. Normal dose and schedule may be given in patients with creatinine clearances of 20 ml/min or greater. In patients whose creatinine clearance is less than 20 ml/min, it is recommended that a dose of 200 mg once daily should not be exceeded. The dose and regimen for patients who are maintained on chronic ambulatory peritoneal dialysis or haemodialysis should follow the same recommendation as that for patients with creatinine clearances of less than 20 ml/min.

Contra-indications: Patients with known hypersensitivity to cephalosporin antibiotics.

Special warnings and precautions for use: Cefixime should be given with caution to patients who have shown hypersensitivity to other drugs. Cephalosporins should be given with caution to penicillin-sensitive patients, as there is some evidence of partial cross-allergenicity between the penicillins and cephalosporins.

Patients have had severe reactions (including anaphylaxis) to both classes of drugs. If an allergic effect occurs with cefixime, the drug should be discontinued and the patient treated with appropriate agents if necessary.

Suprax should be administered with caution in patients with markedly impaired renal function (See *Dosage in renal impairment*).

Treatment with broad spectrum antibiotics alters the normal flora of the colon and may permit overgrowth of clostridia. Studies indicate that a toxin produced by *Clostridium difficile* is a primary cause of antibiotic-associated diarrhoea. Pseudomembraneous colitis is associated with the use of broad-spectrum antibiotics (including macrolides, semi-synthetic penicillins, lincosamides and cephalosporins); it is therefore important to consider its diagnosis in patients who develop diarrhoea in association with the use of antibiotics. Symptoms of pseudomembraneous colitis may occur during or after antibiotic treatment. Management of pseudomembraneous colitis should include sigmoidoscopy, appropriate bacteriologic studies, fluids, electrolytes and protein supplementation. If the colitis does not improve after the drug has bee discontinued, or if the symptoms are severe, oral vancomycin is the drug of choice for antibiotic-associated pseudomembraneous colitis produced by *C.difficile*. Other causes of colitis should be excluded.

Interactions with other medicaments and other forms of interaction: A false positive reaction for glucose in the urine may occur with Benedict's or Fehling's solutuions or with copper sulphate test tablets, but not with tests based on enzymatic glucose oxidase reactions.

A false positive direct Coombs test has been reported during treatment with cephalosporin antibiotics, therefore it should be recognised that a positive Coombs test may be due to the drug.

In common with other cephalosporins, increases in prothrombin times have been noted in a few patients. Care should therefore be taken in patients receiving anticoagulation therapy.

Pregnancy and lactation: Reproduction studies have been performed in mice and rats at doses up to 400 times the human dose and have revealed no evidence of impaired fertility or harm to the foetus due to cefixime. In the rabbit, at doses up to 4 times the human dose, there was no evidence of a teratogenic effect; there was a high incidence of abortion and maternal death which is an expected consequence of the known sensitivity of rabbits to antibiotic-induced changes in the population of the microflora of the intestine. There are no adequate and well-controlled studies in pregnant women. Suprax should therefore not be used in pregnancy or in nursing mothers unless considered essential by the physician.

Effects on ability to drive and use machines: None.

Undesirable effects: Suprax is generally well tolerated. The majority of adverse reactions observed in clinical trials were mild and self limiting in nature.

Gastrointestinal disturbances: The most frequent side effects seen with cefixime are diarrhoea and stool changes; diarrhoea has been more commonly associated with higher doses. Some cases of moderate to severe diarrhoea have been reported; this has occasionally warranted cessation of therapy. Suprax should be discontinued if marked diarrhoea occurs. Other gastrointestinal side effects seen less frequently are nausea, abdominal pain dyspepsia, vomiting and flatulence. Pseudomembraneous colitis has been reported (see above).

Central nervous system: Headache and dizziness.

Hypersensitivity reactions: Allergies in the form of rash, pruritus, urticaria, drug fever and arthralgia have been observed. These reactions usually subsided upon discontinuation of therapy. Rarely, erythema multiforme, Steven Johnson Syndrome and toxic epidermal necrolysis have been reported.

Haematological and clinical chemistry: Thrombocytopenia, leukopenia and eosinophilia have been reported. These reactions were infrequent and reversible. Mild transient changes in liver and renal function tests have been observed.

Miscellaneous: Other possible reaction include genital pruritus and vaginitis.

Overdose: There is no experience with overdoses with cefixime. Adverse reactions seen at dose levels up to 2 g cefixime in normal subjects did not differ from the profile seen in patients treated at the recommended doses. Gastric lavage may be indicated in overdosage. No specific antidote exists. Cefixime is not removed from the circulation in significant quantities by dialysis.

Pharmacological properties

Pharmacodynamic properties: Cefixime is an oral third generation cephalosporin which has marked in-vitro bactericidal activity against a wide variety of Gram-positive and Gram-negative organisms.

Clinical efficacy has been demonstrated in infections caused by commonly occurring pathogens including *Streptococcus pneumoniae, Streptococcus pyogenes, Escherichia coli, Proteus mirabilis, Klebsiella* species, *Haemophilus influenza* (beta-lactamase positive and negative), *Branhamella catarrhalis* (beta-lactamase positive and negative) and *Enterobacter* species. It is highly stable in the presence of beta-lactamase enzymes.

Most strains of enterococci (*Streptococcus faecalis*, group D *Streptococci*) and *Staphylococci* (including coagulase positive and negative strains and methicillin-resistant strains) are resistant to cefixime. In addition, most strains of *Pseudomonas, Bacteroides fragilis, Listeria monocytogenes* and *Clostridia* are resistant to cefixime

Pharmacokinetic properties: The absolute oral bioavailability of cefixime is in the range of 22–54%. Absorption is not significantly modified by the presence of food. Cefixime may therefore be given without regard to meals.

From *in-vitro* studies, serum or urine concentrations of 1 mcg/ml or greater were considered to be adequate for most common pathogens against which cefixime is active. Typically, the peak serum levels following the recommended adult or paediatric doses are between 1.5 and 3 mcg/ml. Little or no accumulation of cefixime occurs following multiple dosing.

The pharmacokinetics of cefixime in healthy elderly (age >64 years) and young volunteers (11–35) compared the administration of 400 mg doses once daily for 5 days. Mean C_{max} and AUC values were slightly greater in the elderly. Elderly patients may be given the same dose as the general population.

Cefixime is predominantly eliminated as unchanged drug in the urine. Glomerular filtration is considered the predominant mechanism. Metabolites of cefixime have not been isolated from human serum or urine.

Serum protein binding is well characterised for human and animal sera; cefixime is almost exclusively bound to the albumin fraction, the mean free fraction being approximately 30%. Protein binding of cefixime is only concentration dependant in human serum at very high concentrations which are not seen following clinical dosing.

Transfer of 14C labelled cefixime from lactating rats to their nursing offspring through breast milk was quantitatively small (approximately 1.5% of the mothers' body content of cefixime in the pup). No data are available on secretion of cefixime in human breast milk. Placetal transfer of cefixime was small in pregnant rats dosed with labelled cefixime.

Preclinical safety data: There are no pre-clinical data of relevance to the prescriber which are additional to that already included in other sections of the Summary of Product Characteristics.

Pharmaceutical particulars

List of excipients: Tablets 200 mg: Tablet cores: cellulose microcrystalline, pregelatinised starch, calcium phosphate dibasic and magnesium stearate.

Tablet coating: light mineral oil, hydroxypropylmethylcellulose, sodium lauryl sulphate and titanium dioxide.

Powder for Paediatric Oral Suspension: sucrose, xantham gum, sodium benzoate and strawberry flavour

Incompatibilities: None.

Shelf life: Tablets 200 mg: 3 years. *Powder for Paediatric Oral Suspension:* 3 years unopened.
2 weeks after reconstitution.

Special precautions for storage: Tablets 200 mg: Store at controlled room temperature (15–25°C).

Powder for Paediatric Oral Suspension: Store unreconstituted product at controlled room temperature (15–25°C). To reconstitute, add 25 ml of water (37.5 ml bottle) or 50 ml of water (75 ml bottle) in two portions shaking after each addition. After reconstitution, the suspension may be stored at room temperature (below 25°C) for 14 days without significant loss of potency. Do not freeze. Keep bottles tightly closed and shake well before use. Discard any unused portion after 14 days. Dilution of the suspension is not recommended

Nature and contents of container: Tablets 200 mg: Vingl oclar/aluminium foil laminate blister packs – pack of 7. Powder for Peadiatric Oral Suspension: Type III amber glass bottles closed with polypropylene screw caps with a pulp backed vinyl-coated aluminium foil liner. The bottles may be supplied with a simple double ended plastic spoon capable of measuring 3.75 and 5.0 ml of the suspension–pack sizes of 37.5 and 75 ml.

Instructions for use/handling: None stated.

Marketing authorisation numbers

Tablets 200 mg: 0012/0316
Powder for Paediatric Oral Suspension: 0012/0318

Date of approval/revision of SPC July 1998

Legal category POM

TAXOTERE* ▼

Qualitative and quantitative composition Single-dose vials of Taxotere containing 20 mg of docetaxel (anhydrous) in 0.5 ml polysorbate 80 and 80 mg of docetaxel (anhydrous) in 2.0 ml polysorbate 80

The viscous solution contains 40 mg/ml docetaxel (anhydrous).

Pharmaceutical form Concentrate and solvent for infusion.

Clinical particulars

Therapeutic indications: Taxotere (docetaxel) monotherapy is indicated for the treatment of patients with locally advanced or metastatic breast cancer after failure of cytotoxic therapy. Previous chemotherapy should have included an anthracycline or an alkylating agent.

The use of docetaxel should be confined to units specialised in the administration of cytotoxic chemotherapy and it should only be administered under the supervision of a qualified oncologist.

Posology and method of administration: Recommended dosage: The recommended dosage of docetaxel monotherapy is 100 mg/m² administered as a one-hour infusion every three weeks (see *Instructions for use/handling*). Patients should be observed closely especially during the first and second infusion of docetaxel because of the risk of hypersensitivity reactions (see *Special warnings and precautions for use*). A premedication consisting of an oral corticosteroid, such as dexamethasone 16 mg per day (e.g. 8 mg bid) for 3 days starting 1 day prior to docetaxel administration, unless contra-indicated, can reduce the incidence and severity of fluid retention as well as the severity of hypersensitivity reactions.

Dosage adjustments during treatment: Docetaxel should be administered when the neutrophil count is ≥1,500 cells/mm³. Patients who experienced either febrile neutropenia, neutrophil <500 cells/mm³ for more than one week, severe or cumulative cutaneous reactions or severe peripheral neuropathy during docetaxel therapy should have the dosage of docetaxel reduced from 100 mg/m² to 75 mg/m². If the patient continues to experience these reactions at 75 mg/m², the dosage should either be decreased from 75 mg/m² to 55 mg/m² or the treatment should be discontinued.

Special populations: Patients with hepatic impairment: Based on pharmacokinetic data, in patients who have both elevations of transaminase (ALT and/or AST) greater than 1.5 times the upper limit of the normal range (ULN) and alkaline phosphatase greater than 2.5 times the ULN, the recommended dose of docetaxel is 75 mg/m² (see *Special warnings and special precautions for use* and *Pharmacokinetic properties*). For those patients with serum bilirubin >ULN and/or ALT and AST >3.5 times the ULN associated with alkaline phosphatase >6 times the ULN, no dose-reduction can be recommended and docetaxel should not be used unless strictly indicated. *Children:* The safety and effectiveness of docetaxel in children have not been established. *Elderly:* Based on a population pharmacokinetic analysis, there are no special instructions for the use in elderly.

Contra-indications: Docetaxel is contra-indicated in patients who have a history of severe hypersensitivity reactions to the drug or polysorbate 80. Docetaxel should not be used in patients with baseline neutrophil count of <1,500 cells/mm³. Docetaxel must not be used in pregnant or breast-feeding women. Docetaxel should not be used in patients with severe liver impairment since there is no data available (see *Special warnings and special precautions for use* and *Posology and method of administration*).

Special warnings and special precautions for use: A premedication consisting of an oral corticosteroid such as dexamethasone 16 mg per day (e.g. 8 mg BID) for 3 days starting one day prior to docetaxel administration, unless contraindicated, can reduce the incidence and severity of fluid retention as well as the severity of hypersensitivity reactions. (see *Posology and method of administration*). Severe hypersensitivity reactions characterised by hypotension or bronchospasm or generalised rash/erythema have occurred in 5.3% of the patients receiving docetaxel.

Haematology: Neutropenia is the most frequent adverse reaction of docetaxel. Neutrophil nadirs occurred at a median of 7 days but this interval may be shorter in heavily pretreated patients. Frequent monitoring of complete blood counts should be conducted on all patients receiving docetaxel. Patients should be retreated with docetaxel when neutrophils recover to a level ≥1,500 cells/mm³ (See *Posology and method of administration*). In the case of severe neutropenia (<500 cells/mm³ for seven days or more) during a course of docetaxel therapy, a reduction in dose for subsequent courses of therapy or the use of appropriate symptomatic measures are recommended.

Hypersensitivity reactions: Patients should be observed closely for hypersensitivity reactions especially during the first and second infusions. As hypersensitivity reactions may occur within a few minutes following the initiation of the infusion of docetaxel, facilities for the treatment of hypotension and bronchospasm should be available. If hypersensitivity reactions occur, minor symptoms such as flushing or localised cutaneous reactions do not require interruption of therapy. However, severe reactions, such as severe hypotension, bronchospasm or generalised rash/erythema require immediate discontinuation of docetaxel and appropriate therapy. Patients who have developed severe hypersensitivity reactions should not be rechallenged with docetaxel.

Cutaneous reactions: Localised skin erythema of the extremities (palms of the hands and soles of the feet) with oedema followed by desquamation has been observed. Severe symptoms such as eruptions followed by desquamation which lead to interruption or discontinuation of docetaxel treatment were reported in 5.9% of the patients (see *Posology and method of administration*). Bullous epidermolysis has not been observed.

Fluid retention: A premedication consisting of an oral corticosteroid such as dexamethasone 16 mg per day (e.g. 8 mg BID) for 3 days starting one day prior to docetaxel administration, unless contraindicated, can reduce the incidence and severity of fluid retention as well as the severity of hypersensitivity reactions (see *Posology and method of administration*). Patients with severe fluid retention such as pleural effusion, pericardial effusion and ascites should be monitored closely.

Patients with liver impairment: In patients treated with docetaxel at 100 mg/m² who have serum transaminase levels (ALT and /or AST) greater than 1.5 times the ULN concurrent with serum alkaline phosphatase levels greater than 2.5 times the ULN, there is a higher risk of developing severe adverse reactions such as toxic deaths including sepsis and gastrointestinal haemorrhage which can be fatal, febrile neutropenia, infections, thrombocytopenia, stomatitis and asthenia. Therefore, the recommended dose of docetaxel in patients with elevated liver function test (LFTs) is 75 mg/m² and LFTs should be conducted at baseline and before each cycle (see *Posology and method of administration*). For patients with serum bilirubin levels> ULN and/or ALT and AST >3.5 times the ULN concurrent with serum alkaline phosphatase levels >6 times the ULN, no dose-reduction can be recommended and docetaxel should not be used unless strictly indicated.

Nervous system: The development of severe peripheral neurotoxicity has been observed in 4.1% of patients and requires a reduction of dose (see *Posology and method of administration*).

Others: Contraceptive measures must be taken during and for at least three months after cessation of therapy.

Interaction with other medicaments and other forms of interaction: There have been no formal clinical studies to evaluate drug interactions of docetaxel. *In vitro* studies have shown that the metabolism of docetaxel may be modified by the concomitant administration of compounds which induce, inhibit or are metabolised by (and thus may inhibit the enzyme competitively) cytochrome P450-3A such as cyclosporin, terfenadine, ketoconazole, erythromycin and troleandomycin. As a result, caution should be exercised when treating patients with these drugs as concomitant therapy since there is a potential for a significant interaction.

Docetaxel is highly protein bound (>95%). Although the possible *in vivo* interaction of docetaxel with concomitantly administered medication has not been investigated formally, *in vitro* interactions with tightly protein-bound drugs such as erythromycin, diphenhydramine, propranolol, propafenone, phenytoin, salicylate, sulfamethoxazole and sodium valproate did not affect protein binding of docetaxel. In addition, dexamethasone did not affect protein binding of docetaxel. Docetaxel did not influence the binding of digoxin.

Pregnancy and lactation: There is no information on the use of docetaxel in pregnant women. Docetaxel has been shown to be both embryotoxic and foetotoxic in rabbits and rats, and to reduce fertility in rats. As with other cytotoxic drugs, docetaxel may cause foetal harm when administered to pregnant women. Therefore, docetaxel must not be used during pregnancy. Women of childbearing age receiving docetaxel should be advised to avoid becoming pregnant, and to inform the treating physician immediately should this occur.

Docetaxel is a lipophilic substance but it is not known whether it is excreted in human milk. Consequently, because of the potential for adverse reactions in nursing infants, breast feeding must be discontinued for the duration of docetaxel therapy.

Effects on ability to drive and use machines: Docetaxel is unlikely to affect the ability to drive or operate machines.

Undesirable effects: Data on the adverse reactions considered to be possibly or probably related to the administration of docetaxel have been obtained from 1312 patients with normal LFTs at baseline who received an initial planned dose of 100 mg/m² over a one-hour infusion regardless of the premedication received. Patients were enrolled in 36 clinical trials conducted in Europe and North America (514 with breast carcinoma and 798 with various other tumour types).

Haematology: The most frequent adverse reaction to docetaxel (in patients who did not receive G-CSF) was neutropenia which was reversible and not cumulative. The median day to nadir was 7 days and the median duration of severe neutropenia (<500 cells/mm³) was 7 days. Severe neutropenia occurred in 56.4% of cycles (76.4% of the patients) and lasted for more than 7 days in 3.5 % of evaluable cycles. Fever was associated with neutropenia (<500 cells/mm³) in 11.8% of the patients (3% of the cycles) and the incidence of severe infections associated with neutrophil counts <500 cells/mm³ was 4.6% of the patients (1.2% of the cycles). Infectious episodes occurred in 20% of the patients (6% of the cycles) and were severe (including sepsis and pneumonia) in 5.7% of the patients (1.4% of the cycles) and were fatal in 1.7% of the patients. Thrombocytopenia (<100,000 cells/mm³) has been reported in 7.8% of the patients. Bleeding episodes were reported in 2.4% of the patients and were rarely associated with severe thrombocytopenia (<50,000 cells/mm³). Anaemia (<11 g/dl) was observed in 90.4% of the patients and was severe (<8 g/dl) in 8.9% of the cases.

Hypersensitivity reactions: Hypersensitivity reactions (HSRs) have occurred in 25.9% of patients (9.4% of the cycles) generally within a few minutes following the start of the infusion of docetaxel and were usually mild to moderate. The most frequently reported symptoms were flushing, rash with or without pruritus, chest tightness, back pain, dyspnoea and drug fever or chills. Severe reactions characterised by hypotension and/or bronchospasm or generalised rash/erythema were observed in 5.3% of patients. They resolved after discontinuing the infusion and instituting appropriate therapy.

Cutaneous: Reversible cutaneous reactions have been observed in 56.6% of the patients and were generally considered as mild to moderate. 73% of these events were reversible within 21 days. The cutaneous reactions were characterised by a rash including localised eruptions mainly on feet, hands, but also on arms, face or thorax, and frequently associated with pruritus. Eruptions generally occurred within one week after the docetaxel infusion, recovered before the next infusion and were not disabling. Less frequently (5.9% of the patients), severe symptoms such as eruptions followed by desquamation which rarely lead to interruption or discontinuation of docetaxel treatment were reported. Nail disorders occurred in 27.9% of the patients and were characterised by hypo- or hyperpigmentation and sometimes pain and onycholysis (2.6% of the patients).

Fluid retention: Fluid retention has been reported in 64.1% (6.5% severe) of patients receiving the recommended premedication compared with 81.6% (22.4% severe) in patients without premedication. Events such as peripheral oedema and less frequently pleural effusion, pericardial effusion, ascites, lacrymation with or without conjunctivitis and weight gain have been reported. The peripheral oedema usually starts at the lower extremities and may become generalised with a weight gain of 3 kgs or more. Fluid retention is cumulative in incidence and severity. The onset of moderate and severe retention is delayed (median cumulative dose: 818.9 mg/m²) in patients with premedication compared with patients without premedication (median cumulative dose: 489.7 mg/m²); however, it has been reported in some patients during the early courses of therapy. The median cumulative dose to treatment discontinuation was more than 1,000 mg/m² in patients receiving the recommended premedication. The median time to fluid retention reversibility was 16.4 weeks (range 0 to 42 weeks) in patients receiving the recommended premedication. Fluid retention has not been accompanied by acute episodes of oliguria or hypotension. Dehydration has been reported rarely in association with fluid retention.

Gastrointestinal: Gastrointestinal effects such as nausea, vomiting, diarrhoea, and abdominal pain were seen in 40.5%, 24.5%, 40.6% and 7.3% of the patients treated respectively with an incidence of severe reactions of 4%, 3%, 4%, and 1%, respectively. Anorexia was reported in 16.8% of the patients and was infrequently severe. Constipation was reported in 9.3% (0.2% severe) of the patients. Stomatitis and oesophagitis were reported in 41.8% (5.3% severe) and 1% (0.4% severe) of the patients, respectively. Taste perversion has been reported in 10.1% of the patients (0.07% severe). Gastrointestinal bleeding has been seen in 1.4% of the patients (0.3% severe). Rare occurrences of gastrointestinal perforation and neutropenic entero-colitis have been reported.

Neurologic: Mild to moderate neuro-sensory signs characterised by paresthesia, dysesthesia or pain including burning were reported in 45.9% of patients and were considered severe in 4.1% of the cases. Neuro-motor events mainly characterised by weakness were reported in 13.8% of patients and were severe in 4% of the patients. The events were spontaneously reversible within 3 months in 35.3% of patients with neurotoxicity for whom data is available.

Cardiovascular: Hypotension occurred in 3.8% of the patients and required therapy in 0.7% of the patients. Dysrhythmia occurred in 4.1% of the patients and was severe in 0.7% of the patients. Other meaningful cardiovascular events included hypertension (2.4%) or heart failure (0.46%); the relationship of these findings to the administration of docetaxel has not been clearly defined. Various thromboembolic events have been rarely reported. Rare cases of myocardial unfarction have been reported.

Infusion site reactions: Infusion site reactions were generally mild and occurred in 5.6% of the patients, and consisted of hyperpigmentation, inflammation, redness or dryness of the skin, phlebitis or extravasation and swelling of the vein.

Hepatic: Increases in serum levels of AST, ALT, bilirubin and alkaline phosphatase greater than 2.5 times the ULN were observed in less than 5% of the patients.

Others: Alopecia was observed in a total of 79% of patients but was considered severe in about 67% of the patients. Alopecia was reversible in 13% of the patients for whom data is available; the median recovery time was 22 weeks following the initial hair loss. Asthenia was observed in 62.6% of patients and was severe in 11.2% of the patients. Arthralgias and myalgias were observed in 8.6% and 20% of the patients, respectively and were generally considered mild to moderate. Dyspnoea was reported in 16.1% (2.7% severe) of the patients and was frequently associated with acute hypersensitivity reactions, respiratory infections, and pulmonary metastasis. Generalised or localised pain has been observed in 16.5% of the patients and was severe in 0.8% of patients. Chest pain was seen in 4.5% of patients (0.4% severe) without any cardiac or respiratory involvement.

Overdose: There were two reports of overdose. One patient received 150 mg/m² and the other received 200 mg/m² of docetaxel as a one hour infusion. They both recovered after experiencing severe neutropenia, mild asthenia, cutaneous reactions and mild paresthesia.

In case of overdose, the patient should be kept in a specialised unit and vital functions closely monitored. There is no known antidote for docetaxel overdose. The primary anticipated complications of overdose would consist of bone marrow suppression, peripheral neurotoxicity and mucositis.

Pharmacological properties

Pharmacodynamic properties: Pharmaco-therapeutic group: Antineoplastic agents.

Preclinical data: Docetaxel is an antineoplastic agent which acts by promoting the assembly of tubulin into stable microtubules and inhibits their disassembly which leads to a marked decrease of free tubulin. The binding of docetaxel to microtubules does not alter the number of protofilaments. Docetaxel has been shown *in vitro* to disrupt the microtubular network in cells which is essential for vital mitotic and interphase cellular functions. Docetaxel was found to be cytotoxic *in vitro* against various murine and human tumour cell lines and against freshly excised human tumour cells in clonogenic assays. Docetaxel achieves high intracellular concentrations with a long cell residence time. In addition, docetaxel was found to be active on some but not all cell lines overexpressing the *p*-glycoprotein which is encoded by the multidrug resistance gene. *In vivo*, docetaxel is schedule independent and has a broad spectrum of experimental antitumour activity against advanced murine and human grafted tumours.

Clinical data: Breast cancer: Six phase II studies were conducted in patients with locally advanced or metastatic breast carcinoma. A total of 117 patients had received no prior chemotherapy (previously untreated) and 111 patients had received prior chemotherapy (previously treated) which included 83 patients who had progressive disease during anthracycline therapy (anthracycline refractory). In these clinical trials, docetaxel was administered as a 100 mg/m² dose given as a one-hour infusion every 3 weeks.

The overall response rate (ORR) was 56% in the anthracycline resistant patients with a 4.4% complete response rate (CR). A 46% ORR was observed in the anthracycline refractory patients with 7.3% CR. The median duration of response was 27 weeks in the anthracycline resistant patients and 28 weeks in the anthracycline refractory patients. The median survival time was 11 months in the anthracycline-resistant patients. There was a high response rate in patients with visceral metastases, 53.1% in the 49 anthracycline resistant patients. In anthracycline resistant patients, a significant response rate of 40% was seen in patients with liver metastases and a 63.2% response rate was observed in patients with soft tissue disease. Two randomised Phase III comparative studies, involving a totoal of 326 alkylating of 392 anthracycline failure metastatic breast cancer patients, have been performed with docetaxel at the recommended dose and regimen of 100 mg/m² administered every 3 weeks.

In patients failing alkylating agent containing regimens, docetaxel was compared to doxorubicin (75 mg/m² every 3 weeks). Without affecting overall survival time (docetaxel 15 months vs doxorubicin 14 months, p=0.38) or time to progression (docetaxel 27 weeks vs doxorubicin 23 weeks, p=0.54), docetaxel increased response rate (52% versus 37%, p=0.01) and shortened time to response (12 weeks vs 23 weeks, p=0.007). Three docetaxel patients (2%) discontinued the treatment due to fluid retention, whereas 15 doxorubicin patients (9%) discontinued due to cardiac toxicity (three fatal congestive heart failures).

In patients failing anthracycline-containing regimens, docetaxel was compared to the combination of mitomycin C and vinblastine (12 mg/m² every 6 weeks and 6 mg/m² every 3 weeks). Docetasel increased response rate (33% vs 12%, $p<0.01$), prolonged time to progression (19 weeks vs 11 weeks, $p=0.0004$) and prolonged overall survival (11.4 months vs 8.7 months, $p=0.01$).

During these Phase III studies, the safety profile of docetaxel was consistent with the safety profile observed in Phase II studies (see *Undesirable effects*).

Pharmacokinetic properties: The pharmacokinetics of docetaxel have been evaluated in cancer patients after administration of 20–115 mg/m² in Phase I studies. The kinetic profile of docetaxel is dose independent and consistent with a three-compartment pharmacokinetic model with half lives for the α, β and γ phases of 4 min, 36 min and 11.1 h, respectively. The late phase is due, in part, to a relatively slow efflux of docetaxel from the peripheral compartment. Following the administration of a 100 mg/m² dose given as a one-hour infusion a mean peak plasma level of 3.7 µg/ml was obtained with a corresponding AUC of 4.6 h•µg/ml. Mean values for total body clearance and *steady-state* volume of distribution were 21 l/h/m² and 113 l, respectively. Interindividual variation in total body clearance was approximately 50%. Docetaxel is more than 95% bound to plasma proteins. A study of ^{14}C-docetaxel has been conducted in three cancer patients. Docetaxel was eliminated in both the urine and faeces following cytochrome P450-mediated oxidative metabolism of the tert-butyl ester group, within seven days, the urinary and faecal excretion accounted for about 6% and 75% of the administered radioactivity, respectively. About 80% of the radioactivity recovered in faeces is excreted during the first 48 hours as one major inactive metabolite and 3 minor inactive metabolites and very low amounts of unchanged drug. A population pharmacokinetic analysis has been performed with docetaxel in 577 patients. Pharmacokinetic parameters estimated by the model were very close to those estimated from Phase I studies. The pharmacokinetics of docetaxel were not altered by the age or sex of the patient. In a small number of patients ($n=23$) with clinical chemistry data suggestive of mild to moderate liver function impairment (ALT, AST $\geq$1.5 times the ULN associated with alkaline phosphatase $\geq$2.5 times the ULN), total clearance was lowered by 27% on average (see *Posology and method of administration*). Docetaxel clearance was not modified in patients with mild to moderate fluid retention and there is no data available in patients with severe fluid retention.

Preclinical safety data: The carcinogenic potential of docetaxel has not been studied. Docetaxel has been shown to be mutagenic in the *in vitro* micronucleus and chromosome aberration test in CHO-K1 cells and in the *in vivo* micronucleus test in the mouse. However, it did not induce mutagenicity in the Ames test or the CHO/HGPRT gene mutation assay. These results are consistent with the pharmacological activity of docetaxel.

Adverse effects on the testis observed in rodent toxicity studies suggest that docetaxel may impair male fertility.

Pharmaceutical particulars

List of excipients: Each ml of docetaxel solution contains 40 mg docetaxel anhydrous and 1040 mg polysorbate 80, each ml of solvent contains 13% ethanol in water for injections.

Incompatibilities: None known.

Shelf life: Vials of Taxotere concentrate and solvent for solution for infusion should be stored under refrigeration and protected from bright light. The shelf life under these conditions is 12 months for Taxotere 20 mg and 15 months for Taxotere 80 mg. Freezing does not adversely affect the product.

Special precautions for storage: Vials should be stored under refrigeration and protected from bright light. Please note: A new formulation is expected. Please refer to the package insert for details of shelf life and storage conditions.

Nature and contents of container: Taxotere 20 mg: Each blister carton contains one single-dose of Taxotere (docetaxel) vial equivalent to 20 mg docetaxel (anhydrous) in 0.5 ml polysorbate 80 (Fill: 23.6 mg/0.59 ml) and one single-dose solvent for Taxotere vial containing 1.83 ml 13% ethanol in water for injections.

Taxotere 80 mg: Each blister carton contains one single-dose TAXOTERE (docetaxel) vial equivalent to 80 mg docetaxel (anhydrous) in 2 ml polysorbate 80 (Fill: 94.4 mg/2.36 ml) and one single-dose solvent for Taxotere vial containing 7.33 ml 13% ethanol in water for injections

The Taxotere 20 mg vial is a 7 ml clear glass vial with a green flip-off cap. The 80 mg vial is a 15 ml clear glass vial with a red flip-off cap.

Both Taxotere 20 mg and 80 mg vials contain a solution of docetaxel in polysorbate 80 at a concentration of 40 mg/ml.

Taxotere 20 mg: Each Taxotere 20 mg vial contains 0.59 ml of the 40 mg/ml solution of docetaxel equivalent to 23.6 mg docetaxel.

Taxotere 80 mg: Each Taxotere 80 mg vial contains 2.36 ml of the 40 mg/ml solution of docetaxel equivalent to 94.4 mg docetaxel.

These volumes have been established during the development of Taxotere to compensate for liquid loss during preparation of the premix due to foaming, adhesion to the walls of the vial and "dead-volume". This overfill ensures that after dilution with the entire contents of the accompanying solvent for Taxotere vial, there is a minimum extractable premix volume of 2 or 8 ml respectively, containing 10 mg/ml docetaxel which correspond to the labeled amount per vial.

Solvent for Taxotere: The solvent for Taxotere 20 vial is a 7 ml clear glass vial and for Taxotere 80 mg a 15 ml clear glass vial with a transparent colourless flip-off cap.

The solvent for Taxotere contains a 13% w/w solution of ethanol in water for injections.

Each solvent for Taxotere 20 mg vial contains 1.83 ml, and those for Taxotere 80 mg contain 7.33 ml. These volumes have been established based on the fill volume of the Taxotere vial. The addition of the entire contents of the solvent vial to the contents of the Taxotere vial ensures a premix concentration of 10 mg/ml docetaxel.

Instructions for use/handling, and disposal (if appropriate):

Recommendations for safe handling: Taxotere is an antineoplastic agent and, as with other potentially toxic compounds, caution should be exercised when preparing and handling Taxotere solutions. The use of latex gloves is recommended.

If Taxotere concentrate, premix solution or infusion solution should come into contact with skin, wash immediately and thoroughly with soap and water. If Taxotere concentrate, premix solution or infusion solution should come into contact with mucous membranes, wash immediately and thoroughly with water.

Preparation for intravenous administration

Preparation of Taxotere premix solution (10 mg docetaxel/ml): If the vials are stored under refrigeration, allow the required number of Taxotere boxes stand at room temperature for 5 minutes.

Using a syringe fitted with a needle, aseptically withdraw the entire contents of the solvent for Taxotere vial.

Inject the entire contents of the syringe into the corresponding Taxotere vial.

Remove the syringe and needle and shake the mixture manually for 15 seconds.

Allow the premix vial to stand for 5 minutes at room temperature and then check that the solution is homogenous and clear (foaming is normal even after 5 minutes due to the presence of polysorbate 80 in the formulation).

The premix solution contains 10 mg/ml docetaxel and should be used immediately to prepare the infusion solution.

Preparation of the infusion solution: More than one premix vial may be necessary to obtain the required dose for the patient. Based on the required dose for the patient expressed in mg, aseptically withdraw the corresponding premix volume containing 10 mg/ml docetaxel from the appropriate number of premix vials using graduated syringes fitted with a needle. For example, a dose of 140 mg docetaxel would require 14 ml docetaxel premix solution.

Inject the required premix volume into a 250 ml infusion bag or bottle containing either 5% glucose solution or 0.9% sodium chloride solution. If a dose greater than 200 mg of docetaxel is required, use a larger volume of the infusion vehicle so that a concentration of 0.74 mg/ml docetaxel is not exceeded.

Mix the infusion bag or bottle manually using a rocking motion.

The Taxotere infusion solution should be aseptically administered intravenously within 4 hours (including the 1 hour infusion time) under room temperature and normal lighting conditions. As with all parenteral products, Taxotere premix solution and infusion solution should be visually inspected prior to use, solutions containing a precipitate should be discarded.

Disposal: All materials that have been utilised for dilution and administration should be disposed of according to standard procedures.

Marketing authorisation number

Taxotere 20 mg EU/1/95/002/001
Taxotere 80 mg EU/1/95/002/002

Date of approval/revision of SPC July 1998

Legal category POM

ZIMOVANE*

Presentation

Zimovane: White, film-coated tablets impressed 'ZM'. Each tablet contains 7.5 mg zopiclone. The tablets also contain lactose, hydroxypropyl methycellulose, microcrystalline cellulose and sodium equivalent to a maximum of 0.2 mg per tablet.

Zimovane LS (low strength): Blue film coated tablets impressed Z. each tablet contains 3.75 mg zopiclone. The tablets also contain lactose, hydroxypropyl methycellulose, microcrystalline cellulose and sodium equivalent to 0.1 mg per tablet.

Uses

Pharmacology: Zopiclone is a non-benzodiazepine hypnotic agent, a member of the cyclopyrrolone group of compounds which is structurally unrelated to other hypnotics and tranquillisers. It rapidly initiates and sustains sleep without reduction of total REM sleep and with preservation of slow wave sleep. Negligible residual effects are seen the following morning. Its pharmacological properties include hypnotic, sedative, anxiolytic, anticonvulsant and muscle-relaxant actions. These are related to its high affinity and specific agonist action at central receptors belonging to the GABA macromolecular receptor complex modulating the opening of the chloride ion channel. However, it has been shown that zopiclone and other cyclopyrrolones act on a different site to those of benzodiazepines inducing different conformational changes in the receptor complex.

Zopiclone has a short elimination half life of approximately 5 hours, with no significant accumulation of drug substance or metabolites on repeated dosage.

Indications: Zimovane tablets are indicated for the short term treatment of insomnia, including difficulties in falling asleep, nocturnal awakening and early awakening, transient, situational or chronic insomnia, and insomnia secondary to psychiatric disturbances, in situations where the insomnia is debilitating or is causing severe distress for the patient.

Long term continuous use is not recommended. A course of treatment should employ the lowest effective dose .

Treatment duration: Transient insomnia 2-5 days. Short term insomnia 2-3 weeks. A single course of treatment should not continue for longer than 4 weeks including any tapering off.

Dosage and administration Each tablet should be swallowed whole without sucking, chewing or breaking.

Adults: The recommended dose is 7.5 mg zopiclone (1 Zimovane tablet) by the oral route shortly before retiring.

Elderly: A lower dose of 3.75 mg zopicone (1 Zimovane LS tablet) should be employed to start treatment in the elderly. Depending on effectiveness and acceptability, the dosage subsequently may be increased if clinically necessary.

Patients with hepatic insufficiency: As elimination of zopiclone may be reduced in patients with hepatic dysfunction a lower dose of 3.75 mg zopiclone nightly is recommended. The standard dose of 7.5 mg zopiclone may be used with caution in some cases, depending on effectiveness and acceptability.

Renal insufficiency: Accumulation of zopiclone or its metabolites has not been seen during treatment of insomnia in patients with renal insufficiency. However it is recommended that patients with impaired renal function should start treatment with 3.75 mg.

Contra-indications, warnings, etc Zimovane is contra-indicated in patients with myasthenia gravis, respiratory failure, severe sleep apnoea syndrome, severe hepatic insufficiency and those people with a hypersensitivity to zopiclone.

As with all hypnotics Zimovane should not be used in children

Use during pregnancy: Experience of the use of zopiclone during pregnancy in humans is limited although there have been no adverse findings in animals. Use in pregnancy is therefore not recommended. If the product is prescribed to a woman of child bearing potential, she should be advised to contact her physician about stopping the product if she intends to become pregnant, or suspects that she is pregnant.

Moreover, if zopiclone is used during the last three months of pregnancy or during labour, due to the pharmacological action of the product, effects on the neonate, such as hypothermia, hypnotic and respiratory depression can be expected.

Infants born to mothers who took benzodiazepines or benzodiazepine-like agents chronically during the latter stages of pregnancy may have developed physical dependence and may be at some risk of developing withdrawal symptoms in the postnatal period.

Use during lactation: Zopiclone is excreted in breast milk and use in nursing mothers must be avoided.

Use in hepatic insufficiency: A reduced dosage is recommended, see above.

Use in renal insufficiency: A reduced dosage is recommended, see above.

Risk of dependence: Clinical experience to date with Zimovane suggests that the risk of dependence is minimal when the duration of treatment is limited to not more than 4 weeks.

Use of benzodiazepines and benzodiazepine-like agents (even at therapeutic doses) may lead to the development of physical and psychological dependence upon these products. The risk of dependence increases with dose and duration of treatment; it is also greater in patients with a history of alcohol and/ or drug abuse, or those who have marked personality disorders. The decision to use a hypnotic in such patients should be taken only with this clearly in mind. If physical dependence has developed, abrupt termination of treatment will be accompanied by withdrawal symptoms. These may consist of headaches, muscle pain, extreme anxiety, tension, restlessness, confusion and irritability. In severe cases the following symptoms may occur: derealisation, depersonalisation, hyperacusis, numbness and tingling of the extremities, hypersensitivity to light, noise and physical contact, hallucinations or epileptic seizures. Rare cases of abuse have been reported.

Withdrawal: The termination of treatment with Zimovane is unlikely to be associated with withdrawal effects when duration of treatment is limited to 4 weeks. Patients may benefit from tapering of the dose before discontinuation.

Depression: As with other hypnotics, zopiclone does not constitute a treatment for depression. Any underlying cause of the insomnia should also be addressed before symptomatic treatment.

Tolerance: Some loss of efficacy to the hypnotic effect of benzodiazepines and benzodiazepine-like agents may develop after repeated use for a few weeks. However with Zimovane there is an absence of any marked tolerance during treatment periods of up to 4 weeks.

Rebound insomnia is a transient syndrome where the symptoms which led to treatment with a benzodiazepine or benzodiazepine-like agent recur in an enhanced form on discontinuation of therapy. It may be accompanied by other reactions including mood changes, anxiety and restlessness. Since the risk of withdrawal/ rebound phenomena may be increased after prolonged treatment, or abrupt discontinuation of therapy decreasing the dosage in a stepwise fashion may be helpful.

A course of treatment should employ the lowest effective dose for the minimum length of time necessary for effective treatment. See above for guidance on possible treatment regimens. A course of treatment should not continue for longer than 4 weeks including any tapering off.

Amnesia: Amnesia is rare, but anterograde amnesia may occur, especially when sleep is interrupted or when retiring to bed is delayed after taking the tablet. To reduce the frequency of this possible event, patients should ensure that:

– they take the tablet strictly when retiring for the night
– they are able to have a full nights sleep.

Interactions: The sedative effect of zopiclone may be enhanced when used in combination with alcohol. Concomitant use is therefore not recommended. In particular this could affect the patients ability to drive or use machines the next day.

In combination with CNS depressants an enhancement of the central depressive effect may occur. The therapeutic benefit of co-administration with antipsychotics (neuroleptics), hypnotics, anxiolytics/sedatives, antidepressant agents, narcotic analgesics, anti epileptic drugs, anaesthetics and sedative antihistamines should therefore be carefully weighed. Concomitant use of benzodiazepine or benzodiazepine-like agents with narcotic analgesics may enhance their euphoric effect and could lead to an increase in psychic dependence. Compounds which inhibit certain hepatic enzymes (particularly cytochrome P450) may enhance the activity of benzodiazepines and benzodiazepine-like agents.

Adverse effects: A mild bitter or metallic after-taste is the most frequently reported adverse effect. Less commonly, mild gastrointestinal disturbances, including nausea and vomiting, dizziness, headache, drowsiness and dry mouth have occurred.

Psychological and behavioural disturbances, such as irritability, aggressiveness, confusion, depressed mood, anterograde amnesia, hallucinations and nightmares have been reported. Rarely these reactions may be severe and may be more likely to occur in the elderly

Rarely allergic and allied manifestations such as urticaria or rashes have been observed and, more rarely, light headedness and incoordination.

Although residual effects are rare and generally of minor significance, patients should be advised not to drive or operate machinery the day after treatment until it is established that their performance is unimpaired.

Withdrawal and rebound insomnia have occasionally been observed on discontinuation of treatment, mainly in association with prolonged treatment.

Overdosage: Overdose is usually manifested by varying degrees of central nervous system depression ranging from drowsiness to coma according to the quantity ingested. Overdose should not be life-threatening unless combined with other CNS depressants (including alcohol). Symptomatic and supportive treatment in an adequate clinical environment is recommended. Attention should be paid to respiratory and cardiovascular functions. Gastric lavage is only useful when performed soon after ingestion. Haemodialysis is of no value due to the large volume of distribution of zopiclone. Flumazenil may be a useful antidote.

Pharmaceutical precautions Protect from light. Store in a dry place below 30°C.

Legal category POM.

Package quantities Zimovane tablets are available in containers of 100 tablets and blister packs of 28 tablets (OP).

Zimovane LS tablets are available in blister packs of 28 tablets (OP).

Further information Nil.

Product licence numbers

Zimovane	0012/0259
Zimovane LS	0012/0260

**Trade Mark*

Roche Products Limited
40 Broadwater Road
Welwyn Garden City
Hertfordshire AL7 3AY

☎ 01707 366000   0800 3281629

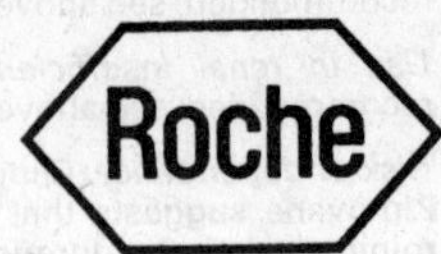

including **Boehringer Mannheim UK Limited**

ANEXATE

Presentation Ampoules containing 500 micrograms flumazenil in 5 ml. The ampoule solution is almost colourless.

Uses
Pharmacological properties: Anexate, an imidazobenzodiazepine, is a specific competitive inhibitor of substances which act via the benzodiazepine receptors, specifically blocking their central effects. The hypnotic-sedative effects of the agonist are rapidly reversed by Anexate and may then reappear gradually within a few hours, depending on the half-life and dose ratio of the agonist and antagonist.

Pharmacokinetics:
Distribution: Flumazenil, a weak lipophilic base, is about 50% bound to plasma proteins. Albumin accounts for two thirds of plasma protein binding. Plasma concentrations of flumazenil decrease with a half-life of 4–11 minutes during the distribution phase.

Metabolism: Flumazenil is extensively metabolised in the liver. The carboxylic acid metabolite is the main metabolite in plasma (free form) and urine (free and conjugated forms). This main metabolite showed no benzodiazepine agonist or antagonist activity in pharmacological tests.

Elimination: Flumazenil is almost completely (99%) eliminated by nonrenal routes. Practically no unchanged flumazenil is excreted in the urine, suggesting complete metabolic degradation of the drug in the body. Elimination of radiolabelled drug is essentially complete within 72 hours, with 90–95% of the radioactivity appearing in urine and 5–10% in the faeces. Elimination is rapid, as shown by a short elimination half-life of 40–80 minutes.

Pharmacokinetics in special clinical situations: In patients with impaired liver function, the elimination half-life of flumazenil is longer and the total body clearance lower than in healthy subjects. The pharmacokinetics of flumazenil are not significantly affected by gender, old age, haemodialysis beginning 1 hour after drug administration or renal failure. Ingestion of food during an intravenous infusion of flumazenil results in a 50% increase in clearance, most likely due to the increased hepatic blood flow that accompanies a meal.

Indications: Anexate is indicated for the complete or partial reversal of the central sedative effects of benzodiazepines. It may therefore be used in anaesthesia and intensive care in the following situations:

Termination of general anaesthesia induced and/or maintained with benzodiazepines.

Reversal of benzodiazepine sedation in short diagnostic and therapeutic procedures.

For the specific reversal of the central effects of benzodiazepines, to allow return to spontaneous respiration and consciousness, in patients in intensive care.

Dosage and administration
Anexate is for slow intravenous injection or infusion. It should only be administered under the supervision of an experienced physician.

Anexate ampoule solution may be diluted with Sodium Chloride Intravenous Infusion BP, Sodium Chloride 0.45% and Dextrose 2.5% Intravenous Infusion BP or Dextrose 5% Intravenous Infusion BP. The resultant infusion solution should be used within 24 hours.

No preparations other than those recommended should be added to the Anexate ampoule or mixed with the Anexate infusion solution.

Anexate may be used concurrently with other resuscitative procedures.

Adults: The recommended initial dose is 200 micrograms administered intravenously over 15 seconds. If the desired level of consciousness is not obtained within 60 seconds a further dose of 100 micrograms can be injected and repeated at 60-second intervals where necessary, up to a maximum total dose of 1 mg or in intensive care situations, 2 mg. The usual dose required is 300–600 micrograms.

If drowsiness recurs, an intravenous infusion of 100–400 micrograms per hour may be employed. The rate of infusion should be individually adjusted to achieve the desired level of arousal.

The individually titrated, slow injections or infusions of Anexate should not produce withdrawal symptoms, even in patients exposed to high doses of benzodiazepines for long periods of time. If, however, unexpected signs of overstimulation occur, an individually titrated dose of diazepam (Valium Roche) or midazolam (Hypnovel) should be given by slow intravenous injection.

If a significant improvement in consciousness or respiratory function is not obtained after repeated doses of Anexate, a non-benzodiazepine aetiology must be assumed.

Use in the elderly: No specific data are available on the use of Anexate in the elderly, but it should be remembered that this population is more sensitive to the effects of benzodiazepines and should be treated with due caution.

Children: There are insufficient data to make dosage recommendations for Anexate in children. It should, therefore, be administered only if the potential benefits to the patient outweigh the possible risks.

Use in renal and hepatic insufficiency: No dosage adjustments are necessary in patients with renal impairment. However, since flumazenil is primarily metabolised in the liver, careful titration of dosage is recommended in patients with impaired hepatic function.

Contra-indications, warnings, etc
Contra-indications: Anexate is contra-indicated in patients with known hypersensitivity to benzodiazepines.

Anexate is contra-indicated in patients who have been given a benzodiazepine for control of a potentially life-threatening condition (e.g. control of intracranial pressure or status epilepticus).

In mixed intoxications with benzodiazepines and tricyclic and/or tetracyclic antidepressants, the toxicity of the antidepressants can be masked by protective benzodiazepine effects. In the presence of autonomic (anticholinergic), neurological (motor abnormalities) or cardiovascular symptoms of severe intoxication with tricyclics/tetracyclics, Anexate should not be used to reverse benzodiazepine effects.

Use in pregnancy and lactation: Like other benzodiazepine compounds, Anexate is expected to cross the placenta and to enter into breast milk, although the total quantities involved would be small. There has been little human usage but animal studies have shown no teratogenic potential. The established medical principle of only administering drugs in early pregnancy when considered absolutely necessary should therefore be observed.

Emergency use of Anexate during lactation is not contra-indicated.

Precautions: In view of the short duration of action of Anexate and the possible need for repeat doses, the patient should remain under close observation until all possible central benzodiazepine effects have subsided.

The use of Anexate is not recommended in epileptic patients who have been receiving benzodiazepine treatment for a prolonged period. Although Anexate exerts a slight intrinsic anticonvulsant effect, its abrupt suppression of the protective effect of a benzodiazepine agonist can give rise to convulsions in epileptic patients.

Anexate should be used with caution in patients with head injury as it may be capable of precipitating convulsions or altering cerebral blood flow in patients receiving benzodiazepines.

Benzodiazepine agonists have a dependence potential when used chronically. Symptoms such as depression, nervousness, rebound insomnia, irritability, sweating and diarrhoea may arise following abrupt cessation of benzodiazepine agonists in patients treated for prolonged periods of time. Rapid injection of Anexate in such patients may trigger these withdrawal symptoms and should therefore be avoided.

When Anexate is used with neuromuscular blocking agents, it should not be injected until the effects of neuromuscular blockade have been fully reversed.

In high-risk patients, the advantages of counteracting the central nervous system depression associated with benzodiazepines should be weighed against the drawbacks of rapid awakening.

The dosage of Anexate should be adjusted individually to the needs of patients suffering from preoperative anxiety or having a history of chronic or episodic anxiety. In anxious patients, particularly those with coronary heart disease, it is preferable to maintain a degree of sedation throughout the early post-operative period rather than bring about complete arousal.

The pain felt by patients in the post-operative period must be taken into account. Following a major intervention, it is preferable to maintain a moderate degree of sedation.

Patients who have received Anexate to reverse the effects of benzodiazepine sedation should be warned not to drive, to operate machinery or to engage in any other physically or mentally demanding activity for at least 24 hours, since the effect of the benzodiazepine may return.

Anexate is not recommended either as a treatment for benzodiazepine dependence or for the management of protracted benzodiazepine abstinence syndromes.

Side-effects and adverse reactions: Anexate is generally well tolerated. In post-operative use, nausea and/or vomiting are occasionally observed, particularly if opiates have also been employed. Flushing has also been noted. If patients are awakened too rapidly, they may become agitated, anxious or fearful. Very rarely, seizures have been reported, particularly in patients known to suffer from epilepsy. Transient increases in blood pressure and heart rate may occur on awakening in intensive care patients.

Any side-effects associated with Anexate usually subside rapidly without the need for special treatment.

Excessive and/or rapidly injected doses of Anexate may induce benzodiazepine withdrawal symptoms such as anxiety attacks, tachycardia, dizziness and sweating in patients on long-term benzodiazepine treatment. Such symptoms may be treated by slow intravenous injection of diazepam or midazolam (see **Dosage and administration**).

Drug interactions: Anexate blocks the central effects of benzodiazepines by competitive interaction at the receptor level; the effects of non-benzodiazepines acting via the benzodiazepine receptor, such as zopiclone, are also blocked by Anexate. However, Anexate is ineffective when unconsciousness is due to other substances.

Interaction with other central nervous system depressants has not been observed. However, particular caution is necessary when using Anexate in cases of intentional overdosage since the toxic effects of other psychotropic drugs (especially tricyclic antidepressants) taken concurrently may increase with the subsidence of the benzodiazepine effect.

The pharmacokinetics of benzodiazepines are unaltered in the presence of Anexate and vice versa.

Treatment of overdosage: Even when given intravenously at doses of 100 mg, no symptoms of overdosage attributable to Anexate have been observed.

Pharmaceutical precautions
Storage: The recommended maximum storage temperature for Anexate ampoules is 30°C.

Diluents: Anexate ampoule solution may be diluted with Sodium Chloride Intravenous Infusion BP, Sodium Chloride 0.45% and Dextrose 2.5% Intravenous Infusion BP or Dextrose 5% Intravenous Infusion BP. The resultant infusion solution should be used within 24 hours.

No preparations other than those recommended should be added to the Anexate ampoule or mixed with the Anexate infusion solution.

Package quantities Anexate ampoules 500 micrograms per 5 ml in packs of 5.

Further information
Availability: Anexate ampoules are available through hospitals, clinics or retail pharmacies.

Product licence number PL 0031/0228

Date of last review June 1998

BEZALIP

Qualitative and quantitative composition Bezafibrate 200 mg

Pharmaceutical form Tablet for oral use. Bezalip is a round film-coated tablet with a white core and is imprinted BM/G6.

Clinical particulars

Therapeutic indications: Bezalip is indicated for use in hyperlipidaemias of Type IIa, IIb, III, IV and V (Fredrickson classification).

Bezalip should be employed only in patients with a fully defined and diagnosed lipid abnormality which is inadequately controlled by dietary means, or by other changes in life-style such as physical exercise and weight reduction, and in whom the long-term risks associated with the condition warrant treatment.

The rationale for the use of Bezalip is to control abnormalities of serum lipids and lipoproteins to reduce or prevent the long term effects which have been shown by many epidemiological studies to be positively and strongly correlated with such hyperlipidaemias.

Posology and method of administration:

Adults: The recommended dosage for Bezalip tablets is three tablets daily, equivalent to 600 mg bezafibrate. The tablets should be swallowed whole with a little fluid after each meal.

Elderly: No specific dosage reduction is necessary in elderly patients.

Children: At present there is inadequate information regarding an appropriate dosage in children.

Renal impairment: In patients with renal insufficiency the dose should be adjusted according to serum creatinine levels or creatinine clearance as shown in the following table.

Serum creatinine (μmol/l)	*Creatinine clearance (ml/min)*	*Dosage (tablets/day)*
Up to 135	Over 60	3
136–225	60–40	2
226–530	40–15	1 every 1 or 2 days
Over 530	Less than 15	1 every 3rd day
Dialysis patients		1 every 3rd day

The response to therapy is normally rapid, although a progressive improvement may occur over a number of weeks. Treatment should be withdrawn if an adequate response has not been achieved within 3 to 4 months.

Contra-indications: Significant hepatic disease (other than fatty infiltration of the liver associated with raised triglyceride values), gall bladder disease with or without cholelithiasis, nephrotic syndrome. Hypersensitivity to bezafibrate.

Special warnings and special precautions for use: See Preclinical safety data.

Interaction with other medicaments and other forms of interaction: Care is required in administering Bezalip to patients taking coumarin-type anti-coagulants, the action of which may be potentiated. The dosage of anti-coagulant should be reduced by up to 50% and readjusted by monitoring blood coagulation.

As bezafibrate improves glucose utilisation the action of antidiabetic medication, including insulin, may be potentiated. Hypoglycaemia has not been observed although increased monitoring of the glycaemic status may be warranted for a brief period after introduction of Bezalip.

Should combined therapy with an ion-exchange resin be considered necessary, there should be an interval of 2 hours between the intake of the resin and Bezalip as the absorption of bezafibrate otherwise may be impaired.

Combination therapy with HMG CoA reductase inhibitors and fibric acid derivatives has been reported to increase the risk of myopathy and should therefore be used with caution. Patients should be monitored for signs of myopathy and increased creatine kinase activity. This combination therapy should not be used in patients with predisposing factors for myopathy (impaired renal function, severe infection, trauma, surgery, disturbances of hormone or electrolyte balance).

MAO-inhibitors (with hepatotoxic potential) should not be administered together with bezafibrate.

Since oestrogens may lead to a rise in lipid levels, the necessity for treatment with Bezalip in patients receiving oestrogens or oestrogen containing preparations should be considered on an individual basis.

Pregnancy and lactation: Although the drug substance has not been shown in animal studies to have any adverse effects on the foetus, it is recommended that Bezalip should not be administered to either pregnant women or to those who are breast feeding.

Effects on ability to drive and use machines: None known.

Undesirable effects: Adverse effects during treatment with Bezalip most frequently are gastro-intestinal in nature, such as loss of appetite, nausea or gastric discomfort. These symptoms generally are transient and do not require withdrawal of therapy. In susceptible patients a slowly increasing dosage over 5 to 7 days may help to avoid such symptoms. More rarely there may be allergic skin reactions such as pruritus or urticaria or general hypersensitivity reactions. Increased hair loss and disturbances of potency have been reported. There have also been reports of marked elevations of creatine kinase, myositis, myopathy and rarely rhabdomyolysis. Patients who develop signs of myotoxicity should be monitored closely and serum creatine kinase levels checked. Treatment with Bezalip should be stopped if myopathy is suspected or if creatine kinase increases to ≥ 10 times the upper limit of normal. All of these adverse effects generally resolve rapidly following withdrawal of therapy.

Rarely headache, dizziness, decreases of haemoglobin, leucocytes, platelets, and single cases of increases in transaminases have been reported. Slight increases in serum creatinine may occur. Special care is needed in patients with renal disease as progressive increases in the serum creatinine level and/or failure to follow the dosage guidelines may result in myotoxicity (rhabdomyolysis).

Bezafibrate may increase the lithogenic index in some patients although studies have shown inconsistent results. There have been isolated reports of the occurrence of gallstones. However, there is no evidence that the administration of Bezalip is associated with an increased frequency of gallstones.

Overdose: The effects of acute overdosage are unknown although no serious biochemical or clinical effects are likely.

Pharmacological properties

Pharmacodynamic properties: Bezafibrate lowers elevated levels of serum cholesterol and triglycerides (i.e. lowers elevated low density lipoprotein and very low density lipoprotein levels, and raises lowered high density lipoprotein levels) by stimulating lipoprotein lipase and hepatic lipase, and by suppressing the activity of 3 HMGCo-A reductase resulting in stimulation of low density lipoprotein receptors on the cell surface.

Studies have shown bezafibrate to be effective in treating hyperlipidaemia in patients with diabetes mellitus. Some cases showed a beneficial reduction in fasting blood glucose.

Significant reductions in serum fibrinogen levels have been observed in hyperfibrinogenaemic patients treated with bezafibrate.

Pharmacokinetic properties: Maximum concentrations of bezafibrate appear around 2 hours after ingestion of Bezalip tablets. The protein-binding of bezafibrate in serum is approximately 95%. The elimination half-life is in the order of 2.1 hours although elimination is markedly slowed in the presence of limited renal function. Elimination may be increased in forced diuresis. The drug substance is non-dialysable (cuprophane filter).

Preclinical safety data: The chronic administration of a high dose of bezafibrate to rats was associated with hepatic tumour formation in females. This dosage was in the order of 30 to 40 times the human dosage. No such effect was apparent at reduced intake levels approximating more closely to the lipid-lowering dosage in humans.

Pharmaceutical particulars

List of excipients: In addition to bezafibrate, the tablets contain maize starch, microcrystalline cellulose, colloidal silicon dioxide, sodium starch glycollate, magnesium stearate, polymethacrylic acid esters, lactose, polyethylene glycol, talc, kaolin, titanium dioxide (E171), polysorbate 80 and sodium citrate dihydrate.

Incompatibilities: Not applicable.

Shelf life: 5 years

Special precautions for storage: Bezalip tablets require no special storage conditions.

Nature and contents of container: Packs of 100 tablets in PVC/Aluminium blister strips.

Instructions for use/handling: Not applicable.

Marketing authorisation number PL 15722/0006

Date of first authorisation/renewal of authorisation 1 January 1997

Date of (partial) revision of the text May 1998

BEZALIP MONO

Qualitative and quantitative composition Bezafibrate 400 mg

Pharmaceutical form Modified release tablet for oral use. Bezalip Mono is a round film-coated tablet with a white core and is imprinted BM/D9.

Clinical particulars

Therapeutic indications: Bezalip Mono is indicated for use in hyperlipidaemias of Type IIa, IIb, III, IV and V (Fredrickson classification).

Bezalip Mono should be employed only in patients with a fully defined and diagnosed lipid abnormality which is inadequately controlled by dietary means, or by other changes in life-style such as physical exercise and weight reduction, and in whom the long-term risks associated with the condition warrant treatment.

The rationale for the use of Bezalip Mono is to control abnormalities of serum lipids and lipoproteins to reduce or prevent the long term effects which have been shown by many epidemiological studies to be positively and strongly correlated with such hyperlipidaemias.

Posology and method of administration:

Adults: The dosage for Bezalip Mono is one tablet daily, equivalent to 400 mg bezafibrate. The tablets should be swallowed whole with a little fluid after a meal either at night or in the morning.

Elderly: No specific dosage reduction is necessary in elderly patients.

Children: At present there is inadequate information regarding an appropriate dosage in children.

Renal impairment: Bezalip Mono is contraindicated in patients with renal impairment with serum creatinine > 135 micromol/l or creatinine clearance < 60 ml/min. Such patients may be treated with conventional Bezalip tablets (200 mg bezafibrate) using an appropriately reduced daily dosage.

The response to therapy is normally rapid, although a progressive improvement may occur over a number of weeks. Treatment should be withdrawn if an adequate response has not been achieved within 3 to 4 months.

Contra-indications: Significant hepatic disease (other than fatty infiltration of the liver associated with raised triglyceride values), gall bladder disease with or without cholelithiasis, nephrotic syndrome or renal impairment (serum creatinine > 135 micromol/l or creatinine clearance < 60 ml/min.) Patients undergoing dialysis. Hypersensitivity to bezafibrate.

Special warnings and special precautions for use: See Preclinical safety data.

Interaction with other medicaments and other forms of interaction: Care is required in administering Bezalip Mono to patients taking coumarin-type anticoagulants, the action of which may be potentiated. The dosage of anti-coagulant should be reduced by up to 50% and readjusted by monitoring blood coagulation.

As bezafibrate improves glucose utilisation the action of antidiabetic medication, including insulin, may be potentiated. Hypoglycaemia has not been observed although increased monitoring of the glycaemic status may be warranted for a brief period after introduction of Bezalip Mono.

Should combined therapy with an ion-exchange resin be considered necessary, there should be an interval of 2 hours between the intake of the resin and Bezalip Mono as the absorption of bezafibrate otherwise may be impaired.

Combination therapy with HMG CoA reductase inhibitors and fibric acid derivatives has been reported to increase the risk of myopathy and should therefore be used with caution. Patients should be monitored for signs of myopathy and increased creatine kinase activity. This combination therapy should not be used in patients with predisposing factors for myopathy (impaired renal function, severe infection, trauma, surgery, disturbances of hormone or electrolyte balance).

MAO-inhibitors (with hepatotoxic potential) should not be administered together with bezafibrate.

Since oestrogens may lead to a rise in lipid levels, the necessity for treatment with Bezalip Mono in patients receiving oestrogens or oestrogen containing preparations should be considered on an individual basis.

Pregnancy and lactation: Although the drug substance has not been shown in animal studies to have any adverse effects on the foetus, it is recommended that Bezalip Mono should not be administered to either pregnant women or to those who are breast feeding.

Effects on ability to drive and use machines: None known.

Undesirable effects: Adverse effects during treatment with Bezalip Mono most frequently are gastro-intestinal in nature, such as loss of appetite, nausea or gastric discomfort. These symptoms generally are transient and do not require withdrawal of therapy. In susceptible patients a slowly increasing dosage over 5 to 7 days may help to avoid such symptoms. More rarely there may be allergic skin reactions such as pruritus or urticaria or general hypersensitivity reactions. Increased hair loss and disturbances of potency have been reported. There have also been reports of marked elevations of creatine kinase, myositis, myopathy and rarely rhabdomyolysis. Patients who develop signs of myotoxicity should be monitored closely and serum creatine kinase levels checked. Treatment with Bezalip Mono should be stopped if myopathy is suspected or if creatine kinase increases to ≥ 10 times the upper limit of normal. All of these adverse effects generally resolve rapidly following withdrawal of therapy.

Rarely headache, dizziness, decreases of haemoglobin, leucocytes, platelets, and single cases of increases in transaminases have been reported. Slight increases in serum creatinine may occur.

Special care is needed in patients with renal disease as progressive increases in the serum creatinine level and/or failure to follow the dosage guidelines may result in myotoxicity (rhabdomyolysis).

Bezafibrate may increase the lithogenic index in some patients although studies have shown inconsistent results. There have been isolated reports of the occurrence of gallstones. However, there is no evidence that the administration of Bezalip Mono is associated with an increased frequency of gallstones.

Overdose: The effects of acute overdosage are unknown although no serious biochemical or clinical effects are likely.

Pharmacological properties

Pharmacodynamic properties: Bezafibrate lowers elevated levels of serum cholesterol and triglycerides (i.e. lowers elevated low density lipoprotein and very low density lipoprotein levels, and raises lowered high density lipoprotein levels) by stimulating lipoprotein lipase and hepatic lipase, and by suppressing the activity of 3 HMGCo-A reductase resulting in stimulation of low density lipoprotein receptors on the cell surface.

Studies have shown bezafibrate to be effective in treating hyperlipidaemia in patients with diabetes mellitus. Some cases showed a beneficial reduction in fasting blood glucose.

Significant reductions in serum fibrinogen levels have been observed in hyperfibrinogenaemic patients treated with bezafibrate.

Pharmacokinetic properties: Maximum serum concentrations of bezafibrate appear around 4 hours after ingestion of Bezalip Mono tablets. The protein-binding of bezafibrate in serum is approximately 95%. The elimination half-life is in the order of 2.1 hours although elimination is markedly slowed in the presence of limited renal function.

Preclinical safety data: The chronic administration of a high dose of bezafibrate to rats was associated with hepatic tumour formation in females. This dosage was in the order of 30 to 40 times the human dosage. No such effect was apparent at reduced intake levels approximating more closely to the lipid-lowering dosage in humans.

Pharmaceutical particulars

List of excipients: Lactose, povidone, sodium lauryl sulphate, hydroxypropyl methylcellulose, colloidal silicon dioxide, magnesium stearate, Eudragit E 30 D, polyethylene glycol, talc, titanium dioxide (E171), polysorbate 80 and sodium citrate dihydrate.

Incompatibilities: Not applicable.

Shelf life: 5 years.

Special precautions for storage: Bezalip Mono requires no special storage conditions.

Nature and contents of container: Calendar packs of 28 tablets in PVC/Aluminium blister strips. HDPE containers of 28 tablets.

Instructions for use/handling: Not applicable.

Marketing authorisation number PL 15722/0013

Date of first authorisation/renewal of authorisation 1 January 1997

Date of (partial) revision of the text May 1998

CELLCEPT 250 mg CAPSULES 

Qualitative and quantitative composition Each capsule contains 250 mg mycophenolate mofetil.

Pharmaceutical form *CellCept capsules:* oblong, blue/brown, branded with black 'CellCept 250' on the capsule cap and 'Company logo' on the capsule body.

Clinical particulars

Therapeutic indications: CellCept is indicated in combination with cyclosporin and corticosteroids for the prophylaxis of acute transplant rejection in patients receiving allogeneic renal or cardiac transplants.

Posology and method of administration: Treatment with CellCept should be initiated and maintained by appropriately qualified transplant specialists.

Use in renal transplant: the initial dose of CellCept should be given orally within 72 hours following transplantation. The recommended dose in renal transplant patients is 1.0 g administered twice daily (2 g daily dose). Although daily doses of both 2 g and 3 g were studied in clinical trials, an efficacy advantage for the 3 g dose could not be established for renal transplant patients. In renal transplant, patients receiving 2 g per day of CellCept had an overall better safety profile than patients receiving 3 g per day.

Use in cardiac transplant: the initial dose of CellCept should be given orally within 5 days following transplantation. The recommended dose in cardiac transplant patients is 1.5 g administered twice daily (3 g daily dose).

Use in children: safety and effectiveness in paediatric patients have not been established. Very limited pharmacokinetic data are available for paediatric renal transplant patients. No data are available for paediatric cardiac transplant patients.

Use in elderly: the recommended dose of 1.0 g administered twice a day for renal transplant patients and 1.5 g twice a day for cardiac transplant patients is appropriate for elderly patients. This recommendation is based on limited numbers of elderly patients treated with CellCept in the pivotal renal (7% n = 73) and cardiac (7% n = 20) transplant trials. Patients in this age group may generally be at increased risk of adverse events compared to younger individuals; this is similarly true for patients receiving CellCept as part of a combination immunosuppressive regimen (see *Undesirable effects*).

Use in renal impairment: in renal transplant patients with severe chronic renal impairment (glomerular filtration rate < 25 ml/min/1.73 m^2), outside of the immediate post-transplant period, doses greater than 1 g administered twice a day should be avoided. These patients should also be carefully observed. No dose adjustments are needed in patients experiencing delayed renal graft function post-operatively (see *Pharmacokinetic properties*).

No data are available for cardiac transplant patients with severe chronic renal impairment.

Use in severe hepatic impairment: no dose adjustments are needed for renal patients with severe hepatic parenchymal disease. No data are available for cardiac patients with severe hepatic parenchymal disease.

Other considerations for use: if neutropenia develops (absolute neutrophil count < 1.3 x 10^3/μl), physicians should perform appropriate diagnostic tests, manage the patients appropriately, and consider interrupting dosing with CellCept.

MPA (mycophenolic acid) is the active metabolite of mycophenolate mofetil. Food has no effect on MPA area under the curve (AUC), but has been shown to decrease Cmax by 40%. It is recommended that CellCept be administered on an empty stomach.

Renal transplant rejection does not lead to changes in MPA pharmacokinetics requiring dosage reduction or interruption of CellCept. Similarly, there is no basis for adjustment of dose following cardiac transplant rejection.

Contra-indications: Allergic reactions to CellCept have been observed. Therefore, CellCept is contra-indicated in patients with a hypersensitivity to mycophenolate mofetil or mycophenolic acid. For information on use in pregnancy and contraceptive requirements (see *Use during pregnancy and lactation*).

Special warnings and special precautions for use: As in patients receiving immunosuppressive regimes involving combinations of drugs, patients receiving CellCept as part of an immunosuppressive regime are at increased risk of developing lymphomas and other malignancies, particularly of the skin (see Undesirable effects). The risk appears to be related to the intensity and duration of immunosuppression rather than to the use of any specific agent.

As usual for patients with increased risk for skin cancer, exposure to sunlight and UV light should be limited by wearing protective clothing and using a sunscreen with a high protection factor.

Oversuppression of the immune system can also increase susceptibility to infection including opportunistic infections, fatal infections and sepsis. In three controlled trials for prevention of renal transplant rejection, patients receiving 2 g per day of CellCept demonstrated an overall better safety profile than did patients receiving 3 g of CellCept. In cardiac transplant patients the overall incidence of opportunistic infections was approximately 10% higher in patients treated with CellCept than in those receiving azathioprine therapy but this did not translate into excess mortality. There were more herpes virus and cytomegalovirus infections in CellCept treated cardiac transplant patients compared to those treated with azathioprine.

Patients receiving CellCept should be monitored for neutropenia. The development of neutropenia may be related to CellCept itself, concomitant medications, viral infections, or some combination of these causes. Patients on CellCept should have complete blood counts weekly during the first month, twice monthly for the second and third months of treatment, then monthly through the first year (See *Posology and method of administration*).

Patients receiving CellCept should be instructed to report immediately any evidence of infection, unexpected bruising, bleeding or any other manifestation of bone marrow depression.

Because CellCept has been associated with an increased incidence of digestive system adverse events, including infrequent cases of gastrointestinal tract ulceration, haemorrhage and perforation, CellCept should be administered with caution in patients with active serious digestive system disease.

Administration of doses greater than 1 g BID to renal transplant patients with severe chronic renal impairment should be avoided and they should be carefully observed. No dose adjustment is recommended for patients with delayed renal graft function post-transplant, however, they should be carefully observed (see *Posology and method of administration*, and *Pharmacokinetic properties*). No data are available for cardiac transplant patients with severe chronic renal impairment.

It is recommended that CellCept not be administered concomitantly with azathioprine because such concomitant administration has not been studied.

In view of the significant reduction in the AUC of MPA by cholestyramine, caution should be used in the concomitant administration of CellCept with drugs that interfere with enterohepatic recirculation because of the potential to reduce the efficacy of CellCept.

Interaction with other medicaments and other forms of interaction: Acyclovir: higher MPAG and acyclovir plasma concentrations were observed when mycophenolate mofetil was administered with acyclovir in comparison to the administration of each drug alone. Because MPAG plasma concentrations are increased in the presence of renal impairment, as are acyclovir concentrations, the potential exists for the two drugs to compete for tubular secretion and thus further increases in concentrations of both drugs may occur.

Antacids with magnesium and aluminum hydroxides: absorption of mycophenolate mofetil was decreased when administered with antacids.

Cholestyramine: following single dose administration of 1.5 g of mycophenolate mofetil to normal healthy subjects pretreated with 4 g TID of cholestyramine for 4 days, there was a 40% reduction in the AUC of MPA.

Cyclosporin A: cyclosporin A pharmacokinetics were unaffected by mycophenolate mofetil.

Ganciclovir: based on the results of a single dose administration study of recommended doses of oral mycophenolate and IV ganciclovir and the known effects of renal impairment on the pharmacokinetics of MMF (see *Special warnings and special precautions for use*) and ganciclovir, it is anticipated that co-administration of these agents (which compete for mechanisms of renal tubular secretion) will result in increases in MPAG and ganciclovir concentration. No substantial alteration of MPA pharmacokinetics are anticipated and MMF dose adjustment is not required. In patients with renal impairment in which MMF and ganciclovir are co-administered the dose recommendations for ganciclovir should be observed and patients monitored carefully.

Oral contraceptives: no pharmacokinetic interaction was observed between mycophenolate mofetil and 1 mg norethisterone/35μg ethinyloestradiol. This single dose study demonstrates the lack of a gross pharmacokinetic interaction, but cannot exclude the possibility of changes in the pharmacokinetics of the oral contraceptive under long term dosing conditions with CellCept which might adversely affect the efficacy of the oral contraceptive.

Trimethoprim/sulphamethoxazole: no effect on the bioavailability of MPA was observed.

Other interactions: co-administration of probenecid with mycophenolate mofetil in monkeys raises plasma AUC of MPAG by 3-fold. Thus, other drugs known to undergo renal tubular secretion may compete with MPAG and thereby raise plasma concentrations of MPAG or the other drug undergoing tubular secretion. Single dose studies of CellCept with ganciclovir and trimethoprim/sulphamethoxazole did not reveal a pharmacokinetic interaction between either of these agents and CellCept. All these types of compounds operate through inhibition of nucleoside synthesis and therefore one cannot exclude a clinical interaction between them.

Use during pregnancy and lactation

Adverse effects on foetal development (including malformations) occurred when pregnant rats and rabbits were dosed during organogenesis (see *Preclinical safety data*). Because there are no adequate and well controlled studies in pregnant women, CellCept should be used in pregnant women only if the potential benefit outweighs the potential risk to the foetus.

It is recommended that CellCept therapy should not be initiated until a negative pregnancy test has been obtained. Patients should be instructed to consult their physician immediately should pregnancy occur.

Effective contraception must be used before beginning CellCept therapy, during therapy, and for six weeks following discontinuation of therapy. Although the results of a single dose drug interaction study with an oral contraceptive suggest the lack of a gross pharmacokinetic interaction, the results cannot exclude the possibility of changes in the pharmacokinetics of the oral contraceptive under long term dosing conditions with CellCept which might adversely affect the efficacy of the oral contraceptive (see *Interaction with other medicaments and other forms of interaction*).

Studies in rats have shown mycophenolate mofetil to be excreted in milk. It is not known whether this drug is excreted in human milk. Because many drugs are excreted in human milk and because of the potential for serious adverse reactions in nursing infants from mycophenolate mofetil, a decision should be made whether to discontinue nursing or to discontinue the drug, taking into account the importance of the drug to the mother.

Effects on ability to drive and use machines: No specific studies have been performed. The pharmacodynamic profile and the reported adverse reactions indicate that an effect is unlikely.

Undesirable effects: The principal adverse reactions associated with the administration of CellCept in combination with cyclosporine and corticosteroids include diarrhoea, leukopenia, sepsis and vomiting and there is evidence of a higher frequency of certain types of infections (see *Special warnings and special precautions for use*).

As in patients receiving immunosuppressive regimes involving combinations of drugs, patients receiving CellCept as part of an immunosuppressive regime are at increased risk of developing lymphomas and other malignancies, particularly of the skin (see *Special warnings and special precautions for use*). Within 3 years post-transplant, lymphoproliferative disease or lymphoma developed in patients receiving CellCept in immunosuppressive regimens in 1.6% of the patients receiving 3 g daily and 0.6% in patients receiving 2 g daily in the controlled studies of prevention of renal rejection compared to the placebo (0%) and azathioprine groups (0.6%). In cardiac transplant patients, the incidence of lymphoproliferative disease was 0.7% in patients receiving CellCept 3 g daily compared to patients receiving azathioprine (2.1%). The incidence of non-melanoma skin cancer in cardiac transplant patients treated with CellCept 3 g per day was 5.5% compared to patients treated with azathioprine (6.9%). Cardiac transplant patients had been followed for a maximum of 3 years with 26% of these followed for less than a year and 34% followed for greater than 2 years. All patients are at increased risk of opportunistic infections, the risk increased with dose (see *Special warnings and special precautions for use*).

Elderly patients, particularly those who are receiving CellCept as part of a combination immunosuppressive regimen, may be at greater increased risk of certain infections (including CMV tissue invasive disease) and possibly gastrointestinal haemorrhage and pulmonary oedema, compared to younger individuals (see *Posology and method of administration*).

Adverse reactions reported in ≥ 10% of patients treated with CellCept in the three Phase III controlled trials for prevention of renal transplant rejection and/or the Phase III controlled cardiac transplant trial are listed in Table 1.

Adverse events, not mentioned in Table 1, reported in ≥ 3% and < 10% in renal transplant and/or cardiac transplant patients are listed in Table 2 on the following page.

Adverse reactions during post marketing experience with CellCept are similar to those seen in the controlled renal and cardiac transplant studies.

Post-marketing experience: Gastro-intestinal: colitis (sometimes caused by cytomegalovirus), pancreatitis.

Disorders of immunosuppression: serious, life-threatening infections such as meningitis and infectious endocarditis have been reported occasionally and there is evidence of a higher frequency of certain types of infections such as tuberculosis and atypical mycobacterial infection.

Overdose: There has been no reported experience of overdosage of mycophenolate mofetil in humans.

At clinically encountered concentrations, MPA and MPAG are not removed by haemodialysis. However, at high MPAG plasma concentrations (> 100µg/ml), small amounts of MPAG are removed. By interfering with enterohepatic circulation of the drug, bile acid sequestrants, such as cholestyramine reduce the MPA AUC.

Table 1: Adverse Events Reported in ≥ 10% of Patients Treated with CellCept in Combination with Cyclosporine and Corticosteroids

Body System	*Events Reported in Both Renal and Cardiac Transplant Studies*	*Events Reported in Renal Transplant Studies Only 991 CellCept treated patients**	*Events Reported in Cardiac Transplant Study MYCS 1864 Only 289 CellCept treated patients***
Body as a Whole	asthenia, fever, headache, infection, pain, (includes abdominal, back and chest), oedema	—	—
Blood and Lymphatic	anaemia, (including hypochromic anaemia), leukocytosis, leukopenia, thrombocytopenia	—	ecchymosis
Urogenital	urinary tract infection	haematuria, renal tubular necrosis	abnormal kidney function, oliguria
Cardiovascular	hypertension	—	arrhythmia, bradycardia, hypotension, cardiac failure, pericardial effusion
Metabolic/Nutritional	hypercholesterolaemia, hyperglycaemia, hyperkalaemia, hypokalaemia	hypophosphataemia	acidosis, bilirubinaemia, elevated BUN, elevated creatinine, elevated enzyme levels (lactic dehydrogenase, SGOT and SGPT), hyperlipaemia, hyperuricaemia, hypervolaemia, hypomagnesaemia, hyponatraemia, weight gain
Gastrointestinal	constipation, diarrhoea, dyspepsia, oral moniliasis, nausea and vomiting	—	flatulence
Respiratory	cough increased, dyspnoea, pharyngitis, pneumonia	bronchitis	asthma, rhinitis, pleural effusion, sinusitis
Skin and Appendages	acne, herpes simplex	—	herpes zoster, rash
Nervous	dizziness, insomnia, tremor	—	anxiety, agitation, confusion, depression, hypertonia, paresthesia, somnolence
Musculoskeletal	—	—	leg cramps, myalgia, myasthaenia
Special Senses	—	—	amblyopia

* (total n=1,483)
** (total n=578)

Pharmacological properties

Pharmacodynamic properties: Pharmacotherapeutic group: immunosuppressant ATC code LO4AA06.

Mycophenolate mofetil is the 2-morpholinoethyl ester of MPA. MPA is a potent, selective, uncompetitive and reversible inhibitor of inosine monophosphate dehydrogenase, and therefore inhibits the *de novo* pathway of guanosine nucleotide synthesis without incorporation into DNA. Because T- and B-lymphocytes are critically dependent for their proliferation on *de novo* synthesis of purines whereas other cell types can utilise salvage pathways, MPA has more potent cytostatic effects on lymphocytes than on other cells.

Pharmacokinetic properties: MPA at clinically relevant concentrations, is 97% bound to plasma albumin.

Following oral administration, mycophenolate mofetil undergoes rapid and extensive absorption and complete presystemic metabolism to the active metabolite, MPA. As evidenced by suppression of acute rejection following renal transplantation, the immunosuppressant activity of CellCept is correlated with MPA concentration. Mycophenolate mofetil is not measurable systemically in plasma following oral administration.

MPA is metabolised principally by glucuronyl transferase to form the phenolic glucoronide of MPA (MPAG), which is not pharmacologically active.

As a result of enterohepatic recirculation, secondary increases in plasma MPA concentration are usually observed at approximately 6–12 hours post-dose. A reduction in the AUC of MPA of approximately 40% is associated with the co-administration of cholestyramine (4 g TID), indicating that there is a significant amount of enterohepatic recirculation.

Negligible amount of drug is excreted as MPA (< 1% of dose) in the urine. Orally administered radiolabelled mycophenolate mofetil resulted in complete recovery of the administered dose; with 93% of the administered dose recovered in the urine and 6% recovered in the faeces. Most (about 87%) of the administered dose is excreted in the urine as MPAG.

The mean bioavailability of oral mycophenolate mofetil, based on MPA AUC, was 94% relative to IV mycophenolate mofetil.

Food had no effect on the extent of absorption (MPA AUC) of mycophenolate mofetil when administered at doses of 1.5 g BID to renal transplant patients. However, MPA Cmax was decreased by 40% in the presence of food.

Immediately post-transplant (< 40 days), mean MPA AUC and Cmax are approximately 50% lower in renal and cardiac transplant patients than that observed in healthy volunteers or in stable renal transplant patients.

In a single dose study (6 subjects per group), mean plasma MPA AUC observed in subjects with severe chronic renal impairment (glomerular filtration rate < 25 ml/min/1.73 m^2) were 28–75% higher relative to the means observed in normal healthy subjects or subjects with lesser degrees of renal impairment. However, the mean single dose MPAG AUC was 3–6 fold higher in subjects with severe renal impairment than in subjects with mild renal impairment or normal healthy subjects, consistent with the known renal elimination of MPAG. Multiple dosing of mycophenolate mofetil in patients with severe chronic renal impairment has not been studied. No data are available for cardiac transplant patients with severe chronic renal impairment.

In patients with delayed graft function post-transplant, mean MPA AUC_{0-12} was comparable to that seen in post-transplant patients without delayed graft function. Mean plasma MPAG AUC_{0-12} was 2–3 fold higher than in post-transplant patients without delayed graft function.

In volunteers with alcoholic cirrhosis, hepatic MPA glucuronidation processes were relatively unaffected by hepatic parenchymal disease. Effects of hepatic disease on this process probably depend on the particular disease. However, hepatic disease with predominantly biliary damage, such as primary biliary cirrhosis, may show a different effect.

Pharmacokinetic behaviour of CellCept in the elderly has not been formally evaluated.

Preclinical safety data: In experimental models, mycophenolate mofetil was not tumourigenic and did not demonstrate mutagenic activity. The highest dose tested in the animal carcinogenicity studies resulted in approximately 2 to 3 times the systemic exposure (AUC or Cmax) observed in renal transplant patients at the recommended clinical dose of 2 g per day and 1.3–2 times the systemic exposure (AUC or Cmax) observed in cardiac transplant patients at the recommended clinical dose of 3 g per day.

Mycophenolate mofetil had no effect on fertility of

Table 2: Adverse Events Reported in ≥ 3% and < 10% of Patients Treated With CellCept in Combination With Cyclosporine and Corticosteroids

Body System	*Events Reported in Both Renal and Cardiac Transplant Studies*	*Events Reported in Renal Transplant Studies Only 991 CellCept treated patients**	*Events Reported in Cardiac Transplant Study 1864 Only 289 CellCept treated patients***
Body as a Whole	enlarged abdomen, cysts (including lymphocele and hydrocele), fever, flu syndrome, facial oedema, haemorrhage, malaise, pelvic pain, hernia	—	cellulitis, neck pain, pallor
Blood and Lymphatic	—	ecchymosis, polycythaemia	petechia, prothrombin increased, thromboplastin time increased
Urogenital	dysuria, impotence, urinary frequency	albuminuria, hydronephrosis, pyelonephritis	haematuria, nocturia, renal failure, urinary incontinence, urinary retention
Cardiovascular	angina pectoris, atrial fibrillation, postural hypotension	hypotension, tachycardia, thrombosis, vasodilatation	arrhythmias (including supraventricular extrasystoles, atrial flutter, supraventricular and ventricular tachycardias), cardiac arrest, congestive heart failure, pulmonary hypertension, syncope, vasospasm, venous pressure increased
Metabolic/Nutritional	alkaline phosphatase increased, dehydration, hypervolaemia, hypocalcinaemia, hypoglycaemia, hypoproteinaemia	acidosis, elevated enzyme levels (gamma glutamyl transpeptidase, lactic dehydrogenase, SGOT and SGPT), elevated creatinine, hypercalcaemia, hyperlipaemia, hyperuricaemia, weight gain	abnormal healing, alkalosis, gout, hypochloraemia, hypophosphataemia, hypoxia, respiratory acidosis, thirst, weight loss
Gastrointestinal	anorexia, gingivitis, gum hyperplasia, gastroenteritis, abnormal liver function, oesophagitis, stomatitis	flatulence, gastrointestinal haemorrhage, gastrointestinal moniliasis, hepatitis, ileus	dysphagia, jaundice, melaena
Respiratory	pulmonary oedema	asthma, pleural effusion, rhinitis, sinusitis	apnoea, atelectasis, bronchitis, epistaxis, haemoptysis, hiccough, neoplasm, pneumothorax, sputum increased, voice alteration
Skin and Appendages	benign neoplasm of skin, skin carcinoma, fungal dermatitis, skin hypertrophy, pruritus, sweating, skin ulcer	alopecia, herpes zoster, hirsutism, rash	haemorrhage
Nervous		anxiety, depression, hypertonia, paresthesia, somnolence	convulsion, emotional lability, hallucinations, neuropathy, thinking abnormal, vertigo
Musculoskeletal	arthralgia	leg cramps, myalgia, myasthenia	—
Special Senses	conjunctivitis	amblyopia, cataract	abnormal vision, deafness, ear pain, eye haemorrhage, tinnitus
Endocrine	diabetes mellitus	parathyroid disorder	Cushing's syndrome, hypothyroidism

* (total n=1,483)
** (total n=578)

male rats at oral doses up to 20 mg/kg/day. The systemic exposure at this dose represents 2 to 3 times the clinical exposure at the recommended clinical dose of 2 g per day in renal transplant patients and 1.3–2 times the clinical exposure at the recommended clinical dose of 3 g per day in cardiac transplant patients. In a female fertility and reproduction study conducted in rats, oral doses of 4.5 mg/kg/day caused malformations (including anophthalmia, agnathia, and hydrocephaly) in the first generation offspring in the absence of maternal toxicity. The systemic exposure at this dose was approximately 0.5 times the clinical exposure at the recommended clinical dose of 2 g per day for renal transplant patients and approximately 0.3 times the clinical exposure at the recommended clinical dose of 3 g per day for cardiac transplant patients. No effects on fertility or reproductive parameters were evident in the dams or in the subsequent generation.

In teratology studies in rats and rabbits, foetal resorptions and malformations occurred in rats at 6 mg/kg/day (including anophthalmia, agnathia, and hydrocephaly) and in rabbits at 90 mg/kg/day (including cardiovascular and renal anomalies, such as ectopia cordis and ectopic kidneys, and diaphragmatic and umbilical hernia), in the absence of maternal toxicity. The systemic exposure at these levels are approximately equivalent to or less than 0.5 times the clinical exposure at the recommended clinical dose of 2 g per day for renal transplant patients and approximately 0.3 times the clinical exposure at the recommended clinical dose of 3 g per day for cardiac transplant patients.

Refer to *Pregnancy and lactation.*

The haematopoietic and lymphoid systems were the primary organs affected in toxicology studies conducted with mycophenolate mofetil in the rat, mouse, dog and monkey. These effects occurred at systemic exposure levels that are equivalent to or less than the clinical exposure at the recommended dose of 2 g per day for renal transplant recipients. Gastrointestinal effects were observed in the dog at systemic exposure levels equivalent to or less than the clinical exposure at the recommended doses. Gastrointestinal and renal effects consistent with dehydration were also observed in the monkey at the highest dose (systemic exposure levels equivalent to or greater than clinical exposure). The nonclinical toxicity profile of mycophenolate mofetil appears to be consistent with adverse events observed in human clinical trials which now provide safety data of more relevance to the patient population (see *Undesirable effects*).

Pharmaceutical particulars

List of excipients: Excipients of CellCept capsules are pregelatinized maize starch, croscarmellose sodium, polyvidone (K-90) and magnesium stearate. The capsule shells contain gelatin, indigo carmine (FP, E132), yellow iron oxide (FP, E172), red iron oxide (FP, E172), titanium dioxide (EP, E171), black iron oxide (FP, E172) potassium hydroxide and shellac.

Incompatibilities: None.

Shelf life: CellCept capsules have a shelf life of three years when stored in opaque polyvinyl chloride blister packs at temperatures not exceeding 30°C.

Special precautions for storage: Store at or below 30°C.

Nature and contents of container: CellCept 250 mg capsules: 1 carton contains 100 capsules (in blister packs of 10), 1 carton contains 300 capsules (in blister packs of 10)

Instructions for use and handling, and disposal (if appropriate): Because mycophenolate mofetil has demonstrated teratogenic effects in rats and rabbits, CellCept capsules should not be opened or crushed. Avoid inhalation or direct contact with skin or mucous membranes of the powder contained in CellCept capsules. If such contact occurs, wash thoroughly with soap and water; rinse eyes with plain water.

Numbers in the community register of medicinal products
EU/1/96/005/001 CellCept (100 capsules)
EU/1/96/005/003 CellCept (300 capsules)

Date of first authorisation/renewal of the authorisation
14 February 1996 (EU/1/96/005/001)
13 May 1997 (EU/1/96/005/003)

Date of revision of the text October 1998

CELLCEPT 500 mg TABLETS 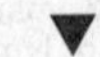

Qualitative and quantitative composition Each tablet contains 500 mg mycophenolate mofetil.

Pharmaceutical form CellCept tablets: Lavender coloured caplet-shaped tablet, branded with black 'CellCept 500' on one side and 'Company logo' on the other.

Clinical particulars

Therapeutic indications: CellCept is indicated in combination with cyclosporin and corticosteroids for the prophylaxis of acute transplant rejection in patients receiving allogeneic renal or cardiac transplants.

Posology and method of administration: Treatment with CellCept should be initiated and maintained by appropriately qualified transplant specialists.

Use in renal transplant: the initial dose of CellCept should be given orally within 72 hours following transplantation. The recommended dose in renal transplant patients is 1.0 g administered twice daily (2 g daily dose). Although daily doses of both 2 g and 3 g were studied in clinical trials, an efficacy advantage for the 3 g dose could not be established for renal transplant patients. In renal transplant, patients receiving 2 g per day of CellCept had an overall better safety profile than patients receiving 3 g per day.

Use in cardiac transplant: the initial dose of CellCept should be given orally within 5 days following transplantation. The recommended dose in cardiac transplant patients is 1.5 g administered twice daily (3 g daily dose).

Use in children: safety and effectiveness in paediatric patients have not been established. Very limited pharmacokinetic data are available for paediatric renal transplant patients. No data are available for paediatric cardiac transplant patients.

Use in elderly: the recommended dose of 1.0 g administered twice a day for renal transplant patients and 1.5 g twice a day for cardiac transplant patients is appropriate for elderly patients. This recommendation is based on limited numbers of elderly patients treated with CellCept in the pivotal renal (7% n = 73) and cardiac (7% n = 20) transplant trials. Patients in this age group may generally be at increased risk of adverse events compared to younger individuals; this is similarly true for patients receiving CellCept as part of a combination immunosuppressive regimen (see *Undesirable effects*).

Use in renal impairment: in renal transplant patients with severe chronic renal impairment (glomerular filtration rate < 25 ml/min/1.73 m^2), outside of the immediate post-transplant period, doses greater than 1 g administered twice a day should be avoided. These patients should also be carefully observed. No dose adjustments are needed in patients experiencing delayed renal graft function post-operatively (see *Pharmacokinetic properties*).

No data are available for cardiac transplant patients with severe chronic renal impairment.

Use in severe hepatic impairment: no dose adjustments are needed for renal patients with severe hepatic parenchymal disease. No data are available for cardiac patients with severe hepatic parenchymal disease.

Other considerations for use: if neutropenia develops (absolute neutrophil count $<1.3\times10^3/\mu l$), physicians should perform appropriate diagnostic tests, manage the patients appropriately, and consider interrupting dosing with CellCept.

MPA (mycophenolic acid) is the active metabolite of mycophenolate mofetil. Food has no effect on MPA area under the curve (AUC), but has been shown to decrease Cmax by 40%. It is recommended that CellCept be administered on an empty stomach.

Renal transplant rejection does not lead to changes in MPA pharmacokinetics requiring dosage reduction or interruption of CellCept. Similarly, there is no basis for adjustment of dose following cardiac transplant rejection.

Contra-indications: Allergic reactions to CellCept have been observed. Therefore, CellCept is contra-indicated in patients with a hypersensitivity to mycophenolate mofetil or mycophenolic acid. For information on use in pregnancy and contraceptive requirements see *Use during pregnancy and lactation.*

Special warnings and special precautions for use: As in patients receiving immunosuppressive regimes involving combinations of drugs, patients receiving CellCept as part of an immunosuppressive regime are at increased risk of developing lymphomas and other malignancies, particularly of the skin (see *Undesirable effects*). The risk appears to be related to the intensity and duration of immunosuppression rather than to the use of any specific agent.

As usual for patients with increased risk for skin cancer, exposure to sunlight and UV light should be limited by wearing protective clothing and using a sunscreen with a high protection factor.

Oversuppression of the immune system can also increase susceptibility to infection including opportunistic infections, fatal infections and sepsis. In three controlled trials for prevention of renal transplant rejection, patients receiving 2 g per day of CellCept demonstrated an overall better safety profile than did patients receiving 3 g of CellCept. In cardiac transplant patients the overall incidence of opportunistic infections was approximately 10% higher in patients treated with CellCept than in those receiving azathioprine therapy but this did not translate into excess mortality. There were more herpes virus and cytomegalovirus infections in CellCept treated cardiac transplant patients compared to those treated with azathioprine.

Patients receiving CellCept should be monitored for neutropenia. The development of neutropenia may be related to CellCept itself, concomitant medications, viral infections, or some combination of these causes. Patients on CellCept should have complete blood counts weekly during the first month, twice monthly for the second and third months of treatment, then monthly through the first year (see *Posology and method of administration*).

Patients receiving CellCept should be instructed to report immediately any evidence of infection, unexpected bruising, bleeding or any other manifestation of bone marrow depression.

Because CellCept has been associated with an increased incidence of digestive system adverse events, including infrequent cases of gastrointestinal tract ulceration, haemorrhage and perforation, CellCept should be administered with caution in patients with active serious digestive system disease.

Administration of doses greater than 1 g BID to renal transplant patients with severe chronic renal impairment should be avoided and they should be carefully observed. No dose adjustment is recommended for patients with delayed renal graft function post-transplant, however, they should be carefully observed (see *Posology and method of administration*, and *Pharmacokinetic properties*). No data are available for cardiac transplant patients with severe chronic renal impairment.

It is recommended that CellCept not be administered concomitantly with azathioprine because such concomitant administration has not been studied.

In view of the significant reduction in the AUC of MPA by cholestyramine, caution should be used in the concomitant administration of CellCept with drugs that interfere with enterohepatic recirculation because of the potential to reduce the efficacy of CellCept.

Table 1: Adverse Events Reported in ≥ 10% of Patients Treated with CellCept in Combination with Cyclosporine and Corticosteroids

Body System	*Events Reported in Both Renal and Cardiac Transplant Studies*	*Events Reported in Renal Transplant Studies Only 991 CellCept treated patients**	*Events Reported in Cardiac Transplant Study MYCS 1864 Only 289 CellCept treated patients***
Body as a Whole	asthenia, fever, headache, infection, pain, (includes abdominal, back and chest), oedema	—	—
Blood and Lymphatic	anaemia, (including hypochromic anaemia), leukocytosis, leukopenia, thrombocytopenia	—	ecchymosis
Urogenital	urinary tract infection	haematuria, renal tubular necrosis	abnormal kidney function, oliguria
Cardiovascular	hypertension	—	arrhythmia, bradycardia, hypotension, cardiac failure, pericardial effusion
Metabolic/Nutritional	hypercholesterolaemia, hyperglycaemia, hyperkalaemia, hypokalaemia	hypophosphataemia	acidosis, bilirubinaemia, elevated BUN, elevated creatinine, elevated enzyme levels (lactic dehydrogenase, SGOT and SGPT), hyperlipaemia, hyperuricaemia, hypervolaemia, hypomagnesaemia, hyponatraemia, weight gain
Gastrointestinal	constipation, diarrhoea, dyspepsia, oral moniliasis, nausea and vomiting	—	flatulence
Respiratory	cough increased, dyspnoea, pharyngitis, pneumonia	bronchitis	asthma, rhinitis, pleural effusion, sinusitis
Skin and Appendages	acne, herpes simplex	—	herpes zoster, rash
Nervous	dizziness, insomnia, tremor	—	anxiety, agitation, confusion, depression, hypertonia, paresthesia, somnolence
Musculoskeletal	—	—	leg cramps, myalgia, myasthaenia
Special Senses	—	—	amblyopia

* (total n=1,483)
** (total n=578)

Interaction with other medicaments and other forms of interaction:

Acyclovir: higher MPAG and acyclovir plasma concentrations were observed when mycophenolate mofetil was administered with acyclovir in comparison to the administration of each drug alone. Because MPAG plasma concentrations are increased in the presence of renal impairment, as are acyclovir concentrations, the potential exists for the two drugs to compete for tubular secretion and thus further increases in concentrations of both drugs may occur.

Antacids with magnesium and aluminum hydroxides: absorption of mycophenolate mofetil was decreased when administered with antacids.

Cholestyramine: following single dose administration of 1.5 g of mycophenolate mofetil to normal healthy subjects pretreated with 4 g TID of cholestyramine for 4 days, there was a 40% reduction in the AUC of MPA.

Cyclosporin A: cyclosporin A pharmacokinetics were unaffected by mycophenolate mofetil.

Ganciclovir: based on the results of a single dose administration study of recommended doses of oral mycophenolate and IV ganciclovir and the known effects of renal impairment on the pharmacokinetics of MMF (see *Special warnings and special precautions for use*) and ganciclovir, it is anticipated that co-administration of these agents (which compete for mechanisms of renal tubular secretion) will result in increases in MPAG and ganciclovir concentration. No substantial alteration of MPA pharmacokinetics are anticipated and MMF dose adjustment is not required. In patients with renal impairment in which MMF and ganciclovir are co-administered the dose recommendations for ganciclovir should be observed and patients monitored carefully.

Oral contraceptives: no pharmacokinetic interaction was observed between mycophenolate mofetil and 1 mg norethisterone/35µg ethinyloestradiol. This single dose study demonstrates the lack of a gross pharmacokinetic interaction, but cannot exclude the possibility of changes in the pharmacokinetics of the oral contraceptive under long term dosing conditions with CellCept which might adversely affect the efficacy of the oral contraceptive.

Trimethoprim/sulphamethoxazole: no effect on the bioavailability of MPA was observed.

Other interactions: co-administration of probenecid with mycophenolate mofetil in monkeys raises plasma AUC of MPAG by 3-fold. Thus, other drugs known to undergo renal tubular secretion may compete with MPAG and thereby raise plasma concentrations of MPAG or the other drug undergoing tubular secretion. Single dose studies of CellCept with ganciclovir and trimethoprim/sulphamethoxazole did not reveal a pharmacokinetic interaction between either of these agents and CellCept. All these types of compounds operate through inhibition of nucleoside synthesis and therefore one cannot exclude a clinical interaction between them.

Use during pregnancy and lactation: Adverse effects on foetal development (including malformations) occurred when pregnant rats and rabbits were dosed during organogenesis (see *Preclinical safety data*). Because there are no adequate and well controlled studies in pregnant women, CellCept should be used in pregnant women only if the potential benefit outweighs the potential risk to the foetus.

It is recommended that CellCept therapy should not be initiated until a negative pregnancy test has been obtained. Patients should be instructed to consult their physician immediately should pregnancy occur.

Effective contraception must be used before beginning CellCept therapy, during therapy, and for six weeks following discontinuation of therapy. Although the results of a single dose drug interaction study with an oral contraceptive suggest the lack of a gross pharmacokinetic interaction, the results cannot exclude the possibility of changes in the pharmacokinetics of the oral contraceptive under long term dosing conditions with CellCept which might adversely affect the efficacy of the oral contraceptive (see *Interaction with other medicinal products*).

Studies in rats have shown mycophenolate mofetil to be excreted in milk. It is not known whether this drug is excreted in human milk. Because many drugs are excreted in human milk and because of the potential for serious adverse reactions in nursing infants from mycophenolate mofetil, a decision should be made whether to discontinue nursing or to discontinue the drug, taking into account the importance of the drug to the mother.

Effects on ability to drive and use machines: No specific studies have been performed. The pharmacodynamic profile and the reported adverse reactions indicate that an effect is unlikely.

Undesirable effects: The principal adverse reactions associated with the administration of CellCept in combination with cyclosporine and corticosteroids include diarrhoea, leukopenia, sepsis and vomiting and there is evidence of a higher frequency of certain types of infections (see *Special warnings and special precautions for use*).

As in patients receiving immunosuppressive regimes involving combinations of drugs, patients receiving CellCept as part of an immunosuppressive regime are at increased risk of developing lymphomas and other malignancies, particularly of the skin (see *Special warnings and special precautions for use*). Within 3 years post-transplant, lymphoproliferative disease or lymphoma developed in patients receiving CellCept in immunosuppressive regimens in 1.6% of the patients receiving 3 g daily and 0.6% in patients receiving 2 g daily in the controlled studies of prevention of renal rejection compared to the placebo (0%) and azathioprine groups (0.6%). In cardiac transplant patients, the incidence of lymphoproliferative disease was 0.7% in patients receiving CellCept 3 g daily compared to patients receiving azathioprine (2.1%). The incidence of non-melanoma skin cancer in cardiac transplant patients treated with CellCept 3 g per day was 5.5% compared to patients treated with azathioprine (6.9%). Cardiac transplant patients had been followed for a maximum of 3 years with 26% of these followed for less than a year and 34% followed for greater than 2 years. All patients are at increased risk of opportunistic infections, the risk increased with dose (see *Special warnings and special precautions for use*).

Elderly patients, particularly those who are receiving CellCept as part of a combination immunosuppressive regimen, may be at greater increased risk of certain infections (including CMV tissue invasive disease) and possibly gastrointestinal haemorrhage and pulmonary oedema, compared to younger individuals (see *Posology and method of administration*).

Adverse reactions reported in ≥ 10% of patients treated with CellCept in the three Phase III controlled trials for prevention of renal transplant rejection and/or the Phase III controlled cardiac transplant trial are listed in Table 1 on the previous page.

Adverse events, not mentioned in Table 1, reported in ≥ 3% and < 10% in renal transplant and/or cardiac transplant patients are listed in Table 2.

Adverse reactions during post marketing experience with CellCept are similar to those seen in the controlled renal and cardiac transplant studies.

Table 2: Adverse Events Reported in ≥ 3% and < 10% of Patients Treated With CellCept in Combination With Cyclosporine and Corticosteroids

Body System	*Events Reported in Both Renal and Cardiac Transplant Studies*	*Events Reported in Renal Transplant Studies Only 991 CellCept treated patients**	*Events Reported in Cardiac Transplant Study 1864 Only 289 CellCept treated patients***
Body as a Whole	enlarged abdomen, cysts (including lymphocele and hydrocele), fever, flu syndrome, facial oedema, haemorrhage, malaise, pelvic pain, hernia	—	cellulitis, neck pain, pallor
Blood and Lymphatic	—	ecchymosis, polycythaemia	petechia, prothrombin increased, thromboplastin time increased
Urogenital	dysuria, impotence, urinary frequency	albuminuria, hydronephrosis, pyelonephritis	haematuria, nocturia, renal failure, urinary incontinence, urinary retention
Cardiovascular	angina pectoris, atrial fibrillation, postural hypotension	hypotension, tachycardia, thrombosis, vasodilatation	arrhythmias (including supraventricular and ventricular extrasystoles, atrial flutter, supraventricular and ventricular tachycardias), cardiac arrest, congestive heart failure, pulmonary hypertension, syncope, vasospasm, venous pressure increased
Metabolic/Nutritional	alkaline phosphatase increased, dehydration, hypervolaemia, hypocalcinaemia, hypoglycaemia, hypoproteinaemia	acidosis, elevated enzyme levels (gamma glutamyl transpeptidase, lactic dehydrogenase, SGOT and SGPT), elevated creatinine, hypercalcaemia, hyperlipaemia, hyperuricaemia, weight gain	abnormal healing, alkalosis, gout, hypochloraemia, hypophosphataemia, hypoxia, respiratory acidosis, thirst, weight loss
Gastrointestinal	anorexia, gingivitis, gum hyperplasia, gastroenteritis, abnormal liver function, oesophagitis, stomatitis	flatulence, gastrointestinal haemorrhage, gastrointestinal moniliasis, hepatitis, ileus	dysphagia, jaundice, melaena
Respiratory	pulmonary oedema	asthma, pleural effusion, rhinitis, sinusitis	apnoea, atelectasis, bronchitis, epistaxis, haemoptysis, hiccough, neoplasm, pneumothorax, sputum increased, voice alteration
Skin and Appendages	benign neoplasm of skin, skin carcinoma, fungal dermatitis, skin hypertrophy, pruritus, sweating, skin ulcer	alopecia, herpes zoster, hirsutism, rash	haemorrhage
Nervous	—	anxiety, depression, hypertonia, paresthesia, somnolence	convulsion, emotional lability, hallucinations, neuropathy, thinking abnormal, vertigo
Musculoskeletal	arthralgia	leg cramps, myalgia, myasthenia	—
Special Senses	conjunctivitis	amblyopia, cataract	abnormal vision, deafness, ear pain, eye haemorrhage, tinnitus
Endocrine	diabetes mellitus	parathyroid disorder	Cushing's syndrome, hypothyroidism

* (total n=1,483)
** (total n=578)

Post-marketing experience: Gastro-intestinal: colitis (sometimes caused by cytomegalovirus), pancreatitis.

Disorders of immunosuppression: serious, life-threatening infections such as meningitis and infectious endocarditis have been reported occasionally and there is evidence of a higher frequency of certain types of infections such as tuberculosis and atypical mycobacterial infection.

Overdose: There has been no reported experience of overdosage of mycophenolate mofetil in humans.
At clinically encountered concentrations, MPA and MPAG are not removed by haemodialysis. However, at high MPAG plasma concentrations (> 100µg/ml), small amounts of MPAG are removed. By interfering with enterohepatic circulation of the drug, bile acid sequestrants, such as cholestyramine reduce the MPA AUC.

Pharmacological properties

Pharmacodynamic properties: Pharmacotherapeutic group: immunosuppressant ATC code LO4AA06

Mycophenolate mofetil is the 2-morpholinoethyl ester of MPA. MPA is a potent, selective, uncompetitive and reversible inhibitor of inosine monophosphate dehydrogenase, and therefore inhibits the *de novo* pathway of guanosine nucleotide synthesis without incorporation into DNA. Because T- and B-lymphocytes are critically dependent for their proliferation on *de novo* synthesis of purines whereas other cell types can utilise salvage pathways, MPA has more potent cytostatic effects on lymphocytes than on other cells.

Pharmacokinetic properties: MPA at clinically relevant concentrations, is 97% bound to plasma albumin.

Following oral administration, mycophenolate mofetil undergoes rapid and extensive absorption and complete presystemic metabolism to the active metabolite, MPA. As evidenced by suppression of acute rejection following renal transplantation, the immunosuppressant activity of CellCept is correlated with MPA concentration. Mycophenolate mofetil is not measurable systemically in plasma following oral administration.

MPA is metabolised principally by glucuronyl transferase to form the phenolic glucoronide of MPA (MPAG), which is not pharmacologically active.

As a result of enterohepatic recirculation, secondary increases in plasma MPA concentration are usually observed at approximately 6–12 hours post-dose. A reduction in the AUC of MPA of approximately 40% is associated with the co-administration of cholestyramine (4 g TID), indicating that there is a significant amount of enterohepatic recirculation.

Negligible amount of drug is excreted as MPA (< 1% of dose) in the urine. Orally administered radiolabelled mycophenolate mofetil resulted in complete recovery of the administered dose; with 93% of the administered dose recovered in the urine and 6% recovered in the faeces. Most (about 87%) of the administered dose is excreted in the urine as MPAG.

The mean bioavailability of oral mycophenolate mofetil, based on MPA AUC, was 94% relative to IV mycophenolate mofetil .

Food had no effect on the extent of absorption (MPA AUC) of mycophenolate mofetil when administered at doses of 1.5 g BID to renal transplant patients. However, MPA Cmax was decreased by 40% in the presence of food.

Immediately post-transplant (< 40 days), mean MPA AUC and Cmax are approximately 50% lower in renal and cardiac transplant patients than that observed in healthy volunteers or in stable renal transplant patients.

In a single dose study (6 subjects per group), mean plasma MPA AUC observed in subjects with severe chronic renal impairment (glomerular filtration rate < 25 ml/min/1.73 m^2) were 28–75% higher relative to the means observed in normal healthy subjects or subjects with lesser degrees of renal impairment. However, the mean single dose MPAG AUC was 3–6 fold higher in subjects with severe renal impairment than in subjects with mild renal impairment or normal healthy subjects, consistent with the known renal elimination of MPAG. Multiple dosing of mycophenolate mofetil in patients with severe chronic renal impairment has not been studied. No data are available for cardiac transplant patients with severe chronic renal impairment.

In patients with delayed graft function post-transplant, mean MPA AUC_{0-12} was comparable to that seen in post-transplant patients without delayed graft function. Mean plasma MPAG AUC_{0-12} was 2–3 fold higher than in post-transplant patients without delayed graft function.

In volunteers with alcoholic cirrhosis, hepatic MPA glucuronidation processes were relatively unaffected by hepatic parenchymal disease. Effects of hepatic disease on this process probably depend on the particular disease. However, hepatic disease with predominantly biliary damage, such as primary biliary cirrhosis, may show a different effect.

Pharmacokinetic behaviour of CellCept in the elderly has not been formally evaluated.

Preclinical safety data: In experimental models, mycophenolate mofetil was not tumorigenic and did not demonstrate mutagenic activity. The highest dose tested in the animal carcinogenicity studies resulted in approximately 2 to 3 times the systemic exposure (AUC or Cmax) observed in renal transplant patients at the recommended clinical dose of 2 g per day and 1.3–2 times the systemic exposure (AUC or Cmax) observed in cardiac transplant patients at the recommended clinical dose of 3 g per day.

Mycophenolate mofetil had no effect on fertility of male rats at oral doses up to 20 mg/kg/day. The systemic exposure at this dose represents 2 to 3 times the clinical exposure at the recommended clinical dose of 2 g per day in renal transplant patients and 1.3–2 times the clinical exposure at the recommended clinical dose of 3 g per day in cardiac transplant patients. In a female fertility and reproduction study conducted in rats, oral doses of 4.5 mg/kg/day caused malformations (including anophthalmia, agnathia, and hydrocephaly) in the first generation offspring in the absence of maternal toxicity. The systemic exposure at this dose was approximately 0.5 times the clinical exposure at the recommended clinical dose of 2 g per day for renal transplant patients and approximately 0.3 times the clinical exposure at the recommended clinical dose of 3 g per day for cardiac transplant patients. No effects on fertility or reproductive parameters were evident in the dams or in the subsequent generation.

In teratology studies in rats and rabbits, foetal resorptions and malformations occurred in rats at 6 mg/kg/day (including anophthalmia, agnathia, and hydrocephaly) and in rabbits at 90 mg/kg/day (including cardiovascular and renal anomalies, such as ectopia cordis and ectopic kidneys, and diaphragmatic and umbilical hernia), in the absence of maternal toxicity. The systemic exposure at these levels are approximately equivalent to or less than 0.5 times the clinical exposure at the recommended clinical dose of 2 g per day for renal transplant patients and approximately 0.3 times the clinical exposure at the recommended clinical dose of 3 g per day for cardiac transplant patients.

Refer to *Pregnancy and lactation.*

The haematopoietic and lymphoid systems were the primary organs affected in toxicology studies conducted with mycophenolate mofetil in the rat, mouse, dog and monkey. These effects occurred at systemic exposure levels that are equivalent to or less than the clinical exposure at the recommended dose of 2 g per day for renal transplant recipients. Gastrointestinal effects were observed in the dog at systemic exposure levels equivalent to or less than the clinical exposure at the recommended doses. Gastrointestinal and renal effects consistent with dehydration were also observed in the monkey at the highest dose (systemic exposure levels equivalent to or greater than clinical exposure). The nonclinical toxicity profile of mycophenolate mofetil appears to be consistent with adverse events observed in human clinical trials which now provide safety data of more relevance to the patient population (see *Undesirable effects*).

Pharmaceutical particulars

List of excipients: Excipients of CellCept tablets are microcrystalline cellulose, polyvidone (K-90), croscarmellose sodium and magnesium stearate. The tablet coating consists of hydroxypropyl methylcellulose, hydroxypropyl cellulose, titanium dioxide (EP, E171), polyethylene glycol 400, indigo carmine aluminium lake (E132), red iron oxide (FP, E172), black iron oxide (FP, E172) and shellac.

Incompatibilities: None.

Shelf life: CellCept tablets have a shelf life of three years when stored in opaque polyvinyl chloride blister packs at temperatures not exceeding 30°C.

Special precautions for storage: Store at or below 30°C. CellCept tablets should be protected from light.

Nature and contents of container: CellCept 500 mg tablets: 1 carton contains 50 tablets (in blister packs of 10)1 carton contains 150 tablets (in blister packs of 10)

Instructions for use and handling, and disposal (if appropriate): Because mycophenolate mofetil has demonstrated teratogenic effects in rats and rabbits, CellCept tablets should not be crushed.

Numbers in the community register of medicinal products

EU/1/96/005/002 CellCept (50 tablets)
EU/1/96/005/004 CellCept (150 tablets)

Date of first authorisation/renewal of authorisation

14 February 1996 (EU/1/96/005/002)
13 May 1997 (EU/1/96/005/004)

CELLCEPT 500 mg powder for concentrate for solution for infusion ▼

Qualitative and quantitative composition Each vial contains the equivalent of 500 mg mycophenolate mofetil (as hydrochloride salt).

Pharmaceutical form Powder for concentrate for solution for infusion.

CellCept 500 mg powder for concentrate for solution for infusion must be reconstituted and further diluted with glucose intravenous infusion 5% prior to administration to the patient. (See *Instructions for use and handling*).

Clinical particulars

Therapeutic indications: CellCept 500 mg powder for concentrate for solution for infusion is indicated in combination with cyclosporin and corticosteroids for the prophylaxis of acute transplant rejection in patients receiving allogeneic renal transplants.

Posology and method of administration: Treatment with CellCept should be initiated and maintained by appropriately qualified transplant specialists.

CAUTION: CELLCEPT I.V. SOLUTION SHOULD NEVER BE ADMINISTERED BY RAPID OR BOLUS INTRAVENOUS INJECTION.

CellCept 500 mg powder for concentrate for solution for infusion is an alternative dosage form to CellCept oral forms (capsules and tablets) that may be administered for up to 14 days. The initial dose of CellCept 500 mg powder for concentrate for solution for infusion should be given within 24 hours following transplantation.

Following reconstitution to a concentration of 6 mg/ml, CellCept 500 mg powder for concentrate for solution for infusion must be administered by slow intravenous infusion over a period of 2 hours by either a peripheral or a central vein. (See *Instructions for use and handling*). Oral administration should be initiated as soon as patients tolerate oral medication.

The recommended dose in renal transplant patients is 1 g administered twice daily (2 g daily dose). Although daily doses of both 2 g and 3 g were studied in clinical trials using CellCept oral, an efficacy advantage for the 3 g dose could not be established for renal transplant patients. In renal transplant, patients receiving 2 g per day of CellCept oral had an overall better safety profile than patients receiving 3 g per day.

Use in children: safety and effectiveness in paediatric patients have not been established. Very limited pharmacokinetic data are available for paediatric renal transplant patients.

Use in elderly: the recommended dose of 1 g administered twice a day is appropriate for elderly patients. This recommendation is based on limited numbers of elderly patients treated with CellCept in the pivotal renal (7% n = 73) transplant trials. Patients in this age group may generally be at increased risk of adverse events compared to younger individuals; this is similarly true for patients receiving CellCept as part of a combination immunosuppressive regimen. (See *Undesirable effects*).

Use in renal impairment: in patients with severe chronic renal impairment (glomerular filtration rate < 25 ml/min/1.73 m²), outside of the immediate post-transplant period, doses greater than 1 g administered twice a day should be avoided. These patients should also be carefully observed. No dose adjustments are needed in patients experiencing delayed graft function post-operatively (see *Pharmacokinetic properties*).

Use in severe hepatic impairment: no dose adjustments are needed for patients with severe hepatic parenchymal disease.

Other considerations for use: if neutropenia develops (absolute neutrophil count < 1.3 x 10³/µl), physicians should perform appropriate diagnostic tests, manage the patients appropriately, and consider interrupting dosing with CellCept.

MPA (mycophenolic acid) is the active metabolite of mycophenolate mofetil. Renal transplant rejection does not lead to changes in MPA pharmacokinetics requiring dosage reduction or interruption of CellCept.

Contra-indications: Allergic reactions to CellCept have been observed. Therefore, CellCept is contra-indicated in patients with a hypersensitivity to mycophenolate mofetil or mycophenolic acid. CellCept 500 mg powder for concentrate for solution for infusion is contra-indicated in patients who are allergic to polysorbate 80. For information on use in pregnancy and contraceptive requirements, see *Pregnancy and lactation.*

Special warnings and special precautions for use: As in patients receiving immunosuppressive regimes involving combinations of drugs, patients receiving CellCept as part of an immunosuppressive regime are at increased risk of developing lymphomas and other malignancies, particularly of the skin (see *Undesirable effects*). The risk appears to be related to the intensity and duration of immunosuppression rather than to the use of any specific agent. As usual for patients with increased risk for skin cancer, exposure to sunlight and UV light should be limited by wearing protective clothing and using a sunscreen with a high protection factor.

Oversuppression of the immune system can also increase susceptibility to infection including opportunistic infections, fatal infections and sepsis. In three controlled trials for prevention of renal transplant rejection, patients receiving 2 g per day of CellCept demonstrated an overall better safety profile than did patients receiving 3 g of CellCept.

Patients receiving CellCept should be monitored for neutropenia. The development of neutropenia may be related to CellCept itself, concomitant medications, viral infections, or some combination of these causes. Patients on CellCept should have complete blood counts weekly during the first month, twice monthly for the second and third months of treatment, then monthly through the first year (see *Posology and method of administration*).

Patients receiving CellCept should be instructed to report immediately any evidence of infection, unexpected bruising, bleeding or any other manifestation of bone marrow depression.

Because CellCept has been associated with an increased incidence of digestive system adverse events, including infrequent cases of gastrointestinal tract ulceration, haemorrhage and perforation. CellCept should be administered with caution in patients with active serious digestive system disease.

Administration of doses greater than 1 g BID to patients with severe chronic renal impairment should be avoided and they should be carefully observed. No dose adjustment is recommended for patients with delayed renal graft function post-transplant, however, they should be carefully observed (see *Posology and method of administration,* and *Pharmacokinetic properties*).

It is recommended that CellCept not be administered concomitantly with azathioprine because such concomitant administration has not been studied.

In view of the significant reduction in the AUC of MPA by cholestyramine, caution should be used in the concomitant administration of CellCept with drugs that interfere with enterohepatic recirculation because of the potential to reduce the efficacy of CellCept. Some degree of enterohepatic recirculation is anticipated following intravenous administration of CellCept.

Interaction with other medicaments and other forms of interaction

Acyclovir: higher MPAG and acyclovir plasma concentrations were observed when mycophenolate mofetil was administered with acyclovir in comparison to the administration of each drug alone. Because MPAG plasma concentrations are increased in the presence of renal impairment, as are acyclovir concentrations, the potential exists for the two drugs to compete for tubular secretion and thus further increases in concentrations of both drugs may occur.

Cholestyramine: following single dose, oral administration of 1.5 g of mycophenolate mofetil to normal healthy subjects pretreated with 4 g TID of cholestyramine for 4 days, there was a 40% reduction in the AUC of MPA.

Cyclosporin A: cyclosporin A pharmacokinetics were unaffected by mycophenolate mofetil.

Ganciclovir: based on the results of a single dose administration study of recommended doses of oral mycophenolate and iv ganciclovir and the known effects of renal impairment on the pharmacokinetics of MMF (see *Special warnings and special precautions for use*) and ganciclovir, it is anticipated that coadministration of these agents (which compete for mechanisms of renal tubular secretion) will result in increases in MPAG and ganciclovir concentration. No substantial alteration of MPA pharmacokinetics are anticipated and MMF dose adjustment is not required. In patients with renal impairment in which MMF and ganciclovir are coadministered the dose recommendations for ganciclovir should be observed and patients monitored carefully.

Oral contraceptives: no pharmacokinetic interaction was observed between mycophenolate mofetil and 1 mg norethisterone/35µg ethinyloestradiol. This single dose study demonstrates the lack of a gross pharmacokinetic interaction, but cannot exclude the possibility of changes in the pharmacokinetics of the oral contraceptive under long term dosing conditions with CellCept which might adversely affect the efficacy of the oral contraceptive.

Trimethoprim/sulphamethoxazole: no effect on the bioavailability of MPA was observed.

Other interactions: co-administration of probenecid with mycophenolate mofetil in monkeys raises plasma AUC of MPAG by 3-fold. Thus, other drugs known to undergo renal tubular secretion may compete with MPAG and thereby raise plasma concentrations of MPAG or the other drug undergoing tubular secretion. Single dose studies of CellCept with ganciclovir and trimethoprim/ sulphamethoxazole did not reveal a pharmacokinetic interaction between either of these agents and CellCept. All these types of compounds operate through inhibition of nucleoside synthesis and therefore one cannot exclude a clinical interaction between them.

Pregnancy and lactation: Adverse effects on foetal development (including malformations) occurred when pregnant rats and rabbits were dosed during organogenesis (see *Preclinical safety data*). Because there are no adequate and well controlled studies in pregnant women, CellCept should be used in pregnant women only if the potential benefit outweighs the potential risk to the foetus.

It is recommended that CellCept therapy should not be initiated until a negative pregnancy test has been obtained. Patients should be instructed to consult their physician immediately should pregnancy occur.

Effective contraception must be used before beginning CellCept therapy, during therapy, and for six weeks following discontinuation of therapy. Although the results of a single dose drug interaction study with an oral contraceptive suggest the lack of a gross pharmacokinetic interaction, the results cannot exclude the possibility of changes in the pharmacokinetics of the oral contraceptive under long term dosing conditions with CellCept which might adversely affect the efficacy of the oral contraceptive (see *Interaction with other medicaments and other forms of interaction*).

Studies in rats have shown mycophenolate mofetil to be excreted in milk. It is not known whether this drug is excreted in human milk. Because many drugs are excreted in human milk and because of the potential for serious adverse reactions in nursing infants from mycophenolate mofetil, a decision should be made whether to discontinue nursing or to discontinue the drug, taking into account the importance of the drug to the mother.

Effects on ability to drive and use machines: No specific studies have been performed. The pharmacodynamic profile and the reported adverse reactions indicate that an effect is unlikely.

Undesirable effects: The principal adverse reactions associated with the administration of CellCept in combination with cyclosporin and corticosteroids include diarrhoea, leucopenia, sepsis and vomiting and there is evidence of a higher frequency of certain types of infections (see *Special warnings and special precautions for use*). The adverse event profile associated with the administration of CellCept 500 mg powder for concentrate for solution for infusion has been shown to be similar to that observed after oral administration.

As in patients receiving immunosuppressive regimes involving combinations of drugs, patients receiving CellCept as part of an immunosuppressive regime are at increased risk of developing lymphomas and other malignancies, particularly of the skin (see *Special warnings and special precautions for use*). Within 3 years post-transplant, lymphoproliferative disease or lymphoma developed in patients receiving CellCept in immunosuppressive regimens in 1.6% of the patients receiving 3 g daily and 0.6% in patients receiving 2 g daily in the controlled studies of prevention of renal rejection compared to the placebo (0%) and azathioprine groups (0.6%). All patients are at increased risk of opportunistic infections, the risk increased with dose (see *Special warnings and special precautions for use*).

Elderly patients, particularly those who are receiving CellCept as part of a combination immunosuppressive regimen, may be at greater increased risk of certain infections (including CMV tissue invasive disease) and possibly gastrointestinal haemorrhage and pulmonary oedema, compared to younger individuals (see *Posology and method of administration*).

The following data refer to the safety experience of oral CellCept. Adverse reactions reported in ≥10% of patients treated with CellCept in the three Phase III controlled trials for prevention of rejection are listed in Table 1.

Adverse events, not mentioned above, reported in ≥3% and <10% in renal transplant patients are listed in Table 2.

Adverse events attributable to peripheral venous infusion were phlebitis and thrombosis, both observed at 4% in patients treated with CellCept 500 mg powder for concentrate for solution for infusion.

Adverse reactions during post marketing experience with CellCept are similar to those seen in the controlled renal transplant studies.

Post-marketing experience: Gastro-intestinal: colitis (sometimes caused by cytomegalovirus), pancreatitis.

Disorders of immunosuppression: serious life-threatening infections such as meningitis and infectious endocarditis have been reported occasionally and there is evidence of a higher frequency of certain types of infections such as tuberculosis and atypical mycobacterial infection.

Overdose: There has been no reported experience of overdosage of mycophenolate mofetil in humans.

At clinically encountered concentrations, MPA and MPAG are not removed by haemodialysis. However, at high MPAG plasma concentrations (>100 µg/ml), small amounts of MPAG are removed. By interfering with enterohepatic circulation of the drug, bile acid sequestrants, such as cholestyramine, reduce the MPA AUC.

Pharmacological properties

Pharmacodynamic properties: Pharmacotherapeutic group: immunosuppressant, ATC code L04AA06

Mycophenolate mofetil is the 2-morpholinoethyl ester of MPA. MPA is a potent, selective, uncompetitive and reversible inhibitor of inosine monophosphate dehydrogenase, and therefore inhibits the *de novo* pathway of guanosine nucleotide synthesis without incorporation into DNA. Because T- and B-lymphocytes are critically dependent for their proliferation on *de novo* synthesis of purines whereas other cell types can utilise salvage pathways, MPA has more potent cytostatic effects on lymphocytes than on other cells.

Pharmacokinetic properties: MPA at clinically relevant concentrations, is 97% bound to plasma albumin.

Following intravenous administration, mycophenolate mofetil undergoes rapid and complete metabolism to the active metabolite, MPA. The parent drug mycophenolate mofetil can be measured systemically during intravenous infusion; however, after oral administration it is below the limit of quantitation (0.4 µg/ml).

MPA is metabolized principally by glucuronyl transferase to form the phenolic glucoronide of MPA (MPAG), which is not pharmacologically active.

As a result of enterohepatic recirculation, secondary increases in plasma MPA concentration are usually observed at approximately 6–12 hours post-dose. A reduction in the AUC of MPA of approximately 40% is associated with the co-administration of cholestyramine (4 g TID), indicating that there is a significant amount of enterohepatic recirculation.

Negligible amount of drug is excreted as MPA (<1% of dose) in the urine. Orally administered radiolabelled mycophenolate mofetil resulted in complete recovery of the administered dose; with 93% of the administered dose recovered in the urine and 6% recovered in faeces. Most (about 87%) of the administered dose is excreted in the urine as MPAG.

Immediately post-transplant (<40 days), mean MPA AUC and Cmax are approximately 50% lower in renal transplant patients than that observed in healthy volunteers or in stable renal transplant patients. MPA AUC values obtained following administration of 1 g BID of CellCept 500 mg powder for concentrate for solution for infusion at the recommended infusion rate to patients in the immediate post-transplant phase are comparable to those observed following oral dosing.

In a single dose study (6 subjects per group), mean plasma MPA AUC observed in subjects with severe chronic renal impairment (glomerular filtration rate <25 ml/min/1.73 m²) were 28–75% higher relative to the means observed in normal healthy subjects or subjects with lesser degrees of renal impairment. However, the mean single dose MPAG AUC was 3–6 fold higher in subjects with severe renal impairment than in subjects with mild renal impairment or normal healthy subjects, consistent with the known renal elimination of MPAG. Multiple dosing of mycophenolate mofetil in patients with severe chronic renal impairment has not been studied.

In patients with delayed graft function post-transplant, mean MPA AUC_{0-12} was comparable to that seen in post-transplant patients without delayed graft function. Mean plasma MPAG AUC_{0-12} was 2–3 fold higher than in post-transplant patients without delayed graft function.

In volunteers with alcoholic cirrhosis, hepatic MPA glucuronidation processes were relatively unaffected by hepatic parenchymal disease. Effects of hepatic disease on this process probably depend on the particular disease. However, hepatic disease with predominantly biliary damage, such as primary biliary cirrhosis, may show a different effect.

Pharmacokinetic behaviour of CellCept in the elderly has not been formally evaluated.

Preclinical safety data: In experimental models, mycophenolate mofetil was not tumourigenic and did not demonstrate mutagenic activity. The highest dose tested in the animal carcinogenicity studies resulted in approximately 2 to 3 times the systemic exposure (AUC or Cmax) observed in renal transplant patients at the recommended clinical dose of 2 g per day.

Mycophenolate mofetil had no effect on fertility of male rats at oral doses up to 20 mg/kg/day. The systemic exposure at this dose represents 2 to 3 times the clinical exposure at the recommended clinical dose of 2 g per day. In a female fertility and reproduction study conducted in rats, oral doses of 4.5 mg/kg/day caused malformations (including anophthalmia, agnathia, and hydrocephaly) in the first generation offspring in the absence of maternal toxicity. The systemic exposure at this dose was approximately 0.5 times the clinical exposure at the recommended clinical dose of 2 g per day. No effects on fertility or reproductive parameters were evident in the dams or in the subsequent generation.

In teratology studies in rats and rabbits, foetal resorptions and malformations occurred in rats at 6 mg/kg/day (including anophthalmia, agnathia, and hydrocephaly) and in rabbits at 90 mg/kg/day (including cardiovascular and renal anomalies, such as ectopia cordis and ectopic kidneys, and diaphragmatic and umbilical hernia), in the absence of maternal toxicity. The systemic exposure at these levels are approximately equivalent to or less than 0.5 times the clinical exposure at the recommended clinical dose of 2 g per day.

Refer to *Pregnancy and lactation*.

The haematopoietic and lymphoid systems were the primary organs affected in toxicology studies conducted with mycophenolate mofetil in the rat, mouse, dog and monkey. These effects occurred at systemic exposure levels that are equivalent to or less than the clinical exposure at the recommended dose of 2 g per day. Gastrointestinal effects were observed in the dog at systemic exposure levels equivalent to or less than the clinical exposure at the recommended dose. Gastrointestinal and renal effects consistent with dehydration were also observed in the monkey at the highest dose (systemic exposure levels equivalent to or greater than clinical exposure). The nonclinical toxicity profile of mycophenolate mofetil appears to be consistent with adverse events observed in human clinical trials which now provide safety data of more relevance to the patient population (see *Undesirable effects)*.

Pharmaceutical particulars

List of excipients: Polysorbate 80, citric acid, hydrochloric acid and sodium chloride.

Incompatibilities: CellCept 500 mg powder for concentrate for solution for infusion infusion solution should not be mixed or administered concurrently via the same catheter with other intravenous drugs or infusion admixtures.

Shelf life: Powder for concentrate for solution for infusion: CellCept 500 mg powder for concentrate for solution for infusion has a shelf-life of three years when stored below 30° C.

Reconstituted solution and infusion solution: if the infusion solution is not prepared immediately prior to administration, the commencement of administration of the infusion solution should be within 3 hours from reconstitution and dilution of the drug product.

Special precautions for storage: Powder for concentrate for solution for infusion: store below 30°C.

Reconstituted solution and infusion solution: store at 15–30°C.

Nature and contents of container: 20 ml type I clear glass vials with grey butyl rubber stopper and aluminium seals with plastic flip-off caps. CellCept 500 mg

Table 1: Adverse Events Reported in ≥ 10% of Renal Transplant Patients Treated with CellCept in Combination with Cyclosporin and Corticosteroids

Body System	Adverse Events
Body as a Whole	asthenia, fever, headache, infection, pain, (includes abdominal, back, and chest), oedema
Blood and Lymphatic	anaemia (including hypochromic anaemia), leucocytosis, leucopenia, thrombocytopenia
Urogenital	urinary tract infection, haematuria, renal tubular necrosis
Cardiovascular	Hypertension
Metabolic/Nutritional	hypercholesterolaemia, hyperglycaemia, hyperkalaemia, hypokalaemia, hypophosphataemia
Gastrointestinal	constipation, diarrhoea, dyspepsia, oral moniliasis, nausea, vomiting
Respiratory	cough increased, dyspnoea, pharyngitis, pneumonia, bronchitis
Skin and Appendages	acne, herpes simplex
Nervous	dizziness, insomnia, tremor

Table 2: Adverse Events Reported in ≥ 3% and < 10% of Renal Transplant Patients Treated with CellCept in Combination with Cyclosporin and Corticosteroids

Body System	Adverse Events
Body as a Whole	enlarged abdomen, cysts (including lymphocele and hydrocele), fever, flu syndrome, facial oedema, haemorrhage, malaise, pelvic pain, hernia
Blood and Lymphatic	Ecchymosis, polycythaemia
Urogenital	dysuria, impotence, urinary frequency, albuminuria, hydronephrosis, pyelonephritis
Cardiovascular	angina pectoris, atrial fibrillation, postural hypotension, hypotension, tachycardia, thrombosis, vasodilatation
Metabolic/Nutritional	alkaline phosphatase increased, dehydration, hypervolaemia, hypocalcinaemia, hypoglycaemia, hypoproteinaemia, acidosis, elevated enzyme levels (gamma glutamyl transpeptidase, lactic dehydrogenase, SGOT and SGPT), elevated creatinine, hypercalcaemia, hyperlipaemia, hyperuricaemia, weight gain
Gastrointestinal	anorexia, gastritis, gastroenteritis, gingivitis, gum hyperplasia, liver function tests abnormal, oesophagitis, flatulence, gastrointestinal haemorrhage, gastrointestinal moniliasis, hepatitis, ileus, stomatitis
Respiratory	lung oedema, asthma, pleural effusion, rhinitis, sinusitis
Skin and Appendages	benign neoplasm of skin, skin carcinoma, fungal dermatitis, skin hypertrophy, pruritus, sweating, skin ulcer, alopecia, herpes zoster, hirsutism, rash
Nervous	anxiety, depression, hypertonia, paresthesia, somnolence
Musculoskeletal	arthralgia, leg cramps, myalgia, myasthenia
Special Senses	conjunctivitis, amblyopia, cataract
Endocrine	diabetes mellitus, parathyroid disorder

powder for concentrate for solution for infusion is available in packs containing 4 vials.

Instructions for use/handling: Preparation of Infusion Solution (6 mg/ml): CellCept 500 mg powder for concentrate for solution for infusion does not contain an antibacterial preservative; therefore, reconstitution and dilution of the product must be performed under aseptic conditions.

CellCept 500 mg powder for concentrate for solution for infusion must be prepared in two steps: the first step is a reconstitution step with glucose intravenous infusion 5% and the second step is a dilution step with glucose intravenous infusion 5%. A detailed description of the preparation is given below:

Step 1 a) Two vials of CellCept 500 mg powder for concentrate for solution for infusion are used for preparing each 1 g dose, Reconstitute the content of each vial by injecting 14 ml of glucose intravenous infusion 5%.

b) Gently shake the vial to dissolve the drug yielding a slightly yellow solution.

c) Inspect the resulting solution for particulate matter and discoloration prior to further dilution. Discard the vial if particulate matter or discoloration is observed.

Step 2 a) Further dilute the content of the two reconstituted vials (approx. 2 x 15 ml) into 140 ml of glucose intravenous infusion 5%. The final concentration of the solution is 6 mg mycophenolate mofetil per ml.

b) Inspect the infusion solution for particulate matter or discoloration. Discard the infusion solution if particulate matter or discoloration is observed.

If the infusion solution is not prepared immediately prior to administration, the commencement of administration of the infusion solution should be within 3 hours from reconstitution and dilution of the drug product. Keep solutions at 15–30°C.

Because mycophenolate mofetil has demonstrated teratogenic effects in rats and rabbits, avoid direct contact of prepared solutions of CellCept 500 mg powder for concentrate for solution for infusion with skin or mucous membranes. If such contact occurs, wash thoroughly with soap and water; rinse eyes with plain water.

Marketing authorisation number EU1/96/005/005

Date of first authorisation/renewal of authorisation 20 October 1998

Date of (partial) revision of the text October 1998

CORO-NITRO PUMP SPRAY (CFC free)

Presentation A metered dose pump spray providing 0.4 mg glyceryl trinitrate per dose. Each bottle contains 200 doses for buccal administration.

Alcohol (75.1 mg ethanol/dose) is present in the formulation.

Uses Treatment and prophylaxis of angina pectoris.

Dosage and administration

Adults: The normal dosage is one or two spray puffs (0.4 to 0.8 mg glyceryl trinitrate) as required for relief of anginal pain or for short term prophylaxis before physical or emotional stress or other factors known to precipitate anginal attacks. Occasionally up to 3 spray puffs (1.2 mg glyceryl trinitrate) may be needed at a single time in severe cases. In no circumstances should this be exceeded.

The valve of the Coro-Nitro Pump Spray must be pressed down three times prior to initial use. This fills the pumping chamber and ensures complete spray capacity. Subsequently the spray can be used immediately unless it has not been used for several days in which case the valve should be pressed 1–2 times prior to use.

Coro-Nitro Pump Spray is for buccal administration and patients must be warned not to inhale the spray. During use the Pump Spray should be held upright, near to the open mouth. Pressure on the valve will release a single dose of 0.4 mg glyceryl trinitrate. The spray should be directed into the mouth preferably onto or under the tongue.

Elderly: As for adults. No special dosage requirements.

Children: Not recommended.

Contra-indications, warnings, etc

Contra-indications: Coro-Nitro Pump Spray is contra-indicated in hypotensive disorders including shock, in cases of significant cerebral trauma, acute myocardial infarction with low left ventricular filling pressure and in patients hypersensitive to glyceryl trinitrate.

Use in pregnancy and lactation: There is inadequate evidence of safety of glyceryl trinitrate in human pregnancy although nitrates have been in wide use for many years without apparent ill consequence, animal studies having shown no adverse effects on the foetus. Use in pregnancy and lactation is not recommended unless considered essential by the patient's physician.

Adverse effects: A number of nitrate related adverse effects may occur including headache, facial flushing, dizziness, nausea, vomiting, feelings of weakness, postural hypotension, reflex tachycardia. The ability to drive or operate machinery may be impaired especially if the patient has been consuming alcohol or is taking other hypotensive medication.

Interactions: The hypotensive effects of other drugs may be potentiated. Concomitant alcohol intake may enhance side effects and should be avoided.

Overdosage: Excessive dosage may promote severe headache, facial flushing, hypotension and fainting and, rarely, cyanosis and methaemoglobinaemia. In some cases the effect of overdose will closely resemble shock. Recovery normally occurs spontaneously. The patient should lie in a supine position with the legs elevated to promote venous return. Symptomatic treatment may be needed if there is severe circulatory or respiratory collapse. Methaemoglobinaemia will respond to methylene blue infusion.

Pharmaceutical precautions Coro-Nitro Pump Spray should stored below 25°C and not close to direct sources of heat. The spray should not be used near naked flames.

Legal category P

Package quantities Each Coro-Nitro Pump Spray will deliver 200 metered doses of 0.4 mg glyceryl trinitrate.

Further information Coro-Nitro Pump Spray may be employed together with other anti-anginal agents when necessary including those used for long term prophylaxis such as isosorbide mononitrate and beta-blockers.

Product licence number PL 15722/0032

Date of preparation May 1998

CYMEVENE CAPSULES

Qualitative and quantitative composition Each capsule contains 250 mg of ganciclovir.

Pharmaceutical form Opaque green hard gelatine capsule printed with "CY 250" on the cap and two partial lines on the body.

Clinical particulars

Therapeutic indications: Cymevene capsules are indicated for the maintenance treatment of CMV retinitis in AIDS patients, where the retinitis is stable following at least 3 weeks of Cymevene intravenous therapy.

Cymevene capsules are also indicated for the prevention of CMV disease in liver transplant recipients.

Posology and method of administration: Cymevene capsules must be taken with food.

For patients with stable CMV retinitis following at least 3 weeks of treatment with intravenous Cymevene therapy, the recommended maintenance dose of Cymevene capsules is 1000 mg three times a day. Alternatively, the dosing regimen may be 500 mg six times a day.

For prevention of CMV disease in liver transplant recipients, the recommended dose is 1000 mg three times a day.

Patients with renal impairment: A dose reduction of Cymevene capsules is required as follows:

Creatinine Clearance (ml/min)	*Dose*
≥ 70	1000 mg three times a day
50 to 69	1500 mg daily
25 to 49	1000 mg daily
10 to 24	500 mg daily
< 10	500 mg three times weekly

To calculate an estimated creatinine clearance:

$$\text{For males} = \frac{(140)\text{–age [years] (body weight [kg])}}{(0.81)\text{ (Serum creatinine [μmol/L])}}$$

For females = 0.85 x male value

Elderly: No studies on the safety or efficacy of Cymevene in elderly patients have been conducted. Since elderly individuals often have reduced renal function, Cymevene should be administered to elderly patients with special consideration of their renal status (see above).

Children: There has been limited clinical experience in treating patients under the age of 12 years. The use of Cymevene capsules in children warrants careful consideration due to the possibility of long-term carcinogenicity and reproductive toxicity. The benefits of treatment should outweigh the risks. Cymevene IS NOT INDICATED FOR THE TREATMENT OF CONGENITAL OR NEONATAL CMV INFECTIONS.

Laboratory monitoring and dosage reductions: Due to the frequency of neutropenia, anaemia and thrombocytopenia in patients receiving orally administered Cymevene, it is recommended that neutrophil counts, haemoglobin levels and platelets counts, are performed every 2 weeks. In patients in whom Cymevene or other nucleoside analogues have previously resulted in leucopenia, or in whom neutrophil counts are less than 1000 cells/mm³ at the beginning of treatment, neutrophil counts should be monitored at least weekly.

Patients with severe neutropenia (< 500 cells/mm³) and/or thrombocytopenia (platelets < 25,000/mm³) require a dose interruption until evidence of marrow recovery is observed (≥ 750 cells/mm³).

As dose reductions are required for patients with renal impairment, serum creatinine or creatinine clearance should be monitored every 2 weeks.

Contra-indications

i) Pregnancy and lactation.

ii) Patients with known hypersensitivity to Cymevene or to acyclovir.

Special warnings and special precautions for use: The clinical toxicity of Cymevene includes leucopenia, anaemia and thrombocytopenia. In preclinical testing ganciclovir caused mutagenicity, teratogenicity and carcinogenicity. It should therefore be considered a potential teratogen and carcinogen in humans.

Cymevene should not be administered if the absolute neutrophil count is less than 500 cells/mm³ or the platelet count is less than 25,000 cells/mm³. Neutropenia, anaemia and thrombocytopenia have been observed in patients treated with Cymevene.

It is considered likely that Cymevene causes temporary or permanent inhibition of spermatogenesis. Animal data also indicate that suppression of fertility in females may occur.

Women of childbearing potential should be advised to use effective contraception during treatment. Male patients should be advised to practise barrier contraception during and for at least 90 days following treatment with Cymevene.

If renal function is impaired, dosage adjustments based on creatinine clearance are required (see *Posology and method of administration*).

Interaction with other medicaments and other forms of interaction: Binding of ganciclovir to plasma proteins is only about 1–2% and drug interactions involving binding site displacement are not anticipated.

Probenecid: It is possible that probenecid, as well as other drugs which inhibit renal tubular secretion or resorption, may reduce renal clearance (22%) of ganciclovir and could increase the plasma half life (45%) of ganciclovir.

Additive toxicity: It is possible that drugs which inhibit replication of rapidly dividing cell populations such as bone marrow, spermatogonia, and germinal layers of skin and gastro-intestinal mucosa might have combined additive toxic effects when used concomitantly with, before or after Cymevene. Because of the possibility of additive toxicity with co-administration of drugs such as dapsone, pentamidine, flucytosine, vincristine, vinblastine, adriamycin, amphotericin B, trimethoprim/sulpha combinations or other nucleoside analogues, combination with Cymevene therapy should be used only if the potential benefits outweigh the risks.

Zidovudine: The amount of zidovudine in the blood may increase (by about 15%) when given concomitantly with ganciclovir.

Since both zidovudine and ganciclovir can cause neutropenia, patients receiving these drugs concomitantly are at an increased risk of developing this condition. Regular monitoring of neutrophil counts should be performed (see *Laboratory monitoring and dosage reductions*).

Didanosine: As ganciclovir can increase the amount of didanosine in the blood (by about 80%), patients must be closely monitored for didanosine toxicity.

There is a decrease in the amount of ganciclovir in the blood (23%) when given 2 hours prior to didanosine, but there is no effect on ganciclovir when the two drugs are given at the same time.

Imipenem-cilastatin: Generalised seizures have been reported in patients taking Cymevene and imipenem-cilastatin concomitantly. Use of these drugs should be avoided.

Pregnancy and lactation: There are no adequate and well-controlled studies in pregnant women.

Teratogenicity has been observed in animal studies. Cymevene should not be given to pregnant women as there is a high likelihood of damage to the developing foetus.

It is not known if ganciclovir is excreted in human milk. Since many drugs are, Cymevene should not be given to lactating mothers. The minimum time interval before nursing can safely be resumed after the last dose of Cymevene is unknown.

Intravenous administration of 90 mg/kg of ganciclovir to female mice prior to mating and continued during gestation and lactation caused hypoplasia of the testes and seminal vesicles in the month old offspring, as well as pathologic changes in the nonglandular region of the stomach.

Effects on ability to drive and use machines: Not known.

Undesirable effects: In three controlled clinical trials, adverse events with orally administered Cymevene (3000 mg daily) occurring at a frequency greater than 1% and thought to be "probably" or "possibly" related to treatment were as follows:

Leucopenia, thrombocytopenia, anaemia, diarrhoea, abdominal pain, dyspepsia, nausea, anorexia, flatulence, vomiting, asthenia, rash, headache, pruritus, fever, abnormal liver function tests, pain and infection.

Adverse events which were thought to be possibly related and occurred in 1% or less of the patients are listed by body systems below.

Body as a whole: cellulitis, laboratory test abnormality, abdomen enlarged, chest pain, chills, drug level increased, malaise.

Digestive system: eructation, mouth ulceration, constipation, dysphagia, faecal incontinence.

Haematologic system: hypochromic anaemia, pancytopenia.

Respiratory system: dyspnoea, cough increased.

Central nervous system: somnolence, dizziness, paraesthesia, abnormal dreams and thoughts, anxiety, euphoria, insomnia, abnormal gait, ataxia, confusion, dry mouth, hypesthesia, manic reaction.

Skin and appendages: alopecia, sweating, acne, maculopapular rash.

Cardiovascular system: deep thrombophlebitis, migraine, vasodilation.

Metabolic and nutritional disorders: increases in creatinine, alkaline phosphatase, SGPT, creatine phosphokinase and lactic dehydrogenase; hypokalemia.

Special senses: abnormal vision, vitreous disorder, eye pain, amblyopia, blindness, conjunctivitis, retinal detachment, retinitis, deafness, taste perversion.

Urogenital system: decrease in creatinine clearance, abnormal kidney function, breast pain, urinary frequency, urinary tract infection.

Musculoskeletal system: myasthenia, myalgia.

Overdose: There have been no reports of overdosage with orally administered Cymevene.

Haemodialysis and hydration may be of benefit in reducing drug plasma levels in patients who receive an overdose of Cymevene.

Pharmacological properties

Ganciclovir (9-[1,3-dihydroxy-2-propoxymethyl] guanine) is a synthetic analogue of guanine which inhibits replication of herpes viruses *in vitro* and *in vivo*. Sensitive human viruses include cytomegalovirus (CMV), herpes simplex virus-1 and -2 (HSV-1 and HSV-2), Epstein-Barr virus (EBV) and varicella zoster virus (VZV). Clinical studies have been limited to assessment of efficacy in patients with CMV infection.

Intracellular ganciclovir is phosphorylated to ganciclovir monophosphate by a cellular deoxyguanosine kinase. Further phosphorylation to ganciclovir triphosphate occurs by several cellular kinases. In CMV-infected cells there is approximately a 10-fold increased concentration of both cellular kinases and ganciclovir triphosphate. Thus, there is a preferential phosphorylation of ganciclovir in virus-infected cells. In such cells ganciclovir triphosphate is metabolised slowly, with 60 to 70% remaining 18 hours after removal of ganciclovir from the extracellular fluid. The antiviral activity of ganciclovir is the result of inhibition of viral DNA synthesis by: (1) competitive inhibition of incorporation of deoxyguanosine triphosphate into DNA by DNA polymerase, and (2) incorporation of ganciclovir triphosphate into viral DNA causing termination of, or very limited, viral DNA elongation.

Emergence of viral resistance has been reported based on *in vitro* sensitivity testing of CMV isolates from patients receiving Cymevene treatment.

Pharmacokinetic properties: The major route of excretion of ganciclovir is via glomerular filtration of unchanged drug. Administration of Cymevene with food increased its bioavailability by approximately 20%. Multiple dose studies with Cymevene capsules indicated that the absolute bioavailability when taken with food was approximately 6%.

Oral doses of 3 g/day yield maximum and minimum plasma concentrations of 1.0 and 0.2μg/ml respectively (corresponding plasma concentrations for IV maintenance therapy of 5 mg/kg/day are 8.0μg/ml and < 0.05μg/ml).

In patients with severe renal impairment, haemodialysis reduced plasma drug levels by 50%.

Pharmaceutical particulars

List of excipients: The capsules contain the following excipients: croscarmellose sodium, magnesium stearate and povidone.

Incompatibilities: None.

Shelf life: 2 years in a high density polyethylene bottle in foil laminate pouches and amber silica glass bottles.

Special precautions for storage: Cymevene capsules should be stored below 30°C.

Nature and contents of container: 180 or 84 capsules in a high density polyethylene bottle with a polypropylene closure, child resistant overcap and with a tamper evident innerseal or an amber silica glass bottle with a tamper evident polypropylene screw closure and polyurethane pad.

Foil laminate pouches. Each strip consists of 4 x 3 capsules. Pack size is either 7 or 14 strips (84 or 168 capsules).

Instructions for use/handling: As Cymevene has shown carcinogenic and mutagenic activity, **caution should be observed in the handling of Cymevene capsules. Avoid inhalation or direct contact of the powder contained in the capsules with the skin or mucous membranes.** If such contact occurs, wash thoroughly with soap and water, rinse eyes thoroughly with plain water.

Cymevene capsules should not be opened or crushed.

Marketing authorisation number PL 0031/0466

Date of first authorisation/renewal of authorisation December 1994

Date of partial revision of the text November 1998

CYMEVENE IV

Qualitative and quantitative composition Ganciclovir 500 mg (as ganciclovir sodium 546 mg).

Pharmaceutical form Sterile, freeze-dried powder for reconstitution with water for injection.

Clinical particulars

Therapeutic indications: Cymevene is indicated for the treatment of life-threatening or sight-threatening cytomegalovirus (CMV) infections in immunocompromised individuals. These states include acquired immunodeficiency syndrome (AIDS), iatrogenic immunosuppression associated with organ transplantation, or chemotherapy for neoplasia.

Cymevene may also be used for the prevention of CMV disease, specifically in those patients receiving immunosuppressive therapy secondary to organ transplantation.

Posology and method of administration: For intravenous infusion following reconstitution with 10 ml water for injection BP. Based on patient weight and therapeutic indication the appropriate calculated dose volume should be removed from the vial (ganciclovir concentration 50 mg/ml) and added to an acceptable infusion fluid (typically 100 ml) for delivery over the course of 1 hour. Infusion concentrations greater than 10 mg/ml are not recommended.

Adults

Treatment of CMV infection: Initial (induction) treatment: 5 mg/kg infused at a constant rate over 1 hour every 12 hours (10 mg/kg/day) for 14 to 21 days.

Long-term (maintenance) treatment: For immunocompromised patients at risk of relapse of CMV retinitis a course of maintenance therapy may be given. Intravenous infusion of 6 mg/kg daily 5 days per week, or 5 mg/kg daily 7 days per week is recommended.

Treatment of disease progression: Indefinite treatment may be required in patients with AIDS, but even with continued maintenance treatment, patients may have progression of retinitis. Any patient in whom the retinitis progresses, either while on maintenance treatment or because treatment with Cymevene has been withdrawn, may be re-treated using the induction treatment regimen.

Prevention of CMV disease: Induction regimen: 5 mg/kg infused every 12 hours (10 mg/kg/day) for 7 to 14 days.

Maintenance regimen: Intravenous infusion of 6 mg/kg daily 5 days per week, or 5 mg/kg 7 days per week is recommended.

For patients with renal insufficiency the induction dose should be modified as follows:

Serum creatinine (micromol/l)	*Dose (mg/kg)*	*Dosing Interval (hours)*
< 124	5.0	12
125–225	2.5	12
226–398	2.5	24
> 398	1.25	24

The optimal maintenance dose for patients with renal insufficiency is not known.

Patients undergoing dialysis should be given 1.25 mg/kg/24 hours. On days when dialysis is performed the dose should be given shortly after the dialysis session.

Elderly

No studies on the efficacy or safety of Cymevene in elderly patients have been conducted. Since elderly individuals often have reduced renal function, Cymevene should be administered to elderly patients with special consideration for their renal status.

Children

There has been limited clinical experience in treating patients under the age of 12 years. Reported adverse events were similar to those seen in adults. However, the use of Cymevene in children warrants careful consideration due to the possibility of long-term carcinogenicity and reproductive toxicity. The benefits of treatment should outweigh the risks. Cymevene is not indicated for the treatment of congenital or neonatal CMV infections.

Laboratory monitoring and dosage reduction

Because of individual patient sensitivity to the myelosuppressive effects of Cymevene regular clinical and haematological assessments are recommended. White blood cell and platelet counts should be performed every two days for the first 14 days of treatment. Patients with a history of marrow sensitivity to ganciclovir or other nucleoside analogues, or with white blood cell counts less than 1000 cells/μl at the beginning of treatment should be monitored daily. During maintenance treatment complete blood counts are recommended weekly, or more frequently if counts are low.

Neutropenia typically occurs during the first or second week of treatment. Severe neutropenia (< 500 cells/μl) requires a dose interruption. For less severe neutropenia a reduction in the total daily dose may be adequate. Cell counts usually normalise within 3 to 7 days after discontinuing the drug or decreasing the dose. As evidence of marrow recovery becomes apparent gradual increases in dose, with careful monitoring of white blood cell counts, may be appropriate.

Contra-indications

i) Pregnancy and lactation.

ii) Patients with known hypersensitivity to Cymevene or to acyclovir.

Special warnings and special precautions for use: The clinical toxicity of Cymevene includes leucopenia and thrombocytopenia. In preclinical testing ganciclovir caused aspermatogenesis, mutagenicity, teratogenicity and carcinogenicity. It should therefore be considered a potential carcinogen and teratogen in humans.

Between approximately 10 and 40% of patients receiving intravenous Cymevene develop neutropenia (neutrophil count less than 1000 cells/μl). Cymevene should, therefore, be used with caution in those patients with a history of cytopenia. In a study of 314 AIDS patients there was no relationship between baseline neutrophil count and the occurrence of neutropenia; therefore, the risk of neutropenia may not be predicted from pre-treatment cell counts. However, Cymevene should not be administered if the absolute neutrophil count falls below 500 cells/μl.

Thrombocytopenia (platelet count less than 50,000/microlitre) was observed in 19% of patients treated with Cymevene. Patients being treated with immunosuppressive drugs were more likely to develop lowered platelet counts than patients with AIDS. Patients with platelet counts less than 100,000/microlitre were also at increased risk of thrombocytopenia.

Because of the mutagenic potential of Cymevene, women of childbearing potential should be advised to use effective contraception during treatment. Likewise, men should be advised to practice barrier contraception for 90 days following treatment.

Administration of Cymevene by intravenous infusion should be accompanied by adequate hydration, since Cymevene is excreted by the kidneys and normal clearance depends upon adequate renal function. If renal function is impaired, dosage adjustments are required. Such adjustments should be based on serum creatinine (see *Posology and method of administration*).

Interaction with other medicaments and other forms of interaction: Binding of ganciclovir to plasma proteins is only about 1–2% and drug interactions involving binding site displacement are not anticipated. It is possible that probenecid, as well as other drugs which inhibit renal tubular secretion or resorption, may reduce renal clearance of ganciclovir and could increase the plasma half-life of ganciclovir. It is also possible that drugs which inhibit replication of rapidly dividing cell populations such as bone marrow, spermatogonia, and germinal layers of skin and gastro-intestinal mucosa might have combined additive toxic effects when used concomitantly with, before, or after Cymevene. Because of the possibility of additive toxicity with co-administration of drugs such as dapsone, pentamidine, flucytosine, vincristine, vinblastine, adriamycin, amphotericin B, trimethoprim/sulpha combinations or other nucleoside analogues, combination with Cymevene therapy should be used only if the potential benefits outweigh the risks.

Patients with AIDS may be receiving, or have received, treatment with zidovudine. Since both zidovudine and Cymevene can result in neutropenia, it is recommended that these two drugs not be given concomitantly during induction treatment with ganciclovir. In addition, data from a small number of patients studied to date indicate that maintenance ganciclovir treatment plus zidovudine at the recommended dose resulted in severe neutropenia in most individuals.

Generalised seizures have been reported in patients taking Cymevene and imipenem-cilastatin concomitantly. These drugs should only be used concomitantly with Cymevene after careful consideration of the risks involved.

Pregnancy and lactation: Teratogenicity has been observed in animal studies. Cymevene should not be given to pregnant women as there is a high likelihood of damage to the developing foetus.

Adverse effects were observed in the offspring of lactating animals. It is not known if ganciclovir is excreted in human milk. However, since many drugs are, Cymevene should not be given to lactating mothers. Nursing should not be resumed until 72 hours after the last dose of Cymevene.

Effects on ability to drive and use machines: None known.

Undesirable effects: Neutropenia (10–40% of patients) and thrombocytopenia (19% of patients) are the most frequently observed side-effects. Anaemia, fever, rash and abnormal liver function tests have been observed in 2% of patients.

Adverse events which were thought to be possibly related and occurred in 1% or less of the patients are listed by body systems below.

Body as a whole: Chills, oedema, infections, malaise.

Cardiovascular system: Arrhythmias, hypertension, hypotension.

Central nervous system: Abnormal thoughts or dreams, ataxia, coma, confusion, dizziness, headache, nervousness, paraesthesia, psychosis, somnolence, tremor.

Digestive system: Nausea, vomiting, anorexia, diarrhoea, haemorrhage, pain.

Haematologic system: Eosinophilia.

Laboratory abnormalities: Decrease in blood glucose.

Respiratory system: Dyspnoea.

Skin and appendages: Alopecia, pruritus, urticaria.

Special senses: Retinal detachment in AIDS patients with CMV retinitis.

Urogenital system: Haematuria, increased serum creatinine, increased blood urea nitrogen (BUN).

Injection site: Inflammation, pain, phlebitis.

Overdose: In the event of overdose, dialysis and hydration may be of benefit in reducing drug plasma levels.

Toxic manifestations seen in animals given very high single intravenous doses of ganciclovir (500 mg/kg) included emesis, hypersalivation, anorexia, bloody diarrhoea, inactivity, cytopenia, abnormal liver function tests and BUN, testicular atrophy and death.

Pharmacological properties

Pharmacodynamic properties: Ganciclovir is a synthetic nucleoside analogue of guanine which inhibits replication of herpes viruses both *in vitro* and *in vivo*. Sensitive human viruses include cytomegalovirus (CMV), herpes simplex virus-1 and -2 (HSV-1 and HSV-2), Epstein-Barr virus (EBV) and varicella zoster virus (VZV).

Intracellular ganciclovir is phosphorylated to ganciclovir monophosphate by a cellular deoxyguanosine kinase. Further phosphorylation occurs by several cellular kinases resulting in ganciclovir triphosphate. In CMV-infected cells there is approximately a 10-fold increased concentration of both cellular kinases and ganciclovir triphosphate. Thus, there is a preferential phosphorylation of ganciclovir in virus-infected cells. In virus-infected cells ganciclovir triphosphate is metabolised slowly, with 60 to 70% remaining 18 hours after removal of ganciclovir from the extracellular fluid. The antiviral activity of ganciclovir is the result of inhibition of viral DNA synthesis by two known modes: (1) ganciclovir triphosphate competitively inhibits dGTP incorporation into DNA by DNA polymerase and (2) incorporation of ganciclovir triphosphate into viral DNA causing termination or very limited viral DNA elongation.

Pharmacokinetic properties: In patients with normal renal function the plasma half-life of ganciclovir following an IV infusion of 5 mg/kg averaged 2.9 hours with a mean systemic clearance of 3.64 ml/min/kg. Twice-daily administration of 5 mg/kg for 14 days did not cause accumulation in plasma. Renal impairment leads to altered kinetics of ganciclovir as indicated below.

	Ganciclovir	
Serum creatinine (micromol/l)	*Systemic plasma clearance (ml/min/kg)*	*Plasma half-life (hours)*
< 124 (n = 32)	3.64	2.9
125–225 (n = 9)	2.00	5.3
226–398 (n = 3)	1.11	9.7
> 398 (n = 5)	0.33	28.5

Metabolism: Ganciclovir is excreted mainly unmetabolised in rats, mice and dogs when administered intravenously. In the monkey, although ganciclovir was the main radioactive component recovered in urine a metabolite having elution characteristics the same as authentic 8-hydroxy ganciclovir accounted for 12% of the radioactivity recovered in the urine of this species following intravenous dosing. No evidence was obtained for cleavage of ganciclovir to guanine in any of the species studied. Pharmacokinetic studies in volunteers were not done because of the toxicological profile of the compound, however, recovery of ganciclovir in urine was studied in four patients. A large fraction (37%–126%) of the intravenously administered dose was recovered unmetabolised in urine.

This metabolite profile in mice, rats, dogs and monkeys paralleled the metabolic profile of acyclovir in these species. Furthermore, in man, acyclovir is excreted mainly unmetabolised in urine.

Preclinical safety data: None stated.

Pharmaceutical particulars

List of excipients: None.

Incompatibilities: The dry powder should not be reconstituted with bacteriostatic water containing parabens, since these are incompatible with ganciclovir sterile powder and may cause precipitation.

Shelf life: 36 months.

Special precautions for storage: The vials should be stored below 30°C. Each infusion solution of ganciclovir should be refrigerated and used within 24 hours of dilution.

Nature and contents of container: 10 ml multidose vials (type I clear glass) with a grey butyl siliconised stopper in quantities of 5 or 25 vials.

Instructions for use/handling: See *Posology and method of administration.*

Marketing authorisation number PL 0031/0465

Date of first authorisation/renewal of authorisation 31 May 1996

Date of (partial) revision of the text February 1998

EUCARDIC ▼

Qualitative and quantitative composition

Each "Eucardic" 3.125 tablet contains 3.125 mg carvedilol.

Each "Eucardic" 6.25 tablet contains 6.25 mg carvedilol.

Each "Eucardic" 12.5 tablet contains 12.5 mg carvedilol.

Each "Eucardic" 25 tablet contains 25 mg carvedilol.

Pharmaceutical form Tablet for oral use

Clinical particulars

Therapeutic indications: Symptomatic chronic heart failure (CHF)

Eucardic is indicated for the treatment of symptomatic CHF (New York Heart Association (NYHA) Classes II and III) as adjunct to standard therapies e.g. diuretics, digoxin, ACE inhibitors. In these patients, addition of Eucardic has been shown to delay the progression of disease.

Patients with NYHA Class II CHF are characterised by slight limitation of physical activity. They are comfortable at rest but ordinary physical activity results in fatigue, palpitation or dyspnoea.

Patients with NYHA Class III CHF are characterised by marked limitation of physical activity. They are comfortable at rest but even less than ordinary activity causes fatigue, palpitation or dyspnoea.

Due to lack of experience, Eucardic should not be initiated in patients with severe (NYHA Class IV) CHF (see *Contra-indications*).

Hypertension: Eucardic is indicated for the treatment of hypertension.

Angina: Eucardic is indicated for the prophylactic treatment of stable angina.

Posology and method of administration: The tablets should be taken with fluid. For CHF patients Eucardic should be given with food.

Symptomatic chronic heart failure

Initiation of therapy with Eucardic in patients with chronic heart failure and its titration to stabilise the patient to the optimal dose should only be under the supervision of a hospital physician.

The dosage must be titrated to individual requirements and patients' clinical status should be monitored for 2–3 hours after initiation and any dose increase during up-titration.

For those patients receiving diuretics and/or digoxin and/or ACE inhibitors, dosing of these other drugs should be stabilised prior to initiation of Eucardic treatment.

Adults

The recommended dose for the initiation of therapy is 3.125 mg twice a day for two weeks. If this dose is tolerated, the dosage should be increased subsequently, at intervals of not less than two weeks, to 6.25 mg twice daily, followed by 12.5 mg twice daily and thereafter 25 mg twice daily. Dosing should be increased to the highest level tolerated by the patient.

The recommended maximum daily dose is 25 mg given twice daily in patients weighing less than 85 kg (187 lbs) and 50 mg twice daily in patients weighing more than 85 kg.

During up-titration of the dose in patients with systolic blood pressure < 100 mmHg, deterioration of renal and/or cardiac functions may occur. Therefore, before each dose increase these patients should be evaluated by the physician for renal function and symptoms of worsening heart failure or vasodilation. Transient worsening of heart failure, vasodilation or fluid retention may be treated by adjusting doses of diuretics or ACE inhibitors or by modifying or temporarily discontinuing Eucardic treatment. Under these circumstances, the dose of Eucardic should not be increased until symptoms of worsening heart failure or vasodilation have been stabilised.

If Eucardic is discontinued for more than two weeks, therapy should be recommenced at 3.125 mg twice daily and up-titrated in line with the above dosing recommendation.

Elderly: As for adults.

Children: Safety and efficacy in children (under 18 years) has not been established.

Hypertension

Once daily dosing is recommended.

Adults: The recommended dose for initiation of therapy is 12.5 mg once a day for the first two days. Thereafter the recommended dosage is 25 mg once a day. Although this is an adequate dose in most patients, if necessary the dose may be titrated up to a recommended daily maximum dose of 50 mg given once a day or in divided doses.

Dose titration should occur at intervals of at least two weeks.

Elderly: An initial dose of 12.5 mg daily is recommended. This has provided satisfactory control in some cases. If the response is inadequate the dose may be titrated up to the recommended daily maximum dose of 50 mg given once a day or in divided doses.

Children: Safety and efficacy in children (under 18 years) has not been established.

Angina: Adults: The recommended dose for initiation of therapy is 12.5 mg twice a day for the first two days. Thereafter, the recommended dosage is 25 mg twice a day.

Elderly: The recommended maximum daily dose is 50 mg given in divided doses.

Children: Safety and efficacy in children (under 18 years) has not been established.

Patients with co-existing hepatic disease

Eucardic is contra-indicated in patients with hepatic dysfunction (see sections *Contra-indications* and *Pharmacokinetic properties*).

Patients with co-existing renal dysfunction

No dose adjustment is anticipated as long as systolic blood pressure is above 100 mmHg (see also sections *Special warnings and precautions for use* and *Pharmacokinetic properties*).

Contra-indications: Due to lack of experience, patients with severe chronic heart failure (NYHA Class IV) should not be initiated on treatment with Eucardic. These patients are characterised by inability to carry on any physical activity without discomfort. Symptoms of cardiac insufficiency may be present even at rest. If any physical activity is undertaken, discomfort is increased.

Patients with obstructive airways disease, liver dysfunction, hypersensitivity to carvedilol or any other constituents of the tablets.

As with other beta-blocking agents: History of bronchospasm or asthma, 2nd and 3rd degree A-V heart block, severe bradycardia (< 50 bpm), cardiogenic shock, sick sinus syndrome (including sino-atrial block), severe hypotension (systolic blood pressure < 85 mmHg), metabolic acidosis and phaeochromocytoma (unless adequately controlled by alpha blockade).

Special warnings and special precautions for use: In chronic heart failure patients, worsening cardiac failure or fluid retention may occur during up-titration of Eucardic. If such symptoms occur, the dose of diuretic should be adjusted and the Eucardic dose should not be advanced until clinical stability resumes. Occasionally it may be necessary to lower the Eucardic dose or temporarily discontinue it. Such episodes do not preclude subsequent successful titration of Eucardic.

Patients who progress to severe (NYHA Class IV) heart failure whilst on therapy should, as with all therapies, have their therapeutic regime reassessed at regular intervals according to the discretion of the physician.

In hypertensive patients who have chronic heart failure controlled with digoxin, diuretics and/or an ACE inhibitor, Eucardic should be used with caution since both digoxin and Eucardic may slow A-V conduction.

As with other drugs with beta-blocking activity, Eucardic may mask the early signs of acute hypoglycaemia in patients with diabetes mellitus. Alternatives to beta-blocking agents are generally preferred in insulin-dependent patients. In patients with diabetes, the use of Eucardic may be associated with worsening control of blood glucose. Therefore, regular monitoring of blood glucose is required in diabetics when Eucardic is initiated or up-titrated and hypoglycaemic therapy adjusted accordingly.

Reversible deterioration of renal function has been observed with Eucardic therapy in chronic heart failure patients with low blood pressure (systolic BP < 100 mmHg), ischaemic heart disease and diffuse vascular disease, and/or underlying renal insufficiency. In CHF patients with these risk factors, renal function should be monitored during up-titration of Eucardic and the drug discontinued or dosage reduced if worsening of renal failure occurs.

Wearers of contact lenses should be advised of the possibility of reduced lacrimation.

Although angina has not been reported on stopping treatment, discontinuation should be gradual (1–2 weeks) particularly in patients with ischaemic heart disease, as Eucardic has beta-blocking activity.

Eucardic may be used in patients with peripheral vascular disease. Pure beta-blockers can precipitate or aggravate symptoms of arterial insufficiency. However as Eucardic also has alpha-blocking properties this effect is largely counterbalanced.

Eucardic, as with other agents with beta-blocking activity, may mask the symptoms of thyrotoxicosis.

If Eucardic induces bradycardia, with a decrease in pulse rate to less than 55 beats per minute, the dosage of Eucardic should be reduced.

Care should be taken in administering Eucardic to patients with a history of serious hypersensitivity reactions and in those undergoing desensitisation therapy as beta-blockers may increase both the sensitivity towards allergens and the seriousness of anaphylactic reactions.

In patients suffering from the peripheral circulatory disorder Raynaud's phenomenon, there may be exacerbation of symptoms.

Patients with a history of psoriasis associated with beta-blocker therapy should be given Eucardic only after consideration of the risk-benefit ratio.

In patients with phaeochromocytoma, an alpha-blocking agent should be initiated prior to the use of any beta-blocking agent. There is no experience of the use of carvedilol in this condition. Therefore, caution should be taken in the administration of Eucardic to patients suspected of having phaeochromocytoma.

Agents with non-selective beta-blocking activity may provoke chest pain in patients with Prinzmetal's variant angina. There is no clinical experience with Eucardic in these patients, although the alpha-blocking activity of Eucardic may prevent such symptoms. However, caution should be taken in the administration of Eucardic to patients suspected of having Prinzmetal's variant angina.

In patients with a tendency to bronchospastic reactions, respiratory distress can occur as a result of a possible increase in airway resistance. The following warnings will be included on the outer packaging and leaflet:

Packaging: Do not take this medicine if you have a history of wheezing due to asthma or other lung diseases.

Leaflet: Do not take this medicine if you have a history of wheezing due to asthma or other lung diseases. Consult your doctor or pharmacist first.

Interaction with other medicaments and other forms of interaction: As with other agents with beta-blocking activity, Eucardic may potentiate the effect of other concomitantly administered drugs that are anti-hypertensive in action (e.g. $alpha_1$-receptor antagonists) or have hypotension as part of their adverse effect profile.

Isolated cases of conduction disturbance (rarely with haemodynamic disruption) have been observed when Eucardic and diltiazem were given concomitantly. Therefore, as with other drugs with beta-blocking activity, careful monitoring of ECG and blood pressure should be undertaken when co-administering calcium channel blockers of the verapamil or diltiazem type, or class I antiarrhythmic drugs. These types of drugs should not be co-administered intravenously in patients receiving Eucardic.

The effects of insulin or oral hypoglycaemics may be intensified. Regular monitoring of blood glucose is therefore recommended.

Trough plasma digoxin levels may be increased by approximately 16% in hypertensive patients co-administered Eucardic and digoxin. Increased monitoring of digoxin levels is recommended when initiating, adjusting or discontinuing Eucardic. Concomitant administration of Eucardic and cardiac glycosides may prolong AV conduction time.

When treatment with Eucardic and clonidine together is to be terminated, Eucardic should be withdrawn first, several days before gradually decreasing the dosage of clonidine.

Care may be required in those receiving inducers of mixed function oxidases e.g. rifampicin, as serum levels of carvedilol may be reduced or inhibitors of mixed function oxidases e.g. cimetidine, as serum levels may be increased.

During general anaesthesia, attention should be paid to the potential synergistic negative inotropic effects of carvedilol and anaesthetic drugs.

Pregnancy and lactation: There is no adequate experience with Eucardic in pregnant women.

Eucardic should not be used in pregnancy or in breast feeding mothers unless the anticipated benefits outweigh the potential risks. There is no evidence from animal studies that Eucardic has any teratogenic effects. Embryotoxicity was observed only after large doses in rabbits. The relevance of these findings for humans is uncertain. Beta blockers reduce placental perfusion which may result in intrauterine foetal death and immature and premature deliveries. In addition, animal studies have shown that carvedilol crosses the placental barrier and is excreted in breast milk and therefore the possible consequences of alpha and beta blockade in the human foetus and neonate should also be borne in mind. With other alpha and beta blocking agents, effects have included perinatal and neonatal distress (bradycardia, hypotension, respiratory depression, hypoglycaemia, hypothermia). There is an increased risk of cardiac and pulmonary complications in the neonate in the postnatal period.

Effects on ability to drive and use machines: As for other drugs which produce changes in blood pressure, patients taking Eucardic should be warned not to drive or operate machinery if they experience dizziness or related symptoms. This applies particularly when starting or changing treatment and in conjunction with alcohol.

Undesirable effects: Adverse events are listed separately for CHF because of differences in the background diseases.

In chronic heart failure

The most commonly reported adverse effect is dizziness. Other common effects include bradycardia, postural hypotension, hypotension, gastrointestinal effects (nausea, diarrhoea and vomiting), oedema (including generalised, peripheral, dependent and genital oedema, oedema of the legs, hypervolaemia and fluid overload), vision abnormalities, thrombocytopenia, hyperglycaemia (in patients with pre-existing diabetes mellitus), weight increase and hypercholesterolaemia.

Infrequently, syncope, A-V block or cardiac failure during up-titration, acute renal failure and renal abnormalities in patients with diffuse vascular disease and/or impaired renal function have also been reported.

The frequency of adverse experiences is not dose dependent, with the exception of dizziness, abnormal vision and bradycardia.

In hypertension and angina

The profile is similar to that observed in chronic heart failure although the incidence of events is generally lower in patients with hypertension or angina treated with Eucardic.

Symptomatic postural hypotension, mainly on the initiation of therapy or when increasing the dose, may occur but the incidence is minimised when the drug is used as recommended. Commonly dizziness, headache, fatigue, gastrointestinal upset (nausea, abdominal pain, diarrhoea; infrequently constipation and vomiting), bradycardia and hypotension (infrequently syncope) have been observed. These effects are usually mild, transient and occur early in the course of treatment. Other common effects have included pain in the extremities and reduced lacrimation and, in predisposed patients, there may be asthma and dyspnoea

Infrequently there may be depressed mood, sleep disturbance, paraesthesia, wheezing, flu-like symptoms, rare or isolated cases of skin reactions (e.g. allergic exanthema, in isolated cases urticaria, pruritus and lichen planus-like reactions). Psoriatic skin lesions may occur or existing lesions may be exacerbated.

Diminished peripheral circulation (cold extremities) or peripheral oedema may occur infrequently. Rarely there may be A-V block, angina pectoris, exacerbation of symptoms in patients suffering from intermittent claudication, Raynaud's phenomenon, or progression of heart failure.

Stuffy nose may occur infrequently.

Isolated cases of changes in serum transaminases, thrombocytopenia and leucopenia have been reported.

There have also been rare cases of sexual impotence, disturbed vision, eye irritation, dryness of the mouth and disturbances of micturition.

Due to the beta-blocking properties it is also possible for latent diabetes mellitus to become manifest, manifest diabetes to be aggravated, and blood glucose counter-regulation to be inhibited.

Overdose: Symptoms and signs

Profound cardiovascular effects such as hypotension and bradycardia would be expected after massive overdose. Heart failure, cardiogenic shock and cardiac arrest may follow. There may also be respiratory problems, bronchospasm, vomiting, disturbed consciousness and generalised seizures.

Treatment

Gastric lavage or induced emesis may be useful in the first few hours after ingestion.

In addition to general procedures, vital signs must be monitored and corrected, if necessary under intensive care conditions.

Patients should be placed in the supine position. Atropine, 0.5 mg to 2 mg i.v. and/or glucagon 1 to 10 mg i.v. (followed by a slow i.v. infusion of 2 to 5 mg/hour if necessary) may be given when bradycardia is present. Pacemaker therapy may be necessary. For excessive hypotension, intravenous fluids may be administered. In addition, norepinephrine may be given, either 5 to 10 micrograms i.v., repeated according to blood pressure response, or 5 micrograms per minute by infusion titrated to blood pressure. Bronchospasm may be treated using salbutamol or other $beta_2$-agonists given as aerosol or, if necessary, by the intravenous route. In the event of seizures, slow i.v. injection of diazepam or clonazepam is recommended.

In cases of severe overdose with symptoms of shock, supportive treatment as described should be continued for a sufficiently long period of time, i.e. until the patient stabilises, since prolonged elimination half life and redistribution of carvedilol from deeper compartments can be expected.

Pharmacological properties

Pharmacodynamic properties: Carvedilol is a vasodilating non-selective beta blocking agent with antioxidant properties. Vasodilation is predominantly mediated through alpha$_1$ receptor antagonism.

Carvedilol reduces the peripheral vascular resistance through vasodilation and suppresses the renin-angiotensin-aldosterone system through beta blockade. The activity of plasma renin is reduced and fluid retention is rare.

Carvedilol has no intrinsic sympathomimetic activity and like propranolol, it has membrane stabilising properties.

Carvedilol is a racemate of two stereoisomers. Beta-blockade is attributed to the S(-) enantiomer; in contrast, both enantiomers exhibit the same α_1-blocking activity.

Carvedilol is a potent antioxidant, a scavenger of reactive oxygen radicals and an anti-proliferative agent. The properties of carvedilol and its metabolites have been demonstrated in *in vitro* and *in vivo* animal studies and *in vitro* in a number of human cell types.

Clinical studies have shown that the balance of vasodilation and beta-blockade provided by carvedilol results in the following effects:

In hypertensive patients, a reduction in blood pressure is not associated with a concomitant increase in total peripheral resistance, as observed with pure beta-blocking agents. Heart rate is slightly decreased. Renal blood flow and renal function are maintained. Peripheral blood flow is maintained, therefore, cold extremities, often observed with drugs possessing beta-blocking activity, are rarely seen.

In patients with stable angina, Eucardic has demonstrated anti-ischaemic and anti-anginal properties. Acute haemodynamic studies demonstrated that Eucardic reduces ventricular pre- and after-load.

In patients with left ventricular dysfunction or chronic heart failure, carvedilol has demonstrated favourable effects on haemodynamics and improvements in left ventricular ejection fraction and dimensions.

Serum lipid profile and electrolytes are not affected.

Pharmacokinetic properties: The absolute bioavailability of carvedilol is approximately 25% in humans. Bioavailability is stereo-selective, 30% for the R-form and 15% for the S-form. Serum levels peak at approximately 1 hour after an oral dose. There is a linear relationship between the dose and serum concentrations. Food does not affect bioavailability or the maximum serum concentration although the time to reach maximum serum concentration is delayed. Carvedilol is highly lipophilic, approximately 98% to 99% is bound to plasma proteins. The distribution volume is approximately 2 l/kg and increased in patients with liver cirrhosis. The first pass effect after oral administration is approximately 60–75%; enterohepatic circulation of the parent substance has been shown in animals.

Carvedilol exhibits a considerable first pass effect. The metabolite pattern reveals intensive metabolism with glucuronidation as one of the major steps. Demethylation and hydroxylation at the phenol ring produce 3 metabolites with beta-receptor blocking activity.

The average elimination half-life ranges from 6 to 10 hours. Plasma clearance is approximately 590 ml/min. Elimination is mainly biliary. The primary route of excretion is via the faeces. A minor portion is eliminated via the kidneys in the form of various metabolites.

The pharmacokinetics of carvedilol are affected by age; plasma levels of carvedilol are approximately 50% higher in the elderly compared to young subjects. In a study in patients with cirrhotic liver disease, the bioavailability of carvedilol was four times greater and the peak plasma level five times higher than in healthy subjects. Since carvedilol is primarily excreted via the faeces, significant accumulation in patients with renal impairment is unlikely. In patients with impaired liver function, bioavailability is raised to as much as 80% due to a reduced first pass effect.

Preclinical safety data: Animal studies revealed no special findings relevant to clinical use (although see *Pregnancy and lactation*).

Pharmaceutical particulars

List of excipients: Lactose, sucrose, povidone, crospovidone, colloidal silicon dioxide, magnesium stearate, yellow iron oxide E172 (6.25 and 12.5 mg tablets) and red iron oxide E172 (3.125 and 12.5 mg tablets).

Incompatibilities: Not applicable.

Shelf life

3.125 mg tablets – 2 years
6.25 mg tablets – 3 years
12.5 mg tablets – 4 years
25 mg tablets – 5 years

Special precautions for storage: The tablets should be stored in a dry place below 25°C and protected from light.

Nature and contents of container: Blister packs, PVC/Aluminium of 28 tablets.

Instructions for use/handling: Not applicable.

Marketing authorisation numbers

"Eucardic" 3.125 tablets PL 15722/0039
"Eucardic" 6.25 tablets PL 15722/0036
"Eucardic" 12.5 tablets PL 15722/0020
"Eucardic" 25 tablets PL 15722/0021

Date of first authorisation/renewal of authorisation

PL 15722/0039, PL 15722/0036–20 July 1998
PL 15722/0020, PL 15722/0021–1 February 1997

Date of (partial) revision of the text October 1998

FANSIDAR

Presentation Round, white tablets with ROCHE and a hexagon imprinted on one face and two break bars on the other, containing 500 mg sulfadoxine and 25 mg pyrimethamine.

Uses

Pharmacological properties: The mode of action of Fansidar is based on the reciprocal potentiation of its two components. Fansidar blocks the action of two enzymes which catalyse consecutive stages in the biosynthesis of folinic acid in malaria parasites. Larger doses of the components of Fansidar are necessary if they are given independently and the effect obtained is inferior to that of the combination.

Fansidar is effective against plasmodial strains which are resistant to chloroquine and/or pyrimethamine and other antifolate preparations.

With Fansidar, the danger of emergence of resistance is reduced. However, in certain malarious areas, particularly South-East Asia and South America, strains of *Plasmodium falciparum* may be encountered which have developed resistance to Fansidar.

Fansidar affects all developmental stages of the parasites. It has prolonged action, yet effective plasma concentrations are rapidly attained after a single dose. Trophozoites and schizonts quickly disappear from the blood. Pre-erythrocytic stages are also affected and the gametocytes, although increased in number, are rendered much less infective for the vector. A protective effect persists for up to two to four weeks depending on the dose given and the immune state of the subject.

Pharmacokinetics:

Absorption: After administration of 1 tablet, peak plasma levels for pyrimethamine (0.21 mg per litre) and for sulfadoxine (63.2 mg per litre) are reached after about four hours (means obtained from 14 test subjects).

Elimination: A relatively long elimination half-life is characteristic of both components. The mean values are 96 hours for pyrimethamine and 184 hours for sulfadoxine. Both pyrimethamine and sulfadoxine are eliminated mainly via the kidneys.

Accumulation: Patients taking 1 tablet a week (recommended adult dose for malaria prophylaxis) can be expected to have mean steady state plasma concentrations of 0.15 mg per litre for pyrimethamine (after about four weeks) and 98.4 mg per litre for sulfadoxine (after about seven weeks).

Protein binding: The following values were determined for binding to plasma protein: pyrimethamine 84.9% and sulfadoxine 91.4%.

Indications: Treatment and prophylaxis of *Plasmodium falciparum* malaria.

Treatment of malaria: Fansidar is indicated for the treatment of *Plasmodium falciparum* malaria when the infection is contracted in an area of chloroquine resistance.

Prophylaxis of malaria: Malaria prophylaxis with Fansidar is indicated for travellers to areas where chloroquine-resistant *Plasmodium falciparum* malaria is endemic. Whenever malaria prophylaxis is prescribed, the malaria situation and in particular, resistance trends at the traveller's destination and any stop-over point must be considered. At present, there is no antimalarial agent which provides absolute protection against malaria, but conscientiously performed drug prophylaxis can usually prevent serious progression of the disease.

Dosage and administration

Curative treatment of malaria: The appropriate amount of the drug is given in one single dose. This dose should not be repeated for at least seven days.

Adults (higher dose for persons over 60 kg)			2 to 3 tablets
Children	10–14 years	(31–45 kg)	2 tablets
	7–9 years	(21–30 kg)	1½ tablets
	4–6 years	(11–20 kg)	1 tablet
	under 4 years	(5–10 kg)	½ tablet

In very severe cases, quinine may be added, preferably parenterally. An adequate supply of fluids and electrolytes should be maintained.

Prophylactic management: The following dose of Fansidar should be taken every seven days:

Adults			1 tablet
Children	9–14 years	(30–45 kg)	¾ tablet
	4–8 years	(11–29 kg)	½ tablet
	under 4 years	(5–10 kg)	¼ tablet

Regular dosage is important for continuous protection to be maintained. Routine measures to protect against mosquito bites should not be omitted.

Fansidar prophylaxis should be started about one week before entering the endemic area in order to assess tolerance; this will enable an alternative drug to be selected in the infrequent case where Fansidar is poorly tolerated.

IMPORTANT: Fansidar prophylaxis should be continued for four to six weeks after returning to a non-malarious area to ensure elimination of possible falciparum infections (malignant malaria). However, as with other prophylactic drugs, infections of benign malaria (vivax and malariae infections) may give rise to clinical attacks up to several months after return, despite regular prophylaxis.

Travellers should be instructed to report to a doctor any fever that occurs during or after their stay in a malarious area.

Use in the elderly: Although no specific studies have been performed to establish the use of Fansidar in the elderly, it has been used extensively and the dosage requirements and side-effects appear to be similar to those of younger adults.

Fansidar tablets are for oral administration.

Contra-indications, warnings, etc

Contra-indications: Patients with known sulphonamide hypersensitivity.

Prophylactic (repeated) use of Fansidar is contra-indicated in patients with severe renal insufficiency, marked liver parenchymal damage or blood dyscrasias.

Treatment must be immediately discontinued upon the appearance of any mucocutaneous signs or symptoms such as pruritus, erythema, rash, urogenital lesions or pharyngitis and a medical practitioner consulted. The possibility of an adverse drug reaction should be considered in patients developing a rash, jaundice, fever or severe generalised malaise during treatment with Fansidar.

Like all other preparations containing sulphonamides, Fansidar is contra-indicated in premature babies and during the first two months of life.

Use in pregnancy and lactation: Foetal damage has been observed in the rat when any drug containing a folate inhibitor, including Fansidar, is administered in early gestation. The damage is caused by the folic acid antagonist, pyrimethamine, a component of Fansidar; the damage can be prevented by the concomitant administration of folinic acid.

However, no such adverse effects attributed to Fansidar have been reported during human clinical use and the preparation is, therefore, not contra-indicated during pregnancy. The usual medical practice of avoiding the use of Fansidar during early pregnancy should be followed unless considered essential by a medical practitioner. Pregnant women should be made aware of the particular risks of contracting malaria during pregnancy, and should be advised not to undertake unnecessary journeys to endemic areas. A folate supplement should be given to pregnant women receiving Fansidar.

Although no cases have been documented to date, there is a possibility that use of Fansidar during pregnancy at term may produce kernicterus in the neonate.

Both pyrimethamine and sulfadoxine are excreted in maternal breast milk. Nursing mothers should not take Fansidar.

Precautions: Excessive exposure to the sun should be avoided.

Regular blood counts are recommended during long-term prophylactic use (over three months) of Fansidar.

Side-effects and adverse reactions: Fansidar is usually well tolerated at the recommended dosage.

As with other drugs containing sulphonamides and/or pyrimethamine, the following side-effects and hypersensitivity reactions may occur:

Skin reactions: Drug rash, pruritus and slight hair loss have been observed. These reactions are usually mild and disappear spontaneously upon withdrawal of the drug. In very rare instances, particularly in hypersensitive patients, cases of erythema multiforme, Stevens-Johnson syndrome and Lyell's syndrome have occurred, some of which have been fatal.

Gastro-intestinal reactions: Feeling of fullness, nausea, rarely vomiting, stomatitis. There have been isolated reports of hepatitis occurring conjointly with administration of Fansidar.

Haematological changes: In rare cases, leucopenia (usually asymptomatic), thrombocytopenia and megaloblastic anaemia have been observed. In extremely rare cases, they take the form of agranulocytosis or purpura. As a rule, all these changes disappear after withdrawal of the drug.

Other side-effects: Fatigue, headache, fever and polyneuritis may occasionally occur.

Pulmonary infiltrates such as eosinophilic or allergic alveolitis have been reported in rare instances. If symptoms such as cough or shortness of breath should occur during Fansidar therapy, the drug should be discontinued.

Adverse reactions occurring after the administration of the sulfadoxine component of Fansidar are not normally more prolonged than those occurring after shorter-acting sulphonamides despite the continued presence of the drug in the body.

Drug interactions: Concurrent administration of other preparations containing folate antagonists (e.g. co-trimoxazole, methotrexate, anticonvulsants) can result in increased impairment of folic acid metabolism which leads to haematological side-effects. Such concomitant therapy should be avoided if possible.

There is evidence which may indicate an increase in incidence and severity of adverse reactions when chloroquine is used with Fansidar, as compared to the use of Fansidar alone.

Treatment of overdosage: Possible symptoms of overdosage include anorexia, nausea, vomiting, signs of excitation, and possibly convulsions and haematological changes (megaloblastic anaemia, leucopenia, thrombocytopenia).

Treatment is symptomatic and may include forced diuresis. Vigorous gastric lavage should be carried out as early as possible after ingestion. Alkalinisation of the urine may aid elimination of the sulfadoxine component of Fansidar. Possible convulsions due to the pyrimethamine component of Fansidar should be watched for and may require anticonvulsant therapy. Hypersensitivity reactions may require treatment with steroids. Calcium folinate may be given to counteract the effects of pyrimethamine on haemopoiesis.

Pharmaceutical precautions *Storage:* No special precautions are required.

Package quantities Fansidar tablets are available in foil strips in packs of 10 and 150.

Product licence number PL 0031/5097R

Date of last review December 1996

FORTOVASE 

Qualitative and quantitative composition One capsule of Fortovase contains 200 mg saquinavir as the free base.

Pharmaceutical form Soft capsule.

The capsule is beige, opaque, with 'ROCHE' and the code '0246' imprinted on the capsule shell.

Clinical particulars

Therapeutic indications: Fortovase in combination with antiretroviral agents is indicated for the treatment of HIV-1 infected adult patients.

Posology and method of administration:

Adults and adolescents over the age of 16 years: The recommended regimen for combination therapy with nucleoside analogues is 1200 mg of Fortovase three times daily within 2 hours after a meal (see *Pharmacokinetic properties* for further information on effect of food). For the recommended dose of the antiretrovirals used in combination therapy, please refer to the Summaries of Product Characteristics of these medicinal products.

For information on special patient groups refer to *Special warnings and special precautions for use.*

Therapy with Fortovase should be initiated by a physician experienced in the management of HIV infection.

Contra-indications: Fortovase is contra-indicated in patients with hypersensitivity to saquinavir or to any of the other components contained in the capsule.

Fortovase increases plasma levels of terfenadine. Fortovase should not be administered with terfenadine because of the potential for serious and/or life-threatening cardiac arrhythmias. As similar interactions are likely with astemizole and cisapride, these drugs should not be administered concurrently with Fortovase (see *Interaction with other medicinal products and other forms of interaction*).

Fortovase is contra-indicated in patients receiving concomitant administration of drugs which significantly (greater than 50%) decrease plasma concentrations of saquinavir e.g. rifampicin.

Fortovase is contra-indicated in patients with severe hepatic impairment.

Special warnings and special precautions for use: Patients should be informed that saquinavir is not a cure for HIV infection and that they may continue to acquire illnesses associated with advanced HIV infection, including opportunistic infections. Patients should also be advised that they may experience undesirable effects associated with co-administered medications.

Considerations when initiating Fortovase therapy: When initiating saquinavir therapy, Fortovase is recommended rather than Saquinavir hard capsules due to the greater bioavailability. For patients taking Saquinavir hard capsules with viral load below the limit of quantification, a switch to Fortovase may be considered. For patients taking Saquinavir hard capsules who have not had an adequate response or are failing therapy, a switch to Fortovase is not advised.

Hepatic impairment: In cases of mild impairment no initial dosage adjustment is necessary at the recommended dose. The use of Fortovase by patients with moderate hepatic impairment has not been studied. In the absence of such studies, caution should be exercised, as increases in saquinavir levels may occur. Although a causal relationship has not been established, there have been reports of exacerbation of chronic liver dysfunction, including portal hypertension, in patients with underlying hepatitis B or C, cirrhosis or other underlying liver abnormalities.

Renal impairment: Renal clearance is only a minor elimination pathway, the principal route of metabolism and excretion for saquinavir being via the liver. Therefore, no initial dose adjustment is necessary for patients with renal impairment. However, patients with severe renal impairment have not been studied and caution should be exercised when prescribing saquinavir in this population.

Young and elderly patients: The safety and efficacy of saquinavir in HIV infected patients younger than 16 years have not been established. Only limited experience is available in patients older than 60 years.

Patients with haemophilia: There have been reports of increased bleeding, including spontaneous skin haematomas and haemarthroses, in haemophiliac patients type A and B treated with protease inhibitors. In some patients additional factor VIII was given. In more than a half of the reported cases, treatment with protease inhibitors was continued or reintroduced if treatment had been discontinued. A causal relationship has been evoked, although the mechanism of action has not been elucidated. Haemophiliac patients should therefore be made aware of the possibility of increased bleeding.

Diabetes mellitus and hyperglycaemia: New onset diabetes mellitus, hyperglycaemia or exacerbation of existing diabetes mellitus has been reported in patients receiving protease inhibitors. In some of these the hyperglycaemia was severe and in some cases was also associated with ketoacidosis. Many patients had confounding medical conditions, some of which required therapy with agents that have been associated with the development of diabetes mellitus or hyperglycaemia.

Lipodystrophy: Combination antiretroviral therapy, including regimens containing a protease inhibitor, is associated with redistribution of body fat in some patients. Protease inhibitors are also associated with metabolic abnormalities such as hypertriglyceridaemia, hypercholesterolaemia, insulin resistance and hyperglycaemia. Clinical examination should include evaluation for physical signs of fat redistribution. Consideration should be given to measurement of serum lipids and blood glucose. The mechanisms of these events and long-term consequences, such as increased risk of cardiovascular disease, are currently unknown.

Interaction with ritonavir: Plasma concentrations of saquinavir increase if co-administered with ritonavir (see *Interactions*). In some cases, co-administration of saquinavir and ritonavir has led to severe adverse events, mainly diabetic ketoacidosis. Therefore, combination therapy of saquinavir and ritonavir should be used with caution.

Interaction with other medicinal products and other forms of interaction: The metabolism of saquinavir is mediated by cytochrome P450, with the specific isoenzyme, CYP3A4, responsible for 90% of the hepatic metabolism. Therefore, drugs that either share this metabolic pathway or modify CYP3A4 activity, may modify the pharmacokinetics of saquinavir. Similarly, saquinavir might also modify the pharmacokinetics of other drugs that share this metabolic pathway.

Several drug interaction studies have been completed with both Fortovase and Saquinavir hard capsules. Results are presented firstly for studies with Fortovase and then for studies with Saquinavir hard capsules. Observations from drug interaction studies with Saquinavir hard capsules may not be predictive for Fortovase.

Interaction studies performed with Fortovase: Indinavir: Co-administration of indinavir with Fortovase (800 mg or 1200 mg single dose) resulted in a 620% or 364% increase in saquinavir plasma AUC, respectively. Currently, there are no safety and efficacy data available from the use of this combination.

Nelfinavir: Concomitant administration of a single 1200 mg dose of Fortovase on the fourth day of multiple nelfinavir dosing (750 mg tid) to 14 HIV infected patients resulted in saquinavir AUC and C_{max} values which were 392% and 179% higher than those seen with saquinavir alone. Concomitant administration of a single 750 mg dose of nelfinavir on the fourth day of multiple Fortovase dosing (1200 mg tid) to the same patients resulted in nelfinavir AUC values which were 18% higher than those seen with nelfinavir alone, C_{max} values remained unchanged. The safety and efficacy of this combination is under investigation.

Ritonavir: In groups of 8 healthy volunteers, concomitant administration of ritonavir (200 mg bid, 300 mg bid, 400 mg bid) and Fortovase 800 mg bid resulted in a respective 1558%, 1968% and 2128% increase in steady-state saquinavir AUC compared to Fortovase monotherapy (800 mg bid). Ritonavir pharmacokinetics was unaffected by the co-administration of Fortovase. A cross study comparison has demonstrated that plasma exposures achieved with Saquinavir hard capsules (400 mg bid) and ritonavir (400 mg bid) are similar to those achieved with Fortovase (400 mg bid) and ritonavir (400 mg bid). In a patient study where saquinavir and ritonavir were used in combination therapy for up to 24 weeks, doses of ritonavir greater than 400 mg bid or doses of both ritonavir and saquinavir greater than 400 mg bid were associated with an increase in adverse events.

Clarithromycin: Concomitant administration of clarithromycin (500 mg bid) and Fortovase (1200 mg tid) to 12 healthy volunteers resulted in steady-state saquinavir AUC and C_{max} values which were 177% and 187% higher than those seen with saquinavir alone. Clarithromycin AUC and C_{max} values were approximately 40% higher than those seen with clarithromycin alone. No dose adjustment is required when the two drugs are co-administered for a limited time at the doses studied.

Terfenadine: Co-administration of terfenadine and Fortovase leads to an increase in plasma terfenadine exposure (AUC) associated with a prolongation of QTc times. Hence, terfenadine is contra-indicated in patients receiving Fortovase. It should be also not be administered with cisapride or astemizole (see *Contra-indications*).

Grapefruit juice: Co-administration of 600 mg saquinavir and quadruple strength grapefruit juice as single administration in healthy volunteers results in a 54% increase in exposure to saquinavir. This increase is not thought to be clinically relevant and no dose adjustment of saquinavir is recommended.

Interaction studies performed with Saquinavir hard capsules.

Zalcitabine and zidovudine: Concomitant use of saquinavir with zalcitabine and/or zidovudine has been studied in adults. Absorption, distribution and elimination of each of the drugs are unchanged when they are used together.

Ketoconazole: Concomitant use of ketoconazole (200 mg once daily) and saquinavir resulted in steady state saquinavir AUC and C_{max} values which were 130% and 147% higher than those seen with saquinavir alone. There was no increase in the elimination half-life or any change in the absorption rate of saquinavir. Ketoconazole pharmacokinetics is not affected by co-administration with saquinavir at a dose of 600 mg three times daily. A similar increase in plasma concentration of saquinavir could occur with other compounds in this class, such as fluconazole, itraconazole and miconazole or with other inhibitors of the CYP3A4 isoenzyme.

Ranitidine: There was an increase in exposure when saquinavir was dosed in the presence of both ranitidine and food, relative to saquinavir dosed with food alone. This resulted in AUC values, which were 67% greater.

Rifampicin and Rifabutin: Rifampicin (600 mg once daily) was shown to decrease plasma concentrations of saquinavir by 80%. Rifabutin also reduces saquinavir plasma concentrations by 40%.

Delavirdine: Co-administration of delavirdine with Saquinavir hard capsules resulted in a 348% increase in saquinavir plasma AUC. Currently there are limited safety and no efficacy data available from the use of this combination. In a small, preliminary study, hepatocellular enzyme elevations occurred in 13% of subjects during the first several weeks of the delavirdine and saquinavir combination (6% Grade 3 or 4). Hepatocellular changes should be monitored frequently if this combination is prescribed.

Nevirapine: Co-administration of nevirapine with Saquinavir hard capsules resulted in a 24% decrease in saquinavir plasma AUC.

Other potential interactions: Although specific studies have not been performed, co-administration with potent sedatives metabolised by CYP3A4 (e.g. midazolam and triazolam) should be avoided due to the potential for prolonged sedation. Other compounds that are substrates of CYP3A4 (e.g. calcium channel blockers, dapsone, quinidine, tacrolimus and ergot derivatives) may have elevated plasma concentrations when co-administered with saquinavir; therefore patients should be monitored for toxicities associated with such drugs. Conversely, co-administration with compounds that are potent inducers of CYP3A4 (e.g. phenobarbital, phenytoin, dexamethasone, carbamazepine) may result in decreased plasma levels of saquinavir.

Use during pregnancy and lactation:
Pregnancy: Evaluation of experimental animal studies does not indicate direct or indirect harmful effects with respect to the development of the embryo or foetus, the course of gestation and peri- and postnatal development. Clinical experience in pregnant women is lacking. Until additional data become available, saquinavir should be given to pregnant women only after special consideration. Also refer to *Preclinical safety data.*

Lactation: There are no laboratory animal or human data available on secretion of saquinavir in breast milk. The potential for adverse reactions to saquinavir in nursing infants cannot be assessed and, therefore, breast-feeding should be discontinued prior to receiving saquinavir. It is recommended that HIV infected women do not breast-feed their infants under any circumstances in order to avoid transmission of HIV.

Effects on ability to drive and use machines: It is not known whether saquinavir has an effect on the ability to drive and to use machines.

Undesirable effects:
Undesirable effects reported with Fortovase: The safety of Fortovase was studied in more than 500 patients who received the drug either alone or in combination with other antiretroviral agents. The majority of adverse events were of mild intensity. The most frequently reported adverse events among patients receiving Fortovase were diarrhoea, nausea, abdominal discomfort and dyspepsia.

Clinical adverse events of moderate or severe intensity considered at least possibly related to study drug or of unknown relationship reported in greater than 2% of 442 patients treated with Fortovase 1200 mg tid plus treatment of choice in an open label safety study with a median duration of treatment of 52 weeks were: diarrhoea (19.9%), nausea (10.6%), abdominal discomfort (8.6%), dyspepsia (8.4%), flatulence (5.7%), headache (5.0%), fatigue (4.7%), vomiting (2.9%), depression (2.7%), abdominal pain (2.3%).

Other adverse events of moderate or severe intensity considered at least possibly related to study drug or of unknown relationship reported in greater than 2% of patients on Fortovase in study NV15355 were: constipation, insomnia, anxiety, libido disorder, taste alteration, musculoskeletal pain and verruca.

Lipodystrophy: Combination antiretroviral therapy, including regimens containing a protease inhibitor, is associated with redistribution of body fat in some patients, including loss of peripheral subcutaneous fat, increased intra-abdominal fat, breast hypertrophy and dorsocervical fat accumulation (buffalo hump). Protease inhibitors are also associated with metabolic abnormalities such as hypertriglyceridaemia, hypercholesterolaemia, insulin resistance and hyperglycaemia.

Fortovase does not alter the pattern, frequency or severity of known major toxicities associated with nucleoside analogues. For comprehensive dose adjustment recommendations and drug-associated adverse reactions for other drugs used in combination, physicians should refer to the Summary of Product Characteristics for each of these medicinal products.

Undesirable effects reported with Fortovase or Saquinavir hard capsules: Serious adverse events at least possibly related to the use of saquinavir (Fortovase and Saquinavir hard capsules) reported from clinical trials are listed below.

Confusion, ataxia and weakness; acute myeloblastic leukaemia; haemolytic anaemia; attempted suicide; Stevens-Johnson syndrome; severe cutaneous reaction associated with increased liver function tests; thrombocytopenia and intracranial haemorrhage; exacerbation of chronic liver disease with Grade 4 elevated liver function test, jaundice, ascites; drug fever; bullous skin eruption and polyarthritis; nephrolithiasis; pancreatitis; intestinal obstruction; portal hypertension; and peripheral vasoconstriction.

Undesirable effects reported with Saquinavir hard capsules: This section describes adverse events reported following Saquinavir hard capsules therapy that have not been listed above. Adverse events (moderate or severe) with an incidence greater than 2% considered at least possibly related to saquinavir seen in a study with Saquinavir hard capsules when given as monotherapy are included: peripheral neuropathy, buccal mucosa ulceration and rash. Serious and non-serious adverse events from Saquinavir hard capsules post-marketing spontaneous reports, for which a causal relationship to saquinavir cannot be excluded, are as follows: myalgia, somnolence, seizures, allergic reactions, hepatitis, diabetes mellitus and abnormal renal function.

Laboratory abnormalities: Marked clinical laboratory abnormalities (change from grade 0 to grade 3 or 4, or change from grade 1 to grade 4) reported in greater than 2% of patients treated with 1200 mg tid in the open label safety study included decreased glucose (6.4%), increased CPK (7.8%), increased gamma glutamyltransferase (5.7%), increased ALT (5.7%), increased AST (4.1%), increased potassium (2.7%) and neutropenia (2.9%).

The following additional marked clinical laboratory abnormalities have been reported following treatment with saquinavir (Fortovase or Saquinavir hard capsules) containing regimens: calcium (high/low), phosphate (low), bilirubin (high), amylase (high), potassium (low), sodium (low/high), haemoglobin (low), platelets (low).

In the safety study there was a 27–33% incidence of greater than or equal to 1 grade shifts in ALT and AST during the 48 week study period. 46% of these were single abnormal values. Only 3–4% of patients had greater than or equal to 3 grade shifts in transaminase levels and less than 0.5% of patients had to discontinue the study for increased liver function tests.

Overdose: Overdosage with Fortovase has not been reported. There are two reports of patients who had overdoses with saquinavir (Saquinavir hard capsules). No sequelae were noted in the first patient after ingesting 8 grams of Saquinavir hard capsules as a single dose. The patient was treated with induction of emesis within 2 to 4 hours after ingestion. The second patient ingested 2.4 grams of Saquinavir hard capsules in combination with 600 mg of ritonavir and experienced pain in the throat that lasted for 6 hours and then resolved.

Pharmacological properties
Pharmacodynamic properties: Pharmaco-therapeutic group: Antiviral agent, ATC code J05AE01

Mechanism of action: The HIV protease carries out specific cleavages of viral precursor proteins in infected cells, as an essential step in the creation of fully formed, infectious virus particles. Saquinavir fits closely into the HIV-1 and HIV-2 protease active sites, *in vitro* acting as a reversible and selective inhibitor, with approximately a 50,000-fold lower affinity for human proteases.

Saquinavir is active at nanomolar concentrations in lymphoblastoid and monocytic lines and in primary cultures of lymphocytes and monocytes infected with laboratory strains or clinical isolates of HIV-1.

Experiments in cell culture show that saquinavir produces an additive to synergistic antiviral effect against HIV-1 in double and triple combination with various reverse transcriptase inhibitors (including zidovudine, zalcitabine, didanosine, lamivudine, stavudine and nevirapine) without enhanced cytotoxicity.

Pharmacodynamic effects: The effects of Fortovase in combination with nucleoside analogues on biological markers, CD4 cell counts and plasma RNA, were evaluated in HIV-1 infected patients.

Study NV15355 is an open-label, randomised, parallel study comparing Fortovase (n = 90) and Saquinavir hard capsules (n = 81) in combination with two nucleoside reverse transcriptase inhibitors of choice in treatment-naive patients. Mean baseline CD4 cell count was 429 cells/mm³, and mean baseline plasma HIV-RNA was 4.8 log_{10} copies/ml. After 16 weeks of treatment, there was a mean viral load suppression of –2.0 log_{10} copies/ml in the Fortovase containing arm compared to –1.6 log_{10} copies/ml in the Saquinavir hard capsules containing arm. The magnitude of the reduction in viral load was limited by the sensitivity of the assay used, especially in the Fortovase arm in which 80% of patients had viral loads below the limit of quantification (<400 copies/ml) at 16 weeks compared to 43% of patients on Saquinavir hard capsules. ($p = 0.001$). At 16 weeks, the increases in CD4 cell counts were 97 and 115 cells/mm³ for the Fortovase and Saquinavir hard capsules arms, respectively.

The clinical benefit of saquinavir (Saquinavir hard capsules) has been established in a randomised, double-blind study (NV14256) in zidovudine pretreated patients (CD4 ≥50, ≤300 cells/mm³). In this study, the combination of saquinavir plus zalcitabine compared to zalcitabine monotherapy prolonged the time to first AIDS-defining illness or death. The combination therapy reduced the risk of a patient having an AIDS-defining illness or dying by 53%. This corresponds to a reduction in the rate of an AIDS-defining illness or death from 29.4% to 16.0% over 18 months. In the three treatment groups, median treatment duration was 11 to 13 months and median follow-up has been 17 months.

Potential for resistance and cross-resistance to saquinavir: Resistance: HIV isolates with reduced susceptibility to saquinavir (4-fold or greater increase in IC50 from baseline; i.e., phenotypic resistance) have been selected *in vitro.* Genotypic analyses of the protease amino acid sequence in these isolates showed several mutations, but only those at positions 48 (glycine to valine = G48V) and 90 (leucine to methionine = L90M) were consistently associated with saquinavir resistance.

Isolates from selected patients with loss of antiviral activity and prolonged (range: 24 to 147 weeks) therapy with Saquinavir hard capsules (alone or in combination with nucleoside analogues) showed reduced susceptibility to saquinavir. Genotypic analysis of these isolates showed that mutations at amino acid positions 48 and/or 90 of the HIV-protease gene were most consistently associated with saquinavir resistance. Mutations at codons 48 and 90 have not been detected in isolates from protease inhibitor naive patients. Other accessory mutations, which occur following changes at positions 48 and/or 90 in the protease gene were also observed at varying but lower frequencies.

In an initial study of 32 patients treated with 8 weeks of Fortovase monotherapy followed by addition of antiretroviral combination therapy, 10 (31%) have shown key genotypic changes (3 L90M, 4 G48V, 3 double mutations) over a period of 4 to 48 weeks (median 32 weeks). The sample included 11 patients from whom viral RNA could not be recovered.

In a study (NV15355) of treatment-naive patients receiving Fortovase in combination with two nucleoside analogues for a period of 16 weeks, 1 of 28 patient isolates showed genotypic changes at codon 71 and 90 in the HIV-protease gene.

Cross-resistance to other antiretrovirals: Cross-resistance between saquinavir and reverse transcriptase inhibitors is unlikely because of their different enzyme targets. HIV isolates resistant to ZDV are sensitive to saquinavir, and conversely, HIV isolates resistant to saquinavir are sensitive to ZDV. Among protease inhibitors variable cross-resistance has been recognised. Analysis of saquinavir-resistant isolates from patients following prolonged (24 to 147 weeks) therapy with Saquinavir hard capsules showed that a proportion of patients had resistance to at least one of four other protease inhibitors (indinavir, nelfinavir, ritonavir, 141W94). However, the majority of patients were sensitive to at least one other protease inhibitor.

Available information from patients who failed or were failing therapy with Saquinavir hard capsules and were subsequently switched to another protease inhibitor suggests that any loss of sensitivity to the second protease inhibitor may be the result of accessory mutations which arise after the primary codon changes at positions 48 and/or 90.

Pharmacokinetic properties: Absorption and bioavailability in adults and effect of food: The absolute bioavailability of saquinavir when administered as Fortovase has not been assessed. In HIV infected patients receiving multiple doses of Fortovase (400–1200 mg tid) a greater than dose-proportional increase in saquinavir plasma concentrations has been observed.

Following multiple dosing of Fortovase (1200 mg tid) in HIV infected patients, the mean steady-state area under the plasma concentration versus time curve (AUC) at week 3 was 7249 ng·h/ml (n = 31) compared to 866 ng·h/ml (n = 10) following multiple dosing with 600 mg tid of Saquinavir hard capsules (Table 1). Preliminary results from a pharmacokinetic substudy showed a mean AUC of 3485 ng·h/ml (n = 11) in patients sampled between weeks 61 to 69 of therapy. While this mean AUC value was lower than that of the week 3 steady-state level for Fortovase (1200 mg tid), it remained several fold higher than the mean AUC value for Saquinavir hard capsules.

Table 1: Mean (%CV) AUC and C_{max} in patients following multiple dosing of saquinavir

	n	AUC_8 (ng·h/ml)	C_{max} (ng/ml)	C_{min} (ng/ml)*
Saquinavir hard capsules 600 mg tid	10	866 (62)	197 (75)	75 (82)
Fortovase 1200 mg tid	31	7249 (85)	2181 (74)	216 (84)

* The observed plasma concentration at 8 hours.

The mean 12-hour AUC after a single 800 mg oral dose of Fortovase in healthy volunteers (n = 12) was increased from 167 ng·h/ml (CV 45%), under fasting conditions, to 1120 ng·h/ml (CV 54%) when saquinavir was given following a heavy breakfast (45 g protein, 76 g carbohydrate, 55 g fat; 961 kcal). The effect of food with Saquinavir hard capsules has been shown to persist for up to 2 hours. The mean 12-hour AUC after a single 1200 mg oral dose of Fortovase in healthy volunteers (n = 12) was increased from 952 ng·h/ml (CV 83%), following a light meal (21 g protein, 50 g carbohydrate, 28 g fat; 524 kcal), to 1388 ng·h/ml (CV 46%) when Fortovase was given following a heavy breakfast (45 g protein, 76 g carbohydrate, 55 g fat; 961 kcal).

HIV infected patients administered Fortovase 1200 mg tid, with the instructions to take Fortovase after a meal or substantial snack, had AUC and maximum plasma concentration (C_{max}) values which were about twice those observed in healthy volunteers receiving the same treatment regimen. The AUC values were 4159 and 8839 ng·h/ml, and C_{max} values were 1420 and 2477 ng/ml for healthy volunteers and patients, respectively.

Distribution in adults: Saquinavir partitions extensively into the tissues. The mean steady-state volume of distribution following intravenous administration of a 12 mg dose of saquinavir was 700l (CV 39%). It has been shown that saquinavir is approximately 97% bound to plasma proteins up to 30 µg/ml. In two patients receiving Saquinavir hard capsules 600 mg three times daily, cerebrospinal fluid concentrations of saquinavir were negligible when compared to concentrations from matching plasma samples.

Metabolism and elimination in adults: In vitro studies using human liver microsomes have shown that the metabolism of saquinavir is cytochrome P450 mediated with the specific isoenzyme, CYP3A4, responsible for more than 90% of the hepatic metabolism. Based on *in vitro* studies, saquinavir is rapidly metabolised to a range of mono- and di-hydroxylated inactive compounds. In a mass balance study using 600 mg 14C-saquinavir (n = 8), 88% and 1% of the orally administered radioactivity, was recovered in faeces and urine, respectively, within 4 days of dosing. In mass balance studies, 13% of circulating saquinavir in plasma was present as unchanged drug after oral administration and the remainder present as metabolites. Following intravenous administration, 66% of circulating saquinavir is present as unchanged drug and the remainder as metabolites, suggesting that saquinavir undergoes extensive first pass metabolism. *In vitro* experiments have shown that the hepatic metabolism of saquinavir becomes saturable at concentrations above 2 µg/ml.

Systemic clearance of saquinavir was high, 1.14 l/h/kg (CV 12%), slightly above the hepatic plasma flow, and constant after intravenous doses of 6, 36 and 72 mg. The mean residence time of saquinavir was 7 hours (n = 8).

Preclinical safety data:

Acute and chronic toxicity: Saquinavir was well tolerated in oral acute and chronic toxicity studies in mice, rats, dogs and marmosets at dose levels that gave maximum plasma exposures (AUC values) approximately 1.5-, 1.0-, 4 to 9- and 3-fold greater, respectively, than those achieved in humans at the recommended dose.

Mutagenesis: Studies, with and without metabolic activation (as appropriate) have shown that saquinavir has no mutagenic or genotoxic activity.

Carcinogenesis: Carcinogenicity studies of saquinavir are ongoing.

Reproductive toxicity: Fertility and reproductive performance were not affected in rats at plasma exposures (AUC values) approximately 50% of those achieved in humans at the recommended dose.

Reproduction studies conducted with saquinavir in rats have shown no embryotoxicity or teratogenicity at plasma exposures (AUC values) approximately 50% of those achieved in humans at the recommended dose or in rabbits at plasma exposures approximately 40% of those achieved at the recommended clinical dose. Distribution studies in these species showed that placental transfer of saquinavir is low (less than 5% of maternal plasma concentrations).

Studies in rats indicated that exposure to saquinavir from late pregnancy through lactation at plasma concentrations (AUC values) approximately 50% of those achieved in humans at the recommended dose had no effect on the survival, growth and development of offspring to weaning.

Pharmaceutical particulars

List of excipients:

Capsule filling: Medium chain mono- and di-glycerides, polyvidone, α-tocopherol.

Capsule shell: Gelatin, glycerol, red and yellow iron oxide (E172), titanium dioxide (E171), and a lubricant coating of medium chain triglycerides and 3-sn-phosphatidylcholine.

Printing ink: Carmine (E120), aluminium chloride, sodium hydroxide, hypromellose, propylene glycol.

Incompatibilities: Not applicable.

Shelf life: 2 years.

Special precautions for storage: Store between 2° and 8°C in the closed original pack.

For patient use, may be stored at or below 25°C for a maximum of 3 months. To ensure this period is not exceeded, the date when the product is first stored at room temperature should be entered in the space provided on the bottle label.

Nature and content of container:

Container: Amber glass bottles with plastic screw closure containing 180 capsules of Fortovase. Packs contain either one bottle (180 capsules) or 3 bottles (540 capsules).

Instructions for use/handling: Not applicable.

Number in the community register of medicinal products
EU/1/98/075/001 (180 capsules)
EU/1/98/075/002 (540 capsules)

Date of first authorisation/renewal of authorisation
20 August 1998

Date of (partial) revision of the text March 1999.

GENTICIN EYE/EAR DROPS

Qualitative and quantitative composition Gentamicin Sulphate Ph. Eur. = 0.3% w/v gentamicin base.

Pharmaceutical form Sterile, isotonic solution in dropper bottles.

Clinical particulars

Therapeutic indications: Genticin eye/ear drops are indicated:

For the treatment of superficial eye and ear infections caused by organisms sensitive to gentamicin.

For prophylaxis against infection in trauma of the eye or ear.

Posology and method of administration: Adults, including the elderly and children

Eyes: 1 or 2 drops should be instilled in the affected eye up to six times a day, or more frequently if required. (Severe infections may require 1 or 2 drops every fifteen to twenty minutes initially, reducing the frequency of instillation gradually as the infection is controlled).

Ears: The area should be cleaned and 2–3 drops instilled in the affected ear three to four times a day and at night, or more frequently if required.

Contra-indications: Hypersensitivity to gentamicin or to any of the ingredients. Cross sensitivity with other aminoglycoside antibiotics may occur. Known or suspected perforation of the ear drum is a contra-indication to use in otitis externa only.

Special warnings and special precautions for use: Long-term continuous topical therapy should be avoided. Prolonged use may lead to skin sensitisation and the emergence of resistant organisms.

In severe infections, topical use of gentamicin should be supplemented with appropriate systemic antibiotic treatment.

Gentamicin may cause irreversible partial or total deafness when given systemically or when applied topically to open wounds or damaged skin. This effect is dose-related and is enhanced by renal and/or hepatic impairment and is more likely in the elderly.

Topical application of aminoglycoside antibiotics into the middle ear carries a theoretical risk of causing hearing loss due to ototoxicity. The benefits of gentamicin therapy should be considered against the risk of infection itself causing hearing loss.

Contact lenses should be removed during the period of treatment of ocular infections.

Interaction with other medicaments and other forms of interaction: None relevant to topical use.

Pregnancy and lactation Safety for use in pregnancy and lactation has not been established. Gentamicin should only be used in pregnancy or lactation when considered essential by the physician, after careful assessment of the potential risks and benefits.

Effects on ability to drive and use machines: Patients should be advised that the use of Genticin in the eye may cause transient blurring of vision. If affected, patients should not drive or operate machinery until vision has cleared.

Undesirable effects: Irritation, burning, stinging, itching and dermatitis may occur. In the event of irritation, sensitisation or super-infection, treatment should be discontinued and appropriate therapy instituted.

Overdose: The oral ingestion of the contents of one bottle is unlikely to cause any significant adverse effect.

Pharmacological properties

Pharmacodynamic properties: Gentamicin is a bactericidal antibiotic which acts by inhibiting protein synthesis.

Pharmacokinetic properties: Topical application of gentamicin can result in some systemic absorption. Treatment of large areas can result in plasma concentrations of up to 1µg/ml.

> 90% Gentamicin is excreted in the urine by glomerular filtration.

< 10% is bound to plasma protein.

$T_{1/2}$ = 2–3 hours in individuals with normal kidney function, but can be increased in cases of renal insufficiency

Preclinical safety data: Not relevant.

Pharmaceutical particulars

List of excipients: Benzalkonium chloride BP, Borax Ph. Eur., Sodium chloride Ph. Eur., Water, purified Ph. Eur.

Incompatibilities: None known.

Shelf life: 3 years. Discard contents 4 weeks after opening.

Special precautions for storage: Store below 25°C. Do not freeze.

Nature and contents of container: Genticin eye/ear drops are available in 10 ml dropper bottles.

Instructions for use/handling: Not applicable.

Marketing authorisation number PL 0031/0380

Date of first authorisation/renewal of authorisation
20 December 1994/ 20 April 1995

Date of (partial) revision of the text October 1997

GENTICIN INJECTABLE

Qualitative and quantitative composition Gentamicin sulphate Ph. Eur. ≡ 4.0% w/v (80 mg) gentamicin base.

Pharmaceutical form Solution for injection.

Each ampoule contains a sterile, clear, colourless to pale yellow liquid. The solution is preservative free.

Clinical particulars

Therapeutic indications: Gentamicin Injectable ampoules are indicated for the treatment of systemic infections due to susceptible bacteria, for example, bacteraemia, septicaemia, urinary-tract infections and severe chest infections.

Posology and method of administration: Genticin is normally administered intramuscularly but may be given intravenously if required.

If intravenous administration is necessary the dose should be given as a bolus injection into the tubing of the giving set or directly into the venous system over a period of 2–3 minutes. Genticin should not be given as a slow infusion or mixed with other drugs before use (see *Incompatibilities*).

With either intramuscular or intravenous administration the following dosage applies for normal renal function:

Adults: 3–4 mg/kg body weight daily in divided doses.

Typical doses: Over 60 kg: 80 mg 8-hourly.

Less than 60 kg: 60 mg 8-hourly.

In cases of impaired renal function a reduction in dosage frequency is recommended. The following table is a guide to recommended dosage schedules:

Blood urea (mg/100 ml)	*Creatinine clearance (GFR) (ml/min)*	*Dose and frequency of administration*
< 40	> 70	80 mg† 8-hourly
40–100	30–70	80 mg† 12-hourly
100–200	10–30	80 mg† daily
> 200	5–10	80 mg† every 48 hours
Twice-weekly intermittent haemodialysis	< 5	80 mg† after dialysis

† 60 mg if body weight < 60 kg.

Urinary tract infections: As above. Alternatively, if renal function is not impaired, 160 mg once daily may be used.

In life-threatening infections the frequency of dosage may need to be increased to 6-hourly and the quantity of each dose may also be increased at the discretion of the clinician up to a total dosage of 5 mg/kg in 24 hours. In such cases it is advisable to monitor gentamicin serum levels.

Elderly: Adjust dosage according to weight and renal function. Periodic serum monitoring is desirable.

Children: In children and in neonates, it can be expected that serum levels will be lower than those found in adults at equivalent dosage per kg body weight.

The recommended paediatric dosage is therefore as follows:

Up to 12 years: 6 mg/kg in 24 hours in three equally divided doses (i.e. 2 mg/kg 8-hourly).

In infants up to 2 weeks this dosage should be given in two equally divided doses (i.e. 3 mg/kg 12-hourly).

Serum levels should preferably be monitored daily.

In neonates, infants and children, subsequent dosage will often need to be increased to achieve therapeutic serum levels. Peak levels should be measured about 1 hour after intramuscular or intravenous injection and should reach 4 microgrammes/ml, but not exceed 10 microgrammes/ml.

Contra-indications: Hypersensitivity to gentamicin, any other ingredient or to other aminoglycosides. Myasthenia gravis.

Special warnings and special precautions for use: Where renal function is impaired through disease or old age the frequency, but not the amount, of each dose should be reduced according to the degree of impairment. Gentamicin is excreted by simple glomerular filtration, and dosage frequency may be predicted by assessing creatinine clearance rates or blood urea and reducing the frequency accordingly.

It is also advisable to check serum levels to confirm that peak (1 hour) levels do not exceed 10 microgrammes/ml and that trough levels (before next injection) do not exceed 2 microgrammes/ml.

Interaction with other medicaments and other forms of interaction: Concurrent use with other potentially nephrotoxic or ototoxic drug substances should be avoided. The potential nephrotoxicity of cephalosporins may be increased in the presence of gentamicin and kidney monitoring is therefore recommended with this combination.

Frusemide and piretanide may potentiate the ototoxicity of gentamicin, and ethacrynic acid, which is ototoxic in its own right, should be avoided with gentamicin.

Ticarcillin has been shown to reduce the gentamicin activity *in vivo* and, if clinically indicated, should be given at different times from gentamicin.

Neuromuscular blockade and respiratory paralysis have occasionally been reported from administration of aminoglycosides to patients who have received curare-type muscle relaxants during anaesthesia.

Bacteriostatic antibiotics may give an antagonistic interaction, but in some cases (e.g. with clindamycin and lincomycin) the disadvantage of antagonism may be outweighed by the addition of activity against anaerobic organisms. Synergistic action has been demonstrated with penicillin. Cross-sensitivity with aminoglycosides may occur.

Pregnancy and lactation: Safety for use in pregnancy and lactation has not been established. Gentamicin crosses the placenta and there is a risk of ototoxicity in the foetus. Gentamicin should only be used where the seriousness of the mother's condition justifies the risk.

Effects on ability to drive and use machines: None.

Undesirable effects: As with all aminoglycosides, at critical levels gentamicin exhibits toxicity. Nephrotoxicity may occur, resulting in a gradual reduction in creatinine clearance after about 2 weeks of treatment. This is rapidly reversed if the drug is withdrawn. Most cases have pre-existing renal disease or have received other nephrotoxic agents.

Vestibular damage or hearing loss may occur, particularly after exposure to ototoxic drugs or in the presence of renal dysfunction. With gentamicin the vestibular mechanism may be affected when peak serum levels of 10 microgrammes/ml or when a trough level of 2 microgrammes/ml are exceeded. This is usually reversible if observed promptly and the dose adjusted. In the patients with normal renal function it is virtually impossible to achieve these levels at standard dosage.

Gentamicin has rarely been associated with pseudomembranous colitis and usually in these cases other antibiotics are also involved.

Overdose: Symptoms include dizziness, vertigo and hearing loss if overdose accidentally given parenterally.

If the reaction is severe consider haemodialysis as treatment.

Pharmacological properties

Pharmacodynamic properties: Gentamicin is a bactericidal antibiotic which acts by inhibiting protein synthesis.

Pharmacokinetic properties: Gentamicin is rapidly absorbed following intramuscular injection, giving peak plasma concentrations after 30 minutes–1 hour. Effective concentrations are still present 4 hours after injection. An injection of 1 mg/kg body weight results in a peak plasma concentration of approximately 4 microgrammes/ml.

> 90% gentamicin is excreted in the urine by glomerular filtration.

< 10% is bound to plasma protein.

$T_{1/2}$ = 2–3 hours in individuals with normal kidney function, but can be increased in individuals with renal insufficiency.

Preclinical safety data: There are no pre-clinical data of relevance to the prescriber which are additional to that already included in other sections of the SPC.

Pharmaceutical particulars

List of excipients: Water for Injection Ph. Eur., Sulphuric acid Ph. Eur.

Incompatibilities: In general, mixing Genticin Injectable with other drugs prior to administration is not advised. In particular the following are incompatible in mixed solution: penicillins, cephalosporins, erythromycin, lipiphysan, heparins and sodium bicarbonate. In the latter case carbon dioxide may be liberated on addition of the two solutions. Normally this will dissolve in the solution, but under some circumstances small bubbles may form.

Dilution in the body will obviate the danger of physical and chemical incompatibility and enable Genticin Injectable to be given concurrently with the drugs listed above either as a bolus injection into the drip tubing with adequate flushing, or at separate sites. However, in the case of carbenicillin and gentamicin they should only be given at separate sites.

Shelf life: 4 years.

Special precautions for storage: Maximum recommended storage temperature 25°C.

Nature and contents of container: Genticin Injectable is available in colourless, Type I glass ampoules containing 2 ml, in boxes of 10 ampoules.

Instructions for use/handling: Not applicable.

Marketing authorisation number PL 0031/0381

Date of first authorisation/renewal of authorisation 20 December 1994

Date of (partial) revision of the text July 1996

GENTISONE HC EAR DROPS

Qualitative and quantitative composition Gentisone HC ear drops is a sterile aqueous suspension in 10 ml dropper bottles containing gentamicin sulphate, equivalent to 0.3% w/v gentamicin base and 1.0% w/v hydrocortisone acetate.

Pharmaceutical form Sterile aqueous suspension.

Clinical particulars

Therapeutic indications: Gentisone HC ear drops are indicated:

1. For the treatment of eczema and infection of the outer ear (otitis externa).
2. For prophylaxis against otitis externa following trauma.
3. For post-operative local use in surgery to infected mastoid cavities.

Posology and method of administration: For all ages

The area should be cleaned and 2–4 drops instilled in the affected ear three to four times a day and at night. Alternatively, wicks medicated with Gentisone HC drops may be placed in the external ear or mastoid cavity.

Contra-indications: Hypersensitivity to gentamicin or to any of the ingredients. Cross sensitivity with other aminoglycoside antibiotics may occur. Known or suspected perforation of the ear drum is a contra-indication to use in otitis externa only.

Special warnings and special precautions for use: Long-term continuous topical therapy should be avoided. Prolonged use may lead to skin sensitisation and the emergence of resistant organisms.

In severe infections, topical use of Gentisone HC should be supplemented with appropriate systemic antibiotic treatment.

Gentamicin may cause irreversible partial or total deafness when given systemically or when applied topically to open wounds or damaged skin. This effect is dose-related and is enhanced by renal and/or hepatic impairment and is more likely in the elderly.

Topical application of aminoglycoside antibiotics into the middle ear carries a theoretical risk of causing hearing loss due to ototoxicity. The benefits of gentamicin therapy should be considered against the risk of infection itself causing hearing loss.

In infants there is a theoretical risk that sufficient steroid may be absorbed to cause adrenal suppression.

Interaction with other medicaments and other forms of interaction: None relevant to topical use.

Pregnancy and lactation: Safety for use in pregnancy and lactation has not been established. Topical administration of any corticosteroid to pregnant animals can cause abnormalities of foetal development. Gentisone HC drops should only be used in pregnancy or lactation when considered essential by the physician, after careful assessment of the potential risks and benefits.

Effects on ability to drive and use machines: Not applicable.

Undesirable effects: In the event of irritation, sensitisation or super-infection, treatment with Gentisone HC should be discontinued and appropriate therapy instituted.

Overdose: Not applicable.

Pharmacological properties

Pharmacodynamic properties: Gentamicin is a bactericidal antibiotic which acts by inhibiting protein synthesis.

Corticosteroids, such as hydrocortisone acetate, are used in pharmacological doses for their anti-inflammatory and immuno-suppressant glucocorticoid properties which suppress the clinical manifestation of disease in a wide range of disorders.

Pharmacokinetic properties: Topical application of gentamicin can result in some systemic absorption. Treatment of large areas can result in plasma concentrations of up to 1μg/ml.

> 90% gentamicin is excreted in the urine by glomerular filtration.

< 10% is bound to plasma protein.

$T_{1/2}$ = 2–3 hours in individuals with normal kidney function, but can be increased in cases of renal insufficiency.

Hydrocortisone acetate is not absorbed through the skin as rapidly as hydrocortisone and therefore has a prolonged action. Some is absorbed systemically, where greater than 90% is protein bound.

> 70% hydrocortisone acetate is metabolised by the liver. The metabolites are excreted in the urine.

Plasma $T_{1/2}$ = $1\frac{1}{2}$ hours.

Preclinical safety data: See *Pregnancy and lactation.*

Pharmaceutical particulars

List of excipients: Benzalkonium chloride (preservative), povidone, polyethylene glycol 4000, sodium chloride, borax, disodium edetate and purified water.

Incompatibilities: None known.

Shelf life: 3 years. Discard contents 4 weeks after opening.

Special precautions for storage: Store below 25°C. Do not freeze or mix with other liquids.

Nature and contents of container: 10 ml dropper bottles.

Instructions for use/handling: Not applicable.

Marketing authorisation number PL 0031/0382

Date of first authorisation 20 December 1994

Date of (partial) revision of the text August 1998

HIVID ▼

Qualitative and quantitative composition Hivid is supplied as film-coated tablets containing 0.375 mg or 0.750 mg zalcitabine.

Pharmaceutical form 0.375 mg and 0.750 mg film-coated tablets for oral administration.

Clinical particulars

Therapeutic indication: Hivid (zalcitabine) is indicated in HIV-infected adults in combination with other antiretroviral drugs.

Posology and method of administration

Recommended dosage: The recommended daily dose of Hivid in combination with other antiretroviral drugs is 0.75 mg administered every 8 hours (2.25 mg total daily dose). Since systemic exposure decreases only slightly with food Hivid may be administered with and without food. The dosage schedule of any other antiretroviral drug should be prescribed as recommended in the complete Product Information for these drugs.

Monitoring of patients: Periodic complete blood counts and clinical chemistry tests should be performed. Serum amylase levels should be monitored in those individuals who have a history of elevated amylase, pancreatitis, ethanol abuse, who are on parenteral nutrition or who are otherwise at high risk of pancreatitis. Careful monitoring for signs or symptoms suggestive of peripheral neuropathy is recommended, particularly in individuals with a low CD_4 cell count who are at a greater risk of developing peripheral neuropathy while on therapy (see *Special warnings and special precautions for use*).

Dose adjustment in particular clinical situations

Renal impairment: Based on sparse data dose adjustment in patients with renal impairment should be considered as follows: estimated creatinine clearance 10 to 40 ml/min–reduce the Hivid dose to 0.750 mg every 12 hours; estimated creatinine clearance < 10 ml/min–reduce the Hivid dose to 0.750 mg once a day.

Hepatic impairment: Recommendations for dose adjustment cannot be given for patients with impaired hepatic function because of limited experience.

Children: Recommendations for the dosage in children younger than 13 years cannot be given since the experience in this age group is limited.

Dosage adjustment in case of undesirable effects during combination therapy

For toxicities that are likely to be associated with Hivid (e.g. peripheral neuropathy, severe oral or oesophageal ulcers, pancreatitis, elevated liver function tests especially in patients with chronic hepatitis B), the Hivid dose should be reduced or Hivid should be interrupted or discontinued as appropriate (see *Special warnings and special precautions for use*). For recipients of combination therapy with Hivid and other antiretroviral agents, dose adjustments or interruption for each drug should be based on the known toxicity profile of the individual drugs. See the complete Product Information for each drug used in combination for a description of known drug associated adverse reactions.

Contra-indications: Hivid is contraindicated in patients with known hypersensitivity to any of the components of the tablets.

Special warnings and special precautions for use: Peripheral neuropathy: The major clinical toxicity of Hivid is peripheral neuropathy. Hivid-related peripheral neuropathy is a sensorimotor neuropathy characterised initially by numbness and burning dysesthesia involving the distal extremities. These symptoms may be followed by sharp shooting pains or severe continuous burning pain if the drug is not withdrawn. The neuropathy may progress to severe pain requiring narcotic analgesics and is potentially irreversible, especially if Hivid is not stopped promptly. In some patients, symptoms of neuropathy may initially progress despite discontinuation of Hivid. With prompt discontinuation of Hivid, the neuropathy is usually slowly reversible.

Patients with moderate to severe peripheral neuropathy, as evidenced by symptoms accompanied by objective findings, are advised to avoid Hivid.

Hivid should be used with caution in patients with a risk of developing peripheral neuropathy: patients with low CD_4 cell counts (CD_4 < 50 cells/mm³) and/or patients receiving Hivid concomitantly with drugs that have the potential to cause peripheral neuropathy (see *Interactions: Drugs that have the potential to cause peripheral neuropathy*). Careful monitoring is strongly recommended for these individuals. If peripheral neuropathy occurs in patients treated with Hivid, the drug should be interrupted or discontinued.

Pancreatitis: Fatal pancreatitis has been observed with the administration of Hivid. Pancreatitis and asymptomatic elevated serum amylase are uncommon occurrences during Hivid therapy.

Caution should be exercised when administering Hivid to any patient with a history of pancreatitis or known risk factor for the development of pancreatitis.

Patients with a history of pancreatitis or a history of elevated serum amylase should be followed more closely while on Hivid therapy. Treatment with Hivid should be interrupted in the setting of a rising serum amylase level associated with dysglycaemia, rising triglyceride level, decreasing serum calcium or other parameters suggestive of impending pancreatitis, until a clinical diagnosis is reached. Treatment with Hivid should also be interrupted if treatment with another drug known to cause pancreatitis (e.g. pentamidine) is required (see also *Drugs that have the potential to cause pancreatitis*).

Hivid should be restarted only after pancreatitis has been ruled out. If clinical pancreatitis develops during Hivid administration, it is recommended that Hivid be permanently discontinued.

Other severe undesirable effects: Infrequent cases of oral and oesophageal ulcer and hypersensitivity reactions (anaphylactic reaction, urticaria without other signs of anaphylaxis) have been reported in individuals receiving Hivid therapy. Interruption of Hivid should be considered in patients who develop oesophageal ulcers which do not respond to specific treatment for opportunistic pathogens.

Infrequent cases of cardiomyopathy and congestive heart failure have been reported in patients receiving Hivid. Treatment with Hivid in patients with baseline cardiomyopathy or history of congestive heart failure should be approached with caution.

Rare occurrences of lactic acidosis in the absence of hypoxemia, and severe hepatomegaly with steatosis have been reported with the use of nucleoside analogues, including zidovidune (ZDV) and Hivid and are potentially life-threatening.

Cases of hepatic failure in association with underlying hepatitis B and Hivid monotherapy have been reported. Treatment with Hivid in patients with pre-existing liver disease, liver enzyme abnormalities, a history of ethanol abuse or hepatitis, should be approached with caution. Hivid should be interrupted or discontinued in the setting of deterioration of liver function tests, hepatic steatosis, progressive hepatomegaly or unexplained lactic acidosis.

Particular clinical situations: Renal Impairment: For patients with renal impairment dose adjustment should be considered (see *Dose adjustment in particular clinical situations – Renal impairment*).

Hepatic impairment: In individuals with pre-existing liver disease or with a history of ethanol abuse, the use of Hivid may be associated with exacerbation of hepatic dysfunction.

Paediatric use: Safety and efficacy of Hivid therapy in HIV-infected children younger than 13 years of age has not been established.

Elderly patients: Specific information about the use of zalcitabine in the elderly is not available. In such patients special attention should be paid to renal and hepatic function information.

Lactose: Hivid contains lactose 151 mg per tablet. This is probably insufficient to be of concern to patients with lactose intolerance.

Information for patients: Patients should be informed that Hivid is not a cure for HIV infection, that they may continue to develop illnesses associated with advanced HIV infection including opportunistic infections. Since it is frequently difficult to determine whether symptoms are a result of drug effect or underlying disease manifestation, patients should be encouraged to report all changes in their condition to their physician. Patients should be informed that the use of Hivid or other antiretroviral drugs do not preclude the ongoing need to maintain practices designed to prevent transmission of HIV.

Patients should be advised of the early symptoms of peripheral neuropathy and pancreatitis and should be instructed to promptly report them to their physician. Since the development of peripheral neuropathy appears to be dose-related to Hivid, patients should follow their physician's instructions regarding the prescribed dose. Women of childbearing age should use effective contraception while using Hivid.

Interaction with other medicaments and other forms of interaction

Nucleoside reverse transcriptase inhibitors: There is no pharmacokinetic interaction between zidovudine and zalcitabine which has been confirmed clinically. No information is available on pharmacokinetic interactions of zalcitabine with didanosine, lamivudine or stavudine.

Zalcitabine has no significant effect on the intracellular phosphorylation of zidovudine, as shown *in vitro* in peripheral blood mononuclear cells or in the lymphoblastoid cell line h1A2v2. Zidovudine, didanosine and stavudine have no significant effect on zalcitabine phosphorylation in peripheral blood mononuclear cells. While competition between zalcitabine and lamivudine for intracellular phosphorylation has been reported, data from the CAESAR study indicate a clinical benefit of lamivudine addition to Hivid + zidovudine therapy.

HIV1 proteinase inhibitors: There is no pharmacokinetic interaction between saquinavir and Hivid. No formal interaction trials with Hivid and proteinase inhibitors other than saquinavir have been conducted. As zalcitabine is mainly excreted as unchanged drug in the urine, there is no rationale to expect an influence of other proteinase inhibitors on the plasma levels of zalcitabine.

Drugs that have the potential to cause peripheral neuropathy: Hivid should be used with caution in patients receiving other medications which have the potential to cause peripheral neuropathy (see *Special warnings and special precautions for use*). Drugs which have been associated with peripheral neuropathy include antiretroviral nucleoside analogues, chloramphenicol, cisplatin, dapsone, disulfiram, ethionamide, glutethimide, gold, hydralazine, iodoquinol, isoniazid, metronidazole, nitrofurantoin, phenytoin, ribavirin and vincristine.

Drugs such as amphotericin, foscarnet and aminoglycosides may increase the risk of developing peripheral neuropathy or other Hivid-associated adverse events by interfering with the renal clearance of zalcitabine (and thereby raising systemic exposure). Patients who require the use of one of these drugs with Hivid should have frequent clinical and laboratory monitoring with dosage adjustment for any significant change in renal function.

Drugs that have the potential to cause pancreatitis: Treatment with Hivid should be interrupted, when the use of a drug that has the potential to cause pancreatitis is required. One death due to fulminant pancreatitis possibly related to Hivid and intravenous pentamidine was reported. If pentamidine is required to treat pneumocystis carinii pneumonia, treatment with Hivid should be interrupted (see *Special warnings and special precautions for use*).

Probenecid/cimetidine/trimethoprim: Concomitant administration of probenecid, cimetidine or trimethoprim decreases the elimination of zalcitabine, most likely by inhibition of renal tubular secretion of zalcitabine. Patients receiving these drugs in combination with zalcitabine should be monitored for signs of toxicity and the dose of zalcitabine reduced if warranted.

Antacid products: Absorption of zalcitabine is moderately reduced (approximately 25%) when co-administered with magnesium/aluminium containing antacid products. The clinical significance of this reduction is not known, hence zalcitabine is not recommended to be ingested simultaneously with magnesium/aluminium containing antacids.

Metoclopramide: Bioavailability is mildly reduced (approximately 10%) when zalcitabine and metoclopramide are co-administered.

Ribavirin: When combined with ribavirin the antiretroviral activity of zalcitabine was impaired under *in vitro* conditions.

Pregnancy and lactation

Use during pregnancy: The safety of Hivid for use in human pregnancy has not been established. A teratogenic effect has been observed in animals at very high exposures to zalcitabine. Neurological and behavioural abnormalities have been observed during foetal development and lactation in offspring of rats treated with zalcitabine for which a no-effect dose was not determined. Therefore Hivid should only be used during pregnancy if the expected benefit justifies the possible risk to the child. Fertile women should not receive Hivid unless they are using effective contraception during the therapy period.

Use during lactation: It is not known whether zalcitabine is excreted in human milk. Women receiving zalcitabine should not breast feed their infants. Some health experts recommend that HIV infected women do not breast feed their infants under any circumstances in order to avoid transmission of HIV.

Effects on ability to drive and use machines: There is no clinical evidence that Hivid may alter the patient's ability to drive or use machines. However, the adverse event profile should be taken into account.

Undesirable effects: The major undesirable effect of Hivid is peripheral neuropathy (see *Special warnings and special precautions for use*).

Other undesirable effects which may occur with Hivid include:

Body as a whole: Asthenia, chest pain, cold extremities, oedema, fatigue, fever, hypersensitivity reactions (see *Special warnings and special precautions for use*), malaise, pain, rigors, weight decrease.

Cardiovascular: Atrial fibrillation, cardiomyopathy, congestive heart failure, hypertension, palpitation, syncope, tachycardia.

Central and peripheral nervous system: Abnormal co-ordination, ataxia, Bell's palsy, dizziness, dysphonia, headache, hyperkinesia, hypokinesia, hypertonia, migraine, neuralgia, neuritis, seizures, stupor, tremor, twitching, vertigo.

Gastrointestinal: Abdominal pain, anorexia, constipation, diarrhoea, dry mouth, dyspepsia, dysphagia, distended abdomen, elevated amylase, eructation, oesophageal pain, oesophagitis, flatulence, gastritis, gastrointestinal haemorrhage, glossitis, gum disorder, haemorrhoids, nausea, oral and oesophageal ulcers, pancreatitis, rectal haemorrhage, rectal ulcers, salivary gland enlargement, stomatitis, tongue ulceration, vomiting.

Haematological: Anaemia, eosinophilia, leukopenia, neutropenia, thrombocytopenia.

Hepatic: Abnormal hepatic function (alkaline phosphatase elevation, SGOT elevation, SGPT elevation), hepatic failure, hepatitis, hepatocellular damage, hepatomegaly, jaundice.

Metabolic and nutritional disorders: Lactic acidosis.

Musculoskeletal: Arthralgia, arthritis, arthropathy, muscle weakness, musculoskeletal pain, myalgia, myositis.

Psychiatric: Agitation, amnesia, anxiety, confusion, dementia, depersonalization, depression, emotional lability, euphoria, impaired concentration, insomnia, manic reaction, somnolence, nervousness.

Respiratory: Coughing, cyanosis, dyspnoea, pharyngitis.

Skin and appendages: Acne, alopecia, bullous eruptions, dermatitis, erythematous papules, flushing, pruritus, rash, sweats, urticaria.

Special senses and vision: Abnormal vision, deafness, ear blockage, eye abnormalities, eye pain, loss of taste, parosmia, taste perversion, tinnitus, xerophthalmia.

Urinary system: Abnormal renal function, acute renal failure, gout, hyperuricaemia, micturition frequency, polyuria, renal calculus, renal cyst, toxic nephropathy.

Overdose: Acute overdose: There is little experience with acute Hivid overdosage and the sequelae are unknown. There is no known antidote for Hivid overdosage. It is not known whether zalcitabine is dialysable by peritoneal dialysis or haemodialysis.

Chronic overdosage: In an initial dose-finding study in which zalcitabine was administered at doses 25 times (0.25 mg/kg every 8 hours) the currently recommended dose, one patient discontinued Hivid after one and one-half weeks of treatment subsequent to the development of a rash and fever. In the early phase I studies, all patients receiving Hivid approximately six times the current total daily recommended dose experienced peripheral neuropathy by week 10.

Eighty percent of the patients who received approximately two times the current total daily recommended dose experienced peripheral neuropathy by week 12.

Pharmacological properties

Pharmacodynamic properties: Virology: Hivid is an antiretroviral agent. Hivid has been shown *in vitro* to act additively or synergistically with zidovudine and saquinavir.

Pharmacotherapeutic group: Antiretroviral agent, ATC code J05AB.

Mechanism of action: Zalcitabine is a synthetic nucleoside analogue of the naturally occurring nucleoside deoxycytidine, in which the 3′-hydroxyl group is replaced by hydrogen. Within cells, zalcitabine is converted to the active metabolite, dideoxycytidine

5'-triphosphate (ddCTP), by the sequential action of cellular enzymes. Dideoxycytidine 5'-triphosphate serves as an alternative substrate to deoxycytidine 5'-triphosphate (dCTP) for HIV reverse transcriptase. Inhibition of HIV replication is attained both by competing for utilization of the natural substrate and by its incorporation into viral DNA. The lack of a 3'-OH group in the incorporated nucleoside analogue prevents the formation of the 5' to 3' phosphodiester linkage essential for DNA chain elongation and therefore the viral DNA growth is terminated.

Comparative studies of the antiviral activity of zalcitabine against HIV-1 and HIV-2 *in vitro* revealed no significant difference in sensitivity between the two viruses when activity was determined by measuring viral cytopathic effect. Hivid has been shown to reduce levels of HIV in infected individuals. A correlation has been established between the reduction of viral load and delay in disease progression and death.

Zalcitabine drug resistance: Current evidence demonstrates that the incidence of resistance to zalcitabine is an infrequent event which occurs late during therapy if combined with zidovudine. Specific phenotypic resistance to zalcitabine is usually associated with the appearance of a point mutation at codon 69 and was reported infrequently during zidovudine/zalcitabine combination therapy. Mutations at five individual codons of the reverse transcriptase gene have been associated with multidrug resistance, including zalcitabine, didanosine and zidovudine. These are A62V, V75I, F77L, F116Y and Q151M. Phenotypic cross-resistance of zalcitabine to zidovudine was never observed in clinical studies with concomitant use of zidovudine + zalcitabine in zidovudine naive patients.

However, in the presence of zidovudine sensitivity to zalcitabine might be reduced due to 215 point mutations ("multidrug resistance"). M41L/T215Y, K70R and T215Y viruses were resistant to zidovudine and sensitive to zalcitabine. 50% inhibitory concentration values for zalcitabine increased 5-fold with M41L/T215Y and T215Y viruses in the presence of zidovudine.

Prior exposure to didanosine, stavudine and lamivudine are reported to select genotypic changes at codons 65, 74, and 184 respectively. These mutations confer reduced sensitivity to zalcitabine *in vitro*.

There is no potential for cross resistance between zalcitabine and HIV protease inhibitors because of the different enzyme targets involved. The use of zalcitabine in combination with zidovudine plus the protease inhibitor saquinavir appears to delay the emergence of saquinavir resistance compared to the combination of only zidovudine plus saquinavir.

Clinical pharmacology: The use of Hivid in combination with other antiretrovirals is based on the clinical results from 4 large, randomised, double-blind trials combining Hivid with zidovudine or saquinavir (ACTG 175, Delta, CPCRA 007 and NV 14256) and activity data from 2 studies investigating Hivid in combination with saquinavir and/or zidovudine (ACTG 229 and NUCA 3002). Zalcitabine displayed in these trials, relatively to other antiretroviral substances, usually stronger effects on viral load than expectation based on CD_4 count would predict. Additional data are available from one further clinical endpoint study (CAESAR) investigating Hivid in combination with zidovudine + lamivudine ± loviride, as well as data from a number of pilot studies evaluating Hivid in combination with other antiretrovirals, including other proteinase inhibitors and other non-nucleoside reverse transcriptase inhibitors.

Clinical Endpoint Studies: Studies ACTG 175, Delta and CPCRA 007 compared rates of disease progression and survival in HIV-1 infected patients treated with zidovudine 200 mg tid given as monotherapy or in combination with Hivid 0.750 mg tid. In these studies, the combination of zidovudine + Hivid was consistently superior to zidovudine monotherapy in terms of delayed disease progression and increased survival. The clinical benefits of zidovudine + Hivid appeared greatest in those patients with no or limited prior zidovudine experience.

NV 14256 was a double-blind study in which 940 patients were randomised to receive either saquinavir or Hivid or saquinavir + Hivid. Compared with saquinavir monotherapy, treatment with saquinavir + Hivid was associated with a 75% reduction in the risk of death (p=0.0001) as well as a 44% reduction in the combined endpoint of progression to AIDS or death (p=0.0043).

Additional Supportive Data: Clinical or activity marker benefit was observed in triple therapy regimens comprising Hivid in combination with zidovudine + saquinavir (ACTG 229), zidovudine + lamivudine ± loviride (CAESAR), and zidovudine + ritonavir (M94-208).

Pharmacokinetic properties: The pharmacokinetics of zalcitabine have been evaluated in studies with HIV-infected patients following 0.01 mg/kg, 0.03 mg/kg and 1.5 mg oral doses, and a 1.5 mg intravenous dose administered as a 1-hour infusion.

Absorption and bioavailability: Following oral administration to HIV-infected patients, the mean absolute bioavailability was > 80% (range 23% to 125%, n=19). The absorption rate of a 1.5 mg oral dose of zalcitabine (n=20) was reduced when administered with food. This resulted in a 39% decrease in mean maximum plasma concentrations (C_{max}) from 25.2ng/ml (range 11.6 to 37.5ng/ml) to 15.5ng/ml (range 9.1 to 23.7ng/ml), and a two-fold increase in time to achieve maximum plasma concentrations from a mean of 0.8 hours under fasting conditions to 1.6 hours when the drug was given with food. The mean extent of absorption (as reflected by AUC) was decreased by 14%. The clinical relevance of this decrease is unknown.

Distribution: The steady-state volume of distribution following i.v. administration of a 1.5 mg dose of zalcitabine averaged 0.534 (± 0.127) l/kg.

The drug was < 4% bound to plasma proteins, indicating that drug interactions involving binding-site displacement are unlikely.

Cerebrospinal fluid obtained 2–3.5 hours following 0.06 mg/kg or 0.09 mg/kg i.v. infusion showed measurable concentrations of zalcitabine. The CSF to plasma concentration ratio ranged from 9–37% (mean 20%), demonstrating penetration of the drug through the blood-brain barrier.

Metabolism and elimination: Zalcitabine is phosphorylated intracellularly to zalcitabine triphosphate, the active substrate for HIV-reverse transcriptase. Concentrations of zalcitabine triphosphate are too low for quantitation following administration of therapeutic doses to humans.

Zalcitabine metabolism in humans has not been fully evaluated. Zalcitabine does not undergo a significant degree of metabolism by the liver. Renal excretion is the primary route of elimination, and accounted for approximately 70% of an orally-administered, radiolabelled dose (i.e. total radioactivity) within 24 hours after dosing. The mean elimination half-life is 2 hours and generally ranges from 1–3 hours in individual patients. Total mean body clearance following an intravenous dose averages 285 ml/min. Less than 10% of a radiolabelled dose of zalcitabine appears in the faeces.

Results from patients with renal impairment (estimated CrCl < 55 ml/min) indicate that the half-life was prolonged (up to 8.5 hours) in these patients compared to those with normal renal function. Maximum plasma concentrations were higher in some patients after single dose.

In patients with normal renal function, the pharmacokinetics of zalcitabine was not altered during three times daily multiple dosing. Accumulation of drug in plasma during this regimen was negligible.

Pharmacokinetics in special clinical situations: In children zalcitabine plasma concentration is lower and the half-life is shorter than in adults given comparable doses, suggesting that zalcitabine may be cleared more rapidly in children than in adults.

Preclinical safety data: Experimental animals are species-specifically rather insensitive to the toxicological potential of zalcitabine: the lowest plasmatic adverse effect levels of zalcitabine are 462 times the human exposure in rats, respectively 1825 times in dogs and 21 times in cynomolgus monkeys.

Carcinogenesis: High doses of zalcitabine, administered for 3 months to B6C3F1 mice (resulting in plasma concentrations over 1000 times those seen in patients taking the recommended doses of Hivid) induced an increased incidence of thymic lymphoma. Although the pathogenesis of the effect is uncertain, a predisposition to chemically induced thymic lymphoma and high rates of spontaneous lymphoreticular neoplasms have previously been noted in this strain of mice. Lymphoma has been identified as a consequence of HIV infection in humans. This most likely represents a consequence of prolonged immunosuppression and not antiviral therapy.

Mutagenesis: Ames tests using seven different tester strains, with and without metabolic activation, were performed with no evidence of mutagenicity. Chinese hamster lung cell tests, with and without metabolic activation, and mouse lymphoma cell tests were performed and there was no evidence of mutagenicity. An unscheduled DNA synthesis assay was performed in rat hepatocytes with no increases in DNA repair. Human peripheral blood lymphocytes were exposed to zalcitabine, with and without metabolic activation, and at 1.5 mcg/ml and higher, dose-related increases in chromosomal aberration were seen. Oral doses of zalcitabine at 2500 and 4500 mg/kg were clastogenic in the mouse micronucleus assay.

Fertility: Fertility and reproductive performance were assessed in rats at plasma concentrations up to 2142 times those achieved with the maximum recommended human dose (MRHD) based on AUC measurements. No adverse effects on rate of conception or general reproductive performance were observed. Plasma concentrations equivalent to or greater than 485 times the MRHD were associated with embryotoxicity.

Embryotoxicity and teratogenicity: Hivid is teratogenic in the tested species (mouse, rat). A variety of structural malformations (limbs, cranio-facial, brain) were induced under very high exposure conditions.

Pre- and post-natal toxicity: In a rat study with treatment during late gestation and lactation, learning and memory were impaired. For these observations, a clear no-effect level has not been established.

Pharmaceutical particulars

List of excipients

Film-coated tablets 0.375 mg: Lactose, Microcrystalline cellulose, Croscarmellose sodium, Red iron oxide (E172), Yellow iron oxide (E172), Black iron oxide (E172), Magnesium stearate, Hydroxypropyl methylcellulose, Polyethylene glycol, Polysorbate 80, Titanium dioxide (E171), Black printing inks.

Film-coated tablets 0.750 mg: Lactose, Microcrystalline cellulose, Croscarmellose sodium, Black iron oxide (E172), Magnesium stearate, Hydroxypropyl methylcellulose, Polyethylene glycol, Polysorbate 80, Titanium dioxide (E171), Black printing inks.

Incompatibilities: None known

Shelf life: Film-coated tablets 0.375 mg 5 years
Film-coated tablets 0.750 mg 5 years

Special precautions for storage: Glass bottles "Store between 15°C and 30°C"

Aluminum blister "Store between 15°C and 25°C, protected from moisture"

Nature and contents of container:
Film-coated tablets 0.375 mg and 0.750 mg

a) Glass bottle with a tight screw closure fitted with a desiccant unit containing 100 film-coated tablets

b) Aluminum blisters with aluminum on both sides

Instructions for use/handling: None

Marketing authorisation numbers

PL 0031/0312 Hivid 0.375 mg tablets
PL 0031/0313 Hivid 0.750 mg tablets

Date of first authorisation/renewal of authorisation

1 September 1994 (PL 0031/0312, PL 0031/0313)

Date of (partial) revision of the text 22 November 1997

HYPNOVEL 10 mg/2 ml

Qualitative and quantitative composition Each 10 mg/2 ml ampoule contains 10 mg of the active ingredient midazolam.

Pharmaceutical form Colourless glass ampoules containing 10 mg of midazolam base as the hydrochloride in 2 ml aqueous solution. The ampoule solution is colourless.

Clinical particulars

Therapeutic indications: As intravenous sedative cover before and during minor medical, dental and surgical procedures such as gastroscopy, endoscopy, cystoscopy, bronchoscopy and cardiac catheterisation.

For sedation by intravenous injection (either continuous infusion or intermittent bolus injection) in critically ill patients in intensive care.

As an intramuscular premedication for patients with physical status ASA I–IV who are to undergo surgical procedures.

As an alternative intravenous agent for the induction of anaesthesia in high risk and elderly patients, especially where cardiovascular stability is of particular importance. Induction is more reliable when heavy opiate premedication has been administered or when Hypnovel is given with a narcotic analgesic such as fentanyl.

Posology and method of administration: Intravenous sedation: One or more intravenous injections over a single operating session.

In most circumstances, the 10 mg/5 ml formulation is more convenient for titration purposes.

Adults

An assessment should be made of the degree of sedation necessary for the planned procedure.

The dose should be titrated against the response of the patient. The desired titration end point will depend upon the procedure. Full sedation will be evident by drowsiness, slurred speech but response to commands will be maintained.

As a guide, it is recommended that 0.4 ml of Hypnovel 10 mg/2 ml solution (equivalent to 2 mg midazolam) be administered intravenously over 30 seconds.

If after 2 minutes, sedation is not adequate, incremental doses of 0.1 to 0.2 ml of Hypnovel 10 mg/2 ml solution (0.5–1 mg midazolam) should be given.

Usual dosage range 2.5–7.5 mg total dose (equivalent to around 0.07 mg/kg body-weight). Dosages greater than 5.0 mg are not usually necessary.

Elderly

THE ELDERLY ARE MORE SENSITIVE TO THE EFFECTS OF BENZODIAZEPINES. IN THESE

PATIENTS DOSES GREATER THAN 3.5MG ARE NOT USUALLY NECESSARY AND LOW DOSES AS LITTLE AS 1–2MG (0.2–0.4ML) MAY BE ADEQUATE. THE INITIAL DOSE SHOULD NOT EXCEED 1–1.5MG (0.2–0.3ML).

Children: Hypnovel has not been evaluated for use as an intravenous sedative in children.

Combination therapy: Where analgesia is provided by a narcotic analgesic, the latter should be administered first, the dose of Hypnovel should then be carefully titrated and low doses 1–2 mg (0.2–0.4 ml) may be adequate. In the elderly, smaller doses as little as 0.5–1 mg (0.1–0.2 ml) may be adequate.

Mode of administration: For the administration of Hypnovel the patient should be placed in a supine position and remain there throughout the procedure. Resuscitation facilities should always be available and a second person, fully trained in the use of such equipment, should always be present. It is recommended that patients should remain under medical supervision until at least 1 hour has elapsed from the time of injection. They should always be accompanied home by a responsible adult.

Patients who have received only Hypnovel for i.v. sedation prior to minor procedures, should be warned not to drive or operate machinery for 12 hours. Where Hypnovel is used concurrently with other central nervous system depressants (e.g. potent analgesics) recovery may be prolonged. Patients should therefore be assessed carefully before being allowed to go home or resume normal activities.

Sedation in the critically ill patient: Hypnovel can be given intravenously by two methods for this purpose, either by continuous infusion or by intermittent bolus dose. Both have their own advantages and disadvantages and the appropriate method of giving Hypnovel will need to be determined for each patient.

The dose of Hypnovel needed to sedate critically ill patients varies considerably between patients. The dose of Hypnovel should be titrated to the desired state of sedation. This will depend on clinical need, physical status, age and concomitant medication.

Hypnovel can also be given in combination with an opioid. The opioid may be used for its analgesic effects or as an antitussive agent to help the patient tolerate the tracheal tube and ventilatory support.

Patients receiving Hypnovel for sedation in the intensive care situation should receive ventilatory support.

Safety of the use of Hypnovel for periods of over 14 days in duration has not been established in clinical trials.

After prolonged i.v. administration of Hypnovel, abrupt discontinuation may be accompanied by withdrawal symptoms, therefore a gradual reduction of Hypnovel is recommended.

Potential drug interactions: The critically ill patient is exposed to many drugs. Because of this, there is a potential for drug interactions. (See *Interaction with other medicaments and other forms of interaction*).

Sedation by intermittent bolus dose in intensive care

Hypnovel only: The exact dose of Hypnovel needs to be titrated to the individual patient response. Small doses of Hypnovel 1.0–2.0 mg can be given, and repeated, until the required degree of sedation is reached.

Hypnovel and an opioid: When Hypnovel and an opioid are used together, the opioid should be given first. Both drugs need to be titrated to the individual patients response and to the level of sedation thought to be necessary. Small doses of Hypnovel 1–2 mg (0.2–0.4 ml) can be given, and repeated, until the required degree of sedation is reached. In the elderly, smaller doses as little as 0.5–1.0 mg (0.1–0.2 ml) may be adequate.

The use of these two groups of drugs can increase the risk of respiratory depression. If the patient is being given ventilatory support, using a mode that depends upon some spontaneous effort by the patient, then the minute volume may decrease.

Sedation by continuous infusion in intensive care

Hypnovel only

Adults and children

Loading dose: For patients already sedated or anaesthetised after an operation, a loading dose of midazolam is unnecessary. In other situations a loading dose of 0.03–0.3 mg/kg is recommended, depending on the level of sedation required. This should be given over a five minute period. The loading dose should be reduced or omitted in hypovolaemic, vasoconstricted or hypothermic patients.

Maintenance dose: A dose between 0.03–0.2 mg/kg/hour is recommended, starting at the lower dose.

The dose should be reduced in hypovolaemic, vasoconstricted or hypothermic patients.

Hypnovel and an opioid: When opioid analgesics are used, the rate of infusion of Hypnovel should be titrated carefully to the sedative needs of the patient. Low doses of Hypnovel 0.01 to 0.1 mg/kg/hour may be used to start.

The use of these two groups of drugs can increase the risk of respiratory depression. If the patient is being given ventilatory support, using a mode that depends upon some spontaneous effort by the patient, then the minute volume may decrease.

Whenever a continuous infusion of Hypnovel is used (with or without an opioid analgesic), its need should be assessed on a daily basis in order to reduce the risk of accumulation and prolonged recovery. Each day the infusion of Hypnovel should be stopped or its rate reduced and the patient seen to recover from its effect. If recovery is prolonged (> 2hours) a lower dose should be used when it is restarted. A sedation score should be used routinely.

When Hypnovel has been given for a number of days and then gradually withdrawn, patients may be awake but show signs of residual sedation for the next 12 to 24 hours. This can cause difficulties because patients may not cough and expectorate well if they are then weaned from ventilatory support. However, while recovering from the effects of Hypnovel, patients may not be sufficiently sedated to tolerate ventilatory support. In such circumstances sedation may be provided with a shorter acting agent while there is recovery from the effects of Hypnovel.

The recommended concentration of a solution for infusion in a critically ill adult patient is 1 mg/ml.

Intravenous induction of anaesthesia: One or more bolus intravenous injections over a single anaesthetic session.

Adults: The dose should be titrated against the individual response of the patient. Hypnovel should be given by slow intravenous injection until there is a loss of eyelid reflex, response to commands and voluntary movements.

In anticipating the required dose of Hypnovel, both the premedication already given and the age of the patient are important. Young, fit unpremedicated patients may need at least 0.3 mg/kg body-weight, whereas patients premedicated with an opiate usually need only 0.2 mg/kg body-weight.

Elderly: THE ELDERLY ARE MORE SENSITIVE TO THE EFFECTS OF BENZODIAZEPINES. INDUCTION MAY BE ADEQUATE WITH 0.1MG/KG BODY-WEIGHT IN PREMEDICATED PATIENTS AND 0.2MG/KG BODY-WEIGHT IN UNPREMEDICATED PATIENTS.

Children over 7 years: Hypnovel has been shown to be an effective agent for induction of anaesthesia in children over 7 years of age, at a dose of 0.15 mg/kg body-weight.

Intramuscular premedication: Adults: A single intramuscular injection of 0.07–0.1 mg/kg body-weight, given 30–60 minutes before anaesthesia, has been shown to be adequate in most cases. The usual dose is about 5 mg.

Atropine or hyoscine hydrobromide may be given concomitantly, bearing in mind that hyoscine hydrobromide will enhance and prolong the sedative and amnesic effects of Hypnovel.

Hypnovel can be combined with atropine or hyoscine hydrobromide in the same syringe to be given as a single intramuscular injection.

Elderly: THE ELDERLY ARE MORE SENSITIVE TO THE EFFECTS OF BENZODIAZEPINES AND IN THESE PATIENTS A LOWER DOSE OF 2.5MG MAY BE ADEQUATE.

Children: Hypnovel has not been evaluated for use as an intramuscular premedicant in children.

Contra-indications: Benzodiazepine sensitivity.

Special warnings and special precautions for use: After prolonged intravenous administration of Hypnovel, abrupt discontinuation may be accompanied by withdrawal symptoms, therefore a gradual reduction of Hypnovel is recommended.

Hypnovel should be given with caution to patients with pulmonary insufficiency, impairment of renal or hepatic function, to elderly or debilitated patients and to patients with myasthenia gravis.

In patients with hepatic impairment there can be a significant prolongation of the elimination half-life of midazolam.

During bolus sedation for operative procedures, extreme caution should be exercised in patients with acute pulmonary insufficiency or respiratory depression.

Disinhibiting effects have been noted, even after a single dose. This possibility should therefore be borne in mind if treating patients with a history of personality disorders.

Interaction with other medicaments and other forms of interaction: When Hypnovel is given along with central nervous system depressants, such as potent analgesics, the sedative effect may be intensified and the possibility of severe respiratory or cardiovascular depression should be considered.

There is a potentially relevant interaction between midazolam and compounds which inhibit certain hepatic enzymes (particularly cytochrome P450 IIIA). Data clearly indicate that these compounds influence the pharmacokinetics of midazolam and may lead to prolonged sedation. At present this interaction is known to occur with cimetidine, erythromycin, diltiazem, verapamil, ketoconazole and itraconazole. There is also a theoretical possibility that, by competitive inhibition of P450 IIIA, midazolam could potentiate the effects of other drugs which are metabolised by this isoenzyme e.g. cyclosporin, nifedipine. Therefore patients receiving the above compounds or others which inhibit P450 IIIA together with midazolam should be monitored carefully for the first few hours after administration of midazolam. (Studies have shown that ranitidine has no influence on the pharmacokinetics of parenterally given midazolam.)

Patients should be instructed to avoid alcohol before and for at least 8 hours after administration of Hypnovel since the individual response cannot be foreseen.

Pregnancy and lactation: Animal experiments have not indicated any teratogenic risk with Hypnovel but evaluation in human pregnancy has not been undertaken. Therefore, Hypnovel should not be used during pregnancy unless this is considered essential by the physician.

The administration of high single doses of benzodiazepines in the last trimester of pregnancy has been reported to produce irregularities in the foetal heart rate, and hypotonia, poor sucking and hypothermia in the neonate. Hypnovel ampoule solution should not, therefore, be used during the last trimester.

Hypnovel may pass into breast milk and caution should be exercised with its use in lactating mothers.

Effects on ability to drive and use machines: Patients who have received Hypnovel alone for intravenous sedation prior to minor procedures should be warned not to drive or operate machinery for 12 hours.

Undesirable effects: Changes in cardiovascular parameters are slight but can include a decrease in mean arterial pressure, cardiac output, stroke volume and systemic vascular resistance. Such changes may be important in patients with impaired myocardial oxygen delivery capacity and hypovolaemia.

Following intravenous application of Hypnovel, respiratory depression and respiratory arrest have occurred. These life-threatening incidents may occur especially in elderly patients or patients with pre-existing respiratory insufficiency, particularly if excessive or too rapidly injected doses are administered.

Paradoxical reactions e.g. agitation, restlessness and disorientation have been reported, although this is rare.

Hallucinations, some of a sexual nature, have been reported.

Other side-effects reported include headache, dizziness and hiccoughs. Anterograde amnesia frequently accompanies the period of peak sedation. Local effects on veins are infrequent. However, pain on injection and thrombophlebitis may occur.

Overdose: The symptoms of overdosage are mainly an intensification of the therapeutic effects (sedation, muscle weakness, profound sleep) or paradoxical excitation. Extreme overdosage may lead to coma, areflexia, cardiopulmonary depression and apnoea requiring appropriate counter measures (ventilation, cardiovascular support). Anexate is a specific intravenous antidote for use in emergency situations. Patients requiring such intervention should be monitored closely in hospital (see separate prescribing information).

Pharmacological properties

Pharmacodynamic properties: Midazolam is a potent imidazobenzodiazepine, forming water-soluble salts which are stable and well tolerated by injection. Midazolam possesses the typical pharmacological properties of the benzodiazepines, namely hypnotic, anxiolytic, muscle-relaxant and anticonvulsant activity. In clinical use the induction of sleep is the main action.

Pharmacokinetic properties: At sedative and anaesthetic doses, given intravenously, the action is rapid in onset and of short duration; anterograde amnesia frequently accompanies the period of peak sedation.

Midazolam is principally cleared by hepatic enzymes (particularly cytochrome P450 IIIA), with a mean elimination half-life of about 2 hours, but this may be prolonged in critically ill patients.

The "second peak" effect, which is known to occur following intravenous diazepam, has not been observed with Hypnovel.

The metabolites of Hypnovel do not contribute significantly to the clinical effects of the drug.

Preclinical safety data: There are no preclinical data of relevance to the prescriber which are additional to that already included in other sections of the SPC.

Pharmaceutical particulars

List of excipients: Sodium chloride, hydrochloric acid, sodium hydroxide, water for injection, nitrogen gas in ampoule.

Incompatibilities: Admixture with Hartmann's solution is not recommended, as the potency of midazolam decreases.

Shelf life: 60 months.

Special precautions for storage: None.

Nature and contents of container: Clear glass 10 ml ampoules.

Instructions for use/handling: Hypnovel ampoule solution is stable, both physically and chemically, for up to 24 hours at room temperature when mixed with 500 ml infusion fluids containing Dextrose 4% with Sodium Chloride 0.18%, Dextrose 5% or Sodium Chloride 0.9%.

Hypnovel ampoule solution is stable, both physically and chemically, for up to 1 hour at room temperature when mixed in the same syringe with Atropine Sulphate Injection 500 micrograms/ml, or Hyoscine Hydrobromide Injection 0.4 mg/ml.

There is no evidence of the adsorption of midazolam onto the plastic of infusion apparatus or syringes.

Marketing authorisation number PL 0031/0126

Date of first authorisation/renewal of authorisation 8 December 1982/22 April 1998

Date of (partial) revision of the text June 1997

HYPNOVEL AMPOULES 10 mg/5 ml

Name of product Hypnovel contains the substance with the approved name midazolam. It is chemically described as 8-chloro-6-(2-fluorophenyl)-1-methyl-*4H*-imidazo [1,5-a][1,4]-benzodiazepine.

Presentation Colourless glass ampoules containing 10 mg of midazolam base as the hydrochloride in 5 ml aqueous solution. The solution in the ampoule is colourless.

Uses
Pharmacological properties: Midazolam is a potent imidazobenzodiazepine, forming water-soluble salts which are stable and well tolerated by injection. Midazolam possesses the typical pharmacological properties of the benzodiazepines, namely hypnotic, anxiolytic, muscle-relaxant and anticonvulsant activity. In clinical use the induction of sleep is the main action.

At sedative and anaesthetic doses, given intravenously, the action is rapid in onset and of short duration; anterograde amnesia frequently accompanies the period of peak sedation.

Midazolam is principally cleared by hepatic enzymes (particularly cytochrome P450 IIIA), with a mean elimination half-life of about 2 hours, but this may be prolonged in critically ill patients.

Indications: As intravenous sedative cover before and during minor medical, dental and surgical procedures such as gastroscopy, endoscopy, cystoscopy, bronchoscopy and cardiac catheterisation.

For sedation by intravenous injection (either continuous infusion or intermittent bolus injection) in critically ill patients in intensive care.

As an alternative intravenous agent for the induction of anaesthesia in high risk and elderly patients, especially where cardiovascular stability is of particular importance. Induction is more reliable when heavy opiate premedication has been administered or when Hypnovel is given with a narcotic analgesic such as fentanyl.

Dosage and administration
Intravenous sedation: One or more intravenous injections over a single operating session.

Adults: An assessment should be made of the degree of sedation necessary for the planned procedure.

The dose should be titrated against the response of the patient. The desired titration end point will depend upon the procedure. Full sedation will be evident by drowsiness and slurred speech but response to commands will be maintained.

As a guide it is recommended that a bolus dose 1 ml Hypnovel 10 mg/5 ml solution (equivalent to 2 mg midazolam) be administered intravenously over 30 seconds. If after 2 minutes, sedation is not adequate, incremental doses of 0.25 to 0.5 ml of Hypnovel 10 mg/5 ml solution (0.5–1 mg midazolam) should be given.

Usual dosage range 2.5–7.5 mg as a total dose (equivalent to around 0.07 mg/kg body-weight). Dosages greater than 5 mg are not usually necessary.

Use in the elderly: The elderly are more sensitive to the effects of benzodiazepines. In these patients, doses greater than 3.5 mg are not usually necessary and low doses as little as 1–2 mg (0.5–1.0 ml) may be adequate. The initial bolus dose should not exceed 1–1.5 mg (0.5–0.75 ml).

Children: Hypnovel has not been evaluated for use as an intravenous sedative in children.

Combination therapy: Where analgesia is provided by a narcotic analgesic, the latter should be administered first, the dose of Hypnovel should then be carefully titrated and low doses 1–2 mg (0.5–1.0 ml) may be adequate. In the elderly, smaller doses as little as 0.5–1 mg (0.25–0.5 ml) may be adequate.

Mode of administration: For the administration of Hypnovel the patient should be placed in a supine position and remain there throughout the procedure. Resuscitation facilities should always be available and a second person, fully trained in the use of such equipment, should always be present. It is recommended that patients should remain under medical supervision until at least 1 hour has elapsed from the time of injection. They should always be accompanied home by a responsible adult.

Patients who have received only Hypnovel for IV sedation prior to minor procedures, should be warned not to drive or operate machinery for 12 hours. Where Hypnovel is used concurrently with other central nervous system depressants (e.g. potent analgesics) recovery may be prolonged. Patients should therefore be assessed carefully before being allowed to go home or resume normal activities.

Sedation in the critically ill patient: Hypnovel can be given intravenously by two methods for this purpose, either by continuous infusion or by intermittent bolus dose. Both have their own advantages and disadvantages and the appropriate method of giving Hypnovel will need to be determined for each patient.

The dose of Hypnovel needed to sedate critically ill patients varies considerably between patients. The dose of Hypnovel should be titrated to the desired state of sedation. This will depend on the clinical need, physical status, age and concomitant medication.

Hypnovel can also be given in combination with an opioid. The opioid may be used for its analgesic effects or as an antitussive agent to help the patient tolerate the tracheal tube and ventilatory support.

Patients receiving Hypnovel for sedation in the intensive care situation should receive ventilatory support.

Safety of the use of Hypnovel for periods of over 14 days in duration has not been established in clinical trials.

After prolonged i.v. administration of Hypnovel, abrupt discontinuation may be accompanied by withdrawal symptoms, therefore a gradual reduction of Hypnovel is recommended.

Potential drug interactions: The critically ill patient is exposed to many drugs. Because of this, there is a potential for drug interactions. (See *Interactions* section under **Contra-indications, warnings, etc.**)

Preparation of intravenous solutions: Hypnovel solution is stable both physically and chemically for up to 24 hours at room temperature when mixed with infusion fluids containing 4% Dextrose with 0.18% Sodium Chloride, 5% Dextrose or 0.9% Sodium Chloride.

Sedation by intermittent bolus dose in intensive care Hypnovel only: The exact dose of Hypnovel needs to be titrated to the individual patient response. Small doses of Hypnovel 1.0–2.0 mg (0.5–1.0 ml) can be given, and repeated, until the required degree of sedation is reached.

Hypnovel and an opioid: When Hypnovel and an opioid are used together, the opioid should be given first. Both drugs need to be titrated to the individual patient's response and to the level of sedation thought to be necessary. Small doses of Hypnovel 1–2 mg can be given, and repeated, until the required degree of sedation is reached. In the elderly, smaller doses as little as 0.5–1.0 mg (0.25–0.5 ml) may be adequate.

The use of these two groups of drugs can increase the risk of respiratory depression. If the patient is being given ventilatory support, using a mode that depends upon some spontaneous effort by the patient, then the minute volume may decrease.

Sedation by continuous infusion in intensive care Hypnovel only

Adults and children: Loading dose: For patients already sedated or anaesthetised after an operation, a loading dose of midazolam is unnecessary. In other situations a loading dose of 0.03–0.3 mg/kg is recommended, depending on the level of sedation required. This should be given over a five minute period. The loading dose should be reduced or omitted in hypovolaemic, vasoconstricted or hypothermic patients.

Maintenance dose: A dose between 0.03–0.2 mg/kg/hour is recommended, starting at the lower dose.

The dose should be reduced in hypovolaemic, vasoconstricted or hypothermic patients.

Hypnovel and an opioid: When opioid analgesics are used, the rate of infusion of Hypnovel should be titrated carefully to the sedative needs of the patient. Low doses of Hypnovel, 0.01 to 0.1 mg/kg/hour may be used to start.

The use of these two groups of drugs can increase the risk of respiratory depression. If the patient is being given ventilatory support, using a mode that depends upon some spontaneous effort by the patient, then the minute volume may decrease.

Whenever a continuous infusion of Hypnovel is used (with or without an opioid analgesic), its need should be assessed on a daily basis in order to reduce the risk of accumulation and prolonged recovery. Each day, the infusion of Hypnovel should be stopped or its rate reduced and the patient seen to recover from its effect. If recovery is prolonged (> 2 hours) a lower dose should be used when it is restarted. A sedation score should be used routinely.

When Hypnovel has been given for a number of days and then gradually withdrawn, patients may be awake but show signs of residual sedation for the next 12 to 24 hours. This can cause difficulties because patients may not cough and expectorate well when weaned from ventilatory support. However, while recovering from the effects of Hypnovel, patients may not be sufficiently sedated to tolerate ventilatory support. In such circumstances sedation may be provided with a shorter acting agent while there is recovery from the effects of Hypnovel.

The recommended concentration of a solution for infusion in a critically ill adult patient is 1 mg/ml.

Intravenous induction of anaesthesia: One or more bolus intravenous injections over a single anaesthetic session.

Adults: The dose should be titrated against the individual response of the patient. Hypnovel should be given by slow intravenous injection until there is a loss of eyelid reflex, response to commands and voluntary movements.

In anticipating the required dose of Hypnovel, both the premedication already given and the age of the patient are important. Young, fit unpremedicated patients may need at least 0.3 mg/kg body-weight, whereas patients premedicated with an opiate usually need only 0.2 mg/kg body-weight.

Use in the elderly: The elderly are more sensitive to the effects of benzodiazepines. Induction may be adequate with 0.1 mg/kg body-weight in premedicated patients and 0.2 mg/kg body-weight in unpremedicated patients.

Children over 7 years: Hypnovel has been shown to be an effective agent for induction of anaesthesia in children over 7 years of age, at a dose of 0.15 mg/kg body-weight.

Contra-indications, warnings, etc
Contra-indications: Benzodiazepine sensitivity.

Use in pregnancy and lactation: Animal experiments have not indicated any teratogenic risk with Hypnovel but evaluation in human pregnancy has not been undertaken. Therefore, Hypnovel should not be used during pregnancy unless this is considered essential by the physician.

The administration of high single doses of benzodiazepines in the last trimester of pregnancy has been reported to produce irregularities in the foetal heart rate, and hypotonia, poor sucking and hypothermia in the neonate. Hypnovel ampoule solution should not, therefore, be used during the last trimester.

Hypnovel may pass into breast milk and caution should be exercised with its use in lactating mothers.

Precautions: After prolonged i.v. administration of Hypnovel, abrupt discontinuation may be accompanied by withdrawal symptoms, therefore a gradual reduction of Hypnovel is recommended.

Hypnovel should be given with caution to patients with pulmonary insufficiency, impairment of renal or hepatic function, to elderly or debilitated patients and to patients with myasthenia gravis. In patients with hepatic impairment there can be a significant prolongation of the elimination half-life of midazolam.

During bolus sedation for operative procedures extreme caution should be exercised in patients with acute pulmonary insufficiency or respiratory depression.

Disinhibiting effects have been noted, even after a single dose. This should therefore be borne in mind if treating patients with a history of personality disorders.

Side-effects and adverse reactions: Changes in cardiovascular parameters are slight but can include a decrease in mean arterial pressure, cardiac output, stroke volume and systemic vascular resistance. Such changes may be important in patients with impaired myocardial oxygen delivery capacity and hypovolaemia.

Following intravenous application of Hypnovel, respiratory depression and respiratory arrest have occurred. These life-threatening incidents may occur especially in elderly patients or patients with pre-existing respiratory insufficiency, particularly if excessive or too rapidly injected doses are administered.

Paradoxical reactions, e.g. agitation, restlessness and disorientation have been reported, although these are rare.

Hallucinations, some of a sexual nature, have been reported.

Other side-effects reported include headache, dizziness and hiccoughs. Anterograde amnesia frequently accompanies the period of peak sedation. Local effects on veins are infrequent. However, pain on injection and thrombophlebitis may occur.

Drug interactions: When Hypnovel is given along with central nervous system depressants, such as potent analgesics, the sedative effect may be intensified and the possibility of severe respiratory or cardiovascular depression should be considered.

There is a potentially relevant interaction between midazolam and compounds which inhibit certain hepatic enzymes (particularly cytochrome P450 IIIA). Data clearly indicate that these compounds influence the pharmacokinetics of midazolam and may lead to prolonged sedation. At present this interaction is known to occur with cimetidine, erythromycin, diltiazem, verapamil, ketoconazole and itraconazole. There is also a theoretical possibility that, by competitive inhibition of P450 IIIA, midazolam could potentiate the effects of other drugs which are metabolised by this isoenzyme e.g. cyclosporin, nifedipine. Therefore patients receiving the above compounds or others which inhibit P450 IIIA together with midazolam should be monitored carefully for the first few hours after administration of midazolam. (Studies have shown that ranitidine has no influence on the pharmacokinetics of parenterally given midazolam.)

Patients should be instructed to avoid alcohol before and for at least 8 hours after administration of Hypnovel since the individual response cannot be foreseen.

Treatment of overdosage: The symptoms of overdosage are mainly an intensification of the therapeutic effects (sedation, muscle weakness, profound sleep) or paradoxical excitation. Extreme overdosage may lead to coma, areflexia, cardiopulmonary depression and apnoea requiring appropriate counter measures (ventilation, cardiovascular support). Anexate is a specific IV antidote for use in emergency situations. Patients requiring such intervention should be monitored closely in hospital (see separate prescribing information).

Pharmaceutical precautions

Additives: Hypnovel ampoule solution is stable, both physically and chemically, for up to 1 hour at room temperature when mixed in the same syringe with Atropine Sulphate Injection 500 micrograms/ml, or Hyoscine Hydrobromide Injection 0.4 mg/ml.

There is no evidence of the adsorption of midazolam onto the plastic of infusion apparatus or syringes.

Legal category UK: CD (Sch.4), POM.

Package quantities Hypnovel ampoules 10 mg/5 ml in packs of 10.

Further information The "second peak" effect, which is known to occur following intravenous diazepam, has not been observed with Hypnovel.

The metabolites of Hypnovel do not contribute significantly to the clinical effects of the drug.

Hypnovel ampoule solution is stable, both physically and chemically, for up to 24 hours at room temperature when mixed with 500 ml infusion fluids containing Dextrose 4% with Sodium Chloride 0.18%, Dextrose 5% or Sodium Chloride 0.9%.

Admixture with Hartmann's solution is not recommended, as the potency of midazolam decreases.

Hypnovel ampoules 10 mg/2 ml are also available, and are recommended especially for use as an intramuscular premedication (see separate prescribing information).

Product licence number PL 0031/0189

Date of last review July 1996

INVIRASE ▼

Qualitative and quantitative composition One capsule of Invirase contains saquinavir mesylate corresponding to 200 mg saquinavir.

Pharmaceutical form Capsules.

Clinical particulars

Therapeutic indications: Invirase in combination with antiretroviral nucleoside analogues is indicated for the treatment of HIV-1 infected adult patients. (See also *Special warnings and special precautions for use*).

Posology and method of administration

Adults and children over the age of 16 years: The recommended regimen for combination therapy with nucleoside analogues is 600 mg of Invirase three times daily within 2 hours after a meal. For the recommended dose of the nucleoside analogues in combination therapy, please refer to the complete prescribing information for these drugs. For information on special patient groups refer to *Special warnings and special precautions for use.*

Dose adjustments

Invirase in combination therapy: For toxicities that may be associated with Invirase the treatment with Invirase should be interrupted. Invirase at doses less than 600 mg tid is not recommended.

Hepatic and/or renal impairment: For information on hepatic and renal impairment refer to *Special warnings and special precautions for use.*

Contra-indications: Invirase is contra-indicated in patients with hypersensitivity to saquinavir or to any of the other components contained in the capsule.

Invirase is contra-indicated in patients receiving terfenadine, astemizole or cisapride (see *Interaction with other medicaments and other forms of interaction*).

Invirase is contra-indicated in patients receiving concomitant administration of drugs which decrease plasma concentrations of saquinavir, e.g. rifampicin, rifabutin or nevirapine (see *Interaction with other medicaments and other forms of interaction*).

Special warnings and special precautions for use: Patients should be informed that saquinavir is not a cure for HIV infection and that they may continue to acquire illnesses associated with advanced HIV infection, including opportunistic infections. Patients should also be advised that they may experience toxicities associated with co-administered medications such as zalcitabine and zidovudine.

In view of the limited and/or variable bioavailability of Invirase, the risk of undertreatment should be considered. Careful consideration should therefore be given to the full regimen of anti-HIV medication.

Hepatic impairment: In cases of mild to moderate impairment no initial dosage adjustment is necessary at the recommended dose. The use of saquinavir by patients with severe hepatic impairment has not been studied. In the absence of such studies, caution should be exercised, as increases in saquinavir levels may occur.

In patients with prior hepatitis B or hepatitis C and/or chronic alcoholism there have been reports of worsening of liver disease and development of portal hypertension after starting saquinavir. Associated symptoms include jaundice, ascites, oedema and, in some cases, oesophageal varices. Several of these patients died. A causal relationship between saquinavir therapy and development of portal hypertension has not been established. Co-administration of saquinavir with drugs known to cause hepatotoxicity should be avoided in these patients.

Renal impairment: Renal clearance is only a minor elimination pathway, the principal route of metabolism and excretion for saquinavir being via the liver. Therefore, no initial dose adjustment is necessary for patients with renal impairment. However, patients with severe renal impairment have not been studied and caution should be exercised when prescribing saquinavir in this population.

Patients with chronic diarrhoea or malabsorption: No information on safety and efficacy of saquinavir is available for patients suffering from chronic diarrhoea or malabsorption. It is unknown whether patients with such conditions could receive subtherapeutic drug levels.

Young and elderly patients: The safety and efficacy of saquinavir in HIV-infected patients (younger than 16 years) have not been established. Only limited experience is available in patients older than 60 years.

Lactose intolerance: Each capsule contains lactose (anhydrous) 63.3 mg. This quantity is probably not sufficient to induce specific symptoms of intolerance.

Patients with haemophilia: There have been reports of increased bleeding, including spontaneous skin haematomas and haemarthroses, in haemophiliac patients type A and B treated with proteinase inhibitors. In some patients additional factor VIII was given. In more than a half of the reported cases, treatment with proteinase inhibitors was continued or reintroduced if treatment had been discontinued. A causal relationship has been evoked, although the mechanism of action has not been elucidated. Haemophiliac patients should therefore be made aware of the possibility of increased bleeding.

Diabetes mellitus and hyperglycaemia: New onset diabetes mellitus, hyperglycaemia or exacerbation of existing diabetes mellitus has been reported in patients receiving proteinase inhibitors. In some of these the hyperglycaemia was severe and in some cases was also associated with ketoacidosis. Many patients had confounding medical conditions, some of which required therapy with agents that have been associated with the development of diabetes mellitus or hyperglycaemia.

Interaction with ritonavir: Plasma concentrations of saquinavir increase if co-administered with ritonavir (see *Interaction with other medicaments and other forms of interaction*). In some cases, co-administration of saquinavir and ritonavir has led to severe adverse reactions, mainly diabetic ketoacidosis. Therefore, combination therapy of saquinavir and ritonavir should be used with caution.

Interaction with other medicaments and other forms of interaction: Concomitant use of saquinavir with zalcitabine and/or zidovudine has been studied in adults. Absorption, distribution and elimination of each of the drugs are unchanged when they are used together.

Ranitidine: There was an increase in exposure when saquinavir was dosed in the presence of both ranitidine and food, relative to saquinavir dosed with food alone. This resulted in AUC values which were 67% higher. This increase is not thought to be clinically relevant and no dose adjustment of saquinavir is recommended.

Grapefruit juice: Co-administration of saquinavir and grapefruit juice as single administration in healthy volunteers results in a 50% and 100% increase in exposure to saquinavir for normal and double strength grapefruit juice, respectively. This increase is not thought to be clinically relevant and no dose adjustment of saquinavir is recommended.

Indinavir: Co-administration of indinavir (800 mg q8h) and single doses of saquinavir (600–1200 mg) resulted in an about fivefold increase in plasma saquinavir AUC. An increase of this magnitude is not expected to influence the safety profile of saquinavir. Hence, no dose adjustment of saquinavir or indinavir are recommended.

Nelfinavir: Co-administration of nelfinavir (750 mg tid x 4 days) with a single dose of 1200 mg saquinavir soft gelatine capsules resulted in an about fourfold increase in saquinavir AUC, while co-administration of multiple doses of saquinavir with single doses of nelfinavir resulted in only an 18% increase in nelfinavir exposure. This increase in saquinavir exposure is not expected to influence the safety profile of Invirase. Hence, no dose adjustments of saquinavir or nelfinavir are recommended.

Nevirapine: Co-administration of nevirapine and saquinavir resulted in a 24% decrease in plasma saquinavir AUC and no change to nevirapine AUC.

Ritonavir: Ritonavir extensively inhibits the metabolism of saquinavir resulting in greatly increased saquinavir plasma concentrations. Compared to steady-state AUC and C_{max} values obtained from 114 patients that received saquinavir 600 mg tid, saquinavir exposures from patients treated with a combination regimen of saquinavir 400 mg bid and ritonavir 400 mg bid increased at least 17-fold and 14-fold based on AUC and C_{max}, respectively. Saquinavir has not been shown to alter the pharmacokinetics of ritonavir following single or multiple oral doses in healthy volunteers. When used in combination therapy, doses greater than 400 mg bid of either ritonavir or saquinavir were associated with an increase in adverse reactions. (See also *Special warnings and special precautions for use*).

Clarithromycin: Co-administration of clarithromycin (500 mg bid) with saquinavir soft gelatine capsules (1200 mg tid) resulted in a 1.8 fold increase in saquinavir plasma AUC, a 45% increase in clarithromycin AUC and a 24% decrease in clarithromycin 14-OH metabolite AUC. No dosage adjustments for either drug is required when the two drugs are co-administered at the dose studied.

Inadvisable associations: Rifampicin (600 mg once daily) was shown to decrease plasma concentrations of saquinavir by 80%. Since this may result in subtherapeutic concentrations of saquinavir, rifampicin should not be administered concomitantly with saquinavir. Rifabutin also reduces saquinavir plasma concentrations by 40%. Other drugs that induce CYP3A4 (e.g. phenobarbital, phenytoin, dexamethasone, carbamazepine) may also reduce saquinavir plasma concentrations. If therapy with such drugs is warranted, physicians should consider using alternatives when a patient is taking Invirase.

Co-administration of terfenadine and saquinavir leads to an increase in plasma terfenadine exposure (AUC) associated with a prolongation of QTc times. Hence, terfenadine is contra-indicated in patients receiving saquinavir (see *Contra-indications*).

Associations requiring precautions for use: Concomitant use of ketoconazole (200 mg once daily) and saquinavir caused a 1.5-fold increase in plasma concentrations of saquinavir, with no increase in the elimination half-life or any change in the absorption rate. Ketoconazole pharmacokinetics are not affected by co-administration with saquinavir at a dose of 600 mg three times daily. No dose adjustment for either drug is required when the two drugs are co-administered at the doses studied.

A similar increase in plasma concentration of saquinavir could occur with other compounds in this class, such as fluconazole, itraconazole and miconazole or with other inhibitors of the CYP3A4 isoenzyme.

Other potential interactions: Co-administration of astemizole or cisapride with drugs which are known to be potent inhibitors of the CYP3A pathway (i.e. ketoconazole, itraconazole, etc.) may lead to elevated plasma concentrations of astemizole or cisapride. Pharmacokinetic interaction studies with Invirase and astemizole or cisapride have not been conducted, and although saquinavir is not a strong inhibitor of CYP3A, physicians should use alternatives to astemizole or cisapride (see *Contra-indications*). Other compounds that are substrates of CYP3A4 (e.g. calcium channel blockers, tacrolimus, dapsone, quinidine, triazolam, midazolam) may have elevated plasma concentrations when co-administered with saquinavir; therefore, patients should be monitored for toxicities associated with such drugs.

It is unknown whether drugs which reduce the gastrointestinal transit time (e.g. metoclopramide and cisapride) could lead to lower saquinavir plasma concentrations.

Pregnancy and lactation:
Pregnancy: Evaluation of experimental animal studies does not indicate direct or indirect harmful effects with respect to the development of the embryo or foetus, the course of gestation and peri- and postnatal development. Clinical experience in pregnant women is lacking. Until additional data become available, saquinavir should be given to pregnant women only after special consideration.

Lactation: There are no laboratory animal or human data available on secretion of saquinavir in breast milk. The potential for adverse reactions to saquinavir in nursing infants cannot be assessed and, therefore, breast-feeding should be discontinued prior to receiving saquinavir. Health experts recommend that HIV-infected women not breast feed their infants under any circumstances in order to avoid transmission of HIV.

Effects on ability to drive and use machines: It is not known whether saquinavir has an effect on the ability to drive and to use machines.

Undesirable effects: Saquinavir does not alter or add to the toxicity profile of zalcitabine and/or zidovudine, when given in combination.

For comprehensive dose adjustment recommendations and drug-associated adverse reactions for either zalcitabine or zidovudine or other drugs used in combination, physicians should refer to the complete product information for each of these drugs.

The most frequently reported adverse events among patients receiving Invirase (excluding those toxicities known to be associated with zidovudine and zalcitabine when used in combinations) were diarrhoea, abdominal discomfort and nausea.

The listing below is based on a pivotal study which included a treatment arm with saquinavir used as single drug (n=327). Adverse events (mild, moderate and severe) with an incidence > 2% considered by the investigator at least remotely related to saquinavir are given.

Skin and appendages: rash (5%), pruritus (3%).

Central and peripheral nervous system: headache (8%), peripheral neuropathy (8%), numbness of extremities (6%), paraesthesia (5%), dizziness (2%).

Gastrointestinal system: diarrhoea (17%), nausea (8%), buccal mucosa ulceration (6%), abdominal discomfort (4%), vomiting (3%), abdominal pain (3%), flatulence (2%).

Body as a whole–general disorders: fatigue (4%), asthenia (2%), fever (2%).

Musculo-skeletal system disorders: pain (3%).

Other adverse effects: Serious adverse events at least possibly related to the use of saquinavir reported from clinical trials are listed below.

Confusion, ataxia and weakness; acute myeloblastic leukaemia; haemolytic anaemia; attempted suicide; Stevens-Johnson syndrome; severe cutaneous reaction associated with increased liver function tests; thrombocytopenia and intracranial haemorrhage; exacerbation of chronic liver disease with Grade 4 elevated liver function test, jaundice, ascites; drug fever; bullous skin eruption and polyarthritis; nephrolithiasis; pancreatitis; intestinal obstruction; portal hypertension; and peripheral vasoconstriction.

These adverse events were reported from a database of > 6000 patients; over 100 of whom had been on saquinavir therapy for > 2 years. Patients received saquinavir either as monotherapy or in combination with a wide variety of other anti-retroviral drugs (nucleoside analogues, non-nucleoside reverse transcriptase inhibitors and proteinase inhibitors).

Serious and non-serious adverse events from post-marketing spontaneous reports, not mentioned above, for which a causal relationship to saquinavir cannot be excluded are listed below:

myalgia, somnolence, depression, seizures, anxiety, allergic reactions, hepatitis, diabetes mellitus and abnormal renal function.

Laboratory abnormalities: The most common marked laboratory abnormalities seen during treatment with saquinavir containing regimens were isolated CPK increase, glucose decrease, glucose increase, raised transaminase values and neutropenia.

Overdose: One patient exceeded the recommended daily dose of saquinavir (1800 mg daily) by taking 8000 mg at once. The patient was treated with induction of emesis within two hours after ingestion of the overdose. The patient did not experience any sequelae. In an exploratory small study, oral dosing with saquinavir at 3600 mg per day has not shown increased toxicity through the first 16 weeks of treatment.

Pharmacological properties

Pharmacodynamic properties: Pharmaco-therapeutic group: Antiviral agent, ATC code J05AE01

Mechanism of action: The HIV proteinase carries out specific cleavages of viral precursor proteins in infected cells, as an essential step in the creation of fully formed, infectious virus particles. These viral precursor proteins contain a type of cleavage site which is recognized only by HIV and closely related viral proteinases. Saquinavir has been designed as a peptide-like structural mimetic of such cleavage sites. As a result, saquinavir fits closely into the HIV-1 and HIV-2 proteinase active sites, *in vitro* acting as a reversible and selective inhibitor, with approximately a 50,000-fold lower affinity for human proteinases.

Unlike nucleoside analogues (zidovudine, etc.), saquinavir acts directly on its viral target enzyme. It does not require metabolic activation. This extends its potential effectiveness into resting cells. Saquinavir is active at nanomolar concentrations in lymphoblastoid and monocytic lines and in primary cultures of lymphocytes and monocytes infected with laboratory strains or clinical isolates of HIV-1.

Experiments in cell culture show that saquinavir produces an additive to synergistic antiviral effect against HIV-1 in double and triple combination with various reverse transcriptase inhibitors (including zidovudine, zalcitabine, didanosine) without enhanced cytotoxicity.

Pharmacodynamic effects: The effects of saquinavir in combination with zalcitabine and zidovudine on biological markers (CD4 cell counts and plasma RNA) were evaluated in HIV-1 infected patients.

In a study (NV14256) with zidovudine pre-treated patients (CD4 $\geq 50 \leq 300$ cells/mm^3), the combination of saquinavir plus zalcitabine compared to zalcitabine monotherapy prolonged the time to first AIDS-defining illness or death.

The combination therapy reduced the risk of a patient having an AIDS-defining illness or dying by 53%. For death alone the combination therapy reduced the risk by 72%. This corresponds to a reduction in the rate of an AIDS-defining illness or death from 29.4% to 16.0% over 18 months. Similarly for death alone, the rate was reduced from 8.6% to 4.1% over 18 months. In the three treatment groups, median treatment duration was 11 to 13 months and median follow-up has been 17 months.

In this study the median CD4 cell count at baseline over all treatment arms was 156 to 176 cells/mm^3. The average change from baseline over 16 weeks (median DAVG16) for saquinavir plus zalcitabine was +26 cells/mm^3 for the CD4 cell count and -0.6 $\log_{10}$ RNA copies/ml of plasma for viral load. The peak mean increase in the CD4 cell count was 47 cells/mm^3 at week 16. The peak mean reduction in viral load was 0.7 $\log_{10}$ RNA copies/ml of plasma at week 12.

Study SV14604 is a randomised, multi-centre, double blind phase III parallel study of zidovudine + zalcitabine, vs. saquinavir + zidovudine, vs. saquinavir + zidovudine + zalcitabine, in untreated/minimally treated HIV infected patients. A fourth treatment arm of zidovudine monotherapy was discontinued; patients originally on zidovudine monotherapy were switched to saquinavir + zidovudine + zalcitabine, constituting a "delayed" triple therapy group.

A total of 3485 patients were treated and had follow up data available (the intent to treat population). Median baseline CD4 across the 3 arms was 199–204 cells/ mm^3, and median baseline HIV RNA was 5.0–5.1 $\log_{10}$ copies/ml. Median duration of study drug treatment was approximately 14 months and the median duration of follow up for AIDS defining events and deaths approximately 17 months.

Progression to first AIDS defining event or death was significantly decreased for patients on saquinavir + zidovudine + zalcitabine with 76 first AIDS defining events/deaths compared to 142 events on zidovudine + zalcitabine (p=0.0001). An exploratory comparison of initial saquinavir + zidovudine + zalcitabine compared to the delayed triple therapy group showed superiority of initial triple therapy including saquinavir with 76 AIDS defining events or deaths on initial triple therapy vs. 116 on the initial zidovudine monotherapy-delayed triple therapy regimen (p=0.001).

Patients receiving triple therapy had greater increases in CD4 count, with a 71 cells/mm^3 median peak increase from baseline compared to a 40 cells/mm^3 median peak increase on zidovudine + zalcitabine. Similarly, reductions in HIV RNA were greater on triple therapy with a -1.5 $\log_{10}$ copies/ml median peak change from baseline compared to a -1.1 $\log_{10}$ copies/ml median peak change on zidovudine + zalcitabine. For both CD4 and HIV RNA, comparisons over 48 weeks between the triple therapy arm and zidovudine + zalcitabine reached statistical significance (p=0.0001).

Monotherapy is not recommended because antiviral activity has not been demonstrated.

Potential for resistance and cross-resistance to saquinavir
Resistance: HIV isolates with reduced susceptibility to saquinavir have been selected after extensive *in vitro* passage using increasing concentrations of the compound. Analysis of the protease amino acid sequence in these isolates shows substitutions at positions 48 (glycine to valine = G48V) and 90 (leucine to methionine = L90M).

Changes to viral sensitivity to drug in culture (= "phenotypic resistance") or in protease amino acid sequence (= "genotypic resistance") have been investigated in clinical trials. Two particular viral protease mutations (L90M or G48V, the former predominating and the combination rare) are found in those saquinavir treated patients with resistant isolates. The overall incidence of genotypic resistance at about one year in a group of phase I/II patients treated in combination with nucleoside analogues (zalcitabine and/or zidovudine), was 38% (15 out of 39 patients). The clinical significance of phenotypic and genotypic changes associated with saquinavir therapy has not been established.

Cross-resistance to other antiretrovirals: Cross-resistance between saquinavir and reverse transcriptase inhibitors is unlikely because of their different enzyme targets. HIV isolates resistant to zidovudine are sensitive to saquinavir, and conversely, HIV isolates resistant to saquinavir are sensitive to zidovudine.

To date, therapy with saquinavir has demonstrated a distinctive and consistent pattern of mutations. Investigations into cross-resistance are in progress.

Pharmacokinetic properties
Absorption and bioavailability in adults and effect of food: In healthy volunteers the extent of absorption (as reflected by AUC) after a 600 mg oral dose of saquinavir was increased from 24ng.h/ml (CV 33%), under fasting conditions, to 161ng.h/ml (CV35%) when saquinavir was given following a heavy breakfast (48 g protein, 60 g carbohydrate, 57 g fat; 1006kcal).

The presence of food also increased the time taken to achieve maximum concentration from 2.4 hours to 3.8 hours and substantially increased the mean maximum plasma concentrations (C_{max}) from 3.0ng/ml to 35.5ng/ml. The effect of food has been shown to persist for up to 2 hours. Therefore, Invirase should be taken within 2 hours after a meal.

Absolute bioavailability averaged 4% (CV 73%, range: 1% to 9%) in 8 healthy volunteers who received a single 600 mg dose (3 x 200 mg) of saquinavir following a heavy breakfast. The low bioavailability is thought to be due to a combination of incomplete absorption and extensive first-pass metabolism. Gastric pH has been shown to be only a minor component in the large increase in bioavailability seen when given with food.

After multiple oral doses (25–600 mg tid) in the presence of food, the increase in exposure (50-fold) was greater than directly proportional to the increase in dose (24-fold). Following multiple dosing (600 mg tid) in HIV-infected patients (n=29), the steady state area under the plasma concentration versus time curve (AUC) was 2.5 times (95% CI 1.6 to 3.8) higher than that observed after a single dose.

HIV-infected patients administered saquinavir 600 mg tid, with the instructions to take saquinavir after a meal or substantial snack, had AUC and maximum plasma concentration (C_{max}) values which were about twice those observed in healthy volunteers receiving the same treatment regimen (see below).

Mean (%CV) AUC and C_{max} in patients and healthy volunteers

	AUC8 (dose interval) in ng·h/ml	*C_{max} in ng/ml*
Healthy volunteers (n=6)	359.0 (46)	90.39 (49)
Patients (n=113)	757.2 (84)	253.3 (99)

Distribution in adults: Saquinavir partitions extensively into the tissues. The mean steady-state volume of distribution following intravenous administration of a 12 mg dose of saquinavir was 700L (CV 39%). Saquinavir shows a high degree of protein binding (approximately 98%) which is independent of concentration over the range 15–700ng/ml. In two patients receiving Invirase 600 mg three times daily, cerebrospinal fluid concentrations of saquinavir were negligible when compared to concentrations from matching plasma samples.

Metabolism and elimination in adults: In vitro studies using human liver microsomes have shown that the metabolism of saquinavir is cytochrome P450 mediated with the specific isoenzyme, CYP3A4, responsible for more than 90% of the hepatic metabolism. Based on *in vitro* studies, saquinavir is rapidly metabolized to a range of mono- and di-hydroxylated inactive compounds. In a mass balance study using 600 mg 14C-saquinavir (n=8), 88% and 1% of the orally administered radioactivity, was recovered in faeces and urine, respectively, within 4 days of dosing. In an additional four subjects administered 10.5 mg 14C-saquinavir intravenously, 81% and 3% of the intravenously administered radioactivity was recovered in faeces and urine, respectively, within 4 days of dosing. In mass balance studies, 13% of circulating saquinavir in plasma was present as unchanged drug after oral adminstration and the remainder present as metabolites. Following intravenous adminstration, 66% of circulating saquinavir is present as unchanged drug and the remainder as metabolites, suggesting that saquinavir undergoes extensive first pass metabolism.

Systemic clearance of saquinavir was high, 1.14 L/h/kg (CV 12%), slightly above the hepatic plasma flow, and constant after intravenous doses of 6, 36 and 72 mg. The mean residence time of saquinavir was 7 hours (n=8).

Preclinical safety data
Acute and chronic toxicity: Oral acute and chronic toxicity and toxicokinetic studies in the mouse, rat, dog and marmoset have demonstrated good tolerance to saquinavir at high plasma exposure to the drug relative to that seen in man.

Mutagenesis: Studies, with and without metabolic activation (as appropriate) have shown that saquinavir has no mutagenic or genotoxic activity.

Carcinogenesis: Carcinogenicity studies of saquinavir are ongoing.

Reproductive toxicity: Refer to *Pregnancy and lactation.*

Pharmaceutical particulars
List of excipients
Capsule filling: lactose (anhydrous), microcrystalline cellulose, povidone, sodium starch glycollate, talc, magnesium stearate.

Capsule shell: gelatine, iron oxide black, red and yellow (E172), indigocarmine (E132), titanium dioxide (E171).

Capsule appearance: light brown and green, opaque; marking "ROCHE" and the code "0245" on each half of the capsule shell.

Incompatibilities: Not applicable.

Shelf life: Three years.

Special precautions for storage: Store in the closed original pack.

Nature and contents of container: Amber glass bottles with plastic screw closure containing 270 capsules of Invirase.

Instructions for use, handling and disposal (if appropriate): Not applicable.

Number in the community register of medicinal products EU/1/96/026/001

Date of first authorisation/renewal of authorisation 4 October 1996

Date of revision of text 24 November 1998

ISMO RETARD

Qualitative and quantitative composition 40 mg isosorbide-5-mononitrate.

Pharmaceutical form Circular, white sugar coated tablets for oral administration.

Clinical particulars
Therapeutic indications: Ismo Retard is indicated for the prophylaxis of angina pectoris.

Posology and method of administration: Dosage: Ismo Retard has been developed to provide a convenient, once daily dosage form of isosorbide mononitrate. It is designed to achieve therapeutic blood concentrations within 30 minutes which persist up to 17 hours. A nitrate free interval of up to 7 hours makes the development of anti-anginal tolerance during chronic therapy unlikely.
The tablets should be taken with fluid and swallowed whole without chewing.

Adults: One tablet daily to be taken in the morning.

Elderly: There is no evidence to suggest an adjustment of dose is necessary. However, caution may be required in elderly patients who are known to be susceptible to the effects of hypotensive medication.

Children: The safety and efficacy of Ismo in children has not been established.

Renal and hepatic impairment: No dosage reduction is necessary.

Contra-indications: Ismo Retard is contra-indicated in patients with a known hypersensitivity to isosorbide mononitrate or isosorbide dinitrate and in cases of marked low blood pressure, shock and acute myocardial infarction with low left ventricular filling pressure.

Special warnings and special precautions for use: Ismo Retard is not indicated for relief of acute anginal attacks. In the event of an acute attack, sublingual or buccal glyceryl trinitrate tablets or spray should be used.

Ismo Retard is contra-indicated in patients with a known hypersensitivity to isosorbide mononitrate or isosorbide dinitrate and in cases of marked low blood pressure, shock and acute myocardial infarction with low left ventricular filling pressure.

In the case of acute myocardial infarction, Ismo Retard should be continued only under strict medical supervision.

Since a rebound phenomenon cannot be excluded, therapy with isosorbide mononitrate should be terminated gradually rather than stopping abruptly.

Interaction with other medicaments and other forms of interaction: The hypotensive effects of other drugs may be potentiated.

Pregnancy and lactation: There is inadequate evidence of safety of isosorbide-5-mononitrate in human pregnancy although nitrates have been in wide use for many years without ill consequence, animal studies having shown no adverse effects on the foetus. There is no information on excretion of isosorbide-5-mononitrate in breast milk. Use in pregnancy and lactation is not recommended unless considered essential by the patient's physician.

Effects on ability to drive and use machines: In theory, the ability to drive or to operate machinery may be impaired in patients experiencing hypotensive side effects.

Undesirable effects: A number of nitrate-related adverse effects may occur during treatment including headache and feelings of dizziness. The incidence of such effects is normally highest at the commencement of treatment and tends to decline with time. The Ismo Starter Pack is provided to assist in minimising such effects initially. In highly sensitive patients hypotension may occur, especially after a high dose. Other reactions, including feelings of weakness, nausea or vomiting may occur occasionally. Side-effects which have been associated with isosorbide dinitrate (e.g. flushing, postural hypotension, dry rash, exfoliative dermatitis) may also occur.

Some patients may develop or experience a worsening of angina.

Overdose – Symptoms and signs: In the event of overdosage the main sign is liable to be hypotension.

Treatment: The stomach should be aspirated to remove any remaining tablets. The patient should be placed in a supine position with the legs elevated to promote venous return. Symptomatic and supportive treatment e.g. plasma expanders and, if necessary, the careful use of vasopressor agents to counterbalance the hypotensive effects may be necessary. Methaemoglobinaemia will normally respond to methylene blue infusion.

Pharmacological properties
Pharmacodynamic properties: The main effect of isosorbide-5-mononitrate is to produce a marked venous vasodilation without a significant effect on the systemic arteries. The venous dilation leads to an accumulation of blood in the capacitance vessels resulting in a reduction of venous return to the heart. This results in a reduction of the ventricular diastolic volume, which produces a reduction in intramural tension (afterload) as well as reductions of filling pressures and pulmonary capillary pressure (preload) and as a result, a reduction in myocardial oxygen requirements from which arises the antianginal effect.

Beta-blocking drugs have a different pharmacological action in angina and may have a complementary effect when co-administered with Ismo Retard.

Administration of isosorbide-5-mononitrate may produce transient hypoxaemia as a result of redistribution of blood flow, with a relative increase in perfusion of poorly supplied areas of the lung. This may cause ischaemia in patients with coronary heart disease. (See *Undesirable effects)*

Pharmacokinetic properties: Isosorbide-5-mononitrate is rapidly and completely absorbed following oral administration. Elimination is by hepatic metabolism to inactive metabolites. The elimination half life is slightly more than 4 hours.

Ismo Retard releases isosorbide-5-mononitrate over several hours. Therapeutic serum levels are present within 30 minutes of a dose. Peak serum concentrations occur between 3 and 4 hours post administration. Pharmacologically active serum concentrations are maintained for up to 17 hours. Simulation studies indicate that accumulation will not occur in hepatically normal patients.

The drug is eliminated solely be the liver and therefore can be used in renal insufficiency.

Anti-anginal tolerance is unlikely to occur during chronic use as the dosage regime provides up to 7 hours daily when isosorbide-5-mononitrate serum concentration is below pharmacologically active values.

Preclinical safety data: No special findings.

Pharmaceutical particulars
List of excipients: Ismo Retard also contains lactose, montanic acid/ethanediol ester, povidone, colloidal silicone dioxide and magnesium stearate. The tablets are covered by a sugar coating which contains polymethacrylic acid esters, talc, sucrose, kaolin, polyethyleneglycol, titanium dioxide, povidone, glucose and montanic acid/ethanediol ester. No azo dyes are used as colouring substances. (The sugar content of each tablet is less than 36 mg).

Incompatibilities: Not applicable.

Shelf life: 5 years.

Special precautions for storage: No special storage of handling precautions apply.

Nature and contents of container: Packs of 100 tablets in blister strips of HDPE containers.

Instructions for use/handling: No special instructions.

Marketing authorisation number PL 15722/0015

Date of last renewal of authorisation 20 September 1994

Date of partial revision of SPC August 1998

ISMO 10

Qualitative and quantitative composition 10 mg isosorbide-5-mononitrate.

Pharmaceutical form Tablet for oral use.

Each tablet is marked Ismo on one face and 10 on the reverse.

Clinical particulars
Therapeutic indications: Ismo products are indicated for use in the treatment and prophylaxis of angina pectoris and as adjunctive therapy in congestive heart failure which does not respond adequately to cardiac glycosides and/or diuretics.

Posology and method of administration:
Adults: The recommended dosage is from 20 to 120 mg isosorbide-5-mononitrate daily in divided doses. The majority of patients will require a dosage in the range of 40 to 60 mg daily in divided doses. The tablets should be taken with fluid and swallowed whole without chewing.

For patients who have not previously received prophylactic nitrate therapy it is recommended that the Ismo Starter Pack be employed. This provides an initial dosage of 10 mg isosorbide-5-mononitrate (1 tablet) daily for 2 days followed by a dosage of 20 mg daily (1 tablet morning and evening) for a further 3 days. Subsequently the daily dosage may be increased to the normal prophylactic level using the Ismo 20 tablets also included in the Starter Pack. Patients already accustomed to chronic nitrate therapy normally may be transferred directly to a therapeutic dose of Ismo.

For those previously treated with isosorbide dinitrate in conventional form the dosage of Ismo should be the same initially. Ismo is effectively twice as potent as sustained release forms of isosorbide dinitrate and patients transferred from such treatment should receive Ismo at half the previous dosage.

Elderly: There is no evidence to suggest an adjustment of dose is necessary. However, caution may be required in elderly patients who are known to be susceptible to the effects of hypotensive medication.

Children: The safety and efficacy of Ismo in children has not been established.

Renal and hepatic impairment: No dosage reduction is necessary.

Contra-indications: Ismo tablets are contra-indicated in patients with a known hypersensitivity to isosorbide-5-mononitrate or isosorbide dinitrate and in cases of marked low blood pressure, shock and acute myocardial infarction with low left ventricular filling pressure.

Special warnings and special precautions for use: Ismo is not indicated for relief of an acute attack, sublingual or buccal glyceryl trinitrate tablets or spray should be used. In the case of acute myocardial infarction, Ismo tablets should be continued only under strict medical supervision. Since a rebound phenomenon cannot be excluded, therapy with isosorbide-5-mononitrate should be terminated gradually rather than stopping abruptly.

Interaction with other medicaments and other forms of interaction: The hypotensive effects of other drugs may be potentiated.

Pregnancy and lactation: There is inadequate evidence of safety of isosorbide-5-mononitrate in human pregnancy although nitrates have been in wide use for many years without ill consequence, animal studies having shown no adverse effects on the foetus. There is no information on excretion of isosorbide-5-mononitrate in breast milk. Use in pregnancy and lactation is not recommended unless considered essential by the patient's physician.

Effects on ability to drive and use machines: In theory, the ability to drive or to operate machinery may be impaired in patients experiencing hypotensive side effects.

Undesirable effects: A number of nitrate-related adverse effects may occur during treatment including headache and feelings of dizziness. The incidence of such effects is normally highest at the commencement of treatment and tends to decline with time. The Ismo Starter Pack is provided to assist in minimising such effects initially. In highly sensitive patients hypotension may occur, especially after a high dose. Other reactions, including feelings of weakness, nausea or vomiting may occur occasionally. Side effects which have been associated with isosorbide dinitrate (e.g. flushing, postural hypotension, dry rash, exfoliative dermatitis) may also occur.

Some patients may develop or experience a worsening of angina.

Overdose:

Symptoms and signs: In the event of overdosage the main sign is liable to be hypotension.

Treatment: The stomach should be aspirated to remove any remaining tablets. The patient should be placed in a supine position with the legs elevated to promote venous return. Symptomatic and supportive treatment e.g. plasma expanders and, if necessary, the careful use of vasopressor agents to counterbalance the hypotensive effects may be necessary. Methaemoglobinaemia will normally respond to methylene blue infusion.

Pharmacological properties

Pharmacodynamic properties: Ismo provides long-term nitrate treatment of angina pectoris and heart failure in a form with complete biological availability due to lack of any significant hepatic first-pass metabolism. This provides consistently uniform blood levels of drug substance and a predictable clinical response. The onset of activity occurs within 20 minutes, and, depending on dosage, is maintained for up to 10 hours.

Beta-blocking drugs have a different pharmacological action in angina and may have a complementary effect when co-administered with Ismo.

The mean effect of isosorbide-5-mononitrate is to produce a marked venous vasodilation without a significant effect on the systemic arteries. The venous dilation leads to an accumulation of blood in the capacitance vessels resulting in a reduction of venous return to the heart. This results in a reduction of the ventricular diastolic volume, which produces a reduction in intramural tension (afterload) as well as reductions of filling pressures and pulmonary capillary pressure (preload) and as a result, a reduction in myocardial oxygen requirements from which arises the antianginal effect.

Administration of isosorbide-5-mononitrate may produce transient hypoxaemia as a result of redistribution of blood flow, with a relative increase in perfusion of poorly supplied areas of the lung. This may cause ischaemia in patients with coronary heart disease.

Pharmacokinetic properties: Isosorbide-5-mononitrate displays 100% bioavailability on oral administration. Consequently, serum levels are predictable, isosorbide-5-mononitrate is rapidly absorbed – peak serum concentrations occuring 1 hour after oral administration. Elimination half life is approximately 5 hours.

The drug is eliminated solely by the liver and therefore can be used in renal insufficiency.

Preclinical safety data: No special findings.

Pharmaceutical particulars

List of excipients: Ismo 10 tablets also contain lactose, microcrystalline cellulose, sodium starch glycollate, povidone, colloidal silicon dioxide and magnesium stearate.

Incompatibilities: Not applicable.

Shelf life: 60 months.

Special precautions for storage: No special storage or handling precautions apply although it is recommended that Ismo products be kept in a cool, dry place in accordance with good pharmaceutical practice.

Nature and contents of container: Ismo Starter Pack: 8 tablets of Ismo 10 and 60 tablets of Ismo 20 in calendarised blister strips.

Ismo 10 – packs of 100 tablets.

Instructions for use/handling: No special instructions.

Marketing authorisation number PL 15722/0014

Date of first authorisation/renewal of authorisation 1 January 1997

Date of (partial) revision of the text August 1998

Ismo is also available in 20 mg and 40 mg tablets

KONAKION AMPOULES

Qualitative and quantitative composition Each Konakion Ampoule contains 1 mg vitamin K_1 (phytomenadione) Ph. Eur. in 0.5 ml.

Pharmaceutical form Amber glass ampoules containing 1 mg phytomenadione in 0.5 ml. The ampoule solution is clear to opalescent, greenish-yellow in colour and contains a polyethoxylated castor oil as a non-ionic surfactant.

Clinical particulars

Therapeutic indications: Konakion is indicated in the treatment of haemorrhage or threatened haemorrhage associated with a low blood level of prothrombin or factor VII. The main indications are:

As an antidote to anticoagulant drugs of the coumarin type.

Prevention and treatment of neonatal haemorrhage.

Posology and method of administration:

Adults: As an antidote to anticoagulant drugs

For potentially fatal and severe haemorrhages: Konakion MM Ampoules are recommended as treatment in this indication (see separate prescribing information).

Less severe haemorrhage: Konakion is given orally in doses of 10–20 mg (1 to 2 tablets). The prothrombin level is estimated 8 to 12 hours later, and if the response has been inadequate, the dose should be repeated. Intramuscular injections of Konakion may also be given in doses of 10–20 mg, repeated if necessary.

Lowering of prothrombin to dangerous level but no haemorrhage: A dose of 5–10 mg Konakion orally may be given to bring the prothrombin level back to within safe limits. In such instances it is not usually necessary to discontinue the anticoagulant.

Adults: Other indications

Doses of 10–20 mg as required.

Elderly: Elderly patients tend to be more sensitive to reversal of anticoagulation with Konakion; dosage in this group should be at the lower end of the ranges recommended.

Children: If, on the recommendation of a physician, a children's dosage is required, then it is suggested that 5–10 mg be given.

Treatment of newborn infants: Prophylactic: 1 mg by intramuscular injection.

Therapeutic: 1 mg by intramuscular injection, repeated at eight-hourly intervals if necessary.

Konakion Ampoules are for intramuscular or intravenous injection.

Konakion Ampoule solution should not be diluted.

Contra-indications: Use in patients with a known hypersensitivity to any of the constituents.

Special warnings and special precautions for use: Konakion Ampoules contain a polyethoxylated castor oil as a non-ionic surfactant. In animal studies, polyethoxylated castor oil can produce severe anaphylactoid reactions associated with histamine release. There is strong circumstantial evidence that similar reactions occurring in patients may have been caused by polyethoxylated castor oil. Polyethoxylated castor oil, when given to patients over a period of several days, can also produce abnormal lipoprotein electrophoretic patterns, alterations in blood viscosity and erythrocyte aggregation.

Large doses of Konakion should be avoided if it is intended to continue with anticoagulant therapy.

Vitamin K_1 is not an antidote to heparin.

Interaction with other medicaments and other forms of interaction: None known.

Pregnancy and lactation: There is no specific evidence regarding the safety of Konakion in pregnancy but, as with most drugs, the administration during pregnancy should only occur if the benefits outweigh the risks.

Effects on ability to drive and use machines: None known.

Undesirable effects: The too rapid intravenous administration of vitamin K_1 has caused reactions, including flushing of the face, sweating, a sense of chest constriction, cyanosis and peripheral vascular collapse.

Repeated intramuscular injections of vitamin K_1 preparations, usually over prolonged periods in patients with hepatic disease, may give rise to local cutaneous and subcutaneous changes.

Overdose: Hypervitaminosis of vitamin K_1 is unknown.

Pharmacological properties

Pharmacodynamic properties: Konakion is a synthetic preparation of vitamin K_1. The presence of vitamin K (i.e. vitamin K_1 itself or substances with vitamin K activity) is essential for the formation within the body of prothrombin, factor VII, factor IX and factor X. Lack of vitamin K leads to increased tendency to haemorrhage. When an antidote to an anticoagulant is necessary it is essential to use vitamin K_1 itself, as vitamin K analogues are much less effective.

Pharmacokinetic properties: The fat-soluble vitamin compound phytomenadione (Vitamin K_1) requires the presence of bile for its absorption from the gastro-intestinal tract. Vitamin K accumulates mainly in the liver but is stored in the body only for short periods of time. Vitamin K does not appear to cross the placenta readily and it is poorly distributed into breast milk. Phytomenadione is rapidly metabolised to more polar metabolites and is excreted in bile and urine as glucuronide and sulphate conjugates.

Preclinical safety data: LD_{50} (i.v.) of Konakion MM (10 mg/ml) in mice: 12.1–17.7 ml/kg.

Pharmaceutical particulars

List of excipients: Polyoxyl 35 castor oil USP, Propylene glycol Ph. Eur., Phenol Ph. Eur., Water for injections Ph. Eur.

Incompatibilities: None known.

Shelf life: The recommended shelf life of Konakion Ampoules is 60 months.

Special precautions for storage: Konakion Ampoule solution should be protected from light; it should not be allowed to freeze. The recommended maximum storage temperature for Konakion Ampoules is 30°C.

Nature and contents of container: Konakion is supplied in 1 ml amber glass ampoules containing 0.6 ml of solution.

Instructions for use/handling: Konakion Ampoules are for intramuscular or intravenous injection. Konakion Ampoule solution should not be diluted.

Marketing authorisation number PL 0031/5023R

Date of first authorisation/renewal of the authorisation 3 July 1985

Date of (partial) revision of the text April 1997

KONAKION MM

Qualitative and quantitative composition Each Konakion MM Ampoule contains 10.0 mg vitamin K_1 (phytomenadione) BP in 1 ml.

Pharmaceutical form Amber glass ampoules containing 10 mg phytomenadione in 1 ml. The ampoule solution is clear to slightly opalescent, pale yellow in colour and contains the active constituent in a mixed micelles vehicle of glycocholic acid and lecithin.

Clinical particulars

Therapeutic indications: Konakion MM is indicated as an antidote to anticoagulant drugs of the coumarin type in the treatment of haemorrhage or threatened haemorrhage, associated with a low blood level of prothrombin or factor VII.

Posology and method of administration:

Adults: As an antidote to anticoagulant drugs

For potentially fatal and severe haemorrhages: Konakion MM therapy should be accompanied by a more immediate effective treatment such as transfusions of whole blood or blood clotting factors. The anticoagulant should be withdrawn and an intravenous injection of Konakion MM given slowly in a dose of 10–20 mg. The prothrombin level should be estimated three hours later and, if the response has been inadequate, the dose should be repeated. Not more than 40 mg of Konakion MM should be given intravenously in 24 hours. Coagulation profiles must be monitored on a daily basis until these have returned to acceptable levels; in severe cases more frequent monitoring is necessary and where there is no immediate efficacy, transfusion of whole blood or blood clotting factors should be used.

Less severe haemorrhage: Oral treatment with Konakion tablets may be used.

Elderly: Elderly patients tend to be more sensitive to reversal of anticoagulation with Konakion MM; dosage in this group should be at the lower end of the ranges recommended.

Instructions for infusion in adults: Konakion MM Ampoules are for intravenous injection and should be diluted with 55 ml of 5% glucose before slowly infusing the product. The solution should be freshly prepared and protected from light. Konakion MM Ampoule solution should not be diluted or mixed with other injectables, but may be injected into the lower part of an infusion apparatus.

Children aged 1 to 18 years: It is advisable that a haematologist is consulted about appropriate investigation and treatment in any child in whom Konakion MM is being considered.

Likely indications for using vitamin K in children are limited and may include:

1. Children with disorders that interfere with absorption of vitamin K (chronic diarrhoea, cystic fibrosis, biliary atresia, hepatitis, coeliac disease).
2. Children with poor nutrition who are receiving broad spectrum antibiotics.
3. Liver disease.
4. Patients receiving anticoagulant therapy with warfarin in whom the INR is increased outside the therapeutic range and therefore are at risk of, or are bleeding, and those with an INR in the therapeutic range who are bleeding.

For patients on warfarin therapy, therapeutic intervention must take into consideration the reason for the child being on warfarin and whether or not anticoagulant therapy has to be continued (e.g. in a child with mechanical heart valve or repeated thromboembolic complications) as vitamin K administration is likely to interfere with anticoagulation with warfarin for 2–3 weeks.

It should be noted that the earliest effect seen with vitamin K treatment is at 4–6 hours and therefore in patients with severe haemorrhage replacement with coagulation factors may be indicated (discuss with haematologist).

Dose of vitamin K: There are few data available regarding use of Konakion MM in children over 1 year. There have been no dose ranging studies in children with haemorrhage. Suggested dosages based on clinical experience are as follows:

Haemorrhage in children: 2–5 mg i.v.

Asymptomatic children at risk of bleeding: 1–5 mg i.v.

Prothrombin levels should be measured 2 to 6 hours later and if the response has not been adequate, the dose may be repeated. Frequent monitoring of vitamin K dependent clotting factors is essential in these patients.

Children on warfarin therapy who need to remain anticoagulated are not included in the above dosage recommendations.

Neonates and babies: Konakion MM Paediatric should be used in these patients. (See separate prescribing information.)

Contra-indications: Use in patients with a known hypersensitivity to any of the constituents.

Special warnings and special precautions for use: When treating patients with severely impaired liver function, it should be borne in mind that one Konakion MM Ampoule 10 mg/1 ml contains 54.6 mg glycocholic acid and this may have a bilirubin displacing effect.

At the time of use, the ampoule contents should be clear. Following incorrect storage, the contents may become turbid or present a phase-separation. In this case the ampoule must no longer be used.

In potentially fatal and severe haemorrhage due to overdosage of coumarin anticoagulants, intravenous injections of Konakion MM must be administered slowly and not more than 40 mg should be given during a period of 24 hours. Konakion MM therapy should be accompanied by a more immediate effective treatment such as transfusion of whole blood or blood clotting factors. When patients with prosthetic heart valves are given transfusions for the treatment of severe or potentially fatal haemorrhages, fresh frozen plasma should be used.

Large doses of Konakion MM (more than 40 mg per day) should be avoided if it is intended to continue with anticoagulant therapy because there is no experience with doses above this maximum of 40 mg per day and higher doses may give rise to unexpected adverse events. Clinical studies have shown a sufficient decrease in the prothrombin time with the recommended dosage. If haemorrhage is severe, a transfusion of fresh whole blood may be necessary whilst awaiting the effect of the vitamin K_1.

Vitamin K_1 is not an antidote to heparin.

Interaction with other medicaments and other forms of interaction: No significant interactions are known other than antagonism of coumarin anticoagulants.

Pregnancy and lactation: There is no specific evidence regarding the safety of Konakion MM in pregnancy but, as with most drugs, the administration during pregnancy should only occur if the benefits outweigh the risks.

Effects on ability to drive and use machines: None.

Undesirable effects: There are only few unconfirmed reports of the occurrence of possible anaphylactoid reactions after intravenous injection of Konakion MM. Very rarely, venous irritation or phlebitis has been reported in association with intravenous administration of Konakion mixed micelle solution. Injection site reactions have been reported after intramuscular injection of Konakion.

Overdose: Hypervitaminosis of vitamin K_1 is unknown.

Pharmacological properties

Pharmacodynamic properties: Konakion MM is a synthetic preparation of vitamin K. The presence of vitamin K (i.e. vitamin K or substances with vitamin K activity) is essential for the formation within the body of prothrombin, factor VII, factor IX and factor X. Lack of vitamin K leads to an increased tendency to haemorrhage. When an antidote to an anticoagulant is necessary it is essential to use vitamin K_1 itself, as vitamin K analogues are much less effective.

In the mixed micelles solution, vitamin K_1 is solubilised by means of a physiological colloidal system, also found in the human body, consisting of lecithin and bile acid. Owing to the absence of organic solvents, the Konakion mixed micelles solution is well tolerated on intravenous administration.

Pharmacokinetic properties: In blood plasma, 90% of vitamin K_1 is bound to lipoproteins. Following an intramuscular dose of 10 mg vitamin K, plasma concentrations of 10–20 mcg/l are produced (normal range 0.4–1.2 mcg/l). Systemic availability following intramuscular administration is about 50% and elimination half-life in plasma is approximately 1.5 - 3 hours.

Preclinical safety data: None applicable.

Pharmaceutical particulars

List of excipients: Glycocholic acid HSE, Sodium hydroxide Ph. Eur., Lecithin (phospholipon 100) HSE, Hydrochloric acid 25% Ph. Eur., Water for injection Ph. Eur.

Incompatibilities: None.

Shelf life: The recommended shelf-life of Konakion MM Ampoules is 36 months.

Special precautions for storage: The recommended maximum storage temperature is 25°C. Do not use if the solution is turbid.

Nature and contents of container: Konakion MM is supplied in amber glass ampoules containing 10 mg phytomenadione in 1 ml. The ampoule solution is clear to slightly opalescent, pale yellow in colour and contains the active constituent in a mixed micelles vehicle of glycocholic acid and lecithin.

Instructions for use/handling: See *Posology and method of administration.*

Marketing authorisation number PL 0031/0254

Date of renewal of authorisation 17 August 1993

Date of (partial) revision of the text August 1998

KONAKION MM PAEDIATRIC

Qualitative and quantitative composition Each ampoule contains 2 mg phytomenadione in 0.2 ml.

Pharmaceutical form The ampoule solution is clear to slightly opalescent, pale yellow in colour and contains the active constituent in a mixed micelles vehicle of glycocholic acid and lecithin.

Clinical particulars

Therapeutic indications: Konakion MM is indicated for the prophylaxis and treatment of haemorrhagic disease of the newborn.

Posology and method of administration:

Neonates and Babies

Prophylaxis: Healthy neonates of 36 weeks gestation and older: 2 mg orally at birth or soon after birth. This should be followed by a second dose of 2 mg at 4–7 days.

Preterm neonates of less than 36 weeks gestation weighing 2.5 kg or greater, and term neonates at special risk: 1 mg IM or IV at birth or soon after birth, the size and frequency of further doses depending on coagulation status.

Preterm neonates of less than 36 weeks gestation weighing less than 2.5 kg: 0.4 mg/kg (equivalent to 0.04 ml/kg) IM or IV at birth or soon after birth. This parenteral dose should not be exceeded (see *Special warnings and special precautions for use*). The frequency of further doses should depend on coagulation status.

Exclusively breast-fed babies: In addition to the doses at birth and at 4–7 days, a further 2 mg oral dose should be given 1 month after birth. Further monthly 2 mg oral doses until formula feeding is introduced have been advised, but no safety or efficacy data exist for these additional doses.

Therapy: Initially 1 mg IV and further doses as required, depending on clinical picture and coagulation status. Konakion therapy may need to be accompanied by a more immediate effective treatment, such as transfusion of whole blood or blood clotting factors to compensate for severe blood loss and delayed response to vitamin K_1.

Contra-indications: Use in patients with a known hypersensitivity to any of the constituents.

Special warnings and special precautions for use: At the time of use, the ampoule contents should be clear. Following incorrect storage, the contents may become turbid or present a phase-separation. In this case the ampoule must no longer be used.

For oral use: After breaking the ampoule open, 0.2 ml of solution should be withdrawn into the oral dispenser until it reaches the mark on the dispenser (0.2 ml = 2 mg vitamin K). Drop the contents of the dispenser directly into the baby's mouth by pressing the plunger.

For parenteral use: Konakion MM paediatric should not be diluted or mixed with other parenteral medications, but may be injected into the lower part of an infusion set.

Parenteral administration to premature babies weighing less than 2.5 kg may increase the risk for the development of kernicterus (bilirubin encephalopathy).

Interaction with other medicaments and other forms of interaction: No significant interactions are known other than antagonism of coumarin anticoagulants.

Pregnancy and lactation: Not applicable.

Effects on ability to drive and use machines: Not applicable.

Undesirable effects: There are only few unconfirmed reports on the occurrence of possible anaphylactoid reactions after IV injection of Konakion MM. Local irritation may occur at the injection site but is unlikely due to the small injection volume. Rarely, injection site reactions may occur which may be severe, including inflammation, atrophy and necrosis.

Overdose: No overdose effects are known.

Pharmacological properties

Pharmacodynamic properties: Konakion MM is a preparation of synthetic phytomenadione (vitamin K_1). The presence of vitamin K_1 is essential for the formation within the body of prothrombin, factor VII, factor IX and factor X, and of the coagulation inhibitors, protein C and protein S.

Vitamin K_1 does not readily cross the placental barrier from mother to child and is poorly excreted in breast milk.

Lack of vitamin K_1 leads to an increased tendency to haemorrhagic disease in the newborn. Vitamin K_1 administration, which promotes synthesis of the above-mentioned coagulation factors by the liver, can reverse an abnormal coagulation status due to vitamin K_1 deficiency.

Pharmacokinetic properties: In the mixed micelle solution, vitamin K_1 is solubilised by means of a physiological colloidal system consisting of lecithin and a bile acid.

Vitamin K_1 is absorbed from the small intestine. Absorption is limited in the absence of bile.

Vitamin K_1 accumulates predominantly in the liver, is up to 90% bound to lipoproteins in the plasma and is stored in the body only for short periods of time.

Vitamin K_1 is transformed to more polar metabolites, such as phytomenadione-2,3-epoxide.

The half-life of vitamin K_1 in plasma is about 1.5 to 3 hours. Vitamin K_1 is excreted in bile and urine as the glucuronide and sulphate conjugates.

Preclinical safety data: None applicable.

Pharmaceutical particulars

List of excipients: Glycocholic acid, lecithin, sodium hydroxide, hydrochloric acid and water.

Incompatibilities: See *Special warnings and special precautions for use.*

Shelf life: 3 years.

Special precautions for storage: Konakion MM Paediatric ampoule solution should be stored below 25°C and be protected from light. The solution should not be frozen. Do not use if the solution is turbid.

Nature and contents of container: Amber glass ampoules containing 2 mg phytomenadione in 0.2 ml. Plastic oral dispensers. Packs of 1, 5 or 10.

Instructions for use/handling: See *Special warnings and special precautions for use.*

Marketing authorisation number PL 0031/0346

Date of first authorisation/renewal of authorisation 20 June 1996

Date of (partial) revision of the text August 1998

KONAKION TABLETS 10 mg

Qualitative and quantitative composition Each Konakion Tablet contains 10 mg vitamin K_1 (phytomenadione) BP.

Pharmaceutical form Round off-white sugar-coated tablets.

Clinical particulars

Therapeutic indications: Konakion is indicated in the treatment of haemorrhage or threatened haemorrhage associated with a low blood level of prothrombin or factor VII. The main indications are:

As an antidote to anticoagulant drugs of the coumarin type.

Posology and method of administration: Konakion tablets are for oral administration and should be chewed or allowed to dissolve slowly in the mouth.

Adults: As an antidote to anticoagulant drugs

For potentially fatal and severe haemorrhages: Konakion intravenous injection (see separate prescribing information).

Less severe haemorrhage: Konakion is given orally in doses of 10 - 20mg (1 to 2 tablets). The prothrombin level is estimated 8 to 12 hours later, and if the response has been inadequate, the dose should be repeated.

Lowering of prothrombin to dangerous level but no haemorrhage: A dose of 5 - 10mg Konakion orally may be given to bring the prothrombin level back to within safe limits. In such instances it is not usually necessary to discontinue the anticoagulant.

Adults: Other indications

Doses of 10 - 20mg as required.

Elderly

Elderly patients tend to be more sensitive to reversal of anticoagulation with Konakion; dosage in this group should be at the lower end of the ranges recommended.

Children

If, on the recommendation of a physician, a children's dosage is required, then it is suggested that 5 - 10mg be given.

Contra-indications: Use in patients with a known hypersensitivity to any of the constituents.

Special warnings and special precautions for use: Large doses of Konakion should be avoided if it is intended to continue with anticoagulant therapy.

Vitamin K_1 is not an antidote to heparin.

Interaction with other medicaments and other forms of interaction: None known.

Pregnancy and lactation: There is no specific evidence regarding the safety of Konakion in pregnancy but, as with most drugs, the administration during pregnancy should only occur if the benefits outweigh the risks.

Effects on ability to drive and use machines: None known.

Undesirable effects: None known.

Overdose: Hypervitaminosis of vitamin K_1 is unknown.

Pharmacological properties

Pharmacodynamic properties: Konakion is a synthetic preparation of vitamin K_1. The presence of vitamin K (i.e. vitamin K_1 itself or substances with vitamin K activity) is essential for the formation within the body of prothrombin, factor VII, factor IX and factor X. Lack of vitamin K leads to increased tendency to haemorrhage. When an antidote to an anticoagulant is necessary it is essential to use vitamin K_1 itself, as vitamin K analogues are much less effective.

Pharmacokinetic properties: The fat-soluble vitamin compound phytomenadione (Vitamin K_1) requires the presence of bile for its absorption from the gastro-intestinal tract. Vitamin K accumulates mainly in the liver but is stored in the body only for short periods of time. Vitamin K does not appear to cross the placenta readily and it is poorly distributed into breast milk. Phytomenadione is rapidly metabolised to more polar metabolites and is excreted in bile and urine as glucuronide and sulphate conjugates.

Preclinical safety data: None stated.

Pharmaceutical particulars

List of excipients: Silicon Dioxide USP, Sucrose Ph. Eur., Glucose Ph. Eur., Skimmed Milk Powder HSE, Cocoa USP, Cocoa Butter BP, Carob Bean Gum FCC, Glycerol Ph. Eur., Rice Starch Ph. Eur., Titanium Dioxide E171, Ethyl Vanillin USP, Acacia Spray Dried Ph. Eur., Paraffin Light Liquid Ph. Eur., Hard Paraffin BP, Talc Ph. Eur., Sodium Carboxymethylcellulose Ph. Eur.

Incompatibilities: None known.

Shelf life: The recommended shelf life of Konakion Tablets is 60 months.

Special precautions for storage: Konakion tablets should be stored in well-closed containers and protected from light.

Nature and contents of container: Konakion Tablets are supplied in white HDPE bottles with tamper evident snap-fit, containing 25 tablets.

Instructions for use/handling: None stated.

Marketing authorisation number PL 0031/5022R

Date of first authorisation/renewal of the authorisation 3 December 1995

Date of (partial) revision of the text April 1996

LARIAM

Name of product Lariam contains the substance with the approved name mefloquine as the hydrochloride. It is chemically known as DL-erythro-2-piperidyl-2, 8-bis (trifluoromethyl)-4-quinolinemethanol hydrochloride.

Presentation Tablets containing 274.09 mg mefloquine hydrochloride, equivalent to 250 mg mefloquine base.

Uses

Pharmacological properties The effectiveness of Lariam in the therapy and prophylaxis of malaria is due essentially to destruction of the asexual blood forms of the malarial pathogens that affect humans (*Plasmodium falciparum, P. vivax, P. malariae, P. ovale*).

Lariam is also effective against malarial parasites resistant to other antimalarials such as chloroquine and other 4-aminoquinoline derivatives, proguanil, pyrimethamine and pyrimethamine-sulfonamide combinations. However, strains of *P. falciparum* resistant to mefloquine have been reported (e.g. in parts of Indochina). Cross-resistance between mefloquine and halofantrine has been observed.

In vitro and *in vivo* studies with mefloquine showed no haemolysis associated with glucose-6-phosphate dehydrogenase deficiency.

Pharmacokinetics: Absorption: The maximum plasma concentration is reached within 6 to 24 hours after a single oral dose of Lariam. The level in micrograms per litre is roughly equivalent to the dose in milligrams (for example, approximately 1000µg/l after a single dose of 1000 mg). The presence of food significantly enhances the rate and extent of absorption.

At a dose of 250 mg once weekly, maximum steady state plasma concentrations of 1000–2000µg/l are reached after 7–10 weeks. The RBC concentration is almost twice as high as the plasma level. Plasma protein binding is about 98%. Clinical experience suggests a minimal suppressive plasma concentration of mefloquine in the order of 600µg/l.

Elimination: The average half-life of mefloquine in Europeans is 21 days. There is evidence that mefloquine is excreted mainly in the bile and faeces. In volunteers, urinary excretion of unchanged mefloquine and its main metabolite accounted for about 9% and 4% of the dose respectively.

Special clinical situations: The pharmacokinetics of mefloquine may be altered in acute malaria. Pharmacokinetic differences have been observed between various ethnic populations. In practice, however, these are of minor importance compared with host immune status and sensitivity of the parasite.

Mefloquine crosses the placenta. Excretion into breast milk appears to be minimal.

Indications: Therapy and prophylaxis of malaria.

Therapy: Lariam is especially indicated for therapy of *P. falciparum* malaria in which the pathogen has become resistant to other antimalarial agents.

Following treatment of *P. vivax* malaria with Lariam, relapse prophylaxis with an 8-amino-quinoline derivative, for example primaquine, should be considered in order to eliminate parasites in the hepatic phase.

Prophylaxis: Malaria prophylaxis with Lariam is particularly recommended for travellers to malarious areas in which multiple resistant *P. falciparum* strains occur. For current advice on geographical resistance patterns and appropriate chemoprophylaxis, current guidelines or the Malaria Reference Laboratory should be consulted, details of which can be found in the British National Formulary (BNF).

Dosage and administration

Curative treatment: The recommended total therapeutic dose of mefloquine for non-immune patients is 20–25 mg/kg. A lower total dose of 15 mg/kg may suffice for partially immune individuals.

The recommended total therapeutic dosages of Lariam tablets relative to bodyweight and immune status are presented in the following table*.

	Non-immune patients	*Partially immune patients*
< 20 kg**	¼ tablet / 2.5–3 kg 1 tablet / 10–12 kg	¼ tablet / 4 kg 1 tablet/16 kg
20–30 kg	2–3 tablets	1¼–2 tablets
> 30–45 kg	3–4 tablets	2–3 tablets
> 45–60 kg	4–5 tablets	3–4 tablets
> 60 kg***	6 tablets	4–6 tablets

* Splitting the total curative dosage into 2–3 doses (e.g. 3 + 1, 3 + 2 or 3 + 2 + 1 tablets) taken 6–8 hours apart may reduce the occurrence or severity of adverse effects.

** Experience with Lariam in infants less than 3 months old or weighing less than 5 kg is limited.

*** There is no specific experience with total dosages of more than 6 tablets in very heavy patients.

A second full dose should be given to patients who vomit less than 30 minutes after receiving the drug. If vomiting occurs 30–60 minutes after a dose, an additional half-dose should be given.

If a full treatment course with Lariam does not lead to improvement within 48–72 hours, alternative treatments should be considered. When breakthrough malaria occurs during Lariam prophylaxis, physicians should carefully evaluate which antimalarial to use for therapy.

Lariam can be given for severe acute malaria after an initial course of intravenous quinine lasting at least 2–3 days. Interactions leading to adverse events can largely be prevented by allowing an interval of at least 12 hours after the last dose of quinine (see *Drug interactions*).

In areas with multi-resistant malaria, initial treatment with artemisinin or a derivative, if available, followed by Lariam is also an option.

Malaria prophylaxis: Prophylaxis of malaria with Lariam should be initiated at least one week and up to 2–3 weeks before arrival in a malarious area. The following dosage schedule is given as a guide:

	Dosage	*Course of prophylaxis*
Adults and children of more than 45 kg body-weight	1 tablet	Stated dose to be given once weekly, always on the same day for a minimum of six weeks.
Children and adults weighing less than 45 kg		First dose at least one week and up to 2–3 weeks before arrival in malarious area. Further doses at weekly intervals during and for four weeks after visiting the malarious area.
5–19 kg	¼ tablet	
20–30 kg	½ tablet	
31–45 kg	¾ tablet	

The maximum recommended duration of administration of Lariam is 12 months.

The tablets should be swallowed whole preferably after a meal with plenty of liquid.

Use in the elderly: No specific adaptation of the usual adult dosage is required for elderly patients.

Contra-indications, warnings, etc

Contra-indications: Prophylactic use in patients with severe impairment of liver function should be regarded for the time being as a contra-indication as no experience has been gained in such patients.

Patients with a history of psychiatric disturbances (including depression) or convulsions should not be prescribed Lariam prophylactically, as it may precipitate these conditions (see *Precautions and Drug interactions*).

Lariam should not be administered to patients with a known hypersensitivity to mefloquine or related compounds, e.g. quinine.

Because of the danger of a potentially fatal prolongation of the QTc interval, halofantrine must not be given simultaneously with or subsequent to Lariam. No data are available where Lariam was given after halofantrine.

Use in pregnancy and lactation: There is too little clinical experience in humans to assess any possible damaging effects of Lariam during pregnancy. However, mefloquine is teratogenic when administered to rats and mice in early gestation. Therefore, Lariam should be used in pregnancy only if there are compelling medical reasons. In the absence of clinical experience, prophylactic use during pregnancy should be avoided as a matter of principle.

Mefloquine is excreted into breast milk in small amounts, the activity of which is unknown. Nursing mothers should be advised not to breast-feed while taking Lariam.

Precautions: Women of childbearing potential travelling to malarious areas in which multiple resistant *P. falciparum* is found and who are receiving Lariam for the treatment and prophylaxis of malaria should take reliable contraceptive precautions for the entire duration of therapy and for three months after the last dose of Lariam. (See *Use in pregnancy and lactation*).

Experience with Lariam in infants less than 3 months old or weighing less than 5 kg is limited.

There is no evidence that dose adjustment is necessary for patients with renal insufficiency. However, since clinical evidence in such patients is limited, caution should be exercised when using Lariam in patients with impaired renal function.

In patients with epilepsy, mefloquine may increase the risk of convulsions. Therefore in such cases Lariam should be used only for curative treatment and only if compelling reasons exist (see *Contra-indications* and *Drug interactions*).

Lariam should be taken with caution in patients suffering from cardiac conduction disorders, since transient cardiac conduction alterations have been observed during curative and preventative use.

Patients should not disregard the possibility that re-infection or recrudescence may occur after effective antimalarial therapy.

Effects on ability to drive and to use machines

Treatment: Mefloquine can cause dizziness or disturbed sense of balance. It is consequently recommended not to drive or to carry out tasks demanding fine co-ordination and spatial discrimination during treatment with mefloquine. Patients should avoid such tasks for at least three weeks following therapeutic use as dizziness, a disturbed sense of balance or neuropsychiatric reactions have been reported up to three weeks after the use of Lariam.

Prophylactic use: Caution should be exercised with regard to driving, piloting aircraft and operating machines, as dizziness, a disturbed sense of balance or neuropsychiatric reactions have been reported during and for up to three weeks after use of Lariam.

Side-effects and adverse reactions: At the doses given for acute malaria, adverse reactions to Lariam may not be distinguishable from symptoms of the disease itself. In a large study of tourists receiving various prophylactic antimalarials, about 22% of the subjects taking Lariam reported adverse events. Because of the long half-life of mefloquine, adverse reactions to Lariam may occur or persist up to several weeks after the last dose.

Patients should be advised to obtain medical advice before the next weekly dose of Lariam, if any concerning or neuropsychiatric symptoms develop. Discontinuation of Lariam should be considered, particularly if neuropsychiatric reactions occur. The need for alternative antimalarial therapy or prophylaxis can then be evaluated.

Common adverse reactions: Nausea, vomiting, dizziness or vertigo, loss of balance, headache, somnolence, sleep disorders (insomnia, abnormal dreams), loose stools or diarrhoea and abdominal pain.

Uncommon adverse reactions:

Psychiatric: Psychiatric reactions sometimes disabling and prolonged have been reported in association with Lariam. These include depression, anxiety, confusion, hallucinations, panic attacks, restlessness, forgetfulness, psychosis and paranoia, emotional instability, aggression and agitation.

Neurological: Convulsions, sensory and motor neuropathies (including paraesthesia), tremor, tinnitus and vestibular disorders, abnormal co-ordination, ataxia and visual disturbances.

Cardiovascular system: Circulatory disturbances (hypotension, hypertension, flushing, syncope), tachycardia or palpitations, bradycardia, irregular pulse, extrasystoles and other transient cardiac conduction alterations.

Skin: Rash, exanthema, erythema, urticaria, pruritus, hair loss, erythema multiforme, Stevens-Johnson syndrome.

Musculo-skeletal system: Muscle weakness, muscle cramps, myalgia, arthralgia.

General symptoms: Asthenia, malaise, fatigue, fever, chills, loss of appetite.

Haematological: Leucopenia or leucocytosis, thrombocytopenia.

Laboratory abnormalities: Transient elevation of transaminases.

Very rare adverse reactions: AV-block and encephalopathy.

Studies *in vitro* and *in vivo* showed no haemolysis associated with G6PD deficiency.

Drug interactions: Concomitant administration of Lariam and other related compounds (e.g. quinine, quinidine and chloroquine) may produce electrocardiographic abnormalities and increase the risk of convulsions. There is evidence that the use of halofantrine after mefloquine causes a significant lengthening of the QTc interval. Clinically significant QTc prolongation has not been found with mefloquine alone (see Dosage and Administration).

This appears to be the only clinically relevant interaction of this kind with Lariam, although theoretically co-administration of other drugs known to alter cardiac conduction (e.g. anti-arrhythmic or β-adrenergic blocking agents, calcium channel blockers, antihistamines or H_1-blocking agents, tricyclic antidepressants and phenothiazines) might also contribute to a prolongation of the QTc interval.

In patients taking an anticonvulsant (e.g. valproic acid, carbamazepine, phenobarbital or phenytoin), the concomitant use of Lariam may reduce seizure control by lowering the plasma levels of the anticonvulsant. Dosage adjustments of antiseizure medication may be necessary in some cases (see *Contra-indications* and *Precautions*).

When Lariam is taken concurrently with oral live typhoid vaccines, attenuation of immunisation cannot be excluded. Vaccinations with oral attenuated live bacteria should therefore be completed at least 3 days before the first dose of Lariam.

No other drug interactions are known. Nevertheless, the effects of Lariam on travellers receiving comedication, particularly those on anticoagulants or antidiabetics, should be checked before departure.

Treatment of overdosage: In cases of overdosage with Lariam, the symptoms mentioned under *Side-effects and adverse reactions* may be more pronounced. Countermeasures: Induce vomiting or perform gastric lavage as appropriate. Monitor cardiac function (if possible by ECG) and neuropsychiatric status for at least 24 hours. Provide symptomatic and intensive supportive treatment as required, particularly for cardiovascular disorders.

Pharmaceutical precautions *Storage* Protect from moisture.

Legal category POM.

Package quantities Tablets (cross-scored) in packs of 8.

Product licence/authorisation number PL 0031/0236

Date of last review May 1997

LEXOTAN

Qualitative and quantitative composition Each 1.5 mg tablet contains 1.5 mg bromazepam.

Each 3 mg tablet contains 3 mg bromazepam.

Pharmaceutical form Tablets for oral administration.

Clinical particulars

Therapeutic indications: Lexotan is indicated for the short-term (2–4 weeks) symptomatic treatment of anxiety that is severe, disabling or subjecting the individual to unacceptable distress, occurring alone or in association with insomnia or short-term psychosomatic, organic or psychotic illness.

Posology and method of administration: The optimum dosage and frequency of administration of Lexotan should be based on the individual patient, the severity of symptoms and previous psychotropic drug history.

Adults: The usual dosage in general practice is from 3 mg to 18 mg daily in divided doses.

In exceptional circumstances, in hospitalised patients, up to the maximum daily dosage of 60 mg in divided doses, may be given.

Elderly and/or debilitated patients: Elderly patients and those with impaired hepatic and/or renal function are more sensitive to the actions of Lexotan; doses should not exceed half those normally recommended.

Children: Lexotan is not for paediatric use.

The patient should be checked regularly at the start of treatment in order to minimise the dosage and/or the frequency of administration to prevent overdose due to accumulation.

These amounts are general recommendations, and dosage should be individually determined. Treatment of outpatients should begin with low doses, gradually increasing to the optimum level. The duration of treatment should be as short as possible. The patient should be reassessed regularly and the need for continued treatment should be evaluated, especially in case the patient is symptom free. The overall treatment generally should not be more than 8–12 weeks, including a tapering off process. In certain cases extension beyond the maximum treatment period may be necessary, if so, it should not take place without re-evaluation of the patient's status with special expertise.

Contra-indications: Patients with known hypersensitivity to benzodiazepines and any of the drug's excipients; severe pulmonary insufficiency, severe hepatic insufficiency, respiratory depression; phobic or obsessional states; chronic psychosis, myasthenia gravis, sleep apnoea syndrome.

Special warnings and special precautions for use: In patients with chronic pulmonary insufficiency dosage may need to be reduced.

Lexotan should not be used alone to treat depression or anxiety associated with depression, since suicide may be precipitated in such patients. Benzodiazepines are not recommended for the primary treatment of psychotic illness.It should be borne in mind that benzodiazepines may induce anterograde amnesia. Anterograde amnesia may occur using therapeutic dosages, the risk increasing at higher dosages. Amnestic effects may be associated with inappropriate behaviour. The condition usually occurs several hours after taking the product and therefore, to reduce the risk, patients should ensure that they will be able to have an uninterrupted sleep of 7 to 8 hours.

In cases of loss or bereavement, psychological adjustment may be inhibited by benzodiazepines.

The use of benzodiazepines and benzodiazepine-like agents may lead to the development of physical and psychological dependence. The risk of dependence increases with dose and duration of treatment. This is particularly so in patients with a history of alcoholism or drug abuse or in patients with marked personality disorders. Regular monitoring in such patients is essential, routine repeat prescriptions should be avoided and treatment should be withdrawn gradually. Once physical dependence has developed, termination of treatment will be accompanied by withdrawal symptoms. These may consist of headaches, muscle pain, extreme anxiety, tension, restlessness, confusion and irritability. In severe cases the following symptoms may occur: derealization, depersonalization, hyperacusis, numbness and tingling of the extremities, hypersensitivity to light, noise and physical contact, hallucinations or epileptic seizures.

Rebound anxiety, a transient syndrome whereby the symptoms that led to treatment with Lexotan recur in an enhanced form, may occur on withdrawal of treatment. It may be accompanied by other reactions including mood changes, anxiety or sleep disturbances and restlessness.

Since the risk of withdrawal phenomena and rebound phenomena is greater after abrupt discontinuation of treatment, it is recommended that the dosage be decreased gradually.

It may be useful to inform the patient when treatment is started that it will be of limited duration and to explain precisely how the dosage will be progressively decreased. It is important that the patient should be aware of the possibility of rebound phenomena that may occur while the drug is being discontinued.

When benzodiazepines with a long duration of action are being used, it is important to warn against changing to a benzodiazepine with a short duration of action as withdrawal symptoms may develop.

Treatment should be kept to a minimum and given only under close medical supervision. Little is known regarding the efficacy or safety of benzodiazepines in long-term use.

Benzodiazepines should be used with extreme caution in patients with a history of alcohol or drug abuse.

Interaction with other medicaments and other forms of interaction: If Lexotan is combined with centrally-acting drugs such as antipsychotics, anxiolytics/ sedatives, antidepressants, hypnotics, anticonvulsants, narcotic analgesics, anaesthetics and sedative antihistamines the sedative effects are likely to be intensified. In the case of narcotic analgesics enhancement of euphoria may also occur, leading to an increase in psychological dependence. The elderly require special supervision.

Concomitant use with alcohol is not recommended due to enhancement of the sedative effect.

When Lexotan is used in conjunction with anticonvulsant drugs, side-effects and toxicity may be more evident, particularly with hydantoins or barbiturates or combinations including them. This requires extra care in adjusting dosage in the initial stages of treatment.

Known inhibitors of hepatic enzymes, e.g. cimetidine, have been shown to reduce the clearance of benzodiazepines and may potentiate their action and known inducers of hepatic enzymes, e.g. rifampicin, may increase the clearance of benzodiazepines.

Cisapride may lead to a temporary increase in the sedative effects of orally administered benzodiazepines due to faster absorption.

Pregnancy and lactation: There is no evidence as to drug safety in human pregnancy, nor is there evidence from animal work that it is free from hazard. Do not use during pregnancy, especially during the first and last trimesters, unless there are compelling reasons.

If the product is prescribed to a woman of child-bearing potential, she should be warned to contact her physician regarding discontinuance of the product if she intends to become or suspects that she is pregnant.

The administration of high doses or prolonged administration of low doses of benzodiazepines in the last trimester of pregnancy has been reported to produce irregularities in the foetal heart rate, and hypotonia, poor sucking, hypothermia and moderate respiratory depression in the neonate.

Moreover, infants born to mothers who took benzodiazepines chronically during the latter stages of pregnancy may have developed physical dependence and may be at some risk for developing withdrawal symptoms in the postnatal period.

Benzodiazepines have been detected in breast milk, therefore the use of Lexotan should be avoided during lactation.

Effects on ability to drive and use machines: Patients should be advised that, like all medicaments of this type, Lexotan may modify patients' performance at skilled tasks. Sedation, amnesia, impaired concentration and impaired muscular function may adversely affect the ability to drive or use machinery.Patients should further be advised that alcohol may intensify any impairment, and should, therefore, be avoided during treatment. If insufficient sleep duration occurs the likelihood of impaired alertness may be increased (see *Interaction with other medicaments and other forms of interaction*).

Undesirable effects: The following undesirable effects may occur: fatigue, drowsiness, muscle weakness, numbed emotions, reduced alertness, confusion, headache, dizziness, ataxia, double vision, vertigo, hypotension and urinary retention. These phenomena occur predominantly at the start of therapy and usually disappear with prolonged administration. Gastrointestinal disturbances, decreased libido and skin reactions have been reported occasionally.

Pre-existing depression may be unmasked during benzodiazepine use.

The elderly are particularly sensitive to the effects of centrally depressant drugs and may experience confusion, especially if organic brain changes are present; the dosage of Lexotan should not exceed one-half that recommended for other adults.

In rare instances, withdrawal following excessive dosages may produce confusional states, psychotic manifestations and convulsions.

Extreme caution should therefore be used in prescribing benzodiazepines to patients with personality disorders.

Paradoxical reactions like restlessness, agitation, irritability, aggressiveness, delusion, rages, nightmares, hallucinations, psychoses, inappropriate behaviour and other adverse behavioural effects are known to occur when using benzodiazepines or benzodiazepine-like agents. Should this occur, the use of the drug should be discontinued. They are more likely to occur in children and elderly patients.

Chronic use (even at therapeutic doses) may lead to the development of physical dependence: discontinuation of therapy may result in withdrawal or rebound phenomena. Psychological dependence may occur. Abuse of benzodiazepines has been reported.

The elderly, and patients with impaired renal and/ or hepatic function, will be particularly susceptible to the adverse effects listed above. It is advisable to review treatment regularly and to discontinue use as soon as possible.

Overdose: Overdose of benzodiazepines is usually manifested by degrees of central nervous system depression ranging from drowsiness to coma. In mild cases, symptoms include drowsiness, mental confusion and lethargy. In most cases it is sufficient to monitor the vital functions and await recovery.

Higher overdoses, especially in combination with other centrally acting drugs, can result in ataxia, hypotonia, hypotension, respiratory depression, rarely coma and very rarely death.

In the management of overdose with any medicinal product, it should be borne in mind that multiple agents may have been taken.

When taken with centrally-acting drugs, especially alcohol, the effects of overdosage are likely to be more severe and, in the absence of supportive measures, may prove fatal.

Following overdose with oral benzodiazepines, vomiting should be induced (within one hour) if the patient is conscious or gastric lavage undertaken with the airway protected if the patient is unconscious. If there is no advantage in emptying the stomach, activated charcoal should be given to reduce the absorption.

The value of dialysis has not been determined. Special attention should be paid to respiratory and cardiac function in intensive care. Flumazenil is a specific IV antidote for use in emergency situations. Patients requiring such intervention should be monitored closely in hospital (see separate prescribing information). Caution should be observed in the use of flumazenil in epileptics treated with benzodiazepines, as antagonism of the benzodiazepine effect in such patients may trigger seizures.

If excitation occurs, barbiturates should not be used.

Pharmacological properties

Pharmacodynamic properties: Lexotan is a pyridylbenzodiazepine compound with anxiolytic properties.

Pharmacokinetic properties:

Absorption: Lexotan is rapidly absorbed from the gastro-intestinal tract. Peak plasma concentrations are usually reached within 2 hours of oral administration of bromazepam. The absolute bioavailability of the unchanged substance is 60%.

Distribution: On average, 70% of bromazepam is bound to plasma proteins. The volume of distribution is between 0.5–1.44L/kg. Steady state plasma concentrations are reached in around 5–9 days.

Metabolism: Bromazepam is metabolized in the liver. Quantitatively, two metabolites predominate: 3-hydroxy-bromazepam and 2-(2-amino-5-bromo-3-hydroxybenzoyl) pyridine. Metabolites of Lexotan do not contribute significantly to the effects of the drug.

Elimination: Bromazepam has an elimination half-life of between approximately 16 and 30 hours, but the half-life may be longer in elderly patients. The metabolites are excreted in the urine, mainly in their conjugated form.

Preclinical safety data: There are no pre-clinical data of relevance to the prescriber which are additional to that already included in other sections of the SmPC.

Pharmaceutical particulars

List of excipients:

Each 1.5 mg tablet contains Microcrystalline Cellulose BP, Lactose BP, Magnesium Stearate BP, Dye Lilac Premix (Talc BP, Lactose BP, Erythrosine lake E127, Indigocarmine lake E132).

Each 3 mg tablet contains Microcrystalline Cellulose BP, Lactose BP, Magnesium Stearate BP, Dye Erythrosine Premix (Talc BP, Lactose BP, Erythrosine lake E127).

Incompatibilities: None known.

Shelf life:

PVDC blister packs: 3 year shelf life, (2 years for professional samples containing 4 or 10 tablets).

HDPE bottles: 5 year shelf life.

Clic-loc containers: 5 year shelf life (professional samples containing 10 tablets).

Special precautions for storage: Lexotan tablets should be protected from light. Lexotan tablets in blister packs should also be stored in a dry place.

Nature and contents of container: PVDC blister packs of 4, 10, 20, 60 or 100 tablets. HDPE bottles of 100 tablets. Clic-loc containers of 10 tablets.

Instructions for use/handling: No special requirements.

Marketing authorisation numbers
1.5 mg tablets: PL 0031/0127
3 mg tablets: PL 0031/0128

Date of first authorisation/renewal of authorisation
15 July 1982/25 June 1998

Date of (partial) revision of the text November 1998

LORON FOR INFUSION

Qualitative and quantitative composition Each ampoule contains 300 mg disodium clodronate.

Pharmaceutical form Clear colourless sterile liquid for use by intravenous infusion after dilution.

Clinical particulars

Therapeutic indications: Loron for Infusion is indicated for the normalisation of serum calcium levels in patients with hypercalcaemia of malignancy in conjunction with full rehydration of patients as appropriate.

Posology and method of administration: Loron for Infusion is a concentrated presentation which must be diluted before use. The only recommended diluent is 0.9% w/v sodium chloride intravenous infusion. No other drugs or nutrients may be added.

Loron for Infusion may be administered either as a single infusion or as multiple infusions. Slow infusion is important for safety. It is recommended that oral or intravenous fluids be administered to establish or maintain full hydration.

Adults

Single infusion: Five ampoules of Loron for Infusion (1500 mg/disodium clodronate) should be added aseptically to 500 ml of sodium chloride intravenous infusion (0.9%). The diluted infusion solution should be administered by slow intravenous infusion over a period of not less than 4 hours.

Multiple infusions: One ampoule of Loron for Infusion (300 mg disodium clodronate) should be added aseptically to 500 ml of sodium chloride intravenous infusion (0.9%). The diluted infusion solution should be administered by slow intravenous infusion over a period of not less than 2 hours on successive days. The duration of treatment by multiple infusion depends on patient response but should not exceed 10 days.

Response: In most cases, an elevated serum calcium level can be lowered to within the normal range after 3–5 days, whichever method of infusion is used. Normocalcaemia may be maintained thereafter with oral administration of Loron 520 or Loron capsules. If hypercalcaemia recurs, the intravenous infusion may be reintroduced.

Elderly: No special dosage recommendations.

Children: Safety and efficacy in children has not been established.

Use in renal impairment: The effect of disodium clodronate in patients with moderate to severe renal impairment (serum creatinine greater than 440 micromol/l) has not been systematically examined in clinical trials. Since disodium clodronate is excreted unchanged by the kidney its use is contra-indicated in these patients. In patients with normal renal function or mild renal impairment (serum creatinine less than 440 micromol/l) serum creatinine should be monitored during therapy.

Contra-indications: Hypersensitivity to disodium clodronate. Pregnancy and lactation. Moderate to severe renal failure (serum creatinine greater than 440 micromol/l). Concomitant use of other bisphosphonates.

Special warnings and special precautions for use: Intravenous infusion of disodium clodronate may be associated with a transient proteinuria immediately after infusion even when the correct dosage and administration recommendations are followed (see *Undesirable effects*). Hypercalcaemia may promote or worsen renal dysfunction and the use of disodium clodronate has normally been demonstrated to improve renal function as the serum calcium concentration is lowered. Nevertheless, care is required with the intravenous route of administration and the recommended dosage must not be exceeded.

It is recommended that appropriate monitoring of renal function with serum creatinine be carried out during treatment with Loron for Infusion. Serum calcium and phosphate should also be monitored periodically. Monitoring of liver enzymes and white cell counts is advised (see *Undesirable effects*).

Interaction with other medicaments and other forms of interaction: No other bisphosphonate drugs should be given with Loron for Infusion. The calcium-lowering action of clodronate can be potentiated by the administration of aminoglycosides either concomitantly or one to several weeks apart. Severe hypocalcaemia has been observed in some cases. Hypomagnesaemia may also occur simultaneously. Patients receiving NSAID's in addition to disodium clodronate have developed renal dysfunction. However, a synergistic action has not been established. There is no evidence from clinical experience that disodium clodronate interacts with other medication, such as steroids, diuretics, calcitonin, non NSAID analgesics, or chemotherapeutic agents.

Pregnancy and lactation: There are insufficient data either from animal studies or from experience in humans of the effects of disodium clodronate on the embryo and foetus. No studies have been conducted on excretion in breast milk. Consequently, disodium clodronate is contraindicated in pregnancy and lactation.

Effects on ability to drive and use machines: No effects.

Undesirable effects: Asymptomatic hypocalcaemia has been noted rarely. A reversible elevation of serum parathyroid hormone may occur. In a small proportion of patients, a mild, reversible increase in serum lactate dehydrogenase and a modest transient leucopenia have been reported although these may have been associated with concurrent chemotherapy. Renal dysfunction, including renal failure, has been reported. Transient proteinuria has been reported immediately after intravenous infusion (see *Special warnings and precautions*). The clinical significance is uncertain. However, chronic proteinurea following infusion has not been observed. Hypersensitivity reactions have been mainly confined to the skin: pruritus, urticaria and rarely exfoliative dermatitis. However, bronchospasm has been precipitated in patients with or without a previous history of asthma.

Overdose: There is no experience of acute overdosage in humans. An overdosage by intravenous infusion, or injection of undiluted infusion concentrate could provoke renal damage and renal function should be monitored. The development of hypocalcaemia is possible for up to 2 or 3 days following the overdosage. Serum calcium should be monitored and oral or parenteral calcium supplementation may be required. Acute overdosage may be associated with gastrointestinal symptoms such as nausea and vomiting. Treatment should be symptomatic.

Pharmacological properties

Pharmacodynamic properties: Disodium clodronate is a bisphosphonate which has a high affinity to bone. It is mainly the portion of the dose adsorbed to bone which is pharmacologically active. The pharmacological effect of disodium clodronate is to suppress osteoclast mediated bone resorption as judged by bone histology and decreases in serum calcium, urine calcium and urinary excretion of hydroxyproline, without adversely affecting mineralisation.

Pharmacokinetic properties: Disodium clodronate is not metabolised. The volume of distribution is approximately 0.3L/kg. Elimination from serum is rapid, 75% of the dose is recovered unchanged in urine within 24 hours.

The elimination kinetics best fit a 3 compartment model. The first two compartments have relatively short half-lives. The third compartment is probably the skeleton. Elimination half life is approximately 12–13 hours.

Preclinical safety data: Disodium clodronate shows relatively little toxicity either on single oral administration or after daily oral administration for a period of up to 6 months. In rats, a dose of 200 mg/kg/day in the chronic toxicity test is at the limit of tolerability. In dogs, 40 mg/kg/day chronically is within the tolerated range.

On daily administration of 500 mg/kg for 6 weeks to rats, signs of renal failure with a clear rise in BUN, and initial liver parenchymal reaction with rises of SGOT, SGPT and AP occurred. No significant haematological changes were found in the toxicological investigations.

Investigations for mutagenic properties did not show any indication of mutagenic potency.

Reproduction toxicology investigations did not provide any indication of peri and post natal disorders, teratogenic damage or disorders of fertility.

It is not known if disodium clodronate passes into the mother's milk or through the placenta.

Pharmaceutical particulars

List of excipients: Loron for Infusion also contains sodium bicarbonate, water for injections and hydrochloric acid.

Incompatibilities: None known.

Shelf life:
Unopened ampoule 2 years
Diluted solution 12 hours

Special precautions for storage: None.

Nature and contents of container: Clear glass ampoules, each containing 10 ml solution.
5 ampoules to a carton.

Instructions for use/handling: None.

Marketing authorisation number PL 0075/0064

Date of first authorisation/renewal of authorisation 11 March 1996

Date of (partial) revision of the text May 1998

LORON CAPSULES

Qualitative and quantitative composition Each Loron capsule contains 400 mg disodium clodronate.

Pharmaceutical form Capsules for oral administration.

Clinical particulars

Therapeutic indications: Loron is indicated for the management of osteolytic lesions, hypercalcaemia and bone pain associated with skeletal metastases in patients with carcinoma of the breast or multiple myeloma. Loron capsules are also indicated for the maintenance of clinically acceptable serum calcium levels in patients with hypercalcaemia of malignancy initially treated with an intravenous infusion of disodium clodronate.

Posology and method of administration:

Adults: The recommended dose is 4 capsules (1600 mg disodium clodronate) daily. If necessary, the dosage may be increased but should not exceed a maximum of 8 capsules (3200 mg disodium clodronate) daily.

The capsules may be taken as a single dose or in two equally divided doses if necessary to improve gastrointestinal tolerance. Loron capsules should be swallowed with a little fluid, but not milk, at least one hour before or one hour after food.

Elderly: No special dosage recommendations.

Children: Safety and efficacy in children has not been established.

Use in renal impairment: In patients with renal insufficiency with creatinine clearance between 10 and 30 ml/min, the daily dose should be reduced to one half the recommended adult dose. Serum creatinine should be monitored during therapy. Disodium clodronate is contra-indicated in patients with creatinine clearance below 10 ml/min.

The oral bioavailability of bisphosphonates is poor. Bioequivalence studies have shown appreciable differences in bioavailability between different oral formulations of disodium clodronate, as well as marked inter and intra patient variability. Dose adjustment may be required if the formulation is changed.

Contra-indications: Hypersensitivity to disodium clodronate. Acute, severe inflammatory conditions of the gastrointestinal tract. Pregnancy and lactation. Renal failure with creatinine clearance below 10 ml/min, except for short term use in the presence of purely functional renal insufficiency caused by elevated serum calcium levels. Concomitant use of other bisphosphonates.

Special warnings and special precautions for use: No information is available on the potential carcinogenicity of disodium clodronate, but patients have been treated in clinical trials for up to 2 years. The duration of the treatment is therefore at the discretion of the physician, according to the status of the underlying malignancy.

Interaction with other medicaments and other forms of interaction: No other bisphosphonate drugs should be given with Loron capsules.

The calcium-lowering action of clodronate can be potentiated by the administration of aminoglycosides either concomitantly or one to several weeks apart. Severe hypocalcaemia has been observed in some cases. Hypomagnesaemia may also occur simultaneously. Patients receiving NSAID's in addition to disodium clodronate have developed renal dysfunction. However, a synergistic action has not been established. There is no evidence from clinical experience that disodium clodronate interacts with other medication, such as steroids, diuretics, calcitonin, non NSAID analgesics, or chemotherapeutic agents. Calcium rich foods, mineral supplements and antacids may impair absorption.

Pregnancy and lactation: There are insufficient data either from animal studies or from experience in humans of the effects of disodium clodronate on the embryo and foetus. No studies have been conducted on excretion in breast milk. Consequently, disodium clodronate is contra-indicated in pregnancy and lactation.

Effects on ability to drive and use machines: No effects.

Undesirable effects: Patients may experience a mild gastrointestinal upset, usually in the form of nausea or mild diarrhoea. The symptoms may respond to the use of a twice daily dosage regime rather than a single dose. It is not normally required to withdraw therapy or to provide medication to control these effects. Asymptomatic hypocalcaemia has been noted rarely. A reversible elevation of serum parathyroid hormone may occur. In a small proportion of patients, a mild, reversible increase in serum lactate dehydrogenase and a modest transient leucopenia have been reported although these may have been associated with concurrent chemotherapy. Renal dysfunction, including renal failure has been reported. Hypersensitivity reactions have been mainly confined to the skin: pruritus, urticaria and rarely exfoliative dermatitis. However, bronchospasm has been precipitated in patients with or without a previous history of asthma.

Overdose:

Symptoms and signs: There is no experience of acute overdosage in humans. The development of hypocalcaemia is possible for up to 2 or 3 days following the overdosage.

Treatment: Serum calcium should be monitored and oral or parenteral calcium supplementation may be required. Acute overdosage may be associated with gastrointestinal symptoms such as nausea and vomiting. Treatment should be symptomatic.

Pharmacological properties

Pharmacodynamic properties: Disodium clodronate is a bisphosphonate which has a high affinity to bone. It is mainly the portion of the dose adsorbed to bone which is pharmacologically active. The pharmacological effect of disodium clodronate is to suppress osteoclast mediated bone resorption as judged by bone histology and decreases in serum calcium, urine calcium and urinary excretion of hydroxyproline, without adversely affecting mineralisation.

Pharmacokinetic properties: Oral bioavailability is in the order of 2%.

Disodium clodronate is not metabolised. The volume of distribution is approximately 0.3L/kg. Elimination from serum is rapid, 75% of the dose is recovered unchanged in urine within 24 hours.

The elimination kinetics best fit a 3 compartment model. The first two compartments have relatively short half-lives. The third compartment is probably the skeleton. Elimination half life is approximately 12–13 hours.

Preclinical safety data: Disodium clodronate shows relatively little toxicity either on single oral administration or after daily oral administration for a period of up to 6 months. In rats, a dose of 200 mg/kg/day in the chronic toxicity test is at the limit of tolerability. In dogs, 40 mg/kg/day chronically is within the tolerated range.

On daily administration of 500 mg/kg for 6 weeks to rats, signs of renal failure with a clear rise in BUN, and initial liver parenchymal reaction with rises of SGOT, SGPT and AP occurred. No significant haematological changes were found in the toxicological investigations.

Investigations for mutagenic properties did not show any indication of mutagenic potency.

Reproduction toxicology investigations did not provide any indication of peri and post natal disorders, teratogenic damage or disorders of fertility.

It is not known if disodium clodronate passes into the mother's milk or through the placenta.

Pharmaceutical particulars

List of excipients: Loron capsules also contain talc, maize starch, magnesium stearate and sodium starch glycollate. The capsule shell is made of gelatin.

Incompatibilities: Not applicable.

Shelf life:
PVC/aluminium blister packs: 5 years
HDPE tubs with LDPE caps: 3 years

Special precautions for storage: None.

Nature and contents of container: PVC/aluminium Blister Packs containing 120 capsules.

HDPE containers with LDPE snap-on tamper evident caps containing 30 or 112 capsules.

Instructions for use/handling: No special instructions

Marketing authorisation number PL 15722/0016

Date of first authorisation/renewal of authorisation 1 January 1997

Date of (partial) revision of the text May 1998

LORON 520

Qualitative and quantitative composition Each Loron 520 tablet contains 520 mg disodium clodronate.

Pharmaceutical form Film-coated tablets for oral administration.

Clinical particulars

Therapeutic indications: Loron is indicated for the management of osteolytic lesions, hypercalcaemia and bone pain associated with skeletal metastases in patients with carcinoma of the breast or multiple myeloma. Loron 520 is also indicated for the maintenance of clinically acceptable serum calcium levels in patients with hypercalcaemia of malignancy initially treated with an intravenous infusion of disodium clodronate.

Posology and method of administration:

Adults: The recommended dose is 2 tablets (1040 mg disodium clodronate) daily. If necessary, the dosage may be increased but should not exceed a maximum of 4 tablets (2080 mg disodium clodronate) daily.

The tablets may be taken as a single dose or in two equally divided doses if necessary to improve gastrointestinal tolerance. Loron tablets should be swallowed with a little fluid, but not milk, at least one hour before or one hour after food.

When changing therapy from Loron capsules (400 mg) to Loron 520 tablets (520 mg), it should be noted that two Loron capsules are equivalent to one Loron 520 tablet. This is due to greater bioavailability of the tablet formulation.

Elderly: No special dosage recommendations.

Children: Safety and efficacy in children has not been established.

Use in renal impairment: In patients with renal insufficiency with creatinine clearance between 10 and 30 ml/min, the daily dose should be reduced to one half the recommended adult dose. Serum creatinine should be monitored during therapy. Disodium clodronate is contra-indicated in patients with creatinine clearance below 10 ml/min.

The oral bioavailability of bisphosphonates is poor. Bioequivalence studies have shown appreciable differences in bioavailability between different oral formulations of disodium clodronate, as well as marked inter and intra patient variability. Dose adjustment may be required if the formulation is changed.

Contra-indications: Hypersensitivity to disodium clodronate. Acute, severe inflammatory conditions of the gastrointestinal tract. Pregnancy and lactation. Renal failure with creatinine clearance below 10 ml/min, except for short term use in the presence of purely functional renal insufficiency caused by elevated serum calcium levels. Concomitant use of other bisphosphonates.

Special warnings and special precautions for use: No information is available on the potential carcinogenicity of disodium clodronate, but patients have been treated in clinical trials for up to 2 years. The duration of the treatment is therefore at the discretion of the physician, according to the status of the underlying malignancy.

It is recommended that appropriate monitoring of renal function with serum creatinine be carried out during treatment. Serum calcium and phosphate should be monitored periodically. Monitoring of liver enzymes and white cells is advised (see side effects).

Interaction with other medicaments and other forms of interaction: No other bisphosphonate drugs should be given with Loron tablets.

The calcium-lowering action of clodronate can be potentiated by the administration of aminoglycosides either concomitantly or one to several weeks apart. Severe hypocalcaemia has been observed in some cases. Hypomagnesaemia may also occur simultaneously. Patients receiving NSAIDs in addition to disodium clodronate have developed renal dysfunction. However, a synergistic action has not been established. There is no evidence from clinical experience that sodium clodronate interacts with other medication, such as steroids, diuretics, calcitonin, non NSAID analgesics, or chemotherapeutic agents. Calcium rich foods, mineral supplements and antacids may impair absorption.

Pregnancy and lactation: There are insufficient data either from animal studies or from experience in humans of the effects of disodium clodronate on the embryo and foetus. No studies have been conducted on excretion in breast milk. Consequently, disodium clodronate is contraindicated in pregnancy and lactation.

Effects on ability to drive and use machines: No known effects which would impair alertness.

Undesirable effects: Patients may experience a mild gastrointestinal upset, usually in the form of nausea or mild diarrhoea. The symptoms may respond to the use of a twice daily dosage regime rather than a single dose. It is not normally required to withdraw therapy or to provide medication to control these effects. Asymptomatic hypocalcaemia has been noted rarely. A reversible elevation of serum parathyroid hormone may occur. In a small proportion of patients, a mild, reversible increase in serum lactate dehydrogenase and a modest transient leucopenia have been reported although these may have been associated with concurrent chemotherapy. Renal dysfunction, including renal failure has been reported. Hypersensitivity reactions have been mainly confined to the skin: pruritus, urticaria and rarely exfoliative dermatitis. However, bronchospasm has been precipitated in patients with or without a previous history of asthma.

Overdose:
Symptoms and signs: There is no experience of acute overdosage in humans. The development of hypocalcaemia is possible for up to 2 or 3 days following the overdosage.

Treatment: Serum calcium should be monitored and oral or parenteral calcium supplementation may be required. Acute overdosage may be associated with gastrointestinal symptoms such as nausea and vomiting. Treatment should be symptomatic.

Pharmacological properties
Pharmacodynamic properties: Disodium clodronate is a bisphosphonate which has a high affinity to bone. It is mainly the portion of the dose adsorbed to bone which is pharmacologically active. The pharmacological effect of disodium clodronate is to suppress osteoclast mediated bone resorption as judged by bone histology and decreases in serum calcium, urine calcium and urinary excretion of hydroxyproline, without adversely affecting mineralisation.

Pharmacokinetic properties: Oral bioavailability is in the order of 2%.

Disodium clodronate is not metabolised. The volume of distribution is approximately 0.3L/kg. Elimination from serum is rapid, 75% of the dose is recovered unchanged in urine within 24 hours.

The elimination kinetics best fit a 3 compartment model. The first two compartments have relatively short half-lives. The third compartment is probably the skeleton. Elimination half life is approximately 12–13 hours.

Preclinical safety data: Disodium clodronate shows relatively little toxicity either on single oral administration or after daily oral administration for a period of up to 6 months. In rats, a dose of 200 mg/kg/day in the chronic toxicity test is at the limit of tolerability. In dogs, 40 mg/kg/day chronically is within the tolerated range.

On daily administration of 500 mg/kg for 6 weeks to rats, signs of renal failure with a clear rise in BUN, and initial liver parenchymal reaction with rises of SGOT, SGPT and AP occurred. No significant haematological changes were found in the toxicological investigations.

Investigations for mutagenic properties did not show any indication of mutagenic potency.

Reproduction toxicology investigations did not provide any indication of peri and post natal disorders, teratogenic damage or disorders of fertility.

It is not known if disodium clodronate passes into the mother's milk or through the placenta.

Pharmaceutical particulars
List of excipients:
Loron 520 tablets also contain:
Core
Disodium clodronate, talc, maize starch, microcrystalline cellulose, magnesium stearate, sodium starch glycollate.
Coating
Methylhydroxypropylcellulose, poly(meth) acrylic acid esters (Eudragit NE 30D), polyoxyethylene alkyl ether (Macrogol 1000), lactose monohydrate, talc, titanium dioxide (E171), polysorbate 80, sodium citrate.

Incompatibilities: Not applicable.

Shelf life: PVC/aluminium blister packs: 5 years.

Special precautions for storage: None

Nature and contents of container: PVC/aluminium blister packs containing 10 or 60 tablets.

Instructions for use/handling: No special instructions.

Marketing authorisation number PL 15722/000029

Date of first authorisation/renewal of authorisation 1 March 1997

Date of (partial) revision of the text May 1998

MABTHERA 100 mg ▼ MABTHERA 500 mg 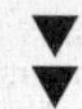

Qualitative and quantitative composition
1 single-use vial contains 100 mg (in 10 ml) of rituximab.

1 single-use vial contains 500 mg (in 50 ml) of rituximab.

Rituximab is a genetically engineered chimeric mouse/human monoclonal antibody representing a glycosylated immunoglobulin with human IgG1 constant regions and murine light-chain and heavy-chain variable regions sequences. The antibody is produced by mammalian (Chinese hamster ovary) cell suspension culture and purified by affinity chromatography and ion exchange, including specific viral inactivation and removal procedures.

Pharmaceutical form Concentrate for solution for infusion.

Clinical particulars
Therapeutic indications: Mabthera is indicated for treatment of patients with stage III–IV follicular lymphoma who are chemoresistant or are in their second or subsequent relapse after chemotherapy.

Posology and method of administration: The recommended dosage of Mabthera used as a single agent for adult patients is 375 mg/m² body surface, administered as an intravenous infusion once weekly for four weeks.

Mabthera infusions should be administered in a hospital environment where full resuscitation facilities are immediately available, and under the close supervision of an experienced oncologist/haematologist.

Premedication consisting of a pain-reliever and an antihistaminic, e.g. paracetamol and diphenhydramine, should always be administered before each infusion of Mabthera. Premedication with corticosteroids should also be considered.

Patients should be closely monitored for the onset of cytokine release syndrome (see *Special warnings and special precautions for use*). Patients who develop evidence of severe reactions, especially severe dyspnoea, bronchospasm or hypoxia should have the infusion interrupted immediately. The patient should then be evaluated for evidence of tumour lysis syndrome including appropriate laboratory tests and, for pulmonary infiltration, with a chest x-ray. The infusion should not be restarted until complete resolution of all symptoms, and normalisation of laboratory values and chest x-ray findings. At this time, the infusion can be initially resumed at not more than one-half the previous rate. If the same severe adverse reactions occur for a second time the decision to stop the treatment should be seriously considered on a case by case basis.

Mild or moderate infusion-related reactions (see *Undesirable effects*) usually respond to a reduction in the rate of infusion. The infusion rate may be increased upon improvement of symptoms.

First infusion: The prepared Mabthera solution should be administered by intravenous infusion through a dedicated line. The recommended initial rate for infusion is 50 mg/hr; after the first 30 minutes, it can be escalated in 50 mg/hr increments every 30 minutes, to a maximum of 400 mg/hr.

Subsequent infusions: Subsequent doses of Mabthera can be infused at an initial rate of 100 mg/hr, and increased by 100 mg/hr increments at 30 minutes intervals, to a maximum of 400 mg/hr.

Retreatment following relapse: Patients who have responded to Mabthera initially have been treated again with Mabthera. Response rate seems to be comparable in these retreated patients.

Contra-indications: Mabthera is contra-indicated in patients with known hypersensitivity to any component of this product or to murine proteins.

Special warnings and special precautions for use: Patients with a high number (>50,000 mm³) of circulating malignant cells or high tumour burden, who may be at higher risk of especially severe cytokine release syndrome, should only be treated with extreme caution and when other therapeutic alternatives have been exhausted. These patients should be very closely monitored throughout the first infusion. Consideration should be given to the use of a reduced infusion rate for the first infusion in these patients.

Severe cytokine release syndrome is characterised by severe dyspnoea, often accompanied by bronchospasm and hypoxia, in addition to fever, chills, rigors, urticaria, and angioedema. This syndrome may be associated with some features of *tumour lysis syndrome* such as hyperuricemia, hyperkalemia, hypocalcemia, acute renal failure, elevated LDH and may be associated with acute respiratory failure and death. The acute respiratory failure may be accompanied by events such as pulmonary interstitial infiltration or oedema, visible on a chest x-ray. The syndrome frequently manifests itself within one or two hours of initiating the first infusion. Patients with a history of pulmonary insufficiency or those with pulmonary tumour infiltration may be at greater risk of poor outcome and should be treated with increased caution. Patients who develop severe cytokine release syndrome should have their infusion interrupted immediately (see *Posology and method of administration*) and should receive aggressive symptomatic treatment. Since initial improvement of clinical symptoms may be followed by deterioration, these patients should be closely monitored until tumour lysis syndrome and pulmonary infiltration have resolved or been ruled out. Further treatment of patients after complete resolution of signs and symptoms has rarely resulted in repeated severe cytokine release syndrome.

Infusion related adverse reactions including cytokine release syndrome (see *Undesirable effects*) accompanied by hypotension and bronchospasm have been observed in 10% of patients treated with Mabthera. These symptoms are usually reversible with interruption of Mabthera infusion and administration of a pain-reliever, an antihistaminic, and, occasionally, oxygen, intravenous saline or bronchodilators, and corticosteroids if required. Please see cytokine release syndrome above for severe reactions.

Anaphylactic and other hypersensitivity reactions have been reported following the intravenous administration of proteins to patients. In contrast to cytokine release syndrome, true hypersensitivity reactions typically occur within minutes after starting infusion. Medications for the treatment of hypersensitivity reactions, e.g., epinephrine, antihistamines and corticosteroids, should be available for immediate use in the event of an allergic reaction during administration of Mabthera. Clinical manifestations of anaphylaxis may appear similar to clinical manifestations of the cytokine release syndrome (described above). Reactions attributed to hypersensitivity have been reported less frequently than those attributed to cytokine release.

Since hypotension may occur during Mabthera infusion, consideration should be given to withholding anti-hypertensive medications 12 hours prior to the Mabthera infusion.

Angina pectoris, or cardiac arrhythmias have occurred in patients treated with Mabthera. Therefore patients with a history of cardiac disease should be monitored closely.

Although Mabthera is not myelosuppressive, caution should be exercised when considering treatment of patients with neutrophils $<1.5\times10^9$/l and/or platelet counts $<75\times10^9$/l, as clinical experience in this population is limited. Mabthera has been used in 21 patients who underwent autologous bone transplantation and other risk groups with a presumable reduced bone marrow function without inducing myelotoxicity.

Periodic monitoring of a complete blood count with platelet count should be considered during therapy with Mabthera.

Do not administer the prepared infusion solutions as an intravenous push or bolus.

Paediatric use: The safety and efficacy of Mabthera in children have not been established.

Interaction with other medicinal products and other forms of interaction: Currently, no data are available on possible drug interactions with Mabthera. Patients with human anti-mouse antibody or human anti-chimeric antibody (HAMA/HACA) titres may have allergic or hypersensitivity reactions when treated with other diagnostic or therapeutic monoclonal antibodies.

The tolerability of simultaneously or sequential combination of Mabthera with agents liable to cause depletion of normal B-cells is not well defined. However, no synergistic toxicity was observed in 40 patients treated with Mabthera in combination with CHOP (*cyclophosphamide, doxorubicin, vincristine, prednisolone*).

Use during pregnancy and lactation:
Pregnancy: Animal reproduction studies have not been conducted with rituximab. It is also not known whether Mabthera can cause foetal harm when administered to a pregnant woman or whether it can affect reproductive capacity. However, since IgG is known to pass the placental barrier, rituximab may cause B-cell depletion in the foetus. For these reasons Mabthera should not be given to a pregnant woman unless the potential benefit outweighs the potential risk.

Due to the long retention time of rituximab in B-cell depleted patients, women of childbearing potential should use effective contraceptive methods during treatment and up to 12 months following Mabthera therapy.

Nursing mothers: Whether rituximab is excreted in human milk is not known. However, because maternal IgG is excreted in human milk, Mabthera should not be given to a nursing woman.

Effects on ability to drive and use machines: It is not known whether rituximab has an effect on the ability to drive and to use machines, although the pharmacological activity and adverse events reported to date do not indicate that such an effect is likely.

Undesirable effects: Patients with high tumour burden defined as single lesions with a diameter >10 cm have an increased incidence of severe (grade 3–4) adverse reactions.

Infusion related adverse reaction: Infusion-related adverse reactions including cytokine release syndrome occured in more than 50% of patients, and were predominantly seen during the first infusion, usually during the first one to two hours. These events mainly comprised fever, chills, and rigours. Other symptoms include flushing, angioedema, nausea, urticaria/rash, fatigue, headache, throat irritation, rhinitis, vomiting, and tumour pain. These symptoms were accompanied by hypotension and bronchospasm in about 10% of the cases. Less frequently, patients experienced an exacerbation of pre-existing cardiac conditions such as angina pectoris or congestive heart failure. The incidence of adverse reactions decreases substantially with subsequent infusions.

Fatal outcomes have been reported for patients who developed severe cytokine release syndrome, occasionally associated with signs and symptoms of tumour lysis syndrome leading to multi-organ failure, respiratory failure, and renal failure (see *Special warnings and special precautions for use*).

Haematologic adverse reaction: Haematologic abnormalities occur in a minority of patients and are usually mild and reversible. Severe thrombocytopenia and neutropenia occurred in 1.3% and 1.9% of patients respectively, and severe anaemia occurred in 1.0% of patients. A single occurrence of transient aplastic anaemia (pure red cell aplasia) and infrequent occurrences of haemolytic anaemia following Mabthera treatment were reported.

Other adverse reaction: Pulmonary adverse reactions, including severe bronchoconstriction and rarely fatalities from respiratory failure, have been reported with Mabthera therapy.

Anaphylaxis has been reported in patients treated with Mabthera (see *Special warnings and special precautions for use*).

Although Mabthera induces B-cell depletion and can be associated with decreased serum immunoglobulins, the incidence of infection does not appear to be greater than expected in this patient population, and serious or opportunistic infections were considerably less than reported with conventional chemotherapy. During treatment and up to one year following therapy, approximately 17% and 16%, respectively, of patients developed infections which were usually common, non opportunistic and mild.

Additional adverse events which have occurred in ≥1% of patients observed in clinical trials are listed below.

Body as a whole: Asthenia, abdominal pain, back pain, chest pain, malaise, abdominal enlargement, pain at infusion site.

Cardiovascular system: Hypertension, bradycardia, tachycardia, arrhythmia, postural hypotension.

Digestive system: Diarrhoea, dyspepsia, anorexia.

Haemic and lymphatic system: Lymphadenopathy.

Metabolic and nutritional disorders: Hyperglycaemia, peripheral oedema, LDH increase, hypocalcaemia.

Musculo-skeletal system: Arthralgia, myalgia, pain, hypertonia.

Nervous system: Dizziness, anxiety, paraesthesia, hypesthesia, agitation, insomnia, nervousness.

Respiratory system: Cough increase, sinusitis, bronchitis, respiratory disease.

Skin and appendages: Night sweats, sweating, herpes simplex, herpes zoster.

Special senses: Lacrimation disorder, conjunctivitis, taste perversion.

Additional severe adverse events occurring in <1% of patients are listed below.

Haemic and lymphatic system: Coagulation disorder.

Respiratory system: Asthma, lung disorder.

Overdose: There has been no experience of overdosage in human clinical trials. However, single doses higher than 500 mg/m² body surface have not been tested.

Pharmacological properties

Pharmacodynamic properties:

Pharmaco-therapeutic group: Antineoplastic agents, ATC Code: L01X X21.

Rituximab binds specifically to the transmembrane antigen, CD20, a non-glycosylated phosphoprotein, located on pre-B and mature B lymphocytes. The antigen is expressed on >95% of all B-cell non-Hodgkin's lymphomas (NHLs).

CD20 is found on both normal and malignant B-cells, but not on haematopoietic stem cells, pro-B-cells, normal plasma cells or other normal tissue. This antigen does not internalise upon antibody binding and is not shed from the cell surface. CD20 does not circulate in the plasma as a free antigen and, thus, does not compete for antibody binding.

The Fab domain of rituximab binds to the CD20 antigen on B lymphocytes and recruits immune effector functions to mediate B-cell lysis via the Fc domain. Possible mechanisms of cell lysis include complement-dependent cytotoxicity (CDC) resulting from C1q binding, and antibody-dependent cellular cytotoxicity (ADCC) mediated by one or more of the Fc γ receptors on the surface of granulocytes, macrophages and NK cells.

Median peripheral B-cell counts declined below normal following completion of the first dose, with recovery beginning after 6 months. B-cell levels returned to normal between 9 and 12 months following completion of therapy.

Clinical laboratory findings: Of 67 patients evaluated for human anti-mouse antibody (HAMA), no responses were noted. Of 355 patients evaluated for HACA, less than 1.0% (3 patients) were positive.

Pharmacokinetic properties: In patients treated with either 125, 250 or 375 mg/m² body surface of Mabthera, given as an intravenous infusion once weekly for four weeks, serum antibody concentrations increased with increasing dose. In patients receiving the 375 mg/m² dose, the mean serum half-life of rituximab was 68.1 hr, the C_{max} was 238.7 µg/ml and the mean plasma clearance was 0.0459 L/hr after the first infusion; after the fourth infusion, the mean values for serum half-life, C_{max} and plasma clearance were 189.9 hr, 480.7 µg/ml and 0.0145 L/hr, respectively. However, variability in serum levels was large.

Rituximab serum concentrations were statistically significantly higher in responding patients compared to non-responding patients just prior to and after the fourth infusion and post treatment. Serum concentrations were negatively correlated with tumour burden. Typically, rituximab was detectable for 3 to 6 months.

Preclinical safety data: Rituximab has shown to be highly specific to the CD20 antigen on B-cells. Toxicity studies in cynomolgus monkeys have shown no other effect than the expected pharmacological depletion of B-cells in peripheral blood and in lymphoid tissue. The recovery of the peripheral B-cells was marked by large intraindividual variability. However, peripheral B-cell recovery usually started two weeks after treatment, and median B-cells counts reached 40% of baseline levels after a 3 month period. No adverse reactions unrelated to the targeted effect were seen, whether in single or in multiple dose studies in the cynomolgus monkey.

No long-term animal studies have been performed to establish the carcinogenic potential of rituximab, or to determine its effects on fertility in males or females. Standard tests to investigate mutagenicity have not been carried out, since such tests are not relevant for this molecule. However, due to its character it is unlikely that rituximab has any mutagenic potential.

Pharmaceutical particulars

List of excipients: Sodium citrate, Polysorbate 80, Sodium chloride, Sodium hydroxide, Hydrochloric acid, Water for injection.

Incompatibilities: No incompatibilities between Mabthera and polyvinyl chloride or polyethylene bags or infusion sets have been observed.

Shelf life: 24 months.

Special precautions for storage: Store vials between 2–8°C. Protect undiluted vials from direct sunlight.

Prepared infusion solutions of Mabthera should be used immediately after dilution and are stable for 12 hours at room temperature. If necessary, the prepared solutions may be stored in the refrigerator (at 2–8°C) and are chemically stable for up to 24 hours. Mabthera does not contain any antimicrobial preservative; therefore, care must be taken to ensure the sterility of the prepared solution.

Nature and content of container: Single-use, preservative-free, clear glass vials with butyl rubber stopper containing 100 mg of rituximab in 10 ml (10 mg/ml). Packs of 2 vials.

Single-use, preservative-free, clear glass vials with butyl rubber stopper containing 500 mg of rituximab in 50 ml (10 mg/ml). Packs of 1 vial.

Instructions for use, handling and disposal (if appropriate): Mabthera is a clear, colourless liquid provided in sterile, preservative-free, non-pyrogenic, single-use vials.

Aseptically withdraw the necessary amount of Mabthera, and dilute to a calculated concentration of 1 to 4 mg/ml rituximab into an infusion bag containing sterile, pyrogen-free 0.9% Sodium Chloride or 5% Dextrose in water. For mixing the solution, gently invert the bag in order to avoid foaming. Care must be taken to ensure the sterility of prepared solutions. Since the drug product does not contain any antimicrobial preservative or bacteriostatic agents, aseptic technique must be observed. Parenteral drug products should be inspected visually for particulate matter and discoloration prior to administration.

Number(s) in the community register of medicinal products
EU/1/98/067/001 (100 mg)
EU/1/98/067/002 (500 mg)

Date of first authorisation/renewal of the authorisation June 1998

Date of revision of text 27th November 1998

MADOPAR CR CAPSULES '125'

Qualitative and quantitative composition Each capsule contains 100.0 mg levodopa and 28.5 mg benserazide hydrochloride (equivalent to 25 mg of the base) in a controlled release formulation.

Pharmaceutical form Modified release capsules.

Clinical particulars

Therapeutic indications: Treatment of all stages of Parkinson's disease. Patients with fluctuations related to levodopa plasma concentrations or timing of dose, e.g. end of dose deterioration or wearing-off effects, are more likely to benefit from switching to Madopar CR.

Posology and method of administration:

Adults, including the elderly: Dosage and administration are very variable and must be titrated to the needs of the individual patient.

Madopar CR capsules must always be swallowed whole, preferably with a little water. They may be taken with or without food but antacid preparations should be avoided.

Patients not currently treated with levodopa: In patients with mild to moderate disease, the initial recommended dose is one capsule of Madopar CR three times daily with meals. Higher doses, in general, of Madopar CR will be required than with conventional levodopa-decarboxylase inhibitor combinations as a result of the reduced bioavailability. The initial dosages should not exceed 600 mg per day of levodopa.

Some patients may require a supplementary dose of conventional Madopar, or Madopar Dispersible, together with the first morning dose of Madopar CR to compensate for the more gradual onset of the CR formulation.

In cases of poor response to Madopar CR at total daily doses of Madopar CR plus any supplementary conventional Madopar corresponding to 1,200 mg levodopa, administration of Madopar CR should be discontinued and alternative therapy considered.

Patients currently treated with levodopa: Madopar CR should be substituted for the standard levodopa-decarboxylase inhibitor preparation by one capsule Madopar CR 125 per 100 mg levodopa. For example, where a patient previously received daily doses of 200 mg levodopa with a decarboxylase inhibitor, then therapy should be initiated with two capsules Madopar CR 125. Therapy should continue with the same frequency of doses as previously.

With Madopar CR, *on average*, a 50% increase in daily levodopa dosage compared with previous therapy has been found to be appropriate. The dosage should be titrated every 2 to 3 days using dosage increments of Madopar CR 125 capsules and a period of up to 4 weeks should be allowed for optimisation of dosage.

Patients already on levodopa therapy should be informed that their condition may deteriorate initially until the optimal dosage regimen has been found. Close medical supervision of the patient is advisable during the initial period whilst adjusting the dosage.

Children: Not to be given to patients under 25 years of age: therefore, no dosage recommendations are made for the administration of Madopar CR to children.

Contra-indications: Madopar must not be given to patients with known hypersensitivity to levodopa or benserazide.

Madopar is contra-indicated in narrow-angle glaucoma (it may be used in wide-angle glaucoma provided that the intra-ocular pressure remains under control); severe psychoneuroses or psychoses; severe endocrine, renal, hepatic or cardiac disorders.

It should not be given in conjunction with, or within 2 weeks of withdrawal of, monoamine oxidase (MAO) inhibitors, except selective MAO-B inhibitors (e.g. selegiline) or selective MAO-A inhibitors (e.g. moclobemide).

It should not be given to patients under 25 years of age.

It should not be given to pregnant women or to women of childbearing potential in the absence of adequate contraception. If pregnancy occurs in a woman taking Madopar, the drug must be discontinued.

Suspicion has arisen that levodopa may activate a malignant melanoma. Therefore, Madopar should not be used in persons who have a history of, or who may be suffering from, a malignant melanoma.

Special warnings and special precautions for use: When other drugs must be given in conjunction with Madopar, the patient should be carefully observed for unusual side-effects or potentiating effects.

In the event of general anaesthesia being required, Madopar therapy should, whenever possible, be discontinued 12–48 hours before surgery.. If therapy is temporarily interrupted, the usual daily dosage may be administered as soon as the patient is able to take oral medication. Whenever therapy has been interrupted for longer periods, dosage should again be adjusted gradually; however, in many cases the patient can rapidly be returned to his previous therapeutic dosage.

If a patient has to undergo emergency surgery, when Madopar has not been withdrawn, anaesthesia with cyclopropane or halothane should be avoided.

There have been occasional reports of a neuroleptic malignant-like syndrome, involving hyperthermia, on abrupt withdrawal of levodopa preparations. Sudden discontinuation of Madopar, without close supervision, or "drug holidays" should therefore be avoided.

Pyridoxine (vitamin B_6) may be given with Madopar since the presence of a decarboxylase inhibitor protects against the peripheral levodopa transformation facilitated by pyridoxine.

Care should be taken when using Madopar in the following circumstances: in endocrine, renal, pulmonary or cardiovascular disease, particularly where there is a history of myocardial infarction or arrhythmia; psychiatric disturbances (e.g. depression); hepatic disorder; peptic ulcer; osteomalacia; where sympathomimetic drugs may be required (e.g. bronchial asthma), due to possible potentiation of the cardiovascular effects of levodopa; where antihypertensive drugs are being used, due to possible increased hypotensive action.

Periodic evaluation of hepatic, haemopoietic, renal and cardiovascular functions is advised.

Patients who improve on Madopar therapy should be advised to resume normal activities gradually as rapid mobilisation may increase the risk of injury.

Patients with diabetes should undergo frequent blood sugar tests and the dosage of antidiabetic agents should be adjusted to blood sugar levels.

Interaction with other medicaments and other forms of interaction: Opioids and drugs which interfere with central amine mechanisms, such as rauwolfia alkaloids (reserpine), tetrabenazine (Nitoman), metoclopramide, phenothiazines, thioxanthenes, butyrophenones, amphetamines and papaverine, should be avoided where possible. If, however, their administration is considered essential, extreme care should be exercised and a close watch kept for any signs of potentiation, antagonism or other interactions and for unusual side-effects.

Combination with other anti-parkinsonian agents (anticholinergics, amantadine, dopamine agonists) is permissible, though both the desired and undesired effects of treatment may be intensified. It may be necessary to reduce the dosage of Madopar or the other substance. Anticholinergics should not be withdrawn abruptly when Madopar therapy is instituted, as levodopa does not begin to take effect for some time.

Levodopa may interfere chemically with several diagnostic laboratory tests including those for glucose, ketone bodies, or catecholamines in urine and for glucose or uric acid in blood. Levodopa therapy has been reported to inhibit the response to protirelin in tests of thyroid function. Coombs' tests may give a false-positive result in patients taking Madopar.

When Madopar CR is given with antacid preparations the bioavailability of levodopa is reduced, in comparison with conventional Madopar.

Pregnancy and lactation: Madopar is contra-indicated in pregnancy and in women of childbearing potential in the absence of adequate contraception since there is evidence of harmful effects in studies in pregnant rabbits and the benserazide component has been found to be associated with skeletal malformations in the rat. If pregnancy occurs in a woman taking Madopar, the drug must be discontinued. Patients taking Madopar should not breast-feed their infants.

Effects on ability to drive and use machines: If drowsiness or psychiatric disturbances should occur, the patient should be warned not to drive or operate machinery.

Undesirable effects: Tolerance to Madopar varies widely between patients and is often related to the rate of dosage increases. Side-effects such as nausea, vomiting, loss of appetite and anorexia, which are frequently observed during the initial stages of levodopa therapy, are much less common in patients treated with Madopar. If such side-effects do occur, they can largely be controlled by taking Madopar with, or immediately after, food and by increasing dosage only slowly. Also, cardiovascular disturbances such as arrhythmias and orthostatic hypotension may occur, but are less frequent than in patients treated with levodopa alone. If experienced, orthostatic disorders usually improve following reduction of the Madopar dose.

Psychiatric disturbances are common in Parkinsonian patients, including those being treated with levodopa. They include mild elation, anxiety, agitation, insomnia, depression, aggression, delusions, hallucinations and "unmasking" of psychoses.

Although there have been rare reports of possible antagonism of levodopa by diazepam, in general diazepam (Valium Roche) and nitrazepam (Mogadon) have been found to be useful in the treatment of anxiety and insomnia, respectively, occurring in Parkinsonism. Depression may be treated with tricyclic antidepressants although isolated cases of hypertensive crisis have been reported with the concomitant use of tricyclic drugs. ECT may be administered if appropriate. MAO inhibitors, except selective MAO-B inhibitors or selective MAO-A inhibitors, must not be used.

Involuntary movements, commonly in the form of oral dyskinesias, often accompanied by "paddling" foot movements, or of the choreo-athetoid type, are common, particularly on long-term administration. These are usually dose-dependent and may disappear or become tolerable after dose adjustment.

Other side-effects which have occasionally been reported with levodopa therapy include diarrhoea, gastro-intestinal bleeding, flushing, sweating, and drowsiness.

Isolated cases of loss or alterations of taste have been reported and there have been rare cases of allergic skin reactions such as pruritus and rash.

On some occasions the urine passed during Madopar treatment may be altered in colour; usually red-tinged, this will turn dark on standing. These changes are due to metabolites and are no cause for concern.

Transient rises in SGOT, SGPT and alkaline phosphatase values have been noted: serum uric acid and blood urea nitrogen levels are occasionally increased. In rare instances, haemolytic anaemia, mild transient leucopenia and thrombocytopenia have been reported.

Overdose: Symptoms of overdosage are qualitatively similar to the side-effects but may be of greater magnitude.

Treatment should include gastric lavage, general supportive measures, intravenous fluids and the maintenance of an adequate airway.

Electrocardiographic monitoring should be instituted and the patient carefully observed for the possible development of arrhythmias. If necessary, anti-arrhythmic therapy should be given and other symptoms treated as they arise.

Pharmacological properties

Pharmacodynamic properties: Madopar is an anti-Parkinsonian agent. Levodopa is the metabolic precursor of dopamine. The latter is severely depleted in the striatum, pallidum and substantia nigra of Parkinsonian patients and it is considered that administration of levodopa raises the level of available dopamine in these centres. However, conversion of levodopa into dopamine by the enzyme dopa decarboxylase also takes place in extracerebral tissues. As a consequence the full therapeutic effect may not be obtained and side-effects occur.

Administration of a peripheral decarboxylase inhibitor, which blocks the extracerebral decarboxylation of levodopa, in conjunction with levodopa has significant advantages; these include reduced gastro-intestinal side-effects, a more rapid response at the initiation of therapy and a simpler dosage regimen. Madopar consists of levodopa and the peripheral decarboxylase inhibitor benserazide in the ratio 4:1 which in clinical trials has been shown to be the most satisfactory combination.

Like every replacement therapy, chronic treatment with Madopar will be necessary.

Pharmacokinetic properties: Madopar CR is a controlled-release form which provides more prolonged, but lower, peak plasma concentrations of levodopa than standard Madopar or other conventional formulations of levodopa.

Absorption: The active ingredients of Madopar CR are released slowly in the stomach and the maximum levodopa plasma concentration is reached approximately 3 hours after ingestion. The plasma concentration-time curve for levodopa shows a longer "half-duration" (= time-span when plasma concentrations are equal to or higher than half the maximum concentration) than that of standard Madopar, which indicates pronounced controlled-release properties. Madopar CR bioavailability is approximately 60% that of standard Madopar. Co-administration of an antacid with Madopar CR reduces the extent of levodopa absorption by 32%.

Distribution: Levodopa crosses the blood-brain barrier by a saturable transport system. It is not bound to plasma proteins. Benserazide does not cross the blood-brain barrier at therapeutic doses. Benserazide is concentrated mainly in the kidneys, lungs, small intestine and liver.

Metabolism: The 2 major routes of metabolism of levodopa are decarboxylation to form dopamine, which in turn is converted to a minor degree to norepinephrine and to a greater extent, to inactive metabolites, and O-methylation, forming 3-O-methyldopa, which has an elimination half-life of approximately 15 hours and accumulates in patients receiving therapeutic doses of Madopar. Decreased peripheral decarboxylation of levodopa when it is administered with benserazide is reflected in higher plasma levels of levodopa and 3-O-methyldopa.

Benserazide is hydroxylated to trihydroxybenzylhydrazine in the intestinal mucosa and the liver.

Elimination: In the presence of the peripheral decarboxylase inhibitor, benserazide, the elimination half-life of levodopa is approximately 1.5 hours. In elderly patients the elimination half-life is slightly (25%) longer. Clearance of levodopa is 430 ml/min. Elimination of levodopa is by biotransformation and excretion of the metabolites in the urine. Urinary recovery of unchanged drug accounts for approximately 7% of the dose.

Benserazide is almost entirely eliminated by metabolism. The metabolites are mainly excreted in the urine and to a small extent in faeces.

Pharmaceutical particulars

List of excipients: Each capsule contains: Hydroxypropyl methylcellulose, Hydrogenated vegetable oil, Calcium phosphate Dibasic Anhydrous, Mannitol, Talc, Povidone, Magnesium stearate and the colouring agents E132, E171 and E172

Incompatibilities: None known.

Shelf life: 3 years.

Special precautions for storage: Recommended maximum storage temperature 25°C. Protect from moisture.

Nature and contents of container: Amber glass bottles with aluminium screw-cap and desiccant containing 100 capsules.

Instructions for use/handling: No special requirements.

Marketing authorisation number PL 0031/0227

Date of first authorisation/renewal of authorisation Last renewal approved 27 April 1994

Date of (partial) revision of the text June 1998

MADOPAR CAPSULES

Qualitative and quantitative composition Each 62.5 capsule contains 50.0 mg levodopa and 14.25 mg benserazide hydrochloride (equivalent to 12.5 mg of the base).

Each 125 capsule contains 100.0 mg levodopa and 28.5 mg benserazide hydrochloride (equivalent to 25 mg of the base).

Each 250 capsule contains 200.0 mg levodopa and 57.0 mg benserazide hydrochloride (equivalent to 50 mg of the base).

Pharmaceutical form Capsules.

Clinical particulars

Therapeutic indications: Parkinsonism–idiopathic post-encephalitic.

Previous neurosurgery is not a contra-indication to Madopar.

Posology and method of administration: Dosage and administration are variable and no more than a guide can be given.

Adults

Patients not previously treated with levodopa: The recommended initial dose is one capsule or dispersible tablet of Madopar 62.5 three or four times daily. If the disease is at an advanced stage, the starting dose should be one capsule or dispersible tablet of Madopar 125 three times daily.

The daily dosage should then be increased by one capsule or dispersible tablet of Madopar 125, or their equivalent, once or twice weekly until a full therapeutic effect is obtained, or side-effects supervene.

In some elderly patients, it may suffice to initiate treatment with one capsule or dispersible tablet of Madopar 62.5 once or twice daily, increasing by one capsule or dispersible tablet every third or fourth day.

The effective dose usually lies within the range of four to eight capsules or dispersible tablets of Madopar 125 (two to four capsules of Madopar 250) daily in divided doses, most patients requiring no more than six capsules or dispersible tablets of Madopar 125 daily.

Optimal improvement is usually seen in one to three weeks but the full therapeutic effect of Madopar may not be apparent for some time. It is advisable, therefore, to allow several weeks to elapse before contemplating dosage increments above the average dose range. If satisfactory improvement is still not achieved, the dose of Madopar may be increased but with caution. It is rarely necessary to give more than ten capsules or dispersible tablets of Madopar 125 (five capsules of Madopar 250) per day.

Treatment should be continued for at least six months before failure is concluded from the absence of a clinical response.

Madopar 62.5 capsules or dispersible tablets may be used to facilitate adjustment of dosage to the needs of the individual patient. Patients who experience fluctuations in response may be helped by dividing the dosage into smaller, more frequent doses with the aid of Madopar 62.5 capsules or dispersible tablets without, however, altering the total daily dose.

Madopar 250 capsules are only for maintenance therapy once the optimal dosage has been determined using Madopar 125 capsules or dispersible tablets.

Patients previously treated with levodopa:

The following procedure is recommended: levodopa alone should be discontinued and Madopar started on the following day. The patient should be initiated on a total of one less Madopar 125 capsule or dispersible tablet daily than the total number of 500 mg levodopa tablets or capsules previously taken (for example, if the patient had previously taken 2 g levodopa daily, then he should start on three capsules or dispersible tablets Madopar 125 daily on the following day). Observe the patient for one week and then, if necessary, increase the dosage in the manner described for new patients.

Patients previously treated with other levodopa/decarboxylase inhibitor combinations: Previous therapy should be withdrawn for 12 hours. In order to minimise the potential for any effects of levodopa withdrawal, it may be beneficial to discontinue previous therapy at night and institute Madopar therapy the following morning. The initial Madopar dose should be one capsule or dispersible tablet of Madopar 62.5 three or four times daily. This dose may then be increased in the manner described for patients not previously treated with levodopa.

Other anti-Parkinsonian drugs may be given with Madopar. Existing treatment with other anti-Parkinsonian drugs, e.g. anticholinergics or amantadine, should be continued during initiation of Madopar therapy. However, as treatment with Madopar proceeds and the therapeutic effect becomes apparent, the dosage of the other drugs may need to be reduced or the drugs gradually withdrawn.

Elderly: Although there may be an age-related decrease in tolerance to levodopa in the elderly, Madopar appears to be well-tolerated and side-effects are generally not troublesome.

Children: Not to be given to patients under 25 years of age: therefore, no dosage recommendations are made for the administration of Madopar to children.

Madopar capsules are for oral administration. They should be taken with, or immediately after, meals.

Contra-indications: Madopar must not be given to patients with known hypersensitivity to levodopa or benserazide.

Madopar is contra-indicated in narrow-angle glaucoma (it may be used in wide-angle glaucoma provided that the intra-ocular pressure remains under control); severe psychoneuroses or psychoses; severe endocrine, renal, hepatic or cardiac disorders.

It should not be given in conjunction with, or within 2 weeks of withdrawal of, monoamine oxidase (MAO) inhibitors, except selective MAO-B inhibitors (e.g. selegiline) or selective MAO-A inhibitors (e.g. moclobemide).

It should not be given to patients under 25 years of age.

It should not be given to pregnant women or to women of childbearing potential in the absence of adequate contraception. If pregnancy occurs in a woman taking Madopar, the drug must be discontinued.

Suspicion has arisen that levodopa may activate a malignant melanoma. Therefore, Madopar should not be used in persons who have a history of, or who may be suffering from, a malignant melanoma.

Special warnings and special precautions for use: When other drugs must be given in conjunction with Madopar, the patient should be carefully observed for unusual side-effects or potentiating effects.

In the event of general anaesthesia being required, Madopar therapy should, whenever possible, be discontinued 12–48 hours before surgery. If therapy is temporarily interrupted, the usual daily dosage may be administered as soon as the patient is able to take oral medication. Whenever therapy has been interrupted for longer periods, dosage should again be adjusted gradually; however, in many cases the patient can rapidly be returned to his previous therapeutic dosage.

If a patient has to undergo emergency surgery, when Madopar has not been withdrawn, anaesthesia with cyclopropane or halothane should be avoided.

There have been occasional reports of a neuroleptic malignant-like syndrome, involving hyperthermia, on abrupt withdrawal of levodopa preparations. Sudden discontinuation of Madopar, without close supervision, or 'drug holidays' should therefore be avoided.

Pyridoxine (vitamin B_6) may be given with Madopar since the presence of a decarboxylase inhibitor protects against the peripheral levodopa transformation facilitated by pyridoxine.

Care should be taken when using Madopar in the following circumstances: in endocrine, renal, pulmonary or cardiovascular disease, particularly where there is a history of myocardial infarction or arrhythmia; psychiatric disturbances (e.g. depression); hepatic disorder; peptic ulcer; osteomalacia; where sympathomimetic drugs may be required (e.g. bronchial asthma), due to possible potentiation of the cardiovascular effects of levodopa; where antihypertensive drugs are being used, due to possible increased hypotensive action.

Periodic evaluation of hepatic, haemopoietic, renal and cardiovascular functions is advised.

Patients with diabetes should undergo frequent blood sugar tests and the dosage of anti-diabetic agents should be adjusted to blood sugar levels.

Patients who improve on Madopar therapy should be advised to resume normal activities gradually as rapid mobilisation may increase the risk of injury.

Interaction with other medicaments and other forms of interaction: Opioids and drugs which interfere with central amine mechanisms, such as rauwolfia alkaloids (reserpine), tetrabenazine (Nitoman), metoclopramide, phenothiazines, thioxanthenes, butyrophenones, amphetamines and papaverine, should be avoided where possible. If, however, their administration is considered essential, extreme care should be exercised and a close watch kept for any signs of potentiation, antagonism or other interactions and for unusual side-effects.

Co-administration of the anticholinergic drug trihexyphenidyl with Madopar reduces the rate, but not the extent, of levodopa absorption.

Combination with other anti-parkinsonian agents (anticholinergics, amantadine, dopamine agonists) is permissible, though both the desired and undesired effects of treatment may be intensified. It may be necessary to reduce the dosage of Madopar or the other substance. Anticholinergics should not be withdrawn abruptly when Madopar therapy is instituted, as levodopa does not begin to take effect for some time.

Levodopa may interfere chemically with several diagnostic laboratory tests including those for glucose, ketone bodies or catecholamines in urine and for glucose or uric acid in blood. Levodopa therapy has been reported to inhibit the response to protirelin in tests of thyroid function. Coombs' tests may give a false-positive result in patients taking Madopar.

Pregnancy and lactation: Madopar is contra-indicated in pregnancy and in women of childbearing potential in the absence of adequate contraception, since there is evidence of harmful effects in studies in pregnant rabbits and the benserazide component has been found to be associated with skeletal malformations in the rat. If pregnancy occurs in a woman taking Madopar, the drug must be discontinued. Patients taking Madopar should not breast-feed their infants.

Effects on ability to drive and use machines: If drowsiness or psychiatric disturbances should occur the patient should be warned not to drive or operate machinery.

Undesirable effects: Tolerance to Madopar varies widely between patients and is often related to the rate of dosage increases. Side-effects such as nausea, vomiting, loss of appetite and anorexia, which are frequently observed during the initial stages of levodopa therapy, are much less common in patients treated with Madopar. If such side-effects do occur, they can largely be controlled by taking Madopar with, or immediately after, food and by increasing dosage only slowly. Also, cardiovascular disturbances such as arrhythmias and orthostatic hypotension may occur, but are less frequent than in patients treated with levodopa alone. If experienced, orthostatic disorders usually improve following reduction of the Madopar dose.

Psychiatric disturbances are common in Parkinsonian patients, including those being treated with levodopa. They include mild elation, anxiety, agitation, insomnia, depression, aggression, delusions, hallucinations, and 'unmasking' of psychoses.

Although there have been rare reports of possible antagonism of levodopa by diazepam, in general diazepam (Valium Roche) and nitrazepam (Mogadon) have been found to be useful in the treatment of anxiety and insomnia, respectively, occurring in Parkinsonism. Depression may be treated with tricyclic antidepressants although isolated cases of hypertensive crisis have been reported with the concomitant use of tricyclic drugs. ECT may be administered if appropriate. MAO inhibitors, except selective MAO-B inhibitors or selective MAO-A inhibitors must not be used.

Involuntary movements, commonly in the form of oral dyskinesias, often accompanied by 'paddling' foot movements, or of the choreo-athetoid type, are common, particularly on long-term administration. These are usually dose-dependent and may disappear or become tolerable after dose adjustment.

With long-term administration, fluctuations in the therapeutic response may be encountered. They include 'freezing' episodes, end-of-dose deterioration and the so-called 'on-off' effect. Patients may be helped by dosage reduction or by giving smaller and more frequent doses.

Other side-effects which have occasionally been reported with levodopa therapy include diarrhoea, gastro-intestinal bleeding, flushing, sweating, and drowsiness.

Isolated cases of loss or alterations of taste have been reported and there have been rare cases of allergic skin reactions such as pruritus and rash.

On some occasions the urine passed during Madopar treatment may be altered in colour; usually red-tinged, this will turn dark on standing. These changes are due to metabolites and are no cause for concern.

Transient rises in SGOT, SGPT and alkaline phosphatase values have been noted. Serum uric acid and blood urea nitrogen levels are occasionally increased. In rare instances, haemolytic anaemia, mild transient leucopenia and thrombocytopenia have been reported.

Overdose: Symptoms of overdosage are qualitatively similar to the side-effects but may be of greater magnitude.

Treatment should include gastric lavage, general supportive measures, intravenous fluids and the maintenance of an adequate airway.

Electrocardiographic monitoring should be instituted and the patient carefully observed for the possible development of arrhythmias. If necessary, anti-arrhythmic therapy should be given and other symptoms treated as they arise.

Pharmacological properties

Pharmacodynamic properties: Madopar is an anti-Parkinsonian agent. Levodopa is the metabolic precursor of dopamine. The latter is severely depleted in the striatum, pallidum and substantia nigra of Parkinsonian patients and it is considered that administration of levodopa raises the level of available dopamine in these centres. However, conversion of levodopa into dopamine by the enzyme dopa decarboxylase also takes place in extracerebral tissues. As a consequence the full therapeutic effect may not be obtained and side-effects occur.

Administration of a peripheral decarboxylase inhibitor, which blocks the extracerebral decarboxylation of levodopa, in conjunction with levodopa has significant advantages; these include reduced gastro-intestinal side-effects, a more rapid response at the initiation of therapy and a simpler dosage regimen. Madopar is a combination of levodopa and benserazide in the ratio 4:1 which in clinical trials has been shown to be the most satisfactory.

Like every replacement therapy, chronic treatment with Madopar will be necessary.

Pharmacokinetic properties:

Absorption: Low levels of endogenous levodopa are detectable in pre-dose blood samples. After oral administration of Madopar, levodopa and benserazide are rapidly absorbed, mainly in the upper regions of the small intestine. Interaction studies indicate that a higher proportion of levodopa is absorbed when administered in combination with benserazide, compared with levodopa administered alone. Maximum plasma concentrations of levodopa are reached approximately one hour after ingestion of Madopar. Bioavailability is approximately 98%.

Distribution: Levodopa crosses the blood-brain barrier by a saturable transport system. It is not bound to plasma proteins. Benserazide does not cross the blood-brain barrier at therapeutic doses. Benserazide is concentrated mainly in the kidneys, lungs, small intestine and liver.

Metabolism: The 2 major routes of metabolism of levodopa are decarboxylation to form dopamine, which in turn is converted to a minor degree to norepinephrine and to a greater extent, to inactive metabolites, and O-methylation, forming 3-O-methyldopa, which has an elimination half-life of approximately 15 hours and accumulates in patients receiving therapeutic doses of Madopar. Decreased peripheral decarboxylation of levodopa when it is administered with benserazide is reflected in higher plasma levels of levodopa and 3-O-methyldopa.

Benserazide is hydroxylated to trihydroxybenzylhydrazine in the intestinal mucosa and the liver.

Elimination: In the presence of the peripheral decarboxylase inhibitor, benserazide, the elimination half-life of levodopa is approximately 1.5 hours. In elderly patients the elimination half-life is slightly (25%) longer. Clearance of levodopa is 430 ml/min. Elimination of levodopa is by biotransformation and excretion of the metabolites in the urine. Urinary recovery of unchanged drug accounts for approximately 7% of the dose.

Benserazide is almost entirely eliminated by metabolism. The metabolites are mainly excreted in the urine and to a small extent in faeces.

Preclinical safety data: See *Pregnancy and lactation.*

Pharmaceutical particulars

List of excipients: Each capsule contains: Microcrystalline cellulose Ph. Eur., Povidone Ph. Eur., Purified talc Ph. Eur., Magnesium stearate Ph. Eur., Mannitol Ph. Eur (62.5 capsule only), Gelatin Ph. Eur., and the colouring agents E132, E171 and E172.

Incompatibilities: None known.

Shelf life: 3 years.

Special precautions for storage: Recommended maximum storage temperature 25°C.

Protect from moisture.

Nature and contents of container: Amber glass bottles with aluminium screw-cap and desiccant containing 100 capsules.

Instructions for use/handling: No special requirements.

Marketing authorisation numbers PL 0031/0125, PL 0031/0073R, PL 0031/0074R

Date of first authorisation/renewal of authorisation March 1995 (62.5) July 1990 (125, 250)

Date of (partial) revision of the text July 1998

MADOPAR DISPERSIBLE

Qualitative and quantitative composition

Madopar 62.5 dispersible tablets: Round, white tablets with ROCHE/62.5 imprinted on one face and a single break bar on the other, containing 50 mg levodopa and 14.25 mg benserazide hydrochloride (equivalent to 12.5 mg of the base).

Madopar 125 dispersible tablets: Round, white tablets with ROCHE/125 imprinted on one face and a single break bar on the other, containing 100 mg levodopa and 28.5 mg benserazide hydrochloride (equivalent to 25 mg of the base).

Pharmaceutical form Madopar 62.5 Dispersible tablets, Madopar 125 Dispersible tablets

Clinical particulars

Therapeutic indications: Parkinsonism–idiopathic, post-encephalitic. Previous neurosurgery is not a contra-indication to Madopar.

Posology and method of administration: Dosage and administration are variable and no more than a guide can be given.

Adults

Patients not previously treated with levodopa: The recommended initial dose is one capsule or dispersible tablet of Madopar 62.5 three or four times daily. If the disease is at an advanced stage, the starting dose should be one capsule or dispersible tablet of Madopar 125 three times daily.

The daily dosage should then be increased by one capsule or dispersible tablet of Madopar 125, or their equivalent, once or twice weekly until a full therapeutic effect is obtained, or side-effects supervene.

In some elderly patients, it may suffice to initiate treatment with one capsule or dispersible tablet of Madopar 62.5 once or twice daily, increasing by one capsule or dispersible tablet every third or fourth day.

The effective dose usually lies within the range of four to eight capsules or dispersible tablets of Madopar 125 (two to four capsules of Madopar 250) daily in divided doses, most patients requiring no more than six capsules or dispersible tablets of Madopar 125 daily.

Optimal improvement is usually seen in one to three weeks but the full therapeutic effect of Madopar may not be apparent for some time. It is advisable, therefore, to allow several weeks to elapse before contemplating dosage increments above the average dose range. If satisfactory improvement is still not achieved, the dose of Madopar may be increased but with caution. It is rarely necessary to give more than ten capsules or dispersible tablets of Madopar 125 (five capsules of Madopar 250) per day.

Treatment should be continued for at least six months before failure is concluded from the absence of a clinical response.

Madopar 62.5 capsules or dispersible tablets may be used to facilitate adjustment of dosage to the needs of the individual patient. Patients who experience fluctuations in response may be helped by dividing the dosage into smaller, more frequent doses with the aid of Madopar 62.5 capsules or dispersible tablets without, however, altering the total daily dose.

Madopar 250 capsules are only for maintenance therapy once the optimal dosage has been determined using Madopar 125 capsules or dispersible tablets.

Patients previously treated with levodopa

The following procedure is recommended: Levodopa alone should be discontinued and Madopar started on the following day. The patient should be initiated on a total of one less Madopar 125 capsule or dispersible tablet daily than the total number of 500 mg levodopa tablets or capsules previously taken (for example, if the patient had previously taken 2 g levodopa daily, then he should start on three capsules or dispersible tablets Madopar 125 daily on the following day). Observe the patient for one week and then, if necessary, increase the dosage in the manner described for new patients.

Patients previously treated with other levodopa/decarboxylase inhibitor combinations: Previous therapy should be withdrawn for 12 hours. In order to minimise the potential for any effects of levodopa withdrawal, it may be beneficial to discontinue previous therapy at night and institute Madopar therapy the following morning. The initial Madopar dose should be one capsule or dispersible tablet of Madopar 62.5 three or four times daily. This dose may then be increased in the manner described for patients not previously treated with levodopa.

Other anti-Parkinsonian drugs may be given with Madopar. Existing treatment with other anti-Parkinsonian drugs, e.g. anticholinergics or amantadine, should be continued during initiation of Madopar therapy. However, as treatment with Madopar proceeds and the therapeutic effect becomes apparent, the dosage of the other drugs may need to be reduced or the drugs gradually withdrawn.

Elderly: Although there may be an age-related decrease in tolerance to levodopa in the elderly, Madopar appears to be well-tolerated and side effects are generally not troublesome.

Children: Not to be given to patients under 25 years of age, therefore, no dosage recommendations are made for the administration of Madopar to children.

Madopar capsules and dispersible tablets are for oral administration. They should be taken with, or immediately after, meals.

Madopar dispersible tablets may be swallowed whole or dispersed in at least 25 ml water per tablet. They may be taken in dilute orange squash (at least 25 ml per tablet) if preferred. However, orange juice should not be used. Madopar dispersible tablets are particularly suitable for patients who dislike taking capsules or have difficulty in swallowing solid dosage forms.

Contra-indications: Madopar must not be given to patients with known hypersensitivity to levodopa or benserazide.

Madopar is contra-indicated in narrow-angle glaucoma (it may be used in wide-angle glaucoma provided that the intra-ocular pressure remains under control); severe psychoneuroses or psychoses; severe endocrine, renal, hepatic or cardiac disorders.

It should not be given in conjunction with, or within 2 weeks of withdrawal of, monoamine oxidase (MAO) inhibitors, except selective MAO-B inhibitors (e.g. selegiline) or selective MAO-A inhibitors (e.g. moclobemide).

It should not be given to patients under 25 years of age.

It should not be given to pregnant women or to women of childbearing potential in the absence of adequate contraception. If pregnancy occurs in a woman taking Madopar, the drug must be discontinued.

Suspicion has arisen that levodopa may activate a malignant melanoma. Therefore, Madopar should not be used in persons who have a history of, or who may be suffering from, a malignant melanoma.

Special warnings and special precautions for use: When other drugs must be given in conjunction with Madopar, the patient should be carefully observed for unusual side-effects or potentiating effects.

In the event of general anaesthesia being required, Madopar therapy should, whenever possible, be discontinued 12–48 hours before surgery. If therapy is temporarily interrupted, the usual daily dosage may be administered as soon as the patient is able to take oral medication. Whenever therapy has been interrupted for longer periods, dosage should again be adjusted gradually; however, in many cases the patient can rapidly be returned to his previous therapeutic dosage.

If a patient has to undergo emergency surgery, when Madopar has not been withdrawn, anaesthesia with cyclopropane or halothane should be avoided. There have been occasional reports of a neuroleptic malignant-like syndrome, involving hyperthermia, on abrupt withdrawal of levodopa preparations. Sudden discontinuation of Madopar, without close supervision, or "drug holidays" should therefore be avoided.

Pyridoxine (vitamin B_6) may be given with Madopar since the presence of a decarboxylase inhibitor protects against the peripheral levodopa transformation facilitated by pyridoxine.

Care should be taken when using Madopar in the following circumstances: In endocrine, renal, pulmonary or cardiovascular disease, particularly where there is a history of myocardial infarction or arrhythmia; psychiatric disturbances (e.g. depression); hepatic disorder; peptic ulcer; osteomalacia; where sympathomimetic drugs may be required (e.g. bronchial asthma), due to possible potentiation of the cardiovascular effects of levodopa; where antihypertensive drugs are being used, due to possible increased hypotensive action.

Periodic evaluation of hepatic, haemopoietic, renal and cardiovascular functions is advised.

Patients with diabetes should undergo frequent blood sugar tests and the dosage of anti-diabetic agents should be adjusted to blood sugar levels.

Patients who improve on Madopar therapy should be advised to resume normal activities gradually as rapid mobilisation may increase the risk of injury.

Interaction with other medicaments and other forms of interaction: Opioids and drugs which interfere with central amine mechanisms, such as rauwolfia alkaloids (reserpine), tetrabenazine (Nitoman), metoclopramide, phenothiazines, thioxanthenes, butyrophenones, amphetamines and papaverine, should be avoided where possible. If, however, their administration is considered essential, extreme care should be exercised and a close watch kept for any signs of potentiation, antagonism or other interactions and for unusual side-effects.

Co-administration of the anticholinergic drug trihexyphenidyl with Madopar reduces the rate, but not the extent, of levodopa absorption.

Combination with other anti-parkinsonian agents (anticholinergics, amantadine, dopamine agonists) is permissible, though both the desired and undesired effects of treatment may be intensified. It may be necessary to reduce the dosage of Madopar or the other substance. Anticholinergics should not be withdrawn abruptly when Madopar therapy is instituted, as levodopa does not begin to take effect for some time.

Levodopa may interfere chemically with several diagnostic laboratory tests including those for glucose, ketone bodies or catecholamines in urine and for glucose or uric acid in blood. Levodopa therapy has been reported to inhibit the response to protirelin in tests of thyroid function. Coombs' tests may give a false-positive result in patients taking Madopar.

Pregnancy and lactation: Madopar is contra-indicated in pregnancy and in women of childbearing potential in the absence of adequate contraception, since there is evidence of harmful effects in studies in pregnant rabbits and the benserazide component has been found to be associated with skeletal malformations in the rat. If pregnancy occurs in a woman taking Madopar, the drug must be discontinued. Patients taking Madopar should not breast-feed their infants.

Effects on ability to drive and use machines: If drowsiness or psychiatric disturbances should occur the patient should be warned not to drive or operate machinery.

Undesirable effects: Tolerance to Madopar varies widely between patients and is often related to the rate of dosage increases. Side-effects such as nausea, vomiting, loss of appetite and anorexia, which are frequently observed during the initial stages of levodopa therapy, are much less common in patients treated with Madopar. If such side-effects do occur, they can largely be controlled by taking Madopar with, or immediately after, food and by increasing dosage only slowly. Also, cardiovascular disturbances such as arrhythmias and orthostatic hypotension may occur, but are less frequent than in patients treated with levodopa alone. If experienced, orthostatic disorders usually improve following reduction of the Madopar dose.

Psychiatric disturbances are common in Parkinsonian patients, including those being treated with levodopa. They include mild elation, anxiety, agitation, insomnia, depression, aggression, delusions, hallucinations and "unmasking" of psychoses.

Although there have been rare reports of possible antagonism of levodopa by diazepam, in general diazepam (Valium Roche) and nitrazepam (Mogadon) have been found to be useful in the treatment of anxiety and insomnia, respectively, occurring in Parkinsonism. Depression may be treated with tricyclic antidepressants although isolated cases of hypertensive crisis have been reported with the concomitant use of tricyclic drugs. ECT may be administered if appropriate. MAO inhibitors, except selective MAO-B inhibitors or selective MAO-A inhibitors must not be used.

Involuntary movements, commonly in the form of oral dyskinesias, often accompanied by "paddling" foot movements, or of the choreo-athetoid type, are common, particularly on long-term administration.

These are usually dose-dependent and may disappear or become tolerable after dose adjustment.

With long-term administration, fluctuations in the therapeutic response may be encountered. They include "freezing" episodes, end-of-dose deterioration and the so-called "on-off" effect. Patients may be helped by dosage reduction or by giving smaller and more frequent doses.

Other side-effects which have occasionally been reported with levodopa therapy include diarrhoea, gastro-intestinal bleeding, flushing, sweating, and drowsiness.

Isolated cases of loss or alterations of taste have been reported and there have been rare cases of allergic skin reactions such as pruritus and rash.

On some occasions the urine passed during Madopar treatment may be altered in colour; usually red-tinged, this will turn dark on standing. These changes are due to metabolites and are no cause for concern.

Transient rises in SGOT, SGPT and alkaline phosphatase values have been noted. Serum uric acid and blood urea nitrogen levels are occasionally increased. In rare instances, haemolytic anaemia, mild transient leucopenia and thrombocytopenia have been reported.

Overdose: Symptoms of overdosage are qualitatively similar to the side-effects but may be of greater magnitude.

Treatment should include gastric lavage, general supportive measures, intravenous fluids and the maintenance of an adequate airway. Electrocardiographic monitoring should be instituted and the patient carefully observed for the possible development of arrhythmias. If necessary, anti-arrhythmic therapy, should be given and other symptoms treated as they arise.

Pharmacological properties

Pharmacodynamic properties: Madopar is an anti-Parkinsonian agent. Levodopa is the metabolic precursor of dopamine. The latter is severely depleted in the striatum, pallidum and substantia nigra of Parkinsonian patients and it is considered that administration of levodopa raises the level of available dopamine in these centres. However, conversion of levodopa into dopamine by the enzyme dopa decarboxylase also takes place in extracerebral tissues. As a consequence the full therapeutic effect may not be obtained and side-effects occur.

Administration of a peripheral decarboxylase inhibitor, which blocks the extracerebral decarboxylation of levodopa, in conjunction with levodopa has significant advantages; these include reduced gastro-intestinal side-effects, a more rapid response at the initiation of therapy and a simpler dosage regimen. Madopar is a combination of levodopa and benserazide in the ratio 4:1 which in clinical trials has been shown to be the most satisfactory.

Like every replacement therapy, chronic treatment with Madopar will be necessary.

Pharmacokinetic properties:

Absorption: Low levels of endogenous levodopa are detectable in pre-dose blood samples. After oral administration of Madopar, levodopa and benserazide are rapidly absorbed, mainly in the upper regions of the small intestine. Interaction studies indicate that a higher proportion of levodopa is absorbed when administered in combination with benserazide, compared with levodopa administered alone. Maximum plasma concentrations of levodopa are reached approximately one hour after ingestion of Madopar. Bioavailability is approximately 98%.

Distribution: Levodopa crosses the blood-brain barrier by a saturable transport system. It is not bound to plasma proteins. Benserazide does not cross the blood-brain barrier at therapeutic doses. Benserazide is concentrated mainly in the kidneys, lungs, small intestine and liver.

Metabolism: The 2 major routes of metabolism of levodopa are decarboxylation to form dopamine, which in turn is converted to a minor degree to norepinephrine and to a greater extent, to inactive metabolites, and O-methylation, forming 3-O-methyldopa, which has an elimination half-life of approximately 15 hours and accumulates in patients receiving therapeutic doses of Madopar. Decreased peripheral decarboxylation of levodopa when it is administered with benserazide is reflected in higher plasma levels of levodopa and 3-O-methyldopa.

Benserazide is hydroxylated to trihydroxybenzylhydrazine in the intestinal mucosa and the liver.

Elimination: In the presence of the peripheral decarboxylase inhibitor, benserazide, the elimination half-life of levodopa is approximately 1.5 hours. In elderly patients the elimination half-life is slightly (25%) longer. Clearance of levodopa is 430 ml/min. Elimination of levodopa is by biotransformation and excretion of the metabolites in the urine. Urinary recovery of unchanged drug accounts for approximately 7% of the dose.

Benserazide is almost entirely eliminated by metabolism. The metabolites are mainly excreted in the urine and to a small extent in faeces.

Preclinical safety data: None stated.

Pharmaceutical particulars

List of excipients: Each dispersible tablet also contains: Anhydrous granular citric acid, starch maize modified, microcrystalline cellulose and magnesium stearate.

Incompatibilities: None known.

Shelf life: 3 years.

Special precautions for storage: Recommended maximum storage temperature 25°C. Protect from moisture.

Nature and contents of container: Amber glass bottles with screw cap and desiccant, containing 100 dispersible tablets.

Instructions for use/handling: No special requirements.

Marketing authorisation numbers PL 0031/0220, PL 0031/0221

Date of first authorisation/renewal of authorisation April 1987

Date of (partial) revision of the text June 1998

MANERIX

Qualitative and quantitative composition

1 film-coated 150 mg tablet contains 150 mg moclobemide.

1 film-coated 300 mg tablet contains 300 mg moclobemide.

Pharmaceutical form Film-coated tablets containing 150 mg or 300 mg of moclobemide.

Clinical particulars

Therapeutic indications: Major depression. Treatment of social phobia.

Posology and method of administration: Manerix tablets are for oral administration. The tablets should be taken at the end of a meal.

Adults: Major depression: The recommended initial dose is 300 mg daily, usually administered in divided doses. The dose may be increased up to 600 mg/day depending on the severity of the depression. The individual response may allow a reduction of the daily dose to 150 mg.

Treatment of social phobia: The recommended dose of moclobemide is 600 mg/day, given in 2 divided doses. The moclobemide dose should be started at 300 mg/day and should be increased to 600 mg/day on day 4. Continuing the 300 mg/day dose for longer than 3 days is not recommended, as the efficacious dose is 600 mg/day. Treatment with 600 mg/day should continue for 8–12 weeks in order to assess the efficacy of the drug. Social phobia may be a chronic condition and it is reasonable to consider continuation of treatment for a responding patient. Patients should be periodically re-evaluated to determine need for further treatment.

Elderly: Elderly patients do not require a special dose adjustment of Manerix.

Children: In view of the lack of clinical data available, Manerix is not recommended for use in children.

Renal/hepatic impairment: Patients with reduced renal function do not require a special dose adjustment of Manerix. When hepatic metabolism is severely impaired by hepatic disease or a drug that inhibits microsomal mono-oxygenase activity (e.g. cimetidine), normal plasma levels are achieved by reducing the daily dose of Manerix to half or one third.

Contra-indications: Manerix is contra-indicated in patients with known hypersensitivity to the drug, in acute confusional states and in patients with phaeochromocytoma.

Manerix should not be co-administered with pethidine or selegiline.

Manerix should not be co-administered with 5-HT re-uptake inhibitors (including those which are tricyclic antidepressants) (see *Special warnings and special precautions for use* and *Interaction with other medicaments and other forms of interaction*). After stopping treatment with 5-HT re-uptake inhibitors a time period equal to 4–5 half lives of the drug or any active metabolite should elapse between stopping therapy and starting therapy with Manerix.

Manerix should not be co-administered with dextromethorphan, contained in many proprietary cough medicines (see *Interaction with other medicaments and other forms of interaction*).

Manerix should not be administered to children for the time being as clinical experience in this category is lacking.

Special warnings and special precautions for use: Manerix is a reversible inhibitor of monoamine oxidase type A (RIMA). It causes less potentiation of tyramine than traditional irreversible MAOIs, and therefore Manerix does not generally necessitate the special dietary restrictions required for these irreversible MAOIs. However, as a few patients may be especially sensitive to tyramine, all patients should be advised to avoid the consumption of large amounts of tyramine rich food (mature cheese, yeast extracts and fermented soya bean products).

Patients should be advised to avoid sympathomimetic agents such as ephedrine, pseudoephedrine and phenylpropanolamine (contained in many proprietary cough and cold medications) (see *Interaction with other medicaments and other forms of interaction*).

Depressive patients with excitation or agitation as the predominant clinical feature should either not be treated with Manerix or only in combination with a sedative (e.g. a benzodiazepine). The sedative should only be used for a maximum of 2 to 3 weeks.

Patients with suicidal tendencies should be closely monitored at the start of treatment.

If a depressive episode is treated in bipolar disorders, manic episodes can be provoked.

Due to the lack of clinical data, patients with concomitant schizophrenia or schizo-affective organic disorders should not be treated with Manerix.

Theoretical pharmacological considerations indicate that MAO inhibitors may precipitate a hypertensive reaction in patients with thyrotoxicosis. As experience with Manerix in this population group is lacking, caution should be exercised before prescribing Manerix.

In patients receiving Manerix, caution should be exercised when co-administering drugs that enhance serotonin in order to prevent precipitation of serotoninergic syndrome (see *Contra-indications* and *Interaction with other medicaments and other forms of interaction*). This is particularly true for clomipramine.

Interaction with other medicaments and other forms of interaction: In animals, Manerix potentiates the effects of opiates. Morphine and fentanyl should be used with caution. A dosage adjustment may be necessary for these drugs.

Cimetidine prolongs the metabolism of Manerix. The normal dose of Manerix should therefore be reduced to half the dose in patients taking cimetidine.

In patients receiving Manerix, additional drugs that enhance serotonin, such as many other antidepressants, particularly in multiple-drug combinations, should be given with caution. This is particularly true for clomipramine. In isolated cases there have been combinations of serious symptoms and signs, including hyperthermia, confusion, hyperreflexia and myoclonus, which are indicative of serotonergic overactivity (see *Contra-indications* and *Special warnings and special precautions for use*). Should such combined symptoms occur, the patient should be closely observed by a physician (and if necessary hospitalised) and appropriate treatment given. Treatment with a tricyclic or other antidepressant could be initiated immediately after withdrawal of Manerix (i.e. without a wash-out period), provided similar caution is observed.

There is, to date, no experience with co-administration of moclobemide and buspirone in humans.

Isolated cases of severe central nervous system adverse reactions have been reported after co-administration of Manerix and dextromethorphan. Since proprietary cough and cold medicines may contain dextromethorphan, they should not be taken without prior consultation with a physician and, if possible, alternatives not containing dextromethorphan should be given (see *Contra-indications*).

The pharmacologic action of systemic regimens of sympathomimetic agents may possibly be intensified and prolonged by concurrent treatment with moclobemide.

Pregnancy and lactation: Reproduction studies in animals have not revealed any risk to the foetus, but the safety of Manerix in human pregnancy has not been established. Therefore the benefits of drug therapy during pregnancy should be weighed against possible risk to the foetus.

Since only a small amount of Manerix passes into breast milk (approximately 1/30 of the maternal dose), the benefits of continuing drug therapy during nursing should be weighed against possible risks to the child.

Effects on ability to drive and use machines: Impairment of performance in activities requiring complete mental alertness (e.g. driving a motor vehicle) is generally not to be expected with Manerix. The individual reaction should however be monitored during early treatment.

Undesirable effects: The following undesirable effects have been observed: sleep disturbances, agitation, feelings of anxiety, restlessness, irritability, dizziness, headache, paraesthesia, dry mouth, visual disturbances, nausea, diarrhoea, constipation, vomiting, oedema and skin reactions such as rash, pruritus, urticaria and flushing. Confusional states have been observed, but these have disappeared rapidly on discontinuation of therapy.

In clinical trials, there was a low incidence of raised liver enzymes without associated clinical sequelae.

Overdose: Experience of overdose in man is so far limited. Signs which have been observed are increasing agitation, aggressiveness and behavioural changes. Treatment of overdose should be aimed primarily at maintenance of the vital functions.

As with other antidepressants, mixed overdoses of moclobemide with other drugs (e.g. other CNS-acting drugs) could be life-threatening. Therefore, patients should be hospitalised and closely monitored so that appropriate treatment may be given.

Pharmacological properties
Pharmacodynamic properties: Manerix is an antidepressant which affects the monoaminergic cerebral neurotransmitter system by means of a reversible inhibition of monoamine oxidase preferentially of type A (RIMA). The metabolism of noradrenaline, dopamine and serotonin (5-HT) is decreased by this effect, and this leads to increased extracellular concentrations of these neuronal transmitters.

Pharmacokinetic properties: Absorption: After oral administration, moclobemide is completely absorbed from the gastrointestinal tract into the portal blood. A hepatic first-pass effect reduces the systemically available dose fraction (bioavailability F). This reduction is more pronounced after single (F: 60%) than after multiple (F: 80%) doses.

Distribution: Due to its lipophilic nature, moclobemide is extensively distributed in the body with an apparent volume of distribution (V_{ss}) of about 1.2 l/kg. Binding of the drug to plasma proteins, mainly albumin, is relatively low (50%). Peak plasma concentrations of the drug are reached within one hour of dosage. After multiple dosing, plasma concentrations of moclobemide increase over the first week of therapy and remain stable thereafter. When the daily dose is increased, there is a more than proportional increase in steady-state concentrations

Metabolism: The drug is almost entirely metabolised before its elimination from the body. Metabolism occurs largely via oxidative reactions on the morpholine moiety of the molecule. Degradation products with pharmacological activity in *in vitro* or animal experiments are present in the systemic circulation in man at very low concentrations only. Approximately 2% of the Caucasian population and 15% of the Asian population have been shown to be slow metabolisers with respect to oxidative hepatic metabolism via the cytochrome P4502C9 isozyme. It was found that the maximum plasma concentration (Cmax) and area under the concentration time curve (AUC) was approximately 1.5 times greater in slow metabolisers compared with extensive metabolisers for the same dose of moclobemide.

Elimination: Moclobemide is rapidly eliminated from the body. Blood clearance is approximately 20–50 1/hour, the elimination half-life one to four hours. Less than 1% of a dose is excreted renally in unchanged form. The metabolites formed are eliminated renally.

Preclinical safety data: Not applicable.

Pharmaceutical particulars
List of excipients: Lactose, maize starch, povidone K30, sodium starch glycollate, magnesium stearate, hydroxypropyl methylcellulose, ethylcellulose, polyethylene glycol 6000, talc and titanium dioxide (E171). The 150 mg tablets also contain yellow iron oxide (E172).

Incompatibilities: Not applicable.

Shelf life: 5 years.

Special precautions for storage: Store in a dry place.

Nature and contents of container: Blister packing.

Pack sizes: 28, 30, 84 and 100 tablets (150 mg tablets), 30 and 60 tablets (300 mg tablets)

Instructions for use/handling: Not applicable.

Marketing authorisation numbers
PL 0031/0275 (150 mg tablets)
PL 0031/0347 (300 mg tablets)

Date of first authorisation/renewal of authorisation
150 mg tablets: First approved 19 June 1991
300 mg tablets: First approved 5 July 1994

Date of (partial) revision of the text March 1998

MOBIFLEX

Name of product Mobiflex contains the substance with the approved name tenoxicam. It is chemically described as 4-hydroxy-2-methyl-N-2-pyridyl-2H-thieno-[2,3-e]-1,2-thiazine-3-carboxamide-1, 1-dioxide.

Presentation Mobiflex Tablets 20 mg–Red-brown, film-coated, pentagonal tablets, imprinted MOBIFLEX on one face, containing 20 mg tenoxicam.

Mobiflex Vials containing 20 mg tenoxicam. Ampoules with 2 ml sterile Water for Injections Ph. Eur.

Uses
Pharmacological properties: Mobiflex is a non-steroidal anti-inflammatory drug which has marked anti-inflammatory and analgesic activity and some anti-pyretic activity. As with other non-steroidal anti-inflammatory drugs, the precise mode of action is unknown, though it is probably multifactorial, involving inhibition of prostaglandin biosynthesis and reduction of leucocyte accumulation at the inflammatory site.

Pharmacokinetics: Mobiflex is long-acting; a single daily dose is effective.

After oral administration, Mobiflex is rapidly and completely absorbed as unchanged drug. Concomitant food reduces the rate, but not the extent, of absorption of Mobiflex. Tenoxicam penetrates well into synovial fluid to give concentrations approximately half those in plasma. The mean plasma elimination half-life is approximately 72 hours.

Following intravenous administration of 20 mg tenoxicam, plasma levels of the drug decline rapidly during the first two hours mainly due to distribution processes. After this short period, no difference in plasma concentrations between intravenous and oral dosing is seen. Following intramuscular injection, levels at or above 90% of the maximally achieved concentrations are reached as early as 15 minutes after a dose, i.e. earlier than after oral dosing. However, again the difference in blood levels between the two routes of administration is restricted to the first two hours after a dose. The bioavailability after an intramuscular dose is complete and indistinguishable from that determined after oral dosing.

With the recommended dosage regimen of 20 mg once daily, steady-state plasma concentrations are reached within 10–15 days, with no unexpected accumulation.

Mobiflex is strongly bound to plasma proteins.

Mobiflex is cleared from the body almost exclusively by metabolism. Approximately two-thirds of the administered dose is excreted in the urine, mainly as the pharmacologically inactive 5-hydroxypyridyl metabolite, and the remainder in the bile, much of it as glucuronide conjugates of hydroxy-metabolites.

No age-specific changes in the pharmacokinetics of Mobiflex have been found although inter-individual variation tends to be higher in elderly persons.

Indications: Mobiflex is indicated for the relief of pain and inflammation in osteoarthritis and rheumatoid arthritis. It is also indicated for the short term management of acute musculoskeletal disorders including strains, sprains and other soft-tissue injuries. IV, IM tenoxicam is also available for these indications in those patients considered unable to take oral tenoxicam.

Dosage and administration
Adults (including the elderly): A single daily dose of 20 mg Mobiflex should be taken orally, at the same time each day. Mobiflex Tablets are for oral administration with water or other fluid. Mobiflex Vials should be given IV or IM. A single daily dose of 20 mg for one to two days initially to be continued with the oral form, with administration at the same time each day. The lyophilisate should be dissolved in 2 ml of the solvent provided (2 ml sterile water for injections). This reconstituted solution should be used immediately. Higher doses should be avoided as they do not usually achieve significantly greater therapeutic effect but may be associated with a higher risk of adverse events.

In acute musculoskeletal disorders treatment should not normally be required for more than 7 days, but in severe cases it may be continued up to a maximum of 14 days.

Use in the elderly: As with other non-steroidal anti-inflammatory drugs, Mobiflex should be used with special caution in elderly patients since they may be less able to tolerate side-effects than younger patients. They are also more likely to be receiving concomitant medication or to have impaired hepatic, renal or cardiovascular function.

Children: There are insufficient data to make a recommendation for administration of Mobiflex to children.

Use in renal and hepatic insufficiency

Creatinine clearance	*Dosage regimen*
Greater than 25 ml/min	Usual dosage but monitor patients carefully (see '*Precautions*')
Less than 25 ml/min	Insufficient data to make dosage recommendations

Because of the high plasma protein-binding of tenoxicam, caution is required when plasma albumin concentrations are markedly reduced (e.g. in nephrotic syndrome) or when bilirubin concentrations are high.

There is insufficient information to make dosage recommendations for Mobiflex in patients with pre-existing hepatic impairment.

Contra-indications, warnings, etc
Contra-indications

1. Active peptic ulceration and a past history of peptic ulceration, gastro-intestinal bleeding (melaena, haematemesis) or severe gastritis.

2. Hypersensitivity to Mobiflex. Mobiflex should also be avoided in cases where the patient has suffered a hypersensitivity reaction (symptoms of asthma, rhinitis, angioedema or urticaria) to other non-steroidal anti-inflammatory drugs, including aspirin, as the potential exists for cross-sensitivity to Mobiflex.

Use in pregnancy and lactation: The safety of Mobiflex during pregnancy and lactation has not been established and the drug should therefore not be given in these conditions.

Although no teratogenic effects were seen in animal studies, Mobiflex, like other non-steroidal anti-inflammatory drugs, is associated with prolonged and delayed parturition and an adverse influence on neonatal viability when administered to animals in late pregnancy. Non-steroidal anti-inflammatory agents are also known to induce closure of the ductus arteriosus in infants.

No information is available on penetration of Mobiflex into milk in humans; animal studies indicate that significant levels may be achieved.

Precautions: Any patient being treated with Mobiflex who presents with symptoms of gastro-intestinal disease should be closely monitored. If peptic ulceration or gastro-intestinal bleeding occurs, Mobiflex should be withdrawn immediately.

In rare cases, non-steroidal anti-inflammatory drugs may cause interstitial nephritis, glomerulonephritis, papillary necrosis and the nephrotic syndrome. Such agents inhibit the synthesis of renal prostaglandin which plays a supportive role in the maintenance of renal perfusion in patients whose renal blood flow and blood volume are decreased. In these patients, administration of a non-steroidal anti-inflammatory drug may precipitate overt renal decompensation, which returns to the pre-treatment state upon withdrawal of the drug. Patients at greatest risk of such a reaction are those with pre-existing renal disease (including diabetics with impaired renal function), nephrotic syndrome, volume depletion, hepatic disease, congestive cardiac failure and those patients receiving concomitant therapy with diuretics or potentially nephrotoxic drugs. Such patients should have their renal, hepatic and cardiac functions carefully monitored.

Occasional elevations of serum transaminases or other indicators of liver function have been reported. In most cases these have been small and transient increases above the normal range. If the abnormality is significant or persistent, Mobiflex should be stopped and follow-up tests carried out. Particular care is required in patients with pre-existing hepatic disease.

Mobiflex reduces platelet aggregation and may prolong bleeding time. This should be borne in mind for patients who undergo major surgery (e.g. joint replacement) and when bleeding time needs to be determined.

Particular care should be taken to regularly monitor elderly patients to detect possible interactions with concomitant therapy and to review renal, hepatic and cardiovascular function which may be potentially influenced by non-steroidal anti-inflammatory drugs.

Adverse eye findings have been reported with non-steroidal anti-inflammatory drugs, therefore it is recommended that patients who develop visual disturbances during treatment with Mobiflex have ophthalmic evaluation.

Side-effects and adverse reactions: For most patients, any side-effects are transient and resolve without discontinuation of treatment.

The most common side-effects relate to the gastro-intestinal tract. They include dyspepsia, nausea, abdominal pain and discomfort, constipation, diarrhoea, flatulence, indigestion, epigastric distress, stomatitis and anorexia. As with other non-steroidal anti-inflammatory drugs, there is a risk of peptic ulceration and gastro-intestinal bleeding, both of which have been reported with Mobiflex. Should this occur, Mobiflex is to be discontinued immediately and appropriate treatment instituted.

As with other non-steroidal anti-inflammatory drugs, peripheral oedema of mild or moderate degree and without clinical sequelae occurred in a small proportion of patients and the possibility of precipitating congestive cardiac failure in elderly patients or those with compromised cardiac function should therefore be borne in mind.

Central nervous system reactions of headache and

dizziness have been reported in a small number of patients. Somnolence, insomnia, depression, nervousness, dream abnormalities, mental confusion, paraesthesias and vertigo have been reported rarely.

Skin reactions of rash and pruritus have been reported. Nail disorders, alopecia, erythema, urticaria and photosensitivity reactions have been reported rarely. As with other non-steroidal anti-inflammatory drugs, Lyell's syndrome and Stevens-Johnson syndrome may develop in rare instances. Vesiculobullous reactions and vasculitis have also been reported rarely. Reversible elevations of blood urea nitrogen and creatinine have been reported (see *Precautions*).

Decreases in haemoglobin, unrelated to gastrointestinal bleeding, have occurred. Anaemia, thrombocytopenia and non-thrombocytopenic purpura, leucopenia and eosinophilia have been reported. Epistaxis has been reported infrequently. Rare cases of agranulocytosis have been reported.

As with most other non-steroidal anti-inflammatory drugs, changes in various liver function parameters have been observed. Some patients may develop raised serum transaminase levels during treatment. Although such reactions are rare, if abnormal liver function tests persist or worsen, if clinical signs and symptoms consistent with liver disease develop or if systemic manifestations occur (e.g. eosinophilia, rash), Mobiflex should be discontinued.

Palpitations and dyspnoea have also been reported rarely. Metabolic abnormalities, such as weight decrease or increase and hyperglycaemia, have occurred rarely.

Swollen eyes, blurred vision and eye irritation have been reported. Ophthalmoscopy and slit-lamp examination have revealed no evidence of ocular changes. Malaise and tinnitus may occur.

Hepatitis has also been reported in isolated cases.

Drug interactions: Antacids may reduce the rate, but not the extent, of absorption of Mobiflex. The differences are not likely to be of clinical significance. No interaction has been found with concomitantly administered cimetidine. In healthy subjects no clinically relevant interaction between Mobiflex and low molecular weight heparin has been observed.

Tenoxicam is highly bound to serum albumin. Although potentiation of warfarin or sulphonylurea compounds such as glibenclamide has not been observed, close monitoring of the effects of anticoagulants or oral hypoglycaemic agents is advised, especially during the initial stages of treatment with Mobiflex. No interaction with digoxin has been observed.

Salicylates can displace tenoxicam from protein-binding sites and so increase the clearance and volume of distribution of Mobiflex. Concurrent treatment with salicylates or other non-steroidal anti-inflammatory drugs should therefore be avoided because of the increased risk of adverse reactions (particularly gastro-intestinal).

Non-steroidal anti-inflammatory drugs have been reported to produce lithium retention. If tenoxicam is prescribed for a patient receiving lithium therapy, the frequency of lithium monitoring should be increased, the patient warned to maintain fluid intake and to be aware of symptoms of lithium intoxication.

Non-steroidal anti-inflammatory drugs may cause sodium, potassium and fluid retention and may interfere with the natriuretic action of diuretic agents. These properties should be kept in mind when treating patients with compromised cardiac function or hypertension since they may be responsible for a worsening of those conditions.

No clinically relevant interaction was found in small numbers of patients receiving treatment with penicillamine or parenteral gold.

Treatment of overdosage: There is no reported experience of serious overdosage with Mobiflex. No specific measures are available; administration of H_2-antagonist drugs may be of benefit. Gastric lavage should be carried out as soon as possible after drug ingestion and the patient should be closely observed and general supportive measures taken as necessary.

Pharmaceutical precautions
Storage: Mobiflex Tablets–The original pack dispenser should be stored in a dry place, otherwise no special storage precautions are necessary.

Mobiflex Vials–The pack should be stored at a temperature below 25°C. Do not freeze as the water ampoule may burst.

Legal category POM–UK.

Package quantities Mobiflex Tablets 20 mg in packs of 28 and 500.

Mobiflex Vials 20 mg in packs of 5 vials together with 5 ampoules containing 2 ml of sterile Water for Injections Ph. Eur. as diluent.

Further information Nil.

Product licence numbers
PL 0031/0200 (Tablets 20 mg)
PL 0031/0330 (Vials 20 mg)
PL 0031/0284 (Ampoules Water for Injections)

Date of last review March 1997

NAPROSYN

Qualitative and quantitative composition Naproxen BP 250 mg.

Pharmaceutical form Round, buff, uncoated tablet embossed "NPR LE 250" on one face and with a breakline on the other.

Clinical particulars
Therapeutic indications: Treatment of rheumatoid arthritis, osteoarthrosis (degenerative arthritis), ankylosing spondylitis, juvenile rheumatoid arthritis, acute gout, acute musculoskeletal disorders and dysmenorrhoea.

Posology and method of administration: Route of administration Oral.

Adults: Rheumatoid arthritis, osteoarthritis and ankylosing spondylitis
500 mg to 1 g taken in 2 doses at 12-hour intervals or alternatively, as a single administration. In the following cases a loading dose of 750 mg or 1 g per day for the acute phase is recommended:

a) In patients reporting severe night-time pain/or morning stiffness.

b) In patients being switched to Naprosyn from a high dose of another anti-rheumatic compound.

c) In osteoarthrosis where pain is the predominant symptom.

Acute gout: 750 mg at once then 250 mg every 8 hours until the attack has passed.

Acute musculoskeletal disorders and dysmenorrhoea: 500 mg initially followed by 250 mg at 6–8 hour intervals as needed, with a maximum daily dose after the first day of 1250 mg.

Elderly: Studies indicate that although total plasma concentration of naproxen is unchanged, the unbound plasma fraction of naproxen is increased in the elderly. The implication of this finding for Naprosyn dosing is unknown. As with other drugs used in the elderly it is prudent to use the lowest effective dose. For the effect of reduced elimination in the elderly refer to Special warnings and special precautions for use.

Children (over 5 years): For juvenile rheumatoid arthritis: 10 mg/kg/day taken in 2 doses at 12-hour intervals.

Contra-indications: Active peptic ulceration or active gastrointestinal bleeding. Hypersensitivity to naproxen or naproxen sodium formulations. Since the potential exists for cross-sensitivity reactions, Naprosyn should not be given to patients in whom aspirin or other non-steroidal anti-inflammatory/analgesic drugs induce the syndrome of asthma, rhinitis or urticaria.

Special warnings and special precautions for use: Episodes of gastro-intestinal bleeding have been reported in patients with naproxen therapy. Naprosyn should be given under close supervision to patients with a history of gastro-intestinal disease.

Serious gastro-intestinal adverse reactions, can occur at any time in patients on therapy with non-steroidal anti-inflammatory drugs. The risk of occurrence does not seem to change with duration of therapy. Studies to date have not identified any subset of patients not at risk of developing peptic ulcer and bleeding. However, elderly and debilitated patients tolerate gastro-intestinal ulceration or bleeding less well than others. Most of the serious gastro-intestinal events associated with non-steroidal anti-inflammatory drugs occurred in this patient population.

The antipyretic and anti-inflammatory activities of Naprosyn may reduce fever and inflammation, thereby diminishing their utility as diagnostic signs.

Bronchospasm may be precipitated in patients suffering from, or with a history of, bronchial asthma or allergic disease.

Sporadic abnormalities in laboratory tests (e.g. liver function tests) have occurred in patients on naproxen therapy, but no definite trend was seen in any test indicating toxicity.

Naproxen decreases platelet aggregation and prolongs bleeding time. This effect should be kept in mind when bleeding times are determined.

Mild peripheral oedema has been observed in a few patients receiving naproxen. Although sodium retention has not been reported in metabolic studies, it is possible that patients with questionable or compromised cardiac function may be at a greater risk when taking Naprosyn.

Use in patients with impaired renal function: As naproxen is eliminated to a large extent (95%) by urinary excretion via glomerular filtration, it should be used with great caution in patients with impaired renal function and the monitoring of serum creatinine and/or creatinine clearance is advised in these patients. Naprosyn is not recommended in patients having a baseline creatinine clearance of less than 20 ml/minute.

Certain patients, specifically those whose renal blood flow is compromised, such as in extracellular volume depletion, cirrhosis of the liver, sodium restriction, congestive heart failure, and pre-existing renal disease, should have renal function assessed before and during Naprosyn therapy. Some elderly patients in whom impaired renal function may be expected, as well as patients using diuretics, may also fall within this category. A reduction in daily dosage should be considered to avoid the possibility of excessive accumulation of naproxen metabolites in these patients.

Use in patients with impaired liver function: Chronic alcoholic liver disease and probably also other forms of cirrhosis reduce the total plasma concentration of naproxen, but the plasma concentration of unbound naproxen is increased. The implication of this finding for Naprosyn dosing is unknown but it is prudent to use the lowest effective dose.

Haematological: Patients who have coagulation disorders or are receiving drug therapy that interferes with haemostasis should be carefully observed if naproxen-containing products are administered.

Patients at high risk of bleeding or those on full anti-coagulation therapy (e.g. dicoumarol derivatives) may be at increased risk of bleeding if given naproxen-containing products concurrently.

Anaphylactic (anaphylactoid) reactions: Hypersensitivity reactions may occur in susceptible individuals. Anaphylactic (anaphylactoid) reactions may occur both in patients with and without a history of hypersensitivity or exposure to aspirin, other non-steroidal anti-inflammatory drugs or naproxen-containing products. They may also occur in individuals with a history of angioedema, bronchospastic reactivity (e.g. asthma), rhinitis and nasal polyps.

Anaphylactoid reactions, like anaphylaxis, may have a fatal outcome.

Steroids: If steroid dosage is reduced or eliminated during therapy, the steroid dosage should be reduced slowly and the patients must be observed closely for any evidence of adverse effects, including adrenal insufficiency and exacerbation of symptoms of arthritis.

Ocular effects: Studies have not shown changes in the eye attributable to naproxen administration. In rare cases, adverse ocular disorders including papillitis, retrobulbar optic neuritis and papilledema, have been reported in users of NSAIDs including naproxen, although a cause-and-effect relationship cannot be established; accordingly, patients who develop visual disturbances during treatment with naproxen-containing products should have an ophthalmological examination.

Combination with other NSAIDs: The combination of naproxen-containing products and other NSAIDs is not recommended, because of the cumulative risks of inducing serious NSAID-related adverse events.

Interaction with other medicaments and other forms of interaction: Concomitant administration of antacid or cholestyramine can delay the absorption of naproxen but does not affect its extent. Concomitant administration of food can delay the absorption of naproxen, but does not affect its extent.

Due to the high plasma protein binding of naproxen, patients simultaneously receiving hydantoins, anticoagulants or a highly protein-bound sulphonamide should be observed for signs of overdosage of these drugs. No interactions have been observed in clinical studies with naproxen and anticoagulants or sulphonylureas, but caution is nevertheless advised since interaction has been seen with other non-steroidal agents of this class.

The natriuretic effect of frusemide has been reported to be inhibited by some drugs of this class.

Inhibition of renal lithium clearance leading to increases in plasma lithium concentrations has also been reported

Naproxen and other non-steroidal anti-inflammatory drugs can reduce the antihypertensive effect of propranolol and other beta-blockers and may increase the risk of renal impairment associated with the use of ACE inhibitors.

Probenecid given concurrently increases naproxen plasma levels and extends its half-life considerably.

Caution is advised where methotrexate is given concurrently because of possible enhancement of its toxicity, since naproxen, among other non-steroidal anti-inflammatory drugs, has been reported to reduce the tubular secretion of methotrexate in an animal model.

NSAID's may exacerbate cardiac failure, reduce GFR and increase plasma cardiac glycoside levels when co-administered with cardiac glycosides.

As with all NSAID's caution is advised when

cyclosporin is co-administered because of the increased risk of nephrotoxicity.

NSAID's should not be used for 8–12 days after mifepristone administration as NSAID's can reduce the effects of mifepristone.

As with all NSAID's, caution should be taken when co-administering with cortico-steroids because of the increased risk of bleeding.

Patients taking quinolones may have an increased risk of developing convulsions.

It is suggested that Naprosyn therapy be temporarily discontinued 48 hours before adrenal function tests are performed, because naproxen may artifactually interfere with some tests for 17-ketogenic steroids. Similarly, naproxen may interfere with some assays of urinary 5-hydroxyindoleacetic acid.

Pregnancy and lactation: Teratology studies in rats and rabbits at dose levels equivalent on a human multiple basis to those which have produced foetal abnormality with certain other non-steroidal anti-inflammatory agents, e.g. aspirin, have not produced evidence of foetal damage with naproxen. As with other drugs of this type naproxen delays parturition in animals (the relevance of this finding to human patients is unknown) and also affects the human foetal cardiovascular system (closure of the ductus arteriosus). Good medical practice indicates minimal drug usage in pregnancy, and the use of this class of therapeutic agent requires cautious balancing of possible benefit against potential risk to the mother and foetus, especially in the first and third trimesters.

The use of Naprosyn should be avoided in patients who are breast-feeding.

Effects on ability to drive and use machines: Some patients may experience drowsiness, dizziness, vertigo, insomnia or depression with the use of Naprosyn. If patients experience these or similar undesirable effects, they should exercise caution in carrying out activities that require alertness.

Undesirable effects: Gastro-intestinal: The more frequent reactions are nausea, vomiting, abdominal discomfort and epigastric distress. More serious reactions which may occur occasionally are gastro-intestinal bleeding, peptic ulceration (sometimes with haemorrhage and perforation), non-peptic gastro-intestinal ulceration and colitis.

Dermatological: Skin rashes, urticaria, angio-oedema. Alopecia, erythema multiforme, Stevens Johnson syndrome, epidermal necrolysis and photosensitivity reactions (including cases in which the skin resembles porphyria cutanea tarda, 'pseudo-porphyria') or epidermolysis bullosa may occur rarely.

Renal: Including but not limited to glomerular nephritis, interstitial nephritis, nephrotic syndrome, haematuria, renal papillary necrosis and renal failure.

CNS: Convulsions, headache, insomnia, inability to concentrate and cognitive dysfunction have been reported.

Haematological: Thrombocytopenia, granulocytopenia including agranulocytosis, aplastic anaemia and haemolytic anaemia may occur rarely.

Other: Tinnitus, hearing impairment, vertigo, mild peripheral oedema. Anaphylactic reactions to naproxen and naproxen sodium formulations have been reported in patients with, or without, a history of previous sensitivity reactions to NSAIDs. Jaundice, fatal hepatitis, visual disturbances, eosinophilic pneumonitis, vasculitis, hyperkalemia, aseptic meningitis and ulcerative stomatitis have been reported rarely.

Overdose: Significant overdosage of the drug may be characterised by drowsiness, heartburn, indigestion, nausea or vomiting. A few patients have experienced seizures, but it is not known whether these were naproxen-related or not. It is not known what dose of the drug would be life-threatening.

Should a patient ingest a large amount of Naprosyn accidentally or purposefully, the stomach may be emptied and usual supportive measures employed. Animal studies indicate that the prompt administration of activated charcoal in adequate amounts would tend to reduce markedly the absorption of the drug.

Haemodialysis does not decrease the plasma concentration of naproxen because of the high degree of protein binding. However, haemodialysis may still be appropriate in a patient with renal failure who has taken naproxen.

Pharmacological properties

Pharmacodynamic properties: Naproxen is a non-steroidal anti-inflammatory analgesic compound with antipyretic properties as has been demonstrated in classical animal test systems. Naproxen exhibits its anti-inflammatory effect even in adrenalectomised animals, indicating that its action is not mediated through the pituitary-adrenal axis.

Naproxen inhibits prostaglandin synthetase (as do other NSAIDs). As with other NSAIDs, however, the exact mechanism of its anti-inflammatory action is not known.

Pharmacokinetic properties: Naproxen is completely absorbed from the gastro-intestinal tract, and peak plasma levels are reached in 2 to 4 hours. Naproxen is present in the blood mainly as unchanged drug, extensively bound to plasma proteins. The plasma half-life is between 12 and 15 hours, enabling a steady state to be achieved within 3 days of initiation of therapy on a twice daily dose regimen. The degree of absorption is not significantly affected by either foods or most antacids. Excretion is almost entirely via the urine, mainly as conjugated naproxen, with some unchanged drug. Metabolism in children is similar to that in adults. Chronic alcoholic liver disease reduces the total plasma concentration of naproxen but the concentration of unbound naproxen increases. In the elderly, the unbound plasma concentration of naproxen is increased although total plasma concentration is unchanged.

Preclinical safety data: None stated.

Pharmaceutical particulars

List of excipients: Povidone, croscarmellose sodium, magnesium stearate, iron oxide E 172, purified water.

Incompatibilities: None stated.

Shelf life: 60 months.

Special precautions for storage: Store below 30°C. Protect from light.

Nature and contents of container: Polypropylene securitainers with LDPE closures or polypropylene bottles with induction seals and polypropylene screw closures or amber glass bottles with metal closures fitted with an expanded polythene wad, containing 50, 60, 120, 250 and 500 tablets.

Clear or opaque PVC blister packaging with aluminium lidding in cartons, containing 2, 4, 56, 60 and 112 tablets.

Instructions for use/handling: None given.

Marketing authorisation number PL 0031/0471

Date of first authorisation/renewal of authorisation 26 April 1996

Date of (partial) revision of the text October 1997

NAPROSYN EC

Qualitative and quantitative composition

Naproxen Ph. Eur 250 mg/tablet.
Naproxen Ph Eur 375 mg/tablet.
Naproxen Ph Eur 500 mg/tablet.

Pharmaceutical form Enteric film-coated tablets.

Clinical particulars

Therapeutic indications: Naprosyn EC is indicated for the treatment of rheumatoid arthritis, osteoarthrosis (degenerative arthritis), ankylosing spondylitis, juvenile rheumatoid arthritis, acute gout, acute musculo-skeletal disorders (such as sprains and strains, direct trauma, lumbosacral pain, cervical spondylitis, tenosynovitis and fibrositis) and dysmenorrhoea.

Posology and method of administration

Adults: Naprosyn EC tablets should be swallowed whole and not broken or crushed.

Therapy should be started at the lowest recommended dose, especially in the elderly.

Rheumatoid arthritis, osteoarthritis and ankylosing spondylitis: The usual dose is 500 mg to 1 g daily taken in 2 doses at 12-hour intervals. Where 1 g per day is needed either one 500 mg tablet twice daily or two 500 mg tablets in a single administration (morning or evening) is recommended. In the following cases a loading dose of 750 mg or 1 g per day for the acute phase is recommended:

a) In patients reporting severe night-time pain/or morning stiffness.

b) In patients being switched to Naprosyn from a high dose of another anti-rheumatic compound.

c) In osteoarthrosis where pain is the predominant symptom.

Acute gout: 750 mg once, then 250 mg every 8 hours until the attack has passed.

Acute musculoskeletal disorders and dysmenorrhoea: 500 mg initially followed by 250 mg at 6–8 hour intervals as needed, with a maximum daily dose after the first day of 1250 mg.

Elderly: Studies indicate that although total plasma concentration of naproxen is unchanged, the unbound plasma fraction of naproxen is increased in the elderly. The implication of this finding for Naprosyn EC dosing is unknown. As with other drugs used in the elderly it is prudent to use the lowest effective dose. For the effect of reduced elimination in the elderly see section Use in patients with impaired renal function.

Children: Naprosyn EC is effective in the treatment of juvenile rheumatoid arthritis in children over 5 years of age at a dose of 10 mg/kg/day taken in 2 doses at 12-hour intervals. Naprosyn EC is not recommended for use in any other indication in children under 16 years of age.

Contra-indications: Active or history of peptic ulceration or active gastrointestinal bleeding. Hypersensitivity to naproxen and naproxen sodium formulations. Since the potential exists for cross-sensitivity reactions, Naprosyn EC should not be given to patients in whom aspirin or other non-steroidal anti-inflammatory/analgesic drugs induce asthma, rhinitis or urticaria.

Special warnings and special precautions for use: Episodes of gastro-intestinal bleeding have been reported in patients with naproxen therapy. Naprosyn EC should be given under close supervision to patients with a history of gastro-intestinal disease.

Serious gastro-intestinal adverse reactions, can occur at any time in patients on therapy with non-steroidal anti-inflammatory drugs. The risk of occurrence does not seem to change with duration of therapy. Studies to date have not identified any subset of patients not at risk of developing peptic ulcer and bleeding. However, elderly and debilitated patients tolerate gastro-intestinal ulceration or bleeding less well than others. Most of the serious gastro-intestinal events associated with non-steroidal anti-inflammatory drugs occurred in this patient population.

The antipyretic and anti-inflammatory activities of Naprosyn EC may reduce fever and inflammation, thereby diminishing their utility as diagnostic signs.

Bronchospasm may be precipitated in patients suffering from, or with a history of, bronchial asthma or allergic disease.

Sporadic abnormalities in laboratory tests (e.g. liver function tests) have occurred in patients on naproxen therapy, but no definite trend indicating toxicity was seen in any test.

Naproxen decreases platelet aggregation and prolongs bleeding time. This effect should be kept in mind when bleeding times are determined.

Mild peripheral oedema has been observed in a few patients receiving naproxen. Although sodium retention has not been reported in metabolic studies, it is possible that patients with questionable or compromised cardiac function may be at a greater risk when taking Naprosyn EC.

Use in patients with impaired renal function: As naproxen is eliminated to a large extent (95%) by urinary excretion via glomerular filtration, it should be used with great caution in patients with impaired renal function and the monitoring of serum creatinine and/or creatinine clearance is advised in these patients. Naprosyn EC is not recommended in patients having a baseline creatinine clearance of less than 20 ml/minute.

Certain patients, specifically those whose renal blood flow is compromised, because of extracellular volume depletion, cirrhosis of the liver, sodium restriction, congestive heart failure, and pre-existing renal disease, should have renal function assessed before and during Naprosyn EC therapy. Some elderly patients in whom impaired renal function may be expected, as well as patients using diuretics, may also fall within this category. A reduction in daily dosage should be considered to avoid the possibility of excessive accumulation of naproxen metabolites in these patients.

Use in patients with impaired liver function: Chronic alcoholic liver disease and probably also other forms of cirrhosis reduce the total plasma concentration of naproxen, but the plasma concentration of unbound naproxen is increased. The implication of this finding for Naprosyn EC dosing is unknown but it is prudent to use the lowest effective dose.

Haematological: Patients who have coagulation disorders or are receiving drug therapy that interferes with haemostasis should be carefully observed if naproxen-containing products are administered.

Patients at high risk of bleeding or those on full anti-coagulation therapy (e.g. dicoumarol derivatives) may be at increased risk of bleeding if given naproxen-containing products.

Anaphylactic (anaphylactoid) reactions: Hypersensitivity reactions may occur in susceptible individuals. Anaphylactic (anaphylactoid) reactions may occur both in patients with and without a history of hypersensitivity or exposure to aspirin, other non-steroidal anti-inflammatory drugs or naproxen-containing products. They may also occur in individuals with a history of angioedema, bronchospastic reactivity (e.g. asthma), rhinitis and nasal polyps.

Anaphylactoid reactions, like anaphylaxis, may have a fatal outcome.

Steroids: If steroid dosage is reduced or eliminated during therapy, the steroid dosage should be reduced slowly and the patients must be observed closely for any evidence of adverse effects, including adrenal insufficiency and exacerbation of symptoms of arthritis.

Ocular effects: Studies have not shown changes in the eye attributable to naproxen administration. In rare cases, adverse ocular disorders including papillitis, retrobulbar optic neuritis and papilledema, have been reported in users of NSAIDs including naproxen, although a cause-and-effect relationship cannot be established; accordingly, patients who develop visual disturbances during treatment with naproxen-containing products should have an ophthalmological examination.

Combination with other NSAIDs: The combination of naproxen-containing products and other NSAIDs is not recommended, because of the cumulative risks of inducing serious NSAID-related adverse events.

Interaction with other medicaments and other forms of interaction: Concomitant administration of antacid or cholestyramine can delay the absorption of naproxen but does not affect its extent. Concomitant administration of food can delay the absorption of naproxen, but does not affect its extent.

Due to the high plasma protein binding of naproxen, patients simultaneously receiving hydantoins, anticoagulants or a highly protein-bound sulphonamide should be observed for signs of overdosage of these drugs. No interactions have been observed in clinical studies with naproxen and anticoagulants or sulphonylureas, but caution is nevertheless advised since interaction has been seen with other non-steroidal agents of this class.

The natriuretic effect of frusemide has been reported to be inhibited by some drugs of this class.

Inhibition of renal lithium clearance leading to increases in plasma lithium concentrations has also been reported

Naproxen and other non-steroidal anti-inflammatory drugs can reduce the antihypertensive effect of propranolol and other beta-blockers and may increase the risk of renal impairment associated with the use of ACE-inhibitors.

Probenecid given concurrently increases naproxen plasma levels and extends its half-life considerably.

Caution is advised where methotrexate is administered concurrently because of possible enhancement of its toxicity, since naproxen, in common with other non-steroidal anti-inflammatory drugs, has been reported to reduce the tubular secretion of methotrexate in an animal model.

NSAIDs may exacerbate cardiac failure, reduce GFR and increase plasma cardiac glycoside levels when co-administered with cardiac glycosides.

As with all NSAIDs caution is advised when cyclosporin is co-administered because of the increased risk of nephrotoxicity.

NSAIDs should not be used for 8–12 days after mifepristone administration as NSAIDs can reduce the effects of mifepristone.

As with all NSAIDs, caution should be taken when co-administering with corticosteroids because of the increased risk of bleeding.

Patients taking quinolones may have an increased risk of developing convulsions.

It is suggested that Naprosyn EC therapy be temporarily discontinued 48 hours before adrenal function tests are performed, because naproxen may artifactually interfere with some tests for 17-ketogenic steroids. Similarly, naproxen may interfere with some assays of urinary 5-hydroxyindoleacetic acid.

Pregnancy and lactation: Teratology studies in rats and rabbits at dose levels equivalent on a human multiple basis to those which have produced foetal abnormality with certain other non-steroidal anti-inflammatory agents, e.g. aspirin, have not produced evidence of foetal damage with naproxen. As with other drugs of this type naproxen delays parturition in animals (the relevance of this finding to human patients is unknown) and also affects the human foetal cardiovascular system (closure of the ductus arteriosus). Good medical practice indicates minimal drug usage in pregnancy, and the use of this class of therapeutic agent requires cautious balancing of possible benefit against potential risk to the mother and foetus, especially in the first and third trimesters.

Naproxen has been found in the milk of lactating mothers. The use of Naprosyn EC should therefore be avoided in patients who are breast-feeding.

Effects on ability to drive and use machines: Some patients may experience drowsiness, dizziness, vertigo, insomnia or depression with the use of Naprosyn. If patients experience these or similar undesirable effects, they should exercise caution in carrying out activities that require alertness.

Undesirable effects: Gastro-intestinal: The more frequent reactions are nausea, vomiting, abdominal discomfort and epigastric distress. More serious reactions which may occur occasionally are gastro-intestinal bleeding, peptic ulceration (sometimes with haemorrhage and perforation), non-peptic gastro-intestinal ulceration and colitis.

Dermatological: Skin rashes, urticaria, angioedema. Alopecia, erythema multiforme, Stevens Johnson syndrome, epidermal necrolysis and photosensitivity reactions (including cases in which the skin resembles porphyria cutanea tarda, 'pseudoporphyria') or epidermolysis bullosa may occur rarely.

Renal: Including but not limited to glomerular nephritis, interstitial nephritis, nephrotic syndrome, haematuria, renal papillary necrosis and renal failure.

CNS: Convulsions, headache, insomnia, inability to concentrate and cognitive dysfunction have been reported.

Haematological: Thrombocytopenia, granulocytopenia including agranulocytosis, aplastic anaemia and haemolytic anaemia may occur rarely.

Other: Tinnitus, hearing impairment, vertigo, mild peripheral oedema. Anaphylactic reactions to naproxen and naproxen sodium formulations have been reported in patients with, or without, a history of previous hypersensitivity reactions to NSAIDs. Jaundice, fatal hepatitis, visual disturbances, eosinophilic pneumonitis, vasculitis, hyperkalemia, aseptic meningitis and ulcerative stomatitis have been reported rarely.

Overdose: Significant overdosage of the drug may be characterised by drowsiness, heartburn, indigestion, nausea or vomiting. A few patients have experienced seizures, but it is not known whether these were naproxen-related or not. It is not known what dose of the drug would be life-threatening.

Should a patient ingest a large amount of Naprosyn EC accidentally or purposefully, the stomach may be emptied and usual supportive measures employed. Animal studies indicate that the prompt administration of activated charcoal in adequate amounts would tend to reduce markedly the absorption of the drug.

Haemodialysis does not decrease the plasma concentration of naproxen because of the high degree of protein binding. However, haemodialysis may still be appropriate in a patient with renal failure who has taken naproxen.

Pharmacological properties

Pharmacodynamic properties: Naproxen has been shown to have anti-inflammatory, analgesic and antipyretic properties when tested in classical animal test systems. It exhibits its anti-inflammatory effect even in adrenalectomised animals, indicating that its action is not mediated through the pituitary-adrenal axis. It inhibits prostaglandin synthetase, as do other non-steroidal anti-inflammatory agents. As with other agents, however, the exact mechanism of its anti-inflammatory action is not known.

Pharmacokinetic properties: Naproxen is completely absorbed from the gastro-intestinal tract, and peak plasma levels are reached in 2 to 4 hours. Naproxen is present in the blood mainly as unchanged drug, extensively bound to plasma proteins. The plasma half-life is between 12 and 15 hours, enabling a steady state to be achieved within 3 days of initiation of therapy on a twice daily dose regimen. The degree of absorption is not significantly affected by either foods or most antacids. Excretion is almost entirely via the urine, mainly as conjugated naproxen, with some unchanged drug. Metabolism in children is similar to that in adults. Chronic alcoholic liver disease reduces the total plasma concentration of naproxen but the concentration of unbound naproxen increases. In the elderly, the unbound plasma concentration of naproxen is increased although total plasma concentration is unchanged.

When naproxen is administered in the enteric-coated form, the peak plasma levels are delayed compared to those seen with standard tablets. However, the mean areas under the plasma concentration-time curves, and hence bioavailability, are equivalent. The tablets, therefore, perform as one would anticipate for a drug which does not disintegrate until it reaches the small intestine, where dissolution is rapid and complete.

Preclinical safety data: No evidence of carcinogenicity was found in rats. Reproduction studies performed in rats, rabbits and mice at doses up to 6 times the human dose revealed no evidence of impaired fertility or harm to the foetus. As with other drugs known to inhibit prostaglandin synthesis, an increased incidence of dystocia and delayed parturition occurred in rats.

Pharmaceutical particulars

List of excipients: The tablets also contain povidone EP, croscarmellose sodium NF, magnesium stearate EP, purified water EP, methacrylic acid copolymer NF, purified talc EP, sodium hydroxide EP, triethyl citrate NF, simethicone emulsion USP and opacode S-1-8106.

Incompatibilities: None known.

Shelf life: 36 months.

Special precautions for storage: Protect from light and store below 30°C.

Nature and contents of container: Polypropylene, polyethylene or glass bottles containing 50, 60, 100 or 250 tablets.

Clear or opaque PVC blister with aluminium lidding in cartons containing 2, 4 or 56 tablets.

Instructions for use/handling: None applicable.

Marketing authorisation numbers

Naprosyn EC 250 PL 0031/0467
Naprosyn EC 375 PL 0031/0468
Naprosyn EC 500 PL 0031/0469

Date of first authorisation 12 July 1991

Date of (partial) revision of the text November 1997

NAPROSYN SUPPOSITORIES

Qualitative and quantitative composition Naproxen BP 500 mg.

Pharmaceutical form White, almost odourless bullet shaped suppository.

Clinical particulars

Therapeutic indications: Treatment of rheumatoid arthritis, osteoarthrosis (degenerative arthritis), ankylosing spondylitis, juvenile rheumatoid arthritis, acute gout, acute musculoskeletal disorders and dysmenorrhoea.

Posology and method of administration

Route of administration: Rectal.

Naprosyn Suppositories are recommended for patients in whom rectal administration may be preferable. One suppository is to be inserted at night. If necessary, another suppository or up to 500 mg oral Naprosyn therapy can be used in the morning.

Adults: Rheumatoid arthritis, osteoarthritis and ankylosing spondylitis

500 mg to 1 g taken in 2 doses at 12 hour intervals. In the following cases a loading dose of 750 mg or 1 g per day for the acute phase is recommended:

a) In patients reporting severe night-time pain/or morning stiffness.

b) In patients being switched to Naprosyn from a high dose of another anti-rheumatic compound.

c) In osteoarthrosis where pain is the predominant symptom.

Acute gout: 750 mg at once then 250 mg every 8 hours until the attack has passed.

Acute musculoskeletal disorders and dysmenorrhoea: 500 mg initially followed by 250 mg at 6–8 hour intervals as needed, with a maximum daily dose after the first day of 1250 mg.

Elderly: Studies indicate that although total plasma concentration of naproxen is unchanged, the unbound plasma fraction of naproxen is increased in the elderly. The implication of this finding for Naprosyn dosing is unknown. As with other drugs used in the elderly it is prudent to use the lowest effective dose. For the effect of reduced elimination in the elderly refer to *Special warnings and special precautions for use.*

Children: For juvenile rheumatoid arthritis: 10 mg/kg/day taken in 2 doses at 12 hour intervals.

Contra-indications: Active peptic ulceration or patients with active gastrointestinal bleeding. Hypersensitivity to naproxen or naproxen sodium formulations. Since the potential exists for cross-sensitivity reactions, Naprosyn should not be given to patients in whom aspirin or other non-steroidal anti-inflammatory/analgesic drugs induce the syndrome of asthma, rhinitis or urticaria.

Special warnings and special precautions for use: Episodes of gastro-intestinal bleeding have been reported in patients with naproxen therapy. Naprosyn should be given under close supervision to patients with a history of gastro-intestinal disease.

Serious gastro-intestinal adverse reactions, can occur at any time in patients on therapy with non-steroidal anti-inflammatory drugs. The risk of occurrence does not seem to change with duration of therapy. Studies to date have not identified any subset of patients not at risk of developing peptic ulcer and bleeding. However, elderly and debilitated patients tolerate gastro-intestinal ulceration or bleeding less well than others. Most of the serious gastro-intestinal events associated with non-steroidal anti-inflammatory drugs occurred in this patient population.

The antipyretic and anti-inflammatory activities of Naprosyn may reduce fever and inflammation, thereby diminishing their utility as diagnostic signs.

Bronchospasm may be precipitated in patients suffering from, or with a history of, bronchial asthma or allergic disease.

Sporadic abnormalities in laboratory tests (e.g. liver function tests) have occurred in patients on naproxen therapy, but no definite trend indicating toxicity was seen in any test indicating toxicity.

Naproxen decreases platelet aggregation and prolongs bleeding time. This effect should be kept in mind when bleeding times are determined.

Mild peripheral oedema has been observed in a few patients receiving naproxen. Although sodium retention has not been reported in metabolic studies, it is possible that patients with questionable or compromised cardiac function may be at a greater risk when taking Naprosyn.

Use in patients with impaired renal function: As naproxen is eliminated to a large extent (95%) by urinary excretion via glomerular filtration, it should be used with great caution in patients with impaired renal function and the monitoring of serum creatinine and/or creatinine clearance is advised in these patients. Naprosyn is not recommended in patients having a baseline creatinine clearance of less than 20 ml/minute.

Certain patients, specifically those whose renal blood flow is compromised, such as in extracellular volume depletion, cirrhosis of the liver, sodium restriction, congestive heart failure, and pre-existing renal disease, should have renal function assessed before and during Naprosyn therapy. Some elderly patients in whom impaired renal function may be expected, as well as patients using diuretics, may also fall within this category. A reduction in daily dosage should be considered to avoid the possibility of excessive accumulation of naproxen metabolites in these patients.

Use in patients with impaired liver function: Chronic alcoholic liver disease and probably also other forms of cirrhosis reduce the total plasma concentration of naproxen, but the plasma concentration of unbound naproxen is increased. The implication of this finding for Naprosyn dosing is unknown but it is prudent to use the lowest effective dose.

Patients who have coagulation disorders or who are receiving drug therapy that interferes with haemostasis should be carefully observed if naproxen-containing products are administered.

Patients at high risk of bleeding or those on full anti-coagulation therapy (e.g. dicoumarol derivatives) may be at increased risk of bleeding if given naproxen-containing products concurrently.

Anaphylactic (anaphylactoid) reactions: Hypersensitivity reactions may occur in susceptible individuals. Anaphylactic (anaphylactoid) reactions may occur both in patients with and without a history of hypersensitivity or exposure to aspirin, other non-steroidal anti-inflammatory drugs or naproxen-containing products. They may also occur in individuals with a history of angioedema, bronchospastic reactivity (e.g. asthma), rhinitis and nasal polyps.

Anaphylactoid reactions, like anaphylaxis, may have a fatal outcome.

Steroids: If steroid dosage is reduced or eliminated during therapy, the steroid dosage should be reduced slowly and the patients must be observed closely for any evidence of adverse effects, including adrenal insufficiency and exacerbation of symptoms of arthritis.

Ocular effects: Studies have not shown changes in the eye attributable to naproxen administration. In rare cases, adverse ocular disorders including papillitis, retrobulbar optic neuritis and papilledema, have been reported in users of NSAIDs including naproxen, although a cause-and-effect relationship cannot be established; accordingly, patients who develop visual disturbances during treatment with naproxen-containing products should have an ophthalmological examination.

Combination with other NSAIDs: The combination of naproxen-containing products and other NSAIDs is not recommended, because of the cumulative risks of inducing serious NSAID-related adverse events.

Interaction with other medicaments and other forms of interaction: Concomitant administration of antacid or cholestyramine can delay the absorption of naproxen but does not affect its extent. Concomitant administration of food can delay the absorption of naproxen, but does not affect its extent.

Due to the high plasma protein binding of naproxen, patients simultaneously receiving hydantoins, anti-coagulants or a highly protein-bound sulphonamide should be observed for signs of overdosage of these drugs. No interactions have been observed in clinical studies with naproxen and anticoagulants or sulphonylureas, but caution is nevertheless advised since interaction has been seen with other non-steroidal agents of this class.

The natriuretic effect of frusemide has been reported to be inhibited by some drugs of this class.

Inhibition of renal lithium clearance leading to increases in plasma lithium concentrations has also been reported

Naproxen and other non-steroidal anti-inflammatory drugs can reduce the antihypertensive effect of propranolol and other beta-blockers and may increase the risk of renal impairment associated with the use of ACE-inhibitors.

Probenecid given concurrently increases naproxen plasma levels and extends its half-life considerably.

Caution is advised where methotrexate is given concurrently because of possible enhancement of its toxicity, since naproxen, among other non-steroidal anti-inflammatory drugs, has been reported to reduce the tubular secretion of methotrexate in an animal model.

NSAIDs may exacerbate cardiac failure, reduce GFR and increase plasma cardiac glycoside levels when co-administered with cardiac glycosides.

As with all NSAIDs caution is advised when cyclosporin is co-administered because of the increased risk of nephrotoxicity.

NSAIDs should not be used for 8–12 days after mifepristone administration as NSAIDs can reduce the effects of mifepristone.

As with all NSAIDs, caution should be taken when co-administering with cortico-steroids because of the increased risk of bleeding.

Patients taking quinolones may have an increased risk of developing convulsions.

It is suggested that Naprosyn therapy be temporarily discontinued 48 hours before adrenal function tests are performed, because naproxen may artifactually interfere with some tests for 17-ketogenic steroids. Similarly, naproxen may interfere with some assays of urinary 5-hydroxyindoleacetic acid.

Pregnancy and lactation: Teratology studies in rats and rabbits at dose levels equivalent on a human multiple basis to those which have produced foetal abnormality with certain other non-steroidal anti-inflammatory agents, e.g. aspirin, have not produced evidence of foetal damage with naproxen. As with other drugs of this type naproxen delays parturition in animals (the relevance of this finding to human patients is unknown) and also affects the human foetal cardiovascular system (closure of the ductus arteriosus). Good medical practice indicates minimal drug usage in pregnancy, and the use of this class of therapeutic agent requires cautious balancing of possible benefit against potential risk to the mother and foetus, especially in the first and third trimesters.

The use of Naprosyn should be avoided in patients who are breast-feeding.

Effects on ability to drive and use machines: Some patients may experience drowsiness, dizziness, vertigo, insomnia or depression with the use of Naprosyn. If patients experience these or similar undesirable effects, they should exercise caution in carrying out activities that require alertness.

Undesirable effects: Gastro-intestinal: The more frequent reactions are nausea, vomiting, abdominal discomfort and epigastric distress. More serious reactions which may occur occasionally are gastro-intestinal bleeding, peptic ulceration (sometimes with haemorrhage and perforation), non-peptic gastro-intestinal ulceration and colitis.

Dermatological: Skin rashes, urticaria, angioedema. Alopecia, erythema multiforme, Stevens Johnson syndrome, epidermal necrolysis and photosensitivity reactions (including cases in which the skin resembles porphyria cutanea tarda, 'pseudoporphyria') or epidermolysis bullosa may occur rarely.

Renal: Including but not limited to glomerular nephritis, interstitial nephritis, nephrotic syndrome, haematuria, renal papillary necrosis and renal failure.

CNS: Convulsions, headache, insomnia, inability to concentrate and cognitive dysfunction have been reported.

Haematological: Thrombocytopenia, granulocytopenia including agranulocytosis, aplastic anaemia and haemolytic anaemia may occur rarely.

Other: Tinnitus, hearing impairment, vertigo, mild peripheral oedema. Anaphylactic reactions to naproxen and naproxen sodium formulations have been reported in patients with, or without, a history of previous sensitivity reactions to NSAIDs. Jaundice, fatal hepatitis, visual disturbances, eosinophilic pneumonitis, vasculitis, hyperkalemia, aseptic meningitis and ulcerative stomatitis have been reported rarely.

Naprosyn suppositories: The following minor side-effects have been reported with the use of Naprosyn Suppositories: rectal discomfort, soreness, burning and itching. Also isolated cases of rectal bleeding, tenesmus and proctitis have been reported. However, the incidence of local side-effects in clinical trials was low.

Overdose: Significant overdosage of the drug may be characterised by drowsiness, heartburn, indigestion, nausea or vomiting. A few patients have experienced seizures, but it is not known whether these were naproxen-related or not. It is not known what dose of the drug would be life-threatening.

Should a patient ingest a large amount of Naprosyn accidentally or purposefully, the stomach may be emptied and usual supportive measures employed. Animal studies indicate that the prompt administration of activated charcoal in adequate amounts would tend to reduce markedly the absorption of the drug.

Haemodialysis does not decrease the plasma concentration of naproxen because of the high degree of protein binding. However, haemodialysis may still be appropriate in a patient with renal failure who has taken naproxen.

Pharmacological properties

Pharmacodynamic properties: Naproxen is a non-steroidal anti-inflammatory analgesic compound with antipyretic properties as has been demonstrated in classical animal test systems. Naproxen exhibits its anti-inflammatory effect even in adrenalectomised animals, indicating that its action is not mediated through the pituitary-adrenal axis.

Naproxen inhibits prostaglandin synthetase (as do other NSAIDs). As with other NSAIDs, however, the exact mechanism of its anti-inflammatory action is not known.

Pharmacokinetic properties: Naproxen is completely absorbed from the gastro-intestinal tract, and peak plasma levels are reached in 2 to 4 hours. Naproxen is present in the blood mainly as unchanged drug, extensively bound to plasma proteins. The plasma half-life is between 12 and 15 hours, enabling a steady state to be achieved within 3 days of initiation of therapy on a twice daily dose regimen. The degree of absorption is not significantly affected by either foods or most antacids. Excretion is almost entirely via the urine, mainly as conjugated naproxen, with some unchanged drug. Metabolism in children is similar to that in adults. Chronic alcoholic liver disease reduces the total plasma concentration of naproxen but the concentration of unbound naproxen increases. In the elderly, the unbound plasma concentration of naproxen is increased although total plasma concentration is unchanged.

Preclinical safety data None stated.

Pharmaceutical particulars

List of excipients: Witepsol.

Incompatibilities: None stated.

Shelf life: 60 months.

Special precautions for storage: Store below 25°C in a dry place. Protect from sunlight and heat.

Nature and contents of container: Strip of polythene lined PVC shells containing 10 suppositories.

Instructions for use/handling: None given.

Marketing authorisation number PL 0031/0474

Date of first authorisation/renewal of authorisation 31 May 1996

Date of (partial) revision of the text October 1997

NAPROSYN S/R

Qualitative and quantitative composition Each white to off white slow release tablet contains naproxen sodium USP 547.638 mg equivalent to naproxen 500.00 mg.

Pharmaceutical form Slow release tablet.

Clinical particulars

Therapeutic indications: Naprosyn S/R is indicated for the treatment of rheumatoid arthritis, osteoarthrosis (degenerative arthritis), ankylosing spondylitis, direct trauma, lumbosacral pain, cervical spondylitis, tenosynovitis and fibrositis.

Posology and method of administration

Route of administration: Oral.

Do not suck or chew tablets.

Adults: One or two tablets once daily.

Elderly: Studies indicate that although total plasma concentration of naproxen is unchanged, the unbound plasma fraction of naproxen is increased in the elderly. The implication of this finding for Naprosyn S/R dosing is unknown. As with other drugs used in the elderly it is prudent to use the lowest effective dose. For the effect of reduced elimination in the elderly refer to *Special warnings and special precautions for use.*

Children: Not recommended for children under 16 years.

Contra-indications: Active peptic ulceration or active gastro-intestinal bleeding. Hypersensitivity to naproxen or naproxen sodium formulations. Since the potential exists for cross-sensitivity reactions, Naprosyn S/R should not be given to patients in whom aspirin or other non-steroidal anti-inflammatory/analgesic drugs induce the syndrome of asthma, rhinitis or urticaria.

Special warnings and special precautions for use: Episodes of gastro-intestinal bleeding have been reported in patients with naproxen therapy. Naprosyn S/R should be given under close supervision to patients with a history of gastro-intestinal disease.

Serious gastro-intestinal adverse reactions can occur at any time in patients on therapy with non-steroidal anti-inflammatory drugs. The risk of occurrence does not seem to change with duration of therapy. Studies to date have not identified any subset of patients not at risk of developing peptic ulcer and bleeding. However, elderly and debilitated patients tolerate gastro-intestinal ulceration or bleeding less well than others. Most of the serious gastro-intestinal events associated with non-steroidal anti-inflammatory drugs occurred in this patient population.

The antipyretic and anti-inflammatory activities of Naprosyn S/R may reduce fever and inflammation, thereby diminishing their utility as diagnostic signs.

Bronchospasm may be precipitated in patients suffering from, or with a history of, bronchial asthma or allergic disease.

Sporadic abnormalities in laboratory tests (e.g. liver function tests) have occurred in patients on naproxen therapy, but no definite trend indicating toxicity was seen in any test indicating toxicity.

Naproxen decreases platelet aggregation and prolongs bleeding time. This effect should be kept in mind when bleeding times are determined.

Mild peripheral oedema has been observed in a few patients receiving naproxen. Although sodium retention has not been reported in metabolic studies, it is possible that patients with questionable or compromised cardiac function may be at a greater risk when taking Naprosyn S/R.

Use in patients with impaired renal function: As naproxen is eliminated to a large extent (95%) by urinary excretion via glomerular filtration, it should be used with great caution in patients with impaired renal function and the monitoring of serum creatinine and/or creatinine clearance is advised in these patients. Naprosyn S/R is not recommended in patients having a baseline creatinine clearance of less than 20 ml/minute.

Certain patients, specifically those whose renal blood flow is compromised, such as in extracellular volume depletion, cirrhosis of the liver, sodium restriction, congestive heart failure, and pre-existing renal disease, should have renal function assessed before and during Naprosyn S/R therapy. Some elderly patients in whom impaired renal function may be expected, as well as patients using diuretics, may also fall within this category. A reduction in daily dosage should be considered to avoid the possibility of excessive accumulation of naproxen metabolites in these patients.

Use in patients with impaired liver function: Chronic alcoholic liver disease and probably also other forms of cirrhosis reduce the total plasma concentration of naproxen, but the plasma concentration of unbound naproxen is increased. The implication of this finding for Naprosyn S/R dosing is unknown but it is prudent to use the lowest effective dose.

Haematological: Patients who have coagulation disorders or are receiving drug therapy that interferes with haemostasis should be carefully observed if naproxen-containing products are administered.

Patients at high risk of bleeding or those on full anti-coagulation therapy (e.g. dicoumarol derivatives) may be at increased risk of bleeding if given naproxen-containing products concurrently.

Anaphylactic (anaphylactoid) reactions: Hypersensitivity reactions may occur in susceptible individuals. Anaphylactic (anaphylactoid) reactions may occur both in patients with and without a history of hypersensitivity or exposure to aspirin, other non-steroidal anti-inflammatory drugs or naproxen-containing products. They may also occur in individuals with a history of angioedema, bronchospastic reactivity (e.g. asthma), rhinitis and nasal polyps.

Anaphylactoid reactions, like anaphylaxis, may have a fatal outcome.

Steroids: If steroid dosage is reduced or eliminated during therapy, the steroid dosage should be reduced slowly and the patients must be observed closely for any evidence of adverse effects, including adrenal insufficiency and exacerbation of symptoms of arthritis.

Ocular effects: Studies have not shown changes in the eye attributable to naproxen administration. In rare cases, adverse ocular disorders including papillitis, retrobulbar optic neuritis and papilledema, have been reported in users of NSAIDs including naproxen, although a cause-and-effect relationship cannot be established; accordingly, patients who develop visual disturbances during treatment with naproxen-containing products should have an ophthalmological examination.

Combination with other NSAIDs: The combination of naproxen-containing products and other NSAIDs is not recommended, because of the cumulative risks of inducing serious NSAID-related adverse events.

Interaction with other medicaments and other forms of interaction: Concomitant administration of antacid or cholestyramine can delay the absorption of naproxen but does not affect its extent. Concomitant administration of food can delay the absorption of naproxen, but does not affect its extent

Due to the high plasma protein binding of naproxen, patients simultaneously receiving hydantoins, anti-coagulants or a highly protein-bound sulphonamide should be observed for signs of overdosage of these drugs. No interactions have been observed in clinical studies with naproxen and anticoagulants or sulphonylureas, but caution is nevertheless advised since interaction has been seen with other non-steroidal agents of this class.

The natriuretic effect of frusemide has been reported to be inhibited by some drugs of this class.

Inhibition of renal lithium clearance leading to increases in plasma lithium concentrations has also been reported

Naproxen and other non-steroidal anti-inflammatory drugs can reduce the antihypertensive effect of propranolol and other beta-blockers and may increase the risk of renal impairment associated with the use of ACE-inhibitors.

Probenecid given concurrently increases naproxen plasma levels and extends its half-life considerably.

Caution is advised where methotrexate is given concurrently because of possible enhancement of its toxicity, since naproxen, among other non-steroidal anti-inflammatory drugs, has been reported to reduce the tubular secretion of methotrexate in an animal model.

NSAID's may exacerbate cardiac failure, reduce GFR and increase plasma cardiac glycoside levels when co-administered with cardiac glycosides.

As with all NSAID's caution is advised when cyclosporin is co-administered because of the increased risk of nephrotoxicity.

NSAID's should not be used for 8-12 days after mifepristone administration as NSAID's can reduce the effects of mifepristone.

As with all NSAID's, caution should be taken when co-administering with cortico-steroids because of the increased risk of bleeding.

Patients taking quinolones may have an increased risk of developing convulsions.

It is suggested that Naprosyn S/R therapy be temporarily discontinued 48 hours before adrenal function tests are performed, because naproxen may artifactually interfere with some tests for 17-ketogenic steroids. Similarly, naproxen may interfere with some assays of urinary 5-hydroxyindoleacetic acid.

Pregnancy and lactation: Teratology studies in rats and rabbits at dose levels equivalent on a human multiple basis to those which have produced foetal abnormality with certain other non-steroidal anti-inflammatory agents, e.g. aspirin, have not produced evidence of foetal damage with naproxen. As with other drugs of this type naproxen delays parturition in animals (the relevance of this finding to human patients is unknown) and also affects the human foetal cardiovascular system (closure of the ductus arteriosus). Good medical practice indicates minimal drug usage in pregnancy, and the use of this class of therapeutic agent requires cautious balancing of possible benefit against potential risk to the mother and foetus, especially in the first and third trimesters.

The use of Naprosyn S/R should be avoided in patients who are breast-feeding.

Effects on ability to drive and use machines: Some patients may experience drowsiness, dizziness, vertigo, insomnia or depression with the use of Naprosyn. If patients experience these or similar undesirable effects, they should exercise caution in carrying out activities that require alertness.

Undesirable effects

Gastro-intestinal: The more frequent reactions are nausea, vomiting, abdominal discomfort and epigastric distress. More serious reactions which may occur occasionally are gastro-intestinal bleeding, peptic ulceration (sometimes with haemorrhage and perforation), non-peptic gastro-intestinal ulceration and colitis.

Dermatological: Skin rashes, urticaria, angio-oedema. Alopecia, erythema multiforme, Stevens Johnson syndrome, epidermal necrolysis and photosensitivity reactions (including cases in which the skin resembles porphyria cutanea tarda, 'pseudoporphyria') or epidermolysis bullosa may occur rarely.

Renal: Including but not limited to glomerular nephritis, interstitial nephritis, nephrotic syndrome, haematuria, renal papillary necrosis and renal failure.

CNS: Convulsions, headache, insomnia, inability to concentrate and cognitive dysfunction have been reported.

Haematological: Thrombocytopenia, granulocytopenia including agranulocytosis, aplastic anaemia and haemolytic anaemia may occur rarely.

Other: Tinnitus, hearing impairment, vertigo, mild peripheral oedema. Anaphylactic reactions to naproxen and naproxen sodium formulations have been reported in patients with, or without, a history of previous sensitivity reactions to NSAIDs. Jaundice, fatal hepatitis, visual disturbances, eosinophilic pneumonitis, vasculitis, hyperkalemia, aseptic meningitis and ulcerative stomatitis have been reported rarely.

Overdose: Significant overdosage of the drug may be characterised by drowsiness, heartburn, indigestion, nausea or vomiting. A few patients have experienced seizures, but it is not known whether these were naproxen-related or not. It is not known what dose of the drug would be life-threatening.

Should a patient ingest a large amount of Naprosyn S/R accidentally or purposefully, the stomach may be emptied and usual supportive measures employed. Animal studies indicate that the prompt administration of activated charcoal in adequate amounts would tend to reduce markedly the absorption of the drug.

Haemodialysis does not decrease the plasma concentration of naproxen because of the high degree of protein binding. However, haemodialysis may still be appropriate in a patient with renal failure who has taken naproxen.

Pharmacological properties

Pharmacodynamic properties: Naproxen sodium is a widely used non-steroidal anti-inflammatory drug. It is a propionic acid derivative in common with ibuprofen, flurbiprofen and ketoprofen.

Its mechanism of action appears to be the inhibition of the enzymatic production of prostaglandins.

Pharmacokinetic properties: Naprosyn S/R is naproxen 500 mg (as the sodium salt) formulated into a sustained release tablet with an immediate release portion. This ensures a rapid initial peak with T_{max} and C_{max} similar to conventional dosage forms. The sustained release portion ensures that therapeutic plasma levels are maintained over a 24 hour period.

Preclinical safety data: None stated.

Pharmaceutical particulars

List of excipients: Talc, citric acid, ammonio methacrylate copolymer type B, ammonio methacrylate copolymer type A, methocrylic acid copolymer type A, polyvidone, crospovidone, microcrystalline cellulose, magnesium stearate, opadry, isopropyl alcohol, acetone, purified water.

Incompatibilities: None.

Shelf life: 24 months.

Special precautions for storage: Store in a dry place below 25°C.

Nature and contents of container: High density polyethylene bottle containing 56 tablets.

Instructions for use/handling: None given.

Marketing authorisation number PL 0031/0473

Date of first authorisation/renewal of authorisation 31 May 1996

Date of (partial) revision of the text October 1997

NEOMERCAZOLE

Qualitative and quantitative composition Each NeoMercazole 5 tablet contains carbimazole BP 5 mg.

Pharmaceutical form Pink, circular biconvex tablet, imprinted with Neo/5 on the obverse and plain on the reverse.

Clinical particulars

Therapeutic indications: NeoMercazole is an anti-thyroid agent. It is indicated in all conditions where reduction of thyroid function is required.

1. Hyperthyroidism.
2. Preparation for thyroidectomy in hyperthyroidism.
3. Preparation for, and as concomitant therapy with, radio-iodine treatment.

Posology and method of administration:

Adults: The initial dose is in the range 20–60 mg, taken as two to three divided doses. This is continued until the patient is euthyroid. Subsequent therapy may then be administered in one of two ways.

Maintenance regimen: Dosage is gradually reduced so as to maintain a euthyroid state. Final dosage is usually in the range 5–15 mg per day, which may be taken as a single daily dose. Therapy should be continued for at least six, and up to eighteen months.

Blocking-replacement regimen: Dosage is maintained at the initial level, i.e. 20–60 mg per day, and supplemental l-thyroxine, 50–150 mcg per day, is administered concomitantly, in order to prevent hypothyroidism. Therapy should be continued for at least six months, and up to eighteen months.

Where a single dosage of less than 20 mg is recommended, it is intended that NeoMercazole 5 should be taken.

Elderly: No special dosage regimen is required, but care should be taken to observe the contra-indications and warnings.

Children: The usual initial daily dose is 15 mg per day.

Contra-indications: NeoMercazole is contra-indicated in patients with a previous history of adverse reactions to carbimazole.

Special warnings and special precautions for use: Patients should be warned about the onset of sore throats, mouth ulcers, pyrexia, or other symptoms which might suggest the early development of bone marrow depression. In such cases it is important that drug treatment is stopped and medical advice sought immediately. In such patients, white blood cell counts should be performed, particularly where there is any clinical evidence of infection. Early withdrawal of the drug will increase the chance of complete recovery.

NeoMercazole should be used with caution in patients with liver disorders.

NeoMercazole should be stopped temporarily at the time of administration of radio-iodine.

Interaction with other medicaments and other forms of interaction: None.

Pregnancy and lactation: Carbimazole crosses the placenta but, provided the mother's dose is within the standard range, and her thyroid status is monitored, there is no evidence of neonatal thyroid abnormalities. Studies have shown that the incidence of congenital malformations is greater in the children of mothers whose hyperthyroidism has remained untreated than in those to whom treatment with carbimazole has been given. However, treatment with carbimazole has been associated very rarely with aplasia cutis in the neonate. The dose of NeoMercazole must be regulated by the patient's clinical condition. The lowest dose possible should be used, and this can often be discontinued three to four weeks before term, in order to reduce the risk of neonatal complications. The blocking-replacement regimen should not be used during pregnancy since very little thyroxine crosses the placenta in the last trimester.

NeoMercazole is secreted in breast milk and, if treatment is continued during lactation, the patient should not continue to breast-feed her baby.

Effects on ability to drive and use machines: None.

Undesirable effects: Adverse reactions usually occur in the first eight weeks of treatment. The most common minor reactions are nausea, headache, arthralgia, mild gastric distress, skin rashes and pruritus. Hair loss has been occasionally reported. These reactions are usually self-limiting and may not require withdrawal of the drug.

Bone marrow depression has been reported and can lead to agranulocytosis. Patients should always be instructed to recognise symptoms which may suggest bone marrow depression, to stop the drug and to seek medical advice immediately. In such patients, white blood cell counts should be performed, particularly where there is any clinical evidence of infection.

Isolated cases of myopathy have been reported. Patients experiencing myalgia after the intake of NeoMercazole should have their creatine phosphokinase levels monitored.

Hepatic disorders, most commonly jaundice, have been reported; in these cases carbimazole should be withdrawn.

Overdose: No symptoms are likely from a single large dose, and so no specific treatment is indicated.

Pharmacological properties

Pharmacodynamic properties: Carbimazole is a thyroid reducing agent.

Pharmacokinetic properties: Carbimazole is rapidly metabolised to methimazole. The mean peak plasma concentration of methimazole is reported to occur one hour after a single dose of carbimazole. The apparent plasma half-life of methimazole is reported as 6.4 hours.

Preclinical safety data: Not relevant.

Pharmaceutical particulars

List of excipients: Each tablet contains Lactose Ph.Eur., Starch Maize Ph.Eur., Gelatin Ph.Eur., Magnesium Stearate Ph.Eur., Sucrose Ph.Eur., Acacia Ph.Eur., Talc Ph.Eur., Red Iron Oxide (E172).

Incompatibilities: None known.

Shelf life: 5 years.

Special precautions for storage: Recommended maximum storage temperature 25°C.

Nature and contents of container: NeoMercazole 5 tablets are available in HDPE bottles with a low density polyethylene tamper evident snap-fit closure. Each bottle contains 100 tablets.

Instructions for use/handling: No special requirements.

Marketing authorisation number PL 0031/0378

Date of first authorisation 20 December 1994

Date of (partial) revision of the text June 1997

NeoMercazole 20 tablets are also available.

NEORECORMON 50,000 MULTIDOSE ▼

Qualitative and quantitative composition

1 vial contains 50,000 international units (IU) corresponding to 415μg epoetin beta (recombinant human erythropoietin) as a powder for solution for injection.

1 ampoule contains 10 ml solvent (water for injection with benzyl alcohol and benzalkonium chloride as preservatives).

1 ml reconstituted solution contains 5000 IU epoetin beta.

Pharmaceutical form Powder and solvent for solution for injection.

Clinical particulars

Therapeutic indications: NeoRecormon 50,000 Multidose is indicated for:

Treatment of anaemia associated with chronic renal failure (renal anaemia) in patients on dialysis.

Treatment of symptomatic renal anaemia in patients not yet undergoing dialysis.

Prevention and treatment of anaemia in adult patients with solid tumours and treated with platinum-based chemotherapy prone to induce anaemia (cisplatin: 75 mg/m²/cycle, carboplatin: 350 mg/m²/cycle).

Increasing the yield of autologous blood from patients in a pre-donation programme. Its use in this indication must be balanced against the reported increased risk of thromboembolic events. Treatment should only be given to patients with moderate anaemia (Hb 10–13 g/dl [6.21 mmol/L–8.07 mmol/L], no iron deficiency), if blood conserving procedures are not available or insufficient when the scheduled major elective surgery requires a large volume of blood (4 or more units of blood for females or 5 or more units for males).

Posology and method of administration: Therapy with NeoRecormon 50,000 Multidose should be initiated by physicians experienced in the above mentioned indications.

This multidose preparation can be used for several patients. To avoid the risk of cross-infection, always follow aseptic techniques and use disposable sterile syringes and needles for each administration. Please check that only one vial of NeoRecormon 50,000 Multidose is in use (i.e. reconstituted) at any one time.

NeoRecormon 50,000 Multidose is supplied as a powder for solution for injection in vials. This is dissolved with the contents of the accompanying solvent ampoule by means of a reconstitution and withdrawal device according to the instructions given in *Instructions for use/handling*. The reconstituted solution has a shelf life of 1 month. Before withdrawal of each dose the rubber seal of the device should be disinfected, preferably with an alcohol spray, to prevent contamination of the contents by repeated needle insertions. Only solutions which are clear or slightly opalescent, colourless and practically free of visible particles may be injected.

As anaphylactoid reactions were observed in isolated cases, it is recommended that the first dose be administered under medical supervision. This product should only be used under consultant supervision usually in a hospital setting.

Treatment of anaemic patients with chronic renal failure: The reconstituted solution can be administered subcutaneously or intravenously. In the case of intravenous administration, the solution should be injected over approx. 2 minutes, e.g. in haemodialysis patients via the arterio-venous fistula at the end of dialysis.

For non-haemodialysed patients, subcutaneous administration should always be preferred in order to avoid puncture of peripheral veins.

The aim of treatment is to increase the packed cell volume to 30-35% whereby the weekly increase should be at least 0.5 vol.% A value of 35% should not be exceeded.

In the presence of hypertension or existing cardiovascular, cerebrovascular or peripheral vascular diseases, the weekly increase in the PCV and the target PCV should be determined individually taking into account the clinical picture. In some patients the optimum PCV may be below 30%.

Treatment with NeoRecormon 50,000 Multidose is divided into two stages.

Correction phase

Subcutaneous administration: The initial dosage is 3 x 20 IU/kg body weight and week. The dosage may be increased every 4 weeks by 3 x 20 IU/kg and week if the increase of the packed cell volume is not adequate (< 0.5% per week).

The weekly dose can also be divided into daily doses.

Intravenous administration: The initial dosage is 3 x 40 IU/kg per week. The dosage may be raised after 4 weeks to 80 IU/kg three times per week - and if further increments are needed they should be at 20 IU/kg, three times per week, at monthly intervals.

For both routes of administration, the maximum dose should not exceed 720 IU/kg and week.

Maintenance phase

To maintain a packed cell volume of between 30 and 35%, the dosage is initially reduced to half of the previously administered amount. Subsequently, the dose is adjusted at intervals of one or two weeks individually for the patient (maintenance dose).

Results of clinical studies in children have shown that, on average, the younger the patient, the higher the NeoRecormon 50,000 Multidose doses required. Nevertheless, the recommended dosing schedule should be followed as the individual response cannot be predicted.

Treatment with NeoRecormon 50,000 Multidose is normally a long-term therapy. It can, however, be interrupted, if necessary, at any time.

Treatment of patients with solid tumours: The reconstituted solution is administered subcutaneously, whereby the weekly dose can be divided into 3 to 7 single doses.

NeoRecormon 50,000 Multidose treatment is indicated if the haemoglobin value is ≤ 13 g/dl (8.1 mmol/l) at the start of chemotherapy. The recommended initial dose is 450 IU/kg body weight and week. If, after 4 weeks, a patient does not show a satisfactory response in terms of haemoglobin values then the dose should be doubled. The therapy should be continued for up to 3 weeks after the end of chemotherapy.

If haemoglobin falls by more than 1 g/dl (0.63 mmol/l) in the first cycle of chemotherapy despite concomitant NeoRecormon 50,000 Multidose therapy, further therapy may not be effective.

An increase in haemoglobin by more than 2 g/dl (1.25 mmol/l) per month or beyond 14 g/dl (8.8 mmol/l) should be avoided. If haemoglobin increases by more than 2 g/dl/month, the NeoRecormon 50,000 Multidose dose should first be reduced by 50%. If values exceed 14 g/dl (8.8 mmol/l) NeoRecormon 50,000 Multidose therapy should be interrupted until a value ≤ 12 g/dl (7.5 mmol/l) is achieved and then restarted with 50% of the previous weekly dose.

Treatment for increasing the amount of autologous blood: The reconstituted solution is administered intravenously over approx. 2 minutes or subcutaneously.

NeoRecormon 50,000 Multidose is administered twice weekly over 4 weeks. On those occasions where the patient's PCV allows blood donation, i.e. PCV ≥ 33%, NeoRecormon 50,000 Multidose is administered at the end of blood donation.

During the entire treatment period, a PCV of 48% should not be exceeded.

The dosage must be determined by the surgical team individually for each patient as a function of the required amount of pre-donated blood and the endogenous red cell reserve:

1 The required amount of pre-donated blood depends on the anticipated blood loss, use, if any, of blood conserving procedures and the physical condition of the patient. This amount should be that quantity which is expected to be sufficient to avoid homologous blood transfusions. The required amount of pre-donated blood is expressed in units whereby one unit in the nomogram is equivalent to 180 ml red cells.

2 The ability to donate blood depends predominantly on the patient's blood volume and baseline PCV. Both variables determine the endogenous red cell reserve, which can be calculated according to the following formula.

Endogenous red cell reserve = blood volume [ml] x (PCV - 33) ÷100

Women: blood volume [ml] = 41 [ml/kg] x body weight [kg] + 1200 [ml]

Men: blood volume [ml] = 44 [ml/kg] x body weight [kg] + 1600 [ml]

(body weight ≥ 45 kg)

The indication for NeoRecormon 50,000 Multidose treatment and, if given, the single dose should be determined from the required amount of pre-donated blood and the endogenous red cell reserve according to the following graphs.

The single dose thus determined is administered twice weekly over 4 weeks. The maximum dose should not exceed 1600 IU/kg b.w and week for intravenous or 1200 IU/kg and week for subcutaneous administration.

Contra-indications: NeoRecormon 50,000 Multidose must not be used in the presence of poorly controlled hypertension and known hypersensitivity to any of the constituents of NeoRecormon 50,000 Multidose or benzoic acid, a metabolite of benzyl alcohol.

In the indication 'increasing the yield of autologous blood', NeoRecormon 50,000 Multidose must not be used in patients who, in the month preceding treatment, have suffered a myocardial infarction or stroke, patients with unstable angina pectoris, or patients who are at risk of deep venous thrombosis such as those with a history of venous thromboembolic disease.

Special warnings and special precautions for use: NeoRecormon 50,000 Multidose should be used with caution in the presence of refractory anaemia with

Female patients
Required amount of pre-donated blood [units]

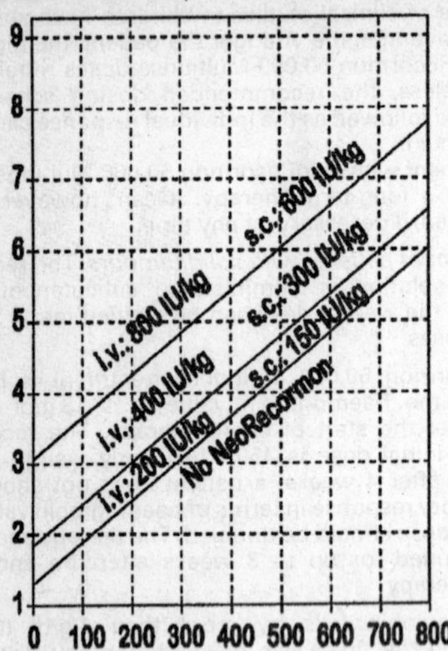

Endogenous red cell reserve [ml]

Male patients
Required amount of pre-donated blood [units]

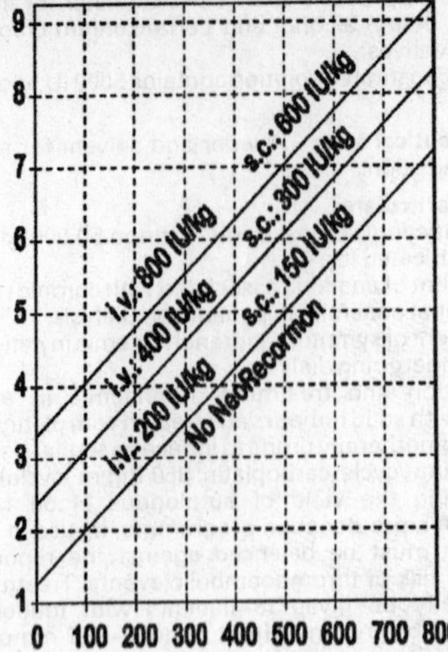

Endogenous red cell reserve [ml]

excess blasts in transformation, epilepsy, thrombocytosis, and chronic liver failure. Folic acid and vitamin B12 deficiencies should be ruled out as they reduce the effectiveness of NeoRecormon 50,000 Multidose.

Severe aluminum overload due to the treatment of renal failure may compromise the effectiveness of NeoRecormon 50,000 Multidose.

The indication for NeoRecormon 50,000 Multidose treatment of nephrosclerotic patients not yet undergoing dialysis should be defined individually as a possible acceleration of progression of renal failure cannot be ruled out with certainty.

Serum potassium levels should be monitored regularly during NeoRecormon 50,000 Multidose therapy. Potassium elevation has been reported in a few uraemic patients receiving NeoRecormon 50,000 Multidose, though causality has not been established. If an elevated or rising potassium level is observed then consideration should be given to ceasing NeoRecormon 50,000 Multidose administration until the level has been corrected.

For the use of NeoRecormon 50,000 Multidose in an autologous pre-donation programme, the official guidelines on principles of blood donation must be considered, in particular:

Only patients with a PCV ≥ 33% (haemoglobin ≥ 11 g/dl [6.9 mmol/l]) should donate;

Special care should be taken with patients below 50 kg weight;

The single volume drawn should not exceed approx. 12% of the patient's estimated blood volume.

Treatment should be reserved for patients in whom it is considered of particular importance to avoid homologous blood transfusion taking into consideration the risk/benefit assessment for homologous transfusions.

Misuse by healthy persons may lead to an excessive increase in packed cell volume. This may be associated with life-threatening complications of the cardiovascular system.

NeoRecormon 50,000 Multidose contains benzyl alcohol as a preservative. Benzyl alcohol has been reported to be associated with an increased incidence of complications in neonates, which are sometimes fatal.

Interaction with other medicaments and other forms of interaction: The clinical results obtained so far do not indicate any interaction of NeoRecormon 50,000 Multidose with other substances.

Animal experiments showed that epoetin beta does not increase the myelotoxicity of mitosis-inhibiting cytostatic drugs like etoposide, cisplatin, cyclophosphamide, and fluorouracil.

Use during pregnancy and lactation: Animal studies revealed that no teratogenic effects occurred under therapeutic conditions. However, NeoRecormon 50,000 Multidose should not be used during pregnancy and lactation, as at present insufficient clinical experience has been gained in these fields.

Effects on ability to drive and use machines: No special instructions are required.

Undesirable effects: Cardiovascular system

Anaemic patients with chronic renal failure: The most frequent adverse reaction during treatment with NeoRecormon 50,000 Multidose is an increase in blood pressure or aggravation of existing hypertension, especially in cases of rapid PCV increases. These increases in blood pressure can be treated with drugs. If blood pressure rises cannot be controlled by drug therapy, a transient interruption of NeoRecormon 50,000 Multidose therapy is recommended. Particularly at beginning of therapy regular monitoring of the blood pressure is recommended including between dialyses. Hypertensive crisis with encephalopathy-like symptoms (e.g. headaches and confused state, sensorimotor disorders - such as speech disturbance or impaired gait – up to tonic-clonic seizures) may occur, also in individual patients with otherwise normal or low blood pressure. This requires the immediate attention of a physician and intensive medical care. Particular attention should be paid to sudden stabbing migraine-like headaches as a possible warning signal.

Patients with solid tumours: Occasionally, there may be an increase in blood pressure, which can be treated with drugs. It is therefore recommended that blood pressure be monitored, in particular in the initial treatment phase. Headache may also occur occasionally.

Blood

Anaemic patients with chronic renal failure: There may be a moderate dose-dependent rise in the platelet count within the normal range during treatment with NeoRecormon 50,000 multidose, especially after intravenous administration. This regresses during the course of therapy. Development of thrombocytosis is very rare. It is recommended that the platelet count is regularly monitored during the first 8 weeks of therapy.

An increase in heparin dose during haemodialysis is frequently required during the course of therapy with NeoRecormon 50,000 Multidose as a result of the increased packed cell volume. Occlusion of the dialysis system is possible if heparinisation is not optimum.

Shunt thromboses may occur, especially in patients who have a tendency to hypotension or whose arteriovenous fistulae exhibit complications (e.g. stenoses, aneurysms). Early shunt revision and thrombosis prophylaxis by administration of acetylsalicylic acid, for example, is recommended in these patients.

In most cases, a fall in serum ferritin values simultaneously with a rise in the packed cell volume is observed. Therefore, oral iron substitution at 200-300 mg Fe^{2+}/day is recommended in all patients with serum ferritin values below 100μg/l or transferrin saturation below 20%. In addition, transient increases in serum potassium and phosphate levels have been observed in isolated cases. These parameters should be monitored regularly.

Patients with solid tumours: In some patients, a fall in iron parameters is observed. Therefore, oral iron substitution of 200-300 mg Fe^{2+}/day is recommended in all patients with serum ferritin values below 100 μg/l or transferrin saturation below 20%. Although no increase in the incidence of thromboembolic events has been observed in clinical trials, platelet counts should be monitored at regular intervals.

Patients in an autologous blood pre-donation programme: There may be an increase in platelet count, mostly within the normal range. Therefore, it is recommended that the platelet count is determined at least once a week. If there is an increase in the platelet count of more than 150 x 10^9/l or if platelets rise above the normal range, treatment with NeoRecormon 50,000 Multidose should be discontinued.

If there are indications of a temporary iron deficiency all patients should be treated orally with 300 mg Fe^{2+}/day from the start of NeoRecormon 50,000 Multidose treatment up to normalisation of ferritin values. If, despite oral iron substitution, iron deficiency (ferritin below or equal to 20μg/l or transferrin saturation below 20%) develops, the administration of intravenous iron should be considered.

Others: Anaphylactoid reactions have been observed in isolated cases.

Overdose: The therapeutic margin of NeoRecormon 50,000 Multidose is very wide. Even at very high serum levels, no symptoms of poisoning have been observed.

Pharmacological properties

Pharmacodynamic properties

Pharmaco-therapeutic group: antianaemic; ATC code: B03XA.

Epoetin beta is identical in its amino acid and carbohydrate composition to erythropoietin that has been isolated from the urine of anaemic patients.

Erythropoietin is a glycoprotein that stimulates the formation of erythrocytes from precursors of the stem cell compartment. It acts as a mitosis stimulating factor and differentiating hormone.

The biological efficacy of epoetin beta has been demonstrated after intravenous and subcutaneous administration in various animal models *in vivo* (normal and uraemic rats, polycythaemic mice, and dogs). After administration of epoetin beta, the number of erythrocytes, the Hb values and reticulocyte counts increase as well as the ^{59}Fe-incorporation rate.

An increased ^{3}H-thymidine incorporation in the erythroid nucleated spleen cells has been found *in vitro* (mouse spleen cell culture) after incubation with epoetin beta.

Investigations in cell cultures of human bone marrow cells showed that epoetin beta stimulates erythropoiesis specifically and does not affect leucopoiesis. Cytotoxic actions of epoetin beta on bone marrow or on human skin cells were not detected. Neither pre-clinical nor clinical investigations have shown any influence of epoetin beta on tumour progression.

After a single dose administration of epoetin beta no effects on the behaviour or locomotor activity of mice and circulatory or respiratory function of dogs were observed.

There are no indications of the development of neutralising antibodies to epoetin beta in humans.

Pharmacokinetic properties: Pharmacokinetic investigations in healthy volunteers and uraemic patients show that the half-life of intravenously administered epoetin beta is between 4 and 12 hours and that the distribution volume corresponds to one to two times the plasma volume. Analogous results have been found in animal experiments in uraemic and normal rats.

After subcutaneous administration of epoetin beta to uraemic patients, the protracted absorption results in a serum concentration plateau, whereby the maximum concentration is reached after an average of 12 - 28 hours. The terminal half-life is higher than after intravenous administration, with an average of 13 - 28 hours.

Bioavailability of epoetin beta after subcutaneous administration is between 23 and 42% as compared with intravenous administration.

Pre-clinical safety data

Acute toxicity: The single intravenous administration of 6000 IU/kg b.w epoetin beta in the dog and in doses of 3; 30; 300; 3000 or 30,000 IU/kg b.w in the rat did not lead to any detectable toxic damage.

Chronic toxicity: Toxic signs were not observed in 3 - month toxicity studies in rats with doses of up to 10,000 IU/kg b.w or in dogs with doses of up to 3000 IU/kg b.w administered daily either subcutaneously or intravenously, with the exception of fibrotic changes of the bone marrow which occurred if the PCV values exceeded 80%. A further study in dogs revealed that the myelofibrosis does not occur if the packed cell volume is kept below 60%. The observation of myelofibrosis is therefore irrelevant to the clinical situation in man.

Carcinogenicity: No effect of epoetin beta was observed on the proliferation of non-haematological normal or malignant cells *in vitro* or transplantable tumours *in vivo.* A carcinogenicity study with homologous erythropoietin in mice did not reveal any signs of proliferative or tumorigenic potential.

Mutagenicity: Epoetin beta did not reveal any genotoxic potential in the Ames test, in the micronucleus test, in the *in vitro* HGPRT test or in a chromosomal aberration test in cultured human lymphocytes.

Reproduction toxicology: Studies on rats and rabbits showed no relevant evidence of embryotoxic, fetotoxic or teratogenic properties. No alteration of fertility was detected. A peri-postnatal toxicity study revealed no adverse effects in pregnant/lactating females and on the development of conceptus and offspring.

Safety of preservatives: Subchronic and chronic toxicity studies have demonstrated a wide safety margin of the selected preservatives.

Pharmaceutical particulars

List of excipients: Urea, sodium chloride, polysorbate 20, sodium dihydrogen phosphate, sodium monohydrogen phosphate, calcium chloride, glycine, leucine, isoleucine, threonine, glutamic acid, phenylalanine. Preservatives: benzyl alcohol, benzalkonium chloride.

Incompatibilities: The following instructions must be observed to avoid incompatibility or loss of activity and to ensure preservation of the product over the period of use:
-Do not use any other solvent other than those supplied,
-Do not mix with other drugs,
-Do not use glass materials for injection. Use only plastic materials.

Shelf life: NeoRecormon 50,000 Multidose is stable for 2 years. The reconstituted solution is stable for 1 month if stored in a refrigerator.

Special precautions for storage: Before and after reconstitution NeoRecormon 50,000 Multidose must be stored at a temperature of +2°C to +8°C (in a refrigerator).

Lyophilisate and preserved solution: NeoRecormon 50,000 Multidose must be stored continuously by the wholesaler/pharmacist in a refrigerator at a temperature of between +2°C to +8°C.

The patient must also store the product continuously in a refrigerator at a temperature of between +2°C and +8°C. For the purpose of ambulatory use the product may be removed from such storage for one single period of a maximum of 5 days at room temperature (up to 25°C).

Reconstituted solution: Leaving the reconstituted solution outside the refrigerator should be limited to the time necessary for preparing the injections.

Nature and content of container: One vial with powder for injection and 1 ampoule with preserved solvent, 1 reconstitution and withdrawal device, 1 needle 21 G2, 1 disposable syringe (10 ml).

Instructions for use/handling: This is a multidose preparation from which different single doses can be withdrawn over a period of 1 month after reconstitution. To avoid the risk of contamination of the contents always observe aseptic techniques (i.e. use disposable sterile syringes and needles to administer each dose) and strictly follow the handling instructions below. Before withdrawing each dose disinfect the rubber seal of the withdrawal device with alcohol to prevent contamination of the contents by repeated needle insertions.

Preparation of NeoRecormon multidose solution

1. Take the vial with the freeze-dried substance out of the package. Write the date of reconstitution and expiry on the label (expiry is 1 month after reconstitution). Remove the plastic cap from the vial and disinfect the rubber seal with alcohol.
2. Take the reconstitution and withdrawal device (which allows sterile air exchange) out of the blister and remove the protective cover from the spike. Attach the device to the vial until the snap lock clicks home.
3. Put the green needle on the syringe contained in the package and remove the needle cover.
4. Hold the OPC (One-Point-Cut) ampoule with the blue point upwards. Shake or tap the ampoule to get any fluid in the stem back into the body of the ampoule. Take hold of the stem and snap off away from you. Withdraw all the solvent into the syringe.
5. Disinfect the rubber seal of the device with alcohol. Penetrate the seal with the needle to a depth of about 1cm and slowly inject the solvent into the vial. Then disconnect the syringe (with needle) from the device.
6. Swirl the vial gently until the powder has dissolved. Do not shake. Check that the solution is clear, colourless and practically free from particles.
7. Put the protective cap on the top of the device as shown in the picture.

Before and after reconstitution NeoRecormon 50,000 Multidose must be stored at +2°C to +8°C (refrigerator).

Preparation of a single injection

8. Before withdrawing each dose disinfect the rubber seal of the device with alcohol.
9. Place a 26G needle onto an appropriate single-use syringe (max.1 ml), remove the needle cover and insert the needle through the rubber seal of the device. Withdraw NeoRecormon solution into the syringe, expel air from the syringe into the vial and adjust the amount of NeoRecormon solution in the syringe to the dose prescribed. Then disconnect the syringe (with needle) from the device.
10. Replace the needle by a new one (the new needle should have the size which you normally use for injections), remove the needle cover and carefully expel air from the needle by holding the syringe vertically and gently pressing the plunger upwards until a bead of liquid appears at the needle tip.
11. For subcutaneous injection, clean the skin at the site of injection using an alcohol wipe. Form a skin fold by pinching the skin between the thumb and the forefinger. Hold the syringe near to the needle and insert the needle into the skin with a quick, firm action. Inject NeoRecormon solution. Withdraw the needle quickly and apply pressure over the injection site with a dry sterile pad.

Number(s) in the community register of medicinal products NeoRecormon 50,000 Multidose: EU/1/97/031/0020.

Date of first authorisation/renewal of authorisation 16th July 1997

Date of revision of the text July 1997

NEORECORMON 10,000 FOR RECO-PEN ▼

Qualitative and quantitative composition 1 cartridge contains 10,000 international units (IU) corresponding to 83μg epoetin beta (recombinant human erythropoietin) as a powder for solution for injection and 1 ml solvent (water for injection with benzyl alcohol and benzalkonium chloride as preservatives).

Pharmaceutical form Powder and solvent for solution for injection.

Clinical particulars

Therapeutic indications: NeoRecormon 10,000 for Reco-Pen is indicated for:

- treatment of anaemia associated with chronic renal failure (renal anaemia) in patients on dialysis.
- treatment of symptomatic renal anaemia in patients not yet undergoing dialysis.
- prevention and treatment of anaemia in adult patients with solid tumours and treated with platinum-based chemotherapy prone to induce anaemia (cisplatin: 75 mg/m²/cycle, carboplatin: 350 mg/m²/cycle).
- increasing the yield of autologous blood from patients in a pre-donation programme. Its use in this indication must be balanced against the reported increased risk of thromboembolic events. Treatment should only be given to patients with moderate anaemia (Hb 10–13 g/dl [6.21–8.07 mmol/L], no iron deficiency), if blood conserving procedures are not available or insufficient when the scheduled major elective surgery requires a large volume of blood (4 or more units of blood for females or 5 or more units for males).

Posology and method of administration: Therapy with NeoRecormon 10,000 for Reco-Pen should be initiated by physicians experienced in the above mentioned indications.

NeoRecormon 10,000 for Reco-Pen is a two-chamber cartridge containing powder for solution for injection and preserved solution. The ready-to-use solution is prepared by inserting the cartridge into the Reco-Pen (for handling instructions see *Instructions for use/handling*). The reconstituted solution has a shelf-life of 1 month.

Only solutions which are clear or slightly opalescent, colourless and practically free of visible particles may be injected.

As anaphylactoid reactions were observed in isolated cases, it is recommended that the first dose be administered under medical supervision. This product should only be used under consultant supervision.

The prepared solution is administered subcutaneously.

Treatment of anaemic patients with chronic renal failure: The aim of treatment is to increase the packed cell volume to 30–35% whereby the weekly increase should be at least 0.5 vol%. A value of 35% should not be exceeded.

In the presence of hypertension or existing cardiovascular, cerebrovascular or peripheral vascular diseases, the weekly increase in the PCV and the target PCV should be determined individually taking into account the clinical picture. In some patients the optimum PCV may be below 30%.

Treatment with NeoRecormon 10,000 for Reco-Pen is divided into two stages.

Correction phase: The initial dosage is 3 x 20 IU/kg body weight and week. The dosage may be increased every 4 weeks by 3 x 20 IU/kg and week if the increase of packed cell volume is not adequate (< 0.5% per week).

The weekly dose can also be divided into daily doses.

The maximum dose should not exceed 720 IU/kg per week.

Maintenance phase: To maintain a packed cell volume of between 30 and 35%, the dosage is initially reduced to half of the previously administered amount. Subsequently, the dose is adjusted at intervals of one or two weeks individually for the patient (maintenance dose).

Results of clinical studies in children have shown that, on average, the younger the patient, the higher the NeoRecormon 10,000 for Reco-Pen doses required. Nevertheless, the recommended dosing schedule should be followed as the individual response cannot be predicted.

Treatment with NeoRecormon 10,000 for Reco-Pen is normally a long-term therapy. It can, however, be interrupted, if necessary, at any time.

Treatment of patients with solid tumours: The reconstituted solution is administered subcutaneously whereby the weekly dose can be divided into 3 to 7 single doses.

NeoRecormon 10,000 for Reco-Pen treatment is indicated if the haemoglobin value is ≤ 13 g/dl (8.1 mmol/l) at the start of chemotherapy. The recommended initial dose is 450 IU/kg body weight and week. If, after 4 weeks, a patient does not show a satisfactory response, in terms of haemoglobin values, then the dose should be doubled. The therapy should be continued for up to 3 weeks after the end of chemotherapy.

If haemoglobin falls by more than 1 g/dl (0.63 mmol/l) in the first cycle of chemotherapy despite concomitant NeoRecormon 10,000 for Reco-Pen therapy, further therapy may not be effective.

An increase in haemoglobin by more than 2 g/dl (1.25 mmol/l) per month or beyond 14 g/dl (8.8 mmol/l) should be avoided. If haemoglobin increases by more than 2 g/dl/month, the NeoRecormon 10,000 for Reco-Pen dose should first be reduced by 50%. If values exceed 14 g/dl (8.8 mmol/l) NeoRecormon 10,000 for Reco-Pen therapy should be interrupted until a value ≤ 12 g/dl (7.5 mmol/l) is achieved and then restarted with 50% of the previous weekly dose.

Treatment for increasing the amount of autologous blood: NeoRecormon 10,000 for Reco-Pen is administered twice weekly over 4 weeks. On those occasions where the patient's PCV allows blood donation, i.e. PCV ≥ 33%, NeoRecormon 10,000 for Reco-Pen is administered at the end of blood donation.

During the entire treatment period, a PCV of 48% should not be exceeded.

The dosage must be determined by the surgical team individually for each patient as a function of the required amount of predonated blood and the endogenous red cell reserve:

1. The required amount of predonated blood depends on the anticipated blood loss, use, if any, of blood conserving procedures and the physical condition of the patient. This amount should be that quantity which is expected to be sufficient to avoid homologous blood transfusions. The required amount of predonated blood is expressed in units whereby one unit in the nomogram is equivalent to 180 ml red cells.

2. The ability to donate blood depends predominantly on the patient's blood volume and baseline PCV. Both variables determine the endogenous red cell reserve, which can be calculated according to the following formula.

Endogenous red cell reserve = blood volume [ml] x (PCV–33) ÷100

Women: blood volume [ml] = 41 [ml/kg] x body weight [kg] + 1200 [ml]

Men:blood volume [ml] = 44 [ml/kg] x body weight [kg] + 1600 [ml]

(body weight ≥ 45 kg)

The indication for NeoRecormon 10,000 for Reco-Pen treatment and, if given, the single dose should be determined from the required amount of predonated blood and the endogenous red cell reserve according to the following graphs. The single dose thus determined is administered twice weekly over 4 weeks. The maximum dose should not exceed 1200 IU/kg b.w. per week.

Contra-indications: NeoRecormon 10,000 for Reco-Pen must not be used in the presence of poorly controllable hypertension, known hypersensitivity to any of the constituents of NeoRecormon 10,000 for Reco-Pen or benzoic acid, a metabolite of benzyl alcohol.

In the indication 'increasing the yield of autologous blood', NeoRecormon 10,000 for Reco-Pen must not be used in patients who, in the month preceding treatment, have suffered a myocardial infarction or stroke, patients with unstable angina pectoris, or patients who are at risk of deep venous thrombosis such as those with a history of venous thromboembolic disease.

Special warnings and special precautions for use: NeoRecormon 10,000 for Reco-Pen should be used with caution in the presence of refractory anaemia with excess blasts in transformation, epilepsy, thrombocytosis, and chronic liver failure. Folic acid and vitamin B12 deficiencies should be ruled out as they reduce the effectiveness of NeoRecormon 10,000 for Reco-Pen.

Severe aluminium overload due to the treatment of renal failure may compromise the effectiveness of NeoRecormon 10,000 for Reco-Pen.

The indication for NeoRecormon 10,000 for Reco-Pen treatment of nephrosclerotic patients not yet undergoing dialysis should be defined individually as a possible acceleration of progression of renal failure cannot be ruled out with certainty.

Serum potassium levels should be monitored regularly during NeoRecormon 10,000 for Reco-Pen therapy. Potassium elevation has been reported in a few uraemic patients receiving NeoRecormon 10,000 for Reco-Pen, though causality has not been established. If an elevated or rising potassium level is observed then consideration should be given to ceasing NeoRecormon 10,000 for Reco-Pen administration until the level has been corrected.

For the use of NeoRecormon 10,000 for Reco-Pen in an autologous predonation programme, the Official guidelines on principles of blood donation must be considered, in particular:

- only patients with a PCV ≥ 33% (haemoglobin ≥ 11 g/dl [6.9 mmol/l]) should donate;
- special care should be taken with patients below 50 kg weight;
- the single volume drawn should not exceed approx. 12% of the patient's estimated blood volume.

Treatment should be reserved for patients in whom it is considered of particular importance to avoid homologous blood transfusion taking into consideration the risk/benefit assessment for homologous transfusions.

Misuse by healthy persons may lead to an excessive increase in packed cell volume. This may be associated with life-threatening complications of the cardiovascular system.

NeoRecormon 10,000 for Reco-Pen contains benzyl alcohol as a preservative. Benzyl alcohol has been reported to be associated with an increased incidence of complications in neonates which are sometimes fatal.

Interactions with other medicaments and other forms of interaction: The clinical results obtained so far do not indicate any interaction of NeoRecormon 10,000 for Reco-Pen with other substances.

Animal experiments revealed that epoetin beta does not increase the myelotoxicity of mitosis-inhibiting cytostatic drugs like etoposide, cisplatin, cyclophosphamide, and fluorouracil.

Pregnancy and lactation: Animal studies revealed that no teratogenic effects occur under therapeutic conditions. However, NeoRecormon 10,000 for Reco-Pen should not be used during pregnancy and lactation, as at present insufficient clinical experience has been gained in these fields.

Effects on ability to drive and use machines: No special instructions are required.

Undesirable effects: Cardiovascular system:

Anaemic patients with chronic renal failure: The most frequent adverse reaction during treatment with NeoRecormon 10,000 for Reco-Pen is an increase in blood pressure or aggravation of existing hypertension, especially in cases of rapid PCV increase These increases in blood pressure can be treated with drugs. If blood pressure rises cannot be controlled by drug therapy, a transient interruption of NeoRecormon 10,000 for Reco-Pen therapy is recommended. Particularly at beginning of therapy, regular monitoring of the blood pressure is recommended, including between dialyses. Hypertensive crisis with encephalopathy-like symptoms (e.g. headaches and confused state, sensorimotor disorders–such as speech disturbance or impaired gait–up to tonic-clonic seizures) may occur, also in individual patients with otherwise normal or low blood pressure. This requires the immediate attention of a physician and intensive medical care. Particular attention should be paid to sudden stabbing migraine-like headaches as a possible warning signal.

Patients with solid tumours: Occasionally, there may be an increase in blood pressure which can be treated with drugs. It is therefore recommended to monitor blood pressure, in particular in the initial treatment phase. Headache may also occur occasionally.

Blood: Anaemic patients with chronic renal failure: There may be a moderate dose-dependent rise in the platelet count within the normal range during treatment with NeoRecormon 10,000 for Reco-Pen, especially after intravenous administration. This regresses during the course of therapy. Development of thrombocytosis is very rare. It is recommended that the platelet count is regularly monitored during the first 8 weeks of therapy.

An increase in heparin dose during haemodialysis is frequently required during the course of therapy with NeoRecormon 10,000 for Reco-Pen as a result of the increased packed cell volume. Occlusion of the dialysis system is possible if heparinisation is not optimum.

Shunt thromboses may occur, especially in patients who have a tendency to hypotension or whose arteriovenous fistulae exhibit complications (e.g. stenoses, aneurysms). Early shunt revision and thrombosis prophylaxis by administration of acetylsalicylic acid, for example, is recommended in these patients.

In most cases, a fall in serum ferritin values simultaneous with a rise in the packed cell volume is observed. Therefore, oral iron substitution of 200–300 mg Fe^{2+}/day is recommended in all patients with serum ferritin values below 100µg/l or transferrin saturation below 20%. In addition, transient increases in serum potassium and phosphate levels have been observed in isolated cases. These parameters should be monitored regularly.

Female patients
Required amount of pre-donated blood [units]

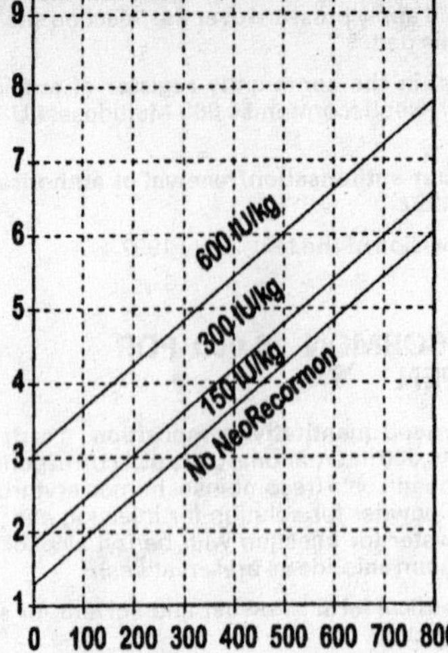

Endogenous red cell reserve [ml]

Male patients
Required amount of pre-donated blood [units]

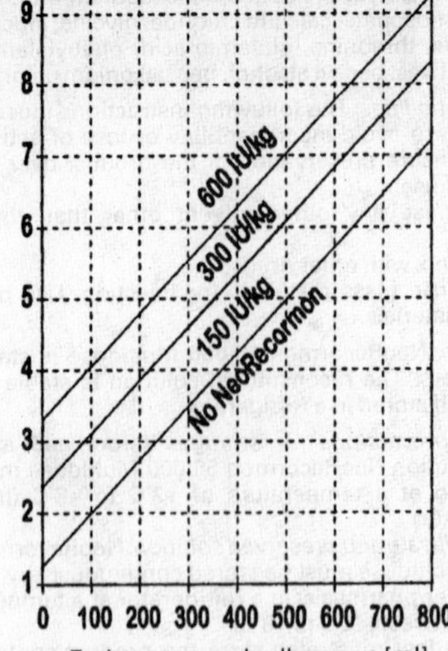

Endogenous red cell reserve [ml]

Patients with solid tumours: In some patients, a fall in serum iron parameters is observed. Therefore, oral iron substitution of 200–300 mg Fe^{2+}/day, is recommended in all patients with serum ferritin values below 100µg/l or transferrin saturation below 20%. Although no increase in the incidence of thromboembolic events has been observed in clinical trials, platelet counts should be monitored at regular intervals.

Patients in an autologous blood predonation programme: There may be an increase in platelet count, mostly within the normal range. Therefore, it is recommended that the platelet count is determined at least once a week. If there is an increase in platelets of more than 150 x 10^9/l or if platelets rise above the normal range, treatment with NeoRecormon 10,000 for Reco-Pen should be discontinued.

As there are indications of a temporary iron deficiency all patients should be treated orally with 300 mg Fe^{2+}/day from the start of NeoRecormon 10,000 for Reco-Pen treatment up to normalisation of ferritin values. If, despite oral iron substitution, iron deficiency (ferritin below or equal to 20µg/l or transferrin saturation below 20%) develops, the additional intravenous administration iron should be considered.

Others: Anaphylactoid reactions have been observed in isolated cases.

Overdose: The therapeutic margin of NeoRecormon 10,000 for Reco-Pen is very wide. Even at very high serum levels, no symptoms of poisoning have been observed.

Pharmacological properties

Pharmacodynamic properties: Pharmaco-therapeutic group: antianaemic; ATC code: B03XA

Epoetin beta is identical in its amino acid and carbohydrate composition to erythropoietin that has been isolated from the urine of anaemic patients.

Erythropoietin is a glycoprotein that stimulates the formation of erythrocytes from precursors of the stem cell compartment. It acts as a mitosis stimulating factor and differentiating hormone.

The biological efficacy of epoetin beta has been demonstrated after intravenous and subcutaneous administration in various animal models *in vivo* (normal and uraemic rats, polycythaemic mice, dogs). After administration of epoetin beta, the number of erythrocytes, the Hb values and reticulocyte counts increase as well as the ^{59}Fe-incorporation rate.

An increased ^{3}H-thymidine incorporation in the erythroid nucleated spleen cells has been found *in vitro* (mouse spleen cell culture) after incubation with epoetin beta.

Investigations in cell cultures of human bone marrow cells showed that epoetin beta stimulates erythropoiesis specifically and does not affect leucopoiesis. Cytotoxic actions of epoetin beta on bone marrow or on human skin cells were not detected. Neither preclinical nor clinical investigations have shown any influence of epoetin beta on tumour progression.

After a single dose administration of epoetin beta no effects on the behaviour or locomotor activity of mice and circulatory or respiratory function of dogs were observed.

There are no indications of development of neutralising antibodies to epoetin beta in humans.

Pharmacokinetic properties: After subcutaneous administration of epoetin beta to uraemic patients, the protracted absorption results in a serum concentration plateau, whereby the maximum concentration is reached after an average of 12–28 hours. The terminal half-life is higher than after intravenous administration, with an average of 13–28 hours.

Bioavailability of epoetin beta after subcutaneous administration is between 23 and 42% as compared with intravenous administration.

Preclinical safety data: Acute toxicity: The single intravenous administration of 6000 IU/kg b.w. epoetin beta in the dog and in doses of 3; 30; 300; 3,000 or 30,000 IU/kg b.w. in the rat did not lead to any detectable toxic damage.

Chronic toxicity: Toxic signs were not observed in 3-month toxicity studies in rats with doses of up to 10,000 IU/kg b.w. or in dogs with doses of up to 3000 IU/kg b.w. administered daily either subcutaneously or intravenously, with the exception of fibrotic changes of the bone marrow which occurred if the PCV values exceeded 80%. A further study in dogs revealed that the myelofibrosis does not occur if the packed cell volume is kept below 60%. The observation of myelofibrosis is therefore irrelevant to the clinical situation in man.

Carcinogenicity: No effect of epoetin beta was observed on the proliferation of non-haematological normal or malignant cells *in vitro* or transplantable tumours *in vivo*. A carcinogenicity study with homologous erythropoietin in mice did not reveal any signs of proliferative or tumorigenic potential.

Mutagenicity: Epoetin beta did not reveal any genotoxic potential in the Ames test, in the micronucleus test, in the *in vitro* HGPRT test or in a chromosomal aberration test in cultured human lymphocytes.

Reproduction toxicology: Studies on rats and rabbits showed no relevant evidence of embryotoxic, fetotoxic or teratogenic properties. No alteration of fertility was detected. A peri-postnatal toxicity study revealed no adverse effects in pregnant/lactating females and on the development of conceptus and offspring.

Safety of preservatives: Subchronic and chronic toxicity studies have demonstrated a wide safety margin of the selected preservatives.

Pharmaceutical particulars

List of excipients: Urea, sodium chloride, polysorbate 20, sodium dihydrogen phosphate, sodium monohydrogen phosphate, calcium chloride, glycine, leucine, isoleucine, threonine, glutamic acid, phenylalanine.

Preservatives: benzyl alcohol, benzalkonium chloride.

Incompatibilities: NeoRecormon 10,000 for Reco-Pen cartridges should only be used with the Reco-Pen.

Shelf life: NeoRecormon: 10,000 for Reco-Pen is stable for 2 years. The reconstituted solution is stable for 1 month if stored in a refrigerator.

Special precautions for storage: Before and after reconstitution NeoRecormon 10,000 for Reco-Pen must be stored at a temperature of +2°C to +8°C. (Refrigerator).

Cartridge: NeoRecormon 10,000 for Reco-Pen must be stored continuously by the wholesaler/pharmacist in a refrigerator at a temperature of between +2°C to +8°C.

The patient must also store the product continuously in a refrigerator at a temperature of between

+2°C and +8°C. For the purpose of ambulatory use the product may be removed from such storage for one single period of maximum 5 days at room temperature (up to 25°C).

Cartridge after insertion into the Reco-Pen: The cooling chain may only be interrupted for administration of the product.

Nature and contents of container: 1 or 3, two-chamber cartridges.

Instructions for use and handling as supplied with the Reco-Pen: The following instructions for use should be read before using NeoRecormon for Reco-Pen.

The Reco-Pen is an injection device for administering NeoRecormon for Reco-Pen. A two-chamber cartridge containing epoetin beta as a freeze-dried substance in one chamber and solvent (clear liquid) in the other chamber is placed in the pen. On assembling the pen, the closed system of the cartridge allows the solvent to flow into the chamber with the powder thus causing it to dissolve. The Reco-Pen with the solution is then ready for use, allowing safe and convenient administration of injections with high dosing accuracy. A single dose of 250 IU to 2500 IU can be administered in steps of 250 IU.

Preparing the pen for first use: Please ask your doctor or pharmacist to demonstrate the Reco-Pen before you use it for the first time.

1 Zero the Reco-Pen by lightly pressing the push button on the top. At the same time turn the push button anti-clockwise (in the opposite direction to that shown by the white arrow on the push button) until it will go no further.

2 Release the push button and slowly turn it clockwise until you hear a click.

3 Unscrew the Reco-Pen.

4 Take a sterile needle from the pack and remove the foil.

5 Thread the needle (still covered with the protective caps) onto the Reco-Pen and turn it until it will go no further.

6 Remove a cartridge from its packaging. Write the date of reconstitution and expiry on the cover inside of the carton (expiry is 1 month after reconstitution). Hold the push button section of the Reco-Pen with the push button pointing downwards and insert the cartridge with the chamber containing the solvent also pointing downwards.

7 Reassemble the Reco-Pen, taking care to hold the window section with the window uppermost as shown in the picture. Make sure that the two parts of the Reco-Pen are completely screwed together until the black dots are lined up. The thread on the pen is deliberately very long to ensure that the epoetin beta is mixed slowly and gently while the pen is being reassembled.

8 Gently tip the Reco-Pen upside down a few times until the solution in the window is clear and the powder has dissolved completely. This takes about 1 minute. Do not shake.

9 Remove the outer and inner protective caps from the sterile needle and set aside. Take care not to unscrew the needle from the Reco-Pen when removing the caps. Do not touch the needle.

10 To ensure that there is no air remaining in the cartridge, hold the Reco-Pen with the needle pointing upwards and tap gently on the window to ensure that air bubbles rise to the top. Slowly depress the push button completely. Liquid should appear at the tip of the needle.

If liquid does not appear, turn the push button clockwise one click in the direction of the white arrow, hold the Reco-Pen with the needle pointing upwards and again depress the push button completely. Large air bubbles should not be visible in the window. Replace the protective caps.

The Reco-Pen is now ready for use. If you are going to inject now, please follow the instructions under 'Setting the dose'. If you do not intend to inject immediately, unscrew the needle (if necessary using the outer protective cap) and dispose of it safely, place the outer protective cap on the Reco-Pen and place the Reco-Pen in a refrigerator.

Setting the dose: Before removing your Reco-Pen storage in the refrigerator, please wash your hands. Clean the rubber surface in the recess of the aluminium closure of the cartridge visible at the tip of the pen with an alcohol wipe. Attach a new needle to the Reco-Pen (already done when preparing for first use) as described in sections 4 and 5.

11 The dose-checking ring (red) is used to check that the right number of clicks has been set. To use the dose-checking ring, turn it so that the black mark between 0 and 4 is lined up with the white mark on the push button.

12 Set the dose prescribed by your doctor by turning the push button clockwise (in the direction indicated by the white arrow). Each click (i.e. quarter turn) corresponds to 250 IU epoetin beta (see table). The table shows the number of clicks required for each dose. Count the number of clicks and check that the white mark on the button is lined up correctly. If you turn the button too many clicks by accident, simply turn it back to the actual number required.

After injection, however, do not turn the button back.

The maximum obtainable single dose is 2500 IU, equivalent to 10 clicks. Do not turn the button by more than 10 clicks since this will result in spontaneous delivery of the excess dose.

When the cartridge is empty (after 40 clicks) you will notice resistance when you try to turn the button further. This indicates that further clicks cannot be set. Do not try to turn the button further otherwise the mechanism will lock and it will not be possible to insert a new cartridge.

Number of clicks	*Selected dose in IU NeoRecormon 10,000 for Reco-Pen*
1	250
2	500
3	750
4	1000
5	1250
6	1500
7	1750
8	2000
9	2250
10	2500

Giving the injection

13 Clean the injection site as shown by your doctor with an alcohol wipe. Remove the protective caps from the needle.

The Reco-Pen is now ready for use.

14 Pinch the skin firmly between your thumb and forefinger. Hold the Reco-Pen as shown and insert the needle into the skin with a quick, firm action. Inject the epoetin beta by slowly depressing the push button until it will go no further. Keep the push button pressed down for 2 to 3 seconds. Withdraw the needle quickly, pulling it straight out and apply pressure to the injection site with a dry gauze pad or cotton wool ball.

After each injection: Place the inner protective cap on the needle, remove it (if necessary using the outer protective cap) and dispose of it safely. The scale of the window section shows the number of remaining clicks (maximum 40). Use this to check on the scale that the correct amount of epoetin beta has been injected and that there is enough liquid left in the cartridge for the next injection. If the cartridge is empty, insert a new one as described in point 15.

Store the Reco-Pen in a refrigerator at + 2°C to + 8°C until the next injection.

Repeat points 11 to 14 at each injection.

Changing the cartridge

15 To change the cartridge first remove the needle. Then zero the Reco-Pen by lightly pressing the push button on the top. At the same time turn the button anti-clockwise (in the opposite direction to that shown by the white arrow on the push button) until it will go no further. Release the push button and slowly turn it clockwise until you hear a click.

16 Unscrew the two parts of the Reco-Pen and remove the empty cartridge. Take a sterile needle from the pack and remove the foil. Thread the needle (still covered with the protective caps) onto the Reco-Pen and turn it until it will go no further. Insert a new cartridge as described in points 5 and 10.

Maintenance: The Reco-Pen needs no maintenance. The exterior can be cleaned by wiping with a damp cloth.

Important note: If you drop the pen please check whether the cartridge is broken and whether the push button still works properly (can be turned and depressed). A damaged Reco-Pen should no longer be used.

Number(s) in the community register of medicinal products
NeoRecormon 10,000 for Reco-Pen (1 cartridge): EU/1/97/031/021
NeoRecormon 10,000 for Reco-Pen (3 cartridges): EU/1/97/031/022

Date of first authorisation/renewal of authorisation 16 July 1997

Date of revision of text July 1997

NEORECORMON SOLUTION FOR INJECTION IN PRE-FILLED SYRINGE ▼

Qualitative and quantitative composition 1 pre-filled syringe contains 500 international units (IU) corresponding to 4.15µg epoetin beta (recombinant human erythropoietin).

1 pre-filled syringe contains 1000 international units (IU) corresponding to 8.3µg epoetin beta (recombinant human erythropoietin).

1 pre-filled syringe contains 2000 international units (IU) corresponding to 16.6µg epoetin beta (recombinant human erythropoietin).

1 pre-filled syringe contains 3000 international units (IU) corresponding to 24.9µg epoetin beta (recombinant human erythropoietin).

1 pre-filled syringe contains 5000 international units (IU) corresponding to 41.5µg epoetin beta (recombinant human erythropoietin).

1 pre-filled syringe contains 10,000 international units (IU) corresponding to 83µg epoetin beta (recombinant human erythropoietin).

Pharmaceutical form Solution for injection. For subcutaneous or intravenous administration.

Clinical particulars

Therapeutic indications: Treatment of anaemia associated with chronic renal failure (renal anaemia) in patients on dialysis.

Treatment of symptomatic renal anaemia in patients not yet undergoing dialysis.

Prevention of anaemia of prematurity in infants with a birth weight of 750 to 1500 g and a gestational age of less than 34 weeks.

Prevention and treatment of anaemia in adult patients with solid tumours and treated with platinum- based chemotherapy prone to induce anaemia (cisplatin: 75 mg/m²/cycle, carboplatin: 350 mg/m²/cycle).

Increasing the yield of autologous blood from patients in a pre-donation programme. Its use in this indication must be balanced against the reported increased risk of thromboembolic events. Treatment should only be given to patients with moderate anaemia (Hb 10–13 g/dl [6.21- 8.07 mmol/l], no iron deficiency), if blood conserving procedures are not available or insufficient when the scheduled major elective surgery requires a large volume of blood (4 or more units of blood for females or 5 or more units for males).

Posology and method of administration: Therapy with NeoRecormon in pre-filled syringe should be initiated by physicians experienced in the above mentioned indications. As hypersensitivity reactions were observed in isolated cases, it is recommended that the first dose be administered under medical supervision.

The NeoRecormon prefilled syringe is ready for use. Only solutions which are clear or slightly opalescent, colourless and practically free of visible particles may be injected.

NeoRecormon in pre-filled syringe is a sterile but unpreserved product. Under no circumstances should more than one dose be administered per syringe.

Treatment of anaemic patients with chronic renal failure: The solution can be administered subcutaneously or intravenously. In the case of intravenous administration, the solution should be injected over approx. 2 minutes, e.g. in haemodialysis patients via the arterio-venous fistula at the end of dialysis.

For non-haemodialysed patients, subcutaneous administration should always be preferred in order to avoid puncture of peripheral veins.

The aim of treatment is to increase the packed cell volume to 30–35% whereby the weekly increase should be at least 0.5 vol%. A value of 35% should not be exceeded.

In the presence of hypertension or existing cardiovascular, cerebrovascular or peripheral vascular diseases, the weekly increase in the PCV and the target PCV should be determined individually taking into account the clinical picture. In some patients the optimum PCV may be below 30%.

Treatment with NeoRecormon in pre-filled syringe is divided into two stages.

1. Correction phase

Subcutaneous administration: The initial dosage is 3 x 20 IU/kg body weight per week. The dosage may be increased every 4 weeks by 3 x 20 IU/kg and week if the increase of packed cell volume is not adequate (< 0.5% per week).

The weekly dose can also be divided into daily doses.

Intravenous administration: The initial dosage is 3 x 40 IU/kg per week. The dosage may be raised after 4 weeks to 80 IU/kg three times per week–and if further increments are needed they should be at 20 IU/kg, three times per week, at monthly intervals.

For both routes of administration, the maximum dose should not exceed 720 IU/kg per week.

2. Maintenance phase

To maintain a packed cell volume of between 30 and 35%, the dosage is initially reduced to half of the previously administered amount. Subsequently, the dose is adjusted at intervals of one or two weeks individually for the patient (maintenance dose).

Results of clinical studies in children have shown that, on average, the younger the patient, the higher the NeoRecormon doses required. Nevertheless, the recommended dosing schedule should be followed as the individual response cannot be predicted.

Treatment with NeoRecormon in pre-filled syringe is normally a long-term therapy. It can, however, be interrupted, if necessary, at any time.

Prevention of anaemia of prematurity: The solution is administered subcutaneously at a dose of 3 x 250 IU/kg b.w. per week. Treatment with NeoRecormon in pre-filled syringe should start as early as possible, preferably by day 3 of life. Premature infants who have already been transfused by the start of treatment with NeoRecormon in pre-filled syringe are not likely to benefit as much as untransfused infants. The treatment should last for 6 weeks.

Treatment of patients with solid tumours: The solution is administered subcutaneously whereby the weekly dose can be divided into 3 to 7 single doses.

Treatment with NeoRecormon in pre-filled syringe is indicated if the haemoglobin value is ≤ 13 g/dl (8.07 mmol/l) at the start of chemotherapy. The recommended initial dose is 450 IU/kg body weight per week. If, after 4 weeks, a patient does not show a satisfactory response in terms of haemoglobin values, then the dose should be doubled. The therapy should be continued for up to 3 weeks after the end of chemotherapy.

If the haemoglobin level falls by more than 1 g/dl (0.62 mmol/l) in the first cycle of chemotherapy despite concomitant therapy with NeoRecormon in pre-filled syringe, further therapy may not be effective. An increase in haemoglobin by more than 2 g/dl (1.24 mmol/l) per month or beyond 14 g/dl (8.79 mmol/l) should be avoided. If haemoglobin increases by more than 2 g/dl/month, the NeoRecormon dose should first be reduced by 50%. If values exceed 14 g/dl (8.79 mmol/l) therapy with NeoRecormon in pre-filled syringe should be interrupted until a value ≤ 12 g/dl (7.45 mmol/l) is achieved and then restarted with 50% of the previous weekly dose.

Treatment for increasing the amount of autologous blood: The solution is administered intravenously over approx. 2 minutes or subcutaneously.

NeoRecormon in pre-filled syringe is administered twice weekly over 4 weeks. On those occasions where the patient's PCV allows blood donation, i.e. PCV ≥ 33%, NeoRecormon in pre-filled syringe is administered at the end of blood donation

During the entire treatment period, a PCV of 48% should not be exceeded.

The dosage must be determined by the surgical team individually for each patient as a function of the required amount of predonated blood and the endogenous red cell reserve:

1. The required amount of predonated blood depends on the anticipated blood loss, use, if any, of blood conserving procedures and the physical condition of the patient. This amount should be that quantity which is expected to be sufficient to avoid homologous blood transfusions. The required amount of predonated blood is expressed in units whereby one unit in the nomogram is equivalent to 180 ml red cells.

2. The ability to donate blood depends predominantly on the patient's blood volume and baseline PCV. Both variables determine the endogenous red cell reserve, which can be calculated according to the following formula.

Endogenous red cell reserve = blood volume [ml] x (PCV–33) ÷100
Women: blood volume [ml] = 41 [ml/kg] x body weight [kg] + 1200 [ml]
Men: blood volume [ml] = 44 [ml/kg] x body weight [kg] + 1600 [ml]
(body weight ≥ 45 kg)

The indication for treatment with NeoRecormon in pre-filled syringe and, if given, the single dose should be determined from the required amount of predonated blood and the endogenous red cell reserve according to the following graphs.

The single dose thus determined is administered twice weekly over 4 weeks. The maximum dose should not exceed 1600 IU/kg b.w. per week for intravenous or 1200 IU/kg per week for subcutaneous administration.

Contra-indications: NeoRecormon in pre-filled syringe must not be used in the presence of poorly controllable hypertension and known hypersensitivity to any of the constituents of the medication.

In the indication 'increasing the yield of autologous blood', NeoRecormon in pre-filled syringe must not be used in patients who, in the month preceding treatment, have suffered a myocardial infarction or stroke, patients with unstable angina pectoris, or patients who are at risk of deep venous thrombosis such as those with a history of venous thromboembolic disease.

Female patients
Required amount of pre-donated blood [units]

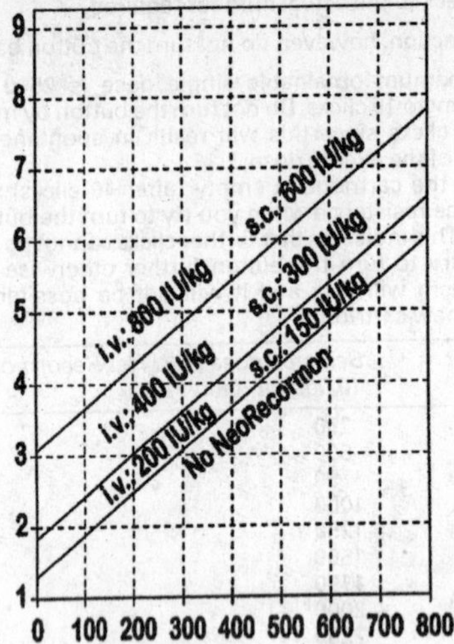

Endogenous red cell reserve [ml]

Male patients
Required amount of pre-donated blood [units]

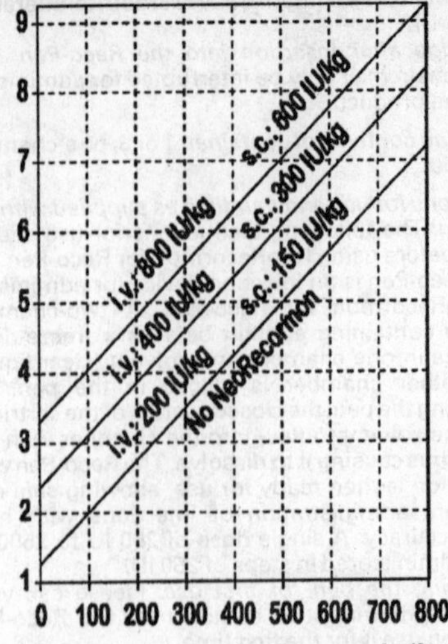

Endogenous red cell reserve [ml]

Special warnings and special precautions for use: NeoRecormon in pre-filled syringe should be used with caution in the presence of refractory anaemia with excess blasts in transformation, epilepsy, thrombocytosis, and chronic liver failure. Folic acid and vitamin B12 deficiencies should be ruled out as they reduce the effectiveness of NeoRecormon in pre-filled syringe.

Severe aluminium overload due to the treatment of renal failure may compromise the effectiveness of NeoRecormon in pre-filled syringe.

The indication for treatment with NeoRecormon in pre-filled syringe of nephrosclerotic patients not yet undergoing dialysis should be defined individually as a possible acceleration of progression of renal failure cannot be ruled out with certainty.

Serum potassium levels should be monitored regularly during therapy with NeoRecormon in pre-filled syringe. Potassium elevation has been reported in a few uraemic patients receiving NeoRecormon in pre-filled syringe, though causality has not been established. If an elevated or rising potassium level is observed then consideration should be given to ceasing administration of NeoRecormon in pre-filled syringe until the level has been corrected.

For the use of NeoRecormon in pre-filled syringe in an autologous predonation programme, the official guidelines on principles of blood donation must be considered, in particular:

only patients with a PCV ≥ 33% (haemoglobin ≥ 11 g/dl [6.83 mmol/l]) should donate;

special care should be taken with patients below 50 kg weight;

the single volume drawn should not exceed approx. 12% of the patient's estimated blood volume.

Treatment should be reserved for patients in whom it is considered of particular importance to avoid homologous blood transfusion taking into consideration the risk/benefit assessment for homologous transfusions.

Misuse by healthy persons may lead to an excessive increase in packed cell volume. This may be associated with life-threatening complications of the cardiovascular system.

Interaction with other medicaments and other forms of interaction: The clinical results obtained so far do not indicate any interaction of NeoRecormon in pre-filled syringe with other substances.

Animal experiments showed that epoetin beta does not increase the myelotoxicity of cytostatic drugs like etoposide, cisplatin, cyclophosphamide, and fluorouracil.

Use during pregnancy and lactation: Animal studies revealed that no teratogenic effects occur under therapeutic conditions. There is no adequate experience in human pregnancy and lactation. NeoRecormon in pre-filled syringe should only be used during pregnancy and lactation if the potential benefit justifies the potential risks.

Effects on ability to drive and use machines: NeoRecormon in pre-filled syringe has no effect on the ability to drive or operate machinery.

Undesirable effects: Cardiovascular system:

Anaemic patients with chronic renal failure: The most frequent adverse reaction during treatment with NeoRecormon in pre-filled syringe is an increase in blood pressure or aggravation of existing hypertension, especially in cases of rapid PCV increase These increases in blood pressure can be treated with drugs. If blood pressure rises cannot be controlled by drug therapy, a transient interruption of therapy with NeoRecormon in pre-filled syringe is recommended. Particularly at beginning of therapy regular monitoring of the blood pressure is recommended including between dialyses. Hypertensive crisis with encephalopathy-like symptoms (e.g. headaches and confused state, sensorimotor disorders–such as speech disturbance or impaired gait–up to tonic-clonic seizures) may occur, also in individual patients with otherwise normal or low blood pressure. This requires the immediate attention of a physician and intensive medical care. Particular attention should be paid to sudden stabbing migraine-like headaches as a possible warning sign.

Patients with solid tumours: Occasionally, there may be an increase in blood pressure which can be treated with drugs. It is therefore recommended to monitor blood pressure, in particular in the initial treatment phase. Headache may also occur occasionally.

Blood anaemic patients with chronic renal failure: There may be a moderate dose-dependent rise in the platelet count within the normal range during treatment with NeoRecormon in pre-filled syringe, especially after intravenous administration. This regresses during the course of continued therapy. Development of thrombocytosis is very rare. It is recommended that the platelet count is regularly monitored during the first 8 weeks of therapy.

An increase in heparin dose during haemodialysis is frequently required during the course of therapy with NeoRecormon in pre-filled syringe as a result of the increased packed cell volume. Occlusion of the dialysis system is possible if heparinisation is not optimum.

Shunt thromboses may occur, especially in patients who have a tendency to hypotension or whose arteriovenous fistulae exhibit complications (e.g. stenoses, aneurysms). Early shunt revision and thrombosis prophylaxis by administration of acetylsalicylic acid, for example, is recommended in these patients.

In most cases, a fall in serum ferritin values simultaneous with a rise in the packed cell volume is observed. Therefore, oral iron substitution at 200–300 mg Fe^{2+}/day is recommended in all patients with serum ferritin values below 100µg/l or transferrin saturation below 20%. In addition, transient increases in serum potassium and phosphate levels have been observed in isolated cases. These parameters should be monitored regularly.

Premature infants: In most cases, a fall in serum ferritin values is observed. Therefore, oral iron treatment should begin as early as possible (by day 14 of life at the latest) with 2 mg Fe^{2+}/day. Iron dosing should be modified according to the serum ferritin level. If serum ferritin is below 100µg/l or if there are other signs of iron deficiency, Fe^{2+} administration should be increased to 5–10 mg Fe^{2+}/day. Iron therapy should be continued until signs of iron deficiency disappear. As there may be a slight rise in platelet count, particularly up to day 12–14 of life, platelets should be monitored regularly.

Patients with solid tumours: In some patients, a fall in serum iron parameters is observed. Therefore, oral iron substitution of 200–300 mg Fe^{2+}/day, is recommended in all patients with serum ferritin values below 100µg/l or transferrin saturation below 20%. Although no increase in the incidence of thromboembolic events has been observed in clinical trials, platelet counts should be monitored at regular intervals.

Patients in an autologous blood predonation programme: There may be an increase in platelet count, mostly within the normal range. Therefore, it is recommended that the platelet count is determined at least once a week. If there is an increase in the platelets of more than 150 x 10^9/l or if platelets rise above the normal range, treatment with NeoRecormon in pre-filled syringe should be discontinued.

Patients in an autologous blood predonation programme have been reported to show a slightly higher frequency of thromboembolic events. However, a causal relationship with treatment with NeoRecormon in pre-filled syringe could not be established.

As there are indications of a temporary iron deficiency all patients should be treated orally with 300 mg Fe^{2+}/day from the start of treatment with NeoRecormon in pre-filled syringe up to normalisation of the ferritin values. If, despite oral iron substitution, iron deficiency (ferritin below or equal to 20µg/l or transferrin saturation below 20%) develops, the addition of intravenous administration of iron should be considered.

Others: Rarely, skin reactions such as rash, pruritus, urticaria or injection site reactions may occur. In isolated cases, anaphylactoid reactions have been reported. However, in controlled clinical studies no increased incidence of hypersensitivity reactions was found.

Overdose: The therapeutic margin of NeoRecormon in pre-filled syringe is very wide. Even at very high serum levels, no symptoms of poisoning have been observed.

Pharmacological properties

Pharmacodynamic properties: Pharmaco-therapeutic group: antianaemic; ATC code: B03XA

Epoetin beta is identical in its amino acid and carbohydrate composition to erythropoietin that has been isolated from the urine of anaemic patients.

Erythropoietin is a glycoprotein that stimulates the formation of erythrocytes from precursors of the stem cell compartment. It acts as a mitosis stimulating factor and differentiating hormone.

The biological efficacy of epoetin beta has been demonstrated after intravenous and subcutaneous administration in various animal models *in vivo* (normal and uraemic rats, polycythaemic mice, dogs). After administration of epoetin beta, the number of erythrocytes, the Hb values and reticulocyte counts increase as well as the ^{59}Fe-incorporation rate.

An increased ^{3}H-thymidine incorporation in the erythroid nucleated spleen cells has been found *in vitro* (mouse spleen cell culture) after incubation with epoetin beta.

Investigations in cell cultures of human bone marrow cells showed that epoetin beta stimulates erythropoiesis specifically and does not affect leucopoiesis. Cytotoxic actions of epoetin beta on bone marrow or on human skin cells were not detected. Neither preclinical nor clinical investigations have shown any influence of epoetin beta on tumour progression.

After a single dose administration of epoetin beta no effects on the behaviour or locomotor activity of mice and circulatory or respiratory function of dogs were observed.

There are no indications of the development of neutralising antibodies to epoetin beta in humans.

Pharmacokinetic properties: Pharmacokinetic investigations in healthy volunteers and uraemic patients show that the half-life of intravenously administered epoetin beta is between 4 and 12 hours and that the distribution volume corresponds to one to two times the plasma volume. Analogous results have been found in animal experiments in uraemic and normal rats.

After subcutaneous administration of epoetin beta to uraemic patients, the protracted absorption results in a serum concentration plateau whereby the maximum concentration is reached after an average of 12–28 hours. The terminal half-life is higher than after intravenous administration, with an average of 13–28 hours.

Bioavailability of epoetin beta after subcutaneous administration is between 23 and 42% as compared with intravenous administration.

Preclinical safety data:

Acute toxicity: The single intravenous administration of 6000 IU/kg b.w. epoetin beta in the dog and in doses of 3; 30; 300; 3000 or 30,000 IU/kg b.w. in the rat did not lead to any detectable toxic damage.

Chronic toxicity: Toxic signs were not observed in 3-month toxicity studies in rats with doses of up to 10,000 IU/kg b.w. or in dogs with doses of up to 3000 IU/kg b.w. administered daily either subcutaneously or intravenously, with the exception of fibrotic changes of the bone marrow which occurred if the PCV values exceeded 80%. A further study in dogs revealed that the myelofibrosis does not occur if the packed cell volume is kept below 60%. The observation of myelofibrosis is therefore irrelevant to the clinical situation in man.

Carcinogenicity: No effect of epoetin beta was observed on the proliferation of non-haematological normal or malignant cells *in vitro* or transplantable tumours *in vivo*. A carcinogenicity study with homologous erythropoietin in mice did not reveal any signs of proliferative or tumorogenic potential.

Mutagenicity: Epoetin beta did not reveal any genotoxic potential in the Ames test, in the micronucleus test, in the *in vitro* HGPRT test or in a chromosomal aberration test in cultured human lymphocytes.

Reproduction toxicology: Studies on rats and rabbits showed no relevant evidence of embryotoxic, fetotoxic or teratogenic properties. No alteration of fertility was detected. A peri-postnatal toxicity study revealed no adverse effects in pregnant/lactating females and on the development of conceptus and offspring.

Pharmaceutical particulars

List of excipients: Urea, sodium chloride, polysorbate 20, sodium dihydrogen phosphate, sodium monohydrogen phosphate, calcium chloride, glycine, leucine, isoleucine, threonine, glutamic acid, phenylalanine and water for injections.

Incompatibilities: To avoid incompatibility or loss of activity, do not mix with other drugs or infusion solutions.

Shelf life: NeoRecormon in pre-filled syringe is stable for 2 years.

Special precautions for storage: NeoRecormon in pre-filled syringe must be stored continuously by the wholesaler/pharmacist in a refrigerator at a temperature between 2°C to 8°C.

The patient must also store the product continuously in a refrigerator at a temperature of between 2°C and 8°C. For the purpose of ambulatory use the product may be removed from such storage for one single period of maximum 3 days at room temperature (up to 25°C).

Nature and contents of container

NeoRecormon 500 IU solution for injection in pre-filled solution: *One pack contains:* 1 or 6 pre-filled syringes with solution for injection and 1 or 6 needles 30G1/2.

NeoRecormon 1000 IU solution for injection in pre-filled syringes: *One pack contains:* 1 or 6 pre-filled syringes with solution for injection and 1 or 6 needles 26G1/2.

NeoRecormon 2000 IU solution for injection in pre-filled syringes: *One pack contains:* 1 or 6 pre-filled syringes with solution for injection and 1 or 6 needles 26G1/2.

NeoRecormon 3000 IU solution for injection in pre-filled syringes: *One pack contains:* 1 or 6 pre-filled syringes with solution for injection and 1 or 6 needles 26G1/2.

NeoRecormon 5000 IU solution for injection in pre-filled syringes: *One pack contains:* 1 or 6 pre-filled syringes with solution for injection and 1 or 6 needles 26G1/2.

NeoRecormon 10,000 IU solution for injection in pre-filled syringes: *One pack contains:* 1 or 6 pre-filled syringes with solution for injection and 1 or 6 needles 26G1/2.

Instructions for use/handling: First wash your hands.

1 Remove one syringe from the pack and check that the solution is clear, colourless and practically free from visible particles. Remove the cap from the syringe.

2 Remove one needle from the pack, fix it on the syringe and remove the protective cap from the needle.

3 Expel air from the syringe and needle by holding the syringe vertically and gently pressing the plunger upwards. Keep pressing the plunger until the amount of NeoRecormon in the syringe is as prescribed.

4 Clean the skin at the site of injection using an alcohol wipe. Form a skin fold by pinching the skin between thumb and forefinger. Hold the syringe barrel near to the needle, and insert the needle into the skin fold with a quick, firm action. Inject the NeoRecormon solution. Withdraw the needle quickly and apply pressure over the injection site with a dry, sterile pad.

Number(s) in the community register of medicinal products

NeoRecormon 500 IU solution for injection in pre-filled syringe: EU/1/97/031/025–026

NeoRecormon 1000 IU solution for injection in pre-filled syringe: EU/1/97/031/027–028

NeoRecormon 2000 IU solution for injection in pre-filled syringe: EU/1/97/031/029–0030

NeoRecormon 3000 IU solution for injection in pre-filled syringe: EU/1/97/031/031–032

NeoRecormon 5000 IU solution for injection in pre-filled syringe: EU/1/97/031/033–034

NeoRecormon 10,000 IU solution for injection in pre-filled syringe: EU/1/97/031/035–036

Date of first authorisation/renewal of authorisation 2 April 1998

Date of revision of the text 3 July 1998

NEOTIGASON

Qualitative and quantitative composition Capsules with brown cap and white body with ROCHE printed in black on both cap and body, containing 10 mg acitretin.

Capsules with brown cap and yellow body with ROCHE printed in black on both cap and body containing 25 mg acitretin.

Pharmaceutical form Capsules for oral administration.

Clinical particulars

Therapeutic indications: Severe extensive psoriasis which is resistant to other forms of therapy.

Palmo-plantar pustular psoriasis.
Severe congenital ichthyosis.
Severe Darier's disease (keratosis follicularis).

Posology and method of administration: Neotigason capsules are for oral administration.

The capsules should be taken once daily with meals or with milk.

There is a wide variation in the absorption and rate of metabolism of Neotigason. This necessitates individual adjustment of dosage. For this reason the following dosage recommendations can serve only as a guide.

Adults: Initial daily dose should be 25 mg or 30 mg for 2 to 4 weeks. After this initial treatment period the involved areas of the skin should show a marked response and/or side-effects should be apparent. Following assessment of the initial treatment period, titration of the dose upwards or downwards may be necessary to achieve the desired therapeutic response with the minimum of side-effects. In general, a daily dosage of 25–50 mg taken for a further 6 to 8 weeks achieves optimal therapeutic results. However, it may be necessary in some cases to increase the dose up to a maximum of 75 mg/day.

In patients with Darier's disease a starting dose of 10 mg may be appropriate. The dose should be increased cautiously as isomorphic reactions may occur.

Therapy can be discontinued in patients with psoriasis whose lesions have improved sufficiently. Relapses should be treated as described above.

Patients with severe congenital ichthyosis and severe Darier's disease may require therapy beyond 3 months. The lowest effective dosage, not exceeding 50 mg/day, should be given.

Continuous use beyond 6 months is contra-indicated as only limited clinical data are available on patients treated beyond this length of time.

Elderly: Dosage recommendations are the same as for other adults.

Children: In view of possible severe side-effects associated with long-term treatment, Neotigason is contra-indicated in children unless, in the opinion of the physician, the benefits significantly outweigh the risks.

The dosage should be established according to bodyweight. The daily dosage is about 0.5 mg/kg. Higher doses (up to 1 mg/kg daily) may be necessary in some cases for limited periods, but only up to a maximum of 35 mg/day. The maintenance dose should be kept as low as possible in view of possible long-term side-effects.

Combination therapy: Other dermatological therapy, particularly with keratolytics, should normally be stopped before administration of Neotigason. However, the use of topical corticosteroids or bland emollient ointment may be continued if indicated.

When Neotigason is used in combination with other types of therapy, it may be possible, depending on the individual patient's response, to reduce the dosage of Neotigason.

Contra-indications: Neotigason is contra-indicated during pregnancy as it is a known human teratogen.

The use of Neotigason is contra-indicated in women who are breast feeding.

Neotigason is contra-indicated in patients with hepatic or renal impairment.

Rare cases of benign intracranial hypertension have been reported after Neotigason and after tetracyclines. Supplementary treatment with antibiotics such as tetracyclines is therefore contra-indicated.

Special warnings and special precautions for use: Neotigason is contra-indicated in women of child-bearing potential unless the following criteria are met:

1. Pregnancy has been excluded before instituting

therapy with Neotigason (negative pregnancy test within 2 weeks prior to therapy).

2. She starts Neotigason therapy only on the second or third day of the next menstrual cycle.

3. Having excluded pregnancy, any woman of childbearing potential who is receiving Neotigason must practice effective contraception for at least one month before treatment, during the treatment period and for at least 2 years following its cessation.

Even female patients who normally do not practice contraception because of a history of infertility should be advised to do so, while taking Neotigason.

4. Contraceptive measures must also be taken in the case of repeated courses of treatment.

5. Any pregnancy occurring during treatment with Neotigason, or in the 2 years following its cessation, carries a high risk of foetal malformation. Therefore, before instituting Neotigason the treating physician must explain clearly and in detail what precautions must be taken. This should include the risks involved and the possible consequences of pregnancy occurring during Neotigason treatment or in the 2 years following its cessation.

6. She is reliable and capable of understanding the risk and complying with effective contraception, and confirms that she has understood the warnings.

In view of the importance of the above precautions, Neotigason Patient Information Leaflets are available to doctors and it is strongly recommended that these be given to all patients.

Patients should not donate blood either during or for at least one year following discontinuation of therapy with Neotigason. Theoretically there would be a small risk to a woman in the first trimester of pregnancy who received blood donated by a patient on Neotigason therapy.

Acitretin has been shown to affect diaphyseal and spongy bone adversely in animals at high doses in excess of those recommended for use in man. Since skeletal hyperostosis and extraosseous calcification have been reported following long-term treatment with etretinate in man, this effect should be expected with acitretin therapy.

Since there have been occasional reports of bone changes in children, including premature epiphyseal closure, skeletal hyperostosis and extraosseous calcification after long-term treatment with etretinate, these effects may be expected with acitretin. Neotigason therapy in children is not, therefore, recommended. If, in exceptional circumstances, such therapy is undertaken the child should be carefully monitored for any abnormalities of musculo-skeletal development.

Any patients complaining of atypical musculoskeletal symptoms on treatment with Neotigason should be promptly and fully investigated to exclude possible acitretin-induced bone changes. If clinically significant bone or joint changes are found, Neotigason therapy should be discontinued.

The effects of UV light are enhanced by retinoid therapy, therefore patients should avoid excessive exposure to sunlight and the unsupervised use of sun lamps.

Liver function and blood lipids (fasting value) should be measured at the start of treatment, after the first month of administration and at 3 monthly intervals thereafter.

In diabetic patients, retinoids can alter glucose tolerance. Blood sugar levels should therefore be checked frequently at the beginning of the treatment period.

Patients should be warned of the possibility of alopecia occurring (see *Side-effects and adverse reactions*).

Interaction with other medicaments and other forms of interaction: Existing data suggest that etretinate is formed from acitretin after ingestion of alcoholic beverages. However, the formation of etretinate without concurrent alcohol intake cannot be excluded. Therefore the post-therapy contraception period in women of childbearing potential must be 2 years.

Patients should be instructed to avoid taking preparations containing high doses of Vitamin A, i.e. more than the recommended dietary allowance of 4,000–5,000 i.u. per day.

An increased risk of hepatitis has been reported following the concomitant use of methotrexate and etretinate. Consequently, the concomitant use of methotrexate and Neotigason should be avoided.

In concurrent treatment with phenytoin, it must be remembered that Neotigason partially reduces the protein binding of phenytoin. The clinical significance of this is as yet unknown.

Interaction studies show acitretin does not interfere with the anti-ovulatory action of the combined oral contraceptives.

Interactions between Neotigason and other substances (e.g. digoxin, cimetidine) have not been observed to date.

Pregnancy and lactation: Neotigason is contra-indicated during pregnancy as it is a known human teratogen.

The use of Neotigason is contra-indicated in women who are breast feeding.

Effects on ability to drive and use machines: None known.

Undesirable effects: Most of the clinical side-effects of Neotigason are dose-related and are usually well-tolerated at the recommended dosages. However, the toxic dose of Neotigason is close to the therapeutic dose and most patients experience some side-effects during the initial period whilst dosage is being adjusted. They are usually reversible with reduction of dosage or discontinuation of therapy.

The skin and mucous membranes are most commonly affected, and it is recommended that patients should be so advised before treatment is commenced. Dryness of the mucous membranes, sometimes with erosion, involving the lips, mouth, conjunctivae and nasal mucosa are seen. Dryness of the skin may be associated with scaling, thinning, erythema (especially of the face) and pruritus. Palmar and plantar exfoliation, epistaxis and epidermal fragility have been reported, as well as paronychia. Granulomatous lesions have occasionally been reported. Dryness of the conjunctivae may lead to mild-to-moderate conjunctivitis and result in intolerance of contact lenses; it may be alleviated by lubrication with artificial tears or topical antibiotics. Hair thinning and frank alopecia may occur, usually noted 4 to 8 weeks after starting therapy, and are reversible following discontinuation of Neotigason. Full recovery usually occurs within 6 months of stopping treatment in the majority of patients.

Rarely, patients may experience photosensitivity reactions.

Non-specific symptoms such as nausea, headache, malaise, drowsiness and sweating have been reported infrequently. Myalgia and arthralgia may occur and be associated with reduced tolerance to exercise.

Benign intracranial hypertension has been reported.

There have been occasional reports of decreased night vision during Neotigason therapy.

Maintenance treatment may result in hyperostosis and extraskeletal calcification, as observed in long-term systemic treatment with other retinoids.

A rise in serum levels of liver enzymes may occur. When significant, dosage reduction or discontinuation of therapy may be necessary. Jaundice and hepatitis have occurred rarely.

Elevation of serum triglycerides above the normal range has been observed, especially where predisposing factors such as a family history of lipid disorders, obesity, alcohol abuse, diabetes mellitus or smoking are present. The changes are dose-related and may be controlled by dietary means (including restriction of alcohol intake) and/or by reduction of dosage of Neotigason.

Overdose: Manifestations of acute Vitamin A toxicity include severe headache, nausea or vomiting, drowsiness, irritability and pruritus. Signs and symptoms of accidental or deliberate overdosage with Neotigason would probably be similar. They would be expected to subside without need for treatment.

Because of the variable absorption of the drug, gastric lavage may be worthwhile within the first few hours after ingestion.

Pharmacological properties

Pharmacodynamic properties: Retinol (Vitamin A) is known to be essential for normal epithelial growth and differentiation, though the mode of this effect is not yet established. Both retinol and retinoic acid are capable of reversing hyperkeratotic and metaplastic skin changes. However, these effects are generally only obtained at dosages associated with considerable local or systemic toxicity. Acitretin, a synthetic aromatic derivative of retinoic acid, has a favourable therapeutic ratio, with a greater and more specific inhibitory effect on psoriasis and disorders of epithelial keratinisation. The usual therapeutic response to acitretin consists of desquamation (with or without erythema) followed by more normal re-epithelialisation.

Acitretin is the main active metabolite of etretinate.

Pharmacokinetic properties: Following oral administration of Neotigason, peak plasma concentrations of acitretin are achieved within 1–6 hours then decline at least 10-fold by 24 hours. Peak levels of the 13-cis acitretin metabolite are lower than those of acitretin, but remain relatively unchanged throughout each dosage interval. During the terminal phase, acitretin and its 13-cis metabolite are interconverted; therefore both compounds are excreted with an elimination half-life of approximately 2 days. Acitretin is highly bound to plasma protein and is excreted via the bile and urine as polar metabolites. Bioavailability is enhanced by food.

IMPORTANT: Etretinate has been detected in the plasma of some patients treated with Neotigason. The levels seen are generally much lower than those occurring during etretinate (Tigason) therapy. Etretinate has a long elimination half-life (approximately 120 days) due to deposition in adipose tissue. Therefore, the 2 year post-therapy contraception period for etretinate is required following Neotigason therapy.

In a study with healthy volunteers, concurrent intake of a single dose of acitretin together with ethanol led to formation of etretinate.

Preclinical safety data: None stated.

Pharmaceutical particulars

List of excipients: Maltodextrin, sodium ascorbate, gelatin, purified water, microcrystalline cellulose, iron oxide black (E172), iron oxide yellow (E172), iron oxide red (E172), titanium dioxide (E171).

Incompatibilities: None.

Shelf life: Neotigason capsules have a shelf-life of 3 years.

Special precautions for storage: The recommended maximum storage temperature is 25°C. Store in a dry place.

Nature and contents of container: All aluminium blisters containing 56 capsules.

PVC/PE/PVDC (Triplex) blisters with aluminium cover foil containing 56 or 60 capsules.

Amber glass bottles with metal screw caps containing 30 or 100 capsules.

Instructions for use/handling: None.

Marketing authorisation numbers

PL 0031/0262 – 10mg capsules.
PL 0031/0263 – 25mg capsules.

Date of first authorisation/renewal of authorisation

8 June 1992

Date of (partial) revision of the text May 1998

PALFIUM

Qualitative and quantitative composition

In terms of the active ingredient: Palfium Tablets 5 mg: Each tablet contains 5 mg dextromoramide as dextromoramide tartrate BP.

Palfium Tablets 10 mg: Each tablet contains 10 mg dextromoramide as dextromoramide tartrate BP.

Pharmaceutical form

Palfium 5 mg tablet is a round, white tablet, scored on one side, for oral use.

Palfium 10 mg tablet is a round, peach tablet, scored on one side, for oral use.

Clinical particulars

Therapeutic indications: Palfium is indicated for the relief of severe pain in inoperable carcinoma and for the relief of other forms of severe and intractable pain.

Posology and method of administration

Adults: The initial dose should not exceed 5 mg. Subsequent doses will depend on the needs of the patient (severity of pain). In cases of severe pain, 10 mg palfium may be required, repeated as necessary to maintain analgesia. The dose required may be influenced by the patient's body weight. Regardless of body weight, however, not more than 20 mg should be given as a single dose. The dose frequency and total daily dosage may vary significantly and should be titrated according to the needs of the individual patient.

In post-operative pain, the initial dose of Palfium in the immediate post-operative period should be restricted, for example to 2.5 mg, as the patient may still be under the influence of circulating anaesthetic agents and pre-medications. For subsequent post-operative care, 5 mg three times daily as required is usually sufficient.

Elderly: A reduced dosage regime may be necessary in elderly patients, as the rate of metabolism of dextromoramide may be reduced.

Children: A paediatric dosage regime has not yet been established. Should the need arise to administer Palfium to a child, the initial dosage should be not more than 0.08 mg per kg of body weight.

Administration: Palfium is as effective orally as by injection, therefore the oral route of administration is preferred. Palfium tablets should be given before meals, if possible.

Contra-indications: Palfium should not be used in patients with respiratory depression or obstructive airways disease or in female patients during childbirth. It is also contra-indicated in patients receiving monoamine oxidase inhibitors and two to three weeks should be allowed to elapse before Palfium is administered to patients who have been treated with these agents.

Special warnings and special precautions for use: In cases where the rate of metabolism of dextromoramide may be reduced, such as in the elderly and in patients with hypothyroidism or chronic hepatic insufficiency, Palfium should be used with caution and it may be advisable to employ a reduced dosage regime.

Interaction with other medicaments and other forms of interaction: There are no known interactions with other medicaments, but Palfium should not be given with monoamine oxidase inhibitors, alcohol or other CNS depressants.

Pregnancy and lactation: There is no evidence from animal studies to suggest that Palfium is harmful to the foetus. As experience in human pregnancy is inadequate, Palfium is not recommended for use during pregnancy. Similarly, there is little experience of the use of Palfium in patients who are breast feeding and no information on excretion of dextromoramide in breast milk.

Effects on ability to drive and use machines: No special instructions are required. Palfium does not normally cloud consciousness or mental activity.

Undesirable effects: Palfium may give rise to dizziness and sweating, especially in the ambulant patient at the start of the treatment. This may be minimised by advising the patient to rest, preferably supine, for a short period after administration of the first few doses. Nausea and vomiting occur only rarely. Continued use of Palfium may lead to tolerance and addiction, as with other potent analgesics.

Overdose: In the event of oral overdose, gastric lavage may be useful in the first few hours after ingestion. If consciousness is impaired and respiration depressed a suitable antagonist such as naloxone may be administered using the appropriate dosage. The circulation should be maintained with intravenous infusion of plasma or suitable electrolyte solutions and assisted ventilation may be necessary until spontaneous breathing is restored.

Pharmacological properties

Pharmacodynamic properties: Dextromoramide is a potent analgesic.

Pharmacokinetic properties: No pharmacokinetic data are available.

Preclinical safety data: No carcinogenicity or teratogenicity studies have been conducted, however, there is no evidence from other animal studies to indicate that dextromoramide tartrate has a harmful effect.

Pharmaceutical particulars

List of excipients: Lactose, microfine cellulose, sodium starch glycollate, colloidal silicon dioxide, magnesium stearate. The 10 mg tablet also contains the colouring agent E110.

Incompatibilities: None known.

Shelf life: 5 years.

Special precautions for storage: None.

Nature and contents of container: PVC/Aluminium foil blister strip containing 20 tablets per strip. Each pack contains 60 tablets (3 x blister strips).

Instructions for use/handling: No special instructions are required for use/handling of the tablets.

Marketing authorisation numbers

Palfium Tablets 5 mg: PL 15722/0004

Palfium Tablets 10 mg: PL 15722/0005

Date of first authorisation/renewal of authorisation

PL 15722/0004: 1 January 1997

PL 15722/0005: 1 March 1997

Date of (partial) revision of the text May 1998

Legal status CD (Sch 2), POM

PALFIUM SUPPOSITORIES

Qualitative and quantitative composition

In terms of the active ingredient: Palfium Suppositories 10 mg: Each suppository contains 10 mg as dextromoramide tartrate BP.

Pharmaceutical form Palfium Suppositories 10 mg are light cream coloured suppositories for rectal administration.

Clinical particulars

Therapeutic indications: Palfium is indicated for the relief of severe pain in inoperable carcinoma and for the relief of other forms of severe and intractable pain.

Posology and method of administration

Adults: One suppository repeated in accordance with the needs of the patient.

Elderly: A reduced dosage regime may be necessary in elderly patients.

Children: Palfium suppositories are not recommended for use in children.

Contra-indications: Palfium should not be used in patients with respiratory depression or obstructive airways disease or in female patients during childbirth. It is also contraindicated in patients receiving monoamine oxidase inhibitors or within two to three weeks of discontinuation of monoamine oxidase inhibitors.

Special warnings and special precautions for use: Reduced dosage may be required in the elderly and in patients with hypothyroidism or hepatic insufficiency.

The labelling must include a warning that the product should not be swallowed.

Interaction with other medicaments and other forms of interaction: There are no known interactions with other medicaments, but Palfium should not be given with monoamine oxidase inhibitors, alcohol or other CNS depressants.

Pregnancy and lactation: There is no evidence from animal studies to suggest that Palfium is harmful to the foetus. As experience in human pregnancy is inadequate, Palfium is not recommended for use during pregnancy. Similarly, there is little experience of the use of Palfium in patients who are breast feeding and no information on excretion of dextromoramide in breast milk.

Effects on ability to drive and use machines: No information is available. Palfium does not normally cloud consciousness or mental activity.

Undesirable effects: Dizziness and sweating may occur, especially at the start of the treatment. Nausea and vomiting are rarely troublesome. Tolerance and dependence may occur.

Overdose: Not applicable.

Pharmacological properties

Pharmacodynamic properties: Dextromoramide is a potent analgesic.

Pharmacokinetic properties: No pharmacokinetic data are available. Based on the pharmacodynamics, it appears that therapeutic blood concentrations are achieved within 30–60 minutes of a rectal dose and that they persist for up to 4 hours.

Preclinical safety data: No carcinogenicity or teratogenicity studies have been conducted, however, there is no evidence from other animal studies to indicate that dextromoramide tartrate has a harmful effect.

Pharmaceutical particulars

List of excipients: Lactose, witepsol H15.

Incompatibilities: None known.

Shelf life: 5 years.

Special precautions for storage: Store in a dry place below 25°C.

Nature and contents of container: Preformed polythene-PVC laminate cavities in a cardboard carton; 10 suppositories per pack.

Instructions for use/handling: No special instructions are required for use/handling of the suppositories.

Marketing authorisation number PL 15722/0003

Date of first authorisation/renewal of authorisation

1 March 1997

Date of (partial) revision of text May 1998

Legal status POM

PULMOZYME

Pulmozyme (dornase alfa) contains the phosphorylated glycosylated recombinant protein human deoxyribonuclease 1.

Qualitative and quantitative composition The active ingredient in Pulmozyme is dornase alfa, which is similar to human DNase isolated from urine. Pulmozyme is a sterile solution for respiratory use at a concentration of 1000 U/ml (1 mg/ml), where 1 Genentech unit/ml = 1 µg/ml. The labelled protein concentration is based solely upon the anhydrous polypeptide content and does not include the mass contribution of the carbohydrate or phosphate.

Pharmaceutical form Pulmozyme is a sterile, clear, colourless solution for respiratory use and is administered by means of a compressed air-driven (jet) nebulizer. Each single-unit ampoule of Pulmozyme will deliver to the nebulizer chamber 2,500 U (2.5 mg) of the active ingredient, dornase alfa.

Clinical particulars

Therapeutic indications: Daily administration of Pulmozyme is indicated in the management of cystic fibrosis patients with an FVC of greater than 40% of predicted and over 5 years of age to improve pulmonary function.

Posology and method of administration: The recommended dose is 2,500 U (corresponding to 2.5 mg) dornase alfa once daily, i.e. inhale the contents of one ampoule of 2.5 ml solution undiluted.

Most patients gain optimal benefit from continuous daily use of Pulmozyme. Studies in which dornase alfa was given on an intermittent regimen indicate that improvement in pulmonary function rapidly subsides on cessation of therapy. Therefore patients should be instructed to take their medication every day.

For patients on Pulmozyme therapy who experience exacerbation of respiratory tract infection, administration of Pulmozyme can be safely continued.

Pulmozyme should be administered using a jet nebulizer. The patient should continue his/her standard regimen of chest physiotherapy. At present, no recommendation can be made as to the optimal time of day for administration of Pulmozyme.

Patients should continue to receive regular medical care when being treated with Pulmozyme. The safety and efficacy of daily administration has not yet been demonstrated in patients under the age of 5 years, or with FVC less than 40% of predicted. Some patients over the age of 21 years may benefit from twice daily therapy.

Contra-indications: Pulmozyme should not be administered to patients with known hypersensitivity to the product or its constituents.

Special warnings and special precautions for use: None.

Interaction with other medicaments and other forms of interaction: There are no known interactions. Pulmozyme should not be mixed with other drugs or solutions in the nebulizer (see *Incompatibilities*). Mixing of Pulmozyme with other drugs or solutions could lead to adverse structural and/or functional changes in Pulmozyme or the admixed compound.

Pulmozyme can be effectively and safely used in conjunction with standard cystic fibrosis therapies such as antibiotics, bronchodilators, digestive enzymes, vitamins, inhaled and systemic corticosteroids, and analgesics.

Pregnancy and lactation: The safety of Pulmozyme has not been established in pregnant women. Studies of dornase alfa in rabbits and rodents show no evidence of impaired fertility, teratogenicity, or effects on development. However, because animal reproduction studies are not always predictive of the human response, Pulmozyme should be used during pregnancy only if clearly needed.

It is not known whether Pulmozyme is excreted in human milk. Because many drugs are excreted in human milk, caution should be exercised when Pulmozyme is administered to a nursing woman. A study performed in lactating cynomolgus monkeys, in which high doses of dornase alfa were given by the intravenous route, low concentrations (<0.1% of the concentrations seen in the serum of pregnant cynomolgus), were measurable in the maternal milk. When used as directed, there is minimal systemic absorption of dornase alfa; little or no measurable concentrations of dornase alfa would be expected in human milk.

Effects on ability to drive and use machines: No effects on the patient's ability to drive and use machines have been reported.

Undesirable effects: Few patients experienced adverse events resulting in permanent discontinuation from dornase alfa, and the discontinuation rate was observed similarly between placebo (2%) and dornase alfa (3%).

In controlled clinical trials directly comparing dornase alfa [up to 2,500 U (2.5 mg) BID] to placebo for up to 6 months, most adverse events were the sequelae of the underlying lung disease. There was no significant difference in the incidence or frequency of adverse events when patients continued treatment for an additional 6 months of open-label therapy. Patients who experience adverse events common to cystic fibrosis can, in general, safely continue administration of Pulmozyme as evidenced by the high percentage of patients completing the clinical trials.

Adverse events frequently seen were pharyngitis (inflammation of the throat), chest pain and voice alteration (hoarseness). Occasionally, laryngitis (inflammation of the larynx), conjunctivitis and skin rash, with and without itchiness, were observed. Upon initiation of dornase alfa therapy, as with any aerosol, pulmonary function may decline and expectoration of sputum may increase.

There have been no reports of anaphylaxis attributed to the administration of dornase alfa. Skin rashes and urticaria have been observed, and have been mild and transient in nature. Less than 5% of patients treated with dornase alfa have developed antibodies to dornase alfa, and none of these patients have developed IgE antibodies to dornase alfa. Improvement in pulmonary function tests has still occurred even after the development of antibodies to dornase alfa.

Overdose: Pulmozyme overdosage has not been established. Single-dose inhalation studies in rats and monkeys at doses up to 180-fold higher than doses routinely used in clinical studies are well tolerated. Oral administration of dornase alfa in doses up to 200 mg/kg are also well tolerated by rats. In clinical studies, CF patients have received up to 20 mg dornase alfa BID for up to six days and 10 mg BID intermittently (2 weeks on/2 weeks off drug) for 168 days. Both dose regimens were shown to be well tolerated.

Pharmacological properties

Pharmacodynamic properties: Recombinant human DNase is a genetically engineered version of a naturally occurring human enzyme which cleaves extracellular DNA.

Retention of viscous purulent secretions in the airways contributes both to reduced pulmonary function and to exacerbations of infection. Purulent secretions contain very high concentrations of extracellular DNA, a viscous polyanion released by degenerating leukocytes, which accumulate in response to infection. *In vitro*, dornase alfa hydrolyses DNA in sputum and greatly reduces the viscoelasticity of cystic fibrosis sputum.

Pharmacokinetic properties: Inhalation studies conducted in rats and non-human primates show a low percentage of dornase alfa systemic absorption, <15% for rats and <2% for monkeys. Consistent with the results of these animal studies, dornase alfa administered to patients as an inhaled aerosol shows low systemic exposure.

Studies in rats and monkeys have shown that, following intravenous administration, dornase alfa was cleared rapidly from the serum. The initial volume of distribution was similar to serum volume in these studies.

Studies in rats indicate that, following aerosol administration the disappearance half-life of dornase alfa from the lungs is 11 hours. Absorption of dornase alfa from the gastrointestinal tract following oral administration to rats is negligible.

DNase is normally present in human serum. Inhalation of up to 40 mg of dornase alfa for up to 6 days did not result in a significant elevation of serum DNase concentration above normal endogenous levels. No increase in serum DNase concentration greater than 10ng/ml was observed. Following administration of 2,500 U (2.5 mg) of dornase alfa twice daily for 24 weeks, mean serum DNase concentrations were no different from the mean pre-treatment baseline value of 3.5±0.1ng/ml; suggesting low systemic absorption or accumulation.

Inhalation of 2,500 U (2.5 mg) dornase alfa results in a mean sputum concentration of dornase alfa of approximately 3 μg/ml within 15 minutes in CF patients. Concentrations of dornase alfa in sputum rapidly decline following inhalation.

No pharmacokinetic data are available in very young or geriatric animals.

Preclinical safety data: Following repeat-daily inhalation exposure for periods of up to 6 months, histopathologic evidence of mild, non-life threatening pulmonary changes were observed in rats and primates at doses to the lungs of 6 to 14 times the clinical dose. The pulmonary changes were reversible following cessation of treatment and were characterized in rodents primarily as an alveolitis and lymphoid hyperplasia. In primates, bronchiolitis and alveolitis were observed in addition to an eosinophilic infiltrate and the presence of hemosiderin-laden macrophages. The treatment-related pulmonary changes are primarily consistent with an expected host response to a foreign protein; evidence of an antibody response to dornase alfa was observed in both species. No evidence of anaphylaxis was observed, despite the presence of significant antibody titers.

High concentrations (up to 10 mg/ml) of dornase alfa in three *in vitro* (Ames, mouse lymphoma, clastogenesis in human PBL) and intravenous doses (up to 10 mg/kg) in one *in vivo* (mouse micronucleus) test systems were shown to be nonmutagenic.

No information regarding carcinogenic potential in animals is currently available. A 2-year inhalation study in rodents is in progress.

Pharmaceutical particulars

List of excipients: The following excipients are contained in a 2.5 ml single-use ampoule of Pulmozyme. Sodium Chloride EP, Calcium Chloride Dihydrate EP, Water for Injection(s) EP.

In this formulation, sodium chloride is used as a tonicity modifier, calcium chloride as a stabiliser, and water for injection(s) is the vehicle. Pulmozyme contains no preservatives; the nominal pH is 6.3.

Incompatibilities: Pulmozyme is an unbuffered aqueous solution and should not be diluted or mixed with other drugs or solutions in the nebulizer bowl. Mixing of this solution could lead to adverse structural and/or functional changes in Pulmozyme or the admixed compound.

Shelf life: Under recommended storage conditions of 2–8°C and protected from strong light, Pulmozyme is stable for up to 24 months.

Special precautions for storage: Pulmozyme should be stored in a refrigerator at 2–8°C and protected from strong light. Avoid exposure to excessive heat. A single brief exposure to elevated temperatures (less than or equal to 24 hours at up to 30°C) does not affect product stability.

Pulmozyme should not be used after the given expiry date.

Pulmozyme ampoules are for single administration only.

Nature and contents of container: Pulmozyme is supplied in single use, low density polyethylene plastic ampoules. The volume in each ampoule is 2.6±0.1 ml. Each ampoule will deliver 2.5 ml of Pulmozyme to the nebulizer chamber.

Instructions for use/handling: The recommended dose for use in patients is one 2,500 U (2.5 mg) single-use ampoule of Pulmozyme inhaled once per day using a recommended nebulizer. Most patients gain optimal benefit from continued daily use of Pulmozyme.

Pulmozyme is provided as a sterile solution for inhalation in single-unit ampoules. At present, only jet nebulizers have been shown to effectively deliver biochemically unaltered dornase alfa. The complete contents of a single ampoule should be placed in the bowl of a jet nebulizer/compressor system, such as the Hudson T Up-draft II/Pulmo-Aide, Airlife Misty/Pulmo-Aide, customised Respirgard/Pulmo-Aide, or Acorn II/Pulmo-Aide. Pulmozyme may also be used in conjunction with a reusable jet nebulizer/compressor system, such as the Pari LL/Inhalierboy, Pari LC/Inhalierboy or Master, Aiolos/2 Aiolos.

Current data indicate that ultrasonic nebulizers are unsuitable for delivery of Pulmozyme because they may inactivate Pulmozyme or have unacceptable aerosol characteristics.

The patient should follow the nebulizer and compressor manufacturers' instructions on the use and maintenance of this equipment.

Containment of the aerosol is not necessary.

Marketing authorisation number PL 0031/0335

Date of first authorisation/renewal of authorisation 12 January 1994

Date of (partial) revision of the text October 1996

RAPILYSIN 10 U ▼

Qualitative/quantitative composition in terms of the active ingredients 1 vial contains 0.56 g reteplase 10 U (INN).

1 prefilled syringe contains 10 ml water for injections.

Potency of reteplase is expressed in units (U) by using a reference standard which is specific for reteplase and is not comparable with units used for other thrombolytic agents.

Pharmaceutical form Powder and solvent for solution for injection.

Clinical particulars

Therapeutic indications: Thrombolytic therapy of acute myocardial infarction (AMI) (within 12 hours after the onset of AMI symptoms).

Posology and method of administration: Reteplase is supplied as a freeze-dried substance in vials. The lyophilizate is reconstituted with the contents of the accompanying syringe (see *Instructions for use and handling*). The reconstituted solution should be used immediately.

Treatment with reteplase should be initiated as soon as possible after the onset of AMI symptoms.

Reteplase is administered as a 10 U bolus dose followed by a second 10 U bolus dose 30 minutes later. Each bolus is administered as a slow intravenous injection over not more than 2 minutes.

The bolus injection is given via an intravenous line. Ensure that the injection is not mistakenly given paravenously. Only clear, colourless solutions should be injected. No other medication should be added to the injection solution.

Heparin and acetylsalicylic acid should be administered concomitantly with and following the administration of reteplase to reduce the risk of rethrombosis. The recommended heparin dose is 5000 I.U. given as a bolus injection prior to reteplase therapy followed by an infusion of 1000 I.U. per hour starting after the second reteplase bolus. Heparin should be administered for at least 24 hours, preferably for 48 (-72) hours, aiming to keep aPTT values 1.5 to 2 times normal.

The initial dose of acetylsalicylic acid prior to thrombolysis should be at least 250 mg (250–350 mg) followed by 75–150 mg/day at least until discharge.

Contra-indications: Because thrombolytic therapy increases the risk of bleeding, reteplase is contraindicated in the following situations:

- known haemorrhagic diathesis
- patients with current concomitant therapy with oral anticoagulants (e.g. warfarin sodium)
- intracranial neoplasm, arteriovenous malformation or aneurysm
- neoplasm with increased bleeding risk
- history of cerebrovascular accident
- recent (< 10 days) prolonged and vigorous external heart massage
- severe uncontrolled hypertension
- active peptic ulceration
- portal hypertension (oesophageal varices)
- severe liver or renal dysfunction
- acute pancreatitis, pericarditis, bacterial endocarditis
- diabetic haemorrhagic retinopathy or other haemorrhagic ophthalmic conditions
- within 3 months of severe bleeding, major trauma or major surgery (e.g. coronary artery bypass graft, intracranial or intraspinal surgery or trauma), obstetric delivery, organ biopsy, previous puncture of noncompressible vessels.

Special warnings and special precautions for use: Reteplase should be used by physicians experienced in the use of thrombolytic treatment and with the facilities to monitor that use.

Each patient being considered for therapy with reteplase should be carefully evaluated.

Bleeding: The most common complication encountered during reteplase therapy is bleeding. The concomitant use of heparin anticoagulation may contribute to bleeding. As fibrin is lysed during reteplase therapy, bleeding from recent puncture sites may occur. Therefore, thrombolytic therapy requires careful attention to all possible bleeding sites (including catheter insertion sites, arterial and venous puncture sites, cutdown sites and needle puncture sites). The use of rigid catheter as well as intramuscular injections and nonessential handling of the patient should be avoided during treatment with reteplase.

Should serious bleeding, in particular cerebral haemorrhage, occur any concomitant heparin should be terminated immediately. In addition, the second bolus of reteplase should not be given if the serious bleeding occurs before it is administered. In general, however, it is not necessary to replace the coagulation factors because of the relatively short half-life of reteplase. Most patients who have bleeding can be managed by interruption of thrombolytic and anticoagulant therapy, volume replacement and manual pressure applied to an incompetent vessel. Protamine should be considered if heparin has been administered within 4 hours of the onset of bleeding. In the patients who fail to respond to these conservative measures, judicious use of transfusion products may be indicated. Transfusions of cryoprecipitate, fibrinogen, fresh frozen plasma and platelets should be considered with clinical and laboratory reassessment after each administration. A target fibrinogen level of 1 g/l is desirable with cryoprecipitate or fibrinogen infusion.

In the following conditions, the risks of reteplase therapy may be increased and should be weighed against the anticipated benefits:

- cerebrovascular disease
- systolic blood pressure at entry > 160 mmHg
- recent gastrointestinal or genitourinary bleeding (within 10 days)
- high likelihood of left heart thrombus e.g. mitral stenosis with atrial fibrillation
- septic thrombophlebitis or occluded arteriovenous cannula at seriously infected site
- advanced age i.e. over 75 years old
- any other conditions in which bleeding constitutes a significant hazard or would be particularly difficult because of its location.

At present, insufficient data in patients with diastolic blood pressure > 100 mmHg prior to thrombolytic therapy are available for reteplase.

Arrhythmias: Coronary thrombolysis may result in arrhythmias associated with reperfusion. It is strongly recommended that antiarrhythmic therapy for bradycardia and/or ventricular tachyarrhythmias (e.g. ventricular tachycardia or fibrillation) is available when reteplase is administered.

Readministration: Since at present there is no experience with readministration of reteplase, readministration is not recommended. However, no antibody formation to the reteplase molecule has been observed.

If an anaphylactoid reaction occurs, the injection should be discontinued immediately and appropriate therapy should be initiated.

Use in children: Safety and effectiveness of reteplase in children have not been established. At present the administration of reteplase in children is not recommended.

Interaction with other medicaments and other forms of interaction: No formal interaction studies with reteplase and drugs commonly administered in patients with AMI have been performed. Retrospective analyses of clinical studies did not reveal any clinical relevant interactions with drugs used concomitantly with reteplase in patients with acute myocardial infarction. Heparin, vitamin K antagonists and drugs that alter platelet function (such as acetylsalicylic acid, dipyridamole) may increase the risk of bleeding if administered prior to, during or after reteplase therapy.

Attention should be paid to this effect especially during periods of low plasma fibrinogen (up to about 2 days after fibrinolytic therapy of AMI).

Use during pregnancy and lactation: No experience in pregnant women is available for reteplase. Except in life-threatening situations Rapilysin 10 U should not be used in pregnant women because animal studies have shown a risk of pregnancy loss; foetal effects have not been studied in animals and there are insufficient data on effects on postnatal development.

It is not known whether reteplase is excreted into breast milk. Breast milk should be discarded within the first 24 hours after thrombolytic therapy.

Effects on ability to drive and use machines: Not applicable.

Undesirable effects:
Haemorrhage: The most frequent adverse drug reaction associated with reteplase treatment is haemorrhage, predominantly at the injection site, occasionally as gastrointestinal, gingival or genitourinary bleeding; haemopericardium, retroperitoneal bleeding, cerebral haemorrhage, epistaxis, eye haemorrhage and ecchymosis were observed rarely (each in less than 1%). Systolic blood pressure over 160 mmHg before thrombolysis with reteplase was associated with greater risk for cerebral bleeding. Blood transfusions were required rarely.

Death and permanent disability are not uncommonly reported in patients who have experienced stroke (including intracranial bleeding) and other serious bleeding episodes.

Cardiovascular: As with other thrombolytic agents the following events have been reported as sequelae of myocardial infarction and/or thrombolytic administration:

- frequently: recurrent ischaemia/angina, hypotension and heart failure/pulmonary oedema
- occasionally: arrhythmias (e.g. AV block, atrial fibrillation/flutter, ventricular tachycardia/fibrillation, electromechanical dissociation (EMD)), cardiac arrest, cardiogenic shock and reinfarction
- rarely: mitral regurgitation, pulmonary embolism, other systemic embolism/cerebral embolism and ventricular septal defect.

These cardiovascular events can be life-threatening and may lead to death.

Nervous system: As with other thrombolytic agents, events related to the nervous system (e.g. epileptic seizure, aphasia, speech disorder, delirium, acute brain syndrome, agitation, confusion, depression, psychosis) have been reported in isolated cases. Ischaemic or haemorrhagic cerebrovascular events may be contributing or underlying conditions.

Hypersensitivity: As with other thrombolytic agents, hypersensitivity reactions (e.g. allergic reactions) have rarely been reported. Serious anaphylaxis/anaphylactoid reactions have been observed in isolated cases. Regarding reteplase, available evidence does not indicate an antibody-mediated origin of these hypersensitivity reactions.

Overdose: In the event of overdosage one might expect depletion of fibrinogen and other blood coagulation components (e.g. coagulation factor V) with a consequent risk of bleeding.

Should serious bleeding, in particular cerebral haemorrhage occur, any concomitant heparin should be terminated immediately. In addition, the second bolus of reteplase should not be given if the serious bleeding occurs before it is administered. In general, however, it is not necessary to replace coagulation factors because of the relatively short half-life of reteplase. Most patients who have bleeding can be managed by interruption of thrombolytic and anticoagulant therapy, volume replacement and manual pressure applied to an incompetent vessel. Protamine should be considered if heparin has been administered within 4 hours of the onset of bleeding. In patients who fail to respond to these conservative measures, judicious use of transfusion products may be indicated. Transfusions of cryoprecipitate, fibrinogen, fresh frozen plasma and platelets should be considered with clinical and laboratory reassessment after each administration. A target fibrinogen level of 1 g/l is desirable with cryoprecipitate or fibrinogen infusion.

Pharmacological properties
Pharmacodynamic properties: Pharmaco-therapeutic group: antithrombotic agent, ATC Code: B 01 A D.

Reteplase is a recombinant plasminogen activator which catalyses the cleavage of endogenous plasminogen to generate plasmin. This plasminogenolysis occurs preferentially in the presence of fibrin. Plasmin in turn degrades fibrin, which is the main component of the matrix of thrombi, thereby exerting its thrombolytic action.

Reteplase (10 + 10 U) dose dependently reduces plasma fibrinogen levels by about 60 to 80%. The fibrinogen level normalises within 2 days. As with other plasminogen activators a rebound phenomenon then occurs during which fibrinogen levels reach a maximum within 9 days and remain elevated for up to 18 days.

Reductions of plasma levels of plasminogen and α_2-antiplasmin normalise within 1 to 3 days. Coagulation factor V, clotting factor VIII, α_2-macroglobulin and C1-esterase inhibitor are only slightly reduced and normalise within 1 to 2 days. Plasminogen activator inhibitor (PAI-1) activity can be reduced to around zero but rapidly normalises within 2 hours showing a rebound phenomenon. Prothrombin activation fragment 1 levels and thrombin-antithrombin III-complexes increase during thrombolysis indicating thrombin production of which the clinical relevance is unknown.

A large comparative mortality trial (INJECT) in approx. 6000 patients showed that reteplase reduced the incidence of heart failure (secondary efficacy criterion) in a significant manner and was at least equally effective in terms of reducing mortality (primary efficacy criterion) when compared to streptokinase. In two clinical trials aiming primarily at patency (RAPID I and II) reteplase was associated with higher early patency rates (primary efficacy criterion), as well as with a lower incidence of heart failure (secondary efficacy criterion) than alteplase (3 hour and "accelerated" dosage regimes). A clinical trial in approximately 15000 patients comparing reteplase with the accelerated dose regimen of alteplase (GUSTO III) (2:1 randomisation reteplase:alteplase) did not show statistically different results for the primary endpoint of 30-day mortality (reteplase 7.47%, alteplase 7.23%, p = 0.61) or for the combined endpoint of 30-day mortality and non-fatal disabling stroke (reteplase 7.89%, alteplase 7.88%, p = 0.99). Overall stroke rates were 1.64% in the reteplase and 1.79% in the alteplase group. In the reteplase group, 49.4% of these strokes were fatal and 27.1% were disabling. In the alteplase group 33.0% were fatal and 39.8% were disabling.

Pharmacokinetic properties: Following intravenous bolus injection of 10 + 10 U in patients with acute myocardial infarction reteplase antigen is distributed in plasma with a dominant half-life ($t_{1/2}\alpha$) of 18 ± 5 min and eliminated with a terminal half-life ($t_{1/2}\beta$) of 5.5 hours ± 12.5 min at a clearance rate of 121 ± 25 ml/min. Reteplase activity is cleared from the plasma at a rate of 283 ± 101 ml/min, resulting in a dominant half-life ($t_{1/2}\alpha$) of 14.6 ± 6.7 min and a terminal half-life ($t_{1/2}\beta$) of 1.6 hours ± 39 min. Only minor amounts of reteplase were immunologically detected in the urine. Exact data of the main elimination routes for reteplase in humans are not available and the consequences of hepatic or renal insufficiency are not known. Experiments in rats indicate that the liver and the kidneys are the main organs of active uptake and lysosomal degradation.

Additional studies in human plasma samples *in vitro* suggest that complexation with C1-inactivator, α_2-antiplasmin and α_2-antitrypsin contributes to the inactivation of reteplase in plasma. The relative contribution of the inhibitors to inactivation of reteplase decreases as follows: C1-inactivator > α_2-antiplasmin > α_2-antitrypsin.

The half-life of reteplase was increased in patients with AMI as compared to healthy volunteers. An additional increase of half-life of activity in patients with myocardial infarction and severely impaired liver and renal function cannot be excluded, but no clinical data of pharmacokinetics of reteplase in these patients are available. Animal data show that, in cases of severely impaired renal function with a pronounced increase in serum creatinine and serum urea, an increase in half-life of reteplase has to be expected. Mild impairment of renal function did not significantly affect the pharmacokinetic properties of reteplase.

Preclinical safety data: Acute toxicity studies have been performed in rats, rabbits and monkeys and subacute toxicity studies were performed in rats, dogs and monkeys. The predominant acute symptom after single high doses of reteplase in rats and rabbits was transient apathy shortly after injection. In cynomolgus monkeys, the sedative effect ranged from slight apathy to unconsciousness, caused by a reversible dose-related drop in blood pressure. There was increased local haemorrhage at the injection site.

Sub acute toxicity studies did not reveal any unexpected adverse events. In dogs, repeated dosing of the human peptide reteplase led to immunologic-allergic reactions. Genotoxicity of reteplase was excluded by a complete battery of tests at different genetic end points *in vitro* and *in vivo.*

Pharmaceutical particulars
List of excipients: Tranexamic acid, di-potassium-hydrogen phosphate, phosphoric acid, sucrose, polysorbate 80.

Incompatibilities: None known to date.

Shelf life: Rapilysin 10 U vials have a shelf-life of 24 months.

When reconstituted as directed, the solution should be used immediately. Chemical stability has been proven for 4 hours.

Special precautions for storage: Rapilysin 10 U should be stored in the original pack at temperatures of 2°C to 25°C. Protect the lyophilizate during extended storage from exposure to light.

Nature and contents of container: 2 vials with powder for solution for injection. 2 syringes with solvent. 2 reconstitution devices and 2 needles 19G1.

Instructions for use/handling:

1. Use aseptic technique throughout.

Remove the protective flip-cap from the vial of Rapilysin 10 U and clean the rubber closure with an alcohol wipe.

2. Open the package containing the reconstitution spike, remove both protective caps from the reconstitution spike.

3. Insert the spike through the rubber closures into the vial of Rapilysin 10U.

4. Take the 10 ml syringe out of the package. Remove the tip cap from the syringe. Connect the syringe to the reconstitution spike and transfer the 10 ml of solvent into the vial of Rapilysin 10U.

5. With the reconstitution spike and syringe still attached to the vial, swirl the vial gently to dissolve the Rapilysin 10U powder. DO NOT SHAKE. The reconstituted preparation results in a clear, colourless solution.

6. Withdraw 10 ml of Rapilysin 10U solution back into the syringe. A small amount of solution may remain in the vial due to overfill.

7. Disconnect the syringe from the reconstitution spike and attach the sterile needle provided. The dose is now ready for intravenous administration.

Marketing authorisation number EU/1/96/018/001

Date of first authorisation/renewal of authorisation 29 August 1996

Date of (partial) revision of the text 5 October 1998

Legal status POM

RIVOTRIL AMPOULES

Qualitative and quantitative composition Each 1 mg/ml ampoule contains 1 mg of the active ingredient clonazepam.

Pharmaceutical form 2 × 1 ml ampoules for injection (active and diluent).

Clinical particulars
Therapeutic indications: Administered intravenously, Rivotril quickly controls status epilepticus in all clinical forms.

Posology and method of administration: Rivotril ampoules are for intravenous administration. For the treatment of status epilepticus, the dose and rate of administration are governed by the response of the patient.

Adults: 1 mg (one ampoule of active substance mixed with one ampoule of diluent) by slow intravenous injection.

Elderly: Care should be taken with the elderly.

Children: 0.5 mg (equivalent to half an ampoule of active substance mixed with half an ampoule of diluent) by slow intravenous injection.

Mode of administration: Intravenous injection of Rivotril should be into a large vein of the antecubital fossa. The injection should be given slowly – in adults, 1 mg over approximately 30 seconds. This will greatly diminish the rare possibility of hypotension or apnoea occurring. Nevertheless, facilities for resuscitation should always be available.

The contents of the diluent ampoule, which contains 1 ml Water for Injection Ph. Eur., *must* be added to the contents of the other ampoule, which contains 1 mg clonazepam in 1 ml, *immediately* before injection.

Rivotril ampoule solution may be diluted when given in intravenous infusions of saline or dextrose, such as are customary in the treatment of status epilepticus.

Thus, up to 3 mg (3 ampoules) in 250 ml of the following solutions is permissible:
Sodium Chloride Injection BP,
Dextrose Injection BP 5% and 10%,
Sodium Chloride and Dextrose Injection BP (0.45% sodium chloride and 2.5% dextrose).

This infusion dilution should be made up freshly and used within 12 hours. The active ingredient clonazepam can be absorbed on PVC. It is therefore recommended either glass containers be used or, if PVC infusion bags are used, that the mixture be infused straight-away over a period of no longer than 2 hours.

Maintenance of stability cannot be guaranteed when Rivotril ampoule solution is diluted.

Contra-indications: Patients with known sensitivity to

benzodiazepines; acute pulmonary insufficiency; respiratory depression.

Special warnings and special precautions for use: Rivotril should be used with caution in patients with chronic pulmonary insufficiency, or with impairment of renal or hepatic function, and in the elderly or the debilitated. In these cases dosage may need to be reduced.

As with all other anti-epileptic drugs, treatment with Rivotril even if of short duration, must not be abruptly interrupted, but must be withdrawn by gradually reducing the dose in view of the risk of precipitating status epilepticus. This precaution must also be taken when withdrawing another drug while the patient is still receiving Rivotril therapy.

In cases of loss or bereavement, psychological adjustment may be inhibited by benzodiazepines.

Interaction with other medicaments and other forms of interaction: Since alcohol can provoke epileptic seizures, irrespective of therapy, patients should be advised not to drink alcohol while under treatment. In combination with Rivotril, alcohol may modify the effects of the drug, compromise the success of therapy or give rise to unpredictable side-effects.

When Rivotril is used in conjunction with other anti-epileptic drugs, side-effects and toxicity may be more evident, particularly with hydantoins or phenobarbitone and combinations including them. This requires extra care in adjusting dosage in the initial stages of treatment. The combination of Rivotril and sodium valproate has, rarely, been associated with the development of absence status epilepticus. Although some patients tolerate and benefit from this combination of drugs, this potential hazard should be borne in mind when its use is considered.

Known inhibitors of hepatic enzymes, e.g. cimetidine, have been shown to reduce the clearance of benzodiazepines and may potentiate their action and known inducers of hepatic enzymes, e.g. rifampicin, may increase the clearance of benzodiazepines.

Pregnancy and lactation: There is little evidence as to the drug safety in human pregnancy nor is there evidence from animal work that it is completely free from hazard. The use of Rivotril during pregnancy or lactation should be avoided unless there are compelling reasons.

The administration of high doses or prolonged administration of low doses of benzodiazepines in the last trimester of pregnancy or during labour has been reported to produce irregularities in the foetal heart rate, and hypotonia, poor sucking and hypothermia in the neonate.

Effects on ability to drive and use machines: As a general rule, epileptic patients are not allowed to drive. Even when adequately controlled on Rivotril, it should be remembered that any increase in dosage or alteration in timings of dosage may modify patients' reactions, depending on individual susceptibility. If a patient is allowed to operate machinery, he should also be warned of these possible effects.

Undesirable effects: The side-effects observed consist of fatigue, somnolence, occasional muscular hypotonia and co-ordination disturbances. Such effects are usually transitory and disappear spontaneously as treatment continues or with dosage reduction. They tend to occur early in treatment and can be greatly reduced, if not avoided, by commencing with low dosages followed by progressive increases.

Rarely respiratory depression may occur with intravenous Rivotril, particularly if other depressant drugs have been administered.

In infants and small children, and particularly those with a degree of mental impairment, Rivotril may give rise to salivary or bronchial hypersecretion with drooling. Supervision of the airway may be required.

As with other benzodiazepines, isolated cases of blood dyscrasias and abnormal liver function tests have been reported.

Rivotril generally has a beneficial effect on behaviour disturbances in epileptic patients. In certain cases, paradoxical effects such as aggressiveness, irritability, agitation, psychotic disorders and activation of new types of seizures may be precipitated. If these occur, the benefit of continuing the drug should be weighed against the adverse effect. The addition to the regimen of another suitable drug may be necessary or, in some cases, it may be advisable to discontinue Rivotril therapy.

Although Rivotril has been given uneventfully to patients with porphyria, rarely it may induce convulsions in these patients.

Overdose: As with other benzodiazepine drugs, overdosage should not present undue problems of management or threat to life. Patients have recovered from overdoses in excess of 60 mg without special treatment. Severe somnolence with muscle hypotonia will be present. Treatment is symptomatic and may include the need to maintain an airway. Gastric lavage may be useful if performed soon after ingestion.

The value of dialysis has not been determined.

Overdosage in non-epileptic patients may be treated with Anexate, a specific IV antidote for use in emergency situations. Patients requiring such intervention should be monitored closely in hospital (see separate prescribing information).

The use of Anexate is not recommended in epileptic patients who have been receiving benzodiazepine treatment for a prolonged period. Although Anexate exerts a slight intrinsic anticonvulsant effect, its abrupt suppression of the protective effect of a benzodiazepine agonist can give rise to convulsions in epileptic patients.

If excitation occurs, barbiturates should not be used.

Pharmacological properties

Pharmacodynamic properties: Rivotril is a benzodiazepine derivative exhibiting marked anticonvulsant properties. These have been demonstrated in the many tests in animals which are employed to establish the anti-epileptic properties of a drug. Animal experiments and electroencephalographic studies in man have shown that Rivotril prevents generalisation of convulsive activity and raises the seizure threshold. In many cases, abnormal electroencephalograms become normal. Rivotril improves both focal seizures and primarily generalised attacks.

Pharmacokinetic properties: Rivotril is widely distributed, then eliminated with a half-life generally between one and two days. Clearance is by metabolism in the liver, by nitro-reduction to the corresponding amine, then acetylation. The metabolites are excreted mainly via the urine. Routine monitoring of plasma concentrations of Rivotril is of unproven value since this does not appear to correlate well with either therapeutic response or side-effects.

Preclinical safety data: There are no preclinical data of relevance to the prescriber.

Pharmaceutical particulars

List of excipients:

Active substance ampoule: Ethanol absolute, glacial acetic acid, benzyl alcohol, propylene glycol, nitrogen pure.

Diluent ampoule: Water for injections.

Incompatibilities: It is recommended that Rivotril is only diluted in accordance with instructions given under posology and method of administration.

Shelf life: 60 months.

Special precautions for storage: Rivotril ampoules (active and diluent) should be protected from light and stored below 30°C.

Nature and contents of container: 2 ml amber glass ampoules.

Twin pack: 1 active, 1 diluent.

Instructions for use/handling: None.

Marketing authorisation number PL 0031/0078R

Date of first authorisation/renewal of authorisation 20 February 1991

Date of (partial) revision of the text July 1997

RIVOTRIL TABLETS

Qualitative and quantitative composition

Rivotril 0.5 mg tablets: Round, dull pinkish-buff tablets with 0.5 imprinted on one face and two break bars on the other, containing 0.5 mg clonazepam.

Rivotril 2 mg tablets: Round, white tablets with 2 imprinted on one face and two break bars on the other, containing 2 mg clonazepam.

Pharmaceutical form Tablets for oral administration.

Clinical particulars

Therapeutic indications:

Tablets: All clinical forms of epileptic disease and seizures in infants, children and adults, especially absence seizures (petit mal) including atypical absence; primary or secondarily generalised tonic-clonic (grand mal), tonic or clonic seizures; partial (focal) seizures with elementary or complex symptomatology; various forms of myoclonic seizures, myoclonus and associated abnormal movements.

Posology and method of administration: The cross-scored 0.5 mg tablets facilitate the administration of lower daily doses in the initial stages of treatment.

Adults: Initial dosage should not exceed 1 mg/day. The maintenance dosage for adults normally falls within the range 4 to 8 mg.

Elderly: The elderly are particularly sensitive to the effects of centrally depressant drugs and may experience confusion. It is recommended that the initial dosage of Rivotril should not exceed 0.5 mg/day.

These are total daily dosages which should be divided into 3 or 4 doses taken at intervals throughout the day. If necessary, larger doses may be given at the discretion of the physician. The maintenance dose should be attained after 2 to 4 weeks of treatment.

Simultaneous administration of more than one antiepileptic drug is a common practice in the treatment of epilepsy and may be undertaken with Rivotril. The dosage of each drug may be required to be adjusted to obtain the optimum effect. If status epilepticus occurs in a patient receiving oral Rivotril, intravenous Rivotril may still control the status. Before adding Rivotril to an existing anticonvulsant regimen, it should be considered that the use of multiple anticonvulsants may result in an increase of undesired effects.

Infants and children: To ensure optimum dosage adjustment, children should be given the 0.5 mg tablets.

Initial dosage should not exceed 0.25 mg/day for infants and small children (1 to 5 years) and 0.5 mg/day for older children. The maintenance dosage normally falls within the ranges:

School children (5 to 12 years) 3 to 6 mg,
Small children (1 to 5 years) 1 to 3 mg,
Infants (0 to 1 year) 0.5 to 1 mg.

In some forms of childhood epilepsy, certain patients may cease to be adequately controlled by Rivotril. Control may be re-established by increasing the dose, or interrupting treatment with Rivotril for 2 or 3 weeks. During the interruption in therapy, careful observation and other drugs may be needed.

Mode of administration: Treatment should be started with low doses. If desired the total dose may be given at night for the first 4 days of treatment. The dose may be increased progressively until the maintenance dose suited to the individual patient has been found.

The dosage of Rivotril must be adjusted to the needs of each individual and depends on the individual response to therapy. The maintenance dosage must be determined according to clinical response and tolerance.

The daily dose should be divided into 3 equal doses. If doses are not equally divided, the largest dose should be given before retiring. Once the maintenance dose level has been reached, the daily amount may be given in a single dose in the evening.

Contra-indications: Patients with known sensitivity to benzodiazepines; or any of the drugs excipients; acute pulmonary insufficiency; severe respiratory insufficiency, sleep apnoea syndrome, myasthenia gravis, severe hepatic insufficiency.

Special warnings and special precautions for use: Rivotril should be used with caution in patients with chronic pulmonary insufficiency, or with impairment of renal or hepatic function, and in the elderly or the debilitated. In these cases dosage may need to be reduced.

As with all other antiepileptic drugs, treatment with Rivotril even if of short duration, must not be abruptly interrupted, but must be withdrawn by gradually reducing the dose in view of the risk of precipitating status epilepticus. This precaution must also be taken when withdrawing another drug while the patient is still receiving Rivotril therapy.

Rivotril may be used only with particular caution in patients with spinal or cerebellar ataxia, in the event of acute intoxication with alcohol or drugs and in patients with severe liver damage (e.g. cirrhosis of the liver).

Benzodiazepines should be used with extreme caution in patients with a history of alcohol or drug abuse.

In infants and small children Rivotril may cause increased production of saliva and bronchial secretion. Therefore special attention must be paid to maintaining patency of the airways.

The dosage of Rivotril must be carefully adjusted to individual requirements in patients with pre-existing disease of the respiratory system (e.g. chronic obstructive pulmonary disease) or liver and in patients undergoing treatment with other centrally acting medications or anticonvulsant (antiepileptic) agents (see *Interaction with other medicaments and other forms of interaction*).

Like all drugs of this type, Rivotril may, depending on dosage, administration and individual susceptibility, modify the patients reactions (e.g. driving ability, behaviour in traffic).

Patients with a history of depression and/or suicide attempts should be kept under close supervision.

In cases of loss or bereavement, psychological adjustment may be inhibited by benzodiazepines.

Interaction with other medicaments and other forms of interaction: Since alcohol can provoke epileptic seizures, irrespective of therapy, patients must under no circumstances drink alcohol while under treatment. In combination with Rivotril, alcohol may modify the effects of the drug, compromise the success of therapy or give rise to unpredictable side-effects.

When Rivotril is used in conjunction with other antiepileptic drugs, side-effects such as sedation and apathy, and toxicity may be more evident, particularly with hydantoins or phenobarbitone and combinations including them. This requires extra care in adjusting dosage in the initial stages of treatment. The combination of Rivotril and sodium valproate has, rarely, been associated with the development of absence status epilepticus. Although some patients tolerate and benefit from this combination of drugs, this potential hazard should be borne in mind when its use is considered.

Known inhibitors of hepatic enzymes, e.g. cimetidine, have been shown to reduce the clearance of benzodiazepines and may potentiate their action and known inducers of hepatic enzymes, e.g. rifampicin, may increase the clearance of benzodiazepines.

In concurrent treatment with phenytoin or primidone, a change, usually a rise in the serum concentration of these two substances has occasionally been observed.

Concurrent use of Rivotril and other centrally acting medications, e.g. other anticonvulsant (antiepileptic) agents, anaesthetics, hypnotics, psychoactive drugs and some analgesics as well as muscle-relaxants may result in mutual potentiation of drug effects. This is especially true in the presence of alcohol. In combination therapy with centrally-acting medications, the dosage of each drug must be adjusted to achieve the optimum effect.

Pregnancy and lactation: From preclinical studies it cannot be excluded that clonazepam possesses the possibility of producing congenital malformations. From epidemiological evaluations there is evidence that anticonvulsant drugs act as teratogens. However, it is difficult to determine from published epidemiological reports which drug or combination of drugs is responsible for defects in the new-born. The possibility also exists that other factors e.g. genetic factors or the epileptic condition itself may be more important than drug therapy in leading to birth defects. Under these circumstances, the drug should only be administered to pregnant women if the potential benefits outweigh the risk to the foetus.

During pregnancy, Rivotril may be administered only if there is a compelling indication. Administration of high doses in the last trimester of pregnancy or during labour can cause hypotonia, mild respiratory depression and poor sucking in the neonate. It should be borne in mind that both pregnancy itself and abrupt discontinuation of the medication can cause exacerbation of epilepsy. Although the active ingredient of Rivotril has been found to pass into the maternal milk in small amounts only, mothers undergoing treatment with this drug should not breastfeed. If there is a compelling indication for Rivotril, breastfeeding should be discontinued.

Infants born to mothers who took benzodiazepines chronically during the latter stages of pregnancy may have developed physical dependence and may be at some risk for developing withdrawal symptoms in the post-natal period.

Effects on ability to drive and use machines: As a general rule, epileptic patients are not allowed to drive. Even when adequately controlled on Rivotril, it should be remembered that any increase in dosage or alteration in timings of dosage may modify patients' reactions, depending on individual susceptibility. Even if taken as directed, clonazepam can slow reactions to such an extent that the ability to drive a vehicle or operate machinery is impaired. This effect is aggravated by consumption of alcohol. Driving, operating machinery and other hazardous activities should therefore be avoided altogether or at least during the first few days of treatment. The decision on this question rests with the patients physician and should be based on the patient's response to treatment and the dosage involved.

Undesirable effects: The side-effects observed consist of fatigue, muscle weakness, dizziness, ataxia, light-headedness, somnolence, occasional muscular hypotonia and co-ordination disturbances. Such effects are usually transitory and disappear spontaneously as treatment continues or with dosage reduction. They tend to occur early in treatment and can be greatly reduced, if not avoided, by commencing with low dosages followed by progressive increases.

Poor concentration, restlessness, confusion and disorientation have been observed. Anterograde amnesia may occur using benzodiazepines at therapeutic dosage, the risk increasing at higher dosages. Amnestic effects may be associated with inappropriate behaviour.

With certain forms of epilepsy, an increase in the frequency of seizures during long-term treatment is possible.

Depression may occur in patients treated with Rivotril, but it may be also associated with the underlying disease.

In rare cases, urticaria, pruritus, transient hairloss, pigmentation changes, nausea, epigastric symptoms, headache, decrease in sexual drive (loss of libido), impotence and urinary incontinence may occur. Isolated cases of reversible development of premature secondary sex characteristics in children (incomplete precocious puberty) have been reported. Allergic reactions and a very few cases of anaphylaxis have been reported to occur with benzodiazepines.

Particularly in long-term or high-dose treatment, reversible disorders such as a slowing or slurring of speech (dysarthria), reduced co-ordination of movements and gait (ataxia) and disorders of vision (double vision, nystagmus) may occur.

Rarely respiratory depression may occur with intravenous Rivotril, particularly if other depressant drugs have been administered. As a rule, this effect can be avoided by careful adjustment of the dose in individual requirements.

Use of benzodiazepines may lead to the development of physical and psychological dependence upon these products. The risk of dependence increases with dose and duration of treatment and is particularly-pronounced in predisposed patients with a history of alcoholism or drug abuse.

Once physical dependence has developed, abrupt termination of treatment will be accompanied by withdrawal symptoms. During long-term treatment, withdrawal symptoms may develop, especially with high doses or if the daily dose is reduced rapidly or abruptly discontinued. The symptoms include tremor, sweating, agitation, sleep disturbances and anxiety, headaches, muscle pain, extreme anxiety, tension, restlessness, confusion, irritability and epileptic seizures which may be associated with the underlying disease. In severe cases the following symptoms may occur: derealisation, depersonalisation. Hyperacusis, numbness and tingling of the extremities, hypersensitivity to light, noise and physical contact or hallucinations. Since the risk of withdrawal symptoms is greater after abrupt discontinuation of treatment, abrupt withdrawal of the drug should therefore be avoided and treatment – even if only of short duration – should be terminated by gradually reducing the daily dose.

In infants and small children, and particularly those with a degree of mental impairment, Rivotril may give rise to salivary or bronchial hypersecretion with drooling. Supervision of the airway may be required.

As with other benzodiazepines, isolated cases of blood dyscrasias and abnormal liver function tests have been reported.

Rivotril generally has a beneficial effect on behaviour disturbances in epileptic patients. In certain cases, paradoxical effects such as aggressiveness, excitability, nervousness, hostility, anxiety, sleep disturbances, nightmares, vivid dreams, irritability, agitation, psychotic disorders and activation of new types of seizures may be precipitated. If these occur, the benefit of continuing the drug should be weighed against the adverse effect. The addition to the regimen of another suitable drug may be necessary or, in some cases, it may be advisable to discontinue Rivotril therapy.

Although Rivotril has been given uneventfully to patients with porphyria, rarely it may induce convulsions in these patients.

Overdose: As with other benzodiazepine drugs, overdosage should not present undue problems of management or threat to life. Patients have recovered from overdoses in excess of 60 mg without special treatment. Severe somnolence with muscle hypotonia will be present. Treatment is symptomatic and may include the need to maintain an airway. Gastric lavage may be useful if performed soon after ingestion.

The symptoms of overdosage or intoxication vary greatly from person to person depending on age, bodyweight and individual response. They range from drowsiness and light-headedness to ataxia, somnolence and stupor, and finally to coma with respiratory depression and circulatory collapse. Serious sequelae are rare unless other drugs or alcohol have been taken concomitantly.

In the management of overdose it should be borne in mind, that multiple agents may have been taken. In addition to monitoring of respiration, pulse rate and blood pressure, IV fluid replacement with general supportive measures is indicated. Hypotension may be treated with sympathomimetic agents.

The value of dialysis has not been determined.

Overdosage in non-epileptic patients may be treated with Anexate, a specific IV antidote for use in emergency situations. Patients requiring such intervention should be monitored closely in hospital (see separate prescribing information).

Warning: The use of Anexate is not recommended in epileptic patients who have been receiving benzodiazepine treatment for a prolonged period. Although Anexate exerts a slight intrinsic anticonvulsant effect, its abrupt suppression of the protective effect of a benzodiazepine agonist can give rise to convulsions in epileptic patients.

If excitation occurs, barbiturates should not be used.

Pharmacological properties

Pharmacodynamic properties: Clonazepam exhibits pharmacological properties which are common to benzodiazepines and include anticonvulsive, sedative, muscle relaxing and anxiolytic effects. Animal data and electroencephalographic investigations in man have shown that clonazepam rapidly suppresses many types of paroxysmal activity including the spike and wave discharge in absences seizures (petit mal), slow spike wave, generalised spike wave, spikes with temporal or other locations as well as irregular spikes and waves.

Generalised EEG abnormalities are more readily suppressed by clonazepam than are focal EEG abnormalities such as focal spikes. Clonazepam has beneficial effects in generalised and focal epilepsies.

Pharmacokinetic properties: Absorption: Clonazepam is quickly and completely absorbed after oral administration of Rivotril. Peak plasma concentrations are reached in most cases within 1–4 hours after an oral dose. Bioavailability is 90% after oral administration.

Routine monitoring of plasma, concentrations of Rivotril is of unproven value since this does not appear to correlate well with either therapeutic response or side-effects.

Distribution: The mean volume of distribution of clonazepam is estimated at about 3 l/kg. Clonazepam must be assumed to cross the placental barrier and has been detected in maternal milk.

Metabolism: The biotransformation of clonazepam involves oxidative hydroxylation and reduction of the 7-nitro group by the liver with formation of 7-amino or 7-acetylamino compounds, which may be further conjugated. The main metabolite is 7-amino-clonazepam.

Within 4–10 days 50–70% of the total radioactivity of a radiolabeled oral dose of clonazepam is excreted in the urine and 10–30% in the faeces, almost exclusively in the form of free or conjugated metabolites. Less than 0.5% appears as unchanged clonazepam in the urine.

Elimination: The elimination half-life is between 20 and 60 hours (mean 30 hours).

Pharmacokinetics in special clinical situations: Based on kinetic criteria no dose adjustment is required in patients with renal failure.

Preclinical safety data: There are no preclinical data of relevance to the prescriber.

Pharmaceutical particulars

List of excipients: Lactose, Maize starch, Talc, Magnesium stearate, Deionised water, Dye iron oxide red E172, Dye iron oxide yellow E172.

Incompatibilities: There are no known incompatibilities with Rivotril tablets.

Shelf life: 60 months.

Special precautions for storage: Rivotril tablets should be protected from light.

Nature and contents of container: Rivotril tablets are available in plastic HDPE bottles with polyethylene snap closures, or amber glass bottles with aluminium screw closures. The bottles contain either 100 or 500 tablets.

Instructions for use/handling: There are no special instructions.

Marketing authorisation numbers
PL 0031/0076R
PL 0031/0077R

Date of first authorisation/renewal of authorisation
PL 0031/0076R 26 July 1983
PL 0031/0077R 26 July 1983

Date of (partial) revision of the text September 1998

ROACCUTANE

Qualitative and quantitative composition Pale red-violet and white capsules imprinted with "R5" in black containing 5 mg of isotretinoin.

Pale red-violet and white capsules imprinted with "ROA 20" in black containing 20 mg isotretinoin.

Pharmaceutical form Capsules.

Clinical particulars

Therapeutic indications: Roaccutane is indicated for the treatment of cystic and conglobate acne and severe acne which has failed to respond to an adequate course of systemic antimicrobial agent.

Posology and method of administration: It is recommended that Roaccutane capsules are given by, or under the supervision of, a consultant dermatologist. The therapeutic response to Roaccutane is dose-related and varies between patients. This necessitates individual adjustment of dosage according to the response of the condition and the patient's tolerance of the drug. In most cases complete or near-complete remission of acne is achieved with a 12- to 16-week course of treatment. It is recommended that repeat courses of treatment should not normally be given.

The daily dosage, to the nearest number of whole capsules, should be taken with food either as a single dose or in two divided doses during the day, whichever is more convenient.

Adults:

Initial dose: All patients initially should receive

Roaccutane 0.5 mg/kg body-weight daily for a period of four weeks, when their responsiveness to the drug will usually be apparent. Acute exacerbation of acne is occasionally seen during the initial period but this subsides, usually within 7–10 days, with continued treatment.

Subsequent dosages: Patients who show early improvement should continue to receive the initial dosage of 0.5 mg/kg body-weight daily for the remainder of the course.

In patients who show little or no initial improvement, and who are tolerating the drug well, dosage should be increased up to 1 mg/kg body-weight daily for the remainder of the course.

In patients who show intolerance to the initial dosage, treatment should be continued with a reduced dosage of 0.1 to 0.2 mg/kg body-weight daily.

Repeated courses of therapy are not normally indicated. With effective treatment, complete clearing of acne is usually achieved and prolonged remission ensues. However, patients whose acne is not completely cleared at the end of treatment can be expected to show continuing improvement for up to several months thereafter. Only if a definite relapse is seen in the post-treatment period should a repeated course be considered.

Concomitant therapy: As a rule, other treatments conventionally used for the treatment of acne, including antibiotics, keratolytics and exfoliants, are not indicated but non-irritant topical preparations may be applied if required.

Elderly: Dosage as for other adults. Older subjects may have a greater risk of drug-induced arthralgia.

Children: Roaccutane is not indicated for the treatment of prepubertal acne.

Roaccutane capsules are for oral administration.

Contra-indications: Hypersensitivity reactions may occur in susceptible individuals. Use of this drug in patients with a known hypersensitivity to isotretinoin and any of the excipients is contra-indicated.

Roaccutane is contra-indicated in hepatic and renal impairment. It should not be given to breast-feeding mothers. Roaccutane is also contra-indicated in hypervitaminosis A, hyperlipidaemia and hypersensitivity to the drug.

Rare cases of benign intracranial hypertension have been reported after Roaccutane and after tetracyclines. Supplementary treatment with tetracyclines is therefore contra-indicated.

Roaccutane is teratogenic; major foetal abnormalities have been reported in humans. Major foetal abnormalities include: hydrocephalus, microcephalus, abnormalities of the external ear (micropinna, small or absent external auditory canals), microphthalmia, cardiovascular abnormalities, facial dysmorphia, thymus gland abnormalities, parathyroid hormone deficiency and cerebellar malformation. There is also a small risk of spontaneous abortion. Roaccutane is therefore contra-indicated in pregnancy. In any women of childbearing potential the risk of its use must be weighed against the expected therapeutic benefit under all circumstances, taking into account the precautions specified below.

Special warnings and special precautions for use: Roaccutane is contra-indicated in a woman of childbearing potential unless she meets the following criteria:

1. Has severe disfiguring cystic acne resistant to standard therapy.
2. Pregnancy should be excluded before instituting therapy with Roaccutane. A negative pregnancy test within two weeks prior to therapy is obtained.
3. Starts Roaccutane therapy only on the second or third day of the next menstrual cycle.
4. Any woman of childbearing potential who is receiving Roaccutane must practise effective contraception for at least four weeks before treatment, during the treatment period and for at least four weeks following its cessation. Even female patients who normally do not practise contraception because of a history of infertility should be advised to do so while taking Roaccutane.
5. Contraceptive measures must also be taken in the case of repeated courses of treatment.
6. Any pregnancy occurring during treatment with Roaccutane, or immediately following its completion, carries the risk of foetal malformation. This would raise the question of the termination of pregnancy for medical reasons. Therefore, before instituting Roaccutane therapy in a woman of childbearing potential the treating physician must explain clearly and in detail what precautions must be taken. This should include the risks involved and the possible consequences of a pregnancy occurring during Roaccutane treatment or in the first four weeks following its completion.
7. The woman is reliable and capable of understanding the risks and complying with effective contraception, and confirms that she has understood the warnings.

In view of the importance of the foregoing precautions, Roaccutane Patient Information Leaflets are available to doctors and it is strongly recommended that these be given to all patients. Wherever practicable a monthly repetition of the pregnancy test is recommended.

Liver function and blood lipids (fasting value) should be measured in all patients at the start of treatment, after the first month of administration and thereafter at 3-monthly intervals before discontinuation of Roaccutane.

Roaccutane may cause depression, psychotic symptoms and rarely suicide attempts and suicide. Particular care needs to be taken in patients with a history of depression and all patients should be monitored for signs of depression and referred for appropriate treatment if necessary.

At the completion of a lifespan study in rats there was an increased incidence of phaeochromocytoma in animals given isotretinoin at dosages of 32 and 8 mg/kg/day, but not 2 mg/kg/day. Since rats are particularly prone to develop this tumour type, the significance of this finding for use of Roaccutane in man is uncertain; nevertheless, repeated courses of treatment are not normally recommended.

Patients should not donate blood either during or for at least four weeks following discontinuation of therapy with Roaccutane. Theoretically there would be a small risk to a woman in the first trimester of pregnancy who received blood donated by a patient on Roaccutane therapy.

Interaction with other medicaments and other forms of interaction: As a rule, other treatments conventionally used for the treatment of acne, including antibiotics, keratolytics and exfoliants, are not indicated nor is concurrent radiation therapy with ultravoilet light or prolonged exposure to strong sunlight indicated but non-irritant topical preparations may be applied if required.

Patients should be instructed to avoid taking preparations containing high doses of vitamin A, i.e. more than the recommended dietary allowance of 4,000–5,000 i.u. per day.

Pregnancy and lactation: Roaccutane is contraindicated in pregnancy and should not be given to breast feeding mothers. It is also contraindicated in women of child bearing potential unless specific criteria are met. (see *Special warnings and special precautions for use*).

Effects on ability to drive and use machines: None.

Undesirable effects: Most of the clinical side effects of Roaccutane are dose related and are usually well tolerated at the recommended dosages. The side effects may recede during continued treatment and have generally proved reversible with reduction of dosage or discontinuation of therapy.

The skin and mucous membranes are most commonly affected. Dryness of the skin may be associated with scaling, thinning, erythema (especially of the face) and pruritus. An increase in epidermal fragility has been reported, and frictional trauma may lead to epidermal blistering. Dryness of the nasal mucosa may be associated with mild epistaxis and dryness of the pharyngeal mucosa with hoarseness. Granulomatous lesions have occasionally been reported. Dryness of the conjunctivae has been reported and may lead to mild to moderate conjunctivitis which may be alleviated by use of topical antibiotics. Decreased tolerance to contact lenses may occur.

Keratitis in association with Roaccutane treatment is a rare event and possibly related to dry eye syndrome. Therefore patients, particularly those with dry eye syndrome, should be monitored for the development of keratitis.

Acne fulminans has been noted to occur in rare cases.

Facial hyperpigmentation may rarely occur in patients treated with Roaccutane.

There have been occasional reports of visual disturbances, including papilloedema and optic neuritis possibly associated with benign intracranial hypertension; also corneal opacities, cataracts, decreased night vision, photophobia and blurred vision. Patients experiencing visual disturbances should be referred for an expert ophthalmological examination and withdrawal of Roaccutane considered.

Isolated cases of hearing deficiency in certain frequencies have been reported.

Hair thinning may occur but is uncommon at dosages below 1 mg/kg/day and is reversible following discontinuation of Roaccutane. Nevertheless, patients should be warned that this is a possibility during treatment. Hirsutism may rarely occur.

There have been occasional reports of allergic vasculitis associated with the administration of Roaccutane. Bronchospasm or asthma-like reactions may rarely occur in susceptible patients, mainly in those with pre-existing asthma, atopic diseases or allergies to various compounds.

Non-specific symptoms such as nausea, headache, malaise, drowsiness and sweating have been reported infrequently. Benign intracranial hypertension has been reported, particularly in association with concomitant antibiotic therapy.

Depression, psychotic symptoms and rarely suicide attempts and suicide have been reported with Roaccutane.

Epileptiform seizures have been reported in patients who are receiving Roaccutane therapy.

Myalgia and arthralgia may occur and may be associated with reduced tolerance to vigorous exercise. Rarely tendinitis may occur. Isolated instances of raised serum CPK values have been reported in patients receiving Roaccutane, particularly those undertaking vigorous physical activity. In these cases the clinical significance is unknown.

There have been occasional reports of menstrual irregularities which return to normal after completion of Roaccutane therapy.

A rise in serum levels of liver enzymes may occur. In a few cases significant increases have occurred, necessitating dosage reduction or discontinuation of Roaccutane. Jaundice and hepatitis have occurred rarely.

Elevation of serum triglycerides and cholesterol above the normal range, usually accompanied by decreases in HDL, has been observed, especially where predisposing factors such as a family history of lipid disorders, obesity, alcohol abuse, diabetes mellitus or smoking are present. The changes are dose-related and may be controlled by dietary means (including restriction of alcohol intake) and/or by reduction of dosage of Roaccutane. Isotretinoin-treated patients with high serum triglycerides (>8 g/l) are at risk of developing pancreatitis.

Rarely hyperuricemia and inflammatory bowel disease (e.g. colitis, ileitis) have been reported.

Isolated cases of paronychia and local or systemic infections due to Gram positive micro-organisms have been reported.

Patients receiving Roaccutane have occasionally experienced problems in the control of their blood sugar. New cases of diabetes have been diagnosed during therapy, although no causal relationship has been established. Rare instances of elevated blood glucose levels have been reported in diabetic patients in whom careful monitoring of glucose levels during treatment is therefore advised.

Isolated cases of thrombocytopenia, thrombocytosis, neutropenia and anaemia have been reported. Lymphadenopathy has been observed in some patients.

Isotretinoin has been shown to affect diaphyseal and spongy bone adversely in animals at high doses in excess of those recommended for use in man. Bone changes, including early epiphyseal closure, have occurred in man after several years administration of Roaccutane in very high doses for disorders of keratinisation. Prospective X-ray examination of some patients treated for severe cystic acne with Roaccutane revealed evidence of skeletal hyperostosis without clinical symptoms.

Haematuria and proteinuria have been associated with Roaccutane treatment and symptoms improve following dose reduction or drug withdrawal. Rarely, patients may experience photosensitivity reactions.

Overdose: Isotretinoin is a derivative of vitamin A and overdosage should be expected to induce symptoms of hypervitaminosis A.

Manifestations of acute vitamin A toxicity include severe headache, nausea or vomiting, drowsiness, irritability and pruritus. Signs and symptoms of accidental or deliberate overdosage with Roaccutane would probably be similar. They would be expected to be reversible and to subside without need for treatment. Because of the variable absorption of the drug, gastric lavage may be worthwhile in the first few hours after ingestion.

Pharmacological properties

Pharmacodynamic properties: Isotretinoin is a stereoisomer of tretinoin (all-*trans*-retinoic acid), an established preparation for topical treatment of acne vulgaris. Taken orally, Roaccutane has marked therapeutic efficacy in severe forms of acne, which are difficult to control with other means. The exact mechanism of action of Roaccutane is not known but clinical improvement is associated with a dose-related suppression of the size and activity of sebaceous glands.

Pharmacokinetic properties: Following oral administration of Roaccutane, peak blood levels of isotretinoin are achieved within 1–4 hours, and decline with a mean elimination half-life of approximately 10–20 hours.

Terminal elimination of the major metabolite, 4-oxo-isotretinoin, is formation rate limited so that its apparent half-life is similar to that for isotretinoin. The parent compound is highly bound to plasma protein and is excreted via bile and kidney as polar metabolites.

Bioavailability is enhanced by administration with food.

Preclinical safety data: None stated.

Pharmaceutical particulars
List of excipients: Soya Bean Oil, Beeswax Yellow, Hydrogenated Soya Bean Oil, Vegetable Oil-Partly Hydrogenated, Gelatin, Glycerol 85%, Karion 83 70%, Titanium Dioxide E171, Canthaxanthin Pigment E16l, 10% RVI Type.

Incompatibilities: None.

Shelf life: 3 years.

Special precautions for storage: Roaccutane capsules should be stored in a well-closed container and protected from light. The recommended maximum storage temperature is 30°C.

Nature and contents of container: Aluminium blister packs, containing 56 capsules.

Amber glass bottles, containing 100 capsules.

Instructions for use/handling: None.

Marketing authorisation numbers PL 0031/0158 – 5 mg, PL 0031/0160 – 20 mg

Date of first authorisation/renewal of authorisation June 1983

Date of (partial) revision of the text March 1998

ROCALTROL

Name of product Rocaltrol contains the substance with the approved name calcitriol and is also known as 1,25-dihydroxycholecalciferol. It is chemically described as (5Z,7E)-9,10-secocholesta-5,7,10 (19)-triene-1a, 3β,25-triol.

Presentation Soft gelatine capsules, one length red opaque and the other white opaque, containing 0.25 mcg calcitriol and the inactive ingredients butylated hydroxyanisole, butylated hydroxytoluene, fractionated coconut oil, gelatin, glycerol, hydrogenated products of partially hydrolysed starch, titanium dioxide E 171 and canthaxanthin E 161.

Soft gelatine capsules, both lengths red opaque, containing 0.5 mcg calcitriol.

Uses
Pharmacological properties: Calcitriol has the greatest biological activity of the known vitamin D metabolites and is normally formed in the kidneys from its immediate precursor, 25-hydroxycholecalciferol. In physiological amounts it augments the intestinal absorption of calcium and phosphate and plays a significant part in the regulation of bone mineralisation. The defective production of calcitriol in chronic renal failure contributes to the abnormalities of mineral metabolism found in that disorder.

Rocaltrol is a synthetic preparation of calcitriol. Oral administration of Rocaltrol to patients with chronic renal failure compensates for impaired endogenous production of calcitriol which is decreased when the glomerular filtration rate falls below 30 ml/min. Consequently, intestinal malabsorption of calcium and phosphate and the resulting hypocalcaemia are improved, thereby reversing the signs and symptoms of bone disease.

In patients with established post-menopausal osteoporosis, Rocaltrol increases calcium absorption, elevates circulating levels of calcitriol and reduces vertebral fracture frequency.

The onset and reversal of the effects of Rocaltrol are more rapid than those of other compounds with vitamin D activity and adjustment of the dose can be achieved sooner and more precisely. The effects of inadvertent overdosage can also be reversed more readily.

Pharmacokinetics: Rocaltrol is efficiently absorbed following an oral dose, and peak serum levels are reached after 4–6 hours. Calcitriol concentrations return to the basal level with a half-life of 3–6 hours, although the duration of pharmacologic activity is approximately 3–5 days. Following oral administration of 1 mcg radiolabelled calcitriol to normal individuals, approximately 10% of the total radioactivity appears in the urine within 24 hours. Biliary excretion and enterohepatic recirculation also occur.

Indications: Rocaltrol is indicated for the correction of the abnormalities of calcium and phosphate metabolism in patients with renal osteodystrophy.

Rocaltrol is also indicated for the treatment of established post-menopausal osteoporosis.

Dosage and administration The dose of Rocaltrol should be carefully adjusted for each patient according to the biological response so as to avoid hypercalcaemia.

The effectiveness of treatment depends in part on an adequate daily intake of calcium, which should be augmented by dietary changes or supplements if necessary. The capsules should be swallowed with a little water.

Oral intermittent (pulse) therapy with Rocaltrol two or three times weekly has been shown to be effective in patients with osteodystrophy refractory to continuous therapy.

Adults
Renal osteodystrophy: The initial daily dose is 0.25 mcg of Rocaltrol. In patients with normal or only slightly reduced calcium levels, doses of 0.25 mcg every other day are sufficient. If no satisfactory response in the biochemical parameters and clinical manifestations of the disease is observed within 2–4 weeks, the dosage may be increased by 0.25 mcg daily at 2–4 week intervals. During this period, serum calcium levels should be determined at least twice weekly. As soon as the serum calcium levels rise to 1 mg/100 ml (250μmol/l) above normal (9 to 11 mg/100 ml, or 2250–2750μmol/l), or serum creatinine rises to > 120μmol/l, treatment with Rocaltrol should be stopped immediately until normocalcemia ensues. Most patients respond to between 0.5 mcg and 1.0 mcg daily. Higher doses may be necessary if barbiturates or anticonvulsant drugs are administered simultaneously.

Post-menopausal osteoporosis: The recommended dose for Rocaltrol is 0.25 mcg twice daily.

Serum calcium and creatinine levels should be determined at 4 weeks, 3 and 6 months and at 6 monthly intervals thereafter.

Use in the elderly: Clinical experience with Rocaltrol in elderly patients indicates that the dosage recommended for use in younger adults may be given without apparent ill-consequence.

Children: Dosage in children has not been established.

Rocaltrol capsules are for oral administration only.

Contra-indications, warnings, etc
Contra-indications: Rocaltrol should not be given to patients with hypercalcaemia or evidence of metastatic calcification. The use of Rocaltrol in patients with known hypersensitivity to calcitriol (or drugs of the same class) and any of the constituent excipients is contra-indicated.

Rocaltrol is contra-indicated if there is evidence of vitamin D toxicity.

Use in pregnancy and lactation: The safety of Rocaltrol during pregnancy has not been established. Studies of reproductive toxicology in animals have not yielded unequivocal findings, and no controlled studies on the effect of exogenous calcitriol on pregnancy and foetal development have been performed in human subjects. Consequently, Rocaltrol should be given only when the potential benefit has been weighed against the possible hazard to the foetus. The usual caution in prescribing any drug for women of child-bearing age should be observed.

It should be assumed that exogenous calcitriol passes into breast milk. Mothers may breastfeed while taking Rocaltrol, provided that the serum calcium levels of the mother and infant are monitored.

Precautions: All other vitamin D compounds and their derivatives, including proprietary compounds or foodstuffs which may be 'fortified' with vitamin D, should be withheld during treatment with Rocaltrol.

Treatment does not obviate the need to control plasma phosphate with phosphate-binding agents. Since Rocaltrol affects phosphate transport in the gut and bone, the dose of phosphate-binding agent may need to be modified.

Side-effects and adverse reactions: The number of adverse effects reported from clinical use of Rocaltrol over a period of 15 years in all indications is very low with each individual effect, including hypercalcemia, occurring rarely.

Hypercalcaemia and hypercalciuria are the major side-effects of Rocaltrol and indicate excessive dosage. Patients with tertiary hyperparathyroidism, renal failure, or on regular haemodialysis are particularly prone to develop hypercalcaemia. The clinical features of hypercalcaemia include anorexia, nausea, vomiting, headache, weakness, apathy and somnolence. More severe manifestations may include thirst, dehydration, polyuria, nocturia, abdominal pain, paralytic ileus and cardiac arrhythmias. Rarely, overt psychosis and metastatic calcification may occur. The relatively short biological half-life of Rocaltrol permits rapid elimination of the compound when treatment is stopped and hypercalcaemia will recede within 2–7 days. This rate of reversal of biological effects is more rapid than when other vitamin D derivatives are used.

In patients with normal renal function, chronic hypercalcemia may be associated with an increase in serum creatinine.

Mild, non-progressive and reversible elevations in levels of liver enzymes (SGOT, SGPT) have been noted in a few patients treated with Rocaltrol, but no pathological changes in the liver have been reported.

Hypersensitivity reactions may occur in susceptible individuals.

Treatment of overdosage: In acute overdosage gastric lavage should be considered as soon after ingestion as possible provided that the drug was taken within the previous 6–8 hours.

Should hypercalcaemia occur, Rocaltrol should be discontinued until plasma calcium levels have returned to normal. A low-calcium diet will speed this reversal. Rocaltrol can then be restarted at a lower dose or given in the same dose but at less frequent intervals than previously. Severe hypercalcaemia may be treated by ensuring adequate hydration, inducing a diuresis where practicable and by general supportive measures. Calcitonin may increase the rate of fall of serum calcium when bone resorption is increased.

In patients treated by intermittent haemodialysis, a low concentration of calcium in the dialysate may also be used.

Pharmaceutical precautions
Storage: Rocaltrol capsules should be protected from heat; the recommended maximum storage temperature is 30°C.

Legal category POM.

Package quantities Rocaltrol capsules 0.25 mcg and 0.5 mcg in packs of 100.

Product licence numbers
PL 0031/0122 (capsules 0.25 mcg)
PL 0031/0123 (capsules 0.5 mcg)

Date of last review September 1997

ROCEPHIN

Trade name of the medicinal product Rocephin is the hydrated disodium salt of ceftriaxone. The free acid has the approved name ceftriaxone and is chemically described as (6R,7R)-7-[2-(2-amino-4-thiazolyl)-(Z)-2-[methoxyimino]-acetamido]-3-[[(2,5-dihydro-6-hydroxy-2-methyl-5-oxo-*as*-triazin-3-yl)thio]methyl]-8-oxo-5-thia-1-azabicyclo-[4,2,0]oct-2-ene-2-carboxylic acid.

Qualitative and quantitative composition Vials containing 250 mg ceftriaxone in the form of a sterile, crystalline powder consisting of 298.3 mg hydrated disodium ceftriaxone. The crystalline powder is for reconstitution with 5 ml Water for Injections BP for intravenous administration or with 1 ml 1% Lignocaine Hydrochloride Injection BP for intramuscular administration.

Vials containing 1 g ceftriaxone in the form of a sterile, crystalline powder consisting of 1.19 g hydrated disodium ceftriaxone. The crystalline powder is for reconstitution with 10 ml Water for Injections BP for intravenous administration or with 3.5 ml 1% Lignocaine Hydrochloride Injection BP for intramuscular administration.

Vials containing 2 g ceftriaxone in the form of a sterile, crystalline powder consisting of 2.39 g hydrated disodium ceftriaxone.

When reconstituted for intramuscular or intravenous injection, the white to yellowish-orange crystalline powder gives a pale yellow to amber solution. The displacement value of 250 mg of Rocephin is 0.194 ml.

Each gram of Rocephin contains approximately 3.6 mmol sodium.

Pharmaceutical form 250 mg, 1 g, 2 g vials.

Clinical particulars
Therapeutic indications: Pneumonia. Septicaemia. Meningitis. Bone, skin and soft tissue infections. Infections in neutropenic patients. Gonorrhoea. Peri-operative prophylaxis of infections associated with surgery.

Treatment may be started before the results of susceptibility tests are known.

Posology and method of administration: Rocephin may be administered by deep intramuscular injection, slow intravenous injection, or as a slow intravenous infusion, after reconstitution of the solution according to the directions given below. Dosage and mode of administration should be determined by the severity of the infection, susceptibility of the causative organism and the patient's condition. Under most circumstances a once-daily dose–or, in the specified indications, a single dose–will give satisfactory therapeutic results.

Adults and children 12 years and over: Standard therapeutic dosage: 1 g once daily.

Severe infections: 2–4 g daily, normally as a single dose every 24 hours.

The duration of therapy varies according to the course of the disease. As with antibiotic therapy in general, administration of Rocephin should be continued for a minimum of 48 to 72 hours after the patient has become afebrile or evidence of bacterial eradication has been obtained.

Acute, uncomplicated gonorrhoea: A single dose of 250 mg intramuscularly should be administered. Simultaneous administration of probenecid is not indicated.

Peri-operative prophylaxis: Usually 1 g as a single

intramuscular or slow intravenous dose. In colorectal surgery, 2 g should be given intramuscularly by slow intravenous injection or by slow intravenous infusion, in conjunction with a suitable agent against anaerobic bacteria.

Elderly: These dosages do not require modification in elderly patients provided that renal and hepatic function are satisfactory (see below).

Neonates, infants and children up to 12 years: The following dosage schedules are recommended for once daily administration:

Neonates: A daily dose of 20–50 mg/kg body weight, not to exceed 50 mg/kg. In the neonate, the intravenous dose should be given over 60 minutes to reduce the displacement of bilirubin from albumin, thereby reducing the potential risk of bilirubin encephalopathy (see *Special warnings and special precautions for use*).

Infants and children of up to 12 years: Standard therapeutic dosage: 20–50 mg/kg body weight once daily.

In severe infections up to 80 mg/kg body weight daily may be given. Doses of 50 mg/kg or over should be given by slow intravenous infusion over at least 30 minutes. Doses greater than 80 mg/kg body weight should be avoided because of the increased risk of biliary precipitates.

Renal and hepatic impairment: In patients with impaired renal function, there is no need to reduce the dosage of Rocephin provided liver function is intact. Only in cases of pre-terminal renal failure (creatinine clearance < 10 ml per minute) should the daily dosage be limited to 2 g or less.

In patients with liver damage there is no need for the dosage to be reduced provided renal function is intact.

In severe renal impairment accompanied by hepatic insufficiency, the plasma concentration of Rocephin should be determined at regular intervals and dosage adjusted.

In patients undergoing dialysis, no additional supplementary dosing is required following the dialysis. Serum concentrations should be monitored, however, to determine whether dosage adjustments are necessary, since the elimination rate in these patients may be reduced.

Contra-indications: Rocephin should not be given to patients with a history of hypersensitivity to cephalosporin antibiotics.

Rocephin should not be given to neonates with jaundice or to those who are hypoalbuminaemic or acidotic or have other conditions, such as prematurity, in which bilirubin binding is likely to be impaired.

Special warnings and special precautions for use: The stated dosage should not be exceeded.

Care is required when administering Rocephin to patients who have previously shown hypersensitivity (especially anaphylactic reaction) to penicillins or other non-cephalosporin beta-lactam antibiotics, as occasional instances of cross-allergenicity between cephalosporins and these antibiotics have been recorded. Anaphylactic shock requires immediate counter measures.

In severe renal impairment accompanied by hepatic insufficiency, dosage reduction is required as outlined under *Posology and method of administration.*

In vivo and *in vitro* studies have shown that ceftriaxone, like some other cephalosporins, can displace bilirubin from serum albumin. Clinical data obtained in neonates have confirmed this finding. Rocephin should therefore not be used in jaundiced new-borns or in those who are hypoalbuminaemic or acidotic, in whom bilirubin binding is likely to be impaired. Particular caution should be exercised in babies born prematurely.

Rocephin may precipitate in the gallbladder and then be detectable as shadows on ultrasound (see *Undesirable effects*). This can happen in patients of any age, but is more likely in infants and small children who are usually given a larger dose of Rocephin on a body weight basis. In children, doses greater than 80 mg/kg body weight should be avoided because of the increased risk of biliary precipitates. There is no clear evidence of gallstones or of acute cholecystitis developing in children or infants treated with Rocephin, and conservative management of ceftriaxone precipitate in the gallbladder is recommended.

Cephalosporins as a class tend to be absorbed onto the surface of the red cell membranes and react with antibodies directed against the drug to produce a positive Coombs' test and occasionally a rather mild haemolytic anaemia. In this respect, there may be some cross-reactivity with penicillins.

Cases of pancreatitis, possibly of biliary obstruction aetiology, have been rarely reported in patients treated with Rocephin. Most patients presented with risk factors for biliary stasis and biliary sludge, e.g. preceding major therapy, severe illness and total parenteral nutrition. A trigger or cofactor role of Rocephin-related biliary precipitation can not be ruled out.

Interaction with other medicaments and other forms of interaction: No impairment of renal function has been observed in man after simultaneous administration of Rocephin with diuretics.

No interference with the action or increase in nephrotoxicity of aminoglycosides has been observed during simultaneous administration with Rocephin.

The ceftriaxone molecule does not contain the N-methylthio-tetrazole substituent which has been associated with a disulfiram-like effect when alcohol is taken during therapy with certain cephalosporins.

In an *in vitro* study, antagonistic effects have been observed with the combination of chloramphenicol and ceftriaxone.

In patients treated with Rocephin, the Coombs' test may rarely become false-positive. Rocephin, like other antibiotics, may result in false-positive tests for galactosaemia. Likewise, non-enzymatic methods for glucose determination in urine may give false-positive results. For this reason, urine-glucose determination during therapy with Rocephin should be done enzymatically.

Pregnancy and lactation: Rocephin has not been associated with adverse effects on foetal development in laboratory animals but its safety in human pregnancy has not been established. Therefore it should not be used in pregnancy unless absolutely indicated. Only minimal amounts of Rocephin are excreted in breast milk. However, caution is advised in nursing mothers.

Effects on ability to drive and use machines: Not applicable.

Undesirable effects: Rocephin has been generally well tolerated. Adverse reactions are usually mild and transient.

The most common side-effects are gastro-intestinal, consisting mainly of loose stools and diarrhoea or, occasionally, nausea and vomiting, stomatitis and glossitis. Cutaneous reactions, including maculopapular rash or exanthema, pruritus, urticaria, oedema and allergic dermatitis have occurred. Isolated cases of severe cutaneous adverse reactions (erythema multiforme, Stevens Johnson Syndrome and Lyell's Syndrome/toxic epidermal necrolysis) have been reported.

Haematological reactions have included anaemia (all grades), haemolytic anaemia, leucopenia, neutropenia, thrombocytopenia, eosinophilia, agranulocytosis and positive Coombs' test. Regular blood counts should be carried out during treatment. Rocephin has rarely been associated with prolongation of prothrombin time.

Headache and dizziness, drug fever, shivering and transient elevations in liver function tests have been reported in a few cases. Other rarely observed adverse reactions include glycosuria, oliguria, haematuria, increase in serum creatinine, mycosis of the genital tract and anaphylactic-type reactions such as bronchospasm.

Very rarely, reversible symptomatic urinary precipitates of calcium ceftriaxone have occurred after Rocephin administration. Patients who are very young, immobilised or who are dehydrated are at increased risk. There have been a few reports of anuria and renal impairment following this reaction.

Shadows which have been mistaken for gallstones, but which are precipitates of calcium ceftriaxone, have been detected by sonograms. These abnormalities are commonly observed after an adult daily dose of two grams per day or more, or its equivalent in children. At doses of two grams a day or above these biliary precipitates may occasionally cause symptoms. Should patients develop symptoms, non-surgical management is recommended and discontinuation of Rocephin should be considered. The evidence suggests biliary precipitates usually disappear once Rocephin has been stopped. The risk of biliary precipitates may be increased by treatment duration greater than 14 days, renal failure, dehydration or total parenteral nutrition. There have been isolated reports of pancreatitis although a causal relationship to ceftriaxone has not been established.

Superinfections with yeasts, fungi or other resistant organisms may occur. A rare side-effect is pseudomembranous colitis which has resulted from infection with *Clostridium difficile* during treatment with Rocephin. Therefore it is important to consider this diagnosis in patients who present with diarrhoea subsequent to the administration of antibacterial agents.

Pain or discomfort may be experienced at the site of intramuscular injection immediately after administration but is usually well tolerated and transient. Local phlebitis has occurred rarely following intravenous administration but can be minimised by slow injection over at least 2–4 minutes.

Overdose: In the case of overdosage, drug concentrations would not be reduced by haemodialysis or peritoneal dialysis. There is no specific antidote. Treatment should be symptomatic.

Pharmacological properties

Pharmacodynamic properties: Rocephin has potent bactericidal activity against a wide range of Gram-positive and, especially, Gram-negative organisms. The spectrum of activity includes both aerobic and some anaerobic species. It has considerable stability against degradation by most bacterial beta-lactamases.

A notable feature of Rocephin is its relatively long plasma elimination half-life of approximately 8 hours, which makes single or once-daily dosage of the drug appropriate for most patients.

Microbiology: Ceftriaxone is usually active against the following micro-organisms *in vitro* and in clinical infections (see *Therapeutic indications*). The list is not exhaustive and focuses on those organisms of particular clinical interest.

Gram-positive aerobes: Staphylococcus aureus (including penicillinase-producing strains), Streptococcus pneumoniae, Streptococcus group A (Streptococcus pyogenes), Streptococcus group B (Streptococcus agalactiae), Streptococcus viridans, Streptococcus bovis.

Note: Methicillin-resistant *Staphylococcus* spp. are resistant to cephalosporins, including ceftriaxone. Most strains of enterococci (e.g. *Enterococcus faecalis*) are resistant. Listeria monocytogenes is also not susceptible to ceftriaxone.

Gram-negative aerobes: Acinetobacter iwoffi (some strains are resistant), *Aeromonas* spp., *Alcaligenes* spp., *Moraxella catarrhalis* (beta-lactamase negative and positive), *Capnocytophaga* spp., *Citrobacter* spp., *Enterobacter* spp. (some strains are resistant), *Escherichia coli,Haemophilus ducreyi,Haemophilus influenzae* (including penicillinase-producing strains), *Haemophilus parainfluenzae,Hafnia alvei,Klebsiella* spp. (including *K. pneumoniae*), *Moraxella* spp., *Morganella morganii* (= *Proteus morganii*), *Neisseria gonorrhoeae* (including penicillinase-producing strains), *Neisseria meningitidis, Pasteurella multocida,Plesimonas shigelloides,Proteus mirabilis,Proteus vulgaris,Providencia* spp., *Salmonella* spp. (including *S. typhi*), *Serratia* spp. (including *S. marcescens*), *Shigella* spp., *Vibrio* spp. (including *V. cholerae*), *Yersinia* spp. (including *Y. enterocolitica*),

Anaerobic organisms: Clostridium spp. (except C. difficile), Fusobacterium spp. (except F. mortiferum and F. varium), Peptococcus spp., Peptostreptococcus spp.

Pharmacokinetic properties: The pharmacokinetics of Rocephin are largely determined by its concentration-dependent binding to serum albumin. The plasma free (unbound) fraction of the drug in man is approximately 5% over most of the therapeutic concentration range, increasing to 15% at concentrations of 300 mg/l. Owing to the lower albumin content, the proportion of free ceftriaxone in interstitial fluid is correspondingly higher than in plasma.

Plasma concentrations: Mean peak concentrations after bolus intravenous injection are about 120 mg/l following a 500 mg dose and about 200 mg/l following a 1 g dose; mean levels of 250 mg/l are achieved after infusion of 2 g over 30 minutes. Intramuscular injection of 500 mg Rocephin in 1% lignocaine produces mean peak plasma concentrations of 40–70 mg/l within 1 hour. Bioavailability after intramuscular injection is 100%.

Excretion: Rocephin is eliminated mainly as unchanged ceftriaxone, approximately 60% of the dose being excreted in the urine (almost exclusively by glomerular filtration) and the remainder via the biliary and intestinal tracts. The total plasma clearance is 10–22 ml/min. The renal clearance is 5–12 ml/min. The elimination half-life in adults is about 8 hours. The half-life is not significantly affected by the dose, the route of administration or by repeated administration.

Pharmacokinetics in special clinical situations: In the first week of life, 80% of the dose is excreted in the urine; over the first month, this falls to levels similar to those in the adult.

In elderly persons aged over 75 years, the average elimination half-life is usually 2 to 3 times longer than in the young adult group. As with all cephalosporins, a decrease in renal function in the elderly may lead to an increase in half-life. Evidence gathered to date with ceftriaxone however, suggests that no modification of the dosage regimen is needed.

In patients with *renal* or *hepatic dysfunction*, the pharmacokinetics of ceftriaxone are only minimally altered and the elimination half-life is only slightly increased. If kidney function alone is impaired, biliary elimination of ceftriaxone is increased; if liver function alone is impaired, renal elimination is increased.

Cerebrospinal fluid: Rocephin crosses non-inflamed and inflamed meninges, attaining concentrations 4–17% of the simultaneous plasma concentration.

Preclinical safety data: There are no preclinical data of relevance to the prescriber which are additional to that already included in other sections of the SPC.

Pharmaceutical particulars
List of excipients: None.

Incompatibilities: Solutions containing Rocephin should not be mixed with or added to solutions containing other agents. In particular, Rocephin is not compatible with calcium-containing solutions such as Hartmann's solution and Ringer's solution. Based on literature reports, ceftriaxone is not compatible with amsacrine, vancomycin, fluconozole, aminoglycosides and labetalol.

Shelf life: Under recommended storage conditions, Rocephin is stable up to 36 months.

Special precautions for storage: The recommended maximum storage temperature is 25°C.

Nature and contents of container: Rocephin 250 mg and 1 g is supplied in 15 ml glass vials with teflonised rubber stoppers and aluminium caps. Packs of 5 vials.

Rocephin 2 g is supplied in 50 ml glass vials with teflonised rubber stoppers and aluminium caps. Packs of 1 vial.

Instructions for use/handling: Preparation of solutions for injection and infusion: The use of freshly prepared solutions is recommended. These maintain potency for at least 6 hours at room temperature in daylight, or 24 hours at 5°C.

Rocephin should not be mixed in the same syringe with any drug other than 1% Lignocaine Hydrochloride Injection BP (for intramuscular injection only).

Intramuscular injection: 250 mg Rocephin should be dissolved in 1 ml of 1% Lignocaine Hydrochloride Injection BP, or 1 g in 3.5 ml of 1% Lignocaine Hydrochloride Injection BP. The solution should be administered by deep intramuscular injection. Dosages greater than 1 g should be divided and injected at more than one site.

Solutions in lignocaine should not be administered intravenously.

Intravenous injection: 250 mg Rocephin should be dissolved in 5 ml of Water for Injections BP or 1 g in 10 ml of Water for Injections BP. The injection should be administered over at least 2–4 minutes, directly into the vein or via the tubing of an intravenous infusion.

Intravenous infusion: 2 g of Rocephin should be dissolved in 40 ml of one of the following calcium-free solutions: Dextrose Injection BP 5% or 10%, Sodium Chloride Injection BP, Sodium Chloride and Dextrose Injection BP (0.45% sodium chloride and 2.5% dextrose), dextran 6% in Dextrose Injection BP 5%, hydroxyethyl starch 6–10% infusions. The infusion should be administered over at least 30 minutes.

Marketing authorisation numbers
Vials 250mg PL 0031/0169
Vials 1g PL 0031/0171
Vials 2g PL 0031/0172

Date of first authorisation/renewal of authorisation
2 September 1988

Date of (partial) revision of the text 17 December 1998

ROFERON-A PRE-FILLED SYRINGE

Qualitative and quantitative composition Roferon-A is supplied in syringes as a ready-to-use solution for injection. Each syringe contains 3 Million International Units (MIU) per 0.5 ml, 4.5 MIU/0.5 ml, 6 MIU/0.5 ml, or 9 MIU/0.5 ml interferon alfa-2a†.

† Contains volume overages.

Pharmaceutical form Syringe containing solution for injection.

Clinical particulars
Therapeutic indications: Roferon-A is indicated for the treatment of:

1) Hairy cell leukaemia.

2) AIDS patients with progressive, asymptomatic Kaposi's sarcoma who have a CD4 count >250/mm³. AIDS patients with CD4 counts <250/mm³, or those with a history of opportunistic infections or constitutional symptoms, are unlikely to respond to Roferon-A therapy and therefore should not be treated (see *Posology and method of administration*).

3) Chronic phase Philadelphia-chromosome positive chronic myelogenous leukaemia. Roferon-A is not an alternative treatment for CML patients who have an HLA-identical relative and for whom allogeneic bone marrow transplantation is planned or possible in the immediate future. It is still unknown whether Roferon-A can be considered as a treatment with a curative potential in this indication.

4) Cutaneous T-cell lymphoma. Interferon alfa-2a (Roferon-A) may be active in patients who have progressive disease and who are refractory to, or unsuitable for, conventional therapy.

5) Adult patients with histologically proven chronic hepatitis B who have markers for viral replication, i.e., those who are positive for HBV-DNA, DNA polymerase or HBeAg.

6) Adult patients with histologically proven chronic hepatitis C who are positive for HCV antibodies and have elevated serum alanine aminotransferase (ALT) without liver decompensation. There is no evidence of long term benefit on clinical and histological grounds.

7) Follicular non-Hodgkin's lymphoma.

8) Advanced renal cell carcinoma.

Posology and method of administration

1. HAIRY CELL LEUKAEMIA
Initial dosage: Three million IU daily, given by subcutaneous or intramuscular injection for 16 - 24 weeks. If intolerance develops, either the daily dose should be lowered to 1.5 million IU or the schedule changed to three times per week, or both.

Maintenance dosage: Three million IU, given three times per week by subcutaneous or intramuscular injection. If intolerance develops, the dose should be lowered to 1.5 million IU three times per week.

Duration of treatment: Patients should be treated for approximately six months before the physician decides whether to continue treatment in responding patients or to discontinue treatment in non-responding patients. Patients have been treated for up to 20 consecutive months. The optimal duration of Roferon-A treatment for hairy cell leukaemia has not been determined.

Note: Subcutaneous administration is recommended for thrombocytopaenic patients (platelet count less than 50×10^9/l) or patients at risk of bleeding.

The minimum effective dose of Roferon-A in hairy cell leukaemia has not been established.

2. AIDS-RELATED KAPOSI'S SARCOMA
Roferon-A is indicated for the treatment of AIDS patients with progressive, asymptomatic Kaposi's sarcoma who have a CD4 count >250/mm³. AIDS patients with CD4 counts <250/mm³, or those with a history of opportunistic infections or constitutional symptoms, are unlikely to respond to Roferon-A therapy and therefore should not be treated. The optimal posology has not yet been well established.

Roferon-A should not be used in conjunction with protease inhibitors. With the exception of zidovudine, there is a lack of safety data for the combination of Roferon-A with reverse transcriptase inhibitors.

Initial dosage: Roferon-A should be given by subcutaneous or intramuscular injection, and escalated to at least 18 million IU daily and if possible to 36 million IU daily for a total of ten to twelve weeks in patients of 18 years or older. The recommended escalation schedule is as follows:

Days 1–3 3 million IU daily
Days 4–6 9 million IU daily
Days 7–9 18 million IU daily and, if tolerated, increase to:
Days 10–84 36 million IU daily

Maintenance dosage: Roferon-A should be given by subcutaneous or intramuscular injection three times per week at the maximum dose which is acceptable to the patient, but not exceeding 36 million IU.

Patients with AIDS-related Kaposi's sarcoma treated with 3 million IU of Roferon-A given daily showed a lower response rate than those treated with the recommended dosage.

Duration of treatment: The evolution of lesions should be documented to determine response to therapy. Patients should be treated for a minimum of 10 weeks and preferably for at least twelve weeks before the physician decides whether to continue treatment in responding patients or to discontinue treatment in non-responding patients. Patients generally showed evidence of response after approximately three months of therapy. Patients have been treated for up to 20 consecutive months. If a response to treatment occurs, treatment should continue at least until there is no further evidence of tumour. The optimal duration of Roferon-A treatment for AIDS-related Kaposi's sarcoma has not been determined.

Note: Lesions of Kaposi's sarcoma frequently reappear when Roferon-A treatment is discontinued.

3. CHRONIC MYELOGENOUS LEUKAEMIA
Roferon-A is indicated for the treatment of patients with chronic phase Philadelphia-chromosome positive chronic myelogenous leukaemia. Roferon-A is not an alternative treatment for CML patients who have an HLA-identical relative and for whom allogeneic bone marrow transplantation is planned or possible in the immediate future.

Roferon-A produces haematological remissions in 60% of patients with chronic phase CML, independent of prior treatment. Two thirds of these patients have complete haematological responses which occur as late as 18 months after treatment start.

In contrast to cytotoxic chemotherapy, interferon alfa-2a is able to generate sustained, ongoing cytogenetic responses beyond 40 months. It is still unknown whether Roferon-A can be considered as a treatment with a curative potential in this indication.

Dosage: It is recommended that Roferon-A should be given by subcutaneous or intramuscular injection for eight to 12 weeks to patients 18 years or more. The recommended schedule is:

Days 1–3 3 million IU daily
Days 4–6 6 million IU daily
Days 7–84 9 million IU daily

Duration of treatment: Patients should be treated for a minimum of eight weeks, preferably for at least twelve weeks before the physician decides whether or not to continue treatment in responding patients or to discontinue treatment in patients not showing any changes in haematological parameters. Responding patients should be treated until complete haematological response is achieved or for a maximum of 18 months. All patients with complete haematologic responses should continue treatment with 9 million IU daily (optimum) or 9 million IU three times a week (minimum) in order to achieve a cytogenetic response in the shortest possible time. The optimal duration of Roferon-A treatment for chronic myelogenous leukaemia has not been determined, although cytogenetic responses have been observed two years after treatment start.

The safety, efficacy and optimal dosage of Roferon-A in children with CML has not yet been established.

4. CUTANEOUS T-CELL LYMPHOMA (CTCL)
Interferon alfa-2a (Roferon-A) may be active in patients with progressive cutaneous T-cell lymphoma and who are refractory to, or unsuitable for conventional therapy.

The optimal dosage has not been established.

Initial dosage: Roferon-A should be given by subcutaneous or intramuscular injection, and escalated to 18 million IU daily for a total of 12 weeks in patients of 18 years or older. The recommended escalation schedule is as follows:

Days 1 to 3 3 million IU daily
Days 4 to 6 9 million IU daily
Days 7 to 84 18 million IU daily

Maintenance dosage: Roferon-A should be given by subcutaneous or intramuscular injection three times per week at the maximum dose which is acceptable to the patient, but not exceeding 18 million IU.

Duration of treatment: Patients should be treated for a minimum of eight weeks and preferably for at least twelve weeks before the physician decides whether to continue treatment in responding patients or to discontinue treatment in non-responding patients. Minimum treatment duration in responding patients should be 12 months in order to maximise the chance to achieve a complete response and improve the chance for a prolonged response. Patients have been treated for up to 40 consecutive months. The optimal duration of Roferon-A treatment for cutaneous T-cell lymphoma has not been determined.

Warning: Objective tumour responses have not been observed in approximately 40% of patients with CTCL. Partial responses are usually seen within 3 months and complete responses within 6 months, although it may occasionally take more than one year to reach the best response.

5. CHRONIC HEPATITIS B
Roferon-A is indicated for the treatment of adult patients with histologically proven chronic hepatitis B who have markers for viral replication, i.e., those who are positive for HBV-DNA, DNA polymerase or HBeAg.

Dosage recommendation: The optimal schedule of treatment has not been established yet. The dose is usually in the range of 2.5 million IU to 5.0 million IU/m² body surface administered subcutaneously three times per week for a period of 4 to 6 months.

The dosage may be adjusted according to the patient's tolerance to the medication. If no improvement has been observed after 3–4 months of treatment, discontinuation of therapy should be considered.

Children: up to 10 million IU/m² has been safely administered to children with chronic hepatitis B. However efficacy of therapy has not been demonstrated.

6. CHRONIC HEPATITIS C
Roferon-A is indicated for the treatment of adult patients with histologically proven chronic hepatitis C who are positive for HCV antibodies and have elevated serum alanine aminotransferase (ALT) without liver decompensation. There is no evidence of long term benefit on clinical and histological grounds.

In responding patients serum ALT will normalize and/or serum HCV-RNA will significantly decrease.

Initial dosage: Roferon-A should be administered at a dose of 3 to 6 million IU by subcutaneous or intramuscular injection three times a week for six months as induction therapy, patient tolerance permitting. In patients who fail to respond after three to four months of treatment, discontinuation of Roferon-A should be considered.

Maintenance dosage: Patients whose serum ALT has normalized require maintenance therapy with 3 million IU Roferon-A three times a week for an additional six months to consolidate the complete response. The optimal duration of treatment has not yet been determined.

Note: The majority of patients who relapse after adequate treatment do so within four months of the end of treatment.

7. FOLLICULAR NON-HODGKINS LYMPHOMA

Roferon-A prolongs disease-free and progression-free survival when used as adjunctive treatment to CHOP-like chemotherapy regimens in patients with advanced (high tumour burden) follicular non-Hodgkin's lymphoma. However, the efficacy of adjunctive interferon treatment on overall long-term survival of these patients has not yet been established.

Dosage recommendation: Roferon-A should be administered concomitantly to a conventional chemotherapy regimen (such as the combination of cyclophosphamide, prednisone, vincristine and doxorubicin) according to a schedule such as 6 million IU/m² given subcutaneously or intramuscularly from day 22 to day 26 of each 28-day cycle.

8. ADVANCED RENAL CELL CARCINOMA

Therapy with Roferon-A in combination with vinblastine induces overall response rates of approximately 17–26%, delays disease progression, and prolongs overall survival in patients with advanced renal cell carcinoma.

Dosage recommendation: Roferon-A should be given by subcutaneous or intramuscular injection at a dose of 3 million IU three times weekly for one week, 9 million IU three times weekly for the following week and 18 million IU three times weekly thereafter. Concomitantly vinblastine should be given intravenously according to the manufacturer's instructions at a dose of 0.1 mg/kg once every 3 weeks.

If the Roferon-A dosage of 18 million IU three times per week is not tolerated the dose may be reduced to 9 million IU three times per week.

Treatment should be given for a minimum of three months, up to a maximum of 12 months or until the development of progressive disease. Patients who achieve a complete response may stop treatment three months after the response is established.

Contra-indications: Roferon-A is contra-indicated in patients with:

1) A history of hypersensitivity to recombinant interferon alfa-2a or any component of the preparation,

2) Patients with severe pre-existing cardiac disease or with any history of cardiac illness. No direct cardiotoxic effect has been demonstrated, but it is likely that acute, self-limiting toxicities (i.e., fever, chills) frequently associated with administration of Roferon-A may exacerbate pre-existing cardiac conditions,

3) Severe renal, hepatic or myeloid dysfunction,

4) Uncontrolled seizure disorders and/or compromised central nervous system function (see *Special warnings and special precautions for use*),

5) Chronic hepatitis with advanced, decompensated hepatic disease or cirrhosis of the liver,

6) Chronic hepatitis who are being or have recently been treated with immunosuppressive agents,

7) Benzyl alcohol which is an excipient in Roferon-A solution for injection has on rare occasions been associated with potentially fatal toxicities in neonates. Therefore, Roferon-A solution for injection should not be used in the neonatal period.

Special warnings and special precautions for use: Roferon-A should be administered under the supervision of a qualified physician experienced in the management of the respective indication. Appropriate management of the therapy and its complications is possible only when adequate diagnostic and treatment facilities are readily available.

Patients should be informed not only of the benefits of therapy but also that they will probably experience adverse reactions.

When mild to moderate renal, hepatic or myeloid dysfunction is present, close monitoring of these functions is required.

In rare cases interferon alpha has been suspected of causing an exacerbation of an underlying autoimmune disease in hepatitis patients. Therefore, when treating hepatitis patients with a history of autoimmune disease caution is recommended. If a deterioration in liver function in these patients develops a determination of autoimmune antibodies should be considered. If necessary treatment should be discontinued.

Careful periodic neuropsychiatric monitoring of all patients is recommended. Suicidal behaviour has been observed rarely in patients receiving Roferon-A. Therapy should be discontinued in patients exhibiting suicidal behaviour.

Extreme caution should be exercised when administering Roferon-A to patients with severe myelosuppression as it has a suppressive effect on the bone marrow, leading to a fall in the white blood count, particularly granulocytes, platelet count and, less commonly, haemoglobin concentration. This can lead to an increased risk of infection or of haemorrhage. It is important to monitor closely these events in patients and periodic complete blood counts should be performed during the course of Roferon-A treatment, both prior to therapy and at appropriate periods during therapy.

In transplant patients (e.g., kidney or bone marrow transplant) therapeutic immunosuppression may be weakened because interferons also exert an immunostimulatory action.

Use of alfa interferon has been rarely associated with exacerbation or provocation of psoriasis.

In rare cases, severe hepatic dysfunction and liver failure have been reported after treatment with alfa interferon.

Hyperglycemia has been observed rarely in patients treated with Roferon-A. All patients who develop symptoms of hyperglycemia should have their blood glucose measured and followed-up accordingly. Patients with diabetes mellitus may require adjustment of their antidiabetic regimen.

The development of different auto-antibodies has been reported during treatment with alfa interferons. Clinical manifestations of autoimmune disease during interferon therapy occur more frequently in subjects predisposed to the development of autoimmune disorders. Autoimmune phenomena such as vasculitis, arthritis, hemolytic anemia, thyroid dysfunction and lupus erythematosus syndrome have been observed rarely in patients receiving Roferon-A. In patients with an underlying or clinical history of autoimmune disorders, monitoring of symptoms suggestive of these disorders, as well as measurement of auto antibodies and TSH level, is recommended.

The use of Roferon-A in children is not recommended as the safety and effectiveness of Roferon-A in children have not been established.

Efficacy in patients with chronic hepatitis B or C who are on haemodialysis or have hemophilia or are coinfected with human immunodeficiency virus has not been demonstrated.

Interaction with other medicaments and other forms of interaction: Since alfa-interferons alter cellular metabolism, the potential to modify the activity of other drugs exists. In a small study, Roferon-A was shown to have an effect on specific microsomal enzyme systems. The clinical relevance of these findings is unknown.

Alfa-interferons may affect the oxidative metabolic process; this should be borne in mind when prescribing concomitant therapy with drugs metabolised by this route. However, as yet no specific information is available.

Roferon-A has been reported to reduce the clearance of theophylline.

As Roferon-A may affect central nervous system functions, interactions could occur following concurrent administration of centrally-acting drugs. The neurotoxic, haematotoxic or cardiotoxic effects of previously or concurrently administered drugs may be increased by interferons.

Pregnancy and lactation: Men and women receiving Roferon-A should practise effective contraception. In pregnancy, Roferon-A should be administered only if the benefit to the woman justifies the potential risk to the foetus. Although animal tests do not indicate that Roferon-A is a teratogen, harm to the foetus from use during pregnancy cannot be excluded. When doses greatly in excess of the recommended clinical dose were administered to pregnant rhesus monkeys in the early to mid-foetal period, an abortifacient effect was observed.

It is not known whether this drug is excreted in human milk. A decision must be taken whether to suspend breast feeding or to discontinue the drug, taking into account the importance of the drug to the mother.

Effects on ability to drive and use machines: Depending on dose and schedule as well as the sensitivity of the individual patient, Roferon-A may have an effect on the speed of reaction which could impair certain operations, e.g., driving, operation of machinery etc.

Undesirable effects: The following data on adverse reactions are based on information derived from the treatment of cancer patients with a wide variety of malignancies and often refractory to previous therapy and suffering from advanced disease, patients with chronic hepatitis B and patients with chronic hepatitis C. Most cancer patients received doses that were significantly higher than the dose now recommended and this probably explains the higher frequency and severity of adverse reactions in this patient group compared with patients with hepatitis B where adverse reactions are usually transient, and patients return to pre-treatment status within 1 to 2 weeks after the end of therapy; increased hair loss may continue for several weeks.

General symptoms: The majority of the patients experienced flu-like symptoms such as fatigue, fever, chills, appetite loss, myalgia, headache, arthralgia and diaphoresis. These acute side-effects can usually be reduced or eliminated by concurrent administration of paracetamol and tend to diminish with continued therapy or dose moderation although continuing therapy can lead to lethargy, weakness and fatigue.

Gastrointestinal tract: About two thirds of cancer patients experienced anorexia and one half nausea. Emesis, taste alterations, mouth dryness, weight loss, diarrhoea and mild or moderate abdominal pain were less frequently observed. Constipation, flatulence, hypermotility or heartburn occurred rarely, and reactivation of peptic ulcer and non-life-threatening gastrointestinal bleeding have been reported in isolated cases.

Alterations of hepatic function shown by an elevation particularly of ALT, but also of alkaline phosphatase, LDH and bilirubin have been observed and generally did not require dose adjustment. In rare cases hepatitis was reported. In hepatitis B patients, changes in transaminases usually signal an improvement in the clinical state of the patient.

Central nervous system: Dizziness, vertigo, visual disturbances, decreased mental status, forgetfulness, depression, drowsiness, confusion, behavioural disturbances such as anxiety and nervousness, and sleep disturbances were uncommon. Suicidal behaviour, severe somnolence, convulsions, coma, cerebrovascular adverse events, transient impotence and ischemic retinopathy were rare complications.

Peripheral nervous system: Paresthesia, numbness, neuropathy, itching and tremor occasionally occurred.

Cardiovascular and pulmonary systems: Disorders were seen in about one fifth of cancer patients and consisted of transient hypotensive and hypertensive episodes, oedema, cyanosis, arrhythmias, palpitations and chest pain. Coughing and mild dyspnea were rarely observed. Rare cases of pulmonary edema, pneumonia, congestive heart failure, cardiorespiratory arrest and myocardial infarction have been reported. Cardiovascular problems are very rarely seen in patients with hepatitis B.

Skin, mucous membranes and adnexa: Re-exacerbation of herpes labialis, rash, pruritus, dryness of skin and mucous membranes, rhinorrhea and epistaxis were reported rarely. Mild to moderate alopecia occurred in up to one fifth of patients, but this was reversible on discontinuation of treatment.

Renal and urinary system: In rare instances, decreased renal function has occurred. Electrolyte disturbances have been seen, generally in association with anorexia or dehydration. Disorders consisted primarily of proteinuria and increased cell count in sediment. Elevation of BUN, serum creatinine and uric acid has been observed in rare cases. Rare cases of acute renal failure have been reported, mainly in cancer patients with renal disease and/or nephrotoxic comedications as concomitant risk factors.

Hematopoietic system: Transient leukopenia occurred variably in about one third to over one half of the patients, but rarely required restriction of dosage. In non-myelosuppressed patients, thrombocytopenia was less frequently seen, and decrease of haemoglobin and hematocrit occurred rarely. In myelosuppressed patients, thrombocytopenia and decreased haemoglobin occurred more frequently. Recovery of severe haematological deviations to pre-treatment levels usually occurred within seven to ten days after discontinuing Roferon-A treatment.

Endocrine disorders: Inconsequential hypocalcemia was reported in about one half of the patients. Hyperglycemia has been observed rarely in patients treated with Roferon-A.

Reactions at injection sites have occurred in patients.

Transient menstrual cycle irregularities including prolonged menstrual periods have been seen in rhesus monkeys administered doses greatly in excess of the recommended clinical dose. The relevance of these findings in man has not been established.

Anti-interferon antibodies: Neutralizing antibodies to proteins may be formed in some subjects following homologous administration. Antibodies to all interferons, whether natural or recombinant, are therefore likely to be found in a certain proportion of patients. In certain clinical conditions (cancer, systemic lupus erythematosus, herpes zoster) antibodies to human leukocyte interferon may also occur spontaneously in patients who have never received exogenous interferons.

In clinical trials where lyophilised Roferon-A which had been stored at 25°C was used, neutralizing antibodies to Roferon-A have been detected in approximately one fifth of patients. In patients with hepatitis C, a trend for responding patients who develop neutralizing antibodies to lose response while still on treatment and to lose it earlier than patients who do not develop such antibodies, has been seen. No other clinical sequelae of the presence of antibodies to Roferon-A have been documented. The clinical significance of the development of antibodies has not been fully clarified.

No data on neutralizing antibodies yet exist from clinical trials in which lyophilized Roferon-A or Roferon-A solution for injection which is stored at 4°C has been used. In a mouse model, the relative immunogenicity of lyophilized Roferon-A increases with time when the material is stored at 25°C – no such increase in immunogenicity is observed when lyophilised Roferon-A is stored at 4°C, the recommended storage conditions.

Overdose: There are no reports of overdosage but repeated large doses of interferon can be associated with profound lethargy, fatigue, prostration and coma. Such patients should be hospitalised for observation and appropriate supportive treatment given.

Patients who experience severe reactions to Roferon-A will usually recover within days after discontinuation of therapy, given appropriate supportive care. Coma has been observed in 0.4% of cancer patients in clinical trials.

Pharmacological properties

Pharmacodynamic properties: Pharmacotherapeutic classification: Immunostimulating Agent/Cytokine. ATC code L03AA04.

Roferon-A has been shown to possess many of the activities of the so-called natural human alfa-interferon preparations. Roferon-A exerts its antiviral effects by inducing a state of resistance to viral infections in cells and by modulating the effector arm of the immune system to neutralize viruses or eliminate virus infected cells. The essential mechanism for the antitumour action of Roferon-A is not yet known. However, several changes are described in human tumoural cells treated with Roferon-A: HT 29 cells show a significant reduction of DNA, RNA and protein synthesis. Roferon-A has been shown to exert antiproliferative activity against a variety of human tumours *in vitro* and to inhibit the growth of some human tumour xenografts in nude mice. A limited number of human tumour cell lines grown *in vivo* in immunocompromised nude mice has been tested for the susceptibility to Roferon-A. *In vivo* antiproliferative activity of Roferon-A has been studied on tumours including breast mucoid carcinoma, adenocarcinoma of the caecum, colon carcinoma and prostatic carcinoma. The degree of antiproliferative activity is variable.

Unlike other human proteins, many of the effects of interferon alfa-2a are partially or completely suppressed when it is tested in other animal species. However, significant antivaccinia virus activity was induced in rhesus monkeys pre-treated with interferon alfa-2a.

Pharmacokinetic properties: The serum concentrations of interferon alfa-2a reflected a large intersubject variation in both healthy volunteers and patients with disseminated cancer. The pharmacokinetics of Roferon-A in animals (monkey, dog and mouse) were similar to those seen in man. The pharmacokinetics of Roferon-A in man were linear over a 3 million to 198 million IU dose range. In healthy man, interferon alfa-2a exhibited an elimination half-life of 3.7–8.5 hours (mean: 5.1 hours), a volume of distribution at steady state of 0.223–0.748 l/kg (mean: 0.4 l/kg) and a total body clearance of 2.14–3.62 ml/min/kg (mean: 2.79 ml/min/kg) after a 36 million IU intravenous infusion. After intramuscular administration of 36 million IU, peak serum concentrations ranged from 1500 to 2580 pg/ml (mean: 2020 pg/ml) at a mean time to peak of 3.8 hours, and after subcutaneous administration of 36 million IU from 1250 to 2320 pg/ml (mean: 1730 pg/ml) at a mean time to peak of 7.3 hours.

The apparent fraction of the dose absorbed after intramuscular or subcutaneous injection is greater than 80%.

The pharmacokinetics of interferon alfa-2a after single intramuscular doses to patients with disseminated cancer and chronic hepatitis B were similar to those found in healthy volunteers. Dose-proportional increases in serum concentrations were observed after single doses up to 198 million IU. There were no changes in the distribution or elimination of interferon alfa-2a during twice daily (0.5–36 million IU), once daily (1–54 million IU), or three times weekly (1–136 million IU) dosing regimens up to 28 days of dosing. Renal catabolism is the major pathway for Roferon-A elimination. Biliary excretion and liver metabolism are considered to be minor pathways of elimination of Roferon-A.

Intramuscular administration of Roferon-A one or more times daily for up to 28 days to some patients with disseminated cancer resulted in peak plasma concentrations of two to four times greater than those seen after single doses. However, multiple dosing caused no changes in its distribution or elimination parameters during several dosage regimens studied.

Preclinical safety data: Because of species specificity of human interferon, only limited toxicological studies have been carried out with Roferon-A. The acute parenteral toxicity of Roferon-A has been studied in mice rats, rabbits and ferrets at doses up to 30 million IU/kg intravenously, and 500 million IU/kg intramuscularly. No treatment-related mortality was noted in any species studied given Roferon-A by any of the routes of administration. With doses greatly exceeding the recommended clinical dose no significant adverse effects were observed except for an abortifacient effect when administered to pregnant rhesus monkeys in the early to mid-foetal period and transient menstrual cycle irregularities including prolonged menstrual periods in non-pregnant monkeys.

Mutagenic effects of Roferon-A have not been observed experimentally.

Pharmaceutical particulars

List of excipients: Ammonium acetate, Sodium Chloride, Benzyl alcohol, Polysorbate 80, Acetic acid, Sodium Hydroxide, Water for Injection.

Incompatibilities: None observed.

Shelf life: 2 years (at 2–8°C).

Special precautions for storage: Store syringes between +2 and +8°C. Protect from light. Do not freeze.

Nature and contents of container: Syringe barrel 1 ml (flint glass), butyl rubber stopper laminated with PTFE (fluororesin D-3), tip cap of butyl rubber and laminated with ETFE (fluororesin D), plunger rod, made of polyethylene, injection needle for subcutaneous injection made of stainless steel, needle hub made of polypropylene. Injection swabs may be supplied with the product.

Each syringe contains 3 MIU/0.5 ml, 4.5 MIU/0.5 ml, 6 MIU/0.5 ml or 9 MIU/0.5 ml interferon alpha-2a in a ready-to-use solution for injection.

Instructions for use/handling: None.

Marketing authorisation numbers

PL 0031/0485 (Roferon-A Prefilled Syringe 3 MIU/0.5 ml)
PL 0031/0486 (Roferon-A Prefilled Syringe 4.5 MIU/0.5 ml)
PL 0031/0487 (Roferon-A Prefilled Syringe 6 MIU/0.5 ml)
PL 0031/0488 (Roferon-A Prefilled Syringe 9 MIU/0.5 ml)

Date of first authorisation/renewal of authorisation
PL 0031/0485–8: 29 July 1996

Date of (partial) revision of text November 1998

ROFERON-A (SOLUTION FOR INJECTION)

Qualitative and quantitative composition Roferon-A is supplied in vials as a ready-to-use solution for injection. Each vial contains 3 Million International Units (MIU) per millilitre, 4.5 MIU/1 ml, 6 MIU/1 ml, 9 MIU/1 ml 18 MIU/1 ml or 18 MIU/3 ml interferon alfa-2a†.

† Contains volume overages of 10% and manufacturing overages.

Pharmaceutical form Vials containing solution for injection.

Clinical particulars

Therapeutic indications: Roferon-A is indicated for the treatment of:

1) Hairy cell leukaemia.

2) AIDS patients with progressive, asymptomatic Kaposi's sarcoma who have a CD4 count >250/mm³. AIDS patients with CD4 counts <250/mm³, or those with a history of opportunistic infections or constitutional symptoms, are unlikely to respond to Roferon-A therapy and therefore should not be treated (see *Posology and method of administration*).

3) Chronic phase Philadelphia-chromosome positive chronic myelogenous leukaemia. Roferon-A is not an alternative treatment for CML patients who have an HLA-identical relative and for whom allogeneic bone marrow transplantation is planned or possible in the immediate future. It is still unknown whether Roferon-A can be considered as a treatment with a curative potential in this indication.

4) Cutaneous T-cell lymphoma. Interferon alfa-2a (Roferon-A) may be active in patients who have progressive disease and who are refractory to, or unsuitable for, conventional therapy.

5) Adult patients with histologically proven chronic hepatitis B who have markers for viral replication, i.e., those who are positive for HBV-DNA, DNA polymerase or HBeAg.

6) Adult patients with histologically proven chronic hepatitis C who are positive for HCV antibodies and have elevated serum alanine aminotransferase (ALT) without liver decompensation. There is no evidence of long term benefit on clinical and histological grounds.

7) Follicular non-Hodgkin's lymphoma.

8) Advanced renal cell carcinoma.

Posology and method of administration

1. HAIRY CELL LEUKAEMIA

Initial dosage: Three million IU daily, given by subcutaneous or intramuscular injection for 16 - 24 weeks. If intolerance develops, either the daily dose should be lowered to 1.5 million IU or the schedule changed to three times per week, or both.

Maintenance dosage: Three million IU, given three times per week by subcutaneous or intramuscular injection. If intolerance develops, the dose should be lowered to 1.5 million IU three times per week.

Duration of treatment: Patients should be treated for approximately six months before the physician decides whether to continue treatment in responding patients or to discontinue treatment in non-responding patients. Patients have been treated for up to 20 consecutive months. The optimal duration of Roferon-A treatment for hairy cell leukaemia has not been determined.

Note: Subcutaneous administration is recommended for thrombocytopenic patients (platelet count less than 50×10^9/l) or patients at risk of bleeding.

The minimum effective dose of Roferon-A in hairy cell leukaemia has not been established.

2. AIDS-RELATED KAPOSI'S SARCOMA

Roferon-A is indicated for the treatment of AIDS patients with progressive, asymptomatic Kaposi's sarcoma who have a CD4 count >250/mm³. AIDS patients with CD4 counts <250/mm³, or those with a history of opportunistic infections or constitutional symptoms, are unlikely to respond to Roferon-A therapy and therefore should not be treated. The optimal posology has not yet been well established.

Roferon-A should not be used in conjunction with protease inhibitors. With the exception of zidovudine, there is a lack of safety data for the combination of Roferon-A with reverse transcriptase inhibitors.

Initial dosage: Roferon-A should be given by subcutaneous or intramuscular injection, and escalated to at least 18 million IU daily and if possible to 36 million IU daily for a total of ten to twelve weeks in patients of 18 years or older. The recommended escalation schedule is as follows:

Days 1-3 3 million IU daily
Days 4-6 9 million IU daily
Days 7-9 18 million IU daily - and, if tolerated, increase to:
Days 10-84 36 million IU daily

Maintenance dosage: Roferon-A should be given by subcutaneous or intramuscular injection three times per week at the maximum dose which is acceptable to the patient, but not exceeding 36 million IU.

Patients with AIDS-related Kaposi's sarcoma treated with 3 million IU of Roferon-A given daily showed a lower response rate than those treated with the recommended dosage.

Duration of treatment: The evolution of lesions should be documented to determine response to therapy. Patients should be treated for a minimum of 10 weeks and preferably for at least twelve weeks before the physician decides whether to continue treatment in responding patients or to discontinue treatment in non-responding patients. Patients generally showed evidence of response after approximately three months of therapy. Patients have been treated for up to 20 consecutive months. If a response to treatment occurs, treatment should continue at least until there is no further evidence of tumour. The optimal duration of Roferon-A treatment for AIDS-related Kaposi's sarcoma has not been determined.

Note: Lesions of Kaposi's sarcoma frequently reappear when Roferon-A treatment is discontinued.

3. CHRONIC MYELOGENOUS LEUKEMIA

Roferon-A is indicated for the treatment of patients with chronic phase Philadelphia-chromosome positive chronic myelogenous leukaemia. Roferon-A is not an alternative treatment for CML patients who have an HLA-identical relative and for whom allogeneic bone marrow transplantation is planned or possible in the immediate future.

Roferon-A produces haematological remissions in 60% of patients with chronic phase CML, independent of prior treatment. Two thirds of these patients have complete haematological responses which occur as late as 18 months after treatment start.

In contrast to cytotoxic chemotherapy, interferon alfa-2a is able to generate sustained, ongoing cytogenetic responses beyond 40 months. It is still unknown whether Roferon-A can be considered as a treatment with a curative potential in this indication.

Dosage: It is recommended that Roferon-A should be given by subcutaneous or intramuscular injection for eight to 12 weeks to patients 18 years or more. The recommended schedule is:

Days 1–3 3 million IU daily
Days 4–6 6 million IU daily
Days 7–84 9 million IU daily

Duration of treatment: Patients should be treated for a minimum of eight weeks, preferably for at least twelve weeks before the physician decides whether or not to continue treatment in responding patients or to discontinue treatment in patients not showing any changes in haematological parameters. Responding patients should be treated until complete haematological response is achieved or for a maximum of 18 months. All patients with complete haematologic responses should continue treatment with 9 million IU daily (optimum) or 9 million IU three times a week (minimum) in order to achieve a cytogenetic response in the shortest possible time. The optimal duration of Roferon-A treatment for chronic myelogenous leukaemia has not been determined, although cytogenetic responses have been observed two years after treatment start.

The safety, efficacy and optimal dosage of Roferon-A in children with CML has not yet been established.

4. CUTANEOUS T-CELL LYMPHOMA (CTCL)

Interferon alfa-2a (Roferon-A) may be active in patients with progressive cutaneous T-cell lymphoma and who are refractory to, or unsuitable for conventional therapy.

The optimal dosage has not been established.

Initial dosage: Roferon-A should be given by subcutaneous or intramuscular injection, and escalated to 18 million IU daily for a total of 12 weeks in patients of 18 years or older. The recommended escalation schedule is as follows:

Days 1 to 3 3 million IU daily
Days 4 to 6 9 million IU daily
Days 7 to 84 18 million IU daily

Maintenance dosage: Roferon-A should be given by subcutaneous or intramuscular injection three times per week at the maximum dose which is acceptable to the patient, but not exceeding 18 million IU.

Duration of treatment: Patients should be treated for a minimum of eight weeks and preferably for at least twelve weeks before the physician decides whether to continue treatment in responding patients or to discontinue treatment in non-responding patients. Minimum treatment duration in responding patients should be 12 months in order to maximise the chance to achieve a complete response and improve the chance for a prolonged response. Patients have been treated for up to 40 consecutive months. The optimal duration of Roferon-A treatment for cutaneous T-cell lymphoma has not been determined.

Warning: Objective tumour responses have not been observed in approximately 40% of patients with CTCL. Partial responses are usually seen within 3 months and complete responses within 6 months, although it may occasionally take more than one year to reach the best response.

5. CHRONIC HEPATITIS B

Roferon-A is indicated for the treatment of adult patients with histologically proven chronic hepatitis B who have markers for viral replication, i.e., those who are positive for HBV-DNA, DNA polymerase or HBeAg.

Dosage recommendation: The optimal schedule of treatment has not been established yet. The dose is usually in the range of 2.5 million IU to 5.0 million IU/m² body surface administered subcutaneously three times per week for a period of 4 to 6 months.

The dosage may be adjusted according to the patient's tolerance to the medication. If no improvement has been observed after 3–4 months of treatment, discontinuation of therapy should be considered.

Children: up to 10 million IU/m² has been safely administered to children with chronic hepatitis B. However efficacy of therapy has not been demonstrated.

6. CHRONIC HEPATITIS C

Roferon-A is indicated for the treatment of adult patients with histologically proven chronic hepatitis C who are positive for HCV antibodies and have elevated serum alanine aminotransferase (ALT) without liver decompensation. There is no evidence of long term benefit on clinical and histological grounds.

In responding patients serum ALT will normalize and/or serum HCV-RNA will significantly decrease.

Initial dosage: Roferon-A should be administered at a dose of 3 to 6 million IU by subcutaneous or intramuscular injection three times a week for six months as induction therapy, patient tolerance permitting. In patients who fail to respond after three to four months of treatment, discontinuation of Roferon-A should be considered.

Maintenance dosage: Patients whose serum ALT has normalized require maintenance therapy with 3 million IU Roferon-A three times a week for an additional six months to consolidate the complete response. The optimal duration of treatment has not yet been determined.

Note: The majority of patients who relapse after adequate treatment do so within four months of the end of treatment.

7. FOLLICULAR NON-HODGKINS LYMPHOMA

Roferon-A prolongs disease-free and progression-free survival when used as adjunctive treatment to CHOP-like chemotherapy regimens in patients with advanced (high tumor burden) follicular non-Hodgkin's lymphoma. However, the efficacy of adjunctive interferon treatment on overall long-term survival of these patients has not yet been established.

Dosage recommendation: Roferon-A should be administered concomitantly to a conventional chemotherapy regimen (such as the combination of cyclophosphamide, prednisone, vincristine and doxorubicin) according to a schedule such as 6 million IU/m² given subcutaneously or intramuscularly from day 22 to day 26 of each 28-day cycle.

8. ADVANCED RENAL CELL CARCINOMA

Therapy with Roferon-A in combination with vinblastine induces overall response rates of approximately 17–26%, delays disease progression, and prolongs overall survival in patients with advanced renal cell carcinoma.

Dosage recommendation: Roferon-A should be given by subcutaneous or intramuscular injection at a dose of 3 million IU three times weekly for one week, 9 million IU three times weekly for the following week and 18 million IU three times weekly thereafter. Concomitantly vinblastine should be given intravenously according to the manufacturer's instructions at a dose of 0.1 mg/kg once every 3 weeks.

If the Roferon-A dosage of 18 million IU three times per week is not tolerated the dose may be reduced to 9 million IU three times per week.

Treatment should be given for a minimum of three months, up to a maximum of 12 months or until the development of progressive disease. Patients who achieve a complete response may stop treatment three months after the response is established.

Contra-indications: Roferon-A is contra-indicated in patients with:

1) A history of hypersensitivity to recombinant interferon alfa-2a or any component of the preparation,

2) Patients with severe pre-existing cardiac disease or with any history of cardiac illness. No direct cardiotoxic effect has been demonstrated, but it is likely that acute, self-limiting toxicities (i.e., fever, chills) frequently associated with administration of Roferon-A may exacerbate pre-existing cardiac conditions,

3) Severe renal, hepatic or myeloid dysfunction,

4) Uncontrolled seizure disorders and/or compromised central nervous system function (see *Special warnings and special precautions for use*),

5) Chronic hepatitis with advanced, decompensated hepatic disease or cirrhosis of the liver,

6) Chronic hepatitis who are being or have recently been treated with immunosuppressive agents,

7) Benzyl alcohol which is an excipient in Roferon-A solution for injection has on rare occasions been associated with potentially fatal toxicities in neonates. Therefore, Roferon-A solution for injection should not be used in the neonatal period.

Special warnings and special precautions for use: Roferon-A should be administered under the supervision of a qualified physician experienced in the management of the respective indication. Appropriate management of the therapy and its complications is possible only when adequate diagnostic and treatment facilities are readily available.

Patients should be informed not only of the benefits of therapy but also that they will probably experience adverse reactions.

When mild to moderate renal, hepatic or myeloid dysfunction is present, close monitoring of these functions is required.

In rare cases interferon alpha has been suspected of causing an exacerbation of an underlying autoimmune disease in hepatitis patients. Therefore, when treating hepatitis patients with a history of autoimmune disease caution is recommended. If a deterioration in liver function in these patients develops a determination of autoimmune antibodies should be considered. If necessary treatment should be discontinued.

Careful periodic neuropsychiatric monitoring of all patients is recommended. Suicidal behaviour has been observed rarely in patients receiving Roferon-A. Therapy should be discontinued in patients exhibiting suicidal behaviour.

Extreme caution should be exercised when administering Roferon-A to patients with severe myelosuppression as it has a suppressive effect on the bone marrow, leading to a fall in the white blood count, particularly granulocytes, platelet count and, less commonly, haemoglobin concentration. This can lead to an increased risk of infection or of haemorrhage. It is important to monitor closely these events in patients and periodic complete blood counts should be performed during the course of Roferon-A treatment, both prior to therapy and at appropriate periods during therapy.

In transplant patients (e.g., kidney or bone marrow transplant) therapeutic immunosuppression may be weakened because interferons also exert an immunostimulatory action.

Use of alfa interferon has been rarely associated with exacerbation or provocation of psoriasis.

In rare cases, severe hepatic dysfunction and liver failure have been reported after treatment with alfa interferon.

Hyperglycemia has been observed rarely in patients treated with Roferon-A. All patients who develop symptoms of hyperglycemia should have their blood glucose measured and followed-up accordingly. Patients with diabetes mellitus may require adjustment of their antidiabetic regimen.

The development of different auto-antibodies has been reported during treatment with alfa interferons. Clinical manifestations of autoimmune disease during interferon therapy occur more frequently in subjects predisposed to the development of autoimmune disorders. Autoimmune phenomena such as vasculitis, arthritis, hemolytic anemia, thyroid dysfunction and lupus erythematosus syndrome have been observed rarely in patients receiving Roferon-A. In patients with an underlying or clinical history of autoimmune disorders, monitoring of symptoms suggestive of these disorders, as well as measurement of auto antibodies and TSH level, is recommended.

The use of Roferon-A in children is not recommended as the safety and effectiveness of Roferon-A in children have not been established.

Efficacy in patients with chronic hepatitis B or C who are on haemodialysis or have hemophilia or are coinfected with human immunodeficiency virus has not been demonstrated.

Interaction with other medicinal products and other forms of interaction: Since alfa-interferons alter cellular metabolism, the potential to modify the activity of other drugs exists. In a small study, Roferon-A was shown to have an effect on specific microsomal enzyme systems. The clinical relevance of these findings is unknown.

Alfa-interferons may affect the oxidative metabolic process; this should be borne in mind when prescribing concomitant therapy with drugs metabolised by this route. However, as yet no specific information is available.

Roferon-A has been reported to reduce the clearance of theophylline.

As Roferon-A may affect central nervous system functions, interactions could occur following concurrent administration of centrally-acting drugs. The neurotoxic, haematotoxic or cardiotoxic effects of previously or concurrently administered drugs may be increased by interferons.

Use during pregnancy and lactation: Men and women receiving Roferon-A should practise effective contraception. In pregnancy, Roferon-A should be administered only if the benefit to the woman justifies the potential risk to the foetus. Although animal tests do not indicate that Roferon-A is a teratogen, harm to the foetus from use during pregnancy cannot be excluded. When doses greatly in excess of the recommended clinical dose were administered to pregnant rhesus monkeys in the early to mid-foetal period, an abortifacient effect was observed.

It is not known whether this drug is excreted in human milk. A decision must be taken whether to suspend breast feeding or to discontinue the drug, taking into account the importance of the drug to the mother.

Effects on ability to drive and use machines: Depending on dose and schedule as well as the sensitivity of the individual patient, Roferon-A may have an effect on the speed of reaction which could impair certain operations, e.g., driving, operation of machinery etc.

Undesirable effects: The following data on adverse reactions are based on information derived from the treatment of cancer patients with a wide variety of malignancies and often refractory to previous therapy and suffering from advanced disease, patients with chronic hepatitis B and patients with chronic hepatitis C. Most cancer patients received doses that were significantly higher than the dose now recommended and this probably explains the higher frequency and severity of adverse reactions in this patient group compared with patients with hepatitis B where adverse reactions are usually transient, and patients return to pre-treatment status within 1 to 2 weeks after the end of therapy; increased hair loss may continue for several weeks.

General symptoms: The majority of the patients

experienced flu-like symptoms such as fatigue, fever, chills, appetite loss, myalgia, headache, arthralgia and diaphoresis. These acute side-effects can usually be reduced or eliminated by concurrent administration of paracetamol and tend to diminish with continued therapy or dose moderation although continuing therapy can lead to lethargy, weakness and fatigue.

Gastrointestinal tract: About two thirds of cancer patients experienced anorexia and one half nausea. Emesis, taste alterations, mouth dryness, weight loss, diarrhoea and mild or moderate abdominal pain were less frequently observed. Constipation, flatulence, hypermotility or heartburn occurred rarely, and reactivation of peptic ulcer and non-life-threatening gastrointestinal bleeding have been reported in isolated cases.

Alterations of hepatic function: Shown by an elevation particularly of ALT, but also of alkaline phosphatase, LDH and bilirubin have been observed and generally did not require dose adjustment. In rare cases hepatitis was reported. In hepatitis B patients, changes in transaminases usually signal an improvement in the clinical state of the patient.

Central nervous system: Dizziness, vertigo, visual disturbances, decreased mental status, forgetfulness, depression, drowsiness, confusion, behavioural disturbances such as anxiety and nervousness, and sleep disturbances were uncommon. Suicidal behaviour, severe somnolence, convulsions, coma, cerebrovascular adverse events, transient impotence and ischemic retinopathy were rare complications.

Peripheral nervous system: Paresthesia, numbness, neuropathy, itching and tremor occasionally occurred.

Cardiovascular and pulmonary systems: Disorders were seen in about one fifth of cancer patients and consisted of transient hypotensive and hypertensive episodes, oedema, cyanosis, arrhythmias, palpitations and chest pain. Coughing and mild dyspnea were rarely observed. Rare cases of pulmonary oedema, pneumonia, congestive heart failure, cardiorespiratory arrest and myocardial infarction have been reported. Cardiovascular problems are very rarely seen in patients with hepatitis B.

Skin, mucous membranes and adnexa: Re-exacerbation of herpes labialis, rash, pruritus, dryness of skin and mucous membranes, rhinorrhea and epistaxis were reported rarely. Mild to moderate alopecia occurred in up to one fifth of patients, but this was reversible on discontinuation of treatment.

Renal and urinary system: In rare instances, decreased renal function has occurred. Electrolyte disturbances have been seen, generally in association with anorexia or dehydration. Disorders consisted primarily of proteinuria and increased cell count in sediment. Elevation of BUN, serum creatinine and uric acid has been observed in rare cases. Rare cases of acute renal failure have been reported, mainly in cancer patients with renal disease and/or nephrotoxic comedications as concomitant risk factors.

Haematopoietic system: Transient leukopenia occurred variably in about one third to over one half of the patients, but rarely required restriction of dosage. In non-myelosuppressed patients, thrombocytopenia was less frequently seen, and decrease of haemoglobin and haematocrit occurred rarely. In myelosuppressed patients, thrombocytopenia and decreased haemoglobin occurred more frequently. Recovery of severe haematological deviations to pre-treatment levels usually occurred within seven to ten days after discontinuing Roferon-A treatment.

Endocrine disorders: Inconsequential hypocalcemia was reported in about one half of the patients. Hyperglycemia has been observed rarely in patients treated with Roferon-A.

Reactions at injection sites have occurred in patients.

Transient menstrual cycle irregularities including prolonged menstrual periods have been seen in rhesus monkeys administered doses greatly in excess of the recommended clinical dose. The relevance of these findings in man has not been established.

Anti-interferon antibodies: Neutralizing antibodies to proteins may be formed in some subjects following homologous administration. Antibodies to all interferons, whether natural or recombinant, are therefore likely to be found in a certain proportion of patients. In certain clinical conditions (cancer, systemic lupus erythematosus, herpes zoster) antibodies to human leukocyte interferon may also occur spontaneously in patients who have never received exogenous interferons.

In clinical trials where lyophilised Roferon-A which had been stored at 25°C was used, neutralizing antibodies to Roferon-A have been detected in approximately one fifth of patients. In patients with hepatitis C, a trend for responding patients who develop neutralizing antibodies to lose response while still on treatment and to lose it earlier than patients who do not develop such antibodies, has been seen. No other clinical sequelae of the presence of antibodies to Roferon-A have been documented. The clinical significance of the development of antibodies has not been fully clarified.

No data on neutralizing antibodies yet exist from clinical trials in which lyophilized Roferon-A or Roferon-A solution for injection which is stored at 4°C has been used. In a mouse model, the relative immunogenicity of lyophilized Roferon-A increases with time when the material is stored at 25°C – no such increase in immunogenicity is observed when lyophilised Roferon-A is stored at 4°C, the recommended storage conditions.

Overdose: There are no reports of overdosage but repeated large doses of interferon can be associated with profound lethargy, fatigue, prostration and coma. Such patients should be hospitalised for observation and appropriate supportive treatment given.

Patients who experience severe reactions to Roferon-A will usually recover within days after discontinuation of therapy, given appropriate supportive care. Coma has been observed in 0.4% of cancer patients in clinical trials.

Pharmacological properties

Pharmacodynamic properties: Pharmacotherapeutic classification: Immunostimulating Agent/Cytokine. ATC code L03AA04.

Roferon-A has been shown to possess many of the activities of the so-called natural human alfa-interferon preparations. Roferon-A exerts its antiviral effects by inducing a state of resistance to viral infections in cells and by modulating the effector arm of the immune system to neutralize viruses or eliminate virus infected cells. The essential mechanism for the antitumour action of Roferon-A is not yet known. However, several changes are described in human tumoural cells treated with Roferon-A: HT 29 cells show a significant reduction of DNA, RNA and protein synthesis. Roferon-A has been shown to exert antiproliferative activity against a variety of human tumours *in vitro* and to inhibit the growth of some human tumour xenografts in nude mice. A limited number of human tumour cell lines grown *in vivo* in immunocompromised nude mice has been tested for the susceptibility to Roferon-A. *In vivo* antiproliferative activity of Roferon-A has been studied on tumours including breast mucoid carcinoma, adenocarcinoma of the caecum, colon carcinoma and prostatic carcinoma. The degree of antiproliferative activity is variable.

Unlike other human proteins, many of the effects of interferon alfa-2a are partially or completely suppressed when it is tested in other animal species. However, significant antivaccinia virus activity was induced in rhesus monkeys pre-treated with interferon alfa-2a.

Pharmacokinetic properties: The serum concentrations of interferon alfa-2a reflected a large intersubject variation in both healthy volunteers and patients with disseminated cancer. The pharmacokinetics of Roferon-A in animals (monkey, dog and mouse) were similar to those seen in man. The pharmacokinetics of Roferon-A in man were linear over a 3 million to 198 million IU dose range. In healthy man, interferon alfa-2a exhibited an elimination half-life of 3.7–8.5 hours (mean: 5.1 hours), a volume of distribution at steady state of 0.223–0.748 l/kg (mean: 0.4 l/kg) and a total body clearance of 2.14–3.62 ml/min/kg (mean: 2.79 ml/min/kg) after a 36 million IU intravenous infusion. After intramuscular administration of 36 million IU, peak serum concentrations ranged from 1500 to 2580 pg/ml (mean: 2020 pg/ml) at a mean time to peak of 3.8 hours, and after subcutaneous administration of 36 million IU from 1250 to 2320 pg/ml (mean: 1730 pg/ml) at a mean time to peak of 7.3 hours.

The apparent fraction of the dose absorbed after intramuscular or subcutaneous injection is greater than 80%.

The pharmacokinetics of interferon alfa-2a after single intramuscular doses to patients with disseminated cancer and chronic hepatitis B were similar to those found in healthy volunteers. Dose-proportional increases in serum concentrations were observed after single doses up to 198 million IU. There were no changes in the distribution or elimination of interferon alfa-2a during twice daily (0.5–36 million IU), once daily (1–54 million IU), or three times weekly (1–136 million IU) dosing regimens up to 28 days of dosing. Renal catabolism is the major pathway for Roferon-A elimination. Biliary excretion and liver metabolism are considered to be minor pathways of elimination of Roferon-A.

Intramuscular administration of Roferon-A one or more times daily for up to 28 days to some patients with disseminated cancer resulted in peak plasma concentrations of two to four times greater than those seen after single doses. However, multiple dosing caused no changes in its distribution or elimination parameters during several dosage regimens studied.

Preclinical safety data: Because of species specificity of human interferon, only limited toxicological studies have been carried out with Roferon-A. The acute parenteral toxicity of Roferon-A has been studied in mice rats, rabbits and ferrets at doses up to 30 million IU/kg intravenously, and 500 million IU/kg intramuscularly. No treatment-related mortality was noted in any species studied given Roferon-A by any of the routes of administration. With doses greatly exceeding the recommended clinical dose no significant adverse effects were observed except for an abortifacient effect when administered to pregnant rhesus monkeys in the early to mid-foetal period and transient menstrual cycle irregularities including prolonged menstrual periods in non-pregnant monkeys.

Mutagenic effects of Roferon-A have not been observed experimentally.

Pharmaceutical particulars

List of excipients: Ammonium acetate, Sodium Chloride, Benzyl alcohol, Polysorbate 80, Acetic acid, Sodium Hydroxide, Water for Injection.

Incompatibilities: None observed.

Shelf life: 2 years (at 2–8°C).

After first withdrawal (18 MIU/3 ml vial only)–30 days at 2 to 8°C and under light protection.

Special precautions for storage: Store vials between +2 and +8°C. Protect from light. Do not freeze.

The 18 MIU/3 ml solution for injection is suitable for multiple-dose use. All other strengths are for single dose use.

Nature and contents of container:

- Vial 2 ml (flint glass), butyl rubber stopper laminated with FPE, aluminium cap (3 MIU/ml, 4.5 MIU/ml, 6 MIU/ml, 9 MIU/ml, 18 MIU/ml).
- Vial 3 ml (flint glass), butyl rubber stopper laminated with FPE, aluminium cap (18 MIU/3 ml).
- An injection kit (1 syringe 2 ml, 1 needle for i.m. injection, 1 needle for s.c. injection) may be supplied with the product.

Instructions for use/handling: Plastic syringes are recommended for administration of Roferon-A solution for injection.

Only the 18 MIU/3 ml vial is suitable for multidose use and is for single patient use only. The top of the vial should be swabbed with disinfectant using an aseptic technique before withdrawal of a dose and the date of first withdrawal should be written in the space provided on the vial label. A new sterile syringe and needle must be used each time a dose is withdrawn from the multidose vial. Used needles and syringes must not be re-inserted into multidose vials. 18 MIU/3 ml multidose vials should be used within 30 days of the first withdrawal.

Marketing authorisation numbers

PL 0031/0400 Roferon-A Solution for injection (vials) 3 MIU/ml
PL 0031/0401 Roferon-A Solution for injection (vials) 4.5 MIU/ml
PL 0031/0402 Roferon-A Solution for injection (vials) 6 MIU/ml
PL 0031/0403 Roferon-A Solution for injection (vials) 9 MIU/ml
PL 0031/0456 Roferon-A Solution for injection (vials) 18 MIU/ml
PL 0031/0404 Roferon-A Solution for injection (vials) 18 MIU/3 ml

Date of first authorisation/renewal of authorisation

PL 0031/0400–0404: 1 September 1995
PL 0031/0456: 12 February 1997

Date of (partial) revision of the text November 98

ROHYPNOL

Qualitative and quantitative composition Each 1 mg tablet contains 1 mg of the active ingredient flunitrazepam.

Pharmaceutical form Rohypnol film-coated tablets 1 mg.

Clinical particulars

Therapeutic indications: Short-term treatment of insomnia when it is severe, disabling or subjecting the individual to unacceptable distress, particularly for patients who have difficulty in falling asleep.

May be employed on an intermittent basis for induction of sleep at unusual times on a short-term or irregular basis.

An underlying cause for insomnia should be sought before deciding upon the use of benzodiazepines for symptomatic relief. Benzodiazepines are not recommended for the primary treatment of psychotic illness.

Posology and method of administration:

Adults: Usual dose 0.5–1 mg; in exceptional circumstances the dose may be increased to 2 mg.

Elderly or debilitated patients: Usual dose 0.5 mg; in exceptional circumstances the dose may be increased to 1 mg. If organic brain changes are present, the dosage of Rohypnol should not exceed 0.5 mg in these patients.

In patients with chronic pulmonary insufficiency

and in patients with chronic renal or hepatic disease, dosage may need to be reduced.

Children: Rohypnol tablets are contra-indicated for use in children.

Treatment should be as short as possible and should be started with the lowest recommended dose. The maximum dose should not be exceeded. Generally the duration of treatment varies from a few days to two weeks with a maximum of four weeks, including the tapering off process. Patients who have taken benzodiazepines for a prolonged time may require a longer period during which doses are reduced. Specialist help may be appropriate. Little is known regarding the efficacy or safety of benzodiazepines in long-term use.

In certain cases, extension beyond the maximum treatment period may be necessary; if so, it should not take place without re-evaluation of the patient's status. Long-term chronic use is not recommended.

The product should be taken just before going to bed. Rohypnol tablets are for oral administration.

Contra-indications: Acute pulmonary insufficiency; respiratory depression; phobic or obsessional states; chronic psychosis; myasthenia gravis; sleep apnoea syndrome; severe hepatic insufficiency; use in children.

Use of this drug is contra-indicated in patients with a known hypersensitivity to flunitrazepam (or other benzodiazepines) and any of the excipients. Hypersensitivity reactions including rash, angioedema and hypotension have been reported on rare occasions in susceptible patients.

Special warnings and special precautions for use: Rohypnol should not be used alone to treat depression or anxiety associated with depression, since suicide may be precipitated in such patients.

In cases of loss or bereavement, psychological adjustment may be inhibited by benzodiazepines.

Use of benzodiazepines may lead to the development of physical and psychological dependence. The dependence potential of the benzodiazepines is low, particularly when limited to short-term use, but this increases when high doses are used, especially when given over long periods. This is particularly so in patients with a history of alcoholism or drug abuse or in patients with marked personality disorders.

Regular monitoring in such patients is essential; routine repeat prescriptions should be avoided and treatment should be withdrawn gradually. Symptoms such as depression, nervousness, extreme anxiety, tension, restlessness, confusion, mood changes, rebound insomnia, irritability, sweating, diarrhoea, headaches and muscle pain have been reported following abrupt cessation of treatment with normal therapeutic doses. In severe cases the following symptoms may occur: derealisation, depersonalisation, hyperacusis, numbness and tingling of the extremities, hypersensitivity to light, noise and physical contact and hallucinations or epileptic seizures. In rare instances, withdrawal following excessive dosages may produce confusional states and psychotic manifestations. Abuse of flunitrazepam has been reported.

Some loss of efficacy to the hypnotic effects of short-acting benzodiazepines may develop after repeated use for a few weeks.

Abnormal psychological reactions to benzodiazepines have been reported. Rare behavioural effects include paradoxical aggressive outbursts, excitement, confusion, restlessness, agitation, irritability, delusion, rages, nightmares, hallucinations, psychoses, inappropriate behaviour and the uncovering of depression with suicidal tendencies. Extreme caution should therefore be used in prescribing benzodiazepines to patients with personality disorders. If any of these reactions occur, use of the drug should be discontinued. These reactions may be quite severe and are more likely to occur in children and the elderly.

Benzodiazepines may induce anterograde amnesia. The condition usually occurs several hours after ingesting the product and therefore, to reduce the risk, patients should ensure that they will be able to have an uninterrupted sleep of 7 to 8 hours.

Interaction with other medicaments and other forms of interaction: Enhancement of the central depressive effect may occur if Rohypnol is combined with centrally-acting drugs such as neuroleptics, tranquillisers, antidepressants, hypnotics, analgesics and anaesthetics, anti-epileptics and sedative anti-histamines. In the case of narcotic analgesics, enhancement of the euphoria may also occur leading to an increase in psychological dependence. The elderly require special supervision.

When Rohypnol is used in conjunction with anti-epileptic drugs, side-effects and toxicity may be more evident, particularly with hydantoins or barbiturates or combinations including them. This requires extra care in adjusting dosage in the initial stages of treatment.

Known inhibitors of hepatic enzymes, e.g. cimetidine, have been shown to reduce the clearance of benzodiazepines and may potentiate their action, and known inducers of hepatic enzymes, e.g. rifampicin, may increase the clearance of benzodiazepines.

Pregnancy and lactation: There is no evidence as to drug safety in human pregnancy, nor is there evidence from animal work that it is free from hazard. Do not use during pregnancy, especially during the first and last trimesters, unless there are compelling reasons.

Administration of benzodiazepines in the last trimester of pregnancy or during labour has been reported to produce irregularities in the foetal heart rate, and hypotonia, poor sucking, hypothermia and moderate respiratory depression in the neonate.

Infants born to mothers who took benzodiazepines chronically during the latter stages of pregnancy may have developed physical dependence and may be at some risk of developing withdrawal symptoms in the postnatal period.

Flunitrazepam has been detected in breast milk. The use of Rohypnol in mothers who are breast-feeding should be avoided.

Effects on ability to drive and use machines: Patients should be advised that, like all medicaments of this type, Rohypnol may modify patients' performance at skilled tasks (driving, operating machinery, etc.) to a varying degree depending upon dosage, administration, sleep pattern and individual susceptibility. Patients should further be advised that alcohol may intensify any impairment and should therefore be avoided during treatment.

Undesirable effects: Adverse effects include drowsiness during the day, numbed emotions, reduced alertness, confusion, fatigue, headache, dizziness, muscle weakness, ataxia and double vision. These phenomena are dose related and are likely to be uncommon with the recommended dosage; they occur predominantly at the start of therapy and usually disappear with repeated administration. The elderly are particularly sensitive to the effects of centrally-depressant drugs.

Other adverse effects are less common and include vertigo, hypotension, gastro-intestinal upsets, skin rashes, changes in libido, and urinary retention. Isolated cases of blood dyscrasias and jaundice have also been reported.

Anterograde amnesia may occur at therapeutic dosages, the risk increasing at higher dosages. Amnesic effects may be associated with inappropriate behaviour.

Pre-existing depression may be unmasked during benzodiazepine use.

Overdose: When taken alone in overdosage, Rohypnol presents few problems in management and should not present a threat to life unless combined with other CNS depressants (including alcohol). In the management of overdose with any medicinal product, it should be borne in mind that multiple agents may have been taken.

Following overdose with oral benzodiazepines, vomiting should be induced if the patient is conscious or gastric lavage undertaken with the airway protected if the patient is unconscious. If there is no advantage in emptying the stomach, activated charcoal should be given to reduce absorption. Special attention should be paid to respiratory and cardiovascular functions in intensive care. Overdose of benzodiazepines is usually manifested by degrees of central nervous system depression ranging from drowsiness to coma. In mild cases, symptoms include drowsiness, mental confusion, dysarthria and lethargy; in more serious cases, symptoms may include ataxia, hypotonia, hypotension, respiratory depression, rarely coma and very rarely death.

Anexate is a specific IV antidote to Rohypnol for use in emergency situations. Patients requiring such intervention should be monitored closely in hospital (see separate prescribing information).

The value of dialysis has not been determined.

If excitation occurs, barbiturates should not be used.

Pharmacological properties

Pharmacodynamic properties: Rohypnol is a full benzodiazepine agonist with a high affinity for the benzodiazepine central site. It has anxiolytic, anticonvulsant and sedative properties, and it causes slowing of psychomotor performance, amnesia, muscle relaxation and sleep induction.

Pharmacokinetic properties: Flunitrazepam is rapidly and almost completely absorbed after oral administration. The distribution half-life of flunitrazepam is about 3 hours; the elimination half-life is variable and may be between 16–35 hours. The onset of effect is rapid and the duration of effect is dose-dependent. Flunitrazepam is almost completely metabolised. The main metabolites are the inactive 7-aminoflunitrazepam and N-desmethyl-flunitrazepam which is less active than the parent compound. The steady state level of the active metabolite is below the minimum effective concentration. The volume of distribution is approximately 3.3–5.5 l/kg. Flunitrazepam is approximately 78% bound to plasma proteins.

Preclinical safety data: None stated.

Pharmaceutical particulars

List of excipients: Lactose, microcrystalline cellulose, magnesium stearate, , hypromellose, ethylcellulose, polyvidone K90, sodium starch glycolate, indigotine, triacetin, titanium dioxide, talc, yellow iron oxide.

Incompatibilities: None.

Shelf life: Rohypnol tablets have a shelf life of 5 years.

Special precautions for storage: Rohypnol tablets should be stored below 25°C in a dry place.

Nature and contents of container: Rohypnol tablets are available in PVC/PVDC blister packs of 30.

Instructions for use/handling: None.

Marketing authorisation numbers PL 0031/0104

Date of first authorisation/renewal of authorisation 17 August 1982

Date of (partial) revision of the text March 1998

SPIROCTAN

Qualitative and quantitative composition

Spiroctan 25 contains 25 mg spironolactone BP
Spiroctan 50 contains 50 mg spironolactone BP
Spiroctan 100 contains 100 mg spironolactone BP

Pharmaceutical form

Spiroctan 25: Light blue coated tablets marked BM B2 and containing 25 mg Spironolactone BP.

Spiroctan 50: Green coated tablets marked BM A8 and containing 50 mg Spironolactone BP.

Spiroctan 100: Light green hard gelatin capsules marked BM A7 and containing 100 mg Spironolactone BP.

Clinical particulars

Therapeutic indications: Spiroctan is recommended for the treatment of congestive cardiac failure, cirrhosis with ascites and oedema, malignant ascites, nephrotic syndrome and also for diagnosis and treatment of primary hyperaldosteronism.

Posology and method of administration:

Adults: Adequate maintenance dosage is usually between 50 and 200 mg daily, depending on the patient's response. This may be increased to 300 to 400 mg daily when necessary. A single dose of 100 mg should not be exceeded.

Elderly: In elderly patients, caution is advised. It is suggested that treatment should begin at the lowest dose, increasing gradually up to the normal adult dose, until the desired response is achieved.

Children: The daily dosage for children is based on an intake of 1.5 to 3.0 mg per kg body weight as shown in the following guidelines.

Age 1 to 3 years (up to approximately 15 kg): One tablet Spiroctan 25 every other day.

Age 4–7 years (up to approximately 23 kg): One tablet Spiroctan 25 each day.

Age 8–12 years (up to approximately 37 kg): One tablet Spiroctan 25 twice daily.

Children should be treated for more than 30 days only if deemed essential.

Spiroctan tablets and capsules should be taken with fluid. For children who cannot swallow solid dosage forms, the tablets may be crushed and taken with food or drink.

Contra-indications: Spiroctan is contraindicated in cases of renal insufficiency (serum creatinine > 180 mol/litre or creatinine clearance < 30 ml/min), acute renal insufficiency, anuria, where hyperkalaemia or hyponatraemia is present, pregnancy, lactation and in patients hypersensitive to spironolactone.

Special warnings and special precautions for use: Although the dose of Spiroctan does not generally need to be reduced in hepatic dysfunction, such patients should be monitored carefully as hepatic coma may be precipitated in susceptible subjects.

Periodic estimation of serum electrolytes is recommended.

Interactions: Potassium supplements should not be administered with Spiroctan except initially in cases of hypokalaemia, and the use of Spiroctan with other potassium-sparing diuretics or ACE inhibitors should be avoided. Combination of spironolactone, ACE inhibitors and loop diuretics may lead to acute renal failure.

The effect of carbenoxolone may be decreased. Acetylsalicylic acid, indomethacin and other inhibitors of prostaglandin synthesis may reduce the inhibiting effects of Spiroctan on aldosterone.

The action of other diuretics may be potentiated. The initial dose should be half that normally administered and the dosage should be adjusted to the patient's needs. Spiroctan may enhance the effect of antihypertensive agents.

Spironolactone may falsely elevate serum digoxin concentration, as determined by radioimmunoassay and can reduce digoxin and renal clearance. Therefore digoxin levels should only be interpreted in conjunction with clinical presentation.

Pregnancy and lactation: Use of Spiroctan during pregnancy is contraindicated. Animal teratogenicity studies have shown evidence of feminisation of the male foetus. As metabolites of spironolactone may be excreted in breast milk, the use of Spiroctan in patients who are breast feeding is not recommended.

Effects on ability to drive and operate machines: Alertness may be impaired.

Undesirable effects: These are infrequent and normally mild. Occasionally central nervous system side effects such as headaches, drowsiness, lethargy or ataxia may occur, and the ability to drive or operate machinery may be impaired. Gastrointestinal effects are possible.

Hyperkalaemia may occur occasionally, especially in patients with renal dysfunction, and a reversible increase in BUN and creatinine may occur even when kidney function is normal. Hyponatraemia and reversible induction or aggravation of hyperchloraemic metabolic acidosis is possible. Occasionally a rise in serum uric acid may occur.

It is theoretically possible that in chronic therapy there may be antiandrogenic effects such as nipple sensitivity and gynaecomastia in men and mastodynia in women. Hirsutism and occasional disorders of menstruation–in rare cases amenorrhoea–have been observed in women. In men there may be occasional disorders of potency. In rare cases there may be irreversible changes in voice pitch. This risk should be considered carefully in patients for whom voice control is important, for example in actors and teachers. There have been isolated cases of skin rashes, alopecia, osteomalacia, hepatotoxicity, hepatitis and agranulocytosis. Rarely eosinophilia (in patients with liver cirrhosis) and thrombocytopenia may occur.

Overdosage: Toxic effects in overdosage are due to hyperkalaemia. Clinical symptoms include irregular pulse, lassitude and muscular weakness, and it may be difficult to differentiate clinically from hypokalaemia. Treatment is by cessation of therapy, administration of potassium-excreting diuretics, use of ion-exchange resins etc.

Pharmacological properties

Pharmacodynamic properties: Spiroctan promotes diuresis by competitive inhibition of aldosterone, a sodium-retaining, potassium-excreting hormone. It acts on the distal portion of the renal tubule, and may be used in conjunction with more proximally acting diuretics.

After initiation of therapy, the diuretic response develops slowly over 2–3 days.

Pharmacokinetic properties: Absorption of spironolactone is proportional to dose up to 100 mg. Thereafter an assumed saturation mechanism is apparent. Spironolactone is rapidly and completely metabolised following administration, and unchanged spironolactone cannot be detected in the urine. The main active metabolites of spironolactone are canrenone, 7' thiomethylspironolactone and sulphur containing metabolites. 10% of a single dose of spironolactone shows antimineralocorticoid activity. This increases to 25% during steady state administration.

The metabolites have a long plasma half-life. Following a single administration of spironolactone, the plasma half-life of canrenone is in the order of 18.5 to 20 hours and that of the other metabolites 15 to 16 hours.

Following oral administration, within 6 days approximately 53% of the dose is excreted in the urine, and approximately 36% in the faeces.

The renal excretion half life is approximately 22 hours.

Preclinical safety data: Spironolactone has been shown to produce tumours in rats when administered at high doses over a long period of time. The significance of these findings with respect to clinical use is not certain. However, the long-term use of spironolactone in young patients requires careful consideration of the benefits and the potential hazard involved. No mutagenic potential was demonstrated in *in-vivo* experiments.

Spironolactone crosses the placental barrier. In animal experiments (rats and dogs) spironolactone shows a feminising effect on male foetuses due to its antiandrogenic properties at doses much higher than those recommended for humans.

Pharmaceutical particulars

List of excipients: Spiroctan tablets also contain lactose, talc, sodium starch glycollate, maize starch, magnesium stearate, sodium lauryl sulphate, agar (only Spiroctan 25 tablets), colloidal silicon dioxide. The sugar coating contains sucrose, kaolin, polyethylene glycol, glucose, titanium dioxide (E171), povidone and montanic acid/ethanediol ester. Both Spiroctan 25 and 50 contain the colouring agent E132. Spiroctan 50 also contains E110 and E104. (The sugar content of each tablet is less than 0.125 g).

Spiroctan 100 capsules contain lactose, maize starch, colloidal silicon dioxide, microcrystalline cellulose, sodium starch glycollate, sodium lauryl sulphate, polyoxyethylene stearate, magnesium stearate, talc, titanium dioxide (E171), gelatin and the colouring agents E104 and E132.

Incompatibilities: Not applicable.

Shelf life

Spiroctan 25 5 years
Spiroctan 50 5 years
Spiroctan 100 5 years

Special precautions for storage: No special storage precautions are necessary. As with all medicines, however, it is recommended that Spiroctan be stored in a cool dry place.

Nature and contents of containers:

Spiroctan 25–Polypropylene tube packs with low density polyethylene caps containing 100 tablets.

Spiroctan 50–Polypropylene tube packs with low density polyethylene caps containing 100 tablets.

Spiroctan 100–PVC/Al blister strips containing 28 capsules.

Instructions for use/handling: None

Marketing authorisation numbers

PL 15722/0007
PL 15722/0008
PL 15722/0009

Date of approval/revision of SPC January 1997

SYNFLEX TABLETS

Qualitative and quantitative composition Naproxen sodium 275 mg (equivalent to naproxen 250 mg).

Pharmaceutical form Pale blue, opaque film-coated tablet.

Clinical particulars

Therapeutic indications: Synflex is indicated for the treatment of musculoskeletal disorders (including sprains and strains, direct trauma, lumbo-sacral pain, cervical spondylitis, fibrositis, bursitis and tendinitis); uterine pain following IUCD insertion, post-operative (including orthopaedic) pain; post-partum pain, rheumatoid arthritis, osteoarthrosis, ankylosing spondylitis, acute gout and dysmenorrhoea.

Synflex is also indicated for the relief of migraine.

Posology and method of administration: Therapy should be started at the lowest recommended dose, especially in the elderly.

Adults: For musculoskeletal disorders and post-operative pain, post IUCD insertion, rheumatoid arthritis, osteoarthrosis and ankylosing spondylitis the recommended dosage is 550 mg twice daily, not more than 1100 mg being taken per day.

For post-partum pain a single dose of 550 mg is recommended.

For dysmenorrhoea and acute gout the recommended dosage is 550 mg initially, followed by 275 mg at 6–8 hour intervals as needed. This represents a maximum dose on the first day of 1375 mg and 1100 mg per day thereafter.

For the relief of migraine, the recommended dose is 825 mg at the first symptom of an impending attack. 275–550 mg can be taken in addition throughout the day, if necessary, but not before half an hour after the initial dose. A total dose of 1375 mg per day should not be exceeded.

Elderly: Studies indicate that although the total plasma concentration of naproxen is unchanged, the unbound plasma fraction of naproxen is increased in the elderly. The implication of this finding for Synflex dosing is unknown. As with other drugs used in the elderly it is prudent to use the lowest effective dose. For the effect of reduced elimination in the elderly, refer to the section *Use in patients with impaired renal function.*

Children: Synflex is not recommended for use in children under sixteen years of age.

Contra-indications: Active or history of peptic ulceration or active gastrointestinal bleeding. Hypersensitivity to naproxen or naproxen sodium formulations. Since the potential exists for cross-sensitivity reactions, Synflex should not be given to patients in whom aspirin or other non-steroidal anti-inflammatory/analgesic drugs induce asthma, rhinitis or urticaria.

Special warnings and special precautions for use: Episodes of gastro-intestinal bleeding have been reported in patients with naproxen or naproxen sodium therapy. Synflex should therefore be given under close supervision to patients with a history of gastro-intestinal disease.

Serious gastro-intestinal adverse reactions can occur, at any time in patients on therapy with non-steroidal anti-inflammatory drugs. The risk of their occurrence does not seem to change with duration of therapy. Studies to date have not identified any subset of patients not at risk of developing peptic ulcer and bleeding, however, elderly and debilitated patients tolerate gastro-intestinal ulceration or bleeding less well than others. Most of the serious gastro-intestinal events associated with non-steroidal anti-inflammatory drugs occurred in this patient population.

The antipyretic and anti-inflammatory activities of Synflex may reduce fever and inflammation, thereby diminishing their usefulness as diagnostic signs.

Bronchospasm may be precipitated in patients suffering from, or with a history of, bronchial asthma or allergic disease.

Sporadic abnormalities in laboratory tests (e.g. liver function tests) have occurred in patients on naproxen or naproxen sodium therapy, but no definite trend was seen in any test indicating toxicity.

Naproxen decreases platelet aggregation and prolongs bleeding time. This effect should be kept in mind when bleeding times are determined.

Mild peripheral oedema has been observed in a few patients receiving naproxen or naproxen sodium. Although sodium retention has not been reported in metabolic studies, it is possible that patients with questionable or compromised cardiac function may be at a greater risk when taking Synflex.

Each Synflex tablet contains approximately 25 mg of sodium (about 1 m Eq). This should be considered in patients whose overall intake of sodium must be markedly restricted.

Use in patients with impaired renal function: As naproxen is eliminated to a large extent (95%) by urinary excretion via glomerular filtration, it should be used with great caution in patients with impaired renal function and the monitoring of serum creatinine and/or creatinine clearance is advised in these patients. Synflex is not recommended in patients having baseline creatinine clearance of less than 20 ml/minute.

Certain patients, specifically those whose renal blood flow is compromised, such as in extracellular volume depletion, cirrhosis of the liver, sodium restriction, congestive heart failure, and pre-existing renal disease, should have renal function assessed before and during Synflex therapy. Some elderly patients in whom impaired renal function may be expected, as well as patients using diuretics, may also fall within this category. A reduction in daily dosage should be considered to avoid the possibility of excessive accumulation of naproxen metabolites in these patients.

Use in patients with impaired liver function: Chronic alcoholic liver disease and probably also other forms of cirrhosis reduce the total plasma concentration of naproxen, but the plasma concentration of unbound naproxen is increased. The implication of this finding for Synflex dosing is unknown but it is prudent to use the lowest effective dose.

Haematological: Patients who have coagulation disorders or are receiving drug therapy that interferes with haemostasis should be carefully observed if naproxen-containing products are administered.

Patients at high risk of bleeding or those on full anti-coagulation therapy (e.g. dicoumarol derivatives) may be at increased risk of bleeding if given naproxen-containing products concurrently.

Anaphylactic (anaphylactoid) reactions: Hypersensitivity reactions may occur in susceptible individuals. Anaphylactic (anaphylactoid) reactions may occur both in patients with and without a history of hypersensitivity or exposure to aspirin, other non-steroidal anti-inflammatory drugs or naproxen-containing products. They may also occur in individuals with a history of angioedema, bronchospastic reactivity (e.g. asthma), rhinitis and nasal polyps.

Anaphylactoid reactions, like anaphylaxis, may have a fatal outcome.

Steroids: If steroid dosage is reduced or eliminated during therapy, the steroid dosage should be reduced slowly and the patients must be observed closely for any evidence of adverse effects, including adrenal insufficiency and exacerbation of symptoms of arthritis.

Ocular effects: Studies have not shown changes in the eye attributable to naproxen administration. In rare cases, adverse ocular disorders including papillitis, retrobulbar optic neuritis and papilledema, have been reported in users of NSAIDs including naproxen, although a cause-and-effect relationship cannot be established; accordingly, patients who develop visual disturbances during treatment with naproxen-containing products should have an ophthalmological examination.

Combination with other NSAIDs: The combination of naproxen-containing products and other NSAIDs is not recommended, because of the cumulative risks of inducing serious NSAID-related adverse events.

Interaction with other medicaments and other forms of interaction: Concomitant administration of antacid or cholestyramine can delay the absorption of naproxen but does not affect its extent. Concomitant administration of food can delay the absorption of naproxen, but does not affect its extent.

Due to the high plasma protein binding of naproxen, patients simultaneously receiving hydantoins, anticoagulants or a highly protein-bound sulfonamide should be observed for signs of overdosage of these drugs. No interactions have been observed in clinical studies with naproxen sodium or naproxen and anticoagulants or sulfonylureas, but caution is nevertheless advised since interaction has been seen with other non-steroidal agents of this class.

The natriuretic effect of frusemide has been reported to be inhibited by some drugs of this class.

Inhibition of renal lithium clearance leading to increases in plasma lithium concentrations has also been reported.

Naproxen and other non-steroidal anti-inflammatory drugs can reduce the antihypertensive effect of propranolol and other beta-blockers and may increase the risk of renal impairment associated with the use of ACE-inhibitors.

Probenecid given concurrently increases naproxen plasma levels and extends its half-life considerably.

Caution is advised where methotrexate is given concurrently because of possible enhancement of its toxicity since naproxen, among other non-steroidal anti-inflammatory drugs, has been reported to reduce the tubular secretion of methotrexate in an animal model.

NSAIDs may exacerbate cardiac failure, reduce GFR and increase plasma cardiac glycoside levels when co-administered with cardiac glycosides.

As with all NSAIDs caution is advised when cyclosporin is co-administered because of the increased risk of nephrotoxicity.

NSAIDs should not be used for 8–12 days after mifepristone administration as NSAIDs can reduce the effects of mifepristone.

As with all NSAIDs, caution should be taken when co-administering with cortico-steroids because of the increased risk of bleeding.

Patients taking quinolones may have an increased risk of developing convulsions.

It is suggested that Synflex therapy be temporarily discontinued 48 hours before adrenal function tests are performed because naproxen may artifactually interfere with some tests for 17-ketogenic steroids. Similarly, naproxen may interfere with some assays of urinary 5-hydroxyindoleacetic acid.

Pregnancy and lactation: Teratology studies in rats and rabbits at dose levels equivalent on a human multiple basis to those which have produced foetal abnormality with certain other non-steroidal anti-inflammatory agents, e.g. aspirin, have not produced evidence of foetal damage with Synflex. As with other drugs of this type Synflex delays parturition in animals (the relevance of this finding to human patients is unknown) and also affects the human foetal cardiovascular system (closure of the ductus arteriosus). Good medical practice indicates minimal drug usage in pregnancy, and use of this class of therapeutic agent requires cautious balancing of possible benefit against potential risk to the mother and foetus especially in the first and third trimesters.

The use of Synflex should be avoided in patients who are breast-feeding.

Effects on ability to drive and use machines: Some patients may experience drowsiness, dizziness, vertigo, insomnia or depression with the use of Synflex. If patients experience these or similar undesirable effects, they should exercise caution in carrying out activities that require alertness.

Undesirable effects:

Gastro-intestinal: The more frequent reactions are nausea, vomiting, abdominal discomfort and epigastric distress. More serious reactions which may occur occasionally are gastro-intestinal bleeding, peptic ulceration (sometimes with haemorrhage and perforation), non-peptic gastro-intestinal ulceration and colitis.

Dermatological: Skin rash, urticaria, angio-oedema. Alopecia, erythema multiforme, Stevens Johnson syndrome, epidermal necrolysis and photosensitivity reactions (including cases in which skin resembles porphyria cutanea tarda "pseudoporphyria") or epidermolysis bullosa may occur rarely.

Renal: Including, but not limited to, glomerular nephritis, interstitial nephritis, nephrotic syndrome, haematuria, renal papillary necrosis and renal failure.

CNS: Convulsions, headache, insomnia, inability to concentrate and cognitive dysfunction have been reported

Haematological: Thrombocytopenia, granulocytopenia including agranulocytosis, aplastic anaemia and haemolytic anaemia may occur rarely.

Other: Tinnitus, hearing impairment, vertigo, mild peripheral oedema. Anaphylactic reactions to naproxen and naproxen sodium formulations have been reported in patients with, or without, a history of previous hypersensitivity reactions to NSAIDs. Jaundice, fatal hepatitis, visual disturbances, eosinophilic pneumonitis, vasculitis, aseptic meningitis, hyperkalemia and ulcerative stomatitis have been reported rarely.

Overdose: Significant overdosage of the drug may be characterised by drowsiness, heartburn, indigestion, nausea or vomiting. A few patients have experienced seizures, but it is not clear whether these were naproxen-related or not. It is not known what dose of the drug would be life-threatening.

Should a patient ingest a large amount of Synflex accidentally or purposefully, the stomach may be emptied and usual supportive measures employed. Animal studies indicate that the prompt administration of activated charcoal in adequate amounts would tend to reduce markedly the absorption of the drug.

Haemodialysis does not decrease the plasma concentration of naproxen because of the high degree of protein binding. However, haemodialysis may still be appropriate in a patient with renal failure who has taken Synflex.

Pharmacological properties

Pharmacodynamic properties: Synflex is a non-steroidal, anti-inflammatory agent. It has analgesic, anti-inflammatory and antipyretic properties.

Pharmacokinetic properties: The sodium salt of naproxen is absorbed more rapidly than naproxen leading to earlier and higher plasma levels of naproxen. This is particularly useful for analgesia, where early availability of the drug in circulation is advantageous.

Typical pharmacokinetic values for naproxen sodium and naproxen are as follows:

Parameter	*2 x 275 mg Naproxen-Na tablet*	*2 x 250 mg Naproxen tablet*	*p. value*
Biol T1/2 (hrs)	13.41	13.43	0.993
T max (min)	56.67	110.0	0.036
Cp max (mcg/ml)	74.67	65.58	0.007
AUC Total (mcg/ml x hr)	1050.9	1006.1	0.478

See also *Special warnings and special precautions for use:* for certain patients, i.e. the elderly and those with impaired renal or liver function.

Preclinical safety data: None stated.

Pharmaceutical particulars

List of excipients: Povidone BP, magnesium stearate BP, microcrystalline cellulose BP, purified water BP, talc BP and opadry.

Incompatibilities: None stated.

Shelf life: 5 years.

Special precautions for storage: Protect from light and moisture.

Nature and contents of container:

a. Opaque high density polyethylene container containing 100 tablets.

b. PVC/foil blister pack containing 60 tablets.

c. Polypropylene securitainers with high density polyethylene lid containing 2 or 4 tablets.

Instructions for use/handling: None stated.

Marketing authorisation number PL 0031/0478

Date of first authorisation/renewal of authorisation 30 May 1996

Date of (partial) revision of the text October 1997

SYNTARIS

Qualitative and quantitative composition Aqueous solution containing flunisolide 0.025% w/v.

Pharmaceutical form Aqueous solution.

Clinical particulars

Therapeutic indications: For the prophylaxis and treatment of perennial and seasonal allergic rhinitis including hay fever.

Posology and method of administration:

Route of administration: Intra-nasal.

Adults (including the elderly): 2 sprays (approximately 25μg) into each nostril twice or 3 times daily. Maximum daily dose should not exceed 6 sprays in each nostril per day.

Children: 5 years and over: One spray into each nostril 3 times daily. Maximum daily dose should not exceed 3 sprays in each nostril per day.

Maintenance dose: After the desired clinical effect is obtained the maintenance dose should be the smallest amount necessary to control the symptoms. Some patients may be maintained on as little as one spray to each nostril per day.

Contra-indications:

1. Untreated fungal, bacterial or viral nasal or ocular infections.

2. Hypersensitivity to the formulation.

Special warnings and special precautions for use: Systemic effects of nasal corticosteroids may occur, particularly at high doses prescribed for prolonged periods. Growth retardation has been reported in children receiving nasal corticosteroids at licensed doses.

It is recommended that the height of children receiving prolonged treatment with nasal corticosteroids is regularly monitored. If growth is slowed, therapy should be reviewed with the aim of reducing the dose of nasal corticosteroid if possible, to the lowest dose at which effective control of symptoms is maintained. In addition consideration should be given to referring the patient to a paediatric specialist.

Treatment with *higher than recommended* doses may result in clinically significant adrenal suppression. If there is evidence for higher than recommended doses being used then additional systemic corticosteroid cover should be considered during periods of stress or elective surgery.

Care must be taken when transferring patients from systemic steroid therapy to Syntaris nasal spray if there is reason to suspect that their adrenal function is impaired.

Because of the inhibitory effect of corticosteroids in wound healing in patients who have experienced recent nasal septal ulcers, recurrent epistaxis, nasal surgery or trauma, a nasal corticosteroid should be used with caution until healing has occurred.

Interaction with other medicaments and other forms of interaction: None known.

Pregnancy and lactation: Not recommended in the first 3 months of pregnancy. If used in the second or third trimester, the expected benefits should be weighed against the potential hazards to the foetus.

Effects on ability to drive and use machines: Not applicable.

Undesirable effects: Glucocorticoids may mask some signs of infection and new infections may appear during their use.

Systemic effects of nasal corticosteroids may occur, particularly when prescribed at high doses for prolonged periods.

Although atrophy of the nasal mucosa have not been observed in clinical trials, the potential for these effects should be considered with prolonged excessive usage.

Adverse reactions noted in clinical trials with Syntaris nasal spray have been consistent with what one would expect when applying topical medication to an already inflamed membrane. The most frequently observed side-effect was aftertaste and a mild transient nasal burning and stinging which was occasionally severe enough to warrant discontinuation of treatment. Other side-effects noted, in order of decreasing prevalence were: nasal irritation, epistaxis, runny and stuffy nose, sore throat, hoarseness, throat irritation and rarely, alteration of smell and/or taste, nasal septal perforation. Rarely, a permanent loss in the sense of smell and/or taste has been reported.

Carcinogenesis: A 22-month study in mice and a 24-month study in rats showed some evidence of tumour formation that was not consistent between the 2 species and is not believed to be biologically meaningful to man.

Overdose: Administration of large amounts of flunisolide over a short period may produce suppression of hypothalamic-pituitary-adrenal function. In such event, Syntaris nasal spray should be reduced immediately to the recommended dosage.

Pharmacological properties

Pharmacodynamic properties: Flunisolide is a synthetic corticosteroid which has been formulated as a topical nasal spray for the treatment of allergic nasal conditions. In animal studies flunisolide has several hundred times the anti-inflammatory, thymolytic and anti-adrenocorticotrophic hormone activities of hydrocortisone. Because of the small dose applied (topically) and low systemic absorption, there is minimal systemic activity.

In controlled clinical trials flunisolide has been shown to be significantly more effective than placebo in the treatment of perennial and seasonal allergic rhinitis.

Pharmacokinetic properties: Flunisolide is rapidly and well absorbed from the gastrointestinal tract. In man peak blood levels after oral administration occurred within one hour, but the systemic availability was estimated to be only 20%. After intra-nasal administration (approximately 100μg) extremely low plasma levels (less than 1ng/ml) were detected within 10–

30 minutes of dosing and these fall to undetectable levels within 4 hours.

In man flunisolide undergoes rapid and extensive first pass metabolism to a 6β-hydroxylated metabolite, which has less than 0.01 times the potency of flunisolide, and is less than 3 times as potent as hydrocortisone.

The plasma half-life of flunisolide is 1.5–2 hours and that of the 6β-hydroxylated metabolite is 2–4 hours. Repeated BD administration of flunisolide by oral inhalation did not result in any cumulative effects. Excretion is via the urine and faeces. Only minor amounts of unchanged free or conjugated flunisolide are excreted in the urine, the major excretory product is the free 6β-hydroxylated metabolite. Animal studies indicate that although a large amount is excreted in the bile, neither flunisolide nor its metabolites appear to enter the entero-hepatic circulation.

Preclinical safety data: None stated.

Pharmaceutical particulars

List of excipients: Propylene glycol, polyethylene glycol, sorbitol, polysorbate, benzalkonium chloride, disodium edetate, citric acid amhydrious, sodium citrate dihydrate, butylated hydroxytolune, purified water.

Incompatibilities: Not applicable.

Shelf life: 30 months.

Special precautions for storage: Store at room temperature below 30°C.

Nature and contents of container: Amber type III glass or white high density polyethylene bottle with a metered pump packaged into an outer carton, containing 24 ml of aqueous solution.

Instructions for use/handling: None stated.

Marketing authorisation number PL 0031/0479

Date of first authorisation/renewal of authorisation 26 April 1996

Date of (partial) revision of the text May 1998

TORADOL

Qualitative and quantitative composition Ketorolac Trometamol 10 mg.

Pharmaceutical form White to creamy white film coated, round tablet, marked "KET 10" on one face, the other face blank.

Clinical particulars

Therapeutic indications: Toradol tablets are indicated for the short-term management of moderate post-operative pain.

Posology and method of administration: Toradol tablets are recommended for short-term use only (up to 7 days) and are not recommended for chronic use.

Adults: 10 mg every 4 to 6 hours as required. Doses exceeding 40 mg per day are not recommended.

Opioid analgesics (e.g. morphine, pethidine) may be used concomitantly, and may be required for optimal analgesic effect in the early postoperative period when pain is most severe. Ketorolac does not interfere with opioid binding and does not exacerbate opioid-related respiratory depression or sedation.

For patients receiving parenteral Toradol, and who are converted to Toradol oral tablets, the total combined daily dose should not exceed 90 mg (60 mg for the elderly, renally-impaired patients and patients less than 50 kg) and the oral component should not exceed 40 mg on the day the change of formulation is made. Patients should be converted to oral treatment as soon as possible.

Elderly: A longer dosing interval, e.g. 6–8 hourly, is advisable in the elderly. The lower end of the dosage range is recommended for patients over 65 years of age.

Children: Toradol is not recommended for use in children under 16 years of age.

Contra-indications:

- a history of peptic ulcer or gastro-intestinal bleeding
- suspected or confirmed cerebrovascular bleeding
- haemorrhagic diatheses, including coagulation disorders
- hypersensitivity to ketorolac trometamol or other NSAIDs and those patients in whom aspirin or other prostaglandin synthesis inhibitors induce allergic reactions (severe anaphylactic-like reactions have been observed in such patients)
- the complete or partial syndrome of nasal polyps, angioedema or bronchospasm
- concurrent treatment with other NSAIDs, oxpentifylline, probenecid or lithium salts
- hypovolaemia from any cause or dehydration
- moderate or severe renal impairment (serum creatinine > 160 micromol/l)
- a history of asthma
- patients who have had operations with a high risk of haemorrhage or incomplete haemostasis
- patients on anticoagulants including low dose heparin (2500–5000 units 12-hourly)
- during pregnancy, labour, delivery or lactation
- children under 16 years of age
- Toradol is contra-indicated as prophylatic analgesia before surgery due to inhibition of platelet aggregation and is contra-indicated intraoperatively because of the increased risk of bleeding
- Toradol is contra-indicated in patients currently receiving aspirin

Special warnings and special precautions for use:

Use in the elderly: Patients over the age of 65 years may be at a greater risk of experiencing adverse events than younger patients. This age-related risk is common to all NSAIDs. Compared to young adults, the elderly have an increased plasma half-life and reduced plasma clearance of ketorolac. A longer dosing interval is advisable (see *Posology and method of administration*).

Gastro-intestinal effects: Toradol can cause gastro-intestinal irritation, ulcers or bleeding in patients with or without a history of previous symptoms. Elderly and debilitated patients are more prone to develop these reactions. The incidence increases with dose and duration of treatment.

In a non-randomised, in-hospital post-marketing surveillance study, increased rates of clinically serious GI bleeding were seen in patients ≤ 65 years of age who received an average daily dose of > 90 mg ketorolac IM as compared to those patients receiving parenteral opioids.

Respiratory effects: Bronchospasm may be precipitated in patients with a history of asthma.

Renal effects: Drugs that inhibit prostaglandin biosynthesis (including non-steroidal anti-inflammatory drugs) have been reported to cause nephrotoxicity, including but not limited to glomerular nephritis, interstitial nephritis, renal papillary necrosis, nephrotic syndrome and acute renal failure. In patients with renal, cardiac or hepatic impairment, caution is required since the use of NSAIDs may result in deterioration of renal function.

As with other drugs that inhibit prostaglandin synthesis, elevations of serum urea, creatinine and potassium have been reported with ketorolac trometamol and may occur after one dose.

Patients with impaired renal function: Since ketorolac trometamol and its metabolites are excreted primarily by the kidney, patients with moderate to severe impairment of renal function (serum creatinine greater than 160 micromol/l) should not receive Toradol. Patients with lesser renal impairment should receive a reduced dose of ketorolac (not exceeding 60 mg/day IM or IV) and their renal status should be closely monitored.

Caution should be observed in patients with conditions leading to a reduction in blood volume and/or renal blood flow, where renal prostaglandins have a supportive role in the maintenance of renal perfusion. In these patients, administration of an NSAID may cause a dose-dependent reduction in renal prostaglandin formation and may precipitate overt renal failure. Patients at greatest risk of this reaction are those who are volume depleted because of blood loss or severe dehydration, patients with impaired renal function, heart failure, liver dysfunction, the elderly and those taking diuretics. Discontinuation of NSAID therapy is typically followed by recovery to the pre-treatment state. Inadequate fluid/blood replacement during surgery, leading to hypovolaemia, may lead to renal dysfunction which could be exacerbated when Toradol is administered. Therefore, volume depletion should be corrected and close monitoring of serum urea and creatinine and urine output is recommended until the patient is normovolaemic. In patients on renal dialysis, ketorolac clearance was reduced to approximately half the normal rate and terminal half-life increased approximately three-fold.

Fluid retention and oedema: Fluid retention and oedema have been reported with the use of Toradol and it should therefore be used with caution in patients with cardiac decompensation, hypertension or similar conditions.

Use in patients with impaired liver function: Patients with impaired hepatic function from cirrhosis do not have any clinically important changes in ketorolac clearance or terminal half-life.

Borderline elevations of one or more liver function tests may occur. These abnormalities may be transient, may remain unchanged, or may progress with continued therapy. Meaningful elevations (greater than 3 times normal) of serum glutamate pyruvate transaminase (SGPT/ALT) or serum glutamate oxaloacetate transaminase (SGOT/AST) occurred in controlled clinical trials in less than 1% of patients. If clinical signs and symptoms consistent with liver disease develop, or if systemic manifestations occur, Toradol should be discontinued.

Haematological effects: Patients with coagulation disorders should not receive Toradol. Patients on anticoagulation therapy may be at increased risk of bleeding if given Toradol concurrently. The concomitant use of ketorolac and prophylactic low-dose heparin (2500–5000 units 12-hourly) has not been studied extensively and may also be associated with an increased risk of bleeding. Patients already on anticoagulants or who require low-dose heparin should not receive ketorolac. Patients who are receiving other drug therapy that interferes with haemostasis should be carefully observed if Toradol is administered. In controlled clinical studies, the incidence of clinically significant postoperative bleeding was less than 1%.

Ketorolac inhibits platelet aggregation and prolongs bleeding time. In patients with normal bleeding function, bleeding times were raised, but not outside the normal range of 2–11 minutes. Unlike the prolonged effects from aspirin, platelet function returns to normal within 24 to 48 hours after ketorolac is discontinued.

In post-marketing experience, postoperative wound haemorrhage has been reported in association with the immediate peri-operative use of Toradol IM/IV. Therefore, ketorolac should not be used in patients who have had operations with a high risk of haemorrhage or incomplete haemostasis. Caution should be used where strict haemostasis is critical, e.g. in cosmetic or day-case surgery. Haematomata and other signs of wound haemorrhage and epistaxis have been reported with the use of Toradol. Physicians should be aware of the pharmacological similarity of ketorolac to other non-steroidal anti-inflammatory drugs that inhibit cyclo-oxygenase and the risk of bleeding, particularly in the elderly.

Toradol is not an anaesthetic agent and possesses no sedative or anxiolytic properties; therefore it is not recommended as a pre-operative medication for the support of anaesthesia when these effects are required.

The risk of clinically serious gastro-intestinal bleeding is dose-dependent. This is particularly true in elderly patients who receive an average daily dose greater than 60 mg/day of Toradol.

Interaction with other medicaments and other forms of interaction: Toradol should not be used with other NSAIDs or in patients receiving aspirin because of the potential for additive side-effects.

Ketorolac is highly bound to human plasma protein (mean 99.2%) and binding is concentration-independent.

Ketorolac did not alter digoxin protein binding. *In vitro* studies indicated that at therapeutic concentrations of salicylate (300 mcg/ml) and above, the binding of ketorolac was reduced from approximately 99.2% to 97.5%. Therapeutic concentrations of digoxin, warfarin, paracetamol, phenytoin and tolbutamide did not alter ketorolac protein binding. Because ketorolac is a highly potent drug and present in low concentrations in plasma, it would not be expected to displace other protein-bound drugs significantly.

There is no evidence in animal or human studies that ketorolac trometamol induces or inhibits the hepatic enzymes capable of metabolising itself or other drugs. Hence Toradol would not be expected to alter the pharmacokinetics of other drugs due to enzyme induction or inhibition mechanisms.

In normovolaemic healthy subjects, ketorolac reduces the diuretic response to frusemide by approximately 20%, so particular care should be taken in patients with cardiac decompensation.

There is an increased risk of renal impairment when ketorolac is administered concurrently with ACE inhibitors, particularly in volume depleted patients.

Caution is advised when methotrexate is administered concurrently, since some prostaglandin synthesis inhibiting drugs have been reported to reduce the clearance of methotrexate, and thus possibly enhance its toxicity.

Probenecid should not be administered concurrently with ketorolac because of increases in ketorolac plasma level and half-life.

Because of an increased tendency to bleeding when oxpentifylline is administered concurrently, this combination should be avoided.

In patients receiving lithium, there is a possible inhibition of renal lithium clearance, increased plasma lithium concentration, and potential lithium toxicity. (See *Contra-indications*).

Pregnancy and lactation: There was no evidence of teratogenicity in rats or rabbits studied at maternally-toxic doses of ketorolac. Prolongation of the gestation period and/or delayed parturition were seen in the rat. Ketorolac and its metabolites have been shown to pass into the foetus and milk of animals. Ketorolac has been detected in human milk at low levels. Safety in human pregnancy has not been established. Ketorolac is therefore contra-indicated during pregnancy, labour or delivery, or in mothers who are breast-feeding.

Effects on ability to drive and use machines: Some

patients may experience drowsiness, dizziness, vertigo, insomnia or depression with the use of Toradol. If patients experience these, or other similar undesirable effects, they should exercise caution in carrying out activities that require alertness.

Undesirable effects: The following side-effects have been reported with Toradol.

Gastro-intestinal: Nausea, dyspepsia, gastro-intestinal pain, gastro-intestinal bleeding, abdominal discomfort, haematemesis, gastritis, oesophagitis, diarrhoea, eructation, constipation, flatulence, fullness, melaena, peptic ulcer, rectal bleeding, stomatitis, vomiting, haemorrhage, perforation, pancreatitis.

Central nervous/musculoskeletal systems: Anxiety, drowsiness, dizziness, headache, sweating, dry mouth, nervousness, paraesthesia, functional disorders, abnormal thinking, depression, euphoria, convulsions, excessive thirst, inability to concentrate, insomnia, stimulation, vertigo, abnormal taste and vision, myalgia, abnormal dreams, hallucinations, hyperkinesia, hearing loss, tinnitus, aseptic meningitis, psychotic reactions.

Renal: Increased urinary frequency, oliguria, acute renal failure, hyponatraemia, hyperkalaemia, haemolytic uraemic syndrome, flank pain (with or without haematuria), raised serum urea and creatinine, interstitial nephritis, urinary retention, nephrotic syndrome.

*Cardiovascular/haematological:*Flushing, bradycardia, pallor, purpura, thrombocytopenia, hypertension, palpitations, chest pain.

Respiratory: Dyspnoea, asthma, pulmonary oedema.

Dermatological: Pruritus, urticaria, Lyell's syndrome, Stevens-Johnson syndrome, exfoliative dermatitis, maculopapular rash.

Hypersensitivity reactions: Anaphylaxis, bronchospasm, laryngeal oedema, hypotension, flushing and rash. Such reactions may occur in patients with or without known sensitivity to Toradol or other non-steroidal anti-inflammatory drugs.

These may also occur in individuals with a history of angioedema, bronchospastic reactivity (e.g. asthma and nasal polyps). Anaphylactoid reactions, like anaphylaxis, may have a fatal outcome (see *Contra-indications*).

Bleeding: Postoperative wound haemorrhage, haematomata, epistaxis, increased bleeding time.

Other: Asthenia, oedema, weight gain, abnormalities of liver function tests, hepatitis, liver failure, fever.

Overdose: Doses of 360 mg given intramuscularly over an 8-hour interval for five consecutive days have caused abdominal pain and peptic ulcers which have healed after discontinuation of dosing. Two patients recovered from unsuccessful suicide attempts. One patient experienced nausea after 210 mg ketorolac, and the other hyperventilation after 300 mg ketorolac.

Pharmacological properties

Pharmacodynamic properties: Ketorolac trometamol is a non-narcotic analgesic. It is a non-steroidal anti-inflammatory agent that exhibits anti-inflammatory and weak antipyretic activity.

Ketorolac trometamol inhibits the synthesis of prostaglandins and is considered a peripherally acting analgesic. It does not have known effects on opiate receptors.

No evidence of respiratory depression has been observed after administration of ketorolac trometamol in controlled clinical trials. Ketorolac trometamol does not cause pupil constriction.

Pharmacokinetic properties: Ketorolac trometamol is rapidly and completely absorbed following oral administration with a peak plasma concentration of 0.87 mcg/ml occurring 50 minutes after a single 10 mg dose. The terminal plasma elimination half-life averages 5.4 hours (S.D. = 1.0) in healthy subjects. In elderly subjects (mean age 72) it is 6.2 hours (S.D. = 1.0). More than 99% of the ketorolac in plasma is protein bound.

The pharmacokinetics of ketorolac in man following single or multiple doses are linear. Steady state plasma levels are achieved after 1 day of Q.I.D. dosing. No changes occurred with chronic dosing. Following a single intravenous dose, the volume of distribution is 0.25 l/kg, the half-life is 5 hours and the clearance 0.55 ml/min/kg. The primary route of excretion of ketorolac and its metabolites (conjugates and the p-hydroxymetabolite) is in the urine (91.4%) and the remainder is excreted in the faeces.

A high fat diet decreased the rate, but not the extent of absorption, while antacid had no effect on ketorolac absorption.

Preclinical safety data: None stated.

Pharmaceutical particulars

List of excipients: Microcrystalline cellulose EP, Spray dried lactose EP, Magnesium stearate EP

Coating suspension: Opadry white YS-1-7002, Purified water

Incompatibilities: None known.

Shelf life: 3 years.

Special precautions for storage: Protect from moisture.

Nature and contents of container: White HDPE bottles with polypropylene screw containers containing 50, 56, 100, 250 or 500 tablets.

Polypropylene securitainers containing 50, 56, 100, 250 or 500 tablets.

Amber or white PVC/aluminium foil blister packs in outer cardboard carton containing 4, 20, 28, 50, 56, 100, 250 or 500 tablets.

Instructions for use/handling: None stated.

Marketing authorisation number PL 0031/0482

Date of first authorisation/renewal of authorisation 31 May 1996

Date of (partial) revision of the text November 1997

TORADOL INJECTION

Qualitative and quantitative composition Toradol contains ketorolac trometamol 10 mg or 30 mg in ampoules of 1 ml. It also contains ethanol, sodium chloride and water.

Pharmaceutical form Toradol is a clear, slightly yellow solution for intramuscular or bolus intravenous injection.

Clinical particulars

Therapeutic indications: Toradol is indicated for the short-term management of moderate to severe acute postoperative pain.

Posology and method of administration: Toradol is for administration by intramuscular or bolus intravenous injection. Bolus intravenous doses should be given over no less than 15 seconds. Toradol should not be used for epidural or spinal administration.

The time to onset of analgesic effect following both IV and IM administration is similar and is approximately 30 minutes, with maximum analgesia occurring within 1 to 2 hours. The median duration of analgesia is generally 4 to 6 hours.

Dosage should be adjusted according to the severity of the pain and the patient response.

The administration of continuous multiple daily doses of ketorolac intramuscularly or intravenously should not exceed 2 days because adverse events may increase with prolonged usage. There has been limited experience with dosing for longer periods since the vast majority of patients have transferred to oral medication, or no longer require analgesic therapy after this time.

Adults: The recommended initial dose of Toradol is 10 mg, followed by 10 to 30 mg every 4 to 6 hours as required. In the initial postoperative period, Toradol may be given as often as every 2 hours if needed. The lowest effective dose should be given. A total daily dose of 90 mg for non-elderly and 60 mg for the elderly, renally-impaired patients and patients less than 50 kg should not be exceeded. The maximum duration of treatment should not exceed 2 days.

Reduce dosage in patients under 50 kg.

Opioid analgesics (e.g. morphine, pethidine) may be used concomitantly, and may be required for optimal analgesic effect in the early postoperative period when pain is most severe. Ketorolac does not interfere with opioid binding and does not exacerbate opioid-related respiratory depression or sedation. When used in association with Toradol IM/IV, the daily dose of opioid is usually less than that normally required. However, opioid side-effects should still be considered, especially in day-case surgery.

For patients receiving parenteral Toradol, and who are converted to Toradol oral tablets, the total combined daily dose should not exceed 90 mg (60 mg for the elderly, renally-impaired patients and patients less than 50 kg) and the oral component should not exceed 40 mg on the day the change of formulation is made. Patients should be converted to oral treatment as soon as possible.

Elderly: For patients over 65 years, the lower end of the dosage range is recommended; a total daily dose of 60 mg should not be exceeded (see *Special warnings and special precautions for use*).

Children: Safety and efficacy in children have not been established. Therefore, Toradol is not recommended for use in children under 16 years of age.

Renal impairment: Contra-indicated in moderate to severe renal impairment; reduce dosage in lesser impairment (not exceeding 60 mg/day IV or IM) (see *Contra-indications*).

Contra-indications:

- a history of peptic ulcer or gastro-intestinal bleeding
- suspected or confirmed cerebrovascular bleeding
- haemorrhagic diatheses, including coagulation disorders
- hypersensitivity to ketorolac trometamol or other NSAIDs and those patients in whom aspirin or other prostaglandin synthesis inhibitors induce allergic reactions (severe anaphylactic-like reactions have been observed in such patients)
- the complete or partial syndrome of nasal polyps, angioedema or bronchospasm
- concurrent treatment with other NSAIDs, oxpentifylline, probenecid or lithium salts
- hypovolaemia from any cause or dehydration
- moderate or severe renal impairment (serum creatinine > 160 micromol/l)
- a history of asthma
- patients who have had operations with a high risk of haemorrhage or incomplete haemostasis
- patients on anticoagulants including low dose heparin (2500–5000 units 12-hourly)
- during pregnancy, labour, delivery or lactation
- children under 16 years of age
- Toradol is contra-indicated as prophylatic analgesia before surgery due to inhibition of platelet aggregation and is contra-indicated intraoperatively because of the increased risk of bleeding
- Toradol is contra-indicated in patients currently receiving aspirin

Special warnings and special precautions for use: Physicians should be aware that in some patients pain relief may not occur until upwards of 30 minutes after IV or IM administration.

Use in the elderly: Patients over the age of 65 years may be at a greater risk of experiencing adverse events than younger patients. This age-related risk is common to all NSAIDs. Compared to young adults, the elderly have an increased plasma half-life and reduced plasma clearance of ketorolac. With Toradol IM/IV, a total daily dose greater than 60 mg is not recommended. With Toradol tablets, a longer dosing interval is advisable (see *Posology and method of administration*).

Gastro-intestinal effects: Toradol can cause gastro-intestinal irritation, ulcers or bleeding in patients with or without a history of previous symptoms. Elderly and debilitated patients are more prone to develop these reactions. The incidence increases with dose and duration of treatment.

In a non-randomised, in-hospital post-marketing surveillance study, increased rates of clinically serious GI bleeding were seen in patients < 65 years of age who received an average daily dose of > 90 mg ketorolac IM as compared to those patients receiving parenteral opioids.

Respiratory effects: Bronchospasm may be precipitated in patients with a history of asthma.

Renal effects: Drugs that inhibit prostaglandin biosynthesis (including non-steroidal anti-inflammatory drugs) have been reported to cause nephrotoxicity, including but not limited to glomerular nephritis, interstitial nephritis, renal papillary necrosis, nephrotic syndrome and acute renal failure. In patients with renal, cardiac or hepatic impairment, caution is required since the use of NSAIDs may result in deterioration of renal function.

As with other drugs that inhibit prostaglandin synthesis, elevations of serum urea, creatinine and potassium have been reported with ketorolac trometamol and may occur after one dose.

Patients with impaired renal function: Since ketorolac trometamol and its metabolites are excreted primarily by the kidney, patients with moderate to severe impairment of renal function (serum creatinine greater than 160 micromol/l) should not receive Toradol. Patients with lesser renal impairment should receive a reduced dose of ketorolac (not exceeding 60 mg/day IM or IV) and their renal status should be closely monitored.

Caution should be observed in patients with conditions leading to a reduction in blood volume and/or renal blood flow, where renal prostaglandins have a supportive role in the maintenance of renal perfusion. In these patients, administration of an NSAID may cause a dose-dependent reduction in renal prostaglandin formation and may precipitate overt renal failure. Patients at greatest risk of this reaction are those who are volume depleted because of blood loss or severe dehydration, patients with impaired renal function, heart failure, liver dysfunction, the elderly and those taking diuretics. Discontinuation of NSAID therapy is typically followed by recovery to the pretreatment state. Inadequate fluid/blood replacement during surgery, leading to hypovolaemia, may lead to renal dysfunction which could be exacerbated when Toradol is administered. Therefore, volume depletion should be corrected and close monitoring of serum urea and creatinine and urine output is recommended until the patient is normovolaemic. In patients on renal dialysis, ketorolac clearance was reduced to approximately half the normal rate and terminal half-life increased approximately three-fold.

Fluid retention and oedema: Fluid retention and oedema have been reported with the use of Toradol and it should therefore be used with caution in patients with cardiac decompensation, hypertension or similar conditions.

Use in patients with impaired liver function: Patients with impaired hepatic function from cirrhosis do not have any clinically important changes in ketorolac clearance or terminal half-life.

Borderline elevations of one or more liver function tests may occur. These abnormalities may be transient, may remain unchanged, or may progress with continued therapy. Meaningful elevations (greater than 3 times normal) of serum glutamate pyruvate transaminase (SGPT/ALT) or serum glutamate oxaloacetate transaminase (SGOT/AST) occurred in controlled clinical trials in less than 1% of patients. If clinical signs and symptoms consistent with liver disease develop, or if systemic manifestations occur, Toradol should be discontinued.

Haematological effects: Patients with coagulation disorders should not receive Toradol. Patients on anticoagulation therapy may be at increased risk of bleeding if given Toradol concurrently. The concomitant use of ketorolac and prophylactic low-dose heparin (2500–5000 units 12-hourly) has not been studied extensively and may also be associated with an increased risk of bleeding. Patients already on anticoagulants or who require low-dose heparin should not receive ketorolac. Patients who are receiving other drug therapy that interferes with haemostasis should be carefully observed if Toradol is administered. In controlled clinical studies, the incidence of clinically significant postoperative bleeding was less than 1%.

Ketorolac inhibits platelet aggregation and prolongs bleeding time. In patients with normal bleeding function, bleeding times were raised, but not outside the normal range of 2–11 minutes. Unlike the prolonged effects from aspirin, platelet function returns to normal within 24 to 48 hours after ketorolac is discontinued.

In post-marketing experience, postoperative wound haemorrhage has been reported in association with the immediate peri-operative use of Toradol IM/IV. Therefore, ketorolac should not be used in patients who have had operations with a high risk of haemorrhage or incomplete haemostasis. Caution should be used where strict haemostasis is critical, e.g. in cosmetic or day-case surgery. Haematomata and other signs of wound haemorrhage and epistaxis have been reported with the use of Toradol. Physicians should be aware of the pharmacological similarity of ketorolac to other non-steroidal anti-inflammatory drugs that inhibit cyclo-oxygenase and the risk of bleeding, particularly in the elderly.

Toradol is not an anaesthetic agent and possesses no sedative or anxiolytic properties; therefore it is not recommended as a pre-operative medication for the support of anaesthesia when these effects are required.

The risk of clinically serious gastro-intestinal bleeding is dose-dependent. This is particularly true in elderly patients who receive an average daily dose greater than 60 mg/day of Toradol.

Interaction with other medicaments and other forms of interaction: Toradol should not be used with other NSAIDs or in patients receiving aspirin because of the potential for additive side-effects.

Ketorolac is highly bound to human plasma protein (mean 99.2%) and binding is concentration-independent.

Ketorolac did not alter digoxin protein binding. *In vitro* studies indicated that at therapeutic concentrations of salicylate (300 mcg/ml) and above, the binding of ketorolac was reduced from approximately 99.2% to 97.5%. Therapeutic concentrations of digoxin, warfarin, paracetamol, phenytoin and tolbutamide did not alter ketorolac protein binding. Because ketorolac is a highly potent drug and present in low concentrations in plasma, it would not be expected to displace other protein-bound drugs significantly.

There is no evidence in animal or human studies that ketorolac trometamol induces or inhibits the hepatic enzymes capable of metabolising itself or other drugs. Hence Toradol would not be expected to alter the pharmacokinetics of other drugs due to enzyme induction or inhibition mechanisms.

In normovolaemic healthy subjects, ketorolac reduces the diuretic response to frusemide by approximately 20%, so particular care should be taken in patients with cardiac decompensation.

There is an increased risk of renal impairment when ketorolac is administered concurrently with ACE inhibitors, particularly in volume depleted patients.

Caution is advised when methotrexate is administered concurrently, since some prostaglandin synthesis inhibiting drugs have been reported to reduce the clearance of methotrexate, and thus possibly enhance its toxicity.

Probenecid should not be administered concurrently with ketorolac because of increases in ketorolac plasma level and half-life.

Because of an increased tendency to bleeding when oxpentifylline is administered concurrently, this combination should be avoided.

In patients receiving lithium, there is a possible inhibition of renal lithium clearance, increased plasma lithium concentration, and potential lithium toxicity. (See *Contra-indications*).

Pregnancy and lactation: There was no evidence of teratogenicity in rats or rabbits studied at maternally-toxic doses of ketorolac. Prolongation of the gestation period and/or delayed parturition were seen in the rat. Ketorolac and its metabolites have been shown to pass into the foetus and milk of animals. Ketorolac has been detected in human milk at low levels. Safety in human pregnancy has not been established. Ketorolac is therefore contra-indicated during pregnancy, labour or delivery, or in mothers who are breast-feeding.

Effects on ability to drive and use machines: Some patients may experience drowsiness, dizziness, vertigo, insomnia or depression with the use of Toradol. If patients experience these, or other similar undesirable effects, they should exercise caution in carrying out activities that require alertness.

Undesirable effects: The following side-effects have been reported with Toradol.

Gastro-intestinal: Nausea, dyspepsia, gastro-intestinal pain, gastro-intestinal bleeding, abdominal discomfort, haematemesis, gastritis, oesophagitis, diarrhoea, eructation, constipation, flatulence, fullness, melaena, peptic ulcer, rectal bleeding, stomatitis, vomiting, haemorrhage, perforation, pancreatitis.

Central nervous/musculoskeletal systems: Anxiety, drowsiness, dizziness, headache, sweating, dry mouth, nervousness, paraesthesia, functional disorders, abnormal thinking, depression, euphoria, convulsions, excessive thirst, inability to concentrate, insomnia, stimulation, vertigo, abnormal taste and vision, myalgia, abnormal dreams, hallucinations, hyperkinesia, hearing loss, tinnitus, aseptic meningitis, psychotic reactions.

Renal: Increased urinary frequency, oliguria, acute renal failure, hyponatraemia, hyperkalaemia, haemolytic uraemic syndrome, flank pain (with or without haematuria), raised serum urea and creatinine, interstitial nephritis, urinary retention, nephrotic syndrome.

Cardiovascular/haematological: Flushing, bradycardia, pallor, purpura, thrombocytopenia, hypertension, palpitations, chest pain.

Respiratory: Dyspnoea, asthma, pulmonary oedema.

Dermatological: Pruritus, urticaria, Lyell's syndrome, Stevens-Johnson syndrome, exfoliative dermatitis, maculopapular rash.

Hypersensitivity reactions: Anaphylaxis, bronchospasm, laryngeal oedema, hypotension, flushing and rash. Such reactions may occur in patients with or without known sensitivity to Toradol or other non-steroidal anti-inflammatory drugs.

These may also occur in individuals with a history of angioedema, bronchospastic reactivity (e.g. asthma and nasal polyps). Anaphylactoid reactions, like anaphylaxis, may have a fatal outcome (see *Contra-indications*).

Bleeding: Postoperative wound haemorrhage, haematomata, epistaxis, increased bleeding time.

Other: Asthenia, oedema, weight gain, abnormalities of liver function tests, hepatitis, liver failure, fever. Injection site pain has been reported in some patients.

Overdose: Doses of 360 mg given intramuscularly over an 8-hour interval for five consecutive days have caused abdominal pain and peptic ulcers which have healed after discontinuation of dosing. Two patients recovered from unsuccessful suicide attempts. One patient experienced nausea after 210 mg ketorolac, and the other hyperventilation after 300 mg ketorolac.

Pharmacological properties

Pharmacodynamic properties: Toradol is a potent analgesic agent of the non-steroidal, anti-inflammatory class (NSAID). It is not an opioid and has no known effects on opioid receptors. Its mode of action is to inhibit the cyclo-oxygenase enzyme system and hence prostaglandin synthesis, and it demonstrates a minimal anti-inflammatory effect at its analgesic dose.

Pharmacokinetic properties:

IM: Following intramuscular administration, ketorolac trometamol was rapidly and completely absorbed, a mean peak plasma concentration of 2.2 mcg/ml occurring an average of 50 minutes after a single 30 mg dose. The influences of age, kidney and liver function on terminal plasma half-life and mean total clearance are outlined in Table 1 above (estimated from a single 30 mg IM dose of ketorolac).

Table 1

Type of subjects	*Total clearance (l/hr/kg) mean (range)*	*Terminal half-life (hrs) mean (range)*
Normal subjects (n = 54)	0.023 (0.010–0.046)	5.3 (3.5–9.2)
Patients with hepatic dysfunction (n = 7)	0.029 (0.013–0.066)	5.4 (2.2–6.9)
Patients with renal impairment (n = 25) (serum creatinine 160–430 micromol/l)	0.016 (0.005–0.043)	10.3 (5.9–19.2)
Renal dialysis patients (n = 9)	0.016 (0.003–0.036)	13.6 (8.0–39.1)
Healthy elderly subjects (n = 13) (mean age 72)	0.019 (0.013–0.034)	7.0 (4.7–8.6)

IV: Intravenous administration of a single 10 mg dose of ketorolac trometamol resulted in a mean peak plasma concentration of 2.4 mcg/ml occurring an average of 5.4 minutes after dosing, with a terminal plasma elimination half-life of 5.1 hours, an average volume of distribution of 0.15 l/kg, and a total plasma clearance of 0.35 ml/min/kg.

The pharmacokinetics of ketorolac in man following single or multiple doses are linear. Steady-state plasma levels are achieved after dosing every 6 hours for one day. No changes in clearance occurred with chronic dosing. The primary route of excretion of ketorolac and its metabolites is renal: 91.4% (mean) of a given dose being found in the urine and 6.1% (mean) in the faeces.

More than 99% of the ketorolac in plasma is protein-bound over a wide concentration range.

Preclinical safety data: An 18-month study in mice with oral doses of ketorolac trometamol at 2 mg/kg/day (0.9 times human systemic exposure at the recommended IM or IV dose of 30 mg qid, based on area-under-the-plasma-concentration curve [AUC]), and a 24-month study in rats at 5 mg/kg/day (0.5 times the human AUC), showed no evidence of tumorigenicity.

Ketorolac trometamol was not mutagenic in the Ames test, unscheduled DNA synthesis and repair, and in forward mutation assays. Ketorolac trometamol did not cause chromosome breakage in the *in vivo* mouse micronucleus assay. At 1590 mcg/ml and at higher concentrations, ketorolac trometamol increased the incidence of chromosomal aberrations in Chinese hamster ovarian cells.

Impairment of fertility did not occur in male or female rats at oral doses of 9 mg/kg (0.9 times the human AUC) and 16 mg/kg (1.6 times the human AUC) of ketorolac trometamol, respectively.

Pharmaceutical particulars

List of excipients: Ethanol, Sodium Chloride, Water

Incompatibilities: Toradol should not be mixed in a small volume (e.g. in a syringe) with morphine sulphate, pethidine hydrochloride, promethazine hydrochloride or hydroxyzine hydrochloride as precipitation of ketorolac will occur.

It is compatible with normal saline, 5% dextrose, Ringer's, lactated Ringer's or Plasmacyte solutions. Compatibility of Toradol with other drugs is unknown.

Shelf life: 24 months.

Special precautions for storage: Store at controlled room temperature (15–30°C) and protect from light. Do not use if particulate matter is present.

Nature and contents of container: Toradol 10 mg and 30 mg is available in single-dose ampoules containing 1 ml of solution in cartons of 1, 5 or 10.

Instructions for use/handling: No special instructions applicable.

Marketing authorisation numbers
PL 0031/0480 (ampoules 10 mg/ml).
PL 0031/0481 (ampoules 30 mg/ml).

Date of first authorisation/renewal of authorisation 8 June 1990

Date of (partial) revision of the text November 1997

TOREM

Qualitative/quantitative composition in terms of the active ingredient Torem 2.5 each contain 2.5 mg torasemide. Torem 5 each contain 5.0 mg torasemide. Torem 10 each contain 10.0 mg torasemide.

Pharmaceutical form Tablets for oral administration.

Pharmacological properties

Pharmacodynamics: Torasemide is a loop diuretic. However, at low doses its pharmacodynamic profile resembles that of the thiazide class regarding the level and duration of diuresis. At higher doses, torasemide induces a brisk diuresis in a dose dependant manner with a high ceiling of effect.

Pharmacokinetics:
Absorption: Torasemide is absorbed rapidly and almost completely after oral administration, and peak serum levels are reached after 1–2 hours.
Serum protein binding: More than 99% of torasemide is bound to plasma proteins.
Distribution: The apparent distribution volume is 16 litres.
Metabolism: Torasemide is metabolised to three metabolites, M1, M3 and M5 by stepwise oxidation, hydroxylation or ring hydroxylation.
Elimination: The terminal half-life of torasemide and its metabolites is 3-4 hours in healthy subjects. Total clearance of torasemide is 40 ml/min and renal clearance about 10 ml/min. About 80% of the dose administered is excreted as torasemide and metabolites into the renal tubule–torasemide 24%, M1 12%, M3 3%, M5 41%.
In the presence of renal failure, elimination half-life of torasemide is unchanged.

Toxicity:
Acute toxicity: Very low toxicity.
Chronic toxicity: The changes observed in toxicity studies in dogs and rats at high doses are attributable to an excess pharmacodynamic action (diuresis). Changes observed were weight reduction, increases in creatinine and urea and renal alterations such as tubular dilatation and interstitial nephritis. All drug induced changes were shown to be reversible.
Teratogenicity: Reproduction toxicology studies in the rat have shown no teratogenic effect, but malformed foetuses have been observed after high doses in pregnant rabbits. No effects on fertility have been seen.
Torasemide showed no mutagenic potential. Carcinogenicity studies in rats and mice showed no tumorigenic potential.

Clinical particulars
Therapeutic indications:
Torem 2.5: Essential hypertension.
Torem 5: Essential hypertension; oedema due to congestive heart failure; hepatic, pulmonary or renal oedema.
Torem 10: Oedema due to congestive heart failure; hepatic, pulmonary or renal oedema.

Contra-indications: Renal failure with anuria; hepatic coma and pre-coma; hypotension; pregnancy and lactation; hypersensitivity to torasemide and sulphonylureas.

Undesirable effects:
Related to diuretic action: As with other diuretics, depending on the dosage and duration of treatment, there may be disturbances of water and electrolyte balance, especially with markedly limited salt intake.
Hypokalaemia (especially if a low potassium diet is being taken, or if vomiting, diarrhoea or excessive use of laxatives takes place, or in cases of hepatic failure); raised serum uric acid, gamma GT, glucose or lipids; aggravation of metabolic acidosis. Raised serum urea and creatinine; dryness of the mouth.
Symptoms and signs of electrolyte and volume depletion, such as headache, dizziness, weakness, loss of appetite and cramps may occur if diuresis is marked, especially at the start of treatment, and in elderly patients. Dose adjustment may be necessary. In patients with urinary outflow obstruction, retention of urine may be precipitated.
Occasional: Gastrointestinal symptoms.
Rare: Paraesthesia in the limbs.
Isolated cases: Thromboembolic complications and circulatory disturbances due to haemoconcentration; decreases in red and white blood cells, and platelets; allergic reactions such as pruritus, rash and photosensitivity; visual disturbance.

Special precautions for use: Hypokalaemia, hyponatraemia, hypovolaemia and disorders of micturition must be corrected before treatment.
On long-term treatment with torasemide, regular monitoring of the electrolyte balance, glucose, uric acid, creatinine and lipids in the blood, is recommended.
Careful monitoring of patients with a tendency to hyperuricaemia and gout is recommended. Carbohydrate metabolism in latent or manifest diabetes mellitus should be monitored.
As for other drugs which produce changes in blood pressure, patients taking torasemide should be warned not to drive or operate machinery if they experience dizziness or related symptoms.

Use during pregnancy and lactation: There are no data from experience in humans of the effect of torasemide on the embryo and foetus. Whilst studies in the rat have shown no teratogenic effect, malformed foetuses have been observed after high doses in pregnant rabbits. No studies have been conducted on excretion in breast milk. Consequently, torasemide is contra-indicated in pregnancy and lactation.

Interactions: When used simultaneously with cardiac glycosides, a potassium and/or magnesium deficiency may increase sensitivity of the cardiac muscle to such drugs. The kaliuretic effect of mineralo-and glucocorticoids and laxatives may be increased.
As with other diuretics, the effect of antihypertensive drugs given concomitantly may be potentiated.
Torasemide, especially at high doses, may potentiate the toxicity of aminoglycoside antibiotics, cisplatin preparations, the nephrotoxic effects of cephalosporins, and the cardio-and neurotoxic effect of lithium. The action of curare-containing muscle relaxants and of theophylline can be potentiated. In patients receiving high doses of salicylates, salicylate toxicity may be increased. The action of anti-diabetic drugs may be reduced.
Sequential or combined treatment, or starting a new co-medication with an ACE inhibitor may result in transient hypotension. This may be minimised by lowering the starting dose of the ACE inhibitor and/or reducing or stopping temporarily the dose of torasemide. Torasemide may decrease arterial responsiveness to pressor agents e.g. adrenaline, noradrenaline.

Posology and method of administration:
Adults:
Essential hypertension: A dose of 2.5 mg torasemide p.o. once daily is recommended. If necessary, the dose may be increased to 5 mg once daily. Studies suggest that doses above 5 mg daily will not lead to further reduction in blood pressure. The maximum effect is exhibited after approximately 12 weeks of continuous treatment.
Oedema: The usual dose is 5 mg p.o. once daily. If necessary, the dose can be increased stepwise up to 20 mg once daily. In individual cases, as much as 40 mg torasemide/day has been administered.
Elderly: No special dosage adjustments are necessary.
Children: There is no experience of torasemide in children.

Overdosage:
Symptoms and signs: No typical picture of intoxication is known. If overdosage occurs, then there may be marked diuresis with the danger of loss of fluid and electrolytes which may lead to somnolence and confusion, hypotension, circulatory collapse. Gastrointestinal disturbances may occur.
Treatment: No specific antidote is known. Symptoms and signs of overdosage require the reduction of the dose or withdrawal of torasemide, and simultaneous replacement of fluid and electrolytes.

Special warnings: Not applicable.

Effects on ability to drive and use machines: As for other drugs which produce changes in blood pressure, patients taking torasemide should be warned not to drive or operate machinery if they experience dizziness or related symptoms.

Pharmaceutical properties
Incompatibilities: Not applicable.

Shelf life:
Torem 2.5–4 years
Torem 5–5 years
Torem 10–4 years

Special precautions for storage: Not applicable.

Nature and contents of containers: Blister packs, PVC/aluminium, containing 14, 28, 100 or 112 tablets.

Marketing authorisation numbers
PL 015722/0023 – Torem 2.5
PL 015722/0024 – Torem 5
PL 015722/0025 – Torem 10

Date of (partial) revision of the text June 1998

VALIUM ROCHE AMPOULES

Qualitative and quantitative composition Valium Roche contains the substance with the approved name diazepam, chemically described as 7-chloro-1,3-dihydro-1-methyl-5-phenyl-2*H*-1,4-benzodiazepin-2-one.

Pharmaceutical form Ampoules containing 10 mg diazepam in 2 ml.

Clinical particulars
Therapeutic indications: Severe acute anxiety or agitation; delirium tremens.
Acute muscle spasm; tetanus.
Acute convulsions including status epilepticus, those due to poisoning, and febrile convulsions.
Pre-operative medication or premedication for a wide variety of procedures, e.g. in dentistry, surgery, radiology, endoscopy, cardiac catheterisation, cardioversion.

Posology and method of administration:
Standard dosage: For optimal effect, the dosage should be carefully individualised.
Adults:
Severe acute anxiety or agitation: 10 mg by IV or IM injection which may be repeated after an interval of not less than 4 hours.
Delirium tremens: 10 to 20 mg IV or IM. Higher doses may be needed, depending on severity of symptoms.
Acute muscle spasm: 10 mg by IV or IM injection which may be repeated after an interval of not less than 4 hours.
Tetanus: Initially an IV dose of 0.1 to 0.3 mg/kg body-weight, repeated at intervals of 1 to 4 hours. Continuous IV infusion of 3 to 10 mg/kg body-weight per 24 hours can also be used. Alternatively, the same dose of oral Valium Roche may be administered by nasoduodenal tube. The selected dose should relate to the severity of the case and in extremely severe cases higher doses have been used.
Status epilepticus, convulsions due to poisoning: 10 to 20 mg IV or IM, repeated if necessary 30–60 minutes later. If indicated, this may be followed by a slow intravenous infusion (maximum dose: 3 mg/kg body-weight over 24 hours).
Pre-operative medication or premedication: 0.2 mg/kg body-weight. The usual adult dose is 10 to 20 mg but higher doses may be necessary according to the clinical response.
Elderly or debilitated patients: Doses should not exceed half those normally recommended.
These patients should be checked regularly at the start of treatment in order to minimize the dosage and/or the frequency of administration to prevent overdose due to accumulation.
Children:
Status epilepticus, convulsions due to poisoning, febrile convulsions: 0.2 to 0.3 mg/kg body-weight IV (or IM) or 1 mg per year of life.
Tetanus: As for adults.
Pre-operative medication or premedication: 0.2 mg/kg body-weight.
Treatment should be kept to a minimum and given only under close medical supervision. Little is known regarding the efficacy or safety of benzodiazepines in long-term use.
In order to reduce the likelihood of untoward effects during intravenous sedation the injection should be given slowly (0.5ml of the solution per half-minute) until the patient becomes drowsy, the eyelids droop and the speech becomes slurred but the patient is still able to respond to requests.
It is strongly recommended that intravenous injections of Valium Roche should be given into a large vein of the antecubital fossa, the patient having been placed in a supine position and kept there throughout the procedure.
If these conditions are adhered to for administration of Valium Roche intravenously the possibility of hypotension or apnoea occurring will be greatly diminished.
Except in emergencies, a second person should always be present during intravenous use and facilities for resuscitation should always be available. It is recommended that patients should remain under medical supervision until at least one hour has elapsed from the time of injection. They should always be accompanied home by a responsible adult, with a warning not to drive or to operate machinery for 24 hours.
Valium Roche ampoule solution should not normally be diluted. An exception to this is when given slowly in large intravenous infusions of normal saline or dextrose, such as are given in the treatment of tetanus and status epilepticus. Not more than 40mg (8ml ampoule solution) should be added to 500ml of infusion solution. The solution should be freshly made up and used within six hours.
Valium Roche ampoule solution should not be mixed with other drugs in the same infusion solution or in the same syringe.
Maintenance of stability cannot be guaranteed if this advice is not followed.
Valium Roche ampoules are for intravenous or intramuscular administration.

Contra-indications: Myasthenia gravis; known sensitivity to benzodiazepines or any of the drugs excipients; severe respiratory insufficiency; respiratory depression; sleep apnoea syndrome; severe hepatic insufficiency; phobic or obsessional states; chronic psychoses.

Special warnings and special precautions for use: Parenteral Valium Roche should not normally be used in patients with organic brain changes (particularly arteriosclerosis) or with chronic pulmonary insufficiency. However, in emergency or when such patients are treated in hospital, Valium Roche may be given parenterally in reduced dosage. For IV administration, the injection should be given slowly.
In patients with chronic pulmonary insufficiency, and in patients with chronic hepatic disease, dosage may need to be reduced. In renal failure the half-life of diazepam is unchanged, therefore no dosage adjustments are required in such patients.
Valium Roche should not be used alone to treat

depression or anxiety associated with depression, since suicide may be precipitated in such patients.

Amnesia may occur. The condition usually occurs several hours after taking the product and therefore, to reduce the risk, patients should ensure that they will be able to have an uninterrupted sleep of 7 to 8 hours.

In cases of loss or bereavement, psychological adjustment may be inhibited by benzodiazepines.

Paradoxical reactions such as restlessness, agitation, irritability, aggressiveness, delusion, rages, nightmares, hallucinations, psychoses, inappropriate behaviour and other adverse behavioural effects are known to occur when using benzodiazepines. Should this occur, the use of the drug should be discontinued. They are more likely to occur in children and in the elderly.

Dependence may occur during benzodiazepine therapy. The risk is more pronounced in patients on long-term therapy and/or on high dosage and is particularly so in predisposed patients with a history of alcohol or drug abuse. Once physical dependence to benzodiazepines has developed, termination of treatment will be accompanied by withdrawal symptoms. These may consist of headache, muscle pain, extreme anxiety, tension, restlessness, confusion and irritability. In severe cases the following symptoms may occur: derealization, depersonalization, hyperacusis, numbness and tingling of the extremities, hypersensitivity to light, noise and physical contact, hallucinations or epileptic seizures.

After prolonged IV administration, abrupt discontinuation may be accompanied by withdrawal symptoms, therefore a gradual reduction in dosage is recommended.

Extreme care must be used when administering injectable Valium Roche, particularly by the IV route, to the elderly, to very ill patients and to those with limited cardiac or pulmonary reserve because of the possibility that apnoea and/or cardiac arrest may occur. Concomitant use of barbiturates, alcohol or other central nervous system depressants increases cardiac or pulmonary depression with increased risk of apnoea. Resuscitative equipment, including that necessary to support respiration, should be readily available.

The benzyl alcohol contained in Valium Roche ampoules may lead to irreversible damage in the newborn, especially in the premature. Therefore, for these patients the ampoules should only be used if no therapeutic alternative is available.

Benzodiazepines should be used with extreme caution in patients with a history of alcohol or drug abuse.

Interaction with other medicaments and other forms of interaction: If Valium Roche is given concomitantly with centrally-acting drugs such as antipsychotics, anxiolytics/sedatives, antidepressants, hypnotics, anti-convulsants, narcotic analgesics, anaesthetics and sedative antihistamines, the sedative effects are likely to be intensified. In the case of narcotic analgesics enhancement of the euphoria may also occur leading to an increase in psychic dependence. Furthermore, if such centrally-depressant drugs are given parenterally in conjunction with intravenous Valium Roche, severe respiratory and cardiovascular depression may occur. The elderly require special supervision.

When intravenous Valium Roche is to be administered concurrently with a narcotic analgesic agent, e.g. in dentistry, it is recommended that Valium Roche be given after the analgesic and that the dose be carefully titrated to meet the patient's needs.

Concomitant use with alcohol is not recommended due to enhancement of the sedative effect.

Pharmacokinetic studies on potential interactions between Valium Roche and anti-epileptic drugs (including valproic acid) have produced conflicting results. Both depression and elevation of drug levels, as well as no change, have been reported. When Valium Roche is used in conjunction with anti-epileptic drugs, side-effects and toxicity may be more evident, particularly with hydantoins or barbiturates or combinations including them. This requires extra care in adjusting dosage in the initial stages of treatment.

Known inhibitors of hepatic enzymes, e.g. cimetidine, fluvoxamine, fluoxetine and omeprazole have been shown to reduce the clearance of benzodiazepines and may potentiate their action and known inducers of hepatic enzymes, e.g. rifampicin, may increase the clearance of benzodiazepines. There have also been reports that the metabolic elimination of phenytoin is affected by diazepam.

Pregnancy and lactation: There is no evidence as to drug safety in human pregnancy, nor is there evidence from animal work that it is free from hazard. Do not use during pregnancy, especially during the first and last trimesters, unless there are compelling reasons.

If the product is prescribed to a woman of child-bearing potential, she should be warned to contact her physician regarding discontinuance of the product if she intends to become or suspects that she is pregnant.

The administration of high doses or prolonged administration of low doses of benzodiazepines in the last trimester of pregnancy or during labour has been reported to produce irregularities in the foetal heart rate, hypotonia, poor sucking, hypothermia and moderate respiratory depression in the neonate. With newborn infants it must be remembered that the enzyme system involved in the breakdown of the drug is not yet fully developed (especially in premature infants).

Moreover, infants born to mothers who took benzodiazepines chronically during the latter stages of pregnancy may have developed physical dependence and may be at some risk for developing withdrawal symptoms in the postnatal period.

Diazepam has been detected in breast milk. The use of Valium Roche should be avoided during lactation.

Effects on ability to drive and use machines: Patients should be advised that, like all medicaments of this type, Valium Roche may modify patients' performance at skilled tasks. Sedation, amnesia, impaired concentration and impaired muscle function may adversely affect the ability to drive or use machinery. If insufficient sleep duration occurs, the likelihood of impaired alertness may be increased. Patients should further be advised that alcohol may intensify any impairment and should, therefore, be avoided during treatment.

Undesirable effects: Intravenous injection may be associated with local reactions, and thrombophlebitis and venous thrombosis may occur. In order to minimise the likelihood of these effects, intravenous injections of Valium Roche should be given into a large vein of the antecubital fossa. Very small veins should not be selected for injection. In particular, intra-arterial injection or extravasation must be strictly avoided.

Apnoea or hypotension may rarely occur following intravenous injection. The incidence may be minimised by not exceeding the recommended rate of administration. Patients should always be managed in the supine position and kept there throughout the procedure.

Circulatory and respiratory depression may follow rapid intravenous administration of Valium Roche.

IM injection can result in local pain, in some cases accompanied by erythema at the site of injection. Tenderness is relatively common.

The most commonly reported undesirable effects are fatigue, drowsiness and muscle weakness; they are usually dose-related. These phenomena occur predominantly at the start of therapy and usually disappear with prolonged administration.

Use (even at therapeutic doses) may lead to the development of physical and psychological dependence (see *Special warnings and special precautions for use*).

Other side effects like confusion, numbed emotions, reduced alertness, anterograde amnesia, ataxia, constipation, depression, diplopia, dysarthria, gastrointestinal disturbances, headache, hypotension, variations in pulse rate, circulatory depression, incontinence, increase or decrease in libido, nausea, dry mouth or hypersalivation, skin reactions, slurred speech, tremor, urinary retention, vertigo, blurred vision and blood dyscrasias have been reported occasionally.

Very rarely, elevated transaminases and alkaline phosphatase, jaundice as well as cases of cardiac arrest have been observed.

The elderly are particularly sensitive to the effects of centrally-depressant drugs and may experience confusion, especially if organic brain changes are present. The dosage of Valium Roche in these patients should not exceed one-half that recommended for other adults.

Paradoxical reactions such as restlessness, agitation, irritability, aggressiveness, delusion, rages, nightmares, hallucinations (some of a sexual nature), psychoses, inappropriate behaviour and other behavioural effects (see *Special warnings and special precautions for use*) have been reported.

Pre-existing depression may be unmasked during benzodiazepine use.

Abuse of benzodiazepines has been reported.

The elderly and patients with impaired hepatic function, will be particularly susceptible to the adverse effects listed above. It is advisable to review treatment regularly and to discontinue use as soon as possible.

Overdose: Overdose of benzodiazepines is usually manifested by central nervous system depression ranging from drowsiness to coma. In mild cases, symptoms include drowsiness, mental confusion and lethargy. In more serious cases, symptoms may include ataxia, hypotonia, hypotension, respiratory depression, coma (rarely) and death (very rarely).

The value of dialysis has not been determined. Special attention should be paid to respiratory and cardiac function in intensive care. Anexate (flumazenil) is a specific IV antidote for use in emergency situations. Patients requiring such intervention should be monitored closely in hospital (see separate prescribing information). Caution should be observed in the use of Anexate in epileptics treated with benzodiazepines.

If excitation occurs, barbiturates should not be used.

Pharmacological properties

Pharmacodynamic properties: Valium Roche has anxiolytic, anticonvulsant and central muscle-relaxant properties. It has little autonomic activity.

Pharmacokinetic properties:

Absorption: On IM injection absorption is complete, though not always more rapid than with oral administration.

Distribution: Diazepam and its metabolites are highly bound to plasma proteins (diazepam 98%). Diazepam and its metabolites cross the blood-brain and placental barriers and are also found in breast milk in concentrations approximately one tenth of those in maternal plasma.

Metabolism: Diazepam is mainly metabolized to the pharmacologically active metabolites such as N-desmethyldiazepam, temazepam and oxazepam.

Elimination: The plasma concentration-time profile of diazepam after IV administration is biphasic, an initial rapid and extensive distribution phase being followed by a prolonged terminal elimination phase (half-life up to 48 hours). The elimination half-life of the active metabolite N-desmethyldiazepam is up to 100 hours. Diazepam and its metabolites are excreted mainly in the urine, predominantly in their conjugated forms. The clearance of diazepam is 20-30 ml/min.

Repeated doses will lead to accumulation of whole drug and metabolites. The latter may take two weeks to reach steady state and can reach higher concentrations than the parent compound.

Pharmacokinetics in special clinical situations: The elimination half-life may be prolonged in the newborn, in the elderly and in patients with liver disease. In renal failure the half-life of diazepam is unchanged.

Intramuscular injection of Valium Roche can lead to a rise in serum creatine phosphokinase activity, with a maximum level occurring between 12 and 24 hours after the injection. This fact should be taken into account in the differential diagnosis of myocardial infarction.

The absorption from intramuscular injection of Valium Roche may be variable, particularly from the gluteal muscles. This route of administration should only be used when oral or intravenous dosing is not possible or advisable.

Preclinical safety data: None stated.

Pharmaceutical particulars

List of excipients: Sodium benzoate, benzoic acid, propylene glycol, 1 M sodium hydroxide, ethanol 94%, benzyl alcohol, water for injection.

Incompatibilities: None.

Shelf life: Valium Roche ampoules have a shelf-life of 3 years.

Special precautions for storage: The recommended maximum storage temperature for Valium Roche ampoules is 30°C. They should be protected from light.

Nature and contents of container: Valium Roche ampoules 10 mg in 2 ml, in packs of 10.

Instructions for use/handling:

Dilution, additives and pharmaceutical precautions: Valium Roche ampoule solutions should not normally be diluted. An exception to this is when given slowly in large intravenous infusions of normal saline or dextrose such as are given in the treatment of tetanus and status epilepticus. Not more than 40 mg (8 ml ampoule solution) should be added to 500 ml of infusion solution. The solution should be freshly made up and used within six hours.

Over 50% of diazepam in solution may be adsorbed onto the walls of plastic containers of infusion solution; these should not therefore be used for diazepam solutions. Adsorption onto plastic drip tubing causes an initial significant reduction of delivered diazepam concentration which then gradually rises over the next few hours. The drip rate should frequently be titrated against the patient's condition.

Bolus injection allows a more accurate and rapid titration of dosage than slow intravenous infusion. It is therefore to be preferred for the management of acute problems.

Valium Roche ampoule solution should not be

mixed with other drugs in the same infusion solution or in the same syringe.

Maintenance of stability cannot be guaranteed if this advice is not followed.

Marketing authorisation number PL 0031/0068R

Date of first authorisation 24 August 1984

Date of (partial) revision of the text October 1998

VALIUM TABLETS

Qualitative and quantitative composition Round, white tablets with ROCHE/2 imprinted on one face and a single break-bar on the other, containing 2 mg diazepam.

Round, pale yellow tablets with ROCHE/5 imprinted on one face and a single break-bar on the other, containing 5 mg diazepam.

Round, pale blue tablets with ROCHE/10 imprinted on one face and a single break-bar on the other, containing 10 mg diazepam.

Pharmaceutical form Valium Tablets 2 mg, 5 mg and 10 mg.

Clinical particulars

Therapeutic indications:

Adults: Short-term (2–4 weeks) symptomatic treatment of anxiety that is severe, disabling or subjecting the individual to unacceptable distress, occurring alone or in association with insomnia or short-term psychosomatic, organic or psychotic illness.

Short-term (2–4 weeks) treatment of conditions where anxiety may be a precipitating or aggravating factor, e.g. tension headaches or migraine attacks.

Symptomatic treatment of acute alcohol withdrawal.

Muscle spasm. As an adjunct to the control of muscle spasm in tetanus.

May be useful in the management of cerebral spasticity in selected cases.

As an adjunct to the management of some types of epilepsy, e.g. myoclonus.

Premedication.

Children: Night terrors and somnambulism.

May be useful in controlling tension and irritability in cerebral spasticity in selected cases.

As an adjunct to the control of muscle spasm in tetanus.

Premedication.

Posology and method of administration:

Standard dosage: For optimal effect, the dosage should be carefully individualized. Treatment should begin at the lowest effective dose appropriate to the particular condition.

Duration of treatment: The duration of treatment should be as short as possible. The patient should be reassessed regularly and the need for continued treatment evaluated, especially if the patient is symptom free. It should not exceed 2–3 months, including the tapering-off period. Extension beyond this period should not take place without reevaluation of the situation. It may be useful to inform the patient when treatment is started that it will be of limited duration and explain precisely how the dosage will be progressively decreased. Moreover, it is important that the patient be aware of the possibility of rebound phenomena, thereby minimizing anxiety over such symptoms should they occur during withdrawal. There is evidence that, in the case of short-acting benzodiazepines, withdrawal phenomena can become manifest within the dosage interval, especially when the dosage is high. When long-acting benzodiazepines such as diazepam are being used, it is important to warn against changing to a short-acting benzodiazepine as withdrawal symptoms may develop.

Anxiety states:

Adults:

Usual dose: 2 mg 3 times daily.

Maximum dose: Up to 30 mg daily in divided doses. Adjusted on an individual basis.

Insomnia associated with anxiety: 5 to 15 mg before retiring.

Treatment should not be continued at the full dose beyond 4 weeks.

Symptomatic relief of acute alcohol withdrawal: 5 to 20 mg, repeated if necessary in 2 to 4 hours.

Night terrors and somnambulism:

Children: 1 to 5 mg at bedtime.

Conditions associated with muscle spasm:

Adults:

Muscle spasm: 2 to 15 mg daily in divided doses.

Management of cerebral spasticity in selected cases: 2 to 60 mg daily in divided doses.

Adjunct to control of muscle spasm in tetanus: 3 to 10 mg/kg body-weight daily by nasoduodenal tube. The selected dose should relate to the severity of the case and in extremely severe cases higher doses have been used. Intravenous Valium is recommended initially (see separate data sheet).

Children:

Control of tension and irritability in cerebral spasticity in selected cases: 2 to 40 mg daily in divided doses.

As an adjunct to the control of muscle spasm in tetanus: As for adults.

Adjunct to the management of some types of epilepsy:

Adults: 2 to 60 mg daily in divided doses.

Premedication:

Adults: 5 to 20 mg.

Children: 2 to 10 mg.

Benzodiazepines should not be given to children without careful assessment of the indication; the duration of treatment must be kept to a minimum.

Elderly:

Elderly or debilitated patients: Doses should not exceed half those normally recommended.

These patients should be checked regularly at the start of treatment in order to minimize the dosage and/or the frequency of administration to prevent overdose due to accumulation.

Impaired hepatic function: Patients with impaired hepatic function should be given a reduced dose.

Little is known regarding the efficacy or safety of benzodiazepines in long-term use.

Valium tablets are for oral administration.

Contra-indications: Patients with known sensitivity to benzodiazepines or any of the drugs excipients; severe pulmonary insufficiency; severe hepatic insufficiency; respiratory depression; phobic or obsessional states; chronic psychosis; myasthenia gravis; sleep apnea syndrome, dependence on other substances including alcohol. An exception to the latter is the management of acute withdrawal reactions.

Valium should not be used alone to treat depression or anxiety associated with depression, since suicide may be precipitated in such patients. Benzodiazepines are not recommended for the primary treatment of psychotic illness.

Special warnings and special precautions for use: In patients with chronic pulmonary insufficiency, and in patients with chronic hepatic disease, dosage may need to be reduced. In renal failure the half-life of diazepam is unchanged, therefore no dosage adjustments are required in such patients.

It should be borne in mind that benzodiazepines may induce anterograde amnesia. Anterograde amnesia may occur using therapeutic dosages, the risk increasing at higher dosages. Amnestic effects may be associated with inappropriate behaviour. The condition usually occurs several hours after taking the product and therefore, to reduce the risk, patients should ensure that they will be able to have an uninterrupted sleep of 7 to 8 hours.

In cases of loss or bereavement, psychological adjustment may be inhibited by benzodiazepines.

Use of benzodiazepines and benzodiazepine-like agents may lead to the development of physical and psychological dependence. The risk of dependence increases with dose and duration of treatment. This is particularly so in patients with a history of alcoholism or drug abuse or in patients with marked personality disorders. Regular monitoring in such patients is essential, routine repeat prescriptions should be avoided and treatment should be withdrawn gradually. Once physical dependence has developed, abrupt termination of treatment will be accompanied by withdrawal symptoms. These may consist of headache, muscle pain, extreme anxiety, tension, restlessness, confusion and irritability. In severe cases, the following symptoms may occur: derealization, depersonalization, hyperacusis, numbness and tingling of the extremities, hypersensitivity to light, noise and physical contact, hallucinations or epileptic seizures.

Paradoxical reactions such as restlessness, agitation, irritability, aggressiveness, delusion, rages, nightmares, hallucinations, psychoses, inappropriate behaviour and other adverse behavioural effects are known to occur when using benzodiazepines. Should this occur, the use of the drug should be discontinued. They are more likely to occur in children and in the elderly.

Some loss of response to the effects of benzodiazepines may develop after repeated use of Valium for a prolonged time.

Rebound anxiety may occur. This is a transient syndrome whereby the symptoms that led to treatment with Valium recur in an enhanced form. This may occur on withdrawal of treatment. It may be accompanied by other reactions including mood changes, anxiety and restlessness.

Since the risk of withdrawal phenomena and rebound phenomena is greater after abrupt discontinuation of treatment, it is recommended that the dosage be decreased gradually.

Interaction with other medicaments and other forms of interaction: If Valium is given concomitantly with centrally-acting drugs such as antipsychotics, anxiolytics/sedatives, antidepressants, hypnotics, anti-convulsants, narcotic analgesics, anaesthetics, and sedative antihistamines, the sedative effects are likely to be intensified. In the case of narcotic analgesics enhancement of the euphoria may also occur leading to an increase in psychic dependence. The elderly require special supervision.

Concomitant use with alcohol is not recommended due to enhancement of the sedative effect.

Pharmacokinetic studies on potential interactions between Valium and anti-epileptic drugs have produced conflicting results. Both depression and elevation of drug levels, as well as no change, have been reported. When Valium is used in conjunction with anti-epileptic drugs, side-effects and toxicity may be more evident, particularly with hydantoins or barbiturates or combinations including them. This requires extra care in adjusting dosage in the initial stages of treatment.

Known inhibitors of hepatic enzymes, e.g. cimetidine, omeprazole, fluvoxamine and fluoxetine have been shown to reduce the clearance of benzodiazepines and may potentiate their action and known inducers of hepatic enzymes, e.g. rifampicin, may increase the clearance of benzodiazepines. There have also been reports that the metabolic elimination of phenytoin is affected by diazepam.

Cisapride may lead to a temporary increase in the sedative effects of orally administered benzodiazepines due to faster absorption.

Pregnancy and lactation: There is no evidence as to drug safety in human pregnancy, nor is there evidence from animal work that it is free from hazard. Do not use during pregnancy, especially during the first and last trimesters, unless there are compelling reasons.

If the product is prescribed to a woman of child-bearing potential, she should be warned to contact her physician regarding discontinuance of the product if she intends to become or suspects that she is pregnant.

The administration of high doses or prolonged administration of low doses of benzodiazepines in the last trimester of pregnancy or during labour has been reported to produce irregularities in the foetal heart rate, hypotonia, poor sucking, hypothermia and moderate respiratory depression in the neonate. With newborn infants it must be remembered that the enzyme system involved in the breakdown of the drug is not yet fully developed (especially in premature infants).

Moreover, infants born to mothers who took benzodiazepines chronically during the latter stages of pregnancy may have developed physical dependence and may be at some risk for developing withdrawal symptoms in the postnatal period.

Diazepam has been detected in breast milk. The use of Valium should be avoided during lactation.

Effects on ability to drive and use machines: Patients should be advised that, like all medicaments of this type, Valium may modify patients' performance at skilled tasks. Sedation, amnesia, impaired concentration and impaired muscle function may adversely affect the ability to drive or use machinery. If insufficient sleep duration occurs, the likelihood of impaired alertness may be increased. Patients should further be advised that alcohol may intensify any impairment and should, therefore, be avoided during treatment.

Undesirable effects: The most commonly reported undesirable effects are fatigue, drowsiness and muscle weakness. These phenomena occur predominantly at the start of therapy and usually disappear with prolonged administration. The following may also occur: ataxia, confusion, constipation, depression, diplopia, dysarthria, gastrointestinal disturbances, headache, hypotension, incontinence, increase or decrease in libido, nausea, dry mouth or hypersalivation, skin reactions, slurred speech, tremor, urinary retention, dizziness and blurred vision; very rarely, elevated transaminases and alkaline phosphatase as well as cases of jaundice have been reported occasionally. The elderly are particularly sensitive to the effects of centrally-depressant drugs and may experience confusion, especially if organic brain changes are present; the dosage of Valium should not exceed one-half that recommended for other adults.

The elderly, and patients with impaired hepatic function, will be particularly susceptible to the adverse effects listed above. It is advisable to review treatment regularly and to discontinue use as soon as possible.

Pre-existing depression may be unmasked during benzodiazepine use.

Chronic use (even at therapeutic doses) may lead to the development of physical and psychological dependence (see *Special warnings and special precautions for use*): discontinuation of the therapy may result in withdrawal or rebound phenomena.

Abuse of benzodiazepines has been reported.

Benzodiazepines may induce anterograde amnesia (see *Special warnings and special precautions for use*).

Paradoxical reactions such as restlessness, agitation, irritability, aggressiveness, delusion, rages, nightmares, hallucinations, psychoses, inappropriate behaviour and other adverse behavioural effects are known to occur when using benzodiazepines (see *Special warnings and special precautions for use*).

Overdose: Overdose of benzodiazepines is usually manifested by central nervous system depression ranging from drowsiness to coma. In mild cases, symptoms include drowsiness, mental confusion and lethargy. In more serious cases, symptoms may include ataxia, hypotonia, hypotension, respiratory depression, coma (rarely) and death (very rarely).

When taken with centrally-acting drugs, especially alcohol, the effects of overdosage are likely to be more severe and, in the absence of supportive measures, may prove fatal.

In the management of overdose with any medicinal product, it should be borne in mind that multiple agents may have been taken. Following overdose with oral benzodiazepines, vomiting should be induced (within 1 hour) if the patient is conscious or gastric lavage undertaken with the airway protected if the patient is unconscious. If there is no advantage in emptying the stomach, activated charcoal should be given to reduce absorption. The value of dialysis has not been determined. Special attention should be paid to respiratory and cardiac function in intensive care. Anexate (flumazenil) is a specific IV antidote for use in emergency situations. Patients requiring such intervention should be monitored closely in hospital (see separate prescribing information). Caution should be observed in the use of Anexate in epileptics treated with benzodiazepines.

If excitation occurs, barbiturates should not be used.

Pharmacological properties

Pharmacodynamic properties: Valium has anxiolytic, anticonvulsant and central muscle-relaxant properties. It has little autonomic activity.

Pharmacokinetic properties:

Absorption: Diazepam is rapidly and completely absorbed from the gastrointestinal tract, peak plasma concentrations appearing 30–90 minutes after oral ingestion.

Distribution: Diazepam and its metabolites are highly bound to plasma proteins (diazepam 98%). Diazepam and its metabolites cross the blood-brain and placental barriers and are also found in breast milk in concentrations approximately one tenth of those in maternal plasma.

Metabolism: Diazepam is mainly metabolized to the pharmacologically active metabolites such as N-desmethyldiazepam, temazepam and oxazepam.

Elimination: The decline in the plasma concentration-time profile after oral administration is biphasic, an initial rapid and extensive distribution phase being followed by a prolonged terminal elimination phase (half-life up to 48 hours). The terminal elimination half-life of the active metabolite N-desmethyldiazepam is up to 100 hours. Diazepam and its metabolites are excreted mainly in the urine, predominantly in their conjugated forms. The clearance of diazepam is 20–30 ml/min.

Repeated doses will lead to accumulation of whole drug and metabolites. The latter may take 2 weeks to reach steady state and can reach higher concentrations than the parent compound.

Pharmacokinetics in special clinical situations: The elimination half-life may be prolonged in the newborn, in the elderly and in patients with liver disease. In renal failure the half-life of diazepam is unchanged.

No clear correlation has been demonstrated between the blood levels of Valium and its clinical effects.

Preclinical safety data: None stated.

Pharmaceutical particulars

List of excipients:

Each 2 mg tablet also contains: Lactose, starch maize white and magnesium stearate.

In addition, each 5 mg tablet also contains dye yellow iron oxide (E172) and each 10 mg tablet also contains indigo carmine (E132).

Incompatibilities: None stated.

Shelf life:

Plastic bottles and PVDC blister packs: 5 years.

Clic-loc containers and mini kegs: 2 years.

Special precautions for storage: Valium tablets should be stored below 30°C and protected from light.

Nature and contents of container: Valium tablets are available in plastic bottles, PVDC and PVC blisters, clic-loc containers and mini-kegs, in packs of 100.

Instructions for use/handling: None.

Marketing authorisation numbers

2mg tablets: PL 0031/5121R
5mg tablets: PL 0031/5122R
10mg tablets: PL 0031/5123R

Date of first authorisation/renewal of authorisation July 1983

Date of (partial) revision of the text December 1998

VASCACE

Qualitative and quantitative composition

One film coated tablet 0.5 mg contains: Cilazapril, anhydrous 0.5 mg, in the form of the monohydrate (cilazapril 0.522 mg).

One film coated tablet 1.0 mg contains: Cilazapril, anhydrous 1.0 mg, in the form of the monohydrate (cilazapril 1.044 mg).

One film coated tablet 2.5 mg contains: Cilazapril, anhydrous 2.5 mg, in the form of the monohydrate (cilazapril 2.61 mg).

One film coated tablet 5.0 mg contains: Cilazapril, anhydrous 5 mg, in the form of the monohydrate (cilazapril 5.22 mg).

Pharmaceutical form Tablets.

Clinical particulars

Therapeutic indications: Vascace is indicated in treatment of all grades of essential hypertension and renovascular hypertension. Vascace is also indicated in the treatment of chronic heart failure, usually as an adjunctive therapy with digitalis and/or diuretics.

Posology and method of administration: Vascace should be administered once-daily. As food intake has no clinically significant influence on absorption, Vascace can be administered before or after a meal. The dose should always be taken at about the same time of day.

Special Dosage Instructions

Essential hypertension: The recommended initial dosage is 1–1.25 mg once a day. Dosage should be adjusted individually in accordance with the blood pressure response until control is achieved. Most patients can be maintained on between 2.5 and 5.0 mg/day. If the blood pressure is not adequately controlled with 5 mg Vascace once daily, a low dose of a non-potassium-sparing diuretic may be administered concomitantly to enhance the anti-hypertensive effect.

Renovascular hypertension: Treatment with Vascace should be initiated with a dose of 0.5 mg or 0.25 mg once daily since these patients may experience more pronounced decreases in blood pressure in response to ACE-inhibitors than patients with essential hypertension. The maintenance dose should be adjusted individually.

Hypertensive patients receiving diuretics: The diuretic should be discontinued two to three days before beginning therapy with Vascace to reduce the likelihood of symptomatic hypotension. It may be resumed later if required. The recommended starting dose in these patients is 0.5 mg once daily.

Chronic heart failure: Vascace can be used as adjunctive therapy with digitalis and/or diuretics in patients with chronic heart failure. Therapy with Vascace should be initiated with a recommended starting dose of 0.5 mg once daily under close medical supervision. The dose should be increased to the lowest maintenance dose of 1 mg daily according to tolerability and clinical status. Further titration within the usual maintenance dose of 1 mg to 2.5 mg daily should be carried out based on patients response, clinical status and tolerability. The usual maximum dose is 5 mg once daily.

Results from clinical trials showed that clearance of cilazaprilat in patients with chronic heart failure is correlated with creatinine clearance. Thus in patients with chronic heart failure and impaired renal function special dosage recommendation as given under 'Impaired Renal Function' should be followed.

Impaired renal function: Reduced dosages may be required for patients with renal impairment, depending on their creatinine clearance see Table 1.

In patients requiring haemodialysis, Vascace should be administered on days when dialysis is not performed and the dosage should be adjusted according to blood pressure response.

Severe hepatic function disorders (including cirrhosis): In the unlikely event that patients with severe hepatic function disorders should require treatment with cilazapril, it should be initiated with caution at a dose of 0.5 mg or 0.25 mg once daily, because significant hypotension may occur.

Elderly: In the treatment of hypertension, Vascace should be initiated with between 0.50 mg and 1.25 mg once daily. Thereafter, the maintenance dose must be adapted to individual response.

In the treatment of chronic heart failure, Vascace should be initiated with a dose of 0.5 mg daily. The maintenance dose of 1 mg to 2.5 mg must be adapted to individual tolerability, response and clinical status.

In elderly patients with chronic heart failure on high diuretic dosage the recommended starting dose of Vascace 0.5 mg must be strictly followed.

Children: Safety and efficacy in children have not been established therefore there is no recommendation for administration of cilazapril to children.

Contra-indications: Vascace is contraindicated in patients who are hypersensitive to the drug cilazapril or other ACE-inhibitors, in patients with ascites and in pregnancy and lactation.

Vascace is also contra-indicated in patients with a history of angioedema after treatment with other ACE-inhibitors.

Special warnings and special precautions for use: (See also *Special Dosage Instructions under Posology and method of administration*).

Vascace should be used with caution in patients with aortic stenosis, hypertrophic cardiomyopathy or outflow obstruction.

In elderly patients with chronic heart failure on high diuretic dosage the recommended starting dose of Vascace 0.5 mg must be strictly followed.

Although the mechanism involved has not been definitely established, there is clinical evidence that haemodialysis with polyacrylonitrile methallyl sulphate high-flux membranes (e.g. AN69), haemofiltration or LDL-apheresis, if performed in patients being treated with ACE-inhibitors, including cilazapril, can lead to the provocation of anaphylaxis/anaphylactoid reactions including life-threatening shock. The above-mentioned procedures must therefore be avoided in such patients.

Symptomatic hypotension: Occasionally, symptomatic hypotension has been reported with ACE-inhibitor therapy, particularly in patients with sodium or volume depletion in connection with conditions such as vomiting, diarrhoea, pre-treatment with diuretics, low sodium diet or after dialysis. In patients with angina pectoris or cerebrovascular disease, treatment with ACE inhibitors should be started under close medical supervision, as excessive hypotension could result in myocardial infarction or cerebrovascular accident.

Patients with chronic heart failure, especially those taking high doses of loop diuretics, may experience a pronounced blood pressure decrease in response to ACE-inhibitors. This should be treated by having the patient rest in the supine position and may require infusion of normal saline or volume expanders. After volume repletion, Vascace therapy may be continued. However, if symptoms persist, the dosage should be reduced or the drug discontinued.

Renal impairment: Reduced dosages may be required for patients with renal impairment, depending on their creatinine clearance (see *Special dosage instructions*). In patients whose renal function depends primarily on the activity of the renin-angiotensin-aldosterone system, such as patients with severe heart failure or with unilateral or bilateral renal artery stenosis, treatment with ACE-inhibitors including Vascace may produce increases in blood urea nitrogen and/or serum creatinine. Although these alterations are usually reversible upon discontinuation of Vascace and/or diuretic therapy, cases of severe renal dysfunction and, rarely, acute renal failure have been reported.

In this patient population, renal function should be monitored during the first weeks of therapy.

For haemodialysis using high-flux polyacrylonitrile (AN69) membranes please see above statement under the heading of *Special warnings and special precautions for use.*

Hepatic impairment: In patients with severe liver function impairment, hypotension may occur.

Serum potassium: Concomitant administration of potassium-sparing diuretics, potassium supplements or potassium containing salt substitutes may lead to increases in serum potassium, particularly in patients with renal impairment. Therefore, if concomitant use for such agents is indicated, their dosage should be reduced when Vascace is initiated and serum potassium and renal function should be monitored carefully.

Surgery anaesthesia: The use of ACE-inhibitors in combination with anaesthetic drugs in surgery that also have blood-pressure-lowering effects, can produce arterial hypotension. If this occurs, volume expansion by means of intravenous infusion or–if resistant to these measures–angiotensin II infusion is indicated.

Interaction with other medicaments and other forms of interaction: Vascace has been administered con-

Table 1: Impaired Renal Function

The following dose schedules are recommended:

Creatinine clearance	*Initial dose of Vascace*	*Maximal dose of Vascace*
> 40 ml/min	1 mg once daily	5 mg once daily
10–40 ml/min	0.5 mg once daily	2.5 mg once daily
< 10 ml/min	0.25–0.5 mg once or twice a week according to blood pressure response	

comitantly with digoxin, nitrates, furosemide, thiazides, oral antidiabetics and H2-receptor blockers. There was no increase in digoxin plasma concentrations and no other clinically significant drug interactions. An additive effect may be observed when Vascace is administered in combination with other blood-pressure-lowering agents.

Potassium-sparing diuretics, potassium supplements or potassium containing salt substitutes administered together with Vascace can lead to increases in serum potassium, particularly in patients with renal impairment (see *Special warnings and special precautions for use*).

As with other ACE-inhibitors, use of Vascace concomitantly with a non-steroidal anti-inflammatory drug (NSAID) may diminish the anti-hypertensive effect of Vascace.

Anaphylactic reactions can occur in patients undergoing desensitisation therapy with wasp or bee venom while receiving an ACE-inhibitor. Cilazapril must therefore be interrupted before the start of desensitisation therapy. Additionally, in this situation, cilazapril must not be replaced by a beta blocker.

Concomitant administration of ACE-inhibitors and anti-diabetic medicines (insulin, oral hypoglycaemic agents) may cause an increased blood glucose lowering effect with the risk of hypoglycaemia. This phenomenon may be more likely to occur during the first weeks of combined treatment and in patients with renal impairment.

The concomitant administration of ACE-inhibitors with lithium may reduce the excretion of lithium. Serum lithium levels should be monitored frequently.

Concomitant administration of allopurinol, cytostatic or immunosuppressive agents, systemic corticosteroids or procainamide with ACE-inhibitors may lead to an increased risk of leucopenia.

Pregnancy and lactation: Vascace is contra-indicated in pregnancy since foetotoxicity has been observed for ACE-inhibitors in animals. Although there is no experience with Vascace, other ACE-inhibitors in human pregnancy have been associated with oligohydramnios and neonatal hypotension and/or anuria. It is not known whether cilazapril passes into human breast milk, but since animal data show the presence of cilazaprilat in rat milk, Vascace should not be administered to nursing mothers.

Effects on ability to drive and use machines: As with other ACE-inhibitors, impairment of performance in activities requiring complete mental alertness (e.g. driving a motor vehicle) is not to be expected with Vascace. However, it should be noted that dizziness may occasionally occur in some people.

Undesirable effects: Headache, dizziness and coughing are the most frequently reported events in patients taking Vascace. Undesirable effects occurring in < 2% of the patients include fatigue, hypotension, dyspepsia, nausea, and rash. In most cases undesirable effects were transient, mild or moderate in degree, and did not require discontinuation of therapy.

Idiosyncratic: ACE-inhibitors have been documented to induce cough in a substantial number of patients. Rarely dyspnoea, sinusitis, rhinitis, glossitis, bronchitis and bronchospasm have been reported.

As with other ACE-inhibitors, angioneurotic oedema has been reported, although rarely, in patients receiving Vascace. Angioedema involving the tongue, glottis or larynx may be **fatal**. If involvement of the face, lips, tongue, glottis and/or larynx occurs Vascace should be discontinued without delay and appropriate therapy instituted without delay when involvement of the face, lips, tongue, glottis and/or larynx occurs and replaced by an agent belonging to another class of drugs. Emergency therapy should be given including, but not necessarily limited to, immediate intramuscular adrenalin (epinephrine) solution 1:1000 (0.3 to 0.5 ml) or slow intravenous adrenalin 1 mg/ml (observing dilution instructions) with control of ECG and blood pressure. The patient should be hospitalised and observed for at least 12 to 24 hours and should not be discharged until complete resolution of symptoms has occurred.

Pancreatitis has been reported rarely in patients treated with ACE-inhibitors (including Vascace); in some cases this has proved fatal.

Laboratory test findings: Clinically relevant changes in laboratory test values possibly or probably related to Vascace treatment have been observed only rarely.

Minor, mostly reversible increases in serum creatinine/urea have been observed in patients treated with Vascace. Such changes are likely to occur in patients with renal artery stenosis or with renal impairment (see *Special warnings and special precautions for use*), but they have also occasionally been observed in patients with normal renal function, particularly in those receiving concomitant diuretics. Isolated cases of acute renal failure have been reported in patients with severe heart failure, renal artery stenosis or renal disorders (see *Precautions*).

In some patients decreases in haemoglobin, haematocrit and/or white blood cell count have been reported, but in no case has a definite causal relationship to Vascace been established.

Overdose: While single doses of up to 160 mg Vascace have been administered to normal healthy volunteers without untoward effects on blood pressure, only a few data on overdose are available in patients.

The most likely symptoms of overdosage are severe hypotension, shock, stupor, bradycardia, electrolyte disturbances and renal failure.

After ingestion of an overdose, the patient should be kept under close supervision, preferably in an intensive care unit. Serum electrolytes and creatinine should be monitored frequently. Therapeutic measures depend on the nature and severity of the symptoms. Measurements to prevent absorption such as gastric lavage, administration of adsorbents and sodium sulphate within 30 minutes after intake, and to hasten elimination should be applied if ingestion is recent. If hypotension occurs, the patient should be placed in the shock position and salt and volume supplementation should be given, rapidly. Treatment with angiotensin II should be considered. Bradycardia or extensive vagal reactions should be treated by administering atropine. The use of a pacemaker may be considered. ACE-inhibitors may be removed from the circulation by haemodialysis. The use of high-flux polyacrylonitrile membranes should be avoided.

Pharmacological properties

Pharmacodynamic properties: Vascace (cilazapril) is a specific, long-acting angiotensin-converting enzyme (ACE) inhibitor which suppresses the renin-angiotensin-aldosterone system and thereby the conversion of the inactive angiotensin I to angiotensin II which is a potent vasoconstrictor. At recommended doses, the effect of Vascace in hypertensive patients and in patients with chronic heart failure is maintained for up to 24 hours.

In patients with normal renal function, serum potassium usually remains within the normal range during Vascace treatment. In patients concomitantly taking potassium-sparing diuretics, potassium levels may rise.

Hypertension: Vascace induces a reduction of both supine and standing systolic and diastolic blood pressure, usually with no orthostatic component. It is effective in all degrees of essential hypertension as well as in renal hypertension. The anti-hypertensive effect of Vascace is usually apparent within the first hour after administration, with maximum effect observed between three and seven hours after dosing. In general the heart rate remains unchanged. Reflex tachycardia is not induced, although small, clinically insignificant alterations of heart rate may occur. In some patients blood pressure reduction may diminish toward the end of the dosage interval.

The initial dosage seldom achieves the desired therapeutic response. Blood pressure should be assessed and dosage adjusted as required. Should the effect of Vascace at the top of the recommended dose be insufficient it can be combined with non-potassium-sparing diuretics.

The anti-hypertensive effect of Vascace is maintained during long-term therapy. No rapid increase in blood pressure has been observed after abrupt withdrawal of Vascace.

In hypertensive patients with moderate to severe renal impairment, the glomerular filtration rate and renal blood flow remained in general unchanged with Vascace despite a clinically significant blood pressure reduction.

As with other ACE-inhibitors, the blood pressure-lowering effect of Vascace in black patients may be less pronounced than in non-blacks. However, racial differences in response are no longer evident when Vascace is administered in combination with hydrochlorothiazide.

Chronic heart failure: In patients with chronic heart failure the renin-angiotensin-aldosterone and the sympathetic nervous systems are generally activated leading to enhanced systemic vasoconstriction and to the promotion of sodium and water retention. By suppressing the renin-angiotensin-aldosterone system, Vascace improves loading conditions in the failing heart by reducing systemic vascular resistance (afterload) and pulmonary capillary wedge pressure (preload) in patients on diuretics and/or digitalis. Furthermore, the exercise tolerance of these patients increases significantly showing an improvement in quality of life. The haemodynamic and clinical effects occur promptly and persist.

Pharmacokinetic properties: Cilazapril is efficiently absorbed and rapidly converted to the active form, cilazaprilat. Ingestion of food immediately prior to Vascace administration, delays and reduces the absorption to a minor extent which, however, is therapeutically irrelevant. The bioavailability of cilazaprilat from oral cilazapril approximates 60% based on urinary recovery data. Maximum plasma concentrations are reached within two hours after administration and are directly related to dosage.

Cilazaprilat is eliminated unchanged by the kidneys, with an effective half-life of nine hours after once-daily dosing with Vascace. In patients with renal impairment, higher plasma concentrations of cilazaprilat are observed than in patients with normal renal function, since drug clearance is reduced when creatinine clearance is lower. There is no elimination in patients with complete renal failure, but haemodialysis reduces concentrations of both cilazapril and cilazaprilat to a limited extent.

In elderly patients whose renal function is normal for age, plasma concentrations of cilazaprilat may be up to 40% higher, and the clearance 20% lower than in younger patients. Similar changes in the pharmacokinetics occur in patients with moderate to severe liver cirrhosis.

In patients with chronic heart failure the clearance of cilazaprilat is correlated with the creatinine clearance. Thus, dosage adjustments beyond those recommended for patients with impaired renal functions (see *Special Dosage Instructions*) should not be necessary.

Preclinical safety data: Please refer to *Pregnancy and lactation.*

Pharmaceutical particulars

List of excipients:

In the tablet core for all strengths: Lactose, Maize starch, Hydroxypropyl methylcellulose 3cp, Talc, Sodium stearyl fumarate.

In the film coat for all strengths: Hydroxypropyl methylcellulose 6cp, Talc, Titanium dioxide E171, Red iron oxide E172 (0.25 mg, 2.5 mg and 5.0 mg only), Yellow iron oxide E172 (1.0 mg and 2.5 mg only).

Incompatibilities: Not applicable.

Shelf life: 3 years.

Special precautions for storage: Protect from heat (below 25°C).

Nature and contents of container:

Glass bottles and aluminium blisters in the following quantities:

0.5mg: 2, 28, 30 or 100 tablets
1.0mg: 2, 28, 30 or 100 tablets
2.5mg: 4, 28, 30, 98 or 100 tablets
5.0mg: 28, 30, 98 or 100 tablets

Marketing authorisation numbers

PL 0031/0244 0.5 mg Tablets
PL 0031/0245 1.0 mg Tablets
PL 0031/0246 2.5 mg Tablets
PL 0031/0247 5.0 mg Tablets

Date of (partial) revision of the text September 1998

VASCACE 0.25 mg

Qualitative and quantitative composition

One film coated tablet 0.25mg contains: Cilazapril, anhydrous 0.25mg, in the form of the monohydrate (cilazapril 0.261mg).

Pharmaceutical form Tablets.

Clinical particulars

Therapeutic indications: Vascace is indicated in treatment of all grades of essential hypertension and renovascular hypertension. Vascace is also indicated in the treatment of chronic heart failure, usually as an adjunctive therapy with digitalis and/or diuretics.

Posology and method of administration: Vascace should be administered once-daily. As food intake has no clinically significant influence on absorption, Vascace can be administered before or after a meal. The dose should always be taken at about the same time of day.

Special Dosage Instructions:

Essential hypertension: The recommended initial dosage is 1–1.25 mg once a day. Dosage should be adjusted individually in accordance with the blood pressure response until control is achieved. Most patients can be maintained on between 2.5 and 5.0 mg/day. If the blood pressure is not adequately controlled with 5 mg Vascace once daily, a low dose of a non-potassium-sparing diuretic may be administered concomitantly to enhance the anti-hypertensive effect.

Renovascular hypertension: Treatment with Vascace should be initiated with a dose of 0.5 mg or 0.25 mg once daily since these patients may experience more pronounced decreases in blood pressure in response to ACE inhibitors than patients with essential hypertension. The maintenance dose should be adjusted individually.

Hypertensive patients receiving diuretics: The diuretic should be discontinued two to three days before beginning therapy with Vascace to reduce the likelihood of symptomatic hypotension. It may be resumed later if required. The recommended starting dose in these patients is 0.5 mg once daily.

Chronic heart failure: Vascace can be used as adjunctive therapy with digitalis and/or diuretics in patients with chronic heart failure. Therapy with Vascace should be initiated with a recommended starting dose of 0.5 mg once daily under close medical supervision. The dose should be increased to the lowest maintenance dose of 1 mg daily according to tolerability and clinical status. Further titration within the usual maintenance dose of 1 mg to 2.5 mg daily should be carried out based on patients response, clinical status and tolerability. The usual maximum dose is 5 mg once daily.

Results from clinical trials showed that clearance of cilazaprilat in patients with chronic heart failure is correlated with creatinine clearance. Thus in patients with chronic heart failure and impaired renal function special dosage recommendation as given under 'Impaired Renal Function' should be followed.

Impaired renal function: Reduced dosages may be required for patients with renal impairment, depending on their creatinine clearance (see Table 1 following).

In patients requiring haemodialysis, Vascace should be administered on days when dialysis is not performed and the dosage should be adjusted according to blood pressure response.

Severe hepatic function disorders (including cirrhosis): In the unlikely event that patients with severe hepatic function disorders should require treatment with cilazapril, it should be initiated with caution at a dose of 0.5 mg or 0.25 mg once daily, because significant hypotension may occur.

Elderly: In the treatment of hypertension, Vascace should be initiated with between 0.50 mg and 1.25 mg once daily. Thereafter, the maintenance dose must be adapted to individual response.

In the treatment of chronic heart failure, Vascace should be initiated with a dose of 0.5 mg daily. The maintenance dose of 1 mg to 2.5 mg must be adapted to individual tolerability, response and clinical status.

In elderly patients with chronic heart failure on high diuretic dosage the recommended starting dose of Vascace 0.5 mg must be strictly followed.

Children: Safety and efficacy in children have not been established therefore there is no recommendation for administration of cilazapril to children.

Contra-indications: Vascace is contra-indicated in patients who are hypersensitive to the drug cilazapril or other ACE inhibitors, in patients with ascites and in pregnancy and lactation.

Vascace is also contra-indicated in patients with a history of angioedema after treatment with other ACE inhibitors.

Special warnings and special precautions for use: (See also *Special Dosage Instructions* under *Posology and method of administration*).

Vascace should be used with caution in patients with aortic stenosis, hypertrophic cardiomyopathy or outflow obstruction.

In elderly patients with chronic heart failure on high diuretic dosage the recommended starting dose of Vascace 0.5 mg must be strictly followed.

Although the mechanism involved has not been definitely established, there is clinical evidence that haemodialysis with polyacrylonitrile methallyl sulphate high-flux membranes (e.g. AN69), haemofiltration or LDL-apheresis, if performed in patients being treated with ACE inhibitors, including cilazapril, can lead to the provocation of anaphylaxis/anaphylactoid reactions including life-threatening shock. The abovementioned procedures must therefore be avoided in such patients.

Symptomatic hypotension: Occasionally, symptomatic hypotension has been reported with ACE inhibitor therapy, particularly in patients with sodium or volume depletion in connection with conditions such as vomiting, diarrhoea, pre-treatment with diuretics, low sodium diet or after dialysis. In patients with angina pectoris or cerebrovascular disease, treatment with ACE inhibitors should be started under close medical supervision, as excessive hypotension could result in myocardial infarction or cerebrovascular accident.

Patients with chronic heart failure, especially those taking high doses of loop diuretics, may experience a pronounced blood pressure decrease in response to ACE inhibitors. This should be treated by having the patient rest in the supine position and may require infusion of normal saline or volume expanders. After volume repletion, Vascace therapy may be continued. However, if symptoms persist, the dosage should be reduced or the drug discontinued.

Renal impairment: Reduced dosages may be required for patients with renal impairment, depending on their creatinine clearance (see *Special Dosage Instructions*). In patients whose renal function depends primarily on the activity of the renin-angiotensin-aldosterone system, such as patients with severe heart failure or with unilateral or bilateral renal artery stenosis, treatment with ACE-inhibitors including Vascace may produce increases in blood urea nitrogen and/or serum creatinine. Although these alterations are usually reversible upon discontinuation of Vascace and/or diuretic therapy, cases of severe renal dysfunction and, rarely, acute renal failure have been reported.

In this patient population, renal function should be monitored during the first weeks of therapy.

For haemodialysis using high-flux polyacrylonitrile ("AN69") membranes please see above statement under the heading of *Special warnings and special precautions for use.*

Hepatic impairment: In patients with severe liver function impairment, hypotension may occur.

Serum potassium: Concomitant administration of potassium-sparing diuretics, potassium supplements or potassium containing salt substitutes may lead to increases in serum potassium, particularly in patients with renal impairment. Therefore, if concomitant use for such agents is indicated, their dosage should be reduced when Vascace is initiated and serum potassium and renal function should be monitored carefully.

Surgery anaesthesia: The use of ACE inhibitors in combination with anaesthetic drugs in surgery that also have blood-pressure-lowering effects, can produce arterial hypotension. If this occurs, volume expansion by means of intravenous infusion or–if resistant to these measures–angiotensin II infusion is indicated.

Interaction with other medicaments and other forms of interaction: Vascace has been administered concomitantly with digoxin, nitrates, furosemide, thiazides, oral antidiabetics and H2-receptor blockers. There was no increase in digoxin plasma concentrations and no other clinically significant drug interactions. An additive effect may be observed when Vascace is administered in combination with other blood-pressure-lowering agents.

Potassium-sparing diuretics, potassium supplements or potassium containing salt substitutes administered together with Vascace can lead to increases in serum potassium, particularly in patients with renal impairment (see *Special warnings and special precautions for use*).

As with other ACE inhibitors, use of Vascace concomitantly with a non-steroidal antiinflammatory drug (NSAID) may diminish the anti-hypertensive effect of Vascace.

Anaphylactic reactions can occur in patients undergoing desensitisation therapy with wasp or bee venom while receiving an ACE inhibitor. Cilazapril must therefore be interrupted before the start of desensitisation therapy. Additionally, in this situation, cilazapril must not be replaced by a beta blocker.

Concomitant administration of ACE inhibitors and anti-diabetic medicines (insulin, oral hypoglycaemic agents) may cause an increase blood glucose lowering effect with the risk of hypoglycaemia. This phenomenon may be more likely to occur during the first weeks of combined treatment and in patients with renal impairment.

The concomitant administration of ACE inhibitors with lithium may reduce the excretion of lithium. Serum lithium levels should be monitored frequently.

Concomitant administration of allopurinol, cytostatic or immunosuppressive agents, systemic corticosteroids or procainamide with ACE inhibitors may lead to an increased risk for leucopenia.

Pregnancy and lactation: Vascace is contra-indicated in pregnancy since foetotoxicity has been observed for ACE inhibitors in animals. Although there is no experience with Vascace, other ACE inhibitors in human pregnancy have been associated with oligohydramnios and neonatal hypotension and/or anuria. It is not known whether cilazapril passes into human breast milk, but since animal data show the presence of cilazaprilat in rat milk, Vascace should not be administered to nursing mothers.

Effects on ability to drive and use machines: As with other ACE inhibitors, impairment of performance in activities requiring complete mental alertness (e.g. driving a motor vehicle) is not to be expected with Vascace. However, it should be noted that dizziness may occasionally occur in some patients.

Table 1: Impaired Renal Function

The following dose schedules are recommended:

Creatinine clearance	*Initial dose of Vascace*	*Maximal dose of Vascace*
> 40 ml/min	1 mg once daily	5 mg once daily
10–40 ml/min	0.5 mg once daily	2.5 mg once daily
< 10 ml/min	0.25–0.5 mg once or twice a week according to blood pressure response	

Undesirable effects: Headache, dizziness and coughing are the most frequently reported events in patients taking Vascace. Undesirable effects occurring in < 2% of the patients include fatigue, hypotension, dyspepsia, nausea, and rash. In most cases undesirable effects were transient, mild or moderate in degree, and did not require discontinuation of therapy.

Idiosyncratic: ACE-inhibitors have been documented to induce cough in a substantial number of patients. Rarely dyspnoea, sinusitis, rhinitis, glossitis, bronchitis and bronchospasm have been reported.

As with other ACE inhibitors, angioneurotic oedema has been reported, although rarely, in patients receiving Vascace. Angioedema involving the tongue, glottis or larynx may be **fatal**. If involvement of the face, lips, tongue, glottis and/or larynx occurs Vascace should be discontinued without delay and appropriate therapy instituted without delay when involvement of the face, lips, tongue, glottis and/or larynx occurs and replaced by an agent belonging to another class of drugs. Emergency therapy should be given including, but not necessarily limited to, immediate intramuscular adrenalin (epinephrine) solution 1:1000 (0.3 to 0.5 ml) or slow intravenous adrenalin 1 mg/ml (observing dilution instructions) with control of ECG and blood pressure. The patient should be hospitalised and observed for at least 12 to 24 hours and should not be discharged until complete resolution of symptoms has occurred.

Pancreatitis has been reported rarely in patients treated with ACE inhibitors (including Vascace); in some cases this has proved fatal.

Laboratory test findings: Clinically relevant changes in laboratory test values possibly or probably related to Vascace treatment have been observed only rarely.

Minor, mostly reversible increases in serum creatinine/urea have been observed in patients treated with Vascace. Such changes are likely to occur in patients with renal artery stenosis or with renal impairment (see *Special warnings and special precautions for use*), but they have also occasionally been observed in patients with normal renal function, particularly in those receiving concomitant diuretics. Isolated cases of acute renal failure have been reported in patients with severe heart failure, renal artery stenosis or renal disorders (see *Special warnings and special precautions for use*).

In some patients decreases in haemoglobin, haematocrit and/or white blood cell count have been reported, but in no case has a definite causal relationship to Vascace been established.

Overdose: While single doses of up to 160 mg Vascace have been administered to normal healthy volunteers without untoward effects on blood pressure, only a few data on overdose are available in patients.

The most likely symptoms of overdosage are severe hypotension, shock, stupor, bradycardia, electrolyte disturbances and renal failure.

After ingestion of an overdose, the patient should be kept under close supervision, preferably in an intensive care unit. Serum electrolytes and creatinine should be monitored frequently. Therapeutic measures depend on the nature and severity of the symptoms. Measurements to prevent absorption such as gastric lavage, administration of adsorbents and sodium sulphate within 30 minutes after intake, and to hasten elimination should be applied if ingestion is recent. If hypotension occurs, the patient should be placed in the shock position and salt and volume supplementation should be given, rapidly. Treatment with angiotensin II should be considered. Bradycardia or extensive vagal reactions should be treated by administering atropine. The use of a pacemaker may be considered. ACE inhibitors may be removed from the circulation by haemodialysis. The use of high-flux polyacrylonitrile membranes should be avoided.

Pharmacological properties

Pharmacodynamic properties: Vascace (cilazapril) is a specific, long-acting angiotensin-converting enzyme (ACE) inhibitor which suppresses the renin-angiotensin-aldosterone system and thereby the conversion of the inactive angiotensin I to angiotensin II which is a potent vasoconstrictor. At recommended doses, the effect of Vascace in hypertensive patients and in patients with chronic heart failure is maintained for up to 24 hours.

In patients with normal renal function, serum potassium usually remains within the normal range during Vascace treatment. In patients concomitantly taking potassium-sparing diuretics, potassium levels may rise.

Hypertension: Vascace induces a reduction of both supine and standing systolic and diastolic blood pressure, usually with no orthostatic component. It is effective in all degrees of essential hypertension as well as in renal hypertension. The anti-hypertensive effect of Vascace is usually apparent within the first hour after administration, with maximum effect observed between three and seven hours after dosing. In general the heart rate remains unchanged. Reflex tachycardia is not induced, although small, clinically insignificant alterations of heart rate may occur. In some patients blood pressure reduction may diminish toward the end of the dosage interval.

The initial dosage seldom achieves the desired therapeutic response. Blood pressure should be assessed and dosage adjusted as required. Should the effect of Vascace at the top of the recommended dose be insufficient it can be combined with non-potassium-sparing diuretics.

The anti-hypertensive effect of Vascace is maintained during long-term therapy. No rapid increase in blood pressure has been observed after abrupt withdrawal of Vascace.

In hypertensive patients with moderate to severe renal impairment, the glomerular filtration rate and renal blood flow remained in general unchanged with Vascace despite a clinically significant blood pressure reduction.

As with other ACE inhibitors, the blood pressure-lowering effect of Vascace in black patients may be less pronounced than in non-blacks. However, racial differences in response are no longer evident when Vascace is administered in combination with hydrochlorothiazide.

Chronic heart failure: In patients with chronic heart failure the renin-angiotensin-aldosterone and the sympathetic nervous systems are generally activated leading to enhanced systemic vasoconstriction and to the promotion of sodium and water retention. By suppressing the renin-angiotensin-aldosterone system, Vascace improves loading conditions in the failing heart by reducing systemic vascular resistance (afterload) and pulmonary capillary wedge pressure (preload) in patients on diuretics and/or digitalis. Furthermore, the exercise tolerance of these patients increases significantly showing an improvement in quality of life. The haemodynamic and clinical effects occur promptly and persist.

Pharmacokinetic properties: Cilazapril is efficiently absorbed and rapidly converted to the active form, cilazaprilat. Ingestion of food immediately prior to Vascace administration, delays and reduces the absorption to a minor extent which, however, is therapeutically irrelevant. The bioavailability of cilazaprilat from oral cilazapril approximates 60% based on urinary recovery data. Maximum plasma concentrations are reached within two hours after administration and are directly related to dosage.

Cilazaprilat is eliminated unchanged by the kidneys, with an effective half-life of nine hours after once-daily dosing with Vascace. In patients with renal impairment, higher plasma concentrations of cilazaprilat are observed than in patients with normal renal function, since drug clearance is reduced when creatinine clearance is lower. There is no elimination in patients with complete renal failure, but haemodialysis reduces concentrations of both cilazapril and cilazaprilat to a limited extent.

In elderly patients whose renal function is normal for age, plasma concentrations of cilazaprilat may be up to 40% higher, and the clearance 20% lower than in younger patients. Similar changes in the pharmacokinetics occur in patients with moderate to severe liver cirrhosis.

In patients with chronic heart failure the clearance of cilazaprilat is correlated with the creatinine clearance. Thus, dosage adjustments beyond those recommended for patients with impaired renal functions (see *Special Dosage Instructions*) should not be necessary.

Preclinical safety data: Please see *Pregnancy and lactation.*

Pharmaceutical particulars

List of excipients: In the tablet core for all strengths: Lactose, Maize starch, Hydroxypropyl methylcellulose 3cp, Talc, Sodium stearyl fumarate.

In the film coat for all strengths: Hydroxypropyl methylcellulose 6cp, Talc, Titanium dioxide E171, Red iron oxide E172.

Incompatibilities: Not applicable.

Shelf life: 3 years.

Special precautions for storage: Protect from heat (below 25°C).

Nature and contents of container: Glass Bottles and Aluminium Blisters in the following quantities: 2, 28, 30 or 100 tablets.

Marketing authorisation number PL 0031/0273

Date of (partial) revision of the text September 1998

VESANOID ▼

Qualitative and quantitative composition 1 capsule contains 10 mg of tretinoin (all-trans retinoic acid).

Pharmaceutical form Capsules.

Clinical particulars

Therapeutic indications: Vesanoid (tretinoin) is indicated for induction of remission in acute promyelocytic leukaemia (APL; FAB classification AML-M3).

This treatment is intended for previously untreated patients as well as patients who relapse after a standard chemotherapy (anthracycline and cytosine arabinoside or equivalent therapies) or patients who are refractory to chemotherapy.

The association of tretinoin with chemotherapy increases the duration of survival and reduces the risk of relapse compared to chemotherapy alone.

Posology and method of administration: A total daily dose of 45 mg/m² body surface divided in 2 equal doses is recommended for oral administration. This is approximately 8 capsules per adult dose.

It is recommended to take the capsules with a meal or shortly thereafter.

There is limited safety and efficacy information on the use of tretinoin in children.

Paediatric patients can be treated with 45 mg/m² unless severe toxicity becomes apparent. Dose reduction should be particularly considered for children with intractable headache.

Treatment should be continued until complete remission has been achieved or up to a maximum of 90 days.

Due to limited information on patients with hepatic and/or renal insufficiency, the dose will be decreased to 25 mg/m² as a precautionary measure.

Full-dose anthracycline-based chemotherapy should be added to the tretinoin regimen as follows (see *Special warnings and special precautions for use*):

- When the leukocyte count at start of therapy is greater than 5 x 10^9/L, chemotherapy should be started together with tretinoin on day one.
- When the leukocyte count at start of therapy is less than 5 x 10^9/L but rapidly increases during tretinoin therapy, chemotherapy should be **immediately** added to the tretinoin regimen if the leukocyte count reaches greater than 6 x 10^9/L by day 5, or greater than 10 x 10^9/L by day 10, or greater than 15 x 10^9/L by day 28.
- All other patients should receive chemotherapy immediately after complete remission is attained.

If chemotherapy is added to tretinoin because of hyperleukocytosis, it is not necessary to modify the dose of tretinoin.

After completion of tretinoin therapy and the first chemotherapy course, consolidation anthracycline-based chemotherapy should be given, for example, a further 2 courses at 4 to 6 week intervals.

In some patients the plasma levels of tretinoin may fall significantly in spite of continued administration.

Contra-indications:

- Known allergy to a product in the class of retinoids.
- Pregnancy.
- Lactation.
- Tetracyclines (see *Interactions*).
- Low-dose progestogens (see *Interactions*).
- Vitamin A (see *Interactions*).

Special warnings and special precautions for use: Tretinoin should be administered to patients with acute promyelocytic leukaemia only under the strict supervision of a physician who is experienced in the treatment of haematological/oncological diseases.

Supportive care appropriate for patients with acute promyelocytic leukaemia, for example prophylaxis for bleeding and prompt therapy for infection, should be maintained during therapy with tretinoin. The patient's haematologic profile, coagulation profile, liver function test results, and triglyceride and cholesterol levels should be monitored frequently.

During clinical trials hyperleukocytosis has been frequently observed (in 75% of the cases), sometimes associated with the "Retinoic Acid Syndrome". Retinoic acid syndrome has been reported in many acute promyelocytic leukaemia patients treated with tretinoin (up to 25% in some centres).

The retinoic acid syndrome is characterised by fever, dyspnoea, acute respiratory distress, pulmonary infiltrates, pleural effusions, hyperleukocytosis, hypotension, oedema, weight gain, hepatic, renal and multi-organ failure.

Untreated, this syndrome can be fatal.

The incidence of the retinoic acid syndrome is diminished when full dose chemotherapy is added to the tretinoin regimen based on the white blood cell count. The current therapeutic treatment recommendations and method of administration are detailed in section *Posology and method of administration.*

Immediate treatment with dexamethasone (10 mg every 12 hours for up to maximum 3 days or until resolution of the symptoms) should be given, if the patient presents any symptom(s) or sign(s) of this syndrome.

There is a risk of thrombosis during the first month of treatment.

Interaction with other medicaments and other forms of interaction: The effect of food on the bioavailability of tretinoin has not been characterised. Since the bioavailability of retinoids, as a class, is known to increase in the presence of food, it is recommended that tretinoin be administered with a meal or shortly thereafter.

As tretinoin is metabolised by the hepatic P-450 system, there is the potential for alteration of pharmacokinetics parameters in patients administered concomitant medications that are also inducers or inhibitors of this system. Medications that generally induce hepatic P-450 enzymes include rifampicin, glucocorticoids, phenobarbital and pentobarbital. Medications that generally inhibit hepatic P-450 enzymes include ketoconazole, cimetidine, erythromycin, verapamil, diltiazem and cyclosporine. There are no data to suggest that co-use with these medications increases or decreases either efficacy or toxicity of tretinoin.

There are no data on a possible pharmacokinetic interaction between tretinoin and daunorubicin or AraC.

Contra-indicated drug associations:

Low-dose progestogens: Tretinoin causes diminution of the contraceptive efficacy of the progestogens.

Tetracyclines: Systemic treatment with retinoids may cause elevation of the intracranial pressure. As tetracyclines may also cause elevation of the intracranial pressure, patients must not be treated with tretinoin and tetracyclines at the same time.

Vitamin A: As with other retinoids, tretinoin must not be administered in combination with vitamin A because symptoms of hypervitaminosis A could be aggravated.

Pregnancy and lactation: All the measures listed below should be considered in relationship to the severity of the disease and the urgency of the treatment.

Pregnancy: Tretinoin is teratogenic. Its use is contra-indicated in pregnant women and women who might become pregnant during the treatment with tretinoin and within one month after cessation of treatment, unless the benefit of tretinoin treatment outweighs the risk of foetal abnormalities due to the severity of the patient's condition and the urgency of treatment.

There is a very high risk for any exposed foetus that a deformed infant will result if pregnancy occurs while taking tretinoin, irrespective of the dose or duration of the treatment.

Therapy with tretinoin should only be started in female patients of child-bearing age if each of the following conditions is met:

-She is informed by her physician of the hazards of becoming pregnant during and one month after treatment with tretinoin.

-She is willing to comply with the mandatory contraception measures: to use a reliable contraception method without interruption during therapy and for one month after discontinuation of treatment with tretinoin.

-Pregnancy tests must be performed at monthly intervals during therapy.

In spite of these precautions, should pregnancy occur during treatment with tretinoin or up to one month after its discontinuation, there is a high risk of severe malformation of the foetus, particularly when tretinoin is given during the first trimester of pregnancy.

Lactation: Nursing must be discontinued if therapy with tretinoin is initiated.

Effects on ability to drive and use machines: The ability to drive or operate machinery might be impaired in patients treated with tretinoin, particularly if they are experiencing dizziness or severe headache.

Undesirable effects: In patients treated with the recommended daily doses of tretinoin the most frequent undesirable effects are consistent with the signs and symptoms of the hypervitaminosis A syndrome (as for other retinoids).

Skin: (> 75% of patients) dryness, erythema, rash, pruritus, hair loss, sweating,

Mucous membranes: (> 75% of patients) cheilitis, dryness of mouth, nose, conjunctiva and other mucous membranes, with or without inflammatory symptoms.

Central nervous system: (> 75% of patients) headache, intra-cranial hypertension, pseudotumor cerebri syndrome (mainly in children), fever, shivering, dizziness, confusion, anxiety, depression, paraesthesias, insomnia, malaise.

Neuro-sensory system: (25%–50% of patients) vision and hearing disorders.

Musculo-skeletal system: (50%–75% of patients) bone pain, chest pain.

Gastrointestinal tract: (> 75% of patients) nausea, vomiting, abdominal pain, diarrhoea, constipation, diminished appetite, pancreatitis.

Metabolic, hepatic and renal dysfunctions: (50%–75% of patients) elevation in serum triglycerides, cholesterol, transaminases (ALAT, ASAT), creatinine.

Respiratory system: (50%–75% of patients) dyspnoea, respiratory insufficiency, pleural effusion, asthma-like syndrome.

Cardiovascular system: (50%–75% of patients) arrhythmias, flushing, oedema. Some cases of thrombosis have also been reported.

These undesirable effects do not seem to represent a permanent or irreversible hazard. The decision to interrupt or continue therapy should be based on an evaluation of the benefit of the treatment versus the severity of the side-effects.

The signs, symptoms and manifestations of the Retinoic Acid Syndrome which could be potentially fatal, as well as its prevention and treatment have been described above (see section *Special warnings and special precautions for use*).

Teratogenicity: See above.

There is limited safety information on the use of tretinoin in children. There have been some reports of increased toxicity in children treated with tretinoin, particularly increased pseudotumor cerebri.

Overdose: No cases of acute overdosage with tretinoin have been reported.

In the event of accidental overdosage of tretinoin, reversible signs of hyper-vitaminosis A (headache, nausea, vomiting) can appear.

The recommended dose in acute promyelocytic leukaemia is one-quarter of the maximum tolerated dose in solid tumour patients and below the maximum tolerated dose in children.

There is no specific treatment in the case of an overdose, however it is important that the patient be treated in a special haematological unit.

Pharmacological properties

Pharmacodynamic properties: Cytostatic-differentiating agent.

Tretinoin is a natural metabolite of retinol and belongs to the class of retinoids, comprising natural and synthetic analogs.

In vitro studies with tretinoin have demonstrated induction of differentiation and inhibition of cell proliferation in transformed haemopoietic cell lines, including human myeloid leukaemia cell lines.

The mechanism of action in acute promyelocytic leukaemia is not known but it may be due to a modification in binding of tretinoin to a nuclear retinoic acid receptor (RAR) given that the α-receptor of retinoic acid is altered by fusion with a protein called PML.

Pharmacokinetic properties: Tretinoin is an endogenous metabolite of vitamin A which is normally present in plasma.

After oral administration, tretinoin is absorbed by the digestive tract and maximum plasma concentrations in healthy volunteers are attained after 3 hours.

There is a large inter-patient and intra-patient variation in plasma levels of tretinoin.

Tretinoin is extensively bound to plasma proteins. Following peak levels, plasma concentrations decline with a mean elimination half life of 0.7 hours. Plasma concentrations return to endogenous levels after 7 to 12 hours following a single 40 mg dose. No accumulation is seen after multiple doses and tretinoin is not retained in body tissues.

After an oral dose of radiolabelled tretinoin, about 60% of the radioactivity was excreted in urine and about 30% in faeces. The metabolites found in urine were formed by oxidation and glucuronidation.

During continuous administration a marked decrease in plasma concentration can occur, possibly due to cytochrome P-450 enzyme induction which increases clearance and decreases bioavailability after oral doses.

At present there are no data on a possible interaction between tretinoin and daunorubicin.

The requirement for dosage adjustment in patients with renal or hepatic insufficiency has not been investigated. As a precautionary measure, the dose will be decreased (see *Posology and method of administration*).

Preclinical safety data: Oral administration of tretinoin to animals indicated that the compound had very low acute toxicity in all species investigated.

In animal experimental tests it was shown that in all investigated species the acute toxicity of tretinoin administered orally is low. After a longer period of administration rats exhibit a dose- and time-dependent bone matrix dissolution, a decrease in erythrocyte count and toxic alterations in kidney and testes.

Dogs mainly exhibited disorders concerning spermatogenesis and hyperplasia of the bone marrow.

Subchronic and chronic toxicity studies in rats indicated that the no effect oral dose was at or below 1 mg/kg/day; in dogs, 30 mg/kg/day was associated with toxic effects including weight loss, dermatological and testicular changes.

Reproduction studies in animals have demonstrated the teratogenic activity of tretinoin.

No evidence of mutagenicity has been found.

Pharmaceutical particulars

List of excipients: 1 capsule contains the following excipients: Yellow beeswax, hydrogenated soybean oil, partially hydrogenated soybean oil, soybean oil.

1 capsule shell contains the following excipients: Gelatin, glycerol, Karion (sorbitol, mannitol, starch), titanium dioxide (E 171), iron oxide yellow (E 172), iron oxide red (E 172).

A capsule is bi-coloured: Orange yellow/reddish brown.

Incompatibilities: None are presently known.

Shelf life: 3 years.

Special precautions for storage: Keep the bottle tightly closed. Protect from light. Store between 5°C and 30°C.

This medicine should not be used after the expiration date (EXP) shown on the outer pack.

Nature and contents of container: Amber glass-bottles of 100 capsules.

Instructions for use/handling: Not applicable.

Marketing authorisation number PL 14878/0006

Date of first authorisation/renewal of authorisation October 1996

Date of (partial) revision of the text Not applicable

VIRACEPT ORAL POWDER 

Qualitative and quantitative composition Viracept 50 mg/g Oral Powder contains 58.45 mg of nelfinavir mesylate corresponding to 50 mg of nelfinavir (as free base) per gram of powder.

Pharmaceutical form Oral Powder

Clinical particulars

Therapeutic indications: Viracept is indicated in combination with antiretroviral nucleoside analogues for the treatment of HIV-1 infected patients with advanced or progressive immunodeficiency.

Combinations of Viracept with antiretroviral nucleoside analogues have been shown to decrease plasma viral load and to increase circulating CD4 lymphocyte counts. Clinical studies are underway to evaluate the clinical benefits of combination regimens.

Refer to *Pharmacodynamic properties.*

Posology and method of administration: Viracept 50 mg/g Oral Powder should preferably be ingested with food.

Patients older than 13 years: Viracept 250 mg Tablets are recommended for adults and older children (see Summary of Product Characteristics for Viracept 250 mg Tablets). The recommended dose of Viracept 50 mg/g Oral Powder is 750 mg three times a day (TID), for patients unable to take tablets.

Patients aged 2 to 13 years: for children, the recommended starting dose is 25–30 mg/kg per dose, TID. For children able to take tablets, Viracept Tablets may be administered instead of the Oral Powder (see Summary of Product Characteristics for Viracept Tablets).

The recommended dose of Viracept Oral Powder to be administered TID to children aged 2 to 13 years is as follows:

Body weight kg	*Number of level 1 g scoops*
7.5 to < 8.5	4
8.5 to < 10.5	5
10.5 to < 12	6
12 to < 14	7
14 to < 16	8
16 to < 18	9
18 to < 23	10
≥ 23	15

The Oral Powder may be mixed with water, milk, formula, soy formula, soy milk, dietary supplements, or pudding. It is recommended that Viracept 50 mg/g Oral Powder mixed in these media be used within 6 hours. Dosing media not recommended, due to taste, includes any acidic food or juice (e.g. orange juice, apple juice or apple sauce). Do not add water to bottles of Viracept 50 mg/g Oral Powder.

Therapy with Viracept should be initiated by a physician experienced in the management of HIV infection.

Renal or hepatic impairment: currently, there are no data specific for these patient populations and therefore specific dosage recommendations cannot be made. Nelfinavir is principally metabolised and eliminated by the liver. Caution should be used when administering Viracept to patients with impaired renal or hepatic function.

Contra-indications: Hypersensitivity to nelfinavir or to any of the excipients.

Viracept is contra-indicated in breastfeeding women.

Viracept should not be administered concurrently with medicinal products with narrow therapeutic windows and which are substrates of CYP3A4. Co-administration may result in competitive inhibition of the metabolism of these medicinal products and create the potential for serious and/or life-threatening adverse events such as cardiac arrhythmias (e.g. terfenadine, astemizole, cisapride, amiodarone, quinidine), prolonged sedation or respiratory depression (e.g. triazolam, midazolam), or other events (e.g. ergot derivatives).

Viracept must not be given with rifampicin. Rifampicin decreases nelfinavir plasma AUC by 82%.

See *Interaction with other medicaments and other forms of interaction.*

Special warnings and special precautions for use: Caution should be used when administering Viracept to patients with impaired renal or hepatic function (see *Posology and method of administration*).

The safety and activity of nelfinavir in children below the age of 2 years have not been established.

Caution is advised whenever Viracept is co-administered with medicinal products which are inducers or inhibitors and/or substrates of CYP3A4; such combinations may require dose adjustment (see *Contra-indications, Interaction with other medicaments and other forms of interaction,* and *Undesirable effects*).

Viracept 50 mg/g Oral Powder contains aspartame as a sweetening agent. Aspartame provides a source of phenylalanine and, therefore, may not be suitable for persons with phenylketonuria.

New onset diabetes mellitus, hyperglycaemia or exacerbation of existing diabetes mellitus has been reported in patients receiving protease inhibitors. In some of these the hyperglycaemia was severe and in some cases also associated with ketoacidosis. Many patients had confounding medical conditions, some of which required therapy with agents that have been associated with the development of diabetes or hyperglycaemia.

There have been reports of increased bleeding, including spontaneous skin haematomas and haemarthroses, in haemophiliac patients type A and B treated with protease inhibitors. In some patients additional factor VIII was given. In more than half of the reported cases, treatment with protease inhibitors was continued or reintroduced if treatment had been discontinued. A causal relationship has been evoked, although the mechanism of action has not been elucidated. Haemophiliac patients should therefore be made aware of the possibility of increased bleeding.

Patients should be instructed that Viracept is not a cure for HIV infection, that they may continue to develop infections or other illnesses associated with HIV disease, and that Viracept has not been shown to reduce the risk of transmission of HIV disease through sexual contact or blood contamination.

Interaction with other medicaments and other forms of interaction: Nelfinavir is metabolised in part via the cytochrome P450 3A system (CYP3A). Caution should be used when co-administering medicinal products that induce CYP3A or potentially toxic medicinal products which are themselves metabolised by CYP3A. Based on *in vitro* data, nelfinavir is unlikely to inhibit other cytochrome P450 isoforms at concentrations in the therapeutic range.

Other antiretrovirals: clinically significant interactions have not been observed between nelfinavir and nucleoside analogues (specifically zidovudine plus lamivudine, stavudine, and stavudine plus didanosine). At present, there is no evidence of inadequate efficacy of zidovudine in the CNS that could be associated with the modest reduction in plasma levels of zidovudine when co-administered with Viracept. Since it is recommended that didanosine be administered on an empty stomach, Viracept should be administered (with food) one hour after or more than 2 hours before didanosine.

Ritonavir: administration of a single 750 mg dose of Viracept following 3 doses of ritonavir 500 mg BID resulted in a 152% increase in nelfinavir plasma area under the plasma concentration-time curve (AUC) and a 156% increase in the elimination half-life of nelfinavir. Administration of a single 500 mg dose of ritonavir following six doses of Viracept 750 mg TID resulted in minimal increase (8%) in ritonavir plasma AUC. The safety of this combination has not been established.

Indinavir: administration of a single 750 mg dose of Viracept following indinavir 800 mg every 8 hours for 7 days resulted in an 83% increase in nelfinavir plasma AUC and a 22% increase in the elimination half-life of nelfinavir. Administration of a single 800 mg dose of indinavir following Viracept 750 mg TID for 7 days resulted in a 51% increase in indinavir plasma AUC concentrations, with a 5-fold increase in trough concentrations measured at 8 hours, but no increase in peak concentrations. The safety of this combination has not been established.

Saquinavir soft gelatin capsule: administration of a single 750 mg dose of Viracept following 4 days of *saquinavir soft gelatin capsule* 1200 mg TID resulted in a 30% increase in nelfinavir plasma AUC. Administration of a single 1200 mg dose of saquinavir soft gelatin capsule following 4 days of Viracept 750 mg TID resulted in a 392% increase in saquinavir plasma AUC.

Metabolic enzyme inducers: rifampicin decreases nelfinavir plasma AUC by 82%. Other potent inducers of CYP3A (e.g. phenobarbital, phenytoin, carbamazepine) may also reduce nelfinavir plasma concentrations. If therapy with such medicinal products is warranted, physicians should consider using alternatives when a patient is taking Viracept.

Co-administration of Viracept and rifabutin results in a 32% decrease in nelfinavir plasma AUC and an approximately 200% increase in rifabutin plasma AUC (see also section 4.4). A dosage reduction of rifabutin to half the standard dose is necessary when Viracept and rifabutin are co-administered.

Metabolic enzyme inhibitors: co-administration of Viracept and a strong inhibitor of CYP3A, ketoconazole, resulted in a 35% increase in nelfinavir plasma AUC. This change is not considered clinically significant and no dose adjustment is needed when ketoconazole and Viracept are co-administered. Based on the metabolic profiles, a clinically relevant drug interaction would not be expected with other specific inhibitors of CYP3A (e.g. fluconazole, itraconazole, clarithromycin, erythromycin); however, the possibility cannot be excluded.

Other potential interactions: Viracept increases terfenadine plasma concentrations; therefore, Viracept should not be administered concurrently with terfenadine because of the potential for serious and/or life-threatening cardiac arrhythmias. Because similar interactions are likely with astemizole and cisapride, Viracept should also not be administered concurrently with these drugs. Although specific studies have not been done, potent sedatives metabolised by CYP3A, such as triazolam or midazolam, should not be co-administered with Viracept due to the potential for prolonged sedation. For other compounds that are substrates for CYP3A (e.g. calcium channel blockers) plasma concentrations may be elevated when co-administered with Viracept; therefore, patients should be monitored for toxicities associated with such medicinal products.

Oral contraceptives: administration of Viracept 750 mg TID and a combination oral contraceptive which included 0.4 mg of norethindrone and 35 µg of 17 α-ethinyl estradiol for 7 days resulted in a 47% decrease in ethinyl estradiol and an 18% decrease in norethindrone plasma AUC. Alternative contraceptive measures should be considered.

Use during pregnancy and lactation: No treatment-related adverse effects were seen in animal reproductive toxicity studies in rats at doses providing systemic exposure comparable to that observed with the clinical dose. Clinical experience in pregnant women is lacking. Until additional data become available, Viracept should be given during pregnancy only after special consideration.

It is recommended that HIV-infected women must not breastfeed their infants under any circumstances in order to avoid transmission of HIV. Studies in lactating rats showed that nelfinavir is excreted in breast milk. There is no data available on nelfinavir excretion into human breast milk. Mothers must be instructed to discontinue breastfeeding if they are receiving Viracept.

Effects on ability to drive and use machines: There is no indication that Viracept affects the ability to drive and use machines.

Undesirable effects: The safety of Viracept was studied in controlled clinical trials with over 800 patients, of which more than half received a dose of 750 mg TID either alone or in combination with nucleoside analogues. Over 4000 patients ≥ 13 years in the expanded access programmes received Viracept at a dose of 750 mg TID. The majority of adverse events were of mild intensity. The most frequently reported adverse event among patients receiving Viracept was diarrhoea.

Across the two phase III, double-blind studies adverse experiences of moderate to severe intensity reported by investigators as at least possibly related to Viracept or of unknown relationship in ≥ 2% of patients treated with the 750 mg TID dose of Viracept (n=200) in combination with nucleoside analogues (for 24 weeks) included the following undesirable effects: diarrhoea (25.9%), flatulence (2.5%), nausea (4.5%), and rash (3.0%). Marked clinical laboratory abnormalities (change from grade 0 to grade 3 or 4, or change from grade 1 to grade 4) reported in ≥ 2% of patients treated with 750 mg TID of Viracept (for 24 weeks) across the same studies included increased creatine kinase (3.9%), and decreased neutrophils (4.5%). Marked increases in transaminases occurred in less than 2% of patients receiving Viracept at the recommended dose and were sometimes accompanied by clinical signs and symptoms of acute hepatitis. Some of these patients were known to be chronic carriers of hepatitis B and/or C viruses. With the exception of diarrhoea, there were no significant differences in the adverse experiences reported by patients treated with Viracept versus the control arms containing zidovudine plus lamivudine or stavudine alone.

Overdose: Human experience of acute overdose with Viracept is limited. There is no specific antidote for overdose with Viracept. If indicated, elimination of unabsorbed nelfinavir should be achieved by emesis or gastric lavage. Administration of activated charcoal may also be used to aid removal of unabsorbed nelfinavir. Since nelfinavir is highly protein bound, dialysis is unlikely to significantly remove it from blood.

Pharmacological properties

Pharmacodynamic properties: Pharmacotherapeutic group: antiviral agent, ATC code: J05A E04

Mechanism of action: HIV protease is an enzyme required for the proteolytic cleavage of the viral polyprotein precursors to the individual proteins found in infectious HIV. The cleavage of these viral polyproteins is essential for the maturation of infectious virus. Nelfinavir reversibly binds to the active site of HIV protease and prevents cleavage of the polyproteins resulting in the formation of immature non-infectious viral particles.

Antiviral activity in vitro: the antiviral activity of nelfinavir *in vitro* has been demonstrated in both HIV acute and chronic infections in lymphoblastoid cell lines, peripheral blood lymphocytes and monocytes/macrophages. Nelfinavir was found to be active against a broad range of laboratory strains and clinical isolates of HIV-1 and the HIV-2 strain ROD. The EC_{95} (95% effective concentration) of nelfinavir ranged from 7 to 111 nM (mean of 58 nM). Nelfinavir demonstrated additive to synergistic effects against HIV in combination with reverse transcriptase inhibitors zidovudine (ZDV), lamivudine (3TC), didanosine (ddI), zalcitabine (ddC) and stavudine (d4T) without enhanced cytotoxicity.

Resistance: HIV isolates with reduced susceptibility to nelfinavir have been selected *in vitro*. Genotypic analysis of a variant which exhibited a nine-fold decrease in sensitivity showed a unique substitution of an aspartic acid (D) to an asparagine (N) in HIV protease at amino acid residue 30 (D30N). Genotypic changes in HIV protease genes obtained from 58 patients enrolled in phase I/II trials were also evaluated. Consistent with the *in vitro* results, the predominant change observed was the D30N substitution. In a subset of these patients followed for up to 44 weeks, this substitution was maintained. Mutations described for other protease inhibitors were either never observed (G48V, V82F/T, I84V) or only rarely (3 of 55 patients) observed (L90M). Sequence analyses were performed on the protease genes derived at 16 weeks from randomly selected patients who received nelfinavir either alone (n=64) or in combination with ZDV and 3TC (n=49) in pivotal trials. The incidence of genotypic resistance to nelfinavir at 16 weeks was significantly reduced when nelfinavir was used in combination with ZDV and 3TC (6%), compared to monotherapy (56%).

Cross-resistance to other antivirals: cross-resistance between nelfinavir and reverse transcriptase inhibitors is unlikely because of the different enzymes targets involved. HIV isolates resistant to nucleoside analogues and non-nucleoside reverse transcriptase inhibitors remain susceptible *in vitro* to nelfinavir. The potential for HIV cross-resistance to other protease inhibitors has been explored with nelfinavir. Six clinical isolates containing the D30N substitution showed no change in sensitivity to saquinavir, ritonavir, indinavir or 141W94 *in vitro*. This lack of cross-resistance was confirmed with an HIV recombinant virus containing the D30N substitution; the recombinant virus exhibited a reduced sensitivity to nelfinavir, yet retained full sensitivity to the other protease inhibitors. In addition, in patients previously treated with ritonavir, indinavir and/or saquinavir five of fourteen clinical isolates with reduced susceptibility to one or more of these protease inhibitors were susceptible to nelfinavir.

Clinical pharmacodynamic data: treatment with nelfinavir alone or in combination with other antiretroviral agents has been documented to reduce viral load and increase CD4 cell counts in HIV-1 seropositive patients. The effects of nelfinavir (alone or combined with other antiretroviral agents) on biological markers of disease activity, CD4 cell count and viral RNA, were evaluated in several studies involving HIV-1 infected patients.

Viracept 750 mg TID in combination with one or more nucleoside analogues was consistently associated with decreases in mean plasma HIV RNA in excess of 1 $\log_{10}$ copies/ml and increases in mean CD4 cell count of 90–100 cells/mm³ which were sustained to at least 24 weeks. Decreases in HIV RNA observed with Viracept monotherapy were less pronounced and of shorter duration.

In a study of 297 HIV-1 seropositive patients receiving zidovudine and lamivudine plus Viracept (2 different doses) or zidovudine and lamivudine alone, the mean decrease in plasma HIV RNA at 24 weeks was 2.15 $\log_{10}$ in patients receiving combination therapy with Viracept 750 mg TID, compared to 1.54 $\log_{10}$ in patients receiving zidovudine and lamivudine alone. At 24 weeks, the percentage of patients whose plasma HIV RNA levels had decreased to below the limit of detection of the assay (<500 copies/ml) were 81% and 18% for the groups treated with Viracept 750 mg TID plus zidovudine and lamivudine or zidovudine and lamivudine, respectively. Mean CD4 cell counts at 24 weeks were increased by 108 and 81 cells/mm³ for the groups treated with Viracept 750 mg TID plus zidovudine and lamivudine or zidovudine and lamivudine, respectively. At 48 weeks, approximately 80% of the patients treated with Viracept 750 mg TID plus zidovudine and lamivudine remained below the level of detection of the assay; CD4 cell counts increased by more than 170 cells/mm³ at 48 weeks in this group.

Pharmacokinetic properties: The pharmacokinetic properties of nelfinavir have been evaluated in healthy volunteers and HIV-infected patients. No substantial differences have been observed between healthy volunteers and HIV-infected patients.

Absorption: after single or multiple oral doses of 500 to 750 mg (two to three 250 mg tablets) with food, peak nelfinavir plasma concentrations were typically achieved in 2 to 4 hours. After multiple dosing with 750 mg every 8 hours for 28 days (steady-state), peak plasma concentrations (C_{max}) averaged 3–4 µg/ml and plasma concentrations prior to the next dose (trough) were 1–3 µg/ml. A greater than dose-proportional increase in nelfinavir plasma concentrations was observed after single doses; however, this was not observed after multiple dosing. The absolute bioavailability has not been determined.

Effect of food on gastrointestinal absorption: maximum plasma concentrations and area under the plasma concentration-time curve were consistently 2 to 3-fold higher under fed conditions compared to fasting. The increased plasma concentrations with food were independent of fat content of the meals.

Distribution: in both animals and humans, the estimated volumes of distribution (2–7 l/kg) exceeded total body water, suggesting extensive penetration of nelfinavir into tissues. Although no studies have been conducted in humans, studies with a single 50 mg/kg dose of ^{14}C-nelfinavir in rats showed that concentrations in the brain were lower than in other tissues, but exceeded the *in vitro* EC_{95} for antiviral activity. Nelfinavir in serum is extensively protein-bound (≥ 98%).

Metabolism: unchanged nelfinavir comprised 82–86% of the total plasma radioactivity after a single oral 750 mg dose of ^{14}C-nelfinavir. One major and several minor oxidative metabolites were found in plasma. The major oxidative metabolite has *in vitro* antiviral activity equal to the parent drug. The plasma levels of this metabolite are approximately 25% of the total plasma nelfinavir-related concentration. *In vitro*, multiple cytochrome P450 isoforms including CYP3A, CYP2C19/C9 and CYP2D6 are responsible for metabolism of nelfinavir.

Elimination: oral clearance estimates after single doses (24–33 l/h) and multiple doses (26–61 l/h) indicate that nelfinavir exhibits medium to high hepatic bioavailability. The terminal half-life in plasma was typically 3.5 to 5 hours. The majority (87%) of an oral 750 mg dose containing ^{14}C-nelfinavir was recovered in the faeces; total faecal radioactivity consisted of nelfinavir (22%) and numerous oxidative metabolites (78%). Only 1–2% of the dose was recovered in urine, of which unchanged nelfinavir was the major component.

Pharmacokinetics in children and the elderly: in children between the ages of 2 and 13 years, the clearance of orally administered nelfinavir is approximately 2 to 3 times higher than in adults, with large intersubject variability. Administration of Viracept Oral Powder or Tablets with food at a dose of approximately 25–30 mg/kg TID achieves steady-state plasma concentrations similar to adult patients receiving 750 mg TID. There are no data available in the elderly.

Preclinical safety data:

Acute and chronic toxicity: oral acute and chronic toxicity studies were conducted in the mouse (500 mg/kg/day), rat (up to 1,000 mg/kg/day) and monkey (up to 800 mg/kg/day). There were increased liver weights and dose-related thyroid follicular cell hypertrophy in rats. Weight loss and general physical decline was observed in monkeys together with general evidence of gastrointestinal toxicity.

Mutagenicity: in vitro and *in vivo* studies with and without metabolic activation have shown that nelfinavir has no mutagenic or genotoxic activity.

Carcinogenicity: carcinogenicity studies of nelfinavir are not completed.

Pharmaceutical particulars

List of excipients: The Oral Powder contains microcrystalline cellulose, maltodextrin, dibasic potassium phosphate, crospovidone, hydroxypropyl methylcellulose, aspartame (E951), sucrose palmitate, and natural and artificial flavour.

Incompatibilities: Viracept Oral Powder should not be mixed with acidic substances due to taste (see *Posology and method of administration*).

Shelf-life: 12 months

Special precautions for storage: Store in the original container at temperatures between 15–30°C.

Nature and contents of container: Viracept 50 mg/g Oral Powder is provided in plastic bottles containing 144 grams of oral powder with a 1 gram polystyrene scoop.

Instructions for use and handling, and disposal (if appropriate): Not applicable

Number(s) in the community register of medicinal products EU/1/97/054/001

Date of first authorisation/renewal of the authorisation January 1998

Date of revision of the text March 1998

VIRACEPT TABLETS ▼

Qualitative and quantitative composition Viracept 250 mg Tablets contain 292.25 mg of nelfinavir mesylate corresponding to 250 mg of nelfinavir (as free base).

Pharmaceutical form Tablets

Clinical particulars

Therapeutic indications: Viracept is indicated in combination with antiretroviral nucleoside analogues for the treatment of HIV-1 infected patients with advanced or progressive immunodeficiency.

Combinations of Viracept with antiretroviral nucleoside analogues has been shown to decrease plasma viral load and to increase circulating CD4 lymphocyte counts. Clinical studies are underway to evaluate the clinical benefits of combination regimens.

Refer to section 5.1 Pharmacodynamic properties.

Posology and method of administration: Viracept Tablets are administered orally and should be ingested with food.

Patients older than 13 years: the recommended dosage of Viracept Tablets is 750 mg (three 250 mg tablets) three times a day (TID) by mouth.

Patients aged 2 to 13 years: for children, the recommended starting dose is 25–30 mg/kg body weight per dose given TID. For children unable to take tablets, Viracept Oral Powder may be administered (see Summary of Product Characteristics for Viracept Oral Powder).

The recommended dose of Viracept Tablets to be administered TID to children aged 2 to 13 years is as follows:

Body weight kg	*Number of tablets**
18 to < 23	2
≥ 23	3

* see Summary of Product Characteristics for Viracept Oral Powder for patients with less than 18 kg body weight.

Therapy with Viracept should be initiated by a physician experienced in the management of HIV infection.

Renal or hepatic impairment: currently, there are no data specific for these patient populations and therefore specific dosage recommendations cannot be made. Nelfinavir is principally metabolised and eliminated by the liver. Caution should be used when administering Viracept to patients with impaired renal or hepatic function.

Contra-indications: Hypersensitivity to nelfinavir or to any of the excipients.

Viracept is contra-indicated in breastfeeding women.

Viracept should not be administered concurrently with medicinal products with narrow therapeutic windows and which are substrates of CYP3A4. Co-administration may result in competitive inhibition of the metabolism of these medicinal products and create the potential for serious and/or life-threatening adverse events such as cardiac arrhythmias (e.g. terfenadine, astemizole, cisapride, amiodarone, quinidine), prolonged sedation or respiratory depression (e.g. triazolam, midazolam), or other events (e.g. ergot derivatives).

Viracept must not be given with rifampicin. Rifampicin decreases nelfinavir plasma AUC by 82%.

See also *Interaction with other medicinal products and other forms of interaction.*

Special warnings and special precautions for use: Caution should be used when administering Viracept to patients with impaired renal or hepatic function (see *Posology and method of administration*).

The safety and activity of nelfinavir in children below the age of 2 years have not been established.

Caution is advised whenever Viracept is co-administered with medicinal products which are inducers or inhibitors and/or substrates of CYP3A4; such combinations may require dose adjustment (see also *Contra-indications, Interaction with other medicaments and other forms of interaction* and *Undesirable effects*).

New onset diabetes mellitus, hyperglycaemia or exacerbation of existing diabetes mellitus has been reported in patients receiving protease inhibitors. In some of these the hyperglycaemia was severe and in some cases also associated with ketoacidosis. Many patients had confounding medical conditions, some of which required therapy with agents that have been associated with the development of diabetes or hyperglycaemia.

There have been reports of increased bleeding, including spontaneous skin haematomas and haemarthroses, in haemophiliac patients type A and B treated with protease inhibitors. In some patients additional factor VIII was given. In more than half of the reported cases, treatment with protease inhibitors was continued or reintroduced if treatment had been discontinued. A causal relationship has been evoked, although the mechanism of action has not been elucidated. Haemophiliac patients should therefore be made aware of the possibility of increased bleeding.

Patients should be instructed that Viracept is not a cure for HIV infection, that they may continue to develop infections or other illnesses associated with HIV disease, and that Viracept has not been shown to reduce the risk of transmission of HIV disease through sexual contact or blood contamination.

Interaction with other medicinal products and other forms of interaction: Nelfinavir is metabolised in part via the cytochrome P450 3A system (CYP3A). Caution should be used when co-administering medicinal products that induce CYP3A or potentially toxic medicinal products which are themselves metabolised by CYP3A. Based on *in vitro* data, nelfinavir is unlikely to inhibit other cytochrome P450 isoforms at concentrations in the therapeutic range.

Other antiretrovirals: clinically significant interactions have not been observed between nelfinavir and nucleoside analogues (specifically zidovudine plus lamivudine, stavudine, and stavudine plus didanosine). At present, there is no evidence of inadequate efficacy of zidovudine in the CNS that could be associated with the modest reduction in plasma levels of zidovudine when co-administered with Viracept. Since it is recommended that didanosine be administered on an empty stomach, Viracept should be administered (with food) one hour after or more than 2 hours before didanosine.

Ritonavir: administration of a single 750 mg dose of Viracept following 3 doses of ritonavir 500 mg BID resulted in a 152% increase in nelfinavir plasma area under the plasma concentration-time curve (AUC) and a 156% increase in the elimination half-life of nelfinavir. Administration of a single 500 mg dose of ritonavir following six doses of Viracept 750 mg TID resulted in minimal increase (8%) in ritonavir plasma AUC. The safety of this combination has not been established.

Indinavir: administration of a single 750 mg dose of Viracept following indinavir 800 mg every 8 hours for 7 days resulted in an 83% increase in nelfinavir plasma AUC and a 22% increase in the elimination half-life of nelfinavir. Administration of a single 800 mg dose of indinavir following Viracept 750 mg TID for 7 days resulted in a 51% increase in indinavir plasma AUC concentrations, with a 5-fold increase in trough concentrations measured at 8 hours, but no increase in peak concentrations. The safety of this combination has not been established.

Saquinavir soft gelatin capsule: administration of a single 750 mg dose of Viracept following 4 days of saquinavir soft gelatin capsule 1200 mg TID resulted in a 30% increase in nelfinavir plasma AUC. Administration of a single 1200 mg dose of saquinavir soft gelatin capsule following 4 days of Viracept 750 mg TID resulted in a 392% increase in saquinavir plasma AUC.

Metabolic enzyme inducers: rifampicin decreases nelfinavir plasma AUC by 82%. Other potent inducers of CYP3A (e.g. phenobarbital, phenytoin, carbamazepine) may also reduce nelfinavir plasma concentrations. If therapy with such medicinal products is warranted, physicians should consider using alternatives when a patient is taking Viracept.

Co-administration of Viracept and rifabutin results in a 32% decrease in nelfinavir plasma AUC and an approximately 200% increase in rifabutin plasma AUC (see also *Special warnings and special precautions for use*). A dosage reduction of rifabutin to half the standard dose is necessary when Viracept and rifabutin are co-administered.

Metabolic enzyme inhibitors: co-administration of Viracept and a strong inhibitor of CYP3A, ketoconazole, resulted in a 35% increase in nelfinavir plasma AUC. This change is not considered clinically significant and no dose adjustment is needed when ketoconazole and Viracept are co-administered. Based on the metabolic profiles, a clinically relevant drug interaction would not be expected with other specific inhibitors of CYP3A (e.g. fluconazole, itraconazole, clarithromycin, erythromycin); however, the possibility cannot be excluded.

Other potential interactions: Viracept increases terfenadine plasma concentrations; therefore, Viracept should not be administered concurrently with terfenadine because of the potential for serious and/or life-threatening cardiac arrhythmias. Because similar interactions are likely with astemizole and cisapride, Viracept should also not be administered concurrently with these drugs. Although specific studies have not been done, potent sedatives metabolised by CYP3A, such as triazolam or midazolam, should not be co-administered with Viracept due to the potential for prolonged sedation. For other compounds that are substrates for CYP3A (e.g. calcium channel blockers) plasma concentrations may be elevated when co-administered with Viracept; therefore, patients should be monitored for toxicities associated with such medicinal products.

Oral contraceptives: administration of Viracept 750 mg TID and a combination oral contraceptive which included 0.4 mg of norethindrone and 35 μg of 17 α-ethinyl estradiol for 7 days resulted in a 47% decrease in ethinyl estradiol and an 18% decrease in norethindrone plasma AUC. Alternative contraceptive measures should be considered.

Use during pregnancy and lactation: No treatment-related adverse effects were seen in animal reproductive toxicity studies in rats at doses providing systemic exposure comparable to that observed with the clinical dose. Clinical experience in pregnant women is lacking. Until additional data become available, Viracept should be given during pregnancy only after special consideration.

It is recommended that HIV-infected women must not breast feed their infants under any circumstances in order to avoid transmission of HIV. Studies in lactating rats showed that nelfinavir is excreted in breast milk. There is no data available on nelfinavir excretion into human breast milk. Mothers must be instructed to discontinue breastfeeding if they are receiving Viracept.

Effects on ability to drive and use machines: There is no indication that Viracept affects the ability to drive and use machines.

Undesirable effects: The safety of Viracept was studied in controlled clinical trials with over 800 patients, of which more than half received a dose of 750 mg TID either alone or in combination with nucleoside analogues. Over 4000 patients ≥ 13 years in the expanded access programmes received Viracept at a dose of 750 mg TID. The majority of adverse events were of mild intensity. The most frequently reported adverse event among patients receiving Viracept was diarrhoea.

Across the two phase III, double-blind studies adverse experiences of moderate to severe intensity reported by investigators as at least possibly related to Viracept or of unknown relationship in ≥ 2% of patients treated with the 750 mg TID dose of Viracept (n=200) in combination with nucleoside analogues (for 24 weeks) included the following undesirable effects: diarrhoea (25.9%), flatulence (2.5%), nausea (4.5%), and rash (3.0%). Marked clinical laboratory abnormalities (change from grade 0 to grade 3 or 4, or change from grade 1 to grade 4) reported in ≥ 2% of patients treated with 750 mg TID of Viracept (for 24 weeks) across the same studies included increased creatine kinase (3.9%), and decreased neutrophils (4.5%). Marked increases in transaminases occurred in less than 2% of patients receiving Viracept at the recommended dose and were sometimes accompanied by clinical signs and symptoms of acute hepatitis. Some of these patients were known to be chronic carriers of hepatitis B and/or C viruses. With the exception of diarrhoea, there were no significant differences in the adverse experiences reported by patients treated with Viracept versus the control arms containing zidovudine plus lamivudine or stavudine alone.

Overdose: Human experience of acute overdose with Viracept is limited. There is no specific antidote for overdose with Viracept. If indicated, elimination of unabsorbed nelfinavir should be achieved by emesis or gastric lavage. Administration of activated charcoal may also be used to aid removal of unabsorbed nelfinavir. Since nelfinavir is highly protein bound, dialysis is unlikely to significantly remove it from blood.

Pharmacological properties

Pharmacodynamic properties: Pharmacotherapeutic group: antiviral agent, ATC code: J05A E04.

Mechanism of action: HIV protease is an enzyme required for the proteolytic cleavage of the viral polyprotein precursors to the individual proteins found in infectious HIV. The cleavage of these viral polyproteins is essential for the maturation of infectious virus. Nelfinavir reversibly binds to the active site of HIV protease and prevents cleavage of the polyproteins resulting in the formation of immature non-infectious viral particles.

Antiviral activity in vitro: the antiviral activity of nelfinavir *in vitro* has been demonstrated in both HIV acute and chronic infections in lymphoblastoid cell lines, peripheral blood lymphocytes and monocytes/macrophages. Nelfinavir was found to be active against a broad range of laboratory strains and clinical isolates of HIV-1 and the HIV-2 strain ROD. The EC_{95} (95% effective concentration) of nelfinavir ranged from 7 to 111 nM (mean of 58 nM). Nelfinavir demonstrated additive to synergistic effects against HIV in combination with reverse transcriptase inhibitors zidovudine (ZDV), lamivudine (3TC), didanosine (ddI), zalcitabine (ddC) and stavudine (d4T) without enhanced cytotoxicity.

Resistance: HIV isolates with reduced susceptibility to nelfinavir have been selected *in vitro.* Genotypic analysis of a variant which exhibited a nine-fold decrease in sensitivity showed a unique substitution of an aspartic acid (D) to an asparagine (N) in HIV protease at amino acid residue 30 (D30N). Genotypic changes in HIV protease genes obtained from 58 patients enrolled in phase I/II trials were also evaluated. Consistent with the *in vitro* results, the predominant change observed was the D30N substitution. In a subset of these patients followed for up to 44 weeks, this substitution was maintained. Mutations described for other protease inhibitors were either never observed (G48V, V82F/T, I84V) or only rarely (3 of 55 patients) observed (L90M). Sequence analyses were performed on the protease genes derived at 16 weeks from randomly selected patients who received nelfinavir either alone (n=64) or in combination with ZDV and 3TC (n=49) in pivotal trials. The incidence of genotypic resistance to nelfinavir at 16 weeks was significantly reduced when nelfinavir was used in combination with ZDV and 3TC (6%), compared to monotherapy (56%).

Cross-resistance to other antivirals: cross-resistance between nelfinavir and reverse transcriptase inhibitors is unlikely because of the different enzyme targets involved. HIV isolates resistant to nucleoside analogues and non-nucleoside reverse transcriptase inhibitors remain susceptible *in vitro* to nelfinavir. The potential for HIV cross-resistance to other protease inhibitors has been explored with nelfinavir. Six clinical isolates containing the D30N substitution showed no change in sensitivity to saquinavir, ritonavir, indinavir or 141W94 *in vitro.* This lack of cross-resistance was confirmed with an HIV recombinant virus containing the D30N substitution; the recombinant virus exhibited a reduced sensitivity to nelfinavir, yet retained full sensitivity to the other protease inhibitors. In addition, in patients previously treated with ritonavir, indinavir and/or saquinavir five of fourteen clinical isolates with reduced susceptibility to one or more of these protease inhibitors were susceptible to nelfinavir.

Clinical pharmacodynamic data: treatment with nelfinavir alone or in combination with other antiretroviral agents has been documented to reduce viral load and increase CD4 cell counts in HIV-1 seropositive patients. The effects of nelfinavir (alone or combined with other antiretroviral agents) on biological markers of disease activity, CD4 cell count and viral RNA, were evaluated in several studies involving HIV-1 infected patients.

Viracept 750 mg TID in combination with one or more nucleoside analogues was consistently associated with decreases in mean plasma HIV RNA in excess of 1 $\log_{10}$ copies/ml and increases in mean CD4 cell count of 90–100 cells/mm³ which were sustained to at least 24 weeks. Decreases in HIV RNA observed with Viracept monotherapy were less pronounced and of shorter duration.

In a study of 297 HIV-1 seropositive patients receiving zidovudine and lamivudine plus Viracept (2 different doses) or zidovudine and lamivudine alone, the mean decrease in plasma HIV RNA at 24 weeks was 2.15 $\log_{10}$ in patients receiving combination therapy with Viracept 750 mg TID, compared to 1.54 $\log_{10}$ in patients receiving zidovudine and lamivudine alone. At 24 weeks, the percentage of patients whose plasma HIV RNA levels had decreased to below the limit of detection of the assay (<500 copies/ml) were 81% and 18% for the groups treated with Viracept 750 mg TID plus zidovudine and lamivudine or zidovudine and lamivudine, respectively. Mean CD4 cell counts at 24 weeks were increased by 108 and 81 cells/mm³ for the groups treated with Viracept 750 mg TID plus zidovudine and lamivudine or zidovudine and lamivudine, respectively. At 48 weeks, approximately 80% of the patients treated with Viracept 750 mg TID plus zidovudine and lamivudine remained below the level of detection of the assay; CD4 cell counts increased by more than 170 cells/mm³ at 48 weeks in this group.

Pharmacokinetic properties: The pharmacokinetic properties of nelfinavir have been evaluated in healthy volunteers and HIV-infected patients. No substantial differences have been observed between healthy volunteers and HIV-infected patients.

Absorption: after single or multiple oral doses of 500 to 750 mg (two to three 250 mg tablets) with food, peak nelfinavir plasma concentrations were typically achieved in 2 to 4 hours. After multiple dosing with 750 mg every 8 hours for 28 days (steady-state), peak plasma concentrations (C_{max}) averaged 3–4 μg/ml and plasma concentrations prior to the next dose (trough) were 1–3 μg/ml. A greater than dose-proportional increase in nelfinavir plasma concentrations was observed after single doses; however, this was not observed after multiple dosing. The absolute bioavailability has not been determined.

Effect of food on gastrointestinal absorption: maximum plasma concentrations and area under the plasma concentration-time curve were consistently 2 to 3-fold higher under fed conditions compared to fasting. The increased plasma concentrations with food were independent of fat content of the meals.

Distribution: in both animals and humans, the estimated volumes of distribution (2–7 l/kg) exceeded total body water, suggesting extensive penetration of nelfinavir into tissues. Although no studies have been conducted in humans, studies with a single 50 mg/kg dose of ^{14}C-nelfinavir in rats showed that concentrations in the brain were lower than in other tissues, but exceeded the *in vitro* EC_{95} for antiviral activity. Nelfinavir in serum is extensively protein-bound (≥ 98%).

Metabolism: unchanged nelfinavir comprised 82–86% of the total plasma radioactivity after a single oral 750 mg dose of ^{14}C-nelfinavir. One major and several minor oxidative metabolites were found in plasma. The major oxidative metabolite has *in vitro* antiviral activity equal to the parent drug. The plasma levels of this metabolite are approximately 25% of the total plasma nelfinavir-related concentration. *In vitro,* multiple cytochrome P450 isoforms including CYP3A, CYP2C19/C9 and CYP2D6 are responsible for metabolism of nelfinavir.

Elimination: oral clearance estimates after single doses (24–33 l/h) and multiple doses (26–61 l/h) indicate that nelfinavir exhibits medium to high hepatic bioavailability. The terminal half-life in plasma was typically 3.5 to 5 hours. The majority (87%) of an oral 750 mg dose containing ^{14}C-nelfinavir was recovered in the faeces; total faecal radioactivity consisted of nelfinavir (22%) and numerous oxidative metabolites (78%). Only 1–2% of the dose was recovered in urine, of which unchanged nelfinavir was the major component.

Pharmacokinetics in children and the elderly: in children between the ages of 2 and 13 years, the clearance of orally administered nelfinavir is approximately 2 to 3 times higher than in adults, with large intersubject variability. Administration of Viracept Oral Powder or Tablets with food at a dose of approximately 25–30 mg/kg TID achieves steady-state plasma concentrations similar to adult patients receiving 750 mg TID. There are no data available in the elderly.

Preclinical safety data:

Acute and chronic toxicity: oral acute and chronic toxicity studies were conducted in the mouse (500 mg/kg/day), rat (up to 1,000 mg/kg/day) and monkey (up to 800 mg/kg/day). There were increased liver weights and dose-related thyroid follicular cell hypertrophy in rats. Weight loss and general physical decline was observed in monkeys together with general evidence of gastrointestinal toxicity.

Mutagenicity: in vitro and *in vivo* studies with and without metabolic activation have shown that nelfinavir has no mutagenic or genotoxic activity.

Carcinogenicity: carcinogenicity studies of nelfinavir are not completed.

Pharmaceutical particulars

List of excipients: Each tablet contains calcium silicate, crospovidone, magnesium stearate, indigo carmine (E132) as powder and aluminium lake.

Incompatibilities: Not applicable

Shelf life: 18 months

Special precautions for storage: Store in the original container at temperatures between 15–30°C.

Nature and contents of container: Viracept Tablets is provided in plastic bottles containing 180 or 270 tablets.

Instructions for use/handling, and disposal (if appropriate): Not applicable

Number(s) in the community register of medicinal products

EU/1/97/054/002 (180 tablets)

EU/1/97/054/003 (270 tablets)

Date of first authorisation/renewal of the authorisation January 1998

Date of revision of the text March 1998

XENICAL ▼

Qualitative and quantitative composition Each hard capsule contains 120 mg orlistat.

Pharmaceutical form Capsule, hard. It is presented as turquoise cap and turquoise body bearing the imprint of "ROCHE XENICAL 120".

Clinical particulars

Therapeutic indications: XENICAL is indicated in conjunction with a mildly hypocaloric diet for the treatment of obese patients with a body mass index (BMI) greater or equal to 30 kg/m², or overweight patients (BMI ≥ 28 kg/m²) with associated risk factors.

Treatment with orlistat should only be started if diet alone has previously produced a weight loss of at least 2.5 kg over a period of 4 consecutive weeks. Treatment with orlistat should be discontinued after 12 weeks if patients have been unable to lose at least 5% of their body weight as measured at the start of drug therapy.

Posology and method of administration:

Adults: The recommended dose of orlistat is one 120 mg capsule which should be taken immediately before, during or up to one hour after each main meal. If a meal is missed or contains no fat, the dose of orlistat should be omitted.

The patient should be on a nutritionally balanced, mildly hypocaloric diet that contains approximately 30% of calories from fat. It is recommended that the diet should be rich in fruit and vegetables. The daily intake of fat, carbohydrate and protein should be distributed over three main meals.

Doses of orlistat above 120 mg three times daily have not been shown to provide additional benefit.

The effect of orlistat results in an increase in faecal fat as early as 24 to 48 hours after dosing. Upon discontinuation of therapy, faecal fat content usually returns to pre-treatment levels, within 48 to 72 hours.

There are no safety and efficacy data beyond 2 years, therefore the duration of treatment with orlistat should not be longer than 2 years.

Special populations: The effect of orlistat in patients with hepatic and/or renal impairment, children and elderly patients has not been studied. Orlistat is not intended to be used in children.

Contra-indications:

- Chronic malabsorption syndrome.
- Cholestasis.
- Breast-feeding.
- Known hypersensitivity to orlistat or any of the excipients contained in the medicinal product.

Orlistat is not recommended for use during pregnancy.

Special warnings and special precautions for use: In clinical trials, the decrease in bodyweight with orlistat treatment was less in type II diabetic patients than in non-diabetic patients. Antidiabetic drug treatment may have to be closely monitored when taking orlistat.

Treatment with orlistat may potentially impair the absorption of fat-soluble vitamins (ADEK).

The vast majority of patients receiving up to two full years of treatment with orlistat in clinical studies had vitamin A, D, E and K and beta-carotene levels that stayed within normal range. In order to ensure adequate nutrition, patients on a weight control diet should be advised to have a diet rich in fruit and vegetables and use of a multivitamin supplement could be considered. If a multivitamin supplement is recommended, it should be taken at least two hours after the administration of orlistat or at bedtime.

Patients should be advised to adhere to the dietary recommendations they are given (see *Posology and method of administration*). The possibility of experiencing gastrointestinal events (see *Undesirable effects*) may increase when orlistat is taken with a diet high in fat (e.g. in a 2000 kcal/day diet, >30% of calories from fat equates to > 67 g of fat). The daily intake of fat should be distributed over three main meals. If orlistat is taken with a meal very high in fat, the possibility of gastrointestinal adverse effects may increase.

Interaction with other medicinal products and other forms of interaction: In the absence of pharmacokinetic interaction studies, the concomitant administration of orlistat with fibrates, acarbose, biguanides or anorectic drugs is not recommended. When warfarin or other anticoagulants are given in combination with orlistat (high dose and long term treatment), international normalised ratio (INR) values should be monitored.

No interactions with digoxin, phenytoin, oral contraceptives, nifedipine GTS, nifedipine slow release, or alcohol have been observed.

+ *Pravastatin:* If orlistat is administered to patients

taking pravastatin, there is an increased risk of (dose-related) pravastatin adverse events, including rhabdomyolysis, due to an increase in pravastatin plasma concentrations. Dose adjustment of pravastatin may be required.

+ *Vitamins and beta-carotene:* Decreases in the absorption of vitamin D, E and beta-carotene should be taken into account (see *Special warnings and special precautions for use*).

Use during pregnancy and lactation: In animal reproductive studies, no teratogenic effect was observed. In the absence of a teratogenic effect in animals, no malformative effect is expected in man. To date, drugs responsible for malformations in man have been found teratogenic in animals when well-conducted studies were performed in two species.

At present, insufficient data are available in pregnant women taking orlistat to enable an evaluation of the potential for orlistat to cause foetal malformations or foetal toxicity. The use of orlistat during pregnancy is therefore not recommended.

As it is not known whether orlistat is secreted into human milk, orlistat is contra-indicated during breast-feeding.

Effects on ability to drive and use machines: No effects on the patient's ability to drive and use machines have been reported.

Undesirable effects: Adverse reactions to orlistat are largely gastrointestinal in nature. During the first year of treatment, commonly observed events were oily spotting from the rectum (27% of patients), flatus with discharge (24% of patients), faecal urgency (22% of patients), fatty/oily stool (20% of patients), oily evacuation (12% of patients), increased defecation (11% of patients) and faecal incontinence (8% of patients). The incidence of adverse events decreased with prolonged use of orlistat.

Other treatment-emergent adverse events that occurred at a frequency of > 2% and with an incidence ≥ 1% above placebo were:

Gastrointestinal system: abdominal pain/discomfort, flatulence, liquid stools, soft stools, rectal pain/discomfort, tooth disorder, gingival disorder.

Respiratory system: upper respiratory infection, lower respiratory infection.

Resistance mechanism: influenza.

Central nervous system: headache.

Reproductive disorders: menstrual irregularity.

Psychiatric disorders: anxiety.

Body as a whole: fatigue.

Urinary system disorders: urinary tract infection.

Overdose: Overdose of orlistat has not been reported. Single doses of 800 mg of orlistat and multiple doses of up to 400 mg tid for 15 days have been studied in normal weight and obese subjects without significant adverse findings. In addition, doses of 240 mg tid have been administered to obese patients for 6 months.

Should a significant overdose of orlistat occur, it is recommended that the patient be observed for 24 hours. Based on human and animal studies, any systemic effects attributable to the lipase-inhibiting properties of orlistat should be rapidly reversible.

Pharmacological properties

Pharmacodynamic properties: Pharmaco-therapeutic group: Anti obesity agent, ATC code A08A B01.

Orlistat is a potent, specific and long-acting inhibitor of gastrointestinal lipases. It exerts its therapeutic activity in the lumen of the stomach and small intestine by forming a covalent bond with the active serine site of the gastric and pancreatic lipases. The inactivated enzyme is thus unavailable to hydrolyse dietary fat, in the form of triglycerides, into absorbable free fatty acids and monoglycerides.

Pooled data from five 2 year studies showed that, after one year of treatment associated with a hypocaloric diet, the percentage of patients taking 120 mg orlistat who lost 10% or more of their body weight was 20% with orlistat 120 mg compared to 8% of patients taking placebo. The mean difference in weight loss with the drug compared to placebo was–3.2 kg. In type II diabetic patients the percentage of responders (≥ 10% of bodyweight loss) was 9% with orlistat as compared to 4% with placebo. The mean difference in weight loss with the drug compared to placebo was–2.1 kg in these patients.

Pharmacokinetic properties:

Absorption: Studies in normal weight and obese volunteers have shown that the extent of absorption of orlistat was minimal. Plasma concentrations of intact orlistat were non-measurable (< 5 ng/ml) eight hours following oral administration of orlistat.

In general, at therapeutic doses, detection of intact orlistat in plasma was sporadic and concentrations were extremely low (< 10 ng/ml or 0.02 μmol), with no evidence of accumulation, which is consistent with minimal absorption.

Distribution: The volume of distribution cannot be determined because the drug is minimally absorbed and has no defined systemic pharmacokinetics. In vitro orlistat is > 99% bound to plasma proteins (lipoproteins and albumin were the major binding proteins). Orlistat minimally partitions into erythrocytes.

Metabolism: Based on animal data, it is likely that the metabolism of orlistat occurs mainly within the gastrointestinal wall. Based on a study in obese patients, of the minimal fraction of the dose that was absorbed systemically, two major metabolites, M1 (4-member lactone ring hydrolysed) and M3 (M1 with N-formyl leucine moiety cleaved), accounted for approximately 42% of the total plasma concentration.

M1 and M3 have an open beta-lactone ring and extremely weak lipase inhibitory activity (1000 and 2500 fold less than orlistat respectively). In view of this low inhibitory activity and the low plasma levels at therapeutic doses (average of 26 ng/ml and 108 ng/ml respectively), these metabolites are considered to be pharmacologically inconsequential.

Elimination: Studies in normal weight and obese subjects have shown that faecal excretion of the unabsorbed drug was the major route of elimination. Approximately 97% of the administered dose was excreted in faeces and 83% of that as unchanged orlistat.

The cumulative renal excretion of total orlistat-related materials was < 2% of the given dose. The time to reach complete excretion (faecal plus urinary) was 3 to 5 days. The disposition of orlistat appeared to be similar between normal weight and obese volunteers. Orlistat, M1 and M3 are all subject to biliary excretion.

Preclinical safety data: Preclinical data reveal no special hazard for humans based on conventional studies of safety pharmacology, repeated dose toxicity, genotoxicity, carcinogenic potential and reproductive toxicology.

Pharmaceutical particulars

List of excipients:

Capsule filling: Microcrystalline cellulose, sodium starch glycollate, povidone, sodium lauryl sulphate and talc.

Capsule shell: Gelatine, indigo carmine (E132), titanium dioxide (E171) and edible printing ink.

Incompatibilities: Not applicable.

Shelf life: 3 years.

Special precautions for storage: Store below 25°C and keep in a dry place.

Nature and contents of container: PVC/PE/PVDC blisters containing 21 and 84 hard capsules.

Instructions for use and handling, and disposal (if appropriate): Not applicable.

Number(s) in the community register of medicinal products

EU/1/98/071/001–Xenical 120 mg, 21 capsule blister pack

EU/1/98/071/003–Xenical 120 mg, 84 capsule blister pack

Date of first authorisation/renewal of authorisation
August 1998

Date of (partial) revision of the text Not applicable

**Trade Mark*

Rybar Laboratories Limited
East Anton
Andover
Hampshire SP10 5RG

☎ 01264 333455   01264 333460

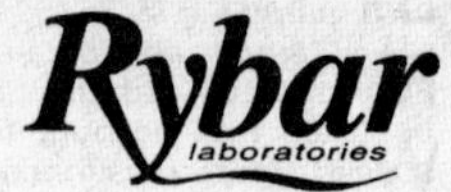

GUAREM* GRANULES

Presentation Sachets, each containing guar gum granules 5 g. The fine pale cream granules, which are tasteless, are readily water-miscible, for the preparation of palatable fluid drinks.

Uses (i) For use in diabetes to help control post-prandial glucose levels, thereby facilitating control, and where appropriate, allowing reduction of insulin or oral hypoglycaemic dosage levels.

(ii) For the relief of the symptoms of the 'dumping syndrome'.

Action: Guar gum is a gel-forming type of carbohydrate which resists digestion and absorption by the human alimentary tract; it contains a high percentage (more than 66%) of a high molecular weight hydrocolloid polysaccharide, a galactomannan composed of galactan and mannan units combined through glycoside linkages.

When added to glucose test meals it reduces post-prandial glycaemia in healthy volunteers and in diabetic patients. Two mechanisms were suggested to account for these effects–that the guar may delay gastric emptying time and so slow the rate of absorption; alternatively, or in addition, the guar may delay the process of absorption within the small intestine.

A study of paracetamol absorption in humans suggests that the effects of guar could simply be due to alterations in the rate of gastric emptying. However, a study of the influence of guar on glucose transport in vitro, using everted sacs prepared from excised rat jejunum suggest that the action of guar is to inhibit glucose transport, and that this effect is probably due to an increase in the thickness of the unstirred solvent layer at the mucosal surface brought about by the higher viscosity of media containing gel-forming polysaccharide gums.

Dosage and administration
Adults including elderly: One 5 g sachet to be taken three times daily with each main meal. The contents of a sachet may be simply sprinkled evenly onto or into food ready for eating and must be accompanied by a drink of 200 ml. Alternatively, the contents can be stirred into 200 ml of a suitable fruit flavoured drink and swallowed promptly.

Guarem should not be ingested as dry granules.

Children (12 and over): As for adults.

Children (under 12): Not recommended.

Contra-indications, warnings, etc
Contra-indications: To avoid the risk of oesophageal obstruction or rupture this product should not be given to patients with a history of oesophageal disease or of difficulty in swallowing.

Precautions: This product should not be ingested as dry granules. It if is taken stirred into food at least a glass of water or other liquid should be drunk. The product can be taken by stirring it into water, juice or milk. During initial therapy, blood glucose levels should be carefully monitored, and concurrent treatment adjusted where necessary, to minimise the danger of hypoglycaemia.

In patients with dumping syndrome, while Guarem may be expected to reduce malabsorption, usual monitoring of nutritional status should be continued.

Interactions: When given simultaneously with Guarem, the absorption of other drugs may be slowed; however the total amounts absorbed and excreted do not appear to be significantly affected. A study with digoxin concluded that long term administration of guar gum will not interfere with adequate digitalisation. When it is important to establish maximum serum levels (e.g. penicillin) administration should precede Guarem by one hour.

Side-effects: Gastro-intestinal disturbances such as flatulence, abdominal pain and diarrhoea are quite common particularly at the commencement of treatment. These side-effects are rarely severe enough to warrant discontinuation of treatment though that may be necessary in some patients.

Use in pregnancy and lactation: There is no experience of the use of this product during pregnancy or lactation.

Overdose: There is no experience of overdosage with this product. From the nature of the product, a feeling of bloating and indigestion may be possible.

Pharmaceutical precautions Store in a cool dry place.

Legal category P

Package quantities Cartons of 50 and 100 sachets.

Further information Each sachet is individually printed with simple and clear administration instructions. The best way to take the product is to stir it into water, juice or milk. If taken in some other way (for example stirred into food) at least a glass of water or other liquid should be drunk.

Product licence number 0237/0023.

**Trade Mark*

Sankyo Pharma UK Limited

Sankyo House
Repton Place
White Lion Road
Little Chalfont
Amersham, Bucks HP7 9LP

☎ 01494 766866   🗋 01494 766557

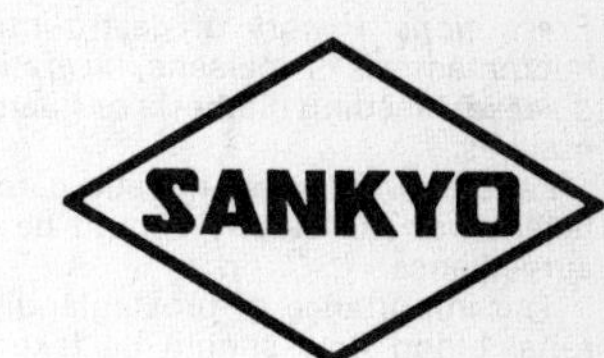

ANACAL* SUPPOSITORIES
ANACAL* RECTAL OINTMENT

Qualitative and quantitative composition
Anacal Suppositories: Each 2 g suppository contains:
Mucopolysaccharide polysulphuric acid ester (Heparinoid) 4.0 mg
Oxypolyethoxydodecane (Lauromacrogol-400) 50.0 mg
Anacal Rectal Ointment:
Mucopolysaccharide polysulphuric acid ester (Heparinoid) 0.2% w/w
Oxypolyethoxydodecane (Lauromacrogol-400) 5.0% w/w.

Pharmaceutical form Suppository/rectal ointment.

Clinical particulars
Therapeutic indications: Anacal Suppositories and Anacal Rectal Ointment are indicated for the treatment of the following conditions: Relief of symptoms associated with haemorrhoids (including perianal haematomas), perianal eczema, pruritus, anal fissure, proctitis, and aftercare of haemorrhoids treated by surgery or injection.

Posology and method of administration
Adults and the elderly: Anacal suppositories: Insert one suppository once or twice daily. *Anacal Rectal Ointment:* To be applied up to four times daily.
Children: Not recommended.

Contra-indications: Anacal Suppositories and Anacal Rectal Ointment are contra-indicated in patients with hypersensitivity to one of the ingredients. Not recommended for use in children.

Special warnings and special precautions for use: Not to be taken orally. If symptoms persist or worsen, seek medical advice.

Interactions with other medicaments and other forms of interaction: None known.

Pregnancy and lactation: There is no evidence to suggest that Anacal Suppositories or Anacal Rectal Ointment should not be used during pregnancy and lactation.

Effects on ability to drive and use machines: None.

Undesirable effects: None known.

Overdose: In the absence of any reports of the accidental ingestion of Anacal, no specific advice is available. General supportive measures may be appropriate.

Pharmacological properties
Pharmacodynamic properties: Mucopolysaccharide polysulphate ester is recognised as having: a weak inhibitory effect on PGE_2 synthesis and an indirect effect on LTB_4 production (based on *in vitro* studies), anti-coagulant activity (as a heparinoid), thrombolytic activity (through potentiation of urokinase activity), anti-exudatory activity (through inhibition of hyaluronidase). Oxypolyethoxydodecane has both topical anaesthetic and anti-pruritic properties.

Pharmacokinetic properties: Radiochemical studies of absorption following *cutaneous* application of mucopolysaccharide polysulphate have shown that between 0.3 and 4% of the mucopolysaccharide administered is absorbed by various tissues (other than the treated area) within the first 8 hours. Typically between 1.7% and 4.6% will be absorbed within 2 to 4 days. Animal studies have also shown that mucopolysaccharide is bound intracellularly within the subcutis. Peak serum concentrations following *cutaneous* application are below the threshold of physiological relevance for coagulation. Mucopolysaccharide is excreted in the urine partly unchanged and partly as depolymerized, shorter chain length molecules.

Pharmaceutical particulars
List of excipients: Anacal Suppositories: Hard Fat.
Anacal Rectal Ointment: Polyethylene highpolymer 1500, Liquid paraffin, Sorbitan monostearate, Methylhydroxybenzoate (E218).

Incompatibilities: None.

Shelf life: 3 years.

Special precautions for storage: Store below 25°C.

Nature and contents of container:
Anacal Suppositories: Aluminium foil strips of 10 suppositories.
Anacal Rectal Ointment: Aluminium tubes of 30 g.

Marketing authorisation numbers
Anacal Suppositories 8265/0005.
Anacal Rectal Ointment 8265/0004.

Date of approval/revision of SPC October 1994.

Legal category P.

HIRUDOID* CREAM
HIRUDOID* GEL

Qualitative and quantitative composition Heparinoid 0.3% w/w (Equivalent to 25 000 Units per 100 g cream or gel).

Pharmaceutical form Topical cream or gel.

Clinical particulars
Therapeutic indications: Hirudoid is indicated for the treatment of superficial thrombophlebitis and the soothing relief of superficial bruising and haematoma.

Posology and method of administration
Adults, the elderly and children over 5 years of age: Hirudoid Cream: Two to six inches (5–15 cm) to be applied up to four times daily to the affected area and gently massaged into the skin. *Hirudoid Gel:* Two to six inches (5–15 cm) to be applied, as a thin layer, up to four times a day to the affected area. Recommended when its cooling effect and rapid action are required.

Contra-indications: Not to be used on large areas of skin, broken skin, sensitive areas of skin or mucous membranes. Not to be used in individuals with a known sensitivity to any active or inactive component of the formulation. Not to be used in childen under 5 years of age.

Special warnings and special precautions for use: For external use only. If symptoms persist or worsen, seek medical advice. Do not exceed the stated dose.

Interactions with other medicaments and other forms of interaction: None known.

Pregnancy and lactation: There is no evidence to suggest that Hirudoid should not be used during pregnancy and lactation.

Effects on ability to drive and use machines: None.

Undesirable effects: None known.

Overdose: In the absence of any reports of the accidental ingestion of Hirudoid, no specific advice is available. General supportive measures may be appropriate.

Pharmacological properties
Pharmacodynamic properties: Heparinoid is recognised as having: a weak inhibitory effect on PGE_2 synthesis and an indirect effect on LTB_4 production (based on *in vitro* studies), anti-coagulant activity (as a heparinoid), thrombolytic activity (through potentiation of urokinase activity), anti-exudatory activity (through inhibition of hyaluronidase).

Pharmacokinetic properties: Radiochemical studies of absorption following cutaneous application of heparinoid (mucopolysaccharide polysulphate) have shown that between 0.3 and 4% of the mucopolysaccharide administered is absorbed by various tissues (other than the treated area) within the first 8 hours. Typically between 1.7% and 4.6% will be absorbed within 2 to 4 days. Animal studies have also shown that mucopolysaccharide is bound intracellularly within the subcutis. Peak serum concentrations following cutaneous application are below the threshold of physiological relevance for coagulation. Mucopolysaccharide is excreted in the urine partly unchanged and partly as depolymerized, shorter chain length molecules.

Pharmaceutical particulars
List of excipients: Hirudoid Cream: Anhydrous eucerine, emulsifying cetostearyl alcohol type A, glycerol, isopropyl alcohol, methyl parahydroxybenzoate (E218), myristyl alcohol, potassium hydroxide, propyl parahydroxybenzoate (E216), purified water, stearic acid, thymol.
Hirudoid Gel: Isopropyl alcohol, perfume oil No 8185, polyacrylic acid, propylene glycol, purified water, sodium hydroxide.

Incompatibilities: None.

Shelf life: 5 years.

Special precautions for storage: Store below 25°C.

Nature and contents of container: Aluminium tubes of 50 g.

Instructions for use/handling: Not applicable.

Marketing authorisation numbers
Hirudoid Cream 8265/0006
Hirudoid Gel 8265/0007.

Date of approval/revision of SPC March 1995.

Legal category P.

MOTIFENE* 75 mg

Presentation Size 2, hard gelatin capsules with a light-blue opaque cap and a colourless, transparent body, marked in white print 'D75M', containing white to cream coloured, round lacquered enteric-coated and sustained-release pellets. Each capsule contains 75 mg of diclofenac sodium; 25 mg as enteric-coated pellets and 50 mg as sustained-release pellets.

Uses
Mode of action: Motifene is a non-steroidal agent with marked analgesic/anti-inflammatory properties. It is an inhibitor of prostaglandin synthetase (cyclo-oxygenase).

Pharmacokinetics: Diclofenac sodium is rapidly absorbed from the gut and is subject to first-pass metabolism. Therapeutic plasma concentrations occur about 1/2 hour after administration of Motifene. The active substance is 99.7% protein bound and the plasma half-life for the terminal elimination phase is 1–2 hours. Approximately 60% of the administered dose is excreted via the kidneys in the form of metabolites and less than 1% in unchanged form. The remainder of the dose is excreted via the bile in metabolised form.

Following rapid gastric passage, the enteric-coated pellet component of Motifene ensures quick availability of the active component in the blood stream. The sustained-release pellets cause a delayed release of the active component, which means one single daily dose is usually sufficient.

Indications: Adults: Rheumatoid arthritis; osteoarthrosis; low back pain; acute musculo-skeletal disorders and trauma such as periarthritis (especially frozen shoulder), tendinitis, tenosynovitis, bursitis, sprains, strains and dislocations; relief of pain in fractures; ankylosing spondylitis; acute gout; control of pain and inflammation in orthopaedic, dental and other minor surgery.

Dosage and administration For oral administration only. The capsules should be swallowed whole with a liberal quantity of liquid.

Adults: One capsule daily. Dose may be increased to two capsules daily if necessary. The first dose should be taken in the morning before breakfast and the second if required 8–12 hours later.

Children: Not for use in children.

Elderly: The pharmacokinetics of Motifene are not impaired to any clinically relevant extent in elderly patients and the standard adult dose may be used. Non-steroidal anti-inflammatory drugs should be used with particular caution in older patients who are generally more prone to adverse reactions.

Contra-indications, warnings, etc
Contra-indications: Active or suspected peptic ulcer or gastro-intestinal bleeding. Previous sensitivity to

Motifene. Patients in whom attacks of asthma, urticaria or acute rhinitis are precipitated by aspirin or other non-steroidal anti-inflammatory agents.

Precautions: History of gastro-intestinal ulceration, haematemesis or melaena, ulcerative colitis, Crohn's disease, bleeding diathesis or haematological abnormalities.

Patients with severe hepatic, cardiac or renal insufficiency or the elderly should be kept under close surveillance.

The importance of prostaglandins in maintaining renal blood flow should be taken into account in patients with impaired cardiac or renal function, those being treated with diuretics or recovering from major surgery.

Patients who experience dizziness or other central nervous system disturbances while taking NSAIDs should refrain from driving or operating machinery.

All patients who are receiving long-term treatment with non-steroidal anti-inflammatory agents should be monitored as a precautionary measure (e.g. renal, hepatic function and blood counts).

Motifene, in common with other NSAIDs, can reversibly inhibit platelet aggregation.

Pregnancy and lactation: Although animal studies have not demonstrated teratogenic effects, Motifene should not be prescribed during pregnancy, unless there are compelling reasons for doing so. If employed, the lowest effective dosage should be used.

Use of prostaglandin synthetase inhibitors may result in premature closure of the ductus arteriosus or uterine inertia. Such drugs are therefore not recommended during the last trimester of pregnancy.

Following oral doses of 50 mg every 8 hours, traces of active substance have been detected in breast milk.

Interactions: Motifene may increase plasma concentrations of lithium and digoxin.

Pharmacodynamic studies have shown no potentiation of oral hypoglycaemic and anticoagulant drugs, but caution and adequate monitoring are nevertheless advised (see statement on platelet aggregation in 'Precautions').

Caution should be exercised if NSAIDs and methotrexate are administered within 24 hours of each other, since NSAIDs may increase methotrexate plasma levels, resulting in increased toxicity.

Concomitant therapy with other systemic NSAIDs may increase the frequency of side-effects.

Various NSAIDs are liable to inhibit the activity of diuretics. Concomitant treatment with potassium-sparing diuretics may be associated with increased serum potassium levels, hence serum potassium should be monitored.

Cyclosporin: Cases of nephrotoxicity have been reported in patients receiving concomitant cyclosporin and NSAIDs including diclofenac. This might be mediated through combined renal antiprostaglandin effects of both the NSAID and cyclosporin.

Side-effects: If serious side-effects occur, Motifene should be withdrawn.

Gastro-intestinal tract: Occasional: epigastric pain, other gastro-intestinal disorders (e.g. nausea, vomiting, diarrhoea). *Rare:* gastro-intestinal bleeding, peptic ulcer. *In isolated cases:* peptic ulcer with perforation, lower gut disorders (e.g. non-specific haemorrhagic colitis and exacerbations of ulcerative colitis).

Central nervous system: Occasional: headache, dizziness or vertigo. *Rare:* drowsiness, tiredness. *In isolated cases:* paraesthesia, memory disturbance, disorientation, disturbances of vision (blurred vision, diplopia), impaired hearing, tinnitus, insomnia, irritability, convulsions, depression, anxiety, nightmares, tremor, psychotic reactions.

Skin: Occasional: rashes or skin eruption. *Rare:* urticaria. *In isolated cases:* bullous eruptions, eczema, erythema multiforme, Stevens-Johnson syndrome, Lyell's syndrome, loss of hair, photosensitivity reactions.

Kidney: In isolated cases: acute renal insufficiency, urinary abnormalities (e.g. haematuria), interstitial nephritis, nephrotic syndrome.

Liver: Rare: Liver function disorders including hepatitis (in isolated cases fulminant) with or without jaundice.

Blood: In isolated cases: thrombocytopenia, leucopenia, agranulocytosis, haemolytic anaemia, aplastic anaemia.

Other organ systems: Rare: oedema, hypersensitivity reactions (e.g. bronchospasm, anaphylactic/anaphylactoid systemic reactions including hypotension).

Overdosage: Management of acute poisoning with NSAIDs essentially consists of supportive and symptomatic measures. There is no typical clinical picture resulting from Motifene overdosage. Absorption should be prevented as soon as possible after overdosage by means of gastric lavage and treatment with activated charcoal. Supportive and symptomatic treatment should be given for complications such as hypotension, renal failure, convulsions, gastro-intestinal irritation, and respiratory depression. Specific therapies such as forced diureses, dialysis or haemoperfusion are probably of no help in eliminating NSAIDs due to their high rate of protein binding and extensive metabolism.

Pharmaceutical precautions Store below 25°C.

Legal category POM.

Package quantities 56 capsules.

Further information Nil.

Product licence number 8265/0003.

Date of approval/revision of SPC July 1994.

MOVELAT* CREAM
MOVELAT* GEL

Qualitative and quantitative composition

Mucopolysaccharide polysulphate (MPS)	0.2% w/w
Salicylic acid	2.0% w/w

Pharmaceutical form Topical cream or gel.

Clinical particulars

Therapeutic indications: Movelat is a mild to moderate anti-inflammatory and analgesic topical preparation for the symptomatic relief of muscular pain and stiffness, sprains and strains and pain due to rheumatic and non-serious arthritic conditions.

Posology and method of administration

Adults, the elderly and children over 12 years of age: *Movelat Cream:* Two to six inches (5–15 cm) to be massaged into the affected area up to four times a day.

Movelat Gel: Two to six inches (5–15 cm) to be applied to the affected area up to four times a day. Children under 12 years of age: Not recommended.

Contra-indications: Not to be used on large areas of skin, broken or sensitive skin or on mucous membranes. Not to be used on children under 12 years of age. Not to be used in individuals with a known sensitivity to any active or inactive component of the formulation. Not to be used in susceptible asthmatic patients in whom salicylates can induce allergic bronchial reactions.

Special warnings and special precautions for use: For external use only. The stated dose should not be exceeded. If the condition persists or worsens, consult a doctor. Although systemic absorption of topical salicylate is much less than for oral dosage forms, the side-effects of salicylates are theoretically possible.

Interactions with other medicaments and other forms of interaction: None known.

Pregnancy and lactation: Do not use during the first trimester or during late pregnancy.

Effects on ability to drive and use machines: None.

Undesirable effects: Allergic skin reactions may occur in individuals sensitive to salicylates.

Overdose: Following accidental ingestion of Movelat, individuals may present with the symptoms of salicylate poisoning (hyperventilation, tinnitus, deafness, vasodilation, sweating). The stomach should be emptied and plasma salicylate, plasma pH and electrolytes should be monitored. Forced alkaline diuresis may be required if the plasma salicylate levels are in excess of 500 mg/litre (3.6 mmol/litre) in adults or 300 mg/litre (2.2 mmol/litre) in children.

Pharmacological properties

Pharmacodynamic properties: Mucopolysaccharide polysulphate ester is recognised as having: a weak inhibitory effect on PGE_2 synthesis and an indirect effect on LTB production (based on *in vitro* studies), anti-coagulant activity (as a heparinoid), thrombolytic activity (through potentiation of urokinase activity), anti-exudatory activity (through inhibition of hyaluronidase). Salicylic acid is employed in the formulation of Movelat for its keratolytic activity.

Pharmacokinetic properties: Radiochemical studies of absorption following cutaneous application of mucopolysaccharide polysulphate have shown that between 0.3 and 4% of the mucopolysaccharide administered is absorbed by various tissues (other than the treated area) within the first 8 hours. Typically between 1.7% and 4.6% will be absorbed within 2 to 4 days. Animal studies have also shown that mucopolysaccharide is bound intracellularly within the subcutis. Peak serum concentrations following cutaneous application are below the threshold of physiological relevance for coagulation.

Mucopolysaccharide is excreted in the urine partly unchanged and partly as depolymerized, shorter chain length molecules. The plasma level of salicylic acid following cutaneous application of Movelat has been shown to remain constant at approximately 0.2 µg/ml even after repeated dosing. The total excretion of salicylate reaches a constant figure of approximately 12 mg/day. Over a seven day period, approximately 6.9% of the administered dose is excreted renally, primarily as salicyluric acid.

Pharmaceutical particulars

List of excipients: Movelat Cream Glycerol Stearic acid, Anhydrous eucerine, Myristyl alcohol, Emulsifying cetostearyl alcohol, Ethanolamine, Thymol, Isopropyl alcohol, Purified water.

Movelat Gel: Isopropyl alcohol, Carbomer, Disodium edetate, Polyethylene glyceryl mono-oleate, Rosemary oil, Purified water.

Incompatibilities: None.

Shelf life: 5 years.

Special precautions for storage: Store below 25°C.

Nature and contents of container: Aluminium tubes of 100 g.

Instructions for use/handling: Not applicable.

Product licence numbers

Movelat Cream	8265/0008.
Movelat Gel	8265/0009.

Date of approval/revision of SPC March 1996.

Legal category P.

**Trade Mark*

Sanofi Winthrop Limited
One Onslow Street
Guildford
Surrey GU1 4YS
☎ 01483 505515 📠 01483 535432

sanofi

AT10*

Presentation A clear, deep straw-coloured, oily solution with a faint nut-like odour containing 250 micrograms/ml Dihydrotachysterol BP.

Uses AT10 is recommended for use in the acute, chronic and latent forms of hypocalcaemic tetany due to hypoparathyroidism where its action is to increase the rate of absorption and utilisation of calcium.

Dosage and administration AT10 is for oral administration only.

Adults including the elderly: In acute cases 3–5 ml may be given on each of the first three days of treatment, followed two or three days later by blood and urinary calcium estimations. The maintenance dose of AT10 is usually in the range of 1–7 ml each week, but the precise amount depends on the results of serum and urinary calcium determinations.

In chronic cases an initial dose of 2 ml of AT10 daily, or on alternate days, may be sufficient to maintain normocalcaemia in moderate cases. The dose of AT10 usually has to be increased during menstruation and periods of unusual activity.

Children: No specific dosage recommendations.

Contra-indications, warnings, etc AT10 is contra-indicated in patients with a hypersensitivity to dihydrotachysterol, patients with hypercalcaemia or hypervitaminosis D and patients with an allergy to nuts (including peanuts). As with calciferol, uncontrolled, prolonged administration of AT10 can result in hypercalcaemia which may lead to nephrocalcinosis. Therefore accurate blood calcium determinations must be made at the beginning of treatment and then periodically until the required maintenance dose has been established. The serum calcium level should subsequently be kept between 2.25–2.5 mmol/litre. Serum phosphate, magnesium and alkaline phosphatase should also be measured periodically to monitor progress. If nausea and vomiting are present, serum calcium levels should be checked.

The Sulkowitch test (for urinary calcium) is a convenient supplement to blood calcium determinations, but it should not be regarded as a substitute, because in hypoparathyroid patients treated with AT10, hypercalcuria can occur in the presence of hypocalcaemia.

Certain individuals, particularly those suffering from sarcoidosis, are very sensitive to the effects of vitamin D and it is advisable to consult a physician in cases of doubt.

Use in pregnancy and lactation: The safety of AT10 in pregnancy is not established. Since there is some evidence that use during pregnancy could lead to foetal damage and hypercalcaemia in the newborn, treatment with AT10 is only justified if potential benefits outweigh possible risks.

Dihydrotachysterol is excreted in breast milk and may cause hypercalcaemia in the suckling infant. AT10 is contra-indicated in breast feeding mothers.

Interactions: Several classes of medicine interact with vitamin D analogues calling for adjustment in the dosage of AT10. Thyroid replacement therapy may increase clearance of dihydrotachysterol; cholestyramine may impair its absorption; thiazide diuretics may enhance the calcaemic response leading to hypercalcaemia; barbiturates, anticonvulsants, rifampicin and isoniazid may reduce the effectiveness of AT10. Hypercalcaemia induced by excessive dosaging of AT10 may enhance the toxic effects of cardiac glycosides.

Side-effects: Side-effects are most likely to be due to overdosage leading to hypercalcaemia, the first signs of which are loss of appetite, listlessness and nausea. More severe manifestations include vomiting, urgency of micturition, polyuria, dehydration, thirst, vertigo, stupor, headache, abdominal cramps and paralysis. The calcium and phosphorus concentrations of serum and urine are increased. With chronic overdosage, calcium may be deposited in many tissues including arteries and the kidneys, leading to hypertension and renal failure. Plasma cholesterol may also be increased.

Overdosage: The symptoms of hypercalcaemia in chronic overdosage will usually respond to withdrawal of medication, bed rest, liberal fluid intake, and the use of laxatives.

In acute overdosage, consideration should be given to recovery of AT10 by emesis or gastric lavage if ingestion is recent. Serum calcium estimations should be helpful in determining management.

In massive overdosage of vitamin D, corticosteroids have been found useful and also neutral phosphate in resistant cases. Several months management may be needed in such cases.

Pharmaceutical precautions Store in well-closed containers protected from heat and light.

Legal category P.

Package quantities AT10 is supplied in bottles containing 15 ml with a 1 ml dropper.

Further information The hypercalcaemic action of AT10 is slower in onset and more prolonged than that of parathyroid hormone, but faster in onset and less persistent in action than calciferol. In patients who have become resistant to large doses of calciferol it may be possible to control blood calcium levels with AT10.

Product licence number 11723/0004.

ADENOCOR*

Qualitative and quantitative composition Adenosine 3 mg/ml.

Pharmaceutical form Injection.

Clinical particulars

Therapeutic indications: Rapid conversion to a normal sinus rhythm of paroxysmal supraventricular tachycardias, including those associated with accessory by-pass tracts (Wolff-Parkinson-White Syndrome).

Diagnostic indications: Aid to diagnosis of broad or narrow complex supraventricular tachycardias. Although Adenocor will not convert atrial flutter, atrial fibrillation or ventricular tachycardia to sinus rhythm, the slowing of AV condition helps diagnosis of atrial activity.

Sensitisation of intra-cavitary electrophysiological investigations.

Posology and method of administration: Adenocor is intended for hospital use only. It should be administered by rapid IV bolus injection according to the ascending dosage schedule below. To be certain the solution reaches the systemic circulation administer either directly into a vein or into an IV line. If given into an IV line it should be injected as proximally as possible, and followed by a rapid saline flush.

Adenocor should only be used when facilities exist for cardiac monitoring. Patients who develop high-level AV block at a particular dose should not be given further dosage increments.

Therapeutic dose
Adult:

Initial dose: 3 mg given as a rapid intravenous bolus (over 2 seconds).

Second dose: If the first dose does not result in elimination of the supraventricular tachycardia within 1 to 2 minutes, 6 mg should be given also as a rapid intravenous bolus.

Third dose: If the second dose does not result in elimination of the supraventricular tachycardia within 1 to 2 minutes, 12 mg should be given also as a rapid intravenous bolus.

Additional or higher doses are not recommended.

Children: No controlled paediatric study has been undertaken. Published uncontrolled studies show similar effects of adenosine in adults and children: effective doses for children were between 0.0375 and 0.25 mg/kg.

Elderly: See dosage recommendations for adults.

Diagnostic dose: The above ascending dosage schedule should be employed until sufficient diagnostic information has been obtained.

Method of administration: Rapid intravenous injection only.

Contra-indications: Adenocor is contra-indicated for patients suffering from:

- Second or third degree AV block (except in patients with a functioning artificial pacemaker).
- Sick sinus syndrome (except in patients with a functional artificial pacemaker).
- Asthma.

Special warnings and special precautions for use:

Special warnings: Due to the possibility of transitory electrophysiological phenomena arising during conversion of the supraventricular tachycardia to normal sinus rhythm, administration should be carried out in hospital with electrocardiographic monitoring.

Since neither the kidney nor the liver are involved in the degradation of exogenous adenosine, Adenocor's efficacy should be unaffected by hepatic or renal insufficiency.

Precautions: Patients with atrial fibrillation/flutter and an accessory by-pass tract may develop increased conduction down the anomalous pathway. Because of the possible risk of torsade de pointes, Adenocor should be used with caution in patients with a prolonged QT interval, whether this is congenital, drug induced or of metabolic origin.

In patients with chronic obstructive pulmonary disease, adenosine may precipitate or aggravate bronchospasm.

Interactions with other medicaments and other forms of interaction: Dipyridamole is a known inhibitor of adenosine uptake and may potentiate the action of Adenocor. Asystole has been reported following concomitant administration. It is suggested that Adenocor should not be administered to patients receiving dipyridamole; if use of Adenocor is essential, dosage should be reduced by a factor of 4 (e.g., initial dosage of 0.5 to 1.0 mg).

Theophylline and other xanthines such as caffeine are known strong inhibitors of adenosine.

Adenocor may interact with drugs tending to impair cardiac conduction.

Pregnancy and lactation: Adenosine is a substance which is naturally present in some form in all cells of the body, therefore, no effect on the foetus would be expected. In the absence of evidence that adenosine does not cause foetal harm, Adenocor should only be used during pregnancy where absolutely necessary.

Effects on ability to drive and use machines: Not applicable.

Undesirable effects: Facial flush, dyspnoea, bronchospasm, a feeling of thoracic constriction, nausea and lightheadedness occur commonly. More rarely observed side-effects have been: feeling of discomfort; sweating; palpitations; hyperventilation, head pressure; apprehension; blurred vision; burning sensation; bradycardia; asystole; chest pains; headache; dizziness; heaviness in arms; arm, back and neck pains; metallic taste. These side-effects were mild, of short duration (usually less than 1 minute) and generally well-tolerated by the patient. Severe bradycardia has been reported and some patients have required temporary pacing. The effects of Adenocor are not blocked by atropine.

One case of worsening of high intracranial pressure has been reported. This was transient (less than 2 minutes) and spontaneously and rapidly reversible. At the time of conversion to normal sinus rhythm, the ECG may show premature ventricular contractions, premature atrial contractions, sinus bradycardia, sinus tachycardia, skipped beats, sinus pause and/or atrioventricular block. The induced bradycardia predisposes to ventricular excitability disorders, including; ventricular fibrillation, and torsade de pointes which justify the recommendations made under *Posology and method of administration.*

Overdose: No cases of overdosage have been reported. As the half life of adenosine in blood is very short, the duration of any effects is expected to be limited.

Pharmacological properties

Pharmacodynamic properties: Antiarrhythmic drug. Adenosine is a purine nucleoside which is present in all cells of the body. Animal pharmacology studies have in several species shown that Adenosine has a negative dromotropic effect on the atrioventricular (AV) node.

In man Adenocor (adenosine) administered by rapid intravenous injection slows conduction through the AV node. This action can interrupt re-entry circuits involving the AV node and restore normal sinus rhythm in patients with paroxysmal supraventricular tachycardias. Once the circuit has been interrupted, the tachycardia stops and normal sinus rhythm is re-established. One acute interruption of the circuit is usually sufficient to arrest the tachycardia.

Since atrial fibrillation and atrial flutter do not involve the AV node as part of a re-entry circuit, Adenosine will not terminate these arrhythmias. By transiently slowing AV conduction, atrial activity is easier to evaluate from ECG recordings and therefore the use of Adenosine can aid the diagnosis of broad or narrow complex tachycardias.

Adenosine may be useful during electrophysiological studies to determine the site of AV block or to determine in some cases of pre-excitation, whether conduction is occurring by an accessory pathway or via the AV node.

Pharmacokinetic properties: Adenosine is impossible to study via classical ADME protocols. It is present in various forms in all cells of the body where it plays an important role in energy production and utilisation systems. An efficient salvage and recycling system exists in the body, primarily in the erythrocytes and blood vessel endothelial cells. The half life *in vitro* is estimated to be <10 seconds. The *in vivo* half life may be even shorter.

Pre-clinical safety data: There are no pre-clinical data of relevance to the prescriber which are additional to that already included in other sections of the SPC.

Pharmaceutical particulars

List of excipients: Sodium Chloride PhEur and Water for Injections PhEur.

Incompatibilities: Compatibility with other medicines is not known.

Shelf life: 36 months.

Special precautions for storage: Do not refrigerate. Any portion of the vial not used at once should be discarded.

Nature and contents of container: Clear, type I glass vials with chlorobutyl rubber closures secured with aluminium caps. Packs of 6 vials in plastic trays in cardboard cartons.

Instructions for use/handling: Any portion of the vial not used at once should be discarded.

Marketing authorisation number PL 11723/0005.

Date of approval/revision of SPC May 1996.

Legal category POM.

ADENOSCAN*

Qualitative and quantitative composition Adenoscan is a sterile solution for intravenous infusion provided in 10 ml clear glass vials containing 30 mg of adenosine.

Pharmaceutical form Sterile solution for intravenous infusion.

Clinical particulars

Therapeutic indications: Intravenous Adenoscan is a coronary vasodilator for use in conjunction with radionuclide myocardial perfusion imaging in patients who cannot exercise adequately or for whom exercise is inappropriate.

Posology and method of administration: Adenoscan is intended for use in hospitals. It should be administered following the same procedure as for exercise testing where facilities for cardiac monitoring and cardio-respiratory resuscitation are available. During administration of Adenoscan continuous ECG control is necessary as life-threatening arrhythmia might occur. Heart rate and blood pressure should be monitored every minute.

Adults

1. Adenoscan should be administered undiluted as a continuous peripheral intravenous infusion at a dose of 140 micrograms/kg/min for six minutes using an infusion pump. Separate venous sites for Adenoscan and radionuclide administration are recommended to avoid an adenosine bolus effect.

2. After three minutes of Adenoscan infusion, the radionuclide is injected to ensure sufficient time for peak coronary blood flow to occur. The optimal vasodilator protocol is achieved with six minutes of Adenoscan infusion.

3. To avoid an adenosine bolus effect, blood pressure should be measured in the arm opposite to the Adenoscan infusion.

The following table is given as a guide for adjustment of the infusion rate of undiluted Adenoscan, in line with bodyweight (total dose 0.84 mg/kg).

Patient weight kg	*Infusion rate ml/min*
45–49	2.1
50–54	2.3
55–59	2.6
60–64	2.8
65–69	3.0
70–74	3.3
75–79	3.5
80–84	3.8
85–89	4.0
90–94	4.2
95–99	4.4
100–104	4.7

Children: In the absence of data, the use of Adenoscan in children cannot be recommended.

Elderly: See dosage recommendations for adults.

Contra-indications: Adenoscan is contra-indicated in patients suffering from:

- Known hypersensitivity to adenosine.
- Second or third degree AV block, sick sinus syndrome except in patients with a functioning artificial pacemaker.
- Long QT syndrome.
- Severe hypotension.
- Unstable angina not successfully stabilised with medical therapy.
- Decompensated states of heart failure.
- Chronic obstructive lung disease with evidence of bronchospasm (e.g. asthma bronchiale).
- Concomitant use of dipyridamole.

Special warnings and special precautions for use: Because it has the potential to cause significant hypotension, Adenoscan should be used with caution in patients with left main coronary stenosis, uncorrected hypovolemia, stenotic valvular heart disease, left to right shunt, pericarditis or pericardial effusion, autonomic dysfunction or stenotic carotid artery disease with cerebrovascular insufficiency. Adenoscan infusion should be discontinued in any patient who develops persistent or symptomatic hypotension. Adenoscan should be used with caution in patients with recent myocardial infarction or severe heart failure. Adenoscan should be used with caution in patients with minor conduction defects (first degree AV block, bundle branch block) that could be transiently aggravated during infusion.

Adenoscan should be used with caution in patients with atrial fibrillation or flutter and especially in those with an accessory by-pass tract since particularly the latter may develop increased conduction down the anomalous pathway.

Rare cases of severe bradycardia have been reported. Some occurred in early post-transplant patients; in the other cases occult sino-atrial disease was present. The occurrence of severe bradycardia should be taken as a warning of underlying disease and should lead to treatment discontinuation.

Severe bradycardia would favour the occurrence of torsade de pointes, especially in patients with prolonged QT intervals. But to date no case of torsades de pointes has been reported when adenosine is continuously infused.

The occurrence of respiratory failure, asystole, angina or severe hypotension should also lead to treatment discontinuation.

In patients with recent heart transplantation (less than 1 year) an increased sensitivity of the heart to adenosine has been observed.

Interaction with other medicaments and other forms of interaction: Dipyridamole inhibits adenosine cellular uptake and metabolism, and potentiates the action of Adenoscan. In one study dipyridamole was shown to produce a 4 fold increase in adenosine actions. It is therefore suggested that Adenoscan should not be administered to patients receiving dipyridamole; if use of Adenoscan is essential, dipyridamole should be stopped 24 hours before hand, or the dose of Adenoscan should be greatly reduced.

Aminophylline, theophylline and other xanthines are competitive adenosine antagonists and should be avoided for 24 hours prior to use of Adenoscan.

Food and drinks containing xanthines (tea, coffee, chocolate and cola) should be avoided for at least 12 hours prior to use of Adenoscan.

Adenosine can safely be co-administered with other cardioactive or vasoactive drugs (see *Pharmacodynamic properties*).

Pregnancy and lactation: It is not known whether Adenoscan can cause harm when administered to pregnant or lactating women. Therefore the use during pregnancy is contra-indicated unless the physician considers the benefits outweigh the risk. Adenoscan should not be used during the lactation period.

Effects on ability to drive and use machines: None known.

Undesirable effects: Effects related to the known pharmacology of adenosine are frequent, but usually self-limiting and of short duration. Flushing, chest pain or pressure and dyspnoea (or the urge to breathe deeply) occur most commonly. Headache, dizziness or feeling lightheaded, abdominal, throat, neck and jaw discomfort have also been reported. Less frequently patients have developed bronchospasm, hypotension, AV block, ST segment depression, arrhythmia (sustained or non-sustained ventricular tachycardia), sweating, nasal congestion, nipple discomfort, nervousness, paraesthesia, tremors, drowsiness, tinnitus, blurred vision, dry mouth, a metallic taste, discomfort in the leg, arm or back, weakness or urinary urgency. Discontinuation of infusion may be necessary if the effect is intolerable.

If sustained second or third degree AV block develops the infusion should be discontinued. If first degree AV block occurs, the patient should be observed carefully as a quarter of patients will progress to a higher degree of block.

Rare cases of severe bradycardia have been reported.

Methylxanthines, such as IV aminophylline have been used to terminate persistent side effects (50–125 mg by slow intravenous injection).

Overdose: No cases of overdosage have been reported. Overdosage would cause severe hypotension, bradycardia or asystole. The half life of adenosine in blood is very short, and side-effects of Adenoscan (when they occur) would quickly resolve when the infusion is discontinued. Administration of IV aminophylline or theophylline may be needed.

Pharmacological properties

Pharmacodynamic properties: Adenosine is a potent vasodilator in most vascular beds, except in renal afferent arterioles and hepatic veins where it produces vasoconstriction. Adenosine exerts its pharmacological effects through activation of purine receptors (cell-surface A_1 and A_2 adenosine receptors). Although the exact mechanism by which adenosine receptor activation relaxes vascular smooth muscle is not known, there is evidence to support both inhibition of the slow inward calcium current reducing calcium uptake, and activation of adenylate cyclase through A_2 receptors in smooth muscle cells. Adenosine may reduce vascular tone by modulating sympathetic neurotransmission. The intracellular uptake of adenosine is mediated by a specific transmembrane nucleoside transport system. Once inside the cell, adenosine is rapidly phosphorylated by adenosine kinase to adenosine monophosphate, or deaminated by adenosine deaminase to inosine. These intracellular metabolites of adenosine are not vasoactive.

Intracoronary Doppler flow catheter studies have demonstrated that intravenous Adenoscan at 140 mcg/kg/min produces maximum coronary hyperaemia (relative to intracoronary papaverine) in approximately 90% of cases within 2–3 minutes of the onset of the infusion. Coronary blood flow velocity returns to basal levels within 1–2 minutes of discontinuing the Adenoscan infusion.

The increase in blood flow caused by Adenoscan in normal coronary arteries is significantly more than that in stenotic arteries. Adenoscan redirects coronary blood flow from the endocardium to the epicardium and may reduce collateral coronary blood flow thereby inducing regional ischaemia.

Continuous infusion of adenosine in man has been shown to produce a mild dose-dependant fall in mean arterial pressure and a dose-related positive chronotropic effect, most likely caused by sympathetic stimulation. The onset of this reflex increase in heart rate occurs later than the negative chronotropic/dromotropic effect. This differential effect is mostly observed after bolus injection thus explaining the potential use of adenosine as a treatment for supraventricular arrhythmias when administered as a bolus or as a coronary vasodilator when administered as an infusion.

Although Adenoscan affects cardiac conduction, it has been safely and effectively administered in the presence of other cardioactive or vasoactive drugs such as beta adrenergic blocking agents, calcium channel antagonists, nitrates, ACE inhibitors, diuretics, digitalis or anti arrhythmics.

Pharmacokinetic properties: It is impossible to study adenosine in classical pharmacokinetic studies. It is present in various forms in all the cells of the body where it plays an important role in energy production and utilisation systems. An efficient salvage and recycling system exists in the body, primarily in erythrocytes and blood vessel endothelial cells. The half life *in vitro* is estimated to be less than 10 seconds. The *in vivo* half life may be even shorter.

Since neither the kidney nor the liver are involved in the degradation of exogenous adenosine, the efficacy of Adenoscan should be unaffected by hepatic or renal insufficiency.

Preclinical safety data: Because adenosine is naturally present in all living cells, studies in animals to evaluate the carcinogenic potential of Adenoscan (adenosine) have not been performed.

Pharmaceutical particulars
List of excipients: Sodium chloride, water for injection.

Incompatibilities: Compatibility with other medicines is not known.

Shelf life: 36 months.

Special precautions for storage: Do not refrigerate. Any portion of the vial not used at once should be discarded.

Nature and contents of container: Type I glass vials with chlorbutyl rubber stoppers, packs with 6 vials containing 10 ml of solution at 3 mg/ml, i.e. 30 mg of adenosine per vial.

Instructions for use/handling: See *Posology and Method of Administration.*

Marketing authorisation number 11723/0086.

Date of approval/revision of SPC February 1997.

Legal category POM.

APROVEL

Qualitative and quantitative composition
Each tablet contains 75 mg, 150 mg or 300 mg irbesartan.

Pharmaceutical Form Tablet.
White to off-white, biconvex, and oval-shaped with a heart debossed on one side and the number 2771 (75 mg), 2772 (150 mg) or 2773 (300 mg) engraved on the other side.

Clinical Particulars
Therapeutic indication
Treatment of essential hypertension

Posology and method of administration: The usual recommended initial and maintenance dose is 150 mg daily, with or without food. Aprovel at a dose of 150 mg once daily generally provides a better 24 hour blood pressure control than 75 mg. However, initiation of therapy with 75 mg could be considered, particularly in haemodialysed patients and in the elderly over 75 years.

In patients insufficiently controlled with 150 mg once daily, the dose of Aprovel can be increased to 300 mg, or other anti-hypersensitive agents can be added. In particular, the addition of a diuretic such as hydrochlorothiazide has been shown to have an additive effect with Aprovel (see *Interactions with other medicinal products and other forms of interaction*).

Renal impairment: no dosage adjustment is necessary in patients with impaired renal function. A lower starting dose (75 mg) should be considered for patients undergoing haemodialysis.

Intravascular volume depletion: volume and/or sodium depletion should be corrected prior to administration of Aprovel.

Hepatic impairment: no dosage adjustment is necessary in patients with mild to moderate hepatic impairment. There is no clinical experience in patients with severe hepatic impairment.

Elderly patients: although consideration should be given to initiating therapy with 75 mg in patients over 75 years of age, dosage adjustment is not usually necessary for the elderly.

Children: safety and efficacy of Aprovel have not been established in children.

Contra-indications
Hypersensitivity to any component of the product (see *List of excipients*).

Pregnancy and lactation (see *Use during pregnancy and lactation.*)

Special warnings and special precautions for use
Intravascular volume depletion: symptomatic hypotension, especially after the first dose, may occur in patients who are volume and/or sodium depleted by vigorous diuretic therapy, dietary salt restriction, diarrhoea or vomiting. Such conditions should be corrected before the administration of Aprovel.

Renovascular hypertension: there is an increased risk of severe hypotension and renal insufficiency when patients with bilateral renal artery stenosis or stenosis of the artery to a single functioning kidney are treated with drugs that affect the renin-angiotensin-aldosterone system. While this is not documented with Aprovel, a similar effect should be anticipated with angiotensin II receptor antagonists.

Renal impairment and kidney transplantation: when Aproval is used in patients with impaired renal function, a periodic monitoring of potassium and creatinine serum levels is recommended. There is no experience regarding the administration of Aprovel in patients with a recent kidney transplantation.

Hyperkalemia: during treatment with other drugs that affect the renin-angiotensin-aldosterone system hyperkalemia may occur, especially in the presence of renal impairment and/or heart failure. While this is not documented with Aprovel, adequate monitoring of serum potassium in patients at risk is recommended (see *Interactions with other medicinal products and other forms of interaction*)

Aortic and mitral valve stenosis, obstructive hypertrophic cardiomyopathy: as with other vasodilators, special caution is indicated in patients suffering from aortic or mitral stenosis, or obstructive hypertrophic cardiomyopathy.

Primary aldosteronism: patients with primary aldosteronism generally will not respond to anti-hypertensive drugs acting through inhibition of the renin-angiotensin system. Therefore, the use of Aprovel is not recommended.

General: in patients whose vascular tone and renal function depend predominantly on the activity of the renin-angiotensin-aldosterone system (e.g. patients with severe congestive heart failure or underlying renal disease, including renal artery stenosis), treatment with other drugs that affect this system has been associated with acute hypotension, azotaemia, oliguria, or rarely acute renal failure. Although the possibility of similar effects are not documented with Aprovel. As with any antihypertensive agent, excessive blood pressure decrease in patients with ischemic cardiopathy or ischemic cardiovascular disease could result in a myocardial infarction or stroke.

Interactions with other medicinal products and other forms of interaction
Diuretics and other antihypertensive agents: other antihypertensive agents may increase the hypotensive effects of irbesartan; however, Aprovel has been safely administered with other antihypertensive agents, such as beta-blockers, long-acting calcium channel blockers, and thiazide diuretics. Prior treatment with high dose diuretics may result in volume depletion and a risk of hypotension when initiating therapy with Aprovel (see *Special warnings and special precautions for use*).

Potassium supplements and potassium-sparing diuretics: based on experience with the use of other drugs that affect the renin-angiotensin system, concomitant use of potassium-sparing diuretics, potassium supplements, salt substitutes containing potassium or other drugs that may increase serum potassium levels (e.g. heparin) may lead to increases in serum potassium (see *Special warnings and special precautions for use*).

Lithium: Reversible increases in serum lithium concentrations and toxicity have been reported during concomitant administration of lithium with angiotensin converting enzyme inhibitors. While this is not documented with Aprovel, the possibility of a similar effect can not be excluded and careful monitoring of serum lithium levels is recommended during concomitant use.

Additional information on drug interactions: The phamacokinetics of digoxin were not altered by co-administration of a 150 mg dose of irbesartan in healthy male volunteers. The pharmacokinetics of irbesartan are not affected co-administration of hydrochlorothiazide. Irbesartan is mainly metabolised by CYP2C9 and to a lesser extent by glucoronidation. Inhibition of the glucuronyl transferase pathway is unlikely to result in clinically significant interactions. In-vitro interactions were observed between irbesartan and warfarin, tolbutamide (CYP2C9 substrates) and nifedipine (CYP2C9 inhibitor). However, no significant pharmacokinetic or pharmacodynamic interactions were observed when irbesartan was co-administered with warfarin in healthy male volunteers. The pharmacokinetics of irbesartan are not affected by co-administration of nifedine. The effects of CYP2C9 inducers such as rifampicin on the pharmacokinetics of irbesartan were not evaluated. Based on *in-vitro* data, no interaction would be expected to occur with drugs whose metabolism is dependent upon cytochrome P450 isoenzymes CYP1A1, CYP1A2, CYP2A6, CYP2B6, CYP2D6, CYP2E1 or CYP3A4.

Use during pregnancy and lactation
Pregnancy: Aprovel is contraindicated during pregnancy. Although there is no experience with Aprovel in pregnant women, *in utero* exposure to ACE inhibitors given to pregnant women during the second and third trimesters has been reported to cause injury and death to the developing foetus.

As for any drug that also acts directly on the renin-angiotensin-aldosterone system, Aprovel, should not be used during pregnancy. If pregnancy is detected during therapy, Aprovel should be discontinued as soon as possible (see *Contra-indications*).

Lactation: Aprovel is contraindicated during lactation. It is not known whether irbesartan is excreted in human milk. Irbesartan is excreted in the milk of lactating rats (see *Contra-indications*).

Effects on ability to drive and use machines: The effect of irbesartan on ability to drive and use machines has not been studied, but based on its pharmacodynamic properties, irbesartan is unlikely to affect this ability. When driving vehicles or operating machines, it should be taken into account that occasionally dizziness or weariness may occur during treatment of hypertension.

Undesirable effects: Undesirable effects in patients receiving Aprovel are generally mild and transient. In placebo-controlled trials in patients with hypertension, the overall incidence of adverse events did not differ between the irbesartan and the placebo groups. Discontinuation due to any clinical or laboratory adverse event was less frequent for irbesartan-treated patients than for placebo-treated patients. The incidence of adverse events was not related to dose (in the recommended dose range), gender, age, race, or duration of treatment.

Clinical adverse events, regardless of whether attributed to therapy, occurring in 1% or more of hypertensive patients with Aprovel in placebo-controlled trials are presented in the following table:

	% of Patients	
	Irbesartan Monotherapy	
Adverse Event	*N=1965*	*Placebo N=641*
respiratory infection[a]	18.4	18.6
headache	12.3	16.7*
musculoskeletal pain[b]	7.3	8.4
dizziness	4.9	5.0
fatigue	4.3	3.7
diarrhoea	3.1	2.2
cough	2.8	2.7
nausea/vomiting	2.1	2.8
musculoskeletal trauma	1.9*	0.5
chest pain	1.8	1.7
dyspepsia/heartburn	1.7	1.1
oedema	1.5	2.3
abdominal pain	1.4	2.0
rash	1.3	2.0
tachycardia	1.2	0.9
anxiety/nervousness	1.1	0.9
UTI	1.1	1.4

[a] Includes upper respiratory infection, sinus abnormality, influenza, pharyngitis and rhinitis.
[b] Includes musculoskeletal pain, musculoskeletal ache, and myalgia.
* Indicates a statistically significant difference between groups ($p < 0.05$).

Adverse events occurred with similar frequency in placebo and irbesartan-treated patients, with the exception of headache, musculoskeletal trauma, and flusing. Headache occurred significantly more often in the placebo group. Musculoskeletal trauma of differing types and causes occurred with significantly higher incidence in the irbesartan group; all reports of musculoskeletal trauma were considered unrelated to irbesartan by the investigators. Flushing occurred in 0.6% of irbesartan patients and in no placebo patients. The occurrence of flushing was not related to dose, was not accompanied by other clinical events, and the relationship with irbesartan therapy is unknown. In over 5500 subjects exposed to irbesartan in clinical trials, there has been no report of angioedema.

No clinically significant changes in laboratory test parameters occurred in controlled clinical trials. Although significant increases in plasma creatine kinase occurred more frequently in irbesartan-treated subjects (1.7% vs 0.7% in placebo-treated subjects), none of these increases were classified as serious, resulted in drug discontinuation, or were associated with identifiable clinical musculoskeletal events. No special monitoring of laboratory parameters is necessary for patients with essential hypertension receiving therapy with Aprovel, when the renal function is normal (see *Special warnings and special precautions for use*).

Overdose: Experience in adults exposed to doses of up to 900 mg/day for 8 weeks revealed no toxicity. The most likely manifestations of overdosage are expected to be hypotension and tachycardia; bradycardia might also occur from overdose. No specific information is available on the treatment of overdosage with Aprovel. The patient should be closely monitored, and the treatment should be symptomatic and supportive. Suggested measures include induction of emesis and/or gastric lavage. Activated charcoal may be useful in the treatment of overdosage. Irbesartan is not removed by haemodialysis.

Pharmacological properties
Pharmacodynamic properties
Pharmaco-therapeutic group: Angiotensin II antagonists, ATC code C09C A.
Irbesartan is a potent, orally active, selective angiotensin II receptor (type AT_1) antagonist. It is expected to block all actions of angiotensin II mediated by the AT_1 receptor, regardless of the source or route of synthesis of angiotensin II. The selective antagonism of the angiotensin II (AT_1) receptors results in increases in plasma renin levels and angiotensin II levels, and a

decrease in plasma aldosterone concentration. Serum potassium levels are not significantly affected by irbesartan alone at the recommended doses. Irbesartan does not inhibit ACE (kininase II), an enzyme which generates angiotensin II and also degrades bradykinin into inactive metabolites. Irbesartan does not require metabolic activation for its activity.

Irbesartan lowers blood pressure with minimal change in heart rate. The decrease in blood pressure is dose-related for once a day doses with a tendency towards plateau at doses above 300 mg. Doses of 150–300 mg once daily lower supine or seated blood pressures at trough (i.e., 24 hours after dosing) by an average of 8-13/5-8 mm Hg (systolic/diastolic) greater than those associated with placebo.

Peak reduction of blood pressure is achieved within 3–6 hours after administration and the blood pressure lowering effect is maintained for at least 24 hours. At 24 hours the reduction of blood pressure was 60–70% of the corresponding peak diastolic and systolic responses at the recommended doses. Once daily dosing with 150 mg produced trough and mean 24 hour responses similar to twice daily dosing on the same total dose.

The blood pressure lowering effect of Aprovel is evident within 1–2 weeks, with the maximal effect occurring by 4–6 weeks after start of therapy. The antihypertensive effects are maintained during long term therapy. After withdrawal of therapy, blood pressure gradually returns toward baseline. Rebound hypertension has not been observed.

The blood pressure lowering effects of irbesartan and thiazide-type diuretics are additive. In patients not adequately controlled by irbesartan alone, the addition of a low dose of hydrochlorothiazide (12.5 mg) to irbesartan once daily results in a further placebo-adjusted blood pressure reduction at trough of 7-10/3-6 mm Hg (systolic/diastolic).

The efficacy of Aprovel is not influenced by age or gender. As is the case with other drugs that affect the renin-angiotensin system, black hypertensive patients have notably less response to irbesartan monotherapy. When irbesartan is administered concomitantly with a low dose of hydrochlorothiazide (e.g., 12.5 mg daily), the antihypertensive response in black patients approaches that of white patients.

There is no clinically important effect on serum uric acid or urinary uric acid secretion.

Pharmacokinetic properties: After oral administration, irbesartan is well absorbed: studies of absolute bioavailability gave values of approximately 60–80%. Concomitant food intake does not significantly influence the bioavailability of irbesartan.

Plasma protein binding is approximately 90%, with negligible binding to cellular blood components. The volume of distribution is 53–93 litres.

Following oral or intravenous administration of ^{14}C irbesartan, 80–85% of the circulating plasma radioactivity is attributable to unchanged irbesartan. Irbesartan is metabolised by the liver via glucuronide conjugation and oxidation. The major circulating metabolite is irbesartan glucoronide (approximately 6%). *In vitro* studies indicate that irbesartan is primarily oxidised by the cytochrome P450 enzyme CYP2C9; isoenzyme CYP3A4 has negligible effect.

Irbesartan exhibits linear and dose proportional pharmacokinetics over the dose range of 10 to 600 mg. A less than proportional increase in oral absorption at doses beyond 600 mg (twice the maximal recommended dose) was observed; the mechanism for this is unknown. Peak plasma concentrations are attained at 1.5–2 hours after oral administration. The total body and renal clearance are 157–176 and 3–3.5 ml/min, respectively. The terminal elimination half-life of irbesartan is 11–15 hours. Steady-rate plasma concentrations are attained within 3 days after initiation of a once-daily dosing regimen. Limited accumulation of irbesartan (<20%) is observed in plasma upon repeated once-daily dosing. In a study, somewhat higher plasma concentrations of irbesartan were observed in female hypertensive patients. However, there was no difference in the half-life and accumulation of irbesartan. No dosage adjustment is necessary in female patients. Irbesartan AUC and C_{max} values were also somewhat greater in elderly subjects (≥65 years) and those of young subjects (18–40 years). However the terminal half-life was not significantly altered. No dosage adjustment is necessary in elderly patients.

Irbesartan and its metabolites are eliminated by both biliary and renal pathways. After either oral or IV administration of ^{14}C irbesartan, about 20% of the radioactivity is recovered in the urine, and the remainder in the faeces. Less than 2% of the dose is excreted in the urine as unchanged irbesartan.

Renal impairment: in patients with renal impairment or those undergoing haemodialysis, the pharmacokinetic parameters of irbesartan are not significantly altered. Irbesartan is not removed by haemodialysis.

Hepatic impairment: in patients with mild to moderate cirrhosis, the pharmacokinetic parameters of irbesartan are not significantly altered. Studies have not been performed in patients with severe hepatic impairment.

Preclinical safety data: There was no evidence of abnormal systemic or target toxicity at clinically relevant doses. In preclinical safety studies, high doses of irbesartan (≥250 mg/kg/day in rats and ≥100 mg/kg/day in macaques) caused a reduction of red blood cell parameters (erythrocytes, haemoglobin, haematocrit). At very high doses (≥500 mg/kg/day), degenerative changes in the kidney (such as interstitial nephritis, tubular distension, basophilic tubules, increased plasma concentrations of urea and creatinine) were induced by irbesartan in the rat and the macaque and are considered secondary to the hypotensive effects of the drug which led to decreased renal perfusion. Furthermore, irbesartan induced hyperplasia/hypertrophy of the juxtaglomerular cells (in rats at ≥250 mg/kg/day, in macaques at ≥10 mg/kg/day). All of these changes were considered to be caused by the pharmacological action of irbesartan. For therapeutic doses of irbesartan in humans, the hyperplasia/hypertrophy of the renal juxtaglomerular cells does not appear to have any relevance.

There was no evidence of mutagenicity, clastogenicity or carcinogenicity.

Animal studies with irbesartan showed transient toxic effects (increased renal pelvic cavitation, hydroureter or subcutaneous oedema) in rat foetuses, which were resolved after birth. In rabbits, abortion or early resorption were noted at doses causing significant maternal toxicity, including mortality. No teratogenic effects were observed in the rat or rabbit.

Pharmaceutical particulars

List of excipients: Microcrystalline cellulose, croscarmellose sodium, lactose monohydrate, magnesium stearate, colloidal hydrated silica, pregelatinised maize starch, and poloxamer 188.

Incompatibilities: None.

Shelf-life: 24 months.

Special precautions for storage: Store in a dry place below 30°C.

Nature and content of container: Aproval tablets are packaged in blister packs containing 28 tablets in PVC/PVDC/Aluminium strips.

Instructions for use, handling and disposal (if appropriate): None.

Marketing authorisation holder: Sanofi Pharma Bristol-Myers Squibb SNC, 174 Avenue de France, F-75013, Paris, France.

Numbers in the community register of medicinal products

Aproval 75 mg	EU/1/97/046/001
Aprovel 150 mg	EU/1/97/046/004
Aprovel 300 mg	EU/1/97/046/007

Date of first authorisation/renewal of the authorisation 27th August 1997

Date of revision of the text December 1998.

Legal category: POM.

BENORAL*

Presentation 1. Benoral Suspension is a white suspension, 10 ml of which contains 4 g Benorylate BP. Benoral Suspension contains sorbitol.

2. Benoral Granules: sachets filled with a white, free-flowing powder which disperses readily in water. The contents of each sachet are equivalent to 2 g Benorylate BP. Benoral Granules contain 550 mg sucrose in each sachet.

3. Benoral Tablets are white, capsule-shaped tablets marked 'benoral' on one side only, each containing 750 mg Benorylate BP.

Uses Benoral is an anti-inflammatory analgesic and antipyretic. It is recommended for the treatment of rheumatoid arthritis, osteoarthritis and painful musculo-skeletal conditions. It may also be used to treat mild to moderate pain due to many other causes and as an antipyretic in febrile conditions.

Dosage and administration Benoral is for oral administration only.

Benoral Suspension may be administered undiluted or taken in hot or cold beverages. Benoral Granules should be stirred into half a glass of water or milk, if preferred and drunk immediately.

Adults (except elderly) The maximum daily dosage of benorylate is 8 g.

Suspension: To treat active rheumatoid arthritis 10 ml of suspension (4 g benorylate) twice daily is normally required.

For osteoarthritis, quiescent rheumatoid arthritis or soft tissue (non-articular) rheumatism 5 ml (2 g benorylate) twice daily may suffice.

For mild to moderate pain and as an antipyretic the normal dosage is 5 ml suspension (2 g benorylate) twice daily.

Tablets: In osteoarthritis, quiescent rheumatoid arthritis and soft tissue rheumatism eight 750 mg tablets (6 g benorylate) per day, in divided doses, are recommended.

Sachets: For acute rheumatic conditions up to four sachets (8 g benorylate) daily in divided doses may be required but three sachets (6 g benorylate) daily are often adequate. For milder rheumatic conditions and for the relief of non-rheumatic pain one sachet (2 g benorylate) twice daily is recommended.

Elderly: In elderly patients, especially those with impaired renal function, symptoms of salicylism may arise at dosages not normally associated with this effect. In elderly patients it is recommended that the adult dose of Benoral be reduced. For example, dose reduction of Benoral Suspension to a 5 ml (2 g benorylate) morning dose with 10 ml (4 g benorylate) at bedtime may be instituted. Further reduction to 5 ml (2 g benorylate) twice daily may be necessary in some cases.

Dose reduction of Benoral Sachets to three sachets (6 g benorylate) daily in divided doses may be instituted. Further reduction to one sachet (2 g benorylate) twice daily may be necessary in some cases.

Children: Benoral is not recommended for children.

Contra-indications, warnings, etc

Contra-indications: Benoral should not be given to patients with active peptic ulcer, nor to patients known to be sensitive to paracetamol or aspirin including those with asthma, or haemophilia and similar coagulation disorders.

The safety of benorylate has not been established in human pregnancy. Whilst there is clinical and epidemiological evidence that its metabolic products, salicylate and paracetamol, are safe in pregnancy, it is also known that benorylate, in high doses, may have an aspirin-like effect on platelet function. As with aspirin therefore, benorylate should be avoided in the last trimester and at term because of a potential risk of contributing to maternal and neonatal bleeding.

Because salicylate is excreted in breast milk, benorylate should also be avoided by breast feeding mothers.

Because of the possible association between Reye's syndrome and aspirin use, Benoral labelling contains the statement 'Do not give to children under 12 unless your doctor tells you to'.

Patients taking Benoral should be advised against taking analgesics containing aspirin or paracetamol.

Precautions: Care is needed in prescribing Benoral for patients with impaired renal or hepatic function and for those with a history of peptic ulcer.

Patients who are taking anticoagulants should have their prothrombin time checked.

Concomitant administration of carbonic anhydrase inhibitors may increase salicylate level and dispose to toxicity, whilst corticosteroids may reduce salicylate level. Salicylate may diminish the diuretic efficiency of frusemide. These possible interactions should be borne in mind in determining respective dosages when initiating or discontinuing concomitant therapy.

Side-effects: Overall tolerance is excellent. Minor disturbances including nausea, constipation or diarrhoea, indigestion or heartburn have occurred from time to time and drowsiness and skin rashes have also been reported. The possibility that gastro-intestinal haemorrhage may be induced by Benoral cannot be excluded. The high salicylate levels obtained with Benoral may give rise to dizziness, tinnitus and deafness. If this happens, the dose should be reduced.

There have been a few reports of blood dyscrasias including thrombocytopenia and agranulocytosis but these were not necessarily causally related to paracetamol.

Overdosage: Symptoms are likely to resemble those caused by paracetamol overdosage or salicylate overdosage. The hazard of paracetamol overdosage is greater in those with non cirrhotic alcohol liver disease. Treatment should be based on the levels of salicylate and paracetamol in the blood. The possibility that overdosage may cause hepatic necrosis due to accumulation of a highly reactive intermediate metabolite of paracetamol, must be considered. Symptoms of paracetamol overdosage in the first 24 hours are pallor, nausea, anorexia and abdominal pain. Liver damage may become apparent 12 to 48 hours after ingestion. Abnormalities of glucose metabolism and acidosis may occur. In severe poisoning, hepatic failure may progress to encephalopathy, coma and death. Cardiac arrhythmia and pancreatitis have been reported. Liver damage is possible in adults who have taken 10 g or more of paracetamol. It is considered that excess quantities of a toxic metabolite (usually adequately detoxified by glutathione when normal doses of paracetamol are ingested), become irreversibly bound to liver tissue. Immediate treatment is essential in the management of paracetamol and salicylate overdose. Despite a lack of significant early symptoms, patients should be referred to hospital urgently for immediate medical attention and any patient who has ingested around 7.5 g or more of paracetamol in the preceding 4 hours should undergo gastric lavage. Administration of oral methionine or intravenous N-acetylsteine which may have a beneficial effect up to at least 48 hours after the overdose, may be required. General supportive measures must be available. Management may also include forced alkaline diuresis and correction of acid-base balance.

Pharmaceutical precautions Nil.

Legal category P.

Package quantities Benoral Suspension – bottles of 300 ml. Benoral Granules – cartons of 60 sachets (OP). Benoral Tablets – bottles of 100.

Further information Benorylate is a prodrug which is metabolised to salicylate and paracetamol by esterases after absorption. It does not give rise to detectable levels of acetylsalicylic acid in the plasma. In chemical terms, 2 g benorylate is equivalent to 1.2 g aspirin and 0.98 g paracetamol.

Product licence numbers
Benoral Suspension 11723/0007
Benoral Granules 11723/0006
Benoral Tablets 11723/0008

CALCIPARINE*

Qualitative and quantitative composition Heparin Calcium PhEur 25,000 IU/ml.

Pharmaceutical form Sterile clear solution of 25,000 International Units of heparin activity per ml as the calcium salt in water for injections.

Clinical particulars
Therapeutic indications: It is indicated for use as an anticoagulant for the prophylaxis and treatment of thromboembolic phenomena, especially myocardial infarction, acute arterial embolism or thrombosis, deep vein thrombosis, thrombophlebitis or pulmonary embolism.

Posology and method of administration: For subcutaneous administration only using a 26-gauge needle. The best site is the subcutaneous tissue of the lateral abdominal wall. The needle should be inserted perpendicularly into a pinched-up fold of skin and held gently but firmly with the skinfold until injection has been completed. Do not rub the site of injection.

Calciparine is not intended for intramuscular use.

Adults:
Prophylaxis: A standard prophylactic dose regimen is 5,000 IU by subcutaneous injection 2 hours before operation, followed by 5,000 IU by subcutaneous injection every 8 to 12 hours for seven days. In patients still confined to bed at the end of this period, the same dosage should be continued until they are ambulant.

The standard prophylactic dose following myocardial infarction is 5,000 IU by subcutaneous injection twice daily for 10 days or until the patient is mobile. In other medical conditions in which there is an associated increased risk of thromboembolic phenomena, the same dosage is recommended.

These standard prophylactic regimens do not require routine control in the absence of contra-indications or conditions listed under special warnings and precautions.

If a myocardial infarction is shown to be anterior and therefore has a risk of mural thrombosis of the left ventricle, a higher dose of 12,500 IU twice daily for at least 10 days is recommended. For this dosage regimen, regular monitoring should be considered.

Treatment: For the treatment of existing thrombosis the standard dose is 0.1 ml Calciparine (2,500 IU) per 10 kg body weight 12 hourly. To enable dosage to be individually adjusted to maintain a coagulation time in a range of 1.5 to 3 times that of control it is recommended that the thrombin clotting time, whole blood clotting time or the activated partial thromboplastin time be measured on blood withdrawn 5 to 7 hours after the first injection and then at intervals until the patient is stabilised. During long term therapy the test should be repeated at least once each week.

Children: Dosage should be individually adjusted according to changes in whole blood clotting time and/or thrombin clotting time and/or APTT. The initial dose should be 0.1 ml Calciparine (2,500 IU) by subcutaneous injection for each 10 kg of body weight. The usual interval between doses is 12 hours, but this also may require individual adjustment.

Other special groups: For both prophylaxis and treatment, higher doses are likely to be required in patients of abnormally high body weight and in those suffering from cancer, diabetes mellitus or other diseases associated with marked hypercoagulability. Lower doses are usually indicated in the elderly and in those with low serum albumin or impaired renal or hepatic function. In such patients coagulation times should be checked frequently and dosage adjusted accordingly.

Use in pregnancy: There is clinical evidence that heparin does not cause foetal damage and may be the anticoagulant of choice when anticoagulation is indicated during pregnancy. However, the risk of maternal bleeding may be increased. Calciparine should be discontinued if peridural anaesthesia is likely. Individual control is essential and the aim should be to maintain plasma heparin levels between 0.1 and 0.4 units/ml, as assessed by anti-XA assay, and a whole blood clotting time of 15 to 20 minutes.

The standard prophylactic dosage of 5,000 IU by subcutaneous injection every 8 hours is a suitable starting dose in the first 3 or 4 months of pregnancy but higher doses are needed as pregnancy progresses, 10,000 IU two or three times daily being usual in the last trimester. Dosage must be reduced during labour and standard prophylactic dosage is suitable post-partum. Heparin is not excreted into breast milk.

Contra-indications: Calciparine is contra-indicated in patients hypersensitive to heparin.

Calciparine is contra-indicated in patients with a condition in which there is an increased danger of haemorrhage. Such conditions include haemorrhagic cerebrovascular accident, haemophilia, thrombocytopenia and other haemorrhagic diatheses (other than disseminated intra-vascular coagulation not induced by heparin): gastric and duodenal ulcer, sub-acute bacterial endocarditis; threatened abortion and major surgery involving the brain, spinal cord and eye.

Calciparine is contra-indicated in patients with a history of thrombocytopenia associated with any heparin.

Calciparine should not be used in patients with advanced renal or hepatic dysfunction, in severe hypertension or patients in shock.

Special warnings and special precautions for use: Special care should be taken in elderly patients, pregnant women and patients with hypertension, history of peptic ulcer or any organic lesion likely to bleed or vascular diseases of the chorio-retina. Patients should be warned of an increased risk of bruising.

Rarely there have been reports of severe thrombocytopenia which may be complicated by venous or arterial thrombotic episodes. In this case treatment should be discontinued. These complications should be considered in patients with thrombocytopenia, thrombosis, worsening of initial thrombosis or disseminated intravascular coagulation occurring during treatment. These reactions may be immuno-allergic in nature and occur mainly between days 5 and 21 of treatment. Platelet count should be measured before treatment and then twice weekly during the first month of treatment; subsequently, monitoring can be performed less frequently.

Interactions with other medicaments and other forms of interaction: Caution should be observed in patients receiving drugs which interfere with platelet aggregation or coagulation, e.g. salicylates, NSAIDs, dextran, systemic corticosteroids, oral anticoagulants (during transfer from heparin to oral anticoagulant therapy, clinical monitoring should be particularly vigilant).

Pregnancy and lactation: There is clinical evidence that heparin does not cause foetal damage and may be the anticoagulant of choice when anticoagulation is indicated during pregnancy. However, the risk of maternal bleeding may be increased. Calciparine should be discontinued if peridural anaesthesia is likely. Heparin is not excreted into breast milk.

Effects on ability to drive and to use machines: None stated.

Undesirable effects: In common with other heparin preparations the following undesirable effects may occur. Hypersensitivity reactions may occur but are rare. Acute thrombocytopenia, usually reversible, has been reported. Platelet counts should be measured in patients under heparin therapy for longer than 5 days and treatment should be stopped in those who develop significant thrombocytopenia.

Rare cases of skin necrosis occurring generally at the injection site have been reported. This may be preceded by the appearance of purpura and erythematous, infiltrated and painful plaques. In this case treatment should be withdrawn immediately.

Overt or concealed haemorrhage from or into any tissue or organ may result from heparin therapy. This can have serious consequences and the presentation may vary.

Raised transaminases, reversible on treatment discontinuation, have been reported.

Osteoporosis and alopecia have been reported after long term treatment. Subcutaneous heparin may lead to a variety of local effects including pain and bruising. Pain and small haematomas may occur at the injection site as may an inflammatory reaction resulting in firm nodules. The nodules disappear after a few days and are not an indication to withdraw treatment. Rarely, priapism, hypoaldosteronism with hyperkalaemia and/or metabolic acidosis have been noted in patients at risk (e.g. diabetes, renal failure). Cutaneous reactions and eosinophilia, which is reversible following treatment discontinuation, have been reported.

Overdosage: Haemorrhage is the major clinical sign of overdosage. In case of bleeding, the platelet count and APTT should be determined. Minor bleeding rarely requires specific therapy, and reducing and/or delaying subsequent doses of Calciparine is usually sufficient.

The anticoagulant effect of heparin can be reversed immediately by intravenous administration of a 1% protamine sulphate solution. The dose of protamine sulphate required for neutralisation should be determined accurately by titrating the patient's plasma.

It is important to avoid overdosage of protamine sulphate because protamine itself has anticoagulant properties. A single dose of protamine sulphate should never exceed 50 mg. Intravenous injection of protamine may cause a sudden fall in blood pressure, bradycardia, dyspnoea and transitory flushing, but these may be avoided or diminished by slow and careful administration.

Pharmacological properties
Pharmacodynamic properties: Heparin calcium is a preparation containing the calcium salt of sulphated polysaccharide acid present in mammalian tissues. It is an anticoagulant which inhibits the clotting of blood *in vitro* and *in vivo*.

No further data are presented here as the pharmacodynamic properties of heparin calcium are well known and it is the subject of a European Pharmacopoeial monograph.

Pharmacokinetic properties: The slow and regular absorption kinetics of Calciparine (or similar calcium heparins) given subcutaneously makes it especially suitable for low dose prophylactic therapy. Calciparine has been used effectively in the routine prophylaxis of postoperative thromboembolism.

No further data are presented here as the properties of heparin calcium are well known. Heparin calcium is the subject of a European Pharmacopoeial monograph.

Preclinical safety data: There is no pre-clinical data of relevance to the prescriber which are additional to that already included in other sections of the SPC.

Pharmaceutical particulars
List of excipients: Calciparine also contains Water for Injection PhEur, Hydrochloric Acid PhEur and Calcium Hydroxide Solution BP.

Incompatibilities: Other preparations should not be mixed with Calciparine.

Shelf life: 48 months.

Special precautions for storage: Store below 25°C but do not freeze.

Nature and contents of container: Unit dose disposable syringe 5,000 IU in 0.2 ml, 7,500 IU in 0.3 ml, 12,500 IU in 0.5 ml and syringe graduated 20,000 IU in 0.8 ml. Ampoule with pre-sterilised plastic syringe 12,500 IU in 0.5 ml and 20,000 IU in 0.8 ml.

Instructions for use/handling: See *Posology and method of administration.*

Marketing authorisation number 11723/0011.

Date of approval/revision of SPC September 1997.

Legal category POM.

CALCIUM RESONIUM*

Presentation Calcium Resonium contains 99.93% calcium polystyrene sulphonate ground and flavoured to a buff-coloured fine powder with a pleasant vanilla odour and sweet taste.

Uses Calcium Resonium is an ion-exchange resin. It is recommended for the treatment of hyperkalaemia associated with anuria or severe oliguria. It is also used to treat hyperkalaemia in patients requiring dialysis and in patients on regular haemodialysis or on prolonged peritoneal dialysis.

Dosage and administration Calcium Resonium is for oral or rectal administration only. The dosage recommendations detailed below are a guide only; the precise requirements should be decided on the basis of regular serum electrolyte determinations.

Adults, including the elderly:
1. *Oral:* Usual dose 15 g three or four times a day. The resin is given by mouth in a little water, or it may be made into a paste with some sweetened vehicle.
2. *Rectal:* In cases where vomiting may make oral administration difficult, the resin may be given rectally as a suspension of 30 g resin in 100 ml 2% Methylcellulose 450 BP (medium viscosity) and 100 ml water, as a daily retention enema. In the initial stages administration by this route as well as orally may help

to achieve a more rapid lowering of the serum potassium level.

The enema should if possible be retained for at least nine hours following which the colon should be irrigated to remove the resin. If both routes are used initially it is probably unnecessary to continue rectal administration once the oral resin has reached the rectum.

Children: 1 g/kg body weight daily in divided doses in acute hyperkalaemia. For maintenance therapy dosage may be reduced to 0.5 g/kg body weight daily in divided doses.

The resin is given orally, preferably with a drink (not a fruit squash because of the high potassium content) or a little jam or honey. When refused by mouth it should be given rectally using a dose at least as great as that which would have been given orally, diluted in the same ratio as described for adults. Following retention of the enema, the colon should be irrigated to ensure adequate removal of the resin.

Neonates: Calcium Resonium should not be given by the oral route. With rectal administration, the minimum effective dosage within the range 0.5 g/kg to 1 g/kg should be employed, diluted as for adults and with adequate irrigation to ensure recovery of the resin.

Contra-indications, warnings, etc

Contra-indications: Calcium Resonium should not be administered orally to neonates and is contraindicated in neonates with reduced gut motility (e.g. post-operatively or drug induced). Calcium Resonium is also contraindicated in patients with hyperparathyroidism, multiple myeloma, sarcoidosis or metastatic carcinoma who may present with renal failure and hypercalcaemia and in the presence of obstructive bowel disease and in use where plasma potassium levels are below 5 mmol/litre and in patients with a history of hypersensitivity to polystyrene sulphonate resins.

Drug interactions: There have been reports of systemic alkalosis following concurrent administration of cation-exchange resins and non-absorbable cation-donating antacids and laxatives such as magnesium hydroxide and aluminium carbonate. Intestinal obstruction due to concretions of aluminium hydroxide has been reported when aluminium hydroxide has been combined with the resins (sodium form). The toxic effects of digitalis on the heart, especially various ventricular arrhythmias and AV nodal dissociation, are likely to be exaggerated if hypokalaemia is allowed to develop. Cation donating agents may reduce the potassium binding effect of Calcium Resonium. Sorbitol added to enemas may cause colonic necrosis.

Precautions: The possibility of severe potassium depletion should be considered and adequate clinical and biochemical control is essential during treatment especially in patients on digitalis.

Administration of the resin should be stopped when the serum potassium falls to 5 mmol/litre. Serum calcium levels should be estimated at weekly intervals to detect the early development of hypercalcaemia, and the dose of resin adjusted to levels at which hypercalcaemia and hypokalaemia are prevented. Like all cation-exchange resins, calcium polystyrene sulphonate is not totally selective for potassium. Hypomagnesemia and/or hypercalcaemia may occur. Accordingly, patients should be monitored for all applicable electrolyte disturbances. In the event of clinically significant constipation, treatment should be discontinued until normal bowel movement is resumed. Magnesium-containing laxatives should not be used. The patient should be positioned carefully when ingesting the resin, in order to avoid aspiration, which may lead to bronchopulmonary complications.

The safety and efficacy of sorbitol and Calcium Resonium has not been established and they should not be used together (see *Interactions*).

In children and neonates, particular care is needed with rectal administration as excessive dosage or inadequate dilution could result in impaction of the resin. Cation donating agents may reduce the potassium binding effectiveness of Calcium Resonium.

Pregnancy and lactation: No data are available regarding the use of polystyrene sulphonate resins in pregnancy and lactation. The administration of Calcium Resonium in pregnancy and during breast feeding therefore, is not advised unless, in the opinion of the physician, the potential benefits outweigh any potential risks.

Side-effects: In accordance with its pharmacological actions, the resin may give rise to sodium retention, hypokalaemia and hypercalcaemia and the related clinical manifestations (see *Warnings and precautions* and *Overdosage*). Gastric irritation, anorexia, nausea, vomiting, constipation and occasionally diarrhoea may occur. Faecal impaction following rectal administration has been reported in children, and gastro-intestinal concretions following oral administration to neonates. Intestinal obstruction has also been reported although this has been extremely rare and, possibly, a reflection of co-existing pathology, excessive dosage or inadequate dilution of the resin.

Some cases of acute bronchitis and/or bronchopneumonia associated with inhalation of particles of calcium polystyrene sulphonate have been described.

Hypercalcaemia has been reported in well-dialysed patients receiving calcium resin, and in the occasional patient with chronic renal failure. Many patients in chronic renal failure have low serum calcium and high serum phosphate, but some, who cannot be screened out beforehand, show a sudden rise in serum calcium to high levels after therapy. The risk emphasises the need for adequate biochemical control.

Overdosage: Biochemical disturbances from overdosage may give rise to clinical signs or symptoms of hypokalaemia, including irritability, confusion, delayed thought processes, muscle weakness, hyporeflexia and eventual paralysis. Apnoea may be a serious consequence of this progression. Electrocardiographic changes may be consistent with hypokalaemia; cardiac arrhythmia may occur. Appropriate measures should be taken to correct serum electrolytes and the resin should be removed from the alimentary tract by appropriate use of laxatives or enemas.

Pharmaceutical precautions Store in a dry place. Suspensions of the resin should be freshly prepared and not stored beyond 24 hours.

Legal category P.

Package quantities HDPE containers of 300 g each containing a plastic scoop which, when filled level, contains approximately 15 g.

Further information Theoretically, each gram of Calcium Resonium should take up 1.3 to 2 mmol of potassium. However, in vivo, the actual amount of potassium bound will be less than this. The sodium content of Calcium Resonium is less than 1 mg/g. Calcium content is about 8% w/w (1.6–2.4 mmol/g).

Product licence number 11723/0010.

CORDARONE* X 100
CORDARONE* X 200

Qualitative and quantitative composition
Cordarone X 100 contain 100 mg of Amiodarone Hydrochloride PhEur.
Cordarone X 200 contain 200 mg of Amiodarone Hydrochloride PhEur.

Pharmaceutical form Tablet.

Clinical particulars Treatment should be initiated and normally monitored only under hospital or specialist supervision. Oral Cordarone X is indicated only for the treatment of severe rhythm disorders not responding to other therapies or when other treatments cannot be used.

Therapeutic indications: Tachyarrhythmias associated with Wolff-Parkinson-White Syndrome.

Atrial flutter and fibrillation when other drugs cannot be used.

All types of tachyarrhythmias of paroxysmal nature including: supraventricular, nodal and ventricular tachycardias, ventricular fibrillation; when other drugs cannot be used.

Tablets are used for stabilisation and long term treatment.

Posology and method of administration:
Adults: It is particularly important that the minimum effective dose be used. In all cases the patient's management must be judged on the individual response and well being. The following dosage regimen is generally effective.

Initial stabilisation: Treatment should be started with 200 mg, three times a day and may be continued for 1 week. The dosage should then be reduced to 200 mg, twice daily for a further week.

Maintenance: After the initial period the dosage should be reduced to 200 mg daily, or less if appropriate. Rarely, the patient may require a higher maintenance dose. The scored 100 mg tablet should be used to titrate the minimum dosage required to maintain control of the arrhythmia. The maintenance dose should be regularly reviewed, especially where this exceeds 200 mg daily.

Changeover from intravenous to oral therapy: As soon as an adequate response has been obtained, oral therapy should be initiated concomitantly at the usual loading dose (200 mg three times a day). Cordarone X Intravenous should than be phased out gradually.

General considerations
Initial dosing: A high dose is needed in order to achieve adequate tissue levels rapidly.

Maintenance: Too high a dose during maintenance therapy can cause side effects which are believed to be related to high tissue levels of amiodarone and its metabolites.

Amiodarone is strongly protein bound and has an average plasma half life of 50 days (reported range 20–100 days). It follows that sufficient time must be allowed for a new distribution equilibrium to be achieved between adjustments of dosage.

It is particularly important that the minimum effective dosage is used and the patient is monitored regularly to detect the clinical features of excess amiodarone dosage. Therapy may then be adjusted accordingly.

Dosage reduction/withdrawal: Side effects slowly disappear as tissue levels fall. Following drug withdrawal, residual tissue bound amiodarone may protect the patient for up to a month. However, the likelihood of recurrence of arrhythmia during this period should be considered. In patients with potentially lethal arrhythmias the long half life is a valuable safeguard as omission of occasional doses does not significantly influence the overall therapeutic effect.

Elderly: As with all patients it is important that the minimum effective dose is used. Whilst there is no evidence that dosage requirements are different for this group of patients they may be more susceptible to bradycardia and conduction defects if too high a dose is employed. Particular attention should be paid to monitoring thyroid function. See *Contra-indications and Warnings.*

Cordarone X is for oral administration.

Contra-indications: Sinus bradycardia and sino-atrial heart block. In patients with severe conduction disturbances (high grade AV block, bifascicular or trifascicular block) or sinus node disease, Cordarone X should be used only in conjunction with a pacemaker.

Evidence or history of thyroid dysfunction. Thyroid function tests should be performed prior to therapy in all patients.

Known hypersensitivity to iodine or to amiodarone. (One 100 mg tablet contains approximately 37.5 mg iodine, one 200 mg tablet contains approximately 75 mg iodine.)

The combination of Cordarone X with drugs which may induce Torsades de Pointes is contra-indicated (see *Interactions* section).

Special warnings and special precautions for use: Too high a dosage may lead to severe bradycardia and to conduction disturbances with the appearance of an idioventricular rhythm, particularly in elderly patients or during digitalis therapy. In these circumstances, Cordarone X treatment should be withdrawn. If necessary beta-adrenostimulants or glucagon may be given.

Oral Cordarone X is not contra-indicated in patients with latent or manifest heart failure but caution should be exercised as, occasionally, existing heart failure may be worsened. In such cases, Cordarone X may be used with other appropriate therapies.

Amiodarone induces ECG changes: QT interval lengthening corresponding to prolonged repolarisation with the possible development of U and deformed T waves; these changes are evidence of its pharmacological action and do not reflect toxicity. Although there have been no literature reports on the potentiation of hepatic adverse effects of alcohol, patients should be advised to moderate their alcohol intake while taking Cordarone X.

Interactions with other medicaments and other forms of interaction: Some of the more important drugs that interact with amiodarone include warfarin, digoxin, phenytoin and any drug which prolongs the QT interval.

Amiodarone raises the plasma concentrations of highly protein bound drugs, for example oral anticoagulants and phenytoin. The dose of warfarin should be reduced accordingly. More frequent monitoring of prothrombin time both during and after amiodarone treatment is recommended. Phenytoin dosage should be reduced if signs of overdosage appear, and plasma levels may be measured.

Administration of Cordarone X to a patient already receiving digoxin will bring about an increase in the plasma digoxin concentration and thus precipitate symptoms and signs associated with high digoxin levels. Monitoring is recommeded and digoxin dosage usually has to be reduced. A synergistic effect on heart rate and atrioventricular conduction is also possible.

Combined therapy with the following drugs which prolong the QT interval is contra-indicated (see *Contra-indications* section) due to the increased risk of Torsades de Pointes; for example:

- Class Ia anti-arrhythmic drugs e.g. quinidine, procainamide, disopyramide
- Class III anti-arrhythmic drugs e.g. sotalol, bretylium
- intravenous erythromycin, co-trimoxazole or pentamidine injection
- anti-psychotics e.g. chlorpromazine, thioridazine, pimozide, haloperidol
- lithium and tricyclic anti-depressants e.g. doxepin, maprotiline, amitriptyline
- certain antihistamines e.g. terfenadine, astemizole

– anti-malarials e.g. quinine, mefloquine, chloroquine, halofantrine.

Combined therapy with the following drugs is not recommended: beta blockers and certain calcium channel inhibitors (diltiazem, verapamil); potentiation of negative chronotropic properties and conduction slowing effects may occur.

Caution should be exercised over combined therapy with the following drugs which may cause hypokalaemia: and/or hypomagnesaemia: diuretics, systemic corticosteroids, tetracosactrin, intravenous amphotericin.

In cases of hypokalaemia, corrective action should be taken and QT interval monitored. In case of Torsades de Pointes antiarrhythmic agents should not be given; pacing may be instituted and IV magnesium may be used.

Caution is advised in patients undergoing general anaesthesia, or receiving high dose oxygen therapy.

Potentially severe complications have been reported in patients taking amiodarone undergoing general anaesthesia: bradycardia unresponsive to atropine, hypotension, disturbances of conduction, decreased cardiac output.

A few cases of adult respiratory distress syndrome, most often in the period immediately after surgery, have been observed. A possible interaction with a high oxygen concentration may be implicated. The anaesthetist should be informed that the patient is taking Cordarone X.

Amiodarone may increase the plasma levels of cyclosporin when used in combination, due to a decrease in the clearance of this drug.

Pregnancy and lactation:

Pregnancy: Although no teratogenic effects have been observed in animals, there are insufficient data on the use of amiodarone during pregnancy in humans to judge any possible toxicity. However, in view of the pharmacological properties of the drug on the foetus and its effect on the foetal thyroid gland, its administration in pregnancy should be avoided.

Lactation: Amiodarone is excreted into the breast milk in significant quantities and breast-feeding is contra-indicated.

Effects on ability to drive and use machines: None stated.

Undesirable effects: Amiodarone can cause serious adverse reactions affecting the lung, liver, thyroid gland, skin and peripheral nervous system (see below). Because these reactions can be delayed, patients on long-term treatment should be carefully supervised.

Pulmonary: Cordarone X can cause pulmonary toxicity (hypersensitivity pneumonitis, alveolar/interstitial pneumonitis or fibrosis, pleuritis, bronchiolitis obliterans organising pneumonia). Sometimes this toxicity can be fatal.

Presenting features can include dyspnoea (which may be severe and unexplained by the current cardiac status), non-productive cough and deterioration in general health (fatigue, weight loss and fever). The onset is usually slow but may be rapidly progressive. Whilst the majority of cases have been reported with long term therapy, a few have occurred soon after starting treatment.

Patients should be carefully evaluated clinically and consideration given to chest X-ray before starting therapy. During treatment, if pulmonary toxicity is suspected, this should be repeated and associated with lung function testing including where possible measurement of transfer factor. Initial radiological changes may be difficult to distinguish from pulmonary venous congestion. Pulmonary toxicity has usually been reversible following early withdrawal of amiodarone therapy, with or without corticosteroid therapy. Clinical symptoms often resolve within a few weeks followed by slower radiological and lung function improvement. Some patients can deteriorate despite discontinuing Cordarone X. A few cases of adult respiratory distress syndrome, most often in the period after surgery, have been observed, resulting sometimes in fatalities (see *Interactions*).

Cardiac: Bradycardia which is generally moderate and dose dependent has been reported. In some cases (sinus node disease, elderly patients) marked bradycardia or more exceptionally sinus arrest has occurred. There have been rare instances of conduction disturbances (sino-atrial block, various degrees of AV block). Because of the long half life of amiodarone, if bradycardia is severe and symptomatic the insertion of a pacemaker should be considered. Amiodarone has a low proarrhythmic effect. However arrhythmia (new occurence or aggravation), followed in some cases by cardiac arrest has been reported; with current knowledge, it is not possible to differentiate a drug effect from the underlying cardiac condition or lack of therapeutic efficacy. This has usually occurred in combination with other precipitating factors particularly other antiarrhythmic agents, hypokalaemia and digoxin.

Hepatic: Amiodarone may be associated with a variety of hepatic effects, including cirrhosis, hepatitis and jaundice. Some fatalities have been reported, mainly following long-term therapy, although rarely they have occurred soon after starting treatment particularly after Cordarone X intravenous. It is advisable to monitor liver function particularly transaminases before treatment and six monthly thereafter.

At the beginning of therapy, elevation of serum transaminases which can be in isolation (1.5 to 3 times normal) may occur. These may return to normal with dose reduction, or sometimes spontaneously.

Isolated cases of acute liver disorders with elevated serum transaminases and/or jaundice may occur; in such cases treatment should be discontinued.

There have been reports of chronic liver disease. Alteration of laboratory tests which may be minimal (transaminases elevated 1.5 to 5 times normal) or clinical signs (possible hepatomegaly) during treatment for longer than 6 months should suggest this diagnosis. Routine monitoring of liver function tests is therefore advised. Abnormal clinical and laboratory test results usually regress upon cessation of treatment. Histological findings may resemble pseudo-alcoholic hepatitis, but they can be variable and include cirrhosis.

Thyroid: Both hyper and hypothyroidism have occurred during, or soon after, amiodarone treatment. Simple monitoring of the usual biochemical tests is confusing because some tests such as free T_4 and free T_3 may be altered where the patient is euthyroid. Clinical monitoring is therefore recommended before start of treatment, then six monthly and should be continued for some months after discontinuation of treatment. This is particularly important in the elderly. In patients whose history indicates an increased risk of thyroid dysfunction, regular assessment is recommended.

Hyperthyroidism: Clinical features such as weight loss, asthenia, restlessness, increase in heart rate, recurrence of the cardiac dysrhythmia, angina or congestive heart failure, should alert the clinician. The diagnosis may be supported by an elevated serum tri-iodothyronine (T_3), a low level of thyroid stimulating hormone (TSH) as measured by high sensitivity methods, and a reduced TSH response to thyrotrophin releasing hormone (TRH). Elevation of reverse T_3 (rT_3) may also be found.

In the case of hyperthyroidism, therapy should be withdrawn. Clinical recovery usually occurs within a few weeks, although severe cases, sometimes resulting in fatalities, have been reported.

Courses of anti-thyroid drugs have been used for the treatment of severe thyroid hyperactivity; large doses may be required initially. These may not always be effective and concomitant high dose corticosteroid therapy (e.g. 1 mg/kg prednisolone) may be required for several weeks.

Hypothyroidism: Clinical features such as weight gain, reduced activity or excessive bradycardia should suggest the diagnosis. This may be supported by an elevated serum TSH level and an exaggerated TSH response to TRH. T_4 and T_3 levels may be low. Thyroid hypofunction usually resolves within 3 months of cessation of therapy; it may be treated cautiously with L-thyroxine. Concomitant use of Cordarone X should be continued only in life threatening situations, when TSH levels may provide a guide to L-thyroxine dosage.

Ophthalmological: Patients on continuous therapy almost always develop microdeposits in the cornea. The deposits are usually only discernible by slit-lamp examinations and may rarely cause subjective symptoms such as visual haloes and blurring of vision. The deposits are considered essentially benign, do not require discontinuation of amiodarone and regress following termination of treatment. Rare cases of impaired visual acuity due to optic neuritis have been reported, although at present, the relationship with amiodarone has not been established. Unless blurred or decreased vision occurs, ophthalmological examination is recommended annually.

Dermatological: Patients taking Cordarone X can become unduly sensitive to sunlight and should be warned of this possibility. In most cases, symptoms are limited to tingling, burning and erythema of sun exposed skin but severe phototoxic reactions with blistering may be seen. Photosensitivity may persist for several months after discontinuation of Cordarone X. Photosensitivity can be minimised by limiting exposure to UV light, wearing suitable protective hats and clothing and by using a broad spectrum sun screening preparation. Rarely, a slate grey or bluish discoloration of light exposed skin, particularly on the face, may occur. Resolution of this pigmentation may be very slow once the drug is discontinued. Other types of skin rashes including isolated cases of exfoliative dermatitis have also been reported. Cases of erythema have been reported during radiotherapy.

Neurological: Peripheral neuropathy can be caused by Cordarone X. Myopathy has occasionally been reported. Both these conditions may be severe although they are usually reversible on drug withdrawal. Nightmares, vertigo, headaches, sleeplessness and paraesthesia may also occur. Tremor and ataxia have also infrequently been reported usually with complete regression after reduction of dose or withdrawal of the drug. Benign intracranial hypertension (pseudo-tumour cerebri) has been reported.

Other: Other unwanted effects occasionally reported include nausea, vomiting, metallic taste (which usually occur with loading dosage and which regress on dose reduction), fatigue, impotence, epididymo-orchitis and alopecia. Isolated cases suggesting a hypersensitivity reaction involving vasculitis, renal involvement with moderate elevation of creatinine levels or thrombocytopenia have been observed. Haemolytic or aplastic anaemia have rarely been reported.

Overdose: Animal studies indicate that amiodarone has a high LD_{50}, hence it is most unlikely that a patient will ingest an acute toxic dose. In such an event gastric lavage may be employed to reduce absorption in addition to general supportive measures. The patient should be monitored; if bradycardia occurs beta-adrenostimulants or glucagon may be given. Spontaneously resolving attacks of ventricular tachycardia may also occur. Due to the pharmacokinetics of amiodarone, adequate and prolonged surveillance of the patient, particularly cardiac status, is recommended. Neither amiodarone nor its metabolites are dialysable.

Pharmacological properties

Pharmacodynamic properties: Amiodarone hydrochloride is an antiarrhythmic.

Pharmacokinetic properties: Amiodarone is strongly protein bound and the plasma half life is usually of the order of 50 days. However there may be considerable inter-patient variation; in individual patients a half life of less than 20 days and a half life of more than 100 days has been reported. High doses of Cordarone X, for example 600 mg/day, should be given initially to achieve effective tissue levels as rapidly as possible. Owing to the long half life of the drug, a maintenance dose of only 200 mg/day, or less is usually necessary. Sufficient time must be allowed for a new distribution equilibrium to be achieved between adjustments of dose.

The long half life is a valuable safeguard for patients with potentially lethal arrhythmias as omission of occasional doses does not significantly influence the protection afforded by Cordarone X.

Preclinical safety data: There are no pre-clinical data of relevance to the prescriber which are additional to that already included in other sections of the SPC.

Pharmaceutical particulars

List of excipients: Lactose, maize starch, polyvidone, colloidal silicon dioxide, magnesium stearate.

Incompatibilities: None stated.

Shelf life: 60 months.

Special precautions for storage: The tablets should be protected from light.

Nature and contents of container: Cordarone X 100 and 200 tablets are supplied in blister packs of **28** and 30 tablets packed in cardboard cartons. The pack size in **bold** is marketed.

Instructions for use/handling: Not applicable.

Marketing authorisation numbers

Cordarone X 100 11723/0012.
Cordarone X 200 11723/0013.

Date of approval/revision of SPC June 1996.

Legal category POM.

CORDARONE* X INTRAVENOUS

Qualitative and quantitative composition Each 3 ml ampoule contains 150 mg Amiodarone Hydrochloride PhEur.

Pharmaceutical form Solution for injection.

Clinical particulars Treatment should be initiated and normally monitored only under hospital or specialist supervision. Intravenous Cordarone X is indicated only for the treatment of severe rhythm disorders not responding to other therapies or when other treatments cannot be used.

Therapeutic indications: Tachyarrhythmias associated with Wolff-Parkinson-White Syndrome.

All types of tachyarrhythmias including: supraventricular, nodal and ventricular tachycardias; atrial flutter and fibrillation; ventricular fibrillation; when other drugs cannot be used. The injection is to be used where a rapid response is required.

Posology and method of administration: Cordarone X Intravenous should only be used when facilities exist for cardiac monitoring, defibrillation, and cardiac pacing.

In children, Cordarone X Intravenous normally should be given under the supervision of a paediatric cardiologist.

IV infusion is preferred to bolus due to the haemodynamic effects sometimes associated with rapid injection.

Cordarone X Intravenous may be used prior to DC conversion.

Repeated or continuous infusion via peripheral veins may lead to local discomfort and inflammation. When repeated or continuous infusion is anticipated, administration by a central venous catheter is recommended.

The standard recommended dose is 5 mg/kg bodyweight given by intravenous infusion over a period of 20 minutes to 2 hours. This should be administered as a dilute solution in 250 ml 5% dextrose. This may be followed by repeat infusion up to 1,200 mg (approximately 15 mg/kg bodyweight) in up to 500 ml 5% dextrose per 24 hours, the rate of infusion being adjusted on the basis of clinical response.

In extreme clinical emergency the drug may, at the discretion of the clinician, be given as a slow injection of 150–300 mg in 10–20 ml 5% dextrose over a minimum of 3 minutes. This should not be repeated for at least 15 minutes.

Patients treated with Cordarone X Intravenous must be closely monitored e.g. in an intensive care unit.

When given by infusion Cordarone X may reduce drop size and, if appropriate, adjustments should be made to the rate of infusion.

Changeover from intravenous to oral therapy: As soon as an adequate response has been obtained, oral therapy should be initiated concomitantly at the usual loading dose (200 mg three times a day). Cordarone X Intravenous should then be phased out gradually.

Elderly: As with all patients it is important that the minimum effective dose is used. Whilst there is no evidence that dosage requirements are different for this group of patients they may be more susceptible to bradycardia and conduction defects if too high a dose is employed. Particular attention should be paid to monitoring thyroid function. See *Contra-indications* and *Warnings*.

Contra-indications: Sinus bradycardia and sino-atrial heart block. In patients with severe conduction disturbances (high grade AV block, bifascicular or trifascicular block) or sinus node disease, Cordarone X should be used only in conjunction with a pacemaker.

Evidence or history of thyroid dysfunction. Thyroid function tests should be performed prior to therapy in all patients.

Severe respiratory failure, circulatory collapse, or severe arterial hypotension; congestive heart failure and cardiomyopathy are also contra-indications when using Cordarone X injection as a bolus injection.

Known hypersensitivity to iodine or to amiodarone. (One ampoule contains approximately 56 mg iodine.)

The combination of Cordarone X with drugs which may induce Torsades de Pointes is contra-indicated (see *Interactions* section).

Special warnings and special precautions for use: Too high a dosage may lead to severe bradycardia and to conduction disturbances with the appearance of an idioventricular rhythm, particularly in elderly patients or during digitalis therapy. In these circumstances, Cordarone X treatment should be withdrawn. If necessary beta-adrenostimulants or glucagon may be given.

Caution should be exercised in patients with hypotension and decompensated cardiomyopathy.

Amiodarone induces ECG changes: QT interval lengthening corresponding to prolonged repolarisation with the possible development of U and deformed T waves; these changes are evidence of its pharmacological action and do not reflect toxicity.

Although there have been no literature reports on the potentiation of hepatic adverse effects of alcohol, patients should be advised to moderate their alcohol intake while taking Cordarone X.

Interaction with other medicaments and other forms of interaction: Some of the more important drugs that interact with amiodarone include warfarin, digoxin, phenytoin and any drug which prolongs the QT interval.

Amiodarone raises the plasma concentrations of highly protein bound drugs, for example oral anticoagulants and phenytoin. The dose of warfarin should be reduced accordingly. More frequent monitoring of prothrombin time both during and after amiodarone treatment is recommended. Phenytoin dosage should be reduced if signs of overdosage appear, and plasma levels may be measured.

Administration of Cordarone X to a patient already receiving digoxin will bring about an increase in the plasma digoxin concentration and thus precipitate symptoms and signs associated with high digoxin levels. Monitoring is recommended and digoxin dosage usually has to be reduced. A synergistic effect on heart rate and atrioventricular conduction is also possible.

Combined therapy with the following drugs which prolong the QT interval is contra-indicated (see *Contra-indications* section) due to the increased risk of Torsades de Pointes; for example:

- Class Ia anti-arrhythmic drugs e.g. quinidine, procainamide, disopyramide
- Class III anti-arrhythmic drugs e.g. sotalol, bretylium
- intravenous erythromycin, co-trimoxazole or pentamidine injection
- anti-psychotics e.g. chlorpromazine, thioridazine, pimozide, haloperidol
- lithium and tricyclic anti-depressants e.g. doxepin, maprotiline, amitriptyline
- certain antihistamines e.g. terfenadine, astemizole
- anti-malarials e.g. quinine, mefloquine, chloroquine, halofantrine.

Combined therapy with the following drugs is not recommended: beta blockers and certain calcium channel inhibitors (diltiazem, verapamil); potentiation of negative chronotropic properties and conduction slowing effects may occur.

Caution should be exercised over combined therapy with the following drugs which may cause hypokalaemia: and/or hypomagnesaemia: diuretics, systemic corticosteroids, tetracosactrin, intravenous amphotericin.

In cases of hypokalaemia, corrective action should be taken and QT interval monitored. In case of Torsades de Pointes antiarrhythmic agents should not be given; pacing may be instituted and IV magnesium may be used.

Caution is advised in patients undergoing general anaesthesia, or receiving high dose oxygen therapy.

Potentially severe complications have been reported in patients taking amiodarone undergoing general anaesthesia: bradycardia unresponsive to atropine, hypotension, disturbances of conduction, decreased cardiac output.

A few cases of adult respiratory distress syndrome, most often in the period immediately after surgery, have been observed. A possible interaction with a high oxygen concentration may be implicated. The anaesthetist should be informed that the patient is taking Cordarone X.

Amiodarone may increase the plasma levels of cyclosporin when used in combination, due to a decrease in the clearance of this drug.

Pregnancy and lactation:

Pregnancy: Although no teratogenic effects have been observed in animals, there are insufficient data on the use of amiodarone during pregnancy in humans to judge any possible toxicity. However, in view of the pharmacological properties of the drug on the foetus and its effect on the foetal thyroid gland, its administration in pregnancy should be avoided.

Lactation: Amiodarone is excreted into the breast milk in significant quantities and breast-feeding is contra-indicated.

Effects on ability to drive and use machines: None stated.

Undesirable effects: Rapid administration of Cordarone X Intravenous has been associated with hot flushes, sweating and nausea. A moderate and transient reduction in blood pressure may occur. Circulatory collapse may be precipitated by too rapid administration or overdosage (atropine has been used successfully in such patients presenting with bradycardia). In cases of respiratory failure, notably in asthmatics, bronchospasm and/or apnoea may also occur. Isolated cases of anaphylactic shock have been reported.

Amiodarone can cause serious adverse reactions affecting the lung, liver, thyroid gland, skin and peripheral nervous system (see below). Because these reactions can be delayed, patients on long-term treatment should be carefully supervised.

Pulmonary: Cordarone X can cause pulmonary toxicity (hypersensitivity pneumonitis, alveolar/interstitial pneumonitis or fibrosis, pleuritis, bronchiolitis obliterans organising pneumonia). Sometimes this toxicity can be fatal.

Presenting features can include dyspnoea (which may be severe and unexplained by the current cardiac status), non-productive cough and deterioration in general health (fatigue, weight loss and fever). The onset is usually slow but may be rapidly progressive. Whilst the majority of cases have been reported with long term therapy, a few have occurred soon after starting treatment.

Patients should be carefully evaluated clinically and consideration given to chest X-ray before starting therapy. During treatment, if pulmonary toxicity is suspected, this should be repeated and associated with lung function testing including where possible measurement of transfer factor. Initial radiological changes may be difficult to distinguish from pulmonary venous congestion. Pulmonary toxicity has usually been reversible following early withdrawal of amiodarone therapy, with or without corticosteroid therapy. Clinical symptoms often resolve within a few weeks followed by slower radiological and lung function improvement. Some patients can deteriorate despite discontinuing Cordarone X. A few cases of adult respiratory distress syndome, most often in the period after surgery, have been observed, resulting sometimes in fatalities (see *Interactions*).

Cardiac: Bradycardia which is generally moderate and dose dependent has been reported. In some cases (sinus node disease, elderly patients) marked bradycardia or more exceptionally sinus arrest has occurred. There have been rare instances of conduction disturbances (sino-atrial block, various degrees of AV block). Because of the long half life of amiodarone, if bradycardia is severe and symptomatic the insertion of a pacemaker should be considered. Amiodarone has a low proarrhythmic effect. However arrhythmia (new occurrence or aggravation), followed in some cases by cardiac arrest has been reported; with current knowledge, it is not possible to differentiate a drug effect from the underlying cardiac condition or lack of therapeutic efficacy. This has usually occurred in combination with other precipitating factors particularly other antiarrhythmic agents, hypokalaemia and digoxin.

Hepatic: Amiodarone may be associated with a variety of hepatic effects, including cirrhosis, hepatitis and jaundice. Some fatalities have been reported, mainly following long-term therapy, although rarely they have occurred soon after starting treatment particularly after Cordarone X Intravenous. It is advisable to monitor liver function particularly transaminases before treatment and six monthly thereafter.

At the beginning of therapy, elevation of serum transaminases which can be in isolation (1.5 to 3 times normal) may occur. These may return to normal with dose reduction, or sometimes spontaneously.

Isolated cases of acute liver disorders with elevated serum transaminases and/or jaundice may occur; in such cases treatment should be discontinued.

There have been reports of chronic liver disease. Alteration of laboratory tests which may be minimal (transaminases elevated 1.5 to 5 times normal) or clinical signs (possible hepatomegaly) during treatment for longer than 6 months should suggest this diagnosis. Routine monitoring of liver function tests is therefore advised. Abnormal clinical and laboratory test results usually regress upon cessation of treatment. Histological findings may resemble pseudo-alcoholic hepatitis, but they can be variable and include cirrhosis.

Thyroid: Both hyper and hypothyroidism have occurred during, or soon after, amiodarone treatment. Simple monitoring of the usual biochemical tests is confusing because some tests such as free T_4 and free T_3 may be altered where the patient is euthyroid. Clinical monitoring is therefore recommended before start of treatment, then six monthly and should be continued for some months after discontinuation of treatment. This is particularly important in the elderly. In patients whose history indicates an increased risk of thyroid dysfunction, regular assessment is recommended.

Hyperthyroidism: Clinical features such as weight loss, asthenia, restlessness, increase in heart rate, recurrence of the cardiac dysrhythmia, angina or congestive heart failure, should alert the clinician. The diagnosis may be supported by an elevated serum T_3, a low level of thyroid stimulating hormone (TSH) as measured by high sensitivity methods, and a reduced TSH response to TRH. Elevation of reverse T_3 (rT_3) may also be found. In the case of hyperthyroidism, therapy should be withdrawn. Clinical recovery usually occurs within a few weeks, although severe cases, sometimes resulting in fatalities, have been reported.

Courses of anti-thyroid drugs have been used for the treatment of severe thyroid hyperactivity; large doses may be required initially. These may not always be effective and concomitant high dose corticosteroid therapy (e.g. 1 mg/kg prednisolone) may be required for several weeks.

Hypothyroidism: Clinical features such as weight gain, reduced activity or excessive bradycardia should suggest the diagnosis. This may be supported by an elevated serum TSH level and an exaggerated TSH response to TRH. T_4 and T_3 levels may be low. Thyroid hypofunction usually resolves within 3 months of cessation of therapy; it may be treated cautiously with L-thyroxine. Concomitant use of Cordarone X should be continued only in life threatening situations, when TSH levels may provide a guide to L-thyroxine dosage.

Ophthalmological: Patients on continuous therapy almost always develop microdeposits in the cornea. The deposits are usually only discernible by slit-lamp examinations and may rarely cause subjective symptoms such as visual haloes and blurring of vision. The deposits are considered essentially benign, do not require discontinuation of amiodarone and regress following termination of treatment. Rare cases of impaired visual acuity due to optic neuritis have been reported, although at present, the relationship with amiodarone has not been established. Unless blurred or decreased vision occurs, ophthalmological examination is recommended annually.

Dermatological: Patients taking Cordarone X can become unduly sensitive to sunlight and should be warned of this possibility. In most cases, symptoms are limited to tingling, burning and erythema of sun exposed skin but severe phototoxic reactions with blistering may be seen. Photosensitivity may persist for several months after discontinuation of Cordarone X. Photosensitivity can be minimised by limiting exposure to UV light, wearing suitable protective hats and clothing and by using a broad spectrum sun screening preparation. Rarely, a slate grey or bluish discoloration of light exposed skin, particularly on the face, may occur. Resolution of this pigmentation may be very slow once the drug is discontinued. Other types of skin rashes including isolated cases of exfoliative dermatitis have also been reported. Cases of erythema have been reported during radiotherapy.

Neurological: Peripheral neuropathy can be caused by Cordarone X. Myopathy has occasionally been reported. Both these conditions may be severe although they are usually reversible on drug withdrawal. Nightmares, vertigo, headaches, sleeplessness and paraesthesia may also occur. Tremor and ataxia have also infrequently been reported usually with complete regression after reduction of dose or withdrawal of the drug. Benign intracranial hypertension (pseudotumour cerebri) has been reported.

Other: Other unwanted effects occasionally reported include nausea, vomiting, metallic taste (which usually occur with loading dosage and which regress on dose reduction), fatigue, impotence, epididymo-orchitis and alopecia. Isolated cases suggesting a hypersensitivity reaction involving vasculitis, renal involvement with moderate elevation of creatinine levels or thrombocytopenia have been observed. Haemolytic or aplastic anaemia have rarely been reported.

Overdose: Animal studies indicate that amiodarone has a high LD_{50}, hence it is most unlikely that a patient will ingest an acute toxic dose. In such an event gastric lavage may be employed to reduce absorption in addition to general supportive measures. The patient should be monitored; if bradycardia occurs beta-adrenostimulants or glucagon may be given. Spontaneously resolving attacks of ventricular tachycardia may also occur. Due to the pharmacokinetics of amiodarone, adequate and prolonged surveillance of the patient, particularly cardiac status, is recommended. Neither amiodarone nor its metabolites are dialysable.

Pharmacological properties

Pharmacodynamic properties: Cordarone X is a product for the treatment of tachyarrhythmias and has complex pharmacological actions. Its effects are anti-adrenergic (partial alpha and beta blockers). It has haemodynamic effects (increased blood flow and systematic/coronary vasodilation). The drug reduces myocardial oxygen consumption and has been shown to have a sparing effect of rat myocardial ATP utilisation, with decreased oxidative processes. Amiodarone inhibits the metabolic and biochemical effects of catecholamines on the heart and inhibits Na^+ and K^+ activated ATP-ase.

Pharmacokinetic properties: Pharmacokinetics of amiodarone are unusual and complex, and have not been completely elucidated. Absorption following oral administration is variable and may be prolonged, with enterohepatic cycling. The major metabolite is desethylamiodarone. Amiodarone is highly protein bound (>95%). Renal excretion is minimal and faecal excretion is the major route. A study in both healthy volunteers and patients after intravenous administration of amiodarone reported that the calculated volumes of distribution and total blood clearance using a two-compartment open model were similar for both groups. Elimination of amiodarone after intravenous injection appeared to be biexponential with a distribution phase lasting about 4 hours. The very high volume of distribution combined with a relatively low apparent volume for the central compartment suggests extensive tissue distribution. A bolus IV injection of 400 mg gave a terminal $T\frac{1}{2}$ of approximately 11 hours.

Preclinical safety data: There are no pre-clinical data of relevance to the prescriber which are additional to that already included in other sections of the SPC.

Pharmaceutical particulars

List of excipients: Benzyl alcohol, polysorbate and water for injections.

Incompatibilities: Cordarone X Intravenous is incompatible with saline and should be administered solely in 5% Dextrose solution. Solutions containing less than 2 ampoules Cordarone X Intravenous in 500 ml Dextrose 5% are unstable and should not be used.

Shelf life: 24 months.

Special precautions for storage: Protect from light.

Nature and contents of container: Each carton contains ten glass ampoules.

Instructions for use/handling: See *Posology and method of administration* section above.

Marketing authorisation number PL 11723/0014.

Date of approval/revision of SPC December 1997.

Legal category POM.

CORGARD* TABLETS

Qualitative and quantitative composition The tablets contain Nadolol 40.0 mg or 80.0 mg.

Pharmaceutical form Pale blue round biconvex tablets.

Clinical particulars

Therapeutic indications: Corgard is indicated in the management of:

Angina pectoris: For the long-term management of patients with angina pectoris by continuous medication.

Hypertension: For the long-term management of essential hypertension, either alone or in combination with other antihypertensive agents, especially thiazide-type diuretics.

Arrhythmias: For the treatment of cardiac tachyarrhythmias.

Migraine: For the prophylactic management of migraine headache. The efficacy of Corgard in the treatment of a migraine attack that has already started has not been established, and Corgard is not indicated for such use.

Thyrotoxicosis: For the relief of the symptoms of hyperthyroidism and the pre-operative preparation of patients for surgery. Nadolol may be used in conjunction with conventional antithyroid therapy.

Posology and method of administration

Adults: Dosage should be titrated gradually with at least a week between increments to assess response; individuals show considerable variation in their response to beta-adrenergic blockade.

Corgard may be given in a once daily dosage without regard to meals. The dosage interval should be increased when creatinine clearance is below 50 ml/min/1.73m².

If Corgard is to be discontinued, reduce dosage over a period of at least two weeks (see Warnings).

Angina pectoris: Initially 40 mg once daily. This may be increased at weekly intervals until an adequate response is obtained or excessive bradycardia occurs. Most patients respond to 160 mg or less daily. The value and safety of daily doses exceeding 240 mg have not been established.

Hypertension: Initially 80 mg once daily. This may be increased by a weekly increment of 80 mg or less until an optimum response is obtained. Many patients respond to 80 mg daily, and most patients respond to 240 mg or less, daily, but higher doses have been required for a few patients. In some patients it is necessary to administer a diuretic, peripheral vasodilator and/or other antihypertensive agents in conjunction with nadolol in order to achieve satisfactory response.

Treatment of hypertension associated with phaeochromocytoma may require the addition of an alpha-blocking agent.

Cardiac tachyarrhythmias: Initially 40 mg once daily. This may be increased if necessary to 160 mg once daily. If bradycardia occurs dosage should be reduced to 40 mg once daily.

Migraine: The initial dose of nadolol is 40 mg once daily. Dosage may be gradually increased in 40 mg increments until optimum migraine prophylaxis is achieved. The usual maintenance dose is 80 to 160 mg administered once daily. After 4 to 6 weeks at the maximum dose if a satisfactory response is not obtained, therapy with nadolol should be withdrawn gradually.

Thyrotoxicosis: The dosage range is 80–160 mg once daily. It has been found that most patients require a dose of 160 mg once daily. Nadolol may be used together with conventional anti-thyroid treatment. For the preparation of patients for partial thyroidectomy, nadolol should be administered in conjunction with potassium iodide for a period of 10 days prior to operation. Nadolol should be administered on the morning of operation. Post-operatively, nadolol dosage should be slowly reduced and then withdrawn following clinical stability.

Children: Safety and effectiveness in children have not been established.

Elderly: In elderly patients a low initial dose should be used so that sensitivity to side-effects may be assessed.

Renal or hepatic impairment: As with all drugs patients with impaired renal or hepatic function should be monitored.

Contra-indications: Like other drugs in this class, nadolol is contra-indicated in bronchial asthma or a history of asthma; sinus bradycardia; 2nd and 3rd degree heart block; cardiogenic shock; right ventricular failure secondary to pulmonary hypertension; congestive heart failure.

Special warnings and special precautions for use: Exacerbation of angina and myocardial infarction have occurred after abrupt discontinuation of therapy with beta-adrenergic blocking agents in patients with angina pectoris or other evidence of coronary artery insufficiency. When discontinuing long-term treatment with nadolol, the dosage should be reduced gradually over a period of at least two weeks and the patient carefully monitored.

Beta-adrenergic blockade carries the potential hazard of precipitating cardiac failure. Should this occur and it is not controlled by digitalisation, nadolol should be withdrawn, consideration being given to the foregoing warning.

Beta-blocking impairs the ability of the heart to respond to stress. It has been the usual practice to recommend withdrawal of beta-blockers several days prior to surgery. However, this may render the patient's blood pressure unstable and difficult to control during anaesthesia and the anaesthetist may wish to advise on discontinuation of therapy. In no circumstances should beta-blockers be discontinued prior to surgery in patients with phaeochromocytoma or thyrotoxicosis. In the event of emergency surgery, the effects of nadolol may be reversed by isoprenaline or noradrenaline. However, such patients may be subject to protracted severe hypotension. General anaesthetics which can cause myocardial depression, such as cyclopropane, trichloroethylene, chloroform and ether, should be avoided if nadolol is continued during surgery.

Nadolol should be administered with caution to patients with chronic obstructive airways disease. Discontinue therapy if condition relapses.

Care should be exercised in the administration of nadolol to diabetic patients since early signs of acute hypoglycaemia may be masked. It may also be necessary to adjust the dosage of hypoglycaemic drugs, or insulin doses.

There have been reports of skin rashes (including a psoriasiform type) and/or ocular changes (conjunctivitis and 'dry eye') associated with the use of beta-adrenergic blocking drugs. The reported incidence is small and in most cases the symptoms have cleared when the treatment was withdrawn. Discontinuance of the drug should be considered if any such reaction is not otherwise explicable. Cessation of the therapy with a beta-adrenergic blocker should be gradual.

Beta-blocking may mask certain signs (e.g. tachycardia) of hyperthyroidism. Patients suspected of developing thyrotoxicosis should be managed carefully to avoid abrupt withdrawal of beta-blockade which might precipitate a thyroid storm.

Precautions: Occasionally, beta-blockade with drugs such as nadolol may produce hypotension and/or marked bradycardia, resulting in vertigo, syncope or orthostatic hypotension.

Nadolol should be used with caution in patients with impaired renal or hepatic function.

Administration in renal failure: In patients with decreased renal function, dosage adjustment is necessary. The recommended dosage intervals are:

Creatinine clearance (ml/min/1.73 m²)		*Dosage interval (Hours)*
Less than	10	40–60
	10–30	24–48
	31–50	24–36
More than	50	24

Interactions with other medicaments and other forms of interaction

General anaesthetics: Those which cause myocardial depression such as chloroform, cyclopropane, trichloroethylene and ether should be avoided as the patient may be subject to protracted severe hypotension.

Myocardial depressants: Myocardial depressants such as lignocaine and procainamide may subject the patient to protracted severe hypotension.

Adrenoceptor stimulants: Beta-adrenoceptor stimulants such as isoprenaline and verapamil, or alpha-adrenoceptor stimulants such as noradrenaline and adrenaline, will reverse the hypotensive effects and increase vasoconstrictor activity.

Catecholamine-depleting drugs: e.g. Reserpine. Excessive reduction in sympathetic drive to the heart might occur. Close observation is advised.

Antihypertensives: e.g. Neurone-blocking drugs, vasodilators, diuretics. Additive hypotensive effect.

Clonidine: If Corgard and clonidine are given concurrently, clonidine should not be discontinued until several days after Corgard withdrawal.

Hypoglycaemics, insulin: Possible dosage adjustment, see Warnings.

Monoamine oxidase inhibitors: Administration of nadolol during and within 2 weeks of administration of adrenergic augmenting psychotropic drugs such as monoamine oxidase inhibitors, should be avoided, although the clinical significance is undetermined.

Pregnancy and lactation: The safety of nadolol in pregnancy has not been established and animal studies have shown some foetotoxicity. Use of any drug in pregnancy or by women of childbearing potential requires that the possible risk to mother and/or foetus be weighed against the expected therapeutic benefit.

Nadolol is excreted in human milk; therefore nursing mothers should only receive nadolol if deemed essential.

Effects on ability to drive and use machines: None known.

Undesirable effects: Most patients tolerate nadolol well. Side-effects resemble those reported with other beta-blocking drugs and rarely require withdrawal of treatment. Those reported infrequently include gastro-intestinal effects, bradycardia, fatigue, light-headedness, cold extremities, insomnia, paraesthesia, dryness of the mouth and alopecia. Cardiac insufficiency, hypotension and AV block have occurred on rare occasions.

Overdose: Excessive bradycardia should be treated initially with atropine. If there is no response, isoprenaline may be administered with caution.

Cardiac failure should be managed by digitalisation and diuretics. Glucagon has also been reported to be useful.

Hypotension may be managed with vasopressors such as adrenaline.

Bronchospasm may be counteracted by isoprenaline and aminophylline.

Pharmacological properties

Pharmacodynamic properties: Nadolol is a beta-adrenergic receptor blocking agent with a prolonged activity, permitting once-daily dosage in angina, hypertension, cardiac arrhythmias, the prophylaxis of migraine, and the relief of hyperthyroid symptoms.

Nadolol is not metabolised. It has no membrane stabilising or intrinsic sympathomimetic activity, and its only effect on the autonomic nervous system is one of beta-adrenergic blockade. Nadolol is nonselective.

Receptor blockade by nadolol results in protection from excessive inappropriate sympathetic activity. Nadolol reduces the number and severity of attacks of angina pectoris by blocking response to catecholamine stimulation and thus lowers the oxygen requirement of the heart at any given level of effort.

Nadolol reduces both supine and erect blood pressure. Like other beta-blockers nadolol exerts an antiarrhythmic action. Nadolol has been shown to reduce the rapid ventricular response which accompanies atrial fibrillation/flutter by slowing conduction through the A-V node. Beta-blockade is of particular value in arrhythmias caused by increased levels of, or sensitivity of the heart to, circulating catecholamines, e.g. arrhythmias associated with phaeochromocytoma, thyrotoxicosis, or exercise. Nadolol is effective in reducing ventricular premature beats in selected patients.

Nadolol exerts an effect in the prophylaxis of migraine by a mechanism which may involve prevention of vasoconstriction in the area served by the internal carotid artery and prevention of excessive adrenergic vasodilation in the external carotid artery.

Nadolol alleviates the symptoms of thyrotoxicosis and provides symptomatic control before and during thyroid surgery.

Beta-blocking agents have been shown in large scale studies to reduce mortality by preventing reinfarction and sudden death in patients surviving their first myocardial infarction.

Pharmacokinetic particulars: About 30 percent of an oral dose of Corgard is absorbed. Peak serum concentrations usually occur in 3 to 4 hours after drug administration. The presence of food in the gastrointestinal tract does not affect the rate or extent of Corgard absorption. Approximately 30 percent of the Corgard present in serum is reversibly bound to plasma protein. Unlike most available beta-blocking agents, Corgard is not metabolised, and is excreted unchanged principally by the kidneys. The serum half-life of therapeutic doses of Corgard is relatively long, ranging from 20 to 24 hours (permitting once daily dosage). A significant correlation between minimum steady-state serum concentrations of Corgard and total oral daily dose has been demonstrated in hypertensive patients; however, the observed dose-response range is wide and proper dosage requires individual titration.

Preclinical safety data: None stated.

Pharmaceutical particulars

List of excipients: The tablets also contain citric acid anhydrous, polyvidone, corn starch, microcrystalline cellulose, magnesium stearate, indigo carmine (E132) and indigo carmine aluminium lake.

Incompatibilities: Not applicable.

Shelf life: 48 months.

Special precautions for storage: Store below 25°C.

Nature and contents of container: Amber glass bottles containing 100 tablets, foil pouches of 100 tablets and blisters in cartons containing 28 tablets.

Instruction for use/handling: None stated.

Marketing authorisation numbers
Corgard tablets 40 mg 11723/0099
Corgard tablets 80 mg 11723/0100

Date of approval/revision of SPC 24 November 1995.

Legal category POM.

CORGARETIC* TABLETS

Qualitative and quantitative composition The 40 mg tablets contain nadolol 40.0 mg and bendrofluazide 5.0 mg. The 80 mg tablets contain nadolol 80.0 mg and bendrofluazide 5.0 mg.

Pharmaceutical form Round biconvex tablet.

Clinical particulars

Therapeutic indications: For the treatment of hypertension. The combination of a diuretic and a beta-blocker may be of particular value in patients whose blood pressure has not been adequately controlled with either component given alone.

Posology and method of administration

Adults: One or two tablets once daily to a maximum of 160 mg nadolol and 10 mg bendrofluazide. For doses of nadolol in excess of 160 mg, the combination product may not be appropriate because an excessive dose of thiazide component may be administered.

Dosage should be titrated gradually with at least a week between increments to assess response; individuals show considerable variation in their response to beta-adrenergic blockade.

Corgaretic may be given in a once daily dosage without regard to meals.

If Corgaretic is to be discontinued, reduce dosage over a period of at least two weeks (see Warnings).

Children: Safety and effectiveness in children have not been established.

Elderly: In elderly patients a low initial dose should be used so that sensitivity to side-effects may be assessed. As with all drugs, patients with impaired renal or hepatic function should be monitored.

Administration in renal failure: Increased blood levels of nadolol occur in the presence of renal failure. Although non-renal elimination does occur, dosage adjustments are necessary in this patient group. The total daily dose of Corgaretic should be reduced or the dose interval increased. Corgaretic, however, would not be appropriate for patients with severe renal impairment since loop diuretics (e.g. frusemide) rather than a thiazide are preferred for such patients.

Method of administration: Oral.

Contra-indications: In bronchial asthma or a history of asthma; sinus bradycardia and 2nd and 3rd degree heart block; cardiogenic shock; right ventricular failure secondary to pulmonary hypertension; congestive heart failure, anuria, past sensitivity to thiazide diuretics or any sulphonamide-derived drugs.

Special warnings and special precautions for use

Warnings: Exacerbation of angina and myocardial infarction have occurred after abrupt discontinuation of therapy with beta-adrenergic blocking agents in patients with angina pectoris or other evidence of coronary artery insufficiency. When discontinuing long-term treatment with nadolol, the dosage should be reduced gradually over a period of at least two weeks and the patient carefully monitored.

Beta-adrenergic blockade carries the potential hazard of precipitating cardiac failure. Should this occur and it is not controlled by digitalisation, nadolol should be withdrawn, consideration being given to the foregoing warning. Beta-blockade impairs the ability of the heart to respond to stress. It has been the usual practice to recommend withdrawal of beta-blockers several days prior to surgery. However, this may render the patient's blood pressure unstable and difficult to control during anaesthesia and the anaesthetist may wish to advise on discontinuation of therapy. In no circumstances should beta-blockers be discontinued prior to surgery in patients with phaeochromocytoma or thyrotoxicosis. In the event of emergency surgery, the effects of nadolol may be reversed by isoprenaline or noradrenaline. However, such patients may be subject to protracted severe hypotension. General anaesthetics which can cause myocardial depression such as cyclopropane, trichloroethylene, chloroform and ether, should be avoided if nadolol is continued during surgery.

Nadolol should be administered with caution to patients with chronic obstructive airways disease. Discontinue therapy if condition relapses.

Diabetic patients should be monitored closely as nadolol may mask the early signs of acute hypoglycaemia and thiazide diuretics can lower insulin tolerance. Therefore dosages of hypoglycaemic drugs or insulin doses may need adjustment.

There have been reports of skin rashes (including a psoriasiform type) and/or ocular changes (conjunctivitis and 'dry eye') associated with the use of beta-adrenergic blocking drugs. The reported incidence is small and in most cases the symptoms have cleared when the treatment was withdrawn. Discontinuance of the drug should be considered if any reaction is not otherwise explicable. Cessation of the therapy with a beta-adrenergic blocker should be gradual.

Beta-blockade may mask certain clinical signs (e.g. tachycardia) of hyperthyroidism. Patients suspected of developing thyrotoxicosis should be managed carefully to avoid abrupt withdrawal of beta-blockade which might precipitate a thyroid storm.

Precautions: Occasionally, beta-blockade with drugs such as nadolol may produce hypotension and/or marked bradycardia, resulting in vertigo, syncope or orthostatic hypotension.

Nadolol should be used with caution in patients with impaired renal or hepatic function (see Dosage and Administration section for dosage adjustment in renal failure).

Periodic determination of serum electrolytes to detect possible imbalance e.g. hyponatraemia, hypochloric alkalosis and hypokalaemia should be performed at regular intervals.

Potassium depletion is a danger to digitalised patients or those with hepatic cirrhosis with ascites. In patients with renal disease, thiazides may precipitate uraemia and cumulative effects of the drug may develop. In patients with impaired renal function, minor alterations of fluid and electrolyte balance may precipitate hepatic coma.

Thiazide diuretics may raise serum uric acid levels, thus exacerbating gout in susceptible patients.

Pathologic changes in the parathyroid gland with hypercalcaemia and hypophosphataemia have been observed in a few patients during prolonged thiazide therapy.

The possibility that thiazides may exacerbate or activate systemic lupus erythematosus has been reported.

Interactions with other medicaments and other forms of interaction

General anaesthetics: Those which cause myocardial depression such as chloroform, cyclopropane, trichloroethylene and ether should be avoided as the patient may be subject to protracted severe hypotension.

Myocardial depressants: Such as lignocaine and procainamide may potentiate the hypotensive action of Nadolol and lead to severe hypotension.

Adrenoceptor stimulants: Beta-adrenoceptor stimulants such as isoprenaline or alpha-adrenoceptor stimulants such as noradrenaline, adrenaline, will reverse the hypotensive effects and increase vasoconstrictor activity. Thiazides may decrease the arterial responsiveness to noradrenaline.

Catecholamine depleting drugs: e.g. reserpine. Excessive reduction in sympathetic drive to the heart might occur. Close observation is advised.

Antihypertensives: e.g. neurone-blocking drugs, vasodilators, diuretics. Additive hypotensive effect.

Hypoglycaemic, insulin: Possible dosage adjustment, see Warnings section.

Clonidine: If nadolol and clonidine are given concurrently, clonidine should not be discontinued until several days after nadolol withdrawal.

Monoamine oxidase inhibitors: Administration of nadolol during and within two weeks of administration of adrenergic augmenting psychotropic drugs such as monoamine oxidase inhibitors, should be avoided, although the clinical significance is undetermined.

Tubocurarine: Thiazides may increase the responsiveness to Tubocurarine.

Pregnancy and lactation: The safety of nadolol in pregnancy has not been established and animal studies have shown some foetotoxicity. The use of diuretics in otherwise healthy pregnant women with or without mild oedema is contra-indicated. The hazards of using thiazides include foetal or neonatal jaundice, thrombocytopenia and possibly other adverse reactions which have occurred in the adult. Nadolol and bendrofluazide are excreted in human milk. Corgaretic is therefore not considered suitable for pregnant patients or nursing mothers.

Effects on ability to drive and use machines: None.

Undesirable effects: Most patients tolerate Corgaretic well.

Nadolol: Side-effects resemble those reported with other beta-blocking drugs and rarely require withdrawal of treatment. Those reported infrequently include gastro-intestinal effects, bradycardia, fatigue, light-headedness, cold extremities, insomnia, paraesthesia, dryness of the mouth and alopecia. Cardiac insufficiency, hypotension and AV block have occurred on rare occasions.

Thiazides: Those reported with the use of thiazides

include hypokalaemia, anorexia, gastric irritation, nausea, vomiting, cramping, diarrhoea, intrahepatic cholestatic jaundice, pancreatitis, dizziness, vertigo, headache, xanthopsia, leucopenia, agranulocytosis, thrombocytopenia, aplastic anaemia, purpura, photosensitivity, rash, urticaria, necrotising angiitis, hyperglycaemia, glycosuria, hyperuricaemia, muscle spasm, weakness and restlessness.

Overdose: Excessive bradycardia should be treated initially with atropine. If there is no response, isoprenaline may be administered with caution.

Cardiac failure should be managed by digitalisation and diuretics. Glucagon has also been reported to be useful.

Hypotension may be managed with vasopressors such as adrenaline.

Bronchospasm may be counteracted by isoprenaline and aminophylline.

Pharmacological properties

Pharmacodynamic properties: Nadolol is a beta-adrenergic receptor blocking agent. It reduces blood pressure and exerts an antiarrhythmic action. It has no membrane stabilising or intrinsic sympathomimetic activity and its only effect on the autonomic nervous system is one of beta-adrenergic blockade. Nadolol is non-selective. It has a low lipid solubility. It can be efficiently removed from the general circulation by haemodialysis.

Bendrofluazide is a thiazide diuretic which interferes with renal tubular electrolyte reabsorption, thereby increasing sodium and water excretion.

Pharmacokinetic properties: About 30 percent of an oral dose of nadolol is absorbed. Peak serum concentrations usually occur in 3 to 4 hours after drug administration. The presence of food in the gastro-intestinal tract does not affect the rate or extent of nadolol absorption. Approximately 30 percent of the nadolol present in serum is reversibly bound to plasma protein. Unlike most available beta-blocking agents, nadolol is not metabolised and is excreted unchanged principally by the kidneys. The serum half-life of therapeutic doses of nadolol is relatively long, ranging from 20 to 24 hours (permitting once daily dosage). A significant correlation between minimum steady-state serum concentrations of Nadolol and total oral daily dose has been demonstrated in hypertensive patients, however, the observed dose-response range is wide and proper dosage requires individual titration.

Bendrofluazide is almost completely absorbed from the gastrointestinal tract. It is extensively metabolised, 30 percent being excreted unchanged in the urine. Its plasma half-life is 3 to 4 hours, its biological half-life being much longer.

Preclinical safety data: None stated.

Pharmaceutical particulars

List of excipients: Microcrystalline Cellulose PhEur, Pregelatinised Maize Starch BP, Povidone K30 BP, Sodium Starch Glycolate BP, Magnesium Stearate PhEur, Blue No 2 Beadlets (E132), lactose anhydrous.

Incompatibilities: None known.

Shelf life: 36 months.

Special precautions for storage: Store below 25°C, avoid excessive heat, protect from moisture and light.

Nature and contents of container: Packs of 100 tablets supplied in either amber glass bottles or HDPE bottles.

Packs of 28 tablets supplied in foil strips or PVC blisters.

Instructions for use/handling: None.

Marketing authorisation numbers
40 mg tablets 11723/0101
80 mg tablets 11723/0102

Date of approval/revision of SPC 28 February 1996.

Legal category POM.

DANOL CAPSULES

Qualitative and quantitative composition
Danol 100 mg Capsules: Danazol 100 mg.
Danol 200 mg Capsules: Danazol 200 mg.

Pharmaceutical form Capsule.

Clinical particulars

Therapeutic indications: Danol capsules are recommended for the treatment of:

(1) Endometriosis, to control pain, pelvic tenderness and other associated symptoms and to resolve or reduce the extent of endometriotic foci. Danol capsules may be used as sole therapy or in preparation for or following surgery.

(2) Dysfunctional uterine bleeding presenting as menorrhagia, to control excessive blood loss and to control associated dysmenorrhoea.

(3) For the treatment of severe cyclical mastalgia with or without nodularity (fibrocystic disease) unresponsive to counselling or simple analgesics, to reduce pain, tenderness and nodularity.

(4) For the control of benign, multiple or recurrent breast cysts in conjunction with aspiration.

(5) Severe symptomatic gynaecomastia, both idiopathic as well as drug induced, to reduce the size of the breast and to control associated pain and tenderness.

(6) Pre-operative thinning of the endometrium prior to hysteroscopic endometrial ablation.

Posology and method of administration

Adults: Danol capsules should be given as a continuous course, dosage being adjusted according to the severity of the condition and the patient's response. In fertile females, Danol capsules should be started during menstruation, preferably on the first day, to avoid exposing a pregnancy to its possible effects. Where doubt exists, appropriate checks should be made to exclude pregnancy before starting medication. Females of child-bearing age should employ non-hormonal contraception throughout the course of treatment.

In endometriosis, the recommended dosage is 200 mg to 800 mg daily in a course of treatment lasting normally six months, although up to nine months may be necessary in some cases. Dosage should be increased if normal cyclical bleeding still persists after two months therapy, a higher dosage (not exceeding 800 mg per day) may also be needed for severe disease.

For dysfunctional bleeding presenting as menorrhagia, the dosage should be 200 mg daily, normally for 3 months.

In severe cyclical mastalgia, dosage normally ranges from 100 mg to 400 mg daily according to the severity of the symptoms, a course of treatment normally lasting 3–6 months.

In benign breast cysts, treatment should commence at a dose of 300 mg daily, a course of treatment normally lasting 3 to 6 months.

In gynaecomastia a six month course of therapy is recommended at a dose of 200 mg daily in adolescents which may be increased to 400 mg daily if no response is obtained after two months. Adults may be given 400 mg daily.

For pre-operative thinning of the endometrium, the usual dose is 400–800 mg daily given as a continuous course normally lasting 3–6 weeks.

Elderly: Danol is not recommended.

Children: Danol is not recommended.

The capsules are for oral administration.

Contra-indications:

1. Pregnancy.
2. Breast feeding:
3. Markedly impaired hepatic, renal or cardiac function.
4. Porphyria.
5. Thromboembolic disease.
6. Androgen dependent tumour.
7. Undiagnosed abnormal genital bleeding.

Special warnings and special precautions for use: Particular care should be observed when using Danol in patients with hepatic or renal disease, hypertension or other cardiovascular disease and in any state which may be exacerbated by fluid retention as well as in diabetes mellitus, polycythaemia, epilepsy, lipoprotein disorder, in those with a history of thrombosis or thromboembolic disease, and in those who have shown marked or persistent androgenic reaction to previous gonadal steroid therapy. Adjustment in concomitant therapy may be called for particularly in patients with hypertension, diabetes mellitus or epilepsy when introducing or discontinuing Danol as well as during Danol treatment.

Caution is advised in patients with migraine.

Until more is known, caution is advised in the use of Danol in the presence of known or suspected malignant disease (see also *Contra-indications*). The presence of carcinoma should be excluded before continuing Danol therapy if breast nodules persist or enlarge during treatment.

In the event of virilisation, Danol should be withdrawn. Androgenic reactions generally prove reversible, but continued use of Danol after evidence of androgenic virilisation increases the risk of irreversible androgenic effects.

In addition to clinical monitoring in all patients, appropriate laboratory monitoring should be considered which may include periodic measurement of hepatic function and haematological state. Danol should be stopped if any clinically significant adverse event arises, and particularly if there is evidence of virilisation, papilloedema, headache, visual disturbances or other signs or symptoms of raised intracranial pressure, jaundice or other indication of significant hepatic disturbance, thrombosis or thromboembolism. The lowest effective dose of Danol should always be sought.

Experience of long term therapy with Danol is limited. Whilst a course of therapy may need to be repeated, care should be observed. The long-term risk of 17-alkylated steroids (including benign hepatic adenomata and peliosis hepatis) and hepatic carcinoma should be considered when danazol, which is chemically related to those compounds, is used for periods longer than those normally recommended.

Interactions with other medicaments and other forms of interaction: (see also *Pharmacological properties, Pharmacodynamic properties*): Anti-convulsant therapy: Danol may affect the plasma level of carbamazepine and possibly the patient's response to this agent and to phenytoin. With phenobarbitone it is likely that similar interaction would occur.

Anti-diabetic therapy: Danol can cause insulin resistance.

Anti-coagulant therapy: Danol can potentiate the action of warfarin.

Anti-hypertensive therapy: Possibly through promotion of fluid retention, Danol can oppose the action of anti-hypertensive agents.

Cyclosporin: Danol can increase the plasma level of cyclosporin.

Concomitant steroids: Although specific instances have not been described, it is likely that interactions will occur between Danol and gonadal steroid therapy.

Migraine therapy: Danol may itself provoke migraine and possibly reduce the effectiveness of medication to prevent that condition.

Ethyl alcohol: Subjective intolerance in the form of nausea and shortness of breath has been reported.

Alpha calcidol: Danol may increase the calcaemic response in primary hypoparathyroidism necessitating a reduction in dosage of this agent.

Interactions with laboratory function tests: Danazol treatment may interfere with laboratory determination of testosterone or plasma proteins.

Pregnancy and lactation: There is epidemiological and toxicological evidence of hazard in human pregnancy. Danazol is known to be associated with the risk of virilisation to the female foetus if administered during human pregnancy. Danazol should not be used during pregnancy. Women of childbearing age should be advised to use an effective, non-hormonal, method of contraception. If the patient conceives during therapy Danazol should be stopped. Danazol has the theoretical potential for androgenic effects in breast-fed infants and therefore either danazol therapy or breast-feeding should be discontinued.

Effects on ability to drive and use machines: No special warning is felt necessary.

Undesirable effects: Side effects: The possible causal relationship between Danol and many of the following events reportedly associated with its use remains to be defined.

Androgenic effects include weight gain, acne and seborrhoea. Hirsutism, hair loss, voice change, which may take the form of hoarseness, sore throat or instability or deepening of pitch may occur. Hypertrophy of the clitoris is rare.

Other possible endocrine effects include menstrual disturbances in the form of spotting, alteration of the timing of the cycle and amenorrhoea. Although cyclical bleeding and ovulation usually return within 60–90 days after Danol, persistent amenorrhoea has occasionally been reported. Flushing, vaginal dryness and irritation and reduction in breast size may reflect a lowering of oestrogen. In the male a modest reduction in spermatogenesis may be evident during treatment. Insulin resistance may be increased in diabetes mellitus but symptomatic hypoglycaemia in non-diabetic patients has also been reported as has an increase in plasma glucagon level.

Danol may aggravate epilepsy and expose the condition in those so predisposed. Cutaneous reactions include rashes, which may be maculopapular, petechial, or purpuric or may take an urticarial form and may be accompanied by facial oedema. Associated fever has also been reported. Rarely, sunsensitive rash has been noted. Inflammatory erythematous nodules, changes in skin pigmentation and exfoliative dermatitis have also been reported.

Musculo-skeletal reactions include backache and muscle cramps which can be severe, creatine phosphokinase level may also rise. Muscle tremors, fasciculation, limb pain, joint pain and joint swelling have also been reported.

Cardiovascular reactions may include exacerbation of hypertension, palpitation and tachycardia.

Benign intracranial hypertension, visual disturbances which may take the form of blurring or difficulty in focusing and in wearing contact lenses or need for temporary alteration in refractive correction have been noted.

Haematological responses include an increase in red cell and platelet count. Reversible erythrocytosis or polycythaemia may be provoked. Eosinophilia, leucopenia and thrombocytopenia have also been noted. Thrombolic events have also been observed.

Hepatic reactions include modest increases in serum transaminase levels and rarely cholestatic jaundice. Rare occurrences of benign hepatic adenomata and peliosis hepatis have been observed with long term use.

Rare cases of pancreatitis have been reported.

Fluid retention may explain the occasional reports of carpal tunnel syndrome. Danol capsules may also provoke migraine.

Possible psychical reactions include increased appetite, emotional lability, anxiety, depressed mood, nervousness and changes in libido. Dizziness, vertigo, nausea, headache, fatigue and epigastric and pleuritic pain have also been noted.

A temporary alteration of lipoproteins in the form of an increase in LDL cholesterol, a decrease in HDL, affecting all subfractions, and a decrease in apolipoproteins AI and AII have been reported with Danol in the female. The clinical significance of these changes is not established.

Other metabolic events have been reported, including induction of amino-levulinic acid (ALA) synthetase, and reduction in thyroid binding globulin, T4, with increased uptake of T3 but without disturbance of thyroid stimulating hormone or free thyroxine index, is also likely during therapy.

Haematuria has rarely been reported with prolonged use in patients with hereditary angioedema.

Overdose: Available evidence suggests that acute overdosage, would be unlikely to give rise to immediate serious reactions.

In the case of acute overdosage, the drug should be removed by emesis or stomach pump (if ingestion is recent) and the patient should be kept under observation in case of any delayed reactions.

Pharmacological properties

Pharmacodynamic properties: Danazol, 17a-pregna-2,4-dien-20-yno(2,3-d)-isoxazol-17-ol, is a synthetic steroid derived from ethisterone. Its pharmacological properties include:

1. Relatively marked affinity for androgen receptors, less marked affinity for progesterone receptors and least affinity for oestrogen receptors. Danazol is a weak androgen but in addition antiandrogenic, progestogenic, antiprogestogenic, oestrogenic and antioestrogenic actions have been observed.

2. Interference with the synthesis of gonadal steroids, possibly by inhibition of the enzymes of steroidogenesis, including 3β hydroxysteroid dehydrogenase, 17β hydroxysteroid dehydrogenase, 17 hydroxylase, 17,20 lyase, 11β hydroxylase, 21 hydroxylase and cholesterol side chain cleavage enzymes, or alternatively by inhibition of the cyclic AMP accumulation usually induced by gonadotrophic hormones in granulosa and luteal cells.

3. Inhibition of the mid-cycle surge of FSH and LH as well as alterations in the pulsatility of LH. Danazol can also reduce the mean plasma levels of these gonadotrophins after the menopause.

4. A wide range of actions on plasma proteins, including increasing prothrombin, plasminogen, antithrombin III, alpha-2 macroglobulin, C1 esterase inhibitor, and erythropoietin and reducing fibrinogen, thyroid binding and sex hormone binding globulins. Danazol increases the proportion and concentration of testosterone carried unbound in plasma. The suppressive effects of danazol on the hypothalmic-pituitary-gonadal axis are reversible, cyclical activity reappearing normally within 60–90 days after therapy.

Pharmacokinetic properties: Danazol is absorbed from the gastrointestinal tract, peak plasma concentrations of 50–80 ng/ml being reached approximately 2–3 hours after dosing. Compared to the fasting state, the bioavailability has been shown to increase 3 fold when the drug is taken with a meal with a high fat content. It is thought that food stimulates bile flow which facilitates the dissolution and absorption of danazol, a highly lipophilic compound.

The apparent plasma elimination half life of danazol in a single dose is approximately 3–6 hours. With multiple doses this may increase to approximately 26 hours.

None of the metabolites of danazol, which have been isolated, exhibits pituitary inhibiting activity comparable to that of danazol.

Few data on excretion routes and rates exist. In the monkey 36% of a radioactive dose was recoverable in the urine and 48% in the faeces within 96 hours.

Preclinical safety data: There are no preclinical data of relevance to the prescriber which are additional to that already included in other sections of the SPC.

Pharmaceutical particulars

List of excipients: Maize starch, lactose, purified talc, magnesium stearate.

Incompatibilities: None.

Shelf life: 60 months.

Special precautions for storage: None.

Nature and contents of container: PVC blister pack compound of polyvinyl chloride (thickness 250 μm) sealed to an aluminium foil (thickness 20 μm). The blister are then packed in a cardboard carton. Pack sizes: 50, 60 and 100 capsules.

Instructions for use/handling: Not applicable.

Marketing authorisation numbers

Danol 100 mg Capsules 11723/0015
Danol 200 mg Capsules 11723/0016

Date of approval/revision of SPC January 1998.

Legal category POM.

DERMALEX* SKIN LOTION

Qualitative and quantitative composition Dermalex Skin Lotion contains Hexachlorophane USP 0.5 w/v.

Pharmaceutical form Skin lotion.

Clinical particulars

Therapeutic indications: For topical application as an antiseptic emollient for use in areas of unbroken skin where infection is likely; including the sacral area and pressure points in the immobile elderly.

Posology and method of administration:

Adults and children over 2 years: Apply sparingly as a routine every 4 to 6 hours and after washing.

Dermalex should not be administered except on medical advice to children under 2 years of age.

Contra-indications: Dermalex Skin Lotion should not be applied to broken skin, open pressure sores, seriously burnt skin or mucous membranes.

Dermalex Skin Lotion is contra-indicated in pregnancy and in nursing mothers.

Dermalex should not be administered except on medical advice to children under two years of age.

Special warnings and special precautions for use: During regular use in the treatment of pressure sores it is inadvisable to apply to areas of the skin in excess of half of the total body surface area.

Interactions with other medicaments and other forms of interaction: It is important to ensure that no barrier creams are used on a patient using Dermalex Skin Lotion.

Pregnancy and lactation: There is evidence of hazard to neonates. It is therefore advised that the product should not be used during pregnancy or by lactating mothers.

Effects on ability to drive and to use machines: None known.

Undesirable effects: None known.

Overdose: No cases of intoxication with Dermalex Skin Lotion due to deliberate or accidental overdosage have been reported to the company. It is considered that overdosage is unlikely to be a problem.

Pharmacological properties

Pharmacodynamic properties: Hexachlorophane is a bisphenol anti-bacterial agent which is particularly effective against gram positive organisms.

Pharmacokinetic properties: Hexachlorophane is absorbed onto the skin and multiple contact results in sustained degerming activity. It is absorbed through the skin but does not accumulate in the blood with continued use.

The majority of hexachlorophane is probably distributed very rapidly in the lipophilic tissue-compartments. A small amount is slowly excreted unchanged in the urine.

The remainder is metabolised by the liver to glucoronide conjugate which is excreted in the bile and the faeces.

Preclinical safety data: There is no pre-clinical data of relevance to the prescriber which are additional to that already included in other sections of the SPC.

Pharmaceutical particulars

List of excipients: Squalane, allantoin, butylated hydroxyanisole, cetyl alcohol, decyloleate, lanoline anhydrous, octylstearate, propyl paraben, stearic acid, carbomer, triethanolomine, methyl paraben, disodium EDTA, sodium lauryl sulphate, sorbitol powder, perfume, water.

Incompatibilities: None known.

Shelf life: 36 months.

Special precautions for storage: To be stored at a temperature not exceeding 25°C.

Nature and contents of container: Blow moulded polyethylene bottle of 60 ml, 100 ml and 250 ml. 60 ml and 100 ml bottles have a polyethylene plug and polyethylene screw cap or a polypropylene screw cap and the 250 ml bottle has a polyethylene or polypropylene dispenser/cap.

Instructions for use/handling: Not applicable.

Marketing authorisation holder: The Dermalex Company Limited.

Marketing authorisation number 1983/5000R

Date of approval/revision of SPC October 1996.

Legal category P.

EPILIM*

Qualitative and quantitative composition

Epilim 500 Enteric Coated: 500 mg Sodium Valproate PhEur.

Epilim 200 Enteric Coated: 200 mg Sodium Valproate PhEur.

Epilim 100 mg Crushable: 100 mg Sodium Valproate PhEur.

Epilim Syrup and Liquid: 200 mg Sodium Valproate PhEur per 5 ml.

Pharmaceutical form

Epilim 500 Enteric Coated: Enteric coated tablets.
Epilim 200 Enteric Coated: Enteric coated tablets.
Epilim 100 mg Crushable: Tablets.
Epilim Syrup: Syrup.
Epilim Liquid: Liquid.

Clinical particulars

Therapeutic indications: In the treatment of generalised, partial or other epilepsy. In women of child bearing age, Epilim should be used only in severe cases or in those resistant to other treatment.

Posology and method of administration: Epilim tablets, syrup and liquid are for oral administration. Daily dosage requirements vary according to age and body weight.

Monotherapy: Usual requirements are as follows:

Adults: Dosage should start at 600 mg daily increasing by 200 mg at three day intervals until control is achieved. This is generally within the dosage range 1000 mg to 2000 mg per day, i.e. 20–30 mg/kg body weight. Where adequate control is not achieved within this range the dose may be further increased to 2500 mg per day.

Children over 20 kg: Initial dosage should be 400 mg/day (irrespective of weight) with spaced increases until control is achieved; this is usually within the range 20–30 mg/kg body weight per day. Where adequate control is not achieved within this range the dose may be increased to 35 mg/kg body weight per day.

Children under 20 kg: 20 mg/kg of body weight per day; in severe cases this may be increased but only in patients in whom plasma valproic acid levels can be monitored. Above 40 mg/kg/day, clinical chemistry and haematological parameters should be monitored.

Use in the elderly: Although the pharmacokinetics of valproate are modified in the elderly, they have limited clinical significance and dosage should be determined by seizure control. The volume of distribution is increased in the elderly and because of decreased binding to serum albumin, the proportion of free drug is increased. This will affect the clinical interpretation of plasma valproic acid levels.

In patients with renal insufficiency: It may be necessary to decrease dosage. Dosage should be adjusted according to clinical monitoring since monitoring of plasma concentrations may be misleading (see *Pharmacokinetic properties*).

In patients where adequate control has been achieved Epilim Chrono formulations are interchangeable with other Epilim conventional or modified release formulations on an equivalent daily dosage basis.

Epilim tablets, syrup and liquid may be given twice daily. Uncoated tablets may be crushed if necessary.

Combined therapy: When starting Epilim in patients already on other anticonvulsants, these should be tapered slowly: initiation of Epilim therapy should then be gradual, with target dose being reached after about 2 weeks. In certain cases it may be necessary to raise the dose by 5 to 10 mg/kg/day when used in combination with anticonvulsants which induce liver enzyme activity, e.g. phenytoin, phenobarbitone and carbamazepine. Once known enzyme inducers have been withdrawn it may be possible to maintain seizure control on a reduced dose of Epilim. When barbiturates are being administered concomitantly and particularly if sedation is observed (particularly in children) the dosage of barbiturate should be reduced.

NB: In children requiring doses higher than 40 mg/kg/day clinical chemistry and haematological parameters should be monitored.

Optimum dosage is mainly determined by seizure control and routine measurement of plasma levels is unnecessary. However, a method for measurement of plasma levels is available and may be helpful where there is poor control or side effects are suspected.

Contra-indications: Hypersensitivity to sodium valproate. Active liver disease, family history of severe hepatic dysfunction, particularly drug related, porphyria.

Special warnings and special precautions for use:

Diabetic patients: Valproate is eliminated mainly through the kidneys, partly in the form of ketone bodies; this may give false positives in the urine testing of possible diabetics (see *Pregnancy and lactation, Undesirable effects*). In addition, care should be taken when treating diabetic patients with Epilim Syrup, as this contains 3.6 g sucrose per 5 ml.

If it is necessary to dilute Epilim Syrup, the recommended diluent is syrup BP, but syrup containing SO_2 as a preservative should not be used. The diluted product will have a 14 day shelf life.

Interactions with other medicaments and other forms of interaction: Caution is advised when using Epilim in combination with newer anti-epileptics whose pharmacodynamics may not be well established.

Valproate has appreciably less enzyme-inducing effect than certain other anticonvulsants, and the efficacy of oral contraceptive agents does not appear to be affected.

Concurrent treatment with Epilim may affect the performance of some drugs and so clinical monitoring is recommended especially at the beginning of combined therapy.

1. The effects of neuroleptics, monoamine oxidase inhibitors, anti-depressants, and benzodiazepines may be potentiated.

2. Phenobarbitone plasma levels may increase and sedation may occur, particularly in children. The dose should be reduced immediately. Clinical monitoring is recommended throughout the first two weeks of combined treatment.

3. Phenytoin plasma levels, particularly of the free form, may increase following an initial decrease in total levels.

4. Primidone plasma levels may increase with exacerbation of adverse effects (such as sedation). The dose should be adjusted when appropriate.

5. The toxic effect of carbamazepine may be potentiated. Dosage should be adjusted when appropriate.

6. The metabolism of lamotrigine may be inhibited and the half life lengthened. Dose should be adjusted (lamotrigine dosage decreased) when appropriate. Co-administration of lamotrigine and Epilim might increase the risk of rash.

7. Zidovudine plasma concentration may be raised leading to increased zidovudine toxicity.

8. Protein-binding of warfarin and other coumarin anticoagulants may be reduced. The prothrombin time should be closely monitored.

Concurrent treatment with some drugs may affect the performance of Epilim and dosage levels might need to be adjusted.

1. Anti-epileptic drugs with enzyme-inducing effects (e.g. phenytoin, phenobarbitone, carbamazepine) may decrease valproate serum concentrations. Adjust dosage according to blood levels.

2. Felbamate may increase valproate serum concentration.

3. Cimetidine (but not ranitidine) and erythromycin may prolong the half-life and reduce clearance of valproate as a result of reduced hepatic metabolism.

4. Melfloquine may increase valproic acid metabolism. It also may have a convulsant effect. Seizures may occur in cases of combined therapy.

5. Cholestyramine may decrease the absorption of valproate.

6. Salicylates, e.g. aspirin, may displace valproate from protein-binding sites.

Pregnancy and lactation: An increased incidence of congenital abnormalities (including facial dysmorphia, neural tube defects and multiple malformations particularly of the limbs) has been demonstrated in offspring born to mothers with epilepsy both untreated and treated, including those treated with sodium valproate.

The incidence of neural tube defects in women receiving valproate during the first trimester has been estimated to be in the region of 1–2%. Folate supplementation has been demonstrated to reduce the incidence of neural tube defects in the offspring of women at high risk. No direct evidence exists of such effects in women receiving anti-epileptic drugs, however there is no reason to contra-indicate folic acid in these women.

The available evidence suggests that anticonvulsant monotherapy is preferred. Dosage should be reviewed before conception and the lowest effective dose used, in divided doses as abnormal pregnancy outcome tends to be associated with higher total daily dosage. Women of child bearing age should be informed of the risks and benefits of continuing anti-epileptic treatment throughout pregnancy. Pregnancies should be carefully screened by alpha-foetoprotein measurement, ultrasound and other techniques if appropriate. There have been rare reports of haemorrhagic syndrome in neonates whose mothers have taken sodium valproate during pregnancy. This haemorrhagic syndrome is related to hypofibrinaemia. Afibrinaemia has also been reported and may be fatal. Hypofibrinaemia is possibly associated with a decrease of coagulation factors. Note however, that haemorrhagic syndrome may also be induced by phenobarbital and other enzyme-inducers. Platelet count, fibrinogen plasma level and coagulation status should be investigated in neonates.

Breast feeding: The concentration of valproic acid found in the breast milk is very low, between 1% and 10% of total maternal plasma levels. There appears to be no contraindication to breast feeding by patients on valproate. The decision to allow the patient to breast feed should be taken with regard to all the known facts.

Effects on ability to drive and to use machines: Not applicable. Use of Epilim may provide seizure control such that the patient may again be eligible to hold a driving licence.

Undesirable effects:

Hepatic: Liver dysfunction, including hepatic failure resulting in fatalities, has occurred in patients whose treatment included valproic acid or sodium valproate. Patients most at risk are children particularly those under the age of three and those with congenital metabolic or degenerative disorders, organic brain disease or severe seizure disorders associated with mental retardation. The incidents mainly occurred during the first 6 months of therapy, the period of maximum risk being 2–12 weeks, and usually involved multiple anticonvulsant therapy. Monotherapy is to be preferred in this group of patients.

Clinical symptoms are more helpful than laboratory investigations in the early stages of hepatic failure. Serious or fatal hepatotoxicity may be preceded by non-specific symptoms, usually of sudden onset, such as loss of seizure control, malaise, weakness, lethargy, oedema, anorexia, vomiting, abdominal pain, drowsiness, jaundice. These are an indication for immediate withdrawal of the drug. Patients should be instructed to report any such signs to the clinician for investigation should they occur. Whilst it is difficult to establish which, if any, investigation is predictive, tests which reflect protein synthesis e.g. prothrombin time may be most relevant.

Routine measurement of liver function should be undertaken before therapy and periodically during the first six months especially in those who seem most at risk, and those with a prior history of liver disease; such patients should have close clinical supervision. Raised liver enzymes are not uncommon during treatment with Epilim and are usually transient or respond to reduction in dosage. Patients with such biochemical abnormalities should be reassessed clinically and tests of liver function including prothrombin time should be monitored until they return to normal. However an abnormally prolonged prothrombin time particularly in association with other relevant abnormalities requires cessation of treatment. Any concomitant use of salicylates should be stopped since they employ the same metabolic pathway.

Metabolic: Hyperammonaemia without changes in liver function tests may occur. Isolated and moderate hyperammonaemia may occur frequently, is usually transient and should not cause treatment discontinuation. However, it may present clinically as vomiting, ataxia and increasing clouding of consciousness. Should these symptoms occur Epilim should be discontinued. Hyperammonaemia associated with neurological symptoms have been reported. In such cases further investigations should be considered. When an abnormality of the urea cycle is suspected (ornithine transcarbamylase deficiency), metabolic investigations should be performed. Oedema has been rarely reported.

Pancreatic: There have been reports of pancreatitis including, rarely, fatalities occurring in patients receiving valproic acid or sodium valproate, usually within the first six months of therapy. Patients experiencing acute abdominal pain should have their pancreatic enzymes including serum amylase estimated; if these levels are elevated treatment should be discontinued.

Renal: There have been isolated reports of a reversible Fanconi's syndrome (a defect in proximal renal tubular function giving rise to glycosuria, amino aciduria, phosphaturia, and uricosuria) associated with valproate therapy, but the mode of action is as yet unclear.

Haematological: Valproic acid inhibits the second stage of platelet aggregation leading to prolongation of bleeding time and frequently to thrombocytopenia. These are usually associated with doses above those recommended and are reversible. Prior to initiation of therapy and also before surgery, clinicians should assure themselves, using the appropriate blood tests, that there is no undue potential for bleeding complications. Spontaneous bruising or bleeding is an indication for withdrawal of medication pending investigations. Red cell hypoplasia, leucopenia and pancytopenia have been reported rarely; the blood picture returned to normal when the drug was discontinued. Isolated reduction of fibrinogen may also occur.

Neurological: Ataxia and tremor have been occasionally reported and appear to be dose-related effects.

Sedation has been reported occasionally, usually when in combination with other anticonvulsants. In monotherapy it occurred early in treatment on rare occasions and is usually transient. Rare cases of lethargy and confusion occasionally progressing to stupor, sometimes with associated hallucinations or convulsions have been reported. Encephalopathy and coma have very rarely been observed. These cases have often been associated with too high a starting dose or too rapid a dose escalation or concomitant use of other anticonvulsants, notably phenobarbitone. They have usually been reversible on withdrawal of treatment or reduction of dosage. Very rare cases of reversible dementia associated with reversible cerebral atrophy have been reported.

An increase in alertness may occur; this is generally beneficial but occasionally aggression, hyperactivity and behavioural deterioration have been reported. Hearing loss, either reversible or irreversible has been reported rarely, though a causal relationship has not been established.

Gastrointestinal: Appetite may increase and an increase in weight is not uncommon. Frequently at the start of treatment minor gastrointestinal irritation and, less commonly, nausea may occur. These problems can usually be overcome by taking Epilim with or after food or by using Enteric Coated Epilim.

Dermatological: Transient hair loss has often been noted in some patients. This effect does not appear to be dose-related and regrowth normally begins within six months, although the hair may become more curly than previously. Cutaneous reactions such as exanthematous rash have been reported rarely. In exceptional cases toxic epidermal necrolysis, Stevens-Johnson syndrome, and erythema multiforme have been reported. Rarely signs of an immune disorder have occurred, therefore caution should be observed when using the drug in patients with features which may suggest systemic lupus erythematosus. The occurrence of vasculitis has occasionally been reported.

Endocrine: There have been isolated reports of irregular periods or amenorrhoea. Very rarely gynaecomastia has occurred.

Overdosage: Cases of accidental and suicidal overdosage have been reported. At plasma concentrations of up to 5 to 6 times the maximum therapeutic levels, there are unlikely to be any symptoms other than nausea, vomiting and dizziness. In massive overdose, i.e., with plasma concentrations 10 to 20 times maximum therapeutic levels there may be serious CNS depression and respiration may be impaired. The symptoms may however be variable and seizures have been reported in the presence of very high plasma levels. Deaths have occurred following large overdoses. Hospital management of overdosage, including induced vomiting, gastric lavage, assisted ventilation and other supportive measures, is recommended. Haemodialysis and haemoperfusion have been used successfully. Intravenous naloxone has also been used sometimes in association with activated charcoal given orally.

Pharmacological properties

Pharmacodynamic properties: Sodium valproate is an anticonvulsant. The most likely mode of action for valproate is potentiation of the inhibitory action of gamma amino-butyric acid (GABA) through an action on the further synthesis or further metabolism of GABA.

Pharmacokinetic properties: The half life of sodium valproate is usually reported to be within the range 8–20 hours. It is usually shorter in children.

In patients with severe renal insufficiency it may be necessary to alter dosage in accordance with free serum valproic acid levels.

The reported effective therapeutic range for plasma valproic acid levels is 40–100 mg/litre (278–694 micromol/litre). This reported range may depend on time of sampling and presence of co-medication. The percentage of free (unbound) drug is usually between 6% and 15% of the total plasma levels. An increased incidence of adverse effects may occur with plasma levels above the effective therapeutic range. The pharmacological (or therapeutic) effects of Epilim may not be clearly correlated with the total or free (unbound) plasma valproic acid levels.

Pre-clinical safety data: Not applicable.

Pharmaceutical particulars

List of excipients:

Enteric coated tablets: Polyvidone, croscarmellose sodium, microcrystalline cellulose, hydrated silica, polyvinylphthalate, lactose, talc, polyethylene glycol, citric acid monohydrate, hydroxypropyl methylcellulose, titanium dioxide (E171), colloidal anhydrous silica, alumina hydrate, sodium alginate, Indigo carmine aluminium lake (E132), carmoisine aluminium lake (E122), beeswax, carnauba wax, polysorbate, water and sorbic acid.

Crushable tablets: Maize starch, kaolin light (natural), silica hydrated, magnesium stearate and purified water†.

Epilim Syrup: Sorbitol powder, sodium methyl hydroxybenzoate, sodium propyl hydroxybenzoate, sodium saccharin, sucrose, flavour IFF cherry 740, Ponceau 4R (E124) and purified water.

Epilim Liquid: Hydroxyethyl cellulose, sorbitol powder, sodium methyl hydroxybenzoate, sodium propyl hydroxybenzoate, saccharin sodium, Ponceau 4R (E124), flavour IFF cherry 740, citric acid anhydrous and purified water.
(† not detected in final formulation.)

Incompatibilities: None.

Shelf life: Epilim Tablets and Syrup: 36 months. Epilim Liquid: 24 months.

Special precautions for storage:
Epilim Tablets: Store in a dry place below 30°C.
Epilim Syrup: Store below 30°C.
Epilim Liquid: Store below 30°C and away from direct sunlight. Epilim Liquid should not be diluted.

Nature and contents of container: Epilim Enteric Coated tablets are supplied in blister packs further packed into a cardboard carton. Pack sizes of 100 and 112 tablets.

Epilim 100 mg Crushable Tablets are supplied in blister packs further packed into a cardboard carton. Pack sizes of 100 and 112 tablets.

Epilim Syrup and Liquid is supplied in amber glass bottles with polypropylene J-cap or aluminium tamper evident cap with extended polyethylene seal and amber polyethylene tetraphthalate bottles with polypropylene tamper evident closure. Bottle size 200 and 300 ml.

Instructions for use/handling: None.

Marketing authorisation numbers
Epilim 500 Enteric Coated 11723/0020.
Epilim 200 Enteric Coated 11723/0018.
Epilim Crushable 11723/0017.
Epilim Syrup 11723/0025.
Epilim Liquid 11723/0024.

Date of approval/revision of SPC September 1997.

Legal category POM.

EPILIM CHRONO*

Qualitative and quantitative composition

Epilim Chrono 200 Controlled Release tablets contain 133.2 mg Sodium Valproate PhEur and 58.0 mg Valproic Acid PhFr equivalent to 200 mg sodium valproate/tablet.

Epilim Chrono 300 Controlled Release tablets contain 199.8 mg Sodium Valproate PhEur and 87.0 mg Valproic Acid PhFr equivalent to 300 mg sodium valproate/tablet.

Epilim Chrono 500 Controlled Release tablets contain 333 mg Sodium Valproate PhEur and 145 mg Valproic Acid PhFr equivalent to 500 mg sodium valproate/tablet.

Pharmaceutical form Controlled release tablets.

Clinical particulars

Therapeutic indications: The treatment of generalised, partial or other epilepsy. In women of childbearing age Epilim should be used only in severe cases or in those resistant to other treatment.

Posology and method of administration: Epilim Chrono Controlled Release tablets are for oral administration.

Epilim Chrono is a controlled release formulation of Epilim which reduces peak concentration and ensures more even plasma concentrations throughout the day.

Epilim Chrono may be given once or twice daily. The tablets should be swallowed whole and not crushed.

Daily dosage requirements vary according to age and body weight.

Monotherapy: Usual requirements are as follows:

Adults: Dosage should start at 600 mg daily increasing by 200 mg at three day intervals until control is achieved. This is generally within the dosage range 1000 mg to 2000 mg per day, i.e. 20–30 mg/kg body weight. Where adequate control is not achieved within this range the dose may be further increased to 2500 mg per day.

Children over 20 kg: Initial dosage should be 400 mg/day (irrespective of weight) with spaced increases until control is achieved; this is usually within the range 20–30 mg/kg body weight per day. Where adequate control is not achieved within this range the dose may be increased to 35 mg/kg body weight per day.

Children under 20 kg: An alternative formulation of Epilim should be used in this group of patients, due to the need for dose titration.

Elderly: Although the pharmacokinetics of valproate are modified in the elderly, they have limited clinical significance and dosage should be determined by seizure control. The volume of distribution is increased in the elderly and because of decreased binding to serum albumin, the proportion of free drug is increased. This will affect the clinical interpretation of plasma valproic acid levels. In patients with renal insufficiency it may be necessary to decrease dosage. Dosage should be adjusted according to clinical monitoring since monitoring of plasma concentrations may be misleading (see *Pharmacokinetic properties*).

In patients where adequate control has been achieved Epilim Chrono formulations are interchangeable with other Epilim conventional or modified release formulations on an equivalent daily dosage basis.

Combined therapy: When starting Epilim in patients already on other anticonvulsants, these should be tapered slowly; initiation of Epilim therapy should then be gradual, with target dose being reached after about 2 weeks. In certain cases it may be necessary to raise the dose by 5 to 10 mg/kg/day when used in combination with anticonvulsants which induce liver enzyme activity, e.g. phenytoin, phenobarbitone and carbamazepine. Once known enzyme inducers have been withdrawn it may be possible to maintain seizure control on a reduced dose of Epilim. When barbiturates are being administered concomitantly and particularly if sedation is observed (particularly in children) the dosage of barbiturate should be reduced.

NB: In children requiring doses higher than 40 mg/kg/day clinical chemistry and haematological parameters should be monitored. Optimum dosage is mainly determined by seizure control and routine measurement of plasma levels is unnecessary. However, a method for measurement of plasma levels is available and may be helpful where there is poor control or side effects are suspected.

Contra-indications: Hypersensitivity to sodium valproate. Active liver disease, family history of severe hepatic dysfunction, particularly drug related, porphyria.

Special warnings and special precautions for use:
Diabetic patients: Valproate is eliminated mainly through the kidneys, partly in the form of ketone bodies; this may give false positives in the urine testing of possible diabetics. (See *Pregnancy and lactation, Undesirable effects*).

Interactions with other medicaments and other forms of interaction: Caution is advised when using Epilim in combination with newer anti-epileptics whose pharmacodynamics may not be well established.

Valproate has appreciably less enzyme-inducing effect than certain other anticonvulsants, and the efficacy of oral contraceptive agents does not appear to be affected.

Concurrent treatment with Epilim may affect the performance of some drugs and so clinical monitoring is recommended especially at the beginning of combined therapy.

1. The effects of neuroleptics, monoamine oxidase inhibitors, anti-depressants, and benzodiazepines may be potentiated.
2. Phenobarbitone plasma levels may increase and sedation may occur, particularly in children. The dose should be reduced immediately. Clinical monitoring is recommended throughout the first two weeks of combined treatment.
3. Phenytoin plasma levels, particularly of the free form, may increase following an initial decrease in total levels.
4. Primidone plasma levels may increase with exacerbation of adverse effects (such as sedation). The dose should be adjusted when appropriate.
5. The toxic effect of carbamazepine may be potentiated. Dosage should be adjusted when appropriate.
6. The metabolism of lamotrigine may be inhibited and the half-life lengthened. Dose should be adjusted (lamotrigine dosage decreased) when appropriate. Co-administration of lamotrigine and Epilim might increase the risk of rash.
7. Zidovudine plasma concentration may be raised leading to increased zidovudine toxicity.
8. Protein-binding of warfarin and other coumarin anticoagulants may be reduced. The prothrombin time should be closely monitored.

Concurrent treatment with some drugs may affect the performance of Epilim and dosage levels might need to be adjusted.

1. Anti-epileptic drugs with enzyme-inducing effects (e.g. phenytoin, phenobarbitone, carbamazepine) may decrease valproate serum concentrations. Adjust dosage according to blood levels.
2. Felbamate may increase valproate serum concentration.
3. Cimetidine (but not ranitidine) and erythromycin may prolong the half-life and reduce clearance of valproate as a result of reduced hepatic metabolism.
4. Melfloquine may increase valproic acid metabolism. It also may have a convulsant effect. Seizures may occur in cases of combined therapy.
5. Cholestyramine may decrease the absorption of valproate.
6. Salicylates, e.g. aspirin, may displace valproate from protein-binding sites.

Pregnancy and lactation: An increased incidence of congenital abnormalities (including facial dysmorphia, neural tube defects and multiple malformations, particularly of the limbs) has been demonstrated in offspring born to mothers with epilepsy both untreated and treated, including those treated with sodium valproate.

The incidence of neural tube defects in women receiving valproate during the first trimester has been estimated to be in the region of 1–2%. Folate supplementation has been demonstrated to reduce the incidence of neural tube defects in the offspring of women at high risk. No direct evidence exists of such effects in women receiving anti-epileptic drugs, however there is no reason to contraindicate folic acid in these women. The available evidence suggests that anticonvulsant monotherapy is preferred. Dosage should be reviewed before conception and the lowest effective dose used, in divided doses, as abnormal pregnancy outcome tends to be associated with higher total daily dosage. Women of child-bearing age should be informed of the risks and benefits of continuing anti-epileptic treatment throughout pregnancy. Pregnancies should be carefully screened by alpha-foetoprotein measurement, ultrasound, and other techniques if appropriate.

There have been rare reports of haemorrhagic syndrome in neonates whose mothers have taken sodium valproate during pregnancy. This haemorrhagic syndrome is related to hypofibrinaemia. Afibrinaemia has also been reported and may be fatal. Hypofibrinaemia is possibly associated with a decrease of coagulation factors. Note however, that haemorrhagic syndrome may also be induced by phenobarbital and other enzyme-inducers.

Platelet count, fibrinogen plasma level and coagulation status should be investigated in neonates.

Breast feeding: The concentration of valproic acid found in the breast milk is very low, between 1% and 10% of total maternal plasma levels. There appears to be no contra-indication to breast feeding by patients on valproate. The decision to allow the patient to breast feed should be taken with regard to all the known facts.

Effects on ability to drive and to use machines: Not applicable. Use of Epilim may provide seizure control such that the patient may be eligible to hold a driving licence.

Undesirable effects: Hepatic: Liver dysfunction, including hepatic failure resulting in fatalities, has occurred in patients whose treatment included valproic acid or sodium valproate. Patients most at risk are children, particularly those under the age of three and those with congenital metabolic or degenerative disorders, organic brain disease or severe seizure disorders associated with mental retardation. The incidents mainly occurred during the first six months of therapy, the period of maximum risk being 2–12 weeks, and usually involved multiple anticonvulsant therapy. Monotherapy is to be preferred in this group of patients.

Clinical symptoms are more helpful than laboratory investigation in the early stages of hepatic failure. Serious or fatal hepatotoxicity may be preceded by non-specific symptoms, usually of sudden onset, such as loss of seizure control, malaise, weakness, lethargy, oedema, anorexia, vomiting, abdominal pain, drowsiness, jaundice. These are an indication for immediate withdrawal of the drug. Patients should be instructed to report any such signs to the clinician for investigation should they occur. Whilst it is difficult to establish which, if any, investigation is predictive, tests which reflect protein synthesis, e.g. prothrombin time, may be most relevant.

Routine measurement of liver function should be undertaken before therapy and periodically during the first six months, especially in those who seem most at risk, and those with a prior history of liver disease; such patients should have close clinical supervision. Raised liver enzymes are not uncommon during treatment with valproate and are usually transient or respond to reduction in dosage.

Patients with such biochemical abnormalities should be reassessed clinically and tests of liver function including prothrombin time, should be monitored until they return to normal. However an abnormally prolonged prothrombin time, particularly in association with other relevant abnormalities requires cessation of treatment. Any concomitant use of salicylates should be stopped, since they employ the same metabolic pathway.

Metabolic: Hyperammonaemia without changes in liver function tests may occur. Isolated and moderate hyperammonaemia may occur frequently, is usually transient and should not cause treatment discontinuation. However, it may present clinically as vomiting, ataxia, and increasing clouding of consciousness. Should these symptoms occur Epilim should be discontinued. Hyperammonaemia associated with neurological symptoms has also been reported. In such cases, further investigations should be considered. When an abnormality of the urea cycle is suspected (Ornithine transcarbamylase deficiency), metabolic investigations should be performed. Oedema has been rarely reported.

Pancreatic: There have been reports of pancreatitis including, rarely, fatalities occurring in patients receiving valproic acid or sodium valproate, usually within the first six months of therapy. Patients experiencing acute abdominal pain should have their pancreatic enzymes including serum amylase estimated; if these levels are elevated treatment should be discontinued.

Haematological: Valproic acid inhibits the second stage of platelet aggregation leading to prolongation of bleeding time and frequently to thrombocytopenia. These are usually associated with doses above those recommended and are reversible. Prior to initiation of therapy and also before surgery, clinicians should assure themselves, using the appropriate blood tests, that there is no undue potential for bleeding complications. Spontaneous bruising or bleeding is an indication for withdrawal of medication pending investigations. Red cell hypoplasia, leucopenia and pancytopenia have been reported rarely; the blood picture returned to normal when the drug was discontinued. Isolated reduction of fibrinogen may also occur.

Neurological: Ataxia and tremor have been occasionally reported and appear to be dose-related effects.

Sedation has been reported occasionally, usually when in combination with other anticonvulsants. In monotherapy it has occurred early in treatment on rare occasions and is usually transient. Rare cases of lethargy and confusion, occasionally progressing to stupor, sometimes with associated hallucinations or convulsions have been reported. Encephalopathy and coma have very rarely been observed. These cases have often been associated with too high a starting dose or too rapid a dose escalation or concomitant use of other anticonvulsants, notably phenobarbitone. They have usually been reversible on withdrawal of treatment or reduction of dosage.

An increase in alertness may occur; this is generally beneficial but occasionally aggression, hyperactivity and behavioural deterioration have been reported. Hearing loss, either reversible or irreversible has been reported rarely, though a causal relationship has not been established.

Gastrointestinal: Appetite may increase and an increase in weight is not uncommon. Frequently at the start of treatment minor gastrointestinal irritation and, less commonly, nausea may occur. These problems can usually be overcome by taking Epilim with or after food or by using Enteric Coated Epilim.

Dermatological: Transient hair loss often has been noted in some patients. This effect does not appear to be dose-related and regrowth normally beings within six months, although the hair may become more curly than previously. Cutaneous reactions such as exanthematous rash have been reported rarely. In exceptional cases toxic epidermal necrolysis, Stevens-Johnson syndrome, and erythema multiforme have been reported.

Rarely, signs of an immune disorder have occurred, therefore caution should be observed when using the drug in patients with features which may suggest systemic lupus erythematosus. The occurrence of vasculitus has occasionally been reported.

Endocrine: There have been isolated reports of irregular periods or amenorrhoea. Very rarely gynaecomastia has occurred.

Overdosage: Cases of accidental and suicidal valproate overdosage have been reported. At plasma concentrations of up to 5 to 6 times the maximum therapeutic levels, there are unlikely to be any symptoms other than nausea, vomiting and dizziness.

In massive overdose, i.e. with plasma concentration 10 to 20 times maximum therapeutic levels, there may be serious CNS depression and respiration may be impaired. The symptoms may however be variable and seizures have been reported in the presence of very high plasma levels. A number of deaths have occurred following large overdoses. Hospital management of overdose including vomiting, gastric lavage, assisted ventilation and other supportive measures is recommended. Haemodialysis and haemoperfusion have been used successfully. Intravenous naloxone has also been used sometimes in association with activated charcoal given orally.

Pharmacological properties

Pharmacodynamic properties: Sodium valproate is an anticonvulsant. The most likely mode of action for valproate is potentiation of the inhibitory action of gamma amino butyric acid (GABA) through an action on the further synthesis or further metabolism of GABA.

Pharmacokinetic properties: The half life of sodium valproate is usually reported to be within the range of 8–20 hours. It is usually shorter in children.

In patients with severe renal insufficiency it may be necessary to alter dosage in accordance with free serum valproic acid levels.

The reported effective therapeutic range for plasma valproic acid levels is 40–100 mg/litre (278–694 micromol/litre). This reported range may depend on time of sampling and presence of co-medication. The percentage of free (unbound) drug is usually between 6% and 15% of total plasma levels. An increased incidence of adverse effects may occur with plasma levels above the effective therapeutic range.

The pharmacological (or therapeutic) effects of Epilim Chrono may not be clearly correlated with the total of free (unbound) plasma valproic acid levels.

Epilim Chrono formulations are controlled release formulations which demonstrate in pharmacokinetic studies less fluctuation in plasma concentration compared with other established conventional and modified release Epilim formulations.

In cases where measurement of plasma levels is considered necessary, the pharmacokinetics of Epilim Chrono make the measurement of plasma levels less dependent upon time of sampling.

The Epilim Chrono formulations are bioequivalent to Epilim Liquid and enteric coated (EC) formulations with respect to the mean areas under the plasma concentration time curves. Steady-state pharmacokinetic data indicate that the peak concentration (Cmax) and trough concentration (Cmin) of Epilim Chrono lie within the effective therapeutic range of plasma levels found in pharmacokinetic studies with Epilim EC.

Pre-clinical safety data: There are no pre-clinical data of relevance to the prescriber which are additional to that already included in other sections of the SPC.

Pharmaceutical particulars

List of excipients: Hydroxypropylmethyl cellulose, ethylcellulose, hydrated silica.

Film coat: Violet coat, containing titanium dioxide (E171), erythrosine BS (E127), indigo carmine (E132), iron oxide black (E172), hydroxypropylmethyl cellulose (E464), polyethylene glycol 400, purified water†. († Not detected in final formulation.)

Incompatibilities: None.

Shelf life: Epilim Chrono tablets have a shelf-life of 36 months.

Special precautions for storage: Store in a dry place below 30°C.

Nature and contents of container: Epilim Chrono Controlled Release tablets are supplied in blister packs further packed into a cardboard carton. Pack size 100 tablets.

Instructions for use/handling: Not applicable.

Marketing authorisation numbers

Epilim Chrono 200 Controlled Release 11723/0078
Epilim Chrono 300 Controlled Release 11723/0021
Epilim Chrono 500 Controlled Release 11723/0079

Date of approval/revision of SPC September 1997.

Legal category POM.

EPILIM* INTRAVENOUS

Presentation Epilim Intravenous. Off-white sterile, freeze dried Sodium Valproate PhEur 400 mg in a clear glass vial supplied with an ampoule of 4 ml of solvent (Water for Injections PhEur).

Uses Epilim Intravenous may be used for epileptic patients who would normally be maintained on oral sodium valproate, and for whom oral therapy is temporarily not possible.

Dosage and administration Daily dosage requirements vary according to age and body weight.

To reconstitute, inject the solvent provided (4 ml) into the vial, allow to dissolve and extract the appropriate dose. Due to displacement of solvent by sodium valproate the concentration of reconstituted sodium valproate is 95 mg/ml.

Each vial of Epilim Intravenous is for single dose injection only. It should be reconstituted immediately prior to use and infusion solutions containing it used within 24 hours. Any unused portion should be discarded.

Epilim Intravenous may be given by direct slow intravenous injection or by infusion using a separate intravenous line in normal saline, dextrose 5%, or dextrose saline.

Patients already satisfactorily treated with Epilim may be continued at their current dosage using continuous or repeated infusion. Other patients may be given a slow intravenous injection over 3–5 minutes, usually 400–800 mg depending on body weight (up to 10 mg/kg) followed by continuous or repeated infusion up to a maximum of 2500 mg/day.

Epilim Intravenous should be replaced by oral Epilim therapy as soon as practicable.

Daily requirement for children is usually in the range 20–30 mg/kg/day and method of administration is as above. Where adequate control is not achieved within this range the dose may be increased up to 40 mg/kg/day but only in patients in whom plasma valproic acid levels can be monitored. Above 40 mg/kg/day clinical chemistry and haematological parameters should be monitored.

Elderly: Although the pharmacokinetics of Epilim are modified in the elderly, they have limited clinical significance and dosage should be determined by seizure control. The volume of distribution is increased in the elderly and because of decreased binding to serum albumin, the proportion of free drug is increased. This will affect the clinical interpretation of plasma valproic acid levels.

Patients with renal insufficiency: It may be necessary to decrease dosage. Dosage should be adjusted according to clinical monitoring since monitoring of plasma concentrations may be misleading.

Combined therapy: When starting Epilim in patients already on other anticonvulsants these should be tapered slowly; initiation of Epilim therapy should then be gradual, with target dose being reached after about 2 weeks. In certain cases it may be necessary to raise the dose by 5 to 10 mg/kg/day when used in combination with anticonvulsants which induce liver enzyme activity, e.g. phenytoin, phenobarbitone, and carbamazepine. Once known enzyme inducers have been withdrawn it may be possible to maintain seizure control on a reduced dose of Epilim. When barbiturates are being administered concomitantly and particularly if sedation is observed (particularly in children) the dosage of barbiturate should be reduced.

NB: In children requiring doses higher than 40 mg/kg/day clinical chemistry and haematological parameters should be monitored.

General considerations: Optimum dosage is mainly determined by seizure control and routine measurement of plasma levels is unnecessary. However, a method for measurement of plasma levels is available and may be helpful where there is poor control or side effects are suspected, see Further Information.

Contra-indications, warnings, etc

Contra-indications: Hypersensitivity to sodium valproate. Active liver disease, family history of severe hepatic dysfunction, particularly drug-related. Porphyria.

Side-effects

Hepatic: Liver dysfunction, including hepatic failure resulting in fatalities, has occurred in patients whose treatment included valproic acid or sodium valproate. Patients most at risk are children particularly those under the age of three and those with congenital metabolic or degenerative disorders, organic brain disease or severe seizure disorders associated with mental retardation. The incidents mainly occurred during the first six months of therapy, the period of maximum risk being 2–12 weeks, and usually involved multiple anticonvulsant therapy. Monotherapy is to be preferred in this group of patients.

Clinical symptoms are more helpful than laboratory investigations in the early stages of hepatic failure. Serious or fatal hepatotoxicity may be preceded by non-specific symptoms, usually of sudden onset, such as loss of seizure control, malaise, weakness, lethargy, oedema, anorexia, vomiting, abdominal pain, drowsiness, jaundice. These are an indication for immediate withdrawal of the drug. Patients should be instructed to report any such signs to the clinician for investigation should they occur. Whilst it is difficult to establish which, if any, investigation is predictive, tests which reflect protein synthesis e.g. prothrombin time may be most relevant.

Routine measurement of liver function should be undertaken before therapy and periodically during the first six months especially in those who seem most at risk and those with a prior history of liver disease; such patients should have close clinical supervision. Raised liver enzymes are not uncommon during treatment with Epilim and are usually transient or respond to reduction in dosage of Epilim. Patients with such biochemical abnormalities should be reassessed clinically and tests of liver function including prothrombin time should be monitored until they return to normal. However an abnormally prolonged prothrombin time particularly in association with other relevant abnormalities requires cessation of treatment. Any concomitant use of salicylates should be stopped, since they employ the same metabolic pathway.

Metabolic: Hyperammonaemia without changes in liver function tests may occur. Isolated and moderate hyperammonaemia may occur frequently, is usually transient and should not cause treatment discontinuation. However, it may present clinically as vomiting, ataxia and increasing clouding of consciousness. Should these symptoms occur Epilim should be discontinued. Hyperammonaemia associated with neurological symptoms has also been reported. In such cases, further investigations should be considered. When an abnormality of the urea cycle is suspected (ornithine transcarbamylase deficiency), metabolic investigations should be performed. Oedema has been rarely reported.

Pancreatic: There have been reports of pancreatitis including rarely, fatalities occurring in patients receiving valproic acid or sodium valproate, usually within the first six months of therapy. Patients experiencing acute abdominal pain should have their serum amylase estimated; if these levels are elevated treatment should be discontinued.

Renal: There have been isolated reports of a reversible Fanconi's syndrome (a defect in proximal renal tubular function giving rise to glycosuria, amino acidura, phosphaturia, and uricosuria) associated with valproate therapy, but the mode of action is as yet unclear.

Haematological: Valproic acid inhibits the second stage of platelet aggregation leading to prolongation of bleeding time and frequently to thrombocytopenia. These are usually associated with doses above those recommended and are reversible. Prior to initiation of therapy and also before surgery, clinicians should assure themselves using the appropriate blood tests, that there is no undue potential for bleeding complications. Spontaneous bruising or bleeding is an indication for withdrawal of medication pending investigations. Red cell hypoplasia, pancytopenia and leucopenia have been reported rarely; the blood picture returned to normal when the drug was discontinued. Isolated reduction of fibrinogen may also occur.

Neurological: Ataxia and tremor have been occasionally reported and appear to be dose-related effects.

Sedation has been reported occasionally, usually when in combination with other anticonvulsants. In monotherapy it occurred early in treatment on rare occasions and is usually transient. Rare cases of lethargy and confusion occasionally progressing to stupor, sometimes with associated hallucinations or convulsions have been reported.

Encephalopathy and coma have very rarely been observed. These cases have often been associated with too high a starting dose or too rapid a dose escalation or concomitant use of other anticonvulsants, notably phenobarbitone. They have usually been reversible on withdrawal of treatment or reduction of dosage. Very rare cases of reversible dementia associated with reversible cerebral atrophy have been reported.

An increase in alertness may occur; this is generally beneficial but occasionally aggression, hyperactivity and behavioural deterioration have been reported.

Hearing loss, either reversible or irreversible has been reported rarely, though a causal relationship has not been established.

Gastrointestinal: Appetite may increase and an increase in weight is not uncommon. Frequently at the start of treatment, minor gastrointestinal irritation, and less commonly, nausea may occur. These problems can usually be overcome by taking Epilim with or after food or by using Enteric Coated Epilim.

Dermatological: Transient hair loss has been noted in some patients. This effect does not appear to be dose-related and regrowth normally begins within six months, although the hair may become more curly than previously. Cutaneous reactions such as exanthematous rash have been reported rarely. In exceptional cases toxic epidermal necrolysis, Stevens-Johnson syndrome, and erythema multiforme have been reported. Rarely signs of an immune disorder have occurred, therefore caution should be observed when using the drug in patients with features which may suggest systemic lupus erythematosus. The occurrence of vasculitis has occasionally been reported.

Endocrine: There have been isolated reports of irregular periods or amenorrhoea. Very rarely gynaecomastia has occurred.

Drug interactions: Caution is advised when using Epilim in combination with newer anti-epileptics whose pharmacodynamics may not be well established.

Valproate has appreciably less enzyme-inducing effect than certain other anticonvulsants, and the efficacy of oral contraceptive agents does not appear to be affected.

Concurrent treatment with Epilim may affect the performance of some drugs and so clinical monitoring is recommended especially at the beginning of combined therapy.

1. The effects of neuroleptics, monoamine oxidase inhibitors, anti-depressants, and benzodiazepines may be potentiated.

2. Phenobarbitone plasma levels may increase and sedation may occur, particularly in children. The dose should be reduced immediately. Clinical monitoring is recommended throughout the first two weeks of combined treatment.

3. Phenytoin plasma levels, particularly of the free form, may increase following an initial decrease in total levels.

4. Primidone plasma levels may increase with exacerbation of adverse effects (such as sedation). The dose should be adjusted when appropriate.

5. The toxic effect of carbamazepine may be potentiated. Dosage should be adjusted when appropriate.

6. The metabolism of lamotrigine may be inhibited and the half-life lengthened. Dose should be adjusted (lamotrigine dosage decreased) when appropriate. Co-administration of lamotrigine and Epilim might increase the risk of rash.

7. Zidovudine plasma concentration may be raised leading to increased zidovudine toxicity.

8. Protein-binding of warfarin and other coumarin anticoagulants may be reduced. The prothrombin time should be closely monitored.

Concurrent treatment with some drugs may affect the performance of Epilim and dosage levels might need to be adjusted.

1. Anti-epileptic drugs with enzyme-inducing effects (e.g. phenytoin, phenobarbitone, carbamazepine) may decrease valproate serum concentrations. Adjust dosage according to blood levels.

2. Felbamate may increase valproate serum concentration.

3. Cimetidine (but not ranitidine) and erythromycin may prolong the half-life and reduce clearance of valproate as a result of reduced hepatic metabolism.

4. Melfloquine may increase valproic acid metabolism. It also may have a convulsant effect. Seizures may occur in cases of combined therapy.

5. Cholestyramine may decrease the absorption of valproate.

6. Salicylates, e.g. aspirin, may displace valproate from protein-binding sites.

Diabetic patients: Epilim is eliminated mainly through the kidneys, partly in the form of ketone bodies; this may give false positives in the urine testing of possible diabetics.

Pregnancy: An increased incidence of congenital abnormalities (including facial dysmorphia, neural tube defects and multiple malformations) particularly of the limbs has been demonstrated in offspring born to mothers with epilepsy both untreated and treated including those treated with sodium valproate.

The incidence of neural tube defects in women receiving valproate during the first trimester has been estimated to be in the region of 1–2%. Folate supplementation has been demonstrated to reduce the incidence of neural tube defects in the offspring of women at high risk. No direct evidence exists of such effects in women receiving anti-epileptic drugs, however there is no reason to contraindicate folic acid in these women.

The available evidence suggests that anticonvulsant monotherapy is preferred. Dosage should be reviewed before conception and the lowest effective dose used, as abnormal pregnancy outcome tends to be associated with higher total daily dosage. Women of childbearing age should be informed of the risks and benefits of continuing anti-epileptic treatment throughout pregnancy. Pregnancies should be carefully screened by alpha-foetoprotein measurement, ultrasound, and other techniques if appropriate.

There have been rare reports of haemorrhagic syndrome in neonates whose mothers have taken sodium valproate during pregnancy. This haemorrhagic syndrome is related to hypofibrinaemia. Afibrinaemia has also been reported and may be fatal. Hypofibrinaemia is possibly associated with a decrease of coagulation factors. Note however, that haemorrhagic syndrome may also be induced by phenobarbital and other enzyme-inducers.

Platelet count, fibrinogen plasma level and coagulation status should be investigated in neonates.

Breast feeding: The concentration of valproic acid found in the breast milk is very low, between 1% and 10% of total maternal plasma levels. Thus there appears to be no contra-indication to breast feeding by patients on Epilim. The decision to allow the patient to breast feed should be taken with regard to all the known facts.

Overdosage: Cases of accidental and suicidal overdosage have been reported. At plasma concentrations of up to 5 to 6 times the maximum therapeutic levels, there are unlikely to be any symptoms other than nausea, vomiting and dizziness.

In massive overdose, i.e. with plasma concentrations 10 to 20 times maximum therapeutic levels there may be serious CNS depression and respiration may be impaired. The symptoms may however be variable and seizures have been reported in the presence of very high plasma levels. Deaths have occurred following large overdoses. Hospital management of overdosage, including induced vomiting, gastric lavage, assisted ventilation and other supportive measures, is recommended. Haemodialysis and haemoperfusion have been used successfully. Intravenous naloxone has also been used sometimes in association with activated charcoal given orally.

Pharmaceutical precautions Epilim Intravenous freeze dried powder should be stored below 25°C; infusion solutions at 2–8°C if stored before use, discarding any remaining after 24 hours. Epilim Intravenous should not be administered via the same IV line as other IV additives. The intravenous solution is suitable for infusion in PVC, polythene, or glass containers.

Legal category POM.

Package quantities Epilim Intravenous is supplied as a pack containing one vial of 400 mg Sodium Valproate PhEur and one ampoule containing 4 ml of solvent.

Further information The half life of sodium valproate is usually reported to be within the range 8–20 hours. It is usually shorter in children.

In patients with severe renal insufficiency it may be necessary to alter dosage in accordance with free serum valproic acid levels.

The reported effective therapeutic range for plasma valproic acid levels is 40–100 mg/litre (278–694 micro mol/litre). This reported range may depend on time of sampling and presence of co-medication. The percentage of free (unbound) drug is usually between 6% and 15% of the total plasma levels. An increased incidence of adverse effects may occur with plasma levels above the effective therapeutic range.

The pharmacological (or therapeutic) effects of Epilim may not be clearly correlated with the total or free (unbound) plasma valproic acid levels.

Product licence numbers

Epilim Intravenous	11723/0022
Water for Injection	11723/0023

FORTAGESIC*

Presentation White tablets with bevelled edges 12.7 mm diameter, marked FORTAGESIC on one side. Each tablet provides Pentazocine BP 15 mg (as the hydrochloride) and Paracetamol PhEur 500 mg. Fortagesic tablets contain sodium metabisulphite.

Uses Fortagesic is a compound analgesic for the relief of moderate pain associated with musculoskeletal disorders or injuries, such as bursitis, sprains, strains, fibrositis, sciatica and osteoarthritis, and for rheumatoid arthritis in patients sensitive to aspirin.

Dosage and administration Fortagesic is for oral administration only.

Adults including the elderly: 2 tablets up to four times daily.

Children: 7–12 years: 1 tablet every three to four hours. Not more than 4 doses to be taken in any 24 hour period. Not recommended for children under 7 years of age.

Contra-indications, warnings, etc

Contra-indications: Fortagesic should not be administered to patients with established respiratory depression, especially in the presence of cyanosis and excessive bronchial secretion and is also contraindicated in the presence of acute alcoholism, head injuries, conditions in which intracranial pressure is raised, acute bronchial asthma, in heart failure, secondary to chronic lung disease and in patients known to be hypersensitive to pentazocine or paracetamol.

Warnings:

Use in pregnancy and lactation: There is epidemiological evidence for the safety of paracetamol in human pregnancy. No such evidence exists for pentazocine (other than during labour) but it has been widely used for many years without apparent ill consequences. In rodents, harmful effects in the foetus have been observed but only at doses high enough to cause maternal toxicity. Pentazocine can readily cross the placental barrier and enter the foetal circulation and has the potential to cause opioid effects including central depression and abstinence syndrome in the foetus and new born infant (see below). It does not appear to have significant adverse effects on uterine function at parturition. Nonetheless, careful consideration should be given to the use of Fortagesic during pregnancy, particularly during the first trimester, or at term.

Special attention should be paid to clinical monitoring of the newborn, particularly premature infants, if pentazocine has been used during labour. Pentazocine is excreted in very small amounts in breast milk. Caution should therefore be observed in administering pentazocine to breast feeding mothers particularly of infants at risk.

Precautions:

Particular caution should be observed in administering Fortagesic to patients with porphyria, since it may provoke an acute attack in susceptible individuals, as well as in its use in patients who are receiving monoamine oxidase inhibitors or who have received them within the preceding 14 days.

Pentazocine can both depress as well as elevate blood pressure possibly through the release of endogenous catecholamines. Particular caution should be observed therefore in using Fortagesic in the presence of phaeochromocytoma, in the acute phase following myocardial infarction when it may increase pulmonary and systemic blood pressure and vascular resistance and in other clinical situations where alteration of vascular resistance or blood pressure might be particularly undesirable. When pentazocine is administered parenterally local effect have been reported at the site of injection.

Caution should be observed in patients with renal or hepatic impairment and in elderly patients, since pentazocine metabolism may be decreased and therefore bioavailability increased. Side effects may be accentuated.

Caution should also be observed in patients with hypothyroidism, adrenocortical insufficiency, prostatic hypertrophy and in patients with inflammatory or obstructive bowel disorders, cholescystitis, pancreatitis or other unidentified abdominal pain.

Caution should also be observed in patients who are prone to seizures. Patients who are taking other opioids or who are opioid-dependent should also be treated cautiously since the weak opioid antagonistic effects of pentazocine may provoke withdrawal symptoms.

Pentazocine may produce sedation, dizziness and occasionally euphoria, so ambulant patients should be warned not to operate machinery or drive if affected.

In chronic usage, care should be exercised to avoid any unnecessary increase in dosage since prolonged use of high doses of pentazocine may produce dependence. Patients with a history of drug abuse should be closely supervised when receiving pentazocine.

Interactions: Monoamine oxidase inhibitors may enhance the opioid effects of pentazocine and the agents may interact through their respective effects on catecholamine breakdown and release. Agents with sedative action including phenothiazines, tricyclic antidepressants and ethyl alcohol can enhance the central depressant effects of pentazocine which are opposed by respiratory stimulants such as doxapram. Tobacco smoking appears to enhance the metabolic clearance rate of pentazocine reducing the clinical effectiveness of a standard dose of pentazocine.

Pentazocine can antagonise the effects of stronger opioid agonists such as diamorphine, morphine and heroin and is itself antagonised by naloxone.

Side-effects: At normal therapeutic doses side-effects are generally of a minor nature. The most frequent side-effects are lightheadedness, dizziness, nausea and vomiting, sedation and sweating. The following side-effects have also been reported.

Cardiovascular: transient hypertension, tachycardia, hypotension, circulatory depression.

Central and peripheral nervous system: hallucinations, disturbance of vision, headache, disorientation, mood changes, nightmares, insomnia, paraesthesia, syncope, euphoria, grand mal convulsions, raised intracranial pressure, confusion, tremor.

Allergic: oedema of the face, flushed skin including facial plethora, dermatitis including pruritus, toxic epidermal necrolysis.

Gastrointestinal: constipation, dry mouth, biliary tract spasm, abdominal pain.

Haematological: depression of white blood cell count especially granulocytes which is usually reversible, moderate transient eosinophilia.

Ophthalmic: miosis.

Respiratory: respiratory depression.

Other: urinary retention, muscle tremor, chills, alterations in rate or strength of uterine contractions during labour.

When pentazocine is administered by injection the following dermatological effects have been observed: soft tissue induration, nodules, cutaneous depression at injection sites, ulceration (sloughing) and severe sclerosis of the skin and subcutaneous tissues (and, rarely underlying muscle), sting on injection.

Abrupt discontinuation of pentazocine in patients receiving large parenteral doses over a prolonged period of time may result in withdrawal symptoms, which can also occur in the newborn following prolonged in utero exposure. The abstinence syndrome of pentazocine is not typical of opiate dependence. Symptoms include mild abdominal cramps, nausea, vomiting, nervousness or restlessness, dizziness, fever and chills, rhinorrhoea and lacrimation but are mild compared with symptoms of opiate withdrawal. Managing the abstinence syndrome of pentazocine has raised few problems. Supportive therapy with tranquillisers may sometimes be required. If problems occur, treatment with pentazocine should be reinstated followed by a slower rate of withdrawal. It should be emphasised that the majority of patients reported to have become dependent on pentazocine had previously been dependent on opiates or had misused other drugs.

Overdose: The symptoms and clinical signs of Fortagesic overdose are likely to resemble those of the individual ingredients. Thus with pentazocine, as with morphine and other opioids, there may be somnolence, respiratory depression and hypotension. Circulatory failure and deepening coma may occur in more severe cases, particularly in patients who have also ingested other CNS depressants such as alcohol, sedatives/hypnotics or antihistamines. Adequate measures to maintain ventilation and general circulatory support should be employed. Gastric lavage and gastric aspiration should be considered where appropriate.

For respiratory depression due to overdosage or unusual sensitivity to pentazocine, parenteral naloxone is a specific and effective antagonist. Initial doses of 0.4 to 2.0 mg of naloxone are recommended, repeated at 2–3 minute intervals if needed, up to a total of 10 mg. Anticonvulsant therapy may be necessary.

With paracetamol overdose, patients may appear well for the first three days, then succumb with liver damage. The hepatic changes produced by overdosage of paracetamol result from the accumulation of a highly active intermediate metabolite in the hepatocytes.

N-acetylcysteine intravenously or methionine orally protects the liver if administered within 10–12 hours of ingesting an overdose.

In managing Fortagesic overdose, consideration should be given to gastric lavage and aspiration.

Pharmaceutical precautions Store below 25°C.

Legal category CD (Sch 3) POM.

Package quantities Fortagesic is supplied in bottles of 100 tablets.

Further information Paracetamol is rapidly and completely absorbed from the gastro-intestinal tract, it is relatively uniformly distributed throughout most body fluids and exhibits variable protein binding. Excretion is almost exclusively renal, in the form of conjugated metabolites.

Pentazocine is a strong opioid analgesic with weak opioid antagonist properties. By mouth, pentazocine has a bioavailability of about 47%. In the plasma it is 50–75% bound to protein and has an elimination half-life of about 4.6 hours. Peak plasma concentrations are obtained in 1 to 3 hours. Pentazocine diffuses across the placenta and appears in cerebro-spinal fluid in concentrations reaching 30–50% of those in plasma. It is metabolised by the liver, only a small proportion of a dose being excreted unchanged in the urine.

Product licence number 11723/0028.

FRANOL*

Presentation Franol Tablets are flat, white tablets with bevelled edges, 8.7 mm in diameter, marked Franol on one side. Each tablet contains 120 mg Theophylline PhEur and 11 mg Ephedrine Hydrochloride PhEur.

Uses Franol Tablets are recommended for the management of bronchospasm in reversible airway-obstruction associated with stable asthma or chronic bronchitis.

Dosage and administration Oral administration only.
Adults: Dosage varies with individual requirements and should be adjusted accordingly. The usual dosage is 3 tablets daily (morning, midday and evening). For the patient who suffers nocturnal attacks, an extra tablet taken at bedtime is recommended.

Elderly: As for adults but see 'Use in special groups'.

Children: Not recommended for children under 12 years of age.

If more than four tablets a day are required, it is advisable to monitor plasma theophylline levels during dose titration to ensure that levels are kept below 20 micrograms/ml.

Contra-indications, warnings, etc
Contra-indications: Franol should not be given to patients who are sensitive to either of its ingredients or to patients with unstable angina, cardiac arrhythmias, severe hypertension, severe coronary artery disease, porphyria or to those receiving other xanthines. Franol should not be used during pregnancy.

Precautions: Avoid or use with special caution in patients with cardiovascular disease, hypertension, agitation, phaeochromocytoma, hyperthyroidism, closed-angle glaucoma, prostatic hypertrophy, peptic ulceration, underlying seizure disorders, patients receiving anti-depressant drugs, or patients on MAO inhibitors within the previous 14 days. Special caution is also needed in the elderly, those with hepatic, renal, or cardiac dysfunction and during lactation. Ephedrine has a potential for tachyphylaxis, and abuse with dependence has been reported.

Potentially serious hypokalaemia can result from the use of $beta_2$ agonists and xanthines in combination particularly when hypoxia is present. The effect may be enhanced by concomitant diuretics or corticosteroids. Care should be observed and serum potassium levels monitored in patients receiving Franol who develop severe asthma, particularly if concomitant diuretic, corticosteroid or $beta_2$ agonist therapy is being employed.

Use in special groups:

Pregnancy: Although caffeine has been implicated as a teratogen, adequate animal teratogenic studies have not been conducted with theophylline nor with ephedrine. The safety of ephedrine and of theophylline, which crosses the placental barrier, have not been established in human pregnancy. Franol should not therefore be prescribed for patients who are pregnant.

Lactation: Theophylline distributes readily into breast milk therefore Franol should be used with caution in nursing women.

Hepatic dysfunction: Theophylline is eliminated primarily by metabolism in the liver. Thus in patients with severe liver disease, theophylline clearance may be decreased. If Franol is used in such patients, dosage may need to be reduced.

Renal dysfunction: Ephedrine is excreted largely unchanged in the urine, therefore Franol should be used with caution in patients with severe renal impairment.

Cardiac dysfunction: Theophylline clearance may be decreased in patients with congestive cardiac failure, acute pulmonary oedema or cor pulmonale, and theophylline may cause arrhythmias or worsen existing arrhythmias, thus caution should be exercised if Franol is used in such patients.

Elderly (over 65 years): Theophylline clearance decreases slightly with age. Elderly patients will tend therefore to have higher serum theophylline levels than younger adults at a given dose. They should be monitored closely for signs of toxicity during dose adjustment.

Others: Theophylline clearance may be increased in heavy smokers, decreased in patients with respiratory infection or those on a high carbohydrate – low protein diet, therefore the dose of Franol may need to be adjusted appropriately in these groups.

Drug interactions: Theophylline clearance may be decreased by concurrent administration of cimetidine, macrolide antibiotics, oral contraceptives, interferons, diltiazem, verapamil and viloxazine. Ciprofloxacin also increases plasma theophylline concentrations and if concomitant use is essential, the dose of theophylline should be reduced and plasma concentrations closely monitored to avoid toxicity. The concomitant use of theophylline and fluvoxamine should usually be avoided. When this is not possible, patients should have their theophylline dose halved and plasma theophylline should be monitored closely. Theophylline clearance may be increased by concurrent administration of barbiturates, carbamazepine, phenytoin, rifampicin, sulphinpyrazone, aminoglutethimide, phenobarbitone and primidone.

The effects of ephedrine are diminished by guanethidine, reserpine, and probably methyldopa, and may be diminished or enhanced by tricyclic anti-depressants. Ephedrine may also diminish the effects of guanethidine and may increase the possibility of arrhythmias in digitalised patients.

Side-effects: Large doses of Franol may give rise to the following side effects: arrhythmias, tachycardia, palpitation, flushing, giddiness, headache, tremor, anxiety, restlessness, insomnia, muscular weakness, nausea, vomiting, dyspepsia, thirst, sweating, difficulty in micturition.

Some patients may exhibit one or more such symptoms with therapeutic doses.

Overdosage: The symptoms and signs of overdosage with Franol are likely to include excessive irritability, sweating, nausea and vomiting, tachycardia, arrhythmias, hypertension, profuse diuresis with fever, flushing and hyperglycaemia, opisthotonus, hallucinations, convulsions and respiratory difficulty. In general the management of overdosage with Franol involves supportive and symptomatic therapy with particular attention being paid to the detection and correction of hypokalaemia, and should include serial assay of plasma potassium and theophylline levels, cardiac monitoring with electro-cardiogram, and maintenance of fluid and electrolyte balance.

Gastric aspiration and lavage may be employed. Convulsions and other CNS stimulation can usually be controlled by intravenous diazepam, or if that fails other anti-convulsants may be used. Marked excitement or hallucinations may be managed with chlorpromazine. Severe hypertension may necessitate the use of an alpha-adrenoreceptor blocking agent and a beta-adrenoreceptor blocking agent may be required to control arrhythmias. Beta 1-receptor agonists such as dopamine should be avoided. Charcoal haemoperfusion may be indicated to remove theophylline, but forced diuresis or peritoneal dialysis are inadequate for this purpose.

Pharmaceutical precautions Store below 25°C.

Legal category P.

Package quantities Franol Tablets are supplied in bottles of 90.

Further information The bronchodilator action of ephedrine is through direct agonism at beta adrenoceptors and, indirectly, through sympathetic amine release. Bronchodilatation with theophylline is attributable to adenosine antagonism or phosphodiesterase inhibition which would be pharmacologically complementary to the action of ephedrine. Theophylline is variably absorbed from the gastrointestinal tract. It is excreted via the urine mainly as 1,3-dimethyluric acid. About 10% is unchanged. Ephedrine is readily absorbed. Its action is evident within one hour. With a plasma elimination half life of about 4 hours, 60–75% is excreted unchanged in the urine.

Product licence number 11723/0035.

FRANOL* PLUS

Presentation Franol Plus Tablets are flat, white tablets with bevelled edges, 8.7 mm in diameter, marked Franol+ on one side. Each tablet contains 120 mg Theophylline PhEur and 15 mg Ephedrine Sulphate USP.

Uses Franol Plus Tablets are recommended for the management of bronchospasm in reversible airway-obstruction associated with stable asthma or chronic bronchitis.

Dosage and administration Oral administration only. *Adults:* Dosage varies with individual requirements and should be adjusted accordingly. The usual dosage is 3 tablets daily (morning, midday and evening). For the patient who suffers from nocturnal attacks, an extra tablet at bedtime is recommended.

Elderly: As for adults but see 'Use in Special Groups'.

Children: Not recommended for children under 12 years of age.

If more than four tablets a day are required, it is advisable to monitor plasma theophylline levels during dose titration to ensure that levels are kept below 20 micrograms/ml.

Contra-indications, warnings, etc

Contra-indications: Franol Plus should not be given to patients who are sensitive to either of its ingredients or to patients with unstable angina, cardiac arrhythmias, severe hypertension, severe coronary artery disease, porphyria or to those receiving other xanthines. Franol Plus should not be used during pregnancy.

Precautions: Avoid or use only with special caution in patients with cardiovascular disease, hypertension, agitation, phaeochromocytoma, hyperthyroidism, closed-angle glaucoma, prostatic hypertrophy, peptic ulceration, underlying seizure disorders, patients receiving anti-depressant drugs, or patients on MAO inhibitors within the previous 14 days. Special caution is also needed in the elderly, those with hepatic, renal, or cardiac dysfunction and during lactation. Ephedrine has a potential for tachyphylaxis, and abuse with dependence has been reported.

Potentially serious hypokalaemia can result from the use of $beta_2$ agonists and xanthines in combination particularly when hypoxia is present. The effect may be enhanced by concomitant diuretics or corticosteroids. Care should be observed and serum potassium levels monitored in patients receiving Franol Plus who develop severe asthma, particularly if concomitant diuretic, corticosteroid or $beta_2$ agonist therapy is being employed.

Use in special groups:

Pregnancy: Although caffeine has been implicated as a teratogen, adequate animal teratogenic studies have not been conducted with theophylline nor with ephedrine. The safety of ephedrine and of theophylline, which crosses the placental barrier, have not been established in human pregnancy. Franol Plus should not therefore be prescribed for patients who are pregnant.

Lactation: Theophylline distributes readily into breast milk therefore Franol Plus should be used with caution in nursing women.

Hepatic dysfunction: Theophylline is eliminated primarily by metabolism in the liver. Thus in patients with severe liver disease, theophylline clearance may be decreased. If Franol Plus is used in such patients, dosage may need to be reduced.

Renal dysfunction: Ephedrine is excreted largely unchanged in the urine, therefore Franol Plus should be used with caution in patients with severe renal impairment.

Cardiac dysfunction: Theophylline clearance may be decreased in patients with congestive cardiac failure, acute pulmonary oedema or cor pulmonale, and theophylline may cause arrhythmias or worsen existing arrhythmias, thus caution should be exercised if Franol Plus is used in such patients.

Elderly (over 65 years): Theophylline clearance decreases slightly with age. Elderly patients will tend therefore to have higher serum theophylline levels than younger adults at a given dose. They should be monitored closely for signs of toxicity during dose adjustment.

Others: Theophylline clearance may be increased in heavy smokers, decreased in patients with respiratory infection or those on a high carbohydrate – low protein diet, therefore the dose of Franol Plus may need to be adjusted appropriately in these groups.

Drug interactions: Theophylline clearance may be decreased by concurrent administration of cimetidine, macrolide antibiotics, oral contraceptives, interferons, diltiazem, verapamil and viloxazine. Ciprofloxacin also increases plasma theophylline concentrations and if concomitant use is essential, the dose of theophylline should be reduced and plasma concentrations closely monitored to avoid toxicity. The concomitant use of theophylline and fluvoxamine should usually be avoided. Where this is not possible, patients should have their theophylline dose halved and plasma theophylline should be monitored closely. Theophylline clearance may be increased by concurrent administration of barbiturates, carbamazepine, phenytoin, rifampicin, sulphinpyrazone, aminoglutethimide, phenobarbitone and primidone. Lithium excretion is accelerated by theophylline.

The effects of ephedrine are diminished by guanethidine, reserpine, and probably methyldopa, and may be diminished or enhanced by tricyclic anti-depressants. Ephedrine may also diminish the effects of guanethidine and may increase the possibility of arrhythmias in digitalised patients.

Side-effects: Large doses of Franol Plus may give rise to the following side effects: arrhythmias, tachycardia, palpitation, flushing, giddiness, headache, tremor, anxiety, restlessness, insomnia, muscular weakness, nausea, vomiting, dyspepsia, thirst, sweating, difficulty in micturition.

Some patients may exhibit one or more such symptoms with therapeutic doses.

Overdosage: The symptoms and signs of overdosage with Franol Plus are likely to include excessive irritability, sweating, nausea and vomiting, tachycardia, arrhythmias, hypertension, profuse diuresis with fever, flushing and hyperglycaemia, opisthotonus, hallucinations, convulsions and respiratory difficulty. In general the management of overdosage with Franol Plus involves supportive and symptomatic therapy with particular attention being paid to the detection and correction of hypokalaemia, and should include serial assay of plasma potassium and theophylline levels, cardiac monitoring with electro-cardiogram, and maintenance of fluid and electrolyte balance.

Gastric aspiration and lavage may be employed. Convulsions and other CNS stimulation can usually be controlled by intravenous diazepam, or if that fails other anti-convulsants may be used. Marked excitement or hallucinations may be managed with chlorpromazine. Severe hypertension may necessitate the use of an alpha-adrenoreceptor blocking agent and a beta-adrenoreceptor blocking agent may be required to control arrhythmias. Beta 1-receptor agonist agents such as dopamine should be avoided. Charcoal haemoperfusion may be indicated to remove theophylline, but forced diuresis or peritoneal dialysis are inadequate for this purpose.

Pharmaceutical precautions Nil.

Legal category P.

Package quantities Franol Plus Tablets are supplied in bottles of 250.

Further information The bronchodilator action of ephedrine is through direct agonism at beta adrenoceptors and, indirectly, through sympathetic amine release. Bronchodilatation with theophylline is attributable to adenosine antagonism or phosphodiesterase inhibition which would be pharmacologically complementary to the action of ephedrine. Theophylline is variably absorbed from the gastrointestinal tract. It is excreted via the urine mainly as 1,3-dimethyluric acid and about 10% is unchanged. Ephedrine is readily absorbed. Its action is evident within one hour. With a plasma elimination half life of about 4 hours, 60–75% is excreted unchanged in the urine.

Product licence number 11723/0034.

GABITRIL* 5 mg
GABITRIL* 10 mg
GABITRIL* 15 mg

Qualitative and quantitative composition

Each Gabitril 5 mg tablet contains: Tiagabine, INN 5 mg (as anhydrous hydrochloride).

Each Gabitril 10 mg tablet contains: Tiagabine, INN 10 mg (as anhydrous hydrochloride).

Each Gabitril 15 mg tablet contains: Tiagabine, INN 15 mg (as anhydrous hydrochloride).

Pharmaceutical form White film-coated scored tablet for oral administration. Gabitril 5, 10 and 15 mg tablets are marked 251, 252 and 253 respectively.

Clinical particulars

Therapeutic indications: Gabitril is an antiepileptic drug indicated as add-on therapy for partial seizures with or without secondary generalisation where control is not achieved by optimal doses of at least one other antiepileptic drug.

Posology and method of administration:

Adults and children over 12 years: Gabitril should be taken orally with meals. The initial dose for those taking enzyme-inducing antiepileptic drugs is 5 mg twice daily for one week followed by weekly increments of 5–10 mg/day.

The following titration schedule is suggested:

Week	*Breakfast*	*Evening meal*	*Total daily dose*
1	5 mg	5 mg	10 mg
2	5 mg	10 mg	15 mg
3	10 mg	10 mg	20 mg
4	15 mg	15 mg	30 mg

The usual maintenance dose is 30–45 mg/day. Doses above 30 mg should be given in three divided doses.

The above regimen is appropriate for patients who are also taking other antiepileptic agents that induce hepatic enzymes (such as phenytoin, carbamazepine, phenobarbitone and primidone); most patients in clinical trials of tiagabine were in this category.

In patients not taking enzyme-inducing drugs, the maintenance dosage initially should be lower at 15–30 mg/day. This is based on population kinetics analysis, which suggested that the clearance of tiagabine in non-induced patients is 60% of that in patients taking enzyme-inducing drugs.

Children under 12 years: There is no experience with Gabitril in children under 12 years of age and as such Gabitril should not be used in this age group.

Use in the elderly: There is limited information available on the use of Gabitril in elderly patients, but pharmacokinetics of tiagabine are unchanged, hence there should be no need for dose modification.

Use in patients with impaired liver function: In patients with mild to moderate hepatic dysfunction (Child Pugh Score 5–9) the initial daily maintenance dosage should be 5–10 mg given once or twice daily. Gabitril should not be used in patients with severely impaired hepatic function.

Contra-indications: Gabitril should not be given to patients with a history of hypersensitivity to tiagabine or one of the excipients.

Special warnings and special precautions for use: Gabitril is eliminated by hepatic metabolism and therefore caution should be exercised when administering the product to patients with impaired hepatic function. Reduced doses and/or dose intervals should be used and patients should be monitored closely for adverse events such as dizziness and tiredness.

Gabitril should not be used in patients with severely impaired hepatic function.

Although Gabitril may slightly prolong the CNS depressant effect of triazolam, this interaction is unlikely to be relevant to clinical practice.

Antiepileptic agents that induce hepatic enzymes (such as phenytoin, carbamazepine, phenobarbitone and primidone) enhance the metabolism of tiagabine. Consequently, patients not taking enzyme-inducing drugs may require doses below the usual dose range.

Although there is no evidence of withdrawal seizures following Gabitril, it is recommended to taper off treatment over a period of 2–3 weeks.

Interaction with other medication and other forms of interaction: Antiepileptic agents that induce hepatic enzymes (such as phenytoin, carbamazepine, phenobarbitone and primidone) enhance the metabolism of tiagabine. The plasma concentration of tiagabine may be reduced by a factor of 1.5–3 by concomitant use of these drugs.

Gabitril does not have any clinically significant effect on the plasma concentrations of phenytoin, carbamazepine, phenobarbitone, warfarin, digoxin, theophylline and hormones from oral contraceptive pills. Gabitril reduces the plasma concentration of valproate by about 10%, and cimetidine increases the bioavailability of tiagabine by about 5%. Neither of these findings are considered clinically important and do not warrant a dose modification.

Pregnancy and lactation: Clinical experience of Gabitril in pregnant women is insufficient to evaluate its safety. Animal experiments do not show an increased incidence of foetal damage. The studies were inadequate to assess the safety of a metabolite excreted uniquely by man. Foetal exposure to the metabolite cannot be excluded although a metabolite has not been detected in human plasma (i.e. <0.1% of maximum tiagabine plasma concentrations). Gabitril should not be used during pregnancy or breast-feeding unless, in the opinion of the physician, the potential benefits of treatment outweigh the potential risks.

Effects on ability to drive and use machines: Gabitril may cause dizziness or other CNS related symptoms especially during initial treatment. Therefore caution should be shown by patients driving vehicles or operating machinery.

Undesirable effects: Adverse events are mainly CNS related.

In placebo controlled parallel group add-on epilepsy trials of Gabitril in combination with other antiepileptic drugs, the adverse events that occurred statistically more frequently with Gabitril than with placebo are tabulated below.

	Gabitril N=493 %	Placebo N=276 %
Dizziness	29	16
Tiredness	22	15
Nervousness (non-specific)	11	4
Tremor	10	4
Diarrhoea	8	3
Concentration difficulties	6	3
Depressed mood	4	1
Emotional lability	4	1
Slowness in speech	2	0

In clinical trials, about 15% of patients receiving Gabitril reported serious adverse events; the causal relationship of these events with Gabitril treatment has not been established and some may be associated with the underlying condition or concomitant treatment. Accidental injury (2.8%) was the only adverse event which occurred with a frequency of more than 1%; others included confusion (1.0%), depression (0.8%), somnolence (0.8%) and psychosis (0.7%). However, none of these adverse events led to the withdrawal of more than 0.2% of patients.

In patients with a history of serious behavioural problems there is a risk of recurrence of these symptoms during treatment with Gabitril, as occurs with certain other antiepileptic drugs.

Although not statistically significant, routine laboratory screening during placebo controlled trials showed a low white blood cell count ($<2.5\times10^9$ per litre) more frequently during Gabitril treatment (4.1%) than placebo (1.5%).

Overdose: Reports on overdosage with Gabitril are few. Symptoms of overdosage are somnolence, dizziness, ataxia or incoordination and, in more severe instances, mute and withdrawn appearance of the patient. In one patient an overdose of about 300 mg of Gabitril in combination with phenytoin resulted in coma. In all episodes of overdosage with Gabitril the patients have recovered within 24 hours without any sequelae.

Standard medical observation and supportive care should be given.

Pharmacological properties

Pharmacodynamic properties: Gabitril is an antiepileptic drug.

Tiagabine is a potent and selective inhibitor of both neuronal and glial GABA uptake, which results in an increase in GABAergic mediated inhibition in the brain.

Tiagabine lacks significant affinity for other neurotransmitter receptor binding sites and/or uptake sites.

Pharmacokinetic properties: Tiagabine is rapidly and virtually completely absorbed from Gabitril tablets, with an absolute bioavailability of 89%. Administration with food results in a decreased rate and not extent of absorption.

The volume of distribution is approximately 1 L/kg.

Plasma protein binding of tiagabine is about 96%.

Renal clearance is negligible. Hepatic metabolism is the principal route for elimination of tiagabine. Less than 2% of the dose is excreted unchanged in urine and faeces. No active metabolites have been identified. Other antiepileptic drugs such as phenytoin, carbamazepine, phenobarbitone and primidone induce hepatic drug metabolism and the hepatic clearance of tiagabine is increased when given concomitantly with these drugs.

There is no evidence that tiagabine causes clinically significant induction or inhibition of hepatic drug metabolising enzymes at clinical doses.

The plasma elimination half-life of tiagabine is 7–9 hours, except in induced patients where it is 2–3 hours.

Absorption and elimination of tiagabine are linear within the therapeutic dose range.

Preclinical safety data: Animal safety data carried out in the rat, mouse and dog gave no clear evidence of specific organ toxicity nor any findings of concern for the therapeutic use of tiagabine. The dog appears to be particularly sensitive to the pharmacological actions of tiagabine as clinical signs such as sedation, insensibility, ataxia and visual impairment reflecting CNS effects were seen at daily doses of 0.5 mg/kg and above in a dose related manner. The results of a wide range of mutagenicity tests showed that tiagabine is unlikely to be genotoxic to humans. Clastogenic activity was seen only at cytotoxic concentrations (> >200-fold human plasma levels) in the *in-vitro* human lymphocyte test in the absence of a metabolising system. In long-term carcinogenicity studies conducted in the rat and mouse, only the rat study revealed slightly increased incidences of hepatocellular adenomas in females and benign Leydig cell tumours in the high-dose (200 mg/kg/day) group only. These changes are considered to be rat-specific and of little clinical importance to humans. In rats treated with 100 mg/kg/day or more, pulmonary macrophages and inflammation were seen at a higher incidence than normal. The significance of this latter finding is unknown.

Pharmaceutical particulars

List of excipients

α-Tocopherol
Macrogol 6000
Lactose, anhydrous
Talc
Hypromellose
Titanium dioxide, E171.

Incompatibilities: None.

Shelf life: 2 years.

Special precautions for storage: Store below 25°C. Do not refrigerate. Keep out of reach of children.

Nature and contents of container: Child resistant, white polyethylene container with white polypropylene screw closure. Available as packs of 50 or 100 Gabitril tablets in 5, 10 or 15 mg strengths.

Instructions for use/handling: No special instructions.

Marketing authorisation holder: Sanofi Winthrop Limited, One Onslow Street, Guildford, Surrey GU1 4YS.

Marketing authorisation numbers

Gabitril 5 mg	PL 11723/0254
Gabitril 10 mg	PL 11723/0255
Gabitril 15 mg	PL 11723/0256

Date of first authorisation/renewal of the authorisation 1 March 1998

Date of (partial) revision of the text November 1997

Legal category POM.

GLURENORM*

Qualitative and quantitative composition Gliquidone HSE 30 mg.

Pharmaceutical form Tablet.

Clinical particulars

Therapeutic indications: Glurenorm tablets are indicated for the treatment of non-insulin dependent diabetics who do not respond adequately to dietary control.

Posology and method of administration: Glurenorm tablets are for oral administration.

Glurenorm should be taken up to half an hour before a meal. The dose and frequency of administration should be adjusted, together with the diet, to obtain the best possible control of the diabetes throughout the day.

Adults (including the elderly): Most patients respond to a total daily dose of 45–60 mg given in two or three divided doses, of which the largest dose is usually taken in the morning with breakfast. The recommended maximum single dose is 60 mg (2 tablets) and the maximum daily dose 180 mg (6 tablets). During stabilisation, dosage adjustment should be based on frequent blood (random and postprandial) and urinary glucose determination.

Stabilisation of previously untreated cases: Normally, treatment should begin with 15 mg (half a tablet) before breakfast and this should be gradually increased by 15 mg increments prior to mealtimes.

Change-over in patients previously treated with other oral antidiabetic agents: Patients can be changed over from other sulphonylureas to Glurenorm without interruption. It is usual to start with 30 mg Glurenorm before breakfast, increasing as necessary by increments of 15 mg at mealtimes. In terms of comparative potency of single doses, 30 mg Glurenorm corresponds approximately to 1000 mg tolbutamide, 5 mg glibenclamide, 250 mg chlorpropamide or 500 mg acetohexamide.

However, in estimating equivalent total daily doses, the half-lives and duration of action of the respective sulphonylureas must be taken into consideration. Thus it will usually be necessary to administer Glurenorm more frequently than a long-acting sulphonylurea.

Change-over in non-insulin dependent diabetics previously treated with insulin: In patients treated with up to 30 IU of insulin daily, change-over to Glurenorm may be attempted with an initial dose of 30 mg accompanied by a simultaneous gradual reduction of the amount of insulin, provided the pancreas still contains some functioning beta cells. Patients who change from insulin to Glurenorm should be strictly supervised and response assessed by frequent and regular blood glucose determinations.

It may be possible to reduce the insulin requirements of patients who require more than 30 IU daily by the concurrent administration of Glurenorm. Blood glucose should be monitored frequently during the change-over period.

Combined treatment: The administration of metformin with Glurenorm to patients who cannot be adequately controlled by Glurenorm alone may achieve satisfactory stabilisation of blood-glucose levels.

Children: Dosage recommendation is not appropriate.

Contra-indications: Do not use for diabetes complicated by acidosis or ketosis nor in patients subject to the stress of surgery or acute infections. Glurenorm should not be used in pregnancy or during breast feeding, nor in patients with severe hepatic or renal failure, or porphyria.

Special warnings and special precautions for use: Patients who miss a meal (particularly the elderly or debilitated) should be warned not to take their dose of Glurenorm, in order to reduce the risk of a hypoglycaemic reaction.

Special care should be observed in the concomitant use of Glurenorm with many other medications because interactions with sulphonylureas are common.

The effect of Glurenorm may be increased by physical exertion.

Interaction with other medicaments and other forms of interaction: The effects of Glurenorm may be increased by physical exertion, alcohol, salicylates, sulphonamides, phenylbutazone, ethionamide, coumarin, anti-coagulants, chloramphenicol, tetracyclines, cyclophosphamide, MAO inhibitors, tuberculostatics and beta-adrenergic blocking agents, azapropazone, co-trimoxazole, miconazole and sulphinpyrazone.

It may be necessary to increase the dose of Glurenorm when any of the following are administered concurrently: oral contraceptives, chlorpromazine, sympathomimetic agents, corticosteroids, thyroid hormones and nicotinic acid preparations, rifampicin, diazoxide and loop or thiazide diuretics.

The effects of barbiturates, vasopressin and oral anti-coagulants are potentiated by the administration of Glurenorm.

Pregnancy and lactation: Glurenorm should not be used in pregnancy or during breast feeding.

Effects on ability to drive and use machines: Not known.

Undesirable effects: Glurenorm is generally well tolerated, but minor skin allergies, gastric upsets and other non-specific symptoms have been noted. Reversible leucopenia has been reported on one occasion and reversible thrombocytopenia twice, but a causal connection with Glurenorm was not established.

Hypoglycaemic reactions are infrequent, but may be accompanied by malaise, impaired concentration and altered consciousness. They may be treated with oral carbohydrate or with intravenous dextrose if the oral route is impractical. Glucagon (1 mg subcutaneously) could also be given.

Overdose: In the conscious patient, hypoglycaemia may be managed by the oral administration of glucose. In the comatose patient, parenteral administration of glucose by intravenous infusion should be instituted. The patients should be kept under observation for further signs of hypoglycaemia. Consideration may be given to the recovery of ingested tablets by gastric lavage.

Pharmacological properties

Pharmacodynamic properties: Glurenorm is a sulphonylurea compound which causes an increase in plasma insulin levels in normal subjects, and in non-insulin dependant diabetic patients there is a corresponding decrease in plasma glucose levels. The onset of activity is normally within one hour of oral dosing, and the optimum effect normally lasts 2–3 hours.

Pharmacokinetic properties: Glurenorm is rapidly absorbed, and quickly attains therapeutic blood levels.

Plasma half-life is approximately 1.4 hours. It is almost completely metabolised in the liver by hydroxylation and demethylation. Only 5% of the pharmacologically inactive metabolites are excreted by the kidneys, the remainder are eliminated in the faeces via the bile. There is thus little risk of hypoglycaemia due to drug accumulation in patients with impaired renal function.

Preclinical safety data: There are no pre-clinical safety data of relevance to the prescriber which are additional to that already included in other sections of the SPC.

Pharmaceutical particulars

List of excipients: Lactose, maize starch, soluble starch, magnesium stearate.

Incompatibilities: Not applicable.

Shelf life: 60 months.

Special precautions for storage: None.

Nature and contents of container: Amber glass bottles with wadless polypropylene screw caps. Pack size of 60 and 100 tablets.

Instructions for use/handling: None.

Marketing authorisation number PL 11723/0037

Date of first authorisation/renewal of authorisation 29th October 1993

Date of (partial) revision of text May 1997

Legal category POM

HEXOPAL* TABLETS 500 mg
HEXOPAL* SUSPENSION
HEXOPAL* FORTE TABLETS

Qualitative and quantitative composition

Hexopal Tablets 500 mg:	Inositol Nicotinate BP 500 mg
Hexopal Suspension:	Inositol Nicotinate BP 1 g/5 ml
Hexopal Forte Tablets:	Inositol Nicotinate BP 750 mg

Pharmaceutical form

Hexopal Tablets 500 mg:	Tablets
Hexopal Suspension:	Suspension
Hexopal Forte Tablets:	Tablet

Clinical particulars

Therapeutic indications: Hexopal is indicated for the symptomatic relief of severe intermittent claudication and Raynaud's phenomenon.

Posology and method of administration: For oral administration.

Adults (including the elderly): The usual dose is 3 g daily (i.e. 2 500 mg tablets three times a day; 5 ml suspension taken three times a day; two Hexopal Forte Tablets twice daily). The dose may be increased to 4 g daily if necessary.

Children: Not recommended.

Contra-indications: Use in patients who have suffered a recent myocardial infarction or are in the acute phase of a cerebrovascular accident.

Use in patients hypersensitive to the active ingredient.

Special warnings and special precautions for use: This product should be used with caution in the presence of cerebrovascular insufficiency or unstable angina.

Interaction with other medicaments and other forms of interaction: None.

Pregnancy and lactation: There is no evidence of the safety of Hexopal in human pregnancy nor is there adequate evidence from animal work that it is free from hazard. The use of Hexopal in pregnancy should therefore be avoided unless there is no safer alternative.

Effects on ability to drive and use machines: None.

Undesirable effects: Side effects are uncommon, but may include flushing, dizziness, headache, nausea, vomiting, syncope, paraesthesia, rash, oedema, and postural hypotension.

Overdose: Despite extensive clinical experience in Britain since 1959, no case of poisoning or overdosage with Hexopal has been reported. In an emergency, it is suggested that the stomach be emptied by gastric lavage and the patient be treated symptomatically.

Pharmacological properties

Pharmacodynamic properties: The mode of action of inositol nicotinate in Raynaud's phenomenon and in intermittent claudication remains to be determined. Inositol nicotinate does not appear to produce general peripheral vasodilation.

Pharmacokinetic properties: Radiolabelled tracer studies indicate that with orally administered inositol nicotinate very low concentrations of nicotinic acid are found in the plasma. These levels appear to be maintained for approximately 24 hours.

Preclinical safety data: There are no preclinical safety data of relevance to the prescriber which are additional to that already included in other sections of the SPC.

Pharmaceutical particulars

List of excipients: Hexopal 500 mg tablets: Soluble starch, Maize starch, Purified talc, Magnesium stearate, Stearic acid, Sodium lauryl sulphate.

Hexopal suspension: Sorbitol solution, Magnesium aluminium silicate, Potassium sorbate, Citric acid (anhydrous), Sorbitol powder, Disodium phosphate dihydrate, Sodium carboxymethyl cellulose, Nipastat, Cetomacrogol 1000, Sodium hydroxide, Purified water.

Hexopal Forte Tablets: Soluble starch, Talc, Magnesium stearate, Maize starch, Stearic acid, Sodium lauryl sulphate.

Incompatibilities: None.

Shelf life:

Hexopal 500 mg tablets:	60 months.
Hexopal suspension:	24 months.
Hexopal Forte Tablets:	60 months.

Special precautions for storage:

Hexopal 500 mg tablets:	Store below 25°C.
Hexopal suspension:	Store at room temperature.
Hexopal Forte Tablets:	Store below 25°C.

Nature and contents of container: Hexopal 500 mg tablets: Amber glass bottle with wadless polypropylene screws caps. Pack size: 100 and 500 tablets. 200 μm white opaque PVC/20 μm aluminium blister pack. Pack size: 100 tablets.

Hexopal suspension: High density polyethylene bottles sealed with low density polyethylene snap-on caps. Pack size: 300 ml.

Hexopal Forte Tablets: Amber glass bottles containing 100, 250 and 500 tablets. 250 μm clear PVC/20 μm aluminium blister pack containing 112 tablets.

Instructions for use/handling: None.

Marketing authorisation numbers

Hexopal 500 mg tablets:	11723/0040
Hexopal suspension:	11723/0039
Hexopal Forte Tablets:	11723/0038

Date of first authorisation/renewal of authorisation

Hexopal 500 mg tablets and suspension:	15 November 1993
Hexopal Forte Tablets:	15 September 1993.

Date of (partial) revision of text April 1998.

Legal category P.

HYPAQUE* 25% AND 45%

Presentation Hypaque is a sterile, almost colourless aqueous solution in clear glass ampoules or infusion bottles containing either 25% w/v or 45% w/v Sodium Diatrizoate BP. Hypaque 25% and 45% contain sodium calcium edetate.

Uses An X-ray radiographic contrast medium suitable for intravenous and retrograde urography, angiography, venography and many other specialised procedures including examination of the gastro-intestinal tract.

Dosage and administration The route of administration of Hypaque, which may be parenteral, oral or rectal, and the volume and concentration employed depend on the procedure being undertaken.

Parenteral administration: suggested strength and quantity according to procedure.

Procedure	*Strength (%)*	*Amount of medium used (ml)*	
		Adults and elderly	*Children*
Urography:			
i.v.	45	0.5–2.0/kg	as adult
infusion	25	4.0/kg	as adult
retrograde	25–45	5–20	as adult
Cystography	10–45	500–1500	100–300
Peripheral arteriography	45	20–40	10–20
Haemorrhoidal portal venography	45	30–40	15–20
Renal cyst puncture	25–45	5–60	5–20
Orbital phlebography	45	2–4	1–2
Intraosseous venography	45	20–45	—
Choledochography:			
percutaneous transhepatic	25–45	15	5
operative	25–45	5–20	5
post-op. 'T' tube	25–45	5–20	5
Hysterosalpingography	45	10	—
Arthrography	25–45	5–20	3–10
Sinography	45	20–40	—
Tube screening (gastric including acute abdomen)	25	5–20	—
Abdominal stab wounds	25	q.s.	q.s.
Dacryocystography	45	1–3	—
Vesiculography	45	1.5–2.0 to a total of 10–12 each side	—
Myography	45	3	—
Duct mammography	25	1–2	—
Discography	45	0.5 max. 2.0	—

Oral or rectal administration in examination of the gastro-intestinal tract: For adults including the elderly, an average dose of 100 ml to 150 ml of a 25–50% solution is suggested when given by mouth or tube. From 500 ml to 1,000 ml of 20–35% solution is suggested as an enema.

For infants or children the dose by mouth or tube may vary from 50 ml to 120 ml of a 10–25% solution, and by enema from 100 ml to 500 ml of a 10–15% solution may be used.

Contra-indications, warnings, etc

Contra-indications: Hypaque should not be used for myelography. Injection of even a small amount into the subarachnoid space may produce convulsions and result in fatality.

Hypaque should not be used in patients with proven or suspected hypersensitivity to iodine-containing contrast media.

Precautions: Particular caution should be exercised in patients with a history of allergy, atopy, asthma, cardiac disease, or a previous adverse reaction with any contrast medium as they may be at higher risk from developing anaphylaxis or cardiovascular collapse. Consideration should be given to the use of low osmolar radiocontrast media in such patients.

Ready availability of emergency resuscitation equipment and familiarity with procedures are prerequisites for the safe use of radiocontrast media.

Recent reports of thyroid storm occurring following the intravascular use of iodinated radio-opaque diagnostic agents in patients with hyperthyroidism or with an autonomously functioning thyroid nodule suggest that this additional risk be evaluated in such patients before use of Hypaque.

In patients with subarachnoid haemorrhage, a rare association between contrast media administration and clinical deterioration, including convulsions and death, has been reported. Therefore, administration of intravascular iodated ionic contrast media to these patients should be undertaken with caution.

Caution should be observed in patients with tuberculosis since it has been suggested that iodine could exacerbate active tuberculosis, although this has not been reported with Hypaque.

Serious, rarely fatal, thromboembolic events causing myocardial infarction and stroke have been reported during angiographic procedures with both ionic and nonionic contrast media. Therefore, meticulous intravascular administration technique is necessary, particularly during angiographic procedures, to minimise thromboembolic events. Numerous factors, including length of procedure, catheter and syringe material, underlying disease state and concomitant medications may contribute to the development of thromboembolic events. For these reasons, meticulous angiographic techniques are recommended including close attention to guidewire and catheter manipulation, use of manifold systems and/ or three-way stopcocks, frequent catheter flushing with heparinised saline solutions and minimising the length of the procedure. The use of plastic syringes in place of glass syringes has been reported to decrease but not eliminate the likelihood of in vitro clotting.

Although Hypaque is not contra-indicated in patients with advanced renal destruction associated with severe uraemia, or in those with severe hepatic disorders, potentially hazardous situations requiring particular care are oliguric renal failure, myeloma and combined renal and hepatic failure. No attempt should be made to dehydrate the uraemic patient, nor should dehydration be carried out in a patient with myeloma. Evidence suggests that, in the latter case, it is dehydration rather than the presence of myeloma protein which has been the cause of adverse effects. Prior purgation should be avoided.

Because of the possibility of inducing a temporary suppression of urine, it is wise to allow an interval of at least 24 hours before repeating excretory or retrograde pyelography in patients with unilateral reduction of normal renal function.

Contrast media may promote sickling in individuals who are homozygous for sickle cell disease when the material is injected intravenously or intra-arterially.

Administration of radio-opaque materials to patients known or suspected of having phaeochromocytoma should be performed with extreme caution. If, in the opinion of the physician, the possible benefits of such procedures outweigh the considered risks, the procedures may be performed; however, the amount of radio-opaque medium injected should be kept to an absolute minimum. The blood pressure should be assessed throughout the procedure and measures for treatment of a hypertensive crisis should be available.

In examinations of the gastro-intestinal tract, Hypaque should be used with caution in infants and debilitated elderly patients because hypovolaemia may develop due to the osmotic activity of the contrast material in the intestines.

Use in pregnancy and lactation: X-ray examinations should be avoided during pregnancy. Animal reproduction studies have not been carried out with Hypaque, and it is not known whether it can cause foetal harm when administered to a pregnant woman. Hypaque can be transferred across the placenta to the foetus, and may also appear in breast milk. Hypaque therefore should only be administered to pregnant women when absolutely necessary. Caution should be observed in its administration to nursing mothers.

Interactions: Organic iodine contrast media are known to remain in the blood serum of patients for periods varying from two days to several years in concentrations sufficient to interfere with tests of thyroid function such as protein-bound iodine determinations. It has been reported that sodium diatrizoate remains in the serum for four days. It is therefore advisable to perform such thyroid function tests before any examination involving the use of Hypaque.

Other tests which may be affected by sodium diatrizoate, and for which an interval of 2 or 3 days should be allowed between administration and testing include:

Blood tests: Diatrizoate salts significantly inhibit all stages of coagulation. The fibrinogen concentration, Factors V, VII and VIII are decreased. Prothrombin time and thromboplastin time are increased.

Platelet aggregation: High levels of plasma diatrizoates inhibit platelet aggregation.

Serum calcium: Diatrizoate salts may decrease serum calcium levels. However, this depletion of serum calcium may also be the result of the addition of chelating agents (edetate disodium) in the preparation of certain contrast media.

Red cell counts: Transitory decreases in red cell counts. Technetium-99m-RBC labelling interference.

Leukocyte counts: Decrease following injection.

Urea nitrogen (BUN): Transitory increase.

Serum creatinine: Transitory increase.

Urine tests: Urine osmolarity and specific gravity may be decreased due to induced diuresis. Diatrizoate in urine cultures may inhibit bacterial growth.

Albumin: crystals of diatrizoic acid may separate out on acidification with mineral acid but these crystals are easily distinguished from the amorphous albumin precipitate. Hypaque does not affect the acetic acid or heat coagulation tests.

Side-effects: Approximately 95 per cent of adverse reactions accompanying the intravascular use of diatrizoate salts are of mild to moderate severity. However, life-threatening reactions and fatalities, including cardiovascular collapse and anaphylactic shock, have occurred.

Adverse reactions to injectable contrast media fall into two categories: chemotoxic reactions and idiosyncratic reactions.

Chemotoxic reactions result from the physicochemical properties of the contrast media, the dose, and the speed of injection. All haemodynamic disturbances and injuries to organs or vessels perfused by the contrast medium are included in this category.

Idiosyncratic reactions occur more frequently in patients 20 to 40 years old and may or may not be dependent on the amount of dose injected, the speed or the mode of injection, and the radiographic procedure. They are subdivided into minor, intermediate, and severe. The minor reactions are self-limiting and of short duration; the severe reactions are life-threatening and treatment is urgent and mandatory.

Most adverse reactions to injectable contrast media appear within one to three minutes after the start of injection, but delayed reactions may occur.

The reported incidence of adverse reactions to contrast media in patients with a history of allergy is twice that of the general population. Patients with a history of previous reactions to a contrast medium are three times more susceptible than other patients. However, sensitivity to contrast media does not appear to increase with repeated examinations.

Adverse reactions are grouped below by system organ class and are listed in decreasing order of occurrence. Significantly more severe reactions are listed before the other reactions regardless of frequency.

Body as a whole: Reported incidences of death range from 6.6 per 1 million (0.00066 percent) to 1 in 10,000 patients (0.01 percent). Most deaths occur during injection or 5 to 10 minutes later, the main feature being cardiac arrest with cardiovascular disease as the main aggravating factor.

Isolated reports of hypotensive collapse and shock following urography are found in the literature. The incidence of shock is estimated to occur in 1 out of 20,000 (0.005 percent) patients.

Greater than 1 in 100 patients: Cardiovascular system: The most frequent adverse reaction to diatrizoate salts is vasodilation (feeling of warmth). The estimated incidence is 49 percent.

Digestive system: Nausea 6 percent, vomiting 3 percent.

Nervous system: Paraesthesia 6 percent, dizziness 5 percent.

Respiratory system: Rhinitis 1 percent, increased cough 2 percent.

Skin and appendages: Urticaria 1 percent. Pain at the injection site is estimated to occur in about 12 percent of the patients undergoing urography. Pain is usually due to extravasation.

Painful hot erythematous swelling above the venipuncture site was estimated to occur in more than one percent of the patients undergoing phlebography.

Special senses: Perversion of taste 11 percent, and numbness.

Urogenital system: Osmotic nephrosis of the proximal tubular cells is estimated to occur in 23 percent of patients following excretory urography.

Less than 1 in 100 patients

Other infrequently reported reactions without accompanying incidence rates are listed below, grouped by organ system.

Body as a whole: Malaria relapse, uraemia, high creatinine and BUN, thrombocytopenia, leukopenia and anaemia.

Cardiovascular system: Cerebral haematomas, haemodynamic disturbances, sinus brachycardia, transient electrocardiographic abnormalities, ventricular fibrillation, and petechiae.

Digestive system: Severe unilateral or bilateral swelling of the parotid and submaxillary glands.

Nervous system: Convulsions, paralysis, coma and agitation.

Respiratory system: Asthma, dyspnoea, laryngeal oedema, pulmonary oedema, bronchospasm and respiratory arrest.

Skin and appendages: Extravasation necrosis, urticaria with or without pruritus, mucocutaneous oedema, and angioneurotic oedema.

Special senses: Bilateral ocular irritation, lacrimation, itching, conjunctival chemosis, infection, and conjunctivitis.

Urogenital: Renal failure, pain.

Pharmaceutical precautions The sterile aqueous solutions are clear and almost colourless. Hypaque solutions should not be re-autoclaved because of the possibility of free amine production. Solutions should be protected from light.

Legal category POM.

Package quantities *Hypaque 25%:* 20 ml ampoules in boxes of 5. Infusion bottles of 250 ml or 350 ml. *Hypaque 45%:* 20 ml ampoules in boxes of 20.

Further information The radio-opacity of sodium diatrizoate is due to the presence of iodine which absorbs X-rays.

Product licence numbers

Hypaque 25% 11723/0041
Hypaque 45% 11723/0042

HYPAQUE* SODIUM POWDER

Qualitative and quantitative composition Active constituents: Sodium Diatrizoate BP 500.0 g.

Pharmaceutical form Powder.

Clinical particulars

Therapeutic indications: Hypaque Sodium Powder is used in the preparation of radiographic contrast media for examination of the gastrointestinal tract and for use in retrograde cystography and micturating urethrography.

Posology and method of administration:

Administration: Hypaque Sodium Powder is used for the preparation of solutions for oral and rectal administration and for introduction into the bladder via a urinary catheter. Hypaque Sodium Powder is not suitable for the preparation of injectable solutions.

Recommended dosage:

(a) Examination of the gastro-intestinal tract:

Adults: For adults an average dose of from 100 to 150 ml of a 25–50% solution is suggested when given by mouth or by tube. From 500 ml to 1,000 ml of 20–35% solution is suggested as an enema.

Children: The oral or tube dose may vary from 50 ml to 120 ml of a 10–25% solution, and as an enema from 100 ml to 500 ml of a 10–15% solution.

Elderly: As for adults, but see *Precautions.*

The solvent may be water, saline or Ringer's solution. For oral use, suitable flavouring such as vanilla or chocolate syrup may be helpful in masking the taste of Hypaque.

(b) Retrograde cystography and micturating urethrography: There is some variation in the strength and quantity of medium employed. However, for urethrography 5 ml to 20 ml of a 25–45% solution is recommended for both adults and children. For cystography the recommendation for adults is 500 ml to 1500 ml of a 10–45% solution, and the recommendation for children is 100 ml–300 ml of a 10–45% solution. To sterilise, 0.012% w/v sodium calcium edetate should be added to the solution which is then autoclaved at 10 lb per sq in (115–116°C) for 30 minutes.

Contra-indications: No specific statement.

Special warnings and special precautions for use: A solution of Hypaque Sodium in water greater than 10% is hypertonic. Therefore, care should be taken when such solutions are used to examine the gastro-intestinal tracts of infants and debilitated elderly patients, since hypovolaemia may develop due to the osmotic activity of the contrast material in the intestines. It is advisable to correct any electrolyte disturbances before using solutions that are extremely hypertonic.

Patients with a history of allergy, especially to iodine, require careful consideration since Hypaque may be absorbed, though in very small amounts, through the intestinal wall.

Caution is advised in patients with tuberculosis since it has been suggested that iodine could exacerbate active tuberculosis, although this has not been reported with Hypaque.

Interaction with other medicaments and other forms of interaction: The presence of sodium diatrizoate in the serum may interfere with tests of thyroid function such as protein bound iodine determinations. It is therefore advisable to perform such thyroid function tests before any examination involving the use of Hypaque.

Pregnancy and lactation: X-ray examinations should be avoided during pregnancy. Animal reproduction studies have not been carried out with Hypaque, and it is not known whether Hypaque can cause foetal harm when administered to a pregnant woman. Hypaque can be transferred across the placenta to the foetus, and may also appear in breast milk. Hypaque therefore should only be administered to pregnant women when absolutely necessary. Caution should be observed in its administration to nursing mothers.

Effects on ability to drive and use machines: No specific statement.

Undesirable effects: Nausea and diarrhoea have been occasionally reported with Hypaque Sodium Powder and dehydration from fluid loss in such cases must be borne in mind. Rarely, the following have been reported: pulmonary oedema following accidental aspiration, colonic overdistension and perforation, mucosal damage due to prolonged contact, and precipitation of the medium as a solid mass in the stomach. Irritation of the urethral and vesicular mucosa has occasionally followed administration into the bladder.

Minor allergic disturbances such as sneezing, rhinorrhoea, lacrimation and pruritus or urticarial rashes may occasionally occur, and should respond to antihistamine treatment.

Overdosage: No specific statement.

Pharmacological properties

Pharmacodynamic properties: Sodium diatrizoate is a radiopaque contrast medium. Its radioopacity is due to the presence of iodine which absorbs X-rays.

Pharmacokinetic properties: Hypaque Sodium Powder is diluted to the required concentration and is administered directly into the area to be visualised. Hence its diagnostic value is independent of its pharmacokinetic properties. Following oral administration to adults, Hypaque passes unchanged through the gastrointestinal tract. A very small amount is absorbed through the intestinal wall, since traces of iodine are excreted by the kidney. Absorption from the gastrointestinal tract occurs to a greater extent in infants.

Preclinical safety data: There are no pre-clinical data of relevance to the prescriber which are additional to that already included in other sections of the SPC.

Pharmaceutical particulars

List of excipients: None.

Incompatibilities: No specific statement.

Shelf life: 60 months.

Storage conditions: None.

Nature and contents of container: Hypaque Sodium Powder is packed in amber round glass bottles with black plastic caps.

Instructions for use/handling: No specific statement.

Marketing authorisation number 11723/0043

Date of approval/revision of SPC July 1996.

Legal category P.

KANNASYN* POWDER

Qualitative and quantitative composition Kanamycin Acid Sulphate PhEur, equivalent to 1 g kanamycin base.

Pharmaceutical form A white or almost white crystalline sterile powder for reconstitution for injection.

Clinical particulars
Therapeutic indications: Kannasyn is recommended for the treatment of infections due to Gram-negative organisms resistant to other antibiotics. It may also be used in the treatment of certain staphylococcal infections due to multiple-resistant strains, and in gonorrhoea.

Posology and method of administration: For intravenous or intramuscular administration.

(i) Intramuscular injections: Kannasyn should be given as a solution containing 250 mg/ml. This can be prepared by dissolving the contents of a 1 g vial in 4 ml of Water for Injections PhEur.

Adults: In acute infections: 1 g daily in two or four equally divided doses. Therapy should normally be limited to six days' treatment, and should not exceed a total of 10 g.

In chronic infections: 3 g weekly (1 g on alternate days) or 1 g twice a day, twice weekly (4 g weekly). The total amount administered should not exceed 50 g.

Children: In acute infections: 15 mg/kg body weight daily in 2–4 equally divided doses for no more than six days.

In chronic infections: There are no specific dosage recommendations.

Elderly: A reduced dosage may be required. See Warnings.

(ii) Intravenous use: This route is recommended only for gravely ill patients with overwhelming infections or with impending cardiovascular collapse. Kannasyn may be given as a solution containing 2.5 mg/ml by slow intravenous infusion at the rate of 3–4 ml per minute. This solution may be prepared by dissolving the contents of a 1 g vial in 400 ml Sodium Chloride Intravenous Infusion BP or Glucose Intravenous Infusion BP.

The dosage for both adults and children is 15–30 mg/kg body weight daily in 2 or 3 divided doses.

Contra-indications: Kannasyn is contra-indicated in patients with a history of hypersensitivity or toxic reaction to kanamycin or other aminoglycosides.

Special warnings and special precautions for use: In cases of impaired renal function, the kidney may be unable to eliminate kanamycin effectively and as a result the serum level will rise quickly. In these conditions reduced doses are necessary to avoid toxic effects. It has been reported that kanamycin is retained in the serum of patients with renal disease for a considerable time. If it is necessary to give the antibiotic to anuric patients, they should not receive increments more frequently than every three to four days and these increments should be one half the loading dose used. The safest procedure, however, is to control the dosage by monitoring the plasma level to prevent it rising above 30 mcg/ml.

Kannasyn should be protected from light. The powder may be stored at room temperature but should be used within three years of assay. Solutions of Kannasyn should be used immediately or stored at 2–8°C for not more than 24 hours.

Kannasyn should always be administered with caution and preferably only in severe or resistant infections caused by organisms known to be sensitive to the compound and blood levels should not be allowed to rise above 30 mcg/ml.

Caution should be observed also in myasthenia gravis because kanamycin has a weak curare-like action.

Interactions with other medicaments and other forms of interaction: The use of potent diuretics such as ethacrynic acid or frusemide with kanamycin should be avoided because they are known to potentiate the toxic action of aminoglycoside antibiotics.

As with other aminoglycoside antibiotics, apnoea and respiratory depression have been reported following the intraperitoneal use of kanamycin because of its curare-like effect. In addition, motor and sensory neuropathy has occurred following local application of kanamycin during spinal surgery. It has also produced slight weakening in muscle strength in a patient with myasthenia gravis. Because of these effects, it has been suggested that kanamycin should not be given intraperitoneally during surgery to patients who have received neuro-muscular blocking agents. Calcium gluconate has been suggested to counteract this curare-like action of kanamycin, but neostigmine appears to be more effective.

It has been shown that calcium can inhibit the antibacterial activity of kanamycin against certain organisms and for this reason the routine prophylactic use of calcium solution with intraperitoneal kanamycin should be discouraged.

It should be noted that prior treatment with streptomycin or viomycin may increase the likelihood of a nephrotoxic reaction with kanamycin.

Concurrent aminoglycosides may increase the risk of ototoxicity as may anti-emetics by masking its development. The dose of concurrent oral anticoagulant may require alteration because kanamycin may affect endogenous vitamin K.

Pregnancy and lactation: Kanamycin should not be used during pregnancy or lactation.

Effects on ability to drive and use machines: There are no specific warnings.

Undesirable effects: Local intolerance to intramuscular injection has sometimes been reported, but it is transient and does not require interruption of therapy. Ecchymoses have also been observed at the site of injection in a few patients. It has been suggested that in concentrations above those achieved in the blood at therapeutic dosage, kanamycin has anticoagulant action which may explain haematomas at the site of injection. Sensitivity rashes appear to be uncommon. Intravenous injections are well tolerated and pain is not a problem. Thrombophlebitis has only been reported once in a patient who was receiving 50 million units of penicillin with the kanamycin.

Particular caution should be observed in those with hearing loss. In common with certain other antibiotics, kanamycin can damage the eighth cranial nerve when used in large doses or for long periods. The resultant hearing loss, which may be permanent, is usually but not always preceded by tinnitus. Vestibular damage is less common. Should tinnitus or other sign of auditory toxicity appear, the dose of kanamycin should be reduced or it should be discontinued.

Hyaline and granular casts are sometimes observed in urine samples collected in the first 16 hours after administration in patients who have been given high doses of kanamycin. In these cases no permanent impairment of renal function occurs and the casts disappear within a few days of stopping treatment. Although nephrotoxic effects have been reported in some studies, serious renal toxicicty is not a frequent problem with the doses now used.

Overdose: In cases of overdosage or toxic reaction, haemodialysis or peritoneal dialysis will aid the removal of kanamycin from the blood.

Pharmacological properties
Pharmacodynamic properties: Kannasyn is recommended for the treatment of infections due to Gram-negative organisms resistant to other antibiotics. It may also be used in the treatment of certain staphylococcal infections due to multiple-resistant strains, and in gonorrhoea.

Pharmacokinetic properties: After intramuscular injection, peak concentrations of kanamycin of about 20 and 30 micrograms per ml are attained in about one hour following doses of 0.5 g and 1 g respectively. A plasma half-life of about 3 hours has been reported.

Kanamycin is rapidly excreted by glomerular filtration and most of a parenteral dose appears in the urine within 24 hours. It has been detected in cord blood and breast milk.

Preclinical safety data: Not applicable.

Pharmaceutical particulars
List of excipients: None.

Incompatibilities: Infusion solutions containing kanamycin have been reported to be incompatible with the following substances: amphotericin, barbiturates, cephalothin sodium, chlorpromazine, electrolytes (Ca^{++}, Mg^{++}, citrate or phosphate ions), heparin, hydrocortisone, methicillin sodium, methohexitone, nitrofurantoin, phenytoin, prochlorperazine, sulphafurazole.

Shelf life: 36 months.

Special precautions for storage: Kannasyn should be protected from light. The powder may be stored at room temperature but should be used within three years of assay. Solutions of Kannasyn should be used immediately or stored at 2–8°C for not more than 24 hours.

Nature and contents of container: Amber glass vials containing 1.43 g Kannasyn each, enclosed in cardboard cartons.

Instructions for use/handling
Intramuscular injection: Prepare by dissolving the contents of a 1 g vial in 4 ml of Water for Injections PhEur.

Intravenous use: Prepare by dissolving the contents of a 1 g vial in 400 ml Sodium Chloride Intravenous Infusion BP or Glucose Intravenous Infusion BP.

Marketing authorisation number 11723/0044.

Date of approval/revision of SPC 12 October 1993.

Legal category POM.

LINGRAINE*

Presentation Lingraine Tablets are light green, biconvex tablets, 6.4 mm in diameter, with no markings. Each tablet contains 2.0 mg Ergotamine Tartrate PhEur. Lingraine Tablets also contain lactose.

Uses Lingraine Tablets are recommended for the relief of migraine and other vascular headaches.

Dosage and administration Lingraine Tablets are for sublingual administration only.

Adults: One tablet to be taken at the first sign of an attack of migraine. If necessary another tablet may be taken half an hour to an hour later. No more than three tablets should be taken in 24 hours and not more than six tablets in any one week.

Elderly: As for adults but see warnings.

Children: Not recommended.

Contra-indications, warnings, etc Since (like other ergot alkaloids) ergotamine tartrate causes contraction of uterine muscle it should not be used during pregnancy. Avoid during breast feeding.

Because ergotamine brings about constriction of peripheral blood vessels Lingraine should not be used in the presence of severe arteriosclerosis, coronary artery disease, thrombophlebitis, Raynaud's syndrome or Buerger's disease. Furthermore, Lingraine should not be used where there is liver or kidney dysfunction, nor in the presence of severe hypertension, hyperthyroidism or porphyria. Concomitant use with beta blockers may increase the risk of peripheral vasoconstriction, whilst with erthromycin, the risk of ergotism.

Side-effects: These are a relatively minor problem if the dose is carefully regulated. Nausea and vomiting are most frequently reported; other side-effects encountered include abdominal pain, leg cramps, vertigo, diarrhoea and, occasionally, increased headache. If such symptoms are profound or accompanied by cardiovascular or neurological disturbances, they are indicative of chronic overdosage (see below).

Pleural and peritoneal fibrosis may occur with excessive use.

Overdosage: Like all the natural amino-acid alkaloids of ergot, ergotamine is a highly toxic substance which may cause chronic or acute poisoning, although the latter is less frequent.

The oral administration of 26 mg over several days has proved fatal, and there have also been deaths from as little as 0.5 mg to 1.5 mg in a single injection.

The principal signs of chronic overdosage are circulatory disturbances, due to vasoconstriction and thrombi-formation, including coldness of the skin, severe muscle pains, and vascular stasis resulting in dry peripheral gangrene. Anginal pain, tachycardia or bradycardia and hypertension or hypotension may occur. Other symptoms include headache, nausea, vomiting, diarrhoea and weakness of the legs. Confusion, drowsiness, hemiplegia and convulsions may also occur.

The main symptoms of acute poisoning consist of nausea, vomiting, diarrhoea, unquenchable thirst, tingling, itching and coldness of the skin, a rapid and weak pulse, confusion and unconsciousness. Treatment: Amyl nitrate inhalations (0.2–0.3 ml) are suggested to counteract arterial spasm.

Pharmaceutical precautions Nil.

Legal category POM.

Package quantities Lingraine Tablets are available in P.P.F.P. laminate strips in boxes of 12 tablets (OP).

Further information Ergotamine is an ergot alkaloid, and acts by antagonism of alpha adrenoceptors.

Product licence number 11723/0045.

MICTRAL* SACHETS

Qualitative and quantitative composition Nalidixic Acid BP 660 mg, Sodium Citrate PhEur 3750 mg, Citric Acid PhEur 250 mg, Sodium Bicarbonate PhEur 250 mg.

Pharmaceutical form Granules which are dissolved in water and suitable for oral administration.

Clinical particulars
Therapeutic indications: For the treatment of cystitis and lower urinary tract infections caused by pathogens sensitive to nalidixic acid.

Posology and method of administration:
Adults: The contents of one sachet should be dissolved in a tumblerful of water and taken three times a day. A 3 day course is normally sufficient.

Elderly: As for adults.

Children and Growing Adolescents: Not recommended.

Mictral sachets are for oral administration.

Contra-indications: Mictral Sachets should not be given to patients with a history of convulsive disorders, nor to patients with renal impairment or porphyria or hypersensitivity to nalidixic acid or related compounds.

Special warnings and special precautions for use: Nalidixic acid is mainly metabolised by the liver and should therefore be used with caution in patients with liver disease.

Caution should be observed in patients with severe cerebral arteriosclerosis or glucose-6-phosphate dehydrogenase deficiency. (Although care should be exercised in treating patients with renal failure, the full dosage of nalidixic acid may be administered in patients with creatinine clearance of more than 20 ml/min and half the normal dosage in patients with creatinine clearance less than this.)

Particular caution is advised in patients with a known allergic disposition. Patients taking nalidixic acid should avoid excessive exposure to sunlight (including sunbathing).

When nalidixic acid is given to patients on anticoagulant therapy, it may be necessary to reduce the anticoagulant dosage.

Caution should be observed and therapy discontinued if patients develop signs or symptoms suggestive of an increase in intracranial pressure, psychosis or other toxic manifestations.

Blood count, renal and liver function should be monitored periodically if treatment is continued for more than two weeks.

Each sachet contains the equivalent of 950 mg (41.3 M Eq) of sodium. This should be taken into account when prescribing for patients for whom sodium restriction is indicated especially the elderly.

Interactions with other medicaments and other forms of interaction: If nalidixic acid is given to patients on anticoagulant therapy, it may be necessary to reduce the anticoagulant dosage because nalidixic acid may interact with anticoagulants by competing for protein binding sites. Monitoring of prothrombin time and appropriate adjustment of the anticoagulant dosage following introduction and withdrawal of Mictral is recommended.

Active proliferation of the organisms is a necessary condition for the antibacterial action of nalidixic acid; the action of Mictral may therefore be inhibited by the presence of other antibacterial substances especially bacteriostatic agents such as tetracycline, chloramphenicol and nitrofurantoin which is antagonistic to nalidixic acid in vitro.

There have been reports of serious gastro-intestinal toxicity following the concomitant use of nalidixic acid and melphalan.

Probenecid may reduce the efficacy of Mictral by inhibiting tubular secretion of nalidixic acid.

It is possible that there will be an increased risk of nephrotoxicity with cyclosporins.

When testing for glycosuria in patients receiving Mictral, glucose specific methods based on glucose oxidase should be used since copper reduction methods may give false-positive results.

Nalidixic acid, in therapeutic doses can interfere with the estimation of urinary 17-ketosteroids and may cause high results in the assay of urinary vanilmandelic acid (Pisano method).

It is recognised that convulsions may occur due to an interaction between quinolones and non-steroidal anti-inflammatory drugs. This has not been observed so far with nalidixic acid.

Pregnancy and lactation: The safety of nalidixic acid during pregnancy has not been established. Therefore it should be used during pregnancy only if the potential benefits outweigh the potential risks, especially during the first trimester (nalidixic acid crosses the placental barrier and has been shown to be taken up by growing cartilage in several animal species) and during the last month of pregnancy because of the potential risk for the neonate. Exposure to maternal nalidixic acid in utero may lead to significant blood levels of nalidixic acid in the neonate immediately after birth.

Since nalidixic acid is excreted in breast milk, it is contraindicated during lactation.

Effects on ability to drive and to use machines: No specific warnings.

Undesirable effects: In keeping with the reduced systemic exposure to nalidixic acid which Mictral therapy entails, it is unlikely that Mictral will give rise to the full spectrum of adverse events reported with conventional oral nalidixic acid therapy, which include:

Central nervous system: Drowsiness, weakness, headache, dizziness and vertigo; subjective visual disturbances such as over-brightness of lights; changed colour perception, difficulty in focusing, decreased visual acuity and double vision, which are infrequent and usually disappear promptly on reducing dosage or stopping therapy.

Toxic psychosis or brief convulsions, which are rare, have usually followed excessive dosage in patients predisposed by epilepsy or cerebral arteriosclerosis and, very rarely, 6th cranial nerve palsy has been observed. The mechanism of these reactions is unknown but following withdrawal of treatment, rapid resolution without sequelae has usually occurred.

Gastro-intestinal: Abdominal pain, nausea, vomiting and diarrhoea.

Allergic: Rash, pruritus, urticaria, angio-oedema, eosinophilia, arthralgia with joint stiffness and swelling and, rarely, anaphylactoid reactions; photosensitivity reactions which include erythema and bullae on exposed surfaces are likely to resolve within 2–8 weeks of stopping therapy but bullae may continue to appear for up to 12 weeks after therapy, with mild skin trauma or exposure to sunlight (see *Warnings*).

Other: Rarely, cholestatis, paraesthesia, metabolic acidosis, thrombocytopenia, leucopenia or haemolytic anaemia, sometimes associated with glucose-6-phosphate dehydrogenase deficiency.

Overdosage: Because of the nature of the product, serious overdose is unlikely. An excessive amount of granules is likely to cause vomiting.

In adults, symptoms of overdose have been noted following single doses of 20 and 25 g. These have included toxic psychosis and convulsions. Occasional reports of metabolic acidosis have occurred in association with overdosage or overdose with concurrent use of probenecid. Vomiting, nausea and lethargy may also occur following overdosage. Reactions are likely to be short-lived because nalidixic acid is normally excreted rapidly.

If systemic absorption has occurred, fluid intake should be promoted; supportive measures such as oxygen and means of artificial respiration should be available. Anti-convulsant therapy may be indicated in a severe case, although it has not been used in the few instances of overdosage that have been reported.

Pharmacological properties

Pharmacodynamic properties: Nalidixic acid is an antibacterial agent which acts by selectively inhibiting bacterial DNA synthesis. The presence of sodium bicarbonate, citric acid and sodium citrate in the formulation is to maintain the urine at optimal pH for nalidixic acid activity and clearance.

Pharmacokinetic properties: Nalidixic acid (0.66 g)+sodium citrate (4 g) was given to healthy male volunteers t.i.d for 3 consecutive days. On day 3 the mean peak plasma concentration of nalidixic acid and hydroxynalidixic acid was 2.8 micrograms/ml and 2.6 micrograms/ml respectively. After undergoing metabolism 80–95% of nalidixic acid and its metabolites were excreted in the urine. The presence of the sodium citrate resulted in the urine of the volunteers becoming more alkaline.

Pre-clinical safety data: Not applicable.

Pharmaceutical particulars

List of excipients: Caster sugar, malic acid, dextrose monohydrate, saccharin sodium, polyvidone, sodium lauryl sulphate, grapefruit flavour 502.107/AP05.51.

Incompatibilities: None.

Shelf life: The shelf-life of this product is 36 months.

Special precautions for storage: Store in a dry place below 25°C.

Nature and contents of container: PPFP sachets containing 7 g of granulate. The sachets are packed into a cardboard carton. Pack sizes of 3 and 9 sachets.

Instructions for use/handling: Not applicable.

Marketing authorisation number PL 11723/0049

Date of approval/revision of SPC June 1997.

Legal category POM.

MODALIM* TABLETS

Qualitative and quantitative composition Each tablet contains 100 mg ciprofibrate.

Pharmaceutical form Tablet.

Clinical particulars

Therapeutic indications: Modalim tablets are recommended for the treatment of primary dyslipoproteinaemias, including types IIa, IIb, III and IV (hypercholesterolaemia, hypertriglyceridaemia and combined forms) – refractory to appropriate dietary treatment. Dietary measures should be continued during therapy.

Posology and method of administration:

Adults: The recommended dosage is one tablet (100 mg ciprofibrate). This dose should not be exceeded (see *Precautions*).

Elderly patients: As for adults, but see *Precautions* and *Warnings*.

Use in case of impaired renal function: In moderate renal impairment it is recommended that dosage be reduced to one tablet every other day. Patients should be carefully monitored. Modalim should not be used in severe renal impairment.

Use in children: Not recommended since safety and efficacy in children has not been established.

Modalim tablets are for oral administration only.

Contra-indications: Modalim is contra-indicated in cases of severe hepatic impairment, cases of severe renal impairment and in pregnancy and lactation.

Special warnings and special precautions for use: Patients should be advised to report unexplained muscle pain, tenderness or weakness immediately.

Doses of 200 mg Modalim per day or greater have been associated with a high risk of rhabdomyolysis. Therefore the daily dose should not exceed 100 mg. Hypoalbuminaemia as seen in nephrotic syndrome, or hypothyroidism may increase the risk of myopathy.

Use with caution in patients with impaired renal or hepatic function. Periodic liver function tests are recommended. Modalim treatment should be halted if liver enzyme abnormalities persist.

Secondary causes of dyslipidaemia, such as hypothyroidism, should be excluded or corrected prior to commencing any lipid lowering drug treatment. If after a period of administration lasting several months, a satisfactory reduction in serum lipid concentrations has not been obtained, additional or different therapeutic measures must be considered.

Interaction with other medicaments and other forms of interaction: Ciprofibrate is highly protein bound and is therefore capable of displacing other drugs from plasma protein binding sites. There is evidence that ciprofibrate potentiates the pharmacological response to warfarin in man. Therefore the dose of anticoagulant therapy should be reduced and then gradually re-adjusted by monitoring prothrombin time. Although there are no data to show that ciprofibrate interacts with other classes of drugs, a possible interaction with oral hypoglycaemic agents and oral contraceptive agents should be considered. As with other fibrates, the concomitant use of ciprofibrate with HMG-CoA reductase inhibitors, or other fibrates, may predispose patients to myopathy.

Pregnancy and lactation: There is no evidence that ciprofibrate is teratogenic but signs of embryotoxicity were observed at high doses in animals. Ciprofibrate is excreted in the breast milk of lactating rats. There are no data on the use of the drug in human pregnancy or lactation. Therefore the use of ciprofibrate is contraindicated during pregnancy and in nursing mothers.

Effects on ability to drive and use machines: Dizziness, drowsiness, or tiredness have only rarely been reported in association with ciprofibrate. It is therefore unlikely to affect the ability to drive or to use machinery.

Undesirable effects: There have been occasional reports of headache, vertigo, rashes and gastrointestinal symptoms including nausea, vomiting, diarrhoea and dyspepsia. Generally these side effects were mild to moderate in nature and occurred early on during treatment, becoming less frequent with continuation of dosing. As with other drugs in this class, a low incidence of impotence and hair loss has been reported.

As with other fibrates, elevation of serum creatine phosphokinase (CPK), myalgia and myopathy including rare cases of rhabdomyolysis have been reported. If symptoms of muscle toxicity develop the serum CPK should be measured immediately. Treatment should be discontinued if CPK levels are greater than ten times the upper limit of the normal range, if levels rise progressively or if there is other evidence of myopathy. In the majority of cases muscle toxicity is reversible when treatment is withdrawn. Isolated cases of pneumonitis or pulmonary fibrosis have been reported. As with other fibrates, abnormal liver function tests have been observed occasionally.

Overdose: Overdosage with ciprofibrate has been reported rarely. Associated adverse events reflect those seen in routine use. There are no specific antidotes to ciprofibrate. Treatment of overdosage should be symptomatic. Gastric lavage and appropriate supportive care may be instituted if necessary. Ciprofibrate is non-dialysable.

Pharmacological properties

Pharmacodynamic properties: Ciprofibrate is a new derivative of phenoxyisobutyric acid which has a marked hypolipidaemic action. It reduces both LDL and VLDL and hence the levels of triglyceride and cholesterol associated with these lipoprotein fractions. It also increases levels of HDL cholesterol.

Ciprofibrate is effective in the treatment of hyperlipidaemia associated with high plasma concentrations of LDL and VLDL (types IIa, IIb, III and IV according to the Fredrickson Classification). In clinical studies ciprofibrate has been shown to be effective in complementing the dietary treatment of such conditions.

Pharmacokinetic properties: Ciprofibrate is readily absorbed in man, with maximum plasma concentrations occurring mainly between one and four hours following an oral dose. Following a single dose of 100 mg, in volunteers, maximum plasma concentration of ciprofibrate was between 21 and 36 micrograms/ml. In patients on chronic therapy, maximum levels from 53 to 165 micrograms/ml have been measured. Terminal elimination half-life in patients on long term therapy varies from 38 to 86 hours. The elimination half-life in subjects with moderate renal insufficiency was slightly increased compared with normal subjects (116.7 h compared with 81.1 h). In subjects with severe renal impairment, a significant increase was noted (171.9 h).

Approximately 30–75% of a single dose administered to volunteers was excreted in the urine in 72 hours, either as unchanged ciprofibrate (20–25% of the total excreted) or as a conjugate. Subjects with moderate renal impairment excreted on average 7.0% of a single dose as unchanged ciprofibrate over 96 hours, compared with 6.9% in normal subjects. In subjects with severe insufficiency this was reduced to 4.7%.

Preclinical safety data: There are no preclinical data of relevance to the prescriber which are additional to that already included in other sections of the SPC.

Pharmaceutical particulars
List of excipients: Maize Starch PhEur, Lactose PhEur, Microcrystalline Cellulose BP, Hydroxypropyl Methylcellulose USP, hydrogenated vegetable oil, Sodium Lauryl Sulphate PhEur.

Incompatibilities: None stated.

Shelf life: 5 years when packed in blister strips (see below).

48 months when packed in amber glass bottles.

Special precautions for storage: There are no special storage precautions.

Nature and contents of container: Clear PVC/Aluminium blister strips in packs of 28 tablets. Amber glass bottles of 100 tablets.

Instructions for use/handling: None stated.

Marketing authorisation number 11723/0050

Date of approval/revision of SPC July 1997.

Legal category POM.

MODECATE*

Qualitative and quantitative composition The product contains Fluphenazine Decanoate BP 25 mg/ml.

Pharmaceutical form Intramuscular injection for administration to human beings.

Clinical particulars
Therapeutic indications: For the treatment and maintenance of schizophrenic patients and those with paranoid psychoses.

While Modecate injection has been shown to be effective in acute states, it is particularly useful in the maintenance treatment of chronic patients who are unreliable at taking their oral medication, and also of those who do not absorb their oral phenothiazine adequately.

Posology and method of administration
Adults: It is recommended that patients be stabilised on the injection in hospital.

Recommended dosage regimes for all indications:
Patients without previous exposure to a depot fluphenazine formulation: Initially 0.5 ml i.e. 12.5 mg (0.25 ml i.e. 6.25 mg for patients over 60) by deep intramuscular injection into the gluteal region.

The onset of action generally appears between 24 and 72 hours after injection and the effects of the drug on psychotic symptoms become significant within 48 to 96 hours. Subsequent injections and the dosage interval are determined in accordance with the patient's response. When administered as maintenance therapy, a single injection may be effective in controlling schizophrenic symptoms for up to four weeks or longer.

It is desirable to maintain as much flexibility in the dose as possible to achieve the best therapeutic response with the least side-effects; most patients are successfully maintained within the dose range 0.5 ml (12.5 mg) to 4.0 ml (100 mg) given at a dose interval of 2 to 5 weeks.

Patients previously maintained on oral fluphenazine: It is not possible to predict the equivalent dose of depot formulation in view of the wide variability of individual response.

Patients previously maintained on depot fluphenazine: Patients who have suffered a relapse following cessation of depot fluphenazine therapy may be restarted on the same dose, although the frequency of injections may need to be increased in the early weeks of treatment until satisfactory control is obtained.

Elderly: Elderly patients may be particularly susceptible to extrapyramidal reactions. Therefore reduced maintenance dosage may be required and a smaller initial dose (see above).

Children: Not recommended for children.

Where a smaller volume of injection is desirable, patients may be transferred directly to the equivalent dose of Modecate Concentrate injection on the basis that 1 ml Modecate Concentrate injection is equivalent to 4 ml Modecate injection.

Note: The dosage should not be increased without close supervision and it should be noted that there is a variability in individual response.

The response to antipsychotic drug treatment may be delayed. If drugs are withdrawn, recurrence of symptoms may not become apparent for several weeks or months.

Route of administration: Intramuscular.

Contra-indications: The product is contra-indicated in the following cases: comatose states; marked cerebral atherosclerosis; phaeochromocytoma; renal failure; liver failure; severe cardiac insufficiency; severely depressed states; existing blood dyscrasias; history of hypersensitivity to any of the ingredients.

Special warnings and special precautions for use: Caution should be exercised with the following: liver disease; cardiac arrhythmias, cardiac disease; thyrotoxicosis; severe respiratory disease; epilepsy, conditions predisposing to epilepsy (e.g. alcohol withdrawal or brain damage); Parkinson's disease; patients who have shown hypersensitivity to other phenothiazines; personal or family history of narrow angle glaucoma; in very hot weather; the elderly, particularly if frail or at risk of hypothermia; hypothyroidism; myasthenia gravis; prostatic hypertrophy.

Interaction with other medicaments and other forms of interaction: The possibility should be borne in mind that phenothiazines may:

1. Increase the central nervous system depression produced by drugs such as alcohol, general anaesthetics, hypnotics, sedatives or strong analgesics.
2. Antagonise the action of adrenaline and other sympathomimetic agents and reverse the blood-pressure-lowering effects of adrenergic-blocking agents such as guanethidine and clonidine.
3. Impair: the anti-parkinsonian effect of L-dopa; the effect of anticonvulsants; metabolism of tricyclic antidepressants; the control of diabetes.
4. Increase the effect of anticoagulants and antidepressants.
5. Interact with lithium.

Anticholinergic effects may be enhanced by anti-parkinsonian or other anticholinergic drugs.

Phenothiazines may enhance: the cardiac-depressant effects of quinidine, the absorption of corticosteroids, digoxin, and neuromuscular blocking agents.

Pregnancy and lactation
Use in pregnancy: The safety for the use of this drug during pregnancy has not been established; therefore, the possible hazards should be weighed against the potential benefits when administering this drug to pregnant patients.

Nursing mothers: Breast feeding is not recommended during treatment with depot fluphenazines, owing to the possibility that fluphenazine may be excreted in the milk of nursing mothers.

Effects on ability to drive and use machines: The use of this drug may impair the mental and physical abilities required for driving a car or operating heavy machinery.

Undesirable effects
Side-effects: Acute dystonic reactions occur infrequently, as a rule within the first 24–48 hours, although delayed reactions may occur. In susceptible individuals they may occur after only small doses. These may include such dramatic manifestations as oculogyric crises and opisthotonos. They are rapidly relieved by intravenous administration of an anti-parkinsonian agent such as procyclidine.

Parkinsonian-like states may occur particularly between the second and fifth days after each injection, but often decrease with subsequent injection. These reactions may be reduced by using smaller doses more frequently, or by the concomitant use of anti-parkinsonian drugs such as benzhexol, benztropine or procyclidine. Anti-parkinsonian drugs should not be prescribed routinely, because of the possible risks of aggravating anti-cholinergic side-effects or precipitating toxic confusional states, or of impairing therapeutic efficacy.

With careful monitoring of the dose the number of patients requiring anti-parkinsonian drugs can be minimised.

Tardive dyskinesia: As with all antipsychotic agents, tardive dyskinesia may appear in some patients on long term therapy or may occur after drug therapy has been discontinued. The risk seems to be greater in elderly patients on high dose therapy, especially females. The symptoms are persistent and in some patients appear to be irreversible.

The syndrome is characterised by rhythmical involuntary movements of the tongue, face, mouth or jaw (e.g. protrusion of tongue, puffing of cheeks, puckering of mouth, chewing movements). Sometimes these may be accompanied by involuntary movements of the extremities. There is no known effective treatment for tardive dyskinesia: anti-parkinsonian agents usually do not alleviate the symptoms of this syndrome. It is suggested that all antipsychotic agents be discontinued if these symptoms appear. Should it be necessary to reinstitute treatment, or increase the dosage of the agent, or switch to a different antipsychotic agent, the syndrome may be masked. It has been reported that fine vermicular movements of the tongue may be an early sign of the syndrome and if the medication is stopped at that time, the syndrome may not develop.

Other undesirable effects: As with other phenothiazines, drowsiness, lethargy, blurred vision, dryness of the mouth, constipation, urinary hesitancy or incontinence, mild hypotension, impairment of judgement and mental skills, and epileptiform attacks are occasionally seen.

Blood dyscrasias have rarely been reported with phenothiazine derivatives. Blood counts should be performed if the patient develops signs of persistent infection. Transient leucopenia and thrombocytopenia have been reported. Antinuclear antibodies and SLE have been reported very rarely.

Jaundice has rarely been reported. Transient abnormalities of liver function tests may occur in the absence of jaundice.

A transient rise in serum cholesterol has been reported rarely in patients on oral fluphenazine.

Abnormal skin pigmentation and lens opacities have sometimes been seen following long-term administration of high doses of phenothiazines.

Phenothiazines are known to cause photosensitivity reactions but this has not been reported for fluphenazine. Skin rashes have occasionally been reported.

Elderly or hypothyroid patients may be particularly susceptible to hypothermia. The hazard of hyperpyrexia may be increased by especially hot or humid weather, or by drugs such as anti-parkinsonian agents, which impair sweating.

Rare occurrences of neuroleptic malignant syndrome (NMS) have been reported in patients on neuroleptic therapy. The syndrome is characterised by hyperthermia, together with some or all of the following: muscular rigidity, autonomic instability (labile blood pressure, tachycardia, diaphoresis), akinesia, and altered consciousness, sometimes progressing to stupor or coma. Leucocytosis, elevated CPK, liver function abnormalities, and acute renal failure may also occur. Neuroleptic therapy should be discontinued immediately and vigorous symptomatic treatment implemented since the syndrome is potentially fatal.

Hormonal effects of phenothiazines include hyperprolactinaemia, which may cause galactorrhoea, gynaecomastia and oligomenorrhoea or amenorrhoea. Sexual function may be impaired.

Oedema has been reported with phenothiazine medication.

Overdose: Overdosage should be treated symptomatically and supportively, extrapyramidal reactions will respond to oral or parenteral anti-parkinsonian drugs such as procyclidine or benztropine. In cases of severe hypotension, all procedures for the management of circulatory shock should be instituted, e.g. vasconstrictors and/or intravenous fluids. However, only the vasoconstrictors metaraminol or noradrenaline should be used, as adrenaline may further lower the blood pressure through interaction with the phenothiazine.

Pharmacological properties
Pharmacodynamic properties: Fluphenazine decanoate is an ester of the potent neuroleptic fluphenazine, a phenothiazine derivative of the piperazine type. The ester is slowly absorbed from the intramuscular site of injection and is then hydrolysed in the plasma to the active therapeutic agent, fluphenazine.

Extrapyramidal reactions are not uncommon, but fluphenazine does not have marked sedative or hypotensive properties.

Pharmacokinetic properties: Plasma level profiles of fluphenazine following intramuscular injection have shown half-lives of plasma clearance ranging from 2.5–16 weeks, emphasising the importance of adjusting dose and interval to the individual requirements of each patient. The slow decline of plasma levels in most patients means that a reasonably stable plasma level can usually be achieved with injections spaced at 2–4 week intervals.

Preclinical safety data: Not applicable.

Pharmaceutical particulars
List of excipients: Benzyl alcohol and sesame oil.

Incompatibilities: None.

Shelf life: 24 months. The in use shelf life for the 10 ml vial is 28 days.

Special precautions for storage: Store below 25°C. Protect from direct sunlight.

Nature and contents of container: Type I Glass ampoules containing 0.5, 1 and 2 ml.

Type I Glass cartridge syringes with Helvoet Pharma rubber plungers and stoppers containing 1 and 2 ml.

Type I Glass vials with pharma-gummi rubber stoppers containing 10 ml.

Instructions for use/handling: For intramuscular administration only.

Marketing authorisation number PL 11723/0103.

Date of approval/revision of SPC March 1996.

Legal category POM.

MODECATE* CONCENTRATE

Qualitative and quantitative composition The product contains Fluphenazine Decanoate BP 100 mg/ml.

Pharmaceutical form Intramuscular injection for administration to human beings.

Clinical particulars

Therapeutic indications: For the treatment and maintenance of schizophrenic patients and those with paranoid psychoses.

While Modecate concentrate injection has been shown to be effective in acute states, it is particularly useful in the maintenance treatment of chronic patients who are unreliable at taking their oral medication, and also of those who do not absorb their oral phenothiazine adequately.

Posology and method of administration

Adults: It is recommended that patients be stabilised on the injection in hospital.

Recommended dosage regimes for all indications:

Patients without previous exposure to a depot fluphenazine formulation: Initially 0.125 ml i.e. 12.5 mg (0.0625 ml i.e. 6.25 mg for patients over 60) by deep intramuscular injection into the gluteal region.

The onset of action generally appears between 24 and 72 hours after injection and the effects of the drug on psychotic symptoms become significant within 48 to 96 hours. Subsequent injections and the dosage interval are determined in accordance with the patient's response. When administered as maintenance therapy, a single injection may be effective in controlling schizophrenic symptoms for up to four weeks or longer.

It is desirable to maintain as much flexibility in the dose as possible to achieve the best therapeutic response with the least side-effects; most patients are successfully maintained within the dose range 0.125 ml (12.5 mg) to 1 ml (100 mg) given at a dose interval of 2 to 5 weeks.

Patients previously maintained on oral fluphenazine: It is not possible to predict the equivalent dose of depot formulation in view of the wide variability of individual response.

Patients previously maintained on depot fluphenazine: Patients who have suffered a relapse following cessation of depot fluphenazine therapy may be restarted on the same dose (as they were receiving formerly), although the frequency of injections may need to be increased in the early weeks of treatment until satisfactory control is obtained.

Elderly: Elderly patients may be particularly susceptible to extrapyramidal reactions. Therefore reduced maintenance dosage may be required and a smaller initial dose (see above).

Children: Not recommended for children.

Where a very small volume/low concentration of fluphenazine is required patients may be transferred to the equivalent dose of Modecate Injection 25 mg/ml on the basis that 1 ml Modecate Concentrate (100 mg/ml) is equivalent to 4 ml Modecate Injection.

Note: The dosage should not be increased without close supervision and it should be noted that there is a variability in individual response.

The response to antipsychotic drug treatment may be delayed. If drugs are withdrawn, recurrence of symptoms may not become apparent for several weeks or months.

Route of administration: Intramuscular.

Contra-indications: The product is contra-indicated in the following cases: comatose states; marked cerebral atherosclerosis; phaeochromocytoma; renal failure; liver failure; severe cardiac insufficiency; severely depressed states; existing blood dyscrasias; history of hypersensitivity to any of the ingredients.

Special warnings and special precautions for use: Caution should be exercised with the following: liver disease; cardiac arrhythmias, cardiac disease; thyrotoxicosis; severe respiratory disease; epilepsy, conditions predisposing to epilepsy (e.g. alcohol withdrawal or brain damage); Parkinson's disease; patients who have shown hypersensitivity to other phenothiazines; personal or family history of narrow angle glaucoma; in very hot weather; the elderly, particularly if frail or at risk of hypothermia; hypothyroidism; myasthenia gravis; prostatic hypertrophy.

Interaction with other medicaments and other forms of interaction: The possibility should be borne in mind that phenothiazines may:

1. Increase the central nervous system depression produced by drugs such as alcohol, general anaesthetics, hypnotics, sedatives or strong analgesics.
2. Antagonise the action of adrenaline and other sympathomimetic agents and reverse the blood-pressure-lowering effects of adrenergic-blocking agents such as guanethidine and clonidine.
3. Impair: the anti-parkinsonian effect of L-dopa; the effect of anticonvulsants; metabolism of tricyclic antidepressants; the control of diabetes.
4. Increase the effect of anticoagulants and antidepressants.
5. Interact with lithium.

Anticholinergic effects may be enhanced by anti-parkinsonian or other anticholinergic drugs.

Phenothiazines may enhance: the cardiac-depressant effects of quinidine, the absorption of corticosteroids, digoxin, and neuromuscular blocking agents.

Pregnancy and lactation

Use in pregnancy: The safety for the use of this drug during pregnancy has not been established; therefore, the possible hazards should be weighed against the potential benefits when administering this drug to pregnant patients.

Nursing mothers: Breast feeding is not recommended during treatment with depot fluphenazines, owing to the possibility that fluphenazine is excreted in the milk of nursing mothers.

Effects on ability to drive and use machines: The use of this drug may impair the mental and physical abilities required for driving a car or operating heavy machinery.

Undesirable effects

Side-effects: Acute dystonic reactions occur infrequently, as a rule within the first 24–48 hours, although delayed reactions may occur. In susceptible individuals they may occur after only small doses. These may include such dramatic manifestations as oculogyric crises and opisthotonos. They are rapidly relieved by intravenous administration of an anti-parkinsonian agent such as procyclidine.

Parkinsonian-like states may occur particularly between the second and fifth days after each injection, but often decrease with subsequent injections. These reactions may be reduced by using smaller doses more frequently, or by the concomitant use of anti-parkinsonian drugs such as benzhexol, benztropine or procyclidine. Anti-parkinsonian drugs should not be prescribed routinely, because of the possible risks of aggravating anti-cholinergic side-effects or precipitating toxic confusional states, or of impairing therapeutic efficacy.

With careful monitoring of the dose the number of patients requiring anti-parkinsonian drugs can be minimised.

Tardive dyskinesia: As with all antipsychotic agents, tardive dyskinesia may appear in some patients on long term therapy or may occur after drug therapy has been discontinued. The risk seems to be greater in elderly patients on high dose therapy, especially females. The symptoms are persistent and in some patients appear to be irreversible.

The syndrome is characterised by rhythmical involuntary movements of the tongue, face, mouth or jaw (e.g. protrusion of tongue, puffing of cheeks, puckering of mouth, chewing movements). Sometimes these may be accompanied by involuntary movements of the extremities. There is no known effective treatment for tardive dyskinesia: anti-parkinsonian agents usually do not alleviate the symptoms of this syndrome. It is suggested that all antipsychotic agents be discontinued if these symptoms appear. Should it be necessary to reinstitute treatment, or increase the dosage of the agent, or switch to a different antipsychotic agent, the syndrome may be masked. It has been reported that fine vermicular movements of the tongue may be an early sign of the syndrome and if the medication is stopped at that time, the syndrome may not develop.

Other undesirable effects: As with other phenothiazines, drowsiness, lethargy, blurred vision, dryness of the mouth, constipation, urinary hesitancy or incontinence, mild hypotension, impairment of judgement and mental skills, and epileptiform attacks are occasionally seen.

Blood dyscrasias have rarely been reported with phenothiazine derivatives. Blood counts should be performed if the patient develops signs of persistent infection. Transient leucopenia and thrombocytopenia have been reported. Antinuclear antibodies and SLE have been reported very rarely.

Jaundice has rarely been reported. Transient abnormalities of liver function tests may occur in the absence of jaundice.

A transient rise in serum cholesterol has been reported rarely in patients on oral fluphenazine.

Abnormal skin pigmentation and lens opacities have sometimes been seen following long-term administration of high doses of phenothiazines.

Phenothiazines are known to cause photosensitivity reactions but this has not been reported for fluphenazine. Skin rashes have occasionally been reported.

Elderly patients may be more susceptible to the sedative and hypotensive effects.

The effects of phenothiazines on the heart are dose-related. ECG changes with prolongation of the QT interval and T-Wave changes have been reported commonly in patients treated with moderate to high dosage; they have been reported to precede serious arrhythmias, including ventricular tachycardia and fibrillation, which have also occurred after overdosage. Sudden, unexpected and unexplained deaths have been reported in hospitalised psychotic patients receiving phenothiazines.

Elderly or hypothyroid patients may be particularly susceptible to hypothermia.

The hazard of hyperpyrexia may be increased by especially hot or humid weather, or by drugs such as anti-parkinsonian agents, which impair sweating.

Rare occurrences of neuroleptic malignant syndrome (NMS) have been reported in patients on neuroleptic therapy. The syndrome is characterised by hyperthermia, together with some or all of the following: muscular rigidity, autonomic instability (labile blood pressure, tachycardia, diaphoresis), akinesia, and altered consciousness, sometimes progressing to stupor or coma. Leucocytosis, elevated CPK, liver function abnormalities, and acute renal failure may also occur. Neuroleptic therapy should be discontinued immediately and vigorous symptomatic treatment implemented since the syndrome is potentially fatal.

Hormonal effects of phenothiazines include hyperprolactinaemia, which may cause galactorrhoea, gynaecomastia and oligomenorrhoea or amenorrhoea. Sexual function may be impaired.

Oedema has been reported with phenothiazine medication.

Overdose: Overdosage should be treated symptomatically and supportively, extrapyramidal reactions will respond to oral or parenteral anti-parkinsonian drugs such as procyclidine or benztropine. In cases of severe hypotension, all procedures for the management of circulatory shock should be instituted, e.g. vasconstrictors and/or intravenous fluids. However, only the vasoconstrictors metaraminol or noradrenaline should be used, as adrenaline may further lower the blood pressure through interaction with the phenothiazine.

Pharmacological properties

Pharmacodynamic properties: Fluphenazine decanoate is an ester of the potent neuroleptic fluphenazine, a phenothiazine derivative of the piperazine type. The ester is slowly absorbed from the intramuscular site of injection and is then hydrolysed in the plasma to the active therapeutic agent, fluphenazine.

Extrapyramidal reactions are not uncommon, but fluphenazine does not have marked sedative or hypotensive properties.

Pharmacokinetic properties: Plasma level profiles of fluphenazine following intramuscular injection have shown half-lives of plasma clearance ranging from 2.5–16 weeks, emphasising the importance of adjusting dose and interval to the individual requirements of each patient. The slow decline of plasma levels in most patients means that a reasonably stable plasma level can usually be achieved with injections spaced at 2–4 week intervals.

Preclinical safety data: Not applicable.

Pharmaceutical particulars

List of excipients: Benzyl alcohol and sesame oil.

Incompatibilities: None.

Shelf life: 24 months.

Special precautions for storage: Store below 25°C. Protect from direct sunlight.

Nature and contents of container: Clear type I glass ampoules containing 0.5 ml (packs of 10) and 1 ml (packs of 5).

Prefilled syringe with neoprene or pharma-gummi rubber plunger and stopper containing 0.5 ml (packs of 10 – unmarketed).

Instructions for use/handling: For intramuscular administration only.

Marketing authorisation number PL 11723/0104.

Date of approval/revision of SPC 21st March 1996.

Legal category POM.

MODITEN* TABLETS

Qualitative and quantitative composition Each 1 mg tablet contains Fluphenazine Hydrochloride BP 1.0 mg.

Each 2.5 mg tablet contains Fluphenazine Hydrochloride BP 2.5 mg.

Each 5 mg tablet contains Fluphenazine Hydrochloride BP 5.0 mg.

Pharmaceutical form Round biconvex coated tablets.

Clinical particulars

Therapeutic indications: As an adjunct to the short-term management of anxiety, severe psychomotor agitation, excitement, violent or dangerously impulsive behaviour.

In schizophrenia; treatment of symptoms and prevention of relapse.

In other psychoses, especially paranoid.

In mania and hypomania.

Posology and method of administration

Adults:

Anxiety and other non-psychotic behavioural disturbances: Initially 1 mg twice daily rising to 2 mg twice daily, if necessary, according to response.

Schizophrenia, mania, hypomania and other psychoses: Initially 2.5–10 mg daily divided into 2 or 3 doses, depending on the severity and duration of symptoms, rising to 20 mg daily, as necessary. Doses exceeding 20 mg daily (10 mg in the elderly) should be used with caution.

Elderly: Elderly patients may be extra susceptible to extrapyramidal reactions. Dosage at the lower end of the range is likely to be sufficient for elderly patients.

Children: Not recommended for children.

Note: The dosage should not be increased without close supervision and it should be noted that there is a variability in individual response.

The response to antipsychotic drug treatment may be delayed. If drugs are withdrawn, recurrence of symptoms may not become apparent for several weeks or months.

Method of administration: Oral.

Contra-indications: The product is contra-indicated in the following: comatose states; marked cerebral atherosclerosis; phaeochromocytoma; renal failure; liver failure; severe cardiac insufficiency; severely depressed states; existing blood dyscrasias; history of hypersensitivity to any of the ingredients.

Special warnings and special precautions for use: Caution should be exercised in patients with the following conditions: liver disease; cardiac arrhythmias, cardiac disease; thyrotoxicosis; severe respiratory disease; epilepsy, conditions predisposing to epilepsy (e.g. alcohol withdrawal or brain damage); Parkinson's disease; patients who have shown hypersensitivity to other phenothiazines; personal or family history of narrow angle glaucoma; in very hot weather; the elderly, particularly if frail or at risk of hypothermia; hypothyroidism; myasthenia gravis; prostatic hypertrophy.

Interaction with other medicaments and other forms of interaction: Phenothiazines may:

1. Increase the central nervous system depression produced by drugs such as alcohol, general anaesthetics, hypnotics, sedatives or strong analgesics.
2. Antagonise the action of adrenaline and other sympathomimetic agents and reverse the blood-pressure-lowering effects of adrenergic-blocking agents such as guanethidine and clonidine.
3. Impair: The anti-parkinsonian effect of L-dopa; the effect of anticonvulsants; metabolism of tricyclic antidepressants; the control of diabetes.
4. Increase the effect of anticoagulants and antidepressants.
5. Interact with lithium.
6. Enhance the cardiac-depressant effects of quinidine; the absorption of corticosteroids, digoxin and neuromuscular blocking agents.

Antacids may impair absorption.

Anticholinergic effects may be enhanced by anti-parkinsonian or other anticholinergic drugs.

Tea and coffee produce insoluble precipitates in vitro but the effect on absorption in man is unclear.

Pregnancy and lactation: Safety for use during pregnancy has not been established; therefore the possible hazards should be weighed against the potential benefits before administration to pregnant patients. Breast feeding is not recommended during treatment as fluphenazine may be excreted in breast milk.

Effects on ability to drive and use machines: May impair the mental and physical abilities required for driving a car or operating heavy machinery.

Undesirable effects: Side effects may include: Extrapyramidal reactions, acute dystonias, oculogyric crises, parkinsonian rigidity, tremor, akathisia, tardive dyskinesia, drowsiness, lethargy, blurred vision, dryness of the mouth, constipation, urinary hesitancy, incontinence, mild hypotension, impairment of judgement and mental skills, epileptiform attacks.

Hormonal effects such as hyperprolactinaemia, which may cause galactorrhoea, gynaecomastia and oligo- or amenorrhoea. Impairment of sexual function.

Hypothermia, particularly in elderly or hypothyroid patients.

Hyperpyrexia in hot/humid weather or when given with anti-parkinsonian agents.

Uncommonly: Blood dyscrasias, transient leucopenia, thrombocytopenia, antinuclear antibodies and SLE.

Jaundice, transient abnormalities of liver function, transient rise in serum cholesterol, abnormal skin pigmentation and lens opacities, skin rashes, neuroleptic malignant syndrome (NMS), oedema.

Acute withdrawal symptoms have been described after abrupt cessation of high doses of phenothiazines. Gradual withdrawal is advisable.

Overdose: Treat symptomatically and supportively. Extrapyramidal reactions will respond to oral or parenteral anti-parkinsonian drugs such as procyclidine or benztropine. In cases of severe hypotension, all procedures for the management of circulatory shock should be instituted, e.g. vasoconstrictors and/or intravenous fluids. However, only the vasoconstrictors metaraminol or noradrenaline should be used, as adrenaline may further lower the blood pressure through interaction with the phenothiazine.

Pharmacological properties

Pharmacodynamic properties: Fluphenazine hydrochloride is a salt of the potent neuroleptic fluphenazine, a phenothiazine derivative of the piperazine type. Extrapyramidal reactions are not uncommon but fluphenazine does not have marked sedative or hypotensive properties.

Pharmacokinetic properties: The plasma half-life of fluphenazine in patients given the hydrochloride by mouth has been shown to be approximately 14.7 hours.

Preclinical safety data: There are no data of relevance to the prescriber which are additional to that already included in other sections of the SPC.

Pharmaceutical particulars

List of excipients: The core tablets also contain: corn starch, lactose, talc, sodium benzoate, acacia powder, magnesium stearate.

The coating solution of the 1.0 mg and 2.5 mg tablets is comprised of Shellac solution, castor oil, talc, polyvidone, chalk, sucrose, erythrosine, titanium dioxide, sodium benzoate, beeswax, carnauba wax, polysorbate and sorbic acid.

The coating solution of the 5.0 mg tablets is comprised of shellac solution, castor oil, talc, polyvidone, sucrose, chalk, beeswax, carnauba wax, polysorbate and sorbic acid.

Incompatibilities: None stated.

Shelf life: 60 months.

Special precautions for storage: Store below 25°C.

Nature and contents of container: Amber glass bottles containing 28, 30, 56, 60, 84, 90, 100 or 500 tablets with one of the following closures:

Wadless polypropylene cap; tin plate cap with pulpboard wad and waxed aluminium facing; black phenolic cap with composition cork wad and tinfoil/melinex lining; roll-on pilfer-proof aluminium cap with polyethylene liner; child-resistant polypropylene cap of the clic-lok type lined with expanded polyethylene with PVDC (saran) facing.

Instructions for use/handling: None stated.

Marketing authorisation numbers

Moditen 5 mg tablets	11723/0107
Moditen 2.5 mg tablets	11723/0106
Moditen 1.0 mg tablets	11723/0105

Date of approval/revision of SPC January 1998.

Legal category POM.

MORCAP SR*

Qualitative and quantitative composition Morphine Sulphate BP 20 mg, 50 mg, 100 mg per capsule.

Pharmaceutical form Modified release capsule.

Clinical particulars

Therapeutic indications: Morcap SR is indicated for the prolonged relief of chronic, moderate to severe pain. Morcap SR is intended for use in patients who require repeated dosing with potent opioid analgesics over a period of more than a few days.

Posology and method of administration (see: *Pharmacology, Warnings* and *Precautions* sections): Morcap SR capsules are to be administered either twice daily (every 12 hours) or once daily (every 24 hours).

Selection of the initial dose of Morcap SR should take into account the following:

(i) the total daily dose, potency and characteristics of previous opioid analgesics (e.g. pure agonists or mixed agonist/antagonist);

(ii) the reliability of the relative potency estimate used to calculate the dose of morphine required (potency estimates vary with the route of administration);

(iii) the degree of opioid tolerance;

(iv) the patient's general medical condition;

(v) concurrent medication;

(vi) type and severity of pain.

The initial dose of Morcap SR in opioid naive patients should be 20 mg every 12 hours or 40 mg every 24 hours.

The first dose of Morcap SR may be taken with the last dose of any immediate-release opioid medication.

For patients who have difficulty swallowing, Morcap SR pellets may be sprinkled onto a small amount of soft foods (such as yoghurt, apple sauce or jam). This should be taken within 30 minutes of sprinkling. The pellets must not be chewed or crushed and the mouth should be rinsed to ensure that all pellets have been swallowed.

MORCAP SR CAPSULES SHOULD BE SWALLOWED WHOLE. THE CAPSULES AND PELLETS SHOULD NOT BE CHEWED OR CRUSHED.

The use of opioid analgesics for the relief of chronic pain, including cancer pain, should be only part of a complete approach to pain control which should include other types of treatment or drug therapy, non-drug measures and psychosocial support.

If signs of excessive opioid effects are observed early in the dosing interval, the next dose should be reduced. If this adjustment leads to inadequate analgesia, that is, 'breakthrough pain' occurs, a supplemental dose of a short acting analgesic may be given. The dosing interval of Morcap SR should not be reduced below every 12 hours. As experience is gained, adjustments can be made to obtain an appropriate balance between pain relief and opioid side effects.

Because of the sustained release properties of Morcap SR, dosage increases should generally be separated by 24 hours.

The peak morphine plasma levels following administration of Morcap SR once daily (every 24 hours) are significantly higher than the peak morphine plasma levels that follow administration of Morcap SR twice daily (every 12 hours). While clinical studies have not shown any difference in morphine related side effects between the dosage regimens, the possibility of increased side effects with the 24 hourly regimen cannot be discounted. Accordingly, close observation is recommended when converting patients from 12 hourly to 24 hourly administration.

For patients currently receiving opioids, the following dosing recommendations should be considered.

Conversion from other oral morphine formulations to Morcap SR: Patients on other oral morphine formulations may be converted to Morcap SR by administering one half of the patient's total daily morphine dose as Morcap SR capsules on an every 12 hours dosing regimen, or by administering the total daily morphine dose as Morcap SR capsules on an every 24 hours dosing regimen. Dose is then adjusted as needed.

Conversion from parenteral morphine or other parenteral or oral opioids to Morcap SR: Morcap SR can be administered as the initial oral morphine drug product. However, in this case, particular care must be exercised in the conversion process. Because of uncertainty about and inter-subject variation in relative estimates of opioid potency and cross tolerance, initial dosing regimens should be conservative, that is, an underestimation of the 24 hour oral morphine requirement is preferred to an overestimate. To this end, initial individual doses of Morcap SR should be estimated conservatively.

Estimates of the relative potency of opioids are only approximate and are influenced by route of administration, individual patient differences, and possibly, by an individual's medical condition.

Consequently, it is difficult to recommend any fixed rule for converting a patient to Morcap SR directly. The following general points should be considered:

Parenteral to oral morphine ratio: Estimates of the oral to parenteral potency of morphine vary. Some authorities suggest that a dose of oral morphine only three times the daily parenteral morphine requirement may be sufficient in chronic use settings.

Other parenteral or oral opioids to oral morphine: Because there are no data on these types of analgesic substitutions, specific recommendations are not possible. Physicians are advised to refer to published relative potency data, keeping in mind that such ratios are only approximate (see Table 1). In general, it is safer to underestimate the daily dose of Morcap SR required and rely upon ad hoc supplementation to deal with inadequate analgesia.

Table 1: Approximate oral opioid potency ratios relative to oral Morphine†

pethidine	1/8	methadone	3–4[2]
papaveretum	2/3	morphine	1
oxycodone	1	dextromoramide	2[1]

[1] Dextromoramide: a single 5 mg dose is equivalent to morphine 15 mg in terms of peak effect but is shorter acting. The overall potency ratio has been adjusted accordingly.

[2] Methadone: a single 5 mg dose is equivalent to morphine 7.5 mg. It has a prolonged plasma half-life, which leads to cumulation when given repeatedly. This means that when given regularly it is several times more potent.

† Adapted from Twycross and Lack, (1989). Oral morphine in advanced cancer. 2nd ed. Beaconsfield.

Conversion from Morcap SR to other Controlled-Release Oral Morphine Formulations.

Morcap SR is not bioequivalent to other controlled-release morphine preparations. Although for a given dose the same amount of morphine is available from Morcap SR as from morphine solution or controlled-release morphine tablets (i.e. AUC is the same), Morcap SR results in reduced maximum and increased minimum plasma morphine concentrations. Conversion from Morcap SR to the same daily dose of other morphine preparations may lead to an initial change in the clinical status of the patient and close observation is recommended.

Conversion from Morcap SR to parenteral opioids: When converting a patient from Morcap SR to parenteral opioids, it is best to assume that the parenteral to oral potency is high. NOTE THAT THIS IS THE CONVERSE OF THE STRATEGY USED WHEN THE DIRECTION OF CONVERSION IS FROM THE PARENTERAL TO ORAL FORMULATIONS. IN BOTH CASES, HOWEVER, THE AIM IS TO ESTIMATE THE NEW DOSE CONSERVATIVELY.

For example, to estimate the required 24 hour dose of morphine for i.m. use, one could employ a conversion of 1 mg of morphine i.m. for every 6 mg of morphine as Morcap SR. Of course, the i.m. 24-hour dose would have to be divided by six and administered every 4 hours. This approach is recommended because it is least likely to cause overdose.

Opioid analgesic agents do not effectively relieve dysesthetic pain, post-herpetic neuralgia, stabbing pains, activity-related pain, and some forms of headache. This does not mean that patients with advanced cancer suffering these types of pain should not be given an adequate trial of opioid analgesics. However, such patients may need to be referred early on for other types of pain therapy. Pain without nociception is usually not opioid-responsive.

Use in children: The use of Morcap SR in children has not been evaluated.

Use in the elderly: Morcap SR should be administered with caution and in reduced dosages in elderly patients.

Contra-indications: Morcap SR should not be given to patients with: known hypersensitivity to morphine, morphine salts or any of the capsule components; acute or severe bronchial asthma; respiratory depression; biliary colic; gastrointestinal obstruction, particularly paralytic ileus; concurrent MAO inhibitors or within 14 days of such therapy (see *Interactions*).

Special warnings and special precautions for use:

Warnings: Impaired respiration: Respiratory depression is the chief hazard of all morphine preparations. Respiratory depression occurs more frequently in elderly and debilitated patients, and in those suffering from conditions accompanied by hypoxia or hypercapnia when even moderate therapeutic doses may significantly decrease pulmonary ventilation.

Morphine should be used with extreme caution in patients with chronic obstructive pulmonary disease or cor pulmonale and in patients having a substantially decreased respiratory reserve, hypoxia, hypercapnia or pre-existing respiratory depression. In such patients, even usual therapeutic doses of morphine may increase airway resistance and decrease respiratory drive to the point of apnoea. Severe pain antagonises the respiratory depressant effects of morphine.

Head injury and increased intracranial pressure: The respiratory depressant effects of morphine with carbon dioxide retention and secondary elevation of cerebrospinal fluid pressure may be markedly exaggerated in the presence of head injury, other intracranial lesions, or a pre-existing increase in intracranial pressure. Morphine produces effects which may obscure neurological signs of further increases in pressure in patients with head injuries. Morphine should only be administered under such circumstances when considered essential and then with extreme caution.

Hypotensive effect: Morcap SR, like all opioid analgesics may cause severe hypotension in an individual whose ability to maintain blood pressure has already been compromised by a reduced blood volume, or a concurrent administration of drugs such as phenothiazines or general anaesthetics (see *Interactions*).

Morcap SR may produce orthostatic hypotension in ambulatory patients. Morcap SR, like all opioid analgesics should be administered with caution to patients in circulatory shock, as vasodilation produced by the drug may further reduce cardiac output and blood pressure.

Gastrointestinal motility: Morcap SR should not be given to patients with gastrointestinal obstruction particularly paralytic ileus as there is a risk of the product remaining in the stomach for an extended period and the subsequent release of a bolus of morphine when normal gut motility is restored.

As with any other solid dose morphine formulation, diarrhoea may reduce morphine absorption.

Drug dependence: Morphine has a potential for physical and psychological dependence. However, this is not a prime concern in the management of terminally ill patients or patients in severe pain. Abrupt cessation or a sudden reduction in dose after prolonged use may result in withdrawal symptoms. If withdrawal is necessary it must be undertaken gradually.

Infants born to mothers who are physically dependent on opioid analgesics may also be physically dependent and may exhibit withdrawal symptoms. These infants may have respiratory depression at birth (see *Precautions*).

Tolerance: Tolerance may develop upon repeated administration of morphine. The dose of Morcap SR may need to be increased to maintain adequate pain relief (see *Posology and method of administration*).

Precautions:

General: Morcap SR is intended for use in patients who require more than several days continuous treatment with a potent opioid analgesic.

As with any potent opioid, it is critical to adjust the dosing regimen of Morcap SR for each patient individually, taking into account the patient's prior analgesic treatment experience. Although it is clearly impossible to enumerate every consideration that is important to the selection of the initial dose of Morcap SR, attention should be given to the points listed under *Posology and method of administration.*

Cordotomy: Patients who are scheduled for cordotomy or other interruption of pain transmission pathways should not receive Morcap SR within 24 hours of the procedure.

Special risk groups: Morcap SR should be administered with caution, and in reduced dosages in elderly or debilitated patients; patients with severe renal or hepatic insufficiency; patients with Addison's disease; myxoedema; hypothyroidism; prostatic hypertrophy or urethral stricture.

Caution should also be exercised in the administration of Morcap SR to patients with CNS depression; toxic psychosis; acute alcoholism or delerium tremens; severe kyphoscoliosis; convulsive disorders; about to undergo biliary surgery and patients with acute pancreatitis secondary to biliary tract disease.

Driving and operating dangerous machinery: Morphine may impair the mental and/or physical abilities needed to perform potentially hazardous activities such as driving a car or operating machinery. Patients must be cautioned accordingly. Patients should also be warned about the potential combined effects of morphine with other CNS depressants, including other opioids, phenothiazines, sedative/hypnotics and alcohol (see *Interactions*).

Interaction with other medicaments and other forms of interaction: CNS Depressants: Morphine should be used with great caution and in reduced dosage in patients concurrently receiving other central nervous system depressants including sedatives, hypnotics, general anaesthetics, phenothiazines, other tranquillisers and alcohol because of the risk of respiratory depression, hypotension and profound sedation or coma. When such combined therapy is contemplated, the dose of one or both agents should be reduced.

Muscle relaxants: Morphine may enhance the neuromuscular blocking action of skeletal relaxants and produce an increased degree of respiratory depression.

Mixed Agonist/Antagonist Opioid Analgesics: From a theoretical perspective, mixed agonist/antagonist opioid analgesics (e.g. pentazocine, and buprenorphine) should NOT be administered to a patient who has received or is receiving a course of therapy with a pure opioid agonist analgesic. In these patients, mixed agonist/antagonist analgesics may reduce the analgesic effect or may precipitate withdrawal symptoms.

Monoamine oxidase inhibitors (MAOIs): MAOIs intensify the effects of morphine and other opioid drugs which can cause anxiety, confusion and significant depression of respiration, sometimes leading to coma. Morphine should not be given to patients taking MAOIs or within 14 days of stopping such treatment.

Cimetidine: There is a report of confusion and severe respiratory depression when a haemodialysis patient was administered morphine and cimetidine.

Diuretics: Morphine reduces the efficacy of diuretics by inducing the release of antidiuretic hormone. Morphine may also lead to acute retention of urine by causing spasm of the sphincter of the bladder, particularly in men with prostatism.

Food: The bioavailability of Morcap SR is not significantly affected by food.

Pregnancy and lactation:

Use in pregnancy: Animal reproduction studies have not been performed using morphine. It is not known whether morphine can cause foetal damage when administered throughout pregnancy or if it can effect reproductive capacity in humans. Pregnant patients should only be given Morcap SR when the benefits clearly outweigh potential risks to the foetus.

Use in labour/delivery and in nursing mothers: Morcap SR is not recommended for use in women during and immediately before labour. The effects of opioid analgesics are unpredictable. They may prolong labour by temporarily reducing the strength, duration and frequency of uterine contractions, or conversely they may tend to shorten labour by increasing the rate of cervical dilatation. Infants born to mothers receiving opioid analgesics during labour should be observed closely for signs of respiratory depression. In such infants a specific opioid antagonist, naloxone hydrochloride, should be available for reversal of narcotic-induced respiratory depression. Morphine is excreted in human milk and breast-feeding is not recommended while a patient is receiving Morcap SR. Withdrawal symptoms have been observed in breast-fed infants when maternal administration of morphine sulphate is stopped.

Effects on ability to drive and use machines: Morphine may impair mental and/or physical ability required for the performance of potentially hazardous tasks (e.g. driving, operating machinery).

Undesirable effects:

Adverse reactions: The adverse reactions caused by morphine are essentially the same as those observed with other oral and parenteral opioid analgesics. They include the following major hazards: respiratory depression, apnoea and to a lesser degree circulatory depression, respiratory arrest, shock and cardiac arrest.

Most common adverse effects: Constipation, light-headedness, dizziness, sedation, nausea, vomiting, sweating, dysphoria and euphoria.

Sedation: Most patients receiving morphine will experience initial drowsiness. This usually disappears in three to five days and is not a cause for concern unless it is excessive, or accompanied with unsteadiness or confusion. Excessive or persistent sedation should be investigated. Factors to be considered should include: concurrent sedative medications, the presence of hepatic or renal insufficiency, exacerbated respiratory failure, tolerance to the dose used especially in older patients, disease severity and the patient's general condition. If the dose of Morcap SR has been reduced and pain is not adequately controlled, the dose may be carefully increased again after a few days.

Dizziness and unsteadiness may be associated with morphine-induced postural hypotension, particularly in elderly or debilitated patients. The dosage should be adjusted according to individual needs but, because of reduced clearance, dosage may be lower in patients over 50 years of age.

Nausea and vomiting: Nausea and vomiting is common after single doses of morphine or as an early undesirable effect of regular opioid therapy. The prescription of a suitable antiemetic should be considered. The frequency of nausea and vomiting usually decreases within a week or so but may persist due to opioid-induced gastric stasis. Metoclopramide is often useful in such patients.

Constipation: Virtually all patients suffer from constipation while taking opioids on a chronic basis. Some patients, particularly elderly, debilitated or bedridden patients may become impacted. Patients must be cautioned accordingly and laxatives, softeners and other appropriate treatments should be initiated at the beginning of opioid therapy.

Other adverse reactions include:

Cardiovascular: Flushing of the face, chills, tachycardia, bradycardia, palpitations, faintness, syncope, hypotension and hypertension.

Central nervous system (CNS): Euphoria, dysphoria, weakness, insomnia, dizziness, confusional symptoms and occasionally hallucinations.

Gastrointestinal: Dry mouth, anorexia, constipation, laryngospasm, colic, taste alterations and biliary colic.

Genitourinary: Urinary retention or hesitancy, reduced libido or potency.

Endocrine: A syndrome of inappropriate antidiuretic hormone secretion characterised by hyponatraemia secondary to decreased free-water excretion may occur (monitoring of electrolytes may be necessary).

Visual disturbances: Blurred vision, nystagmus, diplopia and miosis.

Allergic: Pruritus, urticaria, other skin rashes and oedema.

Withdrawal (abstinence) syndrome: Chronic use of

opioid analgesics may be associated with the development of physical dependence. An abstinence syndrome may be precipitated when opioid administration is suddenly discontinued or opioid antagonists administered.

Withdrawal symptoms that may be observed after discontinuation of opioid use include: body aches, diarrhoea, piloerection, anorexia, nervousness or restlessness, rhinorrhoea, sneezing, tremors or shivering, abdominal colic, nausea, sleep disturbance, unusual increase in sweating and yawning, weakness, tachycardia and unexplained fever. With appropriate dose adjustments and gradual withdrawal these symptoms are usually mild.

Overdose: Symptoms: Acute overdosage with morphine is manifested by respiratory depression, somnolence progressing to stupor or coma, skeletal muscle flaccidity, cold and clammy skin, constricted pupils, and sometimes bradycardia and hypotension.

Treatment: Primary attention should be given to the establishment of a patent airway and institution of assisted or controlled ventilation. The pure opioid antagonist, naloxone hydrochloride, is a specific antidote against respiratory depression which results from opioid overdose. Naloxone (usually 0.4 to 2.0 mg) should be administered intravenously. However, because its duration of action is relatively short, the patient must be carefully monitored until spontaneous respiration is reliably re-established. Morcap SR will continue to release and add to the morphine load for up to 12 hours after administration and the management of morphine overdosage should be modified accordingly. If the response to naloxone is suboptimal or not sustained, additional naloxone may be administered as needed, or given by continuous intravenous infusion to maintain alertness and respiratory function. There is no information available about the cumulative dose of naloxone that may be safely administered.

Naloxone should not be administered in the absence of clinically significant respiratory or circulatory depression secondary to morphine overdosage. Naloxone should be administered cautiously to persons who are known or suspected to be physically dependent on Morcap SR. In such cases, an abrupt or complete reversal of opioid effects may precipitate an acute withdrawal syndrome. The severity of the withdrawal syndrome produced will depend on the degree of physical dependence and the dose of the antagonist administered. If it is necessary to treat serious respiratory depression in the physically dependent patient, the antagonist should be administered with extreme care and by titration with smaller than usual doses of the antagonist.

Supportive measures (including oxygen, vasopressors) should be employed in the management of circulatory shock and pulmonary oedema accompanying overdose as indicated. Cardiac arrest or arrhythmias may require cardiac massage or defibrillation.

Gastric contents may need to be emptied as this can be useful in removing unabsorbed drug, particularly when a sustained-release formulation has been taken. Morphine toxicity may be a result of overdosage but because of the large inter-individual variation in sensitivity to opioids it is difficult to assess the exact dose of any opioid that is toxic or lethal. The toxic effects of morphine tend to be overshadowed by the presence of pain or tolerance. Patients having chronic morphine therapy have been known to take in excess of 3,000 mg/day with no apparent toxic effects being present.

Pharmacological properties

Pharmacodynamic properties: Morphine is an opioid analgesic which exerts an agonist effect at specific, saturable opioid receptors in the CNS and other tissues. Morphine produces diverse pharmacological effects in man including analgesia, suppression of the cough reflex, respiratory depression due to a reduction in the responsiveness of the respiratory centre to carbon dioxide, nausea and emesis through direct stimulation of the chemoreceptor trigger-zone (CTZ), mood changes including euphoria and dysphoria, sedation, mental clouding, alterations in both the endocrine and autonomic nervous systems, and a decrease in gastrointestinal motility leading to constipation.

Pharmacokinetic properties: Morphine is rapidly absorbed from the gastrointestinal tract, nasal mucosa, lung and after subcutaneous (s.c.) and intramuscular (i.m.) injection. When administered orally it is subject to extensive but variable 'first-pass' metabolism and only about 40% of the administered dose reaches the central compartment.

Once absorbed, morphine is distributed to skeletal muscle, kidneys, liver, intestinal tract, lungs, spleen and brain. It crosses the placental membranes and has been found in breast milk. About 30 to 35% of morphine is reversibly protein bound. Although a small fraction of morphine (less than 5%) is demethylated, for all practical purposes, virtually all morphine is converted to glucuronide metabolites including morphine-3-glucuronide and morphine-6-glucuronide. The glucuronide system has very high capacity and is not easily saturated even in disease. Studies in healthy subjects and cancer patients have shown that the glucuronide metabolite to morphine mean molar ratio (based on AUC) are similar following single doses of Morcap SR and morphine sulphate solution, and at steady state for Morcap SR, controlled-release morphine sulphate tablets and morphine sulphate solution. The morphine to morphine-3-glucuronide to morphine-6-glucuronide mean molar ratios (based on AUC) are approximately 1:24:4, similar to those occurring with both morphine sulphate solution and controlled-release morphine tablets following single doses and at steady state.

There has been no evaluation of Morcap SR in patients with impaired hepatic and renal function.

Pharmacokinetic parameters of morphine show considerable inter-subject variation. The average volume of distribution (Vd) is approximately 4 L/kg and the terminal half life is 2 to 4 hours.

Following oral administration the dose normalised extent of absorption (AUC) of morphine from Morcap SR is similar to that obtained from morphine solution or controlled-release tablets. However, the rate of absorption of morphine from Morcap SR is significantly slower.

A single 50 mg oral dose of Morcap SR in 30 healthy male subjects resulted in a mean peak plasma morphine concentration of 8.1 ng/mL (Cmax) at 8.5 hours (Tmax). The extent of absorption was unaffected by food but the Tmax was slightly delayed to 10 hours. However, this is not clinically significant. Morcap SR can be administered with or without food.

When Morcap SR is given on a fixed dosing regimen, steady state is achieved within about two days.

On a 12 hourly dosing schedule Morcap SR at steady state will exhibit a lower mean peak plasma morphine concentration (Cmax) and higher mean trough plasma morphine concentration (Cmin) than the same total daily dose of morphine solution administered on a 4 hourly dosing regimen or controlled-release morphine tablets administered on a 12 hourly dosing regimen. Although there is no clear relationship between analgesic effect or the incidence of adverse reactions and plasma morphine concentrations, the reduced fluctuation in blood morphine concentrations following administration of Morcap SR may reduce adverse reactions and the incidence of breakthrough pain.

Morphine is excreted primarily in the urine as morphine-3-glucuronide and morphine-6-glucuronide. A small amount of the glucuronide metabolites is excreted in the bile and there is some minor enterohepatic cycling. Seven to 10% of administered morphine is excreted in the faeces. Morphine-6-glucuronide has been shown to be pharmacologically active. Because accumulation of this metabolite has been observed in patients with renal disease, caution should be exercised in patients with clinically significant impairment of renal function.

Preclinical safety data: Not applicable.

Pharmaceutical particulars

List of excipients: Sugar spheres (sucrose, maize starch), hypromellose, ethylcellulose, methacrylic acid copolymer, polyethylene glycol, diethyl phthalate, purified talc, gelatin, shellac, black iron oxide (E172), propylene glycol, ammonium hydroxide, potassium hydroxide.

Incompatibilities: None known.

Shelf life: PVC/PVDC Blister strips: 36 months from date of manufacture of product cores.

Blister strips: 30 months from date of manufacture of product cores. HDPE containers: 24 months from date of manufacture of product cores.

Special precautions for storage: Store capsules below 25°C. Protect from light and moisture.

Nature and contents of container: Blister packs of **30** or **60** capsules. HDPE containers of 60 capsules.

The capsules are transparent, contain creamy-white to light-tan sustained release pellets and are identified as follows:

20 mg capsule – coded K 20 with 2 discontinuous black bands.

50 mg capsule – coded K 50 with 3 discontinuous black bands.

100 mg capsule – coded K 100 with 4 discontinuous black bands.

The pack sizes in bold are marketed.

Instructions for use/handling: Take orally with water. No special instructions required.

Marketing authorisation holder: Faulding Pharmaceuticals plc, Spartan Close, Tachbrook Park, Warwick CV34 6RS.

Marketing authorisation numbers

Morcap SR 20 mg 4515/0080
Morcap SR 50 mg 4515/0081
Morcap SR 100 mg 4515/0082

Date of approval/revision of SPC 13/3/98.

Legal category CD (Sch2), POM.

MOTILIUM* SUSPENSION 1 mg/ml MOTILIUM* SUPPOSITORIES 30 mg

Qualitative and quantitative composition

Molitium Suspension 1 mg/ml: Domperidone PhEur 5 mg
Motilium Suppositories 30 mg: Domperidone PhEur 30 mg

Pharmaceutical form

Motilium Suspension 1 mg/ml: Oral suspension
Motilium Suppositories 30 mg: Suppository

Clinical particulars

Therapeutic indications:

Adults (including the elderly): For the acute treatment of nausea and vomiting of any aetiology in adults. The drug is not recommended for chronic use or for the routine prophylaxis of post-operative vomiting.

For up to 12 weeks treatment of nausea and vomiting caused by L-dopa and bromocriptine.

Children: The drug is not recommended for use in children unless indicated for the management of nausea and vomiting following cancer chemotherapy or irradiation.

Posology and method of administration: Dose, route and frequency of administration should be adjusted according to severity and duration of symptoms.

Suspension: Motilium Suspension 1mg/ml is for oral administration.

Adults (including the elderly): 10–20 mg orally at 4–8 hourly intervals.

Children: 0.2–0.4 mg/kg orally at 4–8 hourly intervals.

Suppositories: Adults (including the elderly): 10–60 mg rectally at 4–8 hourly intervals.

Children: 2–12 years: 10–120 mg rectally per day, depending on body weight. Please refer to the table below:

Weight (kg)	*Maximum daily dose*
10.0–15	30 mg
15.5–25	60 mg
25.5–35	90 mg
35.5–45	120 mg

Contra-indications: No specific contra-indications.

Special warnings and special precautions for use: None.

Interaction with other medicaments and other forms of interaction: Whilst adverse interactions have not been reported in general clinical use it is clear that there is a theoretical potential for domperidone to interact with several classes of agent. Domperidone may, therefore, alter the peripheral actions of dopamine agonists such as bromocriptine, including its hypoprolactinaemic action. The actions of domperidone on gastrointestinal function may be antagonised by antimuscarinics and opioid analgesics. Domperidone may enhance the absorption of concomitantly administered drugs, particularly in patients with delayed gastric emptying.

Pregnancy and lactation: Safe use in pregnant women has not been established, although studies in animals have not demonstrated teratogenic effects. It is therefore not advisable to administer domperidone in pregnancy.

Effects on ability to drive and use machines: None.

Undesirable effects: In common with other dopamine antagonists domperidone produces a rise in serum prolactin which may be associated with galactorrhoea, and occasionally with gynaecomastia.

Domperidone does not readily cross the normally functioning blood brain barrier and therefore is less likely to interfere with central dopaminergic function. However, acute extrapyramidal dystonic reactions have been reported.

Overdose: No cases have been reported. There is no specific antidote to domperidone but in the event of overdosage, gastric lavage may be useful.

Phamacological properties

Pharmacodynamic properties: Domperidone is a dopamine antagonist and increases gastro-intestinal motility. It does not reach dopamine receptors in the brain, probably because it is unable to cross the blood brain barrier.

Pharmacokinetic properties: Domperidone is absorbed from the gastro-intestinal tract and metabolised in the liver. It is excreted in the bile mainly as inactive metabolites.

Preclinical safety data: There are no preclinical data of relevance to the prescriber which are additional to that already included in other sections of the SPC.

Pharmaceutical particulars

List of excipients: Suspension: Sorbitol solution 70% non crystallisable, microcrystalline cellulose and sodium carboxymethylcellulose, methyl p-hydroxybenzoate, propyl p-hydroxybenzoate, sodium saccharin, polysorbate 20, sodium hydroxide, purified water.

Suppositories: Polyethylene glycol 4000, polyethylene glycol 400, polyethylene glycol 1000, tartaric acid, butylated hydroxyanisole.

Incompatibilities: None.

Shelf life: 60 months.

Special precautions for storage:
Suspension: None.
Suppositories: Store in a cool place.

Nature and contents of container: Suspension: Amber glass bottles with tamper-proof aluminium screw caps. Bottle sizes of 100 ml and 200 ml.

Suppositories: PVC-PE strips enclosed in cardboard cartons. Pack sizes of 3 and 10 suppositories.

Instructions for use/handling: Not applicable.

Marketing authorisation numbers
Motilium Suspension 1 mg/ml: 11723/0054
Motilium Suppositories 30 mg: 11723/0051

Date of first authorisation/renewal of authorisation
Motilium Suspension 1 mg/ml: 25th July 1997
Motilium Suppositories 30 mg: 18th June 1997

Date of (partial) revision of text August 1997

Legal category POM

MOTILIUM* TABLETS 10 mg

Qualitative and quantitative composition
Domperidone Meleate PhEur 12.72 mg
Equivalent to 10 mg domperidone

Pharmaceutical form Coated tablet.

Clinical particulars

Therapeutic indications:

Adults (including the elderly): 1. For the acute treatment of nausea and vomiting of any aetiology, in adults. The drug is not recommended for chronic use or for the routine prophylaxis of post-operative vomiting.

2. For up to 12 weeks treatment of nausea and vomiting caused by L-dopa and bromocriptine.

3. For the treatment of symptoms of functional dyspepsia.

Children: The drug is not recommended for use in children unless indicated for the management of nausea and vomiting following cancer chemotherapy or irradiation.

Posology and method of administration: Motilium Tablets 10 mg are for oral administration.

Dose, route and frequency of administration should be adjusted according to severity and duration of symptoms.

For the treatment of nausea and vomiting:

Adults (including the elderly): 10–20 mg by mouth at 4–8 hourly intervals.

Children: Not appropriate for children; use suspension.

For the treatment of the symptoms of functional dyspepsia:

Adults (including the elderly): Up to 10–20 mg orally 3 times daily before meals and 10–20 mg at night depending on clinical response.

A course of treatment should not exceed 12 weeks.

Children: Not recommended.

Contra-indications: No specific contra-indications.

Special warnings and special precautions for use: Domperidone tablets 10 mg are not recommended for chronic administration.

Interaction with other medicaments and other forms of interaction: Whilst adverse interactions have not been reported in general clinical use it is clear that there is a theoretical potential for domperidone to interact with several classes of agent. Domperidone may, therefore, alter the peripheral actions of dopamine agonists such as bromocriptine, including its hypoprolactinaemic action. The actions of domperidone on gastrointestinal function may be antagonised by antimuscarinics and opioid analgesics. Domperidone may enhance the absorption of concomitantly administered drugs, particularly in patients with delayed gastric emptying.

Pregnancy and lactation: Safe use in pregnant women has not been established, although studies in animals have not demonstrated teratogenic effects. It is therefore not advisable to administer domperidone in pregnancy. Domperidone is excreted in breast milk but at very low levels.

Effects on ability to drive and use machines: None.

Undesirable effects: In common with other dopamine antagonists domperidone produces a rise in serum prolactin which may be associated with galactorrhoea, and less frequently with gynaecomastia, breast enlargement or soreness; there have been reports of reduced libido.

Domperidone does not readily cross the normally functioning blood brain barrier and therefore is less likely to interfere with central dopaminergic function. However, acute extrapyramidal dystonic reactions including rare instances of oculogyric crises, have been reported with domperidone.

Should treatment of a dystonic reaction be necessary, domperidone should be withdrawn and an anticholinergic anti-parkinsonian drug, or a benzodiazepine should be used.

Occasional rashes and other allergic phenomena, including rare cases of anaphylaxis, have been reported.

Overdose: No cases have been reported. There is no specific antidote to domperidone but in the event of overdosage, gastric lavage may be useful.

Pharmacological properties

Pharmacodynamic properties: Domperidone is a dopamine antagonist and increases gastro-intestinal motility. It does not reach brain dopamine receptors, probably because it is unable to cross the blood brain barrier.

Pharmacokinetic properties: Domperidone is absorbed from the gastro-intestinal tract and metabolised in the liver. It is secreted in the bile mainly as inactive metabolites.

Preclinical safety data: There are no preclinical data of relevance to the prescriber which are additional to that already included in other sections of the SPC.

Phamaceutical particulars

List of excipients: Lactose, maize starch, microcrystalline cellulose, soluble starch, povidone K90, magnesium stearate, silicon dioxide, polysorbate 20, purified water*, hydroxypropyl methylcellulose, propylene glycol.

* not detected in final formulation.

Incompatibilities: None.

Shelf life: 60 months.

Special precautions for storage: Store below 25°C in a dry place.

Nature and contents of container: Blister packs consisting of aluminium foil and PVC genotherm clear glass. Pack sizes of 4, 10, 28, 30 and 100 tablets.

HDPE (Duma) containers. Pack size 500 tablets.

Instructions for use/handling: None.

Marketing authorisation number 11723/0055

Date of first authorisation/renewal of authorisation
2nd January 1994

Date of (partial) revision of text July 1998

Legal category POM

MOTIPRESS* TABLETS
MOTIVAL* TABLETS

Qualitative and quantitative composition

Active constituents – Motipress
Fluphenazine Hydrochloride BP 1.5 mg
Nortriptyline Hydrochloride BP 34.2 mg
(equivalent to 30 mg Nortriptyline base)

Active constituents – Motival
Fluphenazine Hydrochloride BP 0.5 mg
Nortriptyline Hydrochloride BP 11.4 mg
(equivalent to 10.0 mg Nortriptyline base)

Pharmaceutical form
Motipress: Yellow triangular biconvex tablets
Motival: Coral pink triangular biconvex tablets

Clinical particulars

Therapeutic indications: The treatment of patients suffering from mild to moderate mixed anxiety depressive states.

Posology and method of administration

Adults: One Motipress tablet daily preferably before retiring. One Motival tablet three times daily. The course of treatment should be limited to three months. If the patient does not respond after 4 weeks, an alternative treatment should be given.

Children: Not indicated for the treatment of children.

Elderly: Elderly patients should be started on one Motival tablet twice daily. If one tablet three times a day is required subsequently, Motipress may be substituted.

Motipress and Motival tablets are for oral administration.

Contra-indications: Phenothiazines and tricyclic antidepressants have been shown to lower the threshold for electrically induced convulsions in animals; hence, Motipress and Motival are not recommended for patients with a history of epilepsy or brain damage. They are further contra-indicated in patients with blood dyscrasias, severe cardiac insufficiency, renal or liver damage.

It is inadvisable to give monoamine oxidase inhibitors (MAOIs) with Motipress or Motival, nor should they be given in two weeks after cessation of treatment with MAOIs.

Special warnings and precautions for use: Motipress and Motival should be given with caution to patients with glaucoma and to those who have a propensity for urinary retention. Motipress or Motival should be used with caution in patients with cardiac failure, especially when there is evidence of rhythm disturbance, and in patients with recent myocardial infarction.

Interactions with other medicaments and other forms of interaction: Interactions with barbiturates, alcohol and narcotic drugs may occur, so central nervous depressants should be administered with caution. Motipress and Motival may diminish the anti-hypertensive effect of an adrenergic blocking agent and could potentiate the pressor response to locally injected sympathomimetic agents.

Pregnancy and lactation: Do not use during pregnancy, especially in the first and last trimesters unless there are compelling reasons. There is no evidence as to drug safety in human pregnancy, nor are the results of animal studies conclusive. Breast feeding is not recommended for women receiving Motipress and Motival.

Effects on ability to drive and to use machines: The use of Motipress or Motival may impair alertness and abilities required for driving a car or operating machinery.

Undesirable effects: Tardive dyskinesias have been reported in phenothiazine therapy, usually after prolonged courses given at doses adequate to control psychotic illness. Consequently, Motipress and Motival treatment should be limited to three months.

Dryness of the mouth, drowsiness, faintness and constipation. Occasionally tachycardia, nasal congestion, blurred vision and excitement are seen.

Extrapyramidal reactions are unlikely to occur with this dose of fluphenazine alone, and it is probable that the anticholinergic activity of nortriptyline affords protection against such effects.

As with all neuroleptic drugs the presence of unexplained hyperthermia could indicate neuroleptic malignant syndrome. In this event, Motipress, Motival and associated neuroleptic treatment should be discontinued until the origin of the fever has been determined.

Overdose: Overdosage should be treated symptomatically and supportively. If the patient is conscious, prompt gastric lavage, dilution of the stomach contents to delay absorption, or stimulation of vomiting should be attempted. An open airway should be maintained. Extrapyramidal symptoms are amenable to anti-parkinsonian drugs.

In severe hypotension, all the standard procedures for the management of circulatory shock should be instituted, e.g. vasoconstrictors and/or intravenous fluids. If vasocónstrictors are required metaraminol, mephentermine or noradrenaline should be administered but not adrenaline, as this will further lower the blood pressure through interaction with the phenothiazine.

Pharmacological properties

Pharmacodynamic properties: Nortriptyline hydrochloride is a tricyclic antidepressant.

Fluphenazine hydrochloride is a tranquilliser of the phenothiazine type with a piperazine side chain.

Pharmacokinetic properties: Due to the nature of the two active constituents and the large inter and intra subject variability seen in trials, accurate and consistent pharmacokinetic data are not available. This can be illustrated by the fact that studies of nortriptyline hydrochloride have produced half life values ranging from 16 to 38 hours. In the case of Fluphenazine hydrochloride these values have been 10 to 16 hours.

Pharmaceutical particulars

List of excipients: Tablet core: lactose, dicalcium phosphate, corn starch, magnesium stearate, gelatin.

Coating solutions: Motipress: shellac, castor oil, talc, acacia, gelatin, sugar granular, chalk, magnesium carbonate, titanium dioxide, curcumin, polyvidone, sucrose, sodium benzoate, beeswax, carnauba wax, polysorbate and sorbic acid.

Motival: shellac, castor oil, talc, polyvidone, sugar granular, chalk, erythrosine, curcumin, sucrose, titanium dioxide, sodium benzoate, beeswax, carnauba wax, polysorbate and sorbic acid.

Incompatibilities: None known.

Shelf life: 24 months.

Special precautions for storage: Store below 25°C.

Nature and contents of container: Motipress: Packs of 250 tablets supplied in amber glass bottles. Packs of 28 tablets supplied in 250 μm unplasticised PVC/20 μm hard-tempered aluminium (with PVC compatible heat-seal lacquer on the dull side) blister packs further packed into cardboard cartons.

Motival: Packs of 100 and 500 tablets supplied in amber glass bottles with one of the following closures: wadless polypropylene cap; tin plate cap with pulpboard wad and waxed aluminium facing; black phenolic cap with composition cork wad and tin foil/melinex lining; child resistant polypropylene cap of the clik-lock type lined with expanded polyethylene with PVDC (saran) facing. Packs of 30, 84 and 90 tablets supplied in 250 µm unplasticised PVC/20 µm hard-tempered aluminium (with PVC compatible heat-seal lacquer on the dull side) blister packs. Further packed into cardboard cartons.

Instructions for use/handling: None.

Marketing authorisation numbers

Motipress	11723/0109
Motival	11723/0108

Date of approval/revision of SPC November 1995.

Legal category POM.

MYCARDOL* TABLETS

Qualitative and quantitative composition Mycardol Tablets contain 30 mg of Pentaerythritol Tetranitrate BPC.

Pharmaceutical form Tablets.

Clinical particulars

Therapeutic indications: Mycardol tablets are indicated for the management of patients with angina pectoris. They are not recommended as a single measure for the treatment of anginal attacks, but rather as an adjunct to glyceryl trinitrate.

Posology and method of administration: Mycardol tablets are for oral administration.

Adults: The usual dosage is 2 tablets three times a day, though some may need 2 tablets four times daily. If there is nocturnal pain, the last dose should be taken before retiring. The tablets should be taken before meals.

Elderly: As for adults.

Children: Mycardol Tablets are not recommended for children.

Contra-indications: Mycardol should not be used immediately following a coronary thrombosis or in patients with marked anaemia, cerebral haemorrhage or head trauma.

Special warnings and special precautions for use: Care should be taken in treating patients liable to hypotension and those with closed-angle glaucoma. Tolerance to nitrates may occur.

Interactions with other medicaments: Mycardol may potentiate the effect of anti-hypertensive drugs. Tolerance to glyceryl trinitrate may occur during treatment with Mycardol. Alcohol may enhance some effects of Mycardol.

Pregnancy and lactation: There is no evidence of the safety of Mycardol in human pregnancy, nor is there evidence from animal work that it is free from hazard. It should be avoided in pregnancy unless there is no safer alternative.

Effects on ability to drive and use machines: No statement.

Undesirable effects: Side-effects most commonly reported are headaches (8.3% in one study), nausea (4.6%), rash (3.7%), lethargy and drowsiness. They are usually mild and often resolve on reducing the dose.

Overdose: Symptoms of overdose are likely to be similar to those of glyceryl trinitrate: flushing, dizziness, tachycardia, headache, vomiting, restlessness, hypotension, syncope, cyanosis and methaemoglobinaemia, followed by coldness of skin, impairment of respiration and bradycardia. Treatment: gastric lavage, oxygen and assisted ventilation if necessary. Intravenous methylene blue 1–4 mg/kg is given if methaemoglobinaemia is present.

Pharmacological properties

Pharmacodynamic properties: Pentaerythritol tetranitrate has vasodilator activity. It produces coronary vasodilation and increases myocardial perfusion. Its clinical effects may be explained by an improvement in oxygenation of ischaemic areas of the myocardium. Pentaerythritol tetranitrate also produces a decrease in afterload and preload and thereby a reduction in cardiac work. This would reduce the oxygen demand of the myocardium and this could also explain the clinical response.

Pharmacokinetic properties: Following oral administration of radio-labelled pentaerythritol tetranitrate, radioactivity was detected in the blood within 15 minutes, peak levels occurring 4 to 8 hours after the dose. Of the 20 mg and 40 mg doses administered, 32% and 41% respectively were eliminated in the faeces, and 60% and 50% in the urine in 48 hours. The main metabolites of the parent compound are pentaerythritol and the mono-, di- and tri-nitrates. The latter is very active and may contribute substantially to the activity of pentaerythritol tetranitrate.

Pharmaceutical particulars

List of excipients: Mycardol tablets also contain lactose, starch (maize), dextrose monohydrate, alginic acid, stearic acid and talc.

Incompatibilities: No incompatibilities are known.

Shelf life: A shelf life of 60 months is recommended for Mycardol Tablets.

Special precautions for storage: Mycardol Tablets should be stored in a cool place and protected from light.

Nature and contents of container: Amber glass bottles with wadless polypropylene screw caps.

Marketing authorisation number PL 11723/0057.

Date of approval/revision of SPC 18 September 1995.

Legal category P.

NEGRAM*

Presentation Negram Suspension is a deep pink, viscous suspension with a raspberry odour and taste. It contains 300 mg Nalidixic Acid PhEur per 5 ml dose. Negram Suspension contains methyl, propyl and butyl hydroxybenzoate and amaranth (E123).

Negram Tablets are beige, bi-convex tablets, 12.7 mm in diameter, marked 'NEGRAM' on one side. Each tablet contains 500 mg Nalidixic Acid BP.

Uses Negram is recommended for the treatment of acute or chronic infections, especially those of the urinary tract caused by Gram-negative organisms, other than *Pseudomonas* species, sensitive to nalidixic acid. It may also be used for the treatment of selected cases of gastrointestinal Gram-negative infections sensitive to nalidixic acid though relapse rate and treatment failure in gastrointestinal infection may be more common.

Dosage and administration For oral administration only. Nalidixic acid should be taken on an empty stomach, preferably one hour before a meal.

Adults including the elderly: For acute infections, 1 g four times daily for at least seven days, reducing to 0.5 g four times a day for chronic infections.

Children: For those over the age of three months, the maximum recommended dose is 50 mg/kg body weight per day in divided doses. When prolonged treatment is necessary it may be possible to reduce the dose to 30 mg/kg body weight without loss of therapeutic benefit. Nalidixic acid should not be administered to infants less than three months of age.

Contra-indications, warnings, etc

Contra-indications: Negram is contra-indicated for patients with a history of convulsive disorders, porphyria or hypersensitivity to nalidixic acid or related compounds.

Precautions: Particular caution is advised in patients with a known allergic disposition.

Patients taking Negram should avoid excessive exposure to sunlight (including sunbathing).

Negram is mainly metabolised by the liver and should therefore be used with caution in patients with liver disease. Although care should be exercised in treating patients with renal failure, the full dosage of Negram may be administered in patients with creatinine clearance of more than 20 ml/min and half the normal dosage in patients with creatinine clearance less than this.

Caution should be observed in patients with severe cerebral arteriosclerosis or glucose-6-phosphate dehydrogenase deficiency.

When Negram is given to patients on anticoagulant therapy, it may be necessary to reduce the anticoagulant dosage.

Nalidixic acid has been shown to induce lesions in weight-bearing joints of young animals. The relevance of this to man is unknown. The possible risk of late degenerative joint changes in young patients (children and growing adolescents) receiving nalidixic acid preparations should therefore be considered. If symptoms of arthralgia occur, treatment with Negram should be stopped.

Nalidixic acid should not be administered to infants less than three months of age.

Caution should be observed and therapy discontinued if patients develop signs of symptoms suggestive of an increase in intracranial pressure, psychosis or other toxic manifestations.

Blood count, renal and liver function should be monitored periodically if treatment is continued for more than two weeks.

If the clinical response is unsatisfactory or if relapse occurs, therapy should be reviewed in the light of appropriate culture and sensitivity tests. If bacterial resistance to nalidixic acid develops, it does so usually within 48 hours. Cross-resistance between nalidixic acid and other quinolone derivatives such as oxolinic acid and cinoxacin have been observed.

Use in pregnancy and lactation: The safety of nalidixic acid during pregnancy has not been established. Therefore it should be used during pregnancy only if the potential benefits outweigh the potential risks, specially during the first trimester (nalidixic acid crosses the placental barrier and has been shown to be taken up by growing cartilage in several animal species) and during the last month of pregnancy because of the potential risk for the neonate. Exposure to maternal nalidixic acid in utero may lead to significant blood levels of nalidixic acid in the neonate immediately after birth.

Since nalidixic acid is excreted in breast milk, it is contraindicated during lactation.

Interactions: Negram may interact with anticoagulants due to competition for protein binding sites and it may therefore be necessary to reduce the anticoagulant dosage and monitor the prothrombin time during co-administration, until a satisfactory prothrombin ratio is achieved.

There have been reports of serious gastro-intestinal toxicity following the concomitant use of Negram and melphalan.

Nalidixic acid in therapeutic doses can interfere with the estimation of urinary 17-ketosteroids and may cause high results in the assay of urinary vanilmandelic-acid (Pisano method).

When testing for glycosuria in patients receiving Negram, glucose-specific methods based on glucose oxidase should be used because copper reduction methods may give false-positive results.

Active proliferation of the organisms is a necessary condition for the antibacterial activity of nalidixic acid: the action of Negram may therefore be inhibited by the presence of other antibacterial substances especially bacteriostatic agents such as tetracycline, chloramphenicol, and nitrofurantoin which are antagonistic to nalidixic acid in vitro.

Negram also interacts with probenecid, which inhibits the tubular secretion of nalidixic acid. This may reduce the efficacy of the product in the treatment of urinary tract infections.

It is possible that there will be an increased risk of nephrotoxicity with cyclosporin.

It is recognised that convulsions may occur due to an interaction between quinolones and non-steroidal anti-inflammatory drugs. This has not however been observed so far with nalidixic acid.

Side-effects: Reactions reported after oral administration of Negram include:

CNS: drowsiness, weakness, headache, and dizziness and vertigo. Reversible subjective visual disturbances without objective findings have occurred infrequently (generally with each dose during the first few days of treatment). These reactions include overbrightness of lights, change in colour perception, difficulty in focusing, decrease in visual acuity, and double vision. They usually disappear promptly when dosage is reduced or therapy is discontinued. Toxic psychosis or brief convulsions have been reported rarely, usually following excessive doses. In general, the convulsions have occurred in patients with predisposing factors such as epilepsy or cerebral arteriosclerosis. In infants and children receiving therapeutic doses of Negram, increased intracranial pressure with bulging anterior fontanelle, papilloedema, and headache has occasionally been observed. A few cases of 6th cranial nerve palsy have been reported. Although the mechanisms of these reactions are unknown, the signs and symptoms usually disappear rapidly with no sequelae when treatment is discontinued.

Gastro-intestinal: abdominal pain, nausea, vomiting and diarrhoea.

Allergic: rash, pruritus, urticaria, angio-oedema, eosinophilia, arthralgia with joint stiffness and swelling, and rarely, anaphylactoid reaction. Photosensitivity reactions consisting of erythema and bullae on exposed skin surfaces usually resolve completely in 2 weeks to 2 months after Negram is discontinued; however, bullae may continue to appear with successive exposures to sunlight or with mild skin trauma for up to 3 months after discontinuation of the drug. (See Warnings).

Other: rarely cholestasis, paraesthesia, metabolic acidosis, thrombocytopenia, leucopenia, or haemolytic anaemia, sometimes associated with glucose-6-phosphate dehydrogenase deficiency.

Overdosage: In adults, symptoms of overdosage have been noted following single doses of 20 and 25 g. These have included toxic psychosis and convulsions.

Occasional reports of metabolic acidosis have occurred in association with overdosage, use in infants under the age of three months, or overdose with concurrent use of probenecid.

Vomiting and lethargy may also occur following

overdosage. Reactions are likely to be short-lived because nalidixic acid is normally excreted rapidly.

If systemic absorption has occurred, fluid intake should be promoted, supportive measures such as oxygen and means of artificial respiration should be available. Anticonvulsive therapy may be indicated in a severe case, although it has not been used in the few instances of overdosage that have been reported.

Pharmaceutical precautions Nil.

Legal category POM.

Package quantities *Negram Suspension:* Bottles of 150 ml.
Negram Tablets: Boxes of 56 tablets (7 strips of 8 tablets) (OP).

Further information Nalidixic acid acts by selectively inhibiting bacterial DNA synthesis. It is well absorbed following oral administration, and almost all is excreted by the kidneys, about 80% being recovered in the urine. Effective antibacterial concentrations are readily obtainable in the urine: in human volunteers, single 0.5 and 1 g oral doses produce peak urine levels varying from 25 to 250 microgram/ml.

Product licence numbers
Negram Suspenion 11723/0058
Negram Tablets 11723/0059.

OSSOPAN*

Presentation The active ingredient of Ossopan preparations is microcrystalline hydroxyapatite compound (MCHC), which is a source of calcium and phosphorus in a protein base containing trace elements.

Ossopan 800 tablets: Pale buff, film-coated tablets. Each tablet contains 830 mg MCHC, providing 178 mg calcium and 82 mg phosphorus.

Ossopan granules: Coarse, brown granules, with a taste and odour of malt and cocoa. Each sachet contains 3320 mg MCHC, providing 712 mg calcium and 332 mg phosphorus. Each sachet contains approximately 4 grams, equivalent to 4 Ossopan 800 tablets.

Uses Provision of calcium and phosphorus in osteoporosis, rickets and osteomalacia and during lactation.

Dosage and administration
Ossopan 800: 4–8 tablets to be taken daily in divided doses, before meals.

Ossopan granules: One to two sachets daily with or before food.

Contra-indications, warnings, etc
Contra-indications: Hypercalcaemia, hypercalciuria.

Precautions: Care should be exercised in patients with severe immobilisation, e.g. paraplegia, and in patients with a history of renal calcium stone formation.

Interactions: None reported but oral calcium administration may reduce the absorption of concomitant oral tetracycline or fluoride preparations. If concomitant administration is required an interval of at least 2 hours should be observed.

Treatment of overdosage: No cases of intoxication with Ossopan due to deliberate or accidental overdosage have been reported to the Company. It is considered that overdosage is unlikely to be a problem.

Pharmaceutical precautions Tablets: Store in a dry place below 30°C. Granules: Store in a dry place.

Legal category P.

Package quantities
Ossopan 800: packs of 50 tablets.
Ossopan granules: packs containing 28 sachets (OP).

Further information Hydroxyapatite is the complex biological calcium salt which forms the basis of skeletal structure; its overall formula is $Ca_{10}(PO_4)_6(OH)_2$. MCHC contains about 50 per cent hydroxyapatite and X-ray diffraction studies have confirmed the presence and microcrystalline nature of the salt. It also contains many essential trace elements together with natural skeletal protein (collagen), substituent amino acids and glycosaminoglycans. Clinical studies suggest that MCHC may be more readily assimilated than synthetic calcium supplements.

Product licence numbers
Ossopan 800 tablets 0376/0001
Ossopan granules 11723/0062

Product licence holder: Ossopan tablets – Robapharm AG Basel, Switzerland.

OXYPERTINE* CAPSULES

Qualitative and quantitative composition Oxypertine 10 mg.

Pharmaceutical form Capsule.

Clinical particulars
Therapeutic indications: Oxypertine capsules are recommended for the treatment of acute and chronic anxiety states and psychosomatic conditions whether or not accompanied by depressive overlay, tension, apprehension or sleep disturbance.

In chronic anxiety states, treatment should be restricted to short-term courses.

Posology and method of administration
Adults: 10 mg three or four times daily, usually after meals. In certain cases up to 60 mg daily in divided doses may be needed.

Children: Not recommended.

Elderly: Doses lower than those for other adults are recommended.

Oxypertine capsules are for oral administration only.

Contra-indications: Bone marrow depression, closed-angle glaucoma and hypersensitivity to phenothiazines. Because oxypertine can bring about the release of small amounts of catecholamines in experimental animals, it would be wise not to give oxypertine with or within three weeks of the use of monoamine oxidase inhibitors.

Special warnings and special precautions for use: Should be used cautiously in patients with: cardiovascular disease, respiratory disease, phaeochromocytoma, Parkinsonism, epilepsy, acute infections, renal and hepatic impairment, history of jaundice, hypothyroidism, myasthenia gravis and prostatic hypertrophy. Use with caution in very hot and very cold weather. Elderly patients are more susceptible to side-effects and lower doses are recommended.

Interactions with other medicaments and other forms of interaction: Oxypertine can interact with monoamine oxidase inhibitors, leading to CNS excitation and hypertension. Oxypertine may potentiate the central depressant effect of antihypertensives, alcohol and other CNS depressants. There are conflicting reports on the effect of oxypertine on urinary excretion of vanilmandelic acid.

Pregnancy and lactation: There is no information on the use of oxypertine in pregnancy and lactation in humans, although tests on pregnant rabbits (Somers' test) have revealed no teratogenic effects. However, the benefits of using oxypertine during the first trimester of pregnancy should be weighed against the possible risks.

Clinical experience with other phenothiazine derivatives has shown that their use in pregnancy is occasionally associated with extra-pyramidal effects in the neonate, and their use during lactation with drowsiness in the suckling infant.

Effects on ability to drive and to use machines: Patients should be warned to observe caution in car driving and similar activities. If affected by sedation or drowsiness, patients should not drive or operate machinery.

Undesirable effects: Oxypertine would be expected to share the side-effect profiles of phenothiazines. Compared to other phenothiazines, however, oxypertine has fewer sedative, anticholinergic and possibly extra-pyramidal effects. Low doses may produce agitation and hyperactivity, while higher doses are sedative.

Other side-effects reported for either oxypertine or other phenothiazines include gastro-intestinal disturbances, nasal congestion, dry mouth, hypotension, hypothermia, photophobia and photosensitivity, rashes, eosinophilia and other blood dyscrasias, positive LE cell phenomenon, insomnia, dizziness, abnormal liver function tests and jaundice, myalgia and extra-pyramidal signs, disturbances of endocrine function, e.g. hyperglycaemia, hyper-prolactinaemia, menstrual disorders and sexual function. Malignant neuroleptic syndrome, although not reported to date with oxypertine, is a rare but potentially fatal side-effect.

Overdosage: Symptoms and signs include CNS depression, respiratory depression, hypotension, arrhythmias, hypothermia, convulsions and severe Parkinsonism. Treatment is gastric lavage but avoid use of emetics. Hypotension is treated by plasma expanders but adrenaline should be avoided. Treatment of other features is symptomatic and supportive. Dialysis is probably not effective at removing the drug.

Pharmacological properties
Pharmacodynamic properties: It has been reported that oxypertine acts directly on the brain amines and animal studies have shown depletion of brain noradrenaline, serotonin and dopamine.

Pharmacokinetic properties: No pharmacokinetic studies in humans have been performed.

Pharmaceutical particulars
List of excipients: Starch (maize), lactose, magnesium stearate, gelatin, titanium dioxide.

Incompatibilities: None.

Shelf life: 48 months.

Special precautions for storage: Store in a dry place at or below 25°C.

Nature and contents of container: Amber glass bottles with wadless polypropylene screw caps containing 100 capsules.

Instructions for use/handling: No special warnings.

Marketing authorisation number 11723/0185.

Date of approval/revision of SPC March 1996.

Legal category POM.

OXYPERTINE* TABLETS

Qualitative and quantitative composition Oxypertine 40.0 mg.

Pharmaceutical form Tablet.

Clinical particulars
Therapeutic indications: Oxypertine 40 mg tablets are recommended for the treatment of psychotic patients and are particularly useful in withdrawn schizophrenic patients. Oxypertine 40 mg tablets may also be used in acute incidence of mental disturbances such as acute agitation, behavioural disturbances, delirium and acute or subacute psychoses, including the manic phase of manic depressive psychoses.

Posology and method of administration
Adults: The usual dose is 2–3 tablets (80–120 mg) daily in divided doses. This may be varied according to the mental state and clinical response of the patient, but the total daily dosage should not exceed 300 mg.
Children: There are no dose recommendations for children.

Elderly: Doses lower than those for other adults are recommended.

Oxypertine tablets are for oral administration only.

Contra-indications: Bone marrow depression, closed-angle glaucoma and hypersensitivity to phenothiazines. Because oxypertine can bring about the release of small amounts of catecholamines in experimental animals, it would be wise not to give oxypertine with or within three weeks of the use of monoamine oxidase inhibitors.

Special warnings and special precautions for use: Should be used cautiously in patients with: cardiovascular disease, respiratory disease, phaeochromocytoma, Parkinsonism, epilepsy, acute infections, renal and hepatic impairment, history of jaundice, hypothyroidism, myasthenia gravis and prostatic hypertrophy. Use should be cautious in very hot and very cold weather. Elderly patients are more susceptible to side-effects and lower doses are recommended.

Interactions with other medicaments and other forms of interaction: Oxypertine can interact with monoamine oxidase inhibitors, leading to CNS excitation and hypertension. Oxypertine may potentiate the central depressant effect of antihypertensives, alcohol and other CNS depressants. There are conflicting reports on the effect of oxypertine on urinary excretion of vanilmandelic acid.

Pregnancy and lactation: There is no information on the use of oxypertine in pregnancy and lactation in humans. Although tests on pregnant rabbits (Somers' test) have revealed no teratogenic effects of oxypertine, the benefits of using oxypertine in the first trimester of pregnancy should be weighed against the possible risks.

Clinical experience with other phenothiazine derivatives has shown that their use in pregnancy is occasionally associated with extra-pyramidal effects in the neonate, and their use during lactation with drowsiness in the suckling infants.

Effects on ability to drive and to use machines: Patients should be warned to observe caution in car driving and similar activities. If affected by sedation or drowsiness, patients should not drive or operate machinery.

Undesirable effects: Oxypertine would be expected to share the side-effect profiles of phenothiazines. Compared to other phenothiazines, however, oxypertine has fewer sedative, anticholinergic effects and possibly extra-pyramidal effects. Low doses may produce agitation and hyperactivity, while higher doses are sedative.

Other side-effects reported with either oxypertine or with other phenothiazines include gastro-intestinal disturbances, nasal congestion, dry mouth, hypotension, hypothermia, photophobia and photosensitivity, rashes, eosinophilia and other blood dyscrasias, positive LE cell phenomenon, insomnia, dizziness, abnormal liver function tests and jaundice, myalgia and extra-pyramidal signs, disturbances of endocrine function, e.g. hyperglycaemia, hyper-prolactinaemia, menstrual disorders and sexual function. Malignant neuroleptic syndrome, although not reported to date with oxypertine, is a rare but potentially fatal side-effect.

Overdosage: Symptoms and signs include CNS depression, respiratory depression, hypotension, arrhythmias, hypothermia, convulsions and severe Parkinsonism. Treatment is gastric lavage but avoid use of emetics. Hypotension is treated by plasma expanders but adrenaline should be avoided. Treatment of other features is symptomatic and supportive. Dialysis is probably not effective at removing the drug.

Pharmacological properties

Pharmacodynamic properties: It has been reported that oxypertine acts directly on the brain amines and animal studies have shown depletion of brain noradrenaline, serotonin and dopamine.

Pharmacokinetic properties: No pharmacokinetic studies in humans have been performed.

Pharmaceutical particulars

List of excipients: Oxypertine tablets also contain: Magnesium stearate, starch (maize), dibasic calcium phosphate dihydrate, purified talc, pregelatinised starch, lactose, purified water.

Incompatibilities: None.

Shelf life: 36 months.

Special precautions for storage: Store in a dry place at or below 25°C.

Nature and contents of container: Amber glass bottles with wadless polypropylene screw caps containing 250 tablets.

Instructions for use/handling: No special warnings.

Marketing authorisation number 11723/0186.

Date of approval/revision of SPC March 1996.

Legal category POM.

pHiso-Med

Qualitative and quantitative composition Chlorhexidine Gluconate BP 20% w/v.

Pharmaceutical form Solution for topical use.

Clinical particulars

Therapeutic indications:

1. Pre-operative preparation of surgeons' and nurses' hands and the skin of patients.

2. As an antiseptic skin cleanser for routine hand washing and for spots and acne on the face, shoulders and chest.

3. For use in maternity units by nurses and mothers and for bathing babies, as a measure to prevent cross infection.

Posology and method of administration: For topical use only.

Adults:

Pre-operative hand preparation: Wet the hands and forearms, apply about 5 ml of solution and wash for one minute. Thoroughly clean fingernails with a brush or scaper. Rinse, and repeat the wash for two minutes. Rinse thoroughly and dry.

Preparation of patients for elective surgery: Using a sterile swab, the solution is rubbed over the site and surrounding skin for two minutes, adding a little sterile water to work up a lather. Wipe off and dry thoroughly with fresh sterile swabs. Subsequently, at the time of operation, a 0.5% solution of chlorhexidine in alcohol should be applied to the site with sterile gauze swabs. The site and the surrounding skin should be rubbed vigorously for two minutes and until dry.

As an antiseptic skin cleaner: Wet the area to be cleaned, apply 5 ml of solution and wash for one minute. Rinse thoroughly and dry.

Children:

For bathing infants in maternity units: A 1 in 10 dilution of the solution is applied over the body's body with a swab or with the palm of the hand. Rinse thoroughly with warm water and dry in the usual way.

Elderly: No special dosage recommendations.

Contra-indications: None stated.

Special warnings and special precautions for use: Chlorhexidine should not be allowed to come into contact with the brain, meninges or middle ear. During use ensure that the solution is kept away from the eyes and ears. Material which has been in contract with the solution may be stained brown by hypochlorite bleaches.

Interactions with other medicaments and other forms of interaction: None stated.

Pregnancy and lactation: No special warnings.

Effects on ability to drive and use machines: None stated.

Undesirable effects: None stated.

Overdose: If the solution is swallowed, it should be removed from the stomach by gastric lavage, and symptomatic treatment applied as necessary.

Pharmacological properties

Pharmacodynamic properties: Chlorhexidine is a disinfectant effective against a wide range of vegetative Gram positive and Gram negative bacteria. It is more effective against Gram positive than Gram negative bacteria, some species of Pseudomonas and Proteus being relatively less susceptible. Chlorhexidine is most active at a neutral or slightly alkaline pH, but its activity is reduced by blood and other organic matter.

Pharmacokinetic properties: pHiso-Med is intended for topical use only. Pharmacokinetic details are therefore not relevant.

Pre-clinical safety data: There are no pre-clinical data of relevance to the prescriber which are additional to those already in other sections of the SPC.

Pharmaceutical particulars

List of excipients: Aromox C12W – 30%, Solulan 16, Synchrowax HGLC, polyethylene glycol 6000 distearate, Rewoderm LI 420–70, Varonic LI 67, benzyl alcohol, gluconic acid (50% w/w), and purified water.

Incompatibilities: None.

Shelf life: 24 months.

Special precautions for storage: Protect from heat and light.

Nature and contents of container: Polyethylene bottles with polyethylene screw caps, of **150 ml** and 5000 ml capacity.

Instructions for use/handling: Not applicable.

Marketing authorisation number 11723/0060.

Date of approval/revision of SPC November 1996.

Legal category GSL.

PLAQUENIL* TABLETS

Qualitative and quantitative composition Hydroxychloroquine Sulphate BP 200 mg.

Pharmaceutical form Film coated tablet.

Clinical particulars

Therapeutic indications: Treatment of rheumatoid arthritis, juvenile chronic arthritis, discoid and systemic lupus erythematosus, and dermatological conditions caused or aggravated by sunlight.

Posology and method of administration:

Adults (including the elderly): Initially 400 mg daily in divided doses. The dose can be reduced to 200 mg when no further improvement is evident. The maintenance dose should be increased to 400 mg daily if the response lessens. The minimum effective dose should be employed and should not exceed 6.5 mg/kg/day (calculated from ideal body weight and not actual body weight), or 400 mg whichever is smaller.

Children: The minimum effective doses should be employed and should not exceed 6.5 mg/kg/day based on ideal body weight or 400 mg per day, whichever is smaller. The 200 mg tablet is therefore not suitable for use in children with a body weight of less than 33 kg.

Each dose should be taken with a meal or glass of milk.

Hydroxychloroquine is cumulative in action and will require several weeks to exert its beneficial effects, whereas minor side effects may occur relatively early. For rheumatic disease treatment should be discontinued if there is no improvement by 6 months. In light-sensitive diseases, treatment should only be given during periods of maximum exposure to light.

The tablets are for oral administration.

Contra-indications: Hydroxychloroquine sulphate should not be used in patients with pre-existing maculopathy of the eye, nor should it be used in those sensitive to 4-aminoquinolone compounds.

A chemically related compound, chloroquine phosphate, has been found to cause foetal cochlear damage when taken in high doses during pregnancy; therefore Plaquenil should not be used during pregnancy.

Special warnings and special precautions for use: All patients should have an ophthalmological examination before initiating treatment with Plaquenil. Thereafter, ophthalmological examinations must be repeated at least every 6 months. The examination should include testing visual acuity, careful ophthalmoscopy and central visual field testing with a red target. Plaquenil should be discontinued immediately in any patient who develops a pigmentary abnormality, visual field defect, or any other abnormality not explainable by difficulty in accommodation or presense of corneal opacities. Patients should continue to be observed for possible progression of the changes.

The occurrence of retinopathy is very uncommon if the recommended daily dose is not exceeded. The administration of doses in excess of the recommended maximum is likely to increase the risk of retinopathy, and accelerate its onset.

Plaquenil should be used with caution in patients taking medicines which may cause adverse ocular or skin reactions. Caution should also be applied when it is used in patients with hepatic or renal disease, in those taking drugs known to affect those organs, and in patients with severe gastro-intestinal, neurological or blood disorders. Estimation of plasma hydroxychloroquine levels should be undertaken in patients with severely compromised renal or hepatic function and dosage adjusted accordingly.

Although the risk of bone marrow depression is low, periodic blood counts are advisable and Plaquenil should be discontinued if abnormalities develop.

Caution is also advised in patients with a sensitivity to quinine, those with glucose-6-phosphate dehydrogenase deficiency, those with porphyria cutanea tarda which can be exacerbated by hydroxychloroquine and in patients with psoriasis since it appears to increase the risk of skin reactions.

Small children are particularly sensitive to the toxic effects of 4-aminoquinolones; therefore patients should be warned to keep Plaquenil out of the reach of children.

Interaction with other medicaments and other forms of interaction: Hydroxychloroquine sulphate has been reported to increase plasma digoxin levels: serum digoxin levels should be closely monitored in patients receiving combined therapy.

Hydroxychloroquine sulphate may also be subject to several of the known interactions of chloroquine even though specific reports have not appeared. These include: potentiation of its direct blocking action at the neuromuscular junction by aminoglycoside antibiotics; inhibition of its metabolism by cimetidine which may increase plasma concentration of the antimalarial; antagonism of effect of neostigmine and pyridostigmine; reduction of the antibody response to primary immunisation with intradermal human diploid-cell rabies vaccine.

As with chloroquine, antacids may reduce absorption of hydroxychloroquine so it is advised that a 4 hour interval be observed between Plaquenil and antacid dosaging.

Pregnancy and lactation: A chemically related compound, chloroquine phosphate, has been found to cause foetal cochlear damage when taken in high doses during pregnancy; therefore Plaquenil should not be used in pregnancy.

Careful consideration should be given to using hydroxychloroquine during lactation, since it has been shown to be excreted in small amounts in human breast milk.

Effects on ability to drive and use machines: Impaired visual accommodation soon after the start of treatment has been reported and patients should be warned regarding driving or operating machinery. If the condition is not self-limiting, it will resolve on reducing the dose or stopping treatment.

Undesirable effects: Retinopathy with changes in pigmentation and visual field defects can occur, but appears to be uncommon if the recommended daily dose is not exceeded. In its early form it appears reversible on discontinuation of Plaquenil. If allowed to develop, there may be a risk of progession even after treatment withdrawal.

Corneal changes including oedema and opacities have been reported. They are either symptomless or may cause disturbances such as haloes, blurring of vision or photophobia. They may be transient and are reversible on stopping treatment.

Blurring of vision due to a disturbance of accommodation which is dose dependent and reversible may also occur.

Skin rashes sometimes occur; pigmentary changes in skin and mucous membranes, bleaching of hair and hair loss have also been reported. These usually resolve readily on stopping treatment. Isolated cases of exfoliative dermatitis have been reported. Plaquenil can also precipitate or exacerbate porphyria and may precipitate attacks of psoriasis.

Other adverse effects include gastro-intestinal disturbances such as nausea, diarrhoea, anorexia, abdominal cramps and, rarely, vomiting. These symptoms usually resolve immediately on reducing the dose or stopping treatment. Less frequently, muscle weakness, vertigo, tinnitus, nerve deafness, headache, nervousness and emotional upsets have been reported. Rarely, there have been reports of bone-marrow depression, cardiomyopathy, convulsions, neuromyotoxicity, and toxic psychosis. Isolated cases of abnormal liver function tests have been reported: rare cases of fulminant hepatic failure have also been reported.

Overdose: Overdosage with the 4-aminoquinolines is particularly dangerous in infants, as little as 1–2 g have proved fatal.

The symptoms of overdosage may include headache, visual disturbances, cardiovascular collapse and convulsions, followed by sudden and early respiratory and cardiac arrest. Since these effects may appear soon after taking a massive dose, treatment should be prompt and symptomatic. The stomach should be immediately evacuated, either by emesis or by gastric lavage. Finely powdered charcoal in a dose at least five times the overdose may inhibit further absorption if introduced into the stomach by tube following lavage and within 30 minutes of ingestion of the overdose.

Consideration should be given to administration of parenteral diazepam in cases of overdosage; it has been shown to reverse chloroquine cardiotoxicity.

Respiratory support may be needed and the need for intubation or tracheostomy considered. Shock should be treated by the administration of fluid (with plasma expanders if necessary) with central venous pressure monitoring. In severe cases, the administration of dopamine should be considered.

A patient who survives the acute phase and is asymptomatic should be closely observed for at least 6 hours.

Pharmacological properties
Pharmacodynamic properties: Antimalarial agents like chloroquine and hydroxychloroquine have several pharmacological actions which may be involved in their therapeutic effect in the treatment of rheumatic disease, but the role of each is not known. These include interaction with sulphadryl groups, interference with enzyme activity (including phospholipase, NADH – cytochrome C reductase, cholinesterase, proteases and hydrolases), DNA binding, stabilisation of lysosomal membranes, inhibition of prostaglandin formation, inhibition of polymorphonuclear cell chemotaxis and phagocytosis, possible interference with interleukin 1 production from monocytes and inhibition of neutrophil superoxide release.

Pharmacokinetic properties: Hydroxychloroquine has actions, pharmacokinetics and metabolism similar to those of chloroquine. Following oral administration, hydroxychloroquine is rapidly and almost completely absorbed. In one study, mean peak plasma hydroxychloroquine concentrations following a single dose of 400 mg in healthy subjects ranged from 53–208 ng/ml with a mean of 105 ng/ml. The mean time to peak plasma concentration was 1.83 hours. The mean plasma elimination half-life varied, depending on the post-administration period, as folows: 5.9 hours (at C_{max}–10 hours), 26.1 hours (at 10–48 hours) and 299 hours (at 48–504 hours). The parent compound and metabolites are widely distributed in the body and elimination is mainly via the urine, where 3% of the administered dose was recovered over 24 hours in one study.

Preclinical safety data: There are no pre-clinical safety data of relevance to the prescriber, which are additional to that already included in other sections of the SPC.

Pharmaceutical particulars
List of excipients: Lactose, maize starch, magnesium stearate, polyvidone, purified water*, hydroxypropylmethylcellulose, macrogol 400, talc, sunset yellow aluminium lake (E110), titanium dioxide (E171), IMS 74 O.P*.

* Not detected in final formulation.

Incompatibilities: No incompatibilities are known.

Shelf life: 24 months.

Special precautions for storage: Store below 25°C.

Nature and contents of container: Amber glass bottles with a tin plate screw cap containing 100 tablets. HDPE bottle with LDPE cap containing 56 tablets. 200 μm clear PVC/20 μm aluminium foil blister pack containing 56 or 60 tablets.

Instructions for use/handling: None.

Marketing authorisation number PL 11723/0150

Date of first authorisation/renewal of authorisation 27th August 1997

Date of (partial) revision of text Not applicable

Legal category POM

PLAVIX* 75 mg FILM-COATED TABLETS ▼

Qualitative and quantitative composition Clopidogrel hydrogen sulphate 97.875 mg (molar equivalent of 75 mg of clopidogrel base).

Pharmaceutical form Film-coated tablet.

Plavix 75 mg film-coated tablets are pink, round, biconvex, film-coated and engraved with «75» on one side.

Clinical particulars
Therapeutic indications: Reduction of atherosclerotic events (myocardial infarction, stroke, death due to vascular causes) in patients with a history of symptomatic atherosclerotic disease defined by ischaemic stroke (from 7 days until less than 6 months), myocardial infarction (from a few days until less than 35 days) or established peripheral arterial disease.

This indication is based on the results of the CAPRIE study comparing clopidogrel with acetyl salicylic acid (ASA). The slight but statistically significant difference of clopidogrel over ASA was mainly related to patients enrolled due to peripheral arterial disease.

For further information please refer to *Special warnings and special precautions for use* and *Pharmacodynamic properties.*

Posology and method of administration:
• Adults and elderly

Clopidogrel should be given as a single daily dose of 75 mg with or without food.

• Children and adolescents

Safety and efficacy in subjects below the age of 18 have not been established.

Contra-indications: Hypersensitivity to the active substance or any component of the medicinal product.

Severe liver impairment.

Active pathological bleeding such as peptic ulcer or intracranial haemorrhage.

Breast-feeding (see *Use during pregnancy and lactation*).

Special warnings and special precautions for use: In patients with acute myocardial infarction, clopidogrel therapy should not be initiated within the first few days following myocardial infarction.

In view of the lack of data, clopidogrel cannot be recommended in unstable angina, PTCA (stenting), CABG and acute ischaemic stroke (less than 7 days).

As with other anti-platelet agents, clopidogrel should be used with caution in patients who may be at risk of increased bleeding from trauma, surgery or other pathological conditions. If a patient is to undergo elective surgery and an antiplatelet effect is not desired, clopidogrel should be discontinued 7 days prior to surgery.

Clopidogrel prolongs bleeding time and should be used with caution in patients who have lesions with a propensity to bleed (particularly gastrointestinal and intraocular).

Patients should be told that it may take longer than usual to stop bleeding when they take clopidogrel, and that they should report any unusual bleeding to their physician. Patients should inform physicians and dentists that they are taking clopidogrel before any surgery is scheduled and before any new drug is taken.

Therapeutic experience with clopidogrel is limited in patients with renal impairment. Therefore clopidogrel should be used with caution in these patients.

Experience is limited in patients with moderate hepatic disease who may have bleeding diatheses. Clopidogrel should therefore be used with caution in this population.

The concomitant administration of clopidogrel with warfarin is not recommended since it may increase the intensity of bleedings.

In view of the possible increased risk of bleeding, the concomitant administration of clopidogrel with ASA, heparin, or thrombolytics should be undertaken with caution (see *Interaction with other medicinal products and other forms of interaction*).

Drugs that might induce gastrointestinal lesions (such as Non-Steroidal Anti-Inflammatory Drugs) should be used with caution in patients taking clopidogrel (see *Interaction with other medicinal products and other forms of interaction*).

Interaction with other medicinal products and other forms of interaction:

Warfarin: see *Special warnings and special precautions for use.*

Acetylsalicylic acid (ASA): ASA did not modify the clopidogrel-mediated inhibition of ADP-induced platelet aggregation, but clopidogrel potentiated the effect of ASA on collagen-induced platelet aggregation. However, concomitant administration of 500 mg of ASA twice a day for one day did not significantly increase the prolongation of bleeding time induced by clopidogrel intake. The safety of the chronic concomitant administration of ASA and clopidogrel has not been established (see *Special warnings and special precautions for use*).

Heparin: in a clinical study conducted in healthy subjects, clopidogrel did not necessitate modification of the heparin dose or alter the effect of heparin on coagulation. Co-administration of heparin had no effect on the inhibition of platelet aggregation induced by clopidogrel. However, the safety of this combination has not been established and concomitant use should be undertaken with caution (see *Special warnings and special precautions for use*).

Thrombolytics: the safety of the concomitant administration of clopidogrel, rt-PA and heparin was assessed in patients with recent myocardial infarction. The incidence of clinically significant bleeding was similar to that observed when rt-PA and heparin are co-administered with ASA. The safety of the concomitant administration of clopidogrel with other thrombolytic agents has not been established and should be undertaken with caution (see *Special warnings and special precautions for use*).

Non-Steroidal Anti-Inflammatory Drugs (NSAIDs): in a clinical study conducted in healthy volunteers, the concomitant administration of clopidogrel and naproxen increased occult gastrointestinal blood loss. However, due to the lack of interaction studies with other NSAIDs it is presently unclear whether there is an increased risk of gastrointestinal bleeding with all NSAIDs. Consequently, NSAIDs and clopidogrel should be co-administered with caution (see *Special warnings and special precautions for use*).

Other concomitant therapy: a number of other clinical studies have been conducted with clopidogrel and other concomitant medications to investigate the potential for pharmacodynamic and pharmacokinetic interactions. No clinically significant pharmacodynamic interactions were observed when clopidogrel was co-administered with atenolol, nifedipine, or both atenolol and nifedipine. Furthermore, the pharmacodynamic activity of clopidogrel was not significantly influenced by the co-administration of phenobarbital, cimetidine, or oestrogen.

The pharmacokinetics of digoxin or theophylline were not modified by the co-administration of clopidogrel. Antacids did not modify the extent of clopidogrel absorption.

Data from studies with human liver microsomes indicated that the carboxylic acid metabolite of clopidogrel could inhibit the activity of Cytochrome P_{450} 2C9. This could potentially lead to increased plasma levels of drugs such as phenytoin and tolbutamide and the NSAIDs which are metabolised by Cytochrome P_{450} 2C9. Data from the CAPRIE study indicate that phenytoin and tolbutamide can be safely co-administered with clopidogrel.

Use during pregnancy and lactation:
• Pregnancy

Reproduction studies performed in rats and in rabbits revealed no evidence of impaired fertility or harm to the foetus due to clopidogrel. There are, however, no adequate and well-controlled studies in pregnant women. In view of the lack of data, clopidogrel is not recommended during pregnancy.

• Lactation

Studies in rats have shown that clopidogrel and/or its metabolites are excreted in the milk. It is not known whether this medicinal product is excreted in human milk (see *Contra-indications*).

Effects on ability to drive and use machines: No impairment of driving or psychometric performance was observed following clopidogrel administration.

Undesirable effects: Clopidogrel has been evaluated for safety in more than 11,300 patients, including over 7,000 patients treated for 1 year or more. Clopidogrel 75 mg/day was well tolerated compared to ASA 325 mg/day in a large controlled clinical trial (CAPRIE). The overall tolerability of clopidogrel in this study was similar to ASA, regardless of age, gender and race. The clinically relevant adverse effects observed in CAPRIE are discussed below.

Haemorrhagic disorders: in patients treated with either clopidogrel or ASA, the overall incidence of any bleeding was 9.3%. The incidence of severe cases was 1.4% for clopidogrel and 1.6% for ASA. In patients that received clopidogrel, gastrointestinal bleeding occurred at a rate of 2.0%, and required hospitalisation in 0.7%. In patients that received ASA, the corresponding rates were 2.7% and 1.1%, respectively.

The incidence of other bleeding was higher in patients that received clopidogrel compared to ASA (7.3% vs. 6.5%). However, the incidence of severe events was similar in both treatment groups (0.6% vs. 0.4%). The most frequently reported events in both treatment groups were: purpura/bruising/haematoma, and epistaxis. Other less frequently reported events were haematoma, haematuria, and eye bleeding (mainly conjunctival).

The incidence of intracranial bleeding was 0.4% in patients that received clopidogrel and 0.5% for patients that received ASA.

Haematological: severe neutropaenia ($<0.45\times10^9/1$) was observed in 4 patients (0.04%) that received clopidogrel and 2 patients (0.02%) that received ASA. Two of the 9599 patients who received clopidogrel and none of the 9586 patients who received ASA had neutrophil counts of zero. One case of aplastic anaemia occurred on clopidogrel treatment.

The incidence of severe thrombocytopaenia ($<80\times10^9/1$) was 0.2% on clopidogrel and 0.1% on ASA.

Gastrointestinal: the overall, incidence of gastrointestinal events (e.g. abdominal pain, dyspepsia, gastritis and constipation) was significantly lower in patients treated with clopidogrel compared to ASA (27.1% vs. 29.8%). In addition, the number of events resulting in early permanent discontinuation was lower in the clopidogrel group compared to ASA (3.2% vs. 4.0%). However, the incidence of adverse events judged as clinically severe were not statistically different in the groups (3.0% vs. 3.6%). The most frequently reported events in both treatment groups were: abdominal pain, dyspepsia, diarrhoea, and nausea. Other less frequently reported events were constipation, tooth disorder, vomiting, flatulence and gastritis.

Cases of diarrhoea were reported at a significantly higher frequency in patients taking clopidogrel compared to ASA (4.5% vs. 3.4%). The incidence of severe diarrhoea was similar to both treatment groups (0.2% vs. 0.1%). The incidence of peptic, gastric or duodenal ulcers was 0.7% for clopidogrel and 1.2% for ASA.

Skin and appendage disorders: the overall incidence of skin and appendage disorders in patients taking clopidogrel was significantly higher (15.8%) compared to ASA (13.1%). The incidence of severe events was similar in both treatment groups (0.7% vs. 0.5%).

There were significantly more patients with rash in the clopidogrel group compared to the ASA group (4.2% vs. 3.5%). More patients reported pruritus in the clopidogrel group compared to ASA (3.3% vs. 1.6%).

Central and peripheral nervous system disorders: the overall incidence of central and peripheral nervous system disorders (e.g. headache, dizziness, vertigo and paraesthesia) was significantly lower in patients taking clopidogrel compared to ASA (22.3% vs. 23.8%).

Hepatic and biliary disorders: the overall incidence of hepatic and biliary disorders was similar in patients treated with clopidogrel compared to ASA (3.5% vs. 3.4%).

Overdose: One case of deliberate overdosage with clopidogrel has been reported. A 34 year old woman took a single 1,050 mg dose of clopidogrel (equivalent to 14 standard 75 mg tablets). There were no associated undesirable effects. No special therapy was instituted and she recovered without sequelae.

No adverse events were reported after single oral administration of 600 mg (equivalent to 8 standard 75 mg tablets) of clopidogrel to healthy subjects. The bleeding time was prolonged by a factor of 1.7 which is similar to that typically observed with the therapeutic dose of 75 mg per day.

No antidote to the pharmacological activity of clopidogrel has been found. If prompt correction of prolonged bleeding time is required, platelet transfusion may reverse the effects of clopidogrel.

Pharmacological properties

Pharmacodynamic properties:

Pharmacotherapeutical group: platelet aggregation inhibitors excl. Heparin, ATC Code: BO1AC/04.

Clopidogrel selectively inhibits the binding of adenosine diphosphate (ADP) to its platelet receptor, and the subsequent ADP-mediated activation of the GPIIb/IIIa complex, thereby inhibiting platelet aggregation. Biotransformation of clopidogrel is necessary to produce inhibition of platelet aggregation. Clopidogrel also inhibits platelet aggregation induced by other agonists by blocking the amplification of platelet activation by released ADP. Clopidogrel acts by irreversibly modifying the platelet ADP receptor. Consequently, platelets exposed to clopidogrel are affected for the remainder of their lifespan and recovery of normal platelet function occurs at a rate consistent with platelet turnover.

Repeated doses of 75 mg per day produced substantial inhibition of ADP-induced platelet aggregation from the first day; this increased progressively and reached steady state between Day 3 and Day 7. At steady state, the average inhibition level observed with a dose of 75 mg per day was between 40% and 60%. Platelet aggregation and bleeding time gradually returned to baseline values, generally within 5 days after treatment was discontinued.

The safety and efficacy of clopidogrel in preventing vascular ischaemic events have been evaluated in a blinded comparison with ASA (CAPRIE, Clopidogrel versus ASA in Patients at Risk of Ischaemic Events). This study included 19,185 patients with atherothrombosis as manifested by recent myocardial infarction (<35 days), recent ischaemic stroke (between 7 days and 6 months) or established peripheral arterial disease (PAD). Patients were randomised to clopidogrel 75 mg/day or ASA 325 mg/day, and were followed for 1 to 3 years. In the myocardial infarction subgroup, most of the patients received ASA for the first few days following the acute myocardial infarction.

Clopidogrel significantly reduced the incidence of new ischaemic events (combined end point of myocardial infarction, ischaemic stroke and vascular death) when compared to ASA. In the intention to treat analysis, 939 events were observed in the clopidogrel group and 1,020 events with ASA (relative risk reduction (RRR) 8.7%, [95% CI: 0.2 to 16.4]; p=0.045), which corresponds, for every 1000 patients treated for 2 years, to 10 [CI: 0 to 20] additional patients being prevented from experiencing a new ischaemic event. Analysis of total mortality as a secondary endpoint did not show any significant difference between clopidogrel (5.8%) and ASA (6.0%).

In a subgroup analysis by qualifying condition (myocardial infarction, ischaemic stroke, and PAD) the benefit appeared to be strongest (achieving statistical significance at p=0.003) in patients enrolled due to PAD (especially those who also had a history of myocardial infarction) (RRR=23.7%; CI: 8.9 to 36.2) and weaker (not significantly different from ASA) in stroke patients (RRR=7.3%; CI: –5.7 to 18.7). In patients who were enrolled in the trial on the sole basis of a recent myocardial infarction, clopidogrel was numerically inferior, but not statistically different from ASA (RRR=–4.0%; CI: –22.5 to 11.7). In addition, a subgroup analysis by age suggested that the benefit of clopidogrel in patients over 75 years was less than that observed in patients ≤75 years.

Since the CAPRIE trial was not powered to evaluate efficacy of individual subgroups, it is not clear whether the differences in relative risk reduction across qualifying conditions are real, or a result of chance.

Pharmacokinetic properties: After repeated oral doses of 75 mg per day, clopidogrel is rapidly absorbed. However, plasma concentrations of the parent compound are very low and below the quantification limit (0.00025 mg/l) beyond 2 hours. Absorption is at least 50%, based on urinary excretion of clopidogrel metabolites.

Clopidogrel is extensively metabolised by the liver and the main metabolite, which is inactive, is the carboxylic acid derivative which represents about 85% of the circulating compound in plasma. Peak plasma levels of this metabolite (approx. 3 mg/l after repeated 75 mg oral doses) occurred approximately 1 hour after dosing.

Clopidogrel is a prodrug. The active metabolite, a thiol derivative, is formed by oxidation of clopidogrel to 2-oxo-clopidogrel and subsequent hydrolysis. The oxidative step is regulated primarily by Cytochrome P_{450} isoenzymes 2B6 and 3A4 and to a lesser extent by 1A1, 1A2 and 2C19. The active thiol metabolite, which has been isolated *in vitro*, binds rapidly and irreversibly to platelet receptors, thus inhibiting platelet aggregation. This metabolite has not been detected in plasma.

The kinetics of the main circulating metabolite were linear (plasma concentrations increased in proportion to dose) in the dose range of 50 to 150 mg of clopidogrel.

Clopidogrel and the main circulating metabolite bind reversibly *in vitro* to human plasma proteins (98% and 94% respectively). The binding is non-saturable *in vitro* over a wide concentration range.

Following an oral dose of ^{14}C-labelled clopidogrel in man, approximately 50% was excreted in the urine and approximately 46% in the faeces in the 120 hour interval after dosing. The elimination half-life of the main circulating metabolite was 8 hours after single and repeated administration.

After repeated doses of 75 mg clopidogrel per day, plasma levels of the main circulating metabolite were lower in subjects with severe renal disease (creatinine clearance from 5 to 15 ml/min) compared to subjects with moderate renal disease (creatinine clearance from 30 to 60 ml/min) and to levels observed in other studies with healthy subjects. Although inhibition of ADP-induced platelet aggregation was lower (25%) than that observed in healthy subjects, the prolongation of bleeding was similar to that seen in healthy subjects receiving 75 mg of clopidogrel per day. In addition, clinical tolerance was good in all patients.

The pharmacokinetics and pharmacodynamics of clopidogrel were assessed in a single and multiple dose study in both healthy subjects and those with cirrhosis (Child-Pugh class A or B). Daily dosing for 10 days with clopidogrel 75 mg/day was safe and well tolerated. Clopidogrel C_{max} for both single dose and steady state for cirrhotics was many fold higher than in normal subjects. However, plasma levels of the main circulating metabolite together with the effect of clopidogrel on ADP-induced platelet aggregation and bleeding time were comparable between these groups.

Preclinical safety data: During preclinical studies in rat and baboon, the most frequently observed effects were liver changes. These occurred at doses representing at least 25 times the exposure seen in humans receiving the clinical dose of 75 mg/day and were a consequence of an effect on hepatic metabolising enzymes. No effect on hepatic metabolising enzymes were observed in humans receiving clopidogrel at the therapeutic dose.

At very high doses, a poor gastric tolerability (gastritis, gastric erosions and/or vomiting) of clopidogrel was also reported in rat and baboon.

There was no evidence of carcinogenic effect when clopidogrel was administered for 78 weeks to mice and 104 weeks to rats when given at doses up to 77 mg/kg per day (representing at least 25 times the exposure seen in humans receiving the clinical dose of 75 mg/day).

Clopidogrel has been tested in a range of *in vitro* and *in vivo* genotoxicity studies, and showed no genotoxic activity.

Clopidogrel was found to have no effect on the fertility of male and female rats and was not teratogenic in either rats or rabbits. When given to lactating rats, clopidogrel caused a slight delay in the development of the offspring. Specific pharmacokinetic studies performed with radiolabelled clopidogrel have shown that the parent compound or its metabolites are excreted in the milk. Consequently, a direct effect (slight toxicity), or an indirect effect (low palatability) cannot be excluded.

Pharmaceutical particulars

List of excipients

Core: Anhydrous lactose, Modified maize starch, Macrogol 6000, Microcrystalline cellulose, Hydrogenated castor oil.

Coating: Hypromellose, Macrogol 6000, Titanium dioxide (E171), Red iron oxide (E172), Carnauba wax.

Incompatibilities: Not applicable.

Shelf life: Three years.

Special precautions for storage: No special precautions for storage.

Nature and content of container: 28, 50, and 84, tablets packed in blisters in cardboard cartons.

Instruction for use and handling, and disposal (if appropriate): Not applicable.

Marketing authorisation holder: Sanofi Pharma Bristol-Myers Squibb SNC, 174 Avenue de France, F-75013, Paris, France.

Number(s) in the community register of medicinal products

EU/1/98/069/001 – Cartons of 28 tablets
EU/1/98/069/002 – Cartons of 50 tablets
EU/1/98/069/003 – Cartons of 84 tablets

Date of first authorisation/renewal of the authorisation 15.07.98.

Date of revision of the text December 1998.

Legal category POM.

PRIMACOR* INJECTION

Qualitative and quantitative composition Milrinone 1 mg/ml. Clear, colourless to pale yellow liquid.

Pharmaceutical form Injection.

Clinical particulars

Therapeutic indications: Primacor Injection is indicated for the short-term treatment of severe congestive heart failure unresponsive to conventional maintenance therapy, and for the treatment of patients with acute heart failure, including low output states following cardiac surgery.

Posology and method of administration: For intravenous administration.

Adults: Primacor Injection should be given as a loading dose of 50 mcg/kg administered over a period of 10 minutes usually followed by continuous infusion at a dosage titrated between 0.375 mcg/kg/min and 0.75 mcg/kg/min according to a haemodynamic and clinical response, but should not exceed 1.13 mg/kg/day total dose.

The following provides a guide to maintenance infusion delivery rate based upon a solution containing milrinone 200 mcg/ml prepared by adding 40 ml diluent per 10 ml ampoule (400 ml diluent per 100 ml Primacor Injection). 0.45% saline, 0.9% saline or 5% dextrose may be used as diluents.

Primacor Dose (mcg/kg/min)	*Infusion Delivery Rate (ml/kg/hr)*
0.375	0.11
0.400	0.12
0.500	0.15
0.600	0.18
0.700	0.21
0.750	0.22

Solutions of different concentrations may be used according to patient fluid requirements. The duration of therapy should depend upon the patient's response. In congestive cardiac failure, patients have been maintained on the infusion for up to 5 days, although the usual period is 48 to 72 hours. In acute states following cardiac surgery, it is unlikely that treatment need be maintained for more than 12 hours.

Use in patients with impaired renal function: Data obtained from patients with severe renal impairment but without heart failure have demonstrated that the presence of renal impairment significantly increases the terminal elimination half-life of milrinone. For patients with clinical evidence of renal impairment, the following maintenance infusion rates are recommended using the infusion solution described above.

Creatinine Clearance (ml/min/ 1.73m²)	Primacor Injection Dose (mcg/kg/min)	Maintenance Infusion Delivery Rate (ml/kg/hr)
5	0.20	0.06
10	0.23	0.07
20	0.28	0.08
30	0.33	0.10
40	0.38	0.11
50	0.43	0.13

The infusion rate should be adjusted according to haemodynamic response.

Use in elderly patients: Experience so far suggests that no special dosage recommendations are necessary.

Use in children: Safety and effectiveness in children have not been established. Primacor Injection should only be used when the potential benefits outweigh the potential risks.

Contra-indications: Hypersensitivity to milrinone or other ingredients of the preparation.

Special warnings and special precautions for use: The use of Primacor Injection is not recommended immediately following acute myocardial infarction until safety and efficacy have been established in this situation.

Careful monitoring should be maintained during Primacor Injection therapy including blood pressure, heart rate, clinical state, electro-cardiogram, fluid balance, electrolytes and renal function (i.e. serum creatinine).

In patients with severe obstructive aortic or pulmonary valvular disease or hypertrophic subaortic stenosis, Primacor Injection should not be used in place of surgical relief of the obstruction. In these conditions it is possible that a drug with inotropic/vasodilator properties might aggravate outflow obstruction.

Supraventricular and ventricular arrhythmias have been observed in the high risk population treated with Primacor Injection. In some patients an increase in ventricular ectopy including non-sustained ventricular tachycardia has been observed which did not affect patient safety or outcome.

As Primacor Injection produces a slight enhancement in A–V node conduction, there is a possibility of an increased ventricular response rate in patients with uncontrolled atrial flutter/fibrillation. Consideration should therefore be given to digitalisation or treatment with other agents to prolong A-V node conduction time prior to starting Primacor Injection therapy, and to discontinuing the therapy if arrhythmias occur.

The potential for arrhythmia, present in heart failure itself, may be increased by many drugs or a combination of drugs. Patients receiving Primacor Injection should be closely monitored during infusion and the infusion should be stopped if arrhythmias develop.

Milrinone may induce hypotension as a consequence of its vasodilatory activity, therefore caution should be exercised when Primacor Injection is administered to patients who are hypotensive prior to treatment. The rate of infusion should be slowed or stopped in patients showing excessive decreases in blood pressure.

If prior vigorous diuretic therapy is suspected of having caused significant decreases in cardiac filling pressure Primacor Injection should be cautiously administered while monitoring blood pressure, heart rate and clinical symptomatology.

Improvement in cardiac output with resultant diuresis may necessitate a reduction in the dose of diuretic. Potassium loss due to excessive diuresis may necessitate a reduction in the dose of diuretic. Potassium loss due to excessive diuresis may predispose digitalised patients to arrhythmias. Therefore, hypokalaemia should be corrected by potassium supplementation in advance of, or during, the use of Primacor Injection.

Interaction with other medicaments and other forms of interaction: None have been observed during Primacor Injection therapy (but see *Incompatibilities*).

Whilst there is a theoretical potential interaction with calcium channel blockers, there has been no evidence of a clinically significant interaction to date.

Milrinone has a favourable inotropic effect in fully digitalised patients without causing signs of glycoside toxicity.

Pregnancy and lactation: Although animal studies have not revealed evidence of drug-induced foetal damage or other deleterious effects on reproductive function, the safety of milrinone in human pregnancy has not yet been established. It should be used during pregnancy only if the potential benefit justifies the potential risk to the foetus.

Caution should be exercised when Primacor Injection is administered to nursing women, since it is not known whether milrinone is excreted in human milk.

Effects on ability to drive and use machines: Not applicable.

Undesirable effects: Ventricular ectopic activity, supraventricular and ventricular arrhythmias have been reported during treatment with Primacor Injection. An increase in ventricular response rate in patients with atrial fibrillation may occur. The incidence of arrhythmias has not been related to dose or plasma levels of milrinone. These arrhythmias are rarely life threatening. If present, they are often associated with underlying factors such as pre-existing arrhythmias, metabolic abnormalities (e.g. hypokalaemia), abnormal digoxin levels and catheter insertion.

Very rarely cases of Torsades de Pointes have been reported.

Other reported side effects include hypotension, angina/chest pain, headaches, hypokalaemia, tremor, bronchospasm and anaphylactic shock. Thrombocytopenia has been reported with an incidence similar to placebo and has not been definitely related to the administration of Primacor Injection.

Skin reactions such as rash, and abnormality in liver function tests have been observed.

Overdose: Overdose of intravenous Primacor may produce hypotension (because of its vasodilatory effect) and cardiac arrhythmia. If this occurs, Primacor Injection administration should be reduced or temporarily discontinued until the patient's condition stabilises. No specific antidote is known, but general measures for circulatory support should be taken.

Pharmacological properties

Pharmacodynamic properties: Milrinone is a positive inotrope and vasodilator, with little chronotropic activity. It also improves left ventricular diastolic relaxation. It differs in structure and mode of action from the digitalis glycosides, catecholamines or angiotensin converting enzyme inhibitors. It is a selective inhibitor of peak III phosphodiesterase isoenzyme in cardiac and vascular muscle. It produces slight enhancement of A-V node conduction, but no other significant electro-physiological effects.

In clinical studies Primacor Injection has been shown to produce prompt improvements in the haemodynamic indices of congestive heart failure, including cardiac output, pulmonary capillary wedge pressure and vascular resistance, without clinically significant effect on heart rate or myocardial oxygen consumption.

Haemodynamic improvement during intravenous Primacor therapy is accompanied by clinical symptomatic improvement in congestive cardiac failure, as measured by change in New York Heart Association classification.

Pharmacokinetic properties: Following intravenous injections of 12.5 to 125 mcg/kg to congestive heart failure patients, Primacor Injection had a volume of distribution of 0.38 l/kg/hr, a mean terminal elimination half-life of 2.3 hours, and a clearance of 0.13 l/kg/hr. Following intravenous infusions of 0.2 to 0.7 mcg/kg/min to congestive heart failure patients, the drug had a volume of distribution of about 0.45 l/kg, a mean terminal elimination half-life of 2.4 hours, and a clearance of 0.14 l/kg/hr. These pharmacokinetic parameters were not dose-dependent, and the area under the plasma concentration versus time curve following injection was significantly dose-dependent.

The primary route of excretion of milrinone in man is via the urine. The major urinary excretion products of orally administered milrinone in man are milrinone (83%) and its O-glucuronide metabolite (12%). Elimination in normal subjects via the urine is rapid, with approximately 60% recovered within the first two hours following dosing, and approximately 90% recovered within the first eight hours following dosing. The mean renal clearance of milrinone is approximately 0.3 l/min, indicative of active secretion.

Preclinical safety data: There are no preclinical data of relevance to the prescriber which are additional to that already in other sections of the SPC.

Pharmaceutical particulars

List of excipients: Lactic Acid PhEur, Dextrose Anhydrous PhEur, Water for Injection PhEur, Sodium Hydroxide BP.

Incompatibilities: Frusamide or bumetanide should not be administered in intravenous lines containing Primacor Injection since precipitation occurs on admixture. Sodium Bicarbonate Intravenous infusion should not be used for dilution.

Other drugs should not be mixed with Primacor Injection until further compatibility data are available.

Shelf life: 48 months when unopened. A diluted solution of Primacor Injection should be used within 24 hours.

Special precautions for storage: Store below 25°C, avoid freezing.

Nature and contents of container: Type 1 10 ml or 20 ml flint glass ampoules packed in lots of 10.

Instructions for use/handling: Infusion solutions diluted as recommended with 0.45% saline, 0.9% saline or 5% dextrose should be freshly prepared before use. Parenteral drug products should be examined visually and should not be used if particulate matter or discolouration are present.

Marketing authorisation number PL 11723/0064

Date of first authorisation/renewal of authorisation 18 May 1995

Date of (partial) revision of text October 1997

Legal category POM

PROMINAL*

Presentation Prominal Tablets 30 mg are white, biconvex tablets, 6.4 mm in diameter, marked P30 on one side and plain on the other. Each tablet contains 30 mg Methylphenobarbitone PhEur.

Prominal Tablets 60 mg are white, biconvex tablets, 7.9 mm in diameter, marked P60 on one side and plain on the other. Each tablet contains 60 mg Methylphenobarbitone PhEur.

Prominal Tablets 200 mg are white, biconvex tablets, 10.3 mm in diameter, marked P200 on one side and plain on the other. Each tablet contains 200 mg Methylphenobarbitone PhEur.

Prominal Tablets 30 mg, 60 mg and 200 mg contain lactose.

Uses

Indications: Prominal Tablets are recommended for the treatment of epilepsy except absence seizures.

Pharmacology: Barbiturates reversibly depress the activity of all excitable tissues, the central nervous system being exquisitely sensitive to their effects.

Methylphenobarbitone undergoes N-demethylation by hepatic microsomal enzymes, forming phenobarbitone, to which most of its activity in chronic medication can be attributed.

Dosage and administration Prominal is for oral administration only.

Adults: The daily dosage must be determined individually. The average range is 200–400 mg. The maximum daily dose is 600 mg.

Elderly: As for adults but see 'Precautions'.

Children: 5–15 mg/kg/day but see 'Precautions'.

Dosing: Dosage should be adjusted carefully with gradual increments at intervals of two to three weeks until fits are controlled or toxicity supervenes. Plateau-state at a given dosage is only achieved after some weeks of medication. Unless serious toxicity dictates otherwise, any reduction in dosage should proceed very gradually to avoid provoking status epilepticus. Monitoring plasma phenobarbitone levels may be helpful when therapy is switched from phenobarbitone to Prominal or vice versa.

Contra-indications, warnings, etc

Contra-indications: Acute intermittent and variegate porphyria; hypersensitivity or idiosyncrasy to barbiturates, states of debilitation, senility, alcohol or other drug abuse or history of abuse; hyperkinetic children; severe renal or hepatic disease.

Precautions: Prominal should be avoided or used only with particular caution and appropriate supervision in children and the elderly who are likely to be specially sensitive to its effects and may react paradoxically.

Prominal should also be avoided or used with special care in patients with hepatic or renal disease whose ability to excrete phenobarbitone may be impaired. Similar caution should be observed in patients with respiratory insufficiency who may prove specially sensitive to the depressant effects of barbiturate on respiration.

Patients who drive or operate machinery should be warned that Prominal can reduce alertness and impair performance. If affected, patients should not undertake these tasks.

Alcohol should be avoided when taking Prominal since as with other CNS depressants, its depressant effect is likely to be additive to that of the barbiturate. In view of the extensive range of inter-reactions between barbiturates and other drugs (see below) caution is advised whenever Prominal is to be co-administered with another medication.

Vitamin D supplement may be needed during long-term Prominal therapy, since Vitamin D catabolism may be increased. Vitamin K supplement may be needed for neonates exposed to barbiturate (see below).

Abuse and dependence: Prominal, like other barbiturates, may lead to psychical and physical dependence in which tolerance and dose increment may be marked features. Symptoms of chronic intoxication include confusion, poor judgement, irritability, insomnia and somatic complaints. Prominal intake should be reduced with great care and under appropriate supervision. Abrupt cessation may precipitate convulsions and can be fatal. Neonates may also suffer from withdrawal symptoms (see below) even in the face of therapeutic dosaging.

Use in pregnancy: Anticonvulsant drugs are as useful to an epileptic during pregnancy as they are at other times and for the individual epileptic mother the chance of an abnormal baby due to drug treatment is small. However, several reports have appeared in the literature suggesting the possible implication of the epileptic state, anticonvulsants and folic acid deficiency as causative agents in certain congenital abnormalities. Scientific knowledge does not yet permit an adequate definition to be made of the respective roles of these three factors. It is recommended therefore, that if anticonvulsant therapy with Prominal is judged necessary during pregnancy, adequate folic acid supplements should be given and the epilepsy controlled as completely as possible with the lowest effective dose.

Neonates: Barbiturates may be transferred to the foetus in utero, as well as to the suckling neonate. Therefore the possibility of barbiturate effects in the neonate, including respiratory depression, sedation and withdrawal reaction, and of the need to give Vitamin K to counteract possible hypoprothrombinaemia, should be borne in mind.

Interactions with other drugs: Barbiturates can affect the actions of a wide range of other drugs principally through an increase in their disposal by stimulation of hepatic microsomal enzymes with usually a resultant decrease but in some instances, an increase, in their therapeutic effect or toxicity. The interactions may be mutual, the plasma levels and activities of barbiturates being also subject to influence by other drugs. Apart from kinetic and metabolic interactions, there may be an addition of effect, for example, the severe depression that may occur when barbiturates are combined with ethanol or other CNS depressants. For these reasons particular care should be observed when administering Prominal in combination with CNS depressants such as sedatives and antihistamines, coumarin-type anticoagulants, antidepressants, including mono-amine oxidase inhibitors, systemic steroids (including oral contraceptives), anticonvulsants such as phenytoin and valproate, antibiotics such as chloramphenicol, rifampicin, metronidazole, doxycycline and also griseofulvin, antihypertensive agents including beta-blockers such as metoprolol and propranolol, but also frusemide and digoxin, opioids such as pethidine and dextropropoxyphene, and many other agents including theophylline, cimetidine, and some oral hypoglycaemic drugs.

Side-effects: Drowsiness and other evidence of sedation is likely to be the most common side effect, but unsteadiness, vertigo and inco-ordination may occur. Paradoxical excitement, restlessness and confusion may occur in the elderly or in the presence of pain; irritability and hyperexcitability may occur in children. Respiratory depression may also occur even at therapeutic dosage and with chronic medication there may be disorientation, mental confusion, ataxia, depression and dependence.

Allergic reactions particularly affecting the skin are not uncommon, including maculopapular rash, fixed drug eruptions and photosensitivity. Occasionally exfoliative dermatitis, erythema multiforme and toxic epidermal necrolysis have been reported. Megaloblastic anaemia associated with folate deficiency has developed during chronic administration and hypoprothrombinaemia may occur in neonates exposed to the barbiturate. Other reported side effects associated with barbiturate include stomatitis, arthritis, acute interstitial nephritis and hepatitis in patients who may be sensitive to this type of drug.

Overdosage: The signs and symptoms of acute overdosage include varying degrees of cardiorespiratory depression, hypotension, absent bowel sounds, renal failure, hypothermia, CNS depression including coma and areflexia. In this setting, a flat EEG may not indicate irreversible brain damage. The aims in treating poisoning by Prominal are to maintain respiration, treat any shock and prevent further absorption of the drug. Where patients are seen within four hours of taking an overdose, gastric aspiration or lavage may be beneficial in adults, while children who are conscious may be given an emetic (e.g. Ipecacuanha Emetic Mixture Paediatric BP). Severely poisoned patients who continue to deteriorate despite supportive treatment may require additional active measures including forced alkaline diuresis, peritoneal dialysis, haemodialysis and haemoperfusion.

Pharmaceutical precautions Nil.

Legal category CD (Sch 3) POM.

Package quantities Prominal Tablets (30 mg, 60 mg and 200 mg) are supplied in bottles of 100.

Further information Nil.

Product licence numbers

Prominal Tablets 30 mg	11723/0066
Prominal Tablets 60 mg	11723/0067
Prominal Tablets 200 mg	11723/0065

PYROGASTRONE* LIQUID

Qualitative and quantitative composition Active constituents: Carbenoxolone Sodium BP 0.20% w/v, Dried Aluminium Hydroxide EP 3.0% w/v and Potassium Bicarbonate BPC 3.0% w/v.

Pyrogastrone Liquid provides 117 mg (3.0 mmol) potassium and 38.8 mg (1.7 mmol) sodium per 10 ml dose.

Pharmaceutical form A fine, off white powder with a faint odour of liquorice and aniseed.

Clinical particulars

Therapeutic indications: For the treatment of oesophageal inflammation, erosions and ulcers due to hiatus hernia or other conditions causing gastro-oesophageal reflux and for the relief of heartburn, flatulence and other symptoms associated with reflux oesophagitis.

Posology and method of administration:

Adults: 10 ml to be taken three times daily immediately after meals and 20 ml at bedtime. Treatment should be continued for at least six weeks, but up to 12 weeks treatment may be necessary to ensure maximum healing effect.

Elderly: Not recommended for patients over 75 years. Otherwise, as for adults but see *Precautions*.

Children: Not recommended.

Pyrogastrone liquid is for oral administration only.

Contra-indications: Pyrogastrone is contra-indicated in patients over 75 years, in children and in pregnancy. Pyrogastrone should not be administered to patients suffering from cardiac, renal or hepatic failure nor to patients on digitalis glycosides unless serum electrolyte levels are monitored at weekly intervals and measures taken to avoid the development of hypokalaemia. It is contra-indicated in established hypokalaemia.

Special warnings and special precautions for use: Special care should be exercised with patients predisposed to sodium and water retention, potassium loss and hypertension (e.g. those with cardiac, renal or hepatic disease) since carbenoxolone can induce similar changes. Potassium supplements should be considered for those at risk from developing hypokalaemia. Regular monitoring of weight, blood pressure and clinical condition is advisable for all patients. Pyrogastrone should be withdrawn if hypokalaemia or oedema develops or a clinically significant rise in blood pressure occurs. Potassium loss should be corrected by the administration of supplements.

Interactions with other medicaments and other forms of interaction: Pyrogastrone may provoke digitalis glycoside toxicity by inducing hypokalaemia. There is a theoretical possibility of a pharmacodynamic interaction with anti-hypertensive drugs, carbenoxolone possibly making hypertension more difficult to control.

Most classes of diuretics will induce hypokalaemia which may be exacerbated by concomitant administration of carbenoxolone as may the mineralocorticoid effects of steroids.

Although spironolactone and amiloride will antagonise the hypokalaemia induced by carbenoxolone they also inhibit its healing action and therefore, should not be prescribed with Pyrogastrone.

Antacids can interact with a wide variety of medicaments generally through effects on their absorption or excretion. These include:

Analgesics: the absorption of diflunisal is reduced and urinary excretion of aspirin may be increased.

Antiarrhythmics: the urinary excretion of flecainide, mexiletine and quinidine may be reduced.

Antibacterials: the absorption of ciprofloxacin, ofloxacin, pivampicillin, rifampicin and most tetracyclines may be reduced as may the absorption of itraconazole and ketoconazole.

Other agents: the absorption of chloroquine, hydroxychloroquine, phenothiazines, oral iron, dipyridamole and penicillamine may all be reduced whilst excretion of lithium may be increased.

Pregnancy and lactation: Although animal studies have shown no hazard, there is inadequate evidence of the safety of carbenoxolone in human pregnancy. Pyrogastrone should be avoided by patients who are pregnant or are breast-feeding mothers.

Effects on ability to drive and to use machines: None.

Undesirable effects: Pyrogastrone may induce sodium and water retention and potassium loss provoking hypertension and cardiac failure in those so predisposed. If profound hypokalaemia is permitted to develop it may lead to widespread impairment of neuromuscular function and muscle damage. Prolonged hypokalaemia may cause renal damage.

Overdosage: If recently ingested the stomach should be emptied by gastric lavage. Serum electrolytes should be monitored and any dificiency in potassium should be corrected, using the intravenous route if necessary, or slow-release or effervescent tablets of potassium chloride. Should water and sodium retention require correction with a diuretic, careful monitoring of potassium levels is mandatory.

Pharmacological properties

Pharmacodynamic properties: Carbenoxolone sodium is a derivative of enoxolone with marked anti-inflammatory actions. It appears to act locally on the stomach possibly by stimulant actions upon mucin production and the enzyme process involved in cellular regeneration. Aluminium hydroxide is a slow acting antacid. Potassium bicarbonate is an antacid.

Pharmacokinetic properties: Carbenoxolone sodium is absorbed from the gastrointestinal tract, the main site of absorption is the stomach. Absorption is reduced if the gastric pH is above 2. Maximum plasma concentrations are obtained 1 hour after administration in a fasting state but can be delayed for several hours if the dose is taken after food; a second peak appears 2 or 3 hours later probably due to enterohepatic cycling of metabolites. It is bound to proteins in the circulation. Removal of drug from the blood is fairly slow with an elimination half-life of approximately 16 hours. Carbenoxolone is mainly excreted in the faeces via the bile.

Aluminium hydroxide is not generally absorbed from the gastrointestinal tract but patients with renal failure have absorbed aluminium and it has been detected in bone. The hydroxide is converted to chloride in the stomach and reconverted to hydroxide in the intestine. Some insoluble aluminium phosphates are also produced which are excreted in the faeces.

Alginic acid is not absorbed by the body and there is no concentration-effect relationship. It is passed unchanged into the faeces.

Pharmaceutical particulars

List of excipients: Pyrogastrone liquid also contains sucrose, povidone, dispersible cellulose, sodium methylhydroxybenzoate, sodium propylhydroxybenzoate, sodium alginate, Manugel, liquorice/aniseed flavour and water.

Incompatibilities: Not applicable.

Shelf life: The shelf-life of the unopened product is 36 months. The shelf-life of the reconstituted product is 3 months.

Special precautions for storage: Store below 25°C.

Nature and contents of container: The powder is contained in 600 ml glass cylindrical amber glass bottle with a black plastic screw cap. It is reconstituted prior to use with 450 ml of water.

Instructions for use/handling: Not applicable.

Marketing authorisation number 11723/0069.

Date of approval/revision of SPC 15th September 1993.

Legal category POM.

PYROGASTRONE* TABLETS

Presentation Pyrogastrone chewable tablets are white, round, strawberry-flavoured chewable tablets, 22.2 mm in diameter, marked PYROGASTRONE on one side. Each tablet contains:

Carbenoxolone Sodium BP	20 mg
Dried Aluminium Hydroxide PhEur	240 mg
Magnesium Trisilicate PhEur	60 mg

in a base containing 210 mg Sodium Bicarbonate PhEur and 600 mg Alginic Acid BPC.

Each Pyrogastrone chewable tablet contains approximately 59.2 mg (2.6 mmol) sodium.

Uses For the treatment of oesophageal inflammation, erosions and ulcers due to hiatus hernia or other conditions causing gastro-oesophageal reflux and for the relief of heartburn, flatulence and other symptoms associated with reflux oesophagitis.

Dosage and administration For oral administration only.

Adults: 1 tablet to be chewed three times daily immediately after meals and 2 tablets to be chewed at bedtime. The tablets may be followed by a drink of water.

Treatment should be continued for at least six weeks, but up to 12 weeks' treatment may be necessary to ensure maximum healing effect.

Elderly: Not recommended for patients over 75 years. Otherwise, as for adults.

Children: Not recommended.

Contra-indications, warnings, etc
Contra-indications: Pyrogastrone is contra-indicated in patients over 75 years, in children and in pregnancy. Pyrogastrone should not be administered to patients suffering from cardiac, renal or hepatic failure nor to patients on digitalis glycosides unless serum electrolyte levels are monitored at weekly intervals and measures taken to avoid the development of hypokalaemia. It is contra-indicated in established hypokalaemia, patients with a hypersensitivity to carbenoxolone or any of the other ingredients, patients on a low salt diet.

Precautions: Special care should be exercised with patients pre-disposed to sodium and water retention, potassium loss and hypertension (e.g. those with cardiac, renal or hepatic disease) since carbenoxolone can induce similar changes. Potassium supplements should be considered for those at risk from developing hypokalaemia.

Regular monitoring of weight, blood pressure and clinical condition is advisable for all patients. Pyrogastrone should be withdrawn if hypokalaemia or oedema develops or a clinically significant rise in blood pressure occurs. Potassium loss should be corrected by the administration of supplements.

Pregnancy: Although animal studies have shown no hazard, there is inadequate evidence of the safety of carbenoxolone in human pregnancy. Pyrogastrone should be avoided in patients who are pregnant.

Interactions: Pyrogastrone may provoke digitalis glycoside toxicity by inducing hypokalaemia.

There is a theoretical possibility of a pharmacodynamic interaction with anti-hypertensive drugs, carbenoxolone possibly making hypertension more difficult to control.

Most classes of diuretics will induce hypokalaemia which may be exacerbated by concomitant administration of carbenoxolone as may the mineralocorticoid effects of steroids.

Although spironolactone and amiloride will antagonise the hypokalaemia induced by carbenoxolone they also inhibit its healing action and, therefore, should not be prescribed with Pyrogastrone.

Antacids can interact with a wide variety of medications generally through effects on their absorption or excretion. These include:

Analgesics – the absorption of diflunisal is reduced and urinary excretion of aspirin may be increased.

Antiarrhythmics – the urinary excretion of flecainide, mexiletine and quinidine may be reduced.

Antibacterials – the absorption of ciprofloxacin, ofloxacin, pivampicillin, rifampicin and most tetracyclines may be reduced as may the absorption of itraconazole and ketoconazole.

Other agents – the absorption of chloroquine, hydroxychloroquine, phenothiazines, oral iron, dipyridamole and penicillamine may all be reduced whilst excretion of lithium may be increased.

Side-effects: Pyrogastrone may induce sodium and water retention and potassium loss, provoking hypertension and cardiac failure in those so predisposed. If profound hypokalaemia is permitted to develop it may lead to widespread impairment of neuromuscular function and to muscle damage. Prolonged hypokalaemia may cause renal damage.

Overdosage: If recently ingested the stomach should be emptied by gastric lavage. Serum electrolytes should be monitored and any deficiency in potassium should be corrected, using the intravenous route if necessary, or slow-release or effervescent tablets of potassium chloride. Should water and sodium retention require correction with a diuretic, careful monitoring of potassium levels is mandatory.

Pharmaceutical precautions Store in a dry place.

Legal category POM.

Package quantities Boxes containing 25 foil strips of 4 tablets.

Further Information The alginate antacid base of Pyrogastrone forms a clinging viscous foam which has buffering capacity. This relieves symptoms, either by coating the oesophageal wall, by impeding gastro-oesophageal reflux, or the foam may reflux instead of the acid gastric contents. The incorporation of carbenoxolone into the formulation has been shown to exert an additional healing effect on oesophageal ulcers possibly by improving mucus synthesis and/or by increasing the life-span of oesophageal epithelium.

Systemic absorption of carbenoxolone is extensive. There is more than 99.95% binding to plasma proteins. There appears to be enterohepatic circulation which delays clearance. Excretion is mainly via the faeces. Plasma elimination half life increases with age. Aluminium hydroxide is not generally absorbed from the gastrointestinal tract, while alginic acid is not digested and passes unchanged into the faeces.

Product licence number 11723/0068

RESONIUM* A

Presentation Resonium A contains 99.93% sodium polystyrene sulphonate ground and flavoured to a buff-coloured powder with a pleasant vanilla odour and sweet taste.

Uses Resonium A is an ion-exchange resin which is recommended for the treatment of hyperkalaemia associated with anuria or severe oliguria. It is also used to treat hyperkalaemia in patients requiring dialysis and in patients on regular haemodialysis or on prolonged peritoneal dialysis.

Dosage and administration Resonium A is for oral or rectal administration only. The dosage recommendations detailed in this section are a guide only, the precise requirements should be decided on the basis of regular serum electrolyte determinations.

Adults including the elderly:
1. *Oral:* Usual dose 15 g three or four times a day. The resin is given by mouth in a little water, or it may be made into a paste with some sweetened vehicle.
2. *Rectal:* In cases where vomiting may make oral administration difficult, the resin may be given rectally as a suspension of 30 g resin in 100 ml 2% Methylcellulose 450 BP (medium viscosity) and 100 ml water, as a daily retention enema. In the initial stages administration by this route as well as orally may help to achieve a more rapid lowering of the serum potassium level.

The enema should if possible be retained for at least nine hours following which the colon should be irrigated to remove the resin. If both routes are used initially it is probably unnecessary to continue rectal administration once the oral resin has reached the rectum.

Children: 1 g/kg body weight daily in divided doses in acute hyperkalaemia. Dosage may be reduced to 0.5 g/kg body weight in divided doses for maintenance therapy. The resin is given orally, preferably with a drink (not a fruit squash because of the high potassium content) or a little jam or honey. When refused by mouth it should be given rectally, using a dose at least as great as that which would have been given orally, diluted in the same ratio as described for adults. Following retention of the enema, the colon should be irrigated to ensure adequate removal of the resin.

Neonates: Resonium A should not be given by the oral route. With rectal administration, the minimum effective dosage within the range 0.5 g/kg to 1 g/kg should be employed diluted as for adults and with adequate irrigation to ensure recovery of the resin.

Contra-indications, warnings, etc
Contra-indications: Resonium A should not be administered orally to neonates. It should not be administered to neonates with reduced gut motility (e.g. post-operatively or drug induced). Resonium A is also contra-indicated in the presence of obstructive bowel disease, in use where plasma potassium levels are below 5 mmol/litre and in patients with a history of hypersensitivity to polystyrene sulphonate resins.

Precautions: The possibility of severe potassium depletion should be considered and adequate clinical and biochemical control is essential during treatment, especially in patients on digitalis. Administration of the resin should be stopped when the serum potassium level falls to 5 mmol/litre.

Because the resin may bind calcium and magnesium ions, deficiencies of these electrolytes may occur. Accordingly, patients should be monitored for all applicable electrolyte disturbances.

In the event of clinically significant constipation treatment should be discontinued until normal bowel movement has resumed. Magnesium-containing laxatives should not be used.

The patient should be positioned carefully when ingesting the resin, in order to avoid aspiration, which may lead to bronchopulmonary complications.

Sorbitol added to enemas of sodium polystyrene sulphonate has been implicated in cases of colonic necrosis. The safety and efficacy of sorbitol used with sodium polystyrene sulphonate has not been established and they should not be used together.

In children and neonates particular care is needed with rectal administration as excessive dosage or inadequate dilution could result in impaction of the resin. Care should be taken when administering to patients in whom an increase in sodium load may be detrimental (i.e. congestive heart failure, hypertension, renal damage or oedema). In such cases, Calcium Resonium (calcium polystyrene sulphonate) may be used in place of Resonium A.

Interactions: There have been reports of systemic alkalosis following concurrent administration of cation-exchange resins and non-absorbable cation-donating antacids such as magnesium hydroxide and aluminium carbonate. Intestinal obstruction due to concretions of aluminium hydroxide has been reported when aluminium hydroxide has been combined with the resin. The toxic effects of digitalis on the heart, especially various ventricular arrhythmias and AV nodal dissociation, are likely to be exaggerated if hypokalaemia is allowed to develop. Cation donating agents may reduce the potassium binding effect of Resonium A. Sorbitol added to enemas may cause colonic necrosis.

Pregnancy and lactation: No data are available regarding the use of polystyrene sulphonate resins in pregnancy and lactation. The administration of Resonium A in pregnancy and during breast feeding therefore, is not advised unless, in the opinion of the physician, the potential benefits outweigh any potential risks.

Side-effects: In accordance with its pharmacological actions, the resin may give rise to sodium retention, hypokalaemia and hypercalcaemia and the related clinical manifestations (see *Warnings and precautions* and *Overdosage*). Gastric irritation, anorexia, nausea, vomiting, constipation and occasionally diarrhoea may occur. Faecal impaction following rectal administration has been reported in children, and gastro-intestinal concretions following oral administration to neonates, have been reported.

Some cases of acute bronchitis and/or bronchopneumonia associated with inhalation of particles of calcium polystyrene sulphonate have been described. Colonic necrosis has been reported following administration of sodium polystyrene sulphonate in sorbitol as enemas (see also *Interactions*).

Overdosage: Biochemical disturbances from overdosage may give rise to clinical signs or symptoms of hypokalaemia, including irritability, confusion, delayed thought processes, muscle weakness, hyporeflexia and eventual paralysis. Apnoea may be a serious consequence of this progression. Electrocardiographic changes may be consistent with hypokalaemia; cardiac arrhythmia may occur. Hypocalcaemia tetany may occur. Appropriate measures should be taken to correct serum electrolytes and the resin should be removed from the alimentary tract by appropriate use of laxatives or enemas.

Pharmaceutical precautions Suspensions of the resin should be freshly prepared and not stored beyond 24 hours.

Legal category P.

Package quantities Supplied in HDPE containers containing 454 g Resonium A together with a plastic scoop which, when filled level, contains approximately 15 g.

Further information Theoretically, each gram of Resonium A should take up 2.8 to 3.4 mmol of potassium. However, in vivo, the actual amount of potassium bound will be less than this. The sodium content of Resonium A is 4.1 to 4.8 mmol/g.

Product licence number 11723/0070.

SKELID* ▼

Qualitative and quantitative composition Disodium tiludronate 240.00 mg expressed as tiludronic acid 200.00 mg.

Pharmaceutical form Tablet.

Clinical particulars
Therapeutic indications: Treatment of Paget's disease of bone.

Posology and method of administration: Oral route. For use in adults only.

The dosage is 400 mg daily (i.e. 2 tablets) as a single intake for three months (i.e. 12 weeks).

Most patients respond to treatment within the first three months, whether or not they have been previously treated with another bisphosphonate.

Improvements of serum alkaline phosphatase level may last for up to 18 months following discontinuation.

Treatment may be repeated if either biochemical markers (increase in serum alkaline phosphatase with or without an increase in hydroxyprolinuria) or pain suggests relapse. A second course of treatment should be prescribed only after an interval of at least 6 months.

Tablets should be taken in a single dose with a glass of water at least two hours before or after meals.

In the two hours before and after ingestion, patients should refrain from taking food, particularly foods rich in calcium (such as milk and dairy products) and antacid gastric protective agents (cf. interactions).

Contra-indications: Patients with a history of allergy to bisphosphonates; Severe renal failure (creatinine clearance less than 30 ml/min); Juvenile Paget's disease; Pregnancy and breast feeding.

Special warnings and precautions for use: Tiludronate is not metabolised and is excreted unchanged in the urine. Tiludronate should be administered with caution in cases of mild renal failure (creatinine clearance between 60 and 90 ml/min) and moderate renal failure (creatinine clearance between 30 and 60 ml/min) (regularly monitor renal function).

Patients should ensure that their calcium and Vitamin D intake is adequate; calcium metabolism disorders (hypocalcaemia, vitamin D deficiency) should be corrected before initiating treatment.

Interactions with other medicaments and other forms of interaction: Concomitant treatments necessitating additional precautions:

– with calcium salts, gastro-intestinal topical treatments, antacids when administered by the oral route (reduction of gastrointestinal absorption of bisphosphonates).
– with indomethacin (increase of the bioavailability of tiludronic acid).
– tiludronate should not be taken within two hours of these drugs.

The pharmacokinetic parameters of tiludronate are not significantly altered by concomitant treatment with aspirin or diclofenac.

The pharmacokinetic parameters of digoxin are not significantly altered by concomitant treatment with tiludronate.

Concomitant administration of tiludronate and products likely to cause mineralisation disorders is to be avoided.

Pregnancy and lactation

Pregnancy: The administration of tiludronate is contra-indicated in pregnancy (lack of data).

Whereas tiludronate failed to induce harmful effects in reproduction studies delayed skeletal maturation and ossification of the foetus was reported with other bisphosphonates in experimental animals. Data about transplacental transfer of tiludronate in women are lacking.

Breast feeding: The administration of tiludronate is contra-indicated in case of breast feeding (lack of data).

Effects on ability to drive and use machines: No special precaution has to be taken in case of driving or using machines.

Undesirable effects: The adverse effects are mainly gastro-intestinal: stomach pain, nausea, diarrhoea. These effects are slight to moderate and their incidence is dose-related.

In rare cases there have been reports of asthenia, dizziness, headache and skin reactions.

Overdose: In the event of massive overdose, some patients could present with hypocalcaemia and renal failure. Gastric lavage may be useful to remove any unabsorbed tiludronate. Symptomatic treatment of hypocalcaemia (calcium salts by intravenous route, calcium gluconate for example) and/or renal failure should be initiated.

Pharmacological properties

Pharmacodynamic properties: Medicament for the treatment of bone diseases.
(M05 BA Bisphosphonates)

Tiludronate like other bisphosphonates inhibits the bone resorbing activity of osteoclasts.

Tiludronate slows bone remodelling in Paget's disease, as shown by the reduction in serum alkaline phosphatase. In cases of Paget's disease, preliminary studies of biopsies in a small number of patients have shown that tiludronate reduces excessive remodelling due to this disease.

Data concerning possible long-term mineralisation disorders in clinical use are not available. On the other hand, daily long-term administration (6 months to 1 year) of high doses to rats and baboons did not induce osteomalacia.

Pharmacokinetic properties: The absolute bioavailability of tiludronate is low (6% on average) and variable (from 2 to 11%). After repeated administrations of a dose of 400 mg/day, the plasma concentration peaks are very variable (usually between 1 and 5 mg/l and occur 1 to 2 hours after administration). Bioavailability is reduced when administered during or after a meal and greatly reduced in the presence of calcium.

Protein plasma binding is 91% and constant over the therapeutic concentration range. The protein responsible for binding is albumin. Less than 5% is bound to red blood cells. Approximately half of the dose taken undergoes bone fixation.

Tiludronate is excreted in unchanged form by the kidneys. After oral administration of a single dose, the quantities of unchanged tiludronate excreted found after 48 hours are 3.5±1.9%. After treatment withdrawal, the decrease in plasma tiludronate levels is divided into two phases, the second of which is much slower and difficult to determine accurately due to the very low plasma concentrations (half-life greater than 100 hours). The second phase results from bone remodelling and very slow release of tiludronate from the bones.

Preclinical safety data: Single-dose toxicity: after oral administration, tiludronate exhibited moderate acute toxicity in rats (LD50 about 550 mg/kg) and low acute toxicity in mice (LD50≥1000 mg/kg). Lesions were observed in the kidney, stomach and lung.

Repeated-dose toxicity: after repeated oral administration of tiludronate mainly to rats and baboons for up to 1 year, gastritis and renal proximal tubulopathy were observed at doses ≥50 mg/kg/d which were substantially higher than pharmacologically effective doses of 5–10 mg/kg/d leading to inhibition of stimulated bone resorption and increase in bone density or metaphyseal trabeculae.

Genotoxicity and carcinogenesis: *in vitro* and *in vivo* investigations with tiludronate to detect gene mutations, chromosomal aberrations or DNA repair processes showed no effect. There was no evidence of carcinogenicity either in mice treated for 80 weeks with up to 50 mg/kg/d tiludronate or in rats treated with up to 25 mg/kg/d tiludronate for 2 years.

Reproduction toxicity: oral tiludronate in doses up to 375 mg/kg/d did not exert teratogenic or direct embryotoxic effects in rats, mice or rabbits. Up to 75 mg/kg/d tiludronate did not affect fertility or peri- and post-natal development of rats. Nevertheless, considering that delayed skeletal maturation and ossification of the foetus was reported with other bisphosphonates in experimental animals and that data about transplacental transfer in women are lacking tiludronate is contra-indicated in pregnancy.

Pharmaceutical particulars

List of excipients: Sodium lauryl sulphate, methylhydroxypropyl cellulose, crospovidone, magnesium stearate, lactose monohydrate.

Incompatibilities: None.

Shelf life: Three years.

Special precautions for storage: None.

Nature and contents of container: 28 tablets in heat-formed blister packs (polyamide – aluminium – PVC/aluminium).

Marketing authorisation number 11723/0207.

Date of approval/revision of SPC 6 February 1996.

Legal category POM.

SOLPADOL* EFFERVESCENT SOLPADOL CAPLETS*

Presentation

1. White bevelled-edged effervescent tablets, plain on the reverse and scored on the obverse, which effervesce vigorously when placed in water. Each tablet is 25.4 mm in diameter and contains Paracetamol PhEur 500 mg and Codeine Phosphate Hemihydrate PhEur 30 mg.

2. White capsule-shaped tablets marked with SOLPADOL on one side and plain on the reverse. Each tablet contains Paracetamol PhEur 500 mg and Codeine Phosphate Hemihydrate PhEur 30 mg.

Uses Solpadol is an analgesic, the effect being produced by a combination of the peripheral action of paracetamol and the central action of codeine at opioid binding sites. It is recommended for the relief of severe pain.

Dosage and administration Solpadol is for oral administration only.

Adults: 1. *Solpadol effervescent tablets:* Two tablets not more frequently than every 4 hours, up to a maximum of 8 tablets in any 24 hour period. Tablets should be dissolved in at least half a tumblerful of water before taking.

2. *Solpadol Caplets:* Two Caplets not more frequently than every 4 hours, up to a maximum of 8 Caplets in any 24 hour period.

Elderly: A reduced dose may be required – see warnings.

Children: Not recommended for children under 12 years of age.

Contra-indications, warnings, etc

Contra-indications: Hypersensitivity to paracetamol or codeine, or any of the other constituents which is rare. Conditions where morphine and opioids are contra-indicated e.g. acute asthma, respiratory depression, acute alcoholism, head injuries, raised intracranial pressure and following biliary tract surgery; monoamine oxidase inhibitor therapy, concurrent or within 14 days.

Warnings: Patients should be advised not to drive or operate machinery if affected by dizziness or sedation.

Care should be taken in administering the product to any patient whose condition may be exacerbated by opioids, particularly the elderly, who are specially sensitive to their central and gastro-intestinal effects, those on concurrent CNS depressant drugs, those with prostatic hypertrophy and those with inflammatory or obstructive bowel disorders.

Care should also be taken if prolonged therapy is contemplated.

Care is advised in the administration of paracetamol to patient with severe renal or severe hepatic impairment. The hazards of overdose are greater in those with alcoholic liver disease. Patients should be advised not to exceed the recommended dose and not take other paracetamol containing products concurrently.

There is inadequate evidence of the safety of codeine in human pregnancy, but there is epidemiological evidence of the safety of paracetamol. Both substances have been used for many years without apparent adverse effect and animal studies have not shown any hazard. Nonetheless, careful consideration should be given before prescribing Solpadol for pregnant patients. Opioid analgesics may depress neonatal respiration and cause withdrawal effects in neonates of dependent mothers. Paracetamol is excreted in breast milk but not in a clinically significant amount.

Each Solpadol effervescent tablet contains 426.8 mg sodium (18.56 mEq). This sodium content should be taken into account when prescribing for patients for whom sodium restriction is indicated. Each Solpadol Caplet contains less than 1 mg of sodium.

Interactions: Paracetamol may increase the elimination half-life of chloramphenicol. Oral contraceptives may increase its rate of clearance. The speed of absorption of paracetamol may be increased by metoclopramide or domperidone and absorption reduced by cholestyramine. The anticoagulant effect of warfarin and other coumarins may be enhanced by prolonged regular use of paracetamol with increased risk of bleeding; occasional doses have no significant effect. The effects of CNS depressants (including alcohol) may be potentiated by codeine.

Side-effects: Adverse effects to paracetamol are rare, but hypersensitivity including skin rash may occur. There have been reports of blood dyscrasias including thrombocytopenia and agranulocytosis, but these were not necessarily causally related to paracetamol. Codeine can produce typical opioid effects, including constipation, nausea, vomiting, dizziness, light headedness, confusion, drowsiness and urinary retention. The frequency and severity are determined by dosage, duration of treatment and individual sensitivity.

Tolerance and dependence can occur, especially with prolonged high dosage of codeine.

Overdosage: Nausea and vomiting are prominent symptoms of codeine toxicity and there is evidence of circulatory and respiratory depression. Suggested treatment is gastric lavage and catharsis. If CNS depression is severe, assisted ventilation, oxygen and parenteral naloxone may be needed.

Symptoms of paracetamol overdosage in the first 24 hours are pallor, nausea, vomiting, anorexia and abdominal pain. Liver damage may become apparent 12 to 24 hours after ingestion. Abnormalities of glucose metabolism and metabolic acidosis may occur. In severe poisoning, hepatic failure may progress to encephalopathy, coma and death. Acute renal failure with acute tabular necrosis may develop even in the absence of severe liver damage. Cardiac arrhythmias and pancreatitis have been reported.

Liver damage is more likely in adults who have taken 10 g or more of paracetamol. It is considered that excess quantities of a toxic metabolite (usually adequately detoxified by glutathione when normal doses of paracetamol are ingested), become irreversibly bound to liver tissue.

Immediate treatment is essential in the management of paracetamol overdose. Despite a lack of significant early symptoms, patients should be referred to hospital urgently for immediate medical attention and any patient who had ingested around 7.5 g or more of paracetamol in the preceding 4 hours should undergo gastric lavage. Administration of oral methionine or intravenous N-acetylcysteine which may have a beneficial effect up to at least 48 hours after the overdose, may be required. General supportive measures must be available.

Patients in whom oxidative liver enzymes have been induced, including alcoholics and those receiving barbiturates and patients who are chronically malnourished, may be particularly sensitive to the toxic effects of paracetamol in overdosage.

Pharmaceutical precautions Solpadol Caplets and effervescent tablets should be stored below 25°C. Solpadol Caplets should be stored in a dry place.

Legal category POM.

Package quantities Tablets are packed in boxes of 100 tablets (25 laminate strips 4 tablets).

Caplets are packed in foil blisters and supplied in boxes of 100.

Further information Nil

Product licence numbers

Solpadol effervescent tablets	11723/0072
Solpadol Caplets	11723/0071

SOLPADOL* CAPSULES

Qualitative and quantitative composition

Active constituents:

Paracetamol PhEur	500.0 mg
Codeine Phosphate Hemihydrate PhEur	30.0 mg

Pharmaceutical form Capsules.

Clinical particulars

Therapeutic indications: For the relief of severe pain.

Posology and method of administration:

Adults: Two capsules not more frequently than every 4 hours, up to a maximum of 8 capsules in any 24 hour period.

Elderly: As for adults, however, a reduced dose may be required. See *Special warnings and precautions for use.*

Children: Not recommended for children under 12 years of age.

Solpadol capsules are for oral administration.

Contra-indications: Hypersensitivity to paracetamol or codeine which is rare, or hypersensitivity to any of the other constituents. Conditions where morphine and opiods are contra-indicated e.g., acute asthma, respiratory depression, acute alcoholism, head injuries, raised intra-cranial pressure and following biliary tract surgery; monoamine oxidase inhibitor therapy, concurrent or within 14 days.

Special warnings and precautions for use: Care should be observed in administering the product to any patient whose condition may be exacerbated by opioids, particularly the elderly, who may be sensitive to their central and gastro-intestinal effects, those on concurrent CNS depressant drugs, those with prostatic hypertrophy and those with inflammatory or obstructive bowel disorders. Care should also be observed if prolonged therapy is contemplated.

Care is advised in the administration of paracetamol to patients with severe renal or severe hepatic impairment. The hazards of overdose are greater in those with alcoholic liver disease.

Patients should be advised not to exceed the recommended dose and not take other paracetamol containing products concurrently.

Interactions with other medicaments and other forms of interaction: Paracetamol may increase the elimination half-life of chloramphenicol. Oral contraceptives may increase its rate of clearance. The speed of absorption of paracetamol may be increased by metoclopramide or domperidone and absorption reduced by cholestyramine.

The anticoagulant effect of warfarin and other coumarins may be enhanced by prolonged regular use of paracetamol with increased risk of bleeding; occasional doses have no significant effect.

The effects of CNS depressants (including alcohol) may be potentiated by codeine.

Pregnancy and lactation: There is inadequate evidence of the safety of codeine in human pregnancy, but there is epidemiological evidence for the safety of paracetamol. Both substances have been used for many years without apparent ill consequences and animal studies have not shown any hazard. Nonetheless careful consideration should be given before prescribing the products for pregnant patients. Opioid analgesics may depress neonatal respiration and cause withdrawal effects in neonates of dependent mothers.

Paracetamol is excreted in breast milk but not in a clinically significant amount.

Effects on ability to drive and to use machines: Patients should be advised not to drive or operate machinery if affected by dizziness or sedation.

Undesirable effects: Codeine can produce typical opioid effects including constipation, nausea, vomiting, dizziness, light-headedness, confusion, drowsiness and urinary retention. The frequency and severity are determined by dosage, duration of treatment and individual sensitivity. Tolerance and dependence can occur, especially with prolonged high dosage of codeine.

Adverse effects of paracetamol are rare but hypersensitivity including skin rash may occur. There have been reports of blood dyscrasias including thrombocytopenia and agranulocytosis, but these were not necessarily causally related to paracetamol.

Overdose: Nausea and vomiting are prominent symptoms of codeine toxicity and if there is evidence of circulatory and respiratory depression, suggested treatment is gastric lavage and catharsis. If CNS depression is severe, assisted ventilation, oxygen and parenteral naloxone may be needed.

Patients in whom oxidative liver enzymes have been induced, including alcoholics and those receiving barbiturates and patients who are chronically malnourished, may be particularly sensitive to the toxic effects of paracetamol in overdose.

Symptoms of paracetamol overdosage in the first 24 hours are pallor, nausea, vomiting, anorexia and abdominal pain. Liver damage may become apparent 12 to 48 hours after ingestion. Abnormalities of glucose metabolism and metabolic acidosis may occur. In severe poisoning, hepatic failure may progress to encephalopathy, coma and death. Acute renal failure with acute tabular necrosis may develop even in the absence of severe liver damage. Cardiac arrhythmias and pancreatitis have been reported.

Liver damage is likely in adults who have taken 10 g or more of paracetamol. It is considered that excess quantities of a toxic metabolite (usually adequately detoxified by glutathione when normal doses of paracetamol are ingested), become irreversibly bound to liver tissue.

Immediate treatment is essential in the management of paracetamol overdose. Despite a lack of significant early symptoms, patients should be referred to hospital urgently for immediate medical attention and any patient who had ingested around 7.5 g or more of paracetamol in the preceding 4 hours should undergo gastric lavage. Administration of oral methionine or intravenous N-acetylcysteine which may have a beneficial effect up to at least 48 hours after the overdose, may be required. General supportive measures must be available.

Pharmacological properties

Pharmacodynamic properties: Paracetamol is an analgesic which acts peripherally, probably by blocking impulse generation at the bradykinin sensitive chemoreceptors which evoke pain. Although it is a prostaglandin synthetase inhibitor, the synthetase system in the CNS rather than the periphery appears to be more sensitive to it. This may explain paracetamol's lack of appreciable anti-inflammatory activity. Paracetamol also exhibits antipyretic activity.

Codeine is a centrally acting analgesic which produces its effect by its action at opioid-binding sites (μ-receptors) within the CNS. It is a full agonist.

Pharmacokinetic properties: Following oral administration of two capsules (i.e., a dose of paracetamol 1000 mg and codeine phosphate 60 mg) the mean maximum plasma concentrations of paracetamol and codeine phosphate were 17.5 μg/ml and 327 ng/ml respectively. The mean times to maximum plasma concentrations were 1.03 hours for paracetamol 1.10 hours for codeine phosphate.

The mean $AUC_{(0-10)}$ following administration was 48.0 g μml^{-1}.h for paracetamol and 1301 ng/ml^{-1}.h for codeine.

The bioavailabilities of paracetamol and codeine when given as the combination are similar to those when they are given separately.

Pharmaceutical particulars

List of excipients: Maize starch, magnesium stearate, purified talc, indigotine E132, azorubine E122, titanium dioxide E171, gelatin, black iron oxide E172, shellac 1963, industrial methylated spirit, purified water, soya lecithin (food grade), 2-ethoxyethanol 1949, dimethylpolysiloxane 1973.

Incompatibilities: Not applicable.

Shelf life: The shelf life for this product is 36 months in PVC blister packs contained in cardboard cartons.

Special precautions for storage: Store in the original package. Do not store above 25°C.

Nature and contents of container: White, opaque PVC (250 μm)/aluminium foil (20 μm) blister packs contained in cardboard cartons.

Pack sizes of 4, 10, 60 and 100 capsules.

Instructions for use/handling: Not applicable.

Marketing authorisation holder: Sanofi Winthrop Limited, One Onslow Street, Guildford, Surrey GU1 4YS.

Marketing authorisation number PL 11723/0117.

Date of first authorisation/renewal of the authorisation 29th December 1994

Date of (partial) revision of text July 1998

Legal category POM.

STROMBA*

Presentation Stromba Tablets are round, flat, white tablets 9.5 mm in diameter, marked STROMBA on one side and scored in quarters on the other side. Each tablet contains 5 mg Stanozolol BP. Stromba tablets also contain lactose.

Uses

1. For the vascular manifestations of Behcet's disease.

2. For the prevention of spontaneous attacks of proven hereditary angio-oedema.

Dosage and administration Stromba is for oral administration only.

1. Behcet's disease

Adults: 10 mg daily.

2. Hereditary angio-oedema: The initial dosage should be adjusted to control the occurrence of attacks. Thereafter, the dosage may be reduced for maintenance therapy according to patient response.

Adults: Initially 2.5–10 mg daily. Dosage as low as 2.5 mg three times a week has been effective maintenance therapy.

Children: Not suitable for children less than one year old. 1–6 years, initially 2.5 mg daily. 6–12 years, initially 2.5–5 mg daily.

Contra-indications, warnings, etc

Contra-indications: Stromba is not intended for the treatment of loss of appetite, unexplained weight loss or failure to thrive in children. Such cases should be referred to the appropriate centre for investigation.

Because of possible virilising effects on a female foetus, Stromba should not be administered to pregnant women. There are no available data on the excretion of stanozolol in breast milk. Lactating mothers should not breast feed if Stromba treatment is necessary.

Stromba should not be administered to patients with established liver disease. Patients with a history of jaundice should have liver function tests checked prior to commencing treatment.

Stromba should not be used in cases of cancer of the prostate because the condition is androgen-dependent.

Stromba increases ALA synthetase activity and hence porphyrin metabolism. It is therefore not recommended in patients with a history of porphyria as its use may precipitate an acute attack.

Stromba has been used in patients with non-insulin dependent diabetes without adverse consequences. However, it may be advisable to avoid its use in insulin dependent diabetics.

Precautions: Prolonged use in children may lead to premature closure of the epiphyses.

In hereditary angio-oedema:

(a) long-term use of Stromba should be restricted to well established cases who have experienced serious attacks.

(b) Stromba should not be used in pre-menopausal women except in life-threatening situations.

Stromba should be used with caution in the presence of impaired renal or cardiac function as it may encourage sodium and water retention that could result in cardiac failure.

Peliosis hepatis and tumours of the liver have been reported occasionally in patients subject to prolonged treatment with androgenic anabolic steroids. The tumours are not typical of primary hepatocellular carcinoma and in some cases discontinuation of steroids has resulted in tumour regression without other therapy. The possibility that Stromba may induce or enhance the development of peliosis hepatis and hepatic tumours cannot be excluded and this should be considered when long-term treatment is carried out.

Caution should also be observed in treating patients with breast cancer since anabolic steroids may induce hypercalcaemia in this condition. Periodic assessment of liver function, haematocrit and haemoglobin is advised during treatment.

Interactions: Anabolic steroids increase sensitivity to warfarin type anti-coagulants; therefore, the dose of the latter should be decreased by approximately a half in order to maintain the prothrombin time at the desired therapeutic level.

Dosage of oral hypoglycaemic agents may require adjustment when initiating or discontinuing Stromba therapy.

Side-effects: Because of the structural relationship to the male hormones, some androgenic side-effects e.g. acne, hirsutism, amenorrhoea, are to be expected. Because the ratio of anabolic to androgenic properties is high, these effects should be minimal at the recommended dosage and those reported have been generally mild and reversible on stopping treatment. On rare occasions, usually with higher dosage, voice change has been reported; if observed, treatment should be discontinued. Other effects, such as menstrual irregularity, headache, muscle cramp, dyspepsia, skin rash and occasionally hair loss, euphoria and depression have occurred. An increase in haematocrit and haemoglobin level may also occur. There have been occasional reports of cholestatic jaundice, and very rarely, peliosis hepatis and hepatic tumours.

In children, prolonged use may lead to premature closure of the epiphyses.

Stromba may raise levels of aspartate transaminase (AST) and alanine transaminase (ALT) and in some patients these may rise above laboratory normal ranges. These levels return to normal on withdrawing Stromba.

Elevations of creatine phospho-kinase and of alkaline phosphatase have also occasionally been reported.

The use of this preparation may temporarily result in an alteration in the ratio of high and low density lipoproteins. The significance of this is not understood.

Some patients taking Stromba may show increased T3 uptake, decreased T4 levels and a decrease in thyroxine binding globulin although they are clinically euthyroid.

Overdosage: There are no reports of chronic or acute overdosage with Stromba. By analogy with other substances of this type, one would expect chronic overdosage to be associated with the signs and symptoms caused by excessive circulating androgens. It is unlikely that any immediate serious reactions would be seen with a single excessive dose (in animals acute toxicity cannot be measured). In such an event, however, the patient should be kept under observation and liver function monitored, in case of delayed reactions. If large amounts are accidentally ingested treat symptomatically.

Pharmaceutical precautions Nil.

Legal category POM.

Package quantities Calendar packs of 56 tablets (OP).

Further information Stanozolol is an anabolic agent with fibrinolytic properties which are of therapeutic value in modifying the vascular manifestations of Behcet's disease. In patients with hereditary angio-oedema, stanozolol alters the functional level of plasma C1 esterase inhibitor which is depressed in this condition.

Stanozolol given by mouth is readily absorbed into the bloodstream. Within the serum it is highly protein bound. Metabolism is carried out to a large extent in the liver and the conjugated metabolites are excreted in both the faeces and urine.

Product licence number 11723/0073

TICLID* 

Qualitative and quantitative composition
Each tablet contains:
Active ingredient: Ticlopidine Hydrochloride PhEur 250 mg equivalent to ticlopidine base 219.6 mg.

Pharmaceutical form Film coated tablets.

Clinical particulars
Therapeutic indications: Reduction of risk of first and recurrent stroke for patients who have experienced at least one of the following events: complete thromboembolic stroke, minor stroke, reversible ischaemic neurological deficit (RIND), or transient ischaemic attack (TIA) including transient monocular blindness (TMB).

Reduction of risk of major ischaemic accidents, particularly coronary, in patients presenting with chronic arterial disease of the lower limbs at the stage of intermittent claudication.

In view of the risk of serious haematological side effects, the initiation of therapy should be carried out by a clinician in hospital. The prescriber needs to carefully consider the risks and benefits of ticlopidine versus aspirin as the benefit/risk ratio is greater in patients for whom aspirin is not suitable.

Posology and method of administration: The tablets should be taken orally.

Adults: The usual dosage is one tablet twice daily with meals (total daily dose (2×250 mg tablets).

Children, infants and neonates: Not indicated.

Use in the elderly: The major clinical trials were conducted in an elderly population with a mean age of 64 years. Although ticlopidine pharmacokinetics are modified in elderly subjects, the pharmacological and therapeutic activity at a dose of 500 mg per day are unaffected by age.

Use in patients with impaired liver function: As ticlopidine is extensively metabolised by the liver, the drug should be used with caution in patients with impaired liver function, and treatment should be discontinued if hepatitis or jaundice develops.

Use in patients with impaired renal function: There is limited experience in patients with renal impairment. In controlled clinical trials, no unexpected problems have been encountered in patients having mild renal impairment, and there is no experience with dosage adjustment in patients with greater degrees of renal impairment. Nevertheless, for renally impaired patients it may be necessary to reduce the dosage of ticlopidine or discontinue it altogether, if haemorrhagic or haematopoietic problems are encountered.

Contra-indications
- Haemorrhagic diathesis
- Organic lesions which are liable to bleed i.e. active gastroduodenal ulcer or haemorrhagic cerebrovascular accident in the acute phase
- Blood disease involving prolonged bleeding time
- History of allergy to ticlopidine or any of the excipients
- History of leucopenia, thrombocytopenia or agranulocytosis.

Special warnings and special precautions for use:

Haematological and haemorrhagic adverse effects can occur. These may be severe and sometimes fatal consequences have been observed (see *Undesirable effects*).

The haemorrhagic adverse effects can be associated with concomitant administration of anticoagulants or antiplatelet agents such as aspirin and non steroidal anti-inflammatory drugs.

IT IS THEREFORE ESSENTIAL TO COMPLY STRICTLY WITH THE FOLLOWING REQUIREMENTS FOR MONITORING BECAUSE OF THE HAEMATOLOGICAL ADVERSE EFFECTS.

Haematological monitoring: Full blood counts (FBCs) with differential and platelet counts should be performed at the start of treatment and then every two weeks for the first three months of therapy. If treatment is stopped during the first three months of therapy, a full blood count should be taken within 2 weeks of discontinuation of Ticlid.

In the event of neutropenia (<1500 neutrophils/mm^3), or thrombocytopenia (<100,000 platelets/mm^3) treatment should be discontinued and FBCs, with differential and platelet counts, should be monitored until they return to normal.

Clinical monitoring: All patients should be carefully monitored for clinical signs and symptoms of adverse drug reactions specially during the first three months of therapy.

The signs and symptoms possibly related to neutropenia (fever, sore throat, ulcerations in the oral cavity), thrombocytopenia and/or abnormal haemostasis (prolonged or unusual bleeding, bruising, purpura, dark stool) and jaundice (including dark urine, light coloured stool) should be explained to the patient.

All patients should be advised to stop medication and consult their physician immediately if any of the above signs or symptoms occur.

The decision to restart treatment should only be taken according to clinical and laboratory findings.

In the event of suspected thrombotic thrombocytopenic purpura, a specialist should be contacted.

Haemostasis: Ticlopidine should not be used in patients who are at increased risk of bleeding.

The drug should not be given in combination with heparins, oral anticoagulants or antiplatelet drugs (see *Contra-indications, Special warnings and special precautions for use* and *Interaction with other medicaments and other forms of interaction*); however, in exceptional cases of concomitant treatment, close clinical and laboratory monitoring is required, and should include bleeding time.

If the patient is to undergo elective surgery, treatment should, wherever possible, be stopped at least ten days before surgery.

In the event of emergency surgery, platelet transfusions may be given to limit the risk of haemorrhage and prolonged bleeding time.

Use in patients with impaired liver function: As ticlopidine is extensively metabolised by the liver, the drug should be used with caution in patients with impaired liver function, and treatment should be discontinued if hepatitis or jaundice develops.

Use in patients with impaired renal function: There is limited experience in patients with renal impairment. In controlled clinical trials, no unexpected problems have been encountered in patients having mild renal impairment, and there is no experience with dosage adjustment in patients with greater degrees of renal impairment. Nevertheless, for renally impaired patients it may be necessary to reduce the dosage of ticlopidine or discontinue it altogether, if haemorrhagic or haematopoietic problems are encountered.

Interaction with other medicaments and other forms of interaction:
Combinations not recommended:
NSAIDs: Increase of haemorrhagic risk (synergy of platelet antiaggregant activity and NSAIDs' effect on the gastro-duodenal mucous membrane). If such drugs are necessary, close clinical and laboratory monitoring (including bleeding time) is required.

Antiplatelet drugs: Increase of haemorrhagic risk (synergy of platelet antiaggregant activity). If such drugs are necessary, close clinical and laboratory monitoring (including bleeding time) is required.

Oral anticoagulants: Increase of haemorrhagic risk (combination of anticoagulant activity and platelet antiaggregant activity). If such drugs are necessary, close clinical and laboratory monitoring (including bleeding time) is required.

Heparins: Increase of haemorrhagic risk (combination of anticoagulant activity and platelet antiaggregant activity). If such drugs are necessary, close clinical and laboratory monitoring (including bleeding time) is required.

Salicylic derivatives (by extrapolation from acetylsalicylic acid [aspirin]): Increase of haemorrhagic risk (synergy of platelet antiaggregant activity and salicylic derivatives' aggressive effect on the gastro-duodenal mucous membrane). If such drugs are necessary, close clinical and laboratory monitoring (including bleeding time) is required.

Combinations requiring special precautions:
Theophylline: Increase of plasma theophylline levels with risk of overdosage (decrease in total plasma theophylline clearance). Clinical monitoring, and if necessary, plasma theophylline levels are required. Theophylline dosage must be adjusted during and after treatment with ticlopidine.

Digoxin: Co-administration of ticlopidine and digoxin leads to a slight decrease (approximately 15%) in plasma digoxin levels. This should not affect the therapeutic efficacy of digoxin.

Phenobarbital: In healthy volunteers, the inhibitory effects of ticlopidine on platelet aggregation are not affected by chronic administration of phenobarbital.

Phenytoin: In vitro studies demonstrated that ticlopidine does not alter the plasma protein binding of phenytoin. However, the protein binding interactions of ticlopidine and its metabolites have not been studied in vivo. Caution should be exercised in co-administering this drug with ticlopidine and it may be useful to remeasure phenytoin blood concentrations.

Other concomitant therapies:
In clinical studies, ticlopidine was given concomitantly with beta-blockers, calcium-channel blockers and diuretics: no clinically significant adverse interactions were reported.

In vitro studies demonstrate that ticlopidine is reversibly bound to plasma proteins (98%) but that it does not interact with plasma protein binding of propranolol, a basic drug which is also highly protein bound.

In very rare instances, lowering of cyclosporin blood concentration has been reported. Therefore, cyclosporin blood concentration should be monitored in case of co-administration.

Pregnancy and lactation: The safety of ticlopidine in pregnant or nursing women has not been established. Studies in rats have shown that ticlopidine is excreted in the milk. Unless absolutely indicated, ticlopidine should not be prescribed to a pregnant or nursing woman.

Studies have shown that high doses of ticlopidine hydrochloride administered to mice (200 mg per kg per day) and maternal toxic doses in rats (400 mg/kg/d) brought about evidence of foetotoxicity (increase in foetal absorption, inhibition of foetal growth, ossification disorders) in both species. In rabbits, maternal toxic doses of 200 mg ticlopidine hydrochloride per kg per day had no effect on the foetus (see *Preclinical safety data*).

Effects on ability to drive and use machines: There is no evidence available which demonstrates that ticlopidine may interfere with the ability to drive or use machines.

Undesirable effects: The incidence rates of adverse effects are derived from two multicentre controlled clinical trials (CATS and TASS) conducted in 2048 TIA/stroke patients.

Haematological: Full blood counts were closely monitored in two large clinical studies conducted in 2048 TIA/stroke patients treated with ticlopidine. A 2.4% incidence of neutropenia was reported, which includes 0.8% of severe neutropenia (<450 neutrophils/mm^3).

In these clinical trials, as in most of the cases from the post-marketing surveillance studies, most cases of severe neutropenia or agranulocytosis (<300 neutrophils/mm^3) developed within the first three months of ticlopidine treatment, and were not typically accompanied by signs of infection or other clinical signs or symptoms (hence the need for FBC monitoring). In such cases, the bone marrow typically showed a decrease in myeloid precursors.

There have been rare reports of bone marrow aplasia and pancytopenia.

Cases of isolated thrombocytopenia (0.4%) have been reported following ticlopidine treatment.

There have been rare reports of thrombotic thrombocytopenic purpura.

Haemorrhagic: Bleeding disorders occurred in 8.3% of the 2048 TIA/stroke patients referred to above. The most frequent were bruising, ecchymosis, epistaxis, haematuria and petechiae. Peri- and postoperative bleedings have been reported (see *Special warnings and special precautions for use*).

Gastro-intestinal: Gastro-intestinal disturbances may occur as a result of treatment with ticlopidine, particularly diarrhoea (12.5%) and nausea (7%). Diarrhoea is generally mild and transient, and occurs mainly during the first 3 months of treatment. These disturbances usually resolve within 1 to 2 weeks without discontinuation of treatment. Very rare cases of severe diarrhoea with colitis have been reported. If the effect is severe and persistent, therapy should be discontinued.

Cutaneous: Ticlopidine has been associated with skin rashes (5%), particularly maculopapular or urticarial, often accompanied by pruritus. In general, skin rashes occur within the first 3 months of treatment, with a mean time to onset of 11 days. If treatment is discontinued, the symptoms disappear within a few days. These skin rashes may be generalised.

Hepatic: There have been rare reports of hepatitis and cholestatic jaundice during the first months of treatment. The course has generally been favourable after treatment was discontinued.

Immunological: Very rare cases of immunological reactions with different manifestations have been reported; e.g. Quincke oedema, vasculitis, lupus syndrome, hypersensitivity nephropathy.

Altered laboratory findings

– Haematological

Neutropenia and rarely, pancytopenia as well as isolated thrombocytopenia or exceptionally accompanied by haemolytic anaemia, have been associated with ticlopidine treatment (see effects reported under *Haematological* previously).

– Hepatic

In some cases ticlopidine treatment has been accompanied by an increase, either isolated or not, of alkaline phosphatase (7.6%), and transaminases (increased SGOT 3.1%) levels during the first months of treatment (incidence greater than twice the upper limit of normal). Ticlopidine treatment has also been accompanied by a minor elevation of bilirubin.

– Cholesterol

Chronic ticlopidine therapy has been associated with increased serum cholesterol and triglyceride levels (9%). Serum HDL-C, LDL-C, VLDL-C and triglyceride levels may increase 8 to 10% after 1 to 4 months of treatment. No further elevations are seen with continued therapy. The ratios of lipoprotein subfractions (especially the ratio of HDL to LDL) remain unchanged. The data in the clinical studies have shown that the effect does not depend on age, sex, alcohol consumption or diabetes and has no influence on the cardiovascular risk.

Overdose: Based on animal studies, overdosage may cause severe gastro-intestinal intolerance. Following overdosage, induced vomiting, gastric lavage and other general supportive measures are recommended.

Pharmacological properties

Pharmacodynamic properties: Ticlopidine is an inhibitor of platelet aggregation. It causes dose-dependent inhibition of platelet aggregation and release of platelet factors, as well as prolongation of bleeding time. The drug has no significant in vitro activity, but only in vivo activity. However, there is no evidence for a circulating active metabolite.

Ticlopidine interferes with platelet aggregation by inhibiting ADP-dependent binding of fibrinogen to the platelet membrane; it does not involve cyclo-oxygenase inhibition, as does aspirin. Platelet cyclic-AMP does not seem to play a role in its mechanism of action.

Bleeding time with 40 mm Hg cuff pressure maintained, as measured by the Ivy method, is prolonged by more than two-fold over baseline values. The uncuffed bleeding time prolongation is less pronounced.

Upon discontinuation of treatment, bleeding time and other platelet function tests return to normal within one week, in the majority of patients.

Inhibition of platelet aggregation is detected within 2 days of administration with ticlopidine 250 mg bid. The maximum antiplatelet effect is obtained after 5 to 8 days treatment of dosing at 250 mg bid.

At therapeutic dose, ticlopidine inhibits ADP-induced (2.5 mmol/l) platelet aggregation by 50 to 70%. Lower doses are associated with less platelet aggregation inhibition.

Pharmacokinetic properties: After oral administration of a single dose of ticlopidine, a rapid absorption occurs, with peak plasma levels occurring at approximately 2 hours after dosing. Absorption is practically complete. Administration of ticlopidine after meals improves bioavailability.

Steady-state plasma levels are obtained after 7 to 10 days of dosing at 250 mg bid. The average terminal elimination half-life of ticlopidine at steady state is approximately 30 to 50 hours. However, the inhibition of platelet aggregation does not correlate with plasma drug levels.

Ticlopidine is extensively metabolised by the liver. Following an oral dose of radio labelled product, 50 to 60% is recovered in the urine and the rest in the faeces.

Preclinical safety data: Acute toxicity studies of ticlopidine hydrochloride after oral administration in the mouse and the rat reported LD_{50} values of 600–850 mg/kg and 1500–1938 mg/kg body weight respectively. In baboons an oral LD_{50} was reported to be above 5 g/kg body weight. Due to the significant emetic effect, an exact value could not be determined for this species. With increasing effective doses, the symptoms leading to death presented as nervous disorders.

Chronic toxicity studies in the rat and baboon showed that the liver was the organ predominantely affected. However, the results of animal experiments (in rats and baboons: gain in liver weight, increased cytochrome P-450 with slight inhibitory effect on its activity; additionally in rats: hypercholesterolaemia, hepatocyte hypertrophy, endoplasmic reticulum proliferation) cannot generally be applied to humans.

This also applies to the results of specific haematotoxicity studies. No appropriate animal model could be found to explain the changes in human blood counts.

Reproductive toxicology studies in rats, mice and rabbits did not show any evidence of a teratogenic effect of ticlopidine. The highest dose administered to mice (200 mg ticlopidine hydrochloride per kg body weight per day) and maternal toxic doses in rats (400 mg/kg/d) brought about evidence of foetotoxicity (increase in foetal absorption, inhibition of foetal growth, ossification disorders) in both species. In rabbits maternal toxic doses of 200 mg ticlopidine hydrochloride per kg/d had no effect on the foetus.

No effects on fertility were observed.

Ticlopidine hydrochloride demonstrated no evidence of mutagenic or carcinogenic potential.

Pharmaceutical particulars

List of excipients: Microcrystalline cellulose, povidone, citric acid anhydrous, maize starch, magnesium stearate, stearic acid, hypromellose, titanium dioxide (E171), macrogol.

Incompatibilities: None known.

Shelf life: 3 years.

Special precautions for storage: Do not store above 25°C. Store in the original package.

Nature and contents of container: Cartons containing 28, 30, 56 or 60 tablets in PVC/aluminium/polyethylene blisters.

Instructions for use/handling: See *Posology and method of administration.*

Marketing authorisation holder: Sanofi Winthrop Limited, One Onslow Street, Guildford, Surrey GU1 4YS.

Marketing authorisation number 11723/0246.

Date of first authorisation/renewal of the authorisation 21 August 1998.

Date of (partial) revision of the text July 1998.

Legal category POM.

TRIFYBA*

Presentation Trifyba is a light brown particulate powder containing 80% of fibre, derived from the husk of wheat (Testa Triticum Tricum). It is presented as single dose sachets each containing 3.5 g.

Uses Colonic and gastro-intestinal disorders where a high-fibre regimen is indicated including simple constipation, uncomplicated diverticular disease, irritable colon, haemorrhoidal disorders and fissures and other conditions where straining at stool should be avoided.

Dosage and administration

Adults: One sachet two to three times daily.

Children: Half to one sachet once or twice daily depending on age and size.

Trifyba should be taken mixed with food or liquids. For maximum effect adequate fluids should be taken.

Contra-indications, warnings, etc Trifyba is contra-indicated in cases of intestinal obstruction. Some patients may experience transient abdominal distention and flatulence, but this rapidly diminishes and usually disappears within two weeks.

Overdosage: Due to the nature of the preparation, overdosage is unlikely. If it does occur, it should be treated conservatively and the patient given copious fluids by mouth.

Pharmaceutical precautions Nil.

Legal category GSL.

Package quantities Cartons containing 56 sachets.

Further information Trifyba is 80% fibre, and therefore represents a highly concentrated source of fibre. It is classified as an insoluble bulk forming laxative acting by retaining water in a cellular network with consequent improvement in colonic function. Trifyba contains clinically insignificant levels of phytic acid and does not interfere with mineral absorption from the gastrointestinal tract. Trifyba is free from sugar and other additives, contains no starch and can be used for diabetics and others on a calorie restricted diet. Trifyba contains negligible amounts of sodium, a factor of importance in the treatment of patients with cardiac or renal disease. Trifyba contains a small amount of gluten.

Product licence number 5287/0001.

Product licence holder: Labaz Ltd.

**Trade Mark*

Sanofi Winthrop Limited
One Onslow Street
Guildford
Surrey GU1 4YS

☎ 01483 505515 🗋 01483 535432

Bristol-Myers Squibb Pharmaceuticals Ltd
Bristol-Myers Squibb House
141–149 Staines Road
Hounslow, Middlesex, TW3 3JA

☎ 0181 572 7422 🗋 0181 754 3789

APROVEL 

Qualitative and quantitative composition Each tablet contains 75 mg, 150 mg or 300 mg irbesartan.

Pharmaceutical form Tablet.

White to off-white, biconvex, and oval-shaped with a heart debossed on one side and the number 2771 (75 mg), 2772 (150 mg) or 2773 (300 mg) engraved on the other side.

Clinical particulars

Therapeutic indication: Treatment of essential hypertension.

Posology and method of administration: The usual recommended initial and maintenance dose is 150 mg once daily, with or without food. Aprovel at a dose of 150 mg once daily generally provides a better 24 hour blood pressure control than 75 mg. However, initiation of therapy with 75 mg could be considered, particularly in haemodialysed patients and in the elderly over 75 years.

In patients insufficiently controlled with 150 mg once daily, the dose of Aprovel can be increased to 300 mg, or other anti-hypertensive agents can be added. In particular, the addition of a diuretic such as hydrochlorothiazide has been shown to have an additive effect with Aprovel. (See *Interactions with other medicaments and other forms of interaction*)

Renal impairment: No dosage adjustment is necessary in patients with impaired renal function. A lower starting dose (75 mg) should be considered for patients undergoing haemodialysis.

Intravascular volume depletion: Volume and/or sodium depletion should be corrected prior to administration of Aprovel.

Hepatic impairment: No dosage adjustment is necessary in patients with mild to moderate hepatic impairment. There is no clinical experience in patients with severe hepatic impairment.

Elderly patients: Although consideration should be given to initiating therapy with 75 mg in patients over 75 years of age, dosage adjustment is not usually necessary for the elderly.

Children: Safety and efficacy of Aprovel have not been established in children.

Contra-indications: Hypersensitivity to any component of the product (see *List of excipients*)

Pregnancy and lactation: (see *Pregnancy and lactation*).

Special warnings and special precautions for use:

Intravascular volume depletion: Symptomatic hypotension, especially after the first dose, may occur in patients who are volume and/or sodium depleted by vigorous diuretic therapy, dietary salt restriction, diarrhoea or vomiting. Such conditions should be corrected before the administration of Aprovel.

Renovascular hypertension: There is an increased risk of severe hypotension and renal insufficiency when patients with bilateral renal artery stenosis or stenosis of the artery to a single functioning kidney are treated with drugs that affect the renin-angiotensin-aldosterone system. While this is not documented with Aprovel, a similar effect should be anticipated with angiotensin II receptor antagonists.

Renal impairment and kidney transplantation: When Aprovel is used in patients with impaired renal function, a periodic monitoring of potassium and creatinine serum levels is recommended. There is no experience regarding the administration of Aprovel in patients with a recent kidney transplantation.

Hyperkalemia: During treatment with other drugs that affect the renin-angiotensin-aldosterone system hyperkalemia may occur, especially in the presence of renal impairment and/or heart failure. While this is not documented with Aprovel, adequate monitoring of serum potassium in patients at risk is recommended (see *Interaction with other medicaments and other forms of interaction*).

Aortic and mitral valve stenosis, obstructive hypertrophic cardiomyopathy: As with other vasodilators, special caution is indicated in patients suffering from aortic or mitral stenosis, or obstructive hypertrophic cardiomyopathy.

Primary aldosteronism: Patients with primary aldosteronism generally will not respond to anti-hypertensive drugs acting through inhibition of the renin-angiotensin system. Therefore, the use of Aprovel is not recommended.

General: In patients whose vascular tone and renal function depend predominantly on the activity of the renin-angiotensin-aldosterone system (e.g. patients with severe congestive heart failure or underlying renal disease, including renal artery stenosis), treatment with other drugs that affect this system has been associated with acute hypotension, azotaemia, oliguria, or rarely acute renal failure. Although the possibility of similar effects cannot be excluded with angiotensin II receptor antagonists, these effects are not documented with Aprovel. As with any antihypertensive agent, excessive blood pressure decrease in patients with ischemic cardiopathy or ischemic cardiovascular disease could result in a myocardial infarction or stroke.

Interactions with other medicinal products and other forms of interaction:

Diuretics and other antihypertensive agents: Other antihypertensive agents may increase the hypotensive effects of irbesartan; however Aprovel has been safely administered with other antihypertensive agents, such as beta-blockers, long-acting calcium channel blockers, and thiazide diuretics. Prior treatment with high dose diuretics may result in volume depletion and a risk of hypotension when initiating therapy with Aprovel (see *Special warnings and special precautions for use*).

Potassium supplements and potassium-sparing diuretics: Based on experience with the use of other drugs that affect the renin-angiotensin system, concomitant use of potassium-sparing diruetics, potassium supplements, salt substitutes containing potassium or other drugs that may increase serum potassium levels (e.g. heparin) may lead to increases in serum potassium (see *Special warnings and special precautions for use*).

Lithium: Reversible increases in serum lithium concentrations and toxicity have been reported during concomitant administration of lithium with angiotensin converting enzyme inhibitors. While this is not documented with Aprovel, the possibility of a similar effect can not be excluded and careful monitoring of serum lithium levels is recommended during concomitant use.

Additional information on drug interactions: The pharmacokinetics of digoxin were not altered by co-administration of a 150 mg dose of irbesartan in healthy male volunteers. The pharmacokinetics of irbesartan are not affected co-administration of hydrochlorothiazide. Irbesartan is mainly metabolised by CYP2C9 and to a lesser extent by glucuronidation. Inhibition of the glucuronyl transferase pathway is unlikely to result in clinically significant interactions. In-vitro interactions were observed between irbesartan and warfarin, tolbutamide (CYP2C9 substrates) and nifedipine (CYP2C9 inhibitor). However, no significant pharmacokinetic or pharmacodynamic interactions were observed when irbesartan was co-administered with warfarin in healthy male volunteers. The pharmacokinetics of irbesartan are not affected by co-administration of nifedipine. The effects of CYP2C9 inducers such as rifampicin on the pharmacokinetics of irbesartan were not evaluated. Based on *in-vitro* data, no interaction would be expected to occur with drugs whose metabolism is dependent upon cytochrome P450 isoenzymes CYP1A1, CYP1A2, CYP2A6, CYP2B6, CYP2D6, CYP2E1 or CYP3A4.

Pregnancy and lactation:

Pregnancy: Aprovel is contra-indicated during pregnancy. Although there is no experience with Aprovel in pregnant women, *in utero* exposure to ACE inhibitors given to pregnant women during the second and third trimesters has been reported to cause injury and death to the developing foetus.

As for any drug that also acts directly on the renin-angiotensin-aldosterone system, Aprovel, should not be used during pregnancy. If pregnancy is detected during therapy, Aprovel should be discontinued as soon as possible (see *Contra-indications*).

Lactation: Aprovel is contraindicated during lactation. It is not known whether irbesartan is excreted in human milk. Irbesartan is excreted in the milk of lactating rats (see *Contra-indications*).

Effects on ability to drive and use machines: The effect of irbesartan on ability to drive and use machines has not been studied, but based on its pharmacodynamic properties, irbesartan is unlikely to affect this ability. When driving vehicles or operating machines, it should be taken into account that occasionally dizziness or weariness may occur during treatment of hypertension.

Undesirable effects: Undesirable effects in patients receiving Aprovel are generally mild and transient. In placebo-controlled trials in patients with hypertension, the overall incidence of adverse events did not differ between the irbesartan and the placebo groups. Discontinuation due to any clinical or laboratory adverse event was less frequent for irbesartan-treated patients than for placebo-treated patients. The incidence of adverse events was not related to dose (in the recommended dose range), gender, age, race, or duration of treatment.

Clinical adverse events, regardless of whether attributed to therapy, occurring in 1% or more of hypertensive patients with Aprovel in placebo-controlled trials are presented in the following table:

	% of Patients	
Adverse Event	*Irbesartan Monotherapy N=1965*	*Placebo N=641*
respiratory infection[a]	18.4	18.6
headache	12.3	16.7*
musculoskeletal pain[b]	7.3	8.4
dizziness	4.9	5.0
fatigue	4.3	3.7
diarrhoea	3.1	2.2
cough	2.8	2.7
nausea/vomiting	2.1	2.8
musculoskeletal trauma	1.9*	0.5
chest pain	1.8	1.7
dyspepsia/heartburn	1.7	1.1
oedema	1.5	2.3
abdominal pain	1.4	2.0
rash	1.3	2.0
tachycardia	1.2	0.9
anxiety/nervousness	1.1	0.9
UTI	1.1	1.4

[a] Includes upper respiratory infection, sinus abnormality, influenza, pharyngitis, and rhinitis.

[b] Includes musculoskeletal pain, musculoskeletal ache, and myalgia.

* Indicates a statistically significant difference between groups ($p < 0.05$).

Adverse events occurred with similar frequency in placebo and irbesartan-treated patients, with the exception of headache, musculoskeletal trauma, and flushing. Headache occurred significantly more often in the placebo group. Musculoskeletal trauma of differing types and causes occurred with a significantly higher incidence in the irbesartan group; all reports of musculoskeletal trauma were considered unrelated to irbesartan by the investigators. Flushing occurred in 0.6% of irbesartan patients and in no placebo patients. The occurrence of flushing was not related to dose, was not accompanied by other clinical events, and the relationship with irbesartan therapy is unknown. In over 5500 subjects exposed to irbesartan in clinical trials, there has been no report of angioedema.

No clinically significant changes in laboratory test parameters occurred in controlled clinical trials. Although significant increases in plasma creatine kinase occurred more frequently in irbesartan-treated subjects (1.7% vs 0.7% in placebo-treated subjects), none of these increases were classified as serious, resulted in drug discontinuation, or were associated with identifiable clinical musculoskeletal events. No special monitoring of laboratory parameters is necessary for patients with essential hypertension receiving therapy with Aprovel, when the renal function is normal (see *Special warnings and special precautions for use*).

Overdose: Experience in adults exposed to doses of up to 900 mg/day for 8 weeks revealed no toxicity. The most likely manifestations of overdosage are expected to be hypotension and tachycardia; bradycardia might also occur from overdose. No specific information is available on the treatment of overdosage with Aprovel. The patient should be closely monitored, and the treatment should be symptomatic and supportive. Suggested measures include induction of emesis and/or gastric lavage. Activated charcoal may be useful in the treatment of overdosage. Irbesartan is not removed by haemodialysis.

Pharmacological properties
Pharmacodynamic properties:
Pharmaco-therapeutic group: Angiotensin II antagonists, ATC code C09C A.

Irbesartan is a potent, orally active, selective angiotensin II receptor (type AT_1) antagonist. It is expected to block all actions of angiotensin II mediated by the AT_1 receptor, regardless of the source or route of synthesis of angiotensin II. The selective antagonism of the angiotensin II (AT_1) receptors results in increases in plasma renin levels and angiotensin II levels, and a decrease in plasma aldosterone concentration. Serum potassium levels are not significantly affected by irbesartan alone at the recommended doses. Irbesartan does not inhibit ACE (kininase II), an enzyme which generates angiotensin II and also degrades bradykinin into inactive metabolites. Irbesartan does not require metabolic activation for its activity.

Irbesartan lowers blood pressure with minimal change in heart rate. The decrease in blood pressure is dose-related for once a day doses with a tendency towards plateau at doses above 300 mg. Doses of 150-300 mg once daily lower supine or seated blood pressures at trough (i.e., 24 hours after dosing) by an average of 8-13/5-8 mm Hg (systolic/diastolic) greater than those associated with placebo.

Peak reduction of blood pressure is achieved within 3-6 hours after administration and the blood pressure lowering effect is maintained for at least 24 hours. At 24 hours the reduction of blood pressure was 60-70% of the corresponding peak diastolic and systolic responses at the recommended doses. Once daily dosing with 150 mg produced trough and mean 24 hour responses similar to twice daily dosing on the same total dose.

The blood pressure lowering effect of Aprovel is evident within 1-2 weeks, with the maximal effect occurring by 4-6 weeks after start of therapy. The antihypertensive effects are maintained during long term therapy. After withdrawal of therapy, blood pressure gradually returns toward baseline. Rebound hypertension has not been observed.

The blood pressure lowering effects of irbesartan and thiazide-type diuretics are additive. In patients not adequately controlled by irbesartan alone, the addition of a low dose of hydrochlorothiazide (12.5 mg) to irbesartan once daily results in a further placebo-adjusted blood pressure reduction at trough of 7-10/3-6 mm Hg (systolic/diastolic).

The efficacy of Aprovel is not influenced by age or gender. As is the case with other drugs that affect the renin-angiotensin system, black hypertensive patients have notably less response to irbesartan monotherapy. When irbesartan is administered concomitantly with a low dose of hydrochlorothiazide (e.g., 12.5 mg daily), the antihypertensive response in black patients approaches that of white patients.

There is no clinically important effect on serum uric acid or urinary uric acid secretion.

Pharmacokinetic properties: After oral administration, irbesartan is well absorbed: studies of absolute bioavailability gave values of approximately 60-80%. Concomitant food intake does not significantly influence the bioavailability of irbesartan.

Plasma protein binding is approximately 90%, with negligible binding to cellular blood components. The volume of distribution is 53-93 litres.

Following oral or intravenous administration of ^{14}C irbesartan, 80-85% of the circulating plasma radioactivity is attributable to unchanged irbesartan. Irbesartan is metabolised by the liver via glucuronide conjugation and oxidation. The major circulating metabolite is irbesartan glucuronide (approximately 6%). *In vitro* studies indicate that irbesartan is primarily oxidised by the cytochrome P450 enzyme CYP2C9; isoenzyme CYP3A4 has negligible effect.

Irbesartan exhibits linear and dose proportional pharmacokinetics over the dose range of 10 to 600 mg. A less than proportional increase in oral absorption at doses beyond 600 mg (twice the maximal recommended dose) was observed; the mechanism for this is unknown. Peak plasma concentrations are attained at 1.5-2 hours after oral administration. The total body and renal clearance are 157-176 and 3-3.5 ml/min, respectively. The terminal elimination half-life of irbesartan is 11-15 hours. Steady-state plasma concentrations are attained within 3 days after initiation of a once-daily dosing regimen. Limited accumulation of irbesartan (<20%) is observed in plasma upon repeated once-daily dosing. In a study, somewhat higher plasma concentrations of irbesartan were observed in female hypertensive patients. However, there was no difference in the half-life and accumulation of irbesartan. No dosage adjustment is necessary in female patients. Irbesartan AUC and C_{max} values were also somewhat greater in elderly subjects (≥65 years) than those of young subjects (18-40 years). However the terminal half-life was not significantly altered. No dosage adjustment is necessary in elderly patients.

Irbesartan and its metabolites are eliminated by both biliary and renal pathways. After either oral or IV administration of ^{14}C irbesartan, about 20% of the radioactivity is recovered in the urine, and the remainder in the faeces. Less than 2% of the dose is excreted in the urine as unchanged irbesartan.

Renal impairment: In patients with renal impairment or those undergoing haemodialysis, the pharmacokinetic parameters of irbesartan are not significantly altered. Irbesartan is not removed by haemodialysis.

Hepatic impairment: In patients with mild to moderate cirrhosis, the pharmacokinetic parameters of irbesartan are not significantly altered. Studies have not been performed in patients with severe hepatic impairment.

Preclinical safety data: There was no evidence of abnormal systemic or target organ toxicity at clinically relevant doses. In preclinical safety studies, high doses of irbesartan (≥250 mg/kg/day in rats and ≥100 mg/kg/day in macaques) caused a reduction of red blood cell parameters (erythrocytes, haemoglobin, haematocrit). At very high doses (≥500 mg/kg/day), degenerative changes in the kidney (such as interstitial nephritis, tubular distension, basophilic tubules, increased plasma concentrations of urea and creatinine) were induced by irbesartan in the rat and the macaque and are considered secondary to the hypotensive effects of the drug which led to decreased renal perfusion. Furthermore, irbesartan induced hyperplasia/hypertrophy of the juxtaglomerular cells (in rats at ≥250 mg/kg/day, in macaques at ≥10 mg/kg/day). All of these changes were considered to be caused by the pharmacological action of irbesartan. For therapeutic doses of irbesartan in humans, the hyperplasia/hypertrophy of the renal juxtaglomerular cells does not appear to have any relevance.

There was no evidence of mutagenicity, clastogenicity or carcinogenicity.

Animal studies with irbesartan showed transient toxic effects (increased renal pelvic cavitation, hydroureter or subcutaneous oedema) in rat foetuses, which were resolved after birth. In rabbits, abortion or early resorption were noted at doses causing significant maternal toxicity, including mortality. No teratogenic effects were observed in the rat or rabbit.

Pharmaceutical particulars
List of excipients: Microcrystalline cellulose, croscarmellose sodium, lactose monohydrate, magnesium stearate, colloidal hydrated silica, pregelatinised maize starch, and poloxamer 188.

Incompatibilities: None

Shelf-life: 24 months

Special precautions for storage: Store in a dry place below 30°C.

Nature and content of container: Aprovel tablets are packaged in blister packs containing 28 tablets in PVC/PVDC/Aluminium strips.

Instructions for use, handling and disposal (if appropriate): None.

Marketing authorisation holder: Sanofi Pharma Bristol-Myers Squibb SNC, 174 Avenue de France, F-75013 Paris, France.

Numbers in the community register of medicinal products

Aprovel 75 mg	EU/1/97/046/001
Aprovel 150 mg	EU/1/97/046/004
Aprovel 300 mg	EU/1/97/046/007

Date of first authorisation/renewal of the authorisation 27 August 1997

Date of revision of the text December 1998

Legal category: POM

PLAVIX ▼

Qualitative and quantitative compostion Clopidogrel hydrogen sulphate 97.875 mg (molar equivalent of 75 mg of clopidogrel base)

Pharmaceutical form Film-coated tablet.

Plavix 75 mg film-coated tablets are pink, round, biconvex, film-coated and engraved with « 75 » on one side.

Clinical particulars
Therapeutic indications: Reduction of atherosclerotic events (myocardial infarction, stroke, death due to vascular causes) in patients with a history of symptomatic atherosclerotic disease defined by ischaemic stroke (from 7 days until less than 6 months), myocardial infarction (from a few days until less than 35 days) or established peripheral arterial disease.

This indication is based on the results of the CAPRIE study comparing clopidogrel with acetyl salicylic acid (ASA). The slight but statistically significant difference of clopidogrel over ASA was mainly related to patients enrolled due to peripheral arterial disease.

For further information please refer to *Special warnings and special precautions for use* and *Pharmacodynamic properties.*

Posology and method of administration:
Adults and elderly: Clopidogrel should be given as a single daily dose of 75 mg with or without food.

Children and adolescents: Safety and efficacy in subjects below the age of 18 have not been established.

Contra-indications: Hypersensitivity to the active substance or any component of the medicinal product.

Severe liver impairment.

Active pathological bleeding such as peptic ulcer or intracranial haemorrhage.

Breast-feeding (see *Pregnancy and lactation*).

Special warnings and special precautions for use: In patients with acute myocardial infarction, clopidogrel therapy should not be initiated within the first few days following myocardial infarction.

In view of the lack of data, clopidogrel can not be recommended in unstable angina, PTCA (stenting), CABG and acute ischaemic stroke (less than 7 days).

As with other anti-platelet agents, clopidogrel should be used with caution in patients who may be at risk of increased bleeding from trauma, surgery or other pathological conditions. If a patient is to undergo elective surgery and an antiplatelet effect is not desired, clopidogrel should be discontinued 7 days prior to surgery.

Clopidogrel prolongs bleeding time and should be used with caution in patients who have lesions with a propensity to bleed (particularly gastrointestinal and intraocular).

Patients should be told that it may take longer than usual to stop bleeding when they take clopidogrel, and that they should report any unusual bleeding to their physician. Patients should inform physicians and dentists that they are taking clopidogrel before any surgery is scheduled and before any new drug is taken.

Therapeutic experience with clopidogrel is limited in patients with renal impairment. Therefore clopidogrel should be used with caution in these patients.

Experience is limited in patients with moderate hepatic disease who may have bleeding diatheses. Clopidogrel should therefore be used with caution in this population.

The concomitant administration of clopidogrel with warfarin is not recommended since it may increase the intensity of bleedings.

In view of the possible increased risk of bleeding, the concomitant administration of clopidogrel with ASA, heparin, or thrombolytics should be undertaken with caution (see *Interaction with other medicinal products and other forms of interaction*).

Drugs that might induce gastrointestinal lesions (such as Non-Steroidal Anti-Inflammatory Drugs) should be used with caution in patients taking clopidogrel (see *Interaction with other medicinal products and other forms of interaction*).

Interaction with other medicinal products and other forms of interaction:
Warfarin: See *Special warnings and special precautions for use.*

Acetylsalicylic acid (ASA): ASA did not modify the clopidogrel-mediated inhibition of ADP-induced platelet aggregation, but clopidogrel potentiated the effect of ASA on collagen-induced platelet aggregation. However, concomitant administration of 500 mg of ASA twice a day for one day did not significantly increase the prolongation of bleeding time induced by clopidogrel intake. The safety of the chronic concomitant administration of ASA and clopidogrel has not been established (see *Special warnings and special precautions for use*).

Heparin: in a clinical study conducted in healthy subjects, clopidogrel did not necessitate modification of the heparin dose or alter the effect of heparin on coagulation. Co-administration of heparin had no effect on the inhibition of platelet aggregation induced by clopidogrel. However, the safety of this combination has not been established and concomitant use should be undertaken with caution (see *Special warnings and special precautions for use*).

Thrombolytics: the safety of the concomitant administration of clopidogrel, rt-PA and heparin was assessed in patients with recent myocardial infarction. The incidence of clinically significant bleeding was similar to that observed when rt-PA and heparin are co-administered with ASA. The safety of the concomitant administration of clopidogrel with other thrombolytic agents has not been established and should be undertaken with caution (see *Special warnings and special precautions for use*).

Non-Steroidal Anti-Inflammatory Drugs (NSAIDs): in a clinical study conducted in healthy volunteers, the concomitant administration of clopidogrel and naproxen increased occult gastrointestinal blood loss. However, due to the lack of interaction studies with other NSAIDs it is presently unclear whether there is an increased risk of gastrointestinal bleeding with all NSAIDs. Consequently, NSAIDs and clopidogrel should be co-administered with caution (see *Special warnings and special precautions for use*).

Other concomitant therapy: a number of other clinical studies have been conducted with clopidogrel and other concomitant medications to investigate the potential for pharmacodynamic and pharmacokinetic interactions. No clinically significant pharmacodynamic interactions were observed when clopidogrel was co-administered with atenolol, nifedipine, or both atenolol and nifedipine. Furthermore, the pharmacodynamic activity of clopidogrel was not significantly influenced by the co-administration of phenobarbital, cimetidine, or oestrogen.

The pharmacokinetics of digoxin or theophylline were not modified by the co-administration of clopidogrel. Antacids did not modify the extent of clopidogrel absorption.

Data from studies with human liver microsomes indicated that the carboxylic acid metabolite of clopidogrel could inhibit the activity of Cytochrome P_{450} 2C9. This could potentially lead to increased plasma levels of drugs such as phenytoin and tolbutamide and the NSAIDs which are metabolised by Cytochrome P_{450} 2C9. Data from the CAPRIE study indicate that phenytoin and tolbutamide can be safely coadministered with clopidogrel.

Pregnancy and lactation:

Pregnancy: Reproduction studies performed in rats and in rabbits revealed no evidence of impaired fertility or harm to the foetus due to clopidogrel. There are, however, no adequate and well-controlled studies in pregnant women. In view of the lack of data, clopidogrel is not recommended during pregnancy.

Lactation: Studies in rats have shown that clopidogrel and/or its metabolites are excreted in the milk. It is not known whether this medicinal product is excreted in human milk (see *Contra-indications*).

Effects on ability to drive and use machines: No impairment of driving or psychometric performance was observed following clopidogrel administration.

Undesirable effects: Clopidogrel has been evaluated for safety in more than 11,300 patients, including over 7,000 patients treated for 1 year or more. Clopidogrel 75 mg/day was well tolerated compared to ASA 325 mg/day in a large controlled clinical trial (CAPRIE). The overall tolerability of clopidogrel in this study was similar to ASA, regardless of age, gender and race. The clinically relevant adverse effects observed in CAPRIE are discussed below.

Haemorrhagic disorders: In patients treated with either clopidogrel or ASA, the overall incidence of any bleeding was 9.3%. The incidence of severe cases was 1.4% for clopidogrel and 1.6% for ASA. In patients that received clopidogrel, gastrointestinal bleeding occurred at a rate of 2.0%, and required hospitalisation in 0.7%. In patients that received ASA, the corresponding rates were 2.7% and 1.1%, respectively.

The incidence of other bleeding was higher in patients that received clopidogrel compared to ASA (7.3% vs. 6.5%). However, the incidence of severe events was similar in both treatment groups (0.6% vs. 0.4%). The most frequently reported events in both treatment groups were: purpura/bruising/haematoma, and epistaxis. Other less frequently reported events were haematoma, haematuria, and eye bleeding (mainly conjunctival).

The incidence of intracranial bleeding was 0.4% in patients that received clopidogrel and 0.5% for patients that received ASA.

Haematological: Severe neutropaenia ($<0.45\times10^9$/l) was observed in 4 patients (0.04%) that received clopidogrel and 2 patients (0.02%) that received ASA. Two of the 9599 patients who received clopidogrel and none of the 9586 patients who received ASA had neutrophil counts of zero. One case of aplastic anaemia occurred on clopidogrel treatment.

The incidence of severe thrombocytopaenia ($<80\times10^9$/l) was 0.2% on clopidogrel and 0.1% on ASA.

Gastrointestinal: The overall, incidence of gastrointestinal events (e.g. abdominal pain, dyspepsia, gastritis and constipation) was significantly lower in patients treated with clopidogrel compared to ASA (27.1% vs. 29.8%). In addition, the number of events resulting in early permanent discontinuation was lower in the clopidogrel group compared to ASA (3.2% vs. 4.0%). However, the incidence of adverse events judged as clinically severe were not statistically different in the groups (3.0% vs. 3.6%). The most frequently reported events in both treatment groups were: abdominal pain, dyspepsia, diarrhoea, and nausea. Other less frequently reported events were constipation, tooth disorder, vomiting, flatulence and gastritis.

Cases of diarrhoea were reported at a significantly higher frequency in patients taking clopidogrel compared to ASA (4.5% vs. 3.4%). The incidence of severe diarrhoea was similar in both treatment groups (0.2% vs. 0.1%). The incidence of peptic, gastric or duodenal ulcers was 0.7% for clopidogrel and 1.2% for ASA.

Skin and appendage disorders: The overall incidence of skin and appendage disorders in patients taking clopidogrel was significantly higher (15.8%) compared to ASA (13.1%). The incidence of severe events was similar in both treatment groups (0.7% vs. 0.5%).

There were significantly more patients with rash in the clopidogrel group compared to the ASA group (4.2% vs. 3.5%). More patients reported pruritus in the clopidogrel group compared to ASA (3.3% vs. 1.6%).

Central and peripheral nervous system disorders: The overall incidence of central and peripheral nervous system disorders (e.g. headache, dizziness, vertigo and paraesthesia) was significantly lower in patients taking clopidogrel compared to ASA (22.3% vs. 23.8%).

Hepatic and biliary disorders: The overall incidence of hepatic and biliary disorders was similar in patients treated with clopidogrel compared to ASA (3.5% vs. 3.4%).

Overdose: One case of deliberate overdosage with clopidogrel has been reported. A 34 year old woman took a single 1,050 mg dose of clopidogrel (equivalent to 14 standard 75 mg tablets). There were no associated undesirable effects. No special therapy was instituted and she recovered without sequelae.

No adverse events were reported after single oral administration of 600 mg (equivalent to 8 standard 75 mg tablets) of clopidogrel to healthy subjects. The bleeding time was prolonged by a factor of 1.7 which is similar to that typically observed with the therapeutic dose of 75 mg per day.

No antidote to the pharmacological activity of clopidogrel has been found. If prompt correction of prolonged bleeding time is required, platelet transfusion may reverse the effects of clopidogrel.

Pharmacological properties

Pharmacodynamic properties: Pharmacotherapeutical group: platelet aggregation inhibitors excl. Heparin, ATC Code: BO1AC/04.

Clopidogrel selectively inhibits the binding of adenosine diphosphate (ADP) to its platelet receptor, and the subsequent ADP-mediated activation of the GPIIb/IIIa complex, thereby inhibiting platelet aggregation. Biotransformation of clopidogrel is necessary to produce inhibition of platelet aggregation. Clopidogrel also inhibits platelet aggregation induced by other agonists by blocking the amplification of platelet activation by released ADP. Clopidogrel acts by irreversibly modifying the platelet ADP receptor. Consequently, platelets exposed to clopidogrel are affected for the remainder of their lifespan and recovery of normal platelet function occurs at a rate consistent with platelet turnover.

Repeated doses of 75 mg per day produced substantial inhibition of ADP-induced platelet aggregation from the first day; this increased progressively and reached steady state between Day 3 and Day 7. At steady state, the average inhibition level observed with a dose of 75 mg per day was between 40% and 60%. Platelet aggregation and bleeding time gradually returned to baseline values, generally within 5 days after treatment was discontinued.

The safety and efficacy of clopidogrel in preventing vascular ischaemic events have been evaluated in a blinded comparison with ASA (CAPRIE, Clopidogrel versus ASA in Patients at Risk of Ischaemic Events). This study included 19,185 patients with atherothrombosis as manifested by recent myocardial infarction (<35 days), recent ischaemic stroke (between 7 days and 6 months) or established peripheral arterial disease (PAD). Patients were randomised to clopidogrel 75 mg/day or ASA 325 mg/day, and were followed for 1 to 3 years. In the myocardial infarction subgroup, most of the patients received ASA for the first few days following the acute myocardial infarction.

Clopidogrel significantly reduced the incidence of new ischaemic events (combined end point of myocardial infarction, ischaemic stroke and vascular death) when compared to ASA. In the intention to treat analysis, 939 events were observed in the clopidogrel group and 1,020 events with ASA (relative risk reduction (RRR) 8.7%, [95% CI: 0.2 to 16.4]; p = 0.045), which corresponds, for every 1000 patients treated for 2 years, to 10 [CI: 0 to 20] additional patients being prevented from experiencing a new ischaemic event. Analysis of total mortality as a secondary endpoint did not show any significant difference between clopidogrel (5.8%) and ASA (6.0%).

In a subgroup analysis by qualifying condition (myocardial infarction, ischaemic stroke, and PAD) the benefit appeared to be strongest (achieving statistical significance at p = 0.003) in patients enrolled due to PAD (especially those who also had a history of myocardial infarction) (RRR = 23.7%; CI: 8.9 to 36.2) and weaker (not significantly different from ASA) in stroke patients (RRR = 7.3%; CI: -5.7 to 18.7). In patients who were enrolled in the trial on the sole basis of a recent myocardial infarction, clopidogrel was numerically inferior, but not statistically different from ASA (RRR = -4.0%; CI: -22.5 to 11.7). In addition, a subgroup analysis by age suggested that the benefit of clopidogrel in patients over 75 years was less than that observed in patients ≤75 years

Since the CAPRIE trial was not powered to evaluate efficacy of individual subgroups, it is not clear whether the differences in relative risk reduction across qualifying conditions are real, or a result of chance.

Pharmacokinetic properties: After repeated oral doses of 75 mg per day, clopidogrel is rapidly absorbed. However, plasma concentrations of the parent compound are very low and below the quantification limit (0.00025 mg/l) beyond 2 hours. Absorption is at least 50%, based on urinary excretion of clopidogrel metabolites.

Clopidogrel is extensively metabolised by the liver and the main metabolite, which is inactive, is the carboxylic acid derivative which represents about 85% of the circulating compound in plasma. Peak plasma levels of this metabolite (approx. 3 mg/l after repeated 75 mg oral doses) occurred approximately 1 hour after dosing.

Clopidogrel is a prodrug. The active metabolite, a thiol derivative, is formed by oxidation of clopidogrel to 2-oxo-clopidogrel and subsequent hydrolysis. The oxidative step is regulated primarily by Cytochrome P_{450} isoenzymes 2B6 and 3A4 and to a lesser extent by 1A1, 1A2 and 2C19. The active thiol metabolite, which has been isolated *in vitro*, binds rapidly and irreversibly to platelet receptors, thus inhibiting platelet aggregation. This metabolite has not been detected in plasma.

The kinetics of the main circulating metabolite were linear (plasma concentrations increased in proportion to dose) in the dose range of 50 to 150 mg of clopidogrel.

Clopidogrel and the main circulating metabolite bind reversibly *in vitro* to human plasma proteins (98% and 94% respectively). The binding is non-saturable *in vitro* over a wide concentration range.

Following an oral dose of ^{14}C-labelled clopidogrel in man, approximately 50% was excreted in the urine and approximately 46% in the faeces in the 120 hour interval after dosing. The elimination half-life of the main circulating metabolite was 8 hours after single and repeated administration.

After repeated doses of 75 mg clopidogrel per day, plasma levels of the main circulating metabolite were lower in subjects with severe renal disease (creatinine clearance from 5 to 15 ml/min) compared to subjects with moderate renal disease (creatinine clearance from 30 to 60 ml/min) and to levels observed in other studies with healthy subjects. Although inhibition of ADP-induced platelet aggregation was lower (25%) than that observed in healthy subjects, the prolongation of bleeding was similar to that seen in healthy subjects receiving 75 mg of clopidogrel per day. In addition, clinical tolerance was good in all patients.

The pharmacokinetics and pharmacodynamics of clopidogrel were assessed in a single and multiple dose study in both healthy subjects and those with cirrhosis (Child-Pugh class A or B). Daily dosing for 10 days with clopidogrel 75 mg/day was safe and well tolerated. Clopidogrel C_{max} for both single dose and steady state for cirrhotics was many fold higher than in normal subjects. However, plasma levels of the main circulating metabolite together with the effect of clopidogrel on ADP-induced platelet aggregation and bleeding time were comparable between these groups.

Preclinical safety data: During preclinical studies in rat and baboon, the most frequently observed effects were liver changes. These occurred at doses representing at least 25 times the exposure seen in humans receiving the clinical dose of 75 mg/day and were a consequence of an effect on hepatic metabolising enzymes. No effect on hepatic metabolising enzymes were observed in humans receiving clopidogrel at the therapeutic dose.

At very high doses, a poor gastric tolerability (gastritis, gastric erosions and/or vomiting) of clopidogrel was also reported in rat and baboon.

There was no evidence of carcinogenic effect when clopidogrel was administered for 78 weeks to mice and 104 weeks to rats when given at doses up to 77 mg/kg per day (representing at least 25 times the exposure seen in humans receiving the clinical dose of 75 mg/day).

Clopidogrel has been tested in a range of *in vitro* and *in vivo* genotoxicity studies, and showed no genotoxic activity.

Clopidogrel was found to have no effect on the fertility of male and female rats and was not teratogenic in either rats or rabbits. When given to lactating rats, clopidogrel caused a slight delay in the development of the offspring. Specific pharmacokinetic studies performed with radiolabelled clopidogrel have shown that the parent compound or its metabolites are excreted in the milk. Consequently, a direct effect (slight toxicity), or an indirect effect (low palatability) cannot be excluded.

Pharmaceutical particulars
List of excipients:
Core: Anhydrous lactose, Modified maize starch, Macrogol 6000, Microcrystalline cellulose, Hydrogenated castor oil.
Coating: Hypromellose, Macrogol 6000, Titanium dioxide (E171), Red iron oxide (E172), Carnauba wax.

Incompatibilities: Not applicable.

Shelf-life: Three years.

Special precautions for storage: No special precautions for storage.

Nature and content of container: 28, 50, and 84, tablets packed in blisters in cardboard cartons.

Instruction for use and handling, and disposal (if appropriate): Not applicable.

Marketing authorisation holder: Sanofi Pharma Bristol-Myers Squibb SNC, 174 Avenue de France, F-75013 Paris, France.

Number(s) in the community register of medicinal products
EU/1/98/069/001 – Cartons of 28 tablets
EU/1/98/069/002 – Cartons of 50 tablets
EU/1/98/069/003 – Cartons of 84 tablets

Date of first authorisation/renewal of the authorisation 15.07.98

Date of revision of the text December 1998.

Legal category POM

**Trade Mark*

Schering Health Care Limited

The Brow
Burgess Hill
West Sussex RH15 9NE

☎ 01444 232323   🗋 01444 246613

SCHERING

ANDROCUR*

Presentation Each round, white, 9 mm tablet is impressed on one side with 'BV' in a regular hexagon, and is scored on the other. It contains 50 mg cyproterone acetate.
Excipients: lactose, maize starch, povidone 25 000, aerosil, magnesium stearate.

Uses Control of libido in severe hypersexuality and/or sexual deviation in the adult male.

Dosage and administration The daily dose should be divided and taken after the morning and evening meals. The usual dose is 1 tablet twice daily.

Contra-indications, warnings, etc
Contra-indications: Liver diseases. Malignant tumours (other than prostatic cancer, for which cyproterone acetate is indicated – see data sheet for Cyprostat®) and wasting diseases (because of transient catabolic action). A history of, or existing, thrombosis or embolism. Severe diabetes with vascular changes. Sickle cell anaemia. Severe chronic depression. Androcur should not be given to youths under 18 or those whose bone maturation and testicular maturation are incomplete.

Warnings/side-effects: Liver: Direct hepatic toxicity, including jaundice, hepatitis and hepatic failure, which has been fatal in some cases, has been reported in patients treated with 200-300 mg cyproterone acetate. Most reported cases are in men with prostatic cancer. Toxicity is dose-related and develops, usually, several months after treatment has begun. Liver function tests should be performed pre-treatment and whenever any symptoms or signs suggestive of hepatotoxicity occur. If hepatotoxicity is confirmed, cyproterone acetate should normally be withdrawn, unless the hepatotoxicity can be explained by another cause, e.g. metastatic disease, in which case cyproterone acetate should be continued only if the perceived benefit outweighs the risk.

As with other sex steroids, benign and malignant liver changes have been reported in isolated cases. Recognised first-line tests of genotoxicity gave negative results when conducted with cyproterone acetate. However, further tests showed that cyproterone acetate was capable of producing adducts with DNA (and an increase in DNA repair activity) in liver cells from rats and monkeys and also in freshly isolated human hepatocytes. This DNA-adduct formation occurred at exposures that might be expected to occur in the recommended dose regimens for cyproterone acetate. One *in vivo* consequence of cyproterone acetate treatment was the increased incidence of focal, possibly preneoplastic, liver lesions in which cellular enzymes were altered in female rats. The clinical relevance of these findings is presently uncertain. Clinical experience to date would not support an increased incidence of hepatic tumours in man.

In very rare cases, liver tumours may lead to life-threatening intra-abdominal haemorrhage. If severe upper abdominal complaints, liver enlargement or signs of intra-abdominal haemorrhage occur, a liver tumour should be considered in the differential diagnosis.

Inhibition of spermatogenesis: The sperm count and the volume of ejaculate are reduced. Infertility is usual, and there may be azoospermia after eight weeks. There is usually slight atrophy of the seminiferous tubules. Follow-up examinations have shown these changes to be reversible, spermatogenesis usually reverting to its previous state about three to five months after stopping Androcur, or, in some users, up to 20 months. That spermatogenesis can recover even after very long treatment is not yet known. There is evidence that abnormal sperms which might give rise to malformed embryos are produced during treatment with Androcur.

Thromboembolism: In extremely rare cases, the occurrence of thromboembolic events has been reported in temporal association with the use of Androcur. However a causal relationship seems to be questionable.

Tiredness: Fatigue and lassitude are common in the first few weeks but become much less from the third month.

Breathlessness: A sensation of shortness of breath may occur under high-dosed treatment with Androcur, owing to the known stimulatory effect of progesterone and synthetic progestogens on breathing, which is accompanied by hypocapnia and compensatory alkalosis, and is not considered to require treatment.

Gynaecomastia: About one in five patients develops transient or perhaps in some cases permanent enlargement of the mammary glands. In rare cases galactorrhoea and tender benign nodules have been reported. Symptoms mostly subside after discontinuation of treatment or reduction of dosage.

Osteoporosis: Rarely cases of osteoporosis have been reported.

Body weight: During long-term treatment, changes in body weight have been reported, chiefly weight gains.

Other changes that have been reported include reduction of sebum production and consequently improvement of existing acne vulgaris, transient patchy loss and reduced growth of body hair, increased growth of scalp hair, lightening of hair colour and female type of pubic hair growth.

Precautions and special information:

Adrenocortical function: During treatment, adrenocortical function should be supervised, since suppression has been observed.

Diabetes: Androcur can influence carbohydrate metabolism. Parameters of carbohydrate metabolism should be examined carefully in all diabetics before and regularly during treatment. The requirement for oral antidiabetics or insulin can change.

Chronic alcoholism: Alcohol appears to reduce the effect of Androcur, which is of no value in chronic alcoholics.

Haemoglobin: Hypochromic anaemia has been found rarely during long-term treatment, and blood counts before and at regular intervals during treatment are advisable.

Nitrogen balance: A negative nitrogen balance is usual at the start of treatment, but usually does not persist.

Spermatogenesis: A spermatogram should be recorded before starting treatment in patients of procreative age, as a guard against attribution of pre-existing infertility to Androcur at a later stage.

It should be noted that the decline in spermatogenesis is slow, and Androcur should, therefore, not be regarded as a male contraceptive.

Medico-legal considerations: Doctors are advised to ensure that the fully informed consent of the patient to Androcur treatment is obtained and can be verified.

Road safety: The marked lassitude and asthenia that may be experienced, particularly during the first few weeks of treatment, necessitate especial care whilst driving.

Overdosage: There have been no reports of ill-effects from overdosage, which it is, therefore, generally unnecessary to treat. If overdosage is discovered within 2 or 3 hours and is so large that treatment seems desirable, gastric lavage can safely be used. There are no specific antidotes, and treatment should be symptomatic.

Pharmaceutical precautions Shelf-life – Five years.

Legal category POM

Package quantities Original packs containing 56 tablets (4 blister strips of 14 tablets).

Further information Cyproterone acetate acts as an antiandrogen by blocking androgen receptors. It also has progestogenic activity which exerts a negative feedback effect on the hypothalamic receptors, so leading to a reduction in gonadotrophin release, and hence to diminished production of testicular androgens.

Product licence number 0053/0023

BETAFERON* ▼

Qualitative and quantitative composition Interferon beta-1b 0.25 mg (8.0 million IU) per ml when reconstituted.

The potency is determined using a cytopathic effect (CPE) bioassay using the WHO recombinant interferon beta reference standard.

Betaferon is formulated to contain 0.3 mg (9.6 million IU) of interferon beta-1b per vial at a calculated overfill of 20 %.

Interferon beta-1b is a purified, sterile, lyophilised protein that has 165 amino acids. It is produced by recombinant DNA techniques from a strain of *Escherichia coli* that bears a genetically engineered plasmid containing a modified human interferon beta$_{ser17}$-gene. Interferon beta-1b differs structurally from natural human interferon beta by the presence of serine instead of cysteine in position 17, lack of methionine in position 1 and absence of carbohydrate moieties.

Pharmaceutical form Sterile lyophilised white to off-white powder for solution for injection.

Clinical particulars
Therapeutic indications: Betaferon is indicated for the reduction of frequency and degree of severity of clinical relapses, in ambulatory patients (i.e. patients who are able to walk unaided) with relapsing, remitting multiple sclerosis, characterised by at least two attacks of neurological dysfunction over the preceding two year period, followed by complete or incomplete recovery.

Patients receiving Betaferon showed a reduction in frequency (30%) and severity of clinical relapses, as well as the number of hospitalisations due to disease. Furthermore, there was a prolongation of the relapse-free interval.

There is no evidence of an effect of Betaferon on the duration of exacerbations, on symptoms in between exacerbations, or of the progression of the disease. There are also no data on the effect of Betaferon on performance of daily activities or in the social field.

Betaferon has not yet been investigated in patients with progressive MS.

There is no evidence of an effect on disability.

The clinical studies show that not all patients respond to treatment with Betaferon. Furthermore a deterioration in the bouts was observed in some of the patients despite the treatment. There are no clinical criteria that would allow prediction with regard to non-response or deterioration in the individual patient to be treated.

Posology and method of administration: The treatment with Betaferon should be initiated under the supervision of a physician experienced in the treatment of the disease.

The recommended dose of Betaferon is 0.25 mg (8.0 million IU), contained in 1 ml of the reconstituted solution (cf. *Instructions for use, handling and disposal* (if appropriate)), to be injected subcutaneously every other day.

The optimal dose has not been fully clarified.

At the present time, it is not known for how long the patient should be treated. Efficacy of treatment for longer than two years has not been sufficiently demonstrated.

Full clinical assessment should be made at two years in all patients.

A decision for longer-term treatment should be made on an individual basis by the treating physician.

Exposure data for longer than three years are not available.

Treatment is not recommended in patients with less than 2 exacerbations in the previous 2 years.

If the patient fails to respond, for example: there is steady progression of disability for six months, or treatment with at least 3 courses of ACTH or corticosteroids during a one year period is required despite Betaferon therapy, treatment with Betaferon should be stopped.

Efficacy and safety of Betaferon were not investigated in children and adolescents of less than 18 years of age. Therefore, Betaferon should not be administered to this age group.

Contra-indications: Betaferon is contra-indicated in the following conditions:

- Pregnancy (see *Use during pregnancy and lactation*).
- Patients with a history of hypersensitivity to natural or recombinant interferon-β or human albumin.

- Patients with a history of severe depressive disorders and/or suicidal ideation.
- Patients with decompensated liver disease.
- Patients with epilepsy not adequately controlled by treatment.

Serious hypersensitivity reactions (rare but severe acute reactions such as bronchospasm, anaphylaxis and urticaria) may occur. If reactions are severe, Betaferon should be discontinued and appropriate medical intervention instituted.

Special warnings and special precautions for use: Patients to be treated with Betaferon should be informed that depressive disorders and suicidal ideation may be a side effect of the treatment and should report these symptoms immediately to the prescribing physician. In rare cases these symptoms may result in a suicide attempt. Patients exhibiting depressive disorders and suicidal ideation should be monitored closely and cessation of therapy should be considered.

Betaferon should be administered with caution to patients with a history of seizures and of depressive disorders and to those receiving treatment with anti-epileptics (see *Interaction with other medicaments and other forms of interaction*). It should also be used with caution in patients with depressive disorders and to those who suffer from pre-existing cardiac disorders.

Serious hypersensitivity reactions (rare but severe acute reactions such as bronchospasm, anaphylaxis and urticaria) may occur. If reactions are severe, Betaferon should be discontinued and appropriate medical intervention instituted. Other moderate to severe adverse experiences may require modifications of the Betaferon dosage regimen or even discontinuation of the agent.

A full blood count and differential WBC should be obtained prior to initiation of Betaferon and regulary during therapy.

SGOT, SGPT and γ-GT levels should be obtained prior to initiation of Betaferon therapy and regularly during therapy. The occurrence of elevations in serum transaminases should lead to close monitoring and investigation with withdrawal of Betaferon if the levels become significantly increasd or if there are associated symptoms suggesting the development of hepatitis. In the absence of clinical evidence for liver damage and after normalisation of liver enzymes a reintroduction of therapy could be considered with appropriate follow-up of hepatic functions.

There are no data on patients with renal impairment. Renal function should be monitored carefully when such patients receive Betaferon therapy.

In the MS studies, 45 % of the patients developed serum interferon beta-1b neutralising activity on at least one occasion. One third had neutralising activity confirmed by at least two consecutive positive titres. This development of neutralising activity is associated with a reduction in clinical efficacy, becoming evident at 18-24 months.

New adverse events have not been associated with the development of neutralising activity. It has been demonstrated *in vitro* that Betaferon cross reacts with natural interferon beta. However, this has not been investigated *in vivo* and its clinical significance is uncertain.

There are sparse and inconclusive data on patients who have developed neutralising activity and have completed Betaferon therapy.

Injection site necrosis (ISN) has been reported in patients using Betaferon (see *Undesirable effects*). It can be extensive and may involve muscle fascia as well as fat and therefore can result in scar formation. Occasionally debridement and, less often, skin grafting are required and healing may take up to 6 months.

If the patient has multiple lesions Betaferon should be discontinued until healing has occurred. Patients with single lesions may continue on Betaferon provided the necrosis is not too extensive, as some patients have experienced healing of injection site necrosis whilst on Betaferon.

To minimise the risk of injection site necrosis patients should be advised to:
- use an aseptic injection technique
- rotate the injection sites with each dose.

The procedure for the self-administration by the patient should be reviewed periodically especially if injection site reactions have occurred.

Caution should be exercised when administering Betaferon to patients with myelosuppression, anaemia or thrombocytopenia; patients who develop neutropenia should be monitored closely for the development of fever or infection.

Interaction with other medicaments and other forms of interaction: No formal drug interaction studies have been carried out with Betaferon.

The effect of alternate-day administration of 0.25 mg (8.0 million IU) of Betaferon on drug metabolism in MS patients is unknown. Corticosteroid or ACTH treatment of relapses for periods of up to 28 days has been well tolerated in patients receiving Betaferon.

Due to the lack of clinical experience in MS patients use of Betaferon together with immunomodulators other than corticoids or ACTH, is not recommended.

Interferons have been reported to reduce the activity of hepatic cytochrome P450-dependent enzymes in humans and animals. Caution should be exercised when Betaferon is administered in combination with medicinal products that have a narrow therapeutic index and are largely dependent on the hepatic cytochrome P450 system for clearance, e.g. anti-epileptics.

No interaction studies with anti-epileptics have been carried out. Additional caution should be exercised with any co-medication which has an effect on the haematopoietic system.

Pregnancy and lactation: It is not known whether Betaferon can cause fetal harm when administered to a pregnant woman or can affect human reproductive capacity. Spontaneous abortions have been reported in subjects with MS in controlled clinical trials. Recombinant human interferon beta-1b in studies with rhesus monkeys has been proven embryotoxic, causing fetal death in the higher dose range. Therefore, Betaferon is contraindicated during pregnancy and women of childbearing potential should take appropriate contraceptive measures. If the patient becomes pregnant or plans to become pregnant while taking Betaferon, she should be informed of the potential hazards and it should be recommended to discontinue therapy (for preclinical results refer to section *Preclinical safety data*).

It is not known whether interferon beta-1b is excreted in human milk. Because of the potential for serious adverse reactions to Betaferon in nursing infants a decision should be made whether nursing or Betaferon should be discontinued.

Effects on ability to drive and use machines: This has not been investigated.

Central nervous system-related adverse events associated with the use of Betaferon might influence the ability to drive and use machines in susceptible patients.

Undesirable effects: Experience with Betaferon in patients with MS is limited, consequently adverse events with low incidence may not yet have been observed.

Injection site reactions occurred frequently after administration of Betaferon. Redness, swelling, discoloration, inflammation, pain, hypersensitivity, necrosis, and non-specific reactions were significantly associated with 0.25 mg (8.0 million IU) Betaferon treatment. The incidence rate of injection site reactions usually decreased over time.

If the patient experiences any break in the skin, which may be associated with swelling or drainage of fluid from the injection site, the patient should be advised to consult with their physician before continuing injections with Betaferon (see *Special warnings and special precautions for use*).

At the recommended dose, elevations in SGOT, SGPT and γ-GT may occur and there are reports of possible drug-induced hepatitis (see *Special warnings and special precautions for use*).

Leucopenia (lymphopenia, neutropenia) and anaemia have been reported. There have been reports of thrombocytopenia, with profound decreases in platelet count in rare cases.

Low calcium and high uric acid have appeared to be associated with Betaferon administration.

Flu-like symptom complex (fever, chills, myalgia, malaise, or sweating) has been seen frequently. The incidence rate of the symptoms decreased over time.

Serious hypersensitivity reactions (rare but severe acute reactions such as bronchospasm, anaphylaxis and urticaria) may occur. If reactions are severe, Betaferon should be discontinued and appropriate medical intervention instituted.

Menstrual disorders may occur in premenopausal females.

Occasionally, nausea and vomiting may occur.

Alopecia has been reported in rare cases.

Central nervous system (CNS) related adverse events including depression, anxiety, emotional lability, depersonalisation, convulsions, suicide attempts, and confusion have been observed.

Overdose: Interferon beta-1b has been given without serious adverse events compromising vital functions to adult cancer patients at individual doses as high as 5.5 mg (176 million IU) i.v. three times a week.

Pharmacological properties

Pharmacodynamic properties: Pharmacotherapeutic group: Cytokines ATC Code L03 AA.

Interferons belong to the family of cytokines, which are naturally occurring proteins. Interferons have molecular weights ranging from 15,000 to 21,000 daltons. Three major classes of interferons have been identified: alpha, beta, and gamma. Interferon alpha, interferon beta, and interferon gamma have overlapping yet distinct biologic activities. The activities of interferon beta-1b are species-restricted and therefore, the most pertinent pharmacologic information on interferon beta-1b is derived from studies of human cells in culture or in human in vivo studies.

Interferon beta-1b has been shown to possess both antiviral and immunoregulatory activities. The mechanisms by which interferon beta-1b exerts its actions in multiple sclerosis (MS) are not clearly understood. However, it is known that the biologic response-modifying properties of interferon beta-1b are mediated through its interactions with specific cell receptors found on the surface of human cells. The binding of interferon beta-1b to these receptors induces the expression of a number of gene products that are believed to be the mediators of the biological actions of interferon beta-1b. A number of these products have been measured in the serum and cellular fractions of blood collected from patients treated with interferon beta-1b. Interferon beta-1b both decreases the binding affinity and enhances the internalisation and degradation of the interferon-γ receptor. Interferon beta-1b also enhances the suppressor activity of peripheral blood mononuclear cells.

No separate investigations were performed regarding the influence of Betaferon on the cardiovascular system, respiratory system and the function of endocrine organs.

Pharmacokinetic properties: Betaferon serum levels were followed in patients and volunteers by means of a not completely specific bioassay. Maximum serum levels of about 40 IU/ml were found 1–8 hours after subcutaneous injection of 0.5 mg (16.0 million IU) interferon beta-1b. From various studies mean clearance rates and half-lives of disposition phases from serum were estimated to be at most 30 $ml \cdot min^{-1} \cdot kg^{-1}$ and 5 hours, respectively. Every other day Betaferon injections do not lead to serum level increases and pharmacokinetics do not seem to change during therapy.

The absolute bioavailability of subcutaneously administered interferon beta-1b was approximately 50%.

Preclinical safety data: No acute toxicity studies have been carried out. As rodents do not react to human interferon beta, repeated dose studies were carried out with rhesus monkeys. Transitory hyperthermia was observed, as well as a significant rise in lymphocytes and a significant decrease in thrombocytes and segmented neutrophils. No long-term studies have been conducted. Reproduction studies with rhesus monkeys revealed maternal and foetal toxicity, resulting in prenatal mortality. No malformations have been observed in the surviving animals. No investigations on fertility have been conducted. No influence on the monkey oestrous cycle has been observed. Experience with other interferons suggests a potential for impairment of male and female fertility.

In one single genotoxicity study (Ames test), no mutagenic effect has been observed. Carcinogenicity studies have not been performed. An in vitro cell transformation test gave no indication of tumorigenic potential. Local tolerance studies after subcutaneous administration were negative. However, in clinical studies local reactions have been observed following use of Betaferon.

Pharmaceutical particulars

List of excipients: Human albumin PhEur; Dextrose PhEur.

Incompatibilities: None known.

Shelf life: Of the product as packaged for sale: 18 months at 2-8 °C, starting from the date of sterile filtration of the formulated bulk solution. After reconstitution according to directions: up to 3 hours at 2 - 8 °C.

Special precautions for storage: Store at 2 - 8 °C before and after reconstitution.

Nature and contents of container: 3 ml clear glass vial with a 13 mm butyl rubber stopper and aluminium overseal.

Each Betaferon vial is provided with a separate solvent vial containing 2 ml sterile sodium chloride solution (0.54% w/v). The solvent is contained in a 3 ml vial with a 13 mm butyl rubber stopper and aluminium overseal.

Each pack of Betaferon contains either 5 or 15 vials of interferon beta-1b and either 5 or 15 vials of 0.54% sodium chloride solution.

Instructions for use/handling: To reconstitute lyophilised interferon beta-1b for injection, use a sterile syringe and needle to inject 1.2 ml of the supplied solvent (sodium chloride solution, 0.54 % w/v) into the Betaferon vial. Dissolve the powder completely without shaking. Inspect the reconstituted product visually before use. Discard the product before use if it contains particulate matter or is discoloured. The reconstituted solution contains 0.25 mg (8.0 million IU) of interferon beta-1b per ml.

Store all medicinal products properly and keep them out of reach of children.

Marketing authorisation holder: Schering Aktiengesellschaft, D-13342 Berlin

Marketing authorisation numbers EU/1/95/003/001, EU/1/95/003/002

Date of approval/revision of SPC 22 October 1997

Legal category POM

BILISCOPIN* 50 INFUSION

Qualitative and quantitative composition 1 ml Biliscopin contains 105 mg meglumine iotroxate.

Pharmaceutical form Solution for intravenous infusion.

Clinical particulars

Therapeutic indications: Infusion cholecystangiography (infusion cholegraphy).

Intravenous cholegraphy should be performed as the first examination only when there is strong evidence of disease involving the biliary tract. In all other cases for diagnosis – especially in obscure upper abdominal complaints – oral cholegraphy is to be preferred.

Posology and method of administration: The patient should be recumbent during the administration of Biliscopin and kept under close observation for at least 30 minutes (see *Special warnings and special precautions for use*).

Experience shows that contrast medium is tolerated better if it is warmed to body temperature.

Adults: One 100 ml bottle of Biliscopin to be administered by intravenous infusion in not less than 15 minutes. The infusion should always be started at the low rate and increased to the final higher rate after three to five minutes. This technique reduces heterotopic excretion and improves the tolerance.

Children: Because of insufficient experience in the use of Biliscopin in children, optimal paediatric dosages have not been established.

Contra-indications: Severe cardiovascular insufficiency, particularly right ventricular failure or cardiac decompensation. Proven or suspected hypersensitivity to iodine-containing contrast media. Manifest hyperthyroidism. Severe functional disturbance of the liver or kidneys. Monoclonal IgM gammopathy, e.g. macroglobulinaemia (Waldenström's disease).

Special warnings and special precautions for use: For patients with severe impairment of hepatic or renal function, cerebral arteriosclerosis, epileptic conditions, diabetes mellitus requiring drug treatment and/or associated with diabetic complications, pulmonary emphysema, poor general health, latent hyperthyroidism, multiple myeloma or benign nodular goitre the need for examination with X-ray contrast media merits careful consideration. This also applies to patients with a history of allergy, atopy, bronchial asthma, endogenous eczema, cardiac or circulatory insufficiency or a previous adverse reaction with any contrast medium since experience shows that they may be at higher risk from developing anaphylaxis or cardiovascular collapse. Pre-testing does not give a reliable warning of allergic reactions to iodine-containing contrast media.

The patient should be recumbent during the administration of Biliscopin. Thereafter, the patient must be kept under close observation for at least 30 minutes, since about 90% of all severe incidents occur within that time. The patient must not be left unsupervised until the end of the examination. If the administration does not take place on the X-ray table, any patient with a labile circulation should be brought to the X-ray machine sitting or lying down.

Thyroid hyperfunction can increase for some time after the administration of biliary contrast media.

If iodine isotopes are to be administered for the diagnosis of thyroid disease, it should be borne in mind that the capacity of the thyroid tissue to take up iodine will be reduced for eight to ten weeks or more by iodinated biliary contrast media.

Some investigators have reported temporary and reversible changes in liver-function tests after Biliscopin. These changes are not thought to reflect liver damage.

The opinion has been expressed that intravenous infusion cholegraphy should not be performed immediately after negative oral cholegraphy. A large number of radiologists do not share this view – provided that the patient is adequately hydrated and renal function is not impaired.

Particular caution should be exercised in allergic patients who have previously tolerated injectable iodine-containing contrast media without any complication, since they may have become sensitised to these substances. Some radiologists give an antihistamine or a corticoid prophylactically to patients with a history of allergy. As with any contrast medium, the possibility of hypersensitivity must always be considered. If marked side-effects or suspected allergic reactions occur during infusion or injection and persist or even worsen when the administration is interrupted, it is probable that the patient has such a hypersensitivity. Therefore, the investigation must be abandoned. The needle or cannula should be left in the vein for some time in order to maintain access for intravenous therapy. Even relatively minor symptoms, such as itching of the skin, sneezing, violent yawns, tickling in the throat, hoarseness or attacks of coughing may be early signs of a severe reaction and, therefore, merit careful attention.

Interaction with other medicaments and other forms of interaction: Diabetic nephropathy may predispose to renal impairment following intravascular administration of contrast media. This may precipitate lactic acidosis in patients who are taking biguanides. As a precaution biguanides should be stopped 48 hours prior to the contrast medium examination and reinstated only after adequate renal function has been regained.

Hypersensitivity reactions can be aggravated in patients on beta-blockers.

The prevalence of delayed reactions (e.g. fever, rash, flu-like symptoms, joint pain and pruritus) to contrast media is higher in patients who have received interleukin.

Pregnancy and lactation: X-ray examinations should, if possible, be avoided during pregnancy. It has not yet been proved beyond question that Biliscopin may be used without hesitation in pregnant patients. Therefore an examination with a contrast medium during pregnancy should be carried out only if considered absolutely necessary by the physician.

It is not known whether Biliscopin enters the breast milk.

Effects on ability to drive and use machines: Delayed reactions following intravascular administration of iodinated contrast media are rare. Nevertheless, driving or operating machinery is not advisable for the first 24 hours

Undesirable effects: Side effects in association with the use of Biliscopin are usually mild to moderate and temporary.

Nausea, vomiting, erythema, a sensation of pain and a general feeling of warmth are the most frequently recorded reactions on intravascular administration. Such reactions are rare if the recommended rate of administration is adhered to. If they do occur, they can usually be ameliorated quite rapidly by reducing the rate of administration still further or by allowing a brief pause in the procedure. Particularly in patients with (manifest or subclinical) cardiovascular insufficiency or poor general health too rapid an administration may even lead to life-threatening reactions.

Other symptoms which may occur are:

Chills, fever, sweating, headache, dizziness, blanching, weakness, gagging and a feeling of suffocation, gasping, a rise or fall of blood pressure, itching, urticaria, other kinds of skin eruption, oedema, tremor, sneezing and lacrimation. These reactions, which can occur irrespective of the amount administered and the mode of administration, may be the first signs of an incipient state of shock. Administration of the contrast medium must be discontinued immediately and – if necessary – specific therapy instituted intravenously. It is therefore advisable to use a flexible indwelling cannula for the administration of the contrast medium.

Very rarely, severe or even life-threatening incidents, such as severe hypotension and collapse, circulatory failure, ventricular fibrillation, cardiac arrest, pulmonary oedema, anaphylactic shock or other allergic manifestations, convulsions or other cerebral symptoms may occur. In some cases these have proved fatal.

To permit immediate countermeasures to be taken in emergencies, appropriate drugs, an endotracheal tube and a ventilator should be ready to hand.

Experience shows that hypersensitivity reactions occur more frequently in patients with an allergic disposition.

Temporary renal failure may occur in rare cases especially where risk factors exist e.g. patients with: diabetes mellitus, pre-existing renal insufficiency or multiple myeloma; elderly patients or patients receiving large or repeated doses.

In very rare cases also neurological complications such as coma, transient somnolence and convulsions have been described.

Delayed reactions can occasionally occur.

Inadvertent paravenous administration of Biliscopin can cause pain but rarely leads to severe tissue reactions.

Overdose: Since Biliscopin is to be administered intravenously and the recommended dose in adults is equivalent to the pack size, overdosage is unlikely.

Pharmacological properties

Pharmacodynamic properties: Biliscopin, a biliary, iodinated contrast medium, is secreted actively by the hepatocyte. Because of its high hepatocellular transport rate, it leads rapidly to high-grade contrast density in the intra-hepatic and extra-hepatic biliary ducts as well as in the gallbladder. Only when the maximum transport capacity of the liver is exceeded does any appreciable renal elimination occur.

The biliary excretion rate of a contrast medium is determined by the binding to plasma proteins and liver receptor proteins, and also by its transport maximum for the liver, which is particularly high in the case of Biliscopin. In this respect, the biliary contrast media compete with bilirubin and, if present, with drugs as well. For example, biliary elimination of the biliary contrast medium is reduced by an elevated serum bilirubin concentration and/or by liver insufficiency, while heterotopic elimination via the kidney increases simultaneously.

Pharmacokinetic properties: Following intravenous injection, 60 to 90% of the iotroxic acid administered is bound to proteins, depending on the plasma concentration.

At a dose of 70 mg iodine/kg body weight, the mean half-life is about 80 minutes when measured from 30 minutes to 6 hours after the injection. The half-life is prolonged in impaired liver function.

The maximum biliary transport rate for iotroxic acid is 0.35 mg iodine/kg body weight/min in subjects with healthy livers. It is apparently achieved after injection of 30 ml Biliscopin (=5.4 g iodine), is maintained for about 2 hours and does not increase any further under a higher dose. In patients with a post-operative T-drain the maximum iodine concentration in the bile has been shown to be 16±4 mg/ml.

The heterotopic elimination following injection of 30 ml Biliscopin (=5.4 g iodine) within 5 minutes is about 10% of the dose. It increases with more rapid administration, with a higher dose and in the presence of impaired liver function, but can be reduced by slower injection and, in particular, by infusion.

Iotroxic acid is metabolized to only a slight extent by man and animals. Most of the metabolites which do occur are excreted in the urine.

Preclinical safety data: There are no pre-clinical safety data which could be of relevance to the prescriber and which are not already included in other relevant sections of the SPC.

Pharmaceutical particulars

List of excipients: Sodium chloride, Sodium calcium edetate, Sodium hydrogen carbonate, Water for injection

Incompatibilities: Some radiologists give an antihistamine or a corticoid prophylactically to patients with a history of allergy. Because of the possibility of precipitation, contrast medium and prophylactic agents must not be administered mixed together.

Shelf life: Five years

Special precautions for storage: Protect from light, and secondary X-rays.

Nature and contents of container: Clear glass infusion bottles containing 100 ml of Biliscopin.

Available in packs of 10 x 100 ml bottles.

Instructions for use/handling: The infusion bottle should not be attached to the infusion set until immediately before the examination.

Contrast medium solution not used in one examination session must be discarded.

Marketing authorisation number 0053/0110

Date of first authorisation/renewal of authorisation 21st September 1991

Date of approval/revision of the text 9 July 1997

BILOPTIN*

Qualitative and quantitative composition Each capsule contains 500 mg of sodium iopodate.

Pharmaceutical form Capsules

Clinical particulars

Therapeutic indications: Oral contrast medium for cholecystography and cholangiography.

Posology and method of administration: Preparing the patients:

(i) On the day before the X-ray examination patients should be put on a diet of light meals, free from fats and from all foods that tend to cause wind. Tea or coffee (without milk), fruit juice or squash, clear fat-free soup, white bread, lean meat or fish grilled or baked without added fat or oil may be eaten. NONE of the following are allowed: fried food, eggs, fruit, oatmeal, pasta, milk or milk products including butter, margarine, cheese, ice-cream and salad dressings, all vegetables, smoked food or wholemeal or freshly baked bread.

(ii) From 6 p.m on the day before the examination, patients should refrain from eating until after the examination the following day. Tea or coffee (without milk), fruit juice or squash is allowed. Smoking should also be avoided.

(iii) Biloptin capsules should be swallowed whole with a glassful of cold water or squash.

For oral administration in the following dosages:

Routine cholecystography: Biloptin should be taken after the last meal on the evening before examination. Adults and elderly: 6 capsules.

Other examination techniques in adults only

Rapid cholecystography: Six capsules or double dose of twelve capsules.

Cholangiography: Twelve capsules.

Fractionated oral cholecystography: Six capsules 10-12 hours before the examination and another six capsules 3 hours before the examination.

Contra-indications: Manifest hyperthyroidism. Severe impairment of hepatic or renal function.

Special warnings and special precautions for use: Proven or suspected hypersensitivity to iodine-containing contrast media, latent hyperthyroidism and benign nodular goitre.

Interaction with other medicaments and other forms of interaction: If iodine isotopes are to be administered for diagnosing thyroid disease, it should be borne in mind that the capacity of the thyroid tissue to take up iodine will be reduced for 8-10 weeks or more by iodinated biliary X-ray contrast media.

Hypersensitivity reactions can be aggravated in patients on beta-blockers.

The prevalence of delayed reactions (e. g. fever, rash, flulike symptoms, joint pain and pruritus) to contrast media is higher in patients who have received interleukin.

Pregnancy and lactation: Apart from the fact that X-ray examinations should, if possible, be avoided during pregnancy, it must be pointed out that it has not yet been proved beyond question that Biloptin may be used without hesitation in pregnant patients. Therefore, such an examination with a contrast medium during pregnancy should be carried out only if considered absolutely necessary by the physician.

It is not known whether Biloptin enters the breast milk.

Effects on ability to drive and use machines: None stated.

Undesirable effects: Biloptin is well tolerated and side-effects even of a trivial nature, are extraordinarily rare. Sensitive patients may occasionally complain of mild sensations of pressure in the stomach or nausea. Attacks of diarrhoea and vomiting are exceptional. Very few cases of urticaria have been observed. Anaphylactoid reactions ranging to shock are possible. Thyroid hyperfunction can increase for some time after the examination with biliary contrast media.

Overdose: There have been no reports of ill-effects from overdosage and treatment is generally unnecessary. There are no specific antidotes, and further treatment should be symptomatic.

Pharmacological properties

Pharmacodynamic properties: Sodium iopodate is given by mouth as a cholecystographic contrast medium. Following absorption from the gastrointestinal tract, it appears in the bile where the concentration is such that the biliary tract can be examined radiographically.

Pharmacokinetic properties: Sodium iopodate is absorbed from the gastrointestinal tract and maximum concentrations are found in the gall-bladder about 10 hours after ingestion. It is excreted mainly in the urine.

Preclinical safety data: None stated.

Pharmaceutical particulars

List of excipients: Other constituents: Peanut oil (arachis oil), butyl hydroxytoluene, soya lecithin, disodium edetate. Capsule shell: Karion 83, glycerin 85%, gelatin, methylhydroxybenzoate, propylhydroxybenzoate, titanium dioxide (E171), iron oxide, yellow (E172) purified water.

Incompatibilities: None

Shelf life: 3 years.

Special precautions for storage: Store below 30°C. Protect from light and secondary X-rays.

Nature and contents of container: Aluminium blister packs contained within a cardboard outer. Available in packs of 120 capsules.

Instructions for use/handling: None

Marketing authorisation number 0053/5048R

Date of approval/revision of SPC 5 February 1997

Legal category P

CYPROSTAT* 50 mg

Qualitative and quantitative composition Each white, scored tablet contains 50 mg cyproterone acetate.

Pharmaceutical form Tablets.

Clinical particulars

Therapeutic indications: Management of patients with prostatic cancer (1) to suppress 'flare' with initial LHRH analogue therapy, (2) in long-term palliative treatment where LHRH analogues or surgery are contra-indicated, not tolerated, or where oral therapy is preferred, and (3) in the treatment of hot flushes in patients under treatment with LHRH analogues or who have had orchidectomy.

Posology and method of administration:

Adults including the elderly: Dosage for suppression of 'flare' with initial LHRH analogue therapy is 300 mg/day, which may be reduced to 200 mg if the higher dose is not tolerated. For long-term palliative treatment where LHRH analogues or surgery are contra-indicated, not tolerated, or where oral therapy is preferred the dosage is 200–300 mg/day.

For the above two indications the dosage should be divided into 2–3 doses per day and taken after meals.

For the treatment of hot flushes in patients under treatment with LHRH analogues or who have had orchidectomy a 50 mg starting dose, with upward titration if necessary within the range 50–150 mg/day, is recommended. For this indication the dosage should be divided into 1–3 doses per day and taken after meals.

All doses should be taken orally.

Children: Not recommended.

Contra-indications: None.

Special warnings and special precautions for use:

Liver: Direct hepatic toxicity, including jaundice, hepatitis and hepatic failure, which has been fatal in some cases, has been reported in patients treated with 200–300 mg cyproterone acetate. Most reported cases are in men with prostatic cancer. Toxicity is dose-related and develops, usually, several months after treatment has begun. Liver function tests should be performed pre-treatment and whenever any symptoms or signs suggestive of hepatotoxicity occur. If hepatotoxicity is confirmed, cyproterone acetate should normally be withdrawn, unless the hepatotoxicity can be explained by another cause, e.g. metastatic disease, in which case cyproterone acetate should be continued only if the perceived benefit outweighs the risk.

As with other sex steroids, benign and malignant liver changes have been reported in isolated cases.

In very rare cases, liver tumours may lead to life-threatening intra-abdominal haemorrhage. If severe upper abdominal complaints, liver enlargement or signs of intra-abdominal haemorrhage occur, a liver tumour should be considered in the differential diagnosis.

Thromboembolism: Patients with a history of thrombosis may be at risk of recurrence of the disease during Cyprostat therapy.

In patients with a history of thromboembolic processes or suffering from sickle-cell anaemia or severe diabetes with vascular changes, the risk: benefit ratio must be considered carefully in each individual case before Cyprostat is prescribed.

In extremely rare cases, the occurrence of thromboembolic events has been reported in temporal association with the use of Cyprostat. However a causal relationship seems to be questionable.

Chronic depression: It has been found that some patients with severe chronic depression deteriorate whilst taking Cyprostat therapy.

Breathlessness: Shortness of breath may occur. This may be due to the stimulatory effect of progesterone and synthetic progestogens on breathing, which is accompanied by hypocapnia and compensatory alkalosis, and which is not considered to require treatment.

Adrenocortical function: During treatment adrenocortical function should be supervised, since suppression has been observed in children taking cyproterone acetate.

Diabetes: Cyprostat can influence carbohydrate metabolism. Parameters of carbohydrate metabolism should be examined carefully in all diabetics before and regularly during treatment.

Haemoglobin: Hypochromic anaemia has been found rarely during long-term treatment, and blood-counts before and at regular intervals during treatment are advisable.

Nitrogen balance: A negative balance is usual at the start of treatment, but does not persist.

Interaction with other medicaments and other forms of interaction: The requirement for oral antidiabetics or insulin can change.

Pregnancy and lactation: Not applicable.

Effects on ability to drive and use machines: Fatigue and lassitude are common in the first few weeks of therapy but usually become much less from the third month. The marked lassitude and asthenia necessitate especial care when driving or operating machinery.

Undesirable effects:

Inhibition of spermatogenesis: The sperm count and the volume of ejaculate are reduced. Infertility is usual, and there may be azoospermia after 8 weeks. There is usually slight atrophy of seminiferous tubules. Follow-up examinations have shown these changes to be reversible, spermatogenesis usually reverting to its previous state about 3-5 months after stopping Cyprostat, or in some users, up to 20 months. That spermatogenesis can recover even after very long treatment is not yet known. There is evidence that abnormal sperms which might give rise to malformed embryos are produced during treatment with Cyprostat.

Gynaecomastia: Transient, and perhaps in some cases permanent, enlargement of the mammary glands has been reported. In rare cases, galactorrhoea and tender benign nodules have been reported. Symptoms generally subside after discontinuation of treatment or on reduction of dosage, but this should be weighed against the risk from the tumour of using inadequate doses.

Bodyweight: During long-term treatment, changes in bodyweight have been reported. Both increases and decreases have been seen.

Osteoporosis: Rarely cases of osteoporosis have been reported.

Other changes that have been reported include reduction of sebum production leading to dryness of the skin, transient patchy loss and reduced growth of body hair, increased growth of scalp hair, lightening of hair colour and female type of pubic hair growth.

Overdose: There have been no reports of ill-effects of overdosage, which it is, therefore, generally unnecessary to treat. There are no specific antidotes, and treatment should be symptomatic.

Pharmacological particulars

Pharmacodynamic properties: Prostatic carcinoma and its metastases are in general androgen-dependent. Cyproterone acetate exerts a direct anti-androgen action on the tumour and its metastases and in addition it exerts a negative feedback effect on the hypothalamic receptors so leading to a reduction in gonadotrophin release and hence to diminished production of testicular androgens. Cyprostat may be used alone, or in conjunction with surgery or LHRH analogues.

Pharmacokinetic properties: Following oral administration, cyproterone acetate is completely absorbed over a wide dose range. The ingestion of two 50 mg of cyproterone acetate gives maximum serum levels of about 285 ng/ml at about 3 hours. Thereafter, drug serum levels declined during a time interval of typically 24 to 120 h, with a terminal half-life of 43.9 ± 12.8 h. The total clearance of cyproterone acetate from serum is 3.5 ± 1.5 ml/min/kg. Cyproterone acetate is metabolised by various pathways, including hydroxylations and conjugations. The main metabolite in human plasma is the 15β-hydroxy derivative.

Some drug is excreted unchanged with bile fluid. Most of the dose is excreted in the form of metabolites at a urinary to biliary ratio of 3:7. The renal and biliary excretion proceeds with a half-life of 1.9 days. Metabolites from plasma are eliminated at a similar rate (half-life of 1.7 days).

Cyproterone acetate is almost exclusively bound to plasma albumin. About 3.5–4% of total drug levels are present unbound. Because protein binding is non-specific, changes in SHBG (sex hormone binding globulin) levels do not affect the pharmacokinetics of cyproterone acetate.

The absolute bioavailability of cyproterone acetate is almost complete (88% of dose).

Preclinical safety data: Experimental investigations produced corticoid-like effects on the adrenal glands in rats and dogs following higher dosages, which could indicate similar effects in humans at the highest given dose (300 mg/day).

Recognised first-line tests of genotoxicity gave negative results when conducted with cyproterone acetate. However, further tests showed that cyproterone acetate was capable of producing adducts with DNA (and an increase in DNA repair activity) in liver cells from rats and monkeys and also in freshly isolated human hepatocytes. This DNA-adduct formation occurred at exposures that might be expected to occur in the recommended dose regimens for cyproterone acetate. One *in vivo* consequence of cyproterone acetate treatment was the increased incidence of focal, possibly preneoplastic, liver lesions in which cellular enzymes were altered in female rats. The clinical relevance of these findings is presently uncertain. Clinical experience to date would not support an increased incidence of hepatic tumours in man.

Pharmaceutical particulars
List of excipients: Maize starch, Povidone 25 000, Magnesium stearate (E572), Lactose, Aerosil.

Incompatibilities: None known.

Shelf life: 5 years.

Special precautions for storage: None.

Nature and contents of container: Original packs containing 168 tablets (14 blister strips of 12 tablets) or 84 tablets (7 blister strips of 12 tablets).

Instructions for use/handling: Keep out of the reach of children.

Marketing authrosiation number PL 0053/0133

Date of first authorisation/renewal of authorisation 15 February 1982/16 January 1998

Date of (partial) revision of text 12 December 1997.

CYPROSTAT* 100 mg

Qualitative and quantitative composition Each white, scored tablet contains 100 mg cyproterone acetate.

Pharmaceutical form Tablets.

Clinical particulars
Therapeutic indications: Management of patients with prostatic cancer (1) to suppress 'flare' with initial LHRH analogue therapy, (2) in long-term palliative treatment where LHRH analogues or surgery are contra-indicated, not tolerated, or where oral therapy is preferred, and (3) in the treatment of hot flushes in patients under treatment with LHRH analogues or who have had orchidectomy.

Posology and method of administration:
Adults, including the elderly: Dosage for suppression of 'flare' with initial LHRH analogue therapy is 300 mg/day, which may be reduced to 200 mg if the higher dose is not tolerated. For long-term palliative treatment where LHRH analogues or surgery are contra-indicated, not tolerated, or where oral therapy is preferred the dosage is 200-300 mg/day.

For the above two indications the dosage should be divided into 2–3 doses per day and taken after meals.

For the treatment of hot flushes in patients under treatment with LHRH analogues or who have had orchidectomy a 50 mg starting dose, with upward titration if necessary within the range 50–150 mg/day, is recommended. For this indication the dosage should be divided into 1–3 doses per day and taken after meals.

All doses should be taken orally.

Children: Not recommended.

Contra-indications: None.

Special warnings and special precautions for use:
Liver: Direct hepatic toxicity, including jaundice, hepatitis and hepatic failure, which has been fatal in some cases, has been reported in patients treated with 200–300 mg cyproterone acetate. Most reported cases are in men with prostatic cancer. Toxicity is dose-related and develops, usually, several months after treatment has begun. Liver function tests should be performed pre-treatment and whenever any symptoms or signs suggestive of hepatotoxicity occur. If hepatotoxicity is confirmed, cyproterone acetate should normally be withdrawn, unless the hepatotoxicity can be explained by another cause, e.g. metastatic disease, in which case cyproterone acetate should be continued only if the perceived benefit outweighs the risk.

As with other sex steroids, benign and malignant liver changes have been reported in isolated cases.

In very rare cases, liver tumours may lead to life-threatening intra-abdominal haemorrhage. If severe upper abdominal complaints, liver enlargement or signs of intra-abdominal haemorrhage occur, a liver tumour should be considered in the differential diagnosis.

Thromboembolism: Patients with a history of thrombosis may be at risk of recurrence of the disease during Cyprostat therapy.

In patients with a history of thromboembolic processes or suffering from sickle-cell anaemia or severe diabetes with vascular changes, the risk: benefit ratio must be considered carefully in each individual case before Cyprostat is prescribed.

In extremely rare cases, the occurrence of thromboembolic events has been reported in temporal association with the use of Cyprostat. However a causal relationship seems to be questionable.

Chronic depression: It has been found that some patients with severe chronic depression deteriorate whilst taking Cyprostat therapy.

Breathlessness: Shortness of breath may occur. This may be due to the stimulatory effect of progesterone and synthetic progestogens on breathing, which is accompanied by hypocapnia and compensatory alkalosis, and which is not considered to require treatment.

Adrenocortical function: During treatment adrenocortical function should be supervised, since suppression has been observed in children taking cyproterone acetate.

Diabetes: Cyprostat can influence carbohydrate metabolism. Parameters of carbohydrate metabolism should be examined carefully in all diabetics before and regularly during treatment.

Haemoglobin: Hypochromic anaemia has been found rarely during long-term treatment, and blood-counts before and at regular intervals during treatment are advisable.

Nitrogen balance: A negative balance is usual at the start of treatment, but does not persist.

Interaction with other medicaments and other forms of interaction: The requirement for oral antidiabetics or insulin can change.

Pregnancy and lactation: Not applicable.

Effects on ability to drive and use machines: Fatigue and lassitude are common in the first few weeks of therapy but usually become much less from the third month. The marked lassitude and asthenia necessitate especial care when driving or operating machinery.

Undesirable effects:
Inhibition of spermatogenesis: The sperm count and the volume of ejaculate are reduced. Infertility is usual, and there may be azoospermia after 8 weeks. There is usually slight atrophy of seminiferous tubules. Follow-up examinations have shown these changes to be reversible, spermatogenesis usually reverting to its previous state about 3–5 months after stopping Cyprostat, or in some users, up to 20 months. That spermatogenesis can recover even after very long treatment is not yet known. There is evidence that abnormal sperms which might give rise to malformed embryos are produced during treatment with Cyprostat.

Gynaecomastia: Transient, and perhaps in some cases permanent, enlargement of the mammary glands has been reported. In rare cases, galactorrhoea and tender benign nodules have been reported. Symptoms generally subside after discontinuation of treatment or on reduction of dosage, but this should be weighed against the risk from the tumour of using inadequate doses.

Bodyweight: During long-term treatment, changes in bodyweight have been reported. Both increases and decreases have been seen.

Osteoporosis: Rarely cases of osteoporosis have been reported.

Other changes that have been reported include reduction of sebum production leading to dryness of the skin, transient patchy loss and reduced growth of body hair, increased growth of scalp hair, lightening of hair colour and female type of pubic hair growth.

Overdose: There have been no reports of ill-effects of overdosage, which it is, therefore, generally unnecessary to treat. There are no specific antidotes, and treatment should be symptomatic.

Pharmacological particulars
Pharmacodynamic properties: Prostatic carcinoma and its metastases are in general androgen-dependent. Cyproterone acetate exerts a direct anti-androgen action on the tumour and its metastases and in addition it exerts a negative feedback effect on the hypothalamic receptors so leading to a reduction in gonadotrophin release and hence to diminished production of testicular androgens. Cyprostat may be used alone, or in conjunction with surgery or LHRH analogues.

Pharmacokinetic properties: Following oral administration, cyproterone acetate is completely absorbed over a wide dose range. The ingestion of 100 mg of cyproterone acetate gives maximum serum levels of about 239 ng/ml at about 3 hours. Thereafter, drug serum levels declined during a time interval of typically 24 to 120 h, with a terminal half-life of 42.8±9.7 h.. The total clearance of cyproterone acetate from serum is 3.8±2.2 ml/min/kg. Cyproterone acetate is metabolised by various pathways, including hydroxylations and conjugations. The main metabolite in human plasma is the 15β-hydroxy derivative.

Some drug is excreted unchanged with bile fluid. Most of the dose is excreted in the form of metabolites at a urinary to biliary ratio of 3:7. The renal and biliary excretion proceeds with a half-life of 1.9 days. Metabolites from plasma are eliminated at a similar rate (half-life of 1.7 days).

Cyproterone acetate is almost exclusively bound to plasma albumin. About 3.5–4% of total drug levels are present unbound. Because protein binding is non-specific, changes in SHBG (sex hormone binding globulin) levels do not affect the pharmacokinetics of cyproterone acetate.

The absolute bioavailability of cyproterone acetate is almost complete (88% of dose).

Preclinical safety data: Experimental investigations produced corticoid-like effects on the adrenal glands in rats and dogs following higher dosages, which could indicate similar effects in humans at the highest given dose (300 mg/day).

Recognised first-line tests of genotoxicity gave negative results when conducted with cyproterone acetate. However, further tests showed that cyproterone acetate was capable of producing adducts with DNA (and an increase in DNA repair activity) in liver cells from rats and monkeys and also in freshly isolated human hepatocytes. This DNA-adduct formation occurred at exposures that might be expected to occur in the recommended dose regimens for cyproterone acetate. One in vivo consequence of cyproterone acetate treatment was the increased incidence of focal, possibly preneoplastic, liver lesions in which cellular enzymes were altered in female rats. The clinical relevance of these findings is presently uncertain. Clinical experience to date would not support an increased incidence of hepatic tumours in man.

Pharmaceutical particulars
List of excipients: Maize starch, Povidone 25 000, Magnesium stearate (E572), Lactose.

Incompatibilities: None known.

Shelf life: 5 years.

Special precautions for storage: None.

Nature and contents of container: Cartons containing PVC film and aluminium foil blister packs of 42 or 84 tablets.

Instructions for use/handling: Keep out of the reach of children.

Marketing authorisation number PL 0053/0218

Date of first authorisation/renewal of authorisation 5 July 1993/5 November 1998.

Date of (partial) revision of text 25 September 1998

DIANETTE*

Qualitative and quantitative composition Each beige tablet contains 2 milligrams of the anti-androgen, cyproterone acetate and 35 micrograms of the oestrogen, ethinyloestradiol.

Pharmaceutical form Sugar-coated tablets.

Clinical particulars
Therapeutic indications: Dianette is recommended for use in women only for the treatment of (a) severe acne, refractory to prolonged oral antibiotic therapy; (b) moderately severe hirsutism.

Although Dianette also acts as an oral contraceptive, it is not recommended in women solely for contraception, but should be reserved for those women requiring treatment for the androgen-dependent skin conditions described.

Complete remission of acne is to be expected in nearly all cases, often within a few months, but in particularly severe cases treatment for longer may be necessary before the full benefit is seen. It is recommended that treatment be withdrawn when the acne or hirsutism has completely resolved. Repeat courses of Dianette may be given if the condition recurs.

Posology and method of administration:
First treatment course: One tablet daily for 21 days, starting on the first day of the menstrual cycle (the first day of menstruation counting as Day 1).

Subsequent courses: Each subsequent course is started after 7 tablet-free days have followed the preceding course.

When the contraceptive action of Dianette is also to be employed, it is essential that the above instructions be rigidly adhered to. Should bleeding fail to occur during the tablet-free interval, the possibility of pregnancy must be excluded before the next pack is started.

When changing from an oral contraceptive and relying on the contraceptive action of Dianette, follow the instructions given below:

Changing from 21-day combined oral contraceptives: The first tablet of Dianette should be taken on the first day immediately after the end of the previous oral contraceptive course. Additional contraceptive precautions are not required.

Changing from a combined Every Day pill (28 day tablets): Dianette should be started after taking the last active tablet from the Every Day Pill pack. The first Dianette tablet is taken the next day. Additional contraceptive precautions are not then required.

Changing from a progestogen-only pill (POP): The first tablet of Dianette should be taken on the first day of bleeding, even if a POP has already been taken on that day. Additional contraceptive precautions are not then required. The remaining progestogen-only pills should be discarded.

Post-partum and post-abortum use: After pregnancy, Dianette can be started 21 days after a vaginal delivery, provided that the patient is fully ambulant and there are no puerperal complications. Additional

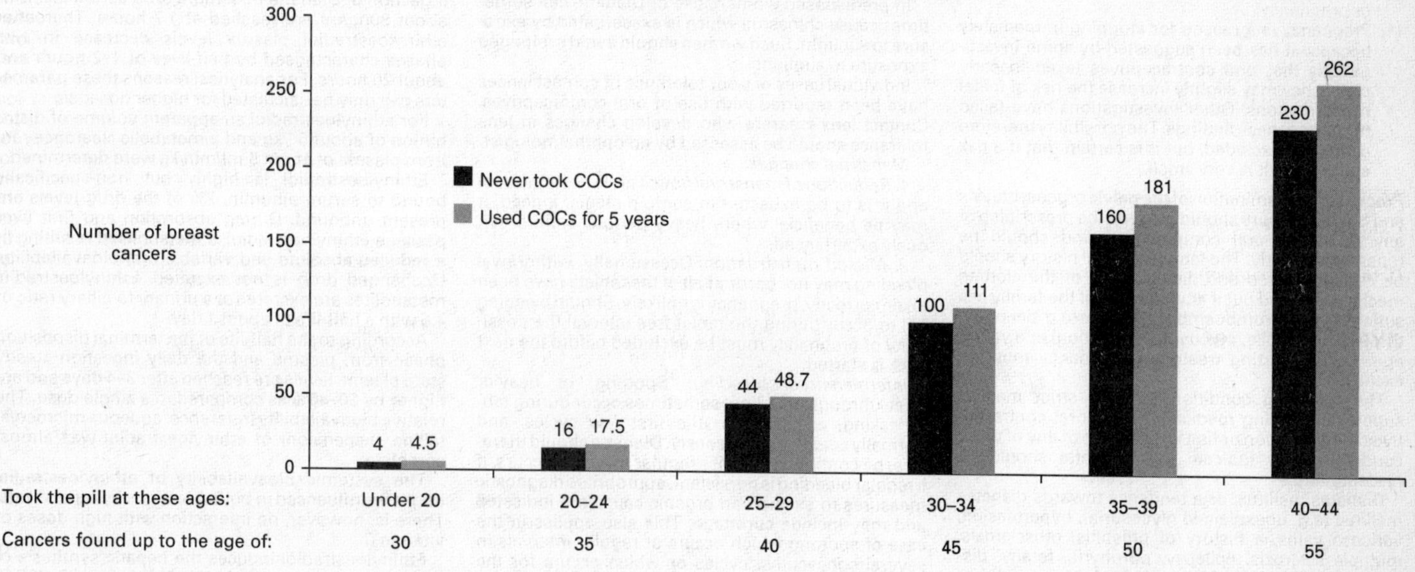

contraceptive precautions will be required for the first 7 days of pill taking. Since the first post-partum ovulation may precede the first bleeding, another method of contraception should be used in the interval between childbirth and the first course of tablets. Lactation is contra-indicated with Dianette. After a first-trimester abortion, Dianette may be started immediately in which case no additional contraceptive precautions are required.

Special circumstances requiring additional contraception:

Incorrect administration: A single delayed tablet should be taken as soon as possible, and if this can be done within 12 hours of the correct time, contraceptive protection is maintained. With longer delays, additional contraception is needed. Only the most recently delayed tablet should be taken, earlier missed tablets being omitted, and additional non-hormonal methods of contraception (except the rhythm or temperature methods) should be used for the next 7 days, while the next 7 tablets are being taken. Additionally, therefore, if tablet(s) have been missed during the last 7 days of a pack, there should be no break before the next pack is started. In this situation, a withdrawal bleed should not be expected until the end of the second pack. Some breakthrough bleeding may occur on tablet taking days but this is not clinically significant. If the patient does not have a withdrawal bleed during the tablet-free interval following the end of the second pack, the possibility of pregnancy must be ruled out before starting the next pack.

Gastro-intestinal upset: Vomiting or diarrhoea may reduce the efficacy of oral contraceptives by preventing full absorption. Tablet-taking from the current pack should be continued. Additional non-hormonal methods of contraception (except the rhythm or temperature methods) should be used during the gastro-intestinal upset and for 7 days following the upset. If these 7 days overrun the end of a pack, the next pack should be started without a break. In this situation, a withdrawal bleed should not be expected until the end of the second pack. If the patient does not have a withdrawal bleed during the tablet-free interval following the end of the second pack, the possibility of pregnancy must be ruled out before starting the next pack. Other methods of contraception should be considered if the gastro-intestinal disorder is likely to be prolonged.

Contra-indications:

1. Pregnancy or lactation
2. Severe disturbances of liver function, jaundice or persistent itching during a previous pregnancy, Dubin-Johnson syndrome, Rotor syndrome, previous or existing liver tumours.
3. Existing or previous arterial or venous thrombotic or embolic processes, conditions which predispose to them e.g. disorders of the clotting processes, valvular heart disease and atrial fibrillation.
4. Sickle-cell anaemia.
5. Mammary or endometrial carcinoma, or a history of these conditions.
6. Severe diabetes mellitus with vascular changes.
7. Disorders of lipid metabolism.
8. History of herpes gestationis.
9. Deterioration of otosclerosis during pregnancy.
10. Undiagnosed abnormal vaginal bleeding.
11. Hypersensitivity to any of the components of Dianette.

Special warnings and special precautions for use:

Warnings: Like many other steroids, Dianette, when given in very high doses and for the majority of the animal's life-span, has been found to cause an increase in the incidence of tumours, including carcinoma, in the liver of rats. The relevance of this finding to humans is unknown.

In rare cases benign and in even rarer cases malignant liver tumours leading in isolated cases to life-threatening intra-abdominal haemorrhage have been observed after the use of hormonal substances such as those contained in Dianette. If severe upper abdominal complaints, liver enlargement or signs of intra-abdominal haemorrhage occur, a liver tumour should be included in the differential diagnosis.

Animal studies have revealed that feminisation of male foetuses may occur if cyproterone acetate is administered during the phase of embryogenesis at which differentiation of the external genitalia occurs. Although the results of these tests are not necessarily relevant to man, the possibility must be considered that administration of Dianette to women after the 45th day of pregnancy could cause feminisation of male foetuses. It follows from this that pregnancy is an absolute contra-indication for treatment with Dianette, and must be excluded before such treatment is begun.

Although its strong anti-androgenic effect is distinctive, Dianette has many properties in common with combined oral contraceptives, which must not be taken during treatment with Dianette. There is a general opinion, based on statistical evidence, that users of combined oral contraceptives experience, more often than non-users, venous thromboembolism, arterial thrombosis, including cerebral and myocardial infarction, and subarachnoid haemorrhage. Full recovery from such disorders does not always occur, and it should be realised that in a few cases they are fatal. How often these disorders occur in users of the modern low-dose pills is not known, but there are reasons for suggesting that they may occur less often than with older pills.

Certain factors may entail some risk of thrombosis, e.g. smoking, obesity, varicose veins, cardiovascular diseases, diabetes and migraine. The risk of arterial thrombosis associated with combined oral contraceptives increases with age, and this risk is aggravated by cigarette-smoking.

In addition, if there is a history in the family of thromboembolic diseases at a young age (e.g. deep vein thrombosis, heart attack or stroke) disturbances of the coagulation system must be ruled out before Dianette is prescribed. The suitability of Dianette should be judged according to the severity of such conditions in the individual case, and should be discussed with the patient before she decides to take it.

Numerous epidemiological studies have been reported on the risks of ovarian, endometrial, cervical and breast cancer in women using combined oral contraceptives. The evidence is clear that combined oral contraceptives offer substantial protection against both ovarian and endometrial cancer.

An increased risk of cervical cancer in long-term users of combined oral contraceptives has been reported in some studies, but there continues to be controversy about the extent to which this is attributable to the confounding effects of sexual behaviour and other factors.

A meta-analysis from 54 epidemiological studies reported that there is a slightly increased relative risk (RR=1.24) of having breast cancer diagnosed in women who are currently using combined oral contraceptives (COCs). The observed pattern of increased risk may be due to an earlier diagnosis of breast cancer in COC users, the biological effects of COCs or a combination of both. The additional breast cancers diagnosed in current users of COCs or in women who have used COCs in the last ten years are more likely to be localised to the breast than those in women who never used COCs.

Breast cancer is rare among women under 40 years of age whether or not they take COCs. Whilst this background risk increases with age, the excess number of breast cancer diagnoses in current and recent COC users is small in relation to the overall risk of breast cancer (see bar chart).

The most important risk factor for breast cancer in COC users is the age women discontinue the COC; the older the age at stopping, the more breast cancers are diagnosed. Duration of use is less important and the excess risk gradually disappears during the course of the 10 years after stopping COC use such that by 10 years there appears to be no excess.

The possible increase in risk of breast cancer should be discussed with the user and weighed against the benefits of COCs taking into account the evidence that they offer substantial protection against the risk of developing certain other cancers (e.g. ovarian and endometrial cancer).

The possibility cannot be ruled out that certain chronic diseases may occasionally deteriorate during the use of Dianette (see *Precautions*).

Reasons for stopping Dianette immediately:

1. Occurrence for the first time, or exacerbation, of migrainous headaches or unusually frequent or unusually severe headaches.
2. Sudden disturbances of vision or hearing or other perceptual disorders.
3. First signs of thrombophlebitis or thromboembolic symptoms (e.g. unusual pains in or swelling of the leg(s), stabbing pains on breathing or coughing for no apparent reason). Feeling of pain and tightness in the chest.
4. Six weeks before an elective major operation (e.g. abdominal, orthopaedic), any surgery to the legs, medical treatment for varicose veins or prolonged immobilisation, e.g. after accidents or surgery. Do not restart until 2 weeks after full ambulation. In case of emergency surgery, thrombotic prophylaxis is usually indicated e.g. subcutaneous heparin.
5. Onset of jaundice, hepatitis, itching of the whole body.
6. Increase in epileptic seizures.
7. Significant rise in blood pressure.
8. Onset of severe depression.

9. Severe upper abdominal pain or liver enlargement.
10. Clear exacerbation of conditions known to be capable of deteriorating during oral contraception or pregnancy.
11. Pregnancy is a reason for stopping immediately because it has been suggested by some investigations that oral contraceptives taken in early pregnancy may slightly increase the risk of foetal malformations. Other investigations have failed to support these findings. The possibility therefore cannot be excluded, but it is certain that if a risk exists at all, it is very small.

Precautions: Examination of the pelvic organs, breasts and blood-pressure should precede the prescribing of any combined oral contraceptive and should be repeated regularly. The family medical history should be carefully noted and disturbances of the clotting mechanism ruled out if any member of the family has suffered from thromboembolic disease (e.g. deep vein thrombosis, stroke, myocardial infarction) at a young age. Before starting treatment pregnancy must be excluded.

The following conditions require strict medical supervision during medication with oral contraceptives. Deterioration or first appearance of any of these conditions may indicate that Dianette should be discontinued:

Diabetes mellitus, or a tendency towards diabetes mellitus (e.g. unexplained glycosuria), hypertension, varicose veins, a history of phlebitis, otosclerosis, multiple sclerosis, epilepsy, porphyria, tetany, disturbed liver function, Sydenham's chorea, renal dysfunction, family history of clotting disorders, obesity, family history of breast cancer and patient history of benign breast disease, history of clinical depression, systemic lupus erythematosus, uterine fibroids, an intolerance to contact lenses, migraine, gall-stones, cardiovascular diseases, chloasma, asthma, or any disease that is prone to worsen during pregnancy.

It should be borne in mind that the use of ultraviolet lamps, for the treatment of acne, or prolonged exposure to sunlight, increases the risk of the deterioration of chloasma.

Some women may experience amenorrhoea or oligomenorrhoea after discontinuation of Dianette, especially when these conditions existed prior to use. Women should be informed of this possibility.

Interaction with other medicaments and other forms of interaction: Hepatic enzyme inducers such as barbiturates, primidone, phenobarbitone, phenytoin, phenylbutazone, rifampicin, carbamazepine and griseofulvin can impair the contraceptive efficacy of Dianette. For women receiving long-term therapy with hepatic enzyme inducers, another method of contraception should be used. The use of antibiotics may also reduce the contraceptive efficacy of Dianette, possibly by altering the intestinal flora.

Women receiving short courses of enzyme inducers and broad spectrum antibiotics should take additional, non-hormonal (except rhythm or temperature method) contraceptive precautions during the time of concurrent medication and for 7 days afterwards. If these 7 days overrun the end of a pack, the next pack should be started without a break. In this situation, a withdrawal bleed should not be expected until the end of the second pack. If the patient does not have a withdrawal bleed during the tablet-free interval following the end of the second pack, the possibility of pregnancy must be ruled out before resuming with the next pack.

The possibility cannot be ruled out that oral tetracyclines, if used in conjunction with Dianette may reduce its contraceptive efficacy, although it has not been shown. When drugs of these classes are being taken it is, therefore, advisable to use additional non-hormonal methods of contraception (except the rhythm or temperature methods) since an extremely high degree of protection must be provided when Dianette is being taken. With rifampicin, additional contraceptive precautions should be continued for 4 weeks after treatment stops, even if only a short course was administered.

The requirement for oral antidiabetics or insulin can change as a result of the effect on glucose tolerance.

Pregnancy and lactation: Contra-indicated.

Animal studies have revealed that feminisation of male foetuses may occur if cyproterone acetate is administered during the phase of embryogenesis at which differentiation of the external genitalia occurs. Although the results of these tests are not necessarily relevant to man, the possibility must be considered that administration of Dianette to women after the 45th day of pregnancy could cause feminisation of male foetuses. It follows from this that pregnancy is an absolute contra-indication for treatment with Dianette, and must be excluded before such treatment is begun.

Effects on ability to drive and use machines: None known.

Undesirable effects: In rare cases, headaches, gastric upsets, nausea, vomiting, breast tenderness, changes in body weight, changes in libido, depressive moods can occur.

In predisposed women, use of Dianette can sometimes cause chloasma which is exacerbated by exposure to sunlight. Such women should avoid prolonged exposure to sunlight.

Individual cases of poor tolerance of contact lenses have been reported with use of oral contraceptives. Contact lens wearers who develop changes in lens tolerance should be assessed by an ophthalmologist.

Menstrual changes:

1. Reduction of menstrual flow: This is not abnormal and it is to be expected in some patients. Indeed, it may be beneficial where heavy periods were previously experienced.

2. Missed menstruation: Occasionally, withdrawal bleeding may not occur at all. If the tablets have been taken correctly, pregnancy is unlikely. Should bleeding fail to occur during the tablet-free interval the possibility of pregnancy must be excluded before the next pack is started.

Intermenstrual bleeding: 'Spotting' or heavier 'breakthrough bleeding' sometimes occur during tablet taking, especially in the first few cycles, and normally cease spontaneously. Dianette should therefore, be continued even if irregular bleeding occurs. If irregular bleeding is persistent, appropriate diagnostic measures to exclude an organic cause are indicated and may include curettage. This also applies in the case of spotting which occurs at regular intervals in several consecutive cycles or which occurs for the first time after long use of Dianette.

Effect on blood chemistry: The use of oral contraceptives may influence the results of certain laboratory tests including biochemical parameters of liver, thyroid, adrenal and renal function, plasma levels of carrier proteins and lipid/lioprotein fractions, parameters of carbohydrate metabolism and parameters of coagulation and fibrinolysis. Laboratory staff should therefore be informed about oral contraceptive use when laboratory tests are requested.

Refer to *Special warnings and special precautions for use* for additional information.

Overdose: Overdose may cause nausea, vomiting and, in females, withdrawal bleeding. There are no specific antidotes and further treatment should be symptomatic.

Pharmacological properties

Pharmacodynamic properties: Dianette blocks androgen-receptors. It also reduces androgen synthesis both by negative feedback effect on the hypothalamo-pituitiary-ovarian systems and by the inhibition of androgen-synthesising enzymes.

Although Dianette also acts as an oral contraceptive, it is not recommended in women solely for contraception, but should be reserved for those women requiring treatment for the androgen-dependent skin conditions described.

Pharmacokinetic properties:

Cyproterone acetate: Following oral administration cyproterone acetate is completely absorbed in a wide dose range. The ingestion of Dianette effects a maximum serum level of 15ng cyproterone acetate/ml at 1.6 hours. Thereafter drug serum levels decrease in two disposition phases characterised by half-lives of 0.8 hours and 2.3 days. The total clearance of cyproterone acetate from serum was determined to be 3.6 ml/min/kg. Cyproterone acetate is metabolised by various pathways including hydroxylations and conjugations. The main metabolite in human plasma is the 15β-hydroxy derivative.

Some dose parts are excreted unchanged with the bile fluid. Most of the dose is excreted in form of metabolites at a urinary to biliary ratio of 3:7. The renal and biliary excretion was determined to proceed with half-life of 1.9 days. Metabolites from plasma were eliminated at a similar rate (half-life of 1.7 days). Cyproterone acetate is almost exclusively bound to plasma albumin. About 3.5–4.0% of total drug levels are present unbound. Because protein binding is non-specific changes in sex hormone binding globulin (SHBG) levels do not affect cyproterone acetate pharmacokinetics.

According to the long half-life of the terminal disposition phase from plasma (serum) and the daily intake cyproterone acetate accumulates during one treatment cycle. Mean maximum drug serum levels increased from 15ng/ml (day 1) to 21ng/ml and 24ng/ml at the end of the treatment cycles 1 and 3 respectively. The area under the concentration versus time profile increased 2.2 fold (end of cycle 1) and 2.4 fold (end of cycle 3). Steady state conditions were reached after about 16 days. During long term treatment cyproterone acetate accumulates over treatment cycles by a factor of 2.

The absolute bioavailability of cyproterone acetate is almost complete (88% of dose). The relative bioavailability of cyproterone acetate from Dianette was 109% when compared to an aqueous microcrystalline suspension.

Ethinyloestradiol: Orally administered ethinyloestradiol is rapidly and completely absorbed. Following ingestion of Dianette maximum drug serum levels of about 80pg/ml are reached at 1.7 hours. Thereafter ethinyloestradiol plasma levels decrease in two phases characterised by half-lives of 1–2 hours and about 20 hours. For analytical reasons these parameters can only be calculated for higher dosages.

For ethinyloestradiol an apparent volume of distribution of about 5 l/kg and a metabolic clearance rate from plasma of about 5 ml/min/kg were determined.

Ethinyloestradiol is highly but non-specifically bound to serum albumin. 2% of the drug levels are present unbound. During absorption and first liver passage ethinyloestradiol is metabolised resulting in a reduced absolute and variable oral bioavailability. Unchanged drug is not excreted. Ethinyloestradiol metabolites are excreted at a urinary to biliary ratio of 4:6 with a half-life of about 1 day.

According to the half-life of the terminal disposition phase from plasma and the daily ingestion steady state plasma levels are reached after 3–4 days and are higher by 30–40% as compared to a single dose. The relative bioavailability (reference: aqueous microcrystalline suspension) of ethinyloestradiol was almost complete.

The systemic bioavailability of ethinyloestradiol might be influenced in both directions by other drugs. There is, however, no interaction with high doses of vitamin C.

Ethinyloestradiol induces the hepatic synthesis of SHBG and corticosteroid binding globulin (CBG) during continuous use. The extent of SHBG induction, however, is dependent upon the chemical structure and dose of the co-administered progestin. During treatment with Dianette SHBG concentrations in serum increased from about 100nmol/l to 300nmol/l and the serum concentrations of CBG were increased from about 50 micrograms/ml to 95 micrograms/ml.

Preclinical safety data: There are no preclinical safety data which could be of relevance to the prescriber and which are not already included in other relevant sections of the SPC.

Pharmaceutical particulars

List of excipients: Lactose, maize starch, povidone, talc, magnesium stearate (E 572), sucrose, macrogol 6,000, calcium carbonate (E 170), titanium dioxide (E 171), glycerol 85%, montan glycol wax, yellow ferric oxide pigment (E 172).

Incompatibilities: None known.

Shelf life: 5 years.

Special precautions for storage: Not applicable.

Nature and contents of container: Outer carton contains aluminium foil and PVC blister memo packs each containing 21 tablets. Each carton contains either 1 or 3 blister memo packs.

Instructions for use/handling: Keep out of the reach of children.

Marketing authorisation number 0053/0190

Date of approval/revision of SPC January 1998

Legal category POM

ECHOVIST*

Qualitative and quantitative composition Each vial contains 3 g granules (1 g granules contains 1 g galactose microparticles). 1 ml aqueous solution for production of the suspension contains 200 mg galactose.

Pharmaceutical form Microcrystalline suspension for transcervical administration.

Clinical particulars

Therapeutic indications: Echo-contrast medium for transcervical administration in contrast-enhanced ultrasound investigation of the female genital tract (hysterosalpingo-contrast sonography). Echovist can be used to enhance gynaecological ultrasound images and assess tubal patency.

Posology and method of administration: To prepare the echo-contrast medium, the galactose solution (13.5 ml) is drawn into a syringe and transferred to the vial containing 3 g of granules using the 'Mini-Spike' supplied. The vial should then be shaken vigorously for about 5 seconds to suspend the granules in solution, producing a homogenous milky-white suspension. The suspension is then drawn up using the 'Mini-Spike', taking care that recognisable air bubbles are removed. The granules and the galactose solution should be at room temperature at the time the suspension is made up. Warming the suspension (e.g. in the hands) or excessive negative pressure on drawing it up should be avoided as this may result in the decrease of the microbubble concentration or development of larger air bubbles.

For transcervical administration in gynaecological investigations the use of an intrauterine balloon catheter is recommended.

Any suspension not used at one examination session must be discarded.

Dosage: For the demonstration of the uterine cavity 2-5 ml of Echovist suspension should be used. In order to demonstrate the Fallopian tubes and to check their patency, additional intermittent administration of doses of 1-2 ml should be given under sonographic control up to a maximum of 30 ml. In general, about 15 ml is normally sufficient.

Contra-indications: Galactosaemia. Intact pregnancy. Pelvic inflammatory disease.

Special warnings and special precautions for use: Aseptic conditions must be observed to reduce the potential risk of ascending infection.

Interaction with other medicaments and other forms of interaction: None so far known.

Pregnancy and lactation: The transcervical administration of Echovist is contraindicated in pregnancy. Since galactose is a natural constituent of milk, there is no contraindication to the use of Echovist during lactation, with the exception of women with galactosaemia.

Effects on ability to drive and use machines: Not applicable.

Undesirable effects: The distension of the uterine cavity and tubes caused by filling with the contrast agent can result in pain which is particularly pronounced in the presence of occluded tubes.

Vasovagal reactions, e.g. outbreaks of sweating, dizziness, nausea and vomiting, may occur in individual cases.

The possibility of ascending genital infection owing to the method itself cannot be ruled out in individual cases.

Overdose: Overdose is unlikely with transcervical administration.

Pharmacological properties

Pharmacodynamic properties: Echovist is an echo-contrast medium for hysterosalpingo-contrast sonography. It consists of a suspension of soluble galactose microparticles in aqueous galactose solution. After transcervical administration this microbubble-microparticle suspension leads to a marked increase of the echo signals from the female genital tract due to the acoustically active inhomogeneities produced.

Pharmacokinetic properties: The galactose and small amount of air in the bubbles are completely absorbed after transcervical administration. The galactose first of all becomes dispersed in the extracellular space and is subjected to glucose metabolism independent of insulin. Galactose is stored above all in the liver through the formation of galactose-1-phosphate or is metabolised and broken down to CO_2 after isomerisation to glucose-1-phosphate. If the plasma galactose level exceeds about 50 mg/100 ml and, therefore, the elimination rate of the liver, galactose is eliminated via the kidneys. The elimination rate in patients with liver disease is about one third lower than in healthy subjects, in whom the plasma galactose level falls by 10% per minute. Total clearance is about 40% lower in patients with liver disease. In the case of liver damage up to 60% of the amount of galactose administered is eliminated via the kidneys, while about 40% is utilised extrahepatically.

Galactose has a half-life of about 10-11 minutes in adults.

Elimination may be substantially prolonged after consumption of alcohol.

Preclinical safety data: Echovist does not pose any risk of acute intoxication even on repeated administration of the diagnostic dose at short intervals of time.

Systemic toxicity studies after repeated daily intravenous administration and after repeated intracardiac (left ventricle) application produced no findings which preclude the usually single transcervical administration in human beings. No unequivocally organ-toxic effects were demonstrable even after very high intravenous dosages.

Studies for embryotoxic and, in particular, teratogenic effects produced no evidence for a teratogenic potential in human beings.

Findings from local tolerance studies on single intravenous, intraarterial, subcutaneous, paravenous intramuscular and, in particular following intrauterine administration, showed that signs of local intolerance are likely only on inadvertent paravenous injection.

No risk of a tumorigenic, mutagenic or sensitising effect to human beings is envisaged on administration of Echovist, since the galactose contained in the medium occurs physiologically and is ingested by human beings with the diet and metabolised, and because no such effects are known for galactose.

Pharmaceutical particulars

List of excipients: Water for injection.

Incompatibilities: None so far known.

Shelf life: Echovist solution and Echovist granulate are both stable for five years.

Special precautions for storage: Not applicable

Nature and contents of container:
Granulate/Galactose solution
Injection vial: Glass type I, siliconized.
Stopper: Chlorinated butyl rubber, grey, fluoropolymer-coated.
Flanged cap: Pure aluminium with polypropylene cover disks.
'Mini-Spike': Plastics.

Combination pack consisting of
1 vial of 20 ml with 3 g granulate
1 vial of 15 ml with 13.5 ml galactose solution
1 'Mini-Spike'

Instructions for use/handling: The ready-to-use suspension has to be prepared according to instructions. Any suspension not used at one examination session must be discarded. Store all drugs properly and keep them out of reach of children.

Marketing authorisation number 0053/0232-3

Date of approval/revision of SPC 22 November 1995

Legal category POM

EUGYNON* 30

Qualitative and quantitative composition Each tablet contains 250 micrograms levonorgestrel and 30 micrograms ethinylestradiol (ethinyloestradiol).

Pharmaceutical form Sugar-coated tablets.

Clinical particulars

Therapeutic indications: Oral contraception and the recognised gynaecological indications for such oestrogen-progestogen combinations.

Posology and method of administration:

First treatment cycle: 1 tablet daily for 21 days, starting on the first day of the menstrual cycle. Contraceptive protection begins immediately.

Subsequent cycles: Tablet taking from the next pack of Eugynon 30 is continued after a 7-day interval, beginning on the same day of the week as the first pack.

Changing from 21-day combined oral contraceptives: The first tablet of Eugynon 30 should be taken on the first day immediately after the end of the previous oral contraceptive course. Additional contraceptive precautions are not required.

Changing from a combined Every Day pill (28 day tablets): Eugynon 30 should be started after taking the last active tablet from the Every Day Pill pack. The first Eugynon 30 tablet is taken the next day. Additional contraceptive precautions are not then required.

Changing from a progestogen-only pill (POP): The first tablet of Eugynon 30 should be taken on the first day of bleeding, even if a POP has already been taken on that day. Additional contraceptive precautions are not then required. The remaining progestogen-only pills should be discarded.

Post-partum and post-abortum use: After pregnancy, oral contraception can be started 21 days after a vaginal delivery, provided that the patient is fully ambulant and there are no puerperal complications. Additional contraceptive precautions will be required for the first 7 days of tablet taking to ensure adequate contraceptive cover if early ovulation has occurred. Since the first post-partum ovulation may precede the first bleeding, another method of contraception should be used in the interval between childbirth and the first course of tablets. After a first-trimester abortion, oral contraception may be started immediately in which case no additional contraceptive precautions are required.

Special circumstances requiring additional contraception

Incorrect administration: A single delayed tablet should be taken as soon as possible, and if this can be done within 12 hours of the correct time, contraceptive protection is maintained. With longer delays, additional contraception is needed. Only the most recently delayed tablet should be taken, earlier missed tablets being omitted, and additional non-hormonal methods of contraception (except the rhythm or temperature methods) should be used for the next 7 days, while the next 7 tablets are being taken. Additionally, therefore, if tablet(s) have been missed during the last 7 days of a pack, there should be no break before the next pack is started. In this situation, a withdrawal bleed should not be expected until the end of the second pack. Some breakthrough bleeding may occur on tablet taking days but this is not clinically significant. If the patient does not have a withdrawal bleed during the tablet-free interval following the end of the second pack, the possibility of pregnancy must be ruled out before starting the next pack.

Gastro-intestinal upset: Vomiting or diarrhoea may reduce the efficacy of oral contraceptives by preventing full absorption. Tablet-taking from the current pack should be continued. Additional non-hormonal methods of contraception (except the rhythm or temperature methods) should be used during the gastro-intestinal upset and for 7 days following the upset. If these 7 days overrun the end of a pack, the next pack should be started without a break. In this situation, a withdrawal bleed should not be expected until the end of the second pack. If the patient does not have a withdrawal bleed during the tablet-free interval following the end of the second pack, the possibility of pregnancy must be ruled out before starting the next pack. Other methods of contraception should be considered if the gastro-intestinal disorder is likely to be prolonged.

Contra-indications:

1. Pregnancy
2. Severe disturbances of liver function, jaundice or persistent itching during a previous pregnancy, Dubin-Johnson syndrome, Rotor syndrome, previous or existing liver tumours.
3. Existing or previous arterial or venous thrombotic or embolic processes, conditions which predispose to them e.g. disorders of the clotting processes, valvular heart disease and atrial fibrillation.
4. Sickle-cell anaemia.
5. Mammary or endometrial carcinoma, or a history of these conditions.
6. Severe diabetes mellitus with vascular changes.
7. Disorders of lipid metabolism.
8. History of herpes gestationis.
9. Deterioration of otosclerosis during pregnancy.
10. Undiagnosed abnormal vaginal bleeding.
11. Hypersensitivity to any of the components of Eugynon 30.

Special warnings and special precautions for use:

Warnings: There is a general opinion, based on statistical evidence, that users of combined oral contraceptives experience, more often than non-users, venous thromboembolism, arterial thrombosis, including cerebral and myocardial infarction, and subarachnoid haemorrhage. Full recovery from such disorders does not always occur, and it should be realised that in a few cases they are fatal. How often these disorders occur in users of the modern low-dose pills is not known, but there are reasons for suggesting that they may occur less often than with older pills.

Certain factors may entail some risk of thrombosis, e.g. smoking, obesity, varicose veins, cardiovascular diseases, diabetes, and migraine. The suitability of a combined oral contraceptive should be judged according to the severity of such conditions in the individual case, and should be discussed with the patient before she decides to take it. The risk of arterial thrombosis associated with combined oral contraceptives increases with age, and this risk is aggravated by cigarette-smoking. The use of combined oral contraceptives by women in the older age-group, especially those who are cigarette smokers, should therefore be discouraged and alternative methods used.

In addition if there is a history in the family of thromboembolic diseases at a young age (e.g. deep vein thrombosis, heart attack or stroke) disturbances of the coagulation system must be ruled out before the pill is prescribed.

Numerous epidemiological studies have been reported on the risks of ovarian, endometrial, cervical and breast cancer in women using combined oral contraceptives. The evidence is clear that combined oral contraceptives offer substantial protection against both ovarian and endometrial cancer.

An increased risk of cervical cancer in long-term users of combined oral contraceptives has been reported in some studies, but there continues to be controversy about the extent to which this is attributable to the confounding effects of sexual behaviour and other factors.

A meta-analysis from 54 epidemiological studies reported that there is a slightly increased relative risk (RR=1.24) of having breast cancer diagnosed in women who are currently using combined oral contraceptives (COCs). The observed pattern of increased risk may be due to an earlier diagnosis of breast cancer in COC users, the biological effects of COCs or a combination of both. The additional breast cancers diagnosed in current users of COCs or in women who have used COCs in the last ten years are more likely to be localised to the breast than those in women who never used COCs.

Breast cancer is rare among women under 40 years of age whether or not they take COCs. Whilst this background risk increases with age, the excess number of breast cancer diagnoses in current and recent

COC users is small in relation to the overall risk of breast cancer (see bar chart).

The most important risk factor for breast cancer in COC users is the age women discontinue the COC; the older the age at stopping, the more breast cancers are diagnosed. Duration of use is less important and the excess risk gradually disappears during the course of the 10 years after stopping COC use such that by 10 years there appears to be no excess.

The possible increase in risk of breast cancer should be discussed with the user and weighed against the benefits of COCs taking into account the evidence that they offer substantial protection against the risk of developing certain other cancers (e.g. ovarian and endometrial cancer).

The possibility cannot be ruled out that certain chronic diseases may occasionally deteriorate during the use of combined oral contraceptives (see *Precautions*).

In rare cases benign and, in even rarer cases, malignant liver tumours leading in isolated cases to life-threatening intra-abdominal haemorrhage have been observed after the use of hormonal substances such as those contained in Eugynon 30. If severe upper abdominal complaints, liver enlargement or signs of intra-abdominal haemorrhage occur, the possibility of a liver tumour should be included in the differential diagnosis.

Reasons for stopping oral contraception immediately:

1. Occurrence for the first time, or exacerbation, of migrainous headaches or unusually frequent or unusually severe headaches.
2. Sudden disturbances of vision or hearing or other perceptual disorders.
3. First signs of thrombophlebitis or thromboembolic symptoms (e.g. unusual pains in or swelling of the leg(s), stabbing pains on breathing or coughing for no apparent reason). Feeling of pain and tightness in the chest.
4. Six weeks before an elective major operation (e.g. abdominal, orthopaedic), any surgery to the legs, medical treatment for varicose veins or prolonged immobilisation, e.g. after accidents or surgery. Do not restart until 2 weeks after full ambulation. In case of emergency surgery, thrombotic prophylaxis is usually indicated e.g. subcutaneous heparin.
5. Onset of jaundice, hepatitis, itching of the whole body.
6. Increase in epileptic seizures.
7. Significant rise in blood pressure.
8. Onset of severe depression.
9. Severe upper abdominal pain or liver enlargement.
10. Clear exacerbation of conditions known to be capable of deteriorating during oral contraception or pregnancy.
11. Pregnancy is a reason for stopping immediately because it has been suggested by some investigations that oral contraceptives taken in early pregnancy may slightly increase the risk of foetal malformations. Other investigations have failed to support these findings. The possibility therefore cannot be excluded, but it is certain that if a risk exists at all, it is very small.

Precautions: Examination of the pelvic organs, breasts and blood-pressure should precede the prescribing of any combined oral contraceptive and should be repeated regularly. The family medical history should be carefully noted and disturbances of the clotting mechanism ruled out if any member of the family has suffered from thromboembolic disease (e.g. deep vein thrombosis, stroke, myocardial infarction) at a young age. Before starting treatment pregnancy must be excluded.

The following conditions require strict medical supervision during medication with oral contraceptives. Deterioration or first appearance of any of these conditions may indicate that use of the oral contraceptive should be discontinued:

Diabetes mellitus, or a tendency towards diabetes mellitus (e.g. unexplained glycosuria), hypertension, varicose veins, a history of phlebitis, otosclerosis, multiple sclerosis, epilepsy, porphyria, tetany, disturbed liver function, Sydenham's chorea, renal dysfunction, family history of clotting disorders, obesity, family history of breast cancer and patient history of benign breast disease, history of clinical depression, systemic lupus erythematosus, uterine fibroids and migraine, gall-stones, cardiovascular diseases, chloasma, asthma, an intolerance to contact lenses, or any disease that is prone to worsen during pregnancy

Some women may experience amenorrhoea or oligomenorrhoea after discontinuation of oral contraceptives, especially when these conditions existed prior to use. Women should be informed of this possibility.

Interaction with other medicaments and other forms of interaction: Hepatic enzyme inducers such as barbiturates, primidone, phenobarbitone, phenytoin, phenylbutazone, rifampicin, carbamazepine and griseofulvin can impair the efficacy of Eugynon 30. For women receiving long-term therapy with hepatic enzyme inducers, another method of contraception should be used. The use of antibiotics may also reduce the efficacy of Eugynon 30, possibly by altering the intestinal flora.

Women receiving short courses of enzyme inducers or broad spectrum antibiotics should take additional, non-hormonal (except rhythm or temperature method) contraceptive precautions during the time of concurrent medication and for 7 days afterwards. If these 7 days overrun the end of a pack, the next pack should be started without a break. In this situation, a withdrawal bleed should not be expected until the end of the second pack. If the patient does not have a withdrawal bleed during the tablet-free interval following the end of the second pack, the possibility of pregnancy must be ruled out before resuming with the next pack. With rifampicin, additional contraceptive precautions should be continued for 4 weeks after treatment stops, even if only a short course was administered.

The requirement for oral antidiabetics or insulin can change as a result of the effect on glucose tolerance.

Pregnancy and lactation: If pregnancy occurs during medication with oral contraceptives, the preparation should be withdrawn immediately (see *Reasons for stopping oral contraception immediately*).

The use of Eugynon 30 during lactation may lead to a reduction in the volume of milk produced and to a change in its composition. Minute amounts of the active substances are excreted with the milk. Mothers who are breast-feeding may be advised instead to use a progestogen-only pill.

Effects on ability to drive and to use machines: None known.

Undesirable effects: In rare cases, headaches, gastric upsets, nausea, vomiting, breast tenderness, changes in body weight, changes in libido, depressive moods can occur.

In predisposed women, use of Eugynon 30 can sometimes cause chloasma which is exacerbated by exposure to sunlight. Such women should avoid prolonged exposure to sunlight.

Individual cases of poor tolerance of contact lenses have been reported with use of oral contraceptives. Contact lens wearers who develop changes in lens tolerance should be assessed by an ophthalmologist.

Menstrual changes:

1. Reduction of menstrual flow: This is not abnormal and it is to be expected in some patients. Indeed, it may be beneficial where heavy periods were previously experienced.

2. Missed menstruation: Occasionally, withdrawal bleeding may not occur at all. If the tablets have been taken correctly, pregnancy is very unlikely. If withdrawal bleeding fails to occur at the end of a second pack, the possibility of pregnancy must be ruled out before resuming with the next pack.

3. Intermenstrual bleeding: 'Spotting' or heavier 'breakthrough bleeding' sometimes occur during tablet taking, especially in the first few cycles, and normally cease spontaneously. Eugynon 30 should therefore, be continued even if irregular bleeding occurs. If irregular bleeding is persistent, appropriate diagnostic measures to exclude an organic cause are indicated and may include curettage. This also applies in the case of spotting which occurs at irregular intervals in several consecutive cycles or which occurs for the first time after long use of Eugynon 30.

4. Effect on blood chemistry: The use of oral contraceptives may influence the results of certain laboratory tests including biochemical parameters of liver, thyroid, adrenal and renal function, plasma levels of carrier proteins and lipid/lipoprotein fractions, parameters of carbohydrate metabolism and parameters of coagulation and fibrinolysis. Laboratory staff should therefore be informed about oral contraceptive use when laboratory tests are requested.

Refer to *Special warnings and special precautions for use* for additional information.

Overdose: Overdosage may cause nausea, vomiting and, in females, withdrawal bleeding.

There are no specific antidotes and treatment should be symptomatic.

Pharmacological particulars

Pharmacodynamic properties: The mode of action includes the inhibition of ovulation by suppression of the mid-cycle surge of luteinising hormone, the inspissation of cervical mucus so as to constitute a barrier to sperm, and the rendering of the endometrium unreceptive to implantation.

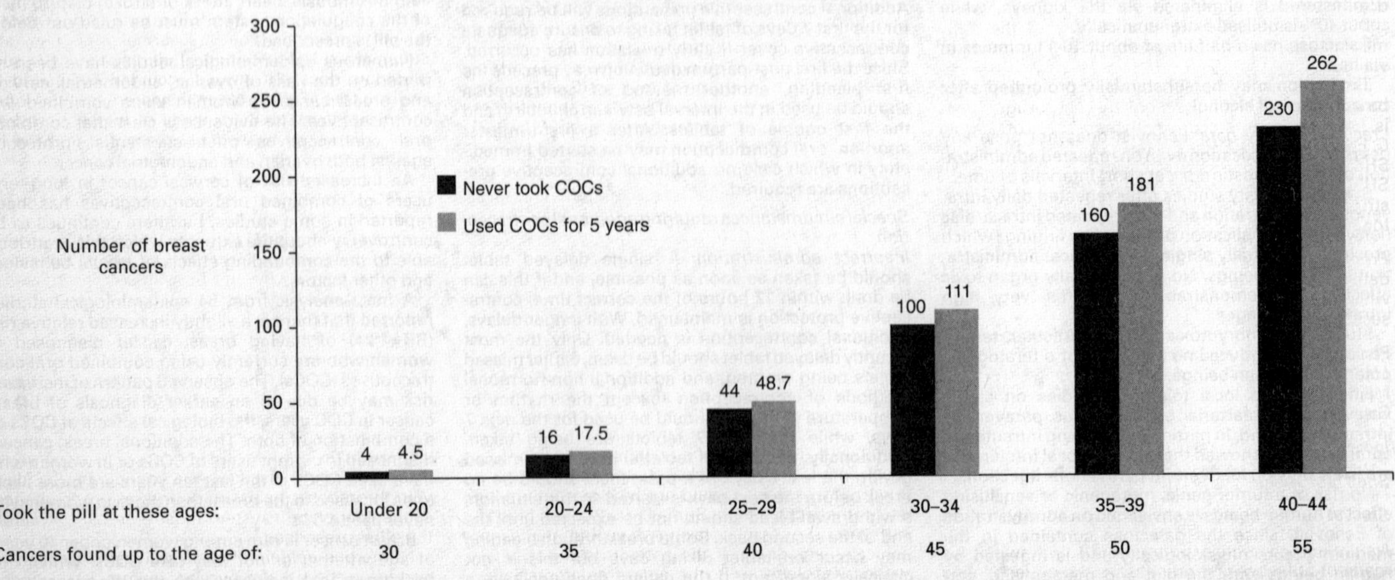

Pharmacokinetic properties: Levonorgestrel.

Orally administered levonorgestrel is rapidly and completely absorbed. Following ingestion of 0.25 mg levonorgestrel together with 0.03 mg ethinylestradiol, maximum drug serum levels of about 5 ng/ml can be expected at 1.0 hour. Thereafter, levonorgestrel serum levels decrease in two phases, characterized by half-lives of 0.5 hours and about 20 hours. For levonorgestrel, a metabolic clearance rate from serum of about 1.5 ml/min/kg was determined. Levonorgestrel is not excreted in unchanged form but as metabolites. Levonorgestrel metabolites are excreted at about equal proportions with urine and faeces. The biotransformation follows the known pathways of steroid metabolism. No pharmacologically active metabolites are known.

Levonorgestrel is bound to serum albumin and to SHBG. Only about 1.5% of the total serum drug levels are present as free steroid, but 65% are specifically bound to SHBG. The relative distribution (free, albumin-bound, SHBG-bound) depends on the SHBG concentrations in the serum. Following induction of the binding protein, the SHBG bound fraction increases while the unbound and the albumin-bound fraction decreases.

Following daily repeated administration, levonorgestrel concentrations in the serum increase by a factor of about 2. Steady-state conditions are reached during the second half of a treatment cycle. The pharmacokinetics of levonorgestrel is influenced by SHBG serum levels. Under treatment with Eugynon 30, an increase in the serum levels of SHBG affects a concomitant increase in the specific binding capacity and therefore also an increase in levonorgestrel serum levels. After 1–3 treatment cycles, there is no further change in the levonorgestrel serum levels to be expected, since the SHBG induction is not increased any more. The absolute bioavailability of levonorgestrel was determined to be almost 100% of the dose administered.

About 0.1% of the maternal dose can be transferred via milk to the nursed infant.

Ethinylestradiol.

Orally administered ethinylestradiol is rapidly and completely absorbed. Following ingestion of 0.25 mg levonorgestrel together with 0.03 mg ethinylestradiol, maximum drug serum levels of about 100 pg/ml can be expected at 1–2 hours. Thereafter, ethinylestradiol serum levels decrease in two phases characterized by half-lives of 1–2 hours and about 20 hours. Because of analytical reasons, these parameters can only be calculated following the administration of higher doses. For ethinylestradiol, an apparent volume of distribution of about 5 l/kg and a metabolic clearance rate from serum of about 5 ml/min/kg were determined. Ethinylestradiol is highly but non-specifically bound to serum albumin. About 2% of drug levels are present unbound. During absorption and first-liver passage, ethinylestradiol is metabolized resulting in a reduced absolute and variable oral bioavailability. Unchanged drug is not excreted. Ethinylestradiol metabolites are excreted at an urinary to biliary ratio of 4:6 with a half-life of about 1 day.

According to the half-life of the terminal disposition phase from serum and the daily ingestion, steady-state serum levels are reached after 3–4 days and are higher by 30–40% as compared to a single dose. The absolute bioavailability of ethinylestradiol is subject to a considerable interindividual variation. Following oral administration, the mean bioavailability was found to be about 40% to 60% of the administered dose.

During established lactation, 0.02% of the daily maternal dose could be transferred to the newborn via milk.

The systemic availability of ethinylestradiol might be influenced in both directions by other drugs. There is, however, no interaction with high doses of vitamin C. Ethinylestradiol induces the hepatic synthesis of SHBG and CBG during continuous use. The extent of SHBG induction, however, depends on the chemical structure and the dose of the co-administered progestogen.

Preclinical safety data: There are no preclinical safety data which could be of relevance to the prescriber and which are not already included in other relevant sections of the SPC.

Pharmaceutical particulars

List of excipients: Lactose, Maize starch, Povidone, Magnesium stearate (E 572), Sucrose, Macrogol 6000, Calcium carbonate (E 170), Talc, Montan glycol wax.

Incompatibilities: None known.

Shelf life: 5 years.

Special precautions for storage: Not applicable.

Nature and contents of container: Deep drawn strips made of polyvinyl chloride film with counter-sealing foil made of aluminium with heat sealable coating.

Presentation: Carton containing memo packs of either 1×21 tablets, 3×21 tablets or 50×21 tablets.

Instructions for use/handling: Keep out of the reach of children.

Marketing authorisation number 0053/0049

Date of first authorisation/renewal of the authorisation 25.9.98.

Date of (partial) revision of the text January 1998.

FEMODENE*

Presentation Each white sugar-coated tablet contains 75 micrograms gestodene and 30 micrograms ethinylestradiol.

Excipients: lactose, maize starch, povidone 25 000, sodium calcium edetate, magnesium stearate, sucrose, povidone 700 000, macrogol 6000, calcium carbonate, talc, montan glycol wax.

Uses Oral contraception and the recognised gynaecological indications for such oestrogen-progestogen combinations. The mode of action includes the inhibition of ovulation by suppression of the mid-cycle surge of luteinising hormone, the inspissation of cervical mucus so as to constitute a barrier to sperm, and the rendering of the endometrium unreceptive to implantation.

Dosage and administration

First treatment cycle: 1 tablet daily for 21 days, starting on the first day of the menstrual cycle. Contraceptive protection begins immediately.

Subsequent cycles: Tablet taking from the next pack of Femodene is continued after a 7-day interval, beginning on the same day of the week as the first pack.

Changing from 21-day combined oral contraceptives: The first tablet of Femodene should be taken on the first day immediately after the end of the previous oral contraceptive course. Additional contraceptive precautions are not required.

Changing from a combined Every Day pill (28 day tablets): Femodene should be started after taking the last active tablet from the Every Day Pill pack. The first Femodene tablet is taken the next day. Additional contraceptive precautions are not then required.

Changing from a progestogen-only pill (POP): The first tablet of Femodene should be taken on the first day of bleeding, even if a POP has already been taken on that day. Additional contraceptive precautions are not then required. The remaining progestogen-only pills should be discarded.

Post-partum and post-abortum use: After pregnancy, oral contraception can be started 21 days after a vaginal delivery, provided that the patient is fully ambulant and there are no puerperal complications. Additional contraceptive precautions will be required for the first 7 days of tablet taking. Since the first post-partum ovulation may precede the first bleeding, another method of contraception should be used in the interval between childbirth and the first course of tablets. After a first-trimester abortion, oral contraception may be started immediately in which case no additional contraceptive precautions are required.

Pregnancy and lactation: If pregnancy occurs during medication with oral contraceptives, the preparation should be withdrawn immediately (see *Reasons for stopping oral contraception immediately*).

The use of Femodene during lactation may lead to a reduction in the volume of milk produced and to a change in its composition. Minute amounts of the active substances are excreted with the milk. Mothers who are breast-feeding may be advised instead to use a progestogen-only pill.

Special circumstances requiring additional contraception

Incorrect administration: A single delayed tablet should be taken as soon as possible, and if this can be done within 12 hours of the correct time, contraceptive protection is maintained. With longer delays, additional contraception is needed. Only the most recently delayed tablet should be taken, earlier missed tablets being omitted, and additional non-hormonal methods of contraception (except the rhythm or temperature methods) should be used for the next 7 days, while the next 7 tablets are being taken. Additionally, therefore, if tablet(s) have been missed during the last 7 days of a pack, there should be no break before the next pack is started. In this situation, a withdrawal bleed should not be expected until the end of the second pack. Some breakthrough bleeding may occur on tablet taking days but this is not clinically significant. If the patient does not have a withdrawal bleed during the tablet-free interval following the end of the second pack, the possibility of pregnancy must be ruled out before starting the next pack.

Gastro-intestinal upset: Vomiting or diarrhoea may reduce the efficacy of oral contraceptives by preventing full absorption. Tablet-taking from the current pack should be continued. Additional non-hormonal methods of contraception (except the rhythm or temperature methods) should be used during the gastro-intestinal upset and for 7 days following the upset. If these 7 days overrun the end of a pack, the next pack should be started without a break. In this situation, a withdrawal bleed should not be expected until the end of the second pack. If the patient does not have a withdrawal bleed during the tablet-free interval following the end of the second pack, the possibility of pregnancy must be ruled out before starting the next pack. Other methods of contraception should be considered if the gastro-intestinal disorder is likely to be prolonged.

Interaction with other drugs: Hepatic enzyme inducers such as barbiturates, primidone, phenobarbitone, phenytoin, phenylbutazone, rifampicin, carbamazepine and griseofulvin can impair the efficacy of Femodene. For women receiving long-term therapy with hepatic enzyme inducers, another method of contraception should be used. The use of antibiotics may also reduce the efficacy of Femodene, possibly by altering the intestinal flora.

Women receiving short courses of enzyme inducers or broad spectrum antibiotics should take additional, non-hormonal (except rhythm or temperature method) contraceptive precautions during the time of concurrent medication and for 7 days afterwards. If these 7 days overrun the end of a pack, the next pack should be started without a break. In this situation, a withdrawal bleed should not be expected until the end of the second pack. If the patient does not have a withdrawal bleed during the tablet-free interval following the end of the second pack, the possibility of pregnancy must be ruled out before resuming with the next pack. With rifampicin, additional contraceptive precautions should be continued for 4 weeks after treatment stops, even if only a short course was administered.

The requirement for oral antidiabetics or insulin can change as a result of the effect on glucose tolerance.

Contra-indications, warnings, etc

Contra-indications:

1. Pregnancy
2. Severe disturbances of liver function, jaundice or persistent itching during a previous pregnancy, Dubin-Johnson syndrome, Rotor syndrome, previous or existing liver tumours
3. Existing or previous arterial or venous thrombotic or embolic processes, conditions which predispose to them, e.g. disorders of the clotting processes, valvular heart disease and atrial fibrillation
4. Sickle-cell anaemia
5. Mammary or endometrial carcinoma, or a history of these conditions
6. Severe diabetes mellitus with vascular changes
7. Disorders of lipid metabolism
8. History of herpes gestationis
9. Deterioration of otosclerosis during pregnancy
10. Undiagnosed abnormal vaginal bleeding
11. Hypersensitivity to any of the components of Femodene.

Warnings: There is a general opinion, based on statistical evidence, that users of combined oral contraceptives experience, more often than non-users, venous thromboembolism, arterial thrombosis, including cerebral and myocardial infarction, and subarachnoid haemorrhage. Full recovery from such disorders does not always occur and it should be realised that in a few cases they are fatal. How often these disorders occur in users of the modern low-dose pills is not known, but there are reasons for suggesting that they may occur less often than with older pills.

Certain factors may entail some risk of thrombosis, e.g. smoking, obesity, varicose veins, cardiovascular diseases, diabetes, and migraine. The suitability of a combined oral contraceptive should be judged according to the severity of such conditions in the individual case, and should be discussed with the patient before she decides to take it. The risk of arterial thrombosis associated with oral contraceptives increases with age, and this risk is aggravated by cigarette-smoking. The use of combined oral contraceptives by women in the older age-group, especially those who are cigarette smokers, should therefore be discouraged and alternative methods used.

In addition if there is a history in the family of thromboembolic diseases at a young age (e.g. deep vein thrombosis, heart attack or stroke) disturbances of the coagulation system must be ruled out before the pill is prescribed.

Numerous epidemiological studies have been reported on the risks of ovarian, endometrial, cervical and breast cancer in women using combined oral

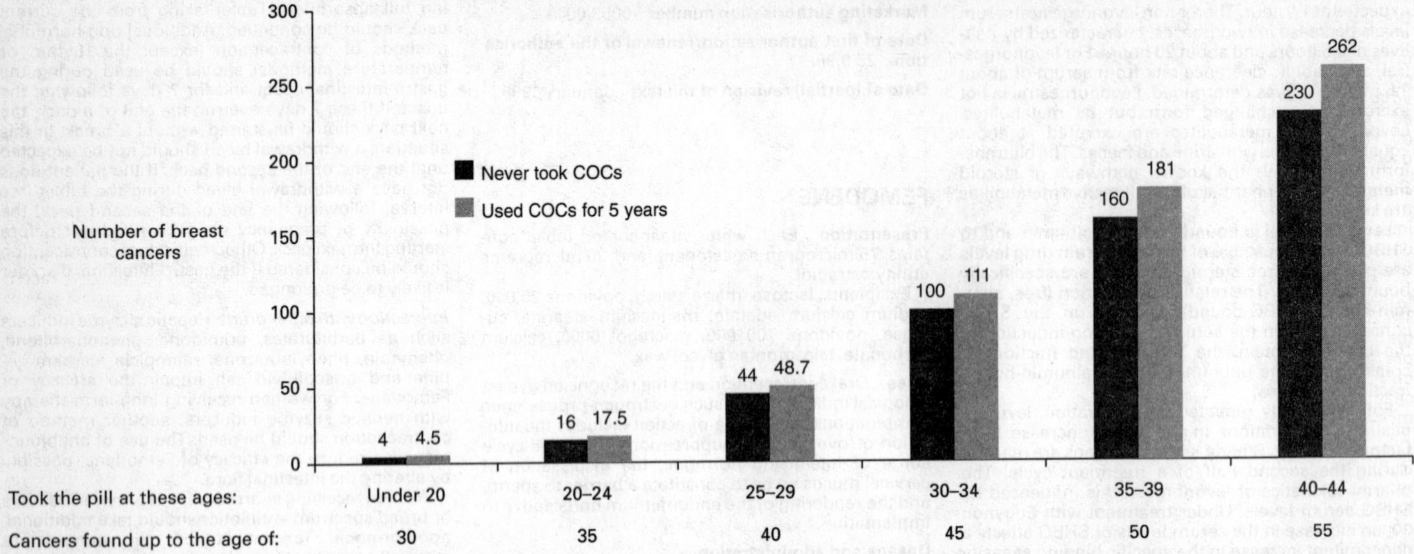

contraceptives. The evidence is clear that combined oral contraceptives offer substantial protection against both ovarian and endometrial cancer.

An increased risk of cervical cancer in long-term users of combined oral contraceptives has been reported in some studies, but there continues to be controversy about the extent to which this is attributable to the confounding effects of sexual behaviour and other factors.

A meta-analysis from 54 epidemiological studies reported that there is a slightly increased relative risk (RR=1.24) of having breast cancer diagnosed in women who are currently using combined oral contraceptives (COCs). The observed pattern of increased risk may be due to an earlier diagnosis of breast cancer in COC users, the biological effects of COCs or a combination of both. The additional breast cancers diagnosed in current users of COCs or in women who have used COCs in the last ten years are more likely to be localised to the breast than those in women who never used COCs.

Breast cancer is rare among women under 40 years of age whether or not they take COCs. Whilst this background risk increases with age, the excess number of breast cancer diagnoses in current and recent COC users is small in relation to the overall risk of breast cancer (see bar chart).

The most important risk factor for breast cancer in COC users is the age women discontinue the COC; the older the age at stopping, the more breast cancers are diagnosed. Duration of use is less important and the excess risk gradually disappears during the course of the 10 years after stopping COC use such that by 10 years there appears to be no excess.

The possible increase in risk of breast cancer should be discussed with the user and weighed against the benefits of COCs taking into account the evidence that they offer substantial protection against the risk of developing certain other cancers (e.g. ovarian and endometrial cancer).

The possibility cannot be ruled out that certain chronic diseases may occasionally deteriorate during the use of combined oral contraceptives (see *Precautions*). The combination of ethinylestradiol and gestodene, like other contraceptive steroids, is associated with an increased incidence of neoplastic nodules in the rat liver, the relevance of which to man is unknown. Malignant liver tumours have been reported on rare occasions in long-term users of oral contraceptives. In rare cases benign and, in even rarer cases, malignant liver tumours leading in isolated cases to life-threatening intra-abdominal haemorrhage have been observed after the use of hormonal substances such as those contained in Femodene. If severe upper abdominal complaints, liver enlargement or signs of intra-abdominal haemorrhage occur, the possibility of a liver tumour should be included in the differential diagnosis.

Reasons for stopping oral contraception immediately:

1. Occurrence for the first time, or exacerbation, of migrainous headaches or unusually frequent or unusually severe headaches
2. Sudden disturbances of vision or hearing or other perceptual disorders
3. First signs of thrombophlebitis or thromboembolic symptoms (e.g. unusual pains in or swelling of the leg(s), stabbing pains on breathing or coughing for no apparent reason). Feeling of pain and tightness in the chest
4. Six weeks before an elective major operation (e.g. abdominal, orthopaedic), any surgery to the legs, medical treatment for varicose veins or prolonged immobilisation, e.g. after accidents or surgery. Do not restart until 2 weeks after full ambulation. In case of emergency surgery, thrombotic prophylaxis is usually indicated e.g. subcutaneous heparin
5. Onset of jaundice, hepatitis, itching of the whole body
6. Increase in epileptic seizures
7. Significant rise in blood pressure
8. Onset of severe depression
9. Severe upper abdominal pain or liver enlargement
10. Clear exacerbation of conditions known to be capable of deteriorating during oral contraception or pregnancy
11. Pregnancy is a reason for stopping immediately because it has been suggested by some investigations that oral contraceptives taken in early pregnancy may slightly increase the risk of foetal malformations. Other investigations have failed to support these findings. The possibility therefore cannot be excluded, but it is certain that if a risk exists at all, it is very small.

Precautions: Examination of the pelvic organs, breasts and blood-pressure should precede the prescribing of any combined oral contraceptive and should be repeated regularly. The family medical history should be carefully noted and disturbances of the clotting mechanism ruled out if any member of the family has suffered from thromboembolic disease (e.g. deep vein thrombosis, stroke, myocardial infarction) at a young age. Before starting treatment pregnancy must be excluded.

The following conditions require strict medical supervision during medication with oral contraceptives. Deterioration or first appearance of any of these conditions may indicate that use of the oral contraceptive should be discontinued:

Diabetes mellitus, or a tendency towards diabetes mellitus (e.g. unexplained glycosuria), hypertension, varicose veins, a history of phlebitis, otosclerosis, multiple sclerosis, epilepsy, porphyria, tetany, disturbed liver function, Sydenham's chorea, renal dysfunction, family history of clotting disorders, obesity, family history of breast cancer and patient history of benign breast disease, history of clinical depression, systemic lupus erythematosus, uterine fibroids, an intolerance of contact lenses, migraine, gall-stones, cardiovascular diseases, chloasma, asthma, or any disease that is prone to worsen during pregnancy.

Some women may experience amenorrhoea or oligomenorrhoea after discontinuation of oral contraceptives, especially when these conditions existed prior to use. Women should be informed of this possibility.

Side-effects: In rare cases headaches, gastric upsets, nausea, vomiting, breast tenderness, changes in bodyweight, changes in libido, depressive moods can occur.

In predisposed women, use of Femodene can sometimes cause chloasma which is exacerbated by exposure to sunlight. Individual cases of poor tolerance of contact lenses have been reported with the use of oral contraceptives. Contact lens wearers who develop changes in lens tolerance should be assessed by an ophthalmologist.

Menstrual changes:

1. Reduction of menstrual flow: This is not abnormal and it is to be expected in some patients. Indeed, it may be beneficial where heavy periods were previously experienced.

2. Missed menstruation: Occasionally, withdrawal bleeding may not occur at all. If the tablets have been taken correctly, pregnancy is very unlikely. If withdrawal bleeding fails to occur at the end of a second pack, the possibility of pregnancy must be ruled out before resuming with the next pack.

Intermenstrual bleeding: 'Spotting' or heavier 'breakthrough bleeding' sometimes occur during tablet taking, especially in the first few cycles, and normally cease spontaneously. Femodene should therefore be continued even if irregular bleeding occurs. If irregular bleeding is persistent, appropriate diagnostic measures to exclude an organic cause are indicated and may include curettage. This also applies in the case of spotting which occurs at irregular intervals in several consecutive cycles or which occurs for the first time after long use of Femodene.

Effect on blood chemistry: The use of oral contraceptives may influence the results of certain laboratory tests including biochemical parameters of liver, thyroid, adrenal and renal function, plasma levels of carrier proteins and lipid/lipoprotein fractions, parameters of carbohydrate metabolism and parameters of coagulation and fibrinolysis. Laboratory staff should therefore be informed about oral contraceptive use when laboratory tests are requested.

Overdosage: Overdosage may cause nausea, vomiting and, in females, withdrawal bleeding. There are no specific antidotes and treatment should be symptomatic.

Pharmaceutical precautions *Shelf-life* – Five years.

Legal category POM

Package quantities Individual packs containing three months' supply (OP)

Further information Nil

Product licence number 0053/0179

FEMODENE* ED

Presentation Each white sugar-coated tablet contains 75 micrograms gestodene and 30 micrograms ethinylestradiol.

In addition, there are 7 white placebo tablets which are larger.

Excipients: lactose, maize starch, povidone 25 000, sodium calcium edetate, magnesium stearate, sucrose, povidone 700 000, macrogol 6000, calcium carbonate, talc, montan glycol wax.

Uses Oral contraception and the recognised gynaecological indications for such oestrogen-progestogen combinations. The mode of action includes the inhibition of ovulation by suppression of the mid-cycle surge of luteinising hormone, the inspissation of cervical mucus so as to constitute a barrier to sperm, and the rendering of the endometrium unreceptive to implantation.

Dosage and administration
First treatment cycle: 1 tablet daily for 28 days, starting in the red sector on the first day of the menstrual cycle. The initial tablet is the one marked with the appropriate day of the week. In the first cycle only, an additional non-hormonal method of contraception (except the rhythm or temperature methods) must be used for the first 14 days of tablet taking.

Subsequent cycles: Tablet-taking is continuous, which means that the next pack of Femodene ED follows immediately without a break. A withdrawal bleed usually occurs when the placebo tablets are being taken.

Changing from another combined oral contraceptive: The first tablet of Femodene ED should be taken from the red sector immediately after the end of the previous oral contraceptive course. In the first cycle only, an additional non-hormonal method of contraception (except the rhythm or temperature methods) must be used for the first 14 days of tablet taking.

Changing from a progestogen-only pill (POP): The first tablet of Femodene ED should be taken from the red sector on the first day of bleeding, even if a POP has already been taken on that day. An additional non-hormonal method of contraception (except the rhythm or temperature methods) must be used for 14 days. The remaining progestogen-only pills should be discarded.

Post-partum and post-abortum use: After pregnancy, Femodene ED can be started 21 days after a vaginal delivery, provided that the patient is fully ambulant and there are no puerperal complications. Additional contraceptive precautions will be required for the first 14 days of tablet taking. Since the first post-partum ovulation may precede the first bleeding, another method of contraception should be used in the interval between childbirth and the first course of tablets. After a first-trimester abortion, oral contraception may be started immediately, in which case additional non-hormonal contraceptive precautions are required (except the rhythm or temperature methods) for the first 14 days of tablet taking in the first cycle of Femodene ED.

Pregnancy and lactation: If pregnancy occurs during medication with oral contraceptives, the preparation should be withdrawn immediately (see 'Reasons for stopping oral contraception immediately').

The use of Femodene ED during lactation may lead to a reduction in the volume of milk produced and to a change in its composition. Minute amounts of the active substances are excreted with the milk. Mothers who are breast-feeding may be advised instead to use a progestogen-only pill.

Special circumstances requiring additional contraception:
Incorrect administration: Errors in taking the 7 placebo tablets (i.e. the first 5 tablets in the red section and the 2 immediately before the red section) can be ignored. A single delayed active (small) tablet should be taken as soon as possible, and if this can be done within 12 hours of the correct time, contraceptive protection is maintained.

With longer delays in taking active tablets, additional contraception is needed. Only the most recently delayed tablet should be taken, earlier missed tablets being omitted, and additional non-hormonal methods of contraception (except the rhythm or temperature methods) should be used for *the next 7 days, while the next 7 active (small) tablets are being taken.* Therefore, if the 7 days additional contraception will extend beyond the Friday just before the red section (i.e. the last active tablet) the user should take the tablets up to and including that Friday, and start a new pack next day with the Saturday tablet in the red section i.e. discard the remaining tablets and go to an appropriate active tablet in the next pack. In this situation, a withdrawal bleed should not be expected until the end of the second pack. Some breakthrough bleeding may occur on tablet taking days but this is not clinically significant. If the patient does not have a withdrawal bleed following the end of the second pack, the possibility of pregnancy must be ruled out before starting the next pack.

Gastro-intestinal upset: Vomiting or diarrhoea may reduce the efficacy of oral contraceptives by preventing full absorption. Tablet taking from the current pack should be continued. Additional non-hormonal methods of contraception (except the rhythm or temperature methods) should be used during the gastro-intestinal upset and for 7 days following the upset. If these 7 days extend beyond the last active (small) tablet (i.e. the Friday just before the red section), any remaining tablets should be discarded and a new pack of Femodene ED started the next day with the Saturday tablet in the red section (i.e an appropriate active (small) tablet). In this situation, a withdrawal bleed should not be expected until the end of the second pack. If the patient does not have a withdrawal bleed at the end of the second pack, the possibility of pregnancy must be ruled out before starting the next pack. Other methods of contraception should be considered if the gastro-intestinal disorder is likely to be prolonged.

Interaction with other drugs: Hepatic enzyme inducers such as barbiturates, primidone, phenobarbitone, phenytoin, phenylbutazone, rifampicin, carbamazepine and griseofulvin can impair the efficacy of Femodene ED. For women receiving long-term therapy with hepatic enzyme inducers, another method of contraception should be used. The use of antibiotics may also reduce the efficacy of Femodene ED, possibly by altering the intestinal flora.

Women receiving short courses of enzyme inducers or broad spectrum antibiotics should take additional, non-hormonal (except rhythm or temperature method) contraceptive precautions during the time of concurrent medication and for 7 days afterwards. If these 7 days extend beyond the last active (small) tablet (i.e. the Friday just before the red section), any remaining tablets should be discarded and a new pack of Femodene ED started the next day with the Saturday tablet in the red section (i.e. an appropriate active (small) tablet). In this situation, a withdrawal bleed should not be expected until the end of the second pack. If the patient does not have a withdrawal bleed at the end of the second pack, the possibility of pregnancy must be ruled out before resuming with the next pack. With rifampicin, additional contraceptive precautions should be continued for 4 weeks after treatment stops, even if only a short course was administered.

The requirement for oral antidiabetics or insulin can change as a result of the effect on glucose tolerance.

Contra-indications, warnings, etc
Contra-indications:
1. Pregnancy
2. Severe disturbances of liver function, jaundice or persistent itching during a previous pregnancy, Dubin-Johnson syndrome, Rotor syndrome, previous or existing liver tumours
3. Existing or previous arterial or venous thrombotic or embolic processes, conditions which predispose to them e.g. disorders of the clotting processes, valvular heart disease and atrial fibrillation
4. Sickle-cell anaemia
5. Mammary or endometrial carcinoma, or a history of these conditions
6. Severe diabetes mellitus with vascular changes
7. Disorders of lipid metabolism
8. History of herpes gestationis
9. Deterioration of otosclerosis during pregnancy
10. Undiagnosed abnormal vaginal bleeding
11. Hypersensitivity to any of the components of Femodene ED.

Warnings: There is a general opinion, based on statistical evidence, that users of combined oral contraceptives experience, more often than non-users, venous thromboembolism, arterial thrombosis, including cerebral and myocardial infarction, and subarachnoid haemorrhage. Full recovery from such disorders does not always occur, and it should be realised that in a few cases they are fatal. How often these disorders occur in users of the modern low-dose pills is not known, but there are reasons for suggesting that they may occur less often than with older pills.

Certain factors may entail some risk of thrombosis, e.g. smoking, obesity, varicose veins, cardiovascular diseases, diabetes, and migraine. The suitability of a combined oral contraceptive should be judged according to the severity of such conditions in the individual case, and should be discussed with the patient before she decides to take it. The risk of arterial thrombosis associated with combined oral contraceptives increases with age, and this risk is aggravated by cigarette-smoking. The use of combined oral contraceptives by women in the older age-group, especially those who are cigarette smokers, should therefore be discouraged and alternative methods used.

In addition if there is a history in the family of thromboembolic diseases at a young age (e.g. deep vein thrombosis, heart attack or stroke) disturbances of the coagulation system must be ruled out before the pill is prescribed.

Numerous epidemiological studies have been reported on the risks of ovarian, endometrial, cervical and breast cancer in women using combined oral contraceptives. The evidence is clear that combined oral contraceptives offer substantial protection against both ovarian and endometrial cancer.

An increased risk of cervical cancer in long-term users of combined oral contraceptives has been reported in some studies, but there continues to be controversy about the extent to which this is attributable to the confounding effects of sexual behaviour and other factors.

A meta-analysis from 54 epidemiological studies reported that there is a slightly increased relative risk (RR=1.24) of having breast cancer diagnosed in women who are currently using combined oral contraceptives (COCs). The observed pattern of increased risk may be due to an earlier diagnosis of breast cancer in COC users, the biological effects of COCs or a combination of both. The additional breast cancers diagnosed in current users of COCs or in women who have used COCs in the last ten years are more likely to be localised to the breast than those in women who never used COCs.

Breast cancer is rare among women under 40 years of age whether or not they take COCs. Whilst this background risk increases with age, the excess number of breast cancer diagnoses in current and recent COC users is small in relation to the overall risk of breast cancer (see bar chart).

The most important risk factor for breast cancer in COC users is the age women discontinue the COC; the older the age at stopping, the more breast cancers are diagnosed. Duration of use is less important and the excess risk gradually disappears during the course of the 10 years after stopping COC use such that by 10 years there appears to be no excess.

The possible increase in risk of breast cancer should be discussed with the user and weighed against the benefits of COCs taking into account the evidence that they offer substantial protection against the risk of developing certain other cancers (e.g. ovarian and endometrial cancer).

The possibility cannot be ruled out that certain chronic diseases may occasionally deteriorate during the use of combined oral contraceptives (see *Precautions*).

The combination of ethinylestradiol and gestodene, like other contraceptive steroids, is associated with an increased incidence of neoplastic nodules in the rat liver, the relevance of which to man is unknown. Malignant liver tumours have been reported on rare occasions in long-term users of oral contraceptives.

In rare cases benign and, in even rarer cases, malignant liver tumours leading in isolated cases to life-threatening intra-abdominal haemorrhage have been observed after the use of hormonal substances such as those contained in Femodene ED. If severe upper abdominal complaints, liver enlargement or signs of intra-abdominal haemorrhage occur, the possibility of a liver tumour should be included in the differential diagnosis.

Reasons for stopping oral contraception immediately:
1. Occurrence for the first time, or exacerbation, of migrainous headaches or unusually frequent or unusually severe headaches
2. Sudden disturbances of vision or hearing or other perceptual disorders
3. First signs of thrombophlebitis or thromboembolic symptoms (e.g. unusual pains in or swelling of the leg(s), stabbing pains on breathing or coughing for no apparent reason). Feeling of pain and tightness in the chest
4. Six weeks before an elective major operation (e.g. abdominal, orthopaedic), any surgery to the legs, medical treatment for varicose veins or prolonged immobilisation, e.g. after accidents or surgery. Do not restart until 2 weeks after full ambulation. In case of emergency surgery, thrombotic prophylaxis is usually indicated e.g. subcutaneous heparin
5. Onset of jaundice, hepatitis, itching of the whole body
6. Increase in epileptic seizures
7. Significant rise in blood pressure
8. Onset of severe depression
9. Severe upper abdominal pain or liver enlargement
10. Clear exacerbation of conditions known to be capable of deteriorating during oral contraception or pregnancy
11. Pregnancy is a reason for stopping immediately because it has been suggested by some investigations that oral contraceptives taken in early pregnancy may slightly increase the risk of foetal malformations. Other investigations have failed to support these findings. The possibility therefore cannot be excluded, but it is certain that if a risk exists at all, it is very small.

Precautions: Examination of the pelvic organs, breasts and blood-pressure should precede the prescribing of any combined oral contraceptive and should be repeated regularly. The family medical history should be carefully noted and disturbances of the clotting mechanism ruled out if any member of the family has suffered from thromboembolic disease (e.g. deep vein thrombosis, stroke, myocardial infarction) at a young age. Before starting treatment pregnancy must be excluded.

The following conditions require strict medical supervision during medication with oral contraceptives. Deterioration or first appearance of any of these

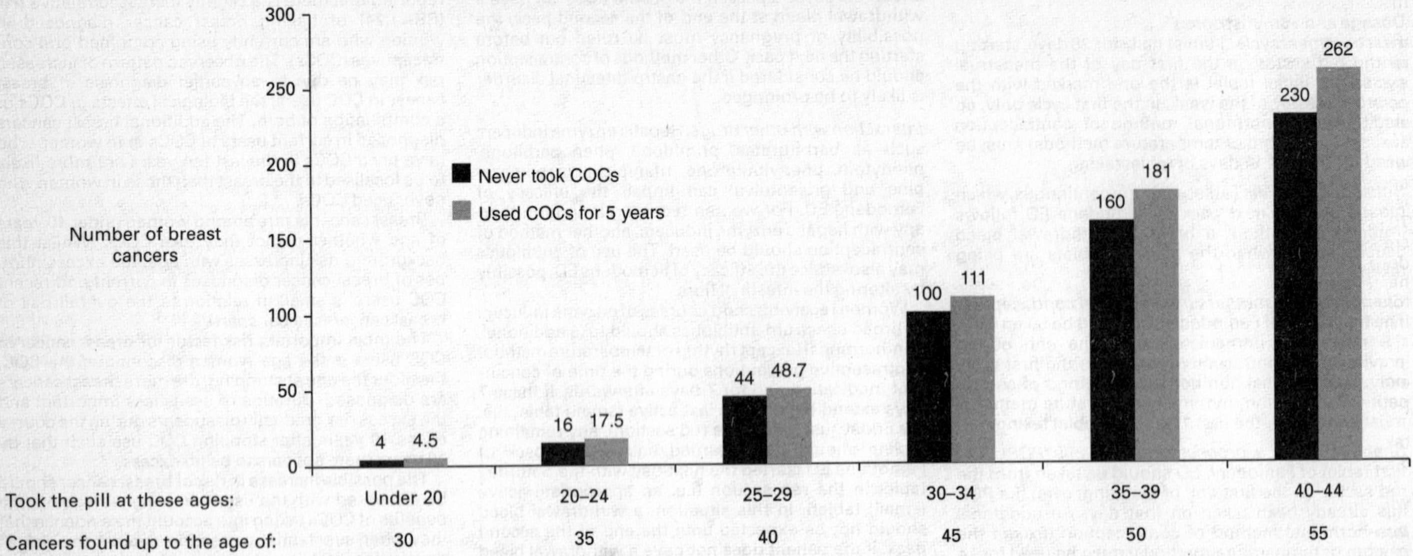

conditions may indicate that use of the oral contraceptive should be discontinued:

Diabetes mellitus, or a tendency towards diabetes mellitus (e.g. unexplained glycosuria), hypertension, varicose veins, a history of phlebitis, otosclerosis, multiple sclerosis, epilepsy, porphyria, tetany, disturbed liver function, Sydenham's chorea, renal dysfunction, family history of clotting disorders, obesity, family history of breast cancer and patient history of benign breast disease, history of clinical depression, systemic lupus erythematosus, uterine fibroids and migraine, gall-stones, cardiovascular diseases, chloasma, asthma, an intolerance of contact lenses, or any disease that is prone to worsen during pregnancy.

Some women may experience amenorrhoea or oligomenorrhoea after discontinuation of oral contraceptives, especially when these conditions existed prior to use. Women should be informed of this possibility.

Side-effects: In rare cases, headaches, gastric upsets, nausea, vomiting, breast tenderness, changes in body weight, changes in libido, depressive moods can occur.

In predisposed women, use of Femodene ED can sometimes cause chloasma which is exacerbated by exposure to sunlight. Such women should avoid prolonged exposure to sunlight.

Individual cases of poor tolerance of contact lenses have been reported with use of oral contraceptives. Contact lens wearers who develop changes in lens tolerance should be assessed by an ophthalmologist.

Menstrual changes:

1. Reduction of menstrual flow: This is not abnormal and it is to be expected in some patients. Indeed, it may be beneficial where heavy periods were previously experienced.

2. Missed menstruation: Occasionally, withdrawal bleeding may not occur at all. If the tablets have been taken correctly, pregnancy is very unlikely. If withdrawal bleeding fails to occur at the end of a second pack, the possibility of pregnancy must be ruled out before resuming with the next pack.

Intermenstrual bleeding: 'Spotting' or heavier 'breakthrough bleeding' sometimes occur during tablet taking, especially in the first few cycles, and normally cease spontaneously. Femodene ED should therefore, be continued even if irregular bleeding occurs. If irregular bleeding is persistent, appropriate diagnostic measures to exclude an organic cause are indicated and may include curettage. This also applies in the case of spotting which occurs at irregular intervals in several consecutive cycles or which occurs for the first time after long use of Femodene ED.

Effect on blood chemistry: The use of oral contraceptives may influence the results of certain laboratory tests including biochemical parameters of liver, thyroid, adrenal and renal function, plasma levels of carrier proteins and lipid/lipoprotein fractions, parameters of carbohydrate metabolism and parameters of coagulation and fibrinolysis. Laboratory staff should therefore be informed about oral contraceptive use when laboratory tests are requested.

Overdosage: Overdosage may cause nausea, vomiting and, in females, withdrawal bleeding. There are no specific antidotes and treatment should be symptomatic.

Pharmaceutical precautions Shelf-life–Five years.

Legal category POM

Package quantities Individual packs containing three months' supply (OP)

Further information Nil

Product licence number 0053/0180

FLUDARA*

Qualitative and quantitative composition Fludarabine phosphate 50 mg per vial.

Pharmaceutical form Fludara is supplied as a sterile lyophilised solid cake.

Clinical particulars

Therapeutic indications: Fludara is indicated for the treatment of patients with B-cell chronic lymphocytic leukaemia (CLL) who have not responded to or whose disease has progressed during or after treatment with at least one standard alkylating-agent containing regimen.

Posology and method of administration: Fludara should be administered under the supervision of a qualified physician experienced in the use of antineoplastic therapy.

It is strongly recommended that Fludara should be only administered intravenously. No cases have been reported in which paravenously administered Fludara led to severe local adverse reactions. However, the unintentional paravenous administration must be avoided.

Adults: The recommended dose is 25 mg fludarabine phosphate/m² body surface given daily for 5 consecutive days in every 28 days by the intravenous route. Each vial is to be made up in 2 ml water for injection. Each ml of the resulting solution will contain 25 mg fludarabine phosphate. Doses should be adjusted for patients with reduced kidney function. If creatinine clearance is between 30 and 70 ml/min, the dose should be reduced by up to 50% and close haematological monitoring should be used to assess toxicity. For further information see *Special warnings and special precautions for use.* Fludara treatment is contra-indicated, if creatinine clearance is <30 ml/min.

The required dose (calculated on the basis of the patient's body surface) is drawn up into a syringe. For intravenous bolus injection this dose is further diluted into 10 ml of 0.9% sodium chloride. Alternatively, the required dose drawn up in a syringe may be diluted into 100 ml 0.9% sodium chloride and infused over approximately 30 minutes.

The optimal duration of treatment has not been clearly established. It is recommended that Fludara be administered up to the achievement of a maximal response (usually 6 cycles) and then the drug should be discontinued.

Children: The safety and effectiveness of Fludara in children has not been established.

Contra-indications: Fludara is contra-indicated in those patients who are hypersensitive to this drug or its components and in renally impaired patients with creatinine clearance < 30 ml/min.

Fludara is contra-indicated during pregnancy and lactation.

Special warnings and special precautions for use: When used at high doses in dose-ranging studies in patients with acute leukaemia, Fludara was associated with severe neurologic effects, including blindness, coma and death. This severe central nervous system toxicity occurred in 36% of patients treated with doses approximately four times greater (96 mg/m²/day for 5–7 days) than the dose recommended for treatment of CLL. Similar severe central nervous system toxicity has been rarely (< 0.2%) reported in patients treated at doses in the range of the dose recommended for CLL. Patients should be closely observed for signs of neurologic side effects.

The effect of chronic administration of Fludara on the central nervous system is unknown. However, patients have received the recommended dose for up to 15 courses of therapy.

Severe bone marrow suppression, notably anaemia, thrombocytopenia and neutropenia, has been reported in patients treated with Fludara. In a Phase I study in solid tumour patients, the median time to nadir counts was 13 days (range, 3–25 days) for granulocytes and 16 days (range, 2–32) for platelets. Most patients had haematologic impairment at baseline either as a result of disease or as a result of prior myelosuppressive therapy. Cumulative myelosuppression may be seen. While chemotherapy-induced myelosuppression is often reversible, administration of fludarabine phosphate requires careful haematologic monitoring.

Fludara is a potent antineoplastic agent with potentially significant toxic side effects. Patients undergoing therapy should be closely observed for signs of haematologic and non-haematologic toxicity. Periodic assessment of peripheral blood counts is recommended to detect the development of anaemia, neutropenia and thrombocytopenia.

Transfusion-associated graft-versus-host disease has been observed rarely (approx. 0.18%) after transfusion of non-irradiated blood in Fludara treated patients. Fatal outcome as a consequence of this disease has been reported with a high frequency. Therefore, patients who require blood transfusion and who are undergoing, or who have received, treatment with Fludara should receive irradiated blood only.

Tumour lysis syndrome associated with Fludara treatment has been reported in CLL patients with large tumour burdens. Since Fludara can induce a response as early as the first week of treatment, precautions should be taken in those patients at risk of developing this complication.

Instances of life-threatening and sometimes fatal autoimmune haemolytic anaemia have been reported to occur during or after treatment with Fludara irrespective of any previous history of autoimmune haemolytic anaemia or Coombs test status. The majority of patients rechallenged with Fludara developed a recurrence in the haemolytic process.

Patients undergoing treatment with Fludara should be closely monitored for signs of autoimmune haemolytic anaemia (decline in haemoglobin linked with haemolysis and positive Coombs test). Discontinuation of therapy with Fludara is recommended in case of haemolysis. Blood transfusion (irradiated, see above) and adrenocorticoid preparations are the most common treatment measures for autoimmune haemolytic anaemia.

The total body clearance of the principle plasma metabolite 2-F-ara-A shows a correlation with creatinine clearance, indicating the importance of the renal excretion pathway for the elimination of the compound. Patients with reduced kidney function demonstrated an increased total body exposure (AUC of 2F-ara-A). Limited clinical data are available in patients with impairment of renal function (creatinine clearance below 70 ml/min). Therefore, if renal impairment is clinically suspected, or in patients over the age of 70 years, creatinine clearance should be measured. If creatinine clearance is between 30 and 70 ml/min, the dose should be reduced by up to 50% and close haematological monitoring should be used to assess toxicity. Fludara treatment is contraindicated, if creatinine clearance is <30 ml/min.

Since there are limited data for the use of Fludara in elderly persons (>75 years), caution should be exercised with the administration of Fludara in these patients.

Females of child-bearing potential or males must take contraceptive measures during and at least for 6 months after cessation of therapy.

During and after treatment with Fludara vaccination with live vaccines should be avoided.

Interaction with other medicaments and other forms of interaction: In a clinical investigation using Fludara in combination with pentostatin (deoxycoformycin) for the treatment of refractory chronic lymphocytic leukaemia (CLL), there was an unacceptably high incidence of fatal pulmonary toxicity. Therefore, the use of Fludara in combination with pentostatin is not recommended.

The therapeutic efficacy of Fludara may be reduced by dipyridamole and other inhibitors of adenosine uptake.

Pregnancy and lactation: There is no experience with the use of Fludara during pregnancy.

Embryotoxicity studies in animals demonstrated an embryotoxic and/or teratogenic potential posing a relevant risk to humans at the envisaged therapeutic dose. Preclinical data in rats demonstrated a transfer of fludarabine phosphate and/or metabolites through the feto-placental barrier.

Fludara should not be used during pregnancy.

Women of child-bearing potential should be advised to avoid becoming pregnant and to inform the treating physician immediately should this occur.

Use during lactation: It is not known whether this drug is excreted in human milk. However, there is evidence from preclinical data that fludarabine phosphate and/or metabolites transfer from maternal blood to milk. Therefore breast-feeding should be discontinued for the duration of Fludara therapy.

Effects on ability to drive and use machines: The effect of treatment with Fludara on the patient's ability to drive or operate machinery has not been evaluated.

Undesirable effects: The most common adverse events include myelosuppression (neutropenia, thrombocytopenia and anaemia), fever, chills and infection. Other commonly reported events include malaise, fatigue, anorexia, nausea, vomiting and weakness. Serious opportunistic infections have occurred in CLL patients treated with Fludara. Fatalities as a consequence of serious adverse events have been reported.

The most frequently reported adverse events and those reactions which are more clearly related to the drug are arranged below according to body system.

Haematopoietic system: Haematologic events (neutropenia, thrombocytopenia, and anaemia) have been reported in the majority of CLL patients treated with Fludara. Myelosuppression may be severe and cumulative.

Clinically significant haemolytic anaemia has been rarely reported in patients receiving Fludara (see *Special warnings and special precautions for use*).

Metabolic: Tumour lysis syndrome has been reported in CLL patients treated with Fludara. This complication may include hyperuricaemia, hyperphosphataemia, hypocalcaemia, metabolic acidosis, hyperkalaemia, haematuria, urate crystalluria, and renal failure. The onset of this syndrome may be heralded by flank pain and haematuria.

Changes of hepatic and pancreatic enzymes are possible.

Nervous system: In rare cases, weakness, agitation, confusion, visual disturbances occurred in CLL patients. Peripheral neuropathy and coma have been observed.

Pulmonary system: Pneumonia has occurred in association with Fludara treatment. Pulmonary hypersensitivity reactions to Fludara characterised by dyspnoea, cough and interstitial pulmonary infiltrate have been observed.

Gastrointestinal system: Gastrointestinal disturbances such as nausea and vomiting, anorexia, diarrhoea, stomatitis and gastrointestinal bleeding have been reported in patients treated with Fludara.

Cardiovascular: Oedema has been reported frequently.

Genitourinary system: Rare cases of haemorrhagic cystitis have been reported in patients treated with Fludara.

Skin: Skin rashes have been reported in patients treated with Fludara.

In extremely rare cases a toxic epidermal necrolysis (Lyell's disease) may develop.

Overdose: High doses of Fludara have been associated with an irreversible central nervous system toxicity characterised by delayed blindness, coma, and death. High doses are also associated with severe thrombocytopenia and neutropenia due to bone marrow suppression. There is no known specific antidote for Fludara overdosage. Treatment consists of drug discontinuation and supportive therapy.

Pharmacological properties

Pharmacodynamic properties: Fludara contains fludarabine phosphate, a fluorinated nucleotide analogue of the antiviral agent vidarabine, 9-β-D-arabinofuranosyladenine (ara-A) that is relatively resistant to deamination by adenosine deaminase.

Fludarabine phosphate is rapidly dephosphorylated to 2F-ara-A which is taken up by cells and then phosphorylated intracellularly by deoxycytidine kinase to the active triphosphate, 2F-ara-ATP. This metabolite has been shown to inhibit ribonucleotide reductase, DNA polymerase α/δ and ε, DNA primase and DNA ligase thereby inhibiting DNA synthesis. Furthermore, partial inhibition of RNA polymerase II and consequent reduction in protein synthesis occur.

While some aspects of the mechanism of action of 2F-ara-ATP are as yet unclear, it is assumed that effects on DNA, RNA and protein synthesis all contribute to inhibition of cell growth with inhibition of DNA synthesis being the dominant factor. In addition, *in vitro* studies have shown that exposure of CLL lymphocytes to 2F-ara-A triggers extensive DNA fragmentation and cell death characteristic of apoptosis.

Pharmacokinetic properties: Plasma and urinary pharmacokinetics of fludarabine (2F-ara-A):

The pharmacokinetics of fludarabine (2F-ara-A) have been studied after intravenous administration by rapid bolus injection and short-term infusion as well as following continuous infusion of fludarabine phosphate (Fludara, 2F-ara-AMP). 2F-ara-AMP is a water-soluble prodrug, which is rapidly and quantitatively dephosphorylated in the human organism to the nucleoside fludarabine (2F-ara-A). After single dose infusion of 25 mg 2F-ara-AMP per m^2 to cancer patients for 30 minutes 2F-ara-A reached mean maximum concentrations in the plasma of 3.5–3.7 μM at the end of the infusion. Corresponding 2F-ara-A levels after the fifth dose showed a moderate accumulation with mean maximum levels of 4.4–4.8 μM at the end of infusion. During a 5-day treatment schedule 2F-ara-A plasma trough levels increased by a factor of about 2. An accumulation of 2F-ara-A over several treatment cycles can be excluded. Postmaximum levels decayed in three disposition phases with an initial half-life of approx. 5 minutes, an intermediate half-life of 1 - 2 hours and a terminal half-life of approx. 20 hours.

An interstudy comparison of 2F-ara-A pharmacokinetics resulted in a mean total plasma clearance (CL) of 79±40 ml/min/m^2 (2.2±1.2 ml/min/kg) and a mean volume of distribution (Vss) of 83±55 l/m^2 (2.4±1.6 l/kg). Data showed a high interindividual variability. Plasma levels of 2F-ara-A and areas under the plasma level time curves increased linearly with the dose, whereas half-lives, plasma clearance and volumes of distribution were independent of the dose indicating a dose linear behaviour.

Occurrence of neutropenia and haematocrit changes indicated that the cytotoxicity of fludarabine phosphate depresses the haematopoiesis in a dose dependent manner.

2F-ara-A elimination is largely by renal excretion. 40 to 60% of the administered i.v. dose was excreted in the urine. Mass balance studies in laboratory animals with ^{3}H-2F-ara-AMP showed a complete recovery of radio-labelled substances in the urine. Another metabolite, 2F-ara-hypoxanthine, which represents the major metabolite in the dog, was not observed in humans. Individuals with impaired renal function exhibit a reduced total body clearance, indicating the need for a dose reduction. *In vitro* investigations with human plasma proteins revealed no pronounced tendency of 2F-ara-A protein binding.

Cellular pharmacokinetics of fludarabine triphosphate:

2F-ara-A is actively transported into leukaemic cells, whereupon it is rephosphorylated to the monophosphate and subsequently to the di- and triphosphate. The triphosphate 2F-ara-ATP is the major intracellular metabolite and the only metabolite known to have cytotoxic activity. Maximum 2F-ara-ATP levels in leukaemic lymphocytes of CLL patients were observed at a median of 4 hours and exhibited a considerable variation with a median peak concentration of approx. 20 μM. 2F-ara-ATP levels in leukaemic cells were always considerably higher than maximum 2F-ara-A levels in the plasma indicating an accumulation at the target sites. *In vitro* incubation of leukaemic lymphocytes showed a linear relationship between extracellular 2F-ara-A exposure (product of 2F-ara-A concentration and duration of incubation) and intracellular 2F-ara-ATP enrichment. 2F-ara-ATP elimination from target cells showed median half-life values of 15 and 23 hours.

No clear correlation was found between 2F-ara-A pharmacokinetics and treatment efficacy in cancer patients.

Preclinical safety data: In acute toxicity studies, single intravenous doses of fludarabine phosphate produced severe intoxication symptoms or death at dosages about two orders of magnitude above the therapeutic dose. As expected for a cytotoxic compound, the bone marrow, lymphoid organs, gastrointestinal mucosa, kidneys and male gonads were affected. In patients, severe side effects were observed closer to the recommended therapeutic dose (factor 3 to 4) and included severe neurotoxicity partly with lethal outcome (cf. *Overdose*).

Systemic toxicity studies following repeated administration of fludarabine phosphate showed also the expected effects on rapidly proliferating tissues above a threshold dose. The severity of morphological manifestations increased with dose levels and duration of dosing and the observed changes were generally considered to be reversible. In principle, the available experience from the therapeutic use of Fludara points to a comparable toxicological profile in humans, although additional undesirable effects such as neurotoxicity were observed in patients (cf. *Undesirable effects*).

The results from animal embryotoxicity studies indicated a teratogenic potential of fludarabine phosphate. In view of the small safety margin between the teratogenic doses in animals and the human therapeutic dose as well as in analogy to other antimetabolites which are assumed to interfere with the process of differentation, the therapeutic use of Fludara is associated with a relevant risk of teratogenic effects in humans (cf. *Pregnancy and lactation*).

Fludarabine phosphate has been shown to induce chromosomal aberrations in an in vitro cytogenetic assay, to cause DNA-damage in a sister chromatid exchange test and to increase the rate of micronuclei in the mouse micronucleus test in vivo, but was negative in gene mutation assays. In view of these results, the known activity of the compound at the DNA-level and in analogy to other antimetabolites, fludarabine phosphate is expected to have a mutagenic potential.

The known activity of fludarabine at the DNA-level and the mutagenicity test results form the basis for the suspicion of a tumorigenic potential. No animal studies which directly address the question of tumorigenicity have been conducted, because the suspicion of an increased risk of second tumours due to Fludara therapy can exclusively be verified by epidemiological data.

According to the results from animal experiments following intravenous administration of fludarabine phosphate, no remarkable local irritation has to be expected at the injection site. Even in case of misplaced injections, no relevant local irritation was observed after paravenous, intraarterial, and intramuscular administration of an aqueous solution containing 7.5 mg fludarabine phosphate/ml.

Pharmaceutical particulars

List of excipients: Each vial of Fludara contains 50 mg of mannitol. Sodium hydroxide is present to adjust the pH to 7.7.

Incompatibilities: Must not be mixed with other drugs.

Shelf life: The shelf life of Fludara stored as a lyophilised solid cake in glass vials is 24 months at up to 30°C. Reconstituted Fludara should be used within 8 hours of reconstitution. Fludara contains no antimicrobial preservative. Care must be taken to assure the sterility of prepared solutions.

Special precautions for storage: Store at room temperature (maximum 30°C).

Nature and contents of container: Fludara is supplied in clear glass single dose vials containing 50 mg fludarabine phosphate.

Instructions for use, handling and disposal (if appropriate): Fludara should be prepared for parenteral use by aseptically adding sterile water for injection. When reconstituted with 2 ml of sterile water for injection, the solid cake should fully dissolve in 15 seconds or less. Each ml of the resulting solution will contain

25 mg of fludarabine phosphate, 25 mg of mannitol, and sodium hydroxide to adjust the pH to 7.7. The pH range for the final product is 7.2–8.2. In clinical studies, the product has been diluted in 100 ml or 125 ml of 5% dextrose injection or 0.9% sodium chloride.

Handling and disposal: Fludara should not be handled by pregnant staff.

Procedures for proper handling and disposal should be observed. Consideration should be given to handling and disposal according to guidelines used for cytotoxic drugs. Any spillage or waste material may be disposed of by incineration.

Caution should be exercised in the handling and preparation of the Fludara solution. The use of latex gloves and safety glasses is recommended to avoid exposure in case of breakage of the vial or other accidental spillage. If the solution comes into contact with the skin or mucous membranes, the area should be washed thoroughly with soap and water. In the event of contact with the eyes, rinse them thoroughly with copious amounts of water. Exposure by inhalation should be avoided.

Marketing authorisation number PL 0053/0239

Date of approval/revision of SPC 12 February 1998

Legal category POM

GASTROGRAFIN*

Qualitative and quantitative composition 1 ml solution contains: 100 mg sodium amidotrizoate (sodium diatrizoate) and 660 mg meglumine amidotrizoate (meglumine diatrizoate).

Pharmaceutical form Aqueous solution for enteral use

Clinical particulars

Therapeutic indications: Gastrografin is designed for investigation of the gastrointestinal tract. It can be used either orally or as an enema. Follow-through examinations with barium can often be improved by combining it with Gastrografin. Gastrografin may be of particular value in the following instances:

1. Suspected partial or complete stenosis
2. Acute haemorrhage
3. Threatening perforation (peptic ulcer, diverticulum)
4. Other acute conditions which are likely to require surgery
5. After resection of the stomach or intestine (danger of perforation or leak)
6. Megacolon
7. Visualisation of a foreign body or tumour before endoscopy
8. Visualisation of a gastrointestinal fistula
9. Before endoscopy.

Further indications: Early diagnosis of a radiologically undetectable perforation or anastomotic defect in the oesophagus.

The treatment of uncomplicated meconium ileus.

Computerised tomography in the abdominal region.

Posology and method of administration: Oral–Adults and children of 10 years of age or over: 60 ml Gastrografin are sufficient for the visualisation of the stomach. Up to 100 ml may be needed for a follow-through examination of the gastrointestinal tract.

For computed tomography, 1 to 1.5 litres of a 3% solution of Gastrografin in water (30 ml/litre).

For elderly or cachectic patients: Dilution with an equal volume of water is recommended.

Children up to 10 years of age: 15–30 ml are usually sufficient. This dose may be diluted with twice its volume of water.

For infants and young children: Dilution of 15–30 ml of the contrast medium with three times its volume of water is recommended.

Rectal–Adults: The contrast medium should be diluted with three to four times its volume of water. Not more than 500 ml of Gastrografin solution should normally be required.

Children: The contrast medium should be diluted with four to five times its volume of water; up to five years of age the weaker dilution should be used.

Gastrografin and Barium Sulphate: Oral and rectal administration.

Adults: 30 ml Gastrografin plus the usual dose of barium should be adequate.

Children: 10 ml Gastrografin may be added to the barium.

For children up to five years of age: from 2–5 ml Gastrografin to 100 ml barium may be preferable.

Further dilution which does not affect the contrast may be used if necessary in cases of pylorospasm or pyloric stenosis.

For the early diagnosis of a perforation or investigation of an anastomosis in the oesophagus or gastrointestinal tract, the patient should drink 100 ml Gastrografin. After 30–60 minutes (later, if the defect is suspected of being in the distal gut), a urine specimen should be taken and 5 ml mixed with 5 drops of concentrated hydrochloric acid. The contrast medium which has undergone renal excretion will appear within two hours as a typical crystal formation in the precipitate.

Technique for the treatment of uncomplicated meconium ileus: Gastrografin can be given by enema to infants for non-operative treatment of uncomplicated meconium ileus in the absence of, e.g. volvulus, gangrene, perforation, peritonitis or atresia, all of which require immediate operation.

A large syringe and soft rubber catheter, No. 8 French, are recommended. The buttocks can be taped tightly together to minimise leakage but a balloon catheter should not be used. The procedure must be carried out slowly and only under fluoroscopic control. Injection should stop as soon as Gastrografin is seen to enter the ileum. Owing to its high osmolarity, Gastrografin may cause the loss of a large amount of fluid into the intestines. An intravenous drip must therefore be set up before the enema is given and plasma should be infused as required. If the Gastrografin is not expelled during the first hour after removal of the rectal catheter, an X-ray should be taken to ensure that overdistension of the bowel as a result of the high osmolarity of Gastrografin has not occurred.

Contra-indications: Hypersensitivity to iodine-containing contrast media. Manifest hyperthyroidism.

Special warnings and special precautions for use: The need for examination merits particularly careful consideration in the case of latent hyperthyroidism, benign nodular goitre, in dehydrated patients and in babies and young children. Disturbances in water or electrolyte balance must first be corrected.

Because of its high osmolality and minimal absorption, Gastrografin should not be administered to infants in higher doses than those recommended above. Caution should be observed in patients with thyroid disease. Aspiration of Gastrografin into the lungs may cause pulmonary oedema. Caution is needed with oesophagotracheal fistulae to avoid passage of the medium into the lungs.

Systemic effects are rare, since Gastrografin is only minimally absorbed from the alimentary tract.

Because of the additives (flavourings and a wetting agent), Gastrografin must not be used intravascularly.

Interaction with other medicaments and other forms of interaction: If iodine isotopes are to be administered for diagnosing thyroid disease, it should be borne in mind that after the administration of iodised contrast media which are excreted via the kidneys, the capacity of the thyroid tissue to take up iodine will be reduced for 2 weeks and sometimes up to 6 weeks.

Hypersensitivity reactions can be aggravated in patients on beta-blockers.

The prevalence of delayed reactions (e.g. fever,rash, flu-like symptoms, joint pain and pruritus) to contrast media is higher in patients who have received interleukin.

Pregnancy and lactation: X-ray examinations should, if possible, be avoided during pregnancy. It has not yet been proved beyond question that Gastrografin may be used without hesitation in pregnant patients. Therefore, an examination with a contrast medium during pregnancy should be carried out only if considered absolutely necessary by the physician.

Effects on ability to drive and to use machines: None known.

Undesirable Effects: Nausea and vomiting occur in exceptional cases. Urticarial skin reactions have occasionally been observed, while anaphylactoid reactions and shock are possible.

Owing to its hypertonicity, Gastrografin may occasionally cause diarrhoea, but this ceases as soon as the intestine has been emptied.

Existing enteritis or colitis may be temporarily exacerbated.

Overdose: There are no specific antidotes to Gastrografin. Treatment should be symptomatic.

Pharmacological properties

Pharmacodynamic properties: Gastrografin does not exert a pharmacological effect. It is an iodine containing contrast medium, iodine being radio-opaque.

Pharmacokinetic properties: Only 3% of amidotrizoic acid, the radio-opaque agent of Gastrografin, is absorbed following oral administration. If a perforation of the gastrointestinal tract is present, Gastrografin finds its way into the abdominal cavity or the surrounding tissue, where it is absorbed and finally excreted via the kidneys.

Preclinical safety data: There are no preclinical data which could be of relevance to the prescriber and which are not already included in other relevant sections of the SPC.

Pharmaceutical particulars

List of excipients: disodium edetate, saccharin sodium, anise oil,polysorbate 80, water for injection.

Incompatibilities: None known.

Shelf life: Three years.

Special precautions for storage: Protect from light and X-rays. Store below 25°C.

Nature and contents of container: Packs of 5 x 100 ml brown glass bottles with pilfer proof screw caps.

Instructions for use/handling: At temperatures below 7°C Gastrografin tends to crystallise, but this can be reversed by gently warming and shaking the bottle. This phenomenon has no effect on the effectiveness or stability of the preparation.

Marketing Authorisation Number PL 0053/5023R

Date of approval/revision of SPC 5 February 1997

Legal category POM

ISOVIST*

Presentation Bottles containing colourless sterile aqueous solutions of various strengths of the non-ionic dimeric contrast medium, iotrolan. Isovist 240 contains 240 mg iodine per ml; Isovist 300 contains 300 mg iodine per ml.

Excipients: Isovist 240: calcium disodium edetate, sodium bicarbonate, sodium chloride, water for injection.

Isovist 300: calcium disodium edetate, sodium chloride, sodium bicarbonate, water for injection.

Uses Isovist is intended for intrathecal use, i.e. radiculography and myelography of all regions, for ventriculography, evaluation of the circulation of cerebrospinal fluid and cisternography by computed tomography, and for use in other body cavities.

Dosage and administration

General information: The patient should attend for myelographic examination fasting but adequately hydrated. Disorders of water and electrolyte balance must be corrected, particularly in patients prone to this type of disorder.

Nervous patients may be given a suitable sedative (e.g. diazepam) prophylactically. No local anaesthesia is required if thin puncture needles are used. If antiemetics are administered, they should not possess neuroleptic properties.

After myelographic investigations–particularly of higher regions–the patient should be confined to bed with head raised for at least 6 hours, and remain passive for 24 hours.

Patients with a known or suspected low seizure threshold must be kept under careful observation for eight hours.

Isovist should not be drawn up into the syringe until immediately before use. Contrast medium not used in one examination must be discarded.

Dosage: The concentration and volume of Isovist chosen depend on the radiological equipment available. If equipment is available that allows films to be taken in all necessary projections without the patient having to move, and with which the injection can be performed under fluoroscopic control, iodine concentrations and volumes of medium at the lower end of the specified range can be used.

Higher concentrations are indicated if it will be necessary to reposition the patient during a myelographic examination, since the medium becomes diluted more quickly as a result of turbulence, and the clarity of detail deteriorates.

Radiculography (excluding the medullary cone)–7–10 ml Isovist 240.

Lumbar myelography (with thoracic transition)–7–12 ml Isovist 240/300.

Thoracic myelography–10–15 ml Isovist 240. 8–12 ml Isovist 300.

Panmyelography (injection in the lumbar region)–10–15 ml Isovist 240/300.

Cervical myelography–Direct (lateral access between C_1/C_2). 8–12 ml Isovist 240. 7–10 ml Isovist 300.

Indirect (injection in the lumbar region). 15 ml Isovist 240. 8–15 ml Isovist 300.

Ventriculography–3–5 ml Isovist 240. 3–5 ml Isovist 300.

CT-cisternography (injection in the lumbar region) –4–12 ml Isovist 240, 4-10 ml Isovist 300

Administration of the contrast medium in myelography: After withdrawal of the volume of cerebrospinal fluid (CSF) needed for examination, the appropriate dose of Isovist is injected. N.B. The more the patient moves after the administration of Isovist, the quicker will the medium mix with the CSF and the density of contrast decrease.

Other body cavities

Indirect lymphography (e.g. lymphoedema)–5–20 ml Isovist 300.

Arthrography 2–15 ml Isovist 240/300

Hysterosalpingography–10–25 ml Isovist 240/300.

Mammary ducts–1–3 ml Isovist 240/300.

Endoscopic retrograde cholangiopancreatography–10–30 ml Isovist 240/300.

Oesophagus–stomach–bowel–10–100 ml Isovist 300.

In the administration of contrast medium for indirect lymphography, multiple simultaneous interstitial (e.g. intracutaneous) injections are to be preferred.

Contra-indications, warnings etc

Contra-indications: Uncontrolled thyrotoxicosis.

Hysterosalpingography must not be carried out during pregnancy or in the presence of acute inflammatory conditions in the pelvic cavity.

Use in pregnancy: X-ray examinations should, if possible, be avoided during pregnancy. It has not yet been proved beyond question that Isovist may be used without hesitation in pregnant patients. Therefore, examination with Isovist during pregnancy should be carried out only if considered essential.

Warnings/side-effects: Epilepsy is a relative contraindication for myelography. If, after careful consideration, myelography is considered necessary, equipment and drugs necessary to treat any convulsion that may occur must be readily available. Neuroleptics or antidepressants should be discontinued 48 hours before the examination, because they lower the seizure threshold. Alcoholics and drug addicts may have a lowered seizure threshold. Anticonvulsants (e.g. phenobarbitone 200 mg i.m.) may be given prophylactically.

Hypersensitivity reactions can be aggravated in patients on beta-blockers. The prevalence of delayed reactions to contrast media is higher in patients who have received interleukin.

Hyperthyroidism may be exacerbated. Iodinated contrast media reduce the capacity of the thyroid gland to take up radio-isotopes of iodine for up to 2 weeks, and sometimes longer. Patients with a history of allergy may be particularly susceptible to hypersensitivity reactions. Such reactions are possible in any patient, but are rare in the recommended indications.

The most frequently reported symptoms are headache, nausea and vomiting. However, experience shows that their incidence is no higher than after the loss of pressure in the subarachnoid space that results from a diagnostic tap of CSF from the spinal canal. In view of this, an effort should be made to remove only as much CSF as is being replaced by the Isovist solution. On the other hand, administration of an amount of Isovist greater than the amount of CSF removed does not lead to an increase in CSF pressure.

Severe side-effects are extremely rare when Isovist is administered in the recommended dosages. Minor side-effects include pain or an increase in existing pain in the back, nape or extremities, and, rarely, very brief non-specific EEG changes. Delayed reactions can occasionally occur. Slight muscular tension or paraesthesia has been reported in rare cases 2-6 hours after administration of the medium.

Severe headaches lasting several days occur rarely. If convulsions occur, give 10 mg diazepam immediately by slow i.v. injection, followed, 20-30 minutes after the subsidence of the convulsions, by 200 mg phenobarbitone i.m. to prevent recurrence, unless this has been given prophylactically. Diazepam should be injected i.v. as a precaution at the first signs of hyperactivity or muscular twitching.

As with other myelographic agents, the CSF cell-count increases somewhat after intrathecal injection of Isovist. Very rarely, headaches, nausea, vomiting, stiffness of the neck and an increased cell-count in the CSF may mimic aseptic meningitis. All symptoms have usually disappeared within a week. Arachnoiditis has not been reported.

Isovist is excreted renally. Therefore, for patients with severe impairment of renal function, proven or suspected hypersensitivity to iodine-containing contrast media, latent hyperthyroidism and benign nodular goitre, the need for examination with Isovist merits careful consideration.

Ready availability of all drugs and equipment for emergency treatment and familiarity with the relevant procedures are prerequisites for the effective management of contrast-medium incidents.

Overdosage: Acute symptoms of poisoning are unlikely with intrathecal administration. Treatment is symptomatic.

Pharmaceutical precautions Protect from light and secondary X-rays. Store below 30°C. Shelf-life–Five years.

Because of possible precipitation, X-ray contrast media and prophylactic agents must not be injected as mixed solutions.

Legal category POM

Package quantities Isovist 240: Box containing 10 bottles of 10 ml. Box containing 10 bottles of 20 ml.

Isovist 300: Box containing 10 bottles of 10 ml.

Further information Isovist is a series of non-ionic, dimeric, water-soluble contrast media with osmolalities close to those of normal body fluids. Isovist 240–270 mosm/kg H_2O at 37°C. Isovist 300–320 mosm/kg H_2O at 37°C.

Product licence numbers
Isovist 240 0053/0201
Isovist 300 0053/0202

LEVOVIST* ▼

Qualitative and quantitative composition 1 g granules contains 999 mg galactose and 1 mg palmitic acid.

Physico–chemical properties

Max. osmolality at 37°C solution	200 mg/ml	1175 mosmol/kg
	300 mg/ml	1965 mosmol/kg
	400 mg/ml	2894 mosmol/kg
"Effective" osmolality at 25°C filtrate	200 mg/ml	910 mosmol/kg
	300 mg/ml	980 mosmol/kg
	400 mg/ml	950 mosmol/kg
Viscosity at 25°C filtrate	200 mg/ml	1.4 mPa.s
	300 mg/ml	1.4 mPa.s
	400 mg/ml	1.4 mPa.s
suspension	200 mg/ml	1.4 mPa.s
	300 mg/ml	3.6 mPa.s
	400 mg/ml	8.0 mPa.s

Pharmaceutical form Sterile granulated powder for injection. For peripheral intravenous administration, after reconstitution with the diluent provided (water for injection) to obtain concentrations of 200, 300 and 400 mg microparticles per ml suspension.

Clinical particulars

Therapeutic indications: One– and two–dimensional Doppler sonographic blood flow imaging in patients, where there is insufficient Doppler signal intensity. B–mode contrast echocardiography.

Posology and method of administration: The suspension has to be prepared according to instructions immediately before administration.

The following dosages are recommended:

Adults:

ONE– AND TWO–DIMENSIONAL DOPPLER SONOGRAPHY

Vascular Doppler sonography: In the case of moderately well detectable but diagnostically unsatisfactory Doppler signals, 10 – 16 ml of the concentration 200 mg/ml.

In the case of weak Doppler signals, e.g. in the presence of small vessels, low blood flow or unfavourable scanning conditions, 5 – 10 ml of the concentration 300 mg/ml.

In the case of very weak or absent Doppler signals, 5 – 8 ml of the concentration 400 mg/ml.

The intravenous injection should be done continuously (approx. 1 – 2 ml/sec.) in order to have homogeneous enhancement effects on the Doppler recording.

A repeat injection of Levovist may be necessary in special cases, e.g. in order to examine several sectional planes. The dose may be increased – particularly by choosing a higher concentration – in order to achieve a stronger effect or longer duration of enhancement. The duration of the increased signal strength is usually 2 – 4 minutes.

Recommended maximum dose: 6 injections of the single dose.

Doppler echocardiography of the right and left heart chambers: 10 – 16 ml of the concentration 200 mg/ml

In patients with very weak or non–detectable Doppler signals and for the clarification of mitral insufficiency: 5 – 10 ml of the concentration 300 mg/ml

Examination only of the right heart chambers: 4 – 10 ml of the concentration 200 mg/ml.

The intravenous injection should be done continuously (approx. 1 – 2 ml/sec.) in order to have homogeneous enhancement effects on the Doppler recording.

A repeat injection of Levovist may be necessary in special cases, e.g. in order to examine several sectional planes. The dose may be increased – particularly by choosing a higher concentration – in order to achieve a stronger effect or longer duration of enhancement. The duration of the increased signal strength is usually 1 – 2 minutes.

Recommended maximum dose: 6 injections of the single dose.

B–MODE CONTRAST ECHOCARDIOGRAPHY: 10 ml of the concentration 300 mg/ml

In cases of unfavourable sound conduction conditions and for stress echocardiography: 5 – 8 ml of the concentration 400 mg/ml

Examination only of the right heart chambers: 4 – 10 ml of the concentration 300 mg/ml

The intravenous injection should be given as bolus. If desired (e.g. for quantitative evaluations), the reproducibility of the quantitatively measurable contrast effects can be improved by an immediately following injection of 5 to 10 ml of physiological saline to ensure that the total dose of contrast medium is applied. In order to be able to add the injection of saline solution without delay, the use of a 3–way connector is recommended.

Recommended maximum dose: 6 injections of the single dose

Contra-indications: Galactosaemia. Use in patients with known or suspected right–to–left shunts.

Use in children is not recommended. There is no experience in patients under 15 years old.

Special warnings and special precautions for use: In patients with severe cardiac insufficiency (e.g. NYHA stage IV), the potential risk of the osmotic load caused by the Levovist injections must be considered carefully before administering.

Interaction with other medicaments and other forms of interaction: None known.

Pregnancy and lactation: No medical objections exist to the peripheral intravenous administration of Levovist as far as the substances contained are concerned. However, no experience is available with the use of Levovist in pregnancy and lactation.

Effects on ability to drive and use machines: Not applicable.

Undesirable effects: Occasionally, transient pain and a sensation of warmth and cold may occur in the area of the injection site during or shortly after the injection.

Sensations of taste, dyspnoea, changes of blood pressure or pulse, nausea and vomiting as well as headache, dizziness and cutaneous manifestations have been reported in individual cases.

Transient, non–specific irritation of the vascular endothelium may occur due to the hyperosmolality of Levovist.

Pain and tissue irritation may occur following accidental paravascular injection.

Overdose: Overdosage is unlikely. Theoretically, the hyperosmolality of the suspension may cause hypervolaemia which would need to be treated by intravenous administration of diuretics (e.g. frusemide) in accordance with symptoms and signs.

Diuresis induced by the osmotic load may affect the serum electrolytes and intravascular volume. These would need to be monitored and controlled as appropriate. Resultant dehydration and possible potassium loss should be treated by oral rehydration or infusion with intravenous fluid and electrolyte replacement.

Pharmacological properties

Pharmacodynamic properties: Levovist is a contrast medium which, after injection into a peripheral vein, leads temporarily to enhanced ultrasound echoes from the heart chambers and blood vessels.

This distinct amplification of the ultrasound echo is caused primarily by micrometre–sized air bubbles, which arise after suspension of the granules in water. Mediated by the palmitic acid additive, they remain stable for several minutes while in transit through the heart and lungs as well as in the subsequent vascular bed before dissolving in the blood stream.

Pharmacokinetic properties: The pharmacokinetic investigation of Levovist was performed with the concentration 400 mg/ml and the injection volumes 35 and 70 ml.

After i.v. administration of Levovist, the galactose microparticles quickly dissolve in the blood stream. The galactose becomes distributed in the extracellular space first of all and is subjected to glucose metabolism independently of insulin. Galactose is stored mainly in the liver through the formation of galactose–1–phosphate or is broken down after isomerisation to glucose–1–phosphate and metabolism to CO_2. Galactose is excreted via the kidneys if the plasma galactose level exceeds 50 mg/100 ml.

The elimination rate is reduced in patients with liver disease, depending on hepatic function, and a correspondingly prolonged elimination half–life should be expected.

Galactose and palmitic acid are physiological substances with rapid metabolism. The plasma half–lives are in the range of 10 – 11 minutes and 1 – 4 minutes, respectively.

Preclinical safety data: The results of animal experiments suggest that an acute adverse reaction to Levovist is unlikely.

Systemic tolerance studies following repeated daily intravenous administration as well as following repeated intercardiac (left ventricle) administration did not result in findings which oppose the intravenous administration to humans. Even after high intravenous doses no organ–toxic findings were observed.

Reproduction toxicological studies produced no

indications of either a teratogenic or an embryotoxic potential. Nor were there any indications of an influence on the fertility.

Local tolerance studies following single intravenous, intra–arterial, subcutaneous, intraperitoneal, paravenous and intramuscular administration indicated that slight symptoms of local intolerance may occur in case of inadvertent paravenous administration.

Although no long–term animal studies or mutagenicity testing have been undertaken on Levovist it is not likely that galactose or palmitic acid possess any mutagenic or carcinogenic potential.

Galactose is a normal constituent of the diet and is readily metabolised. Palmitic acid is contained in human serum (76 – 260 μmol/l).

Pharmaceutical particulars
List of excipients: Water for injection.

Incompatibilities: Not applicable.

Shelf life: 24 months

Special precautions for storage: Protect from light. Store below 30°C.

Nature and contents of container:

Granulate

Injection vial:	glass type 1
Stopper:	chlorinated butyl rubber, grey, fluoropolymer-covered
Flanged cup:	polypropylene covered disk
Container for water	20 ml ampoule made of polyethylene

Equipment

Mini spike:	plastics
Syringe disposable:	20 ml plastic syringe, double scaled

Combination pack consisting of
1 20 ml injection vial containing 4 g granules
1 mini spike
1 20 ml disposable syringe, scaled for 17, 11 and 8 ml
1 plastic ampoule with 20 ml water for injection

Combination pack consisting of
1 20 ml injection vial containing 2.5 g granules
1 mini spike
1 20 ml disposable syringe, scaled for 11, 7 and 5 ml
1 plastic ampoule with 20 ml water for injection

Instructions for use/handling: Adhere strictly to the following instructions for the preparation of the suspension.

Preparation of the ready–for–use Levovist suspension:

Use only the water for injection included in the package.

1. Bend back the tab on the top of the plastic ampoule containing water for injection.

2. Twist to open.

3. Withdraw the appropriate amount of water for injection using the syringe provided.

Injection vial with 4 g granules

Levovist concentration mg micropart./ml	*Volume of water required ml*	*Resulting* total volume ml*
approx 200	17	19.5 ml
approx 300	11	13.5 ml
approx 400	8	10.5 ml

Injection vial with 2.5 g granules

Levovist concentration mg micropart./ml	*Volume of water required ml*	*Resulting* total volume ml*
approx 200	11	12.5 ml
approx 300	7	8.5 ml
approx 400	5	6.5 ml

*Withdrawable volume: approx. 1– 2 ml less.

Remove the plastic cap from the vial containing the granules without disturbing the flanged metal cap. Pierce the rubber stopper with the enclosed mini spike.

4. Attach the syringe to the Luer–Lok–connection of the Sterifix mini spike (yellow cap) and transfer the water to the vial. The air–bleed duct with the sterile filter (white cap) permits pressure compensation without removal of the white cap.

5. Prepare the suspension by immediately shaking vigorously for 5 – 10 seconds by hand. Do not use shaking devices or an ultrasound bath. Leave the suspension to stand for two minutes before use.

6. Withdraw the ready–for–use, homogeneous, milky Levovist suspension through the mini spike into the syringe and administer within 10 minutes of preparation.

Granules and water for injection should be at room temperature before production of the suspension. Warming the suspension up (e.g. by holding the vial enclosed in the hand for a prolonged period) after it has been prepared for injection and excessive low pressure (e.g. on drawing the suspension up) should be avoided. This is necessary to prevent a decrease of the microbubble concentration and the formation of larger air bubbles due to degassing processes.

It is recommended to perform the injection via a flexible indwelling cannula with a sufficient gauge size (e.g. 19 to 20 G). In addition, the use of a Luer–Lok–connection is of practical advantage.

As usual, care must be taken to remove any macroscopically visible air bubbles from the suspension before injection.

Should a slight sedimentation of the microparticles occur during standing time, resuspension of the preparation by gently rotating it immediately before injection is recommended.

Any suspension not used at one examination session must be discarded.

Marketing authorisation numbers

Levovist:	0053/0257
Water for injection:	0053/0258

Date of approval/revision of SPC 17 July 1996

Legal category POM

LOGYNON*

Presentation The memo-pack holds six light brown tablets containing 30 micrograms ethinyloestradiol and 50 micrograms levonorgestrel, five white tablets containing 40 micrograms ethinyloestradiol and 75 micrograms levonorgestrel and ten ochre tablets containing 30 micrograms ethinyloestradiol and 125 micrograms levonorgestrel.

All tablets have a lustrous, sugar coating.

Excipients: lactose, maize starch, povidone 25 000, talc, magnesium stearate, sucrose, povidone 700 000, polyethylene glycol 6000, calcium carbonate, montan glycol wax, titanium dioxide, glycerol, ferric oxide pigment (yellow and red).

Uses Oral contraception and the recognised gynaecological indications for such oestrogen-progestogen combinations. The mode of action includes the inhibition of ovulation by suppression of the mid-cycle surge of luteinising hormone, the inspissation of cervical mucus so as to constitute a barrier to sperm, and the rendering of the endometrium unreceptive to implantation.

Dosage and administration *First treatment cycle:* 1 tablet daily for 21 days, starting on the first day of the menstrual cycle. Contraceptive protection begins immediately.

Subsequent cycles: Tablet taking from the next pack of Logynon is continued after a 7-day interval, beginning on the same day of the week as the first pack.

Changing from 21-day combined oral contraceptives: The first tablet of Logynon should be taken on the first day immediately after the end of the previous oral contraceptive course. Additional contraceptive precautions are not required.

Changing from a combined Every Day pill (28 day tablets): Logynon should be started after taking the last active tablet from the Every Day Pill pack. The first Logynon tablet is taken the next day. Additional contraceptive precautions are not then required.

Changing from a progestogen-only pill (POP): The first tablet of Logynon should be taken on the first day of bleeding, even if a POP has already been taken on that day. Additional contraceptive precautions are not then required. The remaining progestogen-only pills should be discarded.

Post-partum and post-abortum use: After pregnancy, oral contraception can be started 21 days after a vaginal delivery, provided that the patient is fully ambulant and there are no puerperal complications. Additional contraceptive precautions will be required for the first 7 days of tablet taking. Since the first post-partum ovulation may precede the first bleeding, another method of contraception should be used in the interval between childbirth and the first course of tablets. After a first-trimester abortion, oral contraception may be started immediately in which case no additional contraceptive precautions are required.

Pregnancy and lactation: If pregnancy occurs during medication with oral contraceptives, the preparation should be withdrawn immediately.

The use of Logynon during lactation may lead to a reduction in the volume of milk produced and to a change in its composition. Minute amounts of the active substances are excreted with the milk. Mothers who are breast-feeding may be advised instead to use a progestogen-only pill.

Special circumstances requiring additional contraception

Incorrect administration: A single delayed tablet should be taken as soon as possible, and if this can be done within 12 hours of the correct time, contraceptive protection is maintained. With longer delays, additional contraception is needed. Only the most recently delayed tablet should be taken, earlier missed tablets being omitted, and additional non-hormonal methods of contraception (except the rhythm or temperature methods) should be used for the next 7 days, while the next 7 tablets are being taken. Additionally, therefore, if tablet(s) have been missed during the last 7 days of a pack, there should be no break before the next pack is started. In this situation, a withdrawal bleed should not be expected until the end of the second pack. Some breakthrough bleeding may occur on tablet taking days but this is not clinically significant. If the patient does not have a withdrawal bleed during the tablet-free interval following the end of the second pack, the possibility of pregnancy must be ruled out before starting the next pack.

Gastro-intestinal upset: Vomiting or diarrhoea may reduce the efficacy of oral contraceptives by preventing full absorption. Tablet-taking from the current pack should be continued. Additional non-hormonal methods of contraception (except the rhythm or temperature methods) should be used during the gastro-intestinal upset and for 7 days following the upset. If these 7 days overrun the end of a pack, the next pack should be started without a break. In this situation, a withdrawal bleed should not be expected until the end of the second pack. If the patient does not have a withdrawal bleed during the tablet-free interval following the end of the second pack, the possibility of pregnancy must be ruled out before starting the next pack. Other methods of contraception should be considered if the gastro-intestinal disorder is likely to be prolonged.

Interaction with other drugs: Hepatic enzyme inducers such as barbiturates, primidone, phenobarbitone, phenytoin, phenylbutazone, rifampicin, carbamazepine and griseofulvin can impair the efficacy of Logynon. For women receiving long-term therapy with hepatic enzyme inducers, another method of contraception should be used. The use of antibiotics may also reduce the efficacy of Logynon, possibly by altering the intestinal flora.

Women receiving short courses of enzyme inducers or broad spectrum antibiotics should take additional, non-hormonal (except the rhythm or temperature method) contraceptive precautions during the time of concurrent medication and for 7 days afterwards. If these 7 days overrun the end of a pack, the next pack should be started without a break. In this situation, a withdrawal bleed should not be expected until the end of the second pack. If the patient does not have a withdrawal bleed during the tablet-free interval following the end of the second pack, the possibility of pregnancy must be ruled out before resuming with the next pack. With rifampicin, additional contraceptive precautions should be continued for 4 weeks after treatment stops, even if only a short course was administered.

The requirement for oral antidiabetics or insulin can change as a result of the effect on glucose tolerance.

Contra-indications, warnings, etc
Contra-indications:

1. Pregnancy
2. Severe disturbances of liver function, jaundice or persistent itching during a previous pregnancy, Dubin-Johnson syndrome, Rotor syndrome, previous or existing liver tumours
3. Existing or previous arterial or venous thrombotic or embolic processes, conditions which predispose to them e.g. disorders of the clotting processes, valvular heart disease and atrial fibrillation
4. Sickle-cell anaemia
5. Mammary or endometrial carcinoma, or a history of these conditions
6. Severe diabetes mellitus with vascular changes
7. Disorders of lipid metabolism
8. History of herpes gestationis
9. Deterioration of otosclerosis during pregnancy
10. Undiagnosed abnormal vaginal bleeding
11. Hypersensitivity to any of the components of Logynon.

Warnings: There is a general opinion, based on statistical evidence, that users of combined oral contraceptives experience, more often than non-users, venous thromboembolism, arterial thrombosis, including cerebral and myocardial infarction, and subarachnoid haemorrhage. Full recovery from such disorders does not always occur, and it should be realised that in a few cases they are fatal. How often these disorders occur in users of the modern low-dose pills is not known, but there are reasons for suggesting that they may occur less often than with older pills.

Certain factors may entail some risk of thrombosis, e.g. smoking, obesity, varicose veins, cardiovascular diseases, diabetes, and migraine. The suitability of a

Estimated cumulative numbers of breast cancers per 10,000 women diagnosed in 5 years of use and up to 10 years after stopping COCs, compared with numbers of breast cancers diagnosed in 10,000 women who had never used COCs.

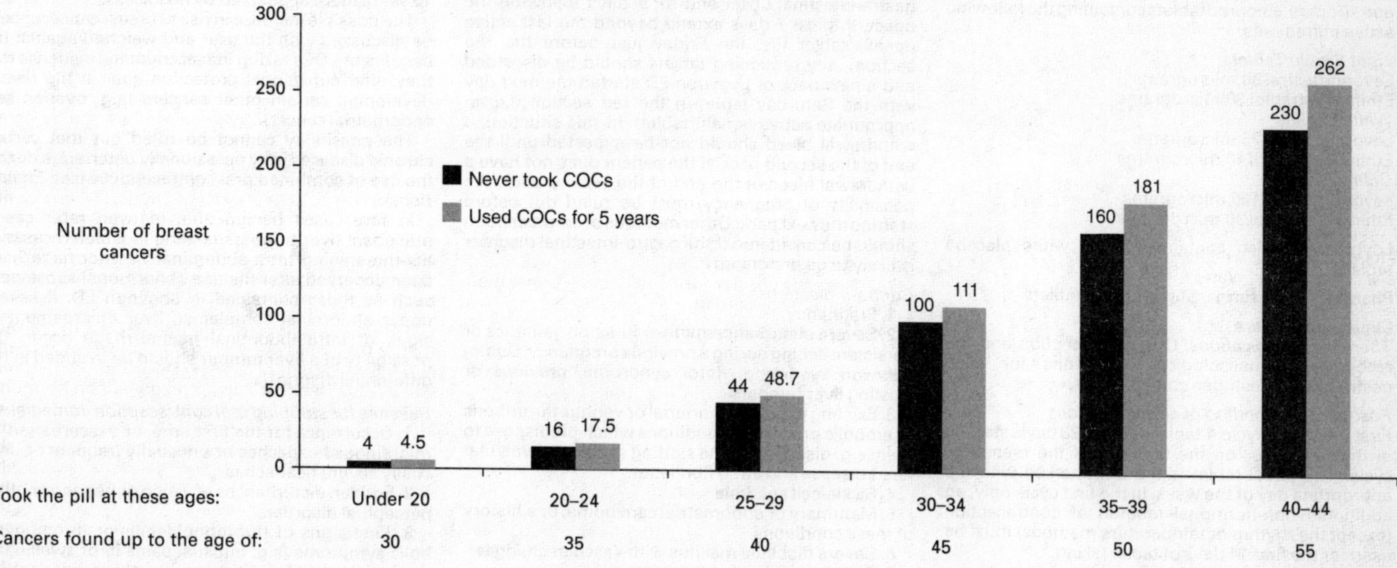

combined oral contraceptive should be judged according to the severity of such conditions in the individual case, and should be discussed with the patient before she decides to take it. The risk of arterial thrombosis associated with combined oral contraceptives increases with age, and this risk is aggravated by cigarette-smoking. The use of combined oral contraceptives by women in the older age-group, especially those who are cigarette smokers, should therefore be discouraged and alternative methods used.

In addition if there is a history in the family of thromboembolic diseases at a young age (e.g. deep vein thrombosis, heart attack or stroke) disturbances of the coagulation system must be ruled out before the pill is prescribed.

Numerous epidemiological studies have been reported on the risks of ovarian, endometrial, cervical and breast cancer in women using combined oral contraceptives. The evidence is clear that combined oral contraceptives offer substantial protection against both ovarian and endometrial cancer.

An increased risk of cervical cancer in long-term users of combined oral contraceptives has been reported in some studies, but there continues to be controversy about the extent to which this is attributable to the confounding effects of sexual behaviour and other factors.

A meta-analysis from 54 epidemiological studies reported that there is a slightly increased relative risk (RR=1.24) of having breast cancer diagnosed in women who are currently using combined oral contraceptives (COCs). The observed pattern of increased risk may be due to an earlier diagnosis of breast cancer in COC users, the biological effects of COCs or a combination of both. The additional breast cancers diagnosed in current users of COCs or in women who have used COCs in the last ten years are more likely to be localised to the breast than those in women who never used COCs.

Breast cancer is rare among women under 40 years of age whether or not they take COCs. Whilst this background risk increases with age, the excess number of breast cancer diagnoses in current and recent COC users is small in relation to the overall risk of breast cancer (see bar chart).

The most important risk factor for breast cancer in COC users is the age women discontinue the COC; the older the age at stopping, the more breast cancers are diagnosed. Duration of use is less important and the excess risk gradually disappears during the course of the 10 years after stopping COC use such that by 10 years there appears to be no excess.

The possible increase in risk of breast cancer should be discussed with the user and weighed against the benefits of COCs taking into account the evidence that they offer substantial protection against the risk of developing certain other cancers (e.g. ovarian and endometrial cancer).

The possibility cannot be ruled out that certain chronic diseases may occasionally deteriorate during the use of combined oral contraceptives (see *Precautions*).

In rare cases benign and, in even rarer cases, malignant liver tumours leading in isolated cases to life-threatening intra-abdominal haemorrhage have been observed after the use of hormonal substances such as those contained in Logynon. If severe upper abdominal complaints, liver enlargement or signs of intra-abdominal haemorrhage occur, the possibility of a liver tumour should be included in the differential diagnosis.

Reasons for stopping oral contraception immediately:

1. Occurrence for the first time, or exacerbation, of migrainous headaches or unusually frequent or unusually severe headaches
2. Sudden disturbances of vision or hearing or other perceptual disorders
3. First signs of thrombophlebitis or thromboembolic symptoms (e.g. unusual pains in or swelling of the leg(s), stabbing pains on breathing or coughing for no apparent reason). Feeling of pain and tightness in the chest
4. Six weeks before an elective major operation (e.g. abdominal, orthopaedic), any surgery to the legs, medical treatment for varicose veins or prolonged immobilisation, e.g. after accidents or surgery. Do not restart until 2 weeks after full ambulation. In case of emergency surgery, thrombotic prophylaxis is usually indicated e.g. subcutaneous heparin
5. Onset of jaundice, hepatitis, itching of the whole body
6. Increase in epileptic seizures
7. Significant rise in blood pressure
8. Onset of severe depression
9. Severe upper abdominal pain or liver enlargement
10. Clear exacerbation of conditions known to be capable of deteriorating during oral contraception or pregnancy
11. Pregnancy is a reason for stopping immediately because it has been suggested by some investigations that oral contraceptives taken in early pregnancy may slightly increase the risk of foetal malformations. Other investigations have failed to support these findings. The possibility therefore cannot be excluded, but it is certain that if a risk exists at all, it is very small.

Precautions: Examination of the pelvic organs, breasts and blood-pressure should precede the prescribing of any combined oral contraceptive and should be repeated regularly. The family medical history should be carefully noted and disturbances of the clotting mechanism ruled out if any member of the family has suffered from thromboembolic disease (e.g. deep vein thrombosis, stroke, myocardial infarction) at a young age. Before starting treatment pregnancy must be excluded.

The following conditions require strict medical supervision during medication with oral contraceptives. Deterioration or first appearance of any of these conditions may indicate that use of the oral contraceptive should be discontinued: diabetes mellitus, or a tendency towards diabetes mellitus (e.g. unexplained glycosuria), hypertension, varicose veins, a history of phlebitis, otosclerosis, multiple sclerosis, epilepsy, porphyria, tetany, disturbed liver function, Sydenham's chorea, renal dysfunction, family history of clotting disorders, obesity, family history of breast cancer and patient history of benign breast disease, history of clinical depression, systemic lupus erythematosus, uterine fibroids and migraine, gall-stones, cardiovascular diseases, chloasma, asthma, an intolerance of contact lenses, or any disease that is prone to worsen during pregnancy

Some women may experience amenorrhoea or oligomenorrhoea after discontinuation of oral contraceptives, especially when these conditions existed prior to use. Women should be informed of this possibility.

Side-effects: In rare cases, headaches, gastric upsets, nausea, vomiting, breast tenderness, changes in body weight, changes in libido, depressive moods can occur.

In predisposed women, use of Logynon can sometimes cause chloasma which is exacerbated by exposure to sunlight. Such women should avoid prolonged exposure to sunlight.

Individual cases of poor tolerance of contact lenses have been reported with use of oral contraceptives. Contact lens wearers who develop changes in lens tolerance should be assessed by an ophthalmologist.

Menstrual changes:

1. *Reduction of menstrual flow:* This is not abnormal and it is to be expected in some patients. Indeed, it may be beneficial where heavy periods were previously experienced.

2. *Missed menstruation:* Occasionally, withdrawal bleeding may not occur at all. If the tablets have been taken correctly, pregnancy is very unlikely. If withdrawal bleeding fails to occur at the end of a second pack, the possibility of pregnancy must be ruled out before resuming with the next pack.

Intermenstrual bleeding: 'Spotting' or heavier 'breakthrough bleeding' sometimes occur during tablet taking, especially in the first few cycles, and normally cease spontaneously. Logynon should therefore, be continued even if irregular bleeding occurs. If irregular bleeding is persistent, appropriate diagnostic measures to exclude an organic cause are indicated and may include curettage. This also applies in the case of spotting which occurs at irregular intervals in several consecutive cycles or which occurs for the first time after long use of Logynon.

Effect on blood chemistry: The use of oral contraceptives may influence the results of certain laboratory tests including biochemical parameters of liver, thyroid, adrenal and renal function, plasma levels of carrier proteins and lipid/lipoprotein fractions, parameters of carbohydrate metabolism and parameters of coagulation and fibrinolysis. Laboratory staff should therefore be informed about oral contraceptive use when laboratory tests are requested.

Overdosage: Overdosage may cause nausea, vomiting and, in females, withdrawal bleeding. There are no specific antidotes and treatment should be symptomatic.

Pharmaceutical precautions Shelf-life – Five years

Legal category POM

Package quantities Individual packs containing three months supply (OP)

Further information Nil

Product licence number 0053/0085

LOGYNON* ED

Qualitative and quantitative composition Calendar pack containing 6 light brown tablets, 5 white tablets and 10 ochre-coloured tablets containing the following active ingredients.

Light Brown Tablets
Levonorgestrel 50 micrograms
Ethinyloestradiol 30 micrograms
White Tablets
Levonorgestrel 75 micrograms
Ethinyloestradiol 40 micrograms
Ochre Tablets
Levonorgestrel 125 micrograms
Ethinyloestradiol 30 micrograms

Loygnon ED also contains 7 large white placebo tablets.

Pharmaceutical form Sugar-coated tablets

Clinical particulars
Therapeutic indications: Oral contraception and the recognised gynaecological indications for such oestrogen-progestogen combinations.

Posology and method of administration:
First treatment cycle: 1 tablet daily for 28 days, starting in the red sector on the first day of the menstrual cycle. The initial tablet is the one marked with the appropriate day of the week. In the first cycle only, an additional non-hormonal method of contraception (except the rhythm or temperature methods) must be used for the first 14 days of tablet taking.

Subsequent cycles: Tablet taking is continuous, which means that the next pack of Logynon ED follows immediately without a break. A withdrawal bleed usually occurs when the white placebo tablets are being taken.

Changing from another combined oral contraceptive: The first tablet of Logynon ED should be taken from the red sector immediately after the end of the previous oral contraceptive course. In the first cycle only, an additional non-hormonal method of contraception (except the rhythm or temperature methods) must be used for the first 14 days of tablet taking.

Changing from a progestogen-only pill (POP): The first tablet of Logynon ED should be taken from the red sector on the first day of bleeding, even if a POP has already been taken on that day. An additional non-hormonal method of contraception (except the rhythm or temperature methods) must be used for 14 days. The remaining progestogen-only pills should be discarded.

Post-partum and post-abortum use: After pregnancy, Logynon ED can be started 21 days after a vaginal delivery, provided that the patient is fully ambulant and there are no puerperal complications. Additional contraceptive precautions will be required for the first 14 days of tablet taking. Since the first post-partum ovulation may precede the first bleeding, another method of contraception should be used in the interval between childbirth and the first course of tablets. After a first-trimester abortion, oral contraception may be started immediately in which case additional non-hormonal methods of contraception (except the rhythm or temperature methods) should be used for the first 14 days of tablet taking in the first cycle of Logynon ED.

Special circumstances requiring additional contraception:
Incorrect administration: Errors in taking the 7 inactive white placebo tablets (i.e. the first 5 tablets in the red section and the 2 immediately before the red section) can be ignored. A single delayed active (small) tablet should be taken as soon as possible, and if this can be done within 12 hours of the correct time, contraceptive protection is maintained.

With longer delays in taking active tablets, additional contraception is needed. Only the most recently delayed tablet should be taken, earlier missed tablets being omitted, and additional non-hormonal methods of contraception (except the rhythm or temperature methods) should be used for *the next 7 days, while the next 7 active (small) tablets are being taken.* Therefore, if the 7 days additional contraception will extend beyond the Friday just before the red section (i.e. the last active tablet) the user should take the tablets up to and including that Friday, and start a new pack next day with the Saturday tablet in the red section i.e. discard the remaining tablets and go to an appropriate active tablet in the next pack. In this situation, a withdrawal bleed should not be expected until the end of the second pack. Some breakthrough bleeding may occur on pill taking days but this is not clinically significant. If the patient does not have a withdrawal bleed following the end of the second pack, the possibility of pregnancy must be ruled out before starting the next pack.

Gastro-intestinal upset: Vomiting or diarrhoea may reduce the efficacy of oral contraceptives by preventing full absorption. Tablet taking from the current pack should be continued. Additional non-hormonal methods of contraception (except the rhythm or temperature methods) should be used during the gastro-intestinal upset and for 7 days following the upset. If these 7 days extend beyond the last active (small) tablet (i.e. the Friday just before the red section), any remaining tablets should be discarded and a new pack of Logynon ED started the next day with the Saturday tablet in the red section (i.e an appropriate active (small) tablet). In this situation, a withdrawal bleed should not be expected until the end of the second pack. If the patient does not have a withdrawal bleed at the end of the second pack, the possibility of pregnancy must be ruled out before starting the next pack. Other methods of contraception should be considered if the gastro-intestinal disorder is likely to be prolonged.

Contra-indications:
1. Pregnancy
2. Severe disturbances of liver function, jaundice or persistent itching during a previous pregnancy, Dubin-Johnson syndrome, Rotor syndrome, previous or existing liver tumours
3. Existing or previous arterial or venous thrombotic or embolic processes, conditions which predispose to them e.g. disorders of the clotting processes, valvular heart disease and atrial fibrillation
4. Sickle-cell anaemia
5. Mammary or endometrial carcinoma, or a history of these conditions
6. Severe diabetes mellitus with vascular changes
7. Disorders of lipid metabolism
8. History of herpes gestationis
9. Deterioration of otosclerosis during pregnancy
10. Undiagnosed abnormal vaginal bleeding
11. Hypersensitivity to any of the components of Logynon ED.

Special warnings and special precautions for use:
Warnings: There is a general opinion, based on statistical evidence, that users of combined oral contraceptives experience, more often than non-users, venous thromboembolism, arterial thrombosis, including cerebral and myocardial infarction, and subarachnoid haemorrhage. Full recovery from such disorders does not always occur, and it should be realised that in a few cases they are fatal. How often these disorders occur in users of the modern low-dose pills is not known, but there are reasons for suggesting that they may occur less often than with older pills.

Certain factors may entail some risk of thrombosis, e.g. smoking, obesity, varicose veins, cardiovascular diseases, diabetes, and migraine. The suitability of a combined oral contraceptive should be judged according to the severity of such conditions in the individual case, and should be discussed with the patient before she decides to take it. The risk of arterial thrombosis associated with combined oral contraceptives increases with age, and this risk is aggravated by cigarette-smoking. The use of combined oral contraceptives by women in the older age-group, especially those who are cigarette smokers, should therefore be discouraged and alternative methods used.

In addition if there is a history in the family of thromboembolic diseases at a young age (e.g. deep vein thrombosis, heart attack or stroke) disturbances of the coagulation system must be ruled out before the pill is prescribed.

Numerous epidemiological studies have been reported on the risks of ovarian, endometrial, cervical and breast cancer in women using combined oral contraceptives. The evidence is clear that combined oral contraceptives offer substantial protection against both ovarian and endometrial cancer.

An increased risk of cervical cancer in long-term users of combined oral contraceptives has been reported in some studies, but there continues to be controversy about the extent to which this is attributable to the confounding effects of sexual behaviour and other factors.

A meta-analysis from 54 epidemiological studies reported that there is a slightly increased relative risk (RR=1.24) of having breast cancer diagnosed in women who are currently using combined oral contraceptives (COCs). The observed pattern of increased risk may be due to an earlier diagnosis of breast cancer in COC users, the biological effects of COCs or a combination of both. The additional breast cancers diagnosed in current users of COCs or in women who have used COCs in the last ten years are more likely to be localised to the breast than those in women who never used COCs.

Breast cancer is rare among women under 40 years of age whether or not they take COCs. Whilst this background risk increases with age, the excess number of breast cancer diagnoses in current and recent COC users is small in relation to the overall risk of breast cancer (see bar chart).

The most important risk factor for breast cancer in COC users is the age women discontinue the COC; the older the age at stopping, the more breast cancers are diagnosed. Duration of use is less important and the excess risk gradually disappears during the course of the 10 years after stopping COC use such that by 10 years there appears to be no excess.

The possible increase in risk of breast cancer should be discussed with the user and weighed against the benefits of COCs taking into account the evidence that they offer substantial protection against the risk of developing certain other cancers (e.g. ovarian and endometrial cancer).

The possibility cannot be ruled out that certain chronic diseases may occasionally deteriorate during the use of combined oral contraceptives (see *Precautions*).

In rare cases benign and, in even rarer cases, malignant liver tumours leading in isolated cases to life-threatening intra-abdominal haemorrhage have been observed after the use of hormonal substances such as those contained in Logynon ED. If severe upper abdominal complaints, liver enlargement or signs of intra-abdominal haemorrhage occur, the possibility of a liver tumour should be included in the differential diagnosis.

Reasons for stopping oral contraception immediately:
1. Occurrence for the first time, or exacerbation, of migrainous headaches or unusually frequent or unusually severe headaches
2. Sudden disturbances of vision or hearing or other perceptual disorders
3. First signs of thrombophlebitis or thromboembolic symptoms (e.g. unusual pains in or swelling of the leg(s), stabbing pains on breathing or coughing for no apparent reason). Feeling of pain and tightness in the chest
4. Six weeks before an elective major operation (e.g. abdominal, orthopaedic), any surgery to the legs, medical treatment for varicose veins or prolonged immobilisation, e.g. after accidents or surgery. Do not restart until 2 weeks after full ambulation. In case of emergency surgery, thrombotic prophylaxis is usually indicated e.g. subcutaneous heparin
5. Onset of jaundice, hepatitis, itching of the whole body
6. Increase in epileptic seizures
7. Significant rise in blood pressure
8. Onset of severe depression
9. Severe upper abdominal pain or liver enlargement
10. Clear exacerbation of conditions known to be capable of deteriorating during oral contraception or pregnancy
11. Pregnancy is a reason for stopping immediately because it has been suggested by some investigations that oral contraceptives taken in early pregnancy may slightly increase the risk of foetal malformations. Other investigations have failed to support these findings. The possibility therefore cannot be excluded, but it is certain that if a risk exists at all, it is very small.

Precautions: Examination of the pelvic organs, breasts and blood-pressure should precede the prescribing of any combined oral contraceptive and should be repeated regularly. The family medical history should be carefully noted and disturbances of the clotting mechanism ruled out if any members of the family have suffered from thromboembolic disease (e.g. deep vein thrombosis, stroke, myocardial infarction) at a young age. Before starting treatment pregnancy must be excluded.

The following conditions require strict medical supervision during medication with oral contraceptives. Deterioration or first appearance of some of these conditions may indicate that use of the oral contraceptive should be discontinued:

Diabetes mellitus, or a tendency towards diabetes mellitus (e.g. unexplained glycosuria), hypertension, varicose veins, a history of phlebitis, otosclerosis, multiple sclerosis, epilepsy, porphyria, tetany, disturbed liver function, Sydenham's chorea (chorea minor), renal dysfunction, family history of clotting disorders, obesity, family history of breast cancer and patient history of benign breast disease, history of clinical depression, systemic lupus erythematosus, uterine fibroids and migraine, gall-stones, cardiovascular diseases, chloasma, asthma, an intolerance of contact lenses, or any disease that is prone to worsen during pregnancy.

Some women may experience amenorrhoea or oligomenorrhoea after discontinuation of oral contraceptives, especially when these conditions existed prior to use. Women should be informed of this possibility.

Interaction with other medicaments and other forms of interaction: Hepatic enzyme inducers such as barbiturates, primidone, phenobarbitone, phenytoin, phenylbutazone, rifampicin, carbamazepine and griseofulvin can impair the efficacy of Logynon ED. For women receiving long-term therapy with hepatic enzyme inducers, another method of contraception should be used. The use of antibiotics may also reduce

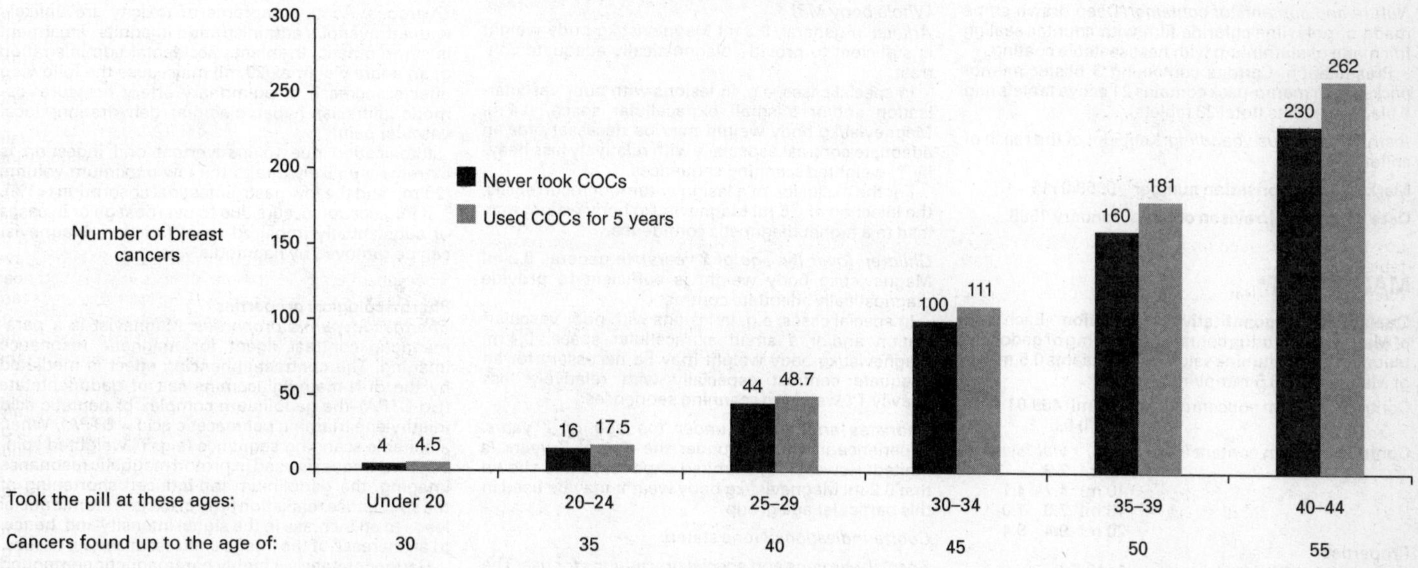

the efficacy of Logynon ED, possibly by altering the intestinal flora.

Women receiving short courses of enzyme inducers or broad spectrum antibiotics should take additional, non-hormonal (except the rhythm or temperature methods) contraceptive precautions during the time of concurrent medication and for 7 days afterwards. If these 7 days extend beyond the last active (small) tablet (i.e. the Friday just before the red section), any remaining tablets should be discarded and a new pack of Logynon ED started the next day with the Saturday tablet in the red section (i.e. an appropriate active (small) tablet). In this situation, a withdrawal bleed should not be expected until the end of the second pack. If the patient does not have a withdrawal bleed at the end of the second pack, the possibility of pregnancy must be ruled out before resuming with the next pack. With rifampicin, additional contraceptive precautions should be continued for 4 weeks after treatment stops, even if only a short course was administered.

The requirement for oral antidiabetics or insulin can change as a result of the effect on glucose tolerance.

Pregnancy and lactation: If pregnancy occurs during medication with oral contraceptives, the preparation should be withdrawn immediately (see 'Reasons for stopping oral contraception immediately').

The use of Logynon ED during lactation may lead to a reduction in the volume of milk produced and to a change in its composition. Minute amounts of the active substances are excreted with the milk. Mothers who are breast-feeding may be advised instead to use a progestogen-only pill.

Effects on ability to drive and to use machines: None known.

Undesirable effects: In rare cases, headaches, gastric upsets, nausea, vomiting, breast tenderness, changes in body weight, changes in libido, depressive moods can occur.

In predisposed women, use of Logynon ED can sometimes cause chloasma which is exacerbated by exposure to sunlight. Such women should avoid prolonged exposure to sunlight.

Individual cases of poor tolerance of contact lenses have been reported with use of oral contraceptives. Contact lens wearers who develop changes in lens tolerance should be assessed by an ophthalmologist.

Menstrual changes:

1. Reduction of menstrual flow: This is not abnormal and it is to be expected in some patients. Indeed, it may be beneficial where heavy periods were previously experienced.

2. Missed menstruation: Occasionally, withdrawal bleeding may not occur at all. If the tablets have been taken correctly, pregnancy is very unlikely. If withdrawal bleeding fails to occur at the end of a second pack, the possibility of pregnancy must be ruled out before resuming with the next pack.

Intermenstrual bleeding: 'Spotting' or heavier 'breakthrough bleeding' sometimes occur during tablet taking, especially in the first few cycles, and normally cease spontaneously. Logynon ED should therefore, be continued even if irregular bleeding occurs. If irregular bleeding is persistent, appropriate diagnostic measures to exclude an organic cause are indicated and may include curettage. This also applies in the case of spotting which occurs at irregular intervals in several consecutive cycles or which occurs for the first time after long use of Logynon ED.

Effect on blood chemistry: The use of oral contraceptives may influence the results of certain laboratory tests including biochemical parameters of liver, thyroid, adrenal and renal function, plasma levels of carrier proteins and lipid/lipoprotein fractions, parameters of carbohydrate metabolism and parameters of coagulation and fibrinolysis. Laboratory staff should therefore be informed about oral contraceptive use when laboratory tests are requested.

Refer to 'Special warnings and special precautions for use' section for additional information.

Overdose: Overdosage may cause nausea, vomiting and, in females, withdrawal bleeding. There are no specific antidotes and treatment should be symptomatic.

Pharmacological particulars

Pharmacodynamic properties: Logynon ED is an oestrogen-progestogen combination which acts by inhibiting ovulation by suppression of the mid-cycle surge of luteinizing hormone, the inspissation of cervical mucus so as to constitute a barrier to sperm, and the rendering of the endometrium unreceptive to implantation.

Pharmacokinetic properties:

Levonorgestrel: Orally administered levonorgestrel is rapidly and completely absorbed. Following ingestion of 0.125 mg levonorgestrel together with 0.03 mg ethinyloestradiol (which represents the combination with the highest levonorgestrel content of the tri-step formulation), maximum drug serum levels of about 4.3ng/ml are reached at 1.0 hour. Thereafter, levonorgestrel serum levels decrease in two phases, characterized by half-lives of 0.4 hours and about 22 hours. For levonorgestrel, a metabolic clearance rate from serum of about 1.5 ml/min/kg was determined. Levonorgestrel is not excreted in unchanged form but as metabolites. Levonorgestrel metabolites are excreted in about equal proportions with urine and faeces. The biotransformation follows the known pathways of steroid metabolism. No pharmacologically active metabolites are known.

Levonorgestrel is bound to serum albumin and to SHBG. Only 1.4% of the total serum drug levels are present as free steroid, but 55% are specifically bound to SHBG. The relative distribution (free, albumin-bound, SHBG-bound) depends on the SHBG concentrations in the serum. Following induction of the binding protein, the SHBG-bound fraction increases while the unbound fractions decrease.

Following daily repeated administration of Logynon ED, levonorgestrel concentrations in the serum increase by a factor of about 4. Steady-state conditions are reached during the second half of a treatment cycle. The pharmacokinetics of levonorgestrel is influenced by SHBG serum levels. Under treatment with Logynon ED, an increase in the serum levels of SHBG by a factor of about 2 occurs during a treatment cycle. Due to the specific binding of levonorgestrel to SHBG, the increase in SHBG levels is accompanied by an almost parallel increase in levonorgestrel serum levels. The absolute bioavailability of levonorgestrel was determined to be almost 100% of the dose administered.

Ethinyloestradiol: Orally administered ethinyloestradiol is rapidly and completely absorbed. Following ingestion of 0.03 mg ethinyloestradiol together with 0.125 mg levonorgestrel, maximum drug serum levels of about 116 pg/ml are reached at 1.3 hours. Thereafter, ethinyloestradiol serum levels decrease in two phases characterized by half-lives of 1–2 hours and about 20 hours. For technical reasons, these parameters can only be calculated following the administration of higher doses. For ethinyloestradiol an apparent volume of distribution of about 5 l/kg and a metabolic clearance rate from serum of about 5 ml/min/kg were determined. Ethinyloestradiol is highly but non-specifically bound to serum albumin. About 2% of drug levels are present unbound. During absorption and first liver passage, ethinyloestradiol is metabolized resulting in a reduced absolute and variable oral bioavailability. Unchanged drug is not excreted. Ethinyloestradiol metabolites are excreted at a urinary to biliary ratio of 4:6 with a half-life of about 1 day.

Due to the half-life of the terminal disposition phase from serum and the daily ingestion, steady-state serum levels are reached after 3-4 days and are higher by 30–40% as compared to a single dose. The absolute bioavailability of ethinyloestradiol is subject to a considerable interindividual variation. Following oral administration, the mean bioavailability was found to be about 40–60% of the administered dose.

During established lactation, 0.02% of the daily maternal dose could be transferred to the newborn via milk.

The systemic availability of ethinyloestradiol might be influenced in both directions by other drugs. There is, however, no interaction with high doses of vitamin C. Ethinyloestradiol induces the hepatic synthesis of SHBG and CBG during continuous use. The extent of SHBG induction, however, depends on the chemical structure and the dose of the co-administered progestogen. During treatment with Logynon ED, SHBG concentrations in the serum increased from about 76 nmol/l to 164 nmol/l and the serum concentrations of CBG increased from about 48 μ g/ml to 111 μ g/ml.

Preclinical safety data: There are no preclinical safety data which could be of relevance to the prescriber and which are not already included in other relevant sections of the SPC.

Pharmaceutical particulars

List of excipients: Excipients included in both active and placebo tablets:

Active tablets	*Placebo tablets*
lactose	lactose
maize starch	maize starch
povidone	povidone
magnesium stearate (E 572)	magnesium stearate (E 572)
sucrose	sucrose
polyethylene glycol 6000	polyethylene glycol 6000
calcium carbonate (E 170)	calcium carbonate (E 170)
talc	talc
montan glycol wax	montan glycol wax
glycerin (E 422)	
titanium dioxide (E171)	
ferric oxide pigment (red and yellow) (E172)	

Incompatibilities: None known.

Shelf life: Five years.

Special precautions for storage: Not applicable.

Nature and contents of container: Deep drawn strips made of polyvinyl chloride film with counter-sealing foil made of aluminium with heat sealable coating.

Presentation: Cartons containing 3 blister memo-packs. Each memo-pack contains 21 active tablets and 7 placebo tablets (total 28 tablets).

Instructions for use/handling: Keep out of the reach of children.

Marketing authorisation number 0053/0115

Date of approval/revison of SPC January 1998

MAGNEVIST*

Qualitative and quantitative composition Each 1 ml of Magnevist solution contains 469.01 mg of gadopentetic acid, dimeglumine salt. This represents 0.5 moles of Magnevist/l (0.5 mmol/ml).

Contrast medium concentration	(mg/ml) 469.01		
	(mol/l) 0.5		
Contrast medium content (g) per		*vial*	*syringe*
	5 ml	2.3	-
	10 ml	4.7	4.7
	15 ml	7.0	7.0
	20 ml	9.4	9.4

Properties	
Osmolarity at 37°C (mosmol/l solution)	1440.0
Osmolality at 37°C (mosmol/kg H_2O)	1960.0
Osmotic pressure at 37°C	
(atm)	49.8
(MPa)	5.06
Density at 20°C (kg/l)	1.210
at 37°C (kg/l)	1.195
Viscosity (mPa.s)	
at 20°C	4.9
at 37°C	2.9
pH	7.0–7.9

Pharmaceutical form Solution for injection.

Clinical particulars

Therapeutic indications: As a paramagnetic contrast medium in cranial, spinal and whole body magnetic resonance imaging (MRI) and for the evaluation of renal function.

Posology and method of administration: The patient should fast for 2 hours prior to examination. The usual precautions for MRI (e.g. exclusion of cardiac pace-makers and other ferro-magnetic objects including vascular clips etc) must be observed.

Magnevist should not be drawn up into the syringe until immediately before use. Likewise, the pre-filled syringes must not be taken from the pack and prepared for the injection until immediately before use. Contrast medium not used in one examination must be discarded.

The required dose of Magnevist should be administered as a single intravenous injection. If required, intravenous bolus administration can be used. Ideally the patient should be recumbent during administration, and should be kept under supervision for at least 30 minutes after the injection.

Contrast-enhanced MRI can start immediately after administration of the medium. The timing of optimal opacification after injection of Magnevist varies depending on the tissue and lesion being examined and the MR sequence used. For example, optimal opacification occurs within 5 minutes in the breast, but with cranial and spinal opacification, it is generally observed within 45 minutes. T_1- weighted scanning sequences are particularly suitable for contrast-enhanced examinations with Magnevist. In the range of field-strengths, from 0.14 tesla up to 1.5 tesla, (resistive or superconductive magnets) the image contrast was found to be independent of the applied field strength.

The recommended doses are given in ml of Magnevist per kg body weight.

Cranial and spinal MRI

Adults: In general, the administration of 0.2 ml Magnevist/kg body weight is sufficient to provide diagnostically adequate contrast.

If a strong clinical suspicion of a lesion persists despite a normal scan, a further injection of 0.2 ml or even 0.4 ml Magnevist/kg body weight within 30 minutes may increase the diagnostic yield.

For the exclusion of metastases or recurrent tumours, injection of 0.6 ml Magnevist/kg body weight may increase the diagnostic yield.

Children (including neonates and infants under the age of 2 years): 0.2 ml Magnevist/kg body weight is sufficient to provide diagnostically adequate contrast.

If a strong clinical suspicion of a lesion persists despite a normal scan, a further injection of 0.2 ml Magnevist /kg body weight within 30 minutes may increase the diagnostic yield.

Whole body MRI

Adults: In general, 0.2 ml Magnevist/kg body weight is sufficient to provide diagnostically adequate contrast.

In special cases, e.g. in lesions with poor vascularisation and/or a small extracellular space, 0.4 ml Magnevist/kg body weight may be necessary for an adequate contrast especially with relatively less heavily T_1-weighted scanning sequences.

For the exclusion of a lesion or tumour recurrences, the injection of 0.6 ml Magnevist/kg body weight may lead to a higher diagnostic confidence.

Children (over the age of 2 years): In general, 0.2 ml Magnevist/kg body weight is sufficient to provide diagnostically adequate contrast.

In special cases, e.g. in lesions with poor vascularisation and/or a small extracellular space, 0.4 ml Magnevist/kg body weight may be necessary for an adequate contrast especially with relatively less heavily T1-weighted scanning sequences.

Neonates and Infants under the age of 2 years: Experience in children under the age of 2 years is limited. However, this limited experience has shown that 0.2 ml Magnevist/kg body weight may be used in this particular age group.

Contra-indications: None stated.

Special warnings and special precautions for use: The decision to use Magnevist must be made after particularly careful evaluation of the risk-benefit-ratio in patients with an allergic disposition, since experience shows that these patients suffer more frequently than others from hypersensitivity reactions.

Magnevist is excreted renally and therefore the need for Magnevist-enhanced MRI requires careful consideration in patients with severely impaired renal function in view of the potential retention of Magnevist that may occur in these cases. No further impairment of renal function or reduction in tolerance to the agent has been observed in such patients. However in severe cases consideration should be given to removing Magnevist by haemodialysis.

Slightly elevated levels of iron and bilirubin (within the normal range in the majority of cases) have been observed in the serum in some patients after administration of Magnevist. However, the elevations were seldom sustained for more than 24 hours and there was always a return to the initial values. The clinical significance of this, if any, is not known, and all patients in whom this effect was observed remained asymptomatic.

The results of serum iron determinations using complexometric methods (e.g. bathophenanthroline) may be reduced for up to 24 hours after the administration of Magnevist because of the free DTPA contained in the contrast-medium solution.

Interactions with other medicaments and other forms of interaction: None stated.

Pregnancy and lactation: There is as yet no evidence of the safety of Magnevist during human pregnancy. With daily dosage in the rat for 10 days of 12.5 times, and in the rabbit for 13 days of at least 7.5 times, the human dose per unit weight, there was slight retardation of foetal growth and ossification.

It is advisable to avoid using Magnevist during pregnancy, unless an enhanced MR investigation is essential, and no suitable alternative is available.

It is known from animal experiments that minimal amounts of Magnevist (less than 0.2% of the administered dose) enter the breast milk. The clinical relevance of this is not known.

Effects on ability to drive and use machinery: None stated.

Undesirable effects: Transient sensations of slight warmth at the injection-site, or of pain have been reported very rarely. Transient disturbances of taste may occur after rapid bolus injections.

Inadvertent paravenous injection of Magnevist may cause pain lasting up to 20 minutes. No other tissue reactions have been observed.

Nausea and vomiting and also dermal and mucosal reactions of allergic type have been observed after the administration of Magnevist.

Patients with an allergic disposition suffer more frequently than others from hypersensitivity reactions. In very rare cases anaphylactoid reactions or shock may occur. Familiarity with the practice of emergency measures is essential for prompt efficient action in the event of contrast medium incidents. Appropriate drugs and instruments (e.g. endotracheal tube and ventilator) must be readily available.

In rare cases convulsions have been observed after the administration of Magnevist. However, a causal relationship seems to be questionable.

Transient headaches, vasodilatation, dizziness, chills and syncope following the administration of Magnevist have occasionally been reported. A causal relationship has not been established.

Overdose: Acute symptoms of toxicity are unlikely with intravenous administration in adults. Treatment is symptomatic. In infants accidental administration of an entire vial (max 20 ml) may cause the following effects: increase of pulmonary artery pressure; osmotic diuresis; hypervolaemia; dehydration; local vascular pain.

Intoxication due to inadvertent oral ingestion is extremely unlikely due to the low maximum volume (20 ml) and the low gastrointestinal absorption (<1%).

If intoxication occurs due to overdosage or in cases of substantially impaired renal function, Magnevist can be removed by haemodialysis.

Pharmacological properties

Pharmacodynamic properties: Magnevist is a paramagnetic contrast agent for magnetic resonance imaging. The contrast-enhancing effect is mediated by the di-N-methylglucamine salt of gadopentetate (Gd-DTPA)–the gadolinium complex of pentetic acid (diethylene triamine pentaacetic acid = DTPA). When a suitable scanning sequence (e.g. T_1-weighted spin-echo technique) is used in proton magnetic resonance imaging, the gadolinium ion-induced shortening of the spin-lattice relaxation time of excited atomic nuclei leads to an increase in the signal intensity and, hence, to an increase of the image contrast of certain tissues.

Gadopentetate is a highly paramagnetic compound which leads to distinct shortening of the relaxation times even in low concentrations. The paramagnetic efficacy, the relaxivity–determined from the influence on the spin-lattice relaxation time of protons in water–is about 3.8 l/mmol/sec at pH 7 and 39°C and displays only slight dependency on the strength of the magnetic field.

DTPA forms a firm complex with the paramagnetic gadolinium ion with extremely high *in-vivo* and *in-vitro* stability (log K = 22-23). The dimeglumine salt of gadopentetate is a highly water-soluble, extremely hydrophilic compound with a distribution coefficient between n-butanol and buffer at pH 7.6 of about 0.0001. The substance does not display any particular protein binding or inhibitory interaction with enzymes (e.g. myocardial Na^+ and K^+ ATPase). Magnevist does not activate the complement system and, therefore, probably has a very low potential for inducing anaphylactoid reactions. No impairment of renal function has been observed.

In higher concentrations and on prolonged incubation, gadopentetate has a slight *in-vitro* effect on erythrocyte morphology. After intravenous administration of Magnevist in man, the reversible process could lead to weak extravascular haemolysis, which might explain the slight increase of serum bilirubin and iron occasionally observed in the first few hours after injection.

The results of the clinical trials do not provide any evidence of an impairment of general well-being or of hepatic, renal or cardiovascular function.

After injection of Magnevist, the resulting opacification of areas with dysfunction of the blood-brain barrier (e.g. glioblastoma) and of intracranial and intraspinal lesions of noncerebral origin provides diagnostic information additional to that obtainable with a plain scan.

Pharmacokinetic properties: Gadopentetate behaves in the organism like other highly hydrophilic biologically inert compounds (e.g mannitol or inulin).

After intravenous administration, the compound quickly diffuses in the extracellular space and is eliminated in unchanged form via the kidneys by glomerular filtration. The portion eliminated extrarenally is extremely small. Seven days after intravenous administration of radioactively labelled gadopentetate, distinctly less than 1% of the dose administered was found in the rest of the body of both the rat and the dog. The relatively highest concentrations of the compound were found in the kidneys in the form of the intact gadolinium complex. The compound penetrates and passes neither an intact blood-brain nor the blood-testis barrier. The slight amount which overcomes the placental barrier is quickly eliminated by the foetus.

The pharmacokinetics observed in man were dose-independent. Up to 0.25 mmol Gd-DTPA/kg body weight (= 0.5 ml Magnevist/kg), the plasma level fell after an early distribution phase lasting a few minutes with a half-life of about 90 minutes, identical to the renal elimination rate. At a dose of 0.1 mmol Gd-DTPA/kg (= 0.2 ml Magnevist/kg body weight), 0.6 mmol Gd-DTPA/l plasma were measured 3 minutes after the injection and 0.24 mmol Gd-DTPA/l plasma 60 minutes p.i.; an average of 83% of the dose was eliminated via the kidneys by 6 hours p.i. About 91% of the dose was recovered in the urine within 24 hours of the injection. By the 5th day, the portion of the dose eliminated with the faeces was less than 1%. No cleavage of the paramagnetic ion or metabolic break-down was demonstrable. The renal clearance of gadopentetate referred to 1.73 m^2 was about 120 ml/min and is therefore comparable to that of inulin or ^{51}Cr-EDTA.

Gadopentetate is completely eliminated via the kidneys even in the presence of impaired renal function (creatinine clearance > 20 ml/min); the plasma half-life increases in relation to the degree of renal insufficiency. An increase in the extrarenal elimination was not observed.

Because the serum half-life is prolonged (up to 30 hours) in the presence of greatly impaired renal function (creatinine clearance < 20 ml/min), gadopentetate should be eliminated by means of extracorporeal haemodialysis.

Preclinical safety data: Experimental systemic tolerance studies following repeated daily intravenous administration produced no findings which object to a single diagnostic administration of Magnevist to human beings.

Reproduction-toxicological studies with Magnevist gave no indication of a teratogenic or other embryotoxic potential following the administration of Magnevist during pregnancy.

Experimental local tolerance studies with Magnevist following single as well as repeated intravenous administration and single intra-arterial administration gave no indication that adverse local effects are to be expected in blood vessels of human beings.

Experimental local tolerance studies following a single paravenous, subcutaneous as well as intramuscular application indicated that slight local intolerance reactions could occur at the administration site after inadvertent paravenous administration.

Studies into genotoxic effects (gene, chromosomal and genome mutation tests) for gadopentetic acid, dimeglumine *in vivo* and *in vitro* gave no indication of a mutagenic potential.

In a tumorigenicity study with Magnevist in rats, no compound-related tumours were observed.

Due to the absence of genotoxic effects and taking into account the pharmacokinetics and the absence of indications of toxic effects on fast-growing tissues as well as the fact that Magnevist was only administered once, there is no evident risk of a tumorigenic effect on humans.

Studies into contact-sensitizing effect gave no indication of a sensitizing potential for Magnevist.

Pharmaceutical particulars

List of excipients: Meglumine, pentetic acid (DTPA), water for injection

Incompatibilities: Not applicable.

Shelf- life: 5 years.

Special precautions for storage: Protect from light.

Nature and contents of container: Glass vials of 5 ml, 10 ml, 15 ml, 20 ml or glass pre-filled syringes containing 10 ml, 15 ml and 20 ml of Magnevist solution.

Instructions for use/handling: Magnevist should not be drawn up into the syringe until immediately before the injection. Likewise, the pre-filled syringes must not be taken from the pack and prepared for the injection until immediately before use. Contrast medium not used in one examination must be discarded.

After preparation, Magnevist remains stable for an examination day. The time indicated does not refer to the physicochemical stability, but to the possibility of microbial contamination.

Marketing authorisation numbers

Vials 0053/0206

Pre-filled syringes 0053/0259

Date of approval/revision of SPC 4 March 1996

Legal category POM

MAGNEVIST* ENTERAL

Presentation Each bottle contains 100 ml of a concentrated colourless aqueous solution of the paramagnetic contrast medium for magnetic resonance imaging, dimeglumine gadopentetate, which is the dimeglumine salt of gadolinium – diethylenetriaminepenta–acetic acid (gadolinium DTPA). A small amount of free DTPA is present to ensure the complete chelation of the gadolinium. 1 ml of Magnevist enteral contains 9.38 mg dimeglumine gadopentetate.

Inactive excipients: sodium citrate dihydrate; diethylenetriaminepenta–acetic acid, sodium hydroxide; mannitol; water.

Uses Demonstration and demarcation of the digestive tract from adjacent normal and pathological tissue structures in MRI. Use of Magnevist enteral leads to positive opacification of the gastrointestinal tract after oral or rectal administration. This permits differentiation of the tract from other tissue structures and organs, providing an improved diagnostic yield from MRI.

Dosage and administration The patient should fast for 4 hours prior to oral administration. A cleansing enema is recommended before rectal administration. The usual precautions for MRI (eg. exclusion of cardiac pacemakers and other ferro–magnetic objects, including vascular clips etc) must be observed.

Magnevist enteral is not recommended for children below 18 years of age owing to the small amount of clinical experience with this age group as yet.

Ensure that the product is clear before use.

Dosage: Magnevist enteral is supplied as a concentrate. The contents of a 100 ml bottle are diluted with 900 ml of tap water immediately before use.

The following guidelines apply to the use of the properly diluted solution in adults:

Oral:

100 – 400 ml for oesophagus and stomach
400 – 600 ml for upper abdomen
600 – 1000 ml for lower abdomen and pelvis
Rectal: 100 – 500 ml

For examinations of the oesophagus, stomach and upper abdomen the total dose of diluted solution should be drunk in about 10 minutes and the MRI examination commenced immediately afterwards. For visualisation of bowel segments in the lower abdomen and pelvis the total dose should be drunk over 30–45 minutes and the examination commenced after waiting a further 15–30 minutes.

Complete filling of the bowel segments in the pelvic region is unlikely within 2 hours of oral administration. Rectal administration is advisable if the rectum and distal segments of the colon are to be demonstrated.

T_1–weighted spin–echo sequences, and gradient–echo sequences are the most suitable for low artefact demonstration. In some cases T_2–weighted spin–echo sequences may be necessary to allow demarcation from the abdominal fatty tissue.

Peristalsis increases with increasing doses of the agent and longer examination sequences and may lead to motion artefacts. This can be substantially reduced or even eliminated by the intravenous administration of spasmolytics.

Contra–indications, warnings, etc. For oral use: suspected ileus. For rectal use: none known.

Use in pregnancy and lactation: There is as yet no evidence of the safety of Magnevist enteral during human pregnancy. Consequently the need for examination merits particularly careful consideration. There have been no studies with Magnevist enteral during lactation. However, since it undergoes minimal enteral absorption it is unlikely that Magnevist enteral enters the breast milk.

Warnings: It is known that larger amounts (50–100 g) of mannitol may exacerbate the symptoms of patients with inflammatory gastrointestinal diseases or pre-existing water/electrolyte imbalances. Although such effects have not been observed with Magnevist enteral (maximum mannitol dose 15 g) they should be borne in mind, particularly in elderly patients.

Procedures involving diathermy (polypectomy etc) should not be performed until at least 48 hours after administration of Magnevist enteral as bacterial decomposition of the mannitol can lead to the production of highly inflammable bowel gases.

Ensure that the product is clear before use.

Side–effects: Gastrointestinal upsets such as thin stools, increased bowel peristalsis, flatulence and diarrhoea may occur due to the large amount of fluid and mannitol in Magnevist enteral. They are generally mild and short–lived. Nausea and vomiting may occur occasionally.

Cutaneous or mucosal hypersensitivity reactions may occur rarely.

Anaphylactoid reactions or shock have not been observed with Magnevist enteral although they have been reported very rarely with intravenous Magnevist. Familiarity with the practice of emergency measures is essential for prompt efficient action in the event of such incidents.

Appropriate drugs and instruments (eg. endotracheal tube and ventilator) must be readily available.

Overdosage: Less than 1% of the usual administered dose of Magnevist enteral is absorbed. Therefore an intoxication due to inadvertent overdosage is unlikely. Treatment is symptomatic.

Pharmaceutical precautions Shelf–life–Three years. Magnevist enteral does not contain a preservative. Therefore it is recommended that the solution should be used immediately after opening the 100 ml bottle.

Legal category POM

Package quantities Bottles of 100 ml

Further information

Osmolality at 37°C : 169 mosm/kg$H_2$0 (dilute solution)
Viscosity at 37°C : 0.75 mPa.s (dilute solution)
Viscosity at 20°C :1.09 mPa.s (dilute solution)
pH 6.5 – 8.0

Product licence number 0053/0229

MICROGYNON* 30

Presentation Each beige sugar-coated tablet contains 150 micrograms levonorgestrel and 30 micrograms ethinyloestradiol.

Excipients: lactose, maize starch, povidone 25 000, talc, magnesium stearate, sucrose, povidone 700 000, macrogol 6000, calcium carbonate, talc, titanium dioxide, glycerin, montan glycol wax, ferric oxide pigment yellow.

Uses Oral contraception and the recognised gynaecological indications for such oestrogen-progestogen combinations. The mode of action includes the inhibition of ovulation by suppression of the mid-cycle surge of luteinising hormone, the inspissation of cervical mucus so as to constitute a barrier to sperm, and the rendering of the endometrium unreceptive to implantation.

Dosage and administration

First treatment cycle: 1 tablet daily for 21 days, starting on the first day of the menstrual cycle. Contraceptive protection begins immediately.

Subsequent cycles: Tablet taking from the next pack of Microgynon 30 is continued after a 7-day interval, beginning on the same day of the week as the first pack.

Changing from 21-day combined oral contraceptives: The first tablet of Microgynon 30 should be taken on the first day immediately after the end of the previous oral contraceptive course. Additional contraceptive precautions are not required.

Changing from a combined Every Day pill (28 day tablets): Microgynon 30 should be started after taking the last active tablet from the Every Day Pill pack. The first Microgynon 30 tablet is taken the next day. Additional contraceptive precautions are not then required.

Changing from a progestogen-only pill (POP): The first tablet of Microgynon 30 should be taken on the first day of bleeding, even if a POP has already been taken on that day. Additional contraceptive precautions are not then required. The remaining progestogen-only pills should be discarded.

Post-partum and post-abortum use: After pregnancy, oral contraception can be started 21 days after a vaginal delivery, provided that the patient is fully ambulant and there are no puerperal complications. Additional contraceptive precautions will be required for the first 7 days of tablet taking. Since the first post-partum ovulation may precede the first bleeding, another method of contraception should be used in the interval between childbirth and the first course of tablets. After a first-trimester abortion, oral contraception may be started immediately, in which case no additional contraceptive precautions are required.

Pregnancy and lactation: If pregnancy occurs during medication with oral contraceptives, the preparation should be withdrawn immediately (see *Reasons for stopping oral contraception immediately*).

The use of Microgynon 30 during lactation may lead to a reduction in the volume of milk produced and to a change in its composition. Minute amounts of the active substances are excreted with the milk. Mothers who are breast-feeding may be advised instead to use a progestogen-only pill.

Special circumstances requiring additional contraception:

Incorrect administration: A single delayed tablet should be taken as soon as possible, and if this can be done within 12 hours of the correct time, contraceptive protection is maintained.

With longer delays, additional contraception is needed. Only the most recently delayed tablet should be taken, earlier missed tablets being omitted, and additional non-hormonal methods of contraception (except the rhythm or temperature methods) should be used for the next 7 days, while the next 7 tablets are being taken. Additionally, therefore, if tablet(s) have been missed during the last 7 days of a pack, there should be no break before the next pack is started. In this situation, a withdrawal bleed should not be expected until the end of the second pack. Some breakthrough bleeding may occur on tablet taking days but this is not clinically significant. If the patient does not have a withdrawal bleed during the tablet-free interval following the end of the second pack, the possibility of pregnancy must be ruled out before starting the next pack.

Gastro-intestinal upset: Vomiting or diarrhoea may

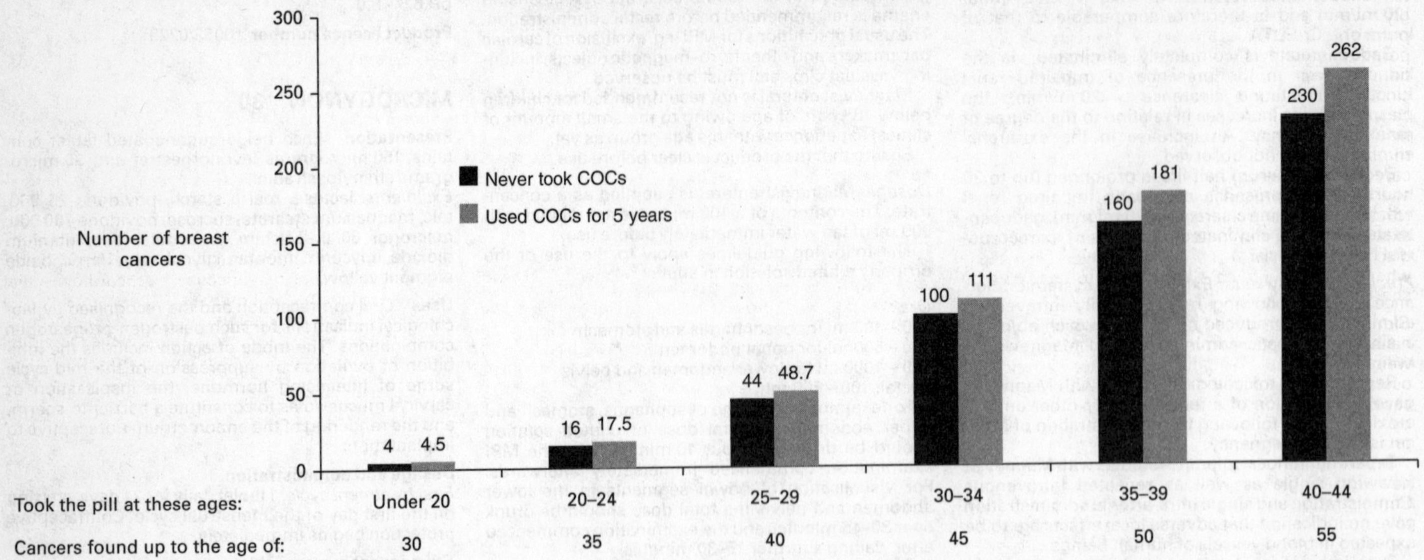

reduce the efficacy of oral contraceptives by preventing full absorption. Tablet-taking from the current pack should be continued. Additional non-hormonal methods of contraception (except the rhythm or temperature methods) should be used during the gastro-intestinal upset and for 7 days following the upset. If these 7 days overrun the end of a pack, the next pack should be started without a break. In this situation, a withdrawal bleed should not be expected until the end of the second pack. If the patient does not have a withdrawal bleed during the tablet-free interval following the end of the second pack, the possibility of pregnancy must be ruled out before starting the next pack. Other methods of contraception should be considered if the gastro-intestinal disorder is likely to be prolonged.

Interaction with other drugs: Hepatic enzyme inducers such as barbiturates, primidone, phenobarbitone, phenytoin, phenylbutazone, rifampicin, carbamazepine and griseofulvin can impair the efficacy of Microgynon 30. For women receiving long-term therapy with hepatic enzyme inducers, another method of contraception should be used. The use of ampicillin and other antibiotics may also reduce the efficacy of Microgynon 30, possibly by altering the intestinal flora. Women receiving short courses of enzyme inducers or broad spectrum antibiotics should take additional, non-hormonal (except rhythm or temperature method) contraceptive precautions during the time of concurrent medication and for 7 days afterwards. If these 7 days overrun the end of a pack, the next pack should be started without a break. In this situation, a withdrawal bleed should not be expected until the end of the second pack. If the patient does not have a withdrawal bleed during the tablet-free interval following the end of the second pack, the possibility of pregnancy must be ruled out before resuming with the next pack. With rifampicin, additional contraceptive precautions should be continued for 4 weeks after treatment stops, even if only a short course was administered.

The requirement for oral antidiabetics or insulin can change as a result of the effect on glucose tolerance.

Contra-indications, warnings, etc

Contra-indications:

1. Pregnancy
2. Severe disturbances of liver function, jaundice or persistent itching during a previous pregnancy, Dubin-Johnson syndrome, Rotor syndrome, previous or existing liver tumours
3. Existing or previous arterial or venous thrombotic or embolic processes, conditions which predispose to them e.g. disorders of the clotting processes, valvular heart disease and atrial fibrillation
4. Sickle-cell anaemia
5. Mammary or endometrial carcinoma, or a history of these conditions
6. Severe diabetes mellitus with vascular changes
7. Disorders of lipid metabolism
8. History of herpes gestationis
9. Deterioration of otosclerosis during pregnancy
10. Undiagnosed abnormal vaginal bleeding
11. Hypersensitivity to any of the components of Microgynon 30.

Warnings: There is a general opinion, based on statistical evidence, that users of combined oral contraceptives experience, more often than non-users, venous thromboembolism, arterial thrombosis, including cerebral and myocardial infarction, and subarachnoid haemorrhage. Full recovery from such disorders does not always occur, and it should be realised that in a few cases they are fatal. How often these disorders occur in users of the modern low-dose pills is not known, but there are reasons for suggesting that they may occur less often than with older pills.

Certain factors may entail some risk of thrombosis, e.g. smoking, obesity, varicose veins, cardiovascular diseases, diabetes, and migraine. The suitability of a combined oral contraceptive should be judged according to the severity of such conditions in the individual case, and should be discussed with the patient before she decides to take it. The risk of arterial thrombosis associated with combined oral contraceptives increases with age, and this risk is aggravated by cigarette-smoking. The use of combined oral contraceptives by women in the older age-group, especially those who are cigarette smokers, should therefore be discouraged and alternative methods used.

In addition if there is a history in the family of thromboembolic diseases at a young age (e.g. deep vein thrombosis, heart attack or stroke) disturbances of the coagulation system must be ruled out before the pill is prescribed.

Numerous epidemiological studies have been reported on the risks of ovarian, endometrial, cervical and breast cancer in women using combined oral contraceptives. The evidence is clear that combined oral contraceptives offer substantial protection against both ovarian and endometrial cancer.

An increased risk of cervical cancer in long-term users of combined oral contraceptives has been reported in some studies, but there continues to be controversy about the extent to which this is attributable to the confounding effects of sexual behaviour and other factors.

A meta-analysis from 54 epidemiological studies reported that there is a slightly increased relative risk (RR=1.24) of having breast cancer diagnosed in women who are currently using combined oral contraceptives (COCs). The observed pattern of increased risk may be due to an earlier diagnosis of breast cancer in COC users, the biological effects of COCs or a combination of both. The additional breast cancers diagnosed in current users of COCs or in women who have used COCs in the last ten years are more likely to be localised to the breast than those in women who never used COCs.

Breast cancer is rare among women under 40 years of age whether or not they take COCs. Whilst this background risk increases with age, the excess number of breast cancer diagnoses in current and recent COC users is small in relation to the overall risk of breast cancer (see bar chart).

The most important risk factor for breast cancer in COC users is the age women discontinue the COC; the older the age at stopping, the more breast cancers are diagnosed. Duration of use is less important and the excess risk gradually disappears during the course of the 10 years after stopping COC use such that by 10 years there appears to be no excess.

The possible increase in risk of breast cancer should be discussed with the user and weighed against the benefits of COCs taking into account the evidence that they offer substantial protection against the risk of developing certain other cancers (e.g. ovarian and endometrial cancer).

The possibility cannot be ruled out that certain chronic diseases may occasionally deteriorate during the use of combined oral contraceptives (see *Precautions*).

In rare cases benign and, in even rarer cases, malignant liver tumours leading in isolated cases to life-threatening intra-abdominal haemorrhage have been observed after the use of hormonal substances such as those contained in Microgynon 30. If severe upper abdominal complaints, liver enlargement or signs of intra-abdominal haemorrhage occur, the possibility of a liver tumour should be included in the differential diagnosis.

Reasons for stopping oral contraception immediately:

1. Occurrence for the first time, or exacerbation, of migrainous headaches or unusually frequent or unusually severe headaches
2. Sudden disturbances of vision or hearing or other perceptual disorders
3. First signs of thrombophlebitis or thromboembolic symptoms (e.g. unusual pains in or swelling of the leg(s), stabbing pains on breathing or coughing for no apparent reason). Feeling of pain and tightness in the chest
4. Six weeks before an elective major operation (e.g. abdominal, orthopaedic), any surgery to the legs, medical treatment for varicose veins or prolonged immobilisation, e.g. after accidents or surgery. Do not restart until 2 weeks after full ambulation. In case of emergency surgery, thrombotic prophylaxis is usually indicated e.g. subcutaneous heparin
5. Onset of jaundice, hepatitis, itching of the whole body
6. Increase in epileptic seizures
7. Significant rise in blood pressure
8. Onset of severe depression
9. Severe upper abdominal pain or liver enlargement
10. Clear exacerbation of conditions known to be capable of deteriorating during oral contraception or pregnancy
11. Pregnancy is a reason for stopping immediately because it has been suggested by some investigations that oral contraceptives taken in early pregnancy may slightly increase the risk of foetal malformations. Other investigations have failed to support these findings. The possibility therefore cannot be excluded, but it is certain that if a risk exists at all, it is very small.

Precautions: Examination of the pelvic organs, breasts and blood-pressure should precede the prescribing of any combined oral contraceptive and should be repeated regularly. The family medical history should be carefully noted and disturbances of the clotting mechanism ruled out if any member of the family has suffered from thromboembolic disease (e.g. deep vein thrombosis, stroke, myocardial infarction) at a young age. Before starting treatment pregnancy must be excluded.

The following conditions require strict medical

supervision during medication with oral contraceptives. Deterioration or first appearance of any of these conditions may indicate that use of the oral contraceptive should be discontinued: diabetes mellitus, or a tendency towards diabetes mellitus (e.g. unexplained glycosuria), hypertension, varicose veins, a history of phlebitis, otosclerosis, multiple sclerosis, epilepsy, porphyria, tetany, disturbed liver function, Sydenham's chorea, renal dysfunction, family history of clotting disorders, obesity, family history of breast cancer and patient history of benign breast disease, history of clinical depression, systemic lupus erythematosus, uterine fibroids and migraine, gall-stones, cardiovascular diseases, chloasma, asthma, an intolerance of contact lenses, or any disease that is prone to worsen during pregnancy. Some women may experience amenorrhoea or oligomenorrhoea after discontinuation of oral contraceptives, especially when these conditions existed prior to use. Women should be informed of this possibility.

Side-effects: In rare cases, headaches, gastric upsets, nausea, vomiting, breast tenderness, changes in body weight, changes in libido, depressive moods can occur. In predisposed women, use of Microgynon 30 can sometimes cause chloasma which is exacerbated by exposure to sunlight. Such women should avoid prolonged exposure to sunlight.

Individual cases of poor tolerance of contact lenses have been reported with use of oral contraceptives. Contact lens wearers who develop changes in lens tolerance should be assessed by an ophthalmologist.

Menstrual changes:

1. Reduction of menstrual flow: This is not abnormal and it is to be expected in some patients. Indeed, it may be beneficial where heavy periods were previously experienced.

2. Missed menstruation: Occasionally, withdrawal bleeding may not occur at all. If the tablets have been taken correctly, pregnancy is very unlikely. If withdrawal bleeding fails to occur at the end of a second pack, the possibility of pregnancy must be ruled out before resuming with the next pack.

Intermenstrual bleeding: 'Spotting' or heavier 'breakthrough bleeding' sometimes occur during tablet taking, especially in the first few cycles, and normally cease spontaneously. Microgynon 30 should therefore be continued even if irregular bleeding occurs. If irregular bleeding is persistent, appropriate diagnostic measures to exclude an organic cause are indicated and may include curettage. This also applies in the case of spotting which occurs at irregular intervals in several consecutive cycles or which occurs for the first time after long use of Microgynon 30.

Effect on blood chemistry: The use of oral contraceptives may influence the results of certain laboratory tests including biochemical parameters of liver, thyroid, adrenal and renal function, plasma levels of carrier proteins and lipid/lipoprotein fractions, parameters of carbohydrate metabolism and parameters of coagulation and fibrinolysis. Laboratory staff should therefore be informed about oral contraceptive use when laboratory tests are requested.

Overdosage: Overdosage may cause nausea, vomiting and, in females, withdrawal bleeding. There are no specific antidotes and treatment should be symptomatic.

Pharmaceutical precautions *Shelf-life:* Five years.

Legal category POM

Package quantities Available in packs containing one months' supply

Product licence number 0053/0064

MICROGYNON* 30 ED

Qualitative and quantitative composition Each memo-pack contains 21 beige active tablets and 7 white placebo tablets which are larger.

Each active tablet contains 150 micrograms levonorgestrel and 30 micrograms ethinylestradiol.

Pharmaceutical form Sugar-coated tablets

Clinical particulars

Therapeutic indications: Oral contraception and the recognised gynaecological indications for such oestrogen-progestogen combinations.

Posology and method of administration:

First treatment cycle: 1 tablet daily for 28 days, starting on the first day of the menstrual cycle. 21 (small) active tablets are taken followed by 7 (larger) placebo tablets. Contraceptive protection begins immediately.

Subsequent cycles: Tablet-taking is continuous, which means that the next pack of Microgynon 30 ED follows immediately without a break. A withdrawal bleed usually occurs when the placebo tablets are being taken.

Changing from 21-day combined oral contraceptives: The first tablet of Microgynon 30 ED should be taken on the first day immediately after the end of the previous oral contraceptive course. Additional contraceptive precautions are not required.

Changing from a combined Every Day pill (28 -day pill): Microgynon 30 ED should be started after taking the last active tablet from the previous Every Day pill pack. The first Microgynon 30 ED tablet is taken the next day. Additional contraceptive precautions are not then required.

Changing from a progestogen-only pill (POP): The first tablet of Microgynon 30 ED should be taken on the first day of bleeding, even if a POP has already been taken on that day. Additional contraceptive precautions are not then required. The remaining progestogen only pills should be discarded.

Post-partum and post-abortum use: After pregnancy, oral contraception can be started 21 days after a vaginal delivery, provided that the patient is fully ambulant and there are no puerperal complications. Additional contraceptive precautions will be required for the first 7 days of tablet taking to ensure adequate contraceptive cover if early ovulation has occurred. Since the first post-partum ovulation may precede the first bleeding, another method of contraception should be used in the interval between childbirth and the first course of tablets. After a first-trimester abortion, oral contraception may be started immediately in which case no additional contraceptive precautions are required.

Special circumstances requiring additional contraception

Incorrect administration: Errors in taking the 7 placebo tablets (i.e. the larger white tablets in the last row)can be ignored.

A single delayed active (small) tablet should be taken as soon as possible, and if this can be done within 12 hours of the correct time, contraceptive protection is maintained.

With longer delays in taking active tablets, additional contraception is needed. Only the most recently delayed tablet should be taken, earlier missed tablets being omitted, and additional non-hormonal methods of contraception (except the rhythm or temperature methods) should be used for *the next 7 days, while the next 7 active (small) tablets are being taken.* Therefore, if the 7 days additional contraception extend beyond the last active (small) tablet, the user should finish taking all the active tablets, discard the placebo tablets and start a new pack of Microgynon 30 ED the next day with an appropriate active (small) tablet. Thus, active tablet follows active tablet with no 7 day break. In this situation, a withdrawal bleed should not be expected until the end of the second pack. Some breakthrough bleeding may occur on tablet taking days but this is not clinically significant. If the patient does not have a withdrawal bleed following the end of the second pack, the possibility of pregnancy must be ruled out before starting the next pack.

Gastro-intestinal upset: Vomiting or diarrhoea may reduce the efficacy of oral contraceptives by preventing full absorption. Tablet-taking from the current pack should be continued. Additional non-hormonal methods of contraception (except the rhythm or temperature methods) should be used during the gastro-intestinal upset and for 7 days following the upset. If these 7 days extend beyond the last active (small) tablet the user should finish taking all the active tablets, discard the placebo tablets and start a new pack of Microgynon 30 ED the next day with an appropriate active (small) tablet. In this situation, a withdrawal bleed should not be expected until the end of the second pack. If the patient does not have a withdrawal bleed at the end of the second pack, the possibility of pregnancy must be ruled out before starting the next pack. Other methods of contraception should be considered if the gastro-intestinal disorder is likely to be prolonged.

Children and the elderly: Microgynon 30 ED is an oral contraceptive and is not applicable in children or the elderly.

Contra-indications:

1. Pregnancy
2. Severe disturbances of liver function, jaundice or persistent itching during a previous pregnancy, Dubin-Johnson syndrome, Rotor syndrome, previous or existing liver tumours
3. Existing or previous arterial or venous thrombotic or embolic processes, conditions which predispose to them e.g. disorders of the clotting processes, valvular heart disease and atrial fibrillation
4. Sickle-cell anaemia
5. Mammary or endometrial carcinoma, or a history of these conditions
6. Severe diabetes mellitus with vascular changes
7. Disorders of lipid metabolism
8. History of herpes gestationis
9. Deterioration of otosclerosis during pregnancy
10. Undiagnosed abnormal vaginal bleeding
11. Hypersensitivity to any of the components of Microgynon 30 ED.

Special warnings and special precautions for use:

Warnings: There is a general opinion, based on statistical evidence, that users of combined oral contraceptives experience, more often than non-users, venous thromboembolism, arterial thrombosis, including cerebral and myocardial infarction, and subarachnoid haemorrhage. Full recovery from such disorders does not always occur, and it should be realised that in a few cases they are fatal. How often these disorders occur in users of the modern low-dose pills is not known, but there are reasons for suggesting that they may occur less often than with older pills.

Certain factors may entail some risk of thrombosis, e.g. smoking, obesity, varicose veins, cardiovascular diseases, diabetes, and migraine. The suitability of a combined oral contraceptive should be judged according to the severity of such conditions in the individual case, and should be discussed with the patient before she decides to take it. The risk of arterial thrombosis associated with combined oral contraceptives increases with age, and this risk is aggravated by cigarette-smoking. The use of combined oral contraceptives by women in the older age-group, especially those who are cigarette smokers, should therefore be discouraged and alternative methods used.

In addition if there is a history in the family of thromboembolic diseases at a young age (e.g. deep vein thrombosis, heart attack or stroke) disturbances of the coagulation system must be ruled out before the pill is prescribed.

Numerous epidemiological studies have been reported on the risks of ovarian, endometrial, cervical and breast cancer in women using combined oral contraceptives. The evidence is clear that combined oral contraceptives offer substantial protection against both ovarian and endometrial cancer.

An increased risk of cervical cancer in long-term users of combined oral contraceptives has been reported in some studies, but there continues to be controversy about the extent to which this is attributable to the confounding effects of sexual behaviour and other factors.

A meta-analysis from 54 epidemiological studies reported that there is a slightly increased relative risk (RR=1.24) of having breast cancer diagnosed in women who are currently using combined oral contraceptives (COCs). The observed pattern of increased risk may be due to an earlier diagnosis of breast cancer in COC users, the biological effects of COCs or a combination of both. The additional breast cancers diagnosed in current users of COCs or in women who have used COCs in the last ten years are more likely to be localised to the breast than those in women who never used COCs.

Breast cancer is rare among women under 40 years of age whether or not they take COCs. Whilst this background risk increases with age, the excess number of breast cancer diagnoses in current and recent COC users is small in relation to the overall risk of breast cancer (see bar chart).

The most important risk factor for breast cancer in COC users is the age women discontinue the COC; the older the age at stopping, the more breast cancers are diagnosed. Duration of use is less important and the excess risk gradually disappears during the course of the 10 years after stopping COC use such that by 10 years there appears to be no excess.

The possible increase in risk of breast cancer should be discussed with the user and weighed against the benefits of COCs taking into account the evidence that they offer substantial protection against the risk of developing certain other cancers (e.g. ovarian and endometrial cancer).

The possibility cannot be ruled out that certain chronic diseases may occasionally deteriorate during the use of combined oral contraceptives (see *Precautions*).

In rare cases benign and, in even rarer cases, malignant liver tumours leading in isolated cases to life-threatening intra-abdominal haemorrhage have been observed after the use of hormonal substances such as those contained in Microgynon 30 ED. If severe upper abdominal complaints, liver enlargement or signs of intra-abdominal haemorrhage occur, the possibility of a liver tumour should be included in the differential diagnosis.

Reasons for stopping oral contraception immediately:

1. Occurrence for the first time, or exacerbation, of migrainous headaches or unusually frequent or unusually severe headaches
2. Sudden disturbances of vision or hearing or other perceptual disorders
3. First signs of thrombophlebitis or thromboembolic symptoms (e.g. unusual pains in or swelling of the leg(s), stabbing pains on breathing or coughing for no apparent reason). Feeling of pain and tightness in the chest

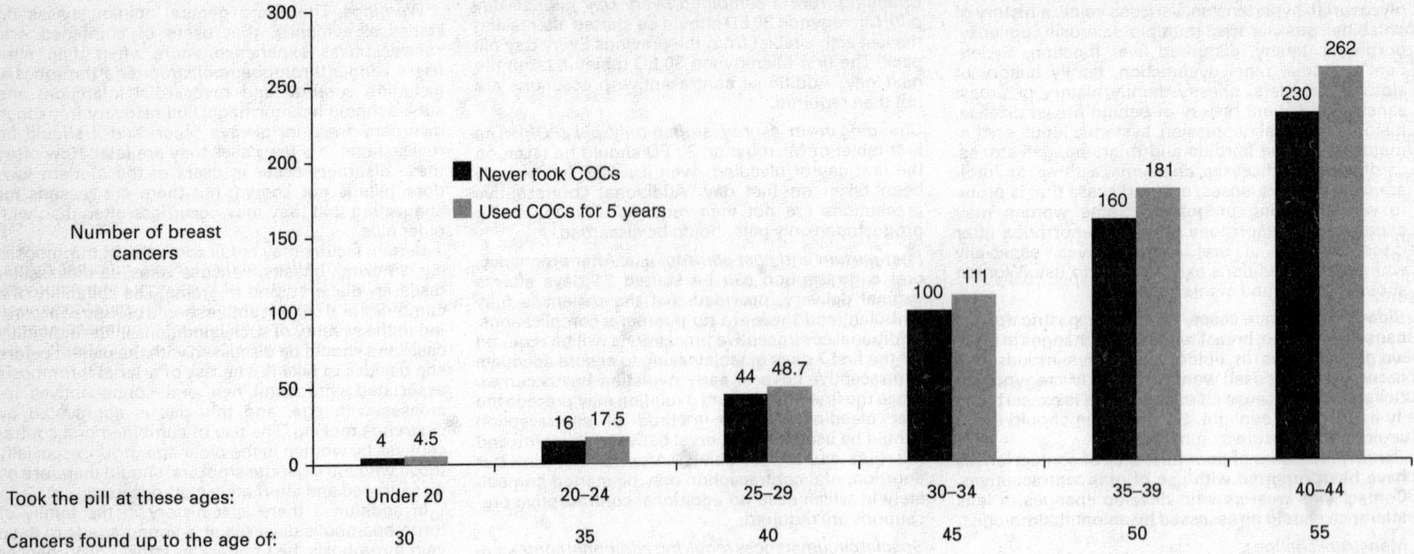

4. Six weeks before an elective major operation (e.g. abdominal, orthopaedic), any surgery to the legs, medical treatment for varicose veins or prolonged immobilisation, e.g. after accidents or surgery. Do not restart until 2 weeks after full ambulation. In case of emergency surgery, thrombotic prophylaxis is usually indicated e.g. subcutaneous heparin
5. Onset of jaundice, hepatitis, itching of the whole body
6. Increase in epileptic seizures
7. Significant rise in blood pressure
8. Onset of severe depression
9. Severe upper abdominal pain or liver enlargement
10. Clear exacerbation of conditions known to be capable of deteriorating during oral contraception or pregnancy
11. Pregnancy is a reason for stopping immediately because it has been suggested by some investigations that oral contraceptives taken in early pregnancy may slightly increase the risk of foetal malformations. Other investigations have failed to support these findings. The possibility therefore cannot be excluded, but it is certain that if a risk exists at all, it is very small.

Precautions: Examination of the pelvic organs, breasts and blood-pressure should precede the prescribing of any combined oral contraceptive and should be repeated regularly. The family medical history should be carefully noted and disturbances of the clotting mechanism ruled out if any member of the family has suffered from thromboembolic disease (e.g. deep vein thrombosis, stroke, myocardial infarction) at a young age. Before starting treatment pregnancy must be excluded.

The following conditions require strict medical supervision during medication with oral contraceptives. Deterioration or first appearance of any of these conditions may indicate that use of the oral contraceptive should be discontinued:

Diabetes mellitus, or a tendency towards diabetes mellitus (e.g. unexplained glycosuria), hypertension, varicose veins, a history of phlebitis, otosclerosis, multiple sclerosis, epilepsy, porphyria, tetany, disturbed liver function, Sydenham's chorea, renal dysfunction, family history of clotting disorders, obesity, family history of breast cancer and patient history of benign breast disease, history of clinical depression, systemic lupus erythematosus, uterine fibroids and migraine, gall-stones, cardiovascular diseases, chloasma, asthma, an intolerance of contact lenses, or any disease that is prone to worsen during pregnancy.

Some women may experience amenorrhoea or oligomenorrhoea after discontinuation of oral contraceptives, especially when these conditions existed prior to use. Women should be informed of this possibility.

Interaction with other medicaments and other forms of interaction: Hepatic enzyme inducers such as barbiturates, primidone, phenobarbitone, phenytoin, phenylbutazone, rifampicin, carbamazepine and griseofulvin can impair the efficacy of Microgynon 30 ED. For women receiving long-term therapy with hepatic enzyme inducers, another method of contraception should be used. The use of ampicillin and other antibiotics may also reduce the efficacy of Microgynon 30 ED, possibly by altering the intestinal flora.

Women receiving short courses of enzyme inducers or broad spectrum antibiotics should take additional, non-hormonal (except rhythm or temperature method) contraceptive precautions during the time of concurrent medication and for 7 days afterwards. If these 7 days extend beyond the last active (small) tablet the user should finish taking all the active tablets, discard the placebo (large) tablets and start a new pack of Microgynon 30 ED the next day with an appropriate active (small) tablet. In this situation, a withdrawal bleed should not be expected until the end of the second pack. If the patient does not have a withdrawal bleed at the end of the second pack, the possibility of pregnancy must be ruled out before resuming with the next pack. With rifampicin, additional contraceptive precautions should be continued for 4 weeks after treatment stops, even if only a short course was administered.

The requirement for oral antidiabetics or insulin can change as a result of the effect on glucose tolerance.

Pregnancy and lactation: If pregnancy occurs during medication with oral contraceptives, the preparation should be withdrawn immediately (see 'Reasons for stopping oral contraception immediately').

The use of Microgynon 30 ED during lactation may lead to a reduction in the volume of milk produced and to a change in its composition. Minute amounts of the active substances are excreted with the milk. Mothers who are breast-feeding may be advised instead to use a progestogen-only pill.

Effects on ability to drive and to use machines: None known.

Undesirable effects: In rare cases, headaches, gastric upsets, nausea, vomiting, breast tenderness, changes in body weight, changes in libido, depressive moods can occur.

In predisposed women, use of Microgynon 30 ED can sometimes cause chloasma which is exacerbated by exposure to sunlight. Such women should avoid prolonged exposure to sunlight.

Individual cases of poor tolerance of contact lenses have been reported with use of oral contraceptives. Contact lens wearers who develop changes in lens tolerance should be assessed by an ophthalmologist.

Menstrual changes:

1. Reduction of menstrual flow: This is not abnormal and it is to be expected in some patients. Indeed, it may be beneficial where heavy periods were previously experienced.

2. Missed menstruation: Occasionally, withdrawal bleeding may not occur at all. If the tablets have been taken correctly, pregnancy is very unlikely. If withdrawal bleeding fails to occur at the end of a second pack, the possibility of pregnancy must be ruled out before resuming with the next pack.

Intermenstrual bleeding: 'Spotting' or heavier 'breakthrough bleeding' sometimes occur during tablet taking, especially in the first few cycles, and normally cease spontaneously. Microgynon 30 ED should therefore, be continued even if irregular bleeding occurs. If irregular bleeding is persistent, appropriate diagnostic measures to exclude an organic cause are indicated and may include curettage. This also applies in the case of spotting which occurs at irregular intervals in several consecutive cycles or which occurs for the first time after long use of Microgynon 30 ED.

Effect on blood chemistry: The use of oral contraceptives may influence the results of certain laboratory tests including biochemical parameters of liver, thyroid, adrenal and renal function, plasma levels of carrier proteins and lipid/lipoprotein fractions, parameters of carbohydrate metabolism and parameters of coagulation and fibrinolysis. Laboratory staff should therefore be informed about oral contraceptive use when laboratory tests are requested.

Refer to 'Special warnings and special precautions for use' section for additional information.

Overdose: Overdosage may cause nausea, vomiting and, in females, withdrawal bleeding.

There are no specific antidotes and treatment should be symptomatic.

Pharmacological particulars

Pharmacodynamic properties: Microgynon 30 ED is an oestrogen-progestogen combination which acts by inhibiting ovulation by suppression of the mid-cycle surge of luteinizing hormone, the inspissation of cervical mucus so as to constitute a barrier to sperm, and the rendering of the endometrium unreceptive to implantation.

Pharmacokinetic properties

Levonorgestrel: Levonorgestrel is absorbed quickly and completely. Maximum active substance levels of approx. 3 ng/ml were reached in serum just one hour after ingestion of Microgynon 30 ED. The serum concentrations subsequently fell in 2 phases with half-lives of around 0.5 hours and 20 hours. The metabolic clearance rate from plasma is approx. 1.5 ml/min/kg.

Levonorgestrel is eliminated not in unchanged form, but in the form of metabolites with a half-life of around one day and in almost equal proportions via the kidney and bile. Biotransformation takes place via the familiar pathways of steroid metabolism. There are no known pharmacologically active products of metabolism.

Levonorgestrel is bound to serum albumin and SHBG. Only around 1.5% of the respective total concentration is present in unbound form, while approx. 65% is bound to SHBG. The relative proportions (free, albumin-bound, SHBG-bound) depend on the concentration of SHBG. After induction of the binding protein, the portion bound to SHBG increases, while the free portion and that bound to albumin decreases.

After daily repeated ingestion, levonorgestrel accumulates by about the factor 2. A steady state is reached during the second half of the treatment cycle. The pharmacokinetics of levonorgestrel are dependent on the concentration of SHBG in plasma. Under treatment with Microgynon 30 ED, an increase in the serum levels of SHBG effect a concomitant increase in the specific binding capacity and therefore also an increase in levonorgestrel serum levels.

The levonorgestrel serum levels do not change any further after 1–3 cycles of use owing to the fact that

SHBG induction is concluded. Compared to a single administration, 3–4 fold higher levonorgestrel serum levels are reached in the steady state.

The absolute bioavailability of levonorgestrel amounts to almost 100%.

Approx. 0.1% of the maternal dose can be passed on to a baby with the breast milk.

Ethinylestradiol: Orally administered ethinylestradiol is absorbed quickly and completely. Ingestion of Microgynon 30 ED leads to maximum plasma levels of approx. 100 pg/ml after 1–2 hours. The substance concentration then falls in 2 phases for which half-lives of around 1–2 hours and about 20 hours have been determined. For technical reasons, these data can only be calculated at higher dosages.

An imaginary distribution volume of around 5 l/kg and a metabolic clearance rate from plasma of approx. 5 ml/min/kg have been determined for ethinylestradiol. Ethinylestradiol is bound non-specifically to serum albumin to the extent of 98%.

Ethinylestradiol is metabolized even during its absorption phase and during its first liver transit, leading to reduced and individually varying oral bioavailability. Ethinylestradiol is eliminated not in unchanged form, but in the form of metabolites with a half-life of around one day. The excretion ratio is 40 (urine) : 60 (bile).

Because of the half-life of the terminal elimination phase from plasma, a steady state characterised by a 30–40% higher plasma substance level becomes established after approx. 5–6 daily administrations.

The absolute bioavailability of ethinylestradiol is subject to considerable interindividual variations. After oral ingestion, it amounts to around 40–60% of the dose.

In women with fully established lactation, around 0.02% of the maternal dose can be passed on to the baby with the breast milk.

Other drugs can have a negative or positive effect on the systemic availability of ethinylestradiol. No interaction with vitamin C takes place. On continuous use, ethinylestradiol induces the hepatic synthesis of CBG and SHBG, the extent of SHBG induction being dependent on the type and dose of the simultaneously administered progestogen.

Preclinical safety data: There are no preclinical safety data which could be of relevance to the prescriber and which are not already included in other relevant sections of the SPC.

Pharmaceutical particulars

List of excipients:

Active tablets: lactose, maize starch, povidone, magnesium stearate (E 572), sucrose, polyethylene glycol 6000, calcium carbonate (E 170), talc, montan glycol wax, titanium dioxide (E 171), ferric oxide pigment yellow (E 172), glycerin (E 422).

Placebo tablets: lactose, maize starch, povidone, magnesium stearate (E 572), sucrose, polyethylene glycol 6000, calcium carbonate (E 170), talc, montan glycol wax.

Incompatibilities: None known.

Shelf life: 5 years.

Special precautions for storage: Not applicable.

Nature and contents of container: Deep drawn strips made of polyvinyl chloride film with counter-sealing foil made of aluminium with heat sealable coating.

Presentation: Each carton contains 1 or 3 blister memo-packs. Each blister memo-pack contains 21 active tablets and 7 placebo tablets.

Instructions for use/handling: Keep out of the reach of children.

Marketing authorisation number 0053/0260

Date of approval/revision of SPC January 1998

Legal category POM.

MIRENA*

Qualitative and quantitative composition Active ingredient: Levonorgestrel 52 mg

Pharmaceutical form Levonorgestrel Intrauterine System

Clinical particulars

Therapeutic indications: Contraception

Posology and method of administration: Intrauterine.

The initial release of levonorgestrel is about 20 micrograms/24 hours. Mirena releases levonorgestrel for five years.

Mirena is intended for use in women of child-bearing age. Clinical trials were conducted in women of 18 years and over.

Postpartum insertions should be postponed until six weeks after delivery.

Contra-indications: Sensitivity to levonorgestrel; known or suspected pregnancy, undiagnosed abnormal genital bleeding; congenital or acquired abnormality of the uterus including fibroids if they distort the uterine cavity; current genital infection; acute or recurrent pelvic inflammatory disease; past attack of bacterial endocarditis or of severe pelvic infection in a woman with an anatomical lesion of the heart or after any prosthetic valve replacement; active or previous severe arterial disease, such as stroke or myocardial infarction; liver tumour; established immunodeficiency; acute malignancies affecting the blood or leukaemias except when in remission; recent trophoblastic disease while hCG levels remain elevated.

Special warnings and special precautions for use: Mirena may be used with caution, or removal of the system should be considered, if any of the following conditions exist or arise for the first time:

Confirmed or suspected hormone dependent neoplasia (including breast cancer), malignancies affecting the blood or leukaemias in remission after specialist consultation; hepatic jaundice or other acute or severe liver disease; severe or multiple risk factors for arterial disease; thrombotic arterial or any current embolic disease; use of chronic corticosteroid therapy; past history of symptomatic functional ovarian cysts.

Mirena produces blood levels of levonorgestrel which are lower than in standard progestogen-only pills and is oestrogen-free. Therefore, the following are less likely to occur or to deteriorate:

Past venous thromboembolism; marked increase in blood pressure; and migraine, crescendo migraine, focal migraine with asymmetrical visual loss or other symptoms which are interpretable as being caused by transient cerebral ischaemia.

In general, women using hormonal contraception should be encouraged to give up smoking.

Patients with congenital or acquired cardiac valve defects may be given antibiotic prophylaxis at the time of IUD insertion or removal to prevent endocarditis.

Women with a previous history of ectopic pregnancy carry a higher risk of a further ectopic pregnancy. The possibility of ectopic pregnancy should be considered in the case of lower abdominal pain–especially in connection with missed periods or if an amenorrhoeic woman starts bleeding.

Irregular bleeding may mask symptoms and signs of endometrial cancer.

Functional ovarian cysts have been diagnosed in about 10-12% of patients, and these are also common with progestin-only contraception. In most cases, the enlarged follicles disappear spontaneously during two to three months' observation. Should this not happen, continued ultrasound monitoring and other diagnostic/therapeutic measures are recommended.

Low-dose levonorgestrel may affect glucose tolerance, and the blood glucose concentration should be monitored in diabetic users of Mirena.

Before insertion, the patient must be informed on the efficacy, risks and side-effects of Mirena. A gynaecological examination, including examination of the breasts and exclusion of a pregnancy, should be performed. Cervical infection and sexually transmitted diseases should be excluded. The position of the uterus and the size of the uterine cavity should be determined. The instructions for insertion should be followed carefully. The patient should be re-examined six weeks after insertion and once a year thereafter, or more frequently if clinically indicated.

Syncope or bradycardia may occur in some women during insertion or removal of an IUD. In the event of early signs of a vasovagal attack, insertion may need to be abandoned or the device removed. The woman should be kept supine, the head lowered and the legs elevated to the vertical position if necessary in order to restore cerebral blood flow. A clear airway must be maintained; an airway should always be at hand. Persistent bradycardia may be controlled with intravenous atropine. If oxygen is available it may be administered.

The possibility of pregnancy should be considered if menstruation does not occur within six weeks of the onset of previous menstruation and expulsion should be excluded. A repeated pregnancy test is not necessary in amenorrhoeic subjects unless indicated by other symptoms.

Pelvic infection: Known risk factors for pelvic inflammatory disease are multiple sexual partners, frequent intercourse and young age. Mirena should be removed if the woman experiences recurrent endometritis or pelvic infection, or if an acute infection does not respond to treatment within a few days.

Expulsion: Symptoms of the partial or complete explusion of any IUD may include bleeding or pain. However, a device can be expelled from the uterine cavity without the woman noticing it. Partial expulsion may decrease the effectiveness of Mirena. As the system decreases menstrual flow, increase of menstrual flow may be indicative of an expulsion.

Perforation: Perforation of the uterine corpus or cervix may occur, most commonly during insertion. If perforation is suspected the system should be removed as soon as possible.

Lost threads: If the retrieval thread is not visible at the cervix on follow-up examination–first exclude pregnancy. The thread may have been drawn up into the uterus or cervical canal and may reappear during the next menstrual period. If pregnancy has been excluded, the thread may usually be located by gently probing with a suitable instrument. If it cannot be found, it may have broken off, or the system may have been expelled. Ultrasound or X-ray may be used to locate Mirena.

Post-coital contraception: Limited experience suggests that Mirena is not suitable for use as a post-coital contraceptive.

Interaction with other medicaments and other forms of interaction: The effect of hormonal contraceptives may be impaired by drugs which induce liver enzymes, including barbiturates, phenytoin, carbamazepine and rifampicin. The influence of these drugs on the efficacy of Mirena has not been studied.

Pregnancy and lactation: Pregnancy: In case of an accidental pregnancy with Mirena *in situ*, the system must be removed and termination of the pregnancy should be considered. Should these procedures not be possible, the woman should be informed about increased risk of spontaneous abortion or premature labour observed during the use of copper and plastic IUDs. Accordingly, such pregnancies should be closely monitored.

Because of the intrauterine administration and the local exposure to the hormone, teratogenicity (especially virilisation) cannot be completely excluded. It can be expected that the systemic hormone exposure of the foetus through the maternal circulation is lower than with any other hormonal contraceptive method. Because of the rareness of pregnancy with Mirena, there is no clinical experience of the outcome.

Lactation: The daily dose and the plasma concentrations of levonorgestrel are lower than with any other hormonal contraceptive method. Concentrations of levonorgestrel have been detected in the breast milk of lactating women. The long-term effects on the nursing infant are unknown.

Effects on ability to drive and use machines: There are no known effects on the ability to drive or use machines.

Undesirable effects:

Side-effects: Side-effects are more common during the first months after the insertion, and subside during prolonged use. Menstrual problems are the most often reported adverse events as described below. The following adverse events have been reported in the order of frequency of occurrence: headache, lower abdominal pain, back pain, skin disorders, vaginal discharge, mastalgia and other benign breast conditions, vaginitis, depression and other mood changes, nausea and oedema. Other adverse events reported include ovarian cysts and pelvic inflammatory disease which may be serious. Weight gain, hair loss or greasy hair, have been reported in individual cases.

The average changes in weight and in blood pressure have been similar to those observed for copper IUD patients.

The rate of ectopic pregnancy has been 0.06 per 100 woman-years. This rate is significantly lower than the rate of 1.2-1.6 estimated for patients not using any contraception. The corresponding figure for the copper IUD is 0.12 per 100 woman-years.

Bleeding patterns: The most common side-effect of Mirena is a change in menstrual bleeding patterns. The changes may include spotting, shorter or longer menstrual periods, or oligo/amenorrhoea.

During the first month of use, users of Mirena have had on average nine days of spotting. However, spotting decreased gradually and the number of days spotting after six months was less than four, which was comparable to the experience with copper IUDs.

During the first month of use, 20% of users experienced prolonged bleeding (more than eight days). For many women, periods became shorter, and during the third month of use, only 3% of users had prolonged bleeding.

Menstrual blood loss is generally reduced during use of Mirena. Scanty blood flow frequently develops into oligo/amenorrhoea. Amenorrhoea is a side-effect that can be positive for some and negative for others. In clinical studies during the first year of use, 17% of women experienced amenorrhoea of at least three months' duration, but the cumulative gross discontinuation rate for amenorrhoea was very low. Amenorrhoea is due to the local effect of levonorgestrel on the endometrium, which-under strong local suppression, does not proliferate in response to oestrogen. Hence, the duration and volume of menstrual bleeding is reduced. The volume of menstrual bleeding was decreased by 88% in menorrhagic women by the end of 3 months use. Reduced bleeding increases the concentration of blood haemoglobin.

Although bleeding patterns may vary from regular scanty menstruation in some women to oligo/amenorrhoea in others, there is no clear difference in follicle development, ovulation or oestradiol and progesterone production in women with different bleeding patterns.

Overdose: Not applicable

Pharmacological properties

Pharmacodynamic properties: Levonorgestrel is a progestin used in gynaecology in various ways: as the progestin component in oral contraceptives, in hormonal replacement therapy or alone for contraception in minipills and subdermal implants. Levonorgestrel can also be administered directly into the uterine cavity as an intrauterine system. This allows a very low daily dosage, as the hormone is released directly into the target organ.

The mechanism of action of Mirena is based on mainly hormonal effects producing the following changes:

- Prevention of proliferation of the endometrium
- Thickening of the cervical mucus thus inhibiting the passage of sperm
- Suppression of ovulation in some women.

The physical presence of the system in the uterus would also be expected to make a minor contribution to its contraceptive effect.

Studies on contraceptive efficacy have suggested a pregnancy rate (Pearl Index) of less than 1 per 100 woman-years.

Mirena may be particularly useful for contraception in patients with excessive menstrual bleeding, as a marked reduction of menstrual flow is noted after three months use. Some users will become amenorrhoeic.

Pharmacokinetic properties: The pharmacokinetics of levonorgestrel itself have been extensively investigated and reported in the literature. One key finding is that the bioavailability of levonorgestrel administered orally is almost 90 per cent. A half life of 20 hours is considered the best estimate although some studies have reported values as short as 9 hours and others as long as 80 hours. Another important finding, although one in agreement with experience with other synthetic steroids, has been marked differences in metabolic clearance rates among individuals, even when administration was by the intravenous route. Levonorgestrel is extensively bound to proteins (mainly sex hormone binding globulin (SHBG)) and extensively metabolised to a large number of inactive metabolites.

The initial release of levonorgestrel from Mirena is 20 micrograms/24 hours, delivered directly into the uterine cavity. Because of the low plasma concentrations, there are only minor effects on the metabolism.

Preclinical safety data: Levonorgestrel is a well established progestogen with anti-oestrogenic activity. The safety profile following systemic administration is well documented. A study in monkeys with intrauterine delivery of levonorgestrel for 12 months confirmed local pharmacological activity with good local tolerance and no signs of systemic toxicity. No embryotoxicity was seen in the rabbit following intrauterine administration of levonorgestrel.

Pharmaceutical particulars

List of excipients: Polydimethylsiloxane elastomer, polydimethylsiloxane tubing, polyethylene, barium sulphate, iron oxide

Incompatibilities: None known

Shelf-life: Three years

Special precautions for storage: Store at a temperature not exceeding +30°C, protected from moisture and direct sunlight.

Nature and contents of container: The system with accessories has been packed into a heat sealed TYVEK sterilisation pouch.

Instructions for use/handling: Mirena is inserted into the uterine cavity within seven days of the onset of menstruation. It can be replaced by a new system at any time of the cycle.

Mirena can also be inserted immediately after first trimester abortion by curettage. Postpartum insertions should be postponed until six weeks after delivery. Special instructions for insertion are in the package.

Mirena is supplied in a sterile pack which should not be opened until required for insertion. Each device should be handled with aseptic precautions. If the seal of the sterile envelope is broken, the device inside should be discarded.

Marketing authorisation number 0053/0265

Date of approval/revision of SPC 30 September 1998

Legal category POM

NEOGEST*

Presentation Each round, dark brown, sugar-coated tablet contains 37.5 micrograms levonorgestrel contained in 75 micrograms norgestrel.

Excipients: lactose, maize starch, povidone 25 000, talc, magnesium stearate, sucrose, povidone 700 000, polyethylene glycol 6000, calcium carbonate, titanium dioxide, ferric oxide pigment (brown), glycerin, montan glycol wax.

Uses Oral contraception

Mode of action: The contraceptive action of Neogest may be explained as follows.

It changes the cervical mucus so that a barrier is formed against the migration of sperm into the uterine cavity. Nidation is impeded because of changes in the structure of the endometrium. As a rule there is no inhibition of ovulation. Evidence suggests that a reduction in corpus-luteum function may also contribute to the contraceptive action.

Dosage and administration *First treatment cycle:* One tablet daily, starting on the first day of the menstrual cycle, at a time of day chosen by the patient. All subsequent tablets must then be taken at this time. The contraceptive effect is likely to be reduced if a tablet is delayed by more than three hours. Additional non-hormonal methods of contraception (except the rhythm or temperature methods) must be used until the first 14 tablets have been taken.

Subsequent cycles: The tablets are taken daily and pack follows pack without interruption, and without regard to bleeding.

Changing from other hormonal contraceptives: When changing over to Neogest from other hormonal contraceptives, non-hormonal contraceptive measures must be employed additionally until 14 consecutive tablets have been taken regularly.

Post-partum and post-abortum use: After pregnancy, Neogest can be started 7 days after a vaginal delivery provided that the patient is fully ambulant and there are no puerperal complications. After a first trimester abortion, Neogest may be started immediately. Additional contraceptive precautions will be required for the first 14 days of pill taking.

Pregnancy and lactation: The administration of Neogest during pregnancy is contraindicated.

If pregnancy occurs during medication with Neogest the preparation is to be withdrawn immediately.

There is no evidence that Neogest diminishes the yield of breast milk. However, minute amounts of the active substance are excreted with the milk.

Special circumstances requiring additional contraception:

Incorrect administration: If a tablet is taken late (i.e. if it is more than 27 hours since the last tablet was taken) or if a tablet is missed, protection against conception may be impaired. Therefore, when such incidents occur, additional, non-hormonal contraceptive methods (except the rhythm or temperature methods) must be employed until 14 consecutive tablets have been taken in the correct manner.

Gastro-intestinal upset: Vomiting or diarrhoea may reduce the effectiveness of the tablets by preventing them from being fully absorbed. If the user vomits shortly after taking her daily Neogest tablet, she can maintain protection against conception by taking a second tablet within 3 hours of the normal time–provided she does not vomit again. For this second intake, the last tablet in the pack should be used.

In the case of repeated vomiting or prolonged diarrhoea, additional, non-hormonal contraceptive methods (except the rhythm or temperature methods) should be continued for a further 14 days after the symptoms have subsided. If the condition reducing the efficacy of the preparation is protracted, other methods of contraception should be considered.

Interaction with other drugs: Hepatic enzyme inducers such as barbiturates, primidone, phenobarbitone, phenytoin, phenylbutazone, rifampicin, carbamazepine and griseofulvin can impair the efficacy of Neogest. For women receiving long-term therapy with hepatic enzyme inducers, another method of contraception should be used. The use of antibiotics may also reduce the efficacy of Neogest, possibly by altering the intestinal flora.

Women receiving short courses of enzyme inducers or broad spectrum antibiotics should take additional non-hormonal (except the rhythm or temperature methods) contraceptive precautions during the time of concurrent medication and for 14 days afterwards. With rifampicin, additional contraceptive precautions should be continued for 4 weeks after treatment stops, even if only a short course was administered.

The requirement for oral antidiabetics or insulin can change as a result of an effect on glucose tolerance in diabetes mellitus.

Contra-indications, warnings etc

Contra-indications:

1. Pregnancy
2. Severe disturbances of liver function
3. Jaundice or persistent itching during a previous pregnancy
4. Dubin-Johnson syndrome
5. Rotor syndrome
6. Previous or existing liver tumours
7. A history of herpes gestationis
8. Mammary carcinoma or a history of this condition
9. Undiagnosed abnormal vaginal bleeding
10. History of or existing thromboembolic processes (e.g. stroke, myocardial infarction)
11. Severe diabetes with vascular changes
12. Sickle-cell anaemia
13. Hypersensitivity to any of the components of Neogest.

Warnings: Diabetes mellitus or tendency towards diabetes mellitus require careful medical supervision.

There is a general opinion, based on statistical evidence, that users of hormonal contraceptives experience, more often than non-users, venous thromboembolism, arterial thrombosis, including cerebral and myocardial infarction, and subarachnoid haemorrhage. Full recovery from such disorders does not always occur, and it should be realised that in a few cases they are fatal.

According to the present state of knowledge, an association between the use of hormonal contraceptives and an increased risk of venous and arterial thromboembolic diseases cannot be ruled out.

The relative risk of arterial thrombosis (e.g. stroke, myocardial infarction) appears to increase further when heavy smoking, increasing age and the use of hormonal contraceptives coincide.

A meta-analysis from 54 epidemiological studies reported that there is a slightly increased relative risk of having breast cancer diagnosed in women who are currently using oral contraceptives (OC). The observed pattern of increased risk may be due to an earlier diagnosis of breast cancer in OC users, the biological effects of OCs or a combination of both. The additional breast cancers diagnosed in current users of OCs or in women who have used OCs in the last 10 years are more likely to be localised to the breast than those in women who never used OCs.

Breast cancer is rare among women under 40 years of age whether or not they take OCs. Whilst the background risk increases with age, the excess number of breast cancer diagnoses in current and recent progestogen-only pill (POP) users is small in relation to the overall risk of breast cancer, possibly of similar magnitude to that associated with combined OCs. However, for POPs, the evidence is based on much smaller populations of users and so is less conclusive than that for combined OCs.

The most important risk factor for breast cancer in POP users is the age women discontinue the POP; the older the age at stopping, the more breast cancers are diagnosed. Duration of use is less important and the excess risk gradually disappears during the course of the 10 years after stopping POP use, such that by 10 years there appears to be no excess.

The evidence suggests that compared with never-users, among 10,000 women who use POPs for up to 5 years but stop by age 20, there would be much less than 1 extra case of breast cancer diagnosed up to 10 years afterwards. For those stopping by age 30 after 5 years use of the POP, there would be an estimated 2–3 extra cases (additional to the 44 cases of breast cancer per 10,000 women in this age group never exposed to oral contraceptives). For those stopping by age 40 after 5 years use, there would be an estimated 10 extra cases diagnosed up to 10 years afterwards (additional to the 160 cases of breast cancer per 10,000 never-exposed women in this age group).

It is important to inform patients that users of all contraceptive pills appear to have a small increase in the risk of being diagnosed with breast cancer, compared with non-users of oral contraceptives, but that this has to be weighed against the known benefits.

If there is a history of ectopic pregnancy or one Fallopian tube is missing, the use of Neogest should be decided on only after carefully weighing the benefits against the risks.

If obscure lower abdominal complaints occur together with an irregular cycle pattern (above all amenorrhoea followed by persistent irregular bleeding), an extrauterine pregnancy must be considered.

In rare cases benign, and in even rarer cases, malignant liver tumours leading in isolated cases to life-threatening intra-abdominal haemorrhage have been observed after the use of hormonal substances such as the one contained in Neogest. If severe upper abdominal complaints, liver enlargement or signs of intra-abdominal haemorrhage occur, a liver tumour should be included in the differential diagnosis.

Reasons for stopping Neogest immediately:

1. Occurrence for the first time, or exacerbation, of migrainous headaches or unusually frequent or unusually severe headaches
2. Sudden disturbances of vision or hearing or other perceptual disorders
3. First signs of thrombophlebitis or thromboembolic symptoms (for example, unusual pains in or swelling of the legs, stabbing pains on breathing or coughing for no apparent reason), feeling of pain and tightness in the chest
4. Six weeks before an elective major operation (e.g. abdominal, orthopaedic) any surgery to the legs, medical treatment for varicose veins or prolonged immobilisation e.g. after accidents or surgery. Do not restart until 2 weeks after full ambulation. In case of emergency surgery, thrombotic prophylaxis is usually indicated e.g. subcutaneous heparin
5. Onset of jaundice, hepatitis, itching of the whole body
6. Significant rise in blood pressure
7. Clear exacerbation of conditions known to be capable of deteriorating during oral contraception or pregnancy
8. Pregnancy.

Pregnancy is a reason for stopping immediately because it has been suggested by some investigations that oral contraceptives taken in early pregnancy may slightly increase the risk of foetal malformations. Other investigations have failed to support these findings. The possibility therefore cannot be excluded, but it is certain that if a risk exists at all it is very small.

Examination of the pelvic organs, breasts and blood pressure should precede the prescribing of Neogest and should be repeated regularly. Before starting treatment, pregnancy must be excluded.

Side-effects: In rare cases, nausea, vomiting, dizziness, headaches, migraine, depressive moods, changes in body weight and libido and allergic reactions can occur. Amenorrhoea and changes in the pattern of the menstrual cycle have also been observed.

Menstrual changes: A usual feature of all progestogen-only oral contraceptives is that they can produce an initial irregularity of the bleeding pattern, but such irregularity tends to decrease with time. Some women may experience amenorrhoea.

For these reasons the possibility of such changes in menstrual rhythm should, as a precaution, be pointed out to the patient before the start of tablet taking.

Missed menstruation: If no menstrual bleeding has occurred within 6 weeks after the last menstrual bleeding, pregnancy must be excluded before tablet taking is continued. If pregnancy has been excluded and the amenorrhoea lasts longer than 3 months or recurs repeatedly, Neogest should be withheld until normal menstrual bleeding has been restored.

Procedure in the event of irregular bleeding: Irregular bleeding is not a medical reason for stopping tablet taking, as long as organic causes for such bleeding and pregnancy can be ruled out and provided it is ensured that the patient is fully compliant.

It is extremely inadvisable to attempt to influence cycle disturbances by the additional administration of an oestrogen. This would only serve to reverse the changes brought about by Neogest in the cervical mucus, thereby seriously reducing the contraceptive effect.

Effect on blood chemistry: The use of oral contraceptives may influence the results of certain laboratory tests including biochemical parameters of liver, thyroid, adrenal and renal function, plasma levels of carrier proteins and lipid/lipoprotein fractions, parameters of carbohydrate metabolism and parameters of coagulation and fibrinolysis.

Overdosage: Acute toxicity studies did not indicate a risk of acute adverse effects in case of inadvertent intake of a multiple of the daily contraceptive dose. In general it is therefore unnecessary to treat overdosage. There are no specific antidotes and any treatment should be symptomatic.

Pharmaceutial precautions *Shelf life:* Five years

Legal category POM

Package quantities Memo-pack containing 35 tablets (OP).

Further information Nil

Product licence number 0053/0062

NERICUR* GEL 5
NERICUR* GEL 10

Presentation Nericur Gel is an aqueous gel containing either 5% or 10% benzoyl peroxide.
Excipients: Carbopol 940, polyoxyethylene 23 lauryl ether, propylene glycol, sodium hydroxide, purified water.

Uses All stages of acne vulgaris. Benzoyl peroxide has a strong antibacterial action against Propionibacterium acnes. It also has keratolytic and sebostatic actions, which cause some dryness and desquamation.

Dosage and administration Treatment should be initiated with Nericur Gel 5%. Once daily, the affected areas should be washed with soap and water and then dried, before Nericur Gel is applied. For stubborn cases treatment may be continued with Nericur Gel 10%, provided that Nericur Gel 5% has been well tolerated. For particularly sensitive skin, Nericur Gel 5% should be applied on alternate days.

For optimal effect, Nericur Gel should be applied in the evening, sufficient time being allowed for it to dry before the patient goes to bed, in order to avoid any bleaching of bed-linen.

Contra-indications, warnings, etc
Contra-indications: Known hypersensitivity to benzoyl peroxide.

Precautions: For external use only. Avoid contact with eyes and mucosae. If the skin is exposed to strong or prolonged sunlight, Nericur Gel should be applied at longer intervals, and a highly protective sun-screening agent should be used. Nericur Gel should only be applied to dry skin, to avoid unnecessary irritation.

Side-effects: As with all keratolytic substances, itching, reddening, burning and a feeling of skin tension may occur. This may be relieved by the use of a moisturising cream or by temporary interruption of use.

In rare cases, a contact dermatitis may occur, in which event treatment should be stopped immediately.

Pharmaceutical precautions Store below 25°C. *Shelf-life:* two years.

Legal category P

Package quantities Tubes containing 30 g (OP).

Further information Nil.

Product licence numbers
Nericur 5 0053/0168
Nericur 10 0053/0169

NERISONE* CREAM, OILY CREAM, OINTMENT

Qualitative and quantitative composition 100 g cream, oily cream or ointment each contains 0.1 g diflucortolone valerate.

Pharmaceutical form Cream, oily cream, ointment.

Clinical particulars
Therapeutic indications: For the topical treatment of corticoid–responsive dermatoses in the absence of infection.

Posology and method of administration
Adults and Children: Initially, 2–3 applications daily according to the severity of the condition. For maintenance, one application daily.

Elderly: Natural thinning of the skin occurs in the elderly. No special precautions are required, however, when Nerisone is used in this group of patients.

Nerisone Cream is suitable for weeping skin conditions. Nerisone Cream has a high water and low fat content. In weeping skin diseases it allows secretions to drain away, thus providing for rapid reduction of swelling and drying up of the skin. Nerisone Cream is also suitable for application to moist, exposed and hairy areas of the body.

If the skin dries out too much under protracted use of Nerisone Cream, the patient should be switched to a form which contains more fat (Nerisone Oily Cream or Nerisone Ointment).

Nerisone Oily Cream is suitable for skin conditions which are neither weeping nor very dry. Such conditions require a base with balanced proportions of fat and water. Nerisone Oily Cream makes the skin slightly greasy without retaining heat or fluid.

Nerisone Ointment is suitable in very dry skin conditions which need an anhydrous fatty base. The occlusive effect of the Nerisone Ointment base promotes the healing process.

Occlusive dressings: An occlusive dressing may be called for in unusually refractory cases and usually under specialist supervision. If an infection develops under the dressing, occlusive treatment must be terminated.

Contra-indications:
- Rosacea and peri-oral dermatitis.
- Acne vulgaris, undiagnosed perianal and genital pruritus, napkin eruptions, viral infections, primary bacterial or fungal infections of the skin.
- Secondary infections in the absence of appropriate anti-infective therapy.

Nerisone is not suitable for the treatment of ophthalmic conditions.

Special warnings and special precautions for use: Long-term continuous therapy with topical corticosteroids should be avoided, irrespective of age. Adrenal suppression can occur, even without occlusion. If used in childhood or on the face, courses should be limited to 5 days and occlusion should not be used.

Nerisone may be applied under an occlusive dressing. However, each dressing should not be left on for more than 24 hours. Although occlusive dressings may be used repeatedly, it should be noted that systemic corticoid absorption is likely to be increased with a consequent increased risk of adrenal suppression. If occlusive treatment is expected to be prolonged, it is advisable to change the dressing every 12 hours.

Nerisone should not be allowed to come into contact with the eyes.

Topical corticosteroids may be hazardous in psoriasis for a number of reasons including rebound relapses following development of tolerance, risk of generalised pustular psoriasis, and local and systemic toxicity due to impaired barrier function of the skin. Careful patient supervision is important in psoriasis.

Infections or secondarily infected dermatoses require additional therapy with antibiotics or chemotherapeutic agents. This treatment can often be topical, but for heavy infections systemic antibacterial therapy may be necessary. If fungal infections are present, a topically active antimycotic should be applied.

Interaction with other medicaments and other forms of interaction: None stated.

Pregnancy and lactation: There is inadequate evidence of safety in human pregnancy. Topical administration of corticosteroids to pregnant animals can cause abnormalities in foetal development including cleft palate and intra-uterine growth retardation. There may, therefore, be a very small risk of such effects on the human foetus and, as a general rule, topical preparations containing corticoids should not be applied during the first trimester of pregnancy. In particular, application to large areas of the body or for prolonged periods must be avoided.

Side effects cannot be excluded in neonates whose mothers have been treated extensively or for a prolonged period of time during pregnancy or while lactating (for example, reduced adrenocortical function, when applied during the last weeks of pregnancy).

Effects on ability to drive and use machines: None stated.

Undesirable effects: In common with all other topical corticoids, side-effects may occur when Nerisone is applied to large areas of the body (10% or more) and for long periods of time (more than four weeks), especially if an occlusive dressing is being used. There may be local signs such as atrophy of the skin, telangiectasia, striae, acneform changes, perioral dermatitis and hypertrichosis, or systemic corticoid effects caused by absorption. In rare cases, allergic skin reactions may occur. Therefore, caution should be exercised when using occlusive dressings, as there is a possibility that natural steroid production may be suppressed.

Overdose: On the basis of results from acute toxicity studies with both diflucortolone valerate and Nerisone preparations, no acute risk of intoxication is to be expected either after a single dermal application of an overdose (application over a large area under conditions favouring resorption) or even after inadvertent oral intake of a whole tube.

Pharmacological properties
Pharmacodynamic properties: Diflucortolone valerate is a topically acting fluoridated corticosteroid which suppresses inflammation in inflammatory and allergic skin conditions and alleviates the subjective complaints such as itching, burning and pain.

Capillary dilatation, intercellular oedema and tissue infiltration regress; capillary proliferation is suppressed. This leads to fading of inflamed skin surfaces.

Pharmacokinetic properties: In order to exert its antiproliferative and anti-inflammatory effects, diflucortolone valerate has to diffuse from the preparation into the living epidermis and into the upper dermis. In vitro penetration studies showed that diflucortolone valerate penetrates human skin rapidly. After application to damaged skin – as a model for diseased skin – the local corticosteroid levels were distinctly higher than in the intact skin.

Once in the skin diflucortolone valerate is partly hydrolysed into the similarly effective diflucortolone. Part of the corticosteroid applied to the skin is percutaneously absorbed, distributed into organs and tissues, metabolised and finally excreted. The extent of percutaneous absorption and the resulting systemic load depend on a series of factors: the vehicle, the exposure conditions (skin area dose, treatment area, duration of treatment), condition of treatment (open/occlusive), the status of the penetration barrier and the localisation of the treated area on the body.

After application of the radiolabelled ointment onto

an intact and a 'stripped' area of skin on the back of 3 volunteers, 0.7% of the dose was percutaneously absorbed during a 7 hour exposure period.

Following percutaneous absorption diflucortolone valerate is hydrolysed very rapidly into diflucortolone and the respective fatty acid. 11-keto-diflucortolone and two further metabolites have been found in the plasma in addition to diflucortolone. Diflucortolone is eliminated from the plasma with a half-life of approximately 4–5 hours, all metabolites together with a half-life of approximately 9 hours (results after i.v. administration). The metabolites are excreted with urine and faeces in a ratio of 75:25.

Preclinical safety data: There are no preclinical safety data which could be of relevance to the prescriber and which are not already included in other relevant sections of the SPC.

Pharmaceutical particulars:
List of excipients:
Nerisone Cream: Polyoxyl–40–stearate [E431]; Stearyl alcohol; Heavy liquid paraffin; White soft paraffin; Disodium edetate dihydrate; Carbopol 934; Sodium hydroxide; Methyl parahydroxybenzoate [E218]; Propyl parahydroxybenzoate [E216]; Purified water.

Nerisone Oily Cream: White beeswax; Heavy liquid paraffin; White soft paraffin; Dehymuls E; Purified water.

Nerisone Ointment: Heavy liquid ointment; White soft paraffin; Lunacera M (microcrystalline wax); Castor oil, hydrogenated.

Incompatibilities: None stated.

Shelf life: 5 years.

Special precautions for storage: Cream: Store below 25°C. Oily cream, ointment: None.

Nature and contents of container: Aluminium tube containing 30 g cream, oily cream or ointment.

Instructions for use/handling: Keep out of reach of children.

Marketing authorisation numbers

Nerisone cream:	0053/0075
Nerisone oily cream:	0053/0073
Nerisone ointment:	0053/0074

Date of approval/revision of the SPC 28 July 1997

NERISONE* FORTE OILY CREAM AND OINTMENT

Qualitative and quantitative composition 100 g oily cream contains 0.3 g diflucortolone valerate, 100 g ointment contains 0.3 g diflucortolone valerate

Pharmaceutical form Oily cream; fatty ointment.

Clinical particulars
Therapeutic indications: Initial and intermittent treatment of severe and recalcitrant corticoid-responsive dermatoses in the absence of infection. These include neurodermatitis (endogenous eczema, atopic dermatitis), lichen planus, discoid lupus erythematosus , severe chronic eczema and psoriasis. Nerisone Forte should not be applied to large areas of the body (more than 10%) in psoriasis (see *Special precautions and special warnings for use*).

Posology and method of administration: Adults and children over the age of four: Initially, Nerisone Forte should be applied 2-3 times a day. Once the clinical picture has improved, the patient should be changed from Nerisone Forte to Nerisone for maintenance therapy. *Elderly:* Natural thinning of the skin occurs in the elderly. No special precautions are required, however, when Nerisone Forte is used in this group of patients.

Nerisone Forte Oily Cream is suitable for skin conditions which are neither weeping nor very dry. It has a base with balanced proportions of water and fat. It makes the skin slightly greasy without retaining heat or fluid.

Nersisone Forte Ointment is suitable for very dry skin conditions. It has an anhydrous fatty base. Its occlusive effect promotes the healing process.

Contra-indications: Acne vulgaris, undiagnosed perianal and genital pruritus, napkin eruptions, viral infections, primary bacterial or fungal infections of the skin. Secondary infections in the absence of appropriate anti-infective therapy.

Nerisone Forte is not suitable for the treatment of ophthalmic conditions.

Infants and children up to the age of 4 years must not be treated with Nerisone Forte.

Nerisone Forte should never be applied to the face.

Special warnings and special precautions for use: Long-term continuous therapy with topical corticosteroids should be avoided, irrespective of age. Adrenal suppression can occur, even without occlusion.

In view of the high efficacy and potency of Nerisone Forte, no more than 60 g a week should be applied, and it is suggested that treatment for one or two weeks should generally be sufficient to obtain control of even the most refractory lesion, after which a change to Nerisone can usually be made if maintenance therapy is necessary.

Since prolonged therapy with potent topical corticosteroids may cause local atrophic changes such as striae, thinning, hypertrichosis and telangiectasia, particularly in skin folds and where occlusive dressings are used, it is recommended that the progress of patients under treatment for more than one week with Nerisone Forte be reviewed weekly, and that repeat prescriptions be written only when the prescribing physician has seen the patient again.

Topical corticosteroids may be hazardous in psoriasis for a number of reasons including rebound relapses following development of tolerance, risk of generalised pustular psoriasis, and local and systemic toxicity due to impaired barrier function of the skin. Careful patient supervision is important in psoriasis.

Since absorption is increased with the use of occlusive dressings, these should not be left on for more than 24 hours. If secondary infection occurs during treatment, the use of occlusive dressings should be stopped until the infection has been eliminated, and appropriate treatment of the infection should be instituted if it persists.

Interaction with other medicaments and other forms of interaction: None known

Pregnancy and lactation: There is inadequate evidence of safety in human pregnancy. Topical administration of corticosteroids to pregnant animals can cause abnormalities of foetal development including cleft palate and intra-uterine growth retardation. There may, therefore, be a very small risk of such effects on the human foetus and, as a general rule, topical preparations containing corticoids should not be applied during the first trimester of pregnancy. In particular, application to large areas of the body or for prolonged periods must be avoided.

Side effects cannot be excluded in neonates whose mothers have been treated extensively or for a prolonged period of time during pregnancy or while lactating (for example, reduced adrenocortical function, when applied during the last weeks of pregnancy).

Effects on ability to drive and use machines: Not applicable.

Undesirable effects: In common with all potent topical corticosteroids, there may be local signs such as atrophy of the skin, striae, thinning, acneform changes, hypertrichosis and systemic effects of the corticoid due to absorption and telangiectasia, particularly in skin folds and where occlusive dressings are used. Side-effects may occur when Nerisone Forte is applied to large areas of the body (10% or more) and for long periods of time (more than 10 days). In rare cases, allergic skin reactions may occur.

Overdose: On the basis of results from acute toxicity studies with both diflucortolone valerate and Nerisone Forte preparations, no acute risk of intoxication is to be expected either after a single dermal application of an overdose (application over a large area under conditions favouring resorption) or even after inadvertent oral intake of a whole tube.

Pharmacological properties
Pharmacodynamic properties: Diflucortolone valerate is a topically acting fluoridated corticosteroid which suppresses inflammation in inflammatory and allergic skin conditions and alleviates the subjective complaints such as itching, burning and pain. Capillary dilatation, intercellular oedema and tissue infiltration regress; capillary proliferation is suppressed. This leads to fading of inflamed skin surfaces.

Pharmacokinetic properties: In order to exert its antiproliferative and anti-inflammatory effects, diflucortolone valerate has to diffuse from the preparation into the living epidermis and into the upper dermis. In vitro penetration studies showed that diflucortolone valerate penetrates human skin rapidly. After application to damaged skin–as a model for diseased skin–the local corticosteroid levels were distinctly higher than in the intact skin.

Once in the skin diflucortolone valerate is partly hydrolysed into the similarly effective diflucortolone. Part of the corticosteroid applied to the skin is percutaneously absorbed, distributed into organs and tissues, metabolised and finally excreted. The extent of percutaneous absorption and the resulting systemic load depend on a series of factors: the vehicle, the exposure conditions (skin area dose, treatment area, duration of treatment), condition of treatment (open/occlusive), the status of the penetration barrier and the localisation of the treated area on the body.

After application of the radiolabelled ointment onto an intact and a 'stripped' area of skin on the back of 3 volunteers, 0.7% of the dose was percutaneously absorbed during a 7 hour exposure period.

Following percutaneous absorption diflucortolone valerate is hydrolysed very rapidly into diflucortolone and the respective fatty acid. 11-keto-diflucortolone and two further metabolites have been found in the plasma in addition to diflucortolone. Diflucortolone is eliminated from the plasma with a half-life of approximately 4-5 hours, all metabolites together with a half-life of approximately 9 hours (results after i.v. administration). The metabolites are excreted with urine and faeces in a ratio of 75:25.

Preclinical safety data: There are no preclinical safety data which could be of relevance to the prescriber and which are not already included in other relevant sections of the SPC.

Pharmaceutical particulars
List of excipients: Oily Cream: white beeswax, liquid paraffin, white soft paraffin, Dehymuls E, purified water. Ointment: liquid paraffin, white soft paraffin, Lunacera M (microcrystalline wax), hydrogenated castor oil.

Incompatibilities: None known.

Shelf life: 5 years.

Special precautions for storage: None.

Nature and contents of container: Aluminium tubes containing 15 g oily cream or ointment

Instructions for use/handling: Keep out of the reach of children.

Marketing authorisation numbers

Oily Cream	0053/0099
Ointment	0053/0100

Date of approval/revision of SPC 1 June 1997

Legal category POM

NORGESTON*

Qualitative and quantitative composition Each tablet contains 30 micrograms levonorgestrel.

Pharmaceutical form Sugar-coated tablets.

Clinical particulars
Therapeutic indications: Oral contraception.

Posology and method of administration: First treatment cycle: One tablet daily, starting on the first day of the menstrual cycle, at a time of day chosen by the patient. All subsequent tablets must then be taken at this time. The contraceptive effect is likely to be reduced if a tablet is delayed by more than three hours. Additional non-hormonal methods of contraception (except the rhythm or temperature methods) must be used until the first 14 tablets have been taken.

Subsequent cycles: The tablets are taken daily and pack follows pack without interruption, and without regard to bleeding.

Changing from other hormonal contraceptives: The first tablet of Norgeston should be taken on the first day immediately after the end of the previous oral contraceptive course. Additional, non-hormonal contraceptive methods (except the rhythm or temperature methods) should be used for the first 14 days of tablet-taking.

Post-partum and post-abortum use: After pregnancy, Norgeston can be started 7 days after a vaginal delivery provided that the patient is fully ambulant and there are no puerperal complications. After a first trimester abortion, Norgeston may be started immediately. Additional contraceptive precautions will be required for the first 14 days of pill-taking.

Special circumstances requiring additional contraception: Incorrect administration: If a tablet is taken late (i.e. if it is more than 27 hours since the last tablet was taken) or if a tablet is missed, protection against conception may be impaired. Therefore, when such incidents occur, additional, non-hormonal contraceptive methods (except the rhythm or temperature methods) must be employed until 14 consecutive tablets have been taken in the correct manner.

Gastro-intestinal upsets: Vomiting or diarrhoea may reduce the effectiveness of the tablets by preventing them from being fully absorbed. If the user vomits shortly after taking her daily Norgeston tablet, she can maintain protection against contraception by taking a second tablet within 3 hours of the normal time–provided she does not vomit again. For this second intake, the last tablet in the pack should be used.

In the case of repeated vomiting or prolonged diarrhoea, additional, non-hormonal contraceptive methods (except the rhythm or temperature method) should be continued for a further 14 days after the symptoms have subsided. If the condition reducing the efficacy of the preparation is protracted, other methods of contraception should be considered.

Contra-indications:

1. Pregnancy
2. Severe disturbances of liver function
3. Jaundice or persistent itching during a previous pregnancy

4. Dubin-Johnson syndrome
5. Rotor syndrome
6. Previous or existing liver tumours
7. A history of herpes of pregnancy
8. Mammary carcinoma or a history of this condition
9. Undiagnosed abnormal vaginal bleeding
10. History of or existing thromboembolic processes (e.g. stroke, myocardial infarction)
11. Severe diabetes with vascular changes
12. Sickle-cell anaemia
13. Hypersensitivity to any of the components of Norgeston.

Special warnings and special precautions for use: Diabetes mellitus or tendency towards diabetes mellitus require careful medical supervision.

There is a general opinion, based on statistical evidence, that users of hormonal contraceptives experience, more often than non-users, venous thromboembolism, arterial thrombosis, including cerebral and myocardial infarction, and subarachnoid haemorrhage. Full recovery from such disorders does not always occur, and it should be realised that in a few cases they are fatal.

According to the present state of knowledge, an association between the use of hormonal contraceptives and an increased risk of venous and arterial thromboembolic diseases cannot be ruled out.

The relative risk of arterial thrombosis (e.g. stroke, myocardial infarction) appears to increase further when heavy smoking, increasing age and the use of hormonal contraceptives coincide.

A meta-analysis from 54 epidemiological studies reported that there is a slightly increased relative risk of having breast cancer diagnosed in women who are currently using oral contraceptives (OC). The observed pattern of increased risk may be due to an earlier diagnosis of breast cancer in OC users, the biological effects of OCs or a combination of both. The additional breast cancers diagnosed in current users of OCs or in women who have used OCs in the last 10 years are more likely to be localised to the breast than those in women who never used OCs.

Breast cancer is rare among women under 40 years of age whether or not they take OCs. Whilst the background risk increases with age, the excess number of breast cancer diagnoses in current and recent progestogen-only pill (POP) users is small in relation to the overall risk of breast cancer, possibly of similar magnitude to that associated with combined OCs. However, for POPs, the evidence is based on much smaller populations of users and so is less conclusive than that for combined OCs.

The most important risk factor for breast cancer in POP users is the age women discontinue the POP; the older the age at stopping, the more breast cancers are diagnosed. Duration of use is less important and the excess risk gradually disappears during the course of the 10 years after stopping POP use, such that by 10 years there appears to be no excess.

The evidence suggests that compared with never-users, among 10,000 women who use POPs for up to 5 years but stop by age 20, there would be much less than 1 extra case of breast cancer diagnosed up to 10 years afterwards. For those stopping by age 30 after 5 years use of the POP, there would be an estimated 2–3 extra cases (additional to the 44 cases of breast cancer per 10,000 women in this age group never exposed to oral contraceptives). For those stopping by age 40 after 5 years use, there would be an estimated 10 extra cases diagnosed up to 10 years afterwards (additional to the 160 cases of breast cancer per 10,000 never-exposed women in this age group).

It is important to inform patients that users of all contraceptive pills appear to have a small increase in the risk of being diagnosed with breast cancer, compared with non-users of oral contraceptives, but that this has to be weighed against the known benefits.

If there is a history of ectopic pregnancy or one Fallopian tube is missing, the use of Norgeston should be decided on only after carefully weighing the benefits against the risks.

If obscure lower abdominal complaints occur together with an irregular cycle pattern (above all amenorrhoea followed by persistent irregular bleeding), an extrauterine pregnancy must be considered.

In rare cases benign, and in even rarer cases, malignant liver tumours leading in isolated cases to life-threatening intra-abdominal haemorrhage have been observed after the use of hormonal substances such as the one contained in Norgeston. If severe upper abdominal complaints, liver enlargement or signs of intra-abdominal haemorrhage occur, a liver tumour should be included in the differential diagnostic considerations.

Reasons for stopping Norgeston immediately

1. Occurrence for the first time, or exacerbation, of migrainous headaches or unusually frequent or unusually severe headaches
2. Sudden disturbances of vision or hearing or other perceptual disorders
3. First signs of thrombophlebitis or thromboembolic symptoms (for example, unusual pains in or swelling of the legs, stabbing pains on breathing or coughing for no apparent reason), feeling of pain and tightness in the chest
4. Six weeks before an elective major operation (e.g. abdominal, orthopaedic) any surgery to the legs, medical treatment for varicose veins or prolonged immobilisation e.g. after accidents or surgery. Do not restart until 2 weeks after full ambulation. In case of emergency surgery, thrombotic prophylaxis is usually indicated e.g. subcutaneous heparin
5. Onset of jaundice, hepatitis, itching of the whole body
6. Significant rise in blood pressure
7. Clear exacerbation of conditions known to be capable of deteriorating during oral contraception or pregnancy
8. Pregnancy.

Pregnancy is a reason for stopping immediately because it has been suggested by some investigations that oral contraceptives taken in early pregnancy may slightly increase the risk of foetal malformations. Other investigations have failed to support these findings. The possibility therefore cannot be excluded, but it is certain that if a risk exists at all it is very small.

Examination of the pelvic organs, breasts and blood pressure should precede the prescribing of Norgeston and should be repeated regularly. Before starting treatment, pregnancy must be excluded.

Interaction with other medicaments and other forms of interaction: Hepatic enzyme inducers such as barbiturates, primidone, phenobarbitone, phenytoin, phenylbutazone, rifampicin, carbamazepine and griseofulvin can impair the efficacy of Norgeston. For women receiving long-term therapy with hepatic enzyme inducers, another method of contraception should be used. The use of antibiotics may also reduce the efficacy of Norgeston, possibly by altering the intestinal flora.

Women receiving short courses of enzyme inducers or broad spectrum antibiotics should take additional non-hormonal (except rhythm or temperature methods) contraceptive precautions during the time of concurrent medication and for 14 days afterwards. With rifampicin, additional contraceptive precautions should be continued for 4 weeks after treatment stops, even if only a short course was administered.

The requirement for oral antidiabetics or insulin can change as a result of an effect on glucose tolerance in diabetes mellitus.

Pregnancy and lactation: The administration of Norgeston during pregnancy is contraindicated.

If pregnancy occurs during medication with Norgeston the preparation is to be withdrawn immediately.

There is no evidence that Norgeston diminishes the yield of breast milk. However, minute amounts of the active substance are excreted with the milk.

Effects on ability to drive and use machines: None known.

Undesirable effects: In rare cases, nausea, vomiting, dizziness, headaches, migraine, depressive moods, changes in body weight and libido and allergic reactions can occur. Amenorrhoea and changes in the pattern of the menstrual cycle have also been observed.

Menstrual changes: A usual, feature of all progestogen-only oral contraceptives is that they can produce an initial irregularity of the bleeding pattern, but such irregularity tends to decrease with time. Some women may experience amenorrhoea.

For these reasons the possibility of such changes in menstrual rhythm should, as a precaution, be pointed out to the patient before the start of tablet-taking.

Missed menstruation: If no menstrual bleeding has occurred within 6 weeks after the last menstrual bleeding, pregnancy must be excluded before tablet-taking is continued. If pregnancy has been excluded and the amenorrhoea lasts longer than 3 months or recurs repeatedly, Norgeston should be withheld until normal menstrual bleeding has been restored.

Procedure in the event of irregular bleeding: Irregular bleeding is not a medical reason for stopping tablet-taking, as long as organic causes for such bleeding and pregnancy can be ruled out provided it is ensured that the patient is fully compliant.

It is extremely inadvisable to attempt to influence cycle disturbances by the additional administration of an oestrogen. This would only serve to reverse the changes brought about by Norgeston in the cervical mucus, thereby seriously reducing the contraceptive effect.

Effect on blood chemistry: The use of oral contraceptives may influence the results of certain laboratory tests including biochemical parameters of liver, thyroid, adrenal and renal function, plasma levels of carrier proteins and lipid/lipoprotein fractions, parameters of carbohydrate metabolism and parameters of coagulation and fibrinolysis. Laboratory staff should therefore be informed about oral contraceptive use when laboratory tests are requested.

Overdose: Acute toxicity studies did not indicate a risk of acute adverse effects in case of inadvertent intake of a multiple of the daily contraceptive dose. In general it is therefore unnecessary to treat overdosage. There are no specific antidotes and further treatment should be symptomatic.

Pharmacological properties

Pharmacodynamic properties: The contraceptive action of Norgeston may be explained as follows: it changes the cervical mucus so that a barrier is formed against the migration of sperm into the uterine cavity; nidation is impeded because of changes in the structure of the endometrium. As a rule there is no inhibition of ovulation. Evidence suggests that a reduction in corpus luteum function may also contribute to the contraceptive action.

Pharmacokinetic properties: As is known from a series of studies comprising various preparations and dosages, levonorgestrel is rapidly and completely absorbed after oral administration. Following ingestion of Norgeston, maximum serum levels of about 0.8 ng/ml were determined at 1 hour. Thereafter, drug serum levels declined biphasically with half-lives of 0.2–0.4 hours and 20 hours. Metabolic clearance rate from serum or plasma accounts for 1.0 to 1.5 ml/min/kg. Levonorgestrel is not excreted in unchanged form but as metabolites, which are eliminated with a half-life of about 1 day. Almost equal dose parts are excreted via the kidney and the liver. The biotransformation follows the known pathways of steroid metabolism. No pharmacologically active metabolites are known.

Levonorgestrel is bound to serum albumin and to SHBG. Only about 1.5% of the respective total serum drug levels are present as free steroid, but about 65% are specifically bound to SHBG. The relative portions (free, albumin-bound, SHBG-bound) depend on the SHBG serum concentrations. Following induction of the carrier protein, the SHBG-bound portion increases while the unbound and albumin-bound portions decrease.

Following daily repeated administration, levonorgestrel accumulates by a factor of approx. 2. Steady-state conditions are reached after about 3–4 days. Levonorgestrel pharmacokinetics is influenced by SHBG serum levels.

Under Norgeston treatment, a slight decline of the SHBG serum levels could occur. The daily ingestion of 0.15 mg levonorgestrel (corresponding to the 5 fold daily dose of Norgeston) led to a 50% decrease in the SHBG serum levels and thus to a 40% reduction in levonorgestrel through levels after 2–3 weeks. A similarly directed effect of Norgeston should account, however, for a decrease of only about 10% in the two parameters. The absolute bioavailability of levonorgestrel from Norgeston was determined to 82% of the dose. About 0.1% of the maternal dose can be transferred to a newborn via milk.

Preclinical safety data: There are no preclinical safety data which could be of relevance to the prescriber and which are not already included in other relevant sections of the SPC.

Pharmaceutical particulars

List of excipients: Lactose, maize starch, povidone, talc, magnesium stearate [E572], sucrose, polyethylene glycol 6000, calcium carbonate [E170], montan glycol wax

Incompatibilities: None known

Shelf life: 5 years

Special precautions for storage: Not applicable.

Nature and contents of container: Norgeston tablets are contained in aluminium foil and PVC blister packs.

These calendar-packs contain 35 tablets.

Instructions for use/handling: Keep out of the reach of children.

Marketing authorisation number 0053/0068

Date of (partial) revision of the text 21 April 1998

NORISTERAT*

Presentation Norethisterone oenanthate in oily solution for intramuscular administration. Ampoules contain 200 mg in 1 ml.

Excipients: benzyl benzoate, castor oil for injection.

Uses Noristerat is a depot contraceptive. It is intended for short-term use when a high level of efficacy independent of possible errors by the patient is required. It has been licensed for short-term use by women whose partners undergo vasectomy, until the vasectomy is effective, and women immunised against rubella, to prevent pregnancy during the period of activity of the virus.

Use after delivery or abortion: Noristerat can generally

be used immediately after delivery or abortion (but see following *'Use during lactation'*).

Use during lactation: Noristerat has not been reported to inhibit milk production, which is an advantage when the mother wishes to breast-feed. However, traces of the hormone appear in the milk, and although considered harmless to a healthy neonate might theoretically, like other steroids, impair the degradation of bilirubin, especially during the first week of life. If the mother has received Noristerat, breast-feeding should therefore be withheld from neonates with severe or persistent jaundice requiring medical treatment.

Dosage and administration 200 mg Noristerat intramuscularly provides contraception for eight weeks. The first injection should be given within the first five days of a menstrual cycle (the first day of menstruation counting as day 1), unless it is given so soon after delivery or abortion that no possibility of pregnancy exists. Provided the injection is carried out according to these instructions, no additional contraceptive cover is required. The injection may be repeated once, after eight weeks. Noristerat must always be injected deep into the gluteal muscles, care being taken that no liquid runs back from the injection site, which could result in loss of efficacy. The viscosity of the liquid at low temperatures is high, necessitating considerable pressure of injection. Therefore it is suggested that the ampoule be immersed in warm water before injection. A needle of at least medium bore should be used, and care taken to ensure that the needle is securely attached to the syringe.

Contra-indications, warnings, etc
Contra-indications:
1. Pregnancy
2. Acute and severe chronic liver disease
3. History, during pregnancy, of idiopathic jaundice or general pruritus or of herpes gestationis
4. History of deterioration of otosclerosis during pregnancy
5. Dubin-Johnson and Rotor syndromes
6. Sickle-cell anaemia
7. Severe diabetes with vascular changes
8. Previous or existing liver tumours
9. Pathologically increased blood pressure
10. Twelve weeks before planned operations and during immobilisation (eg: after accidents)
11. Current thromboembolic disease
12. Disturbances of lipid metabolism
13. Existing or treated breast or endometrial cancer
14. Hypersensitivity to any of the components of Noristerat.

Warnings: Noristerat should not be used in patients with abnormal uterine bleeding until a definite diagnosis has been established and the possibility of genital tract malignancy eliminated.

Although there have been so far no observations of thromboembolic disease during the use of Noristerat, as a precaution it is recommended that this preparation should not be used where there is a history of thromboembolic processes.

No further injection should be given if, during treatment, migrainous headaches occur for the first time or recurrent unusually severe headaches develop, if sudden perceptual disorders occur, if first signs of thrombophlebitis or thromboembolic disease are noted, or if a feeling of pain and tightness in the chest, a significant rise in blood pressure, recurrence of earlier depression or pathological changes of liver function and hormone levels are experienced.

There is a general opinion, based on statistical evidence, that users of hormonal contraceptives experience, more often than non-users, venous thromboembolism, arterial thrombosis, including cerebral and myocardial infarction, and subarachnoid haemorrhage. Full recovery from such disorders does not always occur, and it should be realised that in a few cases they are fatal.

The relative risk of arterial thromboses (e.g. stroke and myocardial infarction) appears to increase further when heavy smoking, increasing age and the use of hormonal contraceptives coincide.

A reduction of glucose tolerance has been observed in some women using progestogens. Consequently, diabetics and women with a tendency to diabetes should be carefully supervised during the use of Noristerat. In the case of diabetes, it may be necessary to reassess the required doses of antidiabetics or insulin.

If there is a history of ectopic pregnancy or one Fallopian tube is missing, the use of Noristerat should be decided on only after carefully weighing the benefits against the risks. If obscure lower abdominal complaints occur together with an irregular cycle pattern (above all amenorrhoea followed by persistent irregular bleeding), an extrauterine pregnancy must be considered.

Like all nortestosterone derivatives used for contraception, Noristerat has slight androgenic activity, and a virilising effect on the external genitalia of a female foetus exposed to Noristerat after the first month of pregnancy cannot be totally ruled out on theoretical grounds. However, no such virilisation has been observed after the few pregnancies that have occurred during the use of Noristerat.

Porphyria and existing impairment of liver function might theoretically be exacerbated by Noristerat. In rare cases benign and, in even rarer cases, malignant liver tumours leading in isolated cases to life-threatening intra-abdominal haemorrhage, have been observed after the use of hormonal substances such as the one contained in Noristerat. If severe upper abdominal complaints, liver enlargement or signs of intra-abdominal haemorrhage occur, a liver tumour should be considered in the differential diagnosis.

In rare cases coughing, dyspnoea and circulatory irregularities may occur during or immediately after the injection. Experience has shown that these reactions can be avoided by injecting Noristerat very slowly.

Precautions: Examination of the pelvic organs, breasts and blood pressure should precede the prescribing of Noristerat. Before starting treatment, pregnancy must be excluded.

Women with a history of severe depressive states, porphyria, disturbed liver function or any disease that is prone to worsen during pregnancy should be carefully observed during medication.

Amenorrhoea: if, when the second injection is due, bleeding has not occurred in the preceding eight weeks the second injection should not be given until pregnancy has been ruled out.

Interaction with other drugs: Some drugs may accelerate the metabolism of Noristerat. Drugs suspected of having this capacity, which may reduce the efficacy of the preparation, include barbiturates, carbamazepine, phenytoin, phenylbutazone, griseofulvin and rifampicin. Reduced substance levels have been observed during the simultaneous use of certain antibiotics (e.g. ampicillin), possibly due to changes in the intestinal flora. The requirement for oral antidiabetics or insulin can change as a result of the effect on glucose tolerance.

Side-effects: Subjective symptoms reported consist mainly of bloating, breast discomfort, headaches, dizziness, depressive moods and transient nausea. Marked increases of weight are rare.

The patient should be informed before starting Noristerat that her menstrual pattern is likely to alter. Menstrual changes in the form of spotting, breakthrough bleeding and delayed menstruation are relatively frequent, and generally do not require treatment. With persistent bleeding however, it may be expedient to administer progestogen/oestrogen tablets e.g. combined oral contraceptives, for 10 days to create a withdrawal bleed 1-4 days later.

Effect on blood chemistry: No influence of Noristerat on basal plasma cortisol, the ACTH test or the metyrapone test has been observed. In the acute dexamethasone suppression test, however, a higher plasma cortisol value than expected was found in 4 out of 10 women, although there were no clinical indications of disturbed adrenocortical function. A shortening of the recalcification time and of the thromboplastin time (Quick's test) were observed in studies of the blood coagulation system.

Overdosage: Acute toxicity studies indicated that even in the case of inadvertent administration of a multiple of the contraceptive dose, no acute toxicity risk is to be expected.

Pharmaceutical precautions Store below 25°C. Protect from light. Shelf-life–Five years

Legal category POM

Package quantities Single packs of 1 ampoule

Further information Nil

Product licence number 0053/0095

NUVELLE*

Qualitative and quantitative composition Each white sugar-coated tablet contains: estradiol valerate 2.0 mg.

Each pink sugar-coated tablet contains: estradiol valerate 2.0 mg and levonorgestrel 75 micrograms.

Pharmaceutical form Sugar coated tablets for oral use.

Clinical particulars
Therapeutic indications: Hormone replacement therapy for the treatment of the climacteric syndrome.

Prevention of postmenopausal osteoporosis in women considered at risk of developing fractures. Epidemiological studies suggest a number of risk factors may contribute to postmenopausal osteoporosis including:

- early menopause (either natural or surgically induced);
- family history of osteoporosis;
- recent corticosteroid therapy;
- a small frame;
- thin;
- cigarette consumption.

For maximum prophylactic benefit treatment should commence as soon as possible after the menopause.

Bone mineral density measurements may help to confirm the presence of low bone mass.

Nuvelle is designed to provide hormone replacement therapy during and after the climacteric. The addition of a progestogen in the second half of each course helps to provide good control of the irregular cycles that are characteristic of the premenopausal phase and opposes the production of endometrial hyperplasia. Whilst ovarian hormone production is little affected, Nuvelle abolishes or improves the characteristic symptoms of the climacteric such as hot flushes, sweating attacks and sleep disorders.

Studies of bone mineral content have shown Nuvelle to be effective in the prevention of progressive bone loss following the menopause.

Nuvelle does not consistently inhibit ovulation and is therefore unsuitable for contraception.

Posology and method of administration:
Adults, including the elderly: If the patient is still menstruating, treatment should begin on the 5th day of menstruation. Patients whose periods are very infrequent or who are postmenopausal may start at any time, provided pregnancy has been excluded. (see Special warnings and special precautions for use).

One white tablet is taken daily for the first 16 days, followed by one pink tablet daily for 12 days. Thus, each pack contains 28 days treatment. Treatment is continuous, which means that the next pack follows immediately without a break. Bleeding usually occurs within the last few days of one pack and the first week of the next.

Contra–indications:
- pregnancy (see *Special warnings and special precautions for use*).
- severe disturbances of liver function
- previous or existing liver tumours
- jaundice or general pruritus during a previous pregnancy
- Dubin–Johnson syndrome
- Rotor syndrome
- active deep venous thrombosis, thromboembolic disorders, or a history of confirmed venous thromboembolism (see also *Special warnings and special precautions for use*)
- sickle–cell anaemia
- suspected or existing hormone–dependent disorders or tumours of the uterus and breast
- undiagnosed irregular vaginal bleeding
- congenital disturbances of lipid metabolism
- a history of herpes gestatiois
- otosclerosis with deterioration in previous pregnancies
- endometriosis
- severe diabetes with vascular changes
- mastopathy.

Special warnings and special precautions for use: Before starting treatment, pregnancy must be excluded. If the expected bleeding fails to occur at about 28–day intervals, treatment should be stopped until pregnancy has been ruled out.

Before starting Nuvelle, patients should have a thorough general medical and gynaecological examination with special emphasis on the body weight, blood pressure, heart, breasts, pelvic organs with an endometrial assessment if indicated, the legs and skin. Follow–up examinations are recommended at least six–monthly during treatment.

At the present time there is some evidence which suggests a slight increase in the relative risk of breast cancer in postmenopausal women receiving long-term hormone replacement therapy. A careful appraisal of the risk/benefit ratio should be undertaken before treating for longer than 5 to 10 years.

Persistent breakthrough bleeding during treatment is an indication for endometrial assessment which may include biopsy.

Treatment should be stopped at once if migrainous or frequent and unusually severe headaches occur for the first time, or if there are other symptoms that are possible prodromata of vascular occlusion.

Treatment should be stopped at once if jaundice or pregnancy occurs, if there is a significant rise in blood pressure, or an increase in epileptic seizures.

Epidemiological studies have suggested that hormone replacement therapy (HRT) is associated with an increased relative risk of developing venous thromboembolism (VTE) i.e. deep vein thrombosis or pulmonary embolism. The studies find a 2–3 fold increase for users compared with non-users which for healthy women amounts to a small risk of one extra case of VTE each year for every 5000 patients taking HRT.

Generally recognised risk factors for VTE include a personal or family history and severe obesity (Body Mass Index >30 kg/m²). In women with these factors the benefits of treatment with HRT need to be carefully weighed against the risks. There is no consensus about the possible role of varicose veins in VTE.

The risk of VTE may be temporarily increased with prolonged immobilisation, major trauma or major surgery. In women on HRT scrupulous attention should be given to prophylactic measures to prevent VTE following surgery. Where prolonged immobilisation is liable to follow elective surgery, particularly abdominal or orthopaedic surgery to the lower limbs, consideration should be given to temporarily stopping HRT 4 weeks earlier, if this is possible.

If venous thromboembolism develops after initiating HRT the drug should be discontinued.

Prolonged exposure to unopposed oestrogens increases the risk of development of endometrial carcinoma. The general consensus of opinion is that the addition of 12 days progestogen towards the end of the cycle, as in Nuvelle, diminishes the possibility of such a risk, and some investigators consider that it might be protective.

Some women are predisposed to cholestasis during steroid therapy. Diseases that are known to be subject to deterioration during pregnancy (e.g. multiple sclerosis, epilepsy, diabetes, benign breast disease, hypertension, cardiac or renal dysfunction, asthma, porphyria, tetany and otosclerosis) and women with a strong family history of breast cancer should be carefully observed during treatment.

Pre-existing fibroids may increase in size under the influence of oestrogens. If this is observed treatment should be discontinued.

In patients with mild chronic liver disease, liver function should be checked every 8–12 weeks.

In rare cases benign and, in even rarer cases, malignant liver tumours leading in isolated cases to life-threatening intra-abdominal haemorrhage have been observed after the use of hormonal substances such as those contained in Nuvelle. If severe upper abdominal complaints, enlarged liver, or signs of intra-abdominal haemorrhage occur, a liver tumour should be included in the differential diagnostic considerations.

Interaction with other medicaments and other forms of interaction: Hormonal contraception should be stopped when treatment with Nuvelle is started and the patient should be advised to take non-hormonal contraceptive precautions.

Drugs which induce hepatic microsomal enzyme systems e.g. barbiturates, phenytoin, rifampicin, accelerate the metabolism of oestrogen/progestogen combinations such as Nuvelle and may reduce their efficacy.

The requirement for oral antidiabetics or insulin can change.

Pregnancy and lactation: Contra-indicated.

Effects on ability to drive and to use machines: None known.

Undesirable effects: During the first few months of treatment, breakthrough bleeding, spotting and breast tenderness or enlargement can occur. These are usually temporary and normally disappear after continued treatment. Other symptoms known to occur are: anxiety; increased appetite; bloating; palpitations; depressive symptoms; headache; migraine; dizziness; dyspepsia; leg pains; oedema; altered libido; nausea; rashes; vomiting; altered weight; chloasma.

Overdose: There have been no reports of ill-effects from overdosage, which it is, therefore, generally unnecessary to treat. There are no specific antidotes, and treatment should be symptomatic.

Pharmacological particulars

Pharmacodynamic properties: Nuvelle contains estradiol valerate (the valeric acid ester of the endogenous female oestrogen, estradiol) and the synthetic progestogen, levonorgestrel. Estradiol valerate provides hormone replacement during and after the climacteric. The addition of levonorgestrel in the second half of each course of tablets helps to provide good cycle control and opposes the development of endometrial hyperplasia.

Most studies show that oral administration of estradiol valerate to post-menopausal women increases serum high density lipoprotein cholesterol (HDL-C) and decreases low density lipoprotein cholesterol (LDL-C). Although epidemiological data are limited such alterations are recognised as potentially protective against the development of arterial disease. A possible attenuation of these effects may occur with the addition of a progestogen. However, at the doses used in Nuvelle, the 12 days of combined therapy with estradiol valerate and levonorgestrel have not been observed to be associated with any unwanted lipid effects.

Pharmacokinetic properties:

1. Levonorgestrel (LNG): Orally administered LNG is rapidly and completely absorbed. Following ingestion of one tablet of Nuvelle maximum drug serum levels of 1.9ng/ml were found at 1.3 hours. Thereafter, LNG serum levels decrease in two disposition phases. The first phase is described by a half-life of 0.5–1.5 hours and the terminal phase by a half-life of 20–27 hours. For LNG, a metabolic clearance rate from serum of about 1.5 ml/min/kg was determined. LNG is not excreted in unchanged form but as metabolites. LNG metabolites are excreted at about equal proportions with urine and faeces. The biotransformation follows the known pathways of steroid metabolism. No pharmacologically active metabolites are known.

LNG is bound to serum albumin and to SHBG. Only about 1.5% of the total serum drug levels are present as free steroid, but 65% are specifically bound to SHBG. The relative distribution (free, albumin-bound, SHBG-bound) depends on the SHBG concentrations in the serum. Following induction of the binding protein, the SHBG bound fraction increases while the unbound and the albumin-bound fraction decrease.

Following daily repeated administration, LNG concentrations in the serum increase by a factor of about 2. Steady-state conditions are reached within a few days. The pharmacokinetics of LNG is influenced by SHBG serum levels. Under treatment with Nuvelle SHBG levels will rise by about 40% during the oestrogen phase and remain constant or slightly decrease thereafter. The absolute bioavailability of LNG was determined to be almost 100% of the dose administered. The relative bioavailability was tested against an aqueous microcrystalline suspension and was found to be complete (108%).

About 0.1% of the maternal dose can be transferred via milk to the nursed infant.

2. Estradiol valerate (E_2 val): E_2 val is completely absorbed from the Nuvelle tablet. During absorption and the first passage through the liver the steroid ester is cleaved into estradiol (E_2) and valeric acid. At the same time E_2 undergoes extensive further metabolism yielding E_2 conjugates, estrone (E_1) and E_1 conjugates. The pharmacologically most active metabolites of E_2 val are E_2 and E_1. Maximum serum levels of 25 pg E_2/ml and 180 pg E_1/ml are reached 5–7 hours after the administration of one Nuvelle tablet.

Mean E_1 serum levels are 10–12 fold higher than mean E_2 serum concentrations. Serum levels of E_1 conjugates are about 25 fold higher than the E_1 serum levels.

E_2 is rapidly metabolised and the metabolic clearance rate has been determined to 30 ml/min/kg. After oral intake of E_2 the half-life of the terminal disposition phase was about 13 hours for E_2. The respective half-life for E_1 serum level decline was about 20 hours. The daily use of Nuvelle will lead to an about 50% increase in E_2 serum levels and to twofold E_1 levels at steady state.

Estradiol is bound to about 97% to serum proteins, about 35% are specifically bound to SHBG. E_2 val is not excreted in unchanged form. The metabolites of estradiol are excreted via urine and bile with a half-life of about 1 day at a ratio of 9:1.

The absolute bioavailability of E_2 from E_2 val is about 3% of oral dose and thus in the same range like oral E_2 (5% of dose).

The relative bioavailability of E_2 val (reference: aqueous microcrystalline suspension) from Nuvelle tablets was complete (111–112%).

Estradiol and its metabolites are excreted into milk only to a minor extent.

Preclinical safety data: There are no preclinical data which could be of relevance to the prescriber and which are not already included in other relevant sections of the SPC.

Pharmaceutical particulars

List of excipients: Nuvelle contains the following excipients: lactose, maize starch, povidone 25 000, povidone 700 000, talcum, magnesium stearate (E572), sucrose, macrogol 6000 (polyethylene glycol 6000), calcium carbonate (E170), glycerol (E422), montan glycol wax, yellow and red ferric iron oxide pigments (E172), titanium dioxide (E171).

Incompatibilities: Not applicable.

Shelf life: 5 years.

Special precautions for storage: None

Nature and contents of container: Packs containing aluminium foil and PVC blister strips of 28 tablets.

Presentation: Carton containing memo-packs of either 1 x 28 tablets or 3 x 28 tablets.

Instructions for use/handling: Not applicable.

Marketing authorisation number 0053/0219

Date of approval/revision of SPC 9 February 1998

Legal category POM

NUVELLE* TS

Qualitative and quantitative composition Nuvelle TS Phase I

Each patch contains 3 mg estradiol (equivalent to 3.1 mg Estradiol Hemihydrate). The nominal average absorption rate from the Phase I patch is 80 micrograms of estradiol per 24 hours.

Nuvelle TS Phase II

Each patch contains 2.5 mg estradiol (equivalent to 2.6 mg Estradiol Hemihydrate) and 1 mg levonorgestrel. The nominal average absorption rate from the Phase II patch is 50 micrograms of estradiol and 20 micrograms of levonorgestrel per 24 hours.

Pharmaceutical form Transdermal patches.

The clear, rectangular shaped phase I patch comprises two layers; a clear polyester backing and a matrix of estradiol in an acrylic adhesive. The clear, rectangular shaped phase II patch comprises two layers; a clear polyester backing and a matrix of estradiol and levonorgestrel in an acrylic adhesive.

Clinical particulars

Therapeutic indications: Hormone replacement therapy (HRT) for the treatment of signs and symptoms of oestrogen deficiency due to the menopause.

Posology and method of administration

Adults: If the patient is still menstruating, treatment should begin any time from the 1st to the 5th day of menstruation. Patients whose periods are very infrequent or who are postmenopausal may start at any time, provided pregnancy has been excluded (see *Special warnings and special precautions for use*).

One cycle of Nuvelle TS therapy consists of four Phase I patches of transdermal estradiol followed by four Phase II patches containing estradiol and levonorgestrel.

One Phase I patch should be applied twice weekly for the first two weeks followed by one Phase II patch twice weekly for the next two weeks. Each used patch is removed after 3 or 4 days and a fresh patch applied to a different site. Thus, two patches are worn consecutively each week and patches are changed on the same days of each week. Recommended application sites are clean, dry and intact areas of skin on the trunk and buttocks. Nuvelle TS should not be applied on or near the breasts. Each pack contains 28 days treatment. Treatment is continuous, which means that the next pack follows immediately without a break. Bleeding usually occurs during the last week of the cycle or within the first few days of the next.

Combined preparations containing an oestrogen and progestogen are only necessary in patients with an intact uterus.

Children: Not recommended for children

Contra-indications: pregnancy and lactation (see *Special warnings and special precautions for use*); severe disturbances of liver function (including porphyria), previous or existing liver tumours, jaundice or general pruritus during a previous pregnancy, Dubin-Johnson syndrome, Rotor syndrome; severe cardiac or severe renal disease; active deep venous thrombosis, thromboembolic disorders, or a history of confirmed venous thromboembolism; sickle-cell anaemia; suspected or existing hormone-dependent disorders or tumours; endometrial cancer and/or cancer of the breast; undiagnosed irregular vaginal bleeding; a history of herpes gestationis; otosclerosis with deterioration in previous pregnancies; hypersensitivity to any of the ingredients.

Special warnings and special precautions for use: Before starting treatment, pregnancy must be excluded. If the expected bleeding fails to occur at about 28-day intervals, treatment should be stopped until pregnancy has been ruled out.

Before starting Nuvelle TS, patients should have a thorough general medical and gynaecological examination with special emphasis on the body weight, blood pressure, heart, pelvic organs with an endometrial assessment if indicated, the legs and skin. Follow-up examinations are recommended at least six-monthly during treatment.

Treatment should be stopped at once if migrainous or frequent and unusually severe headaches occur for the first time, or if there are other symptoms that are possible prodromata of vascular occlusion e.g. sudden visual disturbances.

Treatment should be stopped at once if jaundice, cholestasis, hepatitis or pregnancy occurs, if there is a significant rise in blood pressure, or an increase in epileptic seizures.

There is an increased risk of gall bladder disease in women receiving postmenopausal oestrogens.

Pre-existing fibroids may increase in size under the influence of oestrogens. If this is observed, treatment should be discontinued.

Should endometriosis be reactivated under therapy with Nuvelle TS, therapy should be discontinued.

In patients with mild chronic liver disease, liver function should be checked every 8–12 weeks. Results of liver function tests may be affected by HRT.

Breakthrough bleeding may occasionally occur and can be the result of poor compliance or concurrent antibiotic use. In case of persistent abnormal or excessive vaginal blood loss, adequate diagnostic measurements have to be taken, including an endometrial evaluation with biopsy.

There is an increased risk of endometrial hyperplasia and carcinoma associated with unopposed oestrogen administered long term (for more than one year). However, the appropriate addition of a progestogen to the oestrogen regime statistically lowers the risk.

A meta-analysis from 51 epidemiological studies reported that there is a modest increase in the risk of having breast cancer diagnosed in women who have used HRT for more than five years. The findings may be due to an earlier diagnosis, the biological effects of HRT, or a combination of both. The relative risk increases with duration of treatment (by 2.3% per year of use): see chart below. This is comparable to the increased risk of breast cancer observed in women with every year of delay of natural menopause. The increased risk gradually disappears during the course of the first five years after cessation of HRT. Breast cancers found in women using HRT are more likely to be localised to the breast than those found in non-users. It is important that the increased risk of being diagnosed with breast cancer is discussed with the patient and weighed against the known benefits of HRT.

Between the ages of 50 and 70, about 45 women in every 1000 not using HRT will have breast cancer diagnosed. It is estimated that among those who use HRT for 5 years starting at age 50, 2 extra cases of breast cancer will be detected by age 70 in every 1000 women. For those who use HRT for 10 years there will be 6 extra cases of breast cancer, and for 15 years use 12 extra cases of breast cancer, in every 1,000 women during the 20-year period until age 70.

Regular breast examinations and, where appropriate, mammography should be carried out in women on HRT. Breast status should also be closely monitored in women with a history of, or known breast nodules or fibrocystic breast disease.

Epidemiological studies have suggested that hormone replacement therapy (HRT) is associated with an increased relative risk of developing venous thromboembolism (VTE) i.e. deep vein thrombosis or pulmonary embolism. The studies find a 2-3 fold increase for users compared with non-users which for healthy women amounts to a low risk of one extra case of VTE each year for every 5000 patients taking HRT.

Generally recognised risk factors for VTE include a personal or family history and severe obesity (Body Mass Index >30 kg/m²). In women with these factors the benefits of treatment with HRT need to be carefully weighed against risks. There is no consensus about the possible role of varicose veins in VTE.

The risk of VTE may be temporarily increased with prolonged immobilisation, major trauma or major surgery. In women on HRT scrupulous attention should be given to prophylactic measures to prevent VTE following surgery. Where prolonged immobilisation is liable to follow elective surgery, particularly abdominal or orthopaedic surgery to the lower limbs, consideration should be given to temporarily stopping HRT 4 weeks earlier, if this is possible.

If venous thromboembolism develops after initiating therapy the drug should be discontinued.

Diseases that are known to be subject to deterioration during pregnancy (e.g. multiple sclerosis, epilepsy, diabetes, benign breast disease, hypertension, cardiac or renal dysfunction, asthma, tetany, otosclerosis, systemic lupus erythematosus, and melanoma) and women with a strong family history of breast cancer should be carefully observed during treatment.

Diabetes should be carefully observed when initiating HRT as worsening of glucose tolerance may occur.

Oestrogens may cause fluid retention and therefore patients with cardiac or renal dysfunction should be carefully observed.

Most studies indicate that oestrogen replacement therapy has little effect on blood pressure. Some show that it may decrease blood pressure. In addition studies on combined therapy show that the addition of a progestogen also has little effect on blood pressure. Rarely, idiosyncratic hypertension may occur. When oestrogens are administered to hypertensive women, supervision is necessary and blood pressure should be monitored at regular intervals.

In rare cases benign and in even rarer cases malignant liver tumours leading in isolated cases to life-threatening intra-abdominal haemorrhage have been observed after the use of hormonal substances such as those contained in Nuvelle TS. If severe upper abdominal complaints, enlarged liver, or signs of intra-abdominal haemorrhage occur, a liver tumour should be considered in the differential diagnosis.

Women with severe hypertriglyceridaemia need special surveillance. HRT in these women may be associated with a further increase of triglyceride levels bearing the risk of acute pancreatitis.

Nuvelle TS is not suitable for contraception. Therefore, where applicable, contraception should be practised with non-hormonal methods with the exception of the rhythm and temperature methods.

Interaction with other medicinal products and other forms of interaction: Hormonal contraception should be stopped when treatment with Nuvelle TS is started and the patient should be advised to take non-hormonal contraceptive precautions if required.

Drugs which induce hepatic microsomal enzyme systems e.g. barbiturates, carbamazepine, phenytoin, rifampicin, accelerate the metabolism of oestrogen/progestogen combinations such as Nuvelle TS and may reduce their efficacy.

Transdermal therapy avoids the first pass hepatic pathway and therefore the degree of such interactions may be reduced.

The requirement for oral antidiabetics or insulin can change as a result of the effect on glucose tolerance

There are also some laboratory tests that can be influenced by oestrogens, such as tests for glucose tolerance or thyroid function

Use during pregnancy and lactation: Contra-indicated.

Effects on ability to drive and use machines: None known.

Undesirable effects: During the first few months of treatment, breakthrough bleeding, spotting and breast tenderness or enlargement can occur. These are usually temporary and normally disappear after continued treatment. Occasionally heavy withdrawal bleeding may occur. Other symptoms known to occur are: skin irritation at the application site; increased appetite; bloating; palpitations; anxiety/depressive symptoms; headache; migraine; dizziness; dyspepsia; leg pains; oedema; hypertension; altered libido; nausea; rashes; vomiting; altered weight; chloasma.

Some women are predisposed to cholestasis during steroid therapy.

Overdose: Overdosage is unlikely with this method of administration. There are no specific antidotes, and treatment should be symptomatic. The patch(es) should be removed. The most commonly observed symptoms of overdose with oestrogen therapy are breast tenderness, nausea, vomiting and/or breakthrough bleeding.

Pharmacological properties

Pharmacodynamic properties: Pharmacotherapeutic Group: ATC Code G03FB

Nuvelle TS contains estradiol in the Phase I patch (the endogenous female oestrogen) and a mixture of estradiol and the synthetic progestogen, levonorgestrel in the Phase II patch. Estradiol provides hormone replacement during and after the climacteric. The addition of levonorgestrel in the second half of each cycle helps to provide good cycle control and opposes the development of endometrial hyperplasia. Whilst endogenous ovarian hormone production is little affected, Nuvelle TS abolishes or improves the characteristic symptoms of the climacteric such as hot flushes and sweating attacks. Endometrial protection can be achieved with lower plasma levels of levonorgestrel when administered transdermally than with oral administration.

Most studies show that administration of estradiol to post-menopausal women increases serum high density lipoprotein cholesterol (HDL-C) and decreases low density lipoprotein cholesterol (LDL-C). Although epidemiological data are limited such alterations are recognised as potentially protective against the development of arterial disease. A possible attenuation of these effects may occur with the addition of a progestogen. However, at the doses used in Nuvelle TS, the 14 days of combined therapy with estradiol and levonorgestrel have not been observed to be associated with any unwanted lipid effects.

Pharmacokinetic properties: Following transdermal administration to man, estradiol is metabolised in the liver with the formation of sulphuric-acid and glucuronic acid esters (conjugated oestrogens) which are excreted in the urine. Levonorgestrel is similarly absorbed metabolised by the liver and excreted in the urine and faeces as glucuronide and sulphate conjugates.

A pharmacokinetic study showed that the mean serum estradiol concentrations in the steady state following application of the Nuvelle TS phase I patch were in the range of 150 to 260 pmol/L.

In a further pharmacokinetic study the Nuvelle TS Phase II patch was shown to result in mean plasma concentrations of estradiol in the range of 80 to 140 pmol/L, and levonorgestrel concentrations in the range of 50 to 210 pg/ml.

Preclinical safety data: Estradiol and levonorgestrel have a long history of safe clinical use in humans and

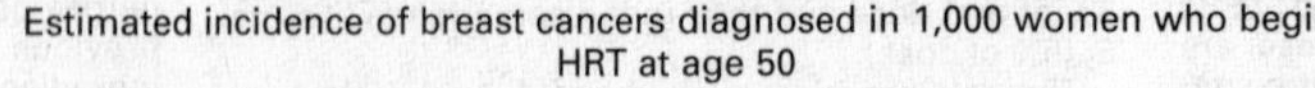

Estimated incidence of breast cancers diagnosed in 1,000 women who begin HRT at age 50

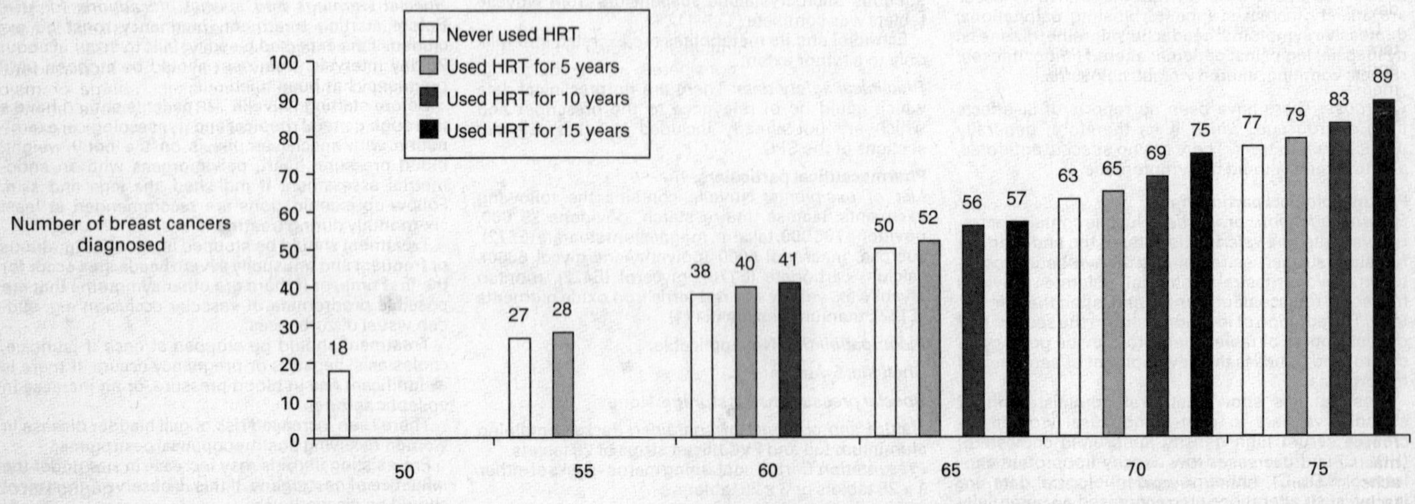

therefore further animal toxicology studies were not considered necessary.

Nuvelle TS contains a number of other constituents including an adhesive copolymer which is unlikely to be absorbed. Therefore neither local or systemic toxicity would be expected. The patches also contain diethyltoluamide as a residual solvent at a low concentration which is unlikely to result in any local or systemic toxicity.

Dermal irritancy studies in human volunteers have confirmed that Nuvelle TS is well tolerated by human skin and does not posess significant sensitising potential.

Pharmaceutical particulars

List of excipients: Acrylic adhesive, diethyltoluamide, polyester backing

Incompatibilities: Not applicable.

Shelf life: Two years.

Special precautions for storage: Keep the patches in their individual packs until just before use.

Store below 25°C. Store all drugs properly and keep them out of the reach of children.

Nature and contents of container: Each one month treatment pack contains four Phase I patches and four Phase II patches and a patient information booklet. Each patch is contained in an individual blister or sachet. Blister packs consist of a PVC/PVdC blister tray with a paper/polyester/aluminium foil lidding. Sachet packs are made from a paper/polyethylene/aluminium/polyethylene laminate.

Where a 12 week pack is available this contains three one month packs and a patient booklet in a carton.

Pack size: Packs of 8 or 24 patches.

Instructions for use and handling: The patch should be used according to the instructions under *Posology and Method of Administration.*

The Phase I patch is covered by a protective metallised polyester which must be removed before use.

The Phase II patch is covered by a protective liner of release coated paper which must be removed before use.

Marketing authorisation holder: Ethical Pharmaceuticals (UK) Ltd, Gemini House, Bartholomew's Walk, Ely, Cambs. CB7 4EA

Marketing authorisation number 10013/0036

Date of revision/approval of the SPC 1 June 1998

PRIMOLUT N*

Presentation Each white, uncoated tablet is impressed with 'AN' in a regular hexagon on one side and contains 5 mg norethisterone BP.

Excipients: lactose, maize starch, magnesium stearate.

Uses Metropathia haemorrhagica. Premenstrual syndrome. Postponement of menstruation. Endometriosis. Menorrhagia. Dysmenorrhoea.

A total dose of about 100-150 mg Primolut N (10-15 mg on each of 10 consecutive days) will produce complete secretory transformation of an endometrium that has been subjected to the proliferative effect of oestrogens.

A particular advantage is that menstruation-like withdrawal bleeding occurs consistently two to three days after Primolut N is stopped.

During treatment with Primolut N the basal body temperature rises, as it does under the influence of endogenous progesterone in the second half of the menstrual cycle.

Dosage and administration The use of Primolut N is restricted to patients in whom there is no possibility of early pregnancy in the cycle concerned.

Metropathia haemorrhagica (dysfunctional uterine bleeding): 1 tablet 3 times daily for 10 days. Bleeding is arrested usually within 1-3 days. A withdrawal bleeding resembling normal menstruation occurs within 2-4 days after discontinuing treatment.

Prophylaxis against recurrence of dysfunctional bleeding: If there are no signs of resumption of normal ovarian function (no rise in the second half of the cycle of the morning temperature, which should be measured daily) recurrence must be anticipated. Cyclical bleeding can be established with 1 tablet twice daily from the 19th to the 26th day of the cycle.

Premenstrual syndrome (including premenstrual mastalgia): Premenstrual symptoms such as headache, migraine, breast discomfort, water retention, tachycardia and psychological disturbances may be relieved by the administration of 2-3 tablets daily from the 19th to the 26th day of the cycle. Treatment should be repeated for several cycles. When treatment is stopped, the patient may remain symptom-free for a number of months.

Postponement of menstruation: In cases of too frequent menstrual bleeding, and in special circumstances (e.g. travel, sports) the postponement of menstruation is possible. 1 tablet Primolut N three times daily, starting 3 days before the expected onset of menstruation. A normal period should occur 2-3 days after the patient has stopped taking tablets.

Endometriosis (pseudo-pregnancy therapy): Long-term treatment is commenced on the 5th day of the cycle with 2 tablets Primolut N daily for the first few weeks. In the event of spotting, the dosage is increased to 4, and, if necessary, 5 tablets daily.

After bleeding has ceased, the initial dose is usually sufficient. Duration of treatment: 4-6 months continuously, or longer if necessary.

*Menorrhagia (*hypermenorrhoea): 1 tablet 2-3 times a day from the 19th to the 26th day of the cycle (counting the first day of menstruation as day 1).

Dysmenorrhoea: Functional or primary dysmenorrhoea is almost invariably relieved by the suppression of ovulation. 1 tablet three times daily for 20 days, starting on the fifth day of the cycle (the first day of menstruation counting as day 1). Treatment should be maintained for three to four cycles followed by treatment-free cycles. A further course of therapy may be employed if symptoms return.

Note: If menstrual bleeding should fail to follow a course of Primolut N, the possibility of pregnancy must be ruled out before a further course is given.

Contra-indications, warnings, etc

Contra-indications: Pregnancy. Severe disturbances of liver function. Dubin-Johnson and Rotor syndromes. Previous or existing liver tumours. History during pregnancy of idiopathic jaundice, severe pruritus or herpes gestationis. Current thromboembolic processes.

Reasons for immediate discontinuation of the tablets: Occurrence for the first time of migrainous headaches or more frequent occurrence of unusually severe headaches, sudden perceptual disorders (e.g. disturbances of vision or hearing), first signs of thrombophlebitis or thromboembolic symptoms, a feeling of pain and tightness in the chest, pending operations (six weeks beforehand), immobilisation (for instance, following accidents), onset of jaundice, hepatitis, general pruritus, significant rise in blood pressure, pregnancy.

Warnings: There is a general opinion, based on statistical evidence that users of combined oral contraceptives experience, more often than non-users, venous thromboembolism, arterial thrombosis, including cerebral and myocardial infarction, and subarachnoid haemorrhage. Full recovery from such disorders does not always occur, and it should be realised that in a few cases they are fatal. Although Primolut N does not contain oestrogen, one should keep the possibility of an increased thromboembolic risk in mind, particularly where there is a history of thromboembolic disease or in the presence of severe diabetes with vascular changes or sickle-cell anaemia.

Primolut N can influence carbohydrate metabolism. Parameters of carbohydrate metabolism should be examined carefully in all diabetics before and regularly during treatment.

In rare cases benign and, in even rarer cases, malignant liver tumours leading in isolated cases to life-threatening intra-abdominal haemorrhage, have been observed after the use of hormonal substances such as the one contained in Primolut N. If severe upper abdominal complaints, liver enlargement or signs of intra-abdominal haemorrhage occur, a liver tumour should be considered in the differential diagnosis.

Side-effects: Rarely occur in doses of 15 mg daily. Amongst those recorded are slight nausea, exacerbation of epilepsy and migraine. With extremely high dosage there may be cholestatic liver changes.

Overdosage: There have been no reports of ill-effects from overdosage and treatment is generally unnecessary.

There are no special antidotes, and treatment should be symptomatic.

Pharmaceutical precautions Shelf-life–Five years.

Legal category POM

Package quantities Packs containing 3 x 10–tablet blisters.

Further information Nil.

Product licence number 0053/5033R

PROGYNOVA* 1MG
PROGYNOVA* 2MG

Presentation Progynova 1 mg: Each beige, sugar-coated tablet contains 1 mg of estradiol valerate.

Progynova 2 mg: Each pale blue, sugar-coated tablet contains 2 mg of estradiol valerate.

Excipients: lactose monohydrate, maize starch, povidone 25 000, talc, magnesium stearate (E572), sucrose, povidone 700 000, macrogol 6000, calcium carbonate (E170), titanium dioxide (E171), glycerol 85% (E422), montan glycol wax, ferric oxide pigment, indigo carmine (E132), purified water.

Uses In menopausal women. In women with a uterus, a progestogen should be added to Progynova for 12 days each month.

Progynova 1 mg and 2 mg: Hormone replacement therapy for the treatment of the climacteric syndrome.

Progynova 2 mg: Prophylaxis of osteoporosis in women at risk of developing fractures.

Epidemiological studies suggest a number of risk factors may contribute to postmenopausal osteoporosis including: early menopause (either natural or surgically induced); family history of osteoporosis; recent corticosteroid therapy; a small frame; thin; cigarette consumption.

Dosage and administration

Progynova 1 mg and Progynova 2 mg:

Climacteric syndrome: One tablet of Progynova 1 mg or Progynova 2 mg to be taken daily.

For maintenance the lowest effective dose should be used.

Progynova 2 mg: Prophylaxis of osteoporosis: One tablet of Progynova 2 mg to be taken daily. For maximum prophylactic benefit, treatment should commence as soon as possible after onset of the menopause. Bone mineral density measurements may help to confirm the presence of low bone mass.

Treatment is continuous which means that the next pack follows immediately without a break.

Contra-indications, warnings, etc

Contra-indications: Pregnancy and lactation, severe disturbances of liver function (including porphyria), previous or existing liver tumours, jaundice or general pruritus during a previous pregnancy, Dubin Johnson syndrome, Rotor syndrome, severe cardiac or severe renal disease; active deep venous thrombosis, thromboembolic disorders, or a history of confirmed venous thromboembolism; suspected or existing hormone-dependent disorders or tumours, tumours of the uterus or breast, congenital disturbances of lipid metabolism; severe diabetes with vascular changes; hypersensitivity to any of the ingredients.

Warnings/side effects: In women with an intact uterus, there is an increased risk of endometrial hyperplasia and carcinoma associated with unopposed oestrogen administered long term (for more than one year). However, the appropriate addition of a progestogen to the oestrogen regimen statistically lowers the risk. Should endometriosis be reactivated under therapy with Progynova, therapy should be discontinued.

Epidemiological studies have suggested that hormone replacement therapy (HRT) is associated with an increased relative risk of developing venous thromboembolism (VTE) i.e. deep vein thrombosis or pulmonary embolism. The studies find a 2–3 fold increase for users compared with non-users which for healthy women amounts to a low risk of one extra case of VTE each year for every 5000 patients taking HRT.

Generally recognised risk factors for VTE include a personal or family history and severe obesity (Body Mass Index >30 kg/m²). In women with these factors the benefits of treatment with HRT need to be carefully weighed against risks. There is no consensus about the possible role of varicose veins in VTE.

The risk of VTE may be temporarily increased with prolonged immobilisation, major trauma or major surgery. In women on HRT scrupulous attention should be given to prophylactic measures to prevent VTE following surgery. Where prolonged immobilisation is liable to follow elective surgery, particularly abdominal or orthopaedic surgery to the lower limbs, consideration should be given to temporarily stopping HRT 4 weeks earlier, if this is possible.

If venous thromboembolism develops after initiating therapy the drug should be discontinued.

During the first few months of treatment, breast tenderness or enlargement can occur. These are usually temporary and normally disappear after continued treatment. Other symptoms known to occur are dyspepsia, flatulence, nausea, vomiting, leg pains, anxiety, depressive symptoms, increased appetite, abdominal pain and bloating, altered weight, oedema, palpitations, altered libido, headache, dizziness, epistaxis, hypertension, rashes, thrombophlebitis, mucous vaginal discharge, general pruritus. Some women are predisposed to cholestasis during steroid therapy.

Diseases that are known to be subject to deterioration during pregnancy (e.g. multiple sclerosis, epilepsy, diabetes, benign breast disease, hypertension, cardiac or renal dysfunction, asthma, migraine, tetany, systemic lupus erythematosus and melanoma) and women with a strong family history of breast cancer should be carefully observed during treatment.

Because of the occurrence of herpes gestationis and the worsening of otosclerosis in pregnancy, it is thought that treatment with female hormones may have similar effects. Patients with these conditions should be carefully monitored. Similarly, patients with sickle-cell anaemia should be monitored because of the increased risk of thrombosis that accompanies this disease.

Precautions and special information: Before starting treatment pregnancy must be excluded. Before starting Progynova, patients should have a thorough general medical and gynaecological examination with special emphasis on the body weight, blood pressure, heart, pelvic organs, the legs and skin. Follow-up examinations are recommended at least six-monthly during treatment.

Treatment should be stopped at once if migrainous or frequent and unusually severe headaches occur for the first time, or if there are any other symptoms that are possible prodromata of vascular occlusion, e.g. sudden visual disturbances.

Treatment should be stopped at once if jaundice, cholestasis, hepatitis or pregnancy occurs or if there is a significant rise in blood-pressure or an increase in epileptic seizures.

In patients with mild chronic liver disease, liver function should be checked every 8–12 weeks. Results of liver function tests may be affected by HRT.

At the present time, there is some evidence which suggests a slight increase in the relative risk of breast cancer in postmenopausal women receiving long-term hormone replacement therapy (more than 5 years). It is not known whether concurrent progestogen use influences this risk.

There is a need for caution when prescribing oestrogens in women who have a history of, or known, breast nodules or fibrocystic disease.

Women on long term therapy should have regular breast examinations and should be instructed in self-examination of the breast. Regular mammographic investigations should be conducted where it is considered appropriate.

There is an increased risk of gall bladder disease in women receiving post menopausal oestrogens.

Patients with pre-existing fibroids should be closely monitored as fibroids may increase in size under the influence of oestrogens. If this is observed, treatment should be discontinued.

Oestrogens may cause fluid retention and therefore patients with renal or cardiac dysfunction should be carefully observed.

Most studies demonstrate that oestrogen replacement therapy has little effect on blood pressure. Some show that it may decrease blood pressure. In addition, studies on combined therapy show that the addition of a progestogen also has little effect on blood pressure. Rarely, idiosyncratic hypertension may occur. When oestrogens are administered to hypersensitive women, supervision is necessary and blood pressure should be monitored at regular intervals.

In rare cases benign, and in even rarer cases, malignant liver tumours leading in isolated cases to life-threatening intra-abdominal haemorrhage have been observed after the use of hormonal substances such as those contained in Progynova. A hepatic tumour should be considered in the differential diagnosis if upper abdominal pain, enlarged liver or signs of intra-abdominal haemorrhage occur.

Diabetes should be carefully observed when initiating HRT as worsening of the glucose tolerance may occur.

In women with a uterus, contraception should be practised with non-hormonal methods.

Interaction with other drugs: Drugs which induce hepatic microsomal enzyme systems e.g barbiturates, carbamazepine, phenytoin, rifampicin accelerate the metabolism of oestrogen products such as Progynova and may reduce their efficacy. The requirement for oral antidiabetics or insulin can change as a result of the effect on glucose tolerance. There are some laboratory tests that can be influenced by oestrogens, such as tests for glucose tolerance, liver function or thyroid function.

Overdosage: Nausea and vomiting may occur with an overdose.

There are no specific antidotes, and treatment should be symptomatic. Withdrawal bleeding may occur in females with a uterus.

Pharmaceutical precautions None.

Shelf-life: Progynova 1 mg – Five years. Progynova 2 mg – Five years.

Legal category POM

Package quantities Carton containing memo-packs of either 1×28 tablets or 3×28 tablets.

Further information Most studies show that oral administration of estradiol valerate to post-menopausal women increases serum high density lipoprotein cholesterol (HDL-C) and decreases low density lipoprotein cholesterol (LDL-C). Although epidemiological data are limited, such alterations are recognised as potentially protective against the development of arterial disease.

Product licence numbers
Progynova 1 mg 0053/0057
Progynova 2 mg 0053/0058

PROGYNOVA *TS
PROGYNOVA *TS FORTE

Qualitative and quantitative composition Estradiol (oestradiol) transdermal systems:

Progynova TS: 12.5 cm² patch contains 3.9 mg of estradiol. Progynova TS forte: 25.0 cm² patch contains 7.8 mg of estradiol.

Nominal average absorption rates of 50 micrograms/day and 100 micrograms/day were calculated for Progynova TS and Progynova TS Forte respectively.

Pharmaceutical form Transdermal delivery system comprising a patch containing estradiol in an acrylate adhesive matrix. The transdermal delivery from a patch is maintained over 7 days.

The active component of the system is estradiol. The remaining components of the system are pharmacologically inactive.

Clinical particulars
Therapeutic indications: Oestrogen replacement therapy for patients with disorders due to natural menopause or surgically induced menopause (only if due to noncarcinomatous diseases) e.g. vasomotor symptoms (hot flushes, sweating), atrophic conditions (such as atrophic vaginitis/vulvitis, and/or atrophic urethritis, trigonitis) caused by deficient endogenous oestrogen production.

Posology and method of administration: Adults (including the elderly): Treatment should be initiated with Progynova TS. If considered necessary, Progynova TS forte should be used. Once treatment is established the lowest effective dose necessary for the relief of symptoms should be used.

Treatment can be given either continuously or on a cyclical basis.

Unopposed oestrogen therapy should not be used unless the patient has had a hysterectomy. Where a progestogen is considered necessary the appropriate dose should be administered for 12 days in every month.

The patches should be applied once weekly on a continuous basis, each used system being removed after 7 days and a fresh system applied to a different site. Recommended application sites are clean, dry and intact areas of skin on the trunk and buttocks. Progynova TS and Progynova TS forte should not be applied on or near the breasts.

The patches may also be prescribed on a cyclical basis. Where this is the preferred option, the patches should be applied weekly for 3 consecutive weeks followed by a 7 day interval, without a patch being applied, before the next course.

Children: Not recommended for children

Contra-indications: Pregnancy; lactation; severe disturbances of liver function (including porphyria); previous or existing liver tumours; Rotor syndrome; Dubin-Johnson syndrome; severe cardiac, severe renal disease; jaundice or general pruritus during a previous pregnancy; existing or previous thromboembolic processes; sickle cell anaemia; severe diabetes with vascular changes; suspected or existing hormone dependent disorders or tumours of the uterus, breast or ovaries; undiagnosed irregular vaginal bleeding, disturbances of lipid metabolism; a history of herpes gestationis; otosclerosis with deterioration in previous pregnancies; endometriosis; hypersensitivity to any of the ingredients.

Special warnings and special precautions for use: Before starting treatment pregnancy must be excluded. Prior to treatment, patients should have a thorough general medical and gynaecological examination with special emphasis on the body weight, blood pressure, heart, pelvic organs with an endometrial assessment if indicated, the legs and skin. Follow-up examinations are recommended at least six-monthly during treatment.

Women on therapy should have regular breast examinations and be instructed in self-breast examination. Regular mammographic investigations should be conducted where considered appropriate.

Treatment should be stopped at once if migrainous or frequent and unusually severe headaches occur for the first time, or if there are other symptoms that are possible prodromata of vascular occlusion, e.g. sudden visual disturbances.

Consideration should be given to discontinuing treatment before operations (6 weeks beforehand) or following immobilisation.

There is an increased risk of gall bladder disease in women receiving postmenopausal oestrogens.

Treatment should be stopped at once if jaundice, cholestasis, hepatitis or pregnancy occurs, or if there is a significant rise in blood pressure, the occurrence of thromboembolic disease or an increase in epileptic seizures.

If there is, repeatedly, persistent skin irritation despite application sites being changed according to directions, consideration should be given to discontinuing transdermal treatment.

Pre-existing fibroids may increase in size during oestrogen therapy. If this is observed treatment should be discontinued. In women with an intact uterus, prolonged exposure to unopposed oestrogens increases the risk of the development of endometrial carcinoma. However, the addition of 12 days progestogen towards the end of the month reduces the possibility of such a risk. If irregular bleeding occurs repeatedly during the use of Progynova TS or Progynova TS forte this should be investigated by endometrial biopsy, if necessary.

At the present time there is some evidence which suggests a slight increase in the relative risk of breast cancer in post-menopausal women receiving long-term hormone replacement therapy. A careful appraisal of the risk/benefit ratio should be undertaken before treating for longer than 5 years. Thromboembolism has been reported in connection with oestrogen replacement therapy but there is no evidence to date that the overall incidence is increased.

Diseases that are known to be subject to deterioration during pregnancy (e.g. multiple sclerosis, epilepsy, diabetes, benign breast disease, varicose veins, hypertension, cardiac, hepatic or renal dysfunction, migraine, asthma, chorea minor, tetany and otosclerosis) and women with a strong family history of breast cancer should be carefully observed during treatment.

In rare cases benign, and in even rarer cases, malignant liver tumours leading in isolated cases to life threatening intra-abdominal haemorrhage have been observed after the use of hormonal substances such as those contained in Progynova TS and Progynova TS forte. A hepatic tumour should be considered in the differential diagnosis if upper abdominal pain, enlarged liver, or signs of intra-abdominal haemorrhage occur.

Interaction with other medicaments and other forms of interaction: Drugs which induce hepatic microsomal enzyme systems, e.g. barbiturates, carbamazepine, phenytoin, rifampicin, accelerate the metabolism of oestrogens, reducing systemic bioavailability and thus, efficacy. However, it is probable that the transdermally applied oestrogens are less affected by such an interaction than oral oestrogens. The requirement for oral antidiabetics or insulin can change as a result of the effect on glucose tolerance.

There are also some laboratory tests that can be influenced by oestrogens, such as the tests for glucose tolerance or thyroid function.

Pregnancy and lactation: Progynova TS and Progynova TS forte are contraindicated during pregnancy and lactation.

Effects on ability to drive and use machines: Not applicable.

Undesirable effects: Hormonal contraception should be stopped when the use of Progynova TS and Progynova TS forte is started and the patient should be advised to take non-hormonal contraceptive precautions if required. During the first few months of treatment, breakthrough bleeding, spotting and breast tenderness or enlargement can occur. These are usually temporary and normally disappear after continued treatment. Other symptoms known to occur are: skin irritation at the application site; in individual cases an allergic contact dermatitis with post-inflammatory pruritus and generalised exanthema; nausea; abdominal pain; bloating; headache; migraine; anxiety/depressive symptoms; dizziness; alterations in body weight; oedema; hypertension; altered libido; changes in vaginal secretion; growth of pre-existing fibroids; chloasma or melasma which may be persistent. Some women are predisposed to cholestasis during steroid therapy.

Overdose: Overdosage is unlikely with this type of application. Nausea, vomiting and withdrawal bleeding may occur in some women. There is no specific antidote and treatment should be symptomatic. The patch(es) should be removed.

Pharmacological properties
Pharmacodynamic properties: The loss of the ovarian function, accompanied by a depletion of oestrogen production, leads to the menopausal syndrome, characterised by vasomotoric-vegetative, and organic symptoms. Hormone replacement therapy aims to eliminate these complaints. Of all physiological oes-

trogens, estradiol is the most potent one with the highest affinity for the oestrogen receptor. In the oestrogen sensitive target organs, in particular uterus, hypothalamus, pituitary, vagina, urethra, breast, bones (osteoclasts) estradiol exerts its effects, as other steroid hormones, by regulating the transcription of a limited number of genes. After diffusion through the cell membrane, estradiol binds with high affinity to the oestrogen receptor. After activation by the estradiol ligand the hormone receptor complex is translocated into the nucleus where it binds to specific DNA sequences (hormone response elements) that enhance the transcription of adjacent genes. The full number of proteins induced by oestrogen is not known but is estimated to be 50 to 100.

After the menopause the production of estradiol in the female is substantially reduced. The remaining estradiol is mainly synthesised from precursors produced in the adrenal cortex, by aromatisation from androstenedione and to a lesser extent from testosterone by the enzyme aromatase thus forming estrone and estradiol, respectively. Estrone is converted into estradiol via the enzyme 17-hydroxysteriod-dehydrogenase. Both enzymes have been found in the liver and in fat and muscle tissue. The estradiol/estrone ratio in postmenopausal women is approximately 0.2 compared to a ratio of >1 in premenopausal women.

Climacteric disturbances can be treated by oestrogen replacement therapy with mean transdermal doses between 25 and 100 micrograms estradiol per day.

Independent of the route of administration, oestrogen doses, which are necessary for improvement of menopausal complaints, exert a dose dependent stimulating effect on mitosis and proliferation of the endometrium. Oestrogen monotherapy increases the frequency of endometrial hyperplasia and thus the risk of endometrial carcinoma. In order to avoid endometrial hyperplasia the sequential administration of a progestin for 10–12 days is recommended in non-hysterectomised postmenopausal women.

Pharmacokinetic properties: The therapy with the once-a-week Progynova TS or Progynova TS forte system is comparable to a continuous low dose intravenous infusion aiming at smooth, stable, plateau-like estradiol serum levels similar to those during the early/mid follicular phase during the reproductive life span. Transdermal administration avoids highly fluctuating estradiol and metabolite levels in the serum seen after oral estradiol substitution and avoids also an inundation of the liver with large amounts of estradiol and its metabolites due to a high presystemic metabolisation of the compound ("first-pass effect") after oral intake. Thus, after transdermal administration of estradiol, no effects on liver protein synthesis have been observed.

During a once-a-week application regimen of Progynova TS or Progynova TS forte, smooth and consistent estradiol and estrone serum level profiles within the desired range are achieved. No accumulation of either substance is observed following multiple 1-week patch applications. The absolute height of the estradiol serum level profile is directly proportional to the area of the patch with mean steady state estradiol serum levels in the range of 35 pg/ml after application of the 12.5 cm² patch and those in the range of approximately 70 pg/ml after application of the 25 cm² patch.

After transdermal administration, the metabolisation of estradiol to estrone and conjugates remains within the physiological range as seen during the early follicular phase in the reproductive life period indicated by an estradiol/estrone serum level ratio of approximately 1. Unphysiologically high estrone levels as a result of the intensive "first pass" metabolisation during oral estradiol hormone replacement therapy, reflected in estradiol/estrone ratios as low as 0.1, are avoided.

The biotransformation and the excretion of the transdermally administered estradiol are the same as that of the endogenous hormone. Estradiol is eliminated from the body with a total serum clearance of approximately 15–30 ml/min/kg by biotransformation mainly in the liver but also extrahepatically, eg. in gut, kidney, skeletal muscles and target organs. These processes involve the formation of estrone, estriol, catecholoestrogens and sulphate and glucuronide conjugates of these compounds, which are all distinctly less oestrogenic or even nonoestrogenic. A certain proportion of estradiol metabolites are excreted in the bile and undergo a so-called enterohepatic circulation. Ultimately estradiol metabolites are mainly excreted as sulphates and glucuronides with the urine.

Preclinical safety data: In primary dermal irritation studies, application of Progynova TS or Progynova TS forte resulted in mild irritation related to mechanical trauma at removal. In sensitisation studies, Progynova TS or Progynova TS forte had no dermal sensitising potential.

The components of the adhesive matrix of Progynova TS or Progynova TS forte (monomer and polymer) have been studied extensively and, at many multiples of the projected human exposure, present a low risk. Additional excipients used in the adhesive matrix are either generally regarded as safe for use in food components or considered acceptable as an inactive ingredient for prescription and topical transdermal products.

The adhesive backing and release liner of Progynova TS or Progynova TS forte were tested in biological test methods and were considered to be compatible with biologic systems.

Pharmaceutical particulars
List of excipients: Ethyl oleate, isopropyl myristate, glycerol monolaurate. The adhesive system is an acrylate copolymer.

Incompatibilities: None so far known.

Shelf life: 3 years.

Special precautions for storage: Do not store unpouched. Apply immediately upon removal from the protective pouch.

Nature and contents of container: Protective pouch containing a Progynova TS patch with a surface area of 12.5 cm² or a Progynova TS forte patch with a surface area of 25 cm². The patches comprise two layers. From the visible surface to the surface attached to the skin these are: a translucent polyethylene film; a drug reservoir of estradiol in an acrylate adhesive matrix; a protective liner of release-coated polyester film is attached to the adhesive surface and must be removed prior to use. The protective pouch contains a desiccant.

Packs containing 4 patches.
Packs containing 12 patches.

Instructions for use/handling: The patch should be used according to the instructions under "Posology and method of administration". Store all drugs properly and keep them out of the reach of children.

Marketing authorisation numbers
Progynova TS: 0053/0241
Progynova TS forte: 0053/0242

Date of approval/revision of SPC 7 April 1997

Legal category POM

PROLUTON*DEPOT

Presentation Hydroxyprogesterone hexanoate BP 250 mg and 500 mg in ampoules for intramuscular injection.

Excipients: Benzyl benzoate, castor oil

Uses Habitual abortion, when associated with proven progesterone-deficiency.

Dosage and administration 250-500 mg Proluton Depot by intramuscular injection at weekly intervals during the first half of pregnancy.

Contra-indications, warnings etc
Contra-indications: A history of herpes gestationis. Previous or existing liver tumours.

Warnings: Many medicinal products, including female sex hormones, have been suspected of being capable of affecting the normal development of a child in the early stages of pregnancy. Many researchers consider that in relation to sex hormones such a suspicion is ill founded but one has to accept that for no medicinal product can teratogenic activity be excluded with absolute certainty. Therefore, the general principle is now widely accepted that inessential use of drugs during pregnancy should be avoided. Following this general principle, Proluton Depot should be used to maintain pregnancy only if it is strictly indicated, i.e. if there is an urgent desire to have a child, and luteal insufficiency is present.

Since Proluton Depot may prevent spontaneous evacuation of a dead foetus (missed abortion) the progress of the pregnancy should be regularly monitored by appropriate means, including immunological tests.

Proluton Depot can influence carbohydrate metabolism. Parameters of carbohydrate metabolism should be examined carefully in all diabetics before and regularly during treatment. The requirement for oral antidiabetics or insulin can change.

In rare cases benign and, in even rarer cases, malignant liver tumours leading in isolated cases to life-threatening intra-abdominal haemorrhage, have been observed after the use of hormonal substances such as the one contained in Proluton Depot. If severe upper abdominal complaints, liver enlargement or signs of intra-abdominal haemorrhage occur, a liver tumour should be considered in the differential diagnosis.

Side-effects: Very rarely, local reactions may occur at the site of injection. In rare cases coughing, dyspnoea and circulatory irregularities may occur during or immediately after the injection. Experience has shown that these reactions can be avoided by injecting very slowly.

Overdosage: There have been no reports of serious ill-effects from overdosage, which is unlikely to occur with intramuscular administration.

Pharmaceutical precautions Protect from light. Shelf-life – Five years.

Legal category POM

Package quantities 250 mg: Packs of 3 ampoules 1 ml

500 mg: Packs of 3 ampoules 2 ml.

Further information Nil

Product licence numbers
Proluton Depot 250 mg 0053/5031R
Proluton Depot 500 mg 0053/5032R

PRO-VIRON*

Qualitative and quantitative composition Each tablet contains 25 mg mesterolone.

Pharmaceutical form Tablets.

Clinical particulars
Therapeutic indications: Androgen deficiency or male infertility when associated with primary or secondary male hypogonadism.

Posology and method of administration: The following dosages are recommended:
Adults: Initially: 3 or 4 tablets daily for several months, followed by maintenance therapy of 2-3 tablets (50-75 mg) daily.
Children: Not recommended in children.

Contra-indications: Pro-Viron is contra-indicated in the presence of prostatic carcinoma since androgens can stimulate the growth of an existing carcinoma.

Previous or existing liver tumours.

Special warnings and special precautions for use: Androgens are not suitable for enhancing muscular development in healthy individuals or for increasing physical ability. Regular examination of the prostate during treatment is advised, in order to exclude prostatic carcinoma. In rare cases benign, and in even rarer cases, malignant liver tumours leading in isolated cases to life-threatening intra-abdominal haemorrhage have been observed after the use of hormonal substances such as the one contained in Pro–Viron. If severe upper abdominal complaints, liver enlargement or signs of intra-abdominal haemorrhage occur, the possibility of a liver tumour should be included in the differential diagnosis.

Frequent or persistent erections of the penis may occur (see *Undesirable effects*).

Interaction with other medicaments and other forms of interaction: None known.

Pregnancy and lactation: Not applicable.

Effects on ability to drive and use machines: None known.

Undesirable effects: If, in individual cases, frequent or persistent erections occur, the dose should be discontinued in order to avoid injury to the penis.

Overdose: There have been no reports of ill-effects from overdosage and treatment is generally unncessary. If overdosage is discovered within two to three hours and is so large that treatment seems desirable, gastric lavage can safely be used.

Pharmacological properties
Pharmacodynamic properties: Pro-Viron is an orally active androgen.The presence of a methyl group at C-1 confers special properties on this steroid which, unlike testosterone and all its derivatives that are used for androgen therapy, is not metabolised to oestrogen.

This difference almost certainly accounts for the observation that, in its usual therapeutic dosage in normal men, Pro-Viron does not significantly depress the release of gonadotrophins from the pituitary. Hence (1) spermatogenesis is unimpaired (2) unlike other androgens, which suppress and therefore replace endogenous androgens, Pro-Viron supplements endogenous androgens.

In contrast to other orally active androgens, liver tolerance is excellent (a fact probably related to the absence of 17-alkyl substitution of the steroid nucleus).

Pharmacokinetic properties: Following oral ingestion mesterolone is rapidly and almost completely absorbed in a wide dose range of 25–100 mg. The intake of Pro-Viron generates maximum serum drug levels of 3.1 ± 1.1 ng/ml after 1.6 ± 0.6 hours. Thereafter, drug levels in serum decrease with a terminal half-life of 12–13 hours. Mesterolone is 98% bound to serum proteins, 40% to albumin and 58% to SHBG (sex hormone binding globulin).

Mesterolone is rapidly inactivated by metabolism.

The metabolic clearance rate from serum accounts for 4.4±1.6 ml•min⁻¹•kg⁻¹. There is no renal excretion of unchanged drug. The main metabolite has been identified as 1α-methyl-androsterone, which–in conjugated form–accounts for 55–70 % of renally excreted metabolites. The ratio of the main metabolite glucuronide to sulphate is about 12:1. A further metabolite 1α-methyl-5α-androstane-3α,17β-diol has been recognized, which accounted for about 3 % of renally eliminated metabolites. No metabolic conversion into oestrogens or corticoids has been observed. 77% of the mesterolone metabolites are excreted via the urine and 13% with the faeces. 50% of the dose is excreted in the urine within 24 hours and 90% within 7 days via the faeces and urine.

The absolute bioavailability of mesterolone is about 3 % of the oral dose.

Preclinical safety data: There are no preclinical data which could be of relevance to the prescriber and which are not already included in other relevant sections of the SPC.

Pharmaceutical particulars

List of excipients: Lactose, maize starch, povidone 25 000 (E1201), methyl parahydroxybenzoate (E218), propyl parahydroxybenzoate (E216), magnesium stearate (E572)

Incompatibilities: None known.

Shelf-life: 5 years.

Special precautions for storage: None.

Nature and contents of container: 3 blister packs of 10 tablets contained in a cardboard outer pack.

Instructions for use/handling: Store all drugs properly and keep them out of reach of children.

Marketing authorisation number 0053/0030

Date of approval/revision of SPC 1 April 1997

Legal category CD (Sch.4, Part I), POM

SCHERING PC4*

Qualitative and quantitative composition Each tablet contains 500 micrograms of norgestrel and 50 micrograms of ethinyloestradiol.

Pharmaceutical form Sugar-coated tablets.

Clinical particulars

Therapeutic indications: Post-coital contraception within 72 hours of unprotected coitus as an occasional emergency measure. Schering PC4 is primarily aimed to prevent implantation of the fertilised ovum in the endometrium.

Posology and method of administration: For oral administration.

The first two tablets should be taken as soon as possible after coitus (up to a maximum of 72 hours afterwards), and the remaining two tablets twelve hours after the first two.

Contra-indications: Pregnancy.

Therapy should not be administered in the following circumstances, as pregnancy may already have occurred:

a) where menstrual bleeding is overdue, and

b) where the patient has already had unprotected intercourse more than 72 hours previously in the present menstrual cycle.

Other contra-indications:

- Thrombotic disorders and a history of these conditions
- Sickle-cell anaemia
- Disorders of lipid metabolism and other conditions in which, in individual cases, there is known or suspected to be a much increased risk of thrombosis
- Acute or severe chronic liver diseases
- Dubin-Johnson syndrome
- Rotor syndrome
- Previous or existing liver tumours
- History during pregnancy of idiopathic jaundice or severe pruritus
- History of herpes gestationis
- Mammary or endometrial carcinoma, or a history of these conditions
- Abnormal vaginal bleeding of unknown cause
- Deterioration of otosclerosis during pregnancy
- Severe diabetes with vascular changes
- Hypersensitivity to any of the components of Schering PC4.

Special warnings and special precautions for use: The repeated use of Schering PC4 within a single monthly cycle is to be avoided.

Schering PC4 does not appear to be as effective as some regularly-used methods of contraception and is suitable only as an occasional emergency measure. Schering PC4 is not effective if started later than 72 hours after coitus and should not be so used.

Vomiting, severe diarrhoea or other causes of malabsorption might impair the efficacy of Schering PC4.

Examination of the pelvic organs, breasts and blood pressure should normally precede the prescribing of any combined oral contraceptive. The following conditions require careful consideration: a history of severe depressive states, diabetes, hypertension, epilepsy, porphyria, tetany, disturbed liver function, gall stones, cardiovascular disease, renal diseases, otosclerosis, obesity and migraine.

The importance of follow-up and the possibility of an early or late onset of the next period should be explained to the patient. The practice of abstinence or careful use of a barrier method until the onset of the next period also should be advised. Follow-up should be carried out 3 weeks after administration of therapy to assess the effectiveness of the method, to discuss future management if a period has not occurred and to counsel the patient about future contraception.

There is a general opinion, based on statistical evidence, that users of combined oral contraceptives (oestrogen-progestogen combinations like Schering PC4) experience, more often than non-users, venous thromboembolism, arterial thrombosis, including cerebral and myocardial infarction, and subarachnoid haemorrhage. Full recovery from such disorders does not always occur and it should be realised that in a few cases they are fatal.

Certain factors may entail some risk of thrombosis e.g. smoking, obesity, varicose veins, cardiovascular diseases, diabetes and migraine. The suitability of Schering PC4 should be judged according to the severity of such conditions in the individual case, and should be discussed with the patient before she decides to take it. The risk of arterial thrombosis associated with combined oral contraceptives increases with age, and this risk is aggravated by cigarette smoking. Therefore the use of Schering PC4 by women in the older age-group, especially those who are cigarette smokers, should therefore be discouraged. Caution is also advised before Schering PC4 is prescribed if there is a history in the family of thromboembolic disease at a young age (e.g. deep vein thrombosis, heart attack or stroke).

Interaction with other medicaments and other forms of interaction: The efficacy of Schering PC4 might be impaired by interaction with concurrently-used drugs including barbiturates, primidone, phenytoin, carbamazepine, phenylbutazone, griseofulvin, rifampicin, ampicillin and other antibiotics.

The requirement for oral antidiabetics or insulin can change as a result of an effect on glucose tolerance.

Pregnancy and lactation: Patients who become pregnant despite post-coital contraception should be carefully evaluated for possible ectopic pregnancy. Since Schering PC4 appears to affect only endometrial implantation, tubal pregnancy may occur at the expected rate and it is thus possible that there will be a relative increase in ectopic pregnancy in patients who become pregnant despite the use of Schering PC4 therapy.

When Schering PC4 is used during lactation, it must be considered that milk production may be reduced. Furthermore, minute amounts of the active substance are eliminated with the milk.

The effect of Schering PC4 on the conceptus in the event of failure to prevent conception is not definitely known. Some investigations have suggested that sex hormones taken in the first trimester of pregnancy may slightly increase the risk of foetal malformations, but numerous other investigations have failed to support these findings. The consensus of opinion amongst teratologists is that even known teratogens will not produce malformations before organogenesis starts, which is much later than the 72 hours after fertilisation to which the use of Schering PC4 is restricted.

Effects on ability to drive and use machines: None known.

Undesirable effects: Nausea and vomiting are common side-effects and the latter may reduce the efficacy of therapy if it occurs within about 2 hours after the ingestion of either dose of tablets, in which event consideration should be given to the taking of more pills.

The concomitant administration of an anti-emetic has been favoured by some practitioners.

The pattern of menstrual bleeding is often temporarily disturbed. Breast discomfort and headaches also may occur.

Overdose: There have been no reports of serious ill-effects from overdosage.

Pharmacological properties

Pharmacodynamic properties: The progestogen/oestrogen combination in Schering PC4 renders the endometrium hostile to implantation of a fertilised ovum.

After use of the preparation, a disturbance of the processes of endometrial differentiation occurs at around the time point of ovulation. The disturbance takes the form primarily of asynchrony between glandular and stromal development. The endometrium offers extremely unfavourable conditions for nidation because of the morphological and enzymatic changes which then take place. The influence on endocrine parameters (progesterone, estradiol) differs. The luteal phase is usually shortened.

Pharmacokinetic properties: Levonorgestrel

Norgestrel is a racemic mixture of levo- and dextrarotatory enantiomers, of which levonorgestrel is the pharmacologically active component. Levonorgestrel is present to 50% in norgestrel. Therefore, the subsequent compound characteristics only refer to levonorgestrel.

Orally administered levonorgestrel is rapidly and completely absorbed. Following ingestion of two coated tablets of Schering PC4, maximum drug serum levels of about 10 ng/ml can be expected at 1.0 hour. Thereafter, levonorgestrel serum levels decrease in two phases, characterised by half-lives of 0.5 hours and about 20 hours. For levonorgestrel, a metabolic clearance rate from serum of about 1.5 ml/min/kg was determined. Levonorgestrel is not excreted in unchanged form but as metabolites. Levonorgestrel metabolites are excreted at about equal proportions with urine and faeces. The biotransformation follows the known pathways of steroid metabolism. No pharmacologically active metabolites are known.

Levonorgestrel is bound to serum albumin and to SHBG (sex hormone binding globulin). Only about 1.5% of the total serum drug levels are present as free steroid, but 65% are specifically bound to SHBG. The relative distribution (free, albumin-bound, SHBG-bound) depends on the SHBG concentrations in the serum. Following induction of the binding protein, the SHBG bound fraction increases while the unbound and the albumin-bound fraction decrease.

Following the ingestion of two coated tablets of Schering PC4 and the same dose 12 hours later about 50% higher levonorgestrel levels can be expected after the second drug administration as compared to the first one. Due to the short treatment period of one day, only a slight increase in the serum levels of SHBG can be expected which has no effect on the pharmacokinetics of levonorgestrel. The absolute bioavailability of levonorgestrel was determined to be almost 100% of the dose administered.

About 0.1% of the maternal dose can be transferred via the breast milk to the nursed infant.

Ethinyloestradiol:

Orally administered ethinyloestradiol is rapidly and completely absorbed. Following the ingestion of two coated tablets of Schering PC4, maximum drug serum levels of about 350 pg/ml can be expected at 1–2 hours. Thereafter, ethinyloestradiol serum levels decrease in two phases characterised by half-lives of 1–2 hours and about 20 hours. Because of analytical reasons, these parameters can only be calculated following the administration of higher doses. For ethinyloestradiol, an apparent volume of distribution of about 5 l/kg and a metabolic clearance rate from serum of about 5 ml/min/kg were determined. Ethinyloestradiol is highly but non-specifically bound to serum albumin. About 2% of drug levels are present unbound. During absorption and first-liver passage, ethinyloestradiol is metabolized resulting in a reduced absolute and variable oral bioavailability. Unchanged drug is not excreted. Ethinyloestradiol metabolites are excreted at an urinary to biliary ratio of 4:6 with a half-life of about 1 day.

The absolute bioavailability of ethinyloestradiol is subject to a considerable interindividual variation. Following oral administration, the mean bioavailability was found to be about 40% to 60% of the administered dose.

During established lactation, 0.02% of the daily maternal dose could be transferred to the newborn via the breast milk.

The systemic availability of ethinyloestradiol might be influenced in both directions by other drugs. There is, however, no interaction with high doses of vitamin C. Ethinyloestradiol induces the hepatic synthesis of SHBG and CBG (corticoid binding globulin) during continuous use. The extent of SHBG induction, however, depends on the chemical structure and the dose of the co-administered progestogen.

Preclinical safety data: For the evaluation of levonorgestrel data from studies with the racemate dl-norgestrel were used as well. The relevance of these data is documented by pharmacological and pharmacokinetic studies.

In animal studies on systemic tolerance with repeated oral administration (including studies for evaluation of a tumorigenic activity) no systemic intolerance reactions which would raise objections to the use of the preparation in therapeutic doses were observed.

In in-vitro and in-vivo studies no indication of a mutagenic potential of both compounds was found.

In reproduction toxicological studies performed

with the combination of drug substances contained in the preparation, no indication of a teratogenic potential was noted. However, Schering PC4 should not be given if menstruation at the end of the previous cycle has not occurred due to the possibility of an existing pregnancy.

Pharmaceutical properties
List of excipients: Lactose, Maize starch, Povidone, Talc, Magnesium Stearate [E572], Sucrose, Polyethylene Glycol 6000, Calcium carbonate [E170], Montan glycol wax.

Incompatibilities: None known.

Shelf life: 5 years.

Special precautions for storage: Not applicable.

Nature and contents of container: Schering PC4 is available in an outer carton containing an aluminium foil and PVC blister pack of 4 tablets.

Instructions for use/handling: Keep out of the reach of children.

Marketing authorisation number 0053/0162

Date of first authorisation/renewal of authorisation 18 January 1984/19 August 1997

Date of (partial) revision of the text 17 July 1995

SCHERIPROCT* OINTMENT AND SUPPOSITORIES

Presentation
Scheriproct ointment: A white ointment containing in 1 g:
Prednisolone hexanoate 1.9 mg
Cinchocaine hydrochloride 5.0 mg
Excipients: polyethylene glycol 400 monoricinoleate, castor oil, hydrogenated castor oil, 2 octyldodecanol, chypre perfume oil.

Scheriproct suppositories: Each white suppository contains:
Prednisolone hexanoate 1.3 mg
Cinchocaine hydrochloride 1.0 mg
Excipient: hard fat

Uses For the symptomatic relief of haemorrhoids and pruritus ani in the short term (5-7 days).

Dosage and administration *Suppositories:* 1 Scheriproct suppository to be inserted daily. In severe cases 1 suppository two to three times daily at the beginning of treatment. The suppositories should be inserted after defaecation.

Ointment: Apply in a thin layer twice daily. In order to obtain a rapid improvement, Scheriproct ointment may be applied three to four times on the first day. The nozzle provided facilitates intra-rectal application.

Contra-indications, warnings etc
Contra-indications: Viral infections. Primary bacterial or fungal infections. Secondary infections of the skin in the absence of appropriate anti-infective therapy. Known sensitivity to local anaesthetics.

Warnings/side-effects: In infants, long-term continuous therapy with topical corticosteroids should be avoided. Occlusion is not appropriate on the perineum. Adrenal suppression can occur, even without occlusion. As with all topical steroids, there is a risk of developing skin atrophy following extensive therapy. The application of unusually large quantities of topical corticoids may result in the absorption of systemically active amounts of corticoid. Infections or secondarily infected dermatoses definitely require additional therapy with antibiotics or chemotherapeutic agents. This treatment can often be topical, but for heavy infections systemic antibacterial therapy may be necessary. If fungal infections are present, a topically active antimycotic should be applied. Allergic skin reactions may occur.

Pregnancy warning: There is inadequate evidence of safety in human pregnancy. Topical administration of corticosteroids to pregnant animals can cause abnormalities of foetal development, including cleft palate and intra-uterine growth retardation. There may therefore be a very small risk of such effects on the human foetus.

Pharmaceutical precautions In order to restore the consistency of suppositories which have become soft owing to warm temperature, they should be put into cold water before the covering is removed.
Suppositories: Store in cool dry conditions.
Ointment: No special storage precautions.
Ointment and Suppositories: Shelf-life – Five years.

Legal category POM

Further information Nil

Package quantities *Suppositories:* Packs of 12 (OP).
Ointment: Tubes of 30 g (OP).

Product licence numbers
Scheriproct Suppositories 0053/5001R
Scheriproct Ointment 0053/5002R

SKINOREN*

Presentation Cream 1 g contains 0.2 g (20%) micronized azelaic acid in an oil-in-water emulsion (approximately 51% water).
Excipients: arlatone 983S, cutina CBS, cetearyl octanoate, propylene glycol, benzoic acid, purified water.

Uses Topical treatment of acne vulgaris.

Dosage and administration Skinoren should be applied to the affected areas twice daily (mornings and evenings), and rubbed in well. Regular use is important.

The duration of use of Skinoren will vary from person to person and also depends on the severity of the acne. In general, a distinct improvement becomes apparent after about 4 weeks. To obtain the best results, Skinoren should be applied over a period of several months but not for more than 6 months.

Patients with sensitive skin should be advised to use Skinoren only once a day (in the evening) for the first week of treatment and then proceed to twice daily applications.

The amount of Skinoren to be applied will depend on the size of the affected area. As a guide, a daily dose of 2 g (1 g per application) will be sufficient for the treatment of the entire facial area (1 g = 4 cm cream).

If other areas of acne, in addition to the face, require treatment, for example the chest and back, a daily dose of 10 g of cream should not, in general, be exceeded.

Before Skinoren is applied, the skin should be thoroughly washed with water alone, or, if necessary, with a mild cleansing agent.

Contra-indications, warnings etc
Contra-indications: Hypersensitivity to propylene glycol.

Precautions: For external use only. Avoid contact with eyes. If Skinoren comes into contact with the eyes, they should immediately be thoroughly irrigated with copious amounts of water.

Side-effects: Local skin irritation (e.g. erythema, scaling, itching or burning) occurs in occasional cases, usually at the start of treatment. However, in the majority of cases, the irritation is mild and regresses as treatment continues. If marked skin irritation persists, the amount of cream per application should be reduced, the frequency of application should be reduced, or the treatment temporarily interrupted until the symptoms regress. Photosensitivity reactions have been reported very rarely during the use of Skinoren.

Use during pregnancy and lactation: There is no evidence of the safety of azelaic acid during human pregnancy or lactation. It is therefore advisable to avoid using Skinoren during pregnancy or lactation unless essential and no suitable alternative treatment is available. Animal studies have however produced no evidence that would suggest any risk to a foetus from use by a pregnant woman.

Pharmaceutical precautions Do not store above 30°C. Shelf-life – Five years.

Legal category POM

Package quantities Tubes containing 30 g.

Further information Azelaic acid inhibits the growth of the propionibacteria involved in the development of acne and their production of acne-promoting fatty acids. Azelaic acid also reduces the multiplication of keratinocytes and their keratinization, and therefore restricts the formation of comedones.

Product licence number 0053/0207

TRAVOGYN*

Qualitative and quantitative composition 1 vaginal tablet contains 300 mg isoconazole nitrate

Pharmaceutical form Vaginal tablet

Clinical particulars
Therapeutic indications: Fungal infections of the vagina including mixed infections with gram-positive bacteria.

Posolgy and method of administration: Two vaginal tablets must be inserted together deep into the vagina. This is best done in a lying position. A suitable time for the application would be in the evening just before going to sleep.
Only one application is required.

Contra-indications: None known.

Special warnings and special precautions for use: Travogyn should not be the treatment of first choice for pure trichomonal infections.

To prevent reinfection, underclothes (preferably cotton), towels and wash cloths (flannels) that have been in contact with the affected area should be changed frequently.

During treatment and in the following week vaginal douching should be avoided.

To prevent reinfection simultaneous prophylactic treatment of the sexual partner should be considered.

Interaction with other medicaments and other forms of interaction: None so far known.

Pregnancy and lactation: In order to avoid any possibility of adverse effects on the foetus, the general principle is now widely accepted that the administration of drugs to women during pregnancy should, as far as possible, be avoided. However, nothing that is known about the effect of isoconazole nitrate, either from animal experiments, or from clinical experience, suggests that Travogyn therapy should not be used during pregnancy.

Because of only slight absorption (less than 10% of the dose administered) and the short duration of therapy, adverse effects on the baby from isoconazole nitrate transferred with the breast milk are unlikely.

Effects on ability to drive and use machines: Not applicable

Undesirable effects: Occasionally, during the first 12 to 24 hours, symptoms of intolerance such as burning or itching of the vagina and vulva may occur.

Overdose: According to the results from single dose toxicity studies, the active ingredient isoconazole can be classified as virtually non-toxic. Acute intoxication is unlikely after a single overdose or inadvertent oral intake of a complete pack.

Pharmacological properties
Pharmacodynamic properties: Isoconazole nitrate, the active constituent of Travogyn, has a fungicidal action upon yeasts and yeast-like fungi (particularly those belonging to *Candida spp* and *Torulopsis glabrata*) in the vulvo-vaginal region, on dermatophytes and upon hyphomycetes. In addition to this antimycotic activity, isoconazole nitrate is also effective against some gram- positive bacteria, including staphylococci, streptococci and micrococci, which may cause secondary infection of inflammatory fungal lesions of the skin. The broad spectrum of action of isoconazole nitrate has been demonstrated in serial dilution tests and in suspension tests.

In serial dilution tests, Travogyn is also effective against trichomonas vaginalis at concentrations of 25 microgram/ml and against *Staphylococcus aureus* after two hours at a concentration of 100 microgram/ml, and after three hours at 10 microgram/ml.

Pharmacokinetic properties: Pharmacokinetic investigations conducted with ^{3}H-labelled isoconazole nitrate in healthy test subjects using a single intravaginal administration of the 100 mg tablet or of two 300 mg tablets demonstrated absorption of 5–10%, on the basis of the elimination with the urine and faeces. This indicates a systemic burden of about 0.2 mg/kg after a single 100 mg tablet and of 1.0 mg/kg after two 300 mg tablets.

The rapid elimination of the ^{3}H activity from the body implies that accumulation of the active substance or its metabolites after repeated administration of the tablets is unlikely.

Preclinical safety data: An animal study has shown that there is a risk of conjunctival irritation after inadvertent contamination of the eye.

Pharmaceutical particulars
List of excipients: Lactose, microcrystalline cellulose (E460), magnesium stearate (E572)

Incompatibilities: None known.

Shelf life: 5 years.

Special precautions for storage: None.
Nature and contents of container: PVC and aluminium foil blister unit packs, each containing two Travogyn tablets 300 mg.
Presentation: Pack size of 1×2 tablets.

Instructions for use/handling: Store all drugs properly and keep them out of reach of children.

Marketing authorisation number 0053/0124

Date of approval/revision of SPC 24 February 1997

Legal category POM

TRIADENE*

Presentation The memo pack holds six beige tablets containing 30 micrograms ethinyloestradiol and 50 micrograms gestodene, five dark brown tablets containing 40 micrograms ethinyloestradiol and

70 micrograms gestodene, and ten white tablets containing 30 micrograms ethinyloestradiol and 100 micrograms gestodene.

All tablets have a lustrous, sugar-coating.

Excipients: lactose, maize starch, povidone 700 000, calcium disodium edetate, magnesium stearate, sucrose, polyethylene glycol 6000, calcium carbonate, talc, montan glycol wax, glycerin, titanium dioxide, brown and yellow ferric oxide pigment.

Uses Oral contraception and the recognised gynaecological indications for such oestrogen-progestogen combinations. The mode of action includes the inhibition of ovulation by suppression of the mid-cycle surge of luteinising hormone, the inspissation of cervical mucus so as to constitute a barrier to sperm, and the rendering of the endometrium unreceptive to implantation.

Dosage and administration

First treatment cycle: 1 tablet daily for 21 days, starting on the first day of the menstrual cycle. Contraceptive protection begins immediately.

Subsequent cycles: Tablet taking from the next pack of Triadene is continued after a 7-day interval, beginning on the same day of the week as the first pack.

Changing from 21-day combined oral contraceptives: The first tablet of Triadene should be taken on the first day immediately after the end of the previous oral contraceptive course. Additional contraceptive precautions are not required.

Changing from a combined Every Day pill (28 day tablets): Triadene should be started after taking the last active tablet from the Every Day Pill pack. The first Triadene tablet is taken the next day. Additional contraceptive precautions are not then required.

Changing from a progestogen-only pill (POP): The first tablet of Triadene should be taken on the first day of bleeding, even if a POP has already been taken on that day. Additional contraceptive precautions are not then required. The remaining progestogen-only pills should be discarded.

Post-partum and post-abortum use: After pregnancy, oral contraception can be started 21 days after a vaginal delivery, provided that the patient is fully ambulant and there are no puerperal complications. Additional contraceptive precautions will be required for the first 7 days of tablet taking. Since the first post-partum ovulation may precede the first bleeding, another method of contraception should be used in the interval between childbirth and the first course of tablets. After a first-trimester abortion, oral contraception may be started immediately in which case no additional contraceptive precautions are required.

Pregnancy and lactation: If pregnancy occurs during medication with oral contraceptives, the preparation should be withdrawn immediately (see *Reasons for stopping oral contraception immediately*).

The use of Triadene during lactation may lead to a reduction in the volume of milk produced and to a change in its composition. Minute amounts of the active substances are excreted with the milk. Mothers who are breast-feeding may be advised instead to use a progestogen-only pill.

Special circumstances requiring additional contraception:

Incorrect administration: A single delayed tablet should be taken as soon as possible, and if this can be done within 12 hours of the correct time, contraceptive protection is maintained. With longer delays, additional contraception is needed. Only the most recently delayed tablet should be taken, earlier missed tablets being omitted, and additional non-hormonal methods of contraception (except the rhythm or temperature methods) should be used for the next 7 days, while the next 7 tablets are being taken. Additionally, therefore, if tablet(s) have been missed during the last 7 days of a pack, there should be no break before the next pack is started. In this situation, a withdrawal bleed should not be expected until the end of the second pack. Some breakthrough bleeding may occur on tablet taking days but this is not clinically significant. If the patient does not have a withdrawal bleed during the tablet-free interval following the end of the second pack, the possibility of pregnancy must be ruled out before starting the next pack.

Gastro-intestinal upset: Vomiting or diarrhoea may reduce the efficacy of oral contraceptives by preventing full absorption. Tablet taking from the current pack should be continued. Additional non-hormonal methods of contraception (except the rhythm or temperature methods) should be used during the gastro-intestinal upset and for 7 days following the upset. If these 7 days overrun the end of a pack, the next pack should be started without a break. In this situation, a withdrawal bleed should not be expected until the end of the second pack. If the patient does not have a withdrawal bleed during the tablet-free interval following the end of the second pack, the possibility of pregnancy must be ruled out before starting the next pack. Other methods of contraception should be considered if the gastro-intestinal disorder is likely to be prolonged.

Interaction with other drugs: Hepatic enzyme inducers such as barbiturates, primidone, phenobarbitone, phenytoin, phenylbutazone, rifampicin, carbamazepine and griseofulvin can impair the efficacy of Triadene. For women receiving long-term therapy with hepatic enzyme inducers, another method of contraception should be used. The use of antibiotics may also reduce the efficacy of Triadene, possibly by altering the intestinal flora.

Women receiving short courses of enzyme inducers or broad spectrum antibiotics should take additional, non-hormonal (except rhythm or temperature method) contraceptive precautions during the time of concurrent medication and for 7 days afterwards. If these 7 days overrun the end of a pack, the next pack should be started without a break. In this situation, a withdrawal bleed should not be expected until the end of the second pack. If the patient does not have a withdrawal bleed during the tablet-free interval following the end of the second pack, the possibility of pregnancy must be ruled out before resuming with the next pack. With rifampicin, additional contraceptive precautions should be continued for 4 weeks after treatment stops, even if only a short course was administered.

The requirement for oral antidiabetics or insulin can change as a result of the effect on glucose tolerance.

Contra-indications, warnings, etc

Contra-indications:

1. Pregnancy
2. Severe disturbances of liver function, jaundice or persistent itching during a previous pregnancy, Dubin-Johnson syndrome, Rotor syndrome, previous or existing liver tumours
3. Existing or previous arterial or venous thrombotic or embolic processes, conditions which predispose to them e.g. disorders of the clotting processes, valvular heart disease and atrial fibrillation
4. Sickle-cell anaemia
5. Mammary or endometrial carcinoma, or a history of these conditions
6. Severe diabetes mellitus with vascular changes
7. Disorders of lipid metabolism
8. History of herpes gestationis
9. Deterioration of otosclerosis during pregnancy
10. Undiagnosed abnormal vaginal bleeding
11. Hypersensitivity to any of the components of Triadene.

Warnings: There is a general opinion, based on statistical evidence, that users of combined oral contraceptives experience, more often than non-users, venous thromboembolism, arterial thrombosis, including cerebral and myocardial infarction, and subarachnoid haemorrhage. Full recovery from such disorders does not always occur, and it should be realised that in a few cases they are fatal. How often these disorders occur in users of the modern low-dose pills is not known, but there are reasons for suggesting that they may occur less often than with older pills.

Certain factors may entail some risk of thrombosis, e.g. smoking, obesity, varicose veins, cardiovascular diseases, diabetes, and migraine. The suitability of a combined oral contraceptive should be judged according to the severity of such conditions in the individual case, and should be discussed with the patient before she decides to take it. The risk of arterial thrombosis associated with combined oral contraceptives increases with age, and this risk is aggravated by cigarette-smoking. The use of combined oral contraceptives by women in the older age-group, especially those who are cigarette smokers, should therefore be discouraged and alternative methods used.

In addition if there is a history in the family of thromboembolic diseases at a young age (e.g. deep vein thrombosis, heart attack or stroke) disturbances of the coagulation system must be ruled out before the pill is prescribed.

Numerous epidemiological studies have been reported on the risks of ovarian, endometrial, cervical and breast cancer in women using combined oral contraceptives. The evidence is clear that combined oral contraceptives offer substantial protection against both ovarian and endometrial cancer.

An increased risk of cervical cancer in long-term users of combined oral contraceptives has been reported in some studies, but there continues to be controversy about the extent to which this is attributable to the confounding effects of sexual behaviour and other factors.

A meta-analysis from 54 epidemiological studies reported that there is a slightly increased relative risk (RR=1.24) of having breast cancer diagnosed in women who are currently using combined oral contraceptives (COCs). The observed pattern of increased risk may be due to an earlier diagnosis of breast cancer in COC users, the biological effects of COCs or a combination of both. The additional breast cancers diagnosed in current users of COCs or in women who have used COCs in the last ten years are more likely to be localised to the breast than those in women who never used COCs.

Breast cancer is rare among women under 40 years of age whether or not they take COCs. Whilst this background risk increases with age, the excess number of breast cancer diagnoses in current and recent COC users is small in relation to the overall risk of breast cancer (see bar chart).

The most important risk factor for breast cancer in COC users is the age women discontinue the COC; the older the age at stopping, the more breast cancers are diagnosed. Duration of use is less important and the excess risk gradually disappears during the course of the 10 years after stopping COC use such that by 10 years there appears to be no excess.

The possible increase in risk of breast cancer should be discussed with the user and weighed against the benefits of COCs taking into account the evidence that they offer substantial protection against the risk of developing certain other cancers (e.g. ovarian and endometrial cancer).

The possibility cannot be ruled out that certain chronic diseases may occasionally deteriorate during the use of combined oral contraceptives (see *Precautions*).

The combination of ethinyloestradiol and gestodene, like other contraceptive steroids, is associated with an increased incidence of neoplastic nodules in the rat liver, the relevance of which to man is unknown. Malignant liver tumours have been reported on rare occasions in long-term users of oral contraceptives.

In rare cases benign and, in even rarer cases, malignant liver tumours leading in isolated cases to life-threatening intra-abdominal haemorrhage have been observed after the use of hormonal substances such as those contained in Triadene. If severe upper abdominal complaints, liver enlargement or signs of intra-abdominal haemorrhage occur, the possibility of a liver tumour should be included in the differential diagnosis.

Reasons for stopping oral contraception immediately:

1. Occurrence for the first time, or exacerbation, of migrainous headaches or unusually frequent or unusually severe headaches
2. Sudden disturbances of vision or hearing or other perceptual disorders
3. First signs of thrombophlebitis or thromboembolic symptoms (e.g. unusual pains in or swelling of the leg(s), stabbing pains on breathing or coughing for no apparent reason). Feeling of pain and tightness in the chest
4. Six weeks before an elective major operation (e.g. abdominal, orthopaedic), any surgery to the legs, medical treatment for varicose veins or prolonged immobilisation, e.g. after accidents or surgery. Do not restart until 2 weeks after full ambulation. In case of emergency surgery, thrombotic prophylaxis is usually indicated e.g. subcutaneous heparin
5. Onset of jaundice, hepatitis, itching of the whole body
6. Increase in epileptic seizures
7. Significant rise in blood pressure
8. Onset of severe depression
9. Severe upper abdominal pain or liver enlargement
10. Clear exacerbation of conditions known to be capable of deteriorating during oral ontraception or pregnancy
11. Pregnancy is a reason for stopping immediately because it has been suggested by some investigations that oral contraceptives taken in early pregnancy may slightly increase the risk of foetal malformations. Other investigations have failed to support these findings. The possibility therefore cannot be excluded, but it is certain that if a risk exists at all, it is very small.

Precautions: Examination of the pelvic organs, breasts and blood-pressure should precede the prescribing of any combined oral contraceptive and should be repeated regularly. The family medical history should be carefully noted and disturbances of the clotting mechanism ruled out if any member of the family has suffered from thromboembolic disease (e.g. deep vein thrombosis, stroke, myocardial infarction) at a young age. Before starting treatment pregnancy must be excluded.

The following conditions require strict medical supervision during medication with oral contraceptives. Deterioration or first appearance of any of these conditions may indicate that use of the oral contraceptive should be discontinued:

Diabetes mellitus, or a tendency towards diabetes mellitus (e.g. unexplained glycosuria), hypertension, varicose veins, a history of phlebitis, otosclerosis, multiple sclerosis, epilepsy, porphyria, tetany, disturbed liver function, Sydenham's chorea, renal dysfunction, family history of clotting disorders, obesity,

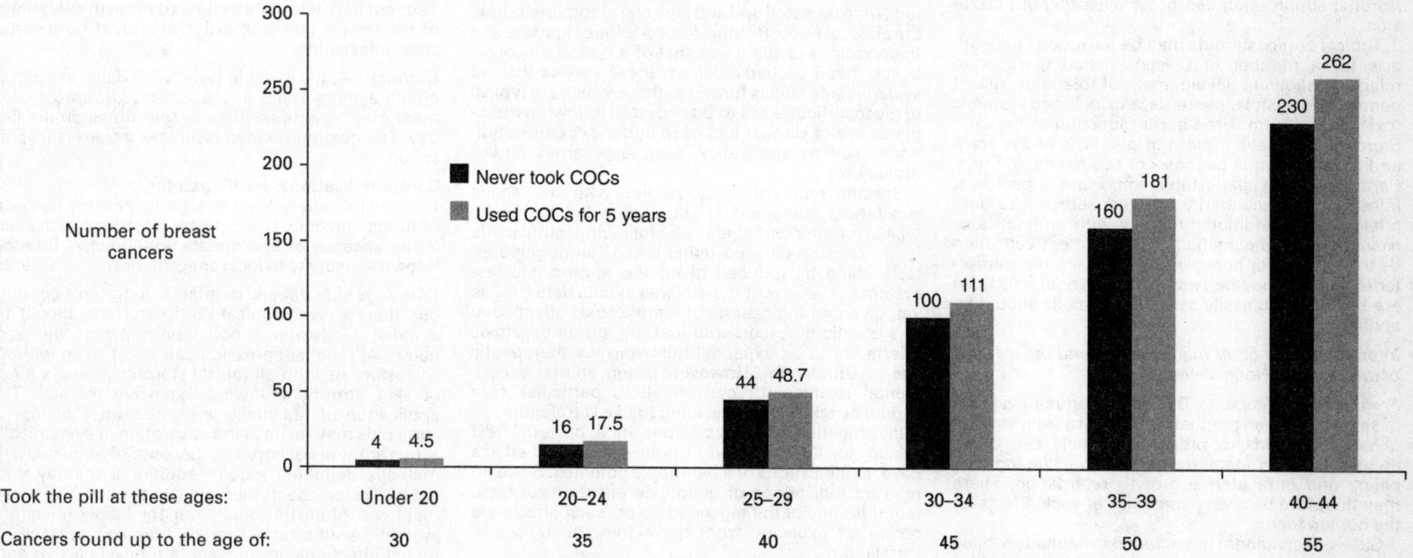

family history of breast cancer and patient history of benign breast disease, history of clinical depression, systemic lupus erythematosus, uterine fibroids and migraine, gall-stones, cardiovascular diseases, chloasma, asthma, an intolerance of contact lenses, or any disease that is prone to worsen during pregnancy.

Some women may experience amenorrhoea or oligomenorrhoea after discontinuation of oral contraceptives, especially when these conditions existed prior to use. Women should be informed of this possibility.

Side-effects: In rare cases, headaches, gastric upsets, nausea, vomiting, breast tenderness, changes in body weight, changes in libido, depressive moods can occur.

In predisposed women, use of Triadene can sometimes cause chloasma which is exacerbated by exposure to sunlight. Such women should avoid prolonged exposure to sunlight.

Individual cases of poor tolerance of contact lenses have been reported with use of oral contraceptives. Contact lens wearers who develop changes in lens tolerance should be assessed by an ophthalmologist.

Menstrual changes:

1. Reduction of menstrual flow: This is not abnormal and it is to be expected in some patients. Indeed, it may be beneficial where heavy periods were previously experienced.

2. Missed menstruation: Occasionally, withdrawal bleeding may not occur at all. If the tablets have been taken correctly, pregnancy is very unlikely. If withdrawal bleeding fails to occur at the end of a second pack, the possibility of pregnancy must be ruled out before resuming with the next pack.

Intermenstrual bleeding: 'Spotting' or heavier 'breakthrough bleeding' sometimes occur during tablet taking, especially in the first few cycles, and normally cease spontaneously. Triadene should therefore, be continued even if irregular bleeding occurs. If irregular bleeding is persistent, appropriate diagnostic measures to exclude an organic cause are indicated and may include curettage. This also applies in the case of spotting which occurs at irregular intervals in several consecutive cycles or which occurs for the first time after long use of Triadene.

Effect on blood chemistry: The use of oral contraceptives may influence the results of certain laboratory tests including biochemical parameters of liver, thyroid, adrenal and renal function, plasma levels of carrier proteins and lipid/lipoprotein fractions, parameters of carbohydrate metabolism and parameters of coagulation and fibrinolysis. Laboratory staff should therefore be informed about oral contraceptive use when laboratory tests are requested.

Overdosage: Overdosage may cause nausea, vomiting and, in females, withdrawal bleeding. There are no specific antidotes and treatment should be symptomatic.

Pharmaceutical precautions Shelf-life – Five years.

Legal category POM

Package quantities Individual packs containing three months' supply (OP)

Further information Nil

Produce licence number 0053/0205

ULTRABASE*

Qualitative and quantitative composition There are no active constituents.

Pharmaceutical form Cream.

Clinical particulars

Therapeutic indications: For general use as:

- an emollient
- a diluent for dermatological preparations and
- a vehicle for various dermatological medicaments.

Additionally, it may be alternated with topical corticosteroids when the latter are being gradually withdrawn, and may be continued alone after complete withdrawal of the topical corticosteroid.

Posology and method of administration: For topical administration as required.

Contra-indications: Hypersensitivity to any of the components of Ultrabase.

Special warnings and special precautions for use: None stated.

Interaction with other medicaments and other forms of interaction: None known.

Pregnancy and lactation: None stated.

Effects on ability to drive and use machines: None known.

Undesirable effects: None known.

Overdose: Not applicable. Ultrabase contains no active ingredients.

Pharmacological properties

Pharmacodynamic properties: Ultrabase has no specific active ingredient, but the cream formulation has good emollient properties.

Pharmacokinetic properties: None stated.

Preclinical safety data: There are no preclinical safety data which could be of relevance to the prescriber and which are not already included in other relevant sections of the SPC.

Pharmaceutical particulars

List of excipients: Polyoxyl 40 stearate [E431], white soft paraffin, liquid paraffin, stearyl alcohol, Carbomer 934, sodium hydroxide, methyl parahydroxybenzoate (methyl paraben) [E218], propyl parahydroxybenzoate (propyl paraben) [E216], disodium edetate [E463], purified water, citrus-rose perfume oil

Incompatibilities: None known.

Shelf life: 5 years.

Special precautions for storage: Not applicable.

Nature and contents of container: This product is available in collapsible aluminium tubes (10 g or 50 g). Also available in polypropylene pump dispensers (500 g).

Instructions for use/handling: Keep out of the reach of children.

Marketing authorisation number 0053/0063

Date of approval/revision of SPC 2 June 1997

Legal category POM

ULTRALANUM* OINTMENT PLAIN AND CREAM PLAIN

Qualitative and quantitative composition

Ointment: Each 100 gm of ointment contains 0.25 gm (0.25%) of fluocortolone monohydrate and 0.25 gm (0.25%) of fluocortolone hexanoate.

Cream: Each 100 gm of cream contains 0.25 gm (0.25%) of fluocortolone pivalate and 0.25 gm (0.25%) of fluocortolone hexanoate.

Pharmaceutical form Ointment and cream

Clinical particulars

Therapeutic indications: Eczema and dermatitis of all types including atopic eczema, photodermatitis and primary irritant and allergic dermatitis, prurigo nodularis and insect bite reactions. Lichen planus, lichen simplex, discoid lupus erythematosus, necrobiosis lipoidica, pretibial myxoedema, erythroderma, psoriasis of the scalp, chronic plaque psoriasis of hands and feet.

Posology and method of administration: Ultralanum is for topical application in children, adults and the elderly as follows:

Initially 2–3 applications daily, according to severity of condition. For maintenance, one application daily.

Skin conditions which are neither weeping nor very dry require a base with balanced proportions of fat and water. Ultralanum Ointment makes the skin slightly greasy without retaining heat or fluid.

Ultralanum Cream has a high water and low fat content. In weeping skin diseases it allows secretions to drain away, thus providing for rapid subsidence and drying up of the skin. Ultralanum Cream is also suitable for application to moist, exposed and hairy areas of the body. If the skin dries out too much under protracted use of Ultralanum Cream, the patient should be switched to Ultralanum Ointment.

Occlusive dressings: An occlusive dressing may be called for in unusually refractory cases in adults and usually under specialist supervision.

If an infection develops under the dressing, occlusive treatment must be terminated.

Contra–indications:

- Rosacea and peri-oral dermatitis.
- Acne vulgaris, undiagnosed perianal and genital pruritus, napkin eruptions, viral infections, primary bacterial or fungal infections of the skin.
- Secondary infections in the absence of appropriate anti–infective therapy.

Not suitable for the treatment of ophthalmic conditions.

Special warnings and special precautions for use: As with all topical steroids, there is a risk of skin atrophy following extensive therapy.

The application of topical steroids may result in the absorption of systemically active amounts of corticoid. If used in childhood or on the face, courses should be limited to 5 days and occlusion should not be used. Long-term continuous therapy should be avoided irrespective of age. Occlusion should be restricted to dermatoses involving limited areas. Adrenal suppression can occur even without occlusion.

Topical corticosteroids may be hazardous in psoriasis for a number of reasons including rebound relapses following development of tolerance, risk of generalised pustular psoriasis, and local and systemic toxicity due to impaired barrier function of the skin. Steroids may have a place in psoriasis of the scalp and chronic plaque psoriasis of the hands and feet. Careful patient supervision is important in psoriasis. Infections or secondarily infected dermatoses definitely require additional therapy with antibiotics or chemotherapeutic agents. This treatment can often be topical, but for heavy infections systemic antibacterial therapy may be necessary. If fungal infections are present, a topically active antimycotic should be applied.

Interaction with other medicaments and other forms of interactions: None stated.

Pregnancy and lactation: There is inadequate evidence of safety in human pregnancy. Topical administration of corticosteroids to pregnant animals can cause abnormalities of foetal development, including cleft palate and intra-uterine growth retardation. There may therefore be a very small risk of such effects on the human foetus.

Side-effects cannot be excluded in neonates whose mothers have been treated extensively or for a prolonged period of time during pregnancy or while lactating (for example, reduced adrenocortical function, when applied during the last weeks of pregnancy).

Effects on ability to drive and use machines: None stated.

Undesirable effects: As with all topical steroids, if Ultralanum is applied to large areas of the body and for long periods of time (more than 4 weeks) there is a risk of local effects, such as telangiectasia, striae, acneform changes, hypertrichosis, perioral dermatitis or skin atrophy. The application of unusually large quantities of topical corticoids may result in the absorption of systemically active amounts of corticoid. Allergic skin reactions may occasionally occur.

Overdose: None stated.

Pharmacological properties
Pharmacodynamic properties: Ultralanum suppresses inflammation in inflammatory and allergic skin conditions and alleviates subjective complaints such as itching, burning and pain. Owing to the different speeds with which the two forms of its corticoid component take effect, Ultralanum is both fast-acting and long-lasting in its effectiveness.

Capillary dilatation, intracellular oedema and tissue infiltration regress and capillary proliferation is suppressed. This leads to fading of inflamed skin surfaces.

Pharmacokinetic properties: A combination of two corticosteroids (steroid alcohol with ester or two different esters of the same steroid) in a dermatological preparation is pharmacokinetically advantageous since a higher skin concentration of corticosteroids can be achieved and maintained over a longer period of time after application of a combination as compared with a single compound. Due to a different lipophilicity the two compounds distribute in a different way into the horny layer and diffuse at different rates through the skin, leading to a rapid onset of action and a longer duration of activity.

Investigations on the time course of the vasoconstriction in volunteers as well as investigations on the percutaneous absorption indicate that fluocortolone and fluocortolone pivalate penetrate more rapidly into and through human skin than fluocortolone hexanoate, giving evidence that the above mentioned principles hold true with the Ultralanum dermatological preparations.

Measurements of drug recovery on the skin surface at the end of the exposure time in healthy skin volunteers as well as in eczema and psoriasis patients overestimate the extent of the percutaneous absorption and are therefore only of limited value for an assessment of the systemic drug load and for risk assessment. Pharmacodynamic investigations of the effect on the pituitary adrenal axis show only a small risk of systemic effects if large areas of the body are not treated over a long time.

Fluocortolone-21-monoesters are hydrolysed, like other 21-esters of corticosteroids most probably already in the skin, usually immediately after percutaneous absorption, into fluocortolone and the corresponding fatty acid. Fluocortolone itself possesses the shortest plasma half-life of all synthetic corticosteroids (approx. 75-90 minutes determined after i.v. administration) comparable to that of endogenous cortisol. Fluocortolone is inactivated in humans via a series of reduction, oxidation and conjugation reactions with glucuronic and sulphonic acid and is excreted as metabolites mainly in the urine.

Preclinical safety data: In systemic tolerance studies following repeated oral and parenteral administration, the effect of fluocortolone, fluocortolone caproate and fluocortolone pivalate was that of a typical glucocorticoid. It can be derived from these results that no systemic side effects further to those which are typical of glucocorticoids are to be expected following therapeutic use of Ultralanum, even under extreme conditions such as application over large areas and/or occlusion.

Specific embryotoxicity studies with the active substances contained in Ultralanum led to results typical of gluococorticoids, i.e. following sufficiently high exposure embryo-lethal and/or teratogenic effects could be induced given the appropriate test systems. A review of the adverse events data has, as yet, given no indications of embryotoxic effects due to systemic glucocorticoid therapy, no embryotoxic effects are to be expected following the therapeutic use of Ultralanum. However, taking animal-experimental results into consideration, particular care should be taken when deciding to use Ultralanum.

Investigation of fluocortolone in a bacterial test system for the detection of point-mutagenic effects gave no indications of a genotoxic potential. Since no relevant indications of genotoxic effects have been found for any of the glucocorticoids, such effects are not to be expected from the active substances in Ultralanum.

Specific tumorigenicity studies have not been carried out with the active substances contained in Ultralanum. On the basis of knowledge concerning the structures, the pharmacological action pattern and the results of systemic tolerance studies with chronic administration, there is no suspicion of tumorigenic potential. Since systemically effective immunosuppressive dosages will not be reached after dermal application of Ultralanum if used as directed, no influence on the occurrence of tumours is to be expected.

Following repeated dermal administration of fluocortolone and the two esters in different combinations and preparations, no substance-related dermal changes were observed.

Pharmaceutical particulars
List of excipients: Each 100 g of ointment contains:

Bleached wax, lanolin, heavy liquid paraffin, white soft paraffin, Amphocerin K.S., purified water, citrus rose perfume oil (PH No: 65803) and Dehymuls E.

Each 100 g of cream contains: Polyoxyl-40-stearate, stearyl alcohol, heavy liquid paraffin, white soft paraffin, disodium edetate dihydrate, Carbopol 934, sodium hydroxide, methyl parahydroxybenzoate, propyl parahydroxybenzoate, purified water and citrus rose perfume oil (PH No. 65803).

Incompatibilities: None so far known.

Shelf-life:
Ointment: 18 months.
Cream: 5 years.

Special precautions for storage:
Ointment: Store below 25°C.
Cream: Not applicable.

Nature and contents of container: Collapsible ointment tubes of pure aluminium lacquered internally. Available in packs of 30 g and 50 g.

Instructions for use/handling: Keep out of reach of children.

Marketing authorisation numbers
Ointment: 0053/5005R
Cream: 0053/5011R

Date of approval/revision of SPC 13 February 1996

Legal category POM

ULTRAPROCT* OINTMENT ULTRAPROCT* SUPPOSITORIES

Presentation
Ultraproct Ointment: A white ointment containing in 1 g:
Fluocortolone pivalate 0.92 mg
Fluocortolone hexanoate 0.95 mg
Cinchocaine hydrochloride 5.00 mg

Excipients: polyethylene glycol 400 monoricinoleate, castor oil, hydrogenated castor oil, 2 octyldodecanol, citrus rose perfume oil.

Ultraproct Suppositories: Each white suppository contains:
Fluocortolone pivalate BP 0.61 mg
Fluocortolone hexanoate BP 0.63 mg
Cinchocaine hydrochloride 1.00 mg

Excipient: solid fat

Uses For the symptomatic relief of haemorrhoids and of pruritus ani in the short term (5-7 days).

Dosage and administration *Suppositories:* 1 Ultraproct Suppository to be inserted daily. In severe cases 1 suppository two to three times daily at the beginning of treatment. The suppositories should be inserted after defaecation.

Ointment: Apply in a thin layer twice daily. In order to obtain a more rapid improvement, Ultraproct Ointment may be applied three or four times on the first day. The nozzle provided facilitates intra-rectal application.

Contra-indications, warnings, etc
Contra-indications: Viral infections. Primary bacterial or fungal infections. Secondary infections of the skin in the absence of appropriate anti-infective therapy. Known sensitivity to local anaesthetics.

Warnings/side-effects: In infants, long-term continuous therapy with topical corticosteroids should be avoided. Occlusion is not appropriate on the perineum. Adrenal suppression can occur even without occlusion. As with all topical steroids, there is a risk of skin atrophy following extensive therapy. The application of unusually large quantities of topical corticoids may result in the absorption of systemically active amounts of corticoid. Secondarily-infected dermatoses definitely require additional therapy with antibiotics or chemotherapeutics agents. This treatment can often be topical but for heavy infections systemic antibacterial therapy may be necessary. If fungal infections are present, a topically active antimycotic should be applied. Allergic skin reactions may occur.

Pregnancy warning: There is inadequate evidence of safety in human pregnancy. Topical administration of corticosteroids to pregnant animals can cause abnormalities of foetal development, including cleft palate and intra-uterine growth retardation. There may therefore be a very small risk of such effects on the human foetus.

Pharmaceutical precautions In order to restore the consistency of suppositories which have become soft owing to warm temperature, they should be put into cold water before the covering is removed.

Shelf-life: Ointment – Three years (do not store above 25°C). Suppositories – Two years (do not store above 25°C).

Legal category POM

Package quantities *Suppositories:* Packs of 12 (OP). *Ointment:* Tubes of 30 g (OP).

Further information Nil

Product licence numbers
Ultraproct Ointment 0053/5008R
Ultraproct Suppositories 0053/5009R

ULTRAVIST*

Presentation Bottles containing colourless, sterile solutions of various strengths of iopromide. Ultravist 150 contains 150 mg iodine per ml, Ultravist 240 contains 240 mg iodine per ml, Ultravist 300 contains 300 mg iodine per ml, Ultravist 370 contains 370 mg iodine per ml.

Excipients: Sodium calcium edetate, trometamol, hydrochloric acid, water for injection.

Uses Non-ionic X-ray contrast media for computed tomography, digital subtraction angiography, intravenous urography, venography, arteriography, visualization of body cavities (e.g. arthrography, hysterosalpingography and fistulography), checking the function of dialysis shunts. Ultravist should not be used for myelography (see *Further information*).

Dosage and administration
Intravenous urography
Adults: The minimum dose is 0.8 ml/kg body weight Ultravist 370, (1 ml/kg Ultravist 300 or 1.3 ml/kg Ultravist 240). These doses should provide adequate filling of the ureters. It may be necessary to increase the dose in individual cases e.g. obesity or impaired renal function.

Children: The poor concentrating ability of the immature nephron of infantile kidneys necessitates the use of relatively high doses of contrast medium, i.e. for Ultravist 300:

Neonates:	4.0 ml/kg body weight
Babies:	3.0 ml/kg body weight
Small children:	1.5 ml/kg body weight

Computed tomography
Cranial CT: The following dosages are recommended for cranial CT:

Ultravist 240:	1.5-2.5 ml/kg body weight
Ultravist 300:	1-2 ml/kg body weight
Ultravist 370:	1-1.5 ml/kg body weight

Whole-body CT: For whole-body computed tomography, the doses of the contrast medium and the rates of administration depend on the organs under investigation, the diagnostic problem and, in particular, the different scan and image-reconstruction times of the scanners in use. Infusion is preferable for slow scanners and injection for fast scanners.

Angiography: The dosage depends on the age, weight, cardiac output and general condition of the patient, the clinical problem, examination technique and the nature and volume of the vascular region to be investigated.

The following dosages may serve as a guide:

Cerebral angiography:
Aortic arch angiography 50-80 ml Ultravist 300/inj.
Selective angiography 6-15 ml Ultravist 300/inj.
Retrograde carotid angiography 30-40 ml Ultravist 300/inj.

Thoracic aortography: 50-80 ml Ultravist 300/inj.

Abdominal aortography: 40-60 ml Ultravist 300/inj.

Bifemoral arteriography: 40-60 ml Ultravist 300/inj.

Peripheral angiography:
Upper extremities:
Arteriography 8-12 ml Ultravist 300/inj.
Venography 50-60 ml Ultravist 240/inj.
15-30 ml Ultravist 300/inj.

Lower extremities:
Arteriography 20-30 ml Ultravist 300/inj.
Venography 50-80 ml Ultravist 240/inj.
30-60 ml Ultravist 300/inj.

Angiocardiography:
Cardiac-ventriculography 40-60 ml Ultravist 370/inj.
Coronary angiography: 5-8 ml Ultravist 370/inj.

Digital subtraction angiography (DSA): I.V. injection of 30–60 ml Ultravist 300 or 370 as a bolus (flow-rate: 8–12 ml/second into the cubital vein; 10–20 ml/second into the vena cava) is recommended for high-contrast demonstrations of the great vessels, of the pulmonary arteries and of the arteries of the neck, head, kidneys and extremities.

Intra-arterial digital subtraction angiography requires smaller volumes and lower iodine concentrations than the intravenous technique.

The more selective the angiography, the lower the dose of contrast medium can be. This method is therefore recommended for patients with impaired renal function. For high-contrast demonstration of the arteries of the head, neck and limbs, several injections of 10–40 ml Ultravist 150, depending on the size of the vessels, are usually given directly or via a catheter. Larger volumes of contrast medium (about 200 ml) may be necessary in some cases to demonstrate the vessels of the lower limbs, particularly if both legs are to be examined.

Dialysis shunt: Ultravist 150 is also suitable for checking the function of a dialysis shunt. About 10 ml of contrast medium is required for this.

Contra-indications, warnings, etc
Contra-indications: Uncontrolled thyrotoxicosis. Hysterosalpingography must not be carried out during pregnancy or in patients with acute inflammatory conditions in the pelvic cavity.

Use in pregnancy: X-ray examinations should, if possible, be avoided during pregnancy. It has not yet been proved beyond question that Ultravist may be used without hesitation in pregnant patients. Therefore, an examination with Ultravist during pregnancy should be carried out only if considered absolutely necessary by the physician. It is not known whether Ultravist enters the breast milk.

Warnings/side-effects: Use with caution in patients with proven or suspected hypersensitivity to iodine containing contrast media. For patients with severe impairment of hepatic or renal function, cardiac or circulatory insufficiency, cerebral arteriosclerosis, epileptic conditions, diabetes mellitus requiring drug treatment and/or associated with diabetic complications, pulmonary emphysema, poor general health, latent hyperthyroidism, multiple myeloma or benign nodular goitre, the need for examination with X-ray contrast media merits careful consideration.

This also applies to patients with a history of allergy, e.g. bronchial asthma, since experience shows that they may exhibit hypersensitivity to drugs. Because of possible precipitation, X-ray contrast media and prophylactic agents against hypersensitivity must not be injected as mixed solutions.

Particular caution should be exercised in allergic patients who have previously tolerated an injectable iodine-containing contrast medium without any complications, because they may become sensitised to these substances in the meantime.

Nonionic contrast media have less anticoagulant activity in vitro than ionic media. Meticulous attention should therefore be paid to angiographic technique. Nonionic media should not be allowed to remain in contact with blood in a syringe, and intravascular catheters should be flushed frequently with physiological saline solution (if necessary with heparin added), to minimise the risk of clotting, which rarely has led to serious thromboembolic complications of the procedures.

The patient should be recumbent during the administration of Ultravist. Thereafter, the patient must be kept under close observation for at least 30 minutes, since about 90% of all severe incidents occur within that time. If the administration does not take place on the X-ray table, any patient with a labile circulation should be brought to the X-ray machine sitting or lying down.

In the case of abdominal angiography, the diagnostic yield is increased if the bowels are emptied of faecal matter and gas. On the two days prior to the examination patients should avoid flatulent food, in particular peas, beans and lentils, salads, fruit, wholemeal and fresh bread and all kinds of uncooked vegetables. On the day before the examination, patients should refrain from eating after 6 p.m. Moreover, it can be appropriate to administer a laxative in the evening.

In babies and young children, however, prolonged fasting and the administration of a laxative before the examination are contraindicated.

Experience shows that pronounced states of excitement, anxiety and pain can be the cause of side-effects or intensify the contrast medium-related reactions. They can be counteracted by calm management of the patient and the use of suitable drugs.

Experience shows that contrast medium is tolerated better if it is warmed to body temperature.

In patients with multiple myeloma, diabetes mellitus requiring drug treatment, polyuria, oliguria or gout and in babies, small children and patients in a very poor state of health, the fluid supply should not be restricted. Existing disturbances of the balance of water and electrolytes must be corrected before the administration of Ultravist.

Premedication with an alpha-blocker is recommended in patients with phaeochromocytoma, because of the risk of blood pressure crises.

Diabetic nephropathy may predispose to renal impairment following intravascular administration of contrast media. This may precipitate lactic acidosis in patients who are taking biguanides. As a precaution biguanides should be stopped 48 hours prior to the examination and reinstated only after control of renal function has been regained.

Hypersensitivity reactions can be aggravated in patients on beta-blockers.

The prevalence of delayed reactions (e.g. fever, rash, flu-like symptoms, joint pain and pruritus) to contrast media is higher in patients who have received interleukin.

If iodine isotopes are to be administered for the diagnosis of thyroid disease, it should be borne in mind that after the administration of iodinated contrast media which are excreted via the kidneys, the capacity of the thyroid tissue to take up iodine will be reduced for two weeks, and sometimes up to six weeks.

Side-effects in association with the intravascular use of iodinated contrast media are usually mild to moderate and temporary, and are less frequent with non-ionic than with ionic preparations. However, severe and life-threatening reactions, even fatal ones, have also been observed.

Nausea, vomiting, erythema, a sensation of pain and a general feeling of warmth are the most frequently recorded reactions on intravascular administration. Subjective complaints such as sensations of warmth or nausea can usually be alleviated quickly by reducing the rate of administration or interrupting the administration briefly.

As with any contrast medium the possibility of hypersensitivity must always be considered.

If marked side-effects or suspected allergic reactions occur during injection and do not disappear, or even get worse, when the injection is briefly interrupted, it is probable that the patient is hypersensitive and the investigation must be abandoned. Even relatively minor symptoms such as itching of the skin, sneezing, violent yawns, tickling in the throat, hoarseness or attacks of coughing may be early signs of a severe reaction and, therefore, merit careful attention. Delayed reactions can occasionally occur. Temporary renal failure may occur in rare cases.

Other symptoms which may occur are: chills, fever, sweating, headache, dizziness, blanching, weakness, gagging and a feeling of suffocation, gasping, a rise or fall of blood pressure, itching, urticaria, other kinds of skin eruption, oedema, cramp, tremor, sneezing and lacrimation. These reactions, which can occur irrespective of the amount administered may be the first signs of an incipient state of shock. Administration of the contrast medium must be discontinued immediately and – if necessary – specific therapy instituted intravenously. It is therefore advisable to use a flexible indwelling cannula for intravenous contrast medium administration. To permit immediate countermeasures to be taken in emergencies, appropriate drugs, an endotracheal tube and a ventilator should be ready to hand. Experience shows that hypersensitivity reactions occur more frequently in patients with an allergic disposition. Some radiologists give an antihistamine or corticosteroid prophylactically to patients with a history of allergy.

Very rarely, severe or even life-threatening side-effects such as severe hypotension and collapse, circulatory failure, ventricular fibrillation, cardiac arrest, pulmonary oedema, anaphylactic shock or other allergic manifestations, convulsions, or other cerebral symptoms may occur. In some cases these have proved fatal.

Ready availability of all drugs and equipment for emergency treatment and familiarity with the respective procedures are prerequisites for the effective management of contrast-medium incidents. Some guidance in the treatment of such incidents is contained in the leaflet supplied with the pack.

Paravascular administration of the contrast medium rarely leads to severe tissue reactions.

Neurological complications such as coma, temporary states of confusion and somnolence, transient paresis, disturbed vision or facial muscle paresis and epileptic fits may occur after cerebral angiography and other procedures in which the contrast medium reaches the brain with the arterial blood. In very rare cases the induction of fits has been observed after intravenous administration of contrast media in epileptics and patients with focal brain damage.

Delayed reactions following intravascular administration of iodinated contrast media are rare. Nevertheless, driving or operating machinery is not advisable for the first 24 hours.

Overdosage: Acute symptoms of poisoning are unlikely with intravascular administration. In special cases, e.g. if renal function is impaired, the contrast medium may be removed by dialysis, and, in cases of intravascular administration of 300 ml or more, the balance of water and electrolytes should be corrected.

Pharmaceutical precautions *Shelf-life:* Ultravist 150: 2 years; Ultravist 240, Ultravist 300 and Ultravist 370: 3 years.

Protect from light and X-rays. Store below 30°C. Because of possible precipitation, X-ray contrast media and prophylactic agents must not be injected as mixed solutions.

Legal category POM

Package quantities
Ultravist 150: Bottles of 50 ml
Ultravist 240: Bottles of 50 ml
Ultravist 300: Bottles of 20 ml, 50 ml, 75 ml, 100 ml and 200 ml
Ultravist 370: Bottles of 30 ml, 50 ml, 75 ml, 100 ml and 200 ml

Further information The Ultravist range consists of non-ionic contrast media with osmotic pressures that are relatively low for contrast media.

Ultravist 150: 0.34 osm/kg H_20 at 37°C
Ultravist 240: 0.48 osm/kg H_20 at 37°C
Ultravist 300: 0.62 osm/kg H_20 at 37°C
Ultravist 370: 0.78 osm/kg H_20 at 37°C

Although it showed excellent neural tolerance in animal studies, the intrathecal administration of iopromide has not been investigated in clinical studies. Ultravist should not therefore be used for myelographic examinations.

Product licence numbers

Ultravist 150	0053/0209
Ultravist 240	0053/0173
Ultravist 300	0053/0174
Ultravist 370	0053/0175

UROGRAFIN*

Presentation Ampoules, vials or bottles containing colourless sterile solutions of varying strengths of meglumine/sodium diatrizoate.

Urografin 150: An intravenous injection or infusion of meglumine diatrizoate 26.1% w/v and sodium diatrizoate 3.9% w/v, containing 146 mg iodine per ml.

Urografin 325: An intravenous injection of meglumine diatrizoate 18% w/v and sodium diatrizoate 40% w/v, containing 325 mg iodine per ml.

Urografin 370: An intravascular injection of meglumine diatrizoate 66% w/v and sodium diatrizoate 10% w/v, containing 370 mg iodine per ml.

Excipients: calcium disodium edetate, water for injection.

Uses X-ray contrast media for the delineation of the vascular and renal systems.

Dosage and administration Experience shows that contrast medium is tolerated better if it is warmed to body temperature.

1. Adults only: Table 1 overleaf shows the medium/media Schering suggest for each investigation. Schering media may be used at the discretion of the radiologist for other established permutations of medium and examination which, for the sake of simplicity, have been omitted from the table.

(Other indications include selective visceral angiography, limb venography, jugular venography, vesiculography, sialography, sinusography, amniography, lypmhangiography, intramuscular urography, operative cholangiography, percutaneous cholangiography, fistulography, oesophageal and anal atresia).

Urografin media are not suitable for myelography.

2. Children and neonates

Intravenous urography: The fact that urograms of infants and young children generally show a lower contrast density than those of adults is explained by the physiologically less effective function of the immature nephron. Relatively high doses of media are therefore indicated. (See Table 2).

Table 2

	Urografin 325/370
Up to 1 year	7–10 ml
1–2 years	10–12 ml
2–6 years	12–15 ml
6–12 years	15–20 ml
over 12 years	adult dose

Drip-infusion urography: Dosage of Urografin 150 should not exceed 4 ml/kg body weight.

Angiocardiography: In neonates up to 5 kg body weight, 8 ml of Urografin 370. Infants over 5 kg body weight, 1 ml/kg body weight up to 25 ml per injection.

Right and left heart catheterisation: 1–1.2 ml/kg body weight of Urografin 370, with a maximum of 15 ml per injection for the right heart and 25 ml per injection for the left heart.

Pulmonary angiography: 0.5–0.6 ml/kg body weight up to 8 ml Urografin 370 per injection.

Contra-indications, warnings, etc

Contra-indications: Proven or suspected hypersensitivity to iodine-containing contrast media, uncontrolled thyrotoxicosis and decompensated cardiac insufficiency.

Hysterosalpingography must not be carried out during pregnancy or in patients with acute inflammatory conditions in the pelvic cavity.

Warnings/side-effects: For patients with severe impairment of hepatic or renal function, cerebral arteriosclerosis, epileptic conditions, diabetes mellitus requiring drug treatment and/or associated with diabetic complications, pulmonary emphysema, poor general health, latent hyperthyroidism, multiple myeloma or benign nodular goitre the need for examination with X-ray contrast media merits careful consideration.

This also applies to patients with a history of allergy, atopy, bronchial asthma, endogenous eczema, cardiac or circulatory insufficiency or a previous adverse reaction with any contrast medium since experience shows that they may be at higher risk from developing anaphylaxis or cardiovascular collapse. Consideration should be given to the use of low osmolar radiocontrast media in such patients.

Particular caution should be exercised in allergic persons who have previously tolerated an injectable iodine-containing contrast medium without any complication because they may have become sensitized to these substances in the meantime.

The patient should be recumbent during the administration of Urografin. Thereafter, the patient must be kept under close observation for at least 30 minutes, since about 90% of all severe incidents occur within that time. If the administration does not take place on the X-ray table, any patient with a labile circulation should be brought to the X-ray machine sitting or lying down.

In patients with multiple myeloma, diabetes mellitus requiring drug treatment, polyuria, oliguria or gout, and in infants, young children and marasmic patients the fluid supply should not be restricted. Existing disturbances of the balance of water and electrolytes must be corrected before the administration of a hypertonic contrast-medium solution.

Premedication with an alpha-blocker is recommended in patients with phaeochromocytoma, because of the risk of hypertensive crisis.

Diabetic nephropathy may predispose to renal impairment following intravascular administration of contrast media. This may precipitate lactic acidosis in patients who are taking biguanides. As a precaution biguanides should be stopped 48 hours prior to the examination and reinstated only after adequate renal function has been regained.

Hypersensitivity reactions can be aggravated in patients on beta-blockers. The prevalence of delayed reactions to contrast media is higher in patients who have received interleukin.

X-ray examinations should if possible be avoided during pregnancy. It has not yet been proved beyond question that Urografin may be used without hesitation in pregnant patients. Therefore, an examination with a contrast medium during pregnancy should be carried out only if considered absolutely necessary by the physician. Renally eliminated contrast media such as Urografin enter the breast milk in only very small amounts. Limited data suggest that the risk to the suckling infant of administering salts of diatrizoic acid to its mother is low.

If iodine isotopes are to be administered for the diagnosis of thyroid disease, it should be borne in mind that after the administration of iodinated contrast media which are excreted via the kidneys, the capacity of the thyroid tissue to take up iodine will be reduced for 2 weeks, and sometimes up to 6 weeks.

Mild subjective symptoms, such as a feeling of heat and nausea, occur very seldom and disappear rapidly when the injection is slowed down or briefly interrupted. Transient pain may occur, in particular during the examination of peripheral vascular regions.

Other symptoms which may occur are: Chills, fever, sweating, headache, dizziness, blanching, weakness, gagging and a feeling of suffocation, gasping, a rise or fall of blood pressure, itching, urticaria, other kinds of skin eruption, oedema, cramp, tremor, sneezing and lacrimation. These reactions, which can occur irrespective of the amount administered and the mode of administration, may be the first signs of incipient shock. Administration of the contrast medium must be discontinued immediately and – if necessary – specific therapy instituted intravenously. It is therefore advisable to use a flexible indwelling cannula for intravenous contrast medium administration. To permit immediate countermeasures to be taken in emergencies, appropriate drugs, an endotracheal tube and a ventilator should be ready to hand.

As with any contrast medium, the possibility of hypersensitivity must always be considered. If marked side-effects or suspected allergic reactions occur during injection and do not disappear, or even get worse, when the injection is briefly interrupted, it is probable that the patient is hypersensitive and the investigation must be abandoned. Even relatively minor symptoms such as itching of the skin, sneezing, violet yawns, tickling in the throat, hoarseness or attacks of coughing may be early signs of a severe reaction and, therefore, merit careful attention. Delayed reactions can occasionally occur.

Very rarely, severe or even life-threatening side-effects such as severe hypotension and collapse, circulatory failure, ventricular fibrillation, cardiac arrest, pulmonary oedema, anaphylactic shock or other allergic manifestations, convulsions, or other cerebral symptoms may occur. In some cases these have proved fatal.

Paravascular administration of the contrast medium rarely leads to severe tissue reactions.

Neurological complications such as coma, temporary states of confusion and somnolence, transient paresis, disturbed vision or facial muscle paresis and epileptic fits may occur after cerebral angiography and other procedures in which the contrast medium reaches the brain with the arterial blood. In very rare cases the induction of fits has been observed after intravenous administration of Urografin in epileptics and patients with focal brain damage. However, a causal relationship seems to be questionable. Temporary renal failure may occur in rare cases.

Ionic iodinated contrast media inhibit blood coagulation in vitro more than non-ionic contrast media. Nevertheless medical personnel performing vascular catheterisation procedures should pay meticulous attention to the angiographic technique and catheter flushing so as to minimise the risk of procedure-related thrombosis and embolisation.

Experience shows that pronounced states of excitement, anxiety and pain can be the cause of side effects or intensify contrast medium-related reactions. They can be counteracted by calm management of the patient and the use of suitable drugs. Delayed reactions following intravascular administration of iodinated contrast media are rare. Nevertheless, driving or operating machinery is not advisable for the first 24 hours.

Ready availability of all drugs and equipment for emergency treatment and familiarity with the respective procedures are prerequisites for the effective management of contrast-medium incidents. Some guidance in the treatment of such incidents is contained in the leaflet supplied with the pack.

Overdosage: Acute symptoms of poisoning are unlikely with intravascular administration. On inadvertent overdosage or in greatly impaired renal function, the contrast medium may be removed by dialysis, and the balance of water and electrolytes should be corrected. Acute toxicity studies do not suggest a risk of acute intoxication.

Table 1

Examination (Adults)	*150*	*325*	*370*
Intravenous urography		Up to 70 ml	Up to 70 ml
High-dose urography		100 ml	
Drip-infusion urography	2–4 ml/kg body wt up to 250 ml		
Retrograde urography	5–10 ml		
Cystography	Up to 500 ml		
Angiocardiography			30–50 ml
Right-heart catheterisation			40–80 ml
Left-heart catheterisation			40–60 ml
Pulmonary angiography			30–40 ml
Coronary arteriography			4–8 ml per artery[a]
Renal arteriography			5–8 ml
Coeliac-axis arteriography			35–80 ml
Thoracic aortography			30–60 ml
Pelvic aortography			20–25 ml
Translumbar abdominal aortography			20–30 ml
Placentography			25 ml
Pelvic venography		25–30 ml	
Venacavography			
Inferior		30–50 ml	
Superior		25–35 ml	
Splenoportography			40–50 ml
Hysterosalpingography			4–7 ml
Arthrography		1–10 ml	

[a]100 ml bottles are available for coronary arteriography.

Pharmaceutical precautions

Storage: Protect from light and secondary X-rays. Shelf-life 5 years. Some radiologists give an antihistamine or a corticoid prophylactically to patients with a history of allergy. However, because of possible precipitation, X-ray contrast media and prophylactic agents must not be injected as mixed solutions.

Legal category POM

Package quantities Urografin 150: Packs of 10 x 10 ml ampoules and 10 x 20 ml ampoules.

Urografin 150 for infusion: Packs of 1 x 250 ml bottles and 1 x 500 ml bottles.

Urograin 325: Packs of 10 x 20 ml ampoules and 10 x 50 ml bottles.

Urografin 370: Packs of 10 x 20 ml ampoules and 10 x 50 ml bottles. In addition packs of 1 x 100 ml bottles.

Further information Nil

Product licence numbers

Urografin 150	0053/5041R
Urografin 150 for infusion	0053/5007R
Urografin 325	0053/5006R
Urografin 370	0053/5044R

**Trade Mark*

Schering-Plough Ltd
Schering-Plough House
Shire Park
Welwyn Garden City
Herts AL7 1TW

 01707 363636 ▯ 01707 363690

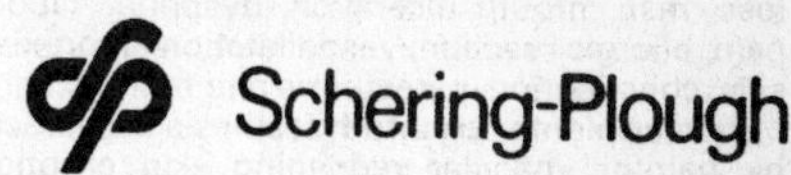

CAELYX* ▼

Qualitative and quantitative composition Each 10 ml vial of Caelyx contains doxorubicin hydrochloride, 2 mg/ml, concentrate for infusion.

Pharmaceutical form Caelyx, a liposome formulation, is doxorubicin hydrochloride encapsulated in liposomes with surface-bound methoxypolyethylene glycol (MPEG). This process is known as pegylation and protects liposomes from detection by the mononuclear phagocyte system (MPS), which increases blood circulation time. Caelyx is a concentrate for infusion presented as a sterile, translucent, red suspension in 10 ml glass vials for single-use intravenous infusion.

Clinical particulars
Therapeutic indications: Caelyx is indicated for AIDS-related Kaposi's sarcoma (KS) in patients with low CD4 counts (< 200 CD4 lymphocytes/mm³) and extensive mucocutaneous or visceral disease.

Caelyx may be used as first-line systemic chemotherapy, or as second line chemotherapy in AIDS-KS patients with disease that has progressed with, or in patients intolerant to, prior combination systemic chemotherapy comprising at least two of the following agents: a vinca alkaloid, bleomycin and doxorubicin (or other anthracycline).

Posology and method of administrtation:
Dosage: Caelyx should be administered intravenously at 20 mg/m² every two-to-three weeks. Intervals shorter than 10 days should be avoided as drug accumulation and increased toxocity cannot be ruled out. Patients should be treated for two-to-three months to achieve a therapeutic response. Treatment should be continued as needed to maintain a therapeutic response.

Administration: Caelyx, diluted in 250 ml 5% Glucose Intravenous infusion, is administered by intravenous infusion over 30 minutes. DO NOT administer as a bolus injection or undiluted solution. It is recommended that the Caelyx infusion line be connected through the side port of an intravenous infusion of 5% Glucose Intravenous Infusion to achieve further dilution and minimise the risk of thrombosis and extravasation. Caelyx must not be given by the intramuscular or subcutaneous route.

Patients with impaired hepatic function: In a small number of patients with impaired hepatic function (bilirubin values up to 4 mg/dl) administered 20 mg/m² of Caelyx, there appeared to be no change in the clearance and terminal half-life of Caelyx. However, until further experience is gained, the Caelyx dosage should be reduced in patients with impaired hepatic function, based on experience with conventional doxorubicin HCl. Prior to Caelyx administration, hepatic function should be evaluated using conventional clinical laboratory tests such as ALT/AST, alkaline phosphatase, and bilirubin. It is recommended that the Caelyx dosage be reduced if the bilirubin is elevated as follows: at serum bilirubin 1.2–3.0 mg/dl, give ½ the normal dose; at > 3 mg/dl, give ¼ the normal dose.

Patients with impaired renal function: As doxorubicin is metabolised by the liver and excreted in the bile, dose modification should not be required with Caelyx.

Patients with splenectomy: As there is no experience with Caelyx in patients with splenectomy, treatment with Caelyx is not recommended.

Paediatric patients: The safety and effectiveness in patients less than 18 years of age have not been established.

Elderly patients: The safety and effectiveness in patients over 60 years of age have not been established.

Contra-indications: Caelyx is contra-indicated in patients who have a history of hypersensitivity reactions to its components or to doxorubicin HCl. Caelyx should not be administered during pregnancy or while breast-feeding.

Caelyx should not be used to treat AIDS-KS that may be effectively treated with local therapy or systemic alfa-interferon.

Special warnings and special precautions for use:
Special warnings
Cardiac risk: All patients receiving Caelyx should routinely undergo frequent ECG monitoring. Transient ECG changes such as T-wave flattening, S-T segment depression and benign arrhythmias are not considered mandatory indications for the suspension of Caelyx therapy. However, reduction of the QRS complex is considered more indicative of cardiac toxicity. If this change occurs, the most definitive test for anthracycline myocardial injury, i.e., endomyocardial biopsy, should be considered.

More specific methods for the evaluation and monitoring of cardiac functions as compared to ECG are a measurement of left ventricular ejection fraction by echocardiography or preferably by Multiple Gated Arteriography (MUGA). These methods should be applied routinely before the initiation of Caelyx therapy and should be repeated periodically during treatment. The evaluation of left ventricular function is considered to be mandatory before each additional administration of Caelyx which exceeds a cumulative dose of 450 mg/m².

Whenever cardiomyopathy is suspected, i.e., the left ventricular ejection fraction has decreased relatively as compared to pre-treatment values and/or (at the same time) left ventricular ejection are lower than a prognostically relevant value (e.g. < 45%), endomyocardial biopsies should be performed and the benefit of continued therapy must be carefully evaluated against the risk of producing irreversible cardiac damage.

Congestive heart failure due to cardiomyopathy may occur suddenly, without prior ECG changes and may also be encountered several weeks after discontinuation of therapy.

The evaluation tests and methods mentioned above concerning the monitoring of cardiac performance during anthracycline therapy should be employed in the following order, ECG monitoring, measurement of left ventricular ejection fraction, endomyocardial biopsy. If a test result indicates possible cardiac injury associated with Caelyx therapy, the benefit of continued therapy must be carefully weighed against the risk of myocardial injury.

Patients with a history of cardiovascular disease should receive Caelyx only when the benefit outweighs the risk to the patient.

Caution should be exercised in patients with impaired cardiac function who receive Caelyx.

Caution should be observed in patients who have received other anthracyclines. The total dose of doxorubicin HCl should also take into account any previous or concomitant) therapy with cardiotoxic compounds such as other anthracyclines/anthraquinones or e.g. 5-FU.

Myelosuppression: Many AIDS-KS patients treated with Caelyx have baseline myelosuppression due to such factors as their HIV disease or numerous concomitant medications. In this population, myelosuppression appears to be the dose-limiting adverse event (see *Undesirable effects*). Because of the potential for bone marrow suppression, periodic blood counts should be performed frequently during the course of Caelyx therapy, and at a minimum, prior to each dose of Caelyx. Persistent severe myelosuppression may result in superinfection or haemorrhage.

Infusion-associated reactions: See *Undesirable effects.*

Special precautions:
Diabetic patients: It should be noted that each vial of Caelyx contains sucrose and is administered in 5% Glucose Intravenous Infusion.

Interaction with other medicaments and other forms of interaction: No formal drug interaction studies have been conducted with Caelyx. Caution should be exercised in the concomitant use of drugs known to interact with doxorubicin HCl. Although not formally studied, Caelyx, like other doxorubicin HCl preparations, may potentiate the toxicity of other anti-cancer therapies. Exacerbation of cyclophosphamide-induced haemorrhage cystitis and enhancement of the hepatotoxicity of 6-mercaptopurine have been reported with doxorubicin HCl. Caution should be exercised when giving any other cytotoxic agents, especially myelotoxic agents, at the same time.

Pregnancy and use during lactation:
Pregnancy: Caelyx is embryotoxic in rats and embryotoxic and abortifacient in rabbits. Teratogenicity cannot be ruled out. There is no experience in pregnant women with Caelyx. Caelyx therefore, should not be administered to pregnant women. Women of child-bearing potential should be advised to avoid pregnancy while they or their male partner are receiving Caelyx and in the six months following discontinuation of Caelyx therapy. (See *Carcinogenesis, Mutagenesis and Reproductive toxicity.*)

Lactation: It is not known whether this drug is excreted in human milk and because of the potential for serious adverse reactions in nursing infants from Caelyx, mothers should discontinue nursing prior to taking this drug.

Effects on the ability to drive and use machines: Although Caelyx should not effect driving performance, in studies to date, dizziness and somnolence were associated infrequently (< 5%) with the administration of Caelyx. Patients who suffer from these effects should avoid driving and operating machinery.

Undesirable effects: Open-label and controlled clinical studies on AIDS-KS patients treated with Caelyx show that myelosuppression was the most frequent side effect considered related to Caelyx occurring in approximately half of the patients.

Leucopenia is the most frequent adverse event experienced with Caelyx in this population; and anaemia and thrombocytopenia can also be expected. These events may occur early on in treatment and are usually transient. In clinical trials patients rarely discontinued treatment due to myelosuppression. Haematological toxicity may require dose reduction or suspension or delay of therapy.

Caelyx treatment should be temporarily suspended in patients when the ANC count is < 1000/mm³ and/or the platelet count is < 50,000/mm³. G-CSF (or GM-CSF) may be given as concomitant therapy to support the blood count when the ANC count is < 1000/mm³. Clinically significant laboratory abnormalities frequently (≥ 5%) occurred in clinical studies with Caelyx. These included increases in alkaline phosphatase; and increases in AST and bilirubin which are believed to be related to the underlying disease and not Caelyx. Reduction in haemoglobin and platelets were less frequently (< 5%) reported. Sepsis related to leucopenia was rarely (< 1%) observed. Some of these abnormalities may have been related to the underlying HIV infection and not Caelyx.

Other frequently (≥ 5%) observed side effects were nausea, asthenia, alopecia, fever, diarrhoea, infusion-associated acute reactions, and stomatitis.

Infusion-associated reactions are characterised by flushing, shortness of breath, facial oedema, headache, chills, back pain, tightness in the chest and throat and/or hypotension. In most cases, the side effect occurs during the first cycle of treatment. Temporarily stopping the infusion or slowing the rate of the infusion resolves these reactions over the course of several hours, regardless of whether any symptomatic treatment is used.

Stomatitis has been reported in patients receiving continuous infusions of conventional doxorubicin HCl and was frequently reported in patients receiving Caelyx. It did not interfere with patients completing therapy and no dosage adjustments are generally required, unless stomatitis is affecting a patient's ability to eat. In this case, the dose interval may be extended by 1–2 weeks or the dose reduced. Respiratory side effects frequently (≥ 5%) occurred in clinical studies of Caelyx and may be related to opportunistic infections in the AIDS population. Opportunistic infections (OI's) are observed in KS patients after administration with Caelyx, and are frequently observed in patients with HIV-induced immunodeficiency. The most frequently observed OI's in clinical studies were candidiasis, cytomegalovirus, herpes simplex, Pneumocystis carinii pneumonia, and myobacterium avium complex.

Other less frequently (< 5%) observed side effects included palmarplantar erythrodysesthesia, oral monoliasis, nausea and vomiting, vomiting, weight loss, rash, mouth ulceration, dyspnoea, abdominal pain, allergic reaction, vasodilatation, anorexia, glossitis, constipation, paresthesia and retinitis.

Palmar-plantar erythrodysesthesia is characterised by painful, macular reddening skin eruptions. In patients experiencing this event, it is generally seen after six or more weeks of treatment. In most patients it clears in one or two weeks, with or without treatment with corticosteroids. It appears to be dose and schedule related and can be reduced by extending the dose interval 1–2 weeks or reducing the dose. This reaction can be severe and debilitating in some patients, however, and may require discontinuation of treatment.

An increased incidence of congestive heart failure is associated with standard doxorubicin therapy. Although, endomyocardial biopsies on nine of ten AIDS-KS patients receiving cumulative doses of Caelyx greater than 460 mg/m² indicate no evidence of anthracycline-induced cardiomyopathy, until further clinical data are available, the risk of developing cardiomyopathy is assumed to be similar to that of standard doxorubicin. The recommended dose of Caelyx for AIDS-KS patients is 20 mg/m² every two-to-three weeks. The cumulative dose at which cardiotoxicity would become a concern (> 400 mg/m²) would require more than 20 courses of Caelyx therapy over 40 to 60 weeks. Although no local necrosis following extravasation has been observed to date, Caelyx should be considered an irritant. Animal studies indicate that administration of doxorubicin HCl as a liposomal formulation reduces the potential for extravasation injury. If any signs or symptoms of extravasation occur (e.g., stinging, erythema) the infusion should be immediately terminated and restarted in another vein. The application of ice over the site of extravasation for approximately 30 minutes may be helpful in alleviating the local reaction. Caelyx must not be given by the intramuscular or subcutaneous route.

Recall of skin reaction due to prior radiotherapy has rarely occurred with Caelyx administration.

Overdose: Acute overdosage with doxorubicin HCl worsens the toxic effects of mucositis, leucopenia and thrombocytopenia. Treatment of acute overdosage of the severely myelosuppressed patient consists of hospitalisation, antibiotics, platelet and granulocyte transfusions and symptomatic treatment of mucositis.

Pharmacological properties

Pharmacodynamic properties: Pharmaco-therapeutic group: Cytotoxic agents (anthracyclines and related substances), ATC code L01DB.

The active ingredient of Caelyx is doxorubicin HCl, a cytotoxic anthracycline antibiotic obtained from *Stretomyces peucetius* var. *caesius.* The exact mechanism of the antitumour activity of doxorubicin is not known. It is generally believed that inhibition of DNA, RNA and protein synthesis is responsible for the majority of the cytotoxic effects. This is probably the result of intercalation of the anthracycline between adjacent base pairs of the DNA double helix thus preventing their unwinding for replication.

Pharmacokinetic properties: Caelyx is a long-circulating pegylated liposomal formulation of doxorubicin HCl that provides greater concentration of doxorubicin in KS tumours than in normal skin. Pegylated liposomes contains surface-grafted segments of the hydrophilic polymer methoxypolyethylene glucol (MPEG). These linear MPEG groups extend from the liposome surface creating a protective coating that reduces interactions between the lipid bilayer membrane and the plasma components. This allows the Caelyx liposomes to circulate for prolonged periods in the blood stream. Pegylated liposomes are small enough (average diameter of approximately 100 nm) to pass intact (extravasate) through defective blood vessels supplying tumours. Evidence of penetration of pegylated liposomes from blood vessels and their entry and accumulation in tumours has been seen in mice with C-26 colon carcinoma tumours and in transgenic mice with KS-like lesions. The pegylated liposomes also have a low permeability lipid matrix and internal aqueous buffer system that combine to keep doxorubicin HCl encapsulated during liposome residence time in circulation.

The plasma pharmacokinetics of Caelyx were evaluated in 23 patients with Kaposi's sarcoma who received single doses of 20 mg/m² administered by a 30-minute infusion. The pharmacokinetic parameters of Caelyx (primarily representing liposome-encapsulated doxorubicin HCl and low levels of unencapsulated doxorubicin HCl) observed after the 20 mg/m² doses are presented in the following table.

The plasma pharmacokinetics of Caelyx in humans differ significantly from those reported in the literature for standard doxorubicin HCl preparations. Caelyx displayed linear pharmacokinetics. Disposition occurred in two phases after Caelyx administration, with a relatively short first phase (~ 5 hours) and a prolonged second phase (~ 55 hours) that accounted for the majority of the area under the curve (AUC). Doxorubicin HCl displays extensive tissue distribution (volume of distribution, 700 to 1100 L/m² and a rapid elimination clearance (24 to 73 L/h/m²). In contrast, the pharmacokinetic profile of Caelyx indicates that Caelyx is confined mostly to the vascular fluid volume and that the clearance of doxorubicin from the blood is dependent upon the liposomal carrier. Doxorubicin becomes available after the liposomes are extravasated and enter the tissue compartment. At equivalent doses, the plasma concentration and AUC values of Caelyx which represent mostly liposome-encapsulated doxorubicin HCl (containing 90% to 95% of the measured doxorubicin) are significantly higher than those achieved with standard doxorubicin HCl preparations. Kaposi's sarcoma lesion and normal skin biopsies were obtained 48 and 96 hours post-infusion. In patients receiving 20 mg/m² Caelyx the concentration of total (liposome encapsulated and unencapsulated) doxorubicin in the KS lesions was a median of 19 (range 3–53) times higher than in normal skin at 48 hours post treatment.

Pharmacokinetic parameters in Caelyx-treated patients

Parameter	*Mean ± Standard Error* 20 mg/m² (n=23)
Maximum Plasma Concentration[a] (μg/ml)	8.34±0.49
Plasma Clearance (L/h/m²)	0.041±0.004
Volume of Distribution (L/m²)	2.72±0.120
AUC (μg/ml h)	590±58.7
λ_1 half-live (hours)	5.2±1.4
λ_2 half-live (hours)	55.0±4.8

[a] Measured at the end of a 30-minute infusion.

Preclinical safety data: In repeat dose studies conducted in animals, the toxicity profile of Caelyx appears very similar to that reported in humans who receive long-term infusions of doxorubicin hydrochloride. With Caelyx, the encapsulation of doxorubicin hydrochloride in pegylated liposomes results in these effects having a differing strength, as follows:

Cardiotoxicity: Studies in rabbits have shown that the cardiotoxicity of Caelyx is reduced compared with conventional doxorubicin HCl preparations.

Dermal toxicity: In studies performed after the repeated administration of Caelyx to rats and dogs, serious dermal inflammations and ulcer formations were observed at clinically relevant dosages. In the study in dogs, the occurrence and severity of these lesions was reduced by lowering the dose or prolonging the intervals between doses. Similar dermal lesions, which are desribed as palmar-plantar erythrodsesthesia were also observed in patients after long-term intravenous infusion (see *Undesirable effects*).

Anaphylactoid response: During repeat dose toxicology studies in dogs, an acute response characterised by hypotension, pale mucous membranes, salivation, emesis and periods of hyperactivity followed by hypoactivity and lethargy was observed following administration of pegylated liposomes (placebo). A similar, but less severe response was also noted in dogs treated with Caelyx and doxorubicin.

The hypotensive response was reduced in magnitude by pretreatment with antihistamines. However, the response was not life-threatening and the dogs recovered quickly upon discontinuation of treatment.

Local toxicity: Subcutaneous tolerance studies indicate that Caelyx, as against doxorubicin HCl, causes slighter local irritation or damage to the tissue after a possible extravasation.

Mutagenicity and carcinogenicity: Although no studies have been conducted with Caelyx, doxorubicin HCl, the pharmacologically active ingredient of Caelyx, is mutagenic and carcinogenic. Pegylated placebo liposomes are neither mutagenic or genotoxic.

Reproductive toxicity: Caelyx resulted in mild moderate ovarian and testicular atrophy in mice after a single dose of 36 mg/kg. Decreased testicular weights and hypospermia were present in rats after repeat doses ≥0.25 mg/kg/day and diffuse degeneration of the semniferous tubules and a marked decrease in spermatogenesis were observed in dogs after repeat doses of 1 mg/kg/day (see *Pregnancy and lactation*).

Pharmaceutical particulars

List of excipients: The following excipients are contained in each vial of product: α-2(2-[1,2-distearoyl-*sn*-glycero(3)phosphooxy]ethylcarbamoyl)-ω-methoxypoly(oxyethylen)-40, sodium salt (MPEG-DSPE) Fully hydrogenated soy phosphatidylcholine (HSPC); Cholesterol NF; Ammonium sulphate ACS; Sucrose PhEur; Histidine PhEur; Water for injections PhEur; Hydrochloric acid PhEur; Sodium hydroxide PhEur.

Incompatibilities: DO NOT MIX WITH OTHER DRUGS.

Shelf-life: Unopened vials of material have a shelf-life of 18 months and should be stored at 2°C to 8°C. After dilution with 5% Glucose Intravenous Infusion, the diluted Caelyx solution should be used immediately. Diluted product not for immediate use should be prepared under aseptic conditions and in line with good pharmaceutical practice should be stored at 2°C to 8°C for no longer than 24 hours. Partially used vials should be discarded.

Special precautions for storage: Store at 2°C to 8°C. Avoid freezing.

Nature and contents of container: The container is a Type 1 glass vial, with a siliconised grey bromobutyl stopper, and an aluminium seal. Caelyx is supplied as a single pack or packs of ten. Each 10 ml vial of Caelyx contains doxorubicin hydrochloride 2 mg/ml; concentrate for infusion.

Instructions for use/handling: DO NOT USE MATERIAL THAT SHOWS EVIDENCE OF PRECIPITATION OR ANY OTHER PARTICULTE MATTER.

Determine the dose of Caelyx to be administered (based upon the recommended dose and the patient's surface area). Take the appropriate volume of Caelyx up into a sterile syringe. Aseptic technique must be strictly observed since no preservative or bacteriostatic agent is present in Caelyx. The appropriate dose of Caelyx must be diluted in 250 ml of 5% Glucose Intravenous prior to administration.

The use of any diluent other than 5% Glucose Intravenous Infusion, or the presence of any bacteriostatic agent such as benzyl alcohol may cause precipitation of Caelyx.

It is recommended that the Caelyx infusion line be connected through the side port of an intravenous infusion of 5% Glucose Intravenous Infusion.

Caution should be exercised in handling Caelyx solution. The use of gloves is required. If Caelyx comes into contact with skin or mucosa, wash immediately and thoroughly with soap and water. Caelyx should be handled and disposed of in a manner consistent with that of other anti-cancer drugs.

Marketing authorisation holder: SP Europe, Rue de Stalle 73, 1180 Brussels, Belgium.

Marketing authorisation numbers
EU/1/96/011/001
EU/1/96/011/002

Date of first authorisation/renewal 21 June 1996

Date of revision of the text 31 October 1996

CLARITYN* TABLETS (Loratadine)

Presentation White, oval tablets plain on one side, and deep score, flask and dish logo with number 10 on the other side. Each tablet contains 10 mg micronised loratadine.

Uses

Mode of action: Clarityn is a long acting tricyclic antihistamine with selective peripheral H_1-receptor antagonistic activity and no central sedative or anticholinergic effects.

Indications: Clarityn Tablets are indicated in adults for the relief of symptoms associated with seasonal and perennial allergic rhinitis, such as sneezing, nasal discharge and itching and ocular itching and burning. Nasal and ocular signs and symptoms are relieved rapidly after oral administration. Clarityn Tablets are also indicated for the relief of symptoms associated with idiopathic chronic urticaria.

Dosage and administration

Adults, including the elderly, and children 12 years of age and over: One 10 mg tablet once daily.

Contra-indications, warnings, etc

Contra-indications: Clarityn Tablets are contra-indicated in patients who have shown hypersensitivity or idiosyncrasy to their components.

Pregnancy and lactation: Clarityn should not be administered during pregnancy. There is no experience of the use of Clarityn in human pregnancy. In animal studies loratadine was not teratogenic, at high doses some embryotoxic effects were observed. Since loratadine is excreted in breast milk it should not be administered to lactating women.

Side effects: During controlled clinical studies the incidence of adverse events, including sedation and anticholinergic effects, observed with 10 mg Clarityn was comparable to that observed with placebo. Other events, fatigue, nausea and headache were reported rarely. Tachycardia and syncope have been reported rarely. Causality has not been established. Spontaneous adverse events reported rarely include: alopecia, anaphylaxis, abnormal hepatic function and supraventricular tachyarrythmias.

Interactions: When administered concurrently with alcohol, Clarityn has no potentiating effects as measured by psychomotor performance studies. Loratadine is metabolised by hepatic cytochromes P450 3A4 and 2D6. Concomitant therapy with drugs which inhibit or are metabolised by either system may therefore elevate plasma concentrations of either drug and adverse reactions might result.

Studies indicate that cimetidine, which inhibits both enzymes, and erythromycin or ketoconazole, which inhibit P450 3A4 each increased loratadine concentrations, although no adverse effects, clinical or electrocardiographic, were observed. Other drugs known to inhibit either P450 3A4 or P450 2D6 are quinidine, fluconazole or fluoxetine.

Overdosage: In the event of overdosage, treatment which should be started immediately is symptomatic and supportive. The patient should be induced to vomit, even if emesis has occurred spontaneously (ipecacuanha is a preferred method), but not in patients with impaired consciousness. Administration of activated charcoal as a slurry with water may be attempted following emesis. If vomiting is unsuccessful or contra-indicated, gastric lavage should be performed. It is not known whether loratadine is dialysable. After emergency treatment, the patient should continue to be under medical supervision.

Pharmaceutical precautions None.

Legal category POM.

Package quantities Blister strips of 10 in OP cartons of 30 tablets.

Further information Nil.

Product licence number PL 0201/0175

Date of revision April 1998.

CLARITYN* SYRUP

Qualitative and quantitative composition Loratadine 1 mg/ml.

Pharmaceutical form Syrup.

Clinical particulars

Therapeutic indications: Clarityn Syrup is indicated in adults for the relief of symptoms associated with seasonal and perennial allergic rhinitis, such as sneezing, nasal discharge and itching and ocular itching and burning. Nasal and ocular signs and symptoms are relieved rapidly after oral administration. Clarityn Syrup is also indicated for the relief of symptoms associated with idiopathic chronic urticaria.

In children over 2 years, Clarityn Syrup is indicated for the symptomatic treatment of seasonal allergic rhinitis and allergic skin conditions such as idiopathic urticaria.

Posology and method of administration: Clarityn Syrup is for oral administration.

Adults, including the elderly and children of 12 years of age or over: 10 mg (two 5 ml spoonsful) of syrup once daily.

Children aged 6 to 12 years of age: 10 mg (two 5 ml spoonsful) of syrup once daily.

Children aged 2 to 5 years: 5 mg (one 5 ml spoonful) of syrup once daily.

Contra-indications: Clarityn Syrup is contra-indicated in patients who have shown hypersensitivity or idiosyncrasy to their components.

Special warnings and precautions for use: Safety and efficacy of Clarityn Syrup in children younger than 2 years of age have not been established.

Interaction with other medicaments and other forms of interaction: When administered concurrently with alcohol, Clarityn Syrup has no potentiating effects as measured by psychomotor performance studies. Loratadine is metabolised by hepatic cytochromes P450 3A4 and 2D6. Concomitant therapy with drugs which inhibit or are metabolised by either system may therefore elevate plasma concentrations of either drug and adverse reactions might result.

Studies indicate that cimetidine, which inhibits both enzymes, and erythromycin or ketoconazole, which inhibit P450 3A4 each increased loratadine concentrations, although no adverse effects, clinical or electrocardiographic, were observed. Other drugs known to inhibit either P450 3A4 or P450 2D6 are quinidine, fluconazole or fluoxetine.

Drug/laboratory test interactions: Antihistamines should be discontinued about four days prior to skin testing procedures, since these drugs may prevent or diminish otherwise positive reactions to dermal reactivity indicators.

Pregnancy and lactation: Clarityn Syrup should not be administered during pregnancy. There is no experience of the use of loratadine in human pregnancy. In animal studies loratadine was not teratogenic, at high doses some embryotoxic effects were observed. Since loratadine is excreted in breast milk it should not be administered to lactating women.

Effects on ability to drive and use machines: Clarityn Syrup has no clinically significant sedative effect at recommended dosage.

Undesirable effects: During controlled clinical studies, the incidence of adverse effects associated with Clarityn Syrup treatment was comparable to that associated with placebo. Clarityn Syrup had no clinically significant sedative or anti-cholinergic properties. Other events, fatigue, nausea and headache were reported rarely.

Tachycardia and syncope have been reported rarely. Causality has not been established. Spontaneous adverse events reported rarely include: alopecia, anaphylaxis, abnormal hepatic function and supraventricular tachyarrythmias.

Overdose: At doses several times higher than the recommended dose, mild sedation was observed. To date, overdosage has not occurred with loratadine. A single acute ingestion of 160 mg in an adult produced no adverse effects.

In the event of overdosage, treatment, which should be started immediately, is symptomatic and supportive. The patient should be induced to vomit, even if emesis has occurred spontaneously (ipecac is a preferred method), but not in patients with impaired consciousness. Administration of activated charcoal as a slurry with water may be attempted following emesis. If vomiting is unsuccessful or contra-indicated, gastric lavage should be performed. Physiologic saline is the lavage solution of choice, particularly in children. Loratadine is not cleared by haemodialysis to any appreciable extent. After emergency treatment, the patient should continue to be medically monitored.

Pharmacological properties

Pharmacodynamic properties: Loratadine is a cyproheptadine derivaive, structurally related to azatadine. It exhibits potent, long acting H_1-antihistamine activity with no central sedative or anticholinergic effects. In man, nasal and other signs and symptoms of allergic rhinitis are relieved rapidly after oral administration.

The sedation profile of 10 mg loratadine daily is comparable to that of placebo and during long term treatment, no clinically significant changes in vital signs, laboratory test values, physical examinations or electrocardiograms were observed. At single oral doses ranging from 10 to 160 mg, wheal suppression occurred within one hour of treatment. Results of studies in paediatric patients demonstrated that single doses of 10 mg loratadine syrup were significantly mor effective than placebo at reducing histamine induced wheals and flares.

Pharmacokinetic properties: Loratadine is well absorbed and is almost totally metabolised. It has a distribution half-life of one hour and an elimination half-life of 15.3 hours. Approximately 81% of the ^{14}C labelled dose is excreted in the urine (40%) and faeces (42%) over a 10 day period. Approximately 27% of the dose is eliminated in the urine during the first 24 hours. Pharmacokinetics in healthy adult volunteers and healthy geriatric volunteers are comparable. Steady state levels of loratadine are reached after the fifth dose.

Loratadine and its active metabolite are excreted in the breast milk of lactating women, only 0.029% of which is detected in the milk 48 hours after dosing. Loratadine is highly bound (97% to 99%) and its active metabolite moderately bound (73% to 76%) to plasma proteins. Bioavailability studies demonstrate the bioequivalence of loratadine administered orally as a capsule, tablet, suspension and solution.

Preclinical safety data: Loratadine was relatively nontoxic when administered orally or intraperitonally in single doses to mice or rats. Oral LD_{50}, values were estimated to be greater than 5000 mg/kg in both species. Rising single doses up to 1280 mg/kg were relatively well tolerated in monkeys. In repeated dose studies, rats were treated orally for periods up to 12 months with doses ranging from 2–240 mg/kg/day; monkeys were treated for up to 17 months with doses ranging from 0.4–90 mg/kg/day.

Anticholergic effects were observed in both species. Evidence of phospholipodosis was also observed; the incidence and severity was dose related and was more pronounced in the rat. It appeared to be reversible.

No evidence of phospholipidosis was observed in man following treatment with 40 mg/kg/day loratadine for 3 months. Studies demonstrate that loradatine is not a cacinogen, mutagen or teratogen.

Pharmaceutical particulars

List of excipients: Propylene glycol PhEur; Glycerin PhEur; Citric Acid Monohydrate PhEur; Sodium Benzoate PhEur; Sucrose, Granulated PhEur; Artificial Peach Flavour; Purified Water PhEur.

Incompatibilties: None known.

Shelf-life: 36 months.

Special precautions for storage: Store in amber glass bottles at 2°C to 30°C.

Nature and contents of container: Type I or Type III amber glass bottle. Tinplate screw on/off cap with HDPE/PE foam/HDPE liner or white polypropylene screw on/off cap with LDPE/PE foam/LDPE liner. Pack size of 100 ml.

Instructions for use/handling: Not applicable.

Marketing authorisation number PL 0201/0173

Date of approval of the text July 1997

Legal category P

DETRUNORM* ▼

Qualitative and quantitative composition

Active ingredients	*Quantity in mg/tablet*
Propiverine Hydrochloride (equivalent to 13.64 mg propiverine)	15.00

Pharmaceutical form Coated tablets.

Clinical particulars

Therapeutic indications: DETRUNORM has been shown to be efficacious in those patients who have either idiopathic bladder instability, or neurogenic bladder (detrusor hyperreflexia) from spinal cord injuries, e.g. transverse lesion paraplegia, for:

- urinary incontinence
- urgency and frequency in unstable bladder conditions

Posology and method of administration: Sugar-coated tablets for oral application.

The recommended daily doses are as follows:

Adults: One sugar-coated tablet (= 15 mg propiverine hydrochloride) two to three times a day. Dosage may be increased to 4 times a day if necessary and tolerated.

Elderly patients: Generally there is no special dosage regime for elderly people. However in elderly and frail patients with diminished body mass it is advisable to start treatment at 15 mg twice daily and increase to 3 times a day as indicated by individual response.

Contra-indications: The drug is contra-indicated in patients being hypersensitive to the preparation and in patients suffering from one of the following disorders:

- obstruction of the bowel
- significant degree of bladder outflow obstruction where urinary retention may be anticipated
- myasthenia gravis
- intestinal atony
- severe ulcerative colitis
- toxic megacolon
- glaucoma
- hepatic disorders
- severe renal disorders

Due to lack of data the drug should not be used in children.

Special warnings and special precautions for use: The drug should be used with caution in patients suffering from:

- autonomic neuropathy

Symptoms that may be aggravated following administration of the drug are:

- hyperthyroidism
- coronary heart disease
- severe congestive heart failure (NYHA IV)
- cardiac arrhythmias
- tachycardias
- prostatic hypertrophy
- hiatus hernia with reflux oesophagitis

Interaction with other medicaments or other forms of interaction: Increased effects due to concomitant medication with tricyclic antidepressants (e.g. imipramine), tranquilisers (e.g. benzodiazipines), anticholinergics, amantadine, neuroleptics (e.g. phenothiazines) and β-sympathomimetics. Decreased effects due to concomitant medication with cholinomimetics. Reduced blood pressure in patients treated with isoniazid.

Pregnancy and lactation: In animal studies, skeletal retardation in the offspring occurred when the drug was administered orally at high doses to pregnant females. The drug was also secreted into the milk of lactating mammals.

DETRUNORM should therefore not be administered to pregnant or nursing women.

Effects on ability to drive and use machines: DETRUNORM may produce drowsiness and blurred vision. The patient should be cautioned regarding activities requiring mental alertness such as operating a motor vehicle or other machinery, performing hazardous work while taking this drug.

Sedative drugs may enahance the drowsiness caused by DEDTRONORM

Undesirable effects: Adverse reactions: following administration of DETRUNORM (propiverine hydrochloride), the symptoms that can be associated with the use of other anticholinergic drugs may occur, frequently: dryness of the mouth, in younger adults blurred vision; seldom: disturbances of gastro-intestinal functioin, decreased blood pressure with drowsiness, slightly increased retention of urine, tiredness; in rare cases: rash due to to idosyncrasy (propiverine hydrochloride) or hypersensitivity (excipients, e.g. colorant), restlessness, heat sensations, tachycardia.

All adverse events are transient and recede after a dose reduction or termination of the therapy after maximum 1–4 days.

In cases of long-term therapy the enzyme pattern of the liver and – in patients at risk of glaucoma – controls of the intraocular pressure are recommended.

Particular attention should be paid to the residual urine volume in cases of urinary tract infections.

Overdose: A maximal dosage of 1 mg/kg body weight-/day should not be exceeded. Ingestion of toxic quantities (greater than 120 mg single dose) may give rise to: restlessness, dizziness, muscular weakness, disorders in speech and vision, dryness of mucosa, vertigo, cardiovascular disorders.

Therapy: Initation of vomiting or gastric lavage using an oiled tube (attention: dryness of mucosa!), followed by symptomatic treatment as in atropine overdose (e.g. physostigmine) with a dosage of 1.0 to 2.0 mg in adults by slow intravenous injection; (may be repeated as necessary to a total of 5 mg); fever should be treated symptomatically with tepid sponging or ice-packs; in cases of pronounced restlessness or excitation, diazepak may be given by intravenous injection up to 10 mg; tachycardia can be treated with propranolol; urinary retention can be treated by catheterisation; in the event of curare-like muscle paralysis, mechanical ventilation may be required.

Pharmacological properties

Pharmacodynamic properties: Pharmacologic group: Spasmolytic, anticholinergic.

Mode of action: Inhibition of calcium influx causing musculotropic spasmolysis.

Inhibition of the efferent connection of the nervous pelvicus due to anticholinergic action.

General: In animal models propiverine hydrochloride causes a dosage dependent decrease of the intravesical pressure and an increase in bladder capacity.

In therapeutic use in man these effects lead to a clinically and urodynamically evalulable improvement of the bladder dysfunctions especially concerning urinary incontinence. In addition dysuria with pollakiuria as well as urge symptoms disappear due to the increased capacity of the bladder and the decrease of micturition rate.

The effect is based on the sum of the pharmacological properties of propiverine and its three active metabolites which are directly musculotropic and anticholinergic.

An analgesic effect has been shown in animal studies in comparison to metamizole, trihexiphenidyl and morphine.

Pharmacokinetic properties: Absorption: After oral administration DETRUNORM is rapidly absorbed from the gastro-intestinal tract. The elimination half-life value is 20 hours. Maximal plasma concentrations are reached after 2.3 hours as an average after single dose of one coated tablet.

The average absolute bioavailability of DETRUNORM is 40.5% (arithm. mean value for $AUC_{0-(p.o.)}/AUC_{0-(i.v.)}$).

Distribution: Propiverine is already intensively metabolised presystemically.

After repeated application (15 mg two or three times a day) steady state is reached after four to five days at a higher concentration level than after single dose application ($C_{average}$ = 61 ng/ml).

The calculated volume of distribution (after 10 mg, 20 mg respecively) of approximately 253 l (125–473 l) indicates, that a large amount of available propiverine is distributed to peripheral compartments.

The protein binding is around 90% for the parent substance and around 60% for the principal metabolite.

Metabolism: The substance has a high pass effect. The main metabolite, the N-oxide of propiverine, is found in the blood at a concentration which greatly exceeds that of the parent substance. Two other metabolites can be detected qualitatively.

Excretion: The elimination of propiverine and its metabolites takes place via the urine, bile and faeces. The parent substance and the principal metabolite are excreted with a total clearance of 141 ml/min, the renal clearance is merely 1 ml/min.

The effect of food and other drugs on bioavailability: None known.

Steady state charcteristics of propiverine following multiple-dose administration (3× 15 mg/6 days of DETRUNORM

Dosage interval [h]	$AUC_{0-t(last)}$ [ngxh/ml]	[%]*	PTF [%]	[%]*	$C_{average}$ [ng/ml]	[%]*
0–8	515	35	57	16	64	64
8–16	460	33	70	25	57	33
16–24	421	36	52	39	52	36

* CV: coefficient of variation
PTF: peak-trough fluctuation

Plasma level of propiverine in healthy volunteers after single and repeated (t.i.d. for 6 days) administration of sugar-coated tablets:

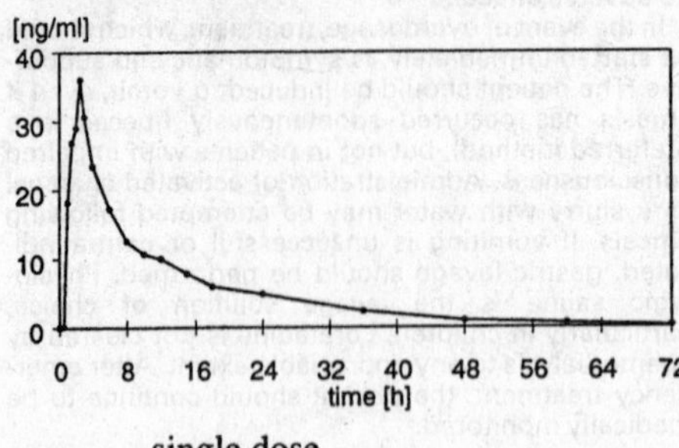

single dose

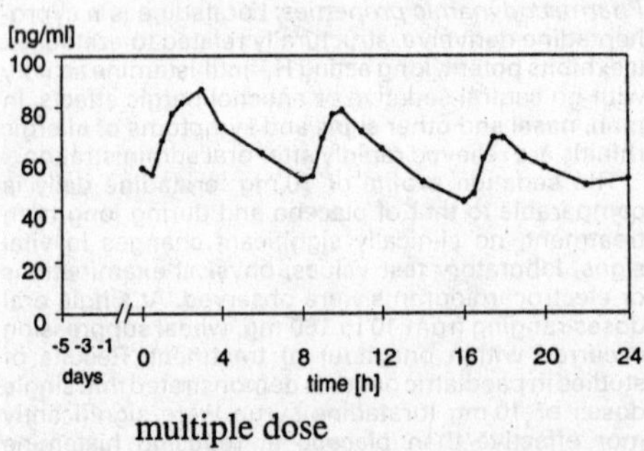

multiple dose

Preclinical safety data: In long term oral dose studies in two mammalian species the main treatment related effect were changes in the liver. These were characterised by hepatic hypertrophy and fatty degeneration. The fatty degeneration was reversible upon cessation of treatment.

In animal studies, skeletal retardation in the offspring occurred when the drug was administered orally at high doses to pregnant females. In lactating propiverine hydrochloride was excreted into the milk.

There was no evidence of mutagenicity. Carcinogenicity studies in rodents revealed three type sof tumours which were considered to be species specific and therefore not of clinical relevance.

Pharmaceutical particulars

List of excipients: Lactose monohydrate, cellulose powder, magnesium stearate, sucrose, talc, heavy kaolin, calcium carbonate, titanium dioxide (E171), acacia, colloidal anhydrous silica, Macrogol 6000, glucose monohydrate, Cochineal red A (E124, lake) yellow beeswax.

Incompatibilities: None known.

Shelf life: Three years.

Special precautions for storage: None.

Nature and contents of container: Strips (Alu – PVC blister foil) in carton with 7 sugar-coated tablets per strip; 28 (4 strips per carton); 56 (8 strips per carton).

Instructions for use/handling: Should be taken orally. No special recommendations necessary.

Marketing authorisation number PL 00201/0248

Date of first authorisation/renewal of authorisation 29 May 1998

Date of (partial) revision of the text 16 April 1998

Legal category POM

DIPROBASE* CREAM

Qualitative and quantitative composition

Chlorocresol BP 0.10% w/w
Cetomacrogol BP 2.25% w/w
Cetostearyl alcohol BP 7.20% w/w
Liquid paraffin BP 6.0% w/w
White soft paraffin BP 15.0% w/w
Phosphoric acid BP 0.002% w/w
Sodium dihydrogen phosphate BP 0.30% w/w
Purified water PhEur to 100.00% w/w

Pharmaceutical form Cream

Clinical particulars

Therapeutic indications: Diprobase Cream is an emollient, moisturising and protective cream for the follow-up treatment with topical steroids or in spacing such treatment. It may also be used as diluent for topical steroids. Diprobase Cream is recommended for the symptomatic treatment of red inflamed, damaged, dry or chapped skin, the protection of raw skin areas and as a pre-bathing emollient for dry/eczematous skin to alleviate drying areas.

Posology and method of administration:

Adults and children: The cream should be applied to the dry skin areas as often as is required and rubbed well into the skin.

Contra-indications: There are no absolute contra-indications to the use of the cream other than hypersensitivity to any of the ingredients.

Special warnings and special precautions for use: None stated

Interactions with other medicaments and other forms of interaction: None stated.

Pregnancy and lactation: None stated.

Effects on ability to drive and use machines: None stated.

Undesirable effects: Rarely, mild skin reactions have been observed.

Overdose: None stated.

Pharmacological properties

Pharmacodynamic properties: Diprobase Cream contains no active ingredients and has no pharmacological action. The ingredients provide emollient, moisturising action or dry or chapped skin.

Pharmacokinetic properties: Not applicable due to topical administration and direct action on the skin.

Preclinical safety data: Not relevant.

Pharmaceutical particulars

List of excipients: Chlorocresol; Cetomacrogol; Cetostearyl alcohol; Liquid paraffin; White soft paraffin; Phosphoric acid; Sodium dihydrogen phosphate; Purified water.

Incompatibilities: None known.

Shelf life: 60 months.

Special precautions for storage: Store below 25°C.

Nature and contents of containers: 50 gm aluminium epoxy lined tubes with plastic caps.

500 gm polypropylene piston pack with polyethylene cap and daplen pump, disc and tube or PVC cap, polypropylene pump, polyolefin disc and HDPE tube.

Instructions for use/handling: Not applicable.

Marketing authorisation number PL 0201/0076

Date of (partial) revision of the text 29 April 1996

Legal category GSL.

DIPROBASE* OINTMENT

Qualitative and quantitative composition

White Soft Paraffin BP 5.0% w/w
Liquid Paraffin BP 95.0% w/w

Pharmaceutical form Ointment

Clinical particulars

Therapeutic indications: Diprobase Ointment is an emollient, moisturising and protective ointment for the follow-up treatment with topical steroids or in spacing such treatment. It may also be used as diluent for topical steroids. Diprobase Ointment is recommended for the symptomatic treatment of red inflamed, damaged, dry or chapped skin, the protection of raw skin areas and as a pre-bathing emollient for dry/eczematous skin to alleviate drying areas.

Posology and method of administration:

Adults and children: The ointment should be thinly applied to cover the affected area completely, massaging gently and thoroughly into the skin. Frequency of application should be established by the physician. Generally, Diprobase Ointment can be used as often as required.

Contra-indications: Hypersensitivity to any of the components of the ointment is a contra-indication to its use.

Special warnings and special precautions for use: None stated

Interactions with other medicaments and other forms of interaction: None stated.

Pregnancy and lactation: None stated.

Effects on ability to drive and use machines: None stated.

Undesirable effects: None stated.

Overdose: None stated.

Pharmacological properties

Pharmacodynamic properties: Diprobase Ointment contains no active ingredients and has no pharmacological action. The ingredients have an emollient action on dry or chapped skin.

Pharmacokinetic properties: Not applicable due to topical administration and direct action on the skin.

Preclinical safety data: Not relevant.

Pharmaceutical particulars
List of excipients: White soft paraffin and liquid paraffin.

Incompatibilities: None known.

Shelf life: 60 months.

Special precautions for storage: Store below 25°C.

Nature and contents of containers: 50 gm epoxy lined aluminium tubes with plastic caps or polypropylene tubes.

Instructions for use/handling: Not applicable.

Marketing authorisation number PL 0201/0075

Date of (partial) revision of the text 29 April 1996

Legal category GSL

DIPROBATH*

Qualitative and quantitative composition Light Liquid Paraffin 46.0% w/w
Isopropyl Myristate 39.0% w/w
Laureth-4 15.0% w/w

Pharmaceutical form Liquid bath emollient.

Clinical particulars
Therapeutic indications: Treatment of dry skin conditions and other hyperkeratoses, including those associated with dermatitis and eczema.

To be diluted in bath water for external application.

Posology and method of administation:
Adults including elderly patients: 25 ml or approximately 2.5 capsful to be diluted in bath of water (100 l approximately). For particularly dry skin the quantity of oil emollient may be doubled.

Children: 10 ml or one capful is sufficient for children's baths.

Frequency and duration of bathing will depend on the type and severity of the conditions, but generally 2 to 3 baths should be taken weekly.

Contra-indications: Known hypersensitivity to any of the ingredients.

Special warnings and precautions for use: As Diprobath deposits a film of oil over the skin, care should be taken to avoid slipping in the bath.

The following warning will appear on the label: 'Take care when entering or leaving the bath which may be more slippery than usual'.

Interactions with other medicaments and other forms of interaction: None known.

Pregnancy and lactation: No special precautions.

Effects on ability to drive and use machines: None known.

Undesirable effects: None known.

Overdose: Not applicable.

Pharmacological properties
Pharmacodynamic properties: Both active ingredients have established emollient properties which are of relevance to use as a bathing emollient.

Pharmacokinetic properties: Pharmacokinetic principles are not involved due to direct topical application.

Preclinical safety data: There are no pre-clinical data of relevance to the prescriber which are additional to that already included in other sections of the SmPC.

Pharmaceutical particulars
List of excipients: Laureth-4.

Incompatibilities: None known.

Shelf life: 24 months.

Special precautions for storage: Store upright at a temperature below 30°C.

Nature and contents of containers: 500 ml natural opaque HDPE single neck container with polypropylene or urea/formaldehyde, steran or expanded polyethylene wadded screw cap.

Instructions for use/handling: Not applicable.

Marketing authorisation number PL 0201/0174

Date of (partial) revision of the text July 1996.

Legal category P

DIPROSALIC* OINTMENT
DIPROSALIC* SCALP APPLICATION

Qualitative and quantitative composition
Ointment: Betamethasone Dipropionate 0.064% w/w*
(* equivalent to 0.05% Betamethasone)
Salicylic Acid 3.00% w/w
Scalp Application: Betamethasone Dipropionate 0.064% w/w*
(* equivalent to 0.05% Betamethasone)
Salicylic Acid 2.00% w/w

Pharmaceutical form Ointment/Scalp application.

Clinical particulars
Therapeutic indications: Betamethasone dipropionate is a synthetic fluorinated corticosteroid. It is active topically and produces a rapid and sustained reponse in those inflammatory dermatoses that are normally responsive to topical corticosteroid therapy, and it is also effective in the less responsive conditions, such as psoriasis of the scalp, chronic plaque psoriasis of the hands and feet, but excluding widespread plaque psoriasis.

Topical salicylic acid softens keratin, loosens cornified epithelium and desquamates the epidermis.

Diprosalic presentations are therefore indicated for the treatment of hyperkeratotic and dry corticosteroid-responsive dermatoses where the cornified epithelium may resist penetration of the steroid. The salicyclic acid constituent of Diprosalic preparations, as a result of its descaling action, allows access of the dermis more rapidly than by applying steroid alone.

Posology and method of administration:
Adults: Once to twice daily. In most cases a thin film should be applied to cover the affected area twice daily.

For some patients adequate maintenance therapy may be achieved with less frequent application.

It is recommended that Diprosalic preparations are prescribed for two weeks, and that treatment is reviewed at that time. The maximum weekly dose should not exceed 60 g.

Children: Dosage in children should be limited to 5 days.

Contra-indications: Rosacea, acne, perioral dermatitis, perianal and genital pruritis. Hypersensitivity to any of the ingredients of the Diprosalic preparations contra-indicates their use as does tuberculous and most viral lesions of the skin, particularly herpes simplex, vacinia, varicella. Diprosalic should not be used in napkin eruptions, fungal or bacterial skin infections without suitable concomitant anti-infective therapy.

Special warnings and special precautions for use: Occlusion must not be used, since under these circumstances the keratolytic action of salicylic acid may lead to enhanced absorption of the steroid.

Local and systemic toxicity is common, especially following long continuous use on large areas of damaged skin, in flexures or with polythene occlusion. If used in children or on the face courses should be limited to five days. Long term continuous therapy should be avoided in all patients irrespective of age.

Topical corticosteroids may be hazardous in psoriasis for a number of reasons, including rebound relapses following development of tolerance, risk of generalised pustular psoriasis and local systemic toxicity due to impaired barrier function of the skin. Careful patient supervision is important.

It is dangerous if Diprosalic presentations come into contact with the eyes. Avoid contact with eyes and mucous membranes.

The systemic absorption of betamethasone dipropionate and salicylic acid may be increased if extensive body surface areas or skin folds are treated for prolonged periods or with excessive amounts of steroids. Suitable precautions should be taken in these circumstances, particularly with infants and children.

Interactions with other medicaments and other forms of interaction: None stated.

Pregnancy and lactation: There is inadequate evidence of safety in human pregnancy. Topical administration of corticosteroids to pregnant animals can cause abnormalities of foetal development, including cleft palate and intrauterine growth retardation. There may therefore be a very small risk of such effects in the human foetus.

Effects on ability to drive and use machines: None stated.

Undesirable effects: Diprosalic skin preparations are generally well tolerated and side-effects are rare. Continuous application without interruption may result in local atrophy of the skin, striae and superficial vascular dilation, particularly on the face.

In addition prolonged use of salicylic acid preparations may cause dermatitis.

Overdose: Excessive prolonged use of topical corticosteroids can suppress pituitary-adrenal functions resulting in secondary adrenal insufficiency which is usually reversible. In such cases appropriate symptomatic treatment is indicated.

With topical preparations containing salicylic acid excessive prolonged use may result in symptoms of salicylism. Treatment is symptomatic.

The steroid content of each tube is so low as to have little or no toxic effect in the unlikely event of accidental oral ingestion.

Pharmacological properties
Pharmacodynamic properties: Diprosalic preparations contain the dipropionate ester of betamethasone which is a glucocorticoid exhibiting the general properties of corticosteroids, and salicyclic acid which has keratolytic properties.

Salicyclic acid is applied topically in the treatment of hyperkeratotic and scaling conditions where its keratolytic action facilitates penetration of the corticosteroid.

In pharmacological doses, corticosteroids are used primarily for their anti-inflammatory and/or immune suppressive effects.

Topical corticosteroids such as betamethasone dipropionate are effective in the treatment of a range of dermatoses because of their anti-inflammatory, anti-pruritic and vasoconstrictive actions. However, while the physiologic, pharmacologic and clinical effects of the corticosteroids are well known, the exact mechanisms of their action in each disease are uncertain.

Pharmacodynamic properties: Salicyclic acid exerts only local action after topical application.

The extent of percutaneous absorption of topical corticosteroids is determined by many factors including vehicle, integrity of the epidermal barrier and the use of occlusive dressings. Topical corticosteroids can be absorbed through intact, normal skin. Inflammation and/or other disease processes in the skin may increase percutaneous absorption.

Occlusive dressings substantially increase the percutaneous absorption of topical corticosteroids.

Once absorbed through the skin, topical corticosteroids enter pharmacokinetic pathways similar to systemically administered corticosteroids. Corticosteroids are bound to plasma proteins in varying degrees, are metabolised primarily in the liver and excreted by the kidneys. Some of the topical corticosteroids and their metabolites are also excreted in the bile.

Preclinical safety data: There are no pre-clinical data of relevance to the prescriber which are additional to that already included in other sections of the SPC.

Pharmaceutical particulars
Lists of excipients:
Ointment: Liquid Paraffin and White Soft Paraffin.
Scalp application: Disodium edetate, hydroxypropyl methylcellulose, sodium hydroxide, isopropyl alcohol, purified water.

Incompatibilities: None stated.

Shelf life:
Ointment: 60 months
Scalp application: 36 months

Special precautions for storage: Store in a cool place.

Nature and contents of containers: Diprosalic Ointment: 30 or 100 gm epoxy-lined aluminimum tubes with plastic caps. Diprosalic Scalp Application: 100 ml polyethylene containers with polypropylene closures.

Instructions for use/handling: Not applicable.

Marketing authorisation numbers
Ointment: PL 0201/0070
Scalp Application: PL 0201/0069

Date of approval/revision of SmPC July 1997

Legal category POM

DIPROSONE* CREAM and OINTMENT

Qualitative and quantitative composition
Betamethasone Dipropionate 0.064% w/w*
(* equivalent to 0.05% Betamethasone)

Pharmaceutical form Cream/Ointment

Clinical particulars
Therapeutic indications: Betamethasone dipropionate is a synthetic fluorinated corticosteroid. It is active topically and produces a rapid and sustained response in eczema and dermatitis of all types, including atopic eczema, photodermatitis, lichen planus, lichen simplex, prurigo nodularis, discoid lupus erythematosus, necrobiosis lipoidica, pretibial myxoedema and erythroderma. It is also effective in the less responsive conditions such as psoriasis of the scalp and chronic plaque psoriasis of the hands and feet, but excluding widespread plaque psoriasis.

Posology and method of administration:
Adults and children: Once to twice daily. In most cases a thin film of Diprosone Cream or Ointment should be applied to cover the affected area twice daily. For some patients adequate maintenance therapy may be achieved with less frequent application.

Diprosone Cream is especially appropriate for moist or weeping surfaces and the ointment for dry, lichenified or scaly lesions but this is not invariably so.

Control over the dosage regimen may be achieved during intermittent and maintenance therapy by using Diprobase Cream or Ointment (PL 0201/0076 and

0201/0075), the base vehicles of Diprosone Cream and Ointment. Such control may be necessary in mild and improving dry skin conditions requiring low dose steroid treatment.

Contra-indications: Rosacea, acne, perioral dermatitis, perianal and genital pruritis. Hypersensitivity to any of the ingredients of the Diprosone preparations contra-indicates their use as does tuberculous and most viral lesions of the skin, particularly herpes simplex, vacinia, varicella. Diprosone should not be used in napkin eruptions, fungal or bacterial skin infections without suitable concomitant anti-infective therapy.

Special warnings and special precautions for use: Local and systemic toxicity is common, especially following long continuous use on large areas of damaged skin, in flexures or with polythene occlusion. If used in children or on the face courses should be limited to 5 days. Long term continuous therapy should be avoided in all patients irrespective of age.

Occlusion must not be used.

Topical corticosteroids may be hazardous in psoriasis for a number of reasons, including rebound relapses following development of tolerance, risk of generalised pustular psoriasis and local systemic toxicity due to impaired barrier function of the skin. Careful patient supervision is important.

Interactions: None stated.

Pregnancy and lactation: There is inadequate evidence of safety in human pregnancy. Topical administration of corticosteroids to pregnant animals can cause abnormalities of foetal development, including cleft palate and intrauterine growth retardation. There may therefore, be a very small risk of such effects in the human foetus.

Effects on ability to drive and use machines: None stated.

Undesirable effects: Diprosone skin preparations are generally well tolerated and side-effects are rare. The systemic absorption of betamethasone dipropionate may be increased if extensive body surface areas or skin folds are treated for prolonged periods or with excessive amounts of steroids. Suitable precautions should be taken in these circumstances, particularly with infants and children.

Continuous application without interruption may result in local atrophy of the skin, striae and superficial vascular dilatation, particularly on the face.

Overdosage: Excessive prolonged use of topical corticosteroids can suppress pituitary-adrenal functions resulting in secondary adrenal insufficiency which is usually reversible. In such cases appropriate symptomatic treatment is indicated.

The steroid content of each tube is so low as to have little or no toxic effect in the unlikely event of accidental oral ingestion.

Pharmacological properties

Pharmacodynamic properties: Diprosone preparations contain the dipropionate ester of betamethasone which is a glucocorticoid exhibiting the general properties of corticosteroids.

In pharmacological doses, corticosteroids are used primarily for their anti-inflammatory and/or immune suppressive effects.

Topical corticosteroids such as betamethsone dipropionate are effective in the treatment of a range of dermatoses because of their anti-inflammatory, antipruritic and vasoconstrictive actions. However, while the physiologic, pharmacologic and clinical effects of the corticosteroids are well known, the exact mechanisms of their action in each disease are uncertain.

Pharmacokinetic properties: The extent of percutaneous absorption of topical corticosteroids is determined by many factors including vehicle, integrity of the epidermal barrier and the use of occlusive dressings.

Topical corticosteroids can be absorbed through intact, normal skin. Inflammation and/or other disease processes in the skin may increase percutaneous absorption. Occlusive dressings substantially increase the percutaneous absorption of topical corticosteroids.

Once absorbed through the skin, topical corticosteroids enter pharmacokinetic pathways similar to systemically administered corticosteroids. Corticosteroids are bound to plasma proteins in varying degrees, are metabolised primarily in the liver and excreted by the kidneys. Some of the topical corticosteroids and their metabolites are also excreted in the bile.

Preclinical safety data: There are no pre-clinical data of relevance to the prescriber which are additional to that already included in other sections of the SPC.

Pharmaceutical particulars

List of excipients: Diprosone Cream: Chlorocresol, Sodium dihydrogen phosphate, Phospatic Acid, White Petrolatum, Mineral Oil, Cetomacrogol 1000, Cetostearyl Alcohol and Purified Water; Diprosone Ointment: Mineral oil and white petrolatum.

Incompatibilties: None known.

Shelf life: 60 months.

Special precautions for storage: Store in a cool place.

Nature and contents of containers: 30 or 100 g epoxy-lined aluminimum tubes with polypropylene caps.

Instructions for use/handling: Not applicable.

Marketing authorisation numbers

Cream: PL 0201/0072
Ointment: PL 0201/0074

Date of approval/revision of SmPC July 1997

Legal category POM

DIPROSONE* LOTION

Qualitative and quantitative composition

Betamethasone 0.064% w/w*
(* equivalent to 0.05% Betamethasone)

Pharmaceutical form Lotion

Clinical particulars

Therapeutic indications: Diprosone Lotion is indicated for eczema and dermatitis of all types effecting the scalp including atopic eczema, photodermatitis, primary irritant and allergic dermatitis, lichen planus, lichen simplex, discoid lupus erythematous, erythroderma.

It is also indicated for psoriasis of the scalp.

Posology and method of administration:

Adults and children: A few drops of Diprosone Lotion should be applied to the affected areas twice daily and massaged gently and thoroughly into the affected area. For some patients adequate maintenance therapy may be achieved with less frequent application.

Contra-indications: Rosacea, acne, perioral dermatitis, perianal and genital pruritis. Hypersensitivity to any of the ingredients of the Diprosone preparations contra-indicates their use as does tuberculous and most viral lesions of the skin, particularly herpes simplex, vacinia, varicella. Diprosone should not be used in napkin eruptions, fungal or bacterial skin infections without suitable concomitant anti-infective therapy.

Special warnings and special precautions for use: Local and systemic toxicity is common, especially following long continuous use on large areas of damaged skin, in flexures or with polythene occlusion. If used in children or on the face courses should be limited to 5 days. Long term continuous therapy should be avoided in all patients irrespective of age.

Occlusion must not be used.

Topical corticosteroids may be hazardous in psoriasis for a number of reasons, including rebound relapses following development of tolerance, risk of generalised pustular psoriasis and local systemic toxicity due to impaired barrier function of the skin. Careful patient supervision is important.

Interactions: None stated.

Pregnancy and lactation: There is inadequate evidence of safety in human pregnancy. Topical administration of corticosteroids to pregnant animals can cause abnormalities of foetal development, including cleft palate and intrauterine growth retardation. There may therefore, be a very small risk of such effects in the human foetus.

Effects on ability to drive and use machines: None stated.

Undesirable effects: Diprosone skin preparations are generally well tolerated and side-effects are rare. The systemic absorption of betamethasone dipropionate may be increased if extensive body surface areas or skin folds are treated for prolonged periods or with excessive amounts of steroids. Suitable precautions should be taken in these circumstances, particularly with infants and children.

Continuous application without interruption may result in local atrophy of the skin, striae and superficial vascular dilatation, particularly on the face.

Overdosage: Excessive prolonged use of topical corticosteroids can suppress pituitary-adrenal functions resulting in secondary adrenal insufficiency which is usually reversible. In such cases appropriate symptomatic treatment is indicated.

The steroid content of each tube is so low as to have little or no toxic effect in the unlikely event of accidental oral ingestion.

Pharmacological properties

Pharmacodynamic properties: Diprosone preparations contain the dipropionate ester of betamethasone which is a glucocorticoid exhibiting the general properties of corticosteroids.

In pharmacological doses, corticosteroids are used primarily for their anti-inflammatory and/or immune suppressive effects.

Topical corticosteroids such as betamethsone dipropionate are effective in the treatment of a range of dermatoses because of their anti-inflammatory, antipruritic and vasoconstrictive actions. However, while the physiologic, pharmacologic and clinical effects of the corticosteroids are well known, the exact mechanisms of their action in each disease are uncertain.

Pharmacokinetic properties: The extent of percutaneous absorption of topical corticosteroids is determined by many factors including vehicle, integrity of the epidermal barrier and the use of occlusive dressings.

Topical corticosteroids can be absorbed through intact, normal skin. Inflammation and/or other disease processes in the skin may increase percutaneous absorption. Occlusive dressings substantially increase the percutaneous absorption of topical corticosteroids.

Once absorbed through the skin, topical corticosteroids enter pharmacokinetic pathways similar to systemically administered corticosteroids. Corticosteroids are bound to plasma proteins in varying degrees, are metabolised primarily in the liver and excreted by the kidneys. Some of the topical corticosteroids and their metabolites are also excreted in the bile.

Preclinical safety data: There are no pre-clinical data of relevance to the prescriber which are additional to that already included in other sections of the SPC.

Pharmaceutical particulars

List of excipients: Carbomer, Isopropyl Alcohol, Sodium Hydroxide and Purified Water.

Incompatibilties: None known.

Shelf life: 36 months.

Special precautions for storage: Store in a cool place.

Nature and contents of containers: Polyethylene containers of 30 or 100 ml with polypropylene closures.

Instructions for use/handling: Not applicable.

Marketing authorisation number PL 0201/0073

Date of approval/revision of SmPC July 1997

Legal category POM

DROGENIL* TABLETS

Qualitative and quantitative composition Flutamide (INN) 250 mg.

Pharmaceutical form Tablets.

Clinical particulars

Therapeutic indications: Treatment of advanced prostatic carcinoma in which suppression of testosterone effects is indicated; as initial treatment in combination with an LHRH agonist, as adjunctive therapy in patients already receiving LHRH agonist therapy; in surgically castrated patients; in the treatment of patients who have not responded to other form of hormonal manipulation or in patients who cannot tolerate such treatment.

In combination with LHRH agonists for the management of locally confined B2–C2 (T2b–T4) prostate carcinoma as initial therapy; bulky primary tumours confined to the prostate (stage B2 or T2b) or extending beyond the capsule (stage C or T3–T4), with or without pelvic node involvement.

Posology and method of administration:

Dosage: One 250 mg tablet three times daily at 8 hour intervals.

Route of administration: Oral.

When used as an initial treatment with an LHRH agonist, a greater reduction in the incidence and severity of the LHRH agonist flare reaction may be achieved if flutamide is introduced before rather than concomitantly with the agonist. It is, therefore, recommended that flutamide one tablet three times daily should be started at least three days prior to initiation of the LHRH agonist and continued thereafter at the same dose.

In the management of locally confined prostatic carcinoma, the recommended dosage is one 250 mg tablet three times a day. DROGENIL should be started at least three days prior to initiation of the LHRH agonist. Administration of DROGENIL and the LHRH agonist should begin eight weeks prior to radiation therapy and continue through the course of radiation therapy (usually approx. 8 weeks) i.e. a total of approximately 16 weeks.

Dosage adjustment in renal or liver insufficiency: In patients with impaired liver function, long-term treatment with flutamide should only be administered after careful assessment of the individual benefits and risks.

Monitoring advice: Flutamide is highly protein bound and will not be removed by dialysis.

Contra-indications: Patients exhibiting sensitivity reactions to flutamide or any component of this preparation.

Special warnings and precautions for use: Hepatic injury: Transaminase abnormalities, cholestatic jaundice, hepatic necrosis, and hepatic encephalopathy have been reported with the use of flutamide. The hepatic conditions were usually reversible after discontinuing therapy or dosage reduction, although there have been occasional reports of a fatal outcome following severe hepatic injury in patients receiving flutamide. Periodic liver function tests should be considered in all patients and performed in patients on long-term treatment. Appropriate laboratory testing should be done at the first symptom/sign of liver dysfunction (e.g., pruritis, dark urine, persistent anorexia, jaundice, right upper quadrant tenderness or unexplained 'flue-like' symptoms). If the patient has laboratory evidence of liver injury or jaundice, in the absence of biopsy-confirmed liver metastases, DROGENIL therapy should be discontinued or the dosage reduced.

In addition, in patients who have not received medical or surgical castration periodic sperm count determinations may be considered during long-term treatment. In such patients, flutamide administration tends to elevate plasma testosterone and estradiol levels. Fluid retention may occur thus the drug should be used with caution in cardiac disease.

Interactions with other medicaments and other forms of interaction: Increases in prothrombin time have been reported in patients receiving long-term warfarin therapy after flutamide monotherapy was initiated. Therefore, close monitoring of prothrombin time is recommended. Adjustment of the anticoagulant dose may be necessary when flutamide is administered concomitantly with warfarin.

Pregnancy and lactation: DROGENIL is indicated only for use in male patients. No studies have been conducted in pregnant or lactating women. Therefore, the possibility that DROGENIL may cause foetal harm if administered to a pregnant woman, or may be present in the breast milk of a lactating woman, must be considered.

Effects on ability to drive and use machines: Flutamide is presumed to be safe, or unlikely to produce an effect.

Undesirable effects: Monotherapy: In clinical studies, the most frequently reported adverse reactions to DROGENIL Tablets are gynecomastia and/or breast tenderness, sometimes accompanied by galactorrhea. These reactions disappear upon discontinuation of treatment or reduction in dosage.

DROGENIL Tablets demonstrate a low potential for cardiovascular liability, and when compared to diethylstilbestrol this liability has been shown to be significantly lower. Less frequent adverse reactions: diarrhoea, nausea, vomiting, increased appetite, insomnia, tiredness, transient abnormal liver function and hepatitis (see *Additional adverse experiences* and *Special warnings*).

Rare adverse reactions: decreased libido, upset stomach, anorexia, ulcer-like pain, heartburn, constipation, oedema, ecchymoses, herpes zoster, pruritis, lupus-like syndrome, headache, dizziness, weakness, malaise, blurred vision, thirst, chest pain, anxiety, depression, lymphoedema.

Reduced sperm counts have been reported rarely.

Combination therapy: In clinical studies, the most frequently reported adverse effects experienced during combination therapy of DROGENIL Tablets with LHRH agonist were hot flushes, decreased libido, impotence, diarrhoea, nausea and vomiting. With the exception of diarrhoea, these adverse experiences are known to occur with LHRH agonist alone, and at comparable frequency.

The high incidence of gynecomastia observed with flutamide monotherapy was reduced greatly in combination therapy. In clinical trials, no significant difference in gynecomastia incidence was observed between the placebo- and the flutamide-LHRH agonist treatment groups.

Rarely, patients experienced anaemia, leukopenia, unspecified gastro-intestinal disorders, anorexia, injection site irritation and rash, oedema, neuromuscular symptoms, jaundice, genitourinary tract symptoms, hypertension, central nervous system adverse events (drowsiness, depression, confusion, anxiety, nervousness) and thrombocytopenia.

Very rarely, pulmonary symptoms, hepatitis and photosensitivity have occurred.

Additional adverse experiences: In addition, the following adverse experiences have been reported during worldwide marketing of DROGENIL Tablets: haemolytic anaemia, macrocytic anaemia, methemoglobinemia, photosensitivity reactions – including erythema, ulcerations, bullous eruptions, and epidermal necrolysis – and change in urine colour to amber or yellow-green appearance, which can be attributed to flutamide and/or its metabolites.

Also observed were cholestatic jaundice, hepatic encephalopathy and hepatic necrosis. The hepatic conditions were usually reversible after discontinuing therapy; however, there have been reports of death following severe hepatic injury associated with use of flutamide.

Two reports of malignant male breast neoplasms in patients dosed with DROGENIL have been reported. One involved aggravation of a pre-existing nodule which was first detected three or four months before initiation of DROGENIL monotherapy in a patient with benign prostatic hypertrophy. After excision, this was diagnosed as a poorly differentiated ductal carcinoma. The other report involved gynecomastia and a nodule noted two and six months, respectively, after initiation of DROGENIL monotherapy for treatment of advanced prostatic carcinoma. Nine months after the initiation of therapy the nodule was excised and diagnosed as a moderately differentiated invasive ductal tumour staged T4NOMO, G3, no metastases had advanced.

Abnormal laboratory test values reported include changes in liver function, elevated blood urea nitrogen (BUN) and rarely, elevated serum creatinine values.

Usually these reactions have not been of sufficient severity to require dosage reduction or discontinuation of therapy.

Overdose: In animal studies with flutamide alone, signs of overdose included hypoactivity, piloerection, slow respiration, ataxia and/or lacrimation, anorexia, tranquilization, emesis and methemoglobinemia.

The single dose of flutamide ordinarily associated with symptoms of overdose of considered to be life-threatening has not been established. One patient survived after taking more than 5 g as a single dose – no adverse effects were observed.

Since flutamide is highly protein bound, dialysis may not be of any use as treatment for overdose.

Pharmacological properties

Pharmacodynamic properties: Flutamide is an anilide, nonsteroidal oral antiandrogen. In animal studies flutamide demonstrates potent antiandrogenic effects. It exerts its antiandrogenic action by inhibiting androgen uptake and/or by inhibiting nuclear binding in target tissues. When flutamide is given in combination with surgical or medical castration, suppression of both testicular and adrenal androgen activity is achieved.

Pharmacokinetic properties: Flutamide is well absorbed following oral ingestion. Studies with radiolabelled flutamide show rapid and extensive conversion to its metabolites which are detectable in plasma up to 8 hours post dosing. Approximately 45% of the administered dose is excreted in urine and 2% in faeces during the first two days. Metabolism removes the radiolabel resulting in apparent slowing of excretion due to retention of the label as tritiated water. Thus excretion and metabolism is essentially complete within two days.

Preclinical safety data: Animal studies to determine tolerance after repeated administration have been performed in monkeys for up to 6 weeks, in rats for up to 52 weeks and in dogs for up to 78 weeks. The daily administered oral doses were up to 90 mg/kg in monkeys, up to 40 mg/kg in dogs and up to 180 mg/kg in rats, corresponding to 1.5 to 18 fold of the dose used in humans. In addition to weight loss and anorexia which occurred in all animal species, vomiting was observed in dogs and monkeys. All other clinical findings showed no abnormalities. The autopsy finding revealed a reduced size of the prostate, testicles and seminal vesicles with suppressed spermatogenesis which correspond to the antiandrogenic effect of flutamide. In addition, an increase in organ weight of the liver in rats and dogs, and increased transaminase levels in dogs were observed without corresponding morphological changes. In rats only, the occurrence of drug-related (but not dose-dependent) adenomas of testicular interstitial cells was observed. This effect is related to the mechanism of action of flutamide and is species-specific. In a long-term study in rats, dose-related increases in mammary gland adenomas or carcinomas were observed.

Mutagenicity: In a range of screening tests flutamide did not show any mutagenic potential.

Reproduction toxicity: The influence of flutamide on fertility and the development of the progeny has been studied in rats; additional teratogenicity studies have been performed in rabbits. The effects were related to the antiandrogenic actions of flutamide. These effects are not relevant to the clinical use of flutamide in prostate cancer.

Pharmaceutical particulars

List of excipients: Lactose, sodium lauryl sulphate, microcrystalline cellulose, starch, silica gel, magnesium stearate.

Incompatibilities: None known.

Shelf life: 60 months.

Special precautions for storage: Store below 25°C. Protect from light.

Nature and contents of container: Calendar packs of 84 tablets OP.

Instructions for use/handling: None.

Marketing authorisation number PL 0201/0062

Date of (partial) revision of the text 23 September 1996

Legal category POM

ELOCON* CREAM
ELOCON* OINTMENT

Qualitative and quantitative composition Mometasone Furoate 0.1% w/w.

Pharmaceutical form Cream/Ointment.

Clinical particulars

Therapeutic indications: Elocon Cream and Ointment are indicated for the treatment of inflammatory and pruritic manifestations of psoriasis (excluding widespread plaque psoriasis) and atopic dermatitis.

Posology and method of administration:

Adults, including elderly patients and children: A thin film of Elocon Cream or Ointment should be applied to the affected areas of skin once daily.

Use of topical corticosteroids in children or on the face should be limited to the least amount compatible with an effective therapeutic regimen and duration of treatment should be no more than 5 days.

Contra-indications: Elocon is contra-indicated in facial rosacea, acne vulgaris, perioral dermatitis, perianal and genital pruritus, napkin eruptions, bacterial (e.g. impetigo), viral (e.g. herpes simplex, herpes zoster and chickenpox) and fungal (e.g. candida or dermatophyte) infections, varicella, tuberculosis, syphilis or post-vaccine reactions. Elocon should not be used in patients who are sensitive to mometasone furoate, or to other corticosteroids.

Special warnings and precautions for use: If irritation or sensitisation develop with the use of Elocon, treatment should be withdrawn and appropriate therapy instituted.

Should an infection develop, use of an appropriate antifungal or antibacterial agent should be instituted. If a favourable response does not occur promptly, the corticosteroid should be discontinued until the infection is adequately controlled.

Local and systemic toxicity is common especially following long continued use on large areas of damaged skin, in flexures and with polythene occlusion. If used in childhood, or on the face, courses should be limited to 5 days and occlusion should not be used. Long term continuous therapy should be avoided in all patients irrespective of age.

Topical steroids may be hazardous in psoriasis for a number of reasons including rebound relapses following development of tolerance, risk of centralised pustular psoriasis and development of local or systemic toxicity due to impaired barrier function of the skin. If used in psoriasis careful patient supervision is important.

Elocon topical preparations are not for ophthalmic use.

Interactions with other medicaments and other forms of interaction: None stated.

Pregnancy and lactation: There is inadequate evidence of safety in human pregnancy. Topical administration of corticosteroids to pregnant animals can cause abnormalities of foetal development including cleft palate and intra-uterine growth retardation. There may therefore be a very small risk of such effects in the human foetus.

It is not known whether topical administration of corticosteroids could result in sufficient systemic absorption to produce detectable quantities in breast milk. Elocon should be administered to nursing mothers only after careful consideration of the benefit/risk relationship.

Effects on ability to drive and use machines: None stated.

Undesirable effects: Local adverse reactions, occasionally reported with Elocon included paresthesia, folliculitis, burning, pruritus, tingling, stinging, allergic contact dermatitis, hypopigmentation, hypertrichosis, secondary infection, striae, acneiform reactions and signs of skin atrophy.

Local adverse reactions reported infrequently with other topical corticosteroids include: irritation, perioral dermatitis, maceration of the skin and miliaria.

Paediatric patients may demonstrate greater susceptibility to topical cosrticosteroid-induced hypothalamic-pituitary-adrenal axis suppression and Cushing's syndrome than mature patients because of a larger skin surface area to body weight ratio. Chronic corticosteroid therapy may interfere with the growth and development of children.

Overdose: None stated.

Pharmacological properties

Pharmacodynamic properties: Mometasone furoate exhibits marked anti-inflammatory activity and marked anti-psoriatic activity in standard animal predictive models.

In the croton oil assay in mice, mometasone was equipotent to betamethasone valerate after single application and about 8 times as potent after five applications.

In guinea pigs, mometasone was approximately twice as potent as betamethasone valerate in reducing m.ovalis-induced epidermal acanthosis (i.e. anti-psoriatic activity) after 14 applications.

Pharmacokinetic properties: Pharmacokinetic studies have indicated that systemic absorption following topical application of mometasone furoate cream 0.1% is minimal, approximately 0.4% of the applied dose in man, the majority of which is excreted within 72 hours following application. Characterisation of metabolites was not feasible owing to the small amounts present in plasma and excreta.

Preclinical safety data: There are no pre-clinical data of relevance to the prescriber which are additional to that already included in other sections of the SPC.

Pharmaceutical particulars

List of excipients: Cream: Hexylene glycol; phosphoric acid; propylene glycolstearate; stearyl alcohol and ceteareth-20; titanium dioxide; aluminium starch octenylsuccinate; white wax; white petrolatum; purified water.

Ointment: Hexylene glycol; phosphoric acid; propylene glycolstearate; white wax; white petrolatum; purified water.

Incompatibilities: None known.

Shelf life: 36 months.

Special precautions for storage: Store between 2 and 30°C.

Nature and contents of container: 30 and 100 gm aluminium tubes with low density polyethylene cap or laminated tubes with high density polyethylene head and polypropylene cap.

Instructions for use/handling: Not applicable.

Marketing authorisation numbers

Elocon Cream PL 0201/0117
Elocon Ointment PL 0201/0118

Date of (partial) revision of the text January 1996

Legal category POM

ELOCON* SCALP LOTION

Qualitative and quantitative composition Mometasone Furoate 0.1% w/w.

Pharmaceutical form Lotion.

Clinical particulars

Therapeutic indications: Elocon Scalp Lotion is indicated for the treatment of inflammatory and pruritic manifestations of psoriasis and seborrhoeic dermatitis of the scalp.

Posology and method of administration:

Adults, including elderly patients and children: A few drops of Elocon Scalp Lotion should be applied to affected scalp sites, once daily; massage gently and thoroughly until the medication disappears.

Use of topical corticosteroids in children should be limited to the least amount compatible with an effective therapeutic regimen and duration of treatment should be no more than 5 days.

Contra-indications: Elocon Scalp Lotion is contraindicated in bacterial (e.g. impetigo), viral (e.g. herpes simplex, herpes zoster and chickenpox) and fungal (e.g. candida or dermatophyte) infections of the scalp. Elocon Scalp Lotion should not be used in patients who are sensitive to mometasone furoate or to other corticosteroids.

Special warmings and precautions for use: If irritation or sensitisation develop with the use of Elocon, treatment should be withdrawn and appropriate therapy instituted.

Should an infection develop, use of an appropriate antifungal or antibacterial agent should be instituted. If a favourable response does not occur promptly, the corticosteroid should be discontinued until the infection is adequately controlled.

Local and systemic toxicity is common especially following long continued use on large areas of damaged skin. If used in childhood, courses should be limited to 5 days. Long term continuous therapy should be avoided in all patients irrespective of age.

Topical steroids may be hazardous in psoriasis for a number of reasons including rebound relapses following development of tolerance, risk of centralised pustular psoriasis and development of local or systemic toxicity due to impaired barrier function of the skin. If used in psoriasis careful patient supervision is important.

Care must be taken to keep the preparation away from the eyes.

Interactions with other medicments and other forms of interaction: None known.

Pregnancy and lactation: There is inadequate evidence of safety in human pregnancy. Topical administration of corticosteroids to pregnant animals can cause abnormalities of foetal development including cleft palate and intra-uterine growth retardation. There may therefore be a very small risk of such effects in the human foetus.

It is not known whether topical administration of corticosteroids could result in sufficient systemic absorption to produce detectable quantities in breast milk. Elocon should be administered to pregnant women or nursing mothers only after careful consideration of the benefit/risk relationship.

Effects on ability to drive and and machines: None known.

Undesirable effects: Local adverse reactions occasionally reported with Elocon included paresthesia, folliculitis, burning, pruritus, tingling, stinging, allergic contact dermatitis, hypopigmentation, hypertrichosis, secondary infection, striae, acneiform reactions and signs of skin atrophy.

Local adverse reactions reported infrequently with other topical corticosteroids include: irritation, perioral dermatitis, maceration of the skin and miliaria.

Paediatric patients may demonstrate greater susceptibility to topical cosrticosteroid-induced hypothalamic-pituitary-adrenal axis suppression and Cushing's syndrome than mature patients because of a larger skin surface area to body weight ratio. Chronic corticosteroid therapy may interfere with the growth and development of children.

Overdose: Excessive prolonged use of topical corticosteroids can suppress pituitary-adrenal function resulting in secondary adrenal insufficiency which is usually reversible. In such cases appropriate symptomatic treatment is indicated.

The steroid content of each container is so low as to have little or no toxic effect in the unlikely event of accidental oral ingestion.

Pharmacological properties

Pharmacodynamic properties: Mometasone furoate exhibits marked anti-inflammatory activity and marked anti-psoriatic activity in standard animal predictive models.

In the croton oil assay in mice, mometasone was equipotent to betamethasone valerate after single application and about 8 times as potent after five applications.

In guinea pigs, mometasone was approximately twice as potent as betamethasone valerate in reducing m.ovalis-induced epidermal acanthosis (i.e. anti-psoriatic activity) after 14 applications.

Pharmacokinetic properties: Pharmacokinetic studies have indicated that systemic absorption following topical application of mometasone furoate cream 0.1% is minimal, approximately 0.4% of the applied dose in man, the majority of which is excreted within 72 hours following application. Characterisation of metabolites was not feasible owing to the small amounts present in plasma and excreta.

Preclinical safety data: There are no pre-clinical data of relevance to the prescriber which are additional to that already included in other sections of the SPC.

Pharmaceutical particulars

List of excipients: Isopropyl alcohol; propylene glycol; hydroxypropyl cellulose; sodium phosphate monomasic monohydrate; phosphoric acid; purified water.

Incompatibilities: None known.

Shelf life: 36 months.

Special precautions for storage: Store below 25°C.

Nature and contents of container: 30 ml white HDPE bottle with LDPE dropper and white HDPE cap.

Instructions for use/handling: Not applicable.

Marketing authorisation number PL 0201/0156

Date of revision of SmPC June 1997

Legal category POM

ETHYOL* (amifostine)

Qualitative and quantitative composition

Composition of amifostine for injection

Name of ingredient	Formulation		Function
	% w/w	mg/vial	
Amifostine	100	500	Active Ingredient

Note: Amifostine is expressed on an anhydrous basis.

Pharmaceutical form Ethyol (amifostine) lypholised powder for Injection is prepared as a sterile lypholised powder requiring reconstitution with 9.7 ml of sterile 0.9% sodium chloride solution before intravenous infusion.

Clinical particulars

Therapeutic indications: Ethyol is indicated to reduce the neutropenia related risk of infection (e.g. neutropenic fever) due to the combination regimen cyclophosphamided and cisplatinum in patients with advanced (FIGO stage III or IV) ovarian carcinoma.

Ethyol is indicated to protect patients with advanced solid tumours of non-germ cell origin from cumulative nephrotoxicity of cisplatin and cisplatin-containing regimens, where unit doses of cisplatin range from 60–120 mg/m², in conjunction with adequate hydration measures.

Posology and method of administration: Prior to intravenous administration, Ethyol for Injection is reconstituted with 9.7 ml of sterile 0.9% sodium chloride solution. The reconstituted solution (500 mg of amifostine/10 ml) may be kept 6 hours at room temperature (up to 25°C) or 24 hours under refrigeration (2°–8°C).

In patients with advanced ovarian carcinoma receiving the combination regimen of cisplatin and cyclophosphamide, the recommended starting dose of Ethyol is 910 mg/m² administered once daily as a 15-minute IV infusion starting within 30 minutes prior to chemotherapy with agents given by short infusion.

If Ethyol is intended to reduce nephrotoxicity associated with cisplatin, then the starting dose of Ethyol should be correlated with the dose and schedule of cisplatin. For cisplatin doses of 100–120 mg/m², the recommended starting dose of Ethyol is 910 mg/m² administered as a 15-minute infusion starting within 30 minutes prior to chemotherapy.

If the dose of cisplatin is less than 100 mg/m², but greater than or equal to 60 mg/m², the recommended starting dose of Ethyol is 740 mg/m² administered as a 15-minute infusion starting within 30 minutes prior to chemotherapy.

The 15-minute infusion for the 740–910 mg/m² dose is reportedly better tolerated than more extended infusion durations. Further reduced infusion times have not been systematically explored.

During the infusion of Ethyol, arterial blood pressure should be monitored.

The infusion of Ethyol should be stopped if the systolic blood pressure decreases significantly from the baseline value as listed in the following guideline:

Guideline for interrupting amifostine infusion due to decrease in systolic blood pressure

	Baseline systolic blood pressure (mm Hg)				
	<100	100–119	120–139	140–179	≥180
Decrease in systolic blood pressure during infusion of amifostine (mm Hg)	20	25	30	40	50

If the blood pressure returns to normal within 5 minutes and the patient is asymptomatic, the infusion may be restarted so that the full dose of Ethyol may be administered. If the full dose of Ethyol cannot be administered, the dose of Ethyol for subsequent cycles should be reduced by 20%. For example, the 910 mg/m² dose would be reduced to 740 mg/m².

It is recommended that antiemetic medication including dexamethasone 20 mg IV and a 5-HT3 antagonist be administered prior to and in conjunction with amifostine especially when used with strongly emetogenic chemotherapy such as cisplatin.

Ethyol should be used under the supervision of physicians experienced in cancer chemotherapy.

Contra-indications: Known sensitivity to aminothiol compounds. Patients who are hypotensive or in a state of dehydration should not receive Ethyol.

As Ethyol is to be administered in conjunction with drugs that are known teratogens and mutagens, therapy should not be administered to pregnant or lactating women.

Due to lack of experience in patients with renal or hepatic impairment, children or patients older than 70 years of age, Ethyol is contra-indicated in these groups.

Special warnings and special precautions for use: Patients should be hydrated adequately prior to Ethyol infusion and kept in a supine position during the infusion of Ethyol reconstituted solution and blood pressure should be monitored during the infusion. Guidelines for interrupting and re-starting amifostine infusion in case of decrease in systolic blood pressure are given (see *Posology and method of administration*). If hypotension occurs, patients should be placed in the Trendelenburg position and be given an infusion of normal saline. It is important that the infusion of the recommended dose (740–910 mg/m²) be given over 15 minutes. The administration of amifostine as a longer infusion is associated with a higher incidence of side effects.

It is recommended that an antiemetic regimen including dexamethasone 20 mg IV and a 5-HT3 antagonist be administered prior and in conjunction with amifostine, especially when used with strongly emetogenic chemotherapy such as cisplatin.

When amifostine is administered with highly emetogenic chemotherapy, the fluid balance of the patient should be monitored carefully.

Antihypertensive therapy should be interrupted 24 hours prior to the administration of amifostine and these patients should be monitored carefully during treatment.

Although reports of clinically relevant hypocalcemia are very rare, calcium serum levels should be monitored in patients at risk of hypocalcemia, such as those with nephrotic syndrome. If necessary, calcium supplements may be administered as needed. Caution should be exercised during treatment of patients receiving hypocalcemic agents.

No experience is available for the usage of Ethyol in children as well as patients older than 70 years. Similarly, use of amifostine in patients with patients with severe hepatic or renal impairment is not documented. Hence Ethyol should not be used in children, the elderly (more than 70 years) or patients with renal or hepatic impairment (see *Contra-indications*).

Interaction with other medicaments and other forms of interaction: Limited experience from interaction studies is available. The rapid clearance of amifostine from the plasma minimises the risk of interaction between amifostine and other drugs.

Special consideration should be given with respect to the concurrent administration of Ethyol with antihypertensive medication or other drugs that could potentiate hypotension.

Pregnancy and lactation: It is not known if amifostine or its metabolites is excreted into human breast milk. Therefore, it is recommended that breast feeding be discontinued prior to the initiation of Ethyol therapy.

While Ethyol has been shown to have dose related embryotoxicity in rats at doses greater than 200 mg/kg, it is not teratogenic. There are no studies in pregnant women. As this drug is administered in conjunction with known teratogenic agents, this therapy should not be administered to pregnant women. If the patient becomes pregnant while receiving this therapy, the patient should be appraised of the potential hazard to the foetus.

Effects on ability to drive and use machines: There is no intrinsic central nervous system toxicity associated with Ethyol administration, but as it is to be administered with chemotherapy and antiemetic regimens, the total therapy regimen might inhibit the patient's ability to competently drive or operate machinery.

Undesirable effects: Hypotension, as manifested by a transient reduction in systolic blood pressure and less frequently by a decrease in diastolic blood pressure, has been reported. The median time to onset was 13 minutes into the 15-minute period of amifostine infusion, and the median duration was 5 minutes. In some cases, the infusion had to be prematurely terminated due to a more pronounced drop in systolic blood pressure. In these cases, the blood pressure returned to normal within 5–15 minutes. Short term and rapidly reversible loss of consciousness has been very rarely reported.

Clinical symptoms of hypotension are quickly reversed by fluid infusion and postural management of the patient. If the blood pressure returns to normal within 5 minutes and the patient is asymptomatic, the infusion may be restarted, so that the full dose of Ethyol can be administered.

Nausea and/or vomiting are frequently reported. Amifostine increased the incidence of mild to moderate nausea/vomiting on day 1 of chemotherapy. However, amifostine does not increase the incidence of delayed nausea and vomiting induced by cisplatin-based chemotherapy. It is recomnmended that an antiemetic regimen including dexamethasone 20 mg IV and a 5-HT3 receptor antagonist be administered prior to and in conjunction with Ethyol.

Other effects which have been described during or following Ethyol infusion are flushing/feeling of warmth, chills/feeling of coldness, dizziness, somnolence, hiccups and sneezing.

Decrease in serum calcium concentrations is a known pharmacological effect of Ethyol. At the recommended doses, no clinically relevant manifestations of hypocalcemia has been reported. However, clinical hypocalcemia has occurred very rarely in patients who received multiple doses of Ethyol within 24 hours.

Allergic reactions, ranging from mild skin rashes to rigors, have occurred in some patients. There has been no reported occurrence of anaphylaxis with Ethyol.

Overdose: In Phase I trials, the maximum single dose of Ethyol administered was 1300 mg/m². No information is available on single doses higher than this in adults. In the setting of a clinical trial, children have received single doses of Ethyol up to 2.7 g/m² with no untoward effects. Multiple doses (up to three times the recommended single dose of 740–910 mg/m²) have been safely administered within a 24-hour period under study conditions. Following the repeated administration of Ethyol at 2 and 4 hours after the initial dose, there has not been any evidence of increased or cumulative side effects, especially nausea and vomiting or hypotension. The most likely symptom of overdosage would be hypotension which should be managed by infusion of normal saline or any other symptomatic treatment. The LD_{50} in mice ranges from 554 mg/kg to 1140 mg/kg.

Pharmacological properties

Pharmacodynamic properties: Ethyol (amifostine; ethanethiol, 2-[(3-amino propyl)amino]-dihydrogen phosphate (ester)) is an organic thiophosphate which, in animal models, selectively protects normal tissues but not tumours against cytoxicity of ionising radiations, DNA-binding chemotherapeutic agents (classical alkylating agents such as cyclophosphamide and non-classical alkylating agents such as mitomycin-C) and platinum analogs.

Ethol is a prodrug that is dephosphorylated to the active metabolite, WR-1065 (free thiol), by alkaline phosphatase and exits the bloodstream rapidly.

Pharmacokinetic properties: Clinical pharmacokinetic studies have shown that amifolstine is rapidly cleared from the plasma with <10% remaining in the plasma 6 minutes after drug administration. Amifostine is rapidly metabolised into the active metabolite WR-1065 (free thiol). WR-33278 (disulfide) is the subsequent inactive metabolite. It is unknown if amifostine crosses the blood placenta barrier.

After a 15 minute infusion of a dose of 910 mg/m², the α-half-life is <1 minute; the elimination half-life of amifostine is <10 minutes.

During a 15 minute infusion of 910 mg/m² the peak plasma concentration of amifostine is approximately 200 μmol/l, the Vd_{ss} is 7 l and the clearance is 2 l/min. Peak plasma concentrations of the active metabolite, WR-1065, during the 15-minute infusion is approximately 35 μmol/l. Measurement of WR-1065 in bone marrow cells 5–8 minutes after the infusion in 3 patients was 82.12 l and 277 μmol/kg.

Less than 4% of amifostine and its metabolites are excreted in urine.

Preclinical safety data (mutagenic and carcinogenic potential): In view of the combination of Ethyol with agents which do have carcinogenic potential of their own, no particular carcinogenic studies were performed. The Ames *salmonella typhimurium* test revealed no mutagenic activity.

Pharmaceutical particulars

List of excipients: Ethyol does not contain any preservative.

Incompatibilities: No known incompatibilities. However it is recommended that no other drug be mixed or administered with the reconstituted Ethyol solution.

Shelf life: Ethyol, lypholised powder for injection is stable for 24 months when stored at room temperature (up to 25°C).

When reconstituted with 9.7 ml of sterile 0.9% sodium chloride solution, the reconstituted Ethyol solution may be kept 6 hours at room temperature (up to 25°C) or 24 hours under refrigeration (2°–8°C).

Special precautions for storage: The lyophilised dosage form is labelled: 'Store at room temperature (up to 25°C)'.

Nature and contents of container: Ethyol (amifostine) lyphilised powder for injection in a 10 ml clear glass vial fitted with a grey rubber stopper sealed with an aluminium seal with a blue flip-off cap. Each vial contains amifostine 500 mg.

Administrative data

Marketing authorisation holder: U.S. Bioscience, Inc., Suite A, 2nd Floor, Gresham House, 53 Clarendon Road, Watford, Hertfordshire WD1 1LA, United Kingdom.

Distributed by: Schering-Plough Ltd, Shire Park, Welwyn Garden City, Hertfordshire AL7 1TW, United Kingdom.

Marketing authorisation number PL 11284/0004

Date of revision of SmPC January 1997

Legal category POM

INTRON A* MULTI-DOSE INJECTION PEN

Qualitative and quantitative composition

Intron A, solution for injection, multi-dose pen: Each carpoule of Intron A, solution for injection, multi-dose pen contains 15 million International Units (IU)/ml (6 doses of 3 million IU for a total deliverable dose of 18 million IU), 25 million IU/ml (6 doses of 5 million IU for a total deliverable dose of 30 million IU) or 50 million IU/ml (6 doses of 10 million IU for a total deliverable dose of 60 million IU) of recombinant interferon alfa-2b.

Pharmaceutical form Solution for injection of Intron A in a delivery system for multiple injections (pen).

For subcutaneous injection.

Clinical particulars

Therapeutic indications:

Chronic Hepatitis B: Treatment of adult patients with histologically proven chronic hepatitis who have serum markers for virus B replication, e.g. those who are positive for HBV-DNA, DNA polymerase, and HBeAg.

Current clinical experience in patients who remain on interferon alfa-2b for 4 to 6 months indicates that therapy can produce clearance of serum HBV-DNA and improvement in liver histology. In patients with loss of HBeAg and HBV-DNA, a significant reduction in morbidity and mortality has been observed.

Chronic hepatitis C: Treatment of adult patients with histologically proven chronic hepatitis who have serum markers for virus C replication, e.g. those who have elevated transminases without liver decompensation and who are positive for serum HCV-RNA or anti-HCV.

Current clinical experience in patients who remain on interferon alfa-2b for 12 months indicates that therapy can produce normalisation of serum ALT, clearance of serum HCV-RNA and improvement in liver histology.

In patients who fail to respond after three to four months of treatment, discontinuation of interferon alfa-2b therapy should be considered.

Hairy cell leukaemia: Treatment of patients with hairy cell leukaemia.

Chronic myelogenous leukaemia: Treatment of adult patients with chronic myelogenous leukaemia.

Clinical experience indicates that a haematologic and cytogenic major/minor response is obtainable in the majority of patients treated. There are no controlled studies demonstrating effects on overall survival.

Multiple myeloma: As maintenance therapy in patients who achieved objective remission (more than 50% reduction in myeloma protein) following initial induction chemotherapy.

Current clinical experience indicates that maintenance therapy with Intron A prolongs the plateau phase; however effects on overall survival have not been conclusively demonstrated.

Follicular lymphoma: Treatment of high tumour burden follicular lymphoma as adjunct to appropriate combination induction chemotherapy such as a CHOP-like regimen. High tumour burden is defined as having at least one of the following: bulky tumour mass (>7 cm), involvement of three or more nodal sites (each >3 cm), systemic symptoms (weight loss >10%, fever >38°C for more than 8 days, or nocturnal sweats), splenomegaly beyond the umbilicus, major organ obstruction or compression syndrome, orbital or epidural involvement, serous effusion, or leukaemia.

Carcinoid tumour: Treatment of carcinoid tumours with lymph node or liver metastases and with 'carcinoid syndrome'.

AIDS-related Kaposi's sarcoma: For patients with progressive asymptomatic Kaposi's sarcoma who have a CD4 count ≥250/mm³, AIDS patients with CD4 counts <250/mm³, or those with a history of opportunistic infections or constitutional symptoms, are unlikely to respond to Intron A therapy and therefore should not be used (see *Special warnings and special precautions for use*).

Malignant melanoma: As adjuvant therapy in patients who are free of disease after surgery but are at high risk of systemic recurrence, e.g., patients with primary or recurrent (clinical or pathological) lymph node involvement.

Posology and method of administration: Intron A, solution for injection, multi-dose pen contains a pre-filled, multi-dose cartridge for subcutaneous administration. It is designed to deliver fixed doses as required using a simple dial mechanism.

The needles provided in the packaging will be used for the Intron A, solution for injection, multi-dose pen only. A new needle is to be use each time the pen delivers a dose.

Each Intron A, solution for injection, multi-dose pen is for individual patient use only.

During the course of treatment with Intron A for any indication, if adverse reactions develop, the dosage should be modified or therapy should be discontinued temporarily until the adverse reactions abate. If persistent or recurrent intolerance develops following adequate dosage adjustment, or disease progresses, the treatment with Intron A should be discontinued. For maintenance dosage regimens administered subcutaneously, at the discretion of the physician, the patient may self-administer the dose.

Chronic active hepatitis B: The recommended dosage is in the range of 5 to 10 million IU administered subcutaneously three times per week (every other day) for a period of four to six months.

If no improvement in serum HBV-DNA is observed after three to four months of treatment (at the 10 million IU dose, if tolerated), interferon alfa-2b therapy should be discontinued.

Chronic hepatitis C: The recommended dose is three million IU administered subcutaneously three times a week (every other day). Most patients who respond demonstrate improvement in ALT levels within three to four months. In these patients therapy should be continued with 3 million IU three times a week (every other day) for 12 months.

The optimal duration of treatment is not yet established. There are no clinical studies directly comparing 12 to 18 months, however, the prolongation of treatment up to 18 months might be usefully considered in some patients.

In patients who fail to respond after three to four months of treatment, discontinuation of interferon alfa-2b should be considered.

Hairy cell leukaemia: The recommended dose is 2 million IU/m² administered subcutaneously three times a week (every other day) for both splenectomised and non-splenectomised patients. For most patients with HCL, normalisation of one or more hematologic variables occurs within one to two months of Intron A treatment. Improvement in all three hematologic variables (granulocyte count, platelet count and haemoglobin level) may require six months or more. This regimen should be maintained unless the disease progresses rapidly or severe intolerance is manifested.

Chronic myelogenous leukaemia: The recommended dosage of Intron A is 4 to 5 million IU/m² administered daily subcutaneously. When the white blood cell count is controlled, the maximum tolerated dose (4 to 10 million IU/m² daily) should be administered to maintain hematologic remission. Intron A treatment should be discontinued after 8 to 12 weeks of treatment if at least a partial hematologic remission or a clinically meaningful cytoreduction has not been achieved.

Multiple myeloma: Maintenance therapy – In patients who are in the plateau phase (more than 50% reduction of myeloma protein) following initial induction chemotherapy, Intron A may be administered as monotherapy, subcutaneously, at a dose of 3 million IU/m² three times a week (every other day).

Follicular lymphoma: Adjunctively with chemotherapy, Intron A may be administered subcutaneously, at a dose of 5 million IU three times a week (every other day) for a duration of 18 months. CHOP-like regimens are advised, but clinical experience is available only with CHVP (combination of cyclophosphamide, doxorubicin, teniposide and prednisolone).

Carcinoid tumour: The usual dose is 5 million IU (3 to 9 million IU) administered subcutaneously three times a week (every other day). Patients with advanced disease may require a daily dose of 5 million IU. The treatment should be temporarily discontinued during and after surgery. Therapy should continue for as long as the patient responds to Intron A treatment.

AIDS-related Kaposi's sarcoma: The optimal dosage is not yet known. Efficacy has been demonstrated at a daily dose of 10 million IU administered subcutaneously. The minimum effective dose is not established. The maximum tolerated daily dose of Intron A is 20 million IU.

If severe adverse reactions develop, the dosage should be modified (50% reduction) or therapy discontinued temporarily until adverse reactions abate.

When disease stabilisation or treatment response occurs, treatment should continue until there is no further evidence of tumour or until discontinuation is required by evidence of a severe opportunistic infection or adverse effect. Intron A therapy has been administered in an outpatient regimen.

Malignant melanoma: As induction therapy, Intron A is administered intravenously at a dose of 20 million IU/m² daily for five days a week for a four-week period; the calculated Intron A dose is added to 50 ml of saline solution and administered as a 20-minute infusion. (The Intron A, solution for injection, multi-dose pen presentations are not suitable for intravenous administration, but may be used for the maintenance regimen.) As maintenance treatment, the recommended dose is 10 million IU/m² administered subcutaneously three days a week (every other day) for 48 weeks.

If severe adverse reactions develop during Intron A treatment, particularly if granulocytes decrease to <500/mm³ or ALT/AST rise to >5× upper limit of normal, treatment should be temporarily discontinued until the adverse reaction abates. Intron A treatment should be restarted at 50% of the previous dose. If intolerance persists after dose adjustment or if granulocytes decrease to <250/mm³ or ALT/AST rise to >10× upper limit of normal, Intron A therapy should be discontinued.

Although the optimal (minimum) dose is unknown, for full clinical benefit, patients should be treated at the recommended dose, with dose modification for toxicity as described.

Contra-indications:

- A history of hypersensitivity to recombinant interferon alfa-2b or any other component of Intron A.
- Severe pre-existing cardiac disease.
- Severe renal or hepatic dysfunction; including that caused by metastases.
- Epilepsy and/or compromised central nervous system (CNS) function (see *Special precautions for use*).
- Chronic hepatitis with decompensated cirrhosis of the liver.
- Chronic hepatitis in patients who are being or have been treated recently with immunosuppressive agents excluding short-term corticosteroid withdrawal.
- Autoimmune hepatitis; or history of autoimmune disease; immunosuppressed transplant recipients.
- Pre-existing thyroid disease unless controlled by conventional treatment.

Special warnings and precautions for use:

For all patients: Acute hypersensitivity reactions (e.g., urticaria, angioedema, bronchoconstriction, anaphylaxis) to Intron A have been observed rarely during Intron A therapy. If such a reaction develops, the drug should be discontinued and appropriate medical therapy instituted immediately. Transient rashes do not necessitate interruption of treatment.

Intron A, solution for injection, multi-dose pen contains m-cresol as preservative; some patients may experience allergic reaction to this ingredient.

Moderate to severe adverse experiences may require modification of the patient's dosage regimen, or in some cases, termination of Intron A therapy. Any patient developing liver function abnormalities during treatment with Intron A should be monitored closely and treatment discontinued if signs and symptoms progress.

Hypotension may occur during Intron A therapy or up to two days post-therapy and may require supportive treatment.

Adequate hydration should be maintained in patients undergoing Intron A therapy since hypotension related to fluid depletion has been seen in some patients. Fluid replacement may be necessary.

While fever may be associated with the flu-like syndrome reported commonly during interferon therapy, other causes of persistent fever should be ruled out.

Paracetamol has been used successfully to alleviate the symptoms of fever and headache which can occur with Intron A therapy. The recommended paracetamol dosage is 500 mg to 1 g given 30 minutes before administration of Intron A. The maximum dosage of paracetamol to be given is 1 g four time daily.

Intron A should be used cautiously in patients with debilitating medical conditions, such as those with a history of pulmonary disease (e.g. chronic obstructive pulmonary disease) or diabetes mellitus prone to ketoacidosis. Caution should be observed also in patients with coagulation disorders (e.g., thrombophlebitis, pulmonary embolism) or severe myelosuppression.

Pulmonary infiltrates, pneumonitis and pneumonia, including fatality, have been observed rarely in interferon alpha treated patients, including those treated with Intron A. The aetiology has not been defined. These symptoms have been reported more frequently when shosaikoto, a Chinese herbal medicine, is administered concomitantly with interferon alfa. Any patient developing fever, cough, dyspnea or other respiratory symptoms should have a chest X-ray taken. If the chest X-ray shows pulmonary infiltrates or there is evidence of pulmonary function impairment, the patient should be monitored closely, and, if appropriate, interferon alfa treatment should be discontinued. While this has been reported more often in patients with oncologic diseases treated with interferon alfa. Prompt discontinuation of interferon alfa administration and treatment with corticosteroids appear to be associated with resolution of pulmonary adverse events.

Ocular adverse events (see *Undesirable effects*) appear to occur after use of the drug for several months, but also have been reported after shorter treatment periods. Any patient complaining of changes in visual acuity or visual fields, or reporting other ophthalmologic symptoms during treatment with Intron A, should have an eye examination. Because the retinal events may have to be differentiated from those seen with diabetic or hypertensive retinopathy, a baseline ocular examination is recommended prior to treatment with interferon in patients with diabetes mellitus or hypertension.

Patients with a pre-existing psychiatric condition or a history of severe psychiatric disorder should not be treated with Intron A.

Severe CNS effects, particularly depression, suicidal ideation and attempted suicide have been observed in some patients during Intron A therapy; in these cases, Intron A therapy should be discontinued. The potential seriousness of these adverse events should be borne in mind by the prescribing physician.

Other CNS effects manifested by confusion and other alterations of mental status have been observed rarely. More significant obtundation and coma have been observed in some patients, usually elderly, treated at higher doses. While these effects are generally reversible, in a few patients full resolution took up to three weeks. Very rarely, seizures have occurred with high doses of Intron A.

Patients with a history of congestive heart failure, myocardial infarction and/or previous or current arrhythmic disorders, who require Intron A therapy, should be closely monitored. Those patients who have pre-existing cardiac abnormalities and/or are in advanced stages of cancer should have electrocardiograms taken prior to and during the course of treatment. Cardiac arrhythmias (primarily supraventricular) usually respond to conventional therapy but may require discontinuation of Intron A therapy.

Because of reports of exacerbating pre-existing psoriatic disease, Intron A should be used in patients with psoriasis only if the potential benefit justifies the potential risk.

Preliminary data may indicate that interferon alpha therapy is associated with an increased rate of graft rejection (liver and kidney transplants).

The development of different auto-antibodies has been reported during treatment with alfa interferons. Clinical manifestations of autoimmune disease during interferon therapy may occur more frequently in patients predisposed to the development of autoimmune disorders.

Treatment with Intron A should be discontinued in patients with chronic hepatitis who develop prolongation of coagulation markers which might indicate liver decompensation.

The efficacy of interferon alfa-2b has not been demonstrated in patients with either chronic hepatitis B or C, with a co-infection with the human immunodeficiency virus (HIV), or undergoing hemodialysis.

Chronic hepatitis C: Infrequently, patients treated for chronic hepatitis C with Intron A developed thyroid abnormalities, either hypothyroid or hyperthyroid. In clinical trials using Intron A therapy, 2.8% patients overall developed thyroid abnormalities. The abnormalities were controlled by conventional therapy for thyroid dysfunction. The mechanism by which Intron A may alter thyroid status is unknown. Prior to initiation of Intron A therapy for the treatment of chronic hepatitis C, serum thyroid-stimulating hormone (TSH) levels should be evaluated. Any thyroid abnormality detected at that time should be treated with conventional therapy. Intron A treatment may be initiated if TSH levels can be maintained in the normal range by medication. If, during the course of Intron A therapy, a patient develops symptoms consistent with possible thyroid dysfunction, TSH levels should be evaluated. In the presence of thyroid dysfunction, Intron A treatment may be continued if TSH levels can be maintained in the normal range of medication. Discontinuation of Intron A therapy has not reversed thyroid dysfunction occurring during treatment.

Concomitant chemotherapy: Administration of Intron A in combination with other chemotherapeutic agents may lead to increased risk of toxicity (severity and duration), which may be life-threatening or fatal as a result of the concomitantly administered drug. The most commonly reported potentially life-threatening or fatal adverse events include mucositis, diarrhoea, neutropenia, renal impairment, and electrolyte disturbance. Because of the risk of increased toxicity, careful adjustments of doses are required for Intron A and for the concomitant chemotherapeutic agents.

AIDS-related Kaposi's sarcoma: Intron A should not be used in conjunction with protease inhibitors. With the exception of zidovudine, there is a lack of safety data for the combination of Intron A with reverse transciptase inhibitors.

Laboratory tests: Standard hematologic tests and blood chemistries (complete blood count and differential, platelet count, electrolytes, liver enzymes, serum protein, serum bilirubin and serum creatinine) should be conducted in all patients prior to and periodically during systemic treatment with Intron A.

During treatment for hepatitis B or C the recommended testing schedule is at weeks 1, 2, 4, 8, 12, 16, and every other month, thereafter, throughout treatment. If ALT flares during Intron A therapy to greater than or equal to 2 times baseline. Intron A therapy may be continued unless signs and symptoms of liver failure are observed. During ALT flare, liver function tests: ALT, prothrombin time, alkaline phosphatase, albumin and bilirubin should be monitored at two-week intervals.

In patients treated for malignant melanoma, liver function and white blood cell (WBC) count and differential should be monitored weekly during the induction phase of therapy and monthly during the maintenance phase of therapy.

Paediatric use: Doses of up to 10 million IU/m² have been administered safely to children with chronic active hepatitis B. However, efficacy of therapy has not been demonstrated. Generally, experience in patients below 18 years of age has been limited, and in such cases the expected benefits should be weighed carefully against potential hazards.

Effect on fertility: Interferon may impair fertility. In studies of interferon use in non-human primates, abnormalities of the menstrual cycle have been observed. Decreased serum estradiol and progesterone concentrations have been reported in women treated with human leukocyte interferon. Therefore, fertile women should not receive Intron A unless they are using effective contraception during the treatment period. Intron A should be used with caution in fertile men.

Interaction with other medicaments and other forms of interaction:
Drug/drug interactions: Narcotics, hypnotics or sedatives should be administered with caution concomitantly with Intron A.

Interactions between Intron A and other drugs have not been fully evaluated. Caution should be exercised when administering Intron A in combination with other potentially myelosuppressive agents.

Interferons may affect the oxidative metabolic process. This should be considered during concomitant therapy with drugs metabolised by this route, such as the xanthine derivatives theophylline or aminophylline. During concomitant therapy with xanthine agents, serum theophylline levels should be monitored and dosage adjusted if necessary.

Use during pregnancy and lactation: Intron A has been shown to have abortifacient effects in *Macaca mulatta* (rhesus monkeys) at 90 and 180 times the recommended intramuscular or subcutaneous dose of 2 million IU/m². Abortion was observed in all dose groups (7.5 million, 15 million and 30 million IU/kg), and was only statistically significant versus control at the mid- and high-dose groups (corresponding to 90 and 180 times the recommended intramuscular or subcutaneous dose of 2 million IU/m²). There are no adequate data in pregnant women. Intron A should be used during pregnancy only if the potential benefit justifies the potential risk to the foetus.

It is not known whether the components of this drug are excreted in human milk. Because of the potential for adverse reactions from Intron A in nursing infants, a decision should be made whether to discontinue nursing or to discontinue the drug, taking into account the importance of the drug to the mother.

Effects on ability to drive and use machines: Patients who develop fatigue, somnolence, or confusion during treatment with Intron A should be cautioned to avoid driving or operating machinery.

Undesirable effects: In clinical trials conducted in a broad range of indications and at a wide rnge of doses, the most commonly reported adverse effects were fever, fatigue, headache and myalgia. Fever and fatigue were reversible within 72 hours of interruption or cessation of treatment and were dose related. In the hepatitis treatment groups these effects were of mild to moderate severity.

Common adverse effects include rigors/chills, anorexia and nausea.

In decreasing order of frequency, less commonly reported effects include vomiting, diarrhoea, arthralgia, asthenia, somnolence, dizziness, dry mouth, alopecia, flu-like symptoms (unspecified), back pain, depression, suicidal attempts, malaise, pain, increased sweating, taste alteration, irritability, insomnia, confusion, impaired concentration and hypotension.

Reported rarely were abdominal pain, rash, nervousness, injection site disorders, paresthesia, herpes simplex, pruritus, eye pain, anxiety, epistaxis, coughing, pharyngitis, pulmonary infiltrates, pneumonitis and pneumonia, impaired consciousness, weight decrease, face oedema, dyspnea, dyspepsia, tachycardia, hypertension, increased appetite, decreased libido, hypoaesthesia, taste perversion, loose stool, gingival bleeding, leg cramps, neuropathy, polyneuropathy, rhabdomyolysis, sometimes serious, and renal insufficiency. Hyperthyroidism or hypothyroidism have also been observed rarely. Hepatotoxicity, including fatality has been observed rarely.

Very rarely following the marketing of Intron A, cases of nephrotic syndrome, renal failure, aggravated diabetes, diabetes/hyperglycaemia, cardiac ischemia, and myocardial infarction have been reported.

Cardiovascular (CVS) adverse reactions, particularly arrhythmia, appeared to be correlated mostly with pre-existing CVS disease and prior therapy with cardiotoxic agents (see *Special warnings and precautions for use*). Transient reversible cardiomyopathy has been reported rarely in patients without prior evidence of cardiac disease.

Retinal haemorrhages, cotton-wool spots, and retinal artery or vein obstruction have been observed rarely in patients treated with interferon alfa, including Intron A (recombinant interferon alfa-2b), powder for solution for injection or solution for injection (see *Special warnings and precautions for use*).

Clinically significant laboratory abnormalities, most frequently occurring at doses greater than 10 Million IU daily, include reduction in granulocyte and white blood cell counts; decreases in haemoglobin level and platelet count; increases in alkaline phosphatase, LDH, serum creatinine and serum urea nitrogen levels. Increase in serum ALT/AST (SGPT/SGOT) levels have been noted as an abnormality in some non-hepatitis subjects and also in some patients with chronic hepatitis B coincident with clearance of viral DNAp.

Overdose: Overdosing has not been reported with Intron A, but as for any pharmacologically active compound, symptomatic treatment with frequent monitoring of vital signs and close observation of the patient is indicated.

Pharmacological properties
Pharmacotherapeutic group:
Immunostimulating agents, cytokines, interferon alfa, ATC code: L03A A04.

Intron A, solution for injection, is a sterile, stable, albumin-free formulation of highly purified interferon alfa-2b produced by recombinant DNA techniques. Recombinant interferon alfa-2b is a water soluble protein with a molecular weight of approximately 19,300 daltons. It is obtained from a clone of *E. coli*, which harbours a genetically engineered plasmid hybrid encompassing an interferon alfa-2 gene from human leukocytes.

The activity of Intron A is expressed in terms of IU, with 1 mg of recombinant interferon alfa-2b protein corresponding to 2.6×10^8 IU. International Units are determined by comparison of the activity of the recombinant interferon alfa-2b with the activity of the international reference preparation of human leukocyte interferon established by the World Health Organisation.

The interferons are a family of small protein molecules with molecular weights of approximately 15,000 to 21,000 daltons. They are produced and secreted by cells in response to viral infections or various synthetic and biological inducers. Three major classes of interferons have been identified: alpha, beta and gamma. These three main classes are themselves not homogeneous and may contain several different molecular species of interferon. More than 14 genetically distinct human alpha interferons have been identified. Intron A has been classified as recombinant interferon alfa-2b.

Pharmacodynamic properties: Interferons exert their cellular activities by binding to specific membrane receptors on the cell surface. Human interferon receptors, as isolated from human lymphoblastoid (Daudi) cells, appear to be highly asymmetric proteins.

They exhibit selectivity for human but not murine interferons, suggesting species specificity. Studies with other interferons have demonstrated species specificity. However, certain monkey species, e.g., Rhesus monkeys, are susceptible to pharmacodynamic stimulation upon exposure to human type 1 interferons.

The results of several studies suggest that, once bound to the cell membrane, interferon initiates a complex sequence of intracellular events that include the induction of certain enzymes. It is thought that this process, at least in part, is responsible for the various cellular responses to interferon, including inhibition of virus replication in virus-infected cells, suppression of cell proliferation and such immunomodulating activities as enhancement of the phagocytic activity of macrophages and augmentation of the specific cytotoxicity of lymphocytes for target cells. Any or all of these activities may contribute to interferon's therapeutic effects.

Recombinant interferon alfa-2b has exhibited antiproliferative effects in studies employing both animal and human cell culture systems as well as human tumour xenografts in animals. It has demonstrated significant immunomodulatory activity *in vitro*.

Recombinant interferon alfa-2b also inhibits viral replication *in vitro* and *in vivo*. Although the exact antiviral mode of action of recombinant interferon alfa-2b is unknown, it appears to alter the host cell metabolism. This action inhibits viral replication or if replication occurs, the progeny virions are unable to leave the cell.

Pharmacokinetic properties: The pharmacokinetics of Intron A were studied in healthy volunteers following single 5 million IU/m² and 10 million IU doses administered subcutaneously, intramuscularly and as a 30-minute intravenous infusion. The mean serum interferon concentrations following subcutaneous and intramuscular injections were comparable. Maximum serum levels occurred three to 12 hours after the lower dose and six to eight hours after the higher dose. The elimination half-lives of interferon injections were approximately two to three hours, and six to seven hours, respectively. Serum levels were below the detection limit 16 and 24 hours, respectively, post-injection. Both subcutaneous and intramuscular administration resulted in bioavailabilities greater than 100%.

After intravenous administration, serum interferon levels peaked (135 to 273 IU/ml) by the end of the infusion, then declined at a slightly more rapid rate than after subcutaneous or intramuscular drug administration, becoming undetectable four hours after the infusion. The elimination half-life was approximately two hours.

Urine levels of interferon were below the detection limit following each of the three routes of administration.

Interferon neutralising factor assays were performed on serum samples of patients who received Intron A in Schering-Plough monitored clinical trials. Interferon neutralising factors are antibodies which neutralise the antiviral activity of interferon. The clinical incidence of neutralising factors developing in cancer patients treated systemically is 2.9% and in chronic hepatitis patients is 6.2%. The detectable titers are low in almost all cases and have not been regularly associated with loss of response or any other autoimmune phenomenon. In patients with hepatitis, no loss of response was observed, apparently due to the low titers.

Preclinical safety data: Although interferon is generally recognised as being species specific, toxicity studies in mice, rats, rabbits and monkeys were conducted. Injections of human recombinant interferon alfa-2b for up to three months have shown no evidence of toxicity.

Results of animal reproduction studies indicate that recombinant interferon alfa-2b was not teratogenic in rats or rabbits, nor did it adversely effect pregnancy, foetal development or reproductive capacity in offspring of treated rats. However, high doses of other forms of interferons alfa and beta are known to produce dose-related anovulatory and abortifacient effects in Rhesus monkeys.

Mutagenicity studies with Intron A revealed no adverse effects.

Pharmaceutical particulars
List of excipients: Sodium phosphate dibasic, sodium phosphate monobasic, edetate disodium, sodium chloride, m-cresol, polysorbate 80, water for injection q.s. and 1.5 ml[1] (deliverable volume from the pen=1.2 ml).

[1] An overfill is required for proper dispensing from the pen delivery system.

Incompatibilities: No other substance or solution should be mixed with Intron A, solution for injection, multi-dose pen.

Shelf life: 12 months when stored at 2° to 8°C.

Special precautions for storage: Intron A, solution for injection, multi-dose pen must be stored at 2° to 8°C (refrigerator) and should not be frozen.

Nature and contents of container:
15 million IU/ml: 1.5 ml carpoule, type I flint glass.
25 million IU/ml: 1.5 ml carpoule, type I flint glass.
50 million IU/ml: 1.5 ml carpoule, type I flint glass.

The pen is packaged in a carton containing disposable needles and alcohol swabs.

Instructions for use and handling, and disposal (if appropriate): As with all parenteral drug products, Intron A should be inspected visually for particulate matter and discolouration prior to administration. Intron A solution for injection is clear and colourless.

Intron A, solution for injection, multi-dose pen is injected subcutaneously after attaching a needle and dialling the prescribed dose.

The multi-dose pen should be at room temperature (≤25°C) before administering each dose. The pen should be removed from the refrigerator approximately 30 minutes before administration to allow the injectable solution to reach room temperature (≤25°C).

Each pen is intended for a maximum two-week use period and then must be discarded. A new needle must be used for each dose. After each use, the needle should be discarded safely and the pen must be returned to the refrigerator immediately. In case the product is left inadvertently at room temperature (≤25°C), a maximum total of 48 hours (two days) of exposure to room temperature (≤25°C) is permitted over the two-week use period.

Marketing authorisation numbers

	UK	*Ireland*
15 miu/ml:	0201/0228	277/50/18
25 miu/ml:	0201/0229	277/50/19
50 miu/ml:	0201/0230	277/50/20

Date of approval/revision of SmPC 16 October 1997

Legal category POM

INTRON A* SOLUTION FOR INJECTION

Qualitative and quantitative composition Each vial of Intron A, solution for injection, contains 25 million International Units (IU) of recombinant interferon alfa-2b in 2.5 ml of solution (10 million IU/ml).

Pharmaceutical form Solution for injection.

Route of administration: Subcutaneous or intravenous injection.

Clinical particulars

Therapeutic indications:

Chronic Hepatitis B: Treatment of adult patients with histologically proven chronic hepatitis who have serum markers for virus B replication, e.g., those who are positive for HBV-DNA, or DNA polymerase, and HBeAg.

Current clinical experience in patients who remain on interferon alfa-2b for 4 to 6 months indicates that therapy can produce clearance of serum HBV-DNA and improvement in liver histology. In patients with loss of HBeAg and HBV-DNA, a significant reduction in morbidity and mortality has been observed.

Chronic hepatitis C: Treatment of adult patients with histologically proven chronic hepatitis who have serum markers for virus C replication, e.g. those who have elevated transminases without liver decompensation and who are positive for serum HCV-RNA or anti-HCV.

Current clinical experience in patients who remain on interferon alfa-2b for 12 months indicates that therapy can produce normalisation of serum ALT, clearance of serum HCV-RNA and improvement in liver histology.

In patients who fail to respond after three to four months of treatment, discontinuation of interferon alfa-2b therapy should be considered.

Hairy cell leukaemia: Treatment of patients with hairy cell leukaemia.

Chronic myelogenous leukaemia: Treatment of adult patients with Philadelphia chromosome or bcr/abl translocation positive chronic myelogenous leukaemia. Clinical experience indicates that a haematologic and cytogenic major/minor response is obtainable in the majority of patients treated. There are no controlled studies demonstrating effects on overall survival.

Multiple myeloma: As maintenance therapy in patients who achieved objective remission (more than 50% reduction in myeloma protein) following initial induction chemotherapy.

Current clinical experience indicates that maintenance therapy with Intron A prolongs the plateau phase; however effects on overall survival have not been conclusively demonstrated.

Follicular lymphoma: Treatment of high tumour burden follicular lymphoma as adjunct to appropriate combination induction chemotherapy such as a CHOP-like regimen. High tumour burden is defined as having at least one of the following: bulky tumour mass (>7 cm), involvement of three or more nodal sites (each >3 cm), systemic symptoms (weight loss >10%, fever >38°C for more than 8 days, or nocturnal sweats), splenomegaly beyond the umbilicus, major organ obstruction or compression syndrome, orbital or epidural involvement, serous effusion, or leukaemia.

Carcinoid tumour: Treatment of carcinoid tumours with lymph node or liver metastases and with 'carcinoid syndrome'.

AIDS-related Kaposi's sarcoma: For patients with progressive asymptomatic Kaposi's sarcoma who have a CD4 count >250/mm³, AIDS patients with CD4 counts <250/mm³, or those with a history of opportunistic infections or constitutional symptoms, are unlikely to respond to Intron A therapy and therefore should not be treated (see *Special warnings and special precautions for use*).

Malignant melanoma: As adjuvant therapy in patients who are free of disease after surgery but are at high risk of systemic recurrence, e.g., patients with primary or recurrent (clincial or pathological) lymph node involvement.

Posology and method of administration:

INTRON A MAY BE ADMINISTERED USING EITHER STERILISED GLASS OR PLASTIC DISPOSABLE SYRINGES.

MULTIDOSE PRESENTATIONS SHOULD BE FOR INDIVIDUAL PATIENT USE ONLY.

During the course of treatment with Intron A for any indication, if adverse reactions develop, the dosage should be modified or therapy should be discontinued temporarily until the adverse reactions abate. If persistent or recurrent intolerance develops following adequate dosage adjustment, or disease progresses, treatment with Intron A should be discontinued. For maintenance dosage regimens administered subcutaneously, at the discretion of the physician, the patient may self-administer the dose.

Chronic active hepatitis B: The recommended dosage is in the range of 5 to 10 million IU administered subcutaneously three times per week (every other day) for a period of four to six months. If no improvement on serum HBV-DNA is observed after three to four months of treatment (at the 10 million IU dose, if tolerated), interferon alfa-2b therapy should be discontinued.

Chronic hepatitis C: The recommended dose is 3 million IU administered subcutaneously three times a week (every other day). Most patients who respond demonstrate improvement in ALT levels within three to four months. In these patients, therapy should be continued with 3 million IU three times a week (every other day) for 12 months.

The optimal duration of treatment is not yet established. There are no clinical studies directly comparing 12 to 18 months, however, the prolongation of treatment up to 18 months might be usefully considered in some patients.

In patients who fail to respond after three to four months of treatment, discontinuation of interferon alfa-2b should be considered.

Hairy cell leukaemia: The recommended dose is 2 million IU/m² administered subcutaneously three times a week (every other day) for both splenectomised and non-splenectomised patients. For most patients with HCL, normalisation of one or more haematologic variables occurs within one to two months of Intron A treatment. Improvement in all three haematologic variables (granulocyte count, platelet count and haemoglobin level) may require six months or more. This regimen should be maintained unless the disease progresses rapidly or severe intolerance is manifested.

Chronic myelogenous leukaemia: The recommended dosage of Intron A is 4 to 5 million IU/m² administered daily subcutaneously. When the white blood cell count is controlled, the maximum tolerated dose (4 to 10 million IU/m² daily) should be administered to maintain haematologic remission. Intron A treatment should be discontinued after 8 to 12 weeks of treatment if at least a partial haematologic remission or a clinically meaningful cytoreduction has not been achieved.

Multiple myeloma: Maintenance therapy – In patients who are in the plateau phase (more than 50% reduction of myeloma protein) following initial induction chemotherapy, Intron A may be administered as monotherapy, subcutaneously, at a dose of 3 million IU/m² three times a week (every other day).

Follicular lymphoma: Adjunctively with chemotherapy, Intron A may be administered subcutaneously, at a dose of 5 million IU three times a week (every other day) for a duration of 18 months. CHOP-like regimens are advised, but clinical experience is available only with CHVP (combination of cyclophosphamide, doxorubicin, teniposide and prednisolone).

Carcinoid tumour: The usual dose is 5 million IU (3 to 9 million IU) administered subcutaneously three times a week (every other day). Patients with advanced disease may require a daily dose of 5 million IU. The treatment should be temporarily discontinued during and after surgery. Therapy should continue for as long as the patient responds to Intron A treatment.

AIDS-related Kaposi's sarcoma: The optimal dosage is not yet known. Efficacy has been demonstrated at a daily dose of 10 million IU administered subcutaneously. The minimum effective dose is not established. The maximum tolerated daily dose of Intron A is 20 million IU.

If severe adverse reactions develop, the dosage should be modified (50% reduction) or therapy discontinued temporarily until the adverse reactions abate.

When disease stabilisation or treatment response occurs, treatment should continue until there is no further evidence of tumour or until discontinuation is required by evidence of a severe opportunistic infection or adverse effect. Intron A therapy has been administered in an outpatient regimen.

Malignant melanoma: As induction therapy, Intron A is administered intravenously at a dose of 20 million IU/m² daily for five days a week for a four-week period; the calculated Intron A dose is added to 50 ml of sterile normal saline solution in a PVC bag or glass bottle for intravenous use, and administered as a 20-minute infusion (see *Instructions for use*). As maintenance treatment, the recommended dose is 10 million IU/m² administered subcutaneously three days a week (every other day) for 48 weeks.

If severe adverse reactions develop during Intron A treatment, particularly if granulocytes decrease to <500/mm³ or ALT/AST rise to >5× upper limit of normal, treatment should be temporarily discontinued until the adverse reaction abates. Intron A treatment should be restarted at 50% of the previous dose. If intolerance persists after dose adjustment or if granulocytes decrease to <250/mm³ or ALT/AST rise to >10× upper limit of normal, Intron A therapy should be discontinued.

Although the optimal (minimum) dose is unknown, for full clinical benefit, patients should be treated at the recommended dose, with dose modification for toxicity as described.

Contra-indications:

- A history of hypersensitivity to recombinant interferon alfa-2b or any other component of Intron A.
- Severe pre-existing cardiac disease.
- Severe renal or hepatic dysfunction; including that caused by metastases.
- Epilepsy and/or compromised central nervous system (CNS) function (see *Special precautions for use*).
- Chronic hepatitis with decompensated cirrhosis of the liver.
- Chronic hepatitis in patients who are being or have been recently treated with immunosuppressive agents excluding short-term corticosteroid withdrawal.
- Autoimmune hepatitis; or history of autoimmune disease; immunosuppressed transplant recipients.
- Pre-existing thyroid disease unless controlled by conventional treatment.

Special warnings and precautions for use:

For all patients: Acute hypersensitivity reactions (e.g., urticaria, angioedema, bronchoconstriction, anaphylaxis) to Intron A have been observed rarely during Intron A therapy. If such a reaction develops, the drug should be discontinued and appropriate medical therapy instituted immediately. Transient rashes do not necessitate interruption of treatment.

Intron A, solution for injection, contains m-cresol as preservative; some patients may experience allergic reaction to this ingredient.

Moderate to severe adverse experiences may require modification of the patient's dosage regimen, or in some cases, termination of Intron A therapy. Any patient developing liver function abnormalities during treatment with Intron A should be monitored closely and treatment discontinued if signs and symptoms progress.

Hypotension may occur during Intron A therapy or up to two days post-therapy and may require supportive treatment.

Adequate hydration should be maintained in patients undergoing Intron A therapy since hypotension related to fluid depletion has been seen in some patients. Fluid replacement may be necessary.

While fever may be associated with the flu-like syndrome reported commonly during interferon therapy, other causes of persistent fever should be ruled out.

Paracetamol has been used successfully to alleviate the symptoms of fever and headache which can occur with Intron A therapy. The recommended paracetamol dosage is 500 mg to 1 g given 30 minutes before administration of Intron A. The maximum dosage of paracetamol to be given is 1 g four time daily.

Intron A should be used cautiously in patients with debilitating medical conditions, such as those with a history of pulmonary disease (e.g. chronic obstructive pulmonary disease) or diabetes mellitus prone to ketoacidosis. Caution should be observed also in patients with coagulation disorders (e.g., thrombophlebitis, pulmonary embolism) or severe myelosuppression.

Pulmonary infiltrates, pneumonitis and pneumonia, including fatality, have been observed rarely in interferon alpha treated patients, including those treated with Intron A. The aetiology has not been defined. These symptoms have been reported more frequently when shosaikoto, a Chinese herbal medicine, is administered concomitantly with interferon alfa. Any patient developing fever, cough, dyspnoea or other respiratory symptoms should have a chest X-ray taken. If the chest X-ray shows pulmonary infiltrates or there is evidence of pulmonary function impairment, the patient should be monitored closely, and, if appropriate, interferon alfa treatment should be discontinued. While this has been reported more often in patients with chronic hepatitis C treated with interferon alfa, it has also been reported in patients with oncologic diseases treated with interferon alfa.

Prompt discontinuation of interferon alfa administration and treatment with corticosteroids appear to be associated with resolution of pulmonary adverse events.

Ocular adverse events (see *Undesirable effects*) appear to occur after use of the drug for several months, but also have been reported after shorter treatment periods. Any patient complaining of changes in visual acuity or visual fields, or reporting other ophthalmologic symptoms during treatment with Intron A, should have an eye examination. Because the retinal events may have to be differentiated from those seen with diabetic or hypertensive retinopathy, a baseline ocular examination is recommended prior to treatment with interferon in patients with diabetes mellitus or hypertension.

Patients with a pre-existing psychiatric condition or a history of severe psychiatric disorder should not be treated with Intron A.

Severe CNS effects, particularly depression, suicidal ideation and attempted suicide have been observed in some patients during Intron A therapy; in these cases, Intron A therapy should be discontinued. The potential seriousness of these adverse events should be borne in mind by the prescribing physician.

Other CNS effects manifested by confusion and other alterations of mental status have been observed rarely. More significant obtundation and coma have been observed in some patients, usually elderly, treated at higher doses. While these effects are generally reversible, in a few patients full resolution took up to three weeks. Very rarely, seizures have occurred with high doses of Intron A.

Patients with a history of congestive heart failure, myocardial infarction and/or previous or current arrhythmic disorders, who require Intron A therapy, should be closely monitored. Those patients who have pre-existing cardiac abnormalities and/or are in advanced stages of cancer should have electrocardiograms taken prior to and during the course of treatment. Cardiac arrhythmias (primarily supraventricular) usually respond to conventional therapy but may require discontinuation of Intron A therapy.

Because of reports of exacerbating pre-existing psoriatic disease, Intron A should be used in patients with psoriasis only if the potential benefit justifies the potential risk.

Preliminary data may indicate that interferon alfa therapy is associated with an increased rate of graft rejection (liver and kidney transplants).

The development of different auto-antibodies has been reported during treatment with alfa interferons. Clinical manifestations of autoimmune disease during interferon therapy may occur more frequently in patients predisposed to the development of autoimmune disorders.

Treatment with Intron A should be discontinued in patients with chronic hepatitis who develop prolongation of coagulation markers which might indicate liver decompensation.

The efficacy of interferon alfa-2b has not been demonstrated in patients with either chronic hepatitis B or C, with a co-infection with the human immunodeficiency virus (HIV), or undergoing haemodialysis.

Chronic hepatitis C: Infrequently, patients treated for chronic hepatitis C with Intron A developed thyroid abnormalities, either hypothyroid or hyperthyroid. In clinical trials using Intron A therapy, 2.8% patients overall developed thyroid abnormalities. The abnormalities were controlled by conventional therapy for thyroid dysfunction. The mechanism by which Intron A may alter thyroid status is unknown. Prior to initiation of Intron A therapy for the treatment of chronic hepatitis C, serum thyroid-stimulating hormone (TSH) levels should be evaluated. Any thyroid abnormality detected at that time should be treated with conventional therapy. Intron A treatment may be initiated if TSH levels can be maintained in the normal range by medication. If, during the course of Intron A therapy, a patient develops symptoms consistent with possible thyroid dysfunction. TSH levels should be evaluated.

In the presence of thyroid dysfunction, Intron A treatment may be continued if TSH levels can be maintained in the normal range of medication. Discontinuation of Intron A therapy has not reversed thyroid dysfunction occurring during treatment.

Concomitant chemotherapy: Administration of Intron A in combination with other chemotherapeutic agents may lead to increased risk of toxicity (severity and duration), which may be life-threatening or fatal as a result of the concomitantly administered drug. The most commonly reported potentially life-threatening or fatal adverse events include mucositis, diarrhoea, neutropenia, renal impairment, and electrolyte disturbance. Because of the risk of increased toxicity, careful adjustments of doses are required for Intron A and for the concomitant chemotherapeutic agents.

AIDS-related Kaposi's sarcoma: Intron A should not be used in conjunction with protease inhibitors. With the exception of zidovudine, there is a lack of safety data for the combination of Intron A with reverse transciptase inhibitors.

Laboratory tests: Standard haematologic tests and blood chemistries (complete blood count and differential, platelet count, electrolytes, liver enzymes, serum protein, serum bilirubin and serum creatinine) should be conducted in all patients prior to and periodically during systemic treatment with Intron A.

During treatment for hepatitis B or C the recommended testing schedule is at weeks 1, 2, 4, 8, 12, 16, and every other month, thereafter, throughout treatment. If ALT flares during Intron A therapy to greater than or equal to 2 times baseline, Intron A therapy may be continued unless signs and symptoms of liver failure are observed. During ALT flare, liver function tests: ALT, prothrombin time, alkaline phosphatase, albumin and bilirubin should be monitored at two-week intervals.

In patients treated for malignant melanoma, liver function and white blood cell (WBC) count and differential should be monitored weekly during the induction phase of therapy and monthly during the maintenance phase of therapy.

Paediatric use: Doses of up to 10 million IU/m² have been administered safely to children with chronic active hepatitis B. However, efficacy of therapy has not been demonstrated. Generally, experience in patients below 18 years of age has been limited, and in such cases the expected benefits should be weighed carefully against potential hazards.

Effect on fertility: Interferon may impair fertility. In studies of interferon use in non-human primates, abnormalities of the menstrual cycle have been observed. Decreased serum estradiol and progesterone concentrations have been reported in women treated with human leukocyte interferon. Therefore, fertile women should not receive Intron A unless they are using effective contraception during the treatment period. Intron A should be used with caution in fertile men.

Interaction with other medicaments and other forms of interaction:
Drug/drug interactions: Narcotics, hypnotics or sedatives should be administered with caution concomitantly with Intron A.

Interactions between Intron A and other drugs have not been fully evaluated. Caution should be exercised when administering Intron A in combination with other potentially myelosuppressive agents.

Interferons may affect the oxidative metabolic process. This should be considered during concomitant therapy with drugs metabolised by this route, such as the xanthine derivatives theophylline or aminophylline. During concomitant therapy with xanthine agents, serum theophylline levels should be monitored and dosage adjusted if necessary.

Use during pregnancy and lactation: Intron A has been shown to have abortifacient effects in *Macaca mulatta* (rhesus monkeys) at 90 and 180 times the recommended intramuscular or subcutaneous dose of 2 million IU/m². Abortion was observed in all dose groups (7.5 million, 15 million and 30 million IU/kg), and was only statistically significant versus control at the mid- and high-dose groups (corresponding to 90 and 180 times the recommended intramuscular or subcutaneous dose of 2 million IU/m²). There are no adequate data in pregnant women. Intron A should be used during pregnancy only if the potential benefit justifies the potential risk to the foetus.

It is not known whether the components of this drug are excreted in human milk. Because of the potential for adverse reactions from Intron A in nursing infants, a decision should be made whether to discontinue nursing or to discontinue the drug, taking into account the importance of the drug to the mother.

Effects on ability to drive and use machines: Patients who develop fatigue, somnolence, or confusion during treatment with Intron A should be cautioned to avoid driving or operating machinery.

Undesirable effects: In clinical trials conducted in a broad range of indications and at a wide range of doses, the most commonly reported adverse effects were fever, fatigue, headache and myalgia. Fever and fatigue were reversible within 72 hours of interruption or cessation of treatment and were dose related. In the hepatitis treatment groups these effects were of mild to moderate severity.

Common adverse effects include rigors/chills, anorexia and nausea.

In decreasing order of frequency, less commonly reported effects include vomiting, diarrhoea, arthralgia, asthenia, somnolence, dizziness, dry mouth, alopecia, flu-like symptoms (unspecified), back pain, depression, suicidal attempts, malaise, pain, increased sweating, taste alteration, irritability, insomnia, confusion, impaired concentration and hypotension.

Reported rarely were abdominal pain, rash, nervousness, injection site disorders, paresthesia, herpes simplex, pruritus, eye pain, anxiety, epistaxis, coughing, pharyngitis, pulmonary infiltrates, pneumonitis and pneumonia, impaired consciousness, weight decrease, face oedema, dyspnoea, dyspepsia, tachycardia, hypertension, increased appetite, decreased libido, hypoaesthesia, taste perversion, loose stool, gingival bleeding, leg cramps, neuropathy, polyneuropathy, rhabdomyolysis, sometimes serious, and renal insufficiency. Hyperthyroidism or hypothyroidism have also been observed rarely. Hepatotoxicity, including fatality has been observed rarely.

Very rarely following the marketing of Intron A, cases of nephrotic syndrome, renal failure, aggravated diabetes, diabetes/hyperglycaemia, cardiac ischemia, and myocardial infarction have been reported.

Cardiovascular (CVS) adverse reactions, particularly arrhythmia, appeared to be correlated mostly with pre-existing CV disease and prior therapy with cardiotoxic agents (see *Special warnings and precautions for use*). Transient reversible cardiomyopathy has been reported rarely in patients without prior evidence of cardiac disease.

Retinal haemorrhages, cotton-wool spots, and retinal artery or vein obstruction have been observed rarely in patients treated with interferon alfa, including Intron A (recombinant interferon alfa-2b). Powder for solution for injection or solution for injection (see *Special warnings and precautions for use*).

Clinically significant laboratory abnormalities, most frequently occurring at doses greater than 10 Million IU daily, include reduction in granulocyte and white blood cell counts; decreases in haemoglobin level and platelet count; increases in alkaline phosphatase, LDH, serum creatinine and serum urea nitrogen levels.

Increase in serum ALT/AST (SGPT/SGOT) levels have been noted as an abnormality in some non-hepatitis subjects and also in some patients with chronic hepatitis B coincident with clearance of viral DNAp.

Overdose: Overdosing has not been reported with Intron A, but as for any pharmacologically active compound, symptomatic treatment with frequent monitoring of vital signs and close observation of the patient is indicated.

Pharmacological properties
Pharmacotherapeutic group:
Immunostimulating agents, cytokines, interferon alfa, ATC code: L03A A04.

Intron A, solution for injection, is a sterile, stable formulation of highly purified interferon alfa-2b produced by recombinant DNA techniques. Recombinant interferon alfa-2b is a water soluble protein with a molecular weight of approximately 19,300 daltons. It is obtained from a clone of *E. coli*, which harbours a genetically engineered plasmid hybrid encompassing an interferon alfa-2 gene from human leukocytes.

The activity of Intron A is expressed in terms of IU, with 1 mg of recombinant interferon alfa-2b protein corresponding to 2.6×10^8 IU. International Units are determined by comparison of the activity of the recombinant interferon alfa-2b with the activity of the international reference preparation of human leukocyte interferon established by the World Health Organisation.

The interferons are a family of small protein molecules with molecular weights of approximately 15,000 to 21,000 daltons. They are produced and secreted by cells in response to viral infections or various synthetic and biological inducers. Three major classes of interferons have been identified: alpha, beta and gamma. These three main classes are themselves not homogeneous and may contain several different molecular species of interferon. More than 14 genetically distinct human alpha interferons have been identified. Intron A has been classified as recombinant interferon alfa-2b.

Pharmacodynamic properties: Interferons exert their cellular activities by binding to specific membrane receptors on the cell surface. Human interferon receptors, as isolated from human lymphoblastoid (Daudi) cells, appear to be highly asymmetric proteins. They exhibit selectivity for human but not murine interferons, suggesting species specificity. Studies with other interferons have demonstrated species specificity. However, certain monkey species, e.g., rhesus monkeys, are susceptible to pharmacodynamic stimulation upon exposure to human type 1 interferons.

The results of several studies suggest that, once bound to the cell membrane, interferon initiates a complex sequence of intracellular events that include the induction of certain enzymes. It is thought that this process, at least in part, is responsible for the various cellular responses to interferon, including inhibition of virus replication in virus-infected cells, suppression of cell proliferation and such immunomodulating activities as enhancement of the phagocytic activity of macrophages and augmentation of the specific cytotoxicity of lymphocytes for target cells. Any or all of these activities may contribute to interferon's therapeutic effects.

Recombinant interferon alfa-2b has exhibited antiproliferative effects in studies employing both animal and human cell culture systems as well as human tumour xenografts in animals. It has demonstrated significant immunomodulatory activity *in vitro*.

Recombinant interferon alfa-2b also inhibits viral replication *in vitro* and *in vivo*. Although the exact antiviral mode of action of recombinant interferon alfa-2b is unknown, it appears to alter the host cell metabolism. This action inhibits viral replication or if replication occurs, the progeny virions are unable to leave the cell.

Pharmacokinetic properties: The pharmacokinetics of Intron A were studied in healthy volunteers following single 5 million IU/m² and 10 million IU doses administered subcutaneously, intramuscularly and as a 30-minute intravenous infusion. The mean serum interferon concentrations following subcutaneous and intramuscular injections were comparable. Maximum serum levels occurred three to 12 hours after the lower dose and six to eight hours after the higher dose. The elimination half-lives of interferon injections were approximately two to three hours, and six to seven hours, respectively. Serum levels were below the detection limit 16 and 24 hours, respectively, post-injection. Both subcutaneous and intramuscular administration resulted in bioavailabilities greater than 100%.

After intravenous administration, serum interferon levels peaked (135 to 273 IU/ml) by the end of the infusion, then declined at a slightly more rapid rate than after subcutaneous or intramuscular drug administration, becoming undetectable four hours after the infusion. The elimination half-life was approximately two hours.

Urine levels of interferon were below the detection limit following each of the three routes of administration.

Interferon neutralising factor assays were performed on serum samples of patients who received Intron A in Schering-Plough monitored clinical trials. Interferon neutralising factors are antibodies which neutralise the antiviral activity of interferon. The clinical incidence of neutralising factors developing in cancer patients treated systemically is 2.9% and in chronic hepatitis patients is 6.2%. The detectable titres are low in almost all cases and have not been regularly associated with loss of response or any other autoimmune phenomenon. In patients with hepatitis, no loss of response was observed, apparently due to the low titres.

Preclinical safety data: Although interferon is generally recognised as being species specific, toxicity studies in mice, rats, rabbits and monkeys were conducted. Injections of human recombinant interferon alfa-2b for up to three months have shown no evidence of toxicity.

Results of animal reproduction studies indicate that recombinant interferon alfa-2b was not teratogenic in rats or rabbits, nor did it adversely effect pregnancy, foetal development or reproductive capacity in offspring of treated rats. However, high doses of other forms of interferons alfa and beta are known to produce dose-related anovulatory and abortifacient effects in Rhesus monkeys.

Mutagenicity studies with Intron A revealed no adverse effects.

Pharmaceutical particulars

List of excipients: Sodium phosphate dibasic, sodium phosphate monobasic, edetate disodium, sodium chloride, m-cresol, polysorbate 80, water for injection.

Incompatibilities: Apart from the saline solution recommended to dilute Intron A before intravenous infusion, no other substance or solution should be mixed with Intron A.

Shelf life:

– Before first use:
  18 months when refrigerated at 2° to 8°C.
– After first use:
  4 weeks maximum when refrigerated at 2° to 8°C. Any solution remaining after 4 weeks must be discarded.

Special precautions for storage: Intron A must be stored at 2° to 8°C (refrigerator) and should not be frozen. For the purpose of transport and/or to facilitate ambulatory use, the solution can be kept at room temperature (up to 25°C) for a period up to seven days before use. Intron A can be put back in the refrigerator at any time during this seven-day period. If the product is not used during the seven-day period, it cannot be put back in the refrigerator for a new storge period and should be discarded.

Nature and contents of container: 25 million IU/ml: 5 ml vial, type I flint glass, containing 2.5 ml fill.

Instructions for use, handling and disposal (if appropriate): Intron A, solution for injection, may be injected directly after withdrawal of the appropriate doses from the vial with a sterile syringe.

Preparation of Intron A for Intravenous Infusion – The infusion should be prepared immediately prior to use. Any size vial may be used to measure the required dose; however, final concentration of interferon in normal saline solution must be not less than 0.3 million IU/ml. The appropriate dose of Intron A should be withdrawn from the vial(s), added to 50 ml of sterile normal saline solution in a PVC bag or glass bottle for intravenous use and administered over 20 minutes.

NO OTHER DRUG CAN BE INFUSED CONCOMITANTLY WITH INTRON A SOLUTION FOR INJECTION.

As with all parenteral drug products, Intron A, solution for injection, should be inspected visually for particulate matter and discolouration prior to administration. Intron A, solution for injection is clear and colourless.

Marketing authorisation numbers
UK: 0201/0213
Ireland: 277/50/14

Date of (partial) revision of SmPC November 1997

Legal category POM

INTRON A* 1, 3, 5, 10 or 18 million IU/ml

Qualitative and quantitative composition Each vial of Intron A, Powder for Solution for Injection, contains 1, 3, 5, 10 or 18 million International Units (IU) of recombinant interferon alfa-2b.

Pharmaceutical form Powder for solution for injection + sterile water for injection.

For subcutaneous or intravenous injection.

Clinical particulars

Therapeutic indications:

Hepatitis B: Treatment of adult patients with chronic hepatitis B, who have markers for virus replication, e.g., those who are positive for HBV-DNA, DNA polymerase of HBeAg. Current clinicl experience in patients who remain on interferon alfa-2b for 4 to 6 months indicates that therapy can produce clearance of serum HBV-DNA and improvement in liver histology. In patients with loss of HBeAg and HBV-DNA, a significant reduction in morbidity and mortality has been observed.

Chronic hepatitis C: Treatment of adult patients with histologically proven chronic hepatitis who have serum markers for virus C replication, e.g. those who have elevated transminases without liver decompensation and who are positive for serum HCV-RNA or anti-HCV.

Current clinical experience in patients who remain on interferon alfa-2b for 12 months indicates that therapy can produce normalisation of serum ALT, clearance of serum HCV-RNA and improvement in liver histology.

In patients who fail to respond after three to four months of treatment, discontinuation of interferon alfa-2b therapy should be considered.

Hairy cell leukaemia: Treatment of patients with hairy cell leukaemia.

Chronic myelogenous leukaemia: Treatment of adult patients with Philadelphia chromosome or bcr/abl translocation positive chronic myelogenous leukaemia. Clinical experience indicates that a haematologic and cytogenic major/minor response is obtainable in the majority of patients treated. There are no controlled studies demonstrating effects on overall survival.

Multiple myeloma: As maintenance therapy in patients who achieved objective remission (more than 50% reduction in myeloma protein) following initial induction chemotherapy.

Current clinical experience indicates that maintenance therapy with Intron A prolongs the plateau phase; however effects on overall survival have not been conclusively demonstrated.

Follicular lymphoma: Treatment of high tumour burden follicular lymphoma as adjunct to appropriate combination induction chemotherapy such as a CHOP-like regimen. High tumour burden is defined as having at least one of the following: bulk tumour mass (>7 cm), involvement of three or more nodal sites (each >3 cm), systemic symptoms (weight loss >10%, fever >38°C for more than 8 days, or nocturnal sweats), splenomegaly beyond the umbilicus, major organ obstruction or compression syndrome, orbital or epidural involvement, serous effusion, or leukaemia.

Carcinoid tumour: Treatment of carcinoid tumours with lymph node or liver metastases and with 'carcinoid syndrome'.

AIDS-related Kaposi's sarcoma: For patients with progressive asymptomatic Kaposi's sarcoma who have a CD4 count >250/mm³, AIDS patients with CD4 counts <250/mm³, or those with a history of opportunistic infections or constitutional symptoms, are unlikely to respond to Intron A therapy and therefore should not be used (see *Special warnings and special precautions for use*).

Malignant melanoma: As adjuvant therapy in patients who are free of disease after surgery but are at high risk of systemic recurrence, e.g., patients with primary or recurrent (clincial or pathoiligical) lymph node involvement.

Posology and method of administration:

INTRON A INJECTION MAY BE ADMINISTERED USING EITHER STERILISED GLASS OR PLASTIC DISPOSABLE SYRINGES.

MULTIDOSE PRESENTATIONS SHOULD BE FOR INDIVIDUAL PATIENT USE ONLY.

During the course of treatment with Intron A for any indication, if adverse reactions develop, the dosage should be modified or therapy should be discontinued temporarily until the adverse reactions abate. If persistent or recurrent intolerance develops following adequate dosage adjustment, or disease progresses, the treatment with Intron A should be discontinued. For maintenance dosage regimens administered subcutaneously, at the discretion of the physician, the patient may self-administer the dose.

Chronic hepatitis B: The recommended dosage is in the range of 5 to 10 million IU administered subcutaneously three times per week (every other day) for a period of four to six months.

If no improvement in serum HBV-DNA is been observed after three to four months of treatment (at the 10 million IU dose, if tolerated), interferon alfa-2b therapy should be discontinued.

Chronic hepatitis C: The recommended dose is three million IU administered subcutaneously three times a week (every other day). Most patients who respond demonstrate improvement in ALT levels within three to four months. In these patients, therapy should be continued with 3 million IU three times a week (every othe day) for 12 months.

The optimal duration of treatment is not yet established. There are no clinical studies directly comparing 12 to 18 months, however, the prolongation of treatment up to 18 months might be usefully considered in some patients.

In patients who fail to respond after three to four months of treatment, discontinuation of interferon alfa-2b should be considered.

Hairy cell leukaemia: The recommended dosage is 2 million IU/m² administered subcutaneously three times a week (every other day) for both splenectomised and non-splenectomised patients. For most patients with HCL, normalisation of one or more haematological variables occurs within one to two months of Intron A treatment. Improvement in all three haematological variables (granulocyte count, platelet count and haemoglobin level) may require six months or more. This regimen should be maintained unless the disease progresses rapidly or severe intolerance is manifested.

Chronic myelogenous leukaemia: The recommended dosage of Intron A Injection is 4 to 5 million IU/m² administered daily subcutaneously. When the white blood cell count is controlled, the maximum tolerated dose (4 to 10 million IU/m² daily) should be administered to maintain haematological remission. Intron A treatment should be discontinued after 8 to 12 weeks of treatment if at least a partial haematological remission or a clinically meaningful cytoreduction has not been achieved.

Multiple myeloma: Maintenance therapy – In patients who are in the plateau phase (more than 50% reduction of myeloma protein) following initial induction chemotherapy, Intron A may be administered as monotherapy, subcutaneously, at a dose of 3 million IU/m² three times a week (every other day).

Follicular lymphoma: Adjunctively with chemotherapy, Intron A Injection may be administered subcutaneously, at a dose of 5 million IU three times a week (every other day) for a duration of 18 months. CHOP-like regimens are advised, but clinical experience is available only with CHVP (combination of cyclophosphamide, doxorubicin, teniposide and prednisolone).

Carcinoid tumour: The usual dose is 5 million IU (3 to 9 million IU) administered subcutaneously three times a week (every other day). Patients with advanced disease may require a daily dose of 5 million IU. The treatment should be temporarily discontinued during and after surgery. Therapy should continue for as long as the patient responds to Intron A treatment.

AIDS-related Kaposi's sarcoma: The optimal dosage is not yet known. Efficacy has been demonstrated at a daily dose of 10 million IU administered subcutaneously. The minimum effective dose is not established. The maximum tolerated daily dose of Intron A is 20 million IU.

If severe adverse reactions develop, the dosage should be modified (50% reduction) or therapy discontinued temporarily until the adverse reactions abate.

When disease stabilisation or treatment response occurs, treatment should continue until there is no further evidence of tumour or until discontinuation is required by evidence of a severe opportunistic infection or adverse effect. Intron A therapy has been administered in an outpatient regimen.

Malignant melanoma: As induction therapy, Intron A is administered intravenously at a dose of 20 million IU/m² daily for five days a week for a four-week period; the calculated Intron A dose is added to 100 ml of saline solution and administered as a 20-minute infusion. As maintenance treatment, the recommended dose is 10 million IU/m^2 administered subcutaneously three days a week (every other day) for 48 weeks.

If severe adverse reactions develop during Intron A treatment, particularly if granulocytes decrease to <500/mm^3 or ALT/AST rise to >5× upper limit of normal, treatment should be temporarily discontinued until the adverse reaction abates. Intron A treatment should be restarted at 50% of the previous dose. If intolerance persists after dose adjustment or if granulocytes decrease to <250/mm^3 or ALT/AST rise to >10× upper limit of normal, Intron A therapy should be discontinued.

Although the optimal (minimum) dose is unknown, for full clinical benefit, patients should be treated at the recommended dose, with dose modification for toxicity as described.

Contra-indications:

- A history of hypersensitivity to recombinant interferon alfa-2b or any other component of Intron A.
- Severe pre-existing cardiac disease.
- Severe renal or hepatic dysfunction; including that caused by metastases.
- Epilepsy and/or compromised central nervous system (CNS) function (see *Special precautions for use*).
- Chronic hepatitis with decompensated cirrhosis of the liver.
- Chronic hepatitis in patients who are being or have been recently treated with immunosuppressive agents excluding short-term corticosteroid withdrawal.
- Autoimmune hepatitis; or history of autoimmune disease; immunosuppressed transplant recipients.
- Pre-existing thyroid disease unless controlled by conventional treatment.

Special warnings and precautions for use:

For all patients: Acute hypersensitivity reactions (e.g., urticaria, angioedema, bronchoconstriction, anaphylaxis) to Intron A have been observed rarely during Intron A therapy. If such a reaction develops, the drug should be discontinued and appropriate medical therapy instituted immediately. Transient rashes do not necessitate interruption of treatment.

Moderate to severe adverse experiences may require modification of the patient's dosage regimen, or in some cases, termination of Intron A therapy. Any patient developing liver function abnormalities during treatment with Intron A should be monitored closely and treatment discontinued if signs and symptoms progress.

Hypotension may occur during Intron A therapy or up to two days post-therapy and may require supportive treatment.

Adequate hydration should be maintained in patients undergoing Intron A therapy since hypotension related to fluid depletion has been seen in some patients. Fluid replacement may be necessary.

While fever may be associated with the flu-like syndrome reported commonly during interferon therapy, other causes of persistent fever should be ruled out.

Paracetamol has been used successfully to alleviate the symptoms of fever and headache which can occur with Intron A therapy. The recommended paracetamol dosage is 500 mg to 1 g given 30 minutes before administration of Intron A. The maximum dosage of paracetamol to be given is 1 g four times daily.

Intron A should be used cautiously in patients with debilitating medical conditions, such as those with a history of pulmonary disease (e.g. chronic obstructive pulmonary disease) or diabetes mellitus prone to ketoacidosis. Caution should be observed also in patients with coagulation disorders (e.g. thrombophlebitis, pulmonary embolism) or severe myelosuppression.

Pulmonary infiltrates, pneumonitis and pneumonia, including fatality, have been observed rarely in interferon alpha treated patients, including those treated with Intron A. The aetiology has not been defined. These symptoms have been reported more frequently when shosaikoto, a Chinese herbal medicine, is administered concomitantly with interferon-alfa.

Any patient developing fever, cough, dyspnea or other respiratory symptoms should have a chest X-ray taken. If the chest X-ray shows pulmonary infiltrates or there is evidence of pulmonary function impairment, the patient should be monitored closely, and, if appropriate, interferon-alfa treatment should be discontinued. While this has been reported more often in patients with chronic hepatitis C treated with interferon-alfa, it has also been reported in patients with oncologic diseases treated with interferon-alfa. Prompt discontinuation of interferon alfa administration and treatment with corticosteroids appear to be associated with resolution of pulmonary adverse events.

Ocular adverse events (see *Undesirable effects*) appear to occur after use of the drug for several months, but also have been reported after shorter treatment periods. Any patient complaining of changes in visual acuity or visual fields, or reporting other ophthalmologic symptoms during treatment with Intron A, should have an eye examination. Because the retinal events may have to be differentiated from those seen with diabetic or hypertensive retinopathy, a baseline ocular examination is recommended prior to treatment with interferon in patients with diabetes mellitus or hypertension.

Patients with a pre-existing psychiatric condition or a history of severe psychiatric disorder should not be treated with Intron A.

Severe CNS effects, particularly depression, suicidal ideation and attempted suicide have been observed in some patients during Intron A therapy; in these cases, Intron A therapy should be discontinued. The potential seriousness of these adverse events should be borne in mind by the prescribing physician.

Other CNS effects manifested by confusion and other alterations of mental status have been observed rarely. More significant obtundation and coma have been observed in some patients, usually elderly, treated at higher doses. While these effects are generally reversible, in a few patients full resolution took up to three weeks. Very rarely, seizures have occurred with high doses of Intron A.

Patients with a history of congestive heart failure, myocardial infarction and/or previous or current arrhythmic disorders, who require Intron A therapy, should be closely monitored. Those patients who have pre-existing cardiac abnormalities and/or are in advanced stages of cancer should have electrocardiograms taken prior to and during the course of treatment. Cardiac arrhythmias (primarily supraventricular) usually respond to conventional therapy but may require discontinuation of Intron A therapy.

Because of reports of exacerbating pre-existing psoriatic disease, Intron A should be used in patients with psoriasis only if the potential benefit justifies the potential risk.

Preliminary data may indicate that interferon alfa therapy is associated with an increased rate of graft rejection (liver and kidney transplants).

The development of different auto-antibodies has been reported during treatment with alfa interferons. Clinical manifestations of autoimmune disease during interferon therapy may occur more freuently in patients predisposed to the development of autoimmune disorders.

Treatment with Intron A should be discontinued in patients with chronic hepatitis who develop prolongation of coagulation markers which might indicate liver decompensation.

The efficacy of interferon alfa-2b has not been demonstrated in patients with either chronic hepatitis B or C, with a co-infection with the human immunodeficiency virus (HIV), or undergoing hemodialysis.

Chronic hepatitis C: Infrequently, patients treated for chronic hepatitis C with Intron A developed thyroid abnormalities, either hypothyroid or hyperthyroid. In clinical trials using Intron A therapy, 2.8% patients overall developed thyroid abnormalities. The abnormalities were controlled by conventional therapy for thyroid dysfunction. The mechanism by which Intron A may alter thyroid status is unknown. Prior to initiation of Intron A therapy for the treatment of chronic hepatitis C, serum thyroid-stimulating hormone (TSH) levels should be evaluated. Any thyroid abnormality detected at that time should be treated with conventional therapy. Intron A treatment may ne initiated if TSH levels can be maintained in the normal range by medication.

If, during the course of Intron A therapy, a patient develops symptoms consistent with possible thyroid dysfunction, TSH levels should be evaluated. In the presence of thyroid dysfunction, Intron A treatment may be continued if TSH levels can be maintained in the normal range of medication. Discontinuation of Intron A therapy has not reversed thyroid dysfunction occurring during treatment.

Concomitant chemotherapy: Administration of Intron A in combination with other chemotherapeutic agents may lead to increased risk of toxicity (severity and duration), which may be life-threatening or fatal as a result of the concomitantly administered drug. The most commonly reported potentially life-threatening or fatal adverse events include mucositis, diarrhoea, neutropenia, renal impairment, and electrolyte disturbance. Because of the risk of increased toxicity, careful adjustments of doses are required for Intron A and for the concomitant chemotherapeutic agents.

AIDS-related Kaposi's sarcoma: Intron A should not be used in conjunction with protease inhibitors. With the exception of zidovudine, there is a lack of safety data for the combination of Intrron A with reverse transciptase inhibitors.

Laboratory tests: Standard haematological tests and blood chemistries (complete blood count and differential, platelet count, electrolytes, liver enzymes, serum protein, serum bilirubin and serum creatinine) should be conducted in all patients prior to and periodically during systemic treatment with Intron A.

During treatment for hepatitis B or C the recommended testing schedule is at weeks 1, 2, 4, 8, 12, 16, and every other month, thereafter, throughout treatment. If ALT flares during Intron A therapy to greater than or equal to 2 times baseline, Intron A therapy may be continued unless signs and symptoms of liver failure are observed.

During ALT flare, liver function tests: ALT, prothrombin time, alkaline phosphatase, albumin and bilirubin should be monitored at two-week intervals.

In patients treated for malignant melanoma, liver function and white blood cell (WBC) count and differential should be monitored weekly during the induction phase of therapy and monthly during the maintenance phase of therapy.

Paediatric use: Doses of up to 10 million IU/m^2 have been administered safely to children with chronic hepatitis B. However, efficacy of therapy has not been demonstrated. Generally, experience in patients below 18 years of age has been limited, and in such cases the expected benefits should be weighed carefully against potential hazards.

Effect on fertility: Interferon may impair fertility. In studies of interferon use in non-human primates, abnormalities of the menstrual cycle have been observed. Decreased serum estradiol and progesterone concentrations have been reported in women treated with human leukocyte interferon. Therefore, fertile women should not receive Intron A unless they are using effective contraception during the treatment period. Intron A should be used with caution in fertile men.

Interaction with other medicaments and other forms of interaction:

Drug/drug interactions: Narcotics, hypnotics or sedatives should be administered with caution concomitantly with Intron A Injection.

Interactions between Intron A and other drugs have not been fully evaluated. Caution should be exercised when administering Intron A in combination with other potentially myelosuppressive agents.

Interferons may affect the oxidative metabolic process. This should be considered during concomitant therapy with drugs metabolised by this route, such as the xanthine derivatives theophylline or aminophylline. During concomitant therapy with xanthine agents, serum theophylline levels should be monitored and dosage adjusted if necessary.

Pregnancy and lactation: Intron A has been shown to have abortifacient effects in *Macaca mulatta* (rhesus monkeys) at 90 and 180 times the recommended intramuscular or subcutaneous dose of 2 million IU/m^2. Abortion was observed in all dose groups (7.5 million, 15 million and 30 million IU/kg), and was only statistically significant versus control at the mid- and high-dose groups (corresponding to 90 and 180 times the recommended intramuscular or subcutaneous dose of 2 million IU/m^2). There are no adequate data in pregnant women. Intron A should be used during pregnancy only if the potential benefit justifies the potential risk to the foetus.

It is not known whether the components of this drug are excreted in human milk. Because of the potential for adverse reactions from Intron A in nursing infants, a decision should be made whether to discontinue nursing or to discontinue the drug, taking into account the importance of the drug to the mother.

Effects on ability to drive and use machines: Patients who develop fatigue, somnolence, or confusion during treatment with Intron A should be cautioned to avoid driving or operating machinery.

Undesirable effects: In clinical trials conducted in a broad range of indications and at a wide range of doses, the most commonly reported adverse effects were fever, fatigue, headache and myalgia. Fever and fatigue were reversible within 72 hours of interruption or cessation of treatment and were dose related. In the hepatitis treatment groups these effects were of mild to moderate severity.

Common adverse effects include rigors/chills, anorexia and nausea.

In decreasing order of frequency, less commonly reported effects include vomiting, diarrhoea, arthralgia, asthenia, somnolence, dizziness, dry mouth, alopecia, flu-like symptoms (unspecified), back pain, depression, suicidal atempts, malaise, pain, increased sweating, taste alteration, irritability, insomnia, confusion, impaired concentration and hypotension.

Reported rarely were abdominal pain, rash, nervousness, injection site disorders, paresthesia, herpes simplex, pruritus, eye pain, anxiety, epistaxis, coughing, pharyngitis, pulmonary infiltrates, pneumonitis and pneumonia, impaired consciousness, weight decrease, face oedema, dyspnea, dyspepsia, tachycardia, hypertension, increased appetite, decreased libido, hypoaesthesia, taste perversion, loose stool, gingival bleeding, leg cramps, neuropathy, polyneuropathy, rhabdomyolysis, sometimes serious, and renal insufficiency.

Hyperthyroidism or hypothyroidism have also been observed rarely. Hepatotoxicity, including fatality has been observed rarely.

Very rarely following the marketing of Intron A, cases of nephrotic syndrome, renal failure, aggravated diabetes, diabetes/hyperglycaemia, cardiac ischemia, and myocardial infarction have been reported.

Cardiovascular (CVS) adverse reactions, particularly arrhythmia, appeared to be correlated mostly with pre-existing CVS disease and prior therapy with cardiotoxic agents (see *Special warnings and precautions for use*). Transient reversible cardiomyopathy has been reported rarely in patients without prior evidence of cardiac disease.

Retinal haemorrhages, cotton-wool spots, and retinal artery or vein obstruction have been observed rarely in patients treated with interferon alfa, including Intron A (recombinant interferon alfa-2b). Powder for Solution for Injection or Solution for Injection (see *Special warnings and precautions for use*).

Clinically significant laboratory abnormalities, most frequently occurring at doses greater than 10 million IU daily, include reduction in granulocyte and white blood cell counts; decreases in haemoglobin level and platelet count; increases in alkaline phosphatase, LDH, serum creatinine and serum urea nitrogen levels. Increase in serum ALT/AST (SGPT/SGOT) levels have been noted as an abnormality in some non-hepatitis subjects and also in some patients with chronic hepatitis B coincident with clearance of viral DNAp.

Overdose: Overdosing has not been reported with Intron A, but as for any pharmacologically active compound, symptomatic treatment with frequent monitoring of vital signs and close observation of the patient is indicated.

Pharmacological properties

Pharmacotherapeutic group:
Immunostimulating agents, cytokines, interferon alfa, ATC code: L03A A04.

Intron A is a sterile, stable, lyophilised formulation of highly purified interferon alfa-2b produced by recombinant DNA techniques. Recombinant interferon alfa-2b is a water soluble protein with a molecular weight of approximately 19,300 daltons. It is obtained from a clone of *E. coli*, which harbours a genetically engineered plasmid hybrid encompassing an interferon alfa-2 gene from human leukocytes.

The activity of Intron A is expressed in terms of IU, with 1 mg of recombinant interferon alfa-2b protein corresponding to 2.6×10^8 IU. International Units are determined by comparison of the activity of the recombinant interferon alfa-2b with the activity of the international reference preparation of human leukocyte interferon established by the World Health Organisation.

The interferons are a family of small protein molecules with molecular weights of approximately 15,000 to 21,000 daltons. They are produced and secreted by cells in response to viral infections or various synthetic and biological inducers. Three major classes of interferons have been identified: alpha, beta and gamma. These three main classes are themselves not homogeneous and may contain several different molecular species of interferon. More than 14 genetically distinct human alpha interferons have been identified. Intron A has been classified as recombinant interferon alfa-2b.

Pharmacodynamic properties: Interferons exert their cellular activities by binding to specific membrane receptors on the cell surface. Human interferon receptors, as isolated from human lymphoblastoid (Daudi) cells, appear to be highly asymmetric proteins.

They exhibit selectivity for human but not murine interferons, suggesting species specificity. Studies with other interferons have demonstrated species specificity. However, certain monkey species, e.g., Rhesus monkeys, are susceptible to pharmacodynamic stimulation upon exposure to human type 1 interferons.

The results of several studies suggest that, once bound to the cell membrane, interferon initiates a complex sequence of intracellular events that include the induction of certain enzymes. It is thought that this process, at least in part, is responsible for the various cellular responses to interferon, including inhibition of virus replication in virus-infected cells, suppression of cell proliferation and such immunomodulating activities as enhancement of the phagocytic activity of macrophages and augmentation of the specific cytotoxicity of lymphocytes for target cells. Any or all of these activities may contribute to interferon's therapeutic effects.

Recombinant interferon alfa-2b has exhibited antiproliferative effects in studies employing both animal and human cell culture systems as well as human tumour xenografts in animals. It has demonstrated significant immunomodulatory activity *in vitro*.

Recombinant interferon alfa-2b also inhibits viral replication *in vitro* and *in vivo*. Although the exact antiviral mode of action of recombinant interferon alfa-2b is unknown, it appears to alter the host cell metabolism. This action inhibits viral replication or if replication occurs, the progeny virions are unable to leave the cell.

Pharmacokinetic properties: The pharmacokinetics of Intron A were studied in healthy volunteers following single 5 million IU/m² and 10 million IU doses administered subcutaneously, intramuscularly and as a 30-minute intravenous infusion. The mean serum interferon concentrations following subcutaneous and intramuscular injections were comparable. Maximum serum levels occurred three to twelve hours after the lower dose and six to eight hours after the higher dose. The elimination half-lives of interferon injections were approximately two to three hours, and six to seven hours, respectively. Serum levels were below the detection limit sixteen and twenty-four hours, respectively, post-injection. Both subcutaneous and intramuscular administration resulted in bioavailabilities greater than 100%.

After intravenous administration, serum interferon levels peaked (135 to 273 IU/ml) by the end of the infusion, then declined at a slightly more rapid rate than after subcutaneous or intramuscular drug administration, becoming undetectable four hours after the infusion. The elimination half-life was approximately two hours.

Urine levels of interferon were below the detection limit following each of the three routes of administration.

Interferon neutralising factor assays were performed on serum samples of patients who received Intron A in Schering-Plough monitored clinical trials. Interferon neutralising factors are antibodies which neutralise the antiviral activity of interferon. The clinical incidence of neutralising factors developing in cancer patients treated systemically is 2.9% and in chronic hepatitis patients is 6.2%. The detectable titres are low in almost all cases and have not been regularly associated with loss of response or any other autoimmune phenomenon. In patients with hepatitis, no loss of response was observed, apparently due to the low titres.

Preclinical safety data: Although interferon is generally recognised as being species specific, toxicity studies in mice, rats, rabbits and monkeys were conducted. Injections of human recombinant interferon alfa-2b for up to three months have shown no evidence of toxicity.

Results of animal reproduction studies indicate that recombinant interferon alfa-2b was not teratogenic in rats or rabbits, nor did it adversely effect pregnancy, foetal development or reproductive capacity in offspring of treated rats. However, high doses of other forms of interferons alfa and beta are known to produce dose-related anovulatory and abortifacient effects in Rhesus monkeys.

Mutagenicity studies with Intron A revealed no adverse effects.

Pharmaceutical particulars

List of excipients:
Powder for solution for injection: glycine, sodium phosphate dibasic, sodium phosphate monobasic and human albumin.

Diluents:
– Sterile water for injection.

Incompatibilities: Apart from the recommended diluent, no other substance or solution should be mixed with Intron A.

Shelf life:
– Non-reconstituted product:
  36 months when stored at 2° to 8°C (refrigerator)
  4 weeks maximum at room temperature (up to 25°C) before use
– Reconstituted solution (single-dose vial)
  12 hours maximum when stored at room temperature (up to 25°C) or 24 hours at 2° to 8°C (refrigerator).

Special precautions for storage: Store refrigerated at 2–8°C. DO NOT FREEZE.

For the purpose of transport and/or to facilitate ambulatory use, the non-reconstituted lyophilised product or the solution product can be kept at room temperature (up to 25°C) for a period up to four weeks before use. If the product is not used during the four-week period, it cannot be put back in the refrigerator for a new storage period and should be discarded.

Container:s
Intron A Powder for Solution for injection:
– 2 ml vial, type I flint glass.

Diluents:
– Sterile water for injection; 2 ml ampoule, type I flint glass.

Instructions for use/handling:
Reconstitution of Intron A, Powder for Solution for Injection, for Parenteral administration: Intron A is supplied as a powder at strengths of 1, 3, 5, 10 and 18 million IU for single-dose use. Single-dose vials must be reconstituted with 1 ml of Sterile Water for Injection. The reconstituted solutions are isotonic for parenteral administration.

Using a sterile syringe and needle, inject 1 ml Sterile Water for Injection into the vial of Intron A. Agitate gently to hasten complete dissolution of the powder. The appropriate dose should then be withdrawn with a sterile syringe and injected.

The reconstituted material, as for all parenteral drug products, should be inspected visually for particulate use matter and discolouratiuon prior to administration.

Preparation of Intron A for Intravenous Infusion: The infusion should be prepared immediately prior to use. The lyophilised powder of Intron A should be reconstituted by adding 1 ml of Sterile Water for Injection to the vial. The calculated amount of interferon for the appropriate dose should then be withdrawn from the vial(s), added to 100 ml of Sterile Normal Saline solution and administered over 20 minutws.

NO OTHER DRUG CAN BE INFUSED CONCOMITANTLY WITHIN INTRON A.

Intravenous (i.v.) administration sets The compatibility of Intron A at a minimum concentration of 1×10^6 IU/ml in normal saline was evaluated in various IV administration sets.

The following intravenous administration sets may be used with Intron A:

Administration Set:	*Manufacturer:*
2C001	Travenol
VI 400	McGaw
Venoset 78	Abbott
Ultipor Blood Transfusion Filter & Administration Set	Pall
Intrafix Air	B. Braun
STK Set Type L76	Aesca
Perfu Pal	Dubernarid Vitrum
Vacoset V34	Baxter
Vacoset V2400	Pharmaseal
Hiplex-Venosteril	—
Venoset	Abbott
Vacoset V-736	McGaw
Vacoset V-717U	McGaw

The following intravenous administration sets are not acceptable and may not be used with Intron A:

Administration Set:	*Manufacturer:*
Versaset V13	Rivero
Addit IV V1444	McGaw
Continue-Flow	Travenol

Marketing authorisation numbers

	UK	*Ireland*
Intron A 1 million IU/ml:	0201/0063	277/50/1
Intron A 3 million IU/ml:	0201/0064	277/50/2
Intron A 5 million IU/ml:	0201/0065	277/50/3
Intron A 10 million IU/ml:	0201/0066	277/50/4
Intron A 18 million IU/ml:	0201/0210	277/50/9

Date of approval September 1998

Legal category POM

LEUCOMAX* ▼

Presentation Leucomax contains molgramostim, a recombinant human granulocyte macrophage-colony stimulating factor (rHuGM-CSF), non-glycosylated with isoleucine at position 100.

Molgramostim is a water-soluble, non-glycosylated protein produced by recombinant techniques. Its activity is expressed in International Units (IU) with 1 million IU corresponding to approximately 90 micrograms of molgramostim protein. Each vial of Leucomax contains the labelled quantity of molgramostim in million IU.

Uses Leucomax is indicated for reduction of risk of infection and to allow better adherence to the chemotherapeutic regimen, by decreasing the severity of cytotoxic chemotherapy-induced neutropenia (see *Precautions, Laboratory tests*).

Leucomax is also indicated for the acceleration of myeloid recovery in patients following autologous or syngeneic bone marrow transplantation. Leucomax has not been shown to improve overall survival or increase time to relapse.

Leucomax is also indicated as adjuvant therapy in ganciclovir (DHPG)-induced neutropenia in patients with AIDS-related cytomegalovirus (CMV) retinitis in order to maintain recommended DHPG dosage.

Dosage and administration Leucomax must be reconstituted before administration (see *Technical instructions*). Leucomax dosing regimens vary according to the indication for therapy. The maximum daily dose should not exceed 0.11×10^6IU/kg/day (10 micrograms/kg/day).

The recommended dosage regimens are:

Cancer chemotherapy: $0.06–0.11 \times 10^6$IU/kg/day (5 to 10 micrograms/kg/day) administered subcutaneously. Treatment should be initiated 24 hours after the last dose of chemotherapy and continued for 7 to 10 days. Dosing may be initiated at 0.06×10⁶IU/kg/day (5 micrograms/kg/day).

Bone marrow transplantation (BMT): 0.11×10⁶IU/kg/day (10 micrograms/kg/day) administered by intravenous infusion over 4 to 6 hours, beginning the day after BMT. Continue until the absolute neutrophil count (ANC) is ≥1×10⁹/l. The maximum duration of treatment is 30 days.

AIDS-related CMV retinitis as adjuvant therapy to ganciclovir (DHPG): 0.06×10⁶ IU/kg (5 micrograms/kg) once daily by subcutaneous injection. After the fifth Leucomax dose has been administered the dose may be titrated to maintain the ANC and WBC count at the desired levels, usually ≥1×10⁹/l and <20×10⁹/l respectively.

Use in children: The safety of Leucomax has been demonstrated in a limited number of patients below the age of 18 years.

Use in the elderly: There are no apparent differences in the safety of Leucomax in elderly patients.

Contra-indications, warnings, etc

Contra-indications: Leucomax is contra-indicated in patients with a history of hypersensitivity to molgramostim or any component of the injectable formulation.

Leucomax should not be used in patients with myeloid malignancies.

Precautions: Leucomax should be used under the supervision of a physician experienced in the treatment of oncologic and haematopoietic disorders or infectious diseases.

The first dose of Leucomax should be administered under medical supervision.

Acute severe, life threatening hypersensitivity reactions, including anaphylaxis, angioedema or bronchoconstriction have occurred in patients receiving Leucomax. If such reactions occur Leucomax should be withdrawn immediately and not reintroduced.

Leucomax has been associated infrequently with pleurisy, or pleural effusion. Pericarditis occurred in 2% (21/1098) and pericardial effusion in <2% (16/1098). If such reactions occur, Leucomax should be withdrawn. Patients with pre-existing pulmonary disease may be predisposed to decreased pulmonary function and dyspnoea, and should be monitored closely when being treated with Leucomax.

In clinical trials, adverse events reported with initiation of dosing were mostly mild to moderate in severity and included rigors, dyspnoea, fever, nausea, vomiting, non-specific chest pain, asthenia, hypotension or flushing. These symptoms, which infrequently required withdrawal of Leucomax were managed symptomatically.

In a few isolated instances, autoimmune disease developed or was exacerbated during rHuGMCSF therapy. Therefore, when administering Leucomax to patients with a history of, or predisposition to autoimmune disease, this should be considered.

Laboratory tests: Standard haematologic tests (full blood count with differential white cell count and platelet count) should be performed and serum albumin levels monitored during therapy with Leucomax.

Because of the potential of receiving higher doses of chemotherapy (i.e. full doses on the prescribed schedule), the patients may be at greater risk of thrombocytopenia and anaemia as consequences of increased chemotherapy doses. Regular monitoring of the platelet count and haematocrit is recommended.

Drug interactions: Since dosing with Leucomax has been associated with a decrease in serum albumin, drugs that are highly bound to serum albumin may require dosage adjustment.

Use in pregnancy and lactation: Safety of Leucomax for use in human pregnancy has not been established. Animal studies have shown reproductive toxicity. In primate models, administration of molgramostim was associated with foetal death and spontaneous abortion at doses of 0.07 and 0.11×10⁶ IU/kg/day (6 and 10 mcg/kg/day).

In the absence of clinical data in pregnancy, the therapeutic benefit to the patient must be weighed against potential risks to the progress of pregnancy.

It is not known whether Leucomax is excreted in human milk. However, because of the potential for adverse effects in infants, nursing is not recommended in women receiving Leucomax.

Side-effects: Since many of the undesirable events reported during Leucomax clinical trials are often associated with underlying or concurrent disease or their treatment, the causal relationship of many of these events to Leucomax cannot be definitively determined. Most adverse reactions were mild to moderate in severity. Rarely were they severe or life threatening.

The most frequently reported undesirable effects across all indications were fever, nausea, dyspnoea, diarrhoea, rash, rigors, injection site reaction (with sc administration), vomiting, fatigue, anorexia, musculoskeletal pain and asthenia.

Less frequently reported events include; non-specific chest pain, stomatitis, headache, increased sweating, abdominal pain, pruritus, dizziness, peripheral oedema, paraesthesia and myalgia.

Serious reactions, which occurred rarely in clinical trials, include: anaphylaxis, bronchospasm, cardiac failure, capillary leak syndrome, cerebrovascular disorders, confusion, convulsions, hypotension, cardiac rhythm abnormalities, intracranial hypertension, pericardial effusion, pericarditis, pleural effusion, pulmonary oedema and syncope.

Laboratory findings – in all patient groups the most frequently occurring changes in laboratory values were decreased platelet count, decreased haemoglobin level, decreased serum albumin level and an increase in eosinophils (absolute count and percent). The causal relationship of these changes to Leucomax cannot be determined definitively.

The frequency of antibodies that bind to molgramostim, measured by enzyme-linked immunosorbent assay (ELISA) and bioassay, was determined to be 1% post treatment. No loss of activity of Leucomax was evident in these patients.

Overdosage: Overdosing has not been reported with Leucomax. As for any pharmacologically active compound, symptomatic treatment with frequent monitoring of vital signs and close observation of the patient is indicated if severe reactions occur.

Pharmaceutical precautions Leucomax sterile lyophilised powder should be stored at 2°C to 8°C and protected from light.

Following reconstitution with sterile water for injection Leucomax solution can be used for 24 hours when refrigerated at 2 to 8°C. Unused Leucomax solution should be discarded.

Technical instructions: Reconstitution of Leucomax – Add 1.0 ml of diluent (sterile water for injection) to the vial of Leucomax. Agitate the vial gently to dissolve the powder completely. This provides the labelled amount of Leucomax as an isotonic solution, which may be used for s.c. administration. When diluted further in accordance with the instructions below, Leucomax may be administered intravenously.

Dilution for i.v. administration – **dilution instructions must be followed carefully to avoid loss of molgramostim as a result of adsorption to the infusion system.**

Reconstitute each of the required number of vials of lyophilised powder to the appropriate strength of molgramostim with 1 ml of sterile water for injection. The reconstituted molgramostim solution may be further diluted in 25 ml, 50 ml or 100 ml infusion bags or bottles of either normal saline solution or 5% dextrose in water. The number and the strength of lyophilised powder vials required must be such that the above infusion admixture solution contains a final concentration of molgramostim of *not less than 0.08×10⁶ IU (7 micrograms) per ml.* The resulting infusion solution is stable for 24 hours when stored in a refrigerator.

Leucomax infusion solution is compatible with the following infusion sets: Travenol 2C0001 and C0334, Intrafix air, Infusionsgerat R, 87 Plus, Souplix, Steriflex, Intrafix Air Euroklappe-ISO, Soluset and Linfosol sets. *Significant adsorption of Leucomax has been observed in a Port-A-Cath (Pharmacia) system, and its use is not recommended.*

For i.v. administration, the use of an in-line, low protein binding 0.2 or 0.22 micrometer filter is recommended. The reconstituted solution is colourless to light yellow and should be inspected visually for discolouration and particulate matter prior to administration.

Further information The excipients contained in Leucomax are mannitol, citric acid, dibasic sodium phosphate, polyethylene glycol and human albumin. Molgramostim has an elimination half-life of one to two hours following intravenous administration and two to three hours following subcutaneous administration.

Legal category POM.

Package quantities Leucomax sterile lyophilised powder is supplied in Type I glass vials with butyl or halobutyl rubber closures and aluminium seal in the following strengths: 1.67×10⁶IU/vial (150 micrograms/vial); 3.33×10⁶IU/vial (300 micrograms/vial); 4.44×10⁶IU/vial (400 micrograms/vial).

Product licence numbers

1.67×10⁶IU/vial (150 mcg/vial) 0201/0150
3.33×10⁶IU/vial (300 mcg/vial) 0201/0181
4.44×10⁶IU/vial (400 mcg/vial) 0201/0151

NASONEX* AQUEOUS NASAL SPRAY ▼

Qualitative and quantitative composition Mometasone furoate 50 micrograms/spray.

Pharmaceutical form Nasal spray suspension.

Clinical particulars

Therapeutic indications: Nasonex Aqueous Nasal Spray is indicated for use in adults and children 12 years of age and older to treat the symptoms of seasonal allergic or perennial rhinitis.

In patients who have a history of moderate to severe symptoms of seasonal allergic rhinitis, prophylactic treatment with Nasonex may be initiated up to four weeks prior to the anticipated start of the pollen season.

Posology and method of administration: After initial priming of the Nasonex Aqueous Nasal Spray pump (usually 6 or 7 actuations, until a uniform spray is observed), each actuation delivers approximately 100 mg of mometasone furoate suspension, containing mometasone fuorate monohydrate equivalent to 50 micrograms mometasone furoate. If the spray pump has not been used for 14 days or longer, it should be reprimed before next use.

Adults (including geriatric patients) and children 12 years of age and older: The usual recommended dose is two sprays (50 micrograms/spray) in each nostril once daily (total dose 200 micrograms). Once symptoms are controlled, dose reduction to one spray in each nostril (total dose 100 micrograms) may be effective for maintenance.

If symptoms are inadequately controlled, the dose may be increased to a maximum daily dose of four sprays in each nostril once daily (total dose 400 micrograms). Dose reduction is recommended following control of symptoms.

Nasonex Aqueous Nasal Spray demonstrated a clinically significant onset of action within 12 hours after the first dose in some patients with seasonal allergic rhinitis; however, full benefit of treatment may not be achieved in the first 48 hours. Therefore, the patient should continue regular use to achieve full therapeutic benefit.

There are no clinical results on use in children under the age of 12 years and therefore Nasonex is not recommended in this age group.

Contra-indications: Hypersensitivity to any ingredients of Nasonex Aqueous Nasal Spray.

Nasonex Aqueous Nasal Spray should not be used in the presence of untreated localised infection involving the nasal mucosa.

Because of the inhibitory effects of corticosteroids on wound healing, patients who have experienced recent nasal surgery or trauma should not use a nasal cortico-steroid until healing has occurred.

Special warnings and precautions for use: Nasonex Aqueous Nasal Spray should be used with caution, if at all, by patients with active or quiescent tuberculous infections of the respiratory tract, or in untreated fungal, bacterial, systemic viral infections or ocular herpes simplex.

Following 12 months of treatment with Nasonex Aqueous Nasal Spray, there was no evidence of atrophy of the nasal mucosa; also, mometasone furoate tended to reverse the nasal mucosa closer to a normal histologic phenotype. As with any long-term treatment, patients using Nasonex Aqueous Nasal Spray over several months or longer should be examined periodically for possible changes in the nasal mucosa. If localised fungal infection of the nose or pharynx develops, discontinuance of Nasonex Aqueous Nasal Spray therapy or appropriate treatment may be required. Persistence of nasopharyngeal irritation may be an indication for discontinuing Nasonex Aqueous Nasal Spray.

Although Nasonex will control the nasal symptoms in most patients, the concomitant use of appropriate additional therapy may provide additional relief of other symptoms, particularly ocular symptoms.

There is no evidence of hypothalamic-pituitary-adrenal (HPA) axis suppression following prolonged treatment with Nasonex Aqueous Nasal Spray. However, patients who are transferred from long-term administation of systemically active corticosteroids to Nasonex Aqueous Nasal Spray require careful attention. Systemic corticosteroid withdrawal in such patients may result in adrenal insufficiency for a number of months until recovery of HPA axis function. If these patients exhibit signs and symptoms of adrenal insufficiency, systemic corticosteroid administration should be resumed and other modes of therapy and appropriate measures instituted.

During transfer from systemic corticosteroids to Nasonex Aqueous Nasal Spray, some patients may experience symptoms of withdrawal from systemically active corticosteroids (e.g. joint and/or muscular pain, lassitude, and depression initially) despite relief from nasal symptoms and will require encouragement to continue with Nasonex Aqueous Nasal Spray therapy. Such transfer may also unmask pre-existing allergic conditions, such as allergic conjunctivitis and eczema, previously suppressed by systemic corticosteroid therapy.

Patients receiving corticosteroids who are potentially immunosuppressed should be warned of the risk of exposure to certain infections (e.g. chickenpox, measles) and of the importance of obtaining medical advice if such exposure occurs.

Following the use of intranasal corticosteroids, instances of nasal septum perforation or increased intraocular pressure have been reported very rarely.

Interaction with other medicaments and other forms of interaction: (See *Special warnings and special precautions for use* with systemic corticosteroids).

A clinical interaction study was conducted with loratadine. No interactions were observed.

Pregnancy and lactation: There are no adequate or well controlled studies in pregnant women. Following intranasal administration of the maximal recommended clinical dose, mometasone plasma concentrations are not measurable; thus foetal exposure is expected to be negligible and the potential for reproductive toxicity, very low.

As with other nasal corticosteroid preparations, Nasonex Aqueous Nasal Spray should not be used in pregnancy or lactation unless the potential benefit to the mother justifies any potential risk to the mother, foetus or infant. Infants born of mothers who received corticosteroids during pregnancy should be observed carefully for hypoadrenalism.

Effects on ability to drive and use machines: None known.

Undesirable effects: Treatment-related adverse events reported in clinical studies include headache (8%), epistaxis (i.e. frank bleeding, blood-tinged mucus, and blood flecks) (8%), pharyngitis (4%), nasal burning (2%), and nasal irritation (2%), and nasal ulceration (1%) which are typically observed with use of a corticosteroid nasal spray. Epistaxis was generally self-limiting and mild in severity, and occurred at a higher incidence compared to placebo (5%), but at a comparable or lower incidence compared to the active control nasal corticosteroids studied (up to 15%). The incidence of all other effects was comparable with that of placebo.

Overdose: Because of the negligible (≤ 0.1%) systemic bioavailability of Nasonex, overdose is unlikely to require any therapy other than observation, followed by initiation of the appropriate prescribed dosage. Inhalation or oral administration of excessive doses of corticosteroids may lead to suppression of HPA axis function.

Pharmacological properties

Pharmacodynamic properties: Mometasone furoate is a topical glucocorticosteroid with local anti-inflammatory properties at doses that are not systemically active.

It is likely that much of the mechanism for the anti-allergic and anti-inflammatory effects of mometasone furoate lies in its ability to inhibit the release of mediators of allergic reactions. Mometasone furoate significantly inhibits the release of leukotrienes from leucocytes of allergic patients.

In cell culture, mometasone furoate demonstrated high potency in inhibition of synthesis and release of IL-1, IL-5, IL-6 and TNFα; it is also a potent inhibitor of leukotriene production. In addition, it is an extremely potent inhibitor of the production of the Th2 cytokines IL-4 and IL-5, from human CD4+ T-cells.

In studies utilising nasal antigen challenge, Nasonex Aqueous Nasal Spray has shown anti-inflammatory activity in both early- and late-phase allergic responses. This has been demonstrated by decreases (vs placebo) in histamine and eosinophil activity and reductions (vs baseline) in eosinophils, neutrophils, and epithelial cell adhesion proteins.

In 28% of the patients with seasonal allergic rhinitis, Nasonex Aqueous Nasal Spray demonstrated a clinically significany onset of action within 12 hours after the first dose. The median (50%) onset time of relief was 35.9 hours.

Pharmacokinetic properties: Mometasone furoate, administered as an aqueous nasal spray, has a negligible (≤ 0.1%) systemic bioavailability and is generally undetectable in plasma, despite the use of a sensitive assay with a lower quantitation limit of 50 pg/ml; thus, there are no relevant pharmacokinetic data for this dosage form. Mometasone furoate suspension is very poorly absorbed from the gastro-intestinal tract, and the small amount that may be swallowed and absorbed undergoes extensive first-pass hepatic metabolism prior to excretion in urine and bile.

Preclinical safety data: No toxicological effects unique to mometasone furoate exposure were demonstrated. All observed effects are typical of this class of compounds and are related to exaggerated pharmacologic effects of glucocorticoids.

Preclinical studies demonstrate that mometasone furoate is devoid of androgenic, antiandrogenic, estrogenic or antiestrogenic activity but, like other glucocorticoids, it exhibits some antiuterotrophic activity and delays vaginal opening in animal modes at high oral doses of 56 mg/kg/day and 280 mg/kg/day.

Like other glucocorticoids, mometasone furoate showed a clastogenic potential *in vitro* at high concentrations. However, no mutagenic effects can be expected at therapeutically relevant doses.

In studies of reproductive function, subcutaneous mometasone furoate, at 15 micrograms/kg prolonged gestation and prolonged and difficult labour occurred with a reduction in offspring survival and body weight or body weight gain. There was no effect on fertility.

Like other glucocorticoids, mometasone furoate is a teratogen in rodents and rabbits. Effects noted were umbilical hernia in rats, cleft palate in mice and gall bladder agenesis, umbilical hernia and flexed front paws in rabbits. There were also reductions in maternal body weight gains, effects on foetal growth (lower foetal body weight and/or delayed ossification) in rats, rabbits and mice and reduced offspring survival in mice.

The carcinogenicity potential of inhaled mometasone furoate (aerosol with CFC propellant and surfactant) at concentrations of 0.25 to 2.0 micrograms/l was investigated in 24-month studies in mice and rats. Typical glucocorticoid-related effects, icluding several non-neoplastic lesions, were observed. No statistically significant dose-response relationship was detected for any of the tumour types.

Pharmaceutical particulars

List of excipients: Dispersible cellulose BP 65 cps (microcrystalline cellulose and carmellose sodium), glycerol, sodium citrate dihydrate, citric acid monohydrate, Polysorbate 80, benzalkonium chloride, phenylethyl alcohol, purified water.

Incompatibilities: None known.

Shelf life: 24 months from date of manufacture. Use within 2 months of first use.

Special precautions for storage: Store between 2° and 25°C.

Nature and contents of container: Nasonex Aqueous Nasal Spray 18 g is contained in a white, high density polyethylene bottle, supplied with a metered-dose, manual polypropylene spray pump actuator which delivers 50 micrograms per acuation.

Instruction for use/handling: Prior to administration of the first dose, shake container well, and actuate pump 6 or 7 times (until a uniform spray is obtained). If pump is not used for 14 days or longer, reprime the pump as before. Shake container well before each use. The bottle should be discarded after 120 actuations or within 2 months of first use.

Marketing authorisation numbers

PL 0201/0216 (UK)
PA 277/77/1 (Ireland)

Date of approval October 1997

Legal category POM

NETILLIN* Injection

Presentation Netillin Injection for parenteral use is an aqueous solution of netilmicin sulphate. Each millilitre contains netilmicin sulphate equivalent to 100 mg, 50 mg or 10 mg of netilmicin base, and is available in ampoules.

Uses Netilmicin sulphate is a semi-synthetic, water-soluble antibiotic of the aminoglycoside group. It is a rapidly acting bactericidal antibiotic which probably acts by inhibiting normal protein synthesis in susceptible organisms. It is active at low concentrations against many strains of a wide variety of pathogenic bacteria including *Escherichia coli, Klebsiella-Enterobacter-Serratia* species, *Citrobacter* species, *Proteus* species (indole-positive and indole-negative), including *Proteus mirabilis, Proteus morganii, Proteus rettgeri, Proteus vulgaris; Pseudomonas aeruginosa,* and *Staphylococcus* species (coagulase-positive and coagulase-negative, including penicillin and methicillin-resistant strains).

Netillin Injection is indicated in: bacteraemia, septicaemia (including neonatal sepsis), serious infections of the respiratory tract, kidney and genitourinary tract infections, skin and soft tissue infections, bone and joint infections, burns, wounds and peri-operative infections, intra-abdominal infections (including peritonitis) and infections of the gastro-intestinal tract.

A single Netillin Injection has been shown to be effective in the treatment of gonorrhoea.

Netillin Injection has also been effective in the treatment of infections caused by organisms resistant to other aminoglycosides, such as kanamycin, gentamicin, tobramycin and amikacin.

Netillin Injection is recommended for prophylactic use.

Dosage and administration The recommended dosage for intramuscular and intravenous administration is identical and should be calculated on mg/kg lean body weight. Netillin Injection should usually be administered intramuscularly. For i.v. administration see Table.

The usual duration of treatment is seven to fourteen days. Longer courses have been well tolerated but it is important that patients treated beyond the usual period be carefully monitored for changes in renal, auditory and vestibular function. Dosage should be reduced if clinically indicated.

Serum levels: The measurement of peak and trough serum levels is of value to assure adequate levels and to avoid potentially toxic levels. Once daily administration of Netillin may lead to transient peak concentrations of 20–30 mcg/ml. Other dosage regimens will result in peak levels generally not exceeding 12 mcg/ml. Prolonged levels above 16 mcg/ml should be avoided. If trough levels are monitored (just prior to next dose) they will usually be 3 mcg/ml or less with the recommended dosage. Trough concentrations above 4 mcg/ml should be avoided.

The regular monitoring of serum levels is particularly important for patients with impaired renal function or where a longer duration of treatment is necessary.

I.V. administration: If i.v. administration is required, the dose may be injected directly into a vein or i.v. tubing over a period of 3 to 5 minutes or administered as an infusion. For infusion in adults, a single dose of Netillin Injection may be diluted in 50 to 200 ml of sterile normal saline or in a sterile solution of dextrose 5% in water; in infants and children the volume of diluent should be dependant on the patients fluid requirements. The solution may be infused over a period of one half to two hours.

Netillin Injection should not be physically pre-mixed with other drugs, but should be administered separately in accordance with the recommended route of administration and dosage schedule. Netillin Injection is physically compatible with the following parenteral solutions: Sterile Water for Injections, Normal Saline, 5% and 10% Dextrose in Water.

Patients with normal renal function:

Adults: Urinary tract or non-life threatening systemic infections: The recommended dose is 4.0–6 mg/kg/day given once daily. The dose may also be given in equal sub doses 12 hourly or 8 hourly. In general within this dose range, lower dosage will be used for urinary tract infections and higher dosage for systemic infections. Dosage should be adjusted for both uses depending on severity of infection and patient condition.

Patients with urinary tract infections may be treated with a single daily dose of 150 mg administered for five days.

Netillin in a single dose of 300 mg may be used in the treatment of gonorrhoea.

Life threatening infections: Dosages up to 7.5 mg/kg/day may be administered in three equal doses every 8 hours. This dosage should be reduced to 6 mg/kg/day or less as soon as clinically indicated, usually within 48 hours.

Children: 6.0–7.5 mg/kg/day (2.0 to 2.5 mg/kg administered every 8 hours).

Infants and neonates: over one week of age: 7.5 to 9.0 mg/kg/day (2.5 to 3.0 mg/kg administered every 8 hours).

Premature or full term neonates: One Week of Age or Less: 6 mg/kg/day (3.0 mg/kg administered every 12 hours).

Patients with impaired renal function: The usual daily dose should be given on the first day as a loading dose (divided into three equal doses every 8 hrs). Dosage must then be adjusted. Whenever possible netilmicin serum concentrations should be monitored and used as the basis for dosage adjustment (see serum levels). If serum levels cannot be measured directly, serum creatinine or creatinine clearance rate may be used as a guide to dosage adjustment, as shown in the Table above.

Haemodialysis: For patients on haemodialysis the recommended dose is 2 mg/kg at the end of each dialysis period. In children a dose of 2–2.5 mg/kg may be administered depending on the severity of infection.

Peritoneal dialysis: Netillin has been used sucessfully in doses of 7.5–10 mg/l at each change of dialysing fluid without elevation of serum levels.

Concomitant therapy: Dosages recommended above for patients with normal or impaired renal function should not be reduced when netilmicin is administered concomitantly with other antibiotics (but see Warnings).

Contra-indications, warnings, etc

Contra-indications: Hypersensitivity to netilmicin contra-indicates its use. A history of hypersensitivity or serious toxic reactions to other aminoglycosides may also be a contra-indication.

Warnings: Patients treated with aminoglycosides

Dosage Adjustment Guide for Patients with Renal Function Impairment
(Daily dose to be divided into three equal doses every 8 hours)

Administer the usual dose on the first day as follows:

1. Adults, urinary tract and systemic infections 4–6 mg/kg/day.
2. Adults, life-threatening infections 7.5 mg/kg/day.
3. Children, 6–7.5 mg/kg/day.
4. Infants and neonates over 1 week of age, 7.5–9 mg/kg/day.
5. Premature or full term neonates one week of age or less, 6 mg/kg/day.

On subsequent days, administer a percent of the usual dose, based on serum creatinine or creatinine clearance rate as follows:

Approx. creatinine clearance rate (ml/min/ 1.73 sq m)	*Serum creatinine level*		*Percent of usual dose*
	mg/100 ml	*S.I. Units µmol/l*	
100	≤1.0	80	100
71–100	1.1–1.3	100–120	80
56–70	1.4–1.6	130–150	65
46–55	1.7–1.9	160–175	55
41–45	2.0–2.2	180–190	50
36–40	2.3–2.5	210–220	40
31–35	2.6–3.0	230–260	35
26–30	3.1–3.5	270–310	30
21–25	3.6–4.0	320–360	25
16–20	4.1–5.1	365–450	20
10–15	5.2–6.6	460–580	15
<10	6.7–8.0	600–700	10

should be under close clinical observation because of the potential toxicity associated with their use. Monitoring of renal and eighth cranial nerve functions is desirable during therapy, particularly for patients with known or suspected reduced renal function.

Evidence of ototoxicity requires dosage adjustment or discontinuance of the drug.

Serum concentration assays of aminoglycosides are of value to assure adequate levels and to avoid potentially toxic levels. Once daily administration of Netillin may lead to transient peak concentrations of 20–30 mcg/ml. Other dosages regimens will result in peak levels not exceeding 12 mcg/ml. Prolonged levels above 16 mcg/ml should be avoided. If trough levels are monitored (just prior to next dose) they will usually be 3 mcg/ml or less with the recommended dosage. Increasing trough concentrations above 4 mcg/ml should be avoided.

In patients with extensive body surface burns, altered pharmocokinetics may result in reduced serum concentrations of aminoglycosides. Measurement of netilmicin serum concentrations is particularly important in these patients as a basis for dosage adjustment.

Concurrent and/or sequential systemic or topical use of other potentially neurotoxic and/or nephrotoxic drugs, such as polymyxin B, colistin, cephaloridine, kanamycin, gentamicin, amikacin, tobramycin, neomycin, streptomycin and vancomycin should be avoided. Advanced age and dehydration may also increase the risk of toxicity.

Increased nephrotoxicity has been reported following concomitant administration of aminoglycoside antibiotics and cephalothin.

Neurotoxic or nephrotoxic antibiotics may be absorbed from body surfaces after local irrigation or application. The potential toxic effect of such antibiotics administered in this fashion should be considered.

The concurrent use of netilmicin with potent diuretics, such as ethacrynic acid or frusemide, should be avoided since these diuretics by themselves may cause ototoxicity. In addition, when administered intravenously, diuretics may enhance aminoglycoside toxicity by altering the antibiotic concentrations in serum and tissue.

Patients should be well hydrated during treatment.

Neuromuscular blockade has been reported in animals receiving netilmicin at doses considerably above those clinically recommended. The possibility of this phenomenon occurring in man should be considered, particularly if aminoglycosides are administered to patients receiving anaesthetics, neuromuscular blocking agents (such as succinylcholine or tubocurarine), or massive transfusions of citrate-anticoagulated blood. If blockade occurs, calcium salts may reverse it.

Aminoglycosides should be used with caution in patients with neuromuscular disorders, such as myasthenia gravis or Parkinsonism, since these drugs theoretically may aggravate muscle weakness because of their potential curare-like effects on the neuromuscular junction.

Elderly patients may have reduced renal function which might not be evident by routine screening tests, such as BUN or serum creatinine. A creatinine clearance determination may be more useful. Monitoring of renal function during netilmicin treatment, as with other aminoglycosides, is particularly important in these patients.

Cross-allergenicity among aminoglycosides has been demonstrated.

Although the *in vitro* mixing of netilmicin and carbenicillin results in a rapid and significant inactivation of netilmicin, this interaction has not been demonstrated in patients with normal renal function who received both drugs by different routes of administration. In patients with severe renal impairment receiving carbenicillin concomitantly with an aminoglycoside, a reduction in aminoglycoside serum half-life has been reported.

Treatment with netilmicin may result in overgrowth of non-susceptible organisms. If this occurs, appropriate therapy is indicated.

Safety for use in pregnancy has not been established.

Netilmicin is not intended for intrathecal use.

Side-effects: Adverse renal effects, generally mild in nature, have been reported infrequently after netilmicin administration. They occur more frequently in patients with a history of renal impairment, in patients treated with larger than the recommended dosage, and are most often reversible. While eighth cranial nerve toxicity has been reported with netilmicin, the incidence is lower and the severity appears milder than with other aminoglycosides. Some clinical studies indicate that at therapeutic dosage, netilmicin may have less effect than other aminoglycosides on eighth cranial nerve function. Adverse effects on both the vestibular and auditory branches of the eighth cranial nerve occur primarily in patients with renal impairment and in patients on high doses and/or prolonged therapy. Symptoms which are often transient may include dizziness, vertigo, tinnitus, roaring in the ears and hearing loss. The latter is usually manifested by diminution of high-tone acuity. Total deafness has not been reported.

Some patients who have had previous ototoxic reactions to other aminoglycosides have been treated safely with Netillin Injection.

Other rarely reported adverse reactions possibly related to netilmicin include: headache, malaise, visual disturbances, disorientation, tachycardia, paraesthesia, rash, chills, fever, fluid retention, vomiting and diarrhoea.

Laboratory abnormalities possibly related to netilmicin include: increased blood sugar, increased alkaline phosphatase, increased SGOT or SGPT; other abnormal liver function studies; decreased haemoglobin, WBCs, and platelets; eosinophilia and increase in prothrombin time.

While local tolerance of Netillin Injection is generally excellent, there has been an occasional report of pain at the injection site or local reaction.

Overdosage: In the event of overdose or toxic reaction, haemodialysis or peritoneal dialysis will aid the removal of netilmicin from the blood.

Pharmaceutical precautions Netillin Injection should be stored at 2°C to 30°C (35.6°F to 86°F). Protect from freezing.

Netillin Injections should not be physically premixed with other drugs, but should be administered separately in accordance with the recommended route of administration and dosage schedule.

Legal category POM.

Package quantities All the presentations of Netillin are colour coded on both cartons and the containers. The 100 mg/ml strength is available in 2 ml (colour coded red), 1.5 ml (brown) and 1 ml (yellow) ampoules. The 50 mg/ml and 10 mg/ml strengths are available in 1 ml (green) and 1.5 ml (blue) ampoules respectively. All ampoules are supplied in packs of ten.

Further information Nil.

Product licence numbers
Netillin Injection 100 mg/ml 3478/0041
Netillin Injection 50 mg/ml 3478/0040
Netillin Injection 10 mg/ml 3478/0039

NITRO-DUR* 0.1 mg/h TRANSDERMAL DRUG DELIVERY SYSTEM
NITRO-DUR* 0.2 mg/h TRANSDERMAL DRUG DELIVERY SYSTEM
NITRO-DUR* 0.4 mg/h TRANSDERMAL DRUG DELIVERY SYSTEM
NITRO-DUR* 0.6 mg/h TRANSDERMAL DRUG DELIVERY SYSTEM

Qualitative and quantitative composition
Active ingredient: Glyceryl trinitrate 37.4% w/w.

Inactive ingredients: Butylacrylate Polymer (Polymer C) 28.4% w/w; Butylacrylate Polymer (Polymer D) 28.4% w/w; Sodium Polyacrylate (Polymer A) 1.4% w/w; Melamine Formaldehyde Resin (Polymer b) 0.3% w/w; Purified Water 4.0% w/w.

Coated onto tan-coloured Saranex* 2014 extruded thermoplastic film 5 cm² (0.1 mg/h); 10.0 cm² (0.2 mg/h); 20 cm² (0.4 mg/h) or 20 cm² (0.6 mg/h).

Adhesive layer covered by PVC Release Liner 5 cm² (0.1 mg/h); 10.0 cm² (0.2 mg/h); 20 cm² (0.4 mg/h) or 30 cm² (0.6 mg/h).

Pharmaceutical form Sustained release transdermal system.

Clinical particulars
Therapeutic indications: For prophylaxis of angina pectoris either alone or in combination with other anti-anginal therapy.

Poslogy and method of administration:
Adults, including elderly patients: The recommended initial dose is one 0.2 mg/h Nitro-Dur patch daily. In some patients dose titration to higher or lower doses may be necessary to achieve optimum therapeutic effect. Nitro-Dur is suitable for continuous or intermittent use. Patients already receiving continuous 24-hour nitrate therapy without signs of nitrate tolerance may continue on this regimen provided clinical response is maintained. Attenuation of effect has however occurred in some patients being treated with sustained release nitrate preparations. In such patients intermittent therapy may be more appropriate. Under these circumstances Nitro-Dur is applied daily for a period of approximately 12 hours. The patch is then removed to provide a nitrate-free interval of 12 hours which may be varied between 8–12 hours to suit individual patients.

Patients experiencing nocturnal angina may benefit from overnight treatment with a nitrate-free interval during the day. In this patient group additional anti-anginal therapy may be needed during the day.

Patients with severe angina may need additional anti-anginal therapy during nitrate-free intervals.

Nitro-Dur Transdermal patches may be applied to any convenient skin area; the recommended site is the chest or outer upper arm. Application sites should be rotated and suitable areas may be shaved if necessary. Nitro-Dur patches should not be applied to the distal part of the extremities.

Children: Not recommended.

Contra-indications: Contra-indicated in patients hypersensitive to nitrates and in patients with marked anaemia. Use is also contra-indicated in severe hypotension, increased cranial pressure and myocardial insufficiency due to valvular or left ventricular outflow tract obstruction.

Special warnings and precautions for use: Nitro-Dur should only be used under careful clinical and/or haemodynamic monitoring in patients with acute myocardial infarction or congestive heart failure. Nitro-Dur is not indicated for the immediate treatment of acute anginal attacks.

Nitro-Dur should be removed before attempting defibrillation or cardioversion, to avoid possibility of electrical arcing, and before diathermy.

The possibility of increased frequency of angina during patch-off periods should be considered. In such cases, the use of concomitant anti-anginal therapy is desirable.

In some patients severe hypotension may occur particularly with upright posture, even with small doses of glyceryl trinitrate. Thus Nitro-Dur should be used with caution in patients who may have volume depletion from diuretic therapy and in patients who have low systolic blood pressure (e.g. below 90 mm Hg).

Paradoxical bradycardia and increased angina may accompany glyceryl-trinitrate-induced hypotension.

Caution should be exercised in patients with arterial

hypoxaemia, due to severe anaemia and patients with hypoxaemia and a ventilation/perfusion imbalance due to lung disease or ischaemic heart failure, as biotransformation of GTN may be reduced.

Interactions with other medicaments and other forms of interaction: Concomitant use of Nitro-Dur with other vasodilating agents, alcohol, anti-hypertensive agents, beta adrenergic blocking agents, ace inhibitors, phenothiazines or calcium channel blocking agents may cause additive hypotensive effects.

Pregnancy and lactation: It is not known whether glyceryl trinitrate in transdermal form can affect reproductive capacity or cause foetal harm. Thus Nitro-Dur should only be administered to pregnant women if the potential benefits to the mother clearly outweighs the potential hazard to the foetus. It is not known whether glyceryl trinitrate is excreted in human milk. Caution should therefore be exercised when Nitro-Dur is administered to nursing mothers.

Effects on ability to drive and use machines: None known.

Undesirable effects: Headache is the most common side-effect, especially at higher doses. Transient episodes of dizziness and light-headedness which may be related to blood pressure change may also occur. Hypotension occurs infrequently but may be severe enough to warrant discontinuation of therapy. Syncope and reflex tachycardia have been reported but are uncommon. Application site irritation may occur but is rarely severe. Hypersensitivity reactions may occur.

Overdose: High doses of glyceryl trinitrate may produce severe hypotension, syncope and methaemoglobinaemia. Increased intracranial pressure with associated cerebral symptoms may occur. Treatment is by removal of the patch or reduction of dose, depending on severity. Thorough scrubbing of underlying skin may reduce absorption more quickly after removal. Any fall in blood pressure or signs of collapse that may occur may be managed by general supportive or resuscitative measures. Adrenaline and related products are ineffective in reversing the severe hypotensive events associated with overdose.

Pharmacological properties

Pharmacodynamic properties: Glyceryl trinitrate, (as other organic nitrates), is a potent dilator of vascular smooth muscle. The effect on veins predominates over that on arteries resulting in decreased cardiac preload. Systemic vascular resistance is relatively unaffected, heart rate is unchanged or slightly increased and pulmonary vascular resistance is consistently reduced.

In normal individuals or those with coronary artery disease (in the absence of heart failure) glyceryl trinitrate decreases cardiac output slightly. Doses which do not alter systemic arterial pressure often produce arteriolar dilatation in the face and neck resulting in flushing. Dilatation of the meningeal arterioles may explain the headache which is often reported. Rapid administration of high doses of glyceryl trinitrate decreases blood pressure and cardiac output resulting in pallor, weakness, dizziness and activation of compensatory sympathetic reflexes. A marked hypotensive effect may occasionally occur especially in the upright position.

Pharmacokinetic properties: Glyceryl trinitrate is rapidly hydrolysed by liver enzymes which are a major factor in bioavailability. Orally administered glyceryl trinitrate is ineffective as a therapeutic agent due to first-pass metabolism and administration has therefore routinely been via the sub-lingual route thus bypassing the hepatic circulation initially. Peak concentrations of glyceryl trinitrate following sub-lingual administration occur within 4 minutes in man with a half-life of 1 to 3 minutes. Transdermal administration, initially with ointment preparations but more recently with sustained-release delivery systems provide an alternative route to bypass the hepatic circulation with longer term concentrations of approximately 200 pg/ml are achieved within approximately 2 h of application of Nitro-Dur and are maintained for 24 h. Rate of absorption is controlled by the skin.

Preclinical safety data: There are no pre-clinical data of relevance to the prescriber which are additional to that already included in other sections of the SPC.

Pharmaceutical particulars

List of excipients: Butylacrylate Polymer (Polymer C); Butylacrylate Polymer (Polymer D); Sodium Polyacrylate (Polymer A); Melamine Formaldehyde Resin (Polymer B); Purified Water.

Coated onto tan-coloured Saranex* 2014 extruded thermoplastic film. Adhesive layer covered by PVC Release Liner.

Incompatibilities: None known.

Shelf life: 24 months.

Special precautions for storage: Store below 30°C. Do not refrigerate.

Nature and contents of container: Sealed pouches consisting of paper lined with polyethylene/foil laminate enclosing individual transdermal patches.

Instruction for use/handling: Nitro-Dur patches are applied after removal from the protective pouch. With the brown lines on the backing cover facing the user, edges are bent away to break open the cover along the brown line. The halves of the cover are peeled off and the patch applied firmly to the skin. Hands should be washed thoroughly after application.

Patients should be advised to dispose of patches carefully to avoid accidental application or use.

Marketing authorisation numbers

Nitro-Dur 0.1 mg/h:	PL 0201/0157
Nitro-Dur 0.2 mg/h:	PL 0201/0158
Nitro-Dur 0.4 mg/h:	PL 0201/0159
Nitro-Dur 0.6 mg/h:	PL 0201/0160

Date of (partial) revision of the text 19 December 1996

Legal category P

OPTIMINE* TABLETS
OPTIMINE* SYRUP

Qualitative and quantitative composition

Tablets:	Azatadine Maleate 1.0 mg
Syrup:	Azatadine Maleate 0.5 mg

Pharmaceutical form Tablets/Syrup.

Clinical particulars

Therapeutic indications: For the symptomatic relief of allergic conditions such as hayfever, vasomotor rhinitis, urticaria, pruritus of allergic origin and allergic reactions associated with insect bites and stings.

Posology and method of administration:

Adults: The elderly and children over 12 years of age – 1 mg (10 ml of syrup or 1 tablet) in the morning and evening in the majority of patients is recommended. In refractory or more severe cases, 2 mg (20 ml of syrup or 2 tablets) twice daily may be used.

Children (6–12 years): 0.5–1.0 mg (5–10 ml syrup or ½ tablet), twice daily.

Children (1–6 years): 0.25 mg azatadine maleate (2.5 ml of syrup) twice daily.

Optimine Syrup may be diluted with syrup BP.

Contra-indications: Monoamine oxidase inhibitors, which are known to intensify or prolong the anticholinergic and sedative action of drugs, should not be used concomitantly with azatadine maleate. Due to the anticholinergic effect of azatadine maleate, the drug should be used with caution in patients with prostatic hypertrophy, urinary retention, glaucoma, stenosing peptic ulcer or pyloroduodenal obstructions.

Special warnings and precautions for use: None known.

Interactions: Patients taking azatadine maleate should be cautioned against ingestion of alcohol. The drug may potentiate central nervous system depressants.

Pregnancy and lactation: Until the safety of azatadine maleate concerning adverse effects on human foetal development has been established, the drug is not recommended for use in pregnant or lactating women.

Effects on ability to drive and use machines: Although drowsiness is infrequent and impairment of psychomotor function is not manifested at the recommended dosage, patients should be cautioned against engaging in mechanical operations requiring mental alertness until individual response to azatadine maleate has been determined.

Undesirable effects: Azatadine maleate is well tolerated and side-effects are generally dose-related and transient. Among these are: weakness, nervousness, dry mouth, increased appetite, anorexia, nausea, headache, drowsiness, dysuria and blurring of vision.

Overdosage: Symptoms may vary from central nervous system depression to stimulation. The latter is particularly likely in children. Atropine-like symptoms may also occur. If vomiting has not occurred spontaneously the patient should be induced to vomit. If unsuccessful, the stomach should be emptied by aspiration and lavage. Stimulants should not be used and vasopressors may be used to treat hypotension.

Pharmacological properties

Pharmacodynamic properties: Azatadine maleate is a H_1-receptor antagonist. It inhibits the response of smooth muscle to histamine and strongly antagonises the action of histamine which is one of the main mediators in allergic reactions; thereby preventing the increased capillary permeability, oedema and/or wheal formation common to many allergic disorders, giving symptomatic relief.

Pharmacokinetic particulars: Azatadine is readily absorbed from the gastro-intestinal tract and is excreted as active drug and metabolites in the urine. Disposition can best be described as a one compartmental model and the plasma half life is approximately 8–9 hours. Metabolism studies show extensive urinary conjugation.

Preclinical safety data: There are no pre-clinical data of relevance to the prescriber which are additional to that already included in other sections of the SPC.

Pharmaceutical particulars

List of excipients:

Tablets: Lactose PhEur; Povidone BP; Corn Starch PhEur and Magnesium Stearate PhEur.

Syrup: Sucrose PhEur; Sorbitol solution PhEur (equivalent to 70% sorbitol); Propylene Glycol PhEur; Methylparaben PhEur; Propylparaben PhEur; alcohol USP; Purified Water PhEur; imitation blackcurrant flavour.

Incompatibilities: None known.

Shelf life:

Tablets: 36 months.

Syrup: 36 months.

Special precautions for storage: None.

Nature and contents of containers:

Tablets: PVC-foil 250 µ blister strips of 14 tablets. The backing for which is made of alu-foil 20 µ.

Syrup: Tyoe III amber glass bottles with metal cap and polyethylene pulp capliner, containing 120 ml syrup.

Instructions for use/handling: Not applicable.

Marketing authorisation numbers

Tablets:	PL 0201/0128
Syrup:	PL 0201/0129

Date of approval/revision of SmPC July 1997

Legal category P.

TEMGESIC INJECTION 1 ml

Qualitative and quantitative composition Buprenorphine hydrochloride 324 µg/ml, equivalent to 300 µg buprenorphine base.

Pharmaceutical form Terminally sterilised solution for injection.

Clinical particulars

Therapeutic indications: As a strong analgesic for the relief of moderate to severe pain.

Posology and method of administration: Administration by i.m. or slow i.v. injection.

Adults and children over 12 years: 1–2 ml (300–600 micrograms of buprenorphine) every 6–8 hours or as required.

Children aged under 12 years: 3–6 micrograms/kg body weight every 6–8 hours. In refractory cases up to 9 micrograms/kg may be administered. There is no clinical experience in infants below the age of 6 months.

There is no evidence that dosage need be modified for the elderly.

Temgesic Injection may be employed in balanced anaesthetic techniques as a pre-medication at a dose of 300 micrograms i.m., or as an analgesic supplement at doses of 300 to 450 micrograms i.v.

Contra-indications: Not to be given to patients who are known to be allergic to Temgesic or other opiates.

Special warnings and precautions for use: Temgesic occasionally causes respiratory depression and, as with other strong centrally acting analgesics, care should be taken when treating patients with impaired respiratory function or patients who are recieving drugs which can cause respiratory depression.

Although volunteer studies have indicated that opiate antagonists may not fully reverse the effects of Temgesic, clinical experience has shown that Naloxone may be of benefit in reversing a reduced respiratory rate. Respiratory stimulants such as Doxapram are also effective. The intensity and duration of action may be affected in patients with impaired liver failure.

Interactions with other medicaments and other forms of interaction: There is no evidence to indicate that therapeutic doses of buprenorphine do not reduce the analgesic efficacy of standard doses of an opioid agonist and that when buprenorphine is employed with the normal therapeutic range, standard doses of opioid agonist may be administered before the effects of the former have ended without compromising analgesia. However, in individuals on high doses of opioids buprenorphine may precipitate abstinence effects due to its properties as a partial agonist.

Controlled human and animal studies indicate that buprenorphine has a substantially lower dependence liability than pure agonist analgesics. In patients abusing opioids in moderate doses substitution with buprenorphine may prevent withdrawal symptoms. In man limited euphorigenic effects have been observed. This has resulted in some abuse of the product and caution should be exercised when prescribing it to patients known to have, or suspected of having, problems with drug abuse.

Temgesic may cause some drowsiness which may

be potentiated by other centrally acting agents, including alcohol, tranquilisers, sedatives and hypnotics. Temgesic should be used with caution in patients receiving monoamine oxidase inhibitors, although animal studies have given no evidence of interactions.

Temgesic has no known effects on diagnostic laboratory tests.

Pregnancy and lactation: Temgesic is not recommended for use during pregnancy. Animal studies indicate that the amounts of buprenorphine excreted in milk are very low and in human use are unlikely to be of clinical significance to the baby. There is indirect evidence in animal studies to suggest that Temgesic may cause a reduction in milk flow during lactation. Although this occurred only at doses well in excess of the human dose, it should be borne in mind when treating lacating women.

Effects on ability to drive and use machines: Ambulant patients should be warned not to drive or operate machinery until they are certain they can tolerate Temgesic.

Undesirable effects: Nausea, vomiting, dizziness, sweating and drowsiness have been reported and may be more frequent in ambulant patients. Hallucinations and other psychotomimetic effects have occurred although more rarely than with agonists/antagonists. Elderly patients would be expected to be more susceptible to these effects. Hypotension leading to syncope may occur. Rashes, headache, urinary retention and blurring of vision have occasionally been reported. Rarely, a serious allergic reaction may occur following a single dose.

Overdose: Supportive measures should be instituted and if appropriate Naxolone or respiratory stimulants can be used. The expected symptoms of overdosage would be drowsiness, nausea and vomiting; marked miosis may occur.

Pharmacological properties

Pharmacodynamic properties: Buprenorphine is a strong analgesic of the partial agonist (mixed agonist/antagonist) class.

Pharmacokinetic properties: Buprenorphine is readily available by i.v. or i.m. routes; the relative bioavailability i.m. to i.v. was 1.07. Peak plasma levels are achieved within a few minutes of i.m. administration and after 10 minutes are not significantly different from those observed after the same dose given i.v.

Preclinical safety data: No preclinical findings of relevance to the prescriber have been reported.

Pharmaceutical particulars

List of excipients: Dextrose anhydrous parenteral, hydrochloride acid and water for injections.

Incompatibilities: None stated.

Shelf life: Five years.

Special precautions for storage: The product, though stable, should be kept cool and protected from light.

Nature and contents of container: Sealed Type I glass ampoules. Pack size: five ampoules.

Instructions for use/handling: Administration by i.m. or slow i.v. injection.

Marketing authorisation number PL 00201/0246

Date of approval/revison of SmPC May 1998

Legal category POM

TEMGESIC SUBLINGUAL TABLETS

Qualitative and quantitative composition Buprenorphine hydrochloride 216 µg/ml, equivalent to 200 µg buprenorphine base.

Pharmaceutical form Sublingual tablets.

Clinical particulars

Therapeutic indications: As a strong analgesic for the relief of moderate to severe pain.

Posology and method of administration: Administration by the sublingual route.

Adults and children over 12: 1–2 tablets (200–400 micrograms) to be dissolved under the tongue every 6–8 hours or as required. The recommended starting dose for moderate to severe pain of the type typically presenting in general practice is 1 to 2 tablets, 8 hourly.

Elderly: There is no evidence that dosage needs to be modified for the elderly.

Children aged 6–12 years:

16–25 kg	(33–55 lb)	½ tablet
25–37.5 kg	(55–82.5 lb)	½–1 tablet
37.5–50 kg	(82.5–110 lb)	1–1½ tablets

There is no clinical experience in infants below the age of 6 months.

Temgesic sublingual may be used in balanced anaesthetic techniques at a dose of 400 micrograms.

Contra-indications: Not to be given to patients who are known to be allergic to Temgesic or other opiates.

Special warnings and precautions for use: Temgesic occasionally causes respiratory depression and, as with other strong centrally acting analgesics, care should be taken when treating patients with impaired respiratory function or patients who are recieving drugs which can cause respiratory depression. Although volunteer studies have indicated that opiate antagonists may not fully reverse the effects of Temgesic, clinical experience has shown that Naloxone may be of benefit in reversing a reduced respiratory rate. Respiratory stimulants such as Doxapram are also effective. The intensity and duration of action may be affected in patients with impaired liver failure.

Interactions with other medicaments and other forms of interaction: There is evidence to indicate that therapeutic doses of buprenorphine do not reduce the analgesic efficacy of standard doses of an opioid agonist and that when buprenorphine is employed with the normal therapeutic range, standard doses of opioid agonist may be administered before the effects of the former have ended without compromising analgesia. However, in individuals on high doses of opioids buprenorphine may precipitate abstinence effects due to its properties as a partial agonist.

Controlled human and animal studies indicate that buprenorphine has a substantially lower dependence liability than pure agonist analgesics. In patients abusing opioids in moderate doses substitution with buprenorphine may prevent withdrawal symptoms. In man limited euphorigenic effects have been observed. This has resulted in some abuse of the product and caution should be exercised when prescribing it to patients known to have, or suspected of having, problems with drug abuse.

Temgesic may cause some drowsiness which may be potentiated by other centrally acting agents, including alcohol, tranquilisers, sedatives and hypnotics. Temgesic should be used with caution in patients receiving monoamine oxidase inhibitors, although animal studies have given no evidence of interactions.

Temgesic has no known effects on diagnostic laboratory tests.

Pregnancy and lactation: Temgesic is not recommended for use during pregnancy. Animal studies indicate that the amounts of buprenorphine excreted in milk are very low and in human use are unlikely to be of clinical significance to the baby. There is indirect evidence in animal studies to suggest that Temgesic may cause a reduction in milk flow during lactation. Although this occurred only at doses well in excess of the human dose, it should be borne in mind when treating lacating women.

Effects on ability to drive and use machines: Ambulant patients should be warned not to drive or operate machinery until they are certain they can tolerate Temgesic.

Undesirable effects: Nausea, vomiting, dizziness, sweating and drowsiness have been reported and may be more frequent in ambulant patients. Hallucinations and other psychotomimetic effects have occurred although more rarely than with agonists/antagonists. Elderly patients would be expected to be more susceptible to these effects. Hypotension leading to syncope may occur. Rashes, headache, urinary retention and blurring of vision have occasionally been reported. Rarely, a serious allergic reaction may occur following a single dose.

Overdose: Supportive measures should be instituted and if appropriate Naxolone or respiratory stimulants can be used. The expected symptoms of overdosage would be drowsiness, nausea and vomiting; marked miosis may occur.

Pharmacological properties

Pharmacodynamic properties: Buprenorphine is a strong analgesic of the partial agonist (mixed agonist/antagonist) class.

Pharmacokinetic properties: Buprenorphine is rapidly absorbed into the buccal mucosa with subsequent slower transfer to the systemic circulation. Any swallowed drug is rapidly metabolised by the gut wall and liver.

Preclinical safety data: None stated.

Pharmaceutical particulars

List of excipients: Lactose, mannitol, maize starch, povidone K30, citric acid anhydrous, magnesium stearate, sodium citrate, purified water and alcohol (96%).

Incompatibilities: None stated.

Shelf life: 36 months.

Special precautions for storage: Not applicable.

Nature and contents of container: Cartons of 50 tablets contained in strips packed in units of 10 tablets each.

Instructions for use/handling: To be dissolved under the tongue and not to be chewed or swallowed.

Marketing authorisation number PL 00201/0245

Date of approval/revison of SmPC May 1998

Legal category POM

TEMGESIC SUBLINGUAL 0.4 mg

Qualitative and quantitative composition Buprenorphine hydrochloride 432 µg/tablet, equivalent to 400 µg buprenorphine base.

Pharmaceutical form Sublingual tablets.

Clinical particulars

Therapeutic indications: As a strong analgesic for the relief of moderate to severe pain.

Posology and method of administration: Administration by the sublingual route.

Adults and children over 12: 200–400 micrograms to be dissolved under the tongue every 6–8 hours or as required. The recommended starting dose for moderate to severe pain of the type typically presenting in general practice is 200–400 micrograms 8 hourly. The tablet should not be chewed or swallowed as this will reduce efficacy.

Elderly: There is no indication that dosage needs to be modified for the elderly.

Children aged 6–12 years:

16–25 kg	(33–55 lb)	100 micrograms
25–37.5 kg	(55–82.5 lb)	100–200 micrograms
37.5–50 kg	(82.5–110 lb)	200–300 micrograms

There is no clinical experience in infants below the age of 6 months.

Temgesic sublingual may be used in balanced anaesthetic techniques at a dose of 400 micrograms.

Contra-indications: Not to be given to patients who are known to be allergic to Temgesic or other opiates.

Special warnings and precautions for use: Temgesic occasionally causes respiratory depression and, as with other strong centrally acting analgesics, care should be taken when treating patients with impaired respiratory function or patients who are recieving drugs which can cause respiratory depression. Although volunteer studies have indicated that opiate antagonists may not fully reverse the effects of Temgesic, clinical experience has shown that Naloxone may be of benefit in reversing a reduced respiratory rate. Respiratory stimulants such as Doxapram are also effective. The intensity and duration of action may be affected in patients with impaired liver failure.

Interactions with other medicaments and other forms of interaction: There is evidence to indicate that therapeutic doses of buprenorphine do not reduce the analgesic efficacy of standard doses of an opioid agonist and that when buprenorphine is employed within the normal therapeutic range, standard doses of opioid agonist may be administered before the effects of the former have ended without compromising analgesia. However, in individuals on high doses of opioids buprenorphine may precipitate abstinence effects due to its properties as a partial agonist.

Controlled human and animal studies indicate that buprenorphine has a substantially lower dependence liability than pure agonist analgesics. In patients abusing opioids in moderate doses substitution with buprenorphine may prevent withdrawal symptoms. In man limited euphorigenic effects have been observed. This has resulted in some abuse of the product and caution should be exercised when prescribing it to patients known to have, or suspected of having, problems with drug abuse.

Temgesic may cause some drowsiness which may be potentiated by other centrally acting agents, including alcohol, tranquilisers, sedatives and hypnotics. Temgesic should be used with caution in patients receiving monoamine oxidase inhibitors, although animal studies have given no evidence of interactions.

Temgesic has no known effects on diagnostic laboratory tests.

Pregnancy and lactation: Temgesic is not recommended for use during pregnancy. Animal studies indicate that the amounts of buprenorphine excreted in milk are very low and in human use are unlikely to be of clinical significance to the baby. There is indirect evidence in animal studies to suggest that Temgesic may cause a reduction in milk flow during lactation. Although this occurred only at doses well in excess of the human dose, it should be borne in mind when treating lacating women.

Effects on ability to drive and use machines: Ambulant patients should be warned not to drive or operate machinery until they are certain they can tolerate Temgesic.

Undesirable effects: Nausea, vomiting, dizziness, sweating and drowsiness have been reported and may be more frequent in ambulant patients. Hallucinations and other psychotomimetic effects have occurred although more rarely than with agonists/

antagonists. Elderly patients would be expected to be more susceptible to these effects. Hypotension leading to syncope may occur. Rashes, headache, urinary retention and blurring of vision have occasionally been reported. Rarely, a serious allergic reaction may occur following a single dose.

Overdose: Supportive measures should be instituted and if appropriate Naxolone or respiratory stimulants can be used. The expected symptoms of overdosage would be drowsiness, nausea and vomiting; marked miosis may occur.

Pharmacological properties
Pharmacodynamic properties: Buprenorphine is a strong analgesic of the partial agonist (mixed agonist/antagonist) class.

Pharmacokinetic properties: Buprenorphine is rapidly absorbed into the buccal mucosa with subsequent slower transfer to the systemic circulation. Any swallowed drug is rapidly metabolised by the gut wall and liver.

Preclinical safety data: None stated.

Pharmaceutical particulars
List of excipients: Lactose, mannitol, maize starch, povidone K30, citric acid anhydrous, magnesium stearate, sodium citrate, purified water and alcohol (96%).

Incompatibilities: None stated.

Shelf life: 36 months.

Special precautions for storage: Not applicable.

Nature and contents of container: Cartons of 50 tablets contained in strips packed in units of 10 tablets each.

Instructions for use/handling: To be dissolved under the tongue and not to be chewed or swallowed.

Marketing authorisation number PL 00201/0244

Date of approval/revison of SmPC May 1998

Legal category POM

TINADERM-M* CREAM

Qualitative and quantitative composition
Tolnaftate 1.0% w/w
Nystatin 100.0% IU

Pharmaceutical form Cream.

Clinical particulars
Therapeutic indications: Tinaderm Cream is recommended in the treatment of cutaneous mycotic infections such as Tinea pedis, Tinea cruris, Tinea corporis, Tinea barbae and Tinea manuum due to *Trichophyton rubrum, T. mentagrophytes, T. tonsurans, Microsporum canis, M. audouini, Epidermophyton floccosum, Candida albicans* and *Tinea versicolor (Malassezia furfur).*

If candida albicans is the primary cause of infections, such conditions as 'athlete's foot' (dermatophytosis), perleche, paronychia, intertrigo, 'nappy rash' and other cutaneous lesions can be successfully treated with Tinaderm-M.

Tinaderm-M is particularly recommended for the treatment of fungal infections localised in intertriginous and other moist areas of the skin where candida infections are present or likely to develop.

Posology and method of administration: A sufficient quantity of Tinaderm-M should be applied to completely cover the affected area two or three times daily until healing is complete. Lesions generally begin to clear during the first treatment week and disappear after 2–3 weeks of treatment. If thickening of skin has occurred, treatment for as long as 4–6 weeks may be required. The concomitant use of a mild keratolytic agent may be indicated in areas where the skin has become hyperkeratotic. Use of wet compresses prior to application of Tinaderm-M aids in the healing of exudative lesions and does not interfere with the fungicidal action of the medication.

Contra-indications: There are no known contra-indications to tolnaftate, however if hypersensitivity to any of the ingredients occurs, treatment should be stopped.

Special warnings and precautions for use: Keep away from eyes and mucous membranes. Mycosis complicated by bacterial infections may require additional antibiotic treatment.

Tinaderm-M is for dermatological use only. If sensitivity occurs, discontinue use.

Interactions with other medicaments and other forms of interaction: None known.

Pregnancy and lactation: Whilst there is no specific evidence of safety of the drug in human pregnancy, both tolnaftate and nystatin have been in widespread topical use for many years without apparent ill consequence.

Effects on ability to drive and use machines: Not applicable.

Undesirable effects: A few cases of mild irritation and sensitisation have been reported.

Overdose: Not applicable.

Pharmacological properties
Pharmacodynamic properties: Tolnaftate is a highly active non-sensitising fungicidal agent that is very effective in the treatment of superficial fungal infections of the skin.

Nystatin, an antibiotic with antifungal activity provides specific therapy for all localised forms of candidiasis.

Pharmacokinetic particulars: Not applicable.

The product is applied topically and systemic absorption is negligible.

Preclinical safety data: There are no pre-clinical data of relevance to the prescriber which are additional to that already included in other sections of this SmPC.

Pharmaceutical particulars
List of excipients: Butylated hydroxytoluene; methylparaben; propylparaben; potassium sorbate; hydrochloric acid; cetomacrogol 1000; cetostearyl alcohol, fractionated coconut oil, perfume no. 66612, purified water.

Incompatibilities: None known.

Shelf life: 36 months.

Special precautions for storage: There are no special precautions for storage.

Nature and contents of container: 10 g or 20 g epoxy resin-lined aluminium tubes with low density polyethylene caps.

Instructions for use/handling: Not applicable.

Marketing authorisation number PL 0201/0071

Date of (partial) revision of the text February 1997

Legal category POM

VIRAFERON*

Qualitative and quantitative composition
Viraferon, solution for injection, multi-dose pen: Each carpoule of Viraferon, solution for injection, multi-dose pen contains 15 million International Units (IU)/ml (6 doses of 3 million IU for a total deliverable dose of 18 million IU), 25 million IU/ml (6 doses of 5 million IU for a total deliverable dose of 30 million IU) or 50 million IU/ml (6 doses of 10 million IU for a total deliverable does of 60 million IU) of recombinant interferon alfa-2b.

Pharmaceutical form Solution for injection of Viraferon in a delivery system for multiple injections (pen).

Clinical particulars
Therapeutic indications:
Chronic hepatitis B: Treatment of adult patients with histologically proven chronic hepatitis who have serum markers for virus B replication, e.g., those who are positive for HBV-DNA, or DNA polymerase, and HBeAg.

Current clinical experience in patients who remain on interferon alfa-2b for 4–6 months indicates that therapy can produce clearance o serum HBV-DNA and improvement in liver histology. In patients with loss of HBeAg and HBV-DNA, a significant reduction in morbidity and mortality has been observed.

Chronic hepatitis C: Treatment of adult patients with histologically proven chronic hepatitis who have serum markers for virus C replication, e.g., those who elevated transminases wihout liver decompensation and who are positive for serum HCV-RNA or anti-HCV.

Current clinical experience in patients who remain on interferon alfa-2b for 12 months indicates that therapy can produce normalistion of serum ALT, clearance of serum HCV-RNA and improvement in liver histology.

In patients who fail to respond after three to four months of treatment, discontinuation of interferon alfa-2b therapy should be considered.

Posology and method of administration: Viraferon, solution for injection, multi-dose pen contains a pre-filled, multi-dose cartridge for subcutaneous administration. It is designed to deliver fixed doses as required using a simple dial mechanism.

The needles provided in the packaging will be used for the Viraferon, solution for injection, multi-dose pen only. A new needle is to be used each time the pen delivers a dose.

Each Viraferon, solution for injection, multi-dose pen is for individual patient use only.

During the course of treatment with Viraferon for any indication, if adverse reactions develop, the dosage should be modified or therapy should be discontinued temporarily until the adverse reactions abate. If persistent or recurrent intolerance develops following adequate dosage adjustment, or disease progresses, the treatment with Viraferon should be discontinued. For maintenance dosage regimens administered subcutaneously, at the discretion of the physician, the patient may self-administer the dose.

Chronic hepatitis B: The recommended dosage is in the range of 5 to 10 million IU adminstered subcutaneously three times per week (every other day) for a period of four to six months.

If no improvement in serum HBV-DNA is observed after three to four months of treatment (at the 10 million IU dose, if tolerated), interferon alfa-2b therapy should be discontinued.

Chronic hepatitis C: The recommended dose is 3 million IU administered subcutaneously three times a week (every other day). Most patients who respond demonstrate improvement in ALT levels within three to four months. In these patients, therapy should be continued with 3 million IU three times a week (every other day) for 12 months.

The optimal duration of treatment is not yet established. There are no clinical studies directly comparing 12 to 18 months, however, the prolongation of treatment up to 18 months might be usefully considered in some patients.

In patients who fail to respond after three to four months of treatment, discontinuation of interferon alfa-2b should be considered.

Contra-indications:
- A history of hypersensitivity to recombinant interferon alfa-2b or any other component of Viraferon
- Severe pre-existing cardiac disease
- Severe renal or hepatic dysfunction; including that caused by metastases
- Epilepsy and/or compromised central nervous system (CNS) function (see *Special precautions for use*)
- Chronic hepatitis with decompensated cirrhosis of the liver
- Chronic hepatitis in patients who are being or have been treated recently with immunosuppressive agents excluding short-term corticosteroid withdrawal
- Autoimmune hepatitis; or history of autoimmune disease; immunosupressed transplant recipients;
- Pre-existing thyroid disease unless it can be controlled with conventional treatment.

Special warnings and special precautions for use:
For all patients: Acute hypersensitivity reactions (e.g., urticaria, angioedema, bronchoconstriction, anaphylaxis) to Viraferon have been observed rarely during Viraferon therapy. If such a reaction develops, the drug should be discontinued and appropriate medical therapy instituted immediately. Transient rashes do not necessitate interruption of treatment.

Viraferon, solution for injection, multi-dose pen contains m-cresol as preservative; some patients may experience allergic reaction to this ingredient.

Moderate to severe adverse experiences may require modification of the patient's dosage regimen, or in some cases, termination of Viraferon therapy. Any patient developing liver function abnormalities during treatment with Viraferon should be monitored closely and treatment discontinued if signs and symptoms progress.

Hypotension may occur during Viraferon therapy or up to two days post-therapy and may require supportive treatment.

Adequate hydration should be maintained in patients undergoing Viraferon therapy since hypotension related to fluid depletion has been seen in some patients. Fluid replacement may be necessary.

While fever may be associated with the flu-like syndrome reported commonly during interferon therapy, other causes of persistent fever should be ruled out.

Paracetamol has been used successfully to alleviate the symptoms of fever and headache which can occur with Viraferon therapy. The recommended paracetamol dosage is 500 mg to 1 g given 30 minutes before administration of Viraferon. The maximum dosage of paracetamol to be given is 1 g four times daily.

Viraferon should be used cautiously in patients with debilitating medical conditions, such as those with a history of pulmonary disease (e.g., chronic obstructive pulmonary disese) or diabetes mellitus prone to ketoacidosis. Caution should be observed also in patients with coagulation disorders (e.g., thrombophlebitis, pulmonary embolism) or severe myelosuppression.

Pulmonary infiltrates, pneumonitis and pneumonia, including fatality, have been observed rarely in interferon alfa treated patients, including those treated with Viraferon. The aetiology has not been defined. These symptoms have been reported more frequently when shosaikoto, a Chinese herbal medicine, is administered concomitantly with interferon alfa. Any patient developing fever, cough, dyspnoea or other respiratory symptoms should have a chest X-ray taken. If the chest X-ray shows pulmonary infiltrates or there is evidence of pulmonary function impairment, the patient should be monitored closely, and, if appropriate, interferon alfa treatment should be discontinued. While this has been reported more often in patients with chronic hepatitis C treated with interferon alfa, it has also been reported in patients with oncologic diseases treated with interferon alfa. Prompt discontinuation of interferon alfa administration and treatment with corticosteroids appear to be associated with resolution of pulmonary adverse events.

Ocular adverse events (see *Undesirable effects*) appear to occur after use of the drug for several months, but also have been reported after shorter treatment periods. Any patient complaining of changes in visual acuity or visual fields, or reporting other ophthalmologic symptoms during treatment with Viraferon, should have an eye examination. Because the retinal events may have to be differentiated from those seen with diabetic or hypertensive retinopathy, a baseline ocular examination is recommended prior to treatment with interferon in patients with diabetes mellitus or hypertension.

Patients with a pre-existing psychiatric condition or a history of severe psychiatric disorder should not be treated with Viraferon.

Severe CNS effects, particularly depression, suicidal ideation and attempted suicide have been observed in some patients during Viraferon therapy; in these cases, Viraferon therapy should be discontinued. The potential seriousness of these adverse events should be borne in mind by the prescribing physician.

Other CNS effects manifested by confusion and other alterations of mental status have been observed rarely. More significant obtundation and coma have been observed in some patients, usually elderly, treated at higher doses. While these effects are generally reversible, in a few patients full resolution took up to three weeks. Very rarely, seizures have occurred with high doses of Viraferon.

Patients with a history of congestive heart failure, myocardial infarction and/or previous or current arrhythmic disorders, who require Viraferon therapy, should be closely monitored. Those patients who have pre-existing cardiac abnormalities and/or are in advanced stages of cancer should have electrocardiograms taken prior to and during the course of treatment. Cardiac arrhythmias (primarily supraventricular) usually respond to conventional therapy but may require discontinuation of Viraferon therapy.

Because of reports of exacerbating pre-existing psoriatic disease, Viraferon should be used in patients with psoriasis only if the potential benefit justifies the potential risk.

Preliminary data may indicate that interferon alfa therapy is associated with an increased rate of graft rejection (liver and kidney transplants).

The development of different auto-antibodies has been reported during treatment with alfa interferons. Clinical manifestations of autoimmune disease during interferon therapy may occur more frequently in patients predisposed to the development of autoimmune disorders.

Treatment with Viraferon should be discontinued in patients with chronic hepatitis who develop prolongation of coagulation markers which might indicate liver decompensation.

The efficacy of interferon alfa-2b has not been demonstrated in patients with either chronic hepatitis B or C, with a co-infection with the human immunodeficiency virus (HIV), or undergoing haemodialysis.

Chronic hepatitis C: Infrequently, patients treated for chronic hepatitis C with Viraferon developed thyroid abnormalities, either hypothyroid or hyperthyroid. In clinical trials using Viraferon therapy, 2.8% patients overall developed thyroid abnormalities. The abnormalities were controlled by conventional therapy for thyroid dysfunction. The mechanism by which Viraferon may alter thyroid status is unknown. Prior to initiation of Viraferon therapy for the treatment of chronic hepatitis C, serum thyroid-stimulating hormone (TSH) levels should be evaluated. Any thyroid abnormality detected at that time should be treated with conventional therapy. Viraferon treatment may be initiated if TSH levels can be maintained in the normal range by medication. If, during the course of Viraferon therapy, a patient develops symptoms consistent with possible thyroid dysfunction, TSH levels should be evaluated. In the presence of thyroid dysfunction, Viraferon treatment may be continued if TSH levels can be maintained in the normal range by medication. DIscontinuation of Viraferon therapy has not reversed thyroid dysfunction occurring during treatment.

Laboratory tests: Standard haematologic tests and blood chemistries (complete blood count and differential, platelet count, electrolytes, liver enzymes, serum protein, serum bilirubin and serum creatinine) should be conducted in all patients prior to and periodically during systemic treatment with Viraferon.

During treatment for hepatitis B or C the recommended testing schedule is at weeks 1, 2, 4, 8, 12, 16, and every other month, thereafter, throughout treatment. If ALT flares during Viraferon therapy to greater than or equal to 2 times baseline, Viraferon therapy may be continued unless signs and symptoms of liver failure are observed. During ALT flare, liver function tests: ALT, prothrombin time, alkaline phosphatase, albumin and bilirubin should be monitored at two-week intervals.

Paediatric use: Doses of up to 10 million IU/m² have been administered safely to children with chronic active hepatitis B. However, efficacy of therapy has not been demonstrated. Generally, experience in patients below 18 years of age has been limited, and in such cases the expected benefits should be weighed carefully against potential hazards.

Effect on fertility: Interferon may impair fertility. In studies of interferon use in non-human primates, abnormalities of the menstrual cycle have been observed. Decreased serum oestradiol and progesterone concentrations have been reported in women treated with human leukocyte interferon. Therefore, fertile women should not receive Viraferon unless they are using effective contraception during the treatment period. Viraferon should be used with caution in fertile men.

Interaction with other medicaments and other forms of interaction:

Drug/drug interactions: Narcotics, hypnotics or sedatives should be administered with caution concomitantly with Viraferon.

Interactions between Viraferon and other drugs have not been fully evaluated. Caution should be exercised when administering Viraferon in combination with other potentially myelosuppressive agents.

Interferons may affect the oxidative metabolic process. This should be considered during concomitant therapy with drugs metabolised by this route, such as the xanthine derivatives theophylline or aminophylline. During concomitant therapy with xanthine agents, serum theophylline levels should be monitored and dosage adjusted if necessary.

Use during pregnancy and lactation: Viraferon has been shown to have abortifacient effects in *Macaca mulatta* (rhesus monkeys) at 90 and 180 times the recommended intramuscular or subcutaneous dose of 2 million IU/m². Abortion was observed in all dose groups (7.5 million, 15 million and 30 million IU/kg), and was statistically significant versus control at the mid- and high-dose groups (corresponding to 90 and 180 times the recommended intramuscular or subcutaneous dose of 2 million IU/m²). There are no adequate in pregnant women. Viraferon should be used during pregnancy only if the potential benefit justifies the potential risk to the foetus.

It is not known whether the components of this drug are excreted in human milk. Because of the potential for adverse reactions from Viraferon in nursing infants, a decision should be made whether to discontinue nursing or to discontinue the drug, taking into account the importance of the drug to the mother.

Effects on ability to drive and use machines: Patients who develop fatigue, somnolence, or confusion during treatment with Viraferon should be cautioned to avoid driving or operating machinery.

Undesirable effects: In clinical trials conducted in a broad range of indciations and at a wide range of doses, the most commonly reported adverse effects were fever, fatigue, headache and myalgia. Fever and fatigue were reversible within 72 hours of interruption or cessation of treatment and were dose related. In the hepatitis treatment groups these effects were of mild to moderate severity.

Common adverse effects include rigors/chills, anorexia and nausea.

In decreasing order of frequency, less commonly reported effects include vomiting, diarrhoea, arthralgia, asthenia, somnolence, dizziness, dry mouth, alopecia, flu-like symptoms (unspecified), back pain, depression, suicidal attempts, malaise, pain, increased sweating, taste alteration, irritability, insomnia, confusion, impaired concentration and hypotension.

Reported rarely were abdominal pain, rash, nervousness, injection site disorders, paresthesia, herpes simplex, pruritus, eye pain, anxiety, epistaxis, coughing, pharyngitis, pulmonary infiltrates, pneumonitis and pneumonia, impaired consciousness, weight decrease, face oedema, dyspnoea, dyspepsia, tachycardia, hypertension, increased appetite, decreased libido, hypoesthesia, taste perversion, loose stool, gingival bleeding, neuropathy, and polyneuropathy, rhabdomyolysis, sometimes serious, and renal insufficiency. Hyperthyroidism or hypothyroidism have also been observed rarely. Hepatotoxicity, including fatality has been observed rarely.

Very rarely following the marketing of Viraferon, cases of nephrotic syndome, renal failure, aggravated diabetes, diabetes/hyperglycaemia, cardiac ischemia, and myocardial infarction have been reported.

Cardiovascular (CVS) adverse reactions, particularly arrhythmia, appeared to be correlated mostly with pre-existing CVS disease and prior therapy with cardiotoxic agents (see *Special warnings and special precautions for use*). Transient reversible cardiomyopathy has been reported rarely in patients without prior evidence of cardiac diasease.

Retinal haemorrhages, cotton wool spots, and retinal artery or vein obstruction have been observed rarely in patients treated with interferon alfa, including Viraferon (recombinant interferon alfa-2b) Powder for solution for injection or Solutin for injection (see *Special warnings and special precautions for use*).

Clinically significant laboratory abnormalities, most frequently occurring at doses greater than 10 million IU daily, include reduction in granulocyte and white blood cell counts; decreases in haemoglobin level and platelet count; increases in alkaline phosphatase, LDH, serum creatinine and serum urea nitrogen levels. Increase in serum ALT/AST (SGOT/SGOT) levels have been noted as an abnormality in some non-hepatitis subjects and also in some patients with chronic hepatitis B coincident with clearance of viral DNAp.

Overdose: Overdosing has not been reported with Viraferon, but as for any pharmacologically active compound, symptomatic treatment with frequent monitoring of vital signs and close observation of the patient is indicated.

Pharmacological properties

Pharmacotherapeutic group:

Immunostimulating agents, cytokines, interferon alfa, ATC code: L03A A04.

Viraferon solution for injection is a sterile, stable, albumin-free formulation of highly purified interferon alfa-2b produced by recombinant DNA techniques. Recombinant interferon alfa-2b is a water soluble protein with a molecular weight of approximately 19,300 daltons. It is obtained from a clone of *E. coli*, which harbours a genetically engineered plasmid hybrid encompassing an interferon alfa-2b gene from human leukocytes.

The activity of Viraferon is expressed in terms of IU, with 1 mg of recombinant interferon alfa-2b protein corresponding to 2×10^8 IU. International Units are determined by comparison of the activity of the recombinant interferon alfa-2b with the activity of the international reference preparation of human leukocyte interferon established by the World Health Organisation.

The interferons are a family of small protein molecules with molecular weights of approximately 15,000 or 21,000 daltons. They are produced and secreted by cells in response to viral infections or various synthetic and biological inducers. Three major classes of interferons have been identified: alpha, beta and gamma. These three main classes are themselves not homogeneous and may contain several different molecular species of interferon. More than 14 genetically distinct human alpha interferons have been identified. Viraferon has been classified as recombinant interferon alfa-2b.

Pharmacodynamic properties: Interferons exert their cellular activities by binding to specific membrane receptors on the cell surface. Human interferon receptors, as isolated from human lymphoblastoid (Daudi) cells, appear to be highly asymmetric proteins. They exhibit selectivity for human but not murine interferons, suggesting species specificity. Studies with other interferons have demonstrated species specificity. However, certain monkey species, e.g., Rhesus monkeys, are susceptible to pharmacodynamic stimulation upon exposure to human type 1 interferons.

The results of several studies suggest that, once bound to the cell membrane, interferon initiates a complex sequence of intracellular events that include the induction of certain enzymes. It is thought that this process, at least in part, is responsible for the various cellular responses to interferon, including inhibition of virus replication in virus-infected cells, suppression of cell proliferation and such immunomodulating activities as enhancement of the phagocytic activity of macrophages and augmentation of the specific cytotoxicity of lymphocytes for target cells. Any or all of these activities may contribute to interferon's therapeutic effects.

Recombinant interferon alfa-2b has exhibited antiproliferative effects in studies employing both animal and human cell culture systems as well as human tumour xenografts in animals. It has demonstrated significant immunomodulatory activity *in vitro*.

Recombinant interferon alfa-2b also inhibits viral replication *in vitro* and *in vivo*. Although the exact antiviral mode of action of recombinant interferon alfa-2b is unknown, it appears to alter the host cell metabolism. This action inhibits viral replication or if replication occurs, the progeny virions are to leave the cell.

Pharacokinetic properties: The pharmacokinetics of Viraferon were studied in healthy volunteers following single 5 million IU/m² and 10 million IU doses administered subcutaneously, intramuscularly and as a 30-minute intravenous infusion. The mean serum interferon concentrations following subcutaneous and intramuscular injections were comparable. Maximum serum levels occurred three to 12 hours after the lower dose and six to eight hours after the higher dose. The elimination half-lives of interferon injections were approximately two to three hours, and six to seven hours, respectively. Serum levels were below the detection limit 16 and 24 hours, respectively, post-injection. Both intramuscular and subcutaneous administration resulted in bioavailabilities greater than 100%.

After intravenous administration, serum interferon levels peaked (135 to 273 IU/ml) by the end of the infusion, then declined at a slightly more rapid rate than after subcutaneous or intramuscular drug administration, becoming undetectable four hours after the infusion. The elimination half-life was approximately two hours.

Urine levels of interferon were below the detection limit following each of the three routes of administration.

Interferon neutralising factor assays were performed on serum samples of patients who received Viraferon in Schering-Plough monitored clinical trials. Interferon neutralising factors are antibodies which neutralise the antiviral activity of interferon. The clinical incidence of neutralising factors developing in cancer patients treated systemically is 2.9% and in hepatitis patients is 6.2%. The detectable titres are low in almost all cases and have not been regularly associated with loss of response or any other autoimmune phenomenon. In patients with hepatitis, no loss of response was observed apparently due to the low titres.

Preclinical safety data: Although interferon is generally recognised to be species specific, toxicity studies in mice, rats, rabbits and monkeys were conducted. Injections of human recombinant interferon alfa-2b for up to three months have shown no evidence of toxicity.

Results of animal reproduction studies indicate that recombinant interferon alfa-2b was not teratogenic in rats or rabbits, nor did it adversely affect pregnancy, foetal development or reproductive capacity in offspring of treated rats. However, high doses of other forms of interfeons alfa and beta are known to produce dose-related anovulatory and abortification effects in Rhesus monkeys.

Mutagenicity studies with Viraferon revealed no adverse effects.

Pharmaceutical particulars

List of excipients: Sodium phosphate dibasic, sodium phosphate monobasic, edetate disodium, sodium chloride, m-cresol, polysorbate 80, water for injection q.s. ad 1.5 ml[1] (deliverable volume from the pen = 1.2 ml).

[1] An overfill is required for proper dispensing from the pen delivery system.

Incompatabilities: No other substance or solution should be mixed with Viraferon, solution for injection, multi-dose pen.

Shelf life: 12 months when stored at 2° to 8°C.

Special precautions for storage: Viraferon, solution for injection, multi-dose pen must be stored at 2° to 8°C (refrigerator) and should not be frozen.

Nature and contents of container:
15 million IU/ml: 1.5 ml carpoule, type I flint glass
25 million IU/ml: 1.5 ml carpoule, type I flint glass
50 million IU/ml: 1.5 ml carpoule, type I flint glass

The pen is packaged in a carton containing disposable needles and alcohol swabs.

Instructions for use and handling, and disposal (if appropriate): As with all parenteral drug products, Viraferon should be inspected visually for particulate matter and discolouration prior to admninistration. Viraferon solution for injection is clear and colourless.

Viraferon, solution for injection, multi-dose pen is injected subcutaneously after attaching a needle and dialling the prescribed dose.

The multi-dose pen should be at room temperature (≤25°C) before administering each dose. The pen should be removed from the refrigerator approximately 30 minutes before administration to allow the injectable solution to reach room temperature (≤25°C).

Each pen is intended for a maximum two-week use period and then must be discarded. A new needle must be used for each dose. After each use, the needle should be discarded safely and the pen must be returned to the refrigerator immediately. In case the product is left inadvertently at room temperature (≤25°C), a maximum total of 48 hours (two days) of exposure to room temperature (≤24°C) is permitted over the two-week use period.

Marketing authorisation numbers
15 MIU/ml: MA 0201/0231
25 MIU/ml: MA 0201/0232
50 MIU/ml: MA 0201/0233

Date of approval 16 October 1997

Legal category POM

VIRAFERON* INJECTABLE SOLUTION

Qualitative and quantitative composition Viraferon Injectable Solution:
Active ingredient: Recombinant interferon alfa-2b, 18 million International Units (IU)/vial (6 million IU/ml).
Inactive ingredients: Sodium phosphate dibasic, sodium phosphate monobasic, edetate disodium, sodium chloride, m-cresol, polysorbate 80, water for injection q.s. ad 3 ml (18 million IU).

Pharmaceutical form Injectable solution.

Clinical particulars
Therapeutic indications:
Hepatitis B: Treatment of adult patients with chronic active hepatitis B, who have markers for viral replication e.g., those who are positive for HBV-DNA, DNA polymerase or HBeAg.

Chronic hepatitis C/non-A, non-B: Reduction of disease activity in adult patients with chronic hepatitis C/non-A, non-B who have elevated liver enzymes without liver decompensation. Studies in these patients demonstrate that Viraferon Injection therapy can produce normalisation of serum ALT, clearance of serum HCV-RNA and improvement in liver histology.

Current clinical experience in patients who remain on Viraferon Injection for 12–18 months indicates that a higher proportion of patients demonstrated a sustained response after longer durations of therapy than those who discontinued therapy after six months.

Posology and method of administration: Viraferon Injection MAY BE ADMINISTERED USING EITHER STERILIZED GLASS OR PLASTIC DISPOSABLE SYRINGES.

MULTIDOSE PRESENTATIONS SHOULD BE FOR INDIVIDUAL PATIENT USE ONLY.

During the course of treatment with Viraferon Injection for any indication, if adverse reactions develop, the dosage should be modified or therapy should be discontinued temporarily until the adverse reactions abate. If persistent or recurrent intolerance develops following adequate dosage adjustment, or disease progresses, the treatment with Viraferon Injection should be discontinued.

For maintenance dosage regimens administered subcutaneously, at the discretion of the physician, the patient may self-administer the dose.

Chronic active hepatitis B: The optimal schedule of treatment has not been established yet. The dosage is usually in the range of 2.5 million IU to 5.0 million IU/m² of body surface administered subcutaneously three times per week for a period of four to six months.

If markers for viral replication or HbeAg do not decrease after one month of therapy, the dose can be escalated. The dosage may be adjusted further according to the patient's tolerance to the medication.

If no improvement has been observed after three to four months of treatment, discontinuation of therapy should be considered.

Chronic hepatitis C/non-A, non-B: The recommended dose is 3 million IU administered subcutaneously three times a week. Most patients who respond demonstrate improvement in ALT levels within 12–16 weeks. In these patients (and in fonction of their tolerance, see *Posology and method of administration*), therapy should be continued with 3 million IU three times a week for up to 18 months. In patients who fail to respond after 12–16 weeks of treatment, discontinuation of Viraferon Injection therapy should be considered.

Contra-indications:
- A history of hypersensitivity to recombinant interferon alfa-2b or any other component of Viraferon Injection;
- severe pre-existing cardiac disease;
- severe renal or hepatic dysfunction;
- epilepsy and/or compromised central nervous system (CNS) function (see *Special warnings and special precautions for use*);
- chronic hepatitis with decompensated hepatic disease or cirrhosis of the liver;
- chronic hepatitis in patients who are being or have been treated recently with immunosuppressive agents excluding short-term corticosteroid withdrawal;
- autoimmune hepatitis; or history of autoimmune disease; immunosupressed transplant recipients;
- pre-existing thyroid disease unless it can be controlled with conventional treatment.

Special warnings and special precautions for use: Efficacy in patients with chronic active hepatitis B co-infected with the human immunodeficiency virus (HIV) has not been demonstrated.

Viraferon should be used cautiously in patients with debilitating medical conditions, such as those with a history of pulmonary disease (e.g. chronic obstructive pulmonary disease) or diabetes mellitus prone to ketoacidosis. Caution should be observed also in patients with coagulation disorders (e.g. thrombophlebitis, pulmonary embolism) or severe myelosuppression.

Acute hypersensitivity reactions (e.g., urticaria, angioedema, broncho-constriction, anaphylaxis) to Viraferon Injection have been observed rarely during Viraferon Injection therapy. If such a reaction develops, the drug should be discontinued and appropriate medical therapy instituted immediately. Transient rashes do not necessitate interruption of treatment.

Moderate to severe adverse experiences may require modification of the patient's dosage regimen, or in some cases, termination of Viraferon Injection therapy. Any patient developing liver function abnormalities during treatment with Viraferon Injection should be monitored closely and treatment discontinued if signs and symptoms progress.

Patients with chronic hepatitis B with evidence of decreasing hepatic synthetic function, such as decreasing albumin levels or prolongation of prothrombin time, who nevertheless meet the criteria for therapy, may be at increased risk of clinical decompensation if a flare of aminotransferases occurs during treatment. In considering these patients for Viraferon therapy, the potential risks must be evaluated against the potential benefits of treatment.

Hypotension may occur during Viraferon Injection therapy or up to two days post-therapy and may require supportive treatment.

Adequate hydration should be maintained in patients undergoing Viraferon Injection therapy since hypotension related to fluid depletion has been seen in some patients. Fluid replacement may be necessary.

Patients with a history of congestive heart failure, myocardial infarction and/or previous or current arrhythmic disorders, who require Viraferon Injection therapy, should be closely monitored. Those patients who have pre-existing cardiac abnormalities and/or are in advanced stages of cancer should have electrocardiograms taken prior to and during the course of treatment. Cardiac arrhythmias (primarily supraventricular) usually respond to conventional therapy but may require discontinuation of Viraferon Injection therapy.

Pulmonary infiltrates, pneumonitis and pneumonia, including fatality, have been observed rarely in interferon-alpha treated patients, including those treated with Viraferon Injection. The etiology has not been defined. These symptoms have been reported more frequently when shosaikoto, a Chinese herbal medicine, is administered concomitantly with interferon-alpha. Any patient developing fever, cough, dyspnea or other respiratory symptoms should have a chest X-ray taken. If the chest X-ray shows pulmonary infiltrates or there is evidence of pulmonary function impairment, the patient should be monitored closely, and, if appropriate, interferon-alpha treatment should be discontinued. While this has been reported more often in patients with chronic hepatitis C/ non-A, non-B treated with interferon-alpha, it has also been reported in patients with oncologic diseases treated with interferon-alpha. Prompt discontinuation of interferon alpha administration and treatment with corticosteroids appear to be associated with resolution of pulmonary adverse events.

Patients with a pre-existing psychiatric condition or a history of severe psychiatric disorder should not be treated with Viraferon Injection.

If severe CNS effects, particularly depression, are observed, Viraferon Injection therapy should be discontinued. CNS effects manifested by depression, confusion and other alterations of mental status have been observed in some patients during Viraferon Injection therapy and suicidal ideation and attempted suicide have been observed rarely. These adverse effects have occurred in patients treated with recommended doses as well as in patients treated with higher Viraferon doses. More significant obtundation and coma have been observed in some patients, usually elderly, treated at higher doses. While these effects are generally reversible, in a few patients full resolution took up to three weeks. Very rarely, seizures have occurred with high doses of Viraferon Injection.

Infrequently, patients treated for chronic hepatitis non-A, non-B/C with Viraferon Injection developed thyroid abnormalities, either hypothyroid or hyperthyroid. In clinical trials < 1% (4/426) developed thyroid abnormalities. The abnormalities were controlled by conventional therapy for thyroid dysfunction. The mechanism by which Viraferon Injection may alter thyroid status is unknown. Prior to initiation of Viraferon Injection therapy for the treatment of chronic hepatitis non-A, non-B/C, serum thyroid-stimulating hormone (TSH) levels should be evaluated. Any thyroid abnormality detected at that time should be treated with conventional therapy. Viraferon Injection treatment may be initiated if TSH levels can be maintained in the normal range by medication. If, during the course of Viraferon Injection therapy, a patient develops symptoms consistent with possible thyroid dysfunction, TSH levels should be evaluated. In the presence of thyroid dysfunction, Viraferon treatment may be continued if TSH levels can be maintained in the normal range by medication. Discontinuation of Viraferon therapy has not reversed thyroid dysfunction occurring during treatment.

Because of reports of exacerbating pre-existing psoriatic disease, Viraferon Injection should be used in patients with psoriasis only if the potential benefit justifies the potential risk.

While fever may be associated with the flu-like syndrome reported commonly during interferon therapy, other causes of persistent fever should be ruled out.

Ocular adverse events (see *Undesirable effects*) appear to occur after use of the drug for several months, but also have been reported after shorter treatment periods. Any patient complaining of changes in visual acuity or visual fields, or reporting other ophthalmologic symptoms during treatment with Viraferon, should have an eye examination. Because the retinal events may have to be differentiated from those seen with diabetic or hypertensive retinopathy, a baseline ocular examination is recommended prior to treatment with interferon in patients with diabetes mellitus or hypertension.

Viraferon Injectable Solution contains m-cresol; some individuals may have an allergic reaction to this ingredient.

Laboratory tests: Standard haematologic tests and blood chemistries (complete blood count and differential, platelet count, electrolytes, liver enzymes, serum protein, serum bilirubin and serum creatinine) should be conducted in all patients prior to and periodically during systemic treatment with Viraferon Injection. In patients treated for hepatitis the recommended testing schedule is at weeks 1, 2, 4, 8, 12, 16, and every other month, thereafter, throughout treatment.

If ALT flares during Viraferon therapy to ≥ 2 times baseline, Viraferon Injection therapy may be continued unless signs and symptoms of liver failure are observed. During ALT flare, liver function tests: ALT, prothrombin time, alkaline phosphatase, albumin and bilirubin should be monitored at two-week intervals.

In patients considered for treatment of hepatitis, a liver biopsy is recommended to document diagnosis and severity of the disease.

Paediatric use: Doses of up to 10 million IU/m² have been administered safely to children with chronic active hepatitis B. However, efficacy of therapy has not been demonstrated. Generally, experience in patients below 18 years of age has been limited, and in such cases the expected benefits should be weighed carefully against potential hazards.

Effect on fertility: Interferon may impair fertility. In studies of interferon use in non-human primates, abnormalities of the menstrual cycle have been observed. Decreased serum estradiol and progesterone concentrations have been reported in women treated with human leukocyte interferon. Therefore, fertile women should not receive Viraferon Injection unless they are using effective contraception during the treatment period. Viraferon Injection should be used with caution in fertile men.

Interaction with other medicaments and other forms of interaction:

Drug/drug interactions: Paracetamol has been used successfully to alleviate the symptoms of fever and headache which can occur with Viraferon Injection therapy. The recommended paracetamol dosage if 500 mg to 1 g given 30 minutes before administration of Viraferon Injection. The maximum dosage of acetaminophen to be given is 1 g four times daily.

Narcotics, hypnotics or sedatives should be administered with caution concomitantly with Viraferon Injection.

Interactions between Viraferon Injection and other drugs have not been fully evaluated. Caution should be exercised when administering Viraferon in combination with other potentially myelosuppressive agents.

Interferons may affect the oxidative metabolic process. This should be considered during concomitant therapy with drugs metabolised by this route, such as the xanthine derivatives theophylline or aminophylline. During concomitant therapy with xanthine agents, serum theophylline levels should be monitored and dosage adjusted if necessary.

Pregnancy and lactation: Viraferon Injection has been shown to have abortifacient effects in *Macaca mulatta* (rhesus monkeys) at 90 and 180 times the recommended intramuscular or subcutaneous dose of 2 million IU/m². Although abortion was observed in all dose groups (7.5 million, 15 million and 30 million IU/kg), it was only statistically significant versus control at the mid- and high-dose groups (corresponding to 90 and 180 times the recommended intramuscular or subcutaneous dose of 2 million IU/m²).

There are no adequate and well controlled studies in pregnant women. Viraferon Injection should be used during pregnancy only if the potential benefit justifies the potential risk to the foetus. It is not known whether the components of this drug are excreted in human milk. Because of the potential for adverse reactions from Viraferon Injection in nursing infants, a decision should be made whether to discontinue nursing or to discontinue the drug, taking into account the importance of the drug to the mother.

Effects on ability to drive and use machines: Not applicable.

Undesirable effects: Systemic administration: The most commonly reported adverse effects were fever, fatigue, headache and myalgia. Fever and fatigue were reversible within 72 hours of interruption or cessation of treatment and were dose related. In the hepatitis treatment groups these effects were of mild to moderate severity.

Common adverse effects include anorexia, nausea and rigors.

Less common adverse effects include vomiting, diarrhoea, arthralgia, asthenia, somnolence, dizziness, dry mouth, alopecia, flu-like symptoms (unspecified), back pain, depression, malaise, pain, increased sweating, taste alteration, irritability, insomnia, confusion, impaired concentration and hypotension.

Rarely reported adverse reactions include abdominal pain, rash, nervousness, injection site disorders, paresthesia, herpes simplex, pruritus, eye pain, anxiety, epistaxis, coughing, pharyngitis, pulmonary infiltrates, pneumonitis and pneumonia, impaired consciousness, weight decrease, face oedema, dyspnea, dyspepsia, tachycardia, hypertension, increased appetite, decreased libido, hypoesthesia, taste perversion, loose stool, gingival bleeding, neuropathy, and polyneuropathy. Hyperthyroidism or hypothyroidism have also been observed rarely. Hepatotoxicity, including fatality has been observed rarely.

Cardiovascular (CVS) adverse reactions, particularly arrhythmia, appeared to be correlated mostly with pre-existing CVS disease and prior therapy with cardiotoxic agents (see *Special warnings and special precautions for use*). Transient reversible cardiomyopathy has been reported rarely in patients without prior evidence of cardiac disease.

Retinal haemorrhages, cotton wool spots, and retinal artery or vein obstruction have been observed rarely in patients treated with interferon alfa, including Viraferon (recombinant interferon alfa-2b) (see *Special warnings and special precautions for use*).

Clinically significant laboratory abnormalities, most frequently occurring at doses greater than 10 million IU daily, include reduction in granulocyte and white blood cell counts; decreases in haemoglobin level and platelet count; increases in alkaline phosphatase, LDH, serum creatinine and serum urea nitrogen levels.

Increase in serum ALT/AST levels have been noted as an abnormality in some non-hepatitis subjects and also in some patients with chronic hepatitis B coincident with clearance of viral DNAp.

Overdose: Overdosing has not been reported with Viraferon Injection, but as for any pharmacologically active compound, symptomatic treatment with frequent monitoring of vital signs and close observation of the patient is indicated.

Pharmacological properties Viraferon Injection is a sterile, stable, formulation of highly purified interferon alfa-2b produced by recombinant DNA techniques. Recombinant interferon alfa-2b is a water soluble protein with a molecular weight of approximately 19,300 daltons. It is obtained from a clone of *E. coli*, which has a genetically engineered plasmid hybridized with an interferon alfa-2b gene from human leukocytes.

The activity of Viraferon Injection is expressed in terms of IU, with 1 mg of recombinant interferon alfa-2b protein corresponding to 2×10^8 IU. International Units are determined by comparison of the activity of the recombinant interferon alfa-2b with the activity of the international reference preparation of human leukocyte interferon established by the World Health Organisation.

The interferons are a family of small protein molecules with molecular weights of approximately 15,000 or 21,000 daltons. They are produced and secreted by cells in response to viral infections or various synthetic and biological inducers. Three major classes of interferons have been identified: alpha, beta and gamma. These three main classes are themselves not homogeneous and may contain several different molecular species of interferon. More than 14 genetically distinct human alpha interferons have been identified. Viraferon Injection has been classified as recombinant interferon alfa-2b.

Pharmacodynamic properties: Interferons exert their cellular activities by binding to specific membrane receptors on the cell surface. Human interferon receptors, as isolated from human lymphoblastoid (Daudi) cells, appear to be highly asymmetric proteins. they exhibit selectivity for human but not murine interferons, suggesting species specificity. Studies with other interferons have demonstrated species specificity.

The results of several studies suggest that, once bound to the cell membrane, interferon initiates a complex sequence of intracellular events that include the induction of certain enzymes. It is thought that this process, at least in part, is responsible for the various cellular responses to interferon, including inhibition of virus replication in virus-infected cells, suppression of cell proliferation and such immunomodulating activities as enhancement of the phagocytic activity of macrophages and augmentation of the specific cytotoxicity of lymphocytes for target cells. Any or all of these activities may contribute to interferon's therapeutic effects.

Recombinant interferon alfa-2b has exhibited antiproliferative effects in studies employing both animal and human cell culture systems as well as human tumour xenografts in animals. It has demonstrated significant immunomodulatory activity *in vitro*.

Recombinant interferon alfa-2b also inhibits viral replication *in vitro* and *in vivo*. Although the exact antiviral mode of action of recombinant interferon alfa-2b is unknown, it appears to alter the host cell metabolism. This action inhibits viral replication or if replication occurs, the progeny virions are to leave the cell. The specific mechanism of action in the treatment of condylomata acuminata is unknown.

Pharacokinetic properties: The pharmacokinetics of Viraferon Injection were studied in healthy volunteers following single 5 million IU/mls2 and 10 million IU doses administered subcutaneously, intramuscularly and as a 30-minute intravenous infusion. The mean serum interferon concentrations following subcutaneous and intramuscular injections were comparable. Maximum serum levels occurred three to 12 hours after the lower dose and six to eight hours after the higher dose. The elimination half-lives of interferon injections were approximately two to three hours, and six to seven hours, respectively. Serum levels were below the detection limit 16 and 24 hours, respectively, post-injection. Both intramuscular and subcutaneous administration resulted in bioavailabilities greater than 100%.

After intravenous administration, serum interferon levels peaked (135 to 273 IU/ml) by the end of the infusion, then declined at a slightly more rapid rate than after subcutaneous or intramuscular drug administration, becoming undetectable four hours after the infusion. The elimination half-life was approximately two hours.

Urine levels of interferon were below the detection limit following each of the three routes of administration.

Interferon neutralising factor assays were performed on serum samples of patients who received Viraferon Injection in Schering-Plough monitored clinical trials. Interferon neutralising factors are antibodies which neutralise the antiviral activity of interferon. The clinical incidence of neutralising factors developing in cancer patients treated systemically is 2.9% and in hepatitis patients is 6.9%. Serum interferon neutralising factors were detected in 0.8% of patients with condylomata acuminata who received Viraferon Injection intralesionally. The detected titres are low in almost all cases and have not been regularly associated with loss of response or any other autoimmune phenomenon. In patients with hepatitis, no loss of response was observed, apparently due to the low titres. No development of neutralising antibodies has been demonstrated in patients who received Viraferon Injection intralesionally in the treatment of basal cell carcinoma.

Preclinical safety data: Although interferon is generally recognised to be species specific, toxicology studies in mice, rats, rabbits and monkeys were conducted. Injections of human recombinant interferon alfa-2b for up to three months have shown no evidence of toxicity.

Results of animal reproduction studies indicate that recombinant interferon alfa-2b was not teratogenic in rats or rabbits, nor did it adversely affect pregnancy, foetal development or reproductive capacity in offspring of treated rats. Furthermore, animal studies have shown that interferons do not cross the placental barrier.

Mutagenicity studies with Viraferon Injection revealed no adverse effects.

Pharmaceutical particulars

List of excipients: Sodium phosphate dibasic, sodium phosphate monobasic, edetate disodium, sodium chloride, m-cresol, polysorbate 80, water for injection.

Incompatabilities: Not applicable.

Shelf life: 18 months when stored at 2° to 8°C. The unopened product may be kept at room temperatures up to 25°C (room temperature) for up to 7 days while in possession of the patient.

Special precautions for storage: Store between 2° to 8°C.

Nature and contents of container: 6 million IU/ml – 18 million IU/vial – 3 mil vial, type I flint glass.

Instructions for use/handling: Following withdrawal of first dose from the vial, the remaining solution is stable for up to four weeks at 2° to 8°C. Any solution remaining after 4 weeks must be discarded.

Marketing authorisation number MA 0201/0214.

Date of first authorisation/revision of SmPC January 1997

Legal category POM

**Trade Mark*

Schwarz Pharma Limited
Schwarz House
East Street
Chesham
Bucks HP5 1DG

☎ 01494 797500 🖷 01494 773934

SCHWARZ
PHARMA

DEPONIT*

Qualitative and quantitative composition Deponit 5: 1 patch contains glyceryl trinitrate 18.7 mg. The average amount of glyceryl trinitrate absorbed from each patch in 24 hours is 5 mg. Deponit 10: 1 patch contains glyceryl trinitrate 37.4 mg. The average amount of glyceryl trinitrate absorbed from each patch in 24 hours is 10 mg.

Pharmaceutical form Transdermal drug delivery system, packaged individually in a sealed sachet.

Clinical particulars
Therapeutic indications: Prophylaxis of angina pectoris alone or in combination with other anti-anginal therapy.

Posology and method of administration:
*Deponit 5 mg: Adults:*Treatment should be initiated with one Deponit 5 daily. If necessary the dosage may be increased to two Deponit 5 Patches.

*Deponit 10 mg: Adults:*Treatment should be initiated with one Deponit 10 daily. If necessary the dosage may be increased to two Deponit 10 Patches.

It is recommended that the patch is applied to the lateral chest wall, the skin should be smooth, unbroken and with few hairs. The replacement patch should be applied to a new area of skin. Allow several days to elapse before applying a fresh patch to the same area of skin. Tolerance may occur during chronic nitrate therapy. Tolerance is likely to be avoided by allowing a patch-free period of 8-12 hours each day, usually at night. Additional anti-anginal therapy with drugs not containing nitro compounds should be considered for the nitrate-free interval.

*Elderly:*No specific information on use in the elderly is available, however there is no evidence to suggest that an alteration in dose is required.

*Children:*The safety and efficacy of Deponit in children has yet to be established.

*Contra-indications:*Hypersensitivity to nitrates, severe hypotension, marked anaemia, increased intracranial pressure, myocardial insufficiency due to obstructions (e.g. in the presence of aortic or mitral stenosis or of constrictive pericarditis).

Special precautions for use: In recent myocardial infarction or acute heart failure, Deponit should be employed only under careful surveillance. As with all anti-anginal nitrate preparations, withdrawal of long-term treatment should be gradual by replacement with decreasing doses of long-acting oral nitrates. Caution should be exercised in patients with hypoxaemia and a ventilation/perfusion imbalance due to lung disease or ischaemic heart failure. If tolerance to glyceryl trinitrate patches develops, the effect of sublingual glyceryl trinitrate on exercise tolerance may be partially diminished. Nitrate therapy may aggravate the angina caused by hypertropic cardiomyopathy.

Interactions: Concomitant treatment with other vasodilators, calcium antagonists, ACE inhibitors, beta blockers, diuretics, antihypertensives, tricyclic antidepressants and major tranquillisers, as well as the consumption of alcohol, may potentiate the hypotensive effect of the preparation. If administered concurrently, Deponit may increase the blood level of dihydroergotamine and lead to coronary vasoconstriction. The possibility that ingestion of acetylsalicylic acid and non-steroidal anti-inflammatory drugs might diminish the therapeutic response to the patch cannot be excluded.

Pregnancy and lactation: Deponit should not be used during pregnancy or lactation unless considered absolutely essential by the physician. It is not known whether the active substance passes into the breast milk. Benefits to the mother must be weighed against risk to the child.

Effects on the ability to drive and use machines: Postural hypotension has been reported rarely following initiation of treatment with glyceryl trinitrate and care is advised when driving or operating machinery.

Undesirable effects: At the beginning of treatment nitrate headaches may occur, but experience has shown that this usually subsides after a few days of continuous use. Slight reddening at the site of application usually disappears without therapeutic measures, after the patch has been removed. Other reported side-effects are facial flushing, faintness, dizziness and postural hypotension which may be associated with reflex-induced tachycardia. Nausea and vomiting may occur rarely.

Overdose: Symptoms - high doses of glyceryl trinitrate are known to cause pronounced systemic side effects, e.g. a marked fall in blood pressure and reflex tachycardia resulting in collapse and syncope. *Treatment* - The effect of Deponit can be rapidly terminated by removing the patch. Any fall in blood pressure or signs of collapse that may occur, may be managed by general resuscitative measures.

Pharmacological properties
Pharmacodynamic properties: The main pharmacological activity of organic nitrates is the relaxation of smooth vascular muscles. The systemic vasodilation induces an increase of venous capacitance. Venous return is reduced. Ventricular volume, filling pressures and diastolic wall tension are diminished (preload reduction). A diminished ventricular radius and reduced wall tension, lower myocardial energy and oxygen consumption, respectively. The dilation of the large arteries near the heart leads to a decrease in both the systemic (reduction of afterload) and the pulmonary vascular resistance. In addition, this relieves the myocardium and lowers oxygen demands. By dilating the large eipicardial coronary arteries, glyceryl trinitrate enhances blood supply to the myocardium, improving its pump function and increasing the oxygen supply. At molecular level, nitrates form nitric oxide (NO), which corresponds to the physical EDRF (endothelium derived relaxing factor). EDRF mediated production of cyclic guanosine monophosphate (CGMP) leads to relaxation of smooth muscle cells.

Pharmacokinetic properties:
General characteristics of the active substance: The transdermal absorption of glyceryl trinitrate circumvents the extensive hepatic first pass metabolism so the bioavailability is about 70% of that achieved after i.v. administration. The steady-state concentration in the plasma depends on the patch dosage and the corresponding rate of absorption. At a rate of absorption of 0.4 mg/h, the steady-state concentration is about 0.2 µg/l on average. Plasma protein binding is about 60%. Glyceryl trinitrate is metabolized to 1,2- and 1,3 dinitroglycerols. The dinitrates exert less vasodilatory activity than glyceryl trinitrate. The contribution to the overall effect is not known. The dinitrates are further metabolized to inactive mononitrates, glyceryl and carbon dioxide. The elimination half-life of glyceryl trinitrate is 2-4 min. The metabolism of glyceryl trinitrate, which is effected in the liver, but also in many other cells, e.g. the red blood cells, includes the separation of one or more nitrate groups. In addition to the metabolism of glyceryl trinitrate, there is a renal excretion of the catabolites.

Characteristics in patients: There is no evidence that a dosage adjustment is required in the elderly or in diseases such as renal failure or hepatic insufficiency.

Preclinical safety data: Glyceryl trinitrate is a well-known active substance, established for more than a hundred years. Thus new preclinical studies have not been carried out with Deponit.

Pharmaceutical particulars
List of excipients: Acrylate/vinyl acetate copolymer, polypropylene.

Incompatibilities: No incompatibilities have so far been demonstrated.

Shelf life: Shelf life of the product as packaged for sale: 2 years.

Special precautions for storage: Store below 25°C.

Nature and contents of container: Multilaminate film/foil pouch with heat-sealed edges. 28 patches per carton.

Instructions for use/handling: The Deponit patch should be removed from the package just before application. After removal of the protective foil, the patch should be applied to unbroken, clean and dry skin that is smooth and with few hairs. The same area of skin should not be used again for some days.

Marketing authorisation numbers

Deponit 5	4438/0036
Deponit 10	4438/0037

Date of approval/revision of SPC January 1997

Legal category P

DIOCTYL* CAPSULES

Presentation Yellow and white soft gelatin capsules containing 100 mg Docusate Sodium USP.

Uses To prevent and treat chronic constipation. As an adjunct in abdominal radiological procedures.

Dosage and administration
Adults and elderly: Up to 500 mg daily in divided doses. Treatment should be commenced with large doses which should be decreased as the condtion of the patient improves.

Children: Not recommended.

The capsules should be swallowed whole with a glass of water.

For use with barium meals: 400 mg to be taken with the barium meal.

Contra-indications, warnings, etc
Contra-indications: Docusate sodium should not be administered when abdominal pain, nausea, vomiting or intestinal obstruction is present. Docusate sodium should not be given to infants under 6 months old.

Interactions: Concurrent administration with mineral oil is contra-indicated. Anthraquinone derivatives should be taken in reduced dose when administered with docusate sodium as it increases their absorption.

Pregnancy and lactation: There is inadequate evidence of the safety of the drug in human pregnancy, and there is no evidence from animal work that it is free from hazard. However it has been in wide use for many years without apparent ill consequence. Therefore Dioctyl should only be used in pregnancy if the benefits outweigh the potential risk. Docusate sodium is excreted in breast milk and should therefore be used with caution in breast-feeding mothers.

Overdose: In rare cases of overdose, excessive loss of water and electrolytes may occur. This should be treated by encouraging the patient to drink plenty of fluid.

Pharmaceutical precautions Dioctyl Capsules should be stored in a dry place below 25°C.

Legal category P

Package quantities Dioctyl Capsules are available in packs of 30 and 100 capsules.

Further information Docusate sodium exerts its clinical effect in the gastro-intestinal tract by means of its physical surfactant properties, by allowing penetration of water and fats into hard, dry faeces. There is some evidence to suggest that docusate sodium is absorbed from the gastro-intestinal tract and that it may enhance absorption of compounds administered concomitantly

Marketing authorisation number 4438/0032

Date of preparation January 1997 (Code: 357).

ELANTAN*

Presentation White tablets with break-score containing the active ingredient isosorbide mononitrate. The tablets are available in three strengths; Elantan 10 (marked E10), Elantan 20 (marked E20) and Elantan 40 (marked E40) containing isosorbide mononitrate 10 mg, 20 mg and 40 mg respectively.

Uses Elantan 10, 20 and 40 are indicated for the prophylaxis of angina pectoris.

Elantan 20 and 40 are indicated as adjunctive therapy in congestive heart failure not responding to cardiac glycosides or diuretics.

Dosage and administration Tablets should be taken unchewed with a little water after meals.

Adults:

Angina prophylaxis: Elantan 10, 20 and 40, one tablet to be taken two to three times a day. The dosage may be increased up to 120 mg per day. For patients not already receiving prophylactic nitrate therapy it is recommended that the initial dose be one tablet of Elantan 10 twice a day.

Congestive heart failure: Elantan 20 and 40, one tablet to be taken two to three times a day. The dosage may be increased up to 120 mg per day.

Elderly: There is no evidence to suggest that an adjustment of the dosage is necessary.

Children: The safety and efficacy of Elantan has yet to be established in children.

Contra-indications, warnings etc.

Contra-indications: This product should not be given to patients with a known sensitivity to nitrates. Elantan should not be used in patients with acute myocardial infarction with low filling pressure, acute circulatory failure (shock, vascular collapse) or very low blood pressure. Elantan should not be used in patients with marked anaemia, head trauma, cerebral haemorrhage, severe hypotension or hypovolaemia.

Interactions: Some of the effects of alcohol may be potentiated by this agent. The effects of Elantan may be potentiated by other hypotensive agents.

Pregnancy and lactation: This product should not be used during pregnancy or in women breast feeding infants unless considered essential by the physician.

Precautions: This preparation may give rise to symptoms of postural hypotension and syncope. These symptoms can largely be avoided if the treatment is started with one tablet of Elantan 10 morning and night. Elantan should be used with caution in patients suffering from hypothyroidism, hypothermia, malnutrition, severe liver or renal disease.

Side-effects: Headaches may occur as a side-effect. It is also a sign of overdose. Usually the headache subsides after a few days.

Overdose: Overdosage may lead to vascular collapse and gastric lavage is indicated in severe cases. Further measures to support the circulation are recommended e.g. elevating the legs and/or treatment with hypertensive agents.

Pharmaceutical precautions None

Legal category
Elantan 10 P
Elantan 20 and 40 POM

Package quantities Elantan 10, 20 and 40 are blister packed in the following pack sizes:
Elantan 10: 56 and 84 tablets.
Elantan 20: 56 and 84 tablets.
Elantan 40: 50, 56, 84 and 100 tablets (50 and 100 tablets to be phased out in 1998).

Further information Nil

Product licence numbers

Elantan 10	04438/0018
Elantan 20	04438/0005
Elantan 40	04438/0008

Date of preparation June 1997 (531).

ELANTAN* LA25

Qualitative and quantitative composition Isosorbide mononitrate 25 mg

Pharmaceutical form Slow release capsules

Clinical particulars

Therapeutic indications: For the prophylaxis of angina pectoris

Posology and method of administration: For oral administration.

Adults: one capsule to be taken in the morning. For patients with higher nitrate requirements the dose may be increased to two capsules taken simultaneously.

Children: the safety and efficacy of Elantan LA25 has yet to be established in children.

Contra-indications: Elantan LA25 should not be used in cases of acute myocardial infarction with low filling pressure, acute circulatory failure, shock, vascular collapse, or very low blood pressure. This product should not be given to patients with a known sensitivity to nitrates, marked anaemia, head trauma, cerebral haemorrhage, severe hypotension or hypovolaemia.

Special warnings and precautions for use: Elantan LA25 should be used with caution in patients who are suffering from hypothyroidism, hypothermia, malnutrition, severe liver disease or severe renal disease. Symptoms of circulatory collapse may arise after first dose, particularly in patients with labile circulation.

Interactions with other medicaments and other forms of interaction: Some of the effects of alcohol and the action of hypotensive agents may be potentiated by this product.

Pregnancy and lactation: There is inadequate evidence of safety of the drug in human pregnancy but nitrates have been used widely in the treatment of angina for many years without apparent ill consequence; animal studies having shown no hazard. Nevertheless it is not advisable to use this drug during pregnancy and lactation.

Effects on ability to drive and use machines: None known.

Undesirable effects: A headache may occur at the start of treatment, but this usually disappears after a few days.

Overdose: Overdosage may lead to vascular collapse and gastric lavage is indicated in severe cases. Further measures to support the circulation are recommended, e.g. elevating the legs and/or treatment with hypertensive agents.

Pharmacological properties

Pharmacodynamic properties: The active ingredient is a coronary vasodilator which reduces venous return.

Pharmacokinetic properties: The pharmacokinetic profile of Elantan LA25 closely follows that of Elantan LA50 (PL 4438/0015). Mean plasma concentration for Elantan LA25 8 hours post dose was shown to be 228 (±53) ng/ml.* Kinetics are approximately linear around the proposed dose range. The extraction rate is zero (F = 1). In patients with cirrhotic disease or cardiac failure or renal failure, pharmacokinetic parameters were similar to those obtained in healthy volunteers.
*Refers to isosorbide mononitrate.

Preclinical safety data: None stated

Pharmaceutical particulars

List of excipients: Lactose, talc, ethyl cellulose, polyethylene glycol, hydroxypropyl cellulose, sucrose, starch, gelatin, titanium dioxide, iron oxide red and iron oxide black.

Incompatibilities: None known.

Shelf life: 3 years.

Special precautions for storage: None.

Nature and contents of container: Cartons of blister strips of PVC and aluminium or of PP and aluminium. Aluminium foil thickness 20μ m or 16μ m. Pack size: 28 capsules.

Instruction for use/handling: None.

Marketing authorisation number 04438/0028

Date of approval/revision of SPC November 1996

Legal category P

ELANTAN* LA50

Presentation Brown and flesh coloured, opaque gelatin capsules containing 50 mg isosorbide mononitrate in a slow release formulation. The capsules also contain gelatin, lactose, ethyl cellulose, talc, hydroxypropyl cellulose, polyethylene glycol, sucrose, corn starch and colours E171 and E172.

Use For the prophylaxis of angina pectoris.

Dosage and administration The capsules are for oral administration and should be swallowed whole.

Adults and elderly: One capsule to be taken in the morning. This may be increased to two capsules if required.

Children: The safety and efficacy of LA50 has yet to be established in children.

Contra-indications, warnings, etc

Contra-indications: Elantan LA50 should not be used in cases of acute myocardial infarction with low filling pressure, acute circulatory failure, severe cerebrovascular insufficiency (shock, vascular collapse), or very low blood pressure. It should not be given to patients with a known sensitivity to nitrates, marked anaemia, head trauma, cerebral haemorrhage, severe hypotension or hypovalaemia.

Interactions: Some of the effects of alcohol and the action of hypotensive agents may be potentiated by this treatment.

Warnings: Elantan LA50 should be used with caution in patients who are suffering from hypothyroidism, hypothermia, malnutrition or severe renal disease. Symptoms of circulatory collapse may arise after the first dose, particularly in patients with labile circulation. A headache may occur at the start of treatment, but this usually disappears after a few days. Symptoms of postural hypotension and syncope may arise in some patients. These effects may be avoided if treatment is started with the lowest possible dose.

Use in pregnancy and lactation: There is inadequate evidence of safety of the drug in human pregnancy but nitrates have been used widely in the treatment of angina for many years, without apparent ill consequence, animal studies having shown no hazard. Nevertheless it is not advisable to use this drug during pregnancy and lactation.

Overdosage: Overdosage may lead to vascular collapse and gastric lavage is indicated in severe cases. Further measures to support the circulation are recommended, e.g elevating the legs, and/or treatment with hypertensive agents.

Pharmaceutical precautions None

Legal category P

Package quantities Elantan LA50 is available in calendar packs of 28 capsules.

Further information Nil

Product licence number 04438/0015

Date of preparation July 1996 (151).

ISOKET* 0.05%

Presentation Isoket 0.05% (Isosorbide dinitrate 0.5 mg/ml) in 50 ml bottles. Isoket 0.05% contains isosorbide dinitrate in sterile isotonic saline, no other additives are present.

Uses The indications for Isoket 0.05% are: Treatment of unresponsive left ventricular failure, secondary to acute myocardial infarction, unresponsive left ventricular failure of various aetiology, severe or unstable angina pectoris, to facilitate or prolong balloon inflation and to prevent or relieve coronary spasm during percutaneous transluminal coronary angioplasty.

Pharmacological actions: Isoket is a vasodilator predominantly of peripheral capacitance veins.

Dosage and administration

Intravenous route: The dose employed must be adjusted according to patient response. In general, a dose of between 2 mg and 12 mg per hour is suitable although doses as high as 20 mg per hour may be necessary.

Intracoronary route: The usual dose is 1 mg given as a bolus injection prior to balloon inflation. Further doses may be given not exceeding 5 mg within a 30 minute period.

Elderly: The dose of nitrates in cardiovascular disease is usually determined by patient response and stabilisation. Clinical experience has not necessitated alternative advice for use in elderly patients.

Children: The safety and efficacy of Isoket 0.05% has not yet been established in children.

Administration:

Intravenous: Isoket 0.05% can be administered undiluted by slow intravenous infusion using a syringe pump. It is compatible with infusion vechicles such as Sodium Chloride injection BP or Dextrose injection BP and can be administered as an admixture if required.

Intracoronary: Isoket 0.05% can be injected directly by this route according to the proposed dosage schedule. Bottles of Isoket are for single use only and should not be regarded as multi-dose containers.

Contra-indications, warnings etc

Contra-indications: These are common to all nitrates: Known hypersensitivity to nitrates, marked anaemia, cerebral haemorrhage, trauma, hypovolaemia and severe hypotension. Use in circulatory collapse or low filling pressure is also contra-indicated. Isoket should not be used in the treatment of cardiogenic shock, unless some means of maintaining an adequate diastolic pressure are undertaken.

Precautions: Isoket should be used with caution in patients who are suffering from hypothyroidism, malnutrition, severe liver or renal disease or hypothermia. Some of the effects of alcohol may be potentiated by this agent. The effects of anti-hypertensive drugs may be enhanced. Close attention to pulse and blood pressure is necessary during the administration of Isoket infusions.

Pregnancy and lactation: No data have been reported which would indicate the possibility of adverse effects resulting from the use of isosorbide dinitrate in pregnancy. Safety in pregnancy however has not been established. Isosorbide dinitrate should only be used in pregnancy and during lactation if, in the opinion of the physician, the possible benefits of treatment outweigh the possible hazards.

Adverse effects: In common with other nitrates, headache, nausea and tachycardia may occur during administration. Whilst sharp falls in systemic arterial pressure can give rise to symptoms of cerebral flow deficiency and decreased coronary perfusion, clinical experience with Isoket has shown that this is not normally a problem. This effect is consistent with the known vasodilatory effects of isosorbide dinitrate which occur predominantly on the venous rather than the arterial side of the circulation.

Treatment of overdosage: General supportive therapy.

Pharmaceutical precautions: Admixtures are stable for approximately 24 hours at room temperature in the recommended containers. Open ampoules or bottles should be used immediately and any unused drug discarded.

Compatibility: Isoket contains isosorbide dinitrate in isotonic saline and is compatible with commonly employed infusion fluids, no incompatibilities have so far been demonstrated. Isoket is compatible with glass infusion bottles and infusion packs made from polyethylene. Isoket may be infused slowly using a syringe pump with a glass or plastic syringe. The use of PVC giving sets and containers should be avoided since significant losses of the active ingredient by absorption can occur.

Legal category POM

Package quantities 50 ml bottle (Isosorbide dinitrate 25 mg/50 ml)

Further information Nil

Product licence number 4438/0017

Date of preparation Aug 1998 (Code: 903).

ISOKET* 0.1%

Qualitative and quantitative composition Isosorbide Dinitrate PhEur 0.1% w/v.

Pharmaceutical form Sterile colourless solution for intravenous infusion.

Clinical particulars

Therapeutic indications:

Intravenous: Isoket is indicated in the treatment of unresponsive left ventricular failure secondary to acute myocardial infarction, unresponsive left ventricular failure of various aetiology and severe or unstable angina pectoris.

Intra-coronary: Isoket is indicated during percutaneous transluminal coronary angioplasty to facilitate prolongation of balloon inflation and to prevent or relieve coronary spasm.

Posology and method of administration: Adults, including the elderly.

Intravenous route: A dose of between 2 mg and 12 mg per hour is usually satisfactory. However, dosages up to 20 mg per hour administered should be adjusted to the patient response.

Intra-coronary route: The usual dose is 1 mg given as a bolus injection prior to balloon inflation. Further doses maybe given not exceeding 5 mg within a 30 minute period.

Children: The safety and efficacy of Isoket has not yet been established in children.

Administration: Isoket is a concentrated solution and should never be injected directly in the form of a bolus except via the intra-coronary route prior to balloon inflation. A dilution of 50% is advocated for intracoronary administration. Isoket can be administered as an intravenous admixture with a suitable vehicle such as Sodium Chloride Injection BP or Dextrose Injection BP. Prepared Isoket admixtures should be given by intravenous infusion or with the aid of a syringe pump incorporating a glass or rigid plastic syringe. During administration the patients blood pressure and pulse should be closely monitored.

Contra-indications: These are common to all nitrates; known hypersensitivity to nitrates, marked anaemia, cerebral haemorrhage, head trauma, hypovolaemia, and severe hypotension. Use in circulatory collapse or low filling pressure is also contraindicated. Isoket should not be used in the treatment of cardiogenic shock, unless some means of maintaining an adequate diastolic pressure is undertaken.

Special warnings and precautions for use: Isoket should be used with caution in patients who are suffering from hypothyroidism, malnutrition, severe liver or renal disease or hypothermia. Close attention to pulse and blood pressure is necessary during the administration of Isoket infusions.

Interaction with other medicaments and other forms of interaction: Some of the effects of alcohol may be potentiated by this agent. The effects of antihypertensive drugs may be enhanced.

Pregnancy and lactation: No data have been reported which would indicate the possibility of adverse effects resulting from the use of isosorbide dinitrate in pregnancy. Safety in pregnancy, however, has not been established. Isosorbide dinitrate should only be used in pregnancy and during lactation if, in the opinion of the physician, the possible benefits of treatment outweigh the possible hazards.

Effects on ability to drive and use machines: None known.

Undesirable effects: In common with other nitrates, headaches, nausea and tachycardia may occur during administration. Whilst sharp falls in systemic arterial pressure can give rise to symptoms of cerebral flow deficiency and decreased coronary perfusion, clinical experience with Isoket has shown that this is not normally a problem.

Overdose: General supportive therapy.

Pharmacological properties

Pharmacodynamic properties: Isosorbide dinitrate is an organic nitrate which, in common with other cardioactive nitrates, is a vasodilator. It produces decreased left and right ventricular end-diastolic pressures to a greater extent than the decrease in systemic arterial pressure, thereby reducing afterload and especially the preload of the heart. Isosorbide dinitrate influences the oxygen supply to ischaemic myocardium by causing the redistribution of blood flow along collateral channels and from epicardial to endocardial regions by selective dilatation of large epicardial vessels. It reduces the requirement of the myocardium for oxygen by increasing venous capacitance, causing a pooling of blood in peripheral veins, thereby reducing ventricular volume and heart wall distension.

Pharmacokinetic properties: Isosorbide dinitrate (ISDN) is eliminated from plasma with a short half-life (about 0.7 H). The metabolic degradation of ISDN occurs via denitration and glucuronidation, like all organic nitrates. The rates of formation of the metabolites has been calculated for isosorbide-5-mononitrate (IS-5-MN) with 0.27 h^{-1}, and isosorbide (IS) with 0.16 h^{-1}. IS-5-MN and IS-2-MN are the primary metabolites which are also pharmacologically active. IS-5-MN is metabolised to isosorbide 5-mononitrate-2-glucuronide (IS-5-MN-2-GLU). The half life of this metabolite (about 2.5 h) is shorter than that of IS-5-MN (about 5.1. h). The half-life of ISDN is the shortest of all and that of IS-2-MN (about 3.2 h) lies in between.

Preclinical safety data: None stated.

Pharmaceutical particulars

List of excipients: Sodium Chloride PhEur. Water for injection PhEur.

Incompatibilities: Isoket contains isosorbide dinitrate in isotonic saline and is compatible with commonly employed infusion fluids, no incompatibilities have so far been demonstrated. Isoket is compatible with glass infusion bottles and infusion packs made from polyethylene. Isoket may be infused slowly using a syringe pump with glass or plastic syringe. The use of PVC giving sets and containers should be avoided since significant losses of the active ingredient by adsorption can occur.

Shelf life: 5 years, as packaged for sale. Admixtures are stable for approximately 24 hours at room temperature in the recommended containers. Open ampoules or bottles should be used immediately and any unused drug discarded.

Special precautions for storage: There are no special precautions for storage of the product as packaged for sale.

Nature and contents of container: Marketed pack sizes, 10 ml glass ampoules, 50 ml glass vials with rubber stoppers.

Instructions for use/handling: Example of admixture preparation; To obtain a dose of 6 mg per hour add 50 ml of Isoket 0.1% to 450 ml of a suitable vehicle, under aseptic conditions. The resultant admixture (500 ml), contains 100 µ g/ml (1 mg/10 ml) isosorbide dinitrate. An infusion rate of 60 ml per hour (equivalent to 60 paediatric microdrops per minute or 20 standard drops per minute), will deliver the required dose of 6 mg per hour. Should it be necessary to reduce fluid intake, 100 ml of Isoket 0.1% may be diluted to 500 ml using a suitable vehicle. The resultant solution now contains 200 µ g/ml (2 mg/10 ml) isosorbide dinitrate. An infusion rate of 30 ml per hour (equivalent to 30 paediatric microdrops per minute or 10 standard drops per minute), will deliver the required dose of 6 mg per hour. A dilution of 50% is advocated to produce a solution containing 0.5 mg/ml where fluid intake is strictly limited.

Marketing authorisation number 04438/0001

Date of approval/revision of SPC January 1997 (Code: 404).

Legal category POM

ISOKET* RETARD

Qualitative and quantitative composition Each tablet contains isosorbide dinitrate 20 mg or 40 mg respectively in a slow release formulation.

Pharmaceutical form Slow release tablets.

Clinical particulars

Therapeutic indications: For the prophylaxis and treatment of angina pectoris.

Posology and method of administration: For oral administration.

Adults: The usual dose is one tablet every 12 hours. No more than four tablets should be taken daily.

Elderly: Clinical experience has not necessitated alternative advice for use in elderly patients.

Children: The safety and efficacy of Isoket Retard has yet to be established.

The tablets should be swallowed without chewing.

Contra-indications: This product should not be given to patients with a known sensitivity to nitrates, very low blood pressure, acute myocardial infarction with low filling pressure, marked anaemia, head trauma, cerebral haemorrhage, acute circulatory failure, severe hypotension or hypovolaemia.

Special warnings and special precautions for use: Isoket Retard should be used with caution in patients who are suffering from hypothyroidism, hypothermia, malnutrition and severe liver or renal disease.

Interactions: Alcohol intake may enhance vasodilation.

Pregnancy and lactation: This product should not be used during pregnancy or lactation unless considered essential by the physician.

Effects on ability to drive and use machines: None known.

Undesirable effects: Cutaneous vasodilation, postural hypotension and dry skin rashes may occur occasionally. Headache may occur at the onset of treatment, but may be minimised by commencing with low doses and gradually increasing the dose. Tolerance may occur.

Overdose: Higher doses may lead to vascular collapse. In rare cases of overdosage, gastric lavage is indicated. Passive exercise of the extremities of the recumbent patient will promote venous return.

Pharmacological properties

Pharmacodynamic properties: Isosorbide dinitrate is an organic nitrate which, in common with other cardioactive nitrates, is a vasodilator. It produces decreased left and right ventricular end-diastolic pressures to a greater extent than the decrease in systemic arterial pressure, thereby reducing afterload and especially the preload of the heart. Isosorbide dinitrate influences the oxygen supply to ischaemic myocardium by causing the redistribution of blood flow along collateral channels and from epicardial to endocardial regions by selective dilatation of large epicardial vessels. It reduces the requirements of the myocardium for oxygen by increasing venous capacitance, causing a pooling of blood in peripheral veins, thereby reducing ventricular volume and heart wall distension.

Pharmacokinetic properties: After administration of one tablet of Isoket Retard 20 at least two peak concentrations of ISDN occurred in the plasma. The initial peak (mean 1.9 ng/ml, range 1.0 to 3.4 ng/ml) occurred during 0.5 to 2 hours and then the mean plasma concentrations declined to 1.3 ng/ml at 3 hours. The concentration then increased again to reach a major peak level (mean 6.2 ng/ml range 1.6 to 12.3 mg/ml) during 4 to 6 hours after dosing. Plasma concentrations of ISDN have been measured after administration of increasing doses in the range 20 to 100 mg as Isoket Retard 20 tablets. Means of peak concentrations of 4.2 ng/ml , 13-1 ng/ml 20.7 ng/ml, 36.8 ng/ml and 34.9 ng/ml were measured after doses of 20 mg, 40 mg, 60 mg, 80 mg and 100 mg respectively.

Pharmaceutical particulars

List of excipients: Lactose, talc, polyvinyl acetate, magnesium stearate, potato starch, sodium sulphate, sodium chloride, purified water and colours; E110 and E104 (Isoket Retard 20), E110 and E124 (Isoket Retard 40).

Incompatibilities: None known.

Shelf life: 5 years.

Special precautions for storage: None.

Nature and contents of container: Cartons of blister strips of polypropylene (PP) and aluminium or of PP/PP. †Pack sizes **50, 56**, 60, 84 and 90 tablets.

†Only those pack sizes marked in bold are currently marketed.

Instructions for use/handling: None.

Marketing authorisation numbers
Isoket Retard 20 04438/0004
Isoket Retard 40 04438/0002

Date of approval/revision of SPC December 1996 (Code: 329).

Legal category P

NITROCINE*

Qualitative and quantitative composition Ampoules containing 10 mg glyceryl trinitrate in 10 ml, or as glass bottles containing 50 mg glyceryl trinitrate in 50 ml.

Pharmaceutical form Isotonic sterile solution.

Clinical particulars
Therapeutic indications:
Surgery: Nitrocine is indicated for:
1. the rapid control of hypertension during cardiac surgery.
2. reducing blood pressure and maintaining controlled hypotension during surgical procedures.
3. controlling myocardial ischaemia during and after cardiovascular surgery.

Unresponsive congestive heart failure: Nitrocine may be used to treat unresponsive congestive heart failure secondary to acute myocardial infarction.

Unstable angina: Nitrocine may be used to treat unstable angina which is refractory to treatment with beta blockers and sublingual nitrates.

Posology and method of administration:
Adults and elderly: The dose of Nitrocine should be adjusted to meet the individual needs of the patient. The recommended dosage range is 10–200 mcg/min but up to 400 mcg/min may be necessary during some surgical procedures.

Children: The safety and efficacy of Nitrocine has not yet been established in children.

Surgery: A starting dose of 25 mcg/min is recommended for the control of hypertension, or to produce hypotension during surgery. This may be increased by increments of 25 mcg/min at 5 minute intervals until the blood pressure is stabilized. Doses between 10–200 mcg/min are usually sufficient during surgery, although doses of up to 400 mcg/min have been required in some cases.

The treatment of perioperative myocardial ischaemia may be started with a dose of 15–20 mcg/min, with subsequent increments of 10–15 mcg/min until the required effect is obtained.

Unresponsive congestive heart failure: The recommended starting dose is 20–25 mcg/min. This may be decreased to 10 mcg/min, or increased in steps of 20–25 mcg/min every 15–30 minutes until the desired effect is obtained.

Unstable angina: An initial dose of 10 mcg/min is recommended with increments of 10 mcg/min being made at approximately 30 minute intervals according to the needs of the patient.

Administration Nitrocine can be administered undiluted by slow intravenous infusion using a syringe pump incorporating a glass or rigid plastic syringe.

Alternatively, Nitrocine may be administered intravenously as an admixture using a suitable vehicle such as Sodium Chloride Injection B.P. or Dextrose Injection B.P.

Prepared admixtures should be given by intravenous infusion or with the aid of a syringe pump to ensure a constant rate of infusion.

During Nitrocine administration there should be close haemodynamic monitoring of the patient.

Example of admixture preparation: To obtain an admixture of GTN at a concentration of 100 mcg/ml, add 50 ml Nitrocine solution (containing 50 mg glyceryl trinitrate) to 450 ml of infusion vehicle to give a final volume of 500 ml.

A dosage of 100 mcg min can be obtained by giving 60 ml of the admixture per hour. This is equivalent to a drip rate of 60 paediatric microdrops per minute or 20 standard drops per minute. At this drip rate the admixture provides enough solution for an infusion time of 8 hours 20 minutes.

For full details it is advisable to consult the dosage chart on the package insert.

Bottles of Nitrocine are for single use only and should not be regarded as multi-dose containers.

Contra-indications: Nitrocine should not be used in the following cases: Known hypersensitivity to nitrates, marked anaemia, severe cerebral haemorrhage, head trauma, uncorrected hypovolaemia or severe hypotension. As the safety of Nitrocine during pregnancy and lactation has not yet been established, it should not be used unless considered absolutely essential.

Special warnings and precautions for use: Close attention to pulse and blood pressure is necessary during the administration of Nitrocine infusions. Nitrocine should be used with caution in patients suffering from hypothyroidism, severe liver or renal disease, hypothermia and malnutrition.

Interaction with other medicaments and other forms of interaction: Unknown.

Pregnancy and lactation: There is no, or inadequate, evidence of safety of the drug in human pregnancy or lactation, but it has been in widespread use for many years without apparent ill consequence, animal studies having shown no hazard. If drug therapy is needed in pregnancy, this product can be used if there is no safer alternative.

Effects on ability to drive and use machines: None stated.

Undesirable effects: In common with other nitrates, headaches and nausea may occur during administration. Other possible adverse reactions include hypotension, tachycardia, retching, diaphoresis, apprehension, restlessness, muscle twitching, retrosternal discomfort, palpitations, dizziness and abdominal pain. Paradoxical bradycardia has also been observed.

Overdose: Mild overdose usually results in hypotension and tachycardia. If arterial systolic blood pressure drops below 90 mmHg and if heart rate increases 10% above its initial value, the infusion should be discontinued to allow a return to pre-treatment levels. If hypotension persists, or in more severe cases, this may be reversed by elevating the legs and/or treatment with hypertensive agents.

Pharmacological properties
Pharmacodynamic properties: Nitroglycerin reduces the tone of vascular smooth muscle. This action is more marked on the venous capacitance vessels than the arterial vessels. There is reduction in venous return to the heart and a lowering of elevated filling pressure. This lowering of filling pressure reduces the left ventricular end diastolic volume and preload. The net effect is a lowering of myocardial oxygen consumption. Systemic vascular resistance, pulmonary vascular pressure and arterial pressure are also reduced by nitroglycerin and there is a net reduction in the afterload. By reducing the preload and afterload, nitroglycerin reduces the workload on the heart. Nitroglycerin affects oxygen supply by redistributing blood flow along collateral channels from the epicardial to endocardial regions.

Pharmacokinetic properties: As with all commonly used organic nitrates the metabolic degradation of nitroglycerin occurs via denitration and glucuronidation. The less active metabolites resulting from this biotransformation can be recovered from the urine within 24 hours. Nitroglycerin is eliminated from plasma with a short half-life of about 2–3 minutes. This rapid disappearance from plasma is consistent with the high systemic clearance values for this drug (up to 3270 L/hour).

Preclinical safety data: None stated.

Pharmaceutical particulars
List of excipients: Glucose, propylene glycol and water for injection.

Incompatibilities: Nitrocine contains nitroglycerin in isotonic sterile solution and is compatible with commonly employed infusion solutions. No incompatibilities have so far been demonstrated.

Nitrocine is compatible with glass infusion bottles and with rigid infusion packs made of polyethylene. Nitrocine may also be infused slowly using a syringe pump with a glass or plastic syringe.

Nitrocine is incompatible with polyvinylchloride (PVC) and severe losses of glyceryl trinitrate (over 40%) may occur if this material is used. Contact with polyvinylchloride bags should be avoided. Polyurethane also induces a loss of the active ingredient.

Shelf life:
Glass ampoules 60 months
Glass vials 36 months

Special precautions for storage: None.

Nature and contents of container: Glass ampoules 10 ml. Glass, rubber stoppered vials 50 ml.

Instructions for use/handling: Bottles of Nitrocine are for single use only and should not be regarded as multi-dose containers.

Administration data
Marketing authorisation holder: Schwarz Pharma Ltd, Schwarz House, East Street, Chesham, Bucks HP5 1DG.

Marketing authorisation number PL 04438/0006

Date of first authorisation 25th August 1982

Date of (partial) revision of the text May 1997 (638)

Legal category POM

PERDIX*

Qualitative and quantitative composition
Each Perdix 7.5 mg tablet contains moexipril hydrochloride 7.5 mg.

Each Perdix 15 mg tablet contains moexipril hydrochloride 15 mg.

Pharmaceutical form Film-coated tablets

Clinical particulars
Therapeutic indications: For the treatment of hypertension as monotherapy. As second line therapy for the treatment of hypertension in combination with diuretics or calcium antagonists, e.g. hydrochlorothiazide or nifedipine.

Posology and method of administration:
Initial therapy: In patients with uncomplicated essential hypertension not on diuretic therapy, the recommended initial dose is 7.5 mg once daily. Dosage should be adjusted according to blood pressure response. The maintenance dose is 7.5–15 mg moexipril daily administered in a single dose. Some patients may benefit from a further increase to 30 mg/day. Doses over 30 mg have been used, but do not appear to give a greater effect. If blood pressure is not controlled with Perdix alone, a low dose of a diuretic may be added. Hydrochlorothiazide 12.5 mg has been shown to provide an additive effect. With concomitant diuretic therapy, it may be possible to reduce the dose of Perdix.

Diuretic treated patients: In hypertensive patients who are currently being treated with a diuretic, symptomatic hypotension may occur occasionally following the initial dose of Perdix. The diuretic should be discontinued, if possible, for two to three days before beginning therapy with Perdix to reduce the likelihood of hypotension (see *Warnings*). The dosage of Perdix should be adjusted according to blood pressure response. If the patient's blood pressure is not controlled with Perdix alone, diuretic therapy may be resumed as described above. If the diuretic cannot be discontinued or the diuretic has recently been withdrawn, an initial dose of 3.75 mg (half 7.5 mg tablet) should be used under medical supervision for at least two hours and until blood pressure has stabilized for at least an additional hour (see *Warnings* and *Precautions*). Concomitant administration of Perdix with potassium supplements, potassium salt substitutes, or potassium-sparing diuretics may lead to increases of serum potassium (see *Precautions*).

Nifedipine treated patients: As add-on therapy, Perdix has been investigated in combination with nifedipine. If Perdix is used as add-on therapy to nifedipine, the starting dose of Perdix should be 3.75 mg (half 7.5 mg tablet).

Elderly patients: In elderly patients, an initial dosage of 3.75 mg (half 7.5 mg tablet) once daily is recommended followed by titration to the optimal response.

Children: Not recommended. Safety and efficacy in children has not been established.

Renal failure: In patients with creatinine clearance ≤ 40 ml/min, an initial dose of 3.75 mg of moexipril (half 7.5 mg tablet) is recommended.

Hepatic cirrhosis: In patients with hepatic cirrhosis, an initial dose of 3.75 mg of moexipril (half 7.5 mg tablet) is recommended.

Afro-Caribbean patients: Where Perdix is used as a single agent in hypertension, Afro-Caribbean patients may show a reduced therapeutic response.

Contra-indications: Perdix is contra-indicated in patients who are hypersensitive to this product and in patients with a history of angioedema related to previous treatment with an angiotensin converting enzyme inhibitor. Perdix is contra-indicated in pregnancy since fetotoxicity has been observed for ACE inhibitors in animals. Although there is no experience with Perdix, other ACE inhibitors in human pregnancy have been associated with oligohydramnios and neonatal hypotension and/or anuria. It is not known whether moexipril passes into human breastmilk, but since animal data indicate that moexipril and its metabolites are present in rat milk Perdix should not be given to nursing mothers.

Special warnings and precautions for use:
Warnings; Angioedema involving the extremities, face, lips, mucous membranes, tongue, glottis or larynx has been reported in patients treated with ACE inhibitors. If angioedema involves the tongue, glottis or larynx, airway obstruction may occur and be fatal. If laryngeal stridor or angioedema of the face, lips mucous membranes, tongue, glottis or extremities occur, treatment with Perdix should be discontinued and appropriate therapy instituted immediately. Where there is involvement of the tongue, glottis, or larynx, likely to cause airway obstruction, appropriate therapy, e.g. subcutaneous epinephrine solution 1:1000 (0.3 ml to 0.5 ml) should be promptly administered (see *Precautions*).

Hypotension: Perdix can cause symptomatic hypotension. Like other ACE inhibitors, Perdix has been only rarely associated with hypotension in hypertensive patients receiving monotherapy. Symptomatic hypotension is most likely to occur in patients who have been volume–and/or salt-depleted as a result of prolonged diurectic therapy, dietary salt restriction, dialysis, diarrhoea, or vomiting. Volume and/or salt depletion should be corrected before initiating therapy with Perdix. If hypotension occurs, the patient should be placed in a supine position and, if necessary, treated with intravenous infusion of physiological saline. Perdix treatment usually can be continued following restoration of blood pressure and volume.

Neutropenia/agranulocytosis: ACE inhibitors have been shown to cause agranulocytosis and bone marrow depression, rarely in uncomplicated patients, but more frequently in patients with renal impairment, especially if they also have a collagen-vascular disease such as systemic lupus erythematosus or scleroderma. Available data from clinical trials of Perdix are insufficient to show that Perdix does not cause agranulocytosis at similar rates. Monitoring of white blood cell counts should be considered in patients with collagen-vascular disease, especially if the disease is associated with impaired renal function.

Precautions:
Impaired renal function: As a consequence of inhibiting the renin-angiotensin-aldosterone system, changes in renal function may be anticipated in susceptible individuals. In hypertensive patients with renal artery stenosis in a solitary kidney or bilateral renal artery stenosis, increases in blood urea nitrogen and serum creatinine may occur. Experience with other angiotensin converting enzyme inhibitors suggests that these increases are usually reversible upon discontinuation of ACE inhibitor and/or diuretic therapy. In such patients, renal function should be monitored during the first few weeks of therapy. Some hypertensive patients with no apparent pre-existing renal vascular disease have developed increases in blood urea nitrogen and serum creatinine, usually minor and transient, especially when Perdix has been given concomitantly with a diuretic. This is more likely to occur in patients with pre-existing renal impairment. Dosage reduction of Perdix and/or discontinuation of the diurectic may be required. Evaluation of the hypertensive patient should always include assessment of renal function. Impaired renal function decreases total clearance of moexiprilat and approximately doubles AUC.

Hyperkalemia: In clinical trials, hyperkalemia (serum potassium greater than 10% above the upper limit of normal) has occurred in approximately 2.6% of hypertensive patients receiving Perdix. In most cases, these were isolated values which resolved despite continued therapy. In clinical trials, 0.1% of patients (two patients) were discontinued from therapy due to an elevated serum potassium. Risk factors for the development of hyperkalemia include renal insufficiency, diabetes mellitus and the concomitant use of potassium-sparing diuretics, potassium supplements and/or potassium-containing salt substitutes, which should be used cautiously, if at all, with Perdix (see *Precautions*).

Hepatic cirrhosis: Since Perdix is primarily metabolized by hepatic and gut wall esterases to its active moiety, moexiprilat, patients with impaired liver function could develop elevated plasma levels of unchanged Perdix. In a study in patients with alcoholic or biliary cirrhosis, the extent of hydrolysis was unaffected, although the rate was slowed. In these patients, the apparent total body clearance of moexiprilat was decreased and the plasma AUC approximately doubled.

Surgery/anaesthesia: In patients undergoing surgery or during anaesthesia with agents that produce hypotension, Perdix will block the angiotensin II formation that could otherwise occur secondary to compensatory renin release. Hypotension that occurs as a result of this mechanism can be corrected by volume expansion.

Interactions:
Diuretics: Excessive reductions in blood pressure, especially in patients in whom diuretic therapy was recently instituted, have been reported with ACE inhibitors. The possibility of hypotensive effects with Perdix can be minimized by discontinuing diuretic therapy or increasing salt intake for several days before initiation of treatment with Perdix. If this is not possible, the starting dose should be reduced (see also *Posology and method of administration* and *Special warnings and precautions for use*).

Nifedipine: The co-administration of nifedipine with Perdix gives rise to an enhanced antihypertensive effect.

Potassium supplements and potassium-sparing diuretics: Perdix can attenuate potassium loss caused by thiazide diuretics. Potassium-sparing diuretics (spironolactone, triamterene, amiloride, and others) or potassium supplements have been shown to increase the risk of hyperkalemia when used concomitantly with ACE inhibitors. Therefore, if concomitant use of such agents is indicated, they should be given with caution and the patient's serum potassium should be monitored frequently.

Oral anticoagulants: Interaction studies with warfarin failed to identify any clinically important effects on the serum concentrations of the anticoagulants or on their anticoagulant effects.

Lithium: Increased serum lithium levels and symptoms of lithium toxicity have been reported in patients receiving ACE inhibitors during therapy with lithium. These drugs should be co-administered with caution, and frequent monitoring of serum lithium levels is recommended. If a diuretic is also used, the risk of lithium toxicity may be increased.

Other agents: No clinically important pharmacokinetic interactions occurred when Perdix was administered concomitantly with hydrochlorothiazide, digoxin, cimetidine, or nifedipine in healthy volunteers. However, in hypertensive patients, the antihypertensive effect of Perdix was enhanced when given in combination with diuretics, or calcium antagonists.

Use during pregnancy and lactation: There is no experience in man. As it is known from other ACE inhibitors that they can adversely affect the fetus, especially during the second and third trimester, for safety reasons a change to a different antihypertensive drug should be made after pregnancy is confirmed in women who are receiving Perdix (see *Contra-indications*) or in women planning to get pregnant. It is not known whether Perdix is excreted in human milk. As animal data indicate that moexipril and its metabolites are present in rat milk, Perdix should not be administered to a nursing woman.

Effects on ability to drive and use machines: The intake of ACE inhibitors may, as any antihypertensive therapy, induce hypotension with subsequent impairment of reactivity. Alcohol intake may enhance this effect.

Undesirable effects: The most commonly reported undesirable effects (more than 1% of patients treated with Perdix in controlled trials) were cough (4.0%), headache (3.6%), dizziness (3.3%), fatigue (1.2%), flushing (1.2%), and rash (1.0%). Other adverse experiences possibly or probably related, or of uncertain relationship to therapy, reported in controlled or uncontrolled clinical trials occurring in less than 1% of Perdix patients and less frequent clinically significant events which have been attributed to ACE inhibitors include the following:
Cardiovascular: Symptomatic hypotension, postural hypotension, or syncope was seen in <1% of patients; these reactions led to discontinuation of therapy in controlled trials in 2 patients (0.1%) who had received Perdix monotherapy and in 1 patient (0.05%) who had received Perdix with hydrochlorothiazide. Other reports included chest pain, angina/myocardial infarction, palpitations, rhythm disturbances, cerebrovascular accident.

Renal: Of hypertensive patients with no apparent pre-existing renal disease, 0.8% of patients receiving Perdix alone and 1.5% of patients receiving Perdix with hydrochlorothiazide have experienced increases in serum creatinine to at least 140% of their baseline values.

Gastrointestinal: Abdominal pain, dyspepsia, constipation, nausea, vomiting, diarrhoea, appetite/weight change, dry mouth, pancreatitis, hepatitis.

Respiratory: Upper respiratory infection, pharyngitis, sinusitis/rhinitis, bronchospasm, dyspnea.

Urogenital: Renal insufficiency.

Dermatologic: Apparent hypersensitivity reactions manifested by urticaria, pruritus, photosensitivity.

Neurological and psychiatric: Drowsiness, sleep disturbances, nervousness, mood changes, anxiety.

Other: Angioedema, taste disturbances, tinnitus, sweating, flu syndrome, malaise, arthralgia, myalgia.

Clinical laboratory test findings:
Creatinine and blood urea nitrogen: As with other ACE inhibitors, minor increases in blood urea nitrogen or serum creatinine, reversible upon discontinuation of therapy, were observed in approximately 1% of patients with essential hypertension who were treated with PERDIX. Increases are more likely to occur in patients receiving concomitant diuretics or in patients with compromised renal function.

Potassium: Since moexipril decreases aldosterone secretion, elevation of serum potassium can occur. Potassium supplements and potassium-sparing diuretics should be given with caution and the patient's serum potassium should be monitored frequently.

Other: Clinically important changes in standard laboratory tests were rarely associated with Perdix administration. Elevations of liver enzymes and uric acid have been reported. In trials, less than 1% of moexipril-treated patients discontinued Perdix treatment because of laboratory abnormalities.

Overdose: Symptoms and treatment. To date, no case of overdosage has been reported. Signs and symptoms expected in cases of overdosage would be related to hypotension and should be relieved by intravenous infusion of isotonic saline solution.

Pharmacological properties
Pharmacodynamic properties: In animals as well as in humans, interactions between the renin-angiotesin-aldosterone system and the kallikrein-kinin system provide an important biochemical basis for blood pressure homeostasis. In hypertension the normal feedback mechanism formed by the renin-angiotensin system (RAS) may be dysfunctional, resulting in a self-perpetuating hypertensive condition. Angiotensin converting enzyme (ACE) inhibitors were developed to interrupt this system and thereby to lower blood pressure. Perdix potently inhibits ACE and by this the formation of angiotensin II, the active agent of the RAS, thus blocking its vasoconstrictor and sodium-retaining effects with a consequent reduction in blood pressure. Since ACE is identical is kininase II, an enzyme that degrades the potent vasodilator bradykinin, inhibition of ACE leads to an additional, nonrenin-mediated reduction in systemic blood pressure. The antihypertensive effects of ACE inhibitors are accompanied by a reduction in peripheral vascular resistance.

Pharmacokinetic properties: The prodrug moexipril is rapidly absorbed and deesterified to the active metabolite moexiprilat. The pharmacokinetic parameters for moexipril and moexiprilat were similar after both, single and multiple does of meoxipril and appear to be dose-proportional. Moexipril and moexiprilat are moderately bound to plasma proteins, predominately albumin. Therefore, concurrently administered drugs are unlikely to interfere with the binding of moexipril and moexiprilat in any clinically significant way. Metabolites of moexipril present in the diketopiperazine derivatives of moexipril and moexiprilat. Both, moexipril and moexiprilat are eliminated in the urine, and moexiprilat is eliminated in the faeces. The pharmacokinetic profile of moexipril and moexiprilat should allow the same dosage recommendation in patients with mild to moderate renal dysfunction (Cl_{cr}>40 ml/min) as in patients with normal renal function. With severe renal dysfunction, dosage reduction is recommended. In patients with liver cirrhosis, the pharmacokinetics of moexipril and moexiprilat were significantly altered as compared with normal subjects. In such patients, therapy with Perdix should be started with 3.75 mg (half 7.5 mg tablet). There were no apparent pharmacokinetic drug interactions with HCTZ, digoxin, cimetidine, warfarin or nifedipine.

Preclinical safety data:
Acute toxicity: Findings of the acute toxicity studies in animals do not raise questions as to the safety of moexipril HCL as well as the main metabolite moexiprilat under the conditions of proposed clinical usage.

Subacute/chronic toxicity: Subacute and chronic toxicity studies in rats and dogs with repeated oral administration of moexipril HCL up to 12 months, revealed mainly heart and kidney as target organs. The effects are completely comparable with those of other ACE inhibitors and can be interpreted as results of highly exaggerated pharmacological activity. First unspecific drug-related side-effects after long-term administration were seen at 75 mg/kg, i.e. a dose which corresponds 150 times the maximum recommended total daily dose in humans when compared on the basis of body weight.

Reproduction studies: Studies in rats and rabbits including all segments of reproduction revealed no direct effects of moexipril HCL on fertility, reproduction and abnormalities in F_1–or F_2-pups. Regarding precautions in women of child bearing potential and use during pregnancy and lactation see 4.3 and 4.6.

Mutagenicity: As conclusion of different 'in vitro' and on 'in vivo' mutagencity studies, the mutagenic potential of moexipril HCL for human beings should be extremely low.

Carcinogenicity: Neither the long term toxicity studies in rats and dogs nor special carcinogenicity studies in mice and rats over 78 and 104 weeks respectively, indicated neoplastigenic properties of moexipril HCL. Therefore, it can be concluded that the carcinogenic risk for human beings will be extremely low.

Pharmaceutical particulars
List of excipients: Lactose, crospovidone, light magnesium oxide, gelatine, magnesium stearate, methyl hydroxypropylcellulose, hydroxypropylcellulose, titanium dioxide, polyethyleneglycol 6000, ferric oxide, purified water (not present in the finished product).

Incompatibilities: No incompatibilities have so far been demonstrated.

Shelf life: 3 years

Special precautions for storage: Store in a dry place below 25°C.

Nature and contents of container: Calendar packs containing 28 tablets, 14 per Al/Al blister pack.

Instruction for use/handling: No special instruction necessary.

Marketing authorisation numbers 4438/0033 and 0034

Date of approval/revision of SPC December 1996

Legal category POM

TYLEX* CAPSULES
TYLEX* EFFERVESCENT

Qualitative and quantitative composition Each capsule and effervescent tablet contains 500 mg of paracetamol PhEur and 30 mg of codeine phosphate PhEur.

Pharmaceutical form

Capsules.

Effervescent tablets.

Clinical particulars

Therapeutic indications: For the relief of severe pain.

Posology and method of administration:

Adults: The capsules and effervescent tablets are given orally. The effervescent tablets should be dissolved in at least half a tumbleful of water before taking. The usual dose is one or two capsules/effervescent tablets every four hours as required. *The total daily dose should not exceed 240 mg of codeine phosphate* (i.e. not more than four doses (8 capsules/tablets) per 24 hours should be taken).

Elderly: A reduced dose may be required.

Children: Use in children under 12 years of age is not recommended.

Dosage should be adjusted according to the severity of the pain and the response of the patient. However, it should be kept in mind that tolerance to codeine can develop with continued use and that the incidence of untoward effects is dose related. Doses of codeine higher than 60 mg fail to give commensurate relief of pain but merely prolong analgesia and are associated with an appreciably increased incidence of undesirable side effects.

Contra-indications: Tylex should not to be administered to patients who have previously exhibited hypersensitivity to either paracetamol or codeine, or to any of its excipients.

Tylex is not recommended for children under the age of 12 years.

Special warnings and special precautions for use: Because safety and effectiveness in the administration of paracetamol with codeine in children under 12 years of age have not been established, such use is not recommended.

Tylex Capsules contain sodium metabisulphite, a sulphite that may cause allergic reactions including anaphylactic symptoms and life threatening or less severe asthmatic episodes in certain susceptible people. The overall prevalence of sulphite sensitivity in the general population is unknown and probably low. Sulphite sensitivity is seen more frequently in asthmatic than non-asthmatic people.

Tylex Effervescent contains 312.9 mg sodium/tablet and this should be taken into account when prescribing for patients for whom sodium restriction is indicated. Tylex Effervescent also contains 25 mg aspartame/tablet and therefore care should be taken in phenylketonuria.

Tylex should be used with caution in patients with head injuries, increased intracranial pressure, acute abdominal conditions, the elderly and debilitated, and those with severe impairment of hepatic or renal function, hypothyroidism, Addison's disease and prostatic hypertrophy or urethral stricture.

Chronic heavy alcohol abusers may be at increased risk of liver toxicity from excessive paracetamol use, although reports of this event are rare. Reports almost invariably involve cases of severe chronic alcoholics and the dosages of paracetamol most often exceed recommended doses and often involve substantial overdose. Professionals should alert their patients who regularly consume large amounts of alcohol not to exceed recommended doses of paracetamol.

At high doses codeine has most of the disadvantages of morphine, including respiratory depression. Codeine can produce drug dependence of the morphine type, and therefore has the potential for being abused. Codeine may impair the mental/or physical abilities required for the performance of potentially hazardous tasks.

Patients should be advised that immediate medical advice should be sought in the event of an overdose, because of the risk of delayed, serious liver damage. They should be advised not to exceed the recommended dose, not to take other paracetamol-containing products concurrently, to consult their doctor if symptoms persist and to keep the product out of the reach of children.

Interaction with other medicaments and other forms of interaction: Patients receiving other central nervous system depressants (including other opioid analgesics, tranquillisers, sedative hypnotics and alcohol) concomitantly with Tylex may exhibit an additive depressant effect. When such therapy is contemplated, the dose of one or both agents should be reduced.

Concurrent use of MAO inhibitors or tricyclic antidepressants with codeine may increase the effect of either the antidepressant or codeine. Concurrent use of anticholinergics and codeine may produce paralytic ileus.

The speed of absorption of paracetamol may be increased by metoclopramide or domperidone and absorption reduced by cholestyramine.

The anti-coagulant effect of warfarin and other coumarins may be enhanced by prolonged regular daily use of paracetamol with increased risk of bleeding; occasional doses have no significant effect.

Pregnancy and lactation: Tylex is not recommended during pregnancy or lactation since safety in pregnant women or nursing mothers has not been established.

Effects on the ability to drive and use machines: Patients should be advised not to drive or operate machinery if affected by dizziness or sedation.

Undesirable effects: The most frequently observed reactions include light headedness, dizziness, sedation, shortness of breath, nausea and vomiting. These effects seem more prominent in ambulatory than non-ambulatory patients and some of these adverse reactions may be alleviated if the patient lies down. Other adverse reactions include allergic reactions, (including skin rash), euphoria, dysphoria, constipation, abdominal pain and pruritus.

In clinical use of paracetamol-containing products, there have been a few reports of blood dyscrasias including thrombocytopenia and agranulocytosis but these were not necessarily causally related to paracetamol.

Overdose: Symptoms of paracetamol overdosage in the first 24 hours are pallor, nausea, vomiting, anorexia and abdominal pain. Liver damage may become apparent 12 to 48 hours after ingestion. Abnormalities of glucose metabolism and metabolic acidosis may occur. In severe poisoning, hepatic failure may progress to encephalopathy, coma and death. Acute renal failure with acute tubular necrosis may develop even in the absence of severe liver damage. Cardiac arrhythmias and pancreatitis have been reported. Liver damage is possible in adults who have taken 10 g or more of paracetamol. It is considered that excess quantities of a toxic metabolite (usually adequately detoxified by glutathione when normal doses of paracetamol are ingested), become irreversibly bound to liver tissue.

Immediate treatment is essential in the management of paracetamol overdose. Despite a lack of significant early symptoms, patients should be referred to hospital urgently for immediate medical attention and any patient who has ingested around 7.5 g or more of paracetamol in the preceding 4 hours should undergo gastric lavage. Administration of oral methionine or intravenous N-acetylcysteine which may have a beneficial effect up to at least 48 hours after the overdose, may be required. General supportive measures must be available.

Serious overdose with codeine is characterised by respiratory depression, extreme somnolence progressing to stupor or coma, skeletal muscle flaccidity, cold and clammy skin and sometimes bradycardia and hypotension. In severe overdose with codeine, apnoea, circulatory collapse, cardiac arrest and death may occur. Primary attention should be given to the re-establishment of adequate respiratory exchange through the provision of a patient airway and the institution of controlled ventilation. Oxygen, intravenous fluids, vasopressors and other supportive measures should be employed as indicated. Opioid antagonists may be employed. Gastric lavage should be considered.

Pharmacological properties

Pharmacodynamic properties: Paracetamol has analgesic and antipyretic actions similar to those of aspirin with weak anti-inflammatory effects. Paracetamol is only a weak inhibitor of prostaglandin biosynthesis, although there is some evidence to suggest that it may be more effective against enzymes in the CNS than those in the periphery. This fact may partly account for its well documented ability to reduce fever and to induce analgesia, effects that involve actions on neural tissues. Single or repeated therapeutic doses of paracetamol have no effect on the cardiovascular and respiratory systems. Acid-based changes do not occur and gastric irritation, erosion or bleeding is not produced as may occur after salicylates. There is only a weak effect upon platelets and no effect on bleeding time or the excretion of uric acid.

Codeine is an analgesic with uses similar to those of morphine but has only mild sedative effects. The major effect is on the CNS and the bowel. The effects are remarkably diverse and include analgesia, drowsiness, changes in mood, respiratory depression, decreased gastrointestinal motility, nausea, vomiting and alterations of the endocrine and autonomic nervous systems. The relief of pain is relatively selective, in that other sensory modalities, (touch, vibration, vision, hearing etc.) are not obtunded.

Pharmacokinetic properties: Paracetamol is readily absorbed from the gastro-intestinal tract with peak plasma concentration occurring about 30 minutes to 2 hours after ingestion. It is metabolised in the liver and excreted in the urine mainly as the glucuronide and sulphate conjugates. Less than 5% is excreted as unchanged paracetamol. The elimination half-life varies from about 1 to 4 hours. Plasma-protein binding is negligible at usual therapeutic concentrations but increases with increasing concentrations.

A minor hydroylated metabolite which is usually produced in very small amounts by mixed-function oxidases in the liver and which is usually detoxified by conjugation with liver glutathione may accumulate following paracetamol overdosage and cause liver damage.

Codeine and its salts are absorbed from the gastro-intestinal tract. Ingestion of codeine phosphate produces peak plasma codeine concentrations in about one hour. Codeine is metabolised by O- & N-demethylation in the liver to morphine and norcodeine. Codeine and its metabolites are excreted almost entirely by the kidney, mainly as conjugates with glucuronic acid.

The plasma half-life has been reported to be between 3 and 4 hours after administration by mouth or intravascular injection.

Preclinical safety data: None stated.

Pharmaceutical particulars

List of excipients:

Tylex Capsules: Pregelatinized Starch, Calcium Stearate, Aerosol OT-B (dioctyl sodium sulfosuccinate, sodium benzoate (E211)), Sodium metabisulphite, gelatin capsule, E171, E127, E132, printing ink: Shellac, soya lecithin, 2-ethyoxyethanol, dimethylpolysiloxane, E172.

Tylex Effervescent: Citric Acid Anhydrous, Sodium Bicarbonate, Sodium Carbonate Anhydrous, Aspartame, Blackcurrant Flavour No. 78004-31, Polyethylene Glycol 6000, Magnesium Stearate, Ethanol 96% (not detected in the finished product)

Incompatibilities: None pertinent.

Shelf life:

Tylex Capsules: 60 months.

Tylex Effervescent: 36 months.

Special precautions for storage: Store at or below 25°C. Protect from light. Store Tylex Effervescent in a dry place.

Nature and contents of container:

Tylex Capsules: PVC/aluminium foil blister strips. Marketed pack sizes: 1×8, 3×8, 5×20 capsules.

Tylex Effervescent: Paper/aluminium laminate blister strips. Marketed pack sizes: 4×2 and 15×6 tablets.

Instructions for use/handling: None.

Marketing authorisation numbers

Tylex Capsules PL 04438/0046

Tylex Effervescent PL 04438/0045

Date of (partial) revision of text November 1997.

Legal category POM.

Date of first authorisation March 1996. (*Code 825*)

VIRIDAL 5
VIRIDAL 10
VIRIDAL 20

Qualitative and quantitative composition

Viridal 5: 1 vial of dry substance (47.7 mg) contains: Alprostadil 5 mcg (used as 1:1 clathrate complex with alfadex)

Viridal 10: 1 vial of dry substance (47.8 mg) contains: Alprostadil 10 mcg (used as 1:1 clathrate complex with alfadex)

Viridal 20: 1 vial of dry substance (48.2 mg) contains: Alprostadil 20 mcg (used as 1:1 clathrate complex with alfadex)

Pharmaceutical form Vials containing lyophilised powder for reconstitution with the diluent provided.

Administration devices: 0.9% saline (1 ml) prefilled syringe (PL 4438/0043), Plunger, Injection needle 21 G×2 (0.8×50) for drug preparation (colour code: green), Injection needle 30 G×½ (0.3×13) for injection (colour code: colourless), 2 antiseptic swabs.

Route of administration: For injection into the penile cavernous body.

Clinical particulars

Indications: As an adjunct to the diagnostic evaluation of erectile dysfunction in adult males.

Treatment of erectile dysfunction in adult males.

Posology and method of administration:

Application: The drug solution should be prepared shortly before the injection.

Prior to injection, the dry substance should be dissolved in 1 ml of 0.9% saline. To do this, flip off the lid from the vial. Clean the rubber stopper of the vial using one of the sterile swabs. After fixing needle 21 G×2 (0.8×50) (colour code: green) onto the prefilled syringe the saline is injected into the vial. Shake the vial gently until the powder is completely dissolved. Initially after reconstitution the solution may appear slightly opaque due to the presence of bubbles. This is of no relevance and disappears within a short time to give a clear solution. Once the solution has cleared the whole of the freshly prepared solution is drawn up into the syringe. After pushing the air out of the syringe and getting the correct amount of drug solution, needle 30 G×½ (0.3×13) (colour code: colourless) is fixed onto the syringe and the air has to be pushed out of it prior to intracavernous injection.

Unused solution must be discarded immediately.

Cavernous body self-injection is done with the thin needle (30 G×½ (0.3×13), colour code: colourless) into either the right or the left cavernous body of the penile shaft. Once the needle is in the cavernous body, the injection should be done within 5 to 10 seconds and is very easy if the needle is in the correct position.

Re-evaluation should take place at regular intervals by the physician and he will decide whether correction of the dosage is necessary and also about the duration and frequency of the treatment.

Dosage for injection in the clinic: Injections for diagnostic evaluation and dose titration must be performed by the attending physician. He will determine an individual dose suitable to produce an erectile response for diagnostic purposes.

The recommended starting dose is 2.5 mcg Viridal in patients with primary psychogenic or neurogenic origin of erectile dysfunction. In all other patients 5 mcg Viridal should be used as a starting dose. Dose adjustments may be performed in increments of about 2.5 mcg to 5 mcg Viridal. Most of the patients require between 10 and 20 mcg per injection. Some patients may need to be titrated to higher doses. Doses exceeding 20 mcg should be prescribed with particular care in patients with cardiovascular risk factors. The dose per injection should never exceed 40 mcg.

Dosage for self-injection therapy at home: The patient should only use his optimum individual dosage which has been pre-determined by his physician using the above mentioned procedure. This dose should allow the patient to have an erection at home which should not last longer than one hour. If he experiences prolonged erections beyond 2 hours but less than 4 hours, the patient is recommended to contact his physician to re-establish the dose of the drug. Maximum injection frequency recommended is 2 or 3 times a week with an interval of at least 24 hours between the injections.

Follow-up: After the first injections and at regular intervals thereafter, the physician should re-evaluate the patient. Any local adverse reaction, e.g. haematoma, fibrosis or nodules should be noted and controlled. Following discussion with the patient, an adjustment of dosage may be necessary.

Contra-indications: Hypersensitivity to alprostadil and/or alfadex (ingredients of Viridal). Patients with diseases causing prolonged erections e.g. sickle-cell disease, leukaemia and multiple myeloma should not use Viridal.

Special precautions: Patients, who experience a prolonged erection lasting longer than four hours should contact their physician immediately. Therefore it is recommended that the patient has an emergency telephone number of his attending physician or of a clinic experienced in therapy of erectile dysfunction. Prolonged erection may damage penile erectile tissue and lead to irreversible erectile dysfunction.

Patients with pre-existing scarring, e.g. fibrosis or nodules of the cavernous body or pre-existing penile deviation or Peyronie's disease should be treated with particular care, e.g. more frequent re-evaluation of the patient's condition. This is due to the increased risk of painful erections.

Patients who have to be treated with alpha-adrenergic drugs due to prolonged erections (see: *Overdose*) may in the case of concomitant therapy with monoamino-oxidase-inhibitors, develop a hypertensive crisis.

Other intracavernous drugs e.g. smooth muscle relaxing agents or alpha-adrenergic blocking agents may lead to prolonged erection and must not be used concomitantly.

Patients with blood clotting disorders or patients on therapy influencing blood clotting parameters should be treated with special care, e.g. monitoring of the clotting parameters and advice to the patient to exercise sufficient manual pressure on the injection site. This is because of the increased risk of bleeding.

Sexual stimulation and intercourse can lead to cardiac and/or pulmonary events in patients with coronary heart disease, congestive heart failure or pulmonary disease. Viridal should be used with care in these patient groups and patients should be examined and cleared for stress resistance by a cardiologist before treatment.

To prevent abuse, self-injection therapy with Viridal should not be used by patients with drug addiction and/or disturbances of psychological or intellectual development.

Use of intracavernous alprostadil offers no protection from the transmission of sexually transmitted diseases. Individuals who use alprostadil should be counselled about the protective measures that are necessary to guard against the spread of sexually transmitted diseases, including the human immunodeficiency virus (HIV). In some patients, injection of Viridal can induce a small amount of bleeding at the injection site. In patients infected with blood borne diseases, this could increase the transmission of such diseases to the partner. For this reason we recommend that a condom is used for intercourse after injecting Viridal.

In any condition that precludes safe self injection like poor manual dexterity, poor visual acuity or morbid obesity, the partner should be trained in the injection technique and should perform the injection.

Up to now, there is no clinical experience in patients under 18 and over 75 years of age.

Viridal does not interfere with ejaculation and fertility.

Interactions: Concomitant use of smooth muscle relaxing drugs like papaverine or other drugs inducing erection like alpha-adrenergic blocking agents may lead to prolonged erection and should not be used in parallel with Viridal.

Risks exist when using alpha-adrenergic drugs to terminate prolonged erections in patients with cardiovascular disorders or receiving MAO inhibitors.

The effects of blood pressure lowering and vasodilating drugs may be increased.

Use during pregnancy and lactation: Not applicable.

[Alprostadil did not cause any adverse effects on fertility or general reproductive performance in male and female rats treated with 40–200 mcg/kg/day. The high dose of 200 mcg/kg/day is about 300 times the maximum human recommended dose on a body weight basis (MHRD <1 mcg/kg). Alprostadil was not fetotoxic or teratogenic at doses up to 5000 mcg/kg/day (7500 times the MHRD) in rats, 200 mcg/kg/day (300 times the MHRD) in rabbits and doses up to 20 mcg/kg/day (30 times the MHRD) in guinea pigs or monkeys].

Effects on ability to drive and use machines: Viridal may rarely induce hypotension with subsequent impairment of reactivity.

Undesirable effects: The most frequent adverse effect of Viridal is a burning pain during and after injection due to the injection technique and the feeling of tension occurring with penile erection. Haematomas are frequently seen at the site of injection. There may also be incorrect injections, e.g. subcutaneous or urethral. Further possible local reactions are haemosiderin deposits, reddening and swelling or bleeding of the injection site, ecchymosis, swelling of foreskin or glans, cavernositis or penile infection.

Prolonged erections lasting longer than four hours occur occasionally, but more often during diagnostic and titration-periods than during the period of self injection once the optimum dose has been determined.

Erections lasting longer than six hours are rare after intracavernous injection of Viridal.

Prolonged erection may damage penile erectile structures and lead to irreversible erectile dysfunction.

Adverse effects of long-term treatment are fibrotic nodules, spots or plaques with/without penile angulation associated with the injection site which occur occasionally. Fibrotic tissue alterations of the cavernous body with/without loss of function and with/without penile angulation occur in very rare cases during treatment of up to three years.

Penile deviations can occur.

Systemic circulation effects e.g. hypotension with/without dizziness, cardiac arrhythmias, chest pains, headaches and circulatory collapse after intracavernous injection of Viridal have been reported very rarely.

Overdose

Symptoms: Full rigid erections lasting more than four hours. If the patient experiences a prolonged erection, he is advised to contact his attending physician or a urologic clinic nearby immediately.

Treatment strategy: Treatment of prolonged erection should be done by a physician experienced in the field of erectile dysfunction: If prolonged erection occurs, the following is recommended:

- If the erection has lasted less than six hours: observation of the erection because spontaneous flaccidity frequently occurs.
- If the erection has lasted longer than six hours: cavernous body injection of alpha-adrenergic substances [e.g. phenylephrine or epinephrine (adrenaline)]. Risks exist when using drugs in patients with cardiovascular disorders or receiving MAO inhibitors. All patients should be monitored for cardiovascular effects when these drugs are used to terminate prolonged erections or aspiration of blood from the cavernous body.

Accidental systemic injection of high doses: Single dose rising tolerance studies in healthy volunteers indicated that single intravenous doses of alprostadil from 1 to 120 mcg were well tolerated. Starting with a 40 mcg bolus intravenous dose, the frequency of drug-related adverse events increased in a dose-dependent manner, characterised mainly by facial flushing.

Pharmacological properties

Pharmacodynamic properties: Alprostadil [Prostaglandin E1 (PGE_1)], the active ingredient of Viridal, is an endogenous compound derived from the essential fatty acid dihomo-gamma-linolenic acid. Alprostadil is a potent smooth muscle relaxant that produces vasodilation and occurs in high concentrations in the human seminal fluid. Precontracted isolated preparations of the human corpus cavernosum, corpus spongiosum and cavernous artery were relaxed by alprostadil, while other prostanoids were less effective. Alprostadil has been shown to bind to specific receptors in the cavernous tissue of human and non-human primates.

The binding of alprostadil to its receptors is accompanied by an increase in intracellular cAMP levels. Human cavernosal smooth muscle cells respond to alprostadil by releasing intracellular calcium. Since relaxation of smooth muscle is associated with a reduction of the cytoplasmic free calcium concentration, this effect may contribute to the relaxing activity of this prostanoid.

Intracavernous injection of alprostadil in healthy monkeys resulted in penile elongation and tumescence without rigidity. The cavernous arterial blood flow was increased for a mean duration of 20 min. In contrast, intracavernous application of alprostadil to rabbits and dogs caused no erectile response.

Systemic intravascular administration of alprostadil leads to a vasodilation and reduction of systemic peripheral vascular resistance. A decrease in blood pressure can be observed after administration of high doses. Alprostadil has also been shown in animal and in vitro tests to reduce platelet reactivity and neutrophil activation. Additional alprostadil activity has been reported: increase in fibrinolytic activity of fibroblasts, improvement of erythrocyte deformability and inhibition of erythrocyte aggregation; inhibition of the proliferative and mitotic activity of non-striated myocytes; inhibition of cholesterol synthesis and LDL-receptor activity; and an increase in the supply of oxygen and glucose to ischaemic tissue along with improved tissue utilization of these substrates.

Pharmacokinetic properties: Pharmacokinetics after intracavernous injection; Viridal contains the active ingredient alprostadil (PGE_1) in the form of an inclusion compound (clathrate) with alfadex (α-cyclodextrin). During the preparation of the solution for injection the clathrate complex dissociates into the components of alprostadil and alfadex, therefore the pharmacokinetic behaviour of both compounds is independent of the clathrate structure of the dry substance.

Preliminary information of the pharmacokinetics of alprostadil alfadex following intracavernous injection is available. There are no significant differences between the systemic plasma concentration of alprostadil and its metabolites PGE_0 and 15-keto-PGE_0 after intracavernous injection in patients and after intravenous injection in healthy volunteers. Based on the extremely short half-life of alprostadil and the resulting experimental difficulties the pharmacokinetic parameters of systemic alprostadil were measured under steady-state conditions.

Pharmacokinetics after intravenous infusion; Alprostadil is an endogenous substance with an extremely short half-life. After i.v. infusion of 60 mcg alprostadil over two hours (0.5 mcg/min) in healthy volunteers, maximum plasma levels of about 5 pg/ml above basal values were measured (basal value 1–2 pg/ml). After cessation of the infusion, the alprostadil concentration dropped to basal values, with half-lives of about 0.2 min (α-phase, estimate) and about 8 min (β-phase). Due to the short half-life, steady state concentrations were reached shortly after the onset of the i.v. infusion.

Alprostadil undergoes biotransformation predominantly in the lungs. During the first pass through the lungs 80–90% of alprostadil is metabolized. Enzymatic oxidation of the C15-hydroxy-group followed by reduction of the C13, 14-double-bond produces the main metabolites 15-keto-PGE_1, PGE_0 and 15-keto-PGE_0. The compound 15-keto-PGE_1 has up to now only been detected in vitro in homogenated lung preparations, whereas PGE_0 and 15-keto-PGE_0 were found in plasma. After degradation by β-oxidation and ω-oxidation, the main metabolites are eliminated via urine (88%) and the faeces (12%).

As a result of biotransformation, PGE_0 (13, 14-dihydro-PGE_1) and 15-keto-PGE_0 were detected in plasma. After i.v. infusion of 60 mcg alprostadil over two hours, plasma concentrations of PGE_0 reached values of about 12 pg/ml above basal value (1–2 pg/ml) and those of 15-keto-PGE_0 were 150 pg/ml above basal value of 4–6 pg/ml. Half-lives were about 2 min (α-phase) and 30 min (β-phase) for PGE_0 and 1–2 min and 20 min respectively for 15-keto-PGE_0.

93% of the alprostadil in plasma is bound to macromolecular compartments. The alfadex was found to have a half-life of about seven minutes in rats. It is excreted renally as unchanged alfadex. Studies on the concentration of alprostadil and its metabolites in various organs and tissues of the rat revealed no evidence of accumulation.

Preclinical safety data: Studies on local tolerance following single and repeated intracavernous injections of alprostadil or alprostadil alfadex in rabbits and/or monkeys, in monkeys up to 6 months with daily injection, revealed in general good local tolerance. Possible adverse effects like haematomas and inflammations are more likely related to the injection procedure.

Within the 6 months study in male monkeys, there were no adverse effects of alprostadil alfadex on male reproductive organs. Different mutagenicity studies with alprostadil alfadex revealed no risk of mutagenicity.

Chronic toxicity studies in dogs (6 months, daily intravenous infusion) and monkeys (6 months, daily intracavernous injection) indicate that systemic side effects are unlikely to occur following intracavernous injection of 5 to 40 mcg alprostadil (used as clathrate complex with alfadex).

Pharmaceutical particulars

List of excipients: Lactose, alfadex

Incompatibilities: No incompatibilities have so far been demonstrated.

Shelf life: Shelf life for the product as packaged for sale: Viridal 5 mcg – 24 months, Viridal 10 mcg – 24 months, Viridal 20 mcg – 24 months

Shelf life after reconstitution: For immediate use only.

Special precautions for storage: Store below 25°C.

Nature and contents of container: Cartons containing one colourless glass vial (glass type I), with a rubber stopper, one prefilled (glass type I) glass syringe, two injection needles, 21 G×2 (0.8×50) for drug preparation and 30 G×½ (0.3×13) for injection, two alcohol swabs.

Instructions for use/handling: Fix the needle [21 G×2 (0.8×50) (colour code: green)] onto the prefilled syringe. Clean the rubber stopper of the vial using one of the sterile swabs. Inject the saline out of the prefilled syringe into the vial. Shake the vial to dissolve the dry substance. Initially after reconstitution the solution may appear slightly opaque due to the presence of bubbles. This is of no relevance and disappears within a short time to give a clear solution. Once the solution has cleared draw back into the syringe the whole freshly prepared solution. After pushing the air out of the syringe and getting the correct amount of drug solution, the needle [30 G×½ (0.3×13) (colour code: colourless)] is fixed onto the syringe prior to intracavernous injection.

After preparation of the solution, the injection must be performed using aseptic procedures, using the 30-gauge needle (colour code: colourless) into either the left or right cavernous body of the penile shaft. Care should be taken not to inject into penile vessels or nerves on the upper side of the penis and into the urethra on the under side. The injection should be completed within 5 to 10 seconds and manual pressure should be applied to the injection site for 2 to 3 minutes.

Unused solution must be discarded immediately.

Advice: The vial contains a white dry powder, which forms a compact layer of approximately 3 mm thickness. This layer may show cracks, and sometimes may crumble slightly. If the vial is damaged, then the normally dry content becomes moist and sticky and extensive loss of volume results. If this has happened, do not use the product.

Marketing authorisation holder Schwarz Pharma Ltd, Schwarz House, East Street, Chesham, Bucks HP5 1DG, England.

Marketing authorisation numbers

Viridal 5	PL 4438/0040	PA 271/9/1
Viridal 10	PL 4438/0041	PA 271/9/2
Viridal 20	PL 4438/0042	PA 271/9/3

Date of first authorisation May 1996

Date of (partial) revision of the text November 1997 (634)

Legal category UK-POM

VIRIDAL 10 DUO
VIRIDAL 20 DUO

Qualitative and quantitative composition

Viridal 10 Duo: 1 double-chamber glass cartridge containing dry substance (47.8 mg) composed of alprostadil 10 mcg (used as 1:1 clathrate complex with alfadex) and diluent (1 ml).

Viridal 20 Duo: 1 double-chamber glass cartridge containing dry substance (48.2 mcg) composed of alprostadil 20 mcg (used as 1:1 clathrate complex with alfadex) and diluent (1 ml).

Diluent: 1 ml sterile sodium chloride solution 0.9% (w/v) PhEur.

Pharmaceutical form/route of administration: Double chamber glass cartridge containing lyophilised powder and diluent for reconstitution.

Administration devices: 1 reusable applicator (starter kit), 1 double-chamber cartridge with dry substance and 1 ml 0.9% sterile sodium chloride solution, 1 injection needle 29 G×½ (0.33 mm×12.7 mm), 2 antiseptic swabs.

Route of administration: For injection into the penile cavernous body.

Clinical particulars

Indications: As an adjunct to the diagnostic evaluation of erectile dysfunction in adult males.

Treatment of erectile dysfunction in adult males.

Posology and method of administration: The drug solution should be prepared shortly before the injection.

Prior to injection the needle should be screwed onto the tip of the applicator. After disinfecting the tip of the cartridge with one of the alcohol swabs, the cartridge should be inserted into the applicator. By screwing the thread part clockwise, the cartridge is fixed in the applicator. Then, the dry substance which is inside the front chamber of the cartridge is reconstituted with 1 ml sterile sodium chloride solution 0.9% in the bottom chamber. While holding the device in a vertical position with the needle upwards, the thread part should be screwed slowly until it will not go any further. The solvent will by-pass the upper stopper into the front chamber and dissolve the dry substance within a few seconds. As soon as the dry substance is reconstituted, the larger external and the smaller inner protective cap have to be removed from the needle. The air should then be expelled out of the cartridge and the prescribed dose adjusted precisely.

Unused solution must be discarded immediately.

Viridal Duo is injected into either the right or the left cavernous body of the penile shaft. Once the needle is in the cavernous body, the injection should be done within 5 to 10 seconds and is very easy without much resistance if the needle is in the correct position.

Re-evaluation should take place at regular intervals by the physician and he will decide whether correction of the dosage is necessary and the duration and frequency of the treatment.

Dosage for injection in the clinic: Injections for diagnostic evaluation and dose titration must be performed by the attending physician. He will determine an individual dose suitable to produce an erectile response for diagnostic purposes.

The recommended starting dose is 2.5 mcg alprostadil in patients with primary psychogenic or neurogenic origin of erectile dysfunction. In all other patients 5 mcg alprostadil should be used as a starting dose. Dose adjustments may be performed in increments of about 2.5 mcg to 5 mcg. Most patients require between 10 mcg and 20 mcg per injection. Some patients may need to be titrated to higher doses. Doses exceeding 20 mcg should be prescribed with particular care in patients with cardiovascular risk factors.

The dose per injection should never exceed 40 mcg.

Dosage for self-injection therapy at home: The patient should only use his optimum individual dosage which has been pre-determined by his physician using the above mentioned procedure. This dose should allow him to have an erection at home which should not last longer than one hour. If he experiences prolonged erections beyond 2 hours but less than 4 hours, the patient is recommended to contact his physician to re-establish the dose of the drug. Maximum injection frequency recommended is 2 or 3 times a week with an interval of at least 24 hours between the injections.

Follow-up: After the first injections and at regular intervals thereafter, the physician should re-evaluate the patient. Any local adverse reaction, e.g. haematoma, fibrosis or nodules should be noted and controlled. Following discussion with the patient, an adjustment of dosage may be necessary.

Contra-indications: Hypersensitivity to alprostadil and/or alfadex (ingredients of Viridal Duo).

Patients with diseases causing prolonged erections e.g. sickle-cell disease, leukaemia and multiple myeloma should not use Viridal Duo.

Special precautions: Patients, who experience a prolonged erection lasting longer than four hours should contact their physician immediately. Therefore it is recommended that the patient has an emergency telephone number of his attending physician or of a clinic experienced in therapy of erectile dysfunction. Prolonged erection may damage penile erectile tissue and lead to irreversible erectile dysfunction.

Patients with pre-existing scarring, e.g. fibrosis or nodules of the cavernous body or pre-existing penile deviation or Peyronie's disease should be treated with particular care, e.g. more frequent re-evaluation of the patient's condition. This is due to the increased risk of painful erections.

Patients who have to be treated with alpha-adrenergic drugs due to prolonged erections (see: *Overdose*) may in the case of concomitant therapy with monoamino-oxidase-inhibitors, develop a hypertensive crisis.

Other intracavernous drugs e.g. smooth muscle relaxing agents or alpha-adrenergic blocking agents may lead to prolonged erection and must not be used concomitantly.

Patients with blood clotting disorders or patients on therapy influencing blood clotting parameters should be treated with special care, e.g. monitoring of the clotting parameters and advice to the patient to exercise sufficient manual pressure on the injection site. This is because of the increased risk of bleeding.

Sexual stimulation and intercourse can lead to cardiac and/or pulmonary events in patients with coronary heart disease, congestive heart failure or pulmonary disease. Viridal Duo should be used with care in these patient groups and patients should be examined and cleared for stress resistance by a cardiologist before treatment. To prevent abuse, self-injection therapy with Viridal Duo should not be used by patients with drug addiction and/or disturbances of psychological or intellectual development.

Use of intracavernous alprostadil offers no protection from the transmission of sexually transmitted diseases. Individuals who use alprostadil should be counselled about the protective measures that are necessary to guard against the spread of sexually transmitted diseases, including the human immunodeficiency virus (HIV). In some patients, injection of Viridal Duo can induce a small amount of bleeding at the injection site. In patients infected with blood borne diseases, this could increase the transmission of such diseases to the partner. For this reason we recommend that a condom is used for intercourse after injecting Viridal Duo.

In any condition that precludes safe self injection like poor manual dexterity, poor visual acuity or morbid obesity, the partner should be trained in the injection technique and should perform the injection.

Up to now, there is no clinical experience in patients under 18 and over 75 years of age.

Viridal Duo does not interfere with ejaculation and fertility.

Interactions: Concomitant use of smooth muscle relaxing drugs like papaverine or other drugs inducing erection like alpha-adrenergic blocking agents may lead to prolonged erection and should not be used in parallel with Viridal Duo.

Risks exist when using alpha-adrenergic drugs to terminate prolonged erections in patients with cardiovascular disorders or receiving MAO inhibitors.

The effects of blood pressure lowering and vasodilating drugs may be increased.

Use during pregnancy and lactation: Not applicable.

Alprostadil did not cause any adverse effects on fertility or general reproductive performance in male and female rats treated with 40–200 mcg/kg/day. The high dose of 200 mcg/kg/day is about 300 times the maximum recommended human dose on a body weight basis (MHRD <1 mcg/kg).

Alprostadil was not fetotoxic or teratogenic at doses up to 5000 mcg/kg/day (7500 times the MHRD) in rats, 200 mcg/kg/day (300 times the MHRD) in rabbits and doses up to 20 mcg/kg/day (30 times the MHRD) in guinea pigs or monkeys.

Effects on ability to drive and use machines: Viridal Duo may rarely induce hypotension with subsequent impairment of reactivity.

Undesirable effects: The most frequent adverse effect of Viridal Duo is a burning pain during and after injection due to the injection technique and the feeling of tension occurring with penile erection. Haematomas are frequently seen at the site of injection.

Further possible local reactions are haemosiderin

deposits, reddening and swelling or bleeding of the injection site, ecchymosis, swelling of foreskin or glans, cavernositis or penile infection.

Prolonged erections lasting longer than four hours occur occasionally, but more often during diagnostic and titration-periods than during the period of self injection once the optimum dose has been determined.

Erections lasting longer than six hours are rare after intracavernous injection of Viridal Duo. Prolonged erection may damage penile erectile structures and lead to irreversible erectile dysfunction.

Adverse effects of long-term treatment are fibrotic nodules, spots or plaques with/without penile angulation associated with the injection site which occur occasionally. Fibrotic tissue alterations of the cavernous body with/without loss of function and with/without penile angulation occur in very rare cases during treatment of up to three years.

Penile deviations can occur.

Systemic circulation effects e.g. hypotension with/without dizziness, cardiac arrhythmias, chest pains, headaches and circulatory collapse after intracavernous injection of Viridal Duo have been reported very rarely.

Overdose

Symptoms: Full rigid erections lasting more than four hours.

If the patient experiences a prolonged erection, he is advised to contact his attending physician or a urologic clinic nearby immediately.

Treatment strategy: Treatment of prolonged erection should be done by a physician experienced in the field of erectile dysfunction. If prolonged erection occurs, the following is recommended:

If the erection has lasted less than six hours:

- observation of the erection became spontaneous flaccidity frequently occurs.

If the erection has lasted longer than six hours:

- cavernous body injection of alpha-adrenergic substances (e.g. phenylephrine or epinephrine (adrenaline)). Risks exist when using drugs in patients with cardiovascular disorders or receiving MAO inhibitors. All patients should be monitored for cardiovascular effects when these drugs are used to terminate prolonged erections.

or

- aspiration of blood from the cavernous body.

Accidental systemic injection of high doses: Single dose rising tolerance studies in healthy volunteers indicated that single intravenous doses of alprostadil from 1 to 120 mcg were well tolerated. Starting with a 40 mcg bolus intravenous dose, the frequency of drug-related adverse events increased in a dose-dependent manner, characterised mainly by facial flushing.

Pharmacological (toxicological and pharmacokinetic) properties

Pharmacodynamic properties: Alprostadil [Prostaglandin E1 (PGE_1)], the active ingredient of Viridal Duo, is an endogenous compound derived from the essential fatty acid dihomo-gamma-linolenic acid. Alprostadil is a potent smooth muscle relaxant that produces vasodilation and occurs in high concentrations in the human seminal fluid. Precontracted isolated preparations of the human corpus cavernosum, corpus spongiosum and cavernous artery were relaxed by alprostadil, while other prostanoids were less effective. Alprostadil has been shown to bind to specific receptors in the cavernous tissue of human and non-human primates.

The binding of alprostadil to its receptors is accompanied by an increase in intracellular cAMP levels. Human cavernosal smooth muscle cells respond to alprostadil by releasing intracellular calcium. Since relaxation of smooth muscle is associated with a reduction of the cytoplasmic free calcium concentration, this effect may contribute to the relaxing activity of this prostanoid.

Intracavernous injection of alprostadil in healthy monkeys resulted in penile elongation and tumescence without rigidity. The cavernous arterial blood flow was increased for a mean duration of 20 min. In contrast, intracavernous application of alprostadil to rabbits and dogs caused no erectile response.

Systemic intravascular administration of alprostadil leads to a vasodilation and reduction of systemic peripheral vascular resistance. A decrease in blood pressure can be observed after administration of high doses. Alprostadil has also been shown in animal and in vitro tests to reduce platelet reactivity and neutrophil activation. Additional alprostadil activity has been reported: increase in fibrinolytic activity of fibroblasts, improvement of erythrocyte deformability and inhibition of erythrocyte aggregation; inhibition of the proliferative and mitotic activity of non-striated myocytes; inhibition of cholesterol synthesis and LDL-receptor activity; and an increase in the supply of oxygen and glucose to ischaemic tissue along with improved tissue utilization of these substrates.

Pharmacokinetic properties: Pharmacokinetics after intracavernous injection; Viridal Duo contains the active ingredient alprostadil (PGE_1) in the form of an inclusion compound (clathrate) with alfadex (α-cyclodextrin). During the preparation of the solution for injection the clathrate complex dissociates into the components of alprostadil and alfadex, therefore the pharmacokinetic behaviour of both compounds is independent of the clathrate structure of the dry substance.

Preliminary information of the pharmacokinetics of alprostadil alfadex following intracavernous injection is available. There are no significant differences between the systemic plasma concentration of alprostadil and its metabolites PGE_0 and 15-keto-PGE_0 after intracavernous injection in patients and after intravenous injection in healthy volunteers. Based on the extremely short half-life of alprostadil and the resulting experimental difficulties the pharmacokinetic parameters of systemic alprostadil were measured under steady-state conditions.

Pharmacokinetics after intravenous infusion; Alprostadil is an endogenous substance with an extremely short half-life. After i.v. infusion of 60 mcg alprostadil over two hours (0.5 mcg/min) in healthy volunteers, maximum plasma levels of about 5 pg/ml above basal values were measured (basal value 1–2 pg/ml). After cessation of the infusion, the alprostadil concentration dropped to basal values, with half-lives of about 0.2 min (α-phase, estimate) and about 8 min (β-phase). Due to the short half-life, steady state concentrations were reached shortly after the onset of the i.v. infusion.

Alprostadil undergoes biotransformation predominantly in the lungs. During the first pass through the lungs 80–90% of alprostadil is metabolized. Enzymatic oxidation of the C15-hydroxy-group followed by reduction of the C13–14-double-bond produces the main metabolites 15-keto-PGE_1, PGE_0 and 15-keto-PGE_0. The compound 15-keto-PGE_1 has up to now only been detected in vitro in homogenated lung preparations, whereas PGE_0 and 15-keto-PGE_0 were found in plasma. After degradation by β-oxidation and ω-oxidation, the main metabolites are eliminated via urine (88%) and the faeces (12%).

As a result of biotransformation, PGE_0 (13, 14-dihydro-PGE_1) and 15-keto-PGE_0 were detected in plasma. After i.v. infusion of 60 mcg alprostadil over two hours, plasma concentrations of PGE_0 reached values of about 12 pg/ml above basal value (1–2 pg/ml) and those of 15-keto-PGE_0 were 150 pg/ml above basal value of 4–6 pg/ml. Half-lives were about 2 min (α-phase) and 30 min (β-phase) for PGE_0 and 1–2 min and 20 min respectively for 15-keto-PGE_0.

93% of the alprostadil in plasma is bound to macromolecular compartments. The alfadex was found to have a half-life of about seven minutes in rats. It is excreted renally as unchanged alfadex. Studies on the concentration of alprostadil and its metabolites in various organs and tissues of the rat revealed no evidence of accumulation.

Preclinical safety data: Studies on local tolerance following single and repeated intracavernous injections of alprostadil or alprostadil alfadex in rabbits and/or monkeys, in monkeys up to 6 months with daily injection, revealed in general good local tolerance. Possible adverse effects like haematomas and inflammations are more likely related to the injection procedure.

Within the 6 months study in male monkeys, there were no adverse effects of alprostadil alfadex on male reproductive organs.

Different mutagenicity studies with alprostadil alfadex revealed no risk of mutagenicity.

Chronic toxicity studies in dogs (6 months, daily intravenous infusion) and monkeys (6 months, daily intracavernous injection) indicate that systemic side effects are unlikely to occur following intracavernous injection of 5 to 40 mcg alprostadil (used as clathrate complex with alfadex).

Pharmaceutical particulars

List of excipients:

Powder for injection: lactose, alfadex

Diluent: sodium chloride, water for injection.

Incompatibilities: No incompatibilities have so far been demonstrated.

Shelf life: Shelf life for the product as packaged for sale: 2 years.

Shelf life after reconstitution: For immediate use only.

Special precautions for storage: None.

Nature and contents of container:

1. Cartons containing one colourless glass double-chamber cartridge, one injection needle 29 G×½ (0.33 mm×12.7 mm), two antiseptic swabs and one reusable applicator (starter kit).
2. Cartons containing two colourless glass double-chamber cartridges, two injection needles 29 G×½ (0.33×12.7 mm), four antiseptic swabs and one reusable applicator (starter kit).
3. Cartons containing one, two or six colourless glass double-chamber cartridges and corresponding number of injection needles 29 G×½ (0.33 mm×12.7 mm) and antiseptic swabs without reusable applicator.

Instructions for use/handling: Fix the injection needle onto the front part of the applicator.

Disinfect the tip of the cartridge with one of the sterile swabs. Insert the cartridge into the reusable applicator and fix it by screwing the thread part. Dissolve the drug substance in the front chamber of the cartridge by completely screwing the thread-part into the applicator thus moving both rubber stoppers to the top of the cartridge and allowing the solvent in to the bottom chamber to reach the dry substance via the bypass of the cartridge. Shake slightly until a clear solution is produced.

Expel the air and adjust the prescribed dosage precisely prior to intracavernous injection.

After preparation of the solution, the injection must be performed using aseptic procedures into either the left or right cavernous body of the penile shaft. Care should be taken not to inject into penile vessels or nerves on the upper side of the penis and into the urethra on the under side. The injection should be completed within 5 to 10 seconds and manual pressure should be applied to the injection site for 2 to 3 minutes.

Unused solution must be discarded immediately.

Advice: The content of the front chamber of the cartridge consists of a white, dry powder which forms a compact layer approximately 8 mm in height. The layer may show cracks and crumble slightly.

In case of damage to the cartridge, the usually dry content of the front chamber becomes moist and sticky and extensively loses volume. Viridal Duo must not be used in this case.

The bottom chamber contains the clear, colourless sodium chloride solvent solution.

The dry substance dissolves immediately after addition of the sodium chloride solution. Initially after reconstitution the solution may appear slightly opaque due to the presence of bubbles. This is of no relevance and disappears within a short time to give a clear solution.

Marketing authorisation holder: Shwarz Pharma Ltd, Schwarz House, East Street, Chesham, Bucks HP5 1DG.

Marketing authorisation numbers

Viridal 10 Duo	PL 04438/0049	PA 271/9/4
Viridal 20 Duo	PL 04438/0050	PA 271/9/5

Date of first authorisation/renewal of authorisation

UK 24 May 1997 (644)

ROI 14 November 1997

Date of (partial) revision of the text

UK November 1997

ROI N/A

Legal category UK POM

VIRIDAL 40 DUO

Qualitative and quantitative composition

Viridal 40 Duo: 1 double-chamber glass cartridge containing dry substance (48.8 mg) composed of alprostadil 40 mcg (used as 1:1 clathrate complex with alfadex) and diluent (1 ml).

Diluent: 1 ml sterile sodium chloride solution 0.9% (w/v) PhEur.

Pharmaceutical form Double chamber glass cartridge containing lyophilised powder and diluent for reconstitution.

Administration devices: 1 reusable applicator (starter kit), 1 double-chamber cartridge with dry substance and 1 ml 0.9% sterile sodium chloride solution, 1 injection needle 29 G×½ (0.33 mm×12.7 mm), 2 sterile swabs.

Route of administration: For injection into the penile cavernous body.

Clinical particulars

Therapeutic indications: As an adjunct to the diagnostic evaluation of erectile dysfunction in adult males.

Treatment of erectile dysfunction in adult males.

Posology and method of administration: The drug solution should be prepared shortly before the injection.

Prior to injection the needle should be screwed onto the tip of the applicator. After disinfecting the tip of the cartridge with one of the alcohol swabs, the cartridge should be inserted into the applicator. By screwing the thread part clockwise, the cartridge is fixed in the applicator. Then, the dry substance which is inside the front chamber of the cartridge is reconstituted with 1 ml sterile sodium chloride solution 0.9% in the bottom chamber. While holding the device in a vertical position with the needle upwards, the thread part should be screwed slowly until it will not go any further. The solvent will by-pass the upper stopper into the front chamber and dissolve the dry substance within a few seconds. As soon as the dry substance is reconstituted, the larger external and the smaller inner protective cap have to be removed from the needle. The air should then be expelled out of the cartridge and the prescribed dose adjusted precisely.

Unused solution must be discarded immediately.

Viridal Duo is injected into either the right or the left cavernous body of the penile shaft. Once the needle is in the cavernous body, the injection should be done within 5 to 10 seconds and is very easy without much resistance if the needle is in the correct position.

Re-evaluation should take place at regular intervals by the physician and he will decide whether correction of the dosage is necessary and the duration and frequency of the treatment.

Dosage for injection in the clinic: Injections for diagnostic evaluation and dose titration must be performed by the attending physician. He will determine an individual dose suitable to produce an erectile response for diagnostic purposes.

The recommended starting dose is 2.5 mcg alprostadil in patients with primary psychogenic or neurogenic origin of erectile dysfunction. In all other patients 5 mcg alprostadil should be used as a starting dose. Dose adjustments may be performed in increments of about 2.5 mcg to 5 mcg. Most patients require between 10 mcg and 20 mcg per injection. Some patients may need to be titrated to higher doses. Doses exceeding 20 mcg should be prescribed with particular care in patients with cardiovascular risk factors.

The dose per injection should never exceed 40 mcg.

Dosage for self-injection therapy at home: The patient should only use his optimum individual dosage which has been pre-determined by his physician using the above mentioned procedure. This dose should allow him to have an erection at home which should not last longer than one hour. If he experiences prolonged erections beyond 2 hours but less than 4 hours, the patient is recommended to contact his physician to re-establish the dose of the drug. Maximum injection frequency recommended is 2 or 3 times a week with an interval of at least 24 hours between the injections.

Follow-up: After the first injections and at regular intervals thereafter, the physician should re-evaluate the patient. Any local adverse reactions, e.g. haematoma, fibrosis or nodules should be noted and controlled. Following discussion with the patient, an adjustment of dosage may be necessary.

Contra-indications: Hypersensitivity to alprostadil and/or alfadex (ingredients of Viridal Duo).

Patients with diseases causing prolonged erections e.g. sickle-cell disease, leukaemia and multiple myeloma should not use Viridal Duo.

Special precautions: Patients, who experience a prolonged erection lasting longer than four hours should contact their physician immediately. Therefore it is recommended that the patient has an emergency telephone number of his attending physician or of a clinic experienced in therapy of erectile dysfunction. Prolonged erection may damage penile erectile tissue and lead to irreversible erectile dysfunction.

Patients with pre-existing scarring, e.g. fibrosis or nodules of the cavernous body or pre-existing penile deviation or Peyronie's disease should be treated with particular care, e.g. more frequent re-evaluation of the patient's condition. This is due to the increased risk of painful erections.

Patients who have to be treated with alpha-adrenergic drugs due to prolonged erections (see: *Overdose*) may in the case of concomitant therapy with mono-amino-oxidase-inhibitors, develop a hypertensive crisis.

Other intracavernous drugs e.g. smooth muscle relaxing agents or alpha-adrenergic blocking agents may lead to prolonged erection and must not be used concomitantly.

Patients with blood clotting disorders or patients on therapy influencing blood clotting parameters should be treated with special care, e.g. monitoring of the clotting parameters and advice to the patient to exercise sufficient manual pressure on the injection site. This is because of the increased risk of bleeding.

Sexual stimulation and intercourse can lead to cardiac and/or pulmonary events in patients with coronary heart disease, congestive heart failure or pulmonary disease. Viridal Duo should be used with care in these patient groups and patients should be examined and cleared for stress resistance by a cardiologist before treatment. To prevent abuse, self-injection therapy with Viridal Duo should not be used by patients with drug addiction and/or disturbances of psychological or intellectual development.

Use of intracavernous alprostadil offers no protection from the transmission of sexually transmitted diseases. Individuals who use alprostadil should be counselled about the protective measures that are necessary to guard against the spread of sexually transmitted diseases, including the human immunodeficiency virus (HIV). In some patients, injection of Viridal can induce a small amount of bleeding at the injection site. In patients infected with blood borne diseases, this could increase the transmission of such diseases to the partner. For this reason we recommend that a condom is used for intercourse after injecting Viridal.

In any condition that precludes safe self injection like poor manual dexterity, poor visual acuity or morbid obesity, the partner should be trained in the injection technique and should perform the injection.

Up to now, there is no clinical experience in patients under 18 and over 75 years of age.

Viridal Duo does not interfere with ejaculation and fertility.

Interactions: Concomitant use of smooth muscle relaxing drugs like papaverine or other drugs inducing erection like alpha-adrenergic blocking agents may lead to prolonged erection and should not be used in parallel with Viridal Duo.

Risks exist when using alpha-adrenergic drugs to terminate prolonged erections in patients with cardiovascular disorders or receiving MAO inhibitors.

The effects of blood pressure lowering and vasodilating drugs may be increased.

Use during pregnancy and lactation: Not applicable.

Alprostadil did not cause any adverse effects on fertility or general reproductive performance in male and female rats treated with 40–200 mcg/kg/day. The high dose of 200 mcg/kg/day is about 300 times the maximum recommended human dose on a body weight basis (MHRD <1 mcg/kg).

Alprostadil was not fetotoxic or teratogenic at doses up to 5000 mcg/kg/day (7500 times the MHRD) in rats, 200 mcg/kg/day (300 times the MHRD) in rabbits and doses up to 20 mcg/kg/day (30 times the MHRD) in guinea pigs or monkeys.

Effects on ability to drive and use machines: Viridal Duo may rarely induce hypotension with subsequent impairment of reactivity.

Undesirable effects: The most frequent adverse effect of Viridal Duo is a burning pain during and after injection due to the injection technique and the feeling of tension occurring with penile erection. Haematomas are frequently seen at the site of injection.

Further possible local reactions are haemosiderin deposits, reddening and swelling or bleeding of the injection site, ecchymosis, swelling of foreskin or glans, cavernositis or penile infection.

Prolonged erections lasting longer than four hours occur occasionally, but more often during diagnostic and titration-periods than during the period of self injection once the optimum dose has been determined.

Erections lasting longer than six hours are rare after intracavernous injection of Viridal Duo.

Prolonged erection may damage penile erectile structures and lead to irreversible erectile dysfunction.

Adverse effects of long-term treatment are fibrotic nodules, spots or plaques with/without penile angulation associated with the injection site which occur occasionally. Fibrotic tissue alterations of the cavernous body with/without loss of function and with/without penile angulation occur in very rare cases during treatment of up to three years.

Penile deviations can occur.

Systemic circulation effects e.g. hypotension with/without dizziness, cardiac arrhythmias, chest pains, headaches and circulatory collapse after intracavernous injection of Viridal Duo have been reported very rarely.

Overdose

Symptoms: Full rigid erections lasting more than four hours.

If the patient experiences a prolonged erection, he is advised to contact his attending physician or a urology clinic nearby immediately.

Treatment strategy: Treatment of prolonged erection should be done by a physician experienced in the field of erectile dysfunction. If prolonged erection occurs, the following is recommended:

If the erection has lasted less than six hours:

- observation of the erection because spontaneous flaccidity frequently occurs.

If the erection has lasted longer than six hours:

- cavernous body injection of alpha-adrenergic substances (e.g. phenylephrine or epinephrine (adrenaline)). Risks exist when using drugs in patients with cardiovascular disorders or receiving MAO inhibitors. All patients should be monitored for cardiovascular effects when these drugs are used to terminate prolonged erections.

or

- aspiration of blood from the cavernous body.

Accidental systemic injection of high doses: Single dose rising tolerance studies in healthy volunteers indicated that single intravenous doses of alprostadil from 1 to 120 mcg were well tolerated. Starting with a 40 mcg bolus intravenous dose, the frequency of drug-related adverse events increased in a dose-dependent manner, characterised mainly by facial flushing.

Pharmacological properties

Pharmacodynamic properties: Alprostadil [Prostaglandin E1 (PGE_1)], the active ingredient of Viridal, is an endogenous compound derived from the essential fatty acid dihomogammalinolenic acid. Alprostadil is a potent smooth muscle relaxant that produces vasodilation and occurs in high concentrations in the human seminal fluid. Precontracted isolated preparations of the human corpus cavernosum, corpus spongiosum and cavernous artery were relaxed by alprostadil, while other prostanoids were less effective. Alprostadil has been shown to bind to specific receptors in the cavernous tissue of human and non-human primates.

The binding of alprostadil to its receptors is accompanied by an increase in intracellular cAMP levels. Human cavernosal smooth muscle cells respond to alprostadil by releasing intracellular calcium. Since relaxation of smooth muscle is associated with a reduction of the cytoplasmic free calcium concentration, this effect may contribute to the relaxing activity of this prostanoid.

Intracavernous injection of alprostadil in healthy monkeys resulted in penile elongation and tumescence without rigidity. The cavernous arterial blood flow was increased for a mean duration of 20 min. In contrast, intracavernous application of alprostadil to rabbits and dogs caused no erectile response.

Systemic intravascular administration of alprostadil leads to a vasodilation and reduction of systemic peripheral vascular resistance. A decrease in blood pressure can be observed after administration of high doses. Alprostadil has also been shown in animal and *in vitro* tests to reduce platelet reactivity and neutrophil activation. Additional alprostadil activity has been reported: increase in fibrinolytic activity of fibroblasts, improvement of erythrocyte deformability and inhibition of erythrocyte aggregation; inhibition of the proliferative and mitotic activity of non-striated myocytes; inhibition of cholesterol synthesis and LDL-receptor activity; and an increase in the supply of oxygen and glucose to ischaemic tissue along with improved tissue utilisation of these substrates.

Pharmacokinetic properties:

Pharmacokinetics after intracavernous injection: Viridal Duo contains the active ingredient alprostadil (PGE_1) in the form of an inclusion compound (clathrate) with alfadex (α-cyclodextrin). During the preparation of the solution for injection the clathrate complex dissociates into the components of alprostadil and alfadex, therefore the pharmacokinetic behaviour of both compounds is independent of the clathrate structure of the dry substance.

Preliminary information of the pharmacokinetics of alprostadil alfadex following intracavernous injection is available. There are no significant differences between the systemic plasma concentration of alprostadil and its metabolites PGE_0 and 15-keto-PGE_0 after intracavernous injection in patients and after intravenous injection in healthy volunteers. Based on the extremely short half-life of alprostadil and the resulting experimental difficulties the pharmacokinetic parameters of systemic alprostadil were measured under steady-state conditions.

Pharmacokinetics after intravenous infusion: Alprostadil is an endogenous substance with an extremely short half-life. After i.v. infusion of 60 mcg alprostadil over two hours (0.5 mcg/min) in healthy volunteers, maximum plasma levels of about 5 pg/ml above basal values were measured (basal value 1–2 pg/ml). After cessation of the infusion, the alprostadil concentration dropped to basal values, with half-lives of about 0.2 min (α-phase, estimate) and about 8 min (β-phase). Due to the short half-life, steady state concentrations were reached shortly after the onset of the i.v. infusion.

Alprostadil undergoes biotransformation predominantly in the lungs. During the first pass through the lungs 80–90% of alprostadil is metabolised. Enzymatic oxidation of the C15-hydroxy-group followed by reduction of the C13–14 double-bond produces the main metabolites 15-keto-PGE_1, PGE_0 and 15-keto-PGE_0. The compound 15-keto-PGE_1 has up to now only been detected in vitro in homogenate lung preparations, whereas PGE_0 and 15-keto-PGE_0 were found in plasma. After degradation by β-oxidation and ω-oxidation, the main metabolites are eliminated via urine (88%) and the faeces (12%).

As a result of biotransformation, PGE_0 (13, 14-dihydro-PGE_1) and 15-keto-PGE_0 were detected in plasma. After i.v. infusion of 60 mcg alprostadil over two hours, plasma concentrations of PGE_0 reached values of about 12 pg/ml above basal value (1–2 pg/ml) and those of 15-keto-PGE_0 were 150 pg/ml above basal value of 4–6 pg/ml. Half-lives were about 2 min (α-phase) and 30 min (β-phase) for PGE_0 and 1–2 min and 20 min respectively for 15-keto-PGE_0.

93% of the alprostadil in plasma is bound to macromolecular compartments. The alfadex was found to have a half-life of about seven minutes in rats. It is excreted renally as unchanged alfadex. Studies on the concentration of alprostadil and its metabolites in various organs and tissues of the rat revealed no evidence of accumulation.

Preclinical safety data: Studies on local tolerance following single and repeated intracavernous injections of alprostadil or alprostadil alfadex in rabbits and/or monkeys, in monkeys up to 6 months with daily injection, revealed in general good local tolerance. Possible adverse effects like haematomas and inflammations are more likely related to the injection procedure.

Within the 6 months study in male monkeys, there were no adverse effects of alprostadil alfadex on male reproductive organs.

Different mutagenicity studies with alprostadil alfadex revealed no risk of mutagenicity.

Chronic toxicity studies in dogs (6 months, daily intravenous infusion) and monkeys (6 months, daily intracavernous injection) indicates that systemic side effects are unlikely to occur following intracavernous injection of 5 to 40 mcg alprostadil (used as clathrate complex with alfadex).

Pharmaceutical particulars

List of excipients: Powder for injection: lactose, alfadex

Diluent: sodium chloride, water for injection.

Incompatibilities: No incompatibilities have so far been demonstrated.

Shelf life: Shelf life for the product as packaged for sale: 2 years.

Shelf life after reconstitution: for immediate use only.

Special precautions for storage: None.

Nature and contents of container:

1. Cartons containing one colourless glass double-chamber cartridge, one injection needle 29 G×½ (0.33 mm×12.7 mm), two antiseptic swabs and one reusable applicator (starter kit).
2. **Cartons containing two colourless glass double-chamber cartridges, two injection needles 29 G×½ (0.33×12.7 mm), four antiseptic swabs and one reusable applicator (starter kit).**
3. **Cartons containing** one, two or six **colourless glass double-chamber cartridges and corresponding number of injection needles 29 G×½ (0.33 mm×12.7 mm) and antiseptic swabs without reusable applicator.**

(only the pack sizes in bold text are currently marketed).

Instructions for use/handling: Fix the injection needle onto the front part of the applicator.

Clean the tip of the cartridge with one of the sterile swabs. Insert the cartridge into the reusable applicator and fix it by screwing the thread part. Dissolve the drug substance in the front chamber of the cartridge by completely screwing the thread-part into the applicator thus moving both rubber stoppers to the top of the cartridge and allowing the solvent in to the bottom chamber to reach the dry substance via the bypass of the cartridge. Shake slightly until a clear solution is produced.

Expel the air and adjust the prescribed dosage precisely prior to intracavernous injection.

After preparation of the solution, the injection must be performed using aseptic procedures into either the left or right cavernous body of the penile shaft. Care should be taken not to inject into penile vessels or nerves on the upper side of the penis and into the urethra on the under side. The injection should be completed within 5 to 10 seconds and manual pressure should be applied to the injection site for 2 to 3 minutes.

Unused solution must be discarded immediately.

Advice: The content of the front chamber of the cartridge consists of a white, dry powder which forms a compact layer approximately 8 mm in height. The layer may show cracks and crumble slightly.

In case of damage to the cartridge, the usually dry content of the front chamber becomes moist and sticky and extensively loses volume. Viridal Duo must not be used in this case.

The bottom chamber contains the clear, colourless sodium chloride solvent solution.

The dry substance dissolves immediately after addition of the sodium chloride solution. Initially after reconstitution the solution may appear slightly opaque due to the presence of bubbles. This is of no relevance and disappears within a short time to give a clear solution.

Marketing authorisation number

PL 04438/0051

Date of first authorisation/renewal of authorisation

7 October 1998

Date of (partial) revision of the text

February 1998

Legal category POM

**Trade Mark*

Searle
PO Box 53
Lane End Road
High Wycombe
Bucks HP12 4HL

☎ 01494 521124 🗋 01494 447872

SEARLE

ALDACTIDE*

Presentation
Aldactide 50: Buff, film-coated tablets engraved 'SEARLE 180' on one side containing Spironolactone BP 50 mg and Hydroflumethiazide BP 50 mg.

Aldactide 25: Buff, film-coated tablets engraved 'Searle 101' on one side containing Spironolactone BP 25 mg and Hydroflumethiazide BP 25 mg.

Uses Congestive cardiac failure.

Dosage and administration Administration of Aldactide once daily with a meal is recommended.

Adults: Most patients will require an initial dosage of four tablets Aldactide 25 or two tablets Aldactide 50 daily. The dosage should be adjusted as necessary and may range from one tablet Aldactide 25 to eight tablets Aldactide 25 or four tablets Aldactide 50 daily.

Elderly: It is recommended that treatment is started with the lowest dose and titrated upwards as required to achieve maximum benefit. Care should be taken in severe hepatic and renal impairment which may alter drug metabolism and excretion.

Children: Although clinical trials using Aldactide have not been carried out in children, as a guide, a daily dosage providing 1.5 to 3 mg of spironolactone per kilogram body weight, given in divided doses, may be employed.

Contra-indications, warnings, etc
Contra-indications: Aldactide is contra-indicated in patients with anuria, acute renal insufficiency, rapidly deteriorating or severe impairment of renal function, hyperkalaemia, significant hypercalcaemia, Addison's disease and in patients who are hypersensitive to spironolactone, thiazide diuretics or to other sulphonamide derived drugs.

Aldactide should not be administered with other potassium-conserving diuretics and potassium supplements should not be given routinely with Aldactide as hyperkalaemia may be induced.

Warnings: Carcinogenicity: Spironolactone has been shown to produce tumours in rats when administered at high doses over a long period of time. The significance of these findings with respect to clinical use is not certain. However, the long term use of spironolactone in young patients requires careful consideration of the benefits and the potential hazard involved.

Sulphonamide derivatives, including thiazides, have been reported to exacerbate or activate systemic lupus erythematosus.

Precautions:
Fluid and electrolyte balance: Fluid and electrolyte status should be regularly monitored, particularly in the elderly, in those with significant renal and hepatic impairment and in patients receiving digoxin and drugs with pro-arrhythmic effects.

Hyperkalaemia may occur in patients with impaired renal function or excessive potassium intake and can cause cardiac irregularities which may be fatal. Should hyperkalaemia develop Aldactide should be discontinued, and if necessary, active measures taken to reduce the serum potassium to normal.

Hypokalaemia may develop as a result of profound diuresis, particularly when Aldactide is used concomitantly with loop diuretics, glucocorticoids or ACTH.

Hyponatraemia may be induced, especially when Aldactide is administered in combination with other diuretics.

Hepatic impairment: Caution should be observed in patients with acute or severe liver impairment as vigorous diuretic therapy may precipitate encephalopathy in susceptible patients. Regular estimation of serum electrolytes is essential in such patients.

Reversible hyperchloraemic metabolic acidosis usually in association with hyperkalaemia has been reported to occur in some patients with decompensated hepatic cirrhosis, even in the presence of normal renal function.

Urea and uric acid: Reversible increases in blood urea have been reported, particularly accompanying vigorous diuresis or in the presence of impaired renal function.

Thiazides may cause hyperuricaemia and precipitate attacks of gout in some patients.

Diabetes mellitus: Thiazides may aggravate existing diabetes and the insulin requirements may alter. Diabetes mellitus which has been latent may become manifest during thiazide administration.

Hyperlipidaemia: Caution should be observed as thiazides may raise serum lipids.

Drug Interactions: Spironolactone has been reported to increase serum digoxin concentration and to interfere with certain serum digoxin assays. In patients receiving digoxin and spironolactone the digoxin response should be monitored by means other than serum digoxin concentrations, unless the digoxin assay used has been proven not to be affected by spironolactone therapy. If it proves necessary to adjust the dose of digoxin patients should be carefully monitored for evidence of enhanced or reduced digoxin effect.

Potentiation of the effect of other antihypertensive drugs occurs and their dosage may need to be reduced when Aldactide is added to the treatment regimen, and then adjusted as necessary. Since ACE inhibitors decrease aldosterone production they should not routinely be used with Aldactide particularly in patients with marked renal impairment.

As carbenoxolone may cause sodium retention and thus decrease the effectiveness of Aldactide, concurrent use should be avoided.

Nonsteroidal anti-inflammatory drugs may attenuate the natriuretic efficacy of diuretics due to inhibition of intrarenal synthesis of prostaglandins.

Concurrent use of lithium and thiazides may reduce lithium clearance leading to intoxication. Spironolactone and thiazides may reduce vascular responsiveness to noradrenaline. Caution should be exercised in the management of patients subjected to regional or general anaesthesia while they are being treated with Aldactide.

In fluorimetric assays spironolactone may interfere with the estimation of compounds with similar fluorescence characteristics.

The absorption of a number of drugs including thiazides is decreased when co-administered with cholestyramine and colestipol.

Thiazides co-administered with calcium and/or vitamin D may increase the risk of hypercalcaemia.

Thiazides may delay the elimination of quinidine.

Pregnancy: Spironolactone or its metabolites may, and hydroflumethazide does, cross the placental barrier. With spironolactone feminisation has been observed in male rat foetuses. Thiazides may decrease placental perfusion, increase uterine inertia and inhibit labour. In the foetus or neonate, thiazides may cause jaundice, thrombocytopenia, hypoglycaemia, electrolyte imbalance and death from maternal complications.

The use of Aldactide in pregnant women requires that the anticipated benefit be weighed against the possible hazards to the mother and foetus.

Nursing mothers: Metabolites of spironolactone, and hydroflumethiazide, have been detected in breast milk. If use of Aldactide is considered essential, an alternative method of infant feeding should be instituted.

Adverse effects: Gynaecomastia may develop in association with the use of spironolactone. Development appears to be related to both dosage level and duration of therapy and is normally reversible when the drug is discontinued. In rare instances some breast enlargement may persist. Other adverse reactions reported in association with spironolactone include: gastrointestinal intolerance, drowsiness, lethargy, headache, mental confusion, ataxia, drug fever, skin rashes, mestrual irregularities, breast soreness, impotence and mild androgenic effects.

Adverse reactions reported in association with thiazides include: gastrointestinal upset, skin rashes, photosensitivity, blood dyscrasias, raised serum lipids, aplastic anaemia, purpura, muscle cramps, weakness, restlessness, headache, dizziness, vertigo, jaundice, orthostatic hypotension, impotence, paraesthesia, and rarely pancreatitis, necrotising vasculitis and xanthopsia. Rarely hypercalcaemia has been reported in association with thiazides, usually in patients with pre-existing metabolic bone disease or parathyroid dysfunction.

Overdosage: Acute overdosage may be manifested by drowsiness, mental confusion, nausea, vomiting, dizziness or diarrhoea. Hyponatraemia, hypokalaemia or hyperkalaemia may be induced, or hepatic coma may be precipitated in patients with severe liver disease, but these effects are unlikely to be associated with acute overdosage. Symptoms of hyperkalaemia may manifest as paraesthesia, weakness flaccid paralysis or muscle spasm and may be difficult to distinguish clinically from hypokalaemia. Electrocardiographic changes are the earliest specific signs of potassium disturbances. No specific antidote has been identified. Improvement may be expected after withdrawal of the drug. General supportive measures including replacement of fluids and electrolytes may be indicated.

Pharmaceutical precautions Store in a dry place below 30°C (86°F).

Legal category POM.

Package quantities *Aldactide 50:* Calendar pack of 28 tablets, Securitainer bottles of 100 tablets. *Aldactide 25:* Blister pack of 100 tablets.

Further information Hydroflumethiazide induces diuresis usually within two hours, which lasts for 12-18 hours.

Spironolactone, as a competitive aldosterone antagonist, increases sodium excretion whilst reducing potassium loss at the distal renal tubule. It has a gradual and prolonged action. The renal action of single doses of spironolactone reaches its peak after 7 hours, and activity persists for at least 24 hours.

Product licence numbers
Aldactide 50: 08821/0012
Aldactide 25: 08821/0013

ALDACTONE*

Presentation
Aldactone 100 mg: Buff, film-coated tablets engraved 'SEARLE 134' on one side. Each tablet contains Spironolactone BP 100 mg.

Aldactone 50 mg: Off-white, film-coated tablets engraved 'SEARLE 916'. Each tablet contains Spironolactone BP 50 mg.

Aldactone 25 mg: Buff, film-coated tablets engraved 'SEARLE 39' on one side. Each tablet contains Spironolactone BP 25 mg.

Uses
Congestive cardiac failure.
Hepatic cirrhosis with ascites and oedema.
Malignant ascites.
Nephrotic syndrome.
Diagnosis and treatment of primary aldosteronism.

Dosage and administration Administration of Aldactone once daily with a meal is recommended.

Adults:
Congestive cardiac failure: Usual dose – 100 mg/day. In difficult or severe cases the dosage may be gradually increased up to 400 mg/day. When oedema is controlled, the usual maintenance level is 75–200 mg/day.

Hepatic cirrhosis with ascites and oedema: If urinary Na^+/K^+ ratio is greater than 1.0, 100 mg/day. If the ratio is less than 1.0, 200–400 mg/day. Maintenance dosage should be individually determined.

Malignant ascites: Initial dose usually 100–200 mg/day. In severe cases the dosage may be gradually increased up to 400 mg/day. When oedema is controlled, maintenance dosage should be individually determined.

Nephrotic syndrome: Usual dose – 100–200 mg/day. Spironolactone has not been shown to be anti-inflammatory, nor to affect the basic pathological process. Its use is only advised if glucocorticoids by themselves are insufficiently effective.

Diagnosis and treatment of primary aldosteronism: Aldactone may be employed as an initial diagnostic measure to provide presumptive evidence of primary hyperaldosteronism while patients are on normal diets.

Long test: Aldactone is administered at a daily dosage of 400 mg for three to four weeks.

Correction of hypokalaemia and of hypertension provides presumptive evidence for the diagnosis of primary hyperaldosteronism.

Short test: Aldactone is administered at daily dosage of 400 mg for four days. If serum potassium increases during Aldactone administration but drops when Aldactone is discontinued, a presumptive diagnosis of primary hyperaldosteronism should be considered.

After the diagnosis of hyperaldosteronism has been established by more definitive testing procedures, Aldactone may be administered in doses of 100 mg to 400 mg daily in preparation for surgery. For patients who are considered unsuitable for surgery, Aldactone may be employed for long term maintenance therapy at the lowest effective dosage determined for the individual patient.

Elderly: It is recommended that treatment is started with the lowest dose and titrated upwards as required to achieve maximum benefit. Care should be taken in severe hepatic and renal impairment which may alter drug metabolism and excretion.

Children: Initial daily dosage should provide 3 mg of spironolactone per kilogram body weight, given in divided doses. Dosage should be adjusted on the basis of response and tolerance. If necessary a suspension may be prepared by crushing Aldactone tablets.

Contra-indications, warnings, etc
Contra-indications: Aldactone is contra-indicated in patients with anuria, acute renal insufficiency, rapidly deteriorating or severe impairment of renal function, hyperkalaemia, Addison's disease and in patients who are hypersensitive to spironolactone.

Aldactone should not be administered concurrently with other potassium-conserving diuretics and potassium supplements should not be given routinely with Aldactone as hyperkalaemia may be induced.

Warnings:
Carcinogenicity: Spironolactone has been shown to produce tumours in rats when administered at high doses over a long period of time. The significance of these findings with respect to clinical use is not certain. However, the long term use of spironolactone in young patients requires careful consideration of the benefits and the potential hazard involved.

Precautions:
Fluid and electrolyte balance: Fluid and electrolyte status should be regularly monitored, particularly in the elderly, and in those with significant renal and hepatic impairment.

Hyperkalaemia may occur in patients with impaired renal function or excessive potassium intake and can cause cardiac irregularities which may be fatal. Should hyperkalaemia develop Aldactone should be discontinued, and if necessary, active measures taken to reduce the serum potassium to normal.

Hyponatraemia may be induced, especially when Aldactone is administered in combination with other diuretics.

Reversible hyperchloraemic metabolic acidosis usually in association with hyperkalaemia has been reported to occur in some patients with decompensated hepatic cirrhosis, even in the presence of normal renal function.

Urea: Reversible increases in blood urea have been reported, in association with Aldactone therapy, particularly in the presence of impaired renal function.

Drug interactions: Spironolactone has been reported to increase serum digoxin concentration and to interfere with certain serum digoxin assays. In patients receiving digoxin and spironolactone the digoxin response should be monitored by means other than serum digoxin concentrations, unless the digoxin assay used has been proven not to be affected by spironolactone therapy. If it proves necessary to adjust the dose of digoxin patients should be carefully monitored for evidence of enhanced or reduced digoxin effect.

Potentiation of the effect of antihypertensive drugs occurs and their dosage may need to be reduced when Aldactone is added to the treatment regimen, and then adjusted as necessary. Since ACE inhibitors decrease aldosterone production they should not routinely be used with Aldactone particularly in patients with marked renal impairment.

As carbenoxolone may cause sodium retention and thus decrease the effectiveness of Aldactone, concurrent use should be avoided.

Nonsteroidal anti-inflammatory drugs may attenuate the natriuretic efficacy of diuretics due to inhibition of intrarenal synthesis of prostaglandins.

Spironolactone reduces vascular responsiveness to noradrenaline. Caution should be exercised in the management of patients subjected to regional or general anaesthesia while they are being treated with Aldactone.

In fluorimetric assays spironolactone may interfere with the estimation of compounds with similar fluorescence characteristics.

Pregnancy: Spironolactone or its metabolites may cross the placental barrier. With spironolactone, feminisation has been observed in male rat foetuses. The use of Aldactone in pregnant women requires that the anticipated benefit be weighed against the possible hazards to the mother and foetus.

Nursing mothers: Metabolites of spironolactone, have been detected in breast milk. If use of Aldactone is considered essential, an alternative method of infant feeding should be instituted.

Adverse effects: Gynaecomastia may develop in association with the use of spironolactone. Development appears to be related to both dosage level and duration of therapy and is normally reversible when spironolactone is discontinued. In rare instances some breast enlargement may persist. Other adverse reactions reported in association with spironolactone include: gastrointestinal intolerance, drowsiness, lethargy, headache, mental confusion, ataxia, drug fever, skin rashes, breast soreness, menstrual irregularities, impotence and mild androgenic effects.

Overdosage: Acute overdosage may be manifested by drowsiness, mental confusion, nausea, vomiting, dizziness or diarrhoea. Hyponatraemia or hyperkalaemia may be induced but these effects are unlikely to be associated with acute overdosage. Symptoms of hyperkalaemia may manifest as paraesthesia, weakness, flaccid paralysis or muscle spasm and may be difficult to distinguish clinically from hypokalaemia. Electrocardiographic changes are the earliest specific signs of potassium disturbances. No specific antidote has been identified. Improvement may be expected after withdrawal of the drug. General supportive measures including replacement of fluids and electrolytes may be indicated. For hyperkalaemia, reduce potassium intake, administer potassium-excreting diuretics, intravenous glucose with regular insulin, or oral ion-exchange resins.

Pharmaceutical precautions Store in a dry place below 30°C (86°F).

Legal category POM.

Package quantities *Aldactone 100 mg:* Calendar pack of 28 tablets, blister pack of 100 tablets.
Aldactone 50 mg: Blister pack of 100 tablets.
Aldactone 25 mg: Blister pack of 100 tablets.

Further information Aldactone, as a competitive aldosterone antagonist, increases sodium excretion whilst reducing potassium loss at the distal renal tubule. It has a gradual and prolonged action, maximum response being usually attained after 2–3 days' treatment. Combination of Aldactone with a conventional, more proximally acting diuretic usually enhances diuresis without excessive potassium loss.

Product licence numbers
Aldactone 100 mg: 08821/0009
Aldactone 50 mg: 08821/0010
Aldactone 25 mg: 08821/0011

ARTHROTEC* 50

Qualitative and quantitative composition Each tablet consists of a gastro-resistant core containing 50 mg diclofenac sodium surrounded by an outer mantle containing 200 mcg misoprostol.

Pharmaceutical form White, round, biconvex tablets marked ⚙ on one side and 'SEARLE 1411' on the other side.

Clinical particulars
Therapeutic indications: Arthrotec 50 is indicated for patients who require the non-steroidal anti-inflammatory drug diclofenac together with misoprostol.

The diclofenac component of Arthrotec 50 is indicated for the symptomatic treatment of osteoarthritis and rheumatoid arthritis. The misoprostol component of Arthrotec 50 is indicated for patients with a special need for the prophylaxis of NSAID-induced gastric and duodenal ulceration.

Posology and method of administration:
Adults: One tablet to be taken with food, two or three times daily. Tablets should be swallowed whole, not chewed.

Elderly/renal impairment/hepatic impairment: No adjustment of dosage is necessary in the elderly or in patients with hepatic impairment or mild to moderate renal impairment as pharmacokinetics are not altered to any clinically relevant extent. Nevertheless patients with severe renal or hepatic impairment should be closely monitored (see also *Undesirable effects*).

Children: The safety and efficacy of Arthrotec 50 in children has not been established.

Contra-indications: Arthrotec 50 is contra-indicated in:

- Patients with active gastric or duodenal ulceration or who have active GI bleeding or other active bleedings e.g. cerebrovascular bleedings.
- Pregnant women and in women planning a pregnancy.
- Patients who are lactating or who are breast feeding.
- Patients with a known hypersensitivity to diclofenac, aspirin, other NSAIDs, misoprostol, other prostaglandins, or any other ingredient of the product.
- Patients in whom attacks of asthma, urticaria or acute rhinitis are precipitated by aspirin or other non-steroidal anti-inflammatory agents.

Special warnings and special precautions for use:
Warnings:
Use in pre-menopausal women (see also Contra-indications): Arthrotec 50 should not be used in pre-menopausal women unless they use effective contraception and have been advised of the risks of taking the product if pregnant (see *Pregnancy and Lactation*).

Precautions: Arthrotec 50, in common with other NSAIDs, may decrease platelet aggregation and prolong bleeding time. Extra supervision is recommended in haematopoietic disorders or in conditions with defective coagulation or in patients with a history of cerebrovascular bleeding.

Fluid retention and oedema have been observed in patients taking NSAIDs, including Arthrotec 50. Therefore, Arthrotec 50 should be used with caution in patients with compromised cardiac function and other conditions predisposing to fluid retention.

In patients with renal, cardiac or hepatic impairment caution is required since the use of NSAIDs may result in deterioration of renal function. In the following conditions Arthrotec 50 should be used only in exceptional circumstances and with close clinical monitoring: advanced cardiac failure, advanced kidney failure, advanced liver disease.

Similarly caution is also required in patients with diuretic treatment or otherwise at risk of hypovolaemia. The dose should be kept as low as possible and renal function should be monitored.

Caution is required in patients suffering from ulcerative colitis or Crohn's disease.

All patients who are receiving long-term treatment with NSAIDs should be monitored as a precautionary measure (e.g. renal, hepatic function and blood counts).

Interactions with other medicaments and other forms of interaction: NSAIDs may attenuate the natriuretic efficacy of diuretics due to inhibition of intrarenal synthesis of prostaglandins. Concomitant treatment with potassium-sparing diuretics may be associated with increased serum potassium levels, hence serum potassium should be monitored.

Because of their effect on renal prostaglandins, cyclo-oxygenase inhibitors such as diclofenac can increase the nephrotoxicity of cyclosporin.

Steady state plasma lithium and digoxin levels may be increased and ketoconazole levels may be decreased.

Pharmacodynamic studies with diclofenac have shown no potentiation of oral hypoglycaemic and anticoagulant drugs. However, as interactions have been reported with other NSAIDs, caution and adequate monitoring are nevertheless advised (see statement on platelet aggregation in *Precautions*).

Because of decreased platelet aggregation caution is also advised when using Arthrotec 50 with anticoagulants.

Caution is advised when methotrexate is administered concurrently with NSAIDs because of possible enhancement of its toxicity by the NSAID as a result of increase in methotrexate plasma levels.

Concomitant use with other NSAIDs or with corticosteroids may increase the frequency of side effects generally.

Pregnancy and lactation
Pregnancy: Arthrotec 50 is contraindicated in pregnant women and in women planning a pregnancy as misoprostol may increase uterine tone and contractions in pregnancy which could produce miscarriage. Also diclofenac may cause premature closure of the ductus arteriosus.

Lactation: Arthrotec 50 should not be administered during breast feeding as there are no data on the excretion into breast milk for either misoprostol or diclofenac.

Effects on ability to drive and use machines: Patients who experience dizziness or other central nervous system disturbances while taking NSAIDs should refrain from driving or operating machinery.

Undesirable effects
Common:
General: Headache, dizziness.
Gastrointestinal: Abdominal pain, diarrhoea, nausea, dyspepsia, flatulence, vomiting, gastritis and eructation.
Diarrhoea is usually mild to moderate and transient and can be minimised by taking Arthrotec 50 with food and by avoiding the use of predominantly magnesium-containing antacids.
Skin: Skin rashes.

Infrequent:
General: Tiredness, peripheral oedema.
Gastrointestinal: Peptic ulcer, stomatitis, decrease in haemoglobin associated with GI blood loss, oesophageal lesions.
Liver: Elevations of SGPT, SGOT, alkaline phosphatase or bilirubin.
Female reproductive system: Menorrhagia, intermenstrual bleeding and vaginal bleeding have been reported in pre-menopausal women and vaginal bleeding in post-menopausal women.

Rarely or very rarely:
Blood system: Thrombocytopenia, leucopenia, agranulocytosis, haemolytic anaemia, aplastic anaemia.
Gastrointestinal: Anorexia, dry mouth, bleeding (haematemesis, melaena), perforated ulcer, glossitis, other GI complaints (ulcerative colitis, Crohn's disease), constipation.
Liver: Hepatitis with or without jaundice.
Skin/hypersensitivity: Urticaria, erythema multiforme, photosensitivity reactions, Steven-Johnson's syndrome, Lyell's syndrome (acute toxic epidermal necrolysis), hypersensitivity including bronchospasm and angioedema, purpura including allergic purpura and hair loss.
CNS: Drowsiness, paraesthesia, memory disorders, disorientation, visual disturbances, tinnitus, insomnia, irritability, convulsions, depression, anxiety, nightmares, tremors, psychotic reactions, taste disturbance.
Renal: As a class NSAIDs have been associated with renal pathology including papillary necrosis, interstitial nephritis, nephrotic syndrome and renal failure.
Other: In isolated cases worsening of inflammation associated with infections have been reported in association with NSAID treatment.

Overdose: The toxic dose of Arthrotec 50 has not been determined and there is no experience of overdosage. Intensification of the pharmacological effects may occur with overdosage. Management of acute poisoning with NSAIDs essentially consists of supportive and symptomatic measures. It is reasonable to take measures to reduce absorption of any recently consumed drug by forced emesis, gastric lavage or activated charcoal.

Pharmacological properties
Pharmacodynamic properties: Arthrotec 50 is a non-steroidal, anti-inflammatory drug which is effective in treating the signs and symptoms of arthritic conditions.
This activity is due to the presence of diclofenac which has been shown to have anti-inflammatory and analgesic properties.
Arthrotec 50 also contains the gastroduodenal mucosal protective component misoprostol which is a synthetic prostaglandin E_1 analogue that enhances several of the factors that maintain gastroduodenal mucosal integrity.

Pharmacokinetic properties: The pharmacokinetic profiles of diclofenac and misoprostol administered as Arthrotec 50 are similar to the profiles when the two drugs are administered as separate tablets and there are no pharmacokinetic interactions between the two components.

Preclinical Safety Data: In co-administration studies in animals, the addition of misoprostol did not enhance the toxic effects of diclofenac. The combination was also shown not to be teratogenic or mutagenic. The individual components show no evidence of carcinogenic potential.
Misoprostol in multiples of the recommended therapeutic dose in animals has produced gastric mucosal hyperplasia. This characteristic response to E-series prostaglandins reverts to normal on discontinuation of the compound.

Pharmaceutical particulars
List of excipients: Arthrotec 50 tablets contain: Lactose, microcrystalline cellulose, maize starch, povidone K-30, cellulose acetate phthalate, diethyl phthalate, methylhydroxypropylcellulose, crospovidone, magnesium stearate, hydrogenated castor oil, colloidal anhydrous silica.

Incompatibilities: None known.

Shelf-life: Arthrotec 50 has a shelf-life of 3 years when stored in cold-formed blisters.

Special precautions for storage: Store in a dry place at or below 25°C.

Nature and contents of container: Arthrotec 50 is presented in cold-formed aluminium blisters in pack sizes of 60 and 140 tablets.

Instructions for use/handling: None.

Marketing authorisation holder: Monsanto p.l.c., PO Box 53, Lane End Road, High Wycombe, Bucks HP12 4HL.

Marketing authorisation number 08821/0006

Date of approval/revision of SPC June 1997.

Legal category POM.

ARTHROTEC* 75

Qualitative and quantitative composition Each tablet consists of a gastro-resistant core containing 75 mg diclofenac sodium surrounded by an outer mantle containing 200 mcg misoprostol.

Pharmaceutical form White, round, biconvex tablets marked ⊕ on one side and 'Searle 1421' on the other side.

Clinical particulars
Therapeutic indications: Arthrotec 75 is indicated for patients who require the non-steroidal anti-inflammatory drug diclofenac together with misoprostol.
The diclofenac component of Arthrotec 75 is indicated for the symptomatic treatment of osteoarthritis and rheumatoid arthritis. The misoprostol component of Arthrotec 75 is indicated for patients with a special need for the prophylaxis of NSAID-induced gastric and duodenal ulceration.

Posology and method of administration:
Adults: One tablet to be taken with food, two times daily. Tablets should be swallowed whole, not chewed.
Elderly/renal impairment/hepatic impairment: No adjustment of dosage is necessary in the elderly or in patients with hepatic impairment or mild to moderate renal impairment as pharmacokinetics are not altered to any clinically relevant extent. Nevertheless patients with renal or hepatic impairment should be closely monitored (see also *Undesirable effects*).
Children: The safety and efficacy of Arthrotec 75 in children has not been established.

Contra-indications: Arthrotec 75 is contra-indicated in:
- Patients with active gastric or duodenal ulceration or who have active GI bleeding or other active bleedings e.g. cerebrovascular bleedings.
- Pregnant women and in women planning a pregnancy.
- Patients who are lactating or who are breast feeding.
- Patients with a known hypersensitivity to diclofenac, aspirin, other NSAIDs, misoprostol, other prostaglandins, or any other ingredient of the product.
- Patients in whom attacks of asthma, urticaria or acute rhinitis are precipitated by aspirin or other non-steroidal anti-inflammatory agents.

Special warnings and special precautions for use:
Warnings:
Use in pre-menopausal women (see also Contra-indications): Arthrotec 75 should not be used in pre-menopausal women unless they use effective contraception and have been advised of the risks of taking the product if pregnant (see *Pregnancy and Lactation*).

Precautions: Arthrotec 75, in common with other NSAIDs, may decrease platelet aggregation and prolong bleeding time. Extra supervision is recommended in haematopoietic disorders or in conditions with defective coagulation or in patients with a history of cerebrovascular bleeding.
Fluid retention and oedema have been observed in patients taking NSAIDs, including Arthrotec 75. Therefore, Arthrotec 75 should be used with caution in patients with compromised cardiac function or other conditions predisposing to fluid retention.
In patients with renal, cardiac or hepatic impairment caution is required since the use of NSAIDs may result in deterioration of renal function. In the following conditions Arthrotec 75 should be used only in exceptional circumstances and with close clinical monitoring: advanced cardiac failure, advanced kidney failure, advanced liver disease.
Similarly caution is also required in patients with diuretic treatment or otherwise at risk of hypovolaemia. The dose should be kept as low as possible and renal functions should be monitored.
Caution is required in patients suffering from ulcerative colitis or Crohn's Disease.
All patients who are receiving long-term treatment with NSAIDs should be monitored as a precautionary measure (e.g. renal, hepatic function and blood counts).

Interactions with other medicaments and other forms of interaction: NSAIDs may attenuate the natriuretic efficacy of diuretics due to inhibition of intrarenal synthesis of prostaglandins. Concomitant treatment with potassium-sparing diuretics may be associated with increased serum potassium levels, hence serum potassium should be monitored.
Because of their effect on renal prostaglandins, cyclo-oxygenase inhibitors such as diclofenac can increase the nephrotoxicity of cyclosporin.
Steady state plasma lithium and digoxin levels may be increased and ketoconazole levels may be decreased.
Pharmacodynamic studies with diclofenac have shown no potentiation of oral hypoglycaemic and anticoagulant drugs. However, as interactions have been reported with other NSAIDs, caution and adequate monitoring are nevertheless advised (see statement on platelet aggregation in *Precautions*).
Because of decreased platelet aggregation caution is also advised when using Arthrotec 75 with anti-coagulants.
Caution is advised when methotrexate is administered concurrently with NSAIDs because of possible enhancement of its toxicity by the NSAID as a result of increase in methotrexate plasma levels.
Concomitant use with other NSAIDs or with corticosteroids may increase the frequency of side effects generally.

Pregnancy and lactation:
Pregnancy: Arthrotec 75 is contra-indicated in pregnant women and in women planning a pregnancy as misoprostol may increase uterine tone and contractions in pregnancy which could produce miscarriage. Also diclofenac may cause premature closure of the ductus arteriosus.
Lactation: Arthrotec 75 should not be administered during breast feeding as there are no data on the excretion into breast milk for either misoprostol or diclofenac.

Effects on ability to drive and use machines: Patients who experience dizziness or other central nervous system disturbances while taking NSAIDs should refrain from driving or operating machinery.

Undesirable effects:
Common:
General: Headache, dizziness.
Gastrointestinal: Abdominal pain, diarrhoea, nausea, dyspepsia, flatulence, vomiting, gastritis and eructation.
Diarrhoea is usually mild to moderate and transient and can be minimised by taking Arthrotec 75 with food and by avoiding the use of predominantly magnesium-containing antacids.
Skin: Skin rashes.

Infrequent:
General: Tiredness, peripheral oedema.
Gastrointestinal: Peptic ulcer, stomatitis, decrease in haemoglobin associated with GI blood loss, oesophageal lesions.
Liver: Elevations of SGPT, SGOT, alkaline phosphatase or bilirubin.
Female reproductive system: Menorrhagia, intermenstrual bleeding and vaginal bleeding have been reported in pre-menopausal women and vaginal bleeding in post-menopausal women.

Rarely or very rarely:
Blood system: Thrombocytopenia, leucopenia, agranulocytosis, haemolytic anaemia, aplastic anaemia.
Gastrointestinal: Anorexia, dry mouth, bleeding (haematemesis, melaena), perforated ulcer, glossitis, other GI complaints (ulcerative colitis, Crohn's disease), constipation.
Liver: Hepatitis with or without jaundice.
Skin/hypersensitivity: Urticaria, erythema multiforme, photosensitivity reactions, Steven-Johnson's syndrome, Lyell's syndrome (acute toxic epidermal necrolysis), hypersensitivity including bronchospasm and angioedema, purpura including allergic purpura and hair loss.
CNS: Drowsiness, paraesthesia, memory disorders, disorientation, visual disturbances, tinnitus, insomnia, irritability, convulsions, depression, anxiety, nightmares, tremors, psychotic reactions, taste disturbance.
Renal: As a class NSAIDs have been associated with renal pathology including papillary necrosis, interstitial nephritis, nephrotic syndrome and renal failure.
Other: In isolated cases worsening of inflammation associated with infections have been reported in association with NSAID treatment.

Overdose: The toxic dose of Arthrotec 75 has not been determined and there is no experience of overdosage. Intensification of the pharmacological effects may occur with overdosage. Management of acute poisoning with NSAIDs essentially consists of supportive and symptomatic measures. It is reasonable to take measures to reduce absorption of any recently consumed drug by forced emesis, gastric lavage or activated charcoal.

Pharmacological properties
Pharmacodynamic properties: Arthrotec 75 is a non-steroidal, anti-inflammatory drug which is effective in treating the signs and symptoms of arthritic conditions.

This activity is due to the presence of diclofenac which has been shown to have anti-inflammatory and analgesic properties.

Arthrotec 75 also contains the gastroduodenal mucosal protective component misoprostol which is a synthetic prostaglandin E_1 analogue that enhances several of the factors that maintain gastroduodenal mucosal integrity.

Arthrotec 75 administered BID provides 200 µg less misoprostol than Arthrotec TID whilst providing the same daily dose (150 mg) of diclofenac and may offer a better therapeutic ratio for certain patients.

Pharmacokinetic properties: The pharmacokinetic profiles of diclofenac and misoprostol administered as Arthrotec 75 are similar to the profiles when the two drugs are administered as separate tablets and there are no pharmacokinetic interactions between the two components.

Diclofenac sodium is completely absorbed from the gastrointestinal (GI) tract after fasting oral administration. Only 50% of the absorbed dose is systemically available due to first pass metabolism. Peak plasma levels are achieved in 2 hours (range 1–4 hours), and the area-under the plasma-concentration curve (AUC) is dose proportional within the range of 25 mg to 150 mg. The extent of diclofenac sodium absorption is not significantly affected by food intake.

The terminal half life is approximately 2 hours. Clearance and volume of distribution are about 350 ml/min and 550 ml/kg, respectively. More than 99% of diclofenac sodium is reversibly bound to human plasma ablumin, and this has been shown not to be age dependent.

Diclofenac sodium is eliminated through metabolism and subsequent urinary and biliary excretion of the glucuronide and the sulfate conjugates of the metabolites. Approximately 65% of the dose is excreted in the urine and 35% in the bile. Less than 1% of the parent drug is excreted unchanged.

Misoprostol is rapidly and extensively absorbed, and it undergoes rapid metabolism to its active metabolite, misoprostol acid, which is eliminated with an elimination $t_{\frac{1}{2}}$ of about 30 minutes. No accumulation of misoprostol acid was found in multiple-dose studies, and plasma steady waste was achieved within 2 days. The serum protein binding of misoprostol acid is less than 90%. Approximately 70% of the administered dose is excreted in the urine, mainly as bioligically inactive metabolites.

Single and multiple dose studies have been conducted comparing the pharmacokinetics of Arthrotec 75 with the diclofenac 75 mg and misoprostol 200 mcg components administered separately. Bioequivalence between the two methods of providing diclofenac were demonstrable for AUC and absorption rate (Cmax/AUC). In the steady state comparisons under fasted conditions bioequivalence was demonstrable in terms of AUC. Food reduced the rate and extent of absorption of diclofenac for both Arthrotec 75 and co-administered diclofenac. Despite the virtually identical mean AUCs in the fed, steady state, statistical bioequivalence was not established. This however is due to the broad co-efficients of variation in these studies due to the wide inter-individual variability in time to absorption and the extensive first-pass metabolism that occurs with diclofenac.

Bioequivalence in terms of AUC (0–24h) was demonstrable when comparing steady state pharmacokinetics of Arthrotec 75 given b.i.d. with diclofenac 50 mg/misoprostol 200 mcg given t.i.d., both regimens providing a total daily dose of 150 mg diclofenac.

With respect to administration of misoprostol, bioequivalence was demonstrated after a single dose of Arthrotec 75 or misoprostol administered alone. Under steady state conditions food decreases the misoprostol Cmax after Arthrotec 75 administration and slightly delays absorption, but the AUC is equivalent.

Preclinical safety data: In co-administration studies in animals, the addition of misoprostol did not enhance the toxic effects of diclofenac. The combination was also shown not to be teratogenic or mutagenic. The individual components show no evidence of carcinogenic potential.

Misoprostol in multiples of the recommended therapeutic dose in animals has produced gastric mucosal hyperplasia. This characteristic response to E-series prostaglandins reverts to normal on discontinuation of the compound.

Pharmaceutical particulars
List of excipients: Arthrotec 75 tablets contain: Lactose, microcrystalline cellulose, maize starch, povidone K-30, methylacrylic acid copolymer type C, sodium hydroxide, talc, triethylcitrate, methylhydroxypropylcellulose, crospovidone, magnesium stearate, hydrogenated castor oil, colloidal enhydrous silica.

Incompatibilities: None known.

Shelf life: Arthrotec 75 has a shelf-life of 3 years when stored in cold-formed blisters.

Special precautions for storage: Store in a dry place, at or below 25°C.

Nature and contents of container: Arthrotec 75 is presented in cold formed aluminium blisters in pack sizes of 10 and 60 tablets.

Instructions for use/handling: None.

Marketing authorisation holder: Monsanto p.l.c., Trading as Searle, PO Box 53, Lane End Road, High Wycombe, Bucks HP12 4HL.

Marketing authorisation number 08821/0044.

Date of approval/revision of SPC January 1997.

Legal category POM.

BREVINOR* TABLETS

Qualitative and quantitative composition Each tablet contains 0.5 milligrams Norethisterone BP and 35 micrograms Ethinyloestradiol BP.

Pharmaceutical form Blue, flat, circular, bevel-edged tablet inscribed 'SEARLE' on one side and 'BX' on the other side.

Clinical particulars
Therapeutic indications: Brevinor is indicated for oral contraception, with the benefit of a low intake of oestrogen.

Posology and method of administration:
Oral administration: The dosage of Brevinor for the initial cycle of therapy is 1 tablet taken at the same time each day from the first day of the menstrual cycle. For subsequent cycles, no tablets are taken for 7 days, then a new course is started of 1 tablet daily for the next 21 days. This sequence of 21 days on treatment, seven days off treatment is repeated for as long as contraception is required.

Patients unable to start taking Brevinor tablets on the first day of the menstrual cycle may start treatment on any day up to and including the 5th day of the menstrual cycle.

Patients starting on day 1 of their period will be protected at once. Those patients delaying therapy up to day 5 may not be protected immediately and it is recommended that another method of contraception is used for the first 7 days of tablet-taking. Suitable methods are condoms, caps plus spermicides and intra-uterine devices. The rhythm, temperature and cervical-mucus methods should not be relied upon.

Tablet omissions: Tablets must be taken daily in order to maintain adequate hormone levels and contraceptive efficacy.

If a tablet is missed within 12 hours of the correct dosage time then the missed tablet should be taken as soon as possible, even if this means taking 2 tablets on the same day, this will ensure that contraceptive protection is maintained. If one or more tablets are missed for more than 12 hours from the correct dosage time it is recommended that the patient takes the last missed tablet as soon as possible and then continues to take the rest of the tablets in the normal manner. In addition, it is recommended that extra contraceptive protection, such as a condom, is used for the next 7 days.

Patients who have missed one or more of the last 7 tablets in a pack should be advised to start the next pack of tablets as soon as the present one has finished (i.e. without the normal seven day gap between treatments). This reduces the risk of contraceptive failure resulting from tablets being missed close to a 7 day tablet free period.

Changing from another oral contraceptive: In order to ensure that contraception is maintained it is advised that the first dose of Brevinor tablets is taken on the day immediately after the patient has finished the previous pack of tablets.

Use after childbirth, miscarriage or abortion: Providing the patient is not breast feeding the first dose of Brevinor tablets should be taken on the 21st day after childbirth. This will ensure the patient is protected immediately. If there is any delay in taking the first dose, contraception may not be established until 7 days after the first tablet has been taken. In these circumstances patients should be advised that extra contraceptive methods will be necessary.

After a miscarriage or abortion patients can take the first dose of Brevinor tablets on the next day; in this way they will be protected immediately.

Contra-indications: As with all combined progestogen/oestrogen oral contraceptives, the following conditions should be regarded as contra-indications:

(i) Thrombophlebitis, thrombo-embolic disorders, cerebrovascular disorders, coronary artery disease, myocardial infarction, angina, hyperlipidaemia or a history of these conditions.

(ii) Acute or severe chronic liver disease, including liver tumours, Dubin-Johnson or Rotor syndrome.

(iii) History during pregnancy of idiopathic jaundice, severe pruritus or pemphigoid gestationis.

(iv) Known or suspected breast or genital cancer.

(v) Known or suspected oestrogen-dependent neoplasia.

(vi) Undiagnosed abnormal vaginal bleeding.

(vii) A history of migraines classified as classical focal or crescendo.

(viii) Pregnancy.

Special warnings and special precautions for use: Women taking oral contraceptives require careful observation if they have or have had any of the following conditions: breast nodules; fibrocystic disease of the breast or an abnormal mammogram; uterine fibroids; a history of severe depressive states; varicose veins; sickle-cell anaemia; diabetes; hypertension; cardiovascular disease; migraine; epilepsy; asthma; otosclerosis; multiple sclerosis; porphyria; tetany; disturbed liver functions; gallstones; kidney disease; chloasma; any condition that is likely to worsen during pregnancy. The worsening or first appearance of any of these conditions may indicate that the oral contraceptive should be stopped. Discontinue treatment if there is a gradual or sudden, partial or complete loss of vision or any evidence of ocular changes, onset or aggravation of migraine or development of headache of a new kind which is recurrent, persistent or severe.

Gastro-intestinal upsets, such as vomiting and diarrhoea, may interfere with the absorption of the tablets leading to a reduction in contraceptive efficacy. Patients should continue to take Brevinor, but they should also be encouraged to use another contraceptive method during the period of gastro-intestinal upset and for the next 7 days.

Progestogen/oestrogen preparations should be used with caution in patients with a history of hepatic dysfunction or hypertension.

A statistical association between the use of oral contraceptives and the occurrence of thrombosis, embolism or haemorrhage has been reported. Patients receiving oral contraceptives should be kept under regular surveillance, in view of the possibility of development of conditions such as thromboembolism.

The risk of coronary artery disease in women taking oral contraceptives is increased by the presence of other predisposing factors such as cigarette smoking, hypercholesterolaemia, obesity, diabetes, history of pre-eclamptic toxaemia and increasing age. After the age of thirty-five years, the patient and physician should carefully re-assess the risk/benefit ratio of using combined oral contraceptives as opposed to alternative methods of contraception.

Brevinor should be discontinued at least four weeks before, and for two weeks following, elective operations and during immobilisation. Patients undergoing injection treatment for varicose veins should not resume taking Brevinor until 3 months after the last injection.

Benign and malignant liver tumours have been associated with oral contraceptive use. The relationship between occurrence of liver tumours and use of female sex hormones is not known at present. These tumours may rupture causing intra-abdominal bleeding. If the patient presents with a mass or tenderness in the right upper quadrant or an acute abdomen, the possible presence of a tumour should be considered.

An increased risk of congenital abnormalities, including heart defects and limb defects, has been reported following the use of sex hormones, including oral contraceptives, in pregnancy. If the patient does not adhere to the prescribed schedule, the possibility of pregnancy should be considered at the time of the first missed period and further use of oral contraceptives should be withheld until pregnancy has been ruled out. It is recommended that for any patient who has missed two consecutive periods, pregnancy should be ruled out before continuing the contraceptive regimen. If pregnancy is confirmed the patient should be advised of the potential risks to the foetus and the advisability of continuing the pregnancy should be discussed in the light of these risks. It is advisable to discontinue Brevinor three months before a planned pregnancy.

The risk of arterial thrombosis associated with combined oral contraceptives increases with age, and this risk is aggravated by cigarette smoking. The use of combined oral contraceptives by women in the older age group, especially those who are cigarette smokers, should therefore be discouraged and alternative methods advised.

The use of this product in patients suffering from epilepsy, migraine, asthma or cardiac dysfunction may result in exacerbation of these disorders because of fluid retention. Caution should also be observed in patients who wear contact lenses.

Decreased glucose tolerance may occur in diabetic patients on this treatment, and their control must be carefully supervised.

The use of oral contraceptives has also been associated with a possible increased incidence of gall bladder disease.

Women with a history of oligomenorrhoea or secondary amenorrhoea or young women without regular cycles may have a tendency to remain anovulatory or to become amenorrhoeic after discontinuation of oral contraceptives. Women with these pre-existing problems should be advised of this possibility and encouraged to use other contraceptive methods.

Numerous epidemiological studies have been reported on the risks of ovarian, endometrial, cervical and breast cancer in women using combined oral contraceptives. The evidence is clear that combined oral contraceptives offer substantial protection against both ovarian and endometrial cancer.

An increased risk of cervical cancer in long-term users of combined oral contraceptives has been reported in some studies, but there continues to be controversy about the extent to which this is attributable to the confounding effects of sexual behaviour and other factors.

A meta-analysis from 54 epidemiological studies reported that there is a slightly increased relative risk (RR=1.24) of having breast cancer diagnosed in women who are currently using combined oral contraceptives (COCs). The observed pattern of increased risk may be due to an earlier diagnosis of breast cancer in COC users, the biological effects of COCs or a combination of both. The additional breast cancers diagnosed in current users of COCs or in women who have used COCs in the last ten years are more likely to be localised to the breast than those in women who never used COCs.

Breast cancer is rare among women under 40 years of age whether or not they take COCs. Whilst this background risk increases with age, the excess number of breast cancer diagnoses in current and recent COC users is small in relation to the overall risk of breast cancer (see bar chart).

The most important risk factor for breast cancer in COC users is the age women discontinue the COC; the older the age at stopping, the more breast cancers are diagnosed. Duration of use is less important and the excess risk gradually disappears during the course of the 10 years after stopping COC use such that by 10 years there appears to be no excess.

The possible increase in risk of breast cancer should be discussed with the user and weighed against the benefits of COCs taking into account the evidence that they offer substantial protection against the risk of developing certain other cancers (e.g. ovarian and endometrial cancer).

Interactions with other medicaments and other forms of interaction: Some drugs may modify the metabolism of Brevinor reducing its effectiveness; these include certain sedatives, antibiotics, anti-epileptic and anti-arthritic drugs. During the time such agents are used concurrently, it is advised that mechanical contraceptives also be used.

The results of a large number of laboratory tests have been shown to be influenced by the use of oestrogen containing oral contraceptives, which may limit their diagnostic value. Among these are: biochemical markers of thyroid and liver function; plasma levels of carrier proteins, triglycerides, coagulation and fibrinolysis factors.

Pregnancy and lactation: Contra-indicated in pregnancy.

Patients who are fully breast-feeding should not take Brevinor tablets since, in common with other combined oral contraceptives, the oestrogen component may reduce the amount of milk produced. In addition, active ingredients or their metabolites have been detected in the milk of mothers taking oral contraceptives. The effect of Brevinor on breast-fed infants has not been determined.

Effects on ability to drive and use machines: None.

Undesirable effects: As with all oral contraceptives, there may be slight nausea at first, weight gain or breast discomfort, which soon disappear.

Other side-effects known or suspected to occur with oral contraceptives include gastro-intestinal symptoms, changes in libido and appetite, headache, exacerbation of existing uterine fibroid disease, depression, and changes in carbohydrate, lipid and vitamin metabolism.

Spotting or bleeding may occur during the first few cycles. Usually menstrual bleeding becomes light and occasionally there may be no bleeding during the tablet-free days.

Hypertension, which is usually reversible on discontinuing treatment, has occurred in a small percentage of women taking oral contraceptives.

Overdose: Overdosage may be manifested by nausea, vomiting, breast enlargement and vaginal bleeding. There is no specific antidote and treatment should be symptomatic. Gastric lavage may be employed if the overdose is large and the patient is seen sufficiently early (within four hours).

Pharmacological properties

Pharmacodynamic properties: The mode of action of Brevinor is similar to that of other progestogen/oestrogen oral contraceptives and includes the inhibition of ovulation, the thickening of cervical mucus so as to constitute a barrier to sperm and the rendering of the endometrium unreceptive to implantation. Such activity is exerted through a combined effect on one or more of the following: hypothalamus, anterior pituitary, ovary, endometrium and cervical mucus.

Pharmacokinetic properties: Norethisterone is rapidly and completely absorbed after oral administration, peak plasma concentrations occurring in the majority of subjects between 1 and 3 hours. Due to first-pass metabolism, blood levels after oral administration are 60% of those after i.v. administration. The half life of elimination varies from 5 to 12 hours, with a mean of 7.6 hours. Norethisterone is metabolised mainly in the liver. Approximately 60% of the administered dose is excreted as metabolites in urine and faeces.

Ethinyloestradiol is rapidly and well absorbed from the gastro-intestinal tract but is subject to some first-pass metabolism in the gut-wall. Compared to many other oestrogens it is only slowly metabolised in the liver. Excretion is via the kidneys with some appearing also in the faeces.

Preclinical safety data: The toxicity of norethisterone is very low. Reports of teratogenic effects in animals are uncommon. No carcinogenic effects have been found even in long-term studies.

Long-term continuous administration of oestrogens in some animals increases the frequency of carcinoma of the breast, cervix, vagina and liver.

Pharmaceutical particulars

List of excipients: Brevinor tablets contain: Maize starch, polyvidone, magnesium stearate, lactose and E132.

Incompatibilities: None stated.

Shelf life: The shelf life of Brevinor tablets is 5 years.

Special precautions for storage: Store in a dry place, below 25°C, away from direct sunlight.

Nature and contents of container: Brevinor tablets are supplied in pvc/foil blister packs of 21 and 63 tablets.

Special instructions for use/handling: None.

Marketing authorisation holder: Monsanto p.l.c., PO Box 53, Lane End Road, High Wycombe, Bucks HP12 4HL.

Marketing authorisation number 08821/0037.

Date of approval/revision of SPC February 1998.

Legal category POM.

CYTOTEC*

Presentation White/off-white, hexagonal tablet, scored on both sides, engraved 'SEARLE 1461' on one side. Each tablet contains misoprostol 200 micrograms.

Uses

Indications: Cytotec is indicated for the healing of duodenal ulcer and gastric ulcer including those induced by nonsteroidal anti-inflammatory drugs (NSAID) in arthritic patients at risk, whilst continuing their NSAID therapy. In addition Cytotec can be used for the prophylaxis of NSAID-induced ulcers.

Actions: Cytotec is an analogue of naturally occurring prostaglandin E_1 which promotes peptic ulcer healing and symptomatic relief.

Estimated cumulative numbers of breast cancers per 10,000 women diagnosed in 5 years of use and up to 10 years after stopping COCs, compared with numbers of breast cancers diagnosed in 10,000 women who had never used COCs.

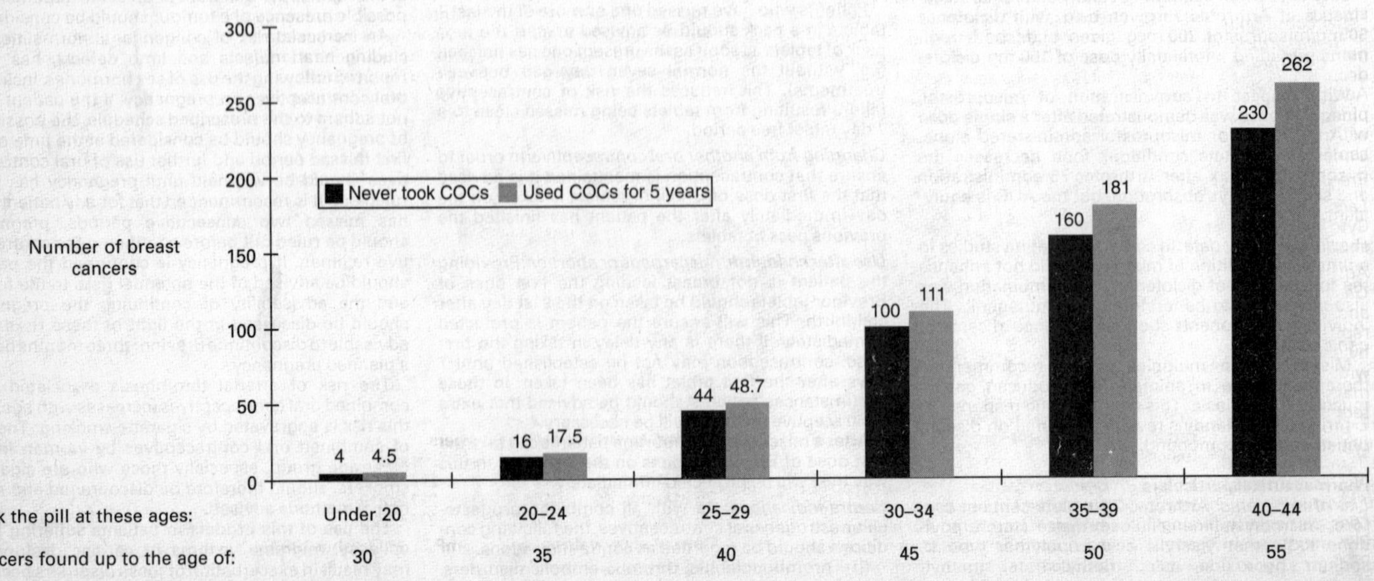

Cytotec protects the gastroduodenal mucosa by inhibiting basal, stimulated and nocturnal acid secretion and by reducing the volume of gastric secretions, the proteolytic activity of the gastric fluid, and increasing bicarbonate and mucus secretion.

Dosage and administration
Adults:
Healing of duodenal ulcer, gastric ulcer and NSAID-induced peptic ulcer: 800 micrograms daily in two or four divided doses taken with breakfast and/or each main meal and at bedtime.

Treatment should be given initially for at least 4 weeks even if symptomatic relief has been achieved sooner. In most patients ulcers will be healed in 4 weeks but treatment may be continued for up to 8 weeks if required. If the ulcer relapses further treatment courses may be given.

Prophylaxis of NSAID-induced peptic ulcer: 200 micrograms twice daily, three times daily or four times daily. Treatment can be continued as required. Dosage should be individualised according to the clinical condition of each patient.

Elderly: The usual dosage may be used.

Renal impairment: Available evidence indicates that no adjustment of dosage is necessary in patients with renal impairment.

Hepatic impairment: Cytotec is metabolised by fatty acid oxidising systems present in organs throughout the body. Its metabolism and plasma levels are therefore unlikely to be affected markedly in patients with hepatic impairment.

Children: Use of Cytotec in children has not yet been evaluated in the treatment of peptic ulceration or NSAID-induced peptic ulcer disease.

Contra-indications, warnings, etc
Contra-indications: Cytotec is contra-indicated in pregnant women and in women planning a pregnancy as it increases uterine tone and contractions in pregnancy which may cause partial or complete expulsion of the products of conception. It is also contra-indicated in patients with a known allergy to prostaglandins.

Warnings
Use in pre-menopausal women (see also Contra-indications): Cytotec should not be used in pre-menopausal women unless the patient requires non-steroidal anti-inflammatory (NSAID) therapy and is at high risk of complications from NSAID-induced ulceration.

In such patients it is advised that Cytotec should only be used if the patient:
—takes effective contraceptive measures
—has been advised of the risks of taking Cytotec if pregnant (see Contra-indications).

Precautions: The results of clinical studies indicate that Cytotec does not produce hypotension at dosages effective in promoting the healing of gastric and duodenal ulcers. Nevertheless, Cytotec should be used with caution in the presence of disease states where hypotension might precipitate severe complications, eg, cerebrovascular disease, coronary artery disease or severe peripheral vascular disease including hypertension.

There is no evidence that Cytotec has adverse effects on glucose metabolism in human volunteers or patients with diabetes mellitus.

Drug interactions: Cytotec is predominantly metabolised via fatty acid oxidising systems and has shown no adverse effect on the hepatic microsomal mixed function oxidase (P450) enzyme system. In specific studies no clinically significant pharmacokinetic interaction has been demonstrated with antipyrine, diazepam and propranolol. In extensive clinical studies no drug interactions have been attributed to Cytotec. Additional evidence shows no clinically important pharmacokinetic or pharmacodynamic interaction with nonsteroidal anti-inflammatory drugs including aspirin, diclofenac and ibuprofen.

Pregnancy: See Contra-indications.

Lactation: It is not known if the active metabolite of Cytotec is excreted in breast milk, therefore Cytotec should not be administered during breast feeding.

Adverse effects:
Gastrointestinal system: Diarrhoea has been reported and is occasionally severe and prolonged and may require withdrawal of the drug. It can be minimised by using single doses not exceeding 200 micrograms with food and by avoiding the use of predominantly magnesium containing antacids when an antacid is required.

Abdominal pain with or without associated dyspepsia or diarrhoea can follow misoprostol therapy.

Other gastrointestinal adverse effects reported include dyspepsia, flatulence, nausea and vomiting.

Female reproductive system: Menorrhagia, vaginal bleeding and intermenstrual bleeding have been reported in pre- and post-menopausal women.

Other adverse events: Skin rashes have been reported. Dizziness has been infrequently reported.

The pattern of adverse events associated with Cytotec is similar when an NSAID is given concomitantly.

Overdosage: Intensification of pharmacological effects may occur with overdose. In the event of overdosage symptomatic and supportive therapy should be given as appropriate. In clinical trials patients have tolerated 1200 micrograms daily for three months without significant adverse effects.

Pharmaceutical precautions Store in a dry place below 30°C (86°F).

Legal category POM.

Package quantities Foil/foil blister pack of 60 (OP).

Further information Cytotec in multiples of the recommended therapeutic dose in animals has produced gastric mucosal hyperplasia. This characteristic response to E prostaglandins reverts to normal on discontinuation of the compound. In patients, histological examination of gastric biopsies taken before and after treatment with misoprostol after up to one year's duration have shown no adverse tissue response attributable to misoprostol.

Inhibition of gastric secretion by Cytotec is achieved by a combination of local and systemic effects. Cytotec is rapidly absorbed following oral administration, with peak plasma levels of the active metabolite (misoprostol acid) occurring after about 30 minutes. The plasma elimination half-life of misoprostol acid is 20–40 minutes. No accumulation of misoprostol acid in plasma occurs after repeated dosing of 400 micrograms twice daily.

Product licence number 08821/0019.

DRAMAMINE*

Qualitative and quantitative composition Each tablet contains 50 mg Dimenhydrinate BP.

Pharmaceutical form Tablet.

Clinical particulars
Therapeutic indications: For OTC pack only: Motion sickness.

For non-OTC packs: Motion sickness, vertigo, nausea and vomiting associated with Meniere's disease and other labyrinthine disorders.

Posology and method of administration: For prevention of motion sickness the first dose should be taken 30 minutes before the journey.

Adults and children over 12 years: 1–2 tablets two or three times daily.

Elderly: Dosage as for adults. The elderly may be more susceptible to anticholinergic side effects.

Children: 1–6 years $\frac{1}{4}$–$\frac{1}{2}$ tablet two or three times daily. 7–12 years $\frac{1}{2}$–1 tablet two or three times daily.

Contra-indications: Dramamine is contra-indicated in patients with a hypersensitivity to dimenhydrinate, diphenhydramine and other antihistamines of similar chemical structure.

Special warnings and precautions for use:
Warnings: For OTC pack only: Warning: May cause drowsiness, if affected do not drive or operate machinery.

Precautions: Dimenhydrinate should be used with caution in patients having conditions which might be aggravated by anticholinergic therapy i.e. with raised intraocular pressure, stenosing peptic ulcer, pyloroduodenal obstruction, prostatic hypertrophy, asthma, hypertension, hyperthyroidism or severe coronary artery disease.

Dimenhydrinate should be used with caution in patients with hepatic or renal failure due to the risk of accumulation in such patients.

Interactions with other medicaments and other forms of interaction: For OTC pack only: Avoid alcoholic drink.

For non-OTC pack: In common with other antihistamines, Dramamine may potentiate the sedative effects of CNS depressants including alcohol, barbiturates, narcotic analgesics, tranquillisers and may enhance the effects of antoicholinergics such as atropine and tricyclic antidepressants. Dramamine may enhance the effect of ephedrine. Monamine oxidase inhibitors may potentiate the anticholinergic and sedative effects of antihistamines.

Dramamine may mask ototoxic symptoms associated with certain antibiotics. Patients should be advised to avoid alcoholic drinks.

Antihistamines may mask the response of the skin to allergenic skin tests.

Pregnancy and lactation:
Pregnancy: For OTC pack only: Use during pregnancy should be on the advice of your doctor.

For non-OTC pack: Reproduction studies in rats and rabbits at doses up to 20 and 25 times the human dose respectively (on a mg/kg basis) have shown no evidence of hazard.

There is inadequate evidence of safety of the use of Dramamine in human pregnancy although it has been in wide use for many years without apparent ill consequences. In view of this Dramamine should be used during pregnancy only if clearly needed.

Lactation: Diphenhydramine, a metabolite of dimenhydrinate, has been detected in breast milk. If a nursing mother is taking Dramamine the infant may exhibit some effects of the drug. In view of this Dramamine should not be administered during breast feeding unless considered essential.

Effects on ability to drive and use machines: In common with other antihistamines Dramamine may cause drowsiness. Patients affected in this way should be advised not to drive or operate machinery.

Undesirable effects: For OTC pack only: When used for the prevention and treatment of motion sickness, sedation is the most commonly reported effect. Occasionally allergy or anaphylaxis have been reported.

For non-OTC pack only: Sedation is the most commonly reported effect. Incoordination and confusion (particularly in the elderly) may also occur. Occasionally allergy and anaphylaxis have been reported. Atropine-like effects such as blurred vision, dry mouth, tachycardia, constipation, urinary hesitancy, tightness of the chest and thickening of secretions may be associated with antihistamines. Other adverse effects which may occur include: tremors, paradoxical excitability (especially in children), skin rash and photosensitivity.

Overdose: Symptoms of overdosage may comprise drowsiness, dizziness and ataxia together with anticholinergic effects such as dry mouth, flushing of the face, dilated pupils, tachycardia, pyrexia, headache and urinary retention.

In massive overdose and in children the central effects of antihistamines may cause convulsions, hallucinations, excitement and respiratory depression. Such symptoms may be delayed. Treatment should consist of gastric aspiration and lavage, administration of activated charcoal and supportive measures. Diazepam may be required for the treatment of convulsions.

Pharmacological properties
Pharmacodynamic properties: The active ingredient of Dramamine, dimehydrinate is the chlorotheophylline salt of diphenhydramine and is an H_1-receptor blocking agent.

Pharmacokinetic properties: An unpublished study of dimenhydrinate 50 mg in 12 volunteers demonstrated mean peak plasma concentrations of 72.1 ng/ml at a mean of 2.29 hours.

Preclinical safety data: In acute toxicity studies in rats and mice (oral, i.p.) LD50s of 149–203 mg/kg (mouse) and 1,320 mg/kg (rat) were determined. Subacute studies in cats (50–100 mg/kg) produced no pathological changes in major body organs and chronic studies in rodents at a mean dose of 22 mg/kg/day showed no abnormalities. Reproduction studies in rats and rabbits at 20–25 times the human dose (mg/kg) have showed no evidence of foetotoxicity.

Pharmaceutical particulars
List of excipients: Dramamine contains lactose, corn starch, pre-gelatinised maize starch and magnesium stearate.

Incompatibilities: None known.

Shelf life: Dramamine tablets have a shelf life of 5 years when packed in foil/PVC blister packs or amber glass bottles and 3 years when packed in HDPE bottles.

Special precautions for storage: Store below 30°C.

Nature and contents of container: OTC pack: Foil/PVC blister strips containing 10 or 12 tablets in a cardboard carton.

Non-OTC pack: 100 PVC tablets packed in foil blister strips or amber glass bottles with screw caps or HDPE bottles with a tamper-evident closure. Bottles are enclosed within a cardboard carton.

Instructions for use/handling: Dramamine may be powdered and dissolved in any acceptable aqueous fluid medium, provided that a concentration of 3 mg/ml is not exceeded. Above this concentration not all of the active constituent may dissolve.

Marketing authorisation holder: Monsanto p.l.c., PO Box 53, Lane End Road, High Wycombe, Bucks HP12 4HL.

Marketing authorisation number 8821/0035.

Date of approval/revision of SPC January 1996.

Legal category P.

EFAMAST 40

Qualitative and quantitative composition

Active Constituent	*Quantity/Dose Unit*
Gamolenic acid provided by Evening Primrose Oil.	40 mg

Pharmaceutical form Soft gelatin capsules.

Clinical particulars
Therapeutic indications: Efamast 40 is indicated for the symptomatic relief of pre-menstrual breast pain (cyclical mastalgia) and non-cyclical mastalgia.

Posology and method of administration
Adults and elderly: 3–4 capsules should be taken orally twice daily, providing a total dose of 6–8 capsules.

It is suggested that patients start treatment at the highest recommended dose.

Some patients may not begin to show a clinical response to treatment for 8–12 weeks due to the gradual onset of action of Efamast 40. Once a clinical response has been achieved, the treatment may be stopped or continued at a lower maintenance dose.

Contra-indications: None known.

Special warnings and precautions for use: Breast pain may occasionally be a sign of breast cancer. The doctor should be satisfied that the patient does not have breast cancer.

Interactions with other medicaments and other Forms of Interaction: Efamast 40 may have the potential to make manifest undiagnosed temporal lobe epilepsy, especially in schizophrenic patients and/or those who are receiving known epileptogenic drugs such as the phenothiazines. Physicians are advised to monitor carefully the effects of Efamast 40 in patients on epileptogenic drugs, or in any individuals with a history of epilepsy.

Pregnancy and lactation:
Pregnancy: No teratogenic effects have been observed in animal studies. However, as with all medicines, caution is advised concerning administration in the first trimester of pregnancy.

Lactation: Efamast 40 may be taken while breast feeding.

Effects on ability to drive and use machines: None.

Undesirable effects: No major adverse effects have been reported. Nausea, indigestion and headache have occurred occasionally. In rare cases, hypersensitivity reactions, including rash, urticaria, pruritus and abdominal pain have been reported. It should be noted that hypersensitivity reactions may require close medical surveillance and that such reactions may occur particularly in patients who have a history of food or other allergies.

Overdose: The only symptom noted in a few cases has been loose stools sometimes accompanied by abdominal pains. No special treatment is required.

There is a high degree of tolerance to evening primrose oil. Up to 25 ml of oil (equivalent to 50 capsules) has been administered daily for one year to children aged 5–12 years, without adverse effects other than occasional loose stools.

Pharmacological properties
Pharmacodynamic properties: Efamast 40 capsules provide an exogenous source of gamolenic acid (GLA), which may be used to restore some subnormal fatty acid levels towards physiologically normal levels.

Clinical studies demonstrate that it improves the symptoms of mastalgia, however the precise pharmacological mode of action is unclear. No undesirable pharmacological effects are known.

Pharmacokinetic properties: The pharmacokinetic profile of evening primrose oil follows that of any normal triglycerides from usual dietary sources. It is approximately 95% absorbed, metabolised in the liver and stored principally in adipose tissue.

There are no unusual pharmacokinetic properties. Gamolenic acid is the unusual fatty acid component of evening primrose oil. It is metablised rapidly to dihomogammalinolenic acid (DGLA) in the body. DGLA levels will fall to pre-treatment levels in approximately two weeks following withdrawal of evening primrose oil.

Preclinical safety data: None of relevance to the prescriber.

Pharmaceutical particulars
List of excipients: D-alpha tocopherol acetate, gelatin, glycerol, water, Opacode S-1-7020 White or Mastercote F11983 White.

Incompatibilities: None known.

Shelf life: 3 years in marketed pack.

Special precautions for storage: Store in a dry place protected from heat.

Nature and contents of container: (1) Marketed pack: PVC/PVDC blister pack (250/40 μm) with lacquered hard temper aluminium foil (20 μm) plus cardboard outer carton.

(2) Sample pack: Blister pack as above, in a plastic wallet.

Instructions for use/handling: For oral administration.

Marketing authorisation holder: Scotia Pharmaceuticals Limited, Stirling, UK FK9 4TZ.

Marketing authorisation number PL 4382/0010.

Date of first authorisation/renewal of the authorisation 24/07/90.

Date of (partial) revision of the text February 1998.

Legal category POM.

EFAMAST 80

Qualitative and quantitative composition

Active Constituent	*Quantity/Dose Unit*
Gamolenic acid provided by Evening Primrose Oil.	80 mg

Pharmaceutical form Soft gelatin capsules.

Clinical particulars
Therapeutic indications: Efamast 80 is indicated for the symptomatic relief of pre-menstrual breast pain (cyclical mastalgia) and non-cyclical mastalgia.

Posology and method of administration
Adults and elderly: 3–4 capsules should be taken orally once daily.

It is suggested that patients start treatment at the highest recommended dose.

Some patients may not begin to show a clinical response to treatment for 8–12 weeks due to the gradual onset of action of Efamast 80. Once a clinical response has been achieved, the treatment may be stopped or continued at a lower maintenance dose.

Contra-indications: None known.

Special warnings and precautions for use: Breast pain may occasionally be a sign of breast cancer. The doctor should be satisfied that the patient does not have breast cancer.

Interactions with other medicaments and other Forms of Interaction: Efamast 80 may have the potential to make manifest undiagnosed temporal lobe epilepsy, especially in schizophrenic patients and/or those who are receiving known epileptogenic drugs such as the phenothiazines. Physicians are advised to monitor carefully the effects of Efamast 80 in patients on epileptogenic drugs, or in any individuals with a history of epilepsy.

Pregnancy and lactation:
Pregnancy: No teratogenic effects have been observed in animal studies. However, as with all medicines, caution is advised concerning administration in the first trimester of pregnancy.

Lactation: Efamast 80 may be taken while breast feeding.

Effects on ability to drive and use machines: None.

Undesirable effects: No major adverse effects have been reported. Nausea, indigestion and headache have occurred occasionally. In rare cases, hypersensitivity reactions, including rash, urticaria, pruritus and abdominal pain have been reported. It should be noted that hypersensitivity reactions may require close medical surveillance and that such reactions may occur particularly in patients who have a history of food or other allergies.

Overdose: The only symptom noted in a few cases has been loose stools sometimes accompanied by abdominal pains. No special treatment is required.

There is a high degree of tolerance to evening primrose oil. Up to 25 ml of oil (equivalent to 36 capsules) has been administered daily for one year to children aged 5–12 years, without adverse effects other than occasional loose stools.

Pharmacological properties
Pharmacodynamic properties: Efamast 80 capsules provide an exogenous source of gamolenic acid (GLA), which may be used to restore some subnormal fatty acid levels towards physiologically normal levels.

Clinical studies demonstrate that it improves the symptoms of mastalgia, however the precise pharmacological mode of action is unclear. No undesirable pharmacological effects are known.

Pharmacokinetic properties: The pharmacokinetic profile of evening primrose oil follows that of any normal triglycerides from usual dietary sources. It is approximately 95% absorbed, metabolised in the liver and stored principally in adipose tissue.

There are no unusual pharmacokinetic properties. Gamolenic acid is the unusual fatty acid component of evening primrose oil. It is metablised rapidly to dihomogammalinolenic acid (DGLA) in the body. DGLA levels will fall to pre-treatment levels in approximately two weeks following withdrawal of evening primrose oil.

Preclinical safety data: None of relevance to the prescriber.

Pharmaceutical particulars
List of excipients:

Capsule contents:	d-alpha Tocopherol Acetate Ph Eur
Capsule shell:	Gelatin Ph Eur, Glycerol Ph Eur
White printing ink:	Opacode S-1-7020 containing shellac, soya lecithin, polydimethylsiloxane and tinanium dioxide or Mastercote F11983 containing hydroxypropylmethylcellulose and titanium dioxide.

Incompatibilities: None known.

Shelf life: 12 months in blister packs.
36 months in HDPE container.

Special precautions for storage: Store below 25°C, in a dry place protected from heat.

Nature and contents of container: Marketed pack: PVC/PVDC blister pack (250/40 μm) with lacquered hard temper aluminium foil (20 μm) plus cardboard outer carton. or HDPE container plus cardboard outer carton.

Instructions for use/handling: No special precautions necessary.

Marketing authorisation holder: Scotia Pharmaceuticals Limited, Scotia House, Castle Business Park, Stirling, UK FK9 4TZ.

Marketing authorisation number PL 04382/0043.

Date of first authorisation/renewal of the authorisation 19 February 1998.

Date of (partial) revision of the text February 1998.

Legal category POM.

ELLESTE DUET* 1 mg

Qualitative and quantitative composition 16 tablets each containing 1 mg oestradiol, 12 tablets each containing 1 mg oestradiol and 1 mg norethisterone acetate.

Pharmaceutical form Coated Tablets.

Clinical particulars
Therapeutic indications: Hormone replacement therapy for the treatment of menopausal symptoms such as sweating and flushes. Prophylaxis and treatment of the postmenopausal sequelae of oestrogen withdrawal, e.g. atrophic vaginitis, atrophic urethritis.

Elleste Duet 1 mg is designed to provide continuous oestrogen and monthly cyclical progestogen therapy after the climacteric. Oestrogen administration is continued without a break in therapy. The addition of a progestogen in the second half of each course helps to provide good control of the irregular cycles that are characteristic of the perimenopausal phase and opposes the production of endometrial hyperplasia.

Posology and method of administration:
Adults: One white tablet to be taken daily for the first 16 days followed by one pale green tablet for the next 12 days. A new cycle should then begin without any break. Therapy may start at any time in patients with established amenorrhoea or who are experiencing long intervals between spontaneous menses. In patients who are menstruating regularly, it is advised that therapy starts on the first day of bleeding. Patients changing from another cyclical preparation should complete the cycle and may then change to Elleste Duet 1 mg without a break in therapy.

Elderly: There are no special dosage requirements for elderly patients.

Children: Not to be used in children.

Contra-indications: Known or suspected pregnancy, lactation.

Active deep venous thrombosis, thromboembolic disorders, or a past history of these conditions (including coronary thrombosis, cerebrovascular accident etc).

Known or suspected cancer of the breast.

Known or suspected oestrogen-dependent neoplasia.

Abnormal genital bleeding, endometriosis.

Severe cardiac or renal disease.

Sickle cell anaemia.

Congenital disturbances of lipid metabolism.

Severe diabetes mellitus with vascular changes.

Acute or chronic liver disease or a history of liver disease when the liver function tests have failed to return to normal. Previous or existing liver tumours. Rotor syndrome or Dubin-Johnson syndrome. Jaundice or general pruritus during previous pregnancy. A history of herpes gestationis, otosclerosis with deterioration in previous pregnancies. Known hypersensitivity to one of the ingredients.

Special warnings and special precautions for use: Before starting treatment, pregnancy must be excluded. If the expected bleeding fails to occur at about 28-day intervals, treatment should be stopped until pregnancy has been ruled out. As Elleste Duet 1 mg is not an oral contraceptive women should be advised to take non-hormonal measures to exclude pregnancy.

Before starting Elleste Duet 1 mg patients should have a thorough general medical and gynaecological examination with special emphasis on the body weight, blood pressure, heart, pelvic organs with an endometrial assessment if indicated, the legs and skin. Follow-up examinations are recommended at least six-monthly during treatment.

Breakthrough bleeding may occasionally occur and can be the result of poor compliance or concurrent antibiotic use. It may however indicate endometrial pathology and therefore any doubt as to its cause is an indication for endometrial evaluation, including biopsy.

Epidemiological evidence suggests that use of hormone replacement therapy (HRT) is associated with an increased relative risk of developing deep vein thrombosis (DVT) or pulmonary embolism (PE). Although this increase in relative risk is about 2–3, for healthy women the excess absolute risk of either of these conditions is about 1 in 5000 per year while taking HRT.

The increased risk of venous thromboembolism (VTE) means that caution should be exercised in using HRT in women who are likely to be at high risk of DVT or PE. Women with severe varicose veins, severe obesity (Body Mass Index >30 kg/m^2), immobilisation for 3 weeks or more, trauma or surgery requiring bed rest, are at increased risk of VTE so that the benefits of treatment with HRT will need to be weighed against risks carefully.

Consideration should be given to discontinuing treatment before elective surgery (6 weeks beforehand).

If venous thromboembolism develops after initiating therapy the drug should be discontinued.

Treatment should be stopped at once if migrainous or frequent and unusually severe headaches occur for the first time, or if there are other symptoms that are possible prodromata of vascular occlusion e.g. sudden visual disturbances.

Treatment should be stopped at once if jaundice, cholestasis, hepatitis, itching of the whole body or pregnancy occurs, or if there is a significant rise in blood pressure, the occurrence of thromboembolic disease or an increase in epileptic seizures.

Pre-existing fibroids may increase in size under the influence of oestrogens, and symptoms associated with endometriosis may be exacerbated. If this is observed, treatment should be discontinued.

There is an increased risk of gall bladder disease in women receiving postmenopausal oestrogens.

In patients with mild chronic liver disease, liver function should be checked every 8–12 weeks.

There is an increased risk of endometrial hyperplasia and carcinoma associated with unopposed oestrogen administered long-term (for more than one year). However, the appropriate addition of a progestogen to the oestrogen regimen statistically lowers the risk.

At the present time there is some evidence which suggests a slight increase in the relative risk of breast cancer in postmenopausal women receiving long-term hormone replacement therapy (more than 5 years). It is not known whether concurrent progestogen use influences this risk. Women on long-term therapy should have regular breast examinations and should be instructed in self-examination of the breast. Regular mammographic investigation should be conducted where it is considered appropriate. Breast status should also be closely monitored in women with a history of known breast nodules or fibrocystic disease.

Women with diseases which may be subject to deterioration during pregnancy or with oestrogen use (e.g. gallstones, porphyria, multiple sclerosis, epilepsy, diabetes, benign breast disease, varicose veins, hypertension, cardiac or renal dysfunction, migraine, asthma, chorea minor, melanoma, systemic lupus erythematosus, tetany and otosclerosis) and women with a strong family history of breast cancer should be carefully observed during treatment.

In rare cases benign, and in even rarer cases malignant liver tumours leading in isolated cases to life-threatening intra-abdominal haemorrhage have been observed after the use of hormonal substances such as those contained in Elleste Duet 1 mg. If severe upper abdominal complaints, enlarged liver, or signs of intra-abdominal haemorrhage occur, a liver tumour should be considered in the differential diagnosis.

Oestrogen may cause fluid retention and therefore patients with cardiac or renal dysfunction should be carefully monitored.

Most studies indicate that oestrogen replacement therapy has little effect on blood pressure. Some show that it may decrease blood pressure. In addition studies on combined therapy show that the addition of a progestogen also has little effect on blood pressure. Rarely, idiosyncratic hypertension may occur. When oestrogens are administered to hypertensive women, supervision is necessary and blood pressure should be monitored at regular intervals.

Interactions with other medicaments and other forms of interaction: Drugs which induce hepatic microsomal enzyme systems e.g. barbiturates, carbamazepine, phenytoin, rifampicin, accelerate the metabolism of oestrogen-progestogen combinations such as Elleste Duet 1 mg and may reduce their efficacy.

The requirements for oral antidiabetics or insulin can change as a result of the effect on glucose tolerance.

Some laboratory tests can be influenced by oestrogens, such as tests for glucose tolerance or thyroid function.

Pregnancy and lactation: Elleste Duet 1 mg is contra-indicated in pregnant or lactating women.

Effects on ability to drive and use machines: No adverse effects on the ability to drive or operate machines have been reported.

Undesirable effects: The following have been reported during treatment with hormone replacement therapy: dyspepsia, flatulence, nausea, vomiting, increased appetite, abdominal pain and bloating, weight gain, breast tension and pain, palpitations, anxiety, depression, dizziness, vertigo, epistaxis, biliary stasis, hypertension, oedema, changes in libido, headaches, urticaria and other rashes, thrombophlebitis, thromboembolic disorders, changes in vaginal secretions, breakthrough vaginal bleeding, general pruitus, alopecia and chloasma or melasma which may be persistent.

Overdose: Overdosage may be manifested by nausea and vomiting. If overdosage is discovered within two or three hours and is so large that treatment seems desirable, gastric lavage can considered. There are no specific antidotes for overdosage and further treatment should be symptomatic.

Pharmacological properties:
Pharmacodynamic properties:
Oestradiol: A naturally occurring oestrogen, active in the development and maintenance of the female sex organs, secondary sex characteristics, control of mammary glands, proliferation of the endometrium, development of the decidua and cyclic changes in the cervix and vagina. Used as a replacement therapy when ovarian function declines.

Norethisterone acetate: Norethisterone acetate is a progestogen added to prevent endometrial hyperplasia and increased risk of endometrial carcinoma which can be induced by unopposed oestrogen use.

Pharmacokinetic properties:
Oestradiol: Readily and fully absorbed from the GI tract when given orally, peak levels are generally observed 3–6 hours after ingestion, but by 24 hours concentrations have returned to baseline.

Oestradiol undergoes first-pass effect in the liver. It is excreted via the kidney in the form of water-soluble esters.

Norethisterone acetate: Norethisterone acetate is absorbed from the GI tract and its effects last for at least 24 hours. Maximum blood concentrations are generally reached 1–4 hours after administration. Norethisterone acetate undergoes first-pass effects with loss of approximately 36% of the dose. Approximately 80% of the dose is excreted in the urine.

Preclinical safety data: No preclinical studies have been conducted for this product, since the safety is well recorded and understood for both oestradiol and norethisterone acetate.

Pharmaceutical particulars
List of excipients: Lactose, maize starch, povidone 25, talc (purified), magnesium stearate, hydroxypropylmethylcellulose (E464), titanium dioxide (E171), polyethylene glycol 400, tartrazine (E102) (oestradiol and norethisterone acetate tablets), lissamine green (E142) (oestradiol and norethisterone acetate tablets).

Incompatibilities: No incompatibilities have been noted.

Shelf life: A shelf life of 36 months is recommended.

Special precautions for storage: Store tablets below 25°C, in a dry place.

Nature and contents of container: Container consists of a UPVC blister and aluminium foil, packed in a cardboard carton. Each blister contains 28 tablets. Two pack sizes are available; cartons containing one blister or cartons containing three blister strips.

Instructions for use/handling: There are no special instructions for handling.

Marketing authorisation holder: Shire Pharmaceutical Contracts Limited, Fosse House, East Anton, Andover, Hampshire SP10 5RG.

Marketing authorisation number 08081/0028.

Date of first authorisation/renewal of authorisation 24th March 1997.

Date of (partial) revision of text July 1997.

Legal category POM.

ELLESTE DUET 2 mg

Qualitative and quantitative composition 16 tablets each containing 2 mg oestradiol, 12 tablets each containing 2 mg oestradiol and 1 mg norethisterone acetate.

Pharmaceutical form Coated tablets.

Clinical particulars
Therapeutic indications: Hormone replacement therapy for the treatment of menopausal symptoms such as sweating and flushes.

Prophylaxis and treatment of the postmenopausal sequelae of oestrogen withdrawal, e.g. atrophic vaginitis, atrophic urethritis and prevention of loss of bone mass which can lead to osteoporosis and fracture.

Elleste Duet 2 mg is designed to provide continuous oestrogen and monthly cyclical progestogen therapy after the climacteric. Oestrogen administration is continued without a break in therapy. The addition of a progestogen in the second half of each course helps to provide good control of the irregular cycles that are characteristic of the premenopausal phase and opposes the production of endometrial hyperplasia.

Posology and method of administration
Adults: One orange tablet is taken daily for the first 16 days, followed by one grey tablet for the next 12 days. A new cycle should then begin without any break. Therapy may start at any time in patients with established amenorrhoea or who are experiencing long intervals between spontaneous menses. In patients who are menstruating, it is advised that therapy starts on the first day of bleeding. Patients changing from another cyclical preparation should complete the cycle and may then change to Elleste Duet 2 mg without a break in therapy.

Elderly: There are no special dosage requirements for elderly patients.

Children: Not to be used in children.

Contra-indications: Known or suspected pregnancy; lactation.

Known or suspected cancer of the breast.

Known or suspected oestrogen-dependent neoplasia.

Abnormal genital bleeding, endometriosis.

Active deep venous thrombosis, thromboembolic disorders, or a past history of these conditions (including coronary thrombosis, cerebrovascular accident etc). Severe cardiac or renal disease. Sickle-cell anaemia. Congenital disturbances of lipid metabolism. Severe diabetes with vascular changes. Acute or chronic liver disease or a history of liver disease when the liver function tests have failed to return to normal. Severe disturbances of liver function (including porphyria). Previous or existing liver tumours. Rotor syndrome or Dubin-Johnson Syndrome. Jaundice or general pruritus during previous pregnancy.

A history of herpes gestationis, otosclerosis with deterioration in previous pregnancies.

Known hypersensitivity to one of the ingredients.

Special warnings and special precautions for use: Before starting treatment, pregnancy must be excluded. If the expected bleeding fails to occur at about 28-day intervals, treatment should be stopped until pregnancy has been ruled out. As Elleste Duet 2 mg is not an oral contraceptive, women should be advised to take non hormonal measures to exclude pregnancy.

Before starting Elleste Duet 2 mg, patients should have a thorough general medical and gynaecological examination with special emphasis on the body weight, blood pressure, heart, pelvic organs with an endometrial assessment if indicated, the legs and skin. Follow-up examinations are recommended at least six-monthly during treatment.

Breakthrough bleeding may occasionally occur and can be the result of poor compliance or concurrent antibiotic use. It may however indicate endometrial pathology and therefore any doubt as to its cause is an indication for endometrial evaluation, including biopsy.

Epidemiological evidence suggests that use of hormone replacement therapy (HRT) is associated with an increased relative risk of developing deep vein thrombosis (DVT) or pulmonary embolism (PE). Althouth this increase in relative risk is about 2–3, for healthy women the excess absolute risk of either of these conditions is about 1 in 5000 per year while taking HRT.

The increased risk of venous thromboembolism (VTE) means that caution should be exercised in using HRT in women who are likely to be at high risk of DVT or PE. Women with severe varicose veins, severe obesity (Body Mass index>30 kg/m²), immobilisation for 3 weeks or more, trauma or surgery requiring bed rest, are at increased risk of VTE so that the benefits of treatment with HRT will need to be weighed against risks carefully.

Consideration should be given to discontinuing treatment before elective surgery (6 weeks before hand).

If venous thromboembolism develops after initiating therapy the drug should be discontinued.

Treatment should be stopped at once if migrainous or frequent and unusually severe headaches occur for the first time, or if there are any other symptoms that are possible prodromata of vascular occlusion eg sudden visual disturbances.

Treatment should also be stopped at once if jaundice, cholestasis, hepatitis, itching of the whole body or pregnancy occurs, or if there is a significant rise in blood pressure, the occurrence of thromboembolic disease or an increase in epileptic seizures.

Pre-existing fibroids may increase in size under the influence of oestrogens, and symptoms associated with endometriosis may be exacerbated. If this is observed, treatment should be discontinued.

There is an increased risk of gall bladder disease in women receiving post menopausal oestrogens.

In patients with mild chronic liver disease, liver function should be checked every 8–12 weeks

There is an increased risk of endometrial hyperplasia and carcinoma associated with unopposed oestrogen administered long-term (for more than one year). However, the appropriate addition of progestogen to the oestrogen regimen statistically lowers the risk.

At the present time there is some evidence which suggests a slight increase in the relative risk of breast cancer in postmenopausal women receiving long-term hormone replacement therapy (more than 5 years). It is not known whether concurrent progestogen use influences this risk. Women on long-term therapy should have regular breast examinations and should be instructed in self examination of the breast. Regular mammographic investigations should be conducted where it is considered appropriate. Breast status should also be closely monitored in women with a history of known breast nodules or fibrocystic disease.

Women with disease which may be subject to deterioration during pregnancy or with oestrogen use (eg gallstones, porphyria, multiple sclerosis, epilepsy, diabetes, benign breast disease, varicose veins, hypertension, cardiac or renal dysfunction, migraine, asthma, chorea minor, melanoma, systemic lupus erythematosus, tetany and otosclerosis) and women with a strong family history of breast cancer should be carefully observed during treatment.

In rare cases benign, and in even rarer cases malignant liver tumours leading in isolated cases to life-threatening intra-abdominal haemorrhage have been observed after the use of hormonal substances such as those contained in Ellests Duet 2 mg. If severe upper abdominal complaints, enlarged liver or signs of intra-abdominal haemorrhage occur, a liver tumour should be considered in the differential diagnosis.

Oestrogen may cause fluid retention and therefore patients with cardiac or renal dysfunction should be carefully monitored.

Most studies indicate that oestrogen replacement therapy has little effect on blood pressure. Some show that it may decrease blood pressure. In addition studies on combined therapy show that the addition of a progestogen also has little effect on blood pressure. Rarely idiosyncratic hypertension may occur. When oestrogens are administered to hypertensive women, supervision is necessary and blood pressure should be monitored at regular intervals.

Interaction with other medicaments and other forms of interaction: Drugs which induce hepatic microsomal enzyme systems e.g. barbiturates, carbamazepine, phenytoin, rifampcin, accelerate the metabolism of oestrogen/progestogen combinations such as Elleste Duet 2 mg and may reduce their efficacy.

The requirement for oral anti-diabetics or insulin can change as a result of the effect on glucose tolerance.

Some laboratory tests can be influenced by oestrogens, such as tests for glucose tolerance or thyroid function.

Use during pregnancy and lactation: Elleste duet 2 mg is contra-indicated in pregnant or lactating women.

Effects on ability to drive and use machines: No adverse effects on the ability to drive or operate machines have been reported.

Undesirable effects: The following have been reported during treatment with hormone replacement therapy: dyspepsia, flatulence, nausea, vomiting, increased appetite, abdominal pain and bloating, weight gain, breast tension and pain, palpitations, anxiety, depression, dizziness, vertigo, epistaxis, biliary stasis, hypertension, oedema, changes in libido, headaches, urticaria and other rashes, thrombophlebitis, thromboembolic disorders, changes in vaginal secretions, breakthrough vaginal bleeding, general pruritus, alopecia and chloasma or melasma which may be persistent.

Overdose: Overdosage may be manifested by nausea and vomiting. If overdosage is discovered within two or three hours and is so large that treatment seems desirable, gastric lavage can be considered. There are no specific antidotes for overdosage, and further treatment should be symptomatic.

Pharmacological properties

Pharmacodynamic properties

Oestradiol: A naturally occurring oestrogen, active in the development and maintenance of the female sex organs, secondary sex characteristics, control of mammary glands, proliferation of the endometrium, development of the decidua and cyclic changes in the cervix and vagina. Used as a replacement therapy when ovarian function declines.

Norethisterone acetate: Norethisterone acetate is a progestrogen added to prevent endometrial hyperplasia and increased risk of endometrial carcinoma which can be induced by unopposed oestrogen use.

Pharmacokinetic properties

Oestradiol: Readily and fully absorbed from the GI tract when given orally, peak levels are generally observed 3–6 hours after ingestion, but by 24 hours concentrations have returned to baseline. Oestradiol undergoes first-pass effect in the liver. It is excreted via the kidney in the form of water-soluble esters.

Norethisterone acetate: Norethisterone acetate is absorbed from GI tract and its effects last for at least 24 hours. Maximum blood concentrations are generally reached 1–4 hours after administration. Norethisterone acetate undergoes first-pass effect with loss of approximately 36% of the dose. Approximately 80% of the dose is excreted in the urine.

Preclinical safety data: No preclinical studies have been conducted for this product since the safety is well recorded and understood for both oestradiol and norethisterone acetate.

Pharmaceutical particulars

List of excipients: Lactose, maize starch, povidone 25, talc (purified), magnesium stearate, hydroxypropylmethyl cellulose (E464), titanium dioxide (E171), polyethylene glycol 400, black iron oxide (E172), (oestradiol and norethisterone acetate tablets), Sunset yellow (E110) (oestradiol only tablets).

Incompatibilities: No incompatibilities have been noted.

Shelf life: A shelf-life of 36 months is recommended.

Special precautions for storage: Store the tablets under 25°C, in a dry place.

Nature and contents of container: Container consists of a UPVC blister and aluminium foil, packed in a cardboard carton. Each blister contains 28 tablets. Two pack sizes are available; cartons containing one blister or cartons containing three blister strips.

Instructions for use/handling: There are no special instructions for handling.

Marketing authorisation holder: Shire Pharmaceutical Contracts Limited, Fosse House, East Anton, Andover, Hampshire, SP10 5RG.

Marketing authorisation number PL 8081/0024.

Date of first authorisation/renewal of authorisation 23rd February 1995

Date of (partial) revision of text April 1997.

Legal category POM.

ELLESTE SOLO 1 MG

Qualitative and quantitative composition Oestradiol 1 mg.

Pharmaceutical form Coated tablets.

Clinical particulars

Therapeutic indications: Hormone replacement therapy for the treatment of menopausal symptoms such as sweating and flushes. The prophylaxis and treatment of the postmenopausal sequelae of oestrogen withdrawal, e.g. atrophic vaginitis, atrophic urethritis.

Posology and method of administration

Adults: One tablet daily to be taken orally. Elleste Solo 1 mg may be taken continuously in hysterectomised women. In women with a uterus, a progestogen should be added for 12–14 days each cycle to oppose the production of an oestrogen-stimulated hyperplasia of the endometrium.

Therapy may start at any time in women with established amenorrhoea or who are experiencing long intervals between spontaneous menses. In women who are menstruating, it is advised that therapy starts on the first day of bleeding.

Elderly: There are no special dosage requirements for elderly patients.

Children: Not to be used in children.

Contra-indications: Known or suspected pregnancy, lactation.

Known or suspected cancer of the breast.

Known or suspected oestrogen-dependent neoplasia.

Abnormal genital bleeding, endometriosis.

Active deep venous thrombosis, thromboembolic disorders, or a past history of these conditions (including coronary thrombosis, cerebrovascular accident etc).

Severe cardiac or renal disease, sickle-cell anaemia.

Congenital disturbances of lipid metabolism. Severe diabetes with vascular changes.

Acute or chronic liver disease or history of liver disease when the liver function tests have failed to return to normal. Severe disturbances of liver function (including porphyria). Previous or existing liver tumours. Rotor Syndrome or Dubin-Johnson Syndrome.

Jaundice or general pruritus during previous pregnancy.

A history of herpes gestationis, otosclerosis with deterioration in previous pregnancies.

Known hypersensitivity to one of the ingredients.

Women with an intact uterus should not be treated with oestrogens unless a progestogen is added.

Special warnings and special precautions for use: Before starting treatment, pregnancy must be excluded. If the expected bleeding fails to occur at about 28-day intervals, treatment should be stopped until pregnancy has been ruled out. As Elleste Solo is not an oral contraceptive, women should be advised to take non hormonal measures to exclude pregnancy.

Before starting Elleste Solo, patients should have a thorough general medical and gynaecological examination with special emphasis on the body weight, blood pressure, heart, pelvic organs with an endometrial assessment if indicated, the legs and skin. Follow-up examinations are recommended at least six-monthly during treatment.

Breakthrough bleeding may occasionally occur and can be the result of poor compliance or concurrent antibiotic use. It may however indicate endometrial pathology and therefore any doubt as to its cause is an indication for endometrial evaluation, including biopsy.

Epidemiological evidence suggests that use of hormone replacement therapy (HRT) is associated with an increased relative risk of developing deep vein thrombosis (DVT) or pulmonary embolism (PE). Although this increase in relative risk is about 2–3, for healthy women the excess absolute risk of either of these conditions is about 1 in 5000 per year while taking HRT.

The increased risk of venous thromboembolism (VTE) means that caution should be exercised in using HRT in women who are likely to be at high risk of DVT or PE. Women with severe varicose veins, severe obesity (Body Mass Index>30 Kg/m²), immobilisation for 3 weeks or more, trauma or surgery requiring bed rest, are at increased risk of VTE so that the benefits of treatment with HRT will need to be weighed against risks carefully.

Consideration should be given to discounting treatment before elective surgery (6 weeks before hand).

If venous thromboembolism develops after initiating therapy the drug should be discontinued.

Treatment should be stopped at once if migrainous or frequent and unusually severe headaches occur for the first time, or if there are any other symptoms that are possible prodromata of vascular occlusion e.g. sudden visual disturbances.

Treatment should also be stopped at once if jaundice, cholestasis, hepatitis, itching of the whole body or pregnancy occurs, or if there is a significant rise in blood pressure, the occurrence of thromboembolic disease or an increase in epileptic seizures.

Pre-existing fibroids may increase in size under the influence of oestrogens, and symptoms associated with endometriosis may be exacerbated. If this is observed, treatment should be discontinued.

There is an increased risk of gall bladder disease in women receiving postmenopausal oestrogens.

In patients with mild chronic liver disease, liver function should be checked every 8–12 weeks.

There is an increased risk of endometrial hyperplasia and carcinoma associated with unopposed oestrogen administered long-term (for more than one year). However, the appropriate addition of a progestogen to the oestrogen regimen statistically lowers the risk.

At the present time there is some evidence which suggests a slight increase in the relative risk of breast cancer in postmenopausal women receiving long-term hormone replacement therapy (more than 5 years). It is not known whether concurrent progestogen use influences this risk. Women on long-term therapy should have regular breast examinations and should be instructed in self examination of the breast. Regular mammographic investigations should be conducted where it is considered appropriate. Breast status should also be closely monitored in women with a history or, or known, breast nodules or fibrocystic disease.

Women with diseases which may be subject to deterioration during pregnancy or with oestrogen use (e.g. gallstones, porphyria, multiple sclerosis, epilepsy, diabetes, benign breast disease, varicose veins, hypertension, cardiac or renal dysfunction, migraine, asthma, chorea minor, melanoma, systemic lupus erythematosus, tetany and otosclerosis) and women with a strong family history of breast cancer should be carefully observed during treatment.

In rare cases benign, and in even rarer cases malignant liver tumours leading in isolated cases to life-threatening intra-abdominal haemorrhage have been observed after the use of hormonal substances such as those contained in Elleste Solo. If severe upper abdominal complaints, enlarged liver or signs of intra-abdominal haemorrhage occur, a liver tumour should be considered in the differential diagnosis.

Oestrogen may cause fluid retention and therefore patients with cardiac or renal dysfunction should be carefully monitored.

Most studies indicate that oestrogen replacement therapy has little effect on blood pressure. Some show that it may decrease blood pressure. Rarely idiosyncratic hypertension may occur. When oestrogens are administered to hypertensive women, supervision is necessary and blood pressure should be monitored at regular intervals.

Interaction with other medicaments and other forms of interaction: Drugs which induce hepatic microsomal enzyme systems e.g. barbiturates, carbamazepine, phenytoin, rifampicin, accelerate the metabolism of oestrogen products such as Elleste Solo and may reduce their efficacy.

The requirement for oral anti-diabetics or insulin can change as a result of the effect of glucose tolerance.

Some laboratory tests can be influenced by oestrogens, such as tests for glucose tolerance or thyroid function.

Use during pregnancy and lactation: Elleste Solo 1 mg is contra-indicated in pregnant or lactating women.

Effects on ability to drive and use machines: No adverse effects on the ability to drive or operate machines have been recorded.

Undesirable effects: The following have been reported during treatment with hormone replacement therapy: dyspepsia, flatulence, nausea, vomiting, increased appetite, abdominal pain and bloating, weight gain, breast tension and pain, palpitations, anxiety, depression, dizziness, vertigo, epistaxis, biliary stasis, hypertension, oedema, changes in libido, headaches, urticaria and other rashes, thrombophlebitis, thromboembolic disorders, changes in vaginal secretions, breakthrough vaginal bleeding, general pruritus, alopecia and chloasma or melasma which may be persistent.

Overdose: Overdosage may be manifested by nausea and vomiting. If overdosage is discovered within two or three hours and is so large that treatment seems desirable, gastric lavage can be considered. There are no specific antidotes for overdosage, and further treatment should be symptomatic.

Pharmacological and pharmacokinetic properties

Pharmacodynamic properties: Oestradiol is a naturally occurring oestrogen, active in the development and maintenance of the female sex organs, secondary sex characteristics, control of mammary glands, proliferation of the endometrium, development of the decidua and cyclic changes in the cervix and vagina. It is used as replacement therapy when ovarian function declines. Oestradiol exerts its effects through interaction with specific receptors in cytoplasm of oestrogen sensitive tissues.

Pharmacokinetic properties: Oestradiol is absorbed from the GI tract. When given orally, peak levels are generally observed 3–6 hours after ingestion, but by 24 hours concentrations have returned to baseline. Oestradiol undergoes first-pass effect in the liver. It is excreted via the kidney in the form of water-soluble esters.

Preclinical safety data: No preclinical studies have been conducted for this product since the safety is well recorded and understood for oestradiol.

Pharmaceutical particulars

List of excipients: Lactose, maize starch, povidone 25, talc (purified), magnesium stearate, hydroxypropylmethyl cellulose (E464), titanium dioxide (E171), polyethylene glycol 400.

Incompatibilities: No incompatibilities have been noted.

Shelf life: A shelf-life of 36 months is recommended.

Special precautions for storage: Store the tablets below 25°C, in a dry place.

Nature and contents of container: Container consists of a UPVC blister and aluminium foil, packed in a cardboard carton. Each blister contains 28 tablets. Two pack sizes are available; cartons containing one blister or cartons containing three blister strips

Instructions for use/handling: There are no special instructions for handling.

Marketing authorisation holder: Shire Pharmaceutical Contracts Limited, Fosse House, East Anton, Andover, Hampshire, SP10 5RG, United Kingdom.

Marketing authorisation number PL 8081/0020

Date of first authorisation/renewal of authorisation 30 September 1994.

Date of (partial) revision of text April 1997.

Legal category POM.

ELLESTE SOLO 2 MG

Qualitative and quantitative composition Oestradiol 2 mg.

Pharmaceutical form Coated tablets.

Clinical particulars

Therapeutic indications: Hormone replacement therapy for the treatment of menopausal symptoms such as sweating and flushes. The prophylaxis and treatment of the postmenopausal sequelae of oestrogen withdrawal, e.g. atrophic vaginitis, atrophic urethritis and prevention of loss of bone mass which can lead to osteoporosis and fractures.

Posology and method of administration

Adults: One tablet daily to be taken orally. Elleste Solo 2 mg may be taken continuously in hysterectomised women. In women with a uterus, a progestogen should be added for 12–14 days each cycle to oppose the production of an oestrogen-stimulated hyperplasia of the endometrium.

Therapy may start at any time in women with established amenorrhoea or who are experiencing long intervals between spontaneous menses. In women who are menstruating, it is advised that therapy starts on the first day of bleeding.

Elderly: There are no special dosage requirements for elderly patients.

Children: Not to be used in children.

Contra-indications: Known or suspected pregnancy, lactation.

Known or suspected cancer of the breast.

Known or suspected oestrogen-dependent neoplasia.

Abnormal genital bleeding, endometriosis.

Active deep venous thrombosis, thromboembolic disorders, or a past history of these conditions (including coronary thrombosis, cerebrovascular accident etc). Severe cardiac or renal disease, sickle-cell anaemia.

Congenital disturbances of lipid metabolism. Severe diabetes with vascular changes.

Acute or chronic liver disease or history of liver disease when the liver function tests have failed to return to normal. Severe disturbances of liver function (including porphyria). Previous or existing liver tumours. Rotor syndrome or Dubin-Johnson Syndrome. Jaundice or general pruritus during previous pregnancy.

A history of herpes gestationis, otosclerosis with deterioration in previous pregnancies.

Known hypersensitivity to one of the ingredients.

Women with an intact uterus should not be treated with oestrogens unless a progestogen is added.

Special warnings and special precautions for use: Before starting treatment, pregnancy must be excluded. If the expected bleeding fails to occur at about 28-day intervals, treatment should be stopped until pregnancy has been ruled out. As Elleste Solo is not an oral contraceptive, women should be advised to take non hormonal measures to exclude pregnancy.

Before starting Elleste Solo, patients should have a thorough general medical and gynaecological examination with special emphasis on the body weight, blood pressure, heart, pelvic organs with an endometrial assessment if indicated, the legs and skin. Follow-up examinations are recommended at least six-monthly during treatment.

Breakthrough bleeding may occasionally occur and can be the result of poor compliance or concurrent antibiotic use. It may however indicate endometrial pathology and therefore any doubt as to its cause is an indication for endometrial evaluation, including biopsy.

Epidemiological evidence suggests that use of hormone replacement therapy (HRT) is associated with an increased relative risk of developing deep vein thrombosis (DVT) or pulmonary embolism (PE). Although this increase in relative risk is about 2–3, for healthy women the excess absolute risk of either of these conditions is about 1 in 5000 per year while taking HRT.

The increased risk of venous thromboembolism (VTE) means that caution should be exercised in using HRT in women who are likely to be at high risk of DVT or PE. Women with severe varicose veins, severe obesity (Body Mass Index>30 Kg/m²), immobilisation for 3 weeks or more, trauma or surgery requiring bed rest, are at increased risk of VTE so that the benefits of treatment with HRT will need to be weighed against risks carefully.

Consideration should be given to discounting treatment before elective surgery (6 weeks before hand).

If venous thromboembolism develops after initiating therapy the drug should be discontinued.

Treatment should be stopped at once if migrainous or frequent and unusually severe headaches occur for the first time, or if there are any other symptoms that are possible prodromata of vascular occlusion e.g. sudden visual disturbances.

Treatment should also be stopped at once if jaundice, cholestasis, hepatitis, itching of the whole body or pregnancy occurs, or if there is a significant rise in blood pressure, the occurrence of thromboembolic disease or an increase in epileptic seizures.

Pre-existing fibroids may increase in size under the influence of oestrogens, and symptoms associated with endometriosis may be exacerbated. If this is observed, treatment should be discontinued.

There is an increased risk of gall bladder disease in women receiving postmenopausal oestrogens.

In patients with mild chronic liver disease, liver function should be checked every 8–12 weeks.

There is an increased risk of endometrial hyperplasia and carcinoma associated with unopposed oestrogen administered long-term (for more than one year). However, the appropriate addition of a progestogen to the oestrogen regimen statistically lowers the risk.

At the present time there is some evidence which suggests a slight increase in the relative risk of breast cancer in postmenopausal women receiving long-term hormone replacement therapy (more than 5 years). It is not known whether concurrent progestogen use influences this risk. Women on long-term therapy should have regular breast examinations and should be instructed in self examination of the breast. Regular mammographic investigations should be conducted where it is considered appropriate. Breast status should also be closely monitored in women with a history of, or known, breast nodules or fibrocystic disease.

Women with diseases which may be subject to deterioration during pregnancy or with oestrogen use (e.g. gallstones, porphyria, multiple sclerosis, epilepsy, diabetes, benign breast disease, varicose veins, hypertension, cardiac or renal dysfunction, migraine, asthma, chorea minor, melanoma, systemic lupus erythematosus, tetany and otosclerosis) and women with a strong family history of breast cancer should be carefully observed during treatment.

In rare cases benign, and in even rarer cases malignant liver tumours leading in isolated cases to life-threatening intra-abdominal haemorrhage have been observed after the use of hormonal substances such as those contained in Elleste Solo. If severe upper abdominal complaints, enlarged liver or signs of intra-abdominal haemorrhage occur, a liver tumour should be considered in the differential diagnosis.

Oestrogen may cause fluid retention and therefore patients with cardiac or renal dysfunction should be carefully monitored.

Most studies indicate that oestrogen replacement therapy has little effect on blood pressure. Some show that it may decrease blood pressure. Rarely idiosyncratic hypertension may occur. When oestrogens are administered to hypertensive women, supervision is necessary and blood pressure should be monitored at regular intervals.

Interaction with other medicaments and other forms of interaction: Drugs which induce hepatic microsomal enzyme systems e.g. barbiturates, carbamazepine, phenytoin, rifampicin, accelerate the metabolism of oestrogen products such as Elleste Solo and may reduce their efficacy.

The requirement for oral anti-diabetics or insulin can change as a result of the effect of glucose tolerance.

Some laboratory tests can be influenced by oestrogens, such as tests for glucose tolerance or thyroid function.

Use during pregnancy and lactation: Elleste Solo 2 mg is contra-indicated in pregnant or lactating women.

Effects on ability to drive and use machines: No adverse effects on the ability to drive or operate machines have been recorded.

Undesirable effects: The following have been reported during treatment with hormone replacement therapy: dyspepsia, flatulence, nausea, vomiting, increased appetite, abdominal pain and bloating, weight gain, breast tension and pain, palpitations, anxiety, depression, dizziness, vertigo, epistaxis, biliary stasis, hypertension, oedema, changes in libido, headaches, urticaria and other rashes, thrombophlebitis, thromboembolic disorders, changes in vaginal secretions, breakthrough vaginal bleeding, general pruritus, alopecia and chloasma or melasma which may be persistent.

Overdose: Overdosage may be manifested by nausea and vomiting. If overdosage is discovered within two or three hours and is so large that treatment seems desirable, gastric lavage can be considered. There are no specific antidotes for overdosage, and further treatment should be symptomatic.

Pharmacological and pharmacokinetic properties

Pharmacodynamic properties: Oestradiol is a naturally occurring oestrogen, active in the development and maintenance of the female sex organs, secondary sex characteristics, control of mammary glands, proliferation of the endometrium, development of the decidua and cyclic changes in the cervix and vagina. It is used as replacement therapy when ovarian function declines. Oestradiol exerts its effects through interaction with specific receptors in cytoplasm of oestrogen sensitive tissues.

Pharmacokinetic properties: Oestradiol is absorbed from the GI tract. When given orally, peak levels are generally observed 3–6 hours after ingestion, but by 24 hours concentrations have returned to baseline. Oestradiol undergoes first-pass effect in the liver. It is excreted via the kidney in the form of water-soluble esters.

Preclinical safety data: No preclinical studies have been conducted for this product since the safety is well recorded and understood for oestradiol.

Pharmaceutical particulars

List of excipients: Lactose, maize starch, povidone 25, talc (purified), magnesium stearate, hydroxypropylmethyl cellulose (E464), titanium dioxide (E171), polyethylene glycol 400, sunset yellow (E110).

Incompatibilities: No incompatibilities have been noted.

Shelf life: A shelf-life of 36 months is recommended.

Special precautions for storage: Store the tablets below 25°C, in a dry place.

Nature and contents of container: Container consists of a UPVC blister and aluminium foil, packed in a cardboard carton. Each blister contains 28 tablets. Two pack sizes are available; cartons containing one blister or cartons containing three blister strips

Instructions for use/handling: There are no special instructions for handling.

Marketing authorisation holder: Shire Pharmaceutical Contracts Limited, Fosse House, East Anton, Andover, Hampshire, SP10 5RG, United Kingdom.

Marketing authorisation number PL 8081/0017

Date of first authorisation/renewal of authorisation 30 September 1994.

Date of (partial) revision of text April 1997.

Legal category POM.

ELLESTE DUET CONTI

Qualitative and quantitative composition Each grey tablet contains:

Oestradiol	2.0 mg
Norethisterone acetate	1.0 mg

Pharmaceutical form Coated tablets.

Clinical particulars

Therapeutic indications: Hormone replacement therapy for the treatment of menopausal symptoms such as night sweats and hot flushes in women who are at least 1 year past their menopause and who have an intact uterus. Treatment of the postmenopausal sequelae of oestrogen withdrawal, including atrophic vaginitis and atrophic urethritis.

Elleste Duet Conti should only be used in women who are at least 1 year past their menopause. If given in the earlier post-menopausal phase the incidence of bleeding is unacceptably high. Administration is continued without a break in therapy. The presence of continuous progestogen is designed to result in the absence of menopausal bleeding whilst also protecting against the production of endometrial hyperplasia.

Posology and method of administration:

Adults, including the elderly: Elleste Duet Conti is only suitable for women who are at least one year past their menopause i.e., at least one year past their last natural menstrual bleed.

One grey tablet is taken daily continuously without a break thus running one packet into the next. The treatment is designed to provide hormone replacement therapy without cyclical bleeding, but bleeding may occur in the first six cycles of use. It can be unpredictable but not excessive. Patients must be warned of this but reassured that this should diminish significantly and finally cease in this time period. If bleeding continues patients should consider discontinuing or changing to sequential therapy.

Before initiation of therapy it is recommended that the patient is fully informed of all likely benefits and potential risks. She should have a full physical and gynaecological examination, with special emphasis on blood pressure, breasts, abdominal and pelvic organs. Endometrial assessment should be carried out if indicated; this may be particularly relevant in patients who are, or who have been, previously treated with oestrogens unopposed by a progestogen. The patient should be asked to keep a diary of any spotting or bleeding that occurs during treatment with Elleste Duet Conti. After the first 6 months, follow up examinations are recommended every 6–12 months and should include examination of the diary.

Since progestogens are only administered to protect against hyperplastic changes of the endometrium, patients without a uterus should be treated with an oestrogen only preparation.

Patients using hormone replacement therapy for the first time: May begin Elleste Duet Conti at any time provided they are at least one year past the menopause and pregnancy has been excluded (see *Special warnings and special precautions for use*).

Patients changing from a sequential combined hormone replacement therapy: In women transferred from sequential HRT, treatment should probably be started at the end of the scheduled bleed. Bleeding may occur in the first six cycles of use. If irregular bleeding continues for more than six months, the patient should discontinue treatment or consider reverting to sequential therapy.

Contra-indications:

1. Known or suspected pregnancy.
2. Known, suspected, or past history of cancer of the breast.
3. Known or suspected oestrogen-dependent neoplasia. Vaginal bleeding or unknown aetiology.
4. Active deep venous thrombosis, thromboembolic disorders, or a history of confirmed venous thromboembolism (see also *Special warnings and special precautions for use*).
5. Acute or chronic liver disease or history of liver disease where the liver function tests have failed to return to normal.
6. Rotor's syndrome or Dubin-Johnson syndrome.
7. Severe cardiac or renal disease.
8. Hypersensitivity to one or more of the ingredients.

Special warnings and special precautions for use: If changing from a sequential combined preparation which generated regular bleeding a pregnancy test is not indicated. Absence of bleeding during Elleste Duet Conti therapy can be expected and is not a cause for anxiety. Elleste Duet Conti does not consistently inhibit ovulation and is therefore, unsuitable for contraception.

Breakthrough bleeding may occasionally occur and can be the result of poor compliance or concurrent antibiotic use. It may however indicate endometrial pathology and therefore any doubt as to its cause is an indication for endometrial evaluation, including biopsy.

Epidemiological studies have suggested that hormone replacement therapy (HRT) is associated with an increased relative risk of developing venous thromboembolism (VTE) i.e. deep vein thrombosis or pulmonary embolism. The studies find a 2–3 fold increase for users compared with non-users which for healthy women amounts to a low risk of one extra case of VTE each year for every 5000 patients taking HRT.

Generally recognised risk factors for VTE include a personal or family history and severe obesity (Body Mass Index >30 kg/m^2). In women with these factors the benefits of treatment with HRT need to be carefully weighed against risks.

The risk of VTE may be temporarily increased with prolonged immobilisation, major trauma or major surgery. In women on HRT scrupulous attention should be given to prophylactic measures to prevent VTE following surgery. Where prolonged immobilisation is liable to follow elective surgery, particularly abdominal or orthopaedic surgery to the lower limbs, consideration should be given to temporarily stopping HRT 4 weeks earlier, if this is possible.

If venous thromboembolism develops after initiating therapy the drug should be discontinued.

Treatment should be stopped at once if migrainous or frequent and unusually severe headaches occur for the first time, or if there are any other symptoms that are possible prodromata of vascular occlusion, e.g. sudden visual disturbances.

Treatment should be stopped at once if jaundice, cholestasis, hepatitis, itching of the whole body or pregnancy occurs, or if there is a significant rise in blood pressure, the occurrence of thromboembolic disease or an increase in epileptic seizures whilst the cause is being investigated.

Pre-existing fibroids may increase in size under the influence of oestrogens, and symptoms associated with endometriosis may be exacerbated. If this is observed, treatment should be discontinued.

There is an increased risk of gall bladder disease in women receiving postmenopausal oestrogens.

In patients with mild chronic liver disease, liver function should be checked every 8–12 weeks.

In the female there is an increased risk of endometrial hyperplasia and carcinoma associated with unopposed oestrogen administered long term (for more than one year). However, the appropriate addition of a progestogen to an oestrogen regimen lowers this additional risk.

At the present time there is some evidence which suggest a slight increase in the relative risk of breast cancer in postmenopausal women receiving long-term hormone replacement therapy (more than 5 years). Women on long-term therapy should be informed of this risk. It is not known whether concurrent progestogen use influences this risk. Women on long-term therapy should have regular breast examination and should be instructed in self-examination of the breast. Regular mammographic investigation should be conducted where it is considered appropriate.

Women with diseases that are known to be subject to deterioration while taking HRT (e.g. gallstones, porphyria, multiple sclerosis, epilepsy, diabetes, benign breast disease, hypertension, cardiac or renal dysfunction, asthma, melanoma, systemic lupus erythematosus, tetany and otosclerosis) and women with a strong family history of breast cancer should be carefully observed during treatment.

In rare cases benign and in even rarer cases malignant liver tumours leading in isolated cases to life-threatening intra-abdominal haemorrhage have been observed after the use of hormonal substances such as those contained in Elleste Duet Conti. If severe upper abdominal complaints, enlarged liver, or signs of intra-abdominal haemorrhage occur, a liver tumour should be considered in the differential diagnosis.

Oestrogens may cause fluid retention and therefore patients with cardiac or renal dysfunction should be carefully observed.

Most studies indicate that oestrogen replacement therapy has little effect on blood pressure. Some show that it may decrease blood pressure. In addition studies on combined therapy show that the addition of a progestogen also has little effect on blood pressure. Rarely, idiosyncratic hypertension may occur. When oestrogens are administered to hypertensive women, supervision is necessary and blood pressure should be monitored at regular intervals.

Glucose tolerance may deteriorate in patients taking oestrogens. Therefore, diabetic patients should be carefully monitored whilst receiving hormone replacement therapy.

Interaction with other medicaments and other forms of interaction: Drugs which induce hepatic microsomal enzyme systems e.g. barbiturates, carbamazepine, phenytoin, rifampicin, accelerate the metabolism of oestrogen-progestogen combinations and therefore may reduce the efficacy of Elleste Duet Conti.

The requirement for oral antidiabetics or insulin can change as a result of the effect of glucose tolerance.

Some laboratory tests can be influenced by oestrogens, such as tests for glucose tolerance or thyroid function.

Pregnancy and lactation: Elleste Duet Conti is contra-indicated in pregnant or lactating women.

Effects on ability to drive and use machines: No adverse effects on the ability to drive or operate machines have been reported.

Undesirable effects: The following additional side effects have been observed with oestrogen/progestogen therapy:

Dermatology – erythema multiforme, erythema nodosum, haemorrhagic eruption, melasma or chloasma which may persist when the drug is discontinued, loss of scalp hair, hirsutism, urticaria and other rashes, general pruritus.

Breasts – enlargement, secretion, tension and pain.

Gastroenterology – jaundice, nausea, vomiting, abdominal pain and bloating, dyspepsia, flatulence, biliary stasis.

Genito-urinary system – breakthrough bleeding, spotting, pre-menstrual-like syndrome, increase in size of uterine fibromyomata, vaginal candidasis, change in cervical erosion and degree of cervical secretion, cystitis-like syndrome, mucous vaginal discharge.

Eyes – steepening of corneal curvature, intolerance to contact lenses.

CNS – headaches, migraine, dizziness, mental confusion, chorea.

Cardiovascular system – thrombophlebitis, hypertension, headaches.

Miscellaneous – reduced carbohydrate intolerance, aggravation of porphyria, changes in libido, leg cramps, weight gain.

Overdose: Overdose may be manifested by nausea and vomiting. If overdosage is discovered within two or three hours and is so large that treatment seems desirable, gastric lavage can be considered. There are no specific antidotes for overdosage, and further treatment should be symptomatic.

Pharmacological and pharmacokinetic properties
Pharmacodynamic properties:
Oestradiol: A naturally occurring oestrogen, active in the development and maintenance of the female sex organs, secondary sex characteristics, control of mammary glands, proliferation of the endometrium, development of the decidua and cyclic changes in the cervix and vagina. Used as a replacement therapy when ovarian function declines.

Norethisterone: Norethisterone acetate is a progestogen added to oppose the stimulation of the endometrium and thereby decrease the increased risk of endometrial hyperplasia and endometrial carcinoma with unopposed oestrogen use in women with an intact uterus.

Pharmacokinetic properties:
Oestradiol: Readily and fully absorbed from the GI tract when given orally, peak levels are generally observed 3–6 hours after ingestion, but by 24 hours concentrations have returned to baseline.

Oestradiol undergoes first-pass effect in the liver. It is excreted via the kidney in the form of water-soluble esters.

Norethisterone acetate: Norethisterone acetate is absorbed from the GI tract and its effects last for at least 24 hours. Maximum blood concentrations are generally reached 1–4 hours after administration. Norethisterone acetate undergoes first-pass effect with loss of approximately 36% of the dose. Approximately 80% of the dose is excreted in the urine.

Preclinical safety data: No preclinical studies have been conducted for this product, since the safety is well recorded and understood for both oestradiol and norethisterone acetate.

Pharmaceutical particulars
List of excipients: Elleste Duet Conti contains the following excipients: lactose, maize starch, povidone, talc (purified), magnesium stearate, hydroxypropylmethyl cellulose (E464), titanium dioxide (E171), polyethylene glycol 400, black iron oxide (E172).

Incompatibilities: Not applicable.

Shelf life: 36 months.

Special precautions for storage: Store below 25°C, in dry conditions.

Nature and contents of container: Container consists of aluminium foil and UPVC blister strips packed in a cardboard carton. Each blister contains 28 tablets. Two pack sizes are available; cartons containing one blister or cartons containing three blister strips.

Instructions for use/handling: Not applicable.

Marketing authorisation holder: Shire Pharmaceutical Contracts Ltd, Fosse House, East Anton, Andover, Hampshire SP10 5RG.

Marketing authorisation number PL 08081/0030.

Date of first authorisation/renewal of authorisation 27 November 1997.

Date of (partial) revision of text October 1997.

Legal category POM.

ELLESTE SOLO MX 40

Qualitative and quantitative composition Elleste Solo MX 40 contains 1.25 mg of oestradiol (Estradiol INN) and each patch delivers approximately 40 micrograms of oestradiol per 24 hours.

Pharmaceutical form Elleste Solo MX is a self adhesive, flexible transdermal patch comprising a layer of clear adhesive sandwiched between a translucent patch and a metallised polyester backing. Elleste Solo MX 40 is a rectangular shape with rounded corners and has an active surface area of 14.25 cm^2.

Clinical particulars
Therapeutic indications: Oestrogen replacement therapy in female patients for the treatment of symptoms of oestrogen deficiency as a result of the natural menopause or oophorectomy.

Posology and method of administration:
Adults: Therapy should be initiated with Elleste Solo MX 40 in women who have menopausal symptoms, who have been oestrogen deficient for a prolonged time or who are likely to be intolerant of high levels of oestradiol. The dosage may be increased if required by using Elleste Solo MX 80. For maintenance therapy the lowest effective dose should be used.

One Elleste Solo MX transdermal patch should be applied twice weekly on a continuous basis. Each patch should be removed after 3 to 4 days and replaced with a new patch applied to a slightly different site. Patches should be applied to clean, dry and intact areas of skin below the waist on the lower back or buttocks. Elleste Solo MX should not be applied on or near the breasts.

Women who are having regular periods should commence therapy within five days of the start of bleeding. Women whose periods have stopped or have become very irregular may commence therapy at any time.

In women with a uterus, a progestogen should be added for 12 to 14 days of each cycle. Most patients will commence bleeding towards the end of the progestogen therapy.

Unopposed oestrogen therapy should not be used unless the patient has undergone a hysterectomy.

Children: Elleste Solo MX is not indicated in children.

Contra-indications: Elleste Solo MX is contra-indicated in women with known or suspected pregnancy, cancer of the breast, genital tract or other oestrogen-dependent neoplasia, undiagnosed vaginal bleeding, endometriosis, severe renal or cardiac disease, acute or chronic liver disease where liver function tests have failed to return to normal, active deep venous thrombosis, thromboembolic disorders, or a history of confirmed venous thromboembolism, Dubin-Johnson syndrome or rotor syndrome.

Special warnings and special precautions for use: It is recommended that the patient should undergo a thorough physical and gynaecological examination before commencing therapy. This should be repeated at regular intervals.

Unopposed oestradiol therapy should not be used in non-hysterectomised women because of the increased risk of endometrial hyperplasia or carcinoma.

At present time there is suggestive evidence of an overall change in the relative risk of breast cancer in post menopausal women receiving oestrogen replacement therapy. While some studies have shown that there may be a small increase in risk with treatment for more than 5 years others have shown no such increase. It is not known whether concurrent progestogen use influences the risk of breast cancer in postmenopausal women taking hormone replacement therapy. A careful appraisal of the risk/benefit ratio should be undertaken before treating for longer than 5 to 10 years.

Women with a history of fibrocystic disease, breast nodules, abnormal mammograms or family history of breast cancer should have regular breast examinations.

Close monitoring of women with a history of uterine fibroids, cholelithiasis, porphyria, epilepsy, migraine, diabetes is necessary as oestrogen therapy may exacerbate or precipitate these conditions. Regular monitoring of blood pressure should be carried out in hypertensive patients.

Certain diseases may be made worse by hormone replacement therapy and patients with these conditions should be closely monitored. These include otosclerosis, multiple sclerosis, systemic lupus erythematosus, thyrotoxicosis, surgically confirmed gall bladder disease and diabetes (worsening of glucose tolerance). In addition pre-existing uterine fibroids may increase in size during oestrogen therapy and symptoms associated with endometriosis may be exacerbated.

Epidemiological studies have suggested that hormone replacement therapy (HRT) is associated with an increased relative risk of developing venous thromboembolism (VTE) i.e. deep vein thrombosis or pulmonary embolism. The studies find a 2–3 fold increase for users compared with non-users which for healthy women amounts to a low risk of one extra case of VTE each year for every 5000 patients taking HRT.

Generally recognised risk factors for VTE include a personal or family history and severe obesity (Body Mass Index >30 kg/m^2). In women with these factors the benefits of treatment with HRT need to be carefully weighed against risks.

The risk of VTE may be temporarily increased with prolonged immobilisation, major trauma or major surgery. In women with HRT scrupulous attention should be given to prophylactic measures to prevent VTE following surgery. Where prolonged immobilisation is liable to follow elective surgery, particularly abdominal or orthopaedic surgery to the lower limbs, consideration should be given to temporarily stopping HRT 4 weeks earlier, if this is possible.

If venous thromboembolism develops after initiating therapy the drug should be discontinued.

Women who may be at risk of pregnancy should be advised to adhere to non-hormonal contraceptive methods.

Interaction with other medicaments and other forms of interaction: None.

Pregnancy and lactation: Elleste Solo MX is contra-indicated.

Effects on ability to drive and use machines: None.

Undesirable effects: Elleste Solo MX is generally well tolerated. The most frequent side effects (reported in 10 to 20% of patients, on at least one occasion, in clinical trials with Elleste Solo MX 80), which do not normally prevent continued treatment include: breast tenderness, headaches and breakthrough bleeding. Some patients experience mild and transient local erythema at the site of application with or without itching; this usually disappears rapidly on removal of the patch. The overall incidence of general patch irritation in clinical studies is less than 5%. In a clinical study 3% of 102 patients showed well defined erythema (Draize scale) 30 minutes after patch removal. No instances of permanent skin damage have been reported. If unacceptable topical side effects do occur discontinuation of treatment should be considered.

Other side effects associated with oestrogen or oestrogen/progestogen treatment which have occasionally been reported (in 1% to 5% of patients in clinical trials with Elleste Solo MX 80) include: abdominal cramps, abdominal bloating, oedema, nausea, migraine and weight changes.

More rarely (less than 1% in clinical trials with Elleste Solo MX 80) dizziness, dysmenorrhoea, leg cramps and visual disturbances and changes in libido or changes in carbohydrate tolerance have been reported with other oestradiol products.

Overdose: This is not likely due to the mode of administration. If it is necessary to stop delivery then the patch can be removed and plasma oestradiol levels will fall rapidly.

Pharmacological properties
Pharmacodynamic properties:
Pharmacotherapeutic group: Natural oestrogen.
Mechanism of action/pharmacodynamic effects: In the female, oestradiol stimulates the accessory reproductive organs and causes development of the secondary sexual characteristics at puberty. It is also responsible for the hypertrophy of the uterus and for the changes in the endometrium during the first half of the menstrual cycle which when acted on by progesterone prepares it for the reception of a fertilised ovum. It furthermore promotes the growth of the ducts of the mammary glands. Large doses inhibit the gonadotropic secretion of the anterior pituitary, thus influencing the normal ovarian cycle.

It is of value in menstrual disorders, ovarian insufficiency, especially at the menopause, and for the treatment of infections of the vagina in children, where it promotes the growth of a cornified and more resistant epithelium; it is also used to terminate lactation, not very successfully, by inhibiting the release of prolactin.

Pharmacokinetic properties:
General characteristics of the active substance:
Absorption: Oestradiol is absorbed from the patch across the stratum corneum and is delivered systemically at a low but constant rate throughout the period of application (3 to 4 days). The estimated delivery of oestradiol is approximately 40 µg/day for Elleste Solo MX 40.

Distribution: Oestrogens circulate in the blood bound to albumin, sex hormone binding globulin (SHBG), cortisol binding globulin and alpha 1-glycoprotein. Following diffusion of free oestrogen into the cells of the target tissues in the hypothalamus, pituitary, vagina, urethra, uterus, breast and liver, binding to specific oestrogen receptors occurs. Very little information is currently available on the distribution of oestradiol following transdermal administration.

Biotransformation: Inactivation of oestrogens in the body is carried out mainly in the liver. Metabolism of 17 β-oestradiol is by oxidation to oestrone, which in turn can be hydrated to form oestriol. There is free interconversion between oestrone and oestradiol. Oestrone and oestriol may then undergo conversion to their corresponding sulphate and glucuronide derivatives for excretion in the urine. Oestrone sulphate has a long biologic half-life because of its enterohepatic recirculation and interconversion to oestrone and oestradiol.

Elimination: The plasma elimination half-life of oestradiol is approximately 1 hour and is independent of the route of administration. The metabolic plasma clearance rate is between 650 and 900 L/day/m^2.

Steady state plasma oestradiol concentrations have been demonstrated in the range of 26 pg/ml to 34 pg/ml for the Elleste Solo MX 40 patch (including baseline levels) and these are maintained throughout the dose interval (for up to four days). Absorption rate may vary between individual patients. After removal of the last patch plasma oestradiol and oestrone concentrations return to baseline values in less than 24 hours.

The median terminal half-life for oestradiol following patch removal has been determined as 5.24 h.

Preclinical safety data: No specific preclinical studies have been conducted on Elleste Solo MX. Supraphysiologically high doses (prolonged overdoses) of oestradiol have been associated with the induction of tumours in oestrogen-dependent target organs in rodent species. Pronounced species differences in toxicology, pharmacology and pharmacodynamics exist.

Pharmaceutical particulars
List of excipients: Diethyltoluamide, Acrylic emulsion (proprietary adhesive), Acrylic emulsion (adhesive thickener).

Backing: Polyester.

Release liner: Siliconised/aluminised/polyester.

Incompatibilities: Not applicable.

Shelf life: The shelf life of the product as packaged for sale is 3 years.

Special precautions for storage: Elleste Solo MX patches should be stored at room temperature (below 25°C) in a dry place.

Nature and contents of container: PVC/PVDC blister tray with paper/polythene/aluminium foil lid containing one transdermal patch. Each carton contains eight patches, sufficient for one 28 day cycle and a patient leaflet.

Instructions for use/handling: Detailed instructions for use are provided in the patient leaflet.

Marketing authorisation holder: Ethical Pharmaceuticals (UK) Ltd, Gemini House, Bartholomew's Walk, Cambridgeshire Business Park, Ely, Cambs CB7 4EA.

Elleste Solo MX is marketed and distributed by Searle Division of Monsanto plc, High Wycombe HP12 4HL.

Marketing authorisation number PL 10013/0032

Date of first authorisation/renewal of authorisation 12 December 1995.

Date of (partial) revision of text October 1997.

Legal category POM.

ELLESTE SOLO MX 80

Qualitative and quantitative composition Elleste Solo MX 80 contains 2.5 mg of oestradiol (Estradiol INN) and each patch delivers approximately 80 micrograms of oestradiol per 24 hours.

Pharmaceutical form Elleste Solo MX 80 is a self adhesive, flexible transdermal patch comprising a layer of clear adhesive sandwiched between a translucent patch and a metallised polyester backing. Elleste Solo MX 80 is a rectangular shape with rounded corners and has an active surface area of 28.5 cm².

Clinical particulars
Therapeutic indications: Oestrogen replacement therapy for the relief of postmenopausal symptoms and for the prevention of osteoporosis in women at risk of developing fractures.

Epidemiological studies suggest a number of individual risk factors contribute to postmenopausal osteoporosis, including:

early menopause (either naturally or sugically); family history of osteoporosis; recent prolonged systemic corticosteroid therapy; a small, thin frame; cigarette use.

If several risk factors are present consideration should be given to oestrogen replacement therapy.

For maximum benefit treatment should commence as soon as possible after the menopause.

Posology and method of administration:
Climacteric symptoms: Therapy should be initiated with Elleste Solo MX 40 in women who have menopausal symptoms, who have been oestrogen deficient for a prolonged time or who are likely to be intolerant of high levels of oestradiol. The dosage may be increased if required by using Elleste Solo MX 80. For maintenance therapy the lowest effective dose should be used.

Prevention of osteoporosis: Treatment should be with Elleste Solo MX 80, as the efficacy of Elleste Solo MX 40 in this indication has yet to be established.

For optimum benefit treatment should continue for 5 to 10 years, protection appears to be effective for as long as treatment continues, however data beyond 10 years is limited. For long term use see also *Special warnings and special precautions for use.*

Dosage schedule (for both indications): One Elleste Solo MX 80 transdermal patch should be applied twice weekly on a continuous basis. Each patch should be removed after 3 to 4 days and replaced with a new patch applied to a slightly different site. Patches should be applied to clean, dry and intact areas of skin below the waist on the lower back or buttocks. Elleste Solo MX should not be applied on or near the breasts.

Women who are having regular periods should commence therapy within five days of the start of bleeding. Women whose periods have stopped or have become very irregular may commence therapy at any time.

In women with a uterus, a progestogen should be added for 12 to 14 days of each cycle. Most patients will commence bleeding towards the end of progestogen therapy.

Unopposed oestrogen therapy should not be used unless the patient has undergone a hysterectomy.

Children: Elleste Solo MX is not indicated in children.

Contra-indications: Elleste Solo MX is contra-indicated in women with known or suspected pregnancy, cancer of the breast, genital tract or other oestrogen-dependent neoplasia, undiagnosed vaginal bleeding, endometriosis, severe renal or cardiac disease, acute or chronic liver disease where liver function tests have failed to return to normal, active deep venous thrombosis, thromboembolic disorders, or a history of confirmed venous thromboembolism (see *Special warnings and special precautions for use*), Dubin-Johnson syndrome or rotor syndrome.

Special warnings and special precautions for use: It is recommended that the patient should undergo a thorough physical and gynaecological examination before commencing therapy. This should be repeated at regular intervals.

Unopposed oestradiol therapy should not be used in non-hysterectomised women because of the increased risk of endometrial hyperplasia or carcinoma.

At present time there is suggestive evidence of an overall change in the relative risk of breast cancer in post menopausal women receiving oestrogen replacement therapy. While some studies have shown that there may be a small increase in risk with treatment for more than 5 years others have shown no such increase. It is not known whether concurrent progestogen use influences the risk of breast cancer in postmenopausal women taking hormone replacement therapy. A careful appraisal of the risk/benefit ratio should be undertaken before treating for longer than 5 to 10 years.

Women with a history of fibrocystic disease, breast nodules, abnormal mammograms or family history of breast cancer should have regular breast examinations.

Certain diseases may be made worse by hormone replacement therapy and patients with these conditions should be closely monitored. These include otosclerosis, multiple sclerosis, systemic lupus erythematosus, cholelithiasis, porphyria, melanoma, epilepsy, migraine, thyrotoxicosis, surgically confirmed gall bladder disease, asthma and diabetes (worsening of glucose tolerance). Pre-existing uterine fibroids may increase in size during oestrogen therapy and symptoms associated with endometriosis may be exacerbated.

Epidemiological studies have suggested that hormone replacement therapy (HRT) is associated with an increased relative risk of developing venous thromboembolism (VTE) i.e. deep vein thrombosis or pulmonary embolism. The studies find a 2–3 fold increase for users compared with non-users which for healthy women amounts to a low risk of one extra case of VTE each year for every 5000 patients taking HRT.

Generally recognised risk factors for VTE include a personal or family history and severe obesity (Body Mass Index >30 kg/m²). In women with these factors the benefits of treatment with HRT need to be carefully weighed against risks.

The risk of VTE may be temporarily increased with prolonged immobilisation, major trauma or major surgery. In women with HRT scrupulous attention should be given to prophylactic measures to prevent VTE following surgery. Where prolonged immobilisation is liable to follow elective surgery, particularly abdominal or orthopaedic surgery to the lower limbs, consideration should be given to temporarily stopping HRT 4 weeks earlier, if this is possible.

If venous thromboembolism develops after initiating therapy the drug should be discontinued.

If jaundice or significant hypertension develop, treatment should be discontinued whilst the cause is investigated. As oestrogens may cause fluid retention, patients with cardiac or renal dysfunction should be closely observed. Regular monitoring of blood pressure should be carried out in hypertensive patients.

Women who may be at risk of pregnancy should be advised to adhere to non-hormonal contraceptive methods.

Interaction with other medicaments and other forms of interaction: Preparations inducing microsomal liver enzymes, e.g. barbiturates, hydantoins, anti-convulsants (including carbamazepine), meprobromate, phenylbutazone, antibiotics (including rifampicin), and activated charcoal may impair the activity of oestrogens. Transdermally applied oestrogens are less likely to be affected by such interactions than oral oestrogens since first pass hepatic metabolism is avoided.

Changes in oestrogen serum concentrations may affect the results of certain endocrine or liver function tests.

Pregnancy and lactation: Elleste Solo MX is contra-indicated.

Effects on ability to drive and use machines: None.

Undesirable effects: Elleste Solo MX is generally well tolerated. The most frequent side effects (reported in 10 to 20% of patients, on at least one occasion, in clinical trials with Elleste Solo MX 80), which do not normally prevent continued treatment include: breast tenderness, headaches and breakthrough bleeding. Some patients experience mild and transient local erythema at the site of application with or without itching; this usually disappears rapidly on removal of the patch. The overall incidence of general patch irritation in clinical studies is less than 5%. In a clinical study 3% of 102 patients showed well defined erythema (Draize scale) 30 minutes after patch removal. No instances of permanent skin damage have been reported. If unacceptable topical side effects do occur discontinuation of treatment should be considered.

Other side effects associated with oestrogen or oestrogen/progestogen treatment have occasionally been reported (in 1% to 5% of patients in clinical trials with Elleste Solo MX 80) include: abdominal cramps, abdominal bloating, oedema, nausea, migraine and weight changes. More rarely (less than 1% in clinical trials with Elleste Solo MX 80) dizziness, dysmenorrhoea, leg cramps and visual disturbances have been reported.

Other side effects which have been rarely reported with oestrogen products include: changes in libido or changes in carbohydrate tolerance, vaginal candidiasis, change in vaginal secretions, cystitis like syndrome, cervical erosion, erythema multiforme, erythema nodosa, haemorrhagic eruptions, chloasma or melasma which may be persistent when the drug is discontinued, steepening of corneal curvature, intolerance to contact lenses, mental depression and chorea minor. Cholestasis may be possible in predisposed patients.

Overdose: This is not likely due to the mode of administration. If it is necessary to stop delivery then the patch can be removed and plasma oestradiol levels will fall rapidly.

Pharmacological properties
Pharmacodynamic properties:

Pharmacotherapeutic group: Natural oestrogen.

Mechanism of action/pharmacodynamic effects: In the female, oestradiol stimulates the accessory reproductive organs and causes development of the secondary sexual characteristics at puberty. It is also responsible for the hypertrophy of the uterus and for the changes in the endometrium during the first half of the menstrual cycle which when acted on by progesterone prepares it for the reception of a fertilised ovum. It furthermore promotes the growth of the ducts of the mammary glands. Large doses inhibit the gonadotropic secretion of the anterior pituitary, thus influencing the normal ovarian cycle.

It is of value in menstrual disorders, ovarian insufficiency, especially at the menopause, and for the treatment of infections of the vagina in children, where it promotes the growth of a cornified and more resistant epithelium; it is also used to terminate lactation, not very successfully, by inhibiting the release of prolactin.

Pharmacokinetic properties: General characteristics of the active substance:

Absorption: Oestradiol is absorbed from the patch across the stratum corneum and is delivered systemically at a low but constant rate throughout the period of application (3 to 4 days). The estimated delivery of oestradiol is approximately 80 micrograms per day for Elleste Solo MX 80.

Distribution: Oestrogens circulate in the blood bound to albumin, sex hormone binding globulin (SHBG), cortisol binding globulin and alpha 1-glycoprotein. Following diffusion of free oestrogen into the cells of the target tissues in the hypothalamus, pituitary, vagina, urethra, uterus, breast and liver, binding to specific oestrogen receptors occurs. Very little information is currently available on the distribution of oestradiol following transdermal administration.

Biotransformation: Inactivation of oestrogens in the body is carried out mainly in the liver. Metabolism of 17 β-oestradiol is by oxidation to oestrone, which in turn can be hydrated to form oestriol. There is free interconversion between oestrone and oestradiol. Oestrone and oestriol may then undergo conversion to their corresponding sulphate and glucuronide derivatives for excretion in the urine. Oestrone sulphate has a long biologic half-life because of its enterohepatic recirculation and interconversion to oestrone and oestradiol.

Elimination: The plasma elimination half-life of oestradiol is approximately 1 hour and is independent of the route of administration. The metabolic plasma clearance rate is between 650 and 900 L/day/m².

Steady state plasma oestradiol concentrations have been demonstrated in the range of 34 to 62 pg/ml for the Elleste Solo MX 80 patch (including baseline levels) and these are maintained throughout the dose interval (for up to four days). Absorption rate may vary between individual patients. After removal of the last patch plasma oestradiol and oestrone concentrations return to baseline values in less than 24 hours. The median terminal half-life for oestradiol following patch removal has been determined as 5.24 h.

Preclinical safety data: No specific preclinical studies have been conducted on Elleste Solo MX. Supraphysiologically high doses (prolonged overdoses) of oestradiol have been associated with the induction of tumours in oestrogen-dependent target organs in rodent species. Pronounced species differences in toxicology, pharmacology and pharmacodynamics exist.

Pharmaceutical particulars
List of excipients: Diethyltoluamide, Acrylic adhesive, Backing: Polyester, Release liner: Aluminised/polyester.

Incompatibilities: Not applicable.

Shelf life: The shelf life of the product as packaged for sale is 3 years.

Special precautions for storage: Elleste Solo MX patches should be stored at room temperature (below 25°C) in a dry place.

Nature and contents of container: PVC/PVDC blister tray with paper/polythene/aluminium foil lid containing one transdermal patch. Each carton contains eight patches, sufficient for one 28 day cycle and a patient leaflet. An additional pack containing two patches may also be available.

Instructions for use/handling: Detailed instructions for use are provided in the patient leaflet.

Marketing authorisation holder: Ethical Pharmaceuticals (UK) Ltd, Gemini House, Bartholomew's Walk, Cambridgeshire Business Park, Ely, Cambs CB7 4EA.

Elleste Solo MX is marketed by Searle a division of Monsanto plc, High Wycombe HP12 4HL.

Marketing authorisation number PL 10013/0021

Date of first authorisation/renewal of authorisation
23 November 1994.

Date of (partial) revision of text October 1997.

Legal category POM.

EPOGAM 40

Qualitative and quantitative composition

Active constituents	*Quantity/dose unit*
Gamolenic acid provided by Evening Primrose Oil	40 mg

Pharmaceutical form Soft gelatin capsules.

Clinical particulars
Therapeutic indications: Epogam is indicated for the symptomatic relief of atopic eczema. All features of the disease may improve but Epogam 40 is particularly effective in relieving the generalised itch of atopic eczema.

Posology and method of administration: For oral administration. When children cannot swallow the capsules the latter may be snipped open and the oil swallowed directly, or mixed with milk, or put on to bread.

Children: Aged 1–12 years; 2–4 capsules twice daily.
Adults: 4–6 capsules twice daily.
Elderly: The usual adult dose.

No formal studies have been carried out in children under the age of 1 year.

Treatment should be started at the highest recommended dose.

Some patients may not begin to show a clinical response to treatment for 8–12 weeks due to the gradual onset of action of Epogam 40. Once a clinical response has been achieved the treatment may be stopped or continued at a lower maintenance dose.

Contra-indications: None known.

Special warnings and special precautions for use: None.

Interaction with other medicaments and other forms of interaction: Epogam 40 may have the potential to make manifest undiagnosed temporal lobe epilepsy, especially in schizophrenic patients and/or those who are receiving known epileptogenic drugs such as the phenothiazines. Physicians are advised to monitor carefully the effects of Epogam 40 in patients on epileptogenic drugs, or in any individuals with a history of epilepsy.

Pregnancy and lactation:
Pregnancy: No teratogenic effects have been observed in animal studies. There is no information available on use during pregnancy in human beings. It should only be used during pregnancy if considered essential by the physician.

Lactation: Epogam 40 may be taken while breast feeding.

Effects on ability to drive and use machines: None.

Undesirable effects: No major adverse effects have been reported. Nausea, indigestion and headache have occurred occasionally. In rare cases, hypersensitivity reactions, including rash, urticaria and pruritus and abdominal pain have been reported. It should be noted that hypersensitivity reactions may require close medical surveillance and that such reactions may occur particularly in patients who have a history of food or other allergies.

Overdose: The only symptom noted in a few cases have been loose stools sometimes accompanied by abdominal pains. No special treatment is required. There is a high degree of tolerance to evening primrose oil. Up to 25 ml of oil (equivalent to 50 capsules) has been administered daily for one year to children aged 5–12 years, without adverse effects other than occasional loose stools.

Pharmacological properties
Pharmacodynamic properties: Epogam 40 capsules provide an exogenous source of gamolenic acid (GLA) which may be used to restore some subnormal fatty acid levels towards physiologically normal levels. Clinical studies demonstrate that it improves the symptoms of atopic eczema, however the precise pharmacological mode of action is unclear. No undesirable pharmacological effects are known.

Pharmacokinetic properties: The pharmacokinetic profile of evening primrose oil follows that of any normal triglycerides from usual dietary sources. It is approximately 95% absorbed, metabolised in the liver and stored principally in adipose tissue.

There are no unusual pharmacokinetic properties. Gamolenic acid is the unusual fatty acid component of evening primrose oil, it is metabolised rapidly to dihomo-gammalinolenic acid (DGLA) in the body. DGLA levels will fall to pretreatment levels in approximately two weeks following withdrawal of evening primrose oil.

Preclinical safety data: None of relevance to the prescriber.

Pharmaceutical particulars
List of excipients: The following excipients are included in Epogam: D-alpha tocopheryl acetate, gelatin, glycerol, Opacode S-1-7020 White or Mastercote F11983 White.

Incompatibilities: None known.

Shelf life: 36 months as packaged for sale.

Special precautions for storage: Store below 25°C, in a dry place, protected from heat.

Nature and contents of containers: (a) HDPE 'Tampertainer' containing 240 Epogam 40 capsules with an LDPE tamper evident closure.

(b) Promotional sample pack containing 12 capsules in PVC/PVDC (250/40) blister pack with lacquered hard temper aluminium foil (20 micron) in a cardboard carton.

Instructions for use/handling: 'Swallow the capsule whole or you can snip the capsule with a pair of scissors. Squeeze the liquid into your mouth and swallow. If you prefer you can mix the oil with a cold drink or put it on to your food'.

Marketing authorisation holder: Scotia Pharmaceuticals Limited, Scotia House, Castle Business Park, Stirling FK9 4TZ, UK.

Marketing authorisation number PL 4382/0005.

Date of first authorisation/renewal of authorisation
13th September 1988/13th September 1993.

Date of (partial) revision of the text August 1997.

Legal category POM.

EPOGAM 80

Qualitative and quantitative composition
Gamolenic acid, 80 mg/capsules, provided by evening primrose oil.

Pharmaceutical form Soft gelatin capsules for oral administration.

Clinical particulars
Therapeutic indications: Epogam 80 is indicated for the symptomatic relief of atopic eczema. All features of the disease may improve, but Epogam 80 is particularly effective in relieving the generalised itch of atopic eczema.

Posology and method of administration: Epogam 80 may be administered to adults, the elderly and children (aged 1–12 years) as specified below:

(i) Adults: 2–3 capsules twice daily, providing a total daily dose of 4–6 capsules.
(ii) The elderly: the usual adult dose.
(iii) Children (aged 1–12 years): 1–2 capsules twice daily, providing a total daily dose of 2–4 capsules.
(iv) No formal studies have been carried out in children under the age of 1 year.

The capsules are not recommended for children or patients who have difficulty in swallowing unless the capsules are pierced or snipped open and the oil swallowed directly or mixed with milk or put onto bread or other food.

It is suggested that patients start treatment at the highest recommended dose.

Some patients may not begin to show a clinical response to treatment for 8–12 weeks due to the gradual onset of action of Epogam 80. Once a clinical reponse has been achieved the treatment may be stopped or continued at a lower maintenance dose.

Contra-indications: None known.

Special warnings and special precautions for use: None.

Interaction with other medicaments and other forms of interaction: Epogam 80 may have the potential to make manifest undiagnosed temporal lobe epilepsy, especially in schizophrenic patients and/or those who are receiving known epileptogenic drugs such as the phenothiazines. Physicians are advised to monitor carefully the effects of Epogam 80 in patients on epileptogenic drugs, or in any individuals with a history of epilepsy.

Pregnancy and lactation:
Pregnancy: No teratogenic effects have been observed in animal studies. However, as with all medicines, caution is advised concerning administration in the first trimester of pregnancy.

Lactation: Epogam 80 may be taken while breast feeding.

Effects on ability to drive and use machines: None.

Undesirable effects: No major adverse effects have been reported. Nausea, indigestion and headache have occurred occasionally. In rare cases, hypersensitivity reactions, including rash, urticaria and pruritus and abdominal pain have been reported. It should be noted that hypersensitivity reactions may require close medical surveillance and that such reactions may occur particularly in patients who have a history of food or other allergies.

Overdose: The only symptoms noted in a few cases have been loose stools sometimes accompanied by abdominal pains. No treatment is required.

There is a high degree of tolerance to evening primrose oil. Up to 25 ml of oil (equivalent to 36 capsules) has been administered daily for one year to children aged 5–12 years, without adverse effects other than occasional loose stools.

Pharmacological properties
Pharmacodynamic properties: Epogam 80 capsules provide an exogenous source of gamolenic acid (GLA) which may be used to restore some subnormal fatty acid levels towards physiologically normal levels. Clinical studies demonstrate that they improve the symptoms of atopic eczema, however the precise pharmacological mode of action is unclear. No undesirable pharmacological effects are known.

Pharmacokinetic properties: The pharmacokinetic profile of evening primrose oil follows that of any normal triglycerides from usual dietary sources. It is approximately 95% absorbed, metabolised in the liver and stored principally in adipose tissue.

There are no unusual pharmacokinetic properties. Gamolenic acid is the unusual fatty acid component of evening primrose oil, it is metabolised rapidly to dihomogammalinolenic acid (DGLA) in the body. DGLA levels will fall to pretreatment levels in approximately two weeks following withdrawal of evening primrose oil.

Preclinical safety data: None of relevance to the prescriber.

Pharmaceutical particulars
List of excipients: dl-alpha tocopheryl acetate PhEur, Gelatin PhEur, Glycerol PhEur, Opacode S-1-7020 White or Mastercote F11983 White.

Incompatibilities: None known.

Shelf life: 3 years.

Special precautions for storage: Store in a dry place, protected from heat.

Nature and contents of containers: High density polyethylene containers.

Instructions for use/handling: None.

Marketing authorisation holder: Scotia Pharmaceuticals Limited, Scotia House, Castle Business Park, Stirling FK9 4TZ, UK.

Marketing authorisation number PL 04382/0027.

Date of first authorisation/renewal of authorisation 7th September 1994.

Date of (partial) revision of the text August 1997.

Legal category POM.

EPOGAM* PAEDIATRIC CAPSULES

Qualitative and quantitative composition

Active constituents	*Quantity/dose unit*
Gamolenic acid (provided by Evening Primrose Oil)	80 mg

Pharmaceutical form Soft gelatin capsules.

Clinical particulars

Therapeutic indications: Epogam Paediatric is indicated for the symptomatic relief of atopic eczema. All features of the disease may improve but Epogam Paediatric is particularly effective in relieving the generalised itch of atopic eczema

Posology and method of administration: These capsules have been specifically designed for children (and also incidentally for older people) who have difficulty swallowing the 40 mg Epogam Capsules. The snip off neck should be cut off and the capsule squeezed to express the contents which may be swallowed directly or mixed with milk or put onto bread or other food.

Children: Aged 1–12 years; 1–2 capsules twice daily, providing a total daily dose of 2–4 capsules.

Adults: 2–3 capsules twice daily, providing a total daily dose of 4–6 capsules.

Elderly: The usual adult dose.

No formal studies have been carried out in children under the age of 1 year.

Treatment should be started at the highest recommended dose.

Some patients may not begin to show a clinical response to treatment for 8–12 weeks due to the gradual onset of action of Epogam Paediatric. Once a clinical response has been achieved the treatment may be stopped or continued at a lower maintenance dose.

Contra-indications: None known.

Special warnings and special precautions for use: None.

Interaction with other medicaments and other forms of interaction: Epogam Paediatric may have the potential to make manifest undiagnosed temporal lobe epilepsy, especially in schizophrenic patients and/or those who are receiving known epileptogenic drugs such as the phenothiazines. Physicians are advised to monitor carefully the effects of Epogam Paediatric in patients on epileptogenic drugs, or in any individuals with a history of epilepsy.

Pregnancy and lactation:

Pregnancy: No teratogenic effects have been observed in animal studies. However, as with all medicines, caution is advised concerning administration in the first trimester of pregnancy.

Lactation: Epogam Paediatric may be taken while breast feeding.

Effects on ability to drive and use machines: None.

Undesirable effects: No frequent major adverse effects have been reported. Nausea, indigestion and headache occur occasionally. In rare cases, hypersensitivity reactions, including rash, urticaria and pruritus and abdominal pain have been reported. It should be noted that hypersensitivity reactions may require close medical surveillance and that such reactions may occur particularly in patients who have a history of food or other allergies.

Overdose: The only symptom noted in a few cases have been loose stools sometimes accompanied by abdominal pains. No special treatment is required.

There is a high degree of tolerance to evening primrose oil. Up to 25 ml of oil (equivalent to 25 capsules) has been administered daily for one year to children aged 5–12 years, without adverse effects other than occasional loose stools.

Pharmacological properties

Pharmacodynamic properties: Epogam Paediatric capsules provide an exogenous source of gamolenic acid (GLA) which may be used to restore some subnormal fatty acid levels towards physiologically normal levels. Clinical studies demonstrate that it improves the symptoms of atopic eczema, however the precise pharmacological mode of action is unclear. No undesirable pharmacological effects are known.

Pharmacokinetic properties: The pharmacokinetic profile of evening primrose oil follows that of any normal triglycerides from usual dietary sources. It is approximately 95% absorbed, metabolised in the liver and stored principally in adipose tissue.

There are no unusual pharmacokinetic properties. Gamolenic acid is the unusual fatty acid component of evening primrose oil, it is metabolised rapidly to dihomo-gammalinolenic acid (DGLA) in the body. DGLA levels will fall to pretreatment levels in approximately two weeks following withdrawal of evening primrose oil.

Preclinical safety data: None of relevance to the prescriber.

Pharmaceutical particulars

List of excipients: The following excipients are included in Epogam: D-alpha tocopheryl acetate, Gelatin, Glycerol, Opacode S-1-7020 White or Mastercote F11983 White.

Incompatibilities: None known.

Shelf life: 36 months as packaged for sale.

Special precautions for storage: Store in a dry place, protected from heat.

Nature and contents of container: (a) HDPE 'Tampertainer' containing 60 or 120 Epogam Paediatric capsules with an LDPE tamper evident closure.

(b) Promotional sample pack containing 4 capsules in PVC/PVDC (250/40) blister pack with lacquered hard tamper aluminium foil (20 micron) in a cardboard carton.

Instructions for use/handling: 'Do not swallow the capsule whole. Snip off the neck of the capsule with a pair of scissors. Squeeze the liquid into your mouth and swallow. If you prefer you can mix the oil with a cold drink or put it onto your bread'.

Marketing authorisation holder: Scotia Pharmaceuticals Limited, Scotia House, Castle Business Park, Stirling FK9 4TZ, UK.

Marketing authorisation number PL 04382/0013

Date of first authorisation/renewal of authorisation 16th March 1990/16th March 1995

Date of (partial) revision of the text August 1997.

Legal category POM.

FEMULEN*

Qualitative and quantitative composition Each tablet contains 500 micrograms ethynodiol diacetate.

Pharmaceutical form White tablet inscribed 'SEARLE' on both sides.

Clinical particulars

Therapeutic indications: Oral contraception.

Posology and method of administration: Starting on the first day of menstruation, one pill every day without a break in medication for as long as contraception is required. Additional contraceptive precautions (such as a condom) should be used for the first 7 days of the first pack. Pills should be taken at the same time each day.

Missed tablets: If a pill is missed within 3 hours of the correct dosage time then the missed pill should be taken as soon as possible; this will ensure that contraceptive protection is maintained. If a pill is taken 3 or more hours late it is recommended that the women takes the last missed pill as soon as possible and then continues to take the rest of the pills in the normal manner. However, to provide continued contraceptive protection it is recommended that an alternative method of contraception, such as a condom, is used for the next 7 days.

Vomiting or diarrhoea: Gastrointestinal upsets, such as vomiting or diarrhoea, may interfere with the absorption of the pill leading to a reduction in contraceptive efficacy. Women should continue to take Femulen, but they should also be advised to use another contraceptive method during the period of gastrointestinal upset and for the next 7 days.

Contra-indications: The contra-indications for progestogen-only oral contraceptives are:

(i) Known, suspected, or a past history of breast, genital or hormone dependent cancer;
(ii) Acute or severe chronic liver diseases including past or present liver tumours, Dubin-Johnson or Rotor syndrome:
(iii) Active liver disease;
(iv) History during pregnancy of idiopathic jaundice or severe pruritus;
(v) Disorders of lipid metabolism;
(vi) Undiagnosed abnormal vaginal bleeding;
(vii) Known or suspected pregnancy;
(viii) Hypersensitivity to any component.

Combined oestrogen/progestogen preparations have been associated with an increase in the risk of thromboembolic and thrombotic disease. Risk has been reported to be related to both oestrogenic and progestogenic activity. In the absence of long term epidemiological studies with progestogen-only oral contraceptives, it is required that the existence, or history of thrombophlebitis, thromboembolic disorders, cerebral vascular disease, myocardial infarction, angina, coronary artery disease, or a haemoglobinopathy be described as a contra-indication to Femulen as it is to oestrogen containing oral contraceptives.

Special warnings and special precautions for use: Women receiving treatment with Femulen should be kept under regular medical surveillance.

Femulen should be discontinued if there is a gradual or sudden, partial or complete loss of vision or any evidence of ocular changes, onset or aggravation of migraine or development of headache of a new kind which is recurrent, persistent or severe, suspicion of thrombosis or infarction, significant rise in blood pressure or if jaundice occurs.

Malignant hepatic tumours have been reported on rare occasions in long-term users of contraceptives. Benign hepatic tumours have also been associated with oral contraceptive usage. A hepatic tumour should be considered in the differential diagnosis when upper abdominal pain, enlarged liver or signs of intra-abdominal haemorrhage occur.

Progestogen-only oral contraceptives may offer less protection against ectopic pregnancy, than against intrauterine pregnancy.

Femulen should be discontinued at least 4 weeks before elective surgery or during periods of prolonged immobilisation. It would be reasonable to resume Femulen two or three weeks after surgery provided the woman is ambulant. However, every woman should be considered individually with regard to the nature of the operation, the extent of immobilisation, the presence of additional risk factors and the chance of unwanted conception.

Caution should be exercised where there is the possibility of an interaction between a pre-existing disorder and a known or suspected side effect. The use of Femulen in women suffering from epilepsy, or with a history of migraine or cardiac or renal dysfunction may result in exacerbation of these disorders because of fluid retention. Caution should also be observed in women who wear contact lenses, women with impaired carbohydrate tolerance, depression, gallstones, a past history of liver disease, varicose veins, hypertension, asthma or any disease that is prone to worsen during pregnancy (e.g. multiple sclerosis, porphyria, tetany and otosclerosis). Progestogen-only oral contraceptives may offer less protection against ectopic pregnancy, than against intrauterine pregnancy.

A meta-analysis from 54 epidemiological studies reported that there is a slightly increased relative risk of having breast cancer diagnosed in women who are currently using oral contraceptives (OC). The observed pattern of increased risk may be due to an earlier diagnosis of breast cancer in OC users, the biological effects of OCs or a combination of both. The additional breast cancers diagnosed in current users of OCs or in women who have used OCs in the last ten years are more likely to be localised to the breast than those in women who never used OCs.

Breast cancer is rare among women under 40 years of age whether or not they take OCs. Whilst the background risk increases with age, the excess number of breast cancer diagnoses in current and recent progesterone-pill only (POP) users is small in relation to the overall risk of breast cancer, possibly of similar magnitude to that associated with combined OCs. However, for POPs, the evidence is based on much smaller populations of users and so is less conclusive than that for combined OCs.

The most important risk factor for breast cancer in POP users is the age women discontinue the POP; the older the age at stopping, the more breast cancers are diagnosed. Duration of use is less important and the excess risk gradually disappears during the course of the 10 years after stopping POP use, such that by 10 years there appears to be no excess.

The evidence suggests that compared with never-users, among 10,000 women who use POPs for up to 5 years but stop by age 20, there would be much less than 1 extra case of breast cancer diagnosed up to 10 years afterwards. For those stopping by age 30 after 5 years use of the POP, there would be an estimated 2–3 extra cases (additional to the 44 cases of breast cancer per 10,000 women in this age group never exposed to oral contraceptives). For those stopping by age 40 after 5 years use, there would be an estimated 10 extra cases diagnosed up to 10 years afterwards (additional to the 160 cases of breast cancer per 10,000 never-exposed women in this age group).

It is important to inform patients that users of all contraceptive pills appear to have a small increase in the risk of being diagnosed with breast cancer, compared with non-users of oral contraceptives, but this has to be weighed against the known benefits.

Interaction with other medicaments and other forms of interaction:

Drug interactions: Some drugs may modify the metabolism of Femulen reducing its effectiveness; these include certain sedatives, antibiotics, anti-epileptic and anti-arthritic drugs. During the time such agents are used concurrently, it is advised that mechanical contraceptives also be used.

Pregnancy and lactation:
Pregnancy: Femulen is contra-indicated in women with suspected pregnancy. Several reports suggest an association between foetal exposure to female sex hormones, including oral contraceptives, and congenital anomalies.

Lactation: There is no evidence that progestogen-only oral contraceptives diminish the yield of breast milk. In a study of nursing mothers taking Femulen, the median percentage of norethisterone, the principal metabolite of ethynodial diacetate given to the mother which was ingested by the infant was 0.02%. No adverse effect of the drug on the infants was noted.

Effects on ability to drive and use machines: None known.

Undesirable effects: Clinical investigations with Femulen indicate that side effects are infrequent and tend to decrease with time. Known or suspected side effects of progestogen-only oral contraceptives include gastrointestinal disorders such as nausea and vomiting, skin disorders including chloasma, breast changes, ocular changes, headache, migraine and depression, appetite and weight changes, change in libido, increase in size of uterine myofibromata, and changes in carbohydrate, lipid or vitamin metabolism. Rarely dizziness, hirsutism and colitis have been reported in users of progestogen-only oral contraceptives.

The use of oral contraceptives has also been associated with a possible increased incidence of gallbladder disease.

Tests of endocrine, hepatic and thyroid function, as well as coagulation tests may be affected by Femulen.

Menstrual pattern: Women taking Femulen for the first time should be informed that they may initially experience menstrual irregularity. This may include amenorrhoea, prolonged bleeding and/or spotting but such irregularity tends to decrease with time. If a women misses two consecutive periods, pregnancy should be ruled out before continuing the contraceptive regimen.

Overdosage: Serious ill effects have not been reported following acute ingestion of large doses of oral contraceptives by young children. Nausea and vomiting may occur and vaginal withdrawal bleeding may present in pre-pubertal girls. There is no specfici antidote and treatment should be symptomatic. Gastric lavage may be employed if the overdose is large and the patient is seen sufficiently early (within four hours).

Pharmacological properties
Pharmacodynamic properties: Femulen does not necessarily inhibit ovulation but it is believed to discourage implantation of the fertilised ovum by altering the endometrium. Cervical mucus viscosity is also changed which may render the passage of sperm less likely.

Pharmacokinetic properties: Ethynodiol diacetate is readily absorbed from the gastrointestinal tract and rapidly metabolised, largely to norethisterone. Following administration of a radiolabelled dose of ethynodiol diacetate about 60% of the radioactivity is stated to be excreted in urine and about 30% in faeces; half life in plasma was about 25 hours.

Preclinical safety data: The toxicity of norethisterone is very low. Reports of teratogenic effects in animals are uncommon. No carcinogenic effects have been found even in long-term studies. In subacute and chronic studies only minimal differences between treated and control animals are observed.

Pharmaceutical particulars
List of excipients: Calcium phosphate dibasic anhydrous, maize starch, polyvinyl pyrrolidine, sodium phosphate dibasic anhydrous, calcium acetate anhydrous, thixcin R (hydrogenated castor oil).

Incompatibilities: None known.

Shelf life: The shelf life of Femulen is 5 years.

Special precautions for storage: Store in a dry place below 30°C.

Nature and contents of container: Femulen tablets are stored in PVC/foil blister packs of 28 and 84 tablets.

Special instructions for use/handling: None.

Marketing authorisation holder: Monsanto plc (Trading as Searle).
PO Box 53, Lane End Road, High Wycombe, Bucks HP12 4HL, England.

Marketing authorisation number PL 08821/0015

Date of first authorisation/renewal of authorisation
First authorised: 25.10.72
Date of renewal: 25.10.97

Date of (partial) revision of the text
October 1997
February 1998

LOMOTIL* TABLETS

Presentation White tablets, engraved 'SEARLE' on one side. Each tablet contains Diphenoxylate Hydrochloride BP 2.5 milligrams with Atropine Sulphate PhEur 25 micrograms.

Uses Adjunctive therapy to appropriate rehydration in diarrhoea.

Control of stool formation after colostomy or ileostomy.

Relief of symptoms in chronic mild ulcerative colitis (see *Warnings)*.

Dosage and administration Caution: The recommended dosage should not be exceeded. Once satisfactory control is achieved, dosage should be reduced to suit the requirements of the individual patient.

Adults: The recommended starting dose is four tablets followed by two tablets every six hours.

Elderly: Consideration should be given to the presence of other disease and concomitant drug therapy (see *Precautions*).

Children: Recommended dosage guide

Under 4 years – not recommended.	
4–8 years	1 tablet three times daily.
9–12 years	1 tablet four times daily.
13–16 years	2 tablets three times daily.

Contra-indications, warnings, etc Lomotil is contra-indicated in patients with a known hypersensitivity to diphenoxylate hydrochloride or atropine, in patients with jaundice, intestinal obstruction, acute ulcerative colitis, and in the treatment of diarrhoea associated with pseudomembranous enterocolitis.

Appropriate fluid and electrolyte therapy should be given to protect against dehydration. If severe dehydration or electrolyte imbalance is present, Lomotil should be withheld until appropriate corrective therapy has been initiated. In some patients with ulcerative colitis, agents which inhibit intestinal motility or delay intestinal transit time have been reported to induce toxic megacolon. Patients with ulcerative colitis should be observed carefully and Lomotil therapy should be discontinued promptly if abdominal distension or other untoward symptoms develop.

Lomotil should be used with extreme caution in patients with advanced hepatorenal disease and in all patients with abnormal liver function since hepatic coma may be precipitated.

Precautions: Because a subtherapeutic dose of atropine is added to Lomotil, atropinic effects may occur in susceptible individuals or in overdosage. Individuals with Down's syndrome appear to have an increased susceptibility to the actions of atropine.

Drug interactions: Since the chemical structure of diphenoxylate hydrochloride resembles that of meperidine hydrochloride, concurrent use with MAO inhibitors could precipitate hypertensive crisis. Close observation is required when these medications are given concomiitantly with diphenoxylate hydrochloride.

Diphenoxylate hydrochloride may potentiate the action of central nervous system depressants such as barbiturates, tranquillisers and alcohol.

Pregnancy: Animal teratology and reproduction studies have demonstrated no adverse effects. The safety of Lomotil in pregnancy has not been established. However, as with all drugs, caution is recommended when used in early pregnancy.

Nursing mothers: Diphenoxylate hydrochloride and atropine sulphate may be excreted in human milk. If a nursing mother is taking Lomotil, the infant may exhibit some effects of the drug.

Adverse effects: Adverse reactions reported include:

Central nervous system: malaise/lethargy/sedation/somnolence, confusion, dizziness, restlessness, depression, euphoria, hallucinations, headache.

Allergic: anaphylaxis, angioedema, urticaria, pruritus.

Gastrointestinal system: paralytic ileus, toxic megacolon, gastrointestinal intolerance such as nausea and vomiting, anorexia, abdominal discomfort.

Atropine effects, such as flushing, dryness of the skin and mucous membranes, tachycardia, hyperthermia and urinary retention may occur, especially in children.

Overdosage: Accidental overdosage may produce narcosis with respiratory depression or atropine poisoning or both, particularly in children. Symptoms of overdosage include dryness of the skin and mucous membranes, flushing, hyperthermia and tachycardia, nystagmus, pinpoint pupils, hypotonic reflexes, lethargy, coma and severe respiratory depression. The onset of symptoms of overdosage may be considerable delayed and respiratory depression may not become evident until as late as 12 to 30 hours after ingestion and may recur in spite of an initial response to narcotic antagonists. Continuous observation should be maintained for at least 48 hours.

If respiratory depression develops, naloxone, a specific antidote, should be administered. The duration of action of naloxone hydrochloride is considerably shorter than that of diphenoxylate hydrochloride and repeated injections of the antidote may be required. Establishment of a patent airway and artificial ventilation may be needed. If the patient is not comatose gastric lavage and administration of a slurry of activated charcoal may be indicated.

Pharmaceutical precautions Store below 30°C (86°F).

Legal category POM.

Package quantities Carton containing blister strips of 100 tablets.

Further information Nil.

Product licence number 08821/0028.

MENOPHASE*

Qualitative and quantitative composition Menophase comprises 6 different formulations:

5 pink tablets containing 12.5 micrograms mestranol;

8 orange tablets containing 25 micrograms mestranol;

2 yellow tablets containing 50 micrograms mestranol;

3 green tablets containing 25 micrograms mestranol and 1 milligram norethisterone;

6 blue tablets containing 30 micrograms mestranol and 1.5 milligrams norethisterone;

4 lavender tablets containing 20 micrograms mestranol and 750 micrograms norethisterone

Tablets are inscribed 'SYNTEX' on one side.

Pharmaceutical form Tablets for oral administration.

Clinical particulars
Therapeutic indications: Menophase is indicated for the treatment of menopausal symptoms and allied disorders. These include hot flushes and sweats, depression, lack of concentration, emotional liability, nervousness, lethargy, insomnia, loss of libido, senile vaginitis, pruritus and dry skin. Menophase is also indicated for the prophylaxis of menopausal osteoporosis in females who are at risk from developing fractures.

Posology and method of administration:
Oral administration: The patient is advised to take her first tablet on a Sunday and thereafter to take one tablet at the same time each day in sequential order round the pack. She starts a new pack the day after she has taken her last lavender tablet from the previous pack. Though menopausal symptoms are likely to improve during the first month of treatment it will be necessary to maintain therapy for 6–12 months. If symptoms recur after discontinuation further courses can be prescribed.

Tablet omissions: Since Menophase is not an oral contraceptive, in the event of a missed tablet the patient should be advised to discard the tablet(s) missed and take only the tablet appropriate to the day of the week.

Contra-indications: Pregnancy (see also *Special warnings and special precautions for use*): Active deep venous thrombosis, thromboembolic disorders, or a history of confirmed venous thromboembolism; benign and malignant liver tumours; severe disturbances of liver function; jaundice or general pruritus during a previous pregnancy; Dubin-Johnson syndrome; Rotor syndrome; cardiovascular or cerebrovascular disorders e.g. thrombophlebitis, thromboembolic processes or a history of these conditions; sickle-cell anaemia; porphyria; existing or previous moderate to severe hypertension; existing or previous breast or uterine cancer or oestrogen-dependent neoplasia; undiagnosed irregular vaginal bleeding; congenital disturbances of lipid metabolism; existing or previous hyperlipoproteinaemia; a history of pemphigoid gestationis or otosclerosis made worse by pregnancy.

Special warnings and special precautions for use: Menophase is not an oral contraceptive. Menophase provides sequential graded doses of hormones; the post-menopausal patient with an intact uterus may therefore experience a small, regular monthly bleed but if forewarned of this possibility, it usually causes no distress. Hormonal contraception should be stopped when Menophase is started and the patient should be advised to take non-hormonal contraceptive precautions during the prescribing period.

Treatment should be stopped at once if jaundice or pregnancy occurs. If pregnancy is confirmed the patient should be told of the potential risk to the foetus and the advisability of continuing the pregnancy should be discussed.

The use of this product in patients suffering from epilepsy, or with a history of hypertension, migraine, asthma or cardiac dysfunction may result in exacerbation of these disorders because of fluid retention; these patients should be kept under special surveillance. Regular monitoring of blood pressure should be carried out in hypertensive patients. Treatment should be discontinued if there is a consistent rise in blood pressure. Because of the possibility of corneal oedema caution should also be observed in patients who wear contact lenses.

Discontinue treatment if there is gradual or sudden, partial or complete loss of vision or any evidence of ocular changes, onset or aggravation of migraine or development of headache of a new kind which is recurrent, persistent or severe.

Diseases known to deteriorate during pregnancy (e.g. multiple sclerosis, epilepsy, diabetes, hypertension, porphyria, tetany and otosclerosis) should be carefully observed during treatment.

Caution should be exercised in treating women with a history of oestrogen related thromboembolic disorders (e.g. during pregnancy) or idiopathic thromboembolic disorders without any obvious risk factors present. In such patients, any inherent abnormality of fibrinolysis or coagulation should be excluded before treatment with Menophase is commenced.

Caution should be observed in patients with severe varicose veins, sickle-cell haemoglobinopathy, untreated polycythaemia or pulmonary hypertension.

Pregnancy must be excluded before starting treatment with Menophase.

Measurement of blood pressure, along with examination of breasts and pelvic organs is advised before and periodically during treatment. Examination of the endometrium may also be considered. Treatment should be discontinued if there is a consistent rise in blood pressure.

Epidemiological studies have suggested that hormone replacement therapy (HRT) is associated with an increased relative risk of developing venous thromboembolism (VTE) i.e. deep vein thrombosis or pulmonary embolism. The studies find a 2–3 fold increase for users compared with non-users which for healthy women amounts to a low risk of one extra case of VTE each year for every 5000 patients taking HRT.

Generally recognised risk factors for VTE include a personal or family history and severe obesity (Body Mass Index >30 kg/m^2). In women with these factors the benefits of treatment with HRT need to be carefully weighed against risks.

The risk of VTE may be temporarily increased with prolonged immobilisation, major trauma or major surgery. In women on HRT scrupulous attention should be given to prophylactic measures to prevent VTE following surgery. Where prolonged immobilisation is liable to follow elective surgery, particularly abdominal or orthopaedic surgery to the lower limbs, consideration should be given to temporarily stopping HRT 4 weeks earlier, if this is possible.

If venous thromboembolism develops after initiating therapy the drug should be discontinued.

Benign and malignant liver tumours have also been associated with long-term oestrogen therapy. The relationship between occurrence of liver tumours and the use of female sex hormones is not known at present. These tumours are very rare but they may rupture, causing intra-abdominal bleeding. If the patient presents with a mass or tenderness in the right upper quadrant or an acute abdomen, the presence of a tumour should be considered.

Decreased glucose tolerance may occur in diabetic patients on this treatment and their control must be carefully supervised. Changes in lipid metabolism may also be observed.

Thyroid hormone binding globulin may be increased, leading to increased circulating total thyroid hormone. Hence, care must be taken in interpreting thyroid function tests.

Caution should be observed in patients with a history of gall stones. Some women are predisposed to cholestasis during steroid therapy. Caution should also be observed in patients with renal dysfunction.

Interaction with other medicaments and other forms of interaction: Menophase may alter the effectiveness of anticonvulsants, antihypertensive agents, betablockers, hypnotics, hypoglycaemic agents, oral anticoagulants, theophylline, tranquillisers, tricyclic antidepressants and vitamins.

Pregnancy and lactation: Contra-indicated in pregnancy.

Effects on ability to drive and use machines: Not applicable.

Undesirable effects: The following symptoms have been reported during treatment: anxiety, increased appetite, bloating, breast symptoms, cardiac symptoms, depression, dizziness, headaches, dyspepsia, leg pains and swelling, altered libido, excessive production of cervical mucus, intermenstrual bleeding, nausea, rashes, vomiting and altered weight.

The following have also been observed: endometrial neoplasia, increase in the size of uterine fibromyomata, endometrial proliferation and aggravation of endometriosis.

Overdose: Overdosage may be manifested by nausea, vomiting, breast enlargement and vaginal bleeding. There is no specific antidote and treatment should be symptomatic. Gastric lavage may be employed if the overdose is large and the patient is seen sufficiently early (within 4 hours).

Pharmacological properties

Pharmacodynamic properties: Mestranol is a synthetic oestrogen which achieves its oestrogenic effect through conversion to ethinyloestradiol. It is active in the development and maintenance of the female sex organs, secondary sex characteristics, control of mammary glands, proliferation of the endometrium, development of the decidua and cyclic changes in the cervix and vagina.

Norethisterone is a progestogen which acts on the endometrium by converting the proliferative phase to a secretory phase and preparing the uterus to receive the fertilised ovum. It also suppresses uterine motility and is responsible for further development of the breasts. It is used in this product to reduce the risk of endometrial hyperplasia which may occur with unopposed long-term oestrogen therapy.

Pharmacokinetic properties: Norethisterone is rapidly and completely absorbed after oral administration, peak plasma concentrations occurring in the majority of subjects between 1 and 3 hours. Due to first-pass metabolism, blood levels after oral administration are 60% of those after i.v. administration. The half life of elimination varies from 5 to 12 hours, with a mean of 7.6 hours. Norethisterone is metabolised mainly in the liver. Approximately 60% of the administered dose is excreted as metabolites in urine and faeces.

Mestranol is rapidly absorbed and extensively metabolised to ethinyloestradiol. Ethinyloestradiol is extensively metabolised, largely in the gastro-intestinal mucosa and to a lesser extent in the liver. Very little is excreted unchanged. The metabolites are excreted in both urine and bile.

Preclinical safety data: The toxicity of norethisterone is very low. Reports of teratogenic effects in animals are uncommon. No carcinogenic effects have been found even in long-term studies.

Long-term continuous administration of oestrogens in some animals increases the frequency of carcinoma of the breast, cervix, vagina and liver.

Pharmaceutical particulars

List of excipients: All of the tablets in the Menophase pack contain: Maize starch, povidone, magnesium stearate and lactose.

The pink tablets also contain E123. The orange tablets contain E110. The yellow tablets contain E104 and E110. The green tablets contain E104 and E132. The blue tablets contain E132. The lavender tablets contain E123 and E132.

Incompatibilities: None stated.

Shelf life: The shelf life of Menophase tablets is 5 years.

Special precautions for storage: Store in a dry place below 25°C away from direct sunlight.

Nature and contents of container: Menophase tablets are supplied in pvc/foil blister packs of 28 tablets.

Instructions for use/handling: None.

Marketing authorisation holder: Monsanto plc, PO Box 53, Lane End Road, High Wycombe, Bucks HP12 4HL.

Marketing authorisation number PL 08821/0038.

Date of first authorisation/renewal of authorisation March 1996

Date of (partial) revision of the text April 1996/ December 1997

NAPRATEC*

Presentation Napratec is a combination pack containing 56 tablets of naproxen and 56 tablets of Cytotec*.

Naproxen is a yellow, oblong tablet engraved SEARLE N.500 with breakline on one side containing 500 mg of Naproxen BP.

Cytotec is a white/off-white hexagonal tablet, scored on both sides, engraved SEARLE 1461 on one side, containing misoprostol 200 micrograms.

Uses

Indications: Napratec combination pack is indicated for patients who require naproxen 500 mg twice daily and Cytotec 200 micrograms twice daily.

Naproxen is indicated for the treatment of rheumatoid arthritis, osteoarthritis (degenerative arthritis) and ankylosing spondylitis.

Cytotec is indicated for the prophylaxis of nonsteroidal anti-inflammatory drug (NSAID)-induced gastroduodenal ulceration.

Actions: Naproxen is a nonsteroidal anti-inflammatory drug (NSAID). Cytotec is an analogue of naturally occurring prostaglandin E_1 which protects the gastroduodenal mucosa against ulcers induced by NSAIDs.

Dosage and administration

Adults: 1 tablet of naproxen and 1 tablet of Cytotec taken together twice daily with food.

Elderly: Studies indicate that although total plasma concentration of naproxen is unchanged, the unbound plasma fraction of naproxen is increased in the elderly.

With Cytotec the usual dosage may be used in the elderly.

Napratec should only be used in those patients for whom 500 mg naproxen twice daily is appropriate and in whom no reduction of naproxen dosage is necessary (see also sections on renal and hepatic impairment).

Renal impairment: As the final pathway for the elimination of naproxen metabolites is largely (95%) by urinary excretion via glomerular filtration, it should be used with great caution in patients with impaired renal function and the monitoring of serum creatinine and/or creatinine clearance is advised in these patients. Naproxen is not recommended in patients having a baseline creatinine clearance of less than 20 ml/minute.

Certain patients, specifically those whose renal blood flow is compromised, such as in extracellular volume depletion, cirrhosis of the liver, sodium restriction, congestive heart failure, and pre-existing renal disease, should have renal function assessed before and during naproxen therapy. Some elderly patients in whom impaired renal function may be expected could also fall within this category. Where there is a possibility of accumulation of naproxen metabolites, such patients may not be suitable to receive naproxen 500 mg twice daily.

With Cytotec no dosage alteration is necessary in patients with impaired renal function.

Hepatic impairment: Chronic alcoholic liver disease and probably also other forms of cirrhosis reduce the total plasma concentration of naproxen, but the plasma concentration of unbound naproxen is increased.

With Cytotec no dosage alteration is necessary in patients with impaired hepatic function.

Children: Napratec is not recommended.

Contra-indications, warnings, etc

Contra-indications

Use in pregnancy and lactation: Napratec is contra-indicated in pregnancy. This is on the basis that Cytotec is contra-indicated in pregnancy or women planning a pregnancy as it increases uterine tone and contractions in pregnancy which may cause partial or complete expulsion of the products of conception.

Teratology studies with naproxen in rats and rabbits at dose levels equivalent on a human multiple basis to those which have produced foetal abnormality with certain other NSAIDs, e.g. aspirin, have not produced evidence of foetal damage with naproxen. As with other drugs of this type, naproxen delays parturition in animals (the relevance of this finding to human patients is unknown) and also affects the human foetal cardiovascular system (closure of the ductus arteriosus).

Napratec should not be administered during breastfeeding.

Napratec is contra-indicated in patients with a known allergy to naproxen, naproxen sodium formulations, or prostaglandins.

As the potential exists with naproxen for cross-sensitivity to aspirin and other nonsteroidal anti-inflammatory drugs, Napratec should not be administered to patients in whom aspirin and other NSAIDs induce asthma, rhinitis, urticaria or angioedema.

As Napratec is a 'prevention pack' it should not be used for treating arthritis in patients with active gastric or duodenal ulceration. Such patients may be treated with a healing dose of Cytotec, 800 micrograms daily in divided doses with meals and the NSAID continued or discontinued at the physician's discretion.

Warnings

Use in pre-menopausal women (see also 'Contra-indications'): Napratec should not be used in pre-menopausal women unless the patient is at high risk of complications from NSAID-induced ulceration. In such patients it is advised that Napratec should only be used if the patient:

- takes effective contraceptive measures
- has been advised of the risks of taking the product if pregnant (see 'Contra-indications').

Precautions: Naproxen in common with other NSAIDs decreases platelet aggregation and prolongs bleeding time. This effect should be considered when bleeding times are determined.

Naproxen may precipitate bronchospasm in patients suffering from, or with a history of, bronchial asthma or allergic disease.

Mild peripheral oedema has been observed in a few

patients receiving naproxen. Although sodium retention has not been reported in metabolic studies, it is possible that patients with questionable or compromised cardiac function may be at a greater risk when taking naproxen.

Sporadic abnormalities in laboratory tests (e.g. liver function tests) have occurred in patients on naproxen, but no definite trend was seen in any test indicating toxicity.

Cytotec should be used with caution in disease states where hypotension might precipitate severe complications, e.g. cerebrovascular disease, coronary artery disease or severe peripheral vascular disease including hypertension.

Drug interactions: Due to the high plasma protein binding of naproxen, patients simultaneously receiving hydantoins, anti-coagulants or a highly protein-bound sulphonamide should be observed for signs of overdosage of these drugs. No interactions have been observed in clinical studies with naproxen and anti-coagulants or sulphonylureas, but caution is nevertheless advised since interaction has been seen with other non-steroidal agents of this class.

NSAIDs may attenuate the natriuretic efficacy of diuretics due to inhibition of intrarenal synthesis of prostaglandins.

NSAIDs including naproxen have been reported to increase steady state plasma lithium levels. It is recommended that these levels are monitored whenever initiating, adjusting or discontinuing naproxen products.

Concomitant administration of naproxen with beta-blockers may reduce their antihypertensive effect.

Probenecid given concurrently increases naproxen plasma levels and extends its plasma half-life considerably.

Caution is advised when methotrexate is administered concurrently because of possible enhancement of its toxicity since naproxen, among other NSAIDs, has been reported to induce the tubular secretion of methotrexate in an animal model.

Naproxen therapy should be temporarily withdrawn before adrenal function tests are performed as it may artificially interfere with some tests for 17-ketogenic steroids. Similarly naproxen may interfere with some assays of urinary 5-hydroxyindoleacetic acid.

Cytotec is predominantly metabolised via fatty acid oxidising systems and has shown no adverse effect on the hepatic microsomal mixed function oxidase (P450) enzyme system. No drug interactions have been attributed to Cytotec, and in specific studies no clinically significant pharmacokinetic or pharmacodynamic interaction has been demonstrated with antipyrine, diazepam, propranolol or NSAIDs.

Adverse effects
Naproxen
Gastrointestinal: The more frequent reactions are nausea, vomiting, abdominal discomfort and epigastric distress. The more serious reaction, colitis, may occasionally occur.

Naproxen also causes gastrointestinal bleeding and gastric and duodenal ulceration, the consequence of which may be haemorrhage and perforation. The inclusion of Cytotec in the combination pack is to prevent naproxen-induced gastric and duodenal ulceration.

Dermatological/hypersensitivity: Skin rashes, urticaria, angio-oedema. Anaphylactic reactions to naproxen and naproxen sodium formulations, eosinophilic pneumonitis, alopecia, erythema multiforme, Stevens Johnson syndrome, epidermal necrolysis, photosensitivity reactions, pseudoporphyria and epidermolysis bullosa may occur rarely.

Central nervous system: Headache, insomnia, inability to concentrate and cognitive dysfunction have been reported.

Haematological: Thrombocytopenia, granulocytopenia, aplastic anaemia, and haemolytic anaemia may occur rarely.

Other: Tinnitus, hearing impairment, vertigo, mild peripheral oedema. Jaundice, fatal hepatitis, nephropathy, haematuria, visual disturbances, vasculitis, aseptic meningitis and ulcerative stomatitis have been reported rarely.

Cytotec
Gastrointestinal: Diarrhoea has been reported and is occasionally severe and prolonged and may require withdrawal of the drug. It can be minimised by taking Cytotec with food and by avoiding the use of predominantly magnesium-containing antacids when an antacid is required. Abdominal pain with or without associated dyspepsia can follow Cytotec therapy. Other gastrointestinal adverse effects reported include dyspepsia, flatulence, nausea and vomiting.

Female reproductive system: Menorrhagia, vaginal bleeding and intermenstrual bleeding have been reported in both pre- and post-menopausal women.

Other adverse effects: Skin rashes have been reported. Dizziness has been infrequently reported.

Overdosage
Naproxen: Significant overdosage of the drug may be characterised by drowsiness, heartburn, indigestion, nausea or vomiting. A few patients have experienced seizures, but it is not clear whether these were naproxen-related or not. It is not known what dose of the drug would be life-threatening.

In the event of overdosage with naproxen, the stomach may be emptied and usual supportive measures employed. Animal studies indicate that the prompt administration of activated charcoal in adequate amounts would tend to reduce markedly the absorption of the drug.

Haemodialysis does not decrease the plasma concentration of naproxen because of the high degree of protein binding. However, haemodialysis may still be appropriate in a patient with renal failure who has taken naproxen.

Cytotec: Intensification of pharmacological and adverse effects may occur with overdose. In the event of overdosage with Cytotec, symptomatic and supportive therapy should be given as appropriate.

Pharmaceutical precautions Store in a dry place below 30°C (86°F).

Legal category POM.

Package quantities Combination pack containing 4×7 day treatment wallets containing 56 naproxen 500 mg tablets in pvc/foil blisters and 56 Cytotec 200 microgram tablets in cold-formed aluminium blisters.

Further information Cytotec in multiples of the recommended therapeutic dose in animals has produced gastric mucosal hyperplasia. This characteristic response to E prostaglandins reverts to normal on discontinuation of the compound. In patients, histological examination of gastric biopsies taken before and after treatment with misoprostol after up to one year's duration have shown no adverse tissue response attributable to misoprostol. Inhibition of gastric secretion by Cytotec is achieved by a combination of local and systemic effects. Cytotec is rapidly absorbed following oral administration, with peak plasma levels of the active metabolite (misoprostol acid) occurring after about 30 minutes. The plasma elimination half-life of misoprostol acid is 20–40 minutes. Increases in the C_{max} and AUC for misoprostol acid have been observed when co-administered with naproxen in a single dose study. These changes are not thought to be clinically significant since the higher values are still well within the variation seen after 200 micrograms misoprostol in other studies. No accumulation of misoprostol acid in plasma occurs after repeated dosing of 400 micrograms twice daily.

Product licence number 08821/0021.

NORIDAY* TABLETS

Qualitative and quantitative composition Each tablet contains 350 micrograms norethisterone.

Pharmaceutical form White, flat, circular, bevel-edged tablet inscribed 'SEARLE' on one side and 'NY' on the other side.

Clinical particulars
Therapeutic indications: Noriday is a progestogen-only oral contraceptive. It is particularly useful for women for whom oestrogens may not be appropriate.

Posology and method of administration:
Oral administration: Starting on the first day of menstruation, one pill every day without a break in medication for as long as contraception is required. Additional contraceptive precautions (such as a condom) should be taken for the first 7 days of the first pack. Pills should be taken at the same time each day.

Missed pills: If a pill is missed within 3 hours of the correct dosage time then the missed pill should be taken as soon as possible; this will ensure that contraceptive protection is maintained. If a pill is taken 3 or more hours late it is recommended that the woman takes the last missed pill as soon as possible and then continues to take the rest of the pills in the normal manner. However, to provide continued contraceptive protection is it recommended that an alternative method of contraception, such as a condom, is used for the next 7 days.

Changing from another oral contraceptive: In order to ensure that contraception is maintained it is advised that the first pill is taken on the day immediately after the patient has finished the previous pack.

Use after childbirth, miscarriage or abortion: The first pill should be taken on the 21st day after childbirth. This will ensure the patient is protected immediately. If there is any delay in taking the first pill, contraception may not be established until 7 days after the first pill has been taken. In these circumstances women should be advised that extra contraceptive methods will be necessary.

After a miscarriage or abortion patients can take the first pill on the next day; in this way they will be protected immediately.

Vomiting and diarrhoea: Gastrointestinal upsets, such as vomiting and diarrhoea, may interfere with the absorption of the pill leading to a reduction in contraceptive efficacy. Women should continue to take Noriday, but they should also be advised to use another contraceptive method during the period of gastrointestinal upset and for the next 7 days.

Contra-indications: The contra-indications for progestogen-only oral contraceptives are:

(i) known, suspected, or a past history of breast, genital or hormone dependent cancer;
(ii) acute or severe chronic liver diseases including past or present liver tumours, Dubin-Johnson or Rotor syndrome;
(iii) active liver disease;
(iv) history during pregnancy of idiopathic jaundice or severe pruritus;
(v) disorders of lipid metabolism;
(vi) undiagnosed abnormal vaginal bleeding;
(vii) known or suspected pregnancy;
(viii) hypersensitivity to any component.

Combined oestrogen/progestogen preparations have been associated with an increase in the risk of thromboembolic and thrombotic disease. Risk has been reported to be related to both oestrogenic and progestogenic activity. In the absence of long term epidemiological studies with progestogen-only oral contraceptives, it is required that the existence, or history of thrombophlebitis, thromboembolic disorders, cerebral vascular disease, myocardial infarction, angina, or coronary artery disease be described as a contra-indication to Noriday as it is to oestrogen containing oral contraceptives.

Special warnings and special precautions for use: Women receiving treatment with Noriday should be kept under regular medical surveillance.

Malignant hepatic tumours have been reported on rare occasions in long-term users of contraceptives. Benign hepatic tumours have also been associated with oral contraceptive usage. A hepatic tumour should be considered in the differential diagnosis when upper abdominal pain, enlarged liver or signs of intra-abdominal haemorrhage occur.

A statistical association between the use of oral contraceptives and the occurrence of thrombosis, embolism or haemorrhage has been reported. Patients receiving oral contraceptives should be kept under regular surveillance, in view of the possibility of development of conditions such as thromboembolism.

The risk of coronary artery disease in women taking oral contraceptives is increased by the presence of other predisposing factors such as cigarette smoking, hypercholesterolaemia, obesity, diabetes, history of pre-eclamptic toxaemia and increasing age. After the age of thirty-five years, the patient and physician should carefully re-assess the risk/benefit ratio of using oral contraceptives as opposed to alternative methods of contraception.

Noriday should be discontinued at least 4 weeks before elective surgery or during periods of prolonged immobilisation. It would be reasonable to resume Noriday 2 weeks after surgery provided the woman is ambulant. However, every woman should be considered individually with regard to the nature of the operation, the extent of immobilisation, the presence of additional risk factors and the chance of unwanted conception.

Noriday should be discontinued if there is a gradual or sudden, partial or complete loss of vision or any evidence of ocular changes, onset or aggravation of migraine or development of headache of a new kind which is recurrent, persistent or severe, suspicion of thrombosis or infarction, significant rise in blood pressure or if jaundice occurs.

Caution should be exercised where there is the possibility of an interaction between a pre-existing disorder and a known or suspected side effect. The use of Noriday in women suffering from epilepsy, or with a history of migraine or cardiac or renal dysfunction may result in exacerbation of these disorders because of fluid retention. Caution should also be observed in women who wear contact lenses, women with impaired carbohydrate tolerance, depression, gallstones, a past history of liver disease, varicose veins, hypertension, asthma or any disease that is prone to worsen during pregnancy (e.g. multiple sclerosis, porphyria, tetany and otosclerosis).

An increased risk of congenital abnormalities, including heart defects and limb defects, has been reported following the use of sex hormones, including oral contraceptives, in pregnancy. If the patient does not adhere to the prescribed schedule, the possibility of pregnancy should be considered at the time of the first missed period and further use of oral contraceptives should be withheld until pregnancy has been ruled out. It is recommended that for any patient who has missed two consecutive periods, pregnancy should be ruled out before continuing the contraceptive regimen. If pregnancy is confirmed the patient should be advised of the potential risks to the foetus and the advisability of continuing the pregnancy should be discussed in the light of these risks. It is advisable to discontinue Noriday three months before a planned pregnancy.

Progestogen-only oral contraceptives may offer less protection against ectopic pregnancy than against intrauterine pregnancy.

A meta-analysis from 54 epidemiological studies reported that there is a slightly increased risk of having breast cancer diagnosed in women who are currently using oral contraceptives (OC). The observed pattern of increased risk may be due to an earlier diagnosis of breast cancer in OC users, the biological effects of OCs or a combination of both. The additional breast cancers diagnosed in current users of OCs or in women who have used OCs in the last ten years are more likely to be localised to the breast than those in women who never used OCs.

Breast cancer is rare among women under 40 years of age whether or not they take OCs. Whilst the background risk increases with age, the excess number of breast cancer diagnoses in current and recent progesterone-only pill (POP) users is small in relation to the overall risk of breast cancer, possibly of similar magnitude to that associated with combined OCs. However, for POPs, the evidence is based on much smaller populations of users and so is less conclusive than that for combined OCs.

The most important risk factor for breast cancer in POP users is the age women discontinue the POP; the older the age at stopping, the more breast cancers are diagnosed. Duration of use is less important and the excess risk gradually disappears during the course of the 10 years after stopping POP use, such that by 10 years there appears to be no excess.

The evidence suggests that compared with never-users, among 10,000 women who use POPs for up to 5 years but stop by age 20, there would be much less than 1 extra case of breast cancer diagnosed up to 10 years afterwards. For those stopping by age 30 after 5 years use of the POP, there would be an estimated 2–3 extra cases (additional to the 44 cases of breast cancer per 10,000 women in this age group never exposed to oral contraceptives). For those stopping by age 40 after 5 years use, there would be an estimated 10 extra cases diagnosed up to 10 years afterwards (additional to the 160 cases of breast cancer per 10,000 never-exposed women in this age group).

It is important to inform patients that users of all contraceptive pills appear to have a small increase in the risk of being diagnosed with breast cancer, compared with non-users of oral contraceptives, but this has to be weighed against the known benefits.

Interaction with other medicaments and other forms of interaction: Some drugs may modify the metabolism of Noriday reducing its effectiveness; these include certain sedatives, antibiotics and anti-epileptics. During the time such agents are used concurrently, it is advised that an alternative method of contraception, such as a condom, is also used.

The serum levels of prednisone, prednisolone, cloprednol and possibly other corticosteroids are considerably increased in those taking oral contraceptives. Both the therapeutic and toxic effects may be expected to increase accordingly.

Pregnancy and lactation: Noriday is contra-indicated in women with suspected pregnancy. Several reports suggest an association between foetal exposure to female sex hormones, including oral contraceptives, and congenital anomalies.

There is no evidence that Noriday tablets diminish the yield of breast milk. Small amounts of steroid materials appear in the milk; their effect on the breast-fed child has not been determined.

Effects on ability to drive and use machines: None known.

Undesirable effects: The incidence of side effects in clinical trials was lower than that experienced with oestrogen-containing oral contraceptives. Side effects which did occur included some cycle irregularity during the first few months of therapy, spotting or breakthrough bleeding, amenorrhoea, breast discomfort, gastrointestinal symptoms, rash, headaches, migraine, depression, fatigue, nervousness, disturbance of appetite and changes in weight and libido.

Hypertension, which is usually reversible on discontinuing treatment, has occurred in a small percentage of women taking oral contraceptives.

Menstrual pattern: Women taking Noriday for the first time should be informed that they may initially experience menstrual irregularity. This may include amenorrhoea, prolonged bleeding and/or spotting but such irregularity tends to decrease with time. If a woman misses two consecutive periods, pregnancy should be ruled out before continuing the contraceptive regimen.

Overdose: Serious ill effects have not been reported following acute ingestion of large doses of oral contraceptives by young children. Overdosage may be manifested by nausea, vomiting, breast enlargement and vaginal bleeding. There is no specific antidote and treatment should be symptomatic. Gastric lavage may be employed if the overdose is large and the patient is seen sufficiently early (within four hours).

Pharmacological properties

Pharmacodynamic properties: Norethisterone administration increases the protein and sialic acid content of cervical mucus which prevents penetration of the mucus by spermatozoa. It causes changes in the structure of the endometrium such that implantation of blastocysts is impaired. It also reduces numbers and height of cilia on cells lining the fallopian tube, which could delay tubal transport of ova.

Pharmacokinetic properties: Norethisterone is rapidly and completely absorbed after oral administration, peak plasma concentrations occurring in the majority of subjects between 1 and 3 hours. Due to first-pass metabolism, blood levels after oral administration are 60% of those after i.v. administration. The half life of elimination varies from 5 to 12 hours, with a mean of 7.6 hours. Norethisterone is metabolised mainly in the liver. Approximately 60% of the administered dose is excreted as metabolites in urine and faeces.

Preclinical safety data: The toxicity of norethisterone is very low. Reports of teratogenic effects in animals are uncommon. No carcinogenic effects have been found even in long-term studies. In subacute and chronic studies only minimal differences between treated and control animals are observed.

Pharmaceutical particulars

List of excipients: Noriday tablets contain: Maize starch, polyvidone, magnesium stearate and lactose.

Incompatibilities: None known.

Shelf life: The shelf life of Noriday tablets is 5 years.

Special precautions for storage: Store in a cool, dry place away from direct sunlight.

Nature and contents of container: Noriday tablets are supplied in pvc/foil blister packs of 28 and 84 tablets. Blister packaging consists of 250 micron PVC and 20 micron aluminium foil.

Instructions for use/handling: None.

Marketing authorisation holder: Monsanto p.l.c. (Trading as Searle), PO Box 53, Lane End Road, High Wycombe, Bucks HP12 4HL.

Marketing authorisation number PL 08821/0036

Date of first authorisation/renewal of authorisation
21 March 1996

Date of (partial) revision of the text
2 January 1996
November 1997
January 1998

NORIMIN* TABLETS

Qualitative and quantitative composition Each tablet contains 1 milligram norethisterone and 35 micrograms ethinyloestradiol.

Pharmaceutical form White round flat tablets with bevel-edged tablet inscribed 'SEARLE' on one side and 'BX' on the other.

Clinical particulars

Therapeutic indications: Norimin is indicated for oral contraception, with the benefit of a low intake of oestrogen.

Posology and method of administration:

Oral administration: The dosage of Norimin for the initial cycle of therapy is 1 tablet taken at the same time each day from the first day of the menstrual cycle. For subsequent cycles, no tablets are taken for 7 days, then a new course is started of 1 tablet daily for the next 21 days. This sequence of 21 days on treatment, seven days off treatment is repeated for as long as contraception is required.

Patients unable to start taking Norimin tablets on the first day of the menstrual cycle may start treatment on any day up to and including the 5th day of the menstrual cycle.

Patients starting on day 1 of their period will be protected at once. Those patients delaying therapy up to day 5 may not be protected immediately and it is recommended that another method of contraception is used for the first 7 days of tablet-taking. Suitable methods are condoms, caps plus spermicides and intra-uterine devices. The rhythm, temperature and cervical-mucus methods should not be relied upon.

Tablet omissions: Tablets must be taken daily in order to maintain adequate hormone levels and contraceptive efficacy.

If a tablet is missed within 12 hours of the correct dosage time then the missed tablet should be taken as soon as possible, even if this means taking 2 tablets on the same day, this will ensure that contraceptive protection is maintained. If one or more tablets are missed for more than 12 hours from the correct dosage time it is recommended that the patient takes the last missed tablet as soon as possible and then continues to take the rest of the tablets in the normal manner. In addition, it is recommended that extra contraceptive protection, such as a condom, is used for the next 7 days.

Patients who have missed one or more of the last 7 tablets in a pack should be advised to start the next pack of tablets as soon as the present one has finished (i.e. without the normal seven day gap between treatments). This reduces the risk of contraceptive failure resulting from tablets being missed close to a 7 day tablet free period.

Changing from another oral contraceptive: In order to ensure that contraception is maintained it is advised that the first dose of Norimin tablets is taken on the day immediately after the patient has finished the previous pack of tablets.

Use after childbirth, miscarriage or abortion: Providing the patient is not breast feeding the first dose of Norimin tablets should be taken on the 21st day after childbirth. This will ensure the patient is protected immediately. If there is any delay in taking the first dose, contraception may not be established until 7 days after the first tablet has been taken. In these circumstances patients should be advised that extra contraceptive methods will be necessary.

After a miscarriage or abortion patients can take the first dose of Norimin tablets on the next day; in this way they will be protected immediately.

Contra-indications: As with all combined progestogen/oestrogen oral contraceptives, the following conditions should be regarded as contra-indications:

(i) Thrombophlebitis, thrombo-embolic disorders, cerebrovascular disorders, coronary artery disease, myocardial infarction, angina, hyperlipidaemia or a history of these conditions.
(ii) Acute or severe chronic liver disease, including liver tumours, Dubin-Johnson or Rotor syndrome.
(iii) History during pregnancy of idiopathic jaundice, severe pruritus or pemphigoid gestationis.
(iv) Known or suspected breast or genital cancer.
(v) Known or suspected oestrogen-dependent neoplasia.
(vi) Undiagnosed abnormal vaginal bleeding.
(vii) A history of migraines classified as classical focal or crescendo.
(viii) Pregnancy.

Special warnings and special precautions for use: Women taking oral contraceptives require careful observation if they have or have had any of the following conditions: breast nodules; fibrocystic disease of the breast or an abnormal mammogram; uterine fibroids; a history of severe depressive states; varicose veins; sickle-cell anaemia; diabetes; hypertension; cardiovascular disease; migraine; epilepsy; asthma; otosclerosis; multiple sclerosis; porphyria; tetany; disturbed liver functions; gallstones; kidney disease; chloasma; any condition that is likely to worsen during pregnancy. The worsening or first appearance of any of these conditions may indicate that the oral contraceptive should be stopped. Discontinue treatment if there is a gradual or sudden, partial or complete loss of vision or any evidence of ocular changes, onset or aggravation of migraine or development of headache of a new kind which is recurrent, persistent or severe.

Gastro-intestinal upsets, such as vomiting and diarrhoea, may interfere with the absorption of the tablets leading to a reduction in contraceptive efficacy. Patients should continue to take Norimin, but they should also be encouraged to use another contraceptive method during the period of gastro-intestinal upset and for the next 7 days.

Progestogen/oestrogen preparations should be used with caution in patients with a history of hepatic dysfunction or hypertension.

A statistical association between the use of oral contraceptives and the occurrence of thrombosis, embolism or haemorrhage has been reported. Patients receiving oral contraceptives should be kept under regular surveillance, in view of the possibility of development of conditions such as thrombo-embolism.

The risk of coronary artery disease in women taking oral contraceptives is increased by the presence of other predisposing factors such as cigarette smoking, hypercholesterolaemia, obesity, diabetes, history of pre-eclamptic toxaemia and increasing age. After the age of thirty-five years, the patient and physician should carefully re-assess the risk/benefit ratio of using combined oral contraceptives as opposed to alternative methods of contraception.

Norimin should be discontinued at least four weeks before, and for two weeks following, elective operations and during immobilisation. Patients undergoing injection treatment for varicose veins should not resume taking Norimin until 3 months after the last injection.

Benign and malignant liver tumours have been associated with oral contraceptive use. The relationship between occurrence of liver tumours and use of female sex hormones is not known at present. These tumours may rupture causing intra-abdominal bleeding. If the patient presents with a mass or tenderness in the right upper quadrant or an acute abdomen, the possible presence of a tumour should be considered.

An increased risk of congenital abnormalities, including heart defects and limb defects, has been reported following the use of sex hormones, including oral contraceptives, in pregnancy. If the patient does not adhere to the prescribed schedule, the possibility of pregnancy should be considered at the time of the first missed period and further use of oral contraceptives should be withheld until pregnancy has been ruled out. It is recommended that for any patient who has missed two consecutive periods, pregnancy should be ruled out before continuing the contraceptive regimen. If pregnancy is confirmed the patient should be advised of the potential risks to the foetus and the advisability of continuing the pregnancy should be discussed in the light of these risks. It is advisable to discontinue Norimin three months before a planned pregnancy.

The risk of arterial thrombosis associated with combined oral contraceptives increases with age, and this risk is aggravated by cigarette smoking. The use of combined oral contraceptives by women in the older age group, especially those who are cigarette smokers, should therefore be discouraged and alternative methods advised.

The use of this product in patients suffering from epilepsy, migraine, asthma or cardiac dysfunction may result in exacerbation of these disorders because of fluid retention. Caution should also be observed in patients who wear contact lenses.

Decreased glucose tolerance may occur in diabetic patients on this treatment, and their control must be carefully supervised.

The use of oral contraceptives has also been associated with a possible increased incidence of gall bladder disease.

Women with a history of oligomenorrhoea or secondary amenorrhoea or young women without regular cycles may have a tendency to remain anovulatory or to become amenorrhoeic after discontinuation of oral contraceptives. Women with these pre-existing problems should be advised of this possibility and encouraged to use other contraceptive methods.

Numerous epidemiological studies have been reported on the risks of ovarian, endometrial, cervical and breast cancer in women using combined oral contraceptives. The evidence is clear that combined oral contraceptives offer substantial protection against both ovarian and endometrial cancer.

An increased risk of cervical cancer in long-term users of combined oral contraceptives has been reported in some studies, but there continues to be controversy about the extent to which this is attributable to the confounding effects of sexual behaviour and other factors.

A meta-analysis from 54 epidemiological studies reported that there is a slightly increased relative risk (RR = 1.24) of having breast cancer diagnosed in women who are currently using combined oral contraceptives (COCs). The observed pattern of increased risk may be due to an earlier diagnosis of breast cancer in COC users, the biological effects of COCs or a combination of both. The additional breast cancers diagnosed in current users of COCs or in women who have used COCs in the last ten years are more likely to be localised to the breast than those in women who never used COCs.

Breast cancer is rare among women under 40 years of age whether or not they take COCs. Whilst this background risk increases with age, the excess number of breast cancer diagnoses in current and recent COC users is small in relation to the overall risk of breast cancer (see bar chart).

The most important risk factor for breast cancer in COC users is the age women discontinue the COC; the older the age at stopping, the more breast cancers are diagnosed. Duration of use is less important and the excess risk gradually disappears during the course of the 10 years after stopping COC use such that by 10 years there appears to be no excess.

The possible increase in risk of breast cancer should be discussed with the user and weighed against the benefits of COCs taking into account the evidence that they offer substantial protection against the risk of developing certain other cancers (e.g. ovarian and endometrial cancer).

Interaction with other medicaments and other forms of interaction: Some drugs may modify the metabolism of Norimin reducing its effectiveness; these include certain sedatives, antibiotics, anti-epileptic and anti-arthritic drugs. During the time such agents are used concurrently, it is advised that mechanical contraceptives also be used.

The results of a large number of laboratory tests have been shown to be influenced by the use of oestrogen containing oral contraceptives, which may limit their diagnostic value. Among these are: biochemical markers of thyroid and liver function; plasma levels of carrier proteins, triglycerides, coagulation and fibrinolysis factors.

Pregnancy and lactation: Contra-indicated in pregnancy.

Patients who are fully breast-feeding should not take Norimin tablets since, in common with other combined oral contraceptives, the oestrogen component may reduce the amount of milk produced. In addition, active ingredients or their metabolites have been detected in the milk of mothers taking oral contraceptives. The effect of Norimin on breast-fed infants has not been determined.

Effects on ability to drive and use machines: Not applicable.

Undesirable effects: As with all oral contraceptives, there may be slight nausea at first, weight gain or breast discomfort, which soon disappear.

Other side-effects known or suspected to occur with oral contraceptives include gastro-intestinal symptoms, changes in libido and appetite, headache, exacerbation of existing uterine fibroid disease, depression, and changes in carbohydrate, lipid and vitamin metabolism.

Spotting or bleeding may occur during the first few cycles. Usually menstrual bleeding becomes light and occasionally there may be no bleeding during the tablet-free days.

Hypertension, which is usually reversible on discontinuing treatment, has occurred in a small percentage of women taking oral contraceptives.

Overdose: Overdosage may be manifested by nausea, vomiting, breast enlargement and vaginal bleeding. There is no specific antidote and treatment should be symptomatic. Gastric lavage may be employed if the overdose is large and the patient is seen sufficiently early (within four hours).

Pharmacological properties

Pharmacodynamic properties: The mode of action of Norimin is similar to that of other progestogen/oestrogen oral contraceptives and includes the inhibition of ovulation, the thickening of cervical mucus so as to constitute a barrier to sperm and the rendering of the endometrium unreceptive to implantation. Such activity is exerted through a combined effect on one or more of the following: hypothalamus, anterior pituitary, ovary, endometrium and cervical mucus.

Pharmacokinetic properties: Norethisterone is rapidly and completely absorbed after oral administration, peak plasma concentrations occurring in the majority of subjects between 1 and 3 hours. Due to first-pass metabolism, blood levels after oral administration are 60% of those after i.v. administration. The half life of elimination varies from 5 to 12 hours, with a mean of 7.6 hours. Norethisterone is metabolised mainly in the liver. Approximately 60% of the administered dose is excreted as metabolites in urine and faeces.

Ethinyloestradiol is rapidly and well absorbed from the gastro-intestinal tract but is subject to some first-pass metabolism in the gut-wall. Compared to many other oestrogens it is only slowly metabolised in the liver. Excretion is via the kidneys with some appearing also in the faeces.

Preclinical safety data: The toxicity of norethisterone is very low. Reports of teratogenic effects in animals are uncommon. No carcinogenic effects have been found even in long-term studies.

Long-term continuous administration of oestrogens in some animals increases the frequency of carcinoma of the breast, cervix, vagina and liver.

Estimated cumulative numbers of breast cancers per 10,000 women diagnosed in 5 years of use and up to 10 years after stopping COCs, compared with numbers of breast cancers diagnosed in 10,000 women who had never used COCs.

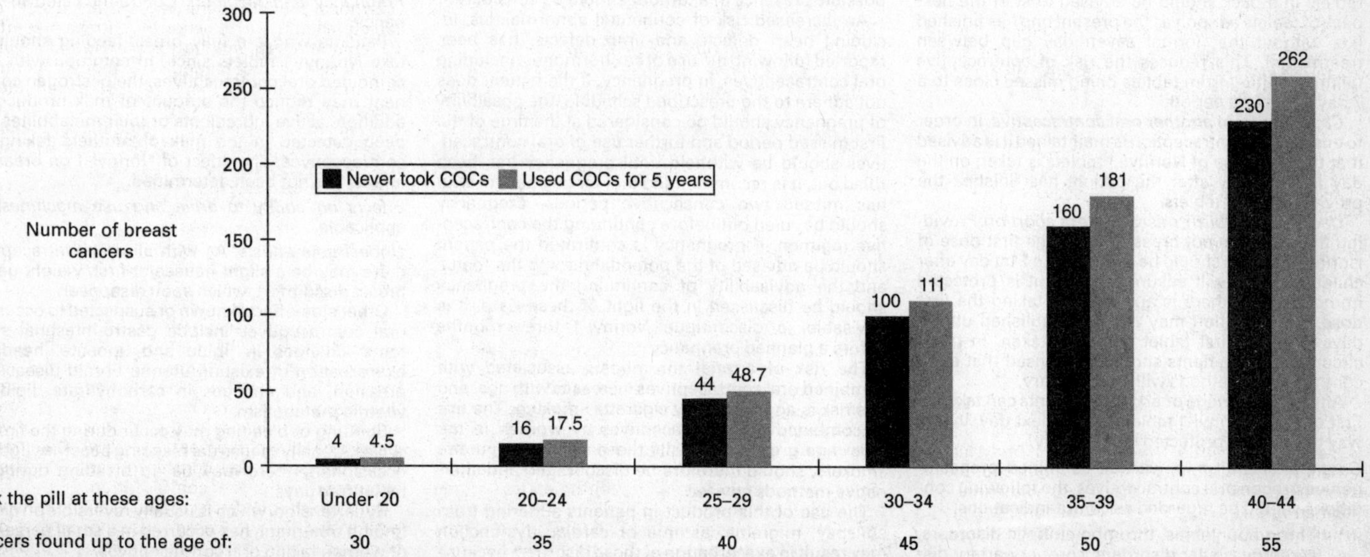

Pharmaceutical particulars

List of excipients: Norimin tablets contain: Maize starch, polyvidone, magnesium stearate and lactose.

Incompatibilities: None stated.

Shelf life: The shelf life of Norimin tablets is 5 years.

Special precautions for storage: Store in a dry place, below 25°C, away from direct sunlight.

Nature and contents of container: Norimin tablets are supplied in pvc/foil blister packs of 21 and 63 tablets.

Instruction for use/handling: None.

Marketing authorisation holder: Monsanto plc (Trading as Searle), PO Box 53, Lane End Road, High Wycombe, Bucks HP12 4HL.

Marketing authorisation number PL 08821/0040.

Date of first authorisation/renewal of authorisation May 1st 1996.

Date of (partial) revision of the text February 1998

NORINYL-1* TABLETS

Qualitative and quantitative composition Each tablet contains 1 milligram norethisterone and 50 micrograms mestranol.

Pharmaceutical form White, flat, circular, bevel-edged tablet inscribed 'SEARLE' on one side and '1' on the other side.

Clinical particulars

Therapeutic indications: Norinyl-1 is indicated for oral contraception, with the benefit of a low intake of oestrogen.

Posology and method of administration:

Oral administration: The dosage of Norinyl-1 for the initial cycle of therapy is 1 tablet taken at the same time each day from the first day of the menstrual cycle. For subsequent cycles, no tablets are taken for 7 days, then a new course is started of 1 tablet daily for the next 21 days. This sequence of 21 days on treatment, seven days off treatment is repeated for as long as contraception is required.

Patients unable to start taking Norinyl-1 tablets on the first day of the menstrual cycle may start treatment on any day up to and including the 5th day of the menstrual cycle.

Patients starting on day 1 of their period will be protected at once. Those patients delaying therapy up to day 5 may not be protected immediately and it is recommended that another method of contraception is used for the first 7 days of tablet-taking. Suitable methods are condoms, caps plus spermicides and intra-uterine devices. The rhythm, temperature and cervical-mucous methods should not be relied upon.

Tablet omissions: Tablets must be taken daily in order to maintain adequate hormone levels and contraceptive efficacy.

If a tablet is missed within 12 hours of the correct dosage time then the missed tablet should be taken as soon as possible, even if this means taking 2 tablets on the same day, this will ensure that contraceptive protection is maintained. If one or more tablets are missed for more than 12 hours from the correct dosage time it is recommended that the patient takes the last missed tablet as soon as possible and then continues to take the rest of the tablets in the normal manner. In addition, it is recommended that extra contraceptive protection, such as a condom, is used for the next 7 days.

Patients who have missed one or more of the last 7 tablets in a pack should be advised to start the next pack of tablets as soon as the present one has finished (i.e. without the normal seven day gap between treatments). This reduces the risk of contraceptive failure resulting from tablets being missed close to a 7 day tablet free period.

Changing from another oral contraceptive: In order to ensure that contraception is maintained it is advised that the first dose of Norinyl-1 tablets is taken on the day immediately after the patient has finished the previous pack of tablets.

Use after childbirth, miscarriage or abortion: Providing the patient is not breast feeding the first dose of Norinyl-1 tablets should be taken on the 21st day after childbirth. This will ensure the patient is protected immediately. If there is any delay in taking the first dose, contraception may not be established until 7 days after the first tablet has been taken. In these circumstances patients should be advised that extra contraceptive methods will be necessary.

After a miscarriage or abortion patients can take the first dose of Norinyl-1 tablets on the next day; in this way they will be protected immediately.

Contra-indications: As with all combined progestogen/oestrogen oral contraceptives, the following conditions should be regarded as contra-indications:

(i) Thrombophlebitis, thrombo-embolic disorders, cerebrovascular disorders, coronary artery disease, myocardial infarction, angina, hyperlipidaemia or a history of these conditions.
(ii) Acute or severe chronic liver disease, including liver tumours, Dubin-Johnson or Rotor syndrome.
(iii) History during pregnancy of idiopathic jaundice, severe pruritus or pemphigoid gestationis.
(iv) Known or suspected breast or genital cancer.
(v) Known or suspected oestrogen-dependent neoplasia.
(vi) Undiagnosed abnormal vaginal bleeding.
(vii) A history of migraines classified as classical focal or crescendo.
(viii) Pregnancy.

Special warnings and special precautions for use: Women taking oral contraceptives require careful observation if they have or have had any of the following conditions: breast nodules; fibrocystic disease of the breast or an abnormal mammogram; uterine fibroids; a history of severe depressive states; varicose veins; sickle-cell anaemia; diabetes; hypertension; cardiovascular disease; migraine; epilepsy; asthma; otosclerosis; multiple sclerosis; porphyria; tetany; disturbed liver functions; gallstones; kidney disease; chloasma; any condition that is likely to worsen during pregnancy. The worsening or first appearance of any of these conditions may indicate that the oral contraceptive should be stopped. Discontinue treatment if there is a gradual or sudden, partial or complete loss of vision or any evidence of ocular changes, onset or aggravation of migraine or development of headache of a new kind which is recurrent, persistent or severe.

Gastro-intestinal upsets, such as vomiting and diarrhoea, may interfere with the absorption of the tablets leading to a reduction in contraceptive efficacy. Patients should continue to take Norinyl-1, but they should also be encouraged to use another contraceptive method during the period of gastro-intestinal upset and for the next 7 days.

Progestogen/oestrogen preparations should be used with caution in patients with a history of hepatic dysfunction or hypertension.

A statistical association between the use of oral contraceptives and the occurrence of thrombosis, embolism or haemorrhage has been reported. Patients receiving oral contraceptives should be kept under regular surveillance, in view of the possibility of development of conditions such as thrombo-embolism.

The risk of coronary artery disease in women taking oral contraceptives is increased by the presence of other predisposing factors such as cigarette smoking, hypercholesterolaemia, obesity, diabetes, history of pre-eclamptic toxaemia and increasing age. After the age of thirty-five years, the patient and physician should carefully re-assess the risk/benefit ratio of using combined oral contraceptives as opposed to alternative methods of contraception.

Norinyl-1 should be discontinued at least four weeks before, and for two weeks following, elective operations and during immobilisation. Patients undergoing injection treatment for varicose veins should not resume taking Norinyl-1 until 3 months after the last injection.

Benign and malignant liver tumours have been associated with oral contraceptive use. The relationship between occurrence of liver tumours and use of female sex hormones is not known at present. These tumours may rupture causing intra-abdominal bleeding. If the patient presents with a mass or tenderness in the right upper quadrant or an acute abdomen, the possible presence of a tumour should be considered.

An increased risk of congenital abnormalities, including heart defects and limb defects, has been reported following the use of sex hormones, including oral contraceptives, in pregnancy. If the patient does not adhere to the prescribed schedule, the possibility of pregnancy should be considered at the time of the first missed period and further use of oral contraceptives should be withheld until pregnancy has been ruled out. It is recommended that for any patient who has missed two consecutive periods, pregnancy should be ruled out before continuing the contraceptive regimen. If pregnancy is confirmed the patient should be advised of the potential risks to the foetus and the advisability of continuing the pregnancy should be discussed in the light of these risks. It is advisable to discontinue Norinyl-1 three months before a planned pregnancy.

The risk of arterial thrombosis associated with combined oral contraceptives increases with age, and this risk is aggravated by cigarette smoking. The use of combined oral contraceptives by women in the older age group, especially those who are cigarette smokers, should therefore be discouraged and alternative methods advised.

The use of this product in patients suffering from epilepsy, migraine, asthma or cardiac dysfunction may result in exacerbation of these disorders because of fluid retention. Caution should also be observed in patients who wear contact lenses.

Decreased glucose tolerance may occur in diabetic patients on this treatment, and their control must be carefully supervised.

The use of oral contraceptives has also been associated with a possible increased incidence of gall bladder disease.

Women with a history of oligomenorrhoea or secondary amenorrhoea or young women without regular cycles may have a tendency to remain anovulatory or to become amenorrhoeic after discontinuation of oral contraceptives. Women with these pre-existing problems should be advised of this possibility and encouraged to use other contraceptive methods.

Numerous epidemiological studies have been reported on the risks of ovarian, endometrial, cervical and breast cancer in women using combined oral contraceptives. The evidence is clear that combined oral contraceptives offer substantial protection against both ovarian and endometrial cancer.

An increased risk of cervical cancer in long-term users of combined oral contraceptives has been reported in some studies, but there continues to be controversy about the extent to which this is attributable to the confounding effects of sexual behaviour and other factors.

A meta-analysis from 54 epidemiological studies reported that there is a slightly increased relative risk (RR = 1.24) of having breast cancer diagnosed in women who are currently using combined oral contraceptives (COCs). The observed pattern of increased risk may be due to an earlier diagnosis of breast cancer in COC users, the biological effects of COCs or a combination of both. The additional breast cancers diagnosed in current users of COCs or in women who have used COCs in the last ten years are more likely to be localised to the breast than those in women who never used COCs.

Breast cancer is rare among women under 40 years of age whether or not they take COCs. Whilst this background risk increases with age, the excess number of breast cancer diagnoses in current and recent COC users is small in relation to the overall risk of breast cancer (see bar chart).

The most important risk factor for breast cancer in COC users is the age women discontinue the COC; the older the age at stopping, the more breast cancers are diagnosed. Duration of use is less important and the excess risk gradually disappears during the course of the 10 years after stopping COC use such that by 10 years there appears to be no excess.

The possible increase in risk of breast cancer should be discussed with the user and weighed against the benefits of COCs taking into account the evidence that they offer substantial protection against the risk of developing certain other cancers (e.g. ovarian and endometrial cancer).

Interaction with other medicaments and other forms of interaction: Some drugs may modify the metabolism of Norinyl-1 reducing its effectiveness; these include certain sedatives, antibiotics, anti-epileptic and anti-arthritic drugs. During the time such agents are used concurrently, it is advised that mechanical contraceptives also be used.

The results of a large number of laboratory tests have been shown to be influenced by the use of oestrogen containing oral contraceptives, which may limit their diagnostic value. Among these are: biochemical markers of thyroid and liver function; plasma levels of carrier proteins, triglycerides, coagulation and fibrinolysis factors.

Pregnancy and lactation: Contra-indicated in pregnancy.

Patients who are fully breast-feeding should not take Norinyl-1 tablets since, in common with other combined oral contraceptives, the oestrogen component may reduce the amount of milk produced. In addition, active ingredients or their metabolites have been detected in the milk of mothers taking oral contraceptives. The effect of Norinyl-1 on breast-fed infants has not been determined.

Effects on ability to drive and use machines: Not applicable.

Undesirable effects: As with all oral contraceptives, there may be a slight nausea at first, weight gain or breast discomfort, which soon disappear.

Other side-effects known or suspected to occur with oral contraceptives include gastro-intestinal symptoms, changes in libido and appetite, headache, exacerbation of existing uterine fibroid disease, depression, and changes in carbohydrate, lipid and vitamin metabolism.

Spotting or bleeding may occur during the first few cycles. Usually menstrual bleeding becomes light and occasionally there may be no bleeding during the tablet-free days.

Hypertension, which is usually reversible on discontinuing treatment, has occurred in a small percentage of women taking oral contraceptives.

Estimated cumulative numbers of breast cancers per 10,000 women diagnosed in 5 years of use and up to 10 years after stopping COCs, compared with numbers of breast cancers diagnosed in 10,000 women who had never used COCs.

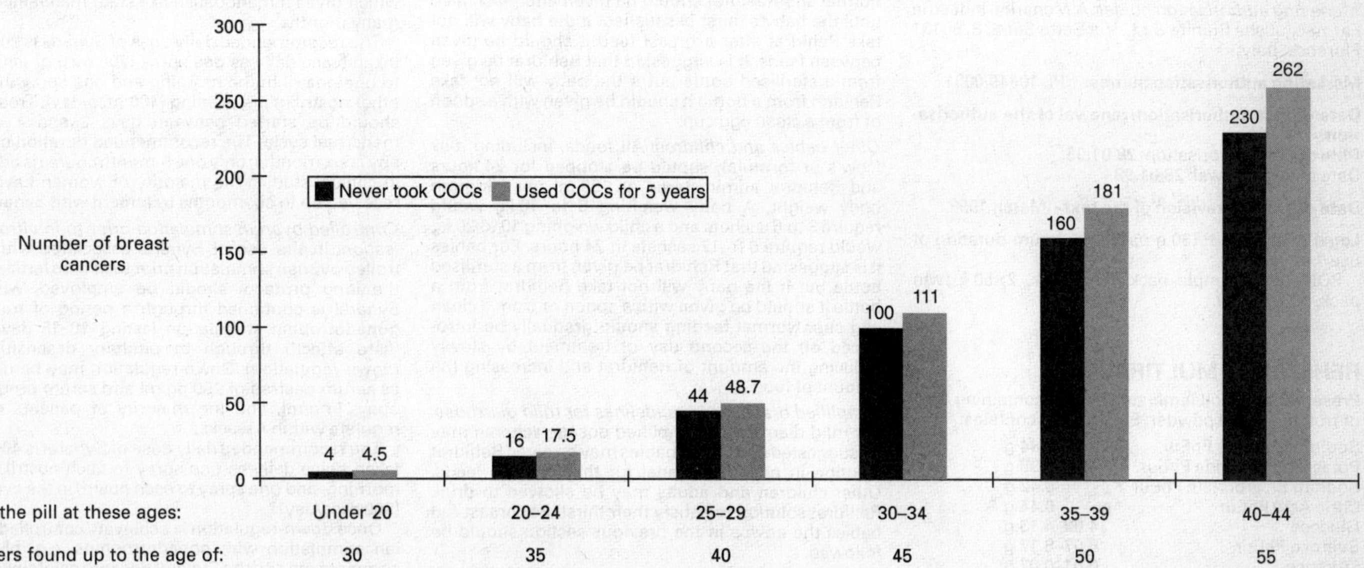

Overdose: Overdosage may be manifested by nausea, vomiting, breast enlargement and vaginal bleeding. There is no specific antidote and treatment should be symptomatic. Gastric lavage may be employed if the overdose is large and the patient is seen sufficiently early (within four hours).

Pharmacological properties

Pharmacodynamic properties: The mode of action of Norinyl-1 is similar to that of other progestogen/oestrogen oral contraceptives and includes the inhibition of ovulation, the thickening of cervical mucus so as to constitute a barrier to sperm and the rendering of the endometrium unreceptive to implantation. Such activity is exerted through a combined effect on one or more of the following: hypothalamus, anterior pituitary, ovary, endometrium and cervical mucus.

Pharmacokinetic properties: Norethisterone is rapidly and completely absorbed after oral administration, peak plasma concentrations occurring in the majority of subjects between 1 and 3 hours. Due to first-pass metabolism, blood levels after oral administration are 60% of those after i.v. administration. The half life of elimination varies from 5 to 12 hours, with a mean of 7.6 hours. Norethisterone is metabolised mainly in the liver. Approximately 60% of the administered dose is excreted as metabolites in urine and faeces.

Mestranol is rapidly absorbed and extensively metabolised to ethinyloestradiol. Ethinyloestradiol is rapidly and well absorbed from the gastro-intestinal tract but is subject to some first-pass metabolism in the gut-wall. Compared to many other oestrogens it is only slowly metabolised in the liver. Excretion is via the kidneys with some appearing also in the faeces.

Preclinical safety data: The toxicity of norethisterone is very low. Reports of teratogenic effects in animals are uncommon. No carcinogenic effects have been found even in long-term studies.

Long-term continuous administration of oestrogens in some animals increases the frequency of carcinoma of the breast, cervix, vagina and liver.

Pharmaceutical particulars

List of excipients: Norinyl-1 tablets contain: Maize starch, polyvidone, magnesium stearate and lactose.

Incompatibilities: None stated.

Shelf life: The shelf life of Norinyl-1 tablets is 5 years.

Special precautions for storage: Store in a dry place below 25°C away from direct sunlight.

Nature and contents of container: Norinyl-1 tablets are supplied in pvc/foil blister packs of 21 and 63 tablets.

Instructions for use/handling: None.

Marketing authorisation holder: Monsanto plc (Trading as Searle), PO Box 53, Lane End Road, High Wycombe, Bucks HP12 4HL.

Marketing authorisation number PPL 08821/0039

Date of first authorisation/renewal of authorisation May 16th 1996

Date of (partial) revision of the text February 1998

POWERGEL

Qualitative and quantitative composition Powergel contains ketoprofen BP 2.5 g/100 g.

Pharmaceutical form Colourless, non-greasy, non-staining gel with an aromatic fragrance for topical application.

Clinical particulars

Therapeutic indications: For local relief of pain and inflammation associated with soft tissue injuries and acute strains and sprains.

Posology and method of administration: Powergel should be applied topically to the affected area two or three times daily. Maximum duration of use should not exceed 7 days if supplied by a pharmacist or 10 days if supplied on prescription. After application Powergel should be rubbed in well to ensure local absorption of ketoprofen.

Adults and elderly: Apply 5 to 10 cm of gel (100–200 mg ketoprofen) with each application.

Children under 12 years of age: Not recommended as experience in children is limited.

Contra-indications: Hypersensitivity to ketoprofen or aspirin or other non-steroidal anti-inflammatory drugs. Severe bronchospasm might be precipitated in these patients and in those suffering from, or with a history of, bronchial asthma or allergic disease. Hence Powergel should not be administered to patients in whom aspirin or other NSAIDs have caused asthma, rhinitis or urticaria.

Special warnings and special precautions for use: Powergel should not be applied to open wounds or lesions of the skin, or near the eyes. Powergel should be used with caution in patients with renal impairment. Keep out of the reach of children.

'P' warning: If symptoms persist after 7 days, consult your doctor.

Interaction with other medicaments and other forms of interaction: No interactions of Powergel with other drugs have been reported. It is however advised to monitor patients under treatment with coumarinic substances.

Pregnancy and lactation: No embryopathic effects have been demonstrated in animals and there is no epidemiological evidence of the safety of ketoprofen in human pregnancy. Therefore, it is recommended to avoid ketoprofen unless considered essential in which case it should be discontinued within one week of expected confinement when NSAIDs might cause premature closure of the ductus arteriosus or persistent pulmonary hypertension in the neonate. They may also delay labour. Trace amounts of ketoprofen are excreted in breast milk after systemic administration.

Effects on ability to drive and use machines: None known.

Undesirable effects: The prolonged use of products for topical administration may cause hypersensitivity phenomena. In such cases the treatment should be discontinued and a suitable alternative therapy instituted. Skin photosensitivity has been reported in isolated cases. Although not known for topical use of ketoprofen, the following adverse events are reported for systemic use: Minor adverse events, frequently transient, consist of gastrointestinal effects such as indigestion, dyspepsia, nausea, constipation, diarrhoea, heartburn and various types of abdominal discomfort. Other minor effects such as headache, dizziness, mild confusion, vertigo, drowsiness, oedema, mood change and insomnia may occur less frequently. Major gastrointestinal adverse events such as peptic ulceration, haemorrhage or perforation may rarely occur. Haematological reactions including thrombocytopenia, hepatic or renal damage, dermatological reactions, bronchospasm and anaphylaxis are exceedingly rare.

Overdose: Considering the low blood levels of ketoprofen by the percutaneous route, no overdosage phenomena have been described yet.

Pharmacological properties

Pharmacodynamic properties: Ketoprofen is an inhibitor of both the cyclooxygenase and lipoxygenase pathways. Inhibition of prostaglandin synthesis provides for potent anti-inflammatory, analgesic and antipyretic effects. Lipoxygenase inhibitors appear to attenuate cell-mediated inflammation and thus retard the progression of tissue destruction in inflamed joints. In addition, ketoprofen is a powerful inhibitor of bradykinin (a chemical mediator of pain and inflammation), it stabilises lysosomal membranes against osmotic damage and prevents the release of lysosomal enzymes that mediate tissue destruction in inflammatory reactions.

Pharmacokinetic properties: Powergel allows the site specific topical delivery of ketoprofen with very low plasma concentrations of drug. Therapeutic levels in the affected tissues provide relief from pain and inflammation, yet will satisfactorily overcome the problem of significant systemic unwanted effects.

Preclinical safety data: There are no preclinical data of relevance to the prescriber which are additional to that already included in other parts of the SPC.

Pharmaceutical particulars

List of excipients: Powergel contains the following excipients: carboxypolymethylene, ethyl alcohol, esters of p-hydroxybenzoic acid, neroli oil, lavender oil, diethanolamine and purified water.

Incompatibilities: Not applicable.

Shelf life: 5 years.

Special precautions for storage: Store below 25°C.

Nature and contents of container: Soft aluminium tube, treated inside with non-toxic epoxy resin. The tubes are packed in cardboard together with a package insert (apart from 30 g sample pack). The following pack sizes are approved:

P: 30 g pack.

POM: 30 g sample pack, 50 g pack, 2×50 g twin pack, 100 g pack.

Instructions for use/handling: Not applicable.

Marketing authorisation holder: A Menarini, Industrie Farmaceutiche Riunite S.r.l., Via Sette Santi, 3, 50131 Florence, Italy.

Marketing authorisation number PL 10649/0001.

Date of first authorisation/renewal of the authorisation
Date of first authorisation: 28.01.93.
Date of last renewal: 28.01.98.

Date of (partial) revision of the text March 1998.

Legal category P (30 g pack, maximum duration of use 7 days).

POM (30 g sample pack, 50 g pack, 2×50 g twin pack, 100 g pack).

REHIDRAT* MULTIPACK

Presentation Foil/laminate sachets containing 14 g of fruit flavoured powder. Each sachet contains:

Sodium Chloride PhEur	0.44 g
Potassium Chloride PhEur	0.38 g
Sodium Bicarbonate PhEur	0.42 g
Citric Acid PhEur	0.44 g
Glucose	4.09–4.13 g
Sucrose PhEur	8.07–8.17 g
Fructose	0.01–0.07 g
Plus flavourings	

Uses Oral electrolyte mixture for the prevention and correction of mild and moderate dehydration in the management of diarrhoea in infants, children and adults.

Maintenance and replacement of fluid and electrolytes following corrective parenteral therapy for dehydration. As a supplement to corrective parenteral therapy for dehydration.

Dosage and administration
General advice: The contents of one 14 g sachet should be dissolved in 250 ml of drinking water. For infants the water should be freshly boiled AND COOLED. The solution should be freshly made immediately prior to use. Any solution remaining should immediately be stored in a fridge where it may be kept and used for a day. If not stored in the fridge, any unused solution should be thrown away after one hour. ADVISE PATIENTS THAT THE SOLUTION SHOULD NOT BE BOILED AFTER RECONSTITUTION, AND THAT IT SHOULD BE USED AT THE RECOMMENDED DILUTION. The degree of dehydration should be assessed. Patients with mild or moderate dehydration may appear almost normal; they may be thirsty and may have normal or slightly diminished skin elasticity or, in children, slightly sunken fontanelle. Urine flow may be reduced. Patients with signs of severe dehydration who are usually too weak to drink will initially require parenteral therapy. Oral therapy should only be instituted when shock is corrected. The volume of reconstituted Rehidrat required will depend on the weight of the patient, using the basic principle of firstly rehydrating the patient by replacing lost fluid and thereafter maintaining fluid replacement in line with the volume of fluid lost from stools or vomiting plus daily requirements. A basic guide is given below:

General guidelines for oral therapy

1. Rehydration – Replacement of fluid and electrolyte losses. Mild or moderate dehydration: 50–120 ml per kilogram body weight orally, usually given in divided doses over 4 to 6 hours. The amounts and rates should be adjusted as needed and tolerated depending on thirst and response to therapy. Adults may need up to 1000 ml per hour. A continuous nasogastric infusion may be used if necessary.

2. Maintenance

Mild to moderate diarrhoea: 100–200 ml per kilogram body weight orally over a period of 24 hours in divided doses.

Continuing diarrhoea: 15 ml per kilogram body weight orally every hour. Observe carefully to confirm adequate maintenance of hydration.

Where nausea or vomiting is present Rehidrat should be administered in small frequent doses, in sips. If vomiting persists appropriate intravenous therapy should be instituted. The patient instruction leaflet included in each carton advises patients to consult their doctor if there is no improvement in 2 days.

Elderly: Administer Rehidrat in amounts appropriate to correct dehydration. Also see *Precautions.*

Babies and children: Diarrhoea can have serious consequences in children under 3 years old. For this age group, the patient instruction leaflet included in each carton, advises that a doctor be consulted.

For bottle fed infants advise mothers to make the feed up for a 24 hour period and to store the reconstituted solution in the refrigerator.

Breast-fed babies: Breast feeding should continue as normal and Rehidrat should be given after each feed until the baby's thirst is satisfied. If the baby will not take Rehidrat after a breast feed it should be given between feeds. It is suggested that Rehidrat be given from a sterilised bottle but if the baby will not take Rehidrat from a bottle it should be given with a spoon or from a clean egg cup.

Other babies and children: All foods, including milk (cow's or formula), should be stopped for 24 hours and Rehidrat administered at 150 ml per kilogram body weight. A baby weighing 5 to 10 kg would require 3 to 6 sachets and a child weighing 10 to 20 kg would require 6 to 12 sachets in 24 hours. For babies it is suggested that Rehidrat be given from a sterilised bottle but if the baby will not take Rehidrat from a bottle it should be given with a spoon or from a clean egg cup. Normal feeding should gradually be introduced on the second day of treatment by slowly reducing the amount of Rehidrat and increasing the amount of food.

Simplified oral dosage guidelines for mild diarrhoea: For mild diarrhoea a simplified dosage scheme may be suggested. Bottle-fed babies may be given Rehidrat solution in quantities usual for their normal feeds. Other children and adults may be allowed to drink Rehidrat solution to satisfy their thirst. For breast-fed babies the advice in the previous section should be followed.

Contra-indications, warnings, etc
Contra-indications: Rehidrat is contra-indicated in patients with renal impairment manifesting as oliguria or anuria, intestinal obstruction, paralytic ileus, intractable vomiting and in patients with severe dehydration which requires parenteral fluid therapy.

Precautions: When Rehidrat is used as a supplement to parenteral fluid therapy, care must be taken not to exceed the total water and electrolyte requirements.

The sugar content of Rehidrat should be considered when treating diabetics.

Administration of oral sugar-electrolyte solutions to patients with sugar malabsorption may worsen diarrhoea.

Drug interactions: Rehidrat should not be mixed or given with electrolyte-containing solutions. Salt or sugar should not be added to Rehidrat.

Adverse effects: Incorrect dilution could result in abnormalities of carbohydrate and electrolyte balance.

Overdosage: Toxicity resulting from overdosage of oral electrolyte solutions is rare. In the event of overdosage hypernatraemia or hyperkalaemia could occur.

Pharmaceutical precautions Store in a dry place below 25°C (77°F).

Legal category P.

Package quantities Boxes of 16 sachets with instructions for use.

Each carton contains a selection of Rehidrat Orange, Rehidrat Blackcurrant and Rehidrat (Lemon & Lime).

Further information When reconstituted, Rehidrat and water solution has the following composition:

	mmol/l
Sodium	50
Potassium	20
Chloride	50
Bicarbonate	20
Citrate	9
Glucose	91–2
Sucrose	94–6
Fructose	<1–2
Total osmolarity	336–337

Product licence number 8821/0034.

SYNAREL NASAL SPRAY*

Qualitative and quantitative composition Solution containing 2 mg/ml of nafarelin (as acetate) supplied in bottles fitted with a metered spray pump that delivers 200 micrograms of nafarelin base per spray.

Pharmaceutical form Nasal spray.

Clinical particulars
Therapeutic indications: The hormonal management of endometriosis, including pain relief and reduction of endometriotic lesions.

Use in controlled ovarian stimulation programmes prior to in-vitro fertilisation, under the supervision of an infertility specialist.

Posology and method of administration

Adult: Synarel is for administration by the intranasal route only.

Experience with the treatment of endometriosis has been limited to women 18 years of age and older.

Endometriosis: In the use of Synarel in endometriosis, the aim is to induce chronic pituitary desensitisation, which gives a menopause-like state maintained over many months.

The recommended daily dose of Synarel is 200 mcg taken twice daily as one spray (200 mcg of nafarelin) to one nostril in the morning and one spray into the other nostril in the evening (400 mcg/day). Treatment should be started between days 2 and 4 of the menstrual cycle. The recommended duration of therapy is six months; only one 6-month course is advised. In clinical studies the majority of women have only received up to six-months treatment with Synarel.

Controlled ovarian stimulation prior to in vitro fertilisation: In the use of Synarel associated with controlled ovarian stimulation prior to *in vitro* fertilisation, the long protocol should be employed, whereby Synarel is continued through a period of transient gonadotrophin stimulation lasting 10–15 days (the 'flare effect') through to pituitary desensitisation (down-regulation). Down-regulation may be defined as serum oestradiol ≤50 pg/ml and serum progesterone ≤1 ng/ml, and the majority of patients down-regulate within 4 weeks.

The recommended daily dose of Synarel is 400 mcg taken twice daily as one spray to each nostril in the morning, and one spray to each nostril in the evening. (800 mcg/day).

Once down-regulation is achieved, controlled ovarian stimulation with gonadotrophins, e.g. hMG, is commenced, and the Synarel dosage maintained until the administration of hCG at follicular maturity (usually a further 8–12 days).

If patients do not down-regulate within 12 weeks of starting Synarel, it is recommended that Synarel therapy be discontinued and the cycle cancelled.

Treatment may begin in either the early follicular phase (day 2) or the mid-luteal phase (usually day 21).

If the use of a nasal decongestant is required at the time of nafarelin administration, it is recommended that the nasal decongestant be used at least 30 minutes after nafarelin dosing.

Sneezing during or immediately after dosing may impair absorption of Synarel. If sneezing occurs upon administration, repeating the dose may be advisable.

Bottles contain either 30 or 60 doses and should not be used for a greater number of doses. The 60 dose-unit bottle is sufficient for 30 days' treatment at 400 mcg (2 sprays) per day, and 15 days' treatment at 800 mcg (4 sprays) per day.

The 30 dose-unit bottle is sufficient for 15 days' treatment at 400 mcg (2 sprays) per day, and 7 days' treatment at 800 mcg (4 sprays) per day. Patients should therefore be advised that continued use after this time may result in delivery of an insufficient amount of nafarelin.

Contra-indications: A small loss of trabecular bone mineral content occurs during 6 months treatment with nafarelin. Although this is mostly reversible within 6 months of stopping treatment, there are no data on the effects of repeat courses on bone loss. Retreatment with Synarel or use for longer than 6 months is, therefore, not recommended. (See Side-effects section on 'Changes in bone density').

Synarel should not be administered to patients who:

1. are hypersensitive to GnRH, GnRH agonist analogues or any of the excipients in Synarel;
2. have undiagnosed vaginal bleeding;
3. are pregnant or may become pregnant whilst taking Synarel (see 'Use in pregnancy and lactation');
4. are breast-feeding.

Special warnings and special precautions for use: When regularly used at the recommended dose, nafarelin inhibits ovulation. Patients should be advised to use non-hormonal, barrier methods of contraception. In the event of missed doses there may be breakthrough ovulation and a potential for conception. If a patient becomes pregnant during treatment, administration of the drug must be discontinued and the patient must be informed of a potential risk to fetal development. NB Synarel treatment will be stopped at least 3 days before fertilised embryos are placed in the uterine cavity.

As with other drugs in this class ovarian cysts have been reported to occur in the first two months of therapy with Synarel. Many, but not all, of these events occurred in patients with polycystic ovarian disease. These cystic enlargements may resolve spontaneously, generally by about four to six weeks of therapy, but in some cases may require discontinuation of drug and/or surgical intervention.

Controlled ovarian stimulation prior to in vitro fertil-

isation: Transient ovarian cyst formation is a recognised complication of GnRH agonist use. These cysts tend to regress spontaneously over a number of weeks and are more common when GnRH agonists are commenced in the follicular phase of the cycle.

There are no clinical data available on the use of Synarel in ovulation induction regimens involving patients with polycystic ovarian syndrome. Caution is advised in this patient group as they are at greater risk of excessive follicular recruitment when undergoing ovulation induction regimens.

Administration of nafarelin in therapeutic doses results in suppression of the pituitary-gonadal system. Normal function is usually restored within 8 weeks after treatment is discontinued. Diagnostic tests of pituitary-gonadal function conducted during the treatment and up to 8 weeks after discontinuation of nafarelin therapy may therefore be misleading.

Interactions with other medicaments and other forms of interaction: Nafarelin would not be expected to participate in pharmacokinetic-based drug-drug interactions because degradation of the compound is primarily by the action of peptidases not cytochrome P-450 enzymes. Additionally, because nafarelin is only about 80% bound to plasma proteins (albumin), drug interactions at the protein-binding level would not be expected to occur.

Rhinitis does not impair nasal absorption of nafarelin. Nasal decongestants used 30 minutes before nafarelin administration decrease absorption.

Pregnancy and lactation: When administered intramuscularly to rats on days 6–15 of pregnancy at doses of 0.4, 1.6 and 6.4 mcg/kg/day (0.6, 2.5 and 10.0 times the intranasal human dose of 400 mcg per day), 4/80 fetuses in the highest dose group had major fetal abnormalities that were not seen in a repeat study in rats. Moreover, studies in mice and rabbits failed to demonstrate an increase in fetal abnormalities. In rats, there was a dose-related increase in fetal mortality, and a decrease in fetal weight with the highest dose. These effects on rat fetal mortality are logical consequences of the alterations in hormonal levels brought about by nafarelin in this species.

Use of nafarelin in human pregnancy has not been studied.

Synarel should not therefore be used during pregnancy or suspected pregnancy. Before starting treatment with Synarel pregnancy must be excluded. If a patient becomes pregnant during treatment, administration of the drug must be discontinued and the patient must be informed of a potential risk to fetal development.

Controlled ovarian stimulation prior to in vitro fertilisation: Pregnancy should be excluded before starting treatment with Synarel, and the medication should be stopped on the day of administration of hCG. Barrier methods of contraception should be employed whilst Synarel is being taken.

It is not known whether or to what extent nafarelin is excreted into human breast milk. The effects, if any on the breast-fed child have not been determined and therefore Synarel should not be used by breast-feeding women.

Effects on ability to drive and use machines: Not applicable.

Undesirable effects: In approximately 0.2% of adult patients, symptoms suggestive of drug sensitivity, such as shortness of breath, chest pain, urticaria, rash and pruritus have occurred.

As would be expected with a drug which lowers serum oestradiol levels to menopausal concentrations the most frequently reported adverse reactions are those related to hypo-oestrogenism.

In controlled studies of nafarelin 400 mcg/day, adverse reactions that were most frequently reported are listed in order of decreasing frequency: hot flushes, changes in libido, vaginal dryness, headaches, emotional lability, acne, myalgia, decreased breast size and irritation of the nasal mucosa.

During post-marketing surveillance, depression, paraesthesia, alopecia, migraine, palpitations, blurred vision have been reported. Emotional lability and depression would be expected with a drug that lowers serum oestradiol to post-menopausal levels.

Changes in bone density: After six months of Synarel treatment there was a reduction in vertebral trabecular bone density and total vertebral mass, averaging about 9% and 4%, respectively. There was very little, if any, decrease in the mineral content of compact bone of the distal radius and second metacarpal. Substantial recovery of bone occurred during the post-treatment period. Total vertebral bone mass, measured by dual photon absorptiometry (DPA), decreased by a mean of about 6% at the end of treatment. Mean total vertebral mass, re-examined by DPA six months after completion of treatment, was 1.4% below pretreatment levels. These changes are similar to those which occur during treatment with other GnRH agonists.

Carcinogenesis/mutagenesis: As seen with other GnRH agonists, nafarelin given parenterally in high doses to laboratory rodents for prolonged periods induced hyperplasia and neoplasia of endocrine organs, including the anterior pituitary (adenoma/carcinoma) of both mice and rats; tumours of the pancreatic islets, adrenal medulla, testes and ovaries occurred only in long-term studies in rats. No metastases of these tumours were observed. Monkeys treated with high doses of nafarelin for one year did not develop any tumours or proliferative changes. Experience in humans is limited but there is no evidence for tumorigenesis of GnRH analogues in human beings.

In vitro studies conducted in bacterial and mammalian systems provided no indication of a mutagenic potential for nafarelin.

Impairment of fertility: Reproduction studies in rats of both sexes have shown full reversibility of fertility suppression when drug treatment was discontinued after continuous administration for up to six months.

Laboratory values: Increased levels of SGOT/SGPT and serum alkaline phosphatase may rarely occur which are reversible on discontinuing treatment.

Overdose: In animals, subcutaneous administration of up to 60 times the recommended human dose (expressed on a mcg/kg basis) had no adverse effects. Orally-administered nafarelin is subject to enzymatic degradation in the gastro-intestinal tract and is therefore inactive. At present there is no clinical experience with overdosage of nafarelin.

Based on studies in monkeys, nafarelin is not absorbed after oral administration.

Pharmacological properties

Pharmacodynamic properties: Nafarelin is a potent agonistic analogue of gonadotrophin releasing hormone (GnRH). Given as a single dose, nafarelin stimulates release of the pituitary gonadotrophins, LH and FSH, with consequent increase of ovarian and testicular steroidogenesis. During repeated dosing this response to stimulation gradually diminishes. Within three to four weeks, daily administration leads to decreased pituitary gonadotrophin secretion and/or the secretion of gonadotrophin secretion and/or the secretion of gonadotrophins with lowered biological activity. There is a consequent suppression of gonadal steroidogenesis and inhibition of functions in tissues that depend on gonadal steroids for their maintenance.

Pharmacokinetic properties: Nafarelin is rapidly absorbed into the circulation after intranasal administration. Maximum plasma concentration is achieved 20 minutes after dosing and the plasma half-life is approximately 4 hours. Bioavailability of the intranasal dose averages 2.8% (range 1.2–5.6%).

Preclinical safety data: This is discussed in 'Undesirable effects'.

Pharmaceutical particulars

List of excipients: Synarel contains: Sorbitol, benzalkonium chloride, glacial acetic acid and water. Sodium hydroxide or hydrochloric acid to adjust pH.

Incompatibilities: None stated.

Shelf life: The shelf life of Synarel is 2 years.

Special precautions for storage: Store upright below 25°C. Avoid heat above 30°C. Protect from light and freezing.

Nature and contents of container: White, high density polyethylene bottles with a 0.1 ml metered spray pump containing 6.5 ml or 10 ml.

PVC-coated glass bottles with an internal conical reservoir in the base and a valois crimp-on pump, containing 4 ml or 8 ml.

Special instructions for use/handling: None.

Marketing authorisation holder: Monsanto p.l.c., PO Box 53, Lane End Road, High Wycombe, Bucks HP12 4HL.

Marketing authorisation number 08821/0042.

Date of approval/revision of SPC May 1996.

Legal category POM.

SYNPHASE*

Qualitative and quantitative composition Synphase consists of 7 blue tablets containing norethisterone 500 micrograms and ethinyloestradiol 35 micrograms, marked 'BX' on one side and 'SEARLE' on the other; 9 white tablets containing norethisterone 1.0 milligram and ethinyloestradiol 35 micrograms inscribed 'SEARLE' on one face and 'BX' on the other; 5 blue tablets containing norethisterone 500 micrograms and ethinyloestradiol 35 micrograms, marked 'BX' on one side and 'SEARLE' on the other.

Pharmaceutical form Tablets for oral administration.

Clinical particulars

Therapeutic indications: Synphase is indicated for oral contraception, with the benefit of a low intake of oestrogen.

Posology and method of administration:

Oral administration: The dosage of Synphase for the initial cycle of therapy is 1 tablet taken at the same time each day from the first day of the menstrual cycle. For subsequent cycles, no tablets are taken for 7 days, then a new course is started of 1 tablet for the next 21 days. This sequence of 21 days on treatment, seven days off treatment is repeated for as long as contraception is required.

Patients unable to start taking Synphase tablets on the first day of the menstrual cycle may start treatment on any day up to and including the 5th day of the menstrual cycle.

Patients starting on day 1 of their period will be protected at once. Those patients delaying therapy up to day 5 may not be protected immediately and it is recommended that another method of contraception is used for the first 7 days of tablet-taking. Suitable methods are condoms, caps plus spermicides and intra-uterine devices.

The rhythm, temperature and cervical-mucus methods should not be relied upon.

Tablet omissions: Tablets must be taken daily in order to maintain adequate hormone levels and contraceptive efficacy.

If a tablet is missed within 12 hours of the correct dosage time then the missed tablet should be taken as soon as possible, even if this means taking 2 tablets on the same day, this will ensure that contraceptive protection is maintained. If one or more tablets are missed for more than 12 hours from the correct dosage time it is recommended that the patient takes the last missed tablet as soon as possible and then continues to take the rest of the tablets in the normal manner. In addition, it is recommended that extra contraceptive protection, such as a condom, is used for the next 7 days.

Patients who have missed one or more of the last 7 tablets in a pack should be advised to start the next pack of tablets as soon as the present one has finished (i.e. without the normal seven day gap between treatments). This reduces the risk of contraceptive failure resulting from tablets being missed close to a 7 day tablet free period.

Changing from another oral contraceptive: In order to ensure that contraception is maintained it is advised that the first dose of Synphase tablets is taken on the day immediately after the patient has finished the previous pack of tablets.

Use after childbirth, miscarriage or abortion: Providing the patient is not breast feeding the first dose of Synphase tablets should be taken on the 21st day after childbirth. This will ensure the patient is protected immediately. If there is any delay in taking the first dose, contraception may not be established until 7 days after the first tablet has been taken. In these circumstances patients should be advised that extra contraceptive methods will be necessary.

After a miscarriage or abortion patients can take the first dose of Synphase tablets on the next day; in this way they will be protected immediately.

Contra-indications: As with all combined progestogen/oestrogen oral contraceptives, the following conditions should be regarded as contra-indications:

(i) Thrombophlebitis, thrombo-embolic disorders, cerebrovascular disorders, coronary artery disease, myocardial infarction, angina, hyperlipidaemia or a history of these conditions.
(ii) Acute or severe chronic liver disease, including liver tumours, Dubin-Johnson or Rotor syndrome.
(iii) History during pregnancy of idiopathic jaundice, severe pruritus or pemphigoid gestationis.
(iv) Known or suspected breast or genital cancer.
(v) Known or suspected oestrogen-dependent neoplasia.
(vi) Undiagnosed abnormal vaginal bleeding.
(vii) A history of migraines classified as classical, focal or crescendo.
(viii) Pregnancy.

Special warnings and special precautions for use: Women taking oral contraceptives require careful observation if they have or have had any of the following conditions: breast nodules; fibrocystic disease of the breast or an abnormal mammogram; uterine fibroids; a history of severe depressive states; varicose veins; sickle-cell anaemia; diabetes; hypertension; cardiovascular disease; migraine; epilepsy; asthma; otosclerosis; multiple sclerosis; porphyria; tetany; disturbed liver functions; gallstones; kidney disease; chloasma; any condition that is likely to worsen during pregnancy. The worsening or first appearance of any of these conditions may indicate that the oral contraceptive should be stopped. Discontinue treatment if there is a gradual or sudden, partial or complete loss of vision or any evidence of ocular changes, onset or aggravation of migraine or development of headache of a new kind which is recurrent, persistent or severe.

Estimated cumulative numbers of breast cancers per 10,000 women diagnosed in 5 years of use and up to 10 years after stopping COCs, compared with numbers of breast cancers diagnosed in 10,000 women who had never used COCs.

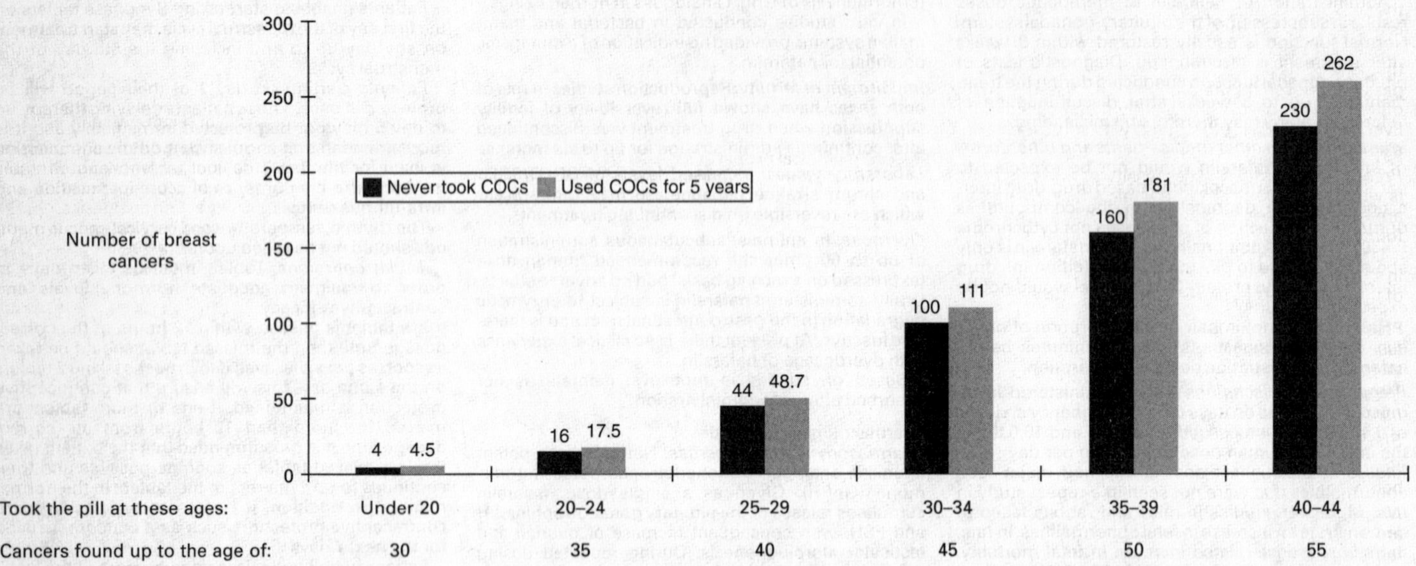

Gastro-intestinal upsets, such as vomiting and diarrhoea, may interfere with the absorption of the tablets leading to a reduction in contraceptive efficacy. Patients should continue to take Synphase, but they should also be encouraged to use another contraceptive method during the period of gastro-intestinal upset and for the next 7 days.

Progestogen/oestrogen preparations should be used with caution in patients with a history of hepatic dysfunction or hypertension.

A statistical association between the use of oral contraceptives and the occurrence of thrombosis, embolism or haemorrhage has been reported. Patients receiving oral contraceptives should be kept under regular surveillance, in view of the possibility of development of conditions such as thrombo-embolism.

The risk of coronary artery disease in women taking oral contraceptives is increased by the presence of other predisposing factors such as cigarette smoking, hypercholesterolaemia, obesity, diabetes, history of pre-eclamptic toxaemia and increasing age. After the age of thirty-five years, the patient and physician should carefully re-assess the risk/benefit ratio of using combined oral contraceptives as opposed to alternative methods of contraception.

Synphase should be discontinued at least four weeks before, and for two weeks following, elective operations and during immobilisation. Patients undergoing injection treatment for varicose veins should not resume taking Synphase until 3 months after the last injection.

Benign and malignant liver tumours have been associated with oral contraceptive use. The relationship between occurrence of liver tumours and use of female sex hormones is not known at present. These tumours may rupture causing intra-abdominal bleeding. If the patient presents with a mass or tenderness in the right upper quadrant or an acute abdomen, the possible presence of a tumour should be considered.

An increased risk of congenital abnormalities, including heart defects and limb defects, has been reported following the use of sex hormones, including oral contraceptives, in pregnancy. If the patient does not adhere to the prescribed schedule, the possibility of pregnancy should be considered at the time of the first missed period and further use of oral contraceptives should be withheld until pregnancy has been ruled out. It is recommended that for any patient who has missed two consecutive periods, pregnancy should be ruled out before continuing the contraceptive regimen. If pregnancy is confirmed the patient should be advised of the potential risks to the foetus and the advisability of continuing the pregnancy should be discussed in the light of these risks. It is advisable to discontinue Synphase three months before a planned pregnancy.

The risk of arterial thrombosis associated with combined oral contraceptives increases with age, and this risk is aggravated by cigarette smoking. The use of combined oral contraceptives by women in the older age group, especially those who are cigarette smokers, should therefore be discouraged and alternative methods advised.

The use of this product in patients suffering from epilepsy, migraine, asthma or cardiac dysfunction may result in exacerbation of these disorders because of fluid retention. Caution should also be observed in patients who wear contact lenses.

Decreased glucose tolerance may occur in diabetic patients on this treatment, and their control must be carefully supervised.

The use of oral contraceptives has also been associated with a possible increased incidence of gall bladder disease.

Women with a history of oligomenorrhoea or secondary amenorrhoea or young women without regular cycles may have a tendency to remain anovulatory or to become amenorrhoeic after discontinuation of oral contraceptives. Women with these pre-existing problems should be advised of this possibility and encouraged to use other contraceptive methods.

Numerous epidemiological studies have been reported on the risks of ovarian, endometrial, cervical and breast cancer in women using combined oral contraceptives. The evidence is clear that combined oral contraceptives offer substantial protection against both ovarian and endometrial cancer.

An increased risk of cervical cancer in long-term users of combined oral contraceptives has been reported in some studies, but there continues to be controversy about the extent to which this is attributable to the confounding effects of sexual behaviour and other factors.

A meta-analysis from 54 epidemiological studies reported that there is a slightly increased relative risk (RR = 1.24) of having breast cancer diagnosed in women who are currently using combined oral contraceptives (COCs). The observed pattern of increased risk may be due to an earlier diagnosis of breast cancer in COC users, the biological effects of COCs or a combination of both. The additional breast cancers diagnosed in current users of COCs or in women who have used COCs in the last ten years are more likely to be localised to the breast than those in women who never used COCs.

Breast cancer is rare among women under 40 years of age whether or not they take COCs. Whilst this background risk increases with age, the excess number of breast cancer diagnoses in current and recent COC users is small in relation to the overall risk of breast cancer (see bar chart).

The most important risk factor for breast cancer in COC users is the age women discontinue the COC; the older the age at stopping, the more breast cancers are diagnosed. Duration of use is less important and the excess risk gradually disappears during the course of the 10 years after stopping COC use such that by 10 years there appears to be no excess.

The possible increase in risk of breast cancer should be discussed with the user and weighed against the benefits of COCs taking into account the evidence that they offer substantial protection against the risk of developing certain other cancers (e.g. ovarian and endometrial cancer).

Interaction with other medicaments and other forms of interaction: Some drugs may modify the metabolism of Synphase reducing its effectiveness; these include certain sedatives, antibiotics, anti-epileptic and anti-arthritic drugs. During the time such agents are used concurrently, it is advised that mechanical contraceptives also be used.

The results of a large number of laboratory tests have been shown to be influenced by the use of oestrogen containing oral contraceptives, which may limit their diagnostic value. Among these are: biochemical markers of thyroid and liver function; plasma levels of carrier proteins, triglycerides, coagulation and fibrinolysis factors.

Pregnancy and lactation: Contra-indicated in pregnancy.

Patients who are fully breast-feeding should not take Synphase tablets since, in common with other combined oral contraceptives, the oestrogen component may reduce the amount of milk produced. In addition, active ingredients or their metabolites have been detected in the milk of mothers taking oral contraceptives. The effect of Synphase on breast-fed infants has not been determined.

Effects on ability to drive and use machines: Not applicable.

Undesirable effects: As with all oral contraceptives, there may be slight nausea at first, weight gain or breast discomfort, which soon disappear.

Other side-effects known or suspected to occur with oral contraceptives include gastro-intestinal symptoms, changes in libido and appetite, headache, exacerbation of existing uterine fibroid disease, depression, and changes in carbohydrate, lipid and vitamin metabolism.

Spotting or bleeding may occur during the first few cycles. Usually menstrual bleeding becomes light and occasionally there may be no bleeding during the tablet-free days.

Hypertension, which is usually reversible on discontinuing treatment, has occurred in a small percentage of women taking oral contraceptives.

Overdose: Overdosage may be manifested by nausea, vomiting, breast enlargement and vaginal bleeding. There is no specific antidote and treatment should be symptomatic. Gastric lavage may be employed if the overdose is large and the patient is seen sufficiently early (within four hours).

Pharmacological properties

Pharmacodynamic properties: The mode of action of Synphase is similar to that of other progestogen/oestrogen oral contraceptives and includes the inhibition of ovulation, the thickening of cervical mucus so as to constitute a barrier to sperm and the rendering of the endometrium unreceptive to implantation. Such activity is exerted through a combined effect on one or more of the following: hypothalamus, anterior pituitary, ovary, endometrium and cervical mucus.

Pharmacokinetic properties: Norethisterone is rapidly and completely absorbed after oral administration, peak plasma concentrations occurring in the majority of subjects between 1 and 3 hours. Due to first-pass metabolism, blood levels after oral administration are 60% of those afer i.v. administration. The half life of elimination varies from 5 to 12 hours, with a mean of 7.6 hours. Norethisterone is metabolised mainly in the liver. Approximately 60% of the administered dose is excreted as metabolites in urine and faeces.

Ethinyloestradiol is rapidly and well absorbed from the gastro-intestinal tract but is subject to some first-pass metabolism in the gut-wall. Compared to many other oestrogens it is only slowly metabolised in the liver. Excretion is via the kidneys with some appearing also in the faeces.

Preclinical safety data: The toxicity of norethisterone is very low. Reports of teratogenic effects in animals are uncommon. No carcinogenic effects have been found even in long-term studies.

Long-term continuous administration of oestrogens in some animals increases the frequency of carcinoma of the breast, cervix, vagina and liver.

Pharmaceutical particulars
List of excipients: Synphase tablets contain: Maize starch, polyvidone, magnesium stearate and lactose. The blue tablets also contain E132.

Incompatibilities: None stated.

Shelf life: The shelf life of Synphase tablets is 5 years.

Special precautions for storage: Store in a dry place below 25°C away from direct sunlight.

Nature and contents of container: Synphase tablets are supplied in pvc/foil blister packs of 21 and 63 tablets.

Instructions for use/handling: None.

Marketing authorisation holder: Monsanto plc (Trading as Searle), PO Box 53, Lane End Road, High Wycombe, Bucks HP12 4HL.

Marketing authorisation number PL 08821/0041.

Date of first authorisation/renewal of authorisation May 10th 1996.

Date of (partial) revision of the text February 1998

UTOVLAN*

Qualitative and quantitative composition Each tablet contains 5 mg Norethisterone BP.

Pharmaceutical form White, flat, circular, bevel-edged tablet inscribed 'SYNTEX' on one side.

Clinical particulars
Therapeutic indications:
At low dose: Dysfunctional uterine bleeding, endometriosis, polymenorrhoea, menorrhagia, metropathia haemorrhagica, postponement of menstruation and premenstrual syndrome.

At high dose: Disseminated carcinoma of the breast.

Posology and method of administration: Oral administration.

Low dose
Dysfunctional uterine bleeding, polymenorrhoea, menorrhagia, dysmenorrhoea and metropathia haemorrhagica: 1 tablet three times daily for 10 days; bleeding usually stops within 48 hours. Withdrawal bleeding resembling true menstruation occurs a few days after the end of treatment. One tablet twice daily, from days 19 to 26 of the two subsequent cycles, should be given to prevent recurrence of the condition.

Endometriosis: 1 tablet three times daily for a minimum treatment period of six months. The dosage should be increased to 4 or 5 tablets a day if spotting occurs. The initial dosage should be resumed when bleeding or spotting stops.

Postponement of menstruation: 1 tablet three times daily, starting three days before the expected onset of menstruation. Menstruation usually follows within three days of finishing the treatment.

Pre-menstrual syndrome: 1 tablet daily from days 16 to 25 of the menstrual cycle.

High dose: For disseminated breast carcinoma the starting dose is 8 tablets (40 mg) per day increasing to 12 tablets (60 mg) if no regression is noted.

Contra-indications: Pregnancy; disturbance of liver function; history during pregnancy of idiopathic jaundice, severe pruritus, or pemphigoid gestationis; undiagnosed irregular vaginal bleeding.

Special warnings and special precautions for use: If menstrual bleeding should fail to follow a course of Utovlan, the possibility of pregnancy must be excluded before a further course is given.

Interaction with other medicaments and other forms of interaction: None.

Pregnancy and lactation: Contra-indicated in pregnancy.

Effects on ability to drive and use machines: None.

Undesirable effects: These rarely occur at the usual dosage level of 15 mg per day. Mild nausea has been reported. High dosage treatment, even over long periods, is well tolerated; transient digestive upsets and jaundice have rarely been reported.

Overdose: Overdosage may be manifested by nausea, vomiting, breast enlargement and later vaginal bleeding. There is no specific antidote and treatment should be symptomatic.

Gastric lavage may be employed if the overdosage is large and the patient is seen sufficiently early (within four hours).

Pharmacological properties
Pharmacodynamic properties: Norethisterone given at intermediate doses (5–10 mg) suppresses ovulation via its effect on the pituitary. The endogenous production of oestrogens and progesterones are also suppressed, and the ectopic endometrium is converted to a decidua resembling that of pregnancy. In carcinoma norethisterone may act by pituitary inhibition or by direct action on tumour deposits.

Pharmacokinetic properties: Norethisterone is rapidly and completely absorbed after oral administration, peak plasma concentration occurring in the majority of subjects between 1 and 3 hours. Due to first-pass metabolism, blood levels after oral administration are 60% of those after i.v. administration. The half life of elimination varies from 5 to 12 hours, with a mean of 7.6 hours. Norethisterone is metabolised mainly in the liver. Approximately 60% of the administered dose is excreted as metabolites in urine and faeces.

Preclinical safety data: The toxicity of norethisterone is very low. Reports of teratogenic effects in animals are uncommon. No carcinogenic effects have been found even in long-term studies.

Pharmaceutical particulars
List of excipients: Utovlan tablets contain: Maize starch, povidone, magnesium stearate and lactose.

Incompatibilities: None stated.

Shelf life: The shelf life of Utovlan tablets is 2 years.

Special precautions for storage: Store in a dry place, below 25°C, away from direct sunlight.

Nature and contents of container: Utovlan tablets are supplied in pvc/foil blister packs of 30 and 90 tablets.

Instructions for use/handling: None.

Marketing authorisation holder: Monsanto p.l.c., PO Box 53, Lane End Road, High Wycombe, Bucks HP12 4HL.

Marketing authorisation number 08821/0043

Date of first authorisation/renewal of authorisation 29 March 1996.

Date of (partial) revision of the text November 1997.

Legal category POM.

ZYDOL* AMPOULES ▼

Qualitative and quantitative composition Each ampoule contains 100 mg tramadol hydrochloride in 2 ml colourless aqueous solution.

Pharmaceutical form Clear glass ampoules containing injectable solution.

Clinical particulars
Therapeutic indications: Management (treatment and prevention) of moderate to severe pain.

Posology and method of administration: As with all analgesic drugs, the dose of Zydol should be adjusted according to the severity of the pain and the clinical response of the individual patient.

Adults and children aged 12 years and over
Parenteral administration: Zydol injection may be administered intramuscularly, by slow intravenous injection, or diluted in solution (see *Pharmaceutical particulars*) for administration by infusion or patient controlled analgesia.

The usual dose is 50 or 100 mg 4–6 hourly by the intravenous or intramuscular route. Dosage should be adjusted according to pain severity and response.

Intravenous injections must be given slowly over 2–3 minutes. For post-operative pain administer a bolus of 100 mg. During the 60 minutes following the initial bolus, further doses of 50 mg may be given every 10–20 minutes, up to a total dose of 250 mg including the initial bolus. Subsequent doses should be 50 mg or 100 mg 4–6 hourly up to a total daily dose of 600 mg.

Elderly: The usual dosages may be used although it should be noted that in volunteers aged over 75 years the elimination half-life of tramadol was increased by 17% following oral administration.

Renal impairment/renal dialysis: The elimination of tramadol may be prolonged. The usual initial dosage should be used. For patients with creatinine clearance <30 ml/min, the dosage interval should be increased to 12 hours. Tramadol is not recommended for patients with severe renal impairment (creatinine clearance <10 ml/min). As tramadol is only removed very slowly by haemodialysis or haemofiltration, post-dialysis administration to maintain analgesia is not usually necessary.

Hepatic impairment: The elimination of tramadol may be prolonged. The usual initial dosage should be used but in severe hepatic impairment the dosage interval should be increased to 12 hours.

Children under 12 years: Not recommended.

Contra-indications: Zydol should not be administered to patients who have previously demonstrated hypersensitivity to it or in cases of acute intoxication with alcohol, hypnotics, centrally acting analgesics, opioids or psychotropic drugs. In common with other opioid analgesics it should not be administered to patients who are receiving monamine oxidase inhibitors or within two weeks of their withdrawal.

Special warnings and special precautions for use:
Warnings: At therapeutic doses, Zydol has the potential to cause withdrawal symptoms. Rarely cases of dependence and abuse have been reported.

At therapeutic doses withdrawal symptoms have been reported at a reporting frequency of 1 in 8,000. Reports of dependence and abuse have been less frequent. Because of this potential the clinical need for continued analgesic treatment should be reviewed regularly.

In patients with a tendency to drug abuse or dependence, treatment should be for short periods and under strict medical supervision.

Zydol is not suitable as a substitute in opioid-dependent patients. Although it is an opioid agonist, Zydol cannot suppress morphine withdrawal symptoms.

Precautions: Zydol should be used with caution in patients with head injury, increased intracranial pressure, severe impairment of hepatic and renal function and in patients prone to convulsive disorders or in shock.

Convulsions have been reported at therapeutic doses and the risk may be increased at doses exceeding the usual upper daily dose limit. Patients with a history of epilepsy or those susceptible to seizures should only be treated with tramadol if there are compelling reasons. The risk of convulsions may increase in patients taking tramadol and concomitant medication that can lower the seizure threshold (see *Interactions with other medicaments and other forms of interaction*).

Care should be taken when treating patients with respiratory depression, or if concomitant CNS depressant drugs are being administered, as the possibility of respiratory depression cannot be excluded in these situations. At therapeutic doses respiratory depression has infrequently been reported.

In one study using a nitrous oxide/opioid (Zydol) anaesthetic technique (with only intermittent administration of enflurane 'as required') Zydol was reported to enhance intra-operative recall. Hence its use during potentially very light planes of general anaesthesia should be avoided.

Two recent studies of Zydol administration during anaesthesia comprising continuous administration of isoflurane did not show clinically significant lightening of anaesthetic depth or intra-operative recall. Therefore providing the current practice of administering continuous, potent (volatile or intravenous) anaesthetic agents is followed, Zydol may be used intra-operatively in the same way as other analgesic agents are routinely used.

Interactions with other medicaments and other forms of interaction: Concomitant administration of Zydol with other centrally acting drugs including alcohol may potentiate CNS depressant effects.

Tramadol may increase the potential for both selective serotonin reuptake inhibitors (SSRIs) and tricyclic antidepressants (TCAs) to cause convulsions (see *Special warnings and special precautions for use* and *Pharmacokinetic properties*). There is a theoretical possibility that tramadol could interact with lithium. There have been no reports of this potential interaction.

Pharmacokinetic studies were conducted to investigate the effects of cimetidine, quinidine and carbamazepine on the pharmacokinetics of tramadol.

Carbamazepine: Simultaneous administration of carbamazepine markedly decreases serum concentrations of tramadol to an extent that a decrease in analgesic effectiveness and a shorter duration of action may occur.

Cimetidine: With the concomitant or previous administration of cimetidine clinically relevant interactions are unlikely to occur. Therefore no alteration of the Zydol dosage regimen is recommended for patients receiving chronic cimetidine therapy.

Quinidine: A study of 12 healthy volunteers has shown that quinidine causes an approximate 25% increase in the tramadol C_{max} and AUC; T_{max} is unaffected. However, the increase in C_{max} and AUC fall within the normal therapeutic range for tramadol, and no dosage adjustment is required.

Pregnancy and lactation:

Pregnancy: Animal studies (rats and rabbits, exposure to tramadol up to 7 times that expected in man) have not revealed teratogenic effects and minimal embryotoxicity (delayed ossification). Fertility, reproductive performance and development of offspring were unaffected. There is inadequate evidence available on the safety of tramadol in human pregnancy, therefore Zydol should not be used in pregnant women.

Lactation: tramadol and its metabolites are found in small amounts in human breast milk. An infant could ingest 0.1% of the dose given to the mother. Zydol should not be administered during breast feeding.

Effects on ability to drive and use machines: Zydol may cause drowsiness and this effect may be potentiated by alcohol and other CNS depressants. Ambulant patients should be warned not to drive or operate machinery if affected.

Undesirable effects: Rapid intravenous administration may be associated with a higher incidence of adverse effects and therefore should be avoided.

Gastrointestinal system: Nausea, vomiting and occasionally dry mouth. Both diarrhoea and constipation have been reported. In controlled clinical trials the incidence of constipation is lower than that of comparator agents.

Central nervous system and psychiatric: Tiredness, fatigue, drowsiness, somnolence, dizziness, headache, confusion, hallucinations and infrequently respiratory depression. Dependence, dysphoria and convulsions have been reported rarely (see *Interactions*).

Physical dependence: Dependence, abuse and withdrawal reactions have been reported. Typical opiate withdrawal reactions include agitation, anxiety, nervousness, insomnia, hyperkinesia, tremor and gastrointestinal symptoms (see *Special warnings and special precautions in use* and *Posology and method of administration*).

Allergic/anaphylactoid reaction: Dyspnoea, wheezing, bronchospasm and worsening of existing asthma.

Other adverse events: Diaphoresis, urticaria and prutitus have been reported. The following have been rarely reported: skin rashes, blurred vision, difficulty passing urine and urinary retention, tachycardia, orthostatic hypotension, increase in blood pressure, bradycardia, flushing syncope and anaphylaxis. Cases of blood dyscrasias have been rarely observed during treatment with tramadol, but causality has not been established.

Overdose: Symptoms of overdosage are typical of other opioid analgesics, and include miosis, vomiting, cardiovascular collapse, sedation and coma, seizures and respiratory depression.

Supportive measures such as maintaining the patency of the airway and maintaining cardiovascular function should be instituted; naloxone should be used to reverse respiratory depression; fits can be controlled with diazepam.

Tramadol is minimally eliminated from the serum by haemodialysis or haemofiltration. Therefore treatment of acute intoxication with Zydol with haemodialysis or haemofiltration alone is not suitable for detoxification.

Pharmacological properties

Pharmacodynamic properties: Zydol is a centrally acting analgesic. It is a non selective pure agonist at mu, delta and kappa opioid receptors with a higher affinity for the mu receptor. Other mechanisms which may contribute to its analgesic effect are inhibition of neuronal reuptake of noradrenaline and enhancement of serotonin release.

Pharmacokinetic properties: After oral administration, tramadol is almost completely absorbed. Mean absolute bioavailability is approximately 70% following a single dose and increases to approximately 90% at steady state. Plasma protein binding of tramadol is approximately 20%. When C14-labelled tramadol was administered to humans, approximately 90% was excreted via the kidneys with the remaining 10% appearing in the faeces.

Tramadol has a linear pharmacokinetic profile within the therapeutic dosage range. The half-life of the terminal elimination phase ($t_{\frac{1}{2}}\beta$) was 6.0±1.5 h in young volunteers. Tramadol pharmacokinetics show little age dependence in volunteers up to the age of 75 years. In volunteers aged 75 years, $t_{\frac{1}{2}}\beta$ was 7.0±1.6 h on oral administration.

Following a single oral dose administration of tramadol 100 mg as capsules or tablets to young helathy volunteers, plasma concentrations were detectable within approximately 15 to 45 minutes with a mean C_{max} of 280 to 308 mcg/L and T_{max} of 1.6 to 2h.

Tramadol is metabolised by the cytochrome P450 isoenzyme CYP2D6. It undergoes biotransformation to a number of metabolites mainly by means of N- and O-demethylation. O-desmethyl tramadol appears to be the most pharmacologically active metabolite, showing analgesic activity in rodents. As humans excrete a higher percentage of unchanged tramadol than animals it is believed that the contribution made by this metabolite to analgesic activity is likely to be less in humans than animals. In humans the plasma concentration of this metabolite is about 25% that of unchanged tramadol.

Since tramadol is eliminated both metabolically and renally, the terminal half-life $t_{\frac{1}{2}}\beta$ may be prolonged in impaired hepatic or renal function. In patients with liver cirrhosis $t_{\frac{1}{2}}\beta$ tramadol was a mean of 13.3±4.9 h; in patients with renal insufficiency (creatinine clearance ≤5 ml/min) it was 11.0±3.2 h.

Preclinical safety data: In single and repeat-dose toxicity studies (rodents and dogs) exposure to tramadol 10 times that expected in man is required before toxicity (hepatotoxicity) is observed. Symptoms of toxicity are typical of opioids and include restlessness, ataxia, vomiting, tremor, dyspnoea and convulsions.

Exposure to tramadol (≥ that expected in man) in lifetime toxicity studies in rodents did not reveal any evidence of carcinogenic hazard, and a battery of in-vitro and in-vivo mutagenicity tests were negative.

Pharmaceutical particulars

List of excipients: Zydol ampoules contain: water for injection, sodium acetate.

Incompatibilities: Precipitation will occur if Zydol injection is mixed in the same syringe with injections of diazepam, diclofenac sodium, indomethacin, midazolam and piroxicam.

Shelf life: Zydol ampoules have a shelf life of 5 years.

Special precautions for storage: Store in a dry place below 30°C (86°F).

Nature and contents of container: Box of 5 ampoules.

Special instructions for use/handling: Zydol injection is physically and chemically compatible for up to 24 hours with 4.2% sodium bicarbonate and Ringer's solution and for up to 5 days with the following infusion solutions:

0.9% sodium chloride
0.18% sodium chloride and 4% glucose
sodium lactate compound
5% glucose
Haemaccel

Marketing authorisation holder: Monsanto plc, trading as Searle, PO Box 53, Lane End Road, High Wycombe, Bucks HP12 4HL.

Marketing authorisation number 08821/0004.

Date of first authorisation/renewal of the authorisation 1 January 1996.

Date of (partial) revision of the text October 1998.

Legal category POM.

ZYDOL* CAPSULES ▼

Qualitative and quantitative composition Each capsule contains 50 mg tramadol hydrochloride.

Pharmaceutical form Green/pale yellow hard gelatine capsules for oral administration.

Clinical particulars

Therapeutic indications: Management (treatment and prevention) of moderate to severe pain.

Posology and method of administration: As with all analgesic drugs, the dose of Zydol should be adjusted according to the severity of the pain and the clinical response of the individual patient.

Adults and children aged 12 years and over
Oral administration:

Acute pain: An initial dose of 100 mg is usually necessary. This can be followed by doses of 50 or 100 mg not more frequently than 4 hourly, and duration of therapy should be matched to clinical need.

Pain associated with chronic conditions: Use an initial dose of 50 mg and then titrate dose according to pain severity. The need for continued treatment should be assessed at regular intervals as withdrawal symptoms and dependence have been reported (see section *Special warnings and special precautions for use*). A total daily dose of 400 mg should not be exceeded except in special clinical circumstances.

Elderly: The usual dosages may be used although it should be noted that in volunteers aged over 75 years the elimination half-life of tramadol was increased by 17% following oral administration.

Renal impairment/renal dialysis: The elimination of tramadol may be prolonged. The usual initial dosage should be used. For patients with creatinine clearance <30 ml/min, the dosage interval should be increased to 12 hours. Tramadol is not recommended for patients with severe renal impairment (creatinine clearance <10 ml/min).

As tramadol is only removed very slowly by haemodialysis or haemofiltration, post-dialysis administration to maintain analgesia is not usually necessary.

Hepatic impairment: The elimination of tramadol may be prolonged. The usual initial dosage should be used but in severe hepatic impairment the dosage interval should be increased to 12 hours.

Children under 12 years: Not recommended.

Contra-indications: Zydol should not be administered to patients who have previously demonstrated hypersensitivity to it or in cases of acute intoxication with alcohol, hypnotics, centrally acting analgesics, opioids or psychotropic drugs. In common with other opioid analgesics it should not be administered to patients who are receiving monoamine oxidase inhibitors or within two weeks of their withdrawal.

Special warnings and special precautions for use

Warnings: At therapeutic doses, Zydol has the potential to cause withdrawal symptoms. Rarely cases of dependence and abuse have been reported.

At therapeutic doses withdrawal symptoms have been reported at a reporting frequency of 1 in 8,000. Reports of dependence and abuse have been less frequent. Because of this potential the clinical need for continued analgesic treatment should be reviewed regularly.

In patients with a tendency to drug abuse or dependence, treatment should be for short periods and under strict medical supervision.

Zydol is not suitable as a substitute in opioid-dependent patients. Although it is an opioid agonist, Zydol cannot suppress morphine withdrawal symptoms.

Precautions: Zydol should be used with caution in patients with head injury, increased intracranial pressure, severe impairment of hepatic and renal function and in patients prone to convulsive disorders or in shock.

Convulsions have been reported at therapeutic doses and the risk may be increased at doses exceeding the usual upper daily dose limit. Patients with a history of epilepsy or those susceptible to seizures should only be treated with tramadol if there are compelling reasons. The risk of convulsions may increase in patients taking tramadol and concomitant medication that can lower the seizure threshold (see *Interactions with other medicaments and other forms of interaction*).

Care should be taken when treating patients with respiratory depression, or if concomitant CNS depressant drugs are being administered, as the possibility of respiratory depression cannot be excluded in these situations. At therapeutic doses respiratory depression has infrequently been reported.

In one study using a nitrous oxide/opioid (Zydol) anaesthetic technique (with only intermittent administration of enflurane 'as required') Zydol was reported to enhance intra-operative recall. Hence its use during potentially very light planes of general anaesthesia should be avoided.

Two recent studies of Zydol administration during anaesthesia comprising continuous administration of isoflurane did not show clinically significant lightening of anaesthetic depth or intra-operative recall. Therefore providing the current practice of administering continuous, potent (volatile or intravenous) anaesthetic agents is followed, Zydol may be used intra-operatively in the same way as other analgesic agents are routinely used.

Interactions with other medicaments and other forms of interaction: Concomitant administration of Zydol with other centrally acting drugs including alcohol may potentiate CNS depressant effects.

Tramadol may increase the potential for both selective serotonin reuptake inhibitors (SSRIs) and tricyclic antidepressants (TCAs) to cause convulsions (see *Special warnings and special precautions for use* and *Pharmacokinetic properties*). There is a theoretical possibility that tramadol could interact with lithium. There have been no reports of this potential interaction.

Pharmacokinetic studies were conducted to investigate the effects of cimetidine, quinidine and carbamazepine on the pharmacokinetics of tramadol.

Carbamazepine: Simultaneous administration of carbamazepine markedly decreases serum concentrations of tramadol to an extent that a decrease in analgesic effectiveness and a shorter duration of action may occur.

Cimetidine: With the concomitant or previous administration of cimetidine clinically relevant interactions are unlikely to occur. Therefore no alteration of the Zydol dosage regimen is recommended for patients receiving chronic cimetidine therapy.

Quinidine: A study of 12 healthy volunteers has shown that quinidine causes an approximate 25% increase in the tramadol C_{max} and AUC; T_{max} is unaffected. However, the increase in C_{max} and AUC fall within the normal therapeutic range for tramadol, and no dosage adjustment is required.

Pregnancy and lactation

Pregnancy: Animal studies (rats and rabbits, exposure to tramadol up to 7 times that expected in man) have not revealed teratogenic effects and minimal embryo-toxicity (delayed ossification). Fertility, reproductive performance and development of offspring were unaffected. There is inadequate evidence available on the safety of tramadol in human pregnancy therefore Zydol should not be used in pregnant women.

Lactation: Tramadol and its metabolites are found in small amounts in human breast milk. An infant could ingest 0.1% of the dose given to the mother. Zydol should not be administered during breast feeding.

Effects on ability to drive and use machines: Zydol may cause drowsiness and this effect may be potentiated by alcohol and other CNS depressants. Ambulant patients should be warned not to drive or operate machinery if affected.

Undesirable effects:

Gastrointestinal system: Nausea, vomiting and occasionally dry mouth. Both diarrhoea and constipation have been reported. In controlled trials the incidence of constipation is lower than that of comparator agents.

Central nervous system and psychiatric: Tiredness, fatigue, drowsiness, somnolence, dizziness, headache, confusion, hallucinations and infrequently respiratory depression. Dependence, dysphoria and convulsions have been reported rarely (see *Interactions*).

Physical dependence: Dependence, abuse and withdrawal reactions have been reported. Typical opiate withdrawal reactions include agitation, anxiety, nervousness, insomnia, hyperkinesia, tremor and gastrointestinal symptoms (see *Special warnings and special precautions in use* and *Posology and method of administration*).

Allergic/anaphylactoid reaction: Dyspnoea, wheezing, bronchospasm and worsening of existing asthma.

Other adverse events: Diaphoresis, urticaria and prutitus have been reported. The following have been rarely reported: skin rashes, blurred vision, difficulty passing urine and urinary retention, tachycardia, orthostatic hypotension, increase in blood pressure, bradycardia, flushing syncope and anaphylaxis. Cases of blood dyscrasias have been rarely observed during treatment with tramadol, but causality has not been established.

Overdose: Symptoms of overdosage are typical of other opioid analgesics, and include miosis, vomiting, cardiovascular collapse, sedation and coma, seizures and respiratory depression.

Supportive measures such as maintaining the patency of the airway and maintaining cardiovascular function should be instituted; naloxone should be used to reverse respiratory depression; fits can be controlled with diazepam.

Tramadol is minimally eliminated from the serum by haemodialysis or haemofiltration. Therefore treatment of acute intoxication with Zydol with haemodialysis or haemofiltration alone is not suitable for detoxification.

Pharmacological properties

Pharmacodynamic properties: Zydol is a centrally acting analgesic. It is a non selective pure agonist at mu, delta and kappa opioid receptors with a higher affinity for the mu receptor. Other mechanisms which may contribute to its analgesic effect are inhibition of neuronal reuptake of noradrenaline and enhancement of serotonin release.

Pharmacokinetic properties: After oral administration, tramadol is almost completely absorbed. Mean absolute bioavailability is approximately 70% following a single dose and increases to approximately 90% at steady state. Plasma protein binding of tramadol is approximately 20%. When C14-labelled tramadol was administered to humans, approximately 90% was excreted via the kidneys with the remaining 10% appearing in the faeces.

Tramadol has a linear pharmacokinetic profile within the therapeutic dosage range. The half-life of the terminal elimination phase ($t_{\frac{1}{2}}\beta$) was 6.0±1.5 h in young volunteers. Tramadol pharmacokinetics show little age dependence in volunteers up to the age of 75 years. In volunteers aged 75 years, $t_{\frac{1}{2}}\beta$ was 7.0±1.6 h on oral administration.

Following a single oral dose administration of tramadol 100 mg as capsules or tablets to young helathy volunteers, plasma concentrations were detectable within approximately 15 to 45 minutes with a mean C_{max} of 280 to 308 mcg/L and T_{max} of 1.6 to 2h.

Tramadol is metabolised by the cytochrome P450 isoenzyme CYP2D6. It undergoes biotransformation to a number of metabolites mainly by means of N- and O-demethylation. O-desmethyl tramadol appears to be the most pharmacologically active metabolite, showing analgesic activity in rodents. As humans excrete a higher percentage of unchanged tramadol than animals it is believed that the contribution made by this metabolite to analgesic activity is likely to be less in humans than animals. In humans the plasma concentration of this metabolite is about 25% that of unchanged tramadol.

Since tramadol is eliminated both metabolically and renally, the terminal half-life $t_{\frac{1}{2}}\beta$ may be prolonged in impaired hepatic or renal function. In patients with liver cirrhosis $t_{\frac{1}{2}}\beta$ tramadol was a mean of 13.3±4.9 h; in patients with renal insufficiency (creatinine clearance ≤5 ml/min) it was 11.0±3.2 h.

Preclinical safety data: In single and repeat-dose toxicity studies (rodents and dogs) exposure to tramadol 10 times that expected in man is required before toxicity (hepatotoxicity) is observed. Symptoms of toxicity are typical of opioids and include restlessness, ataxia, vomiting, tremor, dyspnoea and convulsions.

Exposure to tramadol (≥ that expected in man) in lifetime toxicity studies in rodents did not reveal any evidence of carcinogenic hazard, and a battery of in-vitro and in-vivo mutagenicity tests were negative.

Pharmaceutical particulars

List of excipients: Zydol capsules contain: microcrystalline cellulose, sodium starch glycolate, magnesium stearate, colloidal anhydrous silica. The capsule shell contains: gelatin, and colours E132, E172 and E171.

Incompatibilities: None known.

Shelf life: Zydol capsules have a shelf life of 5 years when stored in PVC/foil or PP/foil blisters.

Special precautions for storage: Store in a dry place below 30°C (86°F).

Nature and contents of container: PVC/foil or PP/foil blister packs of 10, 20 and 100 capsules.

Special instructions for use/handling: None.

Marketing authorisation holder: Monsanto p.l.c., PO Box 53, Lane End Road, High Wycombe, Bucks HP12 4HL.

Marketing authorisation number 08821/0005.

Date of first authorisation/renewal of the authorisation 1st January 1996.

Date of (partial) revision of the text October 1998.

Legal category POM.

ZYDOL* SOLUBLE TABLETS ▼

Qualitative and quantitative composition Each soluble tablet contains 50 mg tramadol hydrochloride.

Pharmaceutical form White, round, flat tablets, scored on one side and engraved 'T4' with manufacturer's logo on the reverse. For oral administration.

Clinical particulars

Therapeutic indications: Management (treatment and prevention) of moderate to severe pain.

Posology and method of administration: As with all analgesic drugs, the dose of Zydol should be adjusted according to the severity of the pain and the clinical response of the individual patient.

Adults and children aged 12 years and over: Oral administration.

Acute pain: An initial dose of 100 mg is usually necessary. This can be followed by doses of 50 or 100 mg not more frequently than 4 hourly and duration of therapy should be matched to clinical need.

Pain associated with chronic conditions: Use an initial dose of 50 mg and then titrate dose according to pain severity. The need for continued treatment should be assessed at regular intervals as withdrawal symptoms and dependence have been reported (see *Special warnings and special precautions for use*). A total daily oral dose of 400 mg should not be exceeded except in special clinical circumstances.

The tablets should be dissolved in at least 50 mls water before administration.

Elderly: The usual dosages may be used although it should be noted that in volunteers aged over 75 years the elimination half-life of tramadol was increased by 17% following oral administration.

Renal impairment/renal dialysis: The elimination of tramadol may be prolonged. The usual initial dosage should be used. For patients with creatinine clearance <30 ml/min, the dosage interval should be increased to 12 hours. Tramadol is not recommended for patients with severe renal impairment (creatinine clearance <10 ml/min).

Hepatic impairment: The elimination of tramadol may be prolonged. The usual initial dosage should be used but in severe hepatic impairment the dosage interval should be increased to 12 hours.

Children under 12 years: Not recommended.

Contra-indications: Zydol should not be administered to patients who have previously demonstrated hypersensitivity to it or in cases of acute intoxication with alcohol, hypnotics, centrally acting analgesics, opioids or psychotropic drugs.

In common with other opioid analgesics it should not be administered to patients who are receiving monamine oxidase inhibitors or within two weeks of their withdrawal.

Special warnings and special precautions for use:

Warnings: At therapeutic doses, Zydol has the potential to cause withdrawal symptoms. Rarely cases of dependence and abuse have been reported.

At therapeutic doses withdrawal symptoms have been reported at a reporting frequency of 1 in 8,000. Reports of dependence and abuse have been less frequent. Because of this potential the clinical need for continued analgesic treatment should be reviewed regularly.

In patients with a tendency to drug abuse or dependence, treatment should be for short periods and under strict medical supervision.

Zydol is not suitable as a substitute in opioid-dependent patients. Although it is an opioid agonist, Zydol cannot suppress morphine withdrawal symptoms.

Precautions: Zydol should be used with caution in patients with head injury, increased intracranial pressure, severe impairment of hepatic and renal function and in patients prone to convulsive disorders or in shock.

Convulsions have been reported at therapeutic doses and the risk may be increased at doses exceeding the usual upper daily dose limit. Patients with a history of epilepsy or those susceptible to seizures should only be treated with tramadol if there are compelling reasons. The risk of convulsions may increase in patients taking tramadol and concomitant medication that can lower the seizure threshold (see *Interactions with other medicaments and other forms of interaction:* Concomitant administration of Zydol with other centrally acting drugs including alcohol may potentiate CNS depressant effects.

Tramadol may increase the potential for both selective serotonin reuptake inhibitors (SSRIs) and tricyclic antidepressants (TCAs) to cause convulsions (see *Special warnings and special precautions for use* and *Pharmacokinetic properties*). There is a theoretical possibility that tramadol could interact with lithium. There have been no reports of this potential interaction.

Pharmacokinetic studies were conducted to investigate the effects of cimetidine, quinidine and carbamazepine on the pharmacokinetics of tramadol.

Carbamazepine: Simultaneous administration of carbamazepine markedly decreases serum concentrations of tramadol to an extent that a decrease in analgesic effectiveness and a shorter duration of action may occur.

Cimetidine: With the concomitant or previous administration of cimetidine clinically relevant interactions are unlikely to occur. Therefore no alteration of the Zydol dosage regimen is recommended for patients receiving chronic cimetidine therapy.

Quinidine: A study of 12 healthy volunteers has shown that quinidine causes an approximate 25% increase in the tramadol C_{max} and AUC; T_{max} is unaffected. However, the increase in C_{max} and AUC fall within the normal therapeutic range for tramadol, and no dosage adjustment is required.

Interactions with other medicaments and other forms of interaction: Concomitant administration of Zydol with other centrally acting drugs including alcohol may potentiate CNS depressant effects.

Tramadol may increase the potential for both selective serotonin reuptake inhibitors (SSRIs) and tricyclic antidepressants (TCAs) to cause convulsions (see *Special warnings and special precautions for use* and *Pharmacokinetic properties*). There is a theoretical possibility that tranadol could interact with lithium. There have been no reports of this potential interaction.

Pharmacokinetic studies were conducted to investigate the effects of cimetidine, quinidine and carbamazepine on the pharmacokinetics of tramadol.

Carbamazepine: Simultaneous administration with carbamazepine marketly decreases serum concentrations of tramadol to an extent that a decrease in analgesic effectiveness and a shorter duration of action may occur.

Cimetidine: With the concomitant or previous administration of cimetidine clinically relevant interactions are unlikely to occur. Therefore no alteration of the Zydol dosage regimen is recommended for patients receiving chronic cimetidine therapy.

Quinidine: A study of 12 healthy volunteers has shown that quinidine causes an approximate 25% increase in the tramadol C_{max} and AUC; T_{max} is unaffected. However, the increase in C_{max} and AUC fall within the normal therapeutic range for tramadol, and no dosage adjustment is required.

Pregnancy and lactation:

Pregnancy: Animal studies (rat and rabbit, exposure to tramadol up to 7 times that expected in man) have not revealed teratogenic effects and minimal embryotoxicity (delayed ossification). Fertility, reproductive performance and development of offspring were unaffected. There is inadequate evidence available on the safety of tramadol in human pregnancy, therefore Zydol should not be used in pregnant women.

Lactation: Tramadol and its metabolites are found in small amounts in human breast milk. An infant could ingest about 0.1% of the dose given to the mother. Zydol should not be administered during breast feeding.

Effects on ability to drive and use machines: Zydol may cause drowsiness and this effect may be potentiated by alcohol and other CNS depressants. Ambulant patients should be warned not to drive or operate machinery if affected.

Undesirable effects:

Gastrointestinal system: Nausea, vomiting and occasionally dry mouth. Both diarrhoea and constipation have been reported. In controlled trials the incidence of constipation is lower than that of comparator agents.

Central nervous system and psychiatric: Tiredness, fatigue, drowsiness, somnolence, dizziness, headache, confusion, hallucinations and infrequently, respiratory depression. Dependence, dysphoria and convulsions have been reported rarely (see *Interactions*).

Physical dependence: Dependence, abuse and withdrawal reactions have been reported. Typical opiate withdrawal reactions include agitation, anxiety, nervousness, insomnia, hyperkinesia, tremor and gastrointestinal symptoms (see *Special warnings and special precautions in use* and *Posology and method of administration*).

Allergic/anaphylactoid reaction: Dyspnoea, wheezing, bronchospasm and worsening of existing asthma.

Other adverse events: Diaphoresis, urticaria and prutitus have been reported. The following have been rarely reported: skin rashes, blurred vision, difficulty passing urine and urinary retention, tachycardia, orthostatic hypotension, increase in blood pressure, bradycardia, flushing syncope and anaphylaxis. Cases of blood dyscrasias have been rarely observed during treatment with tramadol, but causality has not been established.

Overdose: Symptoms of overdosage are typical of other opioid analgesics, and include miosis, vomiting, cardiovascular collapse, sedation and coma, seizures and respiratory depression.

Supportive measures such as maintaining the patency of the airway and maintaining cardiovascular function should be instituted; nalaxone should be used to reverse respiratory depression; fits can be controlled with diazepam.

Tramadol is minimally eliminated from the serum by haemodialysis or haemofiltration. Therefore treatment of acute intoxication with Zydol with haemodialysis or haemofiltration alone is not suitable for detoxification.

Pharmacological properties

Pharmacodynamic properties: Zydol is a centrally acting analgesic. It is a non selective pure agonist at mu, delta and kappa opioid receptors with a higher affinity for the mu receptor. Other mechanisms which may contribute to its analgesic effect are inhibition of neuronal reuptake of noradrenaline and enhancement of serotonin release.

Pharmacokinetic properties: After oral administration, tramadol is almost completely absorbed. Mean absolute bioavailability is approximately 70% following a single dose and increases to approximately 90% at steady state. Plasma protein binding of tramadol is approximately 20%. When C14-labelled tramadol was administered to humans, approximately 90% was excreted via the kidneys with the remaining 10% appearing in the faeces.

Tramadol has a linear pharmacokinetic profile within the therapeutic dosage range. The half-life of the terminal elimination phase ($t_{\frac{1}{2}} \beta$) was 6.0±1.5 h in young volunteers. Tramadol pharmacokinetics show little age dependence in volunteers up to the age of 75 years. In volunteers aged 75 years, $t_{\frac{1}{2}} \beta$ was 7.0±1.6 h on oral administration.

Following a single oral dose administration of tramadol 100 mg as capsules or tablets to young helathy volunteers, plasma concentrations were detectable within approximately 15 to 45 minutes with a mean C_{max} of 280 to 308 mcg/L and T_{max} of 1.6 to 2h.

Tramadol is metabolised by the cytochrome P450 isoenzyme CYP2D6. It undergoes biotransformation to a number of metabolites mainly by means of N- and O-demethylation. O-desmethyl tramadol appears to be the most pharmacologically active metabolite, showing analgesic activity in rodents. As humans excrete a higher percentage of unchanged tramadol than animals it is believed that the contribution made by this metabolite to analgesic activity is likely to be less in humans than animals. In humans the plasma concentration of this metabolite is about 25% that of unchanged tramadol.

Since tramadol is eliminated both metabolically and renally, the terminal half-life $t_{\frac{1}{2}} \beta$ may be prolonged in impaired hepatic or renal function. In patients with liver cirrhosis $t_{\frac{1}{2}} \beta$ tramadol was a mean of 13.3±4.9 h; in patients with renal insufficiency (creatinine clearance ≤5 ml/min) it was 11.0±3.2 h.

Preclinical safety data: In single and repeat-dose toxicity studies (rodents and dogs) exposure to tramadol 10 times that expected in man is required before toxicity (hepatotoxicity) is observed. Symptoms of toxicity are typical of opioids and include restlessness, ataxia, vomiting, tremor, dyspnoea and convulsions.

Exposure to tramadol (≥ that expected in man) in lifetime toxicity studies in rodents did not reveal any evidence of carcinogenic hazard, and a battery of in-vitro and in-vivo mutagenicity tests were negative.

Pharmaceutical particulars

List of excipients: Zydol soluble tablets contain: microcrystalline cellulose, maize starch, saccharin sodium, colloidal anhydrous silica, magnesium stearate, peppermint and aniseed flavouring.

Incompatabilities: None known.

Shelf life: Zydol soluble tablets have a shelf life of 3 years when stored in polypropylene/foil or pvc/pvdc/foil blisters.

Special precautions for storage: Store in a dry place below 25°C.

Nature and contents of container: Polypropylene foil or PVC/PVDC foil blister packs of 10, 20 or 100 tablets.

Special instructions for use/handling: The tablets are formulated to be dissolved in water prior to administration, producing a slightly peppermint/aniseed flavoured oral solution.

Market authorisation holder: Monsanto p.l.c., Trading as Searle, PO Box 53, Lane End Road, High Wycombe, Bucks HP12 4HL.

Marketing authorisation number 8821/0046.

Date of first authorisation/renewal of the authorisation 12th September 1996.

Date of (partial) revision of the text October 1998.

Legal category POM.

ZYDOL SR* ▼

Qualitative and quantitative composition Each slow-release tablet contains 100 mg, 150 mg or 200 mg tramadol hydrochloride.

Pharmaceutical form White, beige or orange biconvex tablets engraved T1, T2 or T3 (for the 100 mg, 150 mg or 200 mg strengths, respectively) on one side and with manufacturer's logo on the other, for oral administration.

Clinical particulars

Therapeutic indications: Management (treatment and prevention) of moderate to severe pain.

Posology and method of administration: As with all analgesic drugs, the dose of Zydol should be adjusted according to the severity of the pain and the clinical response of the individual patient.

Adults and children aged 12 years and over

Oral administration: The usual initial dose is one 100 mg tablet twice daily, morning and evening. If pain relief is insufficient, the dosage may be titrated upwards to one 150 mg or one 200 mg tablet twice daily.

Tablets should be swallowed whole.

Pain associated with chronic conditions: The need for continued treatment should be assessed at regular intervals as withdrawal symptoms and dependence have been reported (see *Special warnings and special precautions for use*).

A total daily oral dose of 400 mg should not be exceeded except in special clinical circumstances.

Elderly: The usual dosages may be used although it should be noted that in volunteers aged over 75 years the elimination half-life of tramadol was increased by 17% following oral administration.

Renal impairment/renal dialysis: As the elimination of tramadol may be prolonged, use of Zydol capsules may be more appropriate. Tramadol is not recommended for patients with severe renal impairment (creatinine clearance < 10 ml/min). As tramadol is only removed very slowly by haemodialysis or haemofiltration, post-dialysis administration to maintain analgesia is not usually necessary.

Hepatic impairment: As the elimination of tramadol may be prolonged use of Zydol capsules may be more appropriate.

Children under 12 years: Not recommended.

Contra-indications: Zydol should not be administered to patients who have previously demonstrated hypersensitivity to it or in cases of acute intoxication with alcohol, hypnotics, centrally acting analgesics, opioids of psychotropic drugs. In common with other opioid analgesics it should not be administered to patients who are receiving monoamine oxidase inhibitors or within two weeks of their withdrawal.

Special warnings and special precautions for use

Warnings: At therapeutic doses, Zydol has the potential to cause withdrawal symptoms. Rarely cases of dependence and abuse have been reported.

At therapeutic doses withdrawal symptoms have been reported at a reporting frequency of 1 in 8,000. Reports of dependence and abuse have been less frequent. Because of this potential the clinical need for continued analgesic treatment should be reviewed regularly.

In patients with a tendency to drug abuse or dependence, treatment should be for short periods and under strict medical supervision.

Zydol is not suitable as a substitute in opioid-dependent patients. Although it is an opioid agonist, Zydol cannot suppress morphine withdrawal symptoms.

Precautions: Zydol should be used with caution in patients with head injury, increased intracranial pressure, severe impairment of hepatic and renal function and in patients prone to convulsive disorders or in shock.

Convulsions have been reported at therapeutic doses and the risk may be increased at doses exceeding the usual upper daily dose limit. Patients with a history of epilepsy or those susceptible to seizures should only be treated with tramadol if there are compelling reasons. The risk of convulsions may increase in patients taking tramadol and concomitant medication that can lower the seizure threshold (see *Interactions with other medicaments and other forms of interaction*).

Care should be taken when treating patients with respiratory depression, or if concomitant CNS depressant drugs are being administered, as the possibility of respiratory depression cannot be excluded in these situations. At therapeutic doses respiratory depression has infrequently been reported.

In one study using a nitrous oxide/opioid (Zydol) anaesthetic technique (with only intermittent administration of enflurane 'as required') Zydol was reported to enhance intra-operative recall. Hence its use during potentially very light planes of general anaesthesia should be avoided.

Two recent studies of Zydol administration during anaesthesia comprising continuous administration of isoflurane did not show clinically significant lightening of anaesthetic depth or intra-operative recall. Therefore providing the current practice of administering continuous, potent (volatile or intravenous) anaesthetic agents is followed, Zydol may be used intra-operatively in the same way as other analgesic agents are routinely used.

Interactions with other medicaments and other forms of interaction: Concomitant administration of Zydol with other centrally acting drugs including alcohol may potentiate CNS depressant effects.

Tramadol may increase the potential for both selective serotonin reuptake inhibitors (SSRIs) and tricyclic antidepressants (TCAs) to cause convulsions (see *Special warnings and special precautions for use* and *Pharmacokinetic properties*). There is a theoretical possibility that tramadol could interact with lithium. There have been no reports of this potential interaction.

Pharmacokinetic studies were conducted to investigate the effects of cimetidine, quinidine and carbamazepine on the pharmacokinetics of tramadol.

Carbamazepine: Simultaneous administration of carbamazepine markedly decreases serum concentrations of tramadol to an extent that a decrease in analgesic effectiveness and a shorter duration of action may occur.

Cimetidine: With the concomitant or previous administration of cimetidine clinically relevant interactions are unlikely to occur. Therefore no alteration of the Zydol dosage regimen is recommended for patients receiving chronic cimetidine therapy.

Quinidine: A study of 12 healthy volunteers has shown that quinidine causes an approximate 25% increase in the tramadol C_{max} and AUC; T_{max} is unaffected. However, the increase in C_{max} and AUC fall within the normal therapeutic range for tramadol, and no dosage adjustment is required.

Pregnancy and lactation

Pregnancy: Animal studies (rats and rabbits, exposure to tramadol up to 7 times that expected in man) have not revealed teratogenic effects and minimal embryotoxicity (delayed ossification). Fertility, reproductive performance and development of offspring were unaffected. There is inadequate evidence available on the safety of tramadol in human pregnancy therefore Zydol should not be used in pregnant women.

Lactation: Tramadol and its metabolites are found in small amounts in human breast milk. An infant could ingest 0.1% of the dose given to the mother. Zydol should not be administered during breast feeding.

Effects on ability to drive and use machines: Zydol may cause drowsiness and this effect may be potentiated by alcohol and other CNS depressants. Ambulant patients should be warned not to drive or operate machinery if affected.

Undesirable effects:

Gastrointestinal system: Nausea, vomiting and occasionally dry mouth. Both diarrhoea and constipation have been reported. In controlled trials the incidence of constipation is lower than that of comparator agents.

Central nervous system and psychiatric: Tiredness, fatigue, drowsiness, somnolence, dizziness, headache, confusion, hallucinations and infrequently respiratory depression. Dependence, dysphoria and convulsions have been reported rarely (see *Interactions*).

Physical dependence: Dependence, abuse and withdrawal reactions have been reported. Typical opiate withdrawal reactions include agitation, anxiety, nervousness, insomnia, hyperkinesia, tremor and gastrointestinal symptoms (see *Special warnings and special precautions in use* and *Posology and method of administration*).

Allergic/anaphylactoid reaction: Dyspnoea, wheezing, bronchospasm and worsening of existing asthma.

Other adverse events: Diaphoresis, urticaria and prutitus have been reported. The following have been rarely reported: skin rashes, blurred vision, difficulty passing urine and urinary retention, tachycardia, orthostatic hypotension, increase in blood pressure, bradycardia, flushing syncope and anaphylaxis. Cases of blood dyscrasias have been rarely observed during treatment with tramadol, but causality has not been established.

Overdose: Symptoms of overdosage are typical of other opioid analgesics, and include miosis, vomiting, cardiovascular collapse, sedation and coma, seizures and respiratory depression.

Supportive measures such as maintaining the patency of the airway and maintaining cardiovascular function should be instituted; naloxone should be used to reverse respiratory depression; fits can be controlled with diazepam.

Tramadol is minimally eliminated from the serum by haemodialysis or haemofiltration. Therefore treatment of acute intoxication with Zydol with haemodialysis or haemofiltration alone is not suitable for detoxification.

Pharmacological properties

Pharmacodynamic properties: Zydol is a centrally acting analgesic. It is a non selective pure agonist at mu, delta and kappa opioid receptors with a higher affinity for the mu receptor. Other mechanisms which may contribute to its analgesic effect are inhibition of neuronal reuptake of noradrenaline and enhancement of serotonin release.

Pharmacokinetic properties: After oral administration, tramadol is almost completely absorbed. Mean absolute bioavailability is approximately 70% following a single dose and increases to approximately 90% at steady state. Plasma protein binding of tramadol is approximately 20%. When C14-labelled tramadol was administered to humans, approximately 90% was excreted via the kidneys with the remaining 10% appearing in the faeces.

Tramadol has a linear pharmacokinetic profile within the therapeutic dosage range. The elimination half life $t_{\frac{1}{2}}\beta$ is 5–7 hrs irrespective of the mode of administration.

In patients over 75 years the elimination half-life of tramadol was increased by 17% following oral administration. The total clearance is 710 ml/min and may be reduced in elderly patients.

Cmax (141±40 ng/ml) is reached 4.9 hrs after oral administration of Zydol SR 100 mg and 4.8 hrs (Cmax 260±62 ng/ml) after oral administration of the 200 mg tablet.

Since tramadol is eliminated both metabolically and renally, the terminal half-life $t_{\frac{1}{2}}\beta$ may be prolonged in impaired hepatic or renal function. In patients with liver cirrhosis $t_{\frac{1}{2}}\beta$ tramadol was a mean of 13.3±4.9; in patients with renal insufficiency (creatinine clearance ≤5 ml/min) it was 11.0±3.2 hrs after capsules.

Preclinical safety data: In single and repeat-dose toxicity studies (rodents and dogs) exposure to tramadol 10 times that expected in man is required before toxicity (hepatotoxicity) is observed.

Symptoms of toxicity are typical of opioids and include restlessness, ataxia, vomiting, tremor, dyspnoea and convulsions.

Exposure to tramadol (≥ that expected in man) in lifetime toxicity studies in rodents did not reveal any evidence of carcinogenic hazard, and a battery of in-vitro and in-vivo mutagenicity tests were negative.

Pharmaceutical particulars

List of excipients: Zydol SR 100 mg tablets contain: microcrystalline cellulose, methylhydroxypropylcellulose, magnesium stearate, colloidal anhydrous silica, lactose, polyethylene glycol 6000, Propylene glycol, talc and titanium dioxide (E171).

Zydol SR 150 mg tablets contain: microcrystalline cellulose, methylhydroxypropylcellulose, magnesium stearate, colloidal anhydrous silica, lactose, polyethylene glycol 6000, Propylene glycol, talc, titanium dioxide (E171), quinoline yellow lake (E104), and red iron oxide (E172).

Zydol SR 200 mg tablets contain: microcrystalline cellulose, methylhydroxypropylcellulose, magnesium stearate, colloidal anhydrous silica, lactose, polyethylene glycol 6000, Propylene glycol, talc, titanium dioxide (E171), quinoline yellow lake (E104), red iron oxide (E172) and brown iron oxide (E172).

Incompatibilities: None known.

Shelf life: Zydol SR 100 mg has a shelf life of 4 years and Zydol SR 150 mg and 200 mg tablets have a shelf life of 3 years when stored in PVC/PVDC/foil blisters.

Special precautions for storage: Store in a dry place below 30°C.

Nature and contents of container: PVC/PVDC/foil blister packs of 2, 4 or 10 tablets (sample/starter packs).

PVC/PVDC/foil blister packs of 30 or 60 tablets.

Special instructions for use/handling: None.

Marketing authorisation holder: Monsanto p.l.c., P.O. Box 53, Lane End Road, High Wycombe, Buckinghamshire, HP12 4HL.

Marketing authorisation numbers

Zydol SR 100 mg	08821/0003
Zydol SR 150mg	08821/0002
Zydol SR 200mg	08821/0001

Date of first authorisation/renewal of the authorisation 1st January 1996.

Date of (partial) revision of the text October 1998.

Legal category POM.

**Trade Mark*

Serono Laboratories (UK) Ltd

99 Bridge Road East
Welwyn Garden City
Hertfordshire AL7 1BG

☎ 01707 331972 🗋 01707 371873

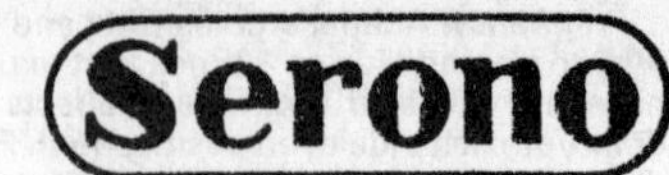

ARES-SERONO GROUP

CUROSURF*

Qualitative and quantitative composition Curosurf is a natural surfactant, prepared from porcine lungs, containing almost exclusively polar lipids, in particular phosphatidylcholine (about 70% of the total phospholipid content) and about 1% of specific low molecular weight hydrophobic proteins SP-B and SP-C.

One 1.5 ml vial contains phospholipid fraction from porcine lung 120 mg. One 3 ml vial contains phospholipid fraction from porcine lung 240 mg.

Composition per ml of suspension: phospholipid fraction from porcine lung 80 mg/ml, equivalent to about 74 mg/ml of total phospholipids and 0.9 mg/ml of low molecular weight hydrophobic proteins.

Pharmaceutical form A white to yellow sterile suspension in single-dose vials for intratracheal administration.

Clinical particulars

Therapeutic indications: Treatment of Respiratory Distress Syndrome (RDS) or hyaline membrane disease in newborn babies with birthweight over 700 g.

Prophylactic use in premature infants between 24 and 31 weeks estimated gestational age at risk from RDS or with evidence of surfactant deficiency.

Posology and method of administration: Curosurf should only be administered by those trained and experienced in the care and resuscitation of preterm infants. It is administered via the intratracheal route in intubated infants undergoing mechanical ventilation for respiratory distress syndrome and whose heart rate and arterial oxygen concentration or oxygen saturation are being continuously monitored. Intubation should not be undertaken merely to administer surfactant.

Curosurf is available in ready to use vials that should be stored in a refrigerator at +2 to +8°C. The vial should be warmed to ambient temperature before use, for example by holding it in the hand for a few minutes, and gently turned upside down, without shaking, in order to obtain a uniform suspension.

The suspension should be withdrawn from the vial using a sterile needle and syringe.

Posology

Prophylaxis: a single dose of 100–200 mg/kg should be administered as soon as possible after birth (preferably within 15 minutes). Further doses of 100 mg/kg can be given 6–12 hours after the first dose and then 12 hours later in babies who have persistent signs of RDS and remain ventilator-dependent (maximum total dose: 300–400 mg/kg).

Rescue treatment: it is advisable to commence the treatment as soon as possible after diagnosing RDS. Therapy with Curosurf starting more than 48 hours after diagnosing RDS has not been investigated. Initially, a single dose of 100–200 mg/kg (1.25–2.5 ml/kg) is advised.

Up to two further doses of 100 mg/kg, administered at about 12 hourly intervals, may also be indicated in infants who remain intubated and in whom RDS is considered responsible for their persisting or deteriorating respiratory status (maximum total dose of 300–400 mg/kg).

Method of administration: Curosurf can be administered either by:

Disconnecting the baby from the ventilator – Disconnect the baby momentarily from the ventilator, administer 1.25 to 2.5 ml/kg of suspension, as a single bolus, directly into the lower trachea via the endotracheal tube. Perform approximately one minute of hand-bagging and then reconnect the baby to the ventilator at the same settings as before administration. Further doses (1.25 ml/kg) that may be required can be administered in the same manner.

OR

Without disconnecting the baby from the ventilator – Administer 1.25 to 2.5 ml/kg of the suspension, as a single bolus, directly into the lower trachea by passing a catheter through the suction port into the endotracheal tube. Further doses (1.25 ml/kg) that may be required can be administered in the same manner.

After administration of Curosurf, pulmonary compliance (chest expansion) can improve rapidly, thus requiring prompt adjustment of the ventilator settings.

The improvement of alveolar gas exchange can result in a rapid increase of arterial oxygen concentration: therefore a rapid adjustment of the inspired oxygen concentration should be made to avoid hyperoxia. In order to maintain proper blood oxygenation values, in addition to periodic haemo-gasanalysis, continuous monitoring of transcutaneous P_aO_2 or oxygen saturation is also advisable.

Contra-indications: No specific contra-indications are yet known.

Special warnings and special precautions of use: The baby's general conditions should be stabilised. Correction of acidosis, hypotension, anaemia, hypoglycaemia and hypothermia is also recommended.

Babies born following very prolonged rupture of the membranes (greater than 3 weeks) may not show optimal response.

Surfactant administration can be expected to reduce the severity of RDS but cannot be expected to eliminate entirely the mortality and morbidity associated with preterm birth, as preterm babies may be exposed to other complications of their immaturity. After administration of Curosurf a transient depression of cerebro-electrical activity has been recorded lasting 2 to 10 minutes. The impact of this is not clear.

Interaction with other medicaments and other forms of interaction: Not known.

Pregnancy and lactation: Not applicable.

Effects on ability to drive and use machines: Not applicable.

Undesirable effects: Pulmonary haemorrhage, the incidence of which increases the more immature the infant is, is a rare and sometimes fatal complication of preterm delivery. No evidence exists of any increased risk of this event following the administration of Curosurf.

No other undesirable effects have been reported.

Overdose: There have been no reports of overdosage following the administration of Curosurf. However, in the unlikely event of accidental overdose, and only if there are clear clinical effects on the infant's respiration, ventilation or oxygenation, as much of the suspension as possible should be aspirated and the baby should be managed with supportive treatment, with particular attention to fluid and electrolyte balance.

Pharmacological properties

Pharmacodynamic properties: Lung surfactant is a mixture of substances, mainly phospholipids and specific proteins, lining the internal surface of alveoli and capable of lowering pulmonary surface tension.

This surface tension lowering activity is essential to stabilise alveoli, and to avoid collapse at end-expiration so that adequate gas exchange is maintained throughout the ventilatory cycle.

Deficiency of lung surfactant, from whatever cause, leads to severe respiratory failure which in preterm babies is known as respiratory distress syndrome (RDS) or hyaline membrane disease (HMD). RDS is a major cause of acute mortality and acute morbidity in the preterm baby and may also be responsible for long term respiratory and neurologic sequelae.

Curosurf was developed to replace this deficiency of endogenous pulmonary surfactant by intratracheal administration of exogenous surfactant.

The surface properties of Curosurf favour its uniform distribution in the lungs and spreading at the air-liquid interfaces in the alveoli. The physiological and therapeutic effects of Curosurf in surfactant deficiency have been documented extensively in various animal models.

In immature rabbit foetuses obtained by hysterectomy and immediately sacrificed the administration of Curosurf caused a marked improvement in lung expansion.

In premature newborn rabbits ventilated with 100% oxygen there was a dramatic improvement of tidal volume and lung-thorax compliance compared to the control animals, after administration of Curosurf via a tracheal cannula.

Also in premature newborn rabbits, treatment with Curosurf (maintaining a standardised tidal volume of about 10 ml/kg) increased the compliance of the lung-thorax system to a level similar to that of mature newborn animals.

Pharmacokinetic properties: Curosurf remains mainly in the lungs following intratracheal administration with a half-life of 14C-labelled dipalmitoyl-phosphatidylcholine of 67 hours in newborn rabbits. Only traces of surfactant lipids can be found in serum and organs other than the lungs 48 hours after administration.

Preclinical safety data: Acute toxicity studies performed in different animal species by intraperitoneal and intratracheal routes did not elicit signs of lung or systemic toxicity, nor mortality.

The subacute intratracheal toxicity study in the dog, rabbit and rat (14 days) showed no clinical effects or haematological changes, nor macroscopic variations. Moreover, Curosurf did not reveal any evidence of direct toxicity in the rat by intraperitoneal route (4 weeks).

Curosurf by the parenteral route in the guinea pig neither elicits active anaphylactic reactions, nor stimulates the production of antibodies detectable by passive cutaneous anaphylactic reaction. No anaphylactic reaction was observed by intratracheal route. Furthermore there is no evidence of dermal sensitising potential (Magnusson and Kligman test).

Curosurf did not show any evidence of mutagenic or clastogenic activity.

Pharmaceutical particulars

List of excipients: Sodium chloride, sodium bicarbonate, water for injections.

Incompatibilities: Not known.

Shelf life: 15 months. This shelf life refers to the unopened and correctly stored product.

Special precautions for storage: The product must be stored in a refrigerator at +2 to +8°C, protected from light, until the moment of use.

Do not use any residual quantity in the vial after the first aspiration.

Warmed vials should not be returned to the refrigerator.

Nature and contents of container: Single dose vials in clear colourless glass, provided with a cap in plastic and aluminium and a chlorobutyl rubber stopper.

Instructions for use/handling: Not applicable.

Marketing authorisation number 3400/0041.

Date of approval/revision of SPC September 1998.

Legal category POM.

GEREF* 50

Qualitative and quantitative composition Each ampoule of lyophilised powder contains sermorelin acetate equivalent to 50 micrograms of sermorelin

Each ampoule of Geref is accompanied by a solvent ampoule containing 0.9% Sodium Chloride Injection BP.

Pharmaceutical form Lyophilised powder for injection after reconstitution with accompanying solvent.

Clinical particulars

Therapeutic indications: For the evaluation of the functional capacity and response of the somatotrophs of the anterior pituitary.

Posology and method of administration: The test should be carried out and interpreted under specialist supervision.

Recommended procedure: A single intravenous injection of 1.0 microgram/kg body weight in the morning following an overnight fast.

Geref should be reconstituted immediately before use with a minimum of 0.5 ml of the accompanying sterile solvent.

Venous blood samples should be drawn 15 minutes before and immediately prior to Geref administration. Venous blood samples are then drawn at 15, 30, 45 and 60 minutes following Geref injection. Samples at 90 and 120 minutes are optional, since in the majority of patients they do not give additional information.

Contra-indications: Use in patients known to be hypersensitive to sermorelin acetate or any of the excipients of Geref.

Special warnings and special precautions for use: Patients already on growth hormone therapy should have therapy discontinued one to two weeks pre-test.

The test should be carried out with particular caution in patients with epilepsy.

Untreated hypothyroidism or use of anti-thyroid medications such as propylthiouracil or high levels of somatostatin at the time of injection may affect the response to Geref.

Obesity, hyperglycaemia and elevated plasma fatty acids are generally associated with poor GH responses to Geref.

Interactions with other medicaments and other forms of interaction: The Geref test should be conducted in the absence of drugs which affect directly the pituitary secretion of somatotrophin. These would include preparations which contain or induce the release of somatostatin, insulin, or glucocorticoids, and cyclo-oxygenase inhibitors such as aspirin and indomethacin.

The somatotrophin levels may be transiently elevated by clonidine, levodopa or insulin-induced hypoglycaemia. The response to Geref may also be reduced by anti-muscarinic agents such as atropine.

Pregnancy and lactation: The product should not be used during pregnancy or lactation.

Effects on ability to drive and use machines: None known.

Undesirable effects: Facial heat, facial flush and injection site pain occasionally occur and usually disappear within a few minutes.

Overdose: No data relating to acute overdosage are available.

Pharmacological properties
Pharmacodynamic properties: The parenteral administration of Geref stimulates growth hormone secretion via direct action on the anterior pituitary gland.

Studies in both animals and man have shown that the N-terminal 29 amino acids possess full biological activity.

Pharmacokinetic properties: Intravenous administration of sermorelin results in dose-related increases in peak blood levels within 5 minutes and maximum elevation in growth hormone 30 to 60 minutes following injection.

Preclinical safety data: Toxicity studies demonstrate the good tolerance of the product, no clinically relevant effects were found at doses up to 100 times the recommended human dose.

Pharmaceutical particulars
List of excipients: Mannitol; Disodium hydrogen phosphate; Sodium dihydrogen phosphate.

Incompatibilities: No known chemical incompatibilities

Shelf life: 24 months.

Special precautions for storage: Store at 2°C to 8°C, protect from light.

Nature and contents of container: Ampoules of colourless neutral glass.

Pack size: 1 ampoule Geref 50 plus 1 ampoule of solvent.

Instructions for use/handling: The injection should be reconstituted immediately prior to use with the solvent provided. Discard any product remaining after use.

Marketing authorisation number PL 3400/0029

Date of first authorisation/renewal of authorisation
First authorisation in UK: 12-09-91

Date of (partial) revision of the text 10-06-97

Legal category POM

GONAL-F* 75 ▼
GONAL-F* 150 ▼

Qualitative and quantitative composition Active ingredient: 75 or 150 IU recombinant human follicle stimulating hormone (follitropin alpha: INN). Follitropin alpha is produced by genetically engineered Chinese Hamster Ovary (CHO) cells and exhibits a specific activity in the range of 7000–14 000 IU–FSH/mg†.

† This range of specific activity is a reflection of the imprecision of the bioassay used to determine potency rather than product variability.

Pharmaceutical form Lyophilised sterile powder for injection after reconstitution with accompanying diluent (Water for Injection). After reconstitution with the diluent provided, Gonal-F has a pH in the range of 6.5 to 7.5.

Clinical particulars
Therapeutic indications: (i) Gonal-F is indicated for anovulation (including polycystic ovarian disease, PCOD) in women who have been unresponsive to treatment with clomiphene citrate.

(ii) Gonal-F is indicated for stimulation of multifollicular development in patients undergoing superovulation for assisted reproductive technologies (ART) such as *in vitro* fertilisation (IVF), gamete intrafallopian transfer (GIFT) and zygote intra-fallopian transfer (ZIFT).

Posology and method of administration: Gonal-F is intended for subcutaneous administration. The powder should be reconstituted immediately prior to use with the diluent provided. In order to avoid the injection of large volumes, up to 3 containers of Gonal-F 75 or Gonal-F 150 may be dissolved in 1 ml of diluent.

Women with anovulation (including PCOD): The object of Gonal-F therapy is to develop a single mature Graafian follicle from which the ovum will be liberated after the administration of hCG.

Gonal-F may be given as a course of daily injections. In menstruating patients treatment should commence within the first 7 days of the menstrual cycle.

Treatment should be tailored to the individual patient's response as assessed by measuring (i) follicle size by ultrasound and/or (ii) oestrogen secretion. A commonly used regimen commences at 75–150 IU FSH daily and is increased preferably by 37.5 IU, or 75 IU at 7 or preferably 14 day intervals if necessary, to obtain an adequate, but not excessive, response. The maximal daily dose is usually not higher than 225 IU FSH. If a patient fails to respond adequately after 4 weeks of treatment, that cycle should be abandoned and the patient should recommence treatment at a higher starting dose than in the abandoned cycle.

When an optimal response is obtained, a single injection of 5000 IU, up to 10000 IU hCG should be adminsitered 24–48 hours after the last Gonal-F injection. The patient is recommended to have coitus on the day of, and the day following, hCG administration.

If an excessive response is obtained, treatment should be stopped and hCG withheld (see *Warnings*). Treatment should recommence in the next cycle at a dosage lower than that of the previous cycle.

Women undergoing ovarian stimulation for multiple follicular development prior to in vitro fertilisation or other assisted reproductive technologies: A commonly used regimen for superovulation involves the administration of 150–225 IU of Gonal-F daily, commencing on days 2 or 3 of the cycle. Treatment is continued until adequate follicular development has been achieved (as assessed by monitoring of serum oestrogen concentrations and/or ultrasound examination), with the dose adjusted according to the patient's response, to usually not higher than 450 IU daily. In general adequate follicular development is achieved on average by the tenth day of treatment (range 5 to 20 days).

A single injection of up to 10 000 IU hCG is administered 24–48 hours after the last Gonal-F injection to induce final follicular maturation.

Down-regulation with a gonadotrophin-releasing hormone (GnRH) agonist is now commonly used in order to suppress the endogenous LH surge and to control tonic levels of LH. In a commonly used protocol, Gonal-F is started approximately 2 weeks after the start of agonist treatment, both being continued until adequate follicular development is achieved. For example, following two weeks of treatment with an agonist, 225 IU Gonal-F are administered for the first 7 days. The dose is then adjusted according to the ovarian response.

Overall experience with IVF indicates that in general the treatment success rate remains stable during the first four attempts and gradually declines thereafter.

The equivalency of the potency of Gonal-F and urinary FSH-containing preparations has not been definitively proven. However, clinical assessment of Gonal-F indicates that its doses, regimens of administration and treatment monitoring procedures should not be different from those currently used for urinary FSH-containing preparations.

Contra-indications: Gonal-F is contra-indicated for safety reasons in:

- pregnancy
- ovarian enlargement or cyst not due to polycystic ovarian disease
- gynaecological haemorrhage of unknown aetiology
- ovarian, uterine or mammary carcinoma
- tumours of the hypothalamus and pituitary gland
- case of prior hypersensitivity to FSH

Gonal-F is contra-indicated when an effective response cannot be obtained, such as:

- primary ovarian failure
- malformations of the sexual organs incompatible with pregnancy
- fibroid tumours of the uterus incompatible with pregnancy.

Special warnings and precautions for use: Before starting treatment, the couple's infertility should be assessed as appropriate and putative contra-indications for pregnancy evaluated. In particular, patients should be evaluated for hypothyroidism, adrenocortical deficiency, hyperprolactinemia and pituitary or hypothalamic tumours, and appropriate specific treatment given.

Patients undergoing stimulation of follicular growth are at an increased risk of developing hyperstimulation in view of the excessive oestrogen response and multiple follicular development. In ART, aspiration of all follicles, prior to ovulation, may however reduce the incidence of hyperstimulation.

Ovarian hyperstimulation syndrome can become a serious medical event characterised by large ovarian cysts which are prone to rupture. Excessive ovarian response seldom gives rise to significant hyperstimulation unless hCG is administered to induce ovulation. It is therefore prudent to withhold hCG in such cases and advise the patient to refrain from coitus for at least 4 days.

Careful monitoring of ovarian response, based on ultrasound is recommended prior to and during stimulation therapy, especially in patients with Polycystic Ovarian Disease (PCOD).

The risk of multiple pregnancy following assisted reproductive technologies is related to the number of oocytes/embryos replaced. In patients undergoing induction of ovulation, the incidence of multiple pregnancies and births is increased compared with natural conception.

To minimise the risk of OHSS or of multiple pregnancy, ultrasound scans as well as oestradiol measurements are recommended. In anovulation the risk of OHSS is increased by a serum oestradiol >900 pg/ml and more than 3 follicles of 14 mm or more in diameter. In ART there is an increased risk of OHSS with a serum oestradiol >3000 pg/ml and 20 or more follicles of 12 mm or more in diameter. When the oestradiol level is >5500 pg/ml and where there are 40 or more follicles in total, it may be necessary to withhold hCG administration.

Adherence to recommended Gonal-F dosage, regimen of administration and careful monitoring of therapy will minimise the incidence of ovarian hyperstimulation and multiple pregnancy (see the chronic low dose protocol in *Posology and method of administration* and *Undesirable effects*).

Pregnancy loss is higher in patients receiving FSH than that in the normal population, but comparable with the rates found in women with other fertility problems.

There have been no reports of hypersensitivity to Gonal-F, however particularly in patients who have a prior history of hypersensitivity to gonadotrophin preparations, there remains the possibility of anaphylactic responses. The first injection of Gonal-F in such patients must be performed under direct medical supervision, with full cardio-pulmonary resuscitation facilities immediately available.

Self-administration of Gonal-F should only be performed by patients who are well-motivated, adequately trained and with access to expert advice.

Interaction with other medications and other forms of interaction: Concomitant use of Gonal-F with other agents used to stimulate ovulation may potentiate the follicular response, whereas concurrent use of GnRH agonist-induced pituitary desensitisation may increase the dosage of Gonal-F needed to elicit an adequate ovarian response.

No drug incompatibilities have been reported for Gonal-F.

Gonal-F should not be administered as a mixture with other drugs in the same injection.

Use during pregnancy and lactation: Gonal-F should not be administered in case of pregnancy and lactation.

Effects on ability to drive and use machines: Gonal-F does not interfere with the patient's ability to drive or use machines.

Undesirable effects: Local reactions at the injection site (pain, redness and bruising), have been reported.

During treatment with Gonal-F the possibility of ovarian hyperstimulation must be taken into consideration. This syndrome occurs with a higher incidence in patients with polycystic ovarian disease. First symptoms of ovarian hyperstimulation are pain in the lower abdominal region, possibly in combination with nausea, vomiting and weight gain. In serious, but rare cases, an ovarian hyperstimulation syndrome with clearly enlarged ovaries, can go hand in hand with possible accumulation of fluid in the abdomen or thorax as well as more serious thromboembolic complications. In rare cases the latter can also be found independently of ovarian hyperstimulation syndrome. Should the above mentioned symptoms occur a careful medical and ultrasound examination is indicated.

When the ovarian response is excessive, treatment

with Gonal-F should be discontinued and the treatment with hCG for ovulation induction must be abandoned. This will reduce the chances of development of ovarian hyperstimulation syndrome.

The incidence of multiple pregnancies is increased by Gonal-F compared with natural conception. The majority of multiple conceptions have been found to be twins. In IVF, it is related to the number of embryos replaced.

In the initial clinical trial, anovulatory patients were treated with Gonal-F using a 'chronic low dose' protocol i.e. starting dose of 75 IU FSH/day, to be maintained for 14 days unless follicular maturity was reached before that time. If after 14 days of 75 IU FSH/day no response was observed, the daily dose was increased by 37.5 IU FSH.

Each subsequent increase in dose could only be effected after seven days of treatment at any dose, and the increment was not to exceed 37.5 IU FSH on each occasion.

One hundred and ten patients were treated with Gonal-F for a total of 252 cycles. One OHSS was reported (0.4%). Eight percent of clinical pregnancies were multiple and 6% of deliveries were multiple.

In rare instances, arterial thromboembolisms have been associated with menotrophin/human chorionic gonadotrophin therapy. This may also occur with Gonal-F/hCG therapy.

Pregnancy wastage by miscarriage or abortion is comparable with the rates in women with other fertility problems. Ectopic pregnancy may occur in women with a history of prior tubal disease.

In the course of clinical studies, 24% of patients have reported one or more, moderate or severe local reactions to Gonal-F injections. Pain was the most frequently reported local reaction. It has been observed mainly during the first few days of therapy, did not require specific treatment and did not lead to any interruption of therapy.

Overdose: The effects of an overdose of Gonal-F are unknown, nevertheless one could expect ovarian hyperstimulation syndrome to occur, which is further described in Special Warnings and Precautions for Use.

Pharmacological properties

Pharmacodynamic properties: Gonal-F is a preparation of follicle stimulating hormone produced by genetically engineered Chinese Hamster Ovary (CHO) cells. The most important effect resulting from parenteral administration of FSH is the development of mature Graafian follicles.

Pharmacokinetic properties: Following intravenous administration, Gonal-F is distributed to the extracellular fluid space with an initial half-life around 2 hours and eliminated from the body with a terminal half-life of about one day. The steady state volume of distribution and total clearance are 10 L and 0.6 L/h, respectively. One-eighth of the Gonal-F dose is excreted in the urine.

Following subcutaneous administration, the absolute bioavailability is about 70%. Following repeated administration, Gonal-F accumulates 3-fold achieving a steady-state within 3–4 days. In women whose endogenous gonadotrophin secretion is suppressed, Gonal-F has nevertheless been shown to effectively stimulate follicular development and steroidogenesis, despite unmeasurable LH levels.

Preclinical safety data: In an extensive range of toxicological, mutagenicity and animal studies (dogs, rats, monkeys), acute and chronic (up to 13 weeks), no significant findings were observed.

Impaired fertility has been reported in rats exposed to pharmacological doses of follitropin alpha (≥40 IU/kg/d) for extended periods, through reduced fecundity.

Given in high doses (≥5 IU/kg/d) follitropin alpha caused a decrease in the number of viable foetuses without being a teratogen, and distocia similar to that observed with urinary hMG.

However, since Gonal-F is contra-indicated in pregnancy, these data are of limited clinical relevance.

Pharmaceutical particulars

List of excipients: Sucrose, sodium dihydrogen phosphate, disodium phosphate, phosphoric acid, sodium hydroxide.

Incompatibilities: There are no known chemical incompatibilities to Gonal-F.

Shelf-life: The lyophilised product is stable for 24 months when stored at or below 25°C, protected from light.

Special precautions for storage: Store at or below 25°C, protected from light.

Nature and contents of container:

Lyophilised powder: Nature: Neutral colourless glass ampoules. Content: Follitropin alpha 75 IU or 150 IU, sucrose, sodium dihydrogen phosphate, disodium hydrogen phosphate, phosphoric acid, sodium hydroxide, nitrogen.

Diluent ampoule: Nature: Neutral colourless glass ampoules. Content: Water for injection 1 ml.

Instructions for use/handling: Gonal-F is for single use only.

To minimise potential losses of FSH due to adsorption onto the syringe, Gonal-F should preferably be administered immediately after reconstitution.

Marketing authorisation holder: Ares-Serono (Europe) Ltd, 24 Gilbert Street, London W1Y 1RJ.

Marketing authorisation numbers

75 IU – Powder for injection 3 ml (1 ampoule) SC	EU/1/95/001/001
75 IU – Powder for injection 3 ml (10 ampoules) SC	EU/1/95/001/004
150 IU – Powder for injection 3 ml (1 ampoule) SC	EU/1/95/001/009
150 IU – Powder for injection 3 ml (10 ampoules) SC	EU/1/95/001/012

Date of first authorisation 20 October 1995

Date of revision of the text April 1997

Legal category POM

METRODIN HIGH PURITY*

Qualitative and quantitative composition Active ingredient: 75 IU or 150 IU human follicle stimulating hormone (urofollitrophin).

Pharmaceutical form Lyophilised sterile powder for injection after reconstitution with accompanying NaCl solvent (sodium chloride solution 0.9%).

Clinical particulars

Therapeutic indications: (i) Metrodin High Purity, followed by chorionic gonadotrophin (hCG), is recommended for the stimulation of follicular development and ovulation in women with hypothalamic-pituitary dysfunction who present with either oligomenorrhoea or amenorrhoea. These women are classified as WHO Group II patients and usually receive clomiphene citrate as primary therapy. They have evidence of endogenous oestrogen production and thus will either spontaneously menstruate or experience withdrawal bleeding after progestagen administration. Polycystic ovarian disease (PCOD) is part of the WHO II classification and is present in the majority of these patients.

(ii) Metrodin High Purity is indicated for stimulation of multifollicular development in patients undergoing superovulation for assisted reproductive technologies (ART) such as *in vitro* fertilisation (IVF), gamete intra-fallopian transfer (GIFT) and zygote intra-fallopian transfer (ZIFT).

(iii) Metrodin High Purity is indicated with concomitant hCG therapy for the stimulation of spermatogenesis in men who have congenital or acquired hypogonadotrophic hypogonadism.

Posology and method of administration: Metrodin High Purity is intended for subcutaneous or intramuscular administration. The powder should be reconstituted immediately prior to use with the diluent provided. In order to avoid the injection of large volumes, up to 5 ampoules of Metrodin High Purity may be dissolved in 1 ml of diluent.

Women with hypothalamic-pituitary dysfunction who present with either oligomenorrhoea or amenorrhoea (WHO Group II): The object of Metrodin High Purity therapy is to develop a single mature Graafian follicle from which the ovum will be liberated after the administration of hCG.

Metrodin High Purity may be given as a course of daily injections. In menstruating patients treatment should commence within the first 7 days of the menstrual cycle.

Treatment should be tailored to the individual patient's response as assessed by measuring (i) follicle size by ultrasound and/or (ii) oestrogen secretion. A commonly used regimen commences at 75–150 IU FSH daily and is increased or decreased by 37.5 IU (up to 75 IU) at 7 or 14 day intervals if necessary, to obtain an adequate, but not excessive, response. If a patient fails to respond adequately after 4 weeks of treatment, that cycle should be abandoned.

When an optimal response is obtained, single intramuscular injection of up to 10,000 IU hCG should be administered 24–48 hours after the last Metrodin High Purity injection. The patient is recommended to have coitus on the day of, and the day following, hCG administration.

If an excessive response is obtained, treatment should be stopped and hCG withheld (see *Warnings*). Treatment should recommence in the next cycle at a dosage lower than that of the previous cycle.

Women undergoing superovulation for in-vitro fertilisation and other assisted reproductive technologies: A regimen for superovulation involves the administration of 150–225 IU of Metrodin High Purity daily, commencing on days 2 or 3 of the cycle. Treatment is continued until adequate follicular development has been achieved (as assessed by monitoring of serum oestrogen concentrations and/or ultrasound examination), with the dose adjusted according to the patient's response, to usually not higher than 450 IU daily.

A single injection of up to 10,000 IU hCG is administered 24–48 hours after the last Metrodin High Purity injection to induce final follicular maturation.

Down-regulation with a GnRH agonist is now commonly used in order to suppress the endogenous LH surge and to control tonic levels of LH. In a commonly used protocol, Metrodin High Purity is started approximately 2 weeks after the start of agonist treatment both being continued until adequate follicular development is achieved. For example, following two-weeks treatment with an agonist, 225 IU Metrodin High Purity are administered (subcutaneous or intramuscular) for the first 7 days. The dose is then adjusted according to the ovarian repsonse.

Men with hypogonadotrophic hypogonadism: Metrodin High Purity should be given, concomitantly, with hCG at the dosage of 150 IU three times a week. This regimen should be continued for a minimum of 4 more months. If after this period, the patient has not responded, the combination treatment (hCG plus Metrodin High Purity 150 IU 3 times a week) may be continued. Current clinical experience indicates that treatment for up to 18 months or more may be necessary to achieve spermatogenesis.

Contra-indications: Metrodin High Purity is contra-indicated in women for safety reasons in:

- cases of prior hypersensitivity to menotrophins (or any excipients used in the formulation)
- pregnancy
- ovarian enlargement or cyst not due to polycystic ovarian syndrome
- gynaecological haemorrhages of unknown aetiology
- ovarian, uterine or mammary carcinoma
- tumours of the hypothalamus and pituitary gland

Metrodin High Purity is also contra-indicated in women when an effective response cannot be obtained, such as:

- primary ovarian failure
- malformations of sexual organs incompatible with pregnancy
- fibroid tumors of the uterus incompatible with pregnancy.

Metrodin High Purity is contra-indicated in men for safety reasons in:

- cases of prior hypersensitivity to menotrophins (or any excipients used in the formulation)

Metrodin High Purity is also contra-indicated in men when an effective response cannot be obtained, such as:

- primary testicular insufficiency.

Special warnings and special precautions for use: Metrodin High Purity may cause local reaction at the injection site. Allergic-type reactions have occasionally been reported, in which lactose intolerance has been suspected, although not proven. It is therefore important to consider the effect of the lactose component of Metrodin High Purity, if administered to lactose-sensitive patients.

Women: Before starting treatment, the couple's infertility should be assessed as appropriate and putative contra-indications for pregnancy evaluated. In particular, patients should be evaluated for hypothyroidism, adrenocortical deficiency, hyperprolactinemia and pituitary or hypothalamic tumours, and appropriate specific treatment given.

Although adherence to recommended Metrodin High Purity dosages will minimise the incidence of ovarian hyperstimulation in patients undergoing ovulation induction, the possibility of hyperstimulation and multiple ovulation should be considered and careful monitoring performed during treatment in order to minimise their occurrence. This syndrome can become a serious medical event characterised by large ovarian cysts which are prone to rupture. Excessive oestrogenic response seldom gives rise of significant hyperstimulation unless hCG is administered to induce ovulation. It is therefore prudent to withhold hCG in such case and advise the patient to refrain from coitus for at least 4 days.

Patients undergoing superovulation are at an increased risk of developing hyperstimulation in view of the excessive oestrogen response and multiple follicular development. Aspiration of all follicles, prior to ovulation, may reduce the incidence of hyperstimulation.

The risk of multiple pregnancy following assisted reproductive technologies is related to the number of oocytes/embryos replaced. In other patients the incidence of multiple pregnancies and births is increased by Metrodin High Purity, as with other agents used to stimulate ovulation; however, the majority of multiple conceptions are twins.

Pregnancy loss is higher than that in the normal population, but comparable with the rates found in women with other fertility problems.

In those patients not undergoing super-ovulation the occurrence of smaller, secondary follicles in the presence of more than one dominant follicle, as visualised by ultrasonography, is reported to be associated with an increased incidence of hyperstimulation.

Men: Elevated endogenous FSH levels are indicative of primary testicular failure. Such patients are unresponsive to Metrodin High Purity/hCG therapy.

Semen analysis is recommended 4 to 6 months after the beginning of treatment in assessing the response.

Interaction with other medicaments and other forms of interaction: No clinically significant adverse drug interactions have been reported during Metrodin High Purity therapy.

Concomitant use of Metrodin High Purity with other agents used to stimulate ovulation may potentiate the follicular response, whereas concurrent use of GnRH agonist-induced pituitary densensitisation may increase the dosage of Metrodin High Purity needed to elicit an adequate ovarian response.

No drug incompatibilities have been reported for Metrodin High Purity. Metrodin High Purity should not be mixed with other drugs in the same syringe.

Use during pregnancy and lactation: Metrodin High Purity should not be administered in case of pregnancy and lactation.

Effects on ability to drive and use machines: Metrodin High Purity does not interfere with the patient's ability to drive or use machines.

Undesirable effects: In clinical trials, headaches have been rarely reported.

Local reactions at the injection site have been reported following urofollitrophin administration.

Women: Fever and arthralgias have been reported following urofollitrophin administration.

Under treatment with Metrodin High Purity the possibility of an ovarian hyperstimulation must be taken into consideration. First symptoms of ovarian hyperstimulation are pain in the lower abdominal region, possibly in combination with nausea, vomiting and weight gain. In serious, but rare cases, an ovarian hyperstimulation syndrome with clearly enlarged ovaries, can go hand in hand with a possible accumulation of fluids in the abdomen or thorax as well as more serious thromboembolic complications. In rare cases the latter can also be found independently of an ovarian hyperstimulation syndrome. Should the above mentioned symptoms occur under treatment with Metrodin High Purity, a careful medical examination is indicated. Treatment with Metrodin High Purity should be discontinued in these cases and the treatment with hCG for ovulation induction should be abandoned.

The incidence of multiple pregnancies is increased by Metrodin High Purity, as with other agents used to stimulate ovulation. The majority of multiple conceptions have been found to be twins. In IVF, it is related to the number of embryos replaced.

In rare instances, arterial thromboembolisms have been associated with menotrophin/human chorionic gonadotrophin therapy. This may also occur with Metrodin High Purity/hCG therapy.

Pregnancy wastage by miscarriage or abortion is comparable with the rates in women with other fertility problems. Ectopic pregnancy may occur in women with a history of prior tubal disease.

Men: Gynecomastia, acne and weight gain may occur occasionally during Metrodin High Purity/hCG therapy. These are known effects of hCG treatment.

Overdose: The effects of an overdose of Metrodin High Purity are unknown, nevertheless one could expect ovarian hyperstimulation syndrome to occur, which is further described in *Special warnings and precautions for use.*

Pharmacological properties

Pharmacodynamic properties:

ATC classification: GO3G AO4.

Women: Metrodin High Purity is a preparation of follicle stimulating hormone (FSH) purified from human menopausal gondaotrophin (hMG). The most important effect resulting from parenteral administration of FSH is the development of mature Graafian follicles.

Men: Metrodin High Purity administered concomitantly with hCG for at least 4 months induces spermatogenesis in men deficient in FSH.

Pharmacokinetic properties: Following a single s.c. or i.m. administration of Metrodin High Purity (150 IU) to male volunteers:

- Peak serum FSH levels were reached 15±7 (s.c.) and 10±4 (i.m.) hours later with an increase of 4.0±2 IU/1 of FSH over baseline values, for both the s.c. and i.m. routes.
- 72 hours after administration, serum FSH levels were still significantly higher than baseline values. The elimination half-life of FSH was estimated to be between 30–40 hrs.

Preclinical safety data: In toxicology and animal studies, no significant findings were observed. Acute toxicology studies were performed in mice and rats at doses exceeding 1500 IU/kg. Subacute toxicology studies in rats and monkeys involved doses up to 100 IU/kg/day for 13 weeks. Metrodin High Purity exhibited no mutagenic activity in a range of mutagenicity studies.

Pharmaceutical particulars

List of excipients: Lactose, sodium hydroxide, hydrochloric acid.

Incompatibilities: There are no known chemical incompatibilities to Metrodin High Purity.

Shelf life: The lyophylised product is stable for two years when stored at or below 25°C, protected from light.

Special precautions for storage: Store at or below 25°C, protected from light.

Nature and contents of containers: Lyophilised powder ampoule:

Nature:	Neutral colourless glass ampoules
Content:	Urofollitrophin 75 IU or 150 IU
Lactose	10 mg

Diluent ampoule:

Nature:	Neutral colourless glass ampoules
Content:	Sodium Chloride (0.9%) in water for injections

Instructions for use/handling: To minimise potential losses of FSH due to adsorption onto the syringe, Metrodin High Purity should preferably be administered immediately after reconstitution. The degree of adsorption which may occur has been shown to have no significant effect on the dose required for clinical efficacy.

Marketing authorisation numbers

Metrodin High Purity 75 IU	3400/0038
Metrodin High Purity 150 IU	3400/0039

Date of approval/revision of SPC July 1998.

Legal category POM.

PERGONAL*

Presentation Pergonal ampoules contain human menopausal gonadotrophin (HMG) in a freeze-dried, sterile powder form (Approved Name: Menotrophin). Each Pergonal ampoule contains:

Human follicle-stimulating hormone (FSH)	75 IU
Human luteinising hormone (LH)	75 IU
Lactose	10 mg

Each Pergonal ampoule is accompanied by a solvent ampoule containing:

Sodium Chloride Injection BP	1 ml

Uses Pergonal is used for the treatment of infertile patients under the guidance of clinicians familiar with infertility problems.

(i) Amenorrhoeic/anovulatory women: Pergonal followed by Chorionic Gonadotrophin (hCG, Profasi*) is indicated for the induction of ovulation in amenorrhoeic patients or anovulatory women with regular or irregular cycles.

(ii) Women undergoing superovulation for assisted conception techniques such as in vitro fertilisation (IVF): Pergonal and Profasi are indicated for the induction of multiple follicular development in patients undergoing an assisted conception technique, such as IVF. The induction of multiple follicular growth is also known as 'superovulation'. Tubal occlusion, unexplained infertility and male subfertility are common indications for IVF.

(iii) Hypogonadotrophic hypogonadism in men: Pergonal with concomitant Profasi therapy is indicated for the stimulation of spermatogenesis in men who have primary or secondary hypogonadotrophic hypogonadism.

Elevated endogenous FSH levels are indicative of primary testicular failure. Such patients are usually unresponsive to Pergonal/Profasi therapy.

Dosage and administration Pergonal is given by intramuscular injection only. In order to avoid the intramuscular injection of large volumes, up to 5 ampoules of Pergonal may be dissolved in 1 ml of solvent.

(i) Amenorrhoeic/anovulatory women: The object is to develop a single mature Graafian follicle with individually tailored doses of Pergonal over several days. Stimulated follicles will not always liberate ova spontaneously, therefore follicular rupture has to be achieved by injecting Profasi, which simulates the normal mid-cycle surge of LH.

Pergonal may be given as a course of daily injections or as injections on alternate days. In menstruating patients treatment should commence within the first 7 days of the menstrual cycle.

Two Pergonal dosage schedules are commonly employed:

Daily therapy: Treatment with Pergonal should be commenced at 2 ampoules daily (Group I patients) or 1 ampoule daily (Group II patients). This dosage may be increased or decreased at approximately weekly intervals until an adequate, but not excessive, response is obtained (see Monitoring). Up to 10,000 IU Profasi should be given 24–48 hours after the last Pergonal injection. Sexual intercourse is recommended on the day of and that following Profasi injection. If a patient fails to respond adequately after treatment for three weeks that cycle should be abandoned.

The dosage in subsequent cycles should be adjusted if necessary depending upon the patient's response to the previous treatment course.

Alternate day therapy: Three equal doses of Pergonal are given on alternate days. This is followed by up to 10,000 IU Profasi one week after the first injection of Pergonal, provided an adequate but not excessive response has been obtained (see 'Monitoring'). Sexual intercourse is recommended on the day of and that following Profasi injection.

The recommended dosage for the initial course of treatment is:

WHO Group I patients (women with little or no evidence of endogenous oestrogen activity)—5 ampoules Pergonal per injection.

WHO Group II patients (women with evidence of some oestrogen activity)—3 ampoules Pergonal per injection.

In both groups of patients, the dosage in subsequent courses should be adjusted if necessary, depending upon the patient's response to the previous course.

Monitoring of Pergonal therapy: The dose of Pergonal required to evoke the desired response is critical and varies both from patient to patient and in the same patient from cycle to cycle. Monitoring of Pergonal therapy is, therefore, essential.

Follicular development may be judged by the concentration of oestrogens measured in blood or urine and/or by ultrasonic visualisation of follicle size—ideally both methods should be used concurrently. Local laboratory normal range of values should be taken into consideration.

Urinary oestrogens: The amount of oestrogen excreted in a 24 hour collection of urine should be estimated at regular intervals throughout treatment. Urinary oestrogen levels between 180 nmol/24 hr (50 microgram/24 hr) and 514 nmol/24 hr (140 microgram/24 hr) generally indicate an optimum response. Values below this therapeutic range may indicate inadequate follicular development. In cases where the levels are in excess of 514 nmol/24 hr or where a very steep rise in oestrogen levels occur there is an increased risk of hyperstimulation. In cycles in which an excessive oestrogen response has occurred, Profasi should be withheld (see 'Warnings') and the patient should refrain from having sexual intercourse for at least the next 4 days.

Plasma oestradiol-17β. The level of plasma oestradiol-17β should be estimated at regular intervals throughout treatment with Pergonal. Levels between 1100 pmol/l (300 pg/ml) and 3000 pmol/l (800 pg/ml) generally indicate an optimum response. Values below this therapeutic range may indicate inadequate follicular development. In cases where the oestradiol-17β level exceeds 3000 pmol/l or where a very steep rise occurs, there is an increased risk of hyperstimulation. Profasi should be withheld (see 'Warnings') and the patient should refrain from having sexual intercourse for at least the next 4 days.

Ultrasound: When monitoring Pergonal therapy by serial ultrasonic visualisation of the follicle size, a follicular diameter of 16–25 mm should indicate the presence of a mature follicle and therefore the optimum time for the administration of Profasi. If the follicular diameter of the dominant follicle is less than 16 mm, further Pergonal may be required.

Profasi should not be given if several mature follicles are visualised as there is a risk of multiple ovulation and the occurrence of hyperstimulation syndrome.

(ii) Women undergoing superovulation for assisted conception techniques such as in vitro fertilisation (IVF): The objective of superovulation is to stimulate multiple follicular growth, thereby increasing the number of eggs available for fertilisation.

A frequently used regimen for superovulation involves pretreatment with Clomiphene Citrate followed by Pergonal and Profasi. A commonly used combined dosage regimen involves the administration of 100 mg Clomiphene Citrate daily on cycle days 2–6. This is followed by Pergonal at a dosage of 2–3 ampoules daily, commencing on day 5 of the cycle and continuing, at a dose dependent upon the patient's response, until adequate follicular development has been achieved.

An alternative regimen using Pergonal and Profasi involves the administration of Pergonal at a dosage of 2–3 ampoules daily, commencing on day 2 or 3 of the cycle. Treatment is continued, with the dose adjusted according to the patient's response, until adequate follicular development has been achieved.

For both regimens, a single injection of up to 10,000 IU Profasi is administered 24–48 hours after the last Pergonal injection to coincide with the expected onset of the (endogenous) LH surge.

Monitoring of superovulation: The administration of Pergonal for superovulation is usually monitored by estimation of plasma oestradiol-17β and ultrasound. One recommendation is that the diameter of at least 3 follicles should be equal to or greater than 15 mm, with the diameter of the leading follicle being 18 mm and the plasma oestradiol-17β level at least 3500 pmol/l (920 pg/ml).

Profasi should not be administered unless there is evidence of adequate follicular development as evidenced by progressively rising oestrogen levels and concomitant follicular growth on ultrasound.

Egg retrieval: Egg retrieval is carried out, either by laparoscopy or ultrasound guided aspiration, about 34–36 hours following Profasi injection. Ideally all follicles should be aspirated at egg retrieval (see 'Warnings').

Further details concerning Pergonal dosage and monitoring for both amenorrhoeic/anovulatory women and superovulation are available on request.

(iii) Hypogonadotrophic hypogonadism in men: Treatment should commence with Profasi at a dosage of 2,000 IU, twice weekly, to bring about the development of secondary sexual characteristics and a testosterone level within the normal range.

If induction of spermatogenesis is required, but the only response to Profasi has been androgenic, therapy should be continued at a dosage of 2,000 IU, twice weekly and Pergonal 1 ampoule, 3 times a week. This regimen should be continued for a minimum of four months.

If, after four months, the patient has not responded with evidence of increased spermatogenesis, therapy may be continued with Profasi 2,000 IU, twice weekly and Pergonal 1–2 ampoules, three times a week.

Although no specific monitoring is required in the male patient, semen analysis is useful in assessing the response to treatment.

Children: Not recommended for use in children.

Elderly: Not recommended for use in the elderly.

Contra-indications, warnings, etc

Contra-indications: Pergonal therapy is precluded in women in whom a satisfactory outcome cannot be expected, e.g. women with tubal occlusion (unless they are undergoing superovulation for IVF), ovarian dysgenesis, absent uterus or premature menopause.

Appropriate treatment should first be given for other endocrine disorders, e.g. hypothyroidism, adrenocortical deficiency, hyperprolactinaemia or pituitary tumour and other possible causes of infertility in either partner. An acceptable semen analysis should be available for those couples undergoing ovulation induction or in vitro fertilisation. However, certain types of male infertility can be successfully treated by assisted conception techniques.

Pergonal is contra-indicated in pregnant and lactating women.

Warnings: Pergonal may occasionally cause local reactions at the injection site. Fever and joint pains have been reported rarely.

Allergic-type reactions have occasionally been reported, in which lactose intolerance has been suspected, although not proven. It is therefore important to consider the effect of the lactose component of Pergonal if administered to lactose-sensitive patients.

Hyperstimulation: Adherence to recommended Pergonal dosages and monitoring schedules will minimise the possibility of ovarian hyperstimulation in amenorrhoeic and anovulatory women. Excessive oestrogenic responses to Pergonal do not generally give rise to significant side effects unless Profasi is given to induce ovulation. Hormone assays will detect an excessive oestrogen response to Pergonal and ultrasound will reveal any excessive follicular development; Profasi administration should be withheld and sexual intercourse should be avoided (see 'Overdosage').

Patients undergoing superovulation may be at an increased risk of developing hyperstimulation in view of the excessive oestrogen response and multiple follicular development. However aspiration of all follicles, prior to ovulation, may reduce the incidence of hyperstimulation syndrome.

Multiple pregnancy: The incidence of multiple births following Pergonal/Profasi therapy in anovulatory and amenorrhoeic women has been variously reported between 10% and 40%. However, the majority of such multiple conceptions are twins: high order multiple births are extremely rare when accurate monitoring is employed.

The incidence of multiple pregnancies following assisted conception techniques, is related to the number of oocytes/embryos replaced.

There have been reports of ectopic pregnancy in women treated with Pergonal who have undergone assisted conception. Women undergoing such procedures may have tubal disease, which is an important predisposing factor for ectopic pregnancy. A causal relationship between ectopic pregnancy and use of Pergonal has not been established.

Pregnancy loss, in both amenorrhoeic/anovulatory patients and women undergoing assisted conception techniques, is higher than that in the normal population, but comparable with the rates found in women with other fertility problems.

The risks of congenital abnormalities are not increased by Pergonal.

Precautions: In amenorrhoeic/anovulatory patients the occurrence of smaller, secondary follicles in the presence of more than one dominant follicle, as visualised by ultrasonography, is reported to be associated with an increased incidence of hyperstimulation syndrome.

Side-effects: Local reaction at injection site; allergic-type reaction possibly due to lactose component; fever and joint pains; hyperstimulation; multiple pregnancy.

No adverse reactions have been reported in men.

Overdosage and treatment: There are no reports of toxic effects occurring as a result of overdosage. However, hyperstimulation syndrome may result from overdosage with Pergonal. Hyperstimulation is generally categorised as mild, moderate or severe and symptoms usually appear 3–6 days after Profasi administration.

Mild hyperstimulation—Symptoms include some abdominal swelling and pain; ovaries enlarged to about 5 cm diameter. Therapy—rest; careful observation and symptomatic relief. Ovarian enlargement declines rapidly.

Moderate hyperstimulation—Symptoms include more pronounced abdominal distension and pain; nausea; vomiting; occasional diarrhoea; ovaries enlarged up to 12 cm diameter. Therapy—bed rest; close observation, in the case of conception occurring, to detect any progression to severe hyperstimulation. Pelvic examination of enlarged ovaries should be gentle in order to avoid rupture of the cysts. Symptoms subside spontaneously over 2–3 weeks.

Severe hyperstimulation—This is a rare but serious complication—symptoms include pronounced abdominal distension and pain; ascites; pleural effusion; decreased blood volume; reduced urine output; electrolyte imbalance and sometimes shock; ovaries enlarge to in excess of 12 cm diameter. Therapy—hospitalisation; treatment should be conservative and concentrate on restoring blood volume and preventing shock. Acute symptoms subside over several days and ovaries return to normal over 20–40 days if conception does not occur—symptoms may be prolonged if conception occurs.

Pharmaceutical precautions Pergonal should be stored below 25°C and protected from light. The injection should be reconstituted immediately prior to use with the solvent provided.

Legal category POM.

Package quantities Boxes containing:
(i) 1 ampoule Pergonal plus 1 ampoule solvent (OP).
(ii) 10 ampoules Pergonal plus 10 ampoules solvent (OP).

Further information One IU of human urinary FSH and one IU of human urinary LH are defined as the activities contained in 0.11388 mg and 0.13369 mg of the 1st International Standard, respectively.

Product licence numbers
Pergonal 3400/0007
Sodium Chloride Injection BP 3400/0024.

PROFASI* 2000, 5000 and 10 000 IU

Qualitative and quantitative composition PROFASI is available in 3 strengths of ampoule containing 2000 IU, 5000 IU and 10 000 IU human chorionic gonadotrophin (hCG).

Pharmaceutical form Powder and solvent for solution for injection.

Clinical particulars
Therapeutic Indications
(i) Anovulatory women: PROFASI is used to induce ovulation in the treatment of anovulatory infertility where its administration forms part of a recognised treatment regimen involving the prior stimulation of follicular maturation and endometrial proliferation.

(ii) Women undergoing superovulation for assisted conception techniques such as in vitro fertilisation (IVF): PROFASI is used as part of a superovulation programme in women undergoing an assisted conception technique. Following follitropin alpha, urofollitrophin or menotrophin treatment, PROFASI is administered to bring about final maturation of the follicles.

(iii) Hypogonadotrophic hypogonadism in men: PROFASI stimulates the interstitial (Leydig) cells of the testes and consequently the secretion of androgens and the development of secondary sexual characteristics. With concomitant urofollitrophin therapy, PROFASI stimulates the induction and maintenance of spermatogenesis.

(iv) Cryptorchidism: PROFASI stimulates the Leydig cells of the testes and effects the secretion of androgens, which leads to the descent of cryptorchid testes.

Posology and Method of Administration: PROFASI is given by subcutaneous or intramuscular injection only.

(i) Anovulatory women: Up to 10 000 IU PROFASI is given in mid-cycle following treatment with clomiphene citrate, follitropin alpha, urofollitrophin or menotrophin, according to a recognised scheme.

(ii) Women undergoing superovulation for assisted conception techniques such as in vitro fertilisation (IVF): Up to 10 000 IU PROFASI is given following the induction of multiple follicular development with follitropin alpha, urofollitrophin or menotrophin, either alone or in combination with clomiphene citrate, according to a recognised treatment scheme.

(iii) Hypogonadotrophic hypogonadism in men: Treatment should commence with PROFASI at a dosage of 2000 IU, twice weekly, if necessary with concomitant urofollitrophin (1 ampoule of 75 IU, three times a week). This regimen should be continued for a minimum of four months.

Although no specific monitoring is required in the male patient, semen analysis is useful in assessing the response to treatment.

(iv) Cryptorchidism: 500–1000 IU PROFASI, dependent upon age, on alternate days for several weeks.

Contraindications: PROFASI is precluded in women in whom stimulation of follicular maturation is not indicated because of the expectations of an unsatisfactory outcome, e.g. women with tubal occlusion unless they are undergoing superovulation for IVF, ovarian dysgenesis, absent uterus or premature menopause.

Appropriate treatment should first be given for other endocrine disorders e.g., hypothyroidism, adrenocortical deficiency, hyperprolactinaemia or pituitary tumour and other possible causes of infertility in either partner. An acceptable semen analysis should be available, however certain types of male infertility can be successfully treated by assisted conception techniques.

In women undergoing ovulation induction, an excessive response to follicular stimulating agents (e.g., clomiphene citrate, follitropin alpha, urofollitrophin or menotrophin) may lead to the development of hyperstimulation syndrome, particularly if PROFASI is given to induce ovulation. PROFASI should be withheld in such cycles.

Special warnings and special precautions for use: The risk of developing hyperstimulation in patients undergoing superovulation for assisted conception may be reduced by aspiration of all follicles prior to ovulation.

The risk of multiple pregnancy following assisted conception techniques, is related to the number of oocytes/embryos replaced. In other patients the incidence of multiple pregnancies and births is increased by gonadotrophin therapy, however, the majority of such multiple pregnancies are twins.

Pregnancy loss, in both anovulatory patients and women undergoing assisted conception techniques, is higher than that found in the normal population but comparable with the rates observed in women with other fertility problems.

In those patients not undergoing superovulation, the occurrence of smaller, secondary follicles in the presence of more than one dominant follicle, as visualised by ultrasonography, is reported to be associated with an increased incidence of hyperstimulation.

Interactions with other medicaments and other forms of interaction: None stated.

Use during pregnancy and lactation: The risk of congenital abnormalities is not increased by PROFASI.

Effects on ability to drive and use machines: PROFASI does not interfere with the patient's ability to drive or use machines.

Undesirable effects: PROFASI may occasionally cause local reactions at the injection site.

In men, high doses of PROFASI may lead to oedema and in such cases the dosage should be considerably reduced.

PROFASI may cause sexual precocity. If signs of

sexual precocity are observed, treatment should be stopped. If continued therapy is considered necessary, a reduced dosage regimen should be instituted.

Hyperstimulation, multiple pregnancy.

Overdose: There are no reports of toxic effects occurring as a result of overdosage. However, hyperstimulation syndrome may result from overdosage with follicle stimulating/ovulation inducing agents. Hyperstimulation is generally categorised as mild, moderate or severe and symptoms usually appear 3–6 days after PROFASI administration.

Mild hyperstimulation: Symptoms may include some abdominal swelling and pain; ovaries enlarged to about 5 cm diameter. Therapy–rest; careful observation and symptomatic relief. Ovarian enlargement declines rapidly.

Moderate hyperstimulation: Symptoms include more pronounced abdominal distension and pain; nausea; vomiting; occasional diarrhoea; ovaries enlarged up to 12 cm diameter. Therapy–bed rest; close observation, in the case of conception occurring, to detect any progression to severe hyperstimulation. Pelvic examination of enlarged ovaries should be gentle, in order to avoid rupture of the cysts. Symptoms subside spontaneously over 2–3 weeks.

Severe hyperstimulation: This is a rare but serious complication. Symptoms include pronounced abdominal distension and pain; ascites; pleural effusion; decreased blood volume; reduced urine output; electrolyte imbalance and sometimes shock; ovaries enlarge to in excess of 12 cm diameter. Therapy–hospitalisation, treatment should be conservative and concentrate on restoring blood volume and preventing shock. Acute symptoms subside over several days and ovaries return to normal over 20–40 days, if conception has not occurred. Symptoms may be prolonged if conception has occurred.

Pharmacological properties

Pharmacodynamic properties: Chorionic gonadotrophin induces ovulation.

Chorionic gonadotrophin has been found in many species to increase both testicular and blood testosterone levels.

The administration of single doses of HCG from 0 to 6000 IU in healthy volunteers (22–24 years old) showed a dose-dependent increase in plasma testosterone levels. At a dose of 6000 IU, plasma progesterone levels remained high for 6 days following injection.

Pharmacokinetic properties: Elimination is essentially renal with chorionic gonadotrophin being excreted in its free form.

Preclinical safety data: There are no pre-clinical data of relevance to the prescriber which are additional to that already included in other sections of the SPC.

Pharmaceutical particulars One IU of chorionic gonadotrophin is defined as the activity contained in 0.001279 mg of the 2nd International Standard.

List of Excipients: PROFASI 2000 IU and 5000 IU contain lactose, dibasic potassium phosphate, monobasic potassium phosphate, sodium hydroxide and acetic acid.

PROFASI 10 000 IU contains mannitol and sodium phosphate buffer.

Solvent contains sodium chloride (0.9%) in water for injections

Incompatibilities: None known

Shelf life: The lyophilised product is stable for 3 years when stored at or below 25°C, protected from light.

Special precautions for storage: PROFASI should be stored below 25°C and protected from light.

Nature and contents of container: PROFASI is provided as a powder in a neutral colourless glass ampoule.

Each PROFASI ampoule is accompanied by a neutral colourless glass solvent ampoule containing Sodium Chloride Injection BP 1 ml.

Package quantities Boxes containing:
3 ampoules of PROFASI 2000 IU with 3 ampoules of solvent.
1 ampoule of PROFASI 5000 IU with 1 ampoule of solvent.
10 ampoules of PROFASI 5000 IU with 10 ampoules solvent.
1 ampoule of PROFASI 10 000 IU with 1 ampoule of solvent.

Instructions for use/handling: The injection should be reconstituted immediately prior to use with the solvent provided.

Marketing authorisation number
PROFASI 2000 PL 3400/0005
PROFASI 5000 PL 3400/0006
PROFASI 10 000 PL 3400/0021
Sodium Chloride Injection BP PL 3400/0024

Date of first authorisation/renewal of authorisation
PROFASI 2000 and 5000
First Authorisation 27 March 1978
Last Renewal 27 May 1993
PROFASI 10 000
First Authorisation 2 October 1992

Date of revision of the text November 98

Legal category POM CD (Sch 4)*
*UK status

REBIF 22 mcg ▼

Qualitative and quantitative composition Rebif (Interferon beta-1a) contains 22 micrograms (6 million IU*) dose of Interferon beta-1a per pre-filled syringe.

* Measured by cytopathic effect (CPE) bioassay against the in-house IFN beta-1a standard which is calibrated against the current international NIH standard (GB-23-902-531).

Pharmaceutical form Solution for injection.

Clinical particulars

Therapeutic indications: Rebif 22 micrograms is indicated for the treatment of ambulatory patients with relapsing-remitting multiple sclerosis (MS) characterised by at least 2 recurrent attacks of neurological dysfunction (relapses) over the preceding 2-year period. Rebif decreases the frequency and severity of relapses over 2 years.

Rebif has not yet been investigated in patients with progressive multiple sclerosis, and should be discontinued in patients who develop progressive multiple sclerosis.

Posology and method of administration: The recommended posology of Rebif is 22 micrograms given three times per week by subcutaneous injection.

Treatment should be initiated under supervision of a physician experienced in the treatment of the disease.

When first starting treatment with Rebif, in order to allow tachyphylaxis to develop thus reducing adverse events, it is recommended that 20% of the total dose (i.e. 4.4 micrograms per injection = 0.1 ml) be administered during the initial 2 weeks of therapy, 50% of total dose (i.e. 11 micrograms per injection = 0.25 ml) be administered in week 3 and 4, and the full dose (22 micrograms = 0.5 ml) from the fifth week onwards.

There is no experience with Rebif in children under 16 years of age with multiple sclerosis and therefore Rebif should not be used in this population.

At the present time, it is not known for how long patients should be treated. Safety and efficacy with Rebif have not been demonstrated beyond 2 years of treatment. Therefore, it is recommended that patients should be evaluated after 2 years of treatment with Rebif and a decision for longer-term treatment be made on an individual basis by the treating physician.

Contra-indications: Interferon beta-1a is contraindicated in patients with a known hypersensitivity to natural or recombinant interferon beta, human serum albumin, or any other component of the formulation.

Interferon beta-1a is contraindicated in pregnant patients (also see *Use during Pregnancy and lactation*), patients with severe depressive disorders and/or suicidal ideation, and in epileptic patients with a history of seizures not adequately controlled by treatment.

Special warnings and special precautions for use: Patients should be informed of the most common adverse events associated with interferon beta administration, including symptoms of the flu-like syndrome (see *Undesirable effects*). These symptoms tend to be most prominent at the initiation of therapy and decrease in frequency and severity with continued treatment.

Interferons should be used with caution in patients with depression. Depression and suicidal ideation are known to occur in increased frequency in the multiple sclerosis population and in association with interferon use. Patients treated with Interferon beta-1a should be advised to immediately report any symptoms of depression and/or suicidal ideation to their prescribing physician. Patients exhibiting depression should be monitored closely during therapy with Interferon beta-1a and treated appropriately. Cessation of therapy with Interferon beta-1a should be considered.

Caution should be exercised when administering Interferon beta-1a to patients with pre-existing seizure disorders. For patients without a pre-existing seizure disorder who develop seizures during therapy with Interferon beta-1a, an aetiological basis should be established and appropriate anti-convulsant therapy instituted prior to resuming Interferon beta-1a treatment.

Patients with cardiac disease, such as angina, congestive heart failure or arrhythmia, should be closely monitored for worsening of their clinical condition during initiation of therapy with Interferon beta-1a. Symptoms of the flu-like syndrome associated with Interferon beta-1a therapy may prove stressful to patients with cardiac conditions.

Injection site necrosis (ISN) has been reported in patients using Rebif (see *Undesirable effects*). To minimise the risk of injection site necrosis patients should be advised to:

- use an aseptic injection technique
- rotate the injection sites with each dose.

The procedure for the self-administration by the patient should be reviewed periodically especially if injection site reactions have occurred.

If the patient experiences any break in the skin, which may be associated with swelling or drainage of fluid from the injection site, the patient should be advised to consult with their physician before continuing injections with Rebif. If the patient has multiple lesions, Rebif should be discontinued until healing has occurred. Patients with single lesions may continue provided that the necrosis is not too extensive.

Patients should be advised about the abortifacient potential of interferon beta (see *Use during pregnancy and lactation* and *Preclinical safety data*).

Laboratory abnormalities are associated with the use of interferons. Therefore, in addition to those laboratory tests, normally required for monitoring patients with multiple sclerosis, complete and differential white blood cell counts, platelet counts and blood chemistries, including liver function tests are recommended during Interferon beta-1a therapy.

Caution should be used, and close monitoring considered when administering Interferon beta-1a to patients with severe renal and hepatic failure and to patients with severe myelosuppression.

Serum neutralising antibodies against Interferon beta-1a may develop. The precise incidence of antibodies is as yet uncertain. Clinical data suggest that after 24 months approximately 24% of patients develop serum antibodies to Interferon beta-1a, sometimes transiently. The presence of antibodies has been shown to attenuate the pharmacodynamic response to Interferon beta-1a (Beta-2 microglobulin and neopterin). The clinical significance of the induction of antibodies has not been fully elucidated, but may be associated with reduced efficacy.

The use of various assays to detect serum antibodies and differing definitions of antibody positivity limits the ability to compare antigenicity among different products.

Interaction with other medicinal products and other forms of interaction: No formal drug interaction studies have been conducted with Rebif (Interferon beta-1a) in humans.

Interferons have been reported to reduce the activity of hepatic cytochrome P450-dependent enzymes in humans and animals. Caution should be exercised when administering Rebif in combination with medicinal products that have a narrow therapeutic index and are largely dependent on the hepatic cytochrome P450 system for clearance, e.g. antiepileptics and some classes of antidepressants.

The interaction of Rebif with corticosteroids or ACTH has not been studied systematically. Clinical studies indicate that multiple sclerosis patients can receive Rebif and corticosteroids or ACTH during relapses.

Use during pregnancy and lactation: Rebif should not be administered in case of pregnancy and lactation.

There are no studies of Interferon beta-1a in pregnant women. At high doses, in monkeys, abortifacient effects were observed with other interferons (see *Preclinical safety data*).

Fertile women receiving Rebif should take appropriate contraceptive measures. Patients planning for pregnancy and those becoming pregnant should be informed of the potential hazards of interferons to the foetus and Rebif should be discontinued.

It is not known whether Rebif is excreted in human milk. Because of the potential for serious adverse reactions in nursing infants, a decision should be made either to discontinue nursing or to discontinue Rebif therapy.

Effects on ability to drive and use machines: Less commonly reported central nervous system-related adverse events associated with the use of interferon beta might influence the patient's ability to drive or use machines (see *Undesirable effects*).

Undesirable effects: The highest incidence of undesirable effects associated with the interferon therapy is related to flu syndrome. The most commonly reported symptoms of the flu syndrome are muscle ache, fever, arthralgia, chills, asthenia, headache, and nausea. Symptoms of the flu syndrome tend to be usually mild and most prominent at the initiation of therapy and decrease in frequency with continued treatment.

Injection site reactions are commonly encountered and are usually mild and reversible. Injection site necrosis has uncommonly been reported. In all cases, the necrosis resolved spontaneously.

Other less common adverse events reported in association with interferon beta include diarrhoea, anorexia, vomiting, insomnia, dizziness, anxiety, rash, vasodilation and palpitation.

The administration of type 1 interferons has rarely

been associated with serious CNS undesirable effects such as depression, suicide, and depersonalisation as well as seizures and arrythmias.

Hypersensitivity reactions may occur.

Laboratory abnormalities such as leukopenia, lymphopenia, thrombocytopenia and elevated AST, ALT, γ-GT and alkaline phosphatase may occur. These are usually mild, asymptomatic and reversible.

In case of severe or persistent undesirable effects, the dose of Rebif may be temporarily lowered or interrupted, at the discretion of the physician.

Overdose: No case of overdose has thus far been described. However, in case of overdosage, patients should be hospitalised for observation and appropriate supportive treatment should be given.

Pharmacological properties
Pharmacodynamic properties: Pharmacotherapeutic group: cytokines, ATC: L03 AA.

Interferons (IFNs) are a group of endogenous glycoproteins endowed with immunomodulatory, antiviral and antiproliferative properties.

Rebif (Interferon beta-1a) is composed of the native amino acid sequence of natural human interferon beta. It is produced in mammalian cells (Chinese Hamster Ovary) and is therefore glycosylated like the natural protein.

The precise mechanism of action of Rebif in multiple sclerosis is still under investigation.

The safety and efficacy of Rebif has been evaluated in patients with relapsing remitting multiple sclerosis at doses ranging from 11 to 44 micrograms (3–12 million IU), administered subcutaneously three times per week. At licensed posology, Rebif has been demonstrated to decrease the incidence (approximately 30% over 2 years) and severity of clinical relapses.

Pharmacokinetic properties: In healthy volunteers after intravenous administration, Interferon beta-1a exhibits a sharp multi-exponential decline, with serum levels proportional to the dose. The initial half-life is in the order of minutes and the terminal half-life is several hours, with the possible presence of a deep compartment. When administered by the subcutaneous or intramuscular routes, serum levels of interferon beta remain low, but are still measurable up to 12 to 24 hours post-dose. Subcutaneous and intramuscular administrations of Rebif produce equivalent exposure to interferon beta. Following a single 60 microgram dose, the maximum peak concentration, as measured by immunoassay, is around 6 to 10 IU/ml, occurring on average around 3 hours after the dose. After subcutaneous administration at the same dose repeated every 48 hours for 4 doses, a moderate accumulation occurs (about 2.5 x for AUC).

Regardless of the route of dosing, pronounced pharmacodynamic changes are associated with the administration of Rebif. After a single dose, intracellular and serum activity of 2-5A synthetase and serum concentrations of beta$_2$-microglobulin and neopterin increase within 24 hours, and start to decline within 2 days. Intramuscular and subcutaneous administrations produce fully superimposable responses. After repeated subcutaneous administration every 48 hours for 4 doses, these biological responses remain elevated, with no signs of tolerance development.

Interferon beta-1a is mainly metabolised and excreted by the liver and the kidneys.

Preclinical safety data: Rebif was tested in toxicology studies of up to 6 months in duration in monkeys and 3 months in rats and caused no overt signs of toxicity except for transient pyrexia.

Rebif has been shown to be neither mutagenic nor clastogenic. Rebif has not been investigated for carcinogenicity.

A study on embryo/foetal toxicity in monkeys showed no evidence of reproductive disturbances. Based on observations with other alpha and beta interferons, an increased risk of abortions cannot be excluded. No information is available on the effects of the Interferon beta-1a on male fertility.

Pharmaceutical particulars
List of excipients: Mannitol, human serum albumin, sodium acetate, acetic acid, sodium hydroxide, water for injections.

Incompatibilities: No incompatibilities have been reported.

Shelf life: 12 months.

Special precautions for storage: Rebif should be stored at 2–8°C in its original container and protected from light. Do not freeze.

Nature and contents of container: Rebif (Interferon beta-1a) is available as a package of 3 or 12 individual doses of Rebif solution for injection (0.5 ml) filled in a 1 ml glass syringe with a stainless steel needle.

Instructions for use, handling and disposal (if appropriate): The solution for injection in a pre-filled syringe is ready for use.

Marketing authorisation holder: ARES-SERONO (Europe) Ltd, 24 Gilbert Street, London W1Y 1RJ, United Kingdom.

Marketing authorisation numbers
EU/1/98/0063/002: Presentation 3 pre-filled syringes
EU/1/98/0063/003: Presentation 12 pre-filled syringes

Date of first authorisation/renewal of authorisation
April 1998

Date of revision of the text April 1998

Legal category POM

SAIZEN* 4 and 10 IU

Qualitative and quantitative composition Saizen vials contain Somatropin (rhGH) in a freeze-dried, sterile powder form.

Each single-use vial of Saizen contains Somatropin PhEur 4 IU (1.33 mg). Each vial is accompanied by an ampoule of solvent containing 1 ml of 0.9% w/v Sodium Chloride Injection BP.

Each multidose vial of Saizen contains Somatropin PhEur 10 IU (3.33 mg). Each vial is accompanied by a sterile solvent vial containing 5 ml saline solvent with benzyl alcohol (0.9% w/v sodium chloride and 0.9% w/v benzyl alcohol).

Pharmaceutical form Powder for injection after reconstitution with accompanying solvent.

Clinical particulars
Therapeutic indications: The treatment of short stature resulting from growth failure caused by decreased or absent secretion of endogenous growth hormone. The diagnosis should be confirmed by appropriate investigations of pituitary function.

Growth failure in patients with gonadal dysgenesis (Turner Syndrome).

Growth failure in prepubertal children due to chronic renal failure (CRF). Treatment should be considered only in children in whom epiphyseal fusion has not yet occurred.

It is recommended that Saizen treatment should be initiated/given under the guidance of a physician experienced in the diagnosis and management of growth disorders.

Posology and method of administration: The lyophilised material should be reconstituted with the solvent provided, using a gentle, swirling motion. Vigorous shaking should be avoided. A slightly cloudy solution may be formed, but this is a normal product characteristic.

The 4 IU vial should be reconstituted with 0.5–1 ml of the accompanying solvent. The calculated dose should be withdrawn and the remainder discarded.

The 10 IU vial is intended for multiple dose use. This should be reconstituted with the accompanying bacteriostatic solvent to a concentration of no more than 10 IU/ml.

Administer by subcutaneous or intramuscular injection to patients with growth failure caused by inadequate secretion of endogenous growth hormone, and by subcutaneous injection to patients with Turner syndrome. The dosage must be individualised for each patient.

1. Treatment of growth failure due to inadequate secretion of normal endogenous growth hormone: The recommended weekly dose is as follows:

0.6 IU/kg or 0.20 mg/kg
12 IU/m² or 4 mg/m²

If response is poor, the weekly dose may be increased to:

0.8 IU/kg or 0.27 mg/kg
20 IU/m² or 7 mg/m²

(a) Subcutaneous injection: The weekly dose can be divided as shown below and is expressed per injection:

3 single doses	0.2 IU/kg or 0.07 mg/kg 4 IU/m² or 1.3 mg/m²
6 single doses	0.1 IU/kg or 0.03 mg/kg 2 IU/m² or 0.7 mg/m²
7 single doses	0.09 IU/kg or 0.03 mg/kg 1.7 IU/m² or 0.6 mg/m²

The injection site should be alternated to prevent lipoatrophy.

(b) Intramuscular injection: The weekly dose should be divided into 3 single injections:

0.2 IU/kg or 0.07 mg/kg
4 IU/m² or 1.3 mg/m²

2. Treatment of growth failure due to gonadal dysgenesis (Turner syndrome): The recommended weekly dose is:

0.6–0.7 IU/kg or 0.20 mg/kg
18 IU/m² or 6 mg/m²

During the second year of treatment, the weekly dose may be increased to:

0.8–1.0 IU/kg or 0.3 mg/kg
24 IU/m² or 8 mg/m²

The weekly dose should be divided in 7 single daily doses corresponding to:

0.1 IU/kg or 0.03 mg/kg
2.6 IU/m² or 0.9 mg/m²

Some patients with Turner syndrome may require higher growth hormone doses even during the first year of treatment to increase their growth velocity sufficiently.

The concomitant treatment with non-androgenic steroids has shown a further improvement in growth velocity.

3. Growth failure in prepubertal children due to chronic renal failure (CRF): 28 IU/m² body surface area, approximately equal to 1.05 IU/kg or 0.35 mg/kg, per week by subcutaneous administration. The weekly dose should be divided into 7 daily doses of 4 IU/m² body surface area, approximately equal to 0.15 IU/kg or 0.05 mg/kg.

Treatment should be continued until the patient has reached a satisfactory adult height or the epiphyses are closed.

Contra-indications: Children in whom epiphyseal fusion has occurred should not be treated with Saizen.

Saizen is also contra-indicated in patients who show recurrence or progression of an underlying intracranial lesion.

Saizen is not recommended for use during pregnancy and lactation.

Special warnings and special precautions for use: Saizen treatment should be carried out under regular medical supervision.

In patients with diabetes mellitus the treatment should be carried out under strict medical control with laboratory monitoring of their diabetic status; adjustment of anti-diabetic therapy may be required.

The possible appearance of hypothyroidism in the course of the therapy with somatropin should be corrected with thyroid hormone in order to obtain a sufficient growth promoting effect.

In patients with endocrine disorders, including growth hormone deficiency, slipped capital femoral epiphyses may occur more frequently. Patients with growth failure due to chronic renal failure should be examined periodically for evidence of progression of renal osteodystrophy. Slipped capital femoral epiphysis or avascular necrosis of the femoral head may be seen in children with advanced renal osteodystrophy and it is uncertain whether these problems are affected by growth hormone therapy. X-rays of the hip should be obtained prior to initiating therapy.

Physicians and parents should be alert to the development of a limp or complaints of hip or knee pain in patients treated with Saizen.

In children with chronic renal failure, renal function should have decreased to below 50% of normal before therapy is instituted. To verify the growth disturbance, growth should have been followed for a year before institution of therapy. Treatment should be discontinued at the time of renal transplantation.

Patients with growth hormone deficiency secondary to a treated intracranial lesion should be examined frequently for recurrence of the underlying disease process.

In case of severe or recurrent headache, visual problems, nausea and/or vomiting, a fundoscopy for papilloedema is recommended. If papilloedema is confirmed a diagnosis of benign intracranial hypertension should be considered and if appropriate the somatropin treatment should be discontinued.

At present there is insufficient evidence to guide clinical decision making in patients with resolved intracranial hypertension. If somatropin treatment is restarted, careful monitoring for symptoms of intracranial hypertension is necessary.

When somatropin is administered subcutaneously at the same site over a long period, local tissue atrophy may result. This can be avoided by rotating the injection site daily.

Benzyl alcohol as a preservative in bacteriostatic sodium chloride solution for injection has been associated with toxicity in newborns. Saizen may be reconstituted with Sodium Chloride Injection BP or sterile Water for Injections for immediate use when administering to newborns.

Interactions with other medicaments and other forms of interaction: In some individuals concomitant corticosteroid therapy may inhibit the growth promoting effects of somatropin. Interactions with other medicines are, at present, unknown. Also see *Precautions* re: insulin-dependent diabetes mellitus.

Pregnancy and lactation: There are no data from either human or animal studies relating to the use of Saizen during pregnancy. In the event of pregnancy occurring, treatment must be discontinued. There is no knowledge regarding the secretion of somatropin into human breast milk.

Effects on ability to drive and use machines: None known.

Undesirable effects: Some patients may experience redness and itching at the site of injection, particularly when the subcutaneous route is used.

In a few children, the use of Saizen has resulted in the transient formation of antibodies which do not appear to be of any clinical significance. In very rare instances, where short stature is due to deletion of the growth hormone gene complex, treatment with growth hormone may induce growth attenuating antibodies.

Intermittent dosage has been associated with the appearance of hypoglycaemia, this has not been reported with the use of uninterrupted, i.e. daily administration.

Some cases of leukaemia have been reported in growth hormone deficient children, untreated as well as treated with growth hormone, and might possibly represent a slightly increased incidence compared with non-growth hormone deficient children. A causal relationship to growth hormone therapy has not been established.

Overdose: Acute overdosage can produce transient hypoglycaemia followed by hyperglycaemia. Long term overdosage may result in the clinical features of acromegaly.

Pharmacological properties

Pharmacodynamic properties: The administration of Saizen stimulates an increase in growth velocity.

Pharmacokinetic properties: Intramuscular (I.M.) administration of 4 IU (1.33 mg)/m² body surface area of Saizen to 12 volunteers produced a peak level after 3 hours (T max). Subcutaneous (S.C.) administration to the same volunteers at the same dosage delayed the mean peak levels to between 4 and 6 hours after administration. The area under the curves for the routes are, however, similar and T max values for Saizen correlate well with those quoted for pituitary growth hormone in the published literature.

Preclinical safety data: The documented toxicological profile and the absence of mutagenic activity in a variety of *in vitro* and *in vivo* preclinical tests demonstrates the good safety profile of Saizen.

Pharmaceutical particulars

List of excipients: Saizen 4 IU – disodium phosphate, sodium dihydrogen phosphate, mannitol, sodium chloride.

Saizen 10 IU – disodium phosphate, sodium dihydrogen phosphate, mannitol.

Incompatibilities: No known chemical incompatibilities.

Shelf life: 24 months.

Special precautions for storage: Store at 2–8°C. Protect from light.

Saizen 4 IU reconstituted with Sodium Chloride Injection BP should be used immediately or within 24 hours when stored at 2–8°C.

Saizen 10 IU reconstituted with saline diluent with benzyl alcohol should be used within 7 days when stored at 2–8°C.

Nature and contents of container: Saizen 4 IU – Each box contains: 1 vial of Saizen 4 IU, 1 ml ampoule Sodium Chloride Injection BP.

Saizen 10 IU – Each box contains: 1 vial of Saizen 10 IU, 5 ml vial saline diluent with benzyl alcohol.

Instructions for use/handling: The lyophilised material should be reconstituted with the solvent provided. Vigorous shaking should be avoided.

Marketing authorisation numbers

Saizen 4 IU	3400/0023
Sodium Chloride Injection BP	3400/0024
Saizen 10 IU	3400/0034
Saline diluent with benzyl alcohol	3400/0035

Date of approval/revision of SPC 3 November 1997.

Legal category CD (Sch 4), POM.

SAIZEN* 24 IU (8 mg) for EASYJECT*

Qualitative and quantitative composition Each vial of Saizen 24 IU (8 mg) contains Somatropin (recombinant human growth hormone).

Reconstitution with the contents of the bacteriostatic solvent cartridge (when used with the Easyject) gives a concentration of 17.5 IU (5.83 mg) per ml.

Pharmaceutical form Powder and solvent for solution for injection: Powder and bacteriostatic solvent (0.3% (w/v) metacresol in water for injections) for parenteral use.

Clinical particulars

Therapeutic indications: Saizen is indicated:

- in the treatment of children with short stature resulting from growth failure caused by decreased or absent secretion of endogenous growth hormone.
- growth failure in girls with gonadal dysgenesis (Turner Syndrome), confirmed by chromosomal analysis.

Posology and method of administration: Saizen 24 IU (8 mg) is intended for multiple dose use.

Saizen dosage should be individualised for each patient based on body surface area (BSA) or on body weight (BW).

It is recommended that Saizen be administered at bedtime according to the following dosage:

Growth failure due to inadequate endogenous growth hormone secretion:

2.1–3.0 IU/m² (0.7–1.0 mg/m²) body surface area (BSA) per day or 0.07–0.10 IU/kg (0.025–0.035 mg/kg) body weight (BW) per day by subcutaneous administration.

Growth failure in girls due to gonadal dysgenesis (Turner Syndrome):

4.3 IU/m² (1.4 mg/m²) body surface area (BSA) per day or 0.14 IU/kg (0.045–0.050 mg/kg) body weight (BW) per day by subcutaneous administration.

Concomitant therapy with non-androgenic anabolic steroids in patients with Turner Syndrome can enhance the growth response.

Duration of treatment: Treatment should be discontinued when the patient has reached a satisfactory adult height, or the epiphyses are fused.

Contra-indications: Saizen should not be used in patients in whom epiphyseal fusion occurred.

Saizen is contraindicated in patients known to be hypersensitive to Somatropin and any of the excipients in the powder for solution for injection or the solvent.

Saizen is contraindicated in patients with active neoplasia.

Saizen should not be used in cases with evidence of any progression or recurrence of an underlying intra-cranial lesion.

Special warnings and special precautions for use: Treatment should be carried out under the regular guidance of a physician who is experienced in the diagnosis and management of growth disorders.

Hypothyroidism may develop during Saizen therapy. Thyroid function tests should be performed periodically during Saizen administration. The possible appearance of hypothyroidism in the course of the therapy with growth hormone should be corrected with thyroid hormone in order to obtain a sufficient growth promoting effect.

Patients with an intra or extracranial neoplasia in remission who are receiving treatment with growth hormone should be examined carefully and at regular intervals by the physician.

Patients with growth hormone deficiency secondary to an intracranial tumour should be examined frequently for progression or recurrence of the underlying disease process.

In case of severe or recurrent headache, visual problems, nausea and/or vomiting, funduscopy for papilloedema is recommended. If papilloedema is confirmed a diagnosis of benign intracranial hypertension (or pseudotumor cerebri) should be considered and if confirmed Saizen treatment should be discontinued. At present there is insufficient evidence to guide clinical decision-making in patients with resolved intracranial hypertension. If growth hormone treatment is restarted, careful monitoring for symptoms of intracranial hypertension is necessary.

Treatment with growth hormone may induce insulin resistance. Patients should be observed for evidence of glucose intolerance.

Saizen should be used with caution in patients with diabetes mellitus or with a family history of diabetes mellitus. Patients with diabetes mellitus may require adjustment of their antidiabetic therapy.

The injection site should be varied to prevent lipoatrophy.

Interaction with other medicinal products and other forms of interaction: Concomitant corticosteroid therapy may inhibit the response to Saizen.

Use during pregnancy and lactation: Not applicable.

There is currently insufficient evidence from human studies on the safety of growth hormone treatment during pregnancy and lactation.

Effects on ability to drive and use machines: Saizen does not interfere with the patient's ability to drive or use machinery.

Undesirable effects: Some patients may experience redness and itching at the site of injection, particularly when the subcutaneous route is used.

Antibodies to Somatropin can form in some patients; the clinical significance of these antibodies is unknown, though to date the antibodies have been of low binding capacity and have not been associated with growth attenuation except in patients with gene deletions. In very rare instances, where short stature is due to deletion of the growth hormone gene complex, treatment with growth hormone may induce growth attenuating antibodies.

Intermittent dosage has been associated with the appearance of hypoglycaemia.

Epiphysiolysis at the site of the hip joint may occur. A child with an unexplained limp should be examined.

Overdose: No cases of acute overdosage have been reported. However, exceeding the recommended doses can cause side effects. Overdosage can lead to hypoglycaemia and subsequently to hyperglycaemia. Long term overdosage could result in signs and symptoms of gigantism and/or acromegaly, consistent with the known effects of excess human growth hormone.

Pharmacological properties

Pharmacodynamic properties: Pharmaco-therapeutic group: Anterior pituitary lobe hormones and analogues, ATC code: HO1A.

Saizen contains recombinant human growth hormone produced by genetically engineered mammalian cells.

It is a peptide of 191 amino acids identical to human pituitary growth hormone with respect to amino acid sequence and composition as well as peptide map, isoelectric point, molecular weight, isomeric structure and bioactivity.

Growth hormone is synthesised in a transformed murine cell line that has been modified by the addition of the gene for pituitary growth hormone.

Saizen is an anabolic and anticatabolic agent which exerts effects not only on growth but also on body composition and metabolism. It interacts with specific receptors on a variety of cell types including myocytes, hepatocytes, adipocytes, lymphocytes and hematopoietic cells. Some, but not all of its effects are mediated through another class of hormones known as somatomedins (IGF-1 and IGF-2).

Depending on the dose, the administration of Saizen elicits a rise in IGF-1, IGFBP-3, non-esterified fatty acids and glycerol, a decrease in blood urea, and decreases in urinary nitrogen, sodium and potassium excretion. The duration of the increase in GH levels may play a role in determining the magnitude of the effects. A relative saturation of the effects of Saizen at high doses is probable. This is not the case for glycemia and urinary C-peptide excretion, which are significantly elevated only after high doses (20 mg).

Pharmacokinetic properties: The pharmacokinetics of Saizen are linear at least up to doses of 8 IU. At higher doses (60 IU/20 mg) some degree of non-linearity cannot be ruled out, however with no clinical relevance.

Following IV administration in healthy volunteers the volume of distribution at steady-state is around 7 L, total metabolic clearance is around 15 L/h while the renal clearance is negligible, and the drug exhibits an elimination half-life of 20 to 35 min.

Following single-dose SC and IM administration of Saizen, the apparent terminal half-life is much longer, around 2 to 4 hours. This is due to a rate limiting absorption process.

Maximum serum growth hormone (GH) concentrations are reached after approximately 4 hours and serum GH levels return to baseline within 24 hours, indicating that no accumulation of GH will occur during repeated administrations.

The absolute bioavailability of both routes is 70–90%.

Preclinical safety data: Preclinical studies were performed on rodents and monkeys with doses up to 40 IU/kg (13.33 mg/kg) in rats and mice and up to 20 IU/kg (6.67 mg/kg) in monkeys for up to 52 weeks. The documented toxicological profile and the absence of mutagenic activity in a variety of *in vitro* and *in vivo* tests demonstrates that administration of Saizen is considered safe.

The local tolerability of Saizen solutions containing 0.3% metacresol when injected in animals was considered good and found suitable for SC or IM administration.

Pharmaceutical particulars

List of excipients:

Powder for solution for injection: Sucrose, Phosphoric acid, Sodium Hydroxide.

Solvent for parenteral use: Metacresol 0.3% (w/v) in water for injections.

Incompatibilities: No incompatibilities of Saizen with other pharmaceutical preparations are known at present.

Shelf life: Saizen 24 IU (8 mg) product in its final packaging has a shelf-life of 2 years.

The reconstituted solution for injection is stable for 21 days.

Special precautions for storage: Saizen 24 IU (8 mg) should be stored at or below 25°C.

Store the reconstituted Saizen 24 IU (8 mg) contained in the cartridge within the Easyject in a refrigerator at 2–8°C, protected from light.

Nature and contents of container: The DIN 2R 3 ml

vials of Saizen 24 IU (8 mg) and the cartridges of the solvent are of neutral glass (Type I).

Saizen 24 IU (8 mg) Easyject is available in the following pack sizes:

1 vial of Saizen 24 IU (8 mg) product, 1 cartridge of bacteriostatic solvent and 1 reconstitution set.

5 vials of Saizen 24 IU (8 mg) product and 5 cartridges of bacteriostatic solvent and 5 reconstitution sets.

Instructions for use/handling: Reconstitution: The powder for solution for injection should be used with the enclosed bacteriostatic solvent (0.3% (w/v) metacresol in water for injections) for parenteral use. The reconstituted solution for injection should be clear with no particles. If the solution contains particles, it must not be injected.

Use with the Easyject: Follow the instruction given in the package leaflet and in the instruction for use provided with each Easyject.

To reconstitute Saizen 24 IU (8 mg), inject the contents the bacteriostatic solvent cartridge into the vial of Saizen 24 IU (8 mg), swirl the vial with a GENTLE rotary motion then leave to stand for up to 5 minutes. Withdraw the reconstituted solution back into the cartridge.

Marketing authorisation number
Saizen 24 IU (8 mg) for Easyject PL 3400/0079
Bacteriostatic Solvent cartridge PL 3400/0076

Date of first authorisation/renewal of authorisation July 1998

Date of (partial) revision of the text July 1998

Legal category POM CD (Sch 4)

SEROPHENE*

Presentation White, round, flat, bevelled tablet, single score on one side and the letter 'S' imprinted on the other, each containing 50 mg Clomiphene Citrate BP.

Uses Serophene is indicated for the induction of ovulation in women with:

(i) hypothalamic-pituitary dysfunction (including polycystic ovarian syndrome (PCOS))

(ii) the induction of multiple follicular development in women undergoing superovulation for assisted conception techniques such as in vitro fertilisation (IVF).

Serophene is prescribable under the supervision of clinicians involved in the treatment of infertility.

Dosage and administration
(i) Hypothalamic pituitary dysfunction (including PCOS): Serophene is given as a 5 day course of tablets, commencing within the first 5 days of spontaneous or progesterone-induced menstrual bleeding. In patients who have not experienced recent uterine bleeding the commencement date is arbitrary.

A suggested dosage schedule is presented in the following table:

	dose mg/day	Result after 1 cycle			Result after 6 cycles—no pregnancy
		ovulation pregnancy	ovulation no pregnancy	no ovulation	
Cycle 1	50	cease therapy	continue to 6 cycles (max)	increase dose (cycle 2)	
Cycle 2	100†	cease therapy	continue to 6 cycles (max)	same dose with hCG may be considered (cycle 3) *or*	reassess patient and consider gonadotrophin therapy
Cycle 3	100† +hCG	cease therapy	continue to 6 cycles (max)	reassess patient and consider gonadotrophin therapy	

† This dose of Serophene should not be exceeded.

If ovulation does not occur naturally, a single subcutaneous or intramuscular injection of up to 10,000 IU Profasi* (Chorionic Gonadotrophin, hCG) may be given 7 to 10 days after the last Serophene tablet to simulate an LH surge.

Sexual intercourse is recommended around the expected time of ovulation (approximately 8–12 days after the last dose of Serophene).

Monitoring of treatment: Patients should be monitored each cycle at least for the first three cycles, ideally using ultrasound, at the expected time of ovulation, to check for ovulation.

Basal body temperature (BBT) charts have been recommended as a monitoring method in the past. However, it is now felt that this method is inappropriate due to inaccuracy, as the temperature rise occurs after ovulation takes place as well as daily negative reinforcement of the couple's problem.

Home monitoring using ovulation predictor kits based on the LH surge, is more accurate and more acceptable to patients than recording of BBT. Sexual intercourse is recommended at the time of the LH surge as this represents the time of ovulation.

The measurement of mid-luteal plasma progesterone may be used to assess the ovulatory response to treatment. On cycle day 21, serum progesterone levels in excess of 30 nmol/l are suggestive of ovulation.

Local laboratory normal range of values should be taken into consideration.

If a patient shows presumptive evidence of ovulation and menstruation does not follow, pregnancy should be excluded before treatment is recommenced.

(ii) Superovulation for an assisted conception technique: The objective of superovulation is to stimulate multiple follicular growth, thereby increasing the number of eggs available for fertilisation.

Serophene is usually administered in combination with gonadotrophins to induce multiple follicular maturation. A commonly used dosage regimen involves the administration of 100 mg (two tablets) Serophene daily on cycle days 2–6, followed by daily gonadotrophins (150–225 IU FSH) commencing on day 5 of the cycle and continuing, at a dose dependent upon the response of the patient, until adequate follicular development has been achieved. (See Pergonal* (Menotrophin Injection BP), Metrodin* High Purity (highly purified urofollitrophin (FSH) injection) and Profasi* Data Sheets for further details).

A single injection of up to 10,000 IU Profasi is administered 24–48 hours after the last gonadotrophin injection to coincide with the expected onset of the (endogenous) LH surge.

Monitoring of superovulation: Superovulation is monitored by estimation of plasma oestradiol-17β and by ultrasonography.

One recommendation is that the diameter of at least 3 follicles should be equal to or greater than 15 mm, with the diameter of the leading follicle 18 mm or more and a plasma oestradiol-17β level greater than 3500 pmol/l.

Profasi should not be administered unless there is evidence of adequate follicular development as evidenced by progressively rising oestrogen levels and concomitant follicular growth on ultrasound.

Egg retrieval: Egg retrieval is carried out, either by laparoscopy or ultrasound guided aspiration, about 34–36 hours following Profasi injection. Ideally, all follicles should be aspirated at egg retrieval (see Warnings).

Further details concerning Serophene dosage and monitoring, are available on request.

Children: Not recommended for use in children.

Elderly: Not recommended for use in the elderly.

Contra-indications, warnings, etc
Contra-indications: Liver disease and liver dysfunction; hereditary defect in bilirubin metabolism; pregnancy; abnormal uterine bleeding; ovarian cysts (except polycystic ovarian syndrome); ovarian endometriosis.

Serophene therapy is precluded in women in whom a satisfactory outcome cannot be expected, e.g., women with tubal occlusion unless thay are undergoing superovulation for IVF, ovarian dysgenesis, absent uterus, premature menopause or hypothalamic pituitary failure.

Serophene is contra-indicated in pregnant and lactating women.

Warnings
Hyperstimulation:
(i) Hypothalamic pituitary dysfunction (including PCOS): Patients receiving Serophene should be instructed to report any abdominal discomfort immediately and undergo appropriate investigations such as ultrasound. Whilst the incidence of clinically significant hyperstimulation is low with the recommended Serophene dosage scheme, the presence of excessive ovarian enlargement may require the dosage scheme to be modified (see Overdosage). Rare occurrences of lutein cyst rupture with intraperitoneal haemorrhage have been reported.

(ii) Superovulation for an assisted conception technique: The incidence of hyperstimulation is minimised in patients undergoing superovulation by the aspiration of all follicles.

Visual symptoms: Clomiphene citrate should be withdrawn if visual disturbances occur, e.g., blurring, spots or flashes (in rare cases scotomata). Patients should not drive or operate machinery if their vision is adversely affected.

Multiple pregnancy: The multiple pregnancy rate in treated patients with hypothalamic pituitary dysfunction or PCOS is approximately 8%, twins representing 90% of this figure.

The multiple pregnancy rate following assisted conception techniques is related to the number of oocytes/embryos replaced.

Although a higher spontaneous abortion rate than that found in the normal population has been reported, this is comparable to the abortion rate in women with other fertility problems. A causal relationship with clomiphene has not been established.

Although Serophene has been shown to be embryotoxic in animals at high doses, there is no evidence to suggest that it increases the incidence of congenital malformations in humans at therapeutic levels. Treatment with Serophene has not been shown to alter the incidence of congenital malformation observed in the offspring of women with fertility problems.

Precautions; Appropriate treatment should first be given for other endocrine disorders, e.g., hypothyroidism, adrenocortical deficiency, hyperprolactinaemia or pituitary tumours and other possible causes of infertility in either partner. An acceptable semen analysis should be available for those couples undergoing ovulation induction.

Side-effects: Side-effects are usually dose-related and generally reversible on drug withdrawal. The following side-effects have been reported:

Ovarian enlargement and abdominal/pelvic discomfort, vasomotor symptoms (hot flushes).

Nausea, vomiting, breast discomfort and visual symptoms have been reported occasionally.

Nervousness, insomnia, headache, dizziness, increased urination, heavier menses, depression, fatigue, skin reactions (dermatitis and urticaria), weight gain and temporary hair loss have been reported rarely.

Convulsions have been reported: patients with a history of seizures may be predisposed.

There have been rare reports of ovarian cancer with fertility drugs; infertility itself is a primary risk factor. Epidemiological data suggests that prolonged use of Serophene may increase this risk. Therefore the recommended duration of treatment should not be exceeded (see Dosage and administration).

Overdosage (and treatment): There is no experience of acute poisoning with Serophene.

Hyperstimulation may occasionally result from an excessive response to clomiphene citrate therapy. Hyperstimulation is categorised as mild, moderate or severe. Generally hyperstimulation will be mild or, very rarely, moderate after clomiphene citrate treatment. Symptoms usually appear 3–6 days after ovulation or Profasi administration.

Mild hyperstimulation—Symptoms may include some abdominal swelling and pain; ovaries enlarged to 5 cm diameter. Therapy—rest; careful observation and symptomatic relief. Ovarian enlargement declines rapidly.

Moderate hyperstimulation—Symptoms include more pronounced abdominal distension and pain; nausea; vomiting; occasional diarrhoea; ovaries enlarged up to 12 cm diameter. Therapy—bed rest; close observation, in the case of conception occurring, to detect any progression to severe hyperstimulation. Pelvic examination should be gentle in order to avoid rupture of the cysts. Symptoms subside spontaneously over 2–3 weeks.

Severe hyperstimulation—A rare but serious complication—symptoms include pronounced abdominal distention and pain; ascites; pleural effusion; decreased blood volume; reduced urine output; electrolyte imbalance and sometimes shock; ovaries enlarged to in excess of 12 cm diameter and may contain cysts. Therapy—hospitalisation, treatment should be conservative concentrating on restoring the blood volume and preventing shock. Acute symptoms subside over several days and ovaries return to normal after 20–40 days if conception does not occur—symptoms may be prolonged if conception has occurred.

Pharmaceutical precautions Serophene should be stored below 25°C and protected from light and moisture.

Legal category POM.

Package quantities Serophene is blister packed in boxes of 10, 30 and 100 tablets (OP).

Further information The mode of action of Serophene at the recommended dose appears to be through competition for available oestrogen receptor sites in the hypothalamus. Oestrogen is displaced from these sites and the hypothalamus perceives an apparent lack of circulating oestrogen. This results in gonadotrophin releasing hormone stimulated secretion of FSH and LH, which initiates the normal menstrual cycle.

Patients with very low baseline levels of endogenous gonadotrophins and oestrogens are usually less responsive to Serophene treatment, and consideration should be given to gonadotrophin therapy.

Clomiphene citrate is readily absorbed from the gastrointestinal tract and slowly excreted through the liver into the bile. The biological half-life is reported to be five days. Enterohepatic recirculation takes place.

There is evidence that some women ovulate spontaneously for some cycles after cessation of Serophene treatment.

Product licence number 3400/0009

UKIDAN*

Qualitative and quantitative composition Ukidan vials contain urokinase in a sterile, white, freeze-dried powder form. Each vial contains 5,000 IU, 25,000 IU or 100,000 IU of urokinase.

Pharmaceutical form Powder for injection after reconstitution with solvent.

Clinical particulars
Therapeutic indications: Ukidan is indicated for the lysis of clots in the following conditions:

(i) Thromboembolic occlusive vascular disease such as deep vein thrombosis (DVT), pulmonary embolism (PE) and peripheral vascular occlusion.

(ii) Hyphaema (haemorrhage into the anterior chamber of the eye).

(iii) Arterio-venous haemodialysis shunts and intravenous cannulae which are blocked by fibrin clots.

Posology and method of administration: Ukidan should be reconstituted with a small amount of sterile Water for Injections or saline and then further diluted with normal saline to the desired volume for administration.
Adults
(i) Thromboembolic Occlusive Vascular Disease:
Deep vein thrombosis: A recommended dosage regimen consists of an initial loading dose of 4,400 IU/kg body weight in 15 ml solution, given over 10 minutes followed by an intravenous infusion of 4,400 IU/kg/hour for 12–24 hours.

Pulmonary embolism: A recommended dosage regimen consists of an initial loading dose of 4,400 IU/kg body weight in 15 ml solution, given over 10 minutes followed by an intravenous infusion of 4,400 IU/kg/hour for 12 hours.

Alternatively, a 50 ml bolus injection of Ukidan into the pulmonary artery, repeated for up to 3 doses, at 24 hour intervals, has been employed. The initial dosage of 15,000 IU/kg body weight may be adjusted if necessary for subsequent injections, dependent upon the plasma fibrinogen concentration produced by the previous injection.

Peripheral vascular occlusion: A recommended dosage regimen involves the infusion of a 2,500 IU/ml solution of Ukidan (500,000 IU in 200 ml) into the clot, using angiography to monitor the progress of treatment. Ukidan should be infused into the clot at a dose rate of 4,000 IU/minute (96 ml/hr) for 2 hours followed by repeat angiography. The catheter is then advanced into the remaining occluded segment and Ukidan infused at 4,000 IU/min for a further 2 hours; this may be repeated up to 4 times if antegrade flow has not occurred. After lysing a channel through the occlusion the catheter is withdrawn until it is proximal to the remaining clot lining the vessel wall. Ukidan is given at a dose rate of 1,000 IU/min (0.4 ml) until the clot has completely lysed. A dose of 500,000 IU given over approximately 8 hours should be sufficient to achieve this.

If the clot is not reduced in length by more than 25% after the initial infusion of 500,000 IU and by an incremental 10% by subsequent infusions of 500,000 IU, consideration should be given to discontinuation of treatment.

After fibrinolytic therapy has been completed, treatment may be continued with suitable anticoagulant therapy.

(ii) Hyphaema: When saline irrigation is unsuccessful in removing the blood clot, Ukidan may be considered for the management of hyphaema, particularly when the clot completely fills the anterior chamber and there is an accompanying rise in intra-ocular pressure. The following general technique is used: an incision of about 3 mm is made inside the temporal limbus of the cornea. 5,000 IU Ukidan is dissolved in Sodium Chloride Injection BP (2 ml) and drawn up into a syringe fitted with a suitable irrigator. The tip of the irrigator is introduced through the incision so as to be over the iris rather than the pupillary space (thus avoiding risk of damage to the lens), with the aperture directed towards the corneal endothelium or parallel to the plane of the iris. The solution is injected and withdrawn repeatedly with minimal pressure. Clot disintegration commonly begins within five minutes, facilitating injection of the solution and aspiration of the clot. The chamber is then washed out with saline. If residual clot remains, a small quantity of the solution (e.g. 0.3 ml) may be left in the anterior chamber to facilitate further dissolution of the clot over the next 24–48 hours.

(iii) Clotted Arterio-Venous Shunts: Generally, 5,000–25,000 IU Ukidan in 2–3 ml Sodium Chloride Injection BP is instilled into the affected limb of the shunt which is then clamped off for 2–4 hours. The lysate is then aspirated. This may be repeated if necessary. For the venous side an infusion of 5,000 IU in 200 ml, run in over 30 minutes, has been used but this may be less satisfactory than the use of more concentrated solutions.

Dosage in the elderly: Initially no dosage alterations are recommended, however, thereafter, the dosage should be adjusted as necessary, according to response.

Dosage in children: Initially no dosage alterations are recommended, however, thereafter, the dosage should be adjusted as necessary, according to response.

Contra-indications: Ukidan is contra-indicated in any situation where bleeding has occurred, or is likely to occur.

Recent surgery (including biopsy): administration of Ukidan for thromboembolic occlusive vascular disease is not recommended for 72 hours following surgery because of the risk of bleeding from the operation site.

Severe hypertension (with systolic bp>200 mmHg and/or diastolic bp>120 mmHg): in patients with severe hypertension, administration of Ukidan carries the risk of cerebral haemorrhage.

Ukidan is contra-indicated in pregnancy and the immediate post-partum period.

Severe hepatic or renal insufficiency.

When used in 'local' situations, the above contra-indications may not be relevant.

Special warnings and special precautions for use: If bleeding occurs following systemic use, the infusion should be stopped immediately. However, this contra-indication is relative. The benefits of the continued use of Ukidan must be weighed against the risks of stopping therapy, for example, in the situation where vascular occlusion can be life-threatening. For treatment of bleeding see *Overdose* section.

When used in the eye, a normal gonioscopy result should be evident.

Systemic Ukidan should be used with caution in patients with gastrointestinal lesions such as peptic ulceration, which may be prone to haemorrhage, and in patients who have had multiple intracardiac and intravascular punctures as a consequence of cardio-pulmonary resuscitation.

Interactions with other medicaments and other forms of interaction: In glucose solution there is a measurable (<10%) reduction in the activity of Ukidan after 8 hours.

Concomitant administration of dextran sulphate may prolong the activity of Ukidan.

Pregnancy and lactation: Ukidan is contra-indicated in pregnancy and the immediate post-partum period.

Effects on ability to drive and use machines: None known.

Undesirable effects: The following side-effects have been associated with Ukidan use in the listed indications.

Hyphaema – none reported;

Arterio-venous shunts – warmth, initial severe pain and dull ache in shunt limb have been reported occasionally;

Thromboembolic occlusive vascular disease – overt bleeding, haemorrhagic complications may occur;

Temporary increase in temperature (when a high yield of lysis degradation products are produced) and haematuria have been reported occasionally.

Overdose: If severe haemorrhage occurs, treatment with Ukidan must be stopped. Aprotinin and synthetic inhibitors such as epsilon-aminocaproic acid, tranexamic acid or p-aminomethylbenzoic acid can be used to inhibit the fibrinolytic action of Ukidan. In serious cases, human fibrinogen, Factor XIII, Cohn-Fraction I, packed red cells or whole blood can be given, as appropriate.

Pharmacological properties
Pharmacodynamic properties: Ukidan is a preparation of urokinase, which is an enzyme extracted from human adult male urine. As Ukidan is of human origin, it is not antigenic in man.

Ukidan brings about the dissolution of blood clots by promoting the activation of plasminogen; the latter is the inactive precursor of plasmin, the proteolytic enzyme responsible for the breakdown of fibrin into small soluble peptides which are dispersible through the blood stream.

Pharmacodynamic properties: Following intravenous administration, urokinase is rapidly cleared from the blood. The *in vivo* half-life of urokinase activity in normal subject is about 10 to 15 minutes.

In cirrhotic patients, the elimination half-life is clearly increased up to about 30 minutes.

In subjects with kidney disease, elimination of endogenous urokinase is markedly decreased, even if the glomerular filtration rate is only moderately impaired.

The liver appears to perform an important function in the metabolism and elimination of urokinase.

The major part of urokinase activity has been found to be excreted in the bile, with peak activity achieved 35 to 60 minutes after injection and falling to unmeasureable levels after 140 to 190 minutes.

Preclinical safety data: Being extracted from human urine, urokinase is species-homologous and is free from inherent toxicity in man.

In animal toxicology studies, single i.v. doses up to 1 MIU/kg were not lethal and did not produce symptoms of intoxication of histological changes in any important organs. With repeated administration in increasing doses, no practical relevant toxic changes or lethal effects were observed.

Pharmaceutical particulars The activity of Ukidan is expressed in International Units (IU), which are approximately equivalent to one Committee on Thrombolytic Agents (CTA) unit.

List of excipients: Mannitol, disodium edetate, disodium hydrogen phosphate.

Incompatibilities: None known.

Shelf life: 24 months.

Special precautions for storage: Ukidan, in the lyophilised form, should be stored below 25°C. When reconstituted, Ukidan is stable for 24 hours when stored below 25°C.

Nature and contents of container: 5 ml vials of colourless neutral glass type 1. The product is packed as single vials.

Instructions for use/handling: The lyophilised material should be reconstituted with a small amount of saline or Water for Injections, and then further diluted with saline.

Product licence numbers
Ukidan 5,000 IU 3400/0001R
Ukidan 25,000 IU 3400/0026R
Ukidan 100,000 IU 3400/0027R

Date of approval/revision of SPC 11 July 1996.

Legal category POM.

**Trade Mark*

Servier Laboratories Limited
Fulmer Hall
Windmill Road
Fulmer, Slough SL3 6HH
☎ 01753 662744 ⎙ 01753 663456

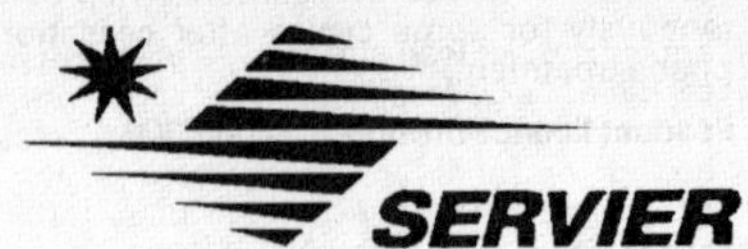

COVERSYL TABLETS

Qualitative and quantitative composition Perindopril tert-butylamine salt 2 mg or 4 mg.

Pharmaceutical form
Coversyl 2 mg: tablet, white, biconvex.
Coversyl 4 mg: tablet, white, oblong, half-scored on one side.

Clinical particulars
Therapeutic indications:
Hypertension: All grades of essential hypertension and renovascular hypertension.

Heart failure: In congestive heart failure Coversyl should be used as an adjunctive therapy with diuretics and, where appropriate, digitalis.

As with other ACE inhibitors, treatment with Coversyl should always be initiated under close medical supervision.

Severe heart failure: In severe heart failure treatment with Coversyl should always be initiated in hospital under close supervision.

Posology and method of administration:
Hypertension: 2 mg once a day is the normal starting dose. Optimum control of blood pressure is achieved by increasing the dose, titrating it against the blood pressure. The usual maintenance dose is 4 mg given once daily.

The maximum daily dose is 8 mg which may be combined with diuretic therapy. Coversyl should be taken before a meal as ingestion of food decreases conversion to perindoprilat.

Congestive heart failure: It is recommended that Coversyl be given with a non-potassium-sparing diuretic and/or digoxin under close medical supervision (in hospital for severe heart failure) with a recommended starting dose of 2 mg taken in the morning. The dose may, in most instances, be increased to 4 mg once daily (once blood pressure acceptability has been demonstrated).

The dose titration of Coversyl may be performed over a two- to four-week period or more rapidly if indicated by the presence of residual signs and symptoms of heart failure. As with other ACE inhibitors, blood pressure and renal function should be monitored closely both before and during treatment with Coversyl. Serum potassium should also be monitored.

In comparative studies versus placebo and other ACE inhibitors, the first administration of 2 mg of Coversyl to patients with mild to moderate heart failure was not associated with any significant reduction of blood pressure as compared to placebo.

However, some patients, other than those with severe heart failure, are considered to be at higher risk when started on an ACE-inhibitor and are recommended for initiation of therapy in hospital. Research data have shown such patients to be: those on multiple or high-dose diuretics (e.g. greater than 80 mg frusemide); patients with hypovolaemia; hyponatraemia (serum sodium less than 130 mmol/l); pre-existing hypotension (systolic blood pressure less than 90 mmHg); patients with unstable cardiac failure; renal impairment (serum creatinine greater than 150 μmol/l); those on high-dose vasodilator therapy; patients aged 70 years and over.

In order to decrease the small possibility of symptomatic hypotension, patients on previous high-dose diuretics should have the diuretic dose reduced before introducing Coversyl. The appearance of hypotension after the initial dose of Coversyl does not preclude subsequent careful dose titration with the drug, following effective treatment of the hypotension.

Combinations with a diuretic: Symptomatic hypotension may occur when Coversyl treatment is initiated in patients receiving diuretic treatment, in particular if diuretic treatment was begun only a short time before. It is therefore recommended to discontinue the diuretic 2–3 days before beginning treatment with Coversyl at the starting dose of 2 mg.

Addition of a diuretic potentiates the anti-hypertensive effects of Coversyl.

If co-treatment with a diuretic is thought necessary in patients on Coversyl therapy, the diuretic should be initiated at the lowest dose.

Potassium sparing diuretics should be avoided or used with extreme caution (see *Warnings*).

Dosage in elderly or in hepatic impairment: Since elderly patients may have renal impairment and/or other organ dysfunction, Coversyl treatment should be initiated at 2 mg daily under close supervision.

Dosage in renal impairment and dialysis: Perindoprilat is excreted by the kidney. Coversyl should therefore be used with caution in patients with renal impairment and the dose adjusted to the degree of renal failure. Normal medical follow-up will include frequent monitoring of potassium and creatinine. The following dosages are recommended:

Creatinine clearance	*Recommended dosage*
Between 30 and 60 ml/min	2 mg per day
Between 15 and 30 ml/min	2 mg every other day
Less than 15 ml/min	2 mg on the day of dialysis On days when the patients are not on dialysis the dose should be tailored to the blood pressure response.

Contra-indications: Patients with a history of hypersensitivity to Coversyl. History of angioneurotic oedema associated with previous other ACE inhibitor therapy.

Pregnancy: Coversyl is contra-indicated in pregnancy and should not be used in women of child-bearing potential, unless protected by effective contraception. Maternal and foetal toxicity has been shown at high doses in rodents and rabbits although not in monkeys.

Neither embryotoxicity nor teratogenicity was observed. Oligohydramnios, neonatal hypotension and anuria have been reported following use of ACE inhibitors in the 2nd and 3rd trimester of pregnancy.

Lactation period: In animals, very little perindopril crosses into maternal milk. No data are available in humans. Coversyl should not be used in nursing mothers.

Special warnings and precautions for use: Renal function should be monitored before and at intervals after treatment.

Hypotension: Symptomatic hypotension was seen rarely in uncomplicated hypertensive patients. Symptomatic hypotension with ACE inhibitors is more likely to occur in patients who have been volume depleted by diuretics, salt restriction, dialysis, diarrhoea or vomiting.

Some patients may experience symptomatic hypotension with the first one or two doses. The occurrence of first dose hypotension does not preclude restarting Coversyl cautiously and subsequent dose titration against the blood pressure after correction of hypovolaemia and hypotension.

Exaggerated hypotensive responses may occur after the initial dose of Coversyl in patients receiving diuretic treatment. The possibilities of such occurrences are reduced by discontinuing diuretic therapy 3 days prior to initiating Coversyl.

In most instances, symptoms are relieved simply by the patient lying down, but volume repletion with oral fluids or intravenous infusion with normal saline may be required.

In some patients with congestive heart failure who have normal or low blood pressure, additional lowering of systemic blood pressure may occur with ACE inhibitors.

It has been reported mainly in patients with severe heart failure with or without associated renal insufficiency. This is more likely in patients on high doses of loop diuretics, or those with hyponatraemia or functional renal impairment.

In these patients, treatment should be started under close medical supervision, preferably in the hospital, with low doses and careful dose titration. If possible, diuretic treatment should be discontinued temporarily.

Similar considerations in terms of initiating therapy with a small dose may apply also to patients with ischaemic heart or cerebrovascular disease in whom severe hypotension could result in a myocardial infarct or cerebrovascular accident. If such hypotension becomes symptomatic, a reduction of dose or discontinuation of Coversyl may become necessary.

However, in comparative studies versus placebo and other ACE inhibitors, the first administration of 2 mg of Coversyl to patients with mild to moderate heart failure was not associated with any significant reduction of blood pressure as compared to placebo.

Patients with renovascular hypertension: Coversyl can be used when surgery is not indicated or prior to surgery. Renal function of patients with renovascular hypertension should be closely monitored.

Patients with renal insufficiency: Renal function of patients with renal failure or insufficiency should be closely monitored. Marked water and sodium depletion (salt-free diet and/or diuretic treatment) or stenosis of the renal arteries stimulate the renin-angiotensin system; blockage of the system by an ACE inhibitor, especially upon initial dosing and during the first 2 weeks of treatment, may lead to an abrupt fall in blood pressure and/or to functional and possibly acute renal failure, although the latter is uncommon and the time interval variable. Discontinuation of Coversyl or discontinuation or reduction of the diuretic may be required.

Patients haemodialysed using high-flux polyacrylonitrile ('AN69') membranes are highly likely to experience anaphylactoid reactions if they are treated with ACE inhibitors. This combination should therefore be avoided, either by use of alternative antihypertensive drugs or alternative membranes for haemodialysis.

Angioedema: Angioedema of the face, extremities, lips, mucous membranes, tongue, glottis and/or larynx may occur in patients treated with ACE inhibitors which especially occurs during the first weeks of treatment.

However, in rare cases severe angioedema may develop after long-term treatment with an angiotensin converting enzyme inhibitor. Treatment should promptly be discontinued and replaced by an agent belonging to another class of drugs.

Angioedema involving the tongue, glottis or larynx may be fatal. Emergency therapy should given including, but not necessarily limited to, immediate subcutaneous epinephrine solution 1:1000 (0.3 to 0.5 ml) or slow intravenous epinephrine 1 mg/ml (observe dilution instructions) with control of ECG and blood pressure. The patient should be hospitalised and observed for at least 12 to 24 hours and should not be discharged until complete resolution of symptoms has occurred.

Cough: During treatment with an ACE inhibitor a dry and non-productive cough may occur which disappears after discontinuation.

Patients with liver insufficiency: Patients with impaired liver function treated with ACE inhibitors primarily metabolised in the liver may develop markedly elevated plasma levels of the drug. Dose adaptation may be necessary, depending on the severity of the liver insufficiency and the way the ACE inhibitor is metabolised.

Elderly: Some elderly patients may be more responsive to an ACE inhibitor than younger patients. Administration of low initial doses and evaluation of the renal function at the beginning of the treatment is recommended.

Children: Coversyl is not recommended in children as paediatric use has not been studied.

Hyperkalaemia: Combination of potassium supplements or potassium-sparing diuretics with Coversyl is not recommended, particularly in patients with renal impairment, since this may lead to a significant increase in plasma potassium. However, if combination with these agents is necessary, caution should be exercised and plasma potassium frequently monitored.

Surgery/anaesthesia: In patients undergoing major surgery or during anaesthesia with agents that produce hypotension, Coversyl blocks angiotensin II formation secondary to compensatory renin release. This may lead to hypotension which can be corrected by volume expansion.

Aortic stenosis/hypertrophic cardiomyopathy: ACE

inhibitors should be used with caution in patients with an obstruction in the outflow tract of the left ventricle.

Neutropenia/agranulocytosis: The risk of neutropenia appears to be dose and type-related and is dependent on patient's clinical status. It is rarely seen in uncomplicated patients but may occur in patients with some degree of renal impairment especially when it is associated with collagen vascular disease e.g. systemic lupus erythematosus, scleroderma and therapy with immunosuppressive agents. It is reversible after discontinuation of the ACE inhibitor.

Proteinuria: It may occur particularly in patients with existing renal function impairment or on relatively high doses of ACE inhibitors.

Interactions with other medicaments and other forms of interaction:
Not recommended association
Potassium sparing diuretics or potassium supplements: ACE inhibitors attenuate diuretic induced potassium loss. Potassium sparing diuretics e.g. spironolactone, triamterene, or amiloride, potassium supplements, or potassium-containing salt substitutes may lead to significant increases in serum potassium. If concomitant use is indicated because of demonstrated hypokalemia they should be used with caution and with frequent monitoring of serum potassium.
Precaution for use
Diurectics: Patients on diurectics and especially those who are volume- and/or salt depleted, may experience an excessive reduction of blood pressure after initiation of therapy with an ACE inhibitor. The possibility of hypotensive effects can be reduced by discontinuation of the diuretic, by increasing volume or salt intake prior to intake and by initiation of therapy with lower doses of the ACE inhibitor. Further increases in dosage should be with caution.

Antidiabetic medicines: Concomitant administration of ACE inhibitors and antidiabetic medicines (insulin, oral hypoglycaemic agents) may cause an increased blood glucose lowering effect with greater risk of hypoglycaemia. This phenomenon may be more likely to occur during the first weeks of combined treatment and in patients with renal impairment.

Lithium: Patients stabilised on lithium therapy who are given an ACE inhibitor concurrently may experience a rise in plasma lithium levels.

Anaesthetic drugs: ACE inhibition may enhance the hypotensive effects of certain anaesthetic drugs.

Narcotic drugs/antipsychotics: Postural hypotension may occur.

Antihypertensive agents: Combination with other antihypertensive agents such as beta-blockers, methyldopa, calcium antagonists or diuretics may increase the antihypertensive efficacy.

Allopurinol, cytostatic or immunosuppressive agents, systemic corticosteroids or procainamide: Concomitant administration with ACE inhibitors may lead to an increased risk for leucopenia.

Take into account
Non-steroidal anti-inflammatory drugs: The administration of a non-steroidal anti-inflammatory agent may reduce the antihypertensive effect of an ACE inhibitor. Furthermore, it has been described that NSAIDs and ACE inhibitors exert an additive effect on the increase in serum potassium, whereas renal function may decrease. These effects are in principle reversible, and occur especially in patients with compromised renal function.

Antacids: Induce decreased bioavailability of ACE inhibitors.

Sympathomimetics: Sympathomimetics may reduce the antihypertensive effects of ACE inhibitors: patients should be carefully monitored to confirm that the desired effect is being obtained.

Pregnancy and lactation: Appropriate and well-controlled studies have not been done in humans. ACE inhibitors cross the placenta and can cause fetal and neonatal morbidity and mortality when administered to pregnant women.

Fetal exposure to ACE inhibitors during the second and third trimesters has been associated with neonatal hypotension, renal failure, face or skull deformities and/or death. Maternal oligohydramnios has also been reported reflecting decreasing renal function in the fetus. Limb contractures, craniofacial deformities, hyplastic lung development and intrauterine growth retardation have been reported in association with oligohydramnios. Infants exposed in utero to ACE inhibitors should be closely observed for hypotension; oliguria and hyperkalemia. Oliguria should be treated with support of blood pressure and renal perfusion. Intrauterine growth retardation, prematurity, patent ductus arteriorus and fetal death have also been reported but it is not clear whether they are related to the ACE inhibition or the underlying maternal disease.

It is not known whether exposure limited to the first trimester can adversely affect fetal outcome. Women who become pregnant while receiving an ACE inhibitor should be informed of the potential hazard to the fetus.

Use during lactation: ACE inhibitors may be excreted in breast milk and their effect on the nursing infant has not been determined. It is recommended that lactating mothers should not breast feed while taking ACE inhibitors.

Effects on ability to drive and use machines: There are no studies on the effects of this medicine on the ability to drive. When driving vehicles or operating machines it should be taken into account that occasionally dizziness or weariness may occur.

Undesirable effects:
Cardiovascular system: Some patients may experience hypotension, usually with the first one or two doses of Coversyl, when the dose is increased, or when a diuretic is also given (see *Posology and method of administration* and *Warnings*).

Renal system: Increases of plasma creatinine and urea may occur but are usually reversible. Proteinuria has been observed in some patients.

Respiratory system: Cough (described as dry and irritating) may sometimes be observed but is usually mild.

Gastro-intestinal tract: Taste impairment, epigastric discomfort, nausea and abdominal pain have been reported. Pancreatitis has been reported rarely in patients treated with ACE inhibitors; in some cases this has proved fatal.

Skin, vessels: Localised skin rashes, pruritus or flushing may occur. Angioneurotic oedema has been reported with Coversyl as with other ACE inhibitors.

Where swelling is confined to the face, lips and mouth, the condition will usually resolve on withdrawal of Coversyl without further treatment although antihistamines may be useful in relieving symptoms.

Where there is involvement of the tongue, glottis or larynx, likely to cause airways obstruction, subcutaneous adrenaline (0.5 ml 1:1000) should be administered promptly. The patient should be closely monitored until swelling has resolved.

Nervous system: Fatigue, asthenia, malaise, headache, disturbances of mood and/or sleep have been reported. Most of these effects occurred on initiating treatment and were transient.

Drug/laboratory parameters: Decreases in haemoglobin and red cells and in platelets have been reported in a few patients with Coversyl as with other inhibitors, but a causal relationship has not been established.

Overdose: To date, no case of overdosage has been reported. Signs and symptoms expected in case of overdosage would be related to hypotension and should be relieved by intravenous infusion of isotonic saline solution. Gastric lavage should be considered. Perindopril is dialysable (70 ml/min).

Pharmacological properties
Pharmacodynamic properties: Perindopril is an inhibitor of the enzyme which converts angiotensin I into angiotensin II (ACE inhibitor).

The converting enzyme of Kininase is an exopeptidase which converts angiotensin I into vasoconstrictive angiotensin II and degrades vasodilatory bradykinin into an inactive heptapeptide. Perindopril acts through its active metabolite, perindoprilat, the other metabolites being inactive.

Systemic hypertension: Efficacy is sustained throughout the 24 hour cycle. Maximum antihypertensive effect is reached 4 to 6 hours after a single perindopril dose.

The decrease in blood pressure is rapidly achieved; in responding patients, normalisation is achieved within 1 month and is sustained.

Discontinuation of treatment does not lead to a rebound effect.

In man, perindopril has been confirmed to demonstrate vasodilatory properties, to restore elastic properties of the arterial blood vessels and to decrease left ventricular hypertrophy.

Pharmacokinetic properties: After oral administration, perindopril is rapidly (peak concentration within 1 hour) and extensively (bioavailability: 65 to 70%) absorbed.

Perindopril is converted into perindoprilat, the active metabolite. The plasma half-life of perindopril is equal to 1 hour. The rate of bioconversion into perindoprilat is approximately 20%. The peak plasma concentration of perindoprilat is achieved within 3 to 4 hours.

Ingestion of food decreases conversion to perindoprilat, hence bioavailability.

The volume of distribution is approximately 0.2 l/kg for unbound perindoprilat. The drug is not extensively bound to protein, the bound fraction is less than 30%, but binding is concentration dependent.

In addition to active perindoprilat, perindopril yields 5 metabolites, all inactive. Perindoprilat is eliminated in the urine, and the half-life of its unbound fraction varies between 3 and 5 hours. Dissociation of the perindoprilat-angiotensin converting enzyme bond yields an 'effective' elimination half-life of 25 hours.

No accumulation of perindopril is observed after repeated administration and the half-life of perindoprilat after repeated administration is equivalent to its active half-life, leading to a state of equilibrium within 4 days.

Elimination of perindopril is slowed in the elderly, and in patients with heart and renal failure. Dosage adjustment is desirable depending on the decrease in creatinine clearance.

Dialysis clearance of perindopril is equal to 70 ml/min.

Preclinical safety date: The target organ is the kidney. In rat, administration of perindopril induces arterial anatomical changes which lead to intra-renal haemodynamic changes and to increase in plasma creatinine levels, these effects being reversible when the treatment is stopped.

Pharmaceutical particulars
List of excipients: Microcrystalline cellulose, lactose, hydrophobic colloidal silica, magnesium stearate.

Incompatibilities: Not applicable.

Shelf life: 2 years.

Special precautions for storage: Store below 25°C.

Nature and contents of container: PVC aluminium blister strip of 30 tablets packaged in carton box.

Instruction for use/handling: Not applicable.

Marketing authorisation holder: Les Laboratoires Servier, 22 rue Garnier, 92200 Neuilly-sur-Seine, France.

Marketing authorisation numbers
Coversyl 2 mg tablet 5815/0001
Coversyl 4 mg tablet 5815/0002

Date of approval/revision of SPC 27 March 1997.

Legal category POM

DIAMICRON*

Qualitative and quantitative composition Gliclazide Tablets BP 80 mg.

Pharmaceutical form Tablets.

Clinical particulars
Therapeutic indications: Non insulin dependent diabetes mellitus.

Posology and method of administration:
Oral administration:
Adults: The total daily dose may vary from 40 to 320 mg taken orally. The dose should be adjusted according to the individual patient's response, commencing with 40–80 mg daily (½–1 tablet) and increasing until adequate control is achieved. A single dose should not exceed 160 mg (2 tablets). When higher doses are required, DIAMICRON* should be taken twice daily and according to the main meals of the day.

In obese patients or those not showing adequate response to DIAMICRON* alone, additional therapy may be required.

Elderly: Plasma clearance of gliclazide is not altered in the elderly and steady state plasma levels can therefore be expected to be similar to those in adults under 65 years. Clinical experience in the elderly to date shows that DIAMICRON* is effective and well tolerated. Care should be exercised, however, when prescribing sulphonylureas in the elderly due to a possible age-related increased risk of hypoglycaemia.

Children: DIAMICRON* as with other sulphonylureas, is not indicated for the treatment of juvenile onset diabetes mellitus.

Contra-Indications: DIAMICRON* should not be used in:
- Juvenile onset diabetes.
- Diabetes complicated by ketosis and acidosis.
- Pregnancy.
- Diabetics undergoing surgery, after severe trauma or during infections.
- Patients known to have hypersensitivity to other sulphonylureas and related drugs.
- Diabetic pre-coma and coma.
- Severe renal or hepatic insufficiency.

Special warnings and precautions for use: Hypoglycaemia: all sulphonylureas drugs are capable of producing moderate or severe hypoglycaemia, particularly in the following conditions:
- in patients controlled by diet alone;
- in cases of accidental overdose;
- when calorie or glucose intake is deficient;
- in patients with hepatic and/or renal impairment: however, in long-term clinical trials, patients with renal insufficiency have been treated satisfactorily, using DIAMICRON* at reduced doses.

In order to reduce the risk of hypoglycaemia it is therefore recommended:
- to initiate treatment for non-insulin dependent diabetics by diet alone, if this is possible;

- to take into account the age of the patient: blood sugar levels not strictly controlled by diet alone might be acceptable in the elderly;
- to adjust the dose of DIAMICRON* according to the blood glucose response and to the 24 hour urinary glucose during the first days of treatment.

Dosage adjustments may be necessary:

- on the occurrence of mild symptoms of hypoglycaemia (sweating, pallor, hunger pangs, tachycardia, sensation of malaise). Such findings should be treated with oral glucose and adjustments made in drug dosage and/or meal patterns;
- on the occurrence of severe hypoglycaemic reactions (coma or neurological impairment, see *Overdosage*);
- loss of control of blood glucose (hyperglycaemia). When a patient stabilised on any diabetic regimen is exposed to stress such as fever, trauma, infection or surgery, a loss of control may occur. At such times, it may be necessary to increase progressively the dosage of DIAMICRON* and if this is insufficient, to discontinue the treatment with DIAMICRON* and to administer insulin. As with other sulphonylureas, hypoglcaemia will occur if the patients' dietary intake is reduced or if they are receiving a larger dose of DIAMICRON* than required.

Care should be exercised in patients with hepatic and/or renal impairment and a small starting dose should be used with careful patient monitoring.

Interactions with other medicaments and other forms of interaction: Care should be taken when giving DIAMICRON* with drugs which are known to alter the diabetic state or potentiate the drug's action.

The hyperglycaemic effect of DIAMICRON* may be potentiated by phenylbutazone salicylates, sulphonamides, coumarin derivatives, MAOIs, beta adrenergic blocking agents, tetracycline compounds, chloramphenicol, clofibrate, disopyramide, miconazole (oral forms) and cimetidine.

It may be diminished by corticosteroids, oral contraceptives, thiazide diuretics, phenothiazine derivatives, thyroid hormones and abuse of laxatives.

Pregnancy and lactation:
Pregnancy: See *Contra-indications.*

Lactation: It has not been established whether gliclazide is transferred to human milk. However, other sulphonylureas have been found in milk and there is no evidence to suggest that gliclazide differs from the group in this respect.

Effects on ability to drive and use machines: Patients should be informed that their concentration may be affected if their diabetes is not satisfactorily controlled, especially at the beginning of treatment (see *Special warnings and precautions*).

Undesirable effects:

- Hypoglycaemia (see *Special warnings and precautions*).
- Abnormalities of hepatic function are not uncommon during DIAMICRON* therapy. There are rare reports of hepatic failure, hepatitis and jaundice following treatment with DIAMICRON*.
- Mild gastro-intestinal disturbances including nausea, dyspepsia, diarrhoea, constipation have been reported but this type of adverse reaction can be avoided if DIAMICRON* is taken during a meal.
- Skin reactions including rash, pruritus, erythema, bullous eruption; blood dyscrasia including anaemia, leucopaenia, thrombocytopaenia and granulocytopaenia have been observed during treatment with DIAMICRON* but are not known to be directly attributable to the drug.

Overdosage: The symptom to be expected with an overdose would be hypoglycaemia. The treatment is gastric lavage and correction of the hypoglycaemia by appropriate means with continual monitoring of the patient's blood sugar until the effect of the drug has ceased.

Pharmacological properties
Pharmacodynamic properties: Gliclazide is an hypoglycaemic sulfonylurea differing from other related compounds by the addition of an azabicyclo octane ring.

In man, apart from having similar hypoglycaemic effect to the other sulphonylureas, gliclazide has been shown to reduce platelet adhesiveness and aggregation and increase fibrinolytic activity. These factors are thought to be implicated in the pathogenesis of long term complications of diabetes mellitus.

Gliclazide primarily enhances the first phase of insulin secretion, but also to a lesser degree its second phase. Both phases are diminished in non-insulin dependent diabetes mellitus.

Pharmacokinetic properties: The drug is well absorbed and its half-life in man is approximately 10–12 hours. Gliclazide is metabolised in the liver, less than 5% of the dose is excreted unchanged in the urine.

Preclinical safety data: No findings in the preclinical testing which could be of relevance for the prescriber.

Pharmaceutical properties
List of excipients: Lactose monohydrate, maize starch, pregelatinized maize starch, talc, magnesium stearate.

Incompatibilities: None.

Shelf life: 5 years

Special storage conditions: None.

Nature and contents of container: Blister strip (PVC/Aluminium) of 20 tablets. 3 stripes per carton.

Instructions for use/handling: Not applicable.

Marketing authorisation number PL 0093/0024

Date of first authorisation/renewal of authorisation 21 December 1979/12 March 1990.

Date of (partial) revision of the text 17 April 1997

Legal category POM.

DOMPERAMOL*

Qualitative and quantitative composition Paracetamol PhEur 500.0 mg. Domperidone Maleate PhEur 12.72 mg*
* equivalent to 10.0 mg of domperidone base.

Pharmaceutical form Coated Tablets.

Clinical particulars
Therapeutic indications: Domperamol is indicated for the symptomatic treatment of migraine.

Posology and method of administration: Domperamol should be taken immediately it is known that a migraine attack has started or is imminent.

Adults (including the elderly): Two tablets not more frequently than every 4 hours up to a maximum of 8 tablets in any 24 hour period.

Children under 12 years: Domperamol is not recommended for use in children.

Domperamol tablets are for oral administration only.

Contra-indications: Hypersensitivity to paracetamol, domperidone or any of the other constituents.

Special warnings and precautions for use: Care is advised in the administration of paracetamol to patients with severe renal or severe hepatic impairment. The hazard of overdose is greater with non-cirrhotic alcoholic liver disease. In the event of an overdose, patients should be advised to seek immediate medical help, even if they feel well, because of the risk of delayed, serious liver damage. Patients should be advised not to take other paracetamol containing products concurrently. Do not exceed the recommended dose. Keep out of reach of children. If symptoms persist consult your doctor. Domperamol tablets are not recommended for chronic administration.

Interactions: Whilst adverse interactions have not been reported in general clinical use, domperidone has the potential to interact with several classes of agents. Domperidone may therefore, alter the peripheral actions of dopamine agonists such as bromocriptine, including its hypoprolactinaemic action. The actions of domperidone on gastrointestinal function may be antagonised by antimuscarinics and opioid analgesics. Domperidone may enhace the absorption of concomitantly administered drugs particularly in patients with delayed gastric emptying.

The speed of absorption of paracetamol may be increased by metoclopramide or domperidone and absorption reduced by cholestyramine. The anticoagulant effect of warfarin and other coumarins may be enhanced by prolonged regular daily use of paracetamol with increased risk of bleeding; occasional doses have no significant effect.

Use in pregnancy and lactation: Epidemiological studies in human pregnancy have shown no ill effects due to paracetamol used in the recommended dosage, but patients should follow the advice of their doctor regarding its use. Paracetamol is excreted in breast milk but not in a clinically significant amount. Domperidone is excreted into breast milk but at very low levels. However, the safe use of domperidone in pregnant women has not been established (although studies in animals have not demonstrated teratogenic effects). It is therefore not advisable to administer Domperamol in pregnancy.

Effects on ability to drive and use machines: No adverse effects on the ability to drive or operate machines have been recorded.

Side effects: In common with other dopamine antagonists domperidone produces a rise in serum prolactin which may be associated with galactorrhoea and less frequently with gynaecomastia, breast enlargement or soreness. There have been reports of reduced libido.

Domperidone does not readily cross the normally functioning blood-brain barrier and is therefore less likely to interfere with the central dopaminergic function. However, acute extra-pyramidal dystonic reactions including rare instances of oculogyric crises have been reported with domperidone. Should treatment of a dystonic reaction be necessary, domperidone should be withdrawn and an anticholinergic, anti-Parkinson drug or a benzodiazepine used.

Occasional rashes and other allergic phenomena have been reported with domperidone.

Adverse effects to paracetamol are rare, but hypersensitivity including skin rash may occur. There have been a few reports of blood dyscrasias including thrombocytopenia and agranulocytosis but these were not necessarily causally related to paracetamol.

Overdosage: Symptoms of paracetamol overdosage in the first 24 hours are pallor, nausea, vomiting, anorexia and abdominal pain. Liver damage may become apparent 12 to 48 hours after ingestion. Abnormalities of glucose metabolism and metabolic acidosis may occur. In severe poisoning, hepatic failure may progress to encephalopathy, coma and death. Acute renal failure with acute tubular necrosis may develop even in the absence of severe liver damage. Cardiac arrhythmias and pancreatitis have been reported. Liver damage is possible in adults who have taken 10 g or more of paracetamol. It is considered that excess quantities of a toxic metabolite (usually adequately detoxified by glutathione when normal doses of paracetamol are ingested), becomes irreversibly bound to liver tissue.

Immediate treatment is essential in the management of paracetamol overdose. Despite a lack of significant early symptoms, patients should be referred to hospital urgently for immediate medical attention and any patient who has ingested 7.5 g or more of paracetamol in the preceding 4 hours should undergo gastric lavage. Administration of oral methionine or intravenous N-acetylcysteine which may have a beneficial effect up to at least 48 hours after the overdose, may be required. General supportive measures must be available.

No cases of overdosage with oral domperidone have been reported. There is no specific antidote to domperidone but in the event of overdosage, gastric lavage may be useful.

Pharmacology
Pharmacodynamic properties: Paracetamol is an antipyretic analgesic. The mechanism of action is dependent on the inhibition of prostaglandin synthesis. This inhibition appears, however, to be on a selective basis. There is some evidence to suggest that it may be more effective against enzymes in the CNS than those in the periphery. Domperidone is a dopamine antagonist and increases gastrointestinal motility. It does not reach brain dopamine receptors, probably because it is unable to cross the blood-brain barrier.

Pharmacokinetic properties: Paracetamol is rapidly and almost completely absorbed from the gastrointestinal tract. The concentration in plasma reaches a peak in 30 to 60 minutes and half-life in plasma is 1 to 4 hours after therapeutic doses. Paracetamol is relatively uniformly distributed throughout most body fluids. Binding of the drug to plasma proteins is variable. Following therapeutic doses 90 to 100% of the drug may be recovered in the urine within the first day. However, practically no paracetamol is excreted unchanged and the bulk is excreted after hepatic conjugation.

Domperidone is absorbed from the gastrointestinal tract and metabolised in the liver. It is secreted in the bile mainly as inactive metabolites.

Pharmaceutical particulars
List of excipients: Pregelatinised starch, Maize starch, Polyvidone (K25), Talc (purified), Stearic acid, Magnesium stearate, Hydroxypropylmethylcellulose, Polyethylene glycol 400, Titanium dioxide E171.

Incompatibilities: Not applicable.

Shelf life: A shelf life of 60 months is recommended.

Special precaution and storage: None.

Nature and contents of container: Domperamol tablets are supplied in packs of 16 tablets packed in white PVC (250 mcg)/aluminium foil (20 mcm) blister packs in cardboard cartons.

Instructions for use/handling: Not applicable.

Market authorisation number 0093/0076

Date of first authorisation 22 July 1997

Date of (partial) revision of text August 1998.

LOCABIOTAL*

Qualitative and quantitative composition Fusafungine. Each metered dose contains 500 mcg of fusafungine.

Pharmaceutical form Solution for oral or nasal inhalation.

Clinical particulars
Therapeutic indications: A topical antibiotic with anti-inflammatory properties for the treatment of infec-

tions and inflammatory conditions of the upper respiratory tract.

Posology and method of administration:

Adults and the elderly: 1 inhalation by mouth and (or) 1 inhalation in each nostril every 4 hours.

Children: 1 inhalation by mouth and (or) 1 inhalation in each nostril every 6 hours.

Administration: By inhalation (via mouth or nose) using the appropriate attachment.

Contra-indications: Hypersensitivity to fusafungine or excipients.

Special warnings and precautions for use: Use with caution in patients with allergic tendencies. Prolonged use may encourage superinfection.

Avoid directing the spray towards the eyes as sprays can cause irritation.

If symptoms and signs do not improve in one week, alternative therapy should be considered.

Interactions with other medicaments and other forms of interaction: There have been no documented reports of any interactions with fusafungine used topically. In particular no interactions have been reported with systemic antibiotics.

Pregnancy and lactation: There are no reports of safety of fusafungine in pregnancy or lactation. From the limited animal studies and the lack of absorption, there is little perceived risk during pregnancy.

Effects on ability to drive and use machines: No evidence of any adverse effect on mental alertness.

Undesirable effects: Side-effects observed are mainly local reactions including coughing, sneezing, dryness of nose or throat, unpleasant taste in mouth and congestion of eyes. Very rarely, general reactions have been observed, particularly in patients with allergic tendencies. These include cutaneous allergy, attack of asthma, urticaria and nausea.

Overdosage: There are no reports of any overdosage and the management should be symptomatic and supportive.

Pharmacological properties

Pharmacodynamic properties: Fusafungine is a topical antibiotic produced by Fusanium Luteritium strain 347, with anti-inflammatory properties. It is bacteriostatic.

Pharmacokinetic properties: Topical use. No systemic absorption of fusafungine has been shown.

Preclinical safety data: Preclinical safety tests which included studies and repeated administration of fusafungine by inhalation and assay of genotoxic potential revealed no findings of relevance to the prescribing clinician.

Pharmaceutical particulars

List of excipients: Flavour composition 14869, Ethanol, Saccharin, Isopropyl myristate.

Incompatibilities: None known.

Shelf life: 24 months.

Special precautions of storage: Store below 25°C.

Nature and contents of container: 15 ml type III glass bottle (plasticised with PVC) sealed with a plastic metered dose pump, containing 2.5 ml solution corresponding to approx. 50 metered doses.

Instructions for use/handling: Before the very first use, press 5 times on the main adapter so as to prime the pump. The bottle must be held upright between the thumb and index finger with the adapter uppermost.

To administer the drug, place the mouth adapter (white) in the mouth, closing the lips around it. Then press firmly and at length on the adapter while inhaling as for normal breathing.

Use the same procedure for nasal administration, after fitting the nasal adapter (yellow) on the bottle.

Marketing authorisation number 00093/0073

Date of first authorisation/renewal of authorisation 9 October 1996

Date of (partial) revision of the text August 1996

Legal category POM

NATRILIX*

Qualitative and quantitative composition Indapamide hemihydrate 2.5 mg

Pharmaceutical form White film-coated lenticular tablets.

Clinical particulars

Therapeutic indications: For the treatment of essential hypertension. Natrilix may be used as sole therapy or combined with other antihypertensive agents.

Posology and method of administration:

Adults: The dosage is one tablet, containing 2.5 mg indapamide hemihydrate, daily, to be taken in the morning. The action of Natrilix is progressive and the reduction in blood pressure may continue and not reach a maximum until several months after the start of therapy. A larger dose than 2.5 mg Natrilix daily is not recommended as there is no appreciable additional antihypertensive effect but a diuretic effect may become apparent. If a single daily tablet of Natrilix does not achieve a sufficient reduction in blood pressure, another antihypertensive agent may be added; those which have been used in combination with Natrilix include beta-blockers, ACE inhibitors, methyldopa, clonidine and other adrenergic blocking agents. The co-administration of Natrilix with diuretics which may cause hypokalaemia is not recommended.

There is no evidence of rebound hypertension on withdrawal of Natrilix.

Elderly: There are no significant changes in the pharmacokinetics of indapamide in the elderly. Numerous clinical studies have shown that it can be used without problems, and, indeed has a particular benefit on systolic blood pressure in the elderly.

Children: There is no experience of the use of this drug in children.

Contra-indications: Natrilix is not recommended in patients with:

- recent cerebrovascular accident,
- severe hepatic failure,
- a known history of allergy to sulphonamide derivatives.

Special warnings and precautions for use:

- Blood potassium and urate levels should be closely monitored:
  - in patients predisposed or sensitive to hypokalaemia (cardiac patients treated with glycosides, elderly, or patients suffering from hyperaldosteronism);
  - in patients suffering from gout.
- In case of an aggravation of pre-existing renal insufficiency, it is recommended to interrupt the treatment with Natrilix.
- In patients with hyperparathyroidism, the treatment with Natrilix should be interrupted on the occurrence of hypercalcaemia.
- Studies in functionally anephric patients for one month undergoing chronic haemodialysis, have not shown evidence of drug accumulation despite the fact that indapamide is not dialysable.
- Although indapamide 2.5 mg daily (one tablet) can be safely administered to hypertensive patients with impaired renal function, the treatment should be discontinued if there are signs of increasing renal insufficiency.

Interactions with other medicaments and other forms of interaction: The concomitant administration of the following medicaments with Natrilix is not recommended:

- Diuretics (risk of electrolyte imbalance);
- Antiarrhythmics such as quinidine derivatives, cardiac glycosides, corticoids or laxatives, in case of hypokalaemia;
- Lithium (increase in blood levels due to a diminished urinary excretion of lithium).

Pregnancy and lactation:

Pregnancy: No teratological effects have been seen in animals but because animal reproduction studies are not always predictive of human response, Natrilix should be used during pregnancy only if clearly needed.

Lactation: It is not known if Natrilix is excreted in human milk.

Because most drugs are excreted in human milk, if use of Natrilix is deemed essential, the patient should stop nursing.

Effects on ability to drive and use machines: There is no evidence of any adverse effect on mental alertness.

Undesirable effects:

- Hypokalaemia, headache, dizziness, fatigue, muscular cramps, nausea, anorexia, diarrhoea, constipation, dyspepsia and cutaneous rash may occur as a result of treatment with Natrilix.
- There have been some rare reports of orthostatic hypotension, palpitations, increase in liver enzymes, blood dyscrasias including thrombocytopaenia, hyponatraemia, metabolic alkaloses, hyperglycaemia, increase in blood urate levels, paraesthesia, erythema multiform, epidermal necrolysis, photosensitivity, impotence, renal insufficiency and reversible acute myopia.
- At the dosage recommended for hypertension, indapamide does not usually adversely influence plasma triglycerides, LDL cholesterol or the LDL-HDL cholesterol ratio. Indapamide does not appear to adversely affect glucose tolerance when used in patients with diabetes and also in non diabetics.

Overdosage: Symptoms of overdosage would be those associated with a diuretic effect: electrolyte disturbances, hypotension and muscular weakness.

Treatment would be symptomatic, directed at correcting the electrolyte abnormalities and gastric lavage or emesis should be considered.

Pharmacological properties

Pharmacodynamic properties: Natrilix (indapamide) is a non-thiazide sulphonamide with an indole ring, belonging to the diuretic family. At the dose of 2.5 mg per day Natrilix exerts a prolonged antihypertensive activity in hypertensive human subjects. Dose-effect studies have demonstrated that, at the dose of 2.5 mg per day, the antihypertensive effect is maximal and the diuretic effect is sub-clinical. At this antihypertensive dose of 2.5 mg per day, Natrilix reduces vascular hyperreactivity to noradrenaline in hypertensive patients and decreases total peripheral resistance and arteriolar resistance.

The implication of an extrarenal mechanism of action in the antihypertensive effect is demonstrated by maintenance of its antihypertensive efficacy in functionally anephric hypertensive patients.

The vascular mechanism of action of Natrilix involves:

- a reduction in the contractility of vascular smooth muscle due to a modification of transmembrane ion exchanges, essentially calcium;
- vasodilatation due to stimulation of the synthesis of prostaglandin PGE 2 and the vasodilator and platelet antiaggregant prostacyclin PG12;
- potentiation of the vasodilator action of bradykynin.

It has also been demonstrated that in the short-, medium- and long-term, in hypertensive patients, Natrilix:

- reduces left ventricular hypertrophy;
- does not appear to alter lipid metabolism: triglycerides, LDL-cholesterol and HDL-cholesterol;
- does not appear to alter glucose metabolism, even in diabetic hypertensive patients. Normalisation of blood pressure and a significant reduction in microalbuminuria have been observed after prolonged administration of Natrilix in diabetic hypertensive subjects.

Lastly, the co-prescription of Natrilix with other antihypertensives (beta-blockers, calcium channel blockers, angiotensin converting enzyme inhibitors) results in an improved control hypertension with an increased percentage of responders compared to that observed with single-agent therapy.

Pharmacokinetic properties: Indapamide is rapidly and completely absorbed after oral administration. Peak blood levels are obtained after 1 to 2 hours.

Indapamide is concentrated in the erythrocytes and is 79% bound to plasma protein and to erythrocytes. It is taken up by the vascular wall in smooth vascular muscle according to its high lipid solubility. 70% of a single oral dose is eliminated by the kidneys and 23% by the gastrointestinal tract. Indapamide is metabolised to a marked degree with 7% of the unchanged product found in the urine during the 48 hours following administration. Elimination half life (β phase) of indapamide is approximately 15–18 hours.

Preclinical safety data: No findings in the preclinical testing which could be of relevance for the prescriber.

Pharmaceutical particulars

List of excipients: Lactose, Maize starch, magnesium stearate, talc, povidone.

Tablet coating: glycerol, white beeswax, sodium lauryl sulphate, methylhydroxy propylcellulose, polyoxyethylene glycol 6000, magnesium stearate, titanium dioxide.

Incompatibilities: None stated.

Shelf life: 5 years.

Special precautions for storage: None.

Nature and contents of container: 30 tablets pack: 1 blister strip (PVC/Aluminium) of 30 tablets per carton. 60 tablets pack: 2 blister strip (PVC/Aluminium) of 30 tablets per carton.

Instruction for use/handling: Not applicable.

Marketing authorisation number PL 0093/0022

Date of first authorisation/renewal of authorisation

Date of grant 20 December 1977

Date of last grant 20 February 1993

Date of (partial) revision of the text March 1998

Legal category POM.

NATRILIX SR*

Qualitative and quantitative composition Indapamide 1.5 mg.

Pharmaceutical form Sustained release coated tablet.

Clinical particulars

Therapeutic indications: Essential hypertension.

Posology and method of administration: Oral administration.

One tablet per 24 hours, preferably in the morning. At higher doses the antihypertensive action of indapamide is not enhanced but the saluretic effect is increased.

Contra-indications: Hypersensitivity to sulphonamides.

Severe renal failure.

Hepatic encephalopathy or severe impairment of liver function.

Hypokalaemia.

Special warnings and special precautions for use:
Warnings: When liver function is impaired, thiazide-related diuretics may cause hepatic encephalopathy. Administration of the diuretic must be stopped immediately if this occurs.

Precautions:
Water and electrolyte balance: Plasma sodium: This must be measured before starting treatment, then at regular intervals subsequently. Any diuretic treatment may cause hyponatraemia, sometimes with very serious consequences. The fall in plasma sodium may be asymptomatic initially and regular monitoring is therefore essential, and should be even more frequent in the elderly and cirrhotic patients (see *Adverse reactions* and *Overdose* sections).

Plasma potassium: Potassium depletion with hypokalaemia is the major risk of thiazide and related diuretics. The risk of onset of hypokalaemia (<3.4 mmol/l) must be prevented in certain high risk populations, i.e. the elderly, malnourished and/or polymedicated, cirrhotic patients with oedema and ascites, coronary artery disease and cardiac failure patients. In this situation, hypokalaemia increases the cardiac toxicity of digitalis preparations and the risks of arrhythmias.

Individuals with a long QT interval are also at risk, whether the origin is congenital or iatrogenic. Hypokalaemia, as well as bradycardia, is then a predisposing factor to the onset of severe arrhythmias, in particular, potentially fatal torsades de pointes.

More frequent monitoring of plasma potassium is required in all the situations indicated above. The first measurement of plasma potassium should be obtained during the first week following the start of treatment. Detection of hypokalaemia requires its correction.

Plasma calcium: Thiazide and related diuretics may decrease urinary calcium excretion and cause a slight and transitory rise in plasma calcium. Frank hypercalcaemia may be due to previously unrecognised hyperparathyroidism. Treatment should be withdrawn before the investigation of parathyroid function.

Blood glucose: Monitoring of blood glucose is important in diabetics, in particular in the presence of hypokalaemia.

Uric acid: Tendency to gout attacks may be increased in hyperuricaemic patients.

Renal function and diuretics: Thiazide and related diuretics are fully effective only when renal function is normal or only minimally impaired (plasma creatinine below levels of the order of 25 mg/l, i.e. 220 µmol/l in an adult). In the elderly, this plasma creatinine must be adjusted in relation to age, weight and gender.

Hypovolaemia, secondary to the loss of water and sodium induced by the diuretic at the start of treatment causes a reduction in glomerular filtration. This may lead to an increase in blood urea and plasma creatinine. This transitory functional renal insufficiency is of no consequence in individuals with normal renal function but may worsen preexisting renal insufficiency.

Athletes: The attention of athletes is drawn to the fact that this drug contains an active ingredient which may give a positive reaction in doping tests.

Interactions with other drugs and other types of interactions
Inadvisable combinations
Lithium: Increased plasma lithium with signs of overdose, as with a salt-free diet (decreased urinary lithium excretion). However, if the use of diuretics is necessary, careful monitoring of plasma lithium and dose adjustment are required.

Non-antiarrhythmic drugs prolonging the QT interval or causing torsade de pointes (astemizol, bepridil, IV-erythromycin, halofantrine, pentamidine, sultopride, terfenadine, vincamine): Torsade de pointes (hypokalaemia is a predisposing factor, the same applying to bradycardia and a preexisting long QT interval). Use substances which do not have the disadvantage of causing torsade de pointes in the presence of hypokalaemia.

Combinations requiring precautions
NSAIDs (systemic), high dose salicylates: Possible decrease in antihypertensive effect of indapamide. Acute renal failure in dehydrated patients (decreased glomerular filtration). Hydrate the patient; monitor renal function at the start of treatment.

Other compounds causing hypokalaemia: amphotericin B (IV), gluco- and mineralocorticoids (systemic), tetracosactide, stimulant laxatives: Increased risk of hypokalaemia (additive effect). Monitoring of plasma potassium and correction if required. Must be particularly borne in mind in case of concomitant digitalis treatment. Use non-stimulant laxatives.

Baclofen: Increased antihypertensive effect. Hydrate the patient; monitor renal function at the start of treatment.

Digitalis preparations: Hypokalaemia predisposing to the toxic effects of digitalis. Monitoring of plasma potassium, ECG and, if necessary, adjust treatment.

Combinations which must be taken into consideration
Potassium-sparing diuretics (amiloride, spironolactone, triamterene): Such rational combinations, useful in certain patients, do not eliminate the possibility of hypokalaemia or, in particular in renal failure and diabetic patients, of hyperkalaemia. Monitor plasma potassium, ECG if required and adjust treatment if necessary.

Angiotensin converting enzyme (ACE) inhibitors: Risk of sudden hypotension and/or acute renal failure when treatment with a converting enzyme inhibitor is started in the presence of preexisting sodium depletion (in particular in individuals with renal artery stenosis).

In hypertension, when prior diuretic treatment may have caused sodium depletion, it is necessary:
- either to stop the diuretic 3 days before starting treatment with the ACE inhibitor, and restart a hypokalaemic diuretic if necessary;
- or give low initial doses of the ACE inhibitor and increase only gradually.

In congestive cardiac failure, start with a very low dose of ACE inhibitor, possibly after a reduction in the dose of the combined hypokalaemic diuretic.

In all cases, monitor renal function (plasma creatinine) during the first weeks of treatment with an ACE inhibitor.

Antiarrhythmic agents causing torsade de pointes: Group Ia antiarrhythmic drugs (quinidine, hydroquinidine, disopyramide), amiodarone, bretylium, sotalol: Torsade de pointes (hypokalaemia is a predisposing factor, the same applying to bradycardia and a preexisting long QT interval). Prevention of hypokalaemia and, if necessary, correction; monitoring of QT interval. In cases of torsade de pointes, do not give antiarrhythmic drugs (management by pacemaker).

Metformin: In the presence of functional renal insufficiency related to diuretics and more particularly to loop diuretics, increased risk of metformin induced lactic acidosis.

Do not use metformin when plasma creatinine exceeds 15 mg/litre (135 µmol/litre) in men and 12 mg/litre (110 µmol/litre) in women.

Iodinated contrast media: In the presence of dehydration caused by diuretics, increased risk of acute renal failure, in particular when large doses of iodinated contrast media are used.

Rehydration before administration of the iodinated compound.

Combinations which must be taken into consideration
Imipramine-like antidepressants (tricyclics), neuroleptics: Antihypertensive effect and risk of orthostatic hypotension increased (additive effect).

Calcium salts: Risk of hypercalcaemia resulting from decreased urinary calcium elimination.

Cyclosporin: Risk of increased plasma creatinine without any change in circulating cyclosporin levels, even in the absence of water/sodium depletion.

Corticosteroids, tetracosactide (systemic): Decreased antihypertensive effect (water/sodium retention due to corticosteroids).

Pregnancy and lactation
Pregnancy: As a general rule, the administration of diuretics should be avoided in pregnant women and should never be used to treat physiological oedema of pregnancy. Diurectics can cause fetoplacental ischaemia, with a risk of impaired fetal growth.

Breast-feeding: Breast-feeding is inadvisable (Indapamide is excreted in human milk).

Effects on ability to drive and use machines: Natrilix SR does not affect vigilance but different reactions in relation to the decrease in blood pressure may occur in individual cases, especially at the start of the treatment or when another antihypertensive agent is added. As a result the ability to drive vehicles or to operate machinery may be impaired.

Undesirable effects: The majority of adverse effects concerning clinical or laboratory parameters are dose-dependent. Thiazide-related diuretics, including indapamide, may cause:

Regarding laboratory parameters: Potassium depletion with hypokalaemia, particularly serious in certain high risk populations (see *Precautions*). During clinical trials, hypokalaemia (plasma potassium ≤3.4 mmol/l) was seen in 10% of patients and <3.2 mmol/l in 4% of patients after 4 to 6 weeks' treatment. After 12 weeks' treatment, the mean fall in plasma potassium was 0.23 mmol/l.

Hyponatraemia with hypovolaemia responsible for dehydration and orthostatic hypotension. Concomitant loss of chloride ions may lead to secondary compensatory metabolic alkalosis: the incidence and degree of this effect are slight.

An increase in plasma uric acid and blood glucose during treatment: appropriateness of these diuretics must be very carefully weighed in patients with gout or diabetes.

Haematological events, very rare: thrombocytopenia, leucopenia, agranulocytosis, aplastic anaemia, haemolytic anaemia.

Hypercalcaemia – extremely rare.

Regarding clinical parameters: In the presence of hepatic insufficiency, possible onset of hepatic encephalopathy (see *Contra-indications* and *Warnings*).

Hypersensitivity reactions, essentially dermatological, in individuals predisposed to allergic and asthmatic manifestations.

Maculopapular rashes, purpura, possible worsening of preexisting acute disseminated lupus erythematosis.

Nausea, constipation, dry mouth, vertigo, fatigue, paraesthesia, headache, occurring rarely and responding in most instances to a dose reduction.

Very rarely, pancreatitis.

Overdose: Indapamide has been found to be free of toxicity at up to 40 mg, i.e. 27 times the therapeutic dose.

Signs of acute poisoning take the form above all of water/electrolyte disturbances (hyponatremia, hypokalaemia). Clinically, possibility of nausea, vomiting, hypotension, cramps, vertigo, drowsiness, confusion, polyuria or oliguria possibly to the point of anuria (by hypovolaemia). Initial measures involve the rapid elimination of the ingested substance(s) by gastric wash-out and/or administration of activated charcoal, followed by restoration of water/electrolyte balance to normal in a specialised centre.

Pharmacological properties
Pharmacodynamic properties: Antihypertensive diuretic. Indapamide is a sulphonamide derivative with an indole ring, pharmacologically related to thiazide diuretics, which acts by inhibiting the reabsorption of sodium in the proximal segment of the distal renal tubule. It increases the urinary excretion of sodium and chlorides and, to a lesser extent, the excretion of potassium and magnesium, thereby increasing urine output and having an antihypertensive action.

Phase II and III studies using monotherapy have demonstrated an antihypertensive effect lasting 24 hours. This was present at doses where the diuretic effect was of mild intensity.

The antihypertensive activity of indapamide is related to an improvement in arterial compliance and a reduction in arteriolar and total peripheral resistance. Indapamide reduces left ventricular hypertrophy.

Thiazide and related diuretics have a plateau therapeutic effect beyond a certain dose, while adverse effects continue to increase. The dose should not be increased if treatment is ineffective.

It has also been shown, in the short, mid and long term in hypertensive patients, that indapamide:
- does not interfere with lipid metabolism: tryglycerides, LDL-cholesterol and HDL-cholesterol;
- does not interfere with carbohydrate metabolism, even in diabetic hypertensive patients.

Pharmacokinetic properties: Indapamide 1.5 mg is supplied in a sustained release dosage based on a matrix system in which the active ingredient is dispersed in a support which allows sustained release of indapamide.

Absorption: The fraction of indapamide released is rapidly and totally absorbed via the gastrointestinal digestive tract.

Eating slightly increases the rapidity of absorption but has no influence on the amount of the drug absorbed.

Peak serum level following a single dose occurs about 12 hours after ingestion, repeated administration reduces the variation in serum levels between 2 doses.

Intra-individual variability exists.

Distribution: Binding of indapamide to plasma proteins is 79%. The plasma elimination half-life is 14 to 24 hours (mean 18 hours). Steady state is achieved after 7 days. Repeated administration does not lead to accumulation.

Metabolism: Elimination is essentially urinary (70% of the dose) and faecal (22%) in the form of inactive metabolites.

High risk individuals: Pharmacokinetic parameters are unchanged in renal failure patients.

Preclinical safety data: The highest doses administered orally to different animal species (40 to 8000 times the therapeutic dose) have shown an exacerbation of the saluretic properties of indapamide. The major symptoms of poisoning in acute toxicity studies with indapamide administered intravenously or intraperitoneally were related to the pharmacological action of indapamide, i.e. bradypnoea and peripheral vasodilation.

Pharmaceutical particulars
List of excipients: Anhydrous colloidal silica, glycerol, hydroxypropylmethylcellulose, lactose, macrogol

6000, magnesium stearate, polyvidone, titanium dioxide.

Incompatibilities: Not applicable.

Shelf life: 2 years.

Special precautions for storage: Store in a dry place at room temperature (15–25°C).

Nature and contents of container: Blister sheet (PVC/Aluminium).

Instructions for use/handling: Not applicable.

Marketing authorisation holder: Les Laboratoires Servier, 905, route de Saran, 45520 Gidy, France.

Marketing authorisation number 05815/0010

Date of approval/revision of SPC January 1996

Legal category POM

NITROMIN SPRAY

Qualitative and quantitative composition Glyceryl Trinitrate 400 micrograms/dose.

Pharmaceutical form Oromucosal spray.

Clinical particulars
Therapeutic indications: For the treatment and prophylaxis of angina pectoris.

Posology and method of administration:
Adult: At the onset of the attack: 1 or 2 sprays (400–800 micrograms). Dose should not exceed more than 3 sprays at any one time.

For prophylaxis: 1–2 sprays (400–800 micrograms) immediately prior to an angina inducing event.

The patient should be in a sitting position. The spray should be held upright and should not be inhaled. After spraying under the tongue the mouth should be closed immediately after each dose.

Elderly: As adult.

Children: Not recommended.

Contra-indications: Hypersensitivity to nitrates. Hypotensive shock. Severe anaemia. Cerebral haemorrhage and brain trauma. Mitral stenosis. Angina caused by hypertrophic obstructive cardiomyopathy.

Special warnings and special precautions for use: Tolerance and cross-tolerance to other nitrates may occur.

Interactions with other medicaments and other forms of interaction: Alcohol may potentiate the hypotensive effects of glyceryl trinitrate.

Nitromin may be employed in conjunction with other nitrate containing products, but care should be taken to avoid excessive total intake. In practical terms this means that sublingual GTN tablets should not be taken in addition to Nitromin for the same anginal attack unless under close medical supervision (this does not apply to long acting nitrate preparations used for attack prevention).

Pregnancy and lactation: There are no specific data available on the use of Nitromin in human pregnancy. Since angina is uncommon in pregnancy it is unlikely that the need for Nitromin would arise. In all cases, the benefit of treatment to the patient must be balanced against any possible hazard to the foetus. There is no information available regarding the excretion of glyceryl trinitrate in breast milk.

Effects on ability to drive and use machines: Nitromin should not impair ability to drive or use machinery, however, patients should be advised not to drive etc. if they feel unwell or faint after using the spray.

Undesirable effects: The following side effects occur in approximately 30–40% of patients: taste disturbance (metallic taste), headache, postural hypotension, flushing and palpitations. These are usually mild and disappear within a few minutes.

Overdose:
Symptoms – flushing, severe headache, a feeling of suffocation, hypotension, fainting. Rarely cyanosis and methaemoglobinaemia. In a few patients a reaction comparable to shock with nausea, vomiting, weakness, sweating and syncope.

Emergency procedures – recovery often occurs without special treatment. Elevate legs to promote venous return.

Antidote – treat methaemoglobinaemia with intravenous methylene blue. Treat symptomatically for serious respiratory and circulatory effects.

Pharmacological properties
Pharmacodynamic properties: Glyceryl Trinitrate relaxes smooth muscle and reduces blood pressure. Its anti-anginal effects are believed to depend on reducing myocardial oxygen demand by means of peripheral vasodilation.

Pharmacokinetic properties: The onset of action following sublingual administration is within 2 minutes. Duration of action is about 30 minutes.

Preclinical safety data: None stated.

Pharmaceutical particulars
List of excipients: Ethanol, Propylene glycol.

Incompatibilities: None known.

Shelf life: Opened and unopened: 36 months.

Special precautions for storage: Store below 25°C. Protect from light and do not expose to temperature above 50°C. Do not pierce or burn after use. Do not spray onto a naked flame or any incandescent material.

Nature and contents of container: Aluminium canister with a metered dosing valve and nozzle. Plastic protective cap. Each 180 dose canister contains 10 g of solution. Each 200 dose canister contains 10.55 g of solution.

Instructions for use/handling: None stated.

Marketing authorisation number PL 00093/0078

Date of first authorisation/renewal of authorisation
2 December 1998

Date of (partial) revision of the text July 1998

**Trade Mark*

Seton Scholl Healthcare plc
Tubiton House
Oldham OL1 3HS

☎ 0161 652 2222 0161 626 9090

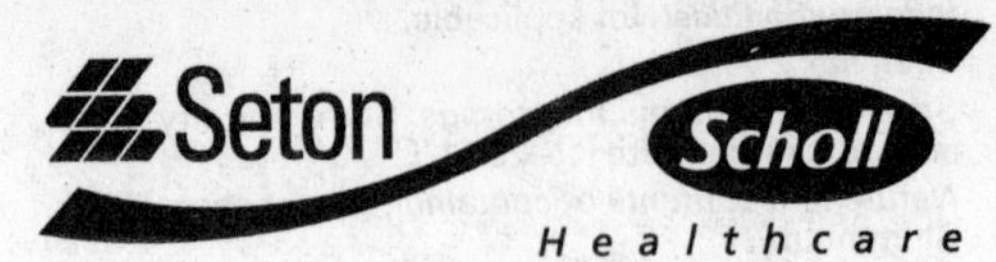

AQUASEPT* SKIN CLEANSER

Qualitative and quantitative composition Triclosan 2.0% w/v.

Pharmaceutical form Clear blue solution.

Clinical particulars
Therapeutic indications: This product has an antibacterial effect and is intended for the following uses:
- Prevention of cross infection
- Prevention of self infection
- Preoperative hand disinfection
- Antiseptic skin cleansing
- Whole body bathing prior to elective surgery
- Whole body bathing to help eliminate the carriage of pathogens

Posology and method of administration:
For preoperative hand disinfection: (100 ml, 250 ml and 500 ml). Wet area to be cleaned. Apply about 5 ml of Aquasept and wash for one minute, paying particular attention to the area around the fingernails and cuticles and between the fingers. Rinse and repeat for two minutes. Rinse thoroughly and dry hands with a sterile towel.

For antiseptic skin cleansing: (100 ml, 250 ml and 500 ml). Wet area to be cleaned and use Aquasept as a liquid soap, washing thoroughly for one minute. Rinse and dry thoroughly.

For whole body bathing: (28.5 ml, 100 ml, 250 ml and 500 ml). In shower or bath, use Aquasept as a liquid soap, paying particular attention to the hair, perineum, groin, axillae and nares. Take two baths or showers on the two days prior to surgery. Approximately 28.5 ml of Aquasept will suffice for one shower or bath.

Contra-indications: None indicated.

Special warnings and precautions for use: For external use only. Avoid contact with eyes. Keep out of the reach of children. Some product excipients may give rise to allergic reactions in some people. In this instance, seek medical advice.

Interactions with other medicaments and other forms of interaction: None stated.

Pregnancy and lactation: None stated.

Effects on ability to drive and use machines: None stated.

Undesirable effects: None stated.

Overdose: Ingestion: Gastric lavage and symptomatic treatment.

Pharmacological properties
Pharmacodynamic properties: Triclosan is a bactericide.

Pharmacokinetic properties: None stated.

Pre-clinical safety data: None stated.

Pharmaceutical particulars
List of excipients: De-ionised water; MEA lauryl sulphate; Cocamide DEA; Cocamidopropyl betaine; Isopropyl Alcohol; Propylene Glycol; Tetrasodium EDTA and Triethanolamide; Chlorocresol; sea fresh perfume; Blue 42051 (E131).

Incompatibilities: None stated.

Shelf life: 36 months.

Special precautions for storage: None stated.

Nature and contents of container: HDPE or HDPP container. Polypropylene wadless screw caps or compression moulded screw caps with steran faced pulpboard liners. Sizes: 28.5 ml, 100 ml, 250 ml and 500 ml.

Instruction for use/handling: Not applicable.

Marketing authorisation number 11314/0096.

Date of approval/revision of SPC September 1997.

Legal category GSL.

ASILONE* SUSPENSION

Qualitative and quantitative composition Asilone Suspension contains, in each 5 ml, Light Magnesium Oxide BP 70.0 mg, Aluminium Hydroxide BP 420.0 mg and Activated Dimethicone 135.0 mg.

Pharmaceutical form Suspension.

Clinical particulars
Therapeutic indications: Anti-flatulent and antacid; for the relief of dyspeptic symptoms of functional or organic origin, including flatulence and associated abdominal distension, heartburn, including heartburn of pregnancy, hiatus hernia, and oesophagitis, symptomatic management of gastritis and peptic ulceration.

Posology and method of administration:
Adults including the elderly: One to two 5 ml spoonfuls after meals and at bedtime or when required, up to a maximum of four times daily.
Use within 28 days of opening.
Children: Not recommended for children under 12 years of age.

Contra-indications: Antacid preparations should not be administered in severe debilitation or renal impairment. Do not use during the first trimester of pregnancy.

Special warnings and precautions for use: Asilone is not recommended in flatulent abdominal distension possibly related to intestinal obstruction.

Interactions with other medicaments and other forms of interaction: Antacids may interfere with the absorption of tetracyclines, rifampicin, warfarin and digoxin if given concomitantly.

Use in pregnancy and lactation: Antacid preparations are not recommended during the first trimester of pregnancy.

Effects on ability to drive and use machines: None stated.

Undesirable effects: Aluminium salts may cause constipation and magnesium salts diarrhoea. However, such bowel disturbances are rare with the formulation of Asilone.

Overdose: No cases of overdosage have been reported with Asilone. The components of Asilone are not expected to cause specific local or systemic toxicity even in acute overdosage in healthy individuals. No special treatment, but symptomatic management only if indicated.

Pharmacological properties
Pharmacodynamic properties: The active ingredients of Asilone Suspension possess antacid and antiflatulent properties which are long established; their actions in a wide variety of gastro-intestinal disorders are well recognised in standard texts. Light magnesium oxide and aluminium hydroxide are potent antacids which increase gastric pH and hence diminish the activity of pepsin in gastric secretion. In addition, aluminium hydroxide has a direct inhibiting effect on pepsin. Silicones are useful anti-foaming agents and the addition of 4-8% of finely divided silicon dioxide increases the anti-foaming activity of dimethicones. Dimethicones activated by silicone dioxide act by changing the surface tension of gas bubbles, thereby causing them to coalesce.

Pharmacokinetic properties: No data on pharmacokinetic studies with Asilone are available. Aluminium hydroxide and activated dimethicone are not generally absorbed. Some magnesium may be absorbed from magnesium oxide in Asilone Suspension, but is generally rapidly excreted in urine.

Pre-clinical safety data: Not stated.

Pharmaceutical particulars
List of excipients: Potassium Sorbate BP; Sodium Saccharin BP; Sorbitol (or Sorbiton Solution 70 % Non Cryst) BP; Flavex Peppermint/Aniseed Flavour L263; Flavex Flavour Modifier No.12; Hydrogen Peroxide (30% v/v) BP; Methyl Parahydroxybenzoate PhEur; Propyl Parahydroxybenzoate PhEur; Purified Water PhEur.

Incompatibilities: None stated.

Shelf life: The product has a shelf life of two years but must be used within 28 days of opening.

Special precautions for storage: Do not freeze.

Nature and contents of container: Bottle of high density polyethylene in blue with a white polypropylene cap or a white polyethylene tamper evident cap with a low density polyethylene inner core liner, containing 500 ml of product.

Marketing authorisation number 11314/0034.

Date of approval/revision of SPC May 1995.

Legal category GSL.

BETADINE* ALCOHOLIC SOLUTION

Presentation A golden brown alcoholic solution containing Povidone Iodine USP 10%w/v.

Uses For use as an antiseptic skin cleanser for major and minor surgical procedures where a quick drying effect is desired. For topical administration.

Dosage and administration
Adults: Apply full strength as an antiseptic skin cleanser.

Children and the elderly: As for adults.
Povidone iodine is not recommended for regular use in neonates and is contra-indicated in very low birth weight infants (below 1500 grams).

Contra-indications, warnings, etc
Contra-indications: Known or suspected iodine hypersensitivity. Regular use is contra-indicated in patients or users with thyroid disorders (in particular nodular colloid goitre, endemic goitre and Hashimoto's thyroiditis).

Interactions: Absorption of iodine from povidone iodine may interfere with thyroid function tests. Contamination with povidone iodine of several types of tests for the detection of occult blood in faeces or blood in urine may produce false-positive results.

Effect on ability to drive and to use machines: None known.

Side effects and adverse reactions: Povidone iodine may produce local skin reactions although it is considered to be less irritant than iodine. The application of povidone iodine to large wounds or severe burns may produce systemic adverse effects such as metabolic acidosis, hypernatraemia, and impairment of renal function.

Use in pregnancy and lactation: Regular use of povidone iodine should be avoided in pregnant or lactating women as absorbed iodine can cross the placental barrier and can be secreted into breast milk. Although no adverse effects have been reported from limited use, caution should be recommended and therapeutic benefit must be balanced against possible effects of the absorption of iodine on foetal thyroid function and development.

Other special precautions and warnings: Special caution is needed when regular applications to broken skin are made to patients with pre-existing renal insufficiency. Regular use should be avoided in patients on concurrent lithium therapy. This preparation is flammable and caution is advised during surgical procedures involving hot wire cautery or diathermy.

Overdose: Excess iodine can produce goitre and hypothyroidism or hyperthyroidism. Systemic absorption of iodine after repeated application of povidone iodine to large areas of wounds or burns may lead to a number of adverse effects: metallic taste in the mouth, increased salivation, burning or pain in the throat or mouth, irritation and swelling of the eyes, skin reactions, gastrointestinal upset and diarrhoea, and difficulty in breathing due to pulmonary oedema. Metabolic acidosis, hypernatraemia and renal impairment may occur. In the case of accidental ingestion of large quantities of Betadine, symptomatic and supportive treatment should be provided with special attention to electrolyte balance and renal and thyroid function.

Pharmaceutical precautions
Storage: Store at or below 25°C. Protect from light.

Legal category P

Package quantities Container of 500 ml.

Further information Betadine Alcoholic Solution has a rapid and prolonged germicidal action and, with repeated use, a cumulative germicidal action. It is active against a wide range of organisms including Gram positive and Gram negative bacteria, fungi, protozoa, viruses, and bacterial spores. In the presence of blood, serum, purulent exudate and necrotic tissue, its activity persists whilst the colour remains.

Product licence number 0223/0010

BETADINE* ANTISEPTIC PAINT

Presentation A golden brown alcoholic solution containing Povidone Iodine USP 10%w/v.

Uses Betadine Antiseptic Paint is a broad spectrum, quick drying antiseptic for the treatment and prevention of infection. It is ideal for herpes simplex, herpes zoster, grazes, abrasions, cuts and wounds or any break in the skin which requires protection from infection. Betadine Antiseptic Paint is effective in the treatment of dermal infections caused by bacteria, fungi, yeasts and viruses (e.g. herpes virus types I and II).

Dosage and administration *Adults and children:* Apply Betadine Antiseptic Paint undiluted as necessary to affected area and allow to dry. Use twice daily and cover with a dressing if desired. Rinse the brush thoroughly after use.

Contra-indications, warnings, etc
Contra-indications: Hypersensitivity to iodine. History of abnormal thyroid function or goitre.

Interactions: None known.

Effect on ability to drive and to use machines: None known.

Side-effects and adverse reactions: Povidone iodine may produce local skin reactions although it is less irritant than iodine. The application of povidone iodine to large wounds or severe burns may produce systemic adverse effects such as metabolic acidosis, hypernatraemia, and impairment of renal function.

Use in pregnancy and lactation: Use in pregnancy and lactation should be limited to minor lesions only and although no adverse effects are anticipated from such limited use, caution is recommended and the therapeutic benefit must be balanced against the possible effect of the absorption of iodine on foetal thyroid development and function.

Other special precautions and warnings: If local irritation or sensitivity develop, then discontinue treatment.

Overdose: In the case of deliberate or accidental ingestion of large quantities of Betadine, symptomatic and supportive treatment should be provided with special attention to electrolyte balance and renal and thyroid function.

Pharmaceutical precautions
Storage: Store at or below 25°C. Protect from light.

Legal category P

Package quantities Glass bottle containing 8 ml with an applicator brush.

Further information Betadine Antiseptic Paint has a rapid and prolonged germicidal action against a wide range of organisms including Gram positive and Gram negative bacteria, fungi, protozoa and viruses. It is also active against bacterial spores. In the presence of blood, serum, purulent exudate and necrotic tissue, its activity persists whilst the golden brown colour remains.

Product licence number 0223/0011

BETADINE CREAM

Presentation A reddish brown cream containing Povidone Iodine USP 5%w/w.

Uses Betadine Cream is a broad spectrum antiseptic for the treatment and prevention of infection in minor cuts, abrasions and small areas of burns. It is also used for the treatment of mycotic and bacterial skin infections and pyodermas.

Dosage and administration
Adults, the elderly and children aged 2 years and over: The affected skin should be cleaned and dried. Apply Betadine Cream to the affected area as required. May be covered with a dressing or bandage.

Contra-indications, warnings etc
Contra-indications: Known or suspected iodine hypersensitivity. Regular use is contra-indicated in patients or users with thyroid disorders (in particular nodular colloid goitre, endemic goitre and Hashimoto's thyroiditis). Not for use in children under 2 years of age.

Interaction: Absorption of iodine from povidone iodine through either intact or damaged skin may interfere with thyroid function tests. Contamination with povidone iodine of several types of tests for the detection of occult blood in faeces or blood in urine may produce false-positive results.

Effect on ability to drive and use machines: None known.

Side effects and adverse reactions: Povidone iodine may produce local skin reactions although it is less irritant than iodine. The application of povidone iodine to large wounds or severe burns may produce systemic adverse effects such as metabolic acidosis, hypernatraemia, and impairment of renal function.

Use in pregnancy and lactation: Regular use of povidone iodine should be avoided in pregnant or lactating women as absorbed iodine can cross the placental barrier and can be secreted into breast milk. Although no adverse effects have been reported from limited use, caution should be recommended and therapeutic benefit must be balanced against possible effects of the absorption of iodine on foetal thyroid function and development.

Other special precautions and warnings: Special caution is needed when regular applications to broken skin are made to patients with pre-existing renal insufficiency. Regular use should be avoided in patients on concurrent lithium therapy. Thyroid function tests should be performed during prolonged use.

Overdose: Excess iodine can produce goitre and hypothyroidism or hyperthyroidism. Systemic absorption of iodine after repeated application of povidone iodine to large areas of wounds or burns may lead to a number of adverse effects: metallic taste in the mouth, increased salivation, burning or pain in the throat or mouth, irritation and swelling of the eyes, skin reactions, gastrointestinal upset and diarrhoea, and difficulty in breathing due to pulmonary oedema. Metabolic acidosis, hypernatraemia and renal impairment may occur. In the case of accidental ingestion of large quantities of Betadine, symptomatic and supportive treatment should be provided with special attention to electrolyte balance and renal and thyroid function.

Pharmaceutical precautions
Storage: Store at or below 25°C.

Legal category GSL

Package quantities Tube of 8 g.

Further information Betadine Cream has a rapid and prolonged germicidal action and, with repeated use, a cumulative germicidal action. It is active against a wide range of organisms including Gram positive and Gram negative bacteria, fungi, protozoa, viruses, and bacterial spores. In the presence of blood, serum, purulent exudate and necrotic tissue, its activity persists whilst the colour remains.

Product licence number 0223/0026

Date of preparation October 1997

BETADINE* DRY POWDER SPRAY

Presentation A pressurised aerosol can containing a brown powder consisting of Povidone Iodine USP 2.5%w/w.

Uses For use as a skin antiseptic for the treatment and prevention of infection in wounds, including ulcers, burns, cuts and other minor injuries.

Dosage and administration
Adults and children over 2 years of age: Shake the can well, spray the required area from a distance of 6-10 inches (15–25 cm) until coated with powder. If necessary, the treated area may be covered with a dressing.

Contra-indications, warnings, etc
Contra-indications: Not to be used in serous cavities. Not for use in infants under 2 years. Hypersensitivity to iodine. History of abnormal thyroid function or goitre.

Warnings: Avoid inhalation or spraying into the eyes. If local irritation or sensitivity develops, then discontinue treatment. Iodine is absorbed through burns and broken skin and, to a lesser extent, through intact skin. Following prolonged application of Betadine Dry Powder Spray to severe burns or large areas of denuded skin, systemic effects such as metabolic acidosis, hypernatraemia, renal impairment and thyroid dysfunction may occur.

Interactions: None known.

Effect on ability to drive and to use machines: None known.

Use in pregnancy and lactation: Use in pregnancy and lactation should be limited to minor lesions only and although no adverse effects are anticipated from such limited use, caution is recommended and the therapeutic benefit must be balanced against the possible effect of the absorption of iodine on foetal thyroid development and function.

Overdose: In the case of deliberate or accidental ingestion of large quantities of Betadine, symptomatic and supportive treatment should be provided with special attention to electrolyte balance and thyroid and renal function.

Pharmaceutical precautions
Storage: Store at or below 25°C away from direct heat and sunlight.

Legal category GSL

Package quantities Aerosol can containing 100 ml.

Further information Betadine Dry Powder Spray has a rapid and prolonged germicidal action and, with repeated use, a cumulative germicidal action. It is active against a wide range of organisms including Gram positive and Gram negative bacteria, fungi, protozoa, viruses, and bacterial spores. In the presence of blood, serum, purulent exudate and necrotic tissue, its activity persists whilst the colour remains.

Product licence number 0223/0013

BETADINE* GARGLE AND MOUTHWASH

Presentation A pleasantly flavoured amber coloured solution containing Povidone Iodine USP 1%w/v.

Uses For the treatment of acute mucosal infections of the mouth and pharynx for example, gingivitis and mouth ulcers. For oral hygiene prior to, during and after dental and oral surgery.

Dosage and administration For oral use, as a gargle and mouthwash. The product should not be swallowed.
Adults and children over 6 years of age: Use undiluted or diluted with an equal volume of warm water. Gargle or rinse with up to 10 ml for up to 30 seconds without swallowing. Repeat up to four times daily, for up to 14 consecutive days, or as directed.

Contra-indications, warnings, etc
Contra-indications: Not for use in children under 6 years of age and in patients with a known or suspected iodine hypersensitivity. Regular use is contra-indicated in patients and users with thyroid disorders (in particular nodular colloid goitre, endemic goitre and Hashimoto's thyroiditis) or in pregnant or lactating women.

Interactions: Absorption of iodine from povidone iodine may interfere with thyroid function tests. Contamination with povidone iodine of several types of tests for the detection of occult blood in faeces or blood in urine may produce false-positive results.

Effect on ability to drive and to use machines: None known.

Side-effects and adverse reactions: Idiosyncratic mucosal irritation and hypersensitivity reactions may occur. Excessive absorption of iodine may produce systemic adverse effects such as metabolic acidosis, hypernatraemia and impairment of renal function.

Use in pregnancy and lactation Regular use of povidone iodine should be avoided in pregnant or lactating women as absorbed iodine can cross the placental barrier and can be secreted into breast milk. Although no adverse effects have been reported from limited use, caution should be recommended and therapeutic benefit must be balanced against possible effects of the absorption of iodine on foetal thyroid function and development. The use of Betadine Gargle and Mouthwash in pregnant and lactating women should be limited to a single treatment session only.

Other special precautions and warnings: Regular use should be avoided as prolonged use may lead to the absorption of a significant amount of iodine. Do not use for more than 14 days. If sores or ulcers in the mouth do not heal within 14 days seek medical or dental advice. Regular use should be avoided in patients on concurrent lithium therapy.

Overdose: Excess iodine can produce goitre and hypothyroidism or hyperthyroidism. Acute overdosage may result in symptoms of metallic taste in the mouth, increased salivation, burning or pain in the throat or mouth, irritation and swelling of the eyes, skin reactions, gastrointestinal upset and diarrhoea, and difficulty in breathing due to pulmonary oedema. Metabolic acidosis, hypernatraemia and renal impairment may occur.

In the case of deliberate or accidental ingestion of large quantities of Betadine, symptomatic and supportive treatment should be provided with special attention to electrolyte balance and renal and thyroid function.

Pharmaceutical precautions
Storage: Store at or below 25°C. Protect from light.

Legal category P

Package quantities Bottle of 250 ml.

Further information Betadine Gargle and Mouthwash does not stain the skin, mucous membranes or teeth, despite its powerful germicidal action. It is effective against a wide spectrum of organisms including Gram positive and Gram negative bacteria, fungi, protozoa, viruses and bacterial spores. In the presence of blood, serum, purulent exudate and necrotic tissue, its activity persists while the colour remains.

Product licence number 0223/0014

BETADINE* OINTMENT

Presentation A golden brown water soluble ointment containing Povidone Iodine USP 10%w/w.

Uses Betadine Ointment is a broad spectrum antiseptic for the treatment or prevention of infection in minor cuts and abrasions, minor surgical procedures and small areas of burns. Treatment of mycotic and bacterial skin infections and pyodermas. Treatment of infections in decubitus and stasis ulcers.

Dosage and administration
For the treatment of infection: Apply once or twice daily or at dressing changes for a maximum of 14 days.

For the prevention of infection: Apply once or twice a week for as long as necessary. The affected skin should be cleaned and dried. Apply Ointment to the affected area. May be covered with a dressing or bandage.

Contra-indications, warnings, etc
Contra-indications: Known or suspected iodine hypersensitivity. Regular use is contra-indicated in patients and users with thyroid disorders (in particular nodular colloid goitre, endemic goitre and Hashimoto's thyroiditis). Not for use in infants under 2 years of age.

Interactions: Absorption of iodine from povidone iodine may interfere with thyroid function tests. Contamination with povidone iodine of several types of tests for the detection of occult blood in faeces or blood in urine may produce false-positive results.

Effect on ability to drive and to use machines: None known.

Side-effects and adverse reactions: Povidone iodine may produce local skin reactions although it is less irritant than iodine. The application of povidone iodine to large wounds or severe burns may produce systemic adverse effects such as metabolic acidosis, hypernatraemia, and impairment of renal function.

Use in pregnancy and lactation: Regular use of povidone iodine should be avoided in pregnant or lactating women as absorbed iodine can cross the placental barrier and can be secreted into breast milk. Although no adverse effects have been reported from limited use, caution should be recommended and therapeutic benefit must be balanced against possible effects of the absorption of iodine on foetal thyroid function and development.

Other special precautions and warnings: Special caution is needed when regular applications to broken skin are made to patients with pre-existing renal insufficiency. Regular use should be avoided in patients on concurrent lithium therapy. Thyroid function tests should be performed during prolonged use.

Overdose: Excess iodine can produce goitre and hypothyroidism or hyperthyroidism. Systemic absorption of iodine after repeated application of povidone iodine to large areas of wounds or burns may lead to a number of adverse effects: metallic taste in the mouth, increased salivation, burning or pain in the throat or mouth, irritation and swelling of the eyes, skin reactions, gastrointestinal upset and diarrhoea, and difficulty in breathing due to pulmonary oedema. Metabolic acidosis, hypernatraemia and renal impairment may occur.

In the case of deliberate or accidental ingestion of large quantities of Betadine, symptomatic and supportive treatment should be provided with special attention to electrolyte balance and renal and thyroid function.

Pharmaceutical precautions
Storage: Store at or below 25°C and protect from light.

Legal category GSL.

Package quantities Tube of 20 g and 80 g.

Further information Betadine Ointment has a rapid and prolonged germicidal action and, with repeated use, a cumulative germicidal action. It is active against a wide range of organisms including Gram positive and Gram negative bacteria, fungi, protozoa, viruses, and bacterial spores. In the presence of blood, serum, purulent exudate and necrotic tissue, its activity persists whilst the colour remains.

Product licence number 0223/0015

BETADINE* SHAMPOO

Presentation A golden brown cleansing and sudsing surfactant solution containing Povidone Iodine USP 4%w/v.

Uses Betadine Shampoo is a broad spectrum antiseptic for the treatment of seborrhoeic conditions of the scalp associated with excessive dandruff, pruritus, scaling, exudation and erythema of the scalp, pityriasis capitis; infected lesions of the scalp–pyodermas (recurrent furunculosis, infective folliculitis and impetigo).

Dosage and administration
Adults, the elderly and children over 12 years: Having first wetted the hair, apply 2 to 3 capfuls of Betadine Shampoo, use warm water to lather. Rinse. Apply again 2 to 3 capfuls of Betadine Shampoo and massage into the scalp with the tips of the fingers. Work up to a golden lather using warm water. Repeat treatment twice weekly until improvement is noted. Afterwards, use Betadine Shampoo once a week.

Children aged 2 to 12 years: As for children over 12 years, substituting 1 or 2 capfuls of Betadine Shampoo.

Contra-indications, warnings, etc
Contra-indications: Known or suspected iodine hypersensitivity. Regular use is contra-indicated in patients and users with thyroid disorders (in particular nodular colloid goitre, endemic goitre and Hashimoto's thyroiditis). Not for use in infants under 2 years.

Interactions: Absorption of iodine from povidone iodine may interfere with thyroid function tests. Contamination with povidone iodine of several types of tests for the detection of occult blood in faeces or blood in urine may produce false-positive results.

Effect on ability to drive and to use machines: None known.

Side-effects and adverse reactions: Povidone iodine may produce local skin reactions although it is considered to be less irritant than iodine.

Use in pregnancy and lactation: Regular use of povidone iodine should be avoided in pregnant or lactating women as absorbed iodine can cross the placental barrier and can be secreted into breast milk. Although no adverse effects have been reported from limited use, caution should be recommended and therapeutic benefit must be balanced against possible effects of the absorption of iodine on foetal thyroid function and development.

Other special precautions and warnings: Special caution is needed when regular applications to broken skin are made to patients with pre-existing renal insufficiency. Regular use should be avoided in patients on concurrent lithium therapy.

Overdose: Excess iodine can produce goitre and hypothyroidism or hyperthyroidism. In the case of deliberate or accidental ingestion of large quantities of Betadine, symptomatic and supportive treatment should be provided with special attention to electrolyte balance and renal and thyroid function.

Pharmaceutical precautions
Storage: Store at or below 25°C and protect from light.

Legal category GSL

Package quantities Plastic bottle containing 250 ml.

Further information Betadine Shampoo has a highly effective germicidal activity. This activity is maintained in the presence of exfoliative debris and infected scalp lesions whilst the colour persists. It does not stain the skin.

Product licence number 0223/0021

BETADINE* SKIN CLEANSER

Presentation A penetrating golden brown sudsing surfactant solution containing Povidone Iodine USP 4%w/v.

Uses Betadine Skin Cleanser is a broad spectrum antiseptic for the treatment of acne vulgaris of the face and neck. For general disinfection of the skin (as a liquid soap).

Dosage and administration
Adults, the elderly, and children over 2 years: Apply directly or with moistened sponge to the affected areas and work up a rich lather. Allow to remain on the skin for 3-5 minutes then rinse off thoroughly with warm water and dry with a clean or sterile towel or gauze. Repeat twice daily.

Infants under 2 years: Limit use to 2–3 days.

Contra-indications, warnings, etc
Contra-indications: Hypersensitivity to iodine. History of abnormal thyroid function, or goitre.

Interactions: None known.

Effect on ability to drive and to use machines: None known.

Side-effects and adverse reactions: Povidone iodine may produce local skin reactions although it is considered to be less irritant than iodine.

Use in pregnancy and lactation: Use in pregnancy and lactation should be limited and although no adverse effects are anticipated from such limited use, caution is recommended and the therapeutic benefit must be balanced against possible effects of the absorption of iodine on foetal thyroid function.

Other special precautions and warnings: If local irritation or sensitivity develops, then discontinue treatment. Do not use on broken skin. Iodine is absorbed through burns and broken skin and, to a lesser extent, through intact skin. Restrict use in infants to 2-3 days.

Overdose: In cases of deliberate or accidental ingestion of large quantities of Betadine, symptomatic and supportive treatment should be provided with special attention to electrolyte balance and renal and thyroid function.

Pharmaceutical precautions
Storage: Store at or below 25°C and protect from light.

Legal category GSL.

Package quantities Plastic bottle containing 250 ml.

Further information Betadine Skin Cleanser has a highly effective germicidal activity. This activity is maintained in the presence of exfoliative debris and infected skin lesions, whilst the colour persists. It does not stain the skin.

Product licence number 0223/0027

BETADINE* STANDARDISED ANTISEPTIC SOLUTION

Presentation A golden brown solution containing Povidone Iodine USP 10%w/v.

Uses For use as a pre-operative and post-operative antiseptic skin cleanser for major and minor surgical procedures. For topical administration.

Dosage and administration
Adults, the elderly and children: Apply full strength as a pre-operative and post-operative antiseptic skin cleanser. Avoid pooling both under the patient and in the skin folds. Wash off excess solution before using occlusive dressings.

Povidone iodine is not recommended for regular use in neonates and is contra-indicated in very low birth weight infants (below 1500 grams).

Contra-indications, warnings, etc
Contra-indications: Known or suspected iodine hypersensitivity. Regular use is contra-indicated in patients and users with thyroid disorders (in particular nodular colloid goitre, endemic goitre and Hashimoto's thyroiditis). Betadine Standardised Antiseptic Solution is not recommended for body cavity irrigation.

Interactions: Absorption of iodine from povidone iodine through either intact or damaged skin may interfere with thyroid function tests. Contamination with povidone iodine of several types of tests for the detection of occult blood in faeces or blood in urine may produce false-positive results.

Effect on ability to drive and to use machines: None known.

Side-effects and adverse reactions: Povidone iodine may produce local skin reactions although it is considered to be less irritant than iodine. The application of povidone iodine to large wounds or severe burns may produce systemic adverse effects such as metabolic acidosis, hypernatraemia, and impairment of renal function.

Use in pregnancy and lactation: Regular use of povidone iodine should be avoided in pregnant or lactating women as absorbed iodine can cross the placental barrier and can be secreted into breast milk. Although no adverse effects have been reported from limited use, caution should be recommended and therapeutic benefit must be balanced against possible effects of the absorption of iodine on foetal thyroid function and development.

Other special precautions and warnings: Special caution is needed when regular applications to broken skin are made to patients with pre-existing renal insufficiency. Regular use should be avoided in patients on concurrent lithium therapy.

Overdose: Excess iodine can produce goitre and hypothyroidism or hyperthyroidism. Systemic absorption of iodine after repeated application of povidone iodine to large areas of wounds or burns may lead to a number of adverse effects: metallic taste in the mouth, increased salivation, burning or pain in the throat or mouth, irritation and swelling of the eyes, pulmonary oedema, skin reactions, gastrointestinal upset and diarrhoea, metabolic acidosis, hypernatraemia and renal impairment.

In the case of deliberate or accidental ingestion of large quantities of Betadine, symptomatic and supportive treatment should be provided with special attention to electrolyte balance and renal and thyroid function.

Pharmaceutical precautions
Storage: Store at or below 25°C and protect from light.

Legal category P

Package quantities Container of 500 ml.

Further information Betadine Standardised Antiseptic Solution has a rapid and prolonged germicidal action and, with repeated use, a cumulative germicidal action. It is active against a wide range of organisms including Gram positive and Gram negative bacteria, fungi, protozoa, viruses, and bacterial spores. In the presence of blood, serum, purulent exudate and necrotic tissue, its activity persists whilst the colour remains.

Product licence number 0223/0012

BETADINE* SURGICAL SCRUB

Presentation A golden brown surfactant solution containing Povidone Iodine USP 7.5%w/v with non-ionic surfactants.

Uses For use as an antiseptic skin cleanser for pre-operative scrubbing and washing by surgeons and theatre staff, and pre-operative preparation of patients' skin.

Dosage and administration
Adults, the elderly and children: Apply full strength as a pre-operative antiseptic skin cleanser.

Povidone iodine is not recommended for regular use in neonates and is contra-indicated in very low birth weight infants (below 1500 grams).

Contra-indications, warnings, etc
Contra-indications: Known or suspected iodine hypersensitivity. Regular use is contra-indicated in patients and users with thyroid disorders (in particular nodular colloid goitre, endemic goitre and Hashimoto's thyroiditis).

Interactions: Absorption of iodine from povidone iodine through either intact or damaged skin may interfere with thyroid function tests. Contamination with povidone iodine of several types of tests for the detection of occult blood in faeces or blood in urine may produce false-positive results.

Effect on ability to drive and to use machines: None known.

Side-effects and adverse reactions: Povidone iodine may produce local skin reactions although it is considered to be less irritant than iodine. The application of povidone iodine to large wounds or severe burns may produce systemic adverse effects such as metabolic acidosis, hypernatraemia, and impairment of renal function.

Use in pregnancy and lactation: Regular use of povidone iodine should be avoided in pregnant or lactating women as absorbed iodine can cross the placental barrier and can be secreted into breast milk. Although no adverse effects have been reported from limited use, caution should be recommended and therapeutic benefit must be balanced against possible effects of the absorption of iodine on foetal thyroid function and development.

Other special precautions and warnings: Special caution is needed when regular applications to broken skin are made to patients with pre-existing renal insufficiency. Regular use should be avoided in patients on concurrent lithium therapy. Betadine Surgical Scrub can permanently discolour white gold jewellery and it is recommended that this type of jewellery should be removed before using Betadine Surgical Scrub.

Overdose: Excess iodine can produce goitre and hypothyroidism or hyperthyroidism. Systemic absorption of iodine after repeated application of povidone iodine to large areas of wounds or burns may lead to a number of adverse effects: metallic taste in the mouth, increased salivation, burning or pain in the throat or mouth, irritation and swelling of the eyes, pulmonary oedema, skin reactions, gastrointestinal upset and diarrhoea, metabolic acidosis, hypernatremia and renal impairment. In the case of deliberate or accidental ingestion of large quantities of Betadine, symptomatic and supportive treatment should be provided with special attention to electrolyte balance and renal and thyroid function.

Pharmaceutical precautions
Storage: Store at or below 25°C and protect from light.

Legal category P

Package quantities Container of 500 ml.

Further information Betadine Surgical Scrub has a rapid and prolonged germicidal action and, with repeated use, a cumulative germicidal action. It is active against a wide range of organisms including Gram positive and Gram negative bacteria, fungi, protozoa, viruses, and bacterial spores. In the presence of blood, serum, purulent exudate and necrotic tissue, its activity persists whilst the colour remains.

Product licence number 0223/0017.

BETADINE* VAGINAL CLEANSING (VC) KIT

Presentation Betadine V.C. Kit consists of V.C. Concentrate, containing 250 ml of Povidone Iodine USP 10% w/v with an applicator squeeze bottle and a plastic vaginal applicator.

Uses For the treatment of vaginitis due to candidal, trichomonal, non-specific or mixed infections, and pre-operative preparation of the vagina.

Dosage and administration
Adults and the elderly: Once a day (preferably in the morning) for a 14 day period, including days of menstruation. Betadine V.C. Concentrate should be diluted 1:10 using the measuring cap, and used according to the patient instruction leaflet provided. The applicators should only be used for the administration of the diluted V.C. Concentrate. May be used in combination with Betadine Vaginal Pessaries or Betadine Vaginal Gel.

Children: Contra-indicated for use in pre-puberty children.

Contra-indications, warnings, etc
Contra-indications: Known or suspected iodine hypersensitivity. Regular use is contra-indicated in patients and users with thyroid disorders (in particular nodular colloid goitre, endemic goitre and Hashimoto's thyroiditis).

Interactions: Absorption of iodine from povidone iodine through either intact or damaged skin may interfere with thyroid function tests. Contamination with povidone iodine of several types of tests for the detection of occult blood in faeces or blood in urine may produce false-positive results.

Effect on ability to drive and to use machines: None known.

Side-effects and adverse reactions: If local irritation, redness or swelling develops, discontinue treatment. Iodine is absorbed from the vagina and following prolonged use, thyroid dysfunction may develop. The product may be spermicidal and should not be used when conception is desired.

Use in pregnancy and lactation: Regular use of povidone iodine should be avoided in pregnant or lactating women as absorbed iodine can cross the placental barrier and can be secreted into breast milk. Although no adverse effects have been reported from limited use, caution should be recommended and therapeutic benefit must be balanced against possible effects of the absorption of iodine on foetal thyroid function and development.

Other special precautions and warnings: Special caution is needed when regular applications to broken skin are made to patients with pre-existing renal insufficiency. Regular use should be avoided in patients on concurrent lithium therapy.

Overdose: Excess iodine can produce goitre and hypothyroidism or hyperthyroidism. In the case of deliberate or accidental ingestion of large quantities of Betadine, symptomatic and supportive treatment should be provided with special attention to electrolyte balance and renal and thyroid function.

Incompatibilities (major): Compatibility with barrier contraceptives has not been established. Therefore this product should not be used with such methods of contraception as their reliability may be affected.

Pharmaceutical precautions
Storage: Store at or below 25°C and protect from light.

Legal category P

Package quantities Carton containing plastic bottle of 250 ml V.C. Concentrate, an empty applicator squeeze bottle and a plastic vaginal applicator.

Further information Betadine V.C. Kit is fungicidal, trichomonacidal and bactericidal to the pathogenic organisms that cause vaginitis. In the presence of blood, serum and necrotic tissue, its activity persists whilst the colour remains. The preparation is water-soluble and does not stain the skin.

Product licence number 0223/0020

BETADINE* VAGINAL GEL

Presentation A golden brown gel containing Povidone Iodine USP 10% w/w.

Uses For the treatment of vaginitis due to candidal, trichomonal, non-specific or mixed infections, and pre-operative preparation of the vagina.

Dosage and administration
Adults and the elderly: Insert an applicator full of gel (5 g) every night for up to 14 days. The regimen may be varied to combine the use of Betadine Vaginal Gel and Betadine Vaginal Pessaries or in combination with the Betadine V.C. Kit using one in the morning and one at night for up to 14 days. If menstruation occurs during treatment, it is important to continue treatment during the days of the period.

Children: Contra-indicated for use in pre-puberty children.

Contra-indications, warnings, etc
Contra-indications: Known or suspected iodine hypersensitivity. Regular use is contra-indicated in patients and users with thyroid disorders (in particular nodular colloid goitre, endemic goitre and Hashimoto's thyroiditis).

Interactions: Absorption of iodine from povidone iodine through either intact or damaged skin may interfere with thyroid function tests. Contamination with povidone iodine of several types of tests for the detection of occult blood in faeces or blood in urine may produce false-positive results.

Effect on ability to drive and to use machines: None known.

Side-effects and adverse reactions: If local irritation, redness or swelling develops, discontinue treatment. Iodine is absorbed from the vagina and following prolonged use, thyroid dysfunction may develop. The product may be spermicidal and should not be used when conception is desired.

Use in pregnancy and lactation: Regular use of povidone iodine should be avoided in pregnant or lactating women as absorbed iodine can cross the placental barrier and can be secreted into breast milk. Although no adverse effects have been reported from limited use, caution should be recommended and therapeutic benefit must be balanced against possible effects of the absorption of iodine on foetal thyroid function and development.

Other special precautions and warnings: Special caution is needed when regular applications to broken skin are made to patients with pre-existing renal insufficiency. Regular use should be avoided in patients on concurrent lithium therapy.

Overdose: Excess iodine can produce goitre and hypothyroidism or hyperthyroidism. In the case of deliberate or accidental ingestion of large quantities of Betadine, symptomatic and supportive treatment should be provided with special attention to electrolyte balance and renal and thyroid function.

Incompatibilities (major): Compatibility with barrier contraceptives has not been established. Therefore this product should not be used with such methods of contraception as their reliability may be affected.

Pharmaceutical precautions
Storage: Store at or below 25°C.

Legal category P

Package quantities 80 g with applicator.

Further information Betadine Vaginal Gel is fungicidal, trichomonacidal and bactericidal to the pathogenic organisms that cause vaginitis. In the presence of blood, serum and necrotic tissue, its activity persists whilst the colour remains. The preparation is water-soluble and does not stain the skin.

Product licence number 0223/0018

BETADINE* VAGINAL PESSARIES

Presentation Golden brown in colour, each contain Povidone Iodine USP 200 mg in a water-soluble base.

Uses For the treatment of vaginitis due to candidal, trichomonal, non-specific or mixed infections, and pre-operative preparation of the vagina.

Dosage and administration
Adults and the elderly: Insert one pessary night and morning for up to 14 days. Each pessary should be wetted with water immediately prior to insertion, thus enabling maximum dispersion of the active constituent and avoiding risk of local irritation.. If menstruation occurs during treatment, it is important to continue treatment during the days of the period.

Children: Contra-indicated for use in pre-puberty children.

Contra-indications, warnings, etc
Contra-indications: Known or suspected iodine hypersensitivity. Regular use is contra-indicated in patients and users with thyroid disorders (in particular nodular colloid goitre, endemic goitre and Hashimoto's thyroiditis).

Interactions: Absorption of iodine from povidone iodine through either intact or damaged skin may interfere with thyroid function tests. Contamination with povidone iodine of several types of tests for the detection of occult blood in faeces or blood in urine may produce false-positive results.

Effect on ability to drive and to use machines: None known.

Side-effects and adverse reactions: If local irritation, redness or swelling develops, discontinue treatment. Iodine is absorbed from the vagina and following prolonged use, thyroid dysfunction may develop. The product may be spermicidal and should not be used when conception is desired.

Use in pregnancy and lactation: Regular use of povidone iodine should be avoided in pregnant or lactating women as absorbed iodine can cross the placental barrier and can be secreted into breast milk. Although no adverse effects have been reported from limited use, caution should be recommended and therapeutic benefit must be balanced against possible effects of the absorption of iodine on foetal thyroid function and development.

Other special precautions and warnings: Special caution is needed when regular applications to broken skin are made to patients with pre-existing renal insufficiency. Regular use should be avoided in patients on concurrent lithium therapy.

Overdose: Excess iodine can produce goitre and hypothyroidism or hyperthyroidism. In the case of deliberate or accidental ingestion of large quantities of Betadine, symptomatic and supportive treatment should be provided with special attention to electrolyte balance and renal and thyroid function.

Incompatibilities (major): Compatibility with barrier contraceptives has not been established. Therefore this product should not be used with such methods of contraception as their reliability may be affected.

Pharmaceutical precautions
Storage: Store at or below 25°C.

Legal category P

Package quantities 28 with applicator (OP).

Further information Betadine Vaginal Pessaries are fungicidal, trichomonacidal and bactericidal to the pathogenic organisms that cause vaginitis. In the presence of blood, serum and necrotic tissue, their activity persists whilst the colour remains. The preparation is water soluble and does not stain the skin.

Product licence number 0223/0019

CARYLDERM LIQUID

Qualitative and quantitative composition Carylderm Liquid contains Carbaril 1.0% w/v.

Pharmaceutical form Liquid.

Clinical particulars
Therapeutic indications: For the eradication of head lice and their eggs.

Posology and method of administration: Adults, the elderly and children aged 6 months and above: For external use only. As this product does not contain alcohol, it may be more suitable for those with asthma and eczema. Keep the head upright and rub Carylderm Liquid well into the roots of the hair and scalp, paying particular attention to the partings, back of the neck, fringes and around the ears. Leave the hair to dry naturally and wash in ordinary shampoo the next day or after 12 hours. After shampoo wash, remove dead eggs with a metal nit comb while the hair is wet. Family members and close contacts should also be treated simultaneously, if infected.

In the event of early re-infestation, Carylderm Liquid should be applied again, provided 7 days have elapsed since the first application.

Not to be used on children under the age of 6 months except under medical supervision.

Contra-indications: Known sensitivity to carbaril.

Special warnings and precautions for use: Avoid contact with eyes. Not to be used on infants under 6 months of age, unless under medical supervision. Use in clinics: nursing staff involved in repeated applications should wear rubber gloves when carrying out treatment. For external use only. Keep out of the reach of children. If Carylderm Liquid is inadvertently swallowed a doctor or casualty department should be contacted at once.

Continued prolonged treatment with Carylderm Liquid should be avoided. It should not be used more than once a week for three weeks at a time.

The feeding of carbaril to rats and mice throughout life led to an increased incidence of benign and malignant tumours only at very high doses. However, a range of *in vivo* and *in vitro* mutagenicity tests have indicated that carbaril is not genotoxic. These findings suggest that the use of carbaril to treat louse infestations is unlikely to pose a significant cancer risk in humans.

Interactions with other medicaments and other forms of interaction: None known.

Pregnancy and lactation: No evidence for safety of this product has been determined in pregnancy and lactation. It is not necessary to contraindicate this product in pregnancy and lactation provided caution is exercised and the directions for use are followed.

Effects on ability to drive and use machines: None stated.

Undesirable effects: None stated.

Overdose: Accidental ingestion: it is unlikely that a toxic dose of carbaril will be ingested. Treatment consists of gastric lavage, assisted respiration and, if necessary in the event of massive ingestion, administration of atropine.

Pharmacological properties
Pharmacodynamic properties: The action of carbamates is to inhibit the acetyl cholinesterases present at synaptic junctions within the insects nervous system.

Pharmacokinetic properties: Carylderm Liquid is applied topically to the affected area.

Preclinical safety data: None stated.

Pharmaceutical particulars
List of excipients: Potassium Citrate PhEur; Citric Acid PhEur; Lanette Wax SX; Propyl Hydroxybenzoate (E217) PhEur; Methyl Hydroxybenzoate (E219) PhEur; Diethylene Glycol; Dimethyl Phthalate BP; Colour Blue 1249 (E131); Bronopol BP; Water.

Incompatibilities: None stated.

Shelf life: Three years.

Special precautions for storage: Store at or below 25°C and do not refrigerate. Protect from sunlight.

Nature and contents of container: Clear or amber glass bottles with polyethylene caps and polypropylene faced wads. The clear glass bottles are contained in cartons. The product is available in bottles containing either 50 or 200 ml of product.

Instruction for use/handling: None stated.

Marketing authorisation number PL 11314/0044

Date of approval/renewal of SPC March 1998

Legal category POM

CARYLDERM* LOTION

Qualitative and quantitative composition Carylderm Lotion contains carbaril 0.5% w/v.

Pharmaceutical form Lotion.

Clinical particulars
Therapeutic indications: Eradication of head louse infestation.

Posology and method of administration:
Adults, the elderly and children aged 6 months and above: For topical external use only.

Rub the lotion gently into the scalp until all the hair and scalp is thoroughly moistened. Allow to dry naturally in a well ventilated room. Do not use a hairdryer or other artificial heat. Live lice will be eradicated after a minimum treatment period of two hours. However the lotion should be left on the head for a period of 10-12 hours to ensure that all eggs are totally eradicated. Shampoo in the normal manner. Rinse and comb the hair while wet to remove the dead lice. In the event of early re-infestation, Carylderm Lotion may be applied again provided 7 days have elapsed since the first application. Residual protective effect is variable of short duration and should not be relied upon. Not to be used on children under six months of age except on medical advice.

Contra-indications: Known sensitivity to carbaril. Not to be used on infants under six months of age except on medical advice.

Special warnings and precautions for use: Avoid contact with the eyes. Do not cover the head until the hair has dried completely. It is advisable that nursing staff involved in repeated applications should wear rubber gloves when carrying out treatment. Carylderm Lotion is for external use only and should be kept out of reach of children. Keep away from exposed flame or lighted objects (e.g. cigarettes, gas and electric fires) during application and while the hair is wet. Continued prolonged treatment with Carylderm Lotion should be avoided. It should not be used more than once a week for three weeks at a time. Alcohol based skin products may cause a stinging sensation on patients with sensitive skin.

The feeding of carbaril to rats and mice throughout life led to an increased incidence of benign and malignant tumours only at very high doses. However, a range of in vivo and in vitro mutagenicity tests have indicated that carbaril is not genotoxic. These findings suggest that use of carbaril to treat louse infestations is unlikely to pose a significant cancer risk in humans.

Interactions with other medicaments and other forms of interaction: None known.

Pregnancy and lactation: No evidence of safety of this product has been determined in pregnancy and lactation. It is not necessary to contraindicate this product in pregnancy and lactation provided caution is exercised and the directions for use are followed. However, as with all medicines, the advice of a doctor should be sought before the product is used.

Effects on ability to drive and use machines: None stated.

Undesirable effects: Very rarely, skin irritation has been reported with carbaril products.

Overdose: Accidental ingestion: gastric lavage, assisted by respiration and, if necessary administration of atropine.

Pharmacological properties
Pharmacodynamic properties: The action of carbamates is to inhibit the acetylcholinesterases present at synaptic junctions within the insects nervous system.

Pharmacokinetic properties: Carylderm Lotion is applied topically to the affected area.

Preclinical safety data: None stated.

Pharmaceutical particulars
List of excipients: Isopropyl Alcohol IPSI BP; D-Limonene 17449 ; Terpineol 18689 BP; Shellsol T; Colour Blue 12401 (E131); Perfume Loxol P6160; Citric Acid PhEur.

Incompatibilities: None stated.

Shelf life: Two years.

Special precautions for storage: Store at or below 25°C. Protect from sunlight.

Nature and contents of container: Clear or amber glass bottles with LDPE caps with HDPE sprinkle plug inserts. The clear glass bottles will be marketed in cartons. Bottles of 50 and 250 ml.

Instructions for use/handling: None stated.

Marketing authorisation number 11314/0053.

Date of approval/revision of SPC July 1998

DERBAC-M* LIQUID

Qualitative and quantitative composition Malathion 0.5% w/w.

Pharmaceutical form Liquid emulsion.

Clinical particulars
Therapeutic indications: For the eradication of head lice, pubic lice and their eggs. For the treatment of scabies.

Posology and method of administration: For topical external use only.

Adults, the elderly and children aged 6 months and over: As this product does not contain alcohol, it may be more suitable for those with asthma or eczema.
Treatment of head lice Rub the liquid into the scalp until all the hair and scalp is thoroughly moistened. Leave the hair to dry naturally in a warm but well ventilated room. After 12 hours, or the next day, if preferred, shampoo the hair in the normal way. Rinse the hair and comb whilst wet to remove dead lice and eggs (nits) using a fine-toothed louse comb.

Treatment of crab lice Apply Derbac-M Liquid to the entire skin surface. Pay particular attention to all hairy areas including beards and moustaches. Avoid any other areas above the neck. Leave on for at least one hour before washing but preferably Derbac-M Liquid should be left on overnight. Wash off in the usual manner.

Treatment of scabies Apply Derbac-M Liquid to the entire skin surface. In adults it may not be necessary to apply above the neck but children under the age of two years should have a thin film of Derbac-M Liquid applied to the scalp, face and ears, avoiding the eyes and mouth. Do not wash off or bathe for 24 hours. If hands or any other parts must be washed during this period, the treatment must be reapplied to those areas immediately. No special sterilisation of clothing is necessary, ordinary laundering or dry-cleaning with hot-iron pressing are sufficient.

The infestation is cleared by the treatment. However, the itching and rash may persist for up to 7 days. An anti-irritant cream can be applied if necessary.

Family members and close contacts should also be treated simultaneously.

Children aged 6 months and under: On medical advice only.

Contra-indications: Known sensitivity to malathion. Not to be used on infants less than 6 months except on medical advice.

Special warnings and precautions for use: Avoid contact with the eyes. For external use only. Keep out of the reach of children. If inadvertently swallowed, a doctor or casualty department should be contacted at once. When Derbac-M Liquid is used by a school nurse or other health officer in the mass treatment of large numbers of children, it is advisable that protective plastic or rubber gloves be worn. Continued prolonged treatment with this product should be avoided. It should be used not more than once a week and for not more than 3 consecutive weeks.

Interactions with other medicaments and other forms of interaction: None stated.

Use in pregnancy and lactation: No known effects in pregnancy and lactation. However, as with all medicines, use with caution.

Effects on ability to drive and use machines: None stated.

Undesirable effects: Very rarely, skin irritation has been reported.

Overdose: It is most unlikely that a toxic dose of malathion will be ingested. Treatment consists of gastric lavage, assisted respiration and, if necessary in the event of massive ingestion, administration of atropine together with pralidoxime.

Pharmacological properties

Pharmacodynamic properties: Derbac-M Liquid contains malathion, a widely used organophosphorous insecticide which is active by cholinesterase inhibition. It is effective against a wide range of insects, but is one of the least toxic organophosphorous insecticides since it is rapidly detoxified by plasma carboxylesterases.

Pharmacokinetic properties: None stated. Derbac-M Liquid is applied topically to the affected area.

Pre-clinical safety data: None stated.

Pharmaceutical particulars

List of excipients: Methyl hydroxybenzoate; propyl hydroxybenzoate; Lanette wax SX; potassium citrate; citric acid; Perfume HT 52; water.

Incompatibilities: None stated.

Shelf life: Two and a half years.

Special precautions for storage: Store at or below 25°C. Protect from sunlight.

Nature and contents of container: Cartoned, clear or amber glass bottles with polyethylene caps and polypropylene faced wads containing either 50 or 200 ml of product.

Instructions for use/handling: None stated.

Marketing authorisation number 11314/0046.

Date of approval/revision of SPC October 1995.

Legal category P.

FULL MARKS LIQUID

Qualitative and quantitive composition Phenothrin 0.5% w/w.

Pharmaceutical form Cutaneous emulsion.

Clinical particulars

Therapeutic indications: For the treatment of head louse infestations.

Posology and method of administration: Adults, the elderly and children aged 6 months and over: For topical external use only. The source of infestation should be sought and treated. Rub the emulsion into the scalp until the hair and scalp are thoroughly moistened. Leave the hair to dry naturally in a warm but well ventilated room. After 12 hours, or the next day, if preferred, shampoo the hair in the normal way. Rinse the hair and comb whilst wet to remove dead lice and eggs (nits) using a nit comb.

Contra-indications: Known sensitivity to pyrethroid insecticides. Not to be used on infants less than 6 months except on medical advice.

Special warnings and precautions for use: Avoid contact with the eyes. For external use only. Keep out of the reach of children. If advertently swallowed, a doctor or casualty department should be contacted at once. When used by a school nurse or other health officer in the mass treatment of large numbers of children, it is advisable that protective plastic or rubber gloves be worn. Continued prolonged treatment with this product should be avoided. It should not be used more than once a week for more than three consecutive weeks. The treatment may affect permed, pre-rinsed or coloured hair.

Interactions with other medicaments and other forms of interaction: None stated.

Pregnancy and lactation: No known effects in pregnancy and lactation. However, as with all medicines, use with caution.

Effects on ability to drive and use machines: None stated.

Undesirable effects: Very rarely, skin irritation has been reported.

Overdose: It is most unlikely that a toxic dose will be ingested. Treatment consists of gastric lavage, assisted respiration and, if necessary in the event of massive ingestion, administratioin of atropine together with pralidoxime.

Pharmacological properties

Pharmacodynamic properties: Phenothrin is a synthetic pyrethroid insecticide, highly effective against human lice but with an exceptionally low mammalian toxicity.

Pharmacokinetic properties: Full Marks Liquid is applied topically to the affected area. A pharmacokinetic study has shown absorption of its active constituent is negligible.

Pre-clinical safety data: None stated.

Pharmaceutical particulars

List of excipients: Potassium Citrate PhEur; Citric Acid Monohydrate PhEur; Emulsifying Wax (Lanette Wax SX) BP; Methylhydroxybenzoate PhEur; Propylhydroxybenzoate PhEur; Perfume HT 52; Diethylene Glycol; Dimethyl Phthalate PhEur; Purified Water PhEur.

Incompatibilities: None stated.

Shelf life: 36 months.

Special precautions for storage: Store below 25°C and do not refrigerate.

Nature and contents of container: Amber glass sirop bottle fitted with a polypropylene tamper evident lined cap containing 50 or 200 ml of product.

Marketing authorisation number PL 11314/0093

Date of approval/renewal of SPC January 1998

Legal category P

FULL MARKS* LOTION

Qualitative and quantitative composition Full Marks Lotion contains Phenothrin 0.2% w/v.

Pharmaceutical form Lotion.

Clinical particulars

Therapeutic indications: For the treatment of head louse and pubic louse infestations.

Posology and method of administration: For topical external use only. The source of infestation should be sought and treated.

Adults, the elderly and children aged 6 months and over:

Treatment of head lice Ensure that the hair is dry before commencing treatment. Sprinkle the lotion on the hair and rub gently onto the head until the entire scalp is moistened. Pay special attention to the back of the neck and the area behind the ears. Take care to avoid the eyes. Allow to dry naturally–use no heat. The hair may be washed with a standard shampoo 2 hours after application. While still wet, comb the hair with an ordinary comb. A fine-toothed louse comb can then be used to remove the dead lice and eggs.

Treatment of pubic lice Application and dosage are as for the head. Apply the lotion to the pubic hair and the hair between the legs and around the anus. Allow to dry naturally using no heat.

Contra-indications: A history of sensitivity to pyrethroid insecticides.

Special warnings and precautions for use: Full Marks Lotion contains isopropyl alcohol which may cause wheezing in asthmatic patients or cause inflammation of the skin in patients with severe eczema. If such events are apparent, patients should use a none alcohol-based formulation. Contains flammable alcohol. Apply and dry with care. Avoid naked flames or lighted objects. Do not use artificial heat (e.g. electric hairdryers). Dry in a well ventilated room. Do not cover the head before the lotion has dried completely. The hair should be dry before retiring to bed.

When Full Marks Lotion is used by a school nurse or other health officer in the mass treatment of large numbers of children, it is advisable that protective plastic or rubber gloves be worn. Children under the age of six months should be treated under medical supervision. This treatment may affect permed, coloured or bleached hair.

Interactions with other medicaments and other forms of interaction: None stated.

Use in pregnancy and lactation: No known effects in pregnancy and lactation. However, as with all medicines, use with caution.

Effects on ability to drive and use machines: None stated.

Undesirable effects: Some patients may experience stinging or inflammation of the skin due to the alcohol content.

Overdose: In the event of deliberate or accidental ingestion, as for ethyl alcohol, empty the stomach by gastric lavage and treat symptomatically.

Pharmacological properties

Pharmacodynamic properties: Phenothrin is a synthetic pyrethroid insecticide, highly effective against human lice but with an exceptionally low mammalian toxicity.

Pharmacokinetic properties: Full Marks Lotion is applied topically to the affected area. A pharmacokinetic study has shown absorption of the active constituent is negligible.

Pre-clinical safety data: None stated.

Pharmaceutical particulars

List of excipients: Herbal green bouquet P15312; isopropanol; purified water.

Incompatibilities: None stated.

Shelf life: Three years.

Special precautions for storage: Store bottle in carton at or below 30°C protected from light.

Nature and contents of container: Cartoned, clear glass or amber bottles with polyethylene caps and polyethylene sprinkler inserts containing either 50 or 200 ml of product.

Instruction for use/handling: None stated.

Marketing authorisation number 11314/0047.

Date of approval/revision of SPC May 1998

Legal category P.

FULL MARKS MOUSSE

Qualititative and quantitative compostiion Phenothrin 0.5% w/w.

Pharmaceutical form Topical mousse.

Clinical particulars

Therapeutic indications: For the treatment of head louse infestations.

Posology and method of administration: Apply the product in a well ventilated room away from naked flames and lighted objects. *Adults, the elderly and children aged 6 months and over:* For topical external use only. The source of infestation should be sought and treated. Family members and close contacts should be inspected and, if found to be infected, treated simultaneoutly. Shake the can well and invert to expel the mousse. Apply sufficient mousse to dry hair at several points on the scalp; massage into the scalp ensuring no part of the scalp is left uncovered. Pay special attention to the temples and crown of the head. Take care to avoid the eyes. Leave on the head for 30 minutes; do not attempt to dry the hair by artificial means (for example, electric hair dryers). Wash hair with normal shampoo. While the hair is still wet, comb with an ordinary comb. A fine-toothed louse comb can then be used to remove the dead or dying lice and eggs. *Infants:* Not to be used on infants under 6 months of age except under medical supervision.

Contra-indications: Known sensitivity to phenothrin.

Special warnings and precautions for use: Children under six months of age should only be treated under medical supervision. Avoid contact with the eyes. When Full Marks Mousse is used by a school nurse or other health officer in the mass treatment of large numbers of children, it is advisable that protective plastic or rubber gloves be worn. Prolonged and repeated application should be avoided. Contains flammable alcohol. Avoid naked flames or lighted objects. Do not use artificial heat (for example, electric hair dryers). Full Marks Mousse contains alcohol which may cause wheezing in asthmatic patients or cause inflammation of the skin in patients with severe eczema. If such effects are apparent, patients should use a none alcohol based formulation. The treatment may affect permed, pre-rinsed, bleached or coloured hair. For external use only.

Interactions with other medicaments and other forms of interaction: None stated.

Pregnancy and lactation: No known effects in pregnancy and lactation. Long term studies have not been performed in humans, therefore as with all medicines,

Full Marks Mousse should be used with caution in pregnant and lactating women.

Effects on ability to drive and use machines: None stated.

Undesirable effects: Very rarely, skin irritation may occur. The treatment may affect pre-rinsed, permed, coloured or bleached hair. The alcohol content of the mousse may cause stinging or inflammation in patients with eczema.

Overdose: This product contains 30% alcohol. In the event of deliberate or accidental consumption, particularly by a child, empty stomach contents by gastric lavage and treat symptomatically as hypoglycaemia may occur.

Pharmacological properties
Pharmacodynamic properties: Phenothrin is a synthetic pyrethroid insecticide, highly effective against human lice but with an exceptionally low mammalian toxicity.

Pharmacokinetic properties: Full Marks Mousse is applied topically to the affected area. A pharmacokinetic study has shown absorption of its active constituent is negligible.

Pre-clinical safety data: Dermal irritation and eye irritation tests carried out in rabbits showed Full Marks Mousse to be a minimal irritant and did not produce positive criteria in any rabbit.

Pharmaceutical particulars
List of excipients: Potassium Citrate PhEur; Citric Acid Anhydrous PhEur; Emulisifying Wax (non-ionic); Purified Water PhEur; Ethanol (denatured); Butane 30.

Incompatibilties: None stated.

Shelf life: 36 months.

Special precautions for storage: Store at or below 25°C. Do not puncture the can or expose to direct sunlight. Avoid naked flames or lighted objects. Do not use artificial heat (for example, electric hair dryers). When empty, dispose of safely as normal household waste.

Nature and contents of container: Aluminium monobloc aerosol cans with a mousse valve assembly, and a vertical foam spout and cap containing either 50 g of product to treat one person or 150 g of product to treat four persons.

Markting authorisation number PL 11314/0102

Date of approval/renewal of SPC April 1998

Legal category P

GASTROCOTE* LIQUID

Qualitative and quantitative composition
Sodium Alginate BP 220 mg; Dried Aluminium Hydroxide BP 80 mg; Magnesium Trisilicate BP 40 mg; Sodium Bicarbonate BP 70 mg.

Pharmaceutical form Oral suspension.

Clinical particulars
Therapeutic indications: Gastrocote Liquid is indicated in heartburn, including heartburn of pregnancy, reflux oesophagitis, especially where associated with hiatus hernia, and in all cases of epigastric distress associated with gastric reflux or regurgitation. It is also indicated for acid indigestion.

Posology and method of administration:
Adults and older children only: One to three 5 ml spoonfuls to be taken four times daily, that is, after main meals and at bedtime.

Infants and young children: Not recommended.

Contra-indications: There are no specific contra-indications to the use of Gastrocote Liquid.

Special warnings and precautions for use: Each 5 ml contains 42 mg sodium (1.8 mmol) which may be important for patients on a restricted salt intake.

Interactions with other medicaments and other forms of interaction: None stated.

Pregnancy and lactation: Indicated for use in pregnancy.

Effects on ability to drive and use machines: No known effects.

Undesirable effects: None stated.

Overdose: Acute overdose is virtually free of hazard. Gastric bloating may be anticipated and, if necessary, should be treated symptomatically.

Pharmacological properties
Pharmacodynamic properties: Alginate antacid products form an alginate foam raft on top of the gastric contents. The antacid components remain entrained in the alginate raft and exert little or no effect on gastric pH.

The presence of the foam raft helps to impede gastro-oesophageal reflux. If reflux is forced the alginate antacid foam enters the oesophagus first coating it with a protective demulcent and antacid layer. This coating process is repeated as the reflux subsides. Any refluxed gastric acid is thus rapidly neutralised, the oesophageal mucosa is protected and any pre-existing oesophagitis or ulceration can heal normally.

Pharmacokinetic properties: There is very little absorption of aluminium hydroxide from the gastrointestinal tract. Only 5% of magnesium is absorbed. However, there is a theoretical possibility of accumulation of aluminium or magnesium in cases of severe renal failure. There is negligible absorption of alginate.

Preclinical safety data: Not applicable.

Pharmaceutical particulars
List of excipients: Aluminium Magnesium Silicate BP; Sunset Yellow FCF (E110); butterscotch liquid flavour; peppermint liquid; Saccharin Sodium BP; Nipacombin SK; Purified water BP.

Incompatibilities: None known.

Shelf life: 24 months unopened, one month after opening.

Special precautions for storage: Store at or below 25°C.

Nature and contents of container: HDPE bottle with tamper evident screw closure or HDPE with screw closure. Bottles of 500 ml.

Instruction for use/handling: Not applicable.

Marketing authorisation number 11314/0062.

Date of approval/revision of SPC July 1996.

Legal category GSL.

GASTROCOTE* TABLETS

Qualitative and quantitative composition Alginic Acid BP 200 mg; Dried Aluminium Hydroxide Gel BP 80 mg; Magnesium Trisilicate BP 40 mg; Sodium Bicarbonate BP 70 mg.

Pharmaceutical form Tablet uncoated.

Clinical particulars
Therapeutic indications: Gastrocote is indicated in heartburn, including heartburn of pregnancy, reflux oesophagitis, particularly where associated with hiatus hernia, and in all cases of epigastric distress associated with gastric reflux or regurgitation. It is also indicated in acid indigestion.

Posology and method of administration:
Adults and older children only: 1 or 2 tablets to be chewed four times a day, that is, after main meals and at bedtime. Not to be given to children under 6 years.
Important The tablets must be well chewed before swallowing.

Contra-indications: There are no specific contra-indications to the use of Gastrocote.

Special warnings and precautions for use: Care should be exercised in treating diabetic patients as the tablets each contain approximately 1 g of sugar. Each tablet also contains 21 mg (0.91 Meq) of sodium which may be important for patients on a low sodium diet. As Gastrocote contains aluminium hydroxide, use with caution in patients with renal dysfunction or on a low phosphate diet.

Interactions with other medicaments and other forms of interaction: None stated.

Pregnancy and lactation: No special warnings required. Gastrocote is indicated in heartburn, including heartburn of pregnancy.

Effects on ability to drive and use machines: None stated.

Undesirable effects: None stated.

Overdose: Overdose is virtually free of hazard although gastric bloating may occur.

Pharmacological properties
Pharmacodynamic properties: Alginate antacid products form an alginate foam raft on top of the gastric contents. The antacid components remain entrained in the alginate raft and exert little or no effect on gastric pH.

The presence of the foam raft helps to impede gastro-oesophageal reflux. If reflux is forced the alginate antacid foam enters the oesophagus first coating it with a protective demulcent and antacid layer. This coating process is repeated as the reflux subsides. Any refluxed gastric acid is thus rapidly neutralised, the oesophageal mucosa is protected and any pre-existing oesophagitis or ulceration can heal normally.

Pharmacokinetic properties: There is very little absorption of aluminium hydroxide from the gastrointestinal tract. Only 5% of magnesium is absorbed. However, there is a theoretical possibility of accumulation of aluminium or magnesium in cases of severe renal failure. There is negligible absorption of alginate.

Pre-clinical safety data: Not applicable.

Pharmaceutical particulars
List of excipients: Powdered Cellulose NF; Carmellose Sodium BP; Butterscotch Flavour; Magnesium Stearate BP; Directly Compressible Sugar NF.

Incompatibilities: None stated.

Shelf life: 60 months.

Special precautions for storage: Store in a cool dry place below 25°C.

Nature and contents of container: Securitainers or high density polyethylene container with tamper evident low density polyethylene lid or blister pack comprised of 20μ aluminium foil and 250μ PVC film. Packs of 100 tablets.

Instructions for use/handling: Not applicable.

Marketing authorisation number 11314/0061

Date of approval/revision of SPC July 1996.

Legal category GSL.

MANUSEPT*

Presentation A clear solution containing 70% v/v Isopropyl Alcohol BP and 0.5% w/v Triclosan.

Uses For the disinfection of physically clean hands. For preoperative disinfection of physically clean hands. For skin disinfection prior to surgery, injection or venepuncture.

Dosage and administration
For the disinfection of physically clean hands: Dispense approximately 3 ml of Manusept into the palm of one hand. Rub both hands, wrists and forearms together vigorously, paying particular attention to the area around the fingernails. Continue rubbing until dry. Repeat this procedure once more for preoperative disinfection.

For the disinfection of intact skin before surgery, injection or venepuncture: Apply a quantity of Manusept with a sterile swab. Rub vigorously until dry. Repeat this procedure once more.

Contra-indications, warnings, etc
Avoid contact with the eyes. For external use only. Do not use in the vicinity of naked flames. Treatment of overdosage: If swallowed, gastric aspiration and lavage avoiding pulmonary aspiration. Apomorphine should not be used.

Pharmaceutical precautions Store at or below normal ambient temperatures.

Legal category GSL.

Package quantities 100 ml, 250 ml and 500 ml.

Further information Triclosan is compatible with soap which can be used to obtain physically clean hands.

Product licence number 11314/0097.

METROTOP*

Qualitative and quantitative composition Metronidazole BP 0.8% w/v.

Pharmaceutical form A colourless aqueous gel.

Clinical particulars
Therapeutic indications: For the treatment of malodour associated with fungating tumours, gravitational ulcers and decubitus ulcers (pressure sores).

Posology and method of administration: For external use only. Studies have shown that offensive odour is usually controlled with the application of Metrotop for one or two weeks. Adults: All wounds should be cleaned thoroughly. Flat wounds require a liberal application of the gel over the complete area. Cavities should be loosely packed with paraffin gauze which has been smeared in the gel. All wounds should be covered with a non-adherent dressing and a pad of lint or gauze. Sticking may occur if the appropriate dressing is not used. Use once or twice daily as necessary. Elderly: No specific instructions. Children: Where necessary, instructions apply as for adults.

Contra-indications: Known hypersensitivity to metronidazole.

Special warnings and precautions for use: The following statements take into the account the possibility that metronidazole may be absorbed after topical application. However, there is no evidence of any significant systemic concentrations of metronidazole following topical applications. Peripheral neuropathy has been reported in association with prolonged use of metronidazole. The elimination half-life of metronidazole remains unchanged in the presence of renal failure. Such patients, however, retain the metabolite of metronidazole. The clinical significance of this is not known at present. However, in patients undergoing dialysis, metronidazole and metabolites are efficiently removed.

Interactions with other medicaments and other forms of interaction: Some potentiation of anticoagulant therapy has been reported when metronidazole has been used with the warfarin type oral anticoagulants. Patients receiving phenobarbitone metabolise metronidazole at a much faster rate than normal, reducing the half-life to approximately 3 hours. Patients are advised not to take alcohol during systemic metronidazole therapy because of the possibility of a disulfiram-like reaction.

Pregnancy and lactation: There is inadequate evidence of the use of metronidazole in pregnancy. Metronidazole gel cannot therefore be recommended during pregnancy or lactation where significant systemic absorption may occur unless the physician considers it essential.

Effects on ability to drive and use machines: None known.

Undesirable effects: No adverse effects have been reported. Systemic metronidazole therapy may occasionally cause an unpleasant taste in the mouth, furred tongue, nausea, vomiting, gastrointestinal disturbance, urticaria, angioedema and anaphylaxis. Drowsiness, dizziness, headache, ataxia, skin rash, pruritus, and darkening of the urine has been reported, but rarely.

Overdose: There is no specific treatment for gross overdosage of metronidazole. Gastric lavage is recommended in cases of accidental ingestion. Uneventful recovery has followed overdosage of up to 12 g taken orally. Metronidazole is readily removed from the plasma by dialysis.

Pharmacological properties
Pharmacodynamic properties: Metronidazole is a potent agent against the anaerobic bacteria which are believed to produce odorous metabolites as a result of localised tissue colonisation. The aim of the product is to provide a high concentration of metronidazole at and around the site of colonisation in a water-miscible base. This form allows surface spread and penetration within the wound accompanied by ease of aseptic application and up to 24 hours duration of action.

Pharmacokinetic properties: There is presently no evidence of any systemic concentrations of metronidazole following topical application.

Pre-clinical safety data: No further data given.

Pharmaceutical particulars
List of excipients: Hypromellose (4500) BP; Benzalkonium Chloride Solution BP; Purified Water BP.

Incompatibilities: None known.

Shelf life: The shelf life shall not exceed 24 months from the date of manufacture.

Special precautions for storage: To be stored between 15° and 25°C. Once opened the contents should be used within 28 days of opening.

Nature and contents of container: Polypropylene tubes each fitted with a plastic screw cap and tamper-evident seal and enclosed within a printed cardboard carton. Single tubes may sometimes be supplied without a carton. Pack sizes: 15 mg (packs of 12) and 30 mg (available in single units).

Instruction for use/handling: None given.

Marketing authorisation number 11314/0090.

Date of approval/revision of SPC December 1997.

Legal category POM.

MEDINOL* PAEDIATRIC PARACETAMOL ORAL SUSPENSION BP 120 mg/5 ml

Presentation A strawberry flavoured sugar and colour free suspension containing 120 mg of Paracetamol BP in each 5 ml dose.

Uses For the relief of pain and feverish conditions.

Dosage and administration To be taken four times daily. Do not repeat dose more frequently than every 4 hours. Do not take more than four doses in 24 hours.

Children 1-5 years: Two 5 ml spoonfuls.

Infants 3 months to 1 year: Half to one 5 ml spoonful.

Infants under 3 months: A 2.5 ml dose is suitable for babies who develop a fever following vaccination at 2 months. In other cases use only under medical supervision. Not to be given to infants under 2 months except on medical advice. If a baby was born prematurely and is less than 3 months old, the doctor should be consulted before use

Contra-indications, warnings, etc
Contra-indications: Use with caution in patients with impaired kidney or liver function.

Drug interactions: Cholestyramine may reduce absorption of paracetamol. Metoclopramide and domperidone may accelerate the absorption of paracetamol. Alcohol, barbiturates, anticonvulsants and tricyclic antidepressants may increase the hepatotoxicity of paracetamol particularly after an overdose.

Side-effects and adverse reactions: If given in therapeutic doses, side effects are rare. Haematological reactions have been reported. Skin reactions and other allergic reactions occur occasionally. Most reports of adverse reactions to paracetamol relate to overdosage with the drug.

Use in pregnancy and lactation: There is epidemiological evidence of the safety of paracetamol in human pregnancy. Medinol may be taken during pregnancy and lactation.

Other special precautions and warnings: If pain and fever persists for more than 3 days, a doctor should be consulted. Prolonged use without medical supervision may be harmful. In case of accidental overdose medical attention should be sought immediately. The stated dose must not be exceeded.

Overdose: An overdose should be treated as soon as possible (within 12 hours) as liver damage from an overdose does not become apparent for 1 to 6 hours after ingestion. Initial symptoms include pallor, nausea, vomiting, anorexia and abdominal pain. Medical attention should be sought. After gastric lavage a suitable antidote such as acetylcysteine or methionine should be given. Acetylcysteine is given by intravenous fluid in an initial dose of 150 mg/kg bodyweight over 15 minutes, followed by 50 mg/kg over 4 hours and then by 100 mg/kg over the next 16 hours. Alternatively, methionine 2.5 g may be given by mouth every 4 hours to a total of four doses. The blood paracetamol levels should be monitored to determine whether further therapy is necessary.

Pharmaceutical precautions
Storage: Store below 25°C. Extremes of temperature should be avoided.

Legal category P.

Package quantities Bottles of 100 ml, 150 ml, 200 ml and 1 litre.

Further information Medinol is suitable for use by diabetics. Medinol is free of animal fat and alcohol so it is suitable for children with specific dietary requirements.

Product licence number 0338/0033

Name and address of product licence holder: Cupal Limited, King Street, Blackburn BB2 2DX.

PRIODERM* LOTION

Qualitative and quantitative composition Prioderm Lotion contains Malathion USP 0.5% w/v.

Pharmaceutical form Topical solution.

Clinical particulars
Therapeutic indications: For the treatment of head louse and pubic louse infestation, and scabies.

Posology and method of administration:
Adults, the elderly and children aged 6 months and above: For topical external use only. The source of infestation should be sought and treated.

For head lice Sprinkle the lotion on the hair and rub gently onto the head until the entire scalp is moistened. Pay special attention to the back of the neck and behind the ears. Take care to avoid the eyes. Allow to dry naturally using no heat.

As all lice and eggs will have been killed, the hair may be shampooed after 2 hours. If a residual effect is required, however, it is recommended that shampooing be carried out after 12 hours.

Whilst still wet, comb the hair with an ordinary comb. A fine toothed louse comb can then be used to remove the dead lice and eggs.

For pubic lice Application and dosage are as for the head. Apply the lotion to the pubic hair and the hair around the legs and around the anus. Allow to dry naturally using no heat. Transient, mild stinging may be experienced due to the alcohol content.

For scabies Use cotton wool to apply the lotion to all parts of the body except the face and scalp. Rub in well and allow to dry naturally. Do not bathe until 12 hours after treatment.

Infants: Infants under the age of 6 months should be treated under medical supervision.

Contra-indications: None stated.

Special warnings and precautions for use: Prioderm Lotion contains isopropyl alcohol which may cause wheezing in asthmatic patients or cause inflammation of the skin in patients with severe eczema.

Contains flammable alcohol. Apply and dry with care. Avoid naked flames or lighted objects. Do not use artificial heat (eg electric hairdryers). Dry in a well ventilated room. Do not cover the head before the lotion has dried completely. The hair should be dry before retiring to bed.

Children under six months should only be treated under medical supervision. When Prioderm Lotion is used by a school nurse or other health officer in the mass treatment of large numbers of children, it is advisable that protective plastic or rubber gloves be worn.

Continued prolonged treatment with this product should be avoided. It should not be used for more than once a week for three weeks at a time.

In the event of contact with the eyes, rinse thoroughly with water. If there is persistent irritation, seek medical advice immediately.

Interactions with other medicaments and other forms of interaction: None stated.

Pregnancy and lactation: There are no known adverse effects in human pregnancy and lactation. However, as with all drugs, it should be used with caution in pregnant and lactating women.

Effects on ability to drive and use machines: None stated.

Undesirable effects: Some patients may experience stinging or inflammation of the skin due to the alcohol content.

Overdose: In the event of deliberate or accidental ingestion, empty stomach contents by gastric lavage and keep patient warm. In the event of massive ingestion, atropine and pralidoxime may be required to counteract cholinesterase inhibition.

Pharmacological properties
Pharmacodynamic properties: Prioderm Lotion contains malathion, a widely used organophosphorous insecticide which is active by cholinesterase inhibition. It is effective against a wide range of insects, but is one of the least toxic organophosphorous insecticides since it is rapidly detoxified by plasma carboxylesterases.

Pharmacokinetic properties: Prioderm Lotion is applied topically to the affected area.

Preclinical safety data: None stated.

Pharmaceutical particulars
List of excipients: Golden delicious perfume P15498; isopropyl myristate; isopropanol.

Incompatibilities: None stated.

Shelf life: Two years.

Special precautions for storage: Store at or below 20°C.

Nature and contents of container: Cartoned, clear glass bottles with polyethylene caps and polyethylene sprinkler inserts or clear soda glass sprinkler bottles with polypropylene caps containing either 55 or 160 ml of product.

Instructions for use/handling: None stated.

Marketing authorisation number 11314/0052.

Date of approval/revision of SPC May 1998.

Legal category P.

PRIPSEN* MEBENDAZOLE TABLETS

Qualitative and quantitative composition Pripsen Mebendazole Tablets contain Mebendazole USP 100 mg.

Pharmaceutical form Tablets.

Clinical particulars
Therapeutic indications: For the treatment of threadworm (enterobiasis) infection.

Posology and method of administration:
Adults, the elderly and children over two years of age: One tablet to be chewed or swallowed whole. The efficacy in threadworm infestations is such that treatment failure will be rare. However, the possibility of re-infection means that some patients may require a second tablet after two weeks, if re-infected. It is strongly recommended that all members of the family are treated at the same time.

Children under two years of age: Not recommended.

Contra-indications: Pregnancy. Mebendazole has not been studied extensively in children under two years of age–for this reason it is not currently recommended for children under two years of age.

Special warnings and precautions for use: Not to be taken during pregnancy or whilst breast feeding. Not recommended for children under two years of age. Keep out of the reach of children. If, after two weeks, there is a need to take the second tablet, following which symptoms persist, then consult a doctor.

Interactions with other medicaments and other forms of interaction: None stated.

Pregnancy and lactation: Mebendazole has shown embryotoxic and teratogenic activity in rats at single oral doses. No such findings have been reported in the rabbit, dog, sheep or horse. Since there is a risk that mebendazole could produce foetal damage if taken during pregnancy, it is contraindicated in pregnant women. No information on secretion into breast milk is available so mothers taking the drug should not breast feed.

Effects on ability to drive and use machines: No known effects.

Undesirable effects: Side effects reported have been minor. Transient abdominal pain and diarrhoea have been reported only rarely in cases of massive infestation and expulsion of worms. (Slight headache and dizziness have been occasionally reported).

Overdose: No cases of overdose have so far been reported with mebendazole but gastric lavage and/or supportive measures would be recommended. Symptoms of acute overdosage would be expected to include gastrointestinal disturbances, abdominal pain, headache, dizziness, pyrexia and convulsions.

Pharmacological properties
Pharmacodynamic properties: Mebendazole is an anthelmintic.

Pharmacokinetic properties: Mebendazole is poorly absorbed from the gastrointestinal tract (5-10%) and undergoes extensive first pass elimination, being metabolised in the liver, eliminated in the bile as unchanged drug and metabolites and excreted in the faeces. Only about 2% of the drug is excreted unchanged or as metabolites in the urine. Mebendazole is highly protein bound.

Pre-clinical safety data: None stated.

Pharmaceutical particulars
List of excipients: sorbitol; Jaffa Orange 61001E; magnesium stearate; povidone; maize starch; Acdisol; sodium saccharin; water.

Incompatibilities: None stated.

Shelf life: Three years.

Special precautions for storage: Store below 25°C in a dry place.

Nature and contents of container: 250 micron white, opaque, rigid, uPVC 20μ aluminium foil blisters in cardboard cartons in packs of two or eight tablets.

Instruction for use/handling: Not applicable

Marketing authorisation holder: Cupal Limited, King Street, Blackburn, Lancashire BB2 2DX.

Marketing authorisation number 0338/0084.

Date of approval/ revision of SPC February 1997.

Legal category P.

PRIPSEN* PIPERAZINE CITRATE ELIXIR

Qualitative and quantitative composition A clear, colourless, orange flavoured liquid containing, in each 5 ml, 750 mg of Piperazine Hydrate (as Citrate) BP.

Pharmaceutical form Oral liquid.

Clinical particulars
Therapeutic indications: To expel enterobiasis (threadworms) and ascariasis (roundworms) from the gastrointestinal tract.

Posology and method of administration:
To expel threadworms: Dosage to be taken daily for 7 days. It may be necessary to repeat the dosage after 7 days for a further 7 days.
Adults, the elderly and children over 12 years of age: Three 5 ml spoonfuls.
Children:
7-12 years of age: Two 5 ml spoonfuls
4-6 years of age: One and a half 5 ml spoonfuls
1-3 years of age: One 5 ml spoonful
Under 1 year of age: On medical advice only

To expel roundworms: Dosage to be taken as a single dose and then repeated after 14 days.
Adults, the elderly and children over 12 years of age: Six 5 ml spoonfuls.
Children: 9-12 years of age: Five 5 ml spoonfuls
6-8 years of age: Four 5 ml spoonfuls
4-5 years of age: Three 5 ml spoonfuls
1-3 years of age: Two 5 ml spoonfuls
Under 1 year of age: On medical advice

Contra-indications: Liver disease, epilepsy, and impaired renal function

Special warnings and precautions for use: Not to be used during pregnancy, unless advised otherwise by a doctor. Not to be used by patients with kidney disease or a history of epilepsy.

Interactions with other medicaments and other forms of interaction: Piperazine potentiates the extrapyramidal effects of chlorpromazine. Care should therefore be taken when giving piperazine to patients taking phenothiazines.

Pregnancy and lactation: The safety of piperazine use in pregnancy has not been established, but foetal toxicity studies in animals and extensive clinical experience have shown rare instances of teratogenicity if used in the first trimester of pregnancy. Therefore, this product should not be taken during pregnancy. Piperazine may be excreted in the breast milk.

Effects on ability to drive and use machines: None known.

Undesirable effects: These are uncommon but the following reactions have been reported: nausea, vomiting, diarrhoea, abdominal pain, headache, paraesthesia and urticaria. These usually disappear rapidly when treatment is stopped. Neurotoxicity has also been reported. Case reports of purpura in a glucose-6-phosphate dehydrogenase deficient individual after piperazine administration appear in the literature.

Overdose: Symptoms are similar to the side effects listed under Undesirable effects and can usually be expected to resolve spontaneously. On severe poisoning the stomach may be emptied by aspiration and lavage. Adequate fluids and routine supportive measures should be given. Convulsions can be controlled by intravenous diazepam or a short-acting barbiturate such as thiopentone sodium.

Pharmacological properties
Pharmacodynamic properties: Pripsen Piperazine Citrate Elixir contains Piperazine Citrate BP equivalent to Piperazine Hydrate BP 750 mg/5 ml. This is an anthelmintic useful for the treatment of enterobiasis and ascariasis infections in children and adults. In ascaris infections, piperazine produces a reversible muscle paralysis and the worms are easily dislodged from the gut by peristaltic motion and expelled in the faeces. Piperazine affects all stages of the parasite in the gut but appears to have little or no effect on larvae in the tissues. Little is known of the effects of piperazine on enterobiasis infections.

Pharmacokinetic properties: None stated.

Pre-clinical safety data: None stated.

Pharmaceutical particulars
List of excipients: Sucrose BP; Alcohol (96%) BP; Soluble Jaffa Essence 7300035E; Citric Acid Monohydrate BP; water.

Incompatibilities: Alkaloidal salts and salts of copper and iron.

Shelf life: Three years.

Special precautions for storage: Store below 25°C.

Nature and contents of container: Amber glass Sirop bottles with white polypropylene closures with EPE liners in cardboard cartons . Bottles of 140 ml.

Instruction for use/handling: Not applicable.

Marketing authorisation holder: Cupal Ltd, King Street, Blackburn BB2 2DX.

Marketing authorisation number 0338/5059R.

Date of approval/revision of SPC February 1995.

Legal category P.

PRIPSEN* PIPERAZINE PHOSPHATE POWDER

Qualitative and quantitative composition Pripsen Powder contains:
Piperazine Phosphate BP 4.0 g
Standardised Senna Pods 15.3 mg (calculated as total sennoside powder).

Pharmaceutical form Powder.

Clinical particulars
Therapeutic indications: For the eradication of enterobiasis (pinworm, threadworm) and ascariasis (roundworm).

Posology and method of administration:
When treating threadworms: Adults and children over 6 years: One sachet. Children aged 1-6 years: 1 level 5 ml spoonful of sachet contents. Infants 3 months–1 year: To be taken only when prescribed by a doctor. 1 level 2.5 ml spoonful of sachet contents. There is no indication that dosage be modified for the elderly.

Pripsen should be stirred into a small glass of milk or water and drunk immediately. It should be taken at bed-time by adults and in the morning by children. The dose should be repeated after 14 days. For children under 10 years of age, only one dual dose should be given in any 28 day period without seeking medical advice.

When treating roundworms: Adults and children over 6 years: One sachet. *Children aged 1-6 years:* 1 level 5 ml spoonful of sachet contents. *Infants 3 months–1 year:* To be taken only when prescribed by a doctor. 1 level 2.5 ml spoonful of sachet contents. There is no indication that dosage be modified for the elderly.

Pripsen should be stirred into a small glass of milk or water and drunk immediately. It should be taken at bed-time by adults and in the morning by children. For children under 10 years of age, only one dual dose should be given in any 28 day period without seeking medical advice.

Additional single prophylactic doses at regular monthly intervals up to three months may be necessary to eliminate the risk of re-infection.

Contra-indications: Pripsen Piperazine Phosphate Powder is contra-indicated in patients suffering from epilepsy, severe bilateral renal dysfunction, hepatic dysfunction, known sensitivity to piperazine, undiagnosed painful abdominal symptoms which may be due to acute appendicitis, and/or other acute surgical conditions, such as intestinal obstruction or acute inflammatory bowel disease, the ileus, and in severe dehydration states with water and electrolyte depletion.

Other special warnings and precautions: The product labelling includes the following:

If you believe you may be pregnant, or are taking a prescribed medicine, consult your doctor before using this product. Do not take Pripsen Piperazine Phosphate Powder if you have kidney disease or have ever suffered from epilepsy. Prolonged use of this product should be avoided.

Interactions with other medicaments and other forms of interaction: Pyrantel pamoate antagonises the mode of action of piperazine and therefore should not be co-administered. Although caution should be exercised when co-administering phenothiazine or tricyclic anti-depressants due to a possible interaction, this has not been shown to be a problem in clinical practice. Concomitant use of Pripsen Piperazine Phosphate Powder with diuretics, cardiac glycosides or adrenocorticosteroids may enhance electrolyte imbalance.

Use in pregnancy and lactation: Isolated instances of foetal malformation have been reported but no causal relationship to piperazine has ever been established. Use in the first trimester of pregnancy is therefore not advised. Unless symptoms warrant immediate treatment, the administration of Pripsen Piperazine Phosphate Powder should be postponed until after parturition. Piperazine is excreted in breast milk but no unwanted effects in the infant have been reported. To minimise the amount of piperazine ingested by the baby, it is recommended that the infant be fed immediately before taking Pripsen Piperazine Phosphate Powder, then eight hours allowed before breast feeding is resumed. During this eight hour period, milk should be expressed and discarded at the usual feeding interval.

Effects on ability to drive and use machines: None known.

Undesirable effects: Unwanted effects resulting from Pripsen Piperazine Phosphate Powder therapy are rare. When such reactions do occur, the most frequent are firstly allergic in nature, such as rash, urticaria, itching or rarely bronchospasm, or secondly mild gastrointestinal disturbances such as nausea, vomiting, colic or diarrhoea. A few cases of neurotoxic reactions have been reported, such as drowsiness, confusion, or clonic contractions if administered in the presence of neurological or renal abnormalities. Others such as dizziness, ataxia, tremors, choreoform movement, hyporeflexia, nystagmus, vertigo and blurred vision have been reported in normal subjects. Isolated cases of Stevens Johnson Syndrome and angioneurotic oedema, including arthralgia and fever have also been reported.

Overdose: Mild symptoms would be expected from overdose of Pripsen Piperazine Phosphate Powder being either gastrointestinal (diarrhoea, nausea, vomiting) or neurological (muscular hypotonia, ataxia and vertigo). General supportive measures including maintenance of an adequate fluid intake should be adopted and, if necessary, anti-convulsant therapy administered. Particular attention should be paid to correcting electrolyte imbalance.

Pharmacological properties
Pharmacodynamic properties: The piperazine in Pripsen Powder is believed to paralyse the worms which are then evacuated by the laxative *action of standardised senna.*

Pharmacokinetic properties: The therapeutic action of Pripsen occurs within the lumen of the gastrointestinal tract, which is independent of any systemic absorption.

Preclinical safety data:
(a) Senna
Single dose toxicity: Senna as crude drug or extracts, as well as sennosides and rhein, showed low acute toxicity in rats and mice after oral treatment.
Repeated dose toxicity: Sennosides showed no specific toxicity when tested at up to 500 mg/kg in dogs for four weeks and up to 100 mg/kg in rats for six months.
Reproductive toxicity: There was no evidence of any embryolethal, teratogenic or fetotoxic actions in rats and rabbits after oral treatment with sennosides. Furthermore, there was no effect on the postnatal development of young rats, on the rearing behaviour of dams or on male and female fertility in rats.
Genotoxicity: Results from in vitro and in vivo genotoxicity studies as well as human and animal pharmacokinetic data indicate no genotoxic risk from senna.
Carcinogenicity: A senna extract given orally for two years was not carcinogenic in male and female rats.
(b) Piperazine phosphate: Piperazine has very low toxicity in mammals and in the doses used clinically there is no specific organ damage or general toxicity. No adequate teratogenicity studies have been conducted but one dose studies did not produce evidence of foetal malformation in the rat and rabbit. No carcinogenicity tests have been performed.

Pharmaceutical particulars
List of excipients: vanilla flavour; caramel flavour; raspberry flavour; saccharin; Hexacol natural carmine.

Incompatibilities: None known.

Shelf life: Two years.

Special precautions for storage: Store at or below 25°C in a dry place.

Nature and contents of container: Sachets comprised of polythene/aluminium foil/paper laminate/surlyn, cut into pairs. One pair of sachets in a cardboard outer carton.

Marketing authorisation number 11314/0029.

Date of approval/revision of SPC December 1994.

Legal category P.

STERIPOD* CHLORHEXIDINE GLUCONATE 0.05% W/V

Presentation Steripod Chlorhexidine Gluconate is a sterile solution of Chlorhexidine Gluconate 0.05% w/v BP in Purified Water BP. The preparation is a clear pale pink pyrogen-free solution supplied in disposable, sealed, blow-moulded, semi-rigid containers made from polyethylene.

Uses Steripod Chlorhexidine Gluconate is a topical antimicrobial cleansing solution for the swabbing of wounds and burns and in obstetrics.

Dosage and administration
Adults and children: Apply undiluted.

Contra-indications, warnings, etc
Contra-indications: Do not use in body cavities or as an enema. The presentation is not suitable for use as an injection. It is contra-indicated in patients who have previously shown a hypersensitivity reaction to chlorhexidine. However, such reactions are rare.

Side-effects and adverse reactions: Generalised allergenic reactions to chlorhexidine have been reported but are extremely rare.

Use in pregnancy and lactation: Although no adverse reactions have been reported, as with all medicines, care should be exercised when administering to pregnant or lactating women.

Other special precautions and warnings: Do not use unless the product is clear or if there is any evidence of leaking prior to breaking the seal. Check for leaks by squeezing the Steripod before use. Discard any surplus. Avoid contact with the eyes, brain, meninges and middle ear. For external use only. If the solution comes into contact with the eyes wash out promptly and thoroughly with water.

Overdose: Chlorhexidine is poorly absorbed following oral ingestion. Do not induce vomiting. Treat with gastric lavage, using milk, egg white, gelatin, or mild soap and employ appropriate supportive measures.

Incompatibilities: Chlorhexidine is incompatible with soaps and other anionic materials. This product will also be incompatible with borates, bicarbonates, carbonates, chlorides, citrates, phosphates and sulphates. Fabrics which have been in contact with chlorhexidine will be stained when bleached with hypochlorite.

Pharmaceutical precautions Steripod Chlorhexidine Gluconate should be stored between 5 and 25°C.

Legal category P

Package quantities Cartons of 25 x 20 ml ampoules.

Further information The Steripod is designed to overcome the inherent disadvantages of sachets. Solution application is more controllable and more easily directed to the desired area. The Steripod opening is designed to reduce the risk of touch contamination, and is opened simply by twisting off the top. Once opened, unlike a sachet, a Steripod will stand upright on a flat surface without loss of solution. Simple instructions on the use of the Steripod are reproduced on the carton.
For safe disposal, empty the contents and incinerate at a minimum of 400°C or landfill at an approved site.

Product licence number 11314/0007

STERIPOD* CHLORHEXIDINE GLUCONATE BP with CETRIMIDE

Qualitative and quantitative composition Chlorhexidine Gluconate BP 0.015% w/v; Cetrimide PhEur 0.15% w/v.

Pharmaceutical form Sterile topical antiseptic solution.

Clinical particulars
Therapeutic indications: For use as a topical antimicrobial cleansing agent for the antiseptic treatment of wounds and burns, and for swabbing.

Posology and method of administration: For topical use only. *Adults, children and the elderly:* use undiluted for topical applications.

Contra-indications: The presentation is not suitable for use as an injection. Avoid contact with the eyes, brain, meninges and middle ear. Steripod Chlorhexidine Gluconate 0.015% with Cetrimide 0.15% is contraindicated in patients who have previously shown a hypersensitivity to chlorhexidine or cetrimide. However, such reactions are extremely rare.

Special warnings and precautions for use: Do not use unless the product is clear, or if there is evidence of leaking prior to breaking the seal. Check for leaks by squeezing the Steripod before use. Discard any surplus.

Interactions with other medicaments and other forms of interaction: None known.

Pregnancy and lactation: Although there is no evidence of any problems regarding the safety of chlorhexidine or cetrimide preparations in expectant mothers, as with all medicinal products, care should be exercised when administering them to pregnant or lactating women.

Effects on ability to drive and use machines: None known.

Undesirable effects: Skin sensitivity to chlorhexidine/cetrimide preparations have been reported. Generalised allergenic reactions to chlorhexidine have been reported but are extremely rare.

Overdose: Chlorhexidine is poorly absorbed following oral ingestion. Treatment: Do not induce vomiting. Treat with gastric lavage using milk, egg white, gelatin, or mild soap and employ appropriate supportive measures.

Pharmacological properties
Pharmacodynamic properties: Not applicable.

Pharmacokinetic properties: Not applicable.

Pre-clincial safety data: Not applicable.

Pharmaceutical particulars
List of excipients: Sodium Hydroxide BP; Water for Injection PhEur.

Incompatibilities: Chlorhexidine is incompatible with soaps and other anionic agents. This product will also be incompatible with borates, bicarbonates, carbonates, chlorides, citrates, phosphates and sulphates. Fabrics which have been in contact with chlorhexidine will be stained when bleached with hypochlorite.

Shelf life: 24 months.

Special precautions for storage: Store between 5 and 25°C.

Nature and contents of container: Disposable blow moulded semi-rigid hermetically sealed ampoule made from low density polyethylene grade LD100 supplied by Exxon, containing 20 ml of product.

Instruction for use/handling: Not applicable.

Marketing authorisation number PL 11314/0005

Date of approval/renewal of SPC August 1997

Legal category P

STER-ZAC* BATH CONCENTRATE

Qualitative and quantitative composition Triclosan 2% w/v.

Pharmaceutical form A clear liquid preparation presented in 28.5 ml and 500 ml.

Clinical particulars
Therapeutic indications: This product has an antibacterial effect in water and is intended for the prevention of cross infection and secondary infection.

Posology and method of administration: For bathing: Add 28.5 ml of Ster-Zac Bath Concentrate to a bathful of water (approximately 140 litres) immediately prior to the patient entering the water.
For washing: Add 1 ml of Ster-Zac Bath Concentrate to 5 litres of water, prior to use. No dosage recommendations are made for administration to the elderly or children.

Contra-indications: Not to be used for pregnant women.

Special warnings and precautions for use: For external use only. Keep out of the reach of children. Avoid contact with the eyes.

Interactions with other medicaments and other forms of interaction: None stated.

Pregnancy and lactation: Not to be used for pregnant women.

Effects on ability to drive and use machines: None stated.

Undesirable effects: Erythema may arise in some patients with allergy problems.

Overdose: If erythema or other skin rashes occur, rinse thoroughly with water. Seek medical advice if the condition worsens.

Pharmacological properties
Pharmacodynamic properties: Triclosan is a bactericide.

Pharmacokinetic properties: None stated.

Pre-clinical safety data: None stated.

Pharmaceutical particulars
List of excipients: Industrial Methylated Spirit BP; Isopropyl Alcohol BP; Dioctyl Sodium Sulphosuccinate 60%; Tetrasodium EDTA and Triethanolamide; Deionised Water.

Incompatibilities: None stated.

Shelf life: 36 months.

Special precautions for storage: Store in a cool place.

Nature and contents of container: High density polyethylene container with either a polypropylene cap or a compression moulded screw cap with a steran faced liner, containing 28.5 ml or 500 ml.

Marketing authorisation number 11314/0098

Date of approval/revision of SPC May 1997

Legal category GSL

STER-ZAC* DC SKIN CLEANSER

Qualitative and quantitative composition Hexachlorophane 3.0% w/v.

Pharmaceutical form A viscous white emulsion presented in 150 ml bottles.

Clinical particulars
Therapeutic indictions: This product has an antibacterial effect and is intended for the pre-operative disinfection of hands.

Posology and method of administration: Moisten the hands. Apply 3–5 ml of product to the hands and massage into the hands, paying particular attention to the area around the fingernails. Wash the hands, wrists and forearms for one minute. Rinse with water. Repeat the above but wash for about two minutes. Rinse thoroughly and dry with a sterile towel.

Contra-indications: Do not use for whole body bathing. Do not apply to burns or badly damaged skin. This product is to be administered to children under 2 years on medical advice only.

Special warnings and precautions for use: For external use only. Keep out of the reach of children. Three adverse drug reactions related to the use of hexachlorophane have been reported to date, including skin and subcutaneous tissue disorders, benign skin neoplasms and granuloma. Some product excipients may give rise to allergic reactions in some people. In this instance, discontinue use and seek medical advice.

Interactions with other medicaments and other forms of interaction: None stated.

Pregnancy and lactation: Not recommended for use on pregnant women.

Effects on ability to drive and use machines: Not applicable.

Undesirable effects: Neurotoxic if used in high concentrations on broken or burned skin.

Overdose: Skin: Remove contaminated clothing, blot off excess product and wash the skin with copious amounts of water, followed by a vegetable oil. Keep patient warm and give supportive treatment. Accidental ingestion: Empty the stomach by lavage, taking care to avoid perforation. Olive oil or another vegetable oil may be added to the water to delay absorption. A small amount of oil may be left in the stomach. Activated charcoal may be useful.

Pharmacological properties
Pharmacodynamic properties: Hexachlorophane is a chlorinated bisphenol antiseptic, more active against Gram positive than Gram negative bacteria, and mainly used for disinfection of skin and hands.

Pharmacokinetic properties: None stated.

Pre-clinical safety data: None stated.

Pharmaceutical particulars
List of excipients: Deionised Water; Sodium Octoxynol-2-Ethane Sulphonate; Polyethylene Glycol 300; Glycerine BP; Propylene Glycol BP; Carbomer; Tetrasodium EDTA and Triethanolamide C12–C18 Fatty Acid Diethanolamide; Chlorocresol BP; Polyethylene Glycol 75 Lanolin; White Soft Paraffin BP; Medicated Bouquet GD 7609.

Incompatibilities: The activity of hexachlorophane has been reported to be reduced by alkaline media and by non-ionic surfactants.

Shelf life: 36 months.

Special precautions for storage: No special storage precautions.

Nature and contents of container: 150 ml bottle of high density polyethylene with polypropylene cap.

Marketing authorisation number PL 11314/0099

Date of approval/renewal of SPC August 1997

Legal category POM

STER-ZAC* POWDER

Presentation A white dusting powder containing 0.33% w/w Hexachlorophane BP.

Uses For the prevention of neo-natal staphylococcal sepsis, as an adjunct for the treatment of recurrent furunculosis, and for the prevention and treatment of pressure sores. For topical administration only.

Dosage and administration
For the prevention of neo-natal staphylococcal sepsis: After ligature of the cord, apply powder by sprinkling on to the perineum, groin, the front of the abdomen and the axillae. After cutting the cord, spray with plastic skin dressing. Dust the cord stump with Ster-Zac Powder, and the adjacent skin. After every napkin change, apply Ster-Zac Powder to the umbilicus, cord, adjacent skin, perineum, groin, axillae and the front of the abdomen. Continue the treatment until the cord stump drops away and the wound is healed.

For the treatment of recurrent furunculosis: Apply Ster-Zac Powder daily to the area of the skin normally subject to furunculosis. For the prevention and treatment of pressure sores. Use Ster-Zac Powder on the areas of skin subject to pressure sores.

Contra-indications, warnings etc
Contra-indictions: Do not use on badly burned or excoriated skin.

Other special precautions and warnings: For external use only. This product is to be administered to children under 2 years of age on medical advice only.

Drug interactions: Hexachlorophane activity can be reduced by contact with non-ionic surfactants.

Side effects and adverse reactions: If hypersensitivity occurs, seek medical advice.

Use in pregnancy and lactation: Not recommended for use on pregnant women. No data available on effects on lactation. Seek medical advice before use.

Overdose: The formulation is unlikely to result in overdosage. If accidentally ingested, treat symptomatically.

Pharmaceutical precautions No special requirements.

Legal category P.

Package quantities Sprinkler tins of 30 g.

Further information May be used on full term and premature infants and low birth weight infants provided that the skin is undamaged.

Product licence number 11314/0100

Legal category POM

SULEO-M* LOTION

Qualitative and quantitative composition Malathion 0.5% w/v.

Pharmaceutical form Lotion.

Clinical particulars

Therapeutic indications: For the eradication of head louse infestation.

Posology and method of administration:
Adults, the elderly and children aged 6 months and over: For topical external use only. Rub the lotion gently into the scalp until all the hair and scalp is thoroughly moistened. Allow to dry naturally in a well ventilated room. Do not use a hairdryer or other artificial heat. Live lice will be eradicated after a minimum treatment period of two hours. However the lotion should be left on the head for a further period of 8-10 hours to ensure that all lice eggs are totally eradicated. Shampoo in the normal manner. Rinse and comb the hair while wet to remove the dead lice. In the event of early re-infestation, Suleo-M Lotion may be applied again provided 7 days have elapsed since the first application. Residual protective effect is variable of short duration and should not be relied upon.

Infants: Infants under the age of six months should be treated under medical supervision.

Contra-indications: Known sensitivity to malathion. Not to be used on infants under six months of age except on medical advice.

Special warnings and precautions for use: Suleo-M Lotion contains isopropyl alcohol which may cause wheezing in asthmatic patients or cause inflammation of the skin in patients with severe eczema. Contains flammable alcohol. Apply and dry with care. Avoid naked flames or lighted objects. Do not use artificial heat (e.g. electric hairdryers). Dry in a well ventilated room. Do not cover the head before the lotion has dried completely. The eyes should be well protected during the application and washing of the hair. In the event of contact with the eyes, rinse thoroughly with water. If there is persistent irritation, medical advice should be sought immediately. When Suleo-M Lotion is used by a school nurse or other health officer in the mass treatment of large numbers of children, it is advisable that protective plastic or rubber gloves be worn. Continuous prolonged treatment with this product should be avoided. It should not be used for more than once a week for three weeks at a time. This treatment may affect permed, coloured or bleached hair.

Interactions with other medicaments and other forms of interaction: None stated.

Use in pregnancy and lactation: No known effects in pregnancy and lactation. However, as with all medicines, use with caution.

Effects on ability to drive and use machines: None stated.

Undesirable effects: Very rarely skin irritation has been reported with malathion products.

Overdose: In the event of deliberate or accidental ingestion, as for ethyl alcohol, empty the stomach by gastric lavage and keep patient warm. In the event of massive ingestion, atropine and pralidoxime may be required to counteract cholinesterase inhibition.

Pharmacological properties
Pharmacodynamic properties: Suleo-M Lotion contains malathion, a widely used organophosphorous insecticide which is active by cholinesterase inhibition. It is effective against a wide range of insects but is one of the least toxic organophosphorous insecticides since it is rapidly detoxified by plasma carboxylesterases.

Pharmacokinetic properties: Suleo-M Lotion is applied topically to the affected area.

Pre-clinical safety data: None stated.

Pharmaceutical particulars
List of excipients: Isopropyl alcohol; D-Limonene 17449; Terpineol 18689; Perfume Loxol P6160; citric acid; Shellsol T.

Incompatibilities: None stated.

Shelf life: Two years.

Special precautions for storage: Store at or below 25°C. Protect from sunlight.

Nature and contents of container: Cartoned, clear or amber glass bottles with low density polyethylene caps and high density polyethylene sprinkler inserts containing either 50 or 200 ml of product.

Instructions for use/handling: None stated.

Marketing authorisation number 11314/0055.

Date of approval/revision of SPC November 1995.

Legal category P.

STERETS TISEPT*

Qualitative and quantitative composition Chlorhexidine Gluconate Solution BP equivalent to Chlorhexidine Gluconate 0.015% w/v; Cetrimide PhEur 0.15% w/v.

Pharmaceutical form Sachets containing a solution of Chlorhexidine Gluconate BP 0.015% w/v with Cetrimide PhEur 0.15% w/v.

Clinical particulars
Therapeutic indications: A broad-spectrum antiseptic with detergent properties for swabbing in obstetrics and during dressing changes. For disinfecting and cleansing traumatic and surgical wounds and burns.

Posology and method of administration: Use without further dilution. For topical application only.

Contra-indications: Sterets Tisept should not come into contact with the brain, eyes, meninges or middle ear. The use of Sterets Tisept is contraindicated in patients who have shown hypersensitivity to chlorhexidine gluconate. However, such reactions are rare.

Special warnings and precautions for use: For external use only. Not for injection. When used in aseptic procedures, the outside of the sachet should be disinfected before opening. Discard any surplus immediately after use.

Interactions with other medicaments and other forms of interaction: Hypochlorite bleaches may cause brown stains to develop in fabrics which have previously been in contact with Sterets Tisept.

Pregnancy and lactation: Although there are no adverse reports for this product in pregnant or lactating mothers, as with all medicines, care should be exercised when administering the product to pregnant or lactating women.

Effects on ability to drive and use machines: None known.

Undesirable effects: Idiosyncratic skin reactions and generalised allergenic reactions to chlorhexidine can occur, but these are rare.

Overdose: Treatment of accidental ingestion: Gastric lavage should be carried out with milk, egg white, gelatine or mild soap.

Pharmacological properties
Pharmacodynamic properties: Chlorhexidine is a disinfectant which is effective against a wide range of vegetative Gram-positive and Gram-negative bacteria; it is more effective aginst Gram-positive than Gram-negative bacteria, some species of Pseudomonas and Proteus being less susceptible. The wide range of organisms against which chlorhexidine is active explains the rationale for presenting it in a solution for swabbing wounds and burns in obstetrics. Cetrimide is a quaternary ammonium disinfectant with properties and uses typical of cationic surfactants. It is used in Sterets Tisept for its surfactant and bactericidal properties.

Pharmacokinetic properties: The British Pharmacopoeia 1993 contains monographs for both chlorhexidine gluconate solution 20% w/v and cetrimide. The pharmacokinetics of the compounds when applied to the skin are well described in the literature.

Pre-clinical safety data: Not applicable.

Pharmaceutical particulars
List of excipients: Sunset Yellow E110; Sodium Hydroxidxe BP; Purified Water PhEur.

Incompatibilities: Sterets Tisept is incompatible with anionic agents.

Shelf life: 36 months unopened.

Special precautions for storage: Store in a cool, dark place. Store sachets in outer container.

Nature and contents of container: Nylon/ethylene propylene copolymer laminate sachets containing either 25 or 100 ml of product, overwrapped in heat sealed polythene/nylon and/or polythene/polyester pouches.

Instructions for use/handling: Not applicable.

Marketing authorisation holder: Seton Prebbles Limited, St John's Road, Bootle L20 8NJ.

Marketing authorisation number PL 0303/0017

Date of approval/renewal of SPC March 1998

Legal category P

STERETS UNISEPT*

Qualitative and quantitative composition Chlorhexidine Gluconate Solution 20% w/v BP 0.05% w/v.

Pharmaceutical form Sterile aqueous solution.

Clinical particulars
Therapeutic indications: Chlorhexidine gluconate is a potent antibacterial agent for general antiseptic pur-

poses. It is bactericidal to a broad spectrum of organisms. Sterets Unisept is recommended for use in obstetrics and for swabbing burns and wounds.

Posology and method of administration: There is no distinction between adults, the elderly and children in terms of the use of this product. Sterets Unisept should be used without further dilution for topical administration only.

Contra-indications: Sterets Unisept should not come into contact with the brain, eyes, meninges or middle ear. The use of Sterets Unisept is contraindicated in patients who have shown hypersensitivity to chlorhexidine gluconate. However, such reactions are rare.

Special warnings and precautions for use: For external use only. Not for injection. When Sterets Unisept is used in aseptic procedures, the outside of the sachet should be disinfected before opening. Discard any surplus immediately after use.

Interactions with other medicaments and other forms of interaction: Hypochlorite bleaches may cause brown stains to develop in fabrics which have previously been in contact with Sterets Unisept solution.

Pregnancy and lactation: Although there are no adverse reports for this product in pregnant or lactating mothers, as with all medicines, care should be exercised when administering the product to pregnant or lactating women.

Effects on ability to drive and use machines: None known.

Undesirable effects: Idiosyncratic skin reactions can occur as can generalised allergenic reactions to chlorhexidine gluconate, but these are rare occurrences.

Overdose: Treatment: Accidental ingestion – Gastric lavage should be carried out with milk, egg white, gelatine or mild soap.

Pharmacological properties

Pharmacodynamic properties: Chlorhexidine is a disinfectant which is effective against a wide range of vegetative Gram-positive and Gram-negative bacteria: it is more effective aginst Gram-positive than Gram-negative bacteria, some species of Pseudomonas and Proteus being less susceptible. The wide range of organisms against which chlorhexidine is active explains the rationale for presenting it in a solution for swabbing wounds and burns in obstetrics.

Pharmacokinetic properties: The British Pharmacopoeia 1993 contains monographs for both Chlorhexidine Gluconate Solution 20% w/v. The pharmacokinetics of the compound when applied to the skin as a topical antiseptic are well understood and described in the literature.

Pre-clinical safety data: Not applicable.

Pharmaceutical particulars

List of excipients: Nonoxynol 10 USNF; Sodium Hydroxidxe BP; Carmoisine Red E122; Purified Water PhEur.

Incompatibilities: Sterets Unisept is incompatible with anionic agents.

Shelf life: 36 months.

Special precautions for storage: Store in a cool, dark place. Store sachets in the outer containers.

Nature and contents of container: Nylon-ethylene-propylene copolymer laminate sachets containing either 25 ml or 100 ml of product overwrapped in heat sealed polythene/nylon and/or polythene/polyester pouches.

Instructions for use/handling: Not applicable.

Marketing authorisation holder: Seton Prebbles Limited, St John's Road, Bootle L20 8NJ.

Marketing authorisation number PL 0303/0016

Date of approval/renewal of SPC March 1998

Legal category P

TRANSVASIN* HEAT RUB

Qualitative and quantitative composition Hexyl Nicotinate 2.0% w/w; Ethyl Nicotinate 2.0% w/w; Tetrahydrofurfuryl Salicylate 14.0% w/w.

Pharmaceutical form Cream.

Clinical particulars

Therapeutic indications: For the relief of rheumatic and muscular pain and the symptoms of sprains and strains.

Posology and method of admnistration: For cutaneous administration only. Massage gently into the affected area until the cream is entirely absorbed. Apply at least twice daily until the symptoms abate. Adults, the elderly, and children: Quantities are not critical. The amount used should be consistent with the directions for use, and will vary with the size of the treated area.

Contra-indications: Sensitivity to the product or any of its ingredients.

Special warnings and precautions for use: Not to be applied to broken or sensitive skin, for example around the eyes or scrotal skin. Avoid use on mucous membranes. For external use only. Transvasin Heat Rub is a rubefacient and, within a few minutes of application, a sensation of warmth is felt, followed by a reddening of the skin. This erythema does not indicate intolerance.

Interactions with other medicaments and other forms of interaction: None known.

Pregnancy and lactation: Although there have been no reports of any adverse effects, as with all medicines, care should be taken when administering to pregnant or lactating women.

Effects on ability to drive and to use machines: None known.

Undesirable effects: Reported effects have taken the form of localised sensitisation reactions and have invariably subsided following withdrawal of medication.

Overdose: As this is a topical application with small amounts of actives, adverse systemic effects are unlikely, even after oral ingestion. Treatment: no specific measures are necessary.

Pharmacological properties

Pharmacodynamic properties: Hexyl nicotinate and ethyl nicotinate are rubefacients. Tetrahydrofurfuryl salicylate is used for musculoskeletal, joint, periarticular and soft tissue disorders.

Pharmacokinetic properties: None stated.

Pre-clinical safety data: There are no pre-clinical data of relevance to the prescriber which are additional to that already included in other sections of the Summary of Product Characteristics.

Pharmaceutical particulars

List of excipients: Purified Water PhEur; Methylhydrobenzoate PhEur; Cetostearyl Alcohol BP; Stearic Acid 1973 BPC; Polysorbate 20 PhEur; Sorbitan Monostearate BP; Perfume.

Incompatibilities: None known.

Shelf Life: 36 months.

Special precautions for storage: Shelf life is valid at temperatures up to 35°C.

Nature and contents of container: Collapsible aluminium tubes with membrane, containing 40 g and 80 g of product. Polyamide-imide lacquer internal coating. Polypropylene piecer cap packed in a cardboard outer.

Instruction for use/handling: Not applicable.

Marketing authorisation number PL 11314/0001

Date of approval/renewal of SPC September 1998

Legal category GSL

**Trade Mark*

Shire Pharmaceuticals Limited

East Anton
Andover
Hampshire SP10 5RG

☎ 01264 333455 🖷 01264 333460

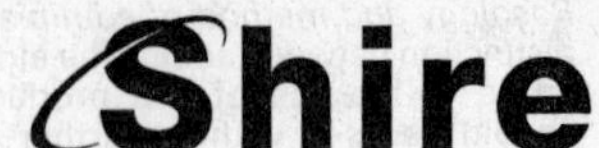

CALCICHEW*

Presentation Round, white slightly speckled, biconvex, chewable tablet with an orange flavour, containing 1250 mg Calcium Carbonate PhEur equivalent to 500 mg calcium.

Uses To be chewed, as a supplemental source of calcium in the correction of dietary deficiencies or when normal requirements are high. As an adjunct to conventional therapy in osteoporosis. Phosphate binding agent in the management of renal failure in patients on renal dialysis.

Dosage and administration
Adults and elderly:
Adjunct to osteoporosis therapy: 2 to 3 tablets daily
Dietary deficiency: 2 to 3 tablets daily.
Osteomalacia: 2 to 6 tablets daily
Phosphate binder: Dose as required by the individual patient depending on serum calcium and phosphate levels. Tablets should be taken just before, during or just after each meal.

Children:
Dietary deficiency: As for adults.
Phosphate binder: As for adults.

Contra-indications, warnings etc.
Contra-indications: Severe hypercalcaemia and hypercalciuria for example in hyperparathyroidism, vitamin D overdose, decalcifying tumours such as plasmacytoma and skeletal metastases, in severe renal failure untreated by renal dialysis, and in osteoporosis due to immobilisation.

Precautions: Patients treated with high doses of vitamin D or who are receiving prolonged calcium treatment, should undergo regulatory measurements of plasma calcium levels which should be interpreted in conjunction with measurements of plasma protein levels.

When used as a phosphate binder in patients on renal dialysis serum phosphate and calcium levels should be monitored regularly.

Interactions: May impair absorption of other drugs, for example, tetracyclines and fluoride preparations. Thiazide diuretics reduce urinary calcium excretion so the risk of hypercalcaemia should be considered. Oral calcium supplementation is aimed at restoring normal serum calcium levels. Although it is extremely unlikely that high enough levels will be achieved to adversely affect digitalised patients, this theoretical possibility should be considered. Vitamin D causes an increase in calcium absorption and plasma calcium levels may continue to rise after stopping vitamin D therapy.

Side effects: Constipation and wind. Rebound acid production.

Hypercalcaemia–although hypercalcaemia would not be expected in patients unless their renal function were impaired, the following symptoms could indicate the possibility of hypercalcaemia: nausea, vomiting, anorexia, constipation, abdominal pain, bone pain, thirst, polyuria, muscle weakness, drowsiness or confusion. Alkalosis with high doses and in patients on renal dialysis. On long term phosphate binding therapy there are rare reports of tissue calcification.

Use in pregnancy and lactation: There is epidemiological and clinical evidence of safety of calcium carbonate in human pregnancy.

Overdosage: There are no reports of overdose. Alkalosis is a theoretical risk.

Pharmaceutical precautions Store below 25°C.

Legal category P

Package quantities Containers of 100 tablets.

Further information Calcichew contains only the following excipients; sorbitol, polyvinylpyrrolidone, orange oil, magnesium stearate, water, isomalt, aspartame, mono, di-fatty acid glycerides.

Product licence number 8557/0003

CALCICHEW* D3

Qualitative and quantitative composition Per tablet: Calcium carbonate 1250 mg equivalent to 500 mg of elemental calcium; cholecalciferol 200 iu (equivalent to 5 micrograms vitamin D_3).

Pharmaceutical form Tablets

Clinical particulars
Therapeutic indications: Calcichew D_3 should be used only as a therapeutic and not as a food supplement when the diet is deficient or when normal requirements of both components are increased. Calcichew D_3 may be used as an adjunct to specific therapy for osteoporosis or as a therapeutic supplement in established osteomalacia, pregnant patients at high risk of needing such a therapeutic supplementation or malnutrition when dietary intake is less than that required.

Posology and method of administration: Orally.
Adults and elderly: Two tablets to be chewed daily
Children: Restrict to over 12 years

Contra-indications: Hypercalcaemia, for example, as a result of hyperparathyroidism (primary or secondary), vitamin D overdosage, decalcifying tumours such as myeloma, bone metastases or sarcoidosis. Severe hypercalciuria, renal stones. Osteoporosis due to immobilisation.

Special warnings and precautions for use: Hypercalcaemia should particularly be avoided in digitalised patients. Patients with mild to moderate renal failure (commonly found in the elderly) or mild hypercalciuria should be supervised carefully with periodic checks of urinary calcium excretion and plasma calcium levels. Urinary calcium excretion should also be measured in patients with a history of renal stones to exclude hypercalciuria.

Interaction with other medicaments and other forms of interaction: Calcium may impair the absorption of tetracyclines, fluoride or iron. At least three hours should intervene between taking Calcichew D_3 and these agents.

Pregnancy and lactation: Normal requirements for calcium and vitamin D are raised during pregnancy and lactation. If supplementation is necessary, it should be given at a different time from iron supplements. Calcium is excreted in breast milk but not sufficiently to produce an adverse effect in the infant. Allowances should be made for vitamin D/calcium from other sources. During pregnancy and lactation therapy should be under medical supervision.

Effects on ability to drive and use machinery: None known

Undesirable effects: Mild gastro-intestinal disturbances (e.g. constipation) can occur with calcium supplements, but are infrequent. Rebound secretion of gastric acid is possible, but unlikely to be clinically significant. Milk-alkali syndrome with hypercalcaemia is a rare possibility in chronically treated individuals.

Overdose: The most serious consequence of acute or chronic overdosage would be hypercalcaemia due to vitamin D toxicity. This is very unlikely unless extreme sensitivity to vitamin D is present, as in normal people over 200 chewable tablets a day would be required to produce a toxic dose. Features of hypercalcaemia include anorexia, nausea, vomiting, weakness, fatigue and headache. With a plasma calcium of over 2.6 mmol per litre, confusion and coma can develop. Polydipsia and polyuria indicate renal damage. Calcium and vitamin D treatment must be stopped and a high fluid intake and low calcium diet given. Corticosteroid and other specialist treatment may be necessary in severe cases.

Pharmacological properties
Pharmacodynamic properties: Calcium carbonate is a well established medicinal item used as an antacid or calcium supplement in deficient states. Vitamin D_3 is a well established medicinal item. Vitamin D compounds are fat-soluble sterols, sometimes considered to be hormones, which are involved in the regulation of calcium and phosphate homeostasis and bone mineralisation.

Pharmacokinetic properties: The pharmacokinetics of calcium and its salts are well established. Calcium carbonate is converted into calcium chloride by gastric acid. Some of the calcium is absorbed from the intestines but about 80% is reconverted to insoluble calcium salts such as the carbonate and stearate, and excreted. The pharmacokinetics of vitamin D substances are well established. These are well absorbed from the gastro-intestinal tract; bile must be present for adequate intestinal absorption. Circulation is via specific gamma-globulins, storage can be long term in the adipose and muscle tissue, excretion Is mainly in the bile and faeces.

Preclinical safety data: Toxic effects would only result from overdosage. Calcium salts by themselves are virtually innocuous in normal subjects. While chronic overdosage with vitamin D is toxic, resulting in hypercalcaemia, the amount present in Calcichew D_3 is too small to represent a practical clinical risk.

Pharmaceutical information
List of excipients: Sorbitol, polyvinylpyrrolidone K30, isomalt, orange oil, magnesium stearate, aspartame and mono, di-fatty acid glycerides.

Incompatibilities: None known

Shelf life: 2 years

Special storage precautions: Maximum storage temperature of 25°C.

Nature and contents of container: Containers of 100 tablets.

Instructions for use/handling: No special conditions.

Marketing authorisation number 8557/0021

Date of approval/revision of SPC January 1998

Legal category P

CALCICHEW* D3 FORTE

Qualitative and quantitative composition Per tablet: Calcium carbonate 1250 mg (equivalent to 500 mg of elemental calcium); cholecalciferol 400 iu (equivalent to 10 micrograms vitamin D_3)

Pharmaceutical form Tablet

Clinical particulars
Therapeutic indications: Calcichew D_3 Forte may be used in: The treatment and prevention of vitamin D/calcium deficiency (characterised by raised serum alkaline phosphatase levels associated with increased bone loss, raised levels of serum PTH and lowered 25-hydroxyvitamin D) particularly in the housebound and institutionalised elderly subjects. The supplementation of vitamin D and calcium as an adjunct to specific therapy for osteoporosis, in pregnancy, in established vitamin D dependent osteomalacia and in other situations requiring therapeutic supplementation of malnutrition.

Posology and method of administration: Oral
Adults and elderly: 2 chewable tablets per day, preferably one tablet morning and evening.
Children: restrict to over 12 years

Contra-indications: Hypercalcaemia, for example as a result of primary hyperparathyroidism, vitamin D overdosage, sarcoidosis or malignant bone diseases such as myeloma, bone metastases. Severe hypercalciuria, renal stones. Osteoporosis due to prolonged immobilisation, for example, paraplegia. Milk alkali syndrome. Severe renal failure.

Special warnings and precautions for use: Patients with mild to moderate renal failure or mild hypercalciuria should be supervised carefully with periodic checks of urinary calcium excretion and plasma calcium levels. Urinary calcium excretion should also be measured in patients with a history of renal stones to exclude hypercalciuria.

Interaction with other medicaments and other forms of interaction: Calcium may impair the absorption of tetracyclines, fluoride or iron. At least 3 hours should intervene between taking Calcichew D_3 Forte and these agents. Thiazide diuretics reduce urinary calcium excretion so the risk of hypercalcaemia should be considered. Hypercalcaemia should particularly be avoided in digitalised patients.

Pregnancy and lactation: Normal requirements for calcium and vitamin D are raised during pregnancy and lactation. If supplementation is necessary, it should be given at a different time from iron supplements. Calcium is excreted in breast milk, but not sufficiently to produce an adverse effect in the infant. Allowances should be made for vitamin D/calcium from other sources. During pregnancy and lactation, therapy should be under medical supervision.

Effects on ability to drive and use machines: None expected.

Undesirable effects: Mild gastrointestinal disturbances, for example, constipation, can occur with calcium supplements, but are infrequent. Rebound secretion of gastric acid is possible, but unlikely to be clinically significant. Milk-alkali syndrome with hypercalcaemia is a rare possibility in chronically treated individuals.

Overdose: The most serious consequence of acute or chronic overdosage would be hypercalcaemia due to vitamin D toxicity. This is very unlikely, as in normal people over 100 chewable tablets a day would be required to produce a toxic dose. Features of hypercalcaemia include anorexia, nausea, vomiting, weakness, fatigue and headache. With a plasma calcium of over 2.6 mmol per litre, confusion and coma can develop. Polydipsia and polyuria indicate renal damage. Calcium and vitamin D treatment must be stopped and a high fluid intake and low calcium diet given. Corticosteroid and other specialist treatment may be necessary in severe cases.

Pharmacological properties
Pharmacological properties: Calcium carbonate is a well established medicinal item used as an antacid or calcium supplement in deficiency states. Vitamin D_3 is a well established medicinal item. Vitamin D compounds are fat-soluble sterols, sometimes considered to be hormones, which are essential for the proper regulation of calcium and phosphate homeostasis and bone mineralisation.

Pharmacokinetic properties: The pharmacokinetics of calcium and its salts are well established. Calcium carbonate is converted to calcium chloride by gastric acid. Some of the calcium is absorbed from the intestines, but about 85% is reconverted to insoluble calcium salts as the carbonate and stearate, and excreted in the faeces. The pharmacokinetics of vitamin D substances are also well established. They are well absorbed from the gastro-intestinal tract; bile must be present for adequate intestinal absorption. Circulation is via specific gamma globulins, storage can be long term in the adipose and muscle tissue, excretion is mainly in the bile and faeces.

Safety data: Toxic effects would only result from overdosage. Calcium salts by themselves are virtually innocuous in normal subjects. While chronic overdosage with vitamin D is toxic, resulting in hypercalcaemia, the amount present in Calcichew D_3 Forte is too small to represent a practical clinical risk.

Pharmaceutical particulars
List of excipients: Sorbitol, povidone, isomalt, lemon flavouring, fatty acid mono- and diglycerides, aspartame, magnesium stearate, sucrose, gelatin, vegetable fat, tocopherol and maize starch.

Incompatibility: Not applicable, oral preparation.

Shelf life: 24 months.

Special storage precautions: Store at a temperature below 25°C and protect against moisture.

Nature and contents of container: White, high density polyethylene bottles. Bottles containing 100 tablets with tamper evident seal.

Instructions for use/handling: No special conditions.

Marketing authorisation number 8557/0029

Date of approval/revision of SPC December 1997

Legal category P

CALCICHEW* FORTE

Presentation Round, white, slightly speckled, flat, bevel-edged, chewable tablets containing 2.5 g Calcium Carbonate PhEur equivalent to 1 g calcium.

Uses To be chewed, as a supplemental source of calcium in the correction of dietary deficiencies or when normal requirements are high. As an adjunct to conventional therapy in osteoporosis. Phosphate binding agent in the management of renal failure in patients on renal dialysis.

Dosage and administration
Adults and elderly:
Adjunct to osteoporosis therapy: 1 tablet daily
Dietary deficiency: 1 tablet daily
Osteomalacia: 1–3 tablets daily
Phosphate binding: Dose as required by the individual patient depending on serum calcium and phosphate levels. Tablets should be taken just before, during or just after each meal.

Children:
Dietary deficiency: As for adults
Phosphate binding: As for adults

Contra-indications, warnings etc.
Contra-indications: Severe hypercalcaemia and hypercalciuria, for example, in hyperparathyroidism, vitamin D overdose, decalcifying tumours such as multiple myeloma, plasmacytoma and skeletal metastases, in severe renal failure untreated by renal dialysis and in osteoporosis due to immobilisation.

Precautions: Patients treated with high doses of vitamin D or who are receiving prolonged calcium treatment, should undergo regulatory measurements of plasma calcium levels which should be interpreted in conjunction with measurements of plasma protein levels. When used as a phosphate binder in patients on renal dialysis serum phosphate and calcium levels should be monitored regularly.

Interactions: May impair absorption of other drugs, for example, tetracyclines and fluoride preparations. Thiazide diuretics reduce urinary calcium excretion so the risk of hypercalcaemia should be considered. Oral calcium supplementation is aimed at restoring normal serum calcium levels, although it is extremely unlikely that high enough levels will be achieved to adversely affect digitalised patients, this theoretical possibility should be considered. Vitamin D causes an increase in calcium absorption and plasma calcium levels may continue to rise after stopping vitamin D therapy.

Side effects: Constipation and wind. Diarrhoea in a small number of patients. Rebound acid production. Hypercalcaemia–although hypercalcaemia would not be expected in patients unless their renal function was impaired. The following symptoms could indicate the possibility of hypercalcaemia: nausea, vomiting, anorexia, constipation, abdominal pain, bone pain, thirst, polyuria, muscle weakness, drowsiness or confusion. Alkalosis with high doses and in patients on renal dialysis. On long term phosphate binding therapy there are rare reports of tissue calcification.

Use in pregnancy and lactation: There is epidemiological and clinical evidence of safety of calcium carbonate in human pregnancy.

Overdosage: There are no reports of overdose. Alkalosis is a theoretical risk.

Pharmaceutical precautions Store below 25°C.

Legal category P

Package quantities Containers of 100 tablets.

Further information Calcichew Forte contains only the following excipients; sorbitol, polyvinylpyrrolidone K30, isomalt, orange oils, magnesium stearate, aspartame, mono, di-fatty acid glycerides.

Product licence number 8557/0022

CALCIDRINK*

Qualitative and quantitative composition Calcium carbonate 2.5 g equivalent to 1 g of calcium.

Pharmaceutical form Dispersible granules.

Clinical particulars
Therapeutic indications: Treatment of calcium deficiency. As an adjunct to conventional therapy in osteoporosis.

Posology and method of administration:
Adults, elderly and children: One sachet to be taken dispersed in water daily.

Contra-indications: Severe hypercalcaemia and hypercalciuria, for example, in primary hyperparathyroidism, vitamin D overdose, osteoporosis due to immobilisation, decalcifying tumours such as plasmacytoma and skeletal metastases. Severe renal failure.

Special warnings and precautions for use: Patients with mild to moderate renal failure or mild calciuria should be supervised carefully with periodic checks of urinary calcium excretion and plasma calcium levels. Urinary calcium excretion should be measured in patients with a history of renal stones to exclude hypercalciuria.

Interaction with other medicaments and other forms of interaction: Calcium may impair the absorption of tetracyclines or fluoride. At least 3 hours should intervene between taking Calcidrink and these agents. Calcium salts can reduce the absorption of bisphosphonates and at least 2 hours should intervene between taking these agents. Thiazide diuretics reduce urinary calcium excretion so the risk of hypercalcaemia should be considered. Hypercalcaemia should particularly be avoided in digitalised patients.

Pregnancy and lactation: There is epidemiological and clinical evidence of safety of calcium carbonate in human pregnancy. Calcium is secreted in breast milk, but not sufficiently to produce an adverse effect in the infant.

Effects on ability to drive and use machines: None expected.

Undesirable effects: Mild gastrointestinal disturbances, for example, constipation, can occur with calcium supplements, but are infrequent. Rebound secretion of gastric acid is possible, but unlikely to be clinically significant. Hypercalcaemia would not normally be expected in patients, even at higher doses, unless there is an underlying cause such as impaired renal function/drug interaction.

Overdose: No cases of intoxication due to calcium overdose are known.

Pharmacological properties
Pharmacodynamic properties: Calcium carbonate is a well established medicinal item.

Pharmacokinetic properties: The pharmacokinetics of calcium and its salts are well established.

Preclinical safety data: Results of preclinical studies are of little relevance for this well established compound.

Pharmaceutical particulars
List of excipients: Citric acid, sugar, glucose, orange oil, saccharin sodium, lecithin, beta carotene, sodium lauryl sulphate, invert sugar, mono, di-fatty acid glycerides and water.

Incompatibilities: Not applicable for an oral preparation.

Shelf life: 36 months.

Special precautions for storage: No special precautions.

Nature and contents of container: Calcidrink is provided in sachets. These are available to pharmacies in boxes of 30.

Instructions for use/handling: The contents of a sachet should be added to a glass of water and stirred before drinking.

Marketing authorisation number: 8557/0018

Date of approval/revision of SPC September 1995

Legal category: P

CALCORT* ▼

Qualitative and quantitative composition
Active ingredient:

1 mg tablet:	deflazacort 1 mg
6 mg tablet:	deflazacort 6 mg
30 mg tablet:	deflazacort 30 mg

Pharmaceutical form

1 mg tablets:	Round, white, uncoated tablets, plain on one face with a 1 on the other face.
6 mg tablets:	Round, white, uncoated tablets, marked with a cross on one face and a 6 on the other face.
30 mg tablets:	Round, white, uncoated tablets, marked with a cross on one face and a 30 on the other face.

Clinical particulars
Therapeutic indications: A wide range of conditions may sometimes need treatment with glucocorticosteroids. The indications include: Anaphylaxis; asthma; severe hypersensitivity reactions. Rheumatoid arthritis; juvenile chronic arthritis; polymyalgia rheumatica. Systemic lupus erythematosus; dermatomyositis; mixed connective tissue disease (other than systemic sclerosis); polyarteritis nodosa; sarcoidosis. Pemphigus; bullous pemphigoid; pyoderma gangrenosum. Minimal change nephrotic syndrome; acute interstitial nephritis. Rheumatic carditis. Ulcerative colitis; Crohn's disease. Uveitis, optic neuritis. Autoimmune haemolytic anaemia, idiopathic thrombocytopenic purpura. Acute and lymphatic leukaemia, malignant lymphoma; multiple myeloma. Immune suppression in transplantation.

Posology and method of administration: Deflazacort is a glucocorticoid derived from prednisolone and 6 mg of deflazacort has approximately the same anti-inflammatory potency as 5 mg prednisone or prednisolone.

Doses vary widely in different diseases and different patients. In more serious and life-threatening conditions, high doses of deflazacort may need to be given. When deflazacort is used long term in relatively benign chronic diseases, the maintenance dose should be kept as low as possible. Dosage may need to be increased during periods of stress or in exacerbation of illness.

The dosage should be individually titrated according to diagnosis, severity of disease and patient response and tolerance. The lowest dose that will produce an acceptable response should be used (see *Warnings and Precautions*).

Adults: For acute disorders, up to 120 mg/day deflazacort may need to be given initially. Maintenance doses in most conditions are within the range 3–18 mg/day. The following regimens are for guidance only:

Rheumatoid arthritis: The maintenance dose is usually within the range 3–18 mg/day. The smallest effective dose should be used and increased if necessary.

Bronchial asthma: In the treatment of an acute attack high doses of 48 to 72 mg/day may be needed, depending on severity, and gradually reduced once the attack has been controlled. For maintenance in chronic asthma, doses should be titrated to the lowest dose that controls symptoms.

Other conditions: The dose of deflazacort depends on clinical need titrated to the lowest effective dose for maintenance. Starting dose may be estimated on the basis of ratio of 5 mg prednisone or prednisolone to 6 mg deflazacort.

Hepatic impairment: In patients with hepatic impairment, blood levels of deflazacort may be increased. Therefore the dose of deflazacort should be carefully monitored and adjusted to the minimum effective dose.

Renal impairment: In renally impaired patients, no special precautions other than those usually adopted in patients receiving glucocorticoid therapy are necessary.

Elderly: In elderly patients, no special precautions other than those usually adopted in patients receiving glucocorticoid therapy are necessary. The common adverse effects of systemic corticosteroids may be associated with more serious consequences in old age (see Warnings and Precautions).

Children: There has been limited exposure of children to deflazacort in clinical trials.

In children, the indications for glucocorticoids are the same as for adults, but it is important that the lowest effective dosage is used. Alternate day administration may be appropriate (see *Warnings and Precautions*).

Doses of deflazacort usually lie in the range 0.25–1.5 mg/kg/day. The following ranges provide general guidance:

Juvenile chronic arthritis: The usual maintenance dose is between 0.25–1.0 mg/kg/day.

Nephrotic syndrome: Initial dose of usually 1.5 mg/kg/day followed by down titration according to clinical need.

Bronchial asthma: On the basis of the potency ratio, the initial dose should be between 0.25–1.0 mg/kg deflazacort on alternate days.

Deflazacort withdrawal: In patients who have received more than physiological doses of systemic corticosteroids (approximately 9 mg per day or equivalent) for greater than 3 weeks, withdrawal should not be abrupt. How dose reduction should be carried out depends largely on whether the disease is likely to relapse as the dose of systemic corticosteroids is reduced. Clinical assessment of disease activity may be needed during withdrawal. If the disease is unlikely to relapse on withdrawal of systemic corticosteroids but there is uncertainty about HPA suppression, the dose of systemic corticosteroids *may* be reduced rapidly to physiological doses. Once a daily dose equivalent to 9 mg deflazacort is reached, dose reduction should be slower to allow the HPA-axis to recover.

Abrupt withdrawal of systemic corticosteroid treatment, which has continued up to 3 weeks is appropriate if it is considered that the disease is unlikely to relapse. Abrupt withdrawal of doses up to 48 mg daily of deflazacort, or equivalent for 3 weeks is unlikely to lead to clinically relevant HPA-axis suppression, in the majority of patients. In the following patient groups, gradual withdrawal of systemic corticosteroid theray should be *considered* even after courses lasing 3 weeks or less:

- Patients who have had repeated courses of systemic corticosteroids, particularly if taken for greater than 3 weeks.
- When a short course has been prescribed within one year of cessation of long-term therapy (months or years).
- Patients who may have reasons for adrenocortical insufficiency other than exogenous corticosteroid therapy.
- Patients receiving doses of systemic corticosteroid greater than 48 mg daily of deflazacort (or equivalent).
- Patients repeatedly taking doses in the evening.

Contra-indications: Systemic infection unless specific anti-infective therapy is employed. Hypersensitivity to deflazacort or any of the ingredients. Patients receiving live virus immunisation.

Special warnings and special precautions for use: A patient information leaflet should be supplied with this product. Undesirable effects may be minimised by using the lowest dose for the minimum period, and by administering the daily requirement as a single morning dose, or, whenever possible, as a single morning dose on alternate days. Frequent patient review is required to appropriately titrate dose against disease activity (see *Dosage* section).

Adrenal suppression: Adrenal cortical atrophy develops during prolonged therapy and may persist for years after stopping treatment. Withdrawal of corticosteroids after prolonged therapy must therefore always be gradual to avoid acute adrenal insufficiency, being tapered off over weeks or months according to the dose and duration of treatment. During prolonged therapy, any intercurrent illness, trauma or surgical procedure will require a temporary increase in dosage; if corticosteroids have been stopped following prolonged therapy they may need to be temporarily reintroduced.

Patients should carry 'Steroid Treatment' cards which give clear guidance on the precautions to be taken to minimise risk and which provide details of prescriber, drug, dosage and the duration of treatment.

Anti-inflammatory/immunosuppressive effects and infections: Suppression of the inflammatory response and immune function increases the susceptibility to infections and their severity. The clinical presentation may often be atypical and serious infections such as septicaemia and tuberculosis may be masked and may reach an advanced stage before being recognised.

Chickenpox is of particular concern since this normally minor illness may be fatal in immunosuppressed patients. Patients (or parents of children) without a definite history of chickenpox should be advised to avoid close personal contact with chickenpox or herpes zoster and, if exposed, they should seek urgent medical attention. Passive immunisation with varicella zoster immunoglobulin (VZIG) is needed by exposed non-immune patients who are receiving systemic corticosteroids or who have used them within the previous 3 months; this should be given within 10 days of exposure to chickenpox. If a diagnosis of chickenpox is confirmed, the illness warrants specialist care and urgent treatment. Corticosteroids should not be stopped and the dose may need to be increased.

Live vaccines should not be given to individuals with impaired responsiveness. The antibody response to other vaccines may be diminished.

Prolonged use of glucocorticoids may produce posterior subcapsular cataracts, glaucoma with possible damage to the optic nerves and may enhance the establishment of secondary ocular infections due to fungi or viruses.

Use in active tuberculosis should be restricted to those cases of fulminating and disseminated tuberculosis in which deflazacort is used for management with appropriate antituberculosis regimen. If glucocorticoids are indicated in patients with latent tuberculosis or tuberculin reactivity, close observation is necessary as reactivation of the disease may occur. During prolonged glucocorticoid therapy, these patients should receive chemoprophylaxis.

Special precautions: The following clinical conditions require special caution and frequent patient monitoring is necessary.

– Cardiac disease or congestive heart failure (except in the presence of active rheumatic carditis), hypertension, thromboembolic disorders. Glucocorticoids can cause salt and water retention and increased excretion of potassium. Dietary salt restriction and potassium supplementation may be necessary.

– Gastritis or oesophagitis, diverticulitis, ulcerative colitis if there is probability of impending perforation, abscess or pyogenic infections, fresh intestinal anastomosis, active or latent peptic ulcer.

– Diabetes mellitus or a family history, osteoporosis, myasthenia gravis, renal insufficiency.

– Emotional instability or psychotic tendency, epilepsy.

– Previous corticosteroid-induced myopathy.

– Liver failure;

– Hypothyroidism and cirrhosis, which may increase glucocorticoid effect.

– Ocular herpes simplex because of possible corneal perforation.

Use in children: Corticosteroids cause dose-related growth retardation in infancy, childhood and adolescence which may be irreversible.

Use in elderly: The common adverse effects of systemic corticosteroids may be associated with more serious consequences in old age, especially osteoporosis, hypertension, hypokalaemia, diabetes, susceptibility to infection and thinning of the skin. Close clinical supervision is required to avoid life-threatening reactions.

Since complications of glucocorticoid therapy are dependent on dose and duration of therapy, the lowest possible dose must be given and a risk/benefit decision must be made as to whether intermittent therapy should be used.

Interactions with other medicaments and other forms of interactions: The same precautions should be exercised as for other glucocorticoids. Deflazacort is metabolised in the liver. It is recommended to increase the maintenance dose of deflazacort if drugs which are liver enzyme inducers are co-administered, e.g. rifampicin, rifabutin, carbamazepine, phenobarbitone, phenytoin, primidone and aminoglutethimide. For drugs which inhibit liver enzymes, e.g. ketoconazole, it may be possible to reduce the maintenance dose of deflazacort.

The desired effects of hypoglycaemic agents (including insulin), anti-hypertensives and diuretics are antagonised by corticosteroids and the hypokalaemic effects of acetazolamide, loop diuretics, thiazide diuretics and carbenoxolone are enhanced.

The efficacy of coumarin anticoagulants may be enhanced by concurrent corticosteroid therapy and close monitoring of the INR or prothrombin time is required to avoid spontaneous bleeding.

The renal clearance of salicylates is increased by corticosteroids and steroid withdrawal may result in salicylate intoxication.

As glucocorticoids can suppress the normal responses of the body to attack by micro-organisms, it is important to ensure that any anti-infective therapy is effective and it is recommended to monitor patients closely. Concurrent use of glucocorticoids and oral contraceptives should be closely monitored as plasma levels of glucocorticoids may be increased. This effect may be due to a change in metabolism or binding to serum proteins. Antacids may reduce bioavailability; leave at least 2 hours between administration of deflazacort and antacids.

Pregnancy: The ability of corticosteroids to cross the placenta varies between individual drugs, however, deflazacort does cross the placenta.

Administration of corticosteroids to pregnant animals can cause abnormalities of foetal development including cleft palate, intra-uterine growth retardation and effects on brain growth and development. There is no evidence that corticosteroids result in an increased incidence of congenital abnormalities, such as cleft palate/lip in man. However, when administered for prolonged periods or repeatedly during pregnancy, corticosteroids may increase the risk of intra-uterine growth retardation. Hypoadrenalism may, in theory, occur in the neonate following prenatal exposure to corticosteroids but usually resolves spontaneously following birth and is rarely clinically important. As with all drugs, corticosteroids should only be prescribed when the benefits to the mother and child outweigh the risks. When corticosteroids are essential however, patients with normal pregnancies may be treated as though they were in the non-gravid state.

Lactation: Corticosteroids are excreted in breast milk, although no data are available for deflazacort. Doses of up to 50 mg daily of deflazacort are unlikely to cause systemic effects in the infant. Infants of mothers taking higher doses than this may have a degree of adrenal suppression but the benefits of breast feeding are likely to outweigh any theoretical risk.

Effects on ability to drive and use machines: On the basis of the pharmacodynamic profile and reported adverse events, it is unlikely that deflazacort will produce an effect on the ability to drive and use machines.

Undesirable effects: The incidence of predictable undesirable effects, including hypothalamic-pituitary-adrenal suppression correlates with the relative potency of the drug, dosage, timing of administration and the duration of treatment (see *Warnings and Precautions*).

Endocrine/metabolic: Suppression of the hypothalamic-pituitary-adrenal axis, growth suppression in infancy, childhood and adolescence, menstrual irregularity and amenorrhoea. Cushingoid facies, hirsutism, weight gain, impaired carbohydrate tolerance with increased requirement for anti-diabetic therapy. Negative protein and calcium balance. Increased appetite.

Anti-inflammatory and immunosuppressive effects: Increased susceptibility and severity of infections with suppression of clinical symptoms and signs, opportunistic infections, recurrence of dormant tuberculosis (see Warnings and Precautions).

Musculoskeletal: Osteoporosis, vertebral and long bone fractures, avascular osteonecrosis, tendon rupture. Proximal myopathy with wasting and weakness, negative nitrogen balance.

Fluid and electrolyte disturbance: Sodium and water retention with hypertension, oedema and heart failure, potassium loss, hypokalaemic alkalosis.

Neuropsychiatric: Headache, vertigo, euphoria, psychological dependence, hypomania or depression, insomnia, restlessness and aggravation of schizophrenia. Increased intra-cranial pressure with papilloedema in children (pseudotumour cerebri), usually after treatment withdrawal. Aggravation of epilepsy.

Ophthalmic: Increased intra-ocular pressure, glaucoma, papilloedema, posterior subcapsular cataracts especially in children, corneal or scleral thinning, exacerbation of ophthalmic viral or fungal diseases.

Gastrointestinal: Dyspepsia, peptic ulceration with perforation and haemorrhage, acute pancreatitis (especially in children), candidiasis.

Dermatological: Impaired healing, skin atrophy, bruising, telangiectasia, striae, acne.

General: Hypersensitivity including anaphylaxis has been reported. Leucocytosis. Thromboembolism. Rare incidence of benign intracranial hypertension.

Withdrawal symptoms and signs: Too rapid a reduction of corticosteroid dosage following prolonged treatment can lead to acute adrenal insufficiency, hypotension and death (see Warnings and Precautions).

A "withdrawal syndrome" may also occur including fever, myalgia, arthralgia, rhinitis, conjunctivitis, painful itchy skin nodules and loss of weight. This may occur in patients even without evidence of adrenal insufficiency.

Overdose: It is unlikely that treatment is needed in cases of acute overdosage. The LD_{50} for the oral dose is greater than 4000 mg/kg in laboratory animals.

Pharmacological properties

Pharmacodynamic properties: Deflazacort is a glucocorticoid. Its anti-inflammatory and immunosuppressive effects are used in treating a variety of diseases and are comparable to other anti-inflammatory steroids. Clinical studies have indicated that the average potency ratio of deflazacort to prednisolone is 0.69–0.89.

Pharmacokinetic properties: Orally administered deflazacort appears to be well absorbed and is immediately converted to plasma esterases to the pharmacologically active metabolite (D–21–OH) which achieves peak plasma concentrations in 1.5 to 2 hours. It is 40% protein-bound and has no affinity for corticosteroid-binding-globulin (transcortin). It's elimination plasma half-life is 1.1 to 1.9 hours. Elimination takes place primarily through the kidneys; 70% of the administered dose is excreted in the urine. The remaining 30% is eliminated in the faeces. Metabolism of D 21–OH is extensive; only 18% of urinary excretion represents D 21–OH. The metabolite of D 21–OH, deflazacort 6-beta–OH, represents one third of the urinary elimination.

Preclinical safety data: Safety studies have been carried out in the rat, dog, mouse and monkey. The findings are consistent with other glucocorticoids at comparable doses. Teratogenic effects demonstrated in rodents and rabbits are typical of those caused by other glucocorticoids. Deflazacort was not found to be carcinogenic in the mouse, but studies in the rat produced carcinogenic findings consistent with the findings with other glucocorticoids.

Pharmaceutical particulars

List of excipients: 6 mg tablets–Microcrystalline Cellulose PhEur, Lactose PhEur, Maize Starch PhEur, Magnesium Stearate PhEur, Sucrose PhEur.

1 mg and 30 mg tablets–Microcrystalline Cellulose, Lactose, Maize Starch and Magnesium Stearate.

Incompatibilities: None reported.

Shelf-life:
1 mg tablets: 3 years
6 and 30 mg tablets: 5 years.

Special precautions for storage: Store in a dry place below 25°C.

Nature and contents of container: Deflazacort will be packed in blister packs of polyvinylchloride and aluminium foil presented in cardboard cartons.
100 tablets per pack–1 mg tablets
60 tablets per pack–6 mg tablets
30 tablets per pack–30 mg tablets.

Instructions for use/handling: No special instructions for use or handling are required.

Marketing authorisation holder: Shire Pharmaceuticals Ltd., East Anton, Andover, Hampshire SP10 5RG.

Marketing authorisation numbers
1 mg tablets: 08557/0036
6 mg tablets: 08557/0037
30 mg tablets: 08557/0038

Date of approval/revision of SPC April 1998.

Legal category POM

CARNITOR* INJECTION 1 g

Presentation Clear colourless or light straw coloured sterile solution containing levocarnitine inner salt 1 g in 5 ml ampoules.

Uses Indicated for the treatment of primary and secondary carnitine deficiency in adults, children, infants and neonates.

Secondary carnitine deficiency in haemodialysis patients: Secondary carnitine deficiency should be suspected in long-term haemodialysis patients who have the following conditions:

1. Severe and persistent muscle cramps and/or hypotensive episodes during dialysis.
2. Lack of energy causing a significant negative effect on the quality of life.
3. Skeletal muscle weakness and/or myopathy.
4. Cardiomyopathy.
5. Anaemia of uraemia unresponsive to or requiring large doses of erythropoietin.
6. Muscle mass loss caused by malnutrition.

Dosage and administration

Adults, children, infants and neonates: For slow intravenous administration over 2–3 minutes.

It is advisable to monitor therapy by measuring free and acyl carnitine levels in both plasma and urine.

The management of inborn errors of metabolism: The dosage required depends upon the specific inborn error of metabolism concerned and the severity of presentation at the time of treatment. However, the following can be considered as a general guide.

In acute decompensation, dosages of up to 100 mg/kg/day in 3–4 divided doses are recommended. Higher doses have been used although an increase in adverse events, primarily diarrhoea, may occur.

Secondary carnitine deficiency in haemodialysis patients: It is strongly recommended that, before initiating therapy with Carnitor, plasma carnitine is measured. Secondary carnitine deficiency is suggested by a plasma ratio of acyl to free carnitine of greater than 0.4 and/or when free carnitine concentrations are lower than 20 micromol per litre.

A dose of 20 mg per kg should be administered as an intravenous bolus at the end of each dialysis session (assuming three sessions per week). The duration of intravenous treatment should be at least three months which is the time usually required to restore normal muscle levels of free carnitine. The overall response should be assessed by monitoring plasma acyl/free carnitine levels and by evaluating the patient's symptoms. When carnitine supplementation has been stopped there will be a progressive decline in carnitine levels. The need for a repeat course of therapy can be assessed by plasma carnitine assays at regular intervals and by monitoring the patient's symptoms.

Haemodialysis–maintenance therapy: If significant clinical benefit has been gained by the first course of intravenous Carnitor then maintenance therapy can be considered using 1 g of Carnitor orally. On the day of dialysis oral Carnitor has to be administered at the end of the session. (See Data Sheet for Carnitor Paediatric Solution 30% and Single Oral Dose 1 g.)

Contra-indications, warnings, etc

Contra-indications: Hypersensitivity to any constituent of the product.

Precautions: There is limited experience of use in patients with primary and secondary systemic carnitine deficiency suffering from renal failure.

Pregnancy and lactation: Reproductive studies were performed in rats and rabbits. There was no evidence of a teratogenic effect in either species. In the rabbit but not in the rat there was a statistically insignificant greater number of post-implantation losses at the highest dose tested (600 mg/kg/ daily) as compared with control animals. The significance of these findings in man is unknown. There is no experience of use in pregnant patients with primary systemic carnitine deficiency.

Taking into account the serious risk if treatment is discontinued, the consequence to a pregnant women who has primary systemic carnitine deficiency requires consideration.

Levocarnitine is a normal component of human milk, use of Carnitor supplementation in nursing mothers has not been studied.

Side-effects: Various mild gastrointestinal complaints have been reported during the long term administration of oral levocarnitine, these include transient nausea and vomiting, abdominal cramps and diarrhoea. Decreasing the dosage often diminishes or eliminates drug related patient body odour or gastrointestinal symptoms when present. Tolerance should be monitored very closely during the first week of the administration and after any dosage increase.

Drug interactions: There are no known interactions.

Overdosage: There have been no reports of toxicity from levocarnitine overdosage. Overdosage should be treated with supportive care.

Pharmaceutical precautions Store at a temperature not exceeding 25°C. Protect from light.

Package quantities The injections are packed in cardboard cartons of five ampoules.

Product licence number 8381/0003

Product licence holder: Sigma-Tau Industrie Farmaceutiche Riunite SpA, Viale Shakespeare, 47-00144, Rome, Italy.

CARNITOR* PAEDIATRIC SOLUTION 30% AND SINGLE ORAL DOSE 1 g

Presentation

Paediatric Solution 30%: Colourless or slightly yellow solution containing levocarnitine 30%.

Single Oral Dose 1 g: A colourless or slightly yellow coloured liquid in a 10 ml amber glass bottle containing levocarnitine inner salt 1 g.

Uses

Paediatric Solution 30%: Indicated for the treatment of primary and secondary carnitine deficiency in children of under 12 years, infants and newborns.

Single Oral Dose 1 g: Indicated for the treatment of primary and secondary carnitine deficiency in adults and children over 12 years of age.

Dosage and administration It is advisable to monitor therapy by measuring free and acyl carnitine levels in both plasma and urine.

The management of inborn errors of metabolism: The dosage required depends upon the specific inborn error of metabolism concerned and the severity of presentation at the time of treatment. However, the following can be considered as a general guide.

An oral dosage of up to 200 mg/kg/day in divided doses (2 to 4) is recommended for chronic use in some disorders, with lower doses sufficing in other conditions. If clinical and biochemical symptoms do not improve, the dose may be increased on a short term basis. Higher doses of up to 400 mg/kg/day may be necessary in acute metabolic decompensation or the i.v. route may be required.

Haemodialysis–Maintenance Therapy: If significant clinical benefit has been gained by a first course of intravenous Carnitor then maintenance therapy can be considered using 1 g per day of Carnitor orally. On the day of the dialysis oral Carnitor has to be administered at the end of the session.

The Paediatric Solution and Single Oral Dose can be drunk directly or diluted further in water or fruit juices.

Contra-indications, warnings, etc.

Contra-indications: Hypersensitivity to any of the constituents of the product.

Precautions: There is limited experience of use in patients with primary and secondary systemic carnitine deficiency suffering from renal failure.

Pregnancy and lactation: Reproductive studies were performed in rats and rabbits. There was no evidence of a teratogenic effect in either species. In the rabbit but not in the rat there was a statistically insignificant greater number of post implantation losses at the highest dose tested (600 mg/kg daily) as compared with control animals.

The significance of these findings in man is unknown. There is no experience of use in pregnant patients with primary systemic carnitine deficiency.

Taking into account the serious consequences in a pregnant woman who has primary systemic carnitine deficiency stopping treatment, the risk to the mother of discontinuing treatment seems greater than the theoretical risk to the foetus if treatment is continued.

Levocarnitine is a normal component of human milk. Use of levocarnitine supplementation in nursing mothers has not been studied.

Side effects: Various mild gastrointestinal complaints have been reported during the long term administration of oral levocarnitine, these include transient nausea and vomiting, abdominal cramps and diarrhoea.

Decreasing the dosage often diminishes or eliminates drug related patient body odour or gastrointestinal symptoms when present. Tolerance should be monitored very closely during the first week of the administration and after any dosage increase.

Drug interactions: There are no known interactions.

Overdosage: There have been no reports of toxicity from levocarnitine overdosage. Overdosage should be treated with supportive care.

Pharmaceutical precautions Store at a temperature not exceeding 25°C in a dry place. Protect from light.

Legal category POM

Package quantities
Paediatric Solution 30%: 20 ml amber glass bottles
Single Oral Dose 1 g: 10 ml amber glass containers in cartons of 10.

Further information Nil.

Product licence numbers

Carnitor Paediatric Solution 30%	8381/0005
Carnitor Oral Dose 1 g	8381/0004

Product licence holder: Sigma Tau Industrie Farmaceutiche Riunite SpA, Viale Shakespeare, 47-00144, Rome, Italy.

CYCLOGEST*

Presentation White pessaries, suitable for vaginal or rectal insertion. Each 1.85 g pessary contains either 200 mg or 400 mg Progesterone PhEur.

Uses Treatment of the symptoms of pre-menstrual syndrome, including pre-menstrual tension and depression.

Treatment of puerperal depression.

Dosage and administration 200 mg daily to 400 mg twice a day, by vaginal or rectal insertion. For pre-menstrual syndrome commence treatment on day 14 of menstrual cycle and continue treatment until onset of menstruation. If symptoms are present at ovulation commence treatment on day 12.

Children: Not applicable.

Elderly: Not applicable.

Contra-indications, warning etc Undiagnosed vaginal bleeding.

Other undesirable effects: Menstruation may occur earlier than expected, or, more rarely, menstruation may be delayed. Soreness, diarrhoea and flatulence may occur with rectal administration. As with other vaginal and rectal preparations, some leakage of the pessary base may occur.

Use in pregnancy and lactation: Due to the indications of the product, it is anticipated that it will not be administered to pregnant women. As progesterone is a natural hormone, it is not expected to have adverse effects, however, no evidence is available to this effect.

Other special warnings and precautions: Use rectally if barrier methods of contraception are used. Use vaginally if patients suffer from colitis or faecal incontinence. Use rectally if patients suffer from vaginal infection (especially moniliasis) or recurrent cystitis. Use rectally in patients who have recently given birth.

Progesterone is metabolised in the liver and should be used with caution in patients with hepatic dysfunction.

Cyclogest contains the hormone progesterone which is present in significant concentrations in women during the second half of the menstrual cycle and during pregnancy. This should be borne in mind when treating patients with conditions that may be hormone-sensitive.

Overdosage: There is a wide margin of safety with Cyclogest pessaries, but overdosage may produce euphoria or dysmenorrhoea.

Pharmaceutical precautions Store below 25°C in a dry place.

Legal category POM

Package quantities Packs of 15 pessaries 200 mg (OP). Packs of 15 pessaries 400 mg (OP).

Further information It is recommended that the diagnosis and evaluation of the treatment of pre-menstrual syndrome be monitored using pre-menstrual charts. The vaginal and rectal absorption of progesterone from Cyclogest are equivalent.

Produce licence numbers

Cyclogest Pessaries 200 mg	2343/0001
Cyclogest Pessaries 400 mg	2343/0002

Product licence holder: L.D. Collins & Co Ltd, Hanwood, Mill Hill, London NW7 4HR

HORMONIN*

Presentation Each pink, round, scored tablet contains: Oestriol USP 0.27 mg; Oestradiol USP 0.6 mg; Oestrone PhEur 1.4 mg.

Uses Hormonin has been designed for replacement therapy in oestrogen-deficiency states, particularly those associated with the menopause such as nocturnal sweating, vasomotor disturbances, atrophic vaginitis and pruritus vulvae.

Prevention of post-menopausal osteoporosis.

Dosage and administration Hormonin may be given continuously or cyclically (three weeks out of four).

Continuous therapy: 1–2 tablets should be taken daily without a break in therapy. In women with an intact uterus the addition of an adequate dose and duration of progestogen (for 12–14 days) in each 28 day cycle is recommended.

Cyclical therapy: Hormonin 1–2 tablets should be taken cyclically (three weeks on followed by one week off). In women with an intact uterus the addition of an adequate dose and duration of progestogen (for 12–14 days) in each 28 day cycle is recommended.

Therapy with Hormonin may be initiated with one tablet daily. This may be increased to 2 tablets daily if symptoms are not fully controlled. For maintenance therapy the lowest effective dose is recommended.

If the patient is not menstruating regularly therapy may be started arbitrarily. If the patient is menstruating regularly, therapy is started on day five of bleeding.

Before therapy commences, the patient should have a complete physical and gynaecological examination with special emphasis on blood pressure, breasts, abdomen and pelvic organs. In women with an intact uterus, endometrial assessments should be carried out whenever possible. Any abnormal bleeding is an indication for endometrial evaluation.

Regular follow-up examinations to include blood pressure and breast examinations are recommended every 6 months, and a complete physical and gynaecological examination every 12 months.

Contra-indications, warnings, etc
Contra-indications: Known or suspected pregnancy and during lactation.

Cardiovascular or cerebrovascular disorders, for example, thrombophlebitis, active deep venous thrombosis or thromboembolic disorders or a history of confirmed venous thromboembolism, moderate to severe hypertension, hyperlipoproteinaemia, or a history of these conditions.

Cancer of the breast.

Known or suspected oestrogen-dependent tumours.

Endometrial hyperplasia, uterine fibromyomata, undiagnosed vaginal bleeding.

Severe liver disease.

Porphyria.

Precautions: In patients with mild hypertension or a history of it, blood pressure should be monitored at regular intervals.

If hypertension develops in patients receiving oestrogens, treatment should be stopped.

Caution should be exercised in prescribing to women with a strong familial history of breast carcinoma, breast nodules or abnormal breast mammograms.

Glucose tolerance may be lowered and may, therefore, increase the need for insulin or other antidiabetic drugs in diabetics.

Thyroid hormone binding globulin may be increased leading to increased circulating total thyroid hormone, therefore care must be taken in interpreting thyroid function tests.

History of gall stones, cholestatic jaundice in pregnancy or jaundice due to oral contraceptives.

If liver function tests become abnormal during oestrogen therapy discontinue treatment.

Endometriosis.

Renal dysfunction. Major depression. Contact lens wearers.

Warnings: Unopposed oestrogens predispose to endometrial neoplasia.

Severe varicose veins–the benefits of oestrogen-containing preparations must be weighed against the possible risks.

Cardiac failure, latent or overt.

Epilepsy, migraine, otosclerosis or a history of these conditions.

Sickle cell haemoglobinopathy, since under certain circumstances, for example infections or anoxia, oestrogen-containing preparations may induce thromboembolic processes in patients with this condition.

Untreated polycythaemia or pulmonary hypertension.

Epidemiological studies have suggested that hormone replacement therapy (HRT) is associated with an increased relative risk of developing venous thromboembolism (VTE) i.e. deep vein thrombosis or pulmonary embolism. The studies find a 2–3 fold increase for users compared with non-users which for healthy women amounts to a low risk of one extra case of VTE each year for every 5000 patients taking HRT.

Generally recognised risk factors for VTE include a personal or family history and severe obesity (Body Mass Index>30 kg/m²). In women with these factors the benefits of treatment with HRT needs to be carefully weighed against risks.

The risk of VTE may be temporarily increased with prolonged immobilisation, major trauma or major surgery. In women on HRT scrupulous attention should be given to prophylactic measures to prevent VTE following surgery. Where prolonged immobilisation is liable to follow elective surgery, particularly abdominal or orthopaedic surgery to the lower limbs, consideration should be given to temporarily stopping HRT 4 weeks earlier, if this is possible.

If venous thromboembolism develops after initiating therapy the drug should be discontinued.

Side-effects: Genito-urinary tract. Endometrial neoplasia, intermenstrual bleeding, increase in the size of uterine fibromyomata, endometrial proliferation or aggravation of endometriosis, excessive production of cervical mucus.

Breast: Tenderness, pain, enlargement, secretion.

Gastro-intestinal tract: Nausea, vomiting, cholelithiasis, cholestatic jaundice.

Cardiovascular system: Hypertension, thrombosis, thrombophlebitis, thromboembolism.

Skin: Erythema nodosum, rash, chloasma, hirsutism, loss of scalp hair.

Eyes: Corneal discomfort if contact lenses are used.

CNS: Headache, migraine, mood changes (elation or depression).

Metabolic: Sodium and water retention, reduced glucose tolerance, and change in body weight.

Pharmaceutical precautions Store in a closed container in a dry place, below 25°C.

Legal category POM

Package quantities Securitainers of 90 tablets.

Further information Nil

Product licence number 0271/5000R

Product licence holder: G.W. Carnrick Co. Ltd., 221-227 High Street, Orpington, Kent BR6 0NZ

HYALGAN* 

Qualitative and quantitative composition Each prefilled syringe contains 20 mg/2 ml of hyaluronic acid sodium salt (Hyalectin*).

Pharmaceutical form Hyalgan is a sterile solution for intra-articular injection for single use only.

Clinical particulars
Therapeutic indications: For the sustained relief of pain in osteoarthritis of the knee.

Posology and method of administration: Adults (including the elderly): The contents of one pre-filled syringe (20 mg/2 ml) to be injected into the affected joint once a week to a total of five injections, using a standard technique. No adjustment of dose is required in elderly patients.

This can be repeated at not less than 6 monthly intervals.

Children: At present there is not enough evidence to recommend a dosage regimen for use in children.

Contra-indications: Hyalectin, the active principle in Hyalgan, is of avian origin. Do not administer to patients with known hypersensitivity to any ingredient of the product or to avian proteins.

Intra-articular injections are contraindicated in cases of infections or skin diseases in the area of the injection site.

Special warnings and precautions for use: Remove joint effusion, if present, before injecting Hyalgan.

Patients should be carefully examined prior to administration to determine signs of acute inflammation and the physician should evaluate whether Hyalgan treatment should be initiated when objective signs of inflammation are present.

As with any invasive joint procedure, it is recommended that care be taken not to overburden the joint immediately following the intra-articular injection.

Use only if the solution is clear.

See also *Instructions for use/handling.*

Interactions with other medicaments and other forms of interaction: Since there is limited experience available, Hyalgan should not be administered simultaneously or mixed with other intra-articular injections.

Do not use concomitantly with disinfectants containing quaternary ammonium salts because hyaluronic acid can precipitate in their presence.

Pregnancy and lactation: No embryotoxicity or teratogenicity has been observed in animal studies. However, there is no experience of the use of Hyalgan in pregnant women and therefore the expected benefit to the mother should be weighed against any potential risk to the foetus.

If Hyalgan is prescribed to a woman of child bearing potential, she should be advised to contact her physician regarding discontinuance of the product if she intends to become, or suspects that she is, pregnant.

Although it is not expected that Hyalgan would be present in human milk, because many drugs are excreted by this route, caution should be exercised when Hyalgan is administered to a nursing mother and the expected benefit to the mother should be weighed against any potential risk to the neonate.

Effects on ability to drive and use machinery: Hyalgan is not expected to have any effect on the patient's ability to drive or operate machinery.

Undesirable effects: Pain, swelling, heat and redness may occur sporadically at the injection site. Such symptoms are transient and usually disappear spontaneously within a few days (usually 1-4). If they should occur, rest the affected joint and apply ice locally.

Isolated cases of an anaphylactic-like reaction have been reported. There were only two cases in approximately 950,000 treated patients (approximately 4,750,000 injections) in post-marketing experience and they had favourable outcomes. No case of anaphylactic-like reactions have been reported during clinical trials.

There is the potential for rare allergic reactions, both local and systemic, to occur. The incidence of this (3 out of 5,376 patients treated with Hyalgan during clinical trials and 3 out of 950,000 patients treated during post-marketing experience), could be attributable to avian proteins, which although present in minimal amounts in Hyalgan, may induce reactivity in patients with a history of avian allergy.

In a 495-patient US multicentre placebo- and naproxen-controlled clinical study, the following adverse events occurred with a frequency greater than 5% in the Hyalgan group (versus placebo): headache 18% (17%), rash 7% (9%), ecchymosis 7% (6%) and pruritus 7% (4%). As these events occurred with equal frequency in the placebo group, there is no proven causality in respect of Hyalgan.

Overdose: Overdosage is unlikely given the route of administration and the single use pack of the drug. No case of overdosage has been reported to date.

Pharmacological properties

Pharmacodynamic properties: Hyalgan is a sterile, non-pyrogenic, viscous, aqueous buffered solution of a defined high molecular weight fraction of highly purified hyaluronic acid sodium salt (Hyalectin). Hyaluronic acid is an important component of the body's extracellular matrix and is present in a particularly high concentration in cartilage and synovial fluid. Endogenous hyaluronic acid provides viscosity and elasticity to synovial fluid, which is fundamental for its lubricating and shock absorbing properties, and it is essential for the correct structure of proteoglycans in articular cartilage. In osteoarthritis there is an insufficient amount of, and a change in the quality of, hyaluronic acid in synovial fluid and cartilage. The intra-articular administration of hyaluronic acid into arthritic joints with degenerating cartilage surfaces and pathologically altered synovial fluid improved joint functions. The observed beneficial effects of exogenous hyaluronic acid may be related to its interactions with various components of the synovial cavity (synoviocytes and chondrocytes).

In controlled clinical studies, treatment cycles with Hyalgan have been shown to ameliorate the symptoms of osteoarthritis for up to 6 months following the end of treatment.

Pharmacokinetic properties: Hyaluronic acid sodium salt (Hyalectin) administered intra-articularly is eliminated from the synovial fluid within 2 to 3 days. Pharmacokinetic studies have shown that it is quickly distributed to the synovial membrane. The highest concentrations of labelled hyaluronic acid have been detected in the synovial fluid and the articular capsule, followed by, in decreasing order, the synovial membrane, the ligaments and the adjacent muscle.

Hyaluronic acid in synovial fluid has been shown to be not significantly metabolised. Animal studies have shown that some degradation occurs in the tissue surrounding the joints, but the major site for metabolisation is the liver and excretion is mainly through the kidneys.

Preclinical safety data: Hyalectin (hyaluronic acid sodium salt) was tested in a standard range of toxicological tests, including mutagenicity and reproductive toxicity studies, and produced negative results throughout.

Pharmaceutical Particulars

List of excipients: Sodium chloride, disodium hydrogen phosphate dodecahydrate, sodium dihydrogen phosphate dihydrate, water for injections.

Incompatibilities: There are currently insufficient data to support the compatibility of Hyalgan with other drugs administered intra-articularly. Therefore the mixing or simultaneous administration with other intra-articular drugs is not recommended.

Shelf life: Hyalgan pre-filled syringes have a shelf life of 36 months when in their original package.

Hyalgan should not be used after the expiry date, printed on the package.

Special storage precautions: Do not use Hyalgan if package is opened or damaged. Store in original packaging (protected from light) below 25°C. DO NOT FREEZE.

Nature and contents of container: Sterile, colourless, Type I borosilicate glass syringes with rubber stoppers on which polypropylene plunger rods are tightened up, containing 2 ml of Hyalgan solution, supplied in packs of 1 pre-filled syringe.

Instructions for use/handling: Hyalgan is for intra-articular injection and is supplied as a single-use, ready to use, sterile solution in a 2 ml pre-filled syringe, and must not be diluted. The contents of the syringe are sterile and must be used immediately once the container has been opened.

Intra-articular injection of Hyalgan should be made using precise, anatomical localisation into the joint cavity of the knee to be treated. The injection site in the knee is determined by that location which is easier to reach. Usually a lateral approach can be followed, but in some cases a medial approach is preferable. Strict aseptic precautions should be observed during the administration. The solution in the pre-filled syringe is ready for use and requires only a sterile disposable needle. To ensure sterility the injection site must be carefully cleansed with antiseptic. Care should be taken to expel any trapped air bubbles from the syringe containing Hyalgan prior to administration.

Joint effusion, if present, should be aspirated by arthrocentesis prior to injection of Hyalgan. The arthrocentesis should be made using a 20 gauge needle and the joint should be aspirated to almost dryness, but not to a degree that would compromise the accuracy of the subsequent Hyalgan injection. An appropriate examination of the joint fluid present should be carried out to exclude bacterial infection, prior to injection.

The intra-articular injection of Hyalgan can be given using the same needle as used for the arthrocentesis by simply detaching the aspirating syringe and attaching the syringe containing the Hyalgan. To make sure the needle is correctly positioned, some synovial fluid should be aspirated prior to the slow injection of Hyalgan. If the patient experiences pain during injection, the procedure may need to be stopped.

For the first 48 hours after the injection, the patient should be advised to rest the treated knee with as little exercise as possible, avoiding any strenuous or prolonged activity. Subsequently, they may gradually return to their normal level of activity.

Discard any unused Hyalgan.

Administrative Data

Name and address of marketing authorisation holder: Fidia S.p.A., Via Ponte della Fabbrica 3/A, 35031 Abano Terme (Padova), Italy

Marketing Authorisation Number PL 04530/0004

Date of First Authorisation/Renewal of Authorisation 14 January 1998

Date of Preparation/Revision of Text November 1997

MIDRID*

Presentation Scarlet capsules, printed with "MOI" in black, containing 65 mg Isometheptene Mucate BP and 325 mg Paracetamol PhEur.

Uses In the treatment of migraine and other vascular headaches. Midrid contains isometheptene mucate, a cerebral vasoconstrictor, which provides prompt relief of migraineous headaches, which stem from dilated cranial vessels. Isometheptene is an indirect adrenergic agent with sympathomimetic properties. The paracetamol in Midrid acts as an analgesic.

Dosage and administration

Adults: 2 capsules at once, then 1 capsule every hour until relief obtained, up to a maximum of 5 capsules within a 12–hour period.

Children: Not recommended.

Contra-indications, warnings, etc.

Contra-indications: Midrid is contra-indicated in severe renal, hepatic or organic heart disease, severe hypertension, glaucoma, and in those patients who are on monoamine-oxidase inhibitor therapy. Porphyria. Hypersensitivity to paracetamol.

Precautions: Cardiovascular disease, diabetes mellitus, hyperthyroidism. Paracetamol should be given with care to patients with impaired liver or kidney function, and to patients taking other drugs that affect the liver. When used in patients with high spinal cord lesions, isometheptene, like other sympathomimetics may cause autonomic dysreflexia.

Patient information leaflet warning: Immediate medical advice should be sought in the event of an overdose, even if you feel well, because of the risk of delayed, serious liver damage.

Label warning: Do not take with any other paracetamol-containing products. Immediate medical advice should be sought in the event of an overdose, even if you feel well.

Interactions: On theoretical grounds care should be taken with patients receiving cardiac glycosides, quinidine, antihypertensives and tricyclic antidepressants. Alcohol reduces liver capacity to deal with paracetamol. Chronic use of paracetamol enhances effect of warfarin. Cholestyramine reduces absorption of paracetamol. May interact with chloramphenicol causing increased plasma levels.

Side-effects: Transient dizziness may appear in hypersensitive patients. This can usually be eliminated by reducing the dose. Circulatory disturbances may occur. Side effects which may be associated with any paracetamol containing preparation are usually mild, though haematological reactions have been reported. Rashes and other allergic reactions occur occasionally. There are isolated reports of thrombocytopenia purpura, methaemoglobinaemia, and agranulocytosis.

Use in pregnancy: There is no evidence of the drug's safety in human pregnancy nor is there evidence from animal work that it is free from hazard. Avoid in pregnancy.

Overdosage: Symptoms of paracetamol overdosage in the first 24 hours are pallor, nausea, vomiting, anorexia, and abdominal pain. Liver damage may become apparent 12 to 48 hours after ingestion. Abnormalities of glucose metabolism and metabolic acidosis may occur. In severe poisoning, hepatic failure may progress to encephalopathy, coma and death. Acute renal failure with acute tubular necrosis may develop even in the absence of severe liver damage. Cardiac arrhythmias have been reported. Prompt treatment is essential in the management of paracetamol overdosage. Any patient who has ingested about 7.5 g or more of paracetamol in the preceding 4 hours should undergo gastric lavage. Specific therapy with an antidote such as acetylcysteine or methionine may be necessary. Treatment should be instituted within 15 hours of ingestion. To assess severity of poisoning, paracetamol levels should be measured.

Acetylcysteine may be given either intravenously or by mouth or methionine may be given by mouth. Cysteamine was also formerly used. In adults, hepatic toxicity has rarely been reported with acute overdoses of less than 10 g.

Pharmaceutical precautions Store below 25°C.

Legal category P

Package quantities Securitainers of 100 capsules. Blister packs of 15 capsules.

Further information Printed Midrid capsules do not contain azo dyes.

Product licence number 0271/5001R.

Product licence holder: G.W. Carnrick Co. Ltd., 221-227 High Street, Orpington, Kent BR6 0NZ.

ROBAXIN* 750

Qualitative and quantitative composition Each white, capsule-shaped tablet contains 750 mg methocarbamol.

Pharmaceutical form Film coated tablet.

Clinical particulars

Therapeutic indications: As a short-term adjunct to the symptomatic treatment of acute musculoskeletal disorders associated with painful muscle spasms.

Posology and method of administration: For oral use.

Dosage: Adults: The usual dose is 2 tablets four times daily but therapeutic response has been achieved with doses as low as 1 tablet three times daily.

Elderly: Half the maximum dose or less may be sufficient to produce a therapeutic response.

Children: Not recommended.

Contra-indications: Hypersensitivity to methocarbamol. Coma or pre-coma states. Known brain damage or epilepsy. Myasthenia gravis.

Special warnings and special precautions for use: Robaxin should be used with caution in patients with renal and hepatic insufficiency.

Interaction with other medicaments and other forms of interaction: This product may potentiate the effects of other central nervous system depressants and stimulants including alcohol, barbiturates, anaesthetics and appetite suppressants. The effects of anticholinergics, eg atropine and some psychotropic drugs may be potentiated by methocarbamol. Little is known about the possibility of interactions with other drugs.

Pregnancy and lactation: There is no evidence of safety in human pregnancy, nor is there any evidence from animal work that it is free from hazard. Do not use during pregnancy, especially the first trimester, or lactation, unless there are compelling reasons to do so.

Effects on ability to drive and use machines: This product may cause drowsiness and patients receiving it should not drive nor operate machinery unless their physical and mental capabilities remain unaffected– especially if other medication capable of causing drowsiness is also being taken.

Undesirable effects: Robaxin may give rise to manifestations of allergy including skin rash, urticaria and angioneurotic oedema. This product may very rarely give rise to restlessness, anxiety, vertigo, tremor, confusion and convulsions. Lightheadedness and dizziness have been reported. Nausea and vomiting have also been reported during the use of Robaxin.

Overdose: Treatment of overdose is gastric lavage with appropriate supportive therapy for 24 hours as methocarbamol is excreted within that time.

Pharmacological properties

Pharmacodynamic properties: Robaxin 750 is used as a short-term adjunct to the symptomatic treatment of acute musculoskeletal disorders associated with painful muscle spasms.

The mechanism of action of methocarbamol in humans has not been established, but may be due to general central nervous system depression. It has no direct action on the contractile mechanism of striated muscle, the motor end plate or the nerve fibre.

Pharmacokinetic properties: Methocarbamol is absorbed from the gastro-intestinal tract and produces peak plasma concentrations after about 1-3 hours. Its activity derives from the intact molecule and only a small proportion is converted to guaiphenesin.

Preclinical safety data: Nothing of note to the prescriber.

Pharmaceutical particulars

List of excipients: Alginic acid, maize starch, povidone, sodium lauryl sulphate, gelatin, magnesium stearate, talc, sepifilm 002, sepisperse white AP 7001, potable mains water.

Incompatibilities: Not applicable.

Shelf life: 60 months

Special precautions for storage: No special storage conditions are necessary.

Nature and contents of container: Polypropylene bottles with HDPE, tamper evident closures containing 100 tablets.

Instructions for use/handling: None

Marketing authorisation holder: A H Robins Company Limited, Huntercombe Lane South, Taplow, Maidenhead, Berkshire SL6 0PH

Marketing authorisation number PL 0100/5026R

Date of first authorisation/renewal of authorisation 19 November 1982 / 19 November 1992

Date of revision of text October 1997

ROBAXIN* INJECTABLE

Qualitative and quantitative composition Each 1 ml of colourless solution contains 100 mg methocarbamol.

Pharmaceutical form Solution for Injection

Clinical particulars

Therapeutic indications: In the treatment of acute painful muscle spasm, due to musculoskeletal disorders or trauma.

Posology and method of administration: For intravenous use.

Dosage: Adults: 10-30 ml dependent on the severity of the condition and therapeutic response. Should not exceed 30 ml per day. Not to be administered for more than three consecutive days.

Elderly: Half the maximum adult dose or less may be sufficient for a therapeutic response in the elderly.

Children: Not recommended.

Rate of administration: Administer by slow intravenous injection or infusion directly into the vein at a maximum rate of 3 ml per minute.

Diluent: May be added to an intravenous drip of sterile, isotonic saline, or sterile 5% dextrose. Dilution should not be greater than 10 ml per 250 ml.

Contra-indications: Hypersensitivity to methocarbamol. Coma or pre-coma states. Known brain damage or epilepsy. Myasthenia gravis.

Special warnings and special precautions for use: Robaxin Injectable should be used with extreme caution in patients with impaired renal function. As the solvent used may cause raised urea levels and acidosis Robaxin should be used with caution in patients with hepatic insufficiency.

Interaction with other medicaments and other forms of interaction: This product may potentiate the effects of other central nervous system depressants and stimulants including alcohol, barbiturates, anaesthetics and appetite suppressants. The effects of anticholinergics, eg atropine and some psychotropic drugs may be potentiated by methocarbamol. Little is known about the possibility of interactions with other drugs.

Pregnancy and lactation: There is no evidence of safety in human pregnancy, nor is there any evidence from animal work that it is free from hazard. Do not use during pregnancy, especially the first trimester, or lactation, unless there are compelling reasons to do so.

Effects on ability to drive and use machines: This product may cause drowsiness and patients receiving it should not drive nor operate machinery unless their physical and mental capabilities remain unaffected– especially if other medication capable of causing drowsiness is also being taken.

Undesirable effects: Robaxin may give rise to manifestations of allergy including skin rash, urticaria and angioneurotic oedema. This product may very rarely give rise to restlessness, anxiety, vertigo, tremor, confusion and convulsions. Lightheadedness and dizziness have been reported. Nausea and vomiting have also been reported during the use of Robaxin.

Overdose: Treatment of overdose is gastric lavage with appropriate supportive therapy for 24 hours as methocarbamol is excreted within that time.

Pharmacological properties

Pharmacodynamic properties: Robaxin Injectable is used in the treatment of acute, painful muscle spasm, due to musculoskeletal disorders or trauma.

The mechanism of action of methocarbamol in humans has not been established, but may be due to general central nervous system depression. It has no direct action on the contractile mechanism of striated muscle, the motor end plate or the nerve fibre.

Pharmacokinetic properties: Half-life of methocarbamol following IV administration is approximately 1 hour. Mean blood levels at 1 hour following 1000 mg IV, 1000 mg as oral solution and 2000 mg as oral tablets were similar.

Preclinical safety data: Nothing of note to the prescriber.

Pharmaceutical particulars

List of excipients: Polyethylene glycol 300, sodium metabisulphite, water for injection

Incompatibilities : Not known

Shelf life: 48 months

Special precautions for storage: No special storage conditions are necessary.

Nature and contents of container: 10 ml ampoules.

Instructions for use/handling: None

Marketing authorisation holder: A H Robins Company Limited, Huntercombe Lane South, Taplow, Maidenhead, Berkshire SL6 0PH

Marketing authorisation number PL 0100/5027R

Date of first authorisation/renewal of authorisation 19 November 1982/19 November 1992

Date of revision of text October 1997

SUPRECUR* INJECTION ▼

Qualitative and quantitative composition Suprecur Injection contains 1.00 mg buserelin as buserelin acetate in 1 ml aqueous solution. 1.00 mg buserelin is equivalent to 1.05 mg buserelin acetate.

Pharmaceutical form Solution for Injection.

Clinical particulars

Therapeutic indications: Pituitary desensitisation in preparation for ovulation induction regimens using gonadotrophins.

Posology and method of administration: The total daily dose is usually in the range 200–500 micrograms given as a single injection by the subcutaneous route. Treatment should start in the early follicular phase (day 1) or, provided the existence of an early pregnancy has been excluded, in the mid-luteal phase (day 21). It should continue at least until down-regulation is achieved. e.g. serum oestradiol < 180 pmol/l and serum progesterone < 3 nmol/l. This will usually take about 1–3 weeks. Doses may have to be adjusted for individuals. Occasionally, patients may require up to 500 micrograms twice daily in order to achieve down-regulation. When down-regulation is achieved, stimulation with gonadotrophin is commenced while the dosage of buserelin is maintained. At the appropriate stage of follicular development, gonadotrophin and buserelin are stopped and hCG is given to induce ovulation.

Treatment monitoring, oocyte transfer and fertilisation techniques are performed according to the normal practice of the individual clinic.

Luteal support with hCG or progesterone should be given as appropriate.

Contra-indications: Hypersensitivity to buserelin, LHRH, or to any of the excipients; pregnancy, lactation, undiagnosed vaginal bleeding; hormone-dependent neoplasms.

Special warnings and precautions for use: Suprecur Injection is for subcutaneous administration ONLY.

Patients known to suffer from depression should be carefully monitored during treatment with Suprecur.

In patients with hypertension, blood pressure must be monitored regularly.

In diabetic patients, blood glucose levels must be checked regularly.

Whenever the treatment is self-administered, it is strongly recommended that initial doses should be administered under close medical supervision due to the possibility of hypersensitivity reactions. Patients should cease injections and seek medical attention should any adverse event occur which may represent an allergic reaction.

Treatment with Suprecur should be initiated only under the supervision of a specialist with experience of the indication.

Induction of ovulation should be carried out under close medical supervision. Risks specific to IVF/ET and related assisted reproduction procedures such as increase in ectopic and multiple pregnancies are unaltered under adjunctive use of buserelin. However, follicle recruitment may be increased especially in patients with polycystic ovarian disorder (PCOD).

Combined use of buserelin with gonadotrophins may bear a higher risk of ovarian hyperstimulation syndrome (OHSS) than the use of gonadotrophins alone. The stimulation cycle should be monitored carefully to identify patients at risk of developing OHSS, hCG should be withheld if necessary.

Possible clinical signs of ovarian hyperstimulation syndrome (OHSS) include: abdominal pain, feeling of abdominal tension, increased abdominal girth, occurrence of ovarian cysts, nausea, vomiting, as well as massive enlargement of the ovaries, dyspnoea, diarrhoea, oliguria, haemoconcentration, hypercoagulability. Pedicle tension or rupture of the ovary may lead to an acute abdomen. Severe thromboembolic events may also occur. Fatal outcome is possible.

Ovarian cysts have been observed in the initial phase of buserelin treatment. No impact on the stimulation cycle has been reported so far.

Interactions with other medicaments and other forms of interaction: During treatment with Suprecur, the effect of antidiabetic agents may be attenuated.

Pregnancy and lactation: Pregnancy must be excluded before starting buserelin and the medication should be stopped on the day of administration of hCG. Buserelin must not be administered to lactating mothers; detectable levels of drug are found in milk.

Effects on ability to drive and use machines: Certain adverse events (e.g. dizziness) may impair the ability to concentrate and react, and therefore constitute a risk in situations where these abilities are of special importance (e.g. operating a vehicle or machinery).

Undesirable effects: After administration of the injection, pain or local reaction at the injection site is possible. Hypersensitivity reactions may also occur. These may become manifest for example, as reddening of the skin, itching, skin rashes (including urticaria) and allergic asthma with dyspnoea as well as, in isolated cases, anaphylactic/anaphylactoid shock.

Side-effects consequent upon the suppression of hormone production occur in most patients. Hot flushes, increased sweating and loss of libido generally occur some weeks after starting treatment and may be severe in some patients. Dryness of the vagina may also be noticed.

Changes in bone density: A decrease in bone mineral, the magnitude of which relates to the duration of therapy, occurs during treatment with buserelin alone. The evidence available indicates that six months' treatment is associated with a decrease in bone mineral density of the spine of 3.5%. These changes are similar to those seen with other agonists. Increased levels of serum alkaline phosphatase may occur.

Combined use of buserelin with gonadotrophins may bear a higher risk of ovarian hyperstimulation syndrome (OHSS) than the use of gonadotrophins alone (see *Special warnings and precautions for use*).

Other adverse events may include:

Frequent: Vaginal discharge, increase or decrease in breast size, breast tenderness, dry skin, acne, increase or decrease in scalp hair, headache, palpitations, nervousness, sleep disturbances, tiredness, drowsiness, dizziness, emotional instability, lower abdominal pain, stomach ache, nausea, vomiting, diarrhoea, constipation, increase or decrease in weight, back pain, pains in the limbs, joint discomfort.

Occasional: Dry eyes (possibly leading to eye irritations in women who wear contact lenses), impaired vision (e.g. blurred vision), feeling of pressure behind the eyes, splitting nails, increase or decrease in body hair, lactation, oedema (of face and extremities), disturbances of memory and concentration, anxiety, depression or worsening of existing depression, increased thirst, change in appetite, paraesthesia, increase in serum liver enzyme levels (e.g. transaminases) increase in serum bilirubin.

Rare: Increase or decrease in blood lipid levels, tinnitus, hearing disorders.

Very rare: Deterioration of blood pressure levels in patients with hypertension, reduction in glucose tolerance which may lead to worsening of control in diabetics, thrombocytopenia, leucopenia.

Isolated cases: Severe hypersensitivity reactions with shock.

Overdose: Overdose may lead to signs and symptoms such as asthenia, headache, nervousness, hot flushes, dizziness, nausea, abdominal pain, oedema of the lower extremities, and mastodynia. Treatment should be symptomatic

Pharmacological properties

Pharmacodynamic properties: Buserelin is a synthetic peptide. It is a super active analogue of natural gonadotrophin releasing hormone (gonadorelin, LHRH or GNRH). After an initial stimulation of gonadotrophin release, it down-regulates the hypothalamic-pituitary-gonadal (HPO) axis such that a decrease in ovarian steroid secretion into the post-menopausal range occurs. The time taken to achieve these levels varies between individuals and with the regimen of administration, so that close monitoring of circulating levels of oestradiol and progesterone should be performed during treatment. This effect provides an appropriate setting for the administration of follicle-stimulating therapy and reduces the incidence of premature ovulation by inhibition of surges in LH.

Pharmacokinetic properties: The bioavailability of buserelin after subcutaneous injection is 100%. Cmax occurs at about 1 hour post-injection. The half-life after injection is about 80 minutes.

Buserelin accumulates preferentially in the liver, kidneys and in the anterior pituitary lobe, the biological target organ. Buserelin circulates in serum predominantly in the intact, active form. Protein binding is about 15%.

Buserelin is inactivated by peptidases (pyroglutamyl peptidase and chymotrypsin-like endopeptidases) in the liver and kidneys. In the pituitary gland, receptor-bound buserelin is inactivated by membrane-located enzymes. Buserelin and inactive buserelin metabolites are excreted via the renal and the biliary route.

Preclinical safety data: No signs of toxicity or histopathological changes were detected in long term pharmacology and toxicology studies with buserelin in rats, dogs, and monkeys; the endocrine effects observed were restricted to the gonads. Pituitary adenoma occurred during long-term treatment in rats, this phenomenon has not been found in dogs and monkeys. There are no indications of a mutagenic or carcinogenic potential.

Pharmaceutical particulars

List of excipients: Sodium Chloride PhEur, Sodium Dihydrogen Phosphate BP, Sodium Hydroxide BP, Benzyl Alcohol BP, Water for Injections PhEur.

Incompatibilities: Not applicable.

Shelf life: Unopened: 36 months (see *Instructions for use/handling*).

Special precautions for storage: Store between 2° and 25°C. Do not freeze. Protect from light.

Nature and contents of container: Box of 2 x 5.5 ml multidose vials each containing 1.05 mg buserelin acetate per 1 ml, corresponding to 1.00 mg buserelin per 1 ml.

Instruction for use/handling: Each vial contains enough material for 10 doses. After finishing the course of treatment, the vial should be disposed of and a new vial started for the next treatment. Do not use if the contents of the vial are cloudy or discoloured. Patients should be instructed on the correct handling of the vial (aseptic technique) by a doctor or nurse.

Marketing authorisation holder: Hoechst Marion Roussel Ltd., Broadwater Park, Denham, Uxbridge, Middlesex UB9 5HP

Marketing authorisation number 13402/0047

Date of approval/revision of SPC December 1997.

Legal category POM.

SUPRECUR* NASAL SPRAY

Presentation Suprecur nasal spray, a colourless to faintly yellowish solution, contains 150 micrograms buserelin as buserelin acetate in one spray dose. 1.50 mg buserelin is equivalent to 1.575 mg buserelin acetate.

The nasal spray also contains citric acid, sodium citrate, sodium chloride and benzalkonium chloride in aqueous solution.

Uses The treatment of endometriosis in cases that do not require surgery as primary therapy.

Pituitary desensitisation in preparation for ovulation induction regimens using gonadotrophins.

Dosage and administration

Endometriosis: The total daily dose is 900 micrograms buserelin, administered as one spray dose in each nostril in the morning, at mid-day and in the evening. The product may be used before or after meals or at other times, provided that uniform intervals are maintained between doses.

The usual duration of treatment is six months and this should not be exceeded.

Only a single course of treatment is recommended.

Pituitary desensitisation prior to ovulation induction: The total intranasal dose for this indication is 600 micrograms buserelin, given in four divided dosages of 150 micrograms (one application in one nostril) spread over the waking hours. Treatment should start in the early follicular phase (day 1) or, provided the existence of an early pregnancy has been excluded in the midluteal phase (day 21). It should continue at least until down-regulation is achieved e.g. serum oestradiol <50 ng/l and serum progesterone <1 microgram/l. This will usually take about 2–3 weeks. In some patients, dosages up to 4 x 300 micrograms may be required to achieve these levels. When down-regulation is achieved, stimulation with gonadotrophin is commenced while the dosage of buserelin is maintained. At the appropriate stage of follicular development, gonadotrophin and buserelin are stopped and hCG is given to induce ovulation.

Treatment monitoring, oocyte transfer and fertilisation techniques are performed according to the normal practice of the individual clinic.

Luteal support with hCG or progesterone should be given as appropriate.

If used correctly, reliable absorption of the active ingredient takes place via nasal mucous membranes. The drug is absorbed even if the patient has a cold; however, in such cases the nose should be blown thoroughly before administration.

If nasal decongestants are being used concurrently, they should be administered at least 30 minutes after the buserelin.

Children: Suprecur is not suitable for use in children.

Elderly: Suprecur is not suitable for use in post-menopausal women.

Contra-indications, warnings etc

Contra-indications: Pregnancy, lactation, undiagnosed vaginal bleeding, hormone dependent neoplasms, hypersensitivity to buserelin acetate, LHRH or benzalkonium chloride.

Precautions and warnings: Patients known to suffer from depression should be carefully monitored during treatment with Suprecur. In patients with hypertension, blood pressure must be checked regularly.

In diabetic patients blood glucose levels must be checked regularly.

Endometriosis: Patients should discontinue oral contraceptives before starting treatment. Where appropriate, alternative, non-hormonal methods of contraception should be used. If treatment is interrupted even for only a few days, ovulation may occur and there is a risk of pregnancy.

Suprecur treatment should be started on the first or second day of menstruation in order to exclude pre-existing pregnancy as far as possible. A pregnancy test is advisable if there is any doubt.

A menstruation-like bleed usually occurs during the first few weeks of treatment. Breakthrough bleeding may also occur during continuing courses of treatment in some patients. Recovery of pituitary-gonadal function usually occurs within 8 weeks of discontinuing treatment.

In the initial treatment with buserelin, ovarian cysts may develop.

Pituitary desensitisation prior to ovulation induction: Induction of ovulation should be carried out under close medical supervision. Risks specific to IVF/ET and related assisted reproduction procedures such as increase in ectopic and multiple pregnancies are unaltered under adjunctive use of buserelin. In addition, follicle recruitment may be increased especially in patients with PCOD.

Combined use of buserelin with gonadotrophins may bear a higher risk of ovarian hyperstimulation syndrome (OHSS) than the use of gonadotrophins alone. The stimulation cycle should be monitored carefully to identify patients at risk of developing OHSS. hCG should be withheld if necessary. Possible clinical signs of ovarian hyperstimulation syndrome (OHSS) include: abdominal pain, feeling of abdominal tension, increased abdominal girth, occurrence of ovarian cysts, nausea, vomiting, as well as massive enlargement of the ovaries, dyspnoea, diarrhoea, oligurea, haemoconcentration, hypercoagulability. Pedicle tension or rupture of the ovary may lead to an acute abdomen. Severe thromboembolic events may also occur. Fatal outcome is possible.

Ovarian cysts have been observed in the initial phase of buserelin treatment. No impact on the stimulation cycle has been reported so far.

Treatment with Suprecur should be initiated only under the supervision of a specialist with experience of the indication.

Interactions: During treatment with buserelin, the effect of antidiabetic agents may be attenuated.

In concomitant treatment with sexual hormones ("add back"), the dosage is to be selected so as to ensure that the overall therapeutic effect is not affected.

Effects on ability to drive and use machines: Certain adverse effects (e.g. dizziness) may impair the patients ability to concentrate and react, and therefore, constitute a risk in those situations where these abilities are of special importance (e.g. operating a vehicle or machinery).

Adverse reactions: As evidence of the biological response to hormone deprivation, patients may experience menopausal-like symptoms and withdrawal bleeding, which are directly related to the pharmacological action of the drug. Symptoms such as hot flushes, increased sweating, dry vagina, dyspareunia, loss of libido occur some weeks after starting treatment and may be severe in some patients. Withdrawal bleeding may occur during the first few weeks of treatment. Breakthrough bleeding may occur during continuing treatment.

Changes in bone density: A decrease in bone mineral, the magnitude of which relates to the duration of therapy, occurs during treatment with buserelin alone. The evidence available indicates that six months' treatment is associated with a decrease in bone mineral density of the spine of 3.5%. These changes are similar to those seen with other agonists. Increased levels of serum alkaline phosphatase may occur. These are reversible on discontinuing treatment.

Other adverse events not directly attributable to the pharmacological effect have been observed. These are changes in breast size (increase/decrease), breast tenderness, splitting nails, acne, dry skin and occasionally vaginal discharge and oedema of the face and extremities (arms and legs).

In addition, vomiting, lactation, stomach ache, lower abdominal pain, paraesthesia may occur, as may dryness of the eyes, leading to eye irritation in wearers of contact lenses.

Buserelin treatment may also lead to:

– changes in scalp and body hair (alopecia, hirsutism),

– deterioration in blood pressure levels in patients with hypertension,

– hypersensitivity reactions, such as reddening of the skin, itching, skin rashes (including urticaria), and allergic asthma with dyspnoea, as well as in isolated cases leading to anaphylactic/anphylactoid shock,

– reduction in glucose tolerance,

– changes in blood lipids, increase in serum levels of liver enzymes (transaminases) increase in bilirubin; thrombopenia and leucopenia,

– headache (of migranous type in rare instances), palpitations, nervousness, sleep disturbances, fatigue (asthenia), drowsiness, disturbances of memory and concentration, emotional instability, feelings of anxiety. In rare cases depression may develop or existing depression may worsen,

– dizziness, tinnitus, hearing disorders, impaired vision (e.g. blurred vision), feeling of pressure behind the eyes,

– nausea, increased thirst, diarrhoea, constipation, changes in appetite, weight changes (increase or decrease),

– back pain, pain in the limbs and joint discomfort,

The nasal spray may irritate the nasal mucosa. This may lead to nosebleeds and hoarseness as well as to disturbances of smell and taste.

Pregnancy and lactation: Suprecur is contra-indicated in pregnancy and lactation, In rats, foetal malformations have been seen after very high doses.

In endometriosis: It is unlikely that pregnancy will occur in the later stages of treatment if the recommended doses are taken regularly. However, if treatment is interrupted even for only a few days, ovulation may occur and the patient may become pregnant. In this event, Suprecur must be withdrawn immediately (see also precautions).

In pituitary desensitisation prior to ovulation induction: Pregnancy should be excluded before starting Suprecur, and the medication should be stopped on the day of administration of hCG.

Buserelin, in small quantities, is excreted in milk. Suprecur should not be prescribed to lactating mothers, although no effects on the child have been observed so far.

Overdose: Overdose may lead to signs and symptoms such as asthenia, headache, nervousness, hot flushes, dizziness, nausea, abdominal pain, oedema of the lower extremities and mastodynia. Treatment should be symptomatic.

Pharmaceutical precautions Store between 2 and 25°C. Do not freeze. Once a bottle has been opened, it may be stored at room temperature for five weeks. Any residual material after this time should be discarded.

Legal category: POM

Package quantities: Cartons containing two bottles and two metered-dose pumps (nebulisers). Each bottle contains 10 g solution.

Further information: Buserelin is an analogue of the hypothalamic peptide LHRH. It competes with its parent molecule for binding sites on the anterior pituitary cells secreting LH and FSH. Initial effects are to increase secretion of the gonadotrophins, but provided that sufficient doses are used with sufficient regularity, the activity of the hypothalamic-pituitary-axis is down-regulated. Ovarian activity will be suppressed and oestradiol levels markedly reduced.

Product licence number: 13402/0048

Product licence holder: Hoechst Marion Roussel Ltd, Broadwater Park, Denham, Uxbridge, Middlesex, UB9 5HP.

SUPREFACT* INJECTION

Qualitative and Quantitative Composition Suprefact injection contains 1.00 mg buserelin as buserelin acetate in 1 ml aqueous solution.

1.00 mg buserelin is equivalent to 1.05 buserelin acetate.

Pharmaceutical Form Injection

Clinical Particulars

Therapeutic indications: For the treatment of advanced prostatic carcinoma (stage C or stage D according to the classification of Murphy *et al*, in Cancer 45, p1889-95, 1980) in which suppression of testosterone is indicated. Buserelin acts by blockade and subsequent down-regulation of pituitary LHRH receptor synthesis. Gonadotrophin release is consequently inhibited. As a result of this inhibition there is a reduced stimulation of testosterone secretion and serum testosterone levels fall to castration range. Before inhibition occurs there is a brief stimulatory phrase during which testosterone levels may rise.

Posology and method of administration: Initiation of therapy: is most conveniently carried out in hospital; 0.5 ml Suprefact injection should be injected subcutaneously at 8 hourly intervals for 7 days.

Maintenance therapy: on the 8th day of treatment the patient is changed to intranasal administration of Suprefact. (see literature for dosage).

Contra-indications: Suprefact should not be used if the tumour is found to be insensitive to hormone manipulation or after surgical removal of the testes. It should not be used in pregnancy. It is contraindicted in cases of known hypersensitivity to benzyl alcohol or buserelin.

Special warnings and precautions for use: Patients known to suffer from depression should be carefully monitored during treatment with Suprefact.

Prostatic carcinoma: Monitoring of the clinical effect of Suprefact is carried out by methods generally used in prostatic carcinoma. Initially serum testosterone levels rise and a clinical effect will not be seen until levels start to fall into therapeutic (castration) range. Disease flare (temporary deterioration of the patient's condition) has been reported at the beginning of treatment. The incidence is variable, but of the order of 10%. Symptoms are usually confined to transient increase in pain, but the exact nature depends on the site of the lesions. Neurological sequelae have been reported where secondary deposits impinge upon the spinal cord or CNS. Disease flare is prevented by the prophylactic use of an anti-androgen, e.g. cyproterone acetate, 300 mg daily. It is recommended that the treatment should be started at least 3 days before the first dose of Suprefact and continued for at least 3 weeks after commencement of the Suprefact therapy.

Once testosterone levels have started to fall below their baseline concentration clinical improvement should start to become apparent. If testosterone levels do not reach the therapeutic range within 4 weeks (6 weeks at the latest) the dose schedule should be checked to be sure that it is being followed exactly. It is unlikely that a patient who is taking the full dose will not show a suppression of testosterone to the therapeutic range. If this is the case, alternative therapy should be considered.

After the initial determination, testosterone levels should be monitored at 3-monthly intervals. A proportion of patients will have tumours that are not sensitive to hormone manipulation. Absence of clinical improvement in the face of adequate testosterone suppression is diagnostic of this condition, which will not benefit from further therapy with buserelin.

In patients with hypertension, blood pressure must be monitored regularly.
In diabetic patients blood glucose levels must be checked regularly.

Interactions with other medicaments and other forms of interaction: During treatment with Suprefact, the effect of antidiabetic agents may be attenuated.

Pregnancy and lactation: Not applicable.

Effects on ability to drive and use machines: Certain adverse effects (eg.dizziness) may impair the ability to concentrate and react, and therefore constitute a risk in situations where these abilities are of special importance (eg. Operating a vehicle or machinery).

Undesirable effects: At the beginning of treatment, a transient rise in the serum testosterone level usually develops and may lead to temporary activation of the tumour with secondary reactions such as:

- occurrence of exacerbation of bone pain in patients with metastases.
- signs of neurological deficit due to tumour compression with eg. muscle weakness in the legs.
- impaired micturition, hydronephrosis or lymphostasis.
- thrombosis with pulmonary embolism.

Such reactions can be largely avoided when an anti-androgen is given concomitantly in the initial phase of buserelin treatment (see Precautions and Warnings). However, even with concomitant anti-androgen therapy, a mild but transient increase in tumour pain as well as a deterioration in general well being may develop in some patients.

Additionally, in most patients, hot flushes and loss of potency or libido (result of hormone deprivation); painless gynaecomastia (occasionally) as well as mild oedemas of the ankles and lower legs may occur.

Buserelin treatment may also lead to:

- changes in scalp or body hair (increase or decrease);
- deterioration in blood pressure levels in patients with hypertension.
- hypersensitivity reactions. These may become manifest as, eg.reddening of the skin, itching, skin rashes (including urticaria) and allergic asthma with dyspnoea as well as, in isolated cases leading to anaphylactic/anaphylactoid shock.
- reduction in glucose tolerance. This may in diabetic patients, lead to a deterioration in metabolic control.
- changes in blood lipids, increase in serum levels of liver enzymes (eg transaminases) increase in bilirubin, thrombopenia and leucopenia.
- headaches, palpitations, nervousness, sleep disturbances, tiredness, drowsiness, disturbances of memory and concentration, emotional instability, feelings of anxiety. In rare cases, depression may develop or existing depression worsen.
- dizziness, tinnitus, hearing disorders, impaired vision (eg. blurred vision), feeling pressure behind the eyes
- nausea, vomiting, increased thirst, diarrhoea, constipation, changes in appetite, weight changes (increase or decrease).
- back pain and pain in the limbs, joint discomfort.

After administration of the injection, pain or local reaction at the injection site is possible.

Overdose: Overdose may lead to signs and symptoms such as asthenia, headache, nervousness, hot flushes, dizziness, nausea, abdominal pain, oedemas of the lower extremities, and mastodynia. Treatment should be symptomatic.

Pharmacological Properties

Pharmacodynamic properties: Buserlin is a synthetic peptide. It is a superactive analogue of natural gonadotrophin releasing hormone (gonadorelin, LHRH or GNRH). After an initial stimulation of gonadotrophin release, it down-regulates the hypothalamic-pituitary-gonadal axis.

Pharmacokinetic properties: Metabolic inactivation by peptidases occurs in the liver and kidney. The drug is also inactivated by pituitary membrane enzymes.

Preclinical safety data: None stated

Pharmaceutical Particulars

List of excipients: Sodium Chloride, Sodium Dihydrogen Phosphate, Sodium Hydroxide, Benzyl Alchol, Water for injections.

Incompatibilities: Not applicable

Shelf life: 3 years

Special precautions for storage: Store between 2° and 25°C. Protect from light.

Nature and contents of container: Box of 1 x 5.5 ml multidose vials containing 1.05 mg buserelin acetate per 1 ml, corresponding to 1.00 mg buserelin per 1 ml.

Pack size: 2 individual cardboard boxes are wrapped together in a clear plastic outer.

Instruction for use/handling: No special instructions

Administration Data

Marketing authorisation holder: Hoechst Marion Roussel Limited, Broadwater Park, Denham, Uxbridge, Middlesex, UB9 5HP

Marketing authorisation number PL 13402/0050

Date of first authorisation/renewal of authorisation 31 December 1997

Date of (partial) revision of the text 15 September 1998

Legal category POM

SUPREFACT* NASAL SPRAY

Qualitative and quantitative composition Suprefact nasal spray contains 100 micrograms buserelin as buserelin acetate in 1 spray dose (100 mg) of aqueous solution containing benzalkonium chloride as preservative.

1.00 mg buserelin is equivalent to 1.05 buserelin acetate.

Pharmaceutical form Nasal spray

Clinical particulars

Therapeutic indications: For the treatment of advanced prostatic carcinoma (stage C or stage D according to the classification of Murphy *et al.* in Cancer, 45, p 1889--95, 1980) in which suppression of testosterone is indicated. Buserelin acts by blockade and subsequent down-regulation of pituitary LHRH receptor synthesis. Gonadotrophin release is consequently inhibited. As a result of this inhibition there is reduced stimulation of testosterone secretion and serum testosterone levels fall to the castration range. Before inhibition occurs there is a brief stimulatory phase during which testosterone levels may rise.

Posology and method of administration: Initiation of therapy: is most conveniently carried out in hospital; 0.5 ml Suprefact injection should be injected subcutaneously at 8 hourly intervals for 7 days.

Maintenance therapy: on the 8th day of treatment the patient is changed to intranasal administration of Suprefact. One spray dose is introduced into each nostril 6 times a day according to the following schedule:

1st dose before breakfast
2nd dose after breakfast
3rd and 4th doses before and after midday meal
5th and 6th doses before and after evening meal.

This dosage regimen is to ensure adequate absorption of the material and to distribute the dose throughout the day.

If used correctly, reliable absorption of the active ingredient takes place via nasal mucous membranes. Suprefact nasal spray is absorbed even if the patient has a cold.

If nasal decongestants are being used concurrently, they should be administered at least 30 minutes after buserelin.

Contra-indications: Suprefact should not be used if the tumour is found to be insensitive to hormone manipulation or after surgical removal of the testes. It should not be used in pregnancy. It is contra-indicated in cases of known hypersensitivity to benzalkonium chloride or buserelin.

Special warnings and special precautions for use: Patients known to suffer from depression should be carefully monitored during treatment with Suprefact.

Monitoring of the clinical effect of Suprefact is carried out by the methods generally used in prostatic carcinoma. Initially serum testosterone levels rise and a clinical effect will not be seen until levels start to fall into the therapeutic (castration) range. Disease flare (temporary deterioration of patient's condition) has been reported at the beginning of treatment. The incidence is variable, but of the order of 10%. Symptoms are usually confined to transient increase in pain, but the exact nature depends on the site of the lesions. Neurological sequelae have been reported where secondary deposits impinge upon the spinal cord or CNS. Disease flare is prevented by the prophylactic use of an anti-androgen, e.g. cyproterone acetate, 300 mg daily. It is recommended that treatment should be started at least 3 days before the first dose of Suprefact and continued for at least 3 weeks after commencement of Suprefact therapy.

Once testosterone levels have started to fall below their baseline concentration clinical improvement should start to become apparent. If testosterone levels do not reach the therapeutic range within 4 weeks (6 weeks at the latest) the dose schedule should be checked to be sure that it is being followed exactly. It is unlikely that a patient who is taking the full dose will not show a suppression of testosterone to the therapeutic range. If this is the case, alternative therapy should be considered.

After the initial determination, testosterone levels should be monitored at 3-monthly intervals. A proportion of patients will have tumours that are not sensitive to hormone manipulation. Absence of clinical improvement in the face of adequate testosterone suppression is diagnostic of this condition, which will not benefit from further therapy with buserelin.

In patients with hypertension, blood pressure must be monitored regularly.

In diabetic patients blood glucose levels must be checked regularly.

Interaction with other medicaments and other forms of interaction: During treatment with Suprefact, the effect of antidiabetic agents may be attenuated.

Pregnancy and lactation: Not applicable.

Effects on ability to drive and use machines: Certain adverse effects (eg dizziness) may impair the ability to concentrate and react, and therefore constitute a risk in situations where these abilities are of special importance (eg operating a vehicle or machinery).

Undesirable effects: At the beginning of treatment, a transient rise in the serum testosterone level usually develops and may lead to temporary activation of the tumour with secondary reactions such as:

- occurrence or exacerbation of bone pain in patients with metastases.
- signs of neurological deficit due to tumour compression with eg. muscle weakness in the legs.
- impaired micturition, hydronephrosis or lymphostasis.
- thrombosis with pulmonary embolism.

Such reactions can be largely avoided when an anti-androgen is given concomitantly in the initial phase of buserelin treatment (see Precautions and Warnings). However, even with concomitant anti-androgen therapy, a mild but transient increase in tumour pain as well as a deterioration in general well-being may develop in some patients.

Additionally, in most patients, hot flushes and loss of potency or libido (result of hormone deprivation); painless gynaecomastia (occasionally) as well as mild oedemas of the ankles and lower legs may occur.

Suprefact treatment may also lead to:

- changes in scalp or body hair (increase or decrease);
- deterioration in blood pressure levels in patients with hypertension
- hypersensitivity reactions. These may become manifest as, eg. reddening of the skin, itching, skin rashes (including urticaria) and allergic asthma with dyspnoea as well as, in isolated cases leading to anaphylactic/anaphylactoid shock.
- reduction in glucose tolerance. This may in diabetic patients, lead to a deterioration of metabolic control.
- changes in blood lipids, increase in serum levels of liver enzymes (eg. transaminases) increase in bilirubin, thrombopenia and leucopenia.
- headaches, palpitations, nervousness, sleep disturbances, tiredness, drowsiness, disturbances of memory and concentration, emotional instability, feelings of anxiety. In rare cases, depression may develop or existing depression worsen
- dizziness, tinnitus, hearing disorders, impaired vision (eg. blurred vision), feeling of pressure behind the eyes.
- nausea, vomiting, increased thirst, diarrhoea, constipation, changes in appetite, weight changes (increase or decrease).
- back pain and pain in the limbs, joint discomfort.

Administration of the nasal spray, may irritate the mucosa in the nasopharynx. This may lead to nose-bleeds and hoarseness as well as to disturbances of taste and smell.

Overdose: Overdose may lead to signs and symptoms such as asthenia, headache, nervousness, hot flushes, dizziness, nausea, abdominal pain, oedemas of the lower extremities, and mastodynia. Treatment should be symptomatic.

Pharmacological properties

Pharmacodynamic properties: Buserelin is a synthetic peptide. It is a superactive analogue of natural gonadotrophin releasing hormone (gonadorelin, LHRH or GNRH). After an initial stimulation of gonadotrophin release, it down-regulates the hypothalamic-pituitary-gonadal axis.

Pharmacokinetic properties: The intra-nasal absorption rate of buserelin is about 3%. Metabolic inactivation by peptides occurs in the liver and kidney. The drug is also inactivated by pituitary membrane enzymes. After intra-nasal administration to humans, buserelin is excreted for more than 8 hours in the urine. Virtually all the serum fraction, and half the urine fraction of buserelin, are present as the parent drug.

The bioavailability of buserelin after nasal administration is not adversely influenced by the presence of rhinitis.

Preclinical Safety Data: None stated

Pharmaceutical particulars

List of excipients: Sodium Chloride, Citric Acid Monohydrate, Sodium Citrate Dihydrate, Benzalkonium Chloride, Water for Injections.

Incompatibilities: Not applicable.

Shelf-life: $2\frac{1}{2}$ years.

Special precautions for storage: Store below 25°C. The spray solution should last for 1 week of treatment. Any residual material after this time should be discarded.

Nature and contents of container: Box of 4 bottles each containing 10 g solution and 4 spray pumps

Instructions for use/handling: How to use the spray bottle.

1. Remove spray cap from bottle.
2. Remove metered dose nebulizer from transparent plastic container and take off both protective caps.
3. Screw nebuliser on to bottle.
4. Before first application only, pump 5-8 times, holding bottle vertical, until the solution has filled the system and a uniform spray is emitted. The preliminary pumping is for the purpose of filling the system and testing the spray. It must not be repeated after the first use, in order to avoid wasting the contents.
5. Keeping the bottle vertical and bending head over it slightly, spray solution into nose. If necessary the nose should be cleaned before applying the solution.
6. After use leave nebulizer on bottle. After replacing protective cap, spray bottle is best stored in its transparent container in an upright position.

Marketing authorisation holder Hoechst Marion Roussel Limited, Broadwater Park, Denham, Uxbridge, Middlesex UB9 5HP

Marketing authorisation number PL 13402/0051

Date of first authorisation/renewal of authorisation 31 December 1997

Date of (partial) revision of the text December 1997

Legal category POM

URISPAS* 200

Qualitative and quantitative composition Each Urispas tablet contains flavoxate hydrochloride 200 mg.

Pharmaceutical form White, sugar-coated tablets overprinted with the name 'URISPAS 200'.

Clinical particulars

Therapeutic indications: Urispas is indicated for the symptomatic relief of dysuria, urgency, nocturia, vesical supra-pubic pain, frequency and incontinence as may occur in cystitis, prostatitis, urethritis, urethrocystitis and urethrotrigonitis.

In addition, the preparation is indicated for the relief of vesico-urethral spasms due to catheterisation, cystoscopy or indwelling catheters; prior to cystoscopy or catheterisation; sequelae of surgical intervention of the lower urinary tract.

Urispas is an antispasmodic, selective to the urinary tract. In animal and human studies, Urispas has been shown to have a direct antispasmodic action on smooth muscle fibres. In addition, animal studies have shown Urispas to have analgesic and local anaesthetic properties.

Where evidence of urinary infection is present, appropriate anti-infective therapy should be instituted concomitantly.

Posology and method of administration: For oral administration.

Adults (including the elderly): The recommended adult dosage is one tablet three times a day for as long as required.

Children: Urispas tablets are not recommended for children under 12 years of age.

Contra-indications: The following obstructive conditions: pyloric or duodenal obstruction, obstructive intestinal lesions or ileus, achalasia, gastro-intestinal haemorrhage and obstructive uropathies of the lower urinary tract.

Special warnings and precautions for use: Urispas should be used with caution in patients with suspected glaucoma.

Interaction with other medicaments and other forms of interaction: None known.

Pregnancy and Lactation: Since there is no evidence of the drug's safety in human pregnancy, nor any evidence from animal work that it is free from hazard, Urispas should be avoided in pregnancy unless there is no safer alternative. It is not known whether flavoxate is excreted in human milk. Because many drugs are excreted in human milk, caution should be exercised when Urispas is administered during breast-feeding.

Effects on ability to drive and use machinery: In the event of drowsiness and blurred vision, the patient should not operate a motor vehicle or machinery.

Undesirable effects: In clinical trials comparing Urispas with other antispasmodic agents, the incidence of side-effects was low. The following adverse reactions have been observed:

Gastro-intestinal: nausea, vomiting, dry mouth, diarrhoea.

CNS: vertigo, headache, mental confusion, especially in the elderly, drowsiness, fatigue and nervousness.

Haematological: leukopenia (one case which was reversible upon discontinuation of the drug).

Cardiovascular: tachycardia and palpitation.

Allergic: urticaria and other dermatoses, eosinophilia and hyperpyrexia.

Ophthalmic: increased ocular tension, blurred vision, disturbance in eye accommodation.

Renal: dysuria.

Overdose: Patients who have taken an overdosage of Urispas should have gastric lavage performed within four hours of the overdosage occurring. If overdosage is extreme, or there is a delay in removing the drug from the stomach, administration of a parasympathomimetic drug should be considered.

Pharmacological properties

Pharmacodynamic properties: Flavoxate hydrochloride (and it's main metabolite MFCA) is an antispasmodic specific to the smooth muscle of the urinary tract.

It's mechanism of action involves intracellular cyclic AMP accumulation and calcium blocking activity. It inhibits bladder contractions induced by various agonists or by electrical stimulation and inhibits the frequency of bladder voiding contractions. It increases bladder volume capacity, reduces the threshold pressure and micturition pressure.

Flavoxate also possesses anaesthetic activity and does not significantly affect cardiac or respiratory functions.

Pharmacokinetic properties: Oral studies in man have indicated that flavoxate is readily absorbed from the intestine and converted almost immediately and, to a large extent, to methyl flavone carboxylic acid, MFCA.

Following an IV dose (equimolar to 100 mg), the following parameters were calculated for flavoxate: T1/2 83.3 mins: apparent volume of distribution 2.89 l/kg. The apparent distribution of MFCA was 0.20 l/kg. No free flavoxate was found in urine (24 hours). However, 47% of the dose was excreted as MFCA.

Following single oral dosing to volunteers of 200 mg and 400 mg flavoxate, almost no free flavoxate was detected in the plasma. The peak level of MFCA was attained at 30-60 mins after the 200 mg dose and at around two hours following the 400 mg dose. The AUC for the 400 mg dose was approximately twice as large as the AUC for the 200 mg dose. About 50% of the dose was excreted as MFCA within 12 hours; most being excreted within the first 6 hours.

After repeated oral dosing (200 mg, TDS, 7 days) the cumulative excretion of metabolites stabilised at 60% of the dose on the third day remaining almost unchanged after one week.

Preclinical safety data: None stated.

Pharmaceutical information

List of excipients: Lactose, sodium starch glycollate, povidone, talc, magnesium stearate, cellulose microcrystalline, purified water, gelatin, sucrose, maize starch, acacia, light magnesium carbonate, titanium dioxide, Opalux AS 7000B, white beeswax, carnauba wax and Opacode S-I-9460 HV Brown.

Incompatibilities: None known.

Shelf life: 3 years.

Special storage precautions: No special precautions are required.

Nature and contents of container: Polypropylene securitainer with polyethylene closure in a pack size of 90 tablets.

Instructions for use/handling: Not applicable.

Name and address of marketing authorisation holder
Shire Pharmaceuticals Limited, East Anton, Andover, Hampshire, SP10 5RG.

Marketing authorisation number PL 08557/0034

Date of first authorisation/renewal of authorisation
30 May 1997

Date of (partial) revision of text March 1998

**Trade Mark*

Smith & Nephew Healthcare Ltd
Healthcare House
Goulton Street
Hull
HU3 4DJ

☎ 01482 222200 🗋 01482 222211

AMETOP* GEL

Qualitative and quantitative composition Amethocaine base 4.0%w/w

Pharmaceutical form Topical, white opalescent gel, each gram containing 40 mg of amethocaine base.

Clinical particulars

Therapeutic indications: Percutaneous local anaesthetic to produce anaesthesia of the skin prior to venepuncture or venous cannulation.

Posology and method of administration:

Adults (including the elderly) and children over 1 month of age: Apply the contents of the tube to the centre of the area to be anaesthetised and cover with an occlusive dressing. The contents expellable from 1 tube (approximately 1 gram) are sufficient to cover and anaesthetise an area of up to 30 sq.cm. (6x5 cm). Smaller areas of anaesthetised skin may be adequate in infants and small children.

Adequate anaesthesia can usually be achieved following a thirty minute application time for venepuncture, and a forty-five minute application time for venous cannulation, after which the gel should be removed with a gauze swab and the site prepared with an antiseptic wipe in the normal manner.

It is not necessary to apply Ametop gel for longer than 30–45 minutes and anaesthesia remains for 4–6 hours in most patients after a single application.

Not recommended for infants under 1 month of age.

Contra-indications: Use in premature babies or in full term infants less than 1 month of age, where the metabolic pathway for amethocaine may not be fully developed.

Known hypersensitivity to local anaesthetics of the ester type.

Do not apply Ametop gel to broken skin, mucous membranes or to the eyes or ears.

Special warnings and special precautions for use: Only apply to intact, normal skin. Not to be taken internally.

Ametop gel, like other local anaesthetics, may be ototoxic and should not be instilled into the middle ear or used for procedures which might involve penetration into the middle ear. Repeated exposure to Ametop gel may increase the risk of sensitisation reactions to amethocaine.

Interaction with other medicaments and other forms of interaction: None known

Pregnancy and lactation: There is no specific information as to the safety of amethocaine in pregnancy, although amethocaine has been in wide use for many years without apparent ill-consequence. It is not known whether amethocaine or its metabolites are secreted in breast milk. Therefore the product is not recommended for use on breast feeding mothers.

Effects on ability to drive and use machines: No adverse effects on the ability to drive or to use hazardous machinery are expected following use of Ametop gel.

Undesirable effects: Slight erythema is frequently seen at the site of application and is due to the pharmacological action of amethocaine in dilating capillary vessels. This may help delineating the anaesthetised area.

Slight oedema or itching are less frequently seen at the site of application. This may be due to the local release of histamine and 5-HT.

More severe erythema, oedema and/or itching confined to the site of application have rarely been reported.

In very rare instances, blistering of the skin at the site of application may be apparent – in these cases, remove the gel immediately and treat the affected area symptomatically.

Overdose: Overdosage with Ametop gel is unlikely to result from application to intact skin. If accidentally ingested systemic toxicity may occur, and signs will be similar to those observed after administration of other local anaesthetics.

Pharmacological properties

Pharmacodynamic properties: Amethocaine is a local anaesthetic and is believed to act by blocking nerve conduction mainly by inhibiting sodium ion flux across the axon membrane. Amethocaine achieves this by acting upon specific receptors that control gating mechanisms responsible for conductance changes in specialised proteinaceous sodium channels.

Blocking sodium ion flux prevents the setting up of an action potential in the nerve axon, thus preventing pain receptors signalling to the central nervous system.

Amethocaine additionally has vasodilatory effects, which commonly results in a localised erythema.

Pharmacokinetic properties: The ester type 'caine' anaesthetics are rapidly metabolised in blood mainly by plasma pseudocholinesterase. A 3.33 μM (1 mcg/ml) concentration of amethocaine was fully metabolised in human plasma within 20 seconds.

In vivo data has demonstrated that Ametop gel is 15±11% bioavailable when administered to intact normal skin, with a mean absorption and elimination half life of 1.23±0.28 hours.

Peak plasma levels of p-(n-butylamino) benzoic acid (BABA), the major metabolite of amethocaine, are between 3–6 hours post dose.

Pharmaceutical particulars

List of excipients: In addition to the active ingredient, Ametop gel contains: Sodium Hydroxide BP, Sodium methyl-p-hydroxybenzoate BP, Sodium propyl-p-hydroxybenzoate BP, Monobasic potassium phosphate USNF, Xanthan gum USNF, Sodium chloride EP, Purified water EP.

Incompatibilities: None known.

Shelf life: The shelf-life shall not exceed 24 months from date of manufacture. Within the recommended shelf life of 2 years at 2–8°C, the product, following dispensing, may be stored for up to 1 month at 25°C at point of use.

Special precautions for storage: Store at 2–8°C. Do not freeze. Protect from heat.

Nature of contents and container: 1.5 g, internally lacquered, aluminium collapsible tubes, designed to deliver 1.0 g of Ametop gel on squeezing.

Instructions for use/handling: As amethocaine can cause contact sensitisation reactions, particularly with repeated contact, healthcare professionals should take care to minimise contact with Ametop gel during application and removal.

Marketing authorisation number PL 14038/0001.

Date of first authorisation/latest revision of SPC

First authorisation: 10 July 1995.
Latest revision: 2nd February 1998.

Legal category P.

CUPLEX* GEL

Qualitative and quantitative composition

Salicylic Acid EP 11% w/w
Lactic Acid EP 4% w/w.

Pharmaceutical form Topical Gel.

Clinical particulars

Therapeutic indications: For the topical treatment of common, juvenile, plantar and mosaic warts; corns and calluses.

Posology and method of administration:

Adults (including the elderly) and children:

1. Every night soak the wart in hot water for 5 minutes.
2. Dry thoroughly.
3. Apply one or two drops of Cuplex Gel to the wart and allow to spread.
4. In the morning, remove elastic film and re-apply.
5. Twice, or three times per week, rub away the wart surface carefully (excessive rubbing will cause stinging when Cuplex Gel is applied) with an emery board or pumice stone, then apply Cuplex gel.

Suitable for all ages except infants.

Contra-indications: Do not apply to facial or anogenital warts. Avoid contact with the eyes. Only apply to the affected area. Keep away from naked flames.

Special warnings and special precautions for use: Warts are contagious and any person suffering from warts should always use their own towel.

Most warts will disappear after 6–12 weeks of treatment with Cuplex Gel, providing instructions are carefully and consistency followed. Where, however, the wart continues to increase in size after 6 weeks treatment, and the patient has not consulted a doctor, the patient should be advised to do so.

Interactions with other medicaments and other forms of interaction: None known.

Pregnancy and lactation: No effects on pregnancy and lactation are anticipated.

Effects on ability to drive and to use machines: No effects are anticipated in the ability to drive and to use machinery.

Undesirable effects: None expected.

Overdose: Overdose is not likely to occur from this topical product.

Pharmacological properties

Pharmacodynamic properties: The active ingredients present in Cuplex gel have no significant systemic effects. There is a long history of safe use of these active ingredients in the local treatment of warts.

Pharmacokinetic properties: Salicylic Acid is absorbed percutaneously in varying amounts dependent on several factors, e.g. Vehicle, dosage, skin area, skin conditions, etc.

Cuplex is used only on very limited skin areas since corns and calluses are skin disease of a very limited extension. The amount of Cuplex applied will thus amount to a max 0.5–1.0 g, corresponding to 0.06–0.1 g salicylic acid applied once or twice daily. Usually the amount is even smaller. Assuming 100% absorption, the amount of salicylic acid absorbed will be so small that detectable plasma concentrations can hardly be found.

Pharmaceutical particulars

List of excipients: Copper (II) acetate, Venice turpentine, Colophony 63 NORD, Collodion, Alcohol.

Incompatibilities: None known.

Shelf life: 24 months from date of manufacture.

Special precautions for storage: Store in a cool place (8–15°C). Highly inflammable.

Nature and contents of container: 5 gram aluminium tube.

Instructions for use/handling: Avoid naked flames.

Marketing authorisation holder: Smith & Nephew Pharmaceuticals Ltd, Hessle Road, Hull HU3 2BN. Distributed in the UK by Smith & Nephew Healthcare Ltd, Goulton Street, Hull HU3 4DJ.

Marketing authorisation number PL 13374/0007.

Date of first authorisation 30.12.93.

Legal category PM.

FLAMAZINE* CREAM 1.0% w/w

Qualitative and quantitative composition Silver sulphadiazine 1.0% w/w.

Pharmaceutical form Topical Cream.

Clinical particulars

Therapeutic indications: Flamazine cream is indicated for the prophylaxis and treatment of infection in burn wounds. Flamazine cream may also be used as an aid to the short-term treatment of infection in leg ulcers and pressure sores, and as an aid to the prophylaxis of infection in skin graft donor sites and extensive abrasions. Flamazine cream is also indicated for the conservative management of finger-tip injuries where pulp, nail loss and/or partial loss of the distal phalanx has occurred.

Posology and method of administration:

Burns: The burn wound should be cleaned and Flamazine cream applied over all the affected areas to a depth of 3–5 mm.

This application is best achieved with a sterile

gloved hand and/or sterile spatula. Where necessary, the cream should be re-applied to any area from which it has been removed by patient activity.

In burns, Flamazine cream should be re-applied at least every 24 hours, or more frequently if the volume of exudate is large.

Hand burns: Flamazine cream can be applied to the burn and the whole hand enclosed in a clear plastic bag or glove which is then closed at the wrist.

The patient should be encouraged to move the hand and fingers. The dressing should be changed when an excessive amount of exudate has accumulated in the bag.

Leg ulcers/pressure sores: The cavity of the ulcer should be filled with Flamazine cream to a depth of at least 3–5 mm. As Flamazine cream can cause maceration of normal skin on prolonged contact, care should be taken to prevent spread onto non-ulcerated areas.

Application of Flamazine cream should be followed by an absorbent pad or gauze dressing, with further application of pressure bandaging as appropriate for the ulcer.

The dressings should normally be changed daily but for wounds which are less exudative, less frequent changes (every 48 hours) may be acceptable. Cleansing and debriding should be performed before application of Flamazine cream.

Flamazine cream is not recommended for use in leg or pressure ulcers that are very exudative.

Finger-tip injuries: Haemostasis of the injury should be achieved prior to the application of a 3–5 mm layer of Flamazine cream. A conventional finger dressing may be used. Alternatively the finger of a plastic or unsterile surgical glove can be used and fixed in place with waterproof adhesive tape. Dressings should be changed every 2–3 days.

Contra-indications: As sulphonamides are known to cause kernicterus, Flamazine cream should not be used at, or near term pregnancy, on premature infants or on newborn infants during the first months of life. Flamazine cream is also contraindicated in patients known to be hypersensitive to silver sulphadiazine or to other components of the preparation such as cetyl alcohol or propylene glycol.

Special warnings and special precautions for use: Flamazine cream should be used with caution in the presence of significant hepatic or renal impairment. Caution of use is required in patients known to be sensitive to systemic sulphonamides and in individuals known to have glucose-6-phosphate dehydrogenase deficiency.

Use of Flamazine cream may delay separation of burn eschar and may alter the appearance of the burn wounds.

Interactions with other medicaments and other forms of interaction: As silver may inactivate enzymatic debriding agents, their concomitant use may be inappropriate.

In large-area burns where serum sulphadiazine levels may approach therapeutic levels, it should be noted that the effects of systemically administered drugs may be altered. This can especially apply to oral hypoglycaemic agents and to phenytoin. In the case of these drugs, it is recommended that blood levels should be monitored as their effects can be potentiated.

Pregnancy and lactation: Safety for use in pregnancy and lactation has not been established. Although animal studies have not shown any hazard, adequate studies in pregnant women have not been performed. Use in pregnancy only if benefit is likely to be greater than the possible risk to the foetus. Since all sulphonamides increase the possibility of kernicterus, caution is required in nursing mothers.

Effects on ability to drive and to use machines: None known.

Undesirable effects: Local reactions such as burning, itching and skin rash may occur in about 2% of patients.

Leucopenia has been reported in 3–5% of burns patients treated with Flamazine cream. This may be a drug-related effect, and often manifests itself 2–3 days after treatment has commenced. It is usually self-limiting and therapy with Flamazine cream does not usually need to be discontinued, although the blood count must be carefully monitored to ensure that it returns to normal within a few days.

Systemic absorption of silver sulphadiazine may very rarely result in any of the adverse reactions attributable to systemic sulphonamide therapy.

Overdose: Not likely to occur with normal usage.

Pharmacological properties

Pharmacodynamic properties: Silver sulphadiazine has bacteriostatic and bactericidal properties. This combination provides a wide spectrum of antimicrobial activity.

Pharmacokinetic properties: There is evidence that in large area wounds and/or after prolonged application, systemic absorption of silver can occur causing clinical argyria. The sulphadiazine readily diffuses across wounds and enters the general circulation. The degree of uptake will significantly depend upon the nature of the wound and the dosing regime. Sulphadiazine is excreted in the urine.

Pharmaceutical particulars

List of excipients: Polysorbate 60 BP, Polysorbate 80 BP, Glycerol Monostearate BP, Cetyl Alcohol, Liquid Paraffin BP, Propylene Glycol BP, Purified Water EP.

Incompatibilities: None known.

Shelf life: 36 months from date of manufacture. The contents of one container are for the treatment of one person. 250 g and 500 g pots should be discarded 24 hours after opening. Tubes of Flamazine should be discarded 7 days after opening.

Special precautions for storage: Store below 25°C. Protect from light.

Nature and contents of container: Flamazine cream is available in polyethylene tubes containing 50 g, and in black polypropylene pots of 250 g and 500 g.

Instructions for use/handling: None.

Marketing authorisation holder: Smith & Nephew Pharmaceuticals Ltd, Hessle Road, Hull HU3 2BN. Distributed in the UK by Smith & Nephew Healthcare Ltd, Goulton Street, Hull HU3 4DJ.

Marketing authorisation number PL 13374/0006.

Date of first authorisation 30 December 1993.

Date of (partial) revision of the text 20 February 1997.

IODOFLEX*

Qualitative and quantitative composition 1 gram unit-dose paste contains: Cadexomer iodine 600 mg equivalent to: Iodine 9 mg PhEur, Cadexomer 591 mg.

Pharmaceutical form Unit-dose paste with gauze backing for topical application.

Clinical particulars

Therapeutic indications: For the treatment of chronic wounds, e.g. leg ulcers.

When applied to wounds, Iodoflex reduces the bacterial count. In chronic leg ulcers it accelerates healing and reduced pain.

For topical application.

Posology and method of administration: In adults and the elderly, Iodoflex is applied to the wound surface and then covered with a dry gauze dressing. The frequency of change depends on the exudation from the wound. Changes should be made when the Iodoflex has become saturated with wound exudate, indicated by loss of colour, usually two to three times a week. If the wound is exudating heavily, daily changes may be needed. Each time the unit-dose paste is changed and at the end of treatment the remaining Iodoflex should be gently removed from the wound surface with a stream of water or saline.

A single application should not exceed 50 g. The total amount of Iodoflex used in one week should not exceed 150 g. The duration of treatment should not exceed 3 months in any single course of treatment.

There is no experience in children, therefore Iodoflex is not recommended.

Contra-indications: As Iodoflex contains 0.9% w/w iodine it should not be used in patients with known or suspected iodine sensitivity. Iodoflex is contra-indicated in Hashimoto's thyroiditis and in cases of non-toxic nodular goitre.

Special warnings and special precautions for use: Iodine may be absorbed systemically, especially when large wounds are treated. Patients with a past history of any thyroid disorder are more susceptible to alterations in thyroid metabolism with chronic Iodoflex therapy. In endemic goitre, there has been isolated reports of hyperthyroidism associated with exogenous iodine.

It has been observed occasionally that an adherent crust can form when Iodoflex is not changed with sufficient frequency.

Interaction with other medicaments and other forms of interaction: There is a potential risk of interaction with lithium.

Pregnancy and lactation: Iodine may cross the placental barrier and is secreted into breast milk. Use of Iodoflex should therefore be avoided in pregnant or lactating women.

Effects on ability to drive and use machines: It is unlikely to have an effect.

Undesirable effects: About 5% of patients treated with Iodoflex experience a transient smarting or pain within the first hour after application. Contact allergy, alteration in thyroid function and local oedema have been reported in rare cases. Minor reddening or swelling around the wound may occur without necessarily being an allergic reaction.

Overdose: There have been no reported overdosages. In case of excessive topical use of Iodoflex, the treatment should be stopped, the area washed and symptomatic treatment introduced.

Pharmacological properties

Pharmacodynamic properties: Iodoflex consists of cadexomer iodine in a macrogol base applied to a polyester gauze carrier. In contact with wound exudate Iodoflex absorbs fluid, removes exudate, pus and debris from the wound surface. One gram of cadexomer iodine can absorb up to 6 ml of fluid. Iodine is physically immobilised within the matrix of the dry cadexomer iodine and is slowly released in an active form during uptake of wound fluid. This mechanism of release provides antibacterial activity both at the wound surface and within the formed gel. There is no evidence of the development of bacterial resistance to iodine. The formed gel can easily be removed without damaging the fragile new epithelium underneath.

Pharmacokinetic properties: Systemically absorbed iodine from Iodoflex is rapidly and almost exclusively excreted into the urine. Cadexomer is biodegradable by amylases, normally present in wound fluid.

Preclinical safety data: In preclinical studies, Iodoflex has been shown not to interfere with normal wound healing. Toxicity studies with daily skin applications of Iodoflex for 6 months in rabbits showed no evidence of local or systemic toxic effect. Iodoflex did not cause sensitisation in animals.

Pharmaceutical particulars

List of excipients: Lanogen 1500 40% consisting in equal part of: Macrogol 300 PhEur, Macrogol 1500 PhEur.

Incompatibilities: No incompatibilities have been encountered in normal use.

Shelf life: 24 months.

Special precautions for storage: This product should be stored below 25°C.

Nature and contents of container: The Iodoflex unit-dose paste is provided with a polyester gauze backing. Each unit of paste is packed in a laminated foil pouch.

The following pack sizes are available:

5 sterile unit-doses of 5 g (6×4 cm) in an outer carton.

3 sterile unit-doses of 10 g (8×6 cm) in an outer carton.

2 sterile unit-doses of 17 g (10×8 cm) in an outer carton.

Instructions for use/handling

1. Clean the wound and let the wound surface stay moist. Dry the surrounding area.
2. Remove the backing gauze and apply Iodoflex directly on the wound surface. Cover with a suitable dressing.
3. Change the dressing when Iodoflex has lost its colour. Irrigate to remove as much remaining Iodoflex as possible.
4. Support bandages or stockings can be applied in conjunction with the use of Iodoflex.

Marketing authorisation number PL 14038/0009.

Date of first authorisation/renewal of authorisation 1 June 1998.

Date of (partial) revision of the text 1 June 1998.

IODOSORB* OINTMENT

Presentation Tubes of sterile cadexomer Iodine (INN) ointment containing Iodine PhEur at a concentration of 0.9% w/w for topical application. The cadexomer Iodine, a modified starch gel microbead, is formulated in an inert ointment base. Each tube is for a single application only.

Uses For the treatment of chronic leg ulcers. When applied to the wound, Iodosorb Ointment absorbs pus and exudate, cleans the wound surface and reduces bacterial count. In chronic ulcers it stimulates granulation, reduces pain and accelerates healing.

The ointment formulation improves the ease of application on awkward wound sites.

Dosage and administration Iodosorb Ointment is applied topically to the wound surface to a depth of approximately 3 mm ($\frac{1}{8}$"). A single application should not exceed 50 g. The total amount of Iodosorb Ointment used in one week must not exceed 150 g. The preparation should be changed approximately three times per week or when the Iodosorb Ointment has become saturated with wound exudate, indicated by a loss of colour. Each time the dressing is changed and at the end of treatment, the remaining Iodosorb should be gently removed from the ulcer surface either with a stream of sterile water or saline, or with a sterile wet swab. The duration of treatment should not exceed 3 months in any single course of treatment. When venous insufficiency is a contributory factor, support bandages or stockings can be applied in conjunction with the use of Iodosorb Ointment.

Contra-indications, warnings, etc
Contra-indications: As Iodosorb Ointment contains 0.9% w/w iodine it should not be used in patients with known or suspected Iodine sensitivity. Iodosorb Ointment is contra-indicated in Hashimoto's Thyroiditis.

In patients with a prior history of Graves Disease it is not recommended to use iodine containing products, which includes Iodosorb Ointment.

The ointment should not be used in the case of non-toxic nodular goitre.

Warnings: Patients with a past history of any thyroid disorder are more susceptible to alteration in thyroid metabolism with chronic Iodosorb therapy.

Iodine is absorbed systemically especially when large wounds are treated.

In endemic goitre there have been isolated reports of hyperthyroidism associated with Iodosorb.

There is a potential for interaction of iodine with the following drugs and therefore co-administration is not recommended, Lithium, Sulphafurazoles and Sulphonylureas.

It has been observed occasionally that an adherent crust can form when the dressing is not changed with significant frequency.

Pregnancy: Iodine can cross the placental barrier and is secreted into milk. Do not use Iodosorb in pregnant or lactating women.

Pharmaceutical precautions Store below 25°C.

Legal category P.

Package quantities Four unit dose tubes containing 10 g of ointment per pack. Two unit dose tubes containing 20 g of ointment per pack.

Further information On contact with wound exudate, the ointment absorbs fluid, removing exudate, pus and debris from the wound surface. Iodine is physically immobilised within the matrix of the ointment and is slowly released in an active form during uptake of wound fluid. This mechanism of release provides antibacterial activity both at the wound surface and within the formed gel. The gel can be removed with a stream of water without damaging the fragile new epithelium.

Product licence number 14038/0008.

IODOSORB* POWDER

Qualitative and quantitative composition 1 g Iodosorb Powder contains Cadexomer iodine 1000 mg equivalent to:

Iodine	9 mg PhEur
Cadexomer	991 mg

Pharmaceutical form Powder for topical application.

Clinical particulars
Therapeutic indications: Treatment of moist wounds including decubitus ulcers and chronic leg ulcers associated with venous disease.

Posology and method of administration: In adults and the elderly, Iodosorb Powder is applied to the wound surface to form a layer 3 mm ($\frac{1}{8}$") deep and covered with a dry dressing of gauze. The dressing should be changed daily, or when all the applied cadexomer iodine has been saturated with wound exudate indicated by loss of colour.

Each time the dressing is changed and at the end of treatment, the remaining cadexomer iodine gel should be gently washed from the ulcer surface either with a gentle stream of sterile water or saline or with a sterile wet swab.

To avoid the risk of cross-contamination, it is recommended that the use of a single sachet of Iodosorb Powder be confined to one patient.

Iodosorb Powder is a dressing for the wound and has no influence on the underlying disturbance of venous function. Where considered appropriate, support bandages or stocking can be applied in conjunction with the use of Iodosorb Powder.

There is no experience in children, therefore, Iodosorb Powder is not recommended.

Contra-indications: Iodosorb Powder contains 0.9% iodine and must not be used in patients with known or suspected iodine sensitivity.

Special warnings and special precautions for use: Iodine is absorbed systemically especially when large wounds are treated. This should be taken into consideration in patients undertaking thyroid function tests.

Interaction with other medicaments and other forms of interaction: No statement.

Pregnancy and lactation: Iodine can cross the placental barrier and is secreted into breast milk. Therefore Iodosorb Powder should not be used in pregnant or lactating women.

Effects on ability to drive and use machines: It is unlikely to have an effect.

Undesirable effects: It has been reported that some patients experience a transient smarting sensation within the first hour after treatment. This can be reduced if the wound surface is left moist before applying Iodosorb Powder. Mild erythema, without sensitisation has been observed occasionally.

It has been observed occasionally that an adherent crust can form when Iodosorb Powder is not changed with significant frequency.

Overdose: There have been no reported overdoses. In case of excessive topical use of Iodosorb Powder, the treatment should be stopped, the area washed and symptomatic treatment introduced.

Pharmacological properties
Pharmacodynamic properties: Iodosorb Powder is a dry yellow-brown powder of modified starch gel microbeads between 0.1 and 0.3 mm in diameter. On contact with wound exudate Iodosorb Powder absorbs 6 times its own weight. Removing pus and debris from the wound surface. Iodine is physically immobilised within the matrix of Iodosorb Powder and is slowly released in an active form during uptake of wound fluid. This mechanism of release provides antibacterial activity both at the wound surface and within the formed gel. This stimulates granulation, reduces pain and accelerates healing.

Pharmacokinetic properties: Not applicable.

Preclinical safety data: In preclinical studies, Iodosorb Powder has shown not to interfere with normal wound healing. Toxicity studies with daily skin application for 3 months showed no evidence of local or systemic toxic effect. Iodosorb Powder did not cause sensitisation in animals.

Pharmaceutical particulars
List of excipients: None.

Incompatibilities: None reported.

Shelf life: 3 years.

Special precautions for storage: Store in a dry place below 25°C.

Nature and contents of container: Unit dose aluminium foil sachets with internal polyethylene laminate. Each sterile sachet containing 3 g Iodosorb Powder. A carton contains 7 sachets.

Instructions for use/handling: Iodosorb Powder is applied topically to the wound surface in a layer approximately 3 mm ($\frac{1}{8}$") deep. It should be changed 2 to 3 times a week or when the Iodosorb Powder has become saturated with wound exudate indicated by a loss of colour.

Each time the dressing is changed and at the end of treatment, the remaining Iodosorb Powder should be gently removed from the wound surface either with sterile water or saline or with a sterile wet swab without damaging the fragile new epithelium. Any remaining Iodosorb Powder can be left in the wound as it will be degraded by amylases in the wound.

Where chronic venous insufficiency is a cause, support bandages or stocking can be used in conjunction with Iodosorb Powder.

Marketing authorisation number PL 14038/0007.

Date of first authorisation/renewal of authorisation 1 June 1998.

Date of (partial) revision of the text 1 June 1998.

SPRILON

Qualitative and quantitative composition

Zinc oxide	12.5% w/w	PhEur
Dimethicone 350	1.04% w/w	PhEur

Pharmaceutical form Aerosol spray ointment.

Clinical particulars
Therapeutic indications: For the prevention and treatment of pressure sores, skin maceration due to faeces or urine, or around fistulae and ileostomies. Protection and treatment of fissures, leg ulcers, moist eczema. Protection of skin beneath plaster casts.

Posology and method of administration: Shake can well. Spray surfaces at right angles from distance of 20 cm (8"). Two to three seconds should be sufficient for the area the size of the buttocks.

Contra-indications: Do not use on patients with known sensitivity to wool fats.

Special warnings and special precautions for use: Protect the eyes. Keep out of the reach of children. DO NOT puncture, incinerate or heat can above 50°C even when empty. Highly flammable.

Interaction: None presently known.

Pregnancy and lactation: Can be used in pregnant and lactating women.

Effects on ability to drive and use machines: Unlikely to product any effect.

Undesirable effects: Skin irritation has been observed on rare occasions.

Overdose: None reported.

Pharmacological properties
Pharmacodynamic properties: Sprilon consists of dimethicone, which has a liquid repellent effect. The zinc oxide ointment base helps moisturise skin. The spray rapidly forms a white, durable, flexible film which, while protecting the skin and assisting healing, allows normal transepidermal water loss.

Pharmacokinetic properties: Not applicable.

Pharmaceutical particulars
List of excipients:

White vaseline	BP
Wool fat	PhEur
Liquid paraffin	PhEur
Cetostearyl alcohol	PhEur
Wool alcohol	PhEur
Dextran CB	In-house spec.
Methylparahydroxy benzoate	PhEur
Propylparahydroxy benzoate	PhEur
Purified water	PhEur
Propellant: butane/propane mix	In-house spec.

Incompatibilities: None presently known.

Shelf life: 3 years.

Special precautions for storage: Highly flammable. Packaging carries appropriate warning.

Nature and contents of container: Aluminium pressurised can with plastic cap containing 115 g of which Sprilon ointment 60 g.

Instructions for use/handling: Spray skin from distance of 20 cm.

Marketing authorisation number PL 14038/0006.

Date of revision of text 1 June 1998.

Date of first authorisation/renewal of authorisation 1 June 1998.

WELLDORM* ELIXIR

Presentation Welldorm Elixir is a clear red syrup, with a pleasant passion-fruit flavour. Welldorm Elixir contains Chloral Hydrate BP 143 mg/5 ml.

Uses Welldorm Elixir is for the short-term treatment of insomnia.

Dosage and administration
Adults: 15–45 ml taken 15–30 minutes before bedtime with water or milk. Dose should not exceed 2 g chloral hydrate per day.

Elderly: Dosage as for adults except in the frail elderly or those with hepatic impairment, where a reduction in dose may be appropriate.

Children: 30–50 mg/kg. Dose should not exceed 1 g chloral hydrate per day.

Contra-indications, warnings, etc Should not be used in patients with marked hepatic or renal impairment, or in patients with severe cardiac disease. Best avoided in the presence of gastritis and in patients who have previously exhibited an idiosyncracy or hypersensitivy to chloral hydrate. Should not be used in patients susceptible to acute attacks of porphyria.

Interactions may occur in patients taking anticoagulants. When chloral hydrate is added to or withdrawn from the drug regimen, or its dosage changed, careful monitoring of the prothrombin time is required.

Patients should be warned that their ability to drive or use machinery may be impaired by drowsiness.

It is contra-indicated in pregnancy and lactation.

Side-effects: Gastric irritation, abdominal distension and flatulence may occur. Excitement, tolerance, allergic skin reactions, headache and ketonuria have occasionally been reported.

Alcohol potentiates the sedative effect. Chloral hydrate followed by intravenous frusemide may result in sweating, hot flushes and variable blood pressure including hypertension due to a hypermetabolic state caused by displacement of thyroid hormone from its bound state. Delerium may occur, especially in the elderly, particularly when used in conjunction with psychotropics or anticholinergics.

Abuse and chronic intoxication: There is a danger of abuse or chronic intoxication and the possibility that habituation may develop. In such patients gastritis and parenchymatous renal injury may develop. After long term use sudden withdrawal may result in delirium.

Overdosage: The signs and symptoms of overdosage

involve the CNS, cardiovascular and respiratory systems. These may include: respiratory depression, arrhythmias, hypothermia, pin-point pupils, hypotension or coma. Gastric irritation may result in vomiting and even gastric necrosis. If the patient survives, icterus due to hepatic damage and albuminuria from renal damage may appear. Serious problems have arisen with doses as little as 4 g and 10 g can be fatal. Overdosage shoud be treated with gastric lavage or inducing vomiting to empty the stomach. Supportive measures must be used. Haemodialysis, and in some cases haemoperfusion, have been reported to be effective in promoting the clearance of trichloroethanol.

Pharmaceutical precautions Syrup BP should be used as a diluent. Welldorm elixir should be stored in a well-stoppered bottle away from direct sunlight.

Legal category POM

Package quantities Welldorm elixir is supplied in bottles containing 150 ml.

Further information Each 5 ml of Welldorm elixir contains approximately 1.65 g of glucose.

Chloral hydrate and its metabolite trichloroethanol act as a central nervous system depressant.

Chloral hydrate leads to a decrease in sleep latency and in the number of awakenings. A near natural sleep is induced and the REM/NON-REM ratio is not altered.

Chloral hydrate is rapidly absorbed from the stomach and starts to act within 30 minutes. It is widely distributed throughout the body and is metabolised to trichloroethanol, also an active hypnotic, and trichloroacetic acid in the erythrocytes, liver and other tissues. It is excreted partly in the urine as trichloroethanol and its glucuronide, urochloralic acid, and as trichloroacetic acid. Significant amounts are also excreted in bile. Trichloroethanol has a plasma half-life of the order of 8 hours. Trichloroacetic acid has a half-life of several days.

Product licence number 13374/0005.

Date of preparation January 1994.

WELLDORM* TABLETS

Presentation An elongated, oval, film coated tablet. The coated tablet has a uniform smooth, film coat, of bluish-purple. Each tablet contains 707 mg chloral betaine, equivalent to 414 mg of chloral hydrate. The tablets are packed in opaque blister strips.

Uses Welldorm Tablets are used for the short-term treatment of insomnia.

Dosage and administration

Adults: The hypnotic dose is one to two tablets taken 15–30 minutes before bedtime with water or milk. Dose should not exceed 2 g of chloral hydrate per day.

Elderly: Dosage as for adults except in the frail elderly or those with hepatic impairment, where a reduction in dose may be appropriate.

Children: Welldorm tablets are not suitable for use in children under the age of 12, for such patients Welldorm Elixir is recommended (please refer to separate data sheet for dosage recommendations).

Contra-indications, warnings, etc Should not be used in patients with marked hepatic or renal impairment, or in patients with severe cardiac disease. Best avoided in the presence of gastritis and in patients who have previously exhibited an idiosyncracy or hypersensitivity to chloral hydrate. Should not be used in patients susceptible to acute attacks of porphyria. Should not be used in pregnancy and lactation.

Interactions may occur in patients taking anticoagulants. When chloral hydrate is added to or withdrawn from the drug regimen, or its dosage changed, careful monitoring of the prothrombin time is required.

Patients should be warned that their ability to drive or use machinery may be impaired by drowsiness.

Side-effects: Gastric irritation, abdominal distension and flatulence may occur. Excitement, tolerance, allergic skin reactions, headache and ketonuria have occasionally been reported.

Alcohol potentiates the sedative effect. Chloral hydrate followed by intravenous frusemide may result in sweating, hot flushes and variable blood pressure including hypertension due to a hypermetabolic state caused by displacement of thyroid hormone from its bound state. Delerium may occur, especially in the elderly, particularly when used in conjunction with psychotropics or anticholinergics.

Abuse and chronic intoxication: There is a danger of abuse or chronic intoxication and the possibility that habituation may develop. In such patients gastritis and parenchymatous renal injury may develop. After long term use sudden withdrawal may result in delirium.

Overdosage: The signs and symptoms of overdosage involve the CNS, cardiovascular and respiratory systems. These may include: respiratory depression, arrhythmias, hypothermia, pin-point pupils, hypotension or coma. Gastric irritation may result in vomiting and even gastric necrosis. If the patient survives, icterus due to hepatic damage and albuminuria from renal damage may appear. Serious problems have arisen with doses as little as 4 g and 10 g can be fatal. Overdosage shoud be treated with gastric lavage or inducing vomiting to empty the stomach. Supportive measures must be used. Haemodialysis, and in some cases haemoperfusion, have been reported to be effective in promoting the clearance of trichloroethanol.

Pharmaceutical precautions The tablets should be stored in a dry place at 15-25°C.

Legal category POM.

Package quantities The tablets are packed in blister strips of 15, two strips (30 tablets) per carton.

Further information Chloral hydrate and its metabolite trichloroethanol act as central nervous system depressants.

Welldorm is a chloral hydrate derivative, which leads to a decrease in sleep latency and in the number of awakenings. A near natural sleep is induced and the REM/NON-REM ratio is not altered.

Chloral hydrate is rapidly absorbed from the stomach, and starts to act within 30 minutes. It is widely distributed throughout the body, and is metabolised to trichloroethanol, also an active hypnotic, and trichloroacetic acid in the erythrocytes, liver and other tissues. It is excreted partly in the urine as trichloroethanol and its glucuronide, urochloralic acid, and as trichloroacetic acid. Significant amounts are also excreted in bile. Trichloroethanol has a plasma half-life of the order of 8 hours. Trichloroacetic acid has a half-life of several days.

Product licence number 13374/0004.

ZIPZOC*

Qualitative and quantitative composition Zipzoc is a sterile rayon stocking impregnated with an ointment containing 20% Zinc Oxide PhEur. Each stocking contains a mean value of 41.5 g ointment.

Pharmaceutical form Medicated stocking for topical application.

Clinical particulars

Therapeutic indications: Treatment of chronic leg ulcers. Where chronic venous insufficiency exists the medicated stocking can be used as a primary contact layer under compression bandaging or hosiery.

Posology and method of administration: For topical application. Zipzoc should be applied to cover the lower leg from the base of the toes to below the knee. All folds should be smoothed out. To protect clothes from Zipzoc a suitable outer bandage should be worn. If chronic venous insufficiency exists, Zipzoc can be used as a primary contact layer under suitable compression bandaging and may be applied for one week. The duration and frequency of application will depend on the clinical circumstances.

Contra-indications: There are no known contra-indications to Zipzoc.

Special warnings and special precautions for use: If arterial insufficiency is an underlying condition then compression bandaging should not be used in conjunction with Zipzoc.

Interaction with other medicaments and other forms of interaction: None known.

Pregnancy and lactation: There is no evidence to suggest Zipzoc should not be used during pregnancy.

Effects on ability to drive and use machines: It is unlikely to have an effect.

Undesirable effects: The skin of leg ulcer patients is easily sensitised to some topical medications. Zipzoc contains no preservatives thereby reducing the risk of skin reactions. Reactions reported include, rash, erythema, itching and maceration of the wound edge. If the outer bandage is inappropriate or the medicated stocking is not changed with sufficient frequency it can cause the stocking to dry out. Because Zipzoc is preservative free it must be changed no less frequently than weekly, to avoid possible risk of infection.

Pharmacological properties

Pharmacodynamic properties: The medicated stocking consists of a tubular rayon gauze impregnated with Zinc Oxide PhEur 20% in an ointment base. Zinc oxide has a soothing and protective effect and has been shown to have a role in wound healing. Zipzoc has no effect on the underlying condition but can be used under appropriate compression bandaging where chronic venous insufficiency is the problem.

Pharmacokinetic properties: Not applicable.

Preclinical safety data: Nothing relevant to add to the prescribing information.

Pharmaceutical particulars

List of excipients: Ointment base consists of: Liquid paraffin PhEur, White soft paraffin BP.

Incompatibilities: None reported.

Shelf life: 2 years.

Special precautions for storage: Store at or below 25°C. Keep all medicines out of reach of children.

Nature and contents of container: Polyethylene aluminium foil laminated pouches, each pouch containing a single medicated stocking. The outer carton will contain either 4 or 10 pouches.

Instructions for use/handling: Zipzoc should be applied to cover the lower leg from the base of the toes to below the knee. All folds should be smoothed out. A suitable outer bandage or dressing should be used to prevent soiling of clothes. If chronic venous insufficiency exists, Zipzac can be used a a primary contact layer under suitable compression bandaging and may be applied for one week.

Marketing authorisation number PL 14038/0010.

Date of first authorisation/renewal of authorisation 1 June 1998.

Legal category P.

**Trade Mark*

SmithKline Beecham Pharmaceuticals
Welwyn Garden City
Hertfordshire AL7 1EY
☎ 01707 325111 🗋 01707 325600

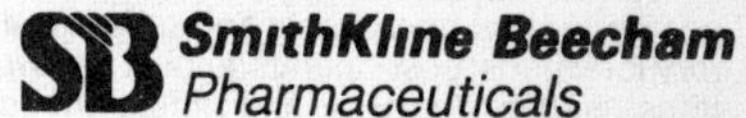

AC VAX*
Meningococcal Polysaccharide vaccine PhEur (groups A and C polysaccharides)

Presentation AC Vax meningococcal meningitis vaccine is a lyophilised preparation of purified polysaccharides from *Neisseria meningitidis* (meningococcus) of groups A and C. It is presented as a white pellet in a glass vial together with a separate ampoule or vial of clear, colourless, sterile diluent. Each 0.5 ml dose of reconstituted vaccine contains 50 micrograms of group A polysaccharide and 50 micrograms of group C polysaccharide dissolved in isotonic sodium chloride (0.9 per cent).

Uses Active immunisation against meningococcal meningitis caused by group A and group C meningococci.

AC Vax is particularly recommended for subjects at risk, for example those living in areas or travelling to countries where the disease is epidemic or highly endemic. It is also recommended in epidemic situations and for close contacts of patients with this disease.

Dosage and administration
Adults and children aged two months and over: 0.5 ml of the reconstituted vaccine administered by deep subcutaneous or intramuscular injection. The vaccine must not be given intravenously under any circumstances.

The vaccine should be reconstituted with the diluent supplied by adding the entire contents of the diluent vial to the vaccine vial.

Contra-indications, warnings, etc
Contra-indications: Do not use in subjects hypersensitive to any component of the vaccine or in those with febrile conditions.

Precautions: AC Vax gives no protection against meningococcal meningitis caused by meningococci belonging to groups other than A and C.

If administered to subjects with impaired immune responses, the vaccine may not induce an effective response.

As with all vaccinations, a solution of 1:1000 adrenaline should be available for injection should an anaphylactic reaction occur.

Use in pregnancy: No studies in animals have been performed. Since the effect of the vaccine on the foetus is not known, it should not be given during pregnancy unless there is a definite risk from groups A and C meningococcal disease.

Adverse reactions: These are mild and short-lasting. Local reactions may consist of erythema, slight induration and tenderness or pain at the site of injection. Febrile reactions and chills have been observed rarely in the first 24 hours after vaccination.

Pharmaceutical precautions AC Vax should be stored between 2°C and 8°C, its shelf life then being four years. The reconstituted vaccine should be used immediately, and certainly within one hour.

Legal category POM.

Package quantities Monodose* vials (OP), each with a separate ampoule of diluent.

Further information One dose of AC Vax will elicit a protective response in over 90 per cent of older children and adults within two to three weeks.

In adults and children over five years of age, immunity will persist for up to five years. In younger children, particularly those below the age of two years, immunity against group C meningococci is unlikely to persist for more than one to two years.

Inactive ingredients in the reconstituted vaccine are lactose and sodium chloride.

Product licence numbers

AC Vax vaccine	10592/0013.
Saline diluent (0.9 per cent)	0002/0194.

ALGITEC* SUSPENSION
ALGITEC* CHEWTAB TABLETS

Presentation A white suspension with an odour of fruit and mint, each 10 ml of which contains 500 mg Sodium Alginate BPC and 200 mg cimetidine.

Circular, off-white, flat-faced chewable tablets with an odour of butterscotch and with a characteristic pattern and 'Algitec' on both sides. Each tablet contains 500 mg Alginic Acid BPC and 200 mg cimetidine.

Uses Algitec combines sodium alginate or alginic acid, which forms a barrier to the reflux of gastric contents, with cimetidine, an H_2-receptor antagonist, which reduces the volume and acidity of gastric juice.

Algitec is indicated in the treatment of gastro-oesophageal reflux disease.

Dosage and administration
Adults only: Oral: 10 ml suspension or one tablet four times a day, after meals and at bedtime, for four to eight weeks. If the response is inadequate, the dosage may be increased to 20 ml suspension or two tablets four times a day. The tablets should be thoroughly chewed and may be followed by a drink of water.

Elderly: The normal adult dosage may be used unless renal function is markedly impaired (see *Precautions* and *Adverse reactions*).

Children: Algitec is not recommended for children.

Contra-indications, warnings, etc
Contra-indication: Hypersensitivity to cimetidine.

Precautions: Because of the need to reduce the dose of cimetidine in patients with marked renal impairment, Algitec is not recommended for such patients.

Cimetidine can prolong the elimination of drugs metabolised by oxidation in the liver. Although pharmacological interactions with a number of drugs, e.g. diazepam, propranolol, have been demonstrated, only those with oral anticoagulants, phenytoin, theophylline and intravenous lignocaine appear, to date, to be of clinical significance. Close monitoring of patients on Algitec receiving oral anticoagulants or phenytoin is recommended and a reduction in the dosage of these drugs may be necessary.

Clinical trials with cimetidine of over six years' continuous treatment and more than 15 years' widespread use have not revealed unexpected adverse reactions related to long-term therapy. The safety of prolonged use is not, however, fully established and care should be taken to observe periodically patients given prolonged treatment.

Cimetidine treatment can mask the symptoms and allow transient healing of gastric cancer. The potential delay in diagnosis should particularly be borne in mind in patients of middle age and over with new or recently changed dyspeptic symptoms.

In patients on drug treatment or with illnesses that could cause falls in blood cell count, the possibility that H_2-receptor antagonism could potentiate this effect should be borne in mind.

Use in pregnancy and lactation: Although tests in animals and clinical evidence have not revealed any hazards from the administration of cimetidine during pregnancy and lactation, both animal and human studies have shown that it does cross the placental barrier and is excreted in milk. As with most drugs, the use of Algitec should be avoided during pregnancy and lactation unless essential.

Adverse reactions: Over 56 million patients have been treated with cimetidine worldwide and adverse reactions have been infrequent. Diarrhoea, dizziness or rash, usually mild and transient, and tiredness have been reported. Gynaecomastia has been reported and is almost always reversible on discontinuing treatment. Biochemical or biopsy evidence of reversible liver damage has been reported occasionally. Reversible confusional states have occurred, usually in elderly or already very ill patients, e.g. those with renal failure. Thrombocytopenia and leucopenia, including agranulocytosis (see *Precautions*), reversible on withdrawal of treatment, have been reported rarely; pancytopenia and aplastic anaemia have been reported very rarely. There have been very rare reports of interstitial nephritis, acute pancreatitis, fever, headache, myalgia, arthralgia, sinus bradycardia, tachycardia and heart block, all reversible on withdrawal of treatment. In common with other H_2-receptor antagonists, there have been very rare reports of anaphylaxis. Alopecia has been reported but no causal relationship has been established. Reversible impotence has also been very rarely reported but no causal relationship has been established at usual therapeutic doses. Isolated increases of plasma creatinine have been of no clinical significance.

Overdosage: Acute overdosage of up to 20 grams of cimetidine has been reported several times with no significant ill effects. Overdosage with sodium alginate or alginic acid presents virtually no hazard, though abdominal bloating may be present. Induction of vomiting and/or gastric lavage may be employed together with symptomatic and supportive therapy.

Pharmaceutical precautions Store the suspension below 25°C but do not refrigerate. Shake the bottle before use. Dilution is not recommended. Store the tablets below 30°C.

Legal category POM.

Package quantities White plastic bottles containing 600 ml suspension, with Patient Information Leaflet. Cartons (OP) containing 120 Chewtab Tablets in six tubes of 20, with Patient Information Leaflet.

Further information Algitec allows the simultaneous use of two distinct and complementary methods, both of proven utility, of treating gastro-oesophageal reflux disease. Alginate and sodium or potassium bicarbonate are converted in the stomach to a viscous frothy gel of alginic acid which floats on the gastric contents to prevent reflux. Should reflux still occur, the gel itself may be refluxed to protect the oesophageal mucosa and allow any inflammation to heal. Cimetidine inhibits gastric secretion of acid and pepsin, reducing both the damaging gastric acidity and the volume available for reflux.

The absorption of cimetidine is not significantly affected by the sodium alginate or alginic acid in Algitec.

Each 10 ml suspension contains 65.8 mg (2.86 mmol) sodium and 1200 mg sorbitol.

Each tablet contains 47 mg (2.05 mmol) sodium, 330 mg lactose and 680 mg sorbitol.

Inactive ingredients include aspartame in the Chewtab Tablets and disodium edetate and parabens in the Suspension.

Product licence numbers

Algitec Suspension	0002/0176.
Algitec Chewtab Tablets	0002/0149.

AMPICLOX* CAPSULES
AMPICLOX* SYRUP
AMPICLOX* NEONATAL SUSPENSION
AMPICLOX* INJECTION
AMPICLOX* NEONATAL INJECTION

Qualitative and quantitative composition
Ampiclox Capsules: 250 mg ampicillin as Ampicillin Trihydrate PhEur and 250 mg cloxacillin as Cloxacillin Sodium PhEur.

Ampiclox Syrup: When reconstituted each 5 ml contains 125 mg ampicillin as Ampicillin Trihydrate PhEur and 125 mg cloxacillin as Cloxacillin Sodium PhEur.

Ampiclox Neonatal Suspension: When reconstituted each 0.6 ml dose contains 60 mg ampicillin as Ampicillin Trihydrate PhEur with 30 mg cloxacillin as Cloxacillin Sodium PhEur.

Ampiclox Injection: 250 mg ampicillin as Ampicillin Sodium PhEur with 250 mg cloxacillin as Cloxacillin Sodium PhEur.

Ampiclox Neonatal Injection: 50 mg ampicillin as Ampicillin Sodium PhEur and 25 mg cloxacillin as Cloxacillin Sodium PhEur.

Pharmaceutical form
Ampiclox Capsules: Black and amethyst capsules.

Ampiclox Syrup: Bottles containing powder for the preparation of 100 ml fruit flavoured syrup.

Ampiclox Neonatal Suspension: Bottles containing powder for the preparation of 10 ml suspension for oral administration. A pipette to measure the 0.6 ml dose is provided. Ampiclox Neonatal Suspension is sugar-free and free from artificial colourings; it contains sodium benzoate.

Ampiclox Injection and Neonatal Injection: Vials containing a sterile powder which on reconstitution is in a suitable form for parenteral administration.

Clinical particulars
Therapeutic indications: Ampiclox is indicated for the

immediate treatment of severe bacterial infections before the infecting organism is identified, and for mixed staphylococcal and Gram negative infections.

Typical indications include: bronchopneumonia, post-influenzal pneumonia and other severe respiratory infections; post-operative chest and wound infections; septic abortion and infections during the puerperium; septicaemia; infections in patients receiving immunosuppressive drugs; prophylaxis in major surgery.

Ampiclox Neonatal Suspension is indicated for the prophylaxis or treatment of bacterial infections in premature babies or neonates, particularly: suspected or confirmed infections; babies born of mothers with infected liquor or whose membranes ruptured more than 48 hours before delivery; babies requiring certain surgical procedures carrying risk of infection such as exchange transfusions; babies born with respiratory distress necessitating endotracheal procedures, when subsequent infection is a possible hazard; babies following difficult delivery, when inhalation of much liquor, mucus or meconium has occurred.

Parenteral usage is indicated where oral dosage is inappropriate.

Posology and method of administration:

ORAL

Adult dosage: one to two capsules or 10-20 ml of syrup every four to six hours.

Children's dosage: Syrup: one month to two years: quarter adult dose; *two to 12 years:* half adult dose.

Neonatal Suspension: 0.6 ml (90 mg) every four hours.

INTRAMUSCULAR/INTRAVENOUS

Adult dosage (including elderly): one to two vials (500 mg) every four to six hours.

Children's dosage: up to two years: quarter adult dose; *two to 10 years:* half adult dose.

Dosage may be further increased where necessary.

Premature babies and neonates dosage: one vial of Neonatal Injection (75 mg) three times a day.

ADMINISTRATION

500 MG VIALS

Intramuscular: Dissolve vial contents in 1.5 ml Water for Injections BP.

Intravenous: Dissolve vial contents in 10 ml Water for Injections BP and administer slowly (three to four minutes). Ampiclox may also be added to infusion fluids or injected, suitably diluted, into the drip tube over a period of three to four minutes.

NEONATAL VIALS

Intramuscular: Add 0.5 ml Water for Injections BP to the vial contents.

Intravenous: Dissolve the vial contents in 2 ml Water for Injections BP and administer slowly (three to four minutes). Ampiclox Neonatal may also be added to infusion fluids or injected, suitably diluted, into the drip tube over a period of three to four minutes.

Contra-indications: Penicillin hypersensitivity; ocular administration. Attention should be paid to possible cross-sensitivity with other beta-lactam antibiotics, e.g. cephalosporins.

Special warnings and special precautions for use: Caution should be observed when administering Ampiclox Neonatal Suspension and Injection to babies whose mothers are hypersensitive to penicillin.

Interaction with other medicaments and other forms of interaction: None known

Pregnancy and lactation: Animal studies have shown no teratogenic effects. The product has been in clinical use since 1968 and the limited number of reported cases of use in human pregnancy has shown no evidence of untoward effect. The use of Ampiclox in pregnancy should be reserved for cases considered essential by the clinician. During lactation, trace quantities of penicillins can be detected in breast milk.

Effects on ability to drive and use machines: None known.

Undesirable effects: Side effects, as with other penicillins, are uncommon and mainly of a mild and transitory nature. Gastrointestinal upsets (e.g. nausea, diarrhoea) and skin rashes have been reported infrequently. An urticarial rash suggests penicillin hypersensitivity; an erythematous-type rash may arise in patients receiving ampicillin who have glandular fever. If a skin rash occurs, treatment should be discontinued. Rarely erythema multiforme and Stevens-Johnson syndrome have been reported. In common with other beta-lactam antibiotics, angioedema and anaphylaxis have been reported. Pseudomembranous colitis has been reported rarely; cholestatic jaundice has been reported rarely with cloxacillin.

Overdose: Problems of overdosage with Ampiclox are unlikely to occur; if encountered they may be treated symptomatically.

Pharmacological properties

Pharmacodynamic properties: Ampiclox is a combination of ampicillin, a broad spectrum antibiotic and cloxacillin, a semi-synthetic beta-lactamase-resistant penicillin with activity against Gram-negative and Gram-positive bacteria including beta-lactamase-producing staphylococci.

Pharmacokinetic properties: Ampicillin has a plasma half-life of approximately one to two hours and is excreted mainly in the bile and urine.

Cloxacillin is excreted in the urine and bile with a serum half-life of approximately 30 minutes.

Preclinical safety data: Not applicable.

Pharmaceutical particulars

List of excipients:

Ampiclox Capsules: Magnesium stearate, gelatin, black iron oxide, titanium dioxide, erythrosine.

Ampiclox Syrup: Methyl polysiloxane, sodium benzoate, sodium citrate, disodium edetate, monoammonium glycyrrhizinate, saccharin sodium, menthol, tutti frutti and blood orange dry flavours, sucrose.

Neonatal Suspension: Sodium saccharin, sodium benzoate, sodium citrate, xanthan gum.

Ampiclox Injection: None.

Ampiclox Neonatal Injection: None.

Incompatibilities: Ampiclox Injection and Neonatal Injection should not be mixed with blood products or other proteinaceous fluids (e.g. protein hydrolysates) or with intravenous lipid emulsions.

If Ampiclox is prescribed concurrently with an aminoglycoside, the antibiotics should not be mixed in the syringe, intravenous fluid container or giving set because loss of activity of the aminoglycoside and possibly precipitation can occur under these conditions.

Shelf-life:

Ampiclox Capsules:	36 months
Ampiclox Syrup:	18 months unopened, (7 days following reconstitution)
Ampiclox Neonatal Suspension:	36 months unopened, (5 days following reconstitution)
Ampiclox Injection:	36 months
Ampiclox Neonatal Injection:	36 months

Special precautions for storage: Ampiclox Capsules, Syrup, Injection, Neonatal Suspension and Neonatal Injection should be stored in a cool dry place. The syrup bottle should be kept tightly closed. Once dispensed, Ampiclox Neonatal Suspension remains stable for five days and Ampiclox Syrup remains stable for seven days, if kept in a cool place. Ampiclox solutions for injection should be used immediately.

Nature and contents of container:

Ampiclox Capsules: Containers of 20 and 100

Ampiclox Syrup: Bottles of 100 ml

Ampiclox Neonatal Suspension: A clear glass bottle containing powder to reconstitute to 10 ml with pipette.

Ampiclox Injection and Neonatal Injection: Clear glass vials supplied in boxes of 10 vials with instructions for use.

Instructions for use/handling: Ampiclox 500 mg Injection may be added to most intravenous fluids (e.g. Water for Injections, sodium chloride 0.9%, glucose 5%, sodium chloride 0.18% with glucose 4%). In intravenous solutions containing glucose or other carbohydrates, Ampiclox should be infused within one hour of preparation. Intravenous solutions of Ampiclox in Water for Injections or sodium chloride 0.9% should be infused within 24 hours of preparation. Full particulars are given in the Package Enclosure Leaflet. Preparation of Ampiclox infusion solutions must be carried out under appropriate aseptic conditions if these extended storage periods are required.

Marketing authorisation holder: Beecham Group plc, SB House, Great West Road, Brentford, Middlesex TW8 9BD.

Trading as SmithKline Beecham Pharmaceuticals Mundells, Welwyn Garden City, Hertfordshire AL7 1EY.

Marketing authorisation numbers

Ampiclox Capsules:	0038/5008R
Ampiclox Syrup:	0038/0115R
Ampiclox Neonatal Suspension:	0038/5009R
Ampiclox Injection:	0038/5003R
Ampiclox Neonatal Injection:	0038/5001R

Date of first authorisation/renewal of authorisation

Ampiclox Capsules:	29.7.97
Ampiclox Syrup:	21.5.93
Ampiclox Neonatal Suspension:	30.7.97
Ampiclox Injection:	24.7.97
Ampiclox Neonatal Injection:	24.7.97

Date of (partial) revision of the text February 1997

Legal category POM.

ANDROPATCH* 2.5 mg ▼

Qualitative and quantitative composition Each Andropatch 2.5 mg System contains 12.2 mg testosterone BP.

Pharmaceutical form Andropatch 2.5 mg is a transdermal drug delivery system consisting of a self-adhesive patch surrounding a central drug reservoir of testosterone dissolved in an alcohol-based gel.

Each Andropatch 2.5 mg System delivers *in vivo* approximately 2.5 mg of testosterone over 24 hours across skin of average permeability. (Active surface area 7.5 cm².)

Clinical particulars

Therapeutic indications: Andropatch 2.5 mg is indicated for testosterone replacement therapy in conditions with a deficiency or an absence of endogenous testosterone associated with primary or secondary hypogonadism.

Posology and method of administration:

Adults and elderly: The usual dose is two Andropatch 2.5 mg Systems applied nightly (approximately 10 pm) and worn for 24 hours, providing approximately 5 mg testosterone per day. The dose can be adjusted up to the equivalent of 7.5 mg nightly or down to 2.5 mg nightly depending on the serum testosterone measured in the morning after application. Measurement of serum testosterone should be repeated taking care to ensure proper system adhesion and correct time of application before the dose is adjusted. Three systems per day may be required for men with a higher body weight (>130 kg). Treatment in non-virilised patients may be initiated with one system applied nightly. The dose should be adjusted as appropriate.

The duration of treatment and frequency of testosterone measurements is determined by the physician.

The adhesive side of the Andropatch 2.5 mg System should be applied to a clean, dry area of the skin on the back, abdomen, upper arms, or thighs. Bony prominences, such as the shoulder and hip areas, and areas that may be subjected to prolonged pressure during sleeping or sitting should be avoided. Application to these sites has been associated with burn-like blister reactions (see *Undesirable effects*). Do not apply to broken or damaged skin. Do not apply to the scrotum. The sites of application should be rotated, with an interval of seven days between applications to the same site. The area selected should not be oily, damaged or irritated.

The system should be applied immediately after opening the pouch and removing the protective release liner. The system should be pressed firmly in place, making sure there is good contact with the skin, especially around the edges.

Children: Andropatch 2.5 mg is not indicated for use in children as there has been no clinical experience of its use below the age of 15.

Contra-indications: Androgens are contra-indicated in men with carcinoma of the breast or known or suspected carcinoma of the prostate, nephrotic syndrome, hypercalcaemia and known hypersensitivity to testosterone.

Andropatch 2.5 mg is contra-indicated in men with known hypersensitivity to other constituents of the patch.

Andropatch 2.5 mg has not been evaluated in women and must not be used in women. Testosterone may be harmful to the foetus.

Special warnings and special precautions for use: Elderly men treated with androgens may be at an increased risk for the development of prostatic hyperplasia.

Elderly men and others with an increased risk of developing prostatic cancer, should be assessed before starting testosterone replacement therapy because testosterone may promote the growth of subclinical prostate cancer.

As in men without testosterone deficiency, patients on testosterone replacement therapy should be periodically evaluated for prostate cancer.

Care should be taken in patients with skeletal metastases due to the risk of hypercalcaemia/hypercalcuria developing from androgen therapy.

If the patient develops an application site reaction, treatment should be reviewed and discontinued if necessary.

Testosterone may cause a rise in blood pressure and Andropatch 2.5 mg should be used with caution in patients with hypertension.

Oedema, with or without congestive heart failure, may result from androgen treatment in patients with pre-existing cardiac, renal, or hepatic disease. In addition to discontinuation of the drug, diuretic therapy may be required.

Andropatch 2.5 mg should be used with caution in patients with ischaemic heart disease, epilepsy and migraine as these conditions may be aggravated.

Interaction with other medicaments and other forms of interaction: When given simultaneously with anticoagulants the anticoagulant effect can increase. Patients receiving oral anticoagulants require close monitoring especially when androgens are started or stopped.

Concurrent administration of oxyphenbutazone and androgens may result in elevated serum levels of oxyphenbutazone.

In diabetic patients, the metabolic effects of androgens may alter blood glucose and, therefore, insulin requirements.

Pregnancy and lactation: Andropatch 2.5 mg therapy has not been evaluated in and must not be used in women under any circumstances. Testosterone may be harmful to the foetus.

Effects on ability to drive and use machines: There is no evidence that Andropatch 2.5 mg will affect the ability of a patient to drive or to use machines.

Undesirable effects: In the majority of cases, transient mild to moderate skin reactions have been observed at the site of application at some time during treatment. These include pruritus; irritation with erythema, induration or burning, rash and allergic contact dermatitis. Burn-like lesions characterised by blisters, skin necrosis, and ulceration that healed over several weeks with scarring in some cases have also been observed.

The burn-like lesions occurred sporadically, usually only at one site, (most commonly over bony prominences or areas that may have been subjected to prolonged pressure during sleeping or sitting). Such lesions should be treated as burns.

As seen with other testosterone treatments, prostate abnormalities, prostate cancer, headache, depression and gastrointestinal bleeding were also observed.

Other known undesirable effects associated with testosterone treatments include hirsuitism, male pattern baldness, seborrhoea, acne, excessive frequency and duration of penile erections, nausea, cholestatic jaundice, increased or decreased libido, anxiety, generalised paraesthaesia. Oligospermia may occur at high doses. Prolonged testosterone administration may cause electrolyte disturbances, e.g. retention of sodium, chloride, potassium, calcium, inorganic phosphates and water.

Overdose: This is not likely due to the mode of administration. Serum testosterone has a half-life of 70 minutes and therefore falls rapidly once the Andropatch 2.5 mg Systems are removed.

Pharmacological properties

Pharmacodynamic properties: Andropatch 2.5 mg delivers physiologic amounts of testosterone producing circulating testosterone concentrations that mimic the normal circadian rhythm of healthy young men.

Testosterone, the primary androgenic hormone is responsible for the normal growth and development of the male sex organs and for maintenance of secondary sex characteristics.

Male hypogonadism results from insufficient secretion of testosterone and is characterised by low serum testosterone concentrations. Symptoms associated with male hypogonadism include the following: impotence and decreased sexual desire; fatigue and loss of energy; mood depression; regression of secondary sexual characteristics.

Androgens promote retention of nitrogen, sodium, potassium and phosphorus, decrease urinary excretion of calcium, increase protein anabolism, decrease protein catabolism, are also responsible for the growth spurt of adolescence and for the eventual termination of linear growth and stimulate the production of red blood cells by enhancing erythropoietin production.

Exogenous administration of androgens inhibits endogenous testosterone release. With large doses of exogenous androgens, spermatogenesis may be suppressed.

Pharmacokinetic properties: Following Andropatch 2.5 mg application to non-scrotal skin, testosterone is continuously absorbed during the 24-hour dosing period. Daily application of two Andropatch 2.5 mg patches at approximately 10 pm results in a serum testosterone concentration profile which mimics the normal circadian variation observed in healthy young men. Maximum concentrations occur in the early morning hours with minimum concentrations in the evening.

In hypogonadal men, application of two Andropatch 2.5 mg Systems to the back, abdomen, thighs or upper arms resulted in average testosterone absorption of 4 to 5 mg over 24 hours. Applications to the chest and shins resulted in greater inter-individual variability and average 24-hour absorption of 3 to 4 mg. The serum testosterone concentration profiles during application were similar for all sites.

Normal range morning serum testosterone concentrations are reached during the first day of dosing. There is no accumulation of testosterone during continuous treatment.

Upon removal of the Andropatch 2.5 mg Systems, serum testosterone concentrations decrease with an apparent half-life of approximately 70 minutes. Hypogonadal concentrations are reached within 24 hours following system removal.

Preclinical safety data: None therapeutically relevant.

Pharmaceutical particulars

List of excipients in drug reservoir: Alcohol USP, Purified Water EP, Glycerin EP, glycerol mono-oleate, methyl laurate, Carbomer 1342 BP, Sodium Hydroxide EP.

Incompatibilities: No specific incompatabilities.

Shelf-life: 24 months.

Special precautions for storage: Store below 25°C. Apply to skin immediately upon removal from the protective pouch. Do not store outside the pouch provided.

Nature and contents of container: Each Andropatch 2.5 mg System contains 12.2 mg testosterone BP for delivery of 2.5 mg testosterone per day. Each Andropatch 2.5 mg System is individually pouched and supplied in cartons of 10, 30 and 60 pouches. The pouch is made from paper, low density polyethylene and aluminium foil.

Instructions for use/handling: Andropatch 2.5 mg may be discarded with household waste in a manner that avoids accidental contact by others.

Damaged systems should not be used.

The drug reservoir may be burst by excessive heat or pressure.

Marketing authorisation holder: SmithKline Beecham plc, SB House, Great West Road, Brentford, Middlesex TW8 9BD.
Trading as SmithKline Beecham Pharmaceuticals Mundells, Welwyn Garden City, Hertfordshire AL7 1EY.

Marketing authorisation number PL 10592/0069

Date of first authorisation/renewal of authorisation 19th July 1996

Date of approval/revision of SPC 16th September 1997

Legal Category POM; CD (Sch. 4)

ANDROPATCH* 5 mg ▼

Qualitative and quantitative composition Each Andropatch System contains 24.3 mg testosterone BP.

Pharmaceutical form Andropatch is a transdermal drug delivery system consisting of a self-adhesive patch surrounding a central drug reservoir of testosterone dissolved in an alcohol-based gel.

Each Andropatch System delivers *in vivo* approximately 5 mg of testosterone over 24 hours across skin of average permeability. (Active surface area 15 cm^2).

Clinical particulars

Therapeutic indications: Andropatch is indicated for testosterone replacement therapy in conditions with a deficiency or an absence of endogenous testosterone associated with primary or secondary hypogonadism.

Posology and method of administration:

Adults and elderly: The usual dose is one Andropatch System applied nightly (approximately 10 pm) and worn for 24 hours, providing approximately 5 mg testosterone per day. The dose can be adjusted up to the equivalent of 7.5 mg nightly or down to 2.5 mg patch nightly depending on the serum testosterone measured in the morning after application. Measurement of serum testosterone should be repeated taking care to ensure proper system adhesion and correct time of application before the dose is adjusted. The equivalent of 7.5 mg per day may be required for men with a higher body weight (>130 kg). Treatment in non-virilised patients may be initiated with one 2.5 mg system applied nightly. The dose should be adjusted as appropriate.

The duration of treatment and frequency of testosterone measurements is determined by the physician.

The adhesive side of the Andropatch System should be applied to a clean, dry area of the skin on the back, abdomen, upper arms, or thighs. Bony prominences, such as the shoulder and hip areas, and areas that may be subjected to prolonged pressure during sleeping or sitting should be avoided. Application to these sites has been associated with burn-like blister reactions (see *Undesirable effects*). Do not apply to broken or damaged skin. Do not apply to the scrotum. The sites of application should be rotated, with an interval of seven days between applications to the same site. The area selected should not be oily, damaged or irritated.

The system should be applied immediately after opening the pouch and removing the protective release liner. The system should be pressed firmly in place, making sure there is good contact with the skin, especially around the edges.

Children: Andropatch is not indicated for use in children as there has been no clinical experience of its use below the age of 15.

Contra-indications: Androgens are contra-indicated in men with carcinoma of the breast or known or suspected carcinoma of the prostate, nephrotic syndrome, hypercalcaemia and known hypersensitivity to testosterone.

Andropatch is contra-indicated in men with known hypersensitivity to other constituents of the patch.

Andropatch has not been evaluated in women and must not be used in women. Testosterone may be harmful to the foetus.

Special warnings and special precautions for use: Elderly men treated with androgens may be at an increased risk for the development of prostatic hyperplasia.

Elderly men and others with an increased risk of developing prostatic cancer, should be assessed before starting testosterone replacement therapy because testosterone may promote the growth of subclinical prostate cancer.

As in men without testosterone deficiency, patients on testosterone replacement therapy should be periodically evaluated for prostate cancer.

Care should be taken in patients with skeletal metastases due to the risk of hypercalcaemia/hypercalcuria developing from androgen therapy.

If the patient develops an application site reaction, treatment should be reviewed and discontinued if necessary.

Testosterone may cause a rise in blood pressure and Andropatch should be used with caution in patients with hypertension.

Oedema, with or without congestive heart failure, may result from androgen treatment in patients with pre-existing cardiac, renal, or hepatic disease. In addition to discontinuation of the drug, diuretic therapy may be required.

Andropatch should be used with caution in patients with ischaemic heart disease, epilepsy and migraine as these conditions may be aggravated.

Interaction with other medicaments and other forms of interaction: When given simultaneously with anticoagulants the anticoagulant effect can increase. Patients receiving oral anticoagulants require close monitoring especially when androgens are started or stopped.

Concurrent administration of oxyphenbutazone and androgens may result in elevated serum levels of oxyphenbutazone.

In diabetic patients, the metabolic effects of androgens may alter blood glucose and, therefore, insulin requirements.

Pregnancy and lactation: Andropatch therapy has not been evaluated in and must not be used in women under any circumstances. Testosterone may be harmful to the foetus.

Effects on ability to drive and use machines: There is no evidence that Andropatch will affect the ability of a patient to drive or to use machines.

Undesirable effects: In the majority of cases, transient mild to moderate skin reactions have been observed at the site of application at some time during treatment. These include pruritus; irritation with erythema, induration or burning, rash and allergic contact dermatitis. Burn-like lesions characterised by blisters, skin necrosis, and ulceration that healed over several weeks with scarring in some cases have also been observed.

The burn-like lesions occurred sporadically, usually only at one site, (most commonly over bony prominences or areas that may have been subjected to prolonged pressure during sleeping or sitting). Such lesions should be treated as burns.

As seen with other testosterone treatments, prostate abnormalities, prostate cancer, headache, depression and gastrointestinal bleeding were also observed.

Other known undesirable effects associated with testosterone treatments include hirsuitism, male pattern baldness, seborrhoea, acne, excessive frequency and duration of penile erections, nausea, cholestatic jaundice, increased or decreased libido, anxiety, generalised paraesthaesia. Oligospermia may occur at high doses. Prolonged testosterone administration may cause electrolyte disturbances, e.g. retention of sodium, chloride, potassium, calcium, inorganic phosphates and water.

Overdose: This is not likely due to the mode of administration. Serum testosterone has a half-life of 70 minutes and therefore falls rapidly once the Andropatch Systems are removed.

Pharmacological properties

Pharmacodynamic properties: Andropatch delivers physiologic amounts of testosterone producing circulating testosterone concentrations that mimic the normal circadian rhythm of healthy young men.

Testosterone, the primary androgenic hormone is responsible for the normal growth and development of the male sex organs and for maintenance of secondary sex characteristics.

Male hypogonadism results from insufficient secretion of testosterone and is characterised by low serum testosterone concentrations. Symptoms associated with male hypogonadism include the following: impotence and decreased sexual desire; fatigue and loss of energy; mood depression; regression of secondary sexual characteristics.

Androgens promote retention of nitrogen, sodium, potassium and phosphorus, decrease urinary excretion of calcium, increase protein anabolism, decrease protein catabolism, are also responsible for the growth spurt of adolescence and for the eventual termination of linear growth and stimulate the production of red blood cells by enhancing erythropoietin production.

Exogenous administration of androgens inhibits endogenous testosterone release. With large doses of exogenous androgens, spermatogenesis may be suppressed.

Pharmacokinetic properties: Following Andropatch application to non-scrotal skin, testosterone is continuously absorbed during the 24-hour dosing period. Daily application of two 2.5 mg or one 5 mg Andropatch patches at approximately 10 pm results in a serum testosterone concentration profile which mimics the normal circadian variation observed in healthy young men. Maximum concentrations occur in the early morning hours with minimum concentrations in the evening.

In hypogonadal men, application of two 2.5 mg or one 5 mg Andropatch Systems to the back, abdomen, thighs or upper arms resulted in average testosterone absorption of 4 to 5 mg over 24 hours. Applications to the chest and shins resulted in greater inter-individual variability and average 24-hour absorption of 3 to 4 mg. The serum testosterone concentration profiles during application were similar for all sites.

Normal range morning serum testosterone concentrations are reached during the first day of dosing. There is no accumulation of testosterone during continuous treatment.

Upon removal of the Andropatch Systems, serum testosterone concentrations decrease with an apparent half-life of approximately 70 minutes. Hypogonadal concentrations are reached within 24 hours following system removal.

Preclinical safety data: None therapeutically relevant.

Pharmaceutical particulars

List of excipients in drug reservoir: Alcohol USP, Purified Water EP, Glycerin EP, glycerol mono-oleate, methyl laurate, Carbomer 1342 BP, Sodium Hydroxide EP.

Incompatibilities: No specific incompatabilities.

Shelf-life: 24 months.

Special precautions for storage: Store below 25°C. Apply to skin immediately upon removal from the protective pouch. Do not store outside the pouch provided.

Nature and contents of container: Each Andropatch System contains 24.3 mg testosterone BP for delivery of 5 mg testosterone per day. Each Andropatch System is individually pouched and supplied in cartons of 5, 15 and 30 pouches. The pouch is made from paper, low density polyethylene and aluminium foil.

Instructions for use/handling: Andropatch may be discarded with household waste in a manner that avoids accidental contact by others.

Damaged systems should not be used.

The drug reservoir may be burst by excessive heat or pressure.

Marketing authorisation holder: SmithKline Beecham plc, SB House, Great West Road, Brentford, Middlesex TW8 9BD.

Trading as SmithKline Beecham Pharmaceuticals Mundells, Welwyn Garden City, Hertfordshire AL7 1EY.

Marketing authorisation number PL 10592/0106

Date of first authorisation/renewal of authorisation 26 August 1997

Date of approval/revision of SPC 26 August 1997

Legal Category POM; CD (Sch. 4)

ASACOL* TABLETS

Qualitative and quantitative composition 400 mg mesalazine (5-aminosalicylic acid) per tablet.

Pharmaceutical form Red-brown, oblong, enteric-coated tablets.

Clinical particulars

Therapeutic indications:

Ulcerative colitis: For the treatment of mild to moderate acute exacerbations. For the maintenance of remission.

Crohn's ileo-colitis: For the maintenance of remission.

Posology and method of administration:

Adults: Oral: Acute disease: Six tablets a day in divided doses, with concomitant corticosteroid therapy where clinically indicated.

Maintenance therapy: Three to six tablets a day in divided doses.

Elderly: The normal adult dosage may be used unless renal function is impaired (see *Special warnings and special precautions for use*).

Children: There is no dosage recommendation.

Contra-indications: A history of sensitivity to salicylates or renal sensitivity to sulphasalazine. Severe renal impairment (GFR less than 20 ml/min). Children under two years of age.

Special warnings and special precautions for use: Use in the elderly should be cautious and subject to patients having normal renal function.

Renal disorder: Mesalazine is excreted rapidly by the kidney, mainly as its metabolite, N-acetyl-5-aminosalicylic acid. In rats, large doses of mesalazine injected intravenously produce tubular and glomerular toxicity. Asacol is best avoided in patients with established renal impairment but, if necessary, it should be used with caution.

Serious blood dyscrasias have been reported very rarely with mesalazine. Haematological investigations should be performed if the patient develops unexplained bleeding, bruising, purpura, anaemia, fever or sore throat. Treatment should be stopped if there is suspicion or evidence of blood dyscrasia.

Interaction with other medicaments and other forms of interaction: Asacol Tablets should not be given with lactulose or similar preparations which lower stool pH and may prevent release of mesalazine.

Pregnancy and lactation: No information is available with regard to teratogenicity; however, negligible quantities of mesalazine are transferred across the placenta and are excreted in breast milk following sulphasalazine therapy. Use of Asacol during pregnancy should be with caution, and only if the potential benefits are greater than the possible hazards. Asacol should, unless essential, be avoided by nursing mothers.

Effects on ability to drive and use machines: Not applicable.

Undesirable effects: The side effects are predominantly gastrointestinal, including nausea, diarrhoea and abdominal pain. Headache has also been reported.

Mesalazine may be associated with an exacerbation of the symptoms of colitis in those patients who have previously had such problems with sulphasalazine. There have been rare reports of leucopenia, neutropenia, agranulocytosis, aplastic anaemia and thrombocytopenia, pancreatitis, hepatitis, allergic lung reactions, lupus erythematosus-like reactions and rash (including urticaria), interstitial nephritis and nephrotic syndrome with oral mesalazine treatment, usually reversible on withdrawal. Renal failure has been reported. Mesalazine-induced nephrotoxicity should be suspected in patients developing renal dysfunction during treatment.

Other side effects observed with sulphasalazine such as depression of sperm count and function, have not been reported with Asacol.

Overdose: Following tablet ingestion, gastric lavage and intravenous transfusion of electrolytes to promote diuresis. There is no specific antidote.

Pharmacological properties

Pharmacodynamic properties: Mesalazine is one of the two components of sulphasalazine, the other being sulphapyridine. It is the latter which is responsible for the majority of the side effects associated with sulphasalazine therapy whilst mesalazine is known to be the active moiety in the treatment of ulcerative colitis.

Pharmacokinetic properties: Asacol Tablets contain 400 mg of available mesalazine. This is released in the terminal ileum and large bowel by the effect of pH. Above pH 7 the Eudragit coat disintegrates and releases the active constituent. Asacol Tablets contain, in a single tablet, an equivalent quantity of mesalazine to that theoretically available from the complete azoreduction of 1 g of sulphasalazine.

Preclinical safety data: There are no preclinical data of relevance to the prescriber which are additional to those already included in other sections of the SPC.

Pharmaceutical particulars

List of excipients: Each tablet contains: lactose, sodium starch glycollate, magnesium stearate, talc, polyvinylpyrrolidone, Eudragit S, dibutylphthalate, iron oxides (E172) and polyethylene glycol.

Incompatibilities: Not applicable.

Shelf-life: Two years.

Special precautions for storage: Store tablets in a dry place at a temperature not exceeding 25°C and protect from direct sunlight.

Nature and contents of container: Tablets in cartons (OP) of 120, each containing 12 opaque PVC blister packs of 10 tablets or cartons (OP) of 90, each containing six opaque PVC blister packs of 15 tablets.

Instructions for use/handling: Do not chew tablets before swallowing.

Marketing authorisation holder: Smith Kline & French Laboratories Ltd., Mundells, Welwyn Garden City, Hertfordshire AL7 1EY.

Trading as:

SmithKline Beecham Pharmaceuticals, Mundells, Welwyn Garden City, Hertfordshire AL7 1EY.

Marketing authorisation number PL 0002/0173

Date of first authorisation/renewal of authorisation 1.2.88 / 19.3.93.

Date of (partial) revision of the text 16.6.98.

Legal category POM.

ASACOL* SUPPOSITORIES 250 mg and 500 mg

Qualitative and quantitative composition Asacol Suppositories contain 250 or 500 mg mesalazine per suppository.

Pharmaceutical form Opaque, beige suppositories, containing 250 mg or 500 mg mesalazine.

Clinical particulars

Therapeutic indications: For the treatment of mild to moderate acute exacerbations of ulcerative colitis.

The suppositories are particularly appropriate in patients with distal disease.

For the maintenance of remission of ulcerative colitis.

Posology and method of administration:

Adults: Suppositories 250 mg: Three to six suppositories a day in divided doses, with the last dose at bedtime.

Suppositories 500 mg: A maximum of three suppositories a day in divided doses, with the last dose at bedtime.

Elderly: The normal adult dosage may be used unless renal function is impaired (see *Special warnings and special precautions for use*).

Children: There is no dosage recommendation.

Contra-indications: A history of sensitivity to salicylates or renal sensitivity to sulphasalazine. Severe renal impairment (GFR <20 ml/min). Children under two years of age.

Special warnings and special precautions for use: Use in the elderly should be cautious and subject to patients having normal renal function.

Renal disorder: Mesalazine is excreted rapidly by the kidney, mainly as its metabolite, N-acetyl-5-aminosalicylic acid. In rats, large doses of mesalazine injected intravenously produce tubular and glomerular toxicity. Asacol is best avoided in patients with established renal impairment but, if necessary, it should be used with caution.

Serious blood dyscrasias have been reported very rarely with mesalazine. Haematological investigations should be performed if the patient develops unexplained bleeding, bruising, purpura, anaemia, fever or sore throat. Treatment should be stopped if there is suspicion or evidence of blood dyscrasia.

Interaction with other medicaments and other forms of interaction: Not applicable.

Pregnancy and lactation: No information is available with regard to teratogenicity; however, negligible quantities of mesalazine are transferred across the placenta and are excreted in breast milk following sulphasalazine therapy. Use of Asacol during pregnancy should be with caution, and only if the potential benefits are greater than the possible hazards. Asacol should, unless essential, be avoided by nursing mothers.

Effects on ability to drive and use machines: Not applicable.

Undesirable effects: The side effects are predominantly gastrointestinal, including nausea, diarrhoea and abdominal pain. Headache has also been reported.

Mesalazine may be associated with an exacerbation of the symptoms of colitis in those patients who have previously had such problems with sulphasalazine. There have been rare reports of leucopenia, neutropenia, agranulocytosis, aplastic anaemia and thrombocytopenia, pancreatitis, hepatitis, allergic lung reactions, lupus erythematosus-like reactions and rash (including urticaria), interstitial nephritis and nephrotic syndrome with oral mesalazine treatment, usually reversible on withdrawal. Renal failure has been reported. Mesalazine-induced nephrotoxicity should be suspected in patients developing renal dysfunction during treatment.

Other side effects observed with sulphasalazine such as depression of sperm count and function, have not been reported with Asacol.

Overdose: There is no specific antidote.

Pharmacological properties
Pharmacodynamic properties: Mesalazine is one of the two components of sulphasalazine, the other being sulphapyridine. It is the latter which is responsible for the majority of the side effects associated with sulphasalazine therapy whilst mesalazine is known to be the active moiety in the treatment of ulcerative colitis. Asacol consists only of this active component which is delivered directly by the suppositories.

Pharmacokinetic properties: The suppository is designed to deliver mesalazine directly to the proposed site of action in the distal bowel.

Preclinical safety data: There are no preclinical data of relevance to the prescriber which are additional to those already included in other sections of the SPC.

Pharmaceutical particulars
List of excipients: Witepsol W45 (Hard Fat).

Incompatibilities: Not applicable.

Shelf-life:
Suppositories 250 mg: Four years.
Suppositories 500 mg: Three years.

Special precautions for storage: Store below 25°C. Protect from light.

Nature and contents of container: Cartoned plastic moulds (OP), each containing 20 suppositories (250 mg) or 10 suppositories (500 mg).

Instructions for use/handling: For rectal administration.

Marketing authorisation holder: Smith Kline & French Laboratories Ltd., Mundells, Welwyn Garden City, Hertfordshire AL7 1EY.
Trading as:
SmithKline Beecham Pharmaceuticals Mundells, Welwyn Garden City, Hertfordshire AL7 1EY.

Marketing authorisation numbers

Asacol Suppositories 250 mg	0002/0158
Asacol Suppositories 500 mg	0002/0195

Date of first authorisation/renewal of authorisation

Asacol Suppositories 250 mg	20.4.88/20.4.98
Asacol Suppositories 500 mg	22.3.90/17.4.97

Date of (partial) revision of the text 29.8.97.

Legal category POM.

ASACOL* FOAM ENEMA

Presentation White, aerosol foam enema, containing 1 g mesalazine per metered dose.

Uses For the treatment of mild to moderate acute exacerbations of ulcerative colitis affecting the distal colon.

Dosage and administration
Route of administration: Rectal.

Adults: For disease affecting the rectosigmoid region, one metered dose 1 g a day for four to six weeks; for disease involving the descending colon, two metered doses 2 g once a day for four to six weeks.

Children: There is no dosage recommendation.

Contra-indications, warnings, etc
Contra-indications: A history of sensitivity to salicylates or renal sensitivity to sulphasalazine. Severe renal impairment (GFR less than 20 ml/min). Children under two years of age.

Precautions: Renal disorder: mesalazine is excreted rapidly by the kidney, mainly as its metabolite, N-acetyl-5-aminosalicylic acid. In rats, large doses of mesalazine injected intravenously produce tubular and glomerular toxicity. Asacol is best avoided in patients with established renal impairment but, if necessary, it should be used with caution.

Serious blood dyscrasias have been reported very rarely with mesalazine. Haematological investigations should be performed if the patient develops unexplained bleeding, bruising, purpura, anaemia, fever or sore throat. Treatment should be stopped if there is suspicion or evidence of blood dyscrasia.

Use in pregnancy and lactation: No information is available with regard to teratogenicity; however, negligible quantities of mesalazine are transferred across the placenta and are excreted in breast milk following sulphasalazine therapy. Use of Asacol during pregnancy should be with caution, and only if, in the opinion of the physician, the potential benefits of treatment are greater than the possible hazards. Asacol should, unless essential, be avoided by nursing mothers.

Elderly: Use in the elderly should be cautious and subject to patients having a normal renal function (see *Precautions*).

Adverse reactions: The side effects are predominantly gastrointestinal, including nausea, diarrhoea and abdominal pain. Headache has also been reported.

Mesalazine may be associated with an exacerbation of the symptoms of colitis in those patients who have previously had such problems with sulphasalazine. There have been rare reports of leucopenia, neutropenia, agranulocytosis, aplastic anaemia and thrombocytopenia, pancreatitis, hepatitis, allergic lung reactions, lupus erythematosus-like reactions and rash (including urticaria), interstitial nephritis and nephrotic syndrome with oral mesalazine treatment, usually reversible on withdrawal. Renal failure has been reported. Mesalazine-induced nephrotoxicity should be suspected in patients developing renal dysfunction during treatment.

Other side effects observed with sulphasalazine such as depression of sperm count and function, have not been reported with Asacol.

Treatment of overdosage: There is no specific antidote.

Pharmaceutical precautions Store the foam enema below 30°C. This is a pressurised canister, containing a flammable propellant. It should be kept away from any flames or sparks, including cigarettes. It should be protected from direct sunlight and must not be pierced or burned even when empty.

Legal category POM.

Package quantities Foam enema in cartoned aerosol can, each carton consisting of one aerosol can containing 14 metered doses, plus 14 disposable applicators and 14 disposable plastic bags.

Further information This Data Sheet supersedes the entry in the ABPI *Data Sheet Compendium 1998-99.*

Mesalazine is one of the two components of sulphasalazine, the other being sulphapyridine. It is the latter which is responsible for the majority of side effects associated with sulphasalazine therapy whilst mesalazine is known to be the active moiety in the treatment of ulcerative colitis. The foam enema is intended to deliver mesalazine directly to the proposed site of action in the colon and rectum.

Inactive ingredients in the foam enema include sodium metabisulphite, disodium edetate, methyl and propyl hydroxybenzoate.

Product licence number PL 0002/0222

AUGMENTIN* 375 MG TABLETS
AUGMENTIN* 625 MG TABLETS
AUGMENTIN* DISPERSIBLE TABLETS 375 MG
AUGMENTIN* 250/62 SF SUSPENSION
AUGMENTIN* 125/31 SF SUSPENSION

Qualitative and quantitative composition
Augmentin 375 mg Tablets: Each tablet contains co-amoxiclav 250/125.

Augmentin 625 mg Tablets: Each tablet contains co-amoxiclav 500/125.

Augmentin Dispersible Tablets 375 mg: Each tablet contains co-amoxiclav 250/125.

Augmentin 250/62 SF Suspension: When reconstituted each 5 ml contains co-amoxiclav 250/62.

Augmentin 125/31 SF Suspension: When reconstituted each 5 ml contains co-amoxiclav 125/31.

In all the above presentations the amoxycillin is present as amoxycillin trihydrate and the clavulanic acid is present as potassium clavulanate.

Pharmaceutical form
Augmentin 375 mg Tablets: White to off-white oval film-coated tablets engraved Augmentin on one side.

Augmentin 625 mg Tablets: White to off-white oval film-coated tablets engraved Augmentin

Augmentin Dispersible Tablets: White round tablets engraved Augmentin.

Augmentin 250/62 SF and 125/31 SF Suspension: Dry powder for reconstitution in water, at time of dispensing, to form an oral sugar-free suspension.

Clinical particulars
Therapeutic indications: Augmentin is an antibiotic agent with a notably broad spectrum of activity against the commonly occurring bacterial pathogens in general practice and hospital. The β-lactamase inhibitory action of clavulanate extends the spectrum of amoxycillin to embrace a wider range of organisms, including many resistant to other β-lactam antibiotics.

Augmentin oral preparations are indicated for short-term treatment of bacterial infections at the following sites when amoxycillin-resistant β-lactamase-producing strains are suspected as the cause. In other situations, amoxycillin alone should be considered.

Upper Respiratory Tract Infections (including ENT) in particular sinusitis, otitis media, recurrent tonsillitis. These infections are often caused by *Streptococcus pneumoniae, Haemophilus influenzae*, Moraxella catarrhalis** and *Streptococcus pyogenes.*

Lower Respiratory Tract Infections in particular acute exacerbations of chronic bronchitis (especially if considered severe), bronchopneumonia. These infections are often caused by *Streptococcus pneumoniae, Haemophilus influenzae** and *Moraxella catarrhalis*.*

Genito-urinary Tract and Abdominal Infections in particular cystitis (especially when recurrent or complicated–excluding prostatitis), septic abortion, pelvic or puerperal sepsis and intra-abdominal sepsis. These infections are often caused by *Enterobacteriaceae** (mainly *Escherichia coli**), *Staphylococcus saprophyticus, Enterococcus* species*.

Skin and Soft Tissue Infections in particular cellulitis, animal bites and severe dental abscess with spreading cellulitis. These infections are often caused by *Staphylococcus aureus*, Streptococcus pyogenes* and *Bacteroides* species*.

A comprehensive list of sensitive organisms is provided in *Pharmacological properties* section.

* Some members of these species of bacteria produce β-lactamase, rendering them insensitive to amoxycillin alone.

Mixed infections caused by amoxycillin-susceptible organisms in conjunction with Augmentin-susceptible β-lactamase-producing organisms may be treated with Augmentin. These infections should not require the addition of another antibiotic resistant to β-lactamases.

Posology and method of administration
Usual dosages for the treatment of infection
Adults and children over 12 years: One Augmentin 375 mg Tablet or Dispersible Tablet three times a day. In severe infections one Augmentin 625 mg Tablet three times a day. Therapy can be started parenterally and continued with an oral preparation.

Children: The usual recommended daily dosage is 25 mg/kg/day* in divided doses every eight hours. The table below presents guidance for children.

Augmention Suspension

Under 1 year	25 mg/kg/day*, for example a 7.5 kg child would require 2 ml Augmentin 125/31 SF Suspension t.d.s.
1–6 years (10–18 kg)	5 ml Augmentin 125/31 SF Suspension t.d.s.
Over 6 years (18–40 kg)	5 ml Augmentin 250/62 SF Suspension t.d.s.

In more serious infections the dosage may be increased up to 50 mg/kg/day in divided doses every eight hours.

* Each 25 mg Augmentin provides co-amoxiclav 20/5.

Augmentin 375 mg and 625 mg Tablets are not recommended in children of 12 years and under.

Dosage in dental infections (e.g. dentoalveolar abscess):
Adults and children over 12 years: One Augmentin Tablet 375 mg three times a day for five days.

Dosage in renal impairment

Adults:
Mild impairment (Creatinine clearance >30 ml/min): No change in dosage.

Moderate impairment (Creatinine clearance 10–30 ml/min): One 375 mg tablet or one 625 mg tablet 12 hourly.

Severe impairment (Creatinine clearance <10 ml/min): Not more than one 375 mg tablet 12 hourly; 625 mg tablets are not recommended.

Children: Similar reductions in dosage should be made for children.

Dosage in hepatic impairment: Dose with caution; monitor hepatic function at regular intervals.

There are, as yet, insufficient data on which to base a dosage recommendation.

Each 375 mg tablet of Augmentin contains 0.63 mmol (25 mg) of potassium.

Administration: Oral: Tablets, dispersible tablets or supsensions. To minimise potential gastrointestinal intolerance, administer at the start of a meal. The absorption of Augmentin is optimised when taken at the start of a meal. Dispersible tablets should be stirred into a little water before taking.

Duration of therapy should be appropriate to the indication and should not exceed 14 days without review.

Contra-indications: Penicillin hypersensitivity. Attention should be paid to possible cross-sensitivity with other β-lactam antibiotics, e.g. cephalosporins.

A previous history of Augmentin- or penicillin-associated jaundice/hepatic dysfunction.

Special warnings and special precautions for use: Changes in liver function tests have been observed in some patients receiving Augmentin. The clinical significance of these changes is uncertain but Augmentin should be used with caution in patients with evidence of hepatic dysfunction.

Cholestatic jaundice, which may be severe, but is usually reversible, has been reported rarely. Signs and symptoms may not become apparent for several weeks after treatment has ceased.

Serious and occasionally fatal hypersensitivity (anaphylactoid) reactions have been reported in patients on penicillin therapy. These reactions are more likely to occur in individuals with a history of penicillin hypersensitivity (see *Contra-indications* section).

Erythematous rashes have been associated with glandular fever in patients receiving amoxycillin.

Prolonged use may also occasionally result in overgrowth of non-susceptible organisms.

Augmentin Suspensions contain 12.5 mg aspartame per 5 ml dose and therefore care should be taken in phenylketonuria.

Interaction with other medicaments and other forms of interaction: Prolongation of bleeding time and prothrombin time have been reported in some patients receiving Augmentin. Augmentin should be used with care in patients on anti-coagulation therapy.

In common with other broad-spectrum antibiotics, Augmentin may reduce the efficacy of oral contraceptives and patients should be warned accordingly.

Concomitant use of allopurinol during treatment with amoxycillin can increase the likelihood of allergic skin reactions. There are no data on the concomitant use of Augmentin and allopurinol.

Pregnancy and lactation: Reproduction studies in animals (mice and rats) with orally and parenterally administered Augmentin have shown no teratogenic effects. There is limited experience of the use of Augmentin in human pregnancy. As with all medicines, use should be avoided in pregnancy, especially during the first trimester, unless considered essential by the physician.

Augmentin may be administered during the period of lactation. With the exception of the risk of sensitisation, associated with the excretion of trace quantities in breast milk, there are no known detrimental effects for the breast-fed infant.

Effects on ability to drive and use machines: None known.

Undesirable effects: Side effects are uncommon and mainly of a mild and transitory nature.

Gastrointestinal reactions: Diarrhoea, indigestion, nausea, vomiting, and mucocutaneous candidiasis have been reported. Antibiotic-associated colitis (including pseudomembranous colitis and haemorrhagic colitis) has been reported rarely. Nausea, although uncommon, is more often associated with higher oral dosages. If gastrointestinal side effects occur with oral therapy they may be reduced by taking Augmentin at the start of meals.

As with other antibiotics the incidence of gastrointestinal side effects may be raised in children under two years. In clinical trials, however, only 4% of children under two years were withdrawn from treatment.

Superficial tooth discolouration has been reported rarely, mostly with the suspension. It can usually be removed by brushing.

Genito-urinary effects: Vaginal itching, soreness and discharge may occur.

Hepatic effects: Moderate and asymptomatic rises in AST and/or ALT and alkaline phosphatases have been reported occasionally. Hepatitis and cholestatic jaundice have been reported rarely. These hepatic reactions have been reported more commonly with Augmentin than with other penicillins.

After Augmentin hepatic reactions have been reported more frequently in males and elderly patients, particularly those over 65 years. The risk increases with duration of treatment longer than 14 days. These reactions have been very rarely reported in children.

Signs and symptoms usually occur during or shortly after treatment but in some cases may not occur until several weeks after treatment has ended. Hepatic reactions are usually reversible but they may be severe and, very rarely, deaths have been reported.

Hypersensitivity reactions: Urticarial and erythematous rashes sometimes occur. Rarely erythema multiforme, Stevens-Johnson syndrome, toxic epidermal necrolysis, bullous exfoliative dermatitis, serum sickness-like syndrome and hypersensitivity vasculitis have been reported. Treatment should be discontinued if one of these disorders occurs. In common with other β-lactam antibiotics angioedema and anaphylaxis have been reported. Interstitial nephritis can occur rarely.

Haematological effects: As with other β-lactams transient leucopenia, thrombocytopenia and haemolytic anaemia have been reported rarely. Prolongation of bleeding time and prothrombin time has also been reported rarely (see *Interaction with other medicaments and other forms of interaction* section).

CNS effects: CNS effects have been seen very rarely. These include reversible hyperactivity, dizziness, headache and convulsions. Convulsions may occur with impaired renal function or in those receiving high doses.

Overdose: Problems of overdosage with Augmentin are unlikely to occur; if encountered gastrointestinal symptoms and disturbance of the fluid and electrolyte balances may be evident. They may be treated symptomatically with attention to the water electrolyte balance. Augmentin may be removed from the circulation by haemodialysis.

Pharmacological properties

Pharmacodynamic properties: Resistance to many antibiotics is caused by bacterial enzymes which destroy the antibiotic before it can act on the pathogen. The clavulanate in Augmentin anticipates this defence mechanism by blocking the β-lactamase enzymes, thus rendering the organisms sensitive to amoxycillin's rapid bactericidal effect at concentrations readily attainable in the body.

Clavulanate by itself has little antibacterial activity; however, in association with amoxycillin as Augmentin, it produces an antibiotic agent of broad spectrum with wide application in hospital and general practice.

Augmentin is bactericidal to a wide range of organisms including:

Gram-positive:

Aerobes: *Enterococcus faecalis**, *Enterococcus faecium**, *Streptococcus pneumoniae*, *Streptococcus pyogenes*, *Streptococcus viridans*, *Staphylococcus aureus**, Coagulase negative staphylococci* (including *Staphylococcus epidermidis**), *Corynebacterium* species, *Bacillus anthracis**, *Listeria monocytogenes*.

Anaerobes: *Clostridium* species, *Peptococcus* species, *Peptostreptococcus*.

Gram-negative:

Aerobes: *Haemophilus influenzae**, *Moraxella catarrhalis* (Branhamella catarrhalis)*, *Escherichia coli**, *Proteus mirabilis**, *Proteus vulgaris**, *Klebsiella* species*, *Salmonella* species*, *Shigella* species*, *Bordetella pertussis*, *Brucella* species, *Neisseria gonorrhoeae**, *Neisseria meningitidis**, *Vibrio cholerae*, *Pasteurella multocida*.

Anaerobes: *Bacteroides* species* including *B. fragilis*.

* Some members of these species of bacteria produce β-lactamase, rendering them insensitive to amoxycillin alone.

Pharmacokinetic properties: The pharmacokinetics of the two components of Augmentin are closely matched. Peak serum levels of both occur about one hour after oral administration. Absorption of Augmentin is optimised at the start of a meal. Both clavulanate and amoxycillin have low levels of serum binding; about 70% remains free in the serum.

Doubling the dosage of Augmentin approximately doubles the serum levels achieved.

Preclinical safety data: Not relevant

Pharmaceutical particulars

List of excipients:

Augmentin 375 mg and 625 mg Tablets: Each tablet contains magnesium stearate, sodium starch glycollate, colloidal silica, microcrystalline cellulose, titanium dioxide (E171), hydroxypropyl methylcellulose, polyethylene glycol and silicone oil.

Augmentin Dispersible Tablets 375 mg: Each tablet contains polyvinylpyrrolidone (cross-linked), silicagel, saccharin sodium, pineapple, strawberry and blood orange dry flavours, magnesium stearate and microcrystalline cellulose.

Augmentin 250/62 and 125/31 SF Suspensions: The powder contains xanthan gum, hydroxypropyl methylcellulose, aspartame, silicon dioxide, colloidal silica, succinic acid, raspberry, orange and golden syrup dry flavours.

Incompatibilities: None

Shelf-life:

Augmentin 375 mg Tablets: Blister pack 36 months; glass bottles 48 months.

Augmentin 625 mg Tablets: Blister pack 24 months; glass bottles 36 months.

Augmentin Dispersible Tablets 375 mg : 24 months.

Augmentin 250/62 SF and 125/31 SF Suspension: Dry powder 18 months. Reconstituted suspensions: seven days

Special precautions for storage:

Augmentin 375 mg and 625 mg Tablets should be stored in a dry place at 25°C or below.

Augmentin Dispersible Tablets 375 mg should be stored in a dry place.

Augmentin 250/62 SF and 125/31 SF Suspensions: the dry powder should be stored in a dry place. Reconstituted suspensions should be kept in a refrigerator (but not frozen) for up to seven days.

Nature and contents of container:

Augmentin 375 mg Tablets: Blister packs of 21 in a carton; also amber glass bottles of 50 and 100.

Augmentin 625 mg Tablets: Blister packs of 21 in a carton; also amber glass bottles of 50.

Augmentin Dispersible Tablets 375 mg: Blister packs of 21 in a carton.

Augmentin 250/62 SF and 125/31 SF Suspensions: Clear glass bottles with aluminium screw caps containing powder for reconstitution to 100 ml.

Instructions for use/handling:

Augmentin 375 mg and 625 mg Tablets: None.

Augmentin Dispersible Tablets 375 mg: The dispersible tablets should be stirred with a little water before taking.

Augmentin 250/62 SF and 125/31 SF Suspensions: At time of dispensing, the dry powder should be reconstituted to form an oral suspension as detailed below:

Strength	*Volume of water to be added to reconstitute*	*Nominal bottle size*	*Final volume of reconstituted oral suspension*
125/31	*92 ml*	*150 ml*	*100 ml*
250/62	*90 ml*	*150 ml*	*100 ml*

Marketing authorisation numbers

Augmentin 375 mg Tablets	0038/0270
Augmentin 625 mg Tablets	0038/0362
Augmentin Dispersible Tablets 375 mg	0038/0272
Augmentin 250/62 SF Suspension	0038/0337
Augmentin 125/31 SF Suspension	0038/0298

Date of approval/revision of SPC November 1997

Legal category POM.

AUGMENTIN* INTRAVENOUS

Qualitative and quantitative composition Vials of sterile powder providing co-amoxiclav 500/100 (600 mg Augmentin) or co-amoxiclav 1000/200 (1.2 g Augmentin). For reconstitution as an intravenous injection or infusion.

The amoxycillin is present as amoxycillin sodium and the clavulanic acid is present as potassium clavulanate.

Pharmaceutical form Sterile powder for injection.

Clinical particulars

Therapeutic indications: Augmentin is an antibiotic agent with a notably broad spectrum of activity against the commonly occurring bacterial pathogens in general practice and hospital. The β-lactamase inhibitory action of clavulanate extends the spectrum of amoxycillin to embrace a wider range of organisms, including many resistant to other β–lactam antibiotics.

Augmentin Intravenous is indicated for short-term treatment of bacterial infections at the following sites when amoxycillin resistant beta-lactamase-producing strains are suspected as the cause. In other situations, amoxycillin alone should be considered.

Upper Respiratory Tract Infections (including ENT) in particular sinusitis, otitis media, recurrent tonsillitis. These infections are often caused by *Streptococcus pneumoniae*, *Haemophilus influenzae**, *Moraxella catarrhalis** and *Streptococcus pyogenes*.

Lower Respiratory Tract Infections in particular acute exacerbations of chronic bronchitis (especially if considered severe), bronchopneumonia. These infections are often caused by *Streptococcus pneumoniae*, *Haemophilus influenzae** and *Moraxella catarrhalis**.

Genito-urinary Tract and Abdominal Infections in particular cystitis (especially when recurrent or complicated–excluding prostatitis), septic abortion, pelvic or puerperal sepsis and intra-abdominal sepsis. These infections are often caused by *Enterobacteriaceae** (mainly *Escherichia coli**), *Staphylococcus saprophyticus*, *Enterococcus* species.*

Skin and Soft Tissue Infections in particular cellulitis, animal bites and severe dental abscess with spreading cellulitis. These infections are often caused by *Staphylococcus aureus**, *Streptococcus pyogenes* and *Bacteroides* species*.

Prophylaxis of wound infection associated with surgical procedures in particular gastrointestinal, pelvic, major head and neck surgery and after limb amputation for infection.

A comprehensive list of sensitive organisms is provided in *Pharmacological properties* section.

* Some members of these species of bacteria produce β-lactamase, rendering them insensitive to amoxycillin alone.

Mixed infections caused by amoxycillin-susceptible organisms in conjunction with Augmentin-susceptible β-lactamase-producing organisms may be treated with Augmentin. These infections should not require the addition of another antibiotic resistant to β-lactamases.

Posology and method of administration
Dosages for the treatment of infection:

Adults and children over 12 years: Usually 1.2 g eight hourly. In more serious infections, increase frequency to six-hourly intervals.

Children 3 months–12 years: Usually 30 mg/kg * Augmentin eight hourly. In more serious infections, increase frequency to six–hourly intervals.

Children 0–3 months: 30 mg/kg* Augmentin every 12 hours in premature infants and in full term infants during the perinatal period, increasing to eight hours thereafter.

* Each 30 mg Augmentin provides co-amoxiclav 25/5.

Adult dosage for surgical prophylaxis: The usual dose is 1.2 g Augmentin Intravenous given at the induction of anaesthesia. Operations where there is a high risk of infection, e.g. colorectal surgery, may require three, and up to four, doses of 1.2 g Augmentin Intravenous in a 24–hour period. These doses are usually given at 0, 8, 16 (and 24) hours. This regimen can be continued for several days if the procedure has a significantly increased risk of infection.

Clear clinical signs of infection at operation will require a normal course of intravenous or oral Augmentin therapy post-operatively.

Dosage in renal impairment
Adults

Mild impairment (creatinine clearance >30 ml/min)	Moderate impairment (creatinine clearance 10-30 ml/min)	Severe impairment (creatinine clearance <10 ml/min)
No change in dosage	1.2 g IV stat., followed by 600 mg IV 12 hourly	1.2 g IV stat., followed by 600 mg IV 24 hourly. Dialysis decreases serum concentrations of Augmentin and an additional 600 mg IV dose may need to be given during dialysis and at the end of dialysis

Children: Similar reductions in dosage should be made for children.

Dosage in hepatic impairment: Dose with caution; monitor hepatic function at regular intervals.

There are, as yet, insufficient data on which to base a dosage recommendation.

Each 1.2 g vial of Augmentin contains 1.0 mmol of potassium and 3.1 mmol of sodium (approx).

Administration: Augmentin Intravenous may be administered either by intravenous injection or by intermittent infusion (see *Instructions for use/handling*). It is not suitable for intramuscular administration.

Duration of therapy should be appropriate to the indication and should not exceed 14 days without review.

Contra-indications: Penicillin hypersensitivity. Attention should be paid to possible cross-sensitivity with other β-lactam antibiotics, e.g. cephalosporins.

A previous history of Augmentin- or penicillin-associated jaundice/hepatic dysfunction.

Special warnings and special precautions for use: Changes in liver function tests have been observed in some patients receiving Augmentin. The clinical significance of these changes is uncertain but Augmentin should be used with caution in patients with evidence of hepatic dysfunction.

Cholestatic jaundice, which may be severe, but is usually reversible, has been reported rarely. Signs and symptoms may not become apparent for several weeks after treatment has ceased.

Serious and occasionally fatal hypersensitivity (anaphylactoid) reactions have been reported in patients on penicillin therapy. These reactions are more likely to occur in individuals with a history of penicillin hypersensitivity (see *Contra-indications*).

Erythematous rashes have been associated with glandular fever in patients receiving amoxycillin.

Prolonged use may also occasionally result in overgrowth of non-susceptible organisms.

During the administration of high doses of Augmentin adequate fluid intake and urinary output should be maintained to minimise the possibility of crystalluria. When present at high concentrations in urine at room temperature, amoxycillin may precipitate in bladder catheters. A regular check on patency should be maintained.

Interaction with other medicaments and other forms of interaction: Prolongation of bleeding time and prothrombin time have been reported in some patients receiving Augmentin. Augmentin should be used with care in patients on anti-coagulation therapy. In common with other broad-spectrum antibiotics, Augmentin may reduce the efficacy of oral contraceptives and patients should be warned accordingly.

Concomitant use of allopurinol during treatment with amoxycillin can increase the likelihood of allergic skin reactions. There are no data on the concomitant use of Augmentin and allopurinol.

Pregnancy and lactation: Reproduction studies in animals (mice and rats) with orally and parenterally administered Augmentin have shown no teratogenic effects. There is limited experience of the use of Augmentin in human pregnancy. As with all medicines, use should be avoided in pregnancy, especially during the first trimester, unless considered essential by the physician.

Augmentin may be administered during the period of lactation. With the exception of the risk of sensitisation, associated with the excretion of trace quantities in breast milk, there are no known detrimental effects for the breast-fed infant.

Effects on ability to drive and use machines: None known.

Undesirable effects: Side effects are uncommon and mainly of a mild and transitory nature.

Gastrointestinal reactions: Diarrhoea, indigestion, nausea, vomiting, and mucocutaneous candidiasis have been reported. Antibiotic-associated colitis (including pseudomembranous colitis and haemorrhagic colitis) has been reported rarely. Nausea, although uncommon, is more often associated with higher oral dosages. If gastrointestinal side effects occur with oral therapy they may be reduced by taking Augmentin at the start of meals. Superficial tooth discolouration has been reported rarely, mostly with the suspension. It can usually be removed by brushing.

Genito-urinary effects: Vaginal itching, soreness and discharge may occur.

Hepatic effects: Moderate and asymptomatic rises in AST and/or ALT and alkaline phosphatases have been reported occasionally. Hepatitis and cholestatic jaundice have been reported rarely. These hepatic reactions have been reported more commonly with Augmentin than with other penicillins.

After Augmentin hepatic reactions have been reported more frequently in males and elderly patients, particularly those over 65 years. The risk increases with duration of treatment longer than 14 days. These reactions have been very rarely reported in children.

Signs and symptoms usually occur during or shortly after treatment but in some cases may not occur until several weeks after treatment has ended. Hepatic reactions are usually reversible but they may be severe and,very rarely, deaths have been reported.

Hypersensitivity reactions: Urticarial and erythematous rashes sometimes occur. Rarely erythema multiforme, Stevens-Johnson syndrome, toxic epidermal necrolysis, bullous exfoliative dermatitis, serum sickness-like syndrome and hypersensitivity vasculitis have been reported. Treatment should be discontinued if one of these disorders occurs. In common with other β-lactam antibiotics angioedema and anaphylaxis have been reported. Interstitial nephritis can occur rarely.

Haematological effects: As with other β-lactams transient leucopenia, thrombocytopenia and haemolytic anaemia have been reported rarely. Prolongation of bleeding time and prothrombin time has also been reported rarely (see *Interactions with other medicaments and other forms of interaction*).

CNS effects: CNS effects have been seen very rarely. These include reversible hyperactivity, dizziness, headache and convulsions. Convulsions may occur with impaired renal function or in those receiving high doses.

Local: Thrombophlebitis at the site of injection has been reported occasionally.

Overdose: Problems of overdosage with Augmentin are unlikely to occur; if encountered gastrointestinal symptoms and disturbance of the fluid and electrolyte balances may be evident. They may be treated symptomatically with attention to the water electrolyte balance. Augmentin may be removed from the circulation by haemodialysis.

Pharmacological properties
Pharmacodynamic properties: Resistance to many antibiotics is caused by bacterial enzymes which destroy the antibiotic before it can act on the pathogen. The clavulanate in Augmentin anticipates this defence mechanism by blocking the β-lactamase enzymes, thus rendering the organisms sensitive to amoxycillin's rapid bactericidal effect at concentrations readily attainable in the body.

Clavulanate by itself has little antibacterial activity; however, in association with amoxycillin as Augmentin, it produces an antibiotic agent of broad spectrum with wide application in hospital and general practice.

Augmentin is bactericidal to a wide range of organisms including:

Gram-positive:

Aerobes: *Enterococcus faecalis*, Enterococcus faecium*, Streptococcus pneumoniae, Streptococcus pyogenes, Streptococcus viridans, Staphylococcus aureus**, Coagulase negative staphylococci* (including *Staphylococcus epidermidis*), Corynebacterium* species, *Bacillus anthracis*, Listeria monocytogenes.*

Anaerobes: *Clostridium* species, *Peptococcus* species, *Peptostreptococcus.*

Gram-negative:

Aerobes: *Haemophilus influenzae*, Moraxella catarrhalis* (Branhamella catarrhalis), Escherichia coli*, Proteus mirabilis*, Proteus vulgaris*, Klebsiella* species*, *Salmonella* species*, *Shigella* species*, *Bordetella pertussis, Brucella* species, *Neisseria gonorrhoeae*, Neisseria meningitidis*, Vibrio cholerae, Pasteurella multocida.*

Anaerobes: *Bacteroides* species* including *B. fragilis.*

* Some members of these species of bacteria produce β-lactamase, rendering them insensitive to amoxycillin alone.

Pharmacokinetic properties: The pharmacokinetics of the two components of Augmentin are closely matched. Both clavulanate and amoxycillin have low levels of serum binding; about 70% remains free in the serum.

Doubling the dosage of Augmentin approximately doubles the serum levels achieved.

Preclinical safety data: Not relevant

Pharmaceutical particulars
List of excipients: None.

Incompatibilities: Augmentin Intravenous should not be mixed with blood products, other proteinaceous fluids such as protein hydrolysates or with intravenous lipid emulsions.

If Augmentin is prescribed concurrently with an aminoglycoside, the antibiotics should not be mixed in the syringe, intravenous fluid container or giving set because loss of activity of the aminoglycoside can occur under these conditions.

Shelf-life: Two years.

Special precautions for storage: Augmentin vials should be stored in a dry place below 25°C.

Nature and contents of container: Clear glass vials (PhEur type III) fitted with butyl rubber bungs and aluminium overseals.

Instructions for use/handling: 600 mg vial: To reconstitute dissolve in 10 ml Water for Injections BP. (Final volume 10.5 ml.)

1.2 g vial: To reconstitute dissolve in 20 ml Water for Injections BP. (Final volume 20.9 ml.)

Augmentin Intravenous should be given by slow intravenous injection over a period of three to four minutes and used within 20 minutes of reconstitution. It may be injected directly into a vein or via a drip tube.

Alternatively, Augmentin Intravenous may be infused in Water for Injections BP or Sodium Chloride Intravenous Injection BP (0.9% w/v). Add, without delay, 600 mg reconstituted solution to 50 ml infusion fluid or 1.2 g reconstituted solution to 100 ml infusion fluid (e.g. using a minibag or in-line burette). Infuse over 30-40 minutes and complete within four hours of reconstitution. For other appropriate infusion fluids, see Package Enclosure Leaflet.

Any residual antibiotic solutions should be discarded.

Augmentin Intravenous is less stable in infusions containing glucose, dextran or bicarbonate. Reconstituted solution should, therefore, not be added to such infusions but may be injected into the drip tubing over a period of three to four minutes.

Marketing authorisation number 0038/0320

Date of approval/revision of SPC February 1997

Legal category POM.

AUGMENTIN-DUO 400/57

Qualitative and quantitative composition Augmentin-Duo 400/57 contains 400 mg amoxycillin and 57 mg clavulanic acid per 5 ml (co-amoxiclav 400/57).

The amoxycillin is present as amoxycillin trihydrate and the clavulanic acid is present as potassium clavulanate.

Pharmaceutical form Dry powder for reconstitution in water, at time of dispensing, to form an oral sugar-free suspension.

Clinical particulars

Therapeutic indications: Augmentin-Duo 400/57 is an antibiotic agent with a notably broad spectrum of activity against the commonly occurring bacterial pathogens in general practice and hospital. The β-lactamase inhibitory action of clavulanate extends the spectrum of amoxycillin to embrace a wider range of organisms, including many resistant to other β-lactam antibiotics.

Augmentin-Duo 400/57, for twice-daily (b.i.d.) oral dosing, is indicated for short-term treatment of bacterial infections at the following sites when amoxycillin-resistant β-lactamase-producing strains are suspected as the cause. In other situations, amoxycillin alone should be considered.

Upper Respiratory Tract Infections (including ENT) in particular sinusitis, otitis media, recurrent tonsillitis. These infections are often caused by *Streptococcus pneumoniae, Haemophilus influenzae*, Moraxella catarrhalis** and *Streptococcus pyogenes.*

Lower Respiratory Tract Infections in particular acute exacerbations of chronic bronchitis (especially if considered severe), bronchopneumonia. These infections are often caused by *Streptococcus pneumoniae, Haemophilus influenzae** and *Moraxella catarrhalis**.

Urinary Tract Infections in particular cystitis (especially when recurrent or complicated – excluding prostatitis). These infections are often caused by *Enterobacteriaceae** (mainly *Escherichia coli**), *Staphylococcus saprophyticus, Enterococcus* species*.

Skin and Soft Tissue Infections in particular cellulitis, animal bites and severe dental abscess with spreading cellulitis. These infections are often caused by *Staphylococcus aureus**, *Streptococcus pyogenes* and *Bacteroides* species*.

A comprehensive list of sensitive organisms is provided in *Pharmacological properties* section.

* Some members of these species of bacteria produce β-lactamase, rendering them insensitive to amoxycillin alone.

Mixed infections caused by amoxycillin-susceptible organisms in conjunction with Augmentin-Duo 400/57-susceptible β-lactamase-producing organisms may be treated with Augmentin-Duo 400/57. These infections should not require the addition of another antibiotic resistant to β-lactamases.

Posology and method of administration: The usual recommended daily dosage is:

25/3.6 mg/kg/day in mild to moderate infections (upper respiratory tract infections e.g. recurrent tonsillitis, lower respiratory infections and skin and soft tissue infections).

45/6.4 mg/kg/day for the treatment of more serious infections (upper respiratory tract infections, e.g. otitis media and sinusitis, lower respiratory tract infections, e.g. bronchopneumonia and urinary tract infections).

The tables below give guidance for children.

Children over 2 years:

25/3.6 mg/kg/day	2–6 years (13–21 kg)	2.5 ml Augmentin-Duo 400/57 Suspension b.i.d.
	7–12 years (22–40 kg)	5.0 ml Augmentin-Duo 400/57 Suspension b.i.d.
45/6.4 mg/kg/day	2–6 years (13–21 kg)	5.0 ml Augmentin-Duo 400/57 Suspension b.i.d.
	7–12 years (22–40 kg)	10.0 ml Augmentin-Duo 400/57 Suspension b.i.d.

Children aged two months to two years: Children under two years should be dosed according to body weight.

Weight (kg)	*25/3.6 mg/kg/day (ml/b.i.d.*)*	*45/6.4 mg/kg/day (ml/b.i.d.*)*
2	0.3	0.6
3	0.5	0.8
4	0.6	1.1
5	0.8	1.4
6	0.9	1.7
7	1.1	2.0
8	1.3	2.3
9	1.4	2.5
10	1.6	2.8
11	1.7	3.1
12	1.9	3.4
13	2.0	3.7
14	2.2	3.9
15	2.3	4.2

* The 35 ml presentation is supplied with a syringe dosing device – See *Nature and contents of container* and *Instructions for use/handling* section.

There is insufficient experience with Augmentin-Duo to make dosage recommendations for children under two months old.

Infants with immature kidney function: For children with immature renal function Augmentin-Duo 400/57 is not recommended.

Renal impairment: For children with a GFR of >30 ml/min. no adjustment in dosage is required. For children with a GFR of <30 ml/min. Augmentin-Duo 400/57 is not recommended.

Hepatic impairment: Dose with caution; monitor hepatic function at regular intervals. There is, as yet, insufficient evidence on which to base a dosage recommendation.

Method of administration: To minimise potential gastrointestinal intolerance, administer at the start of a meal. The absorption of co-amoxiclav is optimised when taken at the start of a meal. Duration of therapy should be appropriate to the indication and should not exceed 14 days without review. Therapy can be started parenterally and continued with an oral preparation.

Contra-indications: Penicillin hypersensitivity. Attention should be paid to possible cross-sensitivity with other β-lactam antibiotics, e.g. cephalosporins. A previous history of co-amoxiclav- or penicillin-associated jaundice/hepatic dysfunction.

Special warnings and special precautions for use: Changes in liver function tests have been observed in some patients receiving co-amoxiclav. The clinical significance of these changes is uncertain but co-amoxiclav should be used with caution in patients with evidence of hepatic dysfunction.

Cholestatic jaundice, which may be severe, but is usually reversible, has been reported rarely. Signs and symptoms may not become apparent for several weeks after treatment has ceased.

In patients with moderate or severe renal impairment Augmentin-Duo 400/57 is not recommended.

Serious and occasionally fatal hypersensitivity (anaphylactoid) reactions have been reported in patients on penicillin therapy. These reactions are more likely to occur in individuals with a history of penicillin hypersensitivity (see *Contra-indications*).

Erythematous rashes have been associated with glandular fever in patients receiving amoxycillin.

Prolonged use may also occasionally result in overgrowth of non-susceptible organisms.

Augmentin-Duo 400/57 contains 12.5 mg aspartame per 5 ml dose and therefore care should be taken in phenylketonuria.

Interaction with other medicaments and other forms of interaction: Prolongation of bleeding time and prothrombin time have been reported in some patients receiving co-amoxiclav. Co-amoxiclav should be used with care in patients on anti-coagulation therapy. In common with other broad-spectrum antibiotics, co-amoxiclav may reduce the efficacy of oral contraceptives and patients should be warned accordingly.

Concomitant use of allopurinol during treatment with amoxycillin can increase the likelihood of allergic skin reactions. There are no data on the concomitant use of co-amoxiclav and allopurinol.

Pregnancy and lactation:

Use in pregnancy: Reproduction studies in animals (mice and rats) with orally and parenterally administered co-amoxiclav have shown no teratogenic effects. There is limited experience of the use of co-amoxiclav in human pregnancy. As with all medicines, use should be avoided in pregnancy, especially during the first trimester, unless considered essential by the physician.

Use in lactation: Co-amoxiclav may be administered during the period of lactation. With the exception of the risk of sensitisation, associated with the excretion of trace quantities in breast milk, there are no known detrimental effects for the breast-fed infant.

Effects on ability to drive and use machines: Adverse effects on the ability to drive or operate machinery have not been observed.

Undesirable effects: Side effects are uncommon and mainly of a mild and transitory nature.

Gastrointestinal reactions: Diarrhoea, indigestion, nausea, vomiting, and mucocutaneous candidiasis have been reported. Antibiotic-associated colitis (including pseudomembranous colitis and haemorrhagic colitis) has been reported rarely. Nausea, although uncommon, is more often associated with higher oral dosages. If gastrointestinal side effects occur with oral therapy they may be reduced by taking co-amoxiclav at the start of meals.

Superficial tooth discolouration has been reported rarely, mostly with the suspension. It can usually be removed by brushing.

Genito-urinary effects: Vaginal itching, soreness and discharge may occur.

Hepatic effects: Moderate and asymptomatic rises in AST and/or ALT and alkaline phosphatases have been reported occasionally. Hepatitis and cholestatic jaundice have been reported rarely. These hepatic reactions have been reported more commonly with co-amoxiclav than with other penicillins.

After co-amoxiclav hepatic reactions have been reported more frequently in males and elderly patients, particularly those over 65 years. The risk increases with duration of treatment longer than 14 days. These reactions have been very rarely reported in children.

Signs and symptoms usually occur during or shortly after treatment but in some cases may not occur until several weeks after treatment has ended. Hepatic reactions are usually reversible but they may be severe and,very rarely, deaths have been reported.

Hypersensitivity reactions: Urticarial and erythematous rashes sometimes occur. Rarely erythema multiforme, Stevens-Johnson syndrome, toxic epidermal necrolysis, bullous exfoliative dermatitis, serum sickness-like syndrome and hypersensitivity vasculitis have been reported. Treatment should be discontinued if one of these disorders occurs. In common with other β-lactam antibiotics angioedema and anaphylaxis have been reported. Interstitial nephritis can occur rarely.

Haematological effects: As with other β-lactams transient leucopenia, thrombocytopenia and haemolytic anaemia have been reported rarely. Prolongation of bleeding time and prothrombin time has also been reported rarely (see *Interaction with other medicaments and other forms of interaction*).

CNS effects: CNS effects have been seen very rarely. These include reversible hyperactivity, dizziness, headache and convulsions. Convulsions may occur with impaired renal function or in those receiving high doses.

Overdose: Problems of overdosage with co-amoxiclav are unlikely to occur. If encountered, gastrointestinal symptoms and disturbance of the fluid and electrolyte balances may be evident. They may be treated symptomatically, with attention to the water/electrolyte balance. Co-amoxiclav may be removed from the circulation by haemodialysis.

Drug abuse and dependence: Drug dependency, addiction and recreational abuse have not been reported as a problem with this compound.

Pharmacological properties Augmentin-Duo 400/57 contains a combination of amoxycillin and clavulanic acid, co-amoxiclav 400/57.

Pharmacodynamic properties:

Microbiology: Amoxycillin is a semi-synthetic antibiotic with a broad spectrum of antibacterial activity against many Gram-positive and Gram-negative micro-organisms. Amoxycillin is, however, susceptible to degradation by β-lactamases and therefore the spectrum of activity of amoxycillin alone does not include organisms which produce these enzymes.

Clavulanic acid is a β-lactam, structurally related to the penicillins, which possesses the ability to inactivate a wide range of β-lactamase enzymes commonly found in micro-organisms resistant to penicillins and cephalosporins. In particular, it has good activity against the clinically important plasmid mediated β-lactamases frequently responsible for transferred drug resistance. It is generally less effective against chromosomally-mediated type 1 β-lactamases.

The presence of clavulanic acid in Augmentin-Duo 400/57 protects amoxycillin from degradation by β-lactamase enzymes and effectively extends the antibacterial spectrum of amoxycillin to include many bacteria normally resistant to amoxycillin and other penicillins and cephalosporins. Thus Augmentin-Duo 400/57 possesses the distinctive properties of a broad spectrum antibiotic and a β-lactamase inhibitor. Augmentin-Duo 400/57 is bactericidal to a wide range of organisms including:

Gram-positive:

Aerobes: *Enterococcus faecalis*, Enterococcus faecium*, Streptococcus pneumoniae, Streptococcus pyogenes, Streptococcus viridans, Staphylococcus aureus**, Coagulase negative *staphylococci** (including *Staphylococcus epidermidis**), *Corynebacterium* species, *Bacillus anthracis**, *Listeria monocytogenes.*

Anaerobes: *Clostridium* species, *Peptococcus* species, *Peptostreptococcus.*

Gram-negative:

Aerobes: *Haemophilus influenzae*, Moraxella catarrhalis* (Branhamella catarrhalis), Escherichia coli*, Proteus mirabilis*, Proteus vulgaris*, Klebsiella* species*, *Salmonella* species*, *Shigella* species*, *Bordetella pertussis, Brucella* species, *Neisseria gonorrhoeae*, Neisseria meningitidis*, Vibrio cholerae, Pasteurella multocida.*

Anaerobes: *Bacteroides* species* including *B. fragilis.*

* Some members of these species of bacteria produce β-lactamase, rendering them insensitive to amoxycillin alone.

Pharmacokinetic properties

Absorption: The two components of Augmentin-Duo 400/57, amoxycillin and clavulanic acid, are each fully dissociated in aqueous solution at physiological pH. Both components are rapidly and well absorbed by the oral route of administration. Absorption of co-amoxiclav is optimised when taken at the start of a meal.

Pharmacokinetics: Pharmacokinetic studies have been performed in children, including one study [25000/382] which has compared co-amoxiclav t.i.d. and b.i.d. All of these data indicate that the elimination pharmacokinetics seen in adults also apply to children with mature kidney function.

The mean AUC values for amoxycillin are essentially the same following twice-a-day dosing with the 875/125 mg tablet or three-times-a-day dosing with the 500/125 mg tablet, in adults. No differences between the 875 mg b.i.d. and 500 mg t.i.d. dosing regimens are seen when comparing the amoxycillin $T_{1/2}$, or C_{max} after normalisation for the different doses of amoxycillin administered. Similarly, no differences are seen for the clavulanate $T_{1/2}$, C_{max} or AUC values after appropriate dose normalisation [Study 360].

The time of dosing of co-amoxiclav relative to the start of a meal has no marked effects on the pharmacokinetics of amoxycillin in adults. In a study of the 875/125 mg tablet [Study 362], the time of dosing relative to ingestion of a meal had a marked effect on the pharmacokinetics of clavulanate. For clavulanate AUC and C_{max}, the highest mean values and smallest inter-subject variabilities were achieved by administering co-amoxiclav at the start of a meal, compared to the fasting state or 30 or 150 minutes after the start of a meal.

The mean C_{max}, T_{max}, $T_{1/2}$ and AUC values for amoxycillin and clavulanic acid are given below for an 875 mg/125 mg dose of co-amoxiclav administered at the start of a meal [Study 362].

Mean pharmacokinetic parameters

Drug administration	*Augmentin Amoxycillin*	*1 g Clavulanic acid*
Dose (mg)	875 mg	125 mg
C_{max} (mg/l)	12.4	3.3
T_{max}* (hours)	1.5	1.3
AUC (mg.h/l)	29.9	6.88
$T_{1/2}$ (hours)	1.36	0.92

* Median values

Amoxycillin serum concentrations achieved with co-amoxiclav are similar to those produced by the oral administration of equivalent doses of amoxycillin alone.

Distribution: Following intravenous administration therapeutic concentrations of both amoxycillin and clavulanic acid may be detected in the tissues and interstitial fluid. Therapeutic concentrations of both drugs have been found in gall bladder, abdominal tissue, skin, fat, and muscle tissues; fluids found to have therapeutic levels include synovial and peritoneal fluids, bile and pus.

Neither amoxycillin nor clavulanic acid is highly protein bound, studies show that about 25% for clavulanic acid and 18% for amoxycillin of total plasma drug content is bound to protein. From animal studies there is no evidence to suggest that either component accumulates in any organ.

Amoxycillin, like most penicillins, can be detected in breast milk. There are no data available on the passage of clavulanic acid into breast milk.

Reproduction studies in animals have shown that both amoxycillin and clavulanic acid penetrate the placental barrier. However, no evidence of impaired fertility or harm to the foetus was detected.

Elimination: As with other penicillins, the major route of elimination for amoxycillin is via the kidney, whereas for clavulanate elimination is by both non-renal and renal mechanisms. Approximately 60-70% of the amoxycillin and approximately 40-65% of the clavulanic acid are excreted unchanged in urine during the first six hours after administration of a single 375 or 625 mg tablet.

Amoxycillin is also partly excreted in the urine as the inactive penicilloic acid in quantities equivalent to 10-25% of the initial dose. Clavulanic acid is extensively metabolised in man to 2,5-dihydro-4-(2-hydroxyethyl)-5-oxo-1H-pyrrole-3-carboxylic acid and 1-amino-4-hydroxy-butan-2-one and eliminated in urine and faeces and as carbon dioxide in expired air.

Preclinical safety data: No further information of relevance.

Pharmaceutical particulars

List of excipients: Xantham gum, aspartame, succinic acid, colloidal silica, hydroxypropyl methylcellulose, orange dry flavour (61071E), orange dry flavour (9/027108), raspberry dry flavour, golden syrup dry flavour, silicon dioxide.

Incompatibilities: None known.

Shelf-life:

Glass bottles: Dry powder: 18 months when stored at temperatures at or below 25°C.

Reconstituted suspensions: seven days when stored in a refrigerator (2-8°C).

Sachets: 18 months when stored at temperatures at or below 25°C.

Special precautions for storage: The dry powder should be stored in well-sealed containers in a dry place.

Nature and contents of container: Clear, glass bottles with aluminium screw caps, containing an off-white dry powder. The 35 ml presentation is supplied in a carton with a polystyrene syringe dosing device.

Single-dose sachets. Four sachets are supplied in a carton.

When reconstituted, an off-white suspension is formed.

Instructions for use/handling:

Glass bottles: At time of dispensing, the dry powder should be reconstituted to form an oral suspension, as detailed below:

Fill weight	*Volume of water to be added to reconstitute*	*Nominal bottle size*	*Final volume of reconstituted oral suspension*
6.3 g	31 ml	90 ml	35 ml
12.6 g	62 ml	150 ml	70 ml

The 35 ml presentation is provided with a syringe dosing device which should be used in place of the aluminium screw cap following reconstitution. This device is used to dose patients under two years according to the schedule in *Posology and method of administration.*

Sachets: Single-dose sachets contain powder for a 2.5 ml dose.

Directions for use: Check that the sachet is intact before use. Cut sachet along dotted line. Empty contents into a glass. Half-fill sachet with water. Pour into the glass, stir well and drink immediately. If two or four sachets have to be taken at once then they can be mixed in the same glass.

Marketing authorisation number 10592/0070

Date of approval/revision of SPC March 1997

Legal category POM.

BACTROBAN* NASAL OINTMENT

Qualitative and quantitative composition Mupirocin 2.0% w/w as mupirocin calcium.

Pharmaceutical form White soft paraffin ointment containing a glycerin ester.

Clinical particulars

Therapeutic indications: The elimination of nasal carriage of staphylococci, including methicillin-resistant *Staphylococcus aureus* (MRSA).

Posology and method of administration:

Dosage: Adults (including the elderly) and children: Bactroban Nasal Ointment should be applied to the anterior nares two to three times a day, as follows:

A small amount of the ointment about the size of a match-head is placed on the little finger and applied to the inside of each nostril. The nostrils are closed by pressing the sides of the nose together; this will spread the ointment throughout the nares. A cotton bud may be used instead of the little finger for the application in particular to infants or patients who are very ill.

Nasal carriage should normally clear within five to seven days of commencing treatment.

Administration: Topical.

Contra-indications: Hypersensitivity to any of the constituents of Bactroban Nasal Ointment.

Special warnings and special precautions for use: As with all topical preparations care should be taken to avoid the eyes.

Interaction with other medicaments and other forms of interaction: The product is not known to interact with other medicaments.

Pregnancy and lactation: Studies in experimental animals have shown mupirocin to be without teratogenic effects. However, there is inadequate evidence of safety to recommend the use of Bactroban Nasal Ointment during pregnancy.

Effects on ability to drive and use machines: None known.

Undesirable effects: During clinical studies some minor adverse effects were noted such as a transient stinging sensation localised to the area of application in about 2% of patients.

Overdose: The toxicity of mupirocin is very low. In the event of overdose symptomatic treatment should be given.

Pharmacological properties

Pharmacodynamic properties: Mupirocin is a novel antibiotic formulated for topical application only. Its spectrum of *in-vitro* antibacterial activity includes *Staphylococcus aureus* (including methycillin-resistant strains), *Staphylococcus epidermidis, Streptococcus* species and certain Gram-negative bacteria, particularly *Haemophilus influenzae* and *Escherichia coli.* Other Gram-negative bacteria are less susceptible and *Pseudomonas aeruginosa* is resistant.

Mupirocin is the major antibacterial compound of a group of structurally related metabolites produced by submerged fermentation of *Ps. Fluorescens.* Mupirocim has a novel mode of action, inhibiting bacterial iso-leucyl transfer-RNA synthetase and thus cross-resistance with other antibiotics is not experienced.

Pharmacokinetic properties: Studies have shown that following topical application of mupirocin there is very little systemic absorption of drug-related material. To mimic possible enhanced systemic penetration of mupirocin by application to damaged skin or a vascular site such as the mucous membrane, intravenous studies have been performed. Mupirocin was rapidly eliminated from the plasma by metabolism to monic acid, which in turn was excreted mainly in the urine.

Preclinical safety data: No further information of relevance.

Pharmaceutical particulars

List of excipients: White soft paraffin and Softisan 649.

Incompatibilities: None known.

Shelf-life: Bactroban Nasal Ointment has a shelf-life of three years.

Special precautions for storage: Store at room temperature (below 25°C).

Nature and contents of container: Lacquered aluminium tube fitted with a nozzle and screw cap containing 3 g ointment.

Instructions for use/handling: None stated.

Marketing authorisation holder: Beecham Group plc, SB House, Great West Road, Brentford, Middlesex TW8 9BD.

Trading as SmithKline Beecham Pharmaceuticals, Mundells, Welwyn Garden City, Hertfordshire AL7 1EY.

Marketing authorisation number PL 0038/0347

Date of first authorisation/renewal of authorisation 7.3.88/15.10.98

Date of (partial) revision of the text June 1997

Legal category POM.

BACTROBAN* OINTMENT

Qualitative and quantitative composition Mupirocin 2.0% w/w.

Pharmaceutical form Ointment in a white, translucent, water-soluble, polyethylene glycol base. For topical administration.

Clinical particulars

Therapeutic indications: Bactroban is a topical antibacterial agent, active against those organisms responsible for the majority of skin infections, e.g. *Staphylococcus aureus,* including methicillin-resistant strains, other staphylococci, streptococci. It is also active against Gram-negative organisms such as *Escherichia coli* and *Haemophilus influenzae.* Bactroban Ointment is used for skin infections, e.g. impetigo, folliculitis, furunculosis.

Posology and method of administration:

Dosage: Adults (including elderly) and children: Bactroban Ointment should be applied to the affected area up to three times a day for up to 10 days.

The area may be covered with a dressing or occluded if desired.

Administration: Topical.

Contra-indications: Hypersensitivity to Bactroban or other ointments containing polyethylene glycols.

This Bactroban Ointment formulation is not suitable for ophthalmic or intranasal use.

Special warnings and special precautions for use: When Bactroban Ointment is used on the face, care should be taken to avoid the eyes.

Polyethylene glycol can be absorbed from open wounds and damaged skin and is excreted by the kidneys. In common with other polyethylene glycol-based ointments, Bactroban Ointment should be used with caution if there is evidence of moderate or severe renal impairment.

Interaction with other medicaments and other forms of interaction: None stated.

Pregnancy and lactation: Studies in experimental animals have shown mupirocin to be without teratogenic effects. However, there is inadequate evidence of safety to recommend the use of Bactroban during pregnancy.

Effects on ability to drive and use machines: None stated.

Undesirable effects: During clinical studies some minor adverse effects, localised to the area of application, were seen such as burning, stinging and itching.

Overdose: The toxicity of mupirocin is very low. In the event of overdose, symptomatic treatment should be given.

Pharmacological properties

Pharmacodynamic properties: Bactroban (mupirocin) potently inhibits bacterial protein and RNA synthesis by inhibition of isoleucyl-transfer RNA synthetase.

Pharmacokinetic properties: After topical application of Bactroban Ointment, mupirocin is only very minimally absorbed systemically and that which is absorbed is rapidly metabolised to the antimicrobially inactive metabolite, monic acid. Penetration of mupirocin into the deeper epidermal and dermal layers of the skin is enhanced in traumatised skin and under occlusive dressings.

Preclinical safety data: None stated.

Pharmaceutical particulars

List of excipients: Polyethylene Glycol 400; Polyethylene Glycol 3350.

Incompatibilities: None stated.

Shelf-life: Bactroban Ointment has a shelf-life of two years.

Special precautions for storage: Store at room temperature (below 25°C).

Nature and contents of container: Original pack of 15 g (sealed tube in a carton) with Patient Information Leaflet.

Instructions for use/handling: No special instructions.

Marketing authorisation number 0038/0319

Date of approval/revision of SPC January 1998

Legal category POM.

DORALESE* TILTAB TABLETS

Qualitative and quantitative composition Indoramin hydrochloride equivalent to 20 mg of indoramin base.

Pharmaceutical form Coated tablets.

Clinical particulars

Therapeutic indications: Conditions for which alpha blockade is indicated.

Management of urinary outflow obstruction due to benign prostatic hyperplasia.

Posology and method of administration:

Hyperplasia: Adults: 20 mg twice daily.

Dosage may be increased in 20 mg increments at two-weekly intervals up to max. 100 mg per day if required.

Elderly: 20 mg at might may be adequate.

Children: Not recommended.

Route of administration: Oral.

Contra-indications: Patients with established heart failure.

Patients already under treatment with a monoamine oxidase inhibitor.

Do not use in patients in established cardiac failure or those under treatment with an MAO inhibitor.

Special warnings and special precautions for use: Incipient cardiac failure should be controlled before treatment with Doralese.

Caution should be observed in prescribing Doralese for patients with hepatic or renal insufficiency.

A few cases of extrapyramidal disorders have been reported in patients treated with Doralese. Caution should be observed in prescribing Doralese in patients with Parkinson's disease.

In animals and in the one reported case of overdose in humans, convulsions have occurred. Due consideration should be given and great caution exercised in the use of Doralese in patients with epilepsy.

Caution should be observed in prescribing Doralese for patients with a history of depression.

Clearance of Doralese may be affected in the elderly. A reduced dose, and/or reduced frequency of dosing may be sufficient in some elderly patients.

Interaction with other medicaments and other forms of interaction: Concomitant use of Doralese with thiazide diurectics, beta-blockers or other antihypertensive drugs may enhance their hypotensive action. Titration of dosage of the latter may therefore be needed.

Alcohol can increase both the rate and extent of absorption of Doralese, but no untoward effects have been reported at recommended doses.

Pregnancy and lactation: Animal experiments indicate no teratogenic effects but Doralese tablets should not be prescribed for pregnant women unless considered essential by the physician.

There are no data available on the excretion of Doralese in human milk but the drug should not be administered during lactation unless in the judgement of the physician such administration is clinically justifiable.

Effects on ability to drive and use machines: Drowsiness is sometimes seen in the initial stages of treatment with Doralese or when dosage is increased too rapidly. If drowsiness occurs, patients should be warned not to drive or operate machinery and to avoid CNS depressants including alcohol.

Undesirable effects: Drowsiness or sedation can occur on starting treatment with Doralese, and also if dosage is increased too rapidly. Less commonly, dry mouth, nasal congestion, weight gain, dizziness, failure of ejaculation and depression have also been noted.

Overdose: Information available at present of the effects of acute overdosage in human beings with Doralese is limited. Effects seen have included deep sedation leading to coma, hypotension and fits. Results of animal work suggest that hypothermia may also occur.

Suggested therapy is along the following lines:

1. Recent ingestion of large numbers of tablets would require gastric lavage or a dose of ipecacuanha to remove any of the product still in the stomach of the conscious patient.
2. Ventilation should be monitored and assisted if necessary.
3. Circulation support and control of hypotension should be maintained.
4. If convulsions occur diazepam may be tried.
5. Temperature should be closely monitored. If hypothermia occurs, rewarming should be carried out very slowly to avoid possible convulsions.

Pharmacological properties

Pharmacodynamic properties: Doralese is an alpha adrenoceptor blocking agent. It acts selectively and competitively on post-synaptic alpha-1 receptors, causing a decrease in peripheral resistance. It also produces relaxation of hyperplastic muscle in the prostate.

Pharmacokinetic properties: Doralese is rapidly absorbed from Doralese tablets and has a half-life of about five hours. There is little accumulation during long-term treatment. When three volunteers and four hypertensive patients were treated with radiolabelled Doralese at doses of 40-60 mg daily for up to three days, plasma concentrations reached a peak one to two hours after administration of single doses. Over 90% of plasma Doralese was protein bound. After two or three days 35% of the radioactivity was excreted in the urine and 46% in the faeces. Extensive first pass metabolism was suggested.

Clearance of Doralese may be affected in the elderly. A reduced dose or reduced frequency of dosing may be sufficient in some elderly patients.

Preclinical safety data: Not applicable.

Pharmaceutical particulars

List of excipients: Lactose, Microcrystalline Cellulose, Amberlite IRP, Magnesium Stearate.

Film-coating: Opadry OY-3736, Purified Water.

Incompatibilities: Not applicable.

Shelf-life: Three years.

Special precautions for storage: Store below 25°C.

Nature and contents of container: Blister packs of 60.

Instructions for use/handling: Not applicable.

Marketing authorisation holder: Smith Kline & French Laboratories Ltd, Mundells, Welwyn Garden City, Hertfordshire AL7 1EY.

Trading as SmithKline Beecham Pharmaceuticals, Mundells, Welwyn Garden City, Hertfordshire AL7 1EY.

Marketing authorisation number PL 0002/0168

Date of first authorisation 21st January 1988

Date of partial revision of the text September 1997

Legal category POM.

DYAZIDE* TABLETS

Qualitative and quantitative composition Each tablet contains 50 mg triamterene and 25 mg hydrochlorothiazide.

Pharmaceutical form Peach-coloured, half-scored, circular tablets bearing the mark SK&F E93.

Clinical particulars

Therapeutic indications: Dyazide is a potassium-conserving diuretic preparation with antihypertensive activity. It is recommended for the treatment of mild to moderate hypertension, alone or in combination with other antihypertensive drugs. It is also indicated in the control of oedema in cardiac failure, cirrhosis of the liver or the nephrotic syndrome and in that associated with corticosteroid treatment.

Posology and method of administration:

Adults only: In hypertension: Initially one tablet a day after the morning meal, thereafter adjusted to the patient's needs. If Dyazide is added to already established therapy with another antihypertensive drug, the dosage of the latter should be reduced, and later adjusted if necessary. If another antihypertensive drug is added to Dyazide therapy, the dosage of the latter will not normally be reduced.

Adults only: In oedema: The usual starting dosage is one Dyazide tablet twice a day after meals. The optimal dosage may be three tablets a day, two after breakfast and one after lunch. Maintenance dosage: Once a diuresis has been established, dosage should be reduced. Usually one tablet a day, or two tablets on alternate days, will suffice.

A dosage of four tablets a day should not be exceeded; at this level adverse reactions such as raised blood urea are more likely.

Elderly: Dosage as above. Dyazide has been widely used and is usually well tolerated in patients over the age of 60 years. The normally occurring reduction in glomerular filtration with age should be borne in mind.

Children: Only limited information is available on the use of Dyazide in children and, therefore, its use in children is not recommended.

Contra-indications: Do not give Dyazide to patients with hyperkalaemia, progressive renal failure, increasing hepatic dysfunction, hypercalcaemia, diabetic ketoacidosis, Addison's disease or known hypersensitivity to either constituent of the product. Potassium supplements, or other potassium-conserving drugs, including ACE inhibitors, should not be given routinely with Dyazide.

Special warnings and special precautions for use: Use Dyazide with caution in patients with hepatic or renal insufficiency, and in those predisposed to gout since both components can elevate uric acid levels. Use with caution with hypotensive agents since an additive effect may result. Since thiazide diuretics can provoke hyperglycaemia and glycosuria, diabetic patients should be treated with care, as should patients with diabetic nephropathy due to an increased risk of hyperkalaemia.

It is advisable to monitor blood urea, serum potassium levels and electrolytes periodically. This is important in the elderly, those with renal impairment and those receiving concomitant treatment with NSAIDs (see *Undesirable effects*).

Triamterene and thiazides reduce excretion of lithium and may thus precipitate intoxication.

Very rare cases of systemic lupus erythematosus (SLE) have been reported associated with Dyazide. Pancreatitis may be aggravated.

Combinations of folate antagonists and triamterene are not advisable in pregnancy or in patients with hepatic cirrhosis because of the increased theoretical risk of folate deficiency developing.

Triamterene may cause a blue fluorescence of the urine under certain light conditions.

Dyazide interfere with some laboratory tests of thyroid and parathyroid functions, and bioassay of folic acid.

Interaction with other medicaments and other forms of interaction: Increased responsiveness to tubocurarine. Use with caution with hypotensive agents. Also use with caution in conjunction with corticosteroids, since an additive effect may result in excess potassium loss, with cardiac glycosides and antiarrhythmic drugs whose toxicity potential is enhanced by hypokalaemia which may result from diuretic treatment, and with carbenoxolone which may antagonise the diurectic action of Dyazide. When used in conjunction with sulphonylureas, the dosage of the hypoglycaemic agent may require upward adjustment. Concomitant treatment with cholestyramine may delay or reduce the absorption of many drugs including diuretics.

It is advisable to monitor blood urea and serum potassium levels periodically in patients receiving concomitant treatment with NSAIDs. Renal failure, reversible on stopping treatment, has been reported very rarely which may be due to a reaction between triamterene and some NSAIDs. Triamterene and thiazides reduce excretion of lithium and may thus precipitate intoxication.

Pregnancy and lactation:

Use in pregnancy and lactation: Animal studies have not suggested foetal abnormalities. Nevertheless, both triamterene and thiazides have been shown to pass through the placenta in humans and also to pass into breast milk. In rare instances, thrombocytopenia, pancreatitis or hypoglycaemia have been reported in newborn infants of mothers treated with thiazides. Dyazide is best avoided in pregnancy unless used for a pre-existing illness and then only after assessing risk versus benifit. It should not be used in breast-feeding mothers.

Effects on ability to drive and use machines: There are no known effects of Dyazide on the ability to drive and operate machinery.

Undesirable effects: Nausea, vomiting, diarrhoea, muscle cramps, weakness, dizziness, headache, dry mouth, thirst, undesirable decreases in blood pressure and rash have been reported. Photosensitivity is rare. Anaphylaxis is a remote possibility.

Minor serum electrolyte changes have been observed infrequently, and marked fluctuations in serum potassium levels are uncommon. Long-term use has confirmed that little change occurs in serum potassium and sodium levels in most patients. Metabolic acidosis occasionally occurs. Electrolyte imbalance may also indicate excessive dosage or be secondary to the condition under treatment. Hyperglycaemia, increased uric acid levels which sometimes lead to gout, and hypercalcaemia that does not lead to tertiary hyperparathyroidism may also occur.

In common with most diuretics, Dyazide may reduce glomerular filtration rate and cause a temporary increase in blood urea and creatinine levels; again this may also indicate excessive dosage or be secondary to the condition under treatment. It can also cause increases in plasma lipid levels.

Renal failure, reversible on stopping treatment, has been reported very rarely and has been due to acute interstitial nephritis or an interaction between triamterene and some NSAIDs.

Triamterene has been found in renal stones both alone and in association with other usual calculus components. There is no evidence that stone formation is increased in patients taking triamterene-containing drugs.

Rare cases of thrombocytopenic purpura and megaloblastic anaemia have been reported with triamterene; thiazides alone have caused jaundice, acute pancreatitis and rarely blood dyscrasias including agranulocytosis, thrombocytopenia and leucopenia.

Overdose: Symptoms of electrolyte imbalance, especially hyperkalaemia, are likely. Symptoms include nausea, vomiting, weakness, lassitude, muscular weakness, hypotension and cardiac arrhythmias. Treatment consists of gastric lavage with careful monitoring of electrolytes and fluid balance. Cardiac rhythm should be monitored and appropriate measures taken to correct hyperkalaemia as necessary. There is no specific antidote. Renal dialysis may be of some benefit in cases of severe overdosage.

Pharmacological properties
Pharmacodynamic properties: The product contains triamterene and hydrochlorothiazide.

Triamterene is a potassium conserving diuretic thought to act by directly inhibiting the exchange of sodium for potassium and hydrogen in the distal renal tubule.

Hydrochorothiazide is a thiazide diuretic which reduces the reabsorption of electrolytes from the renal tubules, thereby increasing the excretion of sodium and chloride ions, and consequently of water. Potassium ions are excreted to a lesser extent.

Pharmacokinetic properties: Onset of diuresis takes place within one hour, peaks at two to three hours and tapers off during the subsequent seven to nine hours.

Triamterene is incompletely but fairly rapidly absorbed from the gastrointestinal tract. It has been estimated to have a plasma half-life of about two hours. It is extensively metabolised and is mainly excreted in the form of metabolities with some unchanged triamterene; variable amounts are also excreted in the bile.

Hydrochlorothiazide is incompletely but fairly rapidly absorbed from the gastro-intestinal tract. It is excreted unchanged in the urine.

Preclinical safety data: No further information of relevance.

Pharmaceutical particulars
List of excipients: Cores: Maize Starch, Vegetable mix (Sterotex HM), Povidone 30, Sodium Lauryl Sulphate, FD&C Yellow No.6 (E110), Purified Water, Coating: Maize Starch, Sodium Starch Glycollate, Magnesium Stearate.

Incompatibilities: Not applicable.

Shelf-life: Dyazide Tablets have a shelf-life of five years.

Special precautions for storage: There are no special storage requirements.

Nature and contents of container: Opaque blister packs containing 30 tablets. Securitainers containing 500 tablets.

Instructions for use/handling: None.

Marketing authorisation holder: Smith Kline and French Laboratories Ltd., Mundells, Welwyn Garden City, Hertfordshire AL7 1EY.
Trading as SmithKline Beecham Pharmaceuticals Mundells, Welwyn Garden City, Hertfordshire AL7 1EY.

Marketing authorisation number PL 0002/0050R

Date of first authorisation 10.4.74

Date of text September 1997

Legal category POM.

DYSPAMET* CHEWTAB TABLETS 200 mg
DYSPAMET* SUSPENSION

Qualitative and quantitative composition Dyspamet Chewtab Tablets contain 200 mg cimetidine per tablet.

Dyspamet Suspension, each 5 ml dose contains 200 mg cimetidine.

Pharmaceutical form White, square, chewable tablets with a surface design consisting of a raised portion towards one side of the tablet and a curved depression over the rest of the surface.

A white vanilla-flavoured suspension.

Clinical particulars
Therapeutic indications: Cimetidine is a histamine H_2-receptor antagonist which rapidly inhibits both basal and stimulated gastric secretion of acid and reduces pepsin output.

Dyspamet is indicated in the treatment of duodenal and benign gastric ulceration, recurrent and stomal ulceration, oesophageal reflux disease and other conditions where reduction of gastric acid by cimetidine has been shown to be beneficial: persistent dyspeptic symptoms with or without ulceration, particularly meal-related upper abdominal pain; the prophylaxis of gastrointestinal haemorrhage from stress ulceration in seriously ill patients; before general anaesthesia in patients thought to be at risk of acid aspiration (Mendelson's) syndrome, particularly obstetric patients during labour; to reduce malabsorption and fluid loss in the short bowel syndrome; and in pancreatic insufficiency to reduce degradation of enzyme supplements. Dyspamet is also recommended in the management of the Zollinger-Ellison syndrome.

Posology and method of administration: Oral: Dyspamet tablets should be chewed thoroughly before swallowing. The total daily dose should not normally exceed 2.4 g. Dosage should be reduced in patients with impaired renal function (see *Special warnings and special precautions for use*).

Adults: The usual dosage is 400 mg twice a day with breakfast and at bedtime. For patients with duodenal or benign gastric ulceration, a single daily dose of 800 mg at bedtime is recommended. Other effective regimens are 200 mg three times a day with meals and 400 mg at bedtime (1.0 g/day) and, if inadequate, 400 mg four times a day (1.6 g/day) also with meals and at bedtime.

Treatment should be given initially for at least four weeks (six weeks in benign gastric ulcer). Most ulcers will have healed by that stage, but those which have not will usually do so after a further course of treatment.

Treatment may be continued for longer periods in those patients who may benefit from reduction of gastric secretion and the dosage may be reduced as appropriate to 400 mg at bedtime or 400 mg in the morning and at bedtime

In patients with benign peptic ulcer disease, relapse may be prevented by continued treatment, usually with 400 mg at bedtime; 400 mg in the morning and at bedtime has also been used.

In oesophageal reflux disease, 400 mg four times a day, with meals and at bedtime, for four to eight weeks is recommended to heal oesophagitis and relieve associated symptoms.

In patients with very high gastric acid secretion (e.g. Zollinger-Ellison syndrome) it may be necessary to increase the dose to 400 mg four times a day, or in occasional cases further.

Since Dyspamet may not give immediate symptomatic relief, antacids can be made available to all patients until symptoms disappear.

In the prophylaxis of haemorrhage from stress ulceration in seriously ill patients, doses of 200-400 mg can be given every four to six hours.

In patients thought to be at risk of acid aspiration syndrome a dose of 400 mg can be given 90-120 minutes before induction of general anaesthesia or, in obstetric practice, at the start of labour. While such a risk persists, a dose of up to 400 mg may be repeated at four-hourly intervals as required up to the usual daily maximum of 2.4 g. The usual precautions to avoid acid aspiration should be taken.

In the short bowel syndrome, e.g. following substantial resection for Crohn's disease, the usual dosage range (see above) can be used according to individual response.

To reduce degradation of pancreatic enzyme supplements, 800-1600 mg a day may be given according to response in four divided doses, one to one and a half hours before meals.

Elderly: The normal adult dosage may be used unless renal function is markedly impaired (see *Special warnings and special precautions for use* and *Undesirable effects*).

Children: Experience in children is less than that in adults. In children more than one year old, cimetidine 25-30 mg/kg body weight per day in divided doses may be administered.

The use of cimetidine in infants under one year old is not fully evaluated; 20 mg/kg body weight per day in divided doses has been used.

Contra-indications: Hypersensitivity to cimetidine

Special warnings and special precautions for use: Dosage should be reduced in patients with impaired renal function according to creatinine clearance. The following dosages are suggested: creatinine clearance of 0 to 15 ml per minute, 200 mg twice a day; 15 to 30 ml per minute, 200 mg three times a day; 30 to 50 ml per minute, 200 mg four times a day; over 50 ml per minute, normal dosage. Cimetidine is removed by haemodialysis, but not to any significant extent by peritoneal dialysis.

Clinical trials with cimetidine of over six years' continuous treatment and more than 15 years' widespread use have not revealed unexpected adverse reactions related to long-term therapy. The safety of prolonged use is not, however, fully established and care should be taken to observe periodically patients given prolonged treatment.

Cimetidine treatment can mask the symptoms and allow transient healing of gastric cancer. This potential delay in diagnosis should particularly be borne in mind in patients of middle age and over with new or recently changed dyspeptic symptoms.

Interaction with other medicaments and other forms of interaction: Cimetidine can prolong the elimination of drugs metabolised by oxidation in the liver. Although pharmacological interactions with a number of drugs, e.g. diazepam, propranolol, have been demonstrated, only those with oral anticoagulants, phenytoin, theophylline and intravenous lignocaine appear, to date, to be of clinical significance. Close monitoring of patients on Dyspamet receiving oral anticoagulants or phenytoin is recommended and a reduction in the dosage of these drugs may be necessary.

In patients on drug treatment or with illnesses that could cause falls in blood cell count, the possibility that H_2-receptor antagonism could potentiate this effect should be borne in mind.

Pregnancy and lactation: Although tests in animals and clinical evidence have not revealed any hazards from the administration of cimetidine during pregnancy or lactation, both animal and human studies have shown that it does cross the placental barrier and is excreted in milk. As with most drugs, the use of Dyspamet should be avoided during pregnancy and lactation unless essential.

Effects on ability to drive and use machines: Not applicable.

Undesirable effects: Over 56 million patients have been treated with cimetidine worldwide and adverse reactions have been infrequent. Diarrhoea, dizziness or rash, usually mild and transient, and tiredness have been reported. Gynaecomastia has been reported and is almost always reversible on discontinuing treatment. Biochemical or biopsy evidence of reversible liver damage has been reported occasionally. Reversible confusional states have occurred, usually in the elderly or already very ill patients, e.g. those with renal failure. Thrombocytopenia and leucopenia, including agranulocytosis (see *Special warnings and special precautions for use*), reversible on withdrawal of treatment, have been reported rarely; pancytopenia and aplastic anaemia have been reported very rarely. There have been very rare reports of interstitial nephritis, acute pancreatitis, fever, headache, myalgia, arthralgia, sinus bradycardia, tachycardia and heart block, all reversible on withdrawal of treatment. In common with other H_2-receptor antagonists, there have been very rare reports of anaphylaxis. Alopecia has been reported but no causal relationship has been established. Reversible impotence has also been very rarely reported but no causal relationship has been established at usual therapeutic doses. Isolated increases of plasma creatinine have been of no clinical significance.

Overdose: Acute overdosage of up to 20 grams cimetidine has been reported several times with no significant ill effects. Induction of vomiting and/or gastric lavage may be employed together with symptomatic and supportive therapy.

Pharmacological properties
Pharmacodynamic properties: Cimetidine is a histamine H_2-receptor antagonist which rapidly inhibits

both basal and stimulated gastric secretion of acid and reduces pepsin output.

Pharmacokinetic properties: Cimetidine is well absorbed after oral administration, metabolised in the liver and excreted mainly through the kidney with a half-life of about two hours. The effects on acid secretion are of longer duration.

Preclinical safety data: Not applicable.

Pharmaceutical particulars
List of excipients:
Chewtab Tablets: Eudragit (E100), sorbitol(E420), lactose, croscarmellose sodium (type A), sodium saccharin, aspartame, magnesium stearate (E572), aniseed and butterscotch flavourings.

Suspension: Microcrystalline cellulose (E460), carboxymethylcellulose sodium (E466), propylene glycol, glycerol (E422), propyl paraben, butyl paraben, titanium dioxide (E171), sodium saccharin, sorbitol (E420), vanilla and cream flavourings.

Incompatibilities: Not applicable.

Shelf-life:
Chewtab Tablets Three years
Suspension Three years

Special precautions for storage: Store the tablets in a dry place.

Store the suspension at a temperature not exceeding 25°C.

Nature and contents of container: Chewtab Tablets, in opaque blister packs of 120 (20×6).

Suspension in white plastic bottles containing 600 ml.

Instructions for use/handling: Dilution of the suspension is not recommended.

Marketing authorisation holder: Smith Kline and French Laboratories Ltd, Mundells, Welwyn Garden City, Hertfordshire AL7 1EY.
Trading as SmithKline Beecham Pharmaceuticals Mundells, Welwyn Garden City, Hertfordshire AL7 1EY.

Marketing authorisation numbers
Chewtab Tablets PL 0002/0148
Suspension PL 0002/0161

Date of first authorisation/renewal of authorisation
Dyspamet Chewtab Tablets 13.7.87/25.7.97.
Dyspamet Suspension 15.9.87/12.1.98.

Date of (partial) revision of the text July 1997

Legal category POM.

ENGERIX B*
Hepatitis B Vaccine (rby)

Presentation Engerix B is a suspension of hepatitis B surface antigen produced by yeast cells using a recombinant DNA technique. It is available as a fine white suspension in the following presentations: adult prefilled syringes (1 ml); adult vials (1 ml); paediatric vials (0.5 ml). Each 1 ml contains 20 micrograms of protein, comprising at least 95% hepatitis B surface antigen, adsorbed on aluminium hydroxide adjuvant, together with thiomersal 1:20,000 as preservative.

Uses Active immunisation against infection caused by hepatitis B virus.

Preference should be given to those at increased risk of infection, primarily those likely to be exposed to blood, blood products or other body fluids.

Immunisation should be considered for the following risk groups:

Parenteral drug abusers.

Those with multiple sexual partners, particularly homosexual and bisexual men and prostitute men and women.

Close family contacts of a case or carrier.

Babies born to mothers who are chronic carriers of the hepatitis B virus or who have had acute hepatitis B during pregnancy.

Haemophiliacs, those receiving regular blood transfusions or blood products, or relatives responsible for the administration of such products.

Patients with chronic renal failure.

Healthcare personnel who have direct contact with blood or blood-stained body fluids or with patients' tissues. This includes doctors, surgeons, dentists, nurses, midwives, laboratory workers and mortuary technicians.

Trainee healthcare workers.

Staff and clients of residential accommodation for the mentally handicapped.

Prisoners.

Long-stay travellers and healthcare personnel going to areas of high prevalence.

Police, ambulance, rescue services and staff of custodial institutions may have certain individuals who are at risk.

In addition, there may be other groups at risk or specific circumstances when immunisation should be given.

It is not known whether responders will need booster doses or whether on exposure to virus natural boosting will occur when anti-HBs titres fall below the protective level of 10 mIU/ml. Until this is clearly known, it would seem wise to recommend a booster dose in those below this 10 mIU/ml level. However, immunity should persist for at least five years after the last dose of vaccine.

Dosage and administration Engerix B is for intramuscular use only, and must not be given intravenously or intradermally. Prior to vaccination, the vaccine should be well shaken and be visually inspected for any colour variations or particulate matter. Once shaken, the vaccine is slightly opaque.

Engerix B must *not* be mixed in the same syringe or injected at the same site as other vaccines.

The immunisation regimen consists of three doses of vaccine, the second dose at one month and the third at six months after the initial dose. Where more rapid immunisation is required, for example with travellers, the third dose may be given at two months after the initial dose, with a booster dose at 12 months. Specific humoral antibodies against the surface antigen of hepatitis B appear in almost 100% of those who have received three doses.

Adults and children over 12 years: 20 micrograms (1 ml) given intramuscularly.

Neonates and children 12 years and under: 10 micrograms (0.5 ml) given intramuscularly.

The vaccine should be administered in the deltoid region, though the antero-lateral thigh is the preferred site for infants. Engerix B should not be administered in the buttock since this may result in a lower immune response.

In patients with severe bleeding tendencies such as haemophiliacs, subcutaneous injection may be considered. In neonates born to HBsAg-positive mothers, hepatitis B immunoglobulin should be given simultaneously with the vaccine at different sites within a few hours of birth. For other subjects at particular risk, similar simultaneous administration may be considered.

Engerix B may be used as a booster in patients previously immunised with other hepatitis B vaccines.

Engerix B can be given concomitantly with BCG, DTP, DT and/or polio vaccine. Engerix B can also be given together with measles-mumps-rubella vaccines, *Haemophilus influenzae* b vaccine and hepatitis A vaccine.

Different injectable vaccines should always be administered at different injection sites.

Contra-indications, warnings, etc
Contra-indications: Hypersensitivity to any component of the vaccine. Severe febrile infections.

Precautions: In patients having renal dialysis, or those who are immunocompromised, response may be impaired and further vaccinations may be necessary.

Because of the prolonged incubation period of hepatitis B, infection may be present at the time of vaccination. If so, Engerix B may be ineffective.

As with all vaccinations, a solution of 1:1000 adrenaline should be available for injection should an anaphylactic reaction occur.

Use in pregnancy: No studies in pregnant animals have been done. Engerix B is not recommended in pregnancy unless there is a definite risk of hepatitis B.

Adverse reactions: These are usually mild. The most common reactions, occurring in up to half of vaccinees, are mild transient local soreness, erythema and induration at the injection site.

Local swelling at the injection site and angioedema have been reported rarely.

Less common systemic complaints, which have been reported include low-grade fever, malaise, fatigue, arthralgia, arthritis, myalgia, headache, dizziness, syncope, nausea, vomiting, diarrhoea, abdominal pain, lymphadenopathy, abnormal liver function tests, and rashes, rarely including urticaria. Thrombocytopenic purpura and severe skin disorders such as erythema multiforme have exceptionally occurred. Very rarely, transient arthralgia, pruritus and urticaria have been reported appearing one week or more after injection.

Neurological manifestations occurring in temporal association have been reported with the vaccine and very rarely include paraesthesia and extremely rarely include paralysis, neuropathy and neuritis (including Guillain-Barré syndrome, optic neuritis and multiple sclerosis). No causal relationship has been established.

Early onset allergic-type reactions have been reported rarely.

Pharmaceutical precautions Engerix B should be stored between 2°C and 8°C, its shelf-life then being three years, and must not be frozen. It should not be diluted. Protect from light.

Legal category POM.

Package quantities Adult prefilled syringes containing 1 ml suspension in packs of one and 10; adult vials containing 1 ml suspension in packs of one, three (OP) and 10; paediatric vials containing 0.5 ml suspension in packs of one.

Further information This Data Sheet supersedes the entry in the *ABPI Compendium of Data Sheets and SPCs* 1996-97.

Inactive ingredients are dried aluminium hydroxide, sodium chloride, sodium monohydrogen phosphate dihydrate, sodium dihydrogen phosphate dihydrate, water for injections, and also thiomersal (see *Presentation*).

Product licence number 10592/0015.

ERVEVAX*
Rubella vaccine, live PhEur (RA27/3 strain)

Presentation Ervevax rubella vaccine is a live attenuated vaccine prepared in human diploid cells. It is presented as a pink pellet in a glass vial; clear, colourless sterile diluent is provided in a separate container. Each 0.5 ml dose of the reconstituted vaccine contains not less than 1,000 $TCID_{50}$ of the RA27/3 live attenuated strain of rubella virus with not more than 25 micrograms (17 IU) neomycin sulphate.

Uses Routine immunisation of pre-pubertal girls against rubella. Also indicated in seronegative women of child-bearing age **who are not pregnant** and in whom the possibility of pregnancy can be excluded for at least one month following vaccination, including *post-partum* mothers, and for immunisation of children aged 12 months and over and adults to prevent transmission of rubella to the at-risk pregnant woman.

Dosage and administration
Adults and children aged 12 months and over: A single dose (0.5 ml) of the reconstituted vaccine administered by deep subcutaneous or intramuscular injection. Do not give intravenously.

The vaccine should be reconstituted using only the sterile Water for Injections supplied. The vaccine is quickly inactivated by alcohol and detergents and care is needed to avoid contact with these substances when sterilising skin before vaccination. Due to minor variations in pH, the colour of the reconstituted vaccine may vary from light orange to light red.

Contra-indications, warnings, etc
Contra-indications: **Never give to pregnant women, or to women of child-bearing age not fully aware of the need to avoid pregnancy for one month after the vaccination, since theoretically the vaccine virus could have an effect on the foetus.**

Acute febrile illness, whether active or expected following exposure to infection (other than rubella).

Ervevax should not be given to subjects with impaired immune responses. These include patients with primary or secondary immunodeficiencies. However, Ervevax can be given to asymptomatic HIV-infected patients without adverse consequences to their illness and may be considered for those who are symptomatic. Do not give to those with known systemic hypersensitivity to this vaccine or to neomycin. Although anaphylactic reactions are rare, facilities for management should always be available.

Precautions: Transmission of vaccine virus to susceptible contacts, whilst accepted as a theoretical possibility, has not been regarded as a significant risk.

Because of the possibility of interference from passive antibodies, the vaccine should not normally be given to subjects who have received blood or human plasma transfusions or human immunoglobulin within the previous three months. If the vaccine is given in these circumstances, serum antibodies should be checked at a later date.

At least three weeks should normally intervene between the administration of any two live vaccines. Ervevax can, however, be given simultaneously with live, oral poliomyelitis vaccine, and with measles and mumps vaccines. In this case the injectable vaccines should be given at different sites.

Adverse reactions: Mild rash, temperature elevation and slight enlargement of the posterior cervical glands, transient arthralgia and arthritis with or without joint effusion, and extremely rarely transient polyneuropathy or thrombocytopenic purpura could occur. Such effects are more common and tend to be more marked in adults than in children. Symptoms, when they do occur, usually begin one to three weeks following vaccination and are normally transient.

Overdosage: Not a problem.

Pharmaceutical precautions Protect from light. The vaccine should be stored between 2°C and 8°C, its shelf-life then being two years (lower temperatures will not harm the vaccine, but may damage the diluent container). At room temperature (20–25°C) the unreconstituted vaccine is stable for up to 10 weeks.

Reconstitution instructions The vaccine should be reconstituted using the sterile Water for Injections provided. For one dose of Ervevax, 0.6 ml of Water for Injections should be withdrawn from the ampoule using a syringe and delivered into the vaccine vial for reconstitution. The reconstituted vaccine should be used immediately, and certainly within one hour.

Legal category POM.

Package quantities Monodose* vials (OP), each with a separate ampoule of sterile diluent. The diluent is Water for Injections PhEur.

Further information Data indicate that satisfactory antibody titres have persisted for up to 20 years so far.

Because of possible interference from persisting maternal antibodies, there is little value in giving the vaccine to infants under one year of age.

Inactive ingredients are human albumin, lactose, sorbitol, dextran 10, amino acids for injection, and also neomycin sulphate (see *Presentation*).

Product licence number 10592/0016.

ESKAZOLE* TABLETS 400 mg

Qualitative and quantitative composition Albendazole 400 mg.

Pharmaceutical form Tablet.

Clinical particulars
Therapeutic indications: Eskazole is a benzimidazole carbamate anthelmintic for use in the treatment of hydatid cysts caused by:

Echinococcosis: Eskazole shows greatest efficacy in the treatment of liver, lung and peritoneal cysts. Experience with bone cysts and those in the heart and central nervous system is limited.

Cystic echinococcosis (caused by *Echinococcus granulosus*): Eskazole is used in patients with cystic echinococcosis:

1. Where surgical intervention is not feasible.
2. Prior to surgical intervention.
3. Post-operatively if pre-operative treatment was too short, if spillage has occurred or if viable material was found at surgery.
4. Following percutaneous drainage of cysts for diagnostic or therapeutic reasons.

Alveolar echinococcosis (caused by *Echinococcus multilocularis*): Eskazole is used in patients with alveolar echinococcosis:

1. In inoperable disease, particularly in cases of local or distant metastasis.
2. Following palliative surgery.
3. Following radical surgery or liver transplantation.

Posology and method of administration:
Route of administration: Oral.

Dosage: Dosages are dependent on the parasite involved, the weight of the patient, and the severity of the infection:

Cystic echinococcosis:
Patients weighing >60 kg: Total daily dose: 800 mg given in two divided doses of 400 mg for a total of 28 days.

Patients weighing <60 kg: Appropriate dosage adjustment is not possible with the 400 mg tablet presentation.

This 28-day treatment period may be repeated after a 14-day period without treatment for a total of three cycles.

Alveolar echinococcosis:
Patients weighing >60 kg: Total daily dose: 800 mg given in two equally divided doses for cycles of 28 days with 14 days between cycles.

Patients weighing <60 kg: Appropriate dosage adjustment is not possible with the 400 mg tablet presentation.

Treatment may need to be prolonged for months or years. Continuous treatment at the same dose has been used for periods of up to 20 months.

Method of administration: Eskazole should be taken with meals.

Cystic echinococcosis:

1. Inoperable and multiple cysts: Up to three 28-day cycles of Eskazole may be given for the treatment of liver, lung and peritoneal cysts. More prolonged treatment may be required for sites such as bone and brain.
2. Pre-operative: Two 28-day cycles should be given where possible prior to surgery. Where surgical intervention is necessary before completion of two cycles, albendazole should be given for as long as possible.
3. Post-operative: Where only a short pre-operative course has been given (less than 14 days) and in cases where emergency surgery is required, Eskazole should be given post-operatively for two 28-day cycles separated by 14 drug-free days.

Additionally, where cysts are found to be viable following pre-surgical treatment or where spillage has occurred, a full two-cycle course should be given.

4. After percutaneous cyst drainage: Treatment as for post-surgery above.

Alveolar echinococcosis: Treatment is normally given in 28-day cycles as for cystic echinococcosis. It may have to be continued for months or even years. Current follow-up suggests that survival times are substantially improved following prolonged treatment. Continuous treatment has been shown in a limited number of patients to lead to apparent cure.

Children: There has been limited experience to date with the use of Eskazole in children under six years of age; therefore, usage in children less than six years is not recommended. In older children under 60 kg body weight, although there is clinical experience, appropriate dosage adjustment is not possible with the 400 mg tablet presentation.

Contra-indications: Albendazole should not be administered during pregnancy or in women thought to be pregnant. Women of childbearing age should be advised to take effective precautions, with non-hormonal contraceptive measures, against conception during and within one month of completion of treatment with Eskazole.

Albendazole is contra-indicated in patients with a known history of hypersensitivity to Eskazole (albendazole or constituents).

Special warnings and precautions for use: Eskazole has been associated with mild to moderate elevations of hepatic enzymes in approximately 16% of patients. These have normalised on discontinuation of treatment.

Liver function tests should be obtained before the start of each treatment cycle and at least every two weeks during treatment. If enzymes are significantly increased (greater than twice the upper limit of normal), Eskazole should be discontinued.

Eskazole may be reinstituted when liver enzymes have returned to normal limits, but laboratory tests should be more frequently obtained during repeat therapy.

Eskazole has been shown to cause occasional reversible modest reductions in total white cell counts.

Blood counts should be performed at the start and every two weeks during each 28-day cycle. Eskazole may be continued if the decrease appears modest and does not progress.

Precautions: In order to avoid administering albendazole during early pregnancy, women of childbearing age should initiate treatment only after a negative pregnancy test. These tests should be repeated at least once before initiating the next cycle.

Interactions with other medicaments and other forms of interactions: Albendazole has been shown to induce liver enzymes of the cytochrome P450 system responsible for its own metabolism. There is therefore a theoretical risk of interaction with theophylline, anticonvulsants, anticoagulants, oral contraceptives and oral hypoglycaemics. Care should therefore be exercised during the introduction of albendazole in patients receiving the above groups of compounds.

Cimetidine and praziquantel have been reported to increase the plasma levels of the albendazole active metabolite.

Pregnancy and lactation:
Pregnancy: Eskazole should not be administered during pregnancy or in women thought to be pregnant (see *Contra-indications*).

Lactation: It is not known whether albendazole or its metabolites are secreted in human breast milk. Thus Eskazole should not be used during lactation unless the potential benefits are considered to outweigh the potential risks associated with treatment.

Effects on ability to drive and use machines: Adverse effects on the ability to drive or operate machinery have not been observed.

Undesirable effects: As with other benzimidazoles, mild to moderate elevations of hepatic enzymes (around 16% of patients in clinical trials) have occurred during treatment with Eskazole.

Gastrointestinal disturbances (abdominal pain, nausea, vomiting) and leucopenia have been associated commonly (>1%) with Eskazole when treating patients with echinococcosis.

Dizziness and headache have been reported commonly.

As with other benzimidazoles, reversible alopecia (thinning of hair, and moderate hair loss) and fever have been associated commonly (>1%) with Eskazole. Pancytopenia has been reported very rarely (<0.01%).

Hypersensitivity reactions including rash, pruritus and urticaria have been reported very rarely.

Overdose: In case of overdosage, symptomatic therapy (gastric lavage) and general supportive measures should be undertaken.

Pharmacological properties
Pharmacodynamic properties: Albendazole is a benzimidazole carbamate with anthelmintic effects against tissue parasites.

Albendazole exhibits larvicidal, ovicidal and vermicidal activity, and it is thought to exert its anthelmintic effect by inhibiting tubulin polymerisation. This causes the disruption of the helminth metabolism, including energy depletion, which immobilises and then kills the susceptible helminth.

Albendazole is effective in the treatment of tissue parasites including cystic echinococcosis and alveolar echinococcosis caused by infestation of *Echinococcus granulosus* and *Echinococcus multilocularis*, respectively.

In the treatment of cysts due to *E. multilocularis*, a minority of patients were considered to be cured and a majority had an improvement or stabilisation of disease due to albendazole.

Pharmacokinetic properties:
Absorption and metabolism: In man, albendazole is poorly absorbed (<5%) following oral administration.

Albendazole rapidly undergoes extensive first-pass metabolism in the liver, and is generally not detected in plasma. Albendazole sulfoxide is the primary metabolite, which is thought to be the active moiety in effectiveness against systemic tissue infections. The plasma half-life of albendazole sulfoxide is 8½ hours.

Following oral administration of a single dose of 400 mg albendazole, the pharmacologically active metabolite, albendazole sulfoxide, has been reported to achieve plasma concentrations from 1.6 to 6.0 micromol/litre when taken with breakfast. The systemic pharmacological effect of albendazole is augmented if the dose is administered with a fatty meal, which enhances the absorption by approximately five-fold.

Excretion: Albendazole sulfoxide and its metabolites appear to be principally eliminated in bile, with only a small proportion appearing in the urine. Elimination from cysts has been shown to occur over several weeks following high and prolonged dosing.

Preclinical safety data: There are no preclinical data of relevance to the prescriber which are additional to that already included in other sections of the SPC.

Pharmaceutical particulars
List of excipients: Lactose; maize starch; sunset yellow lake; sodium lauryl sulphate; polyvinylpyrrolidone; microcrystalline cellulose; sodium saccharin; sodium starch glycollate; vanilla flavour; orange flavour; passion fruit flavour; magnesium stearate; hydroxypropylmethylcellulose; propylene glycol; purified water.

Incompatibilities: None.

Shelf-life: 36 months.

Special precautions for storage: No special storage precautions.

Nature and contents of container: Polypropylene 'securitainer' with polyethylene lid, each pack containing 60 tablets

Instruction for use/handling: No special instructions.

Marketing authorisation number 0002/0202

Date of approval/revision of SPC August 1997

Legal category POM.

FAMVIR* TABLETS

Qualitative and quantitative composition Famciclovir 125, 250, 500, 750 mg.

Pharmaceutical form White, round, film-coated Tiltab tablets containing 125 or 250 mg famciclovir for oral administration. White, oval, film-coated Tiltab tablets containing 500 or 750 mg famciclovir for oral administration.

Clinical particulars
Therapeutic indications: Treatment of herpes zoster (shingles) infections, acute genital herpes infections and suppression of recurrent genital herpes infections in immunocompetent and immunocompromised patients.

Posology and method of administration:
Dosage: Adults:

Herpes zoster infections: One 750 mg tablet once daily for seven days or alternatively three 250 mg tablets once daily for seven days or alternatively one 250 mg tablet three times daily for seven days. If the tablets are taken once a day they should be taken at approximately the same time each day.

In immunocompromised patients, one 500 mg tablet three times daily for 10 days. Treatment should be initiated as early as possible in the course of the disease, promptly after diagnosis.

First-episode genital herpes infections: One 250 mg tablet three times daily for five days.

In immunocompromised patients, one 500 mg tablet twice daily for seven days. Initiation of treatment is recommended as soon as possible after onset of lesions.

Recurrent genital herpes infections: Acute treatment: One 125 mg tablet twice daily for five days. In immunocompromised patients, one 500 mg tablet twice daily for seven days. Initiation of treatment is recommended during the prodromal period or as soon as possible after onset of lesions.

Suppression: One 250 mg tablet twice daily. A dose of 500 mg twice daily has been shown to be efficacious in HIV patients. Therapy should be interrupted periodically at intervals of six to 12 months in order to observe possible changes in the natural history of the disease.

Elderly: Dosage modification is not required unless renal function is impaired.

Renally impaired: As penciclovir is excreted primarily by the kidney, special attention should be given to dosage in patients with impaired renal function (see *Overdose*). The following modifications are recommended:

Immunocompetent patients: For the treatment of herpes zoster and first-episode genital herpes infections:

Creatinine clearance (ml/min/1.73 m²)	*Dosage*
30–59	250 mg twice daily
10–29	250 mg once daily

For the treatment of acute recurrent genital herpes infections:

Creatinine clearance (ml/min/1.73 m²)	*Dosage*
30–59	No dose adjustment necessary
10–29	125 mg once daily

For the suppression of recurrent genital herpes infections:

Creatinine clearance (ml/min/1.73 m²)	*Dosage*
≥ 30	250 mg twice daily
10–29	125 mg twice daily

Immunocompromised patients: For the treatment of herpes zoster infections in immunocompromised patients:

Creatinine clearance (ml/min/1.73 m²)	*Dosage*
≥ 40	500 mg three times daily
30–39	250 mg three times daily
10–29	125 mg three times daily

For the treatment of herpes simplex infections in immunocompromised patients:

Creatinine clearance (ml/min/1.73 m²)	*Dosage*
≥ 40	500 mg twice daily
30–39	250 mg twice daily
10–29	125 mg twice daily

When only serum creatinine is available, a nomogram or the following formula (Cockcroft and Gault) should be used to estimate creatinine clearance.

Formula to estimate creatinine clearance (ml/min/1.73 m²):

$$\frac{[140\text{–age in years}] \times \text{weight (kg)}}{72 \times \text{serum creatinine } (\mu\text{mol/l})}$$

× **either** 88.5 (for males)
or 75.2 (for females)

Renally impaired patients on haemodialysis: Since four hours' haemodialysis results in approximately 75% reduction in plasma concentrations of penciclovir, a dose of famciclovir (250 mg for herpes zoster patients and 125 mg for herpes simplex patients) should be administered immediately following dialysis.

Hepatically impaired: Dosage modification is not required for patients with well compensated chronic liver disease. There is no information on patients with overtly decompensated chronic liver disease; accordingly no precise dose recommendations can be made for this group of patients.

Children: The efficacy and safety of famciclovir has not been investigated in children. Famciclovir should therefore not be used in children unless the potential benefits are considered to justify the potential risks associated with treatment.

Administration: Oral.

For some patients IV penciclovir may be more appropriate than famciclovir (Famvir), the oral prodrug of penciclovir. While the decision on the best patient management and mode of administration should rest with the physician, in severely ill patients initiation of therapy with IV penciclovir should be considered.

Contra-indications: Famvir is contra-indicated in patients with known hypersensitivity to famciclovir or other constituents of Famvir. It is also contra-indicated in those patients who have shown hypersensitivity to penciclovir (Lumavir).

Special warnings and special precautions for use: Special attention should be paid to patients with impaired renal function and dosage adjustment may be necessary (see *Posology and method of administration* and *Overdose*). No special precautions are required for patients with well compensated chronic liver disease or the elderly unless renal function is impaired.

Genital herpes is a sexually transmitted disease; the risk of transmission is increased during acute episodes. Patients should avoid sexual intercourse when symptoms are present even if treatment with an antiviral has been initiated.

During suppressive treatment with famciclovir, the frequency of viral shedding (both symptomatic and asymptomatic) may be reduced. However, the risk of viral transmission remains even during suppressive antiviral therapy and with protected intercourse, i.e. the use of condoms.

Interaction with other medicaments and other forms of interaction: Evidence from preclinical studies has shown no potential for induction of cytochrome P450. Probenecid and other drugs that affect renal physiology could affect plasma levels of penciclovir. In a Phase I study, no drug interactions were observed after co-administration of zidovudine and famciclovir. Oral co-administration of famciclovir (150 mg/kg/day) and 5-fluorouracil (18 mg/kg/day) to rats for seven days at doses five- and three-fold higher, respectively, than those used clinically resulted in reduced systemic exposure to penciclovir and 5-fluorouracil. However, there is no evidence that this finding has any clinical significance.

Pregnancy and lactation: Animal studies have not shown any embryotoxic or teratogenic effects with famciclovir or penciclovir. In a placental transfer study in pregnant rats, foetal tissue was exposed to drug-related material (9.2 mcg penciclovir equivalents/g tissue) following intravenous administration of penciclovir at a high dose (80 mg/kg), which was without embryotoxic/teratogenic effects. Famvir should, therefore, not be used during pregnancy or in nursing mothers unless the potential benefits of treatment outweigh any possible risk.

Studies in rats show that penciclovir is excreted in the breast milk of lactating females given oral famciclovir. There is no information on excretion in human milk.

Effects on ability to drive and use machines: There is no evidence that Famvir will affect the ability of a patient to drive or to use machines.

Undesirable effects: Famciclovir has been well tolerated in human studies. Headache and nausea have been reported in clinical trials. These were generally mild or moderate in nature and occurred at a similar incidence in patients receiving placebo treatment.

In post-marketing experience, in addition to the above, vomiting, dizziness and skin rash, and confusion which was predominantly in the elderly, have been reported rarely. Hallucinations have been reported very rarely.

Famciclovir has also been well tolerated in immunocompromised patients. Undesirable effects reported from clinical studies were similar to those reported in the immunocompetent population. Cases of abdominal pain, fever and rarely granulocytopenia and thrombocytopenia have been observed (granulocytopenia and thrombocytopenia have also been observed in immunocompromised patients not treated with famciclovir).

Overdose: Overdose experience with famciclovir is limited. A report of accidental acute overdosage (10.5 g) was asymptomatic. In a report of chronic use (10 g/day for two years), famciclovir was well tolerated. In the event of an overdose supportive and symptomatic therapy should be given as appropriate.

Acute renal failure has been reported rarely in patients with underlying renal disease where the Famvir dosage has not been appropriately reduced for the level of renal function.

Penciclovir is dialysable and plasma concentrations are reduced by approximately 75% following four hours' haemodialysis.

Pharmacological properties

Pharmacodynamic properties: Famciclovir is the oral form of penciclovir. Famciclovir is rapidly converted *in vivo* into penciclovir, which has *in vivo* and *in vitro* activity against human herpes viruses including *Varicella zoster* virus and *herpes simplex* type 1 and 2.

The antiviral effect of orally administered famciclovir has been demonstrated in several animal models; this effect is due to *in vivo* conversion to penciclovir. In virus-infected cells penciclovir is rapidly and efficiently converted into the triphosphate (mediated via virus-induced thymidine kinase). Penciclovir triphosphate persists in infected cells for more than 12 hours where it inhibits replication of viral DNA and has a half-life of nine, 10 and 20 hours in cells infected with *Varicella zoster, herpes simplex* virus type 1 and *herpes simplex* virus type 2, respectively. In uninfected cells treated with penciclovir, concentrations of penciclovir-triphosphate are only barely detectable. Accordingly, uninfected cells are unlikely to be affected by therapeutic concentrations of penciclovir.

The most common form of resistance encountered with aciclovir among HSV strains is a deficiency in the production of the thymidine kinase (TK) enzyme. Such TK-deficient strains would be expected to be cross-resistant to both penciclovir and aciclovir. However, penciclovir has been shown to be active *in vitro* against a recently isolated aciclovir-resistant *herpes simplex* virus strain which has an altered DNA polymerase.

Results from penciclovir and famciclovir patient studies, including studies of up to four months' treatment with famciclovir, have shown a small overall frequency of penciclovir-resistant isolates: 0.3% in the 981 total isolates tested to date and 0.19% in the 529 virus isolates from immunocompromised patients. The resistant isolates were found at the start of treatment or in a placebo group, with no resistance occurring on or after treatment with famciclovir or penciclovir.

A placebo-controlled study in patients with immunodeficiency due to HIV has shown that famciclovir 500 mg b.i.d. significantly decreased the proportion of days of both symptomatic and asymptomatic HSV shedding.

Pharmacokinetic properties:

General characteristics: Following oral administration, famciclovir is rapidly and extensively absorbed and rapidly converted to the active compound, penciclovir. Bioavailability of penciclovir after oral Famvir is 77%. Mean peak plasma concentrations of penciclovir, following 125, 250 and 500 mg oral doses of famciclovir, were 0.8, 1.6 and 3.3 micrograms/ml, respectively, and occurred at a median time of 45 minutes post-dose. Mean peak plasma concentration of penciclovir, following a 750 mg oral dose of famciclovir, was 4.9 micrograms/ml and occurred at a median time of 50 minutes post-dose. Plasma concentration-time curves of penciclovir are similar following single and repeat (t.i.d. and b.i.d.) dosing. The terminal plasma half-life of penciclovir after both single and repeat dosing with famciclovir is approximately 2.0 hours. There is no accumulation of penciclovir on repeated dosing with famciclovir. Penciclovir and its 6-deoxy precursor are poorly (<20%) bound to plasma proteins.

Famciclovir is eliminated principally as penciclovir and its 6-deoxy precursor which are excreted in urine unchanged. Famciclovir has not been detected in urine. Tubular secretion contributes to the renal elimination of the compound.

Characteristics in patients: Uncomplicated herpes zoster infection does not significantly alter the pharmacokinetics of penciclovir measured after oral administration of Famvir.

Preclinical safety data: Famciclovir has no significant effects on spermatogenesis or sperm morphology and motility in man. At doses greatly in excess of those used therapeutically, impaired fertility was observed in male rats–no such effects being observed in female rats.

At a dose level approximately 50 times the normal therapeutic dose there was an increased incidence of mammary adenocarcinoma in female rats. No such effect was seen in male rats or mice of either sex.

Additionally, famciclovir was found not to be genotoxic in a comprehensive battery of *in vivo* and *in vitro* tests designed to detect gene mutation, chromosomal damage and repairable damage to DNA. Penciclovir, in common with other drugs of this class, has been shown to cause chromosomal damage, but did not induce gene mutation in bacterial or mammalian cell systems, nor was there evidence of increased DNA repair *in vitro*.

These findings are not considered to have any clinical significance.

Pharmaceutical particulars

List of excipients: Hydroxypropyl Cellulose EP, Lactose Anhydrous* NF, Sodium Starch Glycollate BP, Magnesium Stearate EP, Hydroxypropyl Methyl Cellulose EP, Titanium Dioxide EP, Polyethylene Glycol NF.

* Constituent of Famvir 125 and 250 mg tablets only

Incompatibilities: No specific incompatibilities.

Shelf-life: Three years

Special precautions for storage: Famvir 125 and 250 mg tablets–store in a dry place.

Famvir 500 and 750 mg tablets–store at or below 30°C in a dry place.

Nature and contents of container:

Herpes zoster treatment: Famvir is supplied as a shingles patient pack in original blister packs (PVC/PVdC with 20 micron aluminium lidding foil) containing seven x 750 mg tablets or 21×250 mg tablets and as a starter pack of one x 750 mg tablet. For immunocompromised patients Famvir is supplied in blister packs (PVC/PVdC with 20 micron aluminium lidding foil) containing 30×500 mg tablets. Each pack contains a Patient Information Leaflet.

Genital herpes treatment: Famvir is supplied in original blister packs (PVC/PVdC with 20 micron aluminium lidding foil) containing 15 x 250 mg tablets for the treatment of first-episode infection, 10×125 mg tablets for the treatment of acute recurrent infections or 56×250 mg tablets for suppressive treatment. For immunocompromised patients Famvir is supplied in blister packs (PVC/PVdC with 20 micron aluminium lidding foil) containing 14×500 mg tablets for treatment of acute infections or 56×500 mg for suppressive treatment. Each pack contains a Patient Information Leaflet.

Instructions for use/handling: No special instructions

Marketing authorisation holder: SmithKline Beecham plc, SB House, Great West Road, Brentford, Middlesex TW8 9BD.

Trading as SmithKline Beecham Pharmaceuticals Mundells, Welwyn Garden City, Hertfordshire AL7 1EY.

Marketing authorisation numbers

Famvir 125 mg Tablets	PL 10592/0055
Famvir 250 mg Tablets	PL 10592/0035
Famvir 500 mg Tablets	PL 10592/0112
Famvir 750 mg Tablets	PL 10592/0084

Date of first authorisation/renewal of authorisation December 1993

Date of (partial) revision of the text March 1998

Legal Category POM.

FLOXAPEN* SYRUPS FLOXAPEN* CAPSULES

Qualitative and quantitative composition *Floxapen Syrups:* (Flucloxacillin Oral Suspension BP) when reconstituted each 5 ml contains 125 mg or 250 mg flucloxacillin as Flucloxacillin Magnesium BP.

Floxapen Capsules: (Flucloxacillin Capsules BP) containing 250 mg or 500 mg flucloxacillin as Flucloxacillin Sodium BP.

Pharmaceutical form *Floxapen Syrup:* Bottles containing powder for oral suspension.

Floxapen Capsules: Black and caramel capsules overprinted with Floxapen.

Clinical particulars

Therapeutic indications: Floxapen is indicated for the treatment of infections due to sensitive Gram-positive organisms, including infections caused by β-lactamase-producing staphylococci. Typical indications include:

Skin and soft tissue infections:

Boils	Impetigo
Abscesses	Infected wounds
Carbuncles	Infected burns
Furunculosis	Protection for skin grafts
Cellulitis	Otitis media and externa
Infected skin conditions e.g. ulcer, eczema, and acne.	

Respiratory tract infections:

Pneumonia	Pharyngitis
Lung abscess	Tonsillitis
Empyema	Quinsy
Sinusitis	

Other infections caused by Floxapen-sensitive organisms:

Osteomyelitis	Septicaemia
Enteritis	Meningitis
Endocarditis	Urinary Tract Infection

Floxapen is also indicated for use as a prophylactic agent during major surgical procedures when appropriate; for example cardiothoracic and orthopaedic surgery. Parenteral usage is indicated where oral dosage is inappropriate.

Posology and method of administration:

Usual adult dosage (including elderly patients):

Oral – 250 mg four times a day.

Oral doses should be administered half to one hour before meals.

Osteomyelitis, endocarditis – Up to 8 g daily, in divided doses six to eight hourly.

Surgical prophylaxis – 1 to 2 g IV at induction of anaesthesia followed by 500 mg six hourly IV, IM or orally for up to 72 hours.

Usual children's dosage: Two to 10 years: half adult dose

Under two years: quarter adult dose.

Abnormal renal function: In common with other penicillins, Floxapen usage in patients with renal impairment does not usually require dosage reduction. However, in the presence of severe renal failure (creatinine clearance < 10 ml/min) a reduction in dose or an extension of dose interval should be considered. Floxapen is not significantly removed by dialysis and hence no supplementary dosages need to be administered either during, or at the end of the dialysis period.

Contra-indications: Penicillin hypersensitivity

Special warnings and special precautions for use: None known.

Interaction with other medicaments and other forms of interaction: None known.

Pregnancy and lactation: Animal studies have shown no teratogenic effects. The product has been in clinical use since 1970 and the limited number of reported cases of use in human pregnancy have shown no evidence of untoward effect. The use of Floxapen in pregnancy should be reserved for cases considered essential by the clinician.

During lactation trace quantities of penicillins can be detected in breast milk.

Effects on ability to drive and use machines: None known.

Undesirable effects: Side effects, as with other penicillins, are uncommon and mainly of a mild and transitory nature. Gastrointestinal upsets (e.g. nausea, diarrhoea) and skin rashes have been reported. If a skin rash occurs, treatment should be discontinued. Hepatitis and cholestatic jaundice have been reported. These reactions are related neither to the dose nor the route of administration. The onset of these effects may be delayed for up to two months post-treatment: in several cases, the course of the reactions has been protracted and lasted for some months. In very rare cases a fatal outcome has been reported.

Pseudomembranous colitis has been reported rarely and has usually been associated with use of Floxapen in combination with other antibiotics.

In common with other beta-lactam antibiotics angioedema and anaphylaxis have been reported.

Overdose: Problems of overdosage with Floxapen are unlikely to occur; if encountered they may be treated symptomatically.

Pharmacological properties

Pharmacodynamic properties: Floxapen is indicated for the treatment of infections caused by Gram-positive organisms including infections caused by beta-lactamase-producing staphylococci.

Pharmacokinetic properties: Mean pharmacokinetic parameters following administration of magnesium flucloxacillin syrup 125 mg/5 ml at a dose level of 250 mg (10 ml).

Dose	Mean peak serum level µg/ml (S.D)	AUC µg.hr/ml	Urinary excretion 0-6 hr.%dose
250 mg	11.17 (2.01)	12.1	51.5

Flucloxacillin has been reported to have a plasma half life of approximately one hour in healthy subjects.

Flucloxacillin is excreted mainly in the urine and a small amount in the bile.

Preclinical safety data: No further information of relevance to add.

Pharmaceutical particulars

List of excipients:

Floxapen Syrup: Saccharin sodium, xanthan gum, citric acid, sodium citrate, sodium benzoate, blood orange, tutti fruitti and menthol dry flavours, erythrosine CI 45430, quinoline yellow E104, sucrose.

Floxapen Capsules: Magnesium stearate, black iron oxide (E172), titanium dioxide (E171), red iron oxide (E172), yellow iron oxide (E172).

Incompatibilities: None known.

Shelf-life

Floxapen Syrup: three years (following reconstitution: 14 days).

Floxapen Capsules: three years (except in fibreboard drums – 12 months)

Special precautions for storage: Floxapen Syrups should be stored in a dry place.

Once dispensed, Floxapen Syrups (bottles) remain stable for 14 days stored in a refrigerator (5°C).

Floxapen Capsules in Original Packs should be stored in a dry place. Floxapen Capsules in reclosable containers should be stored in a cool, dry place. Fibreboard drums should be kept tightly closed in a cool, dry place.

Nature and contents of container:

Floxapen Syrup 125 mg/5 ml: Clear glass bottles, reconstituted volume of 60 ml or 100 ml.

Floxapen Syrup 250 mg/5 ml: Clear glass bottles, reconstituted volume of 60 ml or 100 ml.

Floxapen Capsules 250 mg: Aluminium canister–20, 50, 100 and 500; Glass bottle with screwcap–20, 50, 100 and 500; Polypropylene tube with polyethylene closure–20, 50, 100 and 500; Aluminium foil–12; Aluminium/PVC/PVdC blister–28; Fibreboard drum with metal or HDPE lid–50,000.

Floxapen Capsules 500 mg: Aluminium canister–50 and 100; Glass bottle with screwcap–50 and 100; Polypropylene tube with polyethylene closure–50 and 100; Aluminium foil–12; Aluminium/PVC/PVdC blister–28.

Instructions for use/handling: None stated.

Marketing authorisation holder: Beecham Group plc, Great West Road, Brentford, Middlesex TW8 9BD.

Trading as SmithKline Beecham Pharmaceuticals Mundells, Welwyn Garden City, Hertfordshire AL7 1EY.

Marketing authorisation number(s)

Floxapen Syrup 125 mg/5 ml:	PL 0038/0309
Floxapen Syrup 250 mg/5 ml:	PL 0038/0310
Floxapen Capsules 250 mg:	PL 0038/5055R
Floxapen Capsules 500 mg:	PL 0038/5056R

Date of renewal of authorisation

Floxapen Syrup 125 mg/5 ml:	20.12.94
Floxapen Syrup 250 mg/5 ml:	20.12.94
Floxapen Capsules 250 mg:	12.12.97
Floxapen Capsules 500 mg:	12.12.97

Date of (partial) revision of the text

Floxapen Syrup 125 mg/5 ml:	May 1997
Floxapen Syrup 250 mg/5 ml:	May 1997
Floxapen Capsules 250 mg:	December 1997
Floxapen Capsules 500 mg:	July 1997

Legal Category POM.

FLOXAPEN* Vials for Injection

Qualitative and quantitative composition Floxapen Vials for Injection (Flucloxacillin Injection BP). Each vial contains 250 mg, 500 mg or 1 g flucloxacillin as Flucloxacillin Sodium BP.

Pharmaceutical form Floxapen Vials for Injection: Vials containing sterile powder for reconstitution.

Clinical particulars

Therapeutic indications: Floxapen is indicated for the treatment of infections due to sensitive Gram-positive organisms, including infections caused by β-lactamase-producing staphylococci. Typical indications include:

Skin and soft tissue infections:

Boils	Impetigo
Abscesses	Infected wounds
Carbuncles	Infected burns
Furunculosis	Protection for skin grafts
Cellulitis	Otitis media and externa
Infected skin conditions e.g. ulcer, eczema, and acne.	

Respiratory tract infections:

Pneumonia	Pharyngitis
Lung abscess	Tonsillitis
Empyema	Quinsy
Sinusitis	

Other infections caused by Floxapen-sensitive organisms:

Osteomyelitis	Septicaemia
Enteritis	Meningitis
Endocarditis	Urinary tract infection

Floxapen is also indicated for use as a prophylactic agent during major surgical procedures when appropriate; for example cardiothoracic and orthopaedic surgery. Parenteral usage is indicated where oral dosage is inappropriate.

Posology and method of administration:

Usual adult dosage (including elderly patients):

Intramuscular – 250 mg four times a day.

Intravenous – 250 mg to 1 g four times a day.

The above systemic dosages may be doubled where necessary.

Osteomyelitis, endocarditis – Up to 8 g daily, in divided doses six to eight hourly.

Surgical prophylaxis 1 to 2 g IV at induction of anaesthesia followed by 500 mg six hourly IV, IM or orally for up to 72 hours.

Floxapen may be administered by other routes in conjunction with systemic therapy. (Proportionately lower doses should be given in children.)

Intrapleural – 250 mg once daily.

By nebuliser – 125 to 250 mg four times a day.

Intra-articular – 250 to 500 mg once daily.

Usual children's dosage: Two to 10 years: half adult dose

Under two years: quarter adult dose.

Abnormal renal function: In common with other penicillins, Floxapen usage in patients with renal impairment does not usually require dosage reduction. However, in the presence of severe renal failure (creatinine clearance < 10 ml/min) a reduction in dose or an extension of dose interval should be considered. Floxapen is not significantly removed by dialysis and hence no supplementary dosages need to be administered either during, or at the end of the dialysis period.

Administration: Routes of administration: intramuscular, intravenous, intrapleural, intra-articular and inhalation.

Intramuscular: Add 1.5 ml Water for Injections BP to 250 mg vial contents.

Intravenous: Dissolve 250-500 mg in 5-10 ml Water for Injections. Administer by slow intravenous injection (three to four minutes). Floxapen may also be added to infusion fluids or injected, suitably diluted, into the drip tube over a period of three to four minutes.

Interpleural: Dissolve 250 mg in 5-10 ml Water for Injections BP.

Intra-articular: Dissolve 250-500 mg in up to 5 ml Water for Injections BP or 0.5% lignocaine hydrochloride solution.

Nebuliser solution: Dissolve 125-250 mg of the vial contents in 3 ml of sterile water.

Contra-indications: Penicillin hypersensitivity. Ocular administration.

Special warnings and special precautions for use: None known.

Interaction with other medicaments and other forms of interaction: None known.

Pregnancy and lactation: Animal studies have shown no teratogenic effects. The product has been in clinical use since 1970 and the limited number of reported cases of use in human pregnancy have shown no evidence of untoward effect. The use of Floxapen in pregnancy should be reserved for cases considered essential by the clinician.

During lactation trace quantities of penicillins can be detected in breast milk.

Effects on ability to drive and use machines: None known.

Undesirable effects: Side effects, as with other penicillins, are uncommon and mainly of a mild and transitory nature. Gastrointestinal upsets (e.g. nausea, diarrhoea) and skin rashes have been reported. If a skin rash occurs, treatment should be discontinued. Hepatitis and cholestatic jaundice have been reported. These reactions are related neither to the dose nor the route of administration. The onset of these effects may be delayed for up to two months post-treatment: in several cases, the course of the reactions has been protracted and lasted for some months. In very rare cases a fatal outcome has been reported.

Pseudomembranous colitis has been reported rarely and has usually been associated with use of Floxapen in combination with other antibiotics.

In common with other beta-lactam antibiotics angioedema and anaphylaxis have been reported.

Overdose: Problems of overdosage with Floxapen are unlikely to occur; if encountered they may be treated symptomatically.

Pharmacological properties

Pharmacodynamic properties: Floxapen is indicated for the treatment of infections caused by Gram-positive organisms including infections caused by beta-lactamase-producing staphylococci.

Pharmacokinetic properties: Flucloxacillin has been reported to have a plasma half life of approximately one hour in healthy subjects.

Flucloxacillin is excreted mainly in the urine and a small amount in the bile.

Preclinical safety data: No further information of relevance to add.

Pharmaceutical particulars

List of excipients: Floxapen Vials for Injection: None

Incompatibilities: If Floxapen is prescribed concurrently with an aminoglycoside, the two antibiotics should not be mixed in the syringe, intravenous fluid container or giving set; precipitation may occur.

Shelf-life: Floxapen Vials for Injection: Three years. After opening, 24 hours.

Special precautions for storage: Floxapen Vials for Injection should be stored in a cool, dry place. Once reconstituted Floxapen solutions should be stored in a refrigerator (2°C-8°C) and used within 24 hours.

Nature and contents of container: Floxapen Vials for Injection 250 mg: Clear glass vials with butyl rubber plug and aluminium seal, boxes of 10.

Floxapen Vials for Injection 500 mg: Clear glass vials with butyl rubber plug and aluminium seal, boxes of 10.

Floxapen Vials for Injection 1 g: Clear glass vials with butyl rubber plug and aluminium seal, boxes of five or 10.

Instructions for use/handling: Floxapen vials are not suitable for multidose use. Any residual Floxapen should be discarded.

Marketing authorisation holder: Beecham Group plc, Great West Road, Brentford, Middlesex TW8 9BD. Trading as SmithKline Beecham Pharmaceuticals Mundells, Welwyn Garden City, Hertfordshire AL7 1EY.

Marketing authorisation number(s)

Floxapen Vials for Injection 250 mg	PL 0038/5051R
Floxapen Vials for Injection 500 mg	PL 0038/5052R
Floxapen Vials for Injection 1 g	PL 0038/5053R

Date of renewal of authorisation

Floxapen Vials for Injection 250 mg	13.01.94
Floxapen Vials for Injection 500 mg	13.01.94
Floxapen Vials for Injection 1 g	13.01.94

Date of (partial) revision of the text

Floxapen Vials for Injection 250 mg	May 1997
Floxapen Vials for Injection 500 mg	May 1997
Floxapen Vials for Injection 1 g	April 1998

Legal Category POM.

FLUARIX*
Influenza vaccine (split virion, inactivated)

Qualitative and quantitative composition Fluarix is an influenza virus vaccine prepared on eggs, purified, inactivated by formaldehyde, split by sodium deoxycholate, containing antigens equivalent to * :

A/Sydney/5/97 (H_3N_2)-like strain: A/Sydney/5/97 (IVR-108)	15 microgram haemagglutinin
A/Beijing/262/95 (H_1N_1)-like strain: A/Beijing/262/95 (X-127)	15 microgram haemagglutinin
B/Beijing/184/93-like strain: B/Harbin/7/94	15 microgram haemagglutinin

The antigen composition and strains for the influenza season 1998-1999 in the Northern Hemisphere are determined by the World Health Organisation (WHO) and the Commission of the European Community.

The volume of a vaccine dose is 0.5 ml
*98/99 season

Pharmaceutical form Suspension for injection.

Clinical particulars

Therapeutic indications: Prophylaxis of influenza, especially in those who run an increased risk of associated complications.

Posology and method of administration:

Posology: Adults and children from 36 months: 0.5 ml.

Children from six months to 35 months: Clinical data are limited. Dosages of 0.25 ml or 0.5 ml have been used. For children who have not previously been infected or vaccinated, a second dose should be given after an interval of at least four weeks.

Method of administration: Immunisation should be carried out by intramuscular or deep subcutaneous injection.

Contra-indications: Hypersensitivity to egg, chicken protein or any constituent of the vaccine.

Immunisation should be postponed in patients with febrile illness or acute infection.

Special warnings and special precautions for use: As with all injectable vaccines, appropriate medical treatment and supervision should always be readily available in case of a rare anaphylactic event following the administration of the vaccine.

The vaccine (Fluarix) should under no circumstances be administered intravascularly.

Antibody response in patients with endogenous or iatrogenic immunosuppression may be insufficient.

The vaccine contains residual amounts of gentamicin, to which hypersensitivity may occur.

Interaction with other medicaments and other forms of interaction: The vaccine (Fluarix) may be given at the same time as other vaccines. Immunisation should be carried out on separate limbs. It should be noted that the adverse reactions may be intensified.

The immunological response may be diminished if the patient is undergoing immunosuppressant treatment.

Following influenza vaccination, false positive results in serology tests using the ELISA method to detect antibodies against HIV1, Hepatitis C and especially HTLV1 have been observed. The Western Blot technique disproves the results. The transient false positive reactions could be due to the IgM response by the vaccine.

Pregnancy and lactation: No relevant animal data are available. In humans, up to now, the data are inadequate to assess teratogenic or foetotoxic risk during pregnancy. In pregnant high-risk patients, the possible risks of clinical infection should be weighed against the possible risks of vaccination.

The vaccine (Fluarix) may be used during lactation.

Effects on ability to drive and use machines: The vaccine is unlikely to produce an effect on the ability to drive and use machines.

Undesirable effects: The following reactions are most common:

Local reactions : redness, swelling, pain, ecchymosis, induration.

Systemic reactions : fever, malaise, shivering, fatigue, headache, sweating, myalgia, arthralgia.

These reactions usually disappear within one to two days without treatment.

The following events are observed rarely: neuralgia, paraesthesia, convulsions, transient thrombocytopenia.

Allergic reactions, in rare cases leading to shock, have been reported.

Vasculitis with transient renal involvement has been reported in very rare cases.

Rarely neurological disorders, such as encephalomyelitis, neuritis and Guillain Barré syndrome have been reported. An increased risk of Guillain Barré syndrome has not been demonstrated with currently used influenza vaccines.

Overdose: Overdosage is unlikely to have any untoward effect.

Pharmacological properties

Pharmacodynamic properties: Seroprotection is generally obtained within two to three weeks. The duration of postvaccinal immunity varies but is usually six to 12 months.

Pharmacokinetic properties: Not applicable.

Preclinical safety data: Not applicable.

Pharmaceutical particulars

List of excipients: Thiomersal, sodium chloride, dodecahydrated sodium hydrogenophosphate, potassium dihydrogenophosphate, potassium chloride, magnesium chloride, Polysorbate 80/Octoxynol 9 (Tween 80/Triton X-100), sucrose, formaldehyde, sodium deoxycholate, traces of gentamicin and water for injections.

Incompatibilities: The vaccine (Fluarix) should not be mixed with other injection fluids.

Shelf-life: The expiry date is indicated on the label and packaging.

The shelf-life is 12 months.

Special precautions for storage: This product should be stored at +2°C to +8°C (in a refrigerator). Do not freeze. Protect from light.

Nature and contents of container: Fluarix is colourless to slightly opalescent and presented in prefilled syringes.

The syringes are made of neutral glass type I, which conforms to European Pharmacopoeia Requirements.

Instructions for use/handling: The vaccine should be allowed to reach room temperature before use. Shake before use.

Vaccines should be inspected visually for any foreign particulate matter and/or variation of physical aspect prior to administration. In the event of either being observed, discard the vaccine.

When a dose of 0.25 ml is indicated, the prefilled syringe should be held in upright position and half of the volume should be eliminated. The remaining volume should be injected.

Marketing authorisation holder: SmithKline Beecham plc, SB House, Great West Road, Brentford, Middlesex TW8 9BD.
Trading as SmithKline Beecham Pharmaceuticals Mundells, Welwyn Garden City, Hertfordshire AL7 1EY.

Marketing authorisation number PL 10592/0118

Date of first authorisation/renewal of authorisation 27 February 1998

Date of revision of the text May 1998

Legal category POM.

HALFAN* TABLETS

Qualitative and quantitative composition Each tablet contains 250 mg halofantrine hydrochloride (233 mg halofantrine as the base).

Pharmaceutical form White to off-white capsule-shaped tablets, with a breakline on one side and enscribed Halfan on the other.

Clinical particulars

Therapeutic indications: Halfan is an antimalarial indicated in the treatment of acute infection with *Plasmodium falciparum* and *P. vivax*. It is schizonticidal and exerts its action at the erythrocytic stage of the life cycle (trophozoite and schizont). It is not effective against exoerythrocytic (hepatic) schizonts or against the merozoite or gametocyte stages of the life cycle of *Plasmodium* species investigated.

Halfan is especially useful for those likely to be infected with chloroquine or multi-drug-resistant strains.

Posology and method of administration: Oral. It is recommended that halofantrine is given on an empty stomach (see *Pharmacokinetic properties*). This is important for all courses of the drug (see *Warnings and precautions*).

All doses are given as halofantrine hydrochloride.

Adults and children of over 37 kilos: A total of six tablets (1500 mg) divided into three doses of two tablets given at six-hourly intervals.

Children of 37 kilos and under: The usual dosage is 24 mg/kg divided into three doses given at six-hourly intervals according to the following scheme:

Weight:

32-37 kg: A total of 4½ tablets (1125 mg) divided into three doses of 1½ tablets given six-hourly.

23-31 kg: A total of three tablets (750 mg) divided into three doses of one tablet given six-hourly.

Less than 23 kg: Appropriate dosage adjustment is not possible with the tablet presentation.

Elderly: There are no studies on the use of Halfan in the elderly.

Note: In cases where the patient has no previous exposure or minimal exposure to malaria, a second course of therapy is recommended one week after the initial treatment. Higher than recommended doses have been shown to increase the likelihood of prolongation of the QTc interval (see *Warnings and precautions*).

Contra-indications: Patients with known hypersensitivity to Halfan. Patients with a known prolonged QTc interval or a family history of congenital QTc prolongation. Pregnancy (see *Pregnancy and lactation*). Do not use for prophylaxis. Unless there are compelling clinical reasons Halfan should not be used in combination with other drugs, e.g. antimalarials (quinine, chloroquine, mefloquine), tricyclic anti-depressants, antipsychotics, some anti-arrhythmic drugs (Vaughan Williams Classes I and III), drugs causing electrolyte disturbance and certain anti-histamines (terfenadine, astemizole), or clinical conditions (e.g. electrolyte abnormalities, particularly hypokalaemia or hypomagnesaemia; thiamine deficiency, ischaemic heart disease, cardiac failure, myocarditis or serious myocardial damage) known to prolong QTc interval, or in patients with known or suspected ventricular dysrhythmias, A–V conduction disorders or unexplained syncopal attacks.

Special warnings and special precautions for use: Halfan has been shown to produce a dose-related prolongation of the QTc interval, which usually is reversible within three to four days. This effect has been associated with serious arrhythmias (sometimes with a fatal outcome), even at the recommended therapeutic dose. Therefore, physicians should take a careful history and consider performing an ECG prior to commencing therapy, as halofantrine is not recommended in patients:

- with known QTc prolongation,
- receiving drugs or having clinical conditions known to prolong the QTc interval,
- with ventricular dysrhythmias, A–V conduction disorders, or unexplained syncopal attacks.

Because of the dose-related nature of the effect on the QTc interval, caution should be taken to avoid increased blood levels that may be associated with higher than recommended doses or increased absorption with fatty foods. It is essential to:

- take the recommended dose on an empty stomach;
- avoid fatty food for 24 hours.

This advice is particularly important during a second course of treatment (see dosage section) as the patient is likely to have improved and be eating normally.

There is no experience with the use of halofantrine in the treatment of patients with cerebral malaria and other complicated malarial conditions. Therefore halofantrine should be used with caution in these conditions.

Interaction with other medicaments and other forms of interaction: An interaction with mefloquine ($t_{\frac{1}{2}}$ 21 days) has been reported to lead to further prolongation of the QT interval (see *Contra-indications* and *Warnings and Precautions*). No interactions with aspirin or paracetamol have been seen.

Pregnancy and lactation: Halfan has been shown to be embryotoxic but not teratogenic in animal tests. Use in women of childbearing age is contra-indicated unless there are compelling clinical grounds.

Animal data suggest that halofantrine may be secreted in breast milk, resulting in reduced rate of weight gain of offspring. Breast feeding should be discontinued whilst the patient is taking Halfan.

Effects on ability to drive and use machines: Not applicable.

Undesirable effects: Diarrhoea, abdominal pain, nausea and vomiting, pruritus and rash have been observed during or following treatment with Halfan. Transient elevation of serum transaminases has been reported. Serious cardiac adverse effects have been reported (see *Contra-indications* and *Special warnings and special precautions for use*). Haemolytic reactions which have compromised renal function have been reported. There have been isolated case reports of anaphylaxis and angioedema. Extremely rarely convulsions have been reported but no causal relationship has been established.

Overdose: There is no experience of acute overdosage with halofantrine. This precludes characterisation of sequelae and assessment of antidotal efficacy at this time. However in case of accidental overdosage, immediate induction of emesis or gastric lavage is recommended in conjunction with appropriate supportive measures which should include ECG monitoring.

Pharmacological properties

Pharmacodynamic properties: Halofantrine hydrochloride is a blood schizonticidal antimalarial agent.

Pharmacokinetic properties: After administration of single doses, Halfan appears in the systemic circulation within one hour. The systemic exposure to halofantrine is increased substantially after a fatty meal. Its elimination half-life from the blood is generally 24 to 48 hours whilst that of its active desbutyl metabolite is approximately twice that time. The major route of elimination is via the faeces.

Preclinical safety data: Refer to *Pregnancy and lactation* section.

Pharmaceutical particulars

List of excipients: Pregelatinised starch; Povidone; Sodium Starch Glycollate; Microcrystalline Cellulose; Purified Talc; Magnesium Stearate; Purified Water.

Incompatibilities: None known.

Shelf-life: Halfan tablet has a shelf-life of three years.

Special precautions for storage: Store in well sealed container at a temperature not exceeding 30°C and protect from light.

Nature and contents of container: Blister pack (OP) of 12 tablets (2×6).

Instructions for use/handling: No special handling instructions.

Marketing authorisation number 0002/0203

Date of approval/revision of SPC 17 April 1997

Legal category POM.

HAVRIX* JUNIOR MONODOSE* VACCINE

Hepatitis A vaccine (HM 175 strain)

Qualitative and quantitative composition

Active ingredient: Hepatitis A virus antigen 720* ELISA units/0.5 ml

Excipients: Aluminium hydroxide gel; 2 Phenoxyethanol; Polysorbate 20 ; Amino acids for injection; Disodium phosphate; Monopotassium phosphate; Sodium chloride; Potassium chloride; Water for injections.

* Calculated overage at release: 10%.

Pharmaceutical form Vaccine for injection.

Clinical particulars

Therapeutic indications: Havrix Junior Monodose vaccine is indicated for active immunisation against HAV infection. The vaccine is particularly indicated for those at increased risk of infection or transmission. It is also indicated for use during outbreaks of hepatitis A infection.

Posology and method of administration: 'Havrix' Junior Monodose vaccine should be injected intramuscularly in the deltoid region. The vaccine should never be administered intravenously.

Dosage:

Children/adolescents (one to 15 years): Primary immunisation consists of a single dose of Havrix Junior Monodose vaccine (720 ELISA units/0.5 ml) given intramuscularly. This provides anti-HAV antibodies for at least one year.

Havrix Junior Monodose confers protection against hepatitis A within two to four weeks.

In order to obtain more persistent immunity for up to 10 years, a booster dose is recommended between six and 12 months following the initial dose.

Patients who have started a course of Havrix Junior Vaccine at a dose of 360 ELISA units/0.5 ml are recommended to complete both the primary course and booster at this dosage.

In the event of a subject being exposed to a high risk of contracting hepatitis A within two weeks of the primary immunisation dose, human normal immunoglobulin may be given simultaneously with Havrix Junior Monodose at different injection sites.

Contra-indications: Hypersensitivity to any component of the vaccine.

Severe febrile illness.

Special warnings and special precautions for use: As with all vaccinations, appropriate medication (e.g. adrenaline) should be readily available for immediate use in case of anaphylaxis.

It is possible that subjects may be in the incubation period of a hepatitis A infection at the time of immunisation. It is not known whether Havrix Junior Monodose will prevent hepatitis A in such cases.

In haemodialysis patients and in subjects with an impaired immune system, adequate anti-HAV antibody titres may not be obtained after the primary immunisation and such patients may therefore require administration of additional doses of vaccine.

Interaction with other medicaments and other forms of interaction: Simultaneous administration of Havrix with normal immunoglobulin does not influence the seroconversion rate to Havrix, however, it may result in a lower antibody titre. A similar effect could be observed with Havrix Junior Monodose.

Preliminary data on the concomitant administration of Havrix, at a dose of 720 ELISA units/ml, with recombinant hepatitis B virus vaccine suggests that there is no interference in the immune response to either antigen. On this basis and since it is an inactivated vaccine interference with immune response is unlikely to occur when Havrix Junior Monodose is administered with other inactivated or live vaccines. When concomitant administration is considered necessary the vaccines must be given at different injection sites.

Havrix Junior Monodose must not be mixed with other vaccines in the same syringe.

Pregnancy and lactation: The effect of Havrix Junior Monodose on foetal development has not been assessed. However, as with all inactivated viral vaccines the risks to the foetus are considered to be negligible. Havrix Junior Monodose should be used during pregnancy only when clearly needed.

The effect on breast-fed infants of the administration of Havrix Junior Monodose to their mothers has not been evaluated in clinical studies. Havrix Junior Monodose should therefore be used with caution in breast-feeding women.

Effects on ability to drive and use machines: Not applicable.

Undesirable effects: These are usually mild and confined to the first few days after vaccination. The most common reactions are mild transient soreness, erythema and induration at the injection site. Less common general complaints, not necessarily related to the vaccination, include headache, fever, malaise, fatigue, nausea, vomiting and loss of appetite and rash. Elevations of serum liver enzymes (usually transient) have been reported occasionally. However, a causal relationship with the vaccine has not been established.

Neurological manifestations occuring in temporal association have been reported extremely rarely with the vaccine and include transverse myelitis, Guillain-Barré syndrome and neuralgic amyotrophy. No causal relationship has been established.

Overdose: Not applicable.

Pharmacological properties

Pharmacodynamic properties: Not applicable.

Pharmacokinetic properties: Not applicable.

Preclinical safety data: Not applicable.

Pharmaceutical particulars

List of excipients: Aluminium hydroxide gel (3% w/w); 2 Phenoxyethanol; Polysorbate 20; Amino acids for injection; Disodium phosphate; Monopotassium phosphate; Sodium chloride; Potassium chloride; Water for injections.

Incompatibilities: Not applicable.

Shelf-life: Havrix Junior Monodose vaccine has a shelf-life of three years from the date of manufacture when stored at 2–8°C.

Special precautions for storage: Store at 2-8°C. Protect from light. Do not freeze.

Nature and contents of container: Prefilled neutral glass syringes (Type 1, PhEur), syringe barrel fitted with needle and rubber shield.

Instructions for use/handling: See Technical Package Leaflet.

Marketing authorisation holder: SmithKline Beecham plc, SB House, Great West Road, Brentford, Middlesex TW8 9BD.

Trading as SmithKline Beecham Pharmaceuticals Mundells, Welwyn Garden City, Hertfordshire AL7 1EY.

Marketing authorisation number PL 10592/0080.

Date of approval/revision of SPC 27th August 1997

Legal Category POM.

HAVRIX* MONODOSE* VACCINE
Hepatitis A vaccine (HM 175 strain)

Qualitative and quantitative composition Each vial contains 1440 ELISA units/1 ml dose of hepatitis A virus antigen.

Pharmaceutical form Vaccine suspension for injection.

Clinical particulars
Therapeutic indications: Active immunisation against infections caused by hepatitis A virus. The vaccine is particularly indicated for those at increased risk of infection or transmission. For example immunisation should be considered for the following risk groups:

- travellers visiting areas of medium or high endemicity, i.e. anywhere outside northern or western Europe, Australia, North America and New Zealand.
- military and diplomatic personnel, haemophiliacs and patients, intravenous drug abusers, homosexual men, laboratory workers working directly with the hepatitis A virus, sanitation workers in contact with untreated sewage.
- close contacts of hepatitis A cases.

Since virus shedding from infected persons may occur for a prolonged period, active immunisation of close contacts may be considered.

Under certain circumstances additional groups could be at increased risk of infection or transmission. Immunisation of such groups should be considered in the light of local circumstances. Such groups might include:

- staff and inmates of residential institutions for the mentally handicapped and other institutions where standards of personal hygiene are poor.
- staff working in day care centres and other settings with children who are not yet toilet trained.
- food packagers or handlers.

In addition there may be other groups at risk or specific circumstances such as an outbreak of hepatitis A infection when immunisation should be given.

Posology and method of administration:
Posology:
Adults (16 years and over): Primary immunisation consists of a single dose of Havrix Monodose vaccine (1440 ELISA units/ml) given intramuscularly. This provides anti-HAV antibodies for at least one year.

Havrix Monodose confers protection against hepatitis A within two to four weeks.

A booster dose is recommended at any time between six and 12 months after the initial dose in order to ensure long-term antibody titres (five to 10 years).

Patients who have started a course of Havrix vaccine at 720 ELISA units/ml are recommended to complete both the primary course and the booster at this dosage.

In the event of a subject being exposed to a high risk of contracting hepatitis A within two weeks of the primary immunisation dose human normal immunoglobulin may be given simultaneously with Havrix Monodose at different injection sites.

Children/adolescents (one to 15 years): Havrix Monodose is not recommended (Havrix Junior Monodose should be used).

Method of administration: Havrix Monodose vaccine should be injected intramuscularly in the deltoid region.

The vaccine should never be administered intravenously.

Contra-indications: Hypersensitivity to any component of the vaccine. Severe febrile illness.

Special warnings and special precautions for use: As for all vaccinations, appropriate medication (e.g. adrenaline) should be readily available for immediate use in case of anaphylaxis.
It is possible that subjects may be in the incubation period of a hepatitis A infection at the time of immunisation. It is not known whether Havrix Monodose will prevent hepatitis A in such cases.

In haemodialysis patients and in subjects with an impaired immune system, adequate anti-HAV antibody titres may not be obtained after the primary immunisation and such patients may therefore require administration of additional doses of vaccine.

Interaction with other medicaments and other forms of interaction: Simultaneous administration of Havrix at a dose of 720 ELISA units/ml with ISG does not influence the seroconversion rate to Havrix, however, it may result in a lower antibody titre. A similar effect could be observed with Havrix Monodose.

Preliminary data on the concomitant administration of Havrix at a dose of 720 ELISA units/ml, with recombinant hepatitis B virus vaccine suggest that there is no interference in the immune response to either antigen. On this basis and since it is an inactivated vaccine interference with immune response is unlikely to occur when Havrix Monodose is administered with other inactivated or live vaccines. When concomitant administration is considered necessary the vaccines must be given at different injection sites.

Havrix Monodose must not be mixed with other vaccines in the same syringe.

Pregnancy and lactation: The effect of Havrix Monodose on foetal development has not been assessed. However, as with all inactivated viral vaccines the risks to the foetus are considered negligible. Havrix Monodose should be used during pregnancy only when clearly needed.

The effect on breast fed infants of the administration of Havrix Monodose to their mothers has not been evaluated in clinical studies. Havrix Monodose should therefore be used with caution in breast feeding women.

Effects on ability to drive and use machines: Not applicable.

Undesirable effects: These are usually mild and confined to the first few days after vaccination. The most common reactions are mild transient soreness, erythema and induration at the injection site. Less common general complaints, not necessarily related to the vaccination, include headache, fever, malaise, fatigue, nausea and loss of appetite and rash. Elevations of serum liver enzymes (usually transient) have been reported occasionally. However, a causal relationship with the vaccine has not been established.

Neurological manifestations occurring in temporal association have been reported extremely rarely with the vaccine and included transverse myelitis, Guillain-Barré syndrome and neurologic amyotrophy. No causal relationship has been established.

Overdose: Not applicable.

Pharmacological properties
Pharmacodynamic properties: Active immunisation against hepatitis A virus

Pharmacokinetic properties: Not applicable to vaccine products.

Preclinical safety data: Not applicable to vaccine products.

Pharmaceutical particulars
List of excipients: Aluminium hydroxide, 2 phenoxyethanol, polysorbate 20, amino acids for injection, disodium phosphate, monopotassium phosphate, sodium chloride, potassium chloride, water for injections and also a trace of neomycin B sulphate (maximum 40 ng, 0.028 IU/ml).

Incompatibilities: Not applicable.

Shelf-life: 36 months.

Special precautions for storage: Store at 2°C-8°C. Protect from light. Do not freeze.

Nature and contents of container: Prefilled neutral glass syringes (Type I, PhEur) syringe barrel fitted with needle and rubber shield containing 1 ml of suspension in packs of one and 10.

Instructions for use/handling: None stated.

Marketing authorisation holder: SmithKline Beecham plc, SB House, Great West Road, Brentford, Middlesex TW8 9BD.
Trading as SmithKline Beecham Pharmaceuticals Mundells, Welwyn Garden City, Hertfordshire AL7 1EY.

Marketing authorisation number PL 10592/0037

Date of first authorisation 18.05.94

Date of text 2.12.97

Legal category POM.

HYCAMTIN* ▼

Qualitative and quantitative composition Each vial contains topotecan hydrochloride equivalent to 4 mg topotecan.

Pharmaceutical form Powder for solution for infusion.

Clinical particulars
Therapeutic indications: Topotecan is indicated for the treatment of patients with metastatic carcinoma of the ovary after failure of first-line or subsequent therapy.

Posology and method of administration: The use of topotecan should be confined to units specialised in the administration of cytotoxic chemotherapy and should only be administered under the supervision of a physician experienced in the use of chemotherapy.
Initial dose: The recommended dose of topotecan is 1.5 mg/m² body surface area/day administered by intravenous infusion over 30 minutes daily for five consecutive days with a three week interval between the start of each course. A minimum of four courses is recommended since median time to response in clinical trials was 7.6–11.6 weeks.

Prior to administration of the first course of topotecan, patients must have a baseline neutrophil count of $\geq 1.5 \times 10^9$/l, and a platelet count of $\geq 100 \times 10^9$/l.

Routine pre-medication for non-haematological adverse events is not required with topotecan.

Topotecan must be reconstituted and further diluted before use (see section *Instructions for use/handling and disposal*).

Subsequent doses: Topotecan should not be re-administered unless the neutrophil count is $\geq 1 \times 10^9$/l, the platelet count is $\geq 100 \times 10^9$/l, and the haemoglobin level is ≥ 9 g/dl (after transfusion if necessary).

Patients who experience severe neutropenia (neutrophil count $< 0.5 \times 10^9$/l) for seven days or more, or severe neutropenia associated with fever or infection, or who have had treatment delayed due to neutropenia, should be treated as follows:

either

be given a reduced dose i.e. 1.25 mg/m²/day (or subsequently down to 1.0 mg/m²/day if necessary)

or

be given G-CSF prophylactically in subsequent courses to maintain dose intensity, starting from day six of the course (the day after completion of topotecan administration). If neutropenia is not adequately managed with G-CSF administration, doses should be reduced.

Doses should be similarly reduced if the platelet count falls below 25×10^9/l. In clinical trials, topotecan was discontinued if the dose had been reduced to 1.0 mg/m² and a further dose reduction was required to manage adverse effects.

Dosage in renally impaired patients: Insufficient data are available to make a recommendation for patients with a creatinine clearance < 20 ml/min. Limited data indicate that the dose should be reduced in patients with moderate renal impairment. The recommended dose in patients with creatinine clearance between 20 and 39 ml/min is 0.75 mg/m² /day.

Contra-indications: Topotecan is contra-indicated in patients who

- have a history of severe hypersensitivity reactions to topotecan and/or its excipients
- are pregnant or breast feeding
- already have severe bone marrow depression prior to starting first course, as evidenced by baseline neutrophils $< 1.5 \times 10^9$/l and/or a platelet count of $\leq 100 \times 10^9$/l.

Special warnings and special precautions for use: Haematological toxicity is dose-related and full blood count including platelets should be monitored regularly.

As expected, patients with poor performance status have a lower response rate and an increased incidence of complications such as fever and infection.

There is no experience of the use of topotecan in patients with severely impaired renal function (creatinine clearance < 20 ml/min) or severely impaired hepatic function (serum bilirubin ≥ 10 mg/dl) due to cirrhosis. Topotecan is not recommended to be used in these patient groups.

A small number of hepatically impaired patients (serum bilirubin ≥ 1.5 ≤ 10 mg/dl) were able to tolerate 1.5 mg/m² for five days every three weeks although a reduction in topotecan clearance was observed. There are insufficient data available to make a dose recommendation for this patient group.

Interaction with other medicinal products and other forms of interaction: No *in vivo* human pharmacokinetic interaction studies have been performed.

Topotecan does not inhibit human P450 enzymes (see *Pharmacokinetic properties*). In a population study, the co-administration of granisetron, ondansetron, morphine or corticosteroids did not appear to have a significant effect on the pharmacokinetics of total topotecan (active and inactive form).

Use during pregnancy and lactation:
Pregnancy: Topotecan is contra-indicated during pregnancy. Topotecan has been shown to be cause embryo-foetal lethality and malformations in preclinical studies.

Lactation: Topotecan is contra-indicated during breast-feeding. Although it is not known whether topotecan is excreted in human breast milk, breast-feeding should be discontinued at the start of therapy.

Effects on ability to drive and use machines: Caution should be observed when driving or operating machinery if fatigue and asthenia persist.

Undesirable effects:
Haematological: In dose-finding studies, the dose-limiting toxicity was found to be haematological. Toxicity was predictable, and reversible. No evidence of cumulative toxicity was seen.

Neutropenia: Severe, (neutrophil count $< 0.5 \times 10^9$/l) during course one was seen in 60% of the patients and with duration ≥ 7 days in 20% and overall in 79% of patients (42% of courses). In association with severe neutropenia, fever or infection occurred in 16% of patients during course one and overall in 21% of patients (7% of courses). Median time to onset of severe neutropenia was nine days and the median duration was seven days. Severe neutropenia lasted beyond seven days in 13% of courses overall.

Among all patients treated in clinical studies (including both those with severe neutropenia and those who did not develop severe neutropenia), 13% (5% of courses) developed fever and 27% (10% of courses) developed infection. In addition, 5% of all patients treated (1% of courses) developed sepsis.

Thrombocytopenia: Severe, (platelets less than 25 x 10^9/l) in 23% of patients (9% of courses); moderate (platelets between 25.0 and 49.9 x 10^9/l) in 20% of patients (13% of courses).

Median time to onset of severe thrombocytopenia was Day 14 and the median duration was five days. Platelet transfusions were given in 4% of courses. Significant sequelae associated with thrombocytopenia were rare.

Anaemia: Moderate to severe (Hb ≤7.9 g/dl) in 36% of patients (15% of courses). Red cell transfusions were given in 54% of patients (23% of courses).

Non-haematological: In clinical trials of 445 ovarian cancer patients, frequently reported non-haematological effects were gastrointestinal such as nausea (68%), vomiting (44%), and diarrhoea (26%), constipation (14%) and stomatitis (20%). Severe (grade 3 or 4) nausea, vomiting, diarrhoea and stomatitis incidence was 6, 4, 3 and 2% respectively.

Mild abdominal pain was also reported amongst 8% of patients.

Fatigue was observed in approximately one-third and asthenia in about one-fifth of patients whilst receiving topotecan. Severe (grade 3 or 4) fatigue and asthenia incidence was 4 and 2% respectively.

Total or pronounced alopecia was observed in 42% of patients and partial alopecia in 17% of patients.

Other severe events occurring in ≥ 1% patients that were recorded as related or possibly related to topotecan treatment were anorexia (1%), malaise (1%) and hyperbilirubinaemia (1%).

Extravasation has been reported rarely. Reactions have been mild and have not generally required specific therapy.

No evidence of significant cardiotoxicity, neurotoxicity or major organ toxicity was observed with topotecan.

Overdose: There is no known antidote for topotecan overdosage. The primary complications of overdosage are anticipated to be bone marrow suppression and mucositis.

Pharmacological properties
Pharmacodynamic properties: Pharmaco-therapeutic group: Antineoplastic and immunomodulating agent: ATC-code: L01X X17

The anti-tumour activity of topotecan involves the inhibition of topoisomerase-I, an enzyme intimately involved in DNA replication as it relieves the torsional strain introduced ahead of the moving replication fork. Topotecan inhibits topoisomerase-I by stabilising the covalent complex of enzyme and strand-cleaved DNA which is an intermediate of the catalytic mechanism. The cellular sequela of inhibition of topoisomerase–I by topotecan is the induction of protein-associated DNA single-strand breaks.

In a comparative study of topotecan and paclitaxel in patients previously treated for ovarian carcinoma with platinum based chemotherapy (n=112 and 114, respectively), the response rate (95% CI) was 20.5% (13, 28) versus 14% (8, 20) and median time to progression 19 weeks versus 15 weeks (hazard ratio 0.7 [0.6, 1.0]), for topotecan and paclitaxel, respectively. Median overall survival was 62 weeks for topotecan versus 53 weeks for paclitaxel (hazard ratio 0.9 [0.6, 1.3]).

The response rate in the whole ovarian carcinoma programme (n=392, all previously treated with cisplatin or cisplatin and paclitaxel) was 16% In patients refractory to, or relapsing within three months after cisplatin therapy (n=186), the response rate was 10%.

These data should be evaluated in the context of the overall safety profile of the drug, in particular to the important haematological toxicity (see *Undesirable effects*).

Pharmacokinetic properties: Following intravenous administration of topotecan at doses of 0.5 to 1.5 mg/m^2 as a 30-minute infusion daily for five days, topotecan demonstrated a high plasma clearance of 62 l/h (SD 22), corresponding to approximately two-thirds of liver blood flow. Topotecan also had a high volume of distribution, about 132 L, (SD 57) and a relatively short half-life of two to three hours. Comparison of pharmacokinetic parameters did not suggest any change in pharmacokinetics over the five days of dosing. Area under the curve increased approximately in proportion to the increase in dose. The binding of topotecan to plasma proteins was low (35%) and distribution between blood cells and plasma was fairly homogeneous.

In a population study, a number of factors including age, weight and ascites had no significant effect on clearance of total topotecan (active and inactive form).

The elimination of topotecan has only been partly investigated in man. A major route of clearance of topotecan was by hydrolysis of the lactone ring to form the ring-opened hydroxy acid. *In vitro* data using human liver microsomes indicate the formulation of small amounts of N-demethylated topotecan. In man, as in animal species, a significant proportion of the dose (generally 20-60%) was excreted in the urine as topotecan or the open ring form. *In vitro*, topotecan did not inhibit human P450 enzymes CYP1A2, CYP2A6, CYP2C8/9, CYP2C19, CYP2D6, CYP2E, CYP3A, or CYP4A nor did it inhibit the human cytosolic enzymes dihydropyrimidine or xanthine oxidase.

Plasma clearance in patients with hepatic impairment (serum bilirubin ≥ 1.5 ≤ 10 mg/dl) decreased to about 67% when compared with a control group of patients. Topotecan half-life was increased by about 30% but no clear change in volume of distribution was observed. Plasma clearance of total topotecan (active and inactive form) in patients with hepatic impairment only decreased by about 10% compared with the control group of patients.

Plasma clearance in patients with renal impairment (creatinine clearance 41–60 ml/min.) decreased to about 67% compared with control patients. Volume of distribution was slightly decreased and thus half-life only increased by 14%. In patients with moderate renal impairment topotecan plasma clearance was reduced to 34% of the value in control patients. Mean half-life increased from 1.9 hours to 4.9 hours.

Preclinical safety data: Resulting from its mechanism of action, topotecan is genotoxic to mammalian cells (mouse lymphoma cells and human lymphocytes) *in vitro* and mouse bone marrow cells *in vivo*. Topotecan was also shown to cause embryo-foetal lethality when given to rats and rabbits.

The carcinogenic potential of topotecan has not been studied

Pharmaceutical particulars
List of excipients: Tartaric acid, mannitol, hydrochloric acid and sodium hydroxide.

Incompatibilities: None known.

Shelf-life: Vials 24 months.

Reconstituted and diluted solutions: The product should be used immediately after reconstitution as it contains no antibacterial preservative. If reconstitution and dilution is performed under strict aseptic conditions (e.g. an LAF bench) the product should be used (infusion completed) within 12 hours at room temperature or 24 hours if stored at 2–8°C after the first breakage.

Special precautions for storage: Before reconstitution the product must be protected from light during long-term storage by being retained in its carton.

Nature and content of container: 5 ml type I flint glass vials, together with 20 mm grey butyl rubber stoppers and 20 mm aluminium seals with plastic flip-off caps. Hycamtin is available in cartons containing 1 vial, 5 vials and 5×5 vials.

Instructions for use/handling and disposal: Topotecan 4 mg vials must be reconstituted with 4 ml Sterile Water for Injection. Further dilution of the appropriate volume of the reconstituted solution with either 0.9% Sodium Chloride Intravenous Infusion or 5% Dextrose Intravenous Infusion is required to a final concentration of between 25 and 50 microgram/ml.

The normal procedures for proper handling and disposal of anticancer drugs should be adopted, namely:

Personnel should be trained to reconstitute the drug.

Pregnant staff should be excluded from working with this drug.

Personnel handling this drug during reconstitution should wear protective clothing including mask, goggles and gloves.

All items for administration or cleaning, including gloves, should be placed in a high-risk, waste disposal bags for high-temperature incineration. Liquid waste may be flushed with large amounts of water.

Accidental contact with the skin or eyes should be treated immediately with copious amounts of water.

Marketing authorisation number EU/1/96/027/001-2

Date of approval/revision of SPC April 1997

Legal category POM.

KYTRIL* INFUSION

Presentation Clear glass ampoules, each containing 3 mg granisetron present as the hydrochloride in 3 ml isotonic saline as a clear, colourless or slightly straw-coloured liquid.

Uses Kytril is indicated for the prevention or treatment of nausea and vomiting induced by cytostatic therapy.

Granisetron is a potent and highly selective 5-hydroxytryptamine (5-HT_3) receptor antagonist with anti-emetic activity.

Dosage and administration *INFUSION:* Kytril ampoules are for intravenous administration only.

Adults: 3 mg Kytril, which should be administered *either* in 15 ml infusion fluid as an intravenous bolus over not less than 30 seconds *or* diluted in 20 to 50 ml infusion fluid and administered over five minutes.

Prevention: In clinical trials, the majority of patients have required only a single dose of Kytril to control nausea and vomiting over 24 hours. Up to two additional doses of 3 mg Kytril may be administered within a 24-hour period. There is clinical experience in patients receiving daily administration for up to five consecutive days in one course of therapy. Prophylactic administration of Kytril should be completed prior to the start of cytostatic therapy.

Treatment: The same dose of Kytril should be used for treatment as for prevention. Additional doses should be administered at least 10 minutes apart.

Maximum daily dosage: Up to three doses of 3 mg Kytril may be administered within a 24-hour period. The maximum dose of Kytril to be administered over 24 hours should not exceed 9 mg.

Concomitant use of dexamethasone: The efficacy of Kytril may be enhanced by the addition of dexamethasone.

Elderly: No special requirements apply to elderly patients.

Children: Prevention: A single dose of 40 mcg/kg body weight (up to 3 mg) should be administered as an intravenous infusion, diluted in 10 to 30 ml infusion fluid and administered over five minutes. Administration should be completed prior to the start of cytostatic therapy.

Treatment: The same dose of Kytril as above should be used for treatment as for prevention.

One additional dose of 40 mcg/kg body weight (up to 3 mg) may be administered within a 24-hour period. This additional dose should be administered at least 10 minutes apart from the initial infusion.

Patients with renal or hepatic impairment: No special requirements apply to those patients with renal or hepatic impairment.

Administration: Adults: To prepare a dose of 3 mg, 3 ml is withdrawn from the ampoule and diluted either to 15 ml with 0.9% w/v Sodium Chloride Injection BP (for bolus administration) or in infusion fluid to a total volume of 20 to 50 ml in any of the following solutions: 0.9% w/v Sodium Chloride Injection BP; 0.18% w/v Sodium Chloride and 4% w/v Glucose Injection BP; 5% w/v Glucose Injection BP; Hartmann's Solution for Injection BP; Sodium Lactate Injection BP; or 10% Mannitol Injection BP (for infusion). No other diluents should be used.

Children: To prepare the dose of 40 mcg/kg the appropriate volume (up to 3 ml) is withdrawn from the ampoule and diluted with infusion fluid (as for adults) to a total volume of 10 to 30 ml.

Contra-indications, warnings, etc.
Contra-indication: Hypersensitivity to granisetron or related substances.

Precautions: As Kytril may reduce lower bowel motility, patients with signs of subacute intestinal obstruction should be monitored following administration of Kytril.

There has been no evidence from human studies that Kytril has any adverse effect on alertness.

Data from two-year carcinogenicity studies have shown an increase in hepatocellular carcinoma and/or adenoma in rats and mice of both sexes given 50 mg/kg (rat dosage reduced to 25 mg/kg/day at week 59). Increases in hepatocellular neoplasia were also detected at 5 mg/kg in male rats. In both species, drug-induced effects (hepatocellular neoplasia) were not observed in the low-dose group (1 mg/kg).

In several *in vitro* and *in vivo* assays, Kytril was shown to be non-genotoxic in mammalian cells.

Drug interactions: In studies in healthy subjects, no evidence of any interaction has been indicated between Kytril and cimetidine or lorazepam. No evidence of drug interactions has been observed in clinical studies.

Use in pregnancy and lactation: Whilst animal studies have shown no teratogenic effects, there is no experience of Kytril in human pregnancy. Therefore Kytril should not be administered to women who are pregnant unless there are compelling clinical reasons. There are no data on the excretion of Kytril in breast milk. Breast feeding should therefore be discontinued during therapy.

Adverse reactions: Kytril has been generally well tolerated in human studies. As reported with other drugs of this class, headache and constipation have been the most frequently noted adverse events, but the majority have been mild or moderate in nature. Rare cases of hypersensitivity reaction, occasionally severe (e.g. anaphylaxis), have been reported. Other allergic reactions including minor skin rashes have also been reported. In clinical trials, transient increases in hepatic transaminases, generally within the normal range, have been seen.

Overdosage: There is no specific antidote for Kytril. In the case of overdosage, symptomatic treatment should be given. One patient has received 10 times the recommended intravenous dose of Kytril The patient reported a slight headache but no other sequelae were observed.

Pharmaceutical precautions Ampoules removed from the pack should be protected from direct sunlight. Do not freeze.

Ideally, intravenous infusions of Kytril should be prepared at the time of administration. After dilution (see **Dosage and administration**) the shelf-life is 24 hours when stored at ambient temperature in normal indoor illumination protected from direct sunlight. It must not be used after 24 hours. If to be stored after preparation, Kytril infusions must be prepared under appropriate aseptic conditions.

As a general precaution, Kytril should not be mixed in solution with other drugs.

Legal category POM.

Package quantities Ampoules in boxes of five and 10.

Further information This Data Sheet supersedes the entry in the ABPI *Data Sheet Compendium* 1998-99.

Kytril is widely distributed with plasma protein binding of approximately 65%. It is rapidly and extensively metabolised mainly by N-demethylation and aromatic ring oxidation followed by conjugation; excretion is both urinary and faecal.

The inactive ingredients in the infusion are sodium chloride and Water for Injections PhEur.

Product licence number PL 10592/0003.

KYTRIL* TABLETS 1 mg and 2 mg

Qualitative and quantitative composition Granisetron hydrochloride equivalent to 1 mg or 2 mg granisetron (free base equivalent).

Pharmaceutical form Kytril is presented as white triangular film-coated tablets containing 1 mg or 2 mg granisetron free base equivalent.

Clinical particulars
Therapeutic indications: Kytril tablets are indicated for the prevention of nausea and vomiting induced by cytostatic therapy.

Posology and method of administration:
Adults: The dose of Kytril is 1 mg twice a day or 2 mg once a day during cytostatic therapy.

The first dose of Kytril should be administered within one hour before the start of cytostatic therapy.

Concomitant use of dexamethasone: The efficacy of Kytril may be enhanced by the addition of dexamethasone.

Maximum dose and duration of treatment: Kytril is also available as ampoules for intravenous administration. The maximum dose of Kytril administered orally and/or intravenously over 24 hours should not exceed 9 mg.

Children: There is insufficient evidence on which to base appropriate dosage regimens for children under 12 years old. Kytril tablets are therefore not recommended in this age group.

Elderly: As for adults.
Renally impaired: As for adults.
Hepatically impaired: As for adults.

Contra-indications: Kytril is contra-indicated in patients hypersensitive to granisetron or related substances.

Special warnings and special precautions for use: As Kytril may reduce lower bowel motility, patients with signs of sub-acute intestinal obstruction should be monitored following administration of Kytril.

Interaction with other medicaments and other forms of interaction: In studies in healthy subjects, no evidence of any interaction has been indicated between Kytril and cimetidine or lorazepam. No evidence of drug interactions has been observed in clinical studies.

Pregnancy and lactation: Whilst animal studies have shown no teratogenic effects, there is no experience of Kytril in human pregnancy. Therefore Kytril should not be administered to women who are pregnant unless there are compelling clinical reasons. There are no data on the excretion of Kytril in breast milk. Breast feeding should therefore be discontinued during therapy.

Effects on ability to drive and use machines: There has been no evidence from human studies that Kytril has any adverse effect on alertness.

Undesirable effects: Kytril has been generally well tolerated in human studies. As reported with other drugs of this class, headache and constipation have been the most frequently noted adverse events, but the majority have been mild or moderate in nature. Rare cases of hypersensitivity reaction, occasionally severe (e.g. anaphylaxis), have been reported. Other allergic reactions including minor skin rashes have also been reported. In clinical trials, transient increases in hepatic transaminases, generally within the normal range, have been seen.

Overdose: There is no specific antidote for Kytril. In the case of overdosage, symptomatic treatment should be given. One patient has received 30 mg of Kytril intravenously. The patient reported a slight headache but no other sequelae were observed.

Pharmacological properties
Pharmacodynamic properties: Kytril is a potent anti-emetic and highly selective antagonist of 5-hydroxytryptamine (5-HT_3) receptors. Radioligand binding studies have demonstrated that Kytril has negligible affinity for other receptor types including 5-HT and dopamine D_2 binding sites.

Kytril is effective orally prophylactically in abolishing the retching and vomiting evoked by cytostatic therapy.

Pharmacokinetic properties:
General characteristics:
Absorption: Absorption of Kytril is rapid and complete, though oral bioavailability is reduced to about 60% as a result of first pass metabolism. Oral bioavailability is generally not influenced by food.

Distribution: Kytril is extensively distributed, with a mean volume of distribution of approximately 3 l/kg; plasma protein binding is approximately 65%.

Biotransformation: Biotransformation pathways involve N-demethylation and aromatic ring oxidation followed by conjugation.

Elimination: Clearance is predominantly by hepatic metabolism. Urinary excretion of unchanged Kytril averages 12% of dose whilst that of metabolites amounts to about 47% of dose. The remainder is excreted in faeces as metabolites. Mean plasma half-life in patients is approximately nine hours, with a wide inter-subject variability.

The pharmacokinetics of Kytril demonstrate no marked deviations from linear pharmacokinetics at oral doses up to 2.5-fold of the recommended clinical dose.

Characteristics in patients: The plasma concentration of Kytril is not clearly correlated with anti-emetic efficacy. Clinical benefit may be conferred even when Kytril is not detectable in plasma.

In elderly subjects after single intravenous doses, pharmacokinetic parameters were within the range found for non-elderly subjects. In patients with severe renal failure, data indicate that pharmacokinetic parameters after a single intravenous dose are generally similar to those in normal subjects. In patients with hepatic impairment due to neoplastic liver involvement, total plasma clearance of an intravenous dose was approximately halved compared to patients without hepatic involvement. Despite these changes, no dosage adjustment is necessary.

Preclinical safety data: Data from two-year carcinogenicity studies have shown an increase in hepatocellular carcinoma and/or adenoma in rats and mice of both sexes given 50 mg/kg (rat dosage reduced to 25 mg/kg/day at week 59). Increases in hepatocellular neoplasia were also detected at 5 mg/kg in male rats. In both species, drug-induced effects (hepatocellular neoplasia) were not observed in the low-dose group (1 mg/kg).

In several *in vitro* and *in vivo* assays, Kytril was shown to be non-genotoxic in mammalian cells.

Pharmaceutical particulars
List of excipients: Microcrystalline Cellulose NF, Sodium Starch Glycollate BP, Hydroxypropyl Methylcellulose 2910 USP, Lactose PhEur, Magnesium Stearate PhEur.

Film coat: Hydroxypropyl Methylcellulose PhEur, Titanium Dioxide PhEur (E171), Polyethylene Glycol NF, Polysorbate 80 PhEur.

Incompatibilities: None.

Shelf-life: Kytril Tablets have a shelf-life of two years.

Special precautions for storage: None.

Nature and contents of container: Kytril is supplied in opaque blister packs packed in cartons containing 5 (2 mg) tablets or 10 (1 mg) tablets.

Instructions for use/handling: None.

Marketing authorisation holder: SmithKline Beecham plc, SB House, Great West Road, Brentford, Middlesex TW8 9BD.
Trading as SmithKline Beecham Pharmaceuticals Mundells, Welwyn Garden City, Hertfordshire AL7 1EY.

Marketing authorisation numbers
Kytril Tablets 1 mg PL 10592/0032.
Kytril Tablets 2 mg PL 10592/0067.

Date of first authorisation/renewal of authorisation
Kytril Tablets 1 mg 4.1.94.
Kytril Tablets 2 mg 26.2.96.

Date of (partial) revision of the text June 1996.

Legal category POM.

KYTRIL* PAEDIATRIC LIQUID

Qualitative and quantitative composition Granisetron hydrochloride equivalent to 200 mcg granisetron (free base equivalent) per 1 ml.

Pharmaceutical form An orange coloured and flavoured clear solution equivalent to 200 mcg of granisetron free base per 1 ml.

Clinical particulars
Therapeutic indications: Kytril Paediatric Liquid is indicated for the prevention of nausea and vomiting induced by cytostatic therapy.

Posology and method of administration:
Children: A single dose of 20 mcg/kg bodyweight (up to 1 mg) twice a day up to five days during cytostatic therapy. The first dose of Kytril should be administered within one hour before the start of cytostatic therapy.

Patients with renal or hepatic impairment: No special requirements apply.

Contra-indications: Hypersensitivity to granisetron, or related substances, or any of the other constituents.

Special warnings and special precautions for use: As Kytril may reduce lower bowel motility, patients with signs of sub-acute intestinal obstruction should be monitored following administration of Kytril.

Interaction with other medicaments and other forms of interaction: In studies in healthy subjects, no evidence of any interaction has been indicated between Kytril and cimetidine or lorazepam. No evidence of drug interactions has been observed in clinical studies.

Pregnancy and lactation: Whilst animal studies have shown no teratogenic effects, there is no experience of Kytril in human pregnancy. Therefore Kytril should not be administered to women who are pregnant unless there are compelling clinical reasons. There are no data on the excretion of Kytril in breast milk. Breast feeding should therefore be discontinued during therapy.

Effects on ability to drive and use machines: There has been no evidence from human studies that Kytril has any adverse effect on alertness.

Undesirable effects: Kytril has been generally well tolerated in human studies. As reported with other drugs of this class, headache and constipation have been the most frequently noted adverse events but the majority have been mild or moderate in nature. Rare cases of hypersensitivity reaction, occasionally severe (e.g. anaphylaxis) have been reported. Other allergic reactions including minor skin rashes have also been reported. In clinical trials transient increases in hepatic transaminases, generally within the normal range, have been seen.

Overdose: There is no specific antidote for Kytril. In the case of overdosage, symptomatic treatment should be given. One patient has received 30 mg of Kytril intravenously. The patient reported a slight headache but no other sequelae were observed.

Pharmacological properties
Pharmacodynamic properties: Kytril is a potent anti-emetic and highly selective antagonist of 5-hydroxytryptamine (5-HT_3) receptors. Radioligand binding studies have demonstrated that Kytril has negligible affinity for other receptor types including 5-HT and dopamine D_2 binding sites.

Kytril is effective orally prophylactically in prevention of the retching and vomiting evoked by cytostatic therapy.

Pharmacokinetic properties:
General characteristics: Absorption: Absorption of Kytril is rapid and complete, though oral bioavailability is reduced to about 60% as a result of first pass metabolism. Oral bioavailability is generally not influenced by food.

Distribution: Kytril is extensively distributed, with a mean volume of distribution of approximately 3 l/kg; plasma protein binding is approximately 65%.

Biotransformation: Biotransformation pathways involve N-demethylation and aromatic ring oxidation followed by conjugation.

Elimination: Clearance is predominantly by hepatic metabolism. Urinary excretion of unchanged Kytril averages 12% of dose whilst that of metabolites amounts to about 47% of dose. The remainder is excreted in faeces as metabolites. Mean plasma half-life in patients is approximately nine hours, with a wide inter-subject variability.

Characteristics in patients: The plasma concentration of Kytril is not clearly correlated with anti-emetic efficacy. Clinical benefit may be conferred even when Kytril is not detectable in plasma.

In elderly subjects after single intravenous doses, pharmacokinetic parameters were within the range found for non-elderly subjects. In patients with severe renal failure, data indicate that pharmacokinetic parameters after a single intravenous dose are generally similar to those in normal subjects. In patients with hepatic impairment due to neoplastic liver involvement, total plasma clearance of an intravenous dose was approximately halved compared to patients without hepatic involvement. Despite these changes, no dosage adjustment is necessary.

In children, after single intravenous doses, pharmacokinetics are similar to those in adults when appropriate parameters (volume of distribution, total plasma clearance) are normalised for body-weight.

Preclinical safety data: Data from two-year carcinogenicity studies have shown an increase in hepatocellular carcinoma and/or adenoma in rats and mice of both sexes given 50 mg/kg (rat dosage reduced to 25 mg/kg/day at week 59). Increases in hepatocellular neoplasia were also detected at 5 mg/kg in male rats. In both species, drug-induced effects (hepatocellular neoplasia) were not observed in the low-dose group (1 mg/kg).

In several *in vitro* and *in vivo* assays, Kytril was shown to be non-genotoxic in mammalian cells.

Pharmaceutical particulars

List of excipients: Sorbitol PhEur; Sodium Benzoate (E211) PhEur; Citric Acid Anhydrous PhEur; Orange Flavour D3798 HSE; Orange Flavour D2362 HSE; F.D. & C Yellow No. 6 (E 110) HSE; Purified Water PhEur.

Incompatibilities: Not applicable.

Shelf-life: Unopened: two years.

After opening for the first time: one month.

Special precautions for storage: Kytril Paediatric Liquid should be stored at or below 30°C and capped after partial use.

Nature and contents of container: Kytril Paediatric Liquid is supplied in a 30 ml amber glass bottle with a child-resistant high-density polyethylene cap with a PVdC faced boxboard wad. The bottle contains 30 ml of solution and is enclosed in an outer carton.

Instructions for use/handling:

Administering the oral solution: *Children:* To administer the dose of 20 mcg/kg, 0.1 ml of solution per one kilogram of body weight should be withdrawn from the bottle up to a maximum of 5 ml per dose.

An oral dosing syringe should be used. When administering the measured dose, insert the syringe tip into the child's mouth and drip the medicine in slowly.

Marketing authorisation number 10592/0077.

Date of approval/revision of SPC March 1996.

Legal category POM.

KYTRIL* AMPOULES 1 mg/1 ml

Qualitative and quantitative composition Ampoule: Granisetron hydrochloride equivalent to 1.0 mg granisetron (free base equivalent).

Pharmaceutical form A glass ampoule containing a sterile, clear solution equivalent to 1 mg of granisetron free base per 1 ml of isotonic saline. The content allows withdrawal of 1 ml. A 15% filling overage is included.

Active constituent: INN: Granisetron.

Clinical particulars

Therapeutic indications: Kytril is indicated for the prevention or treatment of nausea and vomiting induced by cytostatic therapy and for the prevention and treatment of post-operative nausea and vomiting.

Posology and method of administration:

Cytostatic therapy:

Children: Prevention: A single dose of 40 mcg/kg bodyweight (up to 3 mg) should be administered as an intravenous infusion, diluted in 10 to 30 ml infusion fluid and administered over five minutes. Administration should be completed prior to the start of cytostatic therapy.

Treatment: The same dose of Kytril as above should be used for treatment as prevention.

One additional dose of 40 mcg/kg bodyweight (up to 3 mg) may be administered within a 24-hour period if required. This additional dose should be administered at least 10 minutes apart from the initial infusion.

Renally impaired: No special requirements apply.

Hepatically impaired: No special requirements apply.

Post-operative nausea and vomiting:

Adults: For prevention in adults, a single dose of 1 mg of Kytril should be diluted to 5 ml and administered as a slow intravenous injection (over 30 seconds). Administration should be completed prior to induction of anaesthesia.

For the treatment of established post-operative nausea and vomiting in adults, a single dose of 1 mg of Kytril should be diluted to 5 ml and administered by slow intravenous injection (over 30 seconds).

Maximum dose and duration of treatment: Two doses (2 mg) in one day.

Children: There is no experience in the use of Kytril in the prevention and treatment of post-operative nausea and vomiting in children. Kytril is not therefore recommended for the treatment of post-operative nausea and vomiting in this age group.

Elderly: As for adults.

Renally impaired: As for adults.

Hepatically impaired: As for adults.

Contra-indications: Hypersensitivity to granisetron or related substances.

Special warnings and special precautions for use: As Kytril may reduce lower bowel motility, patients with signs of sub-acute intestinal obstruction should be monitored following administration of Kytril.

No special precautions are required for the elderly or renally or hepatically impaired patient.

Interaction with other medicaments and other forms of interaction: In studies in healthy subjects, no evidence of any interaction has been indicated between Kytril and cimetidine or lorazepam. No evidence of drug interactions has been observed in clinical studies conducted.

No specific interaction studies have been conducted in anaesthetised patients, but Kytril has been safely administered with commonly used anaesthetic and analgesic agents. In addition, *in vitro* human microsomal studies have shown that the cytochrome P_{450} sub-family 3A4 (involved in the metabolism of some of the main narcotic analgesic agents) is not modified by Kytril.

Pregnancy and lactation: Whilst animal studies have shown no teratogenic effects, there is no experience of Kytril in human pregnancy. Therefore Kytril should not be administered to women who are pregnant unless there are compelling clinical reasons. There are no data on the excretion of Kytril in breast milk. Breast feeding should therefore be discontinued during therapy.

Effects on ability to drive and use machines: There has been no evidence from human studies that Kytril has any adverse effect on alertness.

Undesirable effects: Kytril has been generally well tolerated in human studies. As reported with other drugs of this class, headache and constipation have been the most frequently noted adverse events but the majority have been mild or moderate in nature. Rare cases of hypersensitivity reaction, occasionally severe (e.g. anaphylaxis) have been reported. Other allergic reactions including minor skin rashes have also been reported. In clinical trials, transient increases in hepatic transaminases, generally within the normal range, have been seen.

Overdose: There is no specific antidote for Kytril. In the case of overdosage, symptomatic treatment should be given. One patient has received 30 mg of Kytril intravenously. The patient reported a slight headache but no other sequelae were observed.

Pharmacological properties

Pharmacodynamic properties: Kytril is a potent anti-emetic and highly selective antagonist of 5-hydroxytryptamine ($5\text{-}HT_3$) receptors. Radioligand binding studies have demonstrated that Kytril has negligible affinity for other receptor types including 5-HT and dopamine D_2 binding sites.

Kytril is effective intravenously, either prophylactically or by intervention, in abolishing the retching and vomiting evoked by administration of cytotoxic drugs or by whole body X-irradiation.

Kytril is effective, intravenously, in the prevention and treatment of post-operative nausea and vomiting.

Pharmacokinetic properties

General characteristics

Distribution: Kytril is extensively distributed, with a mean volume of distribution of approximately 3 l/kg; plasma protein binding is approximately 65%.

Biotransformation: Biotransformation pathways involve N-demethylation and aromatic ring oxidation followed by conjugation.

Elimination: Clearance is predominantly by hepatic metabolism. Urinary excretion of unchanged Kytril averages 12% of dose whilst that of metabolites amounts to about 47% of dose. The remainder is excreted in faeces as metabolites. Mean plasma half-life in patients is approximately nine hours, with a wide inter-subject variability.

Characteristics in patients: The plasma concentration of Kytril is not clearly correlated with antiemetic efficacy. Clinical benefit may be conferred even when Kytril is not detectable in plasma.

In elderly subjects after single intravenous doses, pharmacokinetic parameters were within the range found for non-elderly subjects. In patients with severe renal failure, data indicate that pharmacokinetic parameters after a single intravenous dose are generally similar to those in normal subjects. In patients with hepatic impairment due to neoplastic liver involvement, total plasma clearance of an intravenous dose was approximately halved compared to patients without hepatic involvement. Despite these changes, no dosage adjustment is necessary.

Preclinical safety data: Data from two-year carcinogenicity studies have shown an increase in hepatocellular carcinoma and/or adenoma in rats and mice of both sexes given 50 mg/kg (rat dosage reduced to 25 mg/kg/day at week 59). Increases in hepatocellular neoplasia were also detected at 5 mg/kg in male rats. In both species, drug-induced effects (hepatocellular neoplasia) were not observed in the low-dose group (1 mg/kg).

In several *in vitro* and *in vivo* assays, Kytril was shown to be non-genotoxic in mammalian cells.

Pharmaceutical particulars

List of excipients: Sodium Chloride PhEur, Water for Injection PhEur.

Incompatibilities: As a general precaution, Kytril should not be mixed in solution with other drugs. Prophylactic administration of Kytril should be completed prior to the start of cytostatic therapy or induction of anaesthesia.

Shelf-life: Kytril ampoules have a shelf-life of three years.

Special precautions for storage: Kytril ampoules should be stored protected from light below 30°C. Do not freeze.

Nature and contents of container: Kytril is supplied in clear glass ampoules packaged either individually or in packs of five, with an outer carton.

Instructions for use/handling:

Preparing the infusion:

Children: To prepare the dose of 40 mcg/kg, the appropriate volume is withdrawn and diluted with infusion fluid to a total volume of 10 to 30 ml. Any one of the following solutions may be used: 0.9% w/v Sodium Chloride Injection BP; 0.18% w/v Sodium Chloride and 4% w/v Glucose Injection BP; 5% w/v Glucose Injection BP; Hartmann's Solution for Injection BP; Sodium Lactate Injection BP; or 10% Mannitol Injection BP. No other diluents should be used.

Ideally, intravenous infusions of Kytril should be prepared at the time of administration. After dilution (see above), or when the container is opened for the first time, the shelf-life is 24 hours when stored at ambient temperature in normal indoor illumination protected from direct sunlight. It must not be used after 24 hours. If to be stored after preparation, 'Kytril' infusions must be prepared under appropriate aseptic conditions.

Adults: to prepare a dose of 1 mg, 1 ml should be withdrawn from the ampoule and diluted to 5 ml with 0.9% w/v Sodium Chloride Injection BP. No other diluent should be used.

Marketing authorisation holder: SmithKline Beecham plc, SB House, Great West Road, Brentford, Middlesex TW8 9BD.

Marketing authorisation number PL 10592/0063.

Date of first authorisation/renewal of authorisation 23rd October 1995.

Date of revision of the text January 1997

Legal category POM.

LISKONUM* TABLETS

Qualitative and quantitative composition Liskonum Tablets are available in one strength. Each tablet contains 450 mg lithium carbonate (12.2 mmol Li^+) in controlled-release form.

Pharmaceutical form White, oblong, film-coated tablets, with convex faces and a breakline on both sides.

Clinical particulars

Therapeutic indications: Liskonum is a controlled-release tablet, designed to reduce fluctuations in serum lithium levels and the likelihood of adverse reactions.

It is indicated for the treatment of acute episodes of mania or hypomania and for the prophylaxis of recurrent manic-depressive illness.

Posology and method of administration:

Dosage: Adults only: Liskonum should be given twice a day.

Treatment of acute mania or hypomania: Patients should be started on one or one-and-a-half tablets twice a day. Dosage should then be adjusted to achieve a serum lithium level of 0.8 to a maximum of 1.5 mmol/l. Serum concentration of lithium should be measured after four to seven days' treatment and then at least once a week until dosage has remained constant for four weeks. When the acute symptoms have been controlled, recommendations for prophylaxis should be followed.

Prophylaxis: The usual starting dosage is one tablet twice a day. Dosage should then be adjusted until a serum level of 0.5 to 1.0 mmol/l is maintained. Serum concentration of lithium should be measured after four to seven days' treatment and then every week until dosage has remained constant for four weeks. Frequency of monitoring may then be gradually decreased to a minimum of once every two months, but should be increased following any situation where changes in lithium levels are possible (see *Warnings and precautions*).

Blood samples for measurement of serum lithium concentration should be taken just before a dose is due and not less than 12 hours after the previous dose.

Levels of more than 2 mmol/l *must* be avoided.

Elderly: Use with caution. Start with half a tablet twice a day and adjust serum levels to the lower end of the above ranges (see also *Warnings and precautions*).

The full prophylactic effect of lithium may not be evident for six to 12 months, and treatment should be continued through any recurrence of the illness.

Administration: Oral.

Contra-indications: Do not use in patients with impaired renal function, cardiac disease, or untreated hypothyroidism. Lithium should not be given to patients with low body sodium levels, including, for example, dehydrated patients, those on low sodium diets, or those with Addison's disease.

Special warnings and special precautions for use: Vomiting, diarrhoea, intercurrent infection, fluid deprivation and drugs likely to upset electrolyte balance, such as diuretics, may all reduce lithium excretion and thereby precipitate intoxication; reduction of dosage may be required. In elderly patients, lithium excretion may also be reduced.

The possibility of hypothyroidism and of renal dysfunction arising during prolonged treatment should be borne in mind and periodic assessments made.

Patients should be warned of the symptoms of impending intoxication (see *Undesirable effects*), of the urgency of immediate action should these symptoms appear, and also of the need to maintain a constant and adequate salt and water intake.

Interaction with other medicaments and other forms of interaction: Diuretics should only be used with caution during treatment; thiazides show a paradoxical antidiuretic effect resulting in possible water retention and lithium intoxication. Concomitant use with NSAIDs can increase serum lithium concentrations, possibly resulting in lithium toxicity; serum lithium concentrations should therefore be monitored more frequently if NSAID therapy is initiated or discontinued.

There have been reports of interaction between lithium and some neuroleptics, particularly haloperidol at higher dosages, also between lithium and methyldopa or phenytoin. Fluvoxamine and fluoxetine should be combined with lithium with care.

Pregnancy and lactation: Lithium crosses the placental barrier. In animal studies, lithium has been reported to interfere with fertility, gestation and foetal development. There is epidemiological evidence that the drug may be harmful in human pregnancy. Lithium therapy should not be used during pregnancy, especially during the first trimester, unless considered essential. In certain cases where a severe risk to the patient could exist if treatment were to be stopped, lithium has been continued during pregnancy. If given, however, serum levels should be measured frequently because of the changes in renal function associated with pregnancy and parturition.

Since lithium is secreted in breast milk, bottle feeding is advisable.

Effects on ability to drive and use machines: None.

Undesirable effects: At therapeutic serum levels, mild nausea and diarrhoea, fine tremor of the hands, muscle weakness, vertigo, giddiness, weight gain, oedema and a dazed feeling may occur. Hypothyroidism has been reported. Rarely hyperthyroidism may occur and mild hyperparathyroidism has been reported. Mild polyuria and polydipsia are not infrequent and, occasionally, nephrogenic diabetes insipidus may be present. Histological renal changes, with interstitial fibrosis, have been observed in some patients on long-term treatment; whilst there may be an association with impaired reabsorption, a relationship between these changes and a reduction in glomerular filtration rate or development of renal insufficiency has not been established.

Skin reactions including acne or acneiform eruptions, papular skin disorders, rashes, and exacerbation of psoriasis have been reported.

Intoxication: Vomiting, diarrhoea, drowsiness, lack of co-ordination and/or a coarse tremor of the extremities and lower jaw may occur, especially with serum levels above the therapeutic range. Ataxia, giddiness, blurred vision, dysarthria, tinnitus, muscle hyperirritability, choreoathetoid movements and toxic psychosis have also been described.

If any of the above symptoms appear, treatment should be stopped immediately and arrangements made for serum lithium measurement.

Overdose: Symptoms are similar to those listed in *Undesirable effects* section under intoxication but more marked, particularly those of central nervous system origin. In severe cases, seizures, coma and death may ensue.

Treatment consists of the induction of vomiting and/or gastric lavage together with supportive and symptomatic measures. Particular attention should be paid to maintenance of fluid and electrolyte balance and of adequate renal function. Where convulsions are present, diazepam may be used. Forced alkaline diuresis, peritoneal dialysis or haemodialysis may help eliminate the lithium ion. The latter method is preferable, particularly where serum lithium exceeds 4 mmol/l.

Pharmacological properties

Pharmacodynamic properties: Lithium carbonate is used as a source of lithium ions. The mechanism by which it exerts its effect in affective disorders is not known but may be related to inhibition of neurotransmitter receptor mediated processes involving beta-adrenoceptors. It is used in the treatment of acute episodes of mania or hypomania and for prophylaxis of recurrent manic depressive illness.

Pharmacokinetic properties: Lithium is readily absorbed from the gastrointestinal tract, and is distributed throughout the body over a period of several hours. Lithium is excreted almost exclusively in the kidneys but can also be detected in sweat and saliva. It is not bound to plasma proteins. It crosses the placenta, and is excreted in breast milk. The half-life of non-sustained lithium varies considerably, but generally is considered to be about 12 to 24 hours following a single dose. It is however increased for example in those with renal impairment and with age, and may increase significantly during long-term therapy.

Preclinical safety data: Not applicable

Pharmaceutical particulars

List of excipients: Povidone; Maize Starch; Lactose; Gelatin; Calcium Carboxymethylcellulose; Talcum (E553Cb); Calcium Arachinate; Titanium Dioxide (E171); Magnesium Stearate (E572); Polyethylene Glycol 6000; Eudragit (E12.5).

Incompatibilities: Not applicable.

Shelf-life: Liskonum Tablets have a shelf-life of five years.

Special precautions for storage: Store below 25°C.

Nature and contents of container : Opaque Blister Packs (OP) of 60 (6 x 10) tablets.

Instructions for use/handling: Tablets may be halved but should not be chewed or broken up.

Marketing authorisation number 0002/0083

Date of approval/revision of SPC January 1998

Legal category POM.

MAGNAPEN* CAPSULES
MAGNAPEN* SYRUP
MAGNAPEN* VIALS FOR INJECTION

Qualitative and quantitative composition *Magnapen Capsules* contain 250 mg ampicillin as Ampicillin Trihydrate EP with 250 mg flucloxacillin as Flucloxacillin Sodium BP (co-fluampicil 250/250).

Magnapen Syrup when reconstituted each 5 ml contains 125 mg ampicillin as Ampicillin Trihydrate BP with 125 mg flucloxacillin as Flucloxacillin Magnesium BP (co-fluampicil 125/125).

Magnapen 500 mg Vials contain 250 mg ampicillin as Ampicillin Sodium BP with 250 mg flucloxacillin as Flucloxacillin Sodium BP (co-fluampicil 250/250).

Pharmaceutical form *Capsules:* Black and turquoise capsules overprinted 'Magnapen'.

Syrup: Bottles containing powder for the preparation of 100 ml suspension.

Injection: Vials containing powder for reconstitution for parenteral administration.

Clinical particulars

Therapeutic indications: Magnapen is indicated for the treatment of severe infections where the causative organism is unknown, and for mixed infections involving β-lactamase-producing staphylococci. Typical indications include:

In general practice: Chest infections, ENT infections, skin and soft tissue infections, and infections in patients whose underlying pathology places them at special risk.

In hospital (prior to laboratory results being available): Severe respiratory tract infections, post-operative chest and wound infections; septic abortion, puerperal fever; septicaemia, prophylaxis in major surgery, infections in patients receiving immuno-suppressive therapy.

The spectrum of activity of Magnapen also makes it suitable for the treatment of many mixed infections, particularly those where β-lactamase-producing staphylococci are suspected or confirmed.

Parenteral usage is indicated where oral dosage is inappropriate.

Posology and method of administration:

Usual adult dosage (including elderly patients):

Oral: One capsule or 10 ml syrup four times a day.

Intramuscular/Intravenous: 500 mg four times a day.

Usual children's dosage:

Oral: Under 10 years: 5 ml syrup four times a day*.

Intramuscular/Intravenous: Under two years: quarter adult dose*.

Two to 10 years: half adult dose.

The above dosages for adults and children may be doubled where necessary.

Therapy may be continued for as long as it is indicated by the nature of the infection.

Oral doses should be administered half to one hour before meals.

Administration: Intramuscular: 500 mg Vial: add 1.5 ml Water for Injections BP to vial contents.

Intravenous: Dissolve 500 mg in 10 ml Water for Injections BP. Administer by slow intravenous injection (three to four minutes). Magnapen Injection may be added to infusion fluids or injected, suitably diluted into the drip tube over a period of three to four minutes.

* Ampiclox Neonatal is recommended for the treatment of infections in neonates and premature babies.

Contra-indications: Penicillin hypersensitivity, ocular administration.

Special warnings and special precautions for use: None known.

Interaction with other medicaments and other forms of interaction: None known.

Pregnancy and lactation: Animal studies have shown no teratogenic effects. The product has been in clinical use since 1971 and the limited number of reported cases of use in human pregnancy have shown no evidence of untoward effect. The use of Magnapen in pregnancy should be reserved for cases considered essential by the clinician. During lactation, trace quantities of penicillins can be detected in breast milk.

Effects on ability to drive and use machines: None known.

Undesirable effects: Side effects, as with other penicillins, are uncommon and mainly of a mild and transitory nature. Gastro-intestinal upsets (e.g. nausea, diarrhoea) and skin rashes have been reported. An urticarial rash suggests penicillin hypersensitivity; an erythematous rash may arise in patients receiving ampicillin who have glandular fever. If a skin rash occurs, treatment should be discontinued.

Hepatitis and cholestatic jaundice have been reported in association with flucloxacillin. These reactions are related neither to the dose nor to the route of administration. The onset of these effects may be delayed for up to two months post-treatment: in several cases, the course of the reactions has been protracted and lasted for some months. In very rare cases, a fatal outcome has been reported.

Pseudomembranous colitis has been reported rarely. In common with other β-lactam antibiotics angioedema and anaphylaxis have been reported.

Overdose: Problems of overdosage with Magnapen are unlikely to occur; if encountered they may be treated symptomatically.

Pharmacological properties

Pharmacodynamic properties: Infections encountered in medical practice can be of mixed bacteriology, often including β-lactamase-producing strains. Magnapen provides a broad spectrum of activity, which should be considered when dealing with such infections.

Pharmacokinetic properties: Magnapen is excreted via the kidneys with a plasma half-life of approximately one hour.

Both ampicillin and flucloxacillin have been shown to attain therapeutic serum levels following oral administration of Magnapen and the serum levels achieved are comparable with those which could be expected as a result of administering each penicillin separately.

Preclinical safety data: Not relevant

Pharmaceutical particulars
List of excipients:
Capsules: Magnesium Stearate

Capsule Shells: Gelatin, Black Iron Oxide (E172), Titanium Dioxide (E171), Patent Blue V (E131), Quinoline Yellow (E104)

Syrup: Disodium Edetate, Blood Orange Dry Flavour, Menthol Dry Flavour, Monoammonium Glycyrrhizinate, Sodium Benzoate (E211), Carmellose Sodium Dried, Sodium Citrate Anhydrous, Saccharin Sodium Dried, Sucrose

Injection: None

Incompatibilities: Magnapen should not be mixed with blood products or other proteinaceous fluids (e.g. protein hydrolysates) or with intravenous lipid emulsions.

If Magnapen is prescribed concurrently with an aminoglycoside, the antibiotics should not be mixed in the syringe, intravenous fluid container or giving set because of loss of activity of the aminoglycoside can occur under these conditions.

Shelf-life: Capsules: Two years.

Powder: Three years.

Once dispensed, Magnapen Syrup remains stable for 14 days.

Injection: Three years.

Special precautions for storage: Magnapen Syrup powder should be stored in a dry place.

Once dispensed Magnapen Syrup should be kept in a cool place (15°C)

Magnapen Capsules should be stored in a cool dry place and kept tightly closed. The foil and blister packs should be stored in a dry place at 25°C or below.

Magnapen Vials for Injection should be stored in a cool dry place.

Nature and contents of container:
Capsules: Standard polypropylene tube with a polythene closure or standard aluminium canisters or glass bottles fitted with a screw cap with a waxed pulpboard wad. Pack sizes of 20, 50, 100 or 500.

Aluminium foil pack. Pack size 12 capsules
Aluminium/PVC blister pack with aluminium overseal. Pack size 28 capsules.

Syrup: Clear glass Winchester bottles fitted with 28 mm Flavor–Lok caps. Original pack of 100 ml with Patient Information Leaflet.

Vials: 5 ml glass vials fitted with butyl rubber disc and an aluminium seal. Boxes of 10 vials with instructions for use.

Instructions for use/handling:
Syrup: If dilution of the reconstituted suspension is required, Syrup BP should be used.

Injection: Magnapen solutions for injection should be used immediately.
Magnapen may be added to most intravenous fluids (e.g. Water for Injections, sodium chloride 0.9%, glucose 5%, sodium chloride 0.18% with glucose 4%). In intravenous solutions containing glucose or other carbohydrates, Magnapen should be infused within two hours of preparation. Intravenous solutions of Magnapen in Water for Injections or sodium chloride 0.9% should be infused within 24 hours of preparation. Full particulars are given in the package enclosure leaflet. Preparation of Magnapen infusion solutions must be carried out under appropriate aseptic conditions if these extended storage periods are required.

Marketing authorisation holder: Beecham Group plc, SB House, Great West Road, Brentford, Middlesex TW8 9BD.
Trading as SmithKline Beecham Pharmaceuticals Mundells, Welwyn Garden City, Hertfordshire AL7 1EY.

Marketing authorisation numbers
Capsules: PL 0038/0090R
Syrup: PL 0038/0324
Injection: PL 0038/0089R

Date of first authorisation/renewal of authorisation
Capsules: 22 April 1998
Syrup: 14 May 1996
Injection: 18 December 1997

Date of (partial) revision of the text
Capsules: April 1998
Syrup: April 1996
Injection: December 1997.

PARNATE* TABLETS

Presentation Geranium-red, sugar-coated tablets, marked SKF, each containing 10 mg tranylcypromine present as the sulphate.

Uses Parnate is a non-hydrazine monoamine oxidase inhibitor for the treatment of symptoms of depressive illness especially where phobic symptoms are present or where treatment with other types of antidepressant has failed. It is not recommended for mild depressive states resulting from temporary situational difficulties.

Dosage and administration *Adults only:* Initially, one tablet morning and afternoon. If the response is not adequate after the first week, add a further tablet at midday, and continue for at least a week. A dosage of three tablets a day should only be exceeded with caution. When a satisfactory response has been obtained, dosage may be reduced to a maintenance level, often of one tablet a day.

When given with a tranquilliser, the dosage of Parnate is not affected. When given concurrently with electroconvulsive therapy, the usual dosage is one tablet twice a day during the series and one tablet a day afterwards as maintenance therapy.

Elderly: Use with great caution (see *Contra-indications* and *Precautions* below).

Contra-indications, warnings, etc
Contra-indications: Do not give Parnate less than a week after stopping treatment with any other antidepressant drug including other MAO inhibitors, because of persisting effects, then give half the usual dosage for the first week. Similarly, after stopping Parnate, allow at least two weeks to elapse before starting treatment with any drug or ingesting any food that may interact.

Do not give Parnate with indirectly-acting sympathomimetic amines such as amphetamine, fenfluramine or similar anti-obesity agents, ephedrine or phenylpropanolamine (certain 'cold-cures' may contain such agents), or with levodopa or dopamine, as severe hypertensive reactions may result; with pethidine and closely related narcotic analgesics, and nefopam, as potentiation may occur; with dextromethorphan as a similar reaction has been reported; with other MAO inhibitors, as symptoms of overdosage are possible; or with buspirone, since increased blood pressure may occur.

Reports of hyperactivity, hypertonicity, hyperpyrexia, coma and death have been associated with the use of Parnate in combination with tricyclic antidepressants; tetracyclic antidepressants should also be avoided. The use of clomipramine in patients already on Parnate may be particularly hazardous. Use of MAO inhibitors with or after fluvoxamine or fluoxetine has been reported to produce a serotonin syndrome, sometimes fatal.

Do not use Parnate in patients with actual or suspected cerebrovascular disease or severe cardiovascular disease; in those with actual or suspected phaeochromocytoma, or with hyperthyroidism; or in those with known liver damage or blood dyscrasias.

Dietary precautions: High levels of tyramine in certain foods have been the cause of severe hypertensive reactions in patients on MAO inhibitor therapy (see *Adverse reactions*). Accordingly, patients must be warned to avoid the following: matured cheeses, hydrolysed protein extracts such as Marmite or Bovril, alcoholic drinks, particularly red wines such as Chianti, non-alcoholic beer and lager, and protein foods that are not fresh or whose preparation involved hydrolysis, fermentation, pickling, or 'hanging'; also broad-bean pods, which contain levodopa, and banana skins.

Precautions: Caution should be exercised when giving Parnate with the following: guanethidine, as its action may be antagonised; reserpine, as hyperactivity may occur; methyldopa, as central excitation may result; other hypotensive agents because of possible additive effects; oral hypoglycaemic agents or insulin, as their action may be potentiated; anticholinergic antiparkinsonism drugs, as potentiation has been reported; narcotic analgesics, except pethidine which is contra-indicated (see above), because of possible potentiation; and carbamazepine, which has similarities with tricyclic antidepressants. Although the effects of barbiturates may be enhanced, and this possibility should be borne in mind, they have frequently been given with Parnate, particularly at night. Metrizamide should be avoided in patients on MAO inhibitors since they may lower the seizure threshold. Although MAO inhibitors have been used therapeutically with L-tryptophan, a neuromotor syndrome has been reported with this combination.

Patients should be specifically asked if they are taking any other medication because of the possibility of drug interactions.

Use Parnate with great caution in elderly patients; in those with cardiovascular disease in whom physical activity should be regulated, as the drug may suppress anginal pain; and in epileptic patients, as tranylcypromine has a variable effect on the convulsive threshold in animals. Parnate may aggravate some co-existing symptoms in depression such as anxiety and agitation. Parnate should preferably be withdrawn at least two weeks before elective surgery because of possible drug interaction.

Caution should be exercised in prescribing Parnate for patients with a previous history of dependence on drugs or alcohol.

In common with other drugs acting on the CNS, Parnate may affect ability to drive or operate machinery.

Use in pregnancy and lactation: Do not use in pregnancy, especially during the first and last trimesters, unless there are compelling reasons. There is no evidence as to drug safety in human pregnancy nor is there evidence from animal work that it is free from hazard. Tranylcypromine passes into the milk of lactating dogs.

Adverse reactions: Severe hypertensive reactions may occur, notably in association with foods containing tyramine (see *Dietary precautions*). Such reactions may be presaged by palpitations and unusually frequent headaches; patients should be warned to discontinue the drug if such symptoms occur. As well as a rapid rise in blood pressure, severe occipital headache, which may radiate frontally, is virtually always present, and pain and stiffness in the neck are usual; other features include multiple extrasystoles, often with bradycardia though sometimes with tachycardia, other arrhythmias, substernal pain, nausea and vomiting, sweating, pallor, sometimes followed by flushing, mydriasis and photophobia. Rarely, hypotension may dominate the clinical picture. ECG changes may be seen. The symptoms can mimic subarachnoid haemorrhage or may actually be associated with intracranial bleeding. Exceptionally, hemiparesis, hemiplegia or death has resulted.

Severe hypertensive reactions should be treated at once by reducing the blood pressure; slow intravenous injection of 5 mg phentolamine mesylate should be effective. Injectable or oral chlorpromazine is suitable for milder reactions. Acute symptoms generally subside within 24 hours.

Insomnia is the most frequent side effect; it may usually be overcome by giving the last dose of the day not later than 3 pm, by reducing dosage, or by prescribing a mild hypnotic.

Mild headache, drowsiness, weakness, dizziness, palpitation, transient restlessness, dry mouth, blurred vision, nausea, oedema, weight gain, increased appetite and rash have been reported. Overstimulation, including anxiety and agitation, developing rarely into hypomania, has also been observed; the dosage should be reduced. Hypotension, which may be postural, may occur; it is usually temporary, but if it persists the drug should be stopped. Peripheral neuritis and difficulty in micturition have occurred rarely.

Dependence on Parnate, with tolerance to high doses, has been reported rarely, and can occur in patients without a past history of drug dependence. This should be distinguished from the return of features of the original illness on cessation of treatment.

Liver dysfunction has occurred very rarely, and isolated instances of purpura and blood dyscrasias have been reported.

Overdosage: Signs and symptoms are usually of the type already described as adverse reactions, but may be more intense, may include hyperpyrexia, tremor and convulsions, and may follow a latent period. Treatment consists of the induction of vomiting and/or gastric lavage together with supportive and symptomatic measures. External cooling is recommended for hyperpyrexia. Treat hypotension with fluid replacement; if severe or persistent, noradrenaline may be considered. Hypertension, if it occurs, may be relieved by slow intravenous injection of phentolamine mesylate. Pancuronium with mechanical ventilation may help reverse muscle spasm and pyrexia. Beta-adrenergic receptor blockade has been used successfully.

Pharmaceutical precautions Store in a dry place at a temperature not exceeding 25°C and protect from light.

Legal category POM.

Package quantities Containers of 28 tablets.

Further information It is generally considered that no particular hazard is attached to the use of local anaesthetics containing small amounts of adrenaline in patients receiving Parnate unless cardiovascular disease is present.

Inactive ingredients include sucrose and aluminium lakes of E122 and E124.

Product licence number 0002/5040R.

PARSTELIN* TABLETS

Presentation Leaf-green, sugar-coated tablets, marked SKF, each containing 10 mg tranylcypromine present as the sulphate and 1 mg trifluoperazine present as the hydrochloride.

Uses Parstelin is a combination of a non-hydrazine monoamine oxidase inhibitor and a phenothiazine tranquilliser, for the treatment of symptoms of depressive illness complicated by anxiety.

Dosage and administration *Adults only:* Initially, one tablet morning and afternoon. If the response is not adequate after the first week, add a further tablet at midday, and continue for at least a week. A dosage of three tablets a day should only be exceeded with caution. When a satisfactory response has been obtained, dosage may be reduced to a maintenance level, often of one tablet a day.

Elderly: Use with great caution (see *Contra-indications* and *Precautions* below).

Contra-indications, warnings, etc
Contra-indications: Do not give Parstelin less than a week after stopping treatment with any other antidepressant drug including other MAO inhibitors, because of persisting effects, then give half the usual dosage for the first week. Similarly, after stopping Parstelin, allow at least two weeks to elapse before starting treatment with any drug or ingesting any food that may interact.

Do not give Parstelin with indirectly-acting sympathomimetic amines such as amphetamine, fenfluramine, or similar anti-obesity agents, ephedrine or phenylpropanolamine (certain 'cold-cures' may contain such agents), or with levodopa or dopamine, as severe hypertensive reactions may result; with pethidine and closely related narcotic analgesics, and nefopam, as potentiation may occur; with dextromethorphan as a similar reaction has been reported; with other MAO inhibitors, as symptoms of overdosage are possible; or with buspirone, since increased blood pressure may occur.

Reports of hyperactivity, hypertonicity, hyperpyrexia, coma and death have been associated with the use of tranylcypromine in combination with tricyclic antidepressants; tetracyclic antidepressants should also be avoided. The use of clomipramine in patients already on Parstelin may be particularly hazardous. Use of MAO inhibitors with or after fluvoxamine or fluoxetine has been reported to produce a serotonin syndrome, sometimes fatal.

Do not use Parstelin in patients with actual or suspected cerebrovascular disease or severe cardiovascular disease; in those with actual or suspected phaeochromocytoma, or with hyperthyroidism; in those with existing blood dyscrasias or known liver damage; or in those hypersensitive to the ingredients.

Dietary precautions: High levels of tyramine in certain foods have been the cause of severe hypertensive reactions in patients on MAO inhibitor therapy (see *Adverse reactions*). Accordingly, patients must be warned to avoid the following: matured cheese, hydrolysed protein extracts such as Marmite or Bovril, alcoholic drinks, particularly red wines such as Chianti, non-alcoholic beer and lager, and protein foods that are not fresh or whose preparation involved hydrolysis, fermentation, pickling, or 'hanging'; also broad-bean pods, which contain levodopa, and banana skins.

Precautions: Caution should be exercised when giving Parstelin with the following: guanethidine, as its action may be antagonised; reserpine, as hyperactivity may occur; methyldopa, as central excitation may result; other hypotensive agents because of possible additive effects; oral hypoglycaemic agents or insulin, as their action may be potentiated; anticholinergic antiparkinsonism drugs, as potentiation has been reported; narcotic analgesics, except pethidine which is contra-indicated (see above), because of possible potentiation; and carbamazepine, which has similarities with tricyclic antidepressants. Although the effects of barbiturates may be enhanced, and this possibility should be borne in mind, they have frequently been given with Parstelin, particularly at night. Metrizamide should be avoided in patients on MAO inhibitors since they may lower the seizure threshold. Although MAO inhibitors have been used therapeutically with L-tryptophan, a neuromotor syndrome has been reported with this combination. Potentiation may occur if trifluoperazine is used with other CNS depressants.

Patients should be specifically asked if they are taking any other medication because of the possibility of drug interactions.

Use Parstelin with great caution in elderly patients; in those with cardiovascular disease in whom physical activity should be regulated, as tranylcypromine may suppress anginal pain; and in epileptic patients as tranylcypromine has a variable effect on the convulsive threshold in animals. Tranylcypromine may aggravate some co-existing symptoms in depression such as anxiety and agitation. Parstelin should preferably be withdrawn at least two weeks before elective surgery because of possible drug interaction.

Nausea and vomiting as a sign of organic disease may be masked by the anti-emetic action of trifluoperazine.

Caution should be exercised in prescribing Parstelin for patients with a previous history of dependence on drugs or alcohol.

In common with other drugs acting on the CNS, Parstelin may affect ability to drive or operate machinery.

Use in pregnancy and lactation: Do not use in pregnancy, especially during the first and last trimesters, unless there are compelling reasons. There is no evidence as to drug safety in human pregnancy nor is there evidence from animal work that it is free from hazard. Both tranylcypromine and trifluoperazine pass into the milk of lactating dogs.

Adverse reactions: Severe hypertensive reactions may occur, notably in association with foods containing tyramine (see *Dietary precautions*). Such reactions may be presaged by palpitations and unusually frequent headaches; patients should be warned to discontinue the drug if such symptoms occur. As well as a rapid rise in blood pressure, severe occipital headache, which may radiate frontally, is virtually always present, and pain and stiffness in the neck are usual; other features include multiple extrasystoles, often with bradycardia though sometimes with tachycardia, other arrhythmias, substernal pain, nausea and vomiting, sweating, pallor, sometimes followed by flushing, mydriasis and photophobia. Rarely, hypotension may dominate the clinical picture. ECG changes may be seen. The symptoms can mimic subarachnoid haemorrhage or may actually be associated with intracranial bleeding. Exceptionally, hemiparesis, hemiplegia or death has resulted.

Severe hypertensive reactions should be treated at once by reducing the blood pressure; slow intravenous injection of 5 mg phentolamine mesylate should be effective. Injectable or oral chlorpromazine is suitable for milder reactions. Acute symptoms generally subside within 24 hours.

Insomnia is the most frequent side effect; it may usually be overcome by giving the last dose of the day not later than 3 pm, by reducing dosage, or by prescribing a mild hypnotic.

Mild headache, drowsiness, weakness, dizziness, palpitation, transient restlessness, dry mouth, blurred vision, nausea, oedema, weight gain, increased appetite and rash have been reported. Overstimulation, including anxiety and agitation, developing rarely into hypomania, has also been observed; the dosage should be reduced. Hypotension, which may be postural, may occur; it is usually temporary, but if it persists the drug should be stopped. Peripheral neuritis and difficulty in micturition have occurred rarely.

Dependence on tranylcypromine, with tolerance to high doses, has been reported rarely, and can occur in patients without a past history of drug dependence. This should be distinguished from the return of features of the original illness on cessation of treatment.

Extrapyramidal symptoms due to the trifluoperazine component are very unlikely at the recommended dosage. Extremely rarely, long-term therapy with trifluoperazine in low dosage has been associated with tardive dyskinesia, which can be long-lasting or even irreversible.

Liver dysfunction has occurred very rarely, and isolated instances of purpura and blood dyscrasias have been reported.

Overdosage: Signs and symptoms are usually of the type already described as adverse reactions to tranylcypromine, but may be more intense, may include hyperpyrexia, tremor and convulsions, and may follow a latent period. In the unlikely event of symptoms from the trifluoperazine component, these are extrapyramidal in type. Treatment consists of gastric lavage together with supportive and symptomatic measures. Do not induce vomiting. External cooling is recommended for hyperpyrexia. Treat hypotension with fluid replacement; if severe or persistent, noradrenaline may be considered; adrenaline is contra-indicated. Hypertension, if it occurs, may be relieved by slow intravenous injection of phentolamine mesylate. Pancuronium with mechanical ventilation may help reverse muscle spasm and pyrexia. Beta-adrenergic receptor blockade has been used successfully.

Pharmaceutical precautions Store in a dry place at a temperature not exceeding 25°C and protect from light.

Legal category POM.

Package quantities Containers of 28 tablets.

Further information It is generally considered that no particular hazard is attached to the use of local anaesthetics containing small amounts of adrenaline in patients receiving tranylcypromine unless cardiovascular disease is present.

Inactive ingredients include sucrose and aluminium lake of E110.

Parstelin should normally only be used on the recommendation of a specialist in psychiatry.

Product licence number 0002/5041R.

PENBRITIN* Capsules
PENBRITIN* Syrup
PENBRITIN* Syrup Forte
PENBRITIN* Paediatric Suspension
PENBRITIN* Vials for Injection

Qualitative and quantitative composition *Penbritin Capsules* (Ampicillin Capsules BP): 250 mg or 500 mg ampicillin as Ampicillin Trihydrate EP.

Penbritin Syrups (Ampicillin Oral Suspension BP): When reconstituted each 5 ml contains 125 mg (syrup) or 250 mg (syrup Forte) ampicillin as Ampicillin Trihydrate BP.

Penbritin Paediatric Suspension: When reconstituted each 1.25 ml contains 125 mg ampicillin as Ampicillin Trihydrate EP.

Penbritin Vials for Injection (Ampicillin Sodium BP for Injection): Each vial contains 100 mg, 250 mg, 500 mg or 1 g ampicillin as Ampicillin Sodium EP.

Pharmaceutical form *Penbritin Capsules:* Black and red capsules overprinted 'Penbritin'.

Penbritin Syrups: Bottles containing powder for the preparation of a suspension for oral administration.

Penbritin Paediatric Suspension: Bottles containing powder for the preparation of 25 ml off-white suspension.

Penbritin Vials for Injection: Vials containing sterile powder for injection.

Clinical particulars
Therapeutic indications: Penbritin is a broad-spectrum penicillin, indicated for the treatment of a wide range of bacterial infections caused by ampicillin-sensitive organisms. Typical indications include: ear, nose and throat infections, bronchitis, pneumonia, urinary tract infections, gonorrhoea, gynaecological infections, septicaemia, peritonitis, endocarditis, meningitis, enteric fever, gastro-intestinal infections.

Extraperitoneal application of Penbritin to wounds can be used to prevent infection following abdominal surgery.

Parenteral usage is indicated where oral dosage is inappropriate.

Posology and method of administration:
Usual adult dosage (including elderly patients):
Ear, nose and throat infections: 250 mg four times a day.

Bronchitis: Routine therapy: 250 mg four times a day.

High-dosage therapy: 1 g four times a day.

Pneumonia: 500 mg four times a day.

Urinary tract infections: 500 mg three times a day.

Gonorrhoea: 2 g orally with 1 g probenecid as a single dose. Repeated doses are recommended for the treatment of females.

Gastro-intestinal infections: 500-750 mg three to four times daily.

Enteric: Acute: 1-2 g four times a day for two weeks.

Carriers: 1-2 g four times a day for four to 12 weeks.

Septicaemia, endocarditis, osteomyelitis: 500 mg four to six times a day IM or IV for one to six weeks.

Peritonitis, intra-abdominal sepsis: 500 mg four times a day IM or IV.

Meningitis: Adult dosage: 2 g six-hourly IV.

Children's dosage: 150 mg/kg daily IV in divided doses.

Penbritin may also be administered by other routes of conjunction with systemic therapy.

Intraperitoneal: 500 mg daily in up to 10 ml Water for Injections BP.

Intrapleural: 500 mg daily in 5-10 ml Water for Injections BP.

Intra-articular: 500 mg daily, in up to 5 ml Water for Injections BP or sterile 0.5% procaine hydrochloride solution.

Local use in abdominal surgery: 1 g sterile powder sprinkled into the wound extraperitoneally or into muscle layers to prevent wound infection post-operatively.

Usual children's dosage (under 10 years): Half adult routine dosage.

All recommended dosages are a guide only. In severe infections the above dosages may be increased, or Penbritin given by injection. Oral doses of Penbritin should be taken half to one hour before meals.

Administration: Intramuscular: Add 1.5 ml Water for Injections BP to 250 mg or 500 mg vial contents.

Intravenous: Dissolve 250 mg in 5 ml or 500 mg in 10 ml Water for Injections BP. Administer by slow injection (three to four minutes). Penbritin may also be added to infusion fluids or injected, suitably diluted, into the drip tube over a period of three to four minutes.

Contra-indications: Penicillin hypersensitivity.

Special warnings and special precautions for use: None.

Interaction with other medicaments and other forms of interaction: If Penbritin is prescribed concurrently with an aminoglycoside, the antibiotics should not be mixed in the syringe, intravenous fluid container or giving set because loss of activity of the aminoglycoside can occur under these conditions.

Pregnancy and lactation: Animal studies with Penbritin have shown no teratogenic effects. The product has been in extensive clinical use since 1961 and its use in human pregnancy has been well documented in clinical studies. When antibiotic therapy is required during pregnancy, Penbritin may be considered appropriate.

During lactation, trace quantities of penicillins can be detected in breast milk.

Effects on ability to drive and use machines: None known.

Undesirable effects: Side effects, as with other penicillins, are uncommon and mainly of a mild and transitory nature. Gastro-intestinal upsets (e.g., nausea, diarrhoea) and skin rashes have been reported infrequently. An urticarial rash suggests penicillin hypersensitivity; an erythematous rash may arise in patients receiving ampicillin who have glandular fever. If a skin rash occurs, treatment should be discontinued.

In common with other β-lactam antibiotics angioedema and anaphylaxis have been reported. Pseudomembranous colitis has been reported rarely.

Overdose: Problems of overdosage with Penbritin are unlikely to occur; if encountered they may be treated symptomatically.

Pharmacological properties

Pharmacodynamic properties: Penbritin is a broad spectrum penicillin, indicated for the treatment of a wide range of bacterial infections caused by ampicillin sensitive organisms.

Pharmacokinetic properties: Ampicillin is excreted mainly in the bile and urine with a plasma half-life of one to two hours.

Absorption: The oral administration of 250 mg and 500 mg of ampicillin on a fasting stomach produces maximum serum levels of ± 2 and ± 4 mcg per ml, respectively, after two hours. Bioavailability is 30 to 40%. The absorption of orally administered ampicillin can be diminished by food.

Distribution: Serum protein binding ampicillin is about 20%. Plasma half-life is between one and one and a half hours.

Ampicillin diffuses into most tissues and body fluids. Its presence in therapeutic concentrations has been detected in, among others, bronchial secretions sinuses, saliva, CSF (variable percentage depending on the degree of meningeal inflammation), bile, serous membranes and middle ear.

Crosses the meningeal barrier: There is little ampicillin diffusion into the cerebrospinal fluid, except in cases of inflamed meninges, in which it can reach therapeutic concentrations when administered in high doses and especially by the intravenous route.

Crosses the placenta: Ampicillin diffuses through the placenta.

Passes into mothers' milk: Ampicillin is detected in small quantities in mothers' milk.

Metabolism and excretion: Ampicillin is eliminated chiefly through urine.

Approximately 30% of the dose administered orally and over 60% of the dose administered parenterally are eliminated in active form in urine during the 24 hours which follow the administration of Penbritin. Urinary concentrations are higher following parenteral administration.

A small percentage is eliminated in the bile where high concentrations are found.

Excretion may be delayed in cases of renal failure in accordance with its severity.

Preclinical safety data: No further information of relevance.

Pharmaceutical particulars

List of excipients:

Penbritin Capsules: Magnesium stearate, gelatin, black and red iron oxides (E172), titanium dioxide (E171) and erythrosine (E127).

Penbritin Syrup and Syrup Forte: Sodium benzoate, sodium chloride, apricot dry flavour, caramel dry flavour, peppermint extra dry flavour, methyl polysiloxane, sodium citrate anhydrous, sucrose.

Penbritin Paediatric Suspension: Sodium benzoate, saccharin sodium, sodium carboxymethylcellulose, tutti fruitti dry flavour, peppermint extra dry flavour, sodium citrate anhydrous, sucrose.

Penbritin Vials for Injection: None.

Incompatibilities: Penbritin should not be mixed with blood products or other proteinaceous fluids (e.g. protein hydrolysates) or with intravenous lipid emulsions.

Shelf-life:

Penbritin Capsules: Five years in blister packs only. Three years in all other packs.

Penbritin Syrups: powder three years. Once dispensed Penbritin Syrups remain stable for seven days (stored at 15°C or below) or 15 days (stored in a refrigerator at 5°C or below).

Penbritin Paediatric Suspension: Three years – Once dispensed Penbritin Paediatric Suspension remains stable for seven days if kept in a cool place.

Penbritin Vials for Injection: 36 months.

Special precautions for storage:

Penbritin Capsules: Penbritin should be stored in a cool dry place.

Penbritin Syrups: Penbritin Syrup powder should be stored in a cool dry place. Once dispensed, Penbritin Syrups should be kept in a cool place at 15°C or below (seven days) or in a refrigerator at 5°C or below (15 days).

Penbritin Paediatric Suspension: Penbritin should be stored in a cool dry place. Penbritin Paediatric Suspension, once dispensed should be kept in a cool place (seven days).

Penbritin Vials for Injection: Penbritin should be stored in a cool dry place. Penbritin Solutions for Injection should be stored in a refrigerator (2-8°C) and used within 24 hours.

Nature and contents of container:

Penbritin Capsules: Aluminium canister/Glass bottle fitted with a screw cap/polypropylene tube with a polyethylene closure/aluminium foil pack – 4, 16, 50, 100, 500; Aluminium/PVC blister pack 28.

Penbritin Syrups: White flint glass bottle fitted with a) aluminium Flavor-Lok cap lacquered either rolled-on Duogrip or rolled on pilfer proof or b) Urea Dale Polycone or c) polypropylene wadless cap.100 ml. Powder for reconstitution to 100 ml.

Penbritin Paediatric Suspension: White flint glass bottle fitted with either aluminium Flavor-Lok cap lacquered either rolled on Duogrip or rolled on pilfer proof/Urea Dale Polycone/polypropylene wadless cap–10 ml, 25 ml. A pipette to measure the 1.25 ml dose is provided.

Penbritin Vials for Injection: Clear glass vial (PhEur Type III) fitted with a butyl rubber plug and an aluminium seal–10.

Instructions for use/handling: If dilution of the reconstitution syrup is required, Syrup BP should be used.

Penbritin Vials are not suitable for multidose use. Any residual Penbritin solution should be discarded.

Marketing authorisation holder: Beecham Group plc, SB House, Great West Road, Brentford, Middlesex TW8 9BD.

Trading as SmithKline Beecham Pharmaceuticals Mundells, Welwyn Garden City, Hertfordshire AL7 1EY.

Marketing authorisation numbers

Penbritin Capsules 250 mg PL 0038/5074R
Penbritin Capsules 500 mg PL 0038/5075R
Penbritin Syrup 125 mg/5 ml: PL 0038/0265
Penbritin Syrup Forte 250 mg/5 ml: PL 0038/0266
Penbritin Paediatric Suspension: PL 0038/5066R
Penbritin Vials for Injection 100 mg PL 0038/5059R
Penbritin Vials for Injection 250 mg PL 0038/5060R
Penbritin Vials for Injection 500 mg PL 0038/5061R
Penbritin Vials for Injection 1 g PL 0038/5062R

Date of renewal of authorisation

Penbritin Capsules 250 mg: 04.02.98
Penbritin Capsules 500 mg: 04.02.98
Penbritin Syrup 125 mg/5 ml: 26.11.95
Penbritin Syrup Forte 250 mg/5 ml: 28.11.95
Penbritin Paediatric Suspension: 12.11.97
Penbritin Vials for Injection 100 mg: 13.01.94
Penbritin Vials for Injection 250 mg: 13.01.94
Penbritin Vials for Injection 500 mg: 13.01.94
Penbritin Vials for Injection 1 g: 13.01.94

Date of (partial) revision of the text

Capsules: August 1997
Syrups: July 1995
Paediatric Suspension: July 1997
Vials for Injection: June 1997

Legal category POM.

POLIOMYELITIS VACCINE, LIVE (ORAL) PhEur (TEN DOSE) (Sabin strains)

Presentation Poliomyelitis Vaccine, Live (Oral) PhEur, as supplied by SmithKline Beecham Pharmaceuticals, is a clear liquid, colourless or light yellow to light red, stabilised with molar magnesium chloride. Each dose (3 drops from a 10-dose tube) provides at least 10^6TCID_{50} type 1 (LS-c, 2ab), 10^5TCID_{50} type 2 (P712, Ch, 2ab) and $10^{5.5}TCID_{50}$ type 3 (Leon $12a_1b$) live attenuated strains of poliomyelitis virus grown in monkey kidney cell cultures, and contains not more than 1 microgram (0.7 IU) neomycin sulphate.

Uses Active immunisation against poliomyelitis.

Dosage and administration

Adults and children: For oral use only: NOT FOR INJECTION. Three drops of vaccine from a 10-dose tube constitute one dose which may be given with syrup or on a lump of sugar to mask the bitter salty taste of the magnesium chloride. Do not administer on foods which contain preservatives.

For a complete schedule, three doses of the vaccine should be given at intervals of at least four weeks (see also *Further information*).

Other unvaccinated members of the same household (including adults) should be advised vaccination at the same time as the vaccinee.

The vaccine should be inspected for particulate matter or discolouration before administration.

Since the vaccine contains live attenuated poliomyelitis virus, care should be taken to avoid transfer or spillage. Care should be taken not to contaminate multidose droppers with vaccinee's saliva.

Contra-indications, warnings, etc.

Contra-indications: The vaccine should not be used in the presence of acute febrile illness or intercurrent infection, persistent diarrhoea, vomiting or other gastrointestinal disturbance. (A minor infection is not a contra-indication). The vaccine should also not be given in the presence of impaired immune response including leukaemia, lymphoma, generalised malignancy or treatment with corticosteroids, cytotoxic drugs or irradiation. HIV infection does not contra-indicate immunisation.

Precautions: The vaccine may contain trace amounts of penicillin and streptomycin and neomycin which should not contra-indicate its use except in those with a history of severe anaphylaxis due to either antibiotic.

Contacts of recent vaccinees should be advised to attend to personal hygiene.

Previous vaccination with inactivated Poliomyelitis Vaccine is not a contra-indication.

Diarrhoea or vomiting (including gastrointestinal infections) may interfere with replication ('take' rate).

At least three weeks should normally intervene between the administration of any two live vaccines. Poliomyelitis vaccine can, however, be given simultaneously with measles, mumps and rubella vaccines and with DTP vaccine. In this case the injectable vaccines should be given at different sites.

No data have been generated on the simultaneous administration of OPV with oral typhoid vaccine therefore the theoretical possibility of an interaction between the two products cannot be ruled out.

Poliomyelitis vaccine has been given at the same time as BCG and hepatitis B vaccines.

In some populations and groups of vaccinees lower seroconversion rates have been observed. Due to various non-specific factors all three vaccine viruses may not replicate optimally in the gut of susceptible subjects, even after three doses.

Use in pregnancy: Pregnant women should not be given oral poliomyelitis vaccine unless they are at definite risk from poliomyelitis.

Adverse reactions: Paralysis temporally associated with vaccination has been reported very rarely in recipients or contacts.

Overdosage: Occasional reports of overdosage have been received. Overdosage has not resulted in ill effects.

Pharmaceutical precautions Protect from light and store between 2°C and 8°C. Under these conditions there is no significant loss of virus titre for 12 months.

When tubes of vaccine have been opened there is a risk of contamination with bacteria and moulds which may result in a reduction of vaccine potency. It is good practice, therefore, to discard vaccine remaining in opened 10-dose tubes at the end of the vaccinating session.

Legal category POM.

Package quantities Individual plastic 10-dose dropper tubes.

Further information Current policy recommends that the first dose of oral poliomyelitis vaccine should be given from two months of age. The primary course consists of three separate doses with intervals of one month between each dose, given at the same time as DTP vaccine.

It is currently recommended that a reinforcing dose of poliomyelitis vaccine should be given at school entry and at 15 to 19 years of age. Adults need not be offered a reinforcing dose unless they are at special risk.

Poliomyelitis vaccine has been administered at the same time as BCG and hepatitis B vaccine.

Inactive ingredients are magnesium chloride, polysorbate 80, purified water, and also neomycin sulphate (see *Presentation*).

Product licence number 10592/0017.

POLIOMYELITIS VACCINE, LIVE (ORAL) PhEur (Sabin strains) Monodose* (OPV)

Presentation Poliomyelitis Vaccine, Live (Oral) PhEur, as supplied by SmithKline Beecham Pharmaceuticals, is a clear liquid, colourless or light yellow to light red, stabilised with molar magnesium chloride. Each dose (0.135 ml) provides at least 10^6TCID_{50} type 1 (LS-c, 2ab), 10^5TCID_{50} type 2 (P712, Ch 2ab) and $10^{5.5}TCID_{50}$ type 3 (Leon $12a_1b$) live attenuated strains of poliomyelitis virus grown in monkey kidney cell cultures, and contains not more than 1 microgram (0.7 IU) neomycin sulphate.

Uses Active immunisation against poliomyelitis.

Dosage and administration
Adults and children: For oral use only: NOT FOR INJECTION. Three drops of vaccine from the Monodose* tube constitute one dose which may be given with syrup or on a lump of sugar to mask the bitter salty taste of the magnesium chloride. Do not administer on foods which contain preservatives.

For a complete schedule, three doses of the vaccine should be given at intervals of at least four weeks (see also *Further information*).

Other unvaccinated members of the same household (including adults) should be advised vaccination at the same time as the vaccinee.

The vaccine should be inspected for particulate matter or discolouration before administration.

Since the vaccine contains live attenuated poliomyelitis virus, care should be taken to avoid transfer or spillage.

Both parts of the tube and also the spoon (if used) should be carefully disposed of, e.g. by incineration. Alternatively they may be sterilised by immersing for 30 minutes in 0.1% hypochlorite solution yielding 1000 ppm available chlorine (e.g. 1:10 Milton 1%).

Do not administer directly into the vaccinee's mouth as the tube may slip and cause choking.

Contra-indications, warnings, etc.
Contra-indications: The vaccine should not be used in the presence of acute febrile illness or intercurrent infection, persistent diarrhoea, vomiting or other gastrointestinal disturbance; (a minor infection is not a contra-indication). The vaccine should also not be given in the presence of impaired immune response including leukaemia, lymphoma, generalised malignancy or treatment with corticosteroids, cytotoxic drugs or irradiation.

Precautions: The vaccine may contain trace amounts of penicillin, streptomycin and neomycin which should not contra-indicate its use except in those with a history of severe anaphylaxis due to these antibiotics.

Contacts of recent vaccinees should be advised to attend to strict personal hygiene.

Previous vaccination with inactivated poliomyelitis vaccine is not a contra-indication.

HIV-positive asymptomatic individuals may receive live polio vaccine but excretion of the vaccine virus in the faeces may continue for longer than normal individuals. Household contacts should be warned of this and for the need for strict personal hygiene, including hand-washing after nappy changes for an HIV-positive infant.

For HIV-positive symptomatic individuals, IPV may be used instead of OPV at the discretion of the clinician.

Diarrhoea or vomiting (including gastrointestinal infections) may interfere with replication ('take' rate).

In immunocompetent recipients previous vaccination with inactivated Poliomyelitis Vaccine is not a contra-indication.

At least three weeks should normally intervene between administration of any two live vaccines. Poliomyelitis vaccine can, however, be given simultaneously with measles, mumps and rubella vaccines and with DTP vaccine. In this case the injectable vaccines should be given at different sites.

No data has been generated on the simultaneous administration of OPV with oral typhoid vaccine; therefore the theoretical possibility of an interaction between the two products cannot be ruled out.

Poliomyelitis vaccine has been given at the same time as BCG and Hepatitis B vaccines.

In some populations and groups of vaccinees lower seroconversion rates have been observed. Due to various non-specific factors all three vaccine viruses may not replicate optimally in the gut of susceptible subjects, even after three doses.

Use in pregnancy: Pregnant women should not be given oral poliomyelitis vaccine unless they are at definite risk from poliomyelitis.

Adverse reactions: Paralysis temporally associated with vaccination has been reported very rarely in recipients or contacts.

Overdosage: There have been occasional reports of overdosage but none has resulted in any ill effect.

Pharmaceutical precautions Protect from light and store in a refrigerator between 2°C and 8°C.

Legal category POM.

Package quantities One carton containing 10 individual plastic Monodose* tubes.

Further information Current policy recommends that the first dose of oral poliomyelitis vaccine should be given from two months of age. The primary course consists of three separate doses with intervals of one month between each dose, given at the same time as DTP vaccine.

It is currently recommended that a reinforcing dose of poliomyelitis vaccine should be given at school entry and at 15 to 19 years of age. Adults need not be offered a reinforcing dose unless they are at special risk.

Inactive ingredients are magnesium chloride, amino acid, polysorbate 80, purified water, and also neomycin sulphate (see *Presentation*).

Product licence number 10592/0039.

PRIORIX* ▼

Qualitative and quantitative composition Priorix is a lyophilised mixed preparation of the attenuated Schwarz measles, RIT 4385 mumps (derived from Jeryl Lynn strain) and Wistar RA 27/3 rubella strains of viruses, separately obtained by propagation either in chick embryo tissue cultures (mumps and measles) and MRC_5 human diploid cells (rubella).

Priorix meets the World Health Organisation requirements for manufacture of biological substances and for measles, mumps and rubella vaccines and combined vaccines (live).

Each 0.5 ml dose of the reconstituted vaccine contains not less than $10^{3.0}$ $CCID_{50}$ of the Schwarz measles, not less than $10^{3.7}$ $CCID_{50}$ of the RIT 4385 mumps, and not less than $10^{3.0}$ $CCID_{50}$ of the Wistar RA 27/3 rubella virus strains.

Pharmaceutical form Lyophilised vaccine for reconstitution with the sterile diluent provided.

Clinical particulars
Therapeutic indications: Priorix is indicated for active immunisation against measles, mumps and rubella.

Posology and method of administration:
Posology: A single 0.5 ml dose of the reconstituted vaccine is recommended.

Priorix is recommended for immunisation of children over 12 months of age. It should be given according to the recommended schedule, and may be used for both primary and booster doses.

Method of administration: Priorix is for subcutaneous injection, although it can also be given by intramuscular injection (see *Special warnings and special precautions for use*).

Contra-indications: As with other vaccines, the administration of Priorix should be postponed in subjects suffering from acute severe febrile illness. The presence of a minor infection, however, is not a contra-indication for vaccination.

Priorix is contra-indicated in subjects with known systemic hypersensitivity to neomycin or to any other component of the vaccine (see also *Special warnings and special precautions for use*). A history of contact dermatitis to neomycin is not a contra-indication.

Priorix should not be given to subjects with impaired immune responses. These include patients with primary or secondary immunodeficiencies.

However, measles, mumps, rubella-combined vaccines can be given to asymptomatic HIV-infected persons without adverse consequences to their illness and may be considered for those who are symptomatic.

It is contra-indicated to administer Priorix to pregnant women. Furthermore, pregnancy should be avoided for one month after vaccination (see *Pregnancy and lactation*).

A second dose of measles, mumps, rubella-combined vaccine is contra-indicated in children with a history of thrombocytopenia within six weeks of the first dose.

Special warnings and special precautions for use: Alcohol and other disinfecting agents must be allowed to evaporate from the skin before injection of the vaccine since they can inactivate the attenuated viruses in the vaccine.

Limited protection against measles may be obtained by vaccination up to 72 hours after exposure to natural measles.

Infants below 12 months of age may not respond sufficiently to the measles component of the vaccine, due to the possible persistence of maternal measles antibodies. This should not preclude the use of the vaccine in younger infants (<12 months) since vaccination may be indicated in some situations such as high-risk areas. In these circumstances revaccination at or after 12 months of age should be considered.

As with all injectable vaccines, appropriate medical treatment and supervision should always be readily available in case of a rare anaphylactic event following the administration of the vaccine.

Vaccines produced in chick embryo tissue cultures have been shown not to contain egg proteins in sufficient amounts to elicit hypersensitivity reactions. Persons having egg allergies, that are not anaphylactic in nature, can be considered for vaccination (see *Contra-indications*).

Priorix should be given with caution to persons with a history or family history of allergic diseases or those with a history or family history of convulsions.

Transmission of measles virus from vaccinees to susceptible contacts has never been documented. Pharyngeal excretion of the rubella virus is known to occur about seven to 28 days after vaccination with peak excretion around the 11th day. However there is no evidence of transmission of this excreted vaccine virus to susceptible contacts. Transmission of mumps virus (Urabe strain) from vaccinees to susceptible contacts has been reported.

A limited number of subjects received Priorix intramuscularly. An adequate immune response was obtained for all three components (see *Posology and method of administration*).

PRIORIX SHOULD UNDER NO CIRCUMSTANCES BE ADMINISTERED INTRAVASCULARLY.

Interaction with other medicaments and other forms of interaction: If tuberculin testing has to be done it should be carried out before, or simultaneously with, vaccination since it has been reported that live measles (and possibly mumps) vaccine may cause a temporary depression of tuberculin skin sensitivity. This anergy may last for four to six weeks and tuberculin testing should not be performed within that period after vaccination to avoid false negative results.

Although data on the concomitant administration of Priorix and other vaccines are not yet available, it is generally accepted that measles, mumps and rubella-combined vaccine may be given at the same time as the oral polio vaccine (OPV) or inactivated polio vaccine (IPV), the injectable trivalent diphtheria, tetanus and pertussis vaccines (DTPw/DTPa) and *Haemophilus influenzae* type b (Hib) if separate injection sites are used.

If Priorix cannot be given at the same time as other live attenuated vaccines, an interval of at least three weeks should be left between both vaccinations.

In subjects who have received human gammaglobulins or a blood transfusion, vaccination should be delayed for at least three months because of the likelihood of vaccine failure due to passively acquired mumps, measles and rubella antibodies.

Priorix may be given as a booster dose in subjects who have previously been vaccinated with another measles mumps and rubella-combined vaccine.

Pregnancy and lactation:
Pregnancy: It is contra-indicated to administer Priorix to pregnant women. Furthermore, pregnancy should be avoided for one month after vaccination.

Lactation: There is little human data regarding use in breast-feeding women. Persons can be vaccinated where the benefit outweighs the risk.

Effects on ability to drive and use machines: The vaccine is unlikely to produce an effect on the ability to drive and use machines.

Undesirable effects: In controlled clinical studies, signs and symptoms were actively monitored on more than 5400 vaccinees during a 42-day follow-up period. The vaccinees were also requested to report any clinical events during the study period. The following adverse reactions were reported by the vaccinees in order of frequency.

Local redness–7.2%
Rash–7.1%
Fever–6.4%
Local pain–3.1%
Local swelling–2.6%
Parotid swelling–0.7%
Febrile convulsions–0.1%

During the active monitoring of signs and symptoms, in total, less than 6% of vaccinees had one of the following which were, at least, considered possibly related to the vaccination: nervousness (0.90%), pharyngitis (0.68%), upper respiratory tract infection (0.57%), rhinitis (0.56%), diarrhoea (0.54%), bronchitis (0.52%), vomiting (0.43%), coughing (0.39%), viral infection (0.31%) and otitis media (0.30%).

In comparative studies with other measles, mumps and rubella vaccines, the incidences of local pain, redness and swelling reported with Priorix were low, while the incidences of other adverse reactions were similar.

Overdose: Not applicable.

Pharmacological properties

Pharmacodynamic properties: In clinical studies Priorix has been demonstrated to be highly immunogenic.

Antibodies against measles were detected in 98.0%, against mumps in 96.1% and against rubella in 99.3% of previously seronegative vaccinees.

Subjects followed up to 12 months following vaccination all remained seropositive for anti-measles and anti-rubella antibodies. 88.4% were still seropositive at month 12 for anti-mumps antibody. This percentage is in line with what was observed for other measles, mumps and rubella-combined vaccines (87%).

Pharmacokinetic properties: Not applicable.

Preclinical safety data: Not applicable.

Pharmaceutical particulars

List of excipients: Vaccine: The vaccine contains the following amino acids: L-alanine, L-arginine, glycine, L-histidine, L-isoleucine, L-leucine, L-lysine HC1, L-methionine, L-phenylalanine, L-proline, L-serine, L-threonine, L-tryptophan, L-tyrosine, L-valine, L-aspartic acid, L-cysteine, L-cystine, L-hydroxproline, and human albumin, lactose, mannitol, sorbitol. The vaccine may also contain residual amounts of neomycin 25 micrograms maximum.

Diluent: Water for injection.

Incompatibilities: Priorix should not be mixed with other vaccines in the same syringe.

Shelf-life: The shelf-life of Priorix is two years when the vaccine is stored according to recommendations (see *Special precautions for storage*). The shelf-lives of the vaccine and diluent are not identical, therefore their expiry dates are different. The outer carton bears the earlier of the two expiry dates and this date must be respected. The carton and ALL its contents should be discarded on reaching the outer carton expiry date.

Special precautions for storage: Priorix should be stored in a refrigerator between 2°C and 8°C and protected from light. Do not freeze.
During transport, recommended conditions of storage should be respected, particularly in hot climates.

Nature and contents of container: Priorix is presented as a whitish to slightly pink pellet in a glass vial. The sterile diluent is clear and colourless and presented in a glass prefilled syringe or ampoule. Due to minor variation of its pH, the reconstituted vaccine may vary in colour from light orange to light red without deterioration of the vaccine's potency.

Vials, prefilled syringes and ampoules are made of neutral glass type I, which conforms to European Pharmacopoeia requirements.

Instructions for use/handling: The diluent and reconstituted vaccine should be inspected visually for any foreign particulate matter and/or variation of physical aspects prior to administration. In the event of either being observed, discard the diluent or reconstituted vaccine.

The vaccine must be reconstituted by adding **the entire contents** of the supplied container of diluent to the vial containing the pellet. After the addition of the diluent to the pellet, the mixture should be well shaken until the pellet is completely dissolved in the diluent.

Inject the **entire contents** of the vial.

It is normal practice to administer the vaccine immediately after reconstitution with the diluent provided. However, the vaccine may still be used up to three hours after reconstitution or to the end of the vaccination session whichever is sooner.

Marketing authorisation holder: SmithKline Beecham plc, SB House, Great West Road, Brentford, Middlesex TW8 9BD.
Trading as SmithKline Beecham Pharmaceuticals Mundells, Welwyn Garden City, Hertfordshire AL7 1EY.

Marketing authorisation number 10592/0110

Date of first authorisation/renewal of authorisation
4 December 1997

Legal Category POM.

RELIFEX* TABLETS
RELIFEX* SUSPENSION

Qualitative and quantitative composition

Tablets: Each tablet contains 500 mg nabumetone.

Suspension: Each 5 ml contains 500 mg nabumetone.

Pharmaceutical form

Tablets: Dark red, film-coated tablets marked Relifex on one side and 500 on the other.

Suspension: A white to off-white suspension.

Clinical particulars

Therapeutic indications: Nabumetone is a non-acidic non-steroidal anti-inflammatory agent which is a relatively weak inhibitor of prostaglandin synthesis. However, following absorption from the gastrointestinal tract it is rapidly metabolised in the liver to the principal active metabolite, 6-methoxy-2-naphthylacetic acid (6-MNA), a potent inhibitor of prostaglandin synthesis.

It is indicated for the treatment of osteoarthritis and rheumatoid arthritis requiring anti-inflammatory and analgesic treatment.

Posology and method of administration:
Adults: The recommended daily dose is two tablets or 10 ml suspension (1 g) taken as a single dose at bedtime.

For severe or persistent symptoms, or during acute exacerbations, an additional 500 mg–1 g may be given as a morning dose.

Elderly: In common with many drugs, blood levels may be higher in elderly patients. The recommended daily dose of 1 g should not be exceeded in this age group and in some cases 500 mg may give satisfactory relief.

Children: There are no clinical data to recommend use of Relifex in children.

Administration: Oral.

Contra-indications: Active peptic ulceration. NSAIDs should not be used in patients with a history of recent or recurrent peptic ulceration. Severe hepatic impairment (e.g. cirrhosis). Patients in whom aspirin or other NSAIDs precipitate asthmatic attacks, urticaria or acute rhinitis. Hypersensitivity to the drug.

Special warnings and special precautions for use: It is advisable to avoid the administration of more than one NSAID at a time. Peripheral oedema has been observed in some patients. Relifex should therefore be used with caution in patients with fluid retention, hypertension or heart failure.

Use in patients with impaired renal function: Urine is the major excretion route for the metabolites of Relifex. In patients with impaired renal function (creatinine clearance less than 30 ml/minute), dosage reduction should be considered. It is consistent with good clinical practice that patients with known renal impairment should be monitored regularly during therapy.

Liver function: Fluctuations in some parameters of liver function, particularly alkaline phosphatase, are frequently observed in patients with chronic inflammatory disorders; there is no evidence that Relifex accentuates these changes. However patients with abnormal liver function should be monitored closely.

Interaction with other medicaments and other forms of interaction: As the major circulating metabolite of Relifex is highly protein bound, patients receiving concurrent treatment with oral anti-coagulants, hydantoin anticonvulsants or sulphonylurea hypoglycaemics should be monitored for signs of overdosage of these drugs. Dosages should be adjusted if necessary.

Some NSAIDs are known to increase plasma concentrations of cardiac glycosides, lithium and methotrexate and may decrease the therapeutic efficacy of diuretics and antihypertensives. Such drugs may also induce hyperkalaemia when administered with potassium-sparing diuretics. Interaction studies between Relifex and these other drugs have not been performed; caution in co-administration is therefore recommended.

NSAIDs should not be used eight to 12 days after mifepristone administration, as they could affect the efficacy of mifepristone treatment.

Aluminium hydroxide gel, paracetamol and aspirin have not affected the bioavailability of Relifex in volunteer subjects.

Pregnancy and lactation: Studies in experimental animals have shown no teratogenic potential. As is common with other compounds administered to animals at doses high enough to be maternally toxic, indications of embryotoxicity were noted (studies in the rabbit 300 mg/kg dose). High doses in rats (320 mg/kg) delayed parturition; this effect is considered to be due to inhibition of prostaglandin synthesis. The active metabolite of nabumetone has been found in the milk of lactating animals.

Safety in human pregnancy has not been established. Relifex is not recommended during human pregnancy or in mothers who are breast feeding.

Effects on ability to drive and use machines: None known.

Undesirable effects: Reported gastrointestinal side effects include dry mouth, faecal occult blood, diarrhoea, dyspepsia, nausea, constipation, abdominal pain, flatulence, gastrointestinal bleeding, ulceration and perforation. Headache, dizziness, fatigue, confusion, sedation, depression, insomnia, tinnitus, abnormal vision, oedema, menorrhagia, anaphylaxis and anaphylactoid reaction have also been reported. Skin reactions including rash, pruritus, urticaria, alopecia and photosensitivity reactions may occur.

As with other NSAIDs, severe skin eruptions, e.g. Stevens Johnson syndrome and toxic epidermal necrolysis have been reported very rarely. Blood dyscrasias including leucopenia and thrombocytopenia have also been reported very rarely.

As with other NSAIDs, there have been rare reports of renal adverse effects, including nephrotic syndrome and renal failure.

In clinical trials, increases in doses above 1 g did not lead to an increase in the incidence of side effects. However, the lowest effective dose should always be used.

Overdose: There is no specific antidote. Treatment is with gastric lavage followed by activated charcoal using up to 60 g orally in divided doses with appropriate supportive therapy.

Pharmacological properties

Pharmacodynamic properties: Nabumetone is a non-acidic non-steroidal anti-inflammatory agent which is a relatively weak inhibitor of prostaglandin synthesis. A notable feature of the animal pharmacology is the lack of effect on the gastric mucosa. Following absorption from the gastrointestinal tract nabumetone is rapidly metabolised in the liver to the principal active metabolite, 6-methoxy-2-naphthylacetic acid (6-MNA) a potent inhibitor of prostaglandin synthesis.

Pharmacokinetic properties: Although nabumetone is absorbed essentially intact through the small intestine, extensive metabolism occurs during the first pass through the liver. As a result, concentrations in plasma of nabumetone are barely detectable after oral dosage. Intravenous studies in rats with nabumetone indicate it to be rapidly distributed throughout the body, in keeping with its highly lipophilic character. The active metabolite, 6-MNA, binds strongly to plasma proteins; it is distributed into inflamed tissue and crosses the placenta into foetal tissue. It is found in the milk of lactating females. 6-MNA is eliminated by metabolism, principally conjugation with glucuronic acid, and O-demethylation followed by conjugation, the main route of excretion being the urine. The plasma elimination half-life is about one day in man.

Preclinical safety data: Not applicable.

Pharmaceutical particulars

List of excipients:

Tablets: Sodium starch glycollate; sodium lauryl sulphate; hydroxypropylmethylcellulose; magnesium stearate; microcrystalline cellulose; red carmine; yellow iron oxide; titanium dioxide; talc; polyethylene glycol; saccharin sodium; liquid caramel flavour; purified water

Suspension: Methylcellulose; xanthan gum; sorbitol; sodium benzoate; liquid vanilla flavour; liquid buttermint flavour; monoammonium glycyrrhizinate; glycerin; dilute hydrochloric acid; purified water.

Incompatibilities: Not applicable.

Shelf-life: 36 months.

Special precautions for storage: Tablets: The tablets should be protected from light. Suspension: None.

Nature and contents of container: Tablets: HDPE bottles each containing 8 or 56 tablets. Suspension: HDPE bottles each containing 300 ml

Instructions for use/handling: None.

Marketing authorisation numbers
Tablets 0038/0301
Suspension 0038/0352

Date of approval/revision of SPC September 1996.

Legal category POM.

REQUIP* TABLETS 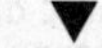

Qualitative and quantitative composition Ropinirole hydrochloride equivalent to 0.25, 1.0, 2.0 or 5.0 mg ropinirole free base.

Pharmaceutical form Film-coated, pentagonal-shaped tablets for oral administration. The tablet strengths are distinguished by colour; 0.25 mg (white), 1.0 mg (green), 2.0 mg (pink) and 5.0 mg (blue).

Clinical particulars

Therapeutic indications: Treatment of idiopathic Parkinson's disease:

Ropinirole may be used alone (without levodopa) in the treatment of idiopathic Parkinson's disease.

Addition of ropinirole to levodopa may be used to control 'on-off' fluctuations and permit a reduction in the total daily dose of levodopa.

Posology and method of administration: Individual dose titration against efficacy and tolerability is recommended.

Ropinirole should be taken three times a day, preferably with meals to improve gastrointestinal tolerance.

Treatment initiation: The initial dose should be 0.25 mg t.i.d. A guide for the titration regimen for the first four weeks of treatment is given in the table below:

	Week			
	1	2	3	4
Unit dose (mg)	0.25	0.5	0.75	1.0
Total daily dose (mg)	0.75	1.5	2.25	3.0

Therapeutic regimen: After the initial titration, weekly increments of up to 3 mg/day may be given. Ropinirole is usually given in divided doses three times per day.

A therapeutic response may be seen between 3 and 9 mg/day, although adjunct therapy patients may require higher doses. If sufficient symptomatic control is not achieved, or maintained, the dose of ropinirole may be increased until an acceptable therapeutic response is established. Doses above 24 mg/day have not been investigated in clinical trials and this dose should not be exceeded.

When ropinirole is administered as adjunct therapy to L-dopa, the concurrent dose of L-dopa may be reduced gradually by around 20% in total.

When switching treatment from another dopamine agonist to ropinirole, the manufacturer's guidance on discontinuation should be followed before initiating ropinirole.

As with other dopamine agonists, ropinirole should be discontinued gradually by reducing the number of daily doses over the period of one week.

In parkinsonian patients with mild to moderate renal impairment (creatinine clearance 30–50 ml/min) no change in the clearance of ropinirole was observed, indicating that no dosage adjustment is necessary in this population.

The use of ropinirole in patients with severe renal (creatinine clearance <30 ml/min) or hepatic impairment has not been studied. Administration of ropinirole to such patients is not recommended.

Elderly: The clearance of ropinirole is decreased in patients over 65 years of age, but the dose of ropinirole for elderly patients can be titrated in the normal manner.

Children: Parkinson's disease does not occur in children. The use of ropinirole in this population has therefore not been studied and it should not be given to children.

Contra-indications: Hypersensitivity to ropinirole.

In light of the results of animal studies and the lack of studies in human pregnancy, ropinirole is contra-indicated in pregnancy, lactation and in women of child-bearing potential unless adequate contraception is used.

Special warnings and special precautions for use: Due to the pharmacological action of ropinirole, patients with severe cardiovascular disease should be treated with caution.

Co-administration of ropinirole with anti-hypertensive and anti-arrhythmic agents has not been studied. As with other dopaminergic drugs, caution should be exercised when these compounds are given concomitantly with ropinirole because of the unknown potential for the occurrence of hypotension, bradycardias or other arrhythmias.

Patients with major psychotic disorders should only be treated with dopamine agonists if the potential benefits outweigh the risks (see also *Interactions*).

Interaction with other medicaments and other forms of interaction: Neuroleptics and other centrally active dopamine antagonists, such as sulpiride or metoclopramide, may diminish the effectiveness of ropinirole and, therefore, concomitant use of these drugs with ropinirole should be avoided.

No pharmacokinetic interaction has been seen between ropinirole and L-dopa or domperidone which would necessitate dosage adjustment of either drug. No interaction has been seen between ropinirole and other drugs commonly used to treat Parkinson's disease but, as is common practice, care should be taken when adding a new drug to a treatment regimen. Ropinirole should not be given with other dopamine agonists.

In a study in parkinsonian patients receiving concurrent digoxin, no interaction was seen which would require dosage adjustment.

It has been established from *in vitro* experiments that ropinirole is metabolised by the cytochrome P450 enzyme CYP1A2. There is, therefore, the potential for an interaction between ropinirole and substrates (such as theophylline) or inhibitors (such as ciprofloxacin, fluvoxamine and cimetidine) of this enzyme. In patients already receiving ropinirole, the dose of ropinirole may need to be adjusted when these drugs are introduced or withdrawn.

Increased plasma concentrations of ropinirole have been observed in patients treated with high doses of oestrogens. In patients already receiving hormone replacement therapy (HRT), ropinirole treatment may be initiated in the normal manner. However, if HRT is stopped or introduced during treatment with ropinirole, dosage adjustment may be required.

No information is available on the potential for interaction between ropinirole and alcohol. As with other centrally active medications, patients should be cautioned against taking ropinirole with alcohol.

Pregnancy and lactation: Ropinirole should not be used during pregnancy. In animal studies, administration of ropinirole to pregnant rats at maternally toxic doses resulted in decreased foetal body weight at 60 mg/kg (approximately three times the AUC of the maximum dose in man), increased foetal death at 90 mg/kg (~x5) and digit malformations at 150 mg/kg (~x9). There was no teratogenic effect in the rat at 120 mg/kg (~x7) and no indication of an effect on development in the rabbit. There have been no studies of ropinirole in human pregnancy.

Ropinirole should not be used in nursing mothers as it may inhibit lactation.

Effects on ability to drive and use machines: No data are available on the effect of ropinirole on the ability to drive or use machinery. Patients should be cautioned about their ability to drive or operate machinery whilst taking ropinirole because of the possibility of somnolence or dizziness.

Undesirable effects: The most common adverse experiences reported by early therapy patients receiving ropinirole in clinical trials, and not seen at an equivalent or greater incidence on placebo, were; nausea, somnolence, leg oedema, abdominal pain, vomiting and syncope.

Similarly, the most common adverse experiences reported in adjunct therapy clinical trials were; dyskinesia, nausea, hallucinations and confusion.

The incidence of postural hypotension, an event commonly associated with dopamine agonists, was not markedly different from placebo in clinical trials with ropinirole. However, decreases in systolic blood pressure have been noted; symptomatic hypotension and bradycardia, occasionally severe, may occur.

Overdose: There have been no incidences of intentional overdose with ropinirole in clinical trials. It is anticipated that the symptoms of ropinirole overdose will be related to its dopaminergic activity.

Pharmacological properties

Pharmacodynamic properties: Ropinirole is a non-ergoline dopamine agonist.

Parkinson's disease is characterised by a marked dopamine deficiency in the nigral striatal system. Ropinirole alleviates this deficiency by stimulating striatal dopamine receptors.

Ropinirole acts in the hypothalamus and pituitary to inhibit the secretion of prolactin.

Pharmacokinetic properties: Oral absorption of ropinirole is rapid and essentially complete. Bioavailability of ropinirole is approximately 50% and average peak concentrations of the drug are achieved at a median time of 1.5 hours post-dose. Wide inter-individual variability in the pharmacokinetic parameters has been seen but, overall, there is a proportional increase in the systemic exposure (C_{max} and AUC) to the drug with an increase in dose, over the therapeutic dose range. Consistent with its high lipophilicity, ropinirole exhibits a large volume of distribution (approx. 8 l/kg) and is cleared from the systemic circulation with an average elimination half-life of about six hours. Plasma protein binding of the drug is low (10-40%). Ropinirole is metabolised primarily by oxidative metabolism and ropinirole and its metabolites are mainly excreted in the urine. The major metabolite is at least 100 times less potent than ropinirole in animal models of dopaminergic function.

No change in the oral clearance of ropinirole is observed following single and repeated oral administration. As expected for a drug being administered approximately every half-life, there is, on average, two-fold higher steady-state plasma concentrations of ropinirole following the recommended t.i.d. regimen compared to those observed following a single oral dose.

Preclinical safety data:

General toxicology: Ropinirole is well tolerated in laboratory animals in the dose range of 15 to 50 mg/kg. The toxicology profile is principally determined by the pharmacological activity of the drug (behavioural changes, hypoprolactinaemia, decrease in blood pressure and heart rate, ptosis and salivation).

Genotoxicity: Genotoxicity was not observed in a battery of *in vitro* and *in vivo* tests.

Carcinogenicity: Two-year studies have been conducted in the mouse and rat at dosages up to 50 mg/kg. The mouse study did not reveal any carcinogenic effect. In the rat, the only drug-related lesions were Leydig cell hyperplasia/adenoma in the testis resulting from the hypoprolactinaemic effect of ropinirole. These lesions are considered to be a species specific phenomenon and do not constitute a hazard with regard to the clinical use of ropinirole.

Pharmaceutical particulars

List of excipients:

Tablet cores: hydrous lactose, microcrystalline cellulose, croscarmellose sodium, magnesium stearate.

The four tablet strengths of ropinirole are distinguished by colour. The composition of the *film coat* therefore varies. All film coats contain hydroxypropyl methylcellulose and polyethylene glycol. The variations are shown in the table below:

Tablet strength (mg) / Tablet Colour	0.25 White	1.0 Green	2.0 Pink	5.0 Blue
Titanium Dioxide	✓	✓	✓	✓
Iron Oxide Yellow		✓	✓	
Iron Oxide Red			✓	
Indigo Carmine Aluminium		✓		✓
Polysorbate 80	✓			
Talc				

Incompatibilities: None known.

Shelf-life: Two years.

Special precautions for storage: This product should be stored in a dry place at or below 25°C and protected from light.

Nature and contents of container:

Tablets 0.25 mg, in opaque PVC/PVdC blister starting pack of 210.

Tablets 1 mg, in 60 ml HPDE bottle of 84.

Tablets 2 mg, in 60 ml HPDE bottle of 84.

Tablets 5 mg, in 60 ml HPDE bottle of 84.

Instructions for use/handling: None.

Marketing authorisation numbers

Requip Tablets 0.25 mg 10592/0085
Requip Tablets 1 mg 10592/0087
Requip Tablets 2 mg 10592/0088
Requip Tablets 5 mg 10592/0089

Date of approval/revision of SPC 12 July 1996

Legal category POM.

SEROXAT* TABLETS 20 mg
SEROXAT* TABLETS 30 mg
SEROXAT* LIQUID 20 mg/10 ml

Qualitative and quantitative composition Each tablet contains paroxetine hydrochloride equivalent to 20 or 30 mg paroxetine free base.

The liquid contains paroxetine hydrochloride equivalent to 20 mg paroxetine free base per 10 ml.

Pharmaceutical form

20 mg tablets: White, film-coated, modified oval, biconvex tablets engraved 'Seroxat 20' on one side and having a breakline on the reverse.

30 mg tablets: Blue, film-coated, modified oval, biconvex tablets engraved 'Seroxat 30' on one side and having a breakline on the reverse.

Liquid: Orange-coloured suspension with the smell of oranges and a sweet taste.

Clinical particulars

Therapeutic indications: Treatment of symptoms of depressive illness of all types including depression accompanied by anxiety. Following an initial satisfactory response, continuation with Seroxat therapy is effective in preventing relapse.

Treatment of symptoms and prevention of relapse of obsessive compulsive disorder (OCD).

Treatment of symptoms and prevention of relapse of panic disorder with or without agoraphobia.

Treatment of symptoms of social anxiety disorder/ social phobia.

Posology and method of administration: For oral administration.

Adults: Depression: The recommended dose is 20 mg daily. In some patients it may be necessary to increase the dose. This should be done gradually by 10 mg increments to a maximum of 50 mg/day according to the patient's response.

Obsessive compulsive disorder: The recommended dose is 40 mg daily. Patients should be started on 20 mg and the dose may be increased weekly in 10 mg increments. Some patients will benefit from having their dose increased up to a maximum of 60 mg/day.

Panic disorder: The recommended dose is 40 mg daily. Patients should be started on 10 mg per day and the dose increased weekly in 10 mg increments according to the patient's response. Some patients may benefit from having their dose increased up to a maximum of 50 mg/day. As is generally recognised, there is the potential for worsening of panic symptomatology during early treatment of panic disorder; a low initial starting dose is therefore recommended.

Social anxiety disorder/social phobia: The recommended dose is 20 mg daily. Patients should be started on 20 mg per day, and if no improvement is seen after at least two weeks, then they may benefit from having their dose increased up to a maximum of 50 mg/day. Dose should be increased in 10 mg increments, at intervals of at least one week, according to the patient's clinical response.

Seroxat has been shown to be effective in 12 week placebo-controlled trials. There is only limited evidence of efficacy after 12 weeks of treatment.

It is recommended that Seroxat be administered once daily in the morning with food. The tablets should be swallowed rather than chewed.

As with all antidepressant drugs, dosage should be reviewed and adjusted if necessary within two to three weeks of initiation of therapy and thereafter as judged clinically appropriate. Patients should be treated for a sufficient period to ensure that they are free from symptoms. This period should be at least four to six months after recovery (UK guidelines and WHO recommendation) for depression and may be even longer for OCD and panic disorder. As with many psychoactive medications, abrupt discontinuation should be avoided (see *Undesirable effects*).

Elderly: Increased plasma concentrations of Seroxat occur in elderly subjects.

Dosing should commence at the adult starting dose and may be increased weekly in 10 mg increments to a maximum of 40 mg per day according to patient's response.

Children: The use of Seroxat in children is not recommended as safety and efficacy have not been established in this population.

Renal/hepatic impairment: Increased plasma concentrations of Seroxat occur in patients with severe renal impairment (creatinine clearance <30 ml/min) or severe hepatic impairment. The recommended dose is 20 mg a day. Incremental dosage, if required, should be restricted to the lower end of the range.

Contra-indications: Known hypersensitivity to Seroxat.

Special warnings and precautions for use: MAO inhibitors: As with most anti-depressants, Seroxat should not be used in combination with MAO inhibitors or within two weeks of terminating treatment with MAO inhibitors. Thereafter treatment should be initiated cautiously and dosage increased gradually until optimal response is reached. MAO inhibitors should not be introduced within two weeks of cessation of therapy with Seroxat.

History of mania: As with all anti-depressants, Seroxat should be used with caution in patients with a history of mania.

Patients receiving oral anticoagulants: Seroxat should be administered with great caution to patients receiving oral anticoagulants (see *Interactions with other medicaments and other forms of interaction*).

Cardiac conditions: Seroxat does not produce clinically significant changes in blood pressure, heart rate and ECG. Nevertheless, as with all psychoactive drugs, caution is advised when treating patients with cardiac conditions.

Epilepsy: As with other antidepressants, Seroxat should be used with caution in patients with epilepsy.

Seizures: Overall, the incidence of seizures is <0.1% in patients treated with Seroxat. Seroxat should be discontinued in any patient who develops seizures.

ECT: There is little clinical experience of concurrent administration of Seroxat with ECT.

Interaction with other medicaments and other forms of interaction: Food/antacids: The absorption and pharmacokinetics of Seroxat are not affected by food or antacids.

Tryptophan: As with other 5-HT reuptake inhibitors, animal studies indicate that an interaction between Seroxat and tryptophan may occur, resulting in a 'serotonin syndrome' suggested by a combination of agitation, restlessness and gastrointestinal symptoms including diarrhoea.

Drug metabolising enzyme inducers/inhibitors: The metabolism and pharmacokinetics of Seroxat may be affected by drugs which induce or inhibit hepatic drug metabolising enzymes. When Seroxat is to be co-administered with a known drug metabolising inhibitor, consideration should be given to using doses at the lower end of the range. No initial dosage adjustment of Seroxat is considered necessary when it is to be co-administered with known drug metabolising enzyme inducers. Any subsequent dosage adjustment should be guided by clinical effect (tolerability and efficacy).

Alcohol: Although Seroxat does not increase the impairment of mental and motor skills caused by alcohol, the concomitant use of Seroxat and alcohol in patients is not advised.

Haloperidol/amylobarbitone/oxazepam: Experience in a limited number of healthy subjects has shown that Seroxat did not increase the sedation and drowsiness associated with haloperidol, amylobarbitone or oxazepam when given in combination.

MAOIs: As with other 5-HT reuptake inhibitors, animal studies indicate that an interaction between Seroxat and monoamine oxidase (MAO) inhibitors may occur (see *Special warnings and precautions for use*).

Lithium: Since there is little clinical experience, and there have been reports of interaction of lithium with other 5-HT reuptake inhibitors, the concurrent administration of Seroxat and lithium should be undertaken with caution. Lithium levels should be monitored.

Phenytoin/anticonvulsants: Co-administration with Seroxat and phenytoin is associated with decreased plasma concentrations of Seroxat and increased adverse experiences. Co-administration of Seroxat with other anticonvulsants may also be associated with an increased incidence of adverse experiences.

Warfarin: Preliminary data suggest that there may be a pharmacodynamic interaction between Seroxat and warfarin which may result in increased bleeding in the presence of unaltered prothrombin times. Seroxat should therefore be administered with great caution to patients receiving oral anticoagulants.

Pregnancy and lactation: Although animal studies have not shown any teratogenic or selective embryotoxic effects, the safety of Seroxat in human pregnancy has not been established and it should not be used during pregnancy or by nursing mothers unless the potential benefit outweighs the possible risk.

Effects on ability to drive and use machines: Clinical experience has shown that therapy with Seroxat is not associated with impairment of cognitive or psychomotor function. However, as with all psychoactive drugs, patients should be cautioned about their ability to drive a car and operate machinery.

Undesirable effects: In controlled trials the most commonly observed adverse events associated with the use of Seroxat and not seen at an equivalent incidence among placebo-treated patients were: nausea, somnolence, sweating, tremor, asthenia, dry mouth, insomnia, sexual dysfunction (including impotence and ejaculation disorders), dizziness, constipation, diarrhoea and decreased appetite. The majority of these adverse experiences decreased in intensity and frequency with continued treatment and did not generally lead to cessation of therapy.

In addition, there have been spontaneous reports of dizziness, vomiting, diarrhoea, restlessness, hallucinations and hypomania. Rash, including urticaria accompanied by pruritus or angioedema, has been reported. Symptoms suggestive of postural hypotension have been reported, often in patients with other risk factors.

Extrapyramidal reactions have been reported infrequently. Most of these have occurred in patients with underlying movement disorders, or who are using neuroleptic medication. Dystonic movements of the face, tongue and eyes have also been reported.

Abnormalities of liver function tests and hyponatraemia have been described rarely. These usually resolve rapidly on discontinuation of Seroxat.

Seroxat is less likely than tricyclic antidepressants to be associated with dry mouth, constipation and somnolence.

Symptoms including dizziness, sensory disturbance (e.g. paraesthesia), anxiety, sleep disturbances (including intense dreams), agitation, tremor, nausea, sweating and confusion have been reported following abrupt discontinuation of Seroxat. They are usually self-limiting and symptomatic treatment is seldom warranted. No particular patient group appears to be at higher risk of these symptoms; it is therefore recommended that when antidepressive treatment is no longer required, gradual discontinuation by dose-tapering or alternate day dosing be considered.

Overdose: A wide margin of safety is evident from available data. Overdose attempts have been reported in patients who took up to 2000 mg alone or in combination with other drugs, including alcohol. Experience of Seroxat in overdose has shown symptoms including nausea, vomiting, tremor, dilated pupils, dry mouth, irritability, sweating and somnolence, but not coma or convulsions.

No specific antidote is known.

Treatment should consist of those general measures employed in the management of overdose with any antidepressant. Early administration of activated charcoal may delay the absorption of Seroxat.

Pharmacological properties

Pharmacodynamic properties: Seroxat is a potent and selective inhibitor of 5-hydroxytryptamine (5-HT, serotonin) reuptake and its antidepressant action and efficacy in the treatment of OCD and panic disorder is thought to be related to its specific inhibition of 5-HT reuptake in brain neurones.

Seroxat is chemically unrelated to the tricyclic, tetracyclic and other available antidepressants.

The principal metabolites of Seroxat are polar and conjugated products of oxidation and methylation, which are readily cleared. In view of their relative lack of pharmacological activity, it is most unlikely that they contribute to the therapeutic effects of Seroxat.

Seroxat inhibits the hepatic cytochrome P450 isozyme responsible for the metabolism of debrisoquine and sparteine. This may lead to enhanced plasma levels of those co-administered drugs which are metabolised by this isozyme. Such drugs may include certain tricyclic antidepressants, phenothiazine neuroleptics and type Ic anti-arrhythmics.

Long-term treatment with Seroxat has shown that antidepressant efficacy is maintained for periods of at least one year.

In a placebo-controlled trial, the efficacy of paroxetine in the treatment of panic disorder has been maintained for at least one year.

Pharmacokinetic properties: Seroxat is well absorbed after oral dosing and undergoes first-pass metabolism.

The elimination half-life is variable but is generally about one day. Steady state systemic levels are attained by seven to 14 days after starting treatment and pharmacokinetics do not appear to change during long-term therapy.

Preclinical safety data: Not applicable.

Pharmaceutical particulars

List of excipients:

Tablet cores: Calcium phosphate (E341), sodium starch glycollate, magnesium stearate (E572).

Tablet film-coat: Hydroxypropyl methylcellulose (E464), titanium dioxide (E171), polyethylene glycol and polysorbate 80 (E433). The coating of the 30 mg tablets also contains indigo carmine (E132).

Liquid: Polacrilin potassium, dispersible cellulose (E460), propylene glycol, glycerol (E422), sorbitol (E420), methyl parahydroxybenzoate (E218), propylparahydroxybenzoate (E216), sodium citrate (E331), citric acid (E330), sodium saccharin (E954), natural orange flavour, natural lemon flavour, yellow colouring (E110), silicone antifoam, purified water.

Incompatibilities: Not applicable

Shelf-life:

Tablets: Two years.

Liquid: Two years.

Special precautions for storage:

Tablets: No special storage precautions are required.

Liquid: Store at 25°C or below.

Nature and contents of container:

Tablets: Available in Original Packs of 30 (two calendar PVC/aluminium or PVC/PVdC aluminium blister strips of 15 tablets).

Liquid: Amber glass bottles containing 150 ml, with white HDPE child-resistant cap with tamper evident seal.

Instruction for use/handling: None.

Marketing authorisation holder: SmithKline Beecham plc, SB House, Great West Road, Brentford, Middlesex TW8 9BD.

Trading as SmithKline Beecham Pharmaceuticals Mundells, Welwyn Garden City, Hertfordshire AL7 1EY.

Marketing authorisation numbers

Seroxat Tablets 20 mg:	10592/0001
Seroxat Tablets 30 mg:	10592/0002
Seroxat Liquid:	10592/0092

Date of first authorisation/renewal of authorisation

Seroxat Tablets 20 mg:	11.12.90 / 09.01.98
Seroxat Tablets 30 mg:	11.12.90 / 09.01.98
Seroxat Liquid:	08.01.97

Date of (partial) revision of the text September 1998

Legal category POM.

TAGAMET* TABLETS 800 mg, 400 mg and 200 mg
TAGAMET* EFFERVESCENT TABLETS 400 mg
TAGAMET* SYRUP
TAGAMET* INJECTION

Qualitative and quantitative composition Each tablet contains 800 mg, 400 mg or 200 mg cimetidine per tablet.

Each effervescent tablet contains 400 mg cimetidine per tablet.

The syrup contains 200 mg cimetidine in each 5 ml dose.

The injection contains 200 mg cimetidine in 2 ml.

Pharmaceutical form

Pale green, oval, film-coated tablets, engraved SK&F T800 on one side.

Pale green, oblong, film-coated tablets, engraved 'TAGAMET' on one side and SK&F 400 on reverse.

Pale green, circular, film-coated tablets, engraved 'TAGAMET' on one side and SK&F 200 on reverse.

White, circular, effervescent tablets with a predominantly orange odour.

A clear, orange-coloured, peach-flavoured syrup.

Ampoules containing 200 mg cimetidine in 2 ml solution.

Clinical particulars

Therapeutic indications: Tagamet is a histamine H_2-

receptor antagonist which rapidly inhibits both basal and stimulated gastric secretion of acid and reduces pepsin output.

Tagamet is indicated in the treatment of duodenal and benign gastric ulceration, including that associated with non-steroidal anti-inflammatory agents, recurrent and stomal ulceration, oesophageal reflux disease and other conditions where reduction of gastric acid by Tagamet has been shown to be beneficial: persistent dyspeptic symptoms with or without ulceration, particularly meal-related upper abdominal pain, including such symptoms associated with non-steroidal anti-inflammatory agents; the prophylaxis of gastrointestinal haemorrhage from stress ulceration in seriously ill patients; before general anaesthesia in patients thought to be at risk of acid aspiration (Mendelson's) syndrome, particularly obstetric patients during labour; to reduce malabsorption and fluid loss in the short bowel syndrome; and in pancreatic insufficiency to reduce degradation of enzyme supplements. Tagamet is also recommended in the management of the Zollinger-Ellison syndrome.

Posology and method of administration: Tagamet is usually given orally, but parenteral dosing may be substituted for all or part of the recommended oral dose in cases where oral dosing is impracticable or considered inappropriate.

The total daily dose by any route should not normally exceed 2.4 g. Dosage should be reduced in patients with impaired renal function (see *Special warnings and special precautions for use*).

Adults: Oral: For patients with duodenal or benign gastric ulceration, a single daily dose of 800 mg at bedtime is recommended. Otherwise the usual dosage is 400 mg twice a day with breakfast and at bedtime. Other effective regimens are 200 mg three times a day with meals and 400 mg at bedtime (1.0 g/day) and, if inadequate, 400 mg four times a day (1.6 g/day) also with meals and at bedtime.

Treatment should be given initially for at least four weeks (six weeks in benign gastric ulcer, eight weeks in ulcer associated with continued non-steroidal anti-inflammatory agents) even if symptomatic relief has been achieved sooner. Most ulcers will have healed by that stage, but those which have not will usually do so after a further course of treatment.

Treatment may be continued for longer periods in those patients who may benefit from reduction of gastric secretion and the dosage may be reduced in those who have responded to treatment, for example to 400 mg at bedtime or 400 mg in the morning and at bedtime.

In patients with benign peptic ulcer disease who have responded to the initial course, relapse may be prevented by continued treatment, usually with 400 mg at bedtime; 400 mg in the morning and at bedtime has also been used.

In oesophageal reflux disease, 400 mg four times a day, with meals and at bedtime, for four to eight weeks is recommended to heal oesophagitis and relieve associated symptoms.

In patients with very high gastric acid secretion (e.g. Zollinger-Ellison syndrome) it may be necessary to increase the dose to 400 mg four times a day, or in occasional cases further.

Since Tagamet may not give immediate symptomatic relief, antacids can be made available to all patients until symptoms disappear.

In the prophylaxis of haemorrhage from stress ulceration in seriously ill patients, doses of 200–400 mg can be given every four to six hours, by oral, nasogastric or parenteral routes. By direct intravenous injection a dose of 200 mg should not be exceeded: see below.

In patients thought to be at risk of acid aspiration syndrome an oral dose of 400 mg can be given 90–120 minutes before induction of general anaesthesia or, in obstetric practice, at the start of labour. While such a risk persists, a dose of up to 400 mg may be repeated (parenterally if appropriate) at four-hourly intervals as required up to the usual daily maximum of 2.4 g. Tagamet Syrup should not be used. The usual precautions to avoid acid aspiration should be taken.

In the short bowel syndrome, e.g. following substantial resection for Crohn's disease, the usual dosage range (see above) can be used according to individual response.

To reduce degradation of pancreatic enzyme supplements, 800–1600 mg a day may be given according to response in four divided doses, one to one and a half hours before meals.

Administration of effervescent tablets: The tablets should be dissolved in a glass of water.

Parenteral: Tagamet may be given intramuscularly or intravenously.

The dose by intramuscular injection is normally 200 mg which may be repeated at four- to six-hourly intervals.

The usual dosage for intravenous administration is 200–400 mg which may be repeated four- to six-hourly.

If direct intravenous injection cannot be avoided, 200 mg should be given **slowly** over at least five minutes, and may be repeated four- to six-hourly. Rapid intravenous injection has been associated with cardiac arrest and arrhythmias. For critically ill patients and patients with cardiovascular impairment, or if a larger dose is needed, the dose should be diluted and given over at least 10 minutes. In such cases infusion is preferable.

For intermittent intravenous infusion, Tagamet may be given at a dosage of 200 mg to 400 mg every four to six hours.

If continuous intravenous infusion is required, Tagamet may be given at an average rate of 50 to 100 mg/hour over 24 hours.

Elderly: The normal adult dosage may be used unless renal function is markedly impaired (see *Special warnings and special precautions for use*).

Children: Experience in children is less than that in adults. In children more than one year old, Tagamet 25–30 mg/kg body weight per day in divided doses may be administered by either the oral or parenteral route.

The use of Tagamet in infants under one year old is not fully evaluated; 20 mg/kg body weight per day in divided doses has been used.

Contra-indications: Hypersensitivity to cimetidine.

Special warnings and special precautions for use: Rapid intravenous injection of cimetidine (less than five minutes) should be avoided as there have been rare associations with cardiac arrest and arrhythmias. Transient hypotension has also been observed, particularly in critically ill patients (see dosage and administration).

Dosage should be reduced in patients with impaired renal function according to creatinine clearance. The following dosages are suggested: creatinine clearance of 0 to 15 ml per minute, 200 mg twice a day; 15 to 30 ml per minute, 200 mg three times a day; 30 to 50 ml per minute, 200 mg four times a day; over 50 ml per minute, normal dosage. Cimetidine is removed by haemodialysis, but not to any significant extent by peritoneal dialysis.

Clinical trials of over six years' continuous treatment and more than 15 years' widespread use have not revealed unexpected adverse reactions related to long-term therapy. The safety of prolonged use is not, however, fully established and care should be taken to observe periodically patients given prolonged treatment.

Tagamet treatment can mask the symptoms and allow transient healing of gastric cancer. The potential delay in diagnosis should particularly be borne in mind in patients of middle age and over with new or recently changed dyspeptic symptoms.

Care should be taken that patients with a history of peptic ulcer, particularly the elderly, being treated with Tagamet and a non-steroidal anti-inflammatory agent are observed regularly.

Each effervescent tablet contains 415 mg sodium which should be included in the daily allowance of patients on sodium-restricted diets. Effervescent tablets contain aspartame which should be taken into account by patients suffering from phenylketonuria.

Interaction with other medicaments and other forms of interaction: Tagamet can prolong the elimination of drugs metabolised by oxidation in the liver. Although pharmacological interactions with a number of drugs, e.g. diazepam, propranolol, have been demonstrated, only those with oral anticoagulants, phenytoin, theophylline and intravenous lignocaine appear, to date, to be of clinical significance. Close monitoring of patients on Tagamet receiving oral anticoagulants or phenytoin is recommended and a reduction in the dosage of these drugs may be necessary.

In patients on drug treatment or with illnesses that could cause falls in blood cell count, the possibility that H_2-receptor antagonism could potentiate this effect should be borne in mind.

Pregnancy and lactation: Although tests in animals and clinical evidence have not revealed any hazards from the administration of Tagamet during pregnancy or lactation, both animal and human studies have shown that it does cross the placental barrier and is excreted in milk. As with most drugs, the use of Tagamet should be avoided during pregnancy and lactation unless essential.

Effects on ability to drive and use machines: Not applicable.

Undesirable effects: Over 56 million patients have been treated with Tagamet worldwide and adverse reactions have been infrequent. Diarrhoea, dizziness or rash, usually mild and transient, and tiredness have been reported. Gynaecomastia has been reported and is almost always reversible on discontinuing treatment. Biochemical or biopsy evidence of reversible liver damage has been reported occasionally. Reversible confusional states have occurred, usually in elderly or already very ill patients, e.g. those with renal failure. Thrombocytopenia and leucopenia, including agranulocytosis (see *Special warnings and special precautions for use*), reversible on withdrawal of treatment, have been reported rarely; pancytopenia and aplastic anaemia have been reported very rarely. There have been very rare reports of interstitial nephritis, acute pancreatitis, fever, headache, myalgia, arthralgia, sinus bradycardia, tachycardia and heart block, all reversible on withdrawal of treatment. In common with other H_2-receptor antagonists, there have been very rare reports of anaphylaxis. Alopecia has been reported but no causal relationship has been established. Reversible impotence has also been very rarely reported but no causal relationship has been established at usual therapeutic doses. Isolated increases of plasma creatinine have been of no clinical significance.

Overdose: Acute overdosage of up to 20 grams has been reported several times with no significant ill effects. Induction of vomiting and/or gastric lavage may be employed together with symptomatic and supportive therapy.

Pharmacological properties

Pharmacodynamic properties: Cimetidine is a histamine H_2-receptor antagonist which rapidly inhibits both basal and stimulated gastric secretion of acid and reduces pepsin output.

Pharmacokinetic properties: Cimetidine is well absorbed after oral administration, metabolised in the liver and excreted mainly through the kidney with a half-life of about two hours. The effects on acid secretion are of longer duration.

Preclinical safety data: Not applicable.

Pharmaceutical particulars

List of excipients:

TAGAMET TABLETS 800 MG, 400 MG AND 200 MG

Each tablet contains maize starch, microcrystalline cellulose (E460), povidone 30, sodium lauryl sulphate, magnesium stearate (E572), sodium starch glycollate, iron oxides (E172), indigo carmine (E132), titanium dioxide (E171), hydroxypropylmethylcellulose (E464), propylene glycol, disodium edetate, talc (E553[b]) and carnauba wax (E903). The sodium contents of the tablets are: 800 mg tablet–1.6 mg sodium, 400 mg tablet–1.0 mg sodium, 200 mg tablet–0.5 mg sodium.

TAGAMET EFFERVESCENT TABLETS 400 MG

Each tablet contains sodium benzoate (E211), monosodium citrate (E331), aspartame, potassium acesulfame, orange flavour, tangerine tetraflavour, polyethylene glycol, citric acid (E330) and sodium bicarbonate (E500). The sodium content per tablet is 415 mg.

TAGAMET SYRUP

The syrup contains saccharin sodium, hydrochloric acid (E507), ethyl alcohol, methyl parahydroxybenzoate (E218), propyl parahydroxybenzoate (E216), propylene glycol, sodium chloride, disodium hydrogen phosphate (E339), sorbitol (E420), sucrose, FD&C Yellow No. 6 (E110), peach flavour, spearmint flavour, Mafco Magnasweet 180, ethylene oxide and propylene oxide polymer and water. The sodium content per 5 ml of syrup is 12.8 mg.

TAGAMET INJECTION

The injection contains hydrochloric acid (E507) and Water for Injections.

Incompatibilities: Not applicable.

Shelf-life: Tablets 800 mg, four years. Tablets 400 mg and 200 mg, five years. Effervescent Tablets, two years. Syrup, three years. Injection, five years.

Special precautions for storage: Store effervescent tablets in a dry place, and replace cap after use. Store syrup below 25°C, and ampoules below 30°C, protected from light.

Nature and contents of container: Tablets 800 mg, in opaque PVC/PVdC calendar packs (OP) of 30 (2 x 15). Tablets 400 mg, in opaque calendar packs (OP) of 60 (4 x 15), ward packs of 1000 (20 x 50). Tablets 200 mg, in opaque blister packs (OP) of 120 (4 x 30). Effervescent Tablets, 400 mg, in containers (OP) of 60 (4 tubes each containing 15 tablets). Syrup in bottles (OP) containing 600 ml. Injection in 2 ml clear glass ampoules in boxes of 20.

Instructions for use/handling: Tagamet has been shown to be compatible with electrolyte and dextrose solutions commonly used for intravenous infusion.

Tagamet Effervescent Tablets 400 mg may be particularly suitable for patients with difficulty in swallowing.

Marketing authorisation holder: Smith Kline & French Laboratories Ltd., Mundells, Welwyn Garden City, Hertfordshire AL7 1EY.

Trading as SmithKline Beecham Pharmaceuticals Mundells, Welwyn Garden City, Hertfordshire AL7 1EY.

Marketing authorisation numbers

Tagamet Tablets 800 mg	PL 0002/0128
Tagamet Tablets 400 mg	PL 0002/0092

Tagamet Tablets 200 mg	PL 0002/0063R
Tagamet Effervescent Tablets 400 mg	PL 0002/0206
Tagamet Syrup	PL 0002/0073R
Tagamet Injection	PL 0002/0059R

Date of first authorisation/renewal of authorisation

Tagamet Tablets 800 mg	18.10.84 / 29.11.95
Tagamet Tablets 400 mg	11.11.81 / 14.7.97
Tagamet Tablets 200 mg	21.5.90 / 14.7.97
Tagamet Effervescent Tablets 400 mg	17.10.90 / 23.6.97
Tagamet Syrup	18.5.90 / 31.5.96
Tagamet Injection	14.2.86 / 4.9.97

Date of (partial) revision of the text August 1998.

Legal category POM.

TIMENTIN* 1.6 G, 3.2 G

Qualitative and quantitative composition
Timentin 1.6 g: Contains 100 mg clavulanic acid with 1.5 g ticarcillin.
Timentin 3.2 g: Contains 200 mg clavulanic acid with 3.0 g ticarcillin.
The clavulanic acid is present as Potassium Clavulanate BP and the ticarcillin as ticarcillin sodium.

Pharmaceutical form Vials containing sterile powder for reconstitution.

Clinical particulars
Therapeutic indications: Timentin is an injectable antibiotic agent with a broad spectrum of bactericidal activity against a wide range of Gram-positive and Gram-negative aerobic and anaerobic bacteria. The presence of clavulanate in the formulation extends the spectrum of activity of ticarcillin to include many β-lactamase-producing bacteria normally resistant to ticarcillin and other β-lactam antibiotics.

Timentin is indicated for the treatment of infections in which susceptible organisms have been detected or are suspected.

Typical indications include: Severe infections in hospitalised patients and proven or suspected infections in patients with impaired or suppressed host defences including: septicaemia, bacteraemia, peritonitis, intra-abdominal sepsis, post-surgical infections, bone and joint infections, skin and soft tissue infections, respiratory tract infections, serious or complicated renal infections (e.g. pyelonephritis), ear, nose and throat infections.

Timentin is bactericidal to a wide range of organisms including:

Gram-positive:

Aerobes: *Staphylococcus* species including *Staphylococcus aureus* and *Staphylococcus epidermidis, Streptococcus* species including *Enterococcus faecalis.*

Anaerobes: *Peptococcus* species, *Peptostreptococcus* species, *Clostridium* species, *Eubacterium* species.

Gram-negative:

Aerobes: *Escherichia coli, Haemophilus* species including *Haemophilus influenzae, Moraxella catarrhalis, Klebsiella* species including *Klebsiella pneumoniae, Enterobacter* species, *Proteus* species including indole-positive strains, *Providentia stuartii, Pseudomonas* species including *Pseudomonas aeruginosa, Serratia* species including *Serratia marcescens, Citrobacter* species, *Acinetobacter* species, *Yersinia enterocolitica*

Anaerobes: *Bacteroides* species *including Bacteroides fragilis, Fusobacterium* species, *Veillonella* species.

Posology and method of administration
Adult dosage (including elderly patients): The usual dosage is 3.2 g Timentin given six to eight hourly. The maximum recommended dosage is 3.2 g four hourly.

Children's dosage: The usual dosage for children is 80 mg Timentin/kg body weight given every six to eight hours.

For premature infants and full-term infants during the perinatal period, the dosage is 80 mg Timentin/kg body weight every 12 hours, increasing to every eight hours thereafter.

Dosage in renal impairment:

Mild impairment (Creatinine Clearance >30 ml/min)	Moderate impairment (Creatinine Clearance 10-30 ml/min)	Severe impairment (Creatinine Clearance <10 ml/min)
3.2 g 8 hourly	1.6 g 8 hourly	1.6 g 12 hourly

Similar reductions in dosage should be made for children.

Administration: Intravenous infusion

Contra-indication: Penicillin hypersensitivity.

Special warnings and special precautions for use: Changes in liver function tests have been observed in some patients receiving Timentin. The clinical significance of these changes is uncertain but Timentin should be used with care in patients with evidence of severe hepatic dysfunction.

For patients with abnormal renal function see *Posology and method of administration.* The sodium intake should be monitored in patients with renal impairment. In treating patients on sodium restriction it should be noted that each gram of ticarcillin contains 5.3 mmol of sodium (approx.). Potassium levels should be monitored and supplementation with potassium provided in appropriate cases.

In rare cases bleeding manifestations have been reported following high dosages of ticarcillin. If bleeding manifestations appear with Timentin, treatment should be discontinued and appropriate therapy instituted unless, in the opinion of the physician, no alternative is available.

Interaction with other medicaments and other forms of interaction: Timentin acts synergistically with aminoglycosides against a number of organisms including *Pseudomonas.* Timentin prescribed concurrently with an aminoglycoside, may therefore be preferred in the treatment of life-threatening infections, particularly in patients with impaired host defences. In such instances the two products should be administered separately, at the recommended dosages.

Pregnancy and lactation: Animal studies with Timentin have shown no teratogenic effects. There is no experience of Timentin in human pregnancy; therefore its use in pregnancy cannot be recommended. During lactation, trace quantities of penicillins can be detected in breast milk.

Effects on ability to drive and use machines: None known.

Undesirable effects: Side effects (gastrointestinal upsets, rash) are uncommon and typical of other injectable penicillins. If a skin rash occurs, treatment should be discontinued.

Hepatitis and cholestatic jaundice have been reported. Hypokalaemia and eosinophilia have been reported rarely. In common with other β-lactam antibiotics angioedema and anaphylaxis have been reported.

Overdose: There is an increased risk of bleeding if ticarcillin is given in excess doses.

Timentin may be removed from the circulation by haemodialysis.

Pharmacological properties
Pharmacodynamic properties: Timentin is an injectable antibiotic, active against a wide range of both Gram-positive and Gram-negative bacteria, including β-lactamase-producing strains.

Resistance to many antibiotics is caused by bacterial enzymes which destroy the antibiotic before it can act on the pathogen. The clavulanate in Timentin anticipates this defence mechanism by blocking the β-lactamase enzymes, thus rendering the organisms sensitive to ticarcillin's rapid bactericidal effect at concentrations readily attainable in the body.

Clavulanate, by itself, has little antibacterial effect; however, in association with ticarcillin, as Timentin it produces an antibiotic agent with a breadth of spectrum suitable for empiric use in a wide range of infections treated parenterally in hospital.

Pharmacokinetic properties: The pharmacokinetics of the two components are closely matched and both components are well distributed in body fluids and tissues. Both clavulanate and ticarcillin have low levels of serum binding; about 20% and 45% respectively.

As with other penicillins the major route of elimination for ticarcillin is via the kidney; clavulanate is also excreted by this route.

Preclinical safety data: Not applicable.

Pharmaceutical particulars
List of excipients: None.

Incompatibilities: Timentin is not compatible with the following:

Proteinaceous fluids (e.g. protein hydrolysates); blood and plasma; intravenous lipids.

If Timentin is prescribed concurrently with an aminoglycoside the antibiotics should not be mixed in the syringe, intravenous fluid container or giving set because loss of activity of the aminoglycoside can occur under these conditions.

Shelf-life: 36 months.

Special precautions for storage: Timentin should be stored in a dry place at temperatures below 25°C.

Nature and contents of container: Clear glass vials with butyl rubber discs and aluminium seals. Supplied as packs of four vials.

Instructions for use/handling: The sterile powder should be dissolved in approximately 10 ml (1.6 g/3.2 g vial) prior to dilution into the infusion container (e.g mini-bag) or in-line burette.

The following approximate infusion volumes are suggested:

	Water for Injections BP	*Glucose Intravenous Infusion BP (5% w/v)*
3.2 g	100 ml	100–150 ml
1.6 g	50 ml	100 ml

Detailed instuctions are given in the Package Enclosure Leaflet.

Each dose of Timentin should be infused intravenously over a period of 30–40 minutes; avoid continuous infusion over longer periods as this may result in subtherapeutic concentrations.

800 mg Timentin has a displacement value of 0.55 ml.

Heat is generated when Timentin dissolves. Reconstituted solutions are normally a pale straw colour.

Timentin presentations are not for multi-dose use or for direct IV or IM injection. Any residual antibiotic solution should be discarded if less than the fully made up vial is used.

Marketing authorisation number 0038/0329

Date of approval/revision of SPC November 1996

Legal category POM.

TRIVAX*-HIB VACCINE ▼
Adsorbed Diphtheria, Tetanus and Pertussis Vaccine BP, DTPer/VAC/Ads (Trivax-AD*) and Haemophilus Type B Conjugate Vaccine (Hib)

Qualitative and quantitative composition Trivax-Hib contains Adsorbed Diphtheria, Tetanus and Pertussis Vaccine BP adsorbed on to aluminium hydroxide. It also contains purified polyribosyl-ribitol-phosphate capsular polysaccharide (PRP) of Hib, covalently bound to tetanus toxoid.

The Trivax-AD* components are prepared from chemically detoxified *Corynebacterium diphtheriae* and *Clostridium tetani* exotoxins, and killed whole *Bordetella pertussis* organisms.

The Hib polysaccharide is prepared from Hib, strain 20 752 and after activation with cyanogen bromide and derivatisation with adipic hydrazide spacer is coupled to tetanus toxoid via carbodiimide condensation. After purification the conjugate is lyophilised in the presence of lactose as a stabiliser.

Trivax-Hib meets the World Health Organisation requirements for manufacture of biological substances of Hib conjugate vaccines and of diphtheria, tetanus, pertussis and combined vaccines.

A 0.5 ml dose of the vaccine contains not less than 30 International units (IU) of diphtheria toxoid, not less than 60 IU of tetanus toxoid and not more than 20,000 million *Bordetella pertussis* organisms with a potency of not less than 4 IU adsorbed on to aluminium hydroxide and 10 micrograms of purified capsular polysaccharide of Hib covalently bound to approximately 30 micrograms tetanus toxoid.

Pharmaceutical form Hib vaccine (lyophilised) for reconstitution with Trivax-AD vaccine (suspension).

Clinical particulars
Therapeutic indications: Trivax-Hib is indicated for active immunisation against diphtheria, tetanus, pertussis and *Haemophilus influenzae* type b in infants and children under 10 years of age.

Posology and method of administration
Posology: The primary immunisation course should start at two months of age, and consists of three doses with an interval of at least one month between each dose.

Each dose consists of 0.5 ml of the vaccine by intramuscular injection.

Method of administration: Intramuscular injection.

Contra-indications: Trivax-Hib should not be administered to subjects with known hypersensitivity to any component of the vaccine, or to subjects that have shown any signs of hypersensitivity after previous administration of diphtheria, tetanus, pertussis or Hib vaccines.

As with other vaccines, the administration of Trivax-Hib should be postponed in subjects suffering from acute severe febrile illness. The presence of a minor non-febrile infection, however, is not a contra-indication to vaccination.

Progressive degenerative neurological disorder.

Severe local reaction to previous dose of the vaccine or one of its components–an area of erythema, swelling and induration involving most of the antero-lateral thigh or a major part of the circumference of the upper arm.

Severe general reaction to a previous dose of the vaccine or one of its components–for example:

a. Prolonged inconsolable crying or screaming for over three hours.
b. A convulsion or temperature >40.5°C occurring

within 72 hours, for which no other cause was found.

c. Hypotonia–hyporesponsive episode occurring within 72 hours.
d. Severe acute neurological illness occurring within 72 hours.
e. Immediate allergic reaction (severe or anaphylactic) to a previous dose of diphtheria, tetanus or pertussis vaccine.

Any child exhibiting a severe local or significant general reaction to a previous dose of a pertussis-containing vaccine should not be given a further dose of pertussis-containing vaccine. However, protection against diphtheria, tetanus and Hib is advisable and can be accomplished by giving Adsorbed Diphtheria and Tetanus Vaccine (CHILD), and a separate dose of Hib.

The vaccine should not be injected intradermally.

Trivax-Hib should not be administered to children aged 10 years and over, adults and the elderly.

Special warnings and precautions for use: Where there is a family or personal history of febrile convulsions, there is an increased risk of these occurring after pertussis immunisation. In such children, immunisation is recommended but advice on prevention of fever should be given at the time of immunisation.

In a recent British study, children with a personal or family history of epilepsy were immunised with pertussis vaccine without any significant adverse events. These children's developmental progress has been normal. In children with a close family history (first degree relatives) of idiopathic epilepsy there may be a risk of developing this condition irrespective of vaccination. Immunisation is recommended for these children. Children whose epilepsy is well controlled may receive pertussis vaccine.

Advice on the prevention of fever should be given.

When there is still an evolving neurological problem, immunisation should be deferred until the condition is stable. When there has been a documented history of cerebral damage in the neonatal period, immunisation should be carried out unless there is evidence of an evolving neurological abnormality. A personal or family history of allergy is not a contra-indication to immunisation with pertussis nor are stable neurological conditions such as cerebral palsy or spina bifida. Where there is doubt, appropriate advice should be sought from a consultant paediatrician, district (Health Board) Immunisation co-ordinator or a consultant in communicable disease control, rather than withholding the vaccine. HIV-positive individuals may receive pertussis vaccine in the absence of contra-indications.

It is good clinical practice that immunisation should be preceded by a review of the medical history (especially with regard to previous immunisation and possible occurrence of undesirable events) and a clinical examination.

As with all vaccinations, a solution of 1:1000 adrenaline should be available for injection should an anaphylactic reaction occur. Recipients of the vaccine should remain under observation until they have been seen to be in good health and not to be experiencing an immediate adverse reaction. It is not possible to specify an exact length of time.

Antipyretic measures may be indicated in those who experience a febrile convulsion following vaccination.

Use of Trivax-Hib in individuals aged 10 years and over may be associated with severe hypersensitivity reactions.

Trivax-Hib should be administered with caution to subjects with thrombocytopenia or a bleeding disorder since bleeding may occur following an intramuscular administration to these subjects. In these subjects Trivax-Hib may be administered by deep subcutaneous injection.

Trivax-Hib should under no circumstances be administered intravenously or intradermally.

Excretion of capsular polysaccharide antigen in the urine has been described following receipt of the Hib vaccine and therefore antigen detection may not have a diagnostic value in suspected Hib disease within one to two weeks of vaccination.

Interactions with other medicaments and other forms of interaction: Trivax-Hib can be administered simultaneously with oral polio.

As with other vaccines it may be expected that in patients receiving immunosuppressive therapy or patients with immunodeficiency, an adequate response may not be achieved.

Pregnancy and lactation: No reproductive studies have been conducted in animals since simultaneous vaccination against diphtheria, tetanus, pertussis and Hib in adults is uncommon. There is no accurate information on the safety of this vaccine in pregnancy therefore this vaccine should not be used in pregnancy or during lactation.

Effects on ability to drive and use machines: There is no information available on the effect of Trivax-Hib on driving and use of machines.

Undesirable effects: Local reactions, particularly erythema, pain and mild swelling at the site of injection, are commonly seen during the 24 hours following vaccination. They normally subside without treatment. A nodule may be found at the site of the injection, especially if the inoculation is introduced into the superficial layers of subcutaneous tissue.

A transient rise in temperature, restlessness, irritability, crying, loss of appetite, vomiting or diarrhoea may sometimes occur a few hours after vaccination, but does not generally call for treatment. Systemic reactions such as headache, malaise and somnolence have been reported. Allergic manifestations including pallor, dyspnoea and collapse have been observed rarely.

Neurological events have occasionally been observed following the administration of pertussis-containing vaccines. The events reported do not appear to constitute a single, identifiable clinical syndrome but include isolated febrile convulsions, infantile spasms, episodes of persistent screaming and severe encephalopathy resulting in permanent brain damage or death. These events cannot be distinguished from those occurring in unvaccinated children of similar age. In the absence of a common, identifiable pathological mechanism, it is not possible to produce a reliable estimate of the incidence of neurological events attributable to pertussis vaccination *per se*.

An increased incidence of reactions may occur due to failure to shake the container and re-suspend the vaccine before withdrawing a dose, to inadvertent intravenous administration, or to an over-rapid injection.

Since combined diphtheria, tetanus and pertussis vaccines are widely used in populations in which sudden illnesses of undefined origin are not uncommon, intercurrent illness bearing a temporal but not a causal relationship to vaccination may be expected.

Any untoward reactions should be reported to the regulatory authorities and to the manufacturer.

Overdose: Not applicable.

Pharmacological properties

Pharmacodynamic properties: Evaluation of pharmacodynamic properties is not required for vaccines.

Pharmacokinetic properties: Evaluation of pharmacokinetic properties is not required for vaccines.

Preclinical safety data: Not applicable.

Relevant Information for vaccines:

Trivax-AD Component: One month after the primary vaccination course 100% of infants vaccinated with Trivax-Hib had antibody titres of ≥ 0.1 IU/ml to tetanus and diphtheria. The vaccine response to the pertussis antigens (PT, FHA, pertactin and agglutinogens II, III) was also 100% i.e. all infants vaccinated at the end of the primary course had a level of antibodies higher than had been present prior to vaccination.

Haemophilus Influenzae Type b component: Titres of ≥ 0.15μg/ml have been obtained in 95-100% of infants one month after the completion of a primary vaccination course. Similar titres are seen following primary immunisation with Trivax-Hib.

Pharmaceutical particulars

List of excipients: Lyophilised Hib vaccine: Lactose.

Trivax-AD vaccine: Aluminium hydroxide, sodium borate, succinic acid, sodium chloride (1.8 mg of elemental sodium per 0.5 ml dose), thiomersal, water for injections.

Incompatibilities: Trivax-Hib should not be mixed with other vaccines in the same syringe, unless specified by the manufacturer.

Shelf-life: The shelf-life of the Trivax-Hib vaccine is two years when stored unopened and unmixed at 2°C to 8°C.

Special precautions for storage: Store between 2°C and 8°C. Protect from light. The Trivax-AD vaccine should not be frozen.

Nature and contents of container: The lyophilised Hib vaccine is presented as a white pellet in a glass vial.

The Trivax-AD vaccine is a suspension supplied in a prefilled syringe made of neutral glass type 1, which conforms to the European Pharmacopoeia. The prefilled syringe contains an overage to compensate for product loss during reconstitution with lyophilised Hib and should not be used on its own.

Instructions for use/handling: The Trivax-AD vaccine and reconstituted Trivax-Hib vaccine should be inspected visually for any foreign particulate matter and/or variation of physical aspect prior to administration. In the event of either being observed, discard the vaccines.

The Hib vaccine must be reconstituted by adding the entire contents of the supplied container of the Trivax-AD vaccine to the vial containing the Hib pellet as follows:

a. Attach the supplied green needle to the prefilled syringe of Trivax-AD.
b. Insert the green needle attached to the prefilled syringe of Trivax-AD through the bung into the Hib vial.
c. Inject the contents of the prefilled syringe of Trivax-AD into the Hib vial.
d. With the needle still inserted, shake the Hib vial vigorously and examine for complete dissolution i.e. a whitish liquid of uniform appearance should be formed.
e. Withdraw the entire mixture back into the syringe.
(f) Replace the green needle with the smaller orange needle supplied and administer the vaccine by intramuscular injection.

After reconstitution, Trivax-Hib should be injected promptly (within one hour).

Disposal should be by incineration at a temperature not less than 1100°C at a registered waste disposal contractor. Trivax-AD vaccine which has been frozen should not be used.

Marketing authorisation number 10592/0083

Date of approval/revision of SPC 4 July 1997

Legal category POM

TWINRIX* ADULT VACCINE ▼ Combined inactivated hepatitis A (720 ELISA units) and rDNA hepatitis B (20 mcg) Vaccine

Qualitative and quantitative composition Twinrix Adult is a combined vaccine formulated by pooling bulk preparations of the purified, inactivated hepatitis A (HA) virus and purified hepatitis B surface antigen (HBsAg), separately adsorbed on to aluminium hydroxide and aluminium phosphate. The HA virus is propagated in MRC_5 human diploid cells. HBsAg is produced by culture, in a selective medium, of genetically engineered yeast cells.

A 1.0 ml dose of vaccine contains not less than 720 ELISA Units of inactivated HA virus and 20 mcg of recombinant HBsAg protein.

Pharmaceutical form Suspension for injection.

Clinical particulars

Therapeutic indications: Twinrix Adult is indicated for use in non-immune adults and adolescents 16 years of age and above who are at risk of both hepatitis A and hepatitis B infection.

Posology and method of administration:

Dosage: A dose of 1.0 ml is recommended for adults and adolescents 16 years of age and above.

Primary vaccination schedule: The standard primary course of vaccination with Twinrix Adult consists of three doses, the first administered at the elected date, the second one month later and the third six months after the first dose. The recommended schedule should be adhered to.

Once initiated, the primary course of vaccination should be completed with the same vaccine.

Booster dose: It is not yet fully established whether immunocompetent individuals who have responded to hepatitis A and/or B vaccination(s) will require booster doses as protection in the absence of detectable antibodies may be ensured by immunological memory.

Long-term antibody persistence data following vaccination with Twinrix Adult are not currently available. However, the anti-HBs and anti-HAV antibody titres observed following a primary vaccination course with the combined vaccine are in the range of what is seen following vaccination with the monovalent vaccines. General guidelines for booster vaccination can therefore be drawn from experience with the monovalent vaccines. These guidelines are based on the assumption that a minimal antibody level is required for protection; protective levels (10 mIU/ml) of anti-HBs will persist in the majority of subjects for five years, with anti-HAV predicted to persist for at least 10 years.

Booster vaccination with the combined vaccine can be recommended five years after initiation of the primary course. If the monovalent vaccines are used as boosters, they can be administered five years after initiation of the primary course for hepatitis B and 10 years after initiation of the primary course for hepatitis A.

Antibody levels of subjects at risk can be assessed at regular intervals and appropriate boosters administered when titres fall below minimal levels.

Method of administration: Twinrix Adult is for intramuscular injection, preferably in the deltoid region.

Exceptionally the vaccine may be administered subcutaneously in patients with thrombocytopenia or bleeding disorders. However, this route of administration may result in suboptimal immune response to the vaccine (see *Warnings and precautions*).

Contra-indications: Twinrix Adult should not be administered to subjects with known hypersensitivity to any constituent of the vaccine, or to subjects having shown signs of hypersensitivity after previous administration of Twinrix Adult or the monovalent hepatitis A or hepatitis B vaccine.

As with other vaccines, the administration of Twinrix Adult should be postponed in subjects suffering from acute severe febrile illness.

Special warnings and special precautions for use: It is possible that subjects may be in the incubation period of a hepatitis A or hepatitis B infection at the time of vaccination. It is not known whether Twinrix Adult will prevent hepatitis A and hepatitis B in such cases.

The vaccine will not prevent infection caused by other agents such as hepatitis C and hepatitis E and other pathogens known to infect the liver.

Twinrix Adult is not recommended for post-exposure prophylaxis (e.g. needle-stick injury).

The vaccine has not been tested in patients with impaired immunity. In haemodialysis patients and persons with an impaired immune system, adequate anti-HAV and anti-HBs antibody titres may not be obtained after the primary immunisation course and such patients may therefore require administration of additional doses of vaccine.

As with all injectable vaccines, appropriate medical treatment and supervision should always be readily available in case of a rare anaphylactic event following the administration of the vaccine.

Since intradermal injection or intramuscular administration into the gluteal muscle could lead to a suboptimal response to the vaccine, these routes should be avoided. However, exceptionally Twinrix Adult can be administered subcutaneously to subjects with thrombocytopenia or bleeding disorders since bleeding may occur following an intramuscular administration to these subjects (see *Posology and method of administration*).

Twinrix Adult should under no circumstances be administered intravascularly.

Interactions with other medicinal products and other forms of interaction: No data on concomitant administration of Twinrix Adult with specific hepatitis A immunoglobulin or hepatitis B immunoglobulin have been generated. However, when the monovalent hepatitis A and hepatitis B vaccines were administered concomitantly with specific immunoglobulins, no influence on seroconversion was observed although it may result in lower antibody titres.

Although the concomitant administration of Twinrix Adult and other vaccines has not specifically been studied, it is anticipated that, if different syringes and other injection sites are used, no interaction will be observed.

It may be expected that in patients receiving immunosuppressive treatment or patients with immunodeficiency, an adequate response may not be achieved.

Use during pregnancy and lactation:
Pregnancy: The effect of Twinrix Adult on foetal development has not been assessed.

However, as with all inactivated vaccines, one does not expect harm to the foetus. Twinrix Adult should be used during pregnancy only when there is a clear risk of hepatitis A and hepatitis B.

Lactation: The effect on breast-fed infants of the administration of Twinrix Adult to their mothers has not been evaluated in clinical studies. Twinrix Adult should therefore be used with caution in breast-feeding women.

Effects on the ability to drive and use machines: The vaccine is unlikely to produce an effect on the ability to drive and use machines.

Undesirable effects: In controlled clinical studies, signs and symptoms were actively monitored in all subjects for four days following the administration of the vaccine. A checklist was used for this purpose. The vaccinees were also requested to report any clinical events occurring during the study period. The most common reactions were those at the site of injection. They included transient pain, redness and swelling. Systemic adverse events seen were fever, headache, malaise, fatigue, nausea and vomiting. These events were transient, only rarely reported and were considered by the subjects as mild.

In a comparative study it was noted that the frequency of solicited adverse events following the administration of Twinrix Adult is not different from the frequency of solicited adverse events following the administration of the monovalent vaccines.

Following widespread use of the monovalent hepatitis A and/or hepatitis B vaccines, the following undesirable events have been reported in temporal association in the days or weeks after vaccination. In many instances, a causal relationship has not been established.

Flu-like symptoms (such as fever, chills, headache, myalgia, arthralgia), fatigue, dizziness.

Rarely reported: paraesthesia, nausea, vomiting, decreased appetite, diarrhoea, abdominal pain, abnormal liver function tests, rash, pruritus, urticaria.

Very rarely reported : allergic reactions mimicking serum sickness, vasculitis, syncope, hypotension, lymphadenopathy, cases of peripheral and/or central neurological disorders, and may include multiple sclerosis, optic neuritis, myelitis, Bell's palsy, polyneuritis such as Guillain-Barré syndrome (with ascending paralysis), meningitis, encephalitis, encephalopathy, thrombocytopenic purpura, erythema exsudativum multiforme.

Overdose: No information available.

Pharmacological properties
Pharmacodynamic properties: Pharmacotherapeutic group: Hepatitis vaccines, ATC code JO7BC.

Twinrix Adult confers immunity against HAV and HBV infection by inducing specific anti-HAV and anti-HBs antibodies.

Protection against hepatitis A and hepatitis B develops within two to four weeks. In the clinical studies, specific humoral antibodies against hepatitis A were observed in approximately 94% of the adults one month after the first dose and in 100% one month after the third dose (i.e. month seven). Specific humoral antibodies against hepatitis B were observed in 70% of the adults after the first dose and approximately 99% after the third dose.

Based on experience with the monovalent vaccines, it is expected that in most vaccinees the antibodies will persist for at least four to five years after the primary vaccination course. To establish long-term protection, booster vaccination with either the monovalent vaccines or the combination vaccine is indicated (see *Posology and method of administration*).

Pharmacokinetic properties: Evaluation of pharmacokinetic properties is not required for vaccines.

Preclinical safety data: Not applicable.

Pharmaceutical particulars
List of excipients: Aluminium hydroxide, aluminium phosphate, aminoacids for injection, formaldehyde, neomycin sulphate, 2-phenoxyethanol, polysorbate 20, sodium chloride, residual tris and phosphate buffer and water for injection.

Incompatibilities: Twinrix Adult should not be mixed with other vaccines in the same syringe.

Shelf-life: The expiry date of the vaccine is indicated on the label and packaging.

Shelf-life is 36 months when stored at +2°C to +8°C.

Special precautions for storage: Twinrix Adult should be stored at +2°C to +8°C.

Do not freeze; discard if the vaccine has been frozen.

Nature and contents of container: Twinrix Adult is presented in a glass prefilled syringe.

The prefilled syringes are made of neutral glass type I, which conforms to European Pharmacopoeia requirements.

The content upon storage may present a fine white deposit with a clear colourless supernatant. Once shaken, the vaccine is slightly opaque.

Instructions for use/handling: The vaccine should be inspected visually for any foreign particulate matter and/or variation of physical aspect prior to administration. Before use of Twinrix Adult, the vaccine should be well shaken to obtain a slightly opaque, white suspension. Discard if the content appears otherwise.

Marketing authorisation numbers

Pack of 1 prefilled syringe	EU/1/96/020/001
Packs 10 prefilled syringes	EU 1/96/020/002

Date of approval/revision of SPC 12 January 1999

Legal category POM.

TWINRIX* PAEDIATRIC VACCINE ▼ Combined inactivated hepatitis A (360 ELISA units) and rDNA hepatitis B (10 mcg) Vaccine

Qualitative and quantitative composition Twinrix Paediatric is a combined vaccine formulated by pooling bulk preparations of the purified, inactivated hepatitis A (HA) virus and purified hepatitis B surface antigen (HBsAg), separately adsorbed on to aluminium hydroxide and aluminium phosphate.

The HA virus is propagated in MRC_5 human diploid cells. HBsAg is produced by culture, in a selective medium, of genetically engineered yeast cells.

A 0.5 ml dose of Twinrix Paediatric contains not less than 360 ELISA Units of inactivated HA virus and 10 mcg of recombinant HBsAg protein.

Pharmaceutical form Suspension for injection.

Clinical particulars
Therapeutic indications: Twinrix Paediatric is indicated for use in non-immune infants, children and adolescents from one year up to and including 15 years who are at risk of both hepatitis A and hepatitis B infection.

Posology and method of administration:
Dosage: The dose of 0.5 ml (360 ELISA Units HA/ 10 mcg HBsAg) is recommended for infants, children and adolescents from one year up to and including 15 years of age.

Primary vaccination schedule: The standard primary course of vaccination withTwinrix Paediatric consists of three doses, the first administered at the elected date, the second one month later and the third six months after the first dose. The recommended schedule should be adhered to. Once initiated, the primary course of vaccination should be completed with the same vaccine.

Booster dose: It is not yet fully established whether immunocompetent individuals who have responded to hepatitis A and/or B vaccination(s) will require booster doses as protection in the absence of detectable antibodies may be ensured by immunological memory.

Long-term antibody persistence data following vaccination with Twinrix Paediatric are not currently available. However, the anti-HBs and anti-HAV antibody titres observed following a primary vaccination course with the combined vaccine are in the range of what is seen following vaccination with the monovalent vaccines. General guidelines for booster vaccination can therefore be drawn from experience with the monovalent vaccines. These guidelines are based on the assumption that a minimal antibody level is required for protection; protective levels (10 mIU/ml) of anti-HBs will persist in the majority of subjects for five years, with anti-HAV predicted to persist for at least 10 years.

Booster vaccination with the combined vaccine can be recommended five years after initiation of the primary course. If the monovalent vaccines are used as boosters, they can be administered five years after initiation of the primary course for hepatitis B and 10 years after initiation of the primary course for hepatitis A.

Antibody levels of subjects at risk can be assessed at regular intervals and appropriate boosters administered when titres fall below minimal levels.

Method of administration: Twinrix Paediatric is for intramuscular injection, preferably in the deltoid region in adolescents and children or in the anterolateral thigh in infants.

Exceptionally, the vaccine may be administered subcutaneously in patients with thrombocytopenia or bleeding disorders. However, this route of administration may result in suboptimal immune response to the vaccine (see *Warnings and precautions*).

Contra-indications: Twinrix Paediatric should not be administered to subjects with known hypersensitivity to any constituent of the vaccine, or to subjects having shown signs of hypersensitivity after previous administration of Twinrix Paediatric or the monovalent hepatitis A or hepatitis B vaccine.

As with other vaccines, the administration of Twinrix Paediatric should be postponed in subjects suffering from acute severe febrile illness.

Special warnings and special precautions for use: It is possible that subjects may be in the incubation period of a hepatitis A or hepatitis B infection at the time of vaccination. It is not known whether Twinrix Paediatric will prevent hepatitis A and hepatitis B in such cases.

The vaccine will not prevent infection caused by other agents such as hepatitis C and hepatitis E and other pathogens known to infect the liver.

Twinrix Paediatric is not recommended for post-exposure prophylaxis (e.g. needlestick injury).

The vaccine has not been tested in patients with impaired immunity. In haemodialysis patients, patients receiving immunosuppressive treatment or patients with an impaired immune system, the anticipated immune response may not be achieved after the primary immunisation course. Such patients may require additional doses of vaccine; nevertheless immunocompromised patients may fail to demonstrate an adequate response.

As with all injectable vaccines, appropriate medical treatment and supervision should always be readily available in case of a rare anaphylactic event following the administration of the vaccine.

Since intradermal injection or intramuscular administration into the gluteal muscle could lead to a suboptimal response to the vaccine, these routes should be avoided. However, exceptionally Twinrix Paediatric can be administered subcutaneously to subjects with thrombocytopenia or bleeding disorders since bleeding may occur following an intramuscular administration to these subjects (see *Posology and method of administration*).

Twinrix paediatric should under no circumstances be administered intravascularly.

Interaction with other medicinal products and other forms of interaction: No data on concomitant administration of Twinrix Paediatric with specific hepatitis A immunoglobulin or hepatitis B immunoglobulin have been generated. However, when the monovalent hepatitis A and hepatitis B vaccines were administered concomitantly with specific immunoglobulins, no influence on seroconversion was observed although it may result in lower antibody titres (see also *Warnings and precautions*).

As the concomitant administration of Twinrix Paediatric and other vaccines has not specifically been studied, it is advised that the vaccine should not be administered at the same time as other vaccines.

Use during pregnancy and lactation:

Pregnancy: The effect of Twinrix Paediatric on foetal development has not been assessed. However, as with all inactivated vaccines, one does not expect harm to the foetus. Twinrix Paediatric should be used during pregnancy only when there is a clear risk of hepatitis A and hepatitis B.

Lactation: The effect on breast-fed infants of the administration of Twinrix Paediatric to their mothers has not been evaluated in clinical studies. Twinrix Paediatric should therefore be used with caution in breast-feeding women.

Effects on the ability to drive and use machines: The vaccine is unlikely to produce an effect on the ability to drive and use machines.

Undesirable effects: During clinical studies, the most common reactions were those at the site of injection (pain, redness and swelling).

Following widespread use of the monovalent hepatitis A and/or hepatitis B vaccines in adults and in children, the following undesirable events have been reported in temporal association in the days or weeks after vaccination. In many instances, a causal relationship has not been established.

Flu-like symptoms (such as fever, chills, headache, myalgia, arthralgia), fatigue, dizziness.

Rarely reported: paraesthesia, nausea, vomiting, decreased appetite, diarrhoea, abdominal pain, abnormal liver function tests, rash, pruritus, urticaria.

Very rarely reported: allergic reactions mimicking serum sickness, vasculitis, syncope, hypotension, lymphadenopathy, cases of peripheral and/or central neurological disorders, and may include multiple sclerosis, optic neuritis, myelitis, Bell's palsy, polyneuritis such as Guillain-Barré syndrome (with ascending paralysis), meningitis, encephalitis, encephalopathy, thrombocytopenic purpura, erythema exsudativum multiforme.

Overdose: No information available.

Pharmacological properties

Pharmacodynamic properties: Pharmacotherapeutic group: Hepatitis vaccines, ATC code JO7BC.

Twinrix Paediatric confers immunity against HAV and HBV infection by inducing specific anti-HA and anti-HBs antibodies.

Protection against hepatitis A and hepatitis B develops within two to four weeks. In the clinical studies, specific humoral antibodies against hepatitis A were observed in approximately 89% of the subjects one month after the first dose and in 100% one month after the third dose (i.e. month seven). Specific humoral antibodies against hepatitis B were observed in approximately 67% of the subjects after the first dose and 100% after the third dose.

Based on experience with the monovalent vaccines, it is expected that in most vaccinees the antibodies will persist for at least four to five years after the primary vaccination course. To establish long-term protection, booster vaccination with either the monovalent vaccines or the combined vaccine is indicated (see *Posology and method of administration*).

Pharmacokinetic properties: Evaluation of pharmacokinetic properties is not required for vaccines.

Preclinical safety data: Not applicable.

Pharmaceutical particulars

List of excipients: Aluminium hydroxide, aluminium phosphate, amino acids for injection, formaldehyde, neomycin sulphate, 2-phenoxyethanol, polysorbate 20, sodium chloride, residual tris and phosphate buffer and water for injection.

Incompatibilities: Twinrix Paediatric should not be mixed with other vaccines in the same syringe.

Shelf-life: The expiry date of the vaccine is indicated on the label and packaging. Shelf-life is 36 months when stored at +2°C to +8°C.

Special precautions for storage: Twinrix Paediatric should be stored at +2°C to +8°C.

Do not freeze; discard if the vaccine has been frozen.

Nature and content of container: Twinrix Paediatric is presented in a glass prefilled syringe.

The prefilled syringes are made of neutral glass type I, which conforms to European Pharmacopoeia requirements.

The content upon storage may present a fine white deposit with a clear colourless supernatant. Once shaken, the vaccine is slightly opaque.

Instructions for use/handling: The vaccine should be inspected visually for any foreign particulate matter and/or variation of physical aspect prior to administration. Before use of Twinrix Paediatric, the vaccine should be well shaken to obtain a slightly opaque, white suspension. Discard if the content appears otherwise.

Marketing authorisation holder: SmithKline Beecham Biologicals S.A., rue de l'Institut 89,1330 Rixensart, Belgium.

Marketing authorisation numbers

Packs of 1 prefilled syringe	EU 1/97/029/001
Packs of 10 prefilled syringes	EU 1/97/029/002

Date of approval/revision of SPC 12 January 1999

Legal category POM.

TYPHERIX*
Vi polysaccharide typhoid vaccine.

Qualitative and quantitative composition Typherix is a clear isotonic colourless solution containing the cell surface Vi polysaccharide extracted from *Salmonella typhi* Ty2 strain.

Typherix complies with WHO and European Pharmacopoeia monograph requirements for Vi polysaccharide typhoid vaccines.

Each 0.5 ml dose of vaccine contains 25 mcg of the Vi polysaccharide of *Salmonella typhi.*

Pharmaceutical form Solution for injection.

Clinical particulars

Therapeutic indications: Active immunisation against typhoid fever for adults and children older than two years of age.

Posology and method of administration:

Posology: A single dose of 0.5 ml containing 25 mcg of the Vi polysaccharide of *Salmonella typhi* is recommended for both children and adults.

Subjects who remain at risk of typhoid fever should be revaccinated using a single dose of vaccine every three years.

Method of administration: Typherix is for **intramuscular** injection.

Typherix should be administered with caution to subjects with thrombocytopenia or bleeding disorders since bleeding may occur following an intramuscular administration to these subjects : following injection, firm pressure should be applied to the site (without rubbing) for at least two minutes.

Typherix should under no circumstances be administered intravascularly.

Contra-indications: Typherix should not be administered to subjects with known hypersensitivity to any component of the vaccine or to subjects having shown signs of hypersensitivity after previous administration.

As with other vaccines, the administration of Typherix should be postponed in subjects suffering from acute severe febrile illness.

Special warnings and special precautions for use: The vaccine protects against typhoid fever caused by *Salmonella typhi.* Protection is not conferred against paratyphoid fever or illness caused by non-invasive Salmonellae.

Typherix has not been evaluated in children under two years of age. Nevertheless, it is known that children under this age may show a suboptimal response to polysaccharide antigen vaccines. The decision to use the vaccine in this age group should be based upon the risk of exposure to disease.

As with all injectable vaccines appropriate medical treatment and supervision should always be readily available in case of a rare anaphylactic reaction following administration of the vaccine.

The importance of scrupulous attention to personal, food and water hygiene must be emphasised for all persons at risk of typhoid fever.

Interaction with other medicaments and other forms of interaction: It may be expected that in patients receiving immunosuppressive treatment or patients with immunodeficiency, an adequate response may not be achieved.

In clinical studies in adults, Typherix has been administered concomitantly in opposite arms with Havrix* Monodose* (1440), SmithKline Beecham's inactivated hepatitis A vaccine.

There was no adverse impact on either the reactogenicity or immunogenicity of the vaccines when they were administered simultaneously in opposite arms.

Although the concomitant administration of Typherix and other vaccines–other than Havrix Monodose (1440) has not specifically been studied, it is anticipated that no interaction will be observed. Different injectable vaccines should always be administered at different injection sites.

Pregnancy and lactation:

Pregnancy: The effect of Typherix on foetal development has not been assessed. However, as with other purified polysaccharide vaccines, no effect is expected.

Typherix should only be used during pregnancy when there is a high risk of infection.

Lactation: The effect on breastfed infants of the administration of Typherix to their mothers has not been evaluated in clinical studies. Typherix should therefore only be used in breastfeeding women, when there is a high risk of infection.

Effects on ability to drive and use machines: The vaccine is unlikely to produce an effect on the ability to drive and use machines.

Undesirable effects: In clinical studies, in the majority of instances, local reactions were usually reported only during the first 48 hours following immunisation. The most common reaction, soreness, has been reported in approximately 7% of vaccinees.

In clinical studies, systemic reactions were also transient; the incidence of the most frequently reported symptoms, fever and headache, did not exceed 9%.

Overdose: Not applicable.

Pharmacological properties

Pharmacodynamic properties: In clinical studies, seroconversion was observed in >95% of recipients when measured at two weeks after administration.

Immunity persists for at least three years.

For individuals who remain at – or who may be reexposed to – risk of typhoid fever, it is recommended that they be revaccinated using a single dose of vaccine every three years.

Pharmacokinetic properties: Evaluation of pharmacokinetic properties is not required for vaccines.

Preclinical safety data: Not applicable.

Pharmaceutical particulars

List of excipients: Sodium chloride, dibasic sodium phosphate, monobasic sodium phosphate, phenol and water for injections.

Incompatibilities: Typherix should not be mixed with other vaccines in the same syringe.

Shelf-life: The expiry date of the vaccine is indicated on the label and packaging.

Shelf-life is 24 months when stored at 2°C to 8°C.

Special precautions for storage: Store at 2°C to 8°C. Protect from light.

Do not freeze.

Nature and contents of container: Typherix is presented as a clear, colourless, liquid vaccine in a glass prefilled syringe.

Glass prefilled syringes are made of neutral glass type I, and comply with European Pharmacopoeia Requirements.

Instructions for use/handling: Vaccines should be inspected for any foreign particulate matter and/or variation of physical aspect. In the event of either being observed, discard the vaccine.

Shake before use.

Marketing authorisation holder: SmithKline Beecham plc, SB House, Great West Road, Brentford, Middlesex TW8 9BD.

Trading as SmithKline Beecham Pharmaceuticals Mundells, Welwyn Garden City, Hertfordshire AL7 1EY.

Marketing authorisation number 10592/0126

Date of first authorisation/renewal of authorisation 5 August 1998

Legal category POM.

VECTAVIR* COLD SORE CREAM

Qualitative and quantitative composition Active constituent: Penciclovir 1% - INN penciclovir.

Pharmaceutical form White cream for topical application.

Clinical particulars

Therapeutic indications: Vectavir Cold Sore Cream is indicated for the treatment of cold sores (herpes labialis).

Posology and method of administration

Adults (including ≥ 16 years of age and the elderly): Vectavir Cold Sore Cream should be applied at approximately two hourly intervals during waking hours. Treatment should be continued for 4 days.

Treatment should be started as early as possible after the first sign of an infection.

Children (under 16 years): No work has been carried out in children.

Contra-indications: Known hypersensitivity to penciclovir or the other constituents of the formulation, e.g. propylene glycol.

Special warnings and special precautions for use: The cream should only be used on cold sores on the lips and around the mouth. It is not recommended for application to mucous membranes. Particular care should be taken to avoid application in or near the eyes.

Severely immunocompromised patients (e.g. AIDS patients or bone marrow transplant recipients) should be encouraged to consult a physician in case oral therapy is indicated.

Interaction with other medicaments and other forms of interaction: Clinical trial experience has not identified any interactions resulting from concomitant administration of topical or systemic drugs with Vectavir Cold Sore Cream.

Pregnancy and lactation: There is unlikely to be any cause for concern regarding adverse effects when the cream is used in pregnant and/or lactating women as systemic absorption of penciclovir following topical administration of Vectavir Cold Sore Cream has been shown to be minimal (see *Pharmacokinetic properties section*).

Animal studies have not shown any embryotoxic or teratogenic effects with penciclovir given intravenously (at doses greater than 1200 times those recommended for clinical use via topical application), nor were there any effects on male and female fertility and general reproductive performance (at doses greater than 1600 times those recommended for clinical use via topical application). Studies in rats show that penciclovir is excreted in the breast milk of lactating females given oral famciclovir (famciclovir; the oral form of penciclovir, is converted *in vivo* to penciclovir). There is no information on excretion of penciclovir in human milk.

Since the safety of penciclovir in human pregnancy has not been established, Vectavir Cold Sore Cream should only be used during pregnancy or in nursing mothers on the advice of a doctor and if the potential benefits are considered to outweigh the potential risks associated with treatment.

Effects on ability to drive and use machines: Adverse effects on the ability to drive or operate machinery have not been observed.

Undesirable effects: Vectavir Cold Sore Cream has been well-tolerated in human studies. Clinical trial experience has shown that there was no difference between Vectavir Cold Sore Cream and placebo in the rate or type of adverse reactions reported. In particular, application site reactions (e.g. transient burning, stinging, numbness) occurred in less than 3% of patients in each group in the pivotal clinical trials.

No cases of photosensitivity were reported in the pivotal clinical trials.

Overdose: No untoward effects would be expected even if the entire contents of a container of Vectavir Cold Sore Cream were ingested orally; penciclovir is poorly absorbed following oral administration. However, some irritation in the mouth could occur. No specific treatment is necessary if accidental oral ingestion occurs.

Pharmacological properties

Pharmacodynamic properties: Penciclovir has demonstrable *in vivo* and *in vitro* activity against herpes simplex viruses (types 1 and 2) and varicella zoster virus. In virus-infected cells penciclovir is rapidly and efficiently converted into a triphosphate (mediated via virus-induced thymidine kinase). Penciclovir triphosphate persists in infected cells for more than 12 hours where it inhibits replication of viral DNA and has a half-life of 9, 10 and 20 hours in cells infected with varicella zoster virus, herpes simplex virus type 1 and herpes simplex virus type 2 respectively. In uninfected cells treated with penciclovir, concentrations of penciclovir triphosphate are only barely detectable. Accordingly, uninfected cells are unlikely to be affected by therapeutic concentrations of penciclovir.

In clinical studies, Vectavir-treated patients healed 30% faster than placebo (up to one day earlier), pain resolution was 25–30% faster (median improvement of up to one day) and infectivity resolved up to 40% faster (one day earlier) than placebo.

Pharmacokinetic properties: Following application of Vectavir Cold Sore Cream in a human volunteer study at a daily dose of 180 mg penciclovir (approximately 67 times the proposed daily clinical dose), to occluded and abraded skin for four days, penciclovir was not quantifiable in plasma and urine.

Pre-clinical safety data

General toxicology: Topical application of 5% Vectavir Cold Sore Cream for four weeks to rats and rabbits was well tolerated. There was no evidence of contact sensitisation in guinea pigs.

A full programme of studies has been conducted using intravenous penciclovir. These studies did not raise any safety concerns regarding topical use of Vectavir Cold Sore Cream. There is a minimal systemic absorption of penciclovir following topical administration.

The results of a wide range of mutagenicity studies *in vitro* and *in vivo* indicate that penciclovir does not pose a genotoxic risk to man.

Pharmaceutical particulars

List of excipients: White soft paraffin, liquid paraffin, cetostearyl alcohol, propylene glycol, cetomacrogol 1000 and purified water

Incompatibilities: No known incompatibilities relevant to topical application of Vectavir Cold Sore Cream.

Shelf-life: Two years.

Special precautions for storage: Store at temperatures not exceeding 30°C. Do not freeze.

Nature and content of container: 2 g aluminium tube.

Instructions for use/handling: Store at room temperatures not exceeding 30°C. Do not freeze.

Marketing authorisation number 10592/0078

Date of approval/revision of SPC August 1996.

Legal category POM.

**Trade Mark*

Solvay Healthcare Limited
Gaters Hill
West End
Southampton SO18 3JD

☎ 01703 472281 🖷 01703 465350

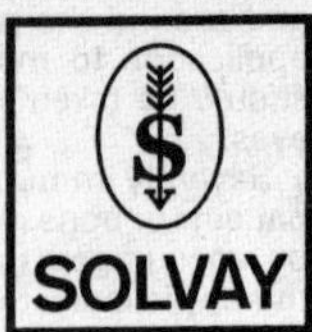

ALGESAL*

Presentation Off white, lavender-scented cream containing diethylamine salicylate 10% w/w. Excipients include glycerol monostearate, ethylene glycol stearate, stearic acid, triethanolamine, liquid and white soft paraffins, microcrystalline wax, Lavandin composition, and purified water.

Uses An analgesic cream for the symptomatic relief of rheumatic and minor musculo-skeletal conditions including lumbago, fibrositis, sciatica, bruises and sprains.

Dosage and administration
Adults (including the elderly) and children over 6 years: Apply three times daily to the affected area, massaging until cream is fully absorbed.

Children under 6 years: Not recommended.

Contra-indications, warnings, etc Algesal should not be used if the surface of the skin is broken. This product contains a salicylate which is related to aspirin.

Use in pregnancy: There is inadequate evidence of safety in human pregnancy, but it has been in wide use for many years without apparent ill consequence. However, it should only be used in pregnancy where there is no safer alternative.

Treatment of overdosage: Adverse systemic effects are unlikely even after accidental oral ingestion. No special measures are necessary.

Pharmaceutical precautions Store at room temperature.

Legal category P.

Package quantities Tube containing 50 g.

Further information Nil.

Product licence number 0512/0066.

COLOFAC* LIQUID

Qualitative and quantitative composition Mebeverine pamoate equivalent to 50 mg mebeverine hydrochloride per 5 ml.

Pharmaceutical form A yellow, banana flavoured, sugar free suspension.

Clinical particulars
Therapeutic indications: For the symptomatic treatment of irritable bowel syndrome and other conditions usually included in this grouping, such as chronic irritable colon, spastic constipation, mucous colitis, spastic colitis. Colofac is effectively used to treat the symptoms of these conditions, such as colicky abdominal pain and cramps, persistent, non-specific diarrhoea (with or without alternating constipation) and flatulence.

For the symptomatic treatment of gastro-intestinal spasm secondary to organic diseases.

Posology and method of administration:
Adults (including the elderly) and children 10 years and over: 15 ml (150 mg) three times a day, preferably 20 minutes before meals.

After a period of several weeks when the desired effect has been obtained, the dosage may be gradually reduced.

Children under 10 years: Not applicable.

Contra-indications: None known.

Special warnings and precautions for use: None.

Interactions with other medicaments and other forms of interaction: None known.

Pregnancy and lactation: Animal experiments have failed to show any teratogenic effects. However, the usual precautions concerning the administration of any drug during pregnancy should be observed.

Effects on ability to drive and use machines: None.

Undesirable effects: None.

Overdose: On theoretical grounds it may be predicted that CNS excitability will occur in cases of overdosage. No specific antidote is known; gastric lavage and symptomatic treatment is recommended.

Pharmacological properties
Pharmacodynamic properties: Mebeverine is a musculotropic antispasmodic with a direct action on the smooth muscle of the gastrointestinal tract, relieving spasm without affecting normal gut motility.

Pharmacokinetic properties: Mebeverine is rapidly and completely absorbed after oral administration in the form of tablets or suspension. Mebeverine is not excreted as such, but metabolised completely. The first step in the metabolism is hydrolysis, leading to veratric acid and mebeverine alcohol. Both veratric acid and mebeverine alcohol are excreted into the urine, the latter partly as the corresponding carboxylic acid and partly as the demethylated carboxylic acid.

Preclinical safety data: None stated.

Pharmaceutical particulars
List of excipients: Microcrystalline cellulose, carboxymethylcellulose sodium, citric acid monohydrate, sodium citrate, polysorbate 20, polyoxyl 40 hydrogenated castor oil, disodium pamoate monohydrate, sodium benzoate, saccharin sodium, banana flavour, simethicone emulsion, purified water.

The sodium content is 20.5 mg/5 ml.

Incompatibilities: Not applicable.

Shelf life: 3 years when stored in the original container.

Special precautions for storage: Store at room temperature, protected from light.

Nature and contents of container: Amber glass bottle with polyethylene tamper evident cap. Each bottle contains 300 ml.

Instructions for use/handling: Shake well before use. Dilution and subsequent storage not recommended. Mebeverine does not produce false positive reactions in standard diagnostic urine tests.

Marketing authorisation number 0512/0061

Date of approval/revision of SPC February 1997

Legal category POM

COLOFAC* TABLETS

Presentation White, round, sugar-coated tablets with no superficial markings each containing 135 mg mebeverine hydrochloride. Excipients include lactose and sucrose.

Uses Mebeverine is a musculotropic antispasmodic with a direct action on the smooth muscle of the gastro-intestinal tract, relieving spasm without affecting normal gut motility. Since this action is not mediated by the autonomic nervous system, anticholinergic side-effects are absent. Mebeverine is suitable for patients with prostatic hypertrophy and glaucoma.

Indications:

1. For the symptomatic treatment of irritable bowel syndrome and other conditions usually included in this grouping such as: chronic irritable colon, spastic constipation, mucous colitis, spastic colitis. Colofac is effectively used to treat the symptoms of these conditions, such as: colicky abdominal pain and cramps, persistent non-specific diarrhoea (with or without alternating constipation) and flatulence.
2. For the symptomatic treatment of gastro-intestinal spasm secondary to organic diseases.

Dosage and administration
Adults (including the elderly) and children 10 years and over: One tablet three times a day, preferably 20 minutes before meals.

After a period of several weeks when the desired effect has been obtained, the dosage may be gradually reduced.

Children under 10 years: Not applicable.

Contra-indications, warnings, etc
Contra-indications: None known.

Warnings: Animal experiments have failed to show any teratogenic effects. However, the usual precautions concerning the administration of any drug during pregnancy should be observed.

Treatment of overdosage: On theoretical grounds it may be predicted that CNS excitability will occur in cases of overdosage. No specific antidote is known; gastric lavage and symptomatic treatment is recommended.

Pharmaceutical precautions Store in a dry place, at room temperature, protected from light.

Legal category POM.

Package quantities Available in packs of 100 (5 strips of 20 blister-packed tablets).

Further information Mebeverine does not produce false positive reactions in standard diagnostic urine tests.

Product licence number 0512/0044

CREON* 10000

Qualitative and quantitative composition Each capsule contains:

10,000	Ph.Eur units lipase
8,000	Ph.Eur units amylase
600	Ph.Eur units protease

Pharmaceutical form Brown/clear capsules containing gastro-resistant granules.

Clinical particulars
Therapeutic indications: For the treatment of pancreatic exocrine insufficiency.

Posology and method of administration: Adults (including the elderly) and children:

Initially one to two capsules with each meal. Dose increases, if required, should be added slowly, with careful monitoring of response and symptomology.

It is important to ensure adequate hydration of patients at all times whilst dosing Creon.

The capsules can be swallowed whole, or for ease of administration they may be opened and the granules taken with fluid or soft food, but without chewing. If the granules are mixed with food it is important that they are taken immediately, otherwise dissolution of the enteric coating may result.

Colonic damage has been reported in patients with cystic fibrosis taking in excess of 10,000 units of lipase/kg/day (see Undesirable effects).

Contra-indications: Substitution with pancreatic enzymes is contra-indicated in the early stages of acute pancreatitis.

Patients with known hypersensitivity to porcine proteins.

Special warnings and special precautions for use: The product is of porcine origin.

Interaction with other medicaments and other forms of interaction: None known

Pregnancy and lactation: There is inadequate evidence of safety in use during pregnancy and lactation. However, as enzymes are not absorbed, it is unlikely that there would be any effect on the nursing infant.

Effect on ability to drive and to use machines: None known

Undesirable effects: Rarely cases of hyper-uricosuria and hyper-uricaemia have been reported with very high doses of pancreatin.

Stricture of the ileo-caecum and large bowel and colitis has been reported in children with cystic fibrosis taking high doses of pancreatic enzyme supplements. To date, Creon has not been implicated in the development of colonic damage. However, unusual abdominal symptoms or changes in abdominal symptoms should be reviewed to exclude the possibility of colonic damage–especially if the patient is taking in excess of 10,000 units of lipase/kg/day.

Overdose: Most cases respond to supportive measures including stopping enzyme therapy, ensuring adequate rehydration.

Pharmacological properties
Pharmacodynamic properties: Replacement therapy in pancreatic enzyme deficiency states. The enzymes have hydrolytic activity on fat, carbohydrates and proteins.

Pharmacokinetic properties: Pharmacokinetic data are

not available as the enzymes act locally in the gastro-intestinal tract. After exerting their action, the enzymes are digested themselves in the intestine.

Preclinical safety data: None stated.

Pharmaceutical particulars
List of excipients: Granules: Polyethylene glycol 4000, liquid paraffin, methylhydroxypropylcellulose phthalate (HP-55), dibutylphthalate, dimethicone 1000.

Capsule shell: gelatin, red, yellow and black iron oxides (E172), titanium dioxide (E171).

Incompatibilities: Not applicable.

Shelf life: 24 months, provided the product is kept in the original undamaged container, at temperatures not exceeding 20°C.

Special precautions for storage: Store below 20°C.

Nature and contents of container: HDPE container with LDPE cap. Containers hold 100 capsules.

Instructions for use/handling: No special instructions.

Marketing authorisation holder: Solvay Pharmaceuticals GmbH, Hans-Böckler-Allee 20, 30173 Hannover, Germany.

Marketing authorisation number 05727/0013

Date of approval/revision of SPC August 1997

Legal category P

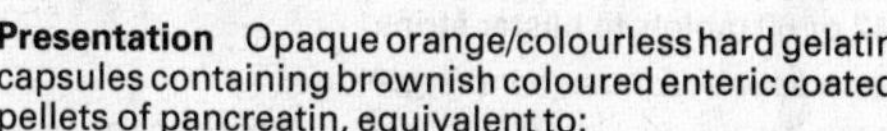

CREON* 25000 ▼

Presentation Opaque orange/colourless hard gelatin capsules containing brownish coloured enteric coated pellets of pancreatin, equivalent to:

25,000	PhEur units of lipase
18,000	PhEur units of amylase
1,000	PhEur units of protease (total).

Uses Replacement therapy in pancreatic enzyme deficiency states.

Indications: For the treatment of pancreatic exocrine insufficiency.

Dosage and administration *Adults (including the elderly) and children:* Initially one capsule with meals. Dose increases, if required, should be added slowly, with careful monitoring of response and symptomatology.

It is important to ensure adequate hydration of patients at all times whilst dosing Creon 25000.

The capsules can be swallowed whole, or for ease of administration they may be opened and the granules taken with fluid or soft food, but without chewing. If the granules are mixed with food it is important that they are taken immediately, otherwise dissolution of the enteric coating may result.

Colonic damage has been reported in patients with cystic fibrosis taking in excess of 10,000 units of lipase/kg/day (see *Warnings*).

Contra-indications, warnings, etc
Contra-indications: Substitution with pancreatic enzymes is contra-indicated in the early stages of acute pancreatitis. Patients with known hypersensitivity to porcine proteins.

Use in pregnancy: There is inadequate evidence of safety in use during pregnancy.

Warnings: The product is of porcine origin. Rarely cases of hyper-uricosuria and hyper-uricaemia have been reported with very high doses of pancreatin.

Perianal irritation, and rarely, inflammation, could occur when large doses are used.

Stricture of the ileo-caecum and large bowel and colitis has been reported in childen with cystic fibrosis taking high doses of pancreatic enzyme supplements. To date, Creon 25000 has not been implicated in the development of colonic damage. However, unusual abdominal symptoms or changes in abdominal symptoms should be reviewed to exclude the possibility of colonic damage – especially if the patient is taking in excess of 10,000 units of lipase/kg/day.

Overdosage: Most cases respond to supportive measures including stopping enzyme therapy and ensuring adequate rehydration.

Pharmaceutical precautions Store below 25°C.

Legal category POM.

Package quantities Available in packs of 100 capsules.

Further information This medicine may be taken by Muslim and Jewish patients.

Marketing authorisation number 5727/0006.

Marketing authorisation holder: Solvay Pharmaceuticals GmbH, Hans-Böckler-Allee 20, 30173 Hannover, Germany.

CREON* SACHETS

Qualitative and quantitative composition Each sachet contains 750 mg pancreatin equivalent to:

20,000	PhEur units of lipase
22,500	PhEur units of amylase
1,125	PhEur units of protease (total).

Pharmaceutical form Sachets containing brownish coloured enteric coated gastro-resistant granules.

Clinical Particulars
Therapeutic indications: For the treatment of pancreatic exocrine insufficiency.

Posology and method of administration: Initially the contents of 1 sachet with meals. Dose increases, if required, should be added slowly, with careful monitoring of response and symptomatology. It is important to ensure adequate hydration of patients at all times whilst dosing Creon.

One Creon sachet contains 20,000 PhEur units of lipase, compared to 8,000 BP units per capsule of Creon. Therefore, two sachets of Creon granules are equivalent to five Creon capsules (1BP unit of lipase=1 PhEur unit).

The contents of each sachet can be taken from a spoon or tipped directly onto the tongue, and then washed down with a drink of water or other fluid. The granules can also be sprinkled on soft food, which should then be swallowed without chewing. If the granules are mixed with food, it is important that they are taken immediately, otherwise dissolution of the enteric coating may result. In order to protect the enteric coating, it is important that the granules are not crushed or chewed.

Colonic damage has been reported in patients with cystic fibrosis taking in excess of 10,000 units of lipase/kg/day (see *Undesirable effects*).

Contra-indications: Substitution with pancreatic enzymes is contra-indicated in the early stages of acute pancreatitis. Patients with known hypersensitivity to porcine proteins.

Special warnings and special precautions for use: The product is of porcine origin.

Interaction with other medicaments and other forms of interaction: None known.

Pregnancy and lactation: There is inadequate evidence of safety in use during pregnancy. There is inadequate evidence of safety in use during lactation. However, as enzymes are not absorbed, it is unlikely that there would be any effect on the nursing infant.

Effects on ability to drive and use machines: None known.

Undesirable effects: Rarely cases of hyper-uricosuria and hyper-uricaemia have been reported with very high doses of pancreatin. Perianal irritation, and rarely, inflammation, could occur when large doses are used.

Stricture of the ileo-caecum and large bowel and colitis has been reported in childen with cystic fibrosis taking high doses of pancreatic enzyme supplements. To date, Creon has not been implicated in the development of colonic damage. However, unusual abdominal symptoms or changes in abdominal symptoms should be reviewed to exclude the possibility of colonic damage – especially if the patient is taking in excess of 10,000 units of lipase/kg/day.

Overdose: Most cases respond to supportive measures including stopping enzyme therapy, ensuring adequate rehydration.

Pharmacological properties
Pharmacodynamic properties: Replacement therapy in pancreatic enzyme deficiency states. The enzymes have hydrolytic activity on fat, carbohydrates and proteins.

Pharmacokinetic properties: Pharmacokinetic data are not available as the enzymes act locally in the gastro-intestinal tract. After exerting their action, the enzymes are digested themselves in the intestine.

Pharmaceutical particulars
List of excipients: Polyethylene glycol 4000, liquid paraffin, methylhydroxypropyl cellulose phthalate (HP-55), dibutyl phthalate, dimethicone 1000.

Incompatibilities: None known.

Shelf life: 2 years in the original undamaged container.

Special precautions for storage: Store at room temperature, protected from heat and moisture.

Nature and contents of container: Unit dose sachets consisting of aluminium/paper composite foil, with an internal coating of LDPE. Available in cartons containing 40 sachets.

Instructions for use/handling: This medicine may be taken by Muslim and Jewish patients.

Marketing authorisation holder: Solvay Pharmaceuticals GmbH, Hans-Böckler-Allee 20, 30173 Hannover, Germany.

Marketing authorisation number 5727/0007

Date of approval/revision of SPC September 1997

Legal category P.

DUPHALAC* (LACTULOSE SOLUTION BP)

Presentation A colourless to brownish yellow, clear or not more than slightly opalescent solution containing lactulose 3.35 g/5 ml. Also contains lactose 0.3 g/5 ml, galactose 0.55 g/5 ml.

Uses The active ingredient, lactulose, is metabolised in the colon by saccharolytic bacteria, producing low molecular weight organic acids, mainly lactic acid which lower the pH of the colonic contents and promote the retention of water by an osmotic effect, thus increasing persistaltic activity.

In patients with hepatic encephalopathy larger doses of lactulose are used; a significant reduction in the pH of the colonic contents results, which reduces markedly the formation and absorption of ammonium ions and other nitrogenous toxins into the portal circulation. Rapid decrements in blood ammonia concentration have been reported following lactulose treatment.

Indications: 1. The relief of constipation.

2. The treatment and prevention of hepatic encephalopathy (Portal systemic encephalopathy): hepatic coma.

Dosage and administration *Constipation:* Initially lactulose may be given twice daily. In due course the dose should be adjusted to the needs of the individual, but the following serves as a guide.

Starting dose	
Adults (including the elderly)	15 ml twice daily
Children 5 to 10 years	10 ml twice daily
Children under 5 years	5 ml twice daily
Babies under 1 year	2.5 ml twice daily

Each dose of Lactulose may, if necessary, be taken with water or fruit juices, etc.

Hepatic encephalopathy
Adults (including the elderly): Initially 30–50 ml. (6–10×5 ml spoonfuls) three times a day. Subsequently adjust the dose to produce two or three soft stools each day.

Children: No dosage recommendations for this indication.

Contra-indications, warnings, etc
Contra-indications: Galactosaemia. In common with other preparations used for the treatment of constipation, lactulose should not be used when there is evidence of gastro-intestinal obstruction.

Precaution: Lactose intolerance.

Use in pregnancy: Wide clinical experience, together with data from animal reproduction studies has not revealed any increase in embryotoxic hazard to the fetus, if used in the recommended dosage during pregnancy. If drug therapy is needed in pregnancy the use of this drug is acceptable.

Side-effects: During the first few days of treatment meteorism and increased flatulence may occur. These symptoms usually disappear with continued therapy. Diarrhoea may occur especially when using higher dosages, e.g. during treatment of portal systemic encephalopathy. Dosage should then be adjusted to obtain two or three formed stools per day.

Treatment of overdosage: No specific antidote. Symptomatic treatment should be given.

Pharmaceutical precautions Store below 20°C. Do not freeze. Dilution and subsequent storage not recommended.

Legal category P.

Package quantities Available in bottles of 300 ml and 500 ml.

Further information Due to lactulose's physiological mode of action it may take up to 48 hours before effects are obtained. However, clinical experience has shown that this medicament does exhibit a 'carry-over' effect which may enable the patient to reduce the effective dose gradually over a period of time.

A maintenance dose of 15 ml per day provides only 58 kJ (14 kcals), and is therefore, unlikely to adversely affect diabetics.

Product licence number 0512/5001R.

DUPHALAC* DRY

Presentation A white to slightly coloured, crystalline powder containing not less than 95% lactulose. Also contains not more than 5% related substances (lactose, galactose).

Uses The active ingredient, lactulose, is metabolised in the colon by the saccharolytic bacteria, producing low molecular weight organic acids, mainly lactic acid, which lower the pH of the colonic contents and promote the retention of water by an osmotic effect, thus increasing peristaltic activity.

In patients with hepatic encephalopathy, larger doses of lactulose are used; a significant reduction in the pH of the colonic content results, which reduces markedly the formation and absorption of ammonium ions and other nitrogenous toxins into the portal circulation. Rapid decrements in blood ammonia concentration have been reported following lactulose treatment.

Indications: 1. The relief of constipation.

2. The treatment and prevention of hepatic encephalopathy (portal systemic encephalopathy): hepatic coma.

Dosage and administration
Constipation: Initially lactulose may be given twice daily. In due course the dose should be adjusted to the needs of the individual, but the following serves as a guide.

Starting dose

Adults (including the elderly)	10 g (1 sachet) twice daily
Children 5 to 10 years	5 g twice daily
Children 5 years and under	Lactulose Solution BP is recommended

The dose can be taken from a spoon or tipped directly onto the tongue and then washed down with a drink of water or other fluid. The crystals may also be sprinkled on food, or mixed with water or other fluids before swallowing.

Hepatic encephalopathy:
Adults (including the elderly): Initially 20–30 g (2–3 sachets) three times daily. Subsequently adjust the dose to produce two or three soft stools each day.

Children: No dosage recommendations for this indication.

Contra-indications, warnings, etc
Contra-indications: Galactosaemia. In common with other preparations used for the treatment of constipation, lactulose should not be used where there is evidence of gastro-intestinal obstruction.

Precaution: Lactose intolerance.

Use in pregnancy: Wide clinical experience, together with data from animal reproduction studies has not revealed any increase in embryotoxic hazard to the fetus, if used in the recommended dosage during pregnancy. If drug therapy is needed in pregnancy the use of this drug is acceptable.

Side-effects: During the first few days of treatment meteorism and increased flatulence may occur. These symptoms usually disappear under continued therapy. Diarrhoea may occur especially when using higher dosages, e.g. during treatment of portal systemic encephalopathy. Dosage should then be adjusted to obtain two or three formed stools per day.

Treatment of overdosage: No specific antidote. Symptomatic treatment should be given.

Pharmaceutical precautions Store at temperatures up to 25°C.

Legal category P.

Package quantities 30 unit dose sachets.

Further information Due to lactulose's physiological mode of action it may take up to 48 hours before effects are obtained. However, clinical experience has shown that this medicament does exhibit a 'carry-over' effect which may enable the patient to reduce the effective dose gradually over a period of time. A maintenance dose of 10 g per day provides only 6kJ (1.44kcals) and is, therefore, unlikely to adversely affect diabetics.

Product licence number 0512/0105.

DUPHASTON*
DUPHASTON-HRT*

Qualitative and quantitative composition Each tablet contains 10 mg Dydrogesterone BP.

Pharmaceutical form Round, white tablet, scored on one side with the imprint '155' on each half of the tablet and imprinted 'S' on the reverse.

Clinical particulars
Therapeutic indications: To counteract the effects of unopposed oestrogen in hormone replacement therapy; pre-menstrual syndrome, endometriosis, dysmenorrhoea, infertility, irregular cycles, dysfunctional bleeding (with added oestrogen), secondary amenorrhoea (with added oestrogen), threatened and habitual abortion (associated with proven progesterone deficiency).

Posology and method of administration
Adults:
Hormone replacement therapy: The standard dose is 10 mg Duphaston daily for the last 14 days of each 28-day oestrogen treatment cycle. The dose may be increased to 10 mg twice daily if either early withdrawal bleeding occurs or if endometrial biopsy reveals inadequate progestational response.

Pre-menstrual syndrome: 10 mg twice daily from day 12 to 26 of the cycle. The dosage may be increased if necessary.

Endometriosis: 10 mg two to three times daily from day 5 to 25 of the cycle, or continuously.

Dysmenorrhoea: 10 mg twice daily from day 5 to 25 of the cycle.

Infertility or irregular cycles: 10 mg twice daily from day 11 to 25 of the cycle. Treatment should be maintained for at least six consecutive cycles. If the patient conceives, it is advisable to continue treatment for the first few months of pregnancy as described under 'habitual abortion'.

Dysfunctional bleeding – to arrest bleeding: 10 mg twice daily together with an oestrogen once daily for five to seven days.

Dysfunctional bleeding – to prevent bleeding: 10 mg twice daily together with an oestrogen once daily from day 11 to 25 of the cycle.

Amenorrhoea: An oestrogen once daily from day 1 to 25 of the cycle, and Duphaston 10 mg twice daily from day 11 to 25 of the cycle.

Threatened abortion: 40 mg at once then 10 mg every eight hours until symptoms remit. If symptoms persist or return during treatment the dose can be increased by one tablet every eight hours. The effective dose must be maintained for a week after symptoms have ceased and can then be gradually decreased unless symptoms return.

Habitual abortion: Treatment should be started as early as possible, preferably before conception. 10 mg should be given twice daily from day 11 to 25 of the cycle until conception and then continuously (10 mg twice daily) until the twentieth week of pregnancy, then dosage may be gradually reduced.

Elderly:
Hormone replacement therapy: Standard adult dosage is recommended.

Children:
Primary dysmenorrhoea: 10 mg twice daily at the discretion of the physician.

Contra-indications: None known.

Special warnings and special precautions for use: None known.

Interaction with other medicaments and other forms of interaction: None known.

Pregnancy and lactation
Pregnancy: There is no known risk in pregnancy. Duphaston is indicated for threatened or habitual abortion, until the twentieth week of pregnancy.

Lactation: Small amounts are expected to be excreted, but exact amounts are unknown. There have been no reports of adverse experiences.

Effects on ability to drive and use machines: None known.

Undesirable effects: Serious side-effects are not expected. Breakthrough bleeding may occur in a few patients. It can, however, be prevented by increasing the dosage. Nausea, breast tenderness, headache, bloated feeling, transient dizziness and skin reactions have occasionally been reported.

Overdose
Symptoms: No reports of ill-effects from overdosage have been reported and remedial action is generally unnecessary.

Treatment: If a large overdosage is discovered within 2–3 hours and treatment seems desirable, gastric lavage is recommended. There are no special antidotes and treatment should be symptomatic.

Pharmacological properties
Pharmacodynamic properties: Dydrogesterone is an orally-active progestogen which produces a complete secretory endometrium in an oestrogen-primed uterus thereby providing protection for oestrogen-induced increased risk of endometrial hyperplasia and/or carcinogenesis. It is indicated in all cases of endogenous progesterone deficiency. Duphaston is non-androgenic, non-oestrogenic, non-thermogenic, non-corticoid and non-anabolic.

Pharmacokinetic properties: After oral administration of labelled dydrogesterone, on average 63% of the dose is excreted into the urine. Within 72 hours excretion is complete. Dydrogesterone is completely metabolised.

The main metabolite of dydrogesterone is 20α-dihydrodydrogesterone (DHD) and is present in the urine predominantly as the glucuronic acid conjugate. A common feature of all metabolites characterised is the retention of the 4,6 diene-3-one configuration of the parent compound and the absence of 17α-hydroxylation. This explains the lack of oestrogenic and androgenic effects of dydrogesterone.

After oral administration of dydrogesterone, plasma concentrations of DHD are substantially higher as compared to the parent drug. The AUC and C_{max} ratios of DHD to dydrogesterone are in the order of 40 and 25, respectively.

Dydrogesterone is rapidly absorbed. The T_{max} values of dydrogesterone and DHD vary between 0.5 and 2.5 hours.

Mean terminal half lives of dydrogesterone and DHD vary between 5 to 7 and 14 to 17 hours, respectively.

Unlike progesterone, dydrogesterone is not excreted in the urine as pregnanediol. It is therefore possible to analyse production of endogenous progesterone even in the presence of dydrogesterone.

Preclinical safety data: Dydrogesterone has been used in several animal models and has been proven to be an entity with low toxicity, not having mutagenic or carcinogenic properties.

No effects were seen in reproduction experiments.

Pharmaceutical particulars
List of excipients: Lactose, maize starch, methylhydroxypropylcellulose, polyethylene glycol 400, silica, magnesium stearate and titanium dioxide (E171).

Incompatibilities: None known.

Shelf life: Five years.

Special precautions for storage: Store in a dry place, at room temperature (25°C), protected from light.

Nature and contents of container: Cartons containing 42 or 60 tablets in blister strips.

Instructions for use/handling: None.

Marketing authorisation number 0512/5004R.

Date of approval/revision of SPC June 1997.

Legal category POM.

FAVERIN*

Presentation Round, biconvex, scored, white film coated tablets imprinted 'S' on one side, '291' on both sides of the score on the reverse. Each tablet contains 50 mg fluvoxamine maleate.

Oval, biconvex, scored, white film coated tablets imprinted 'S' on one side, '313' on both sides of the score on the reverse. Each tablet contains 100 mg fluvoxamine maleate.

Uses The treatment of symptoms of depressive illness. The treatment of symptoms of obsessive-compulsive disorder (OCD).

Dosage and administration The tablets should be swallowed without chewing and with water.

Adults, including the elderly: The effective dosage usually lies between 100 mg and 200 mg, with some patients requiring up to 300 mg per day. The recommended starting dose is 100 mg per day. The dosage should be increased gradually until the effective dosage is achieved, with a maximum of 300 mg per day. A total daily dosage in excess of 100 mg should be given in divided doses. If no improvement of the OCD symptoms is observed within ten weeks, treatment with Faverin should be reconsidered.

Whilst there are no systematic studies to answer the question of how long to continue Faverin treatment, OCD is a chronic condition and it is reasonable to consider continuation beyond ten weeks in responding patients. Dosage adjustments should be made carefully on an individual patient basis, to maintain the patient at the lowest effective dose. The need for treatment should be reassessed periodically. Some clinicians advocate concomitant behavioural psychotherapy for patients who have done well on pharmacotherapy.

Children: There are insufficient data to recommend the use of Faverin in children.

Contra-indications, warnings, etc
Contra-indications: Faverin should not be given with or within two weeks of terminating treatment with monoamine-oxidase inhibitors. A period of 7 days should elapse before starting an MAOI after discontinuation of Faverin.

Faverin is contraindicated in patients with hypersensitivity to any component of the product.

Warnings: As improvement may sometimes be delayed for two or more weeks, patients should be closely monitored during this initial period. The possibility of a suicide attempt is inherent in patients suffering from depressive illness and may persist until significant improvement occurs.

As with other antidepressants, Faverin should be used with caution in patients with a history of epilepsy. If convulsions occur, Faverin therapy should be discontinued.

There is little clinical experience of concurrent administration of Faverin with ECT.

As with most antidepressants Faverin should be discontinued if the patient enters a manic phase.

There have been reports of cutaneous bleeding abnormalities such as ecchymoses and purpura with SSRIs. Caution is advised in patients taking SSRIs particularly in concomitant use with drugs known to affect platelet function (e.g. atypical antipsychotics and phenothiazines, most TCA's, aspirin, NSAIDs) as well as in patients with a history of bleeding disorders.

Driving: Faverin has shown no effect on psychomotor skills associated with driving and operating machinery up to and including 150 mg/day. However, as with all psychoactive drugs, patients should be cautioned about their ability to undertake potentially hazardous tasks such as driving or operating machinery.

Use in pregnancy and lactation: Although studies in animals have not shown any direct teratogenic effect, the safety of Faverin in human pregnancy has not been established. On basic principles, its use during pregnancy and in nursing mothers should be avoided, unless there are compelling reasons.

Hepatic/renal impairment: Patients with hepatic or renal insufficiency should begin treatment with a low dose and be carefully monitored. Rarely treatment with Faverin has been associated with an increase in hepatic enzymes, usually accompanied by symptoms. The drug should be withdrawn in such subjects.

Drug interactions: Faverin can prolong the elimination of drugs metabolised by oxidation in the liver. A clinically significant interaction is possible with drugs with a narrow therapeutic index (e.g. warfarin and other coumarin derivative anticoagulants, carbamazepine, clozapine, phenytoin and theophylline). The concomitant use of Faverin and theophylline should usually be avoided. Where this is not possible, patients should have their theophylline dose halved and plasma theophylline levels should be monitored closely.

In interaction studies, increased plasma levels of propranolol, warfarin and oxidatively metabolised benzodiazepines (e.g. bromazepam) were seen during concurrent administration of Faverin. It may therefore be advisable to lower the dose of these drugs when prescribing Faverin. An increase in previously stable plasma levels of tricyclic antidepressants, when used together with Faverin, has been reported. The combination of these drugs is not recommended. No interactions were seen with digoxin or with atenolol.

Faverin has been used in combination with lithium in the treatment of patients with severe drug-resistant depression. However, lithium (and possibly tryptophan) enhances the serotonergic effects of Faverin and the combination should therefore be used with caution.

There are isolated reports of enhanced serotonergic effects, resembling the neuroleptic malignant syndrome, when Faverin has been combined with lithium or neuroleptic medication.

The effects of alcohol may be potentiated by Faverin.

Side-effects: Many of the symptoms listed below are often associated with the illness and are not necessarily related to treatment.

Frequency >10%:
Digestive: nausea

Frequency 1–10%:
Body: abdominal pain, headache, malaise
Cardiovascular: palpitations/tachycardia
Digestive: anorexia, constipation, diarrhoea, dry mouth, dyspepsia, vomiting
General: asthenia
Nervous system: agitation, anxiety, dizziness, insomnia, nervousness, somnolence, tremor
Skin: sweating

Frequency 0.1–1%:
Cardiovascular: (postural) hypotension
Musculo-skeletal: arthralgia, myalgia
Nervous system: ataxia, confusion, dystonias, hallucinations
Urogenital: abnormal (delayed) ejaculation
Skin: rashes, pruritus

Frequency <0.1%:
Digestive: liver function abnormality
Nervous system: convulsions, mania
Urogenital: galactorrhoea

Particularly in the treatment of obsessive compulsive disorder, asthenia, insomnia and abnormal (delayed) ejaculation have been observed.

Faverin may cause a decrease in heart rate. During treatment, limited changes in repolarisation were observed in the ECG, but no causal relationship could be demonstrated.

Anaphylactoid and photosensitivity reactions have been rarely reported in patients taking Faverin.

Hyponatraemia has been reported in association with other antidepressants, though rarely reported with Faverin.

Withdrawal reactions have been reported with Faverin, these include headache, nausea, paraesthesia, dizziness and anxiety. Abrupt discontinuation of treatment with Faverin should be avoided. The majority of symptoms experienced on withdrawal of Faverin are non-serious and self-limiting.

Haemorrhage: See warnings.

Treatment of overdosage: No specific antidote is known. The stomach should be emptied as soon as possible after tablet ingestion and symptomatic treatment should be given. The use of medicinal charcoal is also recommended.

Pharmaceutical precautions Store below 25°C, protected from light.

Legal category POM.

Package quantities

50 mg tablets:	available in packs of 60.
100 mg tablets:	available in packs of 30.

Further information The mechanism of action of Faverin is thought to be related to its selective serotonin re-uptake inhibition in brain neurones, whilst there is minimum interference with noradrenergic or dopaminergic processes. Faverin is chemically unrelated to other currently available antidepressants.

Faverin is indicated for short-term and maintenance treatment.

Faverin is rapidly and completely absorbed after oral administration. The plasma half-life is approximately 15 hours after a single dose and slightly longer (17–22 hours) during repeated dosing, when steady state plasma levels are usually achieved in 10–14 days. It is transformed in the liver into pharmacologically inactive metabolites which are excreted by the kidney. Seventy-seven per cent of fluvoxamine maleate is bound to plasma proteins.

The pharmacokinetic profile in the elderly is similar to that in the general population.

Product licence numbers

50 mg	0512/0070
100 mg	0512/0072

FEMAPAK* 40

Qualitative and quantitative composition Femapak 40 consists of a pack containing eight Fematrix 40 transdermal patches and a blister strip of 14 Duphaston tablets. Each Fematrix 40 patch contains 1.25 mg estradiol (each patch delivers approximately 40 micrograms of estradiol per 24 hours).

Each Duphaston tablet contains 10 mg Dydrogesterone BP.

Pharmaceutical form Fematrix 40 is a self adhesive, flexible transdermal delivery system comprising a layer of clear adhesive sandwiched between a translucent patch and a metallised polyester backing. Fematrix 40 is a rectangular shape with rounded corners and has an active surface area of 14.25 cm^2.

Duphaston tablets are round and white, marked on one side with an S and on the other scored and marked with 155 on each half of the tablet.

Clinical particulars

Therapeutic indications: Hormone replacement therapy in female patients who have an intact uterus for the treatment of symptoms of oestrogen deficiency as a result of the natural menopause or oophorectomy. Dydrogesterone is provided to counteract the effects of oestrogen during the second two weeks of each cycle.

Posology and method of administration
Adults: Therapy should be initiated with Femapak 40 in women who have menopausal symptoms, who have been oestrogen deficient for a prolonged time or who are likely to be intolerant of high levels of oestradiol. The dosage may be increased if required by using Femapak 80. For maintenance therapy the lowest effective dose should be used.

One Fematrix transdermal patch should be applied twice weekly on a continuous basis. Each patch should be removed after 3 to 4 days and replaced with a new patch applied to a slightly different site. Patches should be applied to clean, dry and intact areas of skin below the waist on the lower back or buttocks. Fematrix should not be applied on or near the breasts.

Women who are having regular periods should commence therapy within five days of the start of bleeding. Women whose periods have stopped or have become very irregular may commence therapy at any time.

During the second two weeks of the cycle, that is from the 15th day after applying the first patch, one Duphaston tablet should be taken each day for the next 14 days. Most patients will commence bleeding towards the end of the Duphaston therapy.

Unopposed oestrogen therapy should not be used unless the patient has undergone a hysterectomy.

Children: Femapak is not indicated in children.

Contra-indications: Femapak is contra-indicated in women with known or suspected pregnancy, cancer of the breast, genital tract or other oestrogen-dependent neoplasia, undiagnosed vaginal bleeding, endometriosis, severe renal or cardiac disease, acute or chronic liver disease where liver function tests have failed to return to normal, active deep venous thrombosis, thromboembolic disorders or a history of confirmed venous thromboembolism (see also *Special warnings and precautions*), Dubin-Johnson syndrome or Rotor syndrome or hypersensitivity to lactose or other ingredients of the tablet.

Special warnings and precautions for use: It is recommended that the patient should undergo a thorough physical and gynaecological examination before commencing therapy. This should be repeated at regular intervals.

Unopposed oestradiol therapy should not be used in non-hysterectomised women because of the increased risk of endometrial hyperplasia or carcinoma.

At the present time there is suggestive evidence of an overall change in the relative risk of breast cancer in post-menopausal women receiving oestrogen replacement therapy. While some studies have shown that there may be a small increase in risk with treatment for more than 5 years others have shown no such increase. It is not known whether concurrent progestogen use influences the risk of breast cancer in post-menopausal women taking hormone replacement therapy. A careful appraisal of the risk/benefit ratio should be undertaken before treating for longer than 5 to 10 years.

Women with a history of fibrocystic disease, breast nodules, abnormal mammograms or family history of breast cancer should have regular breast examinations.

Certain diseases may be made worse by hormone replacement therapy and patients with these conditions should be closely monitored. These include otosclerosis, multiple sclerosis, systemic lupus erythematosus, cholelithiesis, porphyria, melanoma, epilepsy, migraine, thyrotoxicosis, surgically confirmed gall bladder disease, asthma and diabetes (worsening of glucose tolerance). Pre-existing uterine fibroids may increase in size during oestrogen therapy and symptoms associated with endometriosis may be exacerbated.

Epidemiological studies have suggested that hormone replacement therapy (HRT) is associated with an increased relative risk of developing venous thromboembolism (VTE) i.e. deep vein thrombosis or pulmonary embolism. The studies find a 2-3 fold increase for users compared with non-users which for healthy women amounts to a low risk of one extra case of VTE each year for every 5000 patients taking HRT.

Generally recognised risk factors for VTE include a personal or family history and severe obesity (Body Mass Index >30 kg/m^2). In women with these factors, the benefits of treatment with HRT need to be carefully weighed against risks.

The risk of VTE may be temporarily increased with prolonged immobilisation, major trauma or major surgery. In women on HRT, scrupulous attention should be given to prophylactic measures to prevent VTE following surgery. Where prolonged immobilisation is liable to follow elective surgery, particularly abdominal or orthopaedic surgery to the lower limbs, consideration should be given to temporarily stopping HRT 4 weeks earlier, if this is possible.

If venous thromboembolism develops after initiating therapy, the drug should be discontinued.

If jaundice or significant hypertension develop, treatment should be discontinued whilst the cause is investigated.

As oestrogens may cause fluid retention, patients with cardiac or renal dysfunction should be closely observed. Regular monitoring of blood pressure should be carried out in hypertensive patients.

Women of child bearing potential should be advised to adhere to non-hormonal contraceptive methods.

Interactions with other medicaments and other forms of interaction: Preparations inducing microsomal liver enzymes, eg barbiturates, hydantoins, anticonvulsants (including carbamazepine), meprobamate, phenylbutazone, antibiotics (including rifampicin), and activated charcoal may impair the activity of oestrogens. Transdermally applied oestrogens are less likely to be affected by such interactions than oral oestrogens since first pass hepatic metabolism is avoided.

Changes in oestrogen serum concentrations may affect the results of certain endocrine or liver function tests.

Pregnancy and lactation: Femapak is contra-indicated.

Effects on ability to drive and use machines: None.

Undesirable effects: Fematrix is generally well tolerated. The most frequent side effects (reported in 10 to 20% of patients, on at least one occasion, in clinical trials with Fematrix 80) which do not normally prevent continued treatment include: breast tenderness, headaches and breakthrough bleeding. Some patients experience mild and transient local erythema at the site of application with or without itching; this usually disappears rapidly on removal of the patch. The overall incidence of general patch irritation in clinical studies is less than 5%. In a clinical study 3% of 102 patients showed well defined erythema (Draize scale) 30 minutes after patch removal. No instances of permanent skin damage have been reported. If unacceptable topical side effects do occur discontinuation of treatment should be considered.

Other side effects associated with oestrogen or oestrogen/progestogen treatment have occasionally been reported (in 1% to 5% of patients in clinical trials with Fematrix 80) include: abdominal cramps, abdominal bloating, oedema, nausea, migraine and weight changes, additional side effects of dydrogesterone include occasional reports of transient dizziness and skin reactions.

More rarely (less than 1% in clinical trials with Fematrix 80) dizziness, dysmenorrhoea, leg cramps and visual disturbances have been reported.

Other side effects which have been rarely reported with oestrogen products include: changes in libido or changes in carbohydrate tolerance, vaginal candidiasis, change in vaginal secretions, cystitis like syndrome, cervical erosion, erythema multiforme, erythema nodosa, haemorrhagic eruptions, chloasma or melasma which may be persistent, steepening of corneal curvature, intolerance to contact lenses, mental depression and chorea minor. Cholestasis may be possible in predisposed patients.

Overdose: Fematrix 40: This is not likely due to the mode of administration. If it is necessary to stop delivery then the patch can be removed and plasma oestradiol levels will fall rapidly.

Duphaston: Symptoms: No reports of ill effects from overdosage have been recorded and remedial action is generally unnecessary.

Treatment: If a large overdosage is discovered within 2-3 hours and treatment seems desirable, gastric lavage is recommended. There are no special antidotes and treatment should be symptomatic.

Pharmacological properties

Pharmacodynamic properties

Estradiol: In the female, estradiol stimulates the accessory reproductive organs and causes development of the secondary sexual characteristics at puberty. It is also responsible for the hypertrophy of the uterus and for the changes in the endometrium during the first half of the menstrual cycle which when acted on by progesterone prepares it for the reception of a fertilised ovum. It furthermore promotes the growth of the ducts of the mammary glands. Large doses inhibit the gonadotropic secretion of the anterior pituitary, thus influencing the normal ovarian cycle.

It is of value in menstrual disorders, ovarian insufficiency, especially at the menopause, and for the treatment of infections of the vagina in children, where it promotes the growth of a cornified and more resistant epithelium; it is also used to terminate lactation, not very successfully, by inhibiting the release of prolactin.

Dydrogesterone: Dydrogesterone is an orally-active progestogen which produces a complete secretory endometrium in an oestrogen-primed uterus thereby providing protection for oestrogen-induced increased risk of endometrial hyperplasia and/or carcinogenesis. It is indicated in all cases of endogenous progesterone deficiency. Duphaston is non-androgenic, non-oestrogenic, non-corticoid and non-anabolic.

Pharmacokinetic properties

Fematrix: Absorption: Estradiol is absorbed from the patch across the stratum corneum and is delivered systemically at a low but constant rate throughout the period of application (3 to 4 days). The estimated delivery of estradiol is around 40 μmg/day.

Distribution: Oestrogens circulate in the blood bound to albumin, sex hormone binding globulin (SHBG), cortisol binding globulin and alpha1-glycoprotein. Following diffusion of free oestrogen into the cells of the target tissues in the hypothalamus, pituitary, vagina, urethra, uterus, breast and liver, binding to specific oestrogen receptors occurs. Very little information is currently available on the distribution of oestradiol following transdermal administration.

Biotransformation: Inactivation of oestrogens in the body is carried out mainly in the liver. Metabolism of 17β estradiol is by oxidation to oestrone, which in turn can be hydrated to form oestriol. There is free interconversion between oestrone and estradiol. Oestrone and oestriol may then undergo conversion to their corresponding sulphate and glucuronide derivatives for excretion in the urine. Oestrone sulphate has a long biologic half-life because of its enterohepatic recirculation and interconversion to oestrone and oestradiol.

Elimination: The plasma elimination half-life of estradiol is approximately 1 hour and is independent of the route of administration. The metabolic plasma clearance rate is between 650 and 900 L/day /m².

Steady state plasma oestradiol concentrations have been demonstrated in the range of 26 pg/ml to 34 pg/ml for the Fematrix 40 patch and 34 to 62 pg/ml for the Fematrix 80 patch (including baseline levels) and these are maintained throughout the dose interval (for up to four days). Absorption rate may vary between individual patients. After removal of the last patch plasma oestradiol and oestrone concentrations return to baseline values in less than 24 hours.

The median terminal half-life for estradiol following patch removal has been determined as 5.24h.

Dydrogesterone: After oral administration of labelled dydrogesterone on average 63% of the dose is excreted into the urine. Within 72 hours excretion is complete. Dydrogesterone is completely metabolised.

The main metabolite of dydrogesterone is 20 α-dihydrodydrogesterone (DHD) and is present in the urine predominantly as the glucuronic acid conjugate. A common feature of all metabolites characterised is the retention of the 4.6 diene-3-one configuration of the parent compound and the absence of 17 α-hydroxylation. This explains the lack of oestrogenic and androgenic effects of dydrogesterone.

After oral administration of dydrogesterone, plasma concentrations of DHD are substantially higher as compared to the parent drug. The AUC and C_{max} ratios of DHD to dydrogesterone are in the order of 40 and 25, respectively.

Dydrogesterone is rapidly absorbed. The T_{max} values of dydrogesterone and DHD vary between 0.5 and 2.5 hours.

Mean terminal half lives of dydrogesterone and DHD vary between 5 to 7 and 14 to 17 hours, respectively.

Unlike progesterone, dydrogesterone is not excreted in the urine as pregnanediol. It is therefore possible to analyse production of endogenous progesterone even in the presence of dydrogesterone.

Preclinical safety data

Fematrix: No specific preclinical studies have been conducted on Fematrix. Supraphysiologically high doses (prolonged overdoses) of oestradiol have been associated with the induction of tumours in oestrogen-dependent target organs in rodent species. Pronounced species differences in toxicology, pharmacology and pharmacodynamics exist.

Dydrogesterone: Dydrogesterone has been used in several animal models and has been proven to have low toxicity. It does not have mutagenic or carcinogenic properties. No effects were seen in reproduction experiments.

Pharmaceutical particulars

List of excipients:

Fematrix: Diethyltoluamide, Acrylic emulsion (Proprietary adhesive and thickener). Backing: Polyester film (3M Scotchpak 1220). Release liner: Siliconised/Aluminised/Polyester film.

Duphaston: Lactose, maize starch, methylhydroxypropylcellulose, silica, magnesium stearate and titanium dioxide (E171).

Incompatibilities: None known.

Shelf life: The shelf-life of the product as packaged for sale is 3 years.

Special precautions for storage: Femapak 40 should be stored at room temperature below 25°C in a dry place. Duphaston tablets should also be protected from light.

Nature and contents of container:

Fematrix: Blister tray with a foil lid containing one transdermal patch.

Duphaston: Blister strip containing 14 tablets.

Each carton contains eight Fematrix patches and 14 Duphaston HRT tablets sufficient for one 28 day cycle.

Instruction for use/handling: Detailed instructions for use are given in the patient leaflet.

Marketing authorisation holder: Ethical Pharmaceuticals (UK) Limited, Gemini House, Bartholomew's Walk, Cambridgeshire Business Park, Ely, Cambs CB7 4EA.

Marketing authorisation number 10013/0034.

Date of approval/revision of SPC September 1997

Legal category POM

FEMAPAK* 80

Qualitative and quantitative composition Femapak 80 consists of a pack containing eight Fematrix 80 transdermal patches and a blister strip of 14 Duphaston tablets. Each Fematrix 80 patch contains 2.5 mg estradiol (each patch delivers approximately 80 micrograms of estradiol per 24 hours).

Each Duphaston tablet contains 10 mg Dydrogesterone BP.

Pharmaceutical form Fematrix 80 is a self adhesive, flexible transdermal delivery system comprising a layer of clear adhesive sandwiched between a translucent patch and a metallised polyester backing. Fematrix 80 is a rectangular shape with rounded corners and has an active surface area of 28.5 cm².

Duphaston tablets are round and white, marked on one side with an S and on the other scored and marked with 155 on each half of the tablet.

Clinical particulars

Therapeutic indications: Hormone replacement therapy in female patients who have an intact uterus for the treatment of symptoms of oestrogen deficiency as a result of the natural menopause or oophorectomy and for the prevention of osteoporosis in women at risk of developing fractures. Epidemiological studies suggest a number of individual risk factors contribute to post menopausal osteoporosis, including:

Early menopause (either naturally or surgically)
Family history of osteoporosis
Recent prolonged systemic corticosteroid therapy
A small, thin frame
Cigarette use

If several risk factors are present consideration should be given to oestrogen replacement therapy.

For maximum benefit treatment should commence as soon as possible after the menopause.

Dydrogesterone is provided to counteract the effects of estrogen during the second two weeks of each cycle.

Posology and method of administration

Climateric symptoms: Therapy should be initiated with Femapak 40 in women who have menopausal symptoms, who have been oestrogen deficient for a prolonged time or who are likely to be intolerant of high levels of oestradiol. The dosage may be increased if required by using Femapak 80 for maintenance therapy the lowest effective dose should be used.

Prevention of osteoporosis: Treatment should be with Femapak 80, as the efficacy of Femapak 40 in this indication has yet to be established.

For optimum benefit treatment should continue for 5 to 10 years, protection appears to be effective for as long as treatment continues, however, data beyond 10 years is limited. For long term use see also *Precautions and warnings.*

Dosage schedule (for both indications): One Fematrix transdermal patch should be applied twice weekly on a continuous basis. Each patch should be removed after 3 to 4 days and replaced with a new patch applied to a slightly different site. Patches should be applied to clean, dry and intact areas of skin below the waist on the lower back or buttocks. Fematrix should not be applied on or near the breasts.

Women who are having regular periods should commence therapy within five days of the start of bleeding. Women whose periods have stopped or have become very irregular may commence therapy at any time.

During the second two weeks of the cycle, that is from the 15th day after applying the first patch, one Duphaston tablet should be taken each day for the next 14 days. Most patients will commence bleeding towards the end of the Duphaston therapy.

Unopposed oestrogen therapy should not be used unless the patient has undergone a hysterectomy.

Children: Femapak 80 is not indicated in children.

Contra-indications: Femapak 80 is contra-indicated in women with known or suspected pregnancy, cancer of the breast, genital tract or other oestrogen-dependent neoplasia, undiagnosed vaginal bleeding, endometriosis, severe renal or cardiac disease, acute or chronic liver disease where liver function tests have failed to return to normal, active deep venous thrombosis, thromboembolic disorders or a history of confirmed venous thromboembolism (see Special Precautions and Warnings), Dubin-Johnson syndrome or Rotor syndrome or hypersensitivity to lactose or other ingredients of the tablet.

Special warnings and precautions for use: It is recommended that the patient should undergo a thorough physical and gynaecological examination before commencing therapy. This should be repeated at regular intervals.

Unopposed oestradiol therapy should not be used in non-hysterectomised women because of the increased risk of endometrial hyperplasia or carcinoma.

At the present time there is suggestive evidence of an overall change in the relative risk of breast cancer in post-menopausal women receiving oestrogen replacement therapy. While some studies have shown that there may be a small increase in risk with treatment for more than 5 years others have shown no such increase. It is not known whether concurrent progestogen use influences the risk of breast cancer in post-menopausal women taking hormone replacement therapy. A careful appraisal of the risk/benefit ratio should be undertaken before treating for longer than 5 to 10 years.

Women with a history of fibrocystic disease, breast nodules, abnormal mammograms or family history of breast cancer should have regular breast examinations.

Certain diseases may be made worse by hormone replacement therapy and patients with these conditions should be closely monitored. These include otosclerosis, multiple sclerosis, systemic lupus erythematosus, cholelithiasis, porphyria, melanoma, epilepsy, migraine, thyrotoxicosis, surgically confirmed gall bladder disease, asthma and diabetes (worsening of glucose tolerance). Pre-existing uterine fibroids may increase in size during oestrogen therapy and symptoms associated with endometriosis may be exacerbated.

Epidemiological studies have suggested that hormone replacement therapy (HRT) is associated with an increased relative risk of developing venous thromboembolism (VTE) i.e. deep vein thrombosis or pulmonary embolism. The studies find a 2-3 fold increase for users compared with non-users which for healthy women amounts to a low risk of one extra case of VTE each year for every 5000 patients taking HRT.

Generally recognised risk factors for VTE include a personal or family history and severe obesity (Body Mass Index >30 kg/m²). In women with these factors, the benefits of treatment with HRT need to be carefully weighed against risks.

The risk of VTE may be temporarily increased with prolonged immobilisation, major trauma or major surgery. In women on HRT, scrupulous attention should be given to prophylactic measures to prevent VTE following surgery. Where prolonged immobilisation is liable to follow elective surgery, particularly abdominal or orthopaedic surgery to the lower limbs, consideration should be given to temporarily stopping HRT 4 weeks earlier, if this is possible.

If venous thromboembolism develops after initiating therapy, the drug should be discontinued.

If jaundice or significant hypertension develop, treatment should be discontinued whilst the cause is investigated. As oestrogens may cause fluid retention, patients with cardiac or renal dysfunction should be closely observed. Regular monitoring of blood pressure should be carried out in hypertensive patients.

Women who may be at risk of pregnancy should be advised to adhere to non-hormonal contraceptive methods.

Interactions with other medicaments and other forms of interaction: Preparations inducing microsomal liver enzymes, e.g. barbiturates, hydantoins, anti-convulsants (including carbamazepine), meprobromate, phenylbutazone, antibiotics (including rifampicin), and activated charcoal may impair the activity of oestrogens. Transdermally applied oestrogens are less likely to be affected by such interactions than oral oestrogens since first pass hepatic metabolism is avoided.

Changes in oestrogen serum concentrations may affect the results of certain endocrine or liver function tests.

Pregnancy and lactation: Femapak 80 is contra-indicated.

Effects on ability to drive and use machines: None stated.

Undesirable effects: The most frequent side effects (reported in 10 to 20% of patients, on at least one occasion in clinical trials with Fematrix 80) which do not normally prevent continued treatment include: breast tenderness, headaches, and breakthrough bleeding. Some patients experience mild and transient local erythema at the site of patch application with or without itching; this usually disappears rapidly on removal of the patch. The overall incidence of general patch irritation in clinical studies in less than 5%. In a clinical study 3% of 102 patients showed well defined erythema (draize scale) 30 minutes after patch removal. No instances of permanent skin damage have been reported. If unacceptable topical side effects do occur discontinuation of treatment should be considered.

Other side effects associated with estrogen or estrogen/progestogen treatment have occasionally been reported (in 1 to 5% of patients in clinical trials with Fematrix 80) include: abdominal cramps, abdominal bloating, oedema, nausea, migraine and weight changes. More rarely (less than 1% in clinical trials with Fematrix 80) dizziness, dysmenorrhoea, leg cramps and visual disturbances have been reported. Additional side effects of dydrogesterone include occasional reports of transient dizziness and skin reactions.

Other side effects which have been rarely reported with oestrogen products include: changes in libido or changes in carbohydrate tolerance, vaginal candidiasis, change in vaginal secretions, cystitis like syndrome, cervical erosion, erythema multiforme, erythema nodosa, haemeorrhagic eruptions, chloasma or melasma which may be persistent when the drug is discontinued, steepening of corneal curvature, intolerance to contact lenses, mental depression and chorea minor. Cholestatis may be possible in predisposed patients.

Overdose: Fematrix 80: This is not likely due to the mode of administration. If it is necessary to stop delivery then the patch can be removed and plasma estradiol levels will fall rapidly.

Duphaston: Symptoms: No reports of ill effects from overdosage have been recorded and remedial action is generally unnecessary.

Treatment: If a large overdosage is discovered within 2–3 hours and treatment seems desirable, gastric lavage is recommended. There are no special antidotes and treatment should be symptomatic.

Pharmacological properties

Pharmacodynamic properties

Estradiol: In the female, estradiol stimulates the accessory reproductive organs and causes development of the secondary sexual characteristics at puberty. It is also responsible for the hypertrophy of the uterus and for the changes in the endometrium during the first half of the menstrual cycle which when acted on by progesterone prepares it for the reception of a fertilised ovum. It furthermore promotes the growth of the ducts of the mammary glands. Large doses inhibit the gonadotropic secretion of the anterior pituitary, thus influencing the normal ovarian cycle.

It is of value in menstrual disorders, ovarian insufficiency, especially at the menopause, and for the treatment of infections of the vagina in childen, where it promotes the growth of a cornified and more resistant epithelium; it is also used to terminate lactation, not very successfully, by inhibiting the release of prolactin.

Dydrogesterone: Dydrogesterone is an orally-active progestogen which produces a complete secretory endometrium in an oestrogen-primed uterus thereby providing protection for Oestrogen-induced increased risk of endometrial hyperplasia and/or carcinogenesis. It is indicated in all cases of endogenous progesterone deficiency. Duphaston is non-androgenic, non-oestrogenic, non-corticoid and non-anabolic.

Pharmacokinetic properties

Fematrix 80

Absorption: Estradiol is absorbed from the patch across the stratum corneum and is delivered systemically at a low but constant rate throughout the period of application (3 to 4 days). The estimated delivery of estradiol is around 80 μg/day.

Distribution: Oestrogens circulate in the blood bound to albumin, sex hormone binding globulin (SHBG), cortisol binding globulin and alpha 1-glycoprotein. Following diffusion of free oestrogen into the cells of the target tissues in the hypothalamus, pituitary, vagina, urethra, uterus, breast and liver, binding to specific oestrogen receptors occurs. Very little information is currently available on the distribution of estradiol following transdermal administration.

Biotransformation: Inactivation of oestrogens in the body is carried out mainly in the liver. Metabolism of 17β estradiol is by oxidation to oestrone, which in turn can be hydrated to form oestriol. There is free interconversion between oestrone and estradiol. Oestrone and oestriol may then undergo conversion to their corresponding sulphate and glucuronide derivatives for excretion in the urine. Oestrone sulphate has a long biologic half-life because of its enterohepatic recirculation and interconversion to oestrone and estradiol.

Elimination: The plasma elimination half-life of estradiol is approximately 1 hour and is independent of the route of administration. The metabolic plasma clearance rate is between 650 and 900 L/day/m².

Steady state plasma estradiol concentrations have been demonstrated in the range of 34 pg/ml to 62 pg/ml and these are maintained throughout the dose interval (for up to four days). Absorption rate may vary between individual patients. After removal of the last patch plasma estradiol and oestrone concentrations return to baseline values in less than 24 hours. The median terminal half-life for estradiol following patch removal has been determined as 5.24 h.

Dydrogesterone: After oral administration of labelled dydrogesterone on average 63% of the dose is excreted into the urine. Within 72 hours excretion is complete. Dydrogesterone is completely metabolised.

The main metabolite of dydrogesterone is 20 α-dihydrodydrogesterone (DHD) and is present in the urine predominantly as the glucuronic acid conjugate. A common feature of all metabolites characterised is the retention of the 4.6 diene-3-one configuration of the parent compound and the absence of 17 α-hydroxylation. This explains the lack of oestrogenic and androgenic effects of dydrogesterone.

After oral administration of dydrogesterone, plasma concentrations of DHD are substantially higher as compared to the parent drug. The AUC and C_{max} ratios of DHD to dydrogesterone are in the order of 40 and 25, respectively.

Dydrogesterone is rapidly absorbed. The T_{max} values of dydrogesterone and DHD vary between 0.5 and 2.5 hours.

Mean terminal half lives of dydrogesterone and DHD vary between 5 to 7 and 14 to 17 hours, respectively.

Unlike progesterone, dydrogesterone is not excreted in the urine as pregnanediol. It is therefore possible to analyse production of endogenous progesterone even in the presence of dydrogesterone.

Preclinical safety data

Fematrix 80: No specific preclinical studies have been conducted on Fematrix. Supraphysiologically high doses (prolonged overdoses) of oestradiol have been associated with the induction of tumours in oestrogen dependent target organs in rodent species. Pronounced species differences in toxicology, pharmacology and pharmacodynamics exist.

Dydrogesterone: Dydrogesterone has been used in several animal models and has been proven to have low toxicity. It does not have mutagenic or carcinogenic properties. No effects were seen in reproduction experiments.

Pharmaceutical particulars

List of excipients:

Fematrix 80: Diethyltoluamide, Acrylic adhesive). Backing: Polyester film, Release liner: Aluminised/polyester.

Duphaston: Lactose, maize starch, methylhydroxypropylcellulose, silica, magnesium stearate and titanium dioxide (E171).

Incompatibilities: None known.

Shelf life: The shelf-life of the product as packaged for sale is 3 years.

Special precautions for storage: Femapak 80 should be stored at room temperature below 25°C in a dry place. Duphaston tablets should also be protected from light.

Nature and contents of container:

Fematrix 80: Blister tray with a foil lid containing one transdermal patch.

Duphaston: Blister strip containing 14 tablets.

Each carton contains eight Fematrix 80 patches and 14 Duphaston HRT tablets sufficient for one 28 day cycle.

Instruction for use/handling: Detailed instructions for use are given in the patient leaflet.

Marketing authorisation holder: Ethical Pharmaceuticals (UK) Limited, Gemini House, Bartholomew's Walk, Cambridgeshire Business Park, Ely, Cambs CB7 4EA.

Marketing authorisation number 10013/0033.

Date of approval/revision of SPC September 1997.

Legal category POM.

FEMATRIX* 40

Qualitative and quantitative composition Fematrix 40 contains 1.25 mg of oestradiol (Estradiol INN) and each patch delivers approximately 40 micrograms of oestradiol per 24 hours.

Pharmaceutical form Fematrix 40 is a self adhesive, flexible transdermal patch comprising a layer of clear adhesive sandwiched between a translucent patch and a metallised polyester backing. Fematrix 40 is a rectangular shape with rounded corners and has an active surface area of 14.25 cm².

Clinical particulars

Therapeutic indications: Oestrogen replacement therapy in female patients for the treatment of symptoms of oestrogen deficiency as a result of the natural menopause or oophorectomy.

Posology and method of administration

Adults: Therapy should be initiated with Fematrix 40 in women who have menopausal symptoms, who have been oestrogen deficient for a prolonged time or who are likely to be intolerant of high levels of oestradiol. The dosage may be increased if required by using Fematrix 80. For maintenance therapy the lowest effective dose should be used.

One Fematrix transdermal patch should be applied twice weekly on a continuous basis. Each patch should be removed after 3 to 4 days and replaced with a new patch applied to a slightly different site. Patches should be applied to clean, dry and intact areas of skin below the waist on the lower back or buttocks. Fematrix should not be applied on or near the breasts.

Women who are having regular periods should commence therapy within five days of the start of bleeding. Women whose periods have stopped or have become very irregular may commence therapy at any time.

In women with a uterus, a progestogen should be added for 12 to 14 days of each cycle. Most patients will commence bleeding towards the end of the progestogen therapy.

Unopposed oestrogen therapy should not be used unless the patient has undergone a hysterectomy.

Children: Fematrix is not indicated in children.

Contra-indications: Fematrix is contra-indicated in women with known or suspected pregnancy, cancer of the breast, genital tract or other oestrogen-dependent neoplasia, undiagnosed vaginal bleeding, endometriosis, severe renal or cardiac disease, acute or chronic liver disease where liver function tests have failed to return to normal, active deep venous thrombosis, thromboembolic disorders or a history of confirmed venous thromboembolism, Dubin-Johnson syndrome or Rotor syndrome.

Special warnings and precautions for use: It is recommended that the patient should undergo a thorough physical and gynaecological examination before commencing therapy. This should be repeated at regular intervals. Unopposed oestradiol therapy should not be used in non-hysterectomised women because of the increased risk of endometrial hyperplasia or carcinoma.

At present time there is suggestive evidence of an overall change in the relative risk of breast cancer in post menopausal women receiving oestrogen replacement therapy. While some studies have shown that there may be a small increase in risk with treatment for more than 5 years others have shown no such increase. It is not known whether concurrent progestogen use influences the risk of breast cancer in postmenopausal women taking hormone replacement therapy. A careful appraisal of the risk/benefit ratio should be undertaken before treating for longer than 5 to 10 years.

Women with a history of fibrocystic disease, breast nodules, abnormal mammograms or family history of breast cancer should have regular breast examinations.

Close monitoring of women with a history of uterine fibroids, cholelithiasis, porphyria, epilepsy, migraine, diabetes is necessary as oestrogen therapy may exacerbate or precipitate these conditions. Regular monitoring of blood pressure should be carried out in hypertensive patients.

Certain diseases may be made worse by hormone replacement therapy and patients with these conditions should be closely monitored. These include otosclerosis, multiple sclerosis, systemic lupus erythematosus, thyrotoxicosis, surgically confirmed gall bladder disease and diabetes (worsening of glucose tolerance). In addition pre-existing uterine fibroids may increase in size during oestrogen therapy and symptoms associated with endometriosis may be exacerbated.

Epidemiological studies have suggested that hormone replacement therapy (HRT) is associated with an increased relative risk of developing venous thromboembolism (VTE) i.e. deep vein thrombosis or pulmonary embolism. The studies find a 2-3 fold increase for users compared with non-users which for healthy women amounts to a low risk of one extra case of VTE each year for every 5000 patients taking HRT.

Generally recognised risk factors for VTE include a personal or family history and severe obesity (Body Mass Index >30 kg/m²). In women with these factors, the benefits of treatment with HRT need to be carefully weighed against risks.

The risk of VTE may be temporarily increased with prolonged immobilisation, major trauma or major surgery. In women on HRT, scrupulous attention should be given to prophylactic measures to prevent VTE following surgery. Where prolonged immobilisation is liable to follow elective surgery, particularly abdominal or orthopaedic surgery to the lower limbs, consideration should be given to temporarily stopping HRT 4 weeks earlier, if this is possible.

If venous thromboembolism develops after initiating therapy, the drug should be discontinued.

Women who may be at risk of pregnancy should be advised to adhere to non-hormonal contraceptive methods.

Interactions with other medicaments and other forms of interaction: None.

Pregnancy and lactation: Fematrix is contra-indicated.

Effects on ability to drive and use machines: None.

Undesirable effects: Fematrix is generally well tolerated. The most frequent side effects, (reported in 10 to 20% of patients, on at least one occasion, in clinical trials with Fematrix 80) which do not normally prevent continued treatment include: breast tenderness, headaches and breakthrough bleeding . Some patients experience mild and transient local erythema at the site of application with or without itching; this usually disappears rapidly on removal of the patch. The overall incidence of general patch irritation in clinical studies is less than 5%. In a clinical study 3% of 102 patients showed well defined erythema (Draize scale) 30 minutes after patch removal. No instances of permanent skin damage have been reported. If unacceptable topical side effects do occur discontinuation of treatment should be considered.

Other side effects associated with oestrogen or oestrogen/progestogen treatment have occasionally been reported (in 1% to 5% of patients in clinical trials with Fematrix 80) include: abdominal cramps, abdominal bloating, oedema, nausea, migraine and weight changes.

More rarely (less than 1% in clinical trials with Fematrix 80) dizziness, dysmenorrhoea, leg cramps and visual disturbances and changes in libido or changes in carbohydrate tolerance have been reported with other oestradiol products.

Overdose: This is not likely due to the mode of administration. If it is necessary to stop delivery then the patch can be removed and plasma oestradiol levels will fall rapidly.

Pharmacological properties

Pharmacodynamic properties:

Pharmacotherapeutic group: Natural oestrogen.

Mechanism of action/pharmacodynamic effects: In the female, oestradiol stimulates the accessory reproductive organs and causes development of the secondary sexual characteristics at puberty. It is also responsible for the hypertrophy of the uterus and for the changes in the endometrium during the first half of the menstrual cycle which when acted on by progesterone prepares it for the reception of a fertilized ovum. It furthermore promotes the growth of the ducts of the mammary glands. Large doses inhibit the gonadotropic secretion of the anterior pituitary, thus influencing the normal ovarian cycle.

It is of value in menstrual disorders, ovarian insufficiency, especially at the menopause, and for the treatment of infections of the vagina in children, where it promotes the growth of a cornified and more resistant epithelium; it is also used to terminate lactation, not very successfully, by inhibiting the release of prolactin.

Pharmacokinetic properties:

General characteristics of the active substance – Absorption: Oestradiol is absorbed from the patch across the stratum corneum and is delivered systemically at a low but constant rate throughout the period of application (3 to 4 days). The estimated delivery of oestradiol is approximately 40 micrograms per day for Fematrix 40.

Distribution: Oestrogens circulate in the blood bound to albumin, sex hormone binding globulin (SHBG), cortisol binding globulin and alpha-1-glycoprotein. Following diffusion of free oestrogen into the cells of the target tissues in the hypothalamus, pituitary, vagina, urethra, uterus, breast and liver, binding to specific oestrogen receptors occurs. Very little information is currently available on the distribution of oestradiol following transdermal administration.

Biotransformation: Inactivation of oestrogens in the body is carried out mainly in the liver. Metabolism of 17β -oestradiol is by oxidation to oestrone, which in turn can be hydrated to form oestriol. There is free interconversion between oestrone and oestradiol. Oestrone and oestriol may then undergo conversion to their corresponding sulphate and glucuronide derivatives for excretion in the urine. Oestrone sulphate has a long biologic half-life because of its enterohepatic recirculation and interconversion to oestrone and oestradiol.

Elimination: The plasma elimination half-life of oestradiol is approximately 1 hour and is independent of the route of administration. The metabolic plasma clearance rate is between 650 and 900 L/day/m².

Steady state plasma oestradiol concentrations have been demonstrated in the range of 26 pg/ml to 34 pg/ml for the Fematrix 40 patch (including baseline levels) and these are maintained throughout the dose interval (for up to four days). Absorption rate may vary between individual patients. After removal of the last patch plasma oestradiol and oestrone concentrations return to baseline values in less than 24 hours. The median terminal half-life for oestradiol following patch removal has been determined as 5.24h.

Preclinical safety data: No specific preclinical studies have been conducted on Fematrix. Supraphysiologically high doses (prolonged overdoses) of oestradiol have been associated with the induction of tumours in oestrogen-dependent target organs in rodent species. Pronounced species differences in toxicology, pharmacology and pharmacodynamics exist.

Pharmaceutical particulars

List of excipients: Diethyltoluamide, acrylic emulsion (proprietary adhesive), acrylic emulsion (adhesive thickener). Backing: Polyester. Release liner: Siliconised/aluminised/polyester.

Incompatibilities: Not applicable.

Shelf life: The shelf-life of the product as packaged for sale is 3 years.

Special precautions for storage: Fematrix patches should be stored at room temperature (below 25 °C) in a dry place.

Nature and contents of container: PVC/PVDC blister tray with paper/polythene/aluminium foil lid containing one transdermal patch. Each carton contains eight patches, sufficient for one 28 day cycle and a patient leaflet.

Instruction for use/handling: Detailed instructions for use are provided in the patient leaflet.

Marketing authorisation holder: Ethical Pharmaceuticals (UK) Ltd, Gemini House, Bartholomew's Walk, Cambridgeshire Business Park, Ely, Cambs CB7 4EA

Marketing authorisation number 10013/0032

Date of approval/revision of SPC October 1997

Legal category POM

FEMATRIX* 80

Qualitative and quantitative composition Fematrix 80 contains 2.5 mg of oestradiol (Estradiol INN) and each patch delivers approximately 80 micrograms of oestradiol per 24 hours.

Pharmaceutical form Fematrix 80 is a self adhesive, flexible transdermal patch comprising a layer of clear adhesive sandwiched between a translucent patch and a metallised polyester backing. Fematrix 80 is a rectangular shape with rounded corners and has an active surface area of 28.5 cm².

Clinical particulars

Therapeutic indications: Oestrogen replacement therapy for the relief of postmenopausal symptoms and for the prevention of osteoporosis in women at risk of developing fractures.

Epidemiological studies suggest a number of individual risk factors contribute to postmenopausal osteoporosis, including:

early menopause (either naturally or surgically)
family history of osteoporosis
recent prolonged systemic corticosteroid therapy
a small, thin frame
cigarette use

If several risk factors are present consideration should be given to oestrogen replacement therapy.

For maximum benefit treatment should commence as soon as possible after the menopause.

Posology and method of administration

Climacteric symptoms: Therapy should be initiated with Fematrix 40 in women who have menopausal symptoms, who have been oestrogen deficient for a prolonged time or who are likely to be intolerant of high levels of oestradiol. The dosage may be increased if required by using Fematrix 80. For maintenance therapy the lowest effective dose should be used.

Prevention of osteoporosis: Treatment should be with Fematrix 80, as the efficacy of Fematrix 40 in this indication has yet to be established.

For optimum benefit treatment should continue for 5 to 10 years, protection appears to be effective for as long as treatment continues, however data beyond 10 years is limited. For long term use see also Precautions and warnings.

Dosage schedule: One Fematrix 80 transdermal patch should be applied twice weekly on a continuous basis. Each patch should be removed after 3 to 4 days and replaced with a new patch applied to a slightly different site. Patches should be applied to clean, dry and intact areas of skin below the waist on the lower back or buttocks. Fematrix should not be applied on or near the breasts.

Women who are having regular periods should commence therapy within five days of the start of bleeding. Women whose periods have stopped or have become very irregular may commence therapy at any time.

In women with a uterus, a progestogen should be added for 12 to 14 days of each cycle. Most patients will commence bleeding towards the end of the progestogen therapy.

Unopposed oestrogen therapy should not be used unless the patient has undergone a hysterectomy.

Children: Fematrix is not indicated in children.

Contra-indications: Fematrix is contra-indicated in women with known or suspected pregnancy, cancer of the breast, genital tract or other oestrogen-dependent neoplasia, undiagnosed vaginal bleeding, endometriosis, severe renal or cardiac disease, acute or chronic liver disease where liver function tests have failed to return to normal, active deep venous thrombosis, thromboembolic disorders or a history of confirmed venous thromboembolism (see *Special warnings and precautions for use*), Dubin-Johnson syndrome or Rotor syndrome.

Special warnings and precautions for use: It is recommended that the patient should undergo a thorough physical and gynaecological examination before commencing therapy. This should be repeated at regular intervals. Unopposed oestradiol therapy should not be used in non-hysterectomised women because of the increased risk of endometrial hyperplasia or carcinoma.

At present time there is suggestive evidence of an overall change in the relative risk of breast cancer in post-menopausal women receiving oestrogen replacement therapy. While some studies have shown that there may be a small increase in risk with treatment for more than 5 years others have shown no such increase. It is not known whether concurrent progestogen use influences the risk of breast cancer in post-menopausal women taking hormone replacement therapy. A careful appraisal of the risk/benefit ratio should be undertaken before treating for longer than 5 to 10 years.

Women with a history of fibrocystic disease, breast nodules, abnormal mammograms or family history of breast cancer should have regular breast examinations.

Certain diseases may be made worse by hormone replacement therapy and patients with these conditions should be closely monitored. These include otosclerosis, multiple sclerosis, systemic lupus erythematosus, cholelithiasis, porphyria, melanoma, epilepsy, migraine, thyrotoxicosis, surgically confirmed gall bladder disease, asthma and diabetes (worsening of glucose tolerance). Pre-existing uterine fibroids may increase in size during oestrogen therapy and symptoms associated with endometriosis may be exacerbated.

Epidemiological studies have suggested that hormone replacement therapy (HRT) is associated with an increased relative risk of developing venous thromboembolism (VTE) i.e. deep vein thrombosis or pulmonary embolism. The studies find a 2-3 fold increase for users compared with non-users which for healthy women amounts to a low risk of one extra case of VTE each year for every 5000 patients taking HRT.

Generally recognised risk factors for VTE include a personal or family history and severe obesity (Body Mass Index >30 kg/m²). In women with these factors, the benefits of treatment with HRT need to be carefully weighed against risks.

The risk of VTE may be temporarily increased with prolonged immobilisation, major trauma or major surgery. In women on HRT, scrupulous attention should be given to prophylactic measures to prevent VTE following surgery. Where prolonged immobilisation is liable to follow elective surgery, particularly abdominal or orthopaedic surgery to the lower limbs, consideration should be given to temporarily stopping HRT 4 weeks earlier, if this is possible.

If venous thromboembolism develops after initiating therapy, the drug should be discontinued.

If jaundice or significant hypertension develop, treatment should be discontinued whilst the cause is investigated. As oestrogens may cause fluid retention, patients with cardiac or renal dysfunction should be closely observed. Regular monitoring of blood pressure should be carried out in hypertensive patients.

Women who may be at risk of pregnancy should be advised to adhere to non-hormonal contraceptive methods.

Interactions with other medicaments and other forms of interaction: Preparations inducing microsomal liver enzymes, e.g. barbiturates, hydantoins, anti-convulsants (including carbamazepine), meprobromate, phenylbutazone, antibiotics (including rifampicin), and activated charcoal may impair the activity of oestrogens. Transdermally applied oestrogens are less likely to be affected by such interactions than oral oestrogens since first pass hepatic metabolism is avoided.

Changes in oestrogen serum concentrations may affect the results of certain endocrine or liver function tests.

Pregnancy and lactation: Fematrix is contra-indicated.

Effects on ability to drive and use machines: None.

Undesirable effects: Fematrix is generally well tolerated. The most frequent side-effects (reported in 10 to 20% of patients, on at least one occasion, in clinical trials with Fematrix 80), which do not normally prevent continued treatment include: breast tenderness, headaches and breakthrough bleeding. Some patients experience mild and transient local erythema at the site of application with or without itching; this usually disappears rapidly on removal of the patch. The overall incidence of general patch irritation in clinical studies is less than 5%. In a clinical study 3% of 102 patients showed well defined erythema (Draize scale) 30 minutes after patch removal. No instances of permanent skin damage have been reported. If unacceptable topical side-effects do occur discontinuation of treatment should be considered.

Other side-effects associated with oestrogen or oestrogen/progestogen treatment have occasionally been reported (in 1% to 5% of patients in clinical trials with Fematrix 80) include: abdominal cramps, abdominal bloating, oedema, nausea, migraine and weight changes. More rarely (less than 1% in clinical trials with Fematrix 80) dizziness, dysmenorrhoea, leg cramps and visual disturbances have been reported.

Other side effects which have been rarely reported with oestrogen products include: changes in libido or changes in carbohydrate tolerance, vaginal candidiasis, change in vaginal secretions, cystitis like syndrome, cervical erosion, erythema multiforme, erythema nodosa, haemorrhagic eruptions, chloasma or melasma which may be persistent when the drug is discontinued, steepening of corneal curvature, intolerance to contact lenses, mental depression and chorea minor. Cholestasis may be possible in predisposed patients.

Overdose: This is not likely due to the mode of administration. If it is necessary to stop delivery then the patch can be removed and plasma oestradiol levels will fall rapidly.

Pharmacological properties
Pharmacodynamic properties: Pharmacotherapeutic group: Natural oestrogen.

Mechanism of action/pharmacodynamic effects: In the female, oestradiol stimulates the accessory reproductive organs and causes development of the secondary sexual characteristics at puberty. It is also responsible for the hypertrophy of the uterus and for the changes in the endometrium during the first half of the menstrual cycle which when acted on by progesterone prepares it for the reception of a fertilised ovum. It furthermore promotes the growth of the ducts of the mammary glands. Large doses inhibit the gonadotropic secretion of the anterior pituitary, thus influencing the normal ovarian cycle.

It is of value in menstrual disorders, ovarian insufficiency, especially at the menopause, and for the treatment of infections of the vagina in childen, where it promotes the growth of a cornified and more resistant epithelium; it is also used to terminate lactation, not very successfully, by inhibiting the release of prolactin.

Pharmacokinetic properties
General characteristics of the active substance – Absorption: Oestradiol is absorbed from the patch across the stratum corneum and is delivered systemically at a low but constant rate throughout the period of application (3 to 4 days). The estimated delivery of oestradiol is approximately 80 micrograms per day for Fematrix 80.

Distribution: Oestrogens circulate in the blood bound to albumin, sex hormone binding globulin (SHBG), cortisol binding globulin and alpha-1-glycoprotein. Following diffusion of free oestrogen into the cells of the target tissues in the hypothalamus, pituitary, vagina, urethra, uterus, breast and liver, binding to specific oestrogen receptors occurs. Very little information is currently available on the distribution of oestradiol following transdermal administration.

Biotransformation: Inactivation of oestrogens in the body is carried out mainly in the liver. Metabolism of 17β-oestradiol is by oxidation to oestrone, which in turn can be hydrated to form oestriol. There is free interconversion between oestrone and oestradiol. Oestrone and oestriol may then undergo conversion to their corresponding sulphate and glucuronide derivatives for excretion in the urine. Oestrone sulphate has a long biologic half-life because of its enterohepatic recirculation and interconversion to oestrone and oestradiol.

Elimination: The plasma elimination half-life of oestradiol is approximately 1 hour and is independent of the route of administration. The metabolic plasma clearance rate is between 650 and 900 L/day/m2.

Steady state plasma oestradiol concentrations have been demonstrated in the range of 34 to 62 pg/ml for the Fematrix 80 patch (including baseline levels) and these are maintained throughout the dose interval (for up to four days). Absorption rate may vary between individual patients. After removal of the last patch plasma oestradiol and oestrone concentrations return to baseline values in less than 24 hours. The median terminal half-life for oestradiol following patch removal has been determined as 5.24 h.

Preclinical safety data: No specific preclinical studies have been conducted on Fematrix. Supraphysiologically high doses (prolonged overdoses) of oestradiol have been associated with the induction of tumours in oestrogen-dependent target organs in rodent species. Pronounced species differences in toxicology, pharmacology and pharmacodynamics exist.

Pharmaceutical particulars
List of excipients: Diethyltoluamide, Acrylic adhesive, Backing: Polyester. Release liner: Aluminised/polyester.

Incompatibilities: Not applicable.

Shelf life: The shelf-life of the product as packaged for sale is 3 years.

Special precautions for storage: Fematrix patches should be stored at room temperature (below 25°C) in a dry place.

Nature and contents of container: PVC/PVDC blister tray with paper/polythene/aluminium foil lid containing one transdermal patch. Each carton contains eight patches, sufficient for one 28 day cycle and a patient leaflet. An additional pack containing two patches may also be available.

Instruction for use/handling: Detailed instructions for use are provided in the patient leaflet.

Marketing authorisation holder: Ethical Pharmaceuticals (UK) Ltd, Gemini House, Bartholomew's Walk, Cambridgeshire Business Park, Ely, Cambs CB7 4EA.

Marketing authorisation number 10013/0021

Date of approval/revision of SPC October 1997.

Legal category POM.

FEMOSTON*

Qualitative and quantitative composition
Femoston 1/10 mg: This product contains 1 mg estradiol (= 17β-estradiol) per tablet for the first 14 days of a 28-day cycle (white tablets). For the second 14 days of a 28-day cycle, one tablet contains 1 mg estradiol (= 17β-estradiol) and 10 mg dydrogesterone (grey tablets).

Femoston 2/10 mg and Femoston 2/20 mg: These products contain 2 mg estradiol (= 17β-estradiol) per tablet for the first 14 days of a 28-day cycle (orange tablets). For the second 14 days of a cycle of 28 days one tablet contains 2 mg estradiol and 10 mg dydrogesterone (yellow tablets) or 2 mg estradiol and 20 mg dydrogesterone BP (blue tablets).

Pharmaceutical form Film-coated tablets for oral use.

Clinical particulars
Therapeutic indications
Femoston 1/10: For the relief of postmenopausal symptoms in women with a uterus.

Femoston 2/10 and Femoston 2/20: For the relief of postmenopausal symptoms and prevention of osteoporosis in women with a uterus.

Epidemiological studies suggest a number of risk factors may contribute to postmenopausal osteoporisis, including:

- early menopause (either naturally or surgically induced)
- family history of osteoporosis
- recent prolonged corticosteroid therapy
- a small, thin frame
- excessive cigarette consumption

If several risk factors are present consideration should be given to hormone replacement therapy.

Bone mineral density measurements may help to confirm the presence of low bone mass. For maximum prophylactic benefit, treatment should commence as soon as possible after the menopause.

Posology and method of administration: For oral administration.

Postmenopausal symptoms: Initial treatment should be with Femoston 1/10 mg. Femoston 2/10 should be substituted if control of climacteric symptoms is not achieved. The lowest dose compatible with control of symptoms should be used.

One tablet, containing 1 mg or 2 mg estradiol, daily during 14 consecutive days per cycle of 28 days and one tablet, containing 1 mg or 2 mg estradiol and 10 mg dydrogesterone daily during the remaining 14 days has to be taken.

Femoston 2/20 may be prescribed if either early withdrawal bleeding occurs or if endometrial biopsy reveals inadequate progestational response.

Immediately after a 28-day cycle, the next treatment cycle is to be started. Patients should take one tablet a day, according to the sequence indicated on the package. Medication is to be continued without interruption.

If the patient is still menstruating, it is recommended that treatment commences within five days of the start of bleeding.

In patients who had their last period more than approximately 12 months ago, treatment can be started at any time.

Osteoporosis prevention: Treatment should be with Femoston 2/10. Femoston 2/20 may be prescribed if either early withdrawal bleeding occurs or if endometrial biopsy reveals inadequate progestational response.

Contra-indications: Known or suspected carcinoma of the breast, endometrial carcinoma or other hormone dependent neoplasia.

Acute or chronic liver disease.
History of liver disease where the liver function tests have failed to return to normal.
Active deep venous thrombosis, thromboembolic disorders or a history of confirmed venous thromboembolism.
Cerebral vascular accident.
Abnormal genital bleeding of unknown aetiology.
Known or suspected pregnancy.

Special warnings and precautions for use: These relate almost exclusively to the oestrogen component of this product: Physical examination and a complete medical and family history should be taken prior to the initiation of any hormone replacement therapy (HRT) with special reference to blood pressure, palpation of the breasts and the abdomen and a gynaecological examination.

Patients who are, or have previously been, treated with unopposed oestrogens should be examined with special care in order to investigate a possible hyperstimulation of the endometrium before commencing therapy.

As a general rule, HRT should not be prescribed for longer than one year without another physical examination, including gynaecological examination. In case of continuing abnormal and/or irregular bleeding, a diagnostic endometrial biopsy should be performed.

This oestrogen-progestogen combination treatment is not contraceptive. Patients in the peri-menopausal phase should be advised to take *non-hormonal* contraceptive precautions.

Epidemiological studies have suggested that hormone replacement therapy (HRT) is associated with an increased relative risk of developing venous thromboembolism (VTE) i.e. deep vein thrombosis or pulmonary embolism. The studies find a 2-3 fold increase for users compared with non-users which for healthy women amounts to a low risk of one extra case of VTE each year for every 5000 patients taking HRT.

Generally recognised risk factors for VTE include a personal or family history and severe obesity (Body Mass Index >30 kg/m^2). In women with these factors, the benefits of treatment with HRT need to be carefully weighed against risks.

The risk of VTE may be temporarily increased with prolonged immobilisation, major trauma or major surgery. In women on HRT, scrupulous attention should be given to prophylactic measures to prevent VTE following surgery. Where prolonged immobilisation is liable to follow elective surgery, particularly abdominal or orthopaedic surgery to the lower limbs, consideration should be given to temporarily stopping HRT 4 weeks earlier, if this is possible.

If venous thromboembolism develops after initiating therapy, the drug should be discontinued.

Patients with, or developing epilepsy, migraine, diabetes mellitus, cardiac failure, multiple sclerosis, hypertension, porphyria, haemoglobinopathies or otosclerosis should be carefully observed during treatment, as HRT may worsen these conditions. In patients with a past history of liver disease it is advisable to check liver functions on a regular basis.

Special care should be taken in patients with uterine leiomyomata and patients with a history of endometriosis as oestrogens may influence these conditions.

The indications for immediate withdrawal of therapy are:

- deep venous thrombosis
- thromboembolic disorders
- the appearance of jaundice
- the emergence of migraine-type headache
- sudden visual disturbances
- significant increase in blood pressure
- pregnancy

Interaction with other medicaments and other forms of interaction: Oestrogens interact with liver enzyme-inducing drugs with increased metabolism of oestrogens, which may reduce the oestrogen effect. Interactions are documented for the following liver enzyme-inducing drugs: barbiturates, phenytoin, rifampicin, carbamazepine.

No drug interactions are known for dydrogesterone.

Pregnancy and lactation: Known, *or* suspected pregnancy is a contra-indication.

Lactation – this product is not indicated during this period.

Effects on ability to drive and use machines: No effects known.

Undesirable effects: During the first few months of treatment breast tenderness may occur. Nausea, headache, abdominal pain, dysmenorrhoea, bloating, oedema and dizziness have been reported. Symptoms are normally transient. Skin reactions have been reported.

Overdose: There have been no reports of ill-effects from overdosing. If overdosage is discovered within two or three hours and is so large that treatment seems desirable, gastric lavage can safely be used. There is no specific antidote and further treatment should be symptomatic.

Pharmacological properties

Pharmacodynamic properties: Estradiol is chemically and biologically identical to the endogenous human estradiol and is, therefore, classified as a human oestrogen. Estradiol is the primary oestrogen and the most active of the ovarian hormones. The endogenous oestrogens are involved in certain functions of the uterus and accessory organs, including the proliferation of the endometrium and the cyclic changes in the cervix and vagina.

Oestrogens are known to play an important role for bone and fat metabolism. Furthermore, oestrogens also affect the autonomic nervous system and may have indirect positive psychotropic actions.

Dydrogesterone is an orally-active progestogen having an activity comparable to parenterally administered progesterone.

In the context of HRT, dydrogesterone produces a complete secretory endometrium in an oestrogen-primed uterus thereby providing protection for oestrogen induced increased risk of endometrial hyperplasia and/or carcinoma, without androgenic side-effects.

The beneficial effects of 17β-estradiol on lipoprotein, glucose and insulin metabolism are maintained in the presence of dydrogesterone.

Pharmacokinetic properties: Following oral administration, micronised estradiol is readily absorbed, but extensively metabolised. The major unconjugated and conjugated metabolites are oestrone and oestrone sulphate. These metabolites can contribute to the oestrogen activity, either directly or after conversion to estradiol. Oestrone sulphate may undergo enterohepatic circulation. In urine, the major compounds are the glucuronides of oestrone and estradiol.

Oestrogens are secreted in the milk of nursing mothers.

After oral administration of labelled dydrogesterone, on average 63% of the dose is excreted into the urine. Within 72 hours excretion is complete.

In man, dydrogesterone is completely metabolised. The main metabolite of dydrogesterone is 20α-dihydrodydrogesterone (DHD) and is present in the urine predominantly as the glucuronic acid conjugate. A common feature of all metabolites characterised is the retention of the 4,6 diene-3-one configuration of the parent compound and the absence of 17α-hydroxylation. This explains the lack of oestrogenic and androgenic effects of dydrogesterone.

After oral administration of dydrogesterone, plasma concentrations of DHD are substantially higher as compared to the parent drug. The AUC and C_{max} ratios of DHD to dydrogesterone are in the order of 40 and 25, respectively. Dydrogesterone is rapidly absorbed. The T_{max} values of dydrogesterone and DHD vary between 0.5 and 2.5 hours.

Mean terminal half lives of dydrogesterone and DHD vary between 5 to 7 and 14 to 17 hours, respectively.

Dydrogesterone is not excreted in urine as pregnanediol, like progesterone. Analysis of endogenous progesterone production basd on pregnanediol excretion therefore remains possible. No pharmacokinetic interactions occur between estradiol and dydrogesterone.

Preclinical safety data: Supraphysiologically high doses (prolonged overdoses) of estradiol have been associated with the induction of tumours in oestrogen-dependent target organs for all rodent species tested. Pronounced species differences in toxicology, pharmacology and pharmacodynamics exist. The changes observed with dydrogesterone in animal toxicity studies are associated with the effects of progesterone-like compounds.

Doses administered to rats and mice sufficient to produce hormone-mediated changes gave no evidence of carcinogenesis.

Pharmaceutical particulars

List of excipients:

Femoston 1/10 mg: Lactose; methylhydroxypropylcellulose; maize starch; colloidal anhydrous silica; magnesium stearate. Opadry Y-1-7000 white (for 1 mg estradiol only tablet) contains E171. Opadry OY-8243 grey (for combination tablet of 1 mg oestradiol with 10 mg dydrogesterone) contains E171.

Femoston 2/10 mg and 2/20 mg: Lactose; methylhydroxypropylcellulose; maize starch; colloidal anhydrous silica; magnesium stearate. Opadry OY-23000 orange (for 2 mg estradiol only tablet) contains E171. Opadry OY-7915 yellow (for combination tablet of 2 mg oestradiol with 10 mg dydrogesterone). Opadry OY-6535 blue (for combination tablet of 2 mg oestradiol with 20 mg dydrogesterone).

Incompatibilities: Not applicable.

Shelf life: 3 years.

Special precautions for storage: Store below 30°C.

Nature and contents of container: The tablets are packed in blister strips of 28. The blister strips are made of PVC film with a covering aluminium foil. Each carton contains 84 tablets.

Instructions for use/handling: Instructions for use of the blister package are included in the Patient Information Leaflet.

Marketing authorisation numbers

Femoston 1/10 mg	0512/0121
Femoston 2/10 mg	0512/0113
Femoston 2/20 mg	0512/0114

Date of approval/revision of SPC September 1997.

Legal category POM.

INFLUVAC* SUB-UNIT VACCINE

Qualitative and quantitative composition Influvac is an egg-grown, inactivated influenza virus vaccine based on isolated surface antigens of A and B strains of myxovirus influenza. The composition of influenza vaccines is adjusted annually on the basis of the recommendation from the World Health Organisation for the northern hemisphere, and the decision of the European Union (Committee for Proprietary Medicinal Products).

Each 0.5 ml dose contains the haemagglutinin and neuraminidase antigens prepared from the appropriate quantities of the A and B strains currently recommended by the WHO.

Pharmaceutical form Suspension for injection.

Clinical particulars

Therapeutic indications: Prophylaxis of influenza, especially in those who run an increased risk of associated complications.

Posology and method of administration

Adults and children from 36 months: 0.5 ml.

Children from 6 months to 35 months: Clinical data are limited. Dosages of 0.25 ml or 0.5 ml have been used.

For children who have not previously been infected or vaccinated, a second dose should be given after an interval of at least 4 weeks.

Immunisation should be carried out by intramuscular or deep subcutaneous injection.

Contra-indications: Hypersensitivity to eggs, chicken protein or any other constituent of the vaccine. Immunisation should be postponed in patients with febrile illness or acute infection.

Special warnings and special precautions for use: As with all injectable vaccines, appropriate medical treatment and supervision should always be readily available in case of a rare anaphylactic event following the administration of the vaccine.

Influvac should under no circumstances be administered intravascularly.

Antibody response in patients with endogenous or iatrogenic immunosuppression may be insufficient.

The vaccine may contain non-detectable residual amounts of gentamicin. Use with caution in patients known to be hypersensitive to this antibiotic.

Interaction with other medicaments and other forms of interaction: Influvac may be given at the same time as other vaccines. Immunisation should be carried out on separate limbs. It should be noted that the adverse reactions may be intensified.

The immunological response may be diminished if the patient is undergoing immunosuppressant treatment.

Following influenza vaccination, false positive results in serology tests using the ELISA method to detect antibodies against HIV1, Hepatitis C and especially HTLV1 have been observed. The Western Blot technique disproves the results. The transient false positive reactions could be due to the IgM response by the vaccine.

Pregnancy and lactation: No relevant animal data are available. In humans, up to now, the data are inadequate to assess teratogenic or fetotoxic risk during pregnancy. In pregnant high risk patients the possible risks of clinical infection should be weighed against the possible risks of vaccination.

Influvac may be used during lactation.

Effects on ability to drive and use machines: Influvac is unlikely to produce an effect on the ability to drive and use machines.

Undesirable effects: The following reactions are most common:

Local reactions: redness, swelling, pain, ecchymosis, induration.

Systemic reactions: fever, malaise, shivering, fatigue, headache, sweating, myalgia, arthralgia. These reactions usually disappear within 1-2 days without treatment.

The following events are observed rarely: neuralgia, paraesthesia, convulsions, transient thrombocytopenia.

Allergic reactions, in rare cases leading to shock, have been reported.

Vasculitis with transient renal involvement has been reported in very rare cases.

Rarely neurological disorders, such as encephalomyelitis, neuritis and Guillain Barré syndrome have been reported. An increased risk of Guillain Barré syndrome has not been demonstrated with currently used influenza vaccines.

Overdose: Overdosage is unlikely to have any untoward effect.

Pharmacological properties
Pharmacodynamic properties: Seroprotection is generally obtained within 2 to 3 weeks. The duration of postvaccinal immunity varies but is usually 6-12 months.

Pharmacokinetic properties: Not applicable.

Preclinical safety data: Not applicable.

Pharmaceutical particulars
List of excipients: Potassium chloride, potassium dihydrogen phosphate, disodium phosphate dihydrate, sodium chloride, calcium chloride, magnesium chloride hexahydrate, thiomersal and water for injections.

Residues of sucrose, sodium deoxycholate, formaldehyde, cetyltrimethylammonium bromide, polysorbate 80 and traces of gentamicin.

Incompatibilities: Influvac should not be mixed with other injection fluids.

Shelf life: The expiry date is indicated on the label and packaging. The shelf-life is 12 months.

Special precautions for storage: Influvac should be stored at +2°C to +8°C (in a refrigerator). Do not freeze. Protect from light.

Nature and contents of container: Single-dose 0.5 ml pre-filled syringes (glass, type 1), packaged singly or by 10 in a tray.

Instructions for use/handling: Influvac should be allowed to reach room temperature before use. Shake before use.

For administration of an 0.25 ml dose from a syringe, push the front side of the plunger exactly to the edge of the hub (the knurled polypropylene ring); a reproducible volume of vaccine remains in the syringe, suitable for administration.

Marketing authorisation number 0512/0156.

Date of approval/revision of SPC June 1998.

Legal category POM.

MONOTRIM* INJECTION

Qualitative and quantitative composition Trimethoprim 20 mg/ml.

Pharmaceutical form Injection.

Clinical particulars
Therapeutic indications: Treatment of susceptible infections caused by trimethoprim-sensitive microorganisms, particularly infections caused by gram-negative microorganisms.

Posology and method of administration
Route of administration:
1. By direct slow intravenous injection, or
2. Via the tubing (close to the vein) of an established intravenous infusion.

Dosage:
Adults and children over 12 years: 200 mg every 12 hours.

Children under 12 years: The approximate dosage in children is 8 mg trimethoprim per kg body weight per day, divided into two or three equal doses.

In severely ill patients the first doses may be higher or given more frequently.

Advised dosage in patients with reduced kidney function:

Creatinine clearance (ml/sec)	*Plasma creatinine (micromol/l)*		*Dosage advised*
Over 0.45	men	<250	normal
	Women	<175	
0.25-0.45	men	250-600	normal for 3 days then half dose
	Women	175-400	
Under 0.25	men	>600	half the normal dose
	Women	>400	

Trimethoprim is removed by dialysis. However, it should not be administered to dialysis patients unless plasma concentrations can be estimated regularly.

Elderly: As adults.

Contra-indications: Pregnancy, trimethoprim hypersensitivity, blood dyscrasias, severe renal insufficiency where blood levels cannot be monitored.

Special warnings and special precautions for use: Caution should be exercised in the administration of trimethoprim to patients with actual or potential folate deficiency (e.g. elderly) and administration of folate supplement should be considered. Although an effect on folic acid metabolism is possible, interference with haematopoiesis rarely occurs at the recommended dose. If any such change is seen, folinic acid should reverse the effect. Elderly people may be more susceptible and a lower dose may be advisable. Regular haematological tests should be undertaken in long-term treatment.

In neonates, trimethoprim should be used under careful medical supervision.

In patients with impairment of renal function, care should be taken to avoid accumulation.

Interaction with other medicaments and other forms of interaction:

Bone marrow depressants: Trimethoprim may increase the potential for bone marrow aplasia.

Rifampicin may increase the elimination and shorten the elimination half-life of trimethoprim.

Phenytoin and digoxin: The patients should be carefully controlled as trimethoprim may increase the elimination half-life of phenytoin and digoxin.

Cyclosporin may increase the nephrotoxicity of trimethoprim.

Pregnancy and lactation: Pregnancy is a contra-indication. Although trimethoprim is excreted in breast milk, lactation is not a contra-indication for short-term trimethoprim therapy.

Effects on ability to drive and use machinery: Not applicable.

Undesirable effects: Nausea, vomiting and skin rashes have been reported in rare instances. These effects are generally mild and quickly reversible on withdrawal of the drug. Rarely, erythema multiforme and toxic epidermal necrolysis have occured. Aseptic meningitis has been reported. Trimethoprim may affect haematopoiesis.

Overdose: Symptomatic treatment and forced diuresis can be used. In cases of oral overdosage gastric lavage is recommended. Depression of haematopoiesis by trimethoprim can be counteracted by intramuscular administration of calcium folinate.

Pharmacological properties
Pharmacodynamic properties: Trimethoprim is an antimicrobial agent.

Pharmacokinetic properties
Half-life: The half-life is about 10 hours in patients with normal renal function but up to 20-50 hours in anuric patients.

Distribution: Trimethoprim is rapidly and widely distributed to various tissues and fluids, including kidneys, liver, spleen, bronchial secretions, salvia and prostatic tissue and fluid and the tissue concentrations are generally higher than the plasma concentration.

Excretion: Trimethoprim is predominantly excreted in the urine in unchanged form. Urinary concentrations are generally well above the MIC of common pathogens for more than 24 hours after the last dose.

Preclinical safety data: Not relevant (widely used in clinical practice).

Pharmaceutical particulars
List of excipients: Lactic acid, sodium hydroxide, water for injections.

Incompatibilities: Trimethoprim is incompatible with solutions of sulfonamides.

Shelf life: Five years.

Special precautions for storage: Store below 25°C protected from light.

Nature and contents of container: Light-protective cartons of 5 x 5 ml ampoules.

Instructions for use/handling:
Monotrim injection is compatible with the following commonly used infusion fluids:
Dextran 40 intravenous infusion BP 10% W/V
in sodium chloride intravenous infusion 0.9% W/V.
Dextran 70 intravenous infusion BP 6% W/V
in sodium chloride intravenous infusion 0.9% W/V.
Glucose intravenous infusion BP 50 G/L
Fructose intravenous infusion BP 50 G/L
Ringer's injection USP
Sodium chloride intravenous infusion BP 0.9% W/V
Sodium chloride 0.45% W/V and glucose 2.5% W/V intravenous infusion BP
Sodium lactate intravenous infusion BP
Compound sodium lactate intravenous infusion BP

Marketing authorisation holder: A/S GEA Farmaceutisk Fabrik, Holger Danskes Vej 89, DK-2000 Frederiksberg, Denmark.

Marketing authorization number 4012/0008

Date of approval/ revision of SPC 15 June 1998

Legal category POM

MONOTRIM* SUSPENSION

Qualitative and quantitative composition Trimethoprim 10 mg/ml

Pharmaceutical form Suspension

Clinical particulars
Therapeutic indications: Treatment of susceptible infections caused by trimethoprim-sensitive organisms including urinary and respiratory tract infections and for prophylaxis of recurrent urinary tract infections.

Posology and method of administration
Acute infections:
Adults and children over 12 years: 200 mg (20 ml) twice daily.

Children 6 years to 12 years: 100 mg (10 ml) twice daily.

Children 6 months to 5 years: 50 mg (5 ml) twice daily.

Children 6 weeks to 5 months: 25 mg (2.5 ml) twice daily.

The approximate dosage in children is 8 mg trimethoprim per kg body weight per day.

Elderly: Depending on kidney function, see special dosage schedule.

Treatment should continue for at least one week but not last longer than two weeks. The first dose can be doubled.

Long-term treatment and prophylactic therapy:
Adults and children over 12 years: 100 mg (10 ml) at night.

Children 6 years to 12 years: 50 mg (5 ml) at night.

Children 6 months to 5 years: 25 mg (2.5 ml) at night.

The approximate dosage in children is 2 mg trimethoprim per kg body weight per day.

Elderly: Depending on kidney function, see special dosage schedule.

Dosage advised where there is reduced kidney function:

Creatinine clearance (ml/sec)	*Plasma creatinine (micromol/l)*		*Dosage advised*
Over 0.45	men	<250	normal
	women	<175	
0.25-0.45	men	250-600	normal for 3 days then half dose
	women	175-400	
Under 0.25	men	>600	half the normal dose
	women	>400	

Trimethoprim is removed by dialysis. However, it should not be administered to dialysis patients unless plasma concentrations can be estimated regularly.

Contra-indications: Pregnancy, trimethoprim hypersensitivity, blood dyscrasias, severe renal insufficiency where blood levels cannot be monitored.

Special warnings and special precautions for use: Caution should be exercised in the administration of trimethoprim to patients with actual or potential folate deficiency (e.g. elderly) and administration of folate supplement should be considered. Although an effect on folic acid metabolism is possible, interference with haematopoiesis rarely occurs at the recommended dose. If any such change is seen, folinic acid should reverse the effect. Elderly people may be more susceptible and a lower dose may be advisable. Regular haematological tests should be undertaken in long-term treatment.

In neonates, trimethoprim should be used under careful medical supervision.

In patients with impairment of renal function, care should be taken to avoid accumulation.

Interaction with other medicaments and other forms of interaction:

Bone marrow depressants: Trimethoprim may increase the potential for bone marrow aplasia. Rifampicin may increase the elimination and shorten the elimination half-life of trimethoprim. Phenytoin and digoxin: The patients should be carefully controlled as trimethoprim may increase the elimination half-life of phenytoin and digoxin. Cyclosporin may increase the nephrotoxicity of trimethoprim.

Pregnancy and lactation: Pregnancy is a contra-indication. Although trimethoprim is excreted in breast milk, lactation is not a contra-indication for short-term trimethoprim therapy.

Effects on ability to drive and use machines: None known.

Undesirable effects: Nausea, vomiting, and skin rashes have been reported in rare instances. These effects are generally mild and quickly reversible on withdrawal of the drug. Rarely, erythema multiforme and toxic epidermal necrolysis have occurred. Aseptic meningitis has been reported. Trimethoprim may affect haematopoiesis.

Overdose:
Treatment of overdosage: Symptomatic treatment, gastric lavage and forced diuresis can be used. Depression of haematopoiesis by trimethoprim can be counteracted by intramuscular administration of calcium folinate.

Pharmacological properties
Pharmacodynamic properties: Trimethoprim is an antimicrobial agent. The antimicrobial activity is due to selective inhibition of bacterial dihydrofolate reductase.

Trimethoprim is effective in-vitro against most Gram-positive and Gram-negative aerobic organisms, including enterobacteria–E. coli, Proteus, Klebsiella pneumoniae, Streptococcus faecalis, Streptococcus pneumoniae, Haemophilus influenzae, and Staphylococcus aureus.

It is not active against Mycobacterium tuberculosis, Neisseria gonorrhoeae, Pseudomonas aeruginosa, Treponema pallidum, or anaerobic bacteria.

Pharmacokinetic properties
Absorption and half-life: Trimethoprim is absorbed rapidly and almost completely following oral administration and maximal plasma concentrations are reached after 1-2 hours. Peak plasma concentrations of about 1 μg per ml have been reported after a single dose of 100 mg.

The half-life is about 10 hours in patients with normal renal function but up to 20-50 hours in anuric patients.

Distribution: Trimethoprim is rapidly and widely distributed to various tissues and fluids, including kidneys, liver, spleen, bronchial secretions, saliva and prostatic tissue and fluid, and the tissue concentrations are generally higher than the plasma concentration.

Excretion: Trimethoprim is predominantly excreted in the urine in unchanged form. Urinary concentrations are generally well above the MIC of common pathogens for more than 24 hours after the last dose.

Preclinical safety data: Not relevant (widely used in clinical practice).

Pharmaceutical particulars
List of excipients: Microcrystalline cellulose, carboxymethylcellulose sodium, ammonium glycyrrhizinate, methyl parahydroxybenzoate, sorbitol, anise oil, purified water.

Incompatibilities: None known.

Shelf life: 3 years.

Special precautions for storage: Store below 25°C.

Nature and contents of container: Plastic bottle: 100 ml.

Instructions for use/handling: None.

Marketing authorisation holder: A/S GEA Farmaceutisk Fabrik, Holger Danskes Vej 89, DK-2000 Frederiksberg, Denmark.

Marketing authorization number 4012/0002

Date of approval/ revision of SPC January 1996

Legal category POM

MONOTRIM* TABLETS

Qualitative and quantitative composition Trimethoprim 100 mg and 200 mg.

Pharmaceutical form Tablets.

Clinical particulars

Therapeutic indications: Treatment of susceptible infections caused by trimethoprim-sensitive organisms including urinary and respiratory tract infections and for prophylaxis of recurrent urinary tract infections.

Posology and method of administration
Acute infections:
Adults and children over 12 years: 200 mg twice daily.
Children 6 years to 12 years: 100 mg twice daily.
Children 6 months to 5 years: 50 mg twice daily.
The approximate dosage in children is 8 mg trimethoprim per kg body weight per day.
Elderly: Depending on kidney function, see special dosage schedule.

Treatment should continue for at least one week but not last longer than two weeks. The first dose can be doubled.

Long-term treatment and prophylactic therapy:
Adults and children over 12 years: 100 mg at night.
Children 6 years to 12 years: 50 mg at night.
The approximate dosage in children is 2 mg trimethoprim per kg body weight per day.
Elderly: Depending on kidney function, see special dosage schedule.

Dosage advised where there is reduced kidney function:

Creatinine clearance (ml/sec)	*Plasma creatinine (micromol/l)*		*Dosage advised*
Over 0.45	men	<250	normal
	women	<175	
0.25–0.45	men	250–600	normal for 3 days
	women	175–400	then half dose
Under 0.25	men	>600	half the normal dose
	women	>400	

Trimethoprim is removed by dialysis. However, it should not be administered to dialysis patients unless plasma concentrations can be estimated regularly. Route of administration: Oral.

Contra-indications: Pregnancy, trimethoprim hypersensitivity, blood dyscrasias, severe renal insufficiency where blood levels cannot be monitored.

Special warnings and special precautions for use: Caution should be exercised in the administration of trimethoprim to patients with actual or potential folate deficiency (e.g. elderly) and administration of folate supplement should be considered. Although an effect on folic acid metabolism is possible, interference with haematopoiesis rarely occurs at the recommended dose. If any such change is seen, folinic acid should reverse the effect. Elderly people may be more susceptible and a lower dose may be advisable. Regular haematological tests should be undertaken in long-term treatment.

In neonates, trimethoprim should be used under careful medical supervision.

In patients with impairment of renal function, care should be taken to avoid accumulation.

Interaction with other medicaments and other forms of interaction: Bone marrow depressants: Trimethoprim may increase the potential for bone marrow aplasia. Rifampicin may increase the elimination and shorten the elimination half-life of trimethoprim. Phenytoin and digoxin: The patients should be carefully controlled as trimethoprim may increase the elimination half-life of phenytoin and digoxin. Cyclosporin may increase the nephrotoxicity of trimethoprim.

Pregnancy and lactation: Pregnancy is a contra-indication. Although trimethoprim is excreted in breast milk, lactation is not a contra-indication for short-term trimethoprim therapy.

Effects on ability to drive and use machines: None known.

Undesirable effects: Nausea, vomiting, and skin rashes have been reported in rare instances. These effects are generally mild and quickly reversible on withdrawal of the drug. Rarely, erythema multiforme and toxic epidermal necrolysis have occurred. Aseptic meningitis has been reported. Trimethoprim may affect haematopoiesis.

Overdose: Treatment of overdosage: Symptomatic treatment, gastric lavage and forced diuresis can be used. Depression of haematopoiesis by trimethoprim can be counteracted by intramuscular administration of calcium folinate.

Pharmacological properties
Pharmacodynamic properties: Trimethoprim is an antimicrobial agent. The antimicrobial activity is due to selective inhibition of bacterial dihydrofolate reductase.

Trimethoprim is effective *in-vitro* against most Gram-positive and Gram-negative aerobic organisms, including enterobacteria – *E. coli, Proteus, Klebsiella pneumoniae, Streptococcus faecalis, Streptococcus pneumoniae, Haemophilus influenzae*, and *Staphylococcus aureus.*

It is not active against *Mycobacterium tuberculosis, Neisseria gonorrhoeae, Psedomonas aeruginosa, Treponema pallidum*, or anaerobic bacteria.

Pharmacokinetic properties: Absorption and half-life: Trimethoprim is absorbed rapidly and almost completely following oral administration and maximal plasma concentrations are reached after 1–2 hours. Peak plasma concentrations of about 1 μg per ml have been reported after a single dose of 100 mg. The half-life is about 10 hours in patients with normal renal function but up to 20–50 hours in anuric patients.

Distribution: Trimethoprim is rapidly and widely distributed to various tissues and fluids, including kidneys, liver, spleen, bronchial secretions, saliva and prostatic tissue and fluid, and the tissue concentrations are generally higher than the plasma concentration.

Excretion: Trimethoprim is predominantly excreted in the urine in unchanged form. Urinary concentrations are generally well above the MIC of common pathogens for more than 24 hours after the last dose.

Preclinical safety data: Not relevant (widely used in clinical practice).

Pharmaceutical particulars
List of excipients: Lactose monohydrate, potato starch, gelatin, magnesium stearate, talc.

Incompatibilities: None known.

Shelf life: 5 years.

Special precautions for storage: None.

Nature and contents of container: Plastic container. 100 mg: 100 tablets. 200 mg: 100 tablets.

Instructions for use/handling: None.

Marketing authorisation holder: A/S GEA Farmaceutisk Fabrik, Holger Danskes Vej 89, DK-2000 Frederiksberg, Denmark.

Marketing authorisation number 4012/0001/3.

Date of approval/revision of SPC 29 August 1997.

Legal category POM.

PHYSIOTENS* 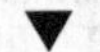

Qualitative and quantitative composition Each tablet contains 200 or 400 micrograms of moxonidine.

Pharmaceutical form Round, biconvex, film-coated tablets. The 200 microgram tablet is light pink imprinted '0.2' on one face. The 400 microgram tablet is dull red imprinted '0.4' on one face.

Clinical particulars
Therapeutic indications: Mild to moderate essential or primary hypertension.

Posology and method of administration
Adults (including the elderly): Treatment should be started with 200 micrograms of Physiotens in the morning. The dose may be titrated after three weeks to 400 micrograms, given as one dose or as divided doses (morning and evening) until a satisfactory response has been achieved. If the response is still unsatisfactory after a further three weeks' treatment, the dosage can be increased up to a maximum of 600 micrograms in divided doses (morning and evening).

A single dose of 400 micrograms of Physiotens and a daily dose of 600 micrograms in divided doses (morning and evening) should not be exceeded.

In patients with moderate renal dysfunction (GFR above 30 ml/min, but below 60 ml/min), the single dose should not exceed 200 micrograms and the daily dose should not exceed 400 micrograms of moxonidine.

The tablets should be taken with a little liquid. As the intake of food has no influence on the pharmacokinetic properties of moxonidine, the tablets may be taken before, during or after the meal.

Children (under 16 years): Physiotens should not be given below the age of 16 years as insufficient therapeutic experience exists in this group.

Contra-indications: Physiotens should not be used in cases of:

- history of angioneurotic oedema
- hypersensitivity to any of the ingredients
- sick sinus syndrome or sino-atrial block
- 2nd or 3rd degree atrioventricular block
- bradycardia (below 50 beats/minute at rest)
- malignant arrhythmia
- severe heart failure
- severe coronary artery disease or unstable angina
- severe liver disease
- severe renal dysfunction (GFR <30 ml/min, serum creatinine concentration >160 μmol/l)

Physiotens should not be used because of lack of therapeutic experience in cases of

- intermittent claudication
- Raynaud's disease
- Parkinson's disease
- epileptic disorders
- glaucoma
- depression
- pregnancy or lactation
- children below 16 years of age

Special warnings and special precautions for use: If Physiotens is used in combination with a beta-blocker and the treatment has to be stopped, the beta-blocker should be stopped first and then Physiotens after a few days have elapsed.

In patients with moderate renal dysfunction (GFR

above 30 but below 60 ml/min, serum creatinine above 105 but below 160 μmol), the hypotensive effect of Physiotens should be closely monitored, especially at the start of treatment.

Due to lack of therapeutic experience, the use of Physiotens concomitantly with alcohol or tricyclic antidepressants should be avoided.

In limited studies no rebound effect of the blood pressure after sudden discontinuation of Physiotens treatment has been detected. Nevertheless, it is advised not to interrupt the intake of Physiotens abruptly. Physiotens should be withdrawn gradually over a period of two weeks.

Interactions with other medicaments and other forms of interaction: Concurrent administration of other antihypertensive agents enhances the hypotensive effect of Physiotens.

The effect of sedatives and hypnotics may be intensified by Physiotens. The sedative effect of benzodiazepines can be enhanced by concurrent administration of Physiotens.

Pregnancy and lactation: As insufficient data are available, Physiotens should not be used during pregnancy. Physiotens should not be used during lactation because it is excreted into breast milk.

Effects on ability to drive and use machines: No data are available to suggest that Physiotens adversely affects the ability to drive or operate machines. However, as somnolence and dizziness have been reported, patients should be cautioned about their ability to undertake potentially hazardous tasks such as driving and operating machinery if so affected.

Undesirable effects: At the start of treatment dry mouth is frequently observed, while headache, asthenia, dizziness, nausea, sleep disturbances and vasodilatation are observed occasionally. Sedation has been reported in less than 1% of patients. The frequency and intensity of these symptoms often decrease in the course of treatment.

Overdose: Oral dosages up to 2.0 mg/day have been tolerated without the occurrence of serious adverse events. Two cases have been reported of accidental overdose with Physiotens by children (2 and 3 years old):

A 2 year old child ingested an unknown quantity of Physiotens. The maximum dosage possibly ingested was 14 mg. The child had the following symptoms: sedation, coma, hypotension, miosis and dyspnoea. Gastric lavage, glucose infusion, mechanically assisted ventilation and rest resulted in the complete disappearance of the symptoms in 11 hours.

A 3 year old child took 3 mg of Physiotens in the morning. The child was hospitalised in the evening for somnolence. There was no hypotension or change in pulse rate. The child was discharged after observation for 24 hours.

Because of the pharmacodynamic properties of Physiotens, the following symptoms can be expected in adults: sedation, hypotension, orthostatic dysregulation, bradycardia, dry mouth. In rare cases emesis and paradoxical hypertension may occur.

No specific antidote is known. Phentolamine (Rogitine) may, depending on the dose, reverse part of the symptoms of moxonidine overdosage. Measures to support blood circulation are recommended.

Pharmacological properties

Pharmacodynamic properties: In different animal models, Physiotens has been shown to be a potent antihypertensive agent. Available experimental data convincingly suggest that the site of the antihypertensive action of Physiotens is the central nervous system (CNS). Within the brainstem, Physiotens has been shown to selectively interact with I_1-imidazoline receptors. These imidazoline-sensitive receptors are concentrated in the rostral ventrolateral medulla, an area critical to the central control of the peripheral sympathetic nervous system. The net effect of this interaction with the I_1-imidazoline receptor appears to result in a reduced activity of sympathetic nerves (demonstrated for cardiac, splanchnic and renal sympathetic nerves).

Physiotens differs from other available centrally acting antihypertensives by exhibiting only low affinity for central α_2-adrenoceptors as compared to I_1-imidazoline receptors; α_2-adrenoceptors are considered to be the molecular target via which sedation and dry mouth, the most common undesired effects of centrally acting antihypertensives, are mediated.

In humans, Physiotens leads to a reduction of systemic vascular resistance and consequently in arterial pressure.

Pharmacokinetic properties: Oral moxonidine treatment of rats and dogs resulted in rapid and almost complete absorption and peak plasma levels within <0.5 hours. Average plasma concentrations were comparable in both species after p.o. and i.v. administration. The elimination half-lives of radioactivity and unchanged compound were estimated to be 1–3 hours. Moxonidine and its two main metabolites (4,5-dehydromoxonidine and a guanidine derivative) were predominantly excreted in the urine. No indication of moxonidine cumulation was observed in either species during chronic toxicity studies after 52 weeks.

In humans, about 90% of an oral dose of moxonidine is absorbed; it is not subject to first-pass metabolism and its bioavailability is 88%. Food intake does not interfere with moxonidine pharmacokinetics. Moxonidine is 10–20% metabolised, mainly to 4,5-dehydromoxonidine and to a guanidine derivative by opening of the imidazoline ring. The hypotensive effect of 4,5-dehydromoxonidine is only 1/10, and that of the guanidine derivative is less than 1/100 of that of moxonidine. The maximum plasma levels of moxonidine are reached 30–180 minutes after the intake of a film-coated tablet.

Only about 7% of moxonidine is bound to plasma protein (Vd_{ss}=1.8±0.4 l/kg). Moxonidine and its metabolites are eliminated almost entirely via the kidneys. More than 90% of the dose is eliminated via the kidneys in the first 24 hours after administration, while only about 1% is eliminated via the faeces. The cumulative renal excretion of unchanged moxonidine is about 50–75%.

The mean plasma elimination half-life of moxonidine is 2.2–2.3 hours, and the renal elimination half-life is 2.6–2.8 hours.

Pharmacokinetics in the elderly: Small differences between the pharmacokinetic properties of moxonidine in the healthy elderly and younger adults are unlikely to be clinically significant. As there is no accumulation of moxonidine, dosage adjustment is unnecessary provided renal function is normal.

Pharmacokinetics in children: No pharmacokinetic studies have been performed in children.

Pharmacokinetics in renal impairment: In moderately impaired renal function (GFR 30–60 ml/min), AUC increased by 85% and clearance decreased to 52%. In such patients the hypotensive effect of Physiotens should be closely monitored, especially at the start of treatment, additionally, single doses should not exceed 200 micrograms and the daily dose should not exceed 400 micrograms.

Preclinical safety data: Chronic oral treatment for 52 weeks of rats (with dosages of 0.12–4 mg/kg) and dogs (with dosages of 0.04–0.4 mg/kg) revealed significant effects of moxonidine only at the highest doses. Slight disturbances of electrolyte balance (decrease of blood sodium and increase of potassium, urea and creatinine) were found in the high dose rats and emesis and salivation only for the high dose dogs. In addition slight increases of liver weight were obvious for both high dose species.

Reproductive toxicology did not show moxonidine effects (at oral doses up to 6.4 mg/kg) on fertility of rats and development of the embryo and foetus. Neither was evidence seen of embryotoxic and teratogenic properties in the rat at oral doses up to 27 mg/kg and the rabbit up to 4.9 mg/kg, nor on peri- and post-natal development in the rat after oral dosage up to 9 mg/kg.

Five different studies also did not show any indication of mutagenic or genotoxic effects of moxonidine. In addition, carcinogenicity studies in rats and mice at oral dose-ranges of 0.1–7.0 mg/kg did not reveal any evidence of carcinogenic potential.

Pharmaceutical particulars

List of excipients: Lactose, povidone, crospovidone, magnesium stearate, hydroxypropylmethyl cellulose, ethyl cellulose, polyethyleneglycol 6000, talc, red ferric oxide (E172), titanium dioxide (E171).

Incompatibilities: Not applicable.

Shelf life: 24 months when stored below 25°C in the original container.

Special precautions for storage: None.

Nature and contents of container: The tablets are packed in blister strips of 14. The blister strips are made of PVC/PVdC or PVC film with covering aluminium foil. Each carton contains 28 tablets.

Instructions for use/handling: No special instructions.

Marketing authorisation numbers:

200 micrograms 0512/0152
400 micrograms 0512/0154

Date of approval/revision of SPC September 1997.

Legal category POM.

SERC* – 8

Presentation A round, flat, white to almost white tablet, imprinted '256' on one face and 'S' on the reverse, each tablet containing 8 mg betahistine dihydrochloride.

Uses Betahistine is an orally effective treatment for Ménière's syndrome, which appears to exert its effect by reducing endolymphatic pressure. It is a histamine analogue which was developed following the successful parenteral use of histamine in patients with Ménière's syndrome. Animal studies have confirmed its specific effect. Clinical experience has demonstrated the efficacy of betahistine on all the principal symptoms of Ménière's syndrome, not only reducing vertiginous episodes and tinnitus but also arresting hearing loss.

Indications: Vertigo, tinnitus and hearing loss associated with Ménière's syndrome.

Dosage and administration *Adults (including the elderly):* Initially 16 mg three times daily, taken preferably with meals. Maintenance doses are generally in the range 24–48 mg daily.

Children: No dosage recommendations are made for children.

Contra-indications, warnings, etc

Contra-indication: Phaeochromocytoma. Hypersensitivity to any component of the product.

Interactions: Although an antagonism beween Serc and antihistamines could be expected on a theoretical basis, no such interactions have been reported.

Other special warnings and precautions: Caution is advised in the treatment of patients with a history of peptic ulcer. Clinical intolerance to Serc in bronchial asthma patients has been shown in a relatively few patients and therefore caution should be exercised when administering betahistine to patients with bronchial asthma.

Use in pregnancy and lactation: High dosage animal tests have shown no teratogenic properties, but the usual precautions should be observed when administering Serc to patients during pregnancy.

Other undesirable effects (frequency and seriousness): Relatively few side effects have been reported. They include gastro-intestinal upset, (including dyspepsia), headache, skin rash and pruritus.

Treatment of overdosage: No specific antidote. Gastric lavage and symptomatic treatment is recommended.

Pharmaceutical precautions Store at room temperature.

Legal category POM.

Package quantities 8 mg: Available in packs of 120 tablets.

Further information Betahistine does not produce false positive reactions in standard diagnostic urine tests.

Product licence number 0512/0076

SERC* – 16

Qualitative and quantitative composition Each tablet contains 16 mg betahistine dihydrochloride.

Pharmaceutical form A round, flat, white to almost white tablet imprinted '267' on one face and 'S' on the reverse.

Clinical particulars

Therapeutic indications: Vertigo, tinnitus and hearing loss associated with Ménière's syndrome.

Posology and method of administration: Adults (including the elderly): Initially 16 mg three times daily taken preferably with meals. Maintenance doses are generally in the range 24-48 mg daily.

Children: No dosage recommendations are made for children.

Contra-indications: Phaeochromocytoma.

Hypersensitivity to any component of the product.

Special warnings and precautions for use: Caution is advised in the treatment of patients with a history of peptic ulcer. Clinical intolerance to Serc in bronchial asthma patients has been shown in a relatively few patients and therefore caution should be exercised when administering betahistine to patients with bronchial asthma.

Interactions with other medicaments and other forms of interaction: Although an antagonism between Serc and antihistamines could be expected on a theoretical basis, no such interactions have been reported.

Pregnancy and lactation: High dosage animal tests have shown no teratogenic properties, but the usual precautions should be observed when administering Serc to patients during pregnancy.

Effects on ability to drive and use machines: It has been shown that at over 4 times the recommended daily dose, betahistine does not affect driving or psychomotor ability.

Undesirable effects: Relatively few side effects have been reported. They include gastro-intestinal upset, (including dyspepsia), headache, skin rash and pruritus.

Overdose:

Symptoms: Nausea.

Treatment: No specific antidote. Gastric lavage and symptomatic treatment is recommended.

Pharmacological properties

Pharmacodynamic properties: The active ingredient is a specific histamine agonist with virtually no H_2-activity. It appears to act on the precapillary sphincter in the stria vascularis of the inner ear, thus reducing the pressure in the endolymphatic space.

Pharmacokinetic properties: Betahistine is rapidly and completely absorbed after oral administration of the drug in tablets. It is excreted almost quantitatively in urine as 2-pyridylacetic acid within 24 hours after administration. No unchanged betahistine has been detected.

Preclinical safety data: There are no pre-clinical data of relevance to the prescriber which are additional to that already included in other sections of the SPC.

Pharmaceutical particulars

List of excipients: Microcrystalline cellulose, mannitol, citric acid monohydrate, colloidal anhydrous silica and talc.

Incompatibilities: None.

Shelf life: 3 years.

Special precautions for storage: Store at room temperature.

Nature and contents of container: Blister strips of 21. The blister strips are made of PVC/PVdC film with covering Aluminium foil. Each carton contains 84 tablets.

Instruction for use/handling: None.

Marketing authorisation number 0512/0088

Date of approval/revision of SPC July 1997

Legal category POM

YUTOPAR* INJECTION

Qualitative and quantitative composition Each ampoule contains 50 mg of ritodrine hydrochloride B.P. (10 mg/ml). Aqueous buffered vehicle contains sodium chloride and sodium metabisulphite.

Pharmaceutical form Clear, sterile aqueous solution.

Clinical particulars

Therapeutic indications:

The management of uncomplicated preterm labour: Yutopar is a betamimetic drug which stimulates beta$_2$-receptors, thereby decreasing uterine contractility. The main purpose of giving Yutopar is to delay delivery for at least 48 hours. No statistically significant effect of the drug on peri-natal mortality has as yet been observed in randomised, placebo-controlled trials. Less effect can be expected if the membranes are ruptured or the dilation of the cervix exceeds 4 cm.

IV therapy: To arrest pre-term labour between 24 and 33 weeks of gestation in patients with no medical or obstetric contra-indication to tocolytic therapy. The most effective use of IV Yutopar is achieved by using the delay in delivery to administer glucocorticosteroids or to implement other measures known to improve peri-natal health.

IM therapy: If intravenous administration is considered to be inappropriate, intramuscular administration may be substituted.

Posology and method of administration

Adults:

IV: To be administered as early as possible after the diagnosis of pre-term labour, and after evaluation of the patient to rule out contra-indications to the use of ritodrine (see contra-indications). The initial dose is 50 micrograms per minute to be gradually increased according to the response by 50 micrograms/minute every 10 minutes until contractions stop, the maternal heart rate reaches 140 beats per minute or a maximum dose of 350 micrograms/minute is reached. The effective dosage usually lies between 150 micrograms and 350 micrograms/minute; the lowest effective dose should be used. If successful, the infusion should be continued for 12 to 48 hours after uterine contractions have ceased. The infusion should be stopped if labour progresses despite treatment at the maximum dose. Careful control of the level of hydration is essential to avoid the risk of maternal pulmonary oedema (see Undesirable Effects). The volume of fluid in which the drug is administered should thus be kept to a minimum. A controlled infusion device, preferably a syringe pump should be used.

If a syringe pump is available, the concentration of the drug infused should be 3 mg/ml (i.e. 15 ml of Yutopar solution should be added to 35 ml of infusion fluid to give a total volume of 50 ml). If a syringe pump is not available, the concentration should be 300 micrograms/ml (150 mg in 500 ml fluid). The recommended infusion fluid is 5% dextrose.

Guidance on infusion rates to achieve the required dose is given in the table below:

I. SYRINGE PUMP

Add 3×5 ml ampoules of Yutopar to 35 ml of 5% w/v dextrose

Dose	*Rate*
50 micrograms/min	1 ml/hour
100 micrograms/min	2 ml/hou
150 micrograms/min	3 ml/hour
200 micrograms/min	4 ml/hour
250 micrograms/min	5 ml/hour
300 micrograms/min	6 ml/hour
350 micrograms/min	7 ml/hour

II. CONTROLLED INFUSION DEVICE

Add 3×5 ml ampoules of Yutopar to 500 ml of 5% w/v dextrose

Dose	*Rate*
50 micrograms/min	10 ml/hour
100 micrograms/min	20 ml/hour
150 micrograms/min	30 ml/hour
200 micrograms/min	40 ml/hour
250 micrograms/min	50 ml/hour
300 micrograms/min	60 ml/hour
350 micrograms/min	70 ml/hour

The maximum recommended dose is 350 micrograms/minute. The dose should be kept to the minimum required to inhibit uterine contractions.

IM: If intravenous administration is considered to be inappropriate, intramuscular administration may be substituted, giving 10 mg intramuscularly every 3 to 8 hours. The intramuscular regime should be continued for 12–48 hours following arrest of labour.

Elderly: Not applicable.

Children: Not applicable.

Contra-indications:

1. Antepartum haemorrhage which demands immediate delivery.
2. Eclampsia and severe pre-eclampsia.
3. Intra-uterine foetal death.
4. Chorioamnionitis.
5. Maternal cardiac disease.
6. Cord compression.

Special warnings and special precautions for use: Maternal pulmonary oedema has been reported in patients treated with ritodrine. Therefore, close monitoring of the patient's state of hydration is advised and if pulmonary oedema develops during administration treatment should be discontinued.

It is advisable to screen patients with potential cardiac risk before deciding on ritodrine treatment.

Yutopar should not be administered to patients with mild to moderate pre-eclampsia, hypertension or hyperthyroidism unless the attending physician considers that the benefits clearly outweigh the risks.

In order to minimise the risk of hypotension associated with tocolytic therapy, special care should be taken to avoid vena caval compression by keeping the patient in the left lateral position throughout the infusion.

Interactions with other medicaments and other forms of interaction: Careful monitoring is required in patients with suspected heart disease and in those receiving drugs which could interact with ritodrine such as monoamine oxidase inhibitors, tricyclic antidepressants, corticosteroids, sympathomimetic amines, beta-adrenergic blocking drugs, anaesthetics used in surgery:

- corticosteroids used concomitantly may increase the risk of pulmonary oedema.
- other sympathomimetic amines may be potentiated when concurrently administered.
- beta-adrenergic blocking drugs inhibit the action of ritodrine; co-administration of these drugs should therefore be avoided.
- anaesthetics used in surgery may potentiate the hypotensive effect of ritodrine.

Monitoring is also needed in patients receiving potassium-depleting diuretics, as intravenous administration of Yutopar has been shown to decrease plasma potassium levels.

In diabetic patients, glucose levels should be closely monitored and insulin requirements adjusted accordingly during intravenous treatment. On oral treatment no alterations have been reported.

Pregnancy and lactation: Animal experiments failed to show a teratogenic effect even in high dosages.

Reproduction studies, in rats and rabbits have revealed no evidence of impaired fertility or harm to the foetus. However, the drug is not recommended during the first 16 weeks of pregnancy.

In a group of children born to ritodrine treated mothers, follow-up of selected variables up to 6 years has not revealed harmful effects on growth, developmental or functional maturation.

Lactation: Not applicable.

Effect on ability to drive and use machines: Not known.

Undesirable effects: Maternal pulmonary oedema has been reported in association with ritodrine usage; in some cases this has proved fatal. Predisposing factors include fluid overload, multiple pregnancy, pre-existing cardiac disease and maternal infection. Close monitoring of the patient's state of hydration is essential. If signs of pulmonary oedema develop (e.g. cough, shortness of breath, haemoptysis), treatment should be discontinued immediately and diuretic therapy instituted.

The maternal pulse rate may progressively increase, usually to a moderate degree. This may lead to palpitations. Any pronounced tachycardia that may arise during intravenous infusion (or oral therapy) with Yutopar disappears after dose reduction or drug withdrawal. Whether the maternal tachycardia is considered acceptable must be determined on a case by case basis, but it is recommended that, in healthy patients, a heart rate of more than 140/min should be avoided. Chest pain or tightness with or without ECG abnormalities, and cardiac arrhythmias have been reported infrequently.

Flushing, sweating, tremor, nausea and vomiting have been reported.

Cases of leucopenia and/or agranulocytosis have been reported with prolonged (i.e. several weeks) intravenous ritodrine treatment. The number of leucocytes returned to normal on drug withdrawal.

Impaired liver function (i.e. increased transaminase levels and hepatitis) has been reported with the use of ritodrine.

Enlargement of the salivary glands and an increased secretion of amylase have been reported infrequently. In most cases, complete recovery occurs within a few days of discontinuation of ritodrine.

Overdose:

Symptoms: The symptoms of overdosage are those of beta-adrenergic stimulation.

Treatment: In cases of overdosage of i.v. Yutopar, discontinue the infusion immediately. A non-selective beta-sympatholytic agent may be given as an antidote.

Pharmacological properties

Pharmacodynamic properties: Ritodrine is beta-sympathomimetic which acts as a uterine relaxant in the management of premature labour. Some chronotropic cardiac effects and peripheral vasodilatation are also seen at therapeutic doses.

Pharmacokinetic properties: On average, 90% of a dose of radioactive ritodrine is excreted in the urine, independent of the route of administration.

The distribution volume after intravenous infusion of 9 mg ritodrine hydrochloride (0.15 mg/minute for 60 minutes), was 0.6-0.9 1/kg, while total body clearance was ca.100 1/hour (N=6 females).

After intramuscular administration of 10 mg, maximum serum levels are 20-33 ng/ml. The mean area under the serum curve (AUC) was 97 ng/ml/hour, and correlated well with that of the intravenous infusion (95 ng/ml/hour).

Preclinical safety data: All toxic effects of ritodrine established by intravenous and oral administration in various animal species, can more or less be ascribed to the beta-adrenergic stimulant properties of the compound. The lowest dose level used (1 mg/kg) was not free from side-effects, such as decreased serum potassium and increased serum glucose, tachycardia, cutaneous vasodilatation. At high dose levels emesis, restlessness and convulsions occurred.

Pharmaceutical particulars

List of excipients: Acetic acid, sodium hydroxide, sodium metabisulphite, sodium chloride, water for injections.

Incompatibilities: The injection fluid should not be mixed with other injection fluids, unless the compatibility is proven.

Shelf life: 36 months when stored below 30°C in the original, undamaged packaging.

Special precautions for storage: None.

Nature and contents of container: Boxes of 10×5 ml colourless glass ampoules containing ritodrine hydrochloride 10 mg/ml.

Instructions for use/handling: If the solution is discoloured or contains any precipitate or particulate matter, parenteral ritodrine should not be used.

Marketing authorisation number 0512/0020R

Date of approval/revision of SPC July 1997

Legal category POM.

YUTOPAR* TABLETS

Presentation Round, flat, yellow tablets with bevelled edges, inscribed 'YUTOPAR' on one face and a breakline on the reverse. Each tablet contains 10 mg ritodrine hydrochloride B.P. Excipients include lactose.

Uses
The management of uncomplicated preterm labour: Yutopar is a betamimetic drug which stimulates $beta_2$-receptors, thereby decreasing uterine contractility. The main purpose of giving Yutopar is to delay delivery for at least 48 hours. No statistically significant effect of the drug on perinatal mortality has as yet been observed in randomised, placebo-controlled trials.

For the maintenance of uterine quiescence following successful parenteral therapy. Oral treatment should not be used initially in an attempt to arrest labour.

Dosage and administration
Adults: One tablet (10 mg) may be given approximately 30 minutes before the termination of intravenous therapy. The usual dosage schedule for the first 24 hours of oral maintenance is one tablet (10 mg) every two hours. Thereafter, the usual dose is one or two tablets (10–20 mg) every four to six hours depending on uterine activity and unwanted effects.

The total daily dose of oral ritodrine should not exceed 120 mg. The treatment may be continued as long as the physician considers it desirable to prolong pregnancy.

Elderly: Not applicable.

Children: Not applicable.

Contra-indications, warnings, etc
Contra-indications:

1. Antepartum haemorrhage which demands immediate delivery.
2. Eclampsia and severe pre-eclampsia.
3. Intra-uterine foetal death.
4. Chorioamnionitis.
5. Maternal cardiac disease.
6. Cord compression.

Precautions: Maternal pulmonary oedema has been reported in patients treated with ritodrine. Therefore, close monitoring of the patient's state of hydration is advised and if pulmonary oedema develops during administration treatment should be discontinued.

Careful monitoring is required in patients with suspected heart disease, or those receiving other drugs, in particular those which could interact with ritodrine such as monoamine oxidase inhibitors, tricyclic anti-depressants, corticosteroids, sympathomimetic amines, beta-adrenergic blocking drugs, anaesthetics used in surgery and potassium-depleting diuretics, as intravenous administration of Yutopar has been shown to decrease plasma potassium levels.

Experiments in animals have shown that even in high dosage Yutopar has no teratogenic properties.

In diabetic patients, glucose levels should be closely monitored and insulin requirements adjusted accordingly during intravenous treatment. On oral treatment no alterations have been reported. It is also advisable to screen patients with potential cardiac risk before deciding on ritodrine treatment.

Yutopar should not be administered to patients with mild to moderate pre-eclampsia, hypertension or hyperthyroidism unless the attending physician considers that the benefits clearly outweigh the risks.

In order to minimise the risk of hypotension associated with tocolytic therapy, special care should be taken to avoid vena caval compression by keeping the patient in the left lateral position throughout the infusion.

Undesirable effects: Maternal pulmonary oedema has been reported in association with ritodrine usage; in some cases this has proved fatal. Predisposing factors include fluid overload, multiple pregnancy, pre-existing cardiac disease and maternal infection. Close monitoring of the patient's state of hydration is essential. If signs of pulmonary oedema develop (e.g. cough, shortness of breath, haemoptysis), treatment should be discontinued immediately and diuretic therapy instituted.

The maternal pulse rate may progressively increase, usually to a moderate degree. This may lead to palpitations. Any pronounced tachycardia that may arise during intravenous infusion (or oral therapy) with Yutopar disappears after dose reduction or drug withdrawal. Whether the maternal tachycardia is considered acceptable must be determined on a case by case basis, but it is recommended that, in healthy patients, a heart rate of more than 140/min should be avoided. Chest pain or tightness with or without ECG abnormalities, and cardiac arrhythmias have been reported infrequently.

Flushing, sweating, tremor, nausea and vomiting have been reported.

Cases of leucopenia and/or agranulocytosis have been reported with prolonged (i.e. several weeks) intravenous ritodrine treatment. The number of leucocytes returned to normal on drug withdrawal.

Impaired liver function (i.e. increased transaminase levels and hepatitis) has been reported with the use of ritodrine.

Enlargement of the salivary glands and an increased secretion of amylase have been reported infrequently. In most cases, complete recovery occurs within a few days of discontinuation of ritodrine.

Treatment of overdosage: In cases of overdosage of Yutopar, a non-selective beta-sympatholytic agent may be given as an antidote.

Pharmaceutical precautions Store in a dry place, not exceeding 30°C.

Legal category POM.

Package quantities Tablets: Packs of 90 tablets each containing 10 mg ritodrine hydrochloride.

Further information Less effect can be expected if the membranes are ruptured or the dilation of the cervix exceeds 4 cm.

Ritodrine does not produce false positive reactions in standard diagnostic urine tests.

Product licence number 0512/0018R

ZUMENON* 1 mg

Qualitative and quantitative composition This product contains 1 mg estradiol hemihydrate PhEur equivalent to 1 mg estradiol per tablet.

Pharmaceutical form White, round, biconvex, film-coated tablets imprinted 'S' on one side and '379' on the other.

Clinical particulars
Therapeutic indications: For the treatment of symptoms of oestrogen deficiency as a result of natural menopause or oophorectomy, eg hot flushes, nocturnal perspiration and atrophic changes in the genito-urinary tract.

In women with a uterus, a progestogen should be added to Zumenon for 10-14 days each month.

Posology and method of administration: One tablet daily without interruption. If clinical response is inadequate, dosage may be increased to two tablets daily, but should be reduced to one tablet daily as soon as practicable.

Treatment of hysterectomized women and post-menopausal women may be started on any convenient day. If the patient is menstruating, treatment is started on day 5 of bleeding.

Contra-indications: Known, suspected or past history of carcinoma of the breast, endometrial carcinoma or other hormone dependent neoplasia.

Acute or chronic liver disease or history of liver disease where the liver function tests have failed to return to normal.

Active deep venous thrombosis, thromboembolic disorders or a history of confirmed venous thrombo-embolism.

Cerebral vascular accident.

Abnormal genital bleeding of unknown aetiology.

Known or suspected pregnancy.

Special warnings and special precautions for use: Physical examination and a complete medical and family history should be taken prior to the initiation of any oestrogen therapy with special reference to blood pressure, palpation of the breasts and the abdomen and a gynaecological examination.

Patients with an intact uterus who are, or have previously been, treated with unopposed oestrogens should be examined with special care in order to investigate a possible hyperstimulation of the endometrium before commencing Zumenon therapy.

As a general rule, oestrogens should not be prescribed for longer than 1 year without another physical examination, including gynaecological examination. In case of continuing abnormal and/or irregular bleeding, a diagnostic endometrial biopsy should be performed.

Patients with or developing epilepsy, migraine, diabetes mellitus, cardiac failure, multiple sclerosis, hypertension, porphyria, haemoglobinopathies or otosclerosis should be carefully observed during treatment, as oestrogens may worsen these conditions. In patients with a past history of liver disease it is advisable to check liver functions on a regular basis.

Special care should be taken in patients with uterine leiomyomata and patients with (a history of) endometriosis as oestrogens may influence these conditions.

The indications for immediate withdrawal of therapy are:-

* deep venous thrombosis
* thromboembolic disorders
* the appearance of jaundice
* the emergence of migraine–type headache
* sudden visual disturbances
* significant increase in blood pressure
* pregnancy

Epidemiological studies have suggested that hormone replacement therapy (HRT) is associated with an increased relative risk of developing venous thromboembolism (VTE) i.e. deep vein thrombosis or pulmonary embolism. The studies find a 2-3 fold increase for users compared with non-users which for healthy women amounts to a low risk of one extra case of VTE each year for every 5000 patients taking HRT.

Generally recognised risk factors for VTE include a personal or family history and severe obesity (Body Mass Index >30 kg/m²). In women with these factors, the benefits of treatment with HRT need to be carefully weighed against risks.

The risk of VTE may be temporarily increased with prolonged immobilisation, major trauma or major surgery. In women on HRT, scrupulous attention should be given to prophylactic measures to prevent VTE following surgery. Where prolonged immobilisation is liable to follow elective surgery, particularly abdominal or orthopaedic surgery to the lower limbs, consideration should be given to temporarily stopping HRT 4 weeks earlier, if this is possible.

If venous thromboembolism develops after initiating therapy, the drug should be discontinued.

Interactions with other medicaments and other forms of interaction: Oestrogens interact with liver enzyme inducing drugs with increased metabolism of oestrogens, which may reduce the oestrogen effect. Interactions are documented for the following liver enzyme inducing drugs: barbiturates, phenytoin, rifampicin, carbamazepine.

Pregnancy and lactation: Known, or suspected pregnancy is a contra-indication to Zumenon therapy.

Lactation: this product is not indicated during this period.

Effects on ability to drive and use machines: No effects known.

Undesirable effects: During the first few months of treatment with Zumenon, breast tenderness may occur. Nausea, headache and oedema occur rarely. Symptoms are normally transient. Furthermore, skin reactions have been reported.

Overdose: There have been no reports of ill-effects from overdosing. If overdosage is discovered within two or three hours and is so large that treatment seems desirable, gastric lavage can safely be used. There is no specific antidote and further treatment should be symptomatic.

Pharmacological properties
Pharmacodynamic properties: Estradiol is chemically and biologically identical to the endogenous human estradiol and is, therefore, classified as a human estrogen. Estradiol is the primary estrogen and the most active of the ovarian hormones. The endogenous estrogens are involved in certain functions of the uterus and accessory organs, including the proliferation of the endometrium and the cyclic changes in the cervix and vagina.

Estrogens are known to play an important role for bone and fat metabolism. Furthermore, estrogens also affect the autonomic nervous system and may have indirect positive psychotropic actions.

Pharmacokinetic properties: Following oral administration, micronised estradiol is readily absorbed, but extensively metabolised. The major unconjugated and conjugated metabolites are estrone and estrone sulphate. These metabolites can contribute to the estrogen activity, either directly or after conversion to estradiol. Estrone sulphate may undergo enterohepatic circulation. In urine, the major compounds are the glucuronides of estrone and estradiol.

Estrogens are secreted in the milk of nursing mothers.

Preclinical safety data: Supraphysiologically high doses (prolonged overdoses) of estradiol have been associated with the induction of tumors in estrogen-dependent target organs for all rodent species tested. Pronounced species differences in toxicology, pharmacology and pharmacodynamics exist.

Pharmaceutical particulars
List of excipients: Lactose, methylhydroxypropyl cellulose, maize starch, colloidal anhydrous silica, magnesium stearate, polyethylene glycol 400, E171.

Incompatibilities: Not applicable

Shelf life: 36 months when stored below 30°C.

Special precautions for storage: None.

Nature and contents of container: The tablets are packed in blister strips of 28. The blister strips are made of PVC film with covering Aluminium foil. Each carton contains 84 tablets.

Instruction for use/handling: Not applicable

Marketing authorisation number 0512/0141

Date of approval/revision of SPC February 1998

Legal category POM

ZUMENON* 2 mg

Qualitative and quantitative composition This product contains 2 mg estradiol hemihydrate PhEur equivalent to 2 mg estradiol per tablet.

Pharmaceutical form Orange, round, biconvex, film-coated tablets imprinted 'S' on one side and '379' on the other.

Clinical particulars

Therapeutic indications: 1. Hormone replacement therapy for the treatment of symptoms of oestrogen deficiency as a result of natural menopause or oophorectomy, eg hot flushes, nocturnal perspiration and atrophic changes in the genito-urinary tract.

2. For the prevention of osteoporosis in women at risk of developing fractures.

Epidemiological studies suggest a number of risk factors may contribute to post-menopausal osteoporosis including: early menopause (either naturally or surgically induced); family history of osteoporosis; recent use of corticosteroids; a small frame; a thin frame; cigarette smoking.

If several of these risk factors are present consideration should be given to hormone replacement therapy.

For maximum prophylactic benefit a treatment should commence as soon as possible after the menopause. Bone mineral density measurements may help to confirm the presence of low bone mass.

In women with a uterus, a progestogen should be added to Zumenon for 10-14 days each month.

Posology and method of administration: Adults (including the elderly):

Climacteric symptoms: Therapy should be initiated with Zumenon 1 mg. The dosage may be increased if required by using Zumenon 2 mg. For maintenance therapy the lowest effective dose should be used.

One tablet daily without interruption. If clinical response is inadequate, dosage may be increased to two tablets daily, but should be reduced to one tablet daily as soon as practicable.

Prevention of osteoporosis: One 2 mg tablet daily without interruption. Treatment should start as soon as possible after the onset of menopause and certainly within 2 or 3 years. Protection appears to be effective for as long as treatment continues, however data beyond 10 years are limited. A careful reappraisal of the risk benefit ratio should be undertaken before treating for longer than 5-10 years. For long term use see also Special warnings and special precautions for use.

Treatment of hysterectomised women and post-menopausal women may be started on any convenient day. If the patient is menstruating, treatment is started on day 5 of bleeding.

Before therapy commences it is recommended that the patient is fully informed of all likely benefits and potential risks. She should have a full physical and gynaecological examination with special emphasis on blood pressure, breasts, abdomen and pelvic organs and an endometrial assessment carried out if indicated. Follow-up examinations are recommended every 6-12 months.

Breakthrough bleeding may occasionally occur in the first few weeks after initiating treatment and will usually settle.

Children: Zumenon is not indicated in children

Contra-indications:

- Known, suspected or past history of carcinoma of the breast, endometrial carcinoma or other hormone dependent neoplasia.
- Acute or chronic liver disease or history of liver disease where the liver function tests have failed to return to normal.
- Active deep venous thrombosis, thromboembolic disorders, or a history of confirmed venous thromboembolism.
- Cerebral vascular accident.
- Abnormal genital bleeding of unknown aetiology.
- Rotor syndrome or Dubin-Johnson syndrome.
- Severe cardiac or renal disease.
- Known or suspected pregnancy.

Special warnings and special precautions for use: Breakthrough bleeding may occasionally occur and can be the result of poor compliance or concurrent antibiotic use. It may however indicate endometrial pathology and therefore any doubt as to the cause of breakthrough bleeding is an indication for endometrial evaluation including endometrial biopsy.

There is an increased risk of endometrial hyperplasia or carcinoma associated with unopposed oestrogen administered long term (for more than 1 year). However, the appropriate addition of a progestogen to an oestrogen regimen lowers this risk.

There is suggestive evidence of a small increased risk of breast cancer with oestrogen replacement therapy used for long term (greater than 5 years). Some studies have reported an increased risk of breast cancer in long term users, others have not shown this relationship. It is not known whether concurrent progestogen use influences the risk of breast cancer in post-menopausal women taking hormone replacement therapy. Women on long-term therapy should have regular breast examinations and should be instructed in self-breast examination. Regular mammographic investigation should be conducted where considered appropriate.

There is need for caution when prescribing oestrogens in women who have a history, or known breast nodules or fibrocystic disease. Breast status should be closely monitored, supported by regular mammography.

Certain diseases may be made worse by hormone replacement therapy and patients with these conditions should be closely monitored. These include otosclerosis, multiple sclerosis, systemic lupus erythematosus, porphyria, melanoma, epilepsy, migraine, asthma, haemoglobinopathies, diabetes mellitus. In patients with a past history of liver disease it is advisable to check liver functions on a regular basis. In addition, pre-existing fibroids may increase in size during oestrogen therapy and symptoms associated with endometriosis may be exacerbated.

Epidemiological studies have suggested that hormone replacement therapy (HRT) is associated with an increased relative risk of developing venous thromboembolism (VTE) i.e. deep vein thrombosis or pulmonary embolism. The studies find a 2-3 fold increase for users compared with non-users which for healthy women amounts to a low risk of one extra case of VTE each year for every 5000 patients taking HRT.

Generally recognised risk factors for VTE include a personal or family history and severe obesity (Body Mass Index >30 kg/m²). In women with these factors, the benefits of treatment with HRT need to be carefully weighed against risks.

The risk of VTE may be temporarily increased with prolonged immobilisation, major trauma or major surgery. In women on HRT, scrupulous attention should be given to prophylactic measures to prevent VTE following surgery. Where prolonged immobilisation is liable to follow elective surgery, particularly abdominal or orthopaedic surgery to the lower limbs, consideration should be given to temporarily stopping HRT 4 weeks earlier, if this is possible.

If venous thromboembolism develops after initiating therapy, the drug should be discontinued.

As oestrogens may cause fluid retention, patients with cardiac or renal dysfunction should be carefully observed.

Zumenon is not an oral contraceptive. Women of child-bearing potential should be advised to use non-hormonal contraceptive methods.

Most studies indicate that oestrogen replacement therapy has little effect on blood pressure and some indicate that oestrogen use may be associated with a small decrease. In addition, most studies on combined therapy indicate that the addition of progestogen also has little effect on blood pressure. Rarely, idiosyncratic hypertension may occur.

When oestrogens are administered to hypertensive women, supervision is necessary and blood pressure should be monitored at regular intervals.

It has been reported that there is an increase in the risk of surgically confirmed gall bladder disease in women receiving post-menopausal oestrogens.

Interactions with other medicaments and other forms of interaction: Oestrogens interact with liver enzyme inducing drugs with increased metabolism of oestrogens, which may reduce the oestrogen effect. Interactions are documented for the following liver enzyme inducing drugs: barbiturates, phenytoin, rifampicin, carbamazepine.

Changes in oestrogen serum concentrations may affect the results of certain endocrine or liver function tests.

Pregnancy and lactation: Known, or suspected pregnancy is a contra-indication to Zumenon therapy.

Lactation: this product is not indicated during this period.

Effects on ability to drive and use machines: No effects known

Undesirable effects: The following side effects have been reported with oestrogen/progestogen therapy:

- Genito-urinary system–Breakthrough bleeding, spotting, change in menstrual flow, dysmenorrhoea, premenstrual-like syndrome, amenorrhoea, increase in size of uterine fibromyomata, vaginal candidiasis, change in cervical erosion and in degree of cervical secretion, cystitis-like syndrome.
- Breasts–Tenderness, enlargement, secretion.
- Gastrointestinal–Nausea, vomiting, abdominal cramps, bloating, cholestatic jaundice.
- Skin–Chloasma or melasma which may persist when drug is discontinued, erythema multiforme, erythema nodosum, haemorrhagic eruption.
- Eyes–Steepening of corneal curvature, intolerance to contact lenses.
- CNS–Headaches, migraine, dizziness, mental depression, chorea.
- Miscellaneous–Increase or decrease in weight, reduced carbohydrate tolerance, aggravation of porphyria, oedema, changes in libido, leg cramps.

Overdose: There have been no reports of ill-effects following overdose. Overdose of oestrogen may cause nausea, and withdrawal bleeding may occur in females.

If overdosage is discovered within two or three hours and is so large that treatment seems desirable, gastric lavage can safely be used. There is no specific antidote and further treatment should be symptomatic.

Pharmacological properties

Pharmacodynamic properties: Estradiol is chemically and biologically identical to the endogenous human estradiol and is, therefore, classified as a human oestrogen. Estradiol is the primary oestrogen and the most active of the ovarian hormones. The endogenous oestrogens are involved in certain functions of the uterus and accessory organs, including the proliferation of the endometrium and the cyclic changes in the cervix and vagina.

Oestrogens are known to play an important role for bone and fat metabolism. Furthermore, oestrogens also affect the autonomic nervous system and may have indirect positive psychotropic actions.

Pharmacokinetic properties: Following oral administration, micronised estradiol is readily absorbed, but extensively metabolised. The major unconjugated and conjugated metabolites are estrone and estrone sulphate. These metabolites can contribute to the oestrogen activity, either directly or after conversion to estradiol. Estrone sulphate may undergo enterohepatic circulation. In urine, the major compounds are the glucuronides of estrone and estradiol.

Oestrogens are secreted in the milk of nursing mothers.

Preclinical safety data: Supraphysiologically high doses (prolonged overdoses) of estradiol have been associated with the induction of tumours in oestrogen-dependent target organs for all rodent species tested. Pronounced species differences in toxicology, pharmacology and pharmacodynamics exist.

Pharmaceutical particulars

List of excipients: Lactose, methylhydroxypropyl cellulose, maize starch, colloidal anhydrous silica, magnesium stearate, methylcellulose, polyethylene glycol 400, quinoline yellow (E104), sunset yellow (E110), ponceau 4R (E124), titanium dioxide (E171).

Incompatibilities: Not applicable

Shelf life: 24 months when stored below 25°C.

Special precautions for storage: None.

Nature and contents of container: The tablets are packed in blister strips of 28. The blister strips are made of PVC film with covering Aluminium foil. Each carton contains 84 tablets.

Instruction for use/handling: Not applicable

Marketing authorisation number 00512/0100

Date of approval/revision of SPC September 1997

Legal category POM

**Trade Mark*

E. R. Squibb & Sons Limited

Bristol-Myers Squibb House
Staines Rd
Hounslow TW3 3JA

☎ 0181 572 7422 🗋 0181 754 3789

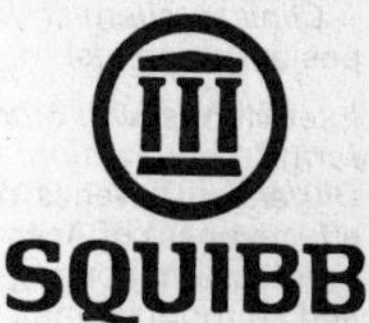

ACEPRIL* TABLETS

Qualitative and quantitative composition Each tablet contains captopril 12.5 mg, 25 mg or 50 mg.

Pharmaceutical form Oral tablet.

Clinical particulars

Therapeutic indications:

Hypertension: Acepril is indicated for the first line treatment of mild to moderate hypertension.

In severe hypertension it should be used where standard therapy is ineffective or inappropriate.

Congestive heart failure: Acepril is indicated for the treatment of congestive heart failure. The drug should be used together with diuretics and, where appropriate digitalis.

Myocardial infarction: Acepril is indicated following myocardial infarction in clinically stable patients with asymptomatic and symptomatic left ventricular dysfunction to improve survival, delay the onset of symptomatic heart failure, reduce hospitalisations for heart failure, and reduce recurrent myocardial infarction and coronary revascularisation procedures.

Determination of cardiac function by radionuclide ventriculography or echocardiography should be undertaken prior to initiation of preventative treatment with Acepril in post myocardial infarction patients.

Diabetic nephropathy: Acepril is indicated for the treatment of diabetic nephropathy (microalbuminuria greater than 30 mg/day) in insulin-dependent diabetics. In these patients, captopril prevents the progression of renal disease and reduces associated clinical events e.g. dialysis, renal transplantation and death.

Posology and method of administration:

Hypertension: Treatment with Acepril should be at the lowest effective dose which should be titrated according to the needs of the patient.

Mild to moderate hypertension: The starting dose is 12.5 mg twice daily. The usual maintenance dose is 25 mg twice daily which can be increased incrementally, at 2–4 week intervals, until a satisfactory response is achieved, to a maximum of 50 mg twice daily.

A thiazide diuretic may be added to Acepril if satisfactory response has not been achieved. The dose of diuretic may be increased at 1-2 week intervals to the level of optimum response or until the maximum dose is reached.

Severe hypertension: In severe hypertension where standard therapy is ineffective or inappropriate because of adverse effects, the starting dose is 12.5 mg b.d. The dosage may be increased incrementally to a maximum of 50 mg t.i.d. Acepril should be used together with other anti-hypertensive agents but the dose of these should be individually titrated. A daily dose of 150 mg of Acepril should not normally be exceeded.

Heart failure: Acepril therapy must be started under close medical supervision. Acepril should be introduced when diuretic therapy (such as frusemide 40-80 mg or equivalent) is insufficient to control symptoms. A starting dose of 6.25 mg or 12.5 mg may minimise a transient hypotensive effect. The possibility of this occurring can be reduced by discontinuing or reducing diuretic therapy if possible, prior to initiating Acepril.

The usual maintenance dose is 25 mg two or three times a day which can be increased incrementally, with intervals of at least two weeks, until a satisfactory response is achieved. The usual maximum dose is 150 mg daily.

Myocardial infarction: Therapy may be initiated as early as three days following a myocardial infarction. After an initial dose of 6.25 mg, captopril therapy should be titrated to a final target dose of 150 mg daily in divided doses over the next several weeks.

Achievement of the target dose of 150 mg should be based on the patient's tolerance to captopril during titration. If symptomatic hypotension occurs, a dosage reduction may be required.

Captopril may be used in patients treated with other post-myocardial infarction therapies, e.g. thrombolytics, aspirin, beta blockers.

Diabetic nephropathy: The recommended daily dose of captopril is 75 to 100 mg in divided doses.

If further blood pressure reduction is required, other antihypertensive agents such as diuretics, beta blockers, centrally acting agents or vasodilators may be used in conjunction with captopril.

Elderly: The dose should be titrated against the blood pressure response and kept as low as possible to achieve adequate control. Since elderly patients may have reduced renal function and other organ dysfunctions, it is suggested that a low dose of Acepril be used initially.

Children: Acepril is not recommended for the treatment of mild to moderate hypertension in children.

Experience in neonates, particularly premature infants, is limited. Because renal function in infants is not equivalent to that of older children and adults, lower doses of Acepril should be used with the patients under close medical supervision.

The starting dose should be 0.3 mg per Kg bodyweight up to a maximum of 6 mg per Kg bodyweight daily in divided doses. The dose should be individualised according to the response and may be given two or three times daily.

Patients with renal impairment: Captopril in divided doses of 75 to 100 mg/day was well tolerated in patients with diabetic nephropathy and mild to moderate renal impairment (creatinine clearance at least 30 ml/min/1.73 m²).

Patients with severely impaired renal function will take longer to reach steady-state captopril levels and will reach higher steady-state levels for a given daily dose than patients with normal renal function. These patients may therefore respond to smaller or less frequent doses.

Therefore, patients with severe renal impairment (creatinine clearance less than 30 ml/min/1.73 m²), the initial daily dose should be 12.5 mg b.d. The dose can then be titrated against the response but adequate time should be allowed between dosage adjustments. When concomitant diuretic therapy is required, a loop diuretic rather than a thiazide diuretic should be the diuretic of choice.

Acepril is readily eliminated by haemodialysis.

Contra-indications: A history of previous hypersensitivity to the product.

Pregnancy: Acepril has been shown to be lethal to rabbit and sheep foetuses. There were no foetotoxic effects to hamster or rat foetuses.

Acepril is contra-indicated in pregnancy and should not be used in women of child bearing potential unless protected by effective contraception.

Exposure of the mother in the second and third trimesters of pregnancy has been associated with oligohydramnios and neonatal hypotension and/or anuria.

Special warnings and special precautions for use:

Precautions: Evaluation of the patient should include assessment of renal function prior to initiation of therapy and at appropriate intervals thereafter (see *Posology and method of administration* section]

Acepril should not be used in patients with aortic stenosis or outflow tract obstruction.

As limited experience has been obtained in the treatment of acute hypertensive crises, the use of Acepril should be avoided in these patients.

Warnings: The incidence of adverse reactions to captopril is principally associated with renal function since the drug is excreted primarily by the kidney. The dose should not exceed that necessary for adequate control and should be reduced in patients with impaired renal function.

Hypotension: With the first one or two doses some patients may experience symptomatic hypotension. In most instances, symptoms are relieved simply by the patient lying down.

In patients with severe and renin dependent hypertension (e.g. renovascular hypertension) or severe congestive heart failure who are receiving large doses of diuretic, exaggerated hypotensive responses have occurred usually within one hour of the initial dose of Acepril. In these patients, by discontinuing diuretic therapy or significantly reducing the diuretic dose for four to seven days prior to initiating Acepril the possibility of this occurrence is reduced. By commencing Acepril therapy with small doses (6.25 mg or 12.5 mg) the duration of any hypotensive effect is lessened. Some patients may benefit from an infusion of saline. The occurrence of first dose hypotension does not preclude subsequent dose titration with Acepril. Hypotension has been occasionally reported in patients on Acepril due to causes of acute volume depletion such as vomiting and diarrhoea.

Serum potassium: Since Acepril decreases aldosterone production, serum potassium is usually maintained in patients on diuretics. Potassium sparing diuretics or potassium supplements should not therefore be used routinely. In patients with marked renal impairment a significant elevation of serum potassium may occur.

Renal: Proteinuria in patients with prior normal renal function is rare.

Where proteinuria has occurred it has usually been in patients with severe hypertension or evidence of prior renal disease. Nephrotic syndrome occurred in some of these patients.

In patients with evidence of prior renal disease, monthly urinary protein estimations (dip stick) are recommended for the first 9 months of therapy.

If repeated determinations show increasing amounts of urinary protein, a 24-hour quantitative determination should be obtained, and if this exceeds 1 g/day, the benefits and risks of continuing Acepril should be evaluated.

In patients with diabetic nephropathy and proteinuria, who received captopril 75 mg/day for a median of 3 years, there was a consistent reduction in proteinuria. It is unknown whether long-term therapy in patients with other types of renal disease would have similar effects.

Although membranous glomerulopathy was found in biopsies taken from some proteinuric patients, a causal relationship to Acepril has not been established.

Some patients with renal disease, particularly those with bilateral renal artery stenosis or unilateral renal artery stenosis in a single functioning kidney, have developed increased concentrations of blood urea and serum creatinine. Acepril dosage reduction and/or discontinuation of diuretic may be required. For some of these patients it may not be possible to normalise blood pressure and maintain adequate renal perfusion.

Recent clinical observations have shown a high incidence of anaphylactoid-like reactions during haemodialysis with high-flux dialysis membranes (e.g. AN69) in patients receiving ACE inhibitors. Therefore, this combination should be avoided.

Haematological: Neutropenia/agranulocytosis, thrombocytopenia and anaemia have been reported in patients receiving Acepril.

In patients with normal renal function and no other complicating factors, neutropenia occurs rarely.

Acepril should be used with extreme caution in patients with collagen vascular disease, immunosuppressant therapy, treatment with allopurinol or procainamide, or a combination of these complicating factors especially if there is pre-existing impaired renal function. Some of these patients developed serious infections which in a few instances did not respond to intensive antibiotic therapy.

If Acepril is used in such patients, it is advised that white blood cell count and differential counts should be performed prior to therapy, every 2 weeks during the first 3 months of Acepril therapy, and periodically thereafter.

During treatment all patients should be instructed to report any sign of infection (e.g. sore throat, fever), when a differential white blood cell count should be performed. Acepril and other concomitant medication should be withdrawn if neutropenia (neutrophils less than 1000/mm³) is detected or suspected.

In most patients neutrophil counts rapidly returned to normal upon discontinuing Acepril.

Surgery/anaesthesia: In patients undergoing major surgery, or during anaesthesia with agents which produce hypotension, captopril will block angiotensin II formation secondary to compensatory renin release.

This may lead to hypotension which can be corrected by volume expansion.

Clinical chemistry: Acepril may cause a false-positive urine test for acetone.

Interactions with other medicinal products and other forms of interaction:
Diuretics: Diuretics potentiate the anti-hypertensive effectiveness of Acepril.

Potassium-sparing diuretics (triamterene, amiloride and spironolactone), or potassium supplements may cause significant increase in serum potassium.

Indomethacin: A reduction of anti-hypertensive effectiveness may occur. This is probably also the case with other non-steroidal anti-inflammatory drugs.

Vasodilators: Acepril has been reported to act synergistically with peripheral vasodilators such as minoxidil. Awareness of this interaction may avert an initial hypotensive response.

Clonidine: It has been suggested that the anti-hypertensive effect of Acepril can be delayed when patients treated with clonidine are changed to Acepril.

Allopurinol and procainamide: There have been reports of neutropenia and/or Stevens-Johnson syndrome in patients on Acepril plus either allopurinol or procainamide. Although a causal relationship has not been established, these combinations should only be used with caution, especially in patients with impaired renal function.

Immunosuppressants: Azathioprine and cyclophosphamide have been associated with blood dyscrasias in patients with renal failure who were also taking Acepril.

Probenecid: The renal clearance of Acepril is reduced in the presence of probenecid.

Lithium: Concomitant use of lithium and ACE-inhibitors may result in an increase of serum lithium concentration.

Hypoglycaemic agents: ACE Inhibitors have been shown to enhance insulin sensitivity. There have been rare reports of hypoglycaemic episodes in diabetic patients treated concomitantly with ACE Inhibitors and antidiabetic medicines (insulin or oral hypoglycaemic agents). This phenomenon may be more likely to occur during the first few weeks of treatment. In such cases a reduction in the dose of the antidiabetic medicine may be required.

Pregnancy and lactation: Acepril has been shown to be lethal to rabbit and sheep foetuses. There were no foetotoxic effects to hamster or rat foetuses.

Acepril is contra-indicated in pregnancy and should not be used in women of child bearing potential unless protected by effective contraception.

Exposure of the mother in the second and third trimesters of pregnancy has been associated with oligohydramnios and neonatal hypotension and/or anuria.

Nursing mothers: Because captopril is excreted in breast milk, Acepril should not be used in nursing mothers.

Effects on ability to drive and use machines: See *Warnings* under *Hypotension* section.

Undesirable effects:
Idiosyncratic: Angioedema involving the extremities, face, lips, mucous membranes, tongue, glottis or larynx has been seen in patients treated with ACE inhibitors, including captopril. In this situation, the ACE inhibitor should be discontinued. Where swelling is confined to the face, lips and mouth the condition will usually resolve without further treatment, although antihistamines may be useful in relieving symptoms. These patients should be followed carefully until the swelling has resolved. However, where there is involvement of the tongue, glottis or larynx, likely to cause airway obstruction, subcutaneous adrenaline (0.5 ml, 1:1,000) should be administered promptly where indicated.

Haematological: Neutropenia, anaemia and thrombocytopenia (see Warnings). Rarely a positive ANA has been reported.

Renal: Proteinuria, elevated blood urea and creatinine, elevated serum potassium and acidosis (see *Warnings*).

Cardiovascular: Hypotension (see *Warnings*), tachycardia.

Skin: Rashes, usually pruritic, may occur. They are usually mild, maculopapular, rarely urticarial and disappear within a few days of dosage reduction, short-term treatment with an antihistamine and/or discontinuing therapy. In a few cases the rash has been associated with fever. Pruritus, flushing, vesicular or bullous rash, and photosensitivity have been reported.

Gastrointestinal: Reversible and usually self-limiting taste impairment has been reported. Weight loss may be associated with the loss of taste. Stomatitis, resembling aphthous ulcers, has been reported. Elevation of liver enzymes has been noted in a few patients. Rare cases of hepatocellular injury and cholestatic jaundice have been reported. Gastric irritation and abdominal pain may occur. Pancreatitis has been reported rarely in patients treated with ACE Inhibitors; in some cases this has proved fatal.

Other: Paraesthesias of the hands, serum sickness, cough, bronchospasm and lymphadenopathy have been reported.

Overdose: In the event of overdosage, blood pressure should be monitored and if hypotension develops volume expansion is the treatment of choice. Captopril is removed by dialysis.

Pharmacological properties

Pharmacodynamic properties: Captopril is a highly specific, competitive inhibitor of angiotensin-I converting enzyme. This enzyme is responsible for the conversion of angiotensin-I to angiotensin-II.

Pharmacokinetic properties:

Total captopril:	t_{MAX}	1 hour
	$t_{\frac{1}{2}}$	8 hours
Free captopril:	t_{MAX}	1 hour
	$t_{\frac{1}{2}}$	1 hour

The absolute bioavailability of an oral dose is approximately 65%.

Preclinical safety data: No further relevant data

Pharmaceutical particulars

List of excipients: Lactose, maize starch, microcrystalline cellulose, stearic acid.

Incompatibilities: None.

Shelf life: 48 Months.

Special precautions for storage: Store below 30°C. Protect from moisture.

Nature and contents of container: The 12.5 mg tablets are available in blister packs of 56 tablets. The 25 mg and 50 mg tablets are available in blister packs of 56 and 84 tablets.

Instructions for use/handling: No special instructions.

Marketing authorisation numbers
12.5 mg: 0034/0298
25 mg: 0034/0299
50 mg: 0034/0300

Date of approval/revision of SPC 5 November 1996

Legal category POM

ACEZIDE* TABLETS

Qualitative and quantitative composition Each tablet contains captopril 50 mg and hydrochlorothiazide 25 mg.

Pharmaceutical form Oral tablet.

Clinical particulars

Therapeutic indications: For the treatment of mild to moderate hypertension in patients who have been stabilised on the individual components given in the same proportions.

Posology and method of administration:
Adults: The usual dose of Acezide is one tablet daily. A daily dose of two tablets should not be exceeded.

Elderly: The dose should be kept as low as possible to achieve adequate blood pressure control. In some patients half a tablet daily may be sufficient.

Children: Safety and effectiveness of Acezide has not been established.

Patients with renal failure: Acezide is not recommended for use in patients with significant renal impairment.

Contra-indications: Acezide is contra-indicated in patients with anuria or hypersensitivity to captopril, thiazides, or any sulphonamide-derived drug.

Pregnancy: Captopril has been shown to be lethal to rabbit and sheep foetuses. There were no foetotoxic effects to hamster or rat foetuses.

Acezide is contra-indicated in pregnancy and should not be used in women of child bearing potential unless protected by effective contraception.

Exposure of the mother in the second and third trimester of pregnancy has been associated with oligohydramnios and neonatal hypertension and/or anuria.

Special warnings and special precautions for use:
Precautions: Acezide should not be used in patients with aortic stenosis or outflow tract obstruction.

Recent clinical observations have shown a high incidence of anaphylactoid-like reactions during haemodialysis with high-flux dialysis membranes (e.g. AN69) in patients receiving ace inhibitors. (see *Contra-indications*).

Interactions with other medicinal products and other forms of interaction:

Diuretics: Potassium-sparing diuretics (triamterene, amiloride and spironolactone), or potassium supplements may cause significant increase in serum potassium.

Indomethacin: A reduction of anti-hypertensive effectiveness may occur. This is probably also the case with other non-steroidal anti-inflammatory drugs.

Vasodilators: Acezide has been reported to act synergistically with peripheral vasodilators such as minoxidil. This may improve blood pressure control and awareness of this interaction may avert an initial hypotensive response.

Clonidine: It has been suggested that the anti-hypertensive effect of captopril can be delayed when patients treated with clonidine are changed to Acezide.

Allopurinol and procainamide: There have been reports of neutropenia and/or Stevens Johnson syndrome in patients on captopril plus either allopurinol or procainamide. Although a causal relationship has not been established, these combinations should only be used with caution, especially in patients with impaired renal function.

Immunosuppressants: Azathioprine and cyclophosphamide have been associated with blood dyscrasias in patients with renal failure who were also taking captopril.

Probenecid: The renal clearance of captopril is reduced in the presence of probenecid.

Pregnancy and lactation: Captopril has been shown to be lethal to rabbit and sheep foetuses. There were no foetotoxic effects to hamster or rat foetuses.

Acezide is contra-indicated in pregnancy and should not be used in women of child bearing potential unless protected by effective contraception.

Exposure of the mother in the second and third trimester of pregnancy has been associated with oligohydramnios and neonatal hypertension and/or anuria.

Acezide should not be used in nursing mothers.

Effects on ability to drive and use machines: Not applicable.

Undesirable effects:
Haematological: Neutropenia/agranulocytosis, thrombocytopenia and anaemia have been reported in patients receiving captopril.

In patients with normal renal function and no other complicating factors, neutropenia occurs rarely.

Captopril should not be used routinely in patients with pre-existing impaired renal function, collagen vascular disease, immunosuppressant therapy, treatment with allopurinol or procainamide, or a combination of these complicating factors. Some of these patients developed serious infections which in a few instances did not respond to intensive antibiotic therapy.

During treatment, all patients should be instructed to report any sign of infection (e.g. persistent sore throat, fever), when a differential white blood cell count should be performed. Acezide and other concomitant medication should be withdrawn if neutropenia (neutrophils less than 1000/mm³) is detected or suspected.

In most patients neutrophil counts rapidly returned to normal upon discontinuing captopril.

Skin: With captopril, rashes, usually pruritic, may occur. They are usually mild, transient and maculopapular, rarely urticarial. In a few cases the rash has been associated with fever and some patients have developed angio-neurotic oedema. Pruritus, flushing, vesicular rash, and photosensitivity have been reported.

With thiazides, purpura, photosensitivity, rash, urticaria, necrotising angiitis, Stevens-Johnson syndrome and other hypersensitivity reactions have been observed.

Gastrointestinal: Reversible and usually self-limiting taste impairment has been reported. Weight loss may be associated with the loss of taste. Stomatitis, resembling aphthous ulcers, has been reported. Elevation of liver enzymes has been noted in a few patients receiving captopril. Rare cases of hepatocellular injury and cholestatic jaundice have been reported. Gastric irritation and abdominal pain may occur. Pancreatitis has been reported rarely in patients treated with ACE Inhibitors; in some cases this has proved fatal.

Other: Paraesthesiae of the hands, serum sickness, cough, bronchospasm and lymphadenopathy have been reported.

With thiazides, dizziness, vertigo, headache, xanthopsia, hyperglycaemia, hypokalaemia, glycosuria, hyperuricaemia, hypercalcaemia, muscle spasm, weakness and restlessness have been reported.

Renal: Proteinuria is a rare complication of captopril therapy.

Some patients with renal disease, particularly those with bilateral renal artery stenoses or unilateral artery stenoses in a single functioning kidney, have developed increased concentrations of blood urea and serum creatinine. Discontinuation of Acezide may be required.

Hepatic: Acezide should be used with caution in patients with impaired hepatic function or progressive liver disease because of the known risks associated with alterations in fluid and electrolyte balance resulting from thiazide treatment in such patients.

Electrolyte imbalance: Patients receiving Acezide should be observed for clinical signs of thiazide-induced fluid or electrolyte imbalance. In such patients periodic determinations of serum electrolytes should be performed. Because captopril reduces the production of aldosterone, its combination with hydrochlorothiazide may minimise diuretic-induced hypokalaemia. However, some patients may still require potassium supplements. Potassium-sparing diuretics should not be used in conjunction with Acezide.

Surgery/anaesthesia: In patients undergoing major surgery, or during anaesthesia with agents which produce hypotension, captopril will block Angiotensin II formation secondary to compensatory renin release. This may lead to hypotension which can be corrected by volume expansion.

Thiazides may decrease the arterial response to noradrenaline. In emergency surgery, pre-anaesthetic and anaesthetic agents should be administered in reduced doses. Thiazides may increase the response to tubocurarine.

Metabolic disorders: Hyperuricaemia may occur, or frank gout be precipitated by thiazides in certain patients. Insulin requirements in diabetic patients may be altered by thiazides and latent diabetes mellitus may emerge. The captopril component of Acezide has been shown to ameliorate these effects of thiazides.

Clinical chemistry: Acezide may cause a false-positive urine test for acetone.

Side effects: Haematological: With thiazides, leucopenia, agranuloooocytosis, thrombocytopenia and aplastic anaemia have occurred. Cardiovascular: tachycardia.

Overdose: In the event of overdosage, blood pressure should be monitored and if hypotension develops volume expansion is the treatment of choice.

Captopril is removed by dialysis.

Pharmacological properties

Pharmacodynamic properties: Captopril inhibits angiotensin converting enzyme which is responsible for the conversation of Angiotensin I to the pressor substance of Angiotensin II.

Hydrochlorothiazide is a diuretic which increases the excretion of sodium and chloride ions. The resulting fall in blood pressure and blood volume results in an increase in Angiotensin II levels which tend to reduce the hypotensive effect.

Pharmacokinetic properties:

Captopril: After oral administration of therapeutic doses of captopril rapid absorption occurs with peak blood levels at about one hour. Average minimal absorption is approximately 75%. In a 24-hour period over 95% of the absorbed dose is eliminated in the urine; 40 to 50% is unchanged drug; most of the remainder is the disulphide dimer of captopril and captopril-cysteine disulphide.

Approximately 25 to 30% of the circulating drug is bound to plasma proteins. The apparent elimination half-life for total radioactivity in blood is probably less than 3 hours. An accurate determination of half-life of unchanged captopril is not, at present, possible but it is probably less than 2 hours. In patients with renal impairment, however, retention of captopril occurs (see dosage and administration).

Hydrochlorothiazide: The mean plasma half-life of hydrochlorothiazide in fasted individuals has been reported to be approximately 2.5 hours. Onset of diuresis occurs in 2 hours and the peak effect at about 4 hours. Its action persists for approximately 6 to 12 hours. Hydrochlorothiazide is eliminated rapidly by the kidney.

Preclinical safety data: No further relevant information.

Pharmaceutical particulars

List of excipients: Lactose, magnesium stearate, maize starch, microcrystalline cellulose, stearic acid.

Incompatibilities: None.

Shelf life: 36 months.

Special precautions for storage: Store below 30°C. Protect from moisture

Nature and contents of container: The tablets are packaged in either PVC/PVDC Blister or Foil Strips.

Instructions for use/handling: No special instructions.

Marketing authorisation number 0034/0301

Date of approval/revision of SPC December 1996

Legal category POM

ADCORTYL* CREAM, AND OINTMENT

Presentation

Cream: White cream containing triamcinolone acetonide 0.1% in an aqueous vanishing cream base.

Other ingredients: Benzyl alcohol, cetyl alcohol, glyceryl monostearate, isopropyl palmitate, polysorbate 60, propylene glycol, water.

Ointment: White almost translucent ointment, containing triamcinolone acetonide 0.1% in Plastibase* (liquid paraffin and polyethylene resin).

Uses

Actions: Triamcinolone acetonide is a potent fluorinated corticosteroid with anti-inflammatory, antipruritic and anti-allergic actions.

Indications: Adcortyl Cream and Ointment are recommended in steroid-responsive conditions which include: atopic eczema, contact eczema, follicular eczema, infantile eczema, otitis externa without frank infection, anogenital eczema, nummular eczema, seborrhoeic or flexural eczema, neurodermatitis, psoriasis of the scalp, chronic plaque psoriasis of the palms and soles and in other selected forms of psoriasis (excluding widespread plaque psoriasis) – 'Precautions'.

Dosage and administration *Adults and children:*

Cream: To be applied to moist, weeping lesions two to four times daily.

Ointment: To be applied to dry, scaly lesions two to four times daily.

Elderly: Corticosteroids should be used sparingly and for short periods of time, as natural thinning of the skin occurs in the elderly.

Contra-indications, warnings, etc

Contra-indications: Contra-indicated in patients with a history of hypersensitivity to the product components. In tuberculous and most viral lesions of the skin, particularly herpes simplex and varicella. The products should not be used in fungal or bacterial skin infections without suitable concomitant anti-infective therapy.

Should not be used for facial rosacea, acne vulgaris, perioral dermatitis or napkin eruptions.

Precautions: Adrenal suppression can occur, with prolonged use of topical corticosteroids or treatment of extensive areas. These effects are more likely to occur in infants and children and if occlusive dressings are used. If used in childhood, or on the face, courses should be limited to 5 days and occlusion should not be used.

Topical corticosteroids may be hazardous in psoriasis for a number of reasons including rebound relapses following development of tolerance, risk of generalised pustular psoriasis and local and systemic toxicity due to impaired barrier function of the skin. Steroids may have a place in psoriasis of the scalp and chronic plaque psoriasis of the hands and feet. Careful patient supervision is important.

Children: In infants, long-term, continuous topical steroid therapy should be avoided. Courses should be limited to 5 days and occlusion should not be used.

Pregnancy: There is inadequate evidence of safety in human pregnancy. Topical administration of corticosteroids to pregnant animals can cause abnormalities of foetal development including cleft palate and intrauterine growth retardation. There may, therefore, be a very small risk of such effects in the human foetus. Caution should be exercised when topical corticosteroids are administered to nursing women.

Side-effects: Triamcinolone acetonide is well tolerated. Where adverse reactions occur they are usually reversible on cessation of therapy. However the following side-effects have been reported usually with prolonged usage:

Dermatological: impaired wound healing, thinning of the skin, petechiae and ecchymoses, facial erythema and telangiectasia, increased sweating, purpura, striae, hirsutism, acneiform eruptions, lupus erythematosus-like lesions and suppressed reactions to skin tests.

These effects may be enhanced with occlusive dressings.

The possibility of the systemic effects which are associated with all steroid therapy should be considered.

Overdosage: Topically applied corticosteroids can be absorbed in sufficient amounts to produce systemic effects (see Side-effects).

In the event of accidental ingestion, the patient should be observed and treated symptomatically.

Pharmaceutical precautions

Storage:

Cream: At room temperature; avoid freezing.

Ointment: At room temperature.

Dilution:

Cream: Cetomacrogol Cream (formula B) BPC or Aqueous Cream BP. Preservative cover may be reduced depending on the diluent. Diluted creams should be stored below 25°C and should be discarded two weeks after dilution.

Ointment: White soft paraffin.

Legal category POM.

Package quantities *Cream:* Tubes of 30 g (OP).
Ointment: Tubes of 30 g (OP).

Further information Nil.

Product licence numbers

Adcortyl Cream 0034/5000R
Adcortyl Ointment 0034/5004R

ADCORTYL* IN ORABASE*

Presentation White to light tan crystalline paste containing triamcinolone acetonide 0.1% in Orabase formulated for adhesion to mucous membrane.

Other ingredients: Gelatin, liquid paraffin, pectin, polyethylene resin, sodium carboxymethylcellulose.

Uses

Actions: Triamcinolone acetonide is a potent fluorinated corticosteroid with anti-inflammatory, antipruritic and anti-allergic actions.

Indications: Adcortyl in Orabase is indicated for aphthous ulcers, ulcerative stomatitis, denture stomatitis, desquamative gingivitis, erosive lichen planus and lesions of the oral mucosa of traumatic origin.

Dosage and administration Adults and children. To be applied to the oral lesion two to four times daily. Apply to the affected area; do not rub in.

Elderly: Corticosteroids should be used sparingly and for short periods of time.

Contra-indications, warnings, etc

Contra-indications: Contra-indicated in patients with a history of hypersensitivity to the product components. In tuberculous and most viral lesions, particularly herpes simplex and varicella. The products should not be used in fungal or bacterial infections without suitable concomitant anti-infective therapy.

Precautions: Adrenal suppression can occur with prolonged use of topical corticosteroids or with occlusion. These effects are more likely to occur in infants and children and courses of treatment in childhood should be limited to 5 days. Dentures may act in the same way as an occlusive dressing.

Pregnancy: There is inadequate evidence of safety in human pregnancy. Topical administration of corticosteroids to pregnant animals can cause abnormalities of foetal development including cleft palate and intrauterine growth retardation. There may, therefore, be a very small risk of such effects in the human foetus.

Side-effects: Triamcinolone acetonide is well tolerated. Where adverse reactions occur they are usually reversible on cessation of therapy.

The possibility of the systemic effects which are associated with all steroid therapy should be considered.

Overdosage: Topically applied corticosteroids can be absorbed in sufficient amounts to produce systemic effects (see side-effects).

In the event of accidental ingestion, the patient should be observed and treated symptomatically.

Pharmaceutical precautions

Storage: At room temperature.

Dilution: Should not be diluted.

Legal category POM.

Package quantities Tubes of 10 g (OP).

Further information Nil.

Product licence number 0034/5006R.

ADCORTYL* INTRA-ARTICULAR/ INTRADERMAL INJECTION 10 MG/ML

Qualitative and quantitative composition Adcortyl Intra-articular/Intradermal Injection contains triamcinolone acetonide 10 mg per ml of sterile suspension.

Pharmaceutical form Sterile aqueous suspension for injection.

Clinical particulars

Therapeutic indications:

Intra-articular use: for alleviating the joint pain, swelling and stiffness associated with rheumatoid arthritis and osteoarthrosis, with an inflammatory component; also for bursitis, epicondylitis, and tenosynovitis.

Intradermal use: for lichen simplex chronicus (neuro-dermatitis), granuloma annulare, lichen planus, keloids, alopecia areata and hypertrophic scars.

Posology and method of administration: Adcortyl is for intra-articular or intramuscular injection. The safety and efficacy of administration by other routes has yet to be established. Strict aseptic precautions should be observed. Since the duration of effect is variable, subsequent doses should be given when symptoms recur and not at set intervals.

Adults: The dose of Adcortyl injection for intra-articular administration, and injection into tendon sheaths and bursae, is dependent on the size of the joint to be treated and on the severity of the condition. Doses of 2.5-5 mg (0.25-0.5 ml) for smaller joints and 5-15 mg (0.5-1.5 ml) for larger joints usually alleviate the symptoms. Triamcinolone acetonide 40 mg/ml (Kenalog) is available to facilitate administration of larger doses. (See Precautions re Achilles tendon).

Intradermal dosage is usually 2-3 mg (0.2-0.3 ml), depending on the size of the lesion. No more than 5 mg (0.5 ml) should be injected at any one site. If several sites are injected the total dosage administered should not exceed 30 mg (3 ml). The injection may be repeated if necessary, at one or two week intervals.

Elderly: Treatment of elderly patients, particularly if long term, should be planned bearing in mind the more serious consequences of the common side effects of corticosteroids in old age, especially osteoporosis, diabetes, hypertension, hypokalaemia, susceptibility to infection and thinning of the skin. Close supervision is required to avoid life-threatening reactions.

Children: Adcortyl is not recommended in children under 6 years. Adcortyl intra-articular/intradermal may be used in older children in suitably adjusted dosages. Growth and development of children on prolonged corticosteroid therapy should be carefully observed.

Contra-indications: Hypersensitivity to any of the ingredients.

Systemic infections unless specific anti-infective therapy is employed.

Administration by intravenous or intrathecal injection.

Special warnings and special precautions for use:
Warnings (intra-articular Injection): Patients should be specifically warned to avoid over-use of joints in which symptomatic benefit has been obtained. Severe joint destruction with necrosis of bone may occur if repeated intra-articular injections are given over a long period of time. Care should be taken if injections are given into tendon sheaths to avoid injection into the tendon itself.

Due to the absence of a true tendon sheath, the Achilles tendon should not be injected with depot corticosteroids.

Precautions: Administration by non-approved routes (see *Posology and method of administration*).

Intra-articular injection should not be carried out in the presence of active infection in or near joints. The preparation should not be used to alleviate joint pain arising from infectious states such as gonococcal or tubercular arthritis.

Undesirable effects may be minimised using the lowest effective dose for the minimum period, and by administering the daily requirement, whenever possible, as a single morning dose on alternate days. Frequent patient review is required to titrate the dose appropriately against disease activity (see *Dosage* section).

Adrenal cortical atrophy develops during prolonged therapy and may persist for years after stopping treatment. Withdrawal of corticosteroids after prolonged therapy must, therefore, always be gradual to avoid acute adrenal insufficiency and should be tapered off over weeks or months according to the dose and duration of treatment. During prolonged therapy any intercurrent illness, trauma or surgical procedure will require a temporary increase in dosage. If corticosteroids have been stopped following prolonged therapy they may need to be reintroduced temporarily. Patients should carry steroid treatment cards which give clear guidance on the precautions to be taken to minimise risk and which provides details of prescriber, drug, dosage and the duration of treatment.

Suppression of the inflammatory response and immune function increases the susceptibility to infections and their severity. The clinical presentation may often be atypical and serious infections such as septicaemia and tuberculosis may be masked and may reach an advanced stage before being recognised.

Chickenpox is of particular concern since this normally minor illness may be fatal in immunosuppressed patients. Patients (or parents of children receiving Adcortyl tablets) without a definite history of chickenpox should be advised to avoid close personal contact with chickenpox or herpes zoster. If exposed they should seek urgent medical attention. Passive immunisation with varicella zoster immunoglobulin (VZIG) is needed by exposed non- immune patients who are receiving systemic corticosteroids or who have used them within 10 days of exposure to chickenpox. If a diagnosis of chickenpox is confirmed, the illness warrants specialist care and urgent treatment. Corticosteroids should not be stopped and the dose may need to be increased.

During corticosteroid therapy antibody response will be reduced and therefore affect the patient's response to vaccines. Live vaccines should not be administered.

Special precautions: Particular care is required when considering use of systemic corticosteroids in patients with the following conditions and frequent patient monitoring is necessary.

Recent intestinal anastomoses, diverticulitis, thrombophlebitis, existing or previous history of severe affective disorders (especially previous steroid psychosis), exanthematous disease, chronic nephritis, or renal insufficiency, metastatic carcinoma, osteoporosis (post-menopausal females are particularly at risk); in patients with an active peptic ulcer (or a history of peptic ulcer). Myasthenia gravis. Latent or healed tuberculosis; in the presence of local or systemic viral infection, systemic fungal infections or in active infections not controlled by antibiotics. In acute psychoses; in acute glomerulonephritis. Hypertension; congestive heart failure; glaucoma (or a family history of glaucoma), previous steroid myopathy or epilepsy. Liver failure.

Corticosteroid effects may be enhanced in patients with hypothyroidism or cirrhosis.

Diabetes may be aggravated, necessitating a higher insulin dosage. Latent diabetes mellitus may be precipitated.

Menstrual irregularities may occur, and this possibility should be mentioned to female patients.

Rare instances of anaphylactoid reactions have occurred in patients receiving corticosteroids, especially when a patient has a history of drug allergies.

All corticosteroids increase calcium excretion

Aspirin should be used cautiously in conjunction with corticosteroids in patients with hypoprothrombinaemia.

Interactions with other medicinal products and other forms of interaction: Barbiturates, phenytoin, rifampicin, rifabutin, carbamazepine, primidone and aminoglutethimide may enhance the metabolic clearance of corticosteroids, resulting in decreased therapeutic effects.

Corticosteroids antagonise the effects of hypoglycaemic agents (including insulin), anti-hypertensives and diuretics. The hypokalaemic effects of acetazolamide, loop diuretics, thiazide diuretics and carbenoxolone are enhanced.

The efficacy of coumarin anticoagulants may be enhanced by concurrent corticosteroid therapy and close monitoring of the INR or prothrombin time is required to avoid spontaneous bleeding.

The renal clearance of salicylates is increased by corticosteroids and steroid withdrawal may result in salicylate intoxication.

Pregnancy and lactation: The ability of corticosteroids to cross the placenta varies between individual drugs, however triamcinolone does cross the placenta.

Administration of corticosteroids to pregnant animals can cause abnormalities of foetal development, including cleft palate, intra-uterine growth retardation and effects on brain growth and development. There is no evidence that corticosteroids result in an increased incidence of congenital abnormalities, such as cleft palate/lip in man. However, when administered for prolonged periods or repeatedly during pregnancy, corticosteroids may increase the risk of intra-uterine growth retardation. Hypoadrenalism may, in theory, occur in the neonate following prenatal exposure to corticosteroids but usually resolves spontaneously following birth and is rarely clinically important. As with all drugs, corticosteroids should only be prescribed when the benefits to the mother and child outweigh the risks. When corticosteroids are essential, however, patients with normal pregnancies may be treated as though they were in the non-gravid state.

Lactation: Corticosteroids may pass into breast milk, although no data are available for triamcinolone. Infants of mothers taking high doses of systemic corticosteroids for prolonged periods may have a degree of adrenal suppression.

Effects on ability to drive and use machines: None known.

Undesirable effects: Where adverse reactions occur they are usually reversible on cessation of therapy. The incidence of predictable side-effects, including hypothalamic-pituitary-adrenal suppression correlate with the relative potency of the drug, dosage, timing of administration and duration of treatment (see *Warnings* and *Precautions*).

Absorption of triamcinolone following Adcortyl injection, especially when given by the intra-articular route, is rare. However, patients should be watched closely for the following adverse reactions which may be associated with any corticosteroid therapy:

Anti-inflammatory and immunosuppressive effects: Increased susceptibility and severity of infections with suppression of clinical symptoms and signs, opportunistic infections, recurrence of dormant tuberculosis (see *Warnings* and *Precautions*).

Fluid and electrolyte disturbances: sodium retention, fluid retention, congestive heart failure in susceptible patients, potassium loss, cardiac arrhythmias or ECG changes due to potassium deficiency, hypokalaemic alkalosis, increased calcium excretion and hypertension.

Musculoskeletal: muscle weakness, fatigue, steroid myopathy, loss of muscle mass, osteoporosis, avascular osteonecrosis, vertebral compression fractures, delayed healing of fractures, aseptic necrosis of femoral and humeral heads, pathological fractures of long bones and spontaneous fractures, tendon rupture.

Gastrointestinal: dyspepsia, peptic ulcer with possible subsequent perforation and haemorrhage, pancreatitis, abdominal distension and ulcerative oesophagitis, candidiasis.

Dermatological: impaired wound healing, thin fragile skin, petechiae and ecchymoses, facial erythema, increased sweating, purpura, striae, hirsutism, acneiform eruptions, lupus erythematous-like lesions and suppressed reactions to skin tests.

Neurological: euphoria, psychological dependence, depression, insomnia, convulsions, increased intracranial pressure with papilloedema (pseudo-tumour cerebri) usually after treatment, vertigo, headache, neuritis or paraesthesias and aggravation of pre-existing psychiatric conditions and epilepsy.

Endocrine: menstrual irregularities and amenorrhoea; development of the Cushingoid state; suppression of growth in childhood and adolescence; secondary adrenocortical and pituitary unresponsiveness, particularly in times of stress (eg. trauma, surgery or illness); decreased carbohydrate tolerance; manifestations of latent diabetes mellitus and increased requirements for insulin or oral hypoglycaemic agents in diabetes, weight gain. Negative protein and calcium balance. Increased appetite.

Ophthalmic: posterior supcapsular cataracts, increased intraocular pressure, glaucoma, exophthalmos, papilloedema, corneal or scleral thinning, exacerbation of ophthalmic viral or fungal diseases.

Others: necrotising angiitis, thrombophlebitis, thromboembolism, leucocytosis, insomnia, syncopal episodes and anaphylactoid reactions, particularly where there is a history of drug allergies.

Withdrawal symptoms and signs: On withdrawal, fever, myalgia, arthralgia, rhinitis, conjunctivitis, painful itchy skin nodules and weight loss may occur. Too rapid a reduction in dose following prolonged treatment can lead to acute adrenal insufficiency, hypotension and death (see *Warnings* and *Precautions*).

Intra-articular injection: Reactions following intra-articular administration have been rare. In a few instances, transient flushing and dizziness have occurred. Pain and other local symptoms may continue for a short time before effective relief is obtained, but an increase in joint discomfort has seldom occurred. Local fat atrophy may occur if the injection is not given into the joint space, but is temporary and disappears within a few weeks to months.

Intradermal injection: Sterile abscesses, hyper- and hypo-pigmentation and subcutaneous and cutaneous atrophy (which usually disappears unless the basic disease process is itself atrophic) have occurred.

Overdose: Not applicable.

Pharmacological properties

Pharmacodynamic properties: Triamcinolone acetonide is a synthetic glucocorticoid with marked anti-inflammatory and anti-allergic actions. Following local injection, relief of pain and swelling and greater freedom of movement are usually obtained within a few hours; such administration avoids the more severe systemic side-effects which may accompany parenteral or oral corticosteroid administration.

Pharmacokinetic properties: Triamcinolone acetonide may be absorbed into the systemic circulation from synovial spaces. However clinically significant systemic levels after intra-articular injection are unlikely to occur except perhaps following treatment of large joints with high doses. Systemic effects do not ordinarily occur with intra-articular injections when the proper techniques of administration and the recommended dosage regimens are observed.

The systemic effects of intradermally administered triamcinolone acetonide have not been extensively studied. The risk of systemic absorption, though minimal, should be taken into consideration especially when repeated intralesional administrations may be necessary.

In common with other corticosteroids, triamcinolone is metabolised largely hepatically but also by the kidney and is excreted in urine. The main metabolic route is 6-beta-hydroxylation; no significant hydrolytic cleavage of the acetonide occurs. In view of the hepatic metabolism and renal excretion of triamcinolone acetonide, functional impairments of the liver or kidney may affect the pharmacokinetics of the drug. This may become clinically significant if large or frequent doses of intradermal or intra-articular triamcinolone acetonide are given.

Preclinical safety data: See *Pregnancy and lactation.*

Pharmaceutical particulars

List of excipients: Benzyl alcohol. polysorbate 80, sodium carboxymethylcellulose, sodium chloride, water.

Incompatibilities: The injection should not be physically mixed with other medicinal products.

Shelf life: 36 months.

Special precautions for storage: In an upright position below 25°C: avoid freezing.

Nature and contents of container: Carton containing glass ampoules 5 x 1 ml or individually cartoned multidose vials of 5 ml.

Instructions for use/handling: No special handling instructions.

Marketing authorisation number 0034/5002R

Date of approval/revision of SPC August 1998

Legal category POM

ADCORTYL* WITH GRANEODIN* CREAM

Quantitative and qualitative composition Containing in each gram the following: triamcinolone acetonide 0.1%, neomycin (as sulphate) 0.25%, gramicidin 0.025%.

Pharmaceutical form Topical Cream.

Clinical particulars

Therapeutic indications: The topical treatment of exudative and/or secondarily infected eczema and dermatitis, including: atopic eczema, contact eczema, follicular eczema, otitis externa, nummular eczema, seborrhoeic eczema, intertrigo, neurodermatitis and infected insect bites.

Posology and method of administration:

Adults and children: Apply to the affected area two to four times daily.

Elderly: Corticosteroids should be used sparingly and for short periods of time, as natural thinning of the skin occurs in the elderly.

If, after about 7 days application, little or no improvement has occurred, cultural isolation of the offending organism should be followed by appropriate local or systemic antimicrobial therapy systemic antimicrobial therapy.

Contra-indications: In tuberculous and most viral lesions of the skin, particularly herpes simplex and varicella. Also in fungal lesions not susceptible to nystatin.

In patients with hypersensitivity to any of the components.

Should not be used for facial rosacea, acne vulgaris or perioral dermatitis.

Should not be applied to the external auditory canal in patients with perforated eardrums.

The products should not be used for extensive areas because of possible risk of systemic absorption and neomycin-induced ototoxicity.

Special warnings and special precautions for use: Adrenal suppression can occur, even without occlusion. The use of occlusive dressings should be avoided because of the increased risk of sensitivity reactions and increased percutaneous absorption. The possibility of sensitivity to neomycin should be taken into consideration.

Steroid-antibiotic combinations should not be continued for more than 7 days in the absence of any clinical improvement, since in this situation occult extension of infection may occur due to the masking effect of the steroid.

Extended or recurrent application may increase the risk of contact sensitisation and should be avoided.

If used on the face, courses should be limited to 5 days and occlusion should not be used.

Children: In infants, long-term continuous topical steroid therapy should be avoided. Courses should be limited to 5 days and occlusion should not be used.

Interactions with other medicinal products and other forms of interaction: Not applicable

Pregnancy and lactation: There is inadequate evidence of safety in human pregnancy. Topical administration of corticosteroids to pregnant animals can cause abnormalities of foetal development including cleft palate and intra-uterine growth retardation. There may, therefore, be a very small risk of such effects in the human foetus. There are theoretical risks of neomycin-induced foetal ototoxicity; therefore the product should be used with caution only when the benefit outweighs the potential risk.

Effects on ability to drive and use machines: Not applicable.

Undesirable effects:

Triamcinolone acetonide: The following side effects have been reported. Usually with prolonged usage: dermatologic–impaired wound healing, thinning of the skin, petechiae and ecchymoses, facial erythema and telangiectasia, increased sweating, purpura, striae, hirsutism, acneiform eruptions, lupus erythematosus-like lesions and suppressed reactions to skin tests. These effects may be enhanced with occlusive dressings.

The possibility of the systemic effects which are associated with all steroid therapy should be considered.

Neomycin: Sensitivity reactions may occur especially with prolonged use. Ototoxicity and nephrotoxicity have been reported. The product should be used with caution and in small amounts in the treatment of skin infections following extensive burns, open lesions and other conditions where absorption of neomycin is possible particularly children and elderly. The product should also be used with care in patients with established hearing loss and those with renal impairment.

Gramicidin: Sensitivity has occasionally been reported.

Overdose: Topically applied corticosteroids can be absorbed in sufficient amounts to produce systemic effects (see *Side effects*).

In the event of accidental ingestion, the patient should be observed and treated symptomatically.

Pharmacological properties

Pharmacodynamic properties: Triamcinolone acetonide is a potent fluorinated corticosteroid with rapid anti-inflammatory, antipruritic and anti-allergic actions.

The combined action of the antibiotics neomycin and gramicidin provides comprehensive antibacterial therapy against a wide range of gram-positive and gram-negative bacteria, including those micro-organisms responsible for most bacterial skin infections.

Pharmacokinetic properties: Not applicable.

Preclinical safety data: No further relevant data

Pharmaceutical particulars

List of excipients: Benzyl alcohol, cetyl alcohol, ethanol, glyceryl monostearate, isopropyl palmitate, polysorbate 60, propylene glycol, water.

Incompatibilities: None known.

Shelf life: 24 months.

Special precautions for storage: Store below 25°C. Avoid freezing.

Nature and contents of container: Aluminium tubes.

Instructions for use/handling: None.

Marketing authorisation number 0034/5015R

Date of approval/revision of SPC 29th August 1996

Legal category POM

AZACTAM* FOR INJECTION

Qualitative and quantitative composition Azactam for Injection vials contain 500 mg, 1 g or 2 g aztreonam.

Pharmaceutical form Sterile powder for reconstitution.

Clinical particulars

Therapeutic indications: The treatment of the following infections caused by susceptible aerobic Gram-negative micro-organisms:

Urinary tract infections: including pyelonephritis and cystitis (initial and recurrent) and asymptomatic bacteriuria, including those due to pathogens resistant to the aminoglycosides, cephalosporins or penicillins.

Gonorrhoea: acute uncomplicated urogenital or anorectal infections due to beta-lactamase producing or non-producing strains of *N. gonorrhoeae.*

Lower respiratory tract infections: including pneumonia, bronchitis and lung infections in patients with cystic fibrosis.

Bacteraemia/septicaemia.

Meningitis caused by *Haemophilus influenza* or *Neisseria meningitidis.* Since Azactam provides only Gram negative cover, it should not be given alone as initial blind therapy, but may be used with an antibiotic active against gram positive organisms until the results of sensitivity tests are known.

Bone and joint infections.

Skin and soft tissue infections: including those associated with postoperative wounds, ulcers and burns.

Intra-abdominal infections: peritonitis.

Gynaecological infections: pelvic inflammatory disease, endometritis and pelvic cellulitis.

Azactam is indicated for adjunctive therapy to surgery in the management of infections caused by susceptible organisms, including abscesses, infections complicating hollow viscus perforations, cutaneous infections and infections of serous surfaces.

Bacteriological studies to determine the causative organism(s) and their sensitivity to aztreonam should be performed. Therapy may be instituted prior to receiving the results of sensitivity tests.

In patients at risk of infections due to non-susceptible pathogens, additional antibiotic therapy should be initiated concurrently with Azactam to provide broad-spectrum coverage before identification and susceptibility testing results of the causative organism(s) are known. Based on these results, appropriate antibiotic therapy should be continued.

Patients with serious *Pseudomonas* infections may benefit from concurrent use of Azactam and an aminoglycoside because of their synergistic action. If such concurrent therapy is considered in these patients, susceptibility tests should be performed *in vitro* to determine the activity in combination. The usual monitoring of serum levels and renal function during aminoglycoside therapy applies.

Posology and method of administration: Intramuscular or intravenous injection, or intravenous infusion.

Adults: The dose range of Azactam is 1 to 8 g daily in equally divided doses. The usual dose is 3 to 4 g daily. The maximum recommended dose is 8 g daily. The dosage and route of administration should be determined by the susceptibility of the causative organisms, severity of infection and the condition of the patient.

Dosage Guide: Adults (see table below)

Type of infection[1]	*Dosage (g)*	*Frequency (hr)*	*Route*
Urinary tract	0.5–1	8–12	IM or IV
Gonorrhoea/cystitis	1	single dose	IM
Cystic Fibrosis	2	6–8	IV
Severe or life-threatening infections	2	6–8	IV
Other infections either	1	8	IM or IV
or	2	12	IV

[1] Because of the serious nature of infections due to *Pseudomonas aeruginosa*, a dose of 2 g every 6 or 8 hours is recommended, at least for initial therapy in systemic infections caused by this organism.

The intravenous route is recommended for patients requiring single doses greater than 1 g, or those with bacterial septicaemia, localised parenchymal abscess (e.g. intra-abdominal abscess), peritonitis, meningitis or other severe systemic or life-threatening infections.

Elderly: In the elderly, renal status is the major determinant of dosage. Estimated creatinine clearance should be used to determine appropriate dosage, since serum creatinine is not an accurate measurement of renal function in these patients.

Elderly patients normally have a creatinine clearance in excess of 30 ml/min and therefore would receive the normal recommended dose. If renal function is below this level, the dosage schedule should be adjusted (see Renal Impairment).

Renal impairment: In patients with impaired renal function, the normal recommended initial dose should be given. This should be followed by maintenance doses as shown in the following table:

Estimated creatinine clearance (ml/min)	*Maintenance dose*
10–30	Half the initial dose
Less than 10	One quarter of the initial dose

The normal dose interval should not be altered.

In patients on haemodialysis, a supplementary one eighth of the initial dose should be given after each dialysis.

Children: The usual dosage for patients older than one week is 30 mg/kg/dose every 6 or 8 hours. For severe infections in patients 2 years of age or older, 50 mg/kg/dose every 6 or 8 hours is recommended. The total daily dose should not exceed 8 g. Dosage information is not yet available for new-borns less than 1 week old.

Reconstitution: Azactam for Injection is supplied in 15 ml vials.

Upon the addition of the diluent the contents should be shaken immediately and vigorously. Vials of reconstituted Azactam are not intended for multi-dose use, and any unused solution from a single dose must be discarded. Depending on the type and amount of diluent, the pH ranges from 4.5 to 7.5, and the colour may vary from colourless to light straw-yellow, which may develop a slight pink tint on standing; however this does not affect the potency.

For intramuscular injection: For each gram of aztreonam add at least 3 ml Water for Injections Ph. Eur. or 0.9% Sodium Chloride Injection B.P. and shake well.

Single-dose vial size	*Volume of diluent to be added*
0.5 g	1.5 ml
1.0 g	3.0 ml

Azactam is given by deep injection into a large muscle mass, such as the upper quadrant of the gluteus maximus or the lateral part of the thigh.

For intravenous injection: To the contents of the vial add 6 to 10 ml of Water for Injections Ph. Eur. and shake well. Slowly inject directly into the vein over a period of 3 to 5 minutes.

For intravenous infusion:
Vials: For each gram of aztreonam add at least 3 ml of Water for Injections Ph. Eur. and shake well.

Dilute this initial solution with an appropriate infusion solution to a final concentration less than 2% w/v (at least 50 ml solution per gram of aztreonam). The infusion should be administered over 20-60 minutes.

Appropriate infusion solutions include:
0.9% Sodium Chloride Injection B.P.
5% Glucose Intravenous Infusion B.P.
5% or 10% Mannitol Intravenous Infusion B.P.
Sodium Lactate Intravenous Infusion B.P.
0.9%, 0.45% or 0.2% Sodium Chloride and 5% Glucose Intravenous Infusion B.P.
Compound Sodium Chloride Injection B.P.C. 1959 (Ringer's Solution for Injection)
Compound Sodium Lactate Intravenous Infusion B.P.
(Hartmann's Solution for Injection).

A volume control administration set may be used to deliver the initial solution of Azactam into a compatible infusion solution being administered. With use of a Y-tube administration set, careful attention should be given to the calculated volume of Azactam solution required so that the entire dose will be infused.

Reconstitution: Intravenous infusion solutions of Azactam for Injection prepared with 0.9% Sodium Chloride Injection B.P. or 5% Glucose Intravenous B.P., in PVC or glass containers, to which clindamycin phosphate, gentamicin sulphate, tobramycin sulphate, or cephazolin sodium have been added at concentrations usually used clinically, are stable for up to 24 hours in a refrigerator (2–8°C). Ampicillin sodium admixtures with aztreonam in 0.9% Sodium Chloride Injection B.P. are stable for 24 hours in a refrigerator (2–8°C); stability in 5% Glucose Intravenous Infusion B.P. is eight hours under refrigeration.

If aztreonam and metronidazole are to be used together, they should be administered separately as a cherry red colour has been observed after storage of solutions containing combinations of the two products.

Contra-indications: Patients with a known hypersensitivity to aztreonam and L-arginine.

Aztreonam is contraindicated in pregnancy. Aztreonam crosses the placenta and enters the foetal circulation.

Special warnings and special precautions for use: Specific studies have not shown significant cross-reactivity between Azactam and antibodies to penicillins or cephalosporins. The incidence of hypersensitivity to Azactam in clinical trials has been low but caution should be exercised in patients with a history of hypersensitivity to beta-lactam antibiotics until further experience is gained.

Experience in patients with impaired hepatic function is limited. Appropriate liver function monitoring in these patients is recommended.

Concurrent therapy with other antimicrobial agents and Azactam is recommended as initial therapy in patients who are at risk of having an infection due to pathogens that are not susceptible to aztreonam.

As with other antibiotics, in the treatment of acute pulmonary exacerbations in patients with cystic fibrosis, while clinical improvement is usually noted, lasting bacterial eradications may not be achieved.

Therapy with Azactam may result in overgrowth of nonsusceptible organisms which may require additional antimicrobial therapy. In comparative studies, the number of patients treated for superinfections was similar to that of the control drugs used.

It is recommended that prothrombin times should be monitored if the patient is on concomitant anticoagulant therapy.

Interactions with other medicinal products and other forms of interaction: Single-dose pharmacokinetic studies have not shown any significant interaction between aztreonam and gentamicin, cephradine, clindamycin or metronidazole.

Unlike broad spectrum antibiotics, aztreonam produces no effects on the normal anaerobic intestinal flora. No disulfuram-like reactions with alcohol ingestion have been reported.

Pregnancy and lactation: Aztreonam is contraindicated in pregnancy. Aztreonam crosses the placenta and enters the foetal circulation.

Aztreonam is excreted in breast milk in concentrations that are less than 1% of those in simultaneously obtained maternal serum. Lactating mothers should refrain from breast feeding during the course of therapy.

Effects on ability to drive and use machines: None known

Undesirable effects: The following side effects have been reported with Azactam therapy:

Dermatological: rash, pruritus, urticaria, erythema, petechia, exfoliative dermatitis, flushing; very rarely toxic epidermal necrolysis.

Haematological: eosinophilia, increases in prothrombin and partial thromboplastin time have occurred. There have been isolated reports of thrombocytopenia, neutropenia, anaemia, bleeding and pancytopenia.

Hepatobiliary: Jaundice and hepatitis: transient elevations of hepatic transaminases and alkaline phosphatase (without overt signs or symptoms of hepatobiliary dysfunction).

Gastrointestinal: Diarrhoea, very rarely pseudomembranous colitis, nausea and/or vomiting, abdominal cramps, mouth ulcer and altered taste.

Local reactions: phlebitis and discomfort at the i.v. injection site: discomfort at the i.m. injection site.

Rare instances of the following events have been reported: vaginitis, candidosis, anaphylaxis, angiooedema, hypotension, weakness, confusion, dizziness, vertigo, sweating, headache, breast tenderness, halitosis, muscle aches, fever, malaise, sneezing and nasal congestion; transient increases in serum creatinine.

Overdose: There have been no reported cases of overdosage.

Pharmacological properties
Pharmacodynamic properties: Aztreonam is a monocyclic beta-lactam antibiotic with potent bactericidal activity against a wide spectrum of gram-negative aerobic pathogens.

Unlike the majority of beta-lactam antibiotics, it is not an inducer *in vitro* of beta-lactamase activity. Aztreonam is usually active *in vitro* against those resistant aerobic organisms whose beta-lactamases hydrolyse other antibiotics.

Pharmacokinetic properties: Single 30-minute i.v. infusions of 0.5 g, 1.0 g and 2.0 g in healthy volunteers produced peak serum levels of 54, 90 and 204 mg/l, and single 3-minute i.v. injections of the same doses produced peak levels of 58, 125 and 242 mg/l. Peak levels of aztreonam are achieved at about one hour after i.m. administration. After identical single i.m. or i.v. doses, the serum concentrations are comparable at 1 hour (1.5 hours from the start of i.v. infusion), with similar slopes of serum concentrations thereafter.

The serum half-life of aztreonam averaged 1.7 hours in subjects with normal renal function, independent of the dose and route. In healthy subjects 60-70% of a single i.m. or i.v. dose was recovered in the urine by 8 hours, and urinary excretion was essentially complete by 12 hours.

Preclinical safety data: Aztreonam was well tolerated in a comprehensive series of preclinical toxicity and safety studies.

Pharmaceutical particulars
List of excipients: L-arginine (780 mg per g of aztreonam).

Incompatibilities: Azactam should not be physically mixed with any other drug, antibiotic or diluent, except those listed in the Posology and Method of Administration section under Reconstitution for Intravenous infusion.

With intermittent infusion of Azactam and another drug via a common delivery tube, the tube should be flushed before and after delivery of Azactam with any appropriate infusion solution compatible with both drug solutions. The drugs should not be delivered simultaneously.

Shelf life:
(a) Product unopened: 36 months
(b) Reconstituted product: 24 hours (2–8°C)

Special precautions for storage:
(a) Storage before reconstitution: Store at room temperature (15–25°C).
(b) Stability after reconstitution: Store at 2–8°C for not more than 24 hours.

Nature and contents of container:
500 mg glass vial pack of 5 x 15 ml
1 g glass vial pack of 5 x 15 ml
2 g glass vial pack of 5 x 15 ml

Instructions for use/handling: Any content of product remaining after use should be discarded.

Marketing authorisation numbers
Azactam for Injection 500 mg vial: PL 0034/0250
Azactam for Injection 1 g vial: PL 0034/0251
Azactam for Injection 2 g vial: PL 0034/0252

Date of first authorisation/renewal of authorisation
15th October 1986 / 22nd November 1991 / 13th August 1998

Date of (partial) revision of the text
12th December 1996

CAPOTEN* TABLETS 12.5 mg, 25 mg and 50 mg

Qualitative and quantitative composition Capoten tablets 12.5 mg: Slightly mottled, white, flat-faced, bevel-edged, capsule-shaped tablets, each containing captopril 12.5 mg. Engraved with 'Squibb' and '450' on one side with a bisecting bar on the other.

Capoten tablets 25 mg: Slightly mottled, white, square, biconvex tablets each containing captopril 25 mg. Engraved with 'Squibb' and '452' on one side and with quadrisect bars on the other.

Capoten tablets 50 mg: Slightly mottled, white, oval, biconvex tablets each containing captopril 50 mg. Engraved with 'Squibb' and '482' on one side with a bisecting bar on the other.

Pharmaceutical form Oral tablet.

Clinical particulars
Therapeutic indications:
Hypertension: Capoten is indicated for the first line treatment of mild to moderate hypertension.

In severe hypertension it should be used where standard therapy is ineffective or inappropriate.

Congestive heart failure: Capoten is indicated for the treatment of congestive heart failure. The drug should be used together with diuretics and, where appropriate digitalis.

Myocardial infarction: Capoten is indicated following myocardial infarction in clinically stable patients with asymptomatic and symptomatic left ventricular dysfunction to improve survival, delay the onset of symptomatic heart failure, reduce hospitalisations for heart failure, and reduce recurrent myocardial infarction and coronary revascularisation procedures.

Determination of cardiac function by radionuclide ventriculography or echocardiography should be undertaken prior to initiation of preventative treatment with Capoten in post myocardial infarction patients.

Diabetic nephropathy: Capoten is indicated for the treatment of diabetic nephropathy (microalbuminuria greater than 30 mg/day) in insulin-dependent diabetics. In these patients, captopril prevents the progression of renal disease and reduces associated clinical events e.g. dialysis, renal transplantation and death.

Posology and method of administration:
Adults:
Hypertension: Treatment with Capoten should be at the lowest effective dose which should be titrated according to the needs of the patient.

Mild to moderate hypertension: The starting dose is 12.5 mg twice daily. The usual maintenance dose is 25 mg twice daily which can be increased incrementally, at 2–4 week intervals, until a satisfactory response is achieved, to a maximum of 50 mg twice daily.

A thiazide diuretic may be added to Capoten if satisfactory response has not been achieved. The dose of diuretic may be increased at 1-2 week intervals to the level of optimum response or until the maximum dose is reached.

Severe hypertension: In severe hypertension where standard therapy is ineffective or inappropriate because of adverse effects, the starting dose is 12.5 mg b.d. The dosage may be increased incrementally to a maximum of 50 mg t.i.d. Capoten should be used together with other anti-hypertensive agents but the dose of these should be individually titrated. A daily dose of 150 mg of Capoten should not normally be exceeded.

Heart failure: Capoten therapy must be started under close medical supervision. Capoten should be introduced when diuretic therapy (such as frusemide 40-80 mg or equivalent) is insufficient to control symptoms. A starting dose of 6.25 mg or 12.5 mg may minimise a transient hypotensive effect. The possibility of this occurring can be reduced by discontinuing or reducing diuretic therapy if possible, prior to initiating Capoten. The usual maintenance dose is 25 mg two or three times a day which can be increased incrementally, with intervals of at least two weeks, until a satisfactory response is achieved. The usual maximum dose is 150 mg daily.

Myocardial infarction: Therapy may be initiated as early as three days following a myocardial infarction. After an initial dose of 6.25 mg, captopril therapy should be titrated to a final target dose of 150 mg daily in divided doses over the next several weeks.

Achievement of the target dose of 150 mg should be based on the patient's tolerance to captopril during titration. If symptomatic hypotension occurs, a dosage reduction may be required.

Captopril may be used in patients treated with other post-myocardial infarction therapies, e.g. thrombolytics, aspirin, beta blockers.

Diabetic nephropathy: The recommended daily dose of captopril is 75 to 100 mg in divided doses.

If further blood pressure reduction is required, other antihypertensive agents such as diuretics, beta blockers, centrally acting agents or vasodilators may be used in conjunction with captopril.

Elderly: The dose should be titrated against the blood pressure response and kept as low as possible to achieve adequate control. Since elderly patients may have reduced renal function and other organ dysfunctions, it is suggested that a low dose of Capoten be used initially.

Children: Capoten is not recommended for the treatment of mild to moderate hypertension in children.

Experience in neonates, particularly premature infants, is limited. Because renal function in infants is not equivalent to that of older children and adults, lower doses of Capoten should be used with the patients under close medical supervision.

The starting dose should be 0.3 mg per Kg bodyweight up to a maximum of 6 mg per Kg bodyweight daily in divided doses. The dose should be individualised according to the response and may be given two or three times daily.

Patients with renal impairment: Captopril in divided doses of 75 to 100 mg/day was well tolerated in patients with diabetic nephropathy and mild to moderate renal impairment (creatinine clearance at least 30 ml/min/1.73 m²).

Patients with severely impaired renal function will take longer to reach steady-state captopril levels and will reach higher steady-state levels for a given daily dose than patients with normal renal function. These patients may therefore respond to smaller or less frequent doses.

Therefore, patients with severe renal impairment (creatinine clearance less than 30 ml/min/1.73 m²), the initial daily dose should be 12.5 mg b.d. The dose can then be titrated against the response but adequate time should be allowed between dosage adjustments. When concomitant diuretic therapy is required, a loop diuretic rather than a thiazide diuretic should be the diuretic of choice.

Capoten is readily eliminated by haemodialysis.

Contra-indications: A history of previous hypersensitivity to the product.

Pregnancy: Capoten has been shown to be lethal to rabbit and sheep foetuses. There were no foetotoxic effects to hamster or rat foetuses.

Capoten is contra-indicated in pregnancy and should not be used in women of child bearing potential unless protected by effective contraception.

Exposure of the mother in the second and third trimesters of pregnancy has been associated with oligohydramnios and neonatal hypertension and/or anuria.

Special warnings and special precautions for use:
Precautions: Evaluation of the patient should include assessment of renal function prior to initiation of therapy and at appropriate intervals thereafter (see *Recommended Dosage and Dosage Schedule*).

Capoten should not be used in patients with aortic stenosis or outflow tract obstruction.

As limited experience has been obtained in the treatment of acute hypertensive crisis, the use of Capoten should be avoided in these patients.

Warnings: The incidence of adverse reactions to captopril is principally associated with renal function since the drug is excreted primarily by the kidney. The dose should not exceed that necessary for adequate control and should be reduced in patients with impaired renal function.

Haematological: Neutropenia/agranulocytosis, thrombocytopenia and anaemia have been reported in patients receiving Capoten

In patients with normal renal function and no other complicating factors, neutropenia occurs rarely.

Capoten should be used with extreme caution in patients with collagen vascular disease, immunosuppressant therapy, treatment with allopurinol or procainamide, or a combination of these complicating factors especially if there is pre-existing impaired renal function. Some of these patients developed serious infections which in a few instances did not respond to intensive antibiotic therapy.

If Capoten is used in such patients, it is advised that white blood cell count and differential counts should be performed prior to therapy, every 2 weeks during the first 3 months of Capoten therapy, and periodically thereafter.

During treatment all patients should be instructed to report any sign of infection (e.g. sore throat, fever), when a differential white blood cell count should be performed. Capoten and other concomitant medication should be withdrawn if neutropenia (neutrophils less than 1000/mm³) is detected or suspected.

In most patients neutrophil counts rapidly returned to normal upon discontinuing Capoten.

Renal: Proteinuria in patients with prior normal renal function is rare.

Where proteinuria has occurred it has usually been in patients with severe hypertension or evidence of prior renal disease. Nephrotic syndrome occurred in some of these patients.

In patients with evidence of prior renal disease, monthly urinary protein estimations (dip stick) are recommended for the first 9 months of therapy. If repeated determinations show increasing amounts of urinary protein, a 24-hour quantitative determination should be obtained, and if this exceeds 1 g/day, the benefits and risks of continuing Capoten should be evaluated.

In patients with diabetic nephropathy and proteinuria, who received captopril 75 mg/day for a median of 3 years, there was a consistent reduction in proteinuria. It is unknown whether long-term therapy in patients with other types of renal disease would have similar effects.

Although membranous glomerulopathy was found in biopsies taken from some proteinuric patients, a causal relationship to Capoten has not been established.

Some patients with renal disease, particularly those with bilateral renal artery stenosis or unilateral renal artery stenosis in a single functioning kidney, have developed increased concentrations of blood urea and serum creatinine. Capoten dosage reduction and/or discontinuation of diuretic may be required. For some of these patients it may not be possible to normalise blood pressure and maintain adequate renal perfusion.

Recent clinical observations have shown a high incidence of anaphylactoid-like reactions during haemodialysis with high-flux dialysis membranes (e.g. AN69) in patients receiving ACE inhibitors. Therefore, this combination should be avoided.

Hypotension: With the first one or two doses some patients may experience symptomatic hypotension. In most instances, symptoms are relieved simply by the patient lying down.

In patients with severe and renin dependent hypertension (e.g. renovascular hypertension) or severe congestive heart failure who are receiving large doses of diuretic, exaggerated hypotensive responses have occurred usually within one hour of the initial dose of Capoten. In these patients, by discontinuing diuretic therapy or significantly reducing the diuretic dose for four to seven days prior to initiating Capoten the possibility of this occurrence is reduced. By commencing Capoten therapy with small doses (6.25 mg or 12.5 mg) the duration of any hypotensive effect is lessened. Some patients may benefit from an infusion of saline. The occurrence of first dose hypotension does not preclude subsequent dose titration with Capoten. Hypotension has been occasionally reported in patients on Capoten due to causes of acute volume depletion such as vomiting and diarrhoea.

Serum potassium: Since Capoten decreases aldosterone production, serum potassium is usually maintained in patients on diuretics. Potassium sparing diuretics or potassium supplements should not therefore be used routinely. In patients with marked renal impairment a significant elevation of serum potassium may occur.

Surgery/anaesthesia: In patients undergoing major surgery, or during anaesthesia with agents which produce hypotension, captopril will block angiotensin II formation secondary to compensatory renin release. This may lead to hypotension which can be corrected by volume expansion.

Clinical chemistry: Capoten may cause a false-positive urine test for acetone.

Interaction with other medicinal products and other forms of interaction:
Diuretics: Diuretics potentiate the anti-hypertensive effectiveness of Capoten.Potassium-sparing diuretics (triamterene, amiloride and spironolactone), or potassium supplements may cause significant increase in serum potassium.

Indomethacin: A reduction of anti-hypertensive effectiveness may occur. This is probably also the case with other non-steroidal anti-inflammatory drugs.

Vasodilators: Capoten has been reported to act synergistically with peripheral vasodilators such as minoxidil. Awareness of this interaction may avert an initial hypotensive response.

Clonidine: It has been suggested that the anti-hypertensive effect of Capoten can be delayed when patients treated with clonidine are changed to Capoten.

Allopurinol and procainamide: There have been reports of neutropenia and/or Stevens-Johnson syndrome in patients on Capoten plus either allopurinol or procainamide. Although a causal relationship has not been established, these combinations should only be used with caution, especially in patients with impaired renal function.

Immunosuppressants: Azathioprine and cyclophosphamide have been associated with blood dyscrasias in patients with renal failure who were also taking Capoten.

Probenecid: The renal clearance of Capoten is reduced in the presence of probenecid.

Lithium: Concomitant use of lithium and ACE-inhibitors may result in an increase of serum lithium concentration.

Hypoglycaemic agents: ACE Inhibitors have been show to enhance insulin sensitivity. There have been rare reports of hypoglycaemic episodes in diabetic patients treated concomitantly with ACE Inhibitors and antidiabetic medicines (insulin or oral hypoglycaemic agents). This phenomenon may be more likely to occur during the first few weeks of treatment. In such cases a reduction in the dose of the antidiabetic medicine may be required.

Pregnancy and lactation:
Pregnancy: See *Contra-indications.*

Nursing mothers: Because captopril is excreted in breast milk, Capoten should not be used in nursing mothers.

Effects on ability to drive and use machines: See warnings under hypotension section.

Undesirable effects:
Idiosyncratic: Angioedema involving the extremities, face, lips, mucous membranes, tongue, glottis or larynx has been seen in patients treated with ACE inhibitors, including captopril. In this situation, the ACE inhibitor should be discontinued. Where swelling is confined to the face, lips and mouth the condition will usually resolve without further treatment, although antihistamines may be useful in relieving symptoms. These patients should be followed carefully until the swelling has resolved. However, where there is involvement of the tongue, glottis or larynx, likely to cause airway obstruction, subcutaneous adrenaline (0.5 ml, 1:1,000) should be administered promptly where indicated.

Haematological: Neutropenia, anaemia and thrombocytopenia (see *Special warnings and special precautions for use*). Rarely a positive ANA has been reported.

Renal: Proteinuria, elevated blood urea and creatinine, elevated serum potassium and acidosis (see *Special warnings and special precautions for use*).

Cardiovascular: Hypotension (see *Special warnings and special precautions for use*), tachycardia.

Skin: Rashes, usually pruritic, may occur. They are usually mild, maculopapular, rarely urticarial and disappear within a few days of dosage reduction, short-term treatment with an antihistamine and/or discontinuing therapy. In a few cases the rash has been associated with fever. Pruritus, flushing, vesicular or bullous rash, and photosensitivity have been reported.

Gastrointestinal: Reversible and usually self-limiting taste impairment has been reported. Weight loss may be associated with the loss of taste. Stomatitis, resembling aphthous ulcers, has been reported. Elevation of liver enzymes has been noted in a few patients. Rare cases of hepatocellular injury and cholestatic jaundice have been reported. Gastric irritation and abdominal pain may occur. Pancreatitis has been reported rarely in patients treated with ACE Inhibitors; in some cases this has proved fatal.

Other: Paraesthesias of the hands, serum sickness, cough, bronchospasm and lymphadenopathy have been reported.

Overdose: In the event of overdosage, blood pressure should be monitored and if hypotension develops volume expansion is the treatment of choice. Captopril is removed by dialysis.

Pharmacological properties
Pharmacodynamic properties: Captopril is a highly specific, competitive inhibitor of angiotensin-I converting enzyme. This enzyme is responsible for the conversion of angiotensin-I to angiotensin-II.

Pharmacokinetic properties:

Total captopril:	t_{MAX}	1 hour
	$t_{\frac{1}{2}}$	8 hours
Free captopril	t_{MAX}	1 hour
	$t_{\frac{1}{2}}$	1 hour

The absolute bioavailability of an oral dose is approximately 65%.

Preclinical safety data: No further relevant data

Pharmaceutical particulars

List of excipients: Lactose, corn starch, microcrystalline cellulose, stearic acid.

Incompatibilites: None.

Shelf life: 48 Months.

Special precautions for storage: Store below 30°C. Protect from moisture

Nature and contents of container: The tablets are packaged in any of the following: amber glass bottles (packs of 100), HDPE bottles (packs of 100), foil strips, PVC/PVDC blisters or PVC/aluminium blisters in packs of 90, 60 or 56's.

Instructions for use/handling: No special instructions.

Marketing authorisation numbers

12.5 mg: 0034/0221
25 mg: 0034/0193
50 mg: 0034/0194

Date of approval/revision of SPC 5 November 1996

Legal category POM

CAPOZIDE* TABLETS

Presentation

Capozide 50 mg/25 mg: White, biconvex, round tablets with possible slight mottling, each containing captopril 50 mg and hydrochlorothiazide 25 mg. Engraved with 'Squibb' and 390 on one side with a bisect bar on the other.

Other ingredients: lactose, magnesium stearate, maize starch, microcrystalline cellulose, stearic acid.

Uses

Actions: Captopril, designated chemically as l-[(2S)-3-mercapto-2-methyl-propionyl]-L-proline, is a specific competitive inhibitor of angiotensin I-converting enzyme, and hydrochlorothiazide is a diuretic-antihypertensive agent.

Captopril and hydrochlorothiazide lower blood pressure by different, though complementary, mechanisms. With diuretic treatment, blood pressure and blood volume fall resulting in a rise in angiotensin II levels which tend to blunt the hypotensive effect. Captopril blocks this rise in angiotensin II. The anti-hypertensive effects of captopril and hydrochlorothiazide are additive.

Indications: For the treatment of mild to moderate hypertension in patients who have been stabilised on the individual components given in the same proportions.

Dosage and administration

Adults: The usual dose of Capozide is one tablet daily. A daily dose of two tablets should not be exceeded.

Elderly: The dose should be kept as low as possible to achieve adequate blood pressure control. In some patients half a tablet daily may be sufficient.

Children: Safety and effectiveness of Capozide has not been established.

Patients with renal failure: Capozide is not recommended for use in patients with significant renal impairment.

Contra-indications, warnings, etc

Contra-indications: Capozide is contra-indicated in patients with anuria or hyper-sensitivity to captopril, thiazides, or any sulphonamide-derived drug.

Pregnancy: Captopril has been shown to be lethal to rabbit and sheep foetuses. There were no foetotoxic effects to hamster or rat foetuses.

Capozide is contra-indicated in pregnancy and should not be used in women of childbearing potential unless protected by effective contraception.

Exposure of the mother in the second and third trimesters of pregnancy has been associated with oligohydramnios and neonatal hypotension and/or anuria.

Precautions: Capozide should not be used in patients with aortic stenosis or outflow tract obstruction.

Warnings

Haematological: Neutropenia/agranulocytosis, thrombocytopenia and anaemia have been reported in patients receiving captopril.

In patients with normal renal function and no other complicating factors, neutropenia occurs rarely.

Captopril should not be used routinely in patients with pre-existing impaired renal function, collagen vascular disease, immunosuppressant therapy, treatment with allopurinol or procainamide, or a combination of these complicating factors. Some of these patients developed serious infections which in a few instances did not respond to intensive antibiotic therapy.

During treatment, all patients should be instructed to report any sign of infection (e.g. persistent sore throat, fever), when a differential white blood cell count should be performed. Capozide and other concomitant medication should be withdrawn if neutropenia (neutrophils less than 1000/mm³) is detected or suspected.

In most patients neutrophil counts rapidly returned to normal upon discontinuing captopril.

Renal: Proteinuria is a rare complication of captopril therapy.

Some patients with renal disease, particularly those with bilateral renal artery stenoses or unilateral renal artery stenoses in a single functioning kidney, have developed increased concentrations of blood urea and serum creatinine. Discontinuation of Capozide may be required.

Recent clinical observations have shown a high incidence of anaphylactoid-like reactions during haemodialysis with high-flux dialysis membranes (e.g. AN69) in patients receiving ACE inhibitors (See *Contra-indications*).

Hepatic: Capozide should be used with caution in patients with impaired hepatic function or progressive liver disease because of the known risks associated with alterations in fluid and electrolyte balance resulting from thiazide treatment in such patients.

Electrolyte imbalance: Patients receiving Capozide, should be observed for clinical signs of thiazide-induced fluid or electrolyte imbalance. In such patients periodic determinations of serum electrolytes should be performed. Because captopril reduces the production of aldosterone, its combination with hydrochlorothiazide may minimise diuretic-induced hypokalaemia. However, some patients may still require potassium supplements. Potassium-sparing diuretics should not be used in conjunction with Capozide.

Nursing mothers: Capozide should not be used in nursing mothers.

Surgery/anaesthesia: In patients undergoing major surgery, or during anaesthesia with agents which produce hypotension, captopril will block angiotensin II formation secondary to compensatory renin release. This may lead to hypotension which can be corrected by volume expansion.

Thiazides may decrease the arterial response to noradrenaline. In emergency surgery, pre-anaesthetic and anaesthetic agents should be administered in reduced doses. Thiazides may increase the response to tubocurarine.

Metabolic disorders: Hyperuricaemia may occur, or frank gout be precipitated by thiazides in certain patients. Insulin requirements in diabetic patients may be altered by thiazides and latent diabetes mellitus may emerge. The captopril component of Capozide has been shown to ameliorate these effects of thiazides.

Clinical chemistry: Capozide may cause a false-positive urine test for acetone.

Side-effects

Haematological: With captopril, neutropenia, anaemia and thrombocytopenia have been reported (see *Warnings*).

With thiazides, leucopenia, agranulocytosis, thrombocytopenia and aplastic anaemia have occurred.

Renal: Proteinuria, elevated blood urea and creatinine, elevated serum potassium and acidosis (see *Warnings*).

Cardiovascular: Hypotension has been reported in volume depleted patients. Tachycardia.

Skin: With captopril, rashes, usually pruritic, may occur. They are usually mild, transient and maculopapular, rarely urticarial. In a few cases the rash has been associated with fever and some patients have developed angio-neurotic oedema. Pruritus, flushing, vesicular rash, and photosensitivity have been reported.

With thiazides, purpura, photosensitivity, rash, urticaria, necrotising angiitis, Stevens-Johnson syndrome and other hypersensitivity reactions have been observed.

Gastro-intestinal: Reversible and usually self-limiting taste impairment has been reported. Weight loss may be associated with the loss of taste. Stomatitis, resembling aphthous ulcers, has been reported. Elevation of liver enzymes has been noted in a few patients receiving captopril. Rare cases of hepatocellular injury and cholestatic jaundice have been reported. Gastric irritation and abdominal pain may occur. Pancreatitis has been reported rarely in patients treated with ACE Inhibitors; in some cases this has proved fatal.

Other: Paraesthesias of the hands, serum sickness, cough, bronchospasm and lymphadenopathy have been reported.

With thiazides, dizziness, vertigo, headache, xanthopsia, hyperglycaemia, hypokalaemia, glycosuria, hyperuricaemia, hypercalcaemia, muscle spasm, weakness and restlessness have been reported.

Overdosage: In the event of overdosage, blood pressure should be monitored and if hypotension develops volume expansion is the treatment of choice.

Captopril is removed by dialysis.

Drug interactions: Diuretics: Potassium-sparing diuretics (triamterene, amiloride and spironolactone), or potassium supplements may cause significant increase in serum potassium. *Indomethacin:* A reduction of anti-hypertensive effectiveness may occur. This is probably also the case with other non-steroidal anti-inflammatory drugs. *Vasodilators:* Capozide has been reported to act synergistically with peripheral vasodilators such as minoxidil. This may improve blood pressure control, and awareness of this interaction may avert an initial hypotensive response. *Clonidine:* It has been suggested that the anti-hypertensive effect of captopril can be delayed when patients treated with clonidine are changed to Capozide. *Allopurinol and procainamide:* There have been reports of neutropenia and/or Stevens-Johnson syndrome in patients on captopril plus either allopurinol or procainamide. Although a causal relationship has not been established, these combinations should only be used with caution, especially in patients with impaired renal function. *Immunosuppressants:* Azathioprine and cyclophosphamide have been associated with blood dyscrasias in patients with renal failure who were also taking captopril. *Probenecid:* The renal clearance of captopril is reduced in the presence of probenecid.

Pharmaceutical precautions Do not store above 30°C (86°F). Keep bottles tightly closed to protect the contents from moisture.

Legal category POM.

Package quantities Capozide: Calendar packs of 28 tablets (OP).

Further information Capozide is designed to aid drug compliance by providing a convenient once daily preparation of captopril combined with hydrochlorothiazide for the treatment of mild to moderate hypertension. Significant anti-hypertensive activity is detectable throughout a 24 hour period following oral therapy.

By combining lower doses than might be required if each component were used alone, side effects, especially the hypokalaemia associated with diuretics, can be minimised.

Product licence number

Capozide Tablets 50 mg/25 mg 0034/0263

CAPOZIDE* LS TABLETS

Qualitative and quantitative compostiion Each tablet contains: Captopril 25 mg and Hydrochlorothiazide 12.5 mg.

Pharmaceutical form Tablets.

Clinical particulars

Therapeutic indications: For the treatment of mild to moderate hypertension in patients who have been stabilised on the individual components given in the same proportions. Capozide LS is particularly suitable for older patients and others requiring lower doses of the components.

Posology and method of administration:

Adults including the elderly: One tablet daily.

Children: Safety and effectiveness of Capozide LS have not been established.

Patients with renal failure: Capozide LS is not recommended for use in patients with significant renal impairment.

Contra-indications: Capozide LS is contra indicated in patients with anuria or hypersensitivity to captopril, thiazides, or any sulphonamide derived drug.

Pregnancy: Captopril has been shown to be lethal to rabbit and sheep foetuses. There were no foetotoxic effects to hamster or rat foetuses.

Capozide ls is contra indicated in pregnancy and should not be used in women of child bearing potential unless protected by effective contraception.

Exposure of the mother in the second and third trimesters of pregnancy has been associated with oligohydramnios and neonatal hypertension and or anuria.

Special warnings and special precautions for use:

Precautions: Capozide LS should not be used in patients with aortic stenosis or outflow tract obstruction.

Warnings:

Haematological: Neutropenia agranulocytosis, thrombocytopenia and anaemia have been reported in patients receiving captopril.

In patients with normal renal function and no other complicating factors, neutropenia occurs rarely.

Captopril should not be used routinely in patients with pre existing impaired renal function, collagen vascular disease, immunosuppressant therapy, treatment with allopurinol or procainamide, or a combination of these complicating factors. Some of these patients developed serious infections which in a few instances did not respond to intensive antibiotic therapy.

During treatment, all patients should be instructed to report any sign of infection (e.g. persistent sore throat, fever), when a differential white blood cell count should be performed. Capozide LS and other concomitant medication should be withdrawn if neutropenia (neutrophils less than 1000 mm³) is detected or suspected.

In most patients neutrophil counts rapidly returned to normal upon discontinuing captopril.

Renal: Proteinuria is a rare complication of captopril therapy.

Some patients with renal disease, particularly those with bilateral renal artery stenoses or unilateral renal artery stenoses in a single functioning kidney, have developed increased concentrations of blood urea and serum creatinine. Discontinuation of Capozide LS may be required.

Renal: Recent clinical observations have shown a high incidence of anaphylactoid like reactions during haemodialysis with high flux dialysis membranes, (e.g. AN69) in patients receiving ACE Inhibitors (see *Contra indications*).

Hepatic: Capozide LS should be used with caution in patients with impaired hepatic function or progressive liver disease because of the known risks associated with alterations in fluid and electrolyte balance resulting from thiazide treatment in such patients.

Electrolyte imbalance: Patients receiving Capozide LS should be observed for clinical signs of thiazide induced fluid or electrolyte imbalance. In such patients periodic determinations of serum electrolytes should be performed. Because captopril reduces the production of aldosterone, its combination with hydrochlorothiazide may minimise diuretic induced hypokalaemia. However, some patients may still require potassium supplements. Potassium sparing diuretics should not be used in conjunction with Capozide LS.

Surgery anaesthesia: In patients undergoing major surgery, or during anaesthesia with agents which produce hypotension, captopril will block angiotensin IIformation secondary to compensatory renin release. This may lead to hypotension which can be corrected by volume expansion.

Thiazides may decrease the arterial response to noradrenaline. In emergency surgery, pre anaesthetic and anaesthetic agents should be administered in reduced doses. Thiazides may increase the response to tubocurarine.

Metabolic disorders: Hyperuricaemia may occur, or frank gout be precipitated by thiazides in certain patients. Insulin requirements in diabetic patients may be altered by thiazides and latent diabetes mellitus may emerge. The captopril component of Capozide LS has been shown to ameliorate these effects of thiazides.

Clinical chemistry: Capozide LS may cause a false positive urine test for acetone.

Interactions with other medicinal products and other forms of interaction:

Diuretics: Potassium sparing diuretics (triamterene, amiloride and spironolactone), or potassium supplements may cause significant increase in serum potassium.

Indomethacin: A reduction of anti hypertensive effectiveness may occur. This is probably also the case with other non steroidal anti inflammatory drugs.

Vasodilators: Capozide LS has been reported to act synergistically with peripheral vasodilators such as minoxidil. This may improve blood pressure control and awareness of this interaction may avert an initial hypotensive response.

Clonidine: It has been suggested that the anti hypertensive effect of captopril can be delayed when patients treated with clonidine are changed to Capozide LS.

Allopurinol and procainamide: There have been reports of neutropenia and or Stevens Johnson syndrome in patients on captopril plus either allopurinol or procainamide. Although a causal relationship has not been established, these combinations should only be used with caution, especially in patients with impaired renal function.

Immunosuppressants: Azathioprine and cyclophosphamide have been associated with blood dyscrasias in patients with renal failure who were also taking captopril.

Probenecid: The renal clearance of captopril is reduced in the presence of probenecid.

Pregnancy and lactation: Captopril has been shown to be lethal to rabbit and sheep foetuses. There were no foetotoxic effects to hamster or rat foetuses.

Capozide LS is contra indicated in pregnancy and should not be used in women of child bearing potential unless protected by effective contraception.

Exposure of the mother in the second and third trimesters of pregnancy has been associated with oligohydramnios and neonatal hypertension and or anuria.

Capozide LS should not be used in nursing mothers.

Effects on ability to drive and use machines: Not applicable.

Undesirable effects:

Haematological: With captopril, neutropenia, anaemia and thrombocytopenia have been reported (see *Warnings*).

With thiazides, leucopenia, agranulocytosis, thrombocytopenia and aplastic anaemia have occurred.

Renal: Proteinuria, elevated blood urea and creatinine, elevated serum potassium and acidosis. (see *Warnings)*

Cardiovascular: Hypotension has been reported in volume depleted patients. Tachycardia.

Skin: With captopril, rashes, usually pruritic, may occur. They are usually mild, transient and maculopapular, rarely urticarial. In a few cases the rash has been associated with fever and some patients have developed angio neurotic oedema. Pruritus, flushing, vesicular rash, and photosensitivity have been reported.

With thiazides, purpura, photosensitivity, rash, urticaria, necrotising angiitis, Stevens Johnson syndrome and other hypersensitivity reactions have been observed.

Gastrointestinal: Reversible and usually self limiting taste impairment has been reported. Weight loss may be associated with the loss of taste. Stomatitis, resembling aphthous ulcers, has been reported. Elevation of liver enzymes has been noted in a few patients receiving captopril. Rare cases of hepatocellular injury and cholestatic jaundice have been reported. Gastric irritation and abdominal pain may occur. Pancreatitis has been reported rarely in patients treated with ACE Inhibitors; in some cases this has proved fatal.

Other: Paraesthesias of the hands, serum sickness, cough, bronchospasm and lymphadenopathy have been reported.

With thiazides, dizziness, vertigo, headache, xanthopsia, hyperglycaemia, hypokalaemia, glycosuria, hyperuricaemia, hypercalcaemia, muscle spasm, weakness and restlessness have been reported.

Overdose: In the event of overdosage, blood pressure should be monitored and if hypotension develops volume expansion is the treatment of choice.

Captopril is removed by dialysis.

Pharmacological properties

Pharmacodynamic properties: Captopril inhibits angiotension converting enzyme which is responsible for the conversion of Angiotensin I to the pressor substance Angiotensin II.

Hydrochloride is a diuretic which increases the excretion of sodium and chloride ions. The resulting fall in blood pressure and blood volume results in an increase in angiotension II levels which tend to reduce the hypotensive effect.

Pharmacokinetic properties:

Captopril: After oral administration of therapeutic doses of captopril rapid absorption occurs with peak blood levels at about one hour. Average minimal absorption is approximately 75%. In a 24 hour period over 95% of the absorbed dose is eliminated in the urine; 40 to 50% is unchanged drug; most of the remainder is the disulphide dimer of captopril and captopril cysteine disulphide.

Approximately 25 to 30% of the circulating drug is bound to plasma proteins. The apparent elimination half life for total radioactivity in blood is probably less than 3 hours. An accurate determination of half life of unchanged captopril is not, at present, possible but it is probably less than 2 hours. In patients with renal impairment, however, retention of captopril occurs (see posology and method of administration).

Hydrochlorothiazide: The mean plasma half life of hydrochlorothiazide in fasted individuals has been reported to be approximately 2.5 hours. Onset of diuresis occurs in 2 hours and the peak effect at about 4 hours. Its action persists for approximately 6 to 12 hours. Hydrochlorothiazide is eliminated rapidly by the kidney.

Pharmaceutical particulars

List of excipients: Lactose, magnesium stearate, maize starch, microcrystalline cellulose, stearic acid.

Incompatibilities: None.

Shelf life: 36 months.

Special precautions for storage: Store below 30°C. Protect from moisture

Nature and contents of container:
PVC/PVDC Blister
Foil strips

Instructions for use/handling: No special instructions.

Marketing authorisation number 0034/0279

Date of approval/revision of SPC March 1995

Legal category POM

ECONACORT* CREAM

Presentation White cream containing 1% w/w econazole nitrate and 1% w/w hydrocortisone.

Other ingredients: Benzoic acid, butylated hydroxyanisole, liquid paraffin, ethoxylated oleic acid glycerides, stearate esters of ethylene glycol and polyoxyethylene glycol, water.

Uses *Actions:* Econazole nitrate is a broad spectrum antifungal and antibiotic agent, active against dermatophytes (*Trichophyton rubrum, Trichophyton mentagrophytes, Epidermophyton floccosum* and *Malassezia furfur*); pathogenic yeasts; *Candida albicans* and other *Candida* species. It is also active against Gram-positive bacteria.

Hydrocortisone is a widely used topical anti-inflammatory agent of value in the treatment of inflammatory skin conditions including atopic and infantile eczema, contact sensitivity reactions and intertrigo.

Indications: Econacort is indicated for the topical treatment of inflammatory dermatoses where infection by susceptible organisms co-exist.

Dosage and administration

Adults and children: To be massaged gently into the affected and surrounding skin area morning and evening. The cream is particularly suitable for moist and weeping lesions.

Elderly: Natural thinning of the skin occurs in the elderly, hence corticosteroids should be used sparingly and for short periods of time.

Contra-indications, warnings, etc

Contra-indications: Hypersensitivity to either of the active ingredients.

In tuberculous and most viral lesions of the skin, particularly herpes simplex, vaccinia and varicella.

Should not be used for facial rosacea, acne vulgaris and perioral dermatitis.

Precautions: Econacort cream should not be used in or near the eyes.

If used in infants and children, or on the face, courses should be limited to 5 days and occlusion should not be used.

Pregnancy: Topical administration of corticosteroids to pregnant animals can cause abnormalities of foetal development including cleft palate and intra-uterine growth retardation. There may, therefore, be a very small risk of such effects in the human foetus.

Side-effects: Econazole nitrate and hydrocortisone are well tolerated. Where adverse reactions occur they are usually reversible on cessation of therapy.

Side-effects of econazole nitrate are limited to occasional local irritation manifested by erythema, burning or stinging sensation, and pruritis, but these may be minimised by the hydrocortisone component.

The possibility of the systemic effects which are associated with all steroid therapy should be considered. These effects may be enhanced with occlusive dressings.

Overdosage: Topically applied corticosteroids can be absorbed in sufficient amounts to produce systemic effects.

In the event of accidental ingestion, the patient should be observed and treated symptomatically.

Pharmaceutical precautions Store below 25°C. Avoid freezing.

Legal category POM.

Package quantities Tubes of 30 g (OP).

Further information Nil.

Product licence number 0034/0249.

ECOSTATIN* CREAM

Presentation

Ecostatin Cream is a white, vanishing-type cream containing 1% w/w econazole nitrate in a cream base.

Other ingredients: Benzoic acid, butylated hydroxyanisole, liquid paraffin, ethoxylated oleic acid glycerides, stearate esters of ethylene glycol and polyoxyethylene, perfume, water.

Uses *Actions:* Econazole nitrate is a broad spectrum antifungal agent, active against dermatophytes (*Trichophyton rubrum, Trichophyton mentagrophytes, Epidermophyton floccosum* and *Malassezia furfur*); pathogenic yeasts; *Candida albicans* and other *Candida* species. Also active against some Gram-positive bacteria, e.g. staphylococci and streptococci.

Indications All fungal skin infections due to dermatophytes (e.g. *Trichophyton* species), yeasts (e.g. *Candida* species), moulds and other fungi. These include ringworm (tinea) infections, athlete's foot, paronychia, pityriasis versicolor, erythrasma, intertrigo, fungal nappy rash, candidal vulvitis and candidal balanitis. Bacterial skin infections due to Gram-positive organisms.

Dosage and administration
Adults and children: Ecostatin Cream should be massaged gently into the affected and surrounding skin area morning and evening. The cream is particularly suitable for moist or weeping lesions.

Clinical improvement usually occurs promptly; however, complete disappearance of the symptoms of the disease may require prolonged treatment. Therapy should continue for several days following both clinical and mycological cure in order to prevent relapse.

Elderly: No specific dosage recommendations.

Contra-indications, warnings, etc
Contra-indications: Patients with a history of sensitivity to any of the components of this preparation.

Precautions: Ecostatin Cream should not be used in or near the eyes. Avoid contact with diaphragms and condoms.

Pregnancy: No specific precautions apply; systemic absorption is likely to be negligible.

Side-effects: Ecostatin Cream is well tolerated. Side-effects are limited to occasional local irritation manifested by erythema, burning or stinging sensations and pruritus.

Pharmaceutical precautions Ecostatin Cream should be stored below 25°C. Avoid freezing.

Legal category P.

Package quantities Tubes of 30 g and 15 g (OP).

Further information Nil.

Product licence number 0034/0231.

ECOSTATIN* PESSARIES AND TWIN PACK

Presentation
Pessaries: White, opaque, oval pessaries each containing 150 mg econazole nitrate in an hydrogonated vegetable oil base. 3 pessary treatment pack.

Other ingredients: Hard fat.

Twin pack: Three Ecostatin pessaries with applicator plus 15 g Ecostatin Cream (containing 1% w/w econazole nitrate).

The Cream also contains: benzoic acid, butylated hydroxyanisole, liquid paraffin, ethoxylated oleic acid glycerides, stearate esters of ethylene glycol and polyoxyethylene, perfume, water.

Uses *Actions:* Econazole nitrate has a broad spectrum of antifungal activity. It is highly active against *Candida albicans* and other *Candida* species and is effective in controlling infections of the vagina and vulva caused by such organisms (thrush).

Indications: Vulvovaginal candidosis. In addition to vaginal treatment the Twin Pack contains cream for topical application to the anogenital area.

Dosage and administration *Adults: Pessaries:* One pessary to be inserted at bedtime for three consecutive nights. Administration should be continued even if menstruation occurs and despite the disappearance of signs and symptoms of the infection.

The pessary should be inserted high into the vagina while the patient is supine.

Cream: The cream is applied twice daily, in the morning and evening, to the anogenital area.

Note: To prevent re-infection with *Candida*, the male consort should be treated concurrently with Ecostatin Cream, applied twice daily to the external genital area during the treatment period.

Although a three day course of therapy usually suffices, it may be necessary to institute a second course of therapy.

Children: Vulvovaginal candidosis is not normally a problem in children, therefore there are no specific dosage recommendations.

Elderly: No specific dosage recommendations or precautions apply.

Contra-indications, warnings, etc
Contra-indications: Patients with a history of sensitivity to any of the components of this preparation.

Precautions: Avoid contact between contraceptive diaphragms and condoms and this product since the rubber may be damaged by the preparation.

Pregnancy: Ecostatin pessaries are effective in the candidal vaginitis associated with pregnancy. Safety of systemic econazole has not been established but percutaneous absorption following topical application is likely to be low. However, as with other agents, Ecostatin should not be used during the first trimester of pregnancy unless the physician deems its use essential for the welfare of the patient. In pregnancy, extra care should be taken in using an applicator to prevent the possibility of mechanical trauma.

Side-effects: Patients may rarely complain of discomfort; this is usually transitory and disappears with continued treatment. Seldom is it necessary to discontinue econazole pessary treatment.

Ecostatin Cream is well tolerated. Side-effects are limited to occasional local irritation manifested by erythema, burning or stinging sensation, and pruritus.

Pharmaceutical precautions *Storage:* Store below 25°C.

Legal category Cream P.
Pessaries POM.

Package quantities *Pessaries:* Pack of three pessaries with applicator (OP).
Twin pack: Three pessaries with applicator plus 15 g cream (OP).

Further information Nil.

Product licence numbers
Ecostatin Pessaries 0034/0233
Ecostatin Cream 0034/0231

ECOSTATIN* -1 PESSARY

Qualitative and quantitative composition Ecostatin-1 Pessary contains Econazole Nitrate 150 mg.

Pharmaceutical form Pessary

Clinical particulars
Therapeutic indications: The treatment of vaginitis due to *Candida albicans* and other yeasts.

Posology and method of administration:
Adults: The recommended dose is one pessary inserted at bedtime. The pessary should be inserted as high as possible into the vagina, using the applicator, with the patient in the supine position.

Although one course of therapy usually suffices, it may be necessary to institute a second course of therapy.

Elderly: No specific dosage recommendations or precautions apply.

Children: Vulvovaginal candidosis is not normally a problem in children, therefore there are no specific dosage recommendations.

Contra-indications: Patients with a known history of sensitivity to any of the components of the preparation.

Special warnings and special precautions for use: Avoid contact between this product and contraceptive diaphragms and condoms since the rubber may be damaged by the preparation. To prevent re-infection with *Candida*, the male consort should be treated concurrently with Ecostatin Cream. Although one course of therapy usually suffices, it may be necessary to institute a second course of therapy.

Interactions with other medicinal products and other forms of interaction: None known.

Pregnancy and lactation: Ecostatin-1 Pessaries are effective in the candidal vaginitis associated with pregnancy. Safety of systemic econazole has not been established but percutaneous absorption following topical application is likely to be low. However, as with other agents, Ecostatin should not be used during the first trimester of pregnancy unless the physician deems its use essential for the welfare of the patient. In pregnancy, extra care should be taken in using an applicator, to prevent the possibility of mechanical trauma.

Effects on ability to drive and use machines: None known.

Undesirable effects: Patients may rarely complain of transitory discomfort.

Overdose: There have been no recorded cases of overdose.

Pharmacological properties
Pharmacodynamic properties: Econazole nitrate has a broad spectrum of antifungal activity. It is highly active against *Candida albicans* and other *Candida* species and is effective in controlling infections of the vagina and vulva caused by such organisms (thrush).

Pharmacokinetic properties: Not applicable.

Pharmaceutical particulars
List of excipients: Colloidal silicon dioxide, hard fat, natural polysaccharides, stearyl heptanoate.

Incompatibilities: None known.

Shelf life: 60 months.

Special precautions for storage: Store below 25°C.

Nature and contents of container: Pre-formed PVC mould packed in a cardboard carton. The carton includes an applicator with directions for use.

Instructions for use/handling: No special instructions apply.

Marketing authorisation number 0034/0266

Date of approval/revision of SPC January 1997

Legal category POM

FLORINEF* TABLETS

Presentation Round, pale pink tablets, scored on one side and engraved Squibb and 429 on reverse, containing 0.1 mg fludrocortisone acetate.

Other ingredients: Dicalcium phosphate, erythrosin, lactose, magnesium stearate, maize starch, sodium benzoate, talc.

Uses *Actions:* Qualitatively, the physiological action of fludrocortisone acetate is similar to hydrocortisone. In very small doses, fludrocortisone maintains life in adrenalectomised animals, enhances the deposition of liver glycogen and produces thymic involution, eosinopenia, retention of sodium and increased urinary excretion of potassium.

Indications: For partial replacement therapy for primary and secondary adrenocortical insufficiency in Addison's disease and for the treatment of salt-losing adrenogenital syndrome.

Dosage and administration
Adult dosage: A daily dosage range of 0.05–0.3 mg Florinef tablets orally. Supplementary parenteral administration of sodium-retaining hormones is not necessary. When an enhanced glucocorticoid effect is desirable, cortisone or hydrocortisone by mouth should be given concomitantly with Florinef tablets.

Children: May be used adjusted to the age and weight of the child according to the severity of the condition (see 'Precautions').

Elderly: No specific dosage recommendations or precautions.

Contra-indications, warnings, etc
Contra-indications: Hypersensitivity to any of the ingredients.

Systemic infections unless specific anti-infective therapy is employed.

Because of its marked effect on sodium retention, the use of Florinef in the treatment of conditions other than those indicated, is not advised.

Since Florinef is a potent mineralocorticoid both the dosage and salt intake should be carefully monitored to avoid the development of hypertension, oedema or weight gain. Periodic checking of serum electrolyte levels is advisable during prolonged therapy.

Precautions: Florinef is a potent mineralocorticoid and is used predominantly for replacement therapy. Although glucocorticoid side effects may occur, these can be reduced by reducing the dosage.

Undesirable effects may be minimised using the lowest effective dose for the minimum period. Frequent patient review is required to titrate the dose appropriately against disease activity (see Dosage section).

Adrenal cortical atrophy develops during prolonged therapy and may persist for years after stopping treatment. Withdrawal of corticosteroids after prolonged therapy must, therefore, always be gradual to avoid acute adrenal insufficiency and should be tapered off over weeks or months according to the dose and duration of treatment. Patients on long-term systemic therapy with Florinef may require supportive corticosteroid therapy in times of stress (such as trauma, surgery or severe illness) both during the treatment period and up to a year afterwards. If corticosteroids have been stopped following prolonged therapy they may need to be reintroduced temporarily.

Patients should carry steroid treatment cards which give clear guidance on the precautions to be taken to minimise risk and which provides details of prescriber, drug, dosage and the duration of treatment.

Anti-inflammatory/immunosuppressive effects: Suppression of the inflammatory response and immune function increases the susceptibility to infections and their severity. The clinical presentation may often be atypical and serious infections such as septicaemia and tuberculosis may be masked and may reach an advanced stage before being recognised.

Chickenpox is of particular concern since this normally minor illness may be fatal in immunosuppressed patients. Patients (or parents of children receiving Florinef tablets) without a definite history of chickenpox should be advised to avoid close personal contact with chickenpox or herpes zoster. If exposed they should seek urgent medical attention. Passive immunisation with varicella zoster immunoglobulin (VZIG) is needed by exposed non-immune patients who are receiving systemic corticosteroids or who have used them within the previous 3 months; this should be given within 10 days of exposure to chickenpox. If a diagnosis of chickenpox is confirmed, the illness warrants specialist care and urgent treatment. Corticosteroids should not be stopped and the dose may need to be increased.

During corticosteroid therapy antibody response will be reduced and therefore affect the patient's response to vaccines. Live vaccines should not be administered.

Special precautions: Particular care is required when considering use of systemic corticosteroids in patients with the following conditions and frequent patient monitoring is necessary.

Recent intestinal anastomoses, diverticulitis, thrombophlebitis, existing or previous history of severe affective disorders (especially previous steroid psychosis), exanthematous disease, chronic nephritis, or renal insufficiency, metastatic carcinoma, osteoporosis (post-menopausal females are particularly at risk); in patients with an active peptic ulcer (or a history of peptic ulcer). Myasthenia gravis. Latent or healed tuberculosis; in the presence of local or systemic viral infection, systemic fungal infections or in active infections not controlled by antibiotics. In acute psychoses; in acute glomerulonephritis. Hypertension; congestive heart failure; glaucoma (or a family history of glaucoma), previous steroid myopathy or epilepsy. Liver failure.

Corticosteroid effects may be enhanced in patients with hypothyroidism or cirrhosis.

Diabetes may be aggravated, necessitating a higher insulin dosage. Latent diabetes mellitus may be precipitated.

Menstrual irregularities may occur, and this possibility should be mentioned to female patients.

Rare instances of anaphylactoid reactions have occurred in patients receiving corticosteroids, especially when a patient has a history of drug allergies.

Aspirin should be used cautiously in conjunction with corticosteroids in patients with hypoprothrombinaemia.

Children: Growth and development of children on prolonged corticosteroid therapy should be carefully observed. Corticosteroids cause dose-related growth retardation in infancy, childhood and adolescence which may be irreversible.

Elderly: The common adverse effects on systemic corticosteroids may be associated with more serious consequences in old age, especially osteoporosis, hypertension, hypokalaemia, diabetes, susceptibility to infection and thinning of the skin. Close clinical supervision is required to avoid life-threatening reactions.

Pregnancy and nursing mothers: It may be decided to continue a pregnancy in a woman requiring replacement mineralocorticoid therapy, despite the risk to the foetus. When corticosteroids are essential however, patients with normal pregnancies may be treated as though they were in the non-gravid state.

There is evidence of harmful effects in pregnancy in animals. There may be a small risk of cleft palate and intra-uterine growth retardation. Hypoadrenalism may occur in the neonate. Patients with pre-eclampsia or fluid retention require close monitoring.

Corticosteroids are found in breast milk.

Infants born of mothers who have received substantial doses of corticosteroids during pregnancy or during breast feeding should be carefully observed for signs of hypoadrenalism. Maternal treatment should be carefully documented in the infant's medical records to assist in follow up.

Drug interactions: Barbiturates, phenytoin, rifampicin, rifabutin, carbamazepine, primidone and aminoglutethimide may enhance the metabolic clearance of corticosteroids, resulting in decreased therapeutic effects.

Corticosteroids antagonise the effects of hypoglycaemic agents (including insulin), anti-hypertensives and diuretics. The hypokalaemic effects of acetazolamide, loop diuretics, thiazide diuretics and carbenoxolone are enhanced.

The efficacy of coumarin anticoagulants may be enhanced by concurrent corticosteroid therapy and close monitoring of the INR or prothombin time is required to avoid spontaneous bleeding.

The renal clearance of salicylates is increased by corticosteroids and steroid withdrawal may result in salicylate intoxication.

Side-effects: Where adverse reactions occur they are usually reversible on cessation of therapy. The incidence of predictable side-effects, including hypothalamic-pituitary-adrenal suppression correlate with the relative potency of the drug, dosage, timing of administration and duration of treatment (see Warnings and Precautions).

Patients should be watched closely for the following adverse reactions which may be associated with any corticosteroid therapy.

Anti-inflammatory and immunosuppressive effects: Increased susceptibility and severity of infections with suppression of clinical symptoms and signs, opportunistic infections, recurrence of dormant tuberculosis (see Warnings and Precautions).

Fluid and electrolyte disturbances: sodium retention, fluid retention, congestive heart failure in susceptible patients, potassium loss, cardiac arrhythmias or ECG changes due to potassium deficiency, hypokalaemic alkalosis, increased calcium excretion and hypertension.

Musculoskeletal: muscle weakness, fatigue, steroid myopathy, loss of muscle mass, osteoporosis, avascular osteonecrosis, vertebral compression fractures, delayed healing of fractures, aseptic necrosis of femoral and humeral heads, pathological fractures of long bones and spontaneous fractures, tendon rupture.

Gastrointestinal: dyspepsia, peptic ulcer with possible subsequent perforation and haemorrhage, pancreatitis, abdominal distension and ulcerative oesophagitis, candidiasis.

Dermatologic: impaired wound healing, thin fragile skin, petechiae and ecchymoses, facial erythema, increased sweating, purpura, striae, hirsutism, acneiform eruptions, lupus erythematous-like lesions and suppressed reactions to skin tests.

Neurological: euphoria, psychological dependence, depression, insomnia, convulsions, increased intracranial pressure with papilloedema (pseudo-tumour cerebri) usually after treatment, vertigo, headache, neuritis or paraesthesias and aggravation of pre-existing psychiatric conditions and epilepsy.

Endocrine/metabolic: menstrual irregularities and amenorrhoea; development of the Cushingoid state; suppression of growth in childhood and adolescence; secondary adrenocortical and pituitary unresponsiveness, particularly in times of stress (e.g. trauma, surgery or illness); decreased carbohydrate tolerance; manifestations of latent diabetes mellitus and increased requirements for insulin or oral hypoglycaemic agents in diabetes, weight gain. Negative protein and calcium balance. Increased appetite.

Ophthalmic: posterior subcapsular cataracts, increased intraocular pressure, glaucoma, exophthalmos, papilloedema, corneal or scleral thinning, exacerbation of ophthalmic viral or fungal diseases.

Others: necrotising angiitis, thrombophlebitis, thrombo-embolism, leucocytosis, insomnia, syncopal episodes and anaphylactoid reactions, particularly where there is a history of drug allergies.

Withdrawal symptoms and signs: On withdrawal, fever, myalgia, arthralgia, rhinitis, conjunctivitis, painful itchy skin nodules and weight loss may occur. Too rapid a reduction in dose following prolonged treatment can lead to acute adrenal insufficiency, hypotension and death (see Warnings and Precautions).

Overdosage: A single large dose should be treated with plenty of water by mouth. Careful monitoring of serum electrolytes is essential, with particular consideration being given to the need for administration of potassium chloride and restriction of dietary sodium intake.

Pharmaceutical precautions *Storage:* Below 25°C.

Legal category POM.

Package quantities Bottles of 56 tablets.

Further information Nil.

Product licence numbers
Florinef Tablets 0.1 mg 0034/5027R.

FUNGILIN* LOZENGE
FUNGILIN* ORAL SUSPENSION
FUNGILIN* ORAL TABLETS

Qualitative and quantitative composition
Fungilin Lozenge: Round, pale yellow, engraved '929' and 'Squibb' containing 10,000 units (10 mg) amphotericin.

Fungilin Oral Suspension: Orange-flavoured, viscous suspension containing 100,000 units (100 mg) amphotericin per ml.

Fungilin Oral Tablets: Yellow to tan, scored one side and engraved 'Squibb' and '430' on reverse, containing 100,000 (100 mg) amphotericin.

Pharmaceutical form
Oral Lozenge
Oral Suspension
Oral Tablets.

Clinical particulars
Therapeutic indications:
Lozenge/Suspension: For the treatment of candidal lesions (thrush) of the oral and perioral areas. The suspension may be used in the treatment of denture stomatitis.

Suspension/Tablets: For the treatment of intestinal candidosis and the suppression of the intestinal reservoir of *C. albicans* which may precipitate cutaneous or vaginal candidosis.

Posology and method of administration:
Adults:
Lozenge: Dissolve one lozenge slowly in the mouth four times a day. Depending on the severity of infection, the dose may be increased to 8 lozenges daily.

To clear the condition fully may require 10-15 days' treatment.

Suspension: For denture stomatitis and oral infections caused by *C. albicans*, 1 ml should be placed in the mouth four times daily; it should be kept in contact with lesions for as long as possible.

For the treatment of suppression of intestinal candidosis, 2 ml four times daily.

Tablets: 1 or 2 tablets four times daily.

Administration of Fungilin for oral and intestinal candidosis should be continued for 48 hours after clinical cure to prevent relapse.

Infants and children:
Lozenge: Not recommended
Suspension: For intestinal and oral candidosis, 1 ml should be dropped into the mouth four times daily. The suspension should be held in contact with oral lesions for as long as possible before swallowing.

For prophylaxis in the newborn, the suggested dose is 1 ml daily.

Tablets: Not recommended

Elderly: No specific dosage recommendations or precautions.

Contra-indications: There are no known contra-indications to the use of these products.

Special warnings and special precautions for use: No specific warnings or precautions apply.

Interactions with other medicinal products and other forms of interaction: None known.

Pregnancy and lactation: No special precautions apply; absorption of amphotericin from the gastro-intestinal tract is negligible.

Effects on ability to drive and use machines: Not applicable.

Undesirable effects: Gastro-intestinal side-effects have occasionally been reported following continuous administration of amphotericin for several months in daily doses in excess of 3 g. These have been mild in nature and have readily cleared on cessation of treatment. No systemic toxic effects or allergic reactions have been associated with its oral use.

Overdose: Since absorption of amphotericin from the gastro-intestinal tract is negligible, overdosage causes no systemic toxicity.

Pharmacological properties
Pharmacodynamic properties:
Actions: Amphotericin is an antifungal antibiotic active against a wide range of yeasts and yeast-like fungi including *Candida albicans*. Extensive clinical experience has not shown problems of toxicity or sensitisation.

Pharmacokinetic properties: Absorption from the gastro-intestinal tract is negligible even with very large doses.

Preclinical safety data: No further relevant information.

Pharmaceutical particulars
List of excipients:
Lozenge: Acacia powder, d-mannitol, flavours, magnesium stearate, polyvinyl alcohol, talc.

Suspension: Citric acid, ethanol, flavours, glycerol, methyl and propyl parahydroxybenzoates, potassium chloride, sodium benzoate, sodium carboxymethylcellulose, sodium phosphate, sodium metabisulphite, water.

Tablets: Ethyl cellulose, lactose, maize starch, magnesium stearate, talc.

Incompatibilities: None known

Shelf life:
Lozenge: 18 months
Suspension: 48 months
Tablets: 24 months

Special precautions for storage:
Lozenge/Tablets: Store below 25°C.

Suspension: Store below 25°C, protect from direct sunlight. Discard any unused suspension 4 days after opening.

Dilution: Fungilin Suspension should not be diluted prior to use; it is formulated to coat and adhere to the oral lesions being treated.

Nature and contents of container:
Lozenge: Aluminium tube, foil or blister pack of 60 lozenges.
Suspension: 12 ml bottles with graduated dropper.
Tablets: Bottles of 56 tablets.

Instructions for use/handling: No special handling instructions.

Marketing authorisation numbers
Lozenge: 0034/5034R
Suspension: 0034/5038R
Tablets: 0034/5039R

Date of approval/revision of SPC
Lozenge: November 1995
Suspension/Tablets January 1996

Legal category POM

FUNGIZONE* INTRAVENOUS

Qualitative and quantitative composition Each vial contains as a yellow, fluffy powder: amphotericin 50,000 units (50 mg).

Pharmaceutical form Powder for Injection

Clinical particulars
Therapeutic indications: Fungizone Intravenous should be administered primarily to patients with progressive, potentially fatal infections. This potent drug should not be used to treat the common forms of fungal disease which show only positive skin or serological tests.

Fungizone Intravenous is specifically intended to treat cryptococcosis (torulosis); North American blastomycosis; the disseminated forms of candidosis, coccidioidomycosis and histoplasmosis; mucormycosis (phycomycosis) caused by species of the genera *Mucor, Rhizopus, Absidia, Entomophthora,* and *Basidiobolus* sporotrichosis (*Sporotrichum schenckii*), aspergillosis (*Aspergillus fumigatus*).

Amphotericin may be helpful in the treatment of American mucocutaneous leishmaniasis but is not the drug of choice in primary therapy.

Posology and method of administration:
Adults and children: Fungizone should be administerd by intravenous infusion over a period of 2-4 hours. Reduction of the infusion rate may reduce the incidence of side-effects. In rare instances infusion times of up to 6 hours may be necessary. Initial daily dose should be 0.25 mg/kg of body weight gradually increasing to a level of 1.0 mg/kg of body weight depending on individual response and tolerance. Within the range of 0.25-1.0 mg/kg the daily dose should be maintained at the highest level which is not accompanied by unacceptable toxicity.

In seriously ill patients the daily dose may be gradually increased up to a total of 1.5 mg/kg. Since amphotericin is excreted slowly, therapy may be given on alternate days in patients on the higher dosage schedule. Several months of therapy are usually necessary; a shorter period of therapy may produce an inadequate response and lead to relapse.

When commencing all new courses of treatment, it is advisable to administer a test dose immediately preceding the first dose. A volume of the infusion containing 1 mg (i.e. 10 ml) should be infused over 20-30 minutes and the patient carefully observed for at least a further 30 minutes. It should be noted that patient responses to the test dose may not be predictive of subsequent severe side effects.

Whenever medication is interrupted for a period longer than seven days, therapy should be resumed by starting with the lowest dosage level, i.e. 0.25 mg/kg of body weight and increased gradually.

CAUTION: Under no circumstances should a total daily dose of 1.5 mg/kg be exceeded. The recommended concentration for intravenous infusion is 10 mg/100 ml.

Elderly: No specific dosage recommendations or precautions.

Preparation of solutions: Reconstitute as follows: An initial concentrate of 5 mg amphotericin per ml is first prepared by rapidly expressing 10 ml sterile water for injection, without a bacteriostatic agent, directly into the lyophilized cake, using a sterile needle (minimum diameter: 20 gauge) and syringe. Shake the vial immediately until the colloidal solution is clear. The infusion solution, providing 10 mg/100 ml is obtained by further dilution (1:50) with 5% Glucose Injection of pH above 4.2. The pH of each container of Glucose Injection should be ascertained before use. Commercial Glucose Injection usually has a pH above 4.2; however, if it is below 4.2 then 1 or 2 ml of buffer should be added to the Glucose Injection before it is used to dilute a concentrated solution of amphotericin. The recommended buffer has the following composition:

Dibasic sodium phosphate (anhydrous) 1.59 g
Monobasic sodium phosphate (anhydrous) 0.96 g
Water for Injections BP q.s. to 100 ml

The buffer should be sterilised before it is added to the Glucose Injection, either by filtration through a bacterial filter, or by autoclaving for 30 mins at 15lb pressure (121°C).

CAUTION: Aseptic technique must be strictly observed in all handling, since no preservative or bacteriostatic agent is present. Do not reconstitute with saline solutions. The use of any diluent other than the ones recommended or the presence of a bacteriostatic agent in the diluent may cause precipitation of the amphotericin. Do not use the initial concentrate or the infusion solution if there is any evidence of precipitation of foreign matter.

An in-line membrane filter may be used for intravenous infusion of amphotericin; however the mean pore diameter of the filter should not be less than 1.0 micron in order to assure passage of the amphotericin dispersion.

Other preparations for injection should not be added to the infusion solution or administered via the cannula being used to administer Fungizone Intravenous.

The use of Fungizone Intravenous by other routes has been documented in the published literature:

Bladder irrigation/instillation (e.g. candiduria): Continuous irrigation with 50 mg Fungizone in 1 litre sterile water each day until urinary cultures are negative. Intermittent use of volumes of 100-400 ml (concentrations of 37.5-200 mcg/ml) has also been reported. The urine should be alkalinized (with potassium citrate) and antifungal ointment applied to the perineal area.

Lung inhalation (e.g. pulmonary aspergillosis): 8-40 mg amphotericin (nebulized in sterile water or 5% Glucose) has been given daily in divided doses. Concurrent eradication of oral and intestinal yeast reservoirs is recommended.

Intrathecal (e.g. coccidiodal meningitis): Current published dosage recommendations are for maintenance 0.25-1.0 mg amphotericin 2-4 times weekly following intitiation with a low dose (0.025 mg) and cautious increases. Amphotericin is irritating when injected into the CSF.

Other: Other uses of solutions prepared using Fungizone Intravenous include local instillations for the treatment of fungal infections of the ear, eye, peritoneum, lung cavities and joint spaces.

Contra-indications: Those patients who are hypersensitive to amphotericin, unless, in the opinion of the physician, the condition requiring treatment is life-threatening and amenable only to such therapy.

Special warnings and special precautions for use: Prolonged therapy with amphotericin is usually necessary. Unpleasant reactions are quite common when the drug is given parenterally at therapeutic dosage levels. Some of these reactions are potentially dangerous. Hence amphotericin should be used parenterally only in hospitalised patients, or those under close clinical observation. If serum creatinine exceeds 260 micromol/l the drug should be discontinued or the dosage markedly reduced until renal function is improved. Weekly blood counts and serum potassium determinations are also advisable. Low serum magnesium levels have also been noted during treatment with amphotericin. Therapy should be discontinued if liver function test results (elevated bromsulphalein, alkaline phosphatase and bilirubin) are abnormal.

Leucoencephalopathy has been reported very occasionally following the use of amphotericin injection in patients who received total body irradiation. Most of these patients received high cumulative doses of amphotericin.

Rapid intravenous infusion, over less than one hour, particularly in patients with renal insufficiency, has been associated with hyperkalaemia and arrhythmias and should therefore be avoided.

Corticosteroids should not be administered concomitantly unless they are necessary to control drug reactions. Other nephrotoxic antibiotics and antineoplastic agents should not be given concomitantly except with great caution.

Interactions with other medicinal products and other forms of interaction: Concomitant administration of nephrotoxic drugs or antineoplastics should be avoided if at all possible.

The hypokalaemia following amphotericin therapy may potentiate the toxicity of digitalis glycosides or enhance the curariform actions of skeletal muscle relaxants.

Corticosteroids may increase the potassium loss due to amphotericin.

Flucytosine toxicity may be enhanced during concomitant administration, possibly due to an increase in its cellular uptake and/or impairment of its renal excretion.

Acute pulmonary reactions have occasionally been observed in patients given amphotericin during or shortly after leukocyte transfusions. It is advisable to separate these infusions as far as possible and to monitor pulmonary function.

Pregnancy and lactation: Safety for use in pregnancy has not been established; therefore it should be used during pregnancy only if the possible benefits to be derived outweigh the potential risks involved.

Effects on ability to drive and use machines: Not applicable.

Undesirable effects: While some patients may tolerate full intravenous doses of amphotericin without difficulty, most will exhibit some intolerance. In patients experiencing adverse reactions these may be made less severe by giving aspirin, antihistamines or anti-emetics. Febrile reactions may be decreased by the intravenous administration of small doses of adrenal corticosteroids, e.g. 25 mg hydrocortisone. This may be administered just prior to or during amphotericin infusion. The dosage and duration of such corticosteroid therapy should be kept to a minimum. Administration of the drug on alternate days may decrease anorexia and phlebitis. Adding a small amount of heparin to the infusion may lessen the incidence of thrombophlebitis and coagulation problems. Extravasation may cause chemical irritation. The adverse reactions that are most commonly observed are: fever (sometimes with shaking chills), headache, anorexia, weight loss, nausea and vomiting, malaise, muscle and joint pains, dyspepsia, cramping epigastric pain, diarrhoea, local venous pain at the injection site with phlebitis and thrombophlebitis, normochromic normocytic anaemia and hypokalaemia. Abnormal renal function including hypokalaemia, azotaemia, hyposthenuria, renal tubular acidosis or nephrocalcinosis, is also commonly observed and usually improves upon interruption of therapy; however, some permanent impairment often occurs, especially in those patients receiving large amounts (over 5 g) of amphotericin.

The following adverse reactions occur less frequently or rarely; anuria (oliguria); cardiovascular toxicity including arrhythmias, ventricular fibrillation, cardiac arrest, hypotension, hypertension; coagulation defects; thrombocytopenia; leucopenia; agranulocytosis; eosinophilia; leucocytosis; melaena or haemorrhagic gastroenteritis; maculopapular rash and pruritus; hearing loss, tinnitus; transient vertigo; blurred vision, or diplopia; encephalopathy (see precautions); peripheral neuropathy, convulsions and other neurologic symptoms; anaphylactoid reactions, acute liver failure and flushing.

Overdose: Amphotericin overdoses can result in cardio-respiratory arrest. If an overdose is suspected, discontinue therapy and monitor the patient's clinical status (e.g., cardio-respiratory, renal, and liver function, haematologic status serum electrolytes) and administer supportive therapy as required. Amphotericin is not haemodialysable. Prior to reinstituting therapy, the patient's condition should be stabilised (including correction of electrolyte deficiencies, etc.)

Pharmacological properties
Pharmacodynamic properties: Amphotericin is a polyene antifungal antibiotic active against a wide range of yeasts and yeast-like fungi including *Candida albicans.* Crystalline amphotericin is insoluble in water; therefore, the antibiotic is solubilised by the addition of sodium desoxycholate to form a mixture which provides a colloidal dispersion for parenteral administration. Amphotericin is fungistatic rather than fungicidal in concentrations obtainable in body fluids. It probably acts by binding to sterols in the fungal cell membrane with a resultant change in membrane permeability which allows leakage of intracellular components. Mammalian cell membranes also contain sterols and it has been suggested that the damage to human and fungal cells may share common mechanisms. No strains of Candida resistant to amphotericin have been reported in clinical use, and although in vitro testing does produce a small number of resistant isolates this occurs only following repeated subcultures.

Pharmacokinetic properties: An initial intravenous infusion of 1 to 5 mg of amphotericin per day, gradually increased to 0.65 mg/kg daily, produces peak plasma concentrations of approximately 2 to 4 mg/l which can persist between doses since the plasma half-life of amphotericin is about 24 hours. It has been reported that amphotericin is highly bound (more than 90%) to plasma proteins and is poorly dialysable.

Amphotericin is excreted very slowly by the kidneys with 2 to 5% of a given dose being excreted in biologically active form. After treatment is discontinued the drug can be detected in the urine for at least seven weeks. The cumulative urinary output over a seven day period amounts to approximately 40% of the amount of drug infused.

Details of tissue distribution and possible metabolic pathways are not known.

Preclinical safety data: No further relevant data.

Pharmaceutical particulars
List of excipients: Other ingredients: desoxycholic acid, phosphoric acid, sodium hydroxide, sodium phosphate, water.

Incompatibilities: None known.

Shelf life: 24 months

Special precautions for storage: Vials of powder for reconstitution should be stored in a refrigerator. The concentrate (5 mg per ml after reconstitution with 10 ml sterile Water for Injections) should be stored protected from light. The absence of any microbial preservative and the risk of contamination during reconstitution mean that the product should be stored for no more than 8 hours at room temperature (25°C) or 24 hours in a refrigerator (2-8°C). Should the need arise and a validated aseptic reconstitution technique is applied, the product is chemically stable when stored for 24 hours at room temperature or one week in a refrigerator. It is not intended as a multidose vial. Any unused material should be discarded. Solutions prepared for intravenous infusion (i.e. 10 mg or less amphotericin per 100 ml) should be used promptly after preparation.

Nature and contents of container: Amber glass vials closed with a grey butyl rubber stopper. Vials of 50 mg

Instructions for use/handling: See *Posology and method of administration.* Aseptic technique must be strictly observed during the preparation of the concentrate, the buffer and the infusion.

Marketing authorisation number 0034/5041R

Date of approval/revision of SPC 24 January 1998

Legal category POM

GRANEODIN* OINTMENT

Qualitative and quantitative composition Soft, slightly opaque, colourless ointment, containing neomycin (as sulphate) 1625 units (0.25%) and gramicidin 0.025% in Plastibase* (liquid paraffin and polyethylene resin).

Pharmaceutical form Ointment

Clinical particulars
Therapeutic indications: Superficial bacterial infections such as impetigo; impetiginised eczema; infected eczema; bacterial infections of the ear (see *Contra-indications*).

Posology and method of administration
Adults and children: To be applied two to four times a day. Any crusts should be removed and the ointment rubbed well in.

Elderly: No specific dosage recommendations or precautions.

If a satisfactory response has not been achieved after 7 days, treatment should be stopped and the organism identified.

In cases of sycosis barbae a longer period of therapy may be necessary to treat the deep infection in the follicle.

Contra-indications: Fungal or viral infections of the skin or for the treatment of deep-seated infections.

Persons with known sensitivity to neomycin.

Should not be applied to the external auditory canal in patients with perforated eardrums.

Should not be used for extensive areas because of possible risk of systemic absorption and neomycin-induced ototoxicity.

Special warnings and special precautions for use: The possibility of sensitivity to neomycin should be taken into consideration during treatment. Since the use of occlusive dressings may increase the risk of sensitivity reactions, such dressings should be avoided.
Children: No specific precautions apply.

Interaction with other medicinal products and other forms of interaction: None stated.

Pregnancy and lactation: There are theoretical risks of neomycin-induced foetal ototoxicity; therefore the product should be used with caution only when the benefit outweighs the potential risk.

Effects on ability to drive and use machines: None stated.

Undesirable effects:
Neomycin: Sensitivity reactions may occur especially with prolonged use. Ototoxicity and nephrotoxicity have been reported. The product should be used with caution and in small amounts in the treatment of skin infections following extensive burns, open lesion and other conditions where absorption of neomycin is possible particularly in children and elderly. The product should also be used with care in patients with established hearing loss and those with renal impairment.

Gramicidin: Sensitivity has occasionally been reported.

Overdose: In the event of accidental ingestion, the patient should be observed and treated symptomatically.

Pharmacological properties
Pharmacodynamic properties:
Actions: Neomycin is active against a wide range of Gram-positive and Gram-negative bacteria, including many of the organisms responsible for bacterial skin infections.

Gramicidin is active against Gram-positive bacteria and supplements the action of neomycin against the many common skin pathogens found in this group.

Pharmacokinetic properties: Not applicable.

Preclinical safety data: No further relevant data.

Pharmaceutical particulars
List of excipients: Liquid paraffin and polyethylene resin.

Incompatibilities: None known.

Shelf life: 48 months

Special precautions for storage:
Storage: Store below 25°C.
Dilution: Not recommended.

Nature and contents of container: Aluminium tubes of 25 g

Instructions for use/handling: Not applicable.

Marketing authorisation number 0034/5042R

Date of approval/revision of SPC 14 October 1996

Legal category POM

HALCIDERM* TOPICAL

Presentation A white topical preparation containing halcinonide 0.1% in a water-miscible base.

Other ingredients: Benzyl alcohol, castor oil, silicone fluid, macrogol ether, propylene glycol, stearates, water, white soft paraffin.

Uses *Actions:* Halcinonide is a potent corticosteroid with rapid anti-inflammatory, antipruritic and anti-allergic actions.

Halciderm is suitable for both wet and dry lesions.

Indications: Halciderm is indicated in acute and chronic corticosteroid-responsive conditions which may include: psoriasis, atopic eczema, contact eczema, follicular eczema, infantile eczema, neurodermatitis, anogenital eczema, nummular eczema, seborrhoeic or flexural eczema, otitis externa without frank infection.

Dosage and administration *Adults:* Halciderm should be applied to the affected area two, or occasionally three, times daily. In long-term therapy, or where lower strength preparations are required, do not dilute but use intermittently.

Children: In infants, long-term continuous topical steroid therapy should be avoided. Courses should be limited to 5 days and occlusion should not be used.

Elderly: Natural thinning of the skin occurs in the elderly; hence corticosteroids should be used sparingly and for short periods of time.

Contra-indications, warnings, etc
Contra-indications: Contra-indicated in patients with a history of hypersensitivity to the product components.

Halciderm is not intended for ophthalmic use, nor should it be applied in the external auditory canal of patients with perforated eardrums.

Halciderm is contra-indicated in tuberculous and most viral lesions of the skin, particularly herpes simplex, vaccinia, varicella. The product should not be used in fungal or bacterial skin infections without suitable concomitant anti-infective therapy.

It should not be used for facial rosacea, acne vulgaris, perioral dermatitis or napkin eruptions.

Precautions: Adrenal suppression can occur with prolonged use of topical corticosteroids or treatment of extensive areas. These effects are more likely to occur in infants and children and if occlusive dressings are used. If used in childhood, or on the face, courses should be limited to 5 days and occlusion should not be used.

Topical corticosteroids may be hazardous in psoriasis for a number of reasons including rebound relapses following development of tolerance, risk of generalised pustular psoriasis and local and systemic toxicity due to impaired barrier function of the skin. Steroids may have a place in psoriasis of the scalp and chronic plaque psoriasis of the hands and feet. Careful patient supervision is important.

Pregnancy: There is inadequate evidence of safety in human pregnancy. Topical administration of corticosteroids to pregnant animals can cause abnormalities of foetal development including cleft palate and intra-uterine growth retardation. There may, therefore, be a very small risk of such effects in the human foetus. Caution should be exercised when topical corticosteroids are administered to nursing women.

Side-effects: Halcinonide is well tolerated. Where adverse reactions occur they are usually reversible on cessation of therapy. However the following side-effects have been reported usually with prolonged usage:

Dermatologic – impaired wound healing, thinning of the skin, petechiae and ecchymoses, facial erythema and telangiectasia, increased sweating, purpura, striae, hirsutism, acneiform eruptions, lupus erythematosus-like lesions and suppressed reaction to skin tests. These effects may be enhanced with occlusive dressings.

Oedema and electrolyte imbalance have not been observed even when high topical dosage has been used. The possibility of the systemic effects which are associated with all steroid therapy should be considered.

Overdosage: Topically applied corticosteroids can be absorbed in sufficient amounts to produce systemic effects (see *Side-effects*).

In the event of accidental ingestion, the patient should be observed and treated symptomatically.

Pharmaceutical precautions *Storage:* Halciderm should be stored below 25°C.

Dilution: Due to special formulation of topical Halciderm, normal dermatological diluents should not be used. For further information consult the manufacturer.

Legal category POM.

Package quantities Tubes containing 30 g.

Further information Halciderm contains halcinonide 0.1%, dissolved in the non-aqueous phase of the formulation.

Product licence number 0034/0160.

HYDREA* CAPSULES

Qualitative and quantitative composition Pink, opaque capsule body with green, opaque cap, printed in black with 'BMS 303' containing 500 mg of hydroxyurea

Pharmaceutical form Hard gelatin capsule.

Clinical particulars
Therapeutic indications: The treatment of chronic myeloid leukaemia.

The treatment of cancer of the cervix in conjunction with radiotherapy.

Posology and method of administration:
Adults: Treatment regimens can be continuous or intermittent. The continuous regimen is particularly suitable for chronic myeloid leukaemia, while the intermittent regimen, with its diminished effect on the bone marrow, is more satisfactory for the management of cancer of the cervix.

Hydrea should be started 7 days before concurrent irradiation therapy. If Hydrea is used concomitantly with radiotherapy, adjustment of radiation dosage is not usually necessary.

An adequate trial period for determining the anti-neoplastic effect of Hydrea is six weeks. Where there is a significant clinical response therapy may be continued indefinitely, provided that the patient is kept under adequate observation and shows no unusual or severe reactions. Therapy should be interrupted if the white cell count drops below 2.5×10^9/L or the platelet count below 100×10^9/L.

Continuous therapy: Hydrea 20-30 mg/kg should be given daily in single doses. Dosage should be based on the patient's actual or ideal weight, whichever is the less. Therapy should be monitored by repeat blood counts.

Intermittent therapy: Hydrea 80 mg/kg in single doses should be given every third day. Using the intermittent regimes the likelihood of WBC depression is diminished, but if low counts are produced, 1 or more doses of Hydrea should be omitted.

Concurrent use of Hydrea with other myelosuppressive agents may require adjustments of dosages.

Children: Because of the rarity of these conditions in children, dosage regimens have not been established.

Elderly: Elderly patients may be more sensitive to the effects of hydroxyurea, and may require a lower dosage regimen.

NB: If the patient prefers, or is unable to swallow capsules, the contents of the capsules may be emptied into a glass of water and taken immediately. The contents of capsules should not be inhaled or allowed to come into contact with the skin or mucous membranes. Spillages must be wiped immediately.

Contra-indications: Marked leucopenia (< 2.5 wbc $\times 10^9$/L), thrombocytopenia ($< 100 \times 10^9$/L), or severe anaemia and those who have previously shown hypersensitivity to Hydrea.

Special warnings and special precautions for use: The complete status of the blood, including bone marrow examination, if indicated, as well as kidney function and liver function should be determined prior to, and repeatedly during, treatment. The determination of haemoglobin level, total leukocyte counts, and platelet counts should be performed at least once a week throughout the course of hydroxyurea therapy. If WBC falls below 2.5×10^9/L or platelet count to $<100 \times 10^9$/L, therapy should be interrupted. Counts should be rechecked after 3 days and treatment resumed when they rise significantly towards normal.

Severe anaemia must be corrected with whole blood replacement before initiating therapy with Hydroxyurea. If, during treatment, anaemia occurs, correct without interrupting Hydrea therapy. Erythrocytic abnormalities; megaloblastic erythropoeisis, which is self-limiting, is often seen early in the course of hydroxyurea therapy. The morphologic change resembles pernicious anaemia, but is not related to vitamin B_{12} or folic acid deficiency. Hydroxyurea may also delay plasma iron clearance and reduce the rate of iron utilization by erythrocytes but it does not appear to alter the red blood cell survival time.

Hydroxyurea should be used with caution in patients with marked renal dysfunction.

In patients receiving long-term therapy with hydroxyurea for myeloproliferative disorders, such as polycythemia, secondary leukaemia has been reported. It is unknown whether this leukaemogenic effect is secondary to hydroxyurea or associated with the patient's underlying disease.

The possibility of an increase in serum uric acid, resulting in the development of gout or, at worst, uric acid nephropathy, should be borne in mind in patients treated with hydroxyurea, especially when used with other cytotoxic agents. It is therefore important to monitor uric acid levels regularly and maintain a high fluid intake during treatment.

Interaction with other medicinal products and other forms of interaction: The myelosuppressive activity may be potentiated by previous or concomitant radiotherapy or cytotoxic therapy.

Pregnancy and lactation: Drugs which affect DNA synthesis, such as hydroxyurea, may be potent mutagenic agents. The physician should carefully consider this possibility before administering this drug to male or female patients who may contemplate conception. Since Hydrea is a cytotoxic agent it has produced a teratogenic effect in some animal species.

In rats and dogs, high doses of hydroxyurea reduced sperm production. Hydroxyurea is excreted in human breast milk.

Hydrea should not normally be administered to patients who are pregnant, or to mothers who are breast feeding, unless the potential benefits outweigh the possible hazards.

When appropriate both male and female patients should be counselled concerning the use of contraceptive measures before and during treatment with Hydrea.

Effects on ability to drive and use machines: Not applicable.

Undesirable effects: Bone-marrow suppression is the major toxic effect of Hydrea, while leucopenia, thrombocytopenia and anaemia may occur in that order. Other side-effects are generally rare, but the following have been reported; anorexia, nausea, vomiting, diarrhoea, constipation, headache, drowsiness, dizziness, stomatitis, alopecia, skin rash, melaena, abdominal pain, disorientations, pulmonary oedema, hallucinations, convulsions, potentiation of the erythema caused by irradiation, skin ulceration, dysuria and impairment of renal tubular function accompanied by elevation in serum uric acid, blood urea nitrogen, and creatinine levels. Fever, chills, malaise, asthenia and elevation of hepatic enzymes have been reported. Acute pulmonary reactions consisting of diffuse pulmonary infiltrates/fibrosis, and dyspnoea have been rarely reported. Skin cancer has also been rarely reported.

In some patients, hyperpigmentation, erythema, atrophy of skin and nails, scaling, violet papules and alopecia have been observed following several years of long-term daily maintenance therapy with hydroxyurea.

Overdose: Immediate treatment consists of gastric lavage, followed by supportive therapy for the cardio-respiratory systems if required. In the long term, careful monitoring of the haemopoietic system is essential and, if necessary, blood should be transfused.

Acute mucocutaneous toxicity has been reported in patients receiving hydroxyurea at a dosage several times greater than that recommended. Soreness, violet erythema, oedema on palms and foot soles followed by scaling of hands and feet, intense generalised hyperpigmentation of skin, and severe acute stomatitis were observed.

Pharmacological properties

Pharmacodynamic properties: Hydroxyurea is an orally active antineoplastic agent. Although the mechanism of action has not yet been clearly defined, hydroxyurea appears to act by interfering with synthesis of DNA.

Pharmacokinetic properties: After oral administration hydroxyurea is readily absorbed from the gastrointestinal tract. Peak plasma concentrations are reached in 2 hours; by 24 hours the serum concentrations are virtually zero. Approximately 80% of an oral or intravenous dose of 7 to 30 mg/kg may be recovered from the urine within 12 hours. Hydroxyurea crosses the blood-brain barrier. Hydroxyurea is well distributed throughout the body.

Preclinical safety data: No further relevant data.

Pharmaceutical particulars

List of excipients: Citric acid, erythrosine, gelatin, indigotine, lactose, magnesium stearate, sodium lauryl sulphate, sodium phosphate, titanium dioxide, yellow iron oxide, opacode S-1-8100 HV black, purified water.

Incompatibilities: None known

Shelf life: Blister packs–24 months
Amber glass bottles–60 months

Special precautions for storage: Store below 25°C. Keep tightly closed.

Nature and contents of container: 100 capsules may be packaged in any of the following: amber glass bottles, PVC/PVDC blisters or PVC/ aluminum blisters.

Instructions for use/handling: Procedures for proper handling and disposal of anticancer drugs should be considered.

Date of approval/revision of SPC 4 January 1997

Legal category POM

KENALOG* INTRA-ARTICULAR / INTRAMUSCULAR INJECTION

Qualitative and quantitaive composition Kenalog Intra-articular / Intramuscular Injection contains triamcinolone acetonide 40 mg per ml of sterile suspension.

Pharmaceutical form Sterile aqueous suspension for injection.

Clinical particulars

Therapeutic indications:

Intra-articular use: for alleviating the joint pain, swelling and stiffness associated with rheumatoid arthritis and osteoarthrosis, with an inflammatory component; also for bursitis, epicondylitis, and tenosynovitis.

Intramuscular use: Where sustained systemic corticosteroid treatment is required: *Allergic states,* e.g. bronchial asthma, seasonal or perennial allergic rhinitis. In seasonal allergies, patients who do not respond to conventional therapy may achieve a remission of symptoms over the entire period with a single intramuscular injection (see *Dosage*); *Endocrine disorders,* e.g. primary or secondary adrenocortical insufficiency. *Collagen disorders,* e.g. during an exacerbation of maintenance therapy of selected cases of SLE or acute rheumatic carditis; *Dermatological diseases,* e.g. pemphigus, severe dermatitis and Stevens Johnson Syndrome; *Rheumatic, Gastrointestinal or Respiratory disorders*–as an adjunctive, short-term therapy; *Haematological disorders,* e.g. acquired (autoimmune) haemolytic anaemia; *Neoplastic diseases,* e.g. palliative management of leukaemia and lymphomas; *Renal disease,* such as acute interstitial nephritis, minimal change nephrotic syndrome or lupus nephritis.

Posology and method of administration: Kenalog is for Intra-articular/Intramuscular Injection. The safety and efficiacy of administration by other routes has yet to be established. Strict aseptic precautions should be observed. Since the duration of effect is variable, subsequent doses should be given when symptoms recur and not at set intervals.

Intra-articular Injection: For intra-articular administration or injection into tendon sheaths and bursae, the dose of Kenalog Injection may vary from 5 mg to 10 mg (0.125–0.25 ml) for smaller joints and up to 40 mg (1.0 ml) for larger joints, depending on the specific disease entity being treated. Single injections into several sites for multiple joint involvement, up to a total of 80 mg, have been given without undue reactions.

It is recommended that, when injections are given into the sheaths of short tendons, Adcortyl Injection (triamcinolone acetonide 10 mg/ml) should be used (see under *Precautions,* re Achilles tendon).

Intramuscular injection: to avoid the danger of subcutaneous fat atrophy, it is important to ensure that deep intramuscular injection is given into the gluteal site. The deltoid should not be used. Alternate sides should be used for subsequent injections.

Adults and children over 12 Years: The suggested initial dose is 40 mg (1.0 ml) injected deeply into the upper, outer quadrant of the gluteal muscle. Subsequent dosage depends on the patient's response and period of relief. Patients with hay fever or pollen asthma who do not respond to conventional therapy may obtain a remission of symptoms lasting throughout the pollen season after a single dose of 40-100 mg given when allergic symptoms appear (see *Warnings* and *Precautions.*)

Elderly: Treatment of elderly patients, particularly if long term, should be planned bearing in mind the more serious consequences of the common side effects of corticosteroids in old age, especially osteoporosis, diabetes, hypertension, susceptibility to infection and thinning of the skin. Close clinical supervision is required to avoid life-threatening reactions.

Children from 6-12 years of age: The suggested initial dose of 40 mg (1.0 ml injected deeply into the gluteal muscle should be scaled according to the severity of symptoms and the age and weight of the child. Kenalog is not recommended for children under six years. Growth and development of children on prolonged corticosteroid therapy should be carefully observed (see *Warnings* and *Precautions*).

Contra-indications: Hypersensitivity to any of the ingredients.

Systemic infections unless specific anti-infective therapy is employed.

Administration by intravenous or intrathecal injection.

Special warnings and special precautions for use:

Warnings – Intra-articular injection: Patients should be specifically warned to avoid over-use of joints in which symptomatic benefit has been obtained. Severe joint destruction with necrosis of bone may occur if repeated intra-articular injections are given over a long period of time. Care should be taken if injections are given into tendon sheaths to avoid injection into the tendon itself.

Due to the absence of a true tendon sheath, the Achilles tendon should not be injected with depot corticosteroids.

Intramuscular injection: During prolonged therapy a liberal protein intake is essential to counteract the tendency to gradual weight loss sometimes associated with negative nitrogen balance and wasting of skeletal muscle.

Precautions: Administration by non-approved routes (see *Posology and method of administration*).

Intra-articular injection should not be carried out in the presence of active infection in or near joints. The preparation should not be used to alleviate joint pain arising from infectious states such as gonococcal or tubercular arthritis.

Undesirable effects may be minimised using the lowest effective dose for the minimum period, and by administering the daily requirement, whenever possible, as a single morning dose on alternate days. Frequent patient review is required to titrate the dose appropriately against disease activity (see dosage section).

Adrenal cortical atrophy develops during prolonged therapy and may persist for years after stopping treatment. Withdrawal of corticosteroids after prolonged therapy must, therefore, always be gradual to avoid acute adrenal insufficiency and should be tapered off over weeks or months according to the dose and duration of treatment. During prolonged therapy any intercurrent illness, trauma or surgical procedure will require a temporary increase in dosage. If corticosteroids have been stopped following prolonged therapy they may need to be reintroduced temporarily.

Patients should carry steroid treatment cards which give clear guidance on the precautions to be taken to minimise risk and which provide details of prescriber, drug, dosage and the duration of treatment.

Suppression of the inflammatory response and immune function increases the susceptibility to infections and their severity. The clinical presentation may often be atypical and serious infections such as septicaemia and tuberculosis may be masked and may reach an advanced stage before being recognised.

Chickenpox is of particular concern since this normally minor illness may be fatal in immunosuppressed patients. Patients (or parents of children receiving Kenalog Injection) without a definite history of chickenpox should be advised to avoid close personal contact with chickenpox or herpes zoster. If exposed they should seek urgent medical attention. Passive immunisation with varicella zoster immunoglobulin (VZIG) is needed by exposed non- immune patients who are receiving systemic corticosteroids or who have used them within the previous 3 months; this should be given within 10 days of exposure to chickenpox. If a diagnosis of chickenpox is confirmed, the illness warrants specialist care and urgent treatment. Corticosteroids should not be stopped and the dose may need to be increased.

During corticosteroid therapy antibody response will be reduced and therefore affect the patient's response to vaccines. Live vaccines should not be administered.

Special precautions: Particular care is required when considering use of systemic corticosteroids in patients with the following conditions and frequent patient monitoring is necessary.

Recent intestinal anastomoses, diverticulitis, thrombophlebitis, existing or previous history of severe affective disorders (especially previous steroid psychosis), exanthematous disease, chronic nephritis, or renal insufficiency, metastatic carcinoma, osteoporosis (post-menopausal females are particularly at risk); in patients with an active peptic ulcer (or a history of peptic ulcer). Myasthenia gravis. Latent or healed tuberculosis; in the presence of local or systemic viral infection, systemic fungal infections or in active infections not controlled by antibiotics. In acute psychoses; in acute glomerulonephritis. Hypertension; congestive heart failure; glaucoma (or a family history of glaucoma), previous steroid myopathy or epilepsy. Liver failure.

Corticosteroid effects may be enhanced in patients with hypothyroidism or cirrhosis.

Diabetes may be aggravated, necessitating a higher insulin dosage. Latent diabetes mellitus may be precipitated.

Menstrual irregularities may occur, and this possibility should be mentioned to female patients.

Rare instances of anaphylactoid reactions have occurred in patients receiving corticosteroids, especially when a patient has a history of drug allergies.

All corticosteroids increase calcium excretion

Aspirin should be used cautiously in conjunction with corticosteroids in patients with hypoprothrombinaemia.

Use in children: Kenalog is not recommended for children under six years. Corticosteroids cause dose-related growth retardation in infancy, childhood and adolescence which may be irreversible, therefore growth and development of children on prolonged corticosteroid therapy should be carefully observed.

Use in elderly: The common adverse effects of systemic corticosteroids may be associated with more serious consequences in old age, especially osteoporosis, hypertension, hypokalaemia, diabetes, susceptibility to infection and thinning of the skin. Close clinical supervision is required to avoid life-threatening reactions.

Interactions with other medicinal products and other forms of interaction: Barbiturates, phenytoin, rifampicin, rifabutin, carbamazepine, primidone and aminoglutethimide may enhance the metabolic clearance of corticosteroids, resulting in decreased therapeutic effects.

Corticosteroids antagonise the effects of hypoglycaemic agents (including insulin), anti-hypertensives and diuretics. The hypokalaemic effects of acetazolamide, loop diuretics, thiazide diuretics and carbenoxolone are enhanced.

The efficacy of coumarin anticoagulants may be enhanced by concurrent corticosteroid therapy and close monitoring of the INR or prothrombin time is required to avoid spontaneous bleeding.

The renal clearance of salicylates is increased by corticosteroids and steroid withdrawal may result in salicylate intoxication.

Pregnancy and lactation: Corticosteroids are not recommended for pregnant patients, particularly in the first trimester, or for nursing mothers, except when the disease for which they are indicated warrants their use. When corticosteroids are essential however, patients with normal pregnancies may be treated as though they were in the non-gravid state.

There is evidence of harmful effects in pregnancy in animals. There may be a small risk of cleft palate and intra-uterine growth retardation. Hypoadrenalism may occur in the neonate. Patients with pre-eclampsia or fluid retention require close monitoring.

Corticosteroids are found in breast milk.

Infants born of mothers who have received substantial doses of corticosteroids during pregnancy or during breast feeding should be carefully observed for signs of hypoadrenalism. Maternal treatment should be carefully documented in the infant's medical records to assist in follow up.

Effects on ability to drive and use machines: None known.

Undesirable effects: Where adverse reactions occur they are usually reversible on cessation of therapy. The incidence of predictable side-effects, including hypothalamic-pituitary-adrenal suppression correlate with the relative potency of the drug, dosage, timing of administration and duration of treatment (see *Warnings* and *Precautions*).

Absorption of triamcinolone following injection by the intra-articular route is rare. However, patients should be watched closely for the following adverse reactions which may be associated with any corticosteroid therapy:

Anti-inflammatory and immunosuppressive effects: Increased susceptibility and severity of infections with suppression of clinical symptoms and signs, opportunistic infections, recurrence of dormant tuberculosis (see *Warnings* and *Precautions*).

Fluid and electrolyte disturbances: sodium retention, fluid retention, congestive heart failure in susceptible patients, potassium loss, cardiac arrhythmias or ECG changes due to potassium deficiency, hypokalaemic alkalosis, increased calcium excretion and hypertension.

Musculoskeletal: muscle weakness, fatigue, steroid myopathy, loss of muscle mass, osteoporosis, avascular osteonecrosis, vertebral compression fractures, delayed healing of fractures, aseptic necrosis of femoral and humeral heads, pathological fractures of long bones and spontaneous fractures, tendon rupture.

Gastrointestinal: dyspepsia, peptic ulcer with possible subsequent perforation and haemorrhage, pancreatitis, abdominal distension and ulcerative oesophagitis, candidiasis.

Dermatological: impaired wound healing, thin fragile skin, petechiae and ecchymoses, facial erythema, increased sweating, purpura, striae, hirsutism, acneiform eruptions, lupus erythematous-like lesions and suppressed reactions to skin tests.

Neurological: euphoria, psychological dependence, depression, insomnia, convulsions, increased intracranial pressure with papilloedema (pseudo-tumour cerebri) usually after treatment, vertigo, headache, neuritis or paraesthesias and aggravation of pre-existing psychiatric conditions and epilepsy.

Endocrine: menstrual irregularities and amenorrhoea; development of the Cushingoid state; suppression of growth in childhood and adolescence; secondary adrenocortical and pituitary unresponsiveness, particularly in times of stress (e.g. trauma, surgery or illness); decreased carbohydrate tolerance; manifestations of latent diabetes mellitus and increased requirements for insulin or oral hypoglycaemic agents in diabetes, weight gain. Negative protein and calcium balance. Increased appetite.

Ophthalmic: posterior supcapsular cataracts, increased intraocular pressure, glaucoma, exophthalmos, papilloedema, corneal or scleral thinning, exacerbation of ophthalmic viral or fungal diseases.

Others: necrotising angiitis, thrombophlebitis, thromboembolism, leucocytosis, insomnia, syncopal episodes and anaphylactoid reactions, particularly where there is a history of drug allergies.

Withdrawal symptoms and signs: On withdrawal, fever, myalgia, arthralgia, rhinitis, conjunctivitis, painful itchy skin nodules and weight loss may occur. Too rapid a reduction in dose following prolonged treatment can lead to acute adrenal insufficiency, hypotension and death (see *Warnings* and *Precautions*).

Intra-articular injection: Reactions following intra-articular administration have been rare. In a few instances, transient flushing and dizziness have occurred. Pain and other local symptoms may continue for a short time before effective relief is obtained, but an increase in joint discomfort has seldom occurred. Local fat atrophy may occur if the injection is not given into the joint space, but is temporary and disappears within a few weeks to months.

Overdose: Not applicable.

Pharmacological properties

Pharmacodynamic properties: Triamcinolone acetonide is a synthetic glucocorticoid with marked anti-inflammatory and anti-allergic actions.

Intra-articular injection: Following local injection, relief of pain and swelling and greater freedom of movement are usually obtained within a few hours.

Intramuscular injection: Provides an extended duration of therapeutic effect and fewer side effects of the kind associated with oral corticosteroid therapy, particularly gastro-intestinal reactions such as peptic ulceration. Studies indicate that, following a single intramuscular dose of 80 mg triamcinolone acetonide, adrenal suppression occurs within 24–48 hours and then gradually returns to normal, usually in approximately three weeks. This finding correlates closely with the extended duration of therapeutic action of triamcinolone acetonide.

Pharmacokinetic properties: Triamcinolone acetonide may be absorbed into the systemic circulation from synovial spaces. However clinically significant systemic levels after intra-articular injection are unlikely to occur except perhaps following treatment of large joints with high doses. Systemic effects do not ordinarily occur with intra-articular injections when the proper techniques of administration and the recommended dosage regimens are observed.

Triamcinolone acetonide is absorbed slowly, though almost completely, following depot administration by deep intramuscular injection; biologically active levels are achieved systemically for prolonged periods (weeks to months). In common with other corticosteroids, triamcinolone is metabolised largely hepatically but also by the kidney and is excreted in urine. The main metabolic route is 6-beta-hydroxylation; no significant hydrolytic cleavage of the acetonide occurs.

In view of the hepatic metabolism and renal excretion of triamcinolone acetonide, functional impairments of the liver or kidney may affect the pharmacokinetics of the drug.

Preclinical safety data: See *Pregnancy and lactation.*

Pharmaceutical particulars

List of excipients: Benzyl alcohol. polysorbate 80, sodium carboxymethylcellulose, sodium chloride, water.

Incompatibilities: The injection should not be physically mixed with other medicinal products.

Shelf life: 36 months

Special precautions for storage: In an upright position below 25°C: avoid freezing.

Nature and contents of container: Carton containing 5 x 1 ml glass vials or individually cartoned 1 ml and 2 ml syringes.

Instructions for use/handling: No special handling instructions.

Marketing authorisation number 0034/5045R

Date of approval/revision of SPC March 1997

Legal category POM

NYSTADERMAL* CREAM

Qualitative and quantitative composition A yellow to light buff cream containing in each gram nystatin 100,000 units and triamcinolone acetonide 0.1% w/w.

Pharmaceutical form Topical cream.

Clinical particulars

Therapeutic indications: Nystadermal Cream is indicated for those cases of cutaneous candidosis where the addition of a corticosteroid to the antifungal antibiotic may be beneficial in controlling the commonly associated inflammation and pruritus.

Nystadermal Cream will also be of benefit in those cases of eczema where *Candida* is either the precipitating cause, or present as a secondary invader.

Posology and method of administration:

Adults and children: To be applied to moist, weeping lesions two to four times daily.

Elderly: Corticosteroids should be used sparingly and for short periods of time, as natural thinning of the skin occurs in the elderly; hence, if, after about 7 days application, little or no improvement has occurred, cultural isolation of the offending organism should be followed by appropriate local or systemic antimicrobial therapy.

Contra-indications: There are no known contra-indications or special precautions for topical application of nystatin.

Corticosteroids are contra-indicated in tuberculous and most viral lesions of the skin, particularly herpes simplex and varicella. The products should not be used in fungal lesions not susceptible to nystatin or bacterial skin infections without suitable concomitant anti-infective therapy.

In patients with hypersensitivity to any of the components.

Should not be used for facial rosacea, acne vulgaris or perioral dermatitis.

Special warnings and special precautions for use: Adrenal suppression can occur, even without occlusion. The use of occlusive dressings should be avoided because of the increased risk of sensitivity reactions and increased percutaneous absorption.

If used in childhood, or on the face, courses should be limited to 5 days and occlusion should not be used.

Children: In infants, long-term continuous topical steroid therapy should be avoided. Courses should be limited to 5 days and occlusion should not be used.

Interactions with other medicinal products and other forms of interaction: None known.

Pregnancy and lactation: There is inadequate evidence of safety in human pregnancy. Topical administration of corticosteroids to pregnant animals can cause abnormalities of foetal development including cleft palate and intra-uterine growth retardation. There may, therefore, be a very small risk of such effects in the human foetus.

Effects on ability to drive and use machines: None known.

Undesirable effects: There have been no substantiated reports of sensitivity associated with topical nystatin.

Triamcinolone acetonide is well tolerated. Where adverse reactions occur they are usually reversible on cessation of therapy. However the following side effects have been reported usually with prolonged usage:

Dermatologic – impaired wound healing, thinning of the skin, petechiae and ecchymoses, facial erythema and telangiectasia, increased sweating, purpura, striae, hirsutism, acneiform eruptions, lupus erythematosus-like lesions and suppressed reactions to skin tests.

These effects may be enhanced with occlusive dressings.

Signs of systemic toxicity such as oedema and electrolyte imbalance have not been observed even when high topical dosage has been used. The possibility of the systemic effects which are associated with all steroid therapy should be considered.

Overdose: Topically applied corticosteroids can be absorbed in sufficient amounts to produce systemic effects (see Side-Effects).

In the event of accidental ingestion, the patient should be observed and treated symptomatically.

Pharmacological properties

Pharmacodynamic properties:

Actions: Triamcinolone acetonide is a potent fluorinated corticosteroid with anti-inflammatory, antipruritic and anti-allergic actions. Nystatin is an antifungal antibiotic active against a wide range of yeasts and yeast-like fungi including *Candida albicans.*

The cream is formulated for use on moist, weeping lesions.

Pharmacokinetic properties: In common with other corticosteroids, triamcinolone is absorbed from sites of local application. When administered under occlusive dressings, or when the skin is broken, a sufficient amount may be absorbed to produce systemic effects.

Nystatin is formulated in oral and topical dosage forms and is not systemically absorbed from any of these preparations.

Preclinical safety data: No further relevant information.

Pharmaceutical particulars

List of excipients: Aluminium hydroxide, antifoam emulsion, benzyl alcohol, macrogol ether, perfume, propylene glycol, sorbitol, titanium dioxide, white soft paraffin, water.

Incompatibilities: None known.

Shelf life: 24 months.

Special precautions for storage: Store below 25°C. Avoid freezing.

Nature and contents of container: Aluminium tubes of 15 g.

Instructions for use/handling: Not applicable.

Marketing authorisation number 0034/0131R.

Date of approval/revision of SPC 29 November 1995.

Legal category POM.

NYSTAN* CREAM, GEL AND OINTMENT

Qualitative and quantitative composition

Cream: Pale buff, containing 100,000 units per gram nystatin in a vanishing-cream base.

Ointment: Yellow to amber, containing 100,000 units per gram nystatin in plastibase.

Gel: Yellow to amber, opaque gel containing 100,000 units nystatin per gram.

Pharmaceutical form Topical cream, gel, ointment.

Clinical particulars

Therapeutic indications: For the treatment of cutaneous and mucocutaneous mycoses, particularly those caused by *Candida albicans.*

Posology and method of administration:

Adults and children: To be applied two to four times daily.

Elderly: No specific dosage recommendations or precautions.

Contra-indications: There are no known contra-indications or special precautions for topical application of nystatin.

Special warnings and special precautions for use:

Children: No specific precautions apply; systemic absorption is negligible.

Interactions with other medicinal products and other forms of interaction: None known.

Pregnancy and lactation: No specific precautions apply; systemic absorption is negligible.

Effects on ability to drive and use machines: None known.

Undesirable effects: There have been no substantiated reports of sensitivity associated with topical nystatin.

Overdose: Since absorption of nystatin from the gastro-intestinal tract is negligible, accidental ingestion causes no systemic toxicity.

Pharmacological properties

Pharmacodynamic properties:

Actions: Nystatin is a polyene, antifungal antibiotic active against a wide range of yeasts and yeast-like fungi, including *Candida albicans.*

Pharmacokinetic properties: Nystatin is formulated in oral and topical dosage forms and is not systemically absorbed from any of these preparations.

Preclinical safety data: No further relevant information.

Pharmaceutical particulars

List of excipients:

Cream: Aluminium hydroxide, antifoam emulsion, benzyl alcohol, macrogol ether, perfume, propylene glycol, sorbitol, titanium dioxide, white soft paraffin, water.

Ointment: Liquid paraffin and polyethylene resin.

Gel: Carbopol, chlorocresol, perfume, potassium phosphates, sodium hydroxide, water.

Incompatibilities: None known.

Shelf life: 48 months.

Special precautions for storage:

Cream and Gel: Store below 25°C. Avoid freezing.

Ointment: Store below 25°C.

Nature and contents of container:

Cream and Ointment: Aluminium tubes of 30 g.

Gel: Aluminium tubes of 30 g.

Instructions for use/handling: Not applicable.

Marketing authorisation numbers

Cream	0034/5058R
Ointment	0034/0161R
Gel	0034/0142R

Date of approval/revision of SPC

Cream	22 November 1995
Ointment	30 November 1995
Gel	28 November 1995

Legal category POM.

NYSTAN* ORAL SUSPENSION NYSTAN* FOR SUSPENSION NYSTAN* TABLETS

Qualitative and quantitative composition

Nystan Oral Suspension: Ready mixed oral suspension containing 100,000 units nystatin per ml.

Nystan for Suspension: Powder for reconstitution to provide oral suspension containing 100,000 units nystatin per ml.

Nystan Tablets: Tablets containing 500,000 units nystatin.

Pharmaceutical form Oral suspension, Granules for the preparation of oral suspension and oral tablets.

Clinical particulars

Therapeutic indications:

Suspension: The prevention and treatment of candidal infections of the oral cavity, oesophagus and intestinal tract. The suspension provides effective prophylaxis against oral candidosis in those born of mothers with vaginal candidosis.

Tablets: Tablets for intestinal candidosis. Also for use in patients who may be susceptible to candidal overgrowth, e.g. patients with malignant disease especially if receiving cytotoxic drugs, and those patients receiving high doses or prolonged courses of antibiotics or corticosteroids.

Posology and method of administration:

Reconstitution of granules for suspension: Add 23 ml water to the bottle and shake vigorously.

Adults: For the treatment of denture sores, and oral infections in adults caused by *C. albicans,* 1 ml of the suspension should be dropped into the mouth four times daily; it should be kept in contact with the affected areas as long as possible.

Tablets: For the treatment of intestinal candidosis 1 tablet four times daily, but this dose may be doubled. For prophylaxis a total daily dosage of 1 million units has been found to suppress the overgrowth of *C. albicans* in patients receiving broad-spectrum antibiotic therapy.

Administration should be continued for 48 hours after clinical cure to prevent relapse.

Children: Suspension: In intestinal and oral candidosis (thrush) in infants and children, 1 ml should be dropped into the mouth four times a day. The longer the suspension is kept in contact with the affected area in the mouth, before swallowing, the greater will be its effect.

For prophylaxis in the newborn the suggested dose is 1 ml once daily.

Elderly: No specific dosage recommendations or precautions.

Contra-indications: Contra-indicated in patients with a history of hypersensitivity to any of the components.

Special warnings and special precautions for use: Nystan Oral Suspension contains sugar. For children with disaccharide intolerance the sugar-free formulation, Nystan For Suspension, is recommended.

Nystan oral preparations should not be used for treatment of systemic mycoses.

Interactions with other medicinal products and other forms of interaction: None known.

Pregnancy and lactation: Animal reproductive studies have not been conducted with nystatin.

It is not known whether nystatin can cause foetal harm when administered to a pregnant woman, however absorption of nystatin from the gastro-intestinal tract is negligible. Nystatin should be prescribed during pregnancy only if the potential benefits to be derived outweigh the possible risks involved.

Nursing mothers: Though gastro-intestinal absorption is insignificant, it is not known whether nystatin is excreted in human breast milk and caution should be exercised when nystatin is prescribed for nursing women.

Effects on ability to drive and use machines: None known.

Undesirable effects: Nystatin is generally well tolerated by all age groups, even during prolonged use. Rarely, oral irritation or sensitisation may occur. Nausea has been reported occasionally during therapy.

Large oral doses of Nystatin have occasionally produced diarrhoea, gastro-intestinal distress, nausea and vomiting. Rash, including urticaria, has been reported rarely. Steven-Johnson Syndrome has been reported very rarely.

Overdose: Since the absorption of nystatin from the gastro-intestinal tract is negligible, overdosage or accidental ingestion causes no systemic toxicity.

Pharmacological properties

Pharmacodynamic properties: Nystatin is an antifungal antibiotic active against a wide range of yeasts and yeast-like fungi, including *Candida albicans.*

Pharmacokinetic properties: Nystatin is formulated in oral and topical dosage forms and is not systemically absorbed from any of these preparations.

Preclinical safety data: No further relevant information.

Pharmaceutical particulars

List of excipients

Nystan Oral Suspension: Ethanol, flavours, glycerin, methyl parahydroxybenzoate, pH adjusters (hydrochloric acid, sodium hydroxide), propyl parahydroxybenzoate, sodium carboxymethylcellulose, sodium phosphate, sucrose, water.

Nystan for Suspension: Methyl parahydroxybenzoate, propyl parahydroxybenzoate, saccharin, saccharin sodium, sodium benzoate, sodium carboxymethylcellulose, water, wood cellulose.

Nystan Tablets: Carnauba wax, castor oil, chalk, iron oxide, lactose, magnesium stearate, maize starch, microcrystalline cellulose, polysorbate 20, polyvidone, shellac, sorbic acid, stearic acid, sucrose, talc, white beeswax.

Incompatibilities: None known.

Shelf life:

Ready-mixed suspension: 36 months.

Granules for suspension: 12 months.

Reconstituted suspension: 7 days.

Tablets: 36 months.

Special precautions for storage:

Nystan Suspension: Store below 25°C.

Nystan for Suspension: Store the dry powder below 25°C.

Tablets: Store below 25°C.

Nature and contents of container:

Nystan Oral Suspension: 30 ml amber glass bottle, packed in a cardboard carton with a graduated, polyethylene dropper.

Nystan For Suspension: 24 ml amber glass bottle, packed in a cardboard carton with a graduated, polyethylene dropper.

Tablets: Amber glass bottle of 56 tablets, packed in a cardboard carton.

Instructions for use/handling:

Suspension: Shake well before use.

Dilution is not recommended as this may reduce therapeutic efficacy.

Marketing authorisation numbers

Nystan Oral Suspension	0034/0130R
Nystan for Suspension	0034/5061R
Nystan Tablets	0034/5063R

Date of approval/revision of SPC

Nystan Oral suspension	28 November 1995
Nystan for Suspension	30 November 1995
Nystan Tablets	12 March 1996

Legal category POM.

NYSTAN* PASTILLES

Presentation Yellow-brown, aniseed flavoured soft pastille providing 100,000 units nystatin per pastille; containing sugar and cinnamon.

Other ingredients: Aniseed oil, cinnamon oil, dextrose monohydrate, gelatin, liquid glucose, pH adjusters (hydrochloric acid/potassium hydroxide), silicone antifoam emulsion, sucrose, water.

Uses *Actions:* Nystatin is an antifungal antibiotic active against a wide range of yeasts and yeast-like fungi, including *Candida albicans.*

Indications: For the treatment of oral candidosis.

Dosage and administration No food or drink should be taken for five minutes before or one hour after consumption of the pastille. The pastilles should be sucked slowly and retained in the mouth for as long as possible in accordance with the doctors instructions.

Adults and children: One pastille to be sucked slowly, four times a day for 7–14 days.

Elderly: No specific dosage recommendations or precautions.

Contra-indications, warnings, etc

Contra-indications: Contra-indicated in patients with a history of hypersensitivity to any of its components.

Precautions: The pastilles contain sugar and should be administered with caution to patients with disaccharide intolerance.

Nystan pastilles should not be used for the treatment of systemic mycoses.

Pregnancy and lactation: Animal reproductive studies have not been conducted with nystatin.

It is not known whether nystatin can cause foetal harm when administered to a pregnant woman, however absorption of nystatin from the gastro-intestinal tract is negligible. Nystatin should be prescribed during pregnancy only if the potential benefits to be derived outweigh the possible risks involved.

Though gastrointestinal absorption is insignificant, it is not known whether nystatin is excreted in human breast milk and caution should be exercised when nystatin is prescribed for nursing women.

Side-effects: Nystatin is generally well tolerated by all age groups, even during prolonged use. Rarely, oral irritation or sensitisation may occur. Nausea has been reported occasionally during therapy.

Large oral doses of nystatin have occasionally produced diarrhoea, gastrointestinal distress, nausea and vomiting. Rash, including urticaria, has been reported rarely. Stevens-Johnson Syndrome has been reported very rarely.

Overdosage: Since the absorption of nystatin from the gastro-intestinal tract is negligible, overdosage causes no systemic toxicity.

Pharmaceutical precautions *Storage:* Store below 25°C.

Legal category POM.

Package quantities Packs of 28 pastilles.

Further information The pastille allows longer contact of the active ingredient nystatin with the mucous membrane than liquid formulations.

Successful treatment of oral candidosis also includes good oral hygiene. Patients with dentures are advised to remove them whilst sucking the pastilles.

Product licence number 0034/0248.

NYSTAN* PESSARIES
NYSTAN* VAGINAL CREAM

Qualitative and quantitative composition

Pessaries: Each pessary contains 100,000 units nystatin.

Cream: Each 4 g application contains 100,000 units nystatin.

Pharmaceutical form

Vaginal tablet.

Cream.

Clinical particulars

Therapeutic indications: The treatment of candidal vaginitis.

Posology and method of administration:

Adults:

Pessaries: 1 or 2 pessaries should be inserted high into the vagina for 14 consecutive nights, or longer, regardless of any intervening menstrual period.

Cream: Insert 1 or 2 applications (of 4 g each) high into the vagina for 14 consecutive nights, or longer, regardless of any intervening menstrual period.

Children:

Cream: Vulvovaginal candidosis is rarely a problem in children. It is suggested that the vaginal cream is the most acceptable formulation for children.

Pessaries: Not recommended for children under 12 years.

Elderly: No specific dosage recommendations or precautions.

Contra-indications: There are no known contra-indications to the use of nystatin.

Special warnings and special precautions for use: Avoid contact between the cream and contraceptive diaphragms and condoms, since the rubber may be damaged by the preparation.

Interactions with other medicinal products and other forms of interaction: None known.

Pregnancy and lactation: There is no evidence that nystatin is absorbed systemically from the vagina. However, as with all drugs, caution should be exercised in pregnancy. Care should be taken while using an applicator to prevent the possibility of mechanical trauma.

Effects on ability to drive and use machines: None known.

Undesirable effects: Nystan is well tolerated and no substantiated sensitivity reactions have been associated with its use. Some transient local discomfort may be experienced.

Overdose: Since the absorption of nystatin from the gastro-intestinal tract is negligible, overdosage or accidental ingestion causes no systemic toxicity.

Pharmacological properties

Pharmacodynamic properties: Nystatin is an antifungal antibiotic active against a wide range of yeasts and yeast-like fungi, including *Candida albicans.*

Pharmacokinetic properties: Nystatin is formulated in oral and topical dosage forms and is not systemically absorbed from any of these preparations.

Preclinical safety data: No further relevant information.

Pharmaceutical particulars

List of excipients

Pessaries: Lactose, magnesium stearate, maize starch, microcrystalline cellulose.

Cream: Aluminium hydroxide, antifoam emulsion, benzyl alcohol, macrogol ether, pH adjusters (hydrochloric acid, sodium hydroxide), propylene glycol, sorbitol, water, white soft paraffin.

Incompatibilities: None known.

Shelf life

Pessaries: 12 months.

Cream: 24 months.

Special precautions for storage:

Pessaries: Store below 25°C.

Cream: Store below 25°C. Avoid freezing.

Nature and contents of container

Pessaries: Foil strip, packed in a carton with an applicator, in packs of 28 pessaries.

Cream: 60 g aluminium tube, packed in a cardboard carton with a vaginal applicator.

Instructions for use/handling: Dilution of the vaginal cream is not recommended as this may reduce therapeutic efficacy.

Marketing authorisation numbers

Pessaries	0034/5062R
Cream	0034/0137R

Date of approval/revision of SPC

Pessaries	6 September 1996
Cream	22 November 1995

Legal category POM

OPHTHAINE* SOLUTION

Qualitative and quantitative composition Ophthaine Solution contains proxymetacaine hydrochloride 0.5%, chlorbutol 0.2%, benzalkonium chloride 0.01%, glycerol, pH modifiers, water.

Pharmaceutical form Sterile, aqueous ophthalmic solution

Clinical particulars

Therapeutic indications: Topical anaesthesia in ophthalmic practice.

Posology and method of administration:

Adults and children: Administered by topical instillation into the eye. The recommended doses are as follows:

Deep anaesthesia: Instil 1 drop every five to ten minutes for 5-7 doses.

Removal of sutures: Instil 1 or 2 drops two or three minutes before removal of stitches.

Removal of foreign bodies: Instil 1 or 2 drops prior to operating.

Tonometry: Instil 1 or 2 drops immediately before measurement.

Elderly: No specific dosage recommendations or precautions.

Contra-indications: Patients with known hypersensitivity to proxymetacaine or any of the other components.

Special warnings and special precautions for use:

Precautions: Ophthaine solution is not intended for long-term use.

Ophthaine Solution is not miscible with fluorescein. However, the eye can be anaesthetised with Ophthaine Solution before fluorescein is administered.

Use cautiously and sparingly in patients with known allergies, cardiac disease, or hyperthyroidism.

Regular and prolonged use of a topical ocular anaesthetic, e.g. in conjunction with contact lens insertion, may cause softening and erosion of the corneal epithelium, which could produce corneal opacification with accompanying loss of vision.

Protection of the eye from irritating chemicals, foreign bodies and rubbing during the period of anaesthesia is very important. Tonometers soaked in sterilising or detergent solutions should be thoroughly rinsed with sterile distilled water prior to use. Patients should be advised to avoid touching the eye until the anaesthesia has worn off.

Interactions with other medicinal products and other forms of interaction: None known.

Pregnancy and lactation: Not applicable.

Effect on ability to drive and use machines: Not applicable.

Undesirable effects: Pupillary dilatation or cycloplegic effects have rarely been observed with Ophthaine Solution. Irritation of the conjunctiva or other toxic reactions attributable to the preparation have occurred only rarely. A severe, immediate-type apparently hyperallergic corneal reaction may rarely occur which includes acute, intense and diffuse epithelial keratitis; a grey ground-glass appearance; sloughing of large areas of necrotic epithelium; corneal filaments and sometimes, iritis with descemetitis.

Overdose: None known.

Pharmacological properties

Pharmacodynamic properties: Proxymetacaine hydrochloride is a rapidly acting local anaesthetic. With a single drop the onset of anaesthesia occurs in an average of 13 seconds and will persist for an average of 15 minutes.

Pharmacokinetic properties: No detectable systemic concentration of proxymetacaine has been recorded in patients following ocular administration of Ophthaine Solution.

Preclinical safety data: Minimal absorption with rapid hydrolysis of proxymetacaine.

Pharmaceutical particulars

List of excipients: Glycerol, pH modifiers, water.

Incompatibilities: None known.

Shelf life: 24 months.

Special precautions for storage: Store in a refrigerator (2-8°C). Do not freeze. Protect from light. If solution shows more than a very pale yellow colour, it should be discarded. The product should not be used one month after first opening the container.

Nature and contents of container: Bottles of 15 ml.

Instructions for use/handling: None.

Marketing authorisation number 0034/5064R

Date of approval/revision of SPC October 1996

Legal category POM

PRONESTYL* TABLETS

Presentation

Tablets: White, engraved Squibb and 754 on one side and scored on reverse, containing 250 mg procainamide hydrochloride.

Other ingredients: Ethylcellulose, lactose, magnesium stearate, maize starch, stearic acid, sucrose.

Uses

Actions: Procainamide is a class I antiarrhythmic agent (Vaughan Williams classification). Abnormal automaticity and excitability are reduced: the former by a slowing of the rate of diastolic phase 4 depolarisation; the latter by a reduction of the rate of rise of phase 0 depolarisation.

Action potention duration is prolonged but the effect on refractory period is greater.

These actions are apparent throughout the myocardium, and are most pronounced within the atria. Abnormal ectopic foci may be suppressed by the slowing of phase 4 depolarisation, while re-entrant tachyarrhythmias may be inhibited both by the reduced excitability of the myocardium and by the prolongation of the refractory period. In those arrhythmias not fully suppressed, procainamide is likely to slow the tachycardia.

Following oral administration therapeutic levels (3–10 mcg/ml) are usually obtained by 30 minutes, with maximal levels occurring after 60 minutes.

Indications: The treatment of atrial tachycardia.

The treatment of symptomatic or potentially malignant ventricular arrhythmias (i.e. extrasystoles or tachycardia).

The treatment or prophylaxis of symptomatic or potentially malignant ventricular arrhythmias following acute myocardial infarction.

Dosage and administration

Children: Pronestyl is not recommended.

Adults: Oral Pronestyl can be used for maintenance therapy once control of arrhythmias is achieved. Intravenous therapy is available for more serious tachyarrhythmias.

Plasma concentrations correlate well with therapeutic and toxic effects; consequently plasma level assays should be carried out if facilities are available. The usual effective antiarrhythmic serum concentration is 3–10 mcg/ml. Toxic manifestations are rare in concentrations less than 12 mcg/ml.

Oral therapy is preferred for treatment of arrhythmias which do not require immediate suppression, and for prevention of recurrence of serious arrhythmias after initial control by cardioversion, by intravenous Pronestyl Injection or by other antiarrhythmic therapy. Ideally, the oral dose and interval of administration should be adjusted for the individual patient, based on clinical assessment of the degree of underlying myocardial disease, the patient's age, and renal function.

As a general guide, for younger patients with normal renal function, an initial total daily oral dose of up to 50 mg/kg of body weight of Pronestyl Tablets may be used, given in divided doses, every three hours, to maintain therapeutic blood levels. For older patients, especially those over 50 years of age, or for patients with renal, hepatic, or cardiac insufficiency, lesser amounts or longer intervals may produce adequate blood levels. The initial total daily dose should be divided for administration at three, four, or six hour intervals as estimated for the patient's needs; then, the dose and interval should be adjusted for the individual.

To provide up to 50 mg per kg of body weight per day:

Patients weighing	
40–50 kg	250 mg 3 hrly to 500 mg 6 hrly
60–70 kg	375 mg 3 hrly to 750 mg 6 hrly
80–90 kg	500 mg 3 hrly to 1 g 6 hrly
More than 100 kg	625 mg 3 hrly to 1.25 g 6 hrly

Atrial arrhythmias: Higher dosages, than for ventricular arrhythmias, may be required (see 'Warnings and precautions').

Elderly: Reduction in dose or increase in dosage interval may be necessary to maintain constant blood levels without accumulation (see Dosage).

Patients with renal or hepatic impairment: Dose reduction or increase in dosage interval may be necessary to produce adequate blood levels without accumulation.

Contra-indications, warnings, etc

Contra-indications: Hypersensitivity to the drug is an absolute contra-indication. In this connection, cross sensitivity to procaine and related drugs must be borne in mind.

Procainamide should not be administered to patients with complete atrioventricular heart block or a high degree of A-V block or bifasicular block unless an electrical pacemaker is operative.

Systemic lupus erythematosus:

'Torsade de Pointes', a variant form of ventricular tachycardia associated with a prolonged QT interval, should not be treated with Pronestyl which may aggravate rather than suppress this arrhythmia.

Warnings and precautions: Myasthenia gravis: Patients with myasthenia gravis may show worsening of symptoms from procainamide due to its procaine-like effect on diminishing acetylcholine release at skeletal muscle motor nerve endings, so that procainamide administration may be hazardous without optimal adjustment of anticholinesterase medications and other precautions.

Digitalis intoxication: Procainamide may further depress conduction and ventricular asystole or fibrillation may result.

If the patient develops first degree heart block, dosage reduction and/or discontinuation of procainamide should be considered.

Caution in patients with congestive heart failure, acute ischaemic heart disease, cardiogenic shock or cardiomyopathy as even slight depression in myocardial contractility may reduce the cardiac output of the damaged heart.

Cardiotoxicity may be reflected by hypotension, excessive widening of the QRS complex or prolongation of the PR interval or the appearance of proarrhythmic effects.

In patients with significant impairment of renal or hepatic function, accumulation of Pronestyl may occur, leading to drug toxicity.

The electrophysiological action of procainamide may be affected by electrolyte imbalance.

Pregnancy and nursing mothers: Safety has not been established; therefore, Pronestyl should be used during pregnancy only if the possible benefits outweigh the potential risks involved. Procainamide crosses the placenta but the extent is unknown. Procainamide is excreted in breast milk; therefore, it should not be given to nursing mothers because of the potential risk of adverse reactions in the infant.

Side-effects: A lupus-like syndrome has been reported after prolonged courses of Pronestyl. The lupus-like syndrome seldom appears in less than two months, but is very common after six months. It is virtually completely reversible and tests for antinuclear factors are usually positive before clinical signs appear. It is perhaps more often observed in patients who are slow acetylators. If long-term treatment is considered desirable, it is advisable to undertake serological tests at no less than monthly intervals and to continue treatment for no longer than absolutely necessary.

Agranulocytosis is a rare side effect of prolonged procainamide therapy. Susceptibility to this is greater in the period following coronary bypass surgery. The patient should be instructed to report any soreness of the mouth, throat, or gums, unexplained fever or any symptoms of upper respiratory tract infection. If any of these should occur, and leucocyte counts indicate cellular depression, Pronestyl therapy should be discontinued, and appropriate treatment should be instituted immediately.

Nausea, vomiting, diarrhoea, abdominal pain, anorexia, bitter taste, mental depression, psychoses with hallucinations, dizziness, headache, pruritus, chills, fever, hepatitis and allergic reactions (such as vasculitis, eosinophilia, skin reactions or angioneurotic oedema) may occur infrequently. They are usually not sufficiently severe to discontinue treatment.

Neutropenia, thrombocytopenia or haemolytic anaemia may rarely be encountered.

As with all other class 1 agents, proarrhythmic effects may occur.

Drug interactions:

Amiodarone: Concomitant use of amiodarone may result in increased plasma procainamide concentrations and subsequent toxicity.

Other antiarrhythmic drugs: Additive effects can occur and dosage reduction may be necessary.

Antihypertensive agents: Procainamide may produce an additive effect and dosage adjustment may be necessary.

Anticholinergic drugs: Additive antivagal effects on A-V nodal conduction may occur.

Neuromuscular blocking agents: Possibly reduce dosage of neuromuscular blocking drugs, as procainamide may reduce acetylcholine release.

Captopril: There have been reports of neutropenia and/or Stevens-Johnson syndrome in patients on procainamide plus captopril. Although a causal relationship has not been established, this combination should only be used with caution, especially in patients with impaired renal function.

Sulphonamides: p-amino benzoic acid is a metabolite of procainamide and can inhibit the action of sulphonamides.

Trimethoprim: The renal clearance of procainamide is reduced by trimethoprim resulting in increased pharmacodynamic response.

Pharmacokinetic interactions: The elimination of procainamide may be decreased by cimetidine or propranolol, and increased by alcohol.

Overdosage: After intravenous administration, but seldom after oral, hypotension may occur. Progressive widening of the QRS or A-V conduction block may be seen as may increased ventricular extrasystoles or even ventricular tachycardia or fibrillation. Procainamide and n-acetyl procainamide are removed by haemodialysis but not by peritoneal dialysis. No specific antidote is known.

Overdosage should be managed by general supportive measures and close observation. Fluid expansion and the infusion of noradrenaline (8 micrograms/ml in Sodium Chloride Injection BP) may be useful for hypotension; insertion of a temporary ventricular pacing system may be beneficial.

Pharmaceutical precautions

Storage: Store below 25°C.

Dispense only in dry, well-sealed containers.

Legal category POM.

Package quantities Bottles of 100.

Further information Procainamide is less readily hydrolysed than procaine and plasma levels decline slowly – about 10–20% per hour. The drug is excreted primarily in the urine, about 10% as free and conjugated p-aminobenzoic acid and about 60% in the unchanged form. The remainder is mainly excreted as n-acetyl procainamide.

The formation of n-acetyl procainamide will depend upon the acetylator status of the patient. As this metabolite also has significant antiarrhythmic activity and a somewhat slower renal clearance than procainamide, both acetylation rate capability and renal function will affect the duration of action.

Product licence number 0034/5066R.

PRONESTYL* SOLUTION FOR INJECTION

Presentation

Solution for Injection: A sterile, aqueous solution containing 100 mg/ml procainamide hydrochloride. Other ingredients: Benzyl alcohol, sodium hydroxide, sodium metabisulphite, water.

Uses

Actions: Procainamide is a class I antiarrhythmic agent (Vaughan Williams classification). Abnormal automaticity and excitability are reduced: the former by a slowing of the rate of diastolic phase 4 depolarisation; the latter by a reduction of the rate of rise of phase 0 depolarisation.

Action potention duration is prolonged but the effect on refractory period is greater.

These actions are apparent throughout the myocardium, and are most pronounced within the atria. Abnormal ectopic foci may be suppressed by the slowing of phase 4 depolarisation, while re-entrant tachyarrhythmias may be inhibited both by the reduced excitability of the myocardium and by the prolongation of the refractory period. In those arrhythmias not fully suppressed, procainamide is likely to slow the tachycardia.

The action of procainamide begins almost immediately after intravenous administration with maximal effects being observed at 30 minutes.

Indications: The treatment of symptomatic or potentially malignant ventricular arrhythmias (i.e. extrasystoles or tachycardia).

The treatment or prophylaxis of symptomatic or potentially malignant ventricular arrhythmias following acute myocardial infarction.

Dosage and administration

Children: Pronestyl is not recommended.

Adults: Intravenous therapy should be reserved for more serious tachyarrhythmias, in which case administration should be under continuous ECG monitoring. Once control is achieved oral Pronestyl can be substituted (see data sheet for Pronestyl Tablets).

Plasma concentrations correlate well with therapeutic and toxic effects; consequently plasma level assays should be carried out if facilities are available. The usual effective antiarrhythmic serum concentration is 3–10 mcg/ml. Toxic manifestations are rare in concentrations less than 12 mcg/ml.

Administration: To initiate therapy, the dose should be diluted in 5% Dextrose Injection BP immediately prior to administration to facilitate control of dosage rate; the dose should be given at a rate no greater than 50 mg per minute under ECG control, and blood pressure must be taken before each dose (see Precautions). Slow administration allows for some initial tissue distribution.

Acute control of tachyarrhythmia: 100 mg may be given every 5 minutes by slow injection, at a rate not exceeding 50 mg in any one minute, until the arrhythmia is suppressed or a maximum dosage of 1 gram has been administered.

Some effects may be seen after the first 100 or 200 mg and it is unusual to require more than 500 to 600 mg to achieve satisfactory antiarrhythmic effects.

Chronic suppression of arrhythmias: An alternative approach to achieving and then maintaining a therapeutic plasma concentration is to infuse 500 to 600 mg of procainamide at a constant rate over a period of 25 to 30 minutes and then change to another infusion for maintenance at a rate of 2 to 6 mg/min (see Table below).

Intravenous therapy should be terminated as soon as the patient's basic cardiac rhythm appears to be stabilized and, if indicated, the patient should be placed on oral antiarrhythmic maintenance therapy.

A period of 3 to 4 hours (one half-life) should elapse after the last intravenous dose of procainamide before administering the first oral dose of procainamide.

Dilutions and rates for intravenous infusions†

Approximate final concentration	*Infusion bottle size (ml)*	*ml of Pronestyl (100 mg/ml) to be added*	*Infusion rate*
0.2% (2 mg/ml)	500 250	10 5	1–3 ml/min
0.4% (4 mg/ml)	500 250	20 10	0.5–1.5 ml/min

†*Caution:* The flow rate of all intravenous infusion solutions must be closely monitored. These dilutions are calculated to deliver 2–6 mg per minute at the infusion rates listed.

Elderly: Reduction in dose or increase in dosage interval may be necessary to maintain constant blood levels without accumulation (see Dosage).

Patients with renal or hepatic impairment: Dose reduction or increase in dosage interval may be necessary to produce adequate blood levels without accumulation.

Contra-indications, warnings, etc

Contra-indications: Hypersensitivity to the drug is an absolute contra-indication. In this connection, cross sensitivity to procaine and related drugs must be borne in mind.

Procainamide should not be administered to patients with complete atrioventricular heart block or a high degree of A-V block or bifasicular block unless an electrical pacemaker is operative.

'Torsade de Pointes', a variant form of ventricular tachycardia associated with a prolonged QT interval, should not be treated with Pronestyl which may aggravate rather than suppress this arrhythmia.

Warnings and precautions: Myasthenia gravis: Patients with myasthenia gravis may show worsening of symptoms from procainamide due to its procaine-like effect on diminishing acetylcholine release at skeletal muscle motor nerve endings, so that procainamide administration may be hazardous without optimal adjustment of anticholinesterase medications and other precautions.

Digitalis intoxication: Procainamide may further depress conduction and ventricular asystole or fibrillation may result.

If the patient develops first degree heart block, dosage reduction and/or discontinuation of procainamide should be considered.

Caution in patients with congestive heart failure, acute ischaemic heart disease, cardiogenic shock or cardiomyopathy as even slight depression in myocardial contractility may reduce the cardiac output of the damaged heart.

Hypotension may occur when Pronestyl is administered intravenously. Patients should be kept in a supine position and blood pressure readings made frequently. If hypotension occurs the rate of injection should be reduced or temporarily discontinued and, if necessary, a vasopressor agent administered cautiously.

Intravenous administration should be monitored by ECG. Excessive widening of the QRS complex or prolongation of the P-R interval suggests the occurrence of myocardial toxicity and Pronestyl administration should be stopped. Cardiotoxicity may also be reflected by the appearance of proarrhythmic effects.

In patients with significant impairment of renal or hepatic function, accumulation of Pronestyl may occur, leading to drug toxicity.

The electrophysiological action of procainamide may be affected by electrolyte imbalance.

Pregnancy and nursing mothers: Safety has not been established: therefore, Pronestyl should be used during pregnancy only if the possible benefits outweigh the potential risks involved. Procainamide crosses the placenta but the extent is unknown. Procainamide is excreted in breast milk; therefore, it should not be given to nursing mothers because of the potential risk of adverse reactions in the infant.

Side-effects: A lupus-like syndrome has been reported after prolonged courses of Pronestyl. The lupus-like syndrome seldom appears in less than two months, but is very common after six months. It is virtually completely reversible and tests for antinuclear factors are usually positive before clinical signs appear. It is perhaps more often observed in patients who are slow acetylators. If long-term treatment is considered desirable, it is advisable to undertake serological tests at no less than monthly intervals and to continue treatment for no longer than absolutely necessary.

Agranulocytosis is a rare side effect of prolonged procainamide therapy. Susceptibility to this is greater in the period following coronary bypass surgery. The patient should be instructed to report any soreness of the mouth, throat, or gums, unexplained fever or any symptoms of upper respiratory tract infection. If any of these should occur, and leucocyte counts indicate cellular depression, Pronestyl therapy should be discontinued, and appropriate treatment should be instituted immediately.

Nausea, vomiting, diarrhoea, abdominal pain, anorexia, bitter taste, mental depression, psychoses with hallucinations, dizziness, headache, pruritus, chills, fever, hepatitis and allergic reactions (such as vasculitis, eosinophilia, skin reactions or angioneurotic oedema) may occur infrequently. They are usually not sufficiently severe to discontinue treatment.

Neutropenia, thrombocytopenia or haemolytic anaemia may rarely be encountered.

As with all other class 1 agents, proarrhythmic effects may occur.

Pronestyl injection contains sodium metabisulphite. This ingredient has been associated with allergic reactions in sensitive individuals.

Drug interactions:

Amiodarone: Concomitant use of amiodarone may result in increased plasma procainamide concentrations and subsequent toxicity. The dosage of intravenous procainamide should be reduced by 20% to 30% during concomitant administration.

Other antiarrhythmic drugs: Additive effects can occur and dosage reduction may be necessary.

Antihypertensive agents: Procainamide may produce an additive effect and dosage adjustment may be necessary.

Anticholinergic drugs: Additive antivagal effects on A-V nodal conduction may occur.

Neuromuscular blocking agents: Possibly reduce dosage of neuromuscular blocking drugs as procainamide may reduce acetylcholine release.

Captopril: There have been reports of neutropenia and/or Stevens-Johnson syndrome in patients on procainamide plus captopril. Although a causal relationship has not been established, this combination should only be used with caution, especially in patients with impaired renal function.

Sulphonamides: p-amino benzoic acid is a metabolite of procainamide and can inhibit the action of sulphonamides.

Trimethoprim: The renal clearance of procainamide is reduced by trimethoprim resulting in increased pharmacodynamic response.

Pharmacokinetic interactions: The elimination of procainamide may be decreased by cimetidine or propranolol, and increased by alcohol.

Overdosage: After intravenous administration, but seldom after oral, hypotension may occur. Progressive widening of the QRS or A-V conduction block may be seen as may increased ventricular extrasystoles or even ventricular tachycardia or fibrillation. Procainamide and n-acetyl procainamide are removed by haemodialysis but not by peritoneal dialysis. No specific antidote is known.

Overdosage should be managed by general supportive measures and close observation. Fluid expansion and the infusion of noradrenaline (8 micrograms/ml in Sodium Chloride Injection BP) may be useful for hypotension; insertion of a temporary ventricular pacing system may be beneficial.

Pharmaceutical precautions

Storage: Store below 25°C.

Legal category POM.

Package quantities Solution 100 mg/ml: 10 ml multidose vials.

Further information Procainamide is less readily hydrolysed than procaine and plasma levels decline slowly – about 10–20% per hour. The drug is excreted primarily in the urine, about 10% as free and conjugated p-aminobenzoic acid and about 60% in the unchanged form. The remainder is mainly excreted as n-acetyl procainamide.

The formation of n-acetyl procainamide will depend upon the acetylator status of the patient. As this metabolite also has significant antiarrhythmic activity and a somewhat slower renal clearance than procainamide, both acetylation rate capability and renal function will affect the duration of action.

Product licence number 0034/5065R.

STARIL* TABLETS

Qualitative and quantitative composition Staril tablets contain 10 mg or 20 mg fosinopril sodium.

Pharmaceutical form Tablets.

Clinical particulars

Therapeutic indications:

Hypertension: Staril is indicated in the treatment of hypertension. Staril may be used alone as initial therapy or in combination with other antihypertensive agents. The antihypertensive effects of Staril and diuretics used concomitantly are approximately additive.

Heart failure: Staril is indicated for the treatment of heart failure in combination with a diuretic. In these patients, Staril improves symptoms and exercise tolerance, reduces severity of heart failure and decreases the frequency of hospitalisation for heart failure.

Posology and method of administration:

Adults and children over 12 years

Hypertensive patients not being treated with diuretics: The dose range is 10 to 40 mg per day administered in a single dose and without regard to meals. The normal starting dose for patients is 10 mg once a day. Dosage may need to be adjusted after approximately 4 weeks according to blood pressure response. No additional blood pressure lowering is achieved with doses greater than 40 mg daily. If blood pressure is not adequately controlled with Staril alone, a diuretic can be added.

Hypertensive patients being treated with concomitant diuretic therapy: The diuretic should preferably be discontinued for several days prior to beginning therapy with Staril to reduce the risk of an excessive hypotensive response. If blood pressure is inadequately controlled after an observation period of approximately 4 weeks, diuretic therapy may be resumed. Alternatively, if diuretic therapy cannot be discontinued, an initial dose of 10 mg of Staril should be used with careful medical supervision for several hours, until blood pressure has stabilised. In diuretic treated hypertensive patients, mean cerebral blood flow is maintained between 4 and 24 hours after Staril, despite significant reduction in blood pressure.

Heart failure: The recommended initial dose is 10 mg once daily, initiated under close medical supervision. If the initial dose is well tolerated patients should be titrated to a dose of up to 40 mg once daily. The appearance of hypotension after the initial dose should not preclude careful dose titration of Staril, following effective management of the hypotension. Staril should be used in conjunction with a diuretic.

Heart failure – high risk patients: It is recommended that treatment is initiated in hospital for patients with severe cardiac failure (NYHA IV) and those at particular risk of first dose hypotension, i.e. patients on multiple or high dose diuretics (e.g. >80 mg frusemide), patients with hypovolaemia, hyponatraemia (serum sodium <130 meq/l), pre-existing hypotension (systolic blood pressure <90 mmHg), patients with unstable cardiac failure and those on high-dose vasodilator therapy.

Children: The paediatric use of Staril has not been established.

Elderly: No dosage reduction is necessary in patients with clinically normal renal and hepatic function as no significant differences in the phamacokinetic parameters or antihypertensive effect of fosinoprilat have been found compared with younger subjects.

Impaired hepatic function: Treatment should be initiated at a dose of 10 mg. Although the rate of hydrolysis may be slowed, the extent of hydrolysis is not appreciably reduced in patients with hepatic impairment. In this group of patients, there is evidence of reduced hepatic clearance of fosinoprilat with compensatory increase in renal excretion.

Renal impairment: Treatment should be initiated at a dose of 10 mg. Depending on the response, the dose should then be titrated to achieve the desired therapeutic effect.

Absorption, bioavailability, protein binding, biotransformation and metabolism are not appreciably altered by reduced renal function. In patients with impaired renal function, the total body clearance of fosinoprilat is approximately 50% slower than that in patients with normal renal function. However, since hepatobiliary elimination compensates at least partially for diminished renal elimination, the body clearance of fosinoprilat is not appreciably different over a wide range of renal insufficiency (creatinine clearances ranging from <10 to 80 ml/min/1.73 m², i.e. including end-stage renal failure).

Clearance of fosinoprilat by haemodialysis and peritoneal dialysis averages 2% and 7%, respectively, of urea clearances.

Contra-indications: A history of hypersensitivity to fosinopril or any of the tablet excipients.

Pregnancy: Staril is contra-indicated in pregnancy. It has been shown to be lethal to rabbit foetuses at doses that were maternally toxic. Oligohydramnios and neonatal hypotension and/or anuria have been reported following use of ACE inhibitors in the second and third trimester of pregnancy.

Nursing mothers: Staril should not be given to nursing mothers as fosinoprilat has been detected in human breast milk.

Special warnings and special precautions for use:

Warnings:

Hypotension: As with all ACE inhibitors, a hypotensive response may be observed. If this occurs it is usually associated with the first dose and in most instances, symptoms are relieved simply by the patient lying down. A transient, hypotensive episode is not a contra-indication to continuing therapy once the patient's blood pressure has been stabilised.

As with other ACE inhibitors, patients at risk of an excessive hypotensive response, sometimes associated with renal dysfunction, include those with: congestive heart failure, renovascular hypertension, renal dialysis, or volume and/or salt depletion of any aetiology. In patients with any one of these risk factors, it may be prudent to discontinue or reduce the dose of diuretic therapy or take other measures to ensure adequate hydration prior to initiating fosinopril treatment. Treatment of these high risk patients should be initiated under careful medical supervision and they should be followed closely, particularly if it becomes necessary to resume or increase the dose of diuretic or Staril.

Impaired renal function: When treated with ACE inhibitors, patients with pre-existing congestive heart failure, renovascular hypertension (especially renal artery stenosis), and salt or volume depletion of any aetiology are at increased risk of developing findings indicative of renal dysfunction, including: increases in BUN and serum creatinine and potassium; proteinuria; changes in urine volume (including oliguria/anuria); and an abnormal urinalysis. Dosage reduction and/or discontinuation of diuretic and/or fosinopril may be required.

Anaphylactoid-like reactions: Recent clinical observations have shown a high incidence of anaphylactoid-like reactions during haemodialysis with high-flux dialysis membranes (e.g. AN69) in patients receiving ACE inhibitors. Therefore, this combination should be avoided. Similar reactions during LDL aphoresis with dextran sulphate absorption have been observed. Rare instances of anaphylactoid reactions during desensitisation treatment (hymenoptera venom) have been recorded with other ACE inhibitors.

Idiosyncratic: Angioedema involving the extremities, face, lips, mucous membranes, tongue, glottis or larynx has been seen in patients treated with ACE inhibitors. If such symptoms occur during treatment with Staril, therapy should be discontinued.

Liver function: Rare potentially fatal cases of cholestatic jaundice and hepatocellular injury have been reported with ACE inhibitors. Patients who develop jaundice or marked elevations of hepatic enzymes should discontinue ACE inhibitor treatment.

Hyperkalaemia: When treated with ACE inhibitors, patients at risk of developing hyperkalaemia include those with renal insufficiency, diabetes mellitus, and those using concomitant potassium-sparing diuretics, potassium supplements and/or potassium-containing salt substitutes.

Neutopenia: ACE inhibitors have been reported rarely to cause agranulocytosis and bone marrow depression; these occur more frequently in patients with renal impairment, especially if they also have a collagen-vascular disease such as systemic lupus erythematosus or scleroderma. Monitoring of white blood cell counts should be considered in such patients.

Surgery/anaesthesia: ACE inhibitors may augment the hypotensive effects of anaesthetics and analgesics. If hypotension occurs in patients undergoing surgery/anaesthesia and concomitantly receiving ACE inhibitors, it can usually be corrected by intravenous administration of fluid.

Precautions:

Pretreatment assessment of renal function: Evaluation of the hypertensive patient should include assessment of renal function prior to initiation of therapy and during treatment where appropriate.

Interactions with other medicinal products and other forms of interaction:

Potassium supplements and potassium-sparing diuretics: Fosinopril can attenuate potassium loss caused by a thiazide diuretic. Potassium-sparing diuretics or potassium supplements can increase the risk of hyperkalaemia. Therefore, if concomitant use of such agents is indicated, they should be given with caution and the patient's serum potassium should be monitored frequently.

Antacids: Antacids may impair absorption of fosinopril. Administration of Staril and antacids should be separated by at least 2 hours.

NSAIDs: Non-steroidal anti-inflammatory drugs may interefere with the anti-hypertensive effect. However, the concomitant use of fosinopril and NSAIDs (including aspirin) is not associated with an increase in clinically significant adverse reactions.

Lithium: Concomitant therapy with lithium may increase the serum lithium concentration.

Other anti-hypertensive agents: Combination with other anti-hypertensive agents such as beta blockers, methyldopa, calcium antagonists, and diuretics may increase the anti-hypertensive efficacy.

Other drugs: In pharmacokinetic studies with nifedipine, propranolol, cimetidine, metoclopramide and propantheline the bioavailability of fosinoprilat was not altered by coadministration of Staril with any one of these drugs.

Staril has been used concomitantly with paracetamol, antihistamines, hypoglycaemic agents, insulin, lipid-lowering agents or oestrogen without evidence of clinically important adverse events.

Laboratory tests: Staril may cause a false low measurement of serum digoxin levels with assays using the charcoal absorption method for digoxin. Other kits which use the antibody coated-tube method may be used.

Pregnancy and lactation: See Contra-indications.

Effect on ability to drive and use machines: Not applicable.

Undesirable effects: In placebo controlled studies, there were no significant differences in clinical adverse experiences.

The most commonly reported side-effects with Staril were dizziness, cough, upper respiratory symptoms, nausea/vomiting, diarrhoea and abdominal pain, palpitations/chest pain, rash/pruritus, musculoskeletal pain/paraesthesia, fatigue and taste disturbance.

As with other ACE-inhibitors, hypotension, including orthostatic hypotension, has been reported in Staril heart failure trials. Pancreatitis has been reported rarely in patients treated with ACE inhibitors; in some cases this has proved fatal.

The incidence and type of side-effects did not differ between elderly and younger patients.

Laboratory test findings showed some modest, usually transient, decreases in haemoglobin and haematocrit values and, infrequently, small increases in blood urea.

Overdose: Blood pressure should be monitored and if hypotension develops, volume expansion is the treatment of choice. Fosinoprilat cannot be removed from the body by dialysis.

Pharmacological properties

Pharmacodynamic properties: Fosinopril, {(4S)-4-Cyclohexyl-1-[(RS)-2-methyl-1-(propionyloxy)propoxy] (4-phenylbutyl)=phosphinoylacetyl}-L-proline; sodium salt, is the ester prodrug of an angiotensin converting enzyme (ACE) inhibitor, fosinoprilat. Angiotensin converting enzyme is a peptidyl dipeptidase enzyme that catalyses a number of peptide conversions. These include the conversion of decapeptide Angiotensin I to the octapeptide, Angiotensin II. Staril also inhibits kininase, the enzyme that degrades bradykinin.

Pharmacokinetic properties: The absolute absorption of fosinopril averaged 36% of an oral dose, and was not affected by the presence of food. Rapid and complete hydrolysis to active fosinoprilat occurs in the gastrointestinal mucosa and liver.

The time to reach C_{max} is independent of dose, achieved in approximately three hours and consistent with peak inhibition of the angiotensin I pressor response 3 to 6 hours following administration.

In hypertensive patients with normal renal and hepatic function who received repeated doses of fosinopril, the effective $T_{\frac{1}{2}}$ for accumulation of fosinoprilat averaged 11.5 hours. In patients with heart failure, the effective $T_{\frac{1}{2}}$ was 14 hours. Fosinoprilat is highly protein bound (> 95%), has a relatively small volume of distribution and negligible binding to cellular components in blood. The elimination of fosinopril is by both hepatic and renal routes. Unlike other ACE-inhibitors, there is compensatory excretion by the alternative route in patients with renal or hepatic insufficiency.

Preclinical safety data: Animal studies indicate a toxicity profile which is an extension of the pharmacological effects of fosinopril. It has shown no evidence of carcinogenicity in rodent studies and no potential for mutagenicity in either *in vitro* or *in vivo* tests.

Pharmaceutical particulars

List of excipients:

Staril Tablets 10 mg: White, flat end, diamond tablets each containing fosinopril sodium 10 mg. Engraved with Squibb and unilog number 158 on one face and a star design on the other.

Staril Tablets 20 mg: White, round biconvex tablets each containing fosinopril sodium 20 mg. Engraved with Squibb and unilog number 609 on one face and a star design on the other.

Other ingredients: Crospovidone, lactose, sodium stearyl fumarate, microcrystalline cellulose, povidone.

Incompatibilities: None known.

Shelf life: 36 months.

Special precautions for storage: Store below 30°C in a dry place.

Nature and contents of container: Cartons containing blister packs of 28 tablets.

Instructions for use/handling: No special handling instructions.

Marketing authorisation numbers
Staril Tablets 10 mg 0034/0293
Staril Tablets 20 mg 0034/0294

Date of approval/revision of SPC November 1995.

Legal category POM.

TRI-ADCORTYL* CREAM
TRI-ADCORTYL* OINTMENT

Qualitative and quantitative composition Containing in each gram the following: Triamcinolone acetonide 0.1%, Neomycin (as sulphate) 0.25%, Gramicidin 0.025%, Nystatin 100,000 units.

Pharmaceutical form
Topical Cream
Topical Ointment

Clinical particulars

Therapeutic indications: The topical treatment of superficial bacterial infections, cutaneous candidosis and dermatological conditions, threatened or complicated by bacterial or candidal superinfections, which are known to respond to topical steroid therapy. These include: atopic eczema, contact eczema, follicular eczema, infantile eczema, otitis externa without frank infection, anogenital pruritus, nummular eczema, post-traumatic infective eczema, seborrhoeic eczema, intertrigo, neurodermatitis and infected insect bites.

Posology and method of administration:

Adults and children: Apply to the affected area two to four times daily.

Elderly: Corticosteroids should be used sparingly and for short periods of time, as natural thinning of the skin occurs in the elderly.

If, after about 7 days application, little or no improvement has occurred, cultural isolation of the offending organism should be followed by appropriate local or systemic antimicrobial therapy.

Contra-indications: In tuberculous and most viral lesions of the skin, particularly herpes simplex and varicella. Also in fungal lesions not susceptible to nystatin.

In patients with hypersensitivity to any of the components.

Should not be used for facial rosacea, acne vulgaris or perioral dermatitis.

Should not be applied to the external auditory canal in patients with perforated eardrums.

The products should not be used for extensive areas because of possible risk of systemic absorption and neomycin-induced ototoxicity.

Special warnings and special precautions for use: Adrenal suppression can occur, even without occlusion. The use of occlusive dressings should be avoided because of the increased risk of sensitivity reactions and increased percutaneous absorption. The possibility of sensitivity to neomycin should be taken into consideration especially in the treatment of patients suffering from leg ulcers.

Steroid-antibiotic combinations should not be continued for more than 7 days in the absence of any clinical improvement, since in this situation occult extension of infection may occur due to the masking effect of the steroid.

Extended or recurrent application may increase the risk of contact sensitisation and should be avoided.

If used on the face, courses should be limited to 5 days and occlusion should not be used.

Children: In infants, long-term continuous topical steroid therapy should be avoided. Courses should be limited to 5 days and occlusion should not be used.

Interactions with other medicinal products and other forms of interaction: Not applicable

Pregnancy and lactation: There is inadequate evidence of safety in human pregnancy. Topical administration of corticosteroids to pregnant animals can cause abnormalities of foetal development including cleft palate and intra-uterine growth retardation. There may, therefore, be a very small risk of such effects in the human foetus. There are theoretical risks of neomycin-induced foetal ototoxicity; therefore the product should be used with caution only when the benefit outweighs the potential risk.

Effects on ability to drive and use machines: Not applicable.

Undesirable effects:

Triamcinolone Acetonide: The following side effects have been reported. Usually with prolonged usage: dermatologic–impaired wound healing, thinning of the skin, petechiae and ecchymoses, facial erythema and telangiectasia, increased sweating, purpura, striae, hirsutism, acneiform eruptions, lupus erythematosus-like lesions and suppressed reactions to skin tests. These effects may be enhanced with occlusive dressings.

The possibility of the systemic effects which are

associated with all steroid therapy should be considered.

Neomycin: Sensitivity reactions may occur especially with prolonged use. Ototoxicity and nephrotoxicity have been reported. The product should be used with caution and in small amounts in the treatment of skin infections following extensive burns, trophic ulceration and other conditions where absorption of neomycin is possible. The product should be used with care in patients with established hearing loss.

Gramicidin: Sensitivity has occasionally been reported.

Nystatin: There have been no substantiated reports of sensitivity associated with topical nystatin.

Overdose: Topically applied corticosteroids can be absorbed in sufficient amounts to produce systemic effects (see *Side effects*).

In the event of accidental ingestion, the patient should be observed and treated symptomatically.

Pharmacological properties

Pharmacodynamic properties: Triamcinolone acetonide is a potent fluorinated corticosteroid with rapid anti- inflammatory, antipruritic and anti-allergic actions.

The combined action of the antibiotics neomycin and gramicidin provides comprehensive antibacterial therapy against a wide range of gram-positive and gram-negative bacteria, including those micro-organisms responsible for most bacterial skin infections.

Nystatin is an antifungal antibiotic, active against a wide range of yeasts and yeast-like fungi, including candida albicans.

Pharmacokinetic properties: Not applicable.

Preclinical safety data: No further relevant data

Pharmaceutical particulars

List of excipients:

Cream: Aluminium hydroxide, antifoam emulsion, benzyl alcohol, ethanol, ethylenediamine, hydrochloric acid, macrogol ether, perfume, polysorbate 60, propylene glycol, sorbitol, titanium dioxide, white soft paraffin, water.

Ointment: Polyethylene resin, liquid paraffin.

Incompatibilities: None known.

Shelf life: Cream: 24 months.
Ointment: 48 months.

Special precautions for storage:
Cream: Store below 25°C. Avoid freezing.
Ointment: Store below 25°C.

Nature and contents of container: Aluminium tubes.

Instruction for use/handling: None.

Marketing authorisation numbers
Cream 0034/5093R
Ointment 0034/5094R

Date of approval/revision of SPC
Cream: October 1995
Ointment: January 1996

Legal category POM

TRI-ADCORTYL* OTIC OINTMENT

Qualitative and quantitative composition Containing in each gram the following: Triamcinolone acetonide 0.1%, Neomycin (as sulphate) 0.25%, Gramicidin 0.025%, Nystatin 100,000 units.

Pharmaceutical form Aural Ointment.

Clinical particulars

Therapeutic indications: For the topical treatment of otitis externa, known to respond to topical steroid therapy, complicated by superficial bacterial or fungal infections.

Posology and method of administration:

Adults and children: Apply a small amount directly from the tube into the aural canal two to four times daily.

Elderly: Corticosteroids should be used sparingly and for short periods of time, as natural thinning of the skin occurs in the elderly.

If, after about 7 days application, little or no improvement has occurred, cultural isolation of the offending organism should be followed by appropriate local or systemic antimicrobial therapy.

Contra-indications: In tuberculous and most viral lesions of the skin, particularly herpes simplex and varicella. Also in fungal lesions not susceptible to nystatin.

In patients with hypersensitivity to any of the components.

Should not be used for facial rosacea, acne vulgaris or perioral dermatitis.

Should not be applied to the external auditory canal in patients with perforated eardrums.

The products should not be used for extensive areas because of possible risk of systemic absorption and neomycin-induced ototoxicity.

Special warnings and special precautions for use: Adrenal suppression can occur, even without occlusion. The use of occlusive dressings should be avoided because of the increased risk of sensitivity reactions and increased percutaneous absorption. The possibility of sensitivity to neomycin should be taken into consideration especially in the treatment of patients suffering from leg ulcers.

Steroid-antibiotic combinations should not be continued for more than 7 days in the absence of any clinical improvement, since in this situation occult extension of infection may occur due to the masking effect of the steroid.

Extended or recurrent application may increase the risk of contact sensitisation and should be avoided.

If used in childhood, or on the face, courses should be limited to 5 days and occlusion should not be used.

Not for ophthalmic use.

Children: In infants, long-term continuous topical steroid therapy should be avoided. Courses should be limited to 5 days and occlusion should not be used.

Interactions with other medicinal products and other forms of interaction: Not applicable

Pregnancy and laction: There is inadequate evidence of safety in human pregnancy. Topical administration of corticosteroids to pregnant animals can cause abnormalities of foetal development including cleft palate and intra-uterine growth retardation. There may, therefore, be a very small risk of such effects in the human foetus. There are theoretical risks of neomycin-induced foetal ototoxicity; therefore the product should be used with caution only when the benefit outweighs the potential risk.

Effects on ability to drive and use machines: Not applicable.

Undesirable effects:

Triamcinolone acetonide: Triamcinolone acetonide is well tolerated. Where adverse reactions occur they are usually reversible on cessation of therapy. However the following side effects have been reported usually with prolonged usage:

Dermatologic–impaired wound healing, thinning of the skin, petechiae and ecchymoses, facial erythema and telangiectasia, increased sweating, purpura, striae, hirsutism, acneiform eruptions, lupus erythematosus-like lesions and suppressed reactions to skin tests.

These effects may be enhanced with occlusive dressings.

Signs of systemic toxicity such as oedema and electrolyte imbalance have not been observed even when high topical dosage has been used. The possibility of the systemic effects which are associated with all steroid therapy should be considered.

Neomycin: Sensitivity reactions may occur especially with prolonged use. Ototoxicity and nephrotoxicity have been reported. The product should be used with caution and in small amounts in the treatment of skin infections following extensive burns, trophic ulceration and other conditions where absorption of neomycin is possible. The product should be used with care in patients with established hearing loss.

Gramicidin: Sensitivity has occasionally been reported.

Nystatin: There have been no substantiated reports of sensitivity associated with topical nystatin.

Overdose: Topically applied corticosteroids can be absorbed in sufficient amounts to produce systemic effects (see *Side effects*).

In the event of accidental ingestion, the patient should be observed and treated symptomatically.

Pharmacological properties

Pharmacodynamic properties: Triamcinolone acetonide is a potent fluorinated corticosteroid with rapid anti- inflammatory, antipruritic and anti-allergic actions.

The combined action of the antibiotics neomycin and gramicidin provides comprehensive antibacterial therapy against a wide range of gram-positive and gram-negative bacteria, including those micro-organisms responsible for most bacterial skin infections.

Nystatin is an antifungal antibiotic, active against a wide range of yeasts and yeast-like fungi, including *candida albicans.*

Pharmacokinetic properties: Not applicable.

Preclinical safety data: No further relevant data

Pharmaceutical particulars

List of excipients: Polylethylene resin and liquid paraffin

Incompatibilites: None known.

Shelf life: 48 months.

Special precautions for storage: Store below 25°C.

Nature and contents of container: Aluminium tubes.

Instructions for use/handling: None.

Marketing authorisation number 0034/5095R

Date of approval/revision of SPC January 1996

Legal category POM

VELOSEF* CAPSULES 250MG AND 500MG
VELOSEF* SYRUP 250MG/5ML

Qualitative and quantitative composition

Capsules 250 mg: Opaque, orange body with opaque blue cap printed Squibb and 113 in white on each half. Each capsule contains 250 mg cephradine.

Capsules 500 mg: Opaque blue printed in white with Squibb and 114 on each half. Each capsule contains 500 mg cephradine.

Syrup 250 mg: When reconstituted contains 250 mg cephradine per 5 ml.

Pharmaceutical form

Oral tablets.

Oral powder for reconstitution.

Clinical particulars

Therapeutic indications: In the treatment of infections of the urinary and respiratory tracts and of the skin and soft tissues. These include:

Upper respiratory infections–pharyngitis, sinusitis, otitis media, tonsillitis, laryngo-tracheo bronchitis.

Lower respiratory infections–acute and chronic bronchitis, lobar and bronchopneumonia.

Urinary tract infections–cystitis, urethritis, pyelonephritis.

Skin and soft tissue infections–abscess, cellulitis, furunculosis, impetigo.

Cephradine has been shown to be effective in reducing the incidence of postoperative infections in patients undergoing surgical procedures associated with a high risk of infection. It is also of value where postoperative infections would be disastrous and where patients have a reduced host resistance to bacterial infection. Protection is best ensured by achieving adequate local tissue concentrations at the time contamination is likely to occur. Thus, cephradine should be administered immediately prior to surgery and continued during the postoperative period.

Bacteriology studies to determine the causative organisms and their sensitivity to cephradine should be performed. Therapy may be instituted prior to receiving the results of the sensitivity test.

Posology and method of administration: Cephradine may be given without regard to meals.

Adults: For urinary tract infections the usual dose is 500 mg four times daily or 1 g twice daily; severe or chronic infections may require larger doses. Prolonged intensive therapy is needed for complications such as prostatitis and epididymitis. For respiratory tract infections and skin and soft tissue infections the usual dose is 250 mg or 500 mg four times daily or 500 mg or 1 g twice daily depending on the severity and site of infections.

Children: The usual dose is from 25 to 50 mg/kg/day total, given in two or four equally divided doses.

For otitis media daily doses from 75 to 100 mg/kg in divided doses every 6 to 12 hours are recommended. Maximum dose 4 g per day.

Elderly: There are no specific dosage recommendations or precautions for use in the elderly except, as with other drugs, to monitor those patients with impaired renal or hepatic function.

All patients, irrespective of age and weight: Larger doses (up to 1 g four times daily) may be given for severe or chronic infections. Therapy should be continued for a minimum of 48-72 hours after the patient becomes asymptomatic or evidence of bacterial eradication has been obtained. In infections caused by haemolytic strains of streptococci, a minimum of 10 days treatment is recommended to guard against the risk of rheumatic fever or glomerulonephritis. In the treatment of chronic urinary tract infections, frequent bacteriological and clinical appraisal is necessary during therapy and may be necessary for several months afterwards. Persistent infections may require treatment for several weeks. Smaller doses than those indicated above should not be used. Doses for children should not exceed doses recommended for adults. As cephradine is available in both injectable and oral form, patients may be changed from the cephradine injectable to cephradine oral at the same dosage level.

Renal impairment dosage:

Patients not on dialysis: The following dosage schedule is suggested as a guideline based on a dosage of 500 mg Q6H and on creatinine clearance. Further modification in the dosage schedule may be required because of the dosage selected and individual variation.

Creatinine Clearance	*Dose*	*Time Interval*
more than 20 ml/min	500 mg	6 hours
5-20 ml/min	250 mg	6 hours
less than 5 ml/min	250 mg	50-70 hours

Patients on chronic, intermittent haemodialysis:

250 mg	At start of haemodialysis
250 mg	6-12 hours after start
250 mg	36-48 hours after start
250 mg	At start of next haemodialysis if >30 hours after previous dose.

Further modification of the dosage schedule may be necessary in children.

Contra-indications: Patients with known hypersensitivity to the cephalosporin antibiotics.

Special warnings and special precautions for use: After treatment with cephradine, a false positive reaction for glucose in the urine may occur with Benedict's or Fehling's solution or with reagent tablets such as Clinitest*, but not with enzyme-based tests such as Clinistix* or Diastix*.

As with all antibiotics, prolonged use may result in overgrowth of non-susceptible organisms.

Interactions with other medicinal products and other forms of interaction: There is evidence of partial cross-allergenicity between the penicillins and the cephalosporins. Therefore cephradine should be used with caution in those patients with known hypersensitivity to penicillins. There have been instances of patients who have had reactions to both drug classes (including anaphylaxis).

Pregnancy and lactation: Although animal studies have not demonstrated any teratogenicity, safety in pregnancy has not been established. Cephradine is excreted in breast milk and should be used with caution in lactating mothers.

Effects on ability to drive and use machines: None known

Undesirable effects: Limited essentially to gastro-intestinal disturbances and on occasion to hypersensitivity phenomena. The latter are more likely to occur in individuals who have previously demonstrated hypersensitivity and those with a history of allergy, asthma, hay fever or urticaria. The majority of reported side-effects have been mild and are rare, and include glossitis, heartburn, dizziness, tightness in the chest, nausea, vomiting, diarrhoea, abdominal pain, vaginitis, candidal overgrowth. Skin and hypersensitivity reactions include urticaria, skin rashes, joint pains, oedema.

As with other cephalosporins, mild transient eosinophilia, leucopenia and neutropenia, positive direct Coombs tests and pseudomembraneous colitis have been reported.

Clinical Chemistry: Elevations of BUN and Serum Creatinine have been reported. In clinical trials, elevations of SGOT, SGPT, total bilirubin and alkaline phosphates were observed.

Overdose: None known.

Pharmacological properties

Pharmacodynamic properties:

Actions: Cephradine is a broad-spectrum, bactericidal antibiotic active against both Gram-positive and Gram-negative bacteria. It is also highly active against most strains of penicillinase-producing Staphylococci.

Microbiology: The following organisms have shown in vitro sensitivity to cephradine.

Gram-positive–Staphylococci (both penicillin sensitive and resistant strains), Streptococci, *Streptococcus pyogenes* (beta haemolytic) and *streptococcus pneumoniae.*

Gram-negative–*Escherichia coli, Klebsiella,* spp, *Proteus mirabilis, Haemophilus influenzae, Shigella* spp., *Salmonella* spp. (including *Salmonella typhi*) and *Neisseria* spp.

Because cephradine is unaffected by penicillinase, many strains of *Escherichia coli* and *Staphylococcus aureus* which produce this enzyme are susceptible to cephradine but resistant to ampicillin.

Pharmacokinetic properties: Cephradine has a high degree of stability to many beta-lactamases. It has a low degree of protein-binding and a large volume of distribution. Therefore, tissue levels are generally found to be high. Oral cephradine can be given twice or four times daily, and is well absorbed.

Human pharmacology: Cephradine is acid stable and is rapidly absorbed following oral administration in the fasting state. Following doses of 250 mg, 500 mg and 1000 mg average peak serum levels of approximately 9, 16.5, and 24.2 micrograms/ml, respectively, were obtained at one hour. The presence of food in the gastrointestinal tract delays the absorption but does not affect the total amount of cephradine absorbed. Measurable serum levels are present six hours after administration. Over 90% of the drug is excreted unchanged in the urine within 6 hours. Peak urine concentrations are approximately 1600 micrograms/ml following a 250 mg dose, 3200 micrograms/ml following a 500 mg dose, and 4000 micrograms/ml following a 1000 mg dose. After 48 hours' administration of 100 mg/kg/day of cephradine for the treatment of otitis media, cephradine has been measured in the middle ear exudate at an average level of 3.6 microgram/ml.

Preclinical safety data: No relevant further data available.

Pharmaceutical particulars

List of excipients:

Capsules 250 mg: Erythrosine, gelatin capsules, indigo carmine, iron oxide, lactose, magnesium stearate, titanium dioxide.

Capsules 500 mg: Gelatin capsules, indigo carmine, lactose, magnesium stearate, titanium dioxide.

Syrup: Citric acid, flavours, guar gum, methylcellulose, sodium citrate, sucrose.

Incompatibilities: None known

Shelf life: Capsules: 36 months.
Syrup: 48 months.

Special precautions for storage:
Capsules: Store below 25°C.
Syrup: Store below 25°C.

After reconstitution; discard unused syrup after 14 days if stored in refrigerator, or seven days at below 25°C.

Nature and contents of container:
Capsules: Blister packs of 20 or 100 capsules.
Syrup: Bottles of 100 ml.

Instructions for use/handling: Not applicable

Marketing authorisation numbers

Velosef Capsules 250 mg	0034/0133R
Velosef Capsules 500 mg	0034/0134R
Velosef Syrup 250 mg/5 ml	0034/0136R

Date of approval/revision of SPC

Capsules:	24 May 1997
Syrup:	4 February 1997

Legal category POM.

VELOSEF* FOR INJECTION

Presentation Velosef for Injection is a sterile powder blend of cephradine and L-arginine. After reconstitution, Velosef for Injection 500 mg and 1.0 g vials provide 500 mg and 1.0 g of cephradine activity, respectively.

Uses *Actions:* Cephradine is a broad-spectrum bactericidal antibiotic active against both Gram-positive and Gram-negative bacteria. It is also highly active against most strains of penicillinase-producing staphylococci.

Microbiology: The following organisms have shown *in vitro* sensitivity to cephradine:

Gram-positive – *Staphylococci* (both penicillin sensitive and resistant strains), *Streptococci, Streptococcus pyogenes* (beta haemolytic) and *Streptococcus pneumoniae.*

Gram-negative – *E. coli, Klebsiella, P. mirabilis, Haemophilus influenzae, Shigella* spp., *Salmonella* spp. (including *Salmonella typhi*) and *Neisseria* spp.

Because cephradine is unaffected by penicillinase, many strains of *E. coli* and *Staphylococcus aureus* which produce this enzyme are susceptible to cephradine but resistant to ampicillin.

Indications: The treatment of infections of the urinary and respiratory tracts and of the skin and soft tissues, bones and joints; also septicaemia and endocarditis. These include:

Upper respiratory infections – pharyngitis, sinusitis, otitis media, tonsillitis, laryngo-tracheo-bronchitis.

Lower respiratory infections – acute and chronic bronchitis, lobar and bronchopneumonia.

Urinary tract infections – cystitis, urethritis, pyelonephritis.

Skin and soft tissue infections – abscess, cellulitis, furunculosis, impetigo.

Velosef has been shown to be effective in reducing the incidence of postoperative infections in patients undergoing surgical procedures associated with a high risk of infection. It is also of value where post-operative infection would be disastrous and where patients have a reduced host resistance to bacterial infection. Protection is best ensured by achieving adequate local tissue concentrations at the time contamination is likely to occur. Thus, Velosef should be administered immediately prior to surgery and continued during the postoperative period.

Bacteriological studies to determine the causative organisms and their sensitivity to cephradine should be performed. Therapy may be instituted prior to receiving the results of the sensitivity test.

Sterile Velosef for injection is indicated primarily for those patients unable to tolerate oral medication. It is also indicated for intravenous use either by direct injection or by intravenous infusion for the treatment of serious and life-threatening infections.

Dosage and administration Intramuscular or intravenous injection and intravenous infusion.

Adults: Treatment: The usual dose range of Velosef for injection is 2-4 g daily in four equally divided doses. This may be increased up to 8 g a day for severe infections, e.g. septicaemia and endocarditis. For the majority of infections, the usual dose is 500 mg q.i.d. in equally spaced doses; severe or chronic infections may require larger doses. Prolonged intensive therapy is needed for complications such as prostatitis and epididymitis. Patients who are severely ill and who require high serum levels of cephradine for treating their infections should be started on intravenous therapy.

Limited experience indicates that intraperitoneal administration of Velosef may be effective after surgery in cases of peritonitis where a surgical drainage system has been established.

Prophylaxis: The recommended dose for surgical prophylaxis is a single, pre-operative 1–2 g IM or IV dose. Subsequent parenteral or oral doses can be administered as appropriate.

Children: The usual dose is 50-100 mg/kg/day total given in four equally divided doses. More serious illnesses (e.g. typhoid fever) may require 200-300 mg/kg/day.

Elderly: There are no specific dosage recommendations or precautions for use in the elderly except, as with other drugs, to monitor those patients with impaired renal or hepatic function.

All patients, regardless of age and weight: Therapy should be continued for a minimum of 48-72 hours after the patient becomes asymptomatic or evidence of bacterial eradication has been obtained. In infections caused by haemolytic strains of streptococci, a minimum of 10 days of treatment is recommended to guard against the risk of rheumatic fever or glomerulonephritis. In the treatment of chronic urinary tract infections, frequent bacteriological and clinical appraisal is necessary during therapy and may be necessary for several months afterwards. Persistent infections may require treatment for several weeks. Smaller doses than those indicated above should not be used. Doses for children should not exceed doses recommended for adults. As Velosef is available in both injectable and oral form, patients may be changed from Velosef injectable to Velosef oral at the same dosage level.

Renal impairment dosage:

Patients not on dialysis: The following dosage schedule is suggested as a guideline based on a dosage of 500 mg Q6H and on creatinine clearance. Further modification in the dosage schedule may be required because of the dosage selected and individual variation.

Creatinine clearance	*Dose*	*Time interval*
more than 20 ml/min	500 mg	6 hours
5–20 ml/min	250 mg	6 hours
less than 5 ml/min	250 mg	50–70 hours

Patients on chronic intermittent haemodialysis:

250 mg	At start of haemodialysis
250 mg	6–12 hours after start
250 mg	36–48 hours after start
250 mg	At start of next haemodialysis >30 hours after previous dose

Further modification of the dosage schedule may be necessary in children.

Reconstitution: For intramuscular use: Aseptically add sterile water for injection or 0.9% sodium chloride injection according to the following table:

Single dose vial size*	*Volume of diluent to be added*
500 mg	2.0 ml
1 g	4.0 ml

* Preparation contains no bactericide and is not intended for multiple dose use.

Shake to effect solution and withdraw the entire contents. Intramuscular solutions should be used within 2 hours at room temperature; when stored in a refrigerator at 5°C, solutions retain full potency for 12 hours. Reconstituted solutions may vary in colour from light to straw yellow; however, this does not affect the potency.

For intravenous use: Velosef for injection may be administered by direct intravenous injection or by infusion. A 3 microgram/ml serum concentration can be maintained for each milligram of cephradine per kg body weight per hour of infusion.

For direct intravenous administration: Suitable intravenous injection solutions are Sterile Water for Injection, 5% Glucose Injection or 0.9% Sodium Chloride Injection.

Aseptically add 5 ml of diluent to the 500 mg vial or 10 ml to the 1 g vial. Shake to effect solution and withdraw the entire contents. The solution may be slowly injected directly into a vein over a 3 to 5 minute period. The solution should be used within 2 hours when kept at room temperature; if stored at 5°C, solutions retain full potency for 12 hours.

For continuous or intermittent intravenous infusion: Suitable intravenous infusion solutions are Sterile Water for Injection (50 mg/ml cephradine solutions are approximately isotonic); 5% or 10% Glucose Injection; 0.9% Sodium Chloride Injection; Sodium Lactate Injection (M/6 sodium lactate); Glucose and Sodium Chloride Injection; Lactated Ringer's Injection; Ringer's Injection; 5% Glucose in Lactated Ringer's Injection; 5% Glucose in Ringer's Injection.

Aseptically add 10 ml of the diluent to the 1 g vial and shake to effect solution. Aseptically transfer the entire contents to the IV infusion diluent. Intravenous infusions prepared remain potent for 12 hours at room temperature or 1 week at 5°C at concentrations up to 10 mg/ml (1%), and for 10 hours at room temperature or 48 hours at 5°C at concentrations up to 50 mg/ml (5%). For prolonged infusion, replace 5% infusions every 10 hours and 1% infusions every 24 hours with freshly-prepared solutions.

N.B. Only cephradine solubilised with arginine may be reconstituted with solutions containing calcium salts, such as Ringer's Solutions.

For further information on compatibilities consult the manufacturer.

Protect solutions of cephradine from concentrated light or direct sunlight.

Contra-indications, warnings, etc
Contra-indications: Patients with known hypersensitivity to the cephalosporin antibiotics.

Precautions: After treatment with Velosef a false positive reaction for glucose in the urine may occur with Benedict's solution or Fehling's solution or with reagent tablets such as Clinitest*, but not with enzyme-based tests such as Clinistix* or Diastix*.

As with all antibiotics, prolonged use may result in overgrowth of non-susceptible organisms.

Administration in renal impairment: A modified dosage schedule in patients with decreased renal function is necessary (see Dosage).

Drug interactions: There is evidence of partial cross-allergenicity between the penicillins and the cephalosporins. Therefore Velosef should be used with caution in those patients with known hypersensitivity to penicillins. There have been instances of patients who have had reactions to both drug classes (including anaphylaxis).

Pregnancy and breast feeding: Although animal studies have not demonstrated any teratogenicity, safety in pregnancy has not been established. Cephradine is excreted in breast milk and should be used with caution in lactating mothers.

Side-effects: Limited essentially to gastro-intestinal disturbances and on occasion to hypersensitivity phenomena. The latter are more likely to occur in individual's who have previously demonstrated hypersensitivity and those with a history of allergy, asthma, hay fever or urticaria. The majority of reported side-effects have been mild and are rare, and include glossitis, heartburn, headache, dizziness, dyspnoea, paraesthesia, nausea, vomiting, diarrhoea, abdominal pain, candidal overgrowth, vaginitis. Skin and hypersensitivity reactions include urticaria, skin rashes, joint pains, oedema.

As with other cephalosporins, mild transient eosinophilia, leucopenia and neutropenia, rarely positive direct Coombs tests and pseudomembranous colitis have been reported.

Clinical chemistry: Elevations of BUN and Serum Creatinine have been reported. In clinical trials, elevations of SGOT, SGPT, total bilirubin and alkaline phosphates were observed.

Injection: As with other parenterally administered antibiotics, transient pain may be experienced at the injection site, but is seldom the cause for discontinuing treatment. Thrombophlebitis has been reported following intravenous injection.

Since sterile abscesses have been reported following accidental subcutaneous injection, the preparation should be administered by deep intramuscular injection.

Pharmaceutical precautions *Storage (before reconstitution):* At room temperature. Not for multidose use.

Legal category POM.

Package quantities *500 mg single-dose vials:* Pack of 5.
1 g single-dose vials: Single-vial pack.

Further information Cephradine has a high degree of stability to beta-lactamases. It has a low degree of protein binding and a large volume of distribution. Therefore, tissue levels are generally found to be high.

Human pharmacology: Following intramuscular administration of a single 0.5 g dose of cephradine to normal volunteers, the average peak serum concentration was 8.41 microgram/ml with the time to peak concentration being 0.93 hours. The serum half-life averaged 1.25 hours. A single 1 g intravenous dose resulted in serum concentrations of 86 microgram/ml at 5 minutes and 12 microgram/ml at 1 hour; these concentrations declined to 1 microgram/ml at 4 hours. Continuous infusion of 500 mg per hour into a 70 kg man maintained a concentration of about 21.4 microgram/ml cephradine activity; this study showed that a serum concentration of approximately 3 microgram/ml can be obtained for each milligram of cephradine administered per kg of body weight per hour of infusion.

Cephradine is excreted unchanged in the urine. The kidneys excrete 57% to 80% of an intramuscular dose in the first six hours; this results in a high urine concentration, e.g. 880 microgram/ml of urine after a 500 mg intramuscular dose. Probenecid slows tubular secretion and almost doubles peak serum concentration.

Assays of bone obtained at surgery have shown that cephradine penetrates bone tissue.

Product licence numbers

Velosef Injection 500 mg	0034/0198
Velosef Injection 1 g	0034/0199

**Trade Mark*

Stafford-Miller Ltd
45 Broadwater Road
Welwyn Garden City
Herts AL7 3SP

☎ 01707 331001 🖷 01707 373370

ALPHOSYL CREAM

Qualitative and quantitative composition

Active ingredients	*Quantity (% w/w)*
Allantoin	2.0
Alcoholic extract of coal tar	5.0

Pharmaceutical form Cream for topical application.

Clinical particulars
Therapeutic indications: For the treatment of psoriasis, its moisturising capability makes it particularly useful on flexures.

Posology and method of administration: Apply liberally 2–4 times daily and rub vigorously into affected areas until the cream is no longer visible.

The dosage schedule is the same for all patients.

The cream can be applied freely, even to the scalp. Where hard scales exist, apply after a hot bath. Several weeks of application may be required for optimum results. After the lesions have been brought under control, continue use to help prevent recurrence.

Contra-indications: Sensitivity to coal tar, acute psoriasis.

Special warnings and special precautions for use: For external use only.

Discontinue use if irritation occurs, or in cases of sensitivity to coal tar.

Interactions with other medicaments and other forms of interaction: None known.

Pregnancy and lactation: Safety in pregnancy and lactation has not been established, it is therefore best avoided in the first trimester of pregnancy.

Effects on ability to drive and use machinery: None known.

Undesirable effects: Skin irritation, acne like eruptions or photosensitivity may occur in some patients who are sensitive to coal tar. These effects resolve when treatment is stopped.

Overdose: Alphosyl Cream is a topical medicine which has no known systemic effects. Overdose may increase the risk of skin irritation and photosensitivity, but is unlikely to have a systemic effect.

Pharmacological properties
Pharmacodynamic properties: Coal tar has keratolytic and keratoplastic properties, allantoin hastens wound healing and is a chemical debrider. Both ingredients act through, as yet, uneluciated mechanisms.

Pharmacokinetic properties: Not applicable.

Preclinical safety data: Not stated.

Pharmaceutical particulars
List of excipients: Beeswax; Cetyl alcohol; Citric acid; Corn oil; Glyceryl monostearate acid stable; Isopropyl palmitate; Mineral oil and lanolin alcohol; Methylparaben; Oleyl alcohol; Propylene glycol; Propyl gallate; Propylparaben; Sorbitan sesquioleate; Squalane; Triethanolamine; Water.

Incompatibilities: None known.

Shelf life: 60 months.

Special precautions for storage: Store at room temperature, do not refrigerate.

Nature of contents of container: Alphosyl Cream is packaged in decorated, collapsible, aluminium tubes with a phenolic/epoxy resin liner and latex end seal. The nozzle is closed with a high density polyethylene screw on cap.

Pack sizes: 100 g.

Legal category P.

Marketing authorisation number PL 0036/5006R.

Date of revision of the SPC 4 June 1996.

ALPHOSYL LOTION

Qualitative and quantitative composition

Active ingredients	*Quantity (% w/w)*
Allantoin	2.0
Alcoholic extract of coal tar	5.0

Pharmaceutical form Lotion for topical application.

Clinical particulars
Therapeutic indications: For the treatment of psoriasis and psoriasis of the scalp.

Posology and method of administration: Apply liberally 2–4 times daily and rub vigorously into affected areas until the lotion is no longer visible.

The dosage schedule is the same for all patients.

Contra-indications: Sensitivity to coal tar, acute psoriasis.

Special warnings and special precautions for use: For external use only.

Discontinue use if irritation occurs, or in cases of sensitivity to coal tar.

Interactions with other medicaments and other forms of interaction: None known.

Pregnancy and lactation: Safety in pregnancy and lactation has not been established, it is therefore best avoided in the first trimester of pregnancy.

Effects on ability to drive and use machinery: None known.

Undesirable effects: Skin irritation, acne like eruptions or photosensitivity may occur in some patients who are sensitive to coal tar. These effects resolve when treatment is stopped.

Overdose: Alphosyl Lotion is a topical medicine which has no known systemic effects. Overdose may increase the risk of skin irritation and photosensitivity, but is unlikely to have a systemic effect.

Pharmacological properties
Pharmacodynamic properties: Coal tar has keratolytic and keratoplastic properties, allantoin hastens wound healing and is a chemical debrider. Both ingredients act through, as yet, uneluciated mechanisms.

Pharmacokinetic properties: Not applicable.

Preclinical safety data: Several animal studies have demonstrated that the non-carcinogenic toxicity profile of medicinal coal tar is acceptable.

Coal tar preparations have been shown to contain chemicals with a known relationship to the development of malignant tumours in experimental models. Animal studies, where coal tar has been applied topically, have consistently given positive results.

However, it is consistently clear that epidemiological studies in man have not confirmed this carcinogenic potential. While isolated case studies have related the use of medicinal coal tar to tumour induction, well controlled retrospective studies have not confirmed the relationship. The individual case reports are not well documented as to causation.

Pharmaceutical particulars
List of excipients: Isopropyl palmitate; Polyoxyethylene (8) stearate; Propylene glycol; Stearic acid; Methyl paraben; Propyl paraben; Water.

Incompatibilities: None known.

Shelf life: 36 months.

Special precautions for storage: Store at room temperature, do not refrigerate.

Nature of contents of container: Alphosyl Lotion is packaged in amber glass bottles, sealed with screw on urea/formaldehyde moulded caps with a polyethylene, polycone insert.

Instructions for use/handling: Rub vigorously into the affected areas until the lotion is no longer visible. Where hard scales exist, apply after a hot bath. Several weeks of application may be required for optimum results. After the lesions have been brought under control, continue use to prevent recurrence.

Marketing authorisation number PL 0036/5008R.

Legal category P.

ALPHOSYL HC CREAM

Qualitative and quantitative composition

Active ingredients	*Quantity (% w/w)*
Allantoin	2.0
Alcoholic extract of coal tar	5.0
Hydrocortisone	0.5

Pharmaceutical form Cream for topical application.

Clinical particulars
Therapeutic indications: For the treatment of psoriasis by topical administration.

Posology and method of administration: For all patients, apply sparingly twice daily to psoriatic plaques and rub in well until the cream is no longer visible.

Not recommended for children under 5 years.

Contra-indications: Tuberculosis or fungal lesions of the skin, herpes simplex, vaccinia or varicella or a history of hypersensitivity to any of the ingredients.

Special warnings and special precautions for use: For external use only, avoid contact with the eyes.

Discontinue use if sensitivity occurs.

Use sparingly.

The following results of steroid use are uncommon at this dosage, however:

- When used over large areas or for prolonged periods systemic side effects can result.
- Under occlusive dressings or in intertriginous areas, topical steroids may cause skin atrophy manifesting as striae, thinning and telangiectasia.
- Viral, bacterial or fungal infection of the skin may be substantially exacerbated by topical steroid treatment unless accompanied by appropriate therapy.
- Wound healing can be significantly retarded.

Interactions with other medicaments and other forms of interaction: None known.

Pregnancy and lactation: Topical administration of corticosteroids to pregnant animals can cause abnormality of foetal development. Topical steroids should not be used extensively in pregnancy, i.e. in large amounts or for long periods because of the risk of teratogenic effects or significant absorption causing suppression of the HPA axis.

Effects on ability to drive and use machinery: None known.

Undesirable effects: Hypersensitivity reactions may occasionally occur.

Overdose: Not applicable.

Pharmacological properties
Pharmacodynamic properties: Coal tar is a standard antipruritic and keratoplastic agent used in the treatment of psoriasis and other skin disorders. Allantoin is a chemical debrider; it stimulates cell proliferation, epithelisation and granulation, and hence hastens wound healing. Steroids are standard in the topical treatment of various skin disorders.

Pharmacokinetic properties: Not applicable.

Preclinical safety data: Several animal studies have demonstrated that the non-carcinogenic toxicity profile of medicinal coal tar is acceptable.

Coal tar preparations have been shown to contain chemicals with a known relationship to the development of malignant tumours in experimental models. Animal studies, where coal tar has been applied topically, have consistently given positive results.

However, it is consistently clear that epidemiological studies in man have not confirmed this carcinogenic potential. While isolated case studies have related the use of medicinal coal tar to tumour induction, well controlled retrospective studies have not confirmed the relationship. The individual case reports are not well documented as to causation.

Pharmaceutical particulars
List of excipients: Beeswax; Cetyl alcohol; Citric acid; Corn oil; Glyceryl monostearate; Isopropyl palmitate; Mineral oil and lanolin alcohol; Methyl paraben; Oleyl alcohol; Propyl gallate; Propyl paraben; PEG 400 dilaurate; Sodium citrate; Squalane; Lecithin; Triethanolamine; Phenylethyl alcohol; Water.

Incompatibilities: None known.

Shelf life: 18 months.

Special precautions for storage: Store between 4°C and 25°C.

Nature of contents of container: Alphosyl HC Cream is packaged in decorated, collapsible, aluminium tubes with a phenolic/epoxy resin liner and latex end seal. The nozzle is closed with a high density polyethylene screw on cap.

Instructions for use/handling: For all patients, apply sparingly twice a day to psoriatic plaques and rub in well until the cream is no longer visible. Alphosyl HC Cream is not recommended for children under 5 years.

Marketing authorisation number PL 0036/0026R.

Legal category POM.

ALPHOSYL '2 IN 1' SHAMPOO

Qualitative and quantitative composition

Active constituent	*% w/w*	*Reference Standard*
Alcoholic extract of coal tar	5.00	HSE

Pharmaceutical form Medicated shampoo.

Clinical particulars

Therapeutic indications: For the treatment of Psoriasis, Seborrhoeic dermatitis, scaling and itching (often associated with eczema), and dandruff.

Posology and method of administration: Adults, children and the elderly: Wet hair thoroughly, then briskly rub a liberal amount of shampoo into the hair and scalp. Rinse thoroughly and repeat the procedure massaging the scalp for several minutes and working the shampoo into a rich lather. Rinse thoroughly.

Dandruff: Once or twice weekly as necessary, or as directed by a physician.

Psoriasis, Seborrhoeic dermatitis, scaling and itching: Use every 2 or 3 days, or as directed by a physician.

Contra-indications: Sensitivity to coal tar.

Special warnings and precautions for use:
For external use only.
Discontinue if irritation develops.
Avoid contact with eyes.
Keep out of reach of children.

Interaction with other medications and other forms of interaction: None known.

Pregnancy and lactation: There is no or inadequate evidence of safety of coal tar in human pregnancy but it has been in wide use for many years without apparent ill consequence. However, use in the first trimester of pregnancy is best avoided.

Effects on ability to drive and use machines: None known.

Undesirable effects: Skin irritation or photosensitivity may occur in some patients who are sensitive to coal tar. Data to determine the frequency of these reactions are not available. These undesirable effects resolve when treatment is stopped.

Overdose: Alphosyl shampoo is a topical medicine which has no known systemic effects. Effects of overdose may increase the rate of skin irritation and photosensitivity but it is unlikely to have a systemic effect.

Pharmacological properties

Pharmacodynamic properties: Coal tar has keratolytic and keratoplastic properties which aids treatment by slowing the excessive epidermal cell turnover.

Pharmacokinetic properties: Not applicable.

Preclinical safety data: Not applicable.

Pharmaceutical particulars

List of excipients: Sodium lauryl sulphate; Ammonium lauryl sulphate; Hexylene Glycolstearate SLS; Lauramide DEA; Herbal Fragrance 41.423; Hydroxy Propyl Methyl Cellulose; Citric acid anhydrous; Guar Hydroxy Propyl Trimonium Chloride; Methyl Parahydroxybenzoate; Propyl Parahydroxybenzoate; Patent Blue V dye; Purified Water.

Incompatibilities: None known.

Shelf life: 24 months.

Special precautions for storage: None.

Nature and contents of container: Alphosyl '2 in 1' shampoo is packaged in white opaque polypropylene bottles with wadded cap and pack sizes; 125, 250 ml.

Instructions for use/handling: None stated.

Marketing authorisation number PL 0036/0052.

Legal category GSL.

Date of first authorisation/renewal of authorisation 13 November 1991.

Date of (partial) revision of text 7 August 1996.

COLIFOAM*

Presentation An aerosol can releasing a white odourless foam containing Hydrocortisone Acetate PhEur 10% w/w.

Uses Anti-inflammatory corticosteroid therapy for the topical treatment of ulcerative colitis, proctosigmoiditis and granular proctitis. For rectal administration.

Dosage and administration One applicatorful inserted into the rectum once or twice daily for two or three weeks and every second day thereafter.

Contra-indications, warnings, etc

Contra-indications: Local contra-indications to the use of intrarectal steroids include obstruction, abscess, perforation, peritonitis, fresh intestinal anastomoses, extensive fistulae, and tuberculous, fungal or viral infections.

Pregnancy: Systemic and topical administration of corticosteroids to pregnant animals can cause abnormalities of foetal development. The relevance of this finding to human beings has not been established, but at present steroids should not be used extensively in pregnancy, that is in large amounts or for prolonged periods.

Warnings: General precautions common to all corticosteroid therapy should be observed during treatment with Colifoam especially in the case of young children. Treatment should be administered with caution in patients with severe ulcerative disease because of their predisposition to perforation of the bowel wall. Although uncommon at this dosage, local irritation may occur. For external use only.

Pharmaceutical precautions Pressurised container containing flammable propellant. Protect from sunlight and do not expose to temperatures above 50°C. Do not spray on a naked flame or any incandescent material. Keep away from sources of ignition–no smoking. Do not pierce or burn even after use. Store below 25°C. Do not refrigerate.

Legal category POM.

Package quantities Aerosol canister containing 20.8 g of foam (approximately 14 applications), plus a plastic applicator.

Further information An illustrated instruction leaflet is enclosed with each pack.

Product licence number 0036/0021.

NYTOL

Qualitative and quantitative composition Nytol contains 25 mg Diphenhydramine Hydrochloride BP per caplet.

Pharmaceutical form Caplets to be taken orally.

Clinical particulars

Therapeutic indication: An aid to the relief of temporary sleep disturbance.

Posology and method of administration: Two caplets to be taken 20 minutes before going to bed, or as directed by a physician. Not recommended for children under 16 years.

Contra-indications: Nytol is contraindicated in patients who are hypersensitive to diphenhydramine and in those with the following conditions: asthma, narrow angle glaucoma, prostatic hypertrophy, stenosing peptic ulcer, pyloroduodenal obstruction or bladder neck obstruction.

Special warnings and precautions for use: Nytol should be used with caution in patients with myasthenia gravis or seizure disorders. Tolerance may develop with continuous use.

Interaction with other drugs and other forms of interaction: Diphenhydramine has additive effects with alcohol and other CNS depressants (hypnotics, sedatives, tranquillisers). Monoamine oxidase (MAO) inhibitors prolong and intensify the anticholinergic effects of Diphenhydramine.

Diphenhydramine should not be used in patients receiving one of these drugs unless directed by a doctor.

Pregnancy and lactation: Diphenhydramine crosses the placenta. Because animal reproduction studies are not always predictive of human response and since there is inadequate experience with use of diphenhydramine in pregnant women, this drug is not recommended during pregnancy.

Diphenhydramine has been detected in milk. Because of higher risks of antihistamines for infants, Nytol is not recommended in nursing mothers.

Effects on ability to drive and use machines: Nytol is a hypnotic and will produce drowsiness or sedation soon after the dose has been taken. This will affect the patient's ability to drive and use machines.

Undesirable effects: Dizziness, drowsiness and grogginess are the undesirable effects most frequently reported by Nytol users. The frequency of these are approximately 6%, 4.5% and 7% respectively. These effects are mild and wear off about 8 hours after taking the medication. Dryness of mouth, nausea and nervousness have also been reported with diphenhydramine. The antihistamines have been reported rarely to cause thrombocytopenia.

Overdose: Overdosage causes CNS depression and CNS stimulation. Treatment should be supportive and directed towards specific symptoms. Convulsions and marked CNS stimulation should be treated with parenteral diazepam.

Pharmacological properties

Diphenhydramine hydrochloride is the active ingredient in Nytol, it is an antihistamine with well known pharmacological activities. As with most of the older antihistamines, diphenhydramine hydrochloride has a pronounced sedative effect. Diphenhydramine hydrochloride has been formulated into Nytol, a caplet for use as an aid to the relief of temporary sleep disturbance.

Pharmacodynamic properties: Diphenhydramine is an ethanolamine-derivative antihistamine. It is an antihistamine with anticholinergic and marked sedative effects. It acts by inhibiting the effects on H1-receptors.

Diphenhydramine is effective in reducing sleep onset (i.e., time to fall asleep) and increasing the depth and quality of sleep.

Pharmacokinetic properties: Diphenhydramine hydrochloride is rapidly absorbed following oral administration. Apparently it undergoes first-pass metabolism in the liver and only about 40–60% of an oral dose reaches systematic circulation as unchanged Diphenhydramine.

It is rapidly distributed throughout the whole body. Peak plasma concentrations are attained within 1–4 hours. The sedative effect also appears to be maximal within 1–3 hours after administration of a single concentration.

It is positively correlated with the plasma drug concentration.

Diphenhydramine is approx 80–85% bound to plasma proteins. Diphenhydramine is rapidly and almost completely metabolised. The drug is metabolised principally to Diphenylmethoxyacetic acid and is also dealkylated.

The metabolites are conjugated with glycine and glutamine and excreted in urine. Only about 1% of a single dose is excreted unchanged in urine.

The elimination half-life ranges from 2.4–9.3 hours in healthy adults. The terminal elimination half-life is prolonged in liver cirrhosis.

Pharmaceutical particulars

List of excipients:

Anhydrous lactose	NF
Stearic acid, powder	NF
Microcrystalline cellulose	PhEur
Silicon dioxide	NF
Maize starch	PhEur

Incompatibilities: None known.

Shelf life: Nytol has shelf life of 4 years in HDPE bottles and, 2 years in blister packs.

Special precaution for storage: Store in a dry place.

Nature and contents of container: High density polyethylene bottles with a polypropylene closure and cotton wool wadding, or an aclar/polyethylene/PVC or PVC/PVDC strip with a heat sealable aluminium foil. Bottles of 16 or 20 caplets and strips of 4, 8, 16, 20 or 24 caplets.

Instructions for use/handling: Not appropriate.

Legal category P.

Marketing authorisation number PL 0036/0050.

Date of first authorisation/renewal of authorisation 21 September 1992.

Date of revision of text July 1998.

NYTOL ONE-A-NIGHT

Qualitative and quantitative composition Nytol One-A-Night contains 50 mg Diphenhydramine Hydrochloride BP per caplet.

Pharmaceutical form Caplets to be taken orally.

Clinical particulars

Therapeutic indication: An aid to the relief of temporary sleep disturbance.

Posology and method of administration: One caplet to be taken 20 minutes before going to bed, or as directed by a physician. Not recommended for children under 16 years.

Contra-indications: Nytol One-A-Night is contraindicated in patients who are hypersensitive to diphenhydramine and in those with the following conditions: asthma, narrow angle glaucoma, prostatic hypertrophy, stenosing peptic ulcer, pyloroduodenal obstruction or bladder neck obstruction.

Special warnings and precautions for use: Nytol One-A-Night should be used with caution in patients with myasthenia gravis or seizure disorders. Tolerance may develop with continuous use.

Interaction with other drugs and other forms of interaction: Diphenhydramine has additive effects with alcohol and other CNS depressants (hypnotics, sedatives, tranquillisers). Monoamine oxidase (MAO) inhibitors prolong and intensify the anticholinergic effects of Diphenhydramine.

Diphenhydramine should not be used in patients receiving one of these drugs unless directed by a doctor.

Pregnancy and lactation: Diphenhydramine crosses the placenta. Because animal reproduction studies are not always predictive of human response and since there is inadequate experience with use of diphenhydramine in pregnant women, this drug is not recommended during pregnancy.

Diphenhydramine has been detected in milk. Because of higher risks of antihistamines for infants, Nytol One-A-Night is not recommended in nursing mothers.

Effects on ability to drive and use machines: Nytol One-A-Night is a hypnotic and will produce drowsiness or sedation soon after the dose has been taken. This will affect the patient's ability to drive and use machines.

Undesirable effects: Dizziness, drowsiness and grogginess are the undesirable effects most frequently reported by Nytol One-A-Night users. The frequency of these are approximately 6%, 4.5% and 7% respectively. These effects are mild and wear off about 8 hours after taking the medication. Dryness of mouth, nausea and nervousness have also been reported with diphenhydramine. The antihistamines have been reported rarely to cause thrombocytopenia.

Overdose: Overdosage causes CNS depression and CNS stimulation. Treatment should be supportive and directed towards specific symptoms. Convulsions and marked CNS stimulation should be treated with parenteral diazepam.

Pharmacological properties
Diphenhydramine hydrochloride is the active ingredient in Nytol One-A-Night, it is an antihistamine with well known pharmacological activities. As with most of the older antihistamines, diphenhydramine hydrochloride has a pronounced sedative effect. Diphenhydramine hydrochloride has been formulated into Nytol One-A-Night, a caplet for use as an aid to the relief of temporary sleep disturbance.

Pharmacodynamic properties: Diphenhydramine is an ethanolamine-derivative antihistamine. It is an antihistamine with anticholinergic and marked sedative effects. It acts by inhibiting the effects on H1-receptors.

Diphenhydramine is effective in reducing sleep onset (i.e., time to fall asleep) and increasing the depth and quality of sleep.

Pharmacokinetic properties: Diphenhydramine hydrochloride is rapidly absorbed following oral administration. Apparently it undergoes first-pass metabolism in the liver and only about 40–60% of an oral dose reaches systematic circulation as unchanged Diphenhydramine.

It is rapidly distributed throughout the whole body. Peak plasma concentrations are attained within 1–4 hours. The sedative effect also appears to be maximal within 1–3 hours after administration of a single dose.

It is positively correlated with the plasma drug concentration.

Diphenhydramine is approx 80–85% bound to plasma proteins. Diphenhydramine is rapidly and almost completely metabolised. The drug is metabolised principally to Diphenylmethoxyacetic acid and is also dealkylated.

The metabolites are conjugated with glycine and glutamine and excreted in urine. Only about 1% of a single dose is excreted unchanged in urine.

The elimination half-life ranges from 2.4–9.3 hours in healthy adults. The terminal elimination half-life is prolonged in liver cirrhosis.

Pharmaceutical particulars
List of excipients:

Anhydrous lactose	USNF
Stearic acid, powder	USP
Microcrystalline cellulose	PhEur
Silicon dioxide	USNF
Maize starch	PhEur

Incompatibilities: None known.

Shelf life: Nytol has shelf life of 2 years in HDPE bottles and PVC/PVDC blister packs and 3 years in Aclar/PE/PVC blister packs.

Special precaution for storage: Store in a dry place.

Nature and contents of container: High density polyethylene bottles with a polypropylene closure and cotton wool wadding, or an aclar/polyethylene/PVC or PVC/PVDC strip with a heat sealable aluminium foil. Bottles of 16 or 20 caplets and strips of 4, 8, 10, 16 or 20 caplets.

Instructions for use/handling: Not appropriate.

Legal category P.

Marketing authorisation number PL 0036/0069.

Date of first authorisation of authorisation 13 February 1995.

Date of revision of text July 1998.

OTOMIZE

Qualitative and quantitative composition Otomize contains: Neomycin Sulphate PhEur 0.5% w/w (3250 IU/ml); Dexamethasone PhEur 0.1% w/w; Glacial Acetic Acid PhEur 2.0% w/w.

Pharmaceutical form: A milky oil-in-water emulsion as a liquid ear spray for application into the external auditory meatus.

Clinical particulars
Therapeutic indications: For the treatment of otitis externa.

Posology and method of administration: Topical spray directly into the ear. Adults, children and the elderly: one metered dose (60 mg) to be administered directly into each affected ear three times daily. Treatment should be continued until two days after symptoms have disappeared. Discontinue treatment if there is no clinical improvement after 7 days.

Contra-indications: The product should not be used in patients with a known sensitivity to neomycin or where a perforated tympanic membrane has been diagnosed or is suspected.

Special warnings and precautions for use: The CSM has warned that when otitis externa is treated topically with preparations containing aminoglycosides, in patients who have a perforation of the tympanic membrane, there is an increased risk of drug-induced deafness. It is therefore important to ensure that there is no perforation in such patients. However, in the presence of a perforation many specialists do use such agents cautiously in patients with otitis media.

Interactions with other medicaments and other forms of interaction: None known.

Pregnancy and lactation: There is inadequate evidence of safety in human pregnancy. Topical administration of corticosteroids to pregnant animals can cause abnormalities of foetal development including cleft palate and intra-uterine growth retardation. There may therefore be a very small risk of such effects in the human foetus.

Effects on ability to drive and use machines: Unresolved ear problems could themselves affect driving ability.

Undesirable effects: Some patients may experience a transient stinging or burning sensation for the first few days of treatment.

Overdose: Overdosage by this route is extremely unlikely.

Pharmacological properties
Pharmacodynamic properties: Neomycin sulphate is an established antibiotic with a well characterised broad spectrum of activity. Dexamethasone is a well established topical anti-inflammatory steroid. Acetic acid functions to produce a low pH to assist in the control of bacterial infection.

Pharmacokinetic properties: Otomize ear spray is applied topically to the external auditory meatus and acts locally. The spray provides excellent distribution and coverage of the surface.

Preclinical safety data: No additional data of relevance.

Pharmaceutical particulars
List of excipients: Ethoxy (2) Stearyl Alcohol; Ethoxy (20) Stearyl Alcohol; Stearyl Alcohol; Methyl Parahydroxybenzoate; Propyl Parahydroxybenzoate; Purified Water.

Incompatibilities: None known.

Shelf life: Shelf life in the product as packaged for sale: 18 months from the date of manufacture.

Shelf life after first opening of the container: Use within one month of first use.

Special precautions for storage: Store upright in a carton up to 25°C.

Nature and contents of container: The product is supplied in an amber glass bottle of 5 ml capacity fitted with a spray device.

Instructions for use/handling: Shake the bottle well before use. Before first use, press actuator down several times to obtain a fine spray. Each press then delivers one metered dose. Do not inhale the spray. Administer spray directly by gently placing nozzle tip into ear opening and pressing down once on the actuator. Use within one month of first use. If there is a period of more than one week since last use, press actuator down a few times before using again.

Legal category POM.

Marketing authorisation number PL 00036/0042.

Date of renewal of authorisation March 1997.

Date of (partial) revision of text March 1998.

PIRITON* SYRUP

Presentation Piriton Syrup is a colourless syrup containing 4 mg Chlorphenamine Maleate BP in 10 ml.

Other ingredients: Sugar, glycerol, alcohol, tingle flavour, peppermint oil, water, and as preservative, a mixture of methyl, ethyl and propyl parahydroxybenzoates.

Uses Piriton Syrup is indicated for symptomatic control of all allergic conditions responsive to antihistamines, including hayfever, vasomotor rhinitis, urticaria, angioneurotic oedema, food allergy, drug and serum reactions, insect bites.

Dosage and administration
Adults: 10 ml every 4 to 6 hours (daily max. 24 mg i.e. 60 ml).

Children aged 6–12 years: 5 ml every 4 to 6 hours (daily max. 12 mg i.e. 30 ml).

Children aged 2–5 years: 2.5 ml every 4 to 6 hours (daily max. 6 mg i.e. 15 ml).

Children aged 1–2 years: 2.5 ml twice daily. Not recommended in children below 1 year.

Elderly: As in adults but such patients are prone to confusional psychosis and other neurological anticholinergic effects.

Contra-indications, warnings, etc
Contra-indications: Piriton Syrup is contra-indicated in patients who are hypersensitive to antihistamines or to any of the syrup ingredients.

The anticholinergic properties of chlorphenamine are intensified by monoamine oxidase inhibitors (MAOIs). Piriton Syrup is therefore contra-indicated in patients who have been treated with MAOIs within the last fourteen days.

Precautions: The anticholinergic properties of chlorphenamine may cause drowsiness, dizziness, blurred vision and psychomotor impairment which may seriously affect patients' ability to drive and use machinery.

Chlorphenamine in common with other drugs having anticholinergic effects, should be used with caution in epilepsy, raised intra-ocular pressure including glaucoma, prostatic hypertrophy; severe hypertension or cardiovascular disease; bronchitis, bronchiectasis and asthma; hepatic disease and thyrotoxicosis. Children and the elderly are more likely to experience the neurological anticholinergic effects.

The effects of alcohol may be increased.

Piriton Syrup contains sugar. It should be administered with care to patients with diabetes mellitus. Long-term use increases the risk of dental caries and it is essential that adequate dental hygiene is maintained.

Drug interactions: Concurrent use of chlorphenamine and hypnotics or anxiolytics may potentiate drowsiness. Concurrent use of alcohol may have a similar effect.

Chlorphenamine inhibits phenytoin metabolism and can lead to phenytoin toxicity.

The anticholinergic effects of chlorphenamine are intensified by MAOIs (see *Contra-indications*).

Pregnancy: There is inadequate evidence of safety in human pregnancy. Piriton Syrup should only be used during pregnancy when clearly needed and when the potential benefits outweigh the potential unknown risks to the foetus. Use during the third trimester may result in reactions in neonates.

Lactation: It is reasonable to assume that chlorphenamine maleate may inhibit lactation and may be secreted in breast milk. The use of Piriton preparations in mothers breast feeding their babies requires that the therapeutic benefits of the drug should be weighed against the potential hazards to the mother and baby.

Side-effects: Sedation varying from slight drowsiness to deep sleep. The following may also occasionally occur; inability to concentrate; lassitude; blurred vision; gastro-intestinal disturbances such as anorexia, dyspepsia, nausea, vomiting, diarrhoea and abdominal pain; hepatitis including jaundice; urinary retention; headaches; dry mouth; dizziness; palpitations; tachycardia; arrhythmias; hypotension; chest tightness; thickening of bronchial secretions; haemolytic anaemia and other blood dyscrasias; allergic reactions including exfoliative dermatitis, photosensitivity and urticaria, twitching, muscular weakness and inco-ordination; tinnitus; depression, irritability and nightmares.

Children and the elderly are more likely to experience the neurological anticholinergic effects.

Overdosage: The estimated lethal dose of chlorphenamine is 25 to 50 mg per kg body weight. Symptoms and signs include sedation, paradoxical stimulation of CNS, toxic psychosis, seizures, apnoea, convulsions, anticholinergic effects, dystonic reactions and cardiovascular collapse including arrhythmias.

Symptomatic and supportive measures should be provided with special attention to cardiac, respiratory, renal and hepatic functions, and fluid and electrolyte balance.

Treatment of overdosage should include gastric lavage or induced emesis using Syrup of Ipecacuanha. Following these measures activated charcoal and cathartics may be administered to minimise absorption.

Hypotension and arrhythmias should be treated vigorously. CNS convulsions may be treated with i.v. diazepam or phenytoin. Haemoperfusion may be used in severe cases.

Pharmaceutical precautions Piriton Syrup should be stored at a temperature not exceeding 25°C and protected from light. Piriton Syrup may be diluted with Syrup BP. The resultant mixture should be used within fourteen days.

Legal category P.

Package quantities Piriton Syrup is supplied in 150 ml amber glass bottles.

Further information Nil.

Product licence number 0036/0088.

PIRITON* TABLETS

Presentation Piriton Tablets are round, biconvex, yellow tablets with a P to one side of the breakline, the reverse face being blank. Each tablet contains 4 mg of the potent antihistamine Chlorphenamine Maleate BP.

Other ingredients: Lactose, maize starch, magnesium stearate, colour, yellow iron oxide (E172).

Uses Piriton Tablets are indicated for symptomatic control of all allergic conditions responsive to antihistamines, including hayfever, vasomotor rhinitis, urticaria, angioneurotic oedema, food allergy, drug and serum reactions, insect bites.

Dosage and administration
Adults: 4 mg 4 to 6 hourly (daily max. 24 mg).

Children aged 6 to 12 years: 2 mg 4 to 6 hourly (daily max. 12 mg).

Elderly: As in adults but such patients are prone to confusional psychosis and other neurological anticholinergic effects.

Contra-indications, warnings, etc
Contra-indications: Piriton Tablets are contra-indicated in patients who are hypersensitive to antihistamines or to any of the other ingredients.

The anticholinergic properties of chlorphenamine are intensified by monoamine oxidase inhibitors (MAOIs). Piriton Tablets are therefore contra-indicated in patients who have been treated with MAOIs within the last fourteen days.

Precautions: The anticholinergic properties of chlorphenamine may cause drowsiness, dizziness, blurred vision and psychomotor impairment which may seriously affect patients ability to drive and use machinery.

Chlorphenamine in common with other drugs having anticholinergic effects, should be used with caution in epilepsy, raised intra-ocular pressure including glaucoma, prostatic hypertrophy; severe hypertension or cardiovascular disease; bronchitis, bronchiectasis and asthma; hepatic disease and thyrotoxicosis. Children and the elderly are more likely to experience the neurological anticholinergic effects.

The effects of alcohol may be increased.

Drug interactions: Concurrent use of chlorphenamine and hypnotics or anxiolytics may potentiate drowsiness. Concurrent use of alcohol may have a similar effect.

Chlorphenamine inhibits phenytoin metabolism and can lead to phenytoin toxicity.

The anticholinergic effects of chlorphenamine are intensified by MAOIs (see *Contra-indications*).

Pregnancy: There is inadequate evidence of safety in human pregnancy. Piriton Tablets should only be used during pregnancy when clearly needed and when the potential benefits outweigh the potential unknown risks to the foetus. Use during the third trimester may result in reactions in neonates.

Lactation: It is reasonable to assume that chlorphenamine maleate may inhibit lactation and may be secreted in breast milk. The use of Piriton preparations in mothers breast feeding their babies requires that the therapeutic benefits of the drug should be weighed against the potential hazards to the mother and baby.

Side-effects: Sedation varying from slight drowsiness to deep sleep. The following may also occasionally occur; inability to concentrate; lassitude; blurred vision; gastro-intestinal disturbances such as anorexia, dyspepsia, nausea, vomiting, diarrhoea and abdominal pain; hepatitis including jaundice; urinary retention; headaches; dry mouth; dizziness; palpitations; tachycardia; arrhythmias; hypotension; chest tightness; thickening of bronchial secretions; haemolytic anaemia and other blood dyscrasias; allergic reactions including exfoliative dermatitis, photosensitivity and urticaria, twitching, muscular weakness and inco-ordination; tinnitus; depression, irritability and nightmares.

Children and the elderly are more likely to experience the neurological anticholinergic effects.

Overdosage: The estimated lethal dose of chlorphenamine is 25 to 50 mg per kg body weight. Symptoms and signs include sedation, paradoxical stimulation of CNS, toxic psychosis, seizures, apnoea, convulsions, anticholinergic effects, dystonic reactions and cardiovascular collapse including arrhythmias.

Symptomatic and supportive measures should be provided with special attention to cardiac, respiratory, renal and hepatic functions, and fluid and electrolyte balance.

Treatment of overdosage should include gastric lavage or induced emesis using Syrup of Ipecacuanha. Following these measures activated charcoal and cathartics may be administered to minimise absorption.

Hypotension and arrhythmias should be treated vigorously, CNS convulsions may be treated with i.v. diazepam or phenytoin. Haemoperfusion may be used in severe cases.

Pharmaceutical precautions Piriton Tablets should be stored below 30°C.

Legal category P.

Package quantities Piriton Tablets are supplied in packs of 500.

Further information Nil.

Product licence number 0036/0090.

PROCTOFOAM

Qualitative and quantitative composition

Hydrocortisone Acetate PhEur	1.0% w/w
Pramoxine Hydrochloride USP	1.0% w/w

Pharmaceutical form Aerosol foam.

Clinical particulars
Therapeutic indications: For the short term (not more than 5-7 days) relief of the symptoms of itching, irritation, discomfort or pain associated with local, non infective anal or perianal conditions.

Posology and method of administration: One applicator full per rectum two or three times daily and after each bowel evacuation (up to a maximum of four times daily). For perianal administration, apply a small quantity on 2 fingers.

Not recommended for use in children.

Contra-indications: Hypersensitivity to pramoxine hydrochloride or to any component of the preparation. Bacterial, viral or fungal infection.

Special warnings and precautions for use: Not for prolonged use. Contact sensitisation to local anaesthetics is common following prolonged application.

Seek medical advice if symptoms worsen, or do not improve within 7 days or if bleeding occurs.

Shake vigorously before use, use at room temperture, keep out of the reach of children. For external use only.

Rectal examination must be performed to exclude serious pathology before initiating treatment with Proctofoam.

Interactions with other medicaments and other forms of interaction: None known.

Pregnancy and lactation: Safety for use in pregnancy and lactation has not been established.

There is inadequate evidence of safety in human pregnancy. Topical administration of corticosteroids to pregnant animals can cause abnormalities to foetal development including cleft palate and intrauterine growth retardation. There may be a very small risk of such effects in the human foetus. No data is available on the use of topical corticosteroids and local anaesthetic agents in nursing mothers. However, the product has been used by nursing mothers for many years without apparent ill consequence.

Effects on ability to drive and use machines: None known.

Undesirable effects: Although uncommon at this dosage, local burning, irritation, allergic dermatitis, secondary infection and skin atrophy may occur. Systemic absorption of topical corticosteroids has produced reversible suppression of the hypothalamic–pituitary–adrenal axis and manifestations of Cushing's Syndrome.

Overdosage: Excess use of topical corticosteroids may produce systemic adverse effects.

Pharmacological properties
Pharmacodynamic properties: Pramoxine hydrochloride is a surface anaesthetic, and thus relieves the pain of anal and perianal conditions.

The use of steroids in inflammatory conditions is well known.

Pharmacokinetic properties: Not applicable.

Preclinical safety data: None stated.

List of excipients

Cetyl Alcohol	PhEur
Emulsifying Wax	NF
Methyl Paraben	PhEur
Polyoxyethylene (10), Stearyl Ether	PhEur
Propylene Glycol	PhEur
Propyl Paraben	PhEur
Triethanolamine	BP
Demineralised Water	PhEur
Propellant HP-70 Consisting of:	
– Isobutane	USNF
– Propane	USNF

Incompatibilities: Compatibility with barrier methods of contraception have not been demonstrated.

Shelf life: 30 months.

Special precautions for storage: Pressurised container containing flammable propellant. Protect from sunlight. Do not expose to temperatures above 5°C. Do not spray on a naked flame or any incandescent material. Keep away from sources of ignition–no smoking. Do not pierce or burn, even after use.

Do not refrigerate.

Nature and contents of container: Aerosol canister containing 20 g of product plus 1.2 g of inert propellant. A 10% overage of product and propellant is included to ensure the required number of doses can be achieved.

Instructions for use/handling

1. Shake the canister vigorously for 30 seconds before each use.
2. Withdraw the plunger slowly until it stops at the catch line.
3. Holding upright, insert the canister top into the applicator tip. Make sure you hold the plunger and applicator body firmly with your fingers.
4. Press down a number of times on the canister top with your fingers. Each press releases a small amount of foam. When the applicator is half full of foam, stop for a few secods until the foam stops expanding.
5. Press down again to complete filling to the fill line.
6. *For internal use*
   Stand with one leg raised on a chair, or lie down on your left side. Insert gently into the back passage and push the plunger fully into the applicator.
7. *For external use*
   Expel a small quantity of foam onto a tissue, pad or two fingers and apply the foam to the affected area.

These instructions are provided on the leaflet with illustrations to assist understanding.

Marketing authorisation number PL 0036/5002R.

Date of first authorisation/renewal of authorisation 14 June 1991.

Date of (partial) revision of the text March 1996.

QUELLADA-M* CREAM SHAMPOO

Qualitative and quantitative composition Malathion USP 1.0% w/w

Pharmaceutical form Cream shampoo

Clinical particulars
Therapeutic indications: For the treatment of head lice and pubic lice infestation. Family members and close contacts should also be treated.

Posology and method of administration: For topical external use only.
As this product does not contain alcohol, it may be more suitable for those with asthma or eczema.

Adults, the elderly and children aged 6 months and over:

For head lice:

1. Wet the hair thoroughly with warm water and apply sufficient shampoo to work up a rich lather and ensure that no part of the scalp is uncovered. Pay special attention to the back of the neck and the area behind the ears. Take care to avoid the eyes.
2. Leave for at least five minutes.
3. Rinse thoroughly with clean warm water and repeat procedure.
4. While hair is still wet, comb with an ordinary comb. A fine-toothed louse comb can then be used to remove the dead lice and eggs.
5. This treatment should be carried out a total of three times at three day intervals.

For pubic lice: Application and dosage are as for the head. Apply the lotion to the pubic hair and the hair between the legs and arms.

Contra-indications: None stated.

Special warnings and precautions for use: As with all shampoos, avoid contact with the eyes. Children under six months should only be treated under medical supervision.

When Quellada-M cream shampoo is used by a school nurse or other health officer in the mass treatment of large numbers of children, it is advisable that protective plastic or rubber gloves be worn. Keep out of the reach of children.

Continued prolonged treatment with this product should be avoided. It should be used for not more than three times at three day intervals then not repeated within a three week period.

Interactions with other medicaments and other forms of interaction: None stated

Pregnancy and lactation: Quellada-M cream shampoo is not known to have any effect on fertility, pregnancy and lactation. Its use in pregnant or lactating women is not recommended unless there is an overdue need.

Effects on ability to drive and use machines: None stated.

Undesirable effects: None stated.

Overdose: In the event of deliberate or accidental ingestion, empty stomach contents by gastric lavage and keep patient warm. In the event of massive ingestion, atropine and pralidoxime may be required to counteract cholinesterase inhibition.

Pharmacological properties
Pharmacodynamic properties: Quellada-M cream shampoo contains malathion, a widely used organophosphorous insecticide which is active by cholinesterase inhibition. It is effective against a wide range of insects, but is one of the least toxic organophosphorous insecticides since it is rapidly detoxified by plasma carboxylesterases.

Pharmacokinetic properties: Quellada-M cream shampoo is applied topically to the affected area.

Preclinical safety data: None stated.

Pharmaceutical particulars
List of excipients: Sodium lauryl sulphate paste; cetostearyl alcohol; lauric diethanolamide; ethoxylated lanolin (50%); methyl hydroxybenzoate; propyl hydroxybenzoate; hydrochloric acid; citric acid (anhydrous); dibasic sodium phosphate; colour yellow (E110); sodium edetate; perfume M&B 1658; purified water.

Incompatibilities: None stated.

Shelf life: 18 months.

Special precautions for storage: Store at or below 20°C.

Nature and contents of container: Boxed, internally lacquered aluminium tube with polyethylene cap containing 40 g of product.

Instructions for use/handling: None stated

Marketing authorisation holder: Ultra Chemical Limited, Tubiton House, Oldham, Lancashire, OL1 3HS.

Marketing authorisation number 14236/0005

Date of approval/revision of SPC July 1995

Legal category P

QUELLADA-M* LIQUID

Qualitative and quantitative composition Malathion 0.5% w/w

Pharmaceutical form Liquid emulsion

Clinical particulars
Therapeutic indications: Eradication of head lice, pubic lice and their eggs. Treatment of scabies.

Posology and method of administration: For topical external use only.

As this product does not contain alcohol, it may be more suitable for those with asthma or eczema.

Adults, the elderly and children aged 6 months and over:
Treatment of headlice: Rub the liquid into the scalp until all the hair and scalp is thoroughly moistened. Leave the hair to dry naturally in a warm but well ventilated room. After 12 hours, or the next day, if preferred, shampoo hair in the normal way. Rinse the hair and comb whilst wet to remove dead lice and eggs (nits) using the louse comb.

Treatment of crab (pubic) lice: Apply Quellada-M liquid to the entire skin surface. Pay particular attention to all hairy areas including beards and moustaches. Avoid any other areas above the neck. Leave on for at least one hour before washing but preferably Quellada-M liquid should be left on overnight. Wash off in the usual manner.

Treatment of scabies: Apply Quellada-M liquid to the entire skin surface. In adults it may not be necessary to apply above the neck but children under the age of two years should have a thin film of Quellada-M liquid applied to the scalp, face and ears, avoiding the eyes and mouth. Do not wash off or bathe for 24 hours. If hands or any other parts must be washed during this period, the treatment must be re-applied to those areas immediately.

No special sterilisation of clothing is necessary, ordinary laundering or dry-cleaning with hot-iron pressing is sufficient. The infestation is cleared by the treatment. However, the itching and rash may persist for up to 7 days. An anti-irritant cream can be applied if necessary. Family members and close contacts should also be treated simultaneously.

Children aged 6 months and under: On medical advice only.

Contra-indications: Known sensitivity to malathion. Not to be used on infants less than 6 months except on medical advice.

Special warnings and precautions for use: Avoid contact with the eyes. For external use only. Keep out of the reach of children. If inadvertently swallowed, a doctor or casualty department should be contacted at once.

When Quellada-M liquid is used by a school nurse or other health officers in the mass treatment of large numbers of children, it is advisable that protective plastic or rubber gloves are worn.

Continued prolonged treatment with this product should be avoided. It should be used not more than once a week and for not more than three consecutive weeks.

Interactions with other medicaments and other forms of interaction: None stated.

Pregnancy and lactation: No known effects in pregnancy and lactation. However, as with all medicines, use with caution.

Effects on ability to drive and use machines: None stated.

Undesirable effects: Very rarely skin irritation has been reported.

Overdose: It is most unlikely that a toxic dose of malathion will be ingested. Treatment consists of gastric lavage, assisted respiration and if necessary in the event of massive ingestion, administration of atropine and pralidoxime.

Pharmacolgical properties
Pharmacodynamic properties: Quellada-M liquid contains malathion, a widely used organophosphorous insecticide which is active by cholinesterase inhibition. It is effective against a wide range of insects, but is one of the least toxic organophosphorous insecticides since it is rapidly detoxified by plasma carboxylesterases.

Pharmacokinetic properties: None stated. Quellada-M liquid is applied topically to the affected area.

Preclinical safety data: None stated.

Pharmaceutical particulars
List of excipients: Methyl hydroxybenzoate; propyl hydroxybenzoate; lanette wax SX,; potassium citrate; citric acid; perfume HT 52; water.

Incompatibilities: None stated.

Shelf life: Two and a half years.

Special precautions for storage: Store at or below 25°C. Protect from sunlight.

Nature and contents of container: Boxed, clear or amber glass bottles with polyethylene caps and polypropylene faced wads containing either 50 ml or 200 ml of product.

Instructions for use/handling: None stated.

Marketing authorisation holder: Ultra Chemical, Tubiton House, Oldham, Lancashire, OL1 3HS

Marketing authorisation number 14236/0004

Date of approval/revision of SPC October 1995

Legal category P

ROZEX CREAM

Qualitative and quantitative composition Metronidazole PhEur 0.75% w/w.

Pharmaceutical form Cream.

Clinical particulars
Therapeutic indications: Indicated in the treatment of inflammatory papules, pustules and erythema of rosacea.

Posology and method of administration: For topical administration only.

The average period of treatment is three to four months. If a clear benefit has been demonstrated, continued therapy for a further three to four months period may be considered by the prescribing physician depending on the severity of the condition. In clinical studies, topical metronidazole therapy for rosacea has been continued for up to 2 years. In the absence of a clear clinical improvement, therapy should be stopped.

Adults: A pea-size amount of cream is applied to the affected areas of skin, twice daily, morning and evening. Areas to be treated should be washed with a mild cleanser before application. Patients may use non-comedogenic and non-astringent cosmetics after application of Rozex cream.

Elderly: The dosage recommended in the elderly is the same as that recommended in adults.

Children: Not recommended. Safety and efficacy have not been established.

Contra-indications: Contraindicated in individuals with a history of hypersensitivity to metronidazole or other ingredients in the formulation.

Special warnings and precautions for use: Contact with eyes and mucous membranes should be avoided.

If a reaction suggesting local irritation occurs patients should be directed to use the medication less frequently, discontinue use temporarily and to seek medical advice if necessary.

Metronidazole is a nitroimidazole and should be used with caution in patients with evidence of, or history of, blood dyscrasia.

Unnecessary and prolonged use of this medication should be avoided.

Exposure of treated sites to ultraviolet or strong sunlight should be avoided during use of metronidazole.

Interactions with other medicaments and other forms of interaction: Interaction with systemic medication is unlikely because absorption of metronidazole following cutaneous application of Rozex cream is low.

Ingestion of alcohol during oral treatment with metronidazole may cause potentiation of the effects of the latter on the central nervous system and may induce a disulfiram-like reaction. Drug interactions are less likely with topical administration but should be kept in mind when Rozex cream is prescribed for patients receiving anticoagulant treatment. Oral metronidazole has been reported to potentiate the anti-coagulant effect of dicoumarin and warfarin, resulting in a prolongation of prothrombin time.

Pregnancy and lactation: There is no experience to date with the use of Rozex Cream in pregnancy. Metronidazole crosses the placental barrier and rapidly enters the foetal circulation. There is inadequate evidence of the safety of metronidazole in human pregnancy. In animals, metronidazole was not teratogenic or embryotoxic unless administered at extremely high doses. Rozex Cream should only be used in pregnancy when there is no safer alternative.

After oral administration, metronidazole is excreted in breast milk in concentrations similar to those found in the plasma, Even though metronidazole blood levels from topical administration are significantly lower than those achieved after oral administration, in nursing mothers, a decision should be made to discontinue nursing or to discontinue the drug, taking into account the importance of the drug to the mother.

Effects on ability to drive and use machines: Not applicable.

Undesirable effects: Because of the minimal absorption of metronidazole and consequently its insignificant plasma concentration after topical administration, the adverse experiences reported with the oral form of the drug have not been reported with Rozex Cream. Adverse reactions reported with Rozex Cream have been only local and mild, and include skin discomfort (burning and stinging), erythema, pruritis, and skin irritation. Rarely, worsening of rosacea has occurred. All individual events occurred in less than 3% of patients.

Overdosage: There is no human experience with overdosage of Rozex Cream. The acute oral toxicity of a gel formulation was determined to be greater than 5 g/kg (the highest dose given) in albino rats. No toxic effects were observed at this dose. This dose is equivalent to the intake of 12 30 g tubes of Rozex Cream for an adult weighing 72 kg and 2 tubes for a child weighing 12 kg.

Pharmacological properties
Pharmacodynamic properties: Metronidazole is an antiprotozoal and antibacterial agent which is active against a wide range of pathogenic micro-organisms. The mechanisms of action of metronidazole in rosacea are unknown but available evidence suggests that the effects may be antibacterial and/or anti-inflammatory.

Pharmacokinetic properties: Metronidazole is rapidly and nearly totally absorbed after oral administration.

The drug is not significantly bound to serum proteins and distributes well to all body compartments with the lowest concentration found in the fat. Metronidazole is excreted primarily in the urine as parent drug, oxidative metabolites and conjugates.

Bioavailability studies with a topical 1 g application of Rozex Cream to the face of normal subjects resulted in mean maximum serum concentrations of 32.9 ng/ml (range 14.8 to 54.4 ng/ml) which is approximately 100 times less than those attained after a single oral dose of 250 mg (mean C_{max}=7248 ng/ml; range 4270–13,970 ng/ml). The peak concentration occurred between 0.25–4 hours after oral dosing, and 6 to 24 hours after cutaneous application of Rozex Cream.

Following topical application of Rozex Cream, serum concentrations of the major metabolite (the hydroxymetabolite 2-hydroxymethylmetronidazole) were below the quantifiable limit of the assay (<9.6 ng/ml) at most of the time points, ranging to a maximum of 17.5 ng/ml peak concentration between 8 and 24 hours after application. In comparison, the peak concentration following a 250 mg oral dose ranged from 626 to 1788 ng/ml between 4 and 12 hours after dosing.

The extent of exposure (Area under the curve, AUC) from a 1 g application of metronidazole administered topically was 1.36% of the AUC of a single oral 250 mg metronidazole dose (mean +912.7 ng.hr/ml and approximately 67,207 ng.ml/hr respectively).

Preclinical safety data: No evidence for a primary dermal irritation was observed in rabbits following a single 24-hour cutaneous application of Rozex Cream to abraded and non-abraded skin, under occlusion.

Metronidazole has shown mutagenic activity in several *in vitro* bacterial assay systems. In addition, a dose-response increase in the frequency of micronuclei was observed in mice after intraperitoneal injection and an increase in chromosome aberrations have been reported in patients with Crohn's disease who were treated with 200 to 1200 mg/day of oral metronidazole for 1 to 24 months. However, the preponderance of evidence from these studies suggests that although metronidazole has a potential for producing mutations, this should not occur in well oxygenated mammalian cells, i.e., under normal aerobic conditions.

The carcinogenicity of metronidazole by the oral route of administration has been evaluated in rats, mice and hamsters. These studies showed that oral metronidazole caused an increased incidence of pulmonary tumours in mice and possibly other tumours, including liver tumours, in the rat. Conversely, two lifetime studies in hamsters produced negative results. Moreover, one study showed a significant enhancement of UV-induced skin tumours in hairless mice treated with metronidazole intraperitoneally (15 μg per g body weight and per day for 28 weeks).

Although the significance of these results to the cutaneous use of metronidazole for the treatment of rosacea is unclear, patients should be advised to avoid or minimise exposure of metronidazole cream-treated sites to sun. After several decades of systemic use, no evidence has been published to suggest that metronidazole is associated with a carcinogenic potential in humans.

Pharmaceutical particulars

List of excipients: Emulsifying Wax, Benzyl alcohol, Isopropyl palmitate, Glycerol, Sorbitol 70% (non-crystallising), Lactic acid and/or Sodium Hydroxide, Purified Water.

Incompatibilities: None known.

Shelf life: Rozex Cream has a shelf life when unopened of 24 months.

Special precautions for storage: Store at a temperature not exceeding 25°C. Do not refrigerate.

Nature and contents of container: Aluminium tubes with epoxy phenolic lining, fitted with white polypropylene screw caps; pack sizes 30 g.

Instructions for use/handling: Replace cap tightly after use.

Marketing authorisation holder: Galderma (UK) Ltd, Leywood House, Woodside Road, Amersham, Buckinghamshire, HP6 6AA.

Marketing authorisation number 10590/0028

Date of first authorisation/renewal of application 18 June 1997

Date of (partial) revision of the text February 1997

Legal category POM.

ROZEX* GEL

Qualitative and quantitative composition Metronidazole PhEur 0.75% w/w.

Pharmaceutical form Gel

Clinical particulars

Therapeutic indications: Indicated in the treatment of inflammatory papules, pustules and erythema of rosacea.

Posology and method of administration: For topical administration only.

Adults: Apply and rub in a film of gel twice daily, morning and evening, to entire affected area after washing.

Elderly: The dosage recommended in the elderly is the same as that recommended in adults.

Children: Not recommended.

Contra-indications: Contraindicated in individuals with a history of hypersensitivity to metronidazole, parabens or other ingredients in the formulation.

Special warnings and special precautions for use: Rozex Gel has been reported to cause lacrimation of the eyes, therefore, contact with the eyes should be avoided. If a reaction suggesting local irritation occurs patients should be directed to use the medication less frequently, discontinue use temporarily or discontinue use until further instructions. Metronidazole is a nitroimidazole and should be used with care in patients with evidence of, or history of, blood dyscrasia. Exposure of treated sites to ultraviolet or strong sunlight should be avoided during use of metronidazole.

Interaction with other medicaments and other forms of interaction: Drug interactions are less likely with topical administration but should be kept in mind when Rozex Gel is prescribed for patients receiving anticoagulant treatment. Oral metronidazole has been reported to potentiate the anti-coagulant effect of dicoumarin and warfarin, resulting in a prolongation of prothrombin time.

Pregnancy and lactation: There is no experience to date with the use of Rozex Gel in pregnancy. Metronidazole crosses the placental barrier and rapidly enters the foetal circulation. There is inadequate evidence of the safety of metronidazole in human pregnancy. In animals, metronidazole was not teratogenic or embryotoxic unless administered at extremely high doses. Rozex Gel should only be used in pregnancy when there is no safer alternative.

After oral administration, metronidazole is excreted in breast milk in concentrations similar to those found in the plasma, metronidazole blood levels from topical administration are significantly lower than those achieved after oral administration. A decision should be made to discontinue nursing or to discontinue the drug, taking into account the importance of the drug to the mother.

Effects on ability to drive and use machines: Not applicable.

Undesirable effects: Because of the minimal absorption of metronidazole and consequently its insignificant plasma concentration after topical administration, the adverse experiences reported with the oral form of the drug have not been reported with Rozex Gel. Adverse reactions reported with Rozex Gel include watery (tearing) eyes if the gel is applied too closely to this area, transient redness and mild dryness, burning and skin irritation.

Overdosage: There is no human experience with overdosage of Rozex Gel. The acute oral toxicity of Rozex Gel was determined to be greater than 5 g/kg (the highest dose given) in albino rats.

Pharmacological properties

Pharmacodynamic properties: Metronidazole is an antiprotozoal and antibacterial agent which is active against a wide range of pathogenic micro-organisms. The mechanisms of action of metronidazole in rosacea are unknown but available evidence suggests that the effects may be antibacterial and/or anti-inflammatory.

Pharmacokinetic properties: Metronidazole is rapidly and nearly totally absorbed after oral administration. The drug is not significantly bound to serum proteins and distributes well to all body compartments with the lowest concentration found in the fat. Metronidazole is excreted primarily in the urine as parent drug, oxidative metabolites and conjugates.

Bioavailability studies with Rozex Gel in rosacea patients treated with 7.5 mg metronidazole applied topically to the face resulted in a maximum serum concentration of 66 nanograms/ml which is approximately 100 times less than those attained after a single oral dose of 250 mg. In most patients at most time points after Rozex Gel application, serum concentrations of metronidazole were below the detectable limits of the assay (25 nanograms/ml).

Preclinical safety data: The toxicity studies conducted with the metronidazole 0.75% topical Gel formulation demonstrate that the product is non-toxic in rats after acute oral administration of 5 g/kg and produced no ocular irritation in rabbit eyes. The formulation produced no observable effects in rabbits after dermal application of 13 mg/kg for 90 days.

No compound-related dermal or systemic effects were observed in a 13-week cutaneous route toxicity study, in which Rozex gel containing Metronidazole 0.75% w/w was applied daily to rabbits at doses ranging between 0.13 and 13 mg/kg.

Metronidazole has shown evidence of carcinogenic activity in a number of studies involving chronic, oral administration in mice and rats but not in studies involving hamsters.

One study showed a significant enhancement of UV induced skin tumours in hairless mice treated with Metronidazole intraperitoneally (15 micrograms per g body weight and per day for 28 weeks). Although the significance of these studies to man is not clear patients should be advised to avoid or minimise exposure of Metronidazole treated sites to sun.

Metronidazole has shown mutagenic activity in several in vitro bacterial assay systems. In addition, a dose-response increase in the frequency of micronuclei was observed in mice after intraperitoneal injection and an increase in chromosome aberrations have been reported in patients with Crohn's disease who were treated with 200 to 1200 mg/day of metronidazole for 1 to 24 months. However, no excess chromosomal aberrations in circulating human lymphocytes have been observed in patients treated for 8 months.

Pharmaceutical particulars

List of excipients: Carbomer (Carbopol 940) BP; Disodium Edetate PhEur; Methyl Hydroxybenzoate PhEur; Propyl Hydroxybenzoate PhEur; Propylene Glycol PhEur; Sodium Hydroxide PhEur; Purified Water PhEur.

Incompatibilities: None known

Shelf life: Rozex Gel has a shelf life when unopened of 36 months.

Special precautions for storage: Store at a temperature not exceeding 25°C, away from direct heat. Do not freeze.

Nature and contents of container: Aluminium tubes with epoxy phenolic lining; white polypropylene or polyethylene screw caps; pack size 30 g.

Instructions for use/handling: Not applicable.

Marketing authorisation holder: Galderma (UK) Ltd, Leywood House, Woodside Road, Amersham, Buckinghamshire, HP6 6AA.

Marketing authorisation number 10590/0016

Date of approval/revision of SPC July 1996

Legal category POM

TARCORTIN*

Presentation Hydrocortisone PhEur 0.5% w/w and refined alcoholic extract of coal tar 5% w/w in a vanishing cream base. It is a light tan, homogeneous cream.

Uses Tarcortin cream is a stimulating antipruritic. It is indicated for sub-acute and chronic eczema, localised neurodermatitis, seborrhoea, dermatitis venenata and psoriasis, excluding widespread plaque psoriasis.

Dosage and administration Tarcortin is applied topically. Apply twice daily or more frequently to the affected area by gentle massage until the cream has vanished into the skin. No dressing is needed. Long term use in children is not advised.

Contra-indications, warnings, etc

Contra-indications: The use of Tarcortin is contra-indicated in the presence of viral or fungal infections, tubercular or syphilitic lesions, and in bacterial infections, unless used in conjunction with appropriate chemotherapy.

Interactions: None known.

Other undesirable effects: The use of coal tar can cause skin irritation, acne-like eruptions and photosensitivity.

Use in pregnancy and lactation: There is inadequate evidence of the safety of topical steroids in human pregnancy. Topical administration of corticosteroids to pregnant animals can cause abnormalities of foetal development, including cleft palate and intra-uterine growth retardation. There may, therefore, be a very small risk of such effects in the human foetus.

Other special warnings and precautions: The cream should be massaged well into the affected area to prevent a temporary discolouration of skin, hair or fabric. Although generally regarded as safe, even for long term administration in adults, there is a potential for overdose in infancy. Extreme caution is required in dermatoses of infancy including napkin eruption. In such patients, courses of treatment should not normally exceed 7 days.

Topical corticosteroids may be hazardous in psoriasis for a number of reasons, including rebound relapse following development of tolerance, risk of generalised pustular psoriasis and local systemic toxicity due to impaired barrier function of the skin. Careful patient supervision is important.

Pharmaceutical precautions Do not refrigerate. Store at room temperature.

Legal category POM

Package quantities Tubes of 100 g.

Product licence number 0036/5007R

**Trade Mark*

STD Pharmaceutical Products Ltd
Fields Yard, Plough Lane
Hereford HR4 0EL

☎ 01432 353684 🖷 01432 342383

FIBRO-VEIN* 3.0%,1.0%,0.5% and 0.2%

Qualitative and quantitative composition
Fibro-vein 3.0%: Sodium Tetradecyl Sulphate BP 3.0% w/v.
Fibro-vein 1.0%: Sodium Tetradecyl Sulphate BP 1.0% w/v
Fibro-vein 0.5%: Sodium Tetradecyl Sulphate BP 0.5% w/v
Fibro-vein 0.2%: Sodium Tetradecyl Sulphate BP 0.2% w/v

Pharmaceutical form Intravenous injection

Clinical particulars

Therapeutic indications: Fibro-vein 3% & 1%; For the treatment of varicose veins of the leg by injection sclerotherapy. Fibro-vein 0.5%; For the treatment of varicose veins and venous flares of the leg by injection sclerotherapy. Fibro-vein 0.2%; For the treatment of minor venules and spider veins (venous flares) by injection sclerotherapy.

Posology and method of administration:
Route of administration: For intravenous administration into the lumen of an isolated segment of emptied vein followed by immediate continuous compression.

Recommended doses and dosage schedules: Adults: Fibro-vein 3.0%; 0.5 to 1.0 ml of 3.0% Fibro-vein injected intravenously at a maximum of 4 sites (maximum 4 ml).

Fibro-vein 1.0%: 0.25 to 1.0 ml of 1.0% Fibro-vein injected intravenously into the lumen of an isolated segment of emptied superficial vein, followed by immediate compression. A maximum of 10 sites (10 ml total) may be injected during one treatment session.

Fibro-vein 0.5%: 0.25 to 1.0 ml of 0.5% Fibro-vein injected intravenously into the lumen of an isolated segment of emptied superficial vein, followed by immediate compression. A maximum of 10 sites (10 ml total) may be injected during one treatment session.

Fibro-vein 0.2%: 0.1 to 1.0 ml of 0.2% Fibro-Vein injected intravenously at a maximum of 10 sites (maximum 10 ml).

The smallest of needles (30 gauge) should be used to perform the injection which should be made slowly so that the blood content of these veins is expelled. In the treatment of spider veins an air block technique may be used.

Children: all strengths: not recommended in children

The elderly: As for adults

Contra-indications:
1. Allergy to sodium tetradecyl sulphate or to any component of the preparation.
2. Patients unable to walk due to any cause.
3. Patients currently taking oral contraceptives.
4. Significant obesity.
5. Acute superficial thrombophlebitis.
6. Local or systemic infection.
7. Varicosities caused by pelvic or abdominal tumours.
8. Uncontrolled systemic disease e.g. diabetes mellitus.
9. Surgical valvular incompetence requiring surgical treatment.

Special warnings and special precautions for use:
1. Fibro-vein should only be administered by practitioners familiar with an acceptable injection technique. Thorough pre-injection assessment for valvular competence and deep vein patency must be carried out. Extreme care in needle placement and slow injection of the minimal effective volume at each injection site are essential for safe and efficient use.
2. A history of allergy should be taken from all patients prior to treatment. Where special caution is indicated a test dose of 0.25 to 0.5 ml Fibro-vein should be given up to 24 hours before any further therapy.
3. Treatment of anaphylaxis may require, depending on the severity of attack, some or all of the following: injection of adrenaline, injection of hydrocortisone, injection of antihistamine, endotracheal intubation with use of a laryngoscope and suction. The treatment of varicose veins by fibro-vein should not be undertaken in clinics where these items are not readily available.
4. Extreme caution in use is required in patients with arterial disease such as severe peripheral atherosclerosis or thromboangiitis obliterans (Buerger's Disease).
5. Special care is required when injecting above and posterior to the medial malleolus where the posterior tibial artery may be at risk.
6. Pigmentation may be more likely to result if blood is extravasated at the injection site (particularly when treating smaller surface veins) and compression is not used.

Interaction with other medicaments and other forms of interaction: Do not use with heparin in the same syringe.

Pregnancy and lactation: Safety for use in pregnancy has not been established. Use only when clearly needed for symptomatic relief and when the potential benefits outweigh the potential hazards to the foetus. It is not known whether sodium tetradecyl sulphate is excreted in human milk. Caution should be exercised when used in nursing mothers.

Effects on ability to drive and to use machines: None known.

Undesirable effects:
1. Local: Pain or burning. Skin pigmentation. Tissue necrosis and ulceration may occur with extravasation. Paraesthesia and anaesthesia may occur if an injection effects a cutaneous nerve.
2. Vascular: Superficial thrombophlebitis. Deep vein thrombosis and pulmonary embolism are very rare. Inadvertent intra-arterial injection is very rare but may lead to gangrene. Most cases have involved the posterior tibial artery above the medial malleolus.
3. Systemic reactions: Allergic reactions are rare, presenting as local or generalised rash, urticaria, nausea or vomiting, asthma, vascular collapse. Anaphylactic shock, which may potentially be fatal, is extremely rare.

Overdose: Not applicable.

Pharmacological properties

Pharmacodynamic properties: Sodium tetradecyl sulphate damages the endothelium cells within the lumen of the injected vein. The object of compression sclerotherapy is then to compress the vein so that the resulting thrombus is kept to the minimum and the subsequent formation of scar tissue within the vein produces a fibrous cord and permanent obliteration. Non-compressed veins permit the formation of a large thrombus and produce less fibrosis within the vein.

Pharmacokinetic properties: Not applicable.

Preclinical safety data: Not applicable

Pharmaceutical particulars

List of excipients: All strengths: Benzyl Alcohol BP, Disodium Hydrogen Phosphate BP, potassium di-hydrogen phosphate analar, Water for Injections BP

Incompatibilities: Do not use with heparin in the same syringe

Shelf life: 36 months

Special precautions for storage: Store below 25° away from direct sunlight.

Nature and contents of containers: Fibro-vein 3.0%: 2 ml ampoules and 5 ml vials; Fibro-vein 1.0%: 2 ml ampoules; Fibro-vein 0.5%: 2 ml ampoules; Fibro-vein 0.2%: 5 ml vials

2 ml ampoules type 1 neutral hydrolytic glass conforming with PhEur requirements for injectable preparations.

5 ml glass vials type 1 neutral hydrolytic glass conforming with PhEur requirements for injectable preparations. Sealed with a chlorobutyl rubber bung and silver aluminium 'tear off' seal conforming with the PhEur requirements

Instructions for use/handling: Each 2 ml glass ampoule is for single use only.

The in use period of each 5 ml multidose vial is a single session of therapy and for use in the treatment of a single patient. Unused vial contents should be discarded immediately afterwards.

Marketing authorisation numbers
Fibro-vein 3.0% 0398/5000R
Fibro-vein 1.0% 0398/0003
Fibro-vein 0.5% 0398/0002
Fibro-vein 0.2% 0398/0004

Date of approval/revision of SPC
Fibro-vein 3.0%: 24 October 1995.
Fibro-vein 1.0%: 17 April 1996.
Fibro-vein 0.5%: 17 April 1996.
Fibro-vein 0.2%: 27 March 1995

Legal category POM

**Trade Mark*

Stiefel Laboratories (UK) Limited

Holtspur Lane
Wooburn Green
High Wycombe
Buckinghamshire HP10 0AU

☎ 01628 524966 01628 810021

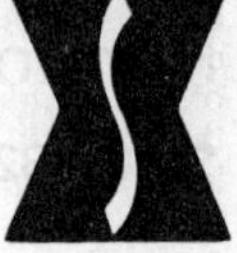

BRĀSIVOL* 1 FINE
BRĀSIVOL* 2 MEDIUM

Presentation Brāsivol is an abrasive cleansing paste in two grades, each containing graded particles of fused synthetic aluminium oxide in a non-irritant soap-detergent base.

Brāsivol No. 1 Fine is an off-white paste containing 38% aluminium oxide.

Brāsivol No. 2 Medium is a light-blue paste containing 52% aluminium oxide.

Excipients: glycerol, polyethylene glycol, stearic acid, lauric acid, myristic acid, quaternium 15, bentonite, sodium lauryl sulphate, colour: fine E172, medium E131, fragrance BV-2, purified water.

Uses Brāsivol is a cleansing and abrading agent which effectively removes debris from blocked pores. It is used in the management of acne vulgaris, either as a sole agent or as an adjunct to other treatment.

Dosage and administration The product is intended for use in adults and children over 12 years of age. The patient should commence treatment with Brāsivol No. 1 Fine. The product should be applied to wetted skin and rubbed gently but firmly over the affected area with a circular motion for 15–20 seconds, then rinsed off thoroughly with water. This routine may be repeated 2 or 3 times daily, replacing ordinary soap and water.

If the condition does not improve after 2 to 3 weeks, the treatment should be repeated using Brāsivol No. 2 Medium in place of Brāsivol No. 1.

Once you have established the most suitable grade for your condition and skin type, continue treatment for 2 to 3 months.

Contra-indications, warnings, etc Brāsivol is contra-indicated in the presence of superficial venules, telangiectasia, cystic acne and rosacea.

Care should be taken to avoid using Brāsivol close to the eyes or mouth and male patients using an electric razor should shave before applying Brāsivol.

A degree of dryness and redness will be seen during the first few days of treatment. Over-enthusiastic use, however, can cause irritation and, if this occurs, treatment should be interrupted for a day or two and then resumed.

There is no experimental evidence of the safety of the drug in human pregnancy but it has been in wide use for many years without ill consequence.

Pharmaceutical precautions Nil.

Legal category GSL.

Package quantities
Brāsivol No. 1 Fine. 75 g.
Brāsivol No. 2 Medium. 75 g.

Further information Brāsivol assists in the treatment of acne by exerting a debrading effect on the skin surface, unblocking the follicles, thus allowing the removal of retained sebum and permitting the sebaceous glands to return to normal size and activity.

Product licence numbers
Brāsivol No. 1 Fine 0174/5000R
Brāsivol No. 2 Medium 0174/5001R

DRICLOR*

Presentation Driclor is a clear colourless alcoholic solution containing Aluminium Chloride Hexahydrate PhEur 20% w/w.

Excipients: ethanol, purified water.

Uses Driclor is indicated for the treatment of hyperhidrosis.

Dosage and administration Apply Driclor last thing at night after drying the affected areas carefully. Wash off in the morning. Do not re-apply the product during the day.

Initially the product may be applied each night until sweating stops during the day. The frequency of application may then be reduced to twice a week or less.

Contra-indications, warnings, etc Ensure that the affected areas to be treated are completely dry before application.

Do not apply Driclor to broken, irritated, or recently shaven skin.

Driclor may cause irritation which may be alleviated by the use of a weak, corticosteroid cream.

Avoid contact with the eyes.

There are no restrictions on the use of Driclor during pregnancy and lactation.

Avoid direct contact with clothing and polished metal surfaces.

Pharmaceutical precautions Store upright in a cool place.
Replace cap tightly after use.
Inflammable – keep away from naked flame.

Legal category P.

Package quantities 60ml in roll-on applicator plastic bottle.

Further information Aluminium chloride hexahydrate acts locally, in the stratum corneum and in the terminal duct, to relieve hyperhidrosis.

Product licence number 0174/0044.

DUOFILM*

Presentation Duofilm is a clear mobile liquid containing:

Salicylic Acid BP 16.7% w/w
Lactic Acid BP 16.7% w/w
in Flexible Collodion BP.

Uses Duofilm is for topical application only and is indicated in the treatment of warts.

Dosage and administration For application to the affected areas on the surface of the skin.

Adults (including the elderly): Apply daily to the affected areas only.

Children under 12: Children over two years are to be treated under supervision, but treatment of infants is not recommended.

Contra-indications, warnings, etc Avoid applying to normal skin.

Duofilm should not be used on the face or anogenital regions.

There are no restrictions on the use of Duofilm during pregnancy and lactation.

Pharmaceutical precautions Store upright in a cool place.
Replace cap tightly after use.
Highly inflammable – keep away from naked flame.

Legal category P.

Package quantities Duofilm is available in an amber screw-capped applicator bottle containing 15 ml.

Further information Lactic acid affects the keratinisation process, reducing the hyperkeratosis which is characteristic of warts. It is caustic, leading to the destruction of the keratotic tissue of the wart and of the causative virus. Salicylic acid is keratolytic, producing desquamation by solubilising the intercellular cement in the stratum corneum.

Product licence number 0174/0025R.

ISOTREX* GEL

Qualitative and quantitative composition Isotretinoin 0.05%.

Pharmaceutical form Gel for cutaneous use.

Clinical particulars
Therapeutic indications: Isotrex Gel is indicated for the topical treatment of mild to moderate inflammatory and non-inflammatory acne vulgaris.

Posology and method of administration: Apply Isotrex Gel sparingly over the whole affected area once or twice daily.

Patients should be advised that 6–8 weeks of treatment may be required before a therapeutic effect is observed.

Paediatric use: The safety and efficacy of Isotrex Gel has not been established in children since acne vulgaris rarely presents in this age group.

Elderly patients: There are no specific recommendations. Acne vulgaris does not present in the elderly.

Contra-indications: Isotrex Gel should not be used in patients with known hypersensitivity to any of the ingredients.

Special warnings and special precautions for use: Contact with the eyes, mouth and mucous membranes and with abraded or eczematous skin should be avoided. Care should be taken not to let the medication accumulate in skin fold areas and in the angles of the nose.

Application to sensitive areas of skin, such as the neck, should be made with caution.

Although tretinoin has not been shown to initiate or promote carcinogenesis in humans, tretinoin applied topically to albino hairless mice had resulted in a dose related acceleration in ultraviolet-β radiation induced cutaneous tumours. The same author also observed the opposite effect in another study of low, non-irritating concentrations of tretinoin. The significance of these findings as related to man is unknown; however, caution should be observed in patients with a personal or family history of cutaneous epithelioma. Exposure to sunlight of areas treated with Isotrex Gel should be avoided or minimised. When exposure to strong sunlight cannot be avoided a sunscreen product and protective clothing should be used. Patients with sunburn should not use Isotrex Gel due to the possibility of increased sensitivity to sunlight. The use of sunlamps should be avoided during treatment.

Interactions with other medicaments and other forms of interaction: Concomitant topical medication should be used with caution during therapy with Isotrex Gel. Particular caution should be exercised when using preparations containing a peeling agent (for example Benzoyl Peroxide) or abrasive cleansers.

Pregnancy and lactation: Category B1. There is inadequate evidence of the safety of topically applied isotretinoin in human pregnancy.

Isotretinoin has been associated with teratogenicity in humans when administered systemically. Reproduction studies conducted in rabbits using Isotrex Gel applied topically at up to 60 times the human dose have, however, revealed no harm to the foetus. The use of Isotrex gel should be avoided during pregnancy.

Use during lactation: Percutaneous absorption of isotretinoin from Isotrex Gel is negligible. It is not known, however, whether isotretinoin is excreted in human milk. Isotrex Gel should not be used during lactation.

Effects on ability to drive and use machines: Isotrex Gel is presumed to be safe or unlikely to produce an effect on ability to drive or use machines.

Undesirable effects: In normal use, Isotrex Gel may cause stinging, burning or irritation; erythema and peeling at the site of application may occur.

If undue irritation occurs, treatment should be interrupted temporarily and resumed once the reaction subsides. If irritation persists, treatment should be discontinued. Reactions will normally resolve on discontinuation of therapy.

Overdosage: Acute overdosage of Isotrex Gel has not been reported to date. Accidental ingestion of Isotrex Gel resulting in overdosage of isotretinoin could be expected to induce symptoms of hypervitaminosis A. These include severe headaches, nausea or vomiting, drowsiness, irritability and pruritus.

Pharmacological properties
Pharmacodynamic properties: Isotretinoin is structurally and pharmacologically related to Vitamin A which regulates epithelial cell growth and differentiation.

The Pharmacological action of isotretinoin remains to be fully elucidated. When used systemically it suppresses sebaceous gland activity and reduces sebum production; it also affects comedogenesis, suppresses *Propionibacterium acnes* and reduces inflammation.

When applied topically, the mode of action of isotretinoin may be comparable with its stereoisomer, tretinoin. Tretinoin stimulates mitosis in the epidermis and reduces intercellular cohesion in the stratum corneum; it contests the hyperkeratosis characteristic of acne vulgaris and aids desquamation, preventing the formation of lesions. Tretinoin also mediates an increased production of less cohesive epidermal sebaceous cells, this appears to promote the initial expulsion and subsequent prevention of comedones.

Animal studies have demonstrated that topical isotretinoin elicits epidermal hyperplasia reduces hyperkeratosis and suppresses sebum production and sebaceous gland size. The anti-inflammatory action of isotretinoin when applied topically has been confirmed in man.

Pharmacokinetic properties: Percutaneous absorption of isotretinoin from the gel is negligible. After applying 30 g per day of isotretinoin 0.05% gel to acne of the face, chest and back for 30 days, HPLC assays for isotretinoin and tretinoin demonstrated non-detectable levels in the plasma samples (0.02 μg/ml). Applying ^{14}C isotretinoin in a cream base on the healthy skin of human volunteers resulted in only 0.03% of the topically applied dose being recovered through estimating the radioactivity of blood, urine and faecal samples.

Preclinical safety data: Not applicable. The relevant information is given in Clinical Paticulars.

Pharmaceutical particulars

List of excipients: Butylated hydroxytoluene; hydroxypropylcellulose; ethanol.

Incompatibilities: Not applicable.

Shelf life: (a) For the product as packaged for sale – Three years.

(b) After first opening the container – Two months.

Special precautions for storage: Store below 25°C.

Nature and contents of container: Aluminium tube of 30 g, fitted with a screw cap.

Instructions for use/handling: There are no special instructions for use or handling of Isotrex Gel.

Marketing authorisation number 0174/0073.

Date of approval/revision of SPC April 1997.

Legal category POM.

ISOTREXIN*

Qualitative and quantitative composition

Active ingredients: Isotretinoin PhEur 0.05% w/w and Erythromycin PhEur 2.00% w/w.

Pharmaceutical form Gel for cutaneous use.

Clinical particulars

Therapeutic indications: Isotrexin is indicated for the topical treatment of mild to moderate acne vulgaris and is effective in treating both inflammatory and non-inflammatory lesions.

Posology and method of administration:

Adults: Apply Isotrexin sparingly over the entire affected area once or twice daily.

Patients should be advised that, in some cases, six to eight weeks of treatment may be required before the full therapeutic effect is observed.

Use in children: Not established for prepubescent children, in whom acne vulgaris rarely presents.

Use in the elderly: No specific recommendations as acne vulgaris does not present in the elderly.

Contra-indications: Isotrexin should not be used in patients with known hypersensitivity to any of the ingredients.

Special warnings and precautions for use: Contact with the mouth, eyes and mucous membranes and with abraded or eczematous skin should be avoided. Application to sensitive areas of skin, such as the neck, should be made with caution. As Isotrexin may cause increased sensitivity to sunlight, deliberate or prolonged exposure to sunlight or sunlamps should be avoided or minimised. Concomitant topical medication should be used with caution because a cumulative irritant effect may occur.

Interactions with other medicaments and other forms of interaction: None known.

Pregnancy and lactation: Category B1. The safety of Isotrexin for use in human pregnancy has not been established. An evaluation of experimental animal studies does not indicate direct or indirect harmful effects with respect to the development of the embryo or foetus, the course of gestation and peri- and postnatal development.

Isotretinoin has been associated with teratogenicity in humans when administered systemically. However, reproduction studies conducted in rabbits using topical isotretinoin applied at up to 60 times the human therapeutic dose have revealed no harm to the foetus. There is no evidence of risk from the erythromycin component in human pregnancy.

The use of Isotrexin should be avoided by women who are pregnant or intending to conceive.

Use during lactation: Percutaneous absorption of isotretinoin from Isotrexin is negligible. However, as it is not known if isotretinoin is excreted in human milk, Isotrexin should not be used during lactation.

Effects on ability to drive and use machines: None.

Undesirable effects: Isotrexin may cause stinging, burning or irritation; erythema and peeling at the site of application may occur. These local effects usually subside with continued treatment. If undue irritation occurs, treatment should be interrupted temporarily and resumed once the reaction subsides. If irritation persists, treatment should be discontinued. Reactions will usually resolve on discontinuation of therapy.

Overdose: Acute overdosage of Isotrexin has not been reported to date. The isotretinoin and erythromycin components are not expected to cause problems on ingestion of the topical gel.

Pharmacological properties

Pharmacodynamic properties: Isotretinoin is structurally and pharmacologically related to vitamin A, which regulates epithelial cell growth and differentiation. The pharmacological action of isotretinoin has not been fully determined. When used systemically, it suppresses sebaceous gland activity and reduces sebum production; it also affects comedogenesis, inhibits follicular keratinisation, suppresses *Propionibacterium acnes* and reduces inflammation. It is thought that topically applied isotretinoin stimulates mitosis in the epidermis and reduces intercellular cohesion in the stratum corneum; contests the hyperkeratosis characteristic of acne vulgaris and aids desquamation, preventing the formation of lesions. It is also thought that it mediates an increased production of less cohesive epidermal sebaceous cells. This appears to promote the initial expulsion and subsequent prevention of comedones.

Studies in animal models have shown similar activity when isotretinoin is applied topically. Inhibition of sebum production by topical isotretinoin has been demonstrated in the ears and flank organs of the Syrian hamster. Application of isotretinoin to the ear for 15 days led to a 50% reduction in sebaceous gland size, and application to the flank organ resulted in a 40% reduction. Topical application of isotretinoin has also been shown to have an effect on the epidermal differentiation of rhino mouse skin. Reduction in the size of the utriculi or superficial cysts leading to normal looking follicles was a predominant feature of isotretinoin treatment and has been used to quantify the antikeratinising effects of isotretinoin.

Isotretinoin has topical anti-inflammatory actions. Topically applied isotretinoin inhibits luekotriene-B_4-induced migration of polymorphonuclear leukocytes, which accounts for topical isotretinoin's anti-inflammatory action. A significant inhibition was produced by topically applied isotretinoin but only a weak inhibition by topical tretinoin. This may account for the reduced rebound effect seen with topical isotretinoin when compared with topical tretinoin.

Erythromycin is a macrolide antibiotic which acts by interfering with bacterial protein synthesis by reversibly binding to ribosomal subunits, thereby inhibiting translocation of aminoacyl transfer-RNA and inhibiting polypeptide synthesis. In the treatment of acne, it is effective through reduction in the population of *Propionibacterium acnes* and through prevention of release of inflammatory mediators by the bacteria. Resistance of *P. acnes* to topical erythromycin can occur, but evidence exists that the combination of erythromycin and isotretinoin in Isotrexin is effective against erythromycin-resistant strains of *P. acnes.*

The isotretinoin component of Isotrexin is very useful in treating the comedonal phase of the disease, while the erythromycin component is effective in the treatment of mild to moderate inflammatory acne vulgaris. Since most cases of acne consist of a combination of comedonal and inflammatory disease, combination topical therapy involving erythromycin and isotretinoin represents a logical approach to treatment.

Pharmacokinetic properties: Percutaneous absorption of isotretinoin and erythromycin from Isotrexin is negligible. In a maximised study of the topical absorption of the two components from Isotrexin in patients suffering from widespread acne, isotretinoin levels were shown to be only slightly raised from baseline levels (isotretinoin is normally present in plasma). Levels remained below 5 ng/ml, and were not increased in the presence of erythromycin when compared to topical isotretinoin alone. The levels of erythromycin were not detectable.

Under conditions of normal use in patients with acne, percutaneous absorption of the active components was negligible.

Preclinical safety data: Isotretinoin and erythromycin, the active ingredients in Isotrexin are well-established pharmacopoeial substances which are regularly used in the topical and systemic treatment of acne vulgaris. Preclinical safety studies have not been conducted on Isotrexin, as an extensive range of toxicological studies has been conducted on isotretinoin and erythromycin as well as their respective topical formulations. A human patch tests for irritation has shown the combination to be comparable to the application of either component alone, with an acceptably low potential for irritation.

Pharmaceutical particulars

List of excipients: Hydroxypropylcellulose USNF; Butylated Hydroxytoluene (BHT) PhEur; Ethanol BP.

Incompatibilities: None known.

Shelf life: (a) For the product packaged for sale – two years.

(b) After first opening the container – comply with expiry date.

Special precautions for storage: Store below 25°C.

Nature and contents of container: Internally lacquered membrane-sealed aluminium tubes fitted with a polypropylene screw-cap, packed into a carton. Pack size 30 grammes.

Instructions for use/handling: None.

Marketing authorisation number 00174/0200.

Date of approval/revision of SPC October 1996.

Legal category POM.

LACTICARE*

Qualitative and quantitative composition Lactic acid 5% w/w, sodium pyrrolidone carboxylate 2.5% w/w.

Pharmaceutical form Lotion for cutaneous use.

Clinical particulars

Therapeutic indications: LactiCare is indicated for the symptomatic relief of hyperkeratotic and other chronic dry skin conditions, and for dry skin conditions caused by low humidity or the use of detergents.

Posology and method of administration: Use as required on affected areas or as directed by a doctor.

Contra-indications: None.

Special warnings and special precautions for use: Keep away from the eyes and mucous membranes. Should contact with the eyes occur, remove with water.

Keep out of reach of children.

Interactions with other medicaments and other forms of interaction: None known.

Pregnancy and lactation: Although there is no experimental evidence to support the safety of the drug during pregnancy and lactation, no adverse effects have been reported.

Effects on ability to drive and use machines: None.

Undesirable effects: Occasionally a transient mild stinging sensation may occur. Should prolonged irritation develop when used on abraded or inflamed skin, discontinue use.

Overdose: Not applicable.

Pharmacological properties

Pharmacodynamic properties: Both lactic acid and sodium pyrrolidone carboxylic acid are hygroscopic. They enhance the ability of the stratum corneum to retain water and counteract the tendency of the skin to dry out. Lactic acid also modulates epidermal keratinisation and increases skin extensibility.

Pharmacokinetic properties: Not applicable.

Preclinical safety data: There are no preclinical data of any relevance additional to that already included in other sections of the SPC.

Pharmaceutical particulars

List of excipients: Carbomer 940; imidurea; dehydroacetic acid; sodium hydroxide; polyethylene glycol ether complex; glyceryl monostearate; cetyl alcohol; isopropyl palmitate; light liquid paraffin; myristyl lactate; antaria essence 73/82; purified water.

Incompatibilities: None.

Shelf life: (a) For the product as packaged for sale – 3 years.

(b) After first opening the container – Comply with expiry date.

Special precautions for storage: None.

Nature and contents of container: High density polyethylene bottle containing 150 ml.

Instructions for use/handling: There are no special instructions for use or handling of LactiCare.

Marketing authorisation number 0174/0038.

Date of approval/revision of SPC 5 April 1995.

Legal category GSL.

OILATUM* CREAM

Qualitative and quantitative composition Arachis oil 21.0% w/w.

Pharmaceutical form Oil in water for cutaneous use.

Clinical particulars
Therapeutic indications: Oilatum Cream is indicated in the treatment of dry, sensitive skin, ichthyosis and similar conditions. The use of Oilatum Cream in such conditions reduces moisture loss from the stratum corneum and thus restores skin flexibility.

Posology and method of administration: Oilatum Cream may be used as often as required. Apply to the affected areas and rub in well.

It is especially effective after washing when the normal acid condition of the skin may be disturbed and when the sebum content of the stratum corneum may be depleted.

The product is suitable for use in adults, children and the elderly.

Contra-indications: None.

Special warnings and special precautions for use: Patients with a known hypersensitivity to any of the ingredients should not use the product.

Interactions with other medicaments and other forms of interaction: None known.

Pregnancy and lactation: There are no restrictions on the use of Oilatum Cream during pregnancy or lactation.

Effects on ability to drive and use machines: None.

Undesirable effects: None.

Overdose: Not applicable.

Pharmacological properties
Pharmacodynamic properties: Arachis oil exerts an emollient effect by forming an occlusive film which reduces trans-epidermal water loss, thus restoring normal skin humidity levels.

Pharmacokinetic properties: Not applicable.

Preclinical safety data: Not applicable.

Pharmaceutical particulars
List of excipients: Polyvinyl pyrrolidone; propylene glycol; glyceryl monostearate; macrogol monostearate; stearic acid; isopropyl palmitate; quaternium 15; potassium sorbate; fragrance 2174 H; purified water.

Incompatibilities: None.

Shelf life: (a) For the product as packaged for sale – Three years.

(b) After first opening the container – Comply with expiry date.

Special precautions for storage: None.

Nature and contents of container: Internally lined aluminium tubes of 40 g and 80 g.

Instructions for use/handling: There are no special instructions for use or handling of Oilatum Cream.

Marketing authorisation number 0174/5014R.

Date of approval/revision of SPC 23 March 1995.

Legal category GSL.

OILATUM* EMOLLIENT

Presentation Oilatum Emollient is a liquid bath additive. Active ingredient: Liquid paraffin 63.4% w/w.

Excipients: acetylated wool alcohols, isopropyl palmitate, macrogol 400 dilaurate, macrogol ester, fragrance floral spice.

Uses Oilatum Emollient is indicated in the treatment of contact dermatitis, atopic dermatitis, senile pruritus, ichthyosis and related dry skin conditions. Oilatum Emollient replaces oil and water and hydrates the keratin. Oilatum Emollient is particularly suitable for infant bathing. The preparation also overcomes the problem of cleansing the skin in conditions where the use of soaps, soap substitutes and colloid or oat-meal baths proves irritating.

Dosage and administration Oilatum Emollient should always be used with water, either added to water or applied to wet skin.

Adult bath: Add 1–3 capfuls to an 8 inch bath of water. Soak for 10–20 minutes. Pat dry.

Infant bath: Add ½–2 capfuls to a basin of water. Apply gently over entire body with a sponge. Pat dry.

Skin cleansing: Rub a small amount of oil into wet skin. Rinse and pat dry.

Where conditions permit, and particularly in cases of extensive areas of dry skin, Oilatum Emollient should be used as a bath oil, ensuring complete coverage by immersion. In addition to the therapeutic benefits, this method of use provides a means of sedating tense patients, particularly relevant in cases of acute pruritic dermatoses where relaxation of tension appears to relieve symptoms.

The product is suitable for use in adults, children and the elderly.

Contra-indications, warnings, etc The patient should be advised to use care to avoid slipping in the bath. If a rash or skin irritation occurs, stop using the product and consult your doctor.

Contains acetylated lanolin alcohols; avoid use in individuals with known lanolin hypersensitivity.

There is no evidence of the safety of Oilatum Emollient in human pregnancy or lactation, but it has been in wide use for many years without ill consequence.

Pharmaceutical precautions Nil.

Legal category GSL.

Package quantities Oilatum Emollient is available in bottles containing 250 ml and 500 ml.

Further information Light liquid paraffin exerts an emollient effect by forming an occlusive film in the stratum corneum. This prevents excessive evaporation of water from the skin surface and aids in the prevention of dryness.

Product licence number 0174/5010R.

OILATUM FRAGRANCE FREE

Presentation Oilatum Fragrance Free is a liquid bath additive. Active ingredient: Liquid Paraffin 63.4% w/w.

Excipients: acetylated wool alcohols, isopropyl palmitate, macrogol 400 dilaurate, macrogol ester.

Uses Oilatum Fragrance Free is indicated in the treatment of contact dermatitis, atopic dermatitis, senile pruritus, ichthyosis and related dry skin conditions. Oilatum Fragrance Free replaces oil and water and hydrates the keratin. Oilatum Fragrance Free is particularly suitable for infant bathing. The preparation also overcomes the problem of cleansing the skin in conditions where the use of soaps, soap substitutes and colloid or oat-meal baths proves irritating.

Dosage and administration Oilatum Fragrance Free should always be used with water, either added to water or applied to wet skin.

Adult bath: Add 1–3 capfuls to an 8 inch bath of water. Soak for 10–20 minutes. Pat dry.

Infant baths: Add ½–2 capfuls to a basin of water. Apply gently over entire body with a sponge. Pat dry.

Skin cleansing: Rub a small amount of oil into wet skin. Rinse and pat dry.

Where conditions permit, and particularly in cases of extensive areas of dry skin, Oilatum Fragrance Free should be used as a bath oil, ensuring complete coverage by immersion. In addition to the therapeutic benefits, this method of use provides a means of sedating tense patients, particularly relevant in cases of acute pruritic dermatoses where relaxation of tension appears to relieve symptoms.

The product is suitable for use in adults, children and the elderly.

Contra-indications, warnings, etc The patient should be advised to use care to avoid slipping in the bath. If a rash or skin irritation occurs, stop using the product and consult your doctor.

Contains acetylated lanolin alcohols; avoid use in individuals with known lanolin hypersensitivity.

There is no evidence of the safety of Oilatum Fragrance Free in human pregnancy or lactation, but it has been in wide use for many years without ill consequence.

Pharmaceutical precautions Nil.

Legal category GSL.

Package quantities Oilatum Fragrance Free is available in bottles containing 500 ml.

Further information Light liquid paraffin exerts an emollient effect by forming an occlusive film in the stratum corneum. This prevents excessive evaporation of water from the skin surface and aids in the prevention of dryness.

Product licence number 0174/0182.

OILATUM* GEL

Presentation Oilatum Gel is an emollient shower gel containing Light Liquid Paraffin BP 70% w/w.

Other ingredients: Polyethylene, macrogol 400 dilaurate, macrogol ester, 2-octadodecanol, macrogol myristyl ether propionate, polyphenylmethylsiloxane copolymer, fragrance floral spice.

Uses Oilatum Gel is indicated in the treatment of contact dermatitis, atopic eczema, senile pruritus, ichthyosis and related dry skin conditions.

Dosage and administration Oilatum Gel should be used as frequently as necessary. Daily application is recommended.

Oilatum Gel should always be applied to wet skin, normally as a shower gel.

Shower as usual. Apply Oilatum Gel to wet skin and massage gently. Rinse briefly and lightly pat the skin dry.

Contra-indications, warnings, etc Use care to avoid slipping in the shower.

Pharmaceutical precautions Store below 25°C.

Legal category GSL.

Package quantities Oilatum Gel is supplied in tubes of 65 g and 125 g.

Further information Oilatum Gel exerts an emollient effect through deposition of an occlusive film of light liquid paraffin on the stratum corneum. This prevents excessive evaporation of moisture from the skin, thus improving hydration, reducing roughness and scaling and relieving discomfort and itching.

Product licence number 0174/0072.

OILATUM* PLUS

Qualitative and quantitative composition Light liquid paraffin 52.5% w/w, benzalkonium chloride 6.0% w/w, triclosan 2.0% w/w.

Pharmaceutical form Solution.

Clinical particulars
Therapeutic indications: For the prophylactic treatment of eczemas at risk from infection.

Posology and method of administration: Oilatum Plus should always be diluted with water. It is an effective cleanser and should not be used with soap.

Adults and children: In an eight inch bath add 2 capfuls, in a four inch bath add 1 capful.

Infants: Add 1 ml (just sufficient to cover the bottom of the cap) and mix well with water.

Not recommended for babies younger than 6 months.

Contra-indications: Patients with a known hypersensitivity to any of the ingredients should not use the product.

Special warnings and special precautions for use: Avoid contact of the undiluted product with the eyes and the skin. If the undiluted product comes into contact with the eye, reddening and watering may occur. Eye irrigation should be performed for 15 minutes and the eye examined under fluorescein stain. If there is persistent irritation or any uptake of fluorescein, the patient should be referred for ophthalmological opinion.

Take care to avoid slipping in the bath.

Interactions with other medicaments and other forms of interaction: None known.

Pregnancy and lactation: There are no restrictions on the use of Oilatum Plus during pregnancy or lactation.

Effects on ability to drive and use machines: None.

Undesirable effects: None known.

Overdosage: Oilatum Plus is intended for topical use only. Ingestion may cause gastro intestinal irritation with vomiting and diarrhoea. Vomiting may result in foam aspiration. In the case of accidental ingestion, give 1 to 2 glasses of milk or water. If a large quantity of the product is ingested, the patient should be observed in hospital and the use of activated charcoal may be considered.

Pharmacological properties
Pharmacodynamic properties: Benzalkonium chloride and triclosan are anti-bacterial agents with proven efficacy against *Straphylococcus aureus*, the principal causative organism in infected eczemas.

Light liquid paraffin is an emollient widely used in the treatment of eczema.

Pharmacokinetic properties: Not applicable.

Preclinical safety data: Not applicable.

Pharmaceutical particulars
List of excipients: Acetylated lanolin alcohols; isopropyl palmitate; oleyl alcohol; polyoxyethylene lauryl ether.

Incompatibilities: None known.

Shelf life: (a) For the product as packaged for sale – Three years.

(b) After first opening the container – Comply with expiry date.

Special precautions for storage: None.

Nature and contents of container: White high density polyethylene bottle containing 500 ml.

Instructions for use/handling: There are no special instructions for use or handling of Oilatum Plus.

Marketing authorisation number 0174/0070.

Date of approval/revision of SPC 30 March 1995.

Legal category GSL.

PANOXYL* Acne Gel 5
PANOXYL* Acne Gel 10

Presentation White viscous gels containing benzoyl peroxide 5 and 10% w/w in an ethanolic base.

Excipients: magnesium aluminium silicate, hypromellose, macrogol lauryl ether, ethanol, citric acid, fragrance 6565A, purified water.

Uses PanOxyl 5 and 10 are each indicated for use in the treatment of acne vulgaris.

Dosage and administration
Adults, the elderly and children over 12 years: Treatment should normally commence with PanOxyl 5. Apply the gel to the affected areas once daily. Washing prior to application greatly enhances the efficacy of the preparation. The reaction of the skin to benzoyl peroxide differs in individual patients, and for this reason the higher percentage of benzoyl peroxide in PanOxyl 10 may be required in order to provide a satisfactory drying and desquamative action.

Children under 12 years: Not recommended.

Contra-indications, warnings, etc Avoid contact with eyes, mouth and mucous membranes. Take care when applying to the neck and other sensitive areas. Do not use in patients with known hypersensitivity to benzoyl peroxide.

In normal use, a mild burning sensation will probably be felt on first application and a moderate reddening and peeling of the skin will occur within a few days. During the first few weeks of treatment a sudden increase in peeling will occur in most patients.

There are no restrictions on the use of PanOxyl 5 and PanOxyl 10 during pregnancy and lactation.

PanOxyl 5 and PanOxyl 10 may bleach dyed fabrics.

Pharmaceutical precautions Store in a cool place.

Legal category P.

Package quantities PanOxyl 5 and PanOxyl 10 are supplied in tubes each containing 40 g.

Further information Benzoyl peroxide has sebostatic and keratolytic activity coupled with antibacterial activity against Propionibacterium acnes, the organism implicated in acne vulgaris. Its use in the treatment of acne is well established.

Product licence numbers
PanOxyl 5 0174/0019R
PanOxyl 10 0174/0020R

PANOXYL* AQUAGEL* 2.5
PANOXYL* AQUAGEL* 5
PANOXYL* AQUAGEL* 10

Presentation White viscous gels containing benzoyl peroxide 2.5, 5 and 10% w/w in an aqueous, non alcoholic base.

Excipients: carbomer, diisopropanolamine, propylene glycol, macrogol lauryl ether, sodium lauryl sulphate, purified water.

Uses PanOxyl Aquagel 2.5, 5 and 10 are each indicated for use in the topical treatment of acne vulgaris.

Dosage and administration Treatment should normally begin with PanOxyl Aquagel 2.5. Apply to the affected areas once daily. Washing prior to application enhances the efficacy of the preparation.

The reaction of the skin to benzoyl peroxide differs in individual patients. The higher concentration in PanOxyl Aquagel 5 or 10 may be required to produce a satisfactory response.

Contra-indications, warnings, etc PanOxyl Aquagel should not be prescribed for patients with a known hypersensitivity to benzoyl peroxide.

Avoid contact with the eyes, mouth and mucous membranes. Care should be taken when applying the product to the neck and other sensitive areas. In normal use, a mild burning sensation will probably be felt on first application and a moderate reddening and peeling of the skin will occur within a few days. During the first weeks of treatment a sudden increase in peeling will occur in most patients, this is not harmful and will normally subside within a day or two if treatment is temporarily discontinued. If excessive irritation, redness or peeling occurs discontinue use.

There are no restrictions on the use of PanOxyl Aquagel during pregnancy and lactation.

These products may bleach dyed fabrics.

Pharmaceutical precautions Store in a cool place.

Legal category P.

Package quantities Tubes of 40 g.

Further information Benzoyl peroxide has sebostatic and keratolytic activity coupled with antibacterial activity against Propionibacterium acnes, the organism implicated in acne vulgaris. Its use in the treatment of acne is well established.

Product licence numbers
PanOxyl Aquagel 2.5 0174/0049
PanOxyl Aquagel 5 0174/0050
PanOxyl Aquagel 10 0174/0051

PANOXYL* CREAM 5
PANOXYL* LOTION 5
PANOXYL* LOTION 10

Presentation Panoxyl 5 is available as a white lotion or cream containing benzoyl peroxide 5% w/w.

Panoxyl 10 is a white lotion containing benzoyl peroxide 10% w/w.

Excipients: macrogol 1000 monostearate, stearic acid, glyceryl monostearate, isopropyl palmitate, propylene glycol, zinc caproate, zinc laurate, zinc myristate, purified water.

Uses Panoxyl 5 and 10 are each indicated for use in the treatment of acne vulgaris.

Dosage and administration Treatment should normally commence with Panoxyl 5. Apply the lotion or cream to the affected areas once daily. Washing with soap and water prior to application greatly enhances the efficacy of the preparation.

The reaction of the skin to benzoyl peroxide differs in individual patients. The higher concentration in Panoxyl 10 may be required to ensure a satisfactory response.

Contra-indications, warnings, etc Panoxyl should not be prescribed for patients with a known hypersensitivity to benzoyl peroxide.

Avoid contact with the eyes, mouth and other mucous membranes. Care should be taken when applying the product to the neck and other sensitive areas. In normal use, a mild burning sensation will probably be felt on first application and a moderate reddening and peeling of the skin will occur within a few days. During the first weeks of treatment a sudden increase in peeling will occur in most patients, this is not harmful and will normally subside within a day or two if treatment is temporarily discontinued.

There are no restrictions on the use of the product during pregnancy and lactation.

Panoxyl may bleach dyed fabrics.

Pharmaceutical precautions Store in a cool place.

Legal category P.

Package quantities Lotion: Bottles of 30 ml.
Cream: Tubes of 40 g.

Further information Benzoyl peroxide has sebostatic and keratolytic activity coupled with antibacterial activity against Propionibacterium acnes, the organism implicated in acne vulgaris. Its use in the treatment of acne is well established.

Product licence numbers
Panoxyl Lotion 5 0174/5003R
Panoxyl Cream 5 0174/5007R
Panoxyl Lotion 10 0174/0034

PANOXYL* WASH 10%

Qualitative and quantitative composition Benzoyl peroxide 10.0% w/w.

Pharmaceutical form Lotion for cutaneous use.

Clinical particulars
Therapeutic indications: Panoxyl Wash 10% is indicated for the treatment of acne vulgaris.

Posology and method of administration
Adults: Wet the affected area with water and wash thoroughly with Panoxyl Wash. Rinse well with warm water, then rinse with cold water. Pat dry with a clean towel. Use once a day.

Elderly patients: There are no specific recommendations. Acne vulgaris does not present in the elderly.

Paediatric use: The product is not intended for use in pre-pubescent children since acne vulgaris rarely presents in this age group.

Contra-indications: Patients with a known hypersensitivity to any of the ingredients should not use the product.

Special warnings and special precautions for use: Avoid contact with the eyes, mouth and other mucous membranes. Care should be taken when applying the product to the neck and other sensitive areas.

The product may bleach dyed fabrics.

Keep out of the reach of children.

Interactions with other medicaments and other forms of interaction: None.

Pregnancy and lactation: There are no restrictions on the use of the product during pregnancy or lactation.

Effects on ability to drive and use machines: None.

Undesirable effects: In normal use, a mild burning sensation will probably be felt on first application and a moderate reddening and peeling of the skin will occur within a few days. During the first few weeks of treatment a sudden increase in peeling will occur in most patients; this is not harmful and will normally subside in a day or two if treatment is temporarily discontinued.

Overdose: Not applicable.

Pharmacological properties
Pharmacodynamic properties: Benzoyl peroxide has antibacterial activity against *Propionibacterium acnes*, the organism implicated in acne vulgaris. It has keratolytic activity and is sebostatic, counteracting the hyperkeratinisation and excessive sebum production associated with acne.

Pharmacokinetic properties: Not applicable.

Preclinical safety data: Not applicable. Benzoyl peroxide has been in widespread use for many years.

Pharmaceutical particulars
List of excipients: Magnesium aluminium silicate; citric acid monohydrate; sodium alkyl aryl polyether sulphonate; sodium dihexyl sulphosuccinate; sodium lauryl sulphoacetate; hydroxypropylmethylcellulose; polyoxyethylene lauryl ether; imidurea; purified water.

Incompatibilities: None.

Shelf life: (a) For the product as packaged – 2 years.
(b) After first opening the container – Comply with expiry date.

Special precautions for storage: Store at room temperature.

Nature and contents of container: Flip top polyethylene bottle containing 150 ml.

Instructions for use/handling: There are no special instructions for use or handling of Panoxyl Wash 10%.

Marketing authorisation number 0174/0048.

Date of approval/revision of SPC 23 March 1995.

Legal category P.

POLYTAR* AF

Presentation Polytar AF is a medicated scalp treatment containing the following active ingredients: Tar blend† 1% w/w, Zinc pyrithione 1% w/w in a shampoo base.

(†Tar blend consists of Pine Tar BP, 30% w/w; Cade Oil BPC, 30% w/w; Coal Tar Solution BP, 10% w/w; Arachis Oil Extract of Coal Tar BP, 30% w/w).

Excipients: coconut diethanolamide, triethanolamine lauryl sulphate, carbomer, hypromellose, octoxinol, glycerol, imidurea, purified water.

Uses Polytar AF is indicated in the topical treatment of scalp disorders such as dandruff, seborrhoeic dermatitis and psoriasis.

Polytar AF has antibacterial and antifungal properties. It is fungicidal against the pathogenic yeasts of the pityrosporum genus which are implicated in dandruff and seborrhoeic dermatitis.

Polytar AF suppresses DNA synthesis in hyperplastic skin; this inhibits mitotic activity and protein synthesis. The product decreases epidermal proliferation and promotes a return to normal keratinisation.

Polytar AF relieves the scaling and pruritus normally associated with seborrhoeic dermatitis and dandruff.

Dosage and administration Adults, children and the elderly: Shake the bottle before use. Wet the hair and massage Polytar AF into the hair, scalp and surrounding skin. Leave for 2–3 minutes, then rinse thoroughly.

Treatment: Use two or three times weekly for at least 3 weeks or until the condition clears.

Prophylaxis for seborrhoeic dermatitis and dandruff: use Polytar AF weekly.

Contra-indications, warnings, etc
Contra-indications: Polytar AF should not be used by patients with known hypersensitivity to any of the ingredients.

Precautions: Avoid contact with the eyes. Tar products may cause skin irritation, rashes and, rarely, photosensitivity. Zinc pyrithione may cause dermatitis, should this occur, Polytar AF should be discontinued.

Pregnancy and lactation: The safety of Polytar AF in human pregnancy or lactation has not been established.

Pharmaceutical precautions Store below 25°C.

Legal category GSL.

Package quantities Polytar AF is available in bottles of 150 ml.

Further information Nil.

Product licence number 0174/0071.

POLYTAR* EMOLLIENT

Presentation Polytar Emollient is a liquid bath additive. The active ingredients are as follows:

Tar blend†	25% w/w
Light Liquid Paraffin	35% w/w

(†Tar blend consists of: Pine Tar BP, 30% w/w; Cade Oil BPC, 30% w/w; Coal Tar Solution BP, 10% w/w; Arachis Oil Extract of Coal Tar BP, 30% w/w.)

Excipients: octoxinol, sorbitan mono-oleate, polysorbate 80, isopropyl palmitate, macrogol 400 dilaurate, purified water.

Uses Polytar Emollient is indicated in the treatment of psoriasis, eczema, atopic and pruritic dermatoses. The use of Polytar Emollient may be combined with ultraviolet radiation and other adjunctive therapy.

Polytar Emollient is also of value in removing loose psoriatic scales and paste following dithranol treatment.

Dosage and administration 15–30 mls (2–4 capfuls) of Polytar Emollient should be added to an 8 inch bath and the patient instructed to soak for 20 minutes.

Contra-indications, warnings, etc Patients should be instructed to guard against slipping when entering or leaving the bath.

Tar products may cause skin irritation, rashes and rarely, photosensitivity. In the event of such a reaction, discontinue use and consult your doctor. Tar products may stain baths and fabrics.

There is no evidence of the safety of Polytar Emollient in human pregnancy but it has been in wide use for many years without apparent ill consequence.

Pharmaceutical precautions Nil.

Legal category GSL.

Package quantities Polytar Emollient is available in bottles of 500 ml.

Further information Tar preparations have keratoplastic and antipruritic activity and are widely used as topical therapy for a range of dermatoses. The use of emollient bath oils in the management of dry and itching skin is well established. Mineral oil exerts its emollient effect by skin absorption.

Polytar Emollient is prescribable on FP10 for the treatment of psoriasis, eczema, atopic and pruritic dermatoses.

Product licence number 0174/5011R.

POLYTAR* LIQUID

Qualitative and quantitative composition Tar Blend 1% w/w. Tar Blend comprises: Pine tar, cade oil, coal tar solution, arachis oil extract of coal tar.

Pharmaceutical form Medicated shampoo.

Clinical particulars

Therapeutic indications: Polytar Liquid is indicated in the treatment of scalp disorders including psoriasis, dandruff, seborrhoea, eczema and pruritus. Polytar Liquid is also of value in the removal of ointments and pastes used in the treatment of psoriasis.

Posology and method of administration: The hair should be wetted and sufficient Polytar Liquid applied to produce an abundant lather. The scalp and adjacent areas should be vigorously massaged with the fingertips. The hair should then be thoroughly rinsed and the procedure repeated.

Polytar Liquid should be used once or twice weekly.

Contra-indications: Patients with a known hypersensitivity to any of the ingredients should not use the product.

Special warnings and special precautions for use: There are no special warnings or precautions.

Interactions with other medicaments and other forms of interaction: There are no known interactions with other medicaments or other forms of interaction.

Pregnancy and lactation: There is no, or inadequate evidence of the safety of Polytar Liquid in human pregnancy and lactation, but it has been in wide use for many years without apparent ill consequence.

Effects on ability to drive and use machines: The use of this product will not affect the ability to drive and to use machines.

Undesirable effects: Tar products may cause skin irritation, rashes and rarely, photosensitivity. If irritation occurs and persists, treatment should be discontinued.

Overdose: The product is intended for external use only. It is applied to the scalp and rinsed off. Use of an excessive quantity is not a cause for concern.

Pharmacological properties

Pharmacodynamic properties: Tars suppress DNA synthesis in hyperplastic skin, inhibiting mitotic activity and protein synthesis. They decrease epidermal proliferation and dermal infiltration and thus promote a return to normal keratinisation.

Tars also have vasoconstrictor, antipruritic and antiseptic properties.

Pharmacokinetic properties: The product is applied topically and acts at the site of application. The potential for systemic absorption from a wash-off shampoo is extremely low.

Preclinical safety data: Tar preparations have been in widespread use for many years and their safety in humans has been established.

Pharmaceutical particulars

List of excipients: Oleyl alcohol; coconut diethanolamide; hexylene glycol; polysorbate 80; triethanolamine lauryl sulphate; sodium chloride; citric acid; octylphenoxypolyethoxy ethanol; imidurea; fragrance 5412; purified water.

Incompatibilities: There are no known incompatibilities.

Shelf life: (a) For the product as packaged for sale – 3 years.

(b) After first opening the container – Comply with expiry date.

Special precautions for storage: There are no special precautions for storage.

Nature and contents of container: High density polyethylene bottles of 150 ml and 250 ml.

Instructions for use/handling: There are no special instructions for use or handling of Polytar Liquid.

Marketing authorisation number 0174/5016R.

Date of approval/revision of SPC 18 September 1995.

Legal category GSL.

POLYTAR PLUS*

Presentation Polytar Plus is a concentrated antiseptic, tar medicated scalp cleanser adjusted to pH 5.5, containing the hair conditioners: Polypeptide and oleyl alcohol and the active ingredient: Tar blend† 1% w/w.

(†Tar blend consists of: Pine Tar BP, 30% w/w; Cade Oil BPC, 30% w/w; Coal Tar Solution BP, 10% w/w; Arachis Oil Extract of Coal Tar BP, 30% w/w.)

Excipients: coconut diethanolamide, hexylene glycol, macrogol oleyl ether, polysorbate 80, triethanolamine lauryl sulphate, citric acid, octoxinol, imidurea, fragrance 5412, purified water.

Uses Polytar Plus is indicated in the treatment of scalp disorders such as dandruff, psoriasis, seborrhoea, eczema and pruritus. Polytar Plus is also of value in the removal of ointments and pastes used in the treatment of psoriasis. Polytar Plus is especially suitable for dry hair.

Dosage and administration

Aduts, children and the elderly: The hair should be wetted and sufficient Polytar Plus applied to produce an abundant lather. The scalp and adjacent areas should be vigorously massaged with the fingertips. The hair should then be thoroughly rinsed and the procedure repeated.

Polytar Plus should be used once or twice weekly.

Contra-indications, warnings, etc Tar products may cause skin irritation, rashes and rarely, photosensitivity. In the event of such a reaction, discontinue use and consult your doctor.

There are no restrictions on the use of Polytar Plus during pregnancy or lactation.

Pharmaceutical precautions Nil.

Legal category GSL.

Package quantities Polytar Plus is available in bottles of 350 ml.

Further information Tars suppress DNA synthesis in hyperplastic skin, this inhibits mitotic activity and protein synthesis. By decreasing epidermal proliferation and dermal infiltration, they promote a return to normal keratinisation. Tars also have vasoconstricting, astringent and antipruritic properties.

Polytar Plus is prescribable on FP10 for psoriasis, eczema and seborrhoea of the scalp and for dandruff.

Product licence number 0174/0037.

SPECTRABAN* LOTION 25

Presentation SpectraBAN Lotion contains Padimate O 3.2% w/w and Para Aminobenzoic Acid USP 5% w/w in an ethanolic base. The product, which is non-greasy and invisible on the skin, is pink in colour.

Excipients: ethanol, carbomer, polyoxyethylene cocoamine, colour E122, oleyl alcohol, fragrance A3012, purified water.

Uses SpectraBAN Lotion is a protective sunscreen lotion indicated in patients at risk from exposure to ultraviolet light within the UVB wavelength range (280–315 nanometres). It is this narrow waveband of ultraviolet light which is responsible for burning and tanning of the skin in man. The product has a UVB Sun Protection Factor 25, thus it should allow 25 times normal exposure to sunlight before burning.

SpectraBAN Lotion is indicated for protection from UV radiation in abnormal cutaneous photosensitivity resulting from genetic disorders or photodermatoses, including those resulting from radiotherapy; chronic or recurrent herpes simplex labialis.

Dosage and administration Apply carefully and evenly to areas to be exposed or protected only by light clothing. Allow to dry before dressing. Allow 45 minutes before swimming or sweat producing exercise. A single application may give day long protection but the product should be re-applied frequently during prolonged sunning or after swimming or excessive sweating.

Contra-indications, warnings, etc Sunscreen preparations occasionally produce a sensitivity reaction. Treatment should be discontinued if a skin rash or irritation develops. Do not apply to broken skin. Avoid contact with the eyes, mouth and other mucous membranes.

The product can stain clothing and other items permanently.

There is no evidence of the safety of the drug in human pregnancy but it has been in wide use for many years without apparent ill consequence.

Pharmaceutical precautions Avoid flame.

Legal category GSL.

Package quantities SpectraBAN Lotion is available in bottles containing 150 ml.

Further information SpectraBAN Lotion is prescribable on FP10.

Product licence number 0174/0035.

STIEDEX* LOTION

Presentation Stiedex Lotion contains desoxymethasone USP 0.25% w/w, Salicylic Acid PhEur 1.0% w/w.

Excipients: Polyol fatty acid ester, 1,2-propylene glycol, ethanol, sodium hydroxide, disodium edetate, purified water.

Uses Stiedex Lotion contains a potent corticosteroid and is indicated for the treatment of psoriasis, particularly of the scalp (but excluding widespread plaque psoriasis), seborrhoeic eczema, chronic lichenified eczema, lichen planus, lichen simplex, non-bullous ichthyosiform erythroderma.

Stiedex Lotion is especially suitable for use in hairy regions such as scalp, cheeks, neck and chest and for skin areas difficult to reach such as the auditory meatus.

Dosage and administration Stiedex Lotion should be applied to the affected areas once or twice daily, preferably morning and/or night. When the skin condition improves, application may be reduced to once daily. In order to prevent recurrence, treatment with Stiedex Lotion should be continued for some days after complete control of the condition. If the lotion is being used on the face or in children, courses should be limited to five days duration.

Contra-indications, warnings, etc *Contra-indications:* Stiedex Lotion is contra-indicated in infants and young children, in facial rosacea, acne vulgaris, perioral dermatitis, perianal and genital pruritis, napkin eruptions, bacterial (e.g. impetigo), viral (e.g. Herpes simplex), and fungal (e.g. Candida or dermatophyte) infections.

Stiedex Lotion contains propylene glycol and should not be used in patients with a known hypersensitivity to this, or any of the other ingredients.

Precautions: The continuous administration of topical steroids over prolonged periods may result in adrenal suppression; in infants and children, this may cause growth retardation. The use of occlusive dressings enhances the absorption of the steroid, and in consequence, systemic effects are more likely to occur. Salicyclic acid may enhance absorption of the steroid or itself be absorbed. Adrenal suppression is unlikely in short courses of treatment or with doses not exceeding 10 g daily.

Long term continuous therapy should be avoided in all patients irrespective of age. The lotion should not be applied to extensive skin surfaces and application under occlusion should be restricted to dermatoses involving limited areas.

The use of topical corticosteroids may be hazardous in psoriasis for a number of reasons including rebound relapses following development of tolerance, risk of generalised pustular psoriasis and local and systemic toxicity due to impaired barrier function of the skin. Careful patient supervision is important if Stiedex Lotion is used in psoriasis.

Prolonged administration of potent corticosteroids has been shown also to cause a thinning in skin collagen and subcutaneous atrophy, resulting in striae, thinning and dilation of superficial blood vessels. These changes are particularly liable to occur on the face.

Percutaneous absorption of salicylic acid due to extensive use could lead to salicylism.

Salicylic acid may alter the permeability of the skin to other substances applied simultaneously. The use of other preparations, cosmetics etc., on skin treated with Stiedex Lotion should be avoided.

Stiedex Lotion should not be applied to or near the eye.

Use in pregnancy: There is inadequate evidence of safety in human pregnancy. Topical administration of corticosteroids to pregnant animals can cause abnormalities of foetal development including cleft palate and intra-uterine growth retardation. There may therefore be a very small risk of such effects in the human foetus.

Pharmaceutical precautions Stiedex Lotion should be protected from heat and stored below 25°C.

Legal category POM.

Package quantities 50 ml.

Further information Nil.

Product licence number 0174/0062.

STIEDEX* LP

Presentation Stiedex LP contains 0.05% w/w desoxymethasone in an oily cream base.

Excipients: isopropyl myristate, wool alcohols ointment, edetic acid, purified water.

Uses Stiedex LP contains a potent corticosteroid and is indicated for the treatment of a wide range of acute inflammatory and allergic conditions, and chronic skin disorders.

Stiedex LP is specifically indicated for the treatment of eczema (including atopic, seborrhoeic and nummular eczema), intertrigo, psoriasis, pompholyx, lichen planus and discoid lupus erythematosus; acute and chronic allergic dermatoses, neurodermatitis; erythroderma, and may also be used in the non-specific treatment of sunburn and insect bites.

Dosage and administration Stiedex LP should be applied sparingly to the affected area and rubbed gently into the skin. Initially, application should be made 2–3 times daily and the frequency of administration reduced as the condition subsides.

Stiedex LP may be applied under an occlusive dressing. The affected area should be thoroughly cleansed prior to administration of cream and dressing to prevent infection.

Contra-indications, warnings, etc

Contra-indications: Stiedex LP is not suitable for infants and young children. Stiedex LP is contra-indicated in facial rosacea, acne vulgaris, perioral dermatitis, perianal and genital pruritus, napkin eruptions, bacterial (e.g. impetigo), viral (e.g. *Herpes simplex*) and fungal (e.g. *Candida* and dermatophyte) infections.

Stiedex LP is contra-indicated in patients with hypersensitivity to the preparation.

Stiedex LP is not suitable for use in the treatment of inflammatory disorders of the eye.

There is inadequate evidence of safety in human pregnancy. Topical administration of corticosteroids to pregnant animals can cause abnormalities of foetal development including cleft palate and intra-uterine growth retardation. There may therefore be a very small risk of such effects in the human foetus.

Precautions: The continuous administration of topical steroids over prolonged periods may result in adrenal suppression; in infants and children, this may cause growth retardation. The use of occlusive dressings enhances the absorption of the active substance, desoxymethasone, and in consequence systemic effects are more likely to occur. Adrenal suppression is unlikely in short courses of treatment or with doses not exceeding 10 g daily.

Prolonged administration of potent corticosteroids has been shown also to cause a reduction in skin collagen and subcutaneous atrophy, resulting in striae, thinning and dilation of superficial blood vessels. These changes are particularly liable to occur on the face.

Pharmaceutical precautions Stiedex LP should be stored in a cool, dry place.

Legal category POM.

Package quantities Stiedex LP is available in tubes of 30 g and 100 g.

Further information Stiedex LP contains no preservative. Stiedex LP may be diluted by admixture with Oily Cream BP.

Product licence number 0174/0053.

STIEMYCIN*

Presentation A clear colourless solution in an amber glass screw-capped applicator bottle. The applicator allows the product to be applied directly to the involved skin.

Each ml contains 20 mg erythromycin base PhEur in an amount equivalent to 20 mg of erythromycin base 1st International Standard, in an ethanol base also containing propylene glycol and Laureth 4.

Uses Stiemycin is indicated for use in the topical treatment of acne vulgaris.

Dosage and administration To be applied to the affected area twice daily after washing.

Contra-indications, warnings, etc Stiemycin is contra-indicated in patients with known sensitivity to any of the ingredients.

Concomitant topical acne therapy should be used with caution because a cumulative irritant effect may occur.

Avoid contact with eyes and other mucous membranes.

This product is for external use only.

There is no evidence of hazard from erythromycin in human pregnancy. It has been in wide use for many years without apparent ill consequence.

Pharmaceutical precautions Store in a cool place.

Legal category POM.

Package quantity 50 ml.

Further information Nil.

Product licence number 0174/0047.

ZEASORB* POWDER

Presentation ZeaSORB is an off-white, highly absorbent, soft, antiseptic dusting powder containing the following:

Chloroxylenol BPC	0.5% w/w
Aluminium dihydroxyallantoinate	0.2% w/w

Excipients: talc, fragrance 6A, microcrystalline cellulose.

Uses Intertrigo, hyperhidrosis, bromidrosis, prevention of tinea pedis and related conditions.

Dosage and administration The affected areas should be dried as thoroughly as possible before applying ZeaSORB Powder. The powder should be smoothed over the surface of the skin, between joints and in folds.

ZeaSORB is intended for use in adults, the elderly and, with supervision, in children. Special care should be taken when using the product in children to avoid inhalation.

Contra-indications, warnings, etc Can be irritant to the eyes. Problems of granuloma have been associated with contact of talc with broken skin. As with all powders, take care to avoid inhalation.

There are no restrictions on the use of ZeaSORB in pregnancy and lactation.

Pharmaceutical precautions Store in a cool dry place.

Legal category P.

Package quantities ZeaSORB Powder is available in sifter-top plastic containers of 50 g.

Further information ZeaSORB Powder is non-caking and remains soft on saturation, preventing irritation.

Product licence number 0174/5015R.

**Trade Mark*

Takeda UK Ltd
3 The Courtyard
Meadowbank
Furlong Road
Bourne End
Bucks SL8 5AJ

☎ 01628 537900/526614   🗋 01628 526615

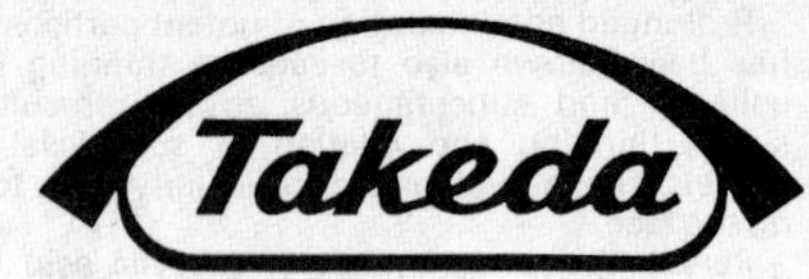

AMIAS* TABLETS ▼

Qualitative and quantitative composition Each tablet contains 2 mg, 4 mg, 8 mg or 16 mg candesartan cilexetil.

Pharmaceutical form Tablets.

Clinical particulars
Therapeutic indications: Essential hypertension.

Posology and method of administration: Dosage: A suggested starting dose of Amias* is 4 mg once daily. The usual maintenance dose is 8 mg once daily. The maximum dose is 16 mg once daily.

Therapy should be adjusted according to blood pressure response. Most of the antihypertensive effect is attained within 4 weeks of initiation of treatment.

Administration: Amias* should be taken once daily with or without food.

Use in the elderly: The starting dose is 4 mg in elderly patients with normal renal and hepatic function. In the presence of renal or hepatic impairment an initial dose of 2 mg is recommended. The dose may be adjusted according to response.

Use in impaired renal function: No dosage adjustment is necessary in patients with mild renal impairment. In patients with moderate to severe renal impairment, an initial dose of 2 mg once daily is recommended. The dose may be adjusted according to response. Due to limited experience, Amias* is not recommended in patients with very severe or end-stage renal impairment ($Cl_{creatinine} < 15$ ml/min).

Use in impaired hepatic function: An initial dose of 2 mg once daily is recommended in patients with mild to moderate hepatic impairment. The dose may be adjusted according to response. There is no experience in patients with severe hepatic impairment.

Concomitant therapy: Addition of a thiazide-type diuretic such as hydrochlorothiazide has been shown to have an additive antihypertensive effect with Amias*.

Use in children: The safety and efficacy of Amias* have not been established in children.

Contra-indications: Hypersensitivity to any component of Amias*.

Pregnancy and lactation (see *Pregnancy and lactation*).

Severe hepatic impairment and/or cholestasis.

Special warnings and special precautions for use: Renal artery stenosis: Other drugs that affect the renin-angiotensin-aldosterone system, i.e. angiotensin converting enzyme (ACE) inhibitors, may increase blood urea and serum creatinine in patients with bilateral renal artery stenosis or stenosis of the artery to a solitary kidney. While this is not reported with Amias*, a similar effect may be anticipated with angiotensin II receptor antagonists.

Intravascular volume depletion: In patients with intravascular volume depletion (such as those receiving high dose diuretics) symptomatic hypotension may occur, as described for other agents acting on the renin-angiotensin-aldosterone system. Therefore, these conditions should be corrected prior to administration of Amias*.

Renal impairment: When Amias* is used in patients with severe renal impairment, periodic monitoring of serum potassium and creatinine levels should be considered. There is limited experience in patients with very severe or end-stage renal impairment ($Cl_{creatinine} <15$ ml/min).

Kidney transplantation: There is no experience regarding the administration of Amias* in patients with a recent kidney transplantation.

Aortic and mitral valve stenosis (obstructive hypertrophic cardiomyopathy): As with other vasodilators, special caution is indicated in patients suffering from haemodynamically relevant aortic or mitral valve stenosis, or obstructive hypertrophic cardiomyopathy.

Primary hyperaldosteronism: Patients with primary hyperaldosteronism will not generally respond to antihypertensive drugs acting through inhibition of the renin-angiotensin-aldosterone system. Therefore, the use of Amias* is not recommended.

Hyperkalaemia: Based on experience with the use of other drugs that affect the renin-angiotensin-aldosterone system, concomitant use of potassium-sparing diuretics, potassium supplements, salt substitutes containing potassium, or other drugs that may increase potassium levels (e.g. heparin) may lead to increases in serum potassium.

General: In patients whose vascular tone and renal function depend predominantly on the activity of the renin-angiotensin-aldosterone system (e.g. patients with severe congestive heart failure or underlying renal disease, including renal artery stenosis), treatment with other drugs that affect this system has been associated with acute hypotension, azotaemia, oliguria or, rarely, acute renal failure. Although the possibility of similar effects cannot be excluded with angiotensin II receptor antagonists, these effects are not reported with Amias*. As with any antihypertensive agent, excessive blood pressure decrease in patients with ischaemic cardiopathy or ischaemic cerebrovascular disease could result in a myocardial infarction or stroke.

Interaction with other medicaments and other forms of interaction: No drug interactions of clinical significance have been identified.

Compounds which have been investigated in clinical pharmacokinetic studies include hydrochlorothiazide, warfarin, digoxin, oral contraceptives (i.e. ethinylestradiol/levonorgestrel), glibenclamide and nifedipine.

Candesartan is eliminated only to a minor extent by hepatic metabolism (CYP2C9). Available interaction studies indicate no effect on CYP2C9 and CYP3A4 but the effect on other cytochrome P450 isoenzymes is presently unknown.

The antihypertensive effect of Amias* may be enhanced by other antihypertensives.

Based on experience with the use of other drugs that affect the renin-angiotensin-aldosterone system, concomitant use of potassium-sparing diuretics, potassium supplements, salt substitutes containing potassium, or other drugs that may increase potassium levels (e.g. heparin) may lead to increases in serum potassium.

Reversible increases in serum lithium concentrations and toxicity have been reported during concomitant administration of lithium with ACE inhibitors. While not reported with Amias* the possibility of a similar effect cannot be excluded and careful monitoring of serum lithium levels is recommended during concomitant use.

The bioavailability of candesartan is not affected by food.

Pregnancy and lactation: Use in pregnancy: There is no experience with the use of Amias* in pregnant women, but animal studies with candesartan cilexetil have demonstrated late foetal and neonatal injury in the kidney. The mechanism is believed to be pharmacologically mediated through effects on the renin-angiotensin-aldosterone system.

In humans, foetal renal perfusion, which is dependent upon the development of the renin-angiotensin-aldosterone system, begins in the second trimester. Thus risk to the foetus increases if Amias* is administered during the second or third trimesters of pregnancy.

Based on the above information, Amias* should not be used in pregnancy. If pregnancy is detected during treatment, Amias* should be discontinued (see *Contra-indications*).

Use in lactation: It is not known whether candesartan is excreted in human milk. However, candesartan is excreted in the milk of lactating rats. Because of the potential for adverse effects on the nursing infant, breast feeding should be discontinued if the use of Amias* is considered essential (see *Contra-indications*).

Effects on ability to drive and use machines: The effect of Amias* on the ability to drive and use machines has not been studied, but based on its pharmacodynamic properties Amias* is unlikely to affect this ability. When driving vehicles or operating machines, it should be taken into account that occasionally dizziness or weariness may occur during treatment of hypertension.

Undesirable effects: In controlled clinical studies adverse events were mild and transient and comparable to placebo. The overall incidence of adverse events showed no association with dose or age. Withdrawals from treatment due to adverse events were similar with candesartan cilexetil (2.4%) and placebo (2.6%).

Clinical adverse events regardless of causal relationship occurring with an incidence of ≥1% on Amias* in double-blind placebo controlled studies are presented in the following table:

	Placebo (n=573) %	*Cand. cil. (n=1388) %*
Headache	10.3	10.4
URTI*	3.8	5.1
Back pain	0.9	3.2
Dizziness	2.3	2.5
Nausea	1.3	1.9
Coughing	1.1	1.6
Influenza-like symptoms	0.8	1.5
Fatigue	1.6	1.5
Abdominal pain	1.3	1.5
Diarrhoea	1.9	1.5
Pharyngitis	0.4	1.1
Peripheral oedema	0.7	1.0
Vomiting	1.2	1.0
Bronchitis	2.2	1.0
Rhinitis	0.4	1.0

*Upper respiratory tract infection

Laboratory findings: In general, there were no clinically important influences of Amias* on routine laboratory variables. Increases in S-ALAT (S-GPT) were reported as adverse events slightly more often with Amias* than with placebo (1.3% vs 0.5%). No routine monitoring of laboratory variables is usually necessary for patients receiving Amias*. However, in patients with severe renal impairment, periodic monitoring of serum potassium and creatinine levels should be considered.

Overdose: Symptoms: Based on pharmacological considerations, the main manifestation of an overdose is likely to be symptomatic hypotension and dizziness. In a case report of an overdose of 160 mg candesartan cilexetil, the patient's recovery was uneventful.

Management: If symptomatic hypotension should occur, symptomatic treatment should be instituted and vital signs monitored. The patient should be placed supine with the legs elevated. If this is not sufficient, plasma volume should be increased by infusion of, for example, isotonic saline solution. Sympathomimetic drugs may be administered if the above-mentioned measures are not sufficient.

Candesartan is unlikely to be removed by haemodialysis.

Pharmacological properties
Pharmacodynamic properties: Pharmaco-therapeutic group: Angiotensin II antagonists, ATC code C09C A.

Angiotensin II is the primary vasoactive hormone of the renin-angiotensin-aldosterone system and plays a significant role in the pathophysiology of hypertension and other cardiovascular disorders. It also has an important role in the pathogenesis of end organ hypertrophy and damage. The major physiological effects of angiotensin II, such as vasoconstriction, aldosterone stimulation, regulation of salt and water homeostasis and stimulation of cell growth, are mediated via the type 1 (AT_1) receptor.

Amias* is a prodrug suitable for oral use. It is rapidly converted to the active drug, candesartan, by ester hydrolysis during absorption from the gastrointestinal tract. Candesartan is an angiotensin II receptor antagonist, selective for AT_1 receptors, with tight binding to and slow dissociation from the receptor. It has no agonist activity.

Candesartan does not inhibit ACE, which converts angiotensin I to angiotensin II and degrades bradykinin. There is no effect on, ACE and no potentiation of bradykinin or substance P. In controlled clinical trials comparing Amias* with ACE inhibitors, the incidence of cough was lower in patients receiving Amias*. Candesartan does not bind to or block other hormone receptors or ion channels known to be important in cardiovascular regulation. The antagonism of the angiotensin II (AT_1) receptors results in dose related increases in plasma renin levels, angiotensin I and angiotensin II levels, and a decrease in plasma aldosterone concentration.

In hypertension, Amias* causes a dose-dependent, long-lasting reduction in arterial blood pressure. The antihypertensive action is due to decreased systemic peripheral resistance, without reflex increase in heart rate. There is no indication of serious or exaggerated first dose hypotension or rebound effect after cessation of treatment.

After administration of a single dose of Amias*, onset of antihypertensive effect generally occurs within 2 hours. With continuous treatment, most of the reduction in blood pressure with any dose is generally attained within four weeks and is sustained during long-term treatment. Amias* once daily provides effective and smooth blood pressure reduction over 24 hours, with little difference between maximum and trough effects during the dosing interval. When Amias* is used together with hydrochlorothiazide, the reduction in blood pressure is additive. Concomitant administration of Amias* with hydrochlorothiazide or amlodipine is well tolerated.

Amias* is similarly effective in patients irrespective of age and gender.

Amias* increases renal blood flow and either has no effect on or increases glomerular filtration rate while renal vascular resistance and filtration fraction are reduced. In hypertensive patients with type II diabetes mellitus, 12 weeks treatment with candesartan cilexetil 8 mg to 16 mg had no adverse effects on blood glucose or lipid profile.

Currently there are no data regarding the effects of candesartan cilexetil on morbidity and mortality in hypertensive patients.

Pharmacokinetic properties: Absorption and distribution: Following oral administration, candesartan cilexetil is converted to the active drug candesartan. The absolute bioavailability of candesartan is approximately 40% after an oral solution of candesartan cilexetil. The relative bioavailability of the tablet formulation compared with the same oral solution is approximately 34% with very little variability. The estimated absolute bioavailability of the tablet is therefore 14%. The mean peak serum concentration (C_{max}) is reached 3-4 hours following tablet intake. The candesartan serum concentrations increase linearly with increasing doses in the therapeutic dose range. No gender related differences in the pharmacokinetics of candesartan have been observed. The area under the serum concentration *versus* time curve (AUC) of candesartan is not significantly affected by food.

Candesartan is highly bound to plasma protein (more than 99%). The apparent volume of distribution of candesartan is 0.1 l/kg.

Metabolism and elimination: Candesartan is mainly eliminated unchanged via urine and bile and only to a minor extent eliminated by hepatic metabolism. The terminal half-life of candesartan is approximately 9 hours. There is no accumulation following multiple doses.

Total plasma clearance of candesartan is about 0.37 ml/min/kg, with a renal clearance of about 0.19 ml/min/kg. The renal elimination of candesartan is both by glomerular filtration and active tubular secretion. Following an oral dose of ^{14}C-labelled candesartan cilexetil, approximately 26% of the dose is excreted in the urine as candesartan and 7% as an inactive metabolite while approximately 56% of the dose is recovered in the faeces as candesartan and 10% as the inactive metabolite.

Pharmacokinetics in special populations: In the elderly (over 65 years) C_{max} and AUC of candesartan are increased by approximately 50% and 80%, respectively in comparison to young subjects. However, the blood pressure response and the incidence of adverse events are similar after a given dose of Amias* in young and elderly patients (see section *Posology and method of administration*).

In patients with mild to moderate renal impairment C_{max} and AUC of candesartan increased during repeated dosing by approximately 50% and 70%, respectively, but $t_{1/2}$ was not altered, compared to patients with normal renal function. The corresponding changes in patients with severe renal impairment were approximately 50% and 110%, respectively. The terminal $t_{1/2}$ of candesartan was approximately doubled in patients with severe renal impairment. The pharmacokinetics in patients undergoing haemodialysis were similar to those in patients with severe renal impairment.

In patients with mild to moderate hepatic impairment, there was a 23% increase in the AUC of candesartan (see *Posology and method of administration*).

Preclinical safety data: There was no evidence of abnormal systemic or target organ toxicity at clinically relevant doses. In preclinical safety studies candesartan had effects on the kidneys and on red cell parameters at high doses in mice, rats, dogs and monkeys. Candesartan caused a reduction of red blood cell parameters (erythrocytes, haemoglobin, haematocrit). Effects on the kidneys (such as interstitial nephritis, tubular distension, basophilic tubules; increased plasma concentrations of urea and creatinine) were induced by candesartan which could be secondary to the hypotensive effect leading to alterations of renal perfusion. Furthermore, candesartan induced hyperplasia/hypertrophy of the juxtaglomerular cells. These changes were considered to be caused by the pharmacological action of candesartan. For therapeutic doses of candesartan in humans, the hyperplasia/hypertrophy of the renal juxtaglomerular cells does not seem to have any relevance.

Foetotoxicity has been observed in late pregnancy (see *Pregnancy and lactation*).

Data from *in vitro* and *in vivo* mutagenicity testing indicates that candesartan will not exert mutagenic or clastogenic activities under conditions of clinical use. There was no evidence of carcinogenicity.

Pharmaceutical particulars

List of excipients: Carmellose calcium, hydroxypropyl cellulose, lactose monohydrate, magnesium stearate, maize starch, polyethylene glycol and iron oxide red E172 (8 mg only).

Incompatibilities: None stated.

Shelf-life: Three years.

Special precautions for storage: Store below 30°C.

Nature and contents of container: Amias* Tablets 2 mg are round white tablets.

Amias* Tablets 4 mg are round white tablets with a single score line on both sides.

Amias* Tablets 8 mg are round pale pink tablets with a single score line on both sides.

Amias* Tablets 16 mg are round white tablets with a single score line on both sides.

2 mg tablet: Polypropylene blister packs of 7 tablets.

4 mg tablet: Polypropylene blister packs of 7 and 28 tablets.

8 mg tablet: Polypropylene blister packs of 28 tablets.

16 mg tablet: Polypropylene blister packs of 28 tablets.

Instructions for use/handling: Not applicable.

Marketing authorisation numbers

Amias Tablets 2 mg–PL 16189/0001
Amias Tablets 4 mg–PL 16189/0002
Amias Tablets 8 mg–PL 16189/0003
Amias Tablets 16 mg–PL 16189/0004

Date of first authorisation/Renewal of authorisation
26 March 1998

Date of (partial) revision of the text 9 January 1998

**Trade Mark*

Trinity Pharmaceuticals Ltd

Tuition House
27/37 St George's Road
London SW19 4EU

☎ 0181 944 9443   🗋 0181 947 9325

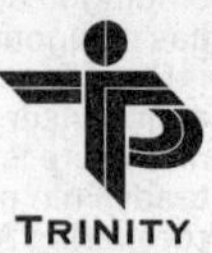

ADIPINE* MR 10
ADIPINE* MR 20

Qualitative and quantitative composition
Adipine MR 10: each modified release tablet contains 10 mg of Nifedipine.
Adipine MR 20: each modified release tablet contains 20 mg of Nifedipine.

Pharmaceutical form Modified release tablets for oral use.

Clinical particulars
Therapeutic indications: Hypertension. Prophylaxis of chronic stable angina pectoris.

Posology and method of administration: The treatment should be as individual as possible according to the seriousness of the disease and the responsiveness of the patient.

Dependent on the respective clinical picture stabilisation with reference to the final dose should be made slowly.

Nifedipine should be taken with a little water.

The recommended starting dose of nifedipine is 10 mg every 12 hours swallowed with water with subsequent titration of dosage according to response. The dose may be adjusted to 40 mg every 12 hours.

The pharmacokinetics of nifedipine are altered in the elderly so that lower maintenance doses of nifedipine may be required compared to younger patients.

Nifedipine is metabolised primarily by the liver and therefore patients with liver dysfunction should be carefully monitored. Patients with renal impairment should not require adjustment of dosage.

Nifedipine is not recommended for use in children.

The simultaneous intake of food delays, but does not reduce overall absorption.

The intervals between the recommended individual maximal daily doses of nifedipine should be not less than 4 hours. Discontinuation of Adipine MR especially from high doses should be made gradually.

Treatment may be continued indefinitely.

Contra-indications: Hypersensitivity to nifedipine or other dihydropyridines because of the theoretical risk of cross reactivity.

Nifedipine should not be used in clinically significant aortic stenosis, unstable angina, or during or within one month of a myocardial infarction.

Nifedipine must not be administered in cases of cardiogenic shock.

Nifedipine should not be used for the treatment of acute attacks of angina.

The safety of nifedipine in malignant hypertension has not been established.

Nifedipine should not be used for secondary prevention of myocardial infarction.

Nifedipine should not be administered concomitantly with rifampicin since effective plasma levels of nifedipine may not be achieved owing to enzyme induction.

Caution is required in cases of markedly low blood-pressure (severe hypotension with less than 90 mm Hg systolic) as well as in cases of cardiac failure.

Special warnings and special precautions for use: None.

Interaction with other medicaments and other forms of interaction: The hypotensive effect of Nifedipine can be increased by other hypotensive drugs as well as by tricyclic antidepressants. When combined with nitrates the effects on blood-pressure and heart rate increase.

When administering Nifedipine and beta receptor blockers at the same time, careful surveillance of the patient is necessary as this might produce a major lowering of the blood-pressure; occasional cardiac failure has also been observed.

Adipine MR is not a beta blocker and therefore gives no protection against the dangers of abrupt beta blocker withdrawal. Any such withdrawal should be a gradual reduction of the dose of the beta blocker preferably over 8 to 10 days. Adipine MR will not prevent possible rebound effects after cessation of other hypertensive therapy.

Certain calcium antagonists may increase the negatively inotropic effect of antiarrhythmics such as amiodarone and quinidine. In this connection, no observations were made with Nifedipine. In individual cases, Nifedipine causes a drop of the quinidine plasma level or after discontinuation of Nifedipine a marked increase of the quinidine plasma level so that in combined therapy the control of the quinidine plasma level is recommended.

Nifedipine may cause an increase of theophylline plasma levels so that the control of the latter is recommended.

Cimetidine and, to a lesser extent, ranitidine may lead to an increase in the Nifedipine plasma level and thus to a more intensive action of Nifedipine.

As with other dihydropyridines, nifedipine should not be taken with grapefruit juice because bioavailability is increased.

The simultaneous administration of nifedipine and digoxin may lead to reduced digoxin clearance and hence an increase in the plasma digoxin. Digoxin levels should be monitored and, if necessary, the digoxin dose reduced.

Nifedipine should not be administered concomitantly with rifampicin since effective plasma levels of nifedipine may not be achieved owing to enzyme induction (see *Contra-indications*).

Pregnancy and lactation: Nifedipine must not be administered during the entire pregnancy as experimental studies have shown foetal deformities. There is no information on humans. Nifedipine penetrates into the mother's milk. As there is no information with respect to possible effects on babies, the child should be weaned, if treatment with Nifedipine should be necessary during the lactation period.

Effects on ability to drive and use machines: The treatment of high blood-pressure with this therapy requires regular medical control. Due to different reactions occurring in individual cases, the ability to drive or of operating machines might be affected. This happens much more at the start of treatment and when changing preparations and is increased by co-administration of alcohol.

Undesirable effects: Especially at the beginning of therapy Nifedipine often might cause temporary headaches and flushing with a sensation of warmth (erythema, erythromelalgia).

Occasionally, tachycardia, palpitations as well as lower leg oedema due to vasodilatation may occur. Furthermore, vertigo and fatigue have been observed. Also occasionally, there may be paraesthesia and a drop in blood-pressure.

In rare cases, treatment with Nifedipine may cause gastro-intestinal disturbances such as nausea, a sensation of fullness and diarrhoea. Furthermore, hypersensitivity reactions of the skin such as pruritis, urticaria and rashes, and in individual cases exfoliative dermatitis, have been observed.

Reductions in the blood count such as anaemia, leucopenia, thrombopenia, thrombocytic purpura after the administration of Nifedipine have been described.

Very rarely, after long-term treatment, alterations of the gingiva (hyperplasia of the gingiva) might occur which disappear completely after stopping treatment.

In individual cases, liver dysfunctions (intrahepatic cholestasis, increases of transaminases) have been observed which disappear after stopping treatment.

Rarely, especially in elderly patients, gynaecomastia has been described in connection with long-term therapy which so far has disappeared in all cases after discontinuation of the treatment.

In individual cases – especially with higher doses – courbature, trembling of the fingers (tremor) as well as a minor temporary alteration of optical perception have been observed.

In individual cases an increase in the blood sugar level in the serum (hyperglycaemia) has been observed. This should be taken into account above all with patients suffering from diabetes mellitus.

Exacerbation of angina pectoris may occur frequently at the start of treatment with sustained release formulations of nifedipine. The occurrence of myocardial infarction has been described although it is not possible to distinguish such an event from the natural couse of ischaemic heart disease.

In dialysis patients with malignant hypertension and hypovolaemia, caution is required as due to vasodilatation a marked drop in the blood-pressure may be produced. Also, during the first weeks of therapy, daily urine volume may be increased.

In case of renal insufficiency during the administration of Nifedipine renal function may be temporarily impaired.

Overdosage:
Symptoms of intoxication: Clouding of consciousness and even coma, a fall in blood pressure, tachycardia, bradycardia, hyperglycaemia, metabolic acidosis, hypoxia and cardiogenic shock with pulmonary oedema have been described.

Therapy for intoxications: The most important therapeutic objectives are the elimination of the drug and the restoration of a stable circulation.

After oral ingestion, a thorough stomach lavage and charcoal instillation if need be, in combination with a lavage of the small intestine are indicated.

Especially, in the case of an overdose with the controlled release preparation, an elimination as complete as possible, including also from the small intestine, should be aimed at in order to avoid the inevitable re-absorption of the drug.

When administering laxatives, however, the reduction of the muscular tone of the intestines and even intestinal atony due to the effect of a calcium antagonist must be taken into account. As haemodialysis is not recommended since Nifedipine cannot be dialysed (high plasma protein bound, relatively low distribution volume) plasmapheresis, however, is recommended.

Bradycardia is symptomatically treated with atropine and/or beta-sympathomimetics, in cases of very serious bradycardia a temporary pacemaker therapy will be necessary.

Low blood-pressure as a consequence of cardiogenic shock and arterial vasodilatation can be treated with calcium (1–2 g of calcium gluconate administered intravenously), dopamine (up to 25 mcg for each kilogram of weight per minute), dobutamine (up to 15 mcg for each kilogram of weight per minute), adrenaline and/or noradrenaline. The dosage of these drugs can be titrated according to the effect obtained on the blood-pressure. The serum-calcium level should be kept at the upper limit of the normal range.

Additional intake of fluid should be monitored carefully to prevent overload.

Pharmacological properties
Pharmacodynamic properties: Nifedipine is a calcium antagonist of the 1,4-dihydro-pyridine type. Calcium antagonists exert an inhibitory effect on the calcium ion inflow through the slow calcium channel in the cell. Nifedipine acts primarily on the smooth muscle cells of the coronary arteries and the peripheral resistance vessels. This effect causes a vasodilatation. Administered in therapeutic doses, Nifedipine has virtually no direct effect on the myocardium.

In the heart, Nifedipine mainly dilates the large coronary arteries. Furthermore, Nifedipine reduces the muscle tone of the conorary arteries, which may produce an improvement in blood circulation. At the same time, Nifedipine, due to vasodilatation, reduces the peripheral resistance (afterload).

At the start of treatment with this calcium antagonist, the heart rate and the cardiac output will be increased by a reflex action. This increase, however, is not sufficient to compensate the vasodilatation.

In long-term treatment with Nifedipine, the cardiac output increases at first and then returns to the initial value. A particularly marked decrease in blood-pressure after the administration of Nifedipine can be observed with concurrent use of anti-hypertensive agents.

Pharmacokinetic properties: The active substance Nifedipine is rapidly and almost completely absorbed from the gastro-intestinal tract after oral administration on an empty stomach. Nifedipine is subject to a 'first pass metabolism' in the liver, resulting in a systemic availability of orally administered Nifedipine of between 50 to 70%. Following administration of a Nifedipine-containing solution maximum serum concentrations are reported to occur after approx. 15 minutes. After the administration of other preparations having an immediate release peak serum concentrations are attained after 15 to 75 minutes.

Approx. 95% of Nifedipine is bound to plasma proteins.

Nifedipine is almost completely metabolised in the liver by oxidative and hydrolytic processes. These metabolites do not show any pharmacodynamic activity.

About 70 to 80% of a Nifedipine dose is excreted in the urine in the form of its metabolites, the main metabolite (M-I) accounts for about 60 to 80% of the administered Nifedipine dose. The rest is excreted in the form of metabolites with the faeces. The unaltered substance is found only in traces (less than 0.1%) in the urine.

The elimination half-life is about 2 to 5 hours.

A cumulation of the substance during permanent therapy with usual doses has not been described.

In cases of reduced hepatic function, the elimination half-life is markedly prolonged and total clearance is reduced. In some cases dose reduction may be necessary.

Bioavailability: A bioavailability study with Adipine MR 20 made in the year 1991 with 24 volunteers showed the following results compared to the reference preparation:

	Test preparation	*Reference preparation*
Maximum steady-state plasma concentration (0–12 h) ($C_{ss,max1}$) (ng/ml):	36.3±12.1	39.8±15.9
Maximum steady-state plasma concentration (12–24 h) ($C_{ss,max2}$) (ng/ml):	39.1±15.4	50.3±19.6
Area under the concentration-time-curve (24 h) (AUC_{ss}) (ng/ml*h):	394.3±165.7	435.6±194.6
Plateau time (0–24 h) (h):	3.67±1.37	3.68±1.97
Peak-trough-fluctuation (0–12 h) (PTF1) (1%):	182.1±40.3	204.6±66.7
Peak-trough-fluctuation (12–24 h) (PTF2) (%):	206.4±48.2	246.6±85.6

Values as mean values ±SD.

Preclinical safety data:

Acute toxicity: Acute toxicity has been studied on various species of animals. No specific sensibility was found.

Subchronic and chronic toxicity: Studies on rats and dogs did not show any toxic effect of Nifedipine.

Tumorigenicity: A long-time study (2 years) on the rat did not yield any indications for oncogenous effects of Nifedipine.

Mutagenicity: The studies in vivo and in vitro were negative without exception so that any mutagenic action in human beings can be excluded sufficiently.

Reproductive toxicology: Experimental studies carried out with three species of animals brought about indications for teratogenous effects (cleft palate, cardiovascular anomalies) in two species of animals. There is no experience with the application to human beings during the first six months of pregnancy. The administration of Nifedipine without detrimental consequences during the last three months has been described for a small number of cases. Nifedipine has a tocolytical effect.

Nifedipine penetrates into the mother's milk. For its administration during the nursing period the experience gathered is not sufficient.

Pharmaceutical particulars

List of excipients: Lactose, microcrystalline cellulose, macrogol 6000, magnesium stearate, maize starch, hydroxypropylmethylcellulose, polysorbate 80 (Tween 80), talc, colourants E171, E172.

Incompatibilities: None known.

Shelf life: 2 years. The medication should not be used after the printed expiration date.

Special precautions for storage: To be kept protected from light.

Store below 25°C.

Note: The active substance Nifedipine is light-sensitive and is protected by special packaging.

When modified release tablets are taken out, they should not be exposed unnecessarily to intensive light for a prolonged period of time.

Nature and contents of container: The modified release tablets are sealed in blister packages made of aluminium foil and PVC film. The blisters are packed, along with the package leaflet, in a folded cardboard box.

Packs containing 56 modified release tablets.

Instructions for use/handling: None.

Marketing authorisation holder: STADA Arzneimittel AG, Stadastrasse 2-18, 61118 Bad Vilbel, FRG.

Marketing authorisation numbers

Adipine MR 10	11204/0038
Adipine MR 20	11204/0005

Date of approval/revision of SPC March 1997.

Legal category POM.

ANGITIL* SR CAPSULES 90, 120, 180 mg
ANGITIL* XL CAPSULES 240, 300 mg (Diltiazem Hydrochloride)

Qualitative and quantitative composition

Angitil SR 90: Diltiazem Hydrochloride PhEur 90 mg.
Angitil SR 120: Diltiazem Hydrochloride PhEur 120 mg.
Angitil SR 180: Diltiazem Hydrochloride PhEur 180 mg.
Angitil XL 240: Diltiazem Hydrochloride PhEur 240 mg.
Angitil XL 300: Diltiazem Hydrochloride PhEur 300 mg.

Pharmaceutical form Sustained-release capsules.

Clinical particulars

Therapeutic indications: For the management of angina pectoris. For the management of mild to moderate hypertension.

Posology and method of administration:

Dosage recommendations: Individual patients' responses to diltiazem may vary, necessitating careful titration. This range of capsule strengths 90 mg, 120 mg, 180 mg, 240 mg, 300 mg facilitates titration to the optimal dose.

The capsules should be swallowed whole and not chewed. Dosage may be taken with or without food.

Angitil SR 90, 120, 180 mg

Angina:

Adults: The usual initial dose is 90 mg twice daily. Dosage may be increased gradually to 120 mg twice daily or 180 mg twice daily if required.

Elderly and patients with renal and hepatic dysfunction: In the elderly, dosage should commence at 90 mg twice daily and the dose carefully titrated as required.

Hypertension:

Adults: The usual initial dose is 90 mg twice daily. Dosage may be increased gradually to 120 mg twice daily or 180 mg twice daily if required.

Elderly and patients with renal and hepatic dysfunction: The starting dose should be one diltiazem 90 mg capsule twice daily increasing to one 120 mg capsule twice daily if clinically indicated.

Angitil XL 240, 300 mg

Adults: For patients new to diltiazem therapy, the usual starting dose is one 240 mg capsule daily.

Patients currently receiving a total daily dose of 180 mg diltiazem (as 90 mg bd) should be given the 240 mg capsule (od). A patient receiving 240 mg/day of diltiazem (as 120 mg bd) should commence treatment on the 240 mg capsule (od), titrating to the 300 mg capsule (od) if required.

Elderly and patients with renal and hepatic dysfunction: For patients new to diltiazem therapy, the usual starting dose is one 90 mg capsule twice daily. If necessary, the dose may be increased gradually but careful monitoring of this group of patients is advised. When 120 mg bd has been demonstrated by titration to be the optimal dose, then it can be switched to 240 mg od.

Children: Diltiazem preparations are not recommended for children. Safety and efficacy in children has not been established.

In order to avoid confusion it is suggested that patients once titrated to an effective dose should remain on this treatment and should not be changed between different presentations.

Contra-indications: Pregnancy and in women of child bearing capacity. Patients with bradycardia (less than 50 bpm), second or third degree heart block, sick sinus syndrome, decompensated cardiac failure, patients with left ventricular dysfunction following myocardial infarction. Concurrent use with dantrolene infusion because of the risk of ventricular fibrillation.

Special warnings and precautions for use: The product should be used with caution in patients with reduced left ventricular function. Patients with mild bradycardia, first degree AV block or prolonged PR interval should be observed closely. Diltiazem is considered unsafe in patients with acute porphyria.

Interactions with other medicaments and other forms of interaction: Due consideration should be given to the possibility of an additive effect when diltiazem is prescribed with drugs which may induce bradycardia or other anti-arrhythmic drugs.

Diltiazem hydrochloride has been used safely in combination with beta-blockers, diuretics, ACE-inhibitors and other antihypertensive agents. It is recommended that patients receiving these combinations should be regularly monitored. Concomitant use with alpha-blockers such as prazosin should be strictly monitored because of the possible synergistic hypotensive effect of this combination.

Patients with pre-existing conduction defects should not receive the combination of diltiazem and beta-blockers.

Case reports have suggested that blood levels of carbamazepine, cyclosporin and theophylline may be increased when given concurrently with diltiazem hydrochoride.

Care should be exercised in patients taking these drugs. In common with other calcium antagonists diltiazem hydrochloride may cause small increases in plasma levels of digoxin.

Concurrent use with H_2-antagonists may increase serum levels of diltiazem.

Treatment with diltiazem has been continued without problem during anaesthesia, but the anaesthetist should be made aware of the treatment regimen.

Pregnancy and lactation: Diltiazem hydrochloride is contra-indicated in pregnant women or women of child-bearing potential, and is not recommended in nursing mothers.

Effects on ability to drive and use machines: None known.

Undesirable effects: Diltiazem is generally well tolerated. Occasional undesirable effects are nausea, headache, allergic skin reactions including erythema multiform and vasculitis have been reported, oedema of the legs, flushing, hypotension and fatigue which disappear on cessation of treatment. Diltiazem may cause depression of atrioventricular nodal conduction and bradycardia. Isolated cases of clinical hepatitis have been reported, which resolved when diltiazem was withdrawn.

Overdose: The clinical symptoms of acute intoxication may include pronounced hypotension or even collapse and sinus bradycardia with or without atrioventricular conduction defects.

The patient should be closely monitored in hospital to exclude arrhythmias or atrioventricular conduction defects. Gastric lavage and osmotic diuresis should be undertaken when considered appropriate. Symptomatic bradycardia and high grade atrioventricular block may respond to atropine, isoprenaline or occasionally temporary cardiac pacing.

Hypotension may require correction with plasma volume expanders, intravenous calcium gluconate and positive inotropic agents. The formulation employs a controlled release system which will continue to release diltiazem for some hours.

Pharmacological properties

Pharmacodynamic properties: Diltiazem is an antianginal agent, calcium antagonist. Diltiazem inhibits transmembrane calcium entry in myocardial muscle fibres and in vascular smooth muscle fibres, thereby decreasing the quantity of intracellular calcium available to the contractile proteins.

Pharmacokinetic properties: Angitil capsules contain slow release forms of microgranules which permit diltiazem hydrochloride to be released along a length of the gastrointestinal tract.

Diltiazem is 80% bound to human plasma proteins (albumin, acid glucoproteins).

The biotransformation routes are:
- Deacetylation
- Oxidative O- and N-demethylation
- Conjugation of the phenolic metabolites.

The primary metabolites, N-demethyldiltiazem and desacetyldiltiazem exert less pharmacological activity than diltiazem. The other metabolites are pharmacologically inactive.

After administration of 180 to 300 mg of Angitil formulation, a peak plasma concentration of 80 to 220 ng/ml, respectively, is obtained after 5.5 hours.

The elimination half-life varies from 6 to 8 hours, depending on the strength.

Pre-clinical safety data: Not applicable.

Pharmaceutical particulars

List of excipients:

Sucrose and maize starch SP microgranules	HSE
Povidone K30	PhEur
Sucrose	PhEur
Ethylcellulose	PhEur
Talc	PhEur
Aquacoat ECD 30	NF
Dibutyl sebacate	HSE
Gelatin	PhEur
Titanium dioxide (E171)	PhEur
Red iron oxide (E172)	PhEur (120 mg, 180 mg only)
Yellow iron oxide (E172)	PhEur (120 mg, 180 mg, 300 mg only)
Black iron oxide (E172)	PhEur (180 mg only)
Indigotine (E132)	PhEur (120 mg only)

Black ink (Shellac, Ethyl alcohol, Isopropyl alcohol, n-Butyl alcohol, Propylene glycol, Water-filtered, Ammonium hydroxide, Potassium hydroxide, Black iron oxide).

Incompatibilities: None known.

Shelf life: 3 years.

Special precautions for storage: Store in a dry place at less than 30°C.

Nature and contents of container: Blister packs (aluminium/PVC) – boxed in cardboard cartons containing 28, 30, 56 or 60 capsules.

Instructions for use/handling: Not applicable.

Administrative data
Marketing authorisation holder: Laboratoires Ethypharm SA, 17–21 Rue Saint Matthieu, 78550 Houdan, France.

Marketing authorisation numbers

Angitil SR 90 mg:	PL 06934/0010
Angitil SR 120 mg:	PL 06934/0011
Angitil SR 180 mg:	PL 06934/0012
Angitil XL 240 mg:	PL 06934/0015
Angitil XL 300 mg:	PL 06934/0013.

Date of first authorisation

Angitil SR 90 mg:	June 5, 1995
Angitil SR 120 mg:	June 5, 1995
Angitil SR 180 mg:	June 5, 1995
Angitil XL 240 mg:	February 25, 1998
Angitil XL 300 mg:	June 5, 1995

Date of (partial) revision of the text
December 1997
March 1998

Legal category POM.

KETOCID* 200

Qualitative and quantitative composition Each capsule contains 200 mg Ketoprofen BP.

Pharmaceutical form Modified release capsule.

Clinical particulars
Therapeutic indications: Ketoprofen is an analgesic, anti-inflammatory and antipyretic; recommended for the treatment of rheumatoid arthritis, osteoarthritis, ankylosing spondylitis and other musculoskeletal conditions including bursitis, capsulitis, synovitis, tendinitis, fibrositis and low back pain. It is also useful to relieve the pain of sciatica, acute gout and dysmenorrhoea.

Posology and method of administration:
Adults: One 200 mg capsule to be taken orally once daily with a little food.

Elderly: As for adult dosage as there is no evidence that the pharmacokinetics of ketoprofen are altered in the elderly.

Children: There are no recommendations for the use of this product in children.

Contra-indications: Ketoprofen should not be given to patients with active peptic ulceration or a history of recurrent peptic ulceration or chronic dyspepsia; known hypersensitivity to ketoprofen, aspirin or other non-steroidal anti-inflammatory agents or with severe renal dysfunction.

Special warnings and precautions for use: Some patients with a history of bronchial asthma or allergic disease may suffer bronchospasm, particularly those with a history of allergy to ketoprofen and related compounds. As non-steroidal anti-inflammatory agents can inhibit renal prostaglandin synthesis and interfere with renal function, care should be taken in patients with renal impairment. NSAIDs have been reported to cause nephrotoxicity in various forms: interstitial nephritis, nephrotic syndrome and renal failure. In patients with renal, cardiac, or hepatic impairment caution is required since the use of NSAIDs may result in deterioration of renal function: the dose should be kept as low as possible and renal function should be monitored. As with other drugs in the same therapeutic category, patients should be advised to take ketoprofen with food, to minimise gastric intolerance.

Interactions with other medicaments and other forms of interaction: The active ingredient, ketoprofen, is highly protein bound. Therefore alteration of the dosage of other protein bound drugs such as anticoagulants, sulphonamides and hydantoins such as phenytoin may be necessary when taken together. Serious interactions have been reported with methotrexate, digoxin, lithium and diuretics. To avoid the risk of increased side effects, ketoprofen should not be given with other non-steroidal anti-inflammatory agents.

Pregnancy and lactation: There is no evidence of teratogenic effects of ketoprofen but as with all drugs, administration during pregnancy should be avoided unless essential. Because ketoprofen interferes with prostaglandin synthesis, there may be premature closure of the ductus arteriosus or persistent pulmonary hypertension in the neonate, or delay in labour if administered within a few days before delivery. Small amounts of ketoprofen are excreted in breast milk so use in nursing mothers should be avoided.

Effects on ability to drive and use machines: Ketoprofen can cause nausea, dizziness, confusion and drowsiness, therefore patients should be warned of these effects and advised to be careful if driving or operating machinery.

Undesirable effects: The most common adverse effects relate to the gastrointestinal tract, mainly indigestion, dyspepsia, heartburn, various types of abdominal discomfort, nausea, constipation and diarrhoea. Other effects such as headache, dizziness, confusion, drowsiness, oedema, change of mood and insomnia occur less commonly. Peptic ulceration, perforation and gastrointestinal haemorrhage may rarely occur. Other rare adverse events reported include haematological reactions such as thrombocytopenia, hepatic or renal damage, dermatological reactions, bronchospasm and anaphylaxis. Should any severe adverse event occur, treatment should be stopped immediately.

Overdose: As with other propionic acid derivatives, ketoprofen demonstrates less toxicity than aspirin or paracetamol. The most likely symptoms of overdosage are drowsiness, abdominal pain and vomiting but hypotension, bronchospasm and gastro-intestinal haemorrhage may occur. Since this is a controlled release (modified release) preparation, continued absorption from capsules in the gastrointestinal tract may be expected. Treatment should be symptomatic and may include gastric washout and the use of activated charcoal.

Pharmacological properties
Pharmacodynamic properites: Ketoprofen is a propionic acid derivative which has analgesic, anti-pyretic and anti-inflammatory properties. It is a strong inhibitor of prostaglandin synthetase.

Pharmacokinetic properties: This controlled release (modified release) ketoprofen formulation is designed to release ketoprofen over a period of time. Following a pharmacokinetic study in volunteers it was found that the average time to achieve maximum plasma concentration was 6.9 hours. The average half-life was found to be 7.4 hours, with a range of 5.5 to 8.0 hours. The average mean residence time was about 14 hours with an average clearance of 2.4 litres per hour. The study carried out over a five day period at the proposed dosage of once daily indicates that there is no accumulation on continued daily dosing. Ketoprofen is very highly bound to plasma protein.

Preclinical safety data: None provided.

Pharmaceutical particulars
List of excipients: Polyethylene Glycol 4000 BP, Ethylcellulose USP, Stearic Acid (purified) USP, Talc PhEur, Eudragit 'RS' HSE.

Neutral pellets: Sucrose PhEur, Corn Starch PhEur.

Ingredients removed during manufacturing process: Ethanol 96% BP, Acetone BP, Purified Water PhEur.

Capsule shell: Erythrosine E127 HSE, Titanium dioxide E171 HSE, Gelatin BP.

Incompatibilities: None reported.

Shelf life: 48 months.

Special precautions for storage: Store in a dry place below 25°C. Protect from light.

Nature and contents of container: Blister packs composed of PVC-PVdC/Aluminium-PVdC, containing 28 capsules.

Instruction for use/handling: Not applicable.

Marketing authorisation number 08829/0041

Date of approval/revision of SPC 23 January 1996.

Legal category POM.

MONOMAX* SR 40
MONOMAX* SR 60

Qualitative and quantitative composition
Monomax SR 40: Isosorbide Mononitrate 40 mg.
Monomax SR 60: Isosorbide Mononitrate 60 mg.

Pharmaceutical form Modified release capsules.

Clinical particulars
Therapeutic indications: For the prophylaxis of angina pectoris.

Posology and method of administration
Dosage recommendations: Dosage may be taken with or without food, and should be swallowed whole and not chewed.

Prophylaxis of angina: Adults: Usual adult dose is 40 mg per day. The daily dose may be increased to 60 mg.

Children: Safety and efficacy in children has not been established.

Elderly: There is no evidence of a need for routine dosage adjustment in the elderly, but special care may be needed in those with increased susceptibility to hypotension or marked hepatic or renal insufficiency.

Contra-indications: This product should not be given to patients with a known sensitivity to nitrates.

Isosorbide-5-Mononitrate should not be used in patients with acute myocardial infarction with low filling pressure, marked anaemia, head trauma, cerebral haemorrhage, severe hypotension or hypovolaemia.

Special warnings and special precautions for use: Isosorbide-5-Mononitrate should be used with caution in patients who are predisposed to closed angle glaucoma.

Isosorbide-5-Mononitrate should be used with caution in patients suffering from hypothyroidism, hypothermia, malnutrition, severe liver or renal disease. Monomax SR capsules are not indicated for relief of acute angina attacks; in the event of an acute attack, sublingual or buccal glyceryl trinitrate tablets/sprays should be used.

Interaction with other medicaments and other forms of interaction: Some of the effects of alcohol may be potentiated by this agent.

Vasodilators, antihypertensives and diuretics may potentiate the hypotension caused by nitrates particularly in the elderly.

There is no evidence of interaction with food.

Pregnancy and lactation: This product should not be used during pregnancy or lactation unless considered essential by the physician.

Effects on ability to drive and use machines: Since postural hypotension with symptoms such as dizziness has been reported, patients should be advised to be careful when driving or operating machinery if they suffer from these symptoms.

Undesirable effects: Side-effects including flushing, postural hypotension and dry skin rashes may occur occasionally. Headache may occur at the onset of treatment but may be minimised by commencing with low doses and gradually increasing the dose.

Using the recommended dosage schedules there is no evidence of development of nitrate tolerance.

Overdose: Treatment should be symptomatic. The main symptom is likely to be hypotension.

Pharmacological properties
Pharamacodynamic properties: Nitrate compounds relax smooth muscle causing dilatation of the veins and arteries, and to a lesser extent of the arterioles. The result is a very marked reduction of preload, accompanied by lowering of right heart pressures and left ventricular and diastolic pressure.

The dimensions of the right and left ventricles and ejection volumes are reduced but the reflex increase of heart rate prevents any reduction of cardiac output. Myocardial oxygen consumption may thus fall by more than 50% in parallel with the reduction of left ventricular preload. At higher doses, afterload is also decreased by arterial and arteriolar dilatation; this also helps to improve cardiac function.

Nitrate compounds exert a dilatory and antispasmodic effect on the coronary vessels; they are effective against both spontaneous and induced spasms.

Pharmacokinetic properties: In man, Isosorbide-5-Mononitrate is absorbed completely and rapidly following oral administration.

Isosorbide-5-Mononitrate is not subject to the 'hepatic first-pass' effect, and provides a low degree of inter-individual variation of blood levels.

Monomax SR capsules have all the pharmackonetic characteristics of a true sustained-release dosage form. Compared with an immediate-release dosage form, the peak plasma concentration obtained is lower and occurs later, while the apparent elimination half-life is unchanged; there is less fluctuation between C_{max} and C_{min}.

The slow continuous diffusion of the active ingredient from the sustained-release microgranules makes it possible, at steady state, to maintain plasma concentrations above the putative effective level of 100 ng/ml for a period of about 16 hours for the 40 mg capsules and 20 hours for the 60 mg capsules.

Preclinical safety data: Isosorbide-5-Mononitrate produces very few toxic effects and is less toxic than isosorbide dinitrate. After chronic adminstration at high doses (60 mg/kg), signs of toxicity have been detected in canine liver and kidneys. Tests conducted have shown no evidence of a teratogenic or mutagenic potential.

Pharmaceutical particulars
List of excipients: Lactose PhEur; sucrose and maize starch microgranules; Shellac FRP; Eudragit L100; Eudragit RS100; Talc PhEur; Gelatin; E171; Ethyl alcohol 95% FRP (ND†); Acetone BP (ND†); E172 (ND†).

† *Not detected in the finished product.*

Incompatibilities: None known.

Shelf life: 2 years.

Special precautions for storage: Store in a dry place below 25°C.

Nature and contents of container: Blister packs (20 µm

aluminium/250 μm PVC) – boxed in cardboard cartons containing 28 capsules.

Instructions for use/handling: Not applicable.

Marketing authorisation numbers
40 mg 8829/0029
60 mg 8829/0030.

Date of approval/revision of SPC 2 April 1996

Legal category POM.

VENTMAX* SR 4 mg
VENTMAX* SR 8 mg

Qualitative and quantitative composition
Ventmax SR 4 mg: Salbutamol sulphate 4.80 mg (equivalent to 4 mg of salbutamol base).
Ventmax SR 8 mg: Salbutamol sulphate 9.60 mg (equivalent to 8 mg of salbutamol base).

Pharmaceutical form Capsule filled with modified-release microgranules.

Clinical particulars
Therapeutic indications: Continuous symptomatic treatment of asthma and other types of reversible obstructive airways disease:

- in patients requiring daily administration of quick-acting beta-2 agonists with a short duration of action;
- and/or with nocturnal symptoms.

N.B.: in asthma, the treatment with Ventmax SR should be combined with an anti-inflammatory treatment, such as inhaled corticosteroids.

Posology and method of administration: Twice-daily administration of Ventmax SR capsules procures a bronchodilator effect which is maintained for about 12 hours after each dose.

Adults: The recommended dose is one 8 mg capsule twice daily.

Elderly patients: It is not necessary to adjust the dose.

Children: In children aged 3 to 12 years, the recommended dose is one 4 mg capsule twice daily.

Contra-indications: History of hypersensitivity to any of the ingredients of the Ventmax SR capsules.

Special warnings and precautions for use:
Warning: Athletes should be advised that this product contains an active substance which may produce a positive dope test reaction.

Precautions for use: In asthma, Ventmax SR is a maintenance treatment reserved, like all long-acting beta-2 agonists, for patients who are not completely controlled by the anti-inflammatory treatments with which it is prescribed concomitantly.

Ventmax SR can be combined on demand with other symptomatic treatments (bronchodilators). If paroxysmal dyspnoea should occur in spite of an adequately followed treatment, it is recommended that a short-acting beta-2 agonist bronchodilator be used to treat such symptoms.

If a patient's consumption of quick and short-acting beta-2 agonists should increase rapidly within a few days, this may be indicative (especially if the peak flow values fall and/or become very irregular), of decompensation of the asthmatic disease, with a possibility of development of a status asthmaticus, and calls for a consultation to re-evaluate the patient's condition. Such decompensation should be treated preferably in a specialised centre.

Interactions with other medicaments and other forms of interaction: Potentially serious hypokalaemia may result from beta-2 agonist therapy. Particular caution is advised in severe asthma as this effect may be potentiated by concomitant treatment with steroids, diuretics and xanthine derivatives such as theophylline. It is recommended that serum potassium levels are monitored in these circumstances.

Non-cardioselective beta-adrenoceptor blocking agents such as propranolol antagonise the effects of salbutamol.

The adverse metabolic effects of high doses of salbutamol may be exacerbated by concomitant administration of high doses of corticosteroids.

Pregnancy and lactation
Pregnancy: Ventmax SR capsules should not be used during pregnancy (especially during the first trimester) unless the benefit for the mother outweighs any possible risk to the foetus. Salbutamol has been used therapeutically for many years in human beings (including its use in the management of premature labour) with no evidence of harmful effects on foetuses or newborn infants. However, as for most drugs, few data have been published on the safety of salbutamol in the early stages of human pregnancy. Animal studies have shown that there are harmful effects on the foetus at very high doses.

Lactation: Since it is possible that salbutamol may be excreted in breast milk, it should not be used during lactation unless the benefit/risk ratio is favourable; it is not known whether salbutamol has harmful effects on newborn infants.

Effects on ability to drive and use machines: Not applicable.

Undesirable effects: Potentially serious hypokalaemia may result from beta-2 agonist therapy. This effect may be potentiated by hypoxia. Particular caution is advised in severe asthma, with monitoring of serum potassium levels.

Like all beta-stimulants, oral salbutamol can produce muscular tremor, predominantly of the extremities. Such tremor seems to be rare in children. Tachycardia may occur at high doses. Digestive disorders (nausea and vomiting) and headaches have been reported.

Overdose
Signs: Intensified tremor, tachycardia, changes in blood pressure, sedation, nervousness.

Treatment: In the event of serious poisoning, the stomach should be emptied and, if necessary, a beta-blocker administered in hospital, with the appropriate caution in patients subject to bronchospasm.

Pharmacological properties
Pharmacodynamic properties: β_2-stimulant bronchodilator.

Salbutamol is a beta-adrenergic receptor agonist, with a selective action focused much more on the beta-2 receptors (of the bronchi, uterus and blood vessels in particular) than on the cardiac beta-1 receptors. Because of this selectivity, cardiac effects are moderate at usual therapeutic doses.

Pharmacokinetic properties: After oral administration, the absolute bioavailability of salbutamol, which varies from one subject to another, is about 40%, owing in particular to a hepatic first-pass effect.

After administration of Ventmax SR, maximum plasma concentrations are reached in 4 to 5 hours. Administering Ventmax SR during a meal does not alter the global bioavailability of the drug, but delays and slightly lowers the peak plasma concentration.

The principal metabolite, a conjugated sulphate, has no effect on the beta receptors.

The apparent elimination half-life is about 12 hours.

The product is eliminated, essentially in the urine (75 to 80%), partly in unchanged form and partly as inactive metabolites.

Preclinical safety data
Carcinogenic and mutagenic potential, impairment of fertility: Salbutamol sulphate has been found to cause a dose-related increase in the incidence of benign leiomyomas of the mesovarium in the rat at oral doses corresponding to 3, 16 and 78 times the maximum oral dose for a 50 kg human. The relevance of these findings to humans is not known. A study in mice, and a lifetime oral study in hamsters, showed no evidence of an oncogenic potential.

In-vitro studies have shown no evidence of mutagenicity.

Oral reproduction studies in rats have shown no evidence of impaired fertility.

Pregnancy: Teratogenic effects: Salbutamol has been shown to be teratogenic in mice when given subcutaneously in doses corresponding to 0.4 times the maximum human oral dose.

There are no adequate and well-controlled studies in pregnant women. A relationship between use of salbutamol and congenital anomalies has not been established.

Pharmaceutical particulars
List of excipients:
Sucrose (European Pharmacopoeia)
Maize starch (European Pharmacopoeia)
Colloidal anhydrous silica (European Pharmacopoeia)
Methacrylic copolymer (USNF 18)
Ethylcellulose (USNF 18)
Dibutyl sebacate
Talc (European Pharmacopoeia)
Gelatin
Titanium dioxide
Black marking ink (Shellac, Ethyl Alcohol, Isopropyl Alcohol, n-Butyl Alcohol, Propylene Glycol, Water-Filtered, Ammonium Hydroxide, Potassium Hydroxide, Black Iron Oxide).

Ventmax SR 4 mg capsules additionally contain Black iron oxide, Yellow iron oxide, Erythrosine and Patient blue V.

Incompatibilities: Not applicable.

Shelf life: 36 months.

Special precautions for storage: Store below 30°C.

Nature and contents of container: Blister packs (250-μm PVC/20-μm aluminium) packed in cardboard boxes containing 28, 30, 56 or 60 capsules.

Instructions for use/handling: Not applicable.

Administrative data
Marketing authorisation holder: Trinity Pharmaceuticals Ltd, Tuition House, 27–37 St George's Road, Wimbledon, London SW19 4EU.

Marketing authorisation number PL 08829/0094, 95 (4 mg, 8 mg respectively).

Date of first authorisation/renewal of authorisation August 22 1997

Date of (partial) revision of the text September 1997

Legal category POM.

VOLSAID* RETARD 75
VOLSAID* RETARD 100

Qualitative and quantitative composition Each controlled release tablet of Volsaid Retard 75 contains 75 mg Diclofenac Sodium BP.

Each controlled release tablet of Volsaid Retard 100 contains 100 mg Diclofenac Sodium BP.

Pharmaceutical form Modified release tablets.

Clinical particulars
Therapeutic indications: Diclofenac sodium is a non-steroidal anti-inflammatory drug (NSAID); recommended for the treatment of rheumatoid arthritis; osteoarthritis; ankylosing spondylitis; acute gout; low back pain, relief of pain in fractures; acute musculo-skeletal disorders and trauma including periarthritis (particularly frozen shoulder), bursitis, tendinitis, tenosynovitis, dislocations, sprains and strains; and the control of pain and inflammation in orthopaedic, dental and other minor surgery.

Posology and method of administration
Adults: Volsaid Retard 75: One tablet to be taken orally once or twice a day, swallowed whole preferably with food.

Volsaid Retard 100: One tablet to be taken orally once a day, swallowed whole preferably with food.

Children: Not suitable for use in children.

Elderly: Care should be used when treating patients who are frail or have a low body weight as they will in general be more susceptible to adverse reactions. The lowest effective dose should be used in these patients. The standard adult dose may be used for other elderly patients.

Contra-indications: Diclofenac sodium should not be given to patients who are hypersensitive to diclofenac sodium, with active or suspected peptic ulcers, gastro-intestinal bleeding and who when taking aspirin or other NSAIDs suffer attacks of asthma, urticaria or acute rhinitis.

Special warnings and precautions for use: Patients with a history of gastro-intestinal ulceration, haematemesis, or melaena, should be carefully observed, and care should be taken when treating patients with ulcerative colitis, Crohn's disease, haematological abnormalities, or bleeding diathesis. Elderly patients and those with renal, hepatic or cardiac impairment should also be carefully monitored as renal function may be reduced by NSAID therapy. Renal function should be monitored and the lowest effective dose used.

In patients with impairment of cardiac or renal function, those recovering from major surgery or those being treated with diuretics, prostaglandins are important for the maintenance of renal blood flow. The possibility of inhibition of prostaglandin synthetase should be considered when giving diclofenac to these patients. On stopping diclofenac, effects on renal function are usually reversible.

Diclofenac should be stopped if liver function tests show abnormalities which persist or worsen, or if liver disease develops of if other symptoms such as eosinophilia or rash occur.

Diclofenac sodium may trigger an attack in patients with hepatic porphyria.

Monitoring of renal function, hepatic function (elevation of liver enzymes may occur) and blood counts should be performed on long-term NSAID patients, as a precautionary measure.

Interactions with other medicaments and other forms of interaction: Diclofenac may increase plasma concentrations of lithium (by the impairment of its excretion from the kidneys) and digoxin.

Methotrexate and NSAIDs should only be administered within 24 hours of each other if given with extreme caution. NSAIDs are reported to increase the plasma levels of methotrexate resulting in increased toxicity.

If other systemic NSAIDs are given concomitantly with diclofenac sodium the frequency of side-effects may be increased.

NSAIDs may increase cyclosporin nephrotoxicity as a result of their effect on renal prostaglandins.

There is an increased risk of convulsions if quinolone antibiotics are given while NSAIDs are being taken, and caution is advised when considering their use.

The activity of diuretics may be inhibited by some

NSAIDs. Increased serum potassium levels may result when diclofenac is given concomitantly with potassium-sparing diuretics. Serum potassium levels should therefore be monitored.

Care is required when giving anticoagulants with NSAIDs as diclofenac may reversibly inhibit platelet aggregation. Monitoring is recommended to ensure the desired response to the anticoagulants is maintained as there are rare reports of increased risk of haemorrhage with combined diclofenac and anticoagulant therapy.

It has been reported that hypo- and hyperglycaemic effects have occurred rarely when diclofenac and oral antidiabetic agents have been given together and adjustment of the hypoglycaemic may be required.

Pregnancy and lactation: Diclofenac sodium should only be used during pregnancy or lactation if considered essential.

Diclofenac sodium is reported to cross the placenta in mice and rats but there have not been any studies reported for humans.

Effects on ability to drive and use machines: Patients should not drive or operate machinery if they experience dizziness or other central nervous system disturbances.

Undesirable effects: Common side-effects include nausea, headache, diarrhoea, epigastric pain, anorexia, dyspepsia, flatulence, abdominal cramps, vertigo and dizziness. Serious effects such as peptic ulcer, gastro-intestinal bleeding and bloody diarrhoea have occasionally been reported, and there are reports of isolated cases of lower gut disorders (exacerbations of ulcerative colitis or Crohn's procotocolitis and non-specific haemorrhagic colitis), glossitis, constipation, pancreatitis, oesophageal lesions and aphthous stomatitis.

Skin rashes and eruptions have occasionally been reported and rarely urticaria. There are also rare reports of erythema multiforme, Stevens-Johnson syndrome, Lyell's syndrome, bullous reactions, eczema, erythroderma, hair loss, photosensitivity reactions and purpura.

Isolated effects on the central nervous system include drowsiness, tiredness, impaired hearing, insomnia, convulsions, irritability, anxiety, depression, psychotic reactions, tremors, memory disturbance, vertigo, disturbance of sensation, disorientation, disturbance of vision, tinnitus, nightmares and taste alterations.

Occasional effects on the kidney include acute renal insufficiency, urinary abnormalities (e.g. haematuria, proteinuria), nephrotic syndrome, papillary necrosis and interstitial nephritis.

Effects on the live include occasional reports of elevation of serum aminotransferase enzymes (ALT, ST) and rarely, liver function disorders including hepatitis with or without jaundice.

Leucopenia, haemolytic anaemia, thrombocytopenia, aplastic anaemia and agranulocytosis have rarely been reported. Other rarely reported reactions include hypersensitivity reactions (anaphylactic/anaphylactoid systemic reactions, hypotension, bronchspasm), oedema, palpitation, impotence, chest pain and hypertension.

Overdose: Gastric lavage and treatment with activated charcoal should be used as soon as possible after overdosage in order to prevent absorption of the drug.

Further treatment is supportive and symptomatic. Complications that might be encountered include renal failure, hypotension, convulsions, respiratory depression, and gastro-intestinal irritation.

Pharmacological properties

Pharmacodynamic properties: Diclofenac sodium is a non-steroidal anti-inflammatory drug (NSAID) with analgesic and antipyretic properties. It is an inhibitor of prostaglandin synthetase.

Pharmacokinetic properties: This extended release diclofenac formulation is designed to release diclofenac over a period of time. Following a pharmacokinetic study with the 100 mg tablet in volunteers, it was found that the average time to reach maximum plasma concentrations was 6.05 hours. The average elimination half-life was found to be 6.75 hours. The average maximum plasma concentrations were found to be 262 ng/ml.

General characteristics of the active substance: Diclofenac sodium is almost totally absorbed after oral administration, and it is subject to significant first-pass metabolism with only approximately 60% of an oral dose reaching the systemic circulation.

Diclofenac sodium is highly protein bound (>99%). It is mainly excreted in the form of metabolites via the urine but also in the bile.

The main metabolite has a minimal anti-inflammatory activity compared to the parent drug.

Characteristics in patients: Plasma concentrations of unchanged diclofenac are not reported to be significantly affected by age, renal or hepatic impairment. The metabolite concentations may be increased by severe renal impairment.

Preclinical safety data: None provided.

Pharmaceutical particulars

List of excipients: Talc PhEur; Ethylcellulose PhEur; Magnesium Stearate PhEur; Povidone PhEur; Stearic Acid USP.

Coating ingredients: Hydroxypropyl methylcellulose PhEur; Ethylcellulose PhEur; Diethylphthalate USP; Titanium Dioxide (E171) PhEur; Polyethylene glycol 4000 BP; Red iron oxide (E172) USP (100 mg tablet only); Yellow iron oxide (E172) USP (100 mg tablet only).

Incompatibilities: None reported.

Shelf life: 18 months.

Special precautions for storage: Store in a dry place below 25°C. Protect from light.

Nature and contents of container: Blister composed of PVC – PVdC/aluminium-PVdC containing 28 and 56 tablets.

Instruction for use/handling: Not applicable.

Marketing authorisation numbers

Volsaid Retard 75	8829/0045
Volsaid Retard 100	8829/0046.

Date of approval/revision of SPC 22 January 1996.

Legal category POM.

***Trade Mark**

Typharm Limited
Unit 26
Newtown Business Park
Albion Close
Poole
Dorset BH12 3LL

☎ 01202 666626 ▯ 01202 666309

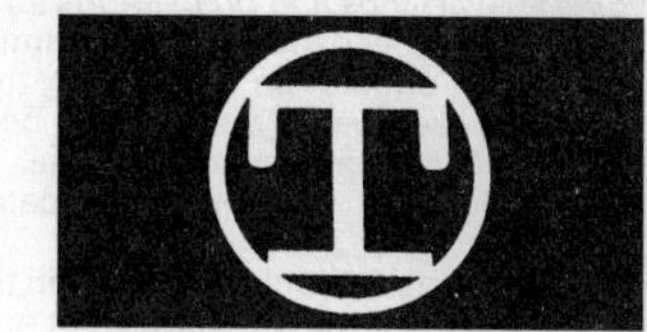

DOCUSOL 100

5 ml of the solution contains docusate sodium USP 12.5 mg.

Pharmaceutical form Oral solution.

Clinical particulars
Therapeutic conditions:
a) To prevent and treat chronic constipation
b) As an adjunct in abdominal radiological procedures.

Posology and method of administration:
Children: One to two 5 ml spoonfuls three times daily.
Infant (over six months): One 5 ml spoonful three times daily.
Docusate sodium may cause an unpleasant aftertaste or burning sensation. This may be minimised by drinking plenty of water after taking the solution.

Contra-indications: Docusol Solution should not be taken in the presence of abdominal pain, nausea or if vomiting occurs.

Special warnings and special precautions for use: Docusol should not be given to infants under six months of age.

Interaction with other medicaments and other forms of interaction: Docusol solution should not be taken concurrently with mineral oil. Anthraquinone derivates should be taken in reduced doses, if administered with Docusol as their absorption is increased.

Effects on ability to drive and use machines: None known.

Undesirable effects: None known.

Overdose: In rare cases of overdose, excessive loss of water and electrolytes should be treated by encouraging the patient to drink plenty of fluid.

Pharmacological properties
Pharmacodynamic properties: Docusate sodium acts as a faecal softener by increasing the penetration of water and fats.

Pharmacokinetic properties: Docusate sodium exerts its effects by means of its physical surfactant properties. However, there is some evidence that it is absorbed from the gastrointestinal tract and excreted in bile.

Pharmaceutical particulars
List of excipients: Sorbitol 70% PhEur, Glycerol 70% PhEur, Povidone BP, Methyl P-Hydroxybenzoate PhEur, Propyl P-hydroxybenzoate PhEur, Sodium acid phosphate PhEur, Sodium phosphate BP, Mandarin flavour, Grapefruit flavour, Purified water.

Incompatibilities: None known.

Shelf life: 3 years.

Special precautions for storage: None.

Nature and contents of container: Glass bottle with a plastic screw with a waxed liner or roll-on pilfer proof aluminium closure. Each bottle contains 100 ml.

Instructions for use/handling: None.

Legal category P

Marketing authorisation number PL 0551/0007

Date of first authorisation/renewal of authorisation 12 March 1995

Date of revision of the text December 1994

DOCUSOL ADULT SOLUTION

Qualitative and quantitative composition 5 ml of the solution contains docusate sodium USP 50 mg.

Pharmaceutical form Oral solution.

Clinical particulars
Therapeutic conditions:
a) To prevent and treat chronic constipation
b) As an adjunct in abdominal radiological procedures.

Posology and method of administration:
Adults: Up to 50 ml to be taken in divided doses daily.
Treatment should be commenced with large doses which should be decreased as the condition of the patient improves.
For barium meals: 40 ml to be taken with the meal.
Elderly: There is no evidence to suggest that an adjustment of the dosage is necessary in the elderly. Docusate sodium may cause an unpleasant aftertaste or burning sensation. This may be minimised by drinking plenty of water after taking the solution.

Contra-indications: Docusol Solution should not be taken in the presence of abdominal pain, nausea or if vomiting occurs.

Interaction with other medicaments and other forms of interaction: Docusol solution should not be taken concurrently with mineral oil. Anthraquinone derivatives should be taken in reduced doses, if administered with Docusol as their absorption is increased.

Pregnancy and lactation: There is inadequate evidence of safety of the drug in human pregnancy, nor is there evidence from animal work that it is free from hazard but it has been in wide use for many years without apparent ill consequence. Use in pregnancy only if the benefits outweigh the potential risks. Docusate sodium is excreted in breast milk and should therefore be used with caution in lactating mothers.

Effects on ability to drive and use machines: None known.

Undesirable effects: None known.

Overdose: In rare cases of overdose, excessive loss of water and electrolytes should be treated by encouraging the patient to drink plenty of fluid.

Pharmacological properties
Pharmacodynamic properties: Docusate sodium acts as a faecal softener by increasing the penetration of water and fats.

Pharmacokinetic properties: Docusate sodium exerts its effects by means of its physical surfactant properties. However, there is some evidence that it is absorbed from the gastrointestinal tract and excreted in bile.

Pharmaceutical particulars
List of excipients: Sorbitol 70% PhEur, Glycerol 70% PhEur, Povidone BP, Methyl P-Hydroxybenzoate PhEur, Propyl P-hydroxybenzoate PhEur, Sodium acid phosphate PhEur, Sodium phosphate BP, Herbmint flavour, Purified water.

Incompatibilities: None known.

Shelf life: 3 years.

Special precautions for storage: None.

Nature and contents of container: Glass bottle with a plastic screw with a waxed liner or roll-on pilfer proof aluminium closure. Each bottle contains 300 ml.

Instructions for use/handling: None.

Legal category P

Marketing authorisation number PL 0551/0006

Date of first authorisation/renewal of authorisation 12 March 1995

Date of revision of the text December 1994

DOCUSOL PAEDIATRIC SOLUTION

Qualitative and quantitative composition 5 ml of the solution contains docusate sodium USP 12.5 mg.

Pharmaceutical form Oral solution.

Clinical particulars
Therapeutic conditions:
a) To prevent and treat chronic constipation
b) As an adjunct in abdominal radiological procedures.

Posology and method of administration:
Children: One to two 5 ml spoonfuls three times daily.
Infant (over six months): One 5 ml spoonful three times daily.
Docusate sodium may cause unpleasant aftertaste or burning sensation. This may be minimised by drinking plenty of water after taking the solution.

Contra-indications: Docusol Solution should not be taken in the presence of abdominal pain, nauses or if vomiting occurs.

Special warnings and special precautions for use: Docusol should not be given to infants under six months of age.

Interaction with other medicaments and other forms of interaction: Docusol solution should not be taken concurrently with mineral oil. Anthraquinone derivatives should be taken in reduced doses, if administered with Docusol as their absorption is increased.

Effects on ability to drive and use machines: None known.

Undesirable effects: None known.

Overdose: In rare cases of overdose, excessive loss of water and electrolytes should be treated by encouraging the patient to drink plenty of fluid.

Pharmacological properties
Pharmacodynamic properties: Docusate sodium acts as a faecal softener by increasing the penetration of water and fats.

Pharmacokinetic properties: Docusate sodium exerts its effects by means of its physical surfactant properties. However, there is some evidence that it is absorbed from the gastrointestinal tract and excreted in bile.

Pharmaceutical particulars
List of excipients: Sorbitol 70% PhEur, Glycerol 70% PhEur, Povidone BP, Methyl P-Hydroxybenzoate PhEur, Propyl P-hydroxybenzoate PhEur, Sodium acid phosphate PhEur, Sodium phosphate BP, Mandarin flavour, Grapefruit flavour, Purified water.

Incompatibilities: None known.

Shelf life: 3 years.

Special precautions for storage: None.

Nature and contents of container: Glass bottle with a plastic screw with a waxed liner or roll-on pilfer proof aluminium closure. Each bottle contains 300 ml.

Instructions for use/handling: None.

Legal category P

Marketing authorisation number PL 0551/0007

Date of first authorisation/renewal of authorisation 12 March 1995

Date of revision of the text December 1994

DOZOL

Qualitative and quantitative composition Each 5 ml contains; Paracetamol PhEur 120 mg and Diphenhydramine HC1 BP 12.5 mg.

Pharmaceutical form Clear amber liquid.

Clinical particulars
Therapeutic indications: For the treatment of mild to moderate pain, including teething pain, headache sore throat, aches and pain.
Symptomatic relief of influenza, feverishness and feverish colds. Controls excessive mucous secretion and eases nasal irritation.

Posology and method of administration:
3 months to under 1 year: 5 ml (1 teaspoonful) 3–4 times daily.
1 year to under 6 years: 5 ml–10 ml (1–2 teaspoonful) 3–4 times daily.
6 years to under 12 years: 10 ml–20 ml (2–4 teaspoonful) 3 times daily.
Allow at least four hours between doses or as directed by your doctor.

Contra-indications: Hypersensitivity to paracetamol and/or other constituents. Large doses of antihistamines may precipitate fits in epileptics.

Special warnings and precautions for use:
(1) Do not exceed the stated dose. Immediate medical advice should be sought in the event of an overdose, even if you feel well, because of the risk of delayed serious liver damage.
(2) Do not take with other paracetamol-containing products.
(3) The product should not be given to children under the age of three months except on doctors advice.
(4) Dose should not be repeated more frequently than 4 hour intervals.
(5) Not more than 4 doses should be taken in any 24 hour period.
(6) Dosage should not be continued for more than 3 days without consulting a doctor.
(7) The product should be administered with caution to patients with known liver or renal impairment. The hazards of overdose are greater in those with alcoholic liver disease.
(8) Keep out of reach of children.

Interaction with other medicaments and other forms of interaction: The speed of absorption of paracetamol may be increased by metoclopramide or domperidone and absorption reduced by cholestyramine.

The anticoagulant effect of warfarin and other coumarins my be enhanced by prolonged regular use of paracetamol with increased risk of bleeding.

Effects of alcohol and other sedatives may be potentiated.

Pregnancy and lactation: Safety in pregnancy has not been established.

Epidemiological studies in human pregnancy have shown no effects due to paracetamol used in the recommended dosage, but patients should follow the advice of their doctor regarding its use. Paracetamol is excreted in breast milk but not in a clinically significantly amount. Available published date do not contraindicate breast feeding.

Effects on ability to drive and use machines: May cause drowsiness. If affected do not drive or operate machinery.

Undesirable effects: Adverse effects of paracetamol are rare hypersensitivity including skin rash may occur.

There have been a few reports of blood dyscrasias including thrombocytopenia and agranulocytosis but these were not necessarily casually related to paracetamol.

Overdose: The features of overdose are: sedation, pallor, nausea, vomiting, diarrhoea, anorexia and abdominal pain; liver damage may become apparent within 12–48 hours. In some children overdose may cause cerebral stimulation resulting in convulsions and hyperpyrexis.

Abnormalities of glucose metabolism and metabolic acidosis may occur. In severe poisoning hepatic failure may progress to encephalopathy, coma and death. Acute renal failure with acute tubular necrosis may develop even in the absence of severe liver damage. Cardiac arrhythmis and pancreatitis have been reported.

Liver damage is likely in adults who have taken 10 g or more of paracetamol. It is considered that excess quantities of a toxic metabolites (usually adequately detoxified by glutathione when normal doses of paracetamol are ingested) become irreversibly bound to liver tissue.

Immediate treatment is essential in the management of paracetamol overdose. Despite a lack of significant early symptoms, patients should be referred to hospital urgently for immediate medical attention and any patient who had ingested around 7.5 g or more of paracetamol in the preceding 4 hours should undergo gastric lavage. Administration of oral methionine or intravenous N-acetyleystrine which may have a beneficial effect up to at least 48 hours after the overdose, may be required. General supportive measures must be available.

Pharmacological properties

Pharmacodynamic properties: Paracetamol is antipyretic an analgesic. Diphenhydramine HC1 is an anthistamine with anticholinergic, anti emetic, anti-allergic and sedative effects.

Pharmacokinetic properties: Paracetamol and Diphenhydramine HC1 are both readily absorbed from the gastro-intestinal tract. Both are widely distributed throughout the body. Both are metabolised in the liver and excreted in the urine. As Dozol is a solution absorption of the actives is rapid following oral ingestion.

Preclinical safety data: Paracetamol and Diphenhydramine HC1 are a well established drug substances whose preclinical profiles have been investigated thoroughly and are established.

Pharmaceutical particulars

List of excipients:

Polyenthylene glycol 4000	BP
Glycerol	BP
Propylene glycol	BP
Sorbitol solution 70%	BP
Lycasin 80/55	Hse
Sodium cyclamate	BP (1968)
Ethanol	BP
Nipasept	Hse
Annatto Extract	Hse
Caramel No 1	Hse
Bright Red Powder	Hse
Water, purified	BP

Incompatibilities: None known.

Shelf life: 3 years from date of manufacture.

Special precautions for storage: Do not refrigerate. Protect from light.

Nature and contents of container: Amber Glass bottles with dic-loc caps with pulp stearing wadding. 100 ml and 30 ml.

Instruction for use/handling: None

Marketing authorisation holder: Ricesteele Manufacturing Limited, Cookstown Industrial Estate, Tallaght, Dublin 24, Ireland.

Marketing authorisation number PL 01648/0004

Date of first authorisation/renewal of authorisation

Date of first grant 20 January 1977
Date of last renewal November 1998

Date of (partial) revision of the text January 1998

EFFERCITRATE* TABLETS

Qualitative and quantitative composition

Active constituents:

Potassium Citrate BP	1.5 g
Citric Acid BP	0.25 g
Other constituents:	
Saccharin Sodium BP	5.0 mg
Lemon Flavour (Givaudan 84260B)	7.5 mg
Lime Flavour (Givaudan 84278B)	7.5 mg
Polyethylene Glycol 6000	100.0 mg
Dioctyl Sodium Sylphosuccinate BPC	1.0 mg
Polyvinylpyrrolidone BPC	65.0 mg
Magnesium Stearate BP	10.0 mg

Pharmaceutical form Effervescent tablets.

Clinical particulars

Therapeutic indications: For the treatment of cystitis and as initial therapy in mild symptomatic cystitis prior to an MSU result. Confirmed bacterial infections should then be treated with an appropriate course of an antibacterial agent.

Posology and method of administration:
Posology:

Adults and children over 6 years: Two tablets dissolved in a glass of water up to three times daily.

Children: 1–6 years: One tablet dissolved in a glass of water up to three times daily.

Under one year: Not recommended.

Elderly: As adult dose.

Sufficient should be given to render and maintain the urine alkaline.

Contra-indications: None.

Special warnings and special precautions for use: Caution should be observed in patients with kidney disease, hypertension of heart disease.

If symptoms persist or worsen, patients should seek medical advice.

Interactions with other medicaments and other forms of interaction: None known.

Pregnancy and lactation: Patients should consult a doctor before taking Effercitrate in pregnancy or lactation.

Effects on ability to drive and use machines: Not applicable.

Undesirable effects: Gastric irritation may occur. The tablets should always be well diluted with water. Gastric effects may be minimised by taking with or after meals.

Overdose: Hyperkalaemia may occur. Below 6.5 mmol/litre poisoning is minimal, moderate up to 8 mmol/litre and severe above 8 mmol/litre. Absolute toxicity is governed by pH and sodium levels. Hyperkalaemia symptoms may be transiently controlled with calcium gluconate, glucose or glucose and insulin, sodium bicarbonate or hypertonic sodium infusions, cationic exchange resins or haemo and peritoneal dialysis. Patients who are digitalised may experience acute digitalis intoxication during potassium removal.

Pharmacological properties

Pharmacodynamic properties: Potassium citrate renders the urine alkaline.

Pharmacokinetic properties: Alkalisation of the urine affects the growth of pathogens. The growth of *ESCH COLI* is inhibited at a pH above 7.5. Alkalised urine is soothing to the epithelium of the bladder and urethra unlike the natural acid urine (symptoms of cystitis).

Preclinical safety data: The active ingredients of Effercitrate tablets are simple compounds with a well established medicinal use and recognised efficacy and an acceptable level of safety.

Pharmaceutical particulars

List of excipients: Saccharin Sodium BP; Lemon Flavour (Givaudan 84260B); Lime Flavour (Givaudan 84278B); Polyethylene Glycol 6000; Dioctyl Sodium Sulphosuccinate BPC; Polyvinylpyrrolidone BPC; Magnesium Stearate BP.

Incompatibilities: None known.

Shelf life: Three years.

Special precautions for storage: Store in a cool dry place below 20°C.

Nature and contents of container: Aluminium tubes with plastic cap containing desiccant of 12 tablets.

Instructions for use/handling: Not applicable.

Marketing authorisation number PL 0551/0002

Date of first authorisation January 1990

Date of revision of text May 1995

GOLDEN* EYE DROPS

Qualitative and quantitative compostion Contain 0.1% w/v propamidine isethionate.

Pharmaceutical form A clear colourless solution practically free from particles.

Clinical particulars

Therapeutic indications: Indicated for the treatment of minor eye and eyelid infections such as conjunctivitis and blepharitis.

Posology and method of administration: For topical ophthalmic administration.

Adults (elderly and children): One or two drops up to four times daily. Medical advice should be obtained if there has been no significant improvement after two days.

Contra-indications:
i. Hypersensitivity to propamidine or any component of the preparation.
ii. Soft or gas permeable contact lenses.

Special warnings and precautions for use:
i. If vision is disturbed or symptoms become worse during therapy, discontinue use and consult a physician.
ii. If there is no significant improvement after two days therapy, discontinue use and consult a physician.

Interaction with other medicaments and other forms of interaction: None known.

Pregnancy and lactation: Safety of use in pregnancy and lactation has not been established. Use during pregnancy and lactation only if considered essential by a physician.

Effects on ability to drive and use machines: May cause transient blurring of vision on instillation. Patients should be warned not to drive or operate machinery unless vision is clear.

Undesirable effects: Hypersensitivity may occur, in which case treatment should be discontinued immediately.

Overdose: Topical overdose not applicable. Oral ingestion of a full 10 ml bottle is unlikely to cause any toxic effects.

Pharmacological properties

Pharmacodynamic properties: Propamidine is a member of the aromatic diamidine class of compounds which possess bacteriostatic properties against a wide range of organisms.

These diamidines exert antibacterial action against pyogenic cocci, antibiotic resistant staphylococci and some gram negative bacilli. The activity of the diamidines is retained in the presence of organic matter such as tissue fluids, pus and serum.

Pharmacokinetic properties: No data available.

Preclinical safety data: Not applicable.

Pharmaceutical particulars

List of excipients: Sodium chloride, benzalkonium chloride solution, purified water.

Incompatibilities: None known.

Shelf life: 48 months unopened and 28 days after opening.

Special precautions for storage: Store below 25°C.

Nature and contents of container: Polypropylene dropper bottle (10 ml) fitted with a low density polyethylene nozzle and a high density polyethylene tamper evident cap.

Instructions for use/handling: Not applicable.

Marketing authorisation number PL 0551/0003

Date of first authorisation/renewal of authorisation 12 March 1992 (renewal).

Date of issue of the text November 1996

GOLDEN* EYE OINTMENT

Qualitative and quantitative composition Contains 0.15% w/w Dibromopropamidine Isethionate BP.

Pharmaceutical form A smooth uniform off white translucent greasy ointment.

Clinical particulars
Therapeutic indications: Indicated for the treatment of minor eye and eyelid infections such as conjunctivitis and blepharitis.

Posology and method of administration: For topical ophthalmic administration.

Adults (elderly and children): Apply topically once or twice daily. Medical advice should be obtained if there has been no significant improvement after two days.

Contra-indications: Hypersensitivity to dibromopropamidine or to any component of the preparation.

Special warnings and precautions for use:
i. If vision is disturbed or symptoms become worse during therapy, discontinue use and consult a physician.
ii. If there is no significant improvement after two days therapy, discontinue use and consult a physician.

Interaction with other medicaments and other forms of interaction: None known.

Pregnancy and lactation: Safety of use in pregnancy and lactation has not been established. Use during pregnancy and lactation only if considered essential by a physician.

Effects on ability to drive and use machines: Eye Ointment will cause blurring of vision on application. Patients should be warned not to drive or operate machinery unless vision is clear.

Undesirable effects: Hypersensitivity may occur, in which case treatment should be discontinued immediately.

Overdose: Topical overdose not applicable. Oral ingestion of a full 5 gram tube is unlikely to cause any toxic effects.

Pharmacological properties
Pharmacodynamic properties: Dibromopropamidine is a member of the aromatic diamidine class of compounds which possess bacteriostatic properties against a wide range of fungi and bacteria.

These diamidines exert antibacterial action against pyogenic cocci, antibiotic resistant staphylococci and some gram negative bacilli. The activity of the diamidines is retained in the presence of organic matter such as pus and blood.

Pharmacokinetic properties: No data available.

Preclinical safety data: Not applicable.

Pharmaceutical particulars
List of excipients: Liquid paraffin and plastibase 30W.

Incompatibilities: None known.

Shelf life: 60 months unopened and 28 days after opening.

Special precautions for storage: Store below 25°C.

Nature and contents of container: A white pigmented, collapsible multi laminate tube (5 gram) incorporating an aluminium foil barrier with inner polyethylene coating with a polyethylene elongated nozzle with a screw cap.

Instruction for use/handling: Not applicable.

Marketing authorisation number PL 0551/0004

Date of first authorisation/renewal of authorisation 17 March 1992 (renewal)

Date of issue of the text November 1996

VERACUR* GEL

Qualitative and quantitative composition
Active constituents: Formaldehyde (as formaldehyde solution BP) 0.75% w/w.

Pharmaceutical form Clear colourless gel.

Clinical particulars
Therapeutic indications: For the treatment of warts, particularly plantar warts (verrucae).

Posology and method of administration:
Adults: Apply directly on to the wart or verruca and cover with a plaster, twice daily. Remove scale and dead tissue from the top of the wart with an emery board or pumice stone.

Correct application technique is essential. Treatment may need to be continued for eight weeks or more.

Children: As adult dose.
Elderly: As adult dose.

Contra-indications: Application to broken skin.

Special warnings and special precautions for use: Do not apply to broken skin. For external use only. Keep out of reach of children.

If required, protect surrounding skin with a thin film of vaseline petroleum jelly before application.

Interaction with other medicaments and other forms of interaction: None known.

Pregnancy and lactation: The safety for use in pregnancy has not been established. Use only when considered essential by a physician.

Effects on ability to drive and use machines: Not applicable.

Undesirable effects: Formaldehyde vapour is irritant to the eyes, nose and respiratory tract and may cause coughing, dysphagia, spasm of the larynx, bronchitis and pneumonia. Asthma has been reported after repeated exposure. Concentrated solutions applied to the skin cause whitening and hardening. Contact dermatitis and sensitivity reactions have occurred after the use of conventional concentrations.

Overdose: Contaminated skin should be washed with soap and water. If accidentally ingested, avoid gastric lavage or emesis, but give water, milk or charcoal. Treat for shock and acidosis if necessary.

Pharmacological properties
Pharmacodynamic properties: Formaldehyde solution is a disinfectant effective against vegetative bacteria, fungi and many viruses.

Pharmacokinetic properties: If ingested, formaldehyde is rapidly metabolised to formic acid in the tissues, especially liver and erythrocytes. The formic acid may then be excreted as carbon dioxide and water excreted in the urine as formate, or metabolised to labile methyl groups.

Preclinical safety data: Formaldehyde solution has a well established medicinal use, recognised efficacy and an acceptable level of safety for topical use at appropriate concentrations.

Pharmaceutical particulars
List of excipients:

Carbopol 940	1.0% w/w
Sodium Hydroxide BP	0.105% w/w
Deionised water	97.30% w/w

Incompatibilities: None known.

Shelf life: Five years.

Special precautions for storage: Store in a cool dry place.

Nature and contents of container: Aluminium tubes, epoxy resin lined, enclosed in cardboard cartons.

Instructions for use/handling: Not applicable.

Marketing authorisation number PL 0551/5000R

Date of first authorisation May 1990

Date of revision of text March 1995

**Trade Mark*

UCB Pharma Limited

Star House
69 Clarendon Road
Watford WD1 1DJ

☎ 01923 211811   🖷 01923 229002

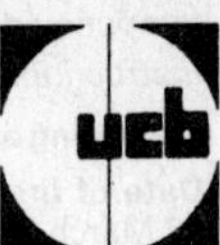

NOOTROPIL* TABLETS 800 mg ▼
NOOTROPIL* TABLETS 1200 mg ▼
NOOTROPIL* SOLUTION 33% ▼

Presentation
Tablets: White, oblong, scored, film coated tablets containing 800 mg or 1200 mg piracetam marked N on either side of the break line.

Solution: A clear and colourless solution containing 333.3 mg piracetam per ml is also available for patients suffering with dysphagia.

Uses Nootropil is indicated for patients suffering from myoclonus of cortical origin, irrespective of aetiology, and should be used in combination with other anti-myoclonic therapies.

Dosage and administration
Adults: The dosage regimen shows an important inter-individual variability, requiring an individualised dose-finding approach: a reasonable protocol would be to introduce piracetam in a dosage of 7.2 g/day, increasing by 4.8 g/day every 3 to 4 days up to a maximum of 20 g/day, given in 2 or 3 divided doses, while keeping other anti-myoclonic drugs unchanged in optimal dosage. If possible, depending upon clinical benefit, an attempt should be made to reduce the dosage of other anti-myoclonic drugs subsequently.

Solution: It is advisable to follow each dose with a drink of water or soft drink to reduce the bitter taste of the solution.

Contra-indications, warnings, etc
Piracetam is contra-indicated in patients with severe renal insufficiency (renal creatinine clearance of less than 20 ml per minute), hepatic impairment and those under 16 years of age.

Pregnancy and lactation: In animal studies piracetam was not teratogenic and had no effect on fertility at the maximal tested dose of 2.7 g/kg/day for the rabbit and 4.8 g/kg/day for rats and mice. Piracetam readily crosses the placental barrier and, very probably, passes into the mother's milk. Since the safety of use in human pregnancy is not established, Nootropil is to be avoided during pregnancy and lactation. Young women using the product should be receiving adequate contraceptive precautions.

Precautions: Abrupt discontinuation of treatment should be avoided as this may, in some myoclonic patients, induce myoclonic or generalised seizures.

As piracetam is almost exclusively excreted by the kidneys, caution should be exercised in treating patients with known renal impairment. In renally impaired and elderly patients, the increase in terminal half-life is directly related to renal function as measured by creatinine clearance. Dosage adjustment is therefore required in those with mild to moderate renal impairment and elderly patients with diminished renal function. The dosage should be modified according to the following scheme if creatinine clearance is between 20 and 60 ml/min or serum creatinine is between 1.25 and 3 mg/100 ml (112–270 μmol/litre).

Creatinine clearance	*Serum creatinine*	*Dosage*
60–40 ml/min	1.25–1.7 mg/100 ml (112–153 μmol/l)	½ usual dose
40–20 ml/min	1.7–3 mg/100 ml (153–270 μmol/l)	¼ usual dose

Side-effects: In placebo-controlled trials covering a range of doses between 1.6 and 15 grams daily undesirable effects reported with an incidence of more than one per cent but less than three per cent are; hyperkinesia, insomnia, weight increase, somnolence, nervousness and depression. Reported effects of less than one per cent are diarrhoea and rash.

Drug interactions: In a single case, confusion, irritability and sleep disorders were reported in concomitant use with thyroid extract (T3+T4). At present, based on a small number of studies, no interaction has been found with the following anti-epileptic medications: clonazepam, carbamazepine, phenytoin, phenobarbitone and sodium valproate. To date, there are no known interactions with other drugs.

Driving: In clinical studies, at dosages between 1.6 and 15 grams per day, hyperkinesia, somnolence, nervousness and depression were reported more frequently in patients on piracetam than on placebo. There is no experience on driving ability in dosages between 15 and 20 grams daily. Caution should therefore be exercised by patients intending to drive or use machinery whilst taking piracetam.

Overdosage: Acute toxicological studies in animals showed lethal doses were obtained in mice (18.2 g/kg and higher) but not in rats and dogs dosed respectively at 21 g/kg or 10 g/kg.

No specific measure is indicated. The pateints' general condition should be closely monitored. Close attention should be given to keeping the patient well hydrated and monitoring the urine flow.

Pharmaceutical precautions The product should be stored at room temperature.

Legal category POM.

Package quantities

Tablets 800 mg:	A box of 90 tablets with 15 tablets to a blister pack.
Tablets 1200 mg:	A box of 56 tablets with 14 tablets to a blister pack.
Solution 33%	Brown glass bottles containing 300 ml of solution.

Further information Piracetam is rapidly and almost completely absorbed, and peak plasma levels are reached within 1.5 hours after administration. The extent of oral bio-availability, assessed from Area Under Curve (AUC), is close to 100% for capsules, tablets and solution. Peak levels and AUC are proportional to the dose given. The volume of distribution of piracetam is 0.7 l/kg and the plasma half-life is 5.0 hours in young adult men. Piracetam crosses the blood-brain and the placental barriers and diffuses across membranes used in renal dialysis. Up to now, no metabolite of piracetam has been found. Piracetam is excreted nearly completely in urine and urinary excretion is dose-independent. Excretion half-life values are consistent with those calculated from plasma/blood data. Clearance of the compound is highly dependent on the renal creatinine clearance and would be expected to diminish in renal insufficiency.

Product licence numbers
Nootropil Tablets 800 mg 8972/0011
Nootropil Tablets 1200 mg 8972/0012
Nootropil Solution 33% 8972/0013

PRESERVEX* TABLETS ▼

Qualitative and quantitative composition

	mg per tablet
Aceclofenac	100.0
Microcrystalline cellulose	89.2
Sodium croscarmellose	6.6
Glyceryl palmitostearate	2.6
Povidone (polyvidone)	6.6
Tablet core weight	205.0
Film coating	
Sepifilm 752 White, composed of:	
Hydroxypropyl methylcellulose	6.2[1]
Polyoxyethylene 40 stearate	0.9[1]
Titanium dioxide	1.9[1]
Total tablet weight	214.0

[1] Approximate quantities.

Pharmaceutical form Preservex tablets 100 mg are presented as white round film-coated tablets, 8 mm in diameter, with an 'A' embosssed on one side.

Clinical particulars
Therapeutic indications: Preservex is indicated for the relief of pain and inflammation in osteoarthritis, rheumatoid arthritis and ankylosing spondylitis.

Posology and method of administration: Preservex tablets are supplied for oral administration and should be swallowed whole with a sufficient quantity of liquid. When Preservex was administered to fasting and fed healthy volunteers only the rate and not the extent of aceclofenac absorption was affected and as such Preservex can be taken with food.

Adults: The recommended dose is 200 mg daily, taken as two separate 100 mg doses, one tablet in the morning and one in the evening.

Children: There are no clinical data on the use of Preservex in children.

Elderly: The pharmacokinetics of Preservex are not altered in elderly patients, therefore it is not considered necessary to modify the dose or dose frequency.

As with other non-steroidal anti-inflammatory drugs (NSAIDs), caution should be exercised in the treatment of elderly patients, who are generally more prone to adverse reactions, and who are more likely to be suffering from impaired renal, cardiovascular or hepatic function and receiving concomitant medication.

Renal insufficiency: There is no evidence that the dosage of Preservex needs to be modified in patients with mild renal impairment, but as with other NSAIDs caution should be exercised (see also Precautions).

Hepatic insufficiency: There is some evidence that the dose of Preservex should be reduced in patients with hepatic impairment and it is suggested that an initial daily dose of 100 mg be used.

Contra-indications: Preservex should not be administered to patients with active or suspected peptic ulcer or gastro-intestinal bleeding.

Preservex should not be given to patients with moderate to severe renal impairment.

Preservex should not be prescribed during pregnancy, unless there are compelling reasons for doing so. The lowest effective dosage should be used.

Preservex should not be administered to patients previously sensitive to aceclofenac or in whom aspirin or NSAIDs precipitate attacks of asthma, acute rhinitis or urticaria or who are hypersensitive to these drugs.

Special warnings and special precautions for use:

Warnings: Gastro-intestinal: Close medical surveillance is imperative in patients with symptoms indicative of gastro-intestinal disorders, with a history suggestive of gastro-intestinal ulceration, with ulcerative colitis or with Crohn's disease, bleeding diathesis or haematological abnormalities.

Gastro-intestinal bleeding or ulcerative perforation, haematemesis and melaena have in general more serious consequences in the elderly. They can occur at any time during treatment, with or without warning symptoms or a previous history. In the rare instances where gastro-intestinal bleeding or ulceration occurs in patients receiving Preservex, the drug should be withdrawn.

Hepatic: Close medical surveillance is also imperative in patients suffering from severe impairment of hepatic function.

Hypersensitivity reactions: As with other NSAIDs, allergic reactions, including anaphylactic/anaphylactoid reactions, can also occur without earlier exposure to the drug.

Precautions:

Renal: Patients with mild renal or cardiac impairment and the elderly should be kept under surveillance, since the use of NSAIDs may result in deterioration of renal function. The lowest effective dose should be used and renal function monitored regularly.

The importance of prostaglandins in maintaining renal blood flow should be taken into account in patients with impaired cardiac or renal function, those being treated with diuretics or recovering from major surgery. Effects on renal function are usually reversible on withdrawal of Preservex.

Hepatic: If abnormal liver function tests persist or worsen, clinical signs or symptoms consistent with liver disease develop or if other manifestations occur (eosinophilia, rash), Preservex should be discontinued. Hepatitis may occur without prodromal symptoms.

Use of Preservex in patients with hepatic porphyria may trigger an attack.

Haematological: Preservex may reversibly inhibit platelet aggregation (see anticoagulants under Interactions).

Long term treatment: All patients who are receiving NSAIDs should be monitored as a precautionary measure e.g. renal function, hepatic function (elevation of liver enzymes may occur) and blood counts.

Interactions:

Lithium and digoxin: Preservex, like many NSAIDs,

may increase plasma concentrations of lithium and digoxin.

Diuretics: Preservex, like other NSAIDs, may inhibit the activity of diuretics. Although it was not shown to affect blood pressure control when co-administered with bendrofluazide, interactions with other diuretics cannot be ruled out. When concomitant administration with potassium-sparing diuretics is employed, serum potassium should be monitored.

Anticoagulants: Like other NSAIDs, Preservex may enhance the activity of anticoagulants. Close monitoring of patients on combined anticoagulant and Preservex therapy should be undertaken.

Antidiabetic agents: Clinical studies have shown that diclofenac can be given together with oral antidiabetic agents without influencing their clinical effect. However, there have been isolated reports of hypoglycaemic and hyperglycaemic effects. Thus with Preservex, consideration should be given to adjustment of the dosage of hypoglycaemic agents.

Methotrexate: Caution should be exercised if NSAIDs and methotrexate are administered within 24 hours of each other, since NSAIDs may increase methotrexate plasma levels, resulting in increased toxicity.

Other NSAIDs and steroids: Concomitant therapy with aspirin, other NSAIDs and steroids may increase the frequency of side effects.

Cyclosporin: Cyclosporin nephrotoxicity may be increased by the effect of NSAIDs on renal prostaglandins.

Quinolone antimicrobials: Convulsions may occur due to an interaction between quinolones and NSAIDs. This may occur in patients with or without a previous history of epilepsy or convulsions. Therefore, caution should be exercised when considering the use of a quinolone in patients who are already receiving a NSAID.

Use during pregnancy and lactation:

Pregnancy: There is no information on the use of Preservex during pregnancy. The regular use of NSAIDs during the last trimester of pregnancy may increase uterine tone and contraction. NSAID use may also result in premature closure of the fetal ductus arteriosus *in utero* and possibly persistent pulmonary hypertension of the new born, delay onset and increase duration of labour.

Animal studies indicate that there was no evidence of teratogenesis in rats although the systemic exposure was low and in rabbits, treatment with aceclofenac (10 mg/kg/day) resulted in a series of morphological changes in some fetuses.

Lactation: There is no information on the secretion of Preservex to breast milk; there was however no notable transfer of radio-labelled (^{14}C) aceclofenac to the milk of lactating rats.

The use of Preservex should therefore be avoided in pregnancy and lactation unless the potential benefits to the mother outweigh the possible risks to the fetus.

Effects of ability to drive and use machines: Patients suffering from dizziness, vertigo, or other central nervous system disorders whilst taking NSAIDs should refrain from driving or handling dangerous machinery.

Undesirable effects: The majority of side-effects observed have been reversible and of a minor nature and include gastro-intestinal disorders (dyspepsia, abdominal pain, nausea and diarrhoea) and occasional occurrence of dizziness. Dermatological complaints including pruritus and rash and abnormal hepatic enzyme levels and raised serum creatinine have occasionally been reported.

If serious side-effects occur, Preservex should be withdrawn.

The following adverse events (described as most frequent ≥5%, occasional <5% or rare cases <0.1%) were reported during all clinical trials.

Gastro-intestinal system disorders: Most frequent: dyspepsia (7.5%), abdominal pain (6.2%). Occasional: nausea (1.5%), diarrhoea (1.5%), flatulence (0.8%), gastritis (0.6%), constipation (0.5%), vomiting (0.5%), ulcerative stomatitis (0.1%). Rare cases: (all <0.1%) pancreatitis, melaena, stomatitis.

Central and peripheral nervous system: Occasional: dizziness (1%), vertigo (0.3%). Rare cases: (all <0.1%) paraesthesia, tremor.

Psychiatric: Rare cases: (all <0.1%) depression, abnormal dreaming, somnolence, insomnia.

Skin and appendages: Occasional: pruritus (0.9%), rash (0.5%), dermatitis (0.2%). Rare cases: (all <0.1%) eczema.

Liver and biliary: Occasional: hepatic enzymes increased (2.5%).

Metabolic: Occasional: BUN increased (0.4%), blood creatinine increased (0.3%). Rare cases: (all <0.1%) alkaline phosphatase increased, hyperkalaemia.

Cardiovascular: Rare cases: (all <0.1%) oedema (dependent), palpitation, leg cramps flushing, purpura.

Respiratory: Rare cases: (all <0.1%) dyspnoea, stridor.

Blood: Rare cases: (all <0.1%) anaemia, granulocytopenia, thrombocytopenia.

Body as a whole, general: Rare cases (all <0.1%) headache, fatigue, face oedema, hot flushes, allergic reaction, weight increase.

Others: Rare cases (all <0.1%) abnormal vision, abnormal taste.

Overdose: Management of acute poisoning with NSAIDs essentially consists of supportive and symptomatic measures.

There are no human data available on the consequences of Preservex overdosage. The therapeutic measures to be taken are: absorption should be prevented as soon as possible after overdosage by means of gastric lavage and treatment with activated charcoal; supportive and symptomatic treatment should be given for complications such as hypotension, renal failure, convulsions, gastro-intestinal irritation, and respiratory depression; specific therapies such as forced diuresis, dialysis or haemoperfusion are probably of no help in eliminating NSAIDs due to their high rate of protein binding and extensive metabolism.

Pharmacological properties

Pharmacodynamic properties: Aceclofenac is a non-steroidal agent with marked anti-inflammatory and analgesic properties.

The mode of action of aceclofenac is largely based on the inhibition of prostaglandin synthesis. Aceclofenac is a potent inhibitor of the enzyme cyclo-oxygenase, which is involved in the production of prostaglandins.

Pharmacokinetic properties: After oral administration, aceclofenac is rapidly and completely absorbed as unchanged drug. Peak plasma concentrations are reached approximately 1.25 to 3.00 hours following ingestion. Aceclofenac penetrates into the synovial fluid, where the concentrations reach approximately 57% of those in plasma. The volume of distribution is approximately 25 L.

The mean plasma elimination half-life is around 4 hours. Aceclofenac is highly protein-bound (>99%). Aceclofenac circulates mainly as unchanged drug. 4'-Hydroxyaceclofenac is the main metabolite detected in plasma. Approximately two-thirds of the administered dose is excreted via the urine, mainly as hydroxymetabolites.

No changes in the pharmacokinetics of aceclofenac have been detected in the elderly.

Preclinical safety data: The results from preclinical studies conducted with aceclofenac are consistent with those expected for NSAIDs. The principal target organ was the gastro-intestinal tract. No unexpected findings were recorded.

Aceclofenac was not considered to have any mutagenic activity in three *in vitro* studies and an *in vivo* study in the mouse.

Aceclofenac was not found to be carcinogenic in either the mouse or rat.

Pharmaceutical particulars

List of excipients: The excipients used in Preservex tablets 100 mg are those commonly recommended for use in pharmaceutical preparations. These are microcrystalline cellulose, sodium croscarmellose, povidone, glyceryl palmitosterate and the film coat, containing partially substituted hydroxypropyl methylcellulose, polyoxyethylene 40 stearate and titanium dioxide.

Incompatibilities: None known.

Shelf life: The shelf-life for this product shall not exceed three years from the date of manufacture.

Special precautions for storage: The tablets are to be stored at 25°C or below.

Nature and contents of container: The immediate container for Preservex tablets 100 mg is a laminated aluminium/aluminium foil pack. Each foil strip contains either 10 or 14 tablets. One, two, four or six foil strips will be provided with a patient information leaflet inside a carton.

Instructions for use/handling: None.

Marketing authorisation holder: Prodesfarma SA, Carrer del Pont Reixat No 5, Apartado PO Box 26, 08960 Sant Just Desvern, Barcelona, Spain.

Marketing authorisation number 08448/0001.

Date of approval/revision of SPC November 1995.

Legal category POM.

ZIRTEK* TABLETS 10mg
ZIRTEK* SOLUTION 1 mg/1 ml

Presentation

Tablets: White, oblong, film-coated tablets containing 10 mg cetirizine dihydrochloride. Each tablet is scored and bears the code Y/Y.

Solution: A clear, colourless, banana flavoured, sugar free solution with a slightly sweet taste containing 1 mg/1 ml cetirizine dihydrochloride.

Uses Cetirizine is a potent antihistamine with a low potential for drowsiness at pharmacologically active doses and with additional anti-allergic properties. It is a selective H_1 antagonist with negligible effects on other receptors and is therefore virtually free from anti-cholinergic and anti-serotonin effects. Cetirizine inhibits the histamine-mediated 'early' phase of the allergic reaction and also reduces the migration of inflammatory cells and the release of mediators associated with the 'late' allergic response. Zirtek is indicated for the treatment of perennial rhinitis, seasonal allergic rhinitis (hay fever) and chronic idiopathic urticaria in adults and children aged 6 years and over, and for seasonal rhinitis (hay fever) in children aged between 2 to 6 years.

Dosage and administration

Tablets

Adults and children 6 years and over: One 10 mg tablet daily.

Solution

Adults and children 6 years and over: Either 10 ml (10 mg) once daily, or 5 ml (5 mg) twice daily.

Children aged between 2 to 6 years: Either 5 ml (5 mg) once daily, or 2.5 ml (2.5 mg) twice daily.

At present there are no data to suggest that the recommended dose needs to be reduced in elderly patients. However, in patients with renal insufficiency dosage should be reduced to half the daily dose of either tablets or drinkable solution.

Contra-indications, warnings, etc

Contra-indications: Zirtek is contra-indicated in patients with a history of hypersensitivity to any constituent in tablet or solution.

Zirtek is contra-indicated in lactating women as the active ingredient, cetirizine, is excreted in breast milk.

Precautions: Studies conducted with healthy volunteers at doses of 20 and 25 mg/day have not revealed effects on alertness or reaction time, however, patients are advised not to exceed the recommended dose if driving or operating machinery.

Pregnancy: No adverse effects have been reported from animal studies. There has been little or no use of Zirtek in pregnancy. As with other drugs the use of Zirtek in pregnancy should be avoided.

Drug interactions: To date, there are no known interactions with any other drugs. Studies with diazepam and cimetidine have revealed no evidence of interactions. As with other antihistamines it is advisable to avoid excessive alcohol consumption.

Side-effects: In objective tests of psychomotor function, the incidence of sedation with cetirizine was similar to that of placebo.

There have been occasional reports of mild and transient side effects such as headaches, dizziness, drowsiness, agitation, dry mouth and gastro-intestinal discomfort. If affected the dose may be taken as 5 mg in the morning and 5 mg in the evening.

Overdosage: Drowsiness can be a symptom of overdosage in adults; in children, agitation can occur. In the case of massive overdosage, gastric lavage should be performed together with the usual supportive measures. To date, there is no specific antidote.

Pharmaceutical precautions Store below 30°C.

Legal category POM.

Package quantities Zirtek tablets are supplied in cartons containing 30 tablets in 3 blister packs of 10.

Zirtek solution is available in 200 ml amber coloured glass bottles.

Further information Peak blood levels of the order of 0.3 micrograms/ml are reached between thirty and sixty minutes after administration of a 10 mg dose of cetirizine. The terminal half-life is approximately 10 hours in adults and 6 hours in children aged between 6 and 12 years and 5 hours in children aged between 2 to 6 years. This data is consistent with the urinary excretion half-life of the drug. The cumulative urinary excretion represents two thirds of the dose given in either adults or children. Consequently, the apparent plasma clearance in children is higher than that measured in adults. Cetirizine is strongly bound to plasma proteins.

Product licence numbers

Tablets 5221/0001

Solution 5221/0002

**Trade Mark*

Warner Lambert Consumer Healthcare

Lambert Court
Chestnut Avenue
Eastleigh
Hampshire SO53 3ZQ

☎ 01703 641400 📠 01703 629726

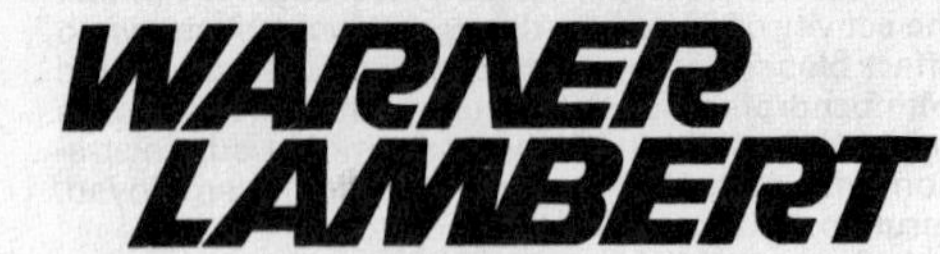

ABIDEC DROPS*

Presentation A clear yellow liquid, with a characteristic odour and taste. Each 0.6 ml contains:

Vitamin A PhEur	4000 units
Vitamin B_1 (Thiamine Hydrochloride PhEur)	1 mg
Vitamin B_2 (Riboflavine PhEur)	400 micrograms
Vitamin B_6 (Pyridoxine Hydrochloride PhEur)	500 micrograms
Vitamin C (Ascorbic Acid PhEur)	50 mg
Vitamin D_2 (Ergocalciferol PhEur)	400 units
Nicotinamide PhEur	5 mg

Uses The prevention of vitamin deficiencies and for the maintenance of normal growth and health during the early years of infancy and childhood; multivitamin supplement.

Dosage and administration
Infants less than one year old: 0.3 ml daily.

Older children: 0.6 ml daily.

Adults: Not appropriate.

Contra-indications, warnings, etc
Contra-indications: Abidec Drops are contra-indicated in individuals with known hypersensitivity to the product or any of it's components.

Interactions with other medicaments and other forms of interaction: None.

Effects on ability to drive and use machines: Unlikely to produce an effect.

Other undesirable effects:
Ascorbic acid (C), Nicotinamide, Pyridoxine (B_6), Riboflavine (B_2) and Thiamine (B_1): These water soluble vitamins are generally non-toxic compounds with a wide margin of safety, the excess amounts being rapidly excreted in the urine. Adverse effects are not anticipated at the quantities present in Abidec Drops.

Ergocalciferol (D_2): The only known adverse effects of Vitamin D occur when excessive doses are taken. Adverse effects are not anticipated at the quantity present in Abidec Drops.

Vitamin A palmitate: Adverse effects are extremely rare at daily doses of less than 9 mg.

Use in pregnancy and lactation: Not appropriate.

Other special warnings and precautions: When prescribing Abidec drops, as with all multi-vitamin preparations, allowance should be made for vitamins obtained from other sources to prevent hypervitaminosis occurring.

Overdosage (symptoms and signs): Abidec Drops contain levels of vitamins which present little risk in overdosage.
Ascorbic acid (C): Ascorbic acid is not stored to a great extent by the body, any excess amounts are eliminated in the urine. Ascorbic acid is thought to become toxic at chronic doses in excess of 6 g.

Ergocalciferol: Excessive doses of Vitamin D, 60,000 units per day, can result in hypercalcaemia and hypercalciuria. Adverse effects of hypercalcaemia may include muscle weakness, apathy, headache, anorexia, nausea and vomiting, hypertension and cardiac arrhythmia's.

Nicotinamide: A single large dose of Nicotinamide is unlikely to have serious ill effects, though transient abnormalities of liver function might occur.

Pyridoxine hydrochloride: Acute doses less than 500 mg per day appear to be safe. Excessive doses may lower serum folate concentrations. Sensory neuropathy has been described with chronic dosing of 200 mg daily.

Riboflavine: Riboflavine has been found to be practically non-toxic.

Thiamine hydrochloride: When taken orally, Thiamine is non-toxic. If large doses are ingested they are not stored by the body but excreted unchanged by the kidneys.

Vitamin A palmitate: Acute administration of high doses of Vitamin A, nausea, vomiting and irritability. In infants acute toxicity can lead to transient hydrocephalus. All these effects disappear within 24 hours of taking retinol.

Treatment: Treatment should be supportive and symptomatic.

Pharmacological particulars:
Ascorbic acid (Vitamin C): Ascorbic acid is a water soluble vitamin and a powerful antioxidant. It is a cofactor in numerous biological processes, such as the metabolism of folic acid, amino acid oxidation and the absorption and transport of iron. It is also required for the formation, maintenance and repair of intercellular cement material. Ascorbic acid is important in the defence against infection, the normal functioning of T-lymphocytes and for effective phagocytic activity of leucocytes. It also protects cells against oxidation damage to essential molecules.

Ergocalciferol (Vitamin D_2): Vitamin D is a regulator of both calcium and phosphate homeostasis.

Nicotinamide: Nicotinamide is an essential component of co-enzymes responsible for proper tissue respiration.

Pyridoxine hydrochloride (Vitamin B_6): Vitamin B_6 is a constituent of the co-enzymes, pyridoxal pyrophosphate and pyridoxamine phosphate, both of which play an important role in protein metabolism.

Riboflavine (Vitamin B_2): Riboflavine is essential for the utilisation of energy from food. It is a component of co-enzymes which play an essential role in oxidative/reductive metabolic reactions. Riboflavine is also necessary for the functioning of pyridoxine and nicotinic acid.

Thiamine hydrochloride (Vitamin B_1): Vitamin B_1 is essential for proper carbohydrate metabolism and plays an essential role in the decarboxylation of alpha keto acids.

Vitamin A palmitate: Vitamin A plays an essential role in the function of the retina, the growth and function of epithelial tissue, bone growth, reproduction and embryonic development.

Pharmacokinetic properties:
Absorption: Vitamin A, B_1, B_2, B_6, C, D_2 and Nicotinamide are well absorbed from the gastro-intestinal tract.

Distribution: The vitamins present in Abidec Drops are widely distributed to all tissues in the body.

Metabolism and elimination: Ascorbic acid (Vitamin C): Ascorbic acid reaches a maximum plasma concentration after 4 hours following oral administration after which there is rapid urinary excretion. Following oral administration 60% of the dose is excreted in 24 hours either as ascorbic acid or it's metabolite dihydroascorbic acid.

Ergocalciferol (Vitamin D_2): Vitamin D circulates in the blood associated with Vitamin D binding protein. It is stored in fat deposits. Ergocalciferol is hydroxylated in the liver and gut to 25-hydroxy cholecalciferol which is then further metabolised in the kidney to the active form 1,25-dihydroxycholecalciferol and other metabolites. Ergocalciferol and it's metabolites are excreted largely in the bile with eventual elimination in the faeces, with only a small amount of some of the metabolites appearing in the urine.

Nicotinamide: Nicotinamide is readily taken up into tissues and utilised for the synthesis of the co-enzyme forms Nicotinamide adenine dinucleotide (NAD) and Nicotinamide adenine dinucleotide phosphate (NADP). Nicotinamide is degraded in the liver and other organs to a number of products that are excreted in the urine, the major metabolites being N-methyl-2-pyridone-5-carboxamide and n-methylnicotinamide.

Pyridoxine hydrochloride (Vitamin B_6): The half life of pyridoxine ranges from 15–20 days. Once absorbed vitamin B_6 is converted to it's active co-enzyme form pyridoxal 5-phosphate. Muscle is the major storage site for pyridoxal 5-phosphate. It is degraded in the liver to 4-pyridoxic acid which is eliminated by the kidneys.

Riboflavine (Vitamin B_2): Following absorption Riboflavine is converted into the coenzymes: flavin mononucleotide (FMN) and flavin adenine dinucleotide (FAD). Riboflavine is not stored in the body tissues to any great extent and amounts in excess of the body's requirements are excreted in the urine largely unchanged.

Thiamine hydrochloride (Vitamin B_1): Thiamine has a plasma half life of 24 hours and is not stored to any great extent in the body. Excess ingested thiamine is excreted in the urine as either the free vitamin or as the metabolite, pyrimidine.

Vitamin A palmitate: Vitamin A palmitate is hydrolysed in the intestinal lumen to retinol which is then absorbed. Retinol circulates in the blood bound to retinol binding protein which protects it from glomerular filtration. The complex circulates to target tissues where the vitamin is released, permeates the cell and binds intracellularly to cellular retinol binding protein. Of the absorbed retinol 20–50% is either conjugated or oxidised to various products and excreted over a matter of days in the urine and faeces, while the remainder is stored. This stored retinol is gradually metabolised by the liver and peripheral tissues.

Pharmaceutical precautions When stored at a temperature not exceeding 25°C and out of direct sunlight, this product is expected to have a shelf life of 2 years.

List of excipients
Sodium hydroxide
Sugar (mineral water grade)
Polysorbate 60
Purified water
Nitrogen (oxygen free)

Legal category GSL

Package quantities 50 ml pack (2×25 ml+2 droppers graduated at 0.3 ml and 0.6 ml). 25 ml pack (1 × 25 ml + 1 dropper graduated at 0.3 ml and 0.6 ml).

Further information Nil.

Product licence number: 15513/0036

ANUSOL* CREAM

Qualitative and quantitative composition Each 100 g of cream contains: Bismuth Oxide 2.14 g, Balsam Peru 1.80 g, Zinc Oxide 10.75 g.

Pharmaceutical form A buff coloured cream.

Clinical particulars
Therapeutic indications: Symptomatic relief of uncomplicated internal and external haemorrhoids, pruritus ani, proctitis and fissures. Also indicated post-operatively in ano-rectal surgical procedures and after incision of thrombosed or sclerosed ano-rectal veins.

Posology and method of administration: Topical.

Adults and elderly (over 65 years): Apply to the affected area at night, in the morning and after each evacuation until the condition is controlled. Thoroughly cleanse the affected area, dry and apply cream. Anusol Cream is prepared in a vanishing cream base and may be gently smoothed onto the affected area without the need to apply a gauze dressing. For internal conditions use rectal nozzle provided and clean it after each use. Not to be taken orally.
Children: Not recommended.

Contra-indications: Known hypersensitivity to any of the constituents.

Special warnings and precautions for use: None known.

Interaction with other medicaments and other forms of interaction: None known.

Pregnancy and lactation: Whilst formal studies on the effect of this product during human pregnancy have not been conducted, there is no epidemiological evidence of adverse effect, either to the pregnant mother or foetus.

Effects on ability to drive and use machines: None known.

Undesirable effects: Rarely, sensitivity reactions. Patients may occasionally experience transient burning on application, especially if the anoderm is not intact.

Overdose: Treatment of a large acute overdose should include gastric lavage, purgation with magnesium sulphate and complete bed rest. If necessary, apply oxygen and give general supportive measures.

Pharmacological properties
Pharmacodynamic properties: Anusol Cream provides antiseptic, astringent and emollient properties which help to relieve discomfort associated with minor ano-rectal conditions. It also provides lubricating properties for use with suppositories.
Bismuth oxide is weakly astringent with supposed antiseptic properties and has a protective action on mucous membranes and raw surfaces. Zinc oxide is an astringent and mild antiseptic and probably owes its actions to the ability of the zinc ion to precipitate protein but other mechanisms may be involved. Zinc oxide is also used to absorb skin moisture and decrease friction and discourage growth of certain bacteria. Balsam Peru has a very mild antiseptic action by virtue of it's content of cinnamic and benzoic acids. It is believed to promote the growth of epithelial cells.

Pharmacokinetic properties: The active ingredients exert their therapeutic effect without being absorbed into the systemic circulation. These observations are supported by evidence from various studies and reviews.

Pre-clinical safety data: The active ingredients of Anusol are well known constituents of medicinal products and their safety profile is well documented

Pharmaceutical particulars
List of excipients: Anusol Cream contains Glycerol monostearate, Liquid paraffin, Propylene glycol, Polysorbate 60, Sorbitan monostearate, Titanium dioxide, Methyl p-hydroxybenzoate, Propyl p-hydroxybenzoate, Purified water.

Incompatibilities: None known.

Shelf life: 3 years when stored in the original packaging.

Special precautions for storage: Store at a temperature not exceeding 25°C.

Nature and contents of container: Pack size 23 g, externally printed and internally lacquered aluminium tube with plastic cap.

Instructions for use/handling: No special requirements.

Marketing authorisation number 15513/0041

Date of approval/revision of SPC 27 March 1996

Legal category: GSL

ANUSOL* OINTMENT

Qualitative and quantitative composition Each 100 g ointment contains:

Zinc Oxide Ph Eur	10.75 g
Bismuth Subgallate BP	2.25 g
Balsam Peru Ph Eur	1.875 g
Bismuth Oxide	0.875 g

Pharmaceutical form A light buff coloured ointment.

Clinical particulars
Therapeutic indications: Symptomatic relief of uncomplicated internal and external haemorrhoids, pruritus ani, proctitis and fissures. Also indicated post operatively in ano-rectal surgical procedures and after incision of thrombosed or sclerosed ano-rectal veins.
Anusol Ointment provides antiseptic, astringent and emollient properties which help to relieve discomfort associated with minor ano-rectal conditions.

Posology and method of administration: Topical.
Adults and elderly (over 65 years): Apply to the affected area at night, in the morning and after each evacuation until the condition is controlled. Thoroughly cleanse the affected area, dry and apply oinment. Anusol Ointment should be applied on a gauze dressing. For internal conditions use rectal nozzle provided and clean it after each use. Not to be taken orally.
Children: Not recommended.

Contra-indications: Known hypersensitivity to any of the constituents.

Special warnings and special precautions for use: None known.

Interaction with other medicaments and other forms of interaction: None known.

Pregnancy and lactation: Whilst formal studies on the effect of this product during pregnancy have not been conducted, there is no epidemiological evidence of adverse effects either to the pregnant mother or foetus.

Effects on ability to drive and use machines: None known.

Undesirable effects: Rarely, sensitivity reactions. Patients may occasionally experience transient burning on application, especially if the anoderm is not intact.

Overdose: Treatment of a large acute overdose should include gastric lavage, purgation with magnesium sulphate and complete bed rest. If necessary, apply oxygen and give general supportive measures.

Pharmacological properties
Pharmacodynamic properties: Anusol Ointment provides antiseptic, astringent and emollient properties which help to relieve discomfort associated with minor ano-rectal conditions.
Bismuth Oxide is weakly astringent with supposed antiseptic properties and has a protective action on mucous membranes and raw surfaces.
Zinc Oxide is an astringent and mild antiseptic and probably owes its actions to the ability of the zinc ion to precipitate protein but other mechanisms may be involved. Zinc Oxide is also used to absorb skin moisture and decrease friction and discourage growth of certain bacteria.
Balsam Peru has a very mild antiseptic action by virtue of its content of cinnamic and benzoic acids. It is believed to promote the growth of epithelial cells.

Pharmacokinetic properties: The active ingredients exert their therapeutic effect without being absorbed into the systemic circulation. These observations are supported by evidence from various studies and reviews.

Pre-clinical safety data: The active ingredients of Anusol are well known constituents of medicinal products and their safety profile is well documented.

Pharmaceutical particulars
List of excipients: Anusol Ointment contains the following excipients:
Magnesium stearate
Cocoa butter
Lanolin anhydrous
Castor oil
Kaolin light
Petroleum Jelly White

Incompatibilities: None known.

Shelf life: Not less than 3 years when stored in the original packing.

Special precautions for storage: Store below 25°C.

Nature and contents of container: Externally printed and internally lacquered 25 g aluminium tube with plastic cap.

Instructions for use/handling: No special requirements.

Marketing authorisation number 15513/0042.

Date of first authorisation/renewal of authorisation 14 March 1997.

ANUSOL* SUPPOSITORIES

Qualitative and quantitative composition Each suppository contains:

Zinc oxide Ph Eur	296 mg
Bismuth subgallate BP 1980	59 mg
Balsam peru Ph Eur	49 mg
Bismuth oxide Ph Eur	24 mg

Pharmaceutical form White or off white suppository.

Clinical particulars
Therapeutic indications: For the relief of internal haemorrhoids and other related ano-rectal conditions.

Posology and method of administration: Anal insertion
Remove wrapper and insert one suppository into the anus at night, in the morning and after each evacuation. Not to be taken orally.
Elderly: (over 65 years): As for adults.
Children: Not recommended.

Contra-indications: History of sensitivity to any of the constituents.

Special warnings and special precautions for use: None known.

Interaction with other medicaments and other forms of interaction: None known.

Pregnancy and lactation: Whilst formal studies on the effect of this product during human pregnancy have not been conducted, there is no epidemiological evidence of adverse effect, either to the pregnant mother or foetus.

Effects on ability to drive and use machines: None known.

Undesirable effects: Rarely, sensitivity reactions. Patients may occasionally experience transient burning on application, especially if the anoderm is not intact.

Overdose: Treatment of a large acute overdose should include gastric lavage, purgation with magnesium sulphate and complete bed rest. If necessary, give oxygen and general supportive measures.

Pharmacological properties
Pharmacodynamic properties: ANUSOL SUPPOSITORIES provides antiseptic, astringent and emollient properties which help to relieve discomfort associated with minor ano-rectal conditions.
Bismuth Oxide, Zinc Oxide and Bismuth Subgallate exert a protective action on mucous membranes and raw surfaces. They are mildly astringent and are reported to have antiseptic properties.
Balsam Peru has protective properties and a very mild antiseptic action by virtue of its content of Cinnamic and Benzoic Acids. It is believed to promote the growth of epithelial cells.

Pharmacokinetic properties: The active ingredients in ANUSOL SUPPOSITORIES exert their therapeutic effect without being absorbed into the systemic circulation. These observations are supported by evidence from various studies and reviews.

Preclinical safety data: The active ingredients of Anusol are well known constituents of medicinal products and their safety profile is well documented.

Pharmaceutical particulars
List of excipients
Suppocire BS2 pastilles
Kaolin light
Titanium Dioxide
Miglyol 812

Incompatibilities: None known.

Shelf life: 3 years.

Special precautions for storage: Store at a temperature not exceeding 25°C.

Nature and contents of container: 12 and 24 pack printed strip pack consisting of white opaque PVC/polyethylene laminated film.

Instructions for use/handling: No special requirements.

Marketing authorisation number 15513/0043.

Date of first authorisation/renewal of authorisation
Date Granted: 15 September 1997.

Date of (partial) revision of the text 15 October 1997.

CALADRYL* LOTION AND CREAM

Presentation
Lotion: A smooth, pink, viscous suspension with a characteristic odour.

Cream: A smooth, pink cream with a characteristic odour.

Composition: Caladryl Lotion and Cream: Zinc oxide 8.0%, Diphenhydramine hydrochloride 1.0%, Racemic camphor 0.1%.

Action: Caladryl combines the cooling and soothing effects of calamine and camphor with the powerful antihistaminic and antipruritic effects of Diphenhydramine hydrochloride.

Uses For relief of irritation associated with urticaria, herpes zoster and other minor skin affections, to alleviate the discomforts of sunburn, prickly heat, insect bites and nettle stings. In infants it may be used for hives.

Dosage and administration Topical application to skin only.

Adults: Apply to affected area three or four times daily.

Elderly (over 65 years): As for adults.

Children and infants of all age groups: As for adults.

Caladryl lotion may be dabbed on the affected part using a pad of cotton wool. The cream may be lightly smoothed on.

Contra-indications, warnings etc Do not use on chicken pox or measles or exudative dermatoses, unless supervised by a doctor. Do not use on extensive areas of the skin except as directed by a doctor. Do not use any other drugs containing Diphenhydramine while using this product.

Pregnancy and lactation: The safety of Caladryl in pregnancy and lactation has not been established. Like any medicine, Caladryl should only be used if the possible benefits outweigh the potential risks involved. Diphenhydramine is known to be absorbed through the skin. Diphenhydramine crosses the placental barrier and is secreted in breast milk.

Precautions and warnings: Caladryl should not be applied to raw, or broken surfaces or mucous membranes as this may result in percutaneous absorption giving rise to systemic effects. Avoid contact with the eyes.
If a burning sensation or rash develops or if the condition persists, treatment should be discontinued. If necessary remove by washing with soap and water.

Side-effects: Rarely, sensitivity, eczematous reactions and photosensitivity have been reported after topical application of antihistamines. If this occurs, treatment should be discontinued.

Overdose: Accidental ingestion or excessive absorption of Caladryl may lead to dose-related signs of Diphenhydramine toxicity. These include drowsiness and sedation with anticholinergic symptoms prevailing. Camphor may produce nausea, vomiting and dizziness. At higher doses, delirium leading to coma, ataxia, increased muscle reflexes and cloniform convulsions may appear.

Treatment of overdose: The stomach should be emptied by lavage and aspiration. In cases of acute poisoning, activated charcoal may be useful. A Sodium sulphate purgative may be given. Convulsions may be controlled with diazepam or Thiopentone sodium. In the case of camphor poisoning, lipid haemodialysis or resin haemoperfusion may be useful.

Pharmaceutical precautions Lotion: Store at a temperature not exceeding 30°C

Cream: Store at a temperature not exceeding 25°C

Legal category P.

Package quantities Lotion: 125 ml. Cream: 42 g.

Further information Nil

Product licence numbers
Lotion: 15513/0063
Cream: 15513/0062

CALGEL* TEETHING GEL

Presentation Calgel Teething Gel contains Lignocaine hydrochloride BP 0.33% w/w and Cetylpyridinium chloride BP 0.1% w/w in a clear yellow, water soluble sugar-free base. It has a herbal flavour.

Uses Calgel Teething Gel is indicated for use in teething. Calgel Teething Gel acts quickly to help relieve teething pain and soothe infants' gums. It also has mild antiseptic properties.

Dosage and administration Calgel Teething Gel is suitable for babies from the age of 3 months. A small quantity of Calgel Teething Gel, approximately one-third of an inch (7.5 mm), should be squeezed onto the tip of a clean finger and rubbed gently onto the affected area of the gum. Application may be repeated after an interval of 20 minutes if necessary, with up to six applications in one day.

Contra-indications, warnings, etc
Contra-indications: None.

Precautions: The recommended dosage should not be exceeded. Keep out of reach of children.

Side-effects: When used according to instructions side effects would not be expected. However, isolated cases of hypersensitivity to lignocaine hydrochloride have been reported in adults and in a child over 12 years following local injection. Hypersensitivity presented in these cases as localised oedema with slight difficulty in breathing or as generalised rash.

Chamomile, a minor ingredient in the herbal flavouring agent, has been documented as causing allergic reactions. Hypersensitivity to Chamomile normally manifests as breathing difficulties in atopic individuals. Anaphylactic reactions have been reported in individuals drinking herbal tea infusions containing Chamomile (herbal tea asthma). Sensitised individuals may demonstrate positive skin reactions to preparations containing Chamomile.

In the event of any unwanted side effects, use should be discontinued and a doctor consulted.

Drug Interactions: No drug interactions with Calgel Teething Gel are known. Drug interactions between intravenously administered Lignocaine and oral Procainamide, oral Phenytoin alone or in combination with Phenobarbitone, Primidone or Carbamazepine, oral Propanolol, and non-potassium sparing diuretics including Bumetanide, Frusemide and Thiazide have been reported. These drug effects are unlikely to be relevant to the use of Calgel Teething Gel.

Toxicity and treatment of overdosage: Suppression of pharyngeal sensation with concomitant effects on swallowing may theoretically result from excessive topical oral use of Calgel Teething Gel. Such an effect has been reported in an adult who gargled and swallowed 5 ml of a 2% Lignocaine hydrochloride solution (equivalent to 100 mg Lignocaine). However, assuming proportionality of body surface area and pharyngeal surface area, this dose would be equivalent to a single dose of 5.4 g of Calgel Teething Gel for a 3 month old child.

It is most unlikely, even with misuse or excessive application of Calgel Teething Gel, that the large amounts of Lignocaine hydrochloride or Cetylpyridinium chloride required to produce clinically-relevant toxic effects would be reached. In the event of overdose, use should be discontinued and a doctor consulted.

Pharmaceutical precautions Store below 25°C.

Legal category GSL.

Package quantities Single packs of 10 g

Further information Calgel Teething Gel is considered to be of low cariogenic potential since the sweetening agents are sorbitol, xylitol and saccharin sodium.

Product licence number 15513/0015

CALPOL* PAEDIATRIC SUSPENSION

Qualitative and quantitative composition CALPOL Paediatric Suspension contains 120 mg Paracetamol in each 5 ml.

Pharmaceutical form Suspension.

Clinical particulars
Therapeutic indications: CALPOL Paediatric Suspension is indicated for the treatment of pain (including teething pain), and as an antipyretic.

Posology and method of administration:
Posology: Children aged 1 to under 6 years: Oral. 5 to 10 ml (120 mg to 240 mg paracetamol). Repeat every 4 hours, if necessary, up to a maximum of 4 doses per 24 hours.

Infants 3 months to under 1 year: Oral. 2.5 to 5 ml (60 mg to 120 mg paracetamol). Repeat every 4 hours, if necessary, up to a maximum of 4 doses per 24 hours.

Infants under 3 months: Oral. A 2.5 ml dose is suitable for babies who develop a fever following vaccination at 2 months. In other cases, use only under medical supervision.

The elderly: In the elderly the rate and extent of paracetamol absorption is normal but plasma half-life is longer and paracetamol clearance is lower than in young adults.

Hepatic/renal dysfunction: Caution should be exercised when administering the product to patients with severe hepatic or renal impairment.

Contra-indications: CALPOL Paediatric Suspension is contra-indicated in patients with known hypersensitivity to paracetamol, or any of the other components.

Special warnings and special precautions for use: CALPOL Paediatric Suspension should be used with caution in moderate to severe renal impairment or severe hepatic impairment.

The hazards of overdose are greater in those with alcoholic liver disease.

The label contains the following statements:
Shake the bottle thoroughly.
Dose 4 times a day.
Keep out of reach of children.
Do not exceed the stated dose.
Do not take more than 4 doses in 24 hours.
Do not repeat doses more frequently than 4 hourly.
Do not give for more than 3 days without consulting a doctor.

As with all medicines, if you are currently taking any medicine consult your doctor or pharmacist before taking this product.

If symptoms persist consult your doctor.
Store below 25°C. Protect from light.
Contains paracetamol.

Immediate advice should be sought in the event of an overdose, even if the child seems well. (label)

Immediate advice should be sought in the event of an overdose, even if the child seems well, because of the risk of delayed, serious liver damage. (leaflet)

Do not give with any other paracetamol containing products.

Interaction with other medicaments and other forms of interaction: The speed of absorption of paracetamol may be increased by metoclopramide or domperidone and absorption reduced by cholestramine.

The anticoagulant effect of warfarin and other coumarins may be enhanced by prolonged regular use of paracetamol with risk of bleeding; occasional doses have no significant effect.

Patients who have taken barbiturates, tricyclic antidepressants and alcohol may show diminished ability to metabolise large doses of paracetamol, the plasma half-life of which can be prolonged.

Alcohol can increase the hepatotoxicity of paracetamol overdosage and may have contributed to the acute pancreatitis reported in one patient who had taken an overdose of paracetamol.

Chronic ingestion of anticonvulsants or oral steroid contraceptives induce liver enzymes and may prevent attainment of therapeutic paracetamol levels by increasing first pass metabolism or clearance.

Pregnancy and lactation: Epidemiological studies in human pregnancy have shown no ill effects due to paracetamol used in the recommended dosage, but patients should follow the advice of the doctor regarding its use.

Paracetamol is excreted in breast milk but not in a clinically significant amount. Available published data do not contra-indicate breast feeding.

Effects on ability to drive and operate machinery: No special comment–unlikely to produce an effect.

Undesirable effects: Paracetamol has been widely used and, when taken at the usual recommended dosage, side effects are mild and infrequent and reports of adverse reactions are rare. Skin rash and other allergic reactions occur rarely.

Most reports of adverse reactions to paracetamol relate to overdosage with the drug.

Isolated cases of thrombocytic purpura, haemolytic anaemia and agranulocytosis have been reported.

Chronic hepatic necrosis has been reported in a patient who took daily therapeutic doses of paracetamol for about a year and liver damage has been reported after daily ingestion of excessive amounts for shorter periods. A review of a group of patients with chronic active hepatitis failed to reveal differences in the abnormalities of liver function in those who were long-term users of paracetamol nor was the control of the disease improved after paracetamol withdrawal.

Nephrotoxic effects following therapeutic doses of paracetamol are uncommon. Papillary necrosis has been reported after prolonged administration.

Overdosage:
Symptoms and signs: Pallor, anorexia, nausea, vomiting and abdominal pain are frequent early symptoms of paracetamol overdosage.

Hepatic necrosis is a dose-related complication of paracetamol overdose. Hepatic enzymes may become elevated and prothrombin time prolonged within 12 to 48 hours but clinical symptoms may not be apparent for 1 to 6 days after ingestion. Toxicity is likely in subjects who have taken single doses of 10 g (150 mg/kg) or more. It is considered that excess quantities of toxic metabolite (usually adequately detoxified by glutathione when normal doses of paracetamol are ingested), become irreversibly bound to liver tissue.

Abnormalities of glucose metabolism and metabolic acidosis may occur. In severe poisoning, hepatic failure may progress to encephalopathy, coma and death. Acute renal failure with acute tubular necrosis may develop even in the absence of severe liver damage. Cardiac arrhythmias and pancreatitis have been reported.

In paracetamol overdosage with liver cell damage, paracetamol half-life is often prolonged from around 2 hours in normal adults to 4 hours or longer. However liver cell damage has been found in patients with a paracetamol half life less than 4 hours. Diminution of $^{14}CO_2$ excretion after ^{14}C-aminopyrine has been reported to correlate better with liver cell damage in paracetamol overdosage than do either plasma paracetamol concentration or half-life, or conventional liver function test measurements.

Treatment: Immediate treatment is essential in the management of paracetamol overdose. Despite a lack of significant early symptoms, patients should be refered to hospital urgently for immediate medical attention and any patient who had ingested around 7.5 g or more of paracetamol in the preceding 4 hours should undergo gastric lavage. Administration of oral methionine or intravenous N-acetylcysteine which may have beneficial effect up to at least 48 hours after overdose, may be required. General supportive measures must be available.

Pharmacological properties
Pharmacodynamic properties: Paracetamol has analgesic and antipyretic effects similar to those of aspirin and is useful in the treatment of mild to moderate pain. It has weak anti-inflammatory effects.

Pharmacokinetic properties: Paracetamol is rapidly and almost completely absorbed from the gastrointestinal tract. Peak plasma concentrations are reached 30-90 minutes post dose and the plasma half-life is in the range of 1 to 3 hours after therapeutic doses. Drug is widely distributed throughout most body fluids. Following therapeutic doses 90-100% of the drug is recovered in the urine within 24 hours almost entirely following hepatic conjugation with glucuronic acid (about 60%), sulphuric acid (about 35%) or cysteine (about 3%). Small amounts of hydroxylated and deacetylated metabolites have also been detected. Children have less capacity for glucuronidation of the drug than do adults. In overdosage there is increased N-hydroxylation followed by glutathione conjugation. When the latter is exhausted, reaction with hepatic proteins is increased leading to necrosis.

Preclinical safety data:
Mutagenicity: There are no studies relating to the mutagenic potential of CALPOL Paediatric Suspension.

In vivo mutagencicity tests of paracetamol in mammals are limited and show conflicting results. Therefore, there is insufficient information to determine whether paracetamol poses a mutagenic risk to man. Paracetamol has been found to be non-mutagenic in bacterial mutagenicity assays, although a clear clastogenic effect has been observed in mammalian cells *in vitro* following exposure to paracetamol (3 and 10 mM for 2 hr).

Carcinogenicity: There are no studies relating to the carcinogenic potential of CALPOL Paediatric Suspension.

There is inadequate evidence to determine the carcinogenic potential of paracetamol in humans. A positive association between the use of paracetamol and cancer of the ureter (but not of other sites in the urinary tract) was observed in a case-control study in which approximate lifetime consumption of paracetamol (whether acute or chronic) was estimated. However, other similar studies have failed to demonstrate a statistically significant association between paracetamol and cancer of the urinary tract, or paracetamol and renal cell carcinoma.

There is limited evidence for the carcinogenicity of paracetamol in experimental animals. Liver cell tumours can be detected in mice and liver and bladder carcinomas can be detected in rats following chronic feeding of 500 mg/kg/day paracetamol.

Teratogenicity: There is no information relating to the teratogenic potential of CALPOL Paediatric Suspension. In humans, paracetamol crosses the placenta and attains concentrations in the foetal circulation similar to those in the maternal circulation. Intermittent maternal ingestion of therapeutic doses of paracetamol are not associated with teratogenic effects in humans.

Paracetamol has been found to be fetotoxic to cultured rat embryo.

Fertility: There is no information relating to the effects of CALPOL Paediatric Suspension. A significant decrease in testicular weight was observed when male Sprague-Dawley rats were given daily high doses of paracetamol (500 mg/kg body weight/day) orally for 70 days.

Pharmaceutical particulars
List of excipients:
Syrup
Sorbitol solution
Glycerol
Xanthan gum
Methyl parahydroxybenzoate
Carmoisine (E122)
Strawberry flavour
Purified water

Incompatibilities: None known.

Shelf life: 36 months.

Special precautions for storage: Store below 25°C. Protect from light.

Nature and contents of container: 5 ml aluminium foil/ polyethylene laminate sachets.

100 ml and 1000 ml amber glassed bottle closed with a two-piece plastic child resistant, tamper evident closure fitted with a polyethylene/polyvinylidine chloride PVDC/polyethylene laminate faced wad
or
a three piece plastic child resistant, tamper evident closure fitted with a polyethylene/polyvinylidenechloride (PVDC)/polyethylene laminate faced wad
or
a polypropylene cap with a Steran or Seran faced wad.

Instructions for use/handling: None applicable.

Marketing authorisation number 15513/0007.

Date of first authorisation/renewal of authorisation 28 April 1997.

Date of revision March 1997.

CALPOL* PAEDIATRIC SUSPENSION SUGAR FREE

Qualitative and quantitative composition CALPOL Paediatric Suspension Sugar Free contains 120 mg Paracetamol in each 5 ml.

Pharmaceutical form Suspension.

Clinical particulars
Therapeutic indications: CALPOL Paediatric Suspension Sugar Free is indicated for the treatment of pain (including teething pain), and as an antipyretic.

Posology and method of administration
Posology:

Children aged 1 to under 6 years: Oral. 5 to 10 ml (120 mg to 240 mg paracetamol). Repeat every 4 hours, if necessary, up to a maximum of 4 doses per 24 hours.

Infants 3 months to under 1 year: Oral. 2.5 to 5 ml (60 mg to 120 mg paracetamol). Repeat every 4 hours, if necessary, up to a maximum of 4 doses per 24 hours.

Infants under 3 months: Oral. A 2.5 ml dose is suitable for babies who develop a fever following vaccination at 2 months. In other cases, use only under medical supervision.

The elderly: In the elderly, the rate and extent of paracetamol absorption is normal but plasma half-life is longer and paracetamol clearance is lower than in young adults.

Contra-indications: CALPOL Paediatric Suspension Sugar Free is contra-indicated in patients with known hypersensitivity to paracetamol, or any of the other components.

Special warnings and special precautions for use: CALPOL Paediatric Suspension Sugar Free should be used with caution in moderate to severe renal impairment or severe hepatic impairment.

The hazards of overdose are greater in those with alcoholic liver disease.

Concomitant use of other paracetamol-containing products with CALPOL Paediatric Suspension Sugar Free could lead to paracetamol overdosage and therefore should be avoided.

The label contains the following statements:
Shake the bottle thoroughly.
Dose 4 times a day.
Keep out of reach of children.
Do not exceed the stated dose.
Do not take more than 4 doses in 24 hours.
Do not repeat doses more frequently than 4 hourly.
Do not give for more than 3 days without consulting a doctor.

As with all medicines, if you are currently taking any medicine consult your doctor or pharmacist before taking this product.
If symptoms persist consult your doctor.
Store below 25°C. Protect from light.
Contains paracetamol.

Immediate advice should be sought in the event of an overdose, even if the child seems well. (label)

Immediate advice should be sought in the event of an overdose, even if the child seems well, because of the risk of delayed, serious liver damage. (leaflet)

Do not give with any other paracetamol containing products.

Interaction with other medicaments and other forms of interaction: The speed of absorption of paracetamol may be increased by metoclopramide or domperidone and absorption reduced by cholestramine.

The anticoagulant effect of warfarin and other coumarins may be enhanced by prolonged regular use of paracetamol with risk of bleeding; occasional doses have no significant effect.

Patients who have taken barbiturates, tricyclic antidepressants and alcohol may show diminished ability to metabolise large doses of paracetamol, the plasma half-life of which can be prolonged.

Alcohol can increase the hepatotoxicity of paracetamol overdosage and may have contributed to the acute pancreatitis reported in one patient who had taken an overdose of paracetamol.

Chronic ingestion of anticonvulsants or oral steroid contraceptives induce liver enzymes and may prevent attainment of therapeutic paracetamol levels by increasing first pass metabolism or clearance.

Pregnancy and lactation: Epidemiological studies in human pregnancy have shown no ill effects due to paracetamol used in the recommended dosage, but patients should follow the advice of the doctor regarding its use.

Paracetamol is excreted in breast milk but not in a clinically significant amount. Available published data do not contraindicate breast feeding.

Effects on ability to drive and use machines: No special comment–unlikely to produce an effect.

Undesirable effects: Paracetamol has been widely used and, when taken at the usual recommended dosage, side effects are mild and infrequent and reports of adverse reactions are rare. Skin rash and other allergic reactions occur rarely.

Most reports of adverse reactions to paracetamol relate to overdosage with the drug.

Isolated cases of thrombocytic purpura, haemolytic anaemia and agranulocytosis have been reported.

Chronic hepatic necrosis has been reported in a patient who took daily therapeutic doses of paracetamol for about a year and liver damage has been reported after daily ingestion of excessive amounts for shorter periods. A review of a group of patients with chronic active hepatitis failed to reveal differences in the abnormalities of liver function in those who were long-term users of paracetamol nor was the control of the disease improved after paracetamol withdrawal.

Nephrotoxic effects following therapeutic doses of paracetamol are uncommon. Papillary necrosis has been reported after prolonged administration.

Overdosage:
Symptoms and signs: Pallor, anorexia, nausea, vomiting and abdominal pain are frequent early symptoms of paracetamol overdosage.

Hepatic necrosis is a dose-related complication of paracetamol overdose. Hepatic enzymes may become elevated and prothrombin time prolonged within 12 to 48 hours but clinical symptoms may not be apparent for 1 to 6 days after ingestion. Toxicity is likely in subjects who have taken single doses of 10 g (150 mg/ kg) or more. It is considered that excess quantities of toxic metabolite (usually adequately detoxified by glutathione when normal doses of paracetamol are ingested, become irreversibly bound to liver tissue.

Abnormalities of glucose metabolism and metabolic acidosis may occur. In severe poisoning, hepatic failure may progress to encephalopathy, coma and death. Acute renal failure with acute tubular necrosis may develop even in the absence of severe liver damage. Cardiac arrhythmias and pancreatitis have been reported.

In paracetamol overdosage with liver cell damage, paracetamol half-life is often prolonged from around 2 hours in normal adults to 4 hours or longer. However liver cell damage has been found in patients with a paracetamol half life less than 4 hours. Diminution of $^{14}CO_2$ excretion after ^{14}C-aminopyrine has been reported to correlate better with liver cell damage in paracetamol overdosage than do either plasma paracetamol concentration or half-life, or conventional liver function test measurements. Renal failure due to acute tubular necrosis may follow paracetamol-induced fulminant hepatic failure. The incidence of this is, however, no more frequent in these patients than in others with fulminant hepatic failure from other causes.

Treatment: Immediate treatment is essential in the management of paracetamol overdose. Despite a lack of significant early symptoms, patients should be refered to hospital urgently for immediate medical attention and any patient who had ingested around 7.5 g or more of paracetamol in the preceding 4 hours should undergo gastric lavage.

Administration of oral methionine or intravenous N-acetylcysteine which may have beneficial effect up to at least 48 hours after overdose, may be required. General supportive measures must be available.

Pharmacological properties
Pharmacodynamic properties: Paracetamol has analgesic and antipyretic effects similar to those of aspirin and is useful in the treatment of mild to moderate pain. It has weak anti-inflammatory effects.

Pharmacokinetic properties: Paracetamol is rapidly and almost completely absorbed from the gastrointestinal tract. Peak plasma concentrations are reached 30-90 minutes post dose and the plasma half-life is in the range of 1 to 3 hours after therapeutic doses. Drug is widely distributed throughout most body fluids. Following therapeutic doses 90-100% of the drug is recovered in the urine within 24 hours almost entirely following hepatic conjugation with glucuronic acid (about 60%), sulphuric acid (about 35%) or cysteine (about 3%). Small amounts of hydroxylated and deacetylated metabolites have also been detected. Children have less capacity for glucuronidation of the drug than do adults. In overdosage there is increased N-hydroxylation followed by glutathione conjugation. When the latter is exhausted, reaction with hepatic proteins is increased leading to necrosis.

Preclinical safety data:
Mutagenicity: There are no studies relating to the mutagenic potential of CALPOL Paediatric Suspension Sugar Free.

In vivo mutagencicity tests of paracetamol in mammals are limited and show conflicting results. Therefore, there is insufficient information to determine whether paracetamol poses a mutagenic risk to man.

Paracetamol has been found to be non-mutagenic in bacterial mutagenicity assays, although a clear clastogenic effect has been observed in mammalian cells *in vitro* following exposure to paracetamol (3 and 10 mM for 2 hr).

Carcinogenicity: There are no studies relating to the carcinogenic potential of CALPOL Paediatric Suspension Sugar Free.

There is inadequate evidence to determine the carcinogenic potential of paracetamol in humans. A positive association between the use of paracetamol and cancer of the ureter (but not of other sites in the urinary tract) was observed in a case-control study in which approximate lifetime consumption of paracetamol (whether acute or chronic) was estimated . However, other similar studies have failed to demonstrate a statistically significant association between paracetamol and cancer of the urinary tract, or paracetamol and renal cell carcinoma.

There is limited evidence for the carcinogenicity of paracetamol in experimental animals. Liver cell tumours can be detected in mice and liver and bladder carcinomas can be detected in rats following chronic feeding of 500 mg/kg/day paracetamol.

Teratogenicity: There is no information relating to the teratogenic potential of CALPOL Paediatric Suspension Sugar Free. In humans, paracetamol crosses the placenta and attains concentrations in the foetal circulation similar to those in the maternal circulation. Intermittent maternal ingestion of therapeutic doses of paracetamol are not associated with teratogenic effects in humans.

Paracetamol has been found to be fetotoxic to cultured rat embryo.

Fertility: There is no information relating to the effects of CALPOL Paediatric Suspension Sugar Free. A significant decrease in testicular weight was observed when male Sprague-Dawley rats were given daily high doses of paracetamol (500 mg/kg body weight/day) orally for 70 days.

Pharmaceutical particulars
List of excipients
Hydrogenated glucose syrup
Sorbitol solution (70% non crystallising)
Glycerol
Dispersible cellulose
Xanthan gum
Methyl hydroxybenzoate
Propyl hydroxybenzoate
Strawberry flavour
Carmoisine (E122)
Purified water

Incompatibilities: None known.

Shelf life: 36 months.

Special precautions for storage: Store below 25°C. Protect from light.

Nature and contents of container: 5 ml paper/foil/surlyn sachets.

100 ml and 1000 ml amber glassed bottle closed with a two-piece plastic child resistant, tamper evident closure fitted with a polyethylene/polvinylidine chloride PVDC/polyethylene laminate faced wad
or
a three piece plastic child resistant, tamper evident closure fitted with a polyethylene/polyvinylidene chloride (PVDC)/polyethylene laminate faced wad
or
a plastic screw cap with a Saran faced wad.

Instructions for use/handling: None applicable.

Marketing authorisation number 15513/0008.

Date of first authorisation/renewal of authorisation 28 April 1997.

Date of revision March 1998.

DRAPOLENE* CREAM

Presentation Drapolene Cream is a pink, water-miscible preparation. Drapolene Cream contains:

Benzalkonium Chloride	0.01% w/w
Cetrimide BP	0.2% w/w

The components benzalkonium chloride and cetrimide are quaternary ammonium compounds used topically for their antiseptic and disinfectant properties. White Soft Paraffin, wool fat and cetyl alcohol are emollient, protective and hydrating. These properties are useful in dry skin conditions.

Uses Drapolene is indicated for the relief of nappy rash and for use as an adjunct to baby care hygiene for the prevention of nappy rash.

Drapolene is indicated for the relief of urinary dermatitis in adults, and as an adjunct to patient care hygiene for the prevention of urinary dermatitis.

Drapolene is indicated for the symptomatic relief of minor burns, limited sunburn and the effects of weather.

Dosage and administration
Babies: The nappy area should be washed then dried thoroughly at each change of nappy. Drapolene Cream should be applied, paying particular attention to folds in the skin.

Adults: The affected area (or the area of application) should be washed and dried thoroughly before applying Drapolene. Regular routine application is advised.

Drapolene should be applied as required for minor burns, sunburn and the effects of weather.

Contra-indications, warnings, etc
Precautions: For external use only. Keep out of the reach of children. It is inadvisable to apply Drapolene Cream to a baby or adult who has an established hypersensitivity to Benzalkonium chloride, Cetrimide or lanolin. Use should be discontinued if an allergic hypersensitivity reaction is suspected.

Side and adverse effects: Allergic hypersensitivity reactions may occur in individuals who are sensitive to one or several components of Drapolene Cream.

Hypersensitivity to lanolin is recognised but rare. In a few individuals, Benzalkonium chloride, used as a preservative in ophthalmic solutions, was associated with oedema and conjunctivitis. Dermatitis as a result of contact allergy to Benzalkonium chloride in plaster of Paris, has also been reported.

Hypersensitivity to Cetrimide is also known to occur, presenting as a localised contact dermatitis. In severe cases the rash may be generalised.

Toxicity and treatment of overdosage: There are no reports of adverse events resulting from excessive application or ingestion of Drapolene Cream..

Pharmaceutical precautions Store below 25°C.

Legal category GSL.

Package quantities Tubs of 200 g, 350 g and tube of 100 g.

Further information Nil

Product licence number 15513/0016

LYCLEAR* CREME RINSE

Presentation Lyclear Creme Rinse contains 1% w/w Permethrin plus 20% w/w Isopropanol in a creme rinse base. It is orange in colour.

Uses Lyclear Creme Rinse is indicated for the treatment of infections with the head louse *Pediculus humanus capitis.*

Dosage and administration
Adults and children 6 months of age and over: Lyclear Creme Rinse should be used after hair has been washed with a mild proprietary shampoo and towelled dry. The bottle should be shaken thoroughly and enough Lyclear Creme Rinse applied to saturate the hair and scalp. Particular attention should be given to the areas behind the ears and at the nape of the neck.

Lyclear Creme Rinse should be left on the hair for 10 minutes before rinsing the hair thoroughly with water. The hair should then be dried in the usual way.

One bottle of Lyclear Creme Rinse is sufficient for shoulder-length hair of average thickness. More may be applied if required and, although no maximum dose has been defined, it is most unlikely that more than two bottles will be required for any one course of treatment.

97–99% of individuals with head lice are successfully treated with a single application of Lyclear Creme Rinse. Residual activity may persist for up to six weeks.

It is not necessary to remove dead eggs or nits except for cosmetic purposes. A fine-toothed comb may be used if desired.

Use in the elderly: Lyclear Creme Rinse is suitable for use in the elderly.

Pharmacology: Permethrin is rapidly absorbed across the insect cuticle. The principal physiological lesion is the induction of electrochemical abnormalities across the membranes of excitable cells, leading to sensory hyperexcitability, inco-ordination and prostration. When presented in an aqueous base the ovicidal activity of permethrin is increased by the addition of an alcohol.

Pharmacokinetics: Permethrin is rapidly metabolised by ester hydrolysis to inactive metabolites which are excreted primarily in the urine. The application of creme rinse to the hair of volunteers for the recommended application time resulted in extremely low or undetectable levels of permethrin metabolites in plasma and urine samples. *In vitro* studies have shown that permethrin levels on hair were not affected by chlorine in concentrations used in swimming pools.

Contra-indications, warnings, etc
Contra-indications: The use of Lyclear Creme Rinse is contra-indicated in individuals with a known hypersensitivity to the product, its components, other pyrethroids or pyrethrins.

Precautions: For external use only. Keep out of reach of children.

Nursing staff who routinely use Lyclear Creme Rinse may wish to wear gloves to avoid any possible irritation to the hands.

Children under 6 months of age should be treated on the advice of a doctor.

Neither Permethrin or Lyclear Creme Rinse are irritants to the eyes. However, should Lyclear Creme Rinse be accidentally introduced into the eyes, rinse immediately with plenty of water.

Side- and adverse effects: Lyclear Creme Rinse is generally well-tolerated with a low potential for inducing skin reactions. In a few individuals erythema, rash, and/or irritation of the scalp has been reported following application of the Creme Rinse, but as an infection with head lice is often associated with such scalp irritation it is difficult in most instances to determine the underlying cause.

If severe or prolonged signs and symptoms of scalp irritation, skin discomfort, or other undesirable effects occur in association with the use of Lyclear Cream Rinse it should be brought to the attention of a doctor or pharmacist.

Use during pregnancy and lactation: Reproduction studies have been performed in mice, rats and rabbits (200–400 mg/kg/day orally) and have revealed no evidence of impaired fertility or harm to the foetus due to Permethrin. There are however, only very limited data on the use of Permethrin in pregnant women. Because animal reproduction studies are not always predictive of the human response, treatment should be considered during pregnancy only if clearly needed.

Studies following oral administration of Permethrin in cattle have indicated that very low concentrations of Permethrin are excreted in milk. However it is not known whether Permethrin is excreted in human milk. Whilst it is unlikely that the concentrations of Permethrin in the milk will present any risk to the infant, consideration should be given to withholding treatment during nursing or temporarily discontinuing nursing.

Drug interactions: No interactions are known.

Toxicity and treatment of overdosage: There are no reports of overdosage with Lyclear Creme Rinse. On the basis of animal and human-volunteer studies, it is extremely unlikely, even with misuse or excessive application, that the amount of Permethrin needed to produce clinically–relevant toxic effects would be reached. The most likely symptoms and signs following repeated, excessive application would be hypersensitivity-type reactions.

Symptomatic treatment is indicated should hypersensitivity-type reactions occur.

Theoretically if swallowed by a small child, alcoholic intoxication may occur due to the Isopropanol content of Lyclear Creme Rinse.

In the event of accidental ingestion of the contents of a bottle by a child, a doctor should be consulted immediately. Gastric lavage should be considered within two hours of ingestion and management should relate to treatment of alcoholic intoxication.

Pharmaceutical precautions Shake well before use. Store below 25°C. Protect from light. Keep out of the reach of children.

Legal category P

Package quantities Plastic bottle of 59 ml.

Further information Permethrin is not affected by the chlorine in swimming baths, so normal swimming activities may continue after use. Lyclear Creme Rinse may be used as normal in asthmatics, however, contact your doctor or pharmacist before commencing treatment if you have any particular concerns.

Product licence number 15513/0019

ORALDENE*

Presentation A clear, red-coloured solution containing hexetidine 0.10% w/v

Uses Oraldene is indicated for use in minor mouth infections including thrush, as an aid in the prevention and treatment of gingivitis and in the management of sore throat and recurrent aphthous ulcers. Also of value in halitosis and pre and post dental surgery.

Dosage and administration
Adults: Oraldene is intended for use solely as a mouthwash. The mouth should be rinsed or the solution may be gargled, undiluted. The mouthwash should not be swallowed in large quantities. Rinse the mouth or gargle with at least 15 ml of Oraldene two or three times a day. Do not swallow

Children: 6 years old and over: As for adults.
5 years old and under: Not recommended.

Contra-indications, warnings, etc None known.

Warnings: Oraldene is not to be taken internally.

Precautions: None applicable.

Side effects: Oraldene mouthwash is generally very well tolerated with a low potential for causing irritation, or sensitisation reactions. Prolonged use of Oraldene mouthwash is also well tolerated.

Patch test of hexetidine containing ointment was negative for irritation or sensitisation potential.

In a few individuals mild irritation (described as sore mouth, burning or itching), of the tongue and / or buccal tissues have been reported. Other side effects which are reported very rarely include transient anaesthesia and taste impairment.

Overdosage:
Alcohol intoxication: There are no reports of overdosage with Oraldene mouthwash.

Hexetidine, at the strength present in Oraldene mouthwash is non-toxic.

Acute alcohol intoxication is extremely unlikely, however, it is theoretically possible that, if a massive dose were swallowed by a small child, alcoholic intoxication may occur due to the ethanol content.

There is no evidence to suggest that repeated, excessive, administration of hexetidine would lead to hypersensitivity-type reactions.

Treatment
Treatment of overdosage is symptomatic, but rarely required. In the event of accidental ingestion of the contents of a bottle by a child, a doctor should be

consulted immediately. Gastric lavage should be considered within two hours of ingestion and management should relate to treatment of alcohol intoxication.

Pharmaceutical precautions: Store away from direct light at a temperature not exceeding 25°C.

Legal category GSL.

Package quantities Oraldene is supplied in clear glass bottles containing 100 ml and 200 ml.

Further information Nil.

Product licence number 15513/0067.

Date of preparation April 1998.

SUDAFED* TABLETS AND ELIXIR

Presentation Each brownish red, biconvex, film coated tablet contains 60 mg Pseudoephedrine hydrochloride BP and is imprinted 'WELLCOME SUDAFED' on one side.

Each 5 ml of red elixir contains 30 mg Pseudoephedrine Hydrochloride BP and has a raspberry flavour.

Uses Sudafed is a decongestant of the mucous membranes of the upper respiratory tract, especially the nasal mucosa and sinuses, and is indicated for the symptomatic relief of conditions such as allergic rhinitis, vasomotor rhinitis, the common cold and influenza.

Dosage and administration
Adults and children over 12 years: 1 tablet or 10 ml elixir every 4–6 hours up to 4 times a day.

Children 6 to 12 years: 5 ml elixir every 4–6 hours up to 4 times a day.

2 to 5 years: 2.5 ml elixir every 4–6 hours up to 4 times a day.

Sudafed Elixir may be diluted 1:1 (1 in 2) or 1:3 (1 in 4) with syrup BP. These dilutions are stable for 4 weeks if stored at 25°C.

Use in the elderly: There have been no specific studies of Sudafed in the elderly. Experience has indicated that normal adult dosage is appropriate.

Hepatic dysfunction: Caution should be exercised when administering Sudafed to patients with severe hepatic impairment.

Renal dysfunction: Caution should be exercised when administering Sudafed to patients with moderate to severe renal impairment.

Pharmacology: Pseudoephedrine has direct and indirect sympathomimetic activity and is an orally effective upper respiratory tract decongestant. Pseudoephedrine is substantially less potent than Ephedrine in producing both tachycardia and elevation in systolic blood pressure and considerably less potent in causing stimulation of the central nervous system.

Contra-indications, warnings, etc
Contra-indications: Sudafed is contra-indicated in individuals with known hypersensitivity to the product or any of its components.

Sudafed is contra-indicated in individuals with severe hypertension or coronary artery disease.

Sudafed is contra-indicated in individuals who are taking or have taken monoamine oxidase inhibitors within the preceding two weeks. The concomitant use of Sudafed and this type of product may occasionally cause a rise in blood pressure.

Precautions: Although Sudafed has virtually no pressor effects in normotensive patients, Sudafed should be used with caution in patients suffering mild to moderate hypertension.

As with other sympathomimetic agents, Sudafed should be used with caution in patients with hypertension, heart disease, diabetes, hyperthyroidism, elevated intraocular pressure and prostatic enlargement.

Caution should be exercised when using the product in the presence of severe hepatic impairment or moderate to severe renal impairment (particularly if accompanied by cardiovascular disease).

Interactions with other medicaments and other forms of interaction: Concomitant use of Sudafed with tricyclic antidepressants, sympathomimetic agents (such as decongestants, appetite suppressants and amphetamine-like psychostimulants) or with monoamine oxidase inhibitors, which interferes with the catabolism of sympathomimetic amines, may occasionally cause a rise in blood pressure.

Because of its Pseudoephedrine content, Sudafed may partially reverse the hypotensive action of drugs which interfere with sympathetic activity including Bretylium, Bethanidine, Guanethidine, Debrisoquine, Methyldopa, alpha- and beta-adrenergic blocking agents.

Side and adverse effects: Serious adverse effects associated with the use of Pseudoephedrine are rare. Symptoms of central nervous system excitation may occur, including sleep disturbances and, rarely, hallucinations have been reported.

Skin rashes, with or without irritation, have occasionally been reported. Urinary retention has been reported occasionally in men receiving Pseudoephedrine; prostatic enlargement could have been an important predisposing factor.

Use in pregnancy and lactation: Although Pseudoephedrine has been in widespread use for many years without apparent ill consequence, there are no specific data on its use during pregnancy. Caution should therefore be exercised by balancing the potential benefit of treatment to the mother against any possible hazards to the developing foetus.

Systemic administration of Pseudoephedrine, up to 50 times the human daily dosage in rats and up to 35 times the human daily dosage in rabbits, did not produce teratogenic effects.

Pseudoephedrine is excreted in breast milk in small amounts but the effect of this on breast-fed infants is not known. It has been estimated that 0.5–0.7% of a single dose of Pseudoephedrine ingested by a mother will be excreted in the breast milk over 24 hours.

Toxicity and treatment of overdosage: As with other sympathomimetic agents, symptoms of overdosage include irritability, restlessness, tremor, convulsions, palpitations, hypertension and difficulty in micturition.

Necessary measures should be taken to maintain and support respiration and control convulsions. Gastric lavage should be performed if indicated. Catheterisation of the bladder may be necessary. If desired, the elimination of Pseudoephedrine can be accelerated by acid diuresis or by dialysis.

Pharmaceutical precautions
Tablets: Store below 30°C. Keep dry. Protect from light. *Elixir:* Store below 25°C. Protect from light.

Legal category P

Package quantities Sudafed Tablets: Container of 100 tablets. Pack containing a blister strip of 12 or 24 tablets. Sudafed Elixir: Bottles of 100 ml and 1 litre.

Product licence numbers
Tablets 15513/0024
Elixir 15513/0023.

SUDAFED* PLUS TABLETS AND SYRUP

Presentation Each tablet contains 2.5 mg Triprolidine Hydrochloride BP and 60 mg Pseudoephedrine Hydrochloride BP. Scored and coded 'WELLCOME M2A'. White in colour.

Each 5 ml of clear, golden-yellow syrup contains 1.25 mg Triprolidine Hydrochloride BP and 30 mg Pseudoephedrine Hydrochloride BP, and has a pleasant flavour.

Uses Symptomatic relief of allergic rhinitis

Dosage and administration
Adults and children over 12 years: 1 tablet or 10 ml every 4–6 hours up to 4 times a day.

Children 6 to 12 years: 5 ml every 4–6 hours up to 4 times a day.

Children 2 to 5 years: 2.5 ml every 4–6 hours up to 4 times a day.

Use in the elderly: No specific studies have been carried out in the elderly, but triprolidine and pseudoephedrine have been widely used in older people.

Hepatic dysfunction: Caution should be exercised when administering Sudafed Plus Tablets or Syrup to patients with severe hepatic impairment.

Renal dysfunction: Caution should be exercised when administering Sudafed Plus Tablets or Syrup to patients with moderate to severe renal impairment.

Pharmacology: Triprolidine provides symptomatic relief in conditions believed to depend wholly or partly upon the triggered release of histamine. It is a potent competitive histamine H1- receptor antagonist of the pyrrolidine class with mild central nervous system depressant properties which may cause drowsiness.

Pseudoephedrine has direct and indirect sympathomimetic activity and is an effective upper respiratory decongestant. Pseudoephedrine is substantially less potent then ephedrine in producing both tachycardia and elevation of systolic blood pressure and considerably less potent in causing stimulation of the central nervous system.

Contra-indications, warnings, etc
Contra-indications: Sudafed Plus is contra-indicated in individuals with known hypersensitivity to pseudoephedrine or triprolidine.

Sudafed Plus is contra-indicated in patients who are taking or have taken monoamine oxidase inhibitors within the preceding two weeks. The concomitant use of pseudoephedrine and this type of product may occasionally cause a rise in blood pressure

Sudafed Plus is contra-indicated in patients with severe hypertension or severe coronary artery disease.

The antibacterial agent furazolidone is known to cause a dose-related inhibition of monoamine oxidase. Although there are no reports of hypertensive crises caused by the concurrent administration of Sudafed Plus and furazolidone, they should not be taken together.

Precautions: Sudafed Plus may cause drowsiness and impair performance in tests of auditory vigilance. Patients should not drive or operate machinery until they have determined their own response.

Although there are no objective data, users of Sudafed Plus should avoid the concomitant use of alcohol or other centrally acting sedatives.

Although pseudoephedine has virtually no pressor effects in patients with normal blood pressure, Sudafed Plus should be used with caution in patients taking antihypertensive agents, tricyclic antidepressants, other sympathomimetic agents, such as decongestants, appetite suppressants and amphetamine-like psychostimulants. The effects of a single dose on the blood pressure of these patients should be observed before recommending repeated or unsupervised treatment.

As with other sympathomimetic agents, caution should be exercised in patients with uncontrolled diabetes, hyperthyroidism, elevated intraocular pressure and prostatic enlargement.

There have been no specific studies of Sudafed Plus in patients with hepatic and/or renal dysfunction. Caution should be exercised in the presence of severe renal or hepatic impairment.

There is insufficient information available to determine whether triprolidine or pseudoephedrine have mutagenic or carcinogenic potential.

Drug interactions: Concomitant use of Sudafed Plus with sympathomimetic agents, such as decongestants, tricyclic antidepressants, appetite suppressants and amphetamine-like psychostimulants, or with monoamine oxidase inhibitors which interfere with the catabolism of sympathomimetic amines, may occasionally cause a rise in blood pressure.

Because of its pseudoephedrine content, Sudafed Plus may partially reverse the hypotensive action of drugs which interfere with sympathetic activity including bretylium, bethanidine, guanethidine, debrisoquine, methyldopa, alpha- and beta-adrenergic blocking agents.

Side- and adverse effects: Central nervous system (CNS) depression or excitation may occur, drowsiness being reported most frequently. Sleep disturbance and, rarely, hallucinations have been reported.

Skin rashes with or without irritation, tachycardia, dryness of mouth, nose and throat have occasionally been reported. Urinary retention has been reported occasionally in men receiving pseudoephedrine; prostatic enlargement could have been an important predisposing factor.

Use in pregnancy and lactation: Although pseudoephedrine and triprolidine have been in widespread use for many years without apparent ill-consequence, there are no specific data on their use during pregnancy. Caution should therefore be exercised by balancing the potential benefit of treatment to the mother against any possible hazards to the developing foetus.

In rats and rabbits systemic administration of triprolidine up to 75 times the human dose did not produce teratogenic effects.

Systemic administration of pseudoephedrine, up to 50 times the human dose in rats and up to 35 times the human dose in rabbits, did not produce teratogenic effects.

No studies have been conducted in animals to determine whether triprolidine or pseudoephedrine have potential to impair fertility. There is no information on the effect of Sudafed Plus on human fertility.

Pseudoephedrine and tripolidine are excreted in breast milk in small amounts but the effect of this on breast-fed infants is not known. It has been estimated that 0.5 to 0.7% of a single dose of pseudoephedrine ingested by a mother will be excreted in the breast milk over 24 hours.

Toxicity and treatment of overdosage: The effects of acute toxicity from Sudafed Plus may include drowsiness, lethargy, dizziness, ataxia, weakness, hypotonicity, respiratory depression, dryness of the skin and mucous membranes, tachycardia, hypertension, hyperpyrexia, hyperactivity, irritability, convulsions and difficulty with micturition.

Necessary measures should be taken to maintain and support respiration and control convulsions. Gastric lavage should be performed up to 3 hours after ingestion if indicated. Catheterisation of the bladder may be necessary. If desired, the elimination of pseudoephedrine can be accelerated by acid diuresis or by dialysis.

Pharmaceutical precautions Tablets: Store below 25°C in a dry place. Protect from light.
Syrup: Store below 25°C Protect from light.

Legal category P.

Package quantities
Sudafed Plus Tablets: Packs of 100 tablets.
Sudafed Plus Syrup: Bottles of 100 ml and 1 litre.

Product licence numbers
Sudafed Plus Tablets: 15513/0029
Sudafed Plus Syrup: 15513/0030

**Trade Mark*

Wellcome UK
The Wellcome Foundation Limited
Stockley Park
Middlesex
UB11 1BT

☎ 0181 990 9000 🗋 0181 990 4321

1990 THE QUEEN'S AWARD FOR TECHNOLOGICAL ACHIEVEMENT TO THE WELLCOME RESEARCH LABORATORIES OF THE WELLCOME FOUNDATION LTD

1991 THE QUEEN'S AWARD FOR EXPORT ACHIEVEMENT

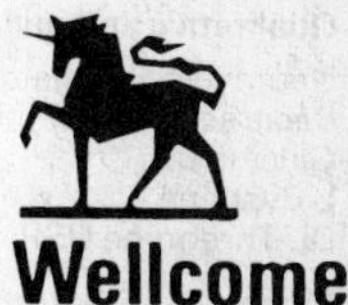

BRETYLATE* INJECTION

Qualitative and quantitative composition Bretylium Tosylate HSE 5.0% w/v.

Pharmaceutical form Injection.

Clinical particulars

Therapeutic indications: Bretylate Injection is indicated primarily for the treatment of ventricular fibrillation and has often proved effective in ventricular fibrillation resistant to direct current countershock, with or without additional use of other anti-arrhythmic drugs such as lignocaine. Consideration should be given at an early stage to the use of Bretylate Injection in resuscitation from ventricular fibrillation.

Bretylate Injection is also indicated for ventricular tachycardia and has proved successful in restoring sinus rhythm where other anti-arrhythmics have failed.

Anti-arrhythmic effectiveness of Bretylate Injection has been demonstrated in:

- Acute myocardial infarction or chronic ischaemic heart disease;
- Ventricular fibrillation complicating severe hypothermia;
- and, ventricular arrhythmias following cardiac surgery.

Posology and method of administration

Adults: For ventricular fibrillation or ventricular tachycardia with associated haemodynamic disturbance, the minimal suggested initial dose is 5 mg/kg bodyweight administered undiluted by rapid intravenous injection. Resuscitation should be continued with further attempts at electrical cardioversion. The anti-fibrillatory effect in responding patients will usually be apparent within 5 to 15 minutes.

If no response is evident after 5 minutes, the dose of bretylium may be repeated or increased to 10 mg/kg by bolus injection. There is little experience with total dosages greater than 40 mg/kg, although with such dosage, adverse effects have not been apparent. In some patients the full anti-arrhythmic effect of Bretylate Injection may require several hours to develop.

If Bretylate Injection is to be used for less serious ventricular rhythm disturbances, it should be given more slowly and in diluted form to reduce the risk of vomiting.

Dilution: Bretylate Injection should be diluted with one of the recommended infusion fluids (see below) in the ratio of 1 part Bretylate Injection added to not less than 4 parts of infusion fluid, i.e. to give a final concentration of not more than 10 mg/ml.

When diluted with either Glucose Intravenous Infusion BP (5% w/v) or Sodium Chloride Intravenous Infusion BP (0.9% w/v) in the ratios recommended, Bretylate Injection is stable for up to 24 hours.

Administration by infusion: The diluted solution (prepared as recommended above) should be infused initially over a period of at least 8 minutes, preferably over 15 to 30 minutes, so as to provide a total dose of 5 to 10 mg/kg bodyweight. If the arrhythmia persists, this initial dose may be repeated at one to two hour intervals.

Once control of the arrhythmia has been established, maintenance therapy using the diluted solution can be given either as a continuous infusion at the rate of 1 to 2 mg per minute, or with a dosage of 5 to 10 mg/kg bodyweight infused over a period of 15 to 30 minutes every 6 hours.

Intramuscular administration: Bretylate Injection has been administered by intramuscular injection. A dose of 5 to 10 mg/kg bodyweight is recommended and this is administered undiluted at intervals of 6 to 8 hours. The site of injection should be varied on repeated injection and not more than 5 ml given into any one site.

Dosage in renal impairment: With repeated bolus doses or continuous intravenous infusions of Bretylate Injection in patients with impaired renal function, it is necessary to reduce the dosage in proportion to the reduction in creatinine clearance. The use of a nomogram is recommended for administration of Bretylate Injection as an infusion to patients with renal impairment, and the literature should be consulted for details.

The following table is intended to be used as a guide for administering Bretylate Injection by continuous infusion.

Creatinine clearance (ml/minute)	*Rate of infusion (mg/hour)*
40–<90	10–40
10–<40	2–10
1–<10	0.6–2

Children: Information on the use of Bretylate Injection as an anti-arrhythmic agent in children is sparse and there are no data on its use in doses in excess of 5 mg/kg/bodyweight.

Use in the elderly: The decision to treat with Bretylate rests on the balance between the expected anti-arrhythmic effect and the disadvantages of inappropriate dosing, taking into account the degree of reduction in cardiac and renal function.

Monitoring: It is recommended that heart rate and blood pressure are monitored during the administration of Bretylate.

Route of administration: Intravenous injection or infusion or intramuscular injection.

Contra-indications: Bretylate Injection is likely to cause a severe hypertensive response in patients with phaeochromocytoma and is therefore contra-indicated in this condition.

Special warnings and precautions for use: Bretylate Injection is not recommended as a prophylactic agent to prevent serious ventricular arrhythmias, but data are conflicting.

Orthostatic hypotension may occur 20 to 30 minutes after acute administration of Bretylate Injection, and in patients with poor cardiac function clinically significant hypotension may occur even in the supine position. An asymptomatic fall in blood pressure usually need not be treated unless the systolic pressure falls below 75 to 80 mm Hg. Hypotension may also be troublesome after cardiac surgery.

Hypovolaemia will augment the hypotensive response to Bretylate Injection. If the blood pressure does not respond to simple postural manoeuvres intravenous fluid should be given. Hypotension requiring such treatment may also respond to vasopressors. Hypersensitivity to infused catecholamines must, however, be anticipated and caution exercised.

Intramuscular administration of bretylium may cause tissue necrosis at the site of injection; this is rare if the site of injection is varied and the injected volume limited to 5 ml.

Interaction with other medicaments and other forms of interaction: Parenteral administration of bretylium may exacerbate ventricular tachyarrhythmias caused by digitalis toxicity.

Hypersensitivity to infused catecholamines would be expected after Bretylate administration because it blocks their normal mechanism of metabolism, namely neuronal uptake and subsequent degradation by monoamine oxidase. For this reason, when it is necessary to increase perfusion pressure to vital organs after bretylium-induced hypotension, noradrenaline or other sympathomimetics should only be given under expert supervision.

The hypotension resulting from adrenergic neurone blockade has been prevented by inhibition of the noradrenaline uptake mechanism, principally by tricyclic antidepressants.

Pregnancy and lactation: There is no reference to the use of bretylium as an anti-arrhythmic in pregnancy in the published literature.

No information is available on the excretion of bretylium into breast milk nor, therefore, on its effects on the breastfed infant.

Effect on ability to drive and use machines: None known.

Undesirable effects: The most common side effect following the administration of bretylium is hypotension, especially in patients whose initial haemodynamic state and/or cardiac function are poor. Hypotension with increased pulmonary vascular resistance has also been reported.

Immediately after commencement of bretylium administration, more ectopic beats may arise, but this effect does not usually lead to serious problems.

Nausea and vomiting may occur following rapid intravenous administration of bretylium.

Moderate increases in blood pressure, heart rate and a positive inotropic effect may occur on commencement of bretylium administration.

Overdose: Bretylium overdose has been reported in a patient with recurrent ventricular fibrillation and tachycardia who was inadvertently given an intravenous bolus of 2 g (approximately 30 mg/kg bodyweight). The authors reported ultimately successful control of the ventricular tachyarrhythmias but the patient exhibited marked hypertension with peak blood pressure of 310/90 mm Hg, followed within an hour or so by marked hypotension refractory to intravenous dobutamine and volume-expansion therapy.

Bretylate can be eliminated by haemodialysis.

Pharmacological properties

Pharmacodynamic properties: Bretylium is a Class III anti-arrhythmic agent. It may produce pharmacological defibrillation, but more usually it facilitates electrical conversion to sinus rhythm in patients with ventricular fibrillation.

Acute administration of bretylium in both animals and man leads to a biphasic cardiovascular response. Monitoring of heart rate and blood pressure is therefore recommended. An initial release of noradrenaline from adrenergic nerve endings is accompanied by an acute rise in systemic arterial pressure and heart rate, followed within 20 to 30 minutes by reduction in vascular resistance, systemic arterial pressure and heart rate. The hypotension caused by Bretylate is orthostatic and was found to occur rarely in recumbent patients with acute myocardial infarction receiving the drug in a coronary care unit.

Pharmacokinetic properties: The anti-arrhythmic effects of a single dose of bretylium last for up to 12 hours. After a single intravenous dose bretylium appears to be eliminated from serum with an elimination half-life of about 13.5 hours. Apart from the particular effect of the drug on ventricular fibrillation, which seems to be exerted within 5 to 15 minutes of initial intravenous bolus administration, the anti-arrhythmic effects of bretylium seem to be related to tissue concentrations rather than serum or plasma concentrations of the drug and the latter are therefore probably not useful indicators during acute treatment.

Preclinical safety data: There are no preclinical data of relevance to the prescriber which are additional to that in other sections of the SmPC.

Pharmaceutical particulars

List of excipients: Water for Injections PhEur.

Incompatibilities: None known.

Shelf life: 60 months.

Special precautions for storage: Store below 25°C. Do not freeze. Protect from light.

Nature and contents of container: Neutral glass ampoules 2 ml and 10 ml. Nominal fill volume. Pack sizes: 2, 10 ml.

Instructions for use/handling: Not applicable.

Marketing authorisation number PL 0003/0038R.

Date of approval/revision of SPC February 1997.

Legal category POM.

CICATRIN* CREAM

Qualitative and quantitative composition

Neomycin Sulphate EP	330,000 units per gram
Bacitracin zinc BP	25,000 units per gram
Glycine BP	1.0% w/w
L-Cysteine	0.2% w/w
DL-Threonine USP	0.1% w/w

Pharmaceutical form Cream.

Clinical particulars
Therapeutic indications: Topical broad-spectrum antibacterial. Superficial bacterial infection of the skin, such as impetigo, varicose ulcers, pressure sores, trophic ulcers and burns.

Posology and method of administration:
Administration and dosage in adults: Before use, the area for application should be cleaned gently. Debris such as pus or crusts should be removed from the affected area.

A thin film of the cream should be applied to the affected area up to three times/day, depending on the clinical condition. Treatment should not be continued for more than 7 days without medical supervision (see *Special warnings and special precautions for use*).

Dosage in children: The adult dose is suitable for use in older children, however in infants dosage should be reduced.

A possibility of increased absorption exists in very young children, thus Cicatrin Cream is not recommended for use in neonates.

Dosage in the elderly: No specific studies have been carried out in the elderly, however, Cicatrin Cream is suitable for use in the elderly (see *Dosage in renal impairment* and *Special warnings and special precautions for use*).

Dosage in renal impairment: Dosage should be reduced in patients with reduced renal function (see *Special warnings and special precautions for use*).

Route of administration: Topical.

Contra-indications: The use of Cicatrin Cream is contra-indicated in patients who have demonstrated allergic hypersensitivity to the product or any of its constituents, or to cross-sensitising substances such as framycetin, kanamycin, gentamycin and other related antibiotics.

The presence of pre-existing nerve deafness is a contra-indication to the use of Cicatrin Cream in circumstances in which significant systemic absorption could occur.

The use of Cicatrin Cream is contra-indicated in circumstances where significant systemic absorption could occur, e.g. application of large amounts, treatment of large areas or chronic wounds, or prolonged treatment.

Cicatrin Cream should not be used on preterm infants and is not recommended for use in neonates.

Cicatrin Cream should not be applied to the eyes.

Special warnings and special precautions for use: Caution should be exercised so that the recommended dosage is not exceeded (see *Administration and dosage* and *Contra-indications*).

Following significant systemic absorption, aminoglycosides such as neomycin can cause irreversible ototoxicity (and exacerbate existing partial nerve deafness); both neomycin sulphate and bacitracin zinc have nephrotoxic potential.

After a treatment course, administration should not be repeated for at least three months.

In neonates and infants, absorption by immature skin may be enhanced and renal function may be immature (see *Contra-indications*).

In renal impairment the plasma clearance of neomycin is reduced, this is associated with an increased risk of ototoxicity; therefore, a reduction in dose should be made that relates to the degree of renal impairment.

As with other antibacterial preparations, prolonged use may result in overgrowth by non-susceptible organisms, including fungi.

Concurrent administration of other aminoglycosides is not recommended.

Interaction with other medicaments and other forms of interaction: Following significant systemic absorption, neomycin sulphate can intensify and prolong the respiratory depressant effect of neuromuscular blocking agents.

Pregnancy and lactation:
Pregnancy: There is little information to demonstrate the possible effect of topically applied neomycin in pregnancy and lactation, therefore the use of Cicatrin is not recommended.

Lactation: No information is available regarding the excretion of the active ingredients in human milk.

Effects on ability to drive and use machines: None known.

Undesirable effects: The incidence of allergic hypersensitivity to neomycin sulphate in the general population is low. However, there is an increased incidence of sensitivity to neomycin in certain selected groups of patients in dermatological practice, particularly those with venous stasis eczema and ulceration.

Allergic hypersensitivity to neomycin following topical application may manifest itself as a reddening and scaling of the affected skin, as an eczematous exacerbation of the lesion, or as a failure of the lesion to heal.

Allergic hypersensitivity, following topical application of bacitracin zinc has been reported but is rare.

Anaphylactic reactions following the topical administration of bacitracin zinc have been reported but are rare.

Overdosage:
Symptoms and signs: No specific symptoms or signs have been associated with excessive use of Cicatrin Cream. However, consideration should be given to significant systemic absorption (see *Special warnings and special precautions for use*).

Management: Use of the product should be stopped and the patient's general status, hearing acuity, renal and neuromuscular functions should be monitored. Blood levels of neomycin sulphate and bacitracin zinc should be determined, and haemodialysis may reduce the serum level of neomycin sulphate.

Pharmacological properties
Pharmacodynamic properties: Not available.

Pharmacokinetic properties: Not applicable.

Preclinical safety data:
A. Mutagenicity: There is insufficient information available to determine whether the active ingredients have mutagenic potential.

B. Carcinogenicity: There is insufficient information available to determine whether the active ingredients have carcinogenic potential.

C. Teratogenicity: There is insufficient information available to determine whether the active ingredients have teratogenic potential.

Neomycin present in maternal blood can cross the placenta and may give rise to a theoretical risk of foetal ototoxicity.

D. Fertility: There is insufficient information available to determine whether any of the active ingredients can affect fertility.

Pharmaceutical particulars
List of excipients: Sorbitan Trioleate, Wool Alcohols, Macrogol (4) Lauryl Ether, Liquid Paraffin, Polysorbate 85, Hard Paraffin, White Soft Paraffin.

Incompatibilities: Cicatrin Cream should not be diluted.

Shelf life: 2 years.

Special precautions for storage: Store below 25°C.

Nature and contents of container: Internally lacquered aluminium collapsible tubes with polypropylene screw caps. Pack size: 15 g and 30 g.

Instructions for use/handling: No special instructions.

Marketing authorisation number
Cream: PL 0003/5082R.

Date of first authorisation/renewal of authorisation 18 January 1991, 18 September 1998.

Date of (partial) revision of the text May 1996.

CICATRIN POWDER

Qualitative and quantitative composition

Neomycin Sulphate	3,300 units
Bacitracin zinc	250 units
Glycine	10 grams
L-Cysteine	2 grams
DL-Threonine	1 gram

Pharmaceutical form Powder.

Clinical particulars
Therapeutic indications: Topical broad-spectrum antibacterial. Superficial bacterial infection of the skin, such as impetigo, varicose ulcers, pressure sores, trophic ulcers and burns.

Posology and method of administration:
Administration and dosage in adults: Before use, the area for application should be cleaned gently. Debris such as pus or crusts should be removed from the affected area.

A light dusting of the powder should be applied to the affected area up to three times/day, depending on the clinical condition. Treatment should not be continued for more than 7 days without medical supervision (see *Special warnings and special precautions for use*).

Dosage in children: The adult dose is suitable for use in older children, however in infants dosage should be reduced.

A possibility of increased absorption exists in very young children, thus Cicatrin Powder is not recommended for use in neonates.

Dosage in the elderly: No specific studies have been carried out in the elderly however, Cicatrin Powder is suitable for use in the elderly (see *Dosage in renal impairment* and *Special warnings and special precautions for use*).

Dosage in renal impairment: Dosage should be reduced in patients with reduced renal function (see *Special warnings and special precautions for use*).

Route of administration: Topical.

Contra-indications: The use of Cicatrin Powder is contra-indicated in patients who have demonstrated allergic hypersensitivity to the product or any of its constituents, or to cross-sensitising substances such as framycetin, kanamycin, gentamycin and other related antibiotics.

The use of Cicatrin Powder is contra-indicated in circumstances where significant systemic absorption could occur, e.g. application of large amounts, treatment of large areas or chronic wounds, or prolonged treatment.

The presence of pre-existing nerve deafness is a contra-indication to the use of Cicatrin Powder in circumstances in which significant systemic absorption could occur.

Cicatrin Powder should not be used on preterm infants and is not recommended for use in neonates.

Cicatrin Powder should not be applied to the eyes.

Special warnings and special precautions for use: Caution should be exercised so that the recommended dosage is not exceeded (see *Administration and dosage* and *Contra-indications*).

Following significant systemic absorption, aminoglycosides such as neomycin can cause irreversible ototoxicity (and exacerbate existing partial nerve deafness); both neomycin sulphate and bacitracin zinc have nephrotoxic potential.

After a treatment course, administration should not be repeated for at least three months.

In neonates and infants, absorption by immature skin may be enhanced and renal function may be immature (see *Contra-indications*).

In renal impairment the plasma clearance of neomycin is reduced, this is associated with an increased risk of ototoxicity; therefore, a reduction in dose should be made that relates to the degree of renal impairment.

As with other antibacterial preparations, prolonged use may result in overgrowth by non-susceptible organisms, including fungi.

Concurrent administration of other aminoglycosides is not recommended.

Interaction with other medicaments and other forms of interaction: Following significant systemic absorption, neomycin sulphate can intensify and prolong the respiratory depressant effect of neuromuscular blocking agents.

Pregnancy and lactation:
Pregnancy: There is little information to demonstrate the possible effect of topically applied neomycin in pregnancy and lactation, therefore the use of Cicatrin is not recommended.

Lactation: No information is available regarding the excretion of the active ingredients in human milk.

Effects on ability to drive and use machines: None known.

Undesirable effects: The incidence of allergic hypersensitivity to neomycin sulphate in the general population is low. However, there is an increased incidence of sensitivity to neomycin in certain selected groups of patients in dermatological practice, particularly those with venous stasis eczema and ulceration.

Allergic hypersensitivity to neomycin following topical application may manifest itself as a reddening and scaling of the affected skin, as an eczematous exacerbation of the lesion, or as a failure of the lesion to heal.

Allergic hypersensitivity, following topical application of bacitracin zinc has been reported but is rare.

Anaphylactic reactions following the topical administration of bacitracin zinc have been reported but are rare.

Overdosage:
Symptoms and signs: No specific symptoms or signs have been associated with excessive use of Cicatrin Powder. However, consideration should be given to significant systemic absorption (see *Special warnings and special precautions for use*).

Management: Use of the product should be stopped and the patient's general status, hearing acuity, renal and neuromuscular functions should be monitored. Blood levels of neomycin sulphate and bacitracin zinc should be determined, and haemodialysis may reduce the serum level of neomycin sulphate.

Pharmacological properties
Pharmacodynamic properties: Not available.

Pharmacokinetic properties: Not applicable.

Preclinical safety data:
A. Mutagenicity: There is insufficient information available to determine whether the active ingredients have mutagenic potential.

B. Carcinogenicity: There is insufficient information available to determine whether the active ingredients have carcinogenic potential.

C. Teratogenicity: There is insufficient information available to determine whether the active ingredients have teratogenic potential.

Neomycin present in maternal blood can cross the placenta and may give rise to a theoretical risk of foetal ototoxicity.

D. Fertility: There is insufficient information available to determine whether any of the active ingredients can affect fertility.

Pharmaceutical particulars
List of excipients: Sterilised Maize Starch.
Incompatibilities: Cicatrin Powder should not be diluted.

Shelf life: 2 years.

Special precautions for storage: Store below 25°C.

Nature and contents of container: Low density polyethylene bottles with nozzle inserts and urea formaldehyde screw caps. Pack size: 15 g and 50 g.

Instructions for use/handling: No special instructions.

Marketing authorisation number PL 0003/5081R.

Date of first authorisation/renewal of authorisation 25.01.91/13.08.96.

DIGIBIND*
Digoxin-specific antibody fragments (Fab)

Presentation Each vial of Digibind contains a sterile, lyophilised, crystalline off-white powder, comprising 38 mg of antigen-binding fragments (Fab) derived from specific anti-digoxin antibodies raised in sheep; approximately 75 mg Sorbitol BP and approximately 28 mg Sodium Chloride BP.

Uses Digibind is indicated for the treatment of known or strongly suspected digoxin or digitoxin toxicity, where measures beyond the withdrawal of the digitalis glycoside and correction of any serum electrolyte abnormality are felt to be necessary.

Dosage and administration
Dosage: The dosage of Digibind varies according to the amount of digoxin (or digitoxin) to be neutralised. The average dose used during clinical testing was 10 vials. When determining the dose for Digibind, the following guidelines should be considered:

Dosage estimates are based on a steady-state volume of distribution of 5 l/kg for digoxin (0.5 l/kg for digitoxin) to convert serum digitalis concentration to the amount of digitalis in the body. These volumes are population averages and vary widely among individuals. Many patients may require higher doses for complete neutralisation. Doses should ordinarily be rounded up to the next whole vial.

Erroneous calculations may result from inaccurate estimates of the amount of digitalis ingested or absorbed or from non steady-state serum digitalis concentrations. Inaccurate serum digitalis concentration measurements are a possible source of error; this is especially so for very high values, since most digoxin assay kits are not designed to measure values above 5 nanogram/ml.

If, after several hours, toxicity has not adequately reversed or appears to recur, re-administration of Digibind at a dose guided by clinical judgement may be required.

Acute ingestion of unknown amount of glycoside: Adults and children over 20 kg: If a patient presents with potentially life-threatening digitalis toxicity after acute ingestion of an unknown amount of digoxin or digitoxin, and neither a serum digoxin concentration nor an estimate of the ingested amount of glycoside is available, 20 vials of Digibind can be administered. This amount will be adequate to treat most life-threatening ingestions in adults and large children.

As an alternative, the physician may consider administering 10 vials of Digibind, observing the patient's response, and following with an additional 10 vials if clinically indicated.

Infants and children ≤ 20 kg: In infants and small children (≤ 20 kg) with potentially life-threatening digitalis toxicity after acute ingestion of an unknown amount of digoxin or digitoxin, when neither a serum concentration nor an estimate of the ingested amount is available, clinical judgement must be exercised to estimate an appropriate number of vials of Digibind to administer.

This estimate should be based on the maximum likely total body load of glycoside and the neutralising capacity of Digibind (one vial of Digibind per 0.5 mg of digoxin or digitoxin). It is important to monitor for volume overload during administration of Digibind.

Acute ingestion of known amount of glycoside: Each vial of Digibind contains 38 mg of purified digoxin-specific Fab fragments which will bind approximately 0.5 mg of digoxin or digitoxin. Thus one can calculate the total number of vials required by dividing the total digitalis body load in mg by 0.5 (see Formula 1).

Formula 1

$$\text{Dose (in number of vials)} = \frac{\text{Total body load (mg)}}{0.5}$$

For toxicity from an acute ingestion, total body load in milligrams will be approximately equal to the amount ingested in milligrams for digitoxin, or the amount ingested in milligrams multiplied by 0.80 (to account for incomplete absorption) for digoxin. Table 1 gives Digibind doses based on an estimate of the number of digoxin tablets (0.25 mg) ingested as a single dose and is applicable to children or adults.

TABLE 1 Approximate Digibind Dose for Reversal of a Single Large Digoxin Overdose

Number of digoxin tablets*	Digibind Dose (number of vials)
25	10
50	20
75	30
100	40
150	60
200	80

* 0.25 mg tablets with 80% bioavailability.

Toxicity during chronic therapy: Adults and children over 20 kg: In adults and children over 20 kg with digitalis toxicity resulting from chronic digoxin or digitoxin therapy and for whom a steady-state serum concentration is not available, a dose of 6 vials of Digibind will usually be adequate to reverse toxicity.

Table 2 (see below) gives dosage estimates in number of vials for adult patients for whom a steady-state serum digoxin concentration is known. The Digibind dose (in number of vials) represented in Table 2 can be approximated using the following formula:

Formula 2

$$\text{Dose (in number of vials)} = \frac{\text{(serum digoxin concentration in ng/ml x weight in kg)}}{100}$$

In patients for whom a steady-state serum digitoxin concentration is known the Digibind dose (in number of vials) can be approximated using the following formula:

Formula 3

$$\text{Dose (in number of vials)} = \frac{\text{serum digitoxin concentration in ng/ml x weight in kg}}{1000}$$

Infants and children ≤ 20 kg: In infants and small children with toxicity resulting from chronic digoxin or digitoxin therapy and for whom a steady-state serum concentration is not available, a dose of one vial of Digibind will usually suffice.

Clinical experience in children has indicated that the calculation of dose of Digibind from steady-state serum digoxin concentration may be carried out as for adults.

Table 3 gives dosage estimates in milligrams for infants and small children based on the steady-state serum digoxin concentration. The Digibind dose represented in Table 3 can be estimated by multiplying the dose (in number of vials) calculated from Formula 2 by the amount of Digibind contained in a vial (38 mg/vial).

Formula 4

Dose (in mg) = 38 x dose (in number of vials)

For very small doses, it may be necessary to dilute the reconstituted vial with sterile isotonic saline to achieve a concentration of 1 mg/ml, and to administer the dose with a tuberculin syringe.

Use in the elderly: Clinical experience has indicated that Digibind is effective and that calculation of dose may be carried out as for adults.

Use in renal impairment: See *Precautions.*

Administration: The contents of each vial to be used should be dissolved in 4 ml of sterile Water for Injection BP, by gentle mixing, thus producing an approximately isosmotic solution with a protein concentration of between 8.5 and 10.5 mg/ml. This may be diluted further to any convenient volume with sterile saline suitable for infusion.

The final solution of Digibind should be infused intravenously over a 30 minute period. Infusion through a 0.22 micron membrane filter is recommended to remove any incompletely dissolved aggregates of Digibind. If cardiac arrest seems imminent, Digibind can be given as a bolus intravenous injection.

Pharmacology: The affinity constant (K_D) of Fab for digoxin is high ($10^{11}M^{-1}$) and greater than that of digoxin for its receptor (Na-K ATPase). The affinity constant of Fab for digitoxin is also high (fifteen fold lower than for digoxin). Digoxin and digitoxin are therefore attracted away from the receptor on heart tissue (and presumably other tissues as well, though this has not been studied) and their rate of elimination is changed from that governed by the kinetics of receptor binding to that governed by the kinetics of access and elimination of Fab.

In dogs, anti-digoxin Fab reverses arrhythmic manifestations of digoxin toxicity much more quickly than does IgG. There is a suggestion that reversal of inotropy with Fab lags behind reversal of cardiac electrophysiological effects.

The plasma elimination (β) half-life of ovine digoxin-specific Fab in the baboon is 9 to 13h and that of the parent IgG antibody is 61h. The total volume of distribution of Digibind in the baboon appears to be about 9 times greater than that of IgG and more ready diffusion of the smaller moiety sufficiently accounts for this.

About 93% of radioactively labelled Fab, injected into baboons, was recovered in the urine within 24h and the corresponding amount of recoverable digoxin-specific IgG was less than 1%. Much of the urinary Fab was not intact; after glomerular filtration, low molecular weight proteins are taken into proximal renal tubular cells and catabolised.

Corresponding information on human patients is sparse, but the close relationship of therapeutic performance to predictions suggest that the animal data will be helpful. The human plasma elimination half-life after intravenous administration of Digibind is about 16 to 20h with good renal function.

Ordinarily, following administration of Digibind, improvements in signs and symptoms of digitalis intoxication begin within 30 minutes.

Contra-indications, warnings, etc
Contra-indications: None known.

TABLE 2: Adult Dose Estimate of Digibind (in number of vials) from Steady-State Serum Digoxin Concentration

Patient Weight (kg)	Serum Digoxin Concentration (ng/ml)						
	1	2	4	8	12	16	20
40	0.5^{v}	1^{v}	2^{v}	3^{v}	5^{v}	7^{v}	8^{v}
60	0.5^{v}	1^{v}	3^{v}	5^{v}	7^{v}	10^{v}	12^{v}
70	1^{v}	2^{v}	3^{v}	6^{v}	9^{v}	11^{v}	14^{v}
80	1^{v}	2^{v}	3^{v}	7^{v}	10^{v}	13^{v}	16^{v}
100	1^{v}	2^{v}	4^{v}	8^{v}	12^{v}	16^{v}	20^{v}

^{v}=vials

TABLE 3: Infants and Small Children Dose Estimates of Digibind (in mg) from Steady-State Serum Digoxin Concentration

Patient Weight (kg)	Serum Digoxin Concentration (ng/ml)						
	1	2	4	8	12	16	20
1	0.4 mg*	1 mg*	1.5 mg*	3 mg	5 mg	6 mg	8 mg
3	1 mg*	2 mg*	5 mg	9 mg	14 mg	18 mg	23 mg
5	2 mg*	4 mg	8 mg	15 mg	23 mg	30 mg	38 mg
10	4 mg	8 mg	15 mg	30 mg	46 mg	61 mg	76 mg
20	8 mg	15 mg	30 mg	61 mg	91 mg	122 mg	152 mg

* Dilution of reconstituted vial to 1 mg/ml may be desirable.

Precautions: Failure to respond to Digibind raises the possibility that the clinical problem is not caused by digitalis intoxication. If there is no response to an adequate dose of Digibind, the diagnosis of digitalis toxicity should be questioned.

Although allergic reactions have been reported rarely, the possibility of anaphylactic, hypersensitive or febrile reactions should be borne in mind. The likelihood of an allergic reaction is distinctly greater where there is a history of allergy to antibiotics or asthma. Since papain is used to cleave the whole antibody into Fab and Fc fragments, and traces of papain or inactivated papain residues may be present in Digibind, patients with known allergies to papain, chymopapain or other papaya extracts would be at particular risk, as would those allergic to ovine proteins. However, as the Fab fragment of the antibody lacks the antigenic determinants of the Fc fragment it should present less of an immunogenic threat to patients than does an intact immunoglobulin molecule.

Many patients with mild or moderate renal dysfunction and some with severe renal dysfunction have been treated successfully with Digibind. There has been no evidence that administration of Digibind to patients with renal dysfunction will exacerbate that dysfunction; the dominant pattern of serial serum creatinine measurements has been one of stable or improved renal function after Digibind administration. The time course and general pattern of therapeutic effect have not been different in patients with severe renal dysfunction, although excretion of the Fab-digoxin complexes from the body is slowed in this situation. A theoretical possibility exists that digoxin could be released after some days from Fab-digoxin complexes which remained in the circulation because their excretion was prevented by renal failure. However, this phenomenon has proved to be rare.

Patients previously dependent on the inotropism of digoxin may develop signs of heart failure when treated with Digibind. After successful management of poisoning, digoxin has had to be reinstituted in some cases. If deemed absolutely necessary, additional inotropic support can be obtained from a non-glycoside inotropic drug such as dopamine or dobutamine, but caution is required as catecholamines and catecholamine analogues can aggravate arrhythmias caused by cardiac glycosides.

Parenteral drug products should be inspected visually for particulate matter and discoloration prior to administration, whenever solution and container permit.

Monitoring and laboratory tests: Patients should have continuous electrocardiographic monitoring during and for at least 24 hours after administration of Digibind.

Presence of the exogenous antibody fragments will interfere with radioimmunoassay measurements of digoxin.

The total serum digoxin concentration may rise precipitously following administration of Digibind, but this will be almost entirely bound to the Fab fragment and therefore not able to react with receptors in the body.

Serum potassium concentrations should be followed carefully, since severe digitalis intoxication can cause life-threatening elevation in serum potassium concentration by shifting it from within the cells. When the effect of digitalis is reversed by Digibind, potassium returns to the cell causing the serum potassium concentrations to fall. It is possible for there to be a total body deficit of potassium in the presence of digitalis toxicity-induced hyperkalaemia and Digibind treatment could result in a significant hypokalaemia.

Side- and adverse effects: Allergic responses of possible or probable attribution to Digibind have been reported rarely. The development of a pruritic rash (either with or without facial flushing and swelling) or shaking or chills without fever, have occurred on the day of treatment. Urticaria and thrombocytopenia have occurred up to 16 days post treatment. There are no reports of any allergic reactions to re-administration of Digibind in the same patient, but there are few instances on which information is available.

Use in pregnancy and lactation: To date there is no evidence that Digibind administered during human pregnancy causes foetal abnormalities; however, the use of Digibind should be considered only if the expected clinical benefit of treatment to the mother outweighs any possible risk to the developing foetus.

Carcinogenesis, mutagenesis, impairment of fertility: There have been no long-term studies performed in animals to evaluate carcinogenic or mutagenic potential or effects on fertility.

Drug interactions: No drug interactions have been identified.

Toxicity and treatment of overdosage: Not relevant.

Pharmaceutical precautions Store at 2 to 8°C. Protect from light. After reconstitution store between 2 and 8°C for up to 4 hours.

Reconstituted product should be used promptly. If it is not used immediately, it may be stored under refrigeration between 2 and 8°C for up to 4 hours. The reconstituted product may be diluted with sterile isotonic saline to a convenient volume.

Legal category POM

Package quantities Single vial of lyophilised powder containing 38 mg of antigen-binding fragments (Fab).

Further information Digoxin-specific antibody Fab fragments have been used successfully to treat a case of lanatoside C intoxication. Reversal of β-methyl digoxin and β-acetyl digoxin-induced arrhythmias by Digibind has been verified in guinea-pigs.

Product licence number 0003/0207

EXOSURF* NEONATAL

Qualitative and quantitative composition Colfosceril Palmitate HSE 108.0 mg or 67.5 mg.

Pharmaceutical form Lyophilised powder, for endotracheal administration after reconstitution.

Clinical particulars

Therapeutic indications: Exosurf Neonatal is indicated for the treatment of newborn infants with or at risk of respiratory distress syndrome, who are undergoing mechanical ventilation and whose heart rate and arterial oxygenation are continuously monitored.

Posology and method of administration:

Recommended doses and dosage schedules: A dose of 5 ml/kg birthweight of reconstituted Exosurf Neonatal should be given via the endotracheal tube. If the baby is still intubated, a second equal dose should be given 12 hours later by the same route. Each dose corresponds to 67.5 mg of colfosceril palmitate per kg birthweight.

Reconstitution: The contents of each vial of Exosurf Neonatal should be reconstituted with the diluent supplied. If this is not available, for the 108 mg vial use 8 ml of water for injections BP (i.e. sterile, preservative-free water) and for the 67.5 mg vial use 5 ml. This gives a white suspension containing 13.5 mg per ml colfosceril palmitate.

Exosurf Neonatal is physically and chemically stable for 24 hours after reconstitution if stored between 2 and 30 degrees centigrade. Exosurf Neonatal contains no antimicrobial preservative. Reconstitution should therefore be performed, either immediately before use, or, if storage is required, under sterile conditions. In either case, any unused suspension should be discarded.

Carry out the preparation as follows:

1. Fill a syringe with the required volume of diluent.
2. Allow the vacuum in the vial of Exosurf Neonatal to draw the diluent into the vial through a needle.
3. Aspirate the resulting suspension back into the syringe and then release the syringe plunger to allow the suspension to return into the Exosurf Neonatal vial.
4. Repeat aspiration and return three or four times to ensure adequate mixing of the vial contents. If the suspension appears to separate, gently shake or swirl the vial to resuspend.
5. Withdraw the required volume of Exosurf Neonatal Suspension from the vial with the tip of the withdrawing needle well below the froth on the surface of the suspension.

Administration: Exosurf Neonatal should be administered only by those trained and experienced in the care and resuscitation of preterm infants.

Exosurf Neonatal can only be administered to endotracheally intubated infants undergoing mechanical ventilation. Infants should not be intubated solely for the administration of Exosurf Neonatal.

The infant's airway should be cleared by suction prior to the administration of Exosurf Neonatal.

Exosurf Neonatal is administered from a syringe into the endotracheal tube via the side-port on a special endotracheal adaptor, without interrupting mechanical ventilation. The part of the endotracheal tube outside the infant should be aligned vertically during administration.

The total dose should be administered at a rate slow enough to allow reconstituted Exosurf Neonatal suspension to pass into the lungs through the endotracheal tube without accumulation. The minimum recommended time for administration of the full dose is 4 minutes.

Dosing should be slowed or interrupted if the infant's skin colour deteriorates, the heart rate slows, arterial oxygen monitors indicate more than transitory depression of arterial oxygen concentration or Exosurf Neonatal accumulates in the endotracheal tube.

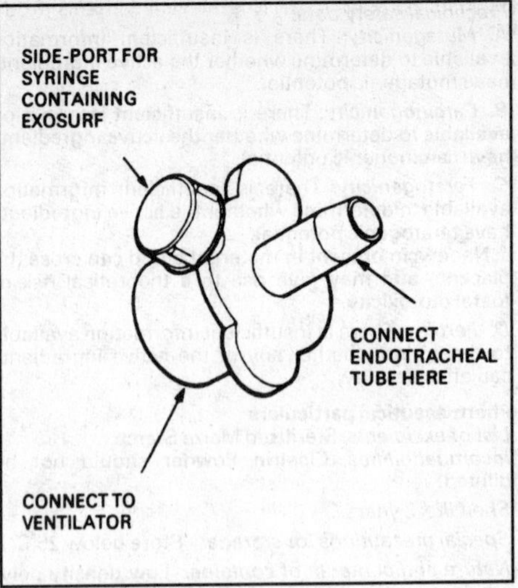

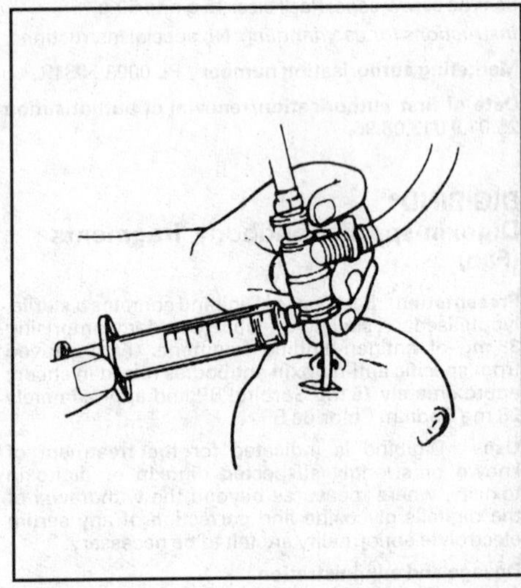

Contra-indications: There are no known contra-indications to treatment with Exosurf Neonatal.

Special warnings and special precautions for use: Exosurf Neonatal should only be administered with adequate facilities for ventilation and monitoring of babies with RDS.

Preterm birth is hazardous, surfactant administration can be expected to diminish the severity of respiratory distress syndrome and hence to diminish complications of the intensive care, especially of the ventilatory support required for the treatment of respiratory distress syndrome, but cannot be expected to eliminate entirely the mortality and morbidity associated with preterm delivery. Infants who but for the administration of surfactant might have died from RDS may be exposed to other complications of their immaturity.

As a consequence of the surfactant properties of Exosurf Neonatal, chest expansion may improve rapidly after dosing. To avoid the risk of pneumothorax and other forms of pulmonary air leak, rapid reduction in peak ventilatory pressure may therefore be necessary.

The improvement in lung mechanics resulting from Exosurf Neonatal administration may result in rapid improvement in arterial oxygen concentration. After any appropriate reduction in ventilator pressure, rapid reduction in inspired oxygen concentration may be needed to avoid hyperoxaemia.

Infants no longer requiring positive pressure ventilation may require treatment for apnoea of prematurity. In clinical trials, infants treated with Exosurf Neonatal had a higher incidence of apnoea, probably as a consequence of earlier ending of positive pressure ventilation. There were no adverse consequences in terms of increased mortality or long-term morbidity associated with this increased incidence.

Problems encountered during dosing in the clinical trials included reflux of Exosurf and changes in arterial oxygen partial pressure (rises and falls of greater than 20 mm Hg). These should be managed by careful attention to the dosing instructions (see *Administration*).

Interaction with other medicaments and other forms of interaction: No specific drug interactions have been identified.

Pregnancy and lactation: Not relevant with this product.

Effects on ability to drive and use machines: Not relevant with this product.

Undesirable effects: Pulmonary haemorrhage, the incidence of which increases the more immature the infant, is a rare but sometimes fatal complication of preterm delivery. In a placebo-controlled trial of single dose Exosurf Neonatal prophylaxis in babies with birth weight 500–700 g, the incidence of pulmonary haemorrhage was significantly increased in the Exosurf group (11% versus 2% in the placebo group). Although no other single trial of Exosurf Neonatal has demonstrated a significant increase in pulmonary haemorrhage, cross study analyses suggest that Exosurf Neonatal administration may be associated with an increase from 1% to 2% in the incidence of pulmonary haemorrhage. As might be expected, this association appears to be more marked the more immature the infant. In an open uncontrolled study of Exosurf Neonatal administration in 11,455 infants the reported incidence of pulmonary haemorrhage was 4%.

Pulmonary haemorrhage after surfactant administration is believed to be a consequence of increased pulmonary blood flow in the presence of a patent ductus arteriosus. Preventative measures, early diagnosis and the treatment of patent ductus arteriosus, especially during the first three days of life, may reduce the incidence of pulmonary haemorrhage.

In occasional infants (approximately three per thousand) Exosurf Neonatal administration has been associated with obstruction of the endotracheal tube by mucous secretions. If endotracheal tube obstruction is suspected this should be treated, according to normal practice, by suction of the tube, or by replacement of the tube if suction is unsuccessful.

Overdosage: There have been no reports of overdosage with Exosurf Neonatal. In case of accidental overdosage, as much as possible of the suspension should be aspirated and the baby should then be managed with supportive treatment, with particular attention to fluid and electrolyte balance.

Pharmacological properties

Pharmacodynamic properties: Exosurf Neonatal is designed to replace deficient surfactant in newborn infants with respiratory distress syndrome. The active component colfosceril palmitate (dipalmitoylphosphatidylcholine) is the major surface active component of natural lung surfactant and acts by forming a stable film that stabilises the terminal airways by lowering the surface tension of the pulmonary fluid lining them. The lowered surface tension prevents alveolar collapse at end-inspiration; the hysteresis effect equalises the distension of adjacent alveoli and hence prevents overdistension which might result in alveolar rupture and pulmonary air leak.

Pharmacokinetic properties: Dipalmitoylphosphatidylcholine is a naturally occurring saturated phospholipid. It can be absorbed from the alveolus into lung tissue then reutilised for further phospholipid synthesis and secretion into the alveolus as new surfactant. Metabolism by the normal metabolic pathways would be followed by incorporation of the products into the body pools.

Preclinical safety data:

A. Mutagenicity: Exosurf Neonatal was non-mutagenic in the Ames Salmonella assay.

B. Carcinogenicity: No studies have been performed in animals to determine whether Exosurf Neonatal has carcinogenic potential.

C. Fertility: The effects of Exosurf Neonatal on fertility have not been studied.

Pharmaceutical particulars

List of excipients: Cetyl alcohol 98% HSE, Hydrochloric acid EP – used to adjust pH, Sodium hydroxide BP – used to adjust pH, Sodium chloride EP, Tyloxapol USP, Water for injections EP.

Incompatibilities: None known.

Shelf life: Exosurf Neonatal Sterile powder, 3 years; Reconstituted Exosurf Neonatal, 24 hours.

Special precautions for storage: Exosurf Neonatal Sterile powder, store below 30°C; Reconstituted Exosurf Neonatal, store between 2 and 30°C.

Nature and contents of container: Neutral glass vials closed with a synthetic bromobutyl rubber stopper secured with an aluminium collar with a plastic flip top cover.

Each pack of Exosurf also contains a vial of water for injection (PL 0003/0284) and five different sizes of sterile endotracheal adaptors for use in administration of the product.

Marketing authorisation number PL 0003/0283.

Date of first authorisation/renewal of authorisation 14.12.90/14.12.95.

FLOLAN

Qualitative and quantitative composition Epoprostenol sodium 0.5 mg.

Pharmaceutical form Freeze-dried powder.

Clinical particulars

Therapeutic indications: Flolan is indicated as an alternative to heparin during renal dialysis, especially when a high risk of bleeding problems due to heparin exists.

Route of administration: By continuous infusion, either intravascularly or into the blood supplying the dialyser.

Posology and method of administration: Flolan is suitable for continuous infusion only, either intravascularly or into the blood supplying the dialyser.

The following schedule of infusion has been found effective in adults:

Prior to dialysis: 5 nanogram/kg/min intravenously.

During dialysis: 5 nanogram/kg/min into the arterial inlet of the dialyser.

The infusion should be stopped at the end of dialysis.

The recommended doses should be exceeded only with appropriate patient monitoring.

Use in children: There is no specific information on the use of Flolan in children.

Use in the elderly: There is no specific information available on the use of Flolan in elderly patients.

Reconstitution: Only the diluent provided for the purpose should be used. The enclosed filter unit must be used once only and then discarded after use.

To reconstitute Flolan, a strict aseptic technique must be used. **Particular care should be taken in calculating dilutions**, and in diluting Flolan the following procedure is recommended:

1. Withdraw approximately 10 ml of the sterile diluent into a sterile syringe.
2. Inject the contents of the syringe into the vial containing Flolan and dissolve the contents completely.
3. Draw up all the Flolan solution into the syringe.
4. Re-inject the entire contents into the residue of the original 50 ml of sterile diluent.
5. Mix well. This solution is now referred to as the ***concentrated solution*** and contains Flolan 10,000 nanograms per millilitre. The ***concentrated solution*** is normally further diluted before use. It may be diluted with physiological saline (0.9%), provided a ratio of 6 volumes of saline to 1 volume of ***concentrated solution*** is not exceeded; e.g. 50 ml of ***concentrated solution*** further diluted with a maximum of 300 ml saline. Other common intravenous fluids are unsatisfactory for the dilution of the ***concentrated solution*** as the required pH is not attained. Flolan solutions are less stable at low pH. For administration using a pump capable of delivering small volume constant infusions, suitable aliquots of concentrated solution may be diluted with sterile physiological saline.
6. Before further dilution, draw up the ***concentrated solution*** into a larger syringe.
7. The filter provided should then be attached to the syringe and the ***concentrated solution*** is dispensed by filtration using firm but not excessive pressure. The typical time taken for filtration of 50 ml of solution is 70 seconds.

When reconstituted and diluted as directed, Flolan infusion solutions have a pH of approximately 10 and will retain 90% of their initial potency for approximately 12 hours at 25°C.

Infusion rate guidance: In general, the infusion rate may be calculated by the following formula:

$$\text{Infusion rate (ml/min)} = \frac{\text{Dosage (ng/kg/min)} \times \text{bodyweight (kg)}}{\text{Concentration of infusion (ng/ml)}}$$

Examples: Flolan may be administered in diluted form (1) or as the ***concentrated solution*** (2) (see Tables below).

Contra-indications: There are no recognised contra-indications to the administration of Flolan in renal dialysis.

Special warnings and special precautions for use: Because of the high pH of the final infusion solutions, care should be taken to avoid extravasation during their administration and consequent risk of tissue damage.

Flolan is a potent vasodilator. The cardiovascular effects during infusion disappear within 30 minutes of the end of administration.

Flolan is not a conventional anticoagulant. Flolan has been successfully used instead of heparin in renal dialysis, but in a small proportion of dialyses clotting has developed in the dialysis circuit, requiring termination of dialysis.

Haemorrhagic complications have not been encountered with Flolan but the possibility should be considered when the drug is administered to patients with spontaneous or drug-induced haemorrhagic diatheses.

Blood pressure and heart rate should be monitored during administration of Flolan. Tachycardia, bradycardia and hypotension may occur during infusions of Flolan.

The effects of Flolan on heart-rate may be masked by concomitant use of drugs which affect cardiovascular reflexes.

If excessive hypotension occurs during administration of Flolan, the dose should be reduced or the infusion discontinued.

The hypotensive effect of Flolan may be enhanced by the use of acetate buffer in the dialysis bath during renal dialysis.

Elevated serum glucose levels have been reported during infusion of Flolan in man but these are not inevitable.

The pack for this product will contain the following statements:

Keep out of reach of children.
Store below 25°C.
Do not freeze.
Protect from light.
Keep dry.
Reconstitute only with the glycine buffer provided.
Prepare immediately prior to use.
Discard any unused solution after 12 hours.

Interaction with other medicaments and other forms of interaction: Flolan may potentiate the action of heparin, and standard anticoagulant monitoring is advisable when Flolan is administered to patients receiving concomitant anticoagulants.

The vasodilator effect of Flolan may augment or be augmented by concomitant use of other vasodilators.

Pregnancy and lactation: In the absence of adequate experience of administration of Flolan to pregnant women, the potential benefit to the mother must be weighed against the unknown risks to the foetus.

There is no information on the use of Flolan during lactation.

Effect on ability to drive and use machines: Not applicable.

Undesirable effects: Facial flushing is commonly seen, even in the anaesthetised patient.

1. *Diluted:* A commonly used dilution is: 10 ml ***concentrated solution*** + 40 ml physiological saline (0.9%).
Resultant concentration = 2,000 nanogram/ml epoprostenol.

		Body weight (kilograms) 30	40	50	60	70	80	90	100
Dosage (ng/kg/min)	1	0.90	1.20	1.50	1.80	2.10	2.40	2.70	3.00
	2	1.80	2.40	3.00	3.60	4.20	4.80	5.40	6.00
	3	2.70	3.60	4.50	5.40	6.30	7.20	8.10	9.00
	4	3.60	4.80	6.00	7.20	8.40	9.60	10.80	12.00
	5	4.50	6.00	7.50	9.00	10.50	12.00	13.50	15.00

Flow rates in mls/hr

2. Using ***concentrated solution,*** i.e. 10,000 ng/ml epoprostenol.

		Body weight (kilograms) 30	40	50	60	70	80	90	100
Dosage (ng/kg/min)	1	0.18	0.24	0.30	0.36	0.42	0.48	0.54	0.60
	2	0.36	0.48	0.60	0.72	0.84	0.96	1.08	1.20
	3	0.54	0.72	0.90	1.08	1.26	1.44	1.62	1.80
	4	0.72	0.96	1.20	1.44	1.68	1.92	2.16	2.40
	5	0.90	1.20	1.50	1.80	2.10	2.40	2.70	3.00

Flow rates in mls/hr

Headache and gastro-intestinal symptoms including nausea, vomiting and abdominal colic have occurred in some conscious individuals.

Jaw pain, dry mouth, lassitude, reddening over the infusion site, chest pain and tightness have been reported with varying frequency.

Bradycardia, accompanied by pallor, nausea, sweating and sometimes abdominal discomfort and orthostatic hypotension, have occurred in healthy volunteers at doses of epoprostenol sodium greater than 5 nanogram/kg/min. Bradycardia associated with a considerable fall in systolic and diastolic blood pressure has followed intravenous administration of a dose of epoprostenol sodium equivalent to 30 nanogram/kg/min in healthy conscious volunteers.

Overdosage: The main feature of overdosage is likely to be hypotension.

Reduce the dose or discontinue the infusion and initiate appropriate supportive measures as necessary; for example, plasma volume expansion and/or adjustment to pump flow.

Pharmacological properties

Pharmacodynamic properties: Epoprostenol is a naturally occurring prostaglandin produced by the intima of blood vessels and is the most potent inhibitor of platelet aggregation known. The inhibition is dose-related unlike many other prostaglandins. It is not metabolised during passage through the pulmonary circulation.

Epoprostenol sodium is a potent vasodilator. The cardiovascular effects disappear within 30 minutes of the end of infusion.

It inhibits platelet aggregation by elevating platelet cyclic adenosine monophosphate. The action is dose-related above 2 nanograms/kg/min. Following intravenous administration significant inhibition of aggregation induced by adenosine diphosphate is observed after intravenous administration of 4 or more nanograms/kg/min. Effects on patelets usually disappear within 30 minutes of discontinuing infusion of epoprostenol sodium.

Higher doses of epoprostenol sodium (20 nanograms/kg/min) disperse circulating platelet aggregates and increase by up to two fold the cutaneous bleeding time.

Epoprostenol sodium reduces platelet procoagulant activity and the release of heparin neutralising factor.

Pharmacokinetic properties: The fate of epoprostenol sodium in man is not fully established. At normal physiological pH and temperature epoprostenol sodium is hydrolysed with a half-life of 2–3 minutes to 6-keto prostaglandin F.

Preclinical safety data: There are no pre-clinical data of relevance to the prescriber which are additional to that already included in other sections of the SPC.

Pharmaceutical particulars

List of excipients: Glycine BP 3.76 mg, Sodium chloride EP 2·932 mg, Mannitol BP 50.0 mg, Sodium hydroxide BP (quantity not fixed; used to adjust pH), Water for injections EP.*

* Water for injections is used during manufacture but is not present in the finished product, but removed during the freeze-drying process.

Incompatibilities: None known.

Shelf life: 2 years, freeze dried powder; 0.5 day, reconstituted solution for injection.

Special precautions for storage: Freeze dried powder: Keep dry. Protect from light. Store below 25°C.

Nature and contents of container: 0.5 mg freeze dried powder is contained in glass vials with synthetic butyl rubber plugs and aluminium collars.

Instructions for use/handling: No special instructions.

Marketing authorisation number PL0003/0151.

Date of first authorisation/renewal of authorisation 18.03.81/13.08.87 and 23.04.91.

Date of (partial) revision of text This is the first SPC 06.03.96.

KEMADRIN* INJECTION

Qualitative and quantitative composition Procyclidine Hydrochloride BP 5 mg per ml (10 mg in each 2 ml ampoule).

Pharmaceutical form Injection.

Clinical particulars

Therapeutic indications: Kemadrin is indicated for the treatment and symptomatic relief of all forms of Parkinson's disease e.g. idiopathic (paralysis agitans), postencephalitic and arteriosclerotic disease.

Kemadrin is also indicated for the control of extrapyramidal symptoms induced by neuroleptic drugs including pseudo-parkinsonism, acute dystonic reactions and akathisia.

Posology and method of administration

The variation in optimum dosage from one patient to another should be taken into consideration by the physician.

Dosage in adults: Parkinson's disease: Treatment is usually started at 2.5 mg procyclidine three times per day, increasing by 2.5 to 5 mg per day at intervals of two or three days until the optimum clinical response is achieved.

The usual maintenance dose to achieve optimal response is 15 to 30 mg procyclidine per day.

Addition of a fourth dose before retiring has been seen to be beneficial in some patients. Doses up to 60 mg procyclidine have been well tolerated, and at the discretion of the attending physician dosing to this level may be appropriate.

In general younger patients or those with postencephalitic parkinsonism may require higher doses for a therapeutic response than older patients and those with arteriosclerotic parkinsonism.

Kemadrin may be combined with levodopa or amantadine in patients who are inadequately controlled on a single agent.

Neuroleptic-induced extrapyramidal symptoms:

Treatment is usually initiated at 2.5 mg procyclidine three times per day increasing by 2.5 mg daily until symptoms are relieved.

The effective maintenance dose is usually 10 to 30 mg procyclidine per day. After a period of 3 to 4 months of therapy, Kemadrin should be withdrawn and the patient observed to see whether the neuroleptic-induced extra-pyramidal symptoms recur.

If this is the case Kemadrin should be reintroduced to avoid debilitating extra-pyramidal symptoms. Cessation of treatment periodically is to be recommended even in patients who appear to require the drug for longer periods.

Kemadrin Injection may be given intramuscularly in doses of 5 to 10 mg, repeated after 20 minutes if necessary, up to a daily maximum of 20 mg procyclidine.

In acute torsion dystonia and paroxysmal dyskinesias, doses of 5 to 10 mg procyclidine intravenously are frequently effective within 5 to 10 minutes. Occasionally, patients may need more than 10 mg procyclidine, and may require up to half an hour to obtain relief.

Dosage in children: The use of Kemadrin in this age group is not recommended.

Dosage in elderly: Elderly patients may be more susceptible than younger adults to the anticholinergic effects of Kemadrin and a reduced dosage may be required (See *Special warnings and special precautions for use*).

Administration: Pharmacokinetic studies have indicated that the mean plasma elimination half life of Kemadrin is sufficient to allow twice daily administration orally or intravenously, if more convenient.

Oral administration may be better tolerated if associated with a meal.

Contra-indications: Kemadrin is contra-indicated in individuals with known hypersensitivity to any component of the preparation, untreated urinary retention, closed angle glaucoma and gastro-intestinal obstruction.

Special warnings and special precautions for use: As with all anticholinergics the benefit/risk ratio should be assessed when prescribing Kemadrin in patients with existing angle-closure (narrow angle) glaucoma or those considered to be predisposed to glaucoma. Cautious prescribing is also indicated in patients predisposed to obstructive disease of the gastrointestinal tract and those with urinary symptoms associated with prostatic hypertrophy.

In a proportion of patients undergoing neuroleptic treatment, tardive dyskinesias will occur. While anticholinergic agents do not cause this syndrome, when given in combination with neuroleptics they may exacerbate the symptoms of tardive dyskinesia or reduce the threshold at which these symptoms appear in predisposed patients. In such individuals subsequent adjustment of neuroleptic therapy or reduction in anticholinergic treatment should be considered.

Patients with mental disorders occasionally experience a precipitation of a psychotic episode when procyclidine is administered for the treatment of the extrapyramidal side effects of neuroleptics.

Elderly patients, especially those on high doses of anticholinergics may be more susceptible to the adverse events associated with such therapy (see *Adverse events*). Specifically, the elderly patient may be particularly vulnerable to Central Nervous System disturbances such as confusion, impairment of cognitive function and memory, disorientation and hallucinations. These effects are usually reversible on reduction or discontinuation of anticholinergic therapy.

There is no specific information available concerning the use of procyclidine hydrochloride in patients with impaired renal or hepatic function. However, since procyclidine is metabolised in the liver and excreted via the urine care should be exercised when administering procyclidine to patients with impairment of renal or hepatic function.

Kemadrin should not be withdrawn abruptly as rebound Parkinsonian symptoms may occur.

Abuse: Kemadrin, along with other anticholinergic drugs, has the potential to be abused. Although the cases of abuse are rare, physicians should exercise caution in prescribing Kemadrin to patients with symptoms that may not be genuine.

Interaction with other medicaments and other forms of interaction: Monoamine oxidase inhibitors or drugs with anticholinergic properties, such as amantadine, antihistamines, phenothiazines, and tricyclic antidepressants, may increase the anticholinergic action of procyclidine.

The use of drugs with cholinergic properties, such as tacrine, may reduce the therapeutic response to Kemadrin.

The concomitant use of procyclidine with some neuroleptics for the treatment of extrapyramidal symptoms has been associated with a reduction in neuroleptic plasma concentrations. However this reduction is unlikely to be associated with a significant reduction in clinical effect.

Anticholinergics, including procyclidine, may reduce the efficacy of levodopa by increasing gastric emptying time, resulting in enhanced gastric degradation.

Procyclidine may potentiate the vagolytic effects of quinidine.

Anticholinergics may reduce the absorption of ketoconazole.

Exposure to high environmental temperature and humidity in association with a phenothiazine/anticholinergic drug regimen has rarely resulted in hyperpyrexia.

Pregnancy and lactation:

Pregnancy: The safety of using Kemadrin during pregnancy has not been established. However, extensive clinical use has not given any evidence that it in any way compromises the normal course of pregnancy. Nevertheless, as with all drugs, use should be considered only when the expected clinical benefit of treatment for the mother outweighs any possible risk to the developing foetus.

Lactation: No information is available on the passage of procyclidine into human breast milk following administration of Kemadrin.

Effects on ability to drive and use machines: Adverse events of a neurological character such as blurred vision, dizziness, confusion and disorientation have been reported with procyclidine. Therefore, if affected, patients should be advised not to drive or operate machinery.

Undesirable effects: The main side effects are those to be expected from any anticholinergic agent. Dry mouth, blurring of vision, constipation, urinary retention are most commonly recorded. Nausea, vomiting, gingivitis, nervousness and rash have occasionally been reported.

The unwanted anticholinergic effects are easily reversed by reducing the dosage.

With high doses of procyclidine dizziness, mental confusion, impaired cognition and memory, disorientation, anxiety, agitation and hallucinations may occur.

Rarely the development of psychotic-like symptoms have been reported in association with procyclidine.

Overdose:

Symptoms and signs: Reports of overdosage are relatively rare and no fatalities are known. Symptoms of overdosage are agitation, restlessness and confusion with severe sleeplessness lasting up to 24 hours or more. Visual and auditory hallucinations have been reported. Most subjects are euphoric but the occasional patient may be anxious and aggressive. The pupils are widely dilated and unreactive to light.

In recorded cases, the disorientation has lasted 1 to 4 days and ended in a recuperative sleep. Tachycardia has also been reported in association with cases of Kemadrin overdose.

Treatment: If procyclidine has been ingested within the previous hour or two (or possibly longer in view of its likely effects on gastric motility) then gastric lavage is probably indicated. Other active measures such as the use of cholinergic agents or haemodialysis are extremely unlikely to be of clinical value although if convulsions occur they should be controlled by injections of diazepam.

Pharmacological, toxicological and pharmacokinetic properties

Pharmacological properties/Pharmacodynamic properties: Procyclidine is a synthetic anticholinergic agent which blocks the excitatory effects of acetylcholine at the muscarinic receptor.

Idiopathic Parkinson's disease is thought to result from degeneration of neurones in the substantia nigra whose axons project and inhibit cells in the corpus striatum. Blockade by neuroleptic drugs of the dopamine released by these terminals produces a similar clinical picture. The cell bodies in the corpus striatum also receive cholinergic innervation which is excitatory. Relief of the Parkinsonian syndrome can be achieved, either by potentiation of the dopaminergic system or blockade of the cholinergic input by anticholinergics. It is by a central action of this latter type by which procyclidine exerts its effect.

Procyclidine is particularly effective in the alleviation of rigidity. Tremor, akinesia, speech and writing difficulties, gait, sialorrhoea and drooling, sweating, oculogyric crises and depressed mood are also beneficially influenced.

Pharmacokinetic properties: Procyclidine is adequately absorbed from the gastro-intestinal tract with a bioavailability of 75% and disappears rapidly from the tissues. The relatively low clearance of 68 ml/min represents a predominantly metabolic change with a small first pass effect. The mean plasma elimination half-life after both oral and intravenous administration is approximately 12 hours.

No detailed information is available on the metabolic fate of procyclidine but very little of the parent compound is excreted in the urine unchanged. When given orally about one fifth of the dose is known to be metabolised in the liver, principally by cytochrome P450 and then conjugated with glucuronic acid. This conjugate has been detected in the urine.

Preclinical safety data:
Fertility: A three generation study in rats dosed at 40 mg/kg/day via the diet before and during pregnancy showed only that the number of viable pups was slightly decreased from the second mating. No other parameters were affected.

Teratogenicity: No teratogenic effects were seen in rats dosed subcutaneously with 10, 30 or 100 mg/kg/day on days 8 to 16 of pregnancy. Maternal bodyweight gain was reduced at doses of 30 or 100 mg/kg/day, and a 10% reduction in foetal weight was seen at 100 mg/kg/day.

Mutagenicity: No data is available regarding the mutagenic potential of procyclidine hydrochloride.

Carcinogenicity: There is no data on the carcinogenic potential of procyclidine hydrochloride.

Pharmaceutical particulars
List of excipients: Lactic acid 10 μg. Lactic acid for pH 3.9 to 4.5 (quantity not fixed). Water for Injections to 2 ml.

Incompatibilities: None known.

Shelf life: 5 years.

Special precautions for storage: Store below 25°C.

Nature and contents of container: 2 ml neutral glass ampoules.

Instructions for use/handling: No special instructions.

Marketing authorisation number PL 0003/5256R

Date of first authorisation MAA: 9 September 1985 (reviewed licence). Renewal: 27th March 1991.

Date of revision of the text November 1998.

KEMADRIN* TABLETS

Qualitative and quantitative composition Procyclidine Hydrochloride BP 5 mg per tablet.

Pharmaceutical form Tablet.

Clinical particulars
Therapeutic indications: Kemadrin is indicated for the treatment and symptomatic relief of all forms of Parkinson's disease e.g. idiopathic (paralysis agitans), postencephalitic and arteriosclerotic disease.

Kemadrin is also indicated for the control of extrapyramidal symptoms induced by neuroleptic drugs including pseudo-parkinsonism, acute dystonic reactions and akathisia.

Posology and method of administration: The variation in optimum dosage from one patient to another should be taken into consideration by the physician.

Dosage in adults: Parkinson's disease: Treatment is usually started at 2.5 mg procyclidine three times per day, increasing by 2.5 to 5 mg per day at intervals of two or three days until the optimum clinical response is achieved.

The usual maintenance dose to achieve optimal response is 15 to 30 mg procyclidine per day.

Addition of a fourth dose before retiring has been seen to be beneficial in some patients. Doses up to 60 mg procyclidine have been well tolerated, and at the discretion of the attending physician dosing to this level may be appropriate.

In general younger patients or those with postencephalitic parkinsonism may require higher doses for a therapeutic response than older patients and those with arteriosclerotic parkinsonism.

Kemadrin may be combined with levodopa or amantadine in patients who are inadequately controlled on a single agent.

Neuroleptic-induced extrapyramidal symptoms: Treatment is usually initiated at 2.5 mg procyclidine three times per day increasing by 2.5 mg daily until symptoms are relieved.

The effective maintenance dose is usually 10 to 30 mg procyclidine per day. After a period of 3 to 4 months of therapy, Kemadrin should be withdrawn and the patient observed to see whether the neuroleptic-induced extra-pyramidal symptoms recur.

If this is the case Kemadrin should be reintroduced to avoid debilitating extra-pyramidal symptoms. Cessation of treatment periodically is to be recommended even in patients who appear to require the drug for longer periods.

Dosage in children: The use of Kemadrin in this age group is not recommended.

Dosage in the elderly: Elderly patients may be more susceptible than younger adults to the anticholinergic effects of Kemadrin and a reduced dosage may be required (See *Special warnings and special precautions for use*).

Administration: Pharmacokinetic studies have indicated that the mean plasma elimination half life of Kemadrin is sufficient to allow twice daily administration orally or intravenously, if more convenient.

Oral administration may be better tolerated if associated with a meal.

Contra-indications: Kemadrin is contra-indicated in individuals with known hypersensitivity to any component of the preparation, untreated urinary retention, closed angle glaucoma and gastro-intestinal obstruction.

Special warnings and special precautions for use: As with all anticholinergics the benefit/risk ratio should be assessed when prescribing Kemadrin in patients with existing angle-closure (narrow angle) glaucoma or those considered to be predisposed to glaucoma. Cautious prescribing is also indicated in patients predisposed to obstructive disease of the gastro-intestinal tract and those with urinary symptoms associated with prostatic hypertrophy.

In a proportion of patients undergoing neuroleptic treatment, tardive dyskinesias will occur. While anticholinergic agents do not cause this syndrome, when given in combination with neuroleptics they may exacerbate the symptoms of tardive dyskinesia or reduce the threshold at which these symptoms appear in predisposed patients. In such individuals subsequent adjustment of neuroleptic therapy or reduction in anticholinergic treatment should be considered.

Patients with mental disorders occasionally experience a precipitation of a psychotic episode when procyclidine is administered for the treatment of the extrapyramidal side effects of neuroleptics.

Elderly patients, especially those on high doses of anticholinergics may be more susceptible to the adverse events associated with such therapy (see *Adverse events*). Specifically, the elderly patient may be particularly vulnerable to Central Nervous System disturbances such as confusion, impairment of cognitive function and memory, disorientation and hallucinations. These effects are usually reversible on reduction or discontinuation of anticholinergic therapy.

There is no specific information available concerning the use of procyclidine hydrochloride in patients with impaired renal or hepatic function. However, since procyclidine is metabolised in the liver and excreted via the urine care should be exercised when administering procyclidine to patients with impairment of renal or hepatic function.

Kemadrin should not be withdrawn abruptly as rebound parkinsonian symptoms may occur.

Abuse: Kemadrin, along with other anticholinergic drugs, has the potential to be abused. Although the cases of abuse are rare, physicians should exercise caution in prescribing Kemadrin to patients with symptoms that may not be genuine.

Interaction with other medicaments and other forms of interaction: Monoamine oxidase inhibitors or drugs with anticholinergic properties, such as amantadine, antihistamines, phenothiazines, and tricyclic antidepressants, may increase the anticholinergic action of procyclidine.

The use of drugs with cholinergic properties, such as tacrine, may reduce the therapeutic response to Kemadrin.

The concomitant use of procyclidine with some neuroleptics for the treatment of extrapyramidal symptoms has been associated with a reduction in neuroleptic plasma concentrations. However this reduction is unlikely to be associated with a significant reduction in clinical effect.

Anticholinergics, including procyclidine, may reduce the efficacy of levodopa by increasing gastric emptying time, resulting in enhanced gastric degradation.

Procyclidine may potentiate the vagolytic effects of quinidine.

Anticholinergics may reduce the absorption of ketoconazole.

Exposure to high environmental temperature and humidity in association with a phenothiazine/anticholinergic drug regimen has rarely resulted in hyperpyrexia.

Pregnancy and lactation:
Pregnancy: The safety of using Kemadrin during pregnancy has not been established. However, extensive clinical use has not given any evidence that it in any way compromises the normal course of pregnancy. Nevertheless, as with all drugs, use should be considered only when the expected clinical benefit of treatment for the mother outweighs any possible risk to the developing foetus.

Lactation: No information is available on the passage of procyclidine into human breast milk following administration of Kemadrin.

Effects on ability to drive and use machines: Adverse events of a neurological character such as blurred vision, dizziness, confusion and disorientation have been reported with procyclidine. Therefore, if affected, patients should be advised not to drive or operate machinery.

Undesirable effects: The main side effects are those to be expected from any anticholinergic agent. Dry mouth, blurring of vision, constipation, urinary retention are most commonly recorded. Nausea, vomiting, gingivitis, nervousness and rash have occasionally been reported.

The unwanted anticholinergic effects are easily reversed by reducing the dosage.

With high doses of procyclidine dizziness, mental confusion, impaired cognition and memory, disorientation, anxiety, agitation and hallucinations may occur.

Rarely the development of psychotic-like symptoms have been reported in association with procyclidine.

Overdose:
Symptoms and signs: Reports of overdosage are relatively rare and no fatalities are known. Symptoms of overdosage are agitation, restlessness and confusion with severe sleeplessness lasting up to 24 hours or more. Visual and auditory hallucinations have been reported. Most subjects are euphoric but the occasional patient may be anxious and aggressive. The pupils are widely dilated and unreactive to light.

In recorded cases, the disorientation has lasted 1 to 4 days and ended in a recuperative sleep.

Tachycardia has also been reported in association with cases of Kemadrin overdose.

Treatment: If procyclidine has been ingested within the previous hour or two (or possibly longer in view of its likely effects on gastric motility) then gastric lavage is probably indicated. Other active measures such as the use of cholinergic agents or haemodialysis are extremely unlikely to be of clinical value although if convulsions occur they should be controlled by injections of diazepam.

Pharmacological, toxicological and pharmacokinetic properties
Pharmacological properties/Pharmacodynamic properties: Procyclidine is a synthetic anticholinergic agent which blocks the excitatory effects of acetylcholine at the muscarinic receptor.

Idiopathic Parkinson's disease is thought to result from degeneration of neurones in the substantia nigra whose axons project and inhibit cells in the corpus striatum. Blockade by neuroleptic drugs of the dopamine released by these terminals produces a similar clinical picture. The cell bodies in the corpus striatum also receive cholinergic innervation which is excitatory.

Relief of the Parkinsonian syndrome can be achieved, either by potentiation of the dopaminergic system or blockade of the cholinergic input by anticholinergics. It is by a central action of this latter type by which procyclidine exerts its effect.

Procyclidine is particularly effective in the alleviation of rigidity. Tremor, akinesia, speech and writing difficulties, gait, sialorrhoea and drooling, sweating, oculogyric crises and depressed mood are also beneficially influenced.

Pharmacokinetic properties: Procyclidine is adequately absorbed from the gastro-intestinal tract with a bioavailability of 75% and disappears rapidly from the tissues. The relatively low clearance of 68 ml/min represents a predominantly metabolic change with a small first pass effect. The mean plasma elimination half-life after both oral and intravenous administration is approximately 12 hours.

No detailed information is available on the metabolic fate of procyclidine but very little of the parent compound is excreted in the urine unchanged. When given orally about one fifth of the dose is known to be metabolised in the liver, principally by cytochrome P450 and then conjugated with glucuronic acid. This conjugate has been detected in the urine.

Preclinical safety data:
Fertility: A three generation study in rats dosed at 40 mg/kg/day via the diet before and during pregnancy

showed only that the number of viable pups was slightly decreased from the second mating. No other parameters were affected.

Teratogenicity: No teratogenic effects were seen in rats dosed subcutaneously with 10, 30 or 100 mg/kg/day on days 8 to 16 of pregnancy. Maternal bodyweight gain was reduced at doses of 30 or 100 mg/kg/day, and a 10% reduction in foetal weight was seen at 100 mg/kg/day.

Mutagenicity: No data is available regarding the mutagenic potential of procyclidine hydrochloride.

Carcinogenicity: There is no data on the carcinogenic potential of procyclidine hydrochloride.

Pharmaceutical particulars

List of excipients: Lactose, Sodium Starch Glycollate, Povidone, Magnesium Stearate.

Incompatibilities: None.

Shelf life: 5 years.

Special precautions for storage: Store below 25°C.

Nature and contents of container: Amber glass bottles with low density polyethylene snap fit closures. Polypropylene containers with polyethylene snap-fit lids. Round enamelled tins with lever lids.

Instructions for use/handling: See *Posology and method of administration.*

Marketing authorisation number PL 0003/5255R

Date of first authorisation 9 September 1985.

Date of revision of the text November 1998.

LAMICTAL* Tablets 50 mg 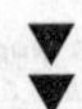
LAMICTAL* Tablets 25 mg ▼

Qualitative and quantitative composition Lamictal tablets containing 50 mg lamotrigine.

Lamictal tablets 50 mg are pale-yellow rounded-square tablets. They are multifaceted on one side and flat with 'LAMICTAL 50' on the other.

Lamictal tablets containing 25 mg lamotrigine.

Lamictal tablets 25 mg are pale-yellow rounded-square tablets. They are multifaceted on one side and flat with 'LAMICTAL 25' on the other.

Pharmaceutical form Tablets.

Clinical particulars

Therapeutic indications: Epilepsy.

Monotherapy in adults and children over 12 years of age:

1. Simple partial seizures.
2. Complex partial seizures.
3. Secondarily generalised tonic-clonic seizures.
4. Primary generalised tonic-clonic seizures.

Monotherapy in children under 12 years of age is not recommended until such time as adequate information is made available from controlled trials in this particular target population.

Add-on therapy in adults and children over 2 years of age:

1. Simple partial seizures.
2. Complex partial seizures.
3. Secondarily generalised tonic-clonic seizures.
4. Primary generalised tonic-clonic seizures.

Lamictal is also indicated for the treatment of seizures associated with Lennox-Gastaut syndrome.

Posology and method of administration:

Administration: Lamictal Tablets should be swallowed whole with a little water.

Lamictal Dispersible tablets may be chewed, dispersed in a small volume of water (at least enough to cover the whole tablet) or swallowed whole with a little water.

To ensure a therapeutic dose is maintained the weight of a child must be monitored and the dose reviewed as weight changes occur. If the doses calculated for children, according to bodyweight, do not equate to whole tablets the dose to be administered is that equal to the lower number of whole tablets.

Dosage in monotherapy: Adults and children over 12 years: The initial Lamictal dose in monotherapy is 25 mg once a day for two weeks, followed by 50 mg once a day for two weeks. Thereafter, the dose should be increased by a maximum of 50 mg–100 mg every 1–2 weeks until the optimal response is achieved. The usual maintenance dose to achieve optimal response is 100–200 mg/day given once a day or as two divided doses. Some patients have required 500 mg/day of Lamictal to achieve the desired response.

Recommended dose escalation of Lamictal for ADULTS AND CHILDREN OVER 12 YEARS on monotherapy

Weeks 1–2	Weeks 3–4	Usual maintenance dose
25 mg (once a day)	50 mg (once a day)	100–200 mg (once a day or two divided doses) To achieve maintenance, doses may be increased by 50–100 mg every 1–2 weeks.

The initial dose and subsequent dose escalation should not be exceeded to minimise the risk of rash (see *Special warnings and special precautions for use*).

Children aged 2 to 12 years: There is insufficient evidence available from appropriate studies in children, upon which to base dosage recommendations for monotherapy use in children under the age of 12 years (see *Therapeutic indications*).

Dosage in add-on therapy: Adults and children over 12 years: In patients taking valproate with/without any other anti-epileptic drug (AED) the initial Lamictal dose is 25 mg every alternate day for two weeks, followed by 25 mg once a day for two weeks. Thereafter, the dose should be increased by a maximum of 25–50 mg every 1–2 weeks until the optimal response is achieved. The usual maintenance dose to achieve optimal response is 100–200 mg/day given once a day or in two divided doses.

In those patients taking enzyme inducing AEDs with/without other AEDs (except valproate) the initial Lamictal dose is 50 mg once a day for two weeks, followed by 100 mg/day given in two divided doses for two weeks. Thereafter, the dose should be increased by a maximum of 100 mg every 1–2 weeks until the optimal response is achieved. The usual maintenance dose to achieve optimal response is 200–400 mg/day given in two divided doses. Some patients have required 700 mg/day of Lamictal to achieve the desired response.

In patients taking AEDs where the pharmacokinetic interaction with lamotrigine is currently not known, the dose escalation as recommended for lamotrigine with concurrent valproate should be used, thereafter, the dose should be increased until optimal response is achieved.

Recommended dose escalation of Lamictal for ADULTS AND CHILDREN OVER 12 YEARS on combined drug therapy

Concomitant medication	Weeks 1–2	Weeks 3–4	Usual maintenance dose
Valproate with/without any other AEDs	12.5 mg (given as 25 mg on alternate days)	25 mg (once a day)	100–200 mg (once a day or two divided doses) To achieve maintenance, doses may be increased by 25–50 mg every 1–2 weeks.
Enzyme inducing AEDs† with/without other AEDs (except valproate)	50 mg (once a day)	100 mg (two divided doses)	200–400 mg (two divided doses) To achieve maintenance, doses may be increased by 100 mg every 1–2 weeks.

† e.g. phenytoin, carbamazepine, phenobarbitone and primidone.

Note: In patients taking AEDs where the pharmacokinetic interaction with lamotrigine is currently not known, the dose escalation as recommended for lamotrigine with concurrent valproate should be used. Thereafter, the dose should be increased until optimal response is achieved.

The initial dose and subsequent dose escalation should not be exceeded to minimise the risk of rash (see *Special warnings and special precautions for use*).

Children aged 2 to 12 years: In patients taking valproate with/without any other anti-epileptic drug (AED), the initial Lamictal dose is 0.2 mg/kg bodyweight/day given once a day for two weeks, followed by 0.5 mg/kg/day given once a day for two weeks. Thereafter, the dose should be increased by a maximum of 0.5–1 mg/kg every 1–2 weeks until the optimal response is achieved. The usual maintenance dose to achieve optimal response is 1–5 mg/kg/day given once a day or in two divided doses.

In those patients taking enzyme inducing AEDs with/without other AEDs (except valproate) the initial Lamictal dose is 2 mg/kg bodyweight/day given in two divided doses for two weeks, followed by 5 mg/kg/day for two weeks. Thereafter, the dose should be increased by a maximum of 2–3 mg/kg every 1–2 weeks until the optimal response is achieved. The usual maintenance dose to achieve optimal response is 5–15 mg/kg/day given in two divided doses.

In patients taking AEDs where the pharmacokinetic interaction with lamotrigine is currently not known, the dose escalation as recommended for lamotrigine with concurrent valproate should be used, thereafter, the dose should be increased until optimal response is achieved.

Recommended dose escalation of Lamictal for children aged 2–12 years on combined drug therapy (total daily dose in mg/kg bodyweight/day)

Concomitant medication	Weeks 1–2	Weeks 3–4	Maintenance dose
Valproate with/without any other AEDs	0.2 mg/kg‡ (once a day)	0.5 mg/kg (once a day)	1-5 mg/kg (once a day or two divided doses) To achieve maintenance, doses may be increased by 0.5–1 mg/kg every 1–2 weeks.
Enzyme inducing AEDs† with/without other AEDs (except valproate)	2 mg/kg (two divided doses)	5 mg/kg (two divided doses)	5–15 mg/kg (two divided doses) To achieve maintenance, doses may be increased by 2–3 mg/kg every 1–2 weeks.

† e.g. phenytoin, carbamazepine, phenobarbitone and primidone.

Note: In patients taking AEDs where the pharmacokinetic interaction with lamotrigine is currently not known, the dose escalation as recommended for lamotrigine with concurrent valproate should be used, thereafter, the dose should be increased until optimal response is achieved.

‡ If the calculated daily dose is 2.5–5 mg, then 5 mg Lamictal may be taken on alternate days for the first two weeks. If the calculated daily dose is less then 2.5 mg, then Lamictal should not be administered.

The initial dose and subsequent dose escalation should not be exceeded to minimise the risk of rash (see *Special warnings and special precautions for use*).

It is likely that patients aged 2–6 years will require a maintenance dose at the higher end of the recommended range.

Children aged less than 2 years: There is insufficient information on the use of Lamictal in children aged less than 2 years.

Elderly: There is limited information on the use of Lamictal in elderly patients. To date, there is no evidence to suggest that the response of this age group differs from that in the young. However, elderly patients should be treated cautiously.

Contra-indications: Lamictal is contraindicated in individuals with known hypersensitivity to lamotrigine.

Lamictal is cleared primarily by metabolism in the liver. No studies have been carried out in patients with significant impairment of hepatic function. Until such data become available, Lamictal cannot be recommended in this condition.

Special warnings and special precautions for use: There have been reports of adverse skin reactions, which have generally occurred within the first 8 weeks after initiation of lamotrigine (Lamictal) treatment. The majority of rashes are mild and self limiting, however, rarely, serious potentially life threatening skin rashes including Stevens-Johnson syndrome (SJS) and toxic epidermal necrolysis (TEN) have been reported (see *Undesirable effects*).

The approximate incidence of serious skin rashes in adults and children over the age of 12 is 1 in 1000. The risk is higher in children under the age of 12 than in adults. Available data from a number of studies suggest the incidence in children under the age of 12 requiring hospitalisation due to rash ranges from 1 in 300 to 1 in 100 (see *Undesirable effects*).

In children, the initial presentation of a rash can be mistaken for an infection, physicians should consider the possibility of a drug reaction in children that develop symptoms of rash and fever during the first eight weeks of therapy.

Additionally the overall risk of rash appears to be strongly associated with:

- High initial doses of lamotrigine and exceeding the recommended dose escalation of lamotrigine therapy (see *Posology and method of administration*).
- Concomitant use of valproate, which increases the mean half-life of lamotrigine nearly two fold (see *Posology and method of administration*).

All patients (adults and children) who develop a rash should be promptly evaluated and lamotrigine withdrawn immediately unless the rash is clearly not drug related.

Rash has also been reported as part of a hypersensitivity syndrome associated with a variable pattern of systemic symptoms including fever, lymphadenopathy, facial oedema and abnormalities of the blood and liver. The syndrome shows a wide spectrum of clinical severity and may, rarely, lead to disseminated intravascular coagulation (DIC) and multiorgan failure. It is important to note that early manifestations of hypersensitivity (e.g. fever, lymphadenopathy) may be present even though rash is not evident. Patients should be warned to seek immediate medical advice if signs and symptoms develop. If such signs and symptoms are present the patient should be evaluated immediately and Lamictal discontinued if an alternative aetiology cannot be established.

As with other AEDs, abrupt withdrawal of Lamictal may provoke rebound seizures. Unless safety concerns (for example rash) require an abrupt withdrawal, the dose of Lamictal should be gradually decreased over a period of 2 weeks.

When concomitant anti-epileptic drugs (AEDs) are withdrawn to achieve Lamictal monotherapy or other anti-epileptic drugs (AEDs) are added-on to Lamictal monotherapy consideration should be given to the effect this may have on lamotrigine pharmacokinetics (see *Interaction with other medicaments and other forms of interaction*).

During clinical experience with lamotrigine used as add-on therapy, there have been, rarely, deaths following rapidly progressive illnesses with status epilepticus, rhabdomyolysis, multiorgan dysfunction and disseminated intravascular coagulation (DIC). The contribution of lamotrigine to these events remains to be established.

Lamictal is a weak inhibitor of dihydrofolate reductase hence there is a possibility of interference with folate metabolism during long-term therapy. However, during prolonged human dosing, lamotrigine did not induce significant changes in the haemoglobin concentration, mean corpuscular volume, or serum or red blood cell folate concentrations up to 1 year or red blood cell folate concentrations for up to 5 years.

In single dose studies in subjects with end-stage renal failure, plasma concentrations of lamotrigine were not significantly altered. However, accumulation of the glucuronide metabolite is to be expected; caution should therefore be exercised in treating patients with renal failure.

Interaction with other medicaments and other forms of interaction: Anti-epileptic agents which induce drug metabolising enzymes (such as phenytoin, carbamazepine, phenobarbitone and primidone) enhance the metabolism of lamotrigine and may increase dose requirements.

Sodium valproate, which competes with lamotrigine for hepatic drug-metabolising enzymes, reduces the metabolism of lamotrigine.

There is no evidence that lamotrigine causes clinically significant induction or inhibition of hepatic oxidative drug-metabolising enzymes. Lamotrigine may induce its own metabolism but the effect is modest and unlikely to have significant clinical consequences.

Although changes in the plasma concentrations of other anti-epileptic drugs have been reported, controlled studies have shown no evidence that lamotrigine affects the plasma concentrations of concomitant anti-epileptic drugs. Evidence from *in vitro* studies indicates that lamotrigine does not displace other anti-epileptic drugs from protein binding sites.

There have been reports of central nervous system events including headache, nausea, blurred vision, dizziness, diplopia and ataxia in patients taking carbamazepine following the introduction of lamotrigine. These events usually resolve when the dose of carbamazepine is reduced.

In a study of 12 female volunteers, lamotrigine did not affect plasma concentrations of ethinyloestradiol and levonorgestrel following the administration of the oral contraceptive pill. However, as with the introduction of other chronic therapy in patients taking oral contraceptives, any change in the menstrual bleeding pattern should be reported to the patient's physician.

Pregnancy and lactation:
Fertility: Administration of Lamictal did not impair fertility in animal reproductive studies. There is no experience of the effect of Lamictal on human fertility.

Teratogenicity: Lamotrigine is a weak inhibitor of dihydrofolate reductase. There is a theoretical risk of human foetal malformations when the mother is treated with a folate inhibitor during pregnancy. However, reproductive toxicology studies with lamotrigine in animals at doses in excess of the human therapeutic dosage showed no teratogenic effects.

Pregnancy: There are insufficient data available on the use of lamotrigine in human pregnancy to evaluate its safety. Lamotrigine should not be used in pregnancy unless, in the opinion of the physician, the potential benefits of treatment to the mother outweigh any possible risks to the developing foetus.

Lactation: Preliminary data indicate that lamotrigine passes into breast milk in concentrations usually of the order of 40-45% of the plasma concentration.

In the small number of infants known to have been breastfed, the dose of lamotrigine received was calculated to be approximately 0.06-0.75 mg/kg/24 hours, and no adverse experiences were reported.

Effects on ability to drive and use machines: Two volunteer studies have demonstrated that the effect of lamotrigine on fine visual motor co-ordination, eye movements, body sway and subjective sedative effects did not differ from placebo.

In clinical trials with lamotrigine adverse events of a neurological character such as dizziness and diplopia have been reported. As there is individual variation in response to all anti-epileptic drug therapy patients should consult their physician on the specific issues of driving and epilepsy.

Undesirable effects: Adverse experiences reported during Lamictal monotherapy trials include headache, tiredness, rash, nausea, dizziness, drowsiness and insomnia.

In double-blind, add-on clinical trials, skin rashes occurred in up to 10% of patients taking lamotrigine and in 5% of patients taking placebo. The skin rashes led to the withdrawal of lamotrigine treatment in 2% of patients. The rash, usually maculopapular in appearance, generally appears within eight weeks of starting treatment and resolves on withdrawal of lamotrigine (see *Special warnings and special precautions for use*).

Rarely, serious potentially life threatening skin rashes, including Stevens-Johnson syndrome and toxic epidermal necrolysis (Lyell Syndrome) have been reported. Although the majority recover on drug withdrawal, some patients experience irreversible scarring and there have been rare cases of associated death (see *Special warnings and special precautions for use*).

The approximate incidence of serious skin rashes in adults and children over the age of 12 is 1 in 1,000. The risk is higher in children under the age of 12 than in adults. Available data from a number of studies suggest the incidence in children under the age of 12 requiring hospitalisation due to rash ranges from 1 in 300 to 1 in 100 (see *Special warnings and special precautions for use*).

In children, the initial presentation of a rash can be mistaken for an infection, physicians should consider the possibility of a drug reaction in children that develop symptoms of rash and fever during the first eight weeks of therapy.

Additionally the overall risk of rash appears to be strongly associated with:

- High initial doses of lamotrigine and exceeding the recommended dose escalation of lamotrigine therapy (see *Posology and method of administration*).
- Concomitant use of valproate, which increases the mean half life of lamotrigine nearly two fold (see *Posology and method of administration*).

All patients (adults and children) who develop a rash should be promptly evaluated and lamotrigine withdrawn immediately unless the rash is clearly not drug related.

Rash has also been reported as part of a hypersensitivity syndrome associated with a variable pattern of systemic symptoms including fever, lymphadenopathy, facial oedema and abnormalities of the blood and liver. The syndrome shows a wide spectrum of clinical severity and may, rarely, lead to disseminated intravascular coagulation (DIC) and multiorgan failure. It is important to note that early manifestations of hypersensitivity (e.g. fever, lymphadenopathy) may be present even though rash is not evident. Patients should be warned to seek immediate medical advice if signs and symptoms develop. If such signs and symptoms are present the patient should be evaluated immediately and Lamictal discontinued if an alternative aetiology cannot be established.

Other adverse experiences reported when lamotrigine is added-on to standard anti-epileptic drug regimens have included diplopia, blurred vision, conjunctivitis, dizziness, drowsiness, headache, unsteadiness, tiredness, gastrointestinal disturbance (including vomiting), irritability/aggression, tremor, agitation, confusion and haematological abnormalities (including neutropenia, leucopenia and thrombocytopenia).

Overdose:
Symptoms and signs: Ingestion of between 1.35 and 4 g lamotrigine has been reported in a few patients. Clinical consequences were not severe, signs and symptoms included nystagmus, ataxia, dizziness, somnolence, headache and vomiting.

A patient who ingested a dose calculated to be between 4 and 5 g lamotrigine was admitted to hospital with coma lasting 8–12 hours followed by recovery over the next 2 to 3 days. A further patient who ingested 5.6 g lamotrigine was found unconscious. Following treatment with activated charcoal for suspected intoxication the patient recovered after sleeping for 16 hours.

Treatment: In the event of overdosage, the patient should be admitted to hospital and given appropriate supportive therapy. Gastric lavage should be performed if indicated.

Pharmacological properties
Pharmacodynamic properties:
Mode of action: The results of pharmacological studies suggest that lamotrigine is a use-dependent blocker of voltage gated sodium channels. It produces a use- and voltage-dependent block of sustained repetitive firing in cultured neurones and inhibits pathological release of glutamate (the amino acid which plays a key role in the generation of epileptic seizures), as well as inhibiting glutamate-evoked bursts of action potentials.

Pharmacodynamics: In tests designed to evaluate the central nervous system effects of drugs, the results obtained using doses of 240 mg lamotrigine administered to healthy volunteers did not differ from placebo, whereas both 1000 mg phenytoin and 10 mg diazepam each significantly impaired fine visual motor coordination and eye movements, increased body sway and produced subjective sedative effects.

In another study, single oral doses of 600 mg carbamazepine significantly impaired fine visual motor co-ordination and eye movements, while increasing both body sway and heart rate, whereas results with lamotrigine at doses of 150 mg and 300 mg did not differ from placebo.

Pharmacokinetic properties: Lamotrigine is rapidly and completely absorbed from the gut with no significant first pass metabolism. Peak plasma concentrations occur approximately 2.5 hours after oral drug administration. Time to maximum concentration is slightly delayed after food but the extent of absorption is unaffected. The pharmacokinetics are linear up to 450 mg, the highest single dose tested. There is considerable inter-individual variation in steady state maximum concentrations but within an individual concentrations vary very little.

Binding to plasma proteins is about 55%. It is very unlikely that displacement from plasma proteins would result in toxicity. The volume of distribution is 0.92 to 1.22 L/kg.

The mean steady state clearance in healthy adults is 39 ± 14 ml/min. Clearance of lamotrigine is primarily metabolic with subsequent elimination of glucuronide-concentrated material in urine. Less than 10% is excreted unchanged in the urine. Only about 2% of drug-related material is excreted in faeces. Clearance and half-life are independent of dose. The mean elimination half-life in healthy adults is 24 to 35 hours. UDP-glucuronyl transferases have been identified as the enzymes responsible for metabolism of lamotrigine. In a study of subjects with Gilbert's syndrome, mean apparent clearance was reduced by 32% compared with normal controls but the values are within the range for the general population.

Lamotrigine induces its own metabolism to a modest extent depending on dose. However, there is no evidence that lamotrigine affects the pharmacokinetics of other AEDs and data suggests that interactions between lamotrigine and drugs metabolised by cytochrome P450 enzymes are unlikely to occur.

The half-life of lamotrigine is greatly affected by concomitant medication. Mean half-life is reduced to approximately 14 hours when given with enzyme-inducing drugs such as carbamazepine and phenytoin and is increased to a mean of approximately 70 hours when co-administered with sodium valproate alone (see *Posology and method of administration*).

Clearance adjusted for bodyweight is higher in children than in adults, with the highest values in children under 5 years. The half-life of lamotrigine is generally shorter in children than in adults with a mean value of approximately 7 hours when given with enzyme-inducing drugs such as carbamazepine and phenytoin, and increasing to mean values of 45 to 50 hours when co-administered with sodium valproate alone (see *Posology and method of administration*).

To date there have been no specific studies of lamotrigine pharmacokinetics in elderly patients with epilepsy. However, a single-dose study in 12 healthy volunteers aged 65 to 76 years and a population analysis of 144 patients including 25 patients aged 65 years and over indicated that no dosage adjustment is required for the elderly.

There is no experience of treatment with lamotrigine of patients with renal failure. Pharmacokinetic studies using single doses in subjects with renal failure indicate that lamotrigine pharmacokinetics are little affected but plasma concentrations of the major glucuronide metabolite increase almost eight-fold due to reduced renal clearance.

Preclinical safety data:
Mutagenicity: The results of a wide range of mutagenicity tests indicate that Lamictal does not present a genetic risk to man.

Carcinogenicity: Lamictal was not carcinogenic in long-term studies in the rat and the mouse.

Pharmaceutical particulars
List of excipients:
Lamictal Tablets: Lactose PhEur, Microcrystalline Cellulose PhEur, Povidone BP, Sodium Starch Glycollate BP, Iron Oxide Yellow (E172) EEC Requirements, Magnesium Stearate PhEur.

Incompatibilities: None reported.

Shelf life: 3 years.

Special precautions for storage: Store below 30°C. Keep dry.

Nature and contents of container:

Lamictal Tablets 50 mg:	PVC/Aluminium foil blister pack containing 42 or 56 tablets
Lamictal Tablets 25 mg:	PVC/Aluminium foil blister pack containing 21, 42 or 56 tablets

Instructions for use/handling: None.

Marketing authorisation numbers

Lamictal Tablets 50 mg:	0003/0273
Lamictal Tablets 25 mg:	0003/0272

Date of first authorisation/renewal of authorisation 27/8/97.

Date of (partial) revision of text August 1997.

LAMICTAL* TABLETS ▼ 100 mg and 200 mg
LAMICTAL* Dispersible 5 mg, 25 mg and 100 mg ▼

Presentation Lamictal Tablets 100 mg are pale-yellow, rounded-square tablets, multifaceted on one side and flat with 'LAMICTAL 100' on the other, each containing 100 mg lamotrigine.

Lamictal Tablets 200 mg are pale-yellow, rounded-square tablets, multifaceted on one side and flat with 'LAMICTAL 200' on the other, each containing 200 mg lamotrigine.

Lamictal Dispersible 5 mg are white, elongated, biconvex tablets, with 'LAMICTAL 5' on one side and scored on the other and contain 5 mg lamotrigine in each tablet.

Lamictal Dispersible 25 mg are white, rounded-square tablets, multifaceted on one side and flat with 'LAMICTAL 25' on the other and contain 25 mg lamotrigine in each tablet.

Lamictal Dispersible 100 mg are white, rounded-square tablets, multifaceted on one side and flat with 'LAMICTAL 100' on the other and contain 100 mg lamotrigine in each tablet.

Uses
Therapeutic indications: Epilepsy.
Monotherapy in adults and children over 12 years of age:

1. simple partial seizures
2. complex partial seizures
3. secondarily generalised tonic-clonic seizures
4. primary generalised tonic-clonic seizures.

Monotherapy in children under 12 years of age is not recommended until such time as adequate information is made available from controlled trials in this particular target population.

Add-on therapy in adults and children over 2 years of age:

1. simple partial seizures
2. complex partial seizures
3. secondarily generalised tonic-clonic seizures.
4. primary generalised tonic-clonic seizures.

Lamictal is also indicated for the treatment of seizures associated with Lennox-Gastaut syndrome.

Mode of action: The results of pharmacological studies suggest that lamotrigine is a use-dependent blocker of voltage gated sodium channels. It produces a use and voltage-dependent block of sustained repetitive firing in cultured neurones and inhibits pathological release of glutamate (the amino acid which plays a key role in the generation of epileptic seizures), as well as inhibiting glutamate-evoked bursts of action potentials.

Pharmacokinetics: Lamotrigine is rapidly and completely absorbed from the gut with no significant first pass metabolism. Peak plasma concentrations occur approximately 2.5 hours after oral drug administration. Time to maximum concentration is slightly delayed after food but the extent of absorption is unaffected. The pharmacokinetics are linear up to 450 mg, the highest single dose tested. There is considerable inter-individual variation in steady state maximum concentrations but within an individual concentrations vary very little.

Binding to plasma proteins is about 55%. It is very unlikely that displacement from plasma proteins would result in toxicity. The volume of distribution is 0.92 to 1.22 l/kg.

The mean steady state clearance in healthy adults is 39 ± 14 ml/min. Clearance of lamotrigine is primarily metabolic with subsequent elimination of glucuronide-concentrated materials in urine. Less than 10% is excreted unchanged in the urine. Only about 2% of drug-related material is excreted in faeces. Clearance and half-life are independent of dose. The mean elimination half-life in healthy adults is 24 to 35 hours. UDP-glucuronyl transferases have been identified as the enzymes responsible for metabolism of lamotrigine. In a study of subjects with Gilbert's syndrome, mean apparent clearance was reduced by 32% compared with normal controls but the values are within the range for the general population.

Lamotrigine induces its own metabolism to a modest extent depending on dose. However, there is no evidence that lamotrigine affects the pharmacokinetics of other AEDs and data suggests that interactions between lamotrigine and drugs metabolised by cytochrome P450 enzymes are unlikely to occur.

The half-life of lamotrigine is greatly affected by concomitant medication. Mean half-life is reduced to approximately 14 hours when given with enzyme-inducing drugs such as carbamazepine and phenytoin and is increased to a mean of approximately 70 hours when co-administered with sodium valproate alone.

Clearance adjusted for bodyweight is higher in children aged 12 years and under than in adults, with the highest values in children under 5 years. The half-life of lamotrigine is generally shorter in children than in adults with a mean value of approximately 7 hours when given with enzyme-inducing drugs such as carbamazepine and phenytoin, and increasing to mean values of approximately 45 to 55 hours when co-administered with sodium valproate alone (see *Posology and method of administration)*.

To date there have been no specific studies of lamotrigine pharmacokinetics in elderly patients with epilepsy. However, a single-dose study in 12 healthy volunteers aged 65 to 76 years and a population analysis of 144 patients including 25 patients aged 65 years and over indicated that no dosage adjustment is required for the elderly.

There is no experience of treatment with lamotrigine of patients with renal failure. Pharmacokinetic studies using single doses in subjects with renal failure indicate that lamotrigine pharmacokinetics are little affected but plasma concentrations of the major glucuronide metabolite increase almost eight-fold due to reduced renal clearance.

Pharmacodynamics: In tests designed to evaluate the central nervous system effects of drugs, the results obtained using doses of 240 mg lamotrigine administered to healthy adult volunteers did not differ from placebo, whereas both 1000 mg phenytoin and 10 mg diazepam each significantly impaired fine visual motor co-ordination and eye movements, increased body sway and produced subjective sedative effects.

In another study, single oral doses of 600 mg carbamazepine significantly impaired fine visual motor co-ordination and eye movements, while increasing both body sway and heart rate, whereas results with lamotrigine at doses of 150 mg and 300 mg did not differ from placebo.

Posology and method of administration
Dosage in monotherapy:
Adults and children over 12 years: The initial Lamictal dose in monotherapy is 25 mg once a day for two weeks, followed by 50 mg once a day for two weeks. Thereafter, the dose should be increased by a maximum of 50 mg–100 mg every 1–2 weeks until the optimal response is achieved. The usual maintenance dose to achieve optimal response is 100–200 mg/day given once a day or as two divided doses. Some patients have required 500 mg/day of Lamictal to achieve the desired response.

Recommended dose escalation of Lamictal for ADULTS AND CHILDREN OVER 12 YEARS on monotherapy

Weeks 1–2	Weeks 3–4	Usual maintenance dose
25 mg (once a day)	50 mg (once a day)	100–200 mg (once a day or two divided doses) To achieve maintenance, doses may be increased by 50–100 mg every 1–2 weeks.

The initial dose and subsequent dose escalation should not be exceeded to minimise the risk of rash (see *Special warnings and special precautions for use*).

Children aged 2 to 12 years: There was insufficient evidence available from appropriate studies in children, upon which to base dosage recommendations for monotherapy use in children under the age of 12 years (see *Uses*).

Dosage in add-on therapy:
Adults and children over 12 years: In patients taking valproate with/without any other anti-epileptic drug (AED) the initial Lamictal dose is 25 mg every alternate day for two weeks, followed by 25 mg once a day for two weeks. Thereafter, the dose should be increased by a maximum of 25–50 mg every 1–2 weeks until the optimal response is achieved. The usual maintenance dose to achieve optimal response is 100–200 mg/day given once a day or in two divided doses.

In those patients taking enzyme inducing AEDs with/without other AEDs (except valproate) the initial Lamictal dose is 50 mg once a day for two weeks, followed by 100 mg/day given in two divided doses for two weeks. Thereafter, the dose should be increased by a maximum of 100 mg every 1–2 weeks until the optimal response is achieved. The usual maintenance dose to achieve optimal response is 200–400 mg/day given in two divided doses. Some patients have required 700 mg/day of Lamictal to achieve the desired response.

In patients taking AEDs where the pharmacokinetic interaction with lamotrigine is currently not known, the dose escalation as recommended for lamotrigine with concurrent valproate should be used, thereafter, the dose should be increased until optimal response is achieved.

Recommended dose escalation of Lamictal for ADULTS AND CHILDREN OVER 12 YEARS on combined drug therapy

Concomitant medication	Weeks 1–2	Weeks 3–4	Usual maintenance dose
Valproate with/without any other AEDs	12.5 mg (given as 25 mg on alternate days)	25 mg (once a day)	100–200 mg (once a day or two divided doses) To achieve maintenance, doses may be increased by 25–50 mg every 1–2 weeks.
Enzyme inducing AEDs† with/without other AEDs (except valproate)	50 mg (once a day)	100 mg (two divided doses)	200–400 mg (two divided doses) To achieve maintenance, doses may be increased by 100 mg every 1–2 weeks.

† e.g. phenytoin, carbamazepine, phenobarbitone and primidone

Note: In patients taking AEDs where the pharmacokinetic interaction with lamotrigine is currently not known, the dose escalation as recommended for lamotrigine with concurrent valproate should be used. Thereafter, the dose should be increased until optimal response is achieved.

The initial dose and subsequent dose escalation should not be exceeded to minimise the risk of rash (see *Special warnings and special precautions for use*).

Children aged 2 to 12 years: In patients taking valproate with/without any other anti-epileptic drug (AED), the initial Lamictal dose is 0.2 mg/kg bodyweight/day given once a day for two weeks, followed by 0.5 mg/kg/day given once a day for two weeks. Thereafter, the dose should be increased by a maximum of 0.5–1 mg/kg every 1–2 weeks until the optimal response is achieved. The usual maintenance dose to achieve optimal response is 1–5 mg/kg/day given once a day or in two divided doses.

In those patients taking enzyme inducing AEDs with/without other AEDs (except valproate) the initial Lamictal dose is 2 mg/kg bodyweight/day given in two divided doses for two weeks, followed by 5 mg/kg/day for two weeks. Thereafter, the dose should be increased by a maximum of 2–3 mg/kg every 1–2 weeks until the optimal response is achieved. The usual maintenance dose to achieve optimal response is 5–15 mg/kg/day given in two divided doses.

In patients taking AEDs where the pharmacokinetic interaction with lamotrigine is currently not known, the dose escalation as recommended for lamotrigine with concurrent valproate should be used, thereafter, the dose should be increased until optimal response is achieved.

Recommended dose escalation of Lamictal for children aged 2–12 years on combined drug therapy (Total daily dose in mg/kg bodyweight/day).

Concomitant medication	*Weeks 1–2*	*Weeks 3–4*	*Maintenance dose*
Valproate with/without any other AEDs	0.2 mg/kg‡ (once a day)	0.5 mg/kg (once a day)	1-5 mg/kg (once a day or two divided doses) To achieve maintenance, doses may be increased by 0.5–1 mg/kg every 1–2 weeks.
Enzyme inducing AEDs† with/without other AEDs (except valproate)	2 mg/kg (two divided doses)	5 mg/kg (two divided doses)	5–15 mg/kg (two divided doses) To achieve maintenance, doses may be increased by 2–3 mg/kg every 1–2 weeks.

† e.g. phenytoin, carbamazepine, phenobarbitone and primidone.

Note: In patients taking AEDs where the pharmacokinetic interaction with lamotrigine is currently not known, the dose escalation as recommended for lamotrigine with concurrent valproate should be used, thereafter, the dose should be increased until optimal response is achieved.

‡ If the calculated daily dose is 2.5–5 mg, then 5 mg Lamictal may be taken on alternate days for the first two weeks. If the calculated daily dose is less then 2.5 mg, then Lamictal should not be administered.

The initial dose and subsequent dose escalation should not be exceeded to minimise the risk of rash (see *Special warnings and special precautions for use*).

It is likely that patients aged 2–6 years will require a maintenance dose at the higher end of the recommended range.

Children aged less than 2 years: There is insufficient information on the use of Lamictal in children aged less than 2 years.

Use in the elderly: There is limited information on the use of Lamictal in elderly patients. To date, there is no evidence to suggest that the response of this age group differs from that in the young. However, elderly patients should be treated cautiously.

Administration: Lamictal tablets should be swallowed whole with a little water.

Lamictal Dispersible Tablets may be chewed or dispersed in a small volume of water (at least enough to cover the whole tablet) or swallowed whole with a little water.

To ensure a therapeutic dose is maintained, the weight of a child must be monitored and the dose reviewed as weight changes occur. If the doses calculated for children, according to bodyweight, do not equate to whole tablets the dose to be administered is that equal to the lower number of whole tablets.

Contra-indications, warnings, etc

Contra-indications: Lamictal is contra-indicated in individuals with known hypersensitivity to lamotrigine.

Lamictal is cleared primarily by metabolism in the liver. No studies have been carried out in patients with significant impairment of hepatic function. Until such data become available Lamictal is contra-indicated in this condition.

Special warnings and special precautions for use: There have been reports of adverse skin reactions, which have generally occurred within the first 8 weeks after initiation of lamotrigine (Lamictal) treatment. The majority of rashes are mild and self limiting. However, rarely, serious potentially life threatening skin rashes including Stevens-Johnson syndrome (SJS) and toxic epidermal necrolysis (TEN) have been reported (see *Undesirable effects*).

The approximate incidence of serious skin rashes in adults and children over the age of 12 is 1 in 1000. The risk is higher in children under the age of 12 than in adults. Available data from a number of studies suggest the incidence in children under the age of 12 requiring hospitalisation due to rash ranges from 1 in 300 to 1 in 100 (see *Undesirable effects*).

In children, the initial presentation of a rash can be mistaken for an infection, physicians should consider the possibility of a drug reaction in children that develop symptoms of rash and fever during the first eight weeks of therapy.

Additionally the overall risk of rash appears to be strongly associated with:

- High initial doses of lamotrigine and exceeding the recommended dose escalation of lamotrigine therapy (see *Posology and method of administration*).
- Concomitant use of valproate, which increases the mean half-life of lamotrigine nearly two fold (see *Posology and method of administration*).

All patients (adults and children) who develop a rash should be promptly evaluated and lamotrigine withdrawn immediately unless the rash is clearly not drug related.

Rash has also been reported as part of a hypersensitivity syndrome associated with a variable pattern of systemic symptoms including fever, lymphadenopathy, facial oedema and abnormalities of the blood and liver. The syndrome shows a wide spectrum of clinical severity and may, rarely, lead to disseminated intravascular coagulation (DIC) and multiorgan failure. It is important to note that early manifestations of hypersensitivity (e.g. fever, lymphadenopathy) may be present even though rash is not evident. Patients should be warned to seek immediate medical advice if signs and symptoms develop. If such signs and symptoms are present the patient should be evaluated immediately and Lamictal discontinued if an alternative aetiology cannot be established.

As with other AEDs, abrupt withdrawal of Lamictal may provoke rebound seizures. Unless safety concerns (for example rash) require an abrupt withdrawal, the dose of Lamictal should be gradually decreased over a period of 2 weeks.

When concomitant anti-epileptic drugs (AEDs) are withdrawn to achieve Lamictal monotherapy or other anti-epileptic drugs (AEDs) are added-on to Lamictal monotherapy consideration should be given to the effect this may have on lamotrigine pharmacokinetics (see *Interaction with other drugs and other forms of interaction*).

During clinical experience with lamotrigine used as add-on therapy, there have been, rarely, deaths following rapidly progressive illnesses with status epilepticus, rhabdomyolysis, multiorgan dysfunction and disseminated intravascular coagulation (DIC). The contribution of lamotrigine to these events remains to be established.

Lamictal is a weak inhibitor of dihydrofolate reductase hence there is a possibility of interference with folate metabolism during long-term therapy. However, during prolonged human dosing, lamotrigine did not induce significant changes in the haemoglobin concentration, mean corpuscular volume, or serum or red blood cell folate concentrations up to 1 year or red blood cell folate concentrations for up to 5 years.

In single dose studies in subjects with end-stage renal failure, plasma concentrations of lamotrigine were not significantly altered. However, accumulation of the glucuronide metabolite is to be expected; caution should therefore be exercised in treating patients with renal failure.

Interaction with other drugs and other forms of interaction: Anti-epileptic agents which induce drug-metabolising enzymes (such as phenytoin, carbamazepine, phenobarbitone and primidone) enhance the metabolism of lamotrigine and may increase dose requirements.

Sodium valproate, which competes with lamotrigine for hepatic drug-metabolising enzymes, reduces the metabolism of lamotrigine.

There is no evidence that lamotrigine causes clinically significant induction or inhibition of hepatic oxidative drug-metabolising enzymes. Lamotrigine may induce its own metabolism but the effect is modest and unlikely to have significant clinical consequences.

Although changes in the plasma concentrations of other anti-epileptic drugs have been reported, controlled studies have shown no evidence that lamotrigine affects the plasma concentrations of concomitant anti-epileptic drugs. Evidence from *in vitro* studies indicates that lamotrigine does not displace other anti-epileptic drugs from protein binding sites.

There have been reports of central nervous system events including headache, nausea, blurred vision, dizziness, diplopia and ataxia in patients taking carbamazepine following the introduction of lamotrigine. These events usually resolve when the dose of carbamazepine is reduced.

In a study of 12 female volunteers, lamotrigine did not affect plasma concentrations of ethinyloestradiol and levonorgestrel following the administration of the oral contraceptive pill. However, as with the introduction of other chronic therapy in patients taking oral contraceptives, any change in the menstrual bleeding pattern should be reported to the patient's physician.

Undesirable effects: Adverse experiences reported during Lamictal monotherapy trials include headache, tiredness, rash, nausea, dizziness, drowsiness and insomnia.

In double-blind, add-on clinical trials, skin rashes occurred in up to 10% of patients taking lamotrigine and in 5% of patients taking placebo. The skin rashes led to the withdrawal of lamotrigine treatment in 2% of patients. The rash, usually maculopapular in appearance, generally appears within eight weeks of starting treatment and resolves on withdrawal of lamotrigine (see *Special warnings and special precautions for use*).

Rarely, serious potentially life threatening skin rashes, including Stevens-Johnson syndrome and toxic epidermal necrolysis (Lyell Syndrome) have been reported. Although the majority recover on drug withdrawal, some patients experience irreversible scarring and there have been rare cases of associated death (see *Special warnings and special precautions for use*).

The approximate incidence of serious skin rashes in adults and children over the age of 12 is 1 in 1,000. The risk is higher in children under the age of 12 than in adults. Available data from a number of studies suggest the incidence in children under the age of 12 requiring hospitalisation due to rash ranges from 1 in 300 to 1 in 100 (see *Special warnings and special precautions for use*).

In children, the initial presentation of a rash can be mistaken for an infection, physicians should consider the possibility of a drug reaction in children that develop symptoms of rash and fever during the first eight weeks of therapy.

Additionally the overall risk of rash appears to be strongly associated with:

- High initial doses of lamotrigine and exceeding the recommended dose escalation of lamotrigine therapy (see *Posology and method of administration*).
- Concomitant use of valproate, which increases the mean half life of lamotrigine nearly two fold (see *Posology and method of administration*).

All patients (adults and children) who develop a rash should be promptly evaluated and lamotrigine withdrawn immediately unless the rash is clearly not drug related.

Rash has also been reported as part of a hypersensitivity syndrome associated with a variable pattern of systemic symptoms including fever, lymphadenopathy, facial oedema and abnormalities of the blood and liver. The syndrome shows a wide spectrum of clinical severity and may, rarely, lead to disseminated intravascular coagulation (DIC) and multiorgan failure. It is important to note that early manifestations of hypersensitivity (e.g. fever, lymphadenopathy) may be present even though rash is not evident. Patients should be warned to seek immediate medical advice if signs and symptoms develop. If such signs and symptoms are present the patient should be evaluated immediately and Lamictal discontinued if an alternative aetiology cannot be established.

Other adverse experiences reported when lamotrigine is added-on to standard anti-epileptic drug regimens have included diplopia, blurred vision, conjunctivitis, dizziness, drowsiness, headache, unsteadiness, tiredness, gastrointestinal disturbance (including vomiting), irritability/aggression, tremor, agitation, confusion and haematological abnormalities (including neutropenia, leucopenia and thrombocytopenia).

Use in pregnancy and lactation:

Fertility: Administration of Lamictal did not impair fertility in animal reproductive studies. There is no experience of the effect of Lamictal on human fertility.

Teratogenicity: Lamotrigine is a weak inhibitor of dihydrofolate reductase. There is a theoretical risk of human foetal malformations when the mother is treated with a folate inhibitor during pregnancy. However, reproductive toxicology studies with lamotrigine in animals at doses in excess of the human therapeutic dosage showed no teratogenic effects.

Pregnancy: There are insufficient data available on the use of lamotrigine in human pregnancy to evaluate its safety. Lamotrigine should not be used in pregnancy unless, in the opinion of the physician, the potential benefits of treatment to the mother outweigh any possible risks to the developing foetus.

Lactation: Preliminary data indicate that lamotrigine passes into breast milk in concentrations usually of the order of 40-45% of the plasma concentration.

In the small number of infants known to have been breastfed, the dose of lamotrigine received was calculated to be approximately 0.06-0.75 mg/kg/24 hours, and no adverse experiences were reported.

Effects on ability to drive and use machines: Two volunteer studies have demonstrated that the effect of lamotrigine on fine visual motor co-ordination, eye movements, body sway and subjective sedative effects did not differ from placebo.

In clinical trials with lamotrigine adverse events of a neurological character such as dizziness and diplopia have been reported. As there is individual variation in response to all anti-epileptic drug therapy patients should consult their physician on the specific issues of driving and epilepsy.

Overdose: Symptoms and signs: Ingestion of between 1.35 and 4 g lamotrigine has been reported in a few patients. Clinical consequences were not severe, signs and symptoms included nystagmus, ataxia, dizziness, somnolence, headache and vomiting.

A patient who ingested a dose calculated to be between 4 and 5 g lamotrigine was admitted to hospital with coma lasting 8-12 hours followed by recovery over the next 2 to 3 days. A further patient who ingested 5.6 g lamotrigine was found unconscious. Following treatment with activated charcoal for suspected intoxication the patient recovered after sleeping for 16 hours.

Treatment: In the event of overdosage, the patient should be admitted to hospital and given appropriate supportive therapy. Gastric lavage should be performed if indicated.

Pharmaceutical precautions Lamictal Tablets (non-dispersible): Store below 30°C. Keep dry.

Lamictal Dispersible: Store below 30°C. Protect from light. Keep dry.

Legal category POM

Package quantities

Lamictal Tablets 100 mg:	Blister pack of 4 x 14 tablets
Lamictal Tablets 200 mg: (Calendar pack)	Blister pack of 4 x 14 tablets
Lamictal Dispersible 5 mg:	Blister pack of 2 x 14 tablets
Lamictal Dispersible 25 mg:	Blister pack of 4 x 14 tablets
Lamictal Dispersible 100 mg:	Blister pack of 4 x 14 tablets

Further information Nil.

Product licence numbers

Lamictal Tablets 100 mg:	0003/0274
Lamictal Tablets 200 mg:	0003/0297
Lamictal Dispersible 5 mg:	0003/0346
Lamictal Dispersible 25 mg:	0003/0347
Lamictal Dispersible 100 mg:	0003/0348

LANOXIN 125 TABLETS

Qualitative and quantitative composition Digoxin PhEur 0.125 mg/tablet.

Pharmaceutical form Tablet.

Clinical particulars

Therapeutic indications: Lanoxin is indicated in the management of chronic cardiac failure. Its therapeutic benefit is greatest in those patients with ventricular dilatation.

Lanoxin is specifically indicated where cardiac failure is accompanied by atrial fibrillation.

Lanoxin is indicated in the management of certain supraventricular arrhythmias, particularly atrial flutter and fibrillation, where its major beneficial effect is reduction of the ventricular rate.

Posology and method of administration:

Route of administration: Oral. The dose of Lanoxin for each patient has to be tailored individually according to age, lean body weight and renal function. Suggested doses are intended only as an initial guide.

Adults and children over 10 years: Rapid oral loading:

750 to 1500 micrograms (0.75 to 1.5 mg) as a single dose.

Where there is less urgency, or a greater risk of toxicity, e.g. in the elderly, the oral loading dose should be given in divided doses 6 hours apart, assessing clinical response before giving each additional dose (see *Special warnings and special precautions for use*).

Slow Oral Loading: 250 to 750 micrograms (0.25 to 0.75 mg) should be given daily for 1 week followed by an appropriate maintenance dose. A clinical response should be seen within one week.

Note: The choice between slow and rapid oral loading depends on the clinical state of the patient and the urgency of the condition.

Maintenance: The maintenance dosage should be based upon the percentage of the peak body stores lost each day through elimination. The following formula has had wide clinical use:

$$\text{Maintenance dose} = \text{Peak body stores} \times \frac{\%\ \text{daily loss}}{100}$$

Where: peak body stores = loading dose; % daily loss = 14 + creatinine clearance (C_{cr})/5.

C_{cr} is creatinine clearance corrected to 70 kg bodyweight or 1.73 m² body surface area. If only serum creatinine (S_{cr}) concentrations are available, a C_{cr} (corrected to 70 kg bodyweight) may be estimated in men as:

$$C_{cr} = \frac{140-\text{age}}{S_{cr}\ (\text{in mg/100 ml})}$$

Note: Where serum creatinine values are obtained in micromol/l, these may be converted to mg/100 ml (mg %) as follows:

$$S_{cr}\ (\text{mg/100 ml}) = \frac{S_{cr}\ (\text{micromol/l}) \times 113.12}{10{,}000} = \frac{S_{cr}\ (\text{micromol/l})}{88.4}$$

Where 113.12 is the molecular weight of creatinine. *For women,* this result should be multiplied by 0.85.

Note: These formulae cannot be used for creatinine clearance in children.

In practice, this will mean that most patients will be maintained on 0.125 to 0.75 mg digoxin daily; however, in those who show increased sensitivity to the adverse effects of digoxin, a dosage of 62.5 microgram (0.0625 mg) daily or less may suffice.

Neonates, infants and children up to 10 years of age (if cardiac glycosides have not been given in the preceding two weeks):

Oral loading dose: This should be administered in accordance with the following schedule:

Pre-term neonates < 1.5 kg	25 microgram/kg over 24 hours
Pre-term neonates 1.5 kg–2.5 kg	30 microgram/kg over 24 hours
Term neonates up to 2 years	45 microgram/kg over 24 hours
2 to 5 years	35 microgram/kg over 24 hours
5 to 10 years	25 microgram/kg over 24 hours

The loading dose should be administered in divided doses with approximately half the total dose given as the first dose and further fractions of the total dose given at intervals of 4 to 8 hours, assessing clinical response before giving each additional dose.

Maintenance: The maintenance dose should be administered in accordance with the following schedule:

Pre-term neonates: daily dose = 20% of 24-hour loading dose

Term neonates and children up to 10 years: daily dose = 25% of 24-hour loading dose

These dosage schedules are meant as guidelines and careful clinical observation and monitoring of serum digoxin levels (see *Monitoring*) should be used as a basis for adjustment of dosage in these paediatric patient groups.

If cardiac glycosides have been given in the two weeks preceding commencement of Lanoxin therapy, it should be anticipated that optimum loading doses of Lanoxin will be less than those recommended above.

Use in the elderly: The tendency to impaired renal function and low lean body mass in the elderly influences the pharmacokinetics of Lanoxin, such that high serum digoxin levels and associated toxicity can occur quite readily, unless dosages of Lanoxin lower than those in non-elderly patients are used. Serum digoxin levels should be checked regularly and hypokalaemia avoided.

Dose recommendations in renal disorder or with diuretic therapy: See *Precautions*.

Monitoring: Serum concentrations of digoxin may be expressed in conventional units of ng/ml or SI units of nmol/l. To convert ng/ml to nmol/l, multiply ng/ml by 1.28.

The serum concentration of digoxin can be determined by radioimmunoassay. Blood should be taken 6 hours or more after the last dose of Lanoxin. There are no rigid guidelines as to the range of serum concentrations that are most efficacious but most patients will benefit, with little risk of toxic symptoms and signs developing, with digoxin concentrations from 0.8 nanogram/ml, ng/ml (1.02 nanomol/litre, nm/l) to 2.0 ng/ml (2.56 nm/l). Above this range, toxic symptoms and signs become more frequent and levels above 3 ng/ml (3.84 nm/l) are quite likely to be toxic. However, in deciding whether a patient's symptoms are due to digoxin, the patient's clinical state together with the serum potassium level and thyroid function are important factors.

Other glycosides, including metabolites of digoxin, can interfere with the assays that are available and one should always be wary of values which do not seem commensurate with the clinical state of the patient.

Contra-indications: Lanoxin is contra-indicated in intermittent complete heart block or second degree atrioventricular block, especially if there is a history of Stokes-Adams attacks.

Lanoxin is contra-indicated in arrhythmias caused by cardiac glycoside intoxication.

Lanoxin is contra-indicated in supraventricular arrhythmias associated with an accessory atrioventricular pathway, as in the Wolff-Parkinson-White syndrome, unless the electrophysiological characteristics of the accessory pathway and any possible deleterious effect of digoxin on these characteristics has been evaluated. If an accessory pathway is known or suspected to be present and there is no history of previous supraventricular arrhythmias, Lanoxin is similarly contra-indicated.

Lanoxin is contra-indicated in Hypertrophic Obstructive Cardiomyopathy, unless there is concomitant atrial fibrillation and heart failure, but even then caution should be exercised if Lanoxin is to be used.

Lanoxin is contra-indicated in patients known to be hypersensitive to digoxin or other digitalis glycosides.

Special warnings and special precautions for use: Arrhythmias may be precipitated by digoxin toxicity, some of which can resemble arrhythmias for which the drug could be advised. For example, atrial tachycardia with varying atrioventricular block requires care as clinically the rhythm resembles atrial fibrillation.

In some cases of sinoatrial disorder (i.e. Sick Sinus Syndrome) digoxin may cause or exacerbate sinus bradycardia or cause sinoatrial block.

Determination of the serum digoxin concentration may be very helpful in making a decision to treat with further digoxin, but toxic doses of other glycosides may cross-react in the assay and wrongly suggest apparently satisfactory measurements. Observations during the temporary withholding of digoxin might be more appropriate.

In cases where cardiac glycosides have been taken in the preceding two weeks, the recommendations for initial dosing of a patient should be reconsidered and a reduced dose is advised.

The dosing recommendations should be reconsidered if patients are elderly or there are other reasons for the renal clearance of digoxin being reduced. A reduction in both initial and maintenance doses should be considered.

Hypokalaemia sensitises the myocardium to the actions of cardiac glycosides.

Hypomagnesaemia and marked hypercalcaemia increase myocardial sensitivity to cardiac glycosides.

Administering Lanoxin to a patient with thyroid disease requires care. Initial and maintenance doses of Lanoxin should be reduced when thyroid function is subnormal. In hyperthyroidism there is relative digoxin resistance and the dose may have to be increased. During the course of treatment of thyrotoxicosis, dosage should be reduced as the thyrotoxicosis comes under control.

Patients with malabsorption syndrome or gastro-intestinal reconstructions may require larger doses of digoxin.

The risk of provoking dangerous arrhythmias with direct current cardioversion is greatly increased in the presence of digitalis toxicity and is in proportion to the cardioversion energy used.

For elective direct current cardioversion of a patient who is taking digoxin, the drug should be withheld for 24 hours before cardioversion is performed. In emergencies, such as cardiac arrest when attempting cardioversion the lowest effective energy should be applied.

Direct current cardioversion is inappropriate in the treatment of arrhythmias thought to be caused by cardiac glycosides.

Many beneficial effects of digoxin on arrhythmias result from a degree of atrioventricular conduction blockage. However, when incomplete atrioventricular block already exists the effects of a rapid progression in the block should be anticipated. In complete heart block the idioventricular escape rhythm may be suppressed.

The administration of digoxin in the period immediately following myocardial infarction is not contra-indicated. However, the possibility of arrhythmias arising in patients who may be hypokalaemic after myocardial infarction and are likely to be cardiologically unstable must be borne in mind. The limitations imposed thereafter on direct current cardioversion must also be remembered.

Although many patients with chronic congestive cardiac failure benefit from acute administration of digoxin, there are some in whom it does not lead to constant, marked or lasting haemodynamic improvement. It is therefore important to evaluate the response of each patient individually when Lanoxin is continued long-term.

Patients with severe respiratory disease may have an increased myocardial sensitivity to digitalis glycosides.

No data are available on whether or not digoxin has mutagenic, carcinogenic or teratogenic effects; however, maternally-administered digoxin has been used to treat foetal tachycardia and congestive heart failure.

There is no information available on the effect of digoxin on human fertility.

Interaction with other medicaments and other forms of interaction: These may arise from effects on the renal excretion, tissue binding, plasma protein binding, distribution within the body, gut absorptive capacity and sensitivity to Lanoxin. Consideration of the possibility of an interaction whenever concomitant therapy is contemplated is the best precaution and a check on serum digoxin concentration is recommended when any doubt exists.

Agents causing hypokalaemia or intracellular potassium deficiency may cause increased sensitivity to Lanoxin; they include diuretics, lithium salts, corticosteroids and carbenoxolone.

Serum levels of digoxin may be *increased* by concomitant administration of the following: amiodarone; captopril; flecainide; prazosin; propafenone; quinidine; spironolactone; tetracycline; erythromycin (and possibly other antibiotics); and propantheline.

Serum levels of digoxin may be *reduced* by concomitant administration of the following: antacids; kaolin-pectin; some bulk laxatives and cholestyramine, diphenoxylate; sulphasalazine; neomycin; rifampicin; cytostatics; phenytoin; metoclopramide; and penicillamine.

Calcium channel blocking agents may either increase or cause no change in serum digoxin levels. Verapamil increases serum digoxin levels. Nifedipine and diltiazem may increase or have no effect on serum digoxin levels. Isradipine causes no change in serum digoxin levels.

Milrinone does not alter steady-state serum digoxin levels.

Pregnancy and lactation: The use of digoxin in pregnancy is not contra-indicated, although the dosage and control may be less predictable in pregnant than in non-pregnant women with some requiring an increased dosage of digoxin during pregnancy. As with all drugs, use should be considered only when the expected clinical benefit of treatment to the mother outweighs any possible risk to the developing foetus.

Although digoxin is excreted in breast milk, the quantities are minute and breast feeding is not contra-indicated.

Effects on ability to drive and use machines: None known.

Undesirable effects:
Non-cardiac: These are principally associated with overdosage but may occur from a temporarily high serum concentration due to rapid absorption. They include anorexia, nausea and vomiting and usually disappear within a few hours of taking the drug. Diarrhoea can also occur. It is inadvisable to rely on nausea as an early warning of excessive digoxin dosage.

Gynaecomastia can occur with long-term administration.

Weakness, apathy, fatigue, malaise, headache, visual disturbances, depression and even psychosis have been reported as adverse central nervous system effects.

Oral digoxin has also been associated with intestinal ischaemia and, rarely, with intestinal necrosis.

Skin rashes of urticarial or scarlatiniform character are rare reactions to digoxin, and may be accompanied by pronounced eosinophilia.

Very rarely, digoxin can cause thrombocytopenia.

Cardiac: Digoxin toxicity can cause various arrhythmias and conduction disturbances. Usually an early sign is the occurrence of ventricular premature contractions; they can proceed to bigeminy or even trigeminy. Atrial tachycardias, frequently an indication for digoxin, may occur with excessive dosage of the drug. Atrial tachycardia with some degree of atrioventricular block is particularly characteristic, and the pulse rate may not necessarily be fast (see also *Precautions*).

Overdose: For symptoms and signs see *Undesirable effects.*

After recent ingestion, such as accidental or deliberate self-poisoning, the load available for absorption may be reduced by gastric lavage.

An overdosage of digoxin of 10 to 15 mg in adults without heart disease and of 6 to 10 mg in children aged 1 to 3 years without heart disease appeared to be the dose resulting in death in half of the patients.

If more than 25 mg of digoxin was ingested by an adult without heart disease, death or progressive toxicity responsive only to digoxin-binding Fab antibody fragments (Digibind) resulted. If more than 10 mg of digoxin was ingested by a child aged 1 to 3 years without heart disease, the outcome was uniformly fatal when Fab fragment treatment was not given.

If hypokalaemia is present, it should be corrected with potassium supplements either orally or intravenously depending on the urgency of the situation. In cases where a large amount of Lanoxin has been ingested, hyperkalaemia may be present due to release of potassium from skeletal muscle. Before administering potassium in digoxin overdose the serum potassium level must be known.

Bradyarrhythmias may respond to atropine but temporary cardiac pacing may be required. Ventricular arrhythmias may respond to lignocaine or phenytoin.

Dialysis is not particularly effective in removing digoxin from the body in potentially life-threatening toxicity.

Rapid reversal of the complications that are associated with serious poisoning by digoxin, digitoxin and related glycosides has followed intravenous administration of digoxin-specific (ovine) antibody fragments (Fab) when other therapies have failed. Digibind is the only specific treatment for digoxin toxicity and is very effective. For details consult the literature supplied with Digibind.

Pharmacological properties
Pharmacodynamic properties: None stated.

Pharmacokinetic properties: None stated.

Preclinical safety data: There are no pre-clinical data of relevance to the prescriber which are additional to that already included in other sections of the SmPC.

Pharmaceutical particulars
List of excipients: Lactose PhEur, Starches PhEur, Hydrolysed Starch HSE, Magnesium Stearate PhEur.

Incompatibilities: None known.

Shelf life: 60 months.

Special precautions for storage: Store below 25°C.

Nature and contents of container: Amber glass bottle with low density polyethylene snap-fit closure. Pack sizes: 28, 50, 500.

Amber glass bottle with a clic-loc child resistant closure. Pack size: 56.

Instructions for use/handling: Not applicable.

Marketing authorisation number PL 0003/0102R.

Date of first authorisation/renewal of authorisation 14 April 1992.

Date of (partial) revision of text September 1997.

LANOXIN INJECTION

Qualitative and quantitative composition Digoxin 0.025% w/v.

Pharmaceutical form Injection.

Clinical particulars
Therapeutic indications: Lanoxin is indicated in the management of chronic cardiac failure. Its therapeutic benefit is greatest in those patients with ventricular dilatation.

Lanoxin is specifically indicated where cardiac failure is accompanied by atrial fibrillation.

Lanoxin is indicated in the management of certain supraventricular arrhythmias, particularly atrial flutter and fibrillation, where its major beneficial effect is reduction of the ventricular rate.

Posology and method of administration: The dose of Lanoxin for each patient has to be tailored individually according to age, lean body weight and renal function. Suggested doses are intended only as an initial guide.

Emergency parenteral loading (in patients who have not been given cardiac glycosides within the preceding two weeks): The loading of parenteral Lanoxin is 500 to 1000 micrograms (0.5 to 1.0 mg) depending on age, lean body weight and renal function.

The loading dose should be administered in divided doses with approximately half the total dose given as the first dose and further fractions of the total dose given at intervals of 4 to 8 hours, assessing clinical response before giving each additional dose. Each dose should be given by intravenous infusion (see *Dilution*) over 10 to 20 minutes.

Neonates, infants and children up to 10 years of age (if cardiac glycosides have not been given in the preceding two weeks): The *intravenous loading dose* in the above groups should be administered in accordance with the following schedule:

Pre-term neonates <1.5 kg	20 microgram/kg over 24 hours
Pre-term neonates 1.5 kg–2.5 kg	30 microgram/kg over 24 hours
Term neonates up to 2 years	35 microgram/kg over 24 hours
2 to 5 years	35 microgram/kg over 24 hours
5 to 10 years	25 microgram/kg over 24 hours

The loading dose should be administered in divided doses with approximately half the total dose given as the first dose and further fractions of the total dose given at intervals of 4 to 8 hours, assessing clinical response before giving each additional dose. Each dose should be given by intravenous infusion (see *Dilution*) over 10 to 20 minutes.

Maintenance: The maintenance dose should be administered in accordance with the following schedule:

Pre-term neonates:
daily dose = 20% of 24-hour loading dose (intravenous or oral)

Term neonates and children up to 10 years:
daily dose= 25% of 24-hour loading dose (intravenous or oral)

These dosage schedules are meant as guidelines and careful clinical observation and monitoring of serum digoxin levels (see *Monitoring*) should be used as a basis for adjustment of dosage in these paediatric patient groups.

If cardiac glycosides have been given in the two weeks preceding commencement of Lanoxin therapy, it should be anticipated that optimum loading doses of Lanoxin will be less than those recommended above.

Use in the elderly: The tendency to impaired renal function and low lean body mass in the elderly influences the pharmacokinetics of Lanoxin, such that high serum digoxin levels and associated toxicity can occur quite readily, unless doses of Lanoxin lower than those in non-elderly patients are used. Serum digoxin levels should be checked regularly and hypokalaemia avoided.

Dose recommendations in renal disorder or with diuretic therapy: See *Precautions.*

Dilution: Lanoxin Injection, 250 micrograms per ml when diluted in the ratio of 1 to 250 (i.e. one 2 ml ampoule containing 500 micrograms added to 500 ml of infusion solution) is known to be compatible with the following infusion solutions and stable for up to 48 hours at room temperature (20 to 25°C);

Sodium Chloride Intravenous Infusion, BP, 0.9% w/v. Sodium Chloride (0.18% w/v) and Glucose (4% w/v) Intravenous Infusion, BP. Glucose Intravenous Infusion, BP, 5% w/v.

Dilution should be carried out either under full aseptic conditions or immediately before use. Any unused solution should be discarded.

Monitoring: Serum concentrations of digoxin may be expressed in conventional units of nanogram/ml or SI Units of nanoMol/L. To convert ng/ml to nmol/L, multiply ng/ml by 1.28.

The serum concentration of digoxin can be determined by radioimmunoassay. Blood should be taken 6 hours or more after the last dose of Lanoxin. There are no rigid guidelines as to the range of serum concentrations that are most efficacious but most patients will benefit, with little risk of toxic symptoms developing, with digoxin concentrations from 0.8 nanogram/ml, (ng/ml) (1.02 nanoMol/litre, nM/L) to 2.0 ng/ml (2.56 nM/L). Above this range toxic symptoms and signs become more frequent and levels above 3 ng/ml (3.84 nM/L) are quite likely to be toxic. However, in deciding whether a patient's symptoms are due to digoxin, the patient's clinical state together with the serum potassium level and thyroid function are important factors.

Other glycosides, including metabolites of digoxin, can interfere with the assays that are available and one should always be wary of values which do not seem commensurate with the clinical state of the patient.

Contra-indications: Lanoxin is contra-indicated in intermittent complete heart block or second degree atrioventricular block, especially if there is a history of Stokes-Adams attacks.

Lanoxin is contra-indicated in arrhythmias caused by cardiac glycoside intoxication.

Lanoxin is contra-indicated in supraventricular arrhythmias associated with an accessory atrioventricular pathway, as in the Wolff-Parkinson-White syndrome, unless the electrophysiological characteristics of the accessory pathway and any possible deleterious effect of digoxin on these characteristics has been evaluated. If an accessory pathway is known or suspected to be present and there is no history of previous supraventricular arrhythmias, Lanoxin is similarly contra-indicated.

Lanoxin is contra-indicated in hypertrophic obstructive cardiomyopathy, unless there is concomitant atrial fibrillation and heart failure, but even then caution should be exercised if digoxin is to be used.

Lanoxin is contra-indicated in patients known to be hypersensitive to digoxin or other digitalis glycosides.

Special warnings and precautions for use: Arrhythmias may be precipitated by digoxin toxicity, some of which can resemble arrhythmias for which the drug could be advised. For example, atrial tachycardia with varying atrioventricular block requires particular care as clinically the rhythm resembles atrial fibrillation.

In some cases of sinoatrial disorder (i.e. Sick Sinus Syndrome) digoxin may cause or exacerbate sinus bradycardia or cause sinoatrial block.

Determination of the serum digoxin concentration may be very helpful in making a decision to treat with further digoxin, but toxic doses of other glycosides may cross-react in the assay and wrongly suggest apparently satisfactory measurements. Observations during the temporary withholding of digoxin might be more appropriate.

In cases where cardiac glycosides have been taken in the preceding two weeks, the recommendations for initial dosing of a patient should be reconsidered and a reduced dose is advised.

The dosing recommendations should be reconsidered if patients are elderly or there are other reasons for the renal clearance of digoxin being reduced. A reduction in both initial and maintenance doses should be considered.

Hypokalaemia sensitises the myocardium to the actions of cardiac glycosides.

Hypomagnesaemia and marked hypercalcaemia increase myocardial sensitivity to cardiac glycosides.

Rapid intravenous injection can cause vasoconstriction producing hypertension and/or reduced coronary flow. A slow injection rate is therefore important in hypertensive heart failure and acute myocardial infarction.

Administering Lanoxin to a patient with thyroid disease requires care. Initial and maintenance doses of Lanoxin should be reduced when thyroid function is subnormal. In hyperthyroidism there is relative digoxin resistance and the dose may have to be increased. During the course of treatment of thyrotoxicosis, dosage should be reduced as the thyrotoxicosis comes under control.

Patients with malabsorption syndrome or gastro-intestinal reconstructions may require larger doses of digoxin.

The risk of provoking dangerous arrhythmias with direct current cardioversion is greatly increased in the presence of digitalis toxicity and is in proportion to the cardioversion energy used.

For elective direct current cardioversion of a patient who is taking digoxin, the drug should be withheld for 24 hours before cardioversion is performed. In emergencies, such as cardiac arrest, when attempting cardioversion the lowest effective energy should be applied.

Direct current cardioversion is inappropriate in the treatment of arrhythmias thought to be caused by cardiac glycosides.

Many beneficial effects of digoxin on arrhythmias result from a degree of atrioventricular conduction blockade. However, when incomplete atrioventricular block already exists the effects of a rapid progression in the block should be anticipated. In complete heart block the idioventricular escape rhythm may be suppressed.

The administration of digoxin in the period immediately following myocardial infarction is not contra-indicated. However, the possibility of arrhythmias arising in patients who may be hypokalaemic after myocardial infarction and are likely to be cardiologically unstable must be borne in mind. The limitations imposed thereafter on direct current-cardioversion must also be remembered.

Although many patients with chronic congestive cardiac failure benefit from acute administration of digoxin, there are some in whom it does not lead to constant, marked or lasting haemodynamic improvement. It is therefore important to evaluate the response of each patient individually when Lanoxin is continued long-term.

The intramuscular route is painful and is associated with muscle necrosis. This route cannot be recommended.

Patients with severe respiratory disease may have an increased myocardial sensitivity to digitalis glycosides.

No data are available on whether or not digoxin has mutagenic, carcinogenic or teratogenic effects; however, maternally-administered digoxin has been used to treat foetal tachycardia and congestive heart failure.

There is no information available on the effect of digoxin on human fertility.

The packs will carry the following statements:
Store below 25°C.
Protect from light.
For intravenous injection under medical supervision.
Keep out of reach of children.

Interaction with other medicaments and other forms of interaction: These may arise from effects on the renal excretion, tissue binding, plasma protein binding, distribution within the body, gut absorptive capacity and sensitivity to Lanoxin. Consideration of the possibility of an interaction whenever concomitant therapy is contemplated is the best precaution and a check on serum digoxin concentration is recommended when any doubt exists.

Agents causing hypokalaemia or intracellular potassium deficiency may cause increased sensitivity to Lanoxin; they include diuretics, lithium salts, corticosteroids and carbenoxolone.

Serum levels of digoxin may be *INCREASED* by concomitant administration of the following: amiodarone; captopril; flecainide; prazosin; propafenone; quinidine; spironolactone; tetracycline; erythromycin (and possibly other antibiotics); and propantheline.

Serum levels of digoxin may be *REDUCED* by concomitant administration of the following: antacids; kaolin-pectin; some bulk laxatives and cholestyramine; diphenoxylate; sulphasalazine; neomycin; rifampicin; cytostatics; phenytoin; metoclopramide; and penicillamine.

Calcium channel blocking agents may either increase or cause no change in serum digoxin levels. Verapamil increases serum digoxin levels. Nifedipine and diltiazem may increase or have no effect on serum digoxin levels. Isradipine causes no change in serum digoxin levels.

Milrinone does not alter steady-state serum digoxin levels.

Pregnancy and lactation: The use of digoxin in pregnancy is not contra-indicated, although the dosage and control may be less predictable in pregnant than in non-pregnant women with some requiring an increased dosage of digoxin during pregnancy. As with all drugs, use should be considered only when the expected clinical benefit of treatment to the mother outweighs any possible risk to the developing foetus.

Although digoxin is excreted in breast milk, the quantities are minute and breast feeding is not contra-indicated.

Effect on ability to drive and use machines: None known.

Undesirable effects: These are principally associated with overdosage but may occur from a temporarily high serum concentration due to rapid absorption. They include anorexia, nausea and vomiting and usually disappear within a few hours of taking the drug.

Diarrhoea can also occur. It is inadvisable to rely on nausea as an early warning of excessive digoxin dosage.

Gynaecomastia can occur with long-term administration.

Weakness, apathy, fatigue, malaise, headache, visual disturbances, depression and even psychosis have been reported as adverse central nervous system effects.

Oral digoxin has also been associated with intestinal ischaemia and, rarely, with intestinal necrosis.

Skin rashes of urticarial or scarlatiniform character are rare reactions to digoxin, and may be accompanied by pronounced eosinophilia.

Very rarely, digoxin can cause thrombocytopenia.

Cardiac: Digoxin toxicity can cause various arrhythmias and conduction disturbances. Usually an early sign is the occurrence of ventricular premature contractions; they can proceed to bigeminy or even trigeminy. Atrial tachycardias, frequently an indication for digoxin, may nevertheless occur with excessive dosage of the drug. Atrial tachycardia with some degree of atrioventricular block is particularly characteristic, and the pulse rate may not necessarily be fast (see also *Precautions*).

Overdosage: For symptoms and signs see *Undesirable effects.*

After recent ingestion, such as accidental or deliberate self-poisoning, the load available for absorption may be reduced by gastric lavage.

An overdosage of digoxin of 10 to 15 mg in adults without heart disease and of 6 to 10 mg in children aged 1 to 3 years without heart disease appeared to be the dose resulting in death in half of the patients. If more than 25 mg of digoxin was ingested by an adult without heart disease, death or progressive toxicity responsive only to digoxin-binding Fab antibody fragments (Digibind) resulted. If more than 10 mg of digoxin was ingested by a child aged 1 to 3 years without heart disease, the outcome was uniformly fatal when Fab fragment treatment was not given.

If hypokalaemia is present, it should be corrected with potassium supplements either orally or intravenously depending on the urgency of the situation. In cases where a large amount of Lanoxin has been ingested, hyperkalaemia may be present due to release of potassium from skeletal muscle. Before administering potassium in digoxin overdose the serum potassium level must be known.

Bradyarrhythmias may respond to atropine but temporary cardiac pacing may be required. Ventricular arrhythmias may respond to lignocaine or phenytoin.

Dialysis is not particularly effective in removing digoxin from the body in potentially life-threatening toxicity.

Rapid reversal of the complications that are associated with serious poisoning by digoxin, digitoxin and related glycosides has followed intravenous administration of digoxin-specific (ovine) antibody fragments (Fab) when other therapies have failed. Digibind is the only specific treatment for digoxin toxicity and is very effective. For details consult the literature supplied with Digibind.

Pharmacological properties

Pharmacokinetic properties: Intravenous administration of a loading dose produces an appreciable pharmacological effect within 5 to 30 minutes; this reaches a maximum in 1 to 5 hours.

Using the oral route, the onset of effect occurs in 0.5 to 2 hours and reaches its maximum at 2 to 6 hours.

The terminal elimination half life of digoxin in patients with normal renal function is 30 to 40 hours. It will be prolonged in patients with impaired renal function, and in anuric patients will be of the order of 100 hours.

Preclinical safety data: There are no pre-clinical data of relevance to the prescriber which are additional to that already included in other sections of the SmPC.

Pharmaceutical particulars

List of excipients:

Ethanol	10.4 v/v
Propylene Glycol	40.0 v/v
Citric Acid Monohydrate	0.075 w/v
Sodium phosphate anhydrous	0.179 w/v
or Sodium phosphate	0.45 w/v
Water for Injections	to 2 ml

Incompatibilities: None known.

Shelf life: 5 years.

Special precautions for storage: Store below 25°C. Protect from light.

Nature and contents of container: Neutral glass ampoules.

Instructions for use/handling: No special instructions.

Marketing authorisation number PL 0003/5259R.

Date of first authorisation/renewal of authorisation 30.08.85 (Reviewed licence)/08.03.91, 22.07.96.

Date of (partial) revision of text July 1996.

LANOXIN PG ELIXIR

Qualitative and quantitative composition Digoxin BP 0.005% w/v.

Pharmaceutical form Liquid.

Clinical particulars

Therapeutic indications: Lanoxin is indicated in the management of chronic cardiac failure. Its therapeutic benefit is greatest in those patients with ventricular dilatation.

Lanoxin is specifically indicated where cardiac failure is accompanied by atrial fibrillation.

Lanoxin is indicated in the management of certain supraventricular arrhythmias, particularly atrial flutter and fibrillation, where its major beneficial effect is reduction of the ventricular rate.

Posology and method of administration: The dose of Lanoxin for each patient has to be tailored individually according to age, lean body weight and renal function. Suggested doses are intended only as an initial guide.

Lanoxin PG Elixir, 50 micrograms in 1 ml, is supplied with a graduated pipette and this should be used for measurement of all doses.

Adults and children over 10 years: Rapid oral loading: 750 to 1500 micrograms (0.75 to 1.5 mg) as a single dose.

Where there is less urgency, or a greater risk of toxicity, e.g. in the elderly, the oral loading dose should be given in divided doses 6 hours apart, assessing clinical response before giving each additional dose (see *Precautions*).

Slow Oral Loading: 250 to 750 micrograms (0.25 to 0.75 mg) should be given daily for 1 week followed by an appropriate maintenance dose. A clinical response should be seen within one week.

Note: The choice between slow and rapid oral loading depends on the clinical state of the patient and the urgency of the condition.

Maintenance: The maintenance dosage should be based upon the percentage of the peak body stores lost each day through elimination. The following formula has had wide clinical use:

$$\text{Maintenance dose} = \text{Peak body stores} \times \frac{\%\ \text{daily loss}}{100}$$

Where: peak body stores = loading dose; % daily loss = 14 + creatinine clearance (C_{cr})/5.

C_{cr} is creatinine clearance corrected to 70 kg bodyweight or 1.73 m^2 body surface area. If only serum creatinine (S_{cr}) concentrations are available, a C_{cr} (corrected to 70 kg bodyweight) may be estimated in men as:

$$C_{cr} = \frac{140\text{–age}}{S_{cr}\ (\text{in mg/100 ml})}$$

Note: Where serum creatinine values are obtained in micromol/l, these may be converted to mg/100 ml (mg %) as follows:

$$S_{cr}\ (\text{mg/100 ml}) = \frac{S_{cr}\ (\text{micromol/L}) \times 113.12}{10{,}000} = \frac{S_{cr}\ (\text{micromol/L})}{88.4}$$

Where 113.12 is the molecular weight of creatinine.

For women, this result should be multiplied by 0.85.

Note: These formulae cannot be used for creatinine clearance in children.

In practice, this will mean that most patients will be maintained on 0.125 to 0.75 mg digoxin daily; however, in those who show increased sensitivity to the adverse effects of digoxin, a dosage of 62.5 microgram (0.0625 mg) daily or less may suffice.

Neonates, infants and children up to 10 years of age (if cardiac glycosides have not been given in the preceding two weeks):

Oral loading dose: This should be administered in accordance with the following schedule:

Pre-term neonates < 1.5 kg	25 microgram/kg over 24 hours
Pre-term neonates 1.5 kg–2.5 kg	30 microgram/kg over 24 hours
Term neonates up to 2 years	45 microgram/kg over 24 hours
2 to 5 years	35 microgram/kg over 24 hours
5 to 10 years	25 microgram/kg over 24 hours

The loading dose should be administered in divided doses with approximately half the total dose given as the first dose and further fractions of the total dose given at intervals of 4 to 8 hours, assessing clinical response before giving each additional dose.

Maintenance: The maintenance dose should be administered in accordance with the following schedule:

Pre-term neonates: daily dose = 20% of 24-hour loading dose

Term neonates and children up to 10 years: daily dose = 25% of 24-hour loading dose

These dosage schedules are meant as guidelines and careful clinical observation and monitoring of serum digoxin levels (see *Monitoring*) should be used as a basis for adjustment of dosage in these paediatric patient groups.

If cardiac glycosides have been given in the two weeks preceding commencement of Lanoxin therapy, it should be anticipated that optimum loading doses of Lanoxin will be less than those recommended above.

Use in the elderly: The tendency to impaired renal function and low lean body mass in the elderly influences the pharmacokinetics of Lanoxin, such that high serum digoxin levels and associated toxicity can occur quite readily, unless doses of Lanoxin lower than those in non-elderly patients are used. Serum digoxin levels should be checked regularly and hypokalaemia avoided.

Dose recommendations in renal disorder or with diuretic therapy: See *Precautions.*

Monitoring: Serum concentrations of digoxin may be expressed in conventional units of ng/ml or SI units of nmol/l. To convert ng/ml to nmol/L, multiply ng/ml by 1.28.

The serum concentration of digoxin can be determined by radioimmunoassay. Blood should be taken 6 hours or more after the last dose of Lanoxin. There are no rigid guidelines as to the range of serum concentrations that are most efficacious but most patients will benefit, with little risk of toxic symptoms and signs developing, with digoxin concentrations from 0.8 nanogram/ml, ng/ml (1.02 nanomol/litre, nm/L) to 2.0 ng/ml (2.56 nm/L). Above this range, toxic symptoms and signs become more frequent and levels above 3 ng/ml (3.84 nm/L) are quite likely to be toxic. However, in deciding whether a patient's symptoms are due to digoxin, the patient's clinical state together with the serum potassium level and thyroid function are important factors.

Other glycosides, including metabolites of digoxin, can interfere with the assays that are available and one should always be wary of values which do not seem commensurate with the clinical state of the patient.

Contra-indications: Lanoxin is contra-indicated in intermittent complete heart block or second degree atrioventricular block, especially if there is a history of Stokes-Adams attacks.

Lanoxin is contra-indicated in arrhythmias caused by cardiac glycoside intoxication.

Lanoxin is contra-indicated in supraventricular arrhythmias associated with an accessory atrioventricular pathway, as in the Wolff-Parkinson-White syndrome, unless the electrophysiological characteristics of the accessory pathway and any possible deleterious effect of digoxin on these characteristics has been evaluated. If an accessory pathway is known or suspected to be present and there is no history of previous supraventricular arrhythmias, Lanoxin is similarly contra-indicated.

Lanoxin is contra-indicated in hypertrophic obstructive cardiomyopathy, unless there is concomitant atrial fibrillation and heart failure, but even then caution should be exercised if Lanoxin is to be used.

Lanoxin is contra-indicated in patients known to be hypersensitive to digoxin or other digitalis glycosides.

Special warnings and special precautions for use: Arrhythmias may be precipitated by digoxin toxicity, some of which can resemble arrhythmias for which the drug could be advised. For example, atrial tachycardia with varying atrioventricular block requires particular care as clinically the rhythm resembles atrial fibrillation.

In some cases of sinoatrial disorder (i.e. Sick Sinus Syndrome) digoxin may cause or exacerbate sinus bradycardia or cause sinoatrial block.

Determination of the serum digoxin concentration may be very helpful in making a decision to treat with further digoxin, but toxic doses of other glycosides may cross-react in the assay and wrongly suggest apparently satisfactory measurements. Observations during the temporary withholding of digoxin might be more appropriate.

In cases where cardiac glycosides have been taken in the preceding two weeks, the recommendations for initial dosing of a patient should be reconsidered and a reduced dose is advised.

The dosing recommendations should be reconsidered if patients are elderly or there are other reasons for the renal clearance of digoxin being reduced. A reduction in both initial and maintenance doses should be considered.

Hypokalaemia sensitises the myocardium to the actions of cardiac glycosides.

Hypomagnesaemia and marked hypercalcaemia increase myocardial sensitivity to cardiac glycosides.

Administering Lanoxin to a patient with thyroid disease requires care. Initial and maintenance doses of Lanoxin should be reduced when thyroid function is subnormal. In hyperthyroidism there is relative digoxin resistance and the dose may have to be increased. During the course of treatment of thyrotoxicosis, dosage should be reduced as the thyrotoxicosis comes under control.

Patients with malabsorption syndrome or gastrointestinal reconstruction may require larger doses of digoxin.

The risk of provoking dangerous arrhythmias with direct current cardioversion is greatly increased in the presence of digitalis toxicity and is in proportion to the cardioversion energy used.

For elective direct current cardioversion of a patient who is taking digoxin, the drug should be withheld for 24 hours before cardioversion is performed. In emergencies, such as cardiac arrest, when attempting cardioversion the lowest effective energy should be applied.

Direct current cardioversion is inappropriate in the treatment of arrhythmias thought to be caused by cardiac glycosides.

Many beneficial effects of digoxin on arrhythmias result from a degree of atrioventricular conduction blockade. However, when incomplete atrioventricular block already exists, the effects of a rapid progression in the block should be anticipated. In complete heart block the idioventricular escape rhythm may be suppressed.

The administration of digoxin in the period immediately following myocardial infarction is not contra-indicated. However, the possibility of arrhythmias arising in patients who may be hypokalaemic after myocardial infarction and are likely to be cardiologically unstable must be borne in mind. The limitations imposed thereafter on direct current cardioversion must also be remembered.

Although many patients with chronic congestive cardiac failure benefit from acute administration of digoxin, there are some in whom it does not lead to constant, marked or lasting haemodynamic improvement. It is therefore important to evaluate the response of each patient individually when Lanoxin is continued long-term.

Patients with severe respiratory diseases may have an increased myocardial sensitivity to digitalis glycosides.

No data are available on whether or not digoxin has mutagenic, carcinogenic or teratogenic effects. However, maternally-administered digoxin has been used to treat foetal tachycardia and congestive heart failure.

There is no information available on the effect of digoxin on human fertility.

Interaction with other medicaments and other forms of interaction: These may arise from effects on the renal excretion, tissue binding, plasma protein binding, distribution within the body, gut absorptive capacity and sensitivity to Lanoxin. Consideration of the possibility of an interaction whenever concomitant therapy is contemplated is the best precaution and a check on serum digoxin concentration is recommended when any doubt exists.

Agents causing hypokalaemia or intracellular potassium deficiency may cause increased sensitivity to Lanoxin; they include diuretics, lithium salts, corticosteroids and carbenoxolone.

Serum levels of digoxin may be *increased* by concomitant administration of the following: amiodarone; captopril; flecainide; prazosin; propafenone; quinidine; spironolactone; tetracycline; erythromycin (and possibly other antibiotics); and propantheline.

Serum levels of digoxin may be *reduced* by concomitant administration of the following: antacids; kaolin-pectin; some bulk laxatives and cholestyramine; diphenoxylate; sulphasalazine; neomycin; rifampicin; cytostatics; phenytoin; metoclopramide; and penicillamine.

Calcium channel blocking agents may either increase or cause no change in serum digoxin levels. Verapamil increases serum digoxin levels. Nifedipine and diltiazem may increase or have no effect on serum digoxin levels. Isradipine causes no change in serum digoxin levels.

Milrinone does not alter steady-state serum digoxin levels.

Pregnancy and lactation: The use of digoxin in pregnancy is not contra-indicated, although the dosage may be less predictable in pregnant than in non-pregnant women with some requiring an increased dosage of digoxin during pregnancy. As with all drugs, use should be considered only when the expected clinical benefit of treatment to the mother outweighs any possible risk to the developing foetus.

Although digoxin is excreted in breast milk, the quantities are minute and breast feeding is not contra-indicated.

Effects on ability to drive and use machines: None known.

Undesirable effects: Non-cardiac: These are principally associated with overdosage but may occur from a temporarily high serum concentration due to rapid absorption. They include anorexia, nausea and vomiting and usually disappear within a few hours of taking the drug. Diarrhoea can also occur. It is inadvisable to rely on nausea as an early warning of excessive digoxin dosage.

Gynaecomastia can occur with long-term administration.

Weakness, apathy, fatigue, malaise, headache, visual disturbances, depression and even psychosis have been reported as adverse central nervous system effects.

Oral digoxin has also been associated with intestinal ischaemia and, rarely, with intestinal necrosis.

Skin rashes of urticarial or scarlatiniform character are rare reactions to digoxin, and may be accompanied by pronounced eosinophilia.

Very rarely, digoxin can cause thrombocytopenia.

Cardiac: Digoxin toxicity can cause various arrhythmias and conduction disturbances. Usually an early sign is the occurrence of ventricular premature contractions; they can proceed to bigeminy or even trigeminy. Atrial tachycardias, frequently an indication for digoxin, may occur with excessive dosage of the drug. Atrial tachycardia with some degree of atrioventricular block is particularly characteristic, and the pulse rate may not necessarily be fast (see also *Precautions*).

Overdose: After symptoms and signs see *Undesirable effects.*

After recent ingestion, such as accidental or deliberate self-poisoning, the load available for absorption may be reduced by gastric lavage.

An overdose of digoxin of 10 to 15 mg in adults without heart disease and of 6 to 10 mg in children aged 1 to 3 years without heart disease appeared to be the dose resulting in death in half of the patients.

If more than 25 mg of digoxin was ingested by an adult without heart disease, death or progressive toxicity responsive only to digoxin-binding Fab antibody fragments (Digibind) resulted. If more than 10 mg of digoxin was ingested by a child aged 1 to 3 years without heart disease, the outcome was uniformly fatal when Fab fragment treatment was not given.

If hypokalaemia is present, it should be corrected with potassium supplements either orally or intravenously depending on the urgency of the situation. In cases where a large amount of Lanoxin has been ingested, hyperkalaemia may be present due to release of potassium from skeletal muscle. Before administering potassium in digoxin overdose the serum potassium level must be known.

Bradyarrhythmias may respond to atropine but temporary cardiac pacing may be required. Ventricular arrhythmias may respond to lignocaine or phenytoin.

Dialysis is not particularly effective in removing digoxin from the body in potentially life-threatening toxicity.

Rapid reversal of the complications that are associated with serious poisoning by digoxin, digitoxin and related glycosides has followed intravenous administration of digoxin-specific (ovine) antibody fragments (Fab) when other therapies have failed. Digibind is the only specific treatment for digoxin toxicity and is very effective. For details consult the literature supplied with Digibind.

Pharmacological properties
Pharmacodynamic properties: None stated.

Pharmacokinetic properties: None stated.

Preclinical safety data: There are no pre-clinical data of relevance to the prescriber which are additional to that in other sections of the SmPC.

Pharmaceutical particulars
List of excipients: Methyl Hydroxybenzoate PhEur, †Sucrose PhEur, †Syrup BP, Anhydrous Sodium Phosphate HSE, Citric Acid Monohydrate PhEur, Quinine Yellow HSE, Ethanol (96%) BP, Propylene Glycol PhEur, Lime Flavour No. 1 NA HSE, Purified Water PhEur.
† These ingredients are alternatives.

Incompatibilities: None known.

Shelf life: 36 months.

Special precautions for storage: Store below 25°C.

Nature and contents of container: Amber glass bottle with a metal roll-on closure and a graduated polyethene dropper assembly plus cap. Pack size: 60 ml.

Instructions for use/handling: Do not dilute.

Marketing authorisation number PL 0003/5260R.

Date of first authorisation/renewal of authorisation 22 November 1991.

Date of (partial) revision of text August 1996.

LANOXIN PG TABLETS

Qualitative and quantitative composition Digoxin PhEur 0.0625 mg/tablet.

Pharmaceutical form Tablet.

Clinical particulars
Therapeutic indications: Lanoxin is indicated in the management of chronic cardiac failure. Its therapeutic benefit is greatest in those patients with ventricular dilatation.

Lanoxin is specifically indicated where cardiac failure is accompanied by atrial fibrillation.

Lanoxin is indicated in the management of certain supraventricular arrhythmias, particularly atrial flutter and fibrillation, where its major beneficial effect is reduction of the ventricular rate.

Posology and method of administration: The dose of Lanoxin for each patient has to be tailored individually according to age, lean body weight and renal function. Suggested doses are intended only as an initial guide.

Adults and children over 10 years: Rapid oral loading: 750 to 1500 micrograms (0.75 to 1.5 mg) as a single dose.

Where there is less urgency, or greater risk of toxicity, e.g. in the elderly, the oral loading dose should be given in divided doses 6 hours apart, assessing clinical response before giving each additional dose (see *Precautions*).

Slow Oral Loading: 250 to 750 micrograms (0.25 to 0.75 mg) should be given daily for 1 week followed by an appropriate maintenance dose. A clinical response should be seen within one week.

Note: The choice between slow and rapid oral loading depends on the clinical state of the patient and the urgency of the condition.

Maintenance: The maintenance dosage should be based upon the percentage of the peak body stores lost each day through elimination. The following formula has had wide clinical use:

$$\text{Maintenance dose} = \text{Peak body stores} \times \frac{\%\ \text{daily loss}}{100}$$

Where: peak body stores = loading dose; % daily loss = 14 + creatinine clearance (C_{cr})/5.

C_{cr} is creatinine clearance corrected to 70 kg bodyweight or 1.73 m² body surface area. If only serum creatinine (S_{cr}) concentrations are available, a C_{cr} (corrected to 70 kg bodyweight) may be estimated in men as:

$$C_{cr} = \frac{140\text{–age}}{S_{cr}\ (\text{in mg/100 ml})}$$

Note: Where serum creatinine values are obtained in micromol/l, these may be converted to mg/100 ml (mg %) as follows:

$$S_{cr}\ (\text{mg/100 ml}) = \frac{S_{cr}\ (\text{micromol/L}) \times 113.12}{10{,}000} = \frac{S_{cr}\ (\text{micromol/L})}{88.4}$$

Where 113.12 is the molecular weight of creatinine.

For women, this result should be multiplied by 0.85.

Note: These formulae cannot be used for creatinine clearance in children.

In practice, this will mean that most patients will be maintained on 0.125 to 0.75 mg digoxin daily; however, in those who show increased sensitivity to the adverse effects of digoxin, a dosage of 62.5 microgram (0.0625 mg) daily or less may suffice.

Neonates, infants and children up to 10 years of age (if cardiac glycosides have not been given in the preceding two weeks):

Oral loading dose: This should be administered in accordance with the following schedule:

Pre-term neonates < 1.5 kg	25 microgram/kg over 24 hours
Pre-term neonates 1.5 kg–2.5 kg	30 microgram/kg over 24 hours
Term neonates up to 2 years	45 microgram/kg over 24 hours
2 to 5 years	35 microgram/kg over 24 hours
5 to 10 years	25 microgram/kg over 24 hours

The loading dose should be administered in divided doses with approximately half the total dose given as the first dose and further fractions of the total dose given at intervals of 4 to 8 hours, assessing clinical response before giving each additional dose.

Maintenance: The maintenance dose should be administered in accordance with the following schedule:

Pre-term neonates: daily dose = 20% of 24-hour loading dose

Term neonates and children up to 10 years: daily dose = 25% of 24-hour loading dose

These dosage schedules are meant as guidelines and careful clinical observation and monitoring of serum digoxin levels (see *Monitoring*) should be used as a basis for adjustment of dosage in these paediatric patient groups.

If cardiac glycosides have been given in the two weeks preceding commencement of Lanoxin therapy, it should be anticipated that optimum loading doses of Lanoxin will be less than those recommended above.

Use in the elderly: The tendency to impaired renal function and low lean body mass in the elderly influences the pharmacokinetics of Lanoxin, such that high serum digoxin levels and associated toxicity can occur quite readily, unless dosages of Lanoxin lower than those in non-elderly patients are used. Serum digoxin levels should be checked regularly and hypokalaemia avoided.

Dose recommendations in renal disorder or with diuretic therapy: See *Precautions.*

Monitoring: Serum concentrations of digoxin may be expressed in conventional units of ng/ml or SI units of nmol/L. To convert ng/ml to nmol/L, multiply ng/ml by 1.28.

The serum concentration of digoxin can be determined by radioimmunoassay. Blood should be taken 6 hours or more after the last dose of Lanoxin. There are no rigid guidelines as to the range of serum concentrations that are most efficacious but most patients will benefit, with little risk of toxic symptoms and signs developing, with digoxin concentrations from 0.8 nanogram/ml, ng/ml (1.02 nanomol/litre, nm/L) to 2.0 ng/ml (2.56 nm/L). Above this range toxic symptoms and signs become more frequent and levels above 3 ng/ml (3.84 nm/L) are quite likely to be toxic. However, in deciding whether a patient's symptoms are due to digoxin, the patient's clinical state together with the serum potassium level and thyroid function are important factors.

Other glycosides, including metabolites of digoxin, can interfere with the assays that are available and one should always be wary of values which do not seem commensurate with the clinical state of the patient.

Route of administration: oral.

Contra-indications: Lanoxin is contra-indicated in intermittent complete heart block or second degree atrioventricular block, especially if there is a history of Stokes-Adams attacks.

Lanoxin is contra-indicated in arrhythmias caused by cardiac glycoside intoxication.

Lanoxin is contra-indicated in supraventricular arrhythmias associated with an accessory atrioventricular pathway, as in the Wolff-Parkinson-White Syndrome, unless the electrophysiological characteristics of the accessory pathway and any possible deleterious effect of digoxin on these characteristics has been evaluated. If an accessory pathway is known or suspected to be present and there is no history of previous supraventricular arrhythmias, Lanoxin is similarly contra-indicated.

Lanoxin is contra-indicated in hypertrophic obstructive cardiomyopathy, unless there is concomitant atrial fibrillation and heart failure, but even then caution should be exercised if Lanoxin is to be used.

Lanoxin is contra-indicated in patients known to be hypersensitive to digoxin or other digitalis glycosides.

Special warnings and precautions for use: Arrhythmias may be precipitated by digoxin toxicity, some of which can resemble arrhythmias for which the drug could be advised. For example, atrial tachycardia with varying atrioventricular block requires care as clinically the rhythm resembles atrial fibrillation.

In some cases of sinoatrial disorder (i.e. Sick Sinus Syndrome) digoxin may cause or exacerbate sinus bradycardia or cause sinoatrial block.

Determination of the serum digoxin concentration may be very helpful in making a decision to treat with further digoxin, but toxic doses of other glycosides may cross-react in the assay and wrongly suggest apparently satisfactory measurements. Observations during the temporary withholding of digoxin might be more appropriate.

In cases where cardiac glycosides have been taken in the preceding two weeks, the recommendations for initial dosing of a patient should be reconsidered and a reduced dose is advised.

The dosing recommendations should be reconsidered if patients are elderly or there are other reasons for the renal clearance of digoxin being reduced. A reduction in both initial and maintenance doses should be considered.

Hypokalaemia sensitises the myocardium to the actions of cardiac glycosides.

Hypomagnesaemia and marked hypercalcaemia increase myocardial sensitivity to cardiac glycosides.

Administering Lanoxin to a patient with thyroid disease requires care. Initial and maintenance doses of Lanoxin should be reduced when thyroid function is subnormal. In hyperthyroidism there is relative digoxin resistance and the dose may have to be increased. During the course of treatment of thyrotoxicosis, dosage should be reduced as the thyrotoxicosis comes under control.

Patients with malabsorption syndrome or gastro-intestinal reconstructions may require larger doses of digoxin.

The risk of provoking dangerous arrhythmias with direct current cardioversion is greatly increased in the presence of digitalis toxicity and is in proportion to the cardioversion energy used.

For elective direct current cardioversion of a patient who is taking digoxin, the drug should be withheld for 24 hours before cardioversion is performed. In emergencies, such as cardiac arrest, when attempting cardioversion the lowest effective energy should be applied. Direct current cardioversion is inappropriate in the treatment of arrhythmias thought to be caused by cardiac glycosides.

Many beneficial effects of digoxin on arrhythmias result from a degree of atrioventricular conduction blockade. However, when incomplete atrioventricular block already exists the effects of a rapid progression in the block should be anticipated. In complete heart block the idioventricular escape rhythm may be suppressed.

The administration of digoxin in the period immediately following myocardial infarction is not contra-indicated. However, the possibility of arrhythmias arising in patients who may be hypokalaemic after myocardial infarction and are likely to be cardiologically unstable must be borne in mind. The limitations imposed thereafter on direct current-cardioversion must also be remembered.

Although many patients with chronic congestive cardiac failure benefit from acute administration of digoxin, there are some in whom it does not lead to constant, marked or lasting haemodynamic improvement. It is therefore important to evaluate the response of each patient individually when Lanoxin is continued long-term.

Patients with severe respiratory disease may have an increased myocardial sensitivity to digitalis glycosides.

No data are available on whether or not digoxin has mutagenic, carcinogenic or teratogenic effects; however, maternally-administered digoxin has been used to treat foetal tachycardia and congestive heart failure.

There is no information available on the effect of digoxin on human fertility.

Interaction with other medicaments and other forms of interaction: These may arise from effects on the renal excretion, tissue binding, plasma protein binding, distribution within the body, gut absorptive capacity and sensitivity to Lanoxin. Consideration of the possibility of an interaction whenever concomitant therapy is contemplated is the best precaution and a check on serum digoxin concentration is recommended when any doubt exists.

Agents causing hypokalaemia or intracellular potassium deficiency may cause increased sensitivity to Lanoxin; they include diuretics, lithium salts, corticosteroids and carbenoxolone.

Serum levels of digoxin may be *increased* by concomitant administration of the following: amiodarone; captopril; flecainide; prazosin; propafenone; quinidine; spironolactone; tetracycline; erythromycin (and possibly other antibiotics); and propantheline.

Serum levels of digoxin may be *reduced* by concomitant administration of the following:

antacids; kaolin-pectin; some bulk laxatives and cholestyramine; diphenoxylate; sulphasalazine; neomycin; rifampicin; cytostatics; phenytoin; metoclopramide; and penicillamine.

Calcium channel blocking agents may either increase or cause no change in serum digoxin levels. Verapamil increases serum digoxin levels. Nifedipine and diltiazem may increase or have no effect on serum digoxin levels. Isradipine causes no change in serum digoxin levels.

Milrinone does not alter steady-state serum digoxin levels.

Pregnancy and lactation: The use of digoxin in pregnancy is not contra-indicated, although the dosage and control may be less predictable in pregnant than in non-pregnant women with some requiring an increased dosage of digoxin during pregnancy. As with all drugs, use should be considered only when the expected clinical benefit of treatment to the mother outweighs any possible risk to the developing foetus.

Although digoxin is excreted in breast milk, the quantities are minute and breast feeding is not contra-indicated.

Effects on ability to drive and use machines: None known.

Undesirable effects:

Non-cardiac: These are principally associated with overdosage but may occur from a temporarily high serum concentration due to rapid absorption. They include anorexia, nausea and vomiting and usually disappear within a few hours of taking the drug. Diarrhoea can also occur. It is inadvisable to rely on nausea as an early warning of excessive digoxin dosage.

Gynaecomastia can occur with long-term administration.

Weakness, apathy, fatigue, malaise, headache, visual disturbances, depression and even psychosis have been reported as adverse central nervous system effects.

Oral digoxin has also been associated with intestinal ischaemia and, rarely, with intestinal necrosis.

Skin rashes of urticarial or scarlatiniform character are rare reactions to digoxin, and may be accompanied by pronounced eosinophilia.

Very rarely, digoxin can cause thrombocytopenia.

Cardiac: Digoxin toxicity can cause various arrhythmias and conduction disturbances. Usually an early sign is the occurrence of ventricular premature contractions; they can proceed to bigeminy or even trigeminy. Atrial tachycardias, frequently an indication for digoxin, may occur with excessive dosage of the drug. Atrial tachycardia with some degree of atrioventricular block is particularly characteristic, and the pulse rate may not necessarily be fast (see also *Precautions*).

Overdose: After recent ingestion, such as accidental or deliberate self-poisoning, the load available for absorption may be reduced by gastric lavage.

An overdosage of digoxin of 10 to 15 mg in adults without heart disease and of 6 to 10 mg in children aged 1 to 3 years without heart disease appeared to be the dose resulting in death in half of the patients. If more than 25 mg of digoxin was ingested by an adult without heart disease, death or progressive toxicity responsive only to digoxin-binding Fab antibody fragments (Digibind) resulted. If more than 10 mg of digoxin was ingested by a child aged 1 to 3 years without heart disease, the outcome was uniformly fatal when Fab fragment treatment was not given.

If hypokalaemia is present, it should be corrected with potassium supplements either orally or intravenously depending on the urgency of the situation. In cases where a large amount of Lanoxin has been ingested, hyperkalaemia may be present due to release of potassium from skeletal muscle. Before administering potassium in digoxin overdose the serum potassium level must be known.

Bradyarrhythmias may respond to atropine but temporary cardiac pacing may be required. Ventricular arrhythmias may respond to lignocaine or phenytoin.

Dialysis is not particularly effective in removing digoxin from the body in potentially life-threatening toxicity.

Rapid reversal of the complications that are associated with serious poisoning by digoxin, digitoxin and related glycosides has followed intravenous administration of digoxin-specific (ovine) antibody fragments (Fab) when other therapies have failed. Digibind is the only specific treatment for digoxin toxicity and is very effective. For details consult the literature supplied with Digibind.

Pharmacological properties

Pharmacodynamic properties: Inhibits the sodium pump of the sarcolema, thereby, probably allowing intracellular accumulation of sodium to displace bound calcium which in turn exert the positive ionotropic effects.

Pharmacokinetic properties: Approximately 63% of Lanoxin is absorbed from the gastrointestinal tract when given as a tablet, but considerable inter-individual variation is seen.

Urinary excretion is 48.5–65.4% of the administered dose at 10 days, with the majority retrieved as the unchanged parent compound. Therapeutic plasma concentrations may range from 0.5 to 0.25 ng/ml, 20–30% is bound to plasma protein. Lanoxin is widely distributed in tissues including heart, brain, kidney, liver and skeletal muscle. Concentrations in myocardium are considerably higher than in plasma. Lanoxin has been detected in plural, cerebrospinal fluid and breast milk. Lanoxin crosses the placenta. Elimination half-life is 1–2 days in normal individuals, but is prolonged in patients with renal failure.

Preclinical safety data: There are no pre-clinical data of relevance to the prescriber which are additional to that already included in other sections of the SmPC.

Pharmaceutical particulars

List of excipients: Lactose PhEur, Starches PhEur, Indigo Carmine HSE, Hydrolysed Starch HSE, Povidone BP, Magnesium Stearate PhEur.

Incompatibilities: None known.

Shelf life: 60 months.

Special precautions for storage: Store below 25°C.

Nature and contents of container: Amber glass bottle with polyethylene snap-fit closure. Pack sizes: 28, 50, 100, 500 tablets.

15 ml amber glass bottle with a clic-loc child resistant closure. Pack size: 56 tablets.

Instructions for use/handling: Not applicable.

Marketing authorisation number PL 0003/0091R.

Date of first authorisation/renewal of authorisation 18/2/92.

Date of (partial) revision of text September 1997.

LANOXIN TABLETS 0.25 mg

Qualitative and quantitative composition Digoxin PhEur 0.25 mg/tablet.

Pharmaceutical form Tablet.

Clinical particulars

Therapeutic indications: Lanoxin is indicated in the management of chronic cardiac failure. Its therapeutic benefit is greatest in those patients with ventricular dilatation.

Lanoxin is specifically indicated where cardiac failure is accompanied by atrial fibrillation.

Lanoxin is indicated in the management of certain supraventricular arrhythmias, particularly atrial flutter and fibrillation, where its major beneficial effect is reduction of the ventricular rate.

Posology and method of administration: The dose of Lanoxin for each patient has to be tailored individually according to age, lean body weight and renal function. Suggested doses are intended only as an initial guide.

Adults and children over 10 years:

Rapid oral loading: 750 to 1500 micrograms (0.75 to 1.5 mg) as a single dose.

Where there is less urgency, or greater risk of toxicity e.g. in the elderly, the oral loading dose should be given in divided doses 6 hours apart, assessing clinical response before giving each additional dose (see *Precautions*).

Slow oral loading: 250 to 750 micrograms (0.25 to 0.75 mg) should be given daily for 1 week followed by an appropriate maintenance dose. A clinical response should be seen within one week.

Note: The choice between slow and rapid oral loading depends on the clinical state of the patient and the urgency of the condition.

Maintenance: The maintenance dosage should be based upon the percentage of the peak body stores lost each day through elimination. The following formula has had wide clinical use:

$$\text{Maintenance dose} = \frac{\text{Peak body stores x \% daily loss}}{100}$$

Where: Peak body stores = loading dose; % daily loss = 14 + creatinine clearance (C_{cr})/5.

C_{cr} is creatinine clearance corrected to 70 kg bodyweight or 1.73 m^2 body surface area. If only serum creatinine (S_{cr}) concentrations are available, a C_{cr} (corrected to 70 kg bodyweight) may be estimated in men as:

$$C_{cr} = \frac{140\text{–age}}{S_{cr} \text{ (in mg/100 ml)}}$$

Note: Where serum creatinine values are obtained in micromol/l, these may be converted to mg/100 ml (mg %) as follows:

$$S_{cr} \text{ (mg/100 ml)} = \frac{S_{cr} \text{ (micromol/L) x 113.12}}{10{,}000} = \frac{S_{cr} \text{ (micromol/L)}}{88.4}$$

Where 113.12 is the molecular weight of creatinine.

For women, this result should be multiplied by 0.85.

Note: These formulae cannot be used for creatinine clearance in children.

In practice, this will mean that most patients will be maintained on 0.125 to 0.75 mg digoxin daily; however, in those who show increased sensitivity to the adverse effects of digoxin, a dosage of 62.5 microgram (0.0625 mg) daily or less may suffice.

Neonates, infants and children up to 10 years of age (if cardiac glycosides have not been given in the preceding two weeks):

Oral loading dose: This should be administered in accordance with the following schedule:

Pre-term neonates < 1.5 kg	25 microgram/kg over 24 hours
Pre-term neonates 1.5 kg to 2.5 kg	30 microgram/kg over 24 hours
Term neonates up to 2 years	45 microgram/kg over 24 hours
2 to 5 years	35 microgram/kg over 24 hours
5 to 10 years	25 microgram/kg over 24 hours

The loading dose should be administered in divided doses with approximately half the total dose given as the first dose and further fractions of the total dose given at intervals of 4 to 8 hours, assessing clinical response before giving each additional dose.

Maintenance: The maintenance dose should be administered in accordance with the following schedule:

Pre-term neonates: daily dose = 20% of 24-hour loading dose.

Term neonates and children up to 10 years: daily dose = 25% of 24-hour loading dose.

These dosage schedules are meant as guidelines and careful clinical observation and monitoring of serum digoxin levels (see *Monitoring*) should be used as a basis for adjustment of dosage in these paediatric patient groups.

If cardiac glycosides have been given in the two weeks preceding commencement of Lanoxin therapy, it should be anticipated that optimum loading doses of Lanoxin will be less than those recommended above.

Use in the elderly: The tendency to impaired renal function and low lean body mass in the elderly influences the pharmacokinetics of Lanoxin, such that high serum digoxin levels and associated toxicity can occur quite readily, unless doses of Lanoxin lower than those in non-elderly patients are used. Serum digoxin levels should be checked regularly and hypokalaemia avoided.

Dose recommendations in renal disorder or with diuretic therapy: See *Precautions*.

Monitoring: Serum concentrations of digoxin may be expressed in conventional units of ng/ml or SI Units of nmol/L. To convert ng/ml to nmol/L, multiply ng/ml by 1.28.

The serum concentration of digoxin can be determined by radioimmunoassay. Blood should be taken 6 hours or more after the last dose of Lanoxin. There are no rigid guidelines as to the range of serum concentrations that are most efficacious but most patients will benefit, with little risk of toxic symptoms developing, with digoxin concentrations from 0.8 nanogram/ml (ng/ml) (1.02 nanomol/litre, nm/L) to 2.0 ng/ml (2.56 nm/L). Above this range toxic symptoms and signs become more frequent and levels above 3.0 ng/ml (3.84 nm/L) are quite likely to be toxic. However, in deciding whether a patient's symptoms are due to digoxin, the patient's clinical state together with the serum potassium level and thyroid function are important factors.

Other glycosides, including metabolites of digoxin, can interfere with the assays that are available and one should always be wary of values which do not seem commensurate with the clinical state of the patient.

Route of administration: Oral.

Contra-indications: Lanoxin is contra-indicated in intermittent complete heart block or second degree atrioventricular block, especially if there is a history of Stokes-Adams attacks.

Lanoxin is contra-indicated in arrhythmias caused by cardiac glycoside intoxication.

Lanoxin is contra-indicated in supraventricular arrhythmias associated with an accessory atrioventricular pathway, as in the Wolff-Parkinson-White Syndrome, unless the electrophysiological characteristics of the accessory pathway and any possible deleterious effect of digoxin on these characteristics have been evaluated. If an accessory pathway is known or suspected to be present and there is no history of previous supraventricular arrhythmias, Lanoxin is similarly contra-indicated.

Lanoxin is contra-indicated in hypertrophic obstructive cardiomyopathy, unless there is concomitant atrial fibrillation and heart failure, but even then caution should be exercised if Lanoxin is to be used.

Lanoxin is contra-indicated in patients known to be hypersensitive to digoxin or other digitalis glycosides.

Special warnings and precautions for use: Arrhythmias may be precipitated by digoxin toxicity, some of which can resemble arrhythmias for which the drug could be advised. For example, atrial tachycardia with varying atrioventricular block requires particular care as clinically the rhythm resembles atrial fibrillation.

In some cases of sinoatrial disorder (i.e. Sick Sinus Syndrome) digoxin may cause or exacerbate sinus bradycardia or cause sinoatrial block.

Determination of the serum digoxin concentration may be very helpful in making a decision to treat with further digoxin, but toxic doses of other glycosides may cross-react in the assay and wrongly suggest apparently satisfactory measurements. Observations during the temporary withholding of digoxin might be more appropriate.

In cases where cardiac glycosides have been taken in the preceding two weeks, the recommendations for initial dosing of a patient should be reconsidered and a reduced dose is advised.

The dosing recommendations should be reconsidered if patients are elderly or there are other reasons for the renal clearance of digoxin being reduced. A reduction in both initial and maintenance doses should be considered.

Hypokalaemia sensitises the myocardium to the actions of cardiac glycosides.

Hypomagnesaemia and marked hypercalcaemia increase myocardial sensitivity to cardiac glycosides.

Administering Lanoxin to a patient with thyroid disease requires care. Initial and maintenance doses of Lanoxin should be reduced when thyroid function is subnormal. In hyperthyroidism there is relative digoxin resistance and the dose may have to be increased. During the course of treatment of thyrotoxicosis, dosage should be reduced as the thyrotoxicosis comes under control.

Patients with malabsorption syndrome or gastro-intestinal reconstructions may require larger doses of digoxin.

The risk of provoking dangerous arrhythmias with direct current cardioversion is greatly increased in the presence of digitalis toxicity and is in proportion to the cardioversion energy used.

For elective direct current cardioversion of a patient who is taking digoxin, the drug should be withheld for 24 hours before cardioversion is performed. In emergencies, such as cardiac arrest, when attempting cardioversion the lowest effective energy should be applied. Direct current cardioversion is inappropriate in the treatment of arrhythmia thought to be caused by cardiac glycosides.

Many beneficial effects of digoxin on arrhythmias result from a degree of atrioventricular conduction blockade. However, when incomplete atrioventricular block already exists the effects of a rapid progression in the block should be anticipated. In complete heart block the idioventricular escape rhythm may be suppressed.

The administration of digoxin in the period immediately following myocardial infarction is not contra-indicated. However, the possibility of arrhythmias arising in patients who may be hypokalaemic after myocardial infarction and are likely to be cardiologically unstable must be borne in mind. The limitations imposed thereafter on direct current cardioversion must also be remembered.

Although many patients with chronic congestive cardiac failure benefit from acute administration of digoxin, there are some in whom it does not lead to constant, marked or lasting haemodynamic improvement. It is therefore important to evaluate the response of each patient individually when Lanoxin is continued long-term.

Patients with severe respiratory disease may have an increased myocardial sensitivity to digitalis glycosides.

No data are available on whether or not digoxin has mutagenic, carcinogenic or teratogenic effects; however, maternally-administered digoxin has been used to treat foetal tachycardia and congestive heart failure.

There is no information available on the effect of digoxin on human fertility.

Interaction with other medicaments and other forms of interaction: These may arise from effects on the renal excretion, tissue binding, plasma protein binding, distribution within the body, gut absorptive capacity and sensitivity to Lanoxin. Consideration of the possibility of an interaction whenever concomitant therapy is contemplated is the best precaution and a check on serum digoxin concentration is recommended when any doubt exists.

Agents causing hypokalaemia or intracellular potassium deficiency may cause increased sensitivity to Lanoxin; they include diuretics, lithium salts, corticosteroids and carbenoxolone.

Serum levels of digoxin may be *increased* by concomitant administration of the following: amiodarone, captopril, flecainide, prazosin, propafenone, quinidine, spironolactone, tetracycline, erythromycin (and possibly other antibiotics), and propantheline.

Serum levels of digoxin may be *reduced* by concomitant administration of the following: antacids, kaolin-pectin, some bulk laxatives and cholestyramine, diphenoxylate, sulphasalazine, neomycin, rifampicin, cytostatics, phenytoin, metoclopramide, and penicillamine.

Calcium channel blocking agents may either increase or cause no change in serum digoxin levels. Verapamil increases serum digoxin levels. Nifedipine and diltiazem may increase or have no effect on serum digoxin levels. Isradipine causes no change in serum digoxin levels.

Milrinone does not alter steady-state serum digoxin levels.

Pregnancy and lactation: The use of digoxin in pregnancy is not contra-indicated, although the dosage and control may be less predictable in pregnant than in non-pregnant women with some requiring an increased dosage of digoxin during pregnancy. As with all drugs, use should be considered only when the expected clinical benefit of treatment to the mother outweighs any possible risk to the developing foetus.

Although digoxin is excreted in breast milk, the quantities are minute and breast feeding is not contra-indicated.

Effect on ability to drive and use machines: None known.

Undesirable effects: Non-cardiac: These are principally associated with overdosage but may occur from a temporarily high serum concentration due to rapid absorption. They include anorexia, nausea and vomiting and usually disappear within a few hours of taking the drug. Diarrhoea can also occur. It is inadvisable to rely on nausea as an early warning of excessive digoxin dosage.

Gynaecomastia can occur with long-term administration.

Weakness, apathy, fatigue, malaise, headache, visual disturbances, depression and even psychosis have been reported as adverse central nervous system effects.

Oral digoxin has also been associated with intestinal ischaemia and, rarely, with intestinal necrosis.

Skin rashes of urticarial or scarlatiniform character are rare reactions to digoxin, and may be accompanied by pronounced eosinophilia.

Very rarely, digoxin can cause thrombocytopenia.

Cardiac: Digoxin toxicity can cause various arrhythmias and conduction disturbances. Usually an early sign is the occurrence of ventricular premature contractions; they can proceed to bigeminy or even trigeminy. Atrial tachycardias, frequently an indication for digoxin, may occur with excessive dosage of the drug. Atrial tachycardia with some degree of atrioventricular block is particularly characteristic, and the pulse rate may not necessarily be fast (see also *Precautions*).

Overdose: After recent ingestion, such as accidental or deliberate self-poisoning, the load available for absorption may be reduced by gastric lavage.

An overdosage of digoxin of 10 to 15 mg in adults without heart disease and of 6 to 10 mg in children aged 1 to 3 years without heart disease appeared to be the dose resulting in death in half of the patients. If more than 25 mg of digoxin was ingested by an adult without heart disease, death or progressive toxicity responsive only to digoxin-binding Fab antibody fragments (Digibind) resulted. If more than 10 mg of digoxin was ingested by a child aged 1 to 3 years without heart disease, the outcome was uniformly fatal when Fab fragment treatment was not given.

If hypokalaemia is present, it should be corrected with potassium supplements either orally or intravenously depending on the urgency of the situation. In cases where a large amount of Lanoxin has been ingested, hyperkalaemia may be present due to release of potassium from skeletal muscle. Before administering potassium in digoxin overdose the serum potassium level must be known.

Bradyarrhythmias may respond to atropine but temporary cardiac pacing may be required. Ventricular arrhythmias may respond to lignocaine or phenytoin.

Dialysis is not particularly effective in removing digoxin from the body in potentially life-threatening toxicity.

Rapid reversal of the complications that are associated with serious poisoning by digoxin, digitoxin and related glycosides has followed intravenous administration of digoxin-specific (ovine) antibody fragments (Fab) when other therapies have failed. Digibind is the only specific treatment for digoxin toxicity and is very effective. For details consult the literature supplied with Digibind.

Pharmacological properties

Pharmacodynamic properties: Inhibits the sodium pump of the sarcolema, thereby, probably allowing intracellular accumulation of sodium to displace bound calcium which in turn exert the positive ionotropic effects.

Pharmacokinetic properties: Approximately 63% of Lanoxin is absorbed from the gastrointestinal tract when given as a tablet, but considerable inter-individual variation is seen.

Urinary excretion is 48.5–65.4% of the administered dose at 10 days, with the majority retrieved as the unchanged parent compound. Therapeutic plasma concentrations may range from 0.5 to 0.25 ng/ml, 20–30% is bound to plasma protein. Lanoxin is widely distributed in tissues including heart, brain, kidney, liver and skeletal muscle. Concentrations in myocardium are considerably higher than in plasma. Lanoxin has been detected in plural, cerebrospinal fluid and breast milk. Lanoxin crosses the placenta, elimination half-life is 1–2 days in normal individuals, but is prolonged in patients with renal failure.

Preclinical safety data: There are no pre-clinical data of relevance to the prescriber which are additional to that already included in other sections of the SmPC.

Pharmaceutical particulars

List of excipients: Lactose PhEur, Maize Starch PhEur, Hydrolysed Starch HSE, Magnesium Stearate PhEur, Rice Starch PhEur.

Incompatibilities: None known.

Shelf life: 60 months.

Special precautions for storage: Store below 25°C.

Nature and contents of container: Amber glass bottle and low-density polyethylene snap fit closures. Pack sizes: 28, 50, 500 tablets.

15 ml amber glass bottle with a clic-loc child resistant closure. Pack size: 56 tablets.

Polypropylene containers with polyethylene snap fit closures. Pack sizes: 1000, 5000 tablets.

Instructions for use/handling: Not applicable.

Marketing authorisation number PL 0003/0090R.

Date of first authorisation/renewal of authorisation 18/02/92.

Date of (partial) revision of text September 1997.

MALOPRIM* TABLETS

Qualitative and quantitative composition Pyrimethamine BP 12.50 mg, Dapsone EP 100 mg.

Pharmaceutical form Tablets.

Clinical particulars

Therapeutic indications: Maloprim is indicated as a causal prophylactic and suppressive agent against malaria caused by *Plasmodium falciparum*. Maloprim is particularly recommended when resistance to pyrimethamine or other anti-folate preparations is known or suspected. It is also effective in chloroquine-resistant areas.

Posology and method of administration:

Route of administration: Oral.

Adults: 1 tablet each week.

Children: over 10 years: 1 tablet each week.

5 to 10 years: ½ tablet each week.

Under 5 years: Formulation not applicable.

The constituents are rapidly absorbed and prophylactic cover can be expected shortly after taking the first dose. Prophylaxis should commence before arrival in an endemic area and be continued once weekly. On returning to a non-malarious area dosage should be maintained for a further four weeks.

The recommended dose must not be exceeded.

Use in the elderly: No specific studies have been carried out in the elderly. However, it may be advisable to monitor renal or hepatic function and if there is serious impairment then caution should be exercised.

Maloprim, at the doses recommended for the prevention of malaria is unlikely to have an adverse effect on older people normally of good health.

Contra-indications: Maloprim should not be given to individuals with a known history of hypersensitivity to sulphonamides, sulphones or pyrimethamine.

Special warnings and special precautions for use: Maloprim should not be used for the treatment of acute attacks of malaria.

Subjects taking malaria prophylaxis should be warned that no antimalarial agent gives complete protection. Further precautionary measures, such as covering exposed areas of the body, application of insect repellents and use of mosquito nets should be advised. Malaria should be considered in the differential diagnosis of any pyrexial illness. Such measures are particularly important in rural areas of East Africa.

Short term usage of Maloprim is unlikely to carry excess risk in patients with renal or hepatic impairment. However, patients with significant kidney or liver disease taking Maloprim for prolonged periods should be monitored regularly for signs of bone marrow depression.

Maloprim may exacerbate folate deficiency in individuals predisposed to this condition through disease or malnutrition. Accordingly, a folic acid supplement should be given to such individuals.

Pyrimethamine was not mutagenic in the Ames test. Chromosome abnormalities have been reported in bone marrow cells from patients with *P.falciparum* malaria given total doses of 200 and 300 mg pyrimethamine. There are no data available on whether or not dapsone has mutagenic potential.

The following statements will appear on packs of this product;

Store below 25°C.

Protect from light.

Keep out of reach of children.

The recommended dose must not be exceeded.

Interaction with other medicaments and other forms of interaction: Maloprim, through its mode of action, may depress folate metabolism in patients already receiving treatment with other folate inhibitors, or agents associated with myelosuppression, including co-trimoxazole, trimethoprim, proguanil and zidovudine.

In vitro data suggest that antacid salts and antidiarrhoeal earths reduce the absorption of pyrimethamine.

Probenecid may reduce renal excretion of dapsone and its metabolites leading to a rise in serum levels.

Rifampicin may shorten the plasma half-life of dapsone.

Pregnancy and lactation: The safety of Maloprim in human pregnancy has not been established. In view of the theoretical risk of foetal malformation with all folate inhibitors, caution should be exercised in the administration of Maloprim during pregnancy, particularly in the first trimester.

Pregnant women should be advised against making unnecessary visits to endemic areas. In addition, consideration should be given to the likelihood of contracting malaria in the area to be visited. Maloprim should only be advised during pregnancy if an unavoidable visit to a hyper-endemic area of known or suspected chloroquine resistant malaria is to be undertaken.

A folate supplement, preferably as folinic acid or calcium folate, should be given to all pregnant women taking Maloprim.

The amount of Maloprim constituents excreted in breast milk is insufficient to contra-indicate its use in lactating mothers, but breast-fed infants should not receive other anti-folate agents.

Effect on ability to drive and use machines: None known.

Undesirable effects: Side effects caused by Maloprim at the recommended doses are rare.

Severe bone marrow depression leading to agranulocytosis or red cell hypoplasia has been reported, particularly in association with doses of one tablet twice weekly.

There have been rare instances of pneumonia, associated with eosinophilic pulmonary infiltration, developing soon after initiation of prophylaxis.

Cyanosis, attributable to methaemoglobinaemia, has been reported, usually following doses higher than those recommended.

Administration of excessive doses over a prolonged period may produce haemolytic or megaloblastic anaemia.

The haemolytic effect of dapsone is dose-related and greater in glucose-6-phosphate dehydrogenase deficiency. The dosage of dapsone as used in Maloprim is insufficient to cause clinically apparent disease in the majority of individuals. However, rare cases of haemoglobinuria have been reported in glucose-6-phosphate dehydrogenase-deficient individuals following Maloprim administration.

Insomnia has been reported when pyrimethamine has been given at weekly doses above those recommended.

Other reactions associated on rare occasions with pyrimethamine or dapsone, usually at higher doses, include: after short-term dosage – rash and other skin disorders; thrombocytopenia; a mononucleosis-like syndrome; jaundice and psychosis; and after long term dosage – motor neuropathy and hypoalbuminaemia.

A dapsone (or sulphone) syndrome, a form of hypersensitivity reaction, has been rarely reported and may occur during the first 6 weeks of therapy. Its most common features are hepatitis (most prominent), fever and rash (often an exfoliative dermatitis), which may be accompanied by hepatosplenomegaly, renal papillary necrosis and by those reactions described in the sections on short- and long-term dosage. Patients usually improve on dapsone withdrawal, however may require steroid treatment. Fatalities have been reported.

Overdose: Acute overdosage: The most commonly observed effects of acute overdosage are methaemoglobinaemia, and in extreme cases, convulsions. There is a possibility of anaemia developing due to the haemolytic effect of dapsone and inhibition of folate metabolism following large doses of pyrimethamine.

In view of the rapid absorption of both constituents of Maloprim, gastric lavage should only be considered within the first 2 hours of ingestion. Oral administration of activated charcoal over several days has been shown to decrease the plasma half-life of dapsone. As there is evidence to suggest enterohepatic circulation of pyrimethamine, this measure may also be of value in its elimination. In addition, adequate fluids should be given to ensure optimal diuresis.

Routine supportive measures, including maintenance of a clear airway and control of convulsions should be given. Methaemoglobinaemia should be treated by oral administration of ascorbic acid, 200 mg three times daily, or by intravenous administration of methylene blue according to the level of methaemoglobin. (Methylene blue should not be given to patients with G-6-PD deficiency.) To counteract possible folate deficiency, calcium folinate should be given for 3 days in a dose of 9 to 15 mg, 6-hourly.

Chronic overdosage: The most likely effects of chronic overdosage are methaemoglobinaemia, haemolytic anaemia and megaloblastic anaemia.

Maloprim administration should be discontinued. Ascorbic acid or methylene blue is of value in the treatment of methaemoglobinaemia. (Methylene blue should not be given to patients with G-6-PD deficiency.) Calcium folinate is of value in the treatment of megaloblastic anaemia.

Pharmacological properties

Pharmacodynamic properties: Pyrimethamine binds to the enzyme dihydrofolate reductase (DHFR), thereby competitively inhibiting the formation of tetrahydrofolic acid, an essential co-factor in nucleic acid synthesis. This, in turn, leads to disruption of nuclear division and protein synthesis. The concentration of pyrimethamine required to inhibit plasmodial DHFR is several orders of magnitude less than that needed to inhibit the corresponding mammalian enzyme.

The antibacterial activity of dapsone is antagonised by para-aminobenzoic acid (PABA). It probably acts by blocking the conversion of PABA to dihydrofolic acid. It is believed that the antimalarial activity is dependent on the same mechanism. Differential activity depends upon the plasmodial requirement for PABA, while mammalian cells use preformed dihydrofolate and tetrahydrofolate. The synergistic effect of the two compounds depends on sequential blockade of the folate pathway.

Pharmacokinetic properties: Following the administration of a single tablet of Maloprim, the plasma half life of pyrimethamine is approximately 80 hours and that of dapsone approximately 25 hours. These figures are comparable with the values obtained when each compound is given individually.

Both compounds undergo entero-hepatic circulation.

The final elimination of the majority of dapsone and its metabolites is via the kidneys, whereas pyrimethamine and its metabolites may be excreted equally in urine and faeces.

Preclinical safety data: At high doses (100 mg/kg 5 times a week for 104 weeks), dapsone has been reported to be carcinogenic in male rats but not female rats, nor in mice of either sex. The clinical significance of this finding is not known. However, cancer mortality among American leprosy patients receiving long-term dapsone therapy was not greater over a 40-year period than that expected from population statistics.

Five intraperitoneal doses of 125 mg pyrimethamine/kg bodyweight, administered over a period of 24 weeks to mice, were associated with an increase in lung tumours. Doses of 62.5 mg and 31.25 mg/kg bodyweight did not induce a statistically significant increase in tumour numbers. Both higher doses were toxic and led to death of more than half of the treated animals before the end of the study period.

Pharmaceutical particulars

List of excipients: Lactose EP, Starches EP, Hydrolysed starch HSE, Magnesium stearate EP (range 0.75 mg to 3.0 mg), Purified water EP.

Incompatibilities: None known.

Shelf life: 60 months.

Special precautions for storage: Store below 25°C. Protect from light.

Nature and contents of container: Vinyl-lacquered aluminium foil strip-packs. Pack size: 30.

Instructions for use/handling: None.

Marketing authorisation number PL 00003/5117R

Date of first authorisation/renewal of authorisation 12 January 1988/12 January 1993.

Date of (partial) revision of text December 1997.

MIGRIL TABLETS

Qualitative and quantitative composition Each tablet contains 2.0 mg Ergotamine Tartrate EP, 50.0 mg Cyclizine Hydrochloride BP and Caffeine BP equivalent to 100 mg Caffeine Hydrate BP.

Pharmaceutical form Tablet.

White, round, biconvex, compression-coated tablets with a pink core, scored and impressed 'Wellcome A4A'.

Clinical particulars

Therapeutic indications: Migril is indicated for the relief of the acute migraine attack.

Posology and method of administration

Adults: Migril should be taken as soon as possible after the first warning of an attack of migraine and repeated if necessary at the prescribed intervals.

The usual initial dose is one tablet.

Additional doses of a half to one tablet may then be required at half-hourly intervals.

No more than 4 tablets (8 mg ergotamine) should be taken in any one attack.

No more than 6 tablets (12 mg ergotamine) should be given in any one week.

Children: There is no absolute contra-indication to the use of Migril in children but its use is not recommended.

Use in the elderly: There are no absolute contra-indications to the use of Migril in the elderly, but see *Contra-indications* and *Precautions*.

Contra-indications: Migril is contra-indicated during pregnancy because of a direct effect of ergotamine on the uterus. In animals, ergotamine has been reported to inhibit implantation, cause peri-natal mortality and foetal retardation.

Migril is contra-indicated during lactation and breast-feeding; it may suppress milk production and may also be excreted in milk at levels high enough to cause pharmacological effects in breast-fed infants.

Migril is contra-indicated in pre-existing vascular disease including coronary disease, obliterative vascular disease, angina, claudication, peripheral ischaemia, Raynaud's syndrome and hypertension.

Migril should not be taken if there is a hypersensitivity to any of its constituents.

Special warnings and special precautions for use: Migril should not be used for migraine prophylaxis because of the risk of inducing ergotism.

The use of ergotamine-containing compounds carries the risk of precipitating arterial constriction and other manifestations of ergotism.

Use the minimum effective dosage of Migril necessary since individual sensitivity to the arterial effects of ergotamine varies considerably.

Discontinue the use of Migril if symptoms of arterial insufficiency develop, including coldness, numbness or tingling of the extremities.

Doses of ergotamine as small as 2 mg have caused signs of arterial insufficiency but this is a very rare occurrence.

Migril should be used with caution in patients with infective hepatitis because of an increased risk of precipitating peripheral ischaemia.

Repeated doses of ergotamine have occasionally been associated with renal artery spasm and loss of renal function.

Alcohol and Migril should not be taken concurrently.

Ergotamine should be used with care when hyperthyroidism, sepsis or anaemia are present.

Interaction with other medicaments and other forms of interaction: The concomitant use of ergot alkaloids and beta-blocking agents increases the risks of peripheral vasoconstriction.

Vomiting and peripheral ischaemia have been reported after concomitant use of ergot alkaloids and the antibiotics erythromycin and oleandomycin.

Pregnancy and lactation: See *Contra-indications*.

Effect on ability to drive and use machines: Cyclizine, in common with other antihistamines, may cause sedation; patients should be cautioned about driving or operating machinery.

Undesirable effects: Habitual use of ergotamine-containing preparations can produce a syndrome of non-migrainous rebound headaches, in which case Migril should be discontinued.

Side-effects seen with Migril are usually due to the ergotamine components of the preparation and are more common if the dosage recommendations are exceeded. They include intermittent claudication, coldness and whiteness of the extremities, dysaesthesia, paraesthesia, formication and precordial pain.

Other side-effects seen with ergotamine include muscle cramps, joint pains, raised blood pressure, pulselessness, cyanosis, thrombophlebitis, peripheral arterial thrombosis, gangrene, abdominal pain, coronary infarction, cerebral thrombosis, nausea, dyspnoea, decreased visual acuity, vertigo and diarrhoea. These effects have mostly occurred following habitual chronic use exceeding the recommended dose; they may occasionally occur however at the therapeutic dose.

Arterial vasospasm severe enough to threaten the viability of the limbs has been reported after routine therapy but it is more normally to be expected after prolonged overdosage.

Overdose:

Acute overdosage: Symptoms: Acute overdosage with an ergotamine-containing preparation is characterised by nausea, vomiting, tachycardia, hypotonia and peripheral ischaemia. Blood pressure may be difficult to measure.

Treatment: If vomiting has not occurred, efforts should be made to clear the stomach contents. General supportive measures should be applied and intravenous vasodilators may be necessary to relieve vasospasm.

Peritoneal dialysis and forced diuresis may help to eliminate ergotamine from the body.

Chronic overdosage: Symptoms: Chronic overdosage with ergotamine-containing preparations usually presents as peripheral ischaemia threatening the viability of the affected limb.

Treatment: Withdraw Migril immediately.

Intravenous vasodilators such as nitroprusside and nitroglycerin may be used to re-establish normal blood flow. Captopril has also been used to reverse the effects of chronic overdosage with ergotamine.

Re-establishment of blood flow may be associated with intense burning sensations in the affected areas but these usually resolve after several weeks.

Pharmacological properties

Pharmacodynamic properties: None stated.

Pharmacokinetic properties: None stated.

Preclinical safety data: No additional data of relevance.

Pharmaceutical particulars

List of excipients: Starches, liquid glucose, amaranth, dioctyl sodium sulphosuccinate or docusate sodium, magnesium stearate, lactose, glucose, gelatin, sodium metabisulphate. Industrial methylated spirit or ethanol, purified water and sulphurous acid solution are all used in the manufacturing process but are not detected in the final formulation.

Incompatibilities: None stated.

Shelf life: 36 months.

Special precautions for storage: Store at 25°C. Keep dry. Protect from light.

Nature and contents of container: Amber glass bottles containing 100 tablets with low density polyethylene snap fit closures.

Instructions for use/handling: None stated.

Marketing authorisation number PL 00003/5114R

Date of first authorisation/renewal of authorisation MAA: 10 December 1991, Renewal: 28 August 1998.

Date of (partial) revision of text August 1996.

OTOSPORIN EAR DROPS

Qualitative and quantitative composition Polymyxin B Sulphate EP 10,000 units per ml, Neomycin Sulphate EP 3,400 units per ml, Hydrocortisone EP 1.0% w/v.

Pharmaceutical form Liquid for topical application to humans.

Clinical particulars

Therapeutic indications: Otosporin Ear Drops are indicated for the treatment of otitis externa due to, or complicated by, bacterial infection.

Route of administration: Topical.

In vitro activity: Otosporin Ear Drops are active against a wide range of bacterial pathogens. The range of activity includes:

Gram-Positive Organisms:

Staphylococcus epidermidis and *Staphylococcus aureus;*

Gram-Negative Organisms:

Enterobacter Spp.
Escherichia Spp.
Haemophilus Spp.
Klebsiella Spp.
Proteus Spp.
Pseudomonas Aeruginosa

Otosporin Ear Drops are not expected to be active against streptococci, including *Streptococcus Pyogenes.*

Hydrocortisone possesses anti-inflammatory, antiallergic and antipruritic activity.

Posology and method of administration

Adults: Following cleansing and drying of the external auditory meatus and canal as appropriate, three drops should be instilled into the affected ear three or four times daily. Alternatively, a gauze wick may be introduced into the external auditory canal and kept saturated with the solution; the wick may be left in place for 24 to 48 hours.

Soap should not be used for cleansing of the external auditory meatus and canal as it may inactivate the antibiotics.

Children: As for adults, but the dose should be reduced in infants. A possibility of increased absorption exists in very young children, thus Otosporin Ear Drops are not recommended in neonates (see *Special warnings and special precautions for use*).

Use in the elderly: As for adults.

Contra-indications: The use of Otosporin Ear Drops is contra-indicated in patients in whom perforation of the tympanic membrane is known or suspected.

The use of Otosporin Ear Drops is contra-indicated in patients who have demonstrated allergic hypersensitivity to any of the components of the preparation or to cross-sensitising substances such as framycetin, kanamycin, gentamicin and other related antibiotics.

The use of Otosporin Ear Drops is contra-indicated in the presence of untreated viral, fungal and tubercular infections.

A possibility of increased absorption exists in very young children, thus Otosporin Ear Drops are not recommended for use in neonates.

Special warnings and special precautions for use: Occasionally, delayed hypersensitivity to corticosteroids may occur. Treatment with topical steroid antibiotic combinations should not be continued for more than seven days in the absence of any clinical improvement, since prolonged use may lead to occult extension of infection due to the masking effect of the steroid. Prolonged use may also lead to skin sensitisation and the emergence of resistant organisms.

All topically active corticosteroids possess the potential to suppress the pituitary-adrenal axis following systemic absorption. Development of adverse systemic effects due to the hydrocortisone component of Otosporin Ear Drops is considered to be unlikely, although the recommended dosage should not be exceeded, particularly in infants.

Prolonged, unsupervised, use should be avoided as it may lead to irreversible partial or total deafness, especially in the elderly and in patients with impaired renal function.

Use in the immediate pre- and post-operative period is not advised as neomycin may rarely cause neuromuscular block; because it potentiates skeletal muscle relaxant drugs, it may cause respiratory depression and arrest.

In neonates and infants, absorption by immature skin may be enhanced and renal function may be immature. (See *Contra-indications.*)

Interaction with other medicaments and other forms of interaction: None known.

Pregnancy and lactation: There is little information to demonstrate the possible effect of topically applied neomycin in pregnancy and lactation. However, neomycin present in maternal blood can cross the placenta and may give rise to a theoretical risk of foetal toxicity thus use of Otosporin Ear Drops is not recommended in pregnancy or lactation.

Effects on ability to drive and use machines: None known.

Undesirable effects: The incidence of allergic hypersensitivity reactions to neomycin sulphate in the general population is low. There is, however, an increased incidence of hypersensitivity to neomycin in certain selected groups of patients in dermatological practice, particularly those with venous stasis eczema and ulceration, and chronic otitis externa.

Allergic hypersensitivity reactions following topical application of polymyxin B sulphate and hydrocortisone are rare.

Allergic hypersensitivity to neomycin following topical use may manifest itself as an eczematous exacerbation with reddening, scaling, swelling and itching or as a failure of the lesion to heal.

Stinging and burning have occasionally been reported when Otosporin Ear Drops gained access to the middle ear.

Otosporin Ear Drops should only be used in the ear and are not suitable for use in the eye.

Overdosage: There is no experience of overdosage with Otosporin.

Pharmacological properties

Pharmacodynamic properties: Otosporin solution is a bactericidal preparation active against all the pathogens commonly found in bacterial infections of the ear. Polymyxin B is bactericidal against a wide range of gram negative bacilli including *Pseudomonas* Spp., *Escherichia* coli, *Enterobacter* Spp., *Klebsiella* Spp., and *Haemophilus influenzae.* It exerts a bactericidal effect by binding to acid phospholipids in the cell wall and membranes of the bacterium, thereby rendering ineffective the osmotic barrier normally provided by the cell membrane. This leads to escape of the cell contents and the death of the organism.

Neomycin sulphate is bactericidal against a wide range of gram positive and negative bacterial pathogens including staphylococci, streptococci, *Escherichia, Enterobacter, Klebsiella, Haemophilus, Proteus, Salmonella* and *Shigella* species. It is also active against some strains of the *Pseudomonas aeruginosa* and against mycobacterium tuberculosis and *Neisseria gonorrhoea.* Neomycin exerts its bactericidal effect by interfering with the protein synthesis of susceptible organisms.

Pharmacokinetic properties: No data are available regarding the pharmacokinetics of this product. However since this is a topical preparation and significant systemic absorption is unlikely to occur, the data are irrelevant.

Systemically absorbed neomycin is predominantly excreted by the kidney and the total amount excreted in the urine varies between 30% and 50%. The pharmacokinetics of systemically absorbed polymyxin B has been described.

Pharmaceutical particulars

List of excipients: Cetostearyl Alcohol EP, Sorbitan Monolaurate BP, Polysorbate 20 EP, Methyl Hydroxybenzoate EP, Dilute Sulphuric Acid BP, Purified Water EP.

Incompatibilities: None known.

Shelf life: 36 months.

Special precautions for storage: Protect from light. Store below 15°C.

Nature and contents of container: Polypropylene bottles with integral nozzles and pilfer proof caps 5 ml or 10 ml pack sizes.

Marketing authorisation number PL 0003/5106R.

Date of first authorisation/renewal of authorisation MAA: 27.12.90.

Date of (partial) revision of the text October 1997.

PENTOSTAM INJECTION

Qualitative and quantitative composition Sodium Stibogluconate BP equivalent to 100 mg pentavalent antimony in each ml.

Pharmaceutical form Injection.

Clinical particulars

Therapeutic indications: Pentostam is indicated for the following diseases: Visceral leishmaniasis (kala azar); Cutaneous leishmaniasis; South American mucocutaneous leishmaniasis.

Pentostam may also be of value in the treatment of leishmaniasis recidivans and diffuse cutaneous leishmaniasis in the New World.

Note: Cutaneous and diffuse cutaneous leishmaniasis caused by *Leishmania aethiopica* infections are unresponsive to treatment with pentavalent antimony compounds, including Pentostam, at conventional dosage, but may respond slowly at higher dosage.

Posology and method of administration

Route of administration: Except where otherwise stated, all doses should be given by the intravenous or intramuscular route.

All dosage recommendations are based on the findings of the WHO Expert Committee on leishmaniasis which met in 1984. There are no special recommendations for different age groups.

Visceral leishmaniasis: 10 to 20 mg Sb^{5+} (0.1 to 0.2 ml Pentostam)/kg bodyweight to a maximum of 850 mg (8.5 ml Pentostam) daily for a minimum period of 20 days. Patients should be examined for evidence of relapse after 2 and 6 months, and in Africa after 12 months.

Cutaneous leishmaniasis NOT caused by L. aethiopica: The dosage regimen outlined for visceral leishmaniasis is recommended. Alternatively, single, non-inflamed nodular lesions known not to be due to *L. braziliensis* may be treated with intralesional injections of 100 to 300 mg Sb^{5+} (1 to 3 ml Pentostam) repeated once or twice if necessary at intervals of 1 to

2 days. Infiltration must be thorough and produce complete blanching of the base of the lesion.

Individuals with cutaneous leishmaniasis due to *L. braziliensis* should be treated systematically for several days after the lesion is healed.

Note: After successful treatment of *L. braziliensis*, anti-leishmania antibody titres decline steadily over 4 to 24 months.

Muco-cutaneous leishmaniasis: Patients with parasitologically confirmed leishmaniasis should be treated with 20 mg Sb^{5+} (0.2 ml Pentostam)/kg bodyweight to a maximum of 850 mg (8.5 ml Pentostam) daily, continuing this dosage for several days longer than it takes to achieve parasitological and clinical cure.

In the event of relapse, a further course should be given for at least twice the previous duration.

Diffuse cutaneous leishmaniasis in the New World and leishmaniasis recidivans: Owing to the rarity of these conditions, precise data on dosage are not available. A dose of 10 to 20 mg Sb^{5+} (0.1 to 0.2 mg Pentostam)/kg bodyweight to a maximum of 850 mg (8.5 ml Pentostam) may be given daily for 2 to 3 weeks. If there is a response, then treatment should be maintained until several days after clinical cure of leishmaniasis recidivans and for several months after clinical and parasitological cure of diffuse cutaneous leishmaniasis.

Use in the elderly: There is little information on the effects of Pentostam on elderly individuals. If treatment of cutaneous leishmaniasis is necessary then local infiltration is preferred. The normal precautions should be strictly adhered to when treating older patients for visceral leishmaniasis.

Contra-indications: Pentostam should not be given to any patient with significantly impaired renal function.

Pentostam should not be given to any patient who has experienced a serious adverse reaction to a previous dose.

Special warnings and special precautions for use: Intravenous injection should be administered very slowly over 5 minutes to reduce the risk of local thrombosis. In the unlikely event of coughing, vomiting or substernal pain occurring, administration should be discontinued immediately. In such cases, extreme care should be taken if Pentostam is re-administered by this route.

Successful treatment of mucocutaneous leishmaniasis may induce severe inflammation around the lesion. In cases of pharyngeal or tracheal involvement, this may be life-threatening. Under such circumstances, corticosteroids may be used.

Very rarely, anaphylactic shock may develop during treatment for which adrenaline injection and appropriate supportive measures should be given immediately.

Pentostam should be used cautiously in patients with heart disease.

Electrocardiographic changes, notably alterations in T wave amplitude, may be expected in the majority of patients given Pentostam and are not of serious significance. Where electrocardiograms have been done in patients receiving doses in excess of 20 mg/kg bodyweight/day, modest increases in the rate-corrected QT interval have been observed. There is no firm evidence of drug-induced arrhythmias in patients receiving Pentostam, but it is recommended that treatment is withdrawn if conduction disturbances occur.

Patients who have recently received other antimonial drugs should be monitored closely for signs of antimony intoxication such as bradycardia and cardiac arrhythmias during administration of Pentostam.

Intercurrent infections, such as pneumonia, should be sought and treated concomitantly.

High concentrations of antimony are found in the livers of animals after repeated dosage with pentavalent antimony. Pentostam should therefore be used with caution in patients with hepatic disease. However, some abnormalities of liver function may be expected in cases of visceral leishmaniasis. In such patients the benefit of pentavalent antimony treatment outweighs the risk. Pentostam may induce mild elevation of hepatic enzymes in serum which later return to normal; in these cases, treatment should not be stopped.

The Pack for this product carries the following statements:

Keep out of reach of children.
Store between 2°C and 25°C.
Protect from light.
Poison

In addition the 100 ml pack will have the following statement:

The contents should not be used more than 1 month after removing the first dose.

Interaction with other medicaments and other forms of interaction: No interactions with Pentostam have been reported.

Pregnancy and lactation: Although no effects on the foetus have been reported, Pentostam should be withheld during pregnancy unless the potential benefits to the patient outweigh the possible risk to the foetus.

Children should not be breast-fed by mothers receiving Pentostam.

Effect on ability to drive and use machines: None known.

Undesirable effects: The majority of side-effects are transitory in nature.

Approximately 1 to 2% of patients complain of nausea, vomiting and/or diarrhoea and a slightly higher number of abdominal pain.

Other common side-effects include anorexia, malaise, myalgia, headache and lethargy.

Transient coughing immediately following injection was reported with varying frequency during several trials.

Intravenous injection of Pentostam may cause transient pain along the course of the vein and eventually thrombosis of that vein.

During some early trials of sodium stibogluconate, pneumonia occurred in a small number of patients treated for visceral leishmaniasis and this occasionally proved fatal. Pneumonia is a feature of the visceral leishmaniasis disease process; however, it has been associated with the toxicity profile of trivalent antimony. It is, therefore, not possible to determine whether these cases were due to the disease or to Pentostam.

Other (rarely reported) side-effects include fever, rigor, sweating, vertigo, facial flushing, worsening of lesions on the cheek, bleeding from the nose or gum, substernal pain, jaundice and rash.

Overdose: The main symptoms of antimony overdosage are gastro-intestinal disturbances (nausea, vomiting and severe diarrhoea). Haemorrhagic nephritis and hepatitis may also occur.

There is only limited information on the use of chelating agents in the treatment of intoxication with antimony compounds. Dimercaprol has been reported to be effective: a dose of 200 mg by intramuscular injection, every six hours until recovery is complete, is suggested.

2,3-dimercaptosuccinic acid (DMSA) may also be effective treatment.

Pharmacological properties

Pharmacodynamic properties: The mode of action of Pentostam is unknown. *In vitro* exposure of amastigotes to 500 mg Sb^{5+}/ml results in a greater than 50% decrease in parasite DNA, RNA protein and purine nucleoside triphosphate levels. It has been postulated that the reduction in ATP (adenosine triphosphate) and GTP (guanosine triphosphate) synthesis contributes to decreased macromolecular synthesis.

Pharmacokinetic properties: Following intravenous or intramuscular administration of sodium stibogluconate, antimony is excreted rapidly via the kidneys, the majority of the dose being detected in the first 12-hour urine collection. This rapid excretion is reflected by a marked fall in serum or whole blood antimony levels to approximately 1 to 4% of the peak level by 8 hours after an intravenous dose. During daily administration, there is a slow accumulation of sodium stibogluconate into the central compartment so that tissue concentrations reach a theoretical maximum level after at least 7 days.

Preclinical safety data: There are no preclinical data of relevance to the prescriber which are additional to that in other sections of the SPC.

Pharmaceutical particulars

List of excipients: Chlorocresol BP, Glucono-delta-lactone HSE, Water for Injections EP.

Incompatibilities: None known.

Shelf life: 36 months.

Special precautions for storage: Store between 2°C and 25°C. Protect from light.

Nature and contents of container: Amber glass vials sealed with synthetic butyl rubber closures and aluminium collars.

Pack sizes: 6 and 100 ml.

Instructions for use/handling: No special instructions.

Marketing authorisation number PL 0003/5105R.

Date of first authorisation/renewal of authorisation
Product Licence of Right: 01.09.72
Reviewed Licence: 13.02.87
Renewal of Product Licence: 20.12.91.

Date of (partial) revision of text 26 November 1996.

SEMPREX* CAPSULES

Presentation Each opaque white capsule contains 8 mg acrivastine. Markings include 'WELLCOME' and a unicorn printed in black, and 'SEMPREX' printed in reddish-brown.

Uses Antihistamine. Semprex is indicated for the symptomatic relief of allergic rhinitis, including hay fever. Semprex is also indicated for chronic idiopathic urticaria, symptomatic dermographism, cholinergic urticaria and idiopathic acquired cold urticaria.

Dosage and administration

Adults, and children over 12 years: One 8 mg capsule three times a day.

Use in the elderly: As yet, no specific studies have been carried out in the elderly. Until further information is available, Semprex should not be given to elderly patients.

Pharmacology: Acrivastine provides symptomatic relief in conditions believed to depend wholly or partly upon the triggered release of histamine.

It is a potent competitive histamine H_1-antagonist which lacks significant anticholinergic effects, and has a low potential to penetrate the central nervous system.

After oral administration of a single dose of 8 mg acrivastine to adults, the onset of action, as determined by the ability to antagonise histamine-induced weals and flares in the skin, is within 1 hour. Peak effects occur at 2 hours, and although activity declines slowly thereafter, significant inhibition of histamine-induced weals and flares still occurs 8 hours after dose.

In patients, relief from the symptoms of allergic rhinitis is apparent within 1 hour after the systemic administration of the drug.

Pharmacokinetics: Acrivastine is well absorbed from the gut. In healthy adult volunteers, the peak plasma concentration (Cmax) is approximately 150 nanogram/ml, occurring at about 1.5 hours (Tmax) after the administration of 8 mg acrivastine. The plasma half-life is approximately 1.5 hours. In multiple dose studies over 6 days, no accumulation of acrivastine was observed.

Contra-indications, warnings, etc Semprex is contra-indicated in individuals with known hypersensitivity to acrivastine or triprolidine. Renal excretion is the principal route of elimination of acrivastine. Until specific studies have been carried out Semprex should not be given to patients with significant renal impairment (creatinine clearance less than 50 ml per minute or serum creatinine greater than 150 micromoles per litre).

Precautions: Most patients do not experience drowsiness with Semprex. Nevertheless, as there is individual variation in response to all medication, it is sensible to caution all patients about engaging in activities requiring mental alertness, such as driving a car or operating machinery, until patients are familiar with their own response to the drug.

It is usual to advise patients not to undertake tasks requiring mental alertness whilst under the influence of alcohol and other CNS depressants. Concomitant administration of acrivastine may, in some individuals, produce additional impairment.

Side- and adverse effects: Reports of drowsiness directly attributable to Semprex are extremely rare. Indeed, for the great majority of patients, treatment with Semprex is not associated with clinically significant anticholinergic or sedative side-effects.

Use in pregnancy and lactation: No data are available on the use of Semprex during pregnancy, therefore caution should be exercised by balancing the potential benefits of treatment against any possible hazard. Systemic administration of acrivastine in animal reproductive studies did not produce embryotoxic or teratogenic effects and did not impair fertility.

There is no information on the levels of acrivastine which may appear in human breast milk after administration of Semprex.

Toxicity and treatment of overdosage: There is no experience of overdosage with Semprex. Appropriate supportive therapy, including gastric lavage, should be initiated if indicated.

Pharmaceutical precautions Protect from light. Keep dry. Store below 30°C.

Legal category POM

Package quantities 84 capsules as 4 blister strips of 21 tablets.

Further information Nil.

Product licence number 0003/0254.

VALOID* TABLETS
VALOID* INJECTION

Presentation Valoid Tablets each contain 50 mg Cyclizine Hydrochloride BP, scored, coded 'WELLCOME T4A', white in colour.

Valoid Injection contains 50 mg cyclizine lactate in each 1 ml ampoule.

Uses Valoid is indicated for the prevention and treatment of nausea and vomiting including motion sickness, nausea and vomiting caused by narcotic analgesics and by general anaesthetics in the post-operative period and radiotherapy, especially for breast cancer since cyclizine does not elevate prolactin levels.

Valoid may be of value in relieving vomiting and attacks of vertigo associated with Meniere's disease and other forms of vestibular disturbance when the oral route cannot be used.

Valoid Injection, by the intravenous route, is also indicated pre-operatively in patients undergoing emergency surgery in order to reduce the hazard of regurgitation and aspiration of gastric contents during induction of general anaesthesia.

Pharmacology: Cyclizine is a histamine H_1-receptor antagonist of the piperazine class which is characterised by a low incidence of drowsiness. It possesses anticholinergic and anti-emetic properties. The exact mechanism by which cyclizine can prevent or suppress both nausea and vomiting from various causes is unknown. Cyclizine increases lower oesophageal sphincter tone and reduces the sensitivity of the labyrinthine apparatus. It may inhibit the part of the midbrain known collectively as the emetic centre.

In healthy adult volunteers the administration of a single oral dose of 50 mg cyclizine resulted in a peak plasma concentration of approximately 70 nanogram/ml occurring at about 2 hours after drug administration. The plasma elimination half-life was approximately 20 hours.

Cyclizine produces its anti-emetic effect within 2 hours and lasts approximately 4 hours.

The N-demethylated derivative, norcyclizine, has been identified as a metabolite of cyclizine.

Norcyclizine has little antihistamine (H_1) activity compared to cyclizine and has a plasma elimination half-life of approximately 20 hours. After a single oral dose of 50 mg cyclizine given to a single adult male volunteer, urine collected over the following 24 hours contained less than 1% of the total dose administered.

Dosage and administration

Valoid Tablets:

Adults and children over 12 years: 1 tablet up to three times daily.

Children 6 to 12 years: ½ tablet, up to three times daily.

Under 6 years: Formulation not applicable.

Valoid Injection

Adults: 50 mg intramuscularly or intravenously up to three times daily. When used intravenously, Valoid should be injected slowly into the bloodstream, with only minimal withdrawal of blood into the syringe.

For the prevention of postoperative nausea and vomiting, administer the first dose by slow intravenous injection 20 minutes before the anticipated end of surgery.

Cyclizine given intravenously, in half the recommended dose, increases the lower oesophageal sphincter tone and thereby reduces the hazard of regurgitation and aspiration of gastric contents if given to patients, undergoing emergency surgery, before induction of general anaesthesia.

Use in the elderly: There have been no specific studies of Valoid in the elderly. Experience has indicated that normal adult dosage is appropriate.

Contra-indications, warnings, etc

Contra-indications: Valoid should not be given to individuals with known hypersensitivity to cyclizine.

Precautions: Although studies designed to detect drowsiness did not reveal sedation in healthy adults who took a single *oral* therapeutic dose (50 mg) of cyclizine, sedation of short duration was reported by subjects receiving intravenous cyclizine. Patients should not drive or operate machinery until they have determined their own response.

Although there are no data available, patients should be cautioned that Valoid may have additive effects with alcohol and other central nervous system depressants, e.g. hypnotics and tranquillisers.

As with other anticholinergic agents, Valoid should be used with caution and appropriate monitoring in patients with glaucoma, obstructive disease of the gastrointestinal tract and in males with possible prostatic hypertrophy. Valoid Injection may have a hypotensive effect.

Cyclizine should be used with caution in patients with severe heart failure. In such patients, cyclizine may cause a fall in cardiac output associated with increases in heart rate, mean arterial pressure and pulmonary wedge pressure.

There have been no specific studies in hepatic and/or renal dysfunction.

Cyclizine was not mutagenic in a full Ames test, including use of S9–microsomes.

No long-term studies have been conducted in animals to determine whether cyclizine has a potential for carcinogenesis.

Side- and adverse effects: Urticaria, drug rash, drowsiness, dryness of the mouth, nose and throat, blurred vision, tachycardia, urinary retention, constipation, restlessness, nervousness, insomnia and auditory and visual hallucinations have been reported, particularly when dosage recommendations have been exceeded. Cholestatic jaundice has occurred in association with cyclizine. Single case reports have been documented of fixed drug eruption, generalised chorea, hypersensitivity hepatitis and agranulocytosis.

A single case of anaphylaxis has been recorded following intravenous administration of cyclizine co-administered with propanidid in the same syringe. An increase in excitatory phenomena (tremor and muscle movements) has been reported when cyclizine has been given before propanidid and methohexitone anaesthesia.

Use in pregnancy and lactation: Some animal studies are interpreted as indicating that cyclizine may be teratogenic.

In a study involving prolonged administration of cyclizine to male and female rats there was no evidence of impaired fertility after continuous treatment for 90 to 100 days. There is no experience of the effect of Valoid on human fertility.

In the absence of any definitive human data, the use of Valoid in pregnancy is not advised.

It is not known whether cyclizine or its metabolite are excreted in human milk.

Drug interactions: Valoid may have additive effects with alcohol and other central nervous system depressants e.g. hypnotics, tranquillisers. Valoid enhances the soporific effect of pethidine. Because of its anticholinergic activity cyclizine may enhance the side-effects of other anticholinergic drugs.

Toxicity and treatment of overdosage: Symptoms: Symptoms of acute toxicity from cyclizine arise from peripheral anticholinergic effects and effects on the central nervous system.

Peripheral anticholinergic symptoms include dry mouth, nose and throat, blurred vision, tachycardia and urinary retention. Central nervous system effects include drowsiness, dizziness, inco-ordination, ataxia, weakness, hyperexcitability, disorientation, impaired judgement, hallucinations, hyperkinesia, extrapyramidal motor disturbances, convulsions, hyperpyrexia and respiratory depression.

An oral dose of 5 mg/kg is likely to be associated with at least one of the clinical symptoms stated above. Younger children are more susceptible to convulsions. The incidence of convulsions, in children less than 5 years, is about 60% when the oral dose ingested exceeds 40 mg/kg.

Treatment: In the management of acute overdosage with Valoid, gastric lavage and supportive measures for respiration and circulation should be performed if necessary. Convulsions should be controlled in the usual way with parenteral anticonvulsant therapy.

Pharmaceutical precautions

Injection: Store below 25°C. Protect from light.
Tablets: Store below 25°C.

Legal category

Injection: POM
Tablets: P

Package quantities

Injection: Box of 5 ampoules
Tablets: Bottle of 100.

Further information Nil.

Product licence numbers

Injection: 0003/5212R
Tablets: 0003/5213R

VALTREX* TABLETS 500 mg

Qualitative and quantitative composition 500 mg of valaciclovir.

Pharmaceutical form Film coated tablets.

Clinical particulars

Therapeutic indications: Valtrex is indicated for the treatment of herpes zoster (shingles).

Valtrex is indicated for the treatment of herpes simplex infections of the skin and mucous membranes, including initial and recurrent genital herpes.

Valtrex is indicated for the suppression (prevention) of recurrent herpes simplex infections of the skin and mucous membranes, including genital herpes.

Posology and method of administration: Route of administration: oral.

Valtrex can prevent lesion development when taken at the first signs and symptoms of an HSV recurrence.

Dosage in adults: Treatment of herpes zoster: 1,000 mg of Valtrex to be taken 3 times daily for 7 days.

Treatment of herpes simplex: 500 mg of Valtrex to be taken twice daily. For recurrent episodes, treatment should be for 5 days. For initial episodes, which can be more severe, treatment may have to be extended to 10 days. Dosing should begin as early as possible. For recurrent episodes of herpes simplex, this should ideally be during the prodromal period or immediately the first signs or symptoms appear.

Suppression (prevention) of herpes simplex infection: For immunocompetent patients the total daily dose is 500 mg. This can be taken as 250 mg twice daily. A dose of 500 mg once daily is also effective, especially in patients with fewer than 10 recurrences per year.

For immunocompromised patients the dose is 500 mg twice daily.

Dosage in children: No data are available.

Dosage in the elderly: Dosage modification is not required unless renal function is significantly impaired (see *Dosage in renal impairment*, below). Adequate hydration should be maintained.

Dosage in renal impairment: The dosage of Valtrex should be modified as follows in patients with significantly impaired renal function.

In patients on haemodialysis, the Valtrex dosage recommended for patients with a creatinine clearance of less than 15 ml/min should be used, but this should be administered after the haemodialysis has been performed.

Dosage in hepatic impairment: Dose modification is not required in patients with mild or moderate cirrhosis (hepatic synthetic function maintained). Pharmacokinetic data in patients with advanced cirrhosis (impaired hepatic synthetic function and evidence of portal-systemic shunting) do not indicate the need for dosage adjustment; however, clinical experience is limited.

Contra-indications, warnings, etc

Contra-indications: Valtrex is contra-indicated in patients known to be hypersensitive to valaciclovir, aciclovir or any components of formulations of Valtrex.

Special warnings and special precautions for use

Use in the elderly: Dosage modification is not required in the elderly unless renal function is significantly impaired (see below). Adequate hydration should be maintained.

Use in renal impairment: The Valtrex dose should be adjusted in patients with significant renal impairment (see *Dosage in renal impairment, Posology and method of administration*).

Interaction with other medicaments and other forms of interaction: No clinically significant interactions have been identified.

Cimetidine and probenecid increase the AUC of aciclovir by reducing its renal clearance: however no dosage adjustment is necessary because of the wide therapeutic index of aciclovir. Other drugs which affect renal physiology could affect plasma levels of aciclovir.

Pregnancy and lactation

Teratogenicity: Valaciclovir was not teratogenic in rats or rabbits.

Subcutaneous administration of aciclovir in internationally accepted tests did not produce teratogenic effects in rats or rabbits. In additional studies in rats, foetal abnormalities were observed at subcutaneous doses that produced plasma levels of 100 µg/ml and maternal toxicity.

Fertility: Valaciclovir did not affect fertility in male or female rats dosed by the oral route.

Pregnancy: There are no data on the use of Valtrex in pregnancy. Valtrex should only be used in pregnancy at the recommended dose and only if the potential benefits of treatment outweigh the potential risk.

However, valaciclovir is broken down in the body to aciclovir, in prospective studies approximately 300 women were exposed to systemic aciclovir during the first trimester of pregnancy. This resulted in no increase in the incidence of birth defects, doses of 800 to 1,000 mg per day were taken. The reported defects show no uniqueness or pattern to suggest a common aetiology.

The daily aciclovir AUC (area under plasma concentration-time curve) following Valtrex 1,000 mg to 3,000 mg would be 2 to 4 times greater than what would be expected with aciclovir 1,000 mg daily.

Lactation: No data are available on valaciclovir excretion in breast milk. Caution is therefore advised if Valtrex is administered to a nursing woman.

A study in lactating rats given radiolabelled valaciclovir orally demonstrated the presence of drug-related substance in milk.

Aciclovir has been detected in breast milk at concentrations ranging from 0.6 to 4.1 times the

Renal Function (CRCL ml/min)	Valtrex Dose Adjustment			
	Herpes Zoster	Herpes Simplex		
		Treatment	Suppression	
			Immuno-competent	Immuno-compromised
15 to 30	1000 mg twice daily	No modification required	No modification required	No modification required
<15	1000 mg once daily	500 mg once daily	250 mg once daily	500 mg once daily

corresponding aciclovir plasma concentrations. *It has been estimated that following administration of 200 mg Zovirax 5 times daily, the mean steady state peak plasma concentration (C^{ss} max) is 3.1 μM (0.7 μg/ml).* This would potentially expose a nursing infant to aciclovir dosages of approximately 1 mg/day. However, Zovirax is used for the treatment of neonatal herpes simplex at intravenous doses of 30 mg/kg bodyweight/day.

Effects on ability to drive and use machines: No special precautions necessary.

Undesirable effects: The adverse reactions reported include headache, skin rashes, including photosensitivity rashes, and gastrointestinal disorders, including nausea, vomiting, diarrhoea and abdominal pain.

Reversible neurological reactions, notably dizziness, confusional states, hallucinations and somnolence have been reported, usually in patients with renal impairment or other predisposing factors.

There have been reports of renal insufficiency, microangiopathic haemolytic anaemia and thrombocytopenia (sometimes in combination) in severely immunocompromised patients receiving high doses (8 g daily) of valaciclovir for prolonged periods in clinical trials. These findings have been observed in patients not treated with valaciclovir who have the same underlying or concurrent conditions.

Overdose: Symptoms and signs: There are at present no data available on overdosage with Valtrex.

A dose, equivalent to the aciclovir exposure from approximately 15 g Valtrex, has been inadvertently administered as a single intravenous dose of aciclovir (up to 80 mg/kg) without adverse effects.

Management: In the event of a symptomatic Valtrex overdose occurring, aciclovir is removable by haemodialysis.

Pharmacological properties

Pharmacodynamic properties: Pharmacotherapeutic group: Valaciclovir, an antiviral, is the L-valine ester of aciclovir. Aciclovir is a purine (guanine) nucleoside analogue.

Mode of action: Valaciclovir is rapidly and almost completely converted in man to aciclovir *and valine,* probably by the enzyme referred to as valaciclovir hydrolase.

Aciclovir is a specific inhibitor of the herpes viruses with *in vitro* activity against herpes simplex viruses (HSV) type 1 and type 2, varicella zoster virus (VZV), cytomegalovirus (CMV), Epstein-Barr Virus (EBV), and human herpes virus 6 (HHV-6). Aciclovir inhibits herpes virus DNA synthesis once it has been phosphorylated to the active triphosphate form.

The first stage of phosphorylation requires the activity of a virus-specific enzyme. In the case of HSV, VZV and EBV this enzyme is the viral thymidine kinase (TK), which is only present in virus infected cells.

Selectivity is maintained in CMV with phosphorylation, at least in part, being mediated through the phosphotransferase gene product of UL97. This requirement for activation of aciclovir by a virus specific enzyme largely explains its selectivity.

The phosphorylation process is completed (conversion from mono- to triphosphate) by cellular kinases. Aciclovir triphosphate competitively inhibits the virus DNA polymerase and incorporation of this nucleoside analogue results in obligate chain termination, halting virus DNA synthesis and thus blocking virus replication.

Extensive monitoring of clinical isolates from patients receiving aciclovir therapy or prophylaxis has revealed that virus with reduced sensitivity to aciclovir is extremely rare in the immunocompetent and is only found infrequently in severely immunocompromised individuals e.g. solid organ or bone marrow transplant recipients, patients receiving chemotherapy for malignant disease and people infected with the human immunodeficiency virus (HIV).

Resistance is normally due to a thymidine kinase deficient phenotype which results in a virus which is profoundly disadvantaged in the natural host. Infrequently, reduced sensitivity to aciclovir has been described as a result of subtle alterations in either the virus thymidine kinase or DNA polymerase. The virulence of these variants resembles that of the wild-type virus.

Pharmacokinetic properties

General characteristics: After oral administration valaciclovir is well absorbed and rapidly and almost completely converted to aciclovir *and valine.* This conversion is probably mediated by an enzyme isolated from human liver referred to as valaciclovir hydrolase.

The bioavailability of aciclovir from 1000 mg valaciclovir is 54%, and is not reduced by food. Mean peak aciclovir concentrations are 10–25 μM (2.2–5.7 μg/ml) following single doses of 250–1000 mg valaciclovir, and occur at a median time of 1.50 hours post dose.

Peak plasma concentrations of valaciclovir are only 4% of aciclovir levels, occur at a median time of 30 to 60 minutes post dose, and are below measurable concentrations 3 hours after dosing. The valaciclovir and aciclovir pharmacokinetic profiles are similar after single and repeat dosing. Binding of valaciclovir to plasma proteins is very low (15%).

The elimination plasma half-life of aciclovir after both single and multiple dosing with valaciclovir is approximately 3 hours. Less than 1% of the administered dose of valaciclovir is recovered in the urine. Valaciclovir is eliminated principally as aciclovir and the known aciclovir metabolite, 9-carboxymethoxymethylguanine (CMMG), in the urine.

Characteristics in patients: Herpes zoster and herpes simplex do not significantly alter the pharmacokinetics of valaciclovir and aciclovir after oral administration of Valtrex.

In patients with HIV infection, the disposition and pharmacokinetic characteristics of aciclovir after oral administration of single or multiple doses of 1000 mg or 2000 mg Valtrex are unaltered compared with healthy subjects.

In transplant recipients receiving valaciclovir 2000 mg 4 times daily, aciclovir peak concentrations are similar to or greater than those in healthy volunteers with comparable doses and renal function. The estimated daily AUCs are appreciably greater.

Preclinical safety data: Mutagenicity: The results of mutagenicity tests *in vitro* and *in vivo* indicate that valaciclovir is unlikely to pose a genetic risk to humans.

Carcinogenicity: Valaciclovir was not carcinogenic in bio-assays performed in mice and rats.

Pharmaceutical particulars

List of excipients

Tablet core: Microcrystalline cellulose, Crospovidone, Povidone K90, Magnesium stearate, Colloidal silicon dioxide.

Film coat: White Colour Concentrate OY-S-28861 containing:
- Hydroxypropylmethylcellulose
- Titanium dioxide
- Polyethylene glycol 400
- Polysorbate 80
- Purified water

Printing ink: Blue printing ink FT124 containing:
- acid brilliant green

Polish: Carnauba wax

Incompatibilities: No data.

Shelf life: Three years.

Special precautions for storage: Store below 30°C.

Nature and contents of container: Tablets are packed into blister packs prepared from unplasticised polyvinyl chloride and aluminium foil.

Pack sizes: 4×500 mg, 10×500 mg, 42×500 mg.

Tablets are packed into polypropylene containers with polyethylene snap-fitting caps. Pack size: 500×500 mg.

Instructions for use/handling: No special instructions for use.

Number in the community register of medicinal products PL 0003/0352.

Date of first authorisation/renewal of authorisation 20 January 1995.

Date of revision of text 11 September 1998.

ZOVIRAX* CREAM

Presentation Zovirax Cream is white and contains 5% w/w aciclovir in an aqueous cream base. It is supplied in tubes containing 2 g or 10 g.

Uses Zovirax Cream is indicated for the treatment of herpes simplex virus infections of the skin including initial and recurrent genital herpes and herpes labialis.

Do not use in eyes.

Dosage and administration Zovirax Cream should be applied five times daily at approximately four hourly intervals, omitting the night time application. Treatment should be continued for 5 days. If, after 5 days, healing is not complete then treatment may be continued for up to an additional 5 days. Zovirax Cream should be applied to the lesion or impending lesion as early as possible after the start of an infection. It is particularly important to start treatment of recurrent episodes during the prodromal period or when lesions first appear.

Use in the elderly: No special comment.

Pharmacology: Aciclovir is an antiviral agent which is highly active *in vitro* against herpes simplex virus (HSV) types I and II and varicella zoster virus. Toxicity to mammalian host cells is low.

Aciclovir is phosphorylated after entry into herpes infected cells to the active compound aciclovir triphosphate. The first step in this process is dependent on the presence of the HSV-coded thymidine kinase. Aciclovir triphosphate acts as an inhibitor of, and substrate for, the herpes-specified DNA polymerase, preventing further viral DNA synthesis without affecting normal cellular processes.

Contra-indications, warnings, etc

Contra-indications: Zovirax Cream is contra-indicated in patients known to be hypersensitive to aciclovir or propylene glycol.

Precautions: In severely immunocompromised patients (e.g. AIDS patients or bone marrow transplant recipients) oral Zovirax dosing should be considered. Such patients should be encouraged to consult a physician concerning the treatment of any infection.

Zovirax Cream is not recommended for application to mucous membranes such as in the mouth, eye or vagina, as it may be irritant.

Particular care should be taken to avoid accidental introduction into the eye.

The results of a wide range of mutagenicity tests *in vitro* and *in vivo* indicate that aciclovir does not pose a genetic risk to man. Aciclovir was not found to be carcinogenic in long-term studies in the rat and the mouse.

Largely reversible adverse effects on spermatogenesis in association with overall toxicity in rats and dogs have been reported only at doses of aciclovir greatly in excess of those employed therapeutically. There has been no experience of the effect of Zovirax Cream on human fertility. Two generation studies in mice did not reveal any effect of (orally administered) aciclovir on fertility. Zovirax Tablets have been shown to have no definite effect upon sperm count, morphology or motility in man.

Side- and adverse effects: Transient burning or stinging following application of Zovirax Cream may occur in some patients. Mild drying or flaking of the skin has occurred in about 5% of patients. Erythema and itching have been reported in a small proportion of patients.

Contact dermatitis has been reported rarely following application. Where sensitivity tests have been conducted, the reactive substances have most often been shown to be components of the cream base rather than aciclovir.

Use in pregnancy and lactation: Systemic administration of aciclovir in internationally accepted standard tests did not produce embryotoxic or teratogenic effects in rats, rabbits or mice.

In a non-standard test in rats, foetal abnormalities were observed, but only following such high subcutaneous doses that maternal toxicity was produced. The clinical relevance of these findings is uncertain.

Experience in humans is limited, so use of Zovirax Cream should be considered only when the potential benefits outweigh the possibility of unknown risks.

Limited human data show that the drug does pass into breast milk following systemic administration.

Drug interactions: Probenecid increases the mean half-life and area under the plasma concentration curve of systemically administered aciclovir. However, this is likely to be of little relevance to the topical application of aciclovir.

Toxicity and treatment of overdosage: No untoward effects would be expected if the entire contents of a Zovirax Cream 10 g tube containing 500 mg of aciclovir were ingested orally. Oral doses of 800 mg five times daily (4 g per day), have been administered for seven days without adverse effects. Single intravenous doses of up to 80 mg/kg have been inadvertently administered without adverse effects. Aciclovir is dialysable.

Pharmaceutical precautions Store below 25°C. Do not refrigerate.

Zovirax Cream contains a specially formulated base and should not be diluted or used as a base for the incorporation of other medicaments.

Legal category POM

Package quantities Tubes of 2 g (OP) and 10 g (OP).

Further information Nil.

Product licence number 0003/0180.

ZOVIRAX* EYE OINTMENT

Qualitative and quantitative composition Aciclovir 3.0% w/w.

Pharmaceutical form Ophthalmic ointment.

Clinical particulars

Therapeutic indications: Treatment of herpes simplex keratitis.

Posology and method of administration: Topical administration to the eye.

Adults: 1 cm ribbon of ointment should be placed inside the lower conjunctival sac five times a day at approximately four hourly intervals, omitting the night time application. Treatment should continue for at least 3 days after healing is complete.

Children: As for adults.

Use in the elderly. As for adults.

Contra-indications: Zovirax Eye Ointment is contra-indicated in patients with a known hypersensitivity to aciclovir.

Special warnings and precautions for use: None.

Interaction with other medicaments and other forms of interaction: Probenecid increases the aciclovir mean half-life and area under the plasma concentration curve of systemically administered aciclovir. Other drugs affecting renal physiology could potentially influence the pharmacokinetics of aciclovir. However, clinical experience has not identified other drug interactions with aciclovir.

Pregnancy and lactation: Experience in humans is limited, so the use of Zovirax Eye Ointment should be considered only when the potential benefits outweigh the possibility of unknown risks. Systemic administration of aciclovir in internationally accepted standard tests did not produce embryotoxic or teratogenic effects in rats, rabbits or mice.

In a non-standard test in rats, foetal abnormalities were observed, but only following such high subcutaneous doses that maternal toxicity was produced. The clinical relevance of these findings is uncertain.

There is no information on the effect of Zovirax Eye Ointment on human female fertility. Two-generation studies in mice did not reveal any effect of (orally administered) aciclovir on fertility.

Limited human data show that the drug does pass into breast milk.

Effect on ability to drive and use machines: Not applicable.

Undesirable effects: For ophthalmic use only.

Transient mild stinging immediately following application may occur in a small proportion of patients. Superficial punctate keratopathy has been reported but has not resulted in patients being withdrawn from therapy, and healing has occurred without apparent sequelae. Local irritation and inflammation such as blepharitis and conjunctivitis have also been reported.

The results of a wide range of mutagenicity tests *in vitro* and *in vivo* indicate that aciclovir does not pose a genetic risk to man. Aciclovir was not found to be carcinogenic in long-term studies in the rat and the mouse. Largely reversible adverse effects on spermatogenesis in association with overall toxicity in rats and dogs have been reported only at doses of aciclovir greatly in excess of those employed therapeutically. Zovirax Tablets have been shown to have no definite effect upon sperm count, morphology or motility in man.

Overdose: No untoward effects would be expected if the entire contents of the tube containing 135 mg of aciclovir were ingested orally. Oral doses of 800 mg five times daily (4 g per day) have been administered for seven days without adverse effects.

Single intravenous doses of up to 80 mg/kg have been inadvertently administered without adverse effects. Aciclovir is dialysable by haemodialysis.

Pharmacological properties

Pharmacodynamic properties: Aciclovir is an antiviral agent which is highly active *in vitro* against herpes simplex (HSV) types I and II, but its toxicity to mammalian cells is low.

Aciclovir is phosphorylated to the active compound aciclovir triphosphate after entry into a herpes infected cell. The first step in this process requires the presence of the HSV coded thymidine kinase. Aciclovir triphosphate acts as an inhibitor of, and substrate for, herpes specified DNA polymerase, preventing further viral DNA synthesis without affecting normal cellular processes.

Pharmacokinetic properties: Aciclovir is rapidly absorbed from the ophthalmic ointment through the corneal epithelium and superficial ocular tissues, achieving antiviral concentrations in the aqueous humor. It has not been possible by existing methods to detect aciclovir in the blood after topical application to the eye. However, trace quantities are detectable in the urine. These levels are not therapeutically significant.

Preclinical safety data: There are no preclinical data of relevance to the prescriber which are additional to that in other sections of the SmPC.

Pharmaceutical particulars

List of excipients: White petroleum USP.

Incompatibilities: None known.

Shelf life: 5 years.

Special precautions for storage: Store below 25°C.

Nature and contents of container: Laminate ophthalmic ointment tubes closed with high-density polyethylene screw caps. Pack size 4.5 g.

Instructions for use/handling: No special instructions.

Marketing authorisation number PL 0003/0150.

Date of first authorisation/renewal of authorisation MAA: 10.06.81, Renewal: 21.10.86, 31.05.91, 16.10.96.

Date of (partial) revision of text This is the first SmPC.

Legal category POM.

ZOVIRAX* TABLETS

Presentation Each blue, film-coated, biconvex, shield-shaped, dispersible tablet is impressed with 'ZOVIRAX 200' on one side and a triangle on the obverse and contains 200 mg aciclovir.

Each pale pink, film-coated, biconvex, shield-shaped, dispersible tablet is impressed with 'ZOVIRAX 400' on one side and a triangle on the obverse and contains 400 mg aciclovir.

Each white, film-coated, biconvex, elongated, dispersible tablet is impressed with 'ZOVIRAX 800' on one side, is scored on the other side and contains 800 mg aciclovir.

Uses Zovirax Tablets are indicated for the treatment of herpes simplex virus infections of the skin and mucous membranes including initial and recurrent genital herpes.

Zovirax Tablets are indicated for the suppression (prevention of recurrences) of recurrent herpes simplex infections in immunocompetent patients.

Zovirax Tablets are indicated for the prophylaxis of herpes simplex infections in immunocompromised patients.

Zovirax Tablets are indicated for the treatment of varicella (chickenpox) and herpes zoster (shingles) infections.

Mode of action: Aciclovir is a synthetic purine nucleoside analogue with *in vitro* and *in vivo* inhibitory activity against human herpes viruses, including herpes simplex virus (HSV) types I and II and varicella zoster virus (VZV).

The inhibitory activity of aciclovir for HSV I, HSV II and VZV is highly selective. The enzyme thymidine kinase (TK) of normal, uninfected cells does not use aciclovir effectively as a substrate, hence toxicity to mammalian host cells is low. However, TK encoded by HSV and VZV converts aciclovir to aciclovir monophosphate, a nucleoside analogue which is further converted to the diphosphate and finally to the triphosphate by cellular enzymes. Aciclovir triphosphate interferes with the viral DNA polymerase and inhibits viral DNA replication with resultant chain termination following its incorporation into the viral DNA.

Prolonged or repeated courses of aciclovir in severely immunocompromised individuals may result in the selection of virus strains with reduced sensitivity, which may not respond to continued aciclovir treatment. Most of the clinical isolates with reduced sensitivity have been relatively deficient in viral TK; however, strains with altered viral TK or viral DNA polymerase have also been reported. *In vitro* exposure of HSV isolates to aciclovir can also lead to the emergence of less sensitive strains. The relationship between the *in vitro*-determined sensitivity of HSV isolates and clinical response to aciclovir therapy is not clear.

Pharmacokinetics: Aciclovir is only partially absorbed from the gut. Mean steady-state peak plasma concentrations ($C^{ss}max$) following doses of 200 mg aciclovir administered four-hourly were 3.1 microMol (0.7 micrograms/ml) and the equivalent trough plasma levels($C^{ss}min$)were1.8 microMol(0.4 micrograms/ml). Corresponding steady-state plasma concentrations following doses of 400 mg and 800 mg aciclovir administered four-hourly were 5.3 microMol (1.2 micrograms/ml) and 8 microMol (1.8 micrograms/ml) respectively, and equivalent trough plasma levels were 2.7 microMol (0.6 micrograms/ml) and 4 microMol (0.9 micrograms/ml).

In adults the terminal plasma half-life after administration of intravenous aciclovir is about 2.9 hours. Most of the drug is excreted unchanged by the kidney. Renal clearance of aciclovir is substantially greater than creatinine clearance, indicating that tubular secretion, in addition to glomerular filtration, contributes to the renal elimination of the drug. 9-carboxymethoxymethylguanine is the only significant metabolite of aciclovir, and accounts for 10–15% of the dose excreted in the urine. When aciclovir is given one hour after 1 gram of probenecid the terminal half-life and the area under the plasma concentration time curve is extended by 18% and 40% respectively.

In adults mean steady-state peak plasma concentrations ($C^{ss}max$) following a one hour infusion of 2.5 mg/kg, 5 mg/kg and 10 mg/kg were 22.7 microMol (5.1 micrograms/ml), 43.6 microMol (9.8 micrograms/ml) and 92 microMol (20.7 micrograms/ml), respectively. The corresponding trough levels ($C^{ss}min$) 7 hours later were 2.2 microMol (0.5 micrograms/ml), 3.1 microMol (0.7 micrograms/ml) and 10.2 microMol (2.3 micrograms/ml), respectively. In children over 1 year of age similar mean peak ($C^{ss}max$) and trough ($C^{ss}min$) levels were observed when a dose of 250 mg/m² was substituted for 5 mg/kg and a dose of 500 mg/m² was substituted for 10 mg/kg. In neonates and young infants (0 to 3 months of age) treated with doses of 10 mg/kg administered by infusion over a one-hour period every 8 hours the $C^{ss}max$ was found to be 61.2 microMol (13.8 micrograms/ml) and $C^{ss}min$ to be 10.1 microMol (2.3 micrograms/ml). The terminal plasma half-life in these patients was 3.8 hours. In the elderly, total body clearance falls with increasing age associated with decreases in creatinine clearance although there is little change in the terminal plasma half-life.

In patients with chronic renal failure the mean terminal half-life was found to be 19.5 hours. The mean aciclovir half-life during haemodialysis was 5.7 hours. Plasma aciclovir levels dropped approximately 60% during dialysis.

Cerebrospinal fluid levels are approximately 50% of corresponding plasma levels. Plasma protein binding is relatively low (9 to 33%) and drug interactions involving binding site displacement are not anticipated.

Dosage and administration

Dosage in adults: Treatment of herpes simplex infections: 200 mg Zovirax should be taken five times daily at approximately four-hourly intervals omitting the night time dose. Treatment should continue for 5 days but in severe initial infections this may have to be extended.

In severely immunocompromised patients (e.g. after marrow transplant) or in patients with impaired absorption from the gut the dose can be doubled to 400 mg Zovirax, or alternatively, intravenous dosing could be considered.

Dosing should begin as early as possible after the start of an infection; for recurrent episodes this should preferably be during the prodromal period or when lesions first appear.

Suppression of herpes simplex infections in immunocompetent patients: 200 mg Zovirax should be taken four times daily at approximately six-hourly intervals.

Many patients may be conveniently managed on a regimen of 400 mg Zovirax twice daily at approximately twelve-hourly intervals.

Dosage titration down to 200 mg Zovirax taken thrice daily at approximately eight-hourly intervals or even twice daily at approximately twelve-hourly intervals, may prove effective.

Some patients may experience break-through infections on total daily doses of 800 mg Zovirax.

Therapy should be interrupted periodically at intervals of six to twelve months, in order to observe possible changes in the natural history of the disease.

Prophylaxis of herpes simplex infections in immunocompromised patients: 200 mg Zovirax should be taken four times daily at approximately six-hourly intervals.

In severely immunocompromised patients (e.g. after marrow transplant) or in patients with impaired absorption from the gut, the dose can be doubled to 400 mg Zovirax, or alternatively, intravenous dosing could be considered.

The duration of prophylactic administration is determined by the duration of the period at risk.

Treatment of varicella and herpes zoster infections: 800 mg Zovirax should be taken five times daily at approximately four-hourly intervals, omitting the night time dose. Treatment should continue for seven days.

In severely immunocompromised patients (e.g. after marrow transplant) or in patients with impaired absorption from the gut, consideration should be given to intravenous dosing.

Dosing should begin as early as possible after the start of an infection; treatment of herpes zoster yields better results if initiated as soon as possible after the onset of the rash. Treatment of chickenpox in immunocompetent patients should begin within 24 hours after onset of the rash.

Dosage in children: Treatment of herpes simplex infections, and prophylaxis of herpes simplex infections in the immunocompromised: Children aged two years and over should be given adult dosages and children below the age of two years should be given ***half*** the adult dose.

Treatment of varicella infections:
6 years and over: 800 mg Zovirax four times daily.
2 to 5 years: 400 mg Zovirax four times daily.
Under 2 years: 200 mg Zovirax four times daily.
Treatment should continue for five days.

No specific data are available on the suppression of *herpes simplex* infections or the treatment of *herpes zoster* infections in immunocompetent children.

Dosage in the elderly: In the elderly, total aciclovir body clearance declines along with creatinine clearance. Adequate hydration of elderly patients taking high oral doses of Zovirax should be maintained. Special attention should be given to dosage reduction in elderly patients with impaired renal function.

Dosage in renal impairment: In the management of *herpes simplex* infections in patients with impaired renal function, the recommended oral doses will not lead to accumulation of aciclovir above levels that have been established by intravenous infusion. However, for patients with severe renal impairment (creatinine clearance less than 10 ml/minute) an adjustment of dosage to 200 mg aciclovir twice daily at approximately twelve-hourly intervals is recommended.

In the treatment of *varicella* and *herpes zoster* infections it is recommended to adjust the dosage to 800 mg aciclovir twice daily at approximately twelve-hourly intervals for patients with severe renal impairment (creatinine clearance less than 10 ml/minute), and to 800 mg aciclovir three times daily at intervals of approximately six to eight hours for patients with moderate renal impairment (creatinine clearance in the range 10 to 25 ml/minute).

Administration: Zovirax Dispersible Tablets may be dispersed in a minimum of 50 ml of water or swallowed whole with a little water. Ensure that patients on high doses of aciclovir are adequately hydrated.

Contra-indications, warnings, etc
Contra-indications: Zovirax Tablets are contra-indicated in patients known to be hypersensitive to aciclovir.

Precautions: The data currently available from clinical studies is not sufficient to conclude that treatment with Zovirax reduces the incidence of chickenpox-associated complications in immunocompetent patients.

The result of a wide range of mutagenicity tests *in vitro* and *in vivo* indicate that aciclovir is unlikely to pose a genetic risk to man. Aciclovir was not found to be carcinogenic in long-term studies in the rat and the mouse. Largely reversible adverse effects on spermatogenesis in association with overall toxicity in rats and dogs have been reported only at doses of aciclovir greatly in excess of those employed therapeutically. Zovirax Tablets have been shown to have no definitive effect upon sperm count, morphology or motility in man.

Side- and adverse effects: Skin rashes have been reported in a few patients receiving Zovirax Tablets; the rashes have resolved on withdrawal of the drug.

Gastrointestinal effects including nausea, vomiting, diarrhoea and abdominal pains have been reported in some patients receiving Zovirax Tablets. In double-blind, placebo-controlled trials the incidence of gastro-intestinal events has not been found to differ between placebo and aciclovir recipients.

Reversible neurological reactions, notably dizziness, confusional states, hallucinations, somnolence and convulsions, have occasionally been reported, usually in patients with renal impairment in whom the dosage was in excess of that recommended or with other predisposing factors.

Occasional reports of accelerated diffuse hair loss have been received. As this type of hair loss has been associated with a wide variety of disease processes and medicines, the relationship of the event to aciclovir therapy is uncertain.

Other events reported rarely in patients receiving oral formulations of Zovirax include headaches, fatigue, mild, transient rises in bilirubin and liver-related enzymes, increases in blood urea and creatinine, small decreases in haematological indices. Hepatitis, jaundice and acute renal failure have been reported on very rare occasions.

Use in pregnancy and lactation: Experience in humans is limited so the use of Zovirax Tablets should be considered only when the potential benefits outweigh the possibility of unknown risks. Systemic administration of aciclovir in internationally accepted standard tests did not produce embryotoxic or teratogenic effects in rats, rabbits or mice.

In a non-standard test in rats, foetal abnormalities were observed, but only following such high subcutaneous doses that maternal toxicity was produced. The clinical relevance of these findings is uncertain.

There is no experience of the effect of Zovirax Tablets on human female fertility. Two-generation studies in mice did not reveal any effects of aciclovir on fertility.

Following oral administration of 200 mg Zovirax five times a day, aciclovir has been detected in breast milk at concentrations ranging from 0.6 to 4.1 times the corresponding plasma levels. These levels would potentially expose nursing infants to aciclovir dosages of up to 0.3 mg/kg/day. Caution is therefore advised if Zovirax is to be administered to a nursing woman.

Drug interactions: Probenecid increases the aciclovir mean half-life and area under the plasma concentration curve. Other drugs affecting renal physiology could potentially influence the pharmacokinetics of aciclovir. However, clinical experience has not identified other drug interactions.

Toxicity and treatment of overdosage: Aciclovir is only partly absorbed in the gastrointestinal tract. It is unlikely that serious toxic effects would occur if a dose of up to 5 g were taken on a single occasion. No data are available on the consequences of the ingestion of higher doses; such an occurrence warrants close observation of the patient.

Single intravenous doses of up to 80 mg/kg have been inadvertently administered without adverse effects. Aciclovir is dialysable by haemodialysis.

Pharmaceutical precautions
Zovirax Tablets 200 mg: Store below 30°C. Protect from light. Keep dry.
Zovirax Tablets 400 mg: Store below 30°C. Protect from light. Keep dry.
Zovirax Tablets 800 mg: Store below 30°C. Protect from light. Keep dry.

Legal category POM

Package quantities

Zovirax Tablets 200 mg:	Pack of 25 tablets (OP)
Zovirax Tablets 400 mg:	Pack of 56 tablets (OP)
Zovirax Tablets 800 mg (Shingles Treatment Pack):	Pack of 35 tablets (OP)

Further information Nil.

Product licence numbers

Zovirax Tablets 200 mg:	0003/0344
Zovirax Tablets 400 mg:	0003/0345
Zovirax Tablets 800 mg:	0003/0299

ZOVIRAX SUSPENSION

Qualitative and quantitative composition Aciclovir 200 mg.

Pharmaceutical form Suspension.

Clinical particulars
Therapeutic indications: Zovirax Suspension is indicated for the treatment of herpes simplex virus infections of the skin and mucous membranes including initial and recurrent genital herpes.

Zovirax Suspension is indicated for the suppression (prevention of recurrences) of recurrent herpes simplex infections in immunocompetent patients.

Zovirax Suspension is indicated for the prophylaxis of herpes simplex infections in immunocompromised patients.

Zovirax Suspension is indicated for the treatment of varicella (chickenpox) and herpes zoster (shingles) infections.

Posology and method of administration
Dosage in adults: Treatment of herpes simplex infections: 200 mg Zovirax should be taken five times daily at approximately four-hourly intervals omitting the night time dose. Treatment should continue for 5 days, but in severe initial infections this may have to be extended.

In severely immunocompromised patients (e.g. after marrow transplant) or in patients with impaired absorption from the gut the dose can be doubled to 400 mg Zovirax or, alternatively, intravenous dosing could be considered.

Dosing should begin as early as possible after the start of an infection; for recurrent episodes this should preferably be during the prodromal period or when lesions first appear.

Suppression of herpes simplex infections in immunocompetent patients: 200 mg Zovirax should be taken four times daily at approximately six-hourly intervals.

Many patients may be conveniently managed on a regimen of 400 mg Zovirax twice daily at approximately twelve-hourly intervals.

Dosage titration down to 200 mg Zovirax taken thrice daily at approximately eight-hourly intervals or even twice daily at approximately twelve-hourly intervals, may prove effective.

Some patients may experience break-through infection on total daily doses of 800 mg Zovirax.

Therapy should be interrupted periodically at intervals of six to twelve months, in order to observe possible changes in the natural history of the disease.

Prophylaxis of herpes simplex infections in immunocompromised patients: 200 mg Zovirax should be taken four times daily at approximately six-hourly intervals.

In severely immunocompromised patients (e.g. after marrow transplant) or in patients with impaired absorption from the gut, the dose can be doubled to 400 mg Zovirax or, alternatively, intravenous dosing could be considered.

The duration of prophylactic administration is determined by the duration of the period at risk.

Treatment of varicella and herpes zoster infections: 800 mg Zovirax should be taken five times daily at approximately four-hourly intervals, omitting the night time dose. Treatment should continue for seven days.

In severely immunocompromised patients (e.g. after marrow transplant) or in patients with impaired absorption from the gut, consideration should be given to intravenous dosing.

Dosing should begin as early as possible after the start of an infection: treatment of herpes zoster yields better results if initiated as soon as possible after the onset of the rash. Treatment of chickenpox in immunocompetent patients should begin within 24 hours after onset of the rash.

Dosage in children:
Treatment of herpes simplex infections, and prophylaxis of herpes simplex infections in the immunocompromised: Children aged two years and over should be given adult dosages and children below the age of two years should be given *half* the adult dose.

Treatment of varicella infections:
6 years and over: 800 mg Zovirax four times daily.
2 to 5 years: 400 mg Zovirax four times daily.
Under 2 years: 200 mg Zovirax four times daily.
Treatment should continue for five days.

Dosing may be more accurately calculated as 20 mg/kg bodyweight (not to exceed 800 mg) Zovirax four times daily.

No specific data are available on the *suppression of herpes simplex* infections or the treatment of *herpes zoster* infections in immunocompetent children.

Zovirax Suspension may be diluted with an equal volume of either Syrup BP or Sorbitol Solution (70%) (non-crystallising) BP. The diluted product is stable for 4 weeks at 25°C but it is recommended that all dilutions are freshly prepared.

Dosage in the elderly: In the elderly, total aciclovir body clearance declines along with creatinine clearance. Adequate hydration of elderly patients taking high oral doses of Zovirax should be maintained. Special attention should be given to dosage reduction in elderly patients with impaired renal function.

Dosage in renal impairment: In the management of *herpes simplex* infections in patients with impaired renal function, the recommended oral doses will not lead to accumulation of aciclovir above levels that have been established by intravenous infusion. However, for patients with severe renal impairment (creatinine clearance less than 10 ml/minute) an adjustment of dosage to 200 mg aciclovir twice daily at approximately twelve-hourly intervals is recommended.

In the treatment of *herpes zoster* infections it is recommended to adjust the dosage to 800 mg aciclovir twice daily at approximately twelve-hourly intervals for patients with severe renal impairment (creatinine clearance less than 10 ml/minute), and to 800 mg aciclovir three times daily at intervals of approximately eight hours for patients with moderate renal impairment (creatinine clearance in the range 10 to 25 ml/minute).

Contra-indications: Zovirax Suspension is contra-indicated in patients known to be hypersensitive to aciclovir.

Special warnings and special precautions for use: The results of a wide range of mutagenicity tests *in vitro* and *in vivo* indicate that aciclovir is unlikely to pose a genetic risk to man. Aciclovir was not found to be carcinogenic in long-term studies in the rat and the mouse. Largely reversible adverse effects on spermatogenesis in association with overall toxicity in rats and dogs have been reported only at doses of aciclovir greatly in excess of those employed therapeutically. Two generation studies in mice did not reveal any effect of aciclovir on fertility. There is no experience of the effect of Zovirax Suspension on human female fertility. Zovirax Suspension has been shown to have no definite effect upon sperm count, morphology or motility in man.

The data currently available from clinical studies is not sufficient to conclude that treatment with Zovirax reduces the incidence of chickenpox-associated complications in immunocompetent patients.

Interaction with other medicaments and other forms of interaction: Probenecid increases the aciclovir mean half-life and area under the plasma concentration curve. Other drugs affecting renal physiology could potentially influence the pharmacokinetics of aciclovir. However, clinical experience has not identified other drug interactions with aciclovir.

Pregnancy and lactation: Limited data are available on the use of aciclovir in pregnancy. Caution should therefore be exercised by balancing the potential benefits of treatment against any possible hazard.

Following oral administration of 200 mg Zovirax five times a day, aciclovir has been detected in breast milk at concentrations ranging from 0.6 to 4.1 times the corresponding plasma levels. These levels would potentially expose nursing infants to aciclovir dosages of up to 0.3 mg/kg/day. Caution is therefore advised if Zovirax is to be administered to a nursing woman.

Effects on ability to drive and use machines: None known.

Undesirable effects: Skin rashes have been reported in a few patients receiving Zovirax Suspension, the rashes have resolved on withdrawal of the drug.

Gastrointestinal effects including nausea, vomiting, diarrhoea and abdominal pains have been reported in some patients receiving Zovirax Suspension. In double-blind, placebo-controlled trials the incidence of gastrointestinal events has not been found to differ between placebo and aciclovir recipients.

Reversible neurological reactions, notably dizziness, confusional states, hallucinations, somnolence and convulsions, have occasionally been reported, usually in patients with renal impairment in whom the dosage was in excess of that recommended or with other predisposing factors.

Occasional reports of accelerated diffuse hair loss have been received. As this type of hair loss has been associated with a wide variety of disease processes and medicines, the relationship of the event to aciclovir therapy is uncertain.

Other events reported rarely in patients receiving oral formulations of Zovirax include headaches, fatigue, mild, transient reversible rises in bilirubin and liver-related enzymes, increases in blood urea and creatinine, small decreases in haematological indices. Hepatitis, jaundice and acute renal failure have been reported on very rare occasions.

Overdose: Aciclovir is only partly absorbed in the gastrointestinal tract. It is unlikely that serious toxic effects would occur if a dose of up to 5 g were taken on a single occasion. No data are available on the consequences of the ingestion of higher doses; such an occurrence warrants close observation of the patient.

Single intravenous doses of up to 80 mg/kg have been inadvertently administered without adverse effects. Aciclovir is dialysable by haemodialysis.

Pharmacological properties

Pharmacodynamic properties: Aciclovir is a synthetic purine nucleoside analogue with *in vitro* and *in vivo* inhibitory activity against human herpes viruses, including herpes simplex virus (HSV) types I and II and varicella zoster virus (VZV).

The inhibitory activity of aciclovir for HSV I, HSV II and VZV is highly selective. The enzyme thymidine kinase (TK) of normal, uninfected cells does not use aciclovir effectively as a substrate, hence toxicity to mammalian host cells is low; however, TK encoded by HSV and VZV converts aciclovir to aciclovir monophosphate, a nucleoside analogue which is further converted to the diphosphate and finally to the triphosphate by cellular enzymes. Aciclovir triphosphate interferes with the viral DNA polymerase and inhibits viral DNA replication with the resultant chain termination following its incorporation into the viral DNA.

Prolonged or repeated courses of aciclovir in severely immunocompromised individuals may result in the selection of virus strains with reduced sensitivity, which may not respond to continued aciclovir treatment. Most of the clinical isolates with reduced sensitivity have been relatively deficient in viral TK, however, strains with altered viral TK or viral DNA polymerase have also been reported. *In vitro* exposure of HSV isolates to aciclovir can also lead to the emergence of less sensitive strains. The relationship between the *in vitro*-determined sensitivity of HSV isolates and clinical response to aciclovir therapy is not clear.

Pharmacokinetic properties: Aciclovir is only partially absorbed from the gut. Mean steady-state peak plasma concentrations (C^{ss}max) following doses of 200 mg aciclovir administered four-hourly were 3.1 microMol (0.7 microgram/ml) and the equivalent trough plasma levels (C^{ss}min) were 1.8 microMol (0.4 microgram/ml). Corresponding steady-state plasma concentrations following doses of 400 mg and 800 mg aciclovir administered four-hourly were 5.3 microMol (1.2 microgram/ml) and 8 microMol (1.8 microgram/ml) respectively, and equivalent trough plasma levels were 2.7 microMol (0.6 microgram/ml) and 4 microMol (0.9 microgram/ml).

In adults the terminal plasma half-life after administration of intravenous aciclovir is about 2.9 hours. Most of the drug is excreted unchanged by the kidney. Renal clearance of aciclovir is substantially greater than creatinine clearance, indicating that tubular secretion, in addition to glomerular filtration, contributes to the renal elimination of the drug.

9-carboxymethoxymethylguanine is the only significant metabolite of aciclovir, and accounts for 10–15% of the dose excreted in the urine. When aciclovir is given one hour after 1 gram of probenecid the terminal half-life and the area under the plasma concentration time curve is extended by 18% and 40% respectively.

In adults, mean steady-state peak plasma concentrations (C^{ss}max) following a one hour infusion of 2.5 mg/kg, 5 mg/kg and 10 mg/kg were 22.7 microMol (5.1 microgram/ml), 43.6 microMol (9.8 microgram/ml) and 92 microMol (20.7 microgram/ml), respectively. The corresponding trough levels (C^{ss}min) 7 hours later were 2.2 microMol (0.5 microgram/ml), 3.1 microMol (0.7 microgram/ml) and 10.2 microMol (2.3 microgram/ml), respectively.

In children over 1 year of age similar mean peak (C^{ss}max) and trough (C^{ss}min) levels were observed when a dose of 250 mg/m^2 was substituted for 5 mg/kg and a dose of 500 mg/m^2 was substituted for 10 mg/kg. In neonates (0 to 3 months of age) treated with doses of 10 mg/kg administered by infusion over a one-hour period every 8 hours the C^{ss}max was found to be 61.2 microMol (13.8 microgram/ml) and C^{ss}min to be 10.1 microMol (2.3 microgram/ml). The terminal plasma half-life in these patients was 3.8 hours.

In the elderly, total body clearance falls with increasing age associated with decreases in creatinine clearance although there is little change in the terminal plasma half-life.

In patients with chronic renal failure the mean terminal half-life was found to be 19.5 hours. The mean aciclovir half-life during haemodialysis was 5.7 hours. Plasma aciclovir levels dropped approximately 60% during dialysis.

Cerebrospinal fluid levels are approximately 50% of corresponding plasma levels. Plasma protein binding is relatively low (9 to 33%) and drug interactions involving binding site displacement are not anticipated.

Preclinical data:

Teratogenicity: Systemic administration of aciclovir in internationally accepted standard tests did not produce embryotoxic or teratogenic effects in rats, rabbits or mice.

In a non-standard test in rats, foetal abnormalities were observed, but only following such high subcutaneous doses that maternal toxicity was produced. The clinical relevance of these findings is undertain.

Pharmaceutical particulars

List of excipients: Sorbitol Solution, 70%, non-crystallising, Glycerol, Dispersible cellulose, Methyl parahydroxybenzoate, Propyl parahydroxybenzoate, Flavour, banana 5708023, Vanillin, Purified water.

Incompatibilities: None known.

Shelf life: 3 years.

Special precautions for storage: Store below 25°C.

Nature and contents of container: Neutral amber glass bottles sealed with polyolefin screw caps or metal roll-on closures fitted with sealing wads of agglomerate cork faced with saran-coated paper or saran-coated expanded polyethylene wads.

This container and these closures are applicable to both pack sizes 25 ml and 125 ml.

The 25 ml pack is a starter pack.

Instructions for use/handling: No special instructions.

Marketing authorisation holder PL 0003/0202.

Date of first authorisation/renewal of authorisation

MAA: 18.10.84
Renewed: 25.01.90
Renewed: 04.03.96

Date of last revision 10.07.98

ZOVIRAX* DOUBLE-STRENGTH SUSPENSION

Presentation Zovirax Double-Strength Suspension is an off-white, viscous suspension with an orange odour and taste and contains 400 mg aciclovir per 5 ml.

Uses Zovirax Double-Strength Suspension is indicated for the treatment of herpes simplex virus infections of the skin and mucous membranes including initial and recurrent genital herpes.

Zovirax Double-Strength Suspension is indicated for the suppression (prevention of recurrences) of recurrent herpes simplex infections in immunocompetent patients.

Zovirax Double-Strength Suspension is indicated for the prophylaxis of herpes simplex infections in immunocompromised patients.

Zovirax Double-Strength Suspension is indicated for the treatment of varicella (chickenpox) and herpes zoster (shingles) infections.

Mode of action: Aciclovir is a synthetic purine nucleoside analogue with *in vitro* and *in vivo* inhibitory activity against human herpes viruses, including herpes simplex virus (HSV) types I and II and varicella zoster virus (VZV).

The inhibitory activity of aciclovir for HSV I, HSV II and VZV is highly selective. The enzyme thymidine kinase (TK) of normal, uninfected cells does not use aciclovir effectively as a substrate, hence toxicity to mammalian host cells is low; however, TK encoded by HSV and VZV converts aciclovir to aciclovir monophosphate, a nucleoside analogue which is further converted to the diphosphate and finally to the triphosphate by cellular enzymes. Aciclovir triphosphate interferes with the viral DNA polymerase and inhibits viral DNA replication with resultant chain termination following its incorporation into the viral DNA.

Prolonged or repeated courses of aciclovir in severely immunocompromised individuals may result in the selection of virus strains with reduced sensitivity, which may not respond to continued aciclovir treatment. Most of the clinical isolates with reduced sensitivity have been relatively deficient in viral TK, however, strains with altered viral TK or viral DNA polymerase have also been reported. *In vitro* exposure of HSV isolates to aciclovir can also lead to the emergence of less sensitive strains. The relationship between the *in vitro*-determined sensitivity of HSV isolates and clinical response to aciclovir therapy is not clear.

Pharmacokinetics: Aciclovir is only partially absorbed from the gut. Mean steady-state peak plasma concentrations (C^{ss}max) following doses of 200 mg aciclovir administered four-hourly were 3.1 microMol (0.7 micrograms/ml) and the equivalent trough plasma levels (C^{ss}min) were 1.8 microMol (0.4 micrograms/ml). Corresponding steady-state plasma concentrations following doses of 400 mg and 800 mg aciclovir administered four-hourly were 5.3 microMol (1.2 micrograms/ml) and 8 microMol (1.8 micrograms/ml) respectively, and equivalent trough plasma levels were 2.7 microMol (0.6 micrograms/ml) and 4 microMol (0.9 micrograms/ml).

In adults the terminal plasma half-life after administration of intravenous aciclovir is about 2.9 hours. Most of the drug is excreted unchanged by the kidney. Renal clearance of aciclovir is substantially greater than creatinine clearance, indicating that tubular secretion, in addition to glomerular filtration, contributes to the renal elimination of the drug. 9-carboxymethoxymethylguanine is the only significant metabolite of aciclovir, and accounts for 10–15% of the dose excreted in the urine. When aciclovir is given one hour after 1 gram of probenecid the terminal half-life and the area under the plasma concentration time curve is extended by 18% and 40% respectively.

In adults, mean steady-state peak plasma concentrations (C^{ss}max) following a one hour infusion of 2.5 mg/kg, 5 mg/kg and 10 mg/kg were 22.7 microMol (5.1 micrograms/ml), 43.6 microMol (9.8 micrograms/ml) and 92 microMol (20.7 micrograms/ml), respectively. The corresponding trough levels (C^{ss}min) 7 hours later were 2.2 microMol (0.5 micrograms/ml), 3.1 microMol (0.7 micrograms/ml) and 10.2 microMol (2.3 micrograms/ml), respectively. In children over 1 year of age similar mean peak (C^{ss}max) and trough (C^{ss}min) levels were observed when a dose of 250 mg/m^2 was substituted for 5 mg/kg and a dose of 500 mg/m^2 was substituted for 10 mg/kg. In neonates and young infants (0 to 3 months of age) treated with doses of 10 mg/kg administered by infusion over a one-hour period every 8 hours the C^{ss}max was found to be 61.2 microMol (13.8 micrograms/ml) and C^{ss}min to be 10.1 microMol (2.3 micrograms/ml). The terminal plasma half-life in these patients was 3.8 hours. In the elderly, total body clearance falls with increasing age associated with decreases in creatinine clearance although there is little change in the terminal plasma half-life.

In patients with chronic renal failure the mean terminal half-life was found to be 19.5 hours. The mean aciclovir half-life during haemodialysis was 5.7 hours. Plasma aciclovir levels dropped approximately 60% during dialysis.

Cerebrospinal fluid levels are approximately 50% of corresponding plasma levels. Plasma protein binding is relatively low (9 to 33%) and drug interactions involving binding site displacement are not anticipated.

Dosage and administration

Dosage in adults: Treatment of herpes simplex infections: 200 mg Zovirax should be taken five times daily at approximately four-hourly intervals omitting the night time dose. Treatment should continue for 5 days, but in severe initial infections this may have to be extended.

In severely immunocompromised patients (e.g. after marrow transplant) or in patients with impaired absorption from the gut the dose can be doubled to 400 mg Zovirax or, alternatively, intravenous dosing could be considered.

Dosing should begin as early as possible after the start of an infection; for recurrent episodes this should preferably be during the prodromal period or when lesions first appear.

Suppression of herpes simplex infections in immunocompetent patients: 200 mg Zovirax should be taken four times daily at approximately six-hourly intervals.

Many patients may be conveniently managed on a regimen of 400 mg Zovirax twice daily at approximately twelve-hourly intervals.

Dosage titration down to 200 mg Zovirax taken thrice daily at approximately eight-hourly intervals or even twice daily at approximately twelve-hourly intervals, may prove effective.

Some patients may experience break-through infections on total daily doses of 800 mg Zovirax.

Therapy should be interrupted periodically at intervals of six to twelve months, in order to observe possible changes in the natural history of the disease.

Prophylaxis of herpes simplex infections in immunocompromised patients: 200 mg Zovirax should be taken four times daily at approximately six-hourly intervals.

In severely immunocompromised patients (e.g. after marrow transplant) or in patients with impaired absorption from the gut, the dose can be doubled to 400 mg Zovirax or, alternatively, intravenous dosing could be considered.

The duration of prophylactic administration is determined by the duration of the period at risk.

Treatment of varicella and herpes zoster infections: 800 mg Zovirax should be taken five times daily at approximately four-hourly intervals, omitting the night time dose. Treatment should continue for seven days.

In severely immunocompromised patients (e.g. after marrow transplant) or in patients with impaired absorption from the gut, consideration should be given to intravenous dosing.

Dosing should begin as early as possible after the start of the infection: treatment of herpes zoster yields better results if initiated as soon as possible after the onset of the rash. Treatment of chickenpox in immunocompetent patients should begin within 24 hours after onset of the rash.

Dosage in children: Treatment of herpes simplex infections and prophylaxis of herpes simplex infections in the immunocompromised: Children aged two years and over should be given adult dosages and children below the age of two years should be given *half* the adult dose.

Treatment of varicella infections:
6 years and over: 800 mg Zovirax four times daily.
2 to 6 years: 400 mg Zovirax four times daily.
Under 2 years: 200 mg Zovirax four times daily.
Treatment should continue for five days.

Dosing may be more accurately calculated as 20 mg/kg bodyweight (not to exceed 800 mg) Zovirax four times daily.

No specific data are available on the suppression of *herpes simplex* infections or the treatment of *herpes zoster* infections in immunocompetent children.

Zovirax Double-Strength Suspension may be diluted with an equal volume of either Syrup BP or Sorbitol Solution (70%) (non-crystallising) BP. The diluted product is stable for 4 weeks at 25°C but it is recommended that all dilutions are freshly prepared.

Dosage in the elderly: In the elderly, the total aciclovir body clearance declines along with creatinine clearance. Adequate hydration of elderly patients taking high oral doses of Zovirax should be maintained. Special attention should be given to dosage reduction in elderly patients with impaired renal function.

Dosage in renal impairment: In the management of *herpes simplex* infections in patients with impaired renal function, the recommended oral doses will not lead to accumulation of aciclovir above levels that have been established by intravenous infusion. However, for patients with severe renal impairment (creatinine clearance less than 10 ml/minute) an adjustment of dosage to 200 mg aciclovir twice daily at approximately twelve-hourly intervals is recommended.

In the treatment of *varicella* and *herpes zoster* infections it is recommended to adjust the dosage to 800 mg aciclovir twice daily at approximately twelve-hourly intervals for patients with severe renal impairment (creatinine clearance less than 10 ml/minute), and to 800 mg aciclovir three times daily at intervals of approximately six to eight hours for patients with moderate renal impairment (creatinine clearance in the range 10 to 25 ml/minute).

Contra-indications, warnings, etc

Contra-indications: Zovirax Double-Strength Suspension is contra-indicated in patients known to be hypersensitive to aciclovir.

Precautions: The data currently available from clinical studies is not sufficient to conclude that treatment with Zovirax reduces the incidence of chickenpox-associated complications in immunocompetent patients.

The result of a wide range of mutagenicity tests *in vitro* and *in vivo* indicate that aciclovir is unlikely to pose a genetic risk to man. Aciclovir was not found to be carcinogenic in long-term studies in the rat and the mouse. Largely reversible adverse effects on spermatogenesis in association with overall toxicity in rats and dogs have been reported only at doses of aciclovir greatly in excess of those employed therapeutically. Zovirax Double-Strength Suspension has been shown to have no definitive effects upon sperm count, morphology or motility in man.

Side- and adverse effects: Skin rashes have been reported in a few patients receiving Zovirax Double-Strength Suspension; the rashes have resolved on withdrawal of the drug.

Gastrointestinal effects including nausea, vomiting, diarrhoea and abdominal pains have been reported in some patients receiving Zovirax Double-Strength Suspension. In double-blind, placebo-controlled trials the incidence of gastrointestinal events has not been found to differ between placebo and aciclovir recipients.

Reversible neurological reactions, notably dizziness, confusional states, hallucinations, somnolence and convulsions, have occasionally been reported, usually in patients with renal impairment in whom the dosage was in excess of that recommended or with other predisposing factors.

Occasional reports of accelerated diffuse hair loss have been received. As this hair loss has been associated with a wide variety of disease processes and medicines, the relationship of the event to aciclovir therapy is uncertain.

Other events reported rarely in patients receiving oral formulations of Zovirax include headaches, fatigue, mild transient reversible rises in bilirubin and liver-related enzymes, increases in blood urea and creatinine and small decreases in haematological indices. Hepatitis, jaundice and acute renal failure have been reported on very rare occasions.

Use in pregnancy and lactation: Experience in humans is limited so the use of Zovirax Double-Strength Suspension should be considered only when the potential benefits outweigh the possibility of unknown risks. Systemic administration of aciclovir in internationally accepted standard tests did not produce embryotoxic or teratogenic effects in rats, rabbits or mice.

In a non-standard test in rats, foetal abnormalities were observed, but only following such high subcutaneous doses that maternal toxicity was produced. The clinical relevance of these findings is uncertain.

There is no experience of the effect of Zovirax Double-Strength Suspension on human female fertility. Two-generation studies in mice did not reveal any effect of aciclovir on fertility.

Following oral administration of 200 mg Zovirax five times a day, aciclovir has been detected in breast milk at concentrations ranging from 0.6 to 4.1 times the corresponding plasma levels. These levels would potentially expose nursing infants to aciclovir dosages of up to 0.3 mg/kg/day. Caution is therefore advised if Zovirax is to be administered to a nursing woman.

Drug interactions: Probenecid increases the aciclovir mean half-life and area under the plasma concentration curve. Other drugs affecting renal physiology could potentially influence the pharmacokinetics of aciclovir. However, clinical experience has not identified other drug interactions with aciclovir.

Toxicity and treatment of overdosage: Aciclovir is only partly absorbed in the gastrointestinal tract. It is unlikely that serious toxic effects would occur if a dose of up to 5 g were taken on a single occasion. No data are available on the consequences of the ingestion of higher doses; such an occurrence warrants close observation of the patient.

Single intravenous doses of up to 80 mg/kg have been inadvertently administered without adverse effects. Aciclovir is dialysable by haemodialysis.

Pharmaceutical precautions
Zovirax Double-Strength Suspension: Store below 30°C.

Legal category POM

Package quantities
Zovirax Double-Strength Suspension
(Chickenpox Treatment Pack): 50 ml bottle (OP)

Further information Nil.

Product licence number
Zovirax Double-Strength Suspension: 0003/0264

Date of revision 20 October 1998.

ZOVIRAX IV 250 mg
ZOVIRAX IV 500 mg

Qualitative and quantitative composition 250 mg Aciclovir OR 500 mg Aciclovir in each vial.

Pharmaceutical form Intravenous injection.

Clinical particulars

Therapeutic indications: Zovirax I.V. is indicated for the treatment of *Herpes simplex* infections in immunocompromised patients and severe initial genital herpes in the non-immunocompromised.

Zovirax I.V. is indicated for the prophylaxis of *Herpes simplex* infections in immunocompromised patients.

Zovirax I.V. is indicated for the treatment of *Varicella zoster* infections.

Zovirax I.V. is indicated for the treatment of herpes encephalitis.

Zovirax I.V. is indicated for the treatment of *Herpes simplex* infections in the neonate and infant up to 3 months of age.

Posology and method of administration:
Route of administration: Slow intravenous infusion.

A course of treatment with Zovirax I.V. usually lasts 5 days, but this may be adjusted according to the patient's condition and response to therapy. Treatment for herpes encephalitis and neonatal *Herpes simplex* infections usually lasts 10 days.

The duration of prophylactic administration of Zovirax I.V. is determined by the duration of the period at risk.

Dosage in adults: Patients with *Herpes simplex* (except herpes encephalitis) or *Varicella zoster* infections should be given Zovirax I.V. in doses of 5 mg/kg bodyweight every 8 hours.

Immunocompromised patients with *Varicella zoster* infections or patients with herpes encephalitis should be given Zovirax I.V. in doses of 10 mg/kg bodyweight every 8 hours provided renal function is not impaired (see *Dosage in renal impairment*).

Dosage in children: The dose of Zovirax I.V. for children aged between 3 months and 12 years is calculated on the basis of body surface area.

Children with *Herpes simplex* (except herpes encephalitis) or *Varicella zoster* infections should be given Zovirax I.V. in doses of 250 mg per square metre of body surface area every 8 hours.

In immunocompromised children with *Varicella zoster* infections or children with herpes encephalitis, Zovirax I.V. should be given in doses of 500 mg per square metre body surface area every 8 hours if renal function is not impaired.

Children with impaired renal function require an appropriately modified dose, according to the degree of impairment.

The dosage of Zovirax I.V. in neonates and infants up to 3 months of age is calculated on the basis of bodyweight.

Neonates and infants up to 3 months of age with *Herpes simplex* infections should be given Zovirax I.V. in doses of 10 mg/kg/bodyweight every 8 hours. Treatment for neonatal herpes simplex infections usually lasts 10 days.

Dosage in the elderly: In the elderly, total aciclovir body clearance declines in parallel with creatinine clearance. Special attention should be given to dosage reduction in elderly patients with impaired creatinine clearance.

Caution is advised when administering Zovirax I.V. to patients with impaired renal function. The following adjustments in dosage are suggested:

Creatinine clearance	Dosage
25 to 50 ml/min	The dose recommended above (5 or 10 mg/kg bodyweight) should be given every 12 hours.
10 to 25 ml/min	The dose recommended above (5 or 10 mg/kg bodyweight) should be given every 24 hours.
0(anuric) to 10 ml/min	In patients receiving continuous ambulatory peritoneal dialysis (CAPD) the dose recommended above (5 or 10 mg/kg bodyweight) should be halved and administered every 24 hours. In patients receiving haemodialysis the dose recommended above (5 or 10 mg/kg bodyweight) should be halved and administered every 24 hours and after dialysis.

Contra-indications: Zovirax I.V. is contra-indicated in patients known to be previously hypersensitive to aciclovir.

Special warnings and special precautions for use: The dose of Zovirax I.V. must be adjusted in patients with impaired renal function in order to avoid accumulation of aciclovir in the body (see *Dosage in renal impairment*).

In patients receiving Zovirax I.V. at higher doses (e.g. for herpes encephalitis), specific care regarding renal function should be taken, particularly when patients are dehydrated or have any renal impairment.

Reconstituted Zovirax I.V. has a pH of approximately 11.0 and should not be administered by mouth.

Zovirax I.V. contains no antimicrobial preservative. Reconstitution and dilution should therefore be carried out under full aseptic conditions immediately before use and any unused solution discarded. The reconstituted or diluted solutions should not be refrigerated.

Other warnings and precautions: The labels shall contain the following statements:

For intravenous infusion only.
Keep out of reach of children.
Store below 25°C.
Prepare immediately for use.
Discard unused solution.

Interaction with other medicaments and other forms of interaction: Probenecid increases the aciclovir mean half-life and area under the plasma concentration time curve. Other drugs affecting renal physiology could potentially influence the pharmacokinetics of aciclovir. However, clinical experience has not identified other drug interactions with aciclovir.

Pregnancy and lactation: Limited data are available on the use of aciclovir during pregnancy. Caution should therefore be exercised by balancing the potential benefits of treatment against any possible hazard.

Following oral administration of 200 mg five times a day, aciclovir has been detected in human breast milk at concentrations ranging from 0.6 to 4.1 times the corresponding plasma levels. These levels would potentially expose nursing infants to aciclovir dosages of up to 0.3 mg/kg bodyweight/day. Caution is therefore advised if Zovirax is to be administered to a nursing woman.

Effect on ability to drive and use machines: None known.

Undesirable effects: Rapid increases in blood urea and creatinine levels may occasionally occur in patients given Zovirax I.V. This is believed to be related to peak plasma levels and the state of hydration of the patient. To avoid this effect the drug should not be given as an intravenous bolus injection but by slow infusion over a one hour period. Adequate hydration of the patient should be maintained.

Renal impairment developing during treatment with Zovirax I.V. usually responds rapidly to rehydration of the patient and/or dosage reduction or withdrawal of the drug. Progression to acute renal failure, however, can occur in exceptional cases.

Severe local inflammatory reactions, sometimes leading to breakdown of the skin, have occurred when Zovirax I.V. has been inadvertently infused into extravascular tissues.

Reversible neurological reactions such as confusion, hallucinations, agitation, tremors, somnolence, psychosis, convulsions and coma have been associated with Zovirax I.V. therapy, usually in medically complicated cases.

Nausea and vomiting have been reported in patients receiving therapy with Zovirax I.V.

Other events reported in patients receiving Zovirax I.V. include reversible increases in bilirubin and liver-related enzymes, rashes and fevers and decreases in haematological indices (anaemia, thrombocytopenia, leucopenia). Hepatitis and jaundice have been reported on very rare occasions.

Overdose: Single and multiple intravenous infusions of up to 100 mg/kg bodyweight aciclovir have been inadvertently administered. Overdosage has resulted in elevations of serum creatinine, blood urea nitrogen and subsequent renal failure. Neurological effects including confusion, hallucinations, agitation, seizures and coma have been described in association with overdosage. Haemodialysis significantly enhances the removal of aciclovir from the blood and may, therefore, be considered an option in the management of overdose of this drug.

Pharmacological properties

Pharmacodynamic properties: Aciclovir is a synthetic purine nucleoside analogue with *in vitro* and *in vivo* inhibitory activity against human herpes viruses, including *Herpes simplex* virus (HSV) types 1 and 2 and *Varicella zoster* virus (VZV), Epstein Barr virus (EBV) and Cytomegalovirus (CMV). In cell culture aciclovir has the greatest antiviral activity against HSV-1, followed (in decreasing order of potency) by HSV-2, VZV, EBV, and CMV.

The inhibitory activity of aciclovir for HSV-1, HSV-2, VZV and EBV is highly selective. The enzyme thymidine kinase (TK) of normal, uninfected cells does not use aciclovir effectively as a substrate, hence toxicity to mammalian host cells is low; however, TK encoded by HSV, VZV and EBV converts aciclovir to aciclovir monophosphate, a nucleoside analogue, which is further converted to the diphosphate and finally to the triphosphate by cellular enzymes. Aciclovir triphosphate interferes with the viral DNA polymerase and inhibits viral DNA replication with resultant chain termination following its incorporation into the viral DNA.

Pharmacokinetic properties: In adults, the terminal plasma half-life of aciclovir after administration of Zovirax I.V. is about 2.9 hours. Most of the drug is excreted unchanged by the kidney. Renal clearance of aciclovir is substantially greater than creatinine clearance, indicating that tubular secretion, in addition to glomerular filtration, contributes to the renal elimination of the drug. 9-carboxymethoxymethylguanine is the only significant metabolite of aciclovir and accounts for 10 to 15% of the dose excreted in the urine.

When aciclovir is given one hour after 1 gram of probenecid the terminal half-life and the area under the plasma concentration time curve, are extended by 18% and 40% respectively.

In adults, mean steady-state peak plasma concentrations ($C^{ss}max$) following a one-hour infusion of 2.5 mg/kg, 5 mg/kg, and 10 mg/kg were 22.7 micromolar (5.1 microgram/ml), 43.6 micromolar (9.8 microgram/ml), and 92 micromolar (20.7 microgram/ml) respectively. The corresponding trough levels ($C^{ss}min$) 7 hours later were 2.2 micromolar (0.5 microgram/ml), 3.1 micromolar (0.7 microgram/ml) and 10.2 micromolar (2.3 microgram/ml) respectively. In children over 1 year of age similar mean peak ($C^{ss}max$) and trough ($C^{ss}min$) levels were observed when a dose of 250 mg/m^2 was substituted for 5 mg/kg and a dose of 500 mg/m^2 was substituted for 10 mg/kg. In neonates (0 to 3 months of age) treated with doses of 10 mg/kg administered by infusion over a one-hour period every 8 hours the $C^{ss}max$ was found to be 61.2 micromolar (13.8 microgram/ml) and the $C^{ss}min$ to be 10.1 micromolar (2.3 microgram/ml).

The terminal plasma half-life in these patients was 3.8 hours. In the elderly, total body clearance falls with increasing age and is associated with decreases in creatinine clearance although there is little change in the terminal plasma half-life.

In patients with chronic renal failure the mean terminal half-life was found to be 19.5 hours. The mean aciclovir half-life during haemodialysis was 5.7 hours. Plasma aciclovir levels dropped approximately 60% during dialysis.

Cerebrospinal fluid levels are approximately 50% of corresponding plasma levels.

Plasma protein binding is relatively low (9 to 33%) and drug interactions involving binding site displacement are not anticipated.

Preclinical safety data: The results of a wide range of mutagenicity tests *in vitro* and *in vivo* indicate that aciclovir is unlikely to pose a genetic risk to man.

Aciclovir was not found to be carcinogenic in long-term studies in the rat and the mouse.

Systemic administration of aciclovir in internationally accepted standard tests did not produce embryotoxic or teratogenic effects in rabbits, rats or mice.

In a non-standard test in rats, foetal abnormalities were observed but only following such high subcutaneous doses that maternal toxicity was produced. The clinical relevance of these findings is uncertain.

Largely reversible adverse effects on spermatogenesis in association with overall toxicity in rats and dogs have been reported only at doses of aciclovir greatly in excess of those employed therapeutically. Two-generation studies in mice did not reveal any effect of (orally administered) aciclovir on fertility.

There is no experience of the effect of Zovirax I.V. on human fertility. Zovirax tablets have been shown to have no definitive effect upon sperm count, morphology or motility in man.

Pharmaceutical particulars

List of excipients: Sodium hydroxide (used to adjust pH).

Incompatibilities: None known.

Shelf life: 60 months.

Special precautions for storage: Store below 25°C.

Nature and contents of container: Neutral glass vials closed with butyl rubber closures secured by aluminium collars.

17 ml-nominal capacity of vial containing 250 mg aciclovir.

20 ml-nominal capacity of vial containing 500 mg aciclovir.

Instructions for use/handling: Reconstitution: Zovirax I.V. should be reconstituted using the following volumes of either Water for Injections BP or Sodium Chloride Intravenous Injection BP (0.9% w/v) to provide a solution containing 25 mg aciclovir per ml:

Formulation	Volume of fluid for reconstitution
250 mg vial	10 ml
500 mg vial	20 ml

From the calculated dose, determine the appropriate number and strength of vials to be used. To reconstitute each vial add the recommended volume of infusion fluid and shake gently until the contents of the vial have dissolved completely.

Administration: The required dose of Zovirax I.V. should be administered by slow intravenous infusion over a one-hour period.

After reconstitution Zovirax I.V. may be administered by a controlled-rate infusion pump.

Alternatively, the reconstituted solution may be further diluted to give an aciclovir concentration of not greater than 5 mg/ml (0.5% w/v) for administration by infusion:

Add the required volume of reconstituted solution to the chosen infusion solution, as recommended below, and shake well to ensure adequate mixing occurs.

For children and neonates, where it is advisable to keep the volume of infusion fluid to a minimum, it is recommended that dilution is on the basis of 4 ml reconstituted solution (100 mg aciclovir) added to 20 ml of infusion fluid.

For adults, it is recommended that infusion bags containing 100 ml of infusion fluid are used, even when this would give an aciclovir concentration substantially below 0.5% w/v. Thus, one 100 ml infusion bag may be used for any dose between 250 mg and 500 mg aciclovir (10 and 20 ml of reconstituted solution) but a second bag must be used for doses between 500 and 1000 mg.

When diluted in accordance with the recommended schedules, Zovirax I.V. is known to be compatible with the following infusion fluids and stable for up to 12 hours at room temperature (15°C to 25°C):

Sodium Chloride Intravenous Infusion BP (0.45% and 0.9% w/v);

Sodium Chloride (0.18% w/v) and Glucose (4% w/v) Intravenous Infusion BP;

Sodium Chloride (0.45% w/v) and Glucose (2.5% w/v) Intravenous Infusion BP;

Compound Sodium Lactate Intravenous Infusion BP (Hartmann's Solution).

Zovirax I.V. when diluted in accordance with the above schedule will give an aciclovir concentration not greater than 0.5% w/v.

Since no antimicrobial preservative is included, reconstitution and dilution must be carried out under full aseptic conditions, immediately before use, and any unused solution discarded.

Should any visible turbidity or crystallisation appear in the solution before or during infusion, the preparation should be discarded.

Marketing authorisation number PL 0003/0159.

Date of first authorisation/renewal of authorisation

MAA:	06.04.82
Renewed Licence:	02.07.87
Renewed Licence:	04.02.92
Renewed Licence:	09.06.97

Date of (partial) revision of text 10 July 1998.

ZYLORIC* TABLETS
ZYLORIC-300* TABLETS

Qualitative and quantitative composition Allopurinol BP 100 mg (Zyloric Tablets), Allopurinol BP 300 mg (Zyloric-300 Tablets).

Pharmaceutical form Tablet.

Clinical particulars

Therapeutic indications: Zyloric is indicated for reducing urate/uric acid formation in conditions where urate/uric acid deposition has already occurred (e.g. gouty arthritis, skin tophi, nephrolithiasis) or is a predictable clinical risk (e.g. treatment of malignancy potentially leading to acute uric acid nephropathy). The main clinical conditions where urate/uric acid deposition may occur are: idiopathic gout; uric acid lithiasis; acute uric acid nephropathy; neoplastic disease and myeloproliferative disease with high cell turnover rates, in which high urate levels occur either spontaneously, or after cytotoxic therapy; certain enzyme disorders which lead to overproduction of urate, for example: hypoxanthine-guanine phosphoribosyltransferase, including Lesch-Nyhan syndrome; glucose-6-phosphatase including glycogen storage disease; phosphoribosylpyrophosphate synthetase, phosphoribosylpyrophosphate amidotransferase; adenine phosphoribosyltransferase. Zyloric is indicated for management of 2,8-dihydroxyadenine (2,8-DHA) renal stones related to deficient activity of adenine phosphoribosyltransferase.

Zyloric is indicated for the management of recurrent mixed calcium oxalate renal stones in the presence of hyperuricosuria, when fluid, dietary and similar measures have failed.

Posology and method of administration: Dosage in adults: Zyloric should be introduced at low dosage e.g. 100 mg/day to reduce the risk of adverse reactions and increased only if the serum urate response is unsatisfactory. Extra caution should be exercised if renal function is poor (see *Dosage in renal impairment*). The following dosage schedules are suggested:

100 to 200 mg daily in mild conditions,
300 to 600 mg daily in moderately severe conditions,
700 to 900 mg daily in severe conditions.

If dosage on a mg/kg bodyweight basis is required, 2 to 10 mg/kg bodyweight/day should be used.

Dosage in children: Children under 15 years: 10 to 20 mg/kg bodyweight/day up to a maximum of 400 mg daily. Use in children is rarely indicated, except in malignant conditions (especially leukaemia) and certain enzyme disorders such as Lesch-Nyhan syndrome.

Dosage in the elderly: In the absence of specific data, the lowest dosage which produces satisfactory urate reduction should be used. Particular attention should be paid to advice in *Dosage in renal impairment* and *Precautions and warnings*.

Dosage in renal impairment: Since allopurinol and its metabolites are excreted by the kidney, impaired renal function may lead to retention of the drug and/or its metabolites with consequent prolongation of plasma half-lives. In severe renal insufficiency, it may be advisable to use less than 100 mg per day or to use single doses of 100 mg at longer intervals than one day.

If facilities are available to monitor plasma oxipurinol concentrations, the dose should be adjusted to maintain plasma oxipurinol levels below 100 micromol/litre (15.2 mg/litre).

Allopurinol and its metabolites are removed by renal dialysis. If dialysis is required two to three times a week consideration should be given to an alternative dosage schedule of 300–400 mg Zyloric immediately after each dialysis with none in the interim.

Dosage in hepatic impairment: Reduced doses should be used in patients with hepatic impairment. Periodic liver function tests are recommended during the early stages of therapy.

Treatment of high urate turnover conditions, e.g. neoplasia, Lesch-Nyhan syndrome: It is advisable to correct existing hyperuricaemia and/or hyperuricosuria with Zyloric before starting cytotoxic therapy. It is important to ensure adequate hydration to maintain optimum diuresis and to attempt alkalinisation of urine to increase solubility of urinary urate/uric acid. Dosage of Zyloric should be at the lower end of the recommended dosage schedule.

If urate nephropathy or other pathology has compromised renal function, the advice given in *Dosage in renal impairment* should be followed.

These steps may reduce the risk of xanthine and/or oxipurinol deposition complicating the clinical situation. See also *Drug interactions* and *Adverse reactions*.

Monitoring advice: The dosage should be adjusted by monitoring serum urate concentrations and urinary urate/uric acid levels at appropriate intervals.

Instructions for use: Zyloric may be taken orally once a day after a meal. It is well tolerated, especially after food. Should the daily dosage exceed 300 mg and gastrointestinal intolerance be manifested, a divided doses regimen may be appropriate.

Contra-indications: Zyloric should not be administered to individuals known to be hypersensitive to allopurinol or to any of the components of the formulation.

Special warnings and special precautions for use: Zyloric should be withdrawn *immediately* when a skin rash or other evidence of sensitivity occurs. Reduced doses should be used in patients with hepatic or renal impairment. Patients under treatment for hypertension or cardiac insufficiency, for example with diuretics or ACE inhibitors, may have some concomitant impairment of renal function and allopurinol should be used with care in this group.

Asymptomatic hyperuricaemia *per se* is generally not considered an indication for use of Zyloric. Fluid and dietary modification with management of the underlying cause may correct the condition.

Acute gouty attacks: Allopurinol treatment should not be started until an acute attack of gout has completely subsided, as further attacks may be precipitated.

In the early stages of treatment with Zyloric, as with uricosuric agents, an acute attack of gouty arthritis may be precipitated. Therefore it is advisable to give prophylaxis with a suitable anti-inflammatory agent or colchicine for at least one month. The literature should be consulted for details of appropriate dosage and precautions and warnings.

If acute attacks develop in patients receiving allopurinol, treatment should continue at the same dosage while the acute attack is treated with a suitable anti-inflammatory agent.

Xanthine deposition: In conditions where the rate of urate formation is greatly increased (e.g. malignant disease and its treatment, Lesch-Nyhan syndrome), the absolute concentration of xanthine in urine could, in rare cases, rise sufficiently to allow deposition in the urinary tract. This risk may be minimised by adequate hydration to achieve optimal urine dilution.

Impaction of uric acid renal stones: Adequate therapy with Zyloric will lead to dissolution of large uric acid renal pelvic stones, with the remote possibility of impaction in the ureter.

Interaction with other medicaments and other forms of interaction

6-mercaptopurine and azathioprine: Azathioprine is metabolised to 6-mercaptopurine which is inactivated by the action of xanthine oxidase. When 6-mercaptopurine or azathioprine is given concurrently with Zyloric, only one-quarter of the usual dose of 6-mercaptopurine or azathioprine should be given because inhibition of xanthine oxidase will prolong their activity.

Vidarabine (adenine arabinoside): Evidence suggests that the plasma half-life of vidarabine is increased in the presence of allopurinol. When the two products are used concomitantly extra vigilance is necessary, to recognise enhanced toxic effects.

Salicylates and uricosuric agents: Oxipurinol, the major metabolite of allopurinol and itself therapeutically active, is excreted by the kidney in a similar way to urate. Hence, drugs with uricosuric activity such as probenecid or large doses of salicylate may accelerate the excretion of oxipurinol. This may decrease the therapeutic activity of Zyloric, but the significance needs to be assessed in each case.

Chlorpropamide: If Zyloric is given concomitantly with chlorpropamide when renal function is poor, there may be an increased risk of prolonged hypoglycaemic activity because allopurinol and chlorpropamide may compete for excretion in the renal tubule.

Coumarin anticoagulants: There is no evidence that interaction between allopurinol and the coumarins seen under experimental conditions has any clinical significance. However, all patients receiving anticoagulants must be carefully monitored.

Phenytoin: Allopurinol may inhibit hepatic oxidation of phenytoin but the clinical significance has not been demonstrated.

Theophylline: Inhibition of the metabolism of theophylline has been reported in normal subjects given relatively high doses of allopurinol (300 mg b.d.) under experimental conditions. The mechanism of the interaction may be explained by xanthine oxidase being involved in the biotransformation of theophylline in man. Although there have been no clinical reports of interaction, theophylline levels should be monitored in patients starting or increasing allopurinol therapy.

Ampicillin/Amoxicillin: An increase in frequency of skin rash has been reported among patients receiving ampicillin or amoxicillin concurrently with allopurinol compared to patients who are not receiving both drugs. The cause of the reported association has not been established. However, it is recommended that in patients receiving allopurinol an alternative to ampicillin or amoxicillin is used where available.

Cyclophosphamide, doxorubicin, bleomycin, procarbazine, mechloroethamine: Enhanced bone marrow suppression by cyclophosphamide and other cytotoxic agents has been reported among patients with neoplastic disease (other than leukaemia), in the presence of allopurinol. However, in a well-controlled study of patients treated with cyclophosphamide, doxorubicin, bleomycin, procarbazine and/or mechloroethamine (mustine hydrochloride) allopurinol did not appear to increase the toxic reaction of these cytotoxic agents.

Cyclosporin: Reports suggest that the plasma concentration of cyclosporin may be increased during concomitant treatment with allopurinol. The possibility of enhanced cyclosporin toxicity should be considered if the drugs are co-administered.

Pregnancy and lactation: There is inadequate evidence of safety of Zyloric in human pregnancy, although it has been in wide use for many years without apparent ill consequence.

Use in pregnancy only when there is no safer alternative and when the disease itself carries risk for the mother or unborn child.

Reports indicate that allopurinol and oxipurinol are excreted in human breast milk. Concentrations of 1.4 mg/litre allopurinol and 53.7 mg/litre oxipurinol have been demonstrated in breast milk from women taking Zyloric 300 mg/day. However, there are no data concerning the effects of allopurinol or its metabolites on the breast-fed baby.

Effects on ability to drive and use machines: None known.

Undesirable effects: Adverse reactions in association with Zyloric are rare in the overall treated population and mostly of a minor nature. The incidence is higher in the presence of renal and/or hepatic disorder.

Skin reactions: These are the most common reactions and may occur at any time during treatment. They may be pruritic, maculopapular, sometimes scaly, sometimes purpuric and rarely exfoliative. Zyloric should be withdrawn *immediately* should such reactions occur. After recovery from mild reactions, Zyloric may, if desired, be re-introduced at a small dose (e.g. 50 mg/day) and gradually increased. If the rash recurs, Zyloric should be *permanently* withdrawn.

Generalised hypersensitivity: Skin reactions associated with exfoliation, fever, lymphadenopathy, arthralgia and/or eosinophilia resembling Stevens-Johnson and/or Lyell syndrome occur rarely. Associated vasculitis and tissue response may be manifested in various ways including hepatitis, interstitial nephritis and, very rarely, epilepsy. If such reactions do occur, it may be at any time during treatment, Zyloric should be withdrawn *immediately and permanently*.

Corticosteroids may be beneficial in overcoming hypersensitivity skin reactions. When generalised hypersensitivity reactions have occurred, renal and/or hepatic disorder has usually been present particularly when the outcome has been fatal.

Angioimmunoblastic lymphadenopathy: Angioimmunoblastic lymphadenopathy has been described rarely following biopsy of a generalised lymphadenopathy. It appears to be reversible on withdrawal of Zyloric.

Granulomatous hepatitis: Very rarely granulomatous hepatitis, without overt evidence of more generalised hypersensitivity, has been described. It appears to be reversible on withdrawal of Zyloric.

Gastrointestinal disorder: In early clinical studies, nausea and vomiting were reported. Further reports suggest that this reaction is not a significant problem and can be avoided by taking Zyloric after meals. Recurrent haematemesis has been reported as an extremely rare event, as has steatorrhoea.

Blood and lymphatic system: Occasional reports have been received of thrombocytopenia, agranulocytosis and aplastic anaemia, particularly in individuals with impaired renal and/or hepatic function, reinforcing the need for particular care in this group of patients.

Miscellaneous: The following complaints have been reported occasionally; fever, general malaise, asthenia, headache, vertigo, ataxia, somnolence, coma, depression, paralysis, paraesthesiae, neuropathy, visual disorder, cataract, macular changes, taste perversion, stomatitis, changed bowel habit, infertility, impotence, diabetes mellitus, hyperlipaemia, furunculosis, alopecia, discoloured hair, angina, hypertension, bradycardia, oedema, uraemia, haematuria, angioedema, gynaecomastia.

Overdose: Ingestion of up to 22.5 g allopurinol without adverse effect has been reported. Symptoms and signs including nausea, vomiting, diarrhoea and dizziness have been reported in a patient who ingested 20 g allopurinol. Recovery followed general supportive measures. Massive absorption of Zyloric may lead to considerable inhibition of xanthine oxidase activity, which should have no untoward effects unless affecting concomitant medication, especially with 6-mercaptopurine and/or azathioprine. Adequate hydration to maintain optimum diuresis facilitates excretion of allopurinol and its metabolites. If considered necessary haemodialysis may be used.

Pharmacological properties

Pharmacodynamic properties: Allopurinol is a xanthine-oxidase inhibitor. Allopurinol and its main metabolite oxipurinol lower the level of uric acid in plasma and urine by inhibition of xanthine oxidase, the enzyme catalysing the oxidation of hypoxanthine to xanthine and xanthine to uric acid. In addition to the inhibition of purine catabolism in some but not all hyperuricaemic patients, de novo purine biosynthesis is depressed via feedback inhibition of hypoxanthine-guanine phosphoribosyltransferase. Other metabolites of allopurinol include allopurinol-riboside and oxipurinol-7 riboside.

Pharmacokinetic properties: Allopurinol is active when given orally and is rapidly absorbed from the upper gastrointestinal tract. Studies have detected allopurinol in the blood 30–60 minutes after dosing. Estimates of bioavailability vary from 67% to 90%. Peak plasma levels of allopurinol generally occur approximately 1.5 hours after oral administration of Zyloric and are much more sustained.

Allopurinol is negligibly bound by plasma proteins and therefore variations in protein binding are not thought to significantly alter clearance. The apparent volume of distribution of allopurinol is approximately 1.6 litre/kg which suggests relatively extensive uptake by tissues. Tissue concentrations of allopurinol have not been reported in humans, but it is likely that allopurinol and oxipurinol will be present in the highest concentrations in the liver and intestinal mucosa where xanthine oxidase activity is high.

Approximately 20% of the ingested allopurinol is excreted in the faeces. Elimination of allopurinol is mainly by metabolic conversion to oxipurinol by xanthine oxidase and aldehyde oxidase, with less than 10% of the unchanged drug excreted in the urine. Allopurinol has a plasma half-life of about 1 to 2 hours.

Oxipurinol is a less potent inhibitor of xanthine oxidase than allopurinol, but the plasma half-life of oxipurinol is far more prolonged. Estimates range from 13 to 30 hours in man. Therefore effective inhibition of xanthine oxidase is maintained over a 24 hour period with a single daily dose of Zyloric. Patients with normal renal function will gradually accumulate oxipurinol until a steady-state plasma oxipurinol concentration is reached. Such patients, taking 300 mg of allopurinol per day will generally have plasma oxipurinol concentrations of 5–10 mg/litre.

Oxipurinol is eliminated unchanged in the urine but has a long elimination half-life because it undergoes tubular reabsorption. Reported values for the elimination half-life range from 13.6 hours to 29 hours. The large discrepancies in these values may be accounted for by variations in study design and/or creatinine clearance in the patients.

Pharmacokinetics in patients with renal impairment: Allopurinol and oxipurinol clearance is greatly reduced in patients with poor renal function resulting in higher plasma levels in chronic therapy. Patients with renal impairment, where creatinine clearance values were between 10 and 20 ml/min, showed plasma oxipurinol concentrations of approximately 30 mg/litre after prolonged treatment with 300 mg allopurinol per day. This is approximately the concentration which would be achieved by doses of 600 mg/day in those with normal renal function. A reduction in the dose of Zyloric is therefore required in patients with renal impairment.

Pharmacokinetics in elderly patients: The kinetics of the drug are not likely to be altered other than due to deterioration in renal function (see *Pharmacokinetics in patients with renal impairment*).

Preclinical data

A. Mutagenicity: Cytogenetic studies show that allopurinol does not induce chromosome aberrations in human blood cells *in vitro* at concentrations up to 100 micrograms/ml and *in vivo* at doses up to 600 mg/day for mean period of 40 months.

Allopurinol does not produce nitraso compounds *in vitro* or affect lymphocyte transformation *in vitro*.

Evidence from biochemical and other cytological investigations strongly suggests that allopurinol has no deleterious effects on DNA at any stage of the cell cycle and is not mutagenic.

B. Carcinogenicity: No evidence of carcinogenicity has been found in mice and rats treated with allopurinol for up to 2 years.

C. Teratogenicity: One study in mice receiving intraperitoneal doses of 50 or 100 mg/kg on days 10 or 13 of gestation resulted in foetal abnormalities, however in a similar study in rats at 120 mg/kg on day 12 of gestation no abnormalities were observed. Extensive studies of high oral doses of allopurinol in mice up to 100 mg/kg/day, rats up to 200 mg/kg/day and rabbits up to 150 mg/kg/day during days 8 to 16 of gestation produced no teratogenic effects.

An *in vitro* study using foetal mouse salivary glands in culture to detect embryotoxicity indicated that allopurinol would not be expected to cause embryotoxicity without also causing maternal toxicity.

Pharmaceutical particulars

List of excipients: Lactose EP, Maize Starch EP, Povidone BP, Magnesium Stearate EP, Purified Water EP.

Incompatibilities: None known.

Shelf life: 5 years.

Special precautions for storage: Store below 25°C. Keep dry.

Nature and contents of container

Zyloric Tablets: Amber glass bottles with low-density polyethylene snap fit closures.

Zyloric-300 Tablets: PVC/aluminium foil blister pack (2 strips of 14 tablets).

Instructions for use/handling: No special instructions.

Marketing authorisation numbers

Zyloric Tablets	PL 0003/5207R
Zyloric-300 Tablets	PL 0003/0092

Date of first authorisation/renewal of authorisation

	Zyloric Tablets	*Zyloric-300 Tablets*
MAA:	20.03.80	14.07.80
Renewal:	06.06.90	18.02.91
Renewal:	14.11.95	25.11.98

Date of (partial) revision of the text This is the first SmPC.

**Trade Mark*

Wyeth Laboratories
incorporating A. H. Robins and Lederle Laboratories
Huntercombe Lane South
Taplow
Maidenhead, Berks SL6 0PH
☎ 01628 604377 🗋 01628 666368

Wyeth

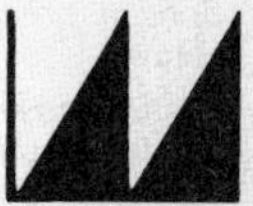

ACHROMYCIN* CAPSULES 250 mg

Presentation *Capsules 250 mg:* Each opaque, orange capsule printed 'Lederle 4874' contains 250 mg tetracycline hydrochloride.

Uses Achromycin is a broad-spectrum antibiotic used for the treatment of infections caused by tetracycline-sensitive organisms.

For example, Achromycin is highly effective in the treatment of infections caused by *Borrellia recurrentis* (relapsing fever), *Calymmatobacterium granulomatis* (granuloma inguinale), *Chlamydia* species (psittacosis, lymphogranuloma venereum, trachoma, inclusion conjunctivitis), *Francisella tularensis* (tularaemia), *Haemophilus ducreyi* (chancroid), *Leptospira* (meningitis, jaundice), *Mycoplasma pneumoniae* (non-gonococcal urethritis) *Pseudomonas mallei* and *pseudomallei* (glanders and melioidosis), *Rickettsiae* (typhus fever, Q fever, rocky mountain spotted fever), *Vibrio* species (cholera). It is also highly effective, alone or in combination with streptomycin, in the treatment of infections due to *Brucella* species (brucellosis), and *Yersinia pestis* (bubonic plague). Severe acne vulgaris.

Other sensitive organisms include: *Actinomyces israelii, Bacillus anthracis* (pneumonia), *Clostridium* species (gas gangrene, tetanus), *Entamoeba histolytica* (dysentery), *Neisseria gonorrhoeae*, and anaerobic species, *Treponema pallidum* and *pertenue* (syphillis and yaws).

Dosage and administration *Adults:* 1 capsule four times a day. This may be increased to 6 or 8 capsules daily in severe infections.

Children: Not recommended for children under 12 years of age. For children above the age of 12 years, the dose is 25–50 mg/kg divided in 2 or 4 equal doses. The maximum dose should not exceed the recommended adult dosage.

Elderly: Achromycin should be used with caution in the treatment of elderly patients where accumulation is a possibility.

Administration: Achromycin should be swallowed whole with plenty of fluid while sitting or standing. Doses should be taken an hour before or two hours after meals and therapy should be continued for up to three days after characteristic symptoms of the infection have subsided.

Contra-indications, warnings, etc.
Contra-indications: A history of hypersensitivity to tetracyclines. Overt renal insufficiency. Children under 12 years of age. Use during pregnancy or during lactation in women breast feeding infants is contra-indicated. (See also *Pregnancy and lactation.*)

Warnings: The use of tetracyclines during tooth development in children under the age of 12 years may cause permanent discolouration. Enamel hypoplasia has also been reported.

Achromycin should be used with caution in patients with renal or hepatic dysfunction or in conjunction with other potentially hepatotoxic or nephrotoxic drugs. Concurrent use with the anaesthetic methoxyflurane increases the risk of kidney failure. The anti-anabolic action of the tetracyclines may cause an increase in BUN.

Lower doses are indicated in cases of renal impairment to avoid excessive systemic accumulation, and if therapy is prolonged, serum level determinations are advisable. Patients who have known liver disease should not receive more than 1 g daily. In long term therapy, periodic laboratory evaluation of organ systems, including haematopoietic, renal and hepatic studies should be performed.

Cross resistance between tetracyclines may develop in micro-organisms and cross-sensitisation in patients. Achromycin should be discontinued if there are signs/symptoms of overgrowth of resistant organisms including candida, enteritis, glossitis, stomatitis, vaginitis, pruritus ani or staphylococcal enterocolitis.

Patients taking oral contraceptives should be warned that if diarrhoea or breakthrough bleeding occur, there is a possibility of contraceptive failure.

Interactions: Achromycin should not be used with penicillins. Tetracyclines depress plasma prothrombin activity and reduced doses of concomitant anticoagulants may be required.

Absorption of Achromycin is impaired by the concomitant administration of iron, calcium, zinc, magnesium and particularly aluminium salts commonly used as antacids.

The concomitant use of tetracyclines may reduce the efficacy of oral contraceptives; an increased incidence of breakthrough bleeding may also be experienced (see statement under Warnings).

Use in pregnancy: Contra-indicated in pregnancy.

Results of animal studies indicate that tetracyclines cross the placenta, are found in foetal tissues, and can have toxic effects on the developing foetus (often related to retardation of skeletal development). Evidence of embryotoxicity has also been noted in animals treated early in pregnancy.

Achromycin therefore, should not be used in pregnancy unless considered essential in which case the maximum daily dose should be 1 g.

The use of drugs of the tetracycline class during tooth development (last half of pregnancy) may cause permanent discolouration of the teeth (yellow-grey-brown). This adverse reaction is more common during long term use of the drugs but has been observed following repeated short term courses. Enamel hypoplasia has also been reported.

Use in lactation: Contra-indicated during lactation in women breast feeding infants.

Tetracyclines have been found in the milk of lactating women who are taking a drug in this class. Permanent tooth discolouration may occur in the developing infant, and enamel hypoplasia has been reported. Therefore, Achromycin should not be administered to lactating women.

Side-effects: Gastro-intestinal disturbances including nausea, vomiting, diarrhoea and rarely dysphagia have been reported. There have been a few cases of oesophagitis and oesophageal ulceration in patients taking oral tetracyclines in solid dose form, usually where medication was taken immediately before retiring or with inadequate fluids. As with all antibiotics, overgrowth of resistant organisms may cause candidiasis, pseudomembranous colitis (*Clostridium difficile* overgrowth), glossitis, stomatitis, vaginitis, or staphylococcal enterocolitis.

In common with other tetracyclines, transient increases in liver function test values, hepatitis, jaundice and hepatic failure have been reported rarely. A few cases of pancreatitis have been reported. Erythematous and maculopapular rashes, photosensitivity, pruritus, bullous dermatoses, exfoliative dermatitis and skin discolouration have occurred occasionally but serious skin reactions are rare. Headache, dizziness, visual disturbances and rarely impaired hearing have been reported with tetracyclines and patients should be warned about the possible hazards of driving or operating machinery during treatment. Bulging fontanelles in infants and benign intracranial hypertension in juveniles and adults have been reported. Treatment should cease if evidence of raised intracranial pressure, such as severe or persistent headache or blurred vision are noted. While the condition and related symptoms usually resolve soon after discontinuation of the tetracycline, the possibility of permanent sequelae exists. There have been isolated cases of myasthenia. Hypersensitivity reactions, including urticaria, angioneurotic oedema, anaphylaxis, anaphylactoid purpura, pericarditis and exacerbation of systemic lupus erythematosus may occur. Renal dysfunction, especially in patients with pre-existing renal impairment, and rarely, acute renal failure or nephritis, have been reported with tetracyclines. Haemolytic anaemia, thrombocytopenia, neutropenia, agranulocytosis, aplastic anaemia and eosinophilia have been reported rarely. When given over prolonged periods, tetracyclines have been reported to produce brown-black discolouration of the thyroid gland. No abnormalities of thyroid function are known to occur.

Overdosage: No specific antidote. Gastric lavage plus oral administration of milk or antacids.

Pharmaceutical precautions Achromycin Capsules should be stored at controlled room temperature (15–30°C) in the original pack.

Legal category POM

Package quantity Bottles of 100

Further information Nil

Product licence number 0095/0041

ACHROMYCIN* OINTMENT 3%

Qualitative and quantitative composition Achromycin Ointment contains 3% tetracycline hydrochloride BP.

Pharmaceutical form A yellow, smooth, homogeneous ointment for topical administration.

Clinical particulars
Therapeutic indications: The treatment of superficial pyogenic infections of the skin. It is indicated for local infections caused by both susceptible Gram-positive and Gram-negative organisms including Streptococci, Staphylococci and the Coli-aerogenes group.

Posology and method of administration:
Adults, including the elderly and children over 8 years: Apply the ointment directly to the involved area, preferably on sterile gauze once or more daily as the condition indicates. In severe local infections, local treatment should be supplemented by oral therapy.

Contra-indications: History of hypersensitivity to tetracycline hydrochloride or to any other component of the preparation.

Special warnings and precautions for use: To reduce the theoretical risk of damage to permanent dentition, topical tetracyclines should not be used in children under 8 years of age, unless other drugs are unlikely to be effective or are contraindicated.

The use of antibiotics may result in overgrowth of non-susceptible organisms. If new infections appear during therapy, appropriate measures should be taken.

Interactions with other medicaments and other forms of interaction: The concomitant use of oral tetracyclines may reduce the efficacy of oral contraceptives; an increased incidence of breakthrough bleeding may also be experienced.

Pregnancy and lactation: The use of drugs of the tetracycline class during tooth development (last half of pregnancy through early childhood) may cause permanent discoloration of the teeth (yellow-grey-brown). This adverse reaction is more common during long-term oral or otherwise systemic use of the drugs and the risk of such effects from topical usage is considered negligible. However, to reduce the theoretical risk of damage to permanent dentition, topical tetracyclines should not be used during the last half of pregnancy or during lactation, unless other drugs are unlikely to be effective or are contraindicated.

Effects on the ability to drive and use machines: None

Undesirable effects: Some patients may be allergic to any of the components. If adverse reaction or idiosyncrasy occurs, discontinue medication.

Achromycin Ointment may cause a yellow staining of clothes. Following extended use, a similar local staining of the skin may occur which disappears on cessation of treatment.

Overdose: Not applicable.

Pharmacological properties
Pharmacodynamic properties: Tetracycline is a broad spectrum antibiotic.

It is active against a large number of Gram-negative and Gram-positive pathogenic bacteria, including some which are resistant to Penicillin.

Pharmacokinetic properties: Topically applied tetracycline preparations are not absorbed into the general circulation to any significant degree.

Pharmceutical particulars
List of excipients: White petroleum jelly, anhydrous lanolin.

Incompatibilities: None.

Shelf life: 5 years.

Special precautions for storage: Store at 25°C or below.

Nature and contents of container: Collapsible aluminium tubes, closed with plastic caps, containing 30 g of the ointment.

Instructions for use/handling: Not applicable.

Marketing authorisation number PL 0095/5031R

Date of revision of text: 26 June 1997.

Legal category POM.

ASENDIS*

Qualitative and quantitative composition
Asendis Tablets 50 mg: Orange, flat, heptagonal-shaped tablets, scored on one side and engraved 'LL50' on the other, each containing 50 mg of amoxapine.

Asendis Tablets 100 mg: Mottled blue, flat, heptagonal-shaped tablets, scored on one side with 'LL100' on the other, each containing 100 mg of amoxapine.

Pharmaceutical form Tablets

Clinical particulars
Therapeutic indications: Asendis is an anti-depressant indicated for the symptomatic treatment of depressive illness.

Posology and method of administration: Adults: Initially 100–150 mg daily increasing slowly according to clinical response up to 300 mg daily, in divided doses or one dose which may be given at night. Usual maintenance dose: 150–250 mg daily.

Elderly: An initial dose of 25 mg twice a day is recommended. If necessary, the dosage may be increased under close supervision after 5 to 7 days to a maximum of 50 mg three times daily. Less than the normal dose may be sufficient to produce a satisfactory clinical response.

Children (under 16 years): Not recommended.

Studies have demonstrated that the initial clinical effect of Asendis can occur within four to seven days. Treatment should be maintained for a minimum period of one month, and current psychiatric practice suggests that several months treatment may be necessary after initial clinical improvement.

Contra-indications: Recent myocardial infarction or coronary artery insufficiency. Heartblock or other cardiac arrhythmias. Mania. Severe liver disease. Use in patients hypersensitive to dibenzoxazepines, or in patients who are currently receiving, or have received, monoamine oxidase inhibitors in the preceding two weeks.

Special warnings and precautions for use: In common with other drugs of this class, caution should be exercised when using in patients with any of the following conditions: urinary retention, narrow angle glaucoma, hyperthyroidism, cardiovascular disorders, blood dyscrasias and hepatic or renal impairment. Asendis should be used with particular caution in patients with a history of epilepsy or recent convulsions.

Psychotic manifestations may be exacerbated during treatment with tri/tetracyclic anti-depressants.

A minority of patients may not improve during the first 2–4 weeks of treatment. Patients should be closely monitored during this period, especially those posing a high suicidal risk.

Concurrent administration with electroconvulsive therapy may increase the hazards associated with such therapy.

Although not indicative of addiction, withdrawal symptoms may occur on abrupt cessation of therapy and include insomnia, irritability, and excessive perspiration.

In common with other anti-depressants, the elderly are more prone to experiencing adverse reactions, especially agitation and confusion, hence the importance of initiating treatment at a lower dose (see Posology and method of administration).

Interactions with other medicaments and other forms of interaction: The drug interactions experienced with Asendis are those that could be expected from a drug of this class and include the following:

Asendis may decrease the anti-hypertensive effect of guanethidine, debrisoquine, bethanidine and possibly clonidine. It would be advisable to review all anti-hypertensive therapy during treatment.

Asendis should not be given with sympathomimetic agents such as adrenaline, ephedrine, isoprenaline, noradrenaline, phenylephrine and phenylpropanolamine.

Asendis may potentiate the effects of drugs having an anticholinergic action, ethchlorvynol, thyroid hormone therapy, and the central nervous depressant action of alcohol.

Barbiturates may increase the metabolism of tri/tetracyclic anti-depressants.

Anaesthetics given during tri/tetracyclic anti-depressant therapy may increase the risk of arrhythmias and hypotension. If surgery is necessary, the anaesthetist should be informed that a patient is being so treated.

Caution should be exercised if Asendis is given concomitantly with Lithium.

Serum levels of several tricyclic anti-depressants have been reported to be significantly increased when cimetidine is administered concurrently; although such an interaction has not been reported to date with Asendis.

Pregnancy and lactation: There are no adequately well controlled studies in pregnant women. Asendis should therefore be used during pregnancy only if the potential benefit justifies the potential risk to the foetus. Asendis like many other systemic drugs is excreted in human milk. The effects of the drug on infants are unknown, and hence the administration to nursing mothers cannot be recommended.

Effects on the ability to drive and use machines: As with many other anti-depressants, Asendis may initially impair alertness. Patients should be warned of the possible hazard when driving or operating machinery.

Undesirable effects: In common with certain other drugs of this class, the following adverse effects have been reported with Asendis. These have been categorised according to incidence.

Incidence greater than 1%: The most frequent types of adverse reactions occurring in clinical trials were sedative and anticholinergic. These included; drowsiness (14%), dry mouth (14%), constipation (12%), and blurred vision (7%).

Less frequently reported reactions:
CNS and neuromuscular: anxiety, insomnia, restlessness, nervousness, palpitations, tremors, confusion, excitement, nightmares, ataxia, alterations in EEG patterns.

Allergic: oedema, skin rash.

Endocrine: elevation of prolactin levels.

Gastrointestinal: nausea.

Other: dizziness, headache, fatigue, weakness, excessive appetite, increased perspiration.

Incidence less than 1%:
Anticholinergic: disturbances of accommodation, mydriasis, urinary retention, nasal stuffiness.

Cardiovascular: hypotension, hypertension, syncope, tachycardia.

Allergic: drug fever, urticaria, photosensitisation, pruritis, rarely vasculitis, hepatitis.

CNS and neuromuscular: tingling, paraesthesia of the extremities, tinnitus, disorientation, seizures, hypomania, numbness, inco-ordination, disturbed concentration, hyperthermia, extrapyramidal symptoms including rarely tardive dyskinesia. Neuroleptic malignant syndrome (see below).

Haematological: leukopenia, agranulocytosis.

Gastrointestinal: epigastric distress, vomiting, flatulence, abdominal pain, peculiar taste, diarrhoea.

Endocrine: increased or decreased libido, impotence, menstrual irregularity, breast enlargement and galactorrhoea in the female, syndrome of inappropriate antidiuretic hormone secretion.

Other: lacrimation, weight loss or gain, altered liver function, painful ejaculation.

Rare cases of Neuroleptic Malignant Syndrome have been reported following the use of Asendis. This syndrome is potentially fatal and presents with symptoms of hyperpyrexia, muscle rigidity, altered mental status, and evidence of autonomic instability. If a patient is diagnosed as suffering from Neuroleptic Malignant Syndrome, the management should include: (1) immediate discontinuation of antipsychotic drugs and other drugs not essential to concurrent therapy (2) symptomatic treatment and monitoring of vital signs and (3) treatment of any concomitant serious medical problems.

Overdose: Toxic manifestations of Asendis overdose differ significantly from those of other tricyclic anti-depressants. The risk of significant cardiotoxicity is low and tends to be limited to sinus tachycardia. However, convulsions may occur frequently (40–50%) in those taking substantial overdoses and status epilepticus is not uncommon. Respiratory and/or metabolic acidosis may develop, usually in association with repeated seizures. Acute renal failure or transient impairment in renal function may develop 2–5 days after substantial overdose of Asendis. There is a rare potential for permanent neurological damage.

There is no specific antidote for Asendis; treatment should be symptomatic and supportive with special attention to prevention or control of seizures. If the patient is conscious, emesis should be induced as soon as possible, followed by gastric lavage. Administration of activated charcoal after gastric lavage may reduce absorption and facilitate drug elimination. An adequate airway should be established in unconscious patients, who may also need full support of vital functions and cardiac monitoring. Convulsions, when they occur, typically begin within 12 hours of ingestion and may respond to standard anti-convulsant therapy such as intravenous diazepam and/or phenytoin. More rigorous treatment is required should status epilepticus develop. Drugs which are known to potentiate respiratory depression should be avoided. Treatment for renal impairment, should it occur, is the same as for non-drug-induced renal dysfunction.

Pharmacological properties
Pharmacodynamic properties: Amoxapine is a tricyclic antidepressant. It has marked anticholinergic and sedative properties, and prevents re-uptake (and hence inactivation) of noradrenaline and serotonin at nerve terminals. Its mode of action in depression is not fully understood.

Pharmacokinetic properties: Amoxapine is readily absorbed from the gastro-intestinal tract. Since amoxapine slows gastro-intestinal transit time, absorption can, however, be delayed, particularly in overdosage.

Amoxapine is metabolised by hydroxylation and excreted in the urine mainly as its metabolites in the conjugated form.

Amoxapine has been reported to have a half life of 8 hours and its major metabolite, 8-hydroxy-amoxapine, a half life of 30 hours. Amoxapine is extensively bound to plasma proteins.

Pre-clinical safety data: There are no pre-clinical data of relevance to the prescriber which are additional to that already included in other sections of the Summary of Product Characteristics.

Pharmaceutical particulars
List of excipients: Dibasic calcium phosphate, maize starch (pregelatinised), corn starch, magnesium stearate, stearic acid and colourings:E104 (50 mg tablet only), E127 (50 mg tablet only) and E132 (100 mg tablet only).

Incompatibilities: None

Shelf life: 36 months

Special precautions for storage: Store below 25°C

Nature and contents of container: Asendis Tablets 50 mg: White polypropylene bottles with white urea screw-on caps of 84 tablets.

Asendis Tablets 100 mg: White polypropylene bottles with white urea screw-on caps of 56 tablets.

Instructions for use/handling: None

Marketing authorisation number
Asendis Tablets 50 mg: PL 00095/0057
Asendis Tablets 100 mg: PL 00095/0058

Date of revision of text December 1997

Legal category POM

ATIVAN* INJECTION

Presentation Ativan injection is a clear, colourless solution containing lorazepam BP at a concentration of 4 mg/ml supplied in 1 ml quantities in clear glass ampoules.

Uses Ativan injection is indicated for: Pre-operative medication or premedication for uncomfortable or prolonged investigations e.g. bronchoscopy, arteriography, endoscopy. The treatment of acute anxiety states, acute excitement or acute mania. The control of status epilepticus.

Dosage and administration *Route of administration:* Ativan injection can be given intravenously or intramuscularly. However, the intravenous route is to be preferred. Care should be taken to avoid injection into small veins and intra-arterial injection.

Absorption from the injection site is considerably slower if the intramuscular route is used and as rapid an effect may be obtained by oral administration of Ativan tablets.

Ativan should not be used for long term chronic treatment.

Preparation of the injection Ativan injection is slightly viscid when cool. To facilitate injection it may be diluted 1:1 with normal Saline or Water for injection BP immediately before administration. If given intramuscularly it should always be diluted.

Ativan injection is presented as a 1 ml solution in a 2 ml ampoule to facilitate dilution.

Ativan injection should not be mixed with other drugs in the same syringe.

Dosage:
1.*Premedication*: *Adults:* 0.05 mg/kg (3.5 mg for an average 70 kg man) By the intravenous route the injection should be given 30–45 minutes before sur-

gery when sedation will be evident after 5–10 minutes and maximal loss of recall will occur after 30–45 minutes. By the intramuscular route the injection should be given 1–1½ hours before surgery when sedation will be evident after 30–45 minutes and maximal loss of recall will occur after 60–90 minutes.

Children: Ativan injection is not recommended in children under 12.

2. *Acute Anxiety: Adults:* 0.025–0.03 mg/kg (1.75–2.1 mg for an average 70 kg man). Repeat 6 hourly.

Children: Ativan injection is not recommended in children under 12.

3. *Status epilepticus: Adults:* 4 mg intravenously

Children: 2 mg intravenously

Elderly: The elderly may respond to lower doses and half the normal adult dose may be sufficient.

Contra-indications, warnings, etc.

Contra-indications:

1. Ativan injection should not be given to patients with a previous history of sensitivity to benzodiazepines or any of the vehicle constituents (polyethylene glycol, propylene glycol, benzyl alcohol), or to patients with acute pulmonary insufficiency.
2. Ativan injection is not recommended for out-patient use unless the patient is accompanied.

Use in pregnancy: Safety for use in pregnancy has not been established. Ativan injection should not be administered during pregnancy or lactation unless in the judgement of the physician such administration is clinically justifiable. Ativan injection is not recommended for use in the first three months of pregnancy. Use during the late phase of pregnancy or at delivery may require ventilation of the infant at birth.

Precautions and warnings:

1. Patients should remain under observation for at least eight hours and preferably overnight.
2. Patients should not drive or operate machinery within 24–48 hours of administration of Ativan injection and should be advised not to take alcohol.
3. The addition of scopolamine to Ativan injection is not recommended, since their combination has been observed to cause an increased incidence of sedation, hallucination and irrational behaviour.
4. The effects of centrally acting cerebral depressant drugs may be potentiated.
5. This product should be used with caution in patients with impairment of renal or hepatic function.
6. The injection should be given slowly except in the control of status epilepticus where rapid injection is required.
7. Airway obstruction may occur in heavily sedated patients and therefore equipment necessary to maintain a patent airway and to support respiration/ventilation should be available.
8. Extreme care must be taken in administering Ativan injection to elderly or very ill patients and to those with limited pulmonary reserve, because of the possibility that apnoea and/or cardiac arrest may occur. Care should also be exercised when administering Ativan injection to a patient with status epilepticus, especially when the patient has received other central nervous system depressants.
9. Elderly patients may require a lower dosage.
10. There is no evidence to support the use of Ativan injection in coma or shock.
11. There is insufficient data regarding obstetrical safety of parenteral Ativan, including use in cesarean section. Respiratory depression, poor sucking and hypothermia in the neonate after delivery have occasionally been reported, especially in infants who are at risk. Such use, therefore, is not recommended.
12. As with all benzodiazepines doctors should be aware of the possibility of dependence and withdrawal symptoms in certain patients. In normal acute usage dependence is unlikely to occur but the risk increases with higher doses and longer-term use and is further increased in patients with a history of alcoholism, drug abuse or in patients with marked personality disorders.

    Symptoms such as anxiety, depression, headache, insomnia, tension and sweating have been reported following abrupt discontinuation of benzodiazepines. Other symptoms such as persistent tinnitus, involuntary movements, paraesthesia, perceptual changes, confusion, convulsions, abdominal and muscle cramps and vomiting may be characteristic of benzodiazepine withdrawal syndrome.
13. The use of benzodiazepines may release suicidal tendencies in depressed patients. Lorazepam should not be used alone to treat depression or anxiety associated with depression. Other rarely reported behavioural effects of the benzodiazepines include paradoxical aggressive outbursts, excitement and confusion.

Side effects: Lorazepam is well tolerated and imbalance or ataxia are signs of excessive dosage. Drowsiness may occur. Occasional confusion, hangover, headache on waking, dizziness, blurred vision, nausea, vomiting, restlessness, depression, crying, sobbing, hallucinations and diplopia have been reported. In addition blood dyscrasias and increased liver enzymes have occasionally been reported. On rare occasions visual disturbances, hypotension, hypertension, gastro-intestinal disturbances and mild transient skin rashes have also been reported.

Overdosage: As with other benzodiazepines, overdosage should not present a threat to life unless combined with other CNS depressants (including alcohol). General supportive measures should be used and the treatment of overdosage is symptomatic. The patient is likely to sleep and a clear airway should be maintained.

Pharmaceutical precautions Store in a refrigerator between 0°C and 4°C. Protect from light.

Legal category POM CD (Sch 4)

Package quantities 10 x 1 ml solution (in 2 ml ampoules) per pack.

Further information Ativan is metabolised by a simple one-step process to a pharmacologically inactive glucuronide. There is minimal risk of accumulation after repeated doses, giving a wide margin of safety. Ativan injection can be administered concurrently with a wide range of other drugs and has minimal effect on blood pressure. Tolerance at the injection site is generally good although, rarely, pain and redness have been reported.

Product licence number 0011/0051

AUDICORT* Ear Drops

Qualitative and quantitative composition

Active Constituent	*per ml*	*Specification reference*
Triamcinolone acetonide	1.0 mg	BP
Neomycin base in propylene glycol equivalent to neomycin base	3.5 mg	HSE

Pharmaceutical form Audicort is a clear, pale yellow to yellow solution for topical application to the ear.

Clinical particulars

Therapeutic indications: Audicort is anti-inflammatory and antibacterial. The preparation is indicated in the treatment of acute and chronic otitis externa due to or complicated by bacterial infection.

Posology and method of administration: Adults and the elderly. After careful cleansing of the ear, administer 2–5 drops of Audicort topically to the ear, usually three or four times daily. If desired, the drops may be used to saturate a gauze or cotton wick placed in the ear. This wick should be kept saturated by instilling 2–5 drops, three to four times a day, and should be replaced every 24–48 hours. Treatment should be reviewed after seven days with continuation of therapy up to 14 days if resolution has not occurred.

Contraindications: Audicort is contraindicated in infants and children and in patients with perforated tympanic membrane. Hypersensitivity to triamcinolone acetonide, neomycin or propylene glycol. The preparation should not be used in the eyes.

Special warnings and special precautions for use: The tympanic membrane should be checked for integrity before Audicort drops are prescribed.

Use of an antibiotic may occasionally result in an overgrowth of non-susceptible micro-organisms, while the presence of an anti-inflammatory steroid may encourage their spread. If superinfection does occur, the drug should be stopped and appropriate therapy instituted.

Unlikely to produce any serious toxic effects if ingested.

Interaction with other medicaments and other forms of interaction: None.

Pregnancy and lactation: Topical administration of corticosteroids to pregnant animals can cause abnormalities of foetal development including cleft palate and intra-uterine growth retardation. There may therefore be a very small risk of such effects in the human foetus. Audicort should only be used in pregnancy when there is no safer alternative.

Although corticosteroids appear in breast milk, the absorption of triamcinolone acetonide from Audicort is expected to be minimal so the risk to the baby is considered to be small.

Effects on ability to drive and operate machines: None

Undesirable effects: Side-effects from triamcinolone and neomycin in otic drops are rare, but neomycin has occasionally been responsible for localised skin sensitisation. Discomfort (stinging) may be experienced by some patients on application of the drops. If local reactions such as irritation or erythema occur, medication should be discontinued.

If absorbed systemically, neomycin is known to be ototoxic. However, during the course of treatment with Audicort, the maximum total exposure to neomycin is 35 mg and this is not thought to pose a significant clinical risk.

Overdose: Overdose of triamcinolone acetonide and neomycin undecylenate otic drops has not been reported. Excess drops can be removed from the ear by gentle washing.

Pharmacological properties

Pharmacodynamic properties:

1. Neomycin (antibiotic) as neomycin undecylenate.
2. Triamcinolone acetonide (corticosteroid with anti-inflammatory action)

Pharmacokinetic properties: Audicort Ear Drops are recommended for topical administration.

Absorption of triamcinolone acetonide by this route of administration is usually minimal. However, when applied topically, particularly to large areas, when the skin is broken, or under occlusive dressings, corticosteroids may be absorbed in sufficient quantities to cause systemic effects.

Absorption of neomycin after topical application is also likely to be minimal. However, absorption has been reported to occur from inflamed skin.

Pharmaceutical particulars

List of excipients:

	Specification Reference
Undecylenic acid	EP
Tromethamine	USP
Disodium edetate	BP
Sodium metabisulphite	BP
Benzoic acid	BP
Water (purified)	BP
Propylene Glycol	BP

Incompatibilities: None

Shelf life: 18 months.

Special precautions for storage: Audicort Ear Drops should be stored in a refrigerator (2–8°C) in the original container. Do not freeze. Excessive heating of the solution should be avoided. Audicort should not be diluted.

Nature and contents of container: Plastic dropper bottles containing 10 ml of solution.

Instructions for use and handling: None

Marketing authorisation number PL 0095/5069R

Date of approval/revision revised November 1996

Legal category POM

AUREOCORT* Ointment

Qualitative and quantitative composition Aureocort Ointment is a topical preparation containing the active ingredients chlortetracycline hydrochloride 3.09% w/w and triamcinolone acetonide 0.1% w/w.

Pharmaceutical form Ointment for topical administration.

Clinical particulars

Therapeutic indications: Aureocort combines the anti-inflammatory action of triamcinolone acetonide with the anti-infective properties of chlortetracycline.

It is indicated in the treatment of secondarily infected atopic dermatitis, contact dermatitis, eczema, neurodermatitis, otitis externa, seborrhoeic dermatitis, varicose eczema and vesiculo–pustular dermatitis. It may also be used in the treatment of infected insect bites.

Posology and method of administration:

Adults, children over 8 years and the elderly: Aureocort Ointment should be applied sparingly to the affected area, either directly or on sterile gauze, two or three times daily.

Please refer to the *Special warnings and precautions for use.*

Contra-indications: The use of Aureocort is contra-indicated in tuberculous, fungal or viral lesions of the skin (herpes simplex, vaccinia and varicella), and primary bacterial infections, e.g. impetigo, pyoderma and furunculosis.

Aureocort Topical preparations are also contra-indicated in patients with a history of hypersensitivity to tetracyclines, corticosteroids, or any other ingredient in the preparation.

Special warnings and precautions for use: To reduce the theoretical risk of damage to permanent dentition by tetracyclines, Aureocort Topical preparations should not be used in children under 8 years of age unless other drugs are unlikely to be effective or are contra-indicated.

Use of antibiotics topically may result in overgrowth of non-susceptible organisms; if new infections appear during therapy, appropriate measures should be taken.

The use of corticosteroids on infected areas should be continuously and carefully observed, bearing in mind the potential spreading of infections (caused by organisms not sensitive to chlortetracycline) by anti-inflammatory corticosteroids. It may be advisable to discontinue corticosteroid therapy and/or initiate alternative antibacterial measures in these circumstances. Generalised dermatological conditions may require systemic corticosteroid therapy.

Steroid-antibiotic combinations should not be continued for more than 7 days in the absence of any clinical improvement, since in this situation, occult extension of infection may occur due to the masking effect of the steroid. Extended or recurrent application may increase the risk of contact sensitisation, and should be avoided. Occlusion should not be used when treating conditions of the face.

Interactions with other medicaments and other forms of interactions: Not applicable.

Pregnancy and lactation: Topical administration of corticosteroids to pregnant rabbits has been reported to cause abnormalities of foetal development, including cleft palate and intrauterine growth retardation at relatively low doses. The relevance of this finding to human beings has not been established. However, topical corticosteroids should not be used extensively (large amounts or for long periods) in early pregnancy. The use of corticosteroid/antibiotic preparations, containing drugs of the tetracyclines class, during tooth development (last half of pregnancy through early childhood) may cause permanent discolouration of the teeth (yellow-grey-brown). This adverse reaction, related only to tetracyclines, is more common during long-term oral or otherwise systemic use of tetracyclines and the risk of such effects from topical usage is considered negligible. However, to reduce the theoretical risk of damage to permanent dentition by tetracyclines, and the risk of any abnormalities of foetal development by corticosteroids, topical corticosteroid / tetracycline combinations should not be used during pregnancy or lactation unless other drugs are unlikely to be effective, or are contra-indicated.

Effects on ability to drive and use machinery: Not applicable.

Undesirable effects: A few patients may be allergic to any of the components. If adverse reaction or idiosyncrasy occurs, medication should be discontinued.

Systemic absorption of corticosteroids may occur if they are used over extensive body areas, with or without occlusive non-permeable dressings. When occlusive non-permeable dressings are used, miliaria, folliculitis and pyoderma may sometimes develop beneath the occlusive material.

Localised atrophy and striae have been reported with the use of corticosteroids by the occlusive technique.

Overdosage: Not applicable.

Pharmacological properties

Pharmacodynamic properties: Aureocort Ointment contains two active ingredients:

(i) Chlortetracycline is a broad spectrum antibiotic. It is active against a large number of gram-positive and gram-negative bacteria, including some which are resistant to penicillin.

(ii) Triamcinolone acetonide is a corticosteroid with anti-inflammatory, anti-pruritis and anti-allergic effects.

Pharmacokinetic properties: Topically applied tetracycline preparations are not absorbed into the general circulation to any significant degree.

Absorption of triamcinolone acetonide from topically applied preparations is usually minimal. However, corticosteroids may be absorbed in sufficient amount to cause systemic effects if applied to large areas, when the skin is broken, or under occlusive dressings.

Pre-clinical safety data: Nothing of note to the prescriber.

Pharmaceutical particulars

List of excipients: White Petroleum Jelly, Anhydrous Lanolin.

Incompatibilities: None known.

Shelf-life: 36 months.

Special precautions for storage: Store at a controlled room temperature (15–30°C) in the original pack.

Nature and contents of container: Collapsible aluminium tubes with crocus yellow, low density polythene caps. Tubes of 15 g.

Marketing authorisation number PL 0095/5076R

Date of approval/revision
First approval 27/12/90
Last revision 19 December 1995

Legal category POM

AUREOMYCIN* Ointment
AUREOMYCIN* Ophthalmic Ointment

Presentation

Aureomycin Ointment 3%: Each gram of yellow ointment contains chlortetracycline hydrochloride 30 mg in a greasy base of anhydrous lanolin and white petroleum jelly.

Aureomycin Ophthalmic Ointment 1%: Each gram of yellow ointment contains 10 mg chlortetracycline hydrochloride in a greasy base of anhydrous lanolin, liquid paraffin and white petroleum jelly.

Uses Aureomycin is a broad-spectrum antibiotic.

Aureomycin Ointment 3%: Aureomycin Ointment 3% is indicated for the treatment of superficial pyogenic infections of the skin caused by susceptible Gram-positive cocci (Streptococci, Staphylococci and Pneumococci) and Gram-negative bacteria (Coli-aerogenes group).

Aureomycin Ophthalmic Ointment 1%: Aureomycin Ophthalmic Ointment 1% is indicated for the treatment of superficial eye infections caused by organisms sensitive to chlortetracycline hydrochloride including trachoma.

Dosage and administration

Adults, children over 8 years, and the elderly:

Aureomycin Ointment 3%: In the treatment of local skin infections apply the preparation directly to the involved area, preferably on sterile gauze once or more daily as the condition warrants. In severe local infection, topical application should be supplemented by systemic antibiotic therapy.

Aureomycin Ophthalmic Ointment 1%: Aureomycin Ophthalmic Ointment should be applied to the infected eye up to three times daily or more frequently if required.

Recommended dosage in the treatment of Trachoma: Trachoma may require oral systemic therapy in addition to topical ophthalmic therapy.

Topical chemotherapy for trachoma must be intensive and prolonged, six weeks being the minimum recommended duration for continuous intensive treatment.

If less frequent or intermittent applications are used, the duration of treatment must be further prolonged. The recommended intermittent applications of chlortetracycline for 5 consecutive days (or once daily for 10 days), each month for six months each year, to be repeated as necessary.

Contra-indications, warnings, etc.

Contra-indications: Aureomycin Topical Preparations are contra-indicated in patients with a history of hypersensitivity to chlortetracycline hydrochloride or any other ingredient in the preparation.

Use in pregnancy and lactation: The use of drugs of the tetracycline class during tooth development (last half of pregnancy through early childhood) may cause permanent discoloration of the teeth (yellow-grey-brown). This adverse reaction is more common during long-term oral or otherwise systemic use of the drugs and the risk of such effects from topical usage is considered negligible.

However, to reduce the theoretical risk of damage to permanent dentition, topical tetracyclines should not be used during the last half of pregnancy or during lactation unless other drugs are unlikely to be effective or are contra-indicated.

Precautions: The use of antibiotics may result in overgrowth of non-susceptible organisms. If new infections appear during therapy, appropriate measures should be taken.

To reduce the theoretical risk of damage to permanent dentition, topical tetracyclines should not be used in children under 8 years of age unless other drugs are unlikely to be effective or are contra-indicated.

Interactions: The concomitant use of oral tetracyclines may reduce the efficacy of oral contraceptives; an increased incidence of breakthrough bleeding may also be experienced.

Side-effects: Some patients may be allergic to any of the components. If adverse reaction or idiosyncrasy occurs, discontinue medication.

Pharmaceutical precautions

Aureomycin Ointment 3%: Store at 25°C or below. The ointment may be diluted with a base of 10% lanolin and white petroleum jelly.

Aureomycin Ophthalmic Ointment 1%: Store at 25°C or below. Dilution of Aureomycin Ophthalmic Ointment is not recommended.

Aureomycin Ointment may cause a yellow staining of clothes. Following extended use a similar local staining of the skin may occur which disappears on cessation of treatment.

Legal category POM

Package quantities
Aureomycin Ointment 3%: Tubes of 30 g
Aureomycin Ophthalmic Ointment 1%: Tubes of 3.5 g

Further information Nil

Product licence numbers
Aureomycin Ointment 3% 0095/5019R
Aureomycin Ophthalmic Ointment 1% 0095/5020R

BEGRIVAC* 98/99

Qualitative and quantitative composition 0.5 ml suspension contains: antigens of influenza virus propagated in embryonated hen eggs, purified, split by tween-ether and inactivated by formaldehyde, equivalent to:

A/Beijing/262/95 (H1N1)–like strain 15 µg HA*
(A/Reass. X-127)
A/Sydney/5/97 (H3N2)–like strain 15 µg HA*
(A/Reass. IVR-108)
B/Beijing/184/93–like strain 15 µg HA*
(B/Harbin/7/94)
* haemagglutinin antigens

The vaccine complies with the WHO recommendation (northern hemisphere) and EU decision for the 98/99 season.

Pharmaceutical form Suspension for injection.

Clinical particulars

Therapeutic indications: Prophylaxis of influenza, especially in those who run an increased risk of associated complications.

Posology and method of administration

Adults and children from 36 months: 0.5 ml.

Children from 6 months to 35 months: Clinical data are limited. Dosages of 0.25 ml or 0.5 ml have been used.

For children who have not previously been infected or vaccinated, a second dose should be given after an interval of at least 4 weeks.

Immunisation should be carried out by intramuscular or deep subcutaneous injection.

Contra-indications: Hypersensitivity to eggs, chicken protein or any constituent of the vaccine. Immunisation should be postponed in patients with febrile illness or acute infection.

Special warnings and special precautions for use: As with all injectable vaccines, appropriate medical treatment and supervision should always be readily available in case of rare anaphylactic event following the administration of the vaccine. Begrivac 98/99 should under no circumstances be administered intravascularly. Antibody response in patients with endogenous or iatrogenic immunosuppression may be insufficient. Begrivac 98/99 may contain residual amounts of polymyxin B, to which hypersensitivity may occur.

Interactions with other medicaments and other forms of interaction: Begrivac 98/99 may be given at the same time as other vaccines. Immunisation should be carried out on separate limbs. It should be noted that the adverse reactions may be intensified. The immunological response may be diminished if the patient is undergoing immunosuppressant treatment.

Following influenza vaccination, false positive results in serology tests using the ELISA method to detect antibodies against HIV1, Hepatitis C and especially HTLV1 have been observed. The Western Blot technique disproves the results. The transient false positive reactions could be due to the IgM response by the vaccine.

Pregnancy and lactation: No relevant animal data are available. In humans, up to now, the data are inadequate to assess teratogenic or fetotoxic risk during pregnancy. In pregnant high risk patients the possible risks of clinical infection should be weighed against the possible risks of vaccination.

Begrivac 98/99 may be used during lactation

Effects on ability to drive and use machines: The vaccine is unlikely to produce an effect on the ability to drive and use machines.

Undesirable effects: The following reactions are most common: *Local reactions*: redness, swelling, pain, ecchymosis, induration. *Systemic reactions*: fever, malaise, shivering, fatigue, headache, sweating, myalgia, arthralgia.

These reactions usually disappear within 1–2 days without treatment.

The following events are observed rarely: neuralgia, paraesthesia, convulsions, transient thrombocytopenia.

Allergic reactions, in rare cases leading to shock, have been reported.

Vasculitis with transient renal involvement has been reported in very rare cases.

Rarely neurological disorders, such as encephalomyelitis, neuritis and Guillain Barré syndrome have been reported. An increased risk of Guillain Barré syndrome has not been demonstrated with currently used influenza vaccines.

Overdose: Overdosage is unlikely to have any untoward effect.

Pharmacological properties
Pharmacodynamic properties: ATC-Code: J07BB01 Seroprotection is generally obtained within 2 to 3 weeks. The duration of postvaccinal immunity varies but is usually 6-12 months.

Pharmacokinetic properties: Not applicable.

Preclinical safety data: Not applicable.

Pharmaceutical particulars
List of excipients: Sodium timerfonate (as preservative), formaldehyde, diethylether, buffer solution (pH 7.2, containing: sodium chloride, potassium chloride, magnesium chloride hexahydrate, disodium hydrogenphosphate dihydrate, potassium dihydrogen phosphate), sucrose, water for injection, in traces: polymyxin B (antimicrobial agent), polysorbate 80.

Incompatibilities: Begrivac 98/99 should not be mixed with other injection fluids.

Shelf life: The expiry date is indicated on the label and packing. The shelf-life is 12 months.

Special precautions for storage: This product should be stored at +2°C to +8°C (in a refrigerator). Do not freeze. Protect from light.

Nature and contents of container: 0.5 ml suspension in prefilled syringe (glass) with needle.
Packs of 1 and 10 pre-filled syringes.

Instructions for use/handling: The vaccine should be allowed to reach room temperature before use.
Shake before use.
For children, when one dose of 0.25 ml is indicated, the pre-filled syringe should be held in upright position and half of the volume should be eliminated. The remaining volume should be injected.

Legal category POM

Product licence number PL 16033/0006

Date of revision of text April 1998

CALCIUM LEUCOVORIN

Presentation *Powder for Injection 15 mg, 30 mg:* Vials containing a lyophilised powder of 15 mg or 30 mg folinic acid as the calcium salt.

Solution for Injection 350 mg in 35 ml (Lederfolin Solution): Vial containing a solution of 350 mg folinic acid as the calcium salt.

Tablets 15 mg: Each yellowish-white scored tablet contains 15 mg folinic acid as the calcium salt.

Uses Calcium leucovorin is the calcium salt of a formyl derivative of tetra-hydrofolic acid, the metabolite of folic acid, and an essential coenzyme for nucleic acid synthesis.

i) *Calcium Leucovorin Rescue:* Calcium leucovorin is used to diminish the toxicity and counteract the action of folic acid antagonists such as methotrexate in cytotoxic therapy. This procedure is commonly known as Calcium Leucovorin Rescue.

ii) *Advanced Colorectal Cancer–Enhancement of 5-Fluorouracil (5-FU) Cytotoxicity:* Calcium leucovorin increases the thymine depleting effects of 5-FU resulting in enhanced cytotoxic activity. Clinical studies in advanced colorectal cancer show greater efficacy for combination regimens of 5-FU with leucovorin compared to 5-FU given alone.

iii) *Treatment of Folate Deficiency:* Calcium leucovorin has also been demonstrated to be effective in producing amelioration of the blood picture in a number of megaloblastic anaemias due to folate deficiency.

Dosage and administration

i) *Calcium Leucovorin Rescue: Adults, Children and the Elderly:* Calcium Leucovorin Rescue therapy should commence 24 hours after the beginning of methotrexate infusion. Dosage regimes vary depending upon the dose of methotrexate administered. In general, the calcium leucovorin should be administered at a dose of 15 mg (approximately 10 mg/m²) every 6 hours for 10 doses either parenterally by intramuscular injection, bolus intravenous injection or intravenous infusion, (refer to (ii) for information concerning use of calcium leucovorin with infusion fluids), or orally using calcium leucovorin tablets. **Do not administer calcium leucovorin intrathecally.**

Where overdosage of methotrexate is suspected, the dose of calcium leucovorin should be equal to or higher than the offending dose of methotrexate and should be administered in the first hour. In the presence of gastrointestinal toxicity, nausea or vomiting, calcium leucovorin should be administered parenterally. **Do not administer calcium leucovorin intrathecally.** Further, oral administration of doses greater than 50 mg is not recommended since the absorption of calcium leucovorin is saturable. In the case of intravenous administration, no more than 160 mg of calcium leucovorin should be injected per minute due to the calcium content of the solution.

In addition to calcium leucovorin administration, measures to ensure the prompt excretion of methotrexate are important as part of Calcium Leucovorin Rescue therapy. These measures include:

a. Alkalinisation of urine so that the urinary pH is greater than 7.0 before methotrexate infusion (to increase solubility of methotrexate and its metabolites).

b. Maintenance of urine output of 1800–2000 cc/m²/24 hr by increased oral or intravenous fluids on days 2, 3 and 4 following methotrexate therapy.

c. Plasma methotrexate concentration, BUN and creatinine should be measured on days 2, 3 and 4.

These measures must be continued until the plasma methotrexate level is less than 10^{-7} molar (0.1μM).

Delayed methotrexate excretion may be seen in some patients. This may be caused by a third space accumulation (as seen in ascites or pleural effusion for example), renal insufficiency or inadequate hydration. Under such circumstances, higher doses of calcium leucovorin or prolonged administration may be indicated. Dosage and administration guidelines for these patients are given in Table 1. Patients who experience delayed early methotrexate elimination are likely to develop reversible renal failure.

Each vial of Calcium Leucovorin Powder for Injection 15 mg or 30 mg should be reconstituted with 3 ml of water for injection to produce a solution for intramuscular or intravenous administration.

ii) *Colorectal Cancer: Enhancement of 5-FU Cytotoxicity: Adults and the Elderly: Administration:* The 350 mg vial of Calcium Leucovorin Solution for Injection (Lederfolin Solution) should be used to administer the high doses of calcium leucovorin required in combination regimens.

When used in combination regimens with 5-FU, calcium leucovorin should only be given by the intravenous route. The agents should not be mixed together.

Each vial of Calcium Leucovorin 350 mg (Lederfolin Solution) contains 1.4 mEq (0.7 mmol) of calcium per vial and it is recommended that the solution is administered over not less than 3–5 minutes.

For intravenous infusion, the 350 mg in 35 ml Solution for Injection (Lederfolin Solution) may be diluted with any of the following infusion fluids before use: Sodium Chloride 0.9%; Glucose 5%; Glucose 10%; Glucose 10% and Sodium Chloride 0.9% Injection; Compound Sodium Lactate Injection.

Calcium leucovorin should not be mixed together with 5-FU in the same infusion.

Dosage: Various combination regimens have been studied and based on the available clinical evidence the following regimen has been found to be effective in advanced colorectal carcinoma:

Calcium leucovorin given at a dose of 200 mg/m² by slow intravenous injection, followed immediately by 5-FU at an initial dose of 370 mg/m² by intravenous injection. The injection of leucovorin should not be given more rapidly than over 3–5 minutes because of the calcium content of the solution. This treatment is repeated daily for 5 consecutive days. Subsequent courses may be given after a treatment-free interval of 21–28 days.

For the above regimen, modification of the 5-FU dosage and the treatment-free interval may be necessary depending on patient condition, clinical response and dose limiting toxicity. A reduction of Calcium leucovorin dosage is not required. The number of repeat cycles used is at the discretion of the clinician.

On the basis of the available data, no specific dosage modifications are recommended in the use of the combination regimen with 5-FU in the elderly. However, particular care should be taken when treating elderly or debilitated patients as these patients are at increased risk of severe toxicity with this therapy (See *Warnings and Precautions*).

Children: There are no data available on the use of this combination in children.

iii) *Treatment of Folate Deficiency: Children up to 12 years of age:* 0.25 mg/kg/day.
Adults and the Elderly: 10–20 mg daily. Oral therapy with one tablet (15 mg) of calcium leucovorin daily is more usual.

Contra-indications, warnings, etc.
Contra-indications: Calcium leucovorin should not be used for the treatment of pernicious anaemia or other megaloblastic anaemias where vitamin B_{12} is deficient.

Warnings and precautions: Calcium leucovorin should only be used with methotrexate or 5-FU under the direct supervision of a clinician experienced in the use of cancer chemotherapeutic agents. When calcium leucovorin has been administered intrathecally following intrathecal overdose of methotrexate, a death has been reported.

Calcium leucovorin should not be given simultaneously with an anti-neoplastic folic acid antagonist, (eg methotrexate), to modify or abort clinical toxicity, as the therapeutic effect of the antagonist may be nullified. Concomitant calcium leucovorin will not however inhibit the antibacterial activity of other folic acid antagonists such as trimethoprim and pyrimethamine.

Folinates given in large amounts may counteract the antiepileptic effect of phenobarbitone, phenytoin and primidone and increase the frequency of seizures in susceptible patients.

Seizures and/or syncope have been reported rarely in cancer patients receiving leucovorin, usually in association with fluoropyrimidine administration, and most commonly in those with CNS metastases or other predisposing factors; however a causal relationship has not been established.

In the combination regimen with 5-FU, the toxicity profile of 5-FU is enhanced by calcium leucovorin. The commonest manifestations are leucopenia, mucositis, stomatitis and/or diarrhoea which may be dose limiting. When calcium leucovorin and 5-FU are used in the treatment of colorectal cancer, the 5-FU dosage must be reduced more in cases of toxicity than when 5-FU is used alone. Toxicities observed in patients treated with the combination are qualitatively similar to those observed in patients treated with 5-FU alone. Gastrointestinal toxicities are observed more commonly and may be more severe or even life threatening. In severe cases, treatment is withdrawal of 5-FU and calcium leucovorin, and supportive intravenous therapy. Elderly or debilitated patients are at a greater risk of severe toxicity with this therapy.

Each vial of Lederfolin Solution contains 4.6 mEq (4.6 mmol) of sodium. This and the use of diluting infusion fluids containing sodium should be borne in mind when treating patients requiring a restricted sodium intake.

Side effects: Adverse reactions to calcium leucovorin are rare, but occasional pyrexial reactions have been reported following parenteral administration.

Hypersensitivity, including anaphylactoid reactions and urticaria, has been reported following administration of both oral and parenteral leucovorin.

Overdosage: There have been no reported sequelae

Table 1: Dosage and Administration Guidelines for Calcium Leucovorin Rescue:

Clinical Situation	*Laboratory Findings*	*Leucovorin Dosage and Duration*
Normal Methotrexate Elimination	Serum methotrexate level approximately 10μM at 24 hours after administration, 1μM at 48 hours and less than 0.2μM at 72 hours.	15 mg PO, IM or IV every 6 hours for 60 hours (10 doses starting at 24 hours after start of methotrexate infusion).
Delayed Late Methotrexate Elimination	Serum methotrexate level remaining above 0.2μM at 72 hours, and more than 0.05μM at 96 hours after administration.	Continue 15 mg PO, IM or IV every 6 hours, until methotrexate level is less than 0.05μM.
Delayed Early Methotrexate Elimination and/or Evidence of Acute Renal Injury	Serum methotrexate level of 50μM or more at 24 hours or 5μM or more at 48 hours after administration, OR; a 100% or greater increase in serum creatinine level at 24 hours after methotrexate administration.	150 mg IV every 3 hours, until methotrexate level is less than 1 micromolar; then 15 mg IV every 3 hours until methotrexate level is less than 0.05μM.

in patients who have received significantly more calcium leucovorin than the recommended dosage. There is no specific antidote. In cases of overdosage, patients should be given appropriate supportive care. Should overdosage of the combination of 5-FU with calcium leucovorin occur, the overdosage instructions for 5-FU should be followed.

Use in pregnancy and lactation: Reproduction studies have been performed in rats and rabbits at doses of at least 50 times the human dose. These studies have revealed no evidence of harm to the foetus due to calcium leucovorin. There are, however, no adequate and well controlled studies in pregnant women. Because animal reproduction studies are not always predictive of human response, calcium leucovorin should only be used in pregnant women if the potential benefit justifies the potential risk to the foetus.

It is not known whether calcium leucovorin is excreted in human milk. Because many drugs are excreted in human milk, caution should be exercised when calcium leucovorin is administered to a nursing mother.

Pharmaceutical precautions Store Calcium Leucovorin Solution for Injection (Lederfolin Solution) under refrigerated conditions (2°–8°C) in original containers. Protect from light.

Store all other presentations at controlled room temperature (15°–30°C) in original containers.

The reconstituted solutions of the Calcium Leucovorin Powder for Injection presentations are intended for immediate administration but may be stored for up to 24 hours under refrigeration (2°–8°C) if necessary.

When the 350 mg in 35 ml Calcium Leucovorin Solution for Injection (Lederfolin Solution) is diluted with the recommended infusion fluids (see *Dosage and Administration*), the resulting solutions are intended for immediate use but may be stored for up to 24 hours under refrigerated conditions (2°–8°C) prior to use if necessary.

Calcium leucovorin should not be mixed together with 5-FU in the same intravenous injection or infusion.

Legal category POM

Package quantities
Powder for Injection 15 mg, 30 mg: Boxes of one vial.
Solution for Injection 350 mg in 35 ml: Boxes of one vial.
Tablets 15 mg: Bottles of 10 tablets.

Further information Further information, particularly on high-dosage regimens in conjunction with methotrexate, is available on request.

Product licence numbers
Powder for Injection 15 mg and 30 mg 0095/0087
Tablets 15 mg 0095/0033
Solution for Injection 350 mg 0095/0274

CRINONE 4% and 8% PROGESTERONE VAGINAL GEL

Qualitative and quantitative composition

Active Ingredient	4% gel mg/dose	% w/w	8% gel mg/dose	% w/w
Progesterone	45	4.0	90	8.0

Pharmaceutical form Vaginal gel.

Clinical particulars
Therapeutic indications: Treatment of disorders associated with progesterone deficiency, such as:

Premenstrual syndrome

Menstrual irregularities, dysmenorrhoea, secondary amenorrhoea

Dysfunctional (anovulatory) uterine bleeding occurring before menopause

Menopausal disorders (in combination with oestrogen therapy)

Infertility due to inadequate luteal phase

For use during in-vitro fertilisation, where infertility is mainly due to tubal, idiopathic or endometriosis linked sterility associated with normal ovulatory cycles

Posology and method of administration: Intravaginal application.

Treatment of progesterone deficiency: one application (1.125 g 4% gel) every other day, preferably in the morning, from day 15 to day 25 of the cycle.

Maintenance therapy can be achieved with an every other day application from day 15 to day 25 of the cycle.

Treatment of menopausal disorders: one application (1.125 g 4% gel) every other day for the last 12 days of each oestrogenic sequence.

Treatment of infertility due to inadequate luteal phase: one application (1.125 g 8% gel) every day, starting after documented ovulation or arbitrarily on the 18th-21st day of the cycle.

When used during in-vitro fertilisation, daily application of Crinone 8% gel should be continued for 30 days if there is laboratory evidence of pregnancy.

Children: Not applicable.

Contra-indications: Known allergy to any of the excipients. Undiagnosed uterine bleeding. Porphyria

Special warnings and special precautions for use: Cautious use in severe hepatic insufficiency. The product should not be used concurrently with other local intravaginal therapy.

Crinone 4%, Vaginal Progesterone Gel, can be prescribed with an oestrogen product as HRT. Epidemiological evidence suggests that the use of HRT is associated with an increased risk of developing deep vein thrombosis (DVT) or pulmonary embolism. The use of Crinone in combination with oestrogen therapy as HRT was not included in these studies. When Crinone is co-prescribed as HRT, the prescribing information for the oestrogen product should be referred to for information about the risks of venous thromboembolism.

Interaction with other medicaments and other forms of interactions: No interaction reported.

Pregnancy and lactation: In case of corpus luteum deficiency, Crinone can be used during the first month of pregnancy.

Do not use during lactation.

Effects on ability to drive and use machines: Drivers and users of machines are warned that risk of somnolence may occur.

Undesirable effects: Rare cases of somnolence. Occasional spotting.

Overdose: Not applicable.

Pharmacological properties
Pharmacodynamic properties: Those of the naturally occurring progesterone with induction of a full secretory endometrium.

Pharmacokinetic properties: The progesterone vaginal gel is based on a polycarbophil delivery system which attaches to the vaginal mucosa and provides a prolonged release of progesterone for at least three days.

Preclinical safety data: In rabbits, Crinone was an eye irritant categorised class IV (minimal effects clearing in less than 24 hours), but not a dermal irritant.

A moderate vaginal irritation was found in rabbits after application of 2.0 ml/day of 8% gel for 5 days.

Pharmaceutical particulars
List of excipients: Glycerin, Light Liquid Paraffin, Hydrogenated Palm Oil Glyceride, Carbomer 974P, Sorbic acid, Polycarbophil, Sodium hydroxide, Purified water.

Incompatibilities: No incompatibilities were found with the usual contraceptive devices.

Shelf life: 36 months.

Special precautions for storage: Store below 25°C.

Nature and contents of container: A single use, one piece, white polyethylene applicator with a twist-off top, designed for intravaginal application.

Each applicator contains 2.6 g of gel and delivers 1.125 g of gel. Each one is wrapped up and sealed in a paper/aluminium/polyethylene foil overwrap.

The applicators are packed in cardboard boxes containing 2 (sample pack) and 6 units of Crinone 4% progesterone vaginal gel, and 15 units of Crinone 8% progesterone vaginal gel.

Instructions for use/handling: Crinone is applied directly from the specially designed sealed applicator into the vagina. Remove the applicator from the sealed wrapper. DO NOT remove the twist-off cap at this time.

1. Grip the applicator firmly by the thick end. Shake down like a thermometer to ensure that the contents are at the thin end.
2. Twist off the tab and discard.
3. The applicator may be inserted while you are in a sitting position or when lying on your back with the knees bent. Gently insert the thin end of applicator well into the vagina.
4. Press the thick end of the applicator firmly to deposit gel. Remove the applicator and discard in a waste container.
5. Crinone coats the vaginal mucosa to provide long-lasting release of progesterone.

Marketing authorisation number
Crinone 4% progesterone vaginal gel PL 11764/0004
Crinone 8% progesterone vaginal gel PL 11764/0005

Date of approval/revision
Last revised March 1998

DETECLO* TABLETS

Presentation Tablets 300 mg: Each blue, film-coated tablet, embossed 'LL' on one side and '5422' on the reverse side, contains:
Tetracycline hydrochloride 115.4 mg
Chlortetracycline hydrochloride 115.4 mg
Demeclocycline hydrochloride 69.2 mg

Uses For the treatment of infections caused by tetracycline-sensitive organisms. For example, Deteclo is highly effective in the treatment of infections caused by *Borrellia recurrentis* (relapsing fever), *Calymmatobacterium granulomatis* (granuloma inguinale), *Chlamydia* species (psittacosis, lymphogranuloma venereum, trachoma, inclusion conjunctivitis), *Francisella tularensis* (tularaemia), *Haemophilus ducreyi* (chancroid), *Leptospira* (meningitis, jaundice), *Mycoplasma pneumoniae* (non-gonococcal urethritis), *Pseudomonas mallei* and *pseudomallei* (glanders and melioidosis), *Rickettsiae* (typhus fever, Q fever, rocky mountain spotted fever), *Vibrio* species (cholera). It is also highly effective, alone or in combination with streptomycin, in the treatment of infections due to *Brucella* species (brucellosis), and *Yersinia pestis* (bubonic plague). Severe acne vulgaris.

Other sensitive organisms include: *Actinomyces israelii*, *Bacillus anthracis* (pneumonia), *Clostridium* species (gas gangrene, tetanus), *Entamoeba histolytica* (dysentery), *Neisseria gonorrhoeae*, and anaerobic species, *Treponema pallidum* and *pertenue* (syphilis and yaws).

Dosage and administration
Dosage: Adults only: One tablet every 12 hours.

This may be increased to 3 or 4 tablets daily for short periods in more severe infections.

Gonorrhoea: 1,200 mg (4 tablets) followed by a similar dose six hours later.

Non-gonococcal urethritis: One tablet twice daily for 10–21 days.

Children: Not recommended for children under 12 years of age.

Elderly: Deteclo should be used with caution in the treatment of elderly patients where accumulation is a possibility.

Administration: Deteclo should be swallowed whole with plenty of fluid while sitting or standing. Deteclo should be taken an hour before or two hours after meals and therapy should be continued for up to three days after characteristic symptoms of the infection have subsided.

Contra-indications, warnings etc
Contra-indications: A history of hypersensitivity to tetracyclines. Overt renal insufficiency. Children under twelve years of age. Use during pregnancy or during lactation in women breast feeding infants is contra-indicated (see also *Pregnancy and lactation*).

Warnings and precautions: Deteclo should be used with caution in patients with renal or hepatic dysfunction or in conjunction with other potentially hepatotoxic or nephrotoxic drugs. Concurrent use with the anaesthetic methoxyflurane increases the risk of kidney failure. The anti-anabolic action of the tetracyclines may cause an increase in BUN.

Lower doses are indicated in cases of renal impairment to avoid excessive systemic accumulation, and if therapy is prolonged, serum level determinations are advisable. Patients who have known liver disease should not receive more than 1 g daily. In long term therapy, periodic laboratory evaluation of organ systems, including haematopoietic, renal and hepatic studies should be performed.

Photoallergic reactions may occur in hypersensitive persons and such patients should be warned to avoid direct exposure to natural or artificial sunlight and to discontinue treatment at the first sign of skin discomfort.

Cross-resistance between tetracyclines may develop in micro-organisms and cross-sensitisation in patients. Deteclo should be discontinued if there are signs/symptoms of overgrowth of resistant organisms including candida, enteritis, glossitis, stomatitis, vaginitis, pruritus ani or staphylococcal enterocolitis.

Patients taking oral contraceptives should be warned that if diarrhoea or breakthrough bleeding occur there is a possibility of contraceptive failure.

Interactions: Deteclo should not be used with penicillins. Tetracyclines depress plasma prothrombin activity and reduced doses of concomitant anticoagulants may be required.

Absorption of Deteclo is impaired by the concomitant administration of iron, calcium, zinc, magnesium and particularly aluminium salts commonly used as antacids.

The concomitant use of tetracyclines may reduce the efficacy of oral contraceptives; an increased incidence of breakthrough bleeding may also be experienced (see statement under *Warnings and Precautions*).

Use in pregnancy: Contra-indicated in pregnancy.

Results of animal studies indicate that tetracyclines cross the placenta, are found in foetal tissues and can have toxic effects on the developing foetus (often related to retardation of skeletal development). Evidence of embryotoxicity has also been noted in animals treated early in pregnancy. Deteclo therefore, should not be used in pregnancy unless considered essential, in which case the maximum daily dose should be 1 g.

The use of drugs of the tetracycline class during tooth development (last half of pregnancy) may cause permanent discolouration of the teeth (yellow-grey-brown). This adverse reaction is more common during long term use of the drugs but has been observed following repeated short term courses. Enamel hypoplasia has also been reported.

Use in lactation: Contra-indicated during lactation in women breast feeding infants.

Tetracyclines have been found in the milk of lactating women who are taking a drug in this class. Permanent tooth discolouration may occur in the developing infant and enamel hypoplasia has been reported. Therefore, Deteclo should not be administered to lactating women.

Use in children: The use of tetracyclines during tooth development in children under the age of 12 years may cause permanent discolouration. Enamel hypoplasia has also been reported.

Side-effects: Gastro-intestinal disturbances including nausea, vomiting, diarrhoea and rarely dysphagia have been reported. There have been a few cases of oesophagitis and oesophageal ulceration in patients taking oral tetracyclines in solid dose form, usually where medication was taken immediately before retiring or with inadequate fluids. As with all antibiotics, overgrowth of resistant organisms may cause candidiasis, pseudomembranous colitis (*Clostridium difficile* overgrowth), glossitis, stomatitis, vaginitis, or staphylococcal enterocolotis. In common with other tetracyclines, transient increases in liver function test values, hepatitis, jaundice and hepatic failure have been reported rarely. A few cases of pancreatitis have been reported. The most commonly reported dermatological reaction is photosensitivity. Erythematous and maculo-papular rashes, photosensitivity, pruritus, bullous dermatoses, exfoliative dermatitis and skin discolouration have occurred occasionally but serious skin reactions are rare. Headache, dizziness, visual disturbances and rarely impaired hearing have been reported with tetracyclines and patients should be warned about the possible hazards of driving or operating machinery during treatment. Bulging fontanelles in infants and benign intracranial hypertension in juveniles and adults have been reported. Treatment should cease if evidence of raised intracranial pressure, such as severe or persistent headache or blurred vision are noted. While the condition and related symptoms usually resolve soon after discontinuation of the tetracycline, the possibility of permanent sequelae exists. There have been isolated cases of myasthenia. Hypersensitivity reactions including urticaria, angioneurotic oedema, anaphylaxis, anaphylactoid purpura, pericarditis and exacerbation of systemic lupus erythematosus may occur. Renal dysfunction, especially in patients with pre-existing renal impairment, and rarely, acute renal failure or nephritis, have been reported with tetracyclines. Haemolytic anaemia, thrombocytopenia, neutropenia, agranulocytosis, aplastic anaemia and eosinophilia have been reported rarely. When given over prolonged periods, tetracyclines have been reported to produce brown-black discolouration of the thyroid gland. No abnormalities of thyroid function are known to occur.

Overdosage: No specific antidote. Gastric lavage plus oral administration of milk or antacids.

Pharmaceutical precautions Store at controlled room temperature (15–30°C) in the original pack or in containers which prevent access of light and moisture.

Legal category POM

Package quantities Bottles of 100 and 500

Further information Deteclo is a unique combination of three effective tetracycline broad-spectrum antibiotics. The ratio of the different tetracyclines has been carefully chosen to ensure that high therapeutic blood levels are rapidly realised and maintained with a reduced potential for side-effects, on a twice daily dosage regime, because of their different rates of absorption and excretion.

Product licence number 0095/5070R

DIAMOX* SODIUM PARENTERAL 500 mg/VIAL

Qualitative and quantitative composition Acetazolamide BP 500 mg/vial.

Pharmaceutical form Powder for solution for injection.

Clinical particulars

Therapeutic indications: Diamox is an enzyme inhibitor which acts specifically on carbonic anhydrase. It is indicated in the treatment of:

i) *Glaucoma:* Diamox is useful in glaucoma (chronic simple (open angle) glaucoma, secondary glaucoma, and perioperatively in acute angle closure glaucoma where delay of surgery is desired in order to lower intraocular pressure) because it acts on inflow, decreasing the amount of aqueous secretion.

ii) *Abnormal retention of fluids:* Diamox is a diuretic whose effect is due to the effect on the reversible hydration of carbon dioxide and dehydration of carbonic acid reaction in the kidney. The result is renal loss of HCO_3^- ion which carries out sodium, water and potassium.

Diamox can be used in conjunction with other diuretics when effects on several segments of the nephron are desirable in the treatment of fluid retaining states.

iii) *Epilepsy:* In conjunction with other anticonvulsants best results with Diamox have been seen in petit mal in children. Good results, however, have been seen in patients, both children and adults, with other types of seizures such as grand mal, mixed seizure patterns, myoclonic jerk patterns etc.

Posology and method of administration: Routes of administration: Intravenous or intramuscular injection. The direct intravenous route is preferred as intramuscular use is limited by the alkaline pH of the solution.

i) *Glaucoma (simple acute congestive and secondary): Adults:* 250–1000 mg per 24 hours, usually in divided doses for amounts over 250 mg daily.

ii) *Abnormal retention of fluid:* Congestive heart failure, drug-induced oedema.

Adults: For diuresis, the starting dose is usually 250–375 mg once daily in the morning. If, after an initial response, the patient fails to continue to lose oedema fluid, do not increase the dose but allow for kidney recovery by omitting a day. Best results are often obtained on a regime of 250–375 mg daily for two days, rest a day, and repeat, or merely giving Diamox every other day. The use of Diamox does not eliminate the need for other therapy, eg. digitalis, bed rest and salt restriction in congestive heart failure and proper supplementation with elements such as potassium in drug-induced oedema.

For cases of fluid retention associated with premenstrual tension, a daily dose (single) of 125–375 mg is suggested.

iii) *Epilepsy: Adults:* 250–1000 mg daily in divided doses.

Children: 8–30 mg/kg in daily divided doses and not to exceed 750 mg/day.

The change from other medication to Diamox should be gradual.

Elderly: Diamox should only be used with particular caution in elderly patients or those with potential obstruction in the urinary tract or with disorders rendering their electrolyte balance precarious or with liver dysfunction.

Contra-indications: Acetazolamide therapy is contra-indicated in situations in which sodium and/or potassium blood serum levels are depressed, in cases of marked kidney and liver disease or dysfunction, suprarenal gland failure, and hyper-chloremic acidosis.

Long-term administration of Diamox acetazolamide is contra-indicated in patients with chronic non-congestive angle-closure glaucoma since it may permit organic closure of the angle to occur while the worsening glaucoma is masked by lowered intraocular pressure.

Diamox should not be used in patients hypersensitive to sulphonamides.

Special warnings and special precautions for use: Increasing the dose does not increase the diuresis and may increase the incidence of drowsiness and/or paraesthesia.

Increasing the dose often results in a decrease in diuresis. Under certain circumstances, however, very large doses have been given in conjunction with other diuretics in order to secure diuresis in complete refractory failure.

When Diamox is prescribed for long-term therapy, special precautions are advisable. The patient should be cautioned to report any unusual skin rash. Periodic blood cell counts and electrolyte levels are recommended. A precipitous drop in formed blood cell elements or the appearance of toxic skin manifestations should call for diminution or cessation of Diamox therapy.

In patients with pulmonary obstruction or emphysema where alveolar ventilation may be impaired, Diamox may aggravate acidosis and should be used with caution.

In patients with a past history of renal calculi, benefit should be balanced against the risks of precipitating further calculi.

The pH of parenteral acetazolamide is 9.1. Care should be taken during intravenous administration of alkaline preparations to avoid extravasation and possible development of skin necrosis.

Interaction with other medicaments and other forms of interaction: Diamox is a sulphonamide derivative. Sulphonamides may potentiate the effects of folic acid antagonists. Possible potentiation of the effects of hypoglycaemics and oral anti-coagulants. Concurrent administration of acetazolamide and aspirin may result in severe acidosis and increase central nervous system toxicity. Adjustment of dose may be required when Diamox is given with cardiac glycosides or hypertensive agents.

When given concomitantly, Diamox modifies the metabolism of phenytoin, leading to increased serum levels of phenytoin. Severe osteomalacia has been noted in a few patients taking acetazolamide in combination with other anticonvulsants. There have been isolated reports of reduced primidone and increased carbamazepine serum levels with concurrent administration of acetazolamide.

Pregnancy and lactation: Acetazolamide has been reported to be teratogenic and embryotoxic in rats, mice, hamsters and rabbits at oral or parenteral doses in excess of ten times those recommended in human beings. Although there is no evidence of these effects in human beings, there are no adequate and well-controlled studies in pregnant women. Therefore, Diamox acetazolamide should not be used in pregnancy, especially during the first trimester.

Diamox has been detected in low levels in the milk of lactating women who have taken Diamox. Although it is unlikely that this will lead to any harmful effects in the infant, extreme caution should be exercised when Diamox is administered to lactating women.

Effects on ability to drive and use machines: Increasing the dose does not increase the diuresis and may increase the incidence of drowsiness and/or paraesthesia. Less commonly, fatigue, dizziness and ataxia have been reported. Disorientation has been observed in a few patients with oedema due to hepatic cirrhosis. Such cases should be under close supervision. Transient myopia has been reported.

These conditions invariably subside upon diminution or discontinuance of the medication.

Undesirable effects: Adverse reactions during short-term therapy are usually non-serious. Those effects which have been noted include: paraesthesia, particularly a 'tingling' feeling in the extremities, some loss of appetite; taste disturbance, polyuria, flushing, thirst, headache, dizziness, fatigue, irritability, depression, reduced libido and occasional instances of drowsiness and confusion. Rarely, photosensitivity has been reported.

During long-term therapy, metabolic acidosis and electrolyte imbalance may occasionally occur. This can usually be corrected by the administration of bicarbonate.

Transient myopia has been reported. This condition invariably subsides upon diminution or discontinuation of the medication.

Gastro-intestinal disturbances such as nausea, vomiting and diarrhoea. Diamox is a sulphonamide derivative and therefore some side-effects similar to those caused by sulphonamides have occasionally been reported. These include fever, agranulocytosis, thrombocytopenia, thrombocytic purpura, leukopenia, and aplastic anaemia, bone marrow depression, pancytopenia, rash (including erythema multiforme, Stevens-Johnson Syndrome, toxic epidermal necrolysis), anaphylaxis, crystalluria, calculus formation, renal and ureteral colic, and renal lesions.

Other occasional adverse reactions include: urticaria, melaena, haematuria, glycosuria, impaired hearing and tinnitus, abnormal liver function and rarely, hepatitis or cholestatic jaundice, flaccid paralysis, and convulsions.

Overdose: No specific antidote. Supportive measures with correction of electrolyte and fluid balance. Force fluids.

Pharmacological properties

Pharmacodynamic properties: Acetazolamide is an inhibitor of carbonic anhydrase. By inhibiting the reaction catalysed by this enzyme in the renal tubules, acetazolamide increases the excretion of bicarbonate and of cations, chiefly sodium and potassium, and so promotes alkaline diuresis.

Continuous administration of acetazolamide is associated with metabolic acidosis and resultant loss of diuretic activity. Therefore the effectiveness of Diamox in diuresis diminishes with continuous use.

By inhibiting carbonic anhydrase in the eye acetazolamide decreases intra-ocular pressure and is therefore useful in the treatment of glaucoma.

Pharmacokinetic properties: Acetazolamide has been estimated to have a plasma half-life of about 4 hours.

It is tightly bound to carbonic anhydrase and accumulates in tissues containing this enzyme, particularly red blood cells and the renal cortex. It is also bound to plasma proteins. It is excreted unchanged in the urine, renal clearance being enhanced in the alkaline urine.

Preclinical safety data: Nothing of note to the prescriber.

Pharmaceutical particulars
List of excipients: Water for injection, sodium hydroxide, hydrochloric acid.

Incompatibilities: None.

Shelf life: 60 months.

Special precautions for storage: Store at controlled room temperature (15°–30°C).

Nature and contents of container: Glass vial with butyl rubber plug and aluminium ring seal.

Pack size: 500 mg vial.

Instructions for use/handling: Reconstitute each vial of DIAMOX Parenteral with at least 5 ml of water for injection prior to use. The reconstituted injection does not contain an antimicrobial preservative. Any unused solution can be stored in a refrigerator for up to 24 hours but any solution not used within this period must be discarded.

The direct intravenous route of administration is preferred. Intramuscular injection may be employed but is painful due to the alkaline pH of the solution.

Marketing authorisation number PL 0095/5073R

Date of approval/revision of SPC September 1998

Legal category POM

DIAMOX* SR

Qualitative and quantitative composition Acetazolamide 250 mg.

Pharmaceutical form Sustained release capsule with a clear body and orange cap printed "WYETH" in black.

Clinical particulars
Therapeutic indications: Glaucoma.

Posology and method of administration: Capsules should be swallowed whole. Do not chew or crush.
Adults: One or two 250 mg capsules a day.
Children: This product is not intended for administration to children.
Elderly: Diamox SR should be used with particular caution in elderly patients or those with potential obstruction in the urinary tract or with disorders rendering their electrolyte balance precarious or with liver dysfunction.

Contra-indications: Diamox SR therapy is contraindicated in situations in which sodium and/or potassium blood serum levels are depressed, in cases of marked kidney and liver dysfunction, suprarenal gland failure and hyperchloraemic acidosis.

Long-term administration of Diamox SR is contraindicated in patients with chronic non-congestive angle-closure glaucoma since it may permit organic closure of the angle to occur while the worsening glaucoma is masked by lowered intraocular pressure.

Diamox SR should not be used in patients hypersensitive to sulphonamides.

Special warnings and special precautions for use: Increasing the dose does not increase the diuresis and may increase the incidence of drowsiness and/or paraesthesia.

When Diamox SR is prescribed for long-term therapy, special precautions are advisable. The patient should be cautioned to report any unusual skin rash. Periodic blood cell counts and electrolyte levels are recommended. A precipitous drop in formed blood cell elements or the appearance of toxic skin manifestations should call for diminution or cessation of Diamox SR therapy.

In patients with pulmonary obstruction or emphysema where alveolar ventilation may be impaired, Diamox SR may aggravate acidosis and should be used with caution.

In patients with a past history of renal calculi, benefit should be balanced against the risks of precipitating further calculi.

Interactions with other medicaments and other forms of interaction: Diamox SR is a sulphonamide derivative. Sulphonamides may potentiate the effects of folic acid antagonists. Possible potentiation of the effects of folic acid antagonists, hypoglycaemics and oral anti-coagulants. Concurrent administration of acetazolamide and aspirin may result in severe acidosis and increase central nervous system toxicity. Adjustment of dose may be required when Diamox SR is given with cardiac glycosides or hypertensive agents.

When given concomitantly, Diamox SR modifies the metabolism of phenytoin, leading to increased serum levels of phenytoin. Severe osteomalacia has been noted in a few patients taking acetazolamide in combination with other anticonvulsants. There have been isolated reports of reduced primidone and increased carbamazepine serum levels with concurrent administration of acetazolamide.

Pregnancy and lactation: Use in pregnancy: Acetazolamide has been reported to be teratogenic and embryotoxic in rats, mice, hamsters and rabbits at oral or parenteral doses in excess of ten times those recommended in human beings. Although there is no evidence of these effects in human beings, there are no adequate and well-controlled studies in pregnant women. Therefore, Diamox SR should not be used in pregnancy, especially during the first trimester.

Use in lactation: Diamox has been detected in low levels in the milk of lactating women who have taken Diamox. Although it is unlikely that this will lead to any harmful effects in the infant, extreme caution should be exercised when Diamox SR is administered to lactating women.

Effects on ability to drive and use machines: Increasing the dose does not increase the diuresis and may increase the incidence of drowsiness and/or paraesthesia. Less commonly, fatigue, dizziness and ataxia have been reported. Disorientation has been observed in a few patients with oedema due to hepatic cirrhosis. Such cases should be under close supervision. Transient myopia has been reported.

These conditions invariably subside upon diminution or discontinuance of the medication.

Undesirable effects: Adverse reactions during short-term therapy are usually non-serious. Those effects which have been noted include: paraesthesia, particularly a 'tingling' feeling in the extremities, some loss of appetite, taste disturbance, polyuria, flushing, thirst, headache, dizziness, fatigue, irritability, depression, reduced libido and occasional instances of drowsiness and confusion. Rarely, photosensitivity has been reported.

During long-term therapy, metabolic acidosis and electrolyte imbalance may occasionally occur. This can usually be corrected by the administration of bicarbonate.

Transient myopia has been reported. This condition invariably subsides upon diminution or discontinuation of the medication.

Gastro-intestinal disturbances such as nausea, vomiting and diarrhoea.

Diamox is a sulphide derivative and therefore some side-effects similar to those caused by sulphonamides have occasionally been reported. These include fever, agranulocytosis, thrombocytopenia, thrombocytic purpura, leukopenia, and aplastic anaemia, bone marrow depression, pancytopenia, rash (including erythema multiforme, Stevens-Johnson Syndrome, toxic epidermal necrolysis), anaphylaxis, crystalluria, calculus formation, renal and ureteral colic and renal lesions.

Other occasional adverse reactions include: urticaria, melaena, haematuria, glycosuria, impaired hearing and tinnitus, abnormal liver function and, rarely, hepatitis or cholestatic jaundice, flaccid paralysis and convulsions.

Overdose: No specific antidote. Supportive measures with correction of electrolyte and fluid balance. Force fluids.

Pharmacological properties
Pharmacodynamic properties: Acetazolamide is a potent inhibiter of the enzyme carbonic anhydrase; the enzyme that catalyses the reversible reaction involving the hydration of carbon dioxide and the dehydration of carbonic acid. In the eye, this inhibitory action of acetazolamide decreases the secretion of the aqueous humor and results in a drop of intraocular pressure and is thus used to treat glaucoma.

Pharmacokinetic properties: Diamox SR is a sustained release formulation designed to obtain a smooth and continuous clinical response. Acetazolamide is readily absorbed after oral administration and binds tightly to plasma proteins as well as to the enzyme carbonic anhydrase. The drug begins to accumulate in tissues in which this enzyme is present notably red blood cells and the renal cortex. It is also bound to plasma proteins.

Peak plasma levels of the drug are reached 1–3 hours after oral administration with whole blood levels reaching peak concentrations approximately one hour later. Plasma levels decay more rapidly than red blood cell or whole blood levels with the elimination frequently being biphasic. The first phase having a half-life in 2 hours and the second phase in 13 hours. This terminal phase half-life corresponds to the leakage from red blood cells.

Acetazolamide is completely cleared by the renal route with the measured unbound renal clearance being some 5–6 times greater than creatinine clearance. Overall, clearance is dependent also on plasma protein binding.

Preclinical safety data: Nothing of note to the prescriber.

Pharmaceutical particulars
List of excipients: Microcrystalline cellulose, sodium lauryl sulphate, purified water; ethylcellulose, hydroxypropylmethyl cellulose, mineral oil light, gelatin, methanol, methylene chloride and opaspray K-I-2506 orange (hydroxypropyl cellulose, E171 and E110).

Incompatibilities: None

Shelf life: Blister packs: 36 months: Polypropylene bottles: 24 months

Special precautions for storage: Store at controlled room temperature (15°–30°C) in the original pack or in well sealed dispensing containers which prevent access of light and moisture.

Nature and contents of container: Blister Packs: 28 capsules/pack

Opaque UPVC/PVDC blister pack heat sealed with aluminium foil and packed in an outer carton.

Polypropylene Bottles: 28, 100 or 500 capsules/bottle

Polypropylene bottles with a heat sealed aluminium induction membrane and a white urea screw cap.

Instructions for use/handling: Not applicable

Marketing authorisation number 0095/0239

Date of approval/revision of SPC July 1998

Legal category POM

DIAMOX* Tablets 250 mg

Qualitative and quantitative composition Acetazolamide BP 250 mg.

Pharmaceutical form and route of administration Diamox Tablets are for oral administration. Each white tablet coded 'Lederle 4395' contains acetazolamide 250 mg.

Clinical particulars
Therapeutic indications: Diamox is an enzyme inhibitor which acts specifically on carbonic anhydrase. It is indicated in the treatment of:

i) *Glaucoma:* Diamox is useful in glaucoma (chronic simple (open angle) glaucoma, secondary glaucoma, and perioperatively in acute angle closure glaucoma where delay of surgery is desired in order to lower intraocular pressure) because it acts on inflow, decreasing the amount of aqueous secretion.

ii) *Abnormal retention of fluids:* Diamox is a diuretic whose effect is due to the effect on the reversible hydration of carbon dioxide and dehydration of carbonic acid reaction in the kidney. The result is renal loss of HCO_3^- ion which carries out sodium, water and potassium.

Diamox can be used in conjunction with other diuretics when effects on several segments of the nephron are desirable in the treatment of fluid retaining states.

iii) *Epilepsy:* In conjunction with other anticonvulsants best results with Diamox have been seen in petit mal in children. Good results, however, have been seen in patients, both children and adults, with other types of seizures such as grand mal, mixed seizure patterns, myoclonic jerk patterns etc.

Posology and method of administration:

i) *Glaucoma (simple acute congestive and secondary): Adults:* 250–1000 mg (1–4 tablets) per 24 hours, usually in divided doses for amounts over 250 mg daily.

ii) *Abnormal retention of fluid:* Congestive heart failure, drug-induced oedema.

Adults: For diuresis, the starting dose is usually 250–375 mg (1–1½ tablets) once daily in the morning. If, after an initial response, the patient fails to continue to lose oedema fluid, do not increase the dose but allow for kidney recovery by omitting a day. Best results are often obtained on a regime of 250–375 mg (1–1½ tablets) daily for two days, rest a day, and repeat, or merely giving the Diamox every other day. The use of Diamox does not eliminate the need for other therapy, eg. digitalis, bed rest and salt restriction in congestive heart failure and proper supplementation with elements such as potassium in drug-induced oedema.

For cases of fluid retention associated with pre-menstrual tension, a daily dose (single) of 125–375 mg is suggested.

iii) *Epilepsy: Adults:* 250–1000 mg daily in divided doses.

Children: 8–30 mg/kg in daily divided doses and not to exceed 750 mg/day.

The change from other medication to Diamox should be gradual.

Elderly: Diamox should only be used with particular caution in elderly patients or those with potential obstruction in the urinary tract or with disorders rendering their electrolyte balance precarious or with liver dysfunction.

Contra-indications: Acetazolamide therapy is contra-indicated in situations in which sodium and/or potassium blood serum levels are depressed, in cases of marked kidney and liver disease or dysfunction, suprarenal gland failure, and hyper-chloremic acidosis.

Long-term administration of Diamox is contra-indicated in patients with chronic non-congestive angle-closure glaucoma since it may permit organic closure of the angle to occur while the worsening glaucoma is masked by lowered intraocular pressure.

Diamox should not be used in patients hypersensitive to sulphonamides.

Special warnings and special precautions for use: Increasing the dose does not increase the diuresis and may increase the incidence of drowsiness and/or paraesthesia.

Increasing the dose often results in a decrease in diuresis. Under certain circumstances, however, very large doses have been given in conjunction with other diuretics in order to secure diuresis in complete refractory failure.

When Diamox is prescribed for long-term therapy, special precautions are advisable. The patient should be cautioned to report any unusual skin rash. Periodic blood cell counts and electrolyte levels are recommended. A precipitous drop in formed blood cell elements or the appearance of toxic skin manifestations should call for diminution or cessation of Diamox therapy.

In patients with pulmonary obstruction or emphysema where alveolar ventilation may be impaired, Diamox may aggravate acidosis and should be used with caution.

In patients with a past history of renal calculi, benefit should be balanced against the risks of precipitating further calculi.

Interaction with other medicaments and other forms of interaction: Diamox is a sulphonamide derivative. Sulphonamides may potentiate the effects of folic acid antagonists. Possible potentiation of the effects of folic acid antagonists, hypoglycaemics and oral anti-coagulants may occur. Concurrent administration of acetazolamide and aspirin may result in severe acidosis and increase central nervous system toxicity. Adjustment of dose may be required when Diamox is given with cardiac glycosides or hypertensive agents.

When given concomitantly, acetazolamide modifies the metabolism of phenytoin, leading to increased serum levels of phenytoin. Severe osteomalacia has been noted in a few patients taking acetazolamide in combination with other anticonvulsants. There have been isolated reports of reduced primidone and increased carbamazepine serum levels with concurrent administration of acetazolamide.

Pregnancy and lactation: Use in pregnancy: Acetazolamide has been reported to be teratogenic and embryotoxic in rats, mice, hamsters and rabbits at oral or parenteral doses in excess of ten times those recommended in human beings. Although there is no evidence of these effects in human beings, there are no adequate and well-controlled studies in pregnant women. Therefore, Diamox should not be used in pregnancy, especially during the first trimester.

Use in lactation: Diamox has been detected in low levels in the milk of lactating women who have taken Diamox. Although it is unlikely that this will lead to any harmful effects in the infant, extreme caution should be exercised when Diamox is administered to lactating women.

Effects on ability to drive and use machines: Increasing the dose does not increase the diuresis and may increase the incidence of drowsiness and/or paraesthesia. Less commonly, fatigue, dizziness and ataxia have been reported. Disorientation has been observed in a few patients with oedema due to hepatic cirrhosis. Such cases should be under close supervision. Transient myopia has been reported.

These conditions invariably subside upon diminution or discontinuance of the medication.

Undesirable effects: Adverse reactions during short-term therapy are usually non-serious. Those effects which have been noted include: paraesthesia, particularly a "tingling" feeling in the extremities; some loss of appetite; taste disturbance, polyuria, flushing, thirst, headache, dizziness, fatigue, irritability, depression, reduced libido and occasional instances of drowsiness and confusion. Rarely, photosensitivity has been reported.

During long-term therapy, metabolic acidosis and electrolyte imbalance may occasionally occur. This can usually be corrected by the administration of bicarbonate.

Transient myopia has been reported. This condition invariably subsides upon diminution or withdrawal of the medication.

Gastro-intestinal disturbances such as nausea, vomiting and diarrhoea.

Diamox is a sulphonamide derivative and therefore some side-effects similar to those caused by sulphonamides have occasionally been reported. These include fever, agranulocytosis, thrombocytopenia, thrombocytic purpura, leukopenia, and aplastic anaemia, bone marrow depression, pancytopenia, rash (including erythema multiforme, Stevens-Johnson Syndrome, toxic epidermal necrolysis), anaphylaxis, crystalluria, calculus formation, renal and ureteral colic, and renal lesions have been reported.

Other occasional adverse reactions include: urticaria, melaena, haematuria, glycosuria, impaired hearing and tinnitus, abnormal liver function and rarely, hepatitis or cholestatic jaundice, flaccid paralysis, and convulsions.

Overdose: No specific antidote. Supportive measures with correction of electrolyte and fluid balance. Force fluids.

Pharmacological properties

Pharmacodynamic properties: Acetazolamide is an inhibitor of carbonic anhydrase. By inhibiting the reaction catalysed by this enzyme in the renal tubules, acetazolamide increases the excretion of bicarbonate and of cations, chiefly sodium and potassium, and so promotes alkaline diuresis.

Continuous administration of acetazolamide is associated with metabolic acidosis and resultant loss of diuretic activity. Therefore the effectiveness of Diamox in diuresis diminishes with continuous use.

By inhibiting carbonic anhydrase in the eye, acetazolamide decreases intra-ocular pressure and is therefore useful in the treatment of glaucoma.

Pharmacokinetic properties: Acetazolamide is fairly rapidly absorbed from the gastro-intestinal tract with peak plasma concentrations occurring about 2 hours after administration by mouth. It has been estimated to have a plasma half-life of about 4 hours. It is tightly bound to carbonic anhydrase and accumulates in tissues containing this enzyme, particularly red blood cells and the renal cortex. It is also bound to plasma proteins. It is excreted unchanged in the urine, renal clearance being enhanced in the alkaline urine.

Pharmaceutical particulars

List of excipients:

Dicalcium phosphate	BP
Corn starch	BP
Magnesium stearate	BP
Sodium starch glycolate	NF
Povidone	USP

Incompatibilities: None.

Shelf life: 48 months.

Special precautions for storage: Diamox Tablets 250 mg should be stored at controlled room temperature (15°–25°C) in either the original pack or in containers which prevent the access of moisture.

Nature and contents of container: Amber glass bottles with metal screw-on caps.

Polypropylene bottles with plastic screw-on caps.

The product is supplied in bottles of 112 and 1000 tablets.

Instructions for use/handling: None.

Marketing authorisation number PL 0095/5075R

Date of approval/revision of SPC July 1998

Legal category POM

DIMOTANE* TABLETS
DIMOTANE* LA
DIMOTANE* ELIXIR

Qualitative and quantitative composition Dimotane Tablets: Tablet containing Brompheniramine Maleate BP 4.0 mg.

Dimotane LA: Tablet containing Brompheniramine Maleate BP 12.0 mg (one-third of active ingredient in coating for immediate release; two-thirds of active ingredient in delayed-release core)

Dimotane Elixir: Elixir containing Brompheniramine Maleate BP 2.0 mg per 5 ml

Pharmaceutical form Dimotane Tablets: Round peach-coloured tablet for oral use. One side is engraved 'AHR', the other side is scored with a breakline.

Dimotane LA: Peach coloured, sugar coated, modified release tablet for oral use

Dimotane Elixir: A clear pale yellow-green liquid with an odour and taste of cola.

Clinical particulars

Therapeutic indications: Antihistamine in the treatment of allergic conditions and reactions such as hayfever and urticaria.

Posology and method of administration:

Dimotane Tablets

Adults and older patients: 1–2 tablets 3 or 4 times daily.

Children 6–12 years: ½–1 tablet 3 or 4 times daily

Under 6 years: Not recommended.

Dimotane LA

Adults and older patients: 1–2 tablets night and morning.

Children 6–12 years: 1 tablet at night on retiring. A further tablet may be taken in the morning if necessary.

Under 6 years: Not recommended.

Dimotane Elixir

Adults and older patients: 10–20 ml 3 or 4 times daily.

Children 6–12 years: 5–10 ml 3 or 4 times daily.

Children 3–6 years: 5 ml 3 or 4 times daily.

Children under 3 years: 0.4–1 mg/kg per 24 hours in four divided doses or at the discretion of the physician.

Contra-indications: Hypersensitivity to any of the ingredients.

Special warnings and special precautions for use: In common with many other antihistamines, brompheniramine has an anticholinergic action and should therefore be used with caution in patients with asthma (especially children), closed-angle glaucoma and prostatic disease.

Brompheniramine maleate may act as a cerebral stimulant in children and the elderly. If this occurs, it is possible that insomnia, nervousness, pyrexia and tremors may occur, and, very rarely, hallucinations and convulsions. It is advisable that children receiving brompheniramine should not be left unattended for long periods. This product should be used with care in epileptic patients.

Interactions with other medicaments and other forms of interaction: This product may potentiate the sedative effects of CNS depressants including alcohol, barbiturates, hypnotics, opioid analgesics, anxiolytics and neuroleptics.

Antihistamines exhibit an additive anticholinergic action with other anticholinergic drugs, such as phenothiazines and tricyclic antidepressants.

Monoamine oxidase inhibitors prolong and intensify the anticholinergic effects of antihistamines.

Pregnancy and lactation: Safety for the use of Dimotane during pregnancy has not been established. Therefore, this product should not be used during pregnancy unless considered essential by the physician.

Effects on the ability to drive and use machines: Drowsiness may occur. Patients receiving brompheniramine should not drive or operate machinery unless it has been shown that their physical and mental capacity remains unaffected.

Undesirable effects: The most common side effect is sedation which may diminish after a few days of treatment.

Anticholinergic effects such as blurred vision, dry mouth, tachycardia and urinary retention may occur.

Other side effects which have been reported rarely are nervousness, urticaria, constipation, pyrexia, dizziness, hallucinations and convulsions.

Overdose: Overdose may be fatal especially in infants and children. The patient may be unconscious, and shows hypotension, coma and occasionally convulsions. Initial excitement is often seen in children.

Management of overdose consists of gastric lavage together with appropriate supportive therapy dependent upon individual symptoms.

Pharmacological properties

Pharmacodynamic properties: Brompheniramine belongs to the alkylamine group of H_1-antihistamines. It competitively antagonises the effects of histamine on H_1 receptors and blocks the constrictor responses to histamine of intestinal and bronchial smooth muscle.

Within the vascular tree, brompheniramine inhibits both the vasoconstrictor and the vasodilator effects of histamine. Secondary to injury, antigens or histamine-releasing pharmacological agents, brompheniramine counteracts both oedema and wheal formation. It also blocks the increased nasal secretion and impaired airflow following nasal histamine challenge.

Single doses of 4–12 mg of brompheniramine have produced CNS depression in terms of subjective sedation and objective impairment of skilled performance which lasts for 5–7 hours.

Pharmacokinetic properties:

(a) General characteristics: Following oral administration, brompheniramine is readily absorbed and distributed into the tissues; peak plasma concentrations are seen at approximately 3 hours after a single oral dose of 10 mg to fasting subjects. Following administration of a controlled release tablet peak plasma levels occur between 3 and 5 hours. An elimination half life of about 25 hours has been reported.

Brompheniramine appears to undergo moderate first pass metabolism.

The major route of elimination is hepatic metabolism with unchanged drug and metabolites being excreted primarily in the urine. Less than 3% is excreted in the faeces.

(b) Characteristics in patients: Effective anti-allergic doses of brompheniramine (8 mg) have produced plasma concentrations of 8–16 microgram/litre over several hours.

Oral brompheniramine 10 mg produced drowsiness in all of a group of adult volunteers, peaking at around 3–4 hours after administration, coinciding with peak plasma concentrations.

Pharmaceutical particulars
List of excipients: Dimotane Tablets: Maize starch, dibasic calcium phosphate dihydrate, magnesium stearate, iron oxide red and iron oxide yellow (E172).

Dimotane LA: Magnesium stearate, sucrose, calcium sulphate, talc, maize starch, zein, stearic acid, glycol monostearate, guar gum, acacia gum, gelatin, carnauba wax, beeswax, titanium dioxide (E171), iron oxide red and iron oxide yellow (E172).

Dimotane Elixir: Sodium benzoate, citric acid anhydrous, sucrose, quinoline yellow (E104), cola flavour, ethanol (96%), water.

Incompatibilities: Incompatibility has been reported with some diatrizoate, iodipamide and iothalamate salts.

Shelf life: Dimotane Tablets, Dimotane Elixir: Three years. Dimotane LA: Four years.

Special precautions for storage: Dimotane Tablets: Store below 25°C. Protect from light. Dimotane LA: Supplied in amber glass bottles, therefore no special storage precautions are required, however the tablets may discolour on exposure to strong sunlight. Dimotane Elixir: None

Nature and contents of container: Dimotane Tablets: Amber glass screw cap bottle containing 28 tablets. Dimotane LA: Amber glass screw cap bottle containing 28 tablets. Dimotane Elixir: Amber glass bottle containing 200 ml

Instructions for use/handling: Not applicable.

Marketing authorisation numbers

Dimotane Tablets	0100/5004
Dimotane LA	0100/5006
Dimotane Elixir	0100/5005

Date of revision of the text January 1998

Legal category P

DIMOTANE* Plus Paediatric DIMOTANE* Plus

Qualitative and quantitative composition Dimotane Plus Paediatric is a liquid preparation containing two active ingredients, Brompheniramine Maleate BP 2.0 mg per 5 ml and Pseudoephedrine Hydrochloride BP 15.0 mg per 5 ml.

This product also contains ethanol and sodium benzoate.

Dimotane Plus is a liquid preparation containing two active ingredients, Brompheniramine Maleate BP 4.0 mg per 5 ml and Pseudoephedrine Hydrochloride BP 30.0 mg per 5 ml.

This product also contains ethanol and sodium benzoate.

Pharmaceutical form Oral liquid.

Clinical particulars
Therapeutic indications: Symptomatic relief of allergic rhinitis.

Posology and method of administration:
Dimotane Plus Paediatric: This product is recommended for paediatric use only:
Children:
6–12 years: 10 ml three times daily.
2–5 years: 5 ml three times daily.
Children under 2 years: not recommended.
The dosage interval should not be less than four hours.
Do not exceed three doses per day.
Dimotane Plus:
Adults and older patients: 10 ml three times daily.
Children 6–12 years: 5 ml three times daily.
Children 2–5 years: 2.5 ml three times daily. Dimotane Plus Paediatric is recommended.
Children under 2 years: not recommended.

The dosage interval should not be less than four hours. Do not exceed three doses per day.

Contra-indications: Hypersensitivity to the active ingredients. Coma or pre-coma states. Known brain disease or epilepsy. Use in patients with acute ischaemic heart disease. Thyrotoxicosis. Glaucoma or urinary retention. Patients currently receiving or who have within two weeks received, monoamine oxidase inhibitors or tricyclic antidepressants. Patients receiving other sympathomimetic drugs. Hypertension or patients receiving antihypertensive therapy.

Special warnings and precautions for use: In common with many other antihistamines, brompheniramine has an atropine-like action and should therefore be used with caution in patients with bronchial asthma, especially children. May act as a cerebral stimulant in children and occasionally in adults. If this occurs it is possible that insomnia, nervousness, hyperpyrexia or tremor may occur and very rarely epileptiform convulsions. Therefore children taking this product should not be left unattended for long periods. Should be used in caution in patients receiving digitalis, adrenergic blockers or non-steroidal anti-inflammatory drugs.

Interactions with other medicaments and other forms of interaction: May potentiate the effects of CNS depressants including alcohol. The effects of anticholinergic drugs may be potentiated.

Pregnancy and lactation: This product should not be used in pregnancy unless considered essential by the physician.

Effects on the ability to drive and use machines: Drowsiness may occur. Patients receiving this product should not drive or operate machinery unless it has been shown that their physical and mental capability remains unaffected.

Undesirable effects: None known

Overdose: Gastric lavage together with appropriate supporting therapy dependent upon individual response to the constituents of the preparation.

Pharmacological properties
Pharmacodynamic properties: Dimotane Plus and Dimotane Plus Paediatric have been formulated to combine an anti-histamine (brompheniramine maleate) and a decongestant (pseudoephedrine hydrochloride) for use in allergic rhinitis.

Pharmacokinetic properties: Dimotane Plus Paediatric is a liquid preparation containing two active ingredients, (Brompheniramine Maleate 2.0 mg/5 ml and Pseudoephedrine Hydrochloride 15.0 mg/5 ml).

Dimotane Plus is a liquid preparation containing two active ingredients, (Brompheniramine Maleate 4.0 mg/5 ml and Pseudoephedrine Hydrochloride 30.0 mg/5 ml).

The pharmacokinetic characteristics of both active ingredients are well documented in the standard reference texts, such as 'Martindale–The Extra Pharmacopoeia, 29th Edition'. The dosage regime complies with the requirements of the text and the BNF for both active ingredients.

Pharmaceutical particulars
List of excipients: Glycerol, sodium carboxymethyl cellulose, saccharin sodium, sodium benzoate, disodium edetate, Lycasin, ethanol, citric acid, purified water, caramel (E150), grape flavour, Hyflo Supercel.

Incompatibilities: None known

Shelf life: Two years.

Special precautions for storage: There are no special storage precautions for this product

Nature and contents of container: This product will be presented in amber glass bottles with screw caps or jay caps. Bottles size 200 ml.

Instructions for use/handling: Not applicable.

Marketing authorisation numbers

Dimotane Plus Paediatric	PL 0100/0086
Dimotane Plus	PL 0100/0085

Date of approval/revision

Dimotane Plus Paediatric:	
First Authorisation	20th August 1985
Last revision	4th October 1995
Dimotane Plus:	
First Authorisation	20th August 1985
Last revision	4th September 1995

Legal Category POM

EFEXOR* ▼

Presentation Efexor Tablets are peach coloured, shield-shaped tablets impressed with the tablet strength and embossed with a 'W' on one side, and plain on the other.

Efexor Tablets are available containing 37.5, 50 or 75 mg of venlafaxine as hydrochloride.

Uses Efexor is indicated for the treatment of depressive illness in both hospitalised patients and outpatients.

Dosage and administration
Adults: The usual recommended dose is 75 mg per day given in two divided doses (37.5 mg twice daily). If, after several weeks, further clinical improvement is required, the dose may be increased to 150 mg per day given in two divided doses (75 mg twice daily).

If, in the judgement of the physician, a higher dose is required, for example in more severely depressed or hospitalised patients, a starting dose of 150 mg per day may be given in two divided doses (75 mg twice daily). The daily dose may then be increased by up to 75 mg every two or three days until the desired response is achieved. The maximum recommended dose is 375 mg per day. The dose should then be gradually reduced to the usual dosage, consistent with patient response and tolerance.

It is recommended that Efexor be taken with food.

Patients with renal or hepatic impairment: For patients with mild renal impairment (GFR >30 ml/minute) or mild hepatic impairment (PT <14 seconds), no change in dosage is necessary.

For patients with moderate renal impairment (GFR 10–30 ml/minute) or moderate hepatic impairment (PT 14–18 seconds), the dose should be reduced by 50%. This dose may be given once daily due to the longer half-lives of venlafaxine and O-desmethylvenlafaxine in these patients.

Insufficient data are available to support the use of Efexor in patients with severe renal impairment (GFR <10 ml/minute) or severe hepatic impairment (PT >18 seconds).

Elderly patients: No adjustment in the usual dosage is recommended for elderly patients. In a trial investigating the kinetics of venlafaxine in the elderly, the half-life (at steady-state conditions) was prolonged by 1–2 hours, mainly in the male subjects. This was apparently due to an 18% reduction in the clearance of venlafaxine and O-desmethylvenlafaxine. The small increase in steady-state plasma levels of venlafaxine and O-desmethylvenlafaxine which resulted, was not judged to be clinically significant; no adjustment in dosage is necessary. However, as with any therapy, caution should be exercised in treating the elderly (eg. due to the possibility of renal impairment. See also dosage recommendations for renal impairment). The lowest effective dose should always be used and patients should be carefully monitored when an increase in the dose is required.

Maintenance/continuation/extended treatment: The physician should periodically re-evaluate the usefulness of long-term treatment with Efexor for the individual patient. It is generally agreed that acute episodes of major depression require several months or longer of sustained therapy. Efexor has been shown to be efficacious during long-term (up to 12 months) treatment.

Discontinuing Efexor: Discontinuation effects are well known to occur with the abrupt withdrawal of other antidepressants. While withdrawal reactions with Efexor have not been systematically evaluated in controlled clinical trials, a retrospective survey of events occurring during taper or following discontinuation of Efexor revealed the following events that occurred at an incidence of at least 5% and at least twice the placebo incidence: fatigue, headache, nausea, dizziness, sleep disturbance and nervousness. Diarrhoea and one hypomanic episode was also reported.

In post-marketing experience, symptoms reported following discontinuation, dose reduction or tapering of venlafaxine at various doses have also included confusion, paraesthesia, sweating, vertigo and vomiting. It is therefore recommended that when discontinuing Efexor after more than one week's therapy, the dose should be gradually reduced over at least one week and the patient monitored in order to minimise the risk of withdrawal reactions.

The period required for discontinuation may depend on the dose, duration of therapy and the individual patient.

Children: Safety and effectiveness in individuals below 18 years of age have not been established and such use is not recommended.

Contra-indications, precautions and warnings etc.
Contra-indications:
1) Known or suspected pregnancy.
2) Insufficient data are available to support the use of Efexor in lactating women. Therefore, such use is contra-indicated.
3) Known hypersensitivity to venlafaxine or any other component of the product.
4) Concomitant use of Efexor with monoamine oxidase inhibitors.
5) Safety and effectiveness in individuals below 18 years of age have not been established and such use is not recommended.

Pregnancy and lactation: The safety of Efexor for use during human pregnancy has not been established. Therefore, the use of Efexor during known or suspected pregnancy is contra-indicated. Patients should be advised to notify their physician if they become pregnant or intend to become pregnant during therapy.

Insufficient data are available to support the use of Efexor in lactating women. Therefore, such use is contra-indicated.

Precautions and warnings:

1) The risk of suicide must be considered in all depressed patients. The smallest quantity of tablets should be prescribed consistent with good patient management in order to reduce the possibility of overdose.
2) During the development of Efexor, 0.2% of patients had a convulsion or event described as possibly having been a seizure. Although this rate was low and all the patients recovered, Efexor (as with all antidepressants) should be introduced with caution in patients with a history of epilepsy and should be discontinued in any patient developing a seizure whilst taking Efexor.
3) During clinical trials, rash developed in 4% of patients given Efexor. Patients should be advised to notify their physician if they develop a rash, urticaria, or a related allergic phenomenon.
4) Three percent (3%) of the 2,181 patients who received Efexor in clinical trials were judged to have clinically significant blood pressure increases. The increases were dose-related. In general, patients treated with 200 mg/day or less, showed minor increases, while in a short-term dose-ranging study, the highest dose (300 to 375 mg/day) was associated with mean increases in supine and diastolic blood pressure of approximately 4 mm Hg by week 4, and 7 mm Hg by week 6. The presence of treated hypertension or elevated blood pressure at baseline did not seem to predispose patients to further increases during Efexor therapy. For patients treated with doses greater than 200 mg/day routine blood pressure monitoring may be advisable.
5) Due to the possibility of drug abuse with CNS active drugs, physicians should evaluate patients for a history of drug abuse and follow such patients closely. Clinical studies have shown no evidence of drug-seeking behaviour, development of tolerance, or dose escalation over time among patients taking Efexor.
6) Efexor has not been evaluated or used to any appreciable extent in patients with a recent history of myocardial infarction or unstable heart disease and, therefore, should be used with caution in these patients. No serious arrhythmias were observed in patients treated with venlafaxine, and mean PR, QRS or QTc intervals were not significantly prolonged. The mean heart rate was increased by approximately 4 beats/minute during treatment.
7) The clearances of venlafaxine and its active metabolite are decreased and half-lives increased in patients with moderate to severe renal impairment or cirrhosis of the liver. Therefore, Efexor should be used with caution in these patients. A lower or less frequent dose may be necessary in such patients as indicated in the Dosage and Administration Section.
8) Although Efexor has been shown not to affect psychomotor, cognitive, or complex behaviour performance in healthy volunteers, any psychoactive drug may impair judgement, thinking or motor skills and therefore patients should be cautioned about their ability to drive a car or operate hazardous machinery.
9) Postural hypotension has been observed occasionally during Efexor treatment. Patients, especially the elderly, should be alerted to the possibility of dizziness or unsteadiness.
10) Women of childbearing potential should employ adequate contraception whilst taking Efexor.

Interactions: Adverse reactions, some serious, have been reported when Efexor therapy has been initiated soon after discontinuation of an MAOI and when an MAOI has been initiated soon after discontinuation of Efexor. Given these reactions as well as the serious sometimes fatal interactions reported with concomitant or immediately consecutive administration of MAOIs and other antidepressants with pharmacological properties similar to Efexor, do not use Efexor in combination with an MAOI or within at least 14 days of discontinuing MAOI treatment. Allow at least 7 days after stopping Efexor before starting an MAOI.

The risk of using Efexor in combination with other CNS-active drugs has not been systematically evaluated, except in the case of lithium and diazepam. Consequently, caution is advised if the concomitant administration of Efexor and other such drugs is required.

In an interaction study, although lithium significantly reduced the renal clearance of venlafaxine, its effect on the renal clearance of the active metabolite, O-desmethylvenlafaxine, was small. Therefore, since the major route of elimination of venlafaxine is via metabolism to O-desmethylvenlafaxine, and not renal excretion, the total clearance values for venlafaxine and its metabolite were not significantly affected. It was also found that venlafaxine itself had no significant effect on the kinetics of lithium.

The pharmacokinetic profiles of venlafaxine and O-desmethylvenlafaxine were not significantly altered by the administration of diazepam. Venlafaxine had no effect on the pharmacokinetic profile of diazepam or on the psychomotor or psychometric effects induced by diazepam.

Cimetidine inhibited the first-pass metabolism of venlafaxine but had no significant effect on the formation or elimination of O-desmethylvenlafaxine, which is present in much greater quantities in the systemic circulation. No dosage adjustment therefore seems necessary when Efexor is coadministered with cimetidine. For elderly patients or patients with hepatic dysfunction, the interaction could potentially be more pronounced. Therefore, clinical monitoring is recommended when Efexor is administered with cimetidine in these patients.

The pharmacokinetic profiles of venlafaxine, O-desmethylvenlafaxine, and ethanol were not altered when venlafaxine and ethanol were administered together to healthy volunteers who consumed alcohol on an occasional basis (equivalent to 3 to 30 ounces of ethanol per month). The administration of venlafaxine in a stable regimen did not potentiate the psychomotor and psychometric effects induced by ethanol in these same social drinkers when they were not receiving venlafaxine.

There is no evidence suggesting incompatibility between treatment with Efexor and treatment with either antihypertensives, (including β-blockers ACE inhibitors and diuretics) or hypoglycaemic agents.

Side-effects: In clinical studies the following adverse events occurred most frequently with Efexor and occurred more frequently than placebo; nausea, headache, insomnia, somnolence, dry mouth, dizziness, constipation, asthenia, sweating and nervousness.

The occurrence of most of these adverse events was dose-related and the majority of them decreased in intensity and frequency over time. They generally did not lead to cessation of treatment.

Other adverse events which occurred less often were, in order of decreasing frequency: anorexia, dyspepsia, abdominal pain, anxiety, impotence, abnormality of accommodation, vasodilation, vomiting, tremor, paraesthesia, abnormal ejaculation/orgasm, chills, hypertension, palpitation, weight gain , agitation, decreased libido.

Clinically significant weight change was seen in less than 1% of patients treated with Efexor in clinical trials.

The adverse events, nausea and impotence are well known to be associated with drugs having serotonergic activity.

The overall incidence of nausea associated with Efexor in placebo-controlled studies was 36% compared to 12% in placebo-treated patients. This incidence decreased with time reducing to a level comparable with placebo after 3 weeks. The nausea experienced was usually mild to moderate, and infrequently resulted in vomiting or withdrawal.

The incidence of nausea is also dose related with a reduced incidence being shown at the usual dose of 75 mg/day. The incidence is likely to increase at the higher end of the dose range, particularly when doses are increased rapidly.

The overall incidence of impotence in clinical trials was 7%.

Treatment with Efexor was associated with an increase in blood pressure in some patients during clinical trials. (See Precautions and warnings)

Postural hypotension has been observed occasionally during Efexor treatment.

Reversible increases of liver enzymes were seen in a small number (0.5%) of patients during clinical trials with Efexor.

Alterations in serum cholesterol have been seen in some patients treated with Efexor. A mean increase of approximately 0.07 mmol/litre from baseline was observed in patients treated with Efexor. The clinical significance of this is not known.

Cases of hyponatraemia have rarely been reported with antidepressants, including SSRIs, usually in the elderly and in patients taking diuretics and/or otherwise volume depleted. Similarly cases of hyponatraemia have rarely been reported with Efexor, usually in the elderly, which have resolved upon discontinuation of the drug.

Withdrawal reactions reported on abrupt cessation, dose reduction or tapering of venlafaxine include fatigue, headache, nausea or vomiting, dizziness, dry mouth, diarrhoea, insomnia, nervousness, confusion, paraesthesia, sweating and vertigo. The majority of symptoms experienced on withdrawal of Efexor are non-serious and self-limiting. (See also Dosage and Administration).

Overdose: In post-marketing experience, electrocardiogram changes (e.g. prolongation of QT interval, bundle branch block, QRS prolongation), sinus and ventricular tachycardia, bradycardia and seizures have been reported in association with overdosage of venlafaxine, usually when in combination with overdose of this drug and/or alcohol. Such events are rare and usually resolve spontaneously.

Management of Overdosage; Ensure an adequate airway, oxygenation and ventilation. Monitoring of cardiac rhythm and vital signs is recommended as are general supportive and symptomatic measures. Use of activated charcoal, induction of emesis or gastric lavage should be considered. No specific antidotes for Efexor are known.

The haemodialysis clearance of venlafaxine and its main active metabolite are low, therefore, they are not considered dialysable.

Pharmaceutical particulars

List of ingredients: The active constituent is venlafaxine as hydrochloride. Other constituents are microcrystalline cellulose, lactose, sodium starch glycollate, magnesium stearate, yellow and brown iron oxide.

Shelf-life: Three years

Special precautions for storage: Store in a dry place at room temperature (at or below 30°C)

Legal category POM

Package quantities

37.5 and 75 mg tablets: Blister packs containing 56 tablets.

50 mg tablets: Blister packs containing 42 tablets.

Further information Efexor is a structurally novel antidepressant which is chemically unrelated to tricyclic, tetracyclic, or other available antidepressant agents. It is a racemate with two active enantiomers.

The mechanism of Efexor's antidepressant action in humans is believed to be associated with its potentiation of neurotransmitter activity in the central nervous system. Preclinical studies have shown that venlafaxine and its major metabolite, O-desmethylvenlafaxine, are potent neuronal serotonin and noradrenaline re-uptake inhibitors (SNRI) and weak inhibitors of dopamine reuptake. In addition, venlafaxine and O-desmethylvenlafaxine reduce β-adrenergic responsiveness in animals after both acute (single dose) and chronic administration. Venlafaxine and its major metabolite appear to be equipotent with respect to their overall action on neurotransmitter re-uptake.

Venlafaxine has virtually no affinity for rat brain muscarinic, histaminergic or adrenergic receptors *in vitro*. Pharmacologic activity at these receptors may be related to various side-effects seen with other antidepressant drugs, such as anticholinergic, sedative and cardiovascular effects.

Pharmacokinetic properties: Venlafaxine is well absorbed and undergoes extensive first-pass metabolism. Mean peak plasma concentrations of venlafaxine range from approximately 33 to 172ng/ml after 25 to 150 mg single doses, and are reached in approximately 2.4 hours. Venlafaxine is extensively metabolised in the liver. O-desmethylvenlafaxine is the major active metabolite of venlafaxine. The mean disposition half-life of venlafaxine and O-desmethylvenlafaxine is approximately 5 and 11 hours, respectively. Mean peak O-desmethyl venlafaxine plasma concentrations range from approximately 61 to 325ng/ml and are reached in approximately 4.3 hours. Plasma concentrations of venlafaxine and O-desmethylvenlafaxine generally correlated well with dose levels. Venlafaxine and O-desmethylvenlafaxine are 27% and 30% bound to plasma proteins respectively. O-desmethylvenlafaxine, other minor venlafaxine metabolites, and non-metabolised venlafaxine are excreted primarily through the kidneys.

Product licence numbers

37.5 mg	0011/0199
50 mg	0011/0200
75 mg	0011/0201

Date of revision of text June 1998

EFEXOR* XL ▼

Qualitative and quantitative composition There are two strengths of Efexor XL capsules, containing 84.8 mg or 169.7 mg of venlafaxine hydrochloride, equivalent to 75 mg or 150 mg of venlafaxine free base, in an extended release formulation. Venlafaxine is chemically defined as (R/S)-1-[(2-dimethylamino)-1-(4-methoxyphenyl)ethyl]cyclohexanol hydrochloride.

Pharmaceutical form Efexor XL 75 mg capsules are opaque peach modified release capsules printed in red with 'W' and '75'. Efexor XL 150 mg capsules are opaque dark orange modified release capsules printed in white with 'W' and '150'.

Clinical particulars

Therapeutic indications: Efexor XL is indicated for the treatment of depressive illness.

Posology and method of administration: The recommended dose for Efexor XL is 75 mg, given once daily. If after 2 weeks further clinical improvement is required, the dose may be increased to 150 mg once daily. If needed, the dose can be further increased up to 225 mg once daily. Dose increments should be made at intervals of approximately 2 weeks or more, but not less than 4 days. Antidepressant activity with the 75 mg dose was observed after 2 weeks of treatment.

Efexor XL should be taken with food. Each capsule should be swallowed whole with fluid. Do not divide, crush, chew, or place the capsule in water. Efexor XL should be administered once daily, at approximately the same time, either in the morning or in the evening.

Depressed patients who are currently being treated with Efexor Tablets may be switched to Efexor XL. For example, a patient receiving Efexor Tablets 37.5 mg b.d. would receive Efexor XL 75 mg o.d. When switching, individual dosage adjustments may be necessary.

Patients with renal or hepatic impairment: The half lives of venlafaxine and O-desmethylvenlafaxine are increased in patients with renal and hepatic impairment.

For patients with mild renal impairment (GFR > 30 ml/minute) or mild hepatic impairment, no change in dosage is necessary.

For patients with moderate renal impairment (GFR 10–30 ml/minute) or moderate hepatic impairment, the dose should be reduced by 50%. For patients requiring a lower daily dose than 75 mg, treatment may be provided with Efexor Tablets.

Insufficient data are available to support the use of Efexor XL in patients with severe renal impairment (GFR < 10 ml/minute) or severe hepatic impairment.

Elderly patients: No adjustment from the usual dosage is recommended for elderly patients. However, as with any therapy, caution should be exercised in treating the elderly (e.g. due to the possibility of renal impairment. See also *Dosage recommendations for renal impairment*). The lowest effective dose should always be used, and patients should be carefully monitored when an increase in the dose is required.

Paediatric use: Safety and effectiveness in individuals below 18 years of age have not been established, and such use is not recommended.

Maintenance/continuation/extended treatment: The physician should periodically re-evaluate the usefulness of long-term Efexor XL treatment for the individual patient. It is generally agreed that acute episodes of major depression require several months or longer of sustained pharmacological therapy.

Venlafaxine has been shown to be efficacious during long-term (up to 12 months) treatment.

Discontinuing Efexor XL: Discontinuation effects are well known to occur with the abrupt withdrawal of other antidepressants. While withdrawal reactions with Efexor XL have not been systematically evaluated in controlled clinical trials, a retrospective survey of events occurring during taper or following discontinuation of Efexor XL revealed the following events that occurred at an incidence of at least 3% and at least twice the placebo incidence: dizziness, dry mouth, insomnia, nausea, nervousness and sweating.

In addition, a retrospective survey of events occurring during taper or following discontinuation of Efexor tablets revealed the following events that occurred at an incidence of at least 5% and at least twice the placebo incidence: fatigue, headache, nausea, dizziness, sleep disturbance and nervousness. Diarrhoea and one hypomanic episode was also reported.

In post-marketing experience, symptoms reported following discontinuation, dose reduction or tapering of venlafaxine at various doses have also included confusion, paraesthesia, sweating, vertigo and vomiting. It is therefore recommended that when discontinuing Efexor XL after more than one week's therapy, the dose should be gradually reduced over at least one week and the patient monitored in order to minimise the risk of withdrawal reactions.

The period required for discontinuation may depend on the dose, duration of therapy and the individual patient.

Contra-indications:

1. Known or suspected pregnancy.
2. Insufficient data are available to support the use of Efexor XL in lactating women. Therefore, such use is contra-indicated.
3. Known hypersensitivity to venlafaxine or any other component of the product.
4. Concomitant use of venlafaxine with monoamine oxidase inhibitors.
5. Paediatric Use–Safety and effectiveness in individuals below 18 years of age have not been established, and such use is not recommended.

Special warnings and precautions for use: Women of childbearing potential should employ adequate contraception whilst taking Efexor XL.

The risk of suicide attempt must be considered in all depressed patients. Prescriptions for Efexor XL should be written for the smallest quantity of capsules consistent with good patient management in order to reduce the possibility of overdose.

In clinical trials with venlafaxine, seizures were reported in 0.2% of all venlafaxine-treated patients. All patients recovered. No seizures occurred in Efexor XL-treated patients during clinical trials. However, as with all antidepressants, Efexor XL should be introduced with care in patients with a history of seizure and should be discontinued in any patient who develops seizures.

During clinical trials, rash developed in 3% of patients treated with venlafaxine. Patients should be advised to notify their physician if they develop a rash, urticaria or related allergic phenomenon.

Clinical studies have shown no evidence of drug-seeking behaviour, development of tolerance, or dose escalation over time among patients taking venlafaxine. However, physicians should evaluate patients for a history of drug abuse, and follow such patients closely, observing them for signs of misuse or abuse of Efexor XL.

The clearances of venlafaxine and its active metabolite are decreased and half-lives increased in patients with moderate to severe renal impairment or cirrhosis of the liver. Therefore, Efexor XL should be used with caution in these patients. A lower daily dose might be necessary in such patients and treatment may be provided with Efexor Tablets as indicated above under '*Posology and method of administration*'.

Venlafaxine has not been evaluated or used to any appreciable extent in patients with a recent history of myocardial infarction or unstable heart disease. Therefore, it should be used with caution in these patients. Clinically significant electrocardiogram findings were observed in 1% of the venlafaxine-treated patients compared with 0.2% of the placebo-treated patients. Clinically significant changes in PR, QRS or QTc intervals were rarely observed in patients treated with venlafaxine during clinical trials. The mean heart rate was increased by approximately 4 beats/minute during treatment with venlafaxine.

Increases in blood pressure have been reported in patients treated with high doses of venlafaxine. Blood pressure monitoring is advisable in patients receiving daily doses of >200 mg.

Interactions with other medicaments and other forms of interaction: Adverse reactions, some serious, have been reported when venlafaxine therapy is initiated soon after discontinuation of an MAOI, and when an MAOI is initiated soon after discontinuation of venlafaxine. Given these reactions as well as the serious, sometimes fatal interactions reported with concomitant or immediately consecutive administration of MAOIs and other antidepressants with pharmacological properties similar to Efexor XL, do not use Efexor XL in combination with an MAOI, or within at least 14 days of discontinuing MAOI treatment. Allow at least 7 days after stopping Efexor XL before starting an MAOI.

The risk of using venlafaxine in combination with other CNS-active drugs has not been systematically evaluated, except in the case of lithium, imipramine and diazepam. Caution is advised if the concomitant administration of Efexor XL and other CNS-active drugs is required.

The pharmacokinetic profiles of venlafaxine and its active metabolite O-desmethylvenlafaxine (ODV) were not altered when Efexor Tablets and diazepam, Efexor Tablets and lithium, or Efexor Tablets and ethanol (0.5 g/kg/day) were administered together to healthy volunteers. Venlafaxine had no effect on the pharmacokinetic profiles of diazepam, lithium or ethanol in these studies. Administration of Efexor Tablets did not affect the psychomotor and psychometric effects induced by diazepam or ethanol.

Venlafaxine did not affect the hepatic metabolism of the tricyclic antidepressant, imipramine or its active metabolite, desipramine. However, the renal clearance of 2-hydroxy desipramine was reduced with coadministration of Efexor Tablets. Imipramine partially inhibited the formation of ODV. However, no dosage adjustment of either drug is necessary when Efexor XL and imipramine are given concomitantly.

Cimetidine inhibited the first-pass metabolism of venlafaxine, but had no apparent effect on the formation or elimination of ODV, which is present in much greater quantities in the systemic circulation. Therefore, no dosage adjustment seems necessary when Efexor XL is coadministered with cimetidine. For elderly patients, or patients with hepatic dysfunction, the interaction could potentially be more pronounced, and for such patients, clinical monitoring is indicated when Efexor XL is administered with cimetidine.

Venlafaxine is primarily metabolised to its equally active metabolite, ODV, by the cytochrome P450 enzyme CYP2D6. However, unlike many other antidepressants, no dosage adjustment is necessary when Efexor XL is administered concomitantly with drugs which inhibit CYP2D6, or when used in patients who are poor CYP2D6 metabolisers, since the total concentration of active compound (venlafaxine and ODV) is not affected.

Venlafaxine is a relatively weak inhibitor of CYP2D6, and does not inhibit CYP1A2, CYP2C9 or CYP3A4. Therefore, Efexor XL is not expected to interact with other drugs metabolised by these hepatic enzymes.

The major elimination pathways for venlafaxine are through CYP2D6 and CYP3A4. Therefore, caution should be used with concomitant intake of drugs which inhibit both of these enzymes. Such interactions have not been studied to date.

Venlafaxine and ODV are 27% and 30% bound to plasma proteins. Therefore, drug interactions due to protein binding of venlafaxine and the major metabolite are not expected.

There is no evidence suggesting incompatibility between treatment with venlafaxine and treatment with either antihypertensives (including β-blockers, ACE inhibitors and diuretics) or hypoglycaemic agents.

There are no clinical studies to evaluate the benefit of combined use of Efexor XL with another antidepressant or electroconvulsive therapy (ECT).

Pregnancy and lactation: The safety of Efexor XL for use during human pregnancy has not been established. Therefore, the use of Efexor XL during known or suspected pregnancy is contra-indicated. Patients should be advised to notify their physician if they become pregnant, or intend to become pregnant during therapy.

Insufficient data are available to support the use of venlafaxine in lactating women. In preclinical studies, venlafaxine and ODV were found to pass into maternal milk. It is not known whether venlafaxine or its metabolites are excreted in human milk. Therefore, such use is contra-indicated.

Effects on ability to drive and use machines: Although venlafaxine has been shown not to affect psychomotor, cognitive or complex behaviour performance in healthy volunteers, any psychoactive drug may impair judgement, thinking or motor skills. Therefore, patients should be cautioned about their ability to drive or operate hazardous machinery.

Undesirable effects: The most commonly observed adverse events associated with the use of venlafaxine in clinical trials, which were not seen at an equivalent incidence in placebo-treated patients, were:- nausea, insomnia, dry mouth, somnolence, dizziness, constipation, sweating, nervousness, asthenia and abnormal ejaculation/orgasm.

Other adverse events occurring in at least 3% of patients and more frequently (greater than 1% difference) with venlafaxine than with placebo, were:- anorexia, abnormal vision/accommodation, impotence, vomiting, tremor, abnormal dreams, vasodilatation, hypertension, rash, agitation, hypertonia and paraesthesia.

The occurrence of most of these adverse events was dose-related, and the majority of them decreased in intensity and frequency over time. They generally did not lead to cessation of treatment.

In clinical studies the incidence of nausea was lower, and the adaptation to nausea appeared to be improved, with Efexor XL compared with Efexor Tablets. A two- to three-fold reduction in the incidence and severity of nausea was observed with Efexor XL when compared with Efexor Tablets in studies with non-depressed subjects.

Of the patients who received venlafaxine in all premarketing trials, 2.2% were judged to have had clinically significant blood pressure increases compared with 0.4% of placebo-treated patients. In studies with Efexor Tablets, the increases in blood pressure were dose-related. In general, patients treated with ≤ 200 mg per day showed minor increases, while in a short-term dose ranging study, the highest dose (300–375 mg/day) was associated with mean increases in supine diastolic blood pressure of approximately 4 mm Hg by week 4, and 7 mm Hg by week 6. The presence of treated hypertension or elevated blood pressure at baseline did not seem to predispose patients to further increases during venlafaxine therapy.

Postural hypotension was observed, and considered clinically significant in 0.4% of patients treated with Efexor Tablets and 0.8% of comparator-treated patients. As with other antidepressants, this effect may be more apparent in the elderly.

Reversible increases in liver enzymes were seen during clinical trials in a small number of patients (0.5%) treated with Efexor Tablets.

Alterations in serum cholesterol are seen in some patients treated with venlafaxine. A mean increase of 0.07 mmol/litre from baseline was observed in patients treated with Efexor Tablets, a change of unknown clinical significance.

Clinically significant weight gain or loss was seen in less than 1% of patients treated with venlafaxine during all premarketing trials.

Cases of hyponatraemia have rarely been reported

with antidepressants including SSRIs, usually in the elderly and in patients taking diuretics or who are otherwise volume depleted. Similarly, cases of hyponatraemia have been reported rarely with Efexor Tablets, usually in the elderly, which have resolved on discontinuation of the drug.

Withdrawal reactions reported on abrupt cessation, dose reduction or tapering of venlafaxine include fatigue, headache, nausea or vomiting, dizziness, dry mouth, diarrhoea, insomnia, nervousness, confusion, parasthesia, sweating and vertigo. The majority of symptoms experienced on withdrawal of Efexor XL are non-serious and self-limiting. (See also *Posology and method of administration*).

Overdose: Among the patients treated with Efexor XL in premarketing evaluations, there were 2 reports of acute overdosage, either alone or in combination with other drugs. One patient took a combination of 6 g of Efexor XL and 2.5 mg of lorazepam. This patient was hospitalised, treated symptomatically, and recovered without any untoward effects. The other patient took 2.85 g of Efexor XL. This patient reported paraesthesia in all four limbs, but recovered without sequelae.

In post-marketing experience with Efexor Tablets, electrocardiogram changes (e.g. prolongation of QT interval, bundle branch block, QRS prolongation), sinus and ventricular tachycardia, bradycardia and seizures have been reported in association with overdosage of Efexor Tablets, either alone or in combination with other drugs and/or alcohol. Such events are rare and usually resolve spontaneously.

Management of Overdosage–Ensure an adequate airway, oxygenation and ventilation. Monitoring of cardiac rhythm and vital signs is recommended. General supportive and symptomatic measures are also recommended. Use of activated charcoal, induction of emesis, or gastric lavage should be considered. No specific antidotes for venlafaxine are known.

The haemodialysis clearance of venlafaxine and its main metabolite, ODV, are low. Therefore, they are not considered dialysable.

Pharmacological properties Venlafaxine is a structurally novel antidepressant which is chemically unrelated to tricyclic, tetracyclic, or other available antidepressants. It is a racemate with two active enantiomers.

Pharmacodynamic properties: The mechanism of venlafaxine's antidepressant action in humans is believed to be associated with its potentiation of neurotransmitter activity in the central nervous system. Preclinical studies have shown that venlafaxine and its major metabolite, ODV, are potent inhibitors of serotonin and noradrenaline reuptake. Venlafaxine also weakly inhibits dopamine uptake. Studies in animals show that tricyclic antidepressants may reduce β-adrenergic responsiveness following chronic administration. In contrast, venlafaxine and ODV reduce β-adrenergic responsiveness after both acute (single dose) and chronic administration. Venlafaxine and ODV are very similar with respect to their overall action on neurotransmitter reuptake.

Venlafaxine has virtually no affinity for rat brain muscarinic cholinergic, H_1-histaminergic or α_1-adrenergic receptors *in vitro*. Pharmacological activity at these receptors may be related to various side effects seen with other antidepressant drugs, such as anticholinergic, sedative and cardiovascular side effects.

Venlafaxine does not possess monoamine oxidase (MAO) inhibitory activity.

In vitro studies revealed that venlafaxine has virtually no affinity for opiate, benzodiazepine, phencyclidine (PCP), or N-methyl-d-aspartic acid (NMDA) receptors. It has no significant central nervous system (CNS) stimulant activity in rodents. In primate drug discrimination studies, venlafaxine showed no significant stimulant or depressant abuse liability.

Pharmacokinetic properties: At least 92% of a single oral dose of venlafaxine is absorbed. After administration of Efexor XL, the peak plasma concentrations of venlafaxine and ODV are attained within 6.0±1.5 and 8.8±2.2 hours, respectively. The rate of absorption of venlafaxine from the Efexor XL capsules is slower than its rate of elimination. Therefore, the apparent elimination half-life of venlafaxine following administration of Efexor XL capsules (15±6 hours) is actually the absorption half-life instead of the true disposition half-life (5±2 hours) observed following administration of an immediate release tablet.

When equal daily doses of venlafaxine were administered as either the immediate release tablet, or the extended release capsule, the exposure (AUC, area under the concentration curve) to both venlafaxine and ODV was similar for the two treatments, and the fluctuation in plasma concentrations was slightly lower following treatment with the Efexor XL capsule. Therefore, the Efexor XL capsule provides a slower rate of absorption, but the same extent of absorption (i.e. AUC), as the Efexor immediate release tablet.

Venlafaxine undergoes extensive first-pass metabolism in the liver, primarily by CYP2D6, to the major metabolite ODV. Venlafaxine is also metabolised to N-desmethylvenlafaxine, catalysed by CYP3A3/4, and to other minor metabolites.

Venlafaxine and its metabolites are excreted primarily through the kidneys. Approximately 87% of a venlafaxine dose is recovered in the urine within 48 hours as either unchanged venlafaxine, unconjugated ODV, conjugated ODV, or other minor metabolites.

Administration of Efexor XL with food has no effect on the absorption of venlafaxine, or on the subsequent formation of ODV.

Subject age and sex do not significantly affect the pharmacokinetics of venlafaxine. No accumulation of venlafaxine or ODV has been observed during chronic administration in healthy subjects.

Preclinical safety data: Studies with venlafaxine in rats and mice revealed no evidence of carcinogenesis. Venlafaxine was not mutagenic in a wide range of *in vitro* and *in vivo* tests.

Pharmaceutical particulars
List of excipients: Microcrystalline cellulose, ethylcellulose, hydroxypropyl methylcellulose, gelatin, red and yellow iron oxides (E172), titanium dioxide (E171) and printing ink.

Incompatibilities: None known

Shelf Life: Three years

Special precautions for storage: Store in a dry place at room temperature (at or below 25°C).

Nature and contents of container: PVC/ACLAR/aluminium foil blister packs of 28 capsules.

Instructions for use/handling: Not applicable

Marketing authorisation numbers
Efexor XL 75 mg PL 00011/0223
Efexor XL 150 mg PL 00011/0224

Date of first authorisation 5 August 1997

Date of (Partial) Revision of the Text June 1998

Legal Category POM.

EQUAGESIC*

Presentation Equagesic tablets are three layer, flat bevel-edged tablets, 12.0 mm in diameter. A white layer is sandwiched between a yellow layer and a pink layer. The yellow face is marked WYETH and the pink face is plain.

Each tablet contains:
Ethoheptazine citrate 75 mg
Meprobamate BP 150 mg
Aspirin BP 250 mg

Uses Equagesic is an analgesic with muscle-relaxant properties indicated for short-term symptomatic treatment of pain occurring in musculoskeletal disorders.

Dosage and administration
Route of administration: Oral

Dosage: Adults: Two tablets three or four times daily as needed for the relief of pain.

Elderly: The elderly may respond to lower doses and half the normal adult dose or less may be sufficient.

Children: Not recommended for children.

Contra-indications, Warnings, etc.
Contra-indications:

1. Equagesic should not be used in patients known to be hypersensitive to the active ingredients or to compounds related to meprobamate such as carisoprodol or carbromal.
2. Meprobamate should not be used in patients with a known propensity for dependence on drugs including alcohol and in patients susceptible to attacks of acute intermittent porphyria.
3. Aspirin should not be used in patients with active peptic ulceration, haemophilia or in renal disease.
4. Equagesic should not be used during lactation.
5. Equagesic should not be used concurrently with coumarin-type anticoagulants.
6. Pregnancy: there is no evidence as to drug safety in human pregnancy nor is there evidence that it is free from hazard. Do not use during pregnancy, especially during the first three months, unless there are compelling reasons.
7. Do not give to children under 12 unless your doctor tells you to, because of a possible association of aspirin with Reye's Syndrome.

Precautions and warnings:

1. This product may cause drowsiness. Patients receiving this medication should not drive or operate machinery unless the drug has been shown not to interfere with physical or mental ability.
2. Meprobamate may increase the effects of concurrently administered central nervous system depressants including alcohol.
3. The concurrent use of CNS depressant drugs should be avoided in hepatic or renal insufficiency.
4. Meprobamate may induce seizures in epileptic patients, and meprobamate withdrawal may precipitate convulsions.
5. Like barbiturates, meprobamate causes induction of liver enzymes, so that the availability and blood levels of drugs given concurrently that are metabolised in the liver may be affected. These include the following: systemic steroids (including oral contraceptives), phenytoin, griseofulvin, rifampicin, phenothiazines (such as chlorpromazine) and tricyclic antidepressants. The clinical importance of the effect of enzyme induction by meprobamate on concurrently administered agents has not been established.
6. Individual response in overdosage with meprobamate is variable but in some cases the symptoms may be severe. It is therefore advisable that caution should be observed in prescribing drugs which contain meprobamate to patients with depression or to others who may be liable to suicidal ideation or intent.
7. Some degree of dependence may occasionally occur with meprobamate in certain cases if dosage recommendations are exceeded with withdrawal symptoms on sudden discontinuation. This is more likely in individuals with emotionally unstable personalities if the drug is taken over long periods, or in others liable to alcohol or other drug dependence. Treatment in these cases should be withdrawn gradually.

   Equagesic is recommended for use for short periods only and therefore the risk of dependence occurring with this product is very small.

Aspirin:

a) Aspirin may prolong labour and contribute to maternal and neonatal bleeding and is best avoided at term. It may precipitate bronchospasm and may induce attacks of asthma in susceptible subjects. Aspirin should only be used with great caution in patients with a history of peptic ulceration.

b) Concomitant administration with certain other medications such as corticosteroids or oral hypoglycaemics may require adjustment of dosage of the various drugs. The action of uricosuric agents may be inhibited.

Overdosage: Meprobamate: Acute poisoning with meprobamate produces coma, shock, vasomotor and respiratory collapse. Very few suicide attempts have proved successful and documented fatal doses have ranged from 12 g to 47.6 g. Recovery has occurred after ingestion of similar large amounts (20–40 g). Gastric lavage is only effective within a short period of drug ingestion as meprobamate is rapidly absorbed from the gastrointestinal tract. Blood concentrations may be reduced by a regime of forced alkaline diuresis or haemodialysis. Respiration may require assistance.

Aspirin: Overdosage with aspirin will result in the appearance of the signs and symptoms of salicylism. Treatment of aspirin poisoning is largely symptomatic and directed towards correction of the acid-base balance and electrolyte balance of the plasma.

Side effects: Drowsiness, dizziness and nausea may be experienced with Equagesic but these symptoms usually disappear as treatment continues. Ataxia, vomiting, hypotension, paraesthesia and paradoxical excitement may also occur.

Hypersensitivity reactions have been reported in about 2% of patients being treated with meprobamate. These reactions include skin rashes, and may arise after one to four doses of the drug. They may be generalised or local, and include urticaria, itchy maculopapular rashes or erythema. Severe systemic reactions with shaking, chills and fever, nausea and vomiting, hypotension and collapse have occasionally occurred.

Blood disorders, including non-thrombocytopenic purpura, and rarely, thrombocytopenia, agranulocytosis, aplastic anaemia and pancytopenia have occurred. Rarely reported reactions, usually occurring as part of a generalised hypersensitivity reaction, include hyperpyrexia, angioneurotic oedema, bronchospasm, oliguria and anuria. Anaphylaxis, erythema multiforme, exfoliative dermatitis, stomatitis, proctitis, Stevens Johnson syndrome and bullous dermatitis have also been reported.

Hypersensitivity reactions to aspirin may manifest themselves as asthma, skin reactions and shock. Aspirin may induce gastrointestinal haemorrhage, which is occasionally severe but in most cases blood loss is not significant.

Pharmaceutical precautions Store in a cool dry place. Keep tightly closed. Where necessary dispense Equagesic tablets into suitable well-closed glass bottles.

Legal category POM CD (Sch 3)

Package quantities Bottles of 100 tablets

Further information Safety and efficacy have not been established beyond short-term use.

Product Licence Number 0011/5009R

HibTITER*

Qualitative and quantitative composition

Active Substance	*Quantity per 0.5 ml dose*
Haemophilus influenzae type b (strain PBCC197) oligosaccharide:	10 µg
conjugated with Diphtheria CRM_{197} protein:	25 µg

HibTITER is a sterile solution of oligosaccharides that are derived via chemical depolymerization from highly purified capsular polysaccharide, polyribosyl-ribitol-phosphate (PRP), isolated from *Haemophilus influenzae* type b. The oligosaccharides are activated selectively and are bound covalently to the CRM_{197} protein. The CRM_{197} protein is a non toxic variant of the diphtheria toxin.

Pharmaceutical form Solution for injection.

Clinical Particulars

Therapeutic indications: HibTITER Haemophilus b vaccine conjugated with (diphtheria CRM_{197} protein) is indicated for the immunisation of infants and children of 2 months to 5 years of age against invasive diseases caused by *Haemophilus influenzae* type b (Hib).

Posology and method of administration:

Posology: A primary series may be started at the age of 2 months or later. It should consist of 3 injections given at intervals of 4 to 8 weeks.

An alternative schedule is of 2 injections given at intervals of 6 to 8 weeks.

For long term protection a booster dose may be administered in the second year of life, especially for those children vaccinated with the two dose schedule.

For children between the age of 6 months and 12 months who have not previously been immunised, a two dose primary series with an interval of 6 to 8 weeks may be sufficient.

For children aged one year or older, not vaccinated previously, a single dose may be administered to achieve protection.

HibTITER may be given to premature infants according to their chronological age.

Method of Administration: HibTITER is for intramuscular injection.

Contra-indications: Hypersensitivity to any component of the vaccine, including diphtheria toxoid.

As with other vaccines, the administration of HibTITER should be postponed in subjects suffering from acute severe febrile illness.

Special warnings and precautions for use: HibTITER is for intramuscular use only. The vaccine should not be injected intradermally or intravenously, since the safety and immunogenicity of these routes have not been evaluated.

As with all injectable vaccines, appropriate medical treatment and supervision should always be readily available in case of a rare anaphylactic event following the administration of the vaccine.

HibTITER will not protect against *H. influenzae* other than b strains or other micro-organisms that cause meningitis or septic disease.

If the vaccine is used in persons deficient in producing antibody, whether due to genetic defect or immunosuppressive therapy, the expected immune response may not be obtained.

Human Immunodeficiency Virus (HIV) infection is not considered as a contra-indication for HibTITER.

Interaction with other medicaments and other forms of interaction: No impairment of the antibody response to the individual antigens has been seen when HibTITER is given at the same time but at separate sites as diphtheria and tetanus toxoid and pertussis vaccine adsorbed plus oral polio vaccine to children of 2 to 20 months of age, or measles, mumps and rubella vaccine to children of 14 to 16 months of age.

Pregnancy and lactation: As HibTITER is not intended for use in adults, information on the safety of the vaccine when used during pregnancy and lactation is not available.

Effects on ability to drive and use machines: Not applicable.

Undesirable effects: Local erythema, warmth or swelling have been reported at the site of injection. As with all injections local pain may occur.

Systemic effects which have been reported following the administration of HibTITER include fever, headache, malaise, irritability, prolonged crying, loss of appetite, vomiting, diarrhoea, restless sleep and hypersensitivity reactions (including anaphylactic reactions and rash).

Erythema multiforme, Guillain-Barré Syndrome and convulsions have been observed following the administration of *Haemophilus influenzae* type b polysaccharide or conjugate vaccines. A cause and effect relationship has not been established.

Overdose: There is no experience with overdosage of HibTITER.

Pharmacological properties

Pharmacotherapeutic group: Haemophilus Influenzae b vaccine, purified antigen conjugated ATC code: J07AG01.

Pharmacodynamic properties: The immune response is predominantly IgG, subclass IgG 1. In addition, a study has shown that when evaluated in an *in vitro* complement-mediated bactericidal assay, 95% and more of the infants sera had bactericidal activity after two and three doses of vaccine, respectively.

Pharmacokinetic properties: The antibody response after each immunisation with HibTITER follows classical T-cell dependent kinetics. No studies have been performed to determine the fate of the HibTITER vaccine at this site of injection or in the circulatory system. However, it is known from human studies that the vaccine and/or its hydrolysis products are partially excreted through the kidneys.

Preclinical safety data: Not applicable.

Pharmaceutical particulars

List of excipients: Sodium chloride, water for injection.

Incompatibilities: No incompatibilities were observed or reported.

Shelf Life: The expiry date of the vaccine is indicated on the label and packaging.

The shelf life is 24 months.

Special precautions for storage: HibTITER should be stored at +2°C to +8°C.

Do not freeze. Discard if the vaccine has been frozen.

Nature and Contents of Container: HibTITER is clear and colourless and presented in a monodose glass vial. Pack sizes of 1 and 10.

Instructions for use, handling and disposal: The vaccine should be inspected visually for any particulate matter and/or variation of physical aspect prior to administration. Before administration the vaccine should be well shaken.

Marketing authorisation number PL 0095 0266

Date of approval/revision of SPC March 1998

Legal category POM

ISOVORIN* ▼ Solution for Injection

Qualitative and quantitative composition Calcium levofolinate (INN: calcium levofolinate) equivalent to 1.00% w/v (10 mg/ml) of levoleucovorin (levofolinic acid).

The product is presented as vials containing the 25 mg, 50 mg or 175 mg of levofolinic acid (as calcium levofolinate) in 2.5 ml, 5 ml or 17.5 ml of solution respectively.

Pharmaceutical form Solution for injection.

Clinical particulars

Therapeutic indications: Calcium Levofolinate Rescue: Calcium levofolinate is used to diminish the toxicity and counteract the action of folic acid antagonists such as methotrexate in cytotoxic therapy. This procedure is known as Calcium Levofolinate Rescue.

Advanced Colorectal Cancer–Enhancement of 5-Fluorouracil (5-FU) Cytotoxicity: Calcium levofolinate increases the thymine depleting effects of 5-FU resulting in enhanced cytotoxic activity. Combination regimens of 5-fluorouracil and levofolinate give greater efficacy compared to 5-FU given alone.

Posology and method of administration: For single use only.

Calcium Levofolinate Rescue: Adults, Children and the Elderly: Calcium Levofolinate Rescue therapy should commence 24 hours after the beginning of methotrexate infusion. Dosage regimes vary depending upon the dose of methotrexate administered. In general, the calcium levofolinate should be administered at a dose of 7.5 mg (approximately 5 mg/m²) every 6 hours for 10 doses by intramuscular injection, bolus intravenous injection or intravenous infusion, (refer to *Posology and method of administration–Colorectal Cancer* for information concerning use of calcium levofolinate with infusion fluids). **Do not administer calcium levofolinate intrathecally.**

Where overdose of methotrexate is suspected, the dose of calcium levofolinate should be at least 50% of the offending dose of methotrexate and should be administered in the first hour. In the case of intravenous administration, no more than 160 mg of calcium levofolinate should be injected per minute due to the calcium content of the solution.

In addition to calcium levofolinate administration, measures to ensure the prompt excretion of methotrexate are important as part of Calcium Levofolinate Rescue therapy. These measures include:

a. Alkalinisation of urine so that the urinary pH is greater than 7.0 before methotrexate infusion (to increase solubility of methotrexate and its metabolites).

b. Maintenance of urine output of 1800-2000 cc/m²/24 hr by increased oral or intravenous fluids on days 2, 3 and 4 following methotrexate therapy.

c. Plasma methotrexate concentration, BUN and creatinine should be measured on days 2, 3 and 4.

These measures must be continued until the plasma methotrexate level is less than 10^{-7} molar (0.1µM).

Delayed methotrexate excretion may be seen in some patients. This may be caused by a third space accumulation (as seen in ascites or pleural effusion for example), renal insufficiency or inadequate hydration. Under such circumstances, higher doses of calcium levofolinate or prolonged administration may be indicated. Dosage and administration guidelines for these patients are given in Table 1. Patients who experience delayed early methotrexate elimination are likely to develop reversible renal failure.

Colorectal Cancer: Enhancement of 5-FU Cytotoxicity: Adults and the elderly:

Administration: The 175 mg in 17.5 ml vial of Calcium Levofolinate Solution for Injection should be used to administer the high doses of calcium levofolinate required in combination regimens.

When used in combination regimens with 5-FU, calcium levofolinate should only be given by the intravenous route. The agents should not be mixed together. Each vial of calcium levofolinate 175 mg contains 0.7 mEq (0.35 mmol) of calcium per vial and it is recommended that the solution is administered over not less than 3 minutes.

For intravenous infusion, the 175 mg in 17.5 ml Solution for Injection may be diluted with any of the following infusion fluids before use: Sodium Chloride 0.9%; Glucose 5%; Glucose 10%; Glucose 10% and Sodium Chloride 0.9% Injection; Compound Sodium Lactate Injection.

Calcium levofolinate should not be mixed together with 5-FU in the same infusion and, because of the risk of degradation, the giving set should be protected from light.

Dosage: Based on the available clinical evidence, the following regimen is effective in advanced colorectal carcinoma:

Calcium levofolinate given at a dose of 100 mg/m² by slow intravenous injection, followed immediately

TABLE 1: Dosage and Administration Guidelines for Calcium Levofolinate Rescue

Clinical Situation	*Laboratory Findings*	*Levofolinate Dosage and Duration*
Normal Methotrexate Elimination	*Serum methotrexate level approximately 10µM at 24 hours after administration, 1µM at 48 hours and less than 0.2µM at 72 hours.*	*7.5 mg IM or IV every 6 hours for 60 hours (10 doses starting at 24 hours after start of methotrexate infusion).*
Delayed Late Methotrexate Elimination	*Serum methotrexate level remaining above 0.2µM at 72 hours, and more than 0.05µM at 96 hours after administration.*	*Continue 7.5 mg IM or IV every 6 hours, until methotrexate level is less than 0.05µM.*
Delayed Early Methotrexate Elimination and/or Evidence of Acute Renal Injury	*Serum methotrexate level of 50µM or more at 24 hours or 5µM or more at 48 hours after administration, OR; a 100% or greater increase in serum creatinine level at 24 hours after methotrexate administration.*	*75 mg IV every 3 hours, until methotrexate level is less than 1µM; then 7.5 mg IV every 3 hours until methotrexate level is less than 0.05µM.*

by 5-FU at an initial dose of 370 mg/m² by intravenous injection. The injection of levofolinate should not be given more rapidly than over 3 minutes because of the calcium content of the solution. This treatment is repeated daily for 5 consecutive days. Subsequent courses may be given after a treatment-free interval of 21-28 days.

For the above regimen, modification of the 5-FU dosage and the treatment-free interval may be necessary depending on patient condition, clinical response and dose limiting toxicity. A reduction of calcium levofolinate dosage is not required. The number of repeat cycles used is at the discretion of the clinician.

On the basis of the available data, no specific dosage modifications are recommended in the use of the combination regimen with 5-FU in the elderly. However, particular care should be taken when treating elderly or debilitated patients as these patients are at increased risk of severe toxicity with this therapy (See *Special warnings and precautions for use*).

Children: There are no data available on the use of this combination in children.

Contra-indications: Calcium levofolinate should not be used for the treatment of pernicious anaemia or other megaloblastic anaemias where vitamin B_{12} is deficient.

Special warnings and precautions for use: Calcium levofolinate should only be used with methotrexate or 5-FU under the direct supervision of a clinician experienced in the use of cancer chemotherapeutic agents. When calcium levofolinate has been administered intrathecally, following intrathecal overdose of methotrexate, a death has been reported.

Interaction with other medicaments and other forms of interaction: Calcium levofolinate should not be given simultaneously with an anti-neoplastic folic acid antagonist, (e.g. methotrexate), to modify or abort clinical toxicity, as the therapeutic effect of the antagonist may be nullified. Concomitant calcium levofolinate will not however inhibit the antibacterial activity of other folic acid antagonists such as trimethoprim and pyrimethamine.

Folinates given in large amounts may counteract the antiepileptic effect of phenobarbitone, phenytoin and primidone and increase the frequency of seizures in susceptible patients.

Seizures and/or syncope have been reported rarely in cancer patients receiving leucovorin, usually in association with fluoropyrimidine administration and most commonly in those with CNS metastases or other predisposing factors; however a causal relationship has not been established.

Pregnancy and lactation: Reproduction studies have been performed in rats and rabbits at doses of at least 50 times the human dose. These studies have revealed no evidence of harm to the foetus due to calcium levofolinate. There are, however, no adequate and well controlled studies in pregnant women. Because animal reproduction studies are not always predictive of human response, calcium levofolinate should only be used in pregnant women if the potential benefit justifies the potential risk to the foetus.

It is not known whether calcium levofolinate is excreted in human milk. Because many drugs are excreted in human milk, caution should be exercised when calcium levofolinate is administered to a nursing mother.

Effects on ability to drive and use machines: None.

Undesirable effects: Adverse reactions to calcium levofolinate are rare but occasional pyrexial reactions have been reported following parenteral administration.

In the combination regimen with 5-FU, the toxicity profile of 5-FU is enhanced by calcium levofolinate. The most common manifestations are leucopenia, mucositis, stomatitis and/or diarrhoea which may be dose limiting. When calcium levofolinate and 5-FU are used in the treatment of colorectal cancer, the 5-FU dosage must be reduced more in cases of toxicity than when 5-FU is used alone. Toxicities observed in patients treated with the combination are qualitatively similar to those observed in patients treated with 5-FU alone. Gastrointestinal toxicities are observed more commonly and may be more severe or even life threatening. In severe cases, treatment is the withdrawal of 5-FU and calcium levofolinate and provision of supportive intravenous therapy. Elderly or debilitated patients are at a greater risk of severe toxicity with this therapy.

Overdose: There have been no reported sequelae in patients who have received significantly more calcium levofolinate than the recommended dosage. There is no specific antidote. In cases of overdose, patients should be given appropriate supportive care. Should overdose of the combination of 5-FU with calcium levofolinate occur, the overdose instructions for 5-FU should be followed.

Pharmacological properties

Pharmacodynamic properties: Levofolinate is the pharmacologically active isomer of 5-formyltetrahydrofolic acid. Levofolinate does not require reduction by the enzyme dihydrofolate reductase in order to participate in reactions utilising folates as a source of 'one carbon' moieties. Levofolinate is actively and passively transported across cell membranes.

Administration of levofolinate can 'rescue' normal cells and thereby prevent toxicity of folic acid antagonists such as methotrexate which act by inhibiting dihydrofolate reductase.

Levofolinate can enhance the therapeutic and toxic effects of fluoropyrimidines used in cancer therapy such as 5-fluorouracil. 5-fluorouracil is metabolised to 5-fluoro-2'-deoxyuridine-5'-monophosphate (FDUMP), which binds to and inhibits thymidylate synthase. Levofolinate is readily converted to another reduced folate, 5, 10-methylenetetrahydrofolate, which acts to stabilise the binding of FDUMP to thymidylate synthase and thereby enhances the inhibition of this enzyme.

Levofolinate is also effective in the treatment of megaloblastic anaemias due to folate deficiencies.

Pharmacokinetic properties: When levofolinate is injected intravenously it is 100% bioavailable.

The pharmacokinetics of levofolinate after intravenous administration of a 15 mg dose were studied in healthy male volunteers. After rapid intravenous administration, serum total tetrahydrofolate (total-THF) concentrations reached a mean peak of 1722ng/ml. Serum levo-5-methyl-THF concentrations reached a mean peak of 275ng/ml and the mean time to peak concentration was 0.9 hours. The mean half-life for total-THF and levo-5-methyl-THF was 5.1 and 6.8 hours respectively.

The distribution and plasma levels of levofolinate following intramuscular administration have not been established.

The distribution in tissue and body fluids and protein binding have not been determined.

In vivo, levofolinate is converted to levo-5-methyltetrahydrofolic acid (levo-5-methyl-THF), the primary circulating form of active reduced folate. Levofolinate and levo-5-methyl-THF are polyglutamated intracellularly by the enzyme folylpolyglutamate synthetase. Folylpolyglutamates are active and participate in biochemical pathways that require reduced folate.

Levofolinate and levo-5-methyl-THF are excreted renally.

Due to the inherent lack of levofolinate toxicity, the influence of impaired renal or hepatic function on levofolinate disposition was not evaluated.

Preclinical safety data: The pre-clinical data raises no concerns for the clinical uses indicated.

Pharmaceutical particulars

List of excipients: Sodium Chloride, Water for Injection, Hydrochloric Acid, Sodium Hydroxide

Incompatibilities: Calcium levofolinate should not be mixed together with 5-FU in the same intravenous injection or infusion.

Shelf life: 24 months.

Special precautions for storage: Store Isovorin Solution for Injection under refrigerated conditions (2–8°C) in original containers. Protect from light.

Discard any unused products.

When Isovorin Solution for Injection is diluted with the recommended infusion fluids, the resulting solutions are intended for immediate use but may be stored for up to 24 hours under refrigerated conditions (2–8°C). Because of the risk of degradation, reconstituted solutions should be protected from light prior to use if necessary.

Nature and contents of container: Type I amber glass vials each containing the equivalent of 25 mg, 50 mg or 175 mg of calcium levofolinate in 2.5 ml, 5 ml or 17.5 ml of solution respectively. Isovorin is packed in boxes of 1 vial.

Instructions for use and handling: See *Posology and method of administration* and *Special precautions for storage*.

Marketing authorisation number PL 0011/0235

Date of approval/revision March 1998

Legal Category POM

LEDERFEN*

Presentation

Lederfen 300 mg Tablets: Light blue, film coated, capsule shaped tablets, each containing 300 mg of fenbufen and engraved 'WY 050' on one side.

Lederfen 300 mg Capsules: Dark blue capsules, each containing 300 mg of fenbufen and printed 'WY 052' on both the cap and body.

Lederfen 450 mg Tablets: Light blue, film coated, lozenge shaped tablets each containing 450 mg of fenbufen and engraved 'WY 051' on one side.

Uses Lederfen is a non-steroidal, anti-inflammatory drug (NSAID) indicated for the symptomatic treatment of rheumatoid arthritis, osteoarthritis, ankylosing spondylitis and acute musculoskeletal disorders.

Dosage and administration

Adults: 300 mg Tablets or Capsules: One in the morning and two at night.

450 mg Tablets: One in the morning and one at night.

Elderly: Clinical studies conducted in elderly patients and patients with mild to moderate renal impairment have shown that the pharmacokinetics of Lederfen are not affected to any clinically relevant extent and the standard adult dose may be used starting with the lowest recommended dose (also see *Precautions*).

Children: Not recommended for administration to children under the age of 14.

Contra-indications, warnings, etc.

Contra-indications: Active or suspected peptic ulcer or a history of peptic ulceration.

Hypersensitivity to propionic acid anti-inflammatory drugs, or aspirin.

Since the potential exists for cross-sensitivity, Lederfen should not be used in patients in whom attacks of asthma, urticaria or acute rhinitis are precipitated by aspirin or other NSAIDs.

Precautions: As with other NSAIDs, Lederfen should be used with great caution in patients with a history of peptic or intestinal ulceration, and only after other forms of treatment have been carefully considered. Gastrointestinal ulceration, haematemesis or melaena may occur with or without warning symptoms or a previous history.

Lederfen should be used with caution in patients with cardiac failure, hypertension, bronchial asthma or a history of bronchial asthema.

It is unnecessary to modify the dosage of Lederfen in mild to moderate renal impairment, however, in common with other NSAIDs, there have been a few reports of deterioration in renal function associated with Lederfen therapy. In view of this, doses in patients with pre-existing renal disease or impaired cardiac or hepatic function should be kept to the minimum necessary to achieve the desired therapeutic effect and renal function should be monitored. Treatment of the elderly should begin with the lowest recommended dose.

Lederfen should not be used concomitantly with other NSAIDs. See *Interactions* Section for precautions on use with other drugs.

Use in Pregnancy and Lactation: Lederfen should not be prescribed during pregnancy or lactation, unless there are compelling reasons for doing so and only after careful consideration of the risk/benefit ratio. If absolutely necessary, the lowest effective dose should be used.

Metabolites of fenbufen have been detected at low concentrations in milk of lactating women. Because of possible adverse effects of prostaglandin-inhibiting drugs on neonates, use in nursing mothers should be avoided.

Warnings and adverse effects: Skin rashes including erythema, maculo-papular, morbilliform and urticaria are the most commonly encountered adverse reactions. Stevens-Johnson syndrome has occasionally been reported. Angioedema, facial oedema, erythema multiforme, epidermal necrolysis, periorbital oedema, vasculitis, purpura, and photosensitivity reactions have all been occasionally reported.

Lederfen treatment should be discontinued immediately on appearance of a rash. Anti-histamine therapy may help any pruritis associated with the rash. The rash is more common in women and in patients with the rare diagnoses of sero-negative rheumatoid arthritis and psoriatic arthritis. If rash does occur, it will most commonly be seen within the second week of therapy but is very unlikely to occur after two weeks of therapy. The median duration of therapy before a rash occurs is ten days. 80% of eruptions will have resolved after one week of discontinuation of therapy and by two weeks nearly 100% of eruptions will have resolved.

NSAIDs have been reported to cause nephrotoxicity in various forms and their use can lead to interstitial nephritis, nephrotic syndrome and renal failure.

In common with other NSAIDs, allergic interstitial lung disorders (allergic alveolitis, or pulmonary eosinophilia) have been reported rarely; these reactions have resolved within 4–6 weeks of discontinuing therapy.

Vomiting, dyspepsia and nausea are the most commonly encountered gastrointestinal effects. Abdominal pain, diarrhoea, gastritis, haematemesis, gastrointestinal haemorrhage, melaena, constipation, stomatitis, ulcerative stomatitis and anorexia have also occasionally been reported.

Oedema, dizziness, depression, sleep disturbances

including vivid dreams, paraesthesia, headache, drowsiness, fatigue, fever and malaise have also occasionally been reported. Increased perspiration and flushing occur rarely. Hypersensitivity reaction such as anaphylaxis and bronchospasm have been reported rarely.

In common with other NSAIDs, disturbances of vision and tinnitus have occasionally been reported.

Slight decreases in blood leucocytes, haemoglobin and haematocrit as well as slight increases in prothrombin time and eosinophils have occasionally been recorded. Haematological effects such as agranulocytosis, thrombocytopenia, granulocytopenia, aplastic anaemia, pancytopenia and haemolytic anaemia have been reported rarely. Transient elevations in values of liver function tests have occurred in some patients. Hepatic disorders including hepatitis and jaundice have been reported rarely.

As Lederfen may induce disturbances of vision or dizziness, patients should be warned not to operate machinery or drive motor vehicles until they know that they are not adversely affected.

Drug interactions: Lederfen is strongly protein bound–prescribers should be aware of the consequences of increased or decreased blood levels of either drug if Lederfen is administered with other protein bound drugs such as sulphonylureas, methotrexate, salicylates, hypoglycaemics etc.

Caution should be exercised if NSAIDs and methotrexate are administered within 24 hours of each other, since NSAIDs may increase methotrexate plasma levels resulting in increased toxicity.

In common with other NSAIDs, Lederfen when administered concurrently with quinolone antibiotics may cause an increased incidence of quinolone CNS side-effects such as convulsions.

Quinolones should not be administered concurrently with Lederfen.

Lederfen produces minor prolongation of prothrombin time in patients taking warfarin. These changes are unlikely to be clinically significant, but patients previously stabilised on oral anticoagulant therapy should be monitored for changes in prothrombin time.

Increases in serum lithium have been reported with some NSAIDs. Serum lithium levels should be monitored if Lederfen is added to therapy for patients previously stabilised on lithium.

Concomitant administration of Lederfen with cardiac glycosides may exacerbate heart failure, reduced glomerular filtration rate and increase plasma-cardiac glycoside concentrations.

The manufacturer of mifepristone recommends that NSAIDs like Lederfen should not be administered until 8–12 days after the administration of mifespristone.

Concomitant administration of Lederfen with cyclosporin may increase the risk of renal toxicity.

Concomitant administration of corticosteroids may increase the risk of gastrointestinal toxicity.

Overdosage: Experience of Lederfen overdosage is limited. There is no specific antidote. Gastric lavage should be performed if appropriate. Otherwise, management should be symptomatic and supportive.

Pharmaceutical precautions Store in the original container at room temperature (below 25°C).

Legal category POM

Package quantities
300 mg Tablets and Capsules: Blister packs of 84 tablets/capsules.
450 mg Tablets: Blister packs of 56 tablets.

Further information Fenbufen is a pro-drug. It is converted into active metabolites following absorption.

Product licence numbers

Lederfen 300 mg Tablets	0095/0081
Lederfen 300 mg Capsules	0095/0043
Lederfen 450 mg Tablets	0095/0092

LEDERMYCIN*

Presentation *Capsules 150 mg:* Each two-piece, hard shell capsule, with a peach coloured body and a dark red cap, printed Lederle 9123 contains 150 mg of demeclocycline hydrochloride.

Uses 1. For the treatment of infections caused by tetracycline-sensitive organisms. For example, Ledermycin is highly effective in the treatment of infections caused by *Borrellia recurrentis* (relapsing fever), *Calymmatobacterium granulomatis* (granuloma inguinale), *Chlamydia* species (psittacosis, lymphogranuloma venereum, trachoma, inclusion conjunctivitis), *Francisella tularensis* (tularaemia), *Haemophilus ducreyi* (chancroid), *Leptospira* (meningitis, jaundice), *Mycoplasma pneumoniae* (non-gonococcal urethritis), *Pseumomonas mallei* and *Pseudomallei* (glanders and melioidosis), *Rickettsiae* (typhus fever, Q fever, rocky mountain spotted fever), *Vibrio* species (cholera). It is also highly effective, alone or in combination with streptomycin, in the treatment of infections due to *Brucella* species (brucellosis), and *Yersinia pestis* (bubonic plague). Severe acne vulgaris.

Other sensitive organisms include: *Actinomyces israelii, Bacillus anthracis* (pneumonia), *Clostridium* species (gas gangrene, tetanus), *Entamoeba histolytica* (dysentery), *Neisseria gonorrhoeae*, and anaerobic species, *Treponema pallidum* and *pertenue* (syphilis and yaws).

2. For the treatment of chronic hyponatraemia associated with the syndrome of inappropriate secretion of antidiuretic hormone (SIADH) secondary to malignant disease, where water restriction is ineffective, and the patient does not have concomitant cirrhosis.

Dosage and administration
1. *For antibiotic use: Adults:* 600 mg daily in two or four divided doses. For primary atypical pneumonia the average daily dose is 900 mg in three divided doses for six days.

Elderly: Use with caution in elderly patients. See Contra-indications and Warnings.

Children: Not recommended for children under 12 years of age.

2. *For the treatment of chronic hyponatraemia due to SIADH: (Adults only)*
Initially: 900–1,200 mg daily in divided doses.
Maintenance dose: 600–900 mg daily in divided doses.

Ledermycin should be swallowed whole with plenty of fluid while sitting or standing. Doses should be taken an hour before or two hours after meals and antibiotic therapy should be continued for one to three days after characteristic symptoms or fever have subsided. The incidence of rheumatic fever or glomerulonephritis following streptococcal infections suggests that therapy of a streptococcal infection should be continued for eight full days even though symptoms have subsided.

Ledermycin therapy in the treatment of chronic hyponatraemia due to SIADH should not be withdrawn without commencing other methods of control.

Contra-indications, warnings, etc.
Contra-indications: A history of hypersensitivity to tetracyclines. Overt renal insufficiency. Children under 12 years of age. Use during pregnancy or during lactation in women breast feeding infants is contra-indicated (see also *Pregnancy and lactation*).

Warnings and Precautions: Ledermycin should be used with caution in patients with renal or hepatic dysfunction, or in conjunction with other potentially hepatotoxic or nephrotoxic drugs. Concurrent use with the anaesthetic methoxyflurane increases the risk of kidney failure. The anti-anabolic action of the tetracyclines may cause an increase in BUN. The treatment of chronic hyponatraemia may necessitate the administration of high doses of Ledermycin for prolonged periods, so increasing the potential for nephrotoxicity (manifested by rises in plasma urea and creatinine) and photo-allergic reactions.

Cross-resistance between tetracyclines may develop in micro-organisms and cross-sensitisation in patients. Ledermycin should be discontinued if there are signs/symptoms of overgrowth of resistant organisms including candida, enteritis, glossitis, stomatitis, vaginitis, pruritus ani or staphylococcal enterocolitis.

Lower doses are indicated in cases of renal impairment to avoid excessive systemic accumulation, and if therapy is prolonged, serum level determinations are advisable. Patients who have known liver disease should not receive more than 1 g daily. In long term therapy, periodic laboratory evaluation of organ systems, including haematopoietic, renal and thepatic studies should be performed.

Ledermycin has the greatest potential of the tetracycline analogues for causing photo-allergic reactions in hypersensitive persons. Such patients should be warned to avoid direct exposure to natural or artificial sunlight and to discontinue therapy at the first sign of skin discomfort.

Patients taking oral contraceptives should be warned that if diarrhoea or breakthrough bleeding occur there is a possibility of contraceptive failure.

Interactions: Ledermycin should not be used with penicillins. Tetracyclines depress plasma prothrombin activity and reduced doses of concomitant anti-coagulants may be required.

Absorption of Ledermycin is impaired by the concomitant administration of iron, calcium, zinc, magnesium and particularly aluminium salts commonly used as antacids.

The concomitant use of tetracyclines may reduce the efficacy of oral contraceptives; an increased incidence of breakthrough bleeding may also be experienced (see statement under *Warnings and Precautions*).

Use in pregnancy: Contra-indicated in pregnancy.

Results of animal studies indicate that tetracyclines cross the placenta, are found in foetal tissues and can have toxic effects on the developing foetus (often related to retardation of skeletal development). Evidence of embryotoxicity has also been noted in animals treated early in pregnancy. Ledermycin, therefore, should not be used in pregnancy unless considered essential.

The use of tetracyclines during tooth development (last half of pregnancy and children to the age of 12 years) may cause permanent discolouration of the teeth. This adverse reaction is more common during long term use of the drugs but has been observed following repeated short term courses. Enamel hypoplasia has also been reported.

Use in lactation: Contra-indicated during lactation in women breast feeding infants.

Tetracyclines have been found in the milk of lactating women who are taking a drug in this class. Permanent tooth discolouration may occur in the developing infant and enamel hypoplasia has been reported. Therefore, Ledermycin should not be administered to lactating women.

Side Effects: Gastro-intestinal disturbances including nausea, vomiting, diarrhoea and rarely dysphagia have been reported. There have been a few cases of oesophagitis and oesophageal ulceration in patients taking oral tetracyclines in solid dose form, usually where medication was taken immediately before retiring or with inadequate fluids. As with all antibiotics, overgrowth of resistant organisms may cause candidiasis, pseudomembranous colitis (*Clostridium difficile* overgrowth), glossitis, stomatitis, vaginitis, or staphylococcal enterocolitis. In common with other tetracyclines, transient increases in liver function test values, hepatitis, jaundice and hepatic failure have been reported rarely. A few cases of pancreatitis have been reported. The most commonly reported dermatological reaction is photosensitivity. Erythematous, and maculo-papular rashes, pruritus, bullous dermatoses, exfoliative dermatitis and skin discolouration have occurred occasionally but serious skin reactions are rare. Headache, dizziness, visual disturbances and rarely impaired hearing have been reported with tetracyclines and patients should be warned about the possible hazards of driving or operating machinery during treatment. Bulging fontanelles in infants and benign intracranial hypertension in juveniles and adults have been reported. Treatment should cease if evidence of raised intracranial pressure, such as severe or persistent headache or blurred vision are noted. While the condition and related symptoms usually resolve soon after discontinuation of the tetracycline, the possibility of permanent sequelae exists. There have been isolated cases of myasthenia. Hypersensitivity reactions, including urticaria, angioneurotic oedema, anaphylaxis, anaphylactoid purpura, pericarditis and exacerbation of systemic lupus erythematosus may occur. Renal dysfunction, especially in patients with pre-existing renal impairment, and rarely, acute renal failure or nephritis, have been reported with tetracyclines. Reversible nephrogenic diabetes insipidus can occur especially if treatment is prolonged and/or at high dosages. Haemolytic anaemia, thrombocytopenia, neutropenia, agranulocytosis, aplastic anaemia and eosinophilia have been reported rarely. When given over prolonged periods, tetracyclines have been reported to produce brown-black discolouration of the thyroid gland. No abnormalities of thyroid function are known to occur.

Overdosage: No specific antidote. Gastric lavage plus oral administration of milk or antacids. Maintain fluid and electrolyte balance.

Pharmaceutical precautions Ledermycin Capsules should be stored at controlled room temperature (below 25°C) in either the original pack or in containers which prevent access of light and moisture.

Legal category POM

Package quantities Bottles of 100

Further information Nil

Product licence number 0095/0052

LEDERSPAN* INJECTION 20 mg/ml
LEDERSPAN* INJECTION 5 mg/ml

Presentation *Suspension 20 mg/ml:* Vials containing a sterile suspension of 20 mg or 100 mg of micronised triamcinolone hexacetonide in 1 ml or 5 ml respectively of an aqueous vehicle with 0.9% benzyl alcohol as preservative.

Suspension 5 mg/ml: Vials containing a sterile suspension of 25 mg of micronised triamcinolone hexacetonide in 5 ml of an aqueous vehicle with 0.9% benzyl alcohol as preservative.

Uses Triamcinolone hexacetonide is a relatively insoluble corticosteroid (0.0003% at 25°C in water). It has a prolonged effect on tissue at the local injection site, the duration usually ranging from a few weeks to several months.

Lederspan 20 mg/ml (for intra-articular and intra-synovial administration): is indicated in the treatment of rheumatoid arthritis; osteoarthritis; synovitis and bursitis; tendinitis and tenosynovitis; and epicondylitis.

Lederspan 5 mg/ml (for intra-lesional and sub-lesional administration): is indicated in the treatment of cystic acne; alopecia areata, nummular and dyshydrotic eczema; granuloma annulare; keloids; lichen planus; discoid lupus erythematosus; localised neurodermatitis.

Dosage and administration *Adults (including the elderly): For intra-articular and intra-synovial use:* 2 mg–30 mg (0.1–1.5 ml), depending on the size of joint (or synovial space) to be injected, the degree of inflammation and the amount of fluid present. In general, large joints (such as knee, hips, shoulder) require 10–30 mg, whereas small joints (such as interphalangeal, metacarpophalangeal) require 2–6 mg. When much synovial fluid is present, aspiration may be performed before administering Lederspan. Subsequent dosage and frequency of injection can best be judged by clinical response. Since Lederspan provides prolonged activity, injections into a single joint or synovial space more frequently than every three to four weeks are not recommended. Repeated intra-articular injections should be as infrequent as possible, consistent with adequate patient care.

Strict asepsis is mandatory during administration. Topical ethyl chloride spray may be used locally before injection. Since micronised triamcinolone hexacetonide has been designed for ease of administration, a small-bore needle (including 24 gauge needles) may be used. The vial should be gently agitated to achieve uniform suspension before each use.

Lederspan triamcinolone hexacetonide 20 mg/ml sterile suspension is formulated to be diluted prior to intra-articular or intra-synovial injection. Sterile suspensions of Lederspan may be diluted with a local anaesthetic such as 1% or 2% lidocaine hydrochloride using formulations which do not contain parabens prior to intra-articular or intra-synovial injections. The optimum dilution for injection into a joint, 1:1, 1:2 or 1:4 should be determined depending on the dose to be administered. This dose is dependent on the size of the joint, degree of inflammation and amount of fluid present.

Lederspan may be administered by Dermojet and the Porton Injector.

For intra-lesional and sub-lesional use: The dosage is 0.5 mg or less per square inch of affected skin. No more than 5 mg should be injected at any one site, and no more than a total dosage of 30 mg should be exceeded regardless of the number of sites injected. If required, the injection can be repeated at one or two week intervals.

Strict asepsis is mandatory during administration. Topical ethyl chloride spray may be used locally before injection. Since micronised triamcinolone hexacetonide has been designed for ease of administration, a small-bore needle (including 24 gauge needles) may be used. The vial should be gently agitated to achieve uniform suspension before each use.

Lederspan triamcinolone hexacetonide 5 mg/ml sterile suspension is formulated to be diluted prior to intra-lesional injection. Sterile suspension of Lederspan may be diluted with a local anaesthetic such as 1% or 2% lidocaine hydrochloride using formulations which do not contain parabens prior to intra-lesional injections. Intra-lesional injections may also be diluted with aqueous vehicles such as Sodium Chloride Injection BP, Dextrose (5% and 10%) in Sodium Chloride for Injection, or Water for Injection BP. These solutions are used as isotonic vehicles. The additional osmotic effect of the drug when added to these vehicles should not be enough to produce any discomfort or tissue irritation when administered. The optimum dilution for intra-lesional use 1:1, 1:2 or 1:4 should be determined by the nature of the lesion, its size, the depth of injection, the volume needed, and the location of the lesion. In general, more superficial injections should be performed with a dilution of 1:4. Certain conditions, such as keloids, require a concentrated suspension (5 mg/ml), with variation in dose and dilution as dictated by the condition of the individual patient. Subsequent dosage, dilution and frequency of injections are best judged by the clinical response.

Lederspan may be administered by Dermojet and the Porton Injector.

Children: Not recommended.

Contra-indications, warnings, etc.
Contra-indications: Although active, latent or questionably healed tuberculosis, ocular herpes simplex and acute psychosis are generally considered to be absolute contra-indications to glucocorticoid therapy, the minimal systemic activity of triamcinolone hexacetonide after local injection might permit cautious use when indicated. The drug should not be used when there is history of hypersensitivity to any of the components of the formulation or when previous injections have produced local atrophy. Infected joints should not be injected with corticosteroids.

As with other glucocorticoid agents, relative contra-indications are active peptic ulcer, acute glomerulonephritis, myasthenia gravis, osteoporosis, fresh intestinal anastomoses, diverticulitis, thrombophlebitis, psychic disturbances, pregnancy, diabetes mellitus, hyperthyroidism, acute coronary artery disease, hypertension, limited cardiac reserve and local or systemic infections, including fungal and exanthematous diseases. The minimal systemic activity of this preparation, however, reduces the risks involved in its use in the presence of these conditions.

Precautions and side-effects: As with all glucocorticoids, an exacerbation of symptoms or 'flare-up' may occur following intra-articular or intra-synovial injections. Local atrophy, burning, flushing, pain and swelling may occur. Other local effects include abscess, erythema, skin discolouration or depigmentation, calcinosis and necrosis at the injection site. Anaphylactic reactions are very rare.

In addition, prolonged and repeated use in weight-bearing joints may result in further joint degeneration. This is probably related to premature use of still-diseased joints following relief of pain and other symptoms. Not more than two or three large joints should be treated simultaneously in the same patient.

Systemic effects are rare with Lederspan due its slow release from the injection site. In addition to those common to all glucocorticoids, some effects particularly associated with triamcinolone therapy are anorexia, myopathy and depression of mood.

In treating conditions such as tendinitis or tenosynovitis, care should be taken that Lederspan is injected into the space between tendon sheath and tendon and not into the tendon itself.

If severe reactions occur or an acute infection develops during therapy, use of the drug should be discontinued and appropriate measures taken.

Use in pregnancy and lactation: Pregnancy: The ability of corticosteroids to cross the placenta varies between individual drugs, however triamcinolone does cross the placenta.

Administration of corticosteroids to pregnant animals can cause abnormalities of foetal development including cleft palate, intra-uterine growth retardation and affects on brain growth and development. There is no evidence that corticosteroids result in an increased incidence of congenital abnormalities, such as cleft palate/lip in man. However, when administered for prolonged periods or repeatedly during pregnancy, corticosteroids may increase the risk of intra-uterine growth retardation. Hypoadrenalism may, in theory, occur in the neonate following prenatal exposure to corticosteroids but usually resolves spontaneously following birth and is rarely clinically important. As with all drugs, corticosteroids should only be prescribed when the benefits to the mother and child outweigh the risks. When corticosteroids are essential however, patients with normal pregnancies may be treated as though they were in the non-gravid state.

Lactation: Corticosteroids may pass into breast milk, although no data are available for triamcinolone. Infants of mothers taking high doses of systemic corticosteroids for prolonged periods may have a degree of adrenal suppression.

Overdose: Overdosage or excessive frequency of intra-lesional injections into the same site may produce local subcutaneous atrophy. If this occurs, recovery may be delayed for several months because of the prolonged action of the drug.

Pharmaceutical precautions Lederspan should be stored at room temperature (15–30°C). Do not freeze. It may be diluted with Water for Injection BP, Sodium Chloride Injection BP, Sodium Chloride and Dextrose Injection BP, Lignocaine Hydrochloride Injection BP, immediately prior to injection.

Fluids containing methyl or propyl hydroxybenzoates or phenol should be avoided since these tend to cause flocculation of the steroid.

Legal category POM

Package quantities
20 mg/ml: Single vials containing 20 mg in 1 ml and 100 mg in 5 ml.
5 mg/ml: Single vials containing 25 mg in 5 ml.

Further information Nil

Product licence numbers
Lederspan 20 mg/ml 0095/0008
Lederspan 5 mg/ml 0095/0009

LOXAPAC*

Presentation *10 mg Capsules:* Two piece, hard shell, opaque capsules with a yellow body and a green cap, printed with script 'Lederle' over 'L2' on one half and '10 mg' on the other in grey ink, containing 10 mg loxapine as loxapine succinate. The capsules have a locking feature.

25 mg Capsules: Two piece, hard shell, opaque capsules with a light green body and a dark green cap, printed with script 'Lederle' over 'L3' on one half and '25 mg' on the other in grey ink, containing 25 mg loxapine as loxapine succinate. The capsules have a locking feature.

50 mg Capsules: Two piece, hard shell, opaque capsules with a blue body and a dark green cap, printed with script 'Lederle' over 'L4' on one half and '50 mg' on the other in grey ink, containing 50 mg loxapine as loxapine succinate. The capsules have a locking feature.

Uses The treatment of acute and chronic psychotic states.

Dosage and administration *Adults:* Initially 20–50 mg/day in two doses. Dosage is then increased over 7–10 days to the range 60–100 mg/day in 2–4 doses, until there is effective control of psychotic symptoms.

Maximum daily dose: 250 mg.

Maintenance doses should be adjusted to the needs of the patient, usually in the range of 20–100 mg/day in divided doses.

Children: Not recommended for use in children.

Contra-indications, warnings, etc.
Contra-indications: Use in comatose or semi-comatose patients or in severe drug-induced depressed states (alcohol, barbiturates, narcotics). In individuals with known hypersensitivity to the drug.

Drug interactions: Loxapac may increase the CNS depression produced by drugs such as alcohol, hypnotics, sedatives, antihistamines, strong analgesics or other anti-psychotics. There have been reports of respiratory depression with concurrent use of loxapine and lorazepam.

The anticholinergic effect of loxapine may be enhanced by other anticholinergic drugs. The possibility of occurrence of heat stroke, severe constipation, paralytic ileus and atropine-like psychoses should be noted. Neuroleptics may impair the anti-parkinsonian effect of l-dopa, while therapeutic efficacy of the neuroleptic may be reduced. Concurrent use of neuroleptics and tricyclic antidepressants may contribute to increased incidence of tardive dyskinesia.

Loxapine may reduce serum levels of phenytoin.

There have been rare reports of patients developing neurotoxicity when treated concurrently with lithium; lithium serum levels were within normal limits and the mechanism of action is unknown.

Precautions: Loxapac may impair mental and/or physical abilities, especially during the first few days of therapy. Therefore, ambulatory patients should be warned about activities requiring alertness, (e.g. operating machinery or vehicles) and about concomitant use of alcohol and other CNS depressants.

Loxapac should be used with extreme caution in patients with a history of convulsive disorders, since it lowers the convulsive threshold. Seizures have been reported in epileptic patients receiving Loxapac at antipsychotic dose levels, and may occur even with maintenance of routine anticonvulsant drug therapy.

Loxapac has an antiemetic effect in animals. Since this effect may also occur in man, Loxapac may mask signs of overdosage of toxic drugs and may obscure conditions such as intestinal obstruction and brain tumour.

Loxapac should be used with caution in patients with cardiovascular disease. Increased pulse rates have been reported in the majority of patients receiving antipsychotic doses; transient hypotension has been reported. In the presence of severe hypotension requiring vasopressor therapy, the preferred drugs may be noradrenaline or angiotensin. Usual doses of adrenaline may be ineffective because of inhibition of its vasopressor effect by Loxapac.

The possibility of ocular toxicity from Loxapac cannot be excluded at this time. Therefore, careful observation should be made for pigmentary retinopathy and lenticular pigmentation, since these have been observed in some patients receiving certain other antipsychotic drugs for prolonged periods.

Because of possible anticholinergic action, the drug should be used cautiously in patients with glaucoma or a tendency to urinary retention, particularly with concomitant administration of anticholinergic type anti-Parkinson medication.

Warnings and adverse effects: CNS effects: Manifestations of adverse effects on the central nervous system other than extrapyramidal effects, have been seen infrequently. Drowsiness usually mild, may occur at the beginning of therapy or when dosage is increased and usually subsides with continued Loxapac therapy. Dizziness, faintness, staggering gait, muscle twitching, weakness, confusional states and seizures have been reported.

Extrapyramidal (Neuromuscular) reactions during the administration of Loxapac have been reported frequently, often during the first few days of treatment. In most patients, these reactions involved Parkinson-like symptoms such as tremor, rigidity, excessive salivation, and a mask like face. Also, akathisia (motor restlessness) has been reported relatively frequently. These symptoms are usually not severe and can be controlled by reduction of dosage or by administration of anti-Parkinson drugs in usual dosage. Dystonias include spasms of muscles of the neck and face, tongue protrusion, and oculogyric choreo-athetoid movements. These reactions sometimes require reduction or temporary withdrawal of Loxapac dosage in addition to appropriate counteractive drugs.

As with all antipsychotic agents, persistent tardive dyskinesia may appear in some patients on long term therapy or may appear after drug therapy has been discontinued. The risk appears to be greater in elderly patients on high-dose therapy, especially females. The symptoms are persistent and in some patients appear to be irreversible. The syndrome is characterised by rhythmical involuntary movement of the tongue, face, mouth or jaw (e.g. protrusion of tongue, puffing of cheeks, puckering of mouth, chewing movements). Sometimes these may be accompanied by involuntary movements of extremities.

There is no known effective treatment for tardive dyskinesia; anti-Parkinson agents usually do not alleviate the symptoms of this syndrome. It is suggested that all antipsychotic agents be discontinued if these symptoms appear.

Should it be necessary to reinstitute treatment, or increase the dose of the agent, or switch to a different antipsychotic agent, the syndrome may be masked. It has been suggested that fine vermicular movements of the tongue may be an early sign of the syndrome, and, if the medication is stopped at that time, the syndrome may not develop.

Cardiovascular effects: Tachycardia, hypotension, hypertension, lightheadedness, and syncope have been reported. A few cases of ECG changes similar to those seen with phenothiazines have been reported. It is not known whether these were related to administration.

Skin: Dermatitis, oedema (puffiness of face), pruritis, and seborrhoea have been reported with Loxapac. The possibility of photosensitivity and/or phototoxicity occurring has not been excluded; skin rashes of uncertain aetiology have been observed in a few patients during hot summer months.

Endocrine effects: Hormonal effects of anti-psychotic neuroleptic drugs include hyperprolactinaemia. Galactorrhoea, hyperprolactinaemia and amenorrhoea have been reported rarely.

Anticholinergic effects: Dry mouth, nasal congestion, constipation, and blurred vision have occurred; these are more likely to occur with concomitant use of anti-Parkinson agents.

Other adverse reactions: Nausea, vomiting, weight gain, weight loss, dyspnoea, ptosis, hyperpyrexia, flushed facies, headache, paraesthesia, and polydipsia have been reported in some patients. Transient abnormalities of liver function tests have been reported rarely. Jaundice has been reported in patients taking neuroleptic medication.

Neuroleptic Malignant Syndrome has been reported rarely following the use of Loxapac. This syndrome is potentially fatal and presents with symptoms of hyperpyrexia, muscle rigidity, altered mental status and evidence of autonomic instability. If a patient is diagnosed as suffering from Neuroleptic Malignant Syndrome, the management should include: (1) immediate discontinuation of antipsychotic drugs and other drugs not essential to concurrent therapy (2) symptomatic treatment and monitoring of vital signs and (3) treatment of any concomitant serious medical problems.

Use in pregnancy and lactation: Loxapac should not be used during pregnancy or lactation unless considered essential by the physician. Studies in animals do not indicate a teratogenic effect but there is no information on uses during human pregnancy. Loxapac crosses the placenta and is excreted in breast milk.

Overdosage: Signs and symptoms of overdosage might be expected to include convulsive seizures and range from mild depression of the CNS and cardiovascular systems to profound hypotension, respiratory depression and unconsciousness. Renal failure has been reported following Loxapac administration. Severe extrapyramidal reactions should be treated with anticholinergic anti-Parkinson agents or diphenhydramine hydrochloride, and anticonvulsant therapy should be initiated as indicated.

The treatment of overdosage would be essentially symptomatic and supportive. Early gastric lavage and extended dialysis might be expected to be beneficial. Centrally acting emetics may have little effect because of the antiemetic action of loxapine. Avoid analeptics, such as picrotoxin and pentylenetetrazole, which may cause convulsions. Severe hypotension might be expected to respond to the administration of levarterenol or phenylephrine. ADRENALINE SHOULD NOT BE USED SINCE ITS USE IN A PATIENT WITH PARTIAL ADRENERGIC BLOCKADE MAY FURTHER LOWER THE BLOOD PRESSURE. Additional measures include oxygen and intravenous fluids.

Pharmaceutical precautions Store at controlled room temperature (15–30°C).

Legal category POM

Package quantities Bottles containing 100 capsules.

Product licence numbers

Loxapac 10 mg Capsules	0095/0036
Loxapac 25 mg Capsules	0095/0037
Loxapac 50 mg Capsules	0095/0038

METHOTREXATE INJECTION

Presentation A clear, yellow, sterile, aqueous, isotonic solution containing Methotrexate Sodium equivalent to 50 mg, 200 mg, 500 mg, 1 g or 5 g of Methotrexate per vial together with sodium chloride and sodium hydroxide or hydrochloric acid to adjust the pH to approximately 8.5. The injection does not contain an antimicrobial preservative.

Uses *Properties:* Methotrexate, a derivative of folic acid, belongs to the class of cytotoxic agents known as antimetabolites. It acts principally during the 'S' phase of cell division, by the competitive inhibition of the enzyme dihydrofolate reductase, thus preventing the reduction of dihydrofolate to tetrahydrofolate, a necessary step in the process of DNA synthesis and cellular replication. Actively proliferating tissues such as malignant cells, bone marrow, foetal cells, buccal and intestinal mucosa, and cells of the urinary bladder are generally more sensitive to the effects of Methotrexate. When cellular proliferation in malignant tissues is greater than in most normal tissues, Methotrexate may impair malignant growth without irreversible damage to normal tissues.

Indications: The treatment of neoplastic disease.

Dosage and administration *Adults and children:* Methotrexate may be given by intramuscular, intravenous (bolus injection or infusion), intrathecal, intra-arterial and intraventricular routes of administration. Dosages are based on the patient's body weight or surface area except in the case of intrathecal or intraventricular administration when a maximum dose of 15 mg is recommended. Doses should be reduced in cases of haematological deficiency and hepatic or renal impairment. Larger doses (greater than 100 mg) are usually given by intravenous infusion over periods not exceeding 24 hours. Part of the dose may be given in an initial rapid intravenous injection.

Methotrexate has been used with beneficial effects in a wide variety of neoplastic diseases, alone and in combination with other cytotoxic agents, hormones, radiotherapy or surgery. Dosage schedules therefore vary considerably, depending on the clinical use, particularly when intermittent high-dose regimes are followed by the administration of Calcium Leucovorin (calcium folinate) to rescue normal cells from toxic effects.

Dosage regimes for Calcium Leucovorin rescue are discussed under Further Information.

Examples of doses of Methotrexate that have been used for particular indications are given below.

Choriocarcinoma and other trophoblastic tumours: Non-metastatic gestational trophoblastic neoplasms have been treated successfully with 0.25–1 mg/kg up to a maximum of 60 mg intramuscularly every 48 hours for four doses, followed by Calcium Leucovorin rescue. This course of treatment is repeated at seven day intervals until levels of urinary chorionic gonadotrophin hormone return to normal. Not less than four courses of treatment are usually necessary. Patients with complications, such as extensive metastases, may be treated with Methotrexate in combination with other cytotoxic drugs.

Methotrexate has also been used in similar doses for the treatment of hydatidiform mole and chorioadenoma destruens.

Leukaemia in children: In acute lymphocytic leukaemia remissions are usually best induced with a combination of corticosteroids and other cytotoxic agents.

Methotrexate 15 mg/m², given parenterally or orally once weekly, in combination with other drugs appears to be the treatment of choice for maintenance of drug-induced remissions.

Meningeal leukaemia in children: Doses up to 15 mg, intrathecally, at weekly intervals, until the CSF appears normal (usually two to three weeks), have been found useful for the treatment of meningeal leukaemia.

Although intravenous doses of the order of 50 mg/m² of Methotrexate do not appreciably penetrate the CSF, larger doses of the order of 500 mg/m² or greater do produce cytotoxic levels of Methotrexate in the CSF. This type of therapy has been used in short courses, followed by administration of Calcium Leucovorin, as initial maintenance therapy to prevent leukaemic invasion of the central nervous system in children with poor prognosis lymphocytic leukaemia.

Lymphoma: Non-Hodgkin's lymphoma, e.g. childhood lymphosarcoma has recently been treated with 3–30 mg/kg (approximately 90–900 mg/m²) of Methotrexate given by intravenous injection and infusion followed by administration of Calcium Leucovorin with the higher doses. Some cases of Burkitt's lymphoma, when treated in the early stages with courses of 15 mg/m² daily orally for five days, have shown prolonged remissions. Combination chemotherapy is also commonly used in all stages of the disease.

Breast cancer: Methotrexate, in intravenous doses of 10–60 mg/m², is commonly included in cyclical combination regimes with other cytotoxic drugs in the treatment of advanced breast cancer. Similar regimes have also been used as adjuvant therapy in early cases following mastectomy and/or radiotherapy.

Osteogenic sarcoma: The use of Methotrexate alone and in cyclical combination regimes has recently been introduced as an adjuvant therapy to the primary treatment of osteogenic sarcoma by amputation with or without prosthetic bone replacement. This has involved the use of intravenous infusions of 20–300 mg/kg (approximately 600–9,000 mg/m²) of Methotrexate followed by Calcium Leucovorin rescue. Methotrexate has also been used as the sole treatment in metastatic cases of osteogenic sarcoma.

Bronchogenic carcinoma: Intravenous infusions of 20–100 mg/m² of Methotrexate have been included in cyclical combination regimes for the treatment of advanced tumours. High doses with Calcium Leucovorin rescue have also been employed as the sole treatment.

Head and neck cancer: Intravenous infusions of 240–1,080 mg/m² with Calcium Leucovorin rescue have been used both as pre-operative adjuvant therapy and in the treatment of advanced tumours. Intra-arterial infusions of Methotrexate have been used in the treatment of head and neck cancers.

Bladder carcinoma: Intravenous injections or infusions of Methotrexate in doses up to 100 mg every one or two weeks have been used in the treatment of bladder carcinoma with promising results, varying from only symptomatic relief to complete though unsustained regressions. The use of high doses of Methotrexate with Calcium Leucovorin rescue is currently being evaluated.

Elderly: Methotrexate should be used with extreme caution in elderly patients, a reduction in dosage should be considered.

Assessment of renal function, liver function and blood elements should be made by history, physical examination and laboratory tests before beginning Methotrexate, periodically during Methotrexate therapy, and before reinstituting Methotrexate after a rest period.

Particular attention should be given to the appearance of liver toxicity by carrying out liver function tests before starting Methotrexate treatment and repeating these at two to four month intervals during therapy. Treatment should not be instituted or should be discontinued if any abnormality of liver function tests, or liver biopsy, is present or develops during therapy.

Such abnormalities should return to normal within two weeks after which treatment may be recommenced at the discretion of the physician.

Children: Safety and effectiveness in children have not been established, other than in cancer chemotherapy.

Contra-indications, warnings, etc

Contra-indications: Profound impairment of renal or hepatic function or haematological impairment. Liver disease including fibrosis, cirrhosis, recent or active hepatitis; active infectious disease; and overt or laboratory evidence of immunodeficiency syndrome(s). Serious cases of anaemia, leucopenia, or thrombocytopenia. Methotrexate is contra-indicated in pregnant patients. Because of the potential for serious adverse reactions from Methotrexate in breast fed infants, breast feeding is contra-indicated in women taking Methotrexate. Patients with a known allergic hypersensitivity to Methotrexate should not receive Methotrexate.

Concomitant administration of folate antagonists such as co-trimoxazole has been reported to cause an acute megaloblastic pancytopenia in rare instances.

Patients receiving other drugs with anti-folate properties (e.g. co-trimoxazole) should not take Methotrexate.

NSAIDs should not be administered prior to, or concomitantly with, high dose Methotrexate.

Warnings: Methotrexate has been shown to be teratogenic; it has been reported to cause foetal death and/or congenital abnormalities. Therefore, it is not recommended in women of childbearing potential unless the benefits can be expected to outweigh the considered risks. If this drug is used during pregnancy for antineoplastic indications, or if the patient becomes pregnant while taking this drug, the patient should be appraised of the potential hazard to the foetus.

Methotrexate should be used with extreme caution in patients with haematological depression, renal impairment, peptic ulcer, ulcerative colitis, ulcerative stomatitis, diarrhoea, debility and in young children and the elderly. (See *Dosage and Administration*).

Patients with pleural effusions or ascites should have these drained if appropriate before treatment or treatment should be withdrawn.

Deaths have been reported with the use of Methotrexate. Serious adverse reactions including deaths have been reported with concomitant administration of Methotrexate (usually in high doses) along with some non-steroidal anti-inflammatory drugs (NSAIDs).

Symptoms of gastro-intestinal toxicity, usually first manifested by stomatitis, indicate interruption of therapy otherwise haemorrhagic enteritis and death from intestinal perforation may occur.

Methotrexate affects spermatogenesis and oogenesis during the period of its administration which may result in decreased fertility. To date, this effect appears to be reversible on discontinuing therapy. Conception should be avoided for at least six months after treatment with Methotrexate has ceased. Patients receiving Methotrexate and their partners should be advised appropriately.

Methotrexate has some immunosuppressive activity and therefore the immunological response to concurrent vaccination may be decreased. In addition, concomitant use of a live vaccine could cause a severe antigenic reaction.

Precautions: Methotrexate should only be used by clinicians who are familiar with the various characteristics of the drug and its mode of action. Before beginning Methotrexate therapy or reinstituting Methotrexate after a rest period, assessment of renal function, liver function and blood elements should be made by history, physical examination and laboratory tests. Patients undergoing therapy should be subject to appropriate supervision so that signs of possible toxic effects or adverse reactions may be detected and evaluated with minimal delay.

It is essential that the following laboratory tests are included regularly (every 2–3 months) in the clinical evaluation and monitoring of patients receiving Methotrexate: complete haematological analysis, urinalysis, renal function tests, liver function tests and, when high doses are administered, determination of plasma levels of Methotrexate.

Particular attention should be given to the appearance of liver toxicity which may occur without correlative changes in liver function tests before starting Methotrexate treatment and repeating these at two to three month intervals during therapy. Treatment should not be instituted, or should be discontinued, if any abnormality in liver function tests or liver biopsy is present or develops during therapy. Such abnormalities should return to normal within two weeks, after which treatment may be recommenced at the discretion of the physician.

When to perform a liver biopsy in rheumatoid arthritis patients has not been established either in terms of a cumulative Methotrexate dose or duration of therapy.

Pleuropulmonary manifestation of rheumatoid arthritis have been reported in the literature. In patients with rheumatoid arthritis, the physician should be specifically alerted to the potential for Methotrexate induced adverse effects in the pulmonary system. Patients should be advised to contact their physicians immediately should they develop a cough or dyspnoea (see *Side effects*).

Haematopoietic suppression caused by Methotrexate may occur abruptly and with apparently safe dosages. Any profound drop in white-cell or platelet counts indicate immediate withdrawal of the drug and appropriate supportive therapy. (See *Side effects*).

It should be noted that intrathecal doses are transported into the cardiovascular system and may give rise to systemic toxicity. Systemic toxicity of Methotrexate may also be enhanced in patients with renal dysfunction, ascites or other effusions due to prolongation of serum half-life.

High doses may cause the precipitation of Methotrexate or its metabolites in the renal tubules. A high fluid throughput and alkalinisation of the urine to pH 6.5–7.0 by oral or intravenous administration of sodium bicarbonate (5x625 mg tablets every three hours) or Diamox* (500 mg orally four times a day) is recommended as a preventive measure.

Malignant lymphomas, may occur in patients receiving low dose methotrexate, in which case therapy must be discontinued. Failure of the lymphoma to show signs of spontaneous regression requires the initiation of cytotoxic therapy.

Carcinogenesis, mutagenesis, and impairment of fertility: Animal carcinogenicity studies have demonstrated Methotrexate to be free of carcinogenic potential. Although Methotrexate has been reported to cause chromosomal damage to animal somatic cells and bone marrow cells in humans, these effects are transient and reversible. In patients treated with Methotrexate, evidence is insufficient to permit conclusive evaluation of any increased risk of neoplasia.

Methotrexate has been reported to cause impairment of fertility, oligospermia, menstrual dysfunction and amenorrhoea in humans, during and for a short period after cessation of therapy. In addition, Methotrexate causes embryotoxicity, abortion and foetal defects in humans. Therefore, the possible risks of effects on reproduction should be discussed with patients of child-bearing potential (See Warnings).

Drug interactions: Methotrexate is extensively protein bound and may be displaced by certain drugs such as salicylates, sulphonamides, diuretics, hypoglycaemics, diphenylhydantoins, tetracyclines, chloramphenicol, p-aminobenzoic acid, and the acidic anti-inflammatory drugs, so causing a potential for increased toxicity when used concurrently. Concomitant use of other drugs with nephrotoxic or hepatotoxic potential (including alcohol) should be avoided.

Caution should be used when NSAIDs and salicylates are administered concomitantly with Methotrexate. These drugs have been reported to reduce the tubular secretion of Methotrexate in an animal model and thereby may enhance its toxicity. Renal tubular transport is also diminished by probenecid and penicillins; use of Methotrexate with these drugs should be carefully monitored.

Patients using constant dosage regimens of NSAIDs have received concurrent doses of Methotrexate without problems observed. Therefore, until more is known about the NSAIDs/Methotrexate interaction, it is recommended that Methotrexate dosage be carefully controlled during treatment with NSAIDs.

Methotrexate should be used with caution in patients taking drugs known to have an antifolate potential including nitrous oxide.

Vitamin preparations containing folic acid or its derivatives may alter response to Methotrexate.

Serum levels of Methotrexate may be increased by etretinate and severe hepatitis has been reported following concurrent use.

Side effects: The most common adverse reactions include ulcerative stomatitis, leucopenia, nausea and abdominal distress. Although very rare, anaphylactic reactions to Methotrexate have occurred. Others reported are eye irritation, malaise, undue fatigue, vasculitis, chills and fever, dizziness, loss of libido/impotence and decreased resistance to infection. Opportunistic infections such as herpes zoster have been reported in relation to or attributed to the use of Methotrexate. In general, the incidence and severity of side effects are considered to be dose-related. Adverse reactions for the various systems are as follows:

Integument: Stevens-Johnson Syndrome, epidermal necrolysis, erythematous rashes, pruritus, urticaria, photosensitivity, pigmentary changes, alopecia, ecchymosis, telangiectasia, acne, furunculosis. Lesions of psoriasis may be aggravated by concomitant exposure to ultraviolet radiation. Skin ulceration has been reported in psoriatic patients. The recall phenomenon has been reported in both radiation and solar damaged skin.

Haematopoietic: Bone marrow depression is most frequently manifested by leukopenia, but thrombocytopenia, anaemia, or any combination may occur. Infection or septicemia and haemorrhage from various sites may result. Hypogammaglobulinaemia has been reported.

Alimentary System: Mucositis (most frequently stomatitis although gingivitis, pharyngitis and even enteritis, intestinal ulceration and bleeding) may occur. In rare cases the effect of Methotrexate on the intestinal mucosa has led to malabsorption or toxic megacolon. Nausea, anorexia and vomiting and/or diarrhoea may also occur.

Hepatic: Hepatic toxicity resulting in significant elevations of liver enzymes, acute liver atrophy, necrosis, fatty metamorphosis, periportal fibrosis or cirrhosis or death may occur, usually following chronic administration.

Urogenital System: Renal failure and uraemia may follow Methotrexate administration, usually in high doses. Vaginitis, vaginal ulcers, cystitis, haematuria and nephropathy have also been reported.

Pulmonary System: Infrequently an acute or chronic interstitial pneumonitis, often associated with blood eosinophilia, may occur and deaths have been reported. Acute pulmonary oedema has also been reported after oral and intrathecal use. Pulmonary fibrosis is rare. A syndrome consisting of pleuritic pain and pleural thickening has been reported following high doses.

In the treatment of rheumatoid arthritis, Methotrexate induced lung disease is a potentially serious adverse drug reaction which may occur acutely at any time during therapy. It is not always fully reversible. Pulmonary symptoms (especially a dry, non productive cough) may require interruption of treatment and careful investigation.

Central Nervous System: Headaches, drowsiness and blurred vision have occurred. Following low doses of Methotrexate, transient subtle cognitive dysfunction, mood alteration, or unusual cranial sensations have been reported occasionally. Aphasia, paresis, hemiparesis, and convulsions have also occurred following administration of higher doses.

There have been reports of leukoencephalopathy following intravenous Methotrexate in high doses, or low doses following cranial-spinal radiation.

Adverse reactions following intrathecal Methotrexate are generally classified into three groups, acute, subacute, and chronic. The acute form is a chemical arachnoiditis manifested by headache, back or shoulder pain, nuchal rigidity, and fever. The subacute form may include paresis, usually transient, paraplegia, nerve palsies, and cerebellar dysfunction. The chronic form is a leukoencephalopathy manifested by irritability, confusion, ataxia, spasticity, occasionally convulsions, dementia, somnolence, coma, and rarely, death. There is evidence that the combined use of cranial radiation and intrathecal Methotrexate increases the incidence of leukoencephalopathy.

Additional reactions related to or attributed to the use of Methotrexate such as osteoporosis, abnormal (usually 'megaloblastic') red cell morphology, precipitation of diabetes, other metabolic changes, and sudden death have been reported.

Overdosage: Calcium Leucovorin is the antidote for neutralising the immediate toxic effects of Methotrexate on the haematopoietic system. It may be administered orally, intramuscularly, or by an intravenous bolus injection or infusion. In cases of accidental overdosage, a dose of Calcium Leucovorin equal to or higher than the offending dose of Methotrexate should be administered within one hour and dosing continued until the serum levels of Methotrexate are below 10^{-7}M. Other supporting therapy such as a blood transfusion and renal dialysis may be required.

In cases of massive overdose, hydration and urinary alkalization may be necessary to prevent precipitation of Methotrexate and/or its metabolites in the renal tubules. Neither haemodialysis nor peritoneal dialysis has been shown to improve Methotrexate elimination.

Following intrathecal overdose, CSF drainage may remove up to 95% of the dose if commenced within 15 minutes of administration, although this falls to 20% after 2 hours. For intrathecal doses over 100 mg ventriculolumbar perfusion should accompany CSF drainage.

Pharmaceutical precautions Parenteral Methotrexate preparations do not contain an antimicrobial preservative. Any unused injection should be discarded.

Parenteral Methotrexate preparations are stable for 24 hours when diluted with the following intravenous infusion fluids: 0.9% Sodium Chloride; Glucose; Sodium Chloride and Glucose; Compound Sodium Chloride (Ringers Injection); Compound Sodium Lactate (Lactated Ringers Injection).

Methotrexate preparations should be stored at controlled room temperature (15°–30°C) and protected from direct sunlight. Other drugs should not be mixed with Methotrexate in the same infusion container.

Handling of cytotoxic drugs: Cytotoxic drugs should only be handled by trained personnel in a designated area. The work surface should be covered with disposable plastic-backed absorbent paper.

Protective gloves and goggles should be worn to avoid the drug accidentally coming into contact with the skin or eyes.

Methotrexate is not vesicant and should not cause harm if it comes in contact with the skin. It should, of course, be washed off with water immediately. Any transient stinging may be treated with bland cream. If there is any danger of systemic absorption of significant quantities of Methotrexate, by any route, Calcium Leucovorin cover should be given.

Cytotoxic preparations should not be handled by pregnant staff.

Any spillage or waste material may be disposed of

by incineration. We do not make any specific recommendations with regard to the temperature of the incinerator.

Legal category POM

Package quantities
Injection 50 mg in 2 ml: Boxes of 1 vial.
Injection 200 mg in 8 ml: Boxes of 1 vial.
Injection 500 mg in 20 ml: Boxes of 1 vial.
Injection 1 g in 40 ml: Boxes of 1 vial.
Injection 5 g in 200 ml: Boxes of 1 vial.

Further information Dosage regimes for Calcium Leucovorin rescue vary, depending upon the dose of Methotrexate administered. In general, up to 150 mg are usually given in divided doses, over 12–24 hours, by intramuscular injection, bolus intravenous injection or intravenous infusion or orally, followed by 12–15 mg intramuscularly, IV, or 15 mg (one tablet) orally, every six hours for the next 48 hours. Rescue therapy is usually started following a delay of 8 to 24 hours from the beginning of the Methotrexate infusion. One tablet (15 mg) of Calcium Leucovorin every six hours for 48–72 hours may be sufficient when lower doses (less than 100 mg) of Methotrexate have been given.

Calcium Leucovorin is available as a vial of powder for injection (15 mg and 30 mg), and as tablets (15 mg) in bottles of 10.

Further information on other formulations of Methotrexate, on results with particular cyclical regimes of combinations of cytotoxic drugs and other aspects of cancer chemotherapy with Methotrexate is available on request.

Product licence numbers
Injection 25 mg/ml 0095/0016

Date of last review November 1998

METHOTREXATE SODIUM TABLETS

Presentation *Tablets 2.5 mg:* Round convex, scored, uncoated, yellow tablets embossed '2.5' and 'MI', containing Methotrexate Sodium equivalent to 2.5 mg of Methotrexate per tablet.

Uses *Properties:* Methotrexate, a derivative of folic acid, belongs to the class of cytotoxic agents known as antimetabolites. It acts principally during the 'S' phase of cell division, by the competitive inhibition of the enzyme dihydrofolate reductase, thus preventing the reduction of dihydrofolate to tetrahydrofolate, a necessary step in the process of DNA synthesis and cellular replication. Actively proliferating tissues such as malignant cells, bone marrow, foetal cells, buccal and intestinal mucosa, and cells of the urinary bladder are generally more sensitive to the effects of Methotrexate. When cellular proliferation in malignant tissues is greater than in most normal tissues, Methotrexate may impair malignant growth without irreversible damage to normal tissues.

The mechanism of action in rheumatoid arthritis is unknown; it may effect immune function. Clarification of the effect of Methotrexate on immune activity and its relation to rheumatoid immunopathogenesis await further investigation.

In psoriasis, the rate of production of epithelial cells in the skin is greatly increased over normal skin. This differential in proliferation rates is the basis for the use of Methotrexate to control the psoriatic process.

Indications: The treatment of neoplastic disease. The treatment of severe cases of uncontrolled psoriasis, unresponsive to conventional therapy.

The treatment of adults with severe, active, classical or definite rheumatoid arthritis who are unresponsive or intolerant to conventional therapy.

Dosage and administration *Adults and children:* Methotrexate may be given by oral, intramuscular, intravenous (bolus injection or infusion), intrathecal, intra-arterial and intraventricular routes of administration. Dosages are based on the patient's body weight or surface area except in the case of intrathecal or intraventricular administration when a maximum dose of 15 mg is recommended. Doses should be reduced in cases of haematological deficiency and hepatic or renal impairment. Larger doses (greater than 100 mg) are usually given by intravenous infusion over periods not exceeding 24 hours. Part of the dose may be given in an initial rapid intravenous injection.

Methotrexate has been used with beneficial effects in a wide variety of neoplastic diseases, alone and in combination with other cytotoxic agents, hormones, radiotherapy or surgery. Dosage schedules therefore vary considerably, depending on the clinical use, particularly when intermittent high-dose regimes are followed by the administration of Calcium Leucovorin (calcium folinate) to rescue normal cells from toxic effects.

Dosage regimes for Calcium Leucovorin rescue are discussed under Further Information.

Examples of doses of Methotrexate that have been used for particular indications are given below.

Choriocarcinoma and other trophoblastic tumours: Non-metastatic gestational trophoblastic neoplasms have been treated successfully with 0.25–1 mg/kg up to a maximum of 60 mg intramuscularly every 48 hours for four doses, followed by Calcium Leucovorin rescue. This course of treatment is repeated at seven day intervals until levels of urinary chorionic gonadotrophin hormone return to normal. Not less than four courses of treatment are usually necessary. Patients with complications, such as extensive metastases, may be treated with Methotrexate in combination with other cytotoxic drugs.

Methotrexate has also been used in similar doses for the treatment of hydatidiform mole and chorioadenoma destruens.

Leukaemia in children: In acute lymphocytic leukaemia remissions are usually best induced with a combination of corticosteroids and other cytotoxic agents.

Methotrexate 15 mg/m², given parenterally or orally once weekly, in combination with other drugs appears to be the treatment of choice for maintenance of drug-induced remissions.

Meningeal leukaemia in children: Doses up to 15 mg, intrathecally, at weekly intervals, until the CSF appears normal (usually two to three weeks), have been found useful for the treatment of meningeal leukaemia.

Although intravenous doses of the order of 50 mg/m² of Methotrexate do not appreciably penetrate the CSF, larger doses of the order of 500 mg/m² or greater do produce cytotoxic levels of Methotrexate in the CSF. This type of therapy has been used in short courses, followed by administration of Calcium Leucovorin, as initial maintenance therapy to prevent leukaemic invasion of the central nervous system in children with poor prognosis lymphocytic leukaemia.

Lymphoma: Non-Hodgkin's lymphoma, e.g. childhood lymphosarcoma has recently been treated with 3–30 mg/kg (approximately 90–900 mg/m²) of Methotrexate given by intravenous injection and infusion followed by administration of Calcium Leucovorin with the higher doses. Some cases of Burkitt's lymphoma, when treated in the early stages with courses of 15 mg/m² daily orally for five days, have shown prolonged remissions. Combination chemotherapy is also commonly used in all stages of the disease.

Breast cancer: Methotrexate, in intravenous doses of 10–60 mg/m², is commonly included in cyclical combination regimes with other cytotoxic drugs in the treatment of advanced breast cancer. Similar regimes have also been used as adjuvant therapy in early cases following mastectomy and/or radiotherapy.

Osteogenic sarcoma: The use of Methotrexate alone and in cyclical combination regimes has recently been introduced as an adjuvant therapy to the primary treatment of osteogenic sarcoma by amputation with or without prosthetic bone replacement. This has involved the use of intravenous infusions of 20–300 mg/kg (approximately 600–9,000 mg/m²) of Methotrexate followed by Calcium Leucovorin rescue. Methotrexate has also been used as the sole treatment in metastatic cases of osteogenic sarcoma.

Bronchogenic carcinoma: Intravenous infusions of 20–100 mg/m² of Methotrexate have been included in cyclical combination regimes for the treatment of advanced tumours. High doses with Calcium Leucovorin rescue have also been employed as the sole treatment.

Head and neck cancer: Intravenous infusions of 240–1,080 mg/m² with Calcium Leucovorin rescue have been used both as pre-operative adjuvant therapy and in the treatment of advanced tumours. Intra-arterial infusions of Methotrexate have been used in the treatment of head and neck cancers.

Bladder carcinoma: Intravenous injections or infusions of Methotrexate in doses up to 100 mg every one or two weeks have been used in the treatment of bladder carcinoma with promising results, varying from only symptomatic relief to complete though unsustained regressions. The use of high doses of Methotrexate with Calcium Leucovorin rescue is currently being evaluated.

Elderly: Methotrexate should be used with extreme caution in elderly patients, a reduction in dosage should be considered.

Assessment of renal function, liver function and blood elements should be made by history, physical examination and laboratory tests before beginning Methotrexate, periodically during Methotrexate therapy, and before reinstituting Methotrexate after a rest period.

Particular attention should be given to the appearance of liver toxicity by carrying out liver function tests before starting Methotrexate treatment and repeating these at two to three month intervals during therapy. Treatment should not be instituted or should be discontinued if any abnormality of liver function tests, or liver biopsy, is present or develops during therapy.

Such abnormalities should return to normal within two weeks after which treatment may be recommenced at the discretion of the physician.

Dosage and administration with reference to psoriasis and rheumatoid arthritis
Adults: It is recommended that a test dose of 5–10 mg should be administered parenterally, one week prior to therapy to detect idiosyncratic adverse reactions.

Psoriasis: In most cases of severe uncontrolled psoriasis, unresponsive to conventional therapy, 10–25 mg orally once a week and adjusted by the patient's response is recommended.

The use of Methotrexate in psoriasis may permit the return to conventional topical therapy which should be encouraged.

Rheumatoid arthritis: In adults with severe, acute, classical or definite rheumatoid arthritis who are unresponsive or intolerant to conventional therapy, 7.5 mg orally once weekly or divided oral doses of 2.5 mg at 12 hour intervals for 3 doses (7.5 mg) as a course once weekly. The schedule may be adjusted gradually to achieve an optimal response but should not exceed a total weekly dose of 20 mg. Once response has been achieved, the schedule should be reduced to the lowest possible effective dose.

Elderly: Methotrexate should be used with extreme caution in elderly patients, a reduction in dosage should be considered.

Children: Safety and effectiveness in children have not been established, other than in cancer chemotherapy.

Contra-indications, warnings, etc
Contra-indications: Profound impairment of renal or hepatic function or haematological impairment. Liver disease including fibrosis, cirrhosis, recent or active hepatitis; active infectious disease; and overt or laboratory evidence of immunodeficiency syndrome(s). Serious cases of anaemia, leucopenia, or thrombocytopenia. Methotrexate is contra-indicated in pregnant patients. Because of the potential for serious adverse reactions from Methotrexate in breast fed infants, breast feeding is contra-indicated in women taking Methotrexate. Patients with a known allergic hypersensitivity to Methotrexate should not receive Methotrexate.

Concomitant administration of folate antagonists such as co-trimoxazole has been reported to cause an acute megaloblastic pancytopenia in rare instances. Patients receiving other drugs with anti-folate properties (e.g. co-trimoxazole) should not take methotrexate.

Warnings: Methotrexate has been shown to be teratogenic; it has been reported to cause foetal death and/or congenital abnormalities. Therefore, it is not recommended in women of childbearing potential unless the benefits can be expected to outweigh the considered risks. If this drug is used during pregnancy for antineoplastic indications, or if the patient becomes pregnant while taking this drug, the patient should be appraised of the potential hazard to the foetus.

Methotrexate should be used with extreme caution in patients with haematological depression, renal impairment, peptic ulcer, ulcerative colitis, ulcerative stomatitis, diarrhoea, debility and in young children and the elderly. (See Dosage and Administration).

Patients with pleural effusions or ascites should have these drained if appropriate before treatment or treatment should be withdrawn.

Deaths have been reported with the use of Methotrexate. Serious adverse reactions including deaths have been reported with concomitant administration of Methotrexate (usually in high doses) along with some non-steroidal anti-inflammatory drugs (NSAIDs).

Symptoms of gastro-intestinal toxicity, usually first manifested by stomatitis, indicate that therapy should be interrupted otherwise haemorrhagic enteritis and death from intestinal perforation may occur.

Methotrexate affects spermatogenesis and oogenesis during the period of its administration which may result in decreased fertility. To date, this effect appears to be reversible on discontinuing therapy. Conception should be avoided for at least six months after treatment with Methotrexate has ceased. Patients receiving Methotrexate and their partners should be advised appropriately.

Methotrexate has some immunosuppressive activity and therefore the immunological response to concurrent vaccination may be decreased. In addition, concomitant use of a live vaccine could cause a severe antigenic reaction.

Precautions: Methotrexate should only be used by clinicians who are familiar with the various characteristics of the drug and its mode of action. Before beginning Methotrexate therapy or reinstituting Methotrexate after a rest period, assessment of renal function, liver function and blood elements should be made by history, physical examination and laboratory tests. Patients undergoing therapy should be subject to appropriate supervision every 2–3 months so that signs of possible toxic effects or adverse reactions may be detected and evaluated with minimal delay.

It is essential that the following laboratory tests are included regularly (every 2–3 months) in the clinical evaluation and monitoring of patients receiving Methotrexate: complete haematological analysis, urinalysis, renal function tests, liver function tests and, when high doses are administered, determination of plasma levels of Methotrexate.

Particular attention should be given to the appearance of liver toxicity which may occur without correlative changes in liver function tests. Treatment should not be instituted, or should be discontinued, if any abnormality in liver function tests or liver biopsy is present or develops during therapy. Such abnormalities should return to normal within two weeks, after which treatment may be recommenced at the discretion of the physician.

When to perform a liver biopsy in rheumatoid arthritis patients has not been established either in terms of a cumulative Methotrexate dose or duration of therapy.

Pleuropulmonary manifestation of rheumatoid arthritis have been reported in the literature. In patients with rheumatoid arthritis, the physician should be specifically alerted to the potential for Methotrexate induced adverse effects in the pulmonary system. Patients should be advised to contact their physicians immediately should they develop a cough or dyspnoea (see *Side effects*).

Haematopoietic suppression caused by Methotrexate may occur abruptly and with apparently safe dosages. Any profound drop in white-cell or platelet counts indicate immediate withdrawal of the drug and appropriate supportive therapy. (See *Side effects*.)

It should be noted that intrathecal doses are transported into the cardiovascular system and may give rise to systemic toxicity. Systemic toxicity of Methotrexate may also be enhanced in patients with renal dysfunction, ascites or other effusions due to prolongation of serum half-life.

High doses may cause the precipitation of Methotrexate or its metabolites in the renal tubules. A high fluid throughput and alkalinisation of the urine to pH 6.5–7.0 by oral or intravenous administration of sodium bicarbonate (5x625 mg tablets every three hours) or Diamox* (500 mg orally four times a day) is recommended as a preventive measure.

Carcinogenesis, mutagenesis, and impairment of fertility: Animal carcinogenicity studies have demonstrated Methotrexate to be free of carcinogenic potential. Although Methotrexate has been reported to cause chromosomal damage to animal somatic cells and bone marrow cells in humans, these effects are transient and reversible. In patients treated with Methotrexate, evidence is insufficient to permit conclusive evaluation of any increased risk of neoplasia.

Methotrexate has been reported to cause impairment of fertility, oligospermia, menstrual dysfunction and amenorrhoea in humans, during and for a short period after cessation of therapy. In addition, Methotrexate causes embryotoxicity, abortion and foetal defects in humans. Therefore, the possible risks of effects on reproduction should be discussed with patients of child-bearing potential (See *Warnings*).

Drug interactions: Methotrexate is extensively protein bound and may be displaced by certain drugs such as salicylates, sulphonamides, diuretics, hypoglycaemics, diphenylhydantoins, tetracyclines, chloramphenicol, p-aminobenzoic acid, and the acidic anti-inflammatory drugs, so causing a potential for increased toxicity when used concurrently. Concomitant use of other drugs with nephrotoxic or hepatotoxic potential (including alcohol) should be avoided.

Caution should be used when NSAIDs and salicylates are administered concomitantly with Methotrexate. These drugs have been reported to reduce the tubular secretion of Methotrexate in an animal model and thereby may enhance its toxicity. Renal tubular transport is also diminished by probenecid and penicillins; use of Methotrexate with these drugs should be carefully monitored.

Patients using constant dosage regimens of NSAIDs have received concurrent doses of Methotrexate without problems observed. Therefore, until more is known about the NSAIDs/Methotrexate interaction, it is recommended that Methotrexate dosage be carefully controlled during treatment with NSAIDs.

Methotrexate should not be used where patients are taking other drugs known to have an antifolate potential including nitrous oxide and co-trimoxazole.

Vitamin preparations containing folic acid or its derivatives may alter response to Methotrexate.

Serum levels of Methotrexate may be increased by etretinate and severe hepatitis has been reported following concurrent use.

Side effects: The most common adverse reactions include ulcerative stomatitis, leucopenia, nausea and abdominal distress. Although very rare, anaphylactic reactions to Methotrexate have occurred. Others reported are eye irritation, malaise, undue fatigue, chills and fever, dizziness, loss of libido/impotence and decreased resistance to infection. Opportunistic infections such as herpes zoster have been reported in relation to or attributed to the use of Methotrexate. In general, the incidence and severity of side effects are considered to be dose-related. Adverse reactions for the various systems are as follows:

Integument: Erythematous rashes, pruritus, urticaria, photosensitivity, pigmentary changes, alopecia, ecchymosis, telangiectasia, acne, furunculosis. Lesions of psoriasis may be aggravated by concomitant exposure to ultraviolet radiation. Skin ulceration has been reported in psoriatic patients. The recall phenomenon has been reported in both radiation and solar damaged skin.

Haematopoietic: Bone marrow depression is most frequently manifested by leukopenia, but thrombocytopenia, anaemia, or any combination may occur. Infection or septicemia and haemorrhage from various sites may result. Hypogammaglobulinaemia has been reported.

Alimentary System: Mucositis (most frequently stomatitis although gingivitis, pharyngitis and even enteritis, intestinal ulceration and bleeding) may occur. In rare cases the effect of Methotrexate on the intestinal mucosa has led to malabsorption or toxic megacolon. Nausea, anorexia and vomiting and/or diarrhoea may also occur.

Hepatic: Hepatic toxicity resulting in significant elevations of liver enzymes, acute liver atrophy, necrosis, fatty metamorphosis, periportal fibrosis or cirrhosis or death may occur, usually following chronic administration.

Urogenital System: Renal failure and uraemia may follow Methotrexate administration, usually in high doses. Vaginitis, vaginal ulcers, cystitis, haematuria and nephropathy have also been reported.

Pulmonary System: Infrequently an acute or chronic interstitial pneumonitis, often associated with blood eosinophilia, may occur and deaths have been reported. Acute pulmonary oedema has also been reported after oral and intrathecal use. Pulmonary fibrosis is rare. A syndrome consisting of pleuritic pain and pleural thickening has been reported following high doses.

In the treatment of rheumatoid arthritis, Methotrexate induced lung disease is a potentially serious adverse drug reaction which may occur acutely at any time during therapy. It is not always fully reversible. Pulmonary symptoms (especially a dry, non productive cough) may require interruption of treatment and careful investigation.

Central Nervous System: Headaches, drowsiness and blurred vision have occurred. Following low doses of Methotrexate, transient subtle cognitive dysfunction, mood alteration, or unusual cranial sensations have been reported occasionally. Aphasia, paresis, hemiparesis, and convulsions have also occurred following administration of higher doses.

There have been reports of leukoencephalopathy following intravenous Methotrexate in high doses, or low doses following cranial-spinal radiation.

Additional reactions related to or attributed to the use of Methotrexate such as osteoporosis, abnormal (usually 'megaloblastic') red cell morphology, precipitation of diabetes, other metabolic changes, and sudden death have been reported.

Overdosage: Calcium Leucovorin is the antidote for neutralising the immediate toxic effects of Methotrexate on the haematopoietic system. It may be administered orally, intramuscularly, or by an intravenous bolus injection or infusion. In cases of accidental overdosage, a dose of Calcium Leucovorin equal to or higher than the offending dose of Methotrexate should be administered within one hour and dosing continued until the serum levels of Methotrexate are below 10^{-7}M. Other supporting therapy such as a blood transfusion and renal dialysis may be required.

Pharmaceutical precautions Methotrexate tablets 2.5 mg should be stored at controlled room temperature (15°–30°C).

Handling of cytotoxic drugs: Cytotoxic drugs should only be handled by trained personnel in a designated area. The work surface should be covered with disposable plastic-backed absorbent paper.

Protective gloves and goggles should be worn to avoid the drug accidentally coming into contact with the skin or eyes.

Methotrexate is not vesicant and should not cause harm if it comes in contact with the skin. It should, of course, be washed off with water immediately. Any transient stinging may be treated with bland cream. If there is any danger of systemic absorption of significant quantities of Methotrexate, by any route, Calcium Leucovorin cover should be given.

Cytotoxic preparations should not be handled by pregnant staff.

Any spillage or waste material may be disposed of by incineration. We do not make any specific recommendations with regard to the temperature of the incinerator.

Legal category POM

Package quantities
Tablets 2.5 mg: Bottles of 100 or 28. Blisters of 28.

Further information Dosage regimes for Calcium Leucovorin rescue vary, depending upon the dose of Methotrexate administered. In general, up to 150 mg are usually given in divided doses, over 12–24 hours, by intramuscular injection, bolus intravenous injection or intravenous infusion or orally, followed by 12–15 mg intramuscularly, IV, or 15 mg (one tablet) orally, every six hours for the next 48 hours. Rescue therapy is usually started following a delay of 8 to 24 hours from the beginning of the Methotrexate infusion. One tablet (15 mg) of Calcium Leucovorin every six hours for 48–72 hours may be sufficient when lower doses (less than 100 mg) of Methotrexate have been given.

Calcium Leucovorin is available as a vial of powder for injection (15 mg and 30 mg), and as tablets (15 mg) in bottles of 10.

Further information on other formulations of Methotrexate, on results with particular cyclical regimes of combinations of cytotoxic drugs and other aspects of cancer chemotherapy with Methotrexate is available on request.

Product licence number
Tablets 2.5 mg 0095/5079R

Date of last review November 1998

MICROVAL*

Qualitative and quantitative composition Each tablet contains 0.03 mg levonorgestrel.

Pharmaceutical form White sugar coated tablets.

Clinical particulars
Therapeutic indication: Oral contraception.

Posology and method of administration:
Adult women only: The tablets are started on the first day of menstruation and taken daily without interruption for as long as contraception is desired. They should be taken at the same time each day, preferably after the evening meal or at bedtime so that the interval between tablets is always about 24 hours. Protection may be reduced when the interval increases beyond 27 hours.

During the first cycle additional contraceptive precautions should be taken for the first 14 days.

If a tablet is not taken at the usual time it should be taken as soon as possible and the next tablet taken at the usual time. If the interval between tablets is more than 27 hours protection may be impaired. The patient should take one tablet as soon as she remembers and thereafter one tablet daily as before but should use additional contraceptive measures until the tablets have been taken regularly for 14 days.

If vomiting occurs shortly after a tablet has been taken contraceptive protection can be maintained by taking another tablet, provided that it is taken within three hours of the normal time. The last tablet in the pack may be used for this purpose. If repeated vomiting or diarrhoea endanger absorption additional contraceptive precautions should be used for 14 days after the symptoms have disappeared.

Irregular spotting or bleeding may occur with a proportion of women initially but menstrual regularity is usually re-established after the first few cycles. Those patients whose menstrual patterns do not become reasonably regular after three to four cycles or who have prolonged bleeding or amenorrhoea lasting for two months should be instructed to return for advice.

Women who change from a combined oral contraceptive to Microval should stop taking the previous product, leave seven clear days and take the first Microval tablet on the eighth day, then continue to take 1 tablet daily. Additional contraceptive precautions should be taken until the fourteenth tablet has been taken.

Microval does not diminish the yield of breast milk and can be used from the seventh post-partum day.

Contra-indications:

1. Patients with established hepatic disease or those in whom there is evidence of persistently abnormal liver function such as the Dubin-Johnson and Rotor syndrome, or those who have a history during pregnancy of idiopathic jaundice or severe pruritus.
2. Patients with a history of infectious hepatitis until

the liver function tests have returned to normal values.
3. Patients with abnormal vaginal bleeding of unknown aetiology.
4. Patients with suspected pregnancy.
5. Although the risk of thromboembolism has not been associated with progestogen-only contraceptives, it is at present required that a history of thromboembolic disorders should be regarded as a contraindication.

Special warnings and pecautions for use:

1. Oral contraceptive medication should be discontinued if there is a gradual or sudden, partial or complete loss of vision, proptosis or diplopia, papilloedema or any evidence of retinal or vascular lesions.
2. Caution should be observed in prescribing oral contraceptives for any patients with a history of migraine, or if migraine is being treated with vasoconstrictor drugs. If migraine worsens or migraine or severe headache develops for the first time during treatment, medication should be discontinued immediately.
3. Women with hypertension who are taking Microval require careful observation and their blood pressure should be monitored regularly.
4. A small fraction of the progestogen has been identified in the milk of mothers receiving the drug. The long-range effects to the nursing infant are currently unknown.
5. Examination of the pelvic organs, breasts and blood pressure should precede prescription of Microval and should be repeated regularly.

Interactions with other medicaments and other forms of interaction: Caution should be observed in prescribing oral contraceptives for patients taking other drugs since various interactions have been reported. Pregnancies have been reported in women taking oral contraceptives concurrently with rifampicin and other antibiotics, anti-epileptic drugs, barbiturates and other sedative drugs.

Steroids affect drug metabolism and the therapeutic or toxic effects of other drugs may be modified. Interactions have been reported between oral contraceptives and tricyclic antidepressants, anti-coagulants and corticosteroids.

Use during pregnacy and lactation: Microval is contraindicated to patients with suspected pregnancy. A small fraction of the progestogen has been identified in the milk of mothers receiving the drug. The long-range effects to the nursing infant are currently unknown.

Effects on ability to drive and use machines: None known.

Undesirable effects: Microval is well tolerated but certain endocrine effects which are also characteristic of ovulatory cycles may occur. Those noted are headache, slight weight gain, nausea, skin disorders, breast tenderness and spotting between periods. The incidence of such effects with Microval is low and tends to decrease as treatment continues.

Overdose: No reports of serious ill-effects from overdosage with oral contraceptives have been reported. In general, therefore, treatment of overdosage is not necessary. If overdosage is, however, discovered within one hour and is so large that treatment seems desirable, gastric lavage or a suitable dose of ipecacuanha can be used. There are no specific antidotes and further treatment should be symptomatic.

Pharmacological properties
Pharmacodynamic properties: Only levonorgestrel is biologically active in the racemic mixture of d-l norgestrel. Levonorgestrel has the same potency as the racemic mixture at half the dosage. Levonorgestrel is a progestogen with some androgenic and anti-oestrogenic properties and no significant oestrogenic activity.

Levonorgestrel appears to exert its contraceptive effects by various methods. These include:

1. An effect on cervical mucus by which sperm do not penetrate through it easily and which appears to affect the capacitation phenomenon.
2. Inhibition of ovulation in some cases.
3. An effect on steroid biosynthesis in corpora lutea.

Pharmacokinetic properties: Studies with C–14 labelled norgestrel in man showed that 21% of the ingested dose was excreted in the urine on the day of administration and a further 20.5% during the following 5 days, after which urinary excretion fell to less than 1% daily, plasma levels of norgestrel were lower and decreased more quickly than those of norethisterone. After 24 hours only 1.2% of the administered dose was present in the plasma. Over 50% of the norgestrel excreted is in the form of the sulphate or glucuronide, the metabolites isolated from the urine are composed completely of the d-forms.

Preclinical safety data: Nothing of relevance to the prescriber.

Pharmaceutical particulars
List of excipients:
Tablet core: lactose, starch, poly-n-vinyl pyrrolidone 25, talc, magnesium stearate.
Coating: sucrose, poly-n-vinyl pyrrolidone K 90, calcium carbonate, polyethylene glycol 6000, talc, carnauba wax, white wax.

Incompatibilities: Not applicable.

Shelf life: 5 years.

Special precautions for storage: Store at, or below 25°C.

Nature and contents of container: Single aluminium foil/PVC blisters containing 35 tablets.

Instructions for use/handling: Not applicable.

Marketing authorisation number PL 0011/0040

Date of revision of text January 1998.

Legal category POM

MINOCIN 50*
MINOCIN* 100 mg Tablets

Presentation *Tablets 50 mg:* Each beige film-coated tablet, embossed M/50 on one face, contains Minocycline hydrochloride equivalent to 50 mg Minocycline base.

Tablets 100 mg: Each orange, film-coated tablet, embossed M/100 on one face, contains Minocycline hydrochloride equivalent to 100 mg Minocycline base.

Uses Minocycline is a broad spectrum antibiotic used for the treatment of infections caused by tetracycline-sensitive organisms. Some tetracycline-resistant strains of Staphylococci are also sensitive.
Typical indications include: Gonorrhoea. Non-gonococcal urethritis. Prostatitis. Acne. Acute and chronic bronchitis. Bronchiectasis. Lung abscess. Pneumonia. Ear, nose and throat infections. Urinary tract infections. Pelvic inflammatory disease (eg salpingitis, oophoritis). Skin and soft tissue infections caused by minocycline sensitive organisms. Ophthalmological infections. Nocardiosis. Prophylactic treatment of asymptomatic meningococcal carriers. Pre- and post-operative prophylaxis of infection.

Dosage and administration *Adults:*

1.1. Routine antibiotic use: 200 mg daily in divided doses.
2. Acne: 50 mg twice daily, for a minimum of 6 weeks.
3. Gonorrhoea: In adult males: 200 mg initially, followed by 100 mg every 12 hours for a minimum of 4 days with post-therapy cultures within 2–3 days. Adult females may require more prolonged therapy.
4. Prophylaxis of asymptomatic meningococcal carriers: 100 mg bid for five days, usually followed by a course of rifampicin.

Children: For children above 12 years of age the recommended dosage for Minocin is one 50 mg tablet every 12 hours. Minocin is not recommended for children under 12 years old.

Elderly: Minocin may be used at the normal recommended dosage in elderly patients even with mild to moderate renal impairment, however caution is advised in patients with severe renal impairment.

Administration: To reduce the risk of oesophageal irritation and ulceration, the tablets should be swallowed whole with plenty of fluid, while sitting or standing. Unlike earlier tetracyclines, absorption of Minocin is not significantly impaired by food or moderate amounts of milk.

Treatment of acne should be continued for a minimum of six weeks. If, after six months, there is no satisfactory response Minocin should be discontinued and other therapies considered. If Minocin is to be continued for longer than six months, patients should be monitored at least three monthly thereafter for signs and symptoms of hepatitis or SLE (see warnings and precautions).

Contra-indications, warnings, etc
Contra-indications: Known hypersensitivity to tetracyclines. Use in pregnancy, lactation, children under the age of 12 years, complete renal failure.

Warnings and precautions: Minocin should be used with caution in patients with hepatic dysfunction and in conjunction with alcohol and other hepatotoxic drugs. Rare cases of auto-immune hepatotoxicity and isolated cases of systemic lupus erythematosus (SLE) and also exacerbation of pre-existing SLE have been reported. If patients develop signs or symptoms of SLE or hepatotoxicity, or suffer exacerbation of pre-existing SLE, minocycline should be discontinued.

Clinical studies have shown that there is no significant drug accumulation in patients with renal impairment when they are treated with Minocin in the recommended doses. In cases of severe renal insufficiency, reduction of dosage and monitoring of renal function may be required.

Cross-resistance between tetracyclines may develop in micro-organisms and cross-sensitisation in patients. Minocin should be discontinued if there are signs/symptoms of overgrowth of resistant organisms, eg enteritis, glossitis, stomatitis, vaginitis, pruritus ani or staphylococcal enteritis.

Patients taking oral contraceptives should be warned that if diarrhoea or breakthrough bleeding occur there is a possibility of contraceptive failure.

Interactions: Minocin should not be used with penicillins. Tetracyclines depress plasma prothrombin activity and reduced doses of concomitant anticoagulants may be necessary.

Absorption of Minocin is impaired by the concomitant administration of antacids, iron, calcium, magnesium, aluminium and zinc salts. Unlike earlier tetracyclines, absorption of Minocin is not significantly impaired by food or moderate amounts of milk.

Use in pregnancy: Results of animal studies indicate that tetracyclines cross the placenta, are found in foetal tissues and can have toxic effects on the developing foetus (often related to retardation of skeletal development). Evidence of embryotoxicity has also been noted in animals treated early in pregnancy. Minocin therefore, should not be used in pregnancy unless considered essential.

The use of drugs of the tetracycline class during tooth development (last half of pregnancy) may cause permanent discolouration of the teeth (yellow-grey-brown). This adverse reaction is more common during long term use of the drugs but has been observed following repeated short term courses. Enamel hypoplasia has also been reported.

Use in lactation: Tetracyclines have been found in the milk of lactating women who are taking a drug in this class. Permanent tooth discolouration may occur in the developing infant and enamel hypoplasia has been reported.

Use in children: The use of tetracyclines during tooth development in children under the age of 12 years may cause permanent discolouration (see above). Enamel hypoplasia has also been reported.

Side-effects: In common with other tetracyclines gastrointestinal disturbances including nausea, anorexia, vomiting and diarrhoea may occur. Dermatological reactions such as erythema multiforme, erythema nodosum, Stevens Johnson syndrome, exfoliative dermatitis, hair loss and photosensitivity have been reported, as well as maculopapular and erythematous rashes and, rarely, fixed drug eruptions. Hypersensitivity reactions can include urticaria, fever, arthralgia, myalgia, arthritis, pulmonary infiltration, wheezing, angioneurotic oedema, anaphylaxis and anaphylactoid purpura. Rarely pericarditis, myocarditis, vasculitis and renal failure including interstitial nephritis have been reported. Cases of systemic lupus erythematosus (SLE) and also exacerbation of pre-existing SLE have been reported.

Headache, lightheadedness, dizziness, vertigo and, rarely, impaired hearing have occurred with Minocin and patients should be warned about the possible hazards of driving or operating machinery during treatment.

As with other tetracyclines bulging fontanelles in infants and benign intracranial hypertension in juveniles and adults have been reported. Treatment should cease if evidence of raised intracranial pressure develops.

Blood: haemolytic anaemia, thrombocytopenia, neutropenia and eosinophilia have been reported with tetracyclines.

In common with other tetracyclines, transient increases in liver function test values and rarely hepatitis and acute liver failure have been reported. Some hepatic reactions have an auto-immune basis, and may occur after several months of Minocin treatment (see dosage and administration). There have been isolated incidences of pancreatitis.

When given over prolonged periods, tetracyclines have been reported to produce brown-black microscopic discolouration of thyroid tissue. Hyperpigmentation of skin, nails or discolouration of teeth and buccal mucosa have been reported occasionally. These are generally reversible on cessation of therapy. Bone discolouration has been reported rarely. There are isolated cases of discolouration of conjunctiva, lacrimal secretions, breast secretions and perspiration. See also Uses in Pregnancy and Lactation.

Overdosage: No specific antidote. Gastric lavage plus appropriate supportive treatment.

Pharmaceutical precautions The product should be stored at controlled room temperature (below 30°C) in the original pack or in containers which prevent access of moisture.

Protect from light.

Legal category POM

Package quantities
50 mg Tablets: Blister packs of 84.
100 mg Tablets: Bottles of 20 and 50.

Further information Nil

Product licence numbers
50 mg Tablets 0095/0062
100 mg Tablets 0095/0006R

Date of last review May 1998

MINOCIN MR*
Minocycline 100 mg Modified Release Capsules

Presentation Minocin MR is a two piece hard shell capsule with an orange body and brown opaque cap, containing a mixture of yellow and off-white round pellets. The capsule is marked in white with Lederle and the number 8560.

Each capsule contains minocycline hydrochloride equivalent to 100 mg minocycline.

Uses Minocin MR capsules are indicated for the treatment of acne.

Dosage and administration *Adults:* One capsule every 24 hours.

Children over 12 years: One capsule every 24 hours.

Elderly: No special dosing requirements.

Administration: To reduce the risk of oesophageal irritation and ulceration, the capsules should be swallowed whole with plenty of fluid, while sitting or standing. Unlike earlier tetracyclines, absorption of Minocin MR is not significantly impaired by food or moderate amounts of milk.

Treatment of acne should be continued for a minimum of six weeks. If, after six months, there is no satisfactory response Minocin MR should be discontinued and other therapies considered. If Minocin MR is to be continued for longer than six months, patients should be monitored at least three monthly thereafter for signs and symptoms of hepatitis or SLE (see warnings and precautions)

Contra-indications, warnings, etc
Contra-indications: Known hypersensitivity to tetracyclines. Use in pregnancy, lactation, children under the age of 12 years, complete renal failure.

Warnings, Precautions: Minocin MR should be used with caution in patients with hepatic dysfunction and in conjunction with alcohol and other hepatotoxic drugs. Rare cases of auto-immune hepatotoxicity and isolated cases of systemic lupus erythmatosus (SLE) and also exacerbation of pre-existing SLE have been reported. If patients develop signs or symptoms of SLE or hepatotoxicity, or suffer exacerbation of pre-existing SLE, minocycline should be discontinued.

Clinical studies have shown that there is no significant drug accumulation in patients with renal impairment when they are treated with Minocin MR in the recommended doses. In cases of severe renal insufficiency, reduction of dosage and monitoring of renal function may be required.

Cross-resistance between tetracyclines may develop in micro-organisms and cross-sensitisation in patients may occur. Minocin MR should be discontinued if there are signs/symptoms of overgrowth of resistant organisms, eg enteritis, glossitis, stomatitis, vaginitis, pruritus ani or staphylococcal enteritis.

Women taking oral contraceptives should be warned that if diarrhoea or breakthrough bleeding occur there is a possibility of contraceptive failure.

Interactions: Minocin MR should not be used with penicillins. Tetracyclines depress plasma prothrombin activity and reduced doses of concomitant anticoagulants may be necessary.

Absorption of Minocin MR is impaired by the concomitant administration of antacids, iron, calcium, magnesium, aluminium and zinc salts. Unlike earlier tetracyclines, absorption of Minocin MR is not significantly impaired by food or moderate amounts of milk.

Use in Pregnancy: Results of animal studies indicate that tetracyclines cross the placenta, are found in foetal tissues and can have toxic effects on the developing foetus (often related to retardation of skeletal development). Evidence of embryotoxicity has also been noted in animals treated early in pregnancy. Minocin MR therefore, should not be used in pregnancy unless considered essential.

The use of drugs of the tetracycline class during tooth development (last half of pregnancy) may cause permanent discolouration of the teeth (yellow-grey-brown). This adverse reaction is more common during long term use of the drugs but has been observed following repeated short term courses. Enamel hypoplasia has also been reported.

Use in Lactation: Tetracyclines have been found in the milk of lactating women who are taking a drug in this class. Permanent tooth discolouration may occur in the developing infant and enamel hypoplasia has been reported.

Use in Children: The use of tetracyclines during tooth development in children under the age of 12 years may cause permanent discolouration (see above). Enamel hypoplasia has also been reported.

Side-effects: In common with other tetracyclines gastrointestinal disturbances including nausea, anorexia, vomiting and diarrhoea may occur. Dermatological reactions such as erythema multiforme, erythema nodosum, Stevens Johnson syndrome, exfoliative dermatitis, hair loss and photosensitivity have been reported, as well as maculopapular and erythematous rashes and, rarely, fixed drug eruptions. Hypersensitivity reactions can include urticaria, fever, arthralgia, myalgia, arthritis, pulmonary infiltration, wheezing, angioneurotic oedema, anaphylaxis and anaphylactoid purpura. Rarely pericarditis, myocarditis, vasculitis and renal failure including interstitial nephritis have been reported. Cases of systemic lupus erythematosus (SLE) and also exacerbation of pre-existing SLE have been reported. (See also *Warnings and precautions*).

Headache, light-headedness, dizziness, vertigo and, rarely, impaired hearing have occurred with Minocin MR and patients should be warned about the possible hazards of driving or operating machinery during treatment.

As with other tetracyclines bulging fontanelles in infants and benign intracranial hypertension in juveniles and adults have been reported. Treatment should cease if evidence of raised intracranial pressure develops.

Blood: haemolytic anaemia, thrombocytopenia, neutropenia and eosinophilia have been reported with tetracyclines.

In common with other tetracyclines, transient increases in liver function test values and rarely hepatitis, and acute liver failure have been reported. Some hepatic reactions have an auto-immune basis, and may occur after several months of Minocin MR treatment (see *Dosage and administration*). There have been isolated incidences of pancreatitis.

When given over prolonged periods, tetracyclines have been reported to produce brown-black microscopic discolouration of thyroid tissue. Hyperpigmentation of skin, nails or discolouration of teeth and buccal mucosa have been reported occasionally. These are generally reversible on cessation of therapy. Bone discolouration has been reported rarely. There are isolated cases of discolouration of conjunctiva, lacrimal secretions, breast secretions and perspiration. See also *Uses in Pregnancy and Lactation.*

Overdosage: No specific antidote. Gastric lavage plus appropriate supportive treatment.

Pharmaceutical precautions The product should be stored at controlled room temperature (15–25°C) in the original container. Protect from light.

Legal category POM

Package quantities Minocin MR is available in calendar packs of 56 capsules.

Further information Minocin MR capsules have been formulated as a 'double pulse' delivery system in which a portion of the minocycline is delivered in the stomach, and a second dose is available for absorption in the duodenum and upper GI tract.

Product licence number 0095/0240

Date of last review May 1998

MINULET*

Presentation Each white sugar coated tablet contains 30 micrograms ethinyloestradiol and 75 micrograms gestodene.

Uses Oral contraception and the recognised gynaecological indications for such oestrogen-progestogen combinations. The mode of action includes the inhibition of ovulation by suppression of the mid-cycle surge of luteinising hormone, the inspissation of cervical mucus so as to constitute a barrier to sperm, and the rendering of the endometrium unreceptive to implantation.

Dosage and administration
First treatment cycle: 1 tablet daily for 21 days, starting with the tablet marked number 1, on the first day of the menstrual cycle. Additional contraception (barriers and spermicides) is not required.

Subsequent cycles: Each subsequent course is started when 7 tablet-free days have followed the preceding course. A withdrawal bleed should occur during the 7 tablet-free days.

Changing from another 21 day combined oral contraceptive: The first tablet of Minulet should be taken on the first day immediately after the end of the previous oral contraceptive course. Additional contraception is not required. A withdrawal bleed should not be expected until the end of the first pack of Minulet.

Changing from an Every Day (ED) 28 day combined oral contraceptive: The first tablet of Minulet should be taken on the day immediately after the day on which the last active pill in the ED pack has been taken. The remaining tablets in the ED pack should be discarded. Additional contraception is not required. A withdrawal bleed should not be expected until the end of the first pack of Minulet.

Changing from a Progestogen-only-Pill (POP): The first tablet of Minulet should be taken on the first day of menstruation even if the POP for that day has already been taken. The remaining tablets in the POP pack should be discarded. Additional contraception is not required.

Post-partum and post-abortum use: After pregnancy combined oral contraception can be started in non-lactating women 21 days after a vaginal delivery, provided that the patient is fully ambulant and there are no puerperal complications.

If the pill is started later than 21 days after delivery, then alternative contraception (barriers and spermicides) should be used until oral contraception is started and for the first 7 days of pill-taking. If unprotected intercourse has taken place after 21 days post partum, then oral contraception should not be started until the first menstrual bleed after childbirth. After a miscarriage or abortion oral contraception may be started immediately.

Special circumstances requiring additional contraception:

Missed Pills: If a tablet is delayed it should be taken as soon as possible and if it is taken within 12 hours of the correct time, additional contraception is not needed. Further tablets should then be taken at the usual time. If the delay exceeds 12 hours, the last missed pill should be taken when remembered, the earlier missed pills left in the pack and normal pill-taking resumed. If one or more tablets are omitted from the 21 days of pill-taking, additional contraception (barriers and spermicides) should be used for the next 7 days of pill-taking. In addition, if one or more pills are missed during the last 7 days of pill-taking, the subsequent pill-free interval should be disregarded and the next pack started the day after taking the last tablet from the previous pack. In this case, a withdrawal bleed should not be expected until the end of the second pack. If the patient does not have a withdrawal bleed at the end of the second pack she must return to her doctor to exclude the possibility of pregnancy.

Gastro-intestinal upset: Vomiting or diarrhoea may reduce the efficacy by preventing full absorption. Additional contraception (barriers and spermicides) should be used during the upset and for the 7 days following the upset. If these 7 days overrun the end of a pack, the next pack should be started without a break. In this case, a withdrawal bleed should not be expected until the end of the second pack. If the patient does not have a withdrawal bleed at the end of the second pack she must return to her doctor to exclude the possibility of pregnancy.

Mild laxatives do not impair contraceptive action.

Interaction with other drugs: Some drugs accelerate the metabolism of oral contraceptives when taken concurrently and these include barbiturates, phenytoin, phenylbutazone and rifampicin. Other drugs suspected of having the capacity to reduce the efficacy of oral contraceptives include ampicillin and other antibiotics. It is, therefore, advisable to use non-hormonal methods of contraception (barriers and spermicides) in addition to the oral contraceptive as long as an extremely high degree of protection is required during treatment with such drugs. The additional contraception should be used while the concurrent medication continues and for 7 days afterwards. If these extra precautions overrun the end of the pack, the next pack should be started without a break. In this case, a withdrawal bleed should not be expected until the end of the second pack. If the patient does not have a withdrawal bleed at the end of the second pack she must return to her doctor to exclude the possibility of pregnancy.

Contra-indications, warnings etc.
Contra-indications:

1. Suspected pregnancy.
2. Thrombotic disorders and a history of these conditions, sickle-cell anaemia, disorders of lipid metabolism and other conditions in which, in individual cases, there is known or suspected to be a much increased risk of thrombosis.
3. Acute or severe chronic liver diseases. Dubin-Johnson syndrome. Rotor syndrome. History,

during pregnancy, of idiopathic jaundice or severe pruritus.
4. History of herpes gestationis.
5. Mammary or endometrial carcinoma, or a history of these conditions.
6. Abnormal vaginal bleeding of unknown cause.
7. Deterioration of otosclerosis during pregnancy.

Warnings:

1. There is a general opinion, based on statistical evidence, that users of combined oral contraceptives experience, more often than non-users, venous thromboembolism, arterial thrombosis, including cerebral and myocardial infarction, and subarachnoid haemorrhage. Full recovery from such disorders does not always occur, and it should be realised that in a few cases they are fatal. How often these disorders occur in users of the modern low-dose pills is not known, but there are reasons for suggesting that they may occur less often than with older pills containing more oestrogen. Certain factors may entail some risk of thrombosis, e.g. smoking, obesity, varicose veins, cardiovascular diseases, diabetes and migraine. The suitability of a combined oral contraceptive should be judged according to the severity of such conditions in the individual case, and should be discussed with the patient before she decides to take it.
2. The risk of arterial thrombosis associated with combined oral contraceptives increases with age, and this risk is aggravated by cigarette smoking. The use of combined oral contraceptives by women in the older age group, especially those who are cigarette smokers, should therefore be discouraged and alternative methods used.
3. The possibility cannot be ruled out that certain chronic diseases may occasionally deteriorate during the use of combined oral contraceptives. (See *Precautions*).
4. The combination of ethinyloestradiol and gestodene, like other contraceptive steroids, is associated with an increased incidence of neoplastic nodules in the rat liver, the relevance of which to man is unknown.
5. Malignant liver tumours have been reported on rare occasions in long-term users of oral contraceptives. Benign hepatic tumours have also been associated with oral contraceptive usage. A hepatic tumour should be considered in the differential diagnosis when upper abdominal pain, enlarged liver or signs of intra-abdominal haemorrhage occur.
6. Numerous epidemiological studies have been reported on the risks of ovarian, endometrial, cervical and breast cancer in women using combined oral contraceptives. The evidence is clear that combined oral contraceptives offer substantial protection against both ovarian and endometrial cancer. An increased risk of cervical cancer in long term users of combined oral contraceptives has been reported in some studies, but there continues to be controversy about the extent to which this is attributable to the confounding effects of sexual behaviour and other factors.
   A meta-analysis from 54 epidemiological studies reported that there is a slightly increased relative risk (RR = 1.24) of having breast cancer diagnosed in women who are currently using combined oral contraceptives (COCs). The observed pattern of increased risk may be due to an earlier diagnosis of breast cancer in COC users, the biological effects of COCs or a combination of both. The additional breast cancers diagnosed in current users of COCs or in women who have used COCs in the last ten years are more likely to be localised to the breast than those in women who never used COCs.
   Breast cancer is rare among women under 40 years of age whether or not they take COCs. Whilst this background risk increases with age, the excess number of breast cancer diagnoses in current and recent COC users is small in relation to the overall risk of breast cancer (see bar chart).
   The most important risk factor for breast cancer in COC users is the age women discontinue the COC; the older the age at stopping, the more breast cancers are diagnosed. Duration of use is less important and the excess risk gradually disappears during the course of the 10 years after stopping COC use such that by 10 years there appears to be no excess.
   The possible increase in risk of breast cancer should be discussed with the user and weighed against the benefits of COCs taking into account the evidence that they offer substantial protection against the risk of developing certain other cancers (e.g. ovarian and endometrial cancer).

Reasons for stopping oral contraception immediately:

1. Occurrence of migraine in patients who have never previously suffered from it. Exacerbation of pre-existing migraine. Any unusually frequent or unusually severe headaches.
2. Any kind of acute disturbance of vision.
3. Suspicion of thrombosis or infarction.
4. Six weeks before elective operations and during immobilisation, e.g. after accidents, etc.
5. Significant rise in blood-pressure.
6. Jaundice.
7. Clear exacerbation of conditions known to be capable of deteriorating during oral contraception or pregnancy.
8. Pregnancy is a reason for stopping immediately because it has been suggested by some investigations that oral contraceptives taken in early pregnancy may slightly increase the risk of foetal malformations. Other investigations have failed to support these findings. The possibility therefore cannot be excluded, but it is certain that if a risk exists at all, it is very small.

Precautions:

1. Examination of the pelvic organs, breasts and blood-pressure should precede the prescribing of any combined oral contraceptive and should be repeated regularly.
2. Before starting treatment, pregnancy must be excluded.
3. The following conditions require careful observation during medication: a history of severe depressive states, varicose veins, diabetes, hypertension, epilepsy, otosclerosis, multiple sclerosis, porphyria, tetany, disturbed liver function, gall-stones, cardiovascular diseases, renal diseases, chloasma, uterine fibroids, asthma, the wearing of contact lenses, or any disease that is prone to worsen during pregnancy. The first appearance or deterioration of any of these conditions may indicate that the oral contraceptive should be stopped.
4. The risk of the deterioration of chloasma, which is often not fully reversible, is reduced by the avoidance of excessive exposure to sunlight.

Side-effects: Occasional side-effects may include nausea, vomiting, headaches, breast tenderness, changed body weight or libido, depressive moods and chloasma.

Menstrual changes:

1. Reduction of menstrual flow: This is not abnormal and it is to be expected in some patients. Indeed, it may be beneficial where heavy periods were previously experienced.
2. Missed menstruation: Occasionally, withdrawal bleeding may not occur at all. If the tablets have been taken correctly, pregnancy is very unlikely, but should be ruled out before a new course of tablets is started.

Intermenstrual bleeding: Very light 'spotting' or heavier 'breakthrough bleeding' may occur during tablet-taking, especially in the first few cycles. It appears to be generally of no significance, except where it indicates errors of tablet-taking, or where the possibility of interaction with other drugs exists (q.v.). However, if irregular bleeding is persistent, an organic cause should be considered.

Effect on adrenal and thyroid glands: Oral contraceptives have no significant influence on adrenocortical function. The ACTH function test for the adrenal cortex remains unchanged. The reduction in corticosteroid excretion and the elevation of plasma corticosteroids are due to an increased cortisol-binding capacity of the plasma proteins.

The response to metyrapone is less pronounced than in untreated women and is thus similar to that during pregnancy.

The radio-iodine uptake shows that thyroid function is unchanged. There is a rise in serum protein-bound iodine, similar to that in pregnancy and during the administration of oestrogens. This is due to the increased capacity of the plasma proteins for binding thyroid hormones, rather than to any change in glandular function. In women taking oral contraceptives, the content of protein-bound iodine in blood serum should therefore, not be used for evaluation of thyroid function.

Effect on blood chemistry: Oral contraceptives may accelerate erythrocyte sedimentation in the absence of any disease. This effect is due to a change in the proportion of the plasma protein fractions. Increases in plasma copper, iron and alkaline phosphatase have also been recorded.

Overdosage: There have been no reports of serious ill-effects from overdosage, even when a considerable number of tablets have been taken by a small child. In general, it is, therefore, unnecessary to treat overdosage. However, if overdosage is discovered within two or three hours and is so large that treatment seems desirable, gastric lavage can be safely used.

There are no specific antidotes and further treatment should be symptomatic.

Pharmaceutical precautions Store in cool, dry conditions. Shelf-life five years.

Legal category POM

Package quantities Individual packs containing 3 months' supply.

Further information NIL

Product licence number 0011/0135

Estimated cumulative numbers of breast cancers per 10,000 women diagnosed in 5 years of use and up to 10 years after stopping COCs, compared with numbers of breast cancers diagnosed in 10,000 women who had never used COCs.

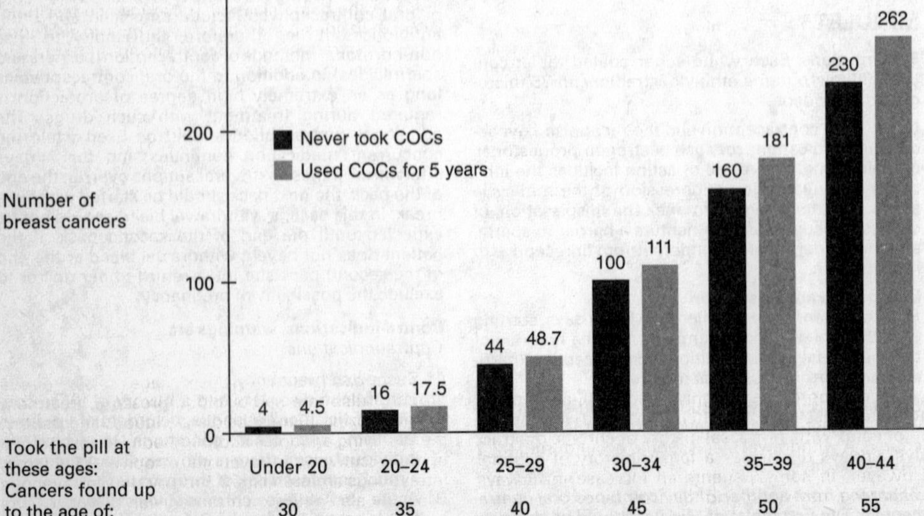

MONOCOR* Tablets

Presentation

Tablets 5 mg: Pink, round, scored, biconvex film-coated tablets marked 'LL' on one side and '5' on reverse, each containing 5 mg bisoprolol fumarate (2:1).

Tablets 10 mg: White, round biconvex film-coated tablets marked 'LL' on one side and '10' on reverse, each containing 10 mg bisoprolol fumarate (2:1).

Uses

Indications: The management of hypertension. The management of angina pectoris.

Mode of action: Monocor is a potent, highly cardioselective B_1-adrenoceptor blocking agent devoid of intrinsic sympathomimetic activity and without relevant membrane stabilising activity.

As with other beta-blocking agents, the mode of action in hypertension is not clear but it is known that Monocor reduces the heart rate and depresses plasma renin activity.

In patients with angina, blocking of cardiac B_1-

receptors causes a diminished cardiac oxygen demand because of the resulting reduced heart action. This makes Monocor effective in eliminating or reducing the symptoms.

Dosage and administration
Adults: The usual adult dose is 10 mg once daily with a maximum recommended dose of 20 mg per day. In some patients, 5 mg per day may be adequate.

It is not necessary to alter the dose in patients with mild to moderate hepatic or renal dysfunction. In patients with severe renal failure (creatinine clearance less than 20 ml/min) or in patients with severe hepatic dysfunction, the dosage should not exceed 10 mg Monocor once daily.

Experience of use of Monocor in renal dialysis patients is limited. However, there is no evidence that the dosage regimen needs to be altered.

Elderly: No dosage adjustment is normally required but 5 mg per day may be adequate in some elderly patients; as for other adults, the dosage may have to be reduced in cases of severe renal or hepatic dysfunction.

Children: There is no paediatric experience with bisoprolol, therefore its use cannot be recommended for children.

Contra-indications, warnings etc
Contra-indications: As with other beta-adrenoceptor antagonists, Monocor should not be used in cases of untreated cardiac failure, cardiogenic shock, sinoatrial block, second or third degree AV block, marked bradycardia (less than 50 beats per minute) or extreme hypotension or severe asthma.

Precautions: Monocor should be used with care in patients with a prolonged PR conduction interval, poor cardiac reserve and peripheral circulatory disturbances, such as Raynaud's phenomena.

In patients suffering ischaemic heart disease treatment should not be discontinued abruptly.

Due to the low affinity of Monocor for B_2-receptors, the drug does not appear to have a hypoglycaemic effect. However, it should be used with caution in diabetic patients since the symptoms of hypoglycaemia (in particular tachycardia) may be masked.

Although Monocor is a highly selective B_1-adrenoceptor blocking agent, it should be used with caution in patients with chronic obstructive airways disease or a family history of asthma. In some asthmatic patients some increase in airways resistance may occur and this may be regarded as a signal to discontinue therapy. Bronchospasm can usually be reversed by commonly used bronchodilators such as salbutamol.

Pregnancy and lactation: No teratogenic effects have been demonstrated in animal studies but the safety of Monocor during human pregnancy has not been established. Like other beta-blockers, the benefits of use during pregnancy should be weighed against the possible hazards to mother and foetus. Beta-blockers administered in late pregnancy may cause bradycardia or hypotension in the foetus/neonate.

Studies in animals suggest that no clinically relevant levels of Monocor reach the breast milk. However, as in pregnancy, caution should be exercised for use during lactation.

Side effects: Monocor is usually well tolerated. The reported side-effects are generally attributable to the pharmacological activity of a beta-blocker and include lassitude, fatigue, dizziness, mild headache, muscle and joint ache, perspiration, aggravation of intermittent claudication or Raynaud's disease, paraesthesia and coldness of the extremities, bronchospasm, oedema and occasional gastro-intestinal side effects such as nausea/vomiting and diarrhoea. A marked decrease in blood pressure and pulse rate or a disturbance of AV conduction may be observed occasionally. As with other beta-blockers, skin rashes, pruritus and dry eyes have been reported although the incidence is low. Sleep disturbances, including vivid dreams, of a type noted with other beta blockers have occasionally been reported. Discontinuation of the drug is recommended if any such reaction is not otherwise explicable.

Drug interactions: Monocor may potentiate the effect of other concurrently administered anti-hypertensive drugs. Concomitant treatment with reserpine, alphamethyldopa and clonidine may cause an exaggerated decrease in heart rate. In particular, if clonidine is to be discontinued this should not be done until Monocor treatment has been discontinued for several days.

Monocor should also be used with care when myocardial depressants, inhibitors of AV conduction such as calcium antagonists of the verapamil and diltiazem type, or Class I antidysrrhythmic agents such as disopyramide are used concurrently.

The intravenous administration of calcium antagonists and antiarrhythmic agents is not recommended during Monocor therapy.

The concurrent use of rifampicin can reduce the elimination half-life of Monocor, although an increase in dose is generally not necessary. The effects of insulin or oral hypoglycaemic agents may be potentiated when used concurrently with Monocor.

Anaesthesia: Prior to anaesthesia, the anaesthetist should be informed if the patient is taking Monocor. In cases of severe ischaemic heart disease the risk/benefit of continuing treatment should be evaluated. Care should be taken when using either cyclopropane or trichloroethylene.

Overdosage: In the case of overdosage or a precipitous drop in pulse rate and/or blood pressure, treatment with Monocor must be discontinued. Excessive bradycardia may be countered by atropine 0.5–2.0 mg intravenously. If necessary this may be followed by a beta stimulant such as orciprenaline by slow intravenous injection. Glucagon may also be useful as a cardiac stimulant in a dose of 1 to 5 mg intravenously.

Pharmaceutical precautions No special requirements.

Legal category POM

Package quantities Calenderised blister packs of 28 tablets in strips of 14.

Further information Monocor is absorbed almost completely from the gastrointestinal tract. Together with the very small first past effect in the liver, this results in a high bioavailability of approximately 90% The drug is cleared equally by the liver and kidneys. The high bioavailability and the dual pathway of clearance lead to predictable blood levels. The long plasma half-life (10–12 hours) provides 24 hour efficacy following a once daily dosage. About 95% of the drug substance is excreted through the kidneys, half of this as unchanged Monocor. There are no active metabolites in man.

Product licence numbers

Tablets 5 mg	0095/0177
Tablets 10 mg	0095/0178

MONOZIDE*10

Presentation White, round, biconvex, film coated tablets marked B-14 on one side and LL on the other, each containing 10 mg bisoprolol fumarate (2:1), and 6.25 mg hydrochlorothiazide.

Uses Management of hypertension.
Mode of Action: Bisoprolol is a potent, highly cardioselective β_1-adrenoreceptor antagonist devoid of intrinsic sympathomimetic activity and without relevant membrane stabilising activity.

As with other β_1-antagonists, the mode of action in hypertension is not clear but it is known that bisoprolol reduces the heart rate and markedly depresses plasma renin activity.

Hydrochlorothiazide is a thiazide diuretic which has an antihypertensive action. It exerts its diuretic effect by inhibiting the resorption of sodium and chloride ions in the loop of Henle and distal tubule. It also appears to decrease peripheral resistance. Hydrochlorothiazide is frequently used in combination with a β-adrenoceptor antagonist where an additional antihypertensive effect is required.

Dosage and administration *Adults:* One tablet daily. No dose reduction is needed in patients with mild to moderate hepatic or renal dysfunction.

Elderly: As for adults.

Children: There is no paediatric experience with bisoprolol and it is not therefore recommended for children.

Contra-indications, warnings, etc.
Contra-indications: As with other β-adrenoceptor antagonist diuretic combinations, Monozide 10 should not be used in cases of untreated or decompensated cardiac failure, cardiogenic shock, sinoatrial block, second or third degree AV block, marked bradycardia (heart rate less than 50 beats/min), extreme hypotension, acute myocardial infarction, and severe asthma. It should not be used in patients with a known allergic hypersensitivity to thiazides or sulphonamides, with severe renal or hepatic failure, as well as in patients with severe hypokalaemia or hyponatraemia.

Precautions: Monozide 10 tablets should be used with care in patients with prolonged PR conduction interval, poor cardiac reserve and peripheral circulatory disturbances, such as Raynaud's phenomenon.

In patients with ischaemic heart disease, treatment should not be withdrawn abruptly.

Since bisoprolol is a highly selective β_1-adrenoceptor antagonist, Monozide 10 may be used with caution in patients with a medical history of chronic obstructive airways disease or a family history of asthma. However, in some patients an increase in airways resistance may occur and this may be regarded as a signal to discontinue therapy. This bronchospasm can usually be reversed by commonly used bronchodilators such as salbutamol.

Due to the low affinity of bisoprolol for β_2-receptors, Monozide 10 does not appear to have a hypoglycaemic effect. However, it should be used with caution in diabetic patients since the symptoms of hypoglycaemia (in particular, tachycardia) may be masked and hydrochlorothiazide may impair glucose tolerance further.

Clinical trials have shown that the low dose of hydrochlorothiazide in this formulation reduces the elevation in uric acid levels normally associated with higher doses of hydrochlorothiazide. However, care should be taken in patients with a predisposition to gout or hyperuricaemia.

The particularly low dose of hydrochlorothiazide in this formulation (6.25 mg) reduces the possibility of significant electrolyte imbalance occurring. However, all patients treated with diuretics should receive periodic monitoring for signs of fluid or electrolyte imbalance. Hypokalaemia can be induced as a result of thiazide therapy and potassium levels should be checked; particularly in older patients, those receiving digitalis preparations for heart failure, those on diets low in potassium and patients suffering from gastro-intestinal complaints.

Pregnancy and lactation: No teratogenic effects have been demonstrated with bisoprolol in animal studies, but thiazide diuretics are not generally recommended for use during pregnancy. Beta-blockers administered in late pregnancy may cause bradycardia or hypotension in the foetus/neonate. Like other anti-hypertensive therapy, the benefits of use during pregnancy should be weighed against the possible hazard to mother and foetus. Whilst clinically relevant levels of bisoprolol may not appear in breast milk, hydrochlorothiazide does appear in the milk and if treatment is essential the patient should stop breast feeding.

Drug interactions: Bisoprolol may potentiate the effect of other concurrently administered antihypertensive drugs. Concomitant treatment with reserpine, α-methlydopa and clonidine may cause an exaggerated decrease in heart rate and blood pressure. In particular, if clonidine is to be discontinued, this should not be done until treatment with Monozide 10 has been discontinued for several days.

Monozide 10 should also be used with care when myocardial depressants, inhibitors of AV conduction such as calcium antagonists of the verapamil and diltiazem type, or class I antidysrhythmic agents such as disopyramide are used concurrently.

The intravenous administration of calcium antagonists and antiarrhythmic agents is not recommended during therapy with Monozide 10.

Lithium should not generally be administered with diuretics as lithium clearance may be significantly reduced.

The concurrent use of rifampicin can reduce the elimination half-life of bisoprolol, although an increase in dose is generally not necessary. The effects of insulin or oral hypoglycaemic agents may be potentiated when used concurrently with bisoprolol.

Anaesthesia: Prior to anaesthesia, the anaesthetist should be informed if the patient is taking Monozide 10. In cases of severe ischaemic heart disease, the risk/benefit of continuing treatment should be evaluated. Care should be taken when using volatile anaesthetics because of an increased hypotensive effect. Hydrochlorothiazide may increase the responsiveness to agents of the tubocurarine type.

Side effects: Monozide 10 is usually well tolerated with reported side effects generally attributable to its pharmacological effects and reflects those of other drugs in the same classes. These include lassitude, fatigue, dizziness, mild headache, muscle and joint ache, perspiration, aggravation of intermittent claudication or Raynaud's disease, paraesthesia and coldness of the extremities, bronchospasm, oedema, pruritus and occasional G.I. side effects such as nausea/vomiting and diarrhoea and sleep disturbances. Occasionally a marked decrease in blood pressure and pulse rate or a disturbance of AV conduction may be observed. Dry eyes noted with other β-blockers have not been reported for patients treated with Monozide 10 but may rarely occur.

Skin rashes, photosensivity, anaphylactic reactions and blood dyscrasias including thrombocytopenia have been associated with hydrochlorothiazide therapy, but occur only rarely. There are no reports of similar reactions associated with Monozide 10 therapy.

Overdosage: In the case of overdosage or a precipitous drop in pulse rate and/or blood pressure, treatment with Monozide 10 must be discontinued. If necessary, the following antidotes should be administered alone or consecutively: intravenous atropine 0.5–2.0 mg, intravenous orciprenaline 0.5 mg by slow intravenous injection; also glucagon may be given at a dose level of 1 to 5 mg.

Pharmaceutical precautions No special requirement.

Legal category POM

Package quantities Calendar packs of 28.

Further information The particularly low dose of hydrochlorothiazide used in this formulation has been shown to reduce the incidence/severity of side effects such as hypokalaemia and hyperuricaemia when compared to therapy using standard doses of the drug (25 mg). When combined with bisoprolol, a potent β_1 selective adrenoceptor antagonist, the tablet provides a convenient combination which should help the patient with its single daily dose, whilst minimising side effects.

Product licence number 0095/0269

MUCAINE* SUSPENSION

Qualitative and quantitative composition Each 5 ml of Mucaine Suspension contains:
Oxethazaine 10 mg
Magnesium Hydroxide BP 100 mg
Aluminium Hydroxide Mixture BP 4.75 ml

Pharmaceutical form Mucaine Suspension is a white oral suspension with the odour and flavour of peppermint.

Clinical particulars
Therapeutic indications: Mucaine is an antacid mixture containing a topical anaesthetic. It is indicated for oesophagitis whatever its cause, including peptic oesophagitis with or without hiatus hernia, radiation oesophagitis and the heartburn of late pregnancy.

Posology and method of administration:
Adults: One to two 5 ml doses should be taken three or four times daily, 15 minutes before meals, and at bedtime, or as required. The dose should not be washed down with a drink.

The elderly: The adult dosage schedule may be used in the elderly.

Children: Not recommended for children.

Contra-indications: The aluminium ion combines with phosphate to form an insoluble complex which is not absorbed. When high doses are given together with a low phosphorus diet, phosphate depletion occurs. Phosphate depletion does not occur in patients on a normal diet. Mucaine is contra-indicated in patients with hypophosphataemia.

The use of magnesium-containing antacids is contraindicated in patients with severe renal impairment because hypermagnesaemia is more likely to occur.

Special warnings and precautions for use: The use of magnesium containing antacids in patients with mild to moderate renal impairment should be carefully observed due to the increased risk of hypermagnesaemia.

In patients with chronic renal failure, hyperaluminaemia may occur.

Interaction with other medicaments and other forms of interaction: The rate and/or extent of absorption of many drugs may be increased or decreased when they are used concurrently with aluminium-magnesium hydroxide-containing antacids. Therefore, as a general rule, medication should not be taken within one to two hours of an antacid, if possible.

This includes: tetracycline, iron salts, chlorpromazine, levodopa, isoniazid, digoxin, H_2-antagonists, indomethacin, nitrofurantoin, and dicoumarol.

Pregnancy and lactation: A rabbit study has shown a dose related reduction in litter size, although the relevance of these findings to man is unknown. There is no evidence of safety of oxethazaine in human pregnancy, therefore the product should not be used during the first trimester of pregnancy or during lactation.

Effects on ability to drive and use machines: None reported.

Undesirable effects: Mucaine is well tolerated. The side effects which have been reported are almost invariably mild and transient in nature, consisting principally of constipation, dryness of the mouth, and nausea. Hypersensitivity reactions including skin eruptions (dermatitis urticaria), pruritus, glossitis and angioedema have been reported on rare occasions.

Overdose: Not reported. Treatment should be symptomatic.

Pharmacological properties
Pharmacodynamic properties: Aluminium Hydroxide Mixture BP has high antacid activity. It is given in conjunction with the antacid magnesium hydroxide which is also a saline laxative. This alleviates any constipatory effect of the aluminium hydroxide mixture. Oxethazaine is a surface anaesthetic of the amide type. It is stable at the levels of acidity or alkalinity found in the upper gastrointestinal tract, and has relatively prolonged action. The relief obtained in the symptomatic treatment of oesophagitis is aided by the physical and antacid properties of the product.

Pharmacokinetic properties: The insoluble aluminium compounds which constitute aluminium hydroxide mixture are incompletely converted to aluminium chloride in the stomach. Some absorption occurs from the gastrointestinal tract, with excretion in the urine. Some of the unabsorbed aluminium hydroxide combines with phosphates present in the gut to form insoluble aluminium phosphates, carbonates and salts of fatty acids. All these salts are excreted in the faeces. Magnesium hydroxide is converted to magnesium chloride. Any absorbed magnesium is usually rapidly excreted in the urine. There is no further information available on oxethazaine.

Preclinical safety data: Nothing of further interest to prescriber.

Pharmaceutical particulars
List of excipients: Alcohol 60 OP, benzoic acid[1], glycerine[1], sodium benzoate[1], ammonia solution (strong), sodium hypochlorite solution[1], peppermint 85599-S, peppermint oil[1], saccharine sodium[1], sorbitol solution[2], water.

[1] Complies with Ph Eur specification
[2] Complies with BPC 1973 specification

Incompatibilities: None known

Shelf life: 24 months

Special precautions for storage: Store in a cool place, discard contents 14 days after opening.

Nature and contents of container: White polypropylene bottles with metal screw cap with liner and tamper-evident seal containing 200 ml.

Instructions for use/handling: None

Marketing authorisation number 0011/5014R

Date of approval/revision of the SPC June 1997

Legal category POM

NIPENT*
(Pentostatin for injection)

Qualitative and quantitative composition One vial contains 10 mg Pentostatin.

Pharmaceutical form Powder for solution for injection/infusion.

Sterile, apyrogenic, lyophilised powder.

Clinical particulars
Therapeutic indications: Pentostatin is indicated as single agent therapy in the treatment of adult patients with hairy cell leukaemia.

Posology and method of administration: Pentostatin is indicated for adult patients.

Administration to patient: It is recommended that patients receive hydration with 500 to 1,000 ml of 5% glucose only or 5% glucose in 0.18% or 0.9% saline or glucose 3.3% in 0.3% saline or 2.5% glucose in 0.45% saline or equivalent before pentostatin administration. An additional 500 ml of 5% glucose only or 5% glucose in 0.18% or 0.9% saline or 2.5% glucose in 0.45% saline or equivalent should be administered after pentostatin is given.

The recommended dosage of pentostatin for the treatment of hairy cell leukaemia is 4 mg/m² in a single administration every other week. Pentostatin may be given intravenously by bolus injection or diluted in a larger volume and given over 20 to 30 minutes. (See *Instruction for use/handling*).

Higher doses are not recommended.

No extravasation injuries were reported in clinical studies.

The optimal duration of treatment has not been determined. In the absence of major toxicity and with observed continuing improvement, the patient should be treated until a complete response has been achieved. Although not established as required, the administration of two additional doses has been recommended following the achievement of a complete response.

All patients receiving pentostatin at 6 months should be assessed for response to treatment. If the patient has not achieved a complete or partial response, treatment with pentostatin should be discontinued.

If the patient has achieved a partial response, pentostatin treatment should be continued in an effort to achieve a complete response. At any time thereafter that a complete response is achieved, two additional doses of pentostatin are recommended. Pentostatin treatment should then be stopped. If the best response to treatment at the end of 12 months is a partial response, it is recommended that treatment with pentostatin be stopped.

Withholding or discontinuation of individual doses may be needed when severe adverse reactions occur. Drug treatment should be withheld in patients with severe rash, and withheld or discontinued in patients showing evidence of nervous system toxicity.

Pentostatin treatment should be withheld in patients with active infection occurring during the treatment but may be resumed when the infection is controlled.

Dosage in patients with cytopenias: No dosage reduction is recommended at the start of therapy with pentosatin in patients with anaemia, neutropenia or thombocytopenia. In addition, dosage reductions are not recommended during treatment in patients with anaemia and thrombocytopenia. Pentostatin should be temporarily withheld if the absolute neutrophil count during treatment falls below 200 cells/mm³ in a patient who had an initial neutrophil count greater than 500 cells/mm³ and may be resumed when the count returns to pre-dose levels.

Renal insufficiency: There is limited experience in patients with impaired renal function (creatinine clearance <60 ml/min). Two patients with impaired renal function (creatinine clearances 50 to 60 ml/min) achieved complete response without unusual adverse events when treated with 2 mg/m². However, given this limited experience, pentostatin is contra-indicated in patients whose creatinine clearance is <60 ml/min.

Liver impairment: Because of limited experience treating patients with abnormal liver function, treatment of such patients should be done with caution.

Administration to elderly patients: The recommended dosage of pentostatin for the treatment of hairy cell leukaemia in the elderly is 4 mg/m² in a single administration every other week. Clinical trials have included patients over 65 years old and no adverse reactions specific to this age group have been reported.

Paediatric use: Hairy cell leukaemia is a disease affecting adults, most commonly in the sixth decade of life. Safety and effectiveness of Nipent in children have not been established.

Contra-indications: Pentostatin is contra-indicated in patients who have demonstrated hypersensitivity to pentostatin.

Pentostatin is contra-indicated in patients with impaired renal function (creatinine clearance <60 ml/min).

Pentostatin is contra-indicated in patients with active infection.

Pentostatin is contra-indicated in pregnancy.

Special warnings and special precautions for use
Warnings: Pentostatin should be administered under the supervision of a physician qualified and experienced in the use of cancer chemotherapeutic agents. The use of doses higher than those specified (see *Administration to patients*) is not recommended. Dose-limiting severe renal, liver, pulmonary and CNS toxicities occurred in Phase 1 studies that used pentostatin at a higher dose (20–50 mg/m²/course) than recommended.

In a clinical investigation in patients with refractory chronic lymphocytic leukaemia using pentostatin at the recommended dose in combination with fludarabine phosphate, four of six patients entered on the study had severe or fatal pulmonary toxicity. The use of pentostatin in combination with fludarabine phosphate is not recommended.

Biochemical studies have demonstrated that pentostatin enhances the effects of vidarabine, a purine nucleoside with anti-viral activity. The combined use of vidarabine and pentostatin may result in an increase in adverse reactions associated with each drug. The therapeutic benefit of the drug combination has not been established.

Patients with hairy cell leukaemia may experience myelosuppression primarily during the first few courses of treatment. Patients with infections prior to pentostatin treatment have in some cases developed worsening of their condition leading to death; whereas others have achieved complete response. Patients with infection should be treated only when the potential benefit of treatment justifies the potential risk to the patient. Efforts should be made to control the infection before treatment is initiated or resumed.

In patients with progressive hairy cell leukaemia, the initial courses of pentostatin treatment were associated with worsening of neutropenia. Therefore, frequent monitoring of complete blood counts during this time is necessary. If severe neutropenia continues beyond the initial cycles, patients should be evaluated for disease status, including a bone marrow examination.

Pentostatin might have harmful effects on the genotype. Therefore, it is recommended that men undergoing treatment with pentostatin should not father a child during treatment or up to six months thereafter. Contraception is to be guaranteed for women of childbearing age. Should pregnancy occur during the treatment, the possibility of a genetic consultation is to be considered.

Bone marrow transplant regimen with high dose cyclophosphamide: Acute pulmonary oedema and hypotension leading to death, have been reported in the literature in patients treated with pentostatin in combination with carmustine, etoposide and high dose cyclophosphamide as part of an ablative regimen for bone marrow transplant. The combination of pentostatin and high dose cyclophosphamide is not recommended.

Elevations in liver function tests occurred during treatment with pentostatin and were generally reversible.

Renal toxicity was observed at higher doses in early studies; however, in patients treated at the recommended dose, elevations in serum creatinine were usually minor and reversible. There were some patients who began treatment with normal renal function who had evidence of mild to moderate toxicity at a final assessment. (See *Administration to patient*).

Rashes, occasionally severe, were commonly reported and may worsen with continued treatment. Withholding of treatment may be required. (See *Administration to patient*).

Extra care should be taken in treating patients beginning therapy with poor performance.

Precautions: Therapy with pentostatin requires regular patient observation and monitoring of haematologic parameters and blood chemistry values. If severe adverse reactions occur, the drug should be withheld (See *Administration to patient*) and appropriate corrective measures should be taken according to the clinical judgement of the physician.

Pentostatin treatment should be withheld or discontinued in patients showing evidence of nervous system toxicity.

Prior to initiating therapy with pentostatin, renal function should be assessed with a serum creatinine and/or a creatinine clearance assay. (See *Pharmacokinetic properties, Administration to patients*). Complete blood counts, serum creatinine, and BUN should be performed before each dose of pentostatin and at appropriate periods during therapy. Severe neutropenia has been observed following the early courses of treatment with pentostatin and therefore frequent monitoring of complete blood counts is recommended during this time. If haematologic parameters do not improve with subsequent courses, patients should be evaluated for disease status, including bone marrow examination. Periodic monitoring of the peripheral blood for hairy cells should be performed to assess the response to treatment.

In addition, bone marrow aspirates and biopsies may be required at 2 to 3 month intervals to assess the response to treatment.

Interaction with other medicaments and other forms of interaction
Allopurinol: Allopurinol and pentostatin are both associated with skin rashes. Based on clinical studies in 25 refractory patients who received both pentostatin and allopurinol, the combined use of pentostatin and allopurinol did not appear to produce a higher incidence of skin rashes than observed with pentostatin alone. There has been a report of one patient who received both drugs and experienced a hypersensitivity vasculitis that resulted in death. It was unclear whether this adverse event and subsequent death resulted from the drug combination.

Vidarabine: Biochemical studies have demonstrated that pentostatin enhances the effects of vidarabine, a purine nucleoside with anti-viral activity. The combined use of vidarabine and pentostatin may result in an increase in adverse reactions associated with each drug. The therapeutic benefit of the drug combination has not been established.

Fludarabine: The combined use of pentostatin and fludarabine phosphate is not recommended because it has been associated with an increased risk of fatal pulmonary toxicity, (See *Warnings*).

Bone marrow transplant regimen with high dose cyclophosphamide: Acute pulmonary oedema and hypotension leading to death, have been reported in the literature in patients treated with pentostatin in combination with carmustine, etoposide and high dose cyclophosphamide as part of an ablative regimen for bone marrow transplant. The combination of pentostatin and high dose cyclophosphamide is not recommended.

Pregnancy and lactation: Pentostatin must not be used during pregnancy. Women of childbearing potential receiving pentostatin should be advised not to become pregnant.

No fertility studies have been conducted in animals. Incompletely reversible seminiferous tubular atrophy and degeneration in rats and in dogs may be indicative of potential effects on male fertility. The possible adverse effects on human fertility have not been determined.

Pentostatin is teratogenic in mice and rats. There are no adequate and well controlled studies in pregnant women. If the patient becomes pregnant while receiving this drug, the patient should be apprised of the potential hazards to the foetus.

It is not known whether pentostatin is excreted in human milk. Because many drugs are excreted in human milk and because of the potential for serious adverse reactions from pentostatin in nursing infants, nursing is not recommended.

Effects on ability to drive and use machines: On the basis of the reported adverse event profile pentostatin is likely to produce minor or moderate adverse effects. Patients should be advised to use caution in driving or using machinery following drug administration.

Undesirable effects: Pentostatin is lymphotoxic. Aside from myelosuppression, pentostatin is immunosuppressive in particular by suppression of the CD_4+ lymphocyte subset. CD_4+ counts smaller than 200 per μl are usually seen during treatment with pentostatin and CD_4+ count suppression can outlast the end of treatment by more than 6 months. With the exception of frequent herpes zoster infections the clinical consequences of the suppression of CD_4+ counts in hairy cell leukaemia are not well understood yet. Long term consequences are not predictable, but currently there is no evidence for higher frequency of secondary malignancies or opportunistic infections.

The following adverse events were reported during clinical studies in patients with hairy cell leukaemia who were refractory to alpha-interferon or were treated as front-line therapy. Most patients experienced an adverse event. The drug association of these adverse events has not been established. However, some of these adverse events can in many cases be attributed to pentostatin administration, whereas others may be associated with the disease itself. 12% of patients withdrew from treatment due to an adverse event.

Adverse events occurring in over 10% of patients treated with pentostatin in front-line therapy for hairy cell leukaemia:

Body as a whole: Abdominal pain, asthenia, chills, fatigue, fever, headache, infection, pain.

Digestive system: Anorexia, diarrhoea, liver damage, nausea, vomiting.

Haemic and lymphatic system: Anaemia, blood dycrasia, leucopenia, thrombocytopenia.

Metabolic and nutritional system: Peripheral oedema.

Nervous system: Somnolence.

Respiratory system: Cough/increased coughing, lung disorder, pneumonia, respiratory disorder.

Skin and appendages: Dry skin, herpes simplex, maculopapular rash, pruritus, rash, skin disorder.

Special senses: Conjunctivitis.

Adverse events occurring in 3 to 10% of patients treated with pentostatin in front-line therapy for hairy cell leukaemia:

Body as a whole: Abscess, allergic reaction, back pain, cellulitis, chest pain, cyst, death, facial oedema, flu syndrome, malaise, moniliasis, neoplasm, photosensitivity reaction, sepsis.

Cardiovascular system: Atrial fibrillation, cardiovascular disorder, congestive heart failure, flushing, haemorrhage, shock.

Digestive system: Constipation, dyspepsia, dysphagia, flatulence, gastrointestinal disorder, gum haemorrhage, jaundice, LFT's abnormal, mouth ulceration, oral moniliasis, rectal disorder, rectal haemorrhage.

Haemic and lymphatic system: Eosinophilia, hypochromic anaemia, pancytopenia, petechia, splenomegaly.

Metabolic and nutritional system: Bilirubinaemia, BUN increased, creatinine increased, oedema, hyperglycaemia, SGOT increased, SGPT increased, weight gain, weight loss.

Musculoskeletal system Arthralgia, bone disorder, joint disorder, myalgia

Nervous system: Abnormal thinking, anxiety, confusion, depersonalisation, depression, dizziness, dry mouth, hypaethesia, insomnia, nervousness, neurologic disorder PNS, tremor, twitching.

Respiratory system Asthma, dyspnoea, lung oedema, pharyngitis, rhinitis, sinusitis, upper respiratory infection.

Skin and appendages Acne, alopecia, exfoliative dermatitis, herpes zoster, skin carcinoma, skin discolouration, sweating/sweating increased, vesiculobullous rash.

Special senses Ear pain, eye disorder, photophobia, taste perversion.

Urogenital system: Dysurea, genitourinary disorder, urinary retention.

Adverse events occurring in over 10% of alpha-interferon refractory patients treated with pentostatin:
Body as a whole: Allergic reaction, chills, fatigue, fever, headache, infection, pain.

Digestive system: Anorexia, diarrhoea, elevated LFTs, nausea, nausea and vomiting.

Haemic and lymphatic system: Anaemia, leucopenia, thrombocytopenia.

Musculoskeletal system Myalgia

Nervous system: Neurologic disorder CNS.

Respiratory system: Cough increased/coughing, lung disorder, upper respiratory infection.

Skin and appendages: Rash, skin disorder

Urogenital system: Genitourinary disorder

Adverse events occurring in 3 to 10% of alpha-interferon refractory patients treated with pentostatin:

Body as a whole: Abdominal pain, asthaenia, back pain, death, chest pain, flu syndrome, malaise, neoplasm, sepsis.

Cardiovascular system: Abnormal electrocardiogram, arrhythmia, haemorrhage, thrombophlebitis.

Digestive system: Constipation, flatulence, stomatitis.

Haemic and lymphatic system: Ecchymosis, lymphadenopathy, petechia.

Metabolic and nutritional system: BUN increased, creatinine increased, LDH increased, peripheral oedema, weight loss.

Musculoskeletal system: Arthralgia.

Nervous system: Abnormal thinking, anxiety, confusion, depression, dizziness, insomnia, nervousness, paraesthesia, somnolence.

Respiratory system: Bronchitis, dyspnoea, epistaxis, lung oedema, pharyngitis, pneumonia, rhinitis, sinusitis.

Skin and appendages: Dry skin, eczema, herpes simplex, herpes zoster, maculopapular rash, pruritus, seborrhoea, skin discolouration, sweating/sweating increased, vesiculobullous rash.

Special senses: Abnormal vision, conjunctivitis, ear pain, eye pain.

Urogenital system: Dysuria, haematuria.

Overdose: No specific antidote for pentostatin overdose is known. Pentostatin administered at higher doses (20–50 mg/m²/course) than recommended was associated with deaths due to severe renal, hepatic, pulmonary and CNS toxicity. In case of overdose, management would include general supportive measures through any period of toxicity that occurs.

Pharmacological properties
Pharmacodynamic properties: LOIX X08.

Pharmacotherapeutic group: Pentostatin is an adenosine deaminase (ADA) inhibitor.

Mechanism of action Pentostatin is a potent transition state inhibitor of the enzyme adenosine deaminase. The greatest activity of ADA is found in cells of the lymphoid system with T-cells having higher activity that B-cells and T-cell malignancies higher ADA activity than B-cell malignancies. Pentostatin inhibition of ADA, as well as direct inhibition of RNA synthesis and increased DNA damage, may contribute to the overall cytotoxic effect of pentostatin. The precise mechanism of pentostatin's anti-tumour effect, however, in hairy cell leukaemia is not known.

Pentostatin has been shown to have activity against a variety of lymphoid malignancies, but is most active against indolent cancers with lower ADA concentration, such as hairy cell leukaemia.

Pharmacokinetic properties: In man, pentostatin pharmacokinetics are linear with plasma concentrations increasing proportionately with dose. Following a single dose of 4 mg/m² of pentostatin infused over 5 minutes, the distribution half-life was 11 minutes and the mean terminal half-life was 5.7 hours, with a range of 2.6 to 10 hours; the mean plasma clearance was 68 ml/min/m², and approximately 90% of the dose was excreted in urine as unchanged pentostatin and/or metabolites as measured by adenosine deaminase inhibitory activity. The plasma protein binding of pentostatin is low, approximately 4%.

A positive correlation was observed between pentostatin clearance and creatinine clearance (CrCl) in patients with creatinine clearance values ranging from 60 ml/min to 130 ml/min. Pentostatin half-life in patients with renal impairment (CrC1<50 ml/min, n=2) was 18 hours, which was much longer than that observed in patients with normal renal function (CrC1>60 ml/min, n=14), about 6 hours.

A tissue distribution and whole-body auto-radiography study in the rat revealed that radioactivity concentrations were highest in the kidneys with very little central nervous system penetration.

Pentostatin penetrates the blood-brain barrier leading to measurable concentrations in the cerebrospinal fluid (CSF).

Pre-clinical safety data:
Acute toxicity: The combined-sex intravenous LD_{10}, LD_{50} and LD_{90} values in mice given formulated pentostatin were 129, 300 and 697 mg/kg (387, 900 and 2091 mg/m²), respectively.

Signs of acute toxicity in rodents and dogs were hypoactivity, dehydration and emaciation. Lymphoid tissue was a principal target of pentostatin in rats and dogs; thymic atrophy and liver damage occurred in mice. There were no gonadal effects in rodents or dogs.

Multi-dose toxicity: Five daily dose IV combined-sex LD_{10}, LD_{50} and LD_{90} values in mice administered bulk pentostatin were 4.9, 6.4 and 8.3 mg/kg (14.8, 19.1 and 24.8 mg/m²), respectively.

Regardless of route or duration of treatment, lymphoid tissue was the primary target of pentostatin in all species examined in toxicology studies. This is consistent with pentostatin's antineoplastic activity in hairy cell leukaemia. Effects of lymphoid tissue may be related to adenosine deaminase inhibition, the major pharmacologic action of pentostatin. Increased serum hepatic enzymes and liver changes in rodents and dogs indicate that the liver is also a target organ at high doses. Testicular changes in rats and dogs may be indicative of potential effects on male fertility. Effects on lymphoid tissue, liver and testes did not resolve completely during observation periods after drug withdrawal. Target organ effects occurring only in rats included alveolar duct metaplasia and/or goblet cell hyperplasia of the bronchioles, lymphoplasmacytic thryroiditis and an increased incidence of spontaneous glomerulonephritis. Published studies, not conducted by the sponsor, indicate that pentostatin has immunosuppressive properties in mice and rats given multiple doses.

Mutagenesis: Pentostatin was not mutagenic in Salmonella typhimurium at concentrations up to 1000 µg/plate or in V79 Chinese hamster lung cells at concentrations up to 3000 µg/ml, in the presence or absence of metabolic activation. Pentostatin was not classtogenic in V79 Chinese Hamster lung cells *in vitro* at concentrations up to 3000 µg/ml. However, pentostatin did increase the frequency of micronucleus formation in mice administered single intravenous injections of formulated pentostatin at 60, 360 and 720 mg/m². The relevance of the positive mouse micronucleus test for man is not known.

Carcinogenicity: The carcinogenic potential of pentostatin has not been evaluated. The possibility that Nipent causes tumours cannot be ruled out.

Pharmaceutical particulars

List of excipients: Mannitol, Sodium hydroxide or Hydrochloric acid.

Incompatibilities: There are no incompatibilities; however, acidic solutions should be avoided.

Shelf-life: 2 years.

The reconstituted solution for injection or reconstituted and further diluted solution for infusion should be used within 8 hours. Immediate administration after reconstitution is recommended. Any remaining solution should be discarded.

Special precautions for storage: Store at 2°C to 8°C.

After reconstitution the solution should not be stored above 25°C.

Nature and contents of container: NIPENT is supplied in single-dose, 10 mg vials packaged in individual cartons. Vials are made from Type I glass.

Instructions for use/handling: Procedures for proper handling and disposal of anti-cancer drugs should be followed.

1. Reconstitution of Nipent should only be carried out by trained personnel in a cytotoxic-designated area.
2. Adequate protective gloves should be worn.
3. The cytotoxic preparation should not be handled by pregnant staff.
4. Adequate care and precautions should be taken in the disposal of items; syringes, needles etc. used to reconstitute cytotoxic drugs.
5. Contaminated surfaces should be washed with copious amounts of water.

Prescribers should refer to national or recognised guidelines on handling cytotoxic agents.

Transfer 5 ml of Sterile Water for Injection to the vial containing NIPENT and mix thoroughly to obtain complete dissolution of a solution yielding 2 mg/ml. Parenteral drug products should be inspected visually for particulate matter and discolouration prior to administration.

NIPENT may be given intravenously by bolus injection or diluted in a larger volume (25 to 50 ml) with 5% Dextrose Injection (5% glucose solution) or 0.9% Sodium Chloride Injection (0.9% saline solution). Dilution of the entire contents of a reconstituted vial with 25 ml or 50 ml provides a pentostatin concentration of 0.33 mg/ml or 0.18 mg/ml, respectively, for the diluted solutions.

NIPENT solution when diluted for infusion with 5% Dextrose Injection (5% glucose solution) or 0.9% Sodium Chloride Injection (0.9% saline solution) does not interact with PVC infusion containers or administration sets at concentrations of 0.18 mg/ml to 0.33 mg/ml.

Marketing authorisation number PL 0019/0176

Date of approval/revision July 1998

NOVANTRONE* INJECTION

Presentation *Novantrone injection (2 mg/ml):* Glass vials containing a sterile, dark blue aqueous isotonic solution of mitozantrone hydrochloride equivalent to 20 mg, 25 mg and 30 mg mitozantrone, together with sodium chloride and a buffer of sodium acetate and acetic acid to approximately pH3.

Uses Novantrone is an antineoplastic agent.

Novantrone is indicated in the treatment of advanced breast cancer, non-Hodgkin's lymphoma and adult acute non-lymphocytic leukaemia.

Novantrone has also been used in the palliation of non-resectable primary hepatocellular carcinoma.

Dosage and administration

Dosage:

1. *Advanced Breast Cancer, Non-Hodgkin's Lymphoma, Hepatoma:*

(a) *Single Agent Dosage:* The recommended initial dosage of Novantrone used as a single agent is 14 mg/m² of body surface area, given as a single intravenous dose which may be repeated at 21–day intervals. A lower initial dosage (12 mg/m² or less) is recommended in patients with inadequate bone marrow reserves) e.g. due to prior chemotherapy or poor general condition.

Dosage modification and the timing of subsequent dosing should be determined by clinical judgement depending on the degree and duration of myelosuppression. For subsequent courses the prior dose can usually be repeated if white blood cell and platelet counts have returned to normal levels after 21 days. The following table is suggested as a guide to dosage adjustment, in the treatment of advanced breast cancer, non-Hodgkin's lymphoma and hepatoma according to haematological nadir (which usually occurs about 10 days after dosing).

Nadir after Prior Dose WBC (per mm³)	Platelets (per mm³)	Time to Recovery	Subsequent dose after adequate haematological recovery
>1,500	AND>50,000	≤21 days	Repeat prior dose after recovery, or increase by 2 mg/m² if myelo suppression is not considered adequate.
>1,500	AND>50,000	>21 days	Withhold until recovery then repeat prior dose.
<1,500	OR <50,000	Any duration	Decrease by 2 mg/m² from prior dose after recovery.
<1,000	OR <25,000	Any duration	Decrease by 4 mg/m² from prior dose after recovery.

(b) *Combination Therapy:* Novantrone has been given as part of combination therapy. In advanced breast cancer, combinations of Novantrone with other cytotoxic agents including cyclophosphamide and 5-fluorouracil or methotrexate and mitomycin C have been shown to be effective. Reference should be made to the published literature for information on dosage modifications and administration. Novantrone has also been used in various combinations for non-Hodgkin's lymphoma, however data are presently limited and specific regimens cannot be recommended.

As a guide, when Novantrone is used in combination chemotherapy with another myelosuppressive agent, the initial dose of Novantrone should be reduced by 2-4 mg/m² below the doses recommended for single agent usage; subsequent dosing, as outlined in the table above, depends on the degree and duration of myelosuppression.

2. *Acute Non-Lymphocytic Leukaemia:*

(a) *Single Agent Dosage in Relapse:* The recommended dosage for remission induction is 12 mg/m² of body surface area, given as a single intravenous dose daily for 5 consecutive days (total of 60 mg/m²). In clinical studies with a dosage of 12 mg/m² daily for 5 days, patients who achieved a complete remission did so as a result of the first induction course.

(b) *Combination Therapy:* Novantrone has been used in combination regimens for the treatment of ANLL. Most clinical experience has been with Novantrone combined with cytosine arabinoside. This combination has been used successfully for primary treatment of ANLL as well as in relapse.

An effective regimen for induction in previously untreated patients has been Novantrone 10-12 mg/m² IV for 3 days combined with cytosine arabinoside 100 mg/m² IV for 7 days (by continuous infusion). This is followed by second induction and consolidation courses as thought appropriate by the treating clinician. In clinical studies, duration of therapy in induction and consolidation courses with Novantrone have been reduced to 2 days and that of cytosine arabinoside to 5 days. However, modification to the above regimen should be carried out by the treating clinician depending on individual patient factors.

Efficacy has also been demonstrated with Novantrone in combination with Etoposide in patients who had relapsed or who were refractory to primary conventional chemotherapy. The use of Novantrone in combination with Etoposide as with other cytotoxics may result in greater myelosuppression than with Novantrone alone.

Reference should be made to the published literature for information on specific dosage regimens. Novantrone should be used by clinicians experienced in the use of chemotherapy regimens. Dosage adjustments should be made by the treating clinician as appropriate, taking into account toxicity, response and individual patient characteristics. As with other cytotoxic drugs, Novantrone should be used with caution in combination therapy until wider experience is available.

(c) *Paediatric Leukaemia:* As experience with Novantrone in paediatric leukaemia is limited, dosage recommendations in this patient population cannot at present be given.

Method of intravenous administration: **NOT FOR INTRATHECAL USE** Syringes containing this product should be labelled *'NOVANTRONE NOT FOR INTRATHECAL USE'*

Care should be taken to avoid contact of Novantrone with the skin, mucous membranes, or eyes: see Pharmaceutical Precautions for further directions on handling. **Vials should be dispensed in the upright position in order to prevent drops of Novantrone collecting in the stopper during preparation and leading to potential aerosolisation of the solution.**

Dilute the required volume of Novantrone injection to at least 50 ml in either of the following intravenous infusions: Sodium Chloride 0.9%, Glucose 5%, or Sodium Chloride 0.18% and Glucose 4%. Use Luer-lock fittings on all syringes and sets. Large bore needles are recommended to minimise pressure and the possible formation of aerosols. The latter may also be reduced by the use of a venting needle. Administer the resulting solution over not less than 3 minutes via the tubing of freely running intravenous infusion of the above fluids. Novantrone should not be mixed with other drugs in the same infusion.

If extravasation occurs the administration should be stopped immediately and restarted in another vein. The non-vesicant properties of Novantrone minimise the possibility of severe local reaction following extravasation.

Contra-indications, warnings etc.

Contra-indications: **NOT FOR INTRATHECAL USE.** Demonstrated hypersensitivity to the drug.

Warnings: Novantrone should be used with caution in patients with myelosuppression (see Dosage section) or poor general condition.

Cases of functional cardiac changes, including congestive heart failure and decreases in left ventricular ejection fraction have been reported. The majority of these cardiac events have occurred in patients who have had prior treatment with anthracyclines, prior mediastinal/thoracic radiotherapy, or with pre-existing heart disease. It is recommended that patients in these categories are treated with Novantrone at full cytotoxic dosage and schedule. However, added caution is required in these patients and careful regular cardiac examinations are recommended from the initiation of treatment.

As experience of prolonged treatment with Novantrone is presently limited, it is suggested that cardiac examinations also be performed in patients without identifiable risk factors during therapy exceeding a cumulative dose of 160 mg/m².

Careful supervision is recommended when treating patients with severe hepatic insufficiency.

The effects of Novantrone on human fertility or pregnancy have not been established. As with other antineoplastic agents, patients and their partners should be advised to avoid conception for at least six months after cessation of therapy. Novantrone should not normally be administered to patients who are pregnant. Novantrone is excreted in human milk and significant concentrations (18 ng/ml) have been reported for 28 days after the last administration. Because of the potential for serious adverse reactions in infants, breast feeding should be discontinued before starting treatment.

Novantrone is mutagenic *in vitro* and *in vivo* in the rat. In the same species there was a possible association between administration of the drug and development of malignant neoplasia. The carcinogenic potential in man is unknown.

There is no experience with the administration of Novantrone other than by the intravenous route. Safety for intrathecal use has not been established.

Precautions: Novantrone is an active cytotoxic drug which should be used by clinicians familiar with the use of antineoplastic agents, and having the facilities for regular monitoring of clinical, haematological and biochemical parameters during and after treatment.

Full blood counts should be undertaken serially during a course of treatment. Dosage adjustments may be necessary based on these counts (see Dosage section).

Side Effects: Some degree of leucopenia is to be expected following recommended doses of Novantrone. With the single dose every 21 days, suppression of WBC count below 1000/mm³ is infrequent; leucopenia is usually transient reaching its nadir at about 10 days after dosing with recovery usually occurring by the 21st day. Thrombocytopenia can occur and anaemia occurs less frequently. Myelosuppression may be more severe and prolonged in patients having had extensive prior chemotherapy or radiotherapy or in debilitated patients.

When Novantrone is used as a single injection given every 21 days in the treatment of advanced breast cancer and lymphomas, the most commonly encountered side effects are nausea and vomiting, although in the majority of cases these are mild and transient. Alopecia may occur, but is most frequently of minimal severity and reversible on cessation of therapy.

Other side effects which have occasionally been reported include allergic reactions, amenorrhoea, anorexia, constipation, diarrhoea, dyspnoea, fatigue and weakness, fever, gastrointestinal bleeding, stomatitis/mucositis/conjunctivitis and non-specific neurological side effects such as somnolence, confusion, anxiety and mild paraesthesia. Tissue necrosis following extravasation has been reported rarely. In patients with leukaemia, the pattern of side effects is generally similar, although there is an increase in both frequency and severity, particularly of stomatitis and mucositis.

Changes in laboratory test values have been observed infrequently e.g. elevated serum creatinine and blood urea nitrogen levels, increased liver enzyme levels (with occasional reports of severe impairment of hepatic function in patients with leukaemia).

Cardiovascular effects, which have occasionally been of clinical significance, include decreased left ventricular ejection fraction, ECG changes and acute arrhythmia. Congestive heart failure has been reported and has generally responded well to treatment with digitalis and/or diuretics. In patients with leukaemia an increase in the frequency of adverse cardiac events has been observed; the direct role of Novantrone in these cases is difficult to assess as most patients had received prior therapy with anthracyclines and since the clinical course in leukaemic patients is often complicated by anaemia, fever, sepsis and intravenous fluid therapy.

Novantrone may impart a blue-green colouration to the urine for 24 hours after administration and patients should be advised that this is to be expected. Blue discolouration of skin and nails has been reported occasionally. Nail dystrophy or reversible blue colouration of the sclerae may be seen very rarely.

Topoisomerase II inhibitors, including Novantrone, in combination with other antineoplastic agents, have been associated with the development of acute leukaemia.

Overdosage: There is no known specific antidote for Novantrone. Haemopoietic, gastrointestinal, hepatic or renal toxicity may be seen depending on dosage given and the physical condition of the patient. In cases of overdosage the patient should be monitored closely and management should be symptomatic and supportive.

Fatalities have occurred on rare occasions as a result of severe leucopenia with infection in patients accidentally given single bolus injections of mitozantrone at over ten times the recommended dosage. Novantrone is extensively tissue-bound and peritoneal dialysis or haemodialysis is unlikely to be effective in managing overdose.

Pharmaceutical precautions Store at controlled room temperature (15°–25°C). Do not freeze.

Novantrone injection does not contain an antimicrobial preservative. Therefore, in accordance with normal practice, dilutions for infusion should be used or discarded within 24 hours. Novantrone dilutions will maintain potency for 24 hours at room temperature in PVC or glass containers.

Novantrone must not be mixed in the same infusion as heparin since a precipitate may form. Because specific compatibility data are not available it is recommended that Novantrone should not be mixed in the same infusion with other drugs.

Handling of Cytotoxic Drugs: Novantrone, in common with other potentially hazardous cytotoxic drugs, should only be handled by adequately trained personnel. Pregnant staff should not be involved in the reconstitution or administration of Novantrone.

Care should be taken to avoid contact of Novantrone with the skin, mucous membranes, or eyes. The use of goggles, gloves and protective gowns is recommended during preparation, administration and disposal and the work surface should be covered with disposable plastic-backed absorbent paper.

Aerosol generation should be minimised. Novantrone can cause staining. Skin accidentally exposed to Novantrone should be rinsed copiously with warm water and if the eyes are involved standard irrigation techniques should be used.

Spillage Disposal: The following clean-up procedure is recommended if Novantrone is spilled on equipment or environmental surfaces. Prepare a 50% solution of fresh concentrated bleach (any recognised proprietary brand containing either sodium or calcium hypochlorite) in water. Wet absorbent tissues in the bleach solution and apply the wetted tissues to the spillage. The spillage is deactivated when the blue colour has been fully discharged. Collect up the tissues with dry tissues. Wash the area with water and soak up the water with dry tissues. Appropriate protective equipment should be worn during the clean-up procedure. All Novantrone contaminated items (eg, syringes, needles, tissues, etc) should be treated as toxic waste and disposed of accordingly. Incineration is recommended.

Legal category POM

Package quantities Novantrone injection is a sterile aqueous solution of mitozantrone hydrochloride, equivalent to 2 mg/ml mitozantrone. It is available in the following vial sizes:
20 mg in 10 ml: packs of 1 vial
25 mg in 12.5 ml: packs of 1 vial
30 mg in 15 ml: packs of 1 vial

Further information Although its mechanism of action has not been determined, Novantrone is a DNA-reactive agent. It has a cytocidal effect on proliferating and non-proliferating cultured human cells, suggesting activity against rapidly proliferating and slow-growing neoplasms.

Animal pharmacokinetic studies in rats, dogs and monkeys given radiolabelled Novantrone indicate rapid, extensive dose proportional distribution into most tissues. Novantrone does not cross the blood-brain barrier to any appreciable extent. Distribution into testes is relatively low. In pregnant rats the placenta is an effective barrier. Plasma concentrations decrease rapidly during the first two hours and slowly thereafter. Animal data established biliary excretion as the major route of elimination. In rats, tissue elimination half-life of radioactivity ranged from 20 days to 25 days as compared with plasma half-life of 12 days. Novantrone is not absorbed significantly in animals following oral administration.

Pharmacokinetic studies in patients following intravenous administration of Novantrone demonstrated a triphasic plasma clearance. Distribution to tissues is rapid and extensive. Elimination of the drug is slow with a mean half-life of 12 days (range 5–18) and persistent tissue concentrations. Similar estimates of half-life were obtained from patients receiving a single dose of Novantrone every 21 days and patients dosed on 5 consecutive days every 21 days.

Novantrone is excreted via the renal and hepatobiliary systems. Only 20–32% of the administered dose was excreted within the first 5 days after dosing (urine 6–11%, faeces 13–25%). Of the material recovered in the urine 65% was unchanged mitozantrone and the remaining 35% is primarily comprised of 2 inactive metabolites and their glucuronide conjugates. Approximately two thirds of the excretion occurred during the first day.

Product licence number 0095/0088

OVRAN*
OVRAN 30*
OVRANETTE*

Presentation Ovran tablets are round, white, sugar coated tablets. Each tablet contains 250 micrograms levonorgestrel (d-norgestrel) BP and 50 micrograms ethinyloestradiol EP.

Ovran 30 tablets are round, white sugar coated tablets, 5.7 mm in diameter. Each tablet contains 250 micrograms levonorgestrel (d-norgestrel) BP and 30 micrograms ethinyloestradiol EP.

Ovranette tablets are round, beige sugar coated tablets, 5.7 mm in diameter. Each tablet contains 150 micrograms levonorgestrel (d-norgestrel) BP and 30 micrograms ethinyloestradiol EP

Uses Oral contraception. Treatment of endometriosis, spasmodic dysmenorrhoea, premenstrual tension, oligomenorrhoea. Treatment of abnormal uterine bleeding such as menorrhagia, metropathia haemorrhagica. Emergency treatment of acute uterine bleeding.

Dosage and administration

First treatment cycle: 1 tablet daily for 21 days, starting with the tablet marked number 1, on the first day of the menstrual cycle. Additional contraception (barriers and spermicides) is not required.

Subsequent cycles: Each subsequent course is started when seven tablet-free days have followed the preceding course. A withdrawal bleed should occur during the 7 tablet-free days.

Changing from another 21 day combined oral contraceptive: The first tablet of Ovran, Ovran 30 or Ovranette should be taken on the first day immediately after the end of the previous oral contraceptive course. Additional contraception is not required. A withdrawal bleed should not be expected until the end of the first pack.

Changing from an Every Day (ED) 28 day combined oral contraceptive: The first tablet of Ovran, Ovran 30 or Ovranette should be taken on the day immediately after the day on which the last active pill in the ED pack has been taken. The remaining tablets in the ED pack should be discarded. Additional contraception is not required. A withdrawal bleed should not be expected until the end of the first pack.

Changing from a Progestogen-only-Pill (POP): The first tablet of Ovran, Ovran 30 or Ovranette should be taken on the first day of menstruation even if the POP for that day has already been taken. The remaining tablets in the POP pack should be discarded. Additional contraception is not required.

Post-partum and post-abortum use: After pregnancy combined oral contraception can be started in non-lactating women 21 days after a vaginal delivery, provided that the patient is fully ambulant and there are no puerperal complications.

If the pill is started later than 21 days after delivery, then alternative contraception (barriers and spermicides) should be used until oral contraception is started and for the first 7 days of pill-taking. If unprotected intercourse has taken place after 21 days post-partum, then oral contraception should not be started until the first menstrual bleed after childbirth.

After a miscarriage or abortion oral contraception may be started immediately.

Other indications: Ovran and Ovranette can be used for the indications listed below, but Ovran usually provides the more convenient dosage unit.

Endometriosis: Treatment should be continuous with 1 Ovran tablet daily. If spotting or breakthrough bleeding occurs it may be necessary to give 2 tablets daily or rarely 3 tablets daily in divided doses.

Spasmodic dysmenorrhoea, premenstrual tension, oligomenorrhoea: Dosage as for oral contraception.

Functional uterine bleeding: When the diagnosis has been established, dosage is similar to the dosage for oral contraception, but in the first one or two cycles, it may be necessary to give 2 Ovran tablets (or in exceptional cases), 3 tablets daily in order to control the regularity of the cycle.

Emergency treatment of acute uterine bleeding: 2 Ovran tablets are given immediately. If bleeding continues, medication is continued at a dose of 4 tablets daily in divided doses. This can usually be reduced to 2 tablets within two to four days. Treatment should continue for 10 days and after this time it can either be discontinued to be followed after seven days by a complete course of 1 tablet daily for 21 days (see *Functional uterine bleeding*) or it can be continued for one to three months to inhibit the menses. In the latter case, it should be possible to reduce the dosage to 1 tablet daily.

Special circumstances requiring additional contraception:

Missed pills: If a tablet is delayed it should be taken as soon as possible and if it is taken within 12 hours of the correct time, additional contraception is not needed. Further tablets should then be taken at the usual time. If the delay exceeds 12 hours, the last missed pill should be taken when remembered, the earlier missed pills left in the pack and normal pill-taking resumed. If one or more tablets are omitted from the 21 days of pill-taking, additional contraception (barriers and spermicides) should be used for the next 7 days of pill-taking. In addition, if one or more pills are missed during the last 7 days of pill-taking, the subsequent pill-free interval should be disregarded and the next pack started the day after taking the last tablet from the previous pack. In this case, a withdrawal bleed should not be expected until the end of the second pack. If the patient does not have a withdrawal bleed at the end of the second pack she must return to her doctor to exclude the possibility of pregnancy.

Gastro-Intestinal Upset: Vomiting or diarrhoea may reduce the efficacy by preventing full absorption. Additional contraception (barriers and spermicides) should be used during the stomach upset and for the 7 days following the upset. If these 7 days overrun the end of a pack, the next pack should be started without a break. In this case, a withdrawal bleed should not be expected until the end of the second pack. If the patient does not have a withdrawal bleed at the end of the second pack she must return to her doctor to exclude the possibility of pregnancy.

Mild laxatives do not impair contraceptive action.

Interaction with other drugs: Some drugs accelerate the metabolism of oral contraceptives when taken concurrently and these include barbiturates, phenytoin, phenylbutazone and rifampicin. Other drugs suspected of having the capacity to reduce the efficacy of oral contraceptives include ampicillin and other antibiotics. It is, therefore, advisable to use non-hormonal methods of contraception (barriers and spermicides) in addition to the oral contraceptive as long as an extremely high degree of protection is required during treatment with such drugs. The additional contraception should be used while the concurrent medication continues and for 7 days afterwards. If these extra precautions overrun the end of the pack, the next pack should be started without a break. In this case, a withdrawal bleed should not be expected until the end of the second pack. If the patient does not have a withdrawal bleed at the end of the second pack she must return to her doctor to exclude the possibility of pregnancy.

Contra-indications, warnings etc.

Contra-indications:

1. Suspected pregnancy.
2. Thrombotic disorders and a history of these conditions, sickle-cell anaemia, disorders of lipid metabolism and other conditions in which, in individual cases, there is known or suspected to be a much increased risk of thrombosis.
3. Acute or severe chronic liver diseases. Dubin-Johnson syndrome. Rotor syndrome. History, during pregnancy, of idiopathic jaundice or severe pruritus.
4. History of herpes gestationis.
5. Mammary or endometrial carcinoma, or a history of these conditions.
6. Abnormal vaginal bleeding of unknown cause.
7. Deterioration of otosclerosis during pregnancy.

Warnings:

1. There is a general opinion, based on statistical evidence, that users of combined oral contraceptives experience, more often than non-users, venous thromboembolism, arterial thrombosis, including cerebral and myocardial infarction, and subarachnoid haemorrhage. Full recovery from such disorders does not always occur, and it should be realised that in a few cases they are fatal. How often these disorders occur in users of the low-dose pills is not known, but there are reasons for suggesting that they may occur less often than with older pills containing more oestrogen. Certain factors may entail some risk of thrombosis, e.g. smoking, obesity, varicose veins, cardiovascular diseases, diabetes and migraine. The suitability of a combined oral contraceptive should be judged according to the severity of such conditions in the individual case, and should be discussed with the patient before she decides to take it.
2. The risk of arterial thrombosis associated with combined oral contraceptives increases with age, and this risk is aggravated by cigarette smoking. The use of combined oral contraceptives by women in the older age group, especially those who are cigarette smokers, should therefore be discouraged and alternative methods used.
3. The possibility cannot be ruled out that certain chronic diseases may occasionally deteriorate during the use of combined oral contraceptives. (See *Precautions*).
4. Malignant liver tumours have been reported on rare occasions in long-term users of oral contraceptives. Benign hepatic tumours have also been associated with oral contraceptive usage. A hepatic tumour should be considered in the differential diagnosis when upper abdominal pain, enlarged liver or signs of intra-abdominal haemorrhage occur.
5. Numerous epidemiological studies have been reported on the risks of ovarian, endometrial, cervical and breast cancer in women using combined oral contraceptives. The evidence is clear that combined oral contraceptives offer substantial protection against both ovarian and endometrial cancer.
   An increased risk of cervical cancer in long term users of combined oral contraceptives has been reported in some studies, but there continues to be controversy about the extent to which this is attributable to the confounding effects of sexual behaviour and other factors.
   A meta-analysis from 54 epidemiological studies reported that there is a slightly increased relative risk (RR=1.24) of having breast cancer diagnosed in women who are currently using combined oral contraceptives (COCs). The observed pattern of increased risk may be due to an earlier diagnosis of breast cancer in COC users, the biological effects of COCs or a combination of both. The additional breast cancers diagnosed in current users of COCs or in women who have used COCs in the last ten years are more likely to be localised to the breast than those in women who never used COCs.
   Breast cancer is rare among women under 40 years of age whether or not they take COCs. Whilst this background risk increases with age, the excess number of breast cancer diagnoses in current and recent COC users is small in relation to the overall risk of breast cancer (see bar chart).
   The most important risk factor for breast cancer in COC users is the age women discontinue the COC; the older the age at stopping, the more breast cancers are diagnosed. Duration of use is less important and the excess risk gradually disappears during the course of the 10 years after stopping COC use such that by 10 years there appears to be no excess.
   The possible increase in risk of breast cancer should be discussed with the user and weighed against the benefits of COCs taking into account the evidence that they offer substantial protection against the risk of developing certain other cancers (e.g. ovarian and endometrial cancer).

Reasons for stopping oral contraception immediately:

1. Occurrence of migraine in patients who have never previously suffered from it. Exacerbation of pre-existing migraine. Any unusually frequent or unusually severe headaches.
2. Any kind of acute disturbance of vision.
3. Suspicion of thrombosis or infarction.
4. Six weeks before elective operations, or treatment of varicose veins by sclerotherapy and during immobilisation, e.g. after accidents, etc.
5. Significant rise in blood-pressure.
6. Jaundice.
7. Clear exacerbation of conditions known to be capable of deteriorating during oral contraception or pregnancy.
8. Pregnancy is a reason for stopping immediately because it has been suggested by some investigations that oral contraceptives taken in early pregnancy may slightly increase the risk of foetal malformations. Other investigations have failed to support these findings. The possibility therefore cannot be excluded, but it is certain that if a risk exists at all, it is very small.

Precautions:

1. Examination of the pelvic organs, breasts and blood-pressure should precede the prescribing of any combined oral contraceptive and should be repeated regularly.
2. Before starting treatment, pregnancy must be excluded.
3. The following conditions require careful observation during medication: a history of severe depressive states, varicose veins, diabetes, hypertension, epilepsy, otosclerosis, multiple sclerosis, porphyria, tetany, disturbed liver function, gall-stones, cardiovascular diseases, renal diseases, chloasma, uterine fibroids, asthma, the wearing of contact lenses, or any disease that is prone to worsen during pregnancy. The first appearance or deterioration of any of these conditions may indicate that the oral contraceptive should be stopped.
4. The risk of the deterioration of chloasma, which is often not fully reversible, is reduced by the avoidance of excessive exposure to sunlight.

Side effects: Occasional side-effects may include nausea, vomiting, headaches, breast tenderness, changed body weight or libido, depressive moods, chloasma and altered serum lipid profile.

Menstrual changes:

1. *Reduction of menstrual flow:* This is not abnormal and it is to be expected in some patients. Indeed, it may be beneficial where heavy periods were previously experienced.
2. *Missed menstruation:* Occasionally, withdrawal bleeding may not occur at all. If the tablets have been taken correctly, pregnancy is very unlikely, but should be ruled out before a new course of tablets is started.

Intermenstrual bleeding: Very light 'spotting' or heavier 'breakthrough bleeding' may occur during tablet-taking, especially in the first few cycles. It appears to be generally of no significance, except where it indicates errors of tablet-taking, or where the possibility of interaction with other drugs exists (q.v.). However, if irregular bleeding is persistent, an organic cause should be considered.

Effect on adrenal and thyroid glands: Oral contraceptives have no significant influence on adrenocortical function. The ACTH function test for the adrenal cortex remains unchanged. The reduction in corticosteroid excretion and the elevation of plasma corticosteroids are due to an increased cortisol-binding capacity of the plasma proteins.

The response to metyrapone is less pronounced than in untreated women and is thus similar to that during pregnancy.

The radio-iodine uptake shows that thyroid function is unchanged. There is a rise in serum protein-bound iodine, similar to that in pregnancy and during the administration of oestrogens. This is due to the increased capacity of the plasma proteins for binding thyroid hormones, rather than to any change in glandular function. In women taking oral contraceptives, the content of protein-bound iodine in blood serum should therefore, not be used for evaluation of thyroid function.

Effect on blood chemistry: Oral contraceptives may accelerate erythrocyte sedimentation in the absence of any disease. This effect is due to a change in the proportion of the plasma protein fractions. Increases in plasma copper, iron and alkaline phosphatase have also been recorded.

Overdosage: There have been no reports of serious ill-effects from overdosage, even when a considerable number of tablets have been taken by a small child. In general, it is, therefore, unnecessary to treat overdosage. However, if overdosage is discovered within two or three hours and is so large that treatment seems desirable, gastric lavage can be safely used.

There are no specific antidotes and further treatment should be symptomatic.

Pharmaceutical precautions Store in cool, dry conditions. Shelf-life: 3 years

Estimated cumulative numbers of breast cancers per 10,000 women diagnosed in 5 years of use and up to 10 years after stopping COCs, compared with numbers of breast cancers diagnosed in 10,000 women who had never used COCs.

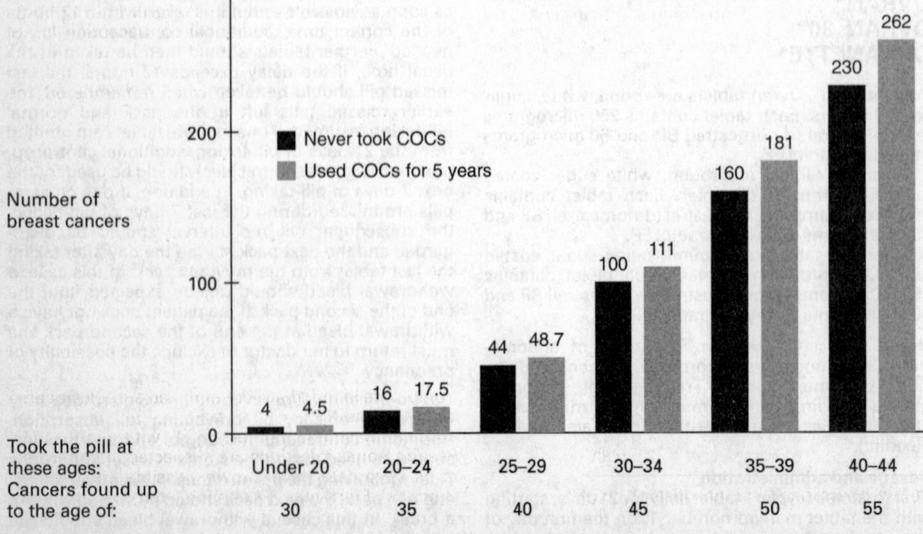

Legal category POM

Package quantities Ovran and Ovran 30 are supplied in memo packs of 21 tablets. Ovranette is supplied in triple packs containing 3 months supply

Further information Pearl Index: Ovran, 0.19, Ovran 30, 0.13. Ovranette, 0.35.

Product licence numbers

Ovran	0011/0015
Ovran 30	0011/0050
Ovranette	0011/0041

PIPRIL* INJECTION

Presentation Vials containing 1 g or 2 g of piperacillin as piperacillin sodium.

Infusion bottles containing 4 g of piperacillin as piperacillin sodium.

Infusion pack containing a 4 g piperacillin infusion bottle, a bottle of Water for Injections BP 50 ml, and a sterile, pyrogen free, transfer needle.

Each 1 g of Pipril contains 1.85 mEq (42.6 mg) of sodium.

Uses Pipril is a broad spectrum bactericidal penicillin antibiotic indicated for the treatment of infections caused by sensitive organisms, and for peri-operative prophylaxis; for example in patients undergoing abdominal surgery, vaginal hysterectomy, caesarean section.

Pipril is highly active against the following clinically important bacteria:

Gram-Negative:
Acinetobacter species
Citrobacter species
Enterobacter species
Escherichia coli
Haemophilus influenzae
Klebsiella pneumoniae and other species
Neisseria gonorrhoeae
Neisseria meningitidis †
Proteus mirabilis
Proteus sp (indole positive)
Providencia species
Pseudomonas aeruginosa and other species
Serratia marcescens and other species
Shigella species †

Anaerobes:
Bacteroides fragilis
Bacteroides species
Clostridium species
Fusobacterium species
Peptococcus species
Peptostreptococcus species
Veillonella species

Gram-Positive:
Streptococcus species
Enterococci
Streptococcus (Diplococcus) *pneumoniae*
B-haemolytic streptococci including Group A *(S. pyogenes)* Group B *(S. agalactiae)*
Staphylococcus aureus ‡
Staphylococcus epidermidis ‡

† While piperacillin is active *in vitro* against these organisms, clinical efficacy has not yet been established.

‡ Methicillin-susceptible, beta-lactamase-negative organisms only.

Because of its broad spectrum of activity, Pipril is indicated for the treatment of the following systemic and/or local infections in which one or more susceptible organisms have been detected or are suspected. Systemic infections including bacterial septicaemia and endocarditis. Urogenital tract infections including gonorrhoea. Respiratory tract infections. Ear, nose and throat and oral cavity infections. Intra-abdominal infections including those of the biliary tract. Gynaecological and obstetric infections. Skin and soft tissue infections including infected wounds and burns. Bone and joint infections. Proven or suspected infections in patients with impaired or suppressed immunological status. Peri-operative prophylaxis.

Dosage and administration Pipril may be given by slow intravenous injection, by intravenous infusion or by intramuscular injection.

For infants and children, intravenous administration of Pipril is recommended.

Intravenous injection: Each gram of Pipril should be reconstituted with at least 5 ml of Water for Injection. The reconstituted solution should be given by slow intravenous injection over three to five minutes.

Intravenous infusion: Each gram of Pipril should be reconstituted with at least 5 ml of Water for Injection. The total dose should then be further diluted to at least 50 ml before infusion over 20–40 minutes. Suitable diluents are listed under Pharmaceutical Precautions.

Intramuscular injection: Each gram of Pipril should be reconstituted with at least 2 ml of Water for Injection or 0.5–1.0% lignocaine. Administration should be by deep intramuscular injection. A single dose in adults should not exceed 2 g. A single dose in children should not exceed 0.5 g.

Adult dosage: Patients with normal renal function: Serious and complicated infections: 200–300 mg/kg/day. The usual dose is therefore 4 g every six or eight hours by IV administration. In life-threatening infections, particularly those caused by Pseudomonas and Klebsiella species a dosage of not less than 16 g/day is recommended.
Mild and uncomplicated infections: 100–150 mg/kg/day. The usual dose is therefore 2 g IV every six or eight hours; 4 g IV every twelve hours or 2 g IM every eight or twelve hours.

For peri-operative prophylaxis: 2 g just prior to surgery (or, in caesarean section, when the umbilical cord is clamped) followed by at least two doses of 2 g at four or six hour intervals within 24 hours of surgery.

Acute gonorrhoea: a single dose of 2 g IM.

Patients with renal insufficiency: In adults with renal impairment, intravenous or intramuscular dosage should be adjusted. Given below are the recommended maximum daily dosages of Pipril according to the degree of renal impairment as assessed by the physician. Regular monitoring is advised to ensure that adequate serum concentrations are achieved.

Duration of therapy: Pipril treatment in acute infections should be continued for three to four days after the disappearance of clinical signs and symptoms of the disease. However, the duration of treatment should be determined by the physician on the basis of the clinical course of infection.

Elderly: Pipril may be used at the same dose levels as adults except in cases of renal impairment when the dosage should be reduced.

Paediatric dosage:
Infants and children (under 12 years of age) with normal renal function:

Less serious and uncomplicated infections: 100–200 mg/kg/day intravenously, in 3 or 4 divided doses.

Serious and complicated infections: 200–300 mg/kg/day, intravenously, in 3 or 4 divided doses.

Neonates:
Dosages for children 0–1 month of age:

<7 days old or >7 days old but less than 2000 g:	150 mg/kg/day intravenously in 3 divided doses.
>7 days old and over 2000 g:	300 mg/kg/day intravenously in 3 or 4 divided doses.

Infants (over 1 month of age) and children (under 12 years) with renal impairment: In paediatric patients with renal impairment, the dosage should be adjusted according to age and degree of that impairment.

Dosages for children over one month of age with renal impairment:

*Creatinine clearance ml/min**	*Urinary tract infection (uncomplicated)*	*Urinary tract infection (complicated)*	*Serious systemic infection*
>40	No adjustment necessary		
20–40	No adjustment	150 mg/kg/day	200 mg/kg/day
<20	75 mg/kg/day	100 mg/kg/day	133 mg/kg/day

* adjusted for body surface, 1.73 M (squared)

Renal function	*Creatinine clearance (ml/min)*	*Serum level (mg %)*	*Maximum daily dosage (in divided doses)*	*Dose schedule*
Mild impairment	40–80	1.5–3.0	16 grams	4 g q 6h
Moderate impairment	20–40	3.1–5.0	12 grams	4 g q 8h
Severe impairment	<20	>5	8 grams	4 g q 12h
Patients on haemodialysis*	—	—	6 grams	2 g q 8h

* Haemodialysis removes 30% to 50% of drug in four hours; an additional dose of 1 g of Pipril should be administered following each dialysis period.

Contra-indications, warnings, etc.
Contra-indications: Penicillin hypersensitivity or severe cephalosporin hypersensitivity.

Precautions: Use with caution in patients with infectious mononucleosis.

Bleeding manifestations have occurred in some patients receiving beta-lactam antibiotics. These reactions have sometimes been associated with abnormalities of coagulation tests such as clotting time, platelet aggregation and prothrombin time and are much more likely to occur in patients with renal failure. If bleeding manifestations occur as a result of antibiotic therapy, the antibiotic should be discontinued and appropriate therapy instituted.

As with other antibiotics, overgrowth of non-susceptible organisms may cause superinfections, especially during prolonged treatment. The possibility of antibiotic-induced pseudomembranous colitis should be considered in cases of severe persistent diarrhoea.

Neuromuscular excitability or convulsions have been known to occur following large intravenous doses of penicillins.

Pipril is a monosodium compound containing 1.85 mEq (42.6 mg) of sodium per gram. This should be borne in mind if used in patients with sodium and fluid retention.

Use in pregnancy and lactation: The product has been in clinical use since 1982 and the limited number of reported cases of use in human pregnancy have shown no evidence of untoward effect. The benefits of use during pregnancy should be weighed against possible hazards to mother and foetus. Piperacillin is licensed for use in neonates.

Piperacillin is excreted in low concentrations in breast milk.

Warnings and side effects: Serious and occasionally fatal anaphylactic reactions have been reported in patients receiving therapy with penicillins. Before initiating therapy with piperacillin, careful inquiry should be made concerning previous hypersensitivity reactions to penicillins, cephalosporins and other allergens. If an allergic reaction occurs during therapy with piperacillin, the antibiotic should be discontinued. Serious hypersensitivity reactions may require adrenaline and other emergency measures.

Side effects are uncommon and typical of the injectable penicillins.

In common with other penicillins, anaphylactic reactions have occasionally been reported in patients receiving piperacillin. Mild allergic reactions such as rash, pruritus, urticaria and fever may occur. These occur more frequently in patients with cystic fibrosis. Rarely, interstitial nephritis and/or renal failure have been reported.

Hepatitis and cholestatic jaundice have been reported rarely with some penicillins, including Pipril. In common with other β-lactam antibiotics, haemolytic anaemia has been reported rarely.

Gastrointestinal disturbances have been reported. Transient increases in liver function test values may be observed.

Transient leucopenia, neutropenia, thrombocytopenia and/or eosinophilia may occur.

Rarely, significant leucopenia may be associated with prolonged therapy.

Dermatological manifestations such as erythema multiforme and Stevens-Johnson syndrome have been reported on rare occasions.

In vitro, Pipril can be inactivated by β-lactamases produced by some strains of gram-negative and gram-positive bacteria.

Prolonged use of an anti-infective may result in the development of superinfection due to organisms resistant to that anti-infective.

Cross-resistance between piperacillin and other β-lactam antibiotics e.g. carbenicillin and ampicillin is possible.

Pain after intramuscular injections (rarely accompanied by induration) has been observed infrequently. This can be minimised by reconstituting Pipril with 0.5–1.0% lignocaine.

Interactions: Pipril acts synergistically with aminoglycosides. Concurrent therapy with both drugs given in full therapeutic doses may be used in the treatment of life-threatening infections or in patients with impaired immune status. Pipril and aminoglycosides should not, however, be mixed in the same solution but administered separately.

Pipril may be used in combination with β-lactamase resistant penicillins in proven or suspected mixed infections involving β-lactamase producing *Staphylococcus aureus.*

Pipril may be administered (separately) with metronidazole in the treatment of mixed aerobic/anaerobic infections.

Cefoxitin should not be given with Pipril when Pseudomonas infections are suspected or confirmed as *in vitro* data have shown possible antagonism. However, Pipril may be administered concomitantly with other β-lactam antibiotics provided that an additive or synergistic antibacterial action is first ascertained through *in vitro* tests where appropriate.

During simultaneous administration of high doses of heparin, oral anticoagulants and other drugs which may affect the blood coagulation system and/or the thrombocyte function, the coagulation parameters should be tested more frequently and monitored regularly.

The ureidopenicillins including piperacillin have been reported to prolong the action of vecuronium. Caution is indicated when piperacillin is used perioperatively with vecuronium and similar neuromuscular blocking agents.

Penicillins may reduce the excretion of methotrexate. Serum levels of methotrexate should be monitored in patients on high dose methotrexate therapy.

Overdosage: Other than general supportive treatment, no specific antidote is known. Excessive serum levels of piperacillin may be reduced by dialysis. In cases of motor excitability or convulsions administration of appropriate anticonvulsant drugs, such as diazepam or barbiturates, may be indicated. Daily doses of piperacillin of 24 grams and above have been administered in man without observation of adverse effects.

Pharmaceutical precautions Pipril should be stored in a dry place at room temperature. Pipril should be freshly prepared prior to administration, any unused solution being discarded.

However, Pipril solutions are chemically stable for at least 24 hours at room temperature or 48 hours at 4°C.

Pipril may be administered in all commonly used intravenous infusion fluids including:

Dextrose 5%, Sodium Chloride 0.9%, Dextrose 5% and Sodium Chloride 0.9%. The above fluids admixed with 40 mEq Potassium Chloride and/or 30 mEq Sodium Bicarbonate. Dextran 6% in Sodium Chloride 0.9%, Dextrose 30%, Mannitol 20%, Water for Injection.

Because of chemical instability, Pipril should not be diluted with solutions containing only sodium bicarbonate.

Pipril should not be added to blood products or protein hydrolysates.

Pipril has also been shown to be compatible over 24 hours at room temperature when mixed with cephazolin sodium, flucloxacillin sodium, cephamandole nafate, or cefoxitin sodium in either Dextrose 5% or Saline 0.9%.

Pipril should not be mixed in the same solution with aminoglycosides and should be administered separately from any drugs unless compatibility is proven.

Legal category POM

Package quantities
Vials containing 1 g or 2 g Pipril boxed singly.
Infusion bottles containing 4 g Pipril, boxed singly.
Pipril 4 g Infusion Packs containing a 4 g infusion bottle, a 50 ml bottle of Water for Injections BP and a transfer needle.

Further information Pipril is widely distributed following parenteral administration into human tissues and body fluids, particularly bile. Pipril penetrates into cerebrospinal fluid in the presence of meningitis. It is not absorbed when given orally. As with other penicillins, Pipril is rapidly excreted, unchanged by glomerular filtration and tubular secretion achieving high urinary concentrations for up to 12 hours after dosing. The binding of piperacillin to human serum protein is low (16%).

Product licence number 0095/0073

PNU-IMUNE*

Qualitative and quantitative composition Each 0.5 ml of Pnu-Imune contains 25µg of antigen to each of the 23 most prevalent or invasive pneumococcal types (see table below).

Antigens present in Pnu-Imune according to Danish Nomenclature [25µg of each per 0.5 ml dose]:

1	2	3	4	5	6B	7F	8	9N	9V	10A	11A
12F	14	15B	17A	18C	19A	19F	20	22F	23F	33F	

Pharmaceutical form Pnu-Imune is a clear, colourless to very light amber sterile solution for injection.

Clinical particulars
Therapeutic indications: Pnu-Imune vaccine consists of a mixture of highly purified capsular polysaccharides from the 23 most prevalent types of *Streptococcus pneumoniae* (pneumococcus) which account for at least 90% of pneumococcal blood isolates. Pnu-Imune is indicated for immunisation against pneumococcal disease caused by those pneumococcal types included in the vaccine.

Adults: Pnu-Imune vaccine should be considered for all those aged over two years in whom pneumococcal infection is likely to be more common and/or dangerous such as immunocompetent individuals who are at increased risk of pneumococcal disease or its complications because of chronic illnesses (e.g., cardiovascular or pulmonary disease, diabetes mellitus, alcoholism or cirrhosis); and for immunocompromised individuals at increased risk of pneumococcal disease or its complications (e.g., splenic dysfunction or anatomical asplenia including sickle cell disease, Hodgkin's disease, lymphoma, multiple myeloma, chronic renal failure, nephrotic syndrome, or conditions such as organ transplantation and Human Immunodeficiency Virus (HIV) associated with immunosuppression).

Children: Not recommended in children less than 2 years.

Posology and method of administration: A single dose of 0.5 ml is given subcutaneously or intramuscularly (preferably in the deltoid muscle or lateral mid-thigh). Intradermal administration should be avoided. The vaccine should not be injected intravenously.

Individuals with HIV should be immunised as early as possible in the disease process.

Pnu-Imune should be inspected visually for particulate matter and discoloration prior to administration.

Simultaneous administration with other vaccines: Pneumococcal vaccine may be given at the same time as influenza vaccine at a different site as there is no antigenic competition. Pnu-Imune, unlike influenza vaccine, is not required annually and therefore the need for simultaneous administration is not always present.

A possible attenuation of the response to Pnu-Imune may be seen in immunocompromised individuals when co-administered with influenza vaccine. This effect has not been seen in clinical studies involving other patient groups.

Re-immunisation: Re-immunisation should be considered after 5 years in individuals at highest risk of pneumococcal infection or where antibody levels are likely to have declined rapidly such as those with no spleen, with splenic dysfunction or with nephrotic syndrome or transplant patients. Re-immunisation before 5 years may cause increased incidence and severity of local reactions.

As antibody levels may decline more rapidly in children, re-immunisation should be carefully considered after 3 to 5 years for children with nephrotic syndrome, asplenia, or sickle cell anaemia who would be 10 years old or younger at the time of re-immunisation.

Persons who received the 14 valent vaccine should not be routinely re-vaccinated with the 23 valent vaccine, as increased coverage is modest and duration of protection is not well defined.

Contra-indications: Hypersensitivity to any component of the vaccine, including thiomersal, a mercury derivative. The occurrence of any type of neurological symptoms or signs following administration of this product is a contra-indication to further use. The vaccine should not be administered to persons with acute febrile illnesses until their temporary symptoms and/or signs have abated.

Persons who have received any pneumococcal vaccine in the last three years.

Persons who are receiving immunosuppressive therapy or who have received it in the last 10 days.

Patients with Hodgkin's Disease who have received extensive chemotherapy and/or nodal irradiation.

Pregnant or lactating women.

Special warnings and special precautions: As with the injection of any biological material, Adrenaline Injection (1:1000) should be available for immediate use should an anaphylactic or other allergic reaction occur.

Pnu-Imune is not an effective agent for prophylaxis against pneumococcal disease caused by types not present in the vaccine.

The expected serum antibody response may not be obtained in patients with impaired immune responsiveness, whether due to the use of immunosuppressive therapy, a genetic defect, HIV infection , or other causes. In order to maximise the benefits of vaccination, patients with HIV should be vaccinated as early as possible in the disease process.

At least 2 weeks should elapse between immunisation and the initiation of chemotherapy or immunosuppressive therapy to allow development of adequate antibody response.

Defer immunisation if acute febrile illness is present.

Patients who have had episodes of pneumococcal pneumonia or other pneumococcal infection may have high levels of pre-existing pneumococcal antibodies that may result in increased reactions to Pnu-Imune, mostly local, but occasionally systemic. Caution should be exercised if such patients are considered for immunisation with Pnu-Imune.

Where required prophylactic antibiotic therapy against pneumococcal infection should not be stopped after immunisation with Pnu-Imune.

Because antibody response to capsular types that most often cause pneumococcal disease in children less than 2 years may be poor, Pnu-Imune vaccine may not be effective and is not generally recommended in this group.

To avoid accidental re-vaccination, a clear note of vaccination should be kept in the patient's records.

Interaction with other medicaments and other forms of interaction: When Pnu-Imune is given with an unrelated vaccine, such as vaccine against influenza virus, there is no antigenic competition.

Pregnancy and lactation: Animal reproduction studies to evaluate teratology and embryotoxicity have not been conducted with Pnu-Imune. It is not known whether Pnu-Imune can cause foetal harm when administered to a pregnant woman or can affect reproduction capacity. Pnu-Imune is not recommended for use in pregnant women.

It is not known whether the vaccine is excreted in human milk. Because many drugs are excreted in human milk, caution should be exercised if Pnu-Imune is administered to a nursing woman.

Effects on ability to drive and use machines: Pnu-Imune is not known to affect the ability to drive or operate machines.

Undesirable effects: Mild side effects, such as erythema and pain at the injection site occur in approximately 50% of persons given pneumococcal vaccine. Fever, myalgia, and severe local reactions have been reported in less than 1% of those vaccinated.

Fever and myalgia are usually confined to the 24 hour period following immunisation. Rash and arthralgia have been reported infrequently.

Although rare, fever over 38.9°C and marked local swelling have been reported with pneumococcal polysaccharide vaccine. Rash, urticaria, arthritis, arthralgia, adenitis, and anaphylactoid reactions have been reported rarely.

Patients with otherwise stabilised idiopathic thrombocytopenic purpura have, on rare occasions, experienced a relapse in their thrombocytopenia, occurring 2 to 14 days after immunisation, and lasting up to 2 weeks.

Reactions of greater severity or extent are unusual. Temporal association of neurological disorders such as paraesthesia and acute radiculoneuropathy, including Guillain-Barre syndrome, have been reported rarely following parenteral injections of biological products including pneumococcal vaccine.

Overdose: There is no experience with overdosage of Pnu-Imune.

Pharmacological properties Pneumococci are surrounded by a polysaccharide capsule, which make the bacteria resistant to attack by white blood cells. However, human blood serum may contain antibodies, which render the bacteria vulnerable to attack. Pnu-Imune vaccine, composed of the purified polysaccharides from bacterial cells, stimulates production of these antibodies and provides active immunity to the 23 types of pneumococcal bacteria represented in the vaccine.

Pharmacodynamic properties: In clinical studies with polyvalent pneumococcal vaccines, more than 90% of all adults showed twofold or greater increase in geometric mean antibody titre for each capsular type contained in the vaccine (data on file, Lederle Laboratories). Patients over the age of 2 years with anatomical or functional asplenia and otherwise intact lymphoid function generally respond to pneumococcal vaccines with a serological conversion comparable to that observed in healthy individuals of the same age.

Most healthy adults, including the elderly, demonstrate at least a twofold rise in type-specific antibodies within 2 to 3 weeks of immunisation. Similar antibody responses have been reported in patients with alcoholic cirrhosis and insulin-dependent diabetes mellitus. In contrast, elderly individuals with chronic pulmonary disease failed to mount a comparable immune response. In immunocompromised patients, the response to immunisation may also be lower. Children under 2 years of age respond poorly to most capsular polysaccharide types. Further, response to some pneumococcal types (e.g., 6A and 14) that are important in paediatric infection is decreased in children less than 5 years of age.

Following immunisation of healthy adults, antibody levels remain elevated for at least 5 years, but in some individuals these may fall to pre-immunisation levels within 10 years. A more rapid decline in antibodies may occur in children, particularly those who have undergone a splenectomy and those with sickle cell disease, in whom antibodies for some types can fall to pre-immunisation levels 3 to 5 years after immunisation. Similar rates of decline can occur in children with nephrotic syndrome.

Patients with AIDS may have an impaired antibody response to pneumococcal vaccine. However, HIV-infected adults show a normal immune response to the 23 valent vaccine when the circulating level of CD4 cells is above 500/μL, but a reduced response when the cell population falls below that threshold.

Pharmacokinetic properties: The capsule of the pneumococcus, despite its lack of toxicity, is the major bacterial structure responsible for the virulence of the organism. The polysaccharide capsule has an antiphagocytic effect, interrupting phagocytic activity elicited by activation of complement and permitting the establishment and progression of infection in the non-immune host. Opsonisation of pneumococci is required for their phagocytosis. Identified as complex polysaccharides, the capsules of the pneumococcus were the first non-protein substances shown to be antigenic in humans, which laid the basis for the subsequent use of pneumococcal capsular polysaccharides as vaccines. Induction of anticapsular polysaccharide antibodies in the host mediate immunity through activation of complement for effective opsonisation. IgM and IgG antibodies confer protection by altering the surface properties of the pneumococcal cell, which facilitates phagocytosis.

Preclinical safety data: Not applicable.

Pharmaceutical particulars
List of excipients: Thiomersal, sodium phosphate buffer.

Incompatibilities: None.

Shelf life: Pnu-Imune may be stored at 2° to 8°C for up to 2 years.

Special precautions for storage: Pnu-Imune should not be frozen. Storage should be under refrigeration, away from the freezer compartment at 2–8°C.

Nature and contents of container: Pnu-Imune is supplied in a 0.5 ml single dose vial for use with a syringe only. (Packs of 1 and 10.)

Instructions for use/handling: There are no special instructions for use/handling.

Marketing authorization number PL 0095/0292

Date of approval/revision 6 January 1997

Legal category POM

PREMARIN* TABLETS

Presentation Premarin Tablets contain naturally conjugated oestrogens.

Premarin Tablets 0.625 mg are maroon, oval, sugar-coated tablets.

Premarin Tablets 1.25 mg are yellow, oval, sugar-coated tablets.

Premarin Tablets 2.5 mg are purple, oval, sugar-coated tablets.

Uses Menopausal and postmenopausal oestrogen therapy in women without a uterus for:

1. vasomotor symptoms such as sweating and flushes.
2. allied disorders of the menopause such as atrophic vaginitis, kraurosis vulvae, atrophic urethritis.
3. prophylaxis of osteoporosis in women at risk of developing fractures.

Dosage and Administration
Adults: Premarin 0.625–1.25 mg daily is the usual starting dose. Continuous administration is recommended. For maintenance, the lowest effective dose should be used.

Vasomotor symptoms: 0.625–1.25 mg daily depending on the response of the individual.

Atrophic vaginitis, kraurosis vulvae, atrophic urethritis: 0.625–1.25 mg daily depending on the response of the individual.

Prophylaxis of osteoporosis: the minimum effective dose is 0.625 mg daily for most patients. Hormone replacement therapy has been found to be effective in the prevention of osteoporosis when started soon after the menopause and used for 5 years and probably up to 10 years. Treatment should start as soon as possible after the onset of the menopause and certainly within 2 to 3 years. Protection appears to be effective for as long as treatment is continued, however data beyond 10 years are limited. A careful re-appraisal of the risk-benefit ratio should be undertaken before treating for longer than 5 to 10 years. For long term use see also Precautions and Warnings.

At present there is no established screening programme for determining women at risk of developing osteoporotic fractures. Epidemiological studies suggest a number of individual risk factors which contribute to the development of postmenopausal osteoporosis. These include: early menopause; family history of osteoporosis; thin, small frame; cigarette use; recent prolonged systemic corticosteroid use.

If several of these risk factors are present in a patient consideration should be given to oestrogen replacement therapy.

Concomitant progestogen use: In women with an intact uterus the addition of a progestogen for 12–14 days per cycle is essential. See also Precautions and Warnings.

For most postmenopausal women therapy may be commenced at any convenient time.

Before therapy commences it is recommended that the patient is fully informed of all likely benefits and potential risks. She should have a full physical and gynaecological examination with special emphasis on blood pressure, breasts, abdomen and pelvic organs, and endometrial assessment carried out if appropriate. Follow-up examinations are recommended every 6–12 months.

Elderly: There are no special dosage requirements for elderly patients, but as with all medicines, the lowest effective dose should be used.

Children: Not recommended.

Contra-indications, warnings etc
Contra-indications:

1. Known or suspected pregnancy.
2. History of, known or suspected cancer of the breast.
3. Known or suspected oestrogen-dependent neoplasia. Undiagnosed abnormal genital bleeding.
4. Active deep vein thrombosis, thromboembolic disorders or a history of confirmed venous thromboembolism.
5. Acute or chronic liver disease or history of liver disease where the liver function tests have failed to return to normal. Rotor syndrome or Dubin-Johnson syndrome.
6. Severe cardiac or renal disease.
7. Hypersensitivity to the components of Premarin tablets.

Pregnancy and lactation: Premarin is contraindicated in the event of known or suspected pregnancy and during lactation.

Warnings and precautions:

1. In the female there is an increased risk of endometrial hyperplasia and carcinoma associated with unopposed oestrogens administered long-term (for more than one year). However, the appropriate addition of a progestogen to an oestrogen regimen lowers this additional risk.
2. There is suggestive evidence of a small increased risk of breast cancer with oestrogen replacement therapy used for long term (greater than 5 years). Some studies have reported an increased risk in long-term users, others, however, have not shown this relationship. It is not known whether concurrent progestogen use influences the risk of breast cancer in post menopausal women taking hormone replacement therapy. Women on long-term therapy should have regular breast examinations, should be instructed in self-breast examination and mammographic investigations conducted where considered appropriate.
   There is a need for caution when prescribing oestrogens in women who have a history of, or known breast nodules or fibrocystic disease. Breast status should be closely monitored, supported by regular mammography.
3. Certain diseases may be made worse by hormone replacement therapy and patients with these conditions should be closely monitored. These include otosclerosis, multiple sclerosis, systemic lupus erythematosis, porphyria, melanoma, epilepsy, migraine and asthma. In addition pre-existing uterine fibroids may increase in size during oestrogen therapy and symptoms associated with endometriosis may be exacerbated.
4. Epidemiological studies have suggested that hormone replacement therapy (HRT) is associated with an increased relative risk of developing venous thromboembolism (VTE) i.e. deep vein thrombosis or pulmonary embolism. The studies find a 2–3 fold increase for users compared with non-users which for healthy women amounts to a low risk of one extra case of VTE each year for every 5000 patients taking HRT.
   Generally recognised risk factors for VTE include a personal or family history and severe obesity (Body Mass Index >30 kg/m^2). In women with these factors the benefit of treatment with HRT need to be carefully weighed against risks. There is no consensus about the possible role of varicose veins in VTE.
   The risk of VTE may be temporarily increased with prolonged immobilisation, major trauma or major surgery. In women on HRT scrupulous attention should be given to prophylactic measures to prevent VTE following surgery. Where prolonged immobilisation is liable to follow elective surgery, particularly abdominal or orthopaedic surgery to the lower limbs, consideration should be given to temporarily stopping HRT 4 weeks earlier, if this is possible.
   If venous thromboembolism develops after initiating therapy the drug should be discontinued.
5. Premarin should be used with caution in patients with a past history of stroke or myocardial infarction.
6. Oestrogens may cause fluid retention and therefore patients with cardiac or renal dysfunction should be carefully observed.
7. If jaundice, migraine-like headaches, visual disturbances, thromboembolic phenomena or a significant increase in blood pressure develop after initiating therapy, the medication should be discontinued while the cause is investigated.
8. Premarin is not an oral contraceptive neither will it restore fertility. If Premarin is administered together with a progestogen to women with an intact uterus of child-bearing potential they should be advised to adhere to non-hormonal contraceptive methods.
9. Most studies indicate that oestrogen replacement therapy has little effect on blood pressure and some indicate that oestrogen use may be associated with a small decrease. In addition, most studies on combined therapy indicate that the addition of a progestogen also has little effect on blood pressure. Rarely, idiosyncratic hypertension may occur.
   When oestrogens are administered to hypertensive women, supervision is necessary and blood pressure should be monitored at regular intervals.
10. Changed oestrogen levels may affect certain endocrine and liver function tests.
11. It has been reported that there is an increase in the risk of surgically confirmed gall bladder disease in women receiving postmenopausal oestrogens.
12. A worsening of glucose tolerance may occur in patients taking oestrogens and therefore diabetic patients should be carefully observed while receiving hormone replacement therapy.
13. As larger doses of oestrogen may increase thyroid binding globulin leading to increased circulating total thyroid hormone, care should be taken in providing oestrogens for patients with thyrotoxicosis.
14. Administration of oestrogens may lead to hypercalcaemia in patients with breast cancer and bone metastases. If this occurs, the drug should be stopped and appropriate measures taken to reduce the calcium level.

Side effects: The following side effects have been reported with oestrogen therapy.

1. Genitourinary system – premenstrual-like syndrome, increase in size of uterine fibromyomata, vaginal candidiasis, change in cervical erosion and in degree of cervical secretion, cystitis-like syndrome.
2. Breasts – Tenderness, enlargement, secretion.
3. Gastrointestinal – Nausea, vomiting, abdominal cramps, bloating, cholestatic jaundice.
4. Skin – Chloasma or melasma which may persist when drug is discontinued, erythema multiforme, erythema nodosum, haemorrhagic eruption, loss of scalp hair, hirsutism.
5. Eyes – Steepening of corneal curvature, intolerance to contact lenses.
6. CNS – Headaches, migraine, dizziness, mental depression, chorea.
7. Miscellaneous – Increase or decrease in weight, reduced carbohydrate tolerance, aggravation of porphyria, oedema, changes in libido, leg cramps.

Acute overdosage: Numerous reports of ingestion of large doses of oestrogen-containing oral contraceptives by young children indicate that acute serious ill effects do not occur. Overdosage of oestrogen may cause nausea, and withdrawal bleeding may occur in females.

Pharmaceutical precautions No special requirements for storage are necessary.

Legal category POM

Package quantities
Premarin 0.625 mg: Triple packs with 3 blister strips of 28 tablets.
Premarin 1.25 mg: Triple packs with 3 blister strips of 28 tablets.
Premarin 2.5 mg: Triple packs with 3 blister strips of 28 tablets.

Further information After the menopause the protective effect that endogenous oestrogens appear to have on the female cardiovascular system is lost, and the risk of women developing cardiovascular disease rises to become similar to that of men.

Most studies show that oral administration of conjugated equine oestrogens to postmenopausal women increase serum high density lipoprotein (HDL-cholesterol) and decrease the potentially atherogenic low density lipoprotein (LDL-cholesterol) levels. This improves the lipid profile and is recognised as a factor contributing to the beneficial effect of conjugated equine oestrogens on the risk of coronary heart disease in postmenopausal women.

Premarin tablets contain the following excipients: lactose, methylcellulose, magnesium stearate, syrup, glucose, glyceryl mono-oleate, polyethylene glycol, carnauba wax, calcium sulphate anhydrous, microcrystalline cellulose.

Product licence numbers
Premarin Tablets 0.625 mg 0011/0165
Premarin Tablets 1.25 mg 0011/0166
Premarin Tablets 2.5 mg 0011/0167

Date of last review June 1998

PREMARIN* VAGINAL CREAM.

Qualitative and quantitative composition Each 1 gram of the cream contains 0.625 mg conjugated oestrogens USP.

Pharmaceutical form Cream for intravaginal or topical administration.

Clinical particulars
Therapeutic indication: Short-term treatment of atrophic vaginitis and postmenopausal atrophic urethritis, Kraurosis vulvae.

Posology and method of administration:

Dosage and administration:
Adults: The usual recommended dose is 1 to 2 g daily administered intravaginally or topically to the vaginal area, depending on the severity of the condition. Administration should be cyclic (e.g. three weeks on and one week off). It should start on the fifth day of bleeding in the patient who is menstruating and arbitrarily if not.

The lowest effective dose which will control symptoms should be used and the need for continuing treatment should be reviewed periodically. Should long-term therapy be considered in women with an intact uterus, an oral progestogen for 10–14 days at the end of each cycle is essential.

Before therapy commences it is recommended that the patient is fully informed of all the likely benefits and potential risks. She should have a full physical and gynaecological examination, with special emphasis on blood pressure, breasts, abdomen and pelvic organs, and endometrial assessment, carried out if appropriate. Follow-up examinations are recommended every 6–12 months. Any break-through bleeding is an indication for endometrial evaluation.

Elderly: There are no special dosage requirements for elderly patients, but as with all medicines, the lowest effective dose should be used.

Children: Not recommended.

Contra-indications:

1. Known or suspected pregnancy.
2. History of, known or suspected cancer of the breast.
3. Known or suspected oestrogen-dependent neoplasia. Undiagnosed abnormal genital bleeding.
4. Active deep vein thrombosis, thromboembolic disorders or a history of confirmed venous thromboembolism.
5. Acute or chronic liver disease or history of liver disease where the liver function tests have failed to return to normal. Rotor syndrome or Dubin-Johnson syndrome.
6. Severe cardiac or renal disease.

Special warnings and precautions for use: Due to oestrogen absorption following the application of Premarin Vaginal Cream, prolonged administration might result in systemic effects. Therefore, the following warnings and precautions should be considered.

1. In the female there is an increased risk of endometrial hyperplasia and carcinoma associated with unopposed oestrogens administered long-term (for more than one year). However, the appropriate addition of a progestogen to an oestrogen regimen lowers this additional risk.
2. There is suggestive evidence of a small increased risk of breast cancer with oestrogen replacement therapy used for long-term (greater than 5 years). Some studies have reported an increased risk in long-term users, others, however, have not shown this relationship. It is not known whether concurrent progestogen use influences the risk of breast cancer in postmenopausal women taking hormone replacement therapy. Women on long-term therapy should have regular breast examinations, should be instructed in self-breast examination and mammographic investigations conducted where considered appropriate.
   There is a need for caution when prescribing oestrogens in women who have a history of, or known breast nodules or fibrocystic disease. Breast status should be closely monitored, supported by regular mammography.
3. Certain diseases may be made worse by hormone replacement therapy and patients with these conditions should be closely monitored. These include otosclerosis, multiple sclerosis, systemic lupus erythematosus, porphyria, melanoma, epilepsy, migraine and asthma. In addition pre-existing uterine fibroids may increase in size during oestrogen therapy and symptoms associated with endometriosis may be exacerbated.
4. Epidemiological studies have suggested that hormone replacement therapy (HRT) is associated with an increased relative risk of developing venous thromboembolism (VTE) i.e. deep vein thrombosis or pulmonary embolism. The studies find a 2–3 fold increase for users compared with non-users which for healthy women amounts to a low risk of one extra case of VTE each year for every 5000 patients taking HRT.
   Generally recognised risk factors for VTE include a personal or family history and severe obesity (Body Mass Index >30 kg/m²). In women with these factors the benefit of treatment with HRT need to be carefully weighed against risks. There is no consensus about the possible role of varicose veins in VTE.
   The risk of VTE may be temporarily increased with prolonged immobilisation, major trauma or major surgery. In women on HRT scrupulous attention should be given to prophylactic measures to prevent VTE following surgery. Where prolonged immobilisation is liable to follow elective surgery, particularly abdominal or orthopaedic surgery to the lower limbs, consideration should be given to temporarily stopping HRT 4 weeks earlier, if this is possible.
   If venous thromboembolism develops after initiating therapy the drug should be discontinued.
5. Premarin Vaginal Cream should be used with caution in patients with a past history of stroke or myocardial infarction.
6. Oestrogens may cause fluid retention and therefore patients with cardiac or renal dysfunction should be carefully observed.
7. If jaundice, migraine-like headaches, visual disturbances, thromboembolic phenomena or a significant increase in blood pressure develop after initiating therapy, the medication should be discontinued while the cause is investigated.
8. Women with an intact uterus of child-bearing potential should be advised to adhere to non-hormonal contraceptive methods.
9. Most studies indicate that oestrogen replacement therapy has little effect on blood pressure and some indicate that oestrogen use may be associated with a small decrease. In addition, most studies on combined therapy indicate that the addition of a progestogen also has little effect on blood pressure. Rarely, idiosyncratic hypertension may occur.
   When oestrogens are administered to hypertensive women, supervision is necessary and blood pressure should be monitored at regular intervals.
10. Changed oestrogen levels may affect certain endocrine and liver function tests.
11. It has been reported that there is an increase in the risk of surgically confirmed gall bladder disease in women receiving postmenopausal oestrogens.
12. A worsening of glucose tolerance may occur in patients taking oestrogens and therefore diabetic patients should be carefully observed while receiving hormone replacement therapy.

Interaction with other medicaments and other forms of interaction: None known.

Pregnancy and lactation: Premarin Vaginal Cream is contraindicated in the event of known or suspected pregnancy and during lactation.

Effects on ability to drive and use machines: Not applicable.

Undesirable effects: (see also *Special warnings and precautions for use*) The following side effects have been reported with oestrogen therapy.

1. Genitourinary system–Premenstrual-like syndrome, increase in size of uterine fibromyomata, vaginal candidiasis, change in cervical erosion and in degree of cervical secretion, cystitis-like syndrome.
2. Breasts–Tenderness, enlargement, secretion.
3. Gastrointestinal–Nausea, vomiting, abdominal cramps, bloating, cholestatic jaundice.
4. Skin–Chloasma or melasma which may persist when drug is discontinued, erythema multiforme, erythema nodosum, haemorrhagic eruption, loss of scalp hair, hirsutism.
5. Eyes–Steepening of corneal curvature, intolerance to contact lenses.
6. CNS–Headaches, migraine, dizziness, mental depression, chorea.
7. Miscellaneous–Increase or decrease in weight, reduced carbohydrate tolerance, aggravation of porphyria, oedema, changes in libido, leg cramps.

Overdose: Numerous reports of ingestion of large doses of oestrogen-containing oral contraceptives by young children indicate that acute serious ill effects do not occur. Overdosage of oestrogen may cause nausea, and withdrawal bleeding may occur in females.

Pharmacological properties
Pharmacodynamic properties: Conjugated oestrogen cream has identical pharmacological actions to endogenous oestrogens. In this preparation the oestrogenic action is utilised to restore levels and thus prevent the symptoms of postmenopausal oestrogen deficiency.

Pharmacokinetic properties: As a topical preparation no information is included.

Preclinical safety data: There are no pre-clinical data of relevance to the prescriber which are additional to that already included in other sections of the SPC.

Pharmaceutical particulars
List of excipients: Mineral oil, glyceryl monostearate, cetyl alcohol, cetyl esters wax, white wax, methyl stearate, sodium lauryl sulphate, phenyl ethyl alcohol, glycerin, propylene glycol monostearate, purified water

Incompatibilities: Not applicable.

Shelf life: 2 years.

Special precautions for storage: Store at room temperature (approx. 25°C).

Nature and contents of container:
Primary container: Aluminium tube with a white screw-on cap, containing 42.5 g of cream.
Secondary container: Cardboard carton.

Instructions for use/handling: Not applicable.

Marketing authorisation number 0011/0163.

Date of approval/revision June 1998

Legal category POM

PREMIQUE*

Presentation Premique is a light blue oval biconvex sugar coated tablet. Each tablet contains conjugated oestrogens 0.625 mg and medroxyprogesterone acetate (MPA) 5.0 mg.

Uses Menopausal and postmenopausal oestrogen therapy in women with an intact uterus for:

1. Vasomotor symptoms associated with oestrogen deficiency.
2. Atrophic vaginitis.
3. Atrophic urethritis.
4. Prevention and management of osteoporosis associated with oestrogen deficiency, in women at risk of developing fractures.

Epidemiological studies suggest a number of individual risk factors which contribute to the development of post-menopausal osteoporosis. These include: early menopause; family history of osteoporosis; thin, small frame; cigarette use; recent prolonged systemic corticosteroid use. If several of the risk factors are present in a patient, consideration should be given to oestrogen replacement therapy.

Dosage and administration
Adults: Premique is taken orally, in a continuous 28-day regimen of one tablet taken daily. There should be no break between packs.

Before therapy commences it is recommended that the patient is fully informed of all likely benefits and potential risks. She should have a full physical and gynaecological examination, with special emphasis on blood pressure, breasts, abdomen, pelvic organs and endometrial assessment carried out if appropriate.

For most postmenopausal women therapy may be commenced at any convenient time although if the patient is still menstruating commencement on first day of bleeding is recommended.

Since progestogens are only administered to reduce the risk of endometrial hyperplasia and endometrial carcinoma, patients without a uterus do not require Premique.

Vasomotor symptoms, atrophic vaginitis, and atrophic urethritis: The usual starting dose is one tablet 0.625 mg/5.0 mg daily.

Prevention and management of osteoporosis: The usual starting dose is one tablet daily. For prevention and treatment of osteoporosis, Premique should be used for at least 5 years and probably up to 10 years. It has been shown that bone mass conservation is sustained only as long as conjugated oestrogen therapy is administered, however data beyond 10 years are limited. Treatment should start as soon as possible after the onset of the menopause and certainly within 2–3 years.

Maintenance/continuation/extended treatment: The continuous regimen of oestrogen plus MPA for 28 days without a break is frequently associated with the development of an atrophic endometrium. However, breakthrough bleeding and spotting may occur in the early stages of Premique therapy. To reduce the likelihood of breakthrough bleeding/spotting occurring and to achieve amenorrhoea a starting dose of 5.0 mg is appropriate.

If breakthrough bleeding persists and endometrial abnormality has been ruled out, cyclic therapy should be considered as an alternative therapy.

Follow-up examinations are recommended every 6–12 months; all patients using Premique should be monitored at least annually for symptoms of endometrial abnormality. For long term use, see also warnings and precautions No.2.

Elderly: There are no special dosage requirements for elderly patients, but, as with all medicines, the lowest effective dose should be used.

Children: Not recommended

Contra-indications, warnings, etc
Contra-indications:

1. Known or suspected pregnancy.
2. Known or suspected cancer of the breast.
3. Known or suspected oestrogen-dependent neoplasia.
4. Undiagnosed abnormal genital bleeding.
5. Active deep vein thrombosis, thromboembolic disorders or a history of confirmed venous thromboembolism.
6. Acute or chronic liver disease where the LFTs have failed to return to normal.
   Rotor or Dubin Johnson syndrome.
7. Severe cardiac or renal disease.
8. Hypersensitivity to any of the components of Premique tablets.

Use in pregnancy and lactation: Premique is contra-indicated in the event of known or suspected pregnancy and during lactation.

Warnings and precautions:

1. In the female there is an increased risk of endometrial hyperplasia and carcinoma associated with the administration of unopposed oestrogens. However, the appropriate addition of a progestogen to an oestrogen regimen lowers this additional risk.
2. There is suggestive evidence of a small increased risk of breast cancer with oestrogen replacement therapy used for long-term (greater than 5 years). Some studies have reported an increased risk for long term users, others, however, have not shown this relationship. It is not known whether concurrent progestogen use influences the risk of breast cancer in post menopausal women taking hormone replacement therapy. Women on long term therapy should have regular breast examinations, should be instructed in self-breast examination and mammographic investigations conducted where considered appropriate.
   There is a need for caution when prescribing oestrogens in women who have a history of or known breast nodules or fibrocystic disease. Breast status should be closely monitored, supported by regular mammography.
3. Epidemiological studies have suggested that hormone replacement therapy (HRT) is associated with an increased relative risk of developing venous thromboembolism (VTE) i.e. deep vein thrombosis or pulmonary embolism. The studies find a 2–3 fold increase for users compared with non-users which for healthy women amounts to a low risk of one extra case of VTE each year for every 5000 patients taking HRT.
   Generally recognised risk factors for VTE include a personal or family history and severe obesity (Body Mass Index >30 kg/m²). In women with these factors the benefits of treatment with HRT need to be carefully weighed against risks. There is no consensus about the possible role of varicose veins in VTE.
   The risk of VTE may be temporarily increased with prolonged immobilisation, major trauma or major surgery. In women on HRT scrupulous attention should be given to prophylactic measures to prevent VTE following surgery. Where prolonged immobilisation is liable to follow elective surgery, particularly abdominal or orthopaedic surgery to the lower limbs, consideration should be given to temporarily stopping HRT 4 weeks earlier, if this is possible.
   If venous thromboembolism develops after initiating therapy the drug should be discontinued.
4. Premique should be used with caution in patients with a past history of stroke or myocardial infarction.
5. If there is any sudden loss of vision, or there is a sudden onset of proptosis, diplopia or migraine, or if thromboembolic phenomena develop after initiating therapy the drug should be discontinued while the cause is investigated.
6. If jaundice develops, therapy should be discontinued.
7. An increase in the risk of surgically confirmed gall bladder disease has been reported in women receiving postmenopausal oestrogens.
8. Certain patients may develop undesirable manifestations of excessive oestrogenic/progestogenic stimulation such as abnormal uterine bleeding, mastodynia, etc. In the event of abnormal vaginal bleeding, adequate diagnostic measures, including endometrial sampling when indicated, should be undertaken to rule out malignancy.
9. Most studies indicate that oestrogen replacement therapy has little effect on blood pressure and some indicate that oestrogen use may be associated with a small decrease. In addition, most studies on combined therapy indicate that the addition of a progestogen has little effect on blood pressure. During trials with Premarin/MPA a few patients had a rise in blood pressure; these changes were mostly judged not to be of clinical significance.
   When oestrogens are administered to hypertensive women, supervision is necessary, and blood pressure should be monitored at regular intervals. If a significant increase in blood pressure develops after initiating therapy, treatment should be discontinued while the cause is investigated. Rarely, idiosyncratic hypertension may occur.
10. Oestrogens/progestogens may cause some degree of fluid retention and therefore patients with cardiac or renal dysfunction should be monitored.
11. Changes in glucose tolerance have been observed in some patients on oestrogen/progestogen therapy. Decreased endogenous insulin levels during hormone replacement therapy have been observed. Diabetic patients should be carefully observed while receiving Premique.
12. Patients should be advised that Premique is not an oral contraceptive, neither will it restore fertility. Women of child-bearing potential should be advised to adhere to non-hormonal contraceptive methods.
13. Patients who have a history of depression should be observed and therapy discontinued if the depression recurs to a serious degree.
14. Certain diseases may be made worse by hormone replacement therapy and patients with these conditions should be closely monitored. These include otosclerosis, multiple sclerosis, systemic lupus erythematosis, porphyria, melanoma, epilepsy, migraine and asthma. In addition pre-existing uterine fibroids may increase in size during oestrogen therapy and symptoms associated with endometriosis may be exacerbated.

Interactions with other medicines: Rifampicin reportedly decreases oestrogenic activity during concomitant use with ethinyloestradiol in oral contraceptives. This effect has been attributed to increased metabolism of oestrogen, presumably by induction of hepatic microsomal enzymes. It is not known whether there are similar effects on conjugated oestrogens. Phenytoin may also decrease oestrogen levels by a similar mechanism.

Changed oestrogen levels may affect certain endocrine and liver function tests.

Side effects: (See also *Warnings and precautions*). The following side-effects have been associated with oestrogen/progestogen therapy:

1. Genitourinary system: PMS-like syndrome, vaginal bleeding, increase in size of uterine fibromyomata.
2. Breasts: Pain, tenderness, enlargement, secretion.
3. Gastrointestinal: Nausea, abdominal cramps, flatulence, bloating, cholelithiasis, cholestatic jaundice.
4. Skin: Alopecia, rash, pruritis, hirsutism. Chloasma or melasma, which may continue after the drug is discontinued.
5. Eyes: Visual disturbance.
6. CNS: Headache, nervousness.
7. Miscellaneous: Increase or decrease in weight, oedema, aggravation of porphyria, reduction in carbohydrate tolerance, leg cramps.

Acute overdosage: Numerous reports of ingestion of large doses of oestrogen/progestogen-containing oral contraceptives by young children indicate that acute serious ill effects have not been observed. Overdosage of oestrogens may cause nausea, and withdrawal bleeding may occur in females.

Should large overdoses occur and medical concerns arise, the standard practices of gastric evacuation, activated charcoal administration, and general supportive therapy may be applicable.

Pharmaceutical precautions Store in a dry place below (25°C).

Legal category POM

Package quantities A 28-day pack containing one wallet holding 28 tablets containing conjugated oestrogens 0.625 mg and medroxyprogesterone acetate 5.0 mg. A carton containing three wallets (3 x 28 days) of tablets.

Further information After the menopause, the protective effect that endogenous oestrogens appear to have on the female cardiovascular system is lost, and the risk of women developing cardiovascular disease rises to become similar to that of men.

A decreased risk of coronary heart disease in postmenopausal women taking oestrogen replacement therapy has been observed. Oral administration of conjugated oestrogens alone to postmenopausal women increased serum high density lipoprotein cholesterol (HDL-C) levels and decreased low density lipoprotein cholesterol (LDL-C) levels. These changes improve the lipid profile and are recognised as a contributory factor to the reduced risk of coronary heart disease in women. Although some of the effects may be modified by the addition of MPA, clinical trial results suggest that the combination of conjugated oestrogens with MPA show similar beneficial effects on lipid parameters to that seen during treatment with conjugated oestrogen therapy alone.

Premique contains the following excipients: calcium phosphate tribasic, calcium sulphate, carnauba wax, microcrystalline cellulose, glyceryl mono-oleate, lactose, magnesium stearate, methyl cellulose, polyethylene glycol, pharmaceutical glaze, sucrose, titanium dioxide (E171) and colour (E132).

Product licence number 0011/0212

PREMIQUE* Cycle

Presentation Premique Cycle is composed of two separate lots of tablets presented in a 28 day calendar pack. Each calendar pack contains 28 conjugated oestrogen tablets and 14 MPA tablets.

The conjugated oestrogen tablets are maroon, biconvex, sugar-coated, and contain 0.625 mg conjugated oestrogens.

The MPA tablets are round, white, imprinted '10' on one side and contain 10.0 mg of the progestogen, medroxyprogesterone acetate (MPA).

Uses Treatment of the following conditions in women with an intact uterus:

1. Vasomotor symptoms associated with oestrogen deficiency.
2. Atrophic vaginitis.
3. Atrophic urethritis.
4. Prevention and management of osteoporosis associated with oestrogen deficiency, in women at risk of developing fractures.

Epidemiological studies suggest a number of individual risk factors which contribute to the development of post-menopausal osteoporosis. These include: early menopause; family history of osteoporosis; thin, small frame; cigarette use; recent prolonged systemic corticosteroid use. If several of the risk factors are present in a patient, consideration should be given to oestrogen replacement therapy.

Dosage and administration
Adults: Premique Cycle is available for oral use in a sequential regimen. That is, 28 days of oestrogen therapy 0.625 mg, with 14 days of MPA tablets taken with the oestrogen tablet on days 15–28. There should be no break between packs.

Before therapy commences it is recommended that the patient is fully informed of all likely benefits and potential risks. She should have a full physical and gynaecological examination, with special emphasis on blood pressure, breasts, abdomen, pelvic organs and endometrial assessment carried out if appropriate.

For most postmenopausal women therapy may be commenced at any convenient time although if the patient is still menstruating commencement on first day of bleeding is recommended.

Since progestogens are only administered to reduce the risk of endometrial hyperplasia and endometrial carcinoma, patients without a uterus will not require Premique Cycle.

Patients should be advised that a regular withdrawal bleed will usually occur at the end of one cycle of Premique Cycle and the beginning of the next.

Vasomotor symptoms, atrophic vaginitis, atrophic urethritis: One oestrogen tablet 0.625 mg daily for 28 days. One MPA tablet is also taken daily on days 15–28.

Prevention and management of osteoporosis: One oestrogen tablet 0.625 mg daily for 28 days. One MPA tablet is taken daily on days 15–28. For prevention and treatment of osteoporosis Premique Cycle should be used for at least 5 years, and probably up to 10 years. It has been shown that bone mass conservation is sustained only as long as conjugated oestrogen therapy is administered, however data beyond 10 years are limited. Treatment should start as soon as possible after the onset of the menopause and certainly within 2–3 years.

Maintenance/continuation/extended treatment: Follow up examinations are recommended every 6–12 months; all patients using Premique Cycle should be monitored at least annually for symptoms of endometrial abnormality. For prevention and treatment of osteoporosis long term treatment is necessary. For long term use, see also Warnings and Precautions No.2.

Elderly: There are no special dosage requirements for elderly patients, but, as with all medicines the lowest effective dose should be used.

Children: Not recommended

Contra-indications, warnings, etc.
Contra-indications:

1. Known or suspected pregnancy.
2. Known or suspected cancer of the breast.
3. Known or suspected oestrogen-dependent neoplasia.
4. Undiagnosed abnormal genital bleeding.
5. Active deep vein thrombosis, thromboembolic disorders or a history of confirmed venous thromboembolism.
6. Acute or chronic liver disease where the LFTs have failed to return to normal. Rotor or Dubin Johnson Syndrome
7. Severe cardiac or renal disease
8. Hypersensitivity to any of the components in the conjugated oestrogen or MPA tablets.

Use in pregnancy and lactation: Premique Cycle is contraindicated in the event of known or suspected pregnancy and during lactation.

Warnings and precautions:

1. In the female there is an increased risk of endometrial hyperplasia and carcinoma associated with the administration of unopposed oestrogens. However, the appropriate addition of a progestogen to an oestrogen regimen lowers this additional risk.
2. There is suggestive evidence of a small increased risk of breast cancer with oestrogen replacement therapy used for long-term (greater than 5 years). Some studies have reported an increased risk for long term users, others, however, have not shown this relationship. It is not known whether concurrent progestogen use influences the risk of breast cancer in post menopausal women taking hormone replacement therapy. Women on long term therapy should have regular breast examinations, should be instructed in self-breast examination and mammographic investigations conducted where considered appropriate.
   There is a need for caution when prescribing oestrogens in women who have a history of or known breast nodules or fibrocystic disease. Breast status should be closely monitored, supported by regular mammography.
3. Epidemiological studies have suggested that hormone replacement therapy (HRT) is associated with an increased relative risk of developing venous thromboembolism (VTE) i.e. deep vein thrombosis or pulmonary embolism. The studies find a 2–3 fold increase for users compared with non-users which for healthy women amounts to a low risk of one extra case of VTE each year for every 5000 patients taking HRT.
   Generally recognised risk factors for VTE include a personal or family history and severe obesity (Body Mass Index >30 kg/m²). In women with these factors the benefits of treatment with HRT need to be carefully weighed against risks. There is no consensus about the possible role of varicose veins in VTE.
   The risk of VTE may be temporarily increased with prolonged immobilisation, major trauma or major surgery. In women on HRT scrupulous attention should be given to prophylactic measures to prevent VTE following surgery. Where prolonged immobilisation is liable to follow elective surgery, particularly abdominal or orthopaedic surgery to the lower limbs, consideration should be given to temporarily stopping HRT 4 weeks earlier, if this is possible.
   If venous thromboembolism develops after initiating therapy the drug should be discontinued.
4. Premique Cycle should be used with caution in patients with a past history of stroke or myocardial infarction.
5. If there is any sudden loss of vision, or there is a sudden onset of proptosis, diplopia or migraine, or if thromboembolic phenomena develop after initiating therapy the drug should be discontinued while the cause is investigated.
6. If jaundice develops, therapy should be discontinued.
7. An increase in the risk of surgically confirmed gall bladder disease has been reported in women receiving postmenopausal oestrogens.
8. Certain patients may develop undesirable manifestations of excessive oestrogenic/progestogenic stimulation, such as abnormal uterine bleeding, mastodynia, etc. In the event of abnormal vaginal bleeding, adequate diagnostic measures, including endometrial sampling when indicated, should be undertaken to rule out malignancy.
9. Most studies indicate that oestrogen replacement therapy has little effect on blood pressure and some indicate that oestrogen use may be associated with a small decrease. In addition, most studies on combined therapy indicate that the addition of a progestogen has little effect on blood pressure. During trials with Premique Cycle a few patients had a rise in blood pressure; these changes were mostly judged not to be of clinical significance.
   When oestrogens are administered to hypertensive women, supervision is necessary, and blood pressure should be monitored at regular intervals.
   If a significant increase in blood pressure develops after initiating therapy treatment should be discontinued while the cause is investigated. Rarely, idiosyncratic hypertension may occur.
10. Oestrogens/progestogens may cause some degree of fluid retention and therefore patients with cardiac or renal dysfunction should be monitored.
11. Changes in glucose tolerance have been observed in some patients on oestrogen/progestogen therapy. Decreased endogenous insulin levels during hormone replacement therapy have been observed. Diabetic patients should be carefully observed while receiving Premique Cycle.
12. Patients should be advised that the resumption of menses associated with hormone replacement therapy is not indicative of fertility. There is no data to support Premique Cycle as an appropriate form of contraception. Women of child-bearing potential taking Premique Cycle require contraception and should be advised to adhere to non-hormonal contraceptive methods.
13. Patients who have a history of depression should be observed and therapy discontinued if the depression recurs to a serious degree.
14. Certain diseases may be made worse by hormone replacement therapy and patients with these conditions should be closely monitored. These include otosclerosis, multiple sclerosis, systemic lupus erythematosus, melanoma, porphyria, epilepsy, migraine and asthma. In addition pre-existing uterine fibroids may increase in size during oestrogen therapy and symptoms associated with endometriosis may be exacerbated.

Interactions with other medicines: Rifampicin reportedly decreases oestrogenic activity during concomitant use with ethinyloestradiol in oral contraceptives. This effect has been attributed to increased metabolism of oestrogen, presumably by induction of hepatic microsomal enzymes. It is not known whether there are similar effects on conjugated oestrogens. Phenytoin may also decrease oestrogen levels by a similar mechanism.

Changed oestrogen levels may affect certain endocrine and liver function tests.

Side effects: The following side-effects have been associated with oestrogen/progestogen therapy.

1. Genitourinary system: PMS-like syndrome, vaginal bleeding, increase in size of uterine fibromyomata.
2. Breasts: Pain, tenderness, enlargement, secretion.
3. Gastrointestinal: Nausea, abdominal cramps, flatulence, bloating, cholelithiasis, cholestatic jaundice.
4. Skin: Alopecia, rash, pruritis, hirsutism. Chloasma or melasma, which may continue after the drug is discontinued.
5. Eyes: Visual disturbance.
6. CNS: Headache, nervousness.
7. Miscellaneous: Increase or decrease in weight, oedema, aggravation of porphyria, reduction in carbohydrate tolerance, leg cramps.

Acute overdosage: Numerous reports of ingestion of large doses of oestrogen/progestogen-containing oral contraceptives by young children indicate that acute serious ill effects have not been observed. Overdosage of oestrogens may cause nausea, and withdrawal bleeding may occur in females. Should large overdoses occur and medical concerns arise, the standard practices of gastric evacuation, activated charcoal administration, and general supportive therapy may be applicable.

Pharmaceutical precautions Store in a dry place below 25°C.

Legal category POM

Package quantities A carton containing three calander packs each containing 28 conjugated oestrogen tablets 0.625 mg and 14 medroxyprogesterone acetate tablets 10.0 mg.

Further information After the menopause, the protective effect that endogenous oestrogens appear to have on the female cardiovascular system is lost, and the risk of women developing cardiovascular disease rises to become similar to that of men.

A decreased risk of coronary heart disease in postmenopausal women taking oestrogen replacement therapy has been observed. Oral administration of conjugated oestrogens alone to postmenopausal women increased serum high density lipoprotein cholesterol (HDL-C) levels and decreased low density lipoprotein cholesterol (LDL-C) levels. These changes improve the lipid profile and are recognised as a contributory factor to the reduced risk of coronary heart disease in women. Although some of the effects may be modified by the addition of MPA, clinical trial results suggest that the combination of conjugated oestrogens with MPA show similar beneficial effects on lipid parameters to that seen during treatment with conjugated oestrogen therapy alone.

Pharmaceutical excipients in the conjugated tablets are: lactose, methylcellulose, magnesium stearate. Coating ingredients are syrup, sucrose, glyceryl mono-oleate, polyethylene glycol, carnauba wax, calcium sulphate, shellac solution, microcrystalline cellulose, titanium dioxide (E171) and colours E110, E132 and E127. Pharmaceutical excipients in the progestogen tablets are: lactose, microcrystalline cellulose, methylcellulose and magnesium stearate.

Product licence number 0011/0205

PREMPAK*-C

Presentation Prempak-C 0.625 consists of 28 maroon tablets containing natural conjugated oestrogens 0.625 mg plus 12 light brown tablets containing norgestrel 0.15 mg.

Prempak-C 1.25 consists of 28 yellow tablets containing natural conjugated oestrogens 1.25 mg plus 12 light brown tablets containing norgestrel 0.15 mg.

Uses Menopausal and postmenopausal oestrogen therapy in women with an intact uterus for:

1. vasomotor symptoms such as sweating and hot flushes
2. allied disorders of the menopause such as atrophic vaginitis, kraurosis vulvae, atrophic urethritis
3. prophylaxis of osteoporosis in women at risk of developing fractures.

Dosage and administration
Adults: Conjugated oestrogens 0.625 mg–1.25 mg daily. One norgestrel tablet should be taken daily from day 17 to day 28 of oestrogen therapy. Continuous oestrogen administration is recommended. For maintenance, the lowest effective dose should be used.

Vasomotor symptoms: 0.625–1.25 mg conjugated oestrogens daily depending on the response of the individual. One norgestrel tablet should be taken daily from day 17 to day 28 of oestrogen therapy.

Atrophic vaginitis, kraurosis vulvae, atrophic urethritis: 0.625–1.25 mg conjugated oestrogens daily depending on the response of the individual. One norgestrel tablet should be taken daily from day 17 to day 28 of oestrogen therapy.

Prophylaxis of osteoporosis: The minimum effective dose is 0.625 mg daily for most patients. One norgestrel tablet should be taken daily from day 17 to day 28 of oestrogen therapy. Hormone replacement therapy has been found to be effective in the prevention of osteoporosis when started soon after the menopause and used for 5 years and probably up to 10 years. Treatment should start as soon as possible after the onset of the menopause and certainly within 2 to 3 years. Protection appears to be effective for as long as treatment is continued, however data beyond 10 years are limited. A careful re-appraisal of the risk-benefit ratio should be undertaken before treating for longer than 5 to 10 years. For long term use see also *Precautions and warnings.*

At present there is no established screening programme for determining women at risk of developing osteoporotic fractures. Epidemiological studies suggest a number of individual risk factors which contribute to the development of postmenopausal osteoporosis. These include: early menopause; family history of osteoporosis; thin, small frame; cigarette use; recent prolonged systemic corticosteroid use.

If several of these risk factors are present in a patient, consideration should be given to oestrogen replacement therapy.

For most postmenopausal women therapy may be commenced at any convenient time although if the patient is still menstruating, commencement on first day of bleeding is recommended. Withdrawal bleeding usually occurs within three to seven days after the last norgestrel tablet.

Since progestogens are only administered to protect against hyperplastic changes of the endometrium, patients without a uterus will not require a progestogen.

Before therapy commences it is recommended that the patient is fully informed of all the likely benefits and potential risks. She should have a full physical and gynaecological examination, with special emphasis on blood pressure, breasts, abdomen and pelvic organs, and endometrial assessment carried out if indicated. Follow-up examinations are recommended every 6–12 months.

Breakthrough bleeding may occasionally occur in the first few weeks after initiating treatment and will usually settle. It can also be the result of poor compliance, or concurrent antibiotic use. It may however indicate endometrial pathology and therefore any doubt as to the cause of breakthrough bleeding is an indication for endometrial evaluation including endometrial biopsy.

Elderly: There are no special dosage requirements for elderly patients, but as with all medicines, the lowest effective dose should be used.

Children: Not recommended.

Contra-indications, warnings etc
Contra-indications:

1. Known or suspected pregnancy.
2. History of, known or suspected cancer of the breast.
3. Known or suspected oestrogen-dependent neoplasia. Undiagnosed abnormal genital bleeding.
4. Active deep vein thrombosis, thromboembolic disorders or a history of confirmed venous thromboembolism.
5. Acute or chronic liver disease or history of liver disease where the liver function tests have failed to return to normal. Rotor syndrome or Dubin-Johnson syndrome.
6. Severe cardiac or renal disease.

Use in pregnancy and lactation: Prempak-C is contra-indicated in the event of known or suspected pregnancy and during lactation.

Warnings and precautions:

1. In the female there is an increased risk of endometrial hyperplasia and carcinoma associated with unopposed oestrogen administered long-term (for more than one year). However, the appropriate addition of a progestogen to an oestrogen regimen lowers this additional risk.
2. There is suggestive evidence of a small increased risk of breast cancer with oestrogen replacement therapy used for long term (greater than 5 years). Some studies have reported an increased risk of breast cancer in long-term users, others however, have not shown this relationship. It is not known whether concurrent progestogen use influences the risk of breast cancer in postmenopausal women taking hormone replacement therapy. Women on long-term therapy should have regular breast examinations, and should be instructed in self-breast examination. Regular mammographic investigations should be conducted where considered appropriate.
   There is a need for caution when prescribing oestrogens in women who have a history of, or known breast nodules, or fibrocystic disease. Breast status should be closely monitored, supported by regular mammography.
3. Certain diseases may be made worse by hormone replacement therapy and patients with these conditions should be closely monitored. These include otosclerosis, multiple sclerosis, systemic lupus erythematosis, porphyria, melanoma, epilepsy, migraine and asthma. In addition pre-existing uterine fibroids may increase in size during oestrogen therapy and symptoms associated with endometriosis may be exacerbated.
4. Epidemiological studies have suggested that hormone replacement therapy (HRT) is associated with an increased relative risk of developing venous thromboembolism (VTE) i.e. deep vein thrombosis or pulmonary embolism. The studies find a 2–3 fold increase for users compared with non-users which for healthy women amounts to a low risk of one extra case of VTE each year for every 5000 patients taking HRT.
   Generally recognised risk factors for VTE include a personal or family history and severe obesity (Body Mass Index >30 kg/m²). In women with these factors the benefits of treatment with HRT need to be carefully weighed against risks. There is no consensus about the possible role of varicose veins in VTE.
   The risk of VTE may be temporarily increased with prolonged immobilisation, major trauma or major surgery. In women on HRT scrupulous attention should be given to prophylactic measures to prevent VTE following surgery. Where prolonged immobilisation is liable to follow elective surgery, particularly abdominal or orthopaedic surgery to the lower limbs, consideration should be given to temporarily stopping HRT 4 weeks earlier, if this is possible.
   If venous thromboembolism develops after initiating therapy the drug should be discontinued.
5. Prempak-C should be used with caution in patients with a past history of stroke or myocardial infarction.
6. Oestrogens may cause fluid retention and therefore patients with cardiac or renal dysfunction should be carefully observed.
7. If jaundice, migraine-like headaches, visual disturbance, thromboembolic phenomena or a significant increase in blood pressure develop after initiating therapy, the medication should be discontinued while the cause is investigated.
8. Prempak-C is not an oral contraceptive neither will it restore fertility. Women of child-bearing potential should be advised to adhere to non-hormonal contraceptive methods.
9. Most studies indicate that oestrogen replacement therapy has little effect on blood pressure and some indicate that oestrogen use may be associated with a small decrease. In addition, most studies on combined therapy indicate that the addition of a progestogen also has little effect on blood pressure. Rarely, idiosyncratic hypertension may occur.
   When oestrogens are administered to hypertensive women, supervision is necessary and blood pressure should be monitored at regular intervals.
10. Changed oestrogen levels may affect certain endocrine and liver function tests.
11. It has been reported that there is an increase in the risk of surgically confirmed gall bladder disease in women receiving postmenopausal oestrogens.
12. A worsening of glucose tolerance may occur in patients taking oestrogens and therefore diabetic patients should be carefully observed while receiving hormone replacement therapy.

Side effects: The following side effects have been reported with oestrogen/progestogen therapy:

1. Genitourinary system: Breakthrough bleeding, spotting, change in menstrual flow, dysmenorrhoea, premenstrual-like syndrome, amenorrhoea, increase in size of uterine fibromyomata, vaginal candidiasis, change in cervical erosion and in degree of cervical secretion, cystitis-like syndrome.
2. Breasts: Tenderness, enlargement, secretion.
3. Gastrointestinal: Nausea, vomiting, abdominal cramps, bloating, cholestatic jaundice.
4. Skin: Chloasma or melasma which may persist when drug is discontinued, erythema multiforme, erythema nodosum, haemorrhagic eruption, loss of scalp hair, hirsutism.
5. Eyes: Steepening of corneal curvature, intolerance to contact lenses.
6. CNS: Headaches, migraine, dizziness, mental depression, chorea.
7. Miscellaneous: Increase or decrease in weight, reduced carbohydrate tolerance, aggravation of porphyria, oedema, changes in libido, leg cramps.

Acute overdosage: Numerous reports of ingestion of large doses of oestrogen-containing oral contraceptives by young children indicate that acute serious ill effects do not occur. Overdosage of oestrogen may cause nausea, and withdrawal bleeding may occur in females.

Pharmaceutical precautions No special requirements for storage are necessary.

Legal category POM

Package quantities Triple packs with 3 blister strips of 28 oestrogen tablets 0.625 mg or 1.25 mg and 12 norgestrel tablets 0.15 mg.

Further information After the menopause the protective effect that endogenous oestrogens appear to have on the female cardiovascular system is lost, and the risk of women developing cardiovascular disease rises to become similar to that of men.

Most studies show that oral administration of conjugated equine oestrogens to postmenopausal women increase serum high density lipoprotein (HDL-cholesterol) and decrease the potentially atherogenic low density lipoprotein (LDL-cholesterol) levels. This improves the lipid profile and is recognised as a factor contributing to the beneficial effect of conjugated equine oestrogens on the risk of coronary heart disease in postmenopausal women. A possible attenuation of these effects may occur with the addition of a progestogen. However epidemiologic data on combined oestrogen and progestogen therapy are limited.

Prempak-C provides oestrogen/progestogen therapy for the menopausal syndrome and associated disorders. The blister strip contains 28 oestrogen tablets. From day 17 to day 28 inclusive each bubble contains in addition one norgestrel 0.15 mg tablet. The two tablets should be taken together for these twelve days.

Product licence numbers

Prempak-C 0.625 0011/0161
Prempak-C 1.25 0011/0162

PROSTAP* 3 Leuprorelin Acetate Depot Injection 11.25 mg.

Qualitative and quantitative composition
Prostap 3 Powder: 11.25 mg leuprorelin acetate (equivalent to 10.72 mg base).

Sterile Vehicle: Each ml contains sodium carboxymethyl cellulose 5 mg, mannitol 50 mg, polysorbate 80 1 mg in water for injection.

Pharmaceutical form and route of administration
Prostap 3 Powder 11.25 mg: A sterile, lyophilised, white, odourless PLA (poly DL-lactic acid) microsphere powder for subcutaneous injection after reconstitution with the sterile vehicle to provide a 3 month depot injection.

Sterile vehicle: Prefilled syringes containing 2 ml of clear, colourless, slightly viscous, sterile vehicle for reconstitution of the powder.

Clinical particulars
Therapeutic indications: Prostap 3 is indicated for use in the management of advanced prostatic cancer.

Posology and method of administration:

Dosage:
Male adults: The usual recommended dose is 11.25 mg presented as a three month depot injection and administered as a single subcutaneous injection at intervals of three months. The majority of patients will respond to this dosage. Prostap therapy should not be discontinued when remission or improvement occurs. As with other drugs administered regularly by injection, the injection site should be varied periodically.

Response to Prostap 3 therapy should be monitored by clinical parameters and by measuring prostate-specific antigen (PSA) serum levels. Clinical studies have shown that testosterone levels increased during the first 4 days of treatment in the majority of non-orchidectomised patients. They then decreased and reached castrate levels by 2–4 weeks. Once attained, castrate levels were maintained as long as drug therapy continued. If a patient's response appears to be sub-optimal, then it would be advisable to confirm that serum testosterone levels have reached or are remaining at castrate levels. Transient increases in acid phosphatase levels sometimes occur early in the treatment period but usually return to normal or near normal values by the 4th week of treatment.

Elderly men: as for adults.

Women and children: the use of Prostap 3 in women and children is not recommended.

Administration: The vial of Prostap 3 microsphere powder should be reconstituted immediately prior to administration by subcutaneous injection. However, the suspension is considered stable for up to 24 hours. Remove flip-cap from vial of Prostap 3 Powder and cap from pre-filled syringe containing 2 ml Sterile Vehicle. Ensure 23 gauge needle is fixed securely by screwing needle hub onto the syringe and inject whole contents of syringe into vial of Prostap 3 Powder using an aseptic technique. Remove the syringe/needle and keep aseptic. Shake the vial gently for 15–20 seconds to produce a uniform cloudy suspension of Prostap. Immediately draw up suspension into syringe taking care to exclude air bubbles. Change the needle on syringe using a 23 gauge needle. Having cleaned an appropriate injection site and ensured that the needle is fixed securely, administer the suspension by subcutaneous injection taking care not to enter a blood vessel. Apply sterile dressing to injection site if required.

The injection should be given as soon as possible after mixing. If any settling of suspension occurs in vial or syringe, re-suspend by gentle shaking and administer immediately.

No other fluid can be used for reconstitution of Prostap 3 Powder.

Contra-indications: There are no known contra-indications to the use of Prostap 3 in men.

The use of Prostap 3 is not indicated in women.

Special warnings and special precautions for use:
Men: In the initial stages of therapy, a transient rise in levels of testosterone, dihydro-testosterone and acid phosphatase may occur. In some cases, this may be associated with a 'flare' or exacerbation of the tumour growth resulting in temporary deterioration of the patient's condition. These symptoms usually subside on continuation of therapy. 'Flare' may manifest itself as systemic or neurological symptoms in some cases.

In order to reduce the risk of flare, an anti-androgen may be administered beginning 3 days prior to leuprorelin therapy and continuing for the first two to three weeks of treatment. This has been reported to prevent the sequelae of an initial rise in serum testosterone.

Patients at risk of ureteric obstruction or spinal cord compression should be considered carefully and closely supervised in the first few weeks of treatment.

These patients should be considered for prophylactic treatment with anti-androgens. Should urological/ neurological complications occur, these should be treated by appropriate specific measures.

If an anti-androgen is used over a prolonged period, due attention should be paid to the contraindications and precautions associated with its extended use.

Whilst the development of pituitary adenomas has been noted in chronic toxicity studies at high doses in some animal species, this has not been observed in long term clinical studies with leuprorelin acetate.

Precautions:
Men: Patients with urinary obstruction and patients with metastatic vertebral lesions should begin Prostap 3 therapy under close supervision for the first few weeks of treatment.

Interaction with other medicaments and other forms of interaction: None have been reported.

Pregnancy and lactation: The use of Prostap 3 is not indicated in women. However, leuprorelin acetate is contraindicated in women who are or may become pregnant while receiving the drug. Leuprorelin acetate should not be used in women who are breast-feeding.

Effects on ability to drive and operate machines: None reported.

Undesirable effects: Many side effects seen during treatment with Prostap 3 are due to the specific pharmacological action or the disease condition itself.

The administration of Prostap is often associated with hot flushes and sometimes sweating. Impotence and decreased libido will be expected with Prostap therapy. Gynaecomastia has been reported occasionally.

In cases where a 'tumour flare' occurs after Prostap therapy, an exacerbation may occur in any symptoms or signs due to disease, for example, bone pain, urinary obstruction etc. These symptoms subside on continuation of therapy.

Adverse events which have been reported include peripheral oedema, fatigue, nausea, headache (occasionally severe), arthralgia, dizziness, insomnia, paraesthesia, visual disturbances, weight changes and irritation at the injection site. Hypersensitivity reactions including rash, pruritis, urticaria and, rarely, wheezing have also been reported. Anaphylactic reactions are rare.

Overdose: There is no clinical experience with the effects of an acute overdose of leuprorelin acetate. In animal studies, doses of up to 500 times the recommended human dose resulted in dyspnoea, decreased activity and local irritation at the injection site. In cases of overdosage, the patients should be monitored closely and management should be symptomatic and supportive.

Pharmacological properties
Pharmacodynamic properties: Prostap 3 contains leuprorelin acetate, a synthetic nonapeptide analogue of naturally occurring gonadotrophin releasing hormone (GnRH) which possesses greater potency than the natural hormone. Leuprorelin acetate is a peptide and is therefore unrelated to the steroids. Chronic administration results in an inhibition of gonadotrophin production and subsequent suppression of ovarian and testicular steroid secretion. This effect is reversible on discontinuation of therapy.

Administration of leuprorelin acetate results in an initial increase in circulating levels of gonadotrophins which leads to a transient increase in gonadal steroid levels in both men and women. Continued administration of leuprorelin acetate results in a decrease of gonadotrophin and sex steroid levels. In men serum testosterone levels, initially raised in response to early luteinising hormone (LH) release, fall to castrate levels in about 2–4 weeks.

Prostap 3 is inactive when given orally.

Pharmacokinetic properties: Leuprorelin acetate is well absorbed after subcutaneous injection. It binds to the luteinising hormone releasing hormone (LHRH) receptors and is rapidly degraded. An initially high plasma level of leuprorelin peaks at around 3 hours after Prostap 3 injection, followed by a decrease to maintenance levels in 7 to 14 days. Prostap 3 provides continuous plasma levels for up to 117 days resulting in suppression of testosterone to below castration level within 4 weeks of the first injection in the majority of patients.

The metabolism, distribution and excretion of leuprorelin acetate in humans have not been fully determined.

Preclinical safety data: Animal studies have shown that leuprorelin acetate has a high acute safety factor. No major overt toxicological problems have been seen during repeated administration. Whilst the development of pituitary adenomas has been noted in chronic toxicity studies at high doses in some animal species, this has not been observed in long-term clinical studies. No evidence of mutagenicity or teratogenicity has been shown. Animal reproductive studies showed increased foetal mortality and decreased foetal weights reflecting the pharmacological effects of this LHRH antagonist.

Pharmaceutical particulars
List of excipients: Poly (D-L lactic acid), Mannitol.

Incompatibilities: No other fluid other than the Sterile Vehicle provided for Prostap 3 can be used for the reconstitution of Prostap 3 Powder.

Shelf life: 36 months unopened. Once reconstituted with Sterile Vehicle, the suspension should be administered immediately.

Special precautions for storage: Store at or below room temperature (25°C), in the original container. Protect from light.

Nature and contents of container: Vials containing 11.25 mg leuprorelin acetate as microsphere powder. Prefilled syringes containing 2 ml of Sterile Vehicle.

Instructions for use and handling: See above.

Marketing authorisation number
Prostap 3: PL 0095/0311
Sterile Vehicle: PL 0095/0220

Date of approval/revision
Last revised December 1996.

PROSTAP* SR

Qualitative and quantitative composition
Prostap SR Powder: 3.75 mg leuprorelin acetate (equivalent to 3.57 mg base).

Sterile Vehicle: Each ml contains sodium carboxymethyl cellulose 5 mg, mannitol 50 mg, polysorbate 80 1 mg in water for injection.

Pharmaceutical form and route of administration
Prostap SR Powder 3.75 mg: A sterile, lyophilised, white odourless PLGA† microsphere powder for subcutaneous or intramuscular injection after reconstitution with the sterile vehicle (4 week depot injection).

†PLGA = Copoly (DL-lactic acid/glycolic acid) 75:25 mol%.

Sterile vehicle: Prefilled syringes containing 1 ml of clear, colourless, slightly viscous, sterile vehicle for reconstitution of the micromicrosphere.

Clinical particulars
Therapeutic indications:

(i) Treatment of advanced prostatic cancer.
(ii) Management of endometriosis, including pain relief and reduction of endometriotic lesions.
(iii) Endometrial preparation prior to intrauterine surgical procedures including endometrial ablation or resection.

Posology and method of administration:

Dosage:
Advanced Prostatic Cancer: The usual recommended dose is 3.75 mg administered as a single subcutaneous or intramuscular injection every month. The majority of patients will respond to a 3.75 mg dose. Prostap therapy should not be discontinued when remission or improvement occurs. As with other drugs administered chronically by injection, the injection site should be varied.

Response to Prostap therapy may be monitored by clinical parameters and by measuring serum levels of testosterone and acid phosphatase. Clinical studies have shown that testosterone levels increased during the first 4 days of treatment in the majority of non-orchidectomised patients. They then decreased and reached castrate levels by 2–4 weeks. Once attained, castrate levels were maintained as long as drug therapy continued. Transient increases in acid phosphatase levels sometimes occur early in the treatment period but usually return to normal or near normal values by the 4th week of treatment.

Endometriosis: The recommended dose is 3.75 mg administered as a single subcutaneous or intramuscular injection every month for a maximum period of 6 months. Treatment should be initiated during the first 5 days of the menstrual cycle.

Endometrial preparation prior to intrauterine surgery: A single 3.75 mg subcutaneous or intramuscular injection 5–6 weeks prior to surgery. Therapy should be initiated during days 3 to 5 of the menstrual cycle.

Elderly: As for adults.

Children: Safety and efficacy in children have not been established.

Administration: The vial of Prostap SR microsphere powder should be reconstituted immediately prior to administration by subcutaneous or intramuscular injection. Remove flip-cap from vial of Prostap SR Powder and cap from prefilled syringe containing 1 ml of Sterile Vehicle. Ensure 23 gauge needle is fixed securely to the syringe and inject whole contents of syringe into vial of Prostap SR Powder using an aseptic technique. Remove the syringe/needle and keep aseptic. Shake vial gently for 15–20 seconds to produce a uniform cloudy suspension of Prostap.

Immediately draw up suspension into syringe taking care to exclude air bubbles. Change the needle on syringe using a 23 gauge needle if the suspension is to be administered subcutaneously or alternatively a 21 gauge needle for intramuscular administration. Having cleaned an appropriate injection site and ensured that the needle is fixed securely, administer the suspension by subcutaneous or intramuscular injection as appropriate taking care not to enter a blood vessel. Apply sterile dressing to injection site if required.

The injection should be given as soon as possible after mixing. If any settling of suspension occurs in vial or syringe, re-suspend by gentle shaking and administer immediately.

No other fluid can be used for reconstitution of Prostap SR Powder.

Contra-indications:
Women: Prostap is contra-indicated in women who are or may become pregnant while receiving the drug. Prostap should not be used in women who are breastfeeding or have undiagnosed abnormal vaginal bleeding.

Men: There are no known contra-indications to the use of Prostap in men.

Special warnings and special precautions for use:
Men: In the initial stages of therapy, a transient rise in levels of testosterone, dihydro-testosterone and acid phosphatase may occur. In some cases, this may be associated with a 'flare' or exacerbation of the tumour growth resulting in temporary deterioration of the patient's condition. These symptoms usually subside on continuation of therapy. 'Flare' may manifest itself as systemic or neurological symptoms in some cases.

In order to reduce the risk of flare, an anti-androgen may be administered beginning 3 days prior to leuprorelin therapy and continuing for the first two to three weeks of treatment. This has been reported to prevent the sequelae of an initial rise in serum testosterone.

Patients at risk of ureteric obstruction or spinal cord compression should be considered carefully and closely supervised in the first few weeks of treatment. These patients should be considered for prophylactic treatment with anti-androgens. Should urological or neurological complications occur, these should be treated by appropriate specific measures.

If an anti-androgen is used over a prolonged period, due attention should be paid to the contra-indications and precautions associated with its extended use.

Whilst the development of pituitary adenomas has been noted in chronic toxicity studies at high doses in some animal species, this has not been observed in long term clinical studies with Prostap.

Women: During the early phase of therapy, sex steroids temporarily rise above baseline because of the physiological effect of the drug. Therefore, an increase in clinical signs and symptoms may be observed during the initial days of therapy, but these will dissipate with continued therapy.

Prostap may cause an increase in uterine cervical resistance, which may result in difficulty in dilating the cervix for intrauterine surgical procedures.

Precautions:
Men: Patients with urinary obstruction and patients with metastatic vertebral lesions should begin Prostap therapy under close supervision for the first few weeks of treatment.

Women: Since menstruation should stop with effective doses of Prostap, the patient should notify her physician if regular menstruation persists.

Interaction with other medicaments and other forms of interaction: None have been reported.

Pregnancy and lactation: Safe use of leuprorelin acetate in pregnancy has not been established clinically. Before starting treatment with Prostap, pregnancy must be excluded.

Prostap should not be used in women who are breastfeeding.

When used monthly at the recommended dose, Prostap usually inhibits ovulation and stops menstruation. Contraception is not ensured, however, by taking Prostap and therefore patients should use non-hormonal methods of contraception during treatment.

Patients should be advised that if they miss successive doses of Prostap, breakthrough bleeding or ovulation may occur with the potential for conception. Patients should be advised to see their physician if they believe they may be pregnant. If a patient becomes pregnant during treatment, the drug must be discontinued. No teratological effect has been demonstrated in rats and rabbits. The patient must be appraised of this evidence and the potential for an unknown risk to the foetus.

Effects on ability to drive and operate machines: None reported.

Undesirable effects: Side effects seen with Prostap are due mainly to the specific pharmacological action, namely increases and decreases in certain hormone levels. Adverse events which have been reported infrequently include peripheral oedema, fatigue, nausea, headache (occasionally severe), arthralgia, dizziness, insomnia, paraesthesia, visual disturbances, weight changes and irritation at the injection site. Hypersensitivity reactions including rash, pruritus, urticaria and, rarely, wheezing have also been reported. Anaphylactic reactions are rare.

Men: In cases where a 'tumour flare' occurs after Prostap therapy, an exacerbation may occur in any symptoms or signs due to disease, for example, bone pain, urinary obstruction etc. These symptoms subside on continuation of therapy.

Impotence and decreased libido will be expected with Prostap therapy.

The administration of Prostap is often associated with hot flushes and sometimes sweating.

Gynaecomastia has been reported occasionally.

Women: Those adverse events occurring most frequently with Prostap are associated with hypo-oestrogenism; the most frequently reported are hot flushes, mood swings including depression (occasionally severe), and vaginal dryness. Oestrogen levels return to normal after treatment is discontinued.

Breast tenderness or change in breast size may occur occasionally. Hair loss has also been reported occasionally.

The induced hypo-oestrogenic state results in a small loss in bone density over the course of treatment, some of which may not be reversible. The extent of bone demineralisation due to hypo-oestrogenaemia is proportional to time and, consequently, is the adverse event responsible for limiting the duration of therapy to 6 months. The generally accepted level of bone loss with LHRH analogues such as Prostap is 5%. In clinical studies the levels varied between 2.3% and 15.7% depending on the method of measurement. During one six-month treatment period, this bone loss should not be important. In patients with major risk factors for decreased bone mineral content such as chronic alcohol and/or tobacco use, strong family history of osteoporosis, or chronic use of drugs that can reduce bone mass such as anticonvulsants or corticosteroids, Prostap therapy may pose an additional risk. In these patients, the risks and benefits must be weighed carefully before therapy with Prostap is instituted.

Overdose: There is no clinical experience with the effects of an acute overdose of Prostap. In animal studies, doses of up to 500 times the recommended human dose resulted in dyspnoea, decreased activity and local irritation at the injection site. In cases of overdosage, the patients should be monitored closely and management should be symptomatic and supportive.

Pharmacological properties

Pharmacodynamic properties: Prostap is a synthetic nonapeptide analogue of naturally occurring gonadotrophin releasing hormone (GnRH) which possesses greater potency than the natural hormone. Prostap is a peptide and is therefore unrelated to the steroids. Chronic administration results in an inhibition of gonadotrophin production and subsequent suppression of ovarian and testicular steroid secretion. This effect is reversible on discontinuation of therapy.

Administration of leuprorelin acetate results in an initial increase in circulating levels of gonadotrophins which leads to a transient increase in gonadal steroid levels in both men and women. Continued administration of leuprorelin acetate results in a decrease of gonadotrophin and sex steroid levels. In men serum testosterone levels, initially raised in response to early luteinising hormone (LH) release, fall to castrate levels in about 2–4 weeks. Oestradiol levels will decrease to postmenopausal levels in premenopausal women within one month of initiating treatment.

The drug is well absorbed from the subcutaneous or intramuscular route, binds to luteinising hormone releasing hormone (LHRH) receptors and is rapidly degraded. In this dose form, an initial high level of leuprorelin in the plasma is achieved within 3 hours followed by a drop over 24–48 hours to maintenance levels of 0.3–0.8 ng/ml and a slow decline thereafter. Effective levels persist for 30–40 days after a single dose. Prostap is inactive when given orally.

Pharmacokinetic properties: Studies submitted show that single intramuscular or subcutaneous doses of leuprorelin acetate over the dose range 3.75 to 15 mg results in detectable levels of leuprorelin for more than 28 days, good bioavailability, a consistent and predictable pharmacokinetic profile, and biological efficacy at plasma levels of less than 0.5 ng/ml. The pharmacokinetic profile is similar to that seen in animal studies using the compound, with an initial high level of drug released from the microcapsules during reconstitution and injection followed by a plateau over a 2–3 week period before levels gradually become undetectable. There appears to be no significant difference between the routes of administration (im vs sc) in biological effectiveness or pharmacokinetics.

The metabolism, distribution and excretion of leuprorelin acetate in humans have not been fully determined.

Pharmaceutical particulars

List of excipients: Gelatin. Copoly (DL-lactic acid/glycolic acid) 75:25 mol%. Mannitol.

Incompatibilities: None reported.

Shelf life: 36 months unopened.

Once reconstituted with Sterile Vehicle, the suspension should be administered immediately.

Special precautions for storage: Store at room temperature (15–25°C), in the original container. Protect from light.

Nature and contents of container: Vials containing 3.75 mg leuprorelin acetate as microsphere powder.

Prefilled syringes containing 1 ml of Sterile Vehicle.

Instructions for use and handling: None.

Marketing authorisation numbers

Prostap SR PL 0095/0218
Sterile Vehicle PL 0095/0220

Date of approval/revision

First approval 11 December 1990
Last revision June 1996

Legal category POM

TAZOCIN*

Qualitative and quantitative composition Tazocin 2.25 g contains 2 active ingredients; piperacillin 2 g and tazobactam 250 mg both present as sodium salts.

Tazocin 4.5 g contains 2 active ingredients; piperacillin 4 g and tazobactam 500 mg both present as sodium salts.

Pharmaceutical form Tazocin, an injectable antibacterial combination for intravenous administration is available as a white to off-white sterile, lyophilised powder for injection packaged in glass vials.

The product contains no excipients or preservatives.

Clinical particulars

Therapeutic indications: Tazocin is indicated for treatment of the following systemic and/or local bacterial infections in which susceptible organisms have been detected or are suspected:

Lower respiratory tract infections; urinary tract infections (complicated and uncomplicated); intra-abdominal infections; skin and skin structure infections; bacterial septicaemia; polymicrobic infections: Tazocin is indicated for polymicrobic infections including those where aerobic and anaerobic organisms are suspected (intra-abdominal, skin and skin structure, lower respiratory tract).

Tazocin, in combination with an aminoglycoside, is indicated for bacterial infections in neutropenic adults or children.

Whilst Tazocin is indicated only for the conditions listed above, infections caused by piperacillin-susceptible organisms are also amenable to Tazocin treatment due to its piperacillin content. Therefore, the treatment of mixed infections caused by piperacillin-susceptible organisms and β-lactamase producing organisms susceptible to Tazocin should not require the addition of another antibiotic.

Tazocin is particularly useful in the treatment of mixed infections and in presumptive therapy prior to the availability of the results of sensitivity tests because of its broad spectrum of activity.

Tazocin acts synergistically with aminoglycosides against certain strains of Pseudomonas aeruginosa. Combined therapy has been successful, especially in patients with impaired host defences. Both drugs should be used in full therapeutic doses. As soon as results of culture and susceptibility tests become available, antimicrobial therapy should be adjusted if necessary.

Piperacillin/tazobactam is highly active against piperacillin-sensitive micro-organisms as well as many β-lactamase producing, piperacillin-resistant micro-organisms.

Gram-negative bacteria: most plasmid mediated β-lactamase producing and non-β-lactamase producing strains of *Escherichia coli, Klebsiella* spp. (including *K. oxytoca, K. pneumoniae*), *Proteus* spp. (including *Proteus vulgaris , Proteus mirabilis*), *Salmonella* spp., *Shigella* spp., *Neisseria gonorrhoeae, Neisseria meningitidis, Moraxella* spp. (including *M . catarrhalis*), *Haemophilus* spp. (including *H. influenzae, H. parinfluenzae*), *Pasteurella multocida, Yersinia* spp., *Campylobacter* spp., *Gardnerella vaginalis.* Many chromosomally mediated β-lactamase producing and non-β-lactamase producing strains of *Enterobacter* spp. (including *E. cloacae, E. aerogenes*), *Citrobacter* spp (including *C. freundii, C. diversus*), *Providencia* spp., *Morganella morganii, Serratia* spp. (including *S. marcescens, S. liquifaciens*), *Pseudomonas aeruginosa* and other *Pseudomonas* spp. (including *P. cepacia, P. fluorescens*), *Xanthamonas maltophilia, Acinetobacter* spp.

Gram-positive bacteria: β-lactamase producing and non-β-lactamase producing strains of streptococci (*S. pneumoniae, S. pyogenes, S. bovis, S. agalactiae, S. viridans*, Group C, Group G), enterococci (*E. faecalis*) , *Staphylococcus aureus* (not methicillin-resistant *S. aureus*), *S. saphrophyticus, S. epidermidis* (coagulase-negative staphylococci), corynebacteria, *Listeria monocytogenes, Norcardia spp.*

Anaerobic bacteria: β-lactamase producing and non-β-lactamase producing anaerobes such as *Bacteroides* spp. (including *B. bivius, B. disiens, B. capillosus, B. melaninogenicus, B. oralis*), the *Bacteroides fragilis* group (including *B. fragilis, B. vulgatus, B. distasonis, B. ovatus, B. thetaiotaomicron, B. uniformis, B. asaccharolyticus*), as well as *Peptostreptococcus* spp., *Fusobacterium* spp., *Eubacterium* group, *Clostridia* spp. (including *C. difficile, C. perfringens*), *Veillonella* spp., and *Actinomyces* spp.

Posology and method of administration Tazocin may be given by slow intravenous injection (3–5 minutes) or by infusion (20–30 minutes)

Neutropenic patients with signs of infection (e.g fever) should receive immediate empirical antibiotic therapy before laboratory results are available.

Adults and children over 12 years: The usual dosage for adults and children over 12 years with normal renal function is 4.5 g Tazocin given every 8 hours.

The total daily dose depends on the severity and localisation of the infection and can vary from 2.25 g to 4.5 g Tazocin administered every 6 or 8 hours.

In neutropenia the recommended dose is 4.5 g Tazocin given every 6 hours in combination with an aminoglycoside.

Children under the age of 12 years: Tazocin is only recommended for the treatment of children with neutropenia.

For children weighing over 50 kg, follow the adult dosing guidance, including the aminoglycoside.

For children with normal renal function and weighing less than 50 kg the dose should be adjusted to 90 mg/kg (80 mg piperacillin/10 mg tazobactam) administered every 6 hours, in combination with an aminoglycoside.

Until further experience is available, Tazocin should not be used in children who do not have neutropenia.

Elderly: Tazocin may be used at the same dose levels as adults except in cases of renal impairment (see below).

Renal insufficiency: In patients with renal insufficiency, the intravenous dose should be adjusted to the degree of actual renal impairment. The suggested daily doses are as follows:

Creatinine Clearance (ml/min)	*Recommended Piperacillin/Tazobactam Dosage*
20–80	12 g/1.5 g/day Divided Doses 4 g/500 mg q 8H
<20	8 g/1 g/day Divided Doses 4 g/500 mg q 12H

For patients on haemodialysis, the maximum daily dose is 8 g/1 g piperacillin/tazobactam. In addition, because haemodialysis removes 30%–50% of piperacillin in 4 hours, one additional dose of 2 g/250 mg piperacillin/tazobactam should be administered following each dialysis period. For patients with renal failure and hepatic insufficiency, measurement of serum levels of Tazocin will provide additional guidance for adjusting dosage.

Renal insufficiency in children weighing < 50 kg: In children weighing less than 50 kg with renal insufficiency the intravenous dosage should be adjusted to the degree of actual renal impairment as follows:

Creatinine Clearance (ml/min)	*Recommended Piperacillin/Tazobactam Dosage*
40–80	90 mg (80 mg piperacillin/10 mg tazobactam)/kg q 6H
20–40	90 mg (80 mg piperacillin/10 mg tazobactam)/kg q 8H
<20	90 mg (80 mg piperacillin/10 mg tazobactam)/kg q 12H

For children weighing <50 kg on haemodialysis the recommended dose is 45 mg/kg q 8H.

Duration of therapy: In acute infections, treatment

with Tazocin should be continued for 48 hours beyond the resolution of clinical symptoms or the fever.

Reconstitution directions: Intravenous injection: Each vial of Tazocin 2.25 g should be reconstituted with 10 ml of one of the following diluents. Each vial of Tazocin 4.5 g should be reconstituted with 20 ml of one of the following diluents: Sterile Water for Injection; Bacteriostatic Water for Injection; Sodium Chloride Injection.

Shake until dissolved. Intravenous injection should be given over 3–5 minutes.

Intravenous infusion: Each vial of Tazocin 2.25 g should be reconstituted with 10 ml of one of the above diluents. Each vial of Tazocin 4.5 g should be reconstituted with 20 ml of one of the above diluents.

The reconstituted solution should be further diluted to at least 50 ml with one of the reconstitution diluents, or with Dextrose 5% in Water or Dextrose 5% and 0.9% Sodium Chloride.

Contra-indications: The use of Tazocin is contra-indicated in patients with a history of allergic reactions to any of the penicillins and/or cephalosporins or β-lactamase inhibitors.

Special warnings and precautions for use: Warnings: Serious and occasionally fatal anaphylactic reactions have been reported in patients receiving therapy with penicillins. These reactions are more apt to occur in persons with a history of sensitivity to multiple allergens.

There have been reports of patients with a history of penicillin hypersensitivity who have experienced severe reactions when treated with a cephalosporin. Before initiating therapy with Tazocin, careful inquiry should be made concerning previous hypersensitivity reactions to penicillins, cephalosporins, and other allergens. If an allergic reaction occurs during therapy with Tazocin, the antibiotic should be discontinued. Serious hypersensitivity reactions may require adrenaline and other emergency measures.

Precautions: While Tazocin possesses the characteristic low toxicity of the penicillin group of antibiotics, periodic assessment of organ system functions including renal, hepatic, and haematopoietic during prolonged therapy is advisable.

Bleeding manifestations have occurred in some patients receiving β-lactam antibiotics. These reactions have sometimes been associated with abnormalities of coagulation tests such as clotting time, platelet aggregation and prothrombin time, and are more likely to occur in patients with renal failure. If bleeding manifestations occur, the antibiotic should be discontinued and appropriate therapy instituted.

In case of severe, persistent diarrhoea, the possibility of antibiotic-induced, life threatening pseudomembranous colitis must be taken into consideration. Therefore, Tazocin must be discontinued immediately in such cases, and suitable therapy be initiated (eg. oral metronidazole or oral vancomycin). Preparations which inhibit peristalsis are contra-indicated.

As with other antibiotics, the possibility of emergence of resistant organisms which might cause superinfections should be kept in mind, particularly during prolonged treatment. Microbiological follow-up may be required to detect any important superinfection. If this occurs, appropriate measures should be taken.

As with other penicillins, patients may experience neuromuscular excitability or convulsions if higher than recommended doses are given intravenously.

Periodic electrolyte determinations should be made in patients with low potassium reserves, and the possibility of hypokalaemia should be kept in mind with patients who have potentially low potassium reserves and who are receiving cytotoxic therapy or diuretics. Modest elevation of indices of liver function may be observed.

Antimicrobials used in high doses for short periods to treat gonorrhoea may mask or delay the symptoms of incubating syphilis. Therefore, prior to treatment, patients with gonorrhoea should also be evaluated for syphilis. Specimens for darkfield examination should be obtained from patients with any suspect primary lesion, and serologic tests should be made for a minimum of 4 months.

Interactions with other medicaments and other forms of interaction: Concurrent administration of probenecid and piperacillin/tazobactam produced a longer half-life and lower renal clearance for both piperacillin and tazobactam. However, peak plasma concentrations of either drug are unaffected. No interaction is found between Tazocin and either vancomycin or tobramycin.

Whenever Tazocin is used concurrently with another antibiotic, especially an aminoglycoside, the drugs must not be mixed in intravenous solutions or administered concurrently due to physical incompatibility.

During simultaneous administration of high doses of heparin, oral anticoagulants and other drugs which may affect the blood coagulation system and/or the thrombocyte function, the coagulation parameters should be tested more frequently and monitored regularly.

The ureidopenicillins including piperacillin have been reported to prolong the action of vecuronium. Caution is indicated when piperacillin is used perioperatively with vecuronium and similar neuromuscular blocking agents.

Penicillins may reduce the excretion of methotrexate. Serum levels of methotrexate should be monitored in patients on high dose methotrexate therapy.

Pregnancy and lactation: Adequate studies on the use of Tazocin during pregnancy and the period of breast feeding are not yet available. Tazocin did not affect fertility in rats and was not teratogenic in mice or rats. Until further experience is available, however, pregnant or nursing women should be treated only if the therapeutic benefit outweighs the risk to the patient and the foetus.

Effects on ability to drive and use machines: Tazocin is not known to affect ability to drive or operate machines.

Undesirable effects: Rarely, significant leucopenia may be associated with prolonged therapy. Rarely, interstitial nephritis and/or renal failure may occur.

Hepatitis and cholestatic jaundice have been reported rarely with some penicillins and β-lactamase inhibitors, including piperacillin/tazobactam.

In common with other β-lactam antibiotics, haemolytic anaemia has been reported rarely with piperacillin and piperacillin/tazobactam.

Many of the patients treated in clinical trials were severely ill and had multiple underlying diseases and physiological impairments, making it difficult to determine causal relationship of adverse experiences to therapy with Tazocin.

Adverse local reactions that were reported as possibly, probably or definitely related to therapy with Tazocin were phlebitis (0.2%) and thrombophlebitis (0.3%).

The most frequently reported systemic adverse clinical reactions that were reported as possibly, probably, or definitely related to Tazocin were diarrhoea (3.8%), rash (0.6%), erythema (0.5%), pruritus (0.5%), vomiting (0.4%), allergic reactions (0.4%), nausea (0.3%), urticaria (0.2%) and superinfection (0.2%).

Additional adverse systemic clinical reactions reported as possibly, probably or definitely drug related occurring in less than 0.1% of the patients were: *Skin and appendages:* skin reactions, eruption, increased sweating, erythema multiforme, eczema, exanthema, maculo-papular rash; *Gastrointestinal:* soft/loose stools, stomatitis, constipation; *Central nervous system:* muscular weakness, hallucination; *Autonomic nervous system:* dry mouth, hypotension; *Musculoskeletal system:* muscle pain; *Vascular (extracardia):* superficial phlebitis; *Body as a whole:* fever, hot flushes, oedema, tiredness; *Local reactions:* injection site inflammation, injection site pain when solution was not prepared according to recommendations.

Adverse laboratory changes without regard to drug relationship that were reported during clinical trials were: *Haematological changes:* transient reduction in the white blood cell count (leukopenia), eosinophilia, thrombocytosis, thrombocytopenia, positive Coombs test; *Clinical chemistry:* hypokalaemia; *Effect on hepatic function:* transient rise in the serum levels of liver enzymes (SGOT, SGPT, alkaline phosphatase), bilirubin; *Effect on renal function:* Rarely increased levels of renal function parameters (urea, creatinine) have been detected in serum.

Overdose: Information on overdose in humans is not available.

Treatment of intoxication: No specific antidote is known.

There is no specific experience with overdose of Tazocin. However, in the event of an emergency, all required intensive medical measures are indicated as in the case of piperacillin.

In case of motor excitability or convulsions, anticonvulsive agents (e.g. diazepam or barbiturates) may be indicated.

In case of severe, anaphylactic reactions, the usual counter-measures are to be initiated.

Pharmacological properties

Pharmacodynamic properties: Piperacillin, a broad spectrum, semisynthetic penicillin active against many gram-positive and gram-negative aerobic and anaerobic bacteria, exerts bactericidal activity by inhibition of both septum and cell wall synthesis. Tazobactam, a triazolylmethyl penicillanic acid sulphone, is a potent inhibitor of many β-lactamases, in particular the plasmid mediated enzymes which commonly cause resistance to penicillins and cephalosporins including third-generation cephalosporins. The presence of tazobactam in the Tazocin formulation enhances and extends the antibiotic spectrum of piperacillin to include many β-lactamase producing bacteria normally resistant to it and other β-lactam antibiotics. Thus, Tazocin combines the properties of a broad spectrum antibiotic and a β-lactamase inhibitor.

Tazocin is highly active against piperacillin-sensitive micro-organisms as well as many β-lactamase producing, piperacillin-resistant micro-orgainisms.

Pharmacokinetic properties: Distribution and plasma levels: Peak piperacillin and tazobactam plasma concentrations are attained immediately after completion of an intravenous infusion or injection. Piperacillin plasma levels produced when given with tazobactam are similar to those attained when equivalent doses of piperacillin are administered alone.

There is a greater proportional (approximately 28%) increase in plasma levels of piperacillin and tazobactam with increasing dose over the dosage range of 250 mg tazobactam/2 g piperacillin to 500 mg tazobactam/4 g piperacillin.

In healthy subjects, Tazocin plasma elimination half-lives ranged from 0.7 to 1.2 hours following single or multiple doses. The half-lives of tazobactam and piperacillin are unaffected by doses or duration of infusion.

Tazobactam and piperacillin are 23% and 21%, respectively, bound to plasma proteins at concentrations up to 100 micrograms/ml.

Tazocin is widely distributed in tissue and body fluids including intestinal mucosa, gallbladder, lung and bile.

Biotransformation: Piperacillin does not undergo biotransformation in humans. Tazobactam is metabolised to a single metabolite which has been found to be micro-biologically inactive.

Excretion: Piperacillin and tazobactam are eliminated by the kidney via glomerular filtration and active secretion. Piperacillin is excreted rapidly as unchanged drug, with 69% of the dose appearing in the urine. Piperacillin is also secreted in the bile. Tazobactam and its metabolite are eliminated primarily by renal excretion, with 80% of the dose appearing as unchanged drug and the remainder of the dose appearing as metabolite.

Impaired Renal Function: The half-lives of piperacillin and tazobactam increase with decreasing creatinine clearance. The increase is two-fold and four-fold for piperacillin and tazobactam, respectively, at creatinine clearance of below 20 ml/min compared to patients with normal function.

Piperacillin and tazobactam are removed from the body during haemodialysis with 31% and 39% of the doses of piperacillin and tazobactam, respectively, recovered in the dialysis fluid. Piperacillin and tazobactam are removed from the body by peritoneal dialysis with 5% and 12% of the dose, respectively, appearing in the dialysate.

Impaired Liver Function: Plasma concentrations of piperacillin and tazobactam are prolonged in hepatically impaired patients. However, dosage adjustments in patients with hepatic impairment are not necessary.

Preclinical safety data: Nothing of note to the prescriber.

Pharmaceutical particulars

List of excipients: Tazocin contains no excipients or preservatives.

Incompatibilities: Tazocin should not be mixed with other drugs in a syringe or infusion bottle since compatibility has not been established. Wherever Tazocin is used concurrently with another antibiotic, the drugs must be administered separately.

Tazocin should be administered through an infusion set separately from any other drugs unless compatibility is proven.

Because of chemical instability, Tazocin should not be used with solutions containing only sodium bicarbonate.

Tazocin should not be added to blood products or albumin hydrolysates.

Shelf life: Vials containing sterile powder for injection : 36 months

Special precautions for storage: Vials containing sterile Tazocin powder for injection should be stored at controlled room temperature (15–25°C) in the original container.

Solution: Vials containing reconstituted solutions for intravenous use are stable for 24 hours when stored under refrigeration (2–8°C).

Diluted solutions prepared for intravenous use are stable for 24 hours when stored under refrigeration (2–8°C) in IV. bags or syringes. Unused solution should be discarded.

Nature and contents of container: Type III glass vial with butyl rubber stopper and light grey aluminium/plastic seal containing Tazocin 2.25 g or Tazocin 4.5 g, boxed singly.

Instruction for use/handling: None.

Marketing authorisation numbers
2.25 g 0095/0252
4.5 g 0095/0254

Date of approval/revision of SPC October 1998

Legal category POM

THIOTEPA Injection

Qualitative and quantitative composition Thiotepa 15 mg.

Pharmaceutical form Sterile powder for injection.

Clinical particulars

Therapeutic indications: Thiotepa (N,N',N' triethylenethiophosphoramide) is a polyfunctional alkylating agent used alone or in combination with other cytotoxic drugs, or in surgery in the treatment of neoplastic diseases. It is believed to exert its cytotoxic effects by the alkylation of DNA.

Posology and method of administration: Thiotepa (15 mg) should be reconstituted with 1.5 ml Water for Injection immediately prior to use. Reconstituted solutions should be clear to slightly opaque. Solutions that are grossly opaque or precipitated should be discarded.

Thiotepa may be given by intravenous, intramuscular and intrathecal routes of injection; it may be given directly into pleural, pericardial or peritoneal cavities and as a bladder instillation.

Use Luer-Lock fittings on all syringes and sets. Large bore needles are recommended to minimise pressure and possible formation of aerosols. The latter may also be reduced by the use of a venting needle.

For intramuscular injection, bladder and intracavitary instillations:

Dosage: Adults and the elderly: Up to 60 mg in single or divided doses. Doses should be reduced in cases of leucopenia as indicated in Table 1. Single dose administration of 90 mg Thiotepa as a bladder instillation is described under 'Bladder cancer'.

Table 1

WBC Count Cells/mm³	*Dose of Thiotepa Adults and Children over 12 years*
6000	60 mg
5000–6000	45 mg
4500–5000	30 mg
4000–4500	20 mg
3500–4000	10 mg
3000–3500	5 mg
below 3000	omit dose

Children: Use in children is not recommended.

Intrathecal injection: Up to a maximum of 10 mg.

It is essential that a complete blood count should be performed 12–24 hours before each dose of Thiotepa. Thrombocytopenia in the absence of leucopenia has been noted.

Dosage schedules of Thiotepa vary widely according to the route of administration and the indication.

Examples of dosage schedules used according to specific tumour types are given below:

Breast cancer: Patients with advanced breast cancer have been treated with Thiotepa as part of a combination regime, given intramuscularly in divided doses of 15–30 mg three times weekly for two weeks; this representing one course of treatment. An interval of six to eight weeks is recommended between courses to allow bone marrow recovery.

An alternative schedule employs Thiotepa as part of a combination regime, given as an initial priming dose of 15 mg intramuscularly or intravenously each day for four days. This may be followed in three weeks by maintenance doses of 15 mg I.M. every 14–21 days.

Bladder cancer: Instillations of Thiotepa have been used to treat multiple superficial tumours of the bladder, resulting in a complete clinical response in about one third of patients. Patients are dehydrated for 8–12 hours prior to treatment. Up to 60 mg Thiotepa dissolved in 60 ml sterile water is instilled into the bladder by catheter once a week for four weeks. During removal of the catheter following instillation, Thiotepa injection is continued to ensure bathing of the prostatic and pendulous urethra . The solution should be retained for up to two hours and the patient should be frequently repositioned to ensure maximum contact with the urothelium.

Patients are generally cytoscoped two weeks after a course of four instillations. If a response is observed a second course of four Thiotepa instillations may be given, generally at a reduced dosage, eg 15–60 mg with intervals of one to two weeks between instillations.

Instillations of Thiotepa have been used prophylactically as an adjunct to surgical resection of superficial tumours of the bladder, resulting in a marked decrease in the recurrence rate. It is recommended that there should be a minimum interval of one week between tumour resection and the commencement of prophylactic instillation of Thiotepa. 30–60 mg Thiotepa dissolved in 60 ml sterile water is instilled into the bladder for two hours and repeated at intervals of one to two weeks for a total of 4–8 instillations. This initial course may be followed by instillations of Thiotepa, 30–60 mg every four to six weeks for one year or longer.

Single dose Thiotepa instillations have been used prophylactically as an adjunct of surgical resection in the treatment of superficial tumours of the bladder. 90 mg Thiotepa dissolved in 100 mg sterile water is instilled into the bladder with the patient in the left lateral position. After 15 minutes the patient is transferred to the right lateral position and after a further 15 minutes the bladder is emptied. It is felt that such single dose administration may decrease the incidence of systemic toxicity by decreasing the extent of systemic absorption of the drug.

Note: Patients who have had previous radiotherapy to the bladder are at increased risk of drug toxicity.

Malignant meningeal disease: Intrathecal injections of Thiotepa have been found to be useful for the palliative treatment of cases of meningeal infiltration by leukaemia and lymphoma. Clinical experience has shown Thiotepa to be effective in carcinomatous involvement of the meninges, but published data is limited. Thiotepa, at a concentration of 1 mg/ml in sterile water is administered by injection through a lumbar theca in doses of up to 10 mg on alternate days until there is clearance of malignant cells from the cerebrospinal fluid (CSF). It is recommended that if no improvement occurs in the CSF after three injections, then treatment should be changed. Not more than four injections should be given on alternate days. Routine blood counts should be performed prior to each dose of Thiotepa.

Ovarian cancer: Ovarian cancer has been treated with Thiotepa as a single agent or as part of a combination regime in a variety of schedules. For example, 15 mg Thiotepa I.V. or I.M. may be given daily for four days initially and then continued with single doses administered once a week or once every two weeks.

Intracavitary instillation of Thiotepa: Instillations of Thiotepa have been used to treat malignant pleural effusions and abdominal ascites. The procedure recommended, is first to aspirate as much fluid as possible and then to instil the dose of Thiotepa, 10–60 mg in 20–60 ml sterile water. This may be repeated once a week or once every two weeks.

Prevention of recurrences of pterygium: A 1:2,000 solution of Thiotepa in sterile Ringer's solution (ie 15 mg powder in 30 ml Ringer's), applied topically as eye drops, every three hours daily for up to six weeks after surgical removal of the pterygium, is effective in reducing the recurrence rate following surgery.

Condyloma acuminata: Thiotepa applied topically or instilled intraurethrally in a gel, has been successfully used to eradicate condyloma acuminata. The drug may be administered by first reconstituting 60 mg Thiotepa with 5 ml sterile water. This is diluted to 15 ml, using a sterile mixture of water and lubricating jelly made to a consistency viscous enough to remain in the urethra and fluid enough to allow easy injection. This therapy may be repeated at weekly intervals.

Contra-indications: Thiotepa administration is contra-indicated in patients with a WBC count below 3,000 and/or platelet count below 100,000.

Special warnings and precautions: Thiotepa must be stored in a refrigerator (2–8°C). The occurrence of a precipitate on reconstitution (with 1.5 ml of Water for Injection) indicates that polymerisation has occurred with the formation of less active constituents and the injection must be discarded.

Reconstituted solutions may be stored in a refrigerator (2–8°C) for 24 hours. However, if a precipitate forms, the solution must be discarded.

Thiotepa may be mixed in the same syringe with procaine hydrochloride 2% or with adrenaline 1 in 1,000 or with both.

Trained personnel should reconstitute Thiotepa in a designated area. Adequate protective gloves and goggles should be worn and the work surface should be covered with plastic-backed absorbent paper. Thiotepa is not a vesicant and should not cause harm if it comes in contact with the skin. It should, of course, be washed off with water immediately. Any transient stinging may be treated with bland cream. The cytotoxic preparation should not be handled by pregnant staff.

Any spillage or waste material may be disposed of by incineration. We do not make any specific recommendations with regard to the temperature of the incinerator.

Thiotepa has been reported to possess mutagenic activity on the basis of bacterial, plant and mammalian mutagenicity tests. It has also been reported to be carcinogenic in mice and rats. These effects are consistent with its activity as an alkylating agent. The carcinogenic potential in humans has not been clearly established.

Thiotepa should only be used by clinicians who are familiar with the various characteristics of cytotoxic drugs and their clinical toxicity. WBC and platelet counts are recommended 12–24 hours before each dose of Thiotepa regardless of route of administration, except when used topically as eye drops or in the treatment of condyloma acuminata. Dosage should be reduced as indicated above, in the presence of a compromised bone marrow, as manifested by a reduced WBC count or platelet count. Safe use in children has not been established.

Interaction with other medicaments and other forms of interaction: See dosage schedules for special tumour types, for usage with concomitant surgery or radiotherapy.

Pregnancy and lactation: Thiotepa is teratogenic and embryotoxic in mice and rats following intraperitoneal administration. In addition, it has been reported to interfere with spermatogenesis and ovarian function in rodent species. The drug therefore, should not normally be administered to patients who are pregnant or to mothers who are breast feeding unless the benefit outweighs the risk to the foetus or child.

Effects on ability to drive and use machines: None.

Undesirable effects: The most serious side-effect is upon the blood forming elements and is a direct consequence of the cytotoxic effect of the drug. In addition, Thiotepa may occasionally cause vomiting, headache and anorexia. Alopecia has been reported as a rare complication of therapy with Thiotepa. Local irritation comparable to a mild radiation cystitis, may follow bladder instillations of Thiotepa, while haemorrhagic cystitis is rare. Depigmentation of periorbital skin has been reported rarely following the use of Thiotepa eye drops.

Overdose: There is no specific antidote. Gastric lavage, forced fluids and general supportive measures are recommended. Blood counts should be carried out to estimate damage to the haematopoietic system and blood transfusions should be given as required.

Pharmacological properties

Pharmacodynamic properties: Thiotepa is an ethyleneimine compound whose antineoplastic effect is related to its alkylating action. It is not a vesicant and may be given by all parenteral routes, as well as directly into tumour masses.

Pharmacokinetic properties: Variable absorption occurs from intramuscular injection sites. Absorption through serous membranes such as the bladder and pleura occurs to some extent. Only traces of unchanged Thiotepa and triethylene phosphoramide are excreted in the urine, together with a large proportion of metabolites.

Preclinical safety data: Nothing of relevance to the prescriber.

Pharmaceutical particulars

List of excipients: Water for Injection

Incompatibilities: None

Shelf life: 18 months

Special precautions for storage: Thiotepa must be stored in a refrigerator (2–8°C). Reconstituted solutions may be stored in a refrigerator (2–8°C) for up to 24 hours.

Nature and contents of container: Flint glass vial with butyl rubber stopper. Pack Size: 15 mg

Instructions for use/handling: See *Special warnings and precautions.*

Marketing authorisation number PL 0095/0234

Date of approval/revision
First approval 22 August 1991
Last revision August 1998

Legal Category POM

TRAXAM* Gel
TRAXAM* Foam

Qualitative and quantitative composition

Active ingredient:

Traxam Gel: Felbinac (Biphenylacetic Acid) 3% w/w.

Traxam Foam: Felbinac (Biphenylacetic Acid) 3.17% w/w.

Pharmaceutical form

Traxam Gel: A clear non-greasy, non staining gel containing 30 mg felbinac in each gram.

Traxam Foam: A 'quick break' foam dispensed from cans which contain a concentrate of 3.17% felbinac in ethanol/aqueous vehicle with butane propellant.

Clinical particulars

Therapeutic indications: Traxam is a topical non-steroidal anti-inflammatory and analgesic drug. It is indicated for the relief of rheumatic pain, the pain of non-serious arthritic conditions and symptoms associated with soft tissue injury such as sprains, strains and contusions.

Traxam Gel may be used as a coupling agent for ultrasound where both treatments are indicated.

Posology and method of administration

Traxam Gel: Rub 1 g of Traxam Gel (approximately 1 inch (2.5 cm) of gel) into the affected area(s) 2 to 4 times a day. If symptoms do not resolve within 14 days, the patient should be reviewed.

The total dose should not exceed 25 g per day irrespective of the number of affected areas.

Elderly: No special dosage recommendations are made for elderly patients.

Children: Safe use of felbinac in early childhood has not been established.

Hands should be washed following application of Traxam Gel unless they are the treatment site.

Traxam Foam: The foam should be dispensed onto the hand and rubbed lightly into the affected area(s). Traxam Foam is formulated to break down into a clear liquid when warmed by contact with the skin.

Gently rub one golf-ball sized (one and a half inches (4 cm) in diameter) quantity of foam into the affected area(s) 2 to 4 times a day.

The total daily dose should not exceed 25 g of foam irrespective of the number of affected areas; a golf ball size quantity of foam weighs approximately 1 gramme.

If symptoms do not resolve, it is advisable to review the patient to assess whether continued treatment is appropriate.

Elderly: No special dosage recommendations are made for elderly patients.

Children: Safe use of felbinac in early childhood has not been established.

Hands should be washed following application of Traxam Foam unless they are the treatment site.

Contra-indications: Hypersensitivity to the ingredients. Patients in whom attacks of asthma, urticaria or acute rhinitis are precipitated by aspirin or other non-steroidal anti-inflammatory drugs.

Special warnings and special precautions for use: Use of Traxam should be limited to intact and non-diseased skin. Contact with mucous membranes and the eyes should be avoided.

Patients should avoid actuation of the Foam aerosol can near their face or eyes. Traxam should not be applied with occlusive dressings at the same site as other topical preparations.

Safe use of Felbinac in early childhood has not been established.

Interactions with other medicaments and other forms of interaction: Felbinac is highly protein bound. However, serum levels following topical application are extremely low and therefore clinical drug interactions are unlikely.

Pregnancy and lactation: Since the safety of felbinac in human pregnancy and lactation has not been established, its use in these circumstances is not recommended. As with other non-steroidal anti-inflammatory agents which inhibit prostaglandin synthesis, dystocia and delayed parturition were observed in animal studies when felbinac was administered subcutaneously late in pregnancy.

Effects on ability to drive and use machines: None.

Undesirable effects: A low incidence of mild local irritation, erythema, dermatitis, pruritus, and paraesthesia, which recovers spontaneously upon cessation of treatment may be expected with Traxam.

Systemic side-effects are rare; hypersensitivity reactions such as widespread rashes including urticaria and bronchospasm have been reported with Traxam.

Gastrointestinal disturbances have been reported occasionally.

Overdose: It is unlikely that Traxam would cause adverse systemic effects even if accidental ingestion should occur. Patients should consult a doctor if ingestion is suspected.

Pharmacological properties

Pharmacodynamic properties: Felbinac is an anti-inflammatory/analgesic agent which has been developed into topical gel and foam formulations for local treatment of pain and inflammation associated with conditions of the musculo-skeletal system.

Pharmacokinetic properties: Clinical pharmacokinetic studies show that a topical dose of 10 g Traxam Gel results in low circulating levels of felbinac in serum (600ng/ml). This is more than 20 times less than the levels recorded following oral administration of a single dose of 600 mg fenbufen.

Traxam Foam administered in a pharmacokinetic study achieves similar low circulating levels of felbinac to Traxam Gel.

Results of distribution studies demonstrate that felbinac is transferred preferentially to a site of inflammation when applied topically.

The metabolism of felbinac is consistent with the known metabolic profile of fenbufen.

Preclinical safety data: Testing of biphenylacetic acid including single and repeat dose studies, foetal toxicity and fertility studies, mutagenic and carcinogenic potential studies showed an acceptable toxicity profile for the active ingredient.

A primary dermal irritation study has shown Traxam Foam to be non-irritant and that it can be safely applied to human skin.

Traxam Foam is irritant to the eye but the irritation subsides within 7 days.

Pharmaceutical particulars

List of excipients: Traxam Gel: Carboxyvinyl polymer, Diisopropanolamine, Ethanol (96%) BP, Purified water BP.

Traxam Foam: Ethanolamine USNF, Ethanol (96%) BP, Purified water BP, Polawax A31, Softigen 767, Butane 40.

Incompatibilities: None.

Shelf life:

Traxam Gel:	36 months
Traxam Foam:	24 months

Special precautions for storage: Traxam Gel and Traxam Foam should be stored below 25°C.

Traxam Foam is packed in a pressurised canister. Protect the canister from sunlight and do not expose to temperatures above 50°C. Extremes of temperature can occur in motor cars. Do not pierce or burn the canister even when empty.

Do not refrigerate Traxam Foam. Do not spray or use near any ignition source (eg. naked flame, open fire) or while smoking.

Nature and contents of container:

Traxam Gel is packed in flurovinyl resin-coated blind ended Aluminium Tubes with plastic caps, LDPE/Aluminium Foil/LDPE laminate tubes with plastic caps or Polyamide-imide or epoxyphenolic coated blind ended aluminium tubes with plastic caps.

Traxam Foam is packed in aluminium monobloc cans with white enamel body, double grinded microflex internal lacquer and colourless overlacquer. Cans are fitted with a valve made of aluminium microflex and diptube and shave foam actuator.

Traxam Gel:	Pack sizes 100 g
Traxam Foam:	Pack sizes 100 g

Instructions for use/handling: Not applicable.

Product licence numbers

Traxam Gel:	PL 0095/0119
Traxam Foam:	PL 0095/0238

Date of approval/revision of the text

Traxam Gel:	July 1998
Traxam Foam:	November 1997

Legal category POM

TRI-MINULET*

Presentation The memo pack holds six beige tablets containing 30 micrograms ethinyloestradiol and 50 micrograms gestodene, five dark brown tablets containing 40 micrograms ethinyloestradiol and 70 micrograms gestodene, and ten white tablets containing 30 micrograms ethinyloestradiol and 100 micrograms gestodene.

All tablets have a lustrous, sugar-coating.

Uses Oral contraception and the recognised gynaecological indications for such oestrogen-progestogen combinations. The mode of action includes the inhibition of ovulation by suppression of the mid-cycle surge of luteinising hormone, the inspissation of cervical mucus so as to constitute a barrier to sperm, and the rendering of the endometrium unreceptive to implantation.

Dosage and administration

First treatment cycle: 1 tablet daily for 21 days, starting with the tablet marked number 1, on the first day of the menstrual cycle.

Additional contraception (barriers and spermicide) is not required.

Subsequent cycles: Each subsequent course is started when seven tablet-free days have followed the preceding course. A withdrawal bleed should occur during the 7 tablet-free days.

Changing from another 21 day combined oral contraceptive: The first tablet of Tri-Minulet should be taken on the first day immediately after the end of the previous oral contraceptive course. Additional contraception is not required. A withdrawal bleed should not be expected until the end of the first pack of Tri-Minulet.

Changing from an Every Day (ED) 28 day combined oral contraceptive: The first tablet of Tri-Minulet should be taken on the day immediately after the day on which the last active pill in the ED pack has been taken. The remaining tablets in the ED pack should be discarded. Additional contraception is not required. A withdrawal bleed should not be expected until the end of the first pack of Tri-Minulet.

Changing from a Progestogen-only-Pill (POP): The first tablet of Tri-Minulet should be taken on the first day of menstruation even if the POP for that day has already been taken. The remaining tablets in the POP pack should be discarded. Additional contraception is not required.

Post-partum and post-abortum use: After pregnancy combined oral contraception can be started in non-lactating women 21 days after a vaginal delivery, provided that the patient is fully ambulant and there are no puerperal complications.

If the pill is started later than 21 days after delivery, then alternative contraception (barriers and spermicides) should be used until oral contraception is started and for the first 7 days of pill-taking. If unprotected intercourse has taken place after 21 days post partum, then oral contraception should not be started until the first menstrual bleed after childbirth.

After a miscarriage or abortion oral contraception may be started immediately.

Special circumstances requiring additional contraception:

Missed pills: If a tablet is delayed it should be taken as soon as possible and if it is taken within 12 hours of the correct time, additional contraception is not needed. Further tablets should then be taken at the usual time. If the delay exceeds 12 hours, the last missed pill should be taken when remembered, the earlier missed pills left in the pack and normal pill-taking resumed. If one or more tablets are omitted from the 21 days of pill-taking, additional contraception (barriers and spermicides) should be used for the next 7 days of pill-taking. In addition, if one or more pills are missed during the last 7 days of pill-taking, the subsequent pill-free interval should be disregarded and the next pack started the day after taking the last tablet from the previous pack. In this case, a withdrawal bleed should not be expected until the end of the second pack. If the patient does not have a withdrawal bleed at the end of the second pack she must return to her doctor to exclude the possibility of pregnancy.

Gastro-intestinal upset: Vomiting or diarrhoea may reduce the efficacy by preventing full absorption. Additional contraception (barriers and spermicides) should be used during the stomach upset and for the 7 days following the upset. If these 7 days overrun the end of a pack, the next pack should be started without a break. In this case, a withdrawal bleed should not be expected until the end of the second pack. If the patient does not have a withdrawal bleed at the end of the second pack she must return to her doctor to exclude the possibility of pregnancy.

Mild laxatives do not impair contraceptive action.

Interaction with other drugs: Some drugs accelerate the metabolism of oral contraceptives when taken concurrently and these include barbiturates, phenytoin, phenylbutazone and rifampicin. Other drugs suspected of having the capacity to reduce the efficacy of oral contraceptives include ampicillin and other antibiotics. It is, therefore, advisable to use non-hormonal methods of contraception (barriers and spermicides) in addition to the oral contraceptive as long as an extremely high degree of protection is required during treatment with such drugs. The additional contraception should be used while the concurrent medication continues and for 7 days afterwards. If these extra precautions overrun the end of the pack, the next pack should be started without a break. In this case, a withdrawal bleed should not be expected until the end of the second pack. If the patient does not have a withdrawal bleed at the end of the second pack she must return to her doctor to exclude the possibility of pregnancy.

Contra-indications, warnings etc.

Contra-indications:

1. Suspected pregnancy.
2. Thrombotic disorders and a history of these conditions, sickle-cell anaemia, disorders of lipid metabolism and other conditions in which, in individual cases, there is known or suspected to be a much increased risk of thrombosis.
3. Acute or severe chronic liver diseases. Dubin-Johnson syndrome. Rotor syndrome. History, during pregnancy, of idiopathic jaundice or severe pruritus.
4. History of herpes gestationis.
5. Mammary or endometrial carcinoma, or a history of these conditions.
6. Abnormal vaginal bleeding of unknown cause.

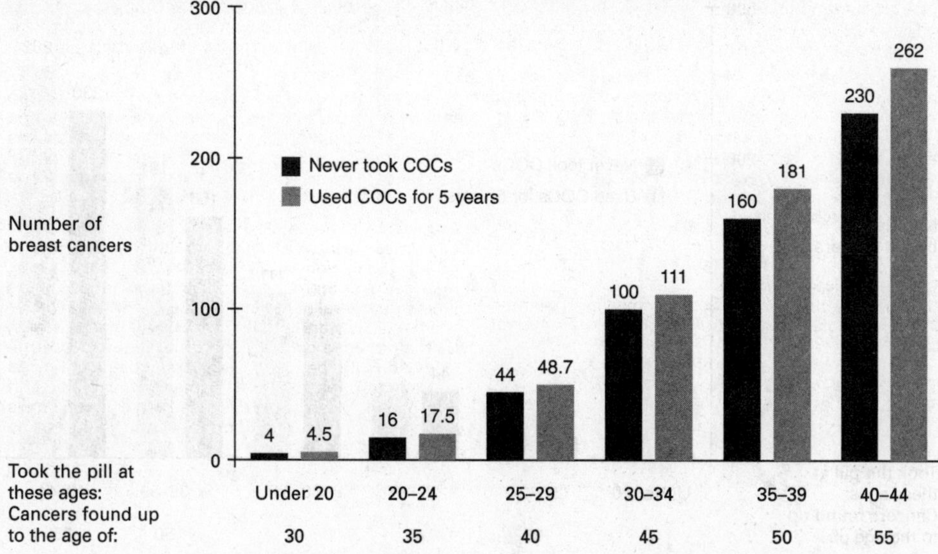

7. Deterioration of otosclerosis during pregnancy.

Warnings:

1. There is a general opinion, based on statistical evidence, that users of combined oral contraceptives experience, more often than non-users, venous thromboembolism, arterial thrombosis, including cerebral and myocardial infarction, and subarachnoid haemorrhage. Full recovery from such disorders does not always occur, and it should be realised that in a few cases they are fatal. How often these disorders occur in users of the modern low-dose pills is not known, but there are reasons for suggesting that they may occur less often than with older pills containing more oestrogen. Certain factors may entail some risk of thrombosis, e.g. smoking, obesity, varicose veins, cardiovascular diseases, diabetes and migraine. The suitability of a combined oral contraceptive should be judged according to the severity of such conditions in the individual case, and should be discussed with the patient before she decides to take it.
2. The risk of arterial thrombosis associated with combined oral contraceptives increases with age, and this risk is aggravated by cigarette smoking. The use of combined oral contraceptives by women in the older age group, especially those who are cigarette smokers, should therefore be discouraged and alternative methods used.
3. The possibility cannot be ruled out that certain chronic diseases may occasionally deteriorate during the use of combined oral contraceptives. (See 'Precautions').
4. The combination of ethinyloestradiol and gestodene, like other contraceptive steroids, is associated with an increased incidence of neoplastic nodules in the rat liver, the relevance of which to man is unknown.
5. Malignant liver tumours have been reported on rare occasions in long-term users of oral contraceptives. Benign hepatic tumours have also been associated with oral contraceptive usage. A hepatic tumour should be considered in the differential diagnosis when upper abdominal pain, enlarged liver or signs of intra-abdominal haemorrhage occur.
6. Numerous epidemiological studies have been reported on the risks of ovarian, endometrial, cervical and breast cancer in women using combined oral contraceptives. The evidence is clear that combined oral contraceptives offer substantial protection against both ovarian and endometrial cancer. An increased risk of cervical cancer in long term users of combined oral contraceptives has been reported in some studies, but there continues to be controversy about the extent to which this is attributable to the confounding effects of sexual behaviour and other factors.
A meta-analysis from 54 epidemiological studies reported that there is a slightly increased relative risk (RR=1.24) of having breast cancer diagnosed in women who are currently using combined oral contraceptives (COCs). The observed pattern of increased risk may be due to an earlier diagnosis of breast cancer in COC users, the biological effects of COCs or a combination of both. The additional breast cancers diagnosed in current users of COCs or in women who have used COCs in the last ten years are more likely to be localised to the breast than those in women who never used COCs.
Breast cancer is rare among women under 40 years of age whether or not they take COCs. Whilst this background risk increases with age, the excess number of breast cancer diagnoses in current and recent COC users is small in relation to the overall risk of breast cancer (see bar chart).
The most important risk factor for breast cancer in COC users is the age women discontinue the COC; the older the age at stopping, the more breast cancers are diagnosed. Duration of use is less important and the excess risk gradually disappears during the course of the 10 years after stopping COC use such that by 10 years there appears to be no excess.
The possible increase in risk of breast cancer should be discussed with the user and weighed against the benefits of COCs taking into account the evidence that they offer substantial protection against the risk of developing certain other cancers (e.g. ovarian and endometrial cancer).

Reasons for stopping oral contraception immediately:

1. Occurrence of migraine in patients who have never previously suffered from it. Exacerbation of pre-existing migraine. Any unusually frequent or unusually severe headaches.
2. Any kind of acute disturbance of vision.
3. Suspicion of thrombosis or infarction.
4. Six weeks before elective operations and during immobilisation, e.g. after accidents, etc.
5. Significant rise in blood-pressure.
6. Jaundice.
7. Clear exacerbation of conditions known to be capable of deteriorating during oral contraception or pregnancy.
8. Pregnancy is a reason for stopping immediately because it has been suggested by some investigations that oral contraceptives taken in early pregnancy may slightly increase the risk of foetal malformations. Other investigations have failed to support these findings. The possibility therefore cannot be excluded, but it is certain that if a risk exists at all, it is very small.

Precautions:

1. Examination of the pelvic organs, breasts and blood-pressure should precede the prescribing of any combined oral contraceptive and should be repeated regularly.
2. Before starting treatment, pregnancy must be excluded.
3. The following conditions require careful observation during medication: a history of severe depressive states, varicose veins, diabetes, hypertension, epilepsy, otosclerosis, multiple sclerosis, porphyria, tetany, disturbed liver function, gall-stones, cardiovascular diseases, renal diseases, chloasma, uterine fibroids, asthma, the wearing of contact lenses, or any disease that is prone to worsen during pregnancy. The first appearance or deterioration of any of these conditions may indicate that the oral contraceptive should be stopped.
4. The risk of the deterioration of chloasma, which is often not fully reversible, is reduced by the avoidance of excessive exposure to sunlight.

Side effects: Occasional side-effects may include nausea, vomiting, headaches, breast tenderness, changed body weight or libido, depressive moods and chloasma.

Menstrual changes:

1. *Reduction of menstrual flow:* This is not abnormal and it is to be expected in some patients. Indeed, it may be beneficial where heavy periods were previously experienced.
2. *Missed menstruation:* Occasionally, withdrawal bleeding may not occur at all. If the tablets have been taken correctly, pregnancy is very unlikely, but should be ruled out before a new course of tablets is started.

Intermenstrual bleeding: Very light 'spotting' or heavier 'breakthrough bleeding' may occur during tablet-taking, especially in the first few cycles. It appears to be generally of no significance, except where it indicates errors of tablet-taking, or where the possibility of interaction with other drugs exists (q.v.). However, if irregular bleeding is persistent, an organic cause should be considered.

Effect on adrenal and thyroid glands: Oral contraceptives have no significant influence on adrenocortical function. The ACTH function test for the adrenal cortex remains unchanged. The reduction in corticosteroid excretion and the elevation of plasma corticosteroids are due to an increased cortisol-binding capacity of the plasma proteins.

The response to metyrapone is less pronounced than in untreated women and is thus similar to that during pregnancy.

The radio-iodine uptake shows that thyroid function is unchanged. There is a rise in serum protein-bound iodine, similar to that in pregnancy and during the administration of oestrogens. This is due to the increased capacity of the plasma proteins for binding thyroid hormones, rather than to any change in glandular function. In women taking oral contraceptives, the content of protein-bound iodine in blood serum should therefore, not be used for evaluation of thyroid function.

Effect on blood chemistry: Oral contraceptives may accelerate erythrocyte sedimentation in the absence of any disease. This effect is due to a change in the proportion of the plasma protein fractions. Increases in plasma copper, iron and alkaline phosphatase have also been recorded.

Overdosage: There have been no reports of serious ill-effects from overdosage, even when a considerable number of tablets have been taken by a small child. In general, it is, therefore, unnecessary to treat overdosage. However, if overdosage is discovered within two or three hours and is so large that treatment seems desirable, gastric lavage can be safely used.

There are no specific antidotes and further treatment should be symptomatic.

Pharmaceutical precautions Store in cool, dry conditions. Shelf-life five years

Legal category POM

Package quantities Individual packs containing 3 months' supply.

Further information NIL

Product licence number 0011/0140

Date of last revision January 1998

TRINORDIOL*

Presentation The memo pack holds six light brown tablets, containing 50 micrograms levonorgestrel BP and 30 micrograms Ethinyloestradiol EP, five white tablets containing 75 micrograms levonorgestrel BP and 40 micrograms Ethinyloestradiol EP and ten ochre tablets containing 125 micrograms levonorgestrel BP and 30 micrograms Ethinyloestradiol EP.

All tablets are round 5.6 mm in diameter with a lustrous sugar coating.

Uses Oral contraception

Dosage and administration

First treatment cycle: 1 tablet daily for 21 days, starting with the tablet marked number 1, on the first day of the menstrual cycle.

Additional contraception (barriers and spermicide) is not required.

Subsequent cycles: Each subsequent course is started when seven tablet-free days have followed the preceding course. A withdrawal bleed should occur during the 7 tablet-free days.

Changing from another 21 day combined oral contraceptive: The first tablet of Trinordiol should be taken on the first day immediately after the end of the previous oral contraceptive course. Additional contraception is not required. A withdrawal bleed should not be expected until the end of the first pack of Trinordiol.

Changing from an Every Day (ED) 28 day combined oral contraceptive: The first tablet of Trinordiol should be taken on the day immediately after the day on which the last active pill in the ED pack has been taken. The remaining tablets in the ED pack should be discarded. Additional contraception is not required. A withdrawal bleed should not be expected until the end of the first pack of Trinordiol.

Changing from a Progestogen-only-Pill (POP): The first tablet of Trinordiol should be taken on the first day of menstruation even if the POP for that day has already been taken. The remaining tablets in the POP pack should be discarded. Additional contraception is not required.

Post-partum and post-abortum use: After pregnancy combined oral contraception can be started in non-lactating women 21 days after a vaginal delivery, provided that the patient is fully ambulant and there are no puerperal complications.

If the pill is started later than 21 days after delivery, then alternative contraception (barriers and spermicides) should be used until oral contraception is started and for the first 7 days of pill-taking. If unprotected intercourse has taken place after 21 days post partum, then oral contraception should not be started until the first menstrual bleed after childbirth.

After a miscarriage or abortion oral contraception may be started immediately.

Special circumstances requiring additional contraception:

Missed pills: If a tablet is delayed it should be taken as soon as possible and if it is taken within 12 hours of the correct time, additional contraception is not needed. Further tablets should then be taken at the usual time. If the delay exceeds 12 hours, the last missed pill should be taken when remembered, the earlier missed pills left in the pack and normal pill-taking resumed. If one or more tablets are omitted from the 21 days of pill-taking, additional contraception (barriers and spermicides) should be used for the next 7 days of pill-taking. In addition, if one or more pills are missed during the last 7 days of pill-taking, the subsequent pill-free interval should be disregarded and the next pack started the day after taking the last tablet from the previous pack. In this case, a withdrawal bleed should not be expected until the end of the second pack. If the patient does not have a withdrawal bleed at the end of the second pack she must return to her doctor to exclude the possibility of pregnancy.

Gastro-intestinal upset: Vomiting or diarrhoea may reduce the efficacy by preventing full absorption. Additional contraception (barriers and spermicides) should be used during the stomach upset and for the 7 days following the upset. If these 7 days overrun the end of a pack, the next pack should be started without a break. In this case, a withdrawal bleed should not be expected until the end of the second pack. If the patient does not have a withdrawal bleed at the end of the second pack she must return to her doctor to exclude the possibility of pregnancy.

Mild laxatives do not impair contraceptive action.

Interaction with other drugs: Some drugs accelerate the metabolism of oral contraceptives when taken concurrently and these include barbiturates, phenytoin, phenylbutazone and rifampicin. Other drugs suspected of having the capacity to reduce the efficacy of oral contraceptives include ampicillin and other antibiotics. It is, therefore, advisable to use non-hormonal methods of contraception (barriers and spermicides) in addition to the oral contraceptive as long as an extremely high degree of protection is required during treatment with such drugs. The additional contraception should be used while the concurrent medication continues and for 7 days afterwards. If these extra precautions overrun the end of the pack, the next pack should be started without a break. In this case, a withdrawal bleed should not be expected until the end of the second pack. If the patient does not have a withdrawal bleed at the end of the second pack she must return to her doctor to exclude the possibility of pregnancy.

Contra-indications, warnings etc.

Contra-indications:

1. Suspected pregnancy.
2. Thrombotic disorders and a history of these conditions, sickle-cell anaemia, disorders of lipid metabolism and other conditions in which, in individual cases, there is known or suspected to be a much increased risk of thrombosis.
3. Acute or severe chronic liver diseases. Dubin-Johnson syndrome. Rotor syndrome. History, during pregnancy, of idiopathic jaundice or severe pruritus.
4. History of herpes gestationis.

Estimated cumulative numbers of breast cancers per 10,000 women diagnosed in 5 years of use and up to 10 years after stopping COCs, compared with numbers of breast cancers diagnosed in 10,000 women who had never used COCs.

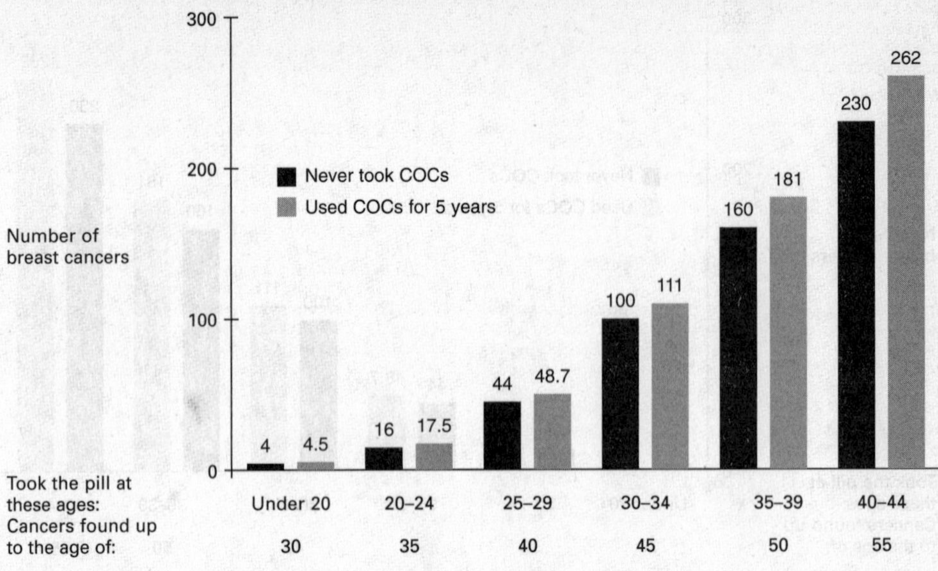

5. Mammary or endometrial carcinoma, or a history of these conditions.
6. Abnormal vaginal bleeding of unknown cause.
7. Deterioration of otosclerosis during pregnancy.

Warnings:

1. There is a general opinion, based on statistical evidence, that users of combined oral contraceptives experience, more often than non-users, venous thromboembolism, arterial thrombosis, including cerebral and myocardial infarction, and subarachnoid haemorrhage. Full recovery from such disorders does not always occur, and it should be realised that in a few cases they are fatal. How often these disorders occur in users of the low-dose pills is not known, but there are reasons for suggesting that they may occur less often than with older pills containing more oestrogen. Certain factors may entail some risk of thrombosis, e.g. smoking, obesity, varicose veins, cardiovascular diseases, diabetes and migraine. The suitability of a combined oral contraceptive should be judged according to the severity of such conditions in the individual case, and should be discussed with the patient before she decides to take it.
2. The risk of arterial thrombosis associated with combined oral contraceptives increases with age, and this risk is aggravated by cigarette smoking. The use of combined oral contraceptives by women in the older age group, especially those who are cigarette smokers, should therefore be discouraged and alternative methods used.
3. The possibility cannot be ruled out that certain chronic diseases may occasionally deteriorate during the use of combined oral contraceptives. (See 'Precautions').
4. Malignant liver tumours have been reported on rare occasions in long-term users of oral contraceptives. Benign hepatic tumours have also been associated with oral contraceptive usage. A hepatic tumour should be considered in the differential diagnosis when upper abdominal pain, enlarged liver or signs of intra-abdominal haemorrhage occur.
5. Numerous epidemiological studies have been reported on the risks of ovarian, endometrial, cervical and breast cancer in women using combined oral contraceptives. The evidence is clear that combined oral contraceptives offer substantial protection against both ovarian and endometrial cancer. An increased risk of cervical cancer in long term users of combined oral contraceptives has been reported in some studies, but there continues to be controversy about the extent to which this is attributable to the confounding effects of sexual behaviour and other factors.
A meta-analysis from 54 epidemiological studies reported that there is a slightly increased relative risk (RR=1.24) of having breast cancer diagnosed in women who are currently using combined oral contraceptives (COCs). The observed pattern of increased risk may be due to an earlier diagnosis of breast cancer in COC users, the biological effects of COCs or a combination of both. The additional breast cancers diagnosed in current users of COCs or in women who have used COCs in the last ten years are more likely to be localised to the breast than those in women who never used COCs.
Breast cancer is rare among women under 40 years of age whether or not they take COCs. Whilst this background risk increases with age, the excess number of breast cancer diagnoses in current and recent COC users is small in relation to the overall risk of breast cancer (see bar chart).
The most important risk factor for breast cancer in COC users is the age women discontinue the COC; the older the age at stopping, the more breast cancers are diagnosed. Duration of use is less important and the excess risk gradually disappears during the course of the 10 years after stopping COC use such that by 10 years there appears to be no excess.
The possible increase in risk of breast cancer should be discussed with the user and weighed against the benefits of COCs taking into account the evidence that they offer substantial protection against the risk of developing certain other cancers (e.g. ovarian and endometrial cancer).

Reasons for stopping oral contraception immediately:

1. Occurrence of migraine in patients who have never previously suffered from it. Exacerbation of pre-existing migraine. Any unusually frequent or unusually severe headaches.
2. Any kind of acute disturbance of vision.
3. Suspicion of thrombosis or infarction.
4. Six weeks before elective operations or treatment of varicose veins by sclerotherapy and during immobilisation, e.g. after accidents, etc.
5. Significant rise in blood-pressure.
6. Jaundice.
7. Clear exacerbation of conditions known to be capable of deteriorating during oral contraception or pregnancy.
8. Pregnancy is a reason for stopping immediately because it has been suggested by some investigations that oral contraceptives taken in early pregnancy may slightly increase the risk of foetal malformations. Other investigations have failed to support these findings. The possibility therefore cannot be excluded, but it is certain that if a risk exists at all, it is very small.

Precautions:

1. Examination of the pelvic organs, breasts and blood-pressure should precede the prescribing of any combined oral contraceptive and should be repeated regularly.
2. Before starting treatment, pregnancy must be excluded.
3. The following conditions require careful observation during medication: a history of severe depressive states, varicose veins, diabetes, hypertension, epilepsy, otosclerosis, multiple sclerosis, porphyria, tetany, disturbed liver function, gall-stones, cardiovascular diseases, renal diseases, chloasma, uterine fibroids, asthma, the wearing of contact lenses, or any disease that is prone to worsen during pregnancy. The first appearance or deterioration of any of these conditions may indicate that the oral contraceptive should be stopped.

4. The risk of the deterioration of chloasma, which is often not fully reversible, is reduced by the avoidance of excessive exposure to sunlight.

Side effects: Occasional side-effects may include nausea, vomiting, headaches, breast tenderness, changed body weight or libido, depressive moods, chloasma and altered serum lipid profile.

Menstrual changes:

1. *Reduction of menstrual flow:* This is not abnormal and it is to be expected in some patients. Indeed, it may be beneficial where heavy periods were previously experienced.
2. *Missed menstruation:* Occasionally, withdrawal bleeding may not occur at all. If the tablets have been taken correctly, pregnancy is very unlikely, but should be ruled out before a new course of tablets is started.

Intermenstrual bleeding: Very light 'spotting' or heavier 'breakthrough bleeding' may occur during tablet-taking, especially in the first few cycles. It appears to be generally of no significance, except where it indicates errors of tablet-taking, or where the possibility of interaction with other drugs exists (q.v.). However, if irregular bleeding is persistent, an organic cause should be considered.

Effect on adrenal and thyroid glands: Oral contraceptives have no significant influence on adrenocortical function. The ACTH function test for the adrenal cortex remains unchanged. The reduction in corticosteroid excretion and the elevation of plasma corticosteroids are due to an increased cortisol-binding capacity of the plasma proteins.

The response to metyrapone is less pronounced than in untreated women and is thus similar to that during pregnancy.

The radio-iodine uptake shows that thyroid function is unchanged. There is a rise in serum protein-bound iodine, similar to that in pregnancy and during the administration of oestrogens. This is due to the increased capacity of the plasma proteins for binding thyroid hormones, rather than to any change in glandular function. In women taking oral contraceptives, the content of protein-bound iodine in blood serum should therefore, not be used for evaluation of thyroid function.

Effect on blood chemistry: Oral contraceptives may accelerate erythrocyte sedimentation in the absence of any disease. This effect is due to a change in the proportion of the plasma protein fractions. Increases in plasma copper, iron and alkaline phosphatase have also been recorded.

Overdosage: There have been no reports of serious ill-effects from overdosage, even when a considerable number of tablets have been taken by a small child. In general, it is, therefore, unnecessary to treat overdosage. However, if overdosage is discovered within two or three hours and is so large that treatment seems desirable, gastric lavage can be safely used.

There are no specific antidotes and further treatment should be symptomatic.

Pharmaceutical precautions Store in cool, dry conditions. Shelf-life five years

Legal category POM

Package quantities Individual packs containing 3 months' supply.

Further information NIL

Product licence number 0011/0066

Date of last review January 1998

VARIDASE TOPICAL 125,000 UNITS PER VIAL

Qualitative and quantitative composition Varidase Topical contains the active ingredients Streptokinase HSE 100,000 IU and Streptodornase HSE 25,000 IU.

Pharmaceutical form Sterile powder for topical use.

Clinical particulars

Therapeutic indications: Varidase Topical is indicated wherever removal of clotted blood, fibrinous or purulent accumulations is required.

It is indicated in the treatment of suppurative surface lesions such as ulcers, pressure sores, amputation sites, diabetic gangrene, radiation necrosis, infected wounds and surgical incisions, until the wound is thoroughly cleansed of clots, fibrinous exudates and pus.

It is also indicated in the treatment of burns and may be used prior to skin grafting.

Varidase Topical can be used to dissolve clots in the bladder or in urinary catheters.

Posology and method of administration:

Adults, children and the elderly: Directions for use in the cleansing of necrotic infected and sloughy wounds.

Reconstitution: Single vial: The contents should be gently mixed with 20 ml of sterile physiological saline or, if unavailable, 20 ml of Water for Injection until the powder is completely dissolved. The resulting clear solution can then be withdrawn into a syringe.

Combi-Pack: Insert one end of the sterile transfer needle into the diluent vial and push the Varidase vial down onto the outer end of the needle.

(Ensure that the transfer needle goes centrally through the upraised circle on the stoppers).

Invert the vials so that the Varidase vial is under the diluent vial and allow the full 20 ml of diluent to run into the Varidase vial to dissolve the powder. Remove the empty diluent vial and discard. If necessary, gently agitate the Varidase vial until the powder is completely dissolved. The resulting clear solution can then be poured from the transfer needle.

As Varidase Topical is packed under vacuum, care should be taken when inserting a needle into the vial.

Excess agitation of the vial should be avoided to prevent frothing and denaturing of the enzymes.

As Varidase Topical does not contain a preservative, multidose use is not recommended.

Standard methods of application: Pre-soak gauze with Varidase Topical solution then apply to the wound. Following application, a semi-occlusive dressing is necessary to prevent drying out of the wound, e.g. a polyethylene film taped on two sides. Alternatively the wound may be packed with dry gauze which is then soaked with Varidase Topical solution and dressed with a semi-occlusive dressing.

Alternative method of application: Where wounds are covered by a thick dry eschar it is usually necessary to cross hatch the eschar into approximately 3–5 mm squares and to a sufficient depth to allow the access of the enzymes to the underlying fibrinous purulent material.

Alternatively, Varidase Topical may be introduced under the eschar, taking care that the solution enters only the cavity beneath and that the volume is not sufficient to cause pain through increased pressure. Introducing Varidase Topical in this way often results in the eschar becoming partly detached thus facilitating its mechanical removal.

Special technique of application: Varidase Topical may be applied in jelly form. This can be prepared by dissolving the contents of one vial in 5 ml of sterile water and mixing the resulting solution thoroughly, but gently, with 15 ml of inert jelly, such as K-Y or carboxymethylcellulose (CMC) jelly. This method can be particularly useful in cases of burns where dressings are not employed.

Frequency of application: Varidase Topical treatment should be repeated once or twice a day. Care should be taken to irrigate the lesion thoroughly with physiological saline to remove loosened material prior to the next application.

Duration of treatment: Treatment should be continued until healthy granulations are present and re-epithelialisation has begun, usually within one to two weeks. In mixed wounds, where granulation has started in some areas, Varidase use can continue until the entire wound is clean and granulating without any harmful effects to the healthy tissues.

Contraindications: Active haemorrhage. Known hypersensitivity to streptokinase and/or streptodornase.

Special warnings and precautions for use: Varidase Topical is intended for local use only. *It should not be used intramuscularly or intravenously.* This product contains streptokinase, which when used systemically is known to be antigenic. However, if used as recommended, there is no evidence to suggest that Varidase Topical is antigenic.

In order to avoid cross-infection, a new vial of Varidase Topical and a separate sterile syringe and needle should be used for each individual patient.

Varidase Topical has been shown to be a sensitiser when administered at relatively low intradermal doses to guinea pigs. The relevance of these findings to humans is considered important only where prolonged repetitive treatment is anticipated. Under such circumstances, the potential to induce allergic reactions may be minimised as described under 'Undesirable effects'.

Interactions with other medicaments and other forms of interaction: The preparation is buffered to physiological pH. The enzymes of Varidase Topical can be inactivated by the concomitant use of other preparations of an acidic or alkaline pH. Aluminium reacts with Varidase Topical. If the reconstituting fluid has a high calcium content, the solution becomes opalescent, but this does not affect the potency of the enzymes.

Pregnancy and lactation: Safe use of Varidase Topical during pregnancy and lactation has not been established. Use in these circumstances should be avoided unless considered essential by the physician.

Effects on the ability to drive and use machines: None known.

Undesirable effects: Allergic reactions to the application of Varidase Topical are infrequent and may be minimised by careful and frequent removal of exudate followed by thorough irrigation using physiological saline prior to retreatment with Varidase Topical. Transient slight burning pain has been reported rarely after application of Varidase Topical.

Overdose: There is no specific antidote. Removal of the preparation by careful washing or by irrigation/suction drainage is recommended.

Pharmacological properties

Pharmacodynamic properties: Streptokinase acts indirectly upon a substrate of fibrin or fibrinogen by activating a fibrinolytic enzyme in human serum. Upon application of streptokinase in situ, the activation of this fibrinolytic system brings about rapid dissolution of blood clots and the fibrinous portion of exudates. Streptodornase liquifies the viscous nucleoprotein of dead cells or pus. Thus the action of the enzymes results in the liquefaction of the two main viscous substances resulting from inflammatory or infectious processes thereby facilitating cleansing and desloughing of wounds.

Varidase Topical has no effect on collagen, living cells or healthy tissue.

Pharmacokinetic properties: There are no published reports concerning the pharmacokinetics of Varidase.

Pharmaceutical particulars

List of excipients: Sodium phosphate monobasic, sodium phosphate dibasic.

Incompatibilities: None known.

Shelf life: 18 months (unopened).

1 day (reconstituted solution stored in a refrigerator at 2–8°C).

Special precautions for storage: The unreconstituted and reconstituted product should be stored in a refrigerator (2–8°C).

Nature and contents of container: 25cc borosilicate Type 1 glass vial with butyl rubber stopper and metal seal with pull tab.

The product is available in:

Boxes containing a single vial of Varidase Topical sterile powder.

Combi-packs containing 1 vial of Varidase Topical sterile powder, 1 vial of Diluent (20 ml of sterile sodium chloride 0.9% solution BP) and 1 sterile transfer needle.

Instructions for use/handling: Refer to section 4.2 ('Posology and method of administration').

Marketing authorisation numbers

Varidase Topical 125,000 units per vial PL 0095/5038R
Diluent for Varidase Topical (Combi-Pack) PL 1502/0006R

Date of approval/revision

Last revised 15 March 1996

Legal category POM

ZOTON* CAPSULES

Presentation

Zoton Capsules 15 mg: Opaque yellow capsules for oral administration. Each capsule contains 15 mg lansoprazole as enteric coated granules.

Zoton Capsules 30 mg: Two tone lilac/purple capsules for oral administration. Each capsule contains 30 mg lansoprazole as enteric coated granules.

Uses Zoton is effective in the treatment of acid-related disorders of the upper gastro-intestinal tract, with the benefit of rapid symptom relief. Zoton is also effective in combination with antibiotics in the eradication of *Helicobacter pylori* (*H. pylori*).

Indications: Healing and long term management of gastro oesophageal reflux disease (GORD).

Healing and maintenance therapy for patients with duodenal ulcer.

Relief of reflux-like symptoms (eg. heartburn) and/or ulcer-like symptoms (eg. upper epigastric pain) associated with acid-related dyspepsia.

Healing of benign gastric ulcer.

Treatment of NSAID-associated benign gastric ulcers, duodenal ulcers and relief of symptoms in patients requiring continued NSAID treatment.

Long term management of pathological hypersecretory conditions including Zollinger-Ellison syndrome.

Zoton is also effective in patients with benign peptic lesions, including reflux oesophagitis, unresponsive to H_2 receptor antagonists.

Eradication of *H. pylori* from the upper gastrointestinal tract when used in combination with appropriate antibiotics in patients with gastritis or duodenal ulcer leading to the healing and prevention of relapse of the ulcer.

Dosage and administration
Dosage:
Gastro oesophageal reflux disease: Zoton 30 mg once daily for 4 weeks. The majority of patients will be healed after the first course. For those patients not fully healed at this time, a further 4 weeks treatment at the same dosage should be given.

For long term management, a maintenance dose of Zoton 15 mg or 30 mg once daily can be used dependant upon patient response.

Duodenal ulcer: The recommended dose is Zoton 30 mg once daily for 4 weeks.

For prevention of relapse, the recommended maintenance dose is Zoton 15 mg once daily.

Acid-related dyspepsia: Zoton 15 mg or 30 mg once daily for 2–4 weeks depending on the severity and persistence of symptoms. Patients who do not respond after 4 weeks, or who relapse shortly afterwards, should be investigated.

Benign gastric ulcer: Zoton 30 mg once daily for 8 weeks.

NSAID-associated benign gastric and duodenal ulcers and relief of symptoms: Zoton 15 mg or 30 mg once daily for 4 or 8 weeks. Most patients will be healed after 4 weeks; for those patients not fully healed, a further 4 weeks treatment can be given.

For patients at particular risk or with ulcers that may be difficult to heal, the higher dose and/or the longer treatment duration should be used.

Hypersecretory conditions: The initial dose should be Zoton 60 mg once daily. The dosage should then be adjusted individually. Treatment should be continued for as long as clinically indicated.

For patients who require 120 mg or more per day, the dose should be divided and administered twice daily.

Eradication of H. pylori: The following combinations have been shown to be effective when given for 7 days;

Zoton 30 mg twice daily plus clarithromycin 250-500 mg twice daily and amoxycillin 1 g twice daily or

Zoton 30 mg twice daily plus clarithromycin 250 mg twice daily and metronidazole 400 mg twice daily or

Zoton 30 mg twice daily plus amoxycillin 1 g twice daily and metronidazole 400 mg twice daily.

The best eradication results are obtained when clarithromycin is combined with either amoxycillin or metronidazole. When used in combination with the recommended antibiotics, Zoton is associated with *H. pylori*-eradication rates of up to 90%.

Eradication of *H. pylori* with any one of the above regimens has been shown to result in the healing of duodenal ulcers, without the need for continued anti-ulcer drug therapy. The risk of reinfection is low, and relapse following successful eradication is, therefore, unlikely.

To achieve the optimal acid inhibitory effect, and hence most rapid healing and symptom relief, Zoton 'once daily' should be administered in the morning before food. Zoton 'twice daily' should be administered once in the morning before food, and once in the evening.

The capsules should be swallowed whole. Do not crush or chew.

Elderly: Dose adjustment is not required in the elderly. The normal daily dosage should be given.

Children: There is no experience with Zoton in children.

Impaired hepatic and renal function: Lansoprazole is metabolised substantially by the liver. Clinical trials in patients with liver disease indicate that metabolism of lansoprazole is prolonged in patients with severe hepatic impairment. However, no dose adjustment is necessary; the recommended dose should not be exceeded.

There is no need to alter the dosage in patients with impaired renal function.

Contra-indications, warnings, etc.
Contra-indications: The use of Zoton is contra-indicated in patients with a history of hypersensitivity to any of the ingredients of Zoton capsules.

Warnings and precautions: In common with other anti-ulcer therapies, the possibility of malignancy should be excluded when gastric ulcer is suspected, as symptoms may be alleviated and diagnosis delayed. Similarly, the possibility of serious underlying disease such as malignancy should be excluded before treatment for dyspepsia commences, particularly in patients of middle age or older who have new or recently changed dyspeptic symptoms.

Before using Zoton with antibiotics to eradicate *H. pylori*, prescribers should refer to the full prescribing information of the respective antibiotics for guidance.

Decreased gastric acidity due to any means, including proton pump inhibitors, increases gastric counts of bacteria normally present in the gastrointestinal tract. Treatment with acid-reducing drugs may lead to a slightly increased risk of gastrointestinal infections such as Salmonella and Campylobacter.

Zoton is not known to affect ability to drive or operate machines.

Use in pregnancy and lactation: There is insufficient experience to recommend the use of Zoton in pregnancy. Animal studies do not reveal any teratogenic effect. Reproduction studies indicate slightly reduced litter survival and weights in rats and rabbits given very high doses of lansoprazole. The use of Zoton in pregnancy should be avoided.

Animal studies indicate that lansoprazole is secreted in breast milk. There is no information on the secretion of lansoprazole into breast milk in humans. The use of Zoton during breast feeding should be avoided unless considered essential.

Side effects: Zoton is well-tolerated, with adverse events generally being mild and transient.

The most commonly reported adverse events are headache, dizziness, fatigue and malaise.

Gastrointestinal effects include diarrhoea, constipation, abdominal pain, dyspepsia, nausea, vomiting, flatulence and dry or sore mouth or throat.

Alterations in liver function test values and, rarely, jaundice or hepatitis, have been reported.

Dermatological reactions include skin rashes, urticaria and pruritus. These generally resolve on discontinuation of drug therapy. Serious dermatological reactions are rare but there have been occasional reports of erythematous or bullous rashes including erythema multiforme. Cases of hair thinning and photosensitivity have also been reported.

Other hypersensitivity reactions include angioedema, wheezing, and very rarely, anaphylaxis. Cases of interstitial nephritis have been reported which have sometimes resulted in renal failure.

Haematological effects (thrombocytopenia, eosinophilia, leucopenia and pancytopenia) have occurred rarely. Bruising, purpura and petechiae have also been reported.

Other reactions include arthralgia, myalgia, depression, peripheral oedema and, rarely, paraesthesia or blurred vision, taste disturbances, vertigo, confusion and hallucinations.

Gynaecomastia and impotence have been raported rarely.

Interactions: Lansoprazole is hepatically metabolised and studies indicate that it is a weak inducer of Cytochrome P450. There is the possibility of interaction with drugs which are metabolised by the liver. Caution should be exercised when oral contraceptives and preparations such as phenytoin, theophylline, or warfarin are taken concomitantly with the administration of Zoton.

No clinically significant effects on NSAIDs or diazepam have been found.

Antacids and sucralfate may reduce the bioavailability of lansoprazole and should, therefore, not be taken within an hour of Zoton.

Animal Toxicology: Gastric tumours have been observed in life-long studies in rats.

An increased incidence of spontaneous retinal atrophy has been observed in life-long studies in rats. These lesions which are common to albino laboratory rats have not been observed in monkeys or dogs or life-long studies in mice. They are considered to be rat specific. No such treatment related changes have been observed in patients treated continuously for long periods.

Overdosage: There is no information on the effect of overdosage. However, Zoton has been given at doses up to 120 mg/day without significant adverse effects. Symptomatic and supportive therapy should be given as appropriate.

Pharmaceutical precautions Zoton Capsules should be stored at room temperature (15–25°C) in a dry place.

Legal category POM

Package quantities
Zoton Capsules 30 mg: Blister packs of 56, 28, 14 or 7 capsules.
Zoton Capsules 15 mg: Blister packs of 56 or 28 capsules.

Further information Lansoprazole is a member of a class of drugs called proton pump inhibitors. Its mode of action is to inhibit specifically the H^+/K^+ ATPase (proton pump) of the parietal cell in the stomach, the terminal step in acid production, thus reducing gastric acidity, a key requirement for healing of acid-related disorders such as gastric ulcer, duodenal ulcer and reflux oesophagitis. A single dose of 30 mg inhibits pentagastrin-stimulated acid secretion by approximately 80%, indicating effective acid inhibition from the first day of dosing.

Lansoprazole exhibits high (80–90%) bioavailability with a single dose. As a result, effective acid inhibition is achieved rapidly. Peak plasma levels occur within 1.5 to 2.0 hours. The plasma elimination half-life ranges from 1 to 2 hours following single or multiple doses in healthy subjects. The plasma protein binding is 97%.

Lansoprazole has a prolonged pharmacological action providing effective acid suppression over 24 hours, thereby promoting rapid healing and symptom relief.

Helicobacter pylori is the cause of the vast majority of cases of non-immune gastritis, and is implicated as the cause of a very high proportion of gastric and duodenal ulcers. There is evidence that *H. pylori* may also be associated with gastric carcinoma.

By reducing gastric acidity, Zoton creates an environment in which appropriate antibiotics can be effective against *H. pylori*. *In-vitro* studies have shown that lansoprazole has a direct antimicrobial effect on *H. pylori*.

The eradication of *H. pylori* results in the cure of a high proportion of patients with peptic ulcer disease, thus reducing the need for long term anti-secretory therapy, and preventing complications such as gastro-intestinal haemorrhage.

Marketing authorisation numbers

Zoton Capsules 15 mg	0095/0302
Zoton Capsules 30 mg	0095/0264

ZOTON* SUSPENSION 30MG

Qualitative and quantitative composition Each single dose sachet contains 30 mg of lansoprazole.

Pharmaceutical form Gastro-resistant granules for oral suspension.

When constituted in water the granules give a pink suspension with a strawberry flavour.

Clinical particulars
Therapeutic indications: Uses: Zoton is effective in the treatment of acid-related disorders of the upper gastro-intestinal tract, with the benefit of rapid symptom relief. Zoton is also effective in combination with antibiotics in the eradication of *Helicobacter pylori* (*H. pylori*).

Zoton Suspension may be particularly useful for patients who have difficulty swallowing, such as the elderly or patients with oesophageal strictures or dysphagia caused by severe oesophagitis.

Indications: Healing and long term management of Gastro Oesophageal Reflux Disease (GORD).

Healing and maintenance therapy for patients with duodenal ulcer.

Relief of reflux-like symptoms (eg. heartburn) and/or ulcer-like symptoms (eg. upper epigastric pain) associated with acid related dyspepsia.

Healing of benign gastric ulcer.

Treatment of NSAID-associated benign gastric ulcers, duodenal ulcers and relief of symptoms in patients requiring continued NSAID treatment.

Long term management of pathological hypersecretory conditions including Zollinger-Ellison syndrome.

Zoton is also effective in patients with benign peptic lesions, including reflux oesophagitis, unresponsive to H_2 receptor antagonists.

Eradication of *H. pylori* from the upper gastrointestinal tract when used in combination with appropriate antibiotics in patients with gastritis or duodenal ulcer leading to the healing and prevention of relapse of the ulcer.

Posology and method of administration: The contents of one sachet should be reconstituted by stirring into 30 mg (2 tablespoons) of tap water, and swallowed immediately.

Dosage: For patients requiring 30 mg lansoprazole daily, Zoton Capsules 30 mg or Zoton Suspension may be used.

For patients requiring 15 mg lansoprazole daily, Zoton Capsules 15 mg should be used.

Gastro oesophageal reflux disease: Zoton 30 mg once daily for 4 weeks. The majority of patients will be healed after the first course. For those patients not fully healed at this time, a further 4 weeks treatment at the same dosage should be given.

For long term management, a maintenance dose of Zoton 15 mg or 30 mg once daily can be used dependant upon patient response.

Duodenal ulcer: Zoton 30 mg once daily for 4 weeks.

For prevention of relapse, the recommended maintenance dose is Zoton Capsules 15 mg once daily.

Acid-related dyspepsia: Zoton 15 mg or 30 mg once daily for 2–4 weeks depending on the severity and persistence of symptoms. Patients who do not respond after 4 weeks, or who relapse shortly afterwards, should be investigated.

Benign gastric ulcer: Zoton 30 mg once daily for 8 weeks.

NSAID-associated benign gastric and duodenal ulcers and relief of symptoms: Zoton 15 mg or 30 mg once daily for 4 or 8 weeks. Most patients will be healed after 4 weeks; for those patients not fully healed, a further 4 weeks treatment can be given.

For patients at particular risk or with ulcers that may

be difficult to heal, the higher dose and/or the longer treatment duration should be used.

Hypersecretory conditions: The initial dose should be Zoton 60 mg once daily. The dosage should then be adjusted individually. Treatment should be continued for as long as clinically indicated.

For patients who require 120 mg or more per day, the dose should be divided and administered twice daily.

Eradication of H. pylori: The following combinations have been shown to be effective when given for 7 days:

Zoton 30 mg twice daily plus clarithromycin 250–500 mg twice daily and amoxycillin 1 g twice daily or

Zoton 30 mg twice daily plus clarithromycin 250 mg twice daily and metronidazole 400 mg twice daily or

Zoton 30 mg twice daily plus amoxycillin 1 g twice daily and metronidazole 400 mg twice daily.

The best eradication results are obtained when clarithromycin is combined with either amoxycillin or metronidazole. When used in combination with the recommended antibiotics, Zoton is associated with *H. pylori*-eradication rates of up to 90%.

Eradication of *H. pylori* with any one of the above regimens has been shown to result in the healing of duodenal ulcers, without the need for continued anti-ulcer drug therapy. The risk of reinfection is low and relapse following successful eradication is, therefore, unlikely.

Zoton should be taken once daily, except when used to eradicate *H. pylori.* To achieve the optimal acid inhibitory effect, and hence most rapid healing and symptom relief, Zoton should be administered in the morning before food.

Elderly: Dose adjustment is not required in the elderly. The normal daily dosage should be given.

Children: There is no experience with Zoton in children.

Impaired hepatic and renal function: Lansoprazole is metabolised substantially by the liver. Clinical trials in patients with liver disease indicate that metabolism of lansoprazole is prolonged in patients with severe hepatic impairment. However, no dose adjustment is necessary; the recommended dose should not be exceeded.

There is no need to alter the dosage in patients with impaired renal function.

Contra-indications: The use of Zoton is contra-indicated in patients with a history of hypersensitivity to any of the ingredients of Zoton Suspension.

Special warnings and precautions for use: In common with other anti-ulcer therapies, the possibility of malignancy should be excluded when gastric ulcer is suspected, as symptoms may be alleviated and diagnosis delayed. Similarly, the possibility of serious underlying disease such as malignancy should be excluded before treatment for dyspepsia commences, particularly in patients of middle age or older who have new or recently changed dyspeptic symptoms.

Before using Zoton with antibiotics to eradicate *H. pylori,* prescribers should refer to the full prescribing information of the respective antibiotics for guidance.

Decreased gastric acidity due to any means, including proton pump inhibitors, increases gastric counts of bacteria normally present in the gastrointestinal tract. Treatment with acid-reducing drugs may lead to a slightly increased rick of gastrointestinal infections such as *Samonella* and *Campylobacter.*

Interactions with other medicaments and other forms of interaction: Lansoprazole is hepatically metabolised and studies indicate that it is a weak inducer of Cytochrome P450. There is the possibility of interaction with drugs which are metabolised by the liver. Caution should be exercised when oral contraceptives and preparations such as phenytoin, theophylline, or warfarin are taken concomitantly with the administration of Zoton.

No clinically significant effects on NSAIDs or diazepam have been found.

Antacids and sucralfate may reduce the bioavailability of lansoprazole and should, therefore, not be taken within an hour of Zoton.

Pregnancy and lactation: There is insufficient experience to recommend the use of Zoton in pregnancy. Animal studies do not reveal any teratogenic effect. Reproduction studies indicate slightly reduced litter survival and weights in rats and rabbits given very high doses of lansoprazole.

The use of Zoton in pregnancy should be avoided.

Animal studies indicate that lansoprazole is secreted in breast milk. There is no information on the secretion of lansoprazole into breast milk in humans.

The use of Zoton during breast feeding should be avoided unless considered essential.

Effects on ability to drive and use machines: Zoton is not known to affect ability to drive or operate machines.

Undesirable effects: Zoton is well-tolerated, with adverse events generally being mild and transient.

The most commonly reported adverse events are headache, dizziness, fatigue and malaise.

Gastrointestinal effects include diarrhoea, constipation, abdominal pain, nausea, vomiting, flatulence and dry or sore mouth or throat.

Alterations in liver function test values and, rarely, jaundice or hepatitis, have been reported.

Dermatological reactions include skin rashes, urticaria and pruritus. These generally resolve on discontinuation of drug therapy. Serious dermatological reactions are rare but there have been occasional reports of erythematous or bullous rashes including erythema multiforme. Cases of hair thinning and photosensitivity have also been reported.

Other hypersensitivity reactions include angioedema, wheezing, and very rarely, anaphylaxis. Cases of interstitial nephritis have been reported which have sometimes resulted in renal failure.

Haematological effects (thrombocytopenia, eosinophilia, leucopenia and pancytopenia) have occurred rarely. Bruising, purpura and petechiae have also been reported.

Other reactions include arthralgia, myalgia, depression, peripheral oedema and, rarely, paraesthesia, blurred vision, taste disturbances, vertigo, confusion and hallucinations.

Gynaecomastia and impotence have been reported rarely.

Overdosage: There is no information on the effect of overdosage. However, Zoton has been given at doses up to 120 mg/day without significant adverse effects. Symptomatic and supportive therapy should be given as appropriate.

Pharmacological properties

Pharmacodynamic properties: Lansoprazole is a member of a class of drugs called proton pump inhibitors. Its mode of action is to inhibit specifically the H^+ / K^+ ATPase (proton pump) of the parietal cell in the stomach, the terminal step in acid production, thus reducing gastric acidity, a key requirement for healing of acid-related disorders such as gastric ulcer, duodenal ulcer and reflux oesophagitis.

It is believed that the parent drug is biotransformed into its active form(s) in the acidic environment of the parietal cell, whereupon it reacts with the sulphydryl group of the H^+ / K^+ ATPase causing inhibition. This inhibition is reversible *in-vitro* by intrinsic and extrinsic reducing agents. Lansoprazole's mode of action differs significantly from the H_2 antagonists which inhibit one of the three pathways involved in stimulation of acid production. A single dose of 30 mg inhibits pentagastrin-stimulated acid secretion by approximately 80%, indicating effective acid inhibition from the first day of dosing.

Lansoprazole has a prolonged pharmacological action providing effective acid suppression over 24 hours, thereby promoting rapid healing and symptom relief.

By reducing gastric acidity, Zoton creates an environment in which appropriate antibiotics can be effective against *H. pylori. In-vitro* studies have shown that lansoprazole has a direct antimicrobial effect on *H. pylori.*

Pharmacokinetic properties: One sachet of Zoton Suspension 30 mg is bioequivalent to one Zoton Capsule 30 mg.

Lansoprazole exhibits high (80-90%) bioavailability with a single dose. As a result, effective acid inhibition is achieved rapidly. Peak plasma levels occurred within 1.5 to 2.0 hours. The plasma elimination half-life ranges from 1 to 2 hours following single or multiple doses in healthy subjects. There is no evidence of accumulation following multiple doses in healthy subjects. The plasma protein binding is 97%.

Following absorption, lansoprazole is extensively metabolised and is excreted by both the renal and biliary route. A study with ^{14}C-labelled lansoprazole indicated that up to 50% of the dose was excreted in the urine. Lansoprazole is metabolised substantially by the liver.

Preclinical safety data: Gastric tumours have been observed in life-long studies in rats.

An increased incidence of spontaneous retinal atrophy has been observed in life-long studies in rats. These lesions which are common to albino laboratory rats have not been observed in monkeys or dogs or life-long studies in mice. They are considered to be rat specific. No such treatment related changes have been observed in patients treated continuously for long periods.

Pharmaceutical particulars

List of Excipients: Enteric Coated Granules:

Magnesium Carbonate[1], Non-pariel Inert Microgranules[4], Purified Sucrose[1], Maize Starch[1], Low Substituted Hydroxypropyl Cellulose (L-HPC-31)[1], Hydroxypropyl Cellulose (HPC-L)[1], Methacrylic Acid Copolymer (Eudragit L30D-55), Talc[1], Polyethylene Glycol 6000 (PEG 6000), Titanium Dioxide[1], Polysorbate 80[1], Colloidal Anhydrous Silica[1], Purified Water[1,5].

Suspending Granules:

Sucrose[2], Mannitol[2], Docusate Sodium[2], Crospovidone[3], Xanthan Gum[3], Strawberry flavour (J2161), Citric Acid[2], Red Iron Oxide (E172)[6], Colloidal Anhydrous Silica[2], Magnesium Stearate[2], Ethanol[5]

[1] Complies with Ph. Eur specification.

[2] Complies with B.P. specification.

[3] Complies with U.S National Formulary specification.

[4] Comprising sucrose and starch.

[5] Used during processing; does not appear in final product.

[6] Complies with the E.U. directives on colours.

Incompatibilities: None known.

Shelf life: 24 months.

Once opened Zoton Suspension should be suspended in water and consumed immediately.

Special precautions for storage: Zoton Suspension sachets should be stored at room temperature (below 25°C) in a dry place.

Nature and contents of container: Sachets consisting of paper, polythene, aluminium foil and ionomer laminate.

28 sachets/carton

Instructions for use/handling: Patients Instructions:

Directions for constituting suspension from sachets:
1. Empty granules from sachet into a glass
2. Add two tablespoons (30 ml) of water
3. Stir well and drink immediately

Marketing authorisation number 0095/0319

Date of first authorisation 28 July 1998

Legal category POM

**Trade Mark*

Yamanouchi Pharma Ltd
Yamanouchi House
Pyrford Road
West Byfleet, Surrey

☎ 01932 345535/342291 🗋 01932 353458

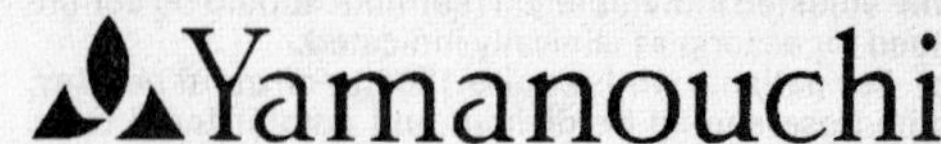

BICILLIN* INJECTION

Qualitative and quantitative composition Procaine Penicillin PhEur 300 mg (300,000 units) and Benzylpenicillin Sodium PhEur 60 mg (100,000 units) per ml upon constitution.

Pharmaceutical form Powder for constitution.

Clinical particulars

Therapeutic indications: For the treatment of infections due to penicillin sensitive organisms.

Posology and method of administration:

Adults and the elderly: Usually 1 ml 24 hourly or 12 hourly, or as directed by the physician.

Children: Over 25 kg – as for adults. Under 25 kg – proportionally to body weight.

In acute uncomplicated gonorrhoea: Up to 12 ml as a single dose, or as directed by the physician.

In early syphilis: 3 ml (4 ml in heavier patients) daily for 10 days, or as directed by the physician.

Contra-indications: Hypersensitivity to penicillin or procaine.

Special warnings and precautions for use: None.

Interaction with other medicaments and other forms of interaction: Probenecid delays the excretion of penicillin.

Pregnancy and lactation: The safety of Bicillin Injection in these circumstances has not been established.

Effects on ability to drive and use machines: None known.

Undesirable effects: Skin reactions may occur but usually resolve on cessation of therapy. Generalised, systemic reactions are rare and usually associated with a history of allergy or penicillin intolerance.

Overdose: General supportive measures.

Pharmacological properties

Pharmacodynamic properties: The penicillin constituents of Bicillin are bactericidal, inhibiting the structural cross linkages in the bacterial cell wall.

Whilst the sodium penicillin component offers an immediate but short acting effect, the procaine penicillin component provides a depot effect, often producing therapeutic blood levels for 24 hours following injection.

Pharmacokinetic properties: After an intramuscular dose of 300,000 units of procaine penicillin, a peak serum concentration of benzylpenicillin of about 1.6 units/ml is attained in 1 to 3 hours falling to 0.4 unit/ml at 6 hours; serum concentrations are lower than those achieved after an equivalent dose of benzylpenicillin.

Preclinical safety data: There is no relevant preclinical safety data.

Pharmaceutical particulars

List of excipients: Polysorbate 80 NF, Sodium Citrate (anhydrous) USP, Citric Acid PhEur.

Incompatibilities: None known.

Shelf life: 5 years.

Special precautions for storage: Not more than 15°C when unconstituted. Upon constitution the preparation is for single-dose use only. It may be kept at 2°C–8°C for up to 24 hours after constitution but must be discarded after the first usage or at the end of that period of 24 hours.

Nature and contents of container: Glass multi-dose injection vial, with rubber stopper and aluminium seal. Each vial contains 1.8 g (1,800,000 units Procaine Penicillin PhEur and 360 mg (600,000 units) Benzylpenicillin Sodium PhEur and on constitution provides 6 ml of an injection containing in each ml 300 mg (300,000 units) Procaine Penicillin PhEur and 60 mg (100,000 units) Benzylpenicillin Sodium PhEur.

Instructions for use/handling: For constitution, add 4.6 ml water for injections to each vial, to produce 6 ml injection, equivalent to Fortified Procaine Penicillin Injection BP.

Marketing authorisation number 0166/0147.

Date of approval/revision of SPC October 1995.

Legal category POM.

CARDENE 20 mg

Qualitative and quantitative composition Nicardipine 20 mg.

Pharmaceutical form Capsules.

Clinical particulars

Therapeutic indications: Cardene is indicated for the prophylaxis of patients with chronic stable angina. For the treatment of hypertension considered to be mild to moderate in severity. Cardene capsules are for oral administration.

Posology and method of administration: Nicardipine should be taken with a little water.

Prophylaxis of chronic stable angina:

Starting dose: 20 mg every 8 hours titrating upwards as required.

Usual effective dose: 30 mg every 8 hours (range of total dose 60 mg–120 mg per day).

Allow at least 3 days before increasing the dose of Cardene to ensure steady state plasma levels have been achieved.

Hypertension:

Starting dose: 20 mg every 8 hours titrating upwards as required.

Usual effective dose: 30 mg every 8 hours (range of total dose 60 mg–120 mg per day).

Use in elderly: Starting dose is 20 mg 3 times a day. Titrate upwards with care as nicardipine may lower systolic pressure more than diastolic pressure in these patients.

Children: Cardene is not recommended in patients under the age of 18.

Contra-indications:

i). Pregnancy and lactation.

ii). Hypersensitivity to nicardipine hydrochloride or other dihydropyridines because of the theoretical risk of cross reactivity.

iii). Because part of the effect of nicardipine is secondary to reduced afterload, the drug should not be given to patients with advanced aortic stenosis. Reduction of diastolic pressure in these patients may worsen rather than improve myocardial infarction.

iv). Cardene should not be used in cardiogenic shock, clinically significant aortic stenosis, unstable angina, and during or within one month of a myocardial infarction.

v). Cardene should not be used for acute attacks of angina.

vi). Cardene should not be used for secondary prevention of myocardial infarction.

Special warnings and special precautions for use: If used in combination with diuretics or beta-blockers, careful titration of Cardene is advised to avoid excessive reduction in blood pressure.

If switching from beta-blockers to Cardene, gradually reduce the beta-blocker dose (preferably over 8–10 days) since nicardipine gives no protection against the dangers of abrupt beta-blocker withdrawal.

Stop Cardene in patients experiencing ischaemic pain within 30 minutes of starting therapy or after increasing the dose.

Use in patients with congestive heart failure or poor cardiac reserve: Haemodynamic studies in patients with heart failure have shown that nicardipine reduces afterload and improves overall haemodynamics. In one study, intravenous nicardipine reduced myocardial contractility in patients with severe heart failure despite increases in cardiac index and ejection fraction noted in the same patients.

Since nicardipine has not been extensively studied in patients with severe left ventricular dysfunction and cardiac failure one must consider that worsening of cardiac failure may occur.

Use in patients with impaired hepatic or renal function: Since Cardene is subject to first pass metabolism, use with caution in patients with impaired liver function or reduced hepatic blood flow. Patients with severe liver disease showed elevated blood levels and the half-life of nicardipine was prolonged. Cardene blood levels may also be elevated in some renally impaired patients. Therefore, the lowest starting dose and extending the dosing interval should be individually considered in these patients.

Use in patients following a stroke (infarction or haemorrhage): Avoid inducing systemic hypotension when administering Cardene to these patients.

Laboratory tests: Transient elevations of alkaline phosphatase, serum bilirubin, SGPT, SGOT and glucose, have been observed. BUN and creatinine may also become elevated. While out-of-range values were seen in T_3, T_4 and TSH, the lack of consistent alterations suggest that any changes were not drug-related.

Treatment with short acting nicardipine may induce an exaggerated fall in blood pressure and reflex tachycardia which can cause cardiovascular complications such as myocardial and cerebrovascular ischaemia.

There has been some concern about increased mortality and morbidity in the treatment of ischaemic heart disease using higher than recommended doses of some other short-acting dihydropyridines.

Interactions with other medicaments and other forms of interaction

Digoxin: Careful monitoring of serum digoxin levels is advised in patients also receiving Cardene as levels may be increased.

Propanolol, Dipyridamole, Warfarin, Quinidine, Naproxen: Therapeutic concentrations of these drugs does not change the *in vitro* plasma protein binding of nicardipine.

Cimetidine: Cimetidine increases nicardipine plasma levels. Carefully monitor patients receiving both drugs.

Fentanyl anaesthesia: Severe hypotension has been reported during fentanyl anaesthesia with concomitant use of a beta-blocker and calcium blockade. Even though such interactions have not been seen in clinical trials, such hypotensive episodes should be vigorously treated with conventional therapy such as intravenous fluids.

Cyclosporin: Monitor cyclosporin plasma levels and reduce dosage accordingly in patients concomitantly receiving nicardipine as elevated cyclosporin levels have been reported.

Rifampicin: Rifampicin can interact with other dihydropyridines to substantially reduce their plasma levels and so rifampicin and nicardipine should be used together with caution.

As with other dihydropyridines, nicardipine should not be taken with grapefruit juice because bioavailability may be increased.

Cardene may be used in combination with beta-blocking and other anti-hypertensive drugs but the possibility of an additive effect resulting in postural hypotension should be considered.

Pregnancy and lactation: See *Contra-indications.*

Effects on ability to drive and use machines: None known.

Undesirable effects: Majority are not serious and are expected consequences of the vasodilator effects of Cardene.

The most frequent side-effects reported are headache, pedal oedema, heat sensation and/or flushing, palpitations, nausea and dizziness.

Other side-effects noted in clinical trials include the following:

Cardiovascular system: as with the use of other short-acting dihydropyridines in patients with ischaemic heart disease, exacerbation of angina pectoris may occur frequently at the start of treatment with nicardipine capsules. The occurrence of myocardial infarction has been reported although it is not possible to distinguish such an event from the natural course of ischaemic heart disease.

Central nervous system: drowsiness, insomnia, tinnitus, paraesthesiae, functional disorders.

Skin: itching, rashes.

Hepato-renal: impairment, frequency of micturition.

Dyspnoea, gastro-intestinal upset and, rarely, depression, impotence and thrombocytopenia, have also been reported.

Overdose: Symptoms may include marked hypotension, bradycardia, palpitations, flushing, drowsiness, confusion and slurred speech. In laboratory animals, overdosage also resulted in reversible hepatic function abnormalities, sporadic focal hepatic necrosis and progressive atrioventricular conduction block.

For treatment of overdose, standard measures including monitoring of cardiac and respiratory functions should be implemented. The patient should be positioned so as to avoid cerebral anoxia. Frequent blood pressure determinations are essential. Vasopressors are clinically indicated for patients exhibiting profound hypotension. Intravenous calcium gluconate may help reverse the effects of calcium entry blockade.

Pharmacological properties

Pharmacodynamic properties: Cardene is a potent calcium antagonist. Pharmacological studies demonstrate its preferential high selectivity for the peripheral vasculature over the myocardium which accounts for its minimal negative inotropic effects. Cardene produces smooth muscle relaxation and marked peripheral vasodilatation.

In man Cardene produces a significant decrease in systemic vascular resistance, the degree of vasodilatation being more predominant in hypertensive patients than in normotensive subjects. Haemodynamic studies in patients with coronary artery disease and normal left ventricular function have shown significant increases in cardiac index and coronary blood flow, with little if any increase in left ventricular end-diastolic pressure.

Electrophysiologic effects: Electrophysiological studies in man show that Cardene does not depress sinus node function or atrial or ventricular conduction in patients with either normal or decreased electrical conduction systems. Refractory periods of the His-Purkinje system were actually shortened slightly by nicardipine and SA conduction time was improved.

Pharmacokinetic properties: Pharmacokinetics and metabolism: Nicardipine is rapidly and completely absorbed with plasma levels detectable 20 minutes following an oral dose. Maximal plasma levels are observed within 30 minutes to two hours (mean Tmax = 1 hour). When given with a high fat meal peak plasma levels are reduced by 30%. Nicardipine is subject to saturable first-pass metabolism and the bioavailability is about 35% following a 30 mg oral dose at steady state.

The pharmacokinetics of Cardene are non-linear due to saturable hepatic first pass metabolism.

Steady-state plasma levels are achieved after about 3 days of dosing at 20 and 30 mg tds and remain relatively constant over 28 days of dosing at 30 mg tds. Considerable intersubject variability in plasma levels is observed. Following dosing to steady state using doses of 30 mg and 40 mg (tds), the terminal plasma half-life of nicardipine averaged 8.6 hours. Nicardipine is highly protein-bound (>99%) in human plasma over a wide concentration range.

Nicardipine does not induce its own metabolism and does not induce hepatic microsomal enzymes.

Preclinical safety data: Please refer to *Pregnancy and lactation.*

Pharmaceutical particulars

List of excipients:

20 mg Capsules: Starch, pregelatinised, Magnesium stearate.

Capsule shell body: Titanium dioxide E171, Gelatin.

Capsule shell cap: Indigotine E132, Titanium dioxide E171, Gelatin.

Incompatibilities: None known.

Shelf life: 60 months.

Special precautions for storage: No special precautions.

Nature and contents of container: 20 mg Capsules: Securitainer packs of 50 and 100. PVC/aluminium foil blister strips of 21, 56, 84, 100 and 200 capsules.

Instructions for use/handling: Not applicable.

Administrative data

Marketing authorisation holder: Yamanouchi Pharma Ltd, Yamanouchi House, Pyrford Road, West Byfleet, Surrey KT14 6RA, United Kingdom.

Marketing authorisation number PL 00166/0181

Date of first authorisation/renewal of authorisation 15 May 1998

Date of (partial) revision of text March 1997.

CARDENE 30 mg

Qualitative and quantitative composition Nicardipine 30 mg.

Pharmaceutical form Capsules.

Clinical particulars

Therapeutic indications: Cardene is indicated for the prophylaxis of patients with chronic stable angina. For the treatment of hypertension considered to be mild to moderate in severity. Cardene capsules are for oral administration.

Posology and method of administration: Nicardipine should be taken with a little water.

Prophylaxis of chronic stable angina:

Starting dose: 20 mg every 8 hours titrating upwards as required.

Usual effective dose: 30 mg every 8 hours (range of total dose 60 mg–120 mg per day).

Allow at least 3 days before increasing the dose of Cardene to ensure steady state plasma levels have been achieved.

Hypertension:

Starting dose: 20 mg every 8 hours titrating upwards as required.

Usual effective dose: 30 mg every 8 hours (range of total dose 60 mg–120 mg per day).

Use in elderly: Starting dose is 20 mg 3 times a day. Titrate upwards with care as nicardipine may lower systolic pressure more than diastolic pressure in these patients.

Children: Cardene is not recommended in patients under the age of 18.

Contra-indications:

i). Pregnancy and lactation.
ii). Hypersensitivity to nicardipine hydrochloride or other dihydropyridines because of the theoretical risk of cross reactivity.
iii). Because part of the effect of nicardipine is secondary to reduced afterload, the drug should not be given to patients with advanced aortic stenosis. Reduction of diastolic pressure in these patients may worsen rather than improve myocardial infarction.
iv). Cardene should not be used in cardiogenic shock, clinically significant aortic stenosis, unstable angina, and during or within one month of a myocardial infarction.
v). Cardene should not be used for acute attacks of angina.
vi). Cardene should not be used for secondary prevention of myocardial infarction.

Special warnings and special precautions for use: If used in combination with diuretics or beta-blockers, careful titration of Cardene is advised to avoid excessive reduction in blood pressure.

If switching from beta-blockers to Cardene, gradually reduce the beta-blocker dose (preferably over 8–10 days) since nicardipine gives no protection against the dangers of abrupt beta-blocker withdrawal.

Stop Cardene in patients experiencing ischaemic pain within 30 minutes of starting therapy or after increasing the dose.

Use in patients with congestive heart failure or poor cardiac reserve: Haemodynamic studies in patients with heart failure have shown that nicardipine reduces afterload and improves overall haemodynamics. In one study, intravenous nicardipine reduced myocardial contractility in patients with severe heart failure despite increases in cardiac index and ejection fraction noted in the same patients.

Since nicardipine has not been extensively studied in patients with severe left ventricular dysfunction and cardiac failure one must consider that worsening of cardiac failure may occur.

Use in patients with impaired hepatic or renal function: Since Cardene is subject to first pass metabolism, use with caution in patients with impaired liver function or reduced hepatic blood flow. Patients with severe liver disease showed elevated blood levels and the half-life of nicardipine was prolonged. Cardene blood levels may also be elevated in some renally impaired patients. Therefore, the lowest starting dose and extending the dosing interval should be individually considered in these patients.

Use in patients following a stroke (infarction or haemorrhage): Avoid inducing systemic hypotension when administering Cardene to these patients.

Laboratory tests: Transient elevations of alkaline phosphatase, serum bilirubin, SGPT, SGOT and glucose, have been observed. BUN and creatinine may also become elevated. While out-of-range values were seen in T_3, T_4 and TSH, the lack of consistent alterations suggest that any changes were not drug-related.

Treatment with short acting nicardipine may induce an exaggerated fall in blood pressure and reflex tachycardia which can cause cardiovascular complications such as myocardial and cerebrovascular ischaemia.

There has been some concern about increased mortality and morbidity in the treatment of ischaemic heart disease using higher than recommended doses of some other short-acting dihydropyridines.

Interactions with other medicaments and other forms of interaction

Digoxin: Careful monitoring of serum digoxin levels is advised in patients also receiving Cardene as levels may be increased.

Propanolol, Dipyridamole, Warfarin, Quinidine, Naproxen: Therapeutic concentrations of these drugs does not change the *in vitro* plasma protein binding of nicardipine.

Cimetidine: Cimetidine increases nicardipine plasma levels. Carefully monitor patients receiving both drugs.

Fentanyl anaesthesia: Severe hypotension has been reported during fentanyl anaesthesia with concomitant use of a beta-blocker and calcium blockade. Even though such interactions have not been seen in clinical trials, such hypotensive episodes should be vigorously treated with conventional therapy such as intravenous fluids.

Cyclosporin: Monitor cyclosporin plasma levels and reduce dosage accordingly in patients concomitantly receiving nicardipine as elevated cyclosporin levels have been reported.

Rifampicin: Rifampicin can interact with other dihydropyridines to substantially reduce their plasma levels and so rifampicin and nicardipine should be used together with caution.

As with other dihydropyridines, nicardipine should not be taken with grapefruit juice because bioavailability may be increased.

Cardene may be used in combination with beta-blocking and other anti-hypertensive drugs but the possibility of an additive effect resulting in postural hypotension should be considered.

Pregnancy and lactation: See *Contra-indications.*

Effects on ability to drive and use machines: None known.

Undesirable effects: Majority are not serious and are expected consequences of the vasodilator effects of Cardene.

The most frequent side-effects reported are headache, pedal oedema, heat sensation and/or flushing, palpitations, nausea and dizziness.

Other side-effects noted in clinical trials include the following:

Cardiovascular system: as with the use of other short-acting dihydropyridines in patients with ischaemic heart disease, exacerbation of angina pectoris may occur frequently at the start of treatment with nicardipine capsules. The occurrence of myocardial infarction has been reported although it is not possible to distinguish such an event from the natural course of ischaemic heart disease.

Central nervous system: drowsiness, insomnia, tinnitus, paraesthesiae, functional disorders.

Skin: itching, rashes.

Hepato-renal: impairment, frequency of micturition.

Dyspnoea, gastro-intestinal upset and, rarely, depression, impotence and thrombocytopenia, have also been reported.

Overdose: Symptoms may include marked hypotension, bradycardia, palpitations, flushing, drowsiness, confusion and slurred speech. In laboratory animals, overdosage also resulted in reversible hepatic function abnormalities, sporadic focal hepatic necrosis and progressive atrioventricular conduction block.

For treatment of overdose, standard measures including monitoring of cardiac and respiratory functions should be implemented. The patient should be positioned so as to avoid cerebral anoxia. Frequent blood pressure determinations are essential. Vasopressors are clinically indicated for patients exhibiting profound hypotension. Intravenous calcium gluconate may help reverse the effects of calcium entry blockade.

Pharmacological properties

Pharmacodynamic properties: Cardene is a potent calcium antagonist. Pharmacological studies demonstrate its preferential high selectivity for the peripheral vasculature over the myocardium which accounts for its minimal negative inotropic effects. Cardene produces smooth muscle relaxation and marked peripheral vasodilatation.

In man Cardene produces a significant decrease in systemic vascular resistance, the degree of vasodilatation being more predominant in hypertensive patients than in normotensive subjects. Haemodynamic studies in patients with coronary artery disease and normal left ventricular function have shown significant increases in cardiac index and coronary blood flow, with little if any increase in left ventricular end-diastolic pressure.

Electrophysiologic effects: Electrophysiological studies in man show that Cardene does not depress sinus node function or atrial or ventricular conduction in patients with either normal or decreased electrical conduction systems. Refractory periods of the His-Purkinje system were actually shortened slightly by nicardipine and SA conduction time was improved.

Pharmacokinetic properties: Pharmacokinetics and metabolism: Nicardipine is rapidly and completely absorbed with plasma levels detectable 20 minutes following an oral dose. Maximal plasma levels are observed within 30 minutes to two hours (mean Tmax = 1 hour). When given with a high fat meal peak plasma levels are reduced by 30%. Nicardipine is subject to saturable first-pass metabolism and the bioavailability is about 35% following a 30 mg oral dose at steady state.

The pharmacokinetics of Cardene are non-linear due to saturable hepatic first pass metabolism.

Steady-state plasma levels are achieved after about 3 days of dosing at 20 and 30 mg tds and remain relatively constant over 28 days of dosing at 30 mg tds. Considerable intersubject variability in plasma levels is observed. Following dosing to steady state using doses of 30 mg and 40 mg (tds), the terminal plasma half-life of nicardipine averaged 8.6 hours. Nicardipine is highly protein-bound (>99%) in human plasma over a wide concentration range.

Nicardipine does not induce its own metabolism and does not induce hepatic microsomal enzymes.

Preclinical safety data: Please refer to *Pregnancy and lactation.*

Pharmaceutical particulars

List of excipients:

30 mg Capsules: Starch, pregelatinised, Magnesium stearate.

Capsule shell body: Indigotine E132, Titanium dioxide E171, Gelatin.

Capsule shell cap: Indigotine E132, Titanium dioxide E171, Gelatin.

Incompatibilities: None known.

Shelf life: 60 months.

Special precautions for storage: No special precautions.

Nature and contents of container: 30 mg Capsules: Securitainer packs of 50 and 100. PVC/aluminium foil blister strips of 21, 56, 60, 84, 100 and 200 capsules.

Instructions for use/handling: Not applicable.

Administrative data

Marketing authorisation holder: Yamanouchi Pharma Ltd, Yamanouchi House, Pyrford Road, West Byfleet, Surrey KT14 6RA.

Marketing authorisation number PL 00166/0182

Date of first authorisation/renewal of authorisation 15 May 1998

Date of (partial) revision of text March 1997.

CARDENE SR 30

Qualitative and quantitative composition Nicardipine 30 mg.

Pharmaceutical form Sustained release capsules.

Clinical particulars

Therapeutic indications: Treatment of mild to moderate hypertension.

Posology and method of administration:

Adults:

Starting dose: 30 mg every 12 hours titrating upwards as required.

Usual effective dose: 45 mg every 12 hours (range 30 to 60 mg every 12 hours).

Individually adjust the dose for each patient. Where appropriate Cardene SR may also be used in combination with beta-blockers and/or diuretics.

Use in the elderly:

Starting dose: 30 mg every 12 hours. Titrate upwards with care as nicardipine may lower systolic pressure more than diastolic pressure in these patients.

Children: Cardene SR is not recommended for use in patients under the age of 18.

Contra-indications:

i). Use in pregnancy and lactation.

ii). Hypersensitivity to nicardipine hydrochloride or other dihydropyridines because of the theoretical risk of cross reactivity.

iii). As part of the effect of nicardipine is secondary to reduced afterload, the drug should not be given to patients with advanced aortic stenosis. Reduction in diastolic pressure in these patients may worsen rather than improve myocardial oxygen balance.

iv). Cardene should not be used in cardiogenic shock, clinically significant aortic stenosis, and during or within one month of a myocardial infarction.

v). Cardene should not be used for the secondary prevention of myocardial infarction.

Special warnings and special precautions for use: If used in combination with diuretics or beta-blockers, careful titration of Cardene SR is advised to avoid excessive reduction in blood pressure.

If switching from beta-blockers to Cardene SR, gradually reduce the beta-blocker dose (preferably over 8–10 days) since nicardipine gives no protection against the dangers of abrupt beta-blocker withdrawal.

Stop Cardene SR in patients experiencing ischaemic pain within 30 minutes of starting therapy or after increasing the dose.

Use in patients with congestive heart failure or poor cardiac reserve: Haemodynamic studies in patients with heart failure have shown that nicardipine reduces afterload and improves overall haemodynamics. In one study, intravenous nicardipine reduced myocardial contractility in patients with severe heart failure despite increases in cardiac index and ejection fraction noted in the same patients.

Since nicardipine has not been extensively studied in patients with severe left ventricular dysfunction and cardiac failure, one must consider that worsening of cardiac failure may occur.

Use in patients with impaired hepatic or renal function: Since Cardene is subject to first pass metabolism, use with caution in patients with impaired liver function or reduced hepatic blood flow. Patients with severe liver disease showed elevated blood levels and the half-life of nicardipine was prolonged. Cardene blood levels may also be elevated in some renally-impaired patients. Therefore, the lowest starting dose and extending the dosing interval should be individually considered in these patients.

Use in patients following a stroke (infarction or haemorrhage): Avoid inducing systemic hypotension when administering Cardene SR to these patients.

Laboratory tests: Transient elevations of alkaline phosphatase, serum bilirubin, SGPT, SGOT and glucose, have been observed. BUN and creatinine may also become elevated. While out-of-range values were seen in T_3, T_4 and TSH, the lack of consistent alterations suggest that any changes were not drug-related.

Treatment with short acting nicardipine may induce an exaggerated fall in blood pressure and reflex tachycardia which can cause cardiovascular complications such as myocardial and cerebrovascular ischaemia.

There has been some concern about increased mortality and morbidity in the treatment of ischaemic heart disease using higher than recommended doses of some other short-acting dihydropyridines.

Interactions with other medicaments and other forms of interaction

Digoxin: Careful monitoring of serum digoxin levels is advised in patients also receiving Cardene as levels may be increased.

Propanolol, Dipyridamole, Warfarin, Quinidine, Naproxen: Therapeutic concentrations of these drugs does not change the *in vitro* plasma protein binding of nicardipine.

Cimetidine: Cimetidine increases nicardipine plasma levels. Carefully monitor patients receiving both drugs.

Fentanyl anaesthesia: Severe hypotension has been reported during fentanyl anaesthesia with concomitant use of a beta-blocker and calcium blockade. Even though such interactions have not been seen in clinical trials, such hypotensive episodes should be vigorously treated with conventional therapy such as intravenous fluids.

Cyclosporin: Monitor cyclosporin plasma levels and reduce dosage accordingly in patients concomitantly receiving nicardipine as elevated cyclosporin levels have been reported.

Rifampicin: Rifampicin can interact with other dihydropyridines to substantially reduce their plasma levels and so rifampicin and nicardipine should be used together with caution.

As with other dihydropyridines, nicardipine should not be taken with grapefruit juice because bioavailability may be increased.

Cardene may be used in combination with beta-blocking and other anti-hypertensive drugs but the possibility of an additive effect resulting in postural hypotension should be considered.

Pregnancy and lactation: See *Contra-indications.*

Effects on ability to drive and use machines: None known.

Undesirable effects: Most are expected consequences of the vasodilator effects of Cardene SR.

The most frequent side-effects reported are headache, pedal oedema, heat sensation and/or flushing, palpitations, nausea and dizziness.

Other side-effects noted in clinical trials include the following:

Cardiovascular system: as with the use of other sustained-release dihydropyridines in patients with ischaemic heart disease, exacerbation of angina pectoris may occur rarely at the start of treatment with Cardene SR. The occurrence of myocardial infarction has been reported although it is not possible to distinguish such an event from the natural course of ischaemic heart disease.

Central nervous system: drowsiness, insomnia, tinnitus, paraesthesiae, functional disorders.

Skin: itching, rashes.

Hepato-renal: impairment, frequency of micturition.

Dyspnoea, gastro-intestinal upset and, rarely, depression, impotence and thrombocytopenia, have also been reported.

Overdose: Symptoms may include marked hypotension, bradycardia, palpitations, flushing, drowsiness, confusion and slurred speech. In laboratory animals, overdosage also resulted in reversible hepatic function abnormalities, sporadic focal hepatic necrosis and progressive atrioventricular conduction block.

Use routine measures (e.g. gastric lavage), including monitoring of cardiac and respiratory functions. Position the patient to avoid cerebral anoxia. Frequent blood pressure determinations are essential. Vasopressors are clinically indicated for patients exhibiting the effects of calcium entry blockade.

Pharmacological properties

Pharmacodynamic properties

Mode of action: Cardene is a potent calcium channel blocker. Pharmacological studies suggest it is highly selective for the peripheral vasculature over the myocardium, accounting for its minimal negative inotropic effects and marked peripheral vasodilatation when used clincally.

In mild to moderate hypertensive patients, Cardene SR has been shown to reduce blood pressure and maintain control over 24 hours, only if the doses are regularly administered exactly 12 hours apart.

Electrophysiological effects: Electrophysiological studies in man show that Cardene does not depress sinus node function or atrial or ventricular conduction in patients with either normal or diseased electrical conduction systems. Refractory periods of the His-Purkinje system were actually shortened slightly by nicardipine and SA conduction time was improved.

Pharmacokinetic properties: Cardene Capsules are completely absorbed with plasma levels detectable 20 minutes following an oral dose. Maximal plasma levels are generally achieved between one and four hours. Cardene SR is subject to saturable first pass metabolism with somewhat lower bioavailability than the standard capsule formulation of nicardipine (about 35% following a 30 mg oral standard capsule at steady state) except at the 60 mg dose. Minimum plasma levels produced by equivalent daily doses are similar. Cardene SR thus exhibits significantly reduced fluctuation in plasma levels in comparison to standard nicardipine capsules.

When Cardene SR is taken with a high fat meal, fluctuation in plasma levels are reduced.

Cardene is extensively metabolised by the liver; none of the metabolites possess significant biological activity.

Preclinical safety data: Please refer to *Pregnancy and lactation.*

Pharmaceutical particulars

List of excipients:

Pregelatinised starch BP, Magnesium stearate BP, Microcrystalline cellulose BP, Starch EP, Lactose EP, Methacrylic acid co-polymer US NF.

Incompatibilities: None known.

Shelf life: 60 months.

Special precautions for storage: Protect from light and excessive humidity. Store below 25°C.

Nature and contents of container:

Blister packs of 56.

Blister packs of 14.

Securitainers of 100.

Instructions for use/handling: No special instructions required.

Administration data

Marketing authorisation holder: Yamanouchi Pharma Ltd, Yamanouchi House, Pyrford Road, West Byfleet, Surrey KT14 6RA.

Marketing authorisation number PL 00166/0183

Date of first authorisation/renewal of authorisation 1 July 1998

Date of (partial) revision of text March 1997.

CARDENE SR 45

Qualitative and quantitative composition Nicardipine 45 mg.

Pharmaceutical form Sustained release capsules.

Clinical particulars

Therapeutic indications: Treatment of mild to moderate hypertension.

Posology and method of administration:

Adults:

Starting dose: 30 mg every 12 hours titrating upwards as required.

Usual effective dose: 45 mg every 12 hours (range 30 to 60 mg every 12 hours).

Individually adjust the dose for each patient. Where appropriate Cardene SR may also be used in combination with beta-blockers and/or diuretics.

Use in the elderly:
Starting dose: 30 mg every 12 hours. Titrate upwards with care as nicardipine may lower systolic pressure more than diastolic pressure in these patients.

Children: Cardene SR is not recommended for use in patients under the age of 18.

Contra-indications:
i). Use in pregnancy and lactation.
ii). Hypersensitivity to nicardipine hydrochloride or other dihydropyridines because of the theoretical risk of cross reactivity.
iii). As part of the effect of nicardipine is secondary to reduced afterload, the drug should not be given to patients with advanced aortic stenosis. Reduction in diastolic pressure in these patients may worsen rather than improve myocardial oxygen balance.
iv). Cardene should not be used in cardiogenic shock, clinically significant aortic stenosis, and during or within one month of a myocardial infarction.
v). Cardene should not be used for the secondary prevention of myocardial infarction.

Special warnings and special precautions for use: If used in combination with diuretics or beta-blockers, careful titration of Cardene SR is advised to avoid excessive reduction in blood pressure.

If switching from beta-blockers to Cardene SR, gradually reduce the beta-blocker dose (preferably over 8–10 days) since nicardipine gives no protection against the dangers of abrupt beta-blocker withdrawal.

Stop Cardene SR in patients experiencing ischaemic pain within 30 minutes of starting therapy or after increasing the dose.

Use in patients with congestive heart failure or poor cardiac reserve: Haemodynamic studies in patients with heart failure have shown that nicardipine reduces afterload and improves overall haemodynamics. In one study, intravenous nicardipine reduced myocardial contractility in patients with severe heart failure despite increases in cardiac index and ejection fraction noted in the same patients.

Since nicardipine has not been extensively studied in patients with severe left ventricular dysfunction and cardiac failure, one must consider that worsening of cardiac failure may occur.

Use in patients with impaired hepatic or renal function: Since Cardene is subject to first pass metabolism, use with caution in patients with impaired liver function or reduced hepatic blood flow. Patients with severe liver disease showed elevated blood levels and the half-life of nicardipine was prolonged. Cardene blood levels may also be elevated in some renally-impaired patients. Therefore, the lowest starting dose and extending the dosing interval should be individually considered in these patients.

Use in patients following a stroke (infarction or haemorrhage): Avoid inducing systemic hypotension when administering Cardene SR to these patients.

Laboratory tests: Transient elevations of alkaline phosphatase, serum bilirubin, SGPT, SGOT and glucose, have been observed. BUN and creatinine may also become elevated. While out-of-range values were seen in T_3, T_4 and TSH, the lack of consistent alterations suggest that any changes were not drug-related.

Treatment with short acting nicardipine may induce an exaggerated fall in blood pressure and reflex tachycardia which can cause cardiovascular complications such as myocardial and cerebrovascular ischaemia.

There has been some concern about increased mortality and morbidity in the treatment of ischaemic heart disease using higher than recommended doses of some other short-acting dihydropyridines.

Interactions with other medicaments and other forms of interaction
Digoxin: Careful monitoring of serum digoxin levels is advised in patients also receiving Cardene as levels may be increased.

Propanolol, Dipyridamole, Warfarin, Quinidine, Naproxen: Therapeutic concentrations of these drugs does not change the *in vitro* plasma protein binding of nicardipine.

Cimetidine: Cimetidine increases nicardipine plasma levels. Carefully monitor patients receiving both drugs.

Fentanyl anaesthesia: Severe hypotension has been reported during fentanyl anaesthesia with concomitant use of a beta-blocker and calcium blockade. Even though such interactions have not been seen in clinical trials, such hypotensive episodes should be vigorously treated with conventional therapy such as intravenous fluids.

Cyclosporin: Monitor cyclosporin plasma levels and reduce dosage accordingly in patients concomitantly receiving nicardipine as elevated cyclosporin levels have been reported.

Rifampicin: Rifampicin can interact with other dihydropyridines to substantially reduce their plasma levels and so rifampicin and nicardipine should be used together with caution.

As with other dihydropyridines, nicardipine should not be taken with grapefruit juice because bioavailability may be increased.

Cardene may be used in combination with beta-blocking and other anti-hypertensive drugs but the possibility of an additive effect resulting in postural hypotension should be considered.

Pregnancy and lactation: See *Contra-indications.*

Effects on ability to drive and use machines: None known.

Undesirable effects: Most are expected consequences of the vasodilator effects of Cardene SR.

The most frequent side-effects reported are headache, pedal oedema, heat sensation and/or flushing, palpitations, nausea and dizziness.

Other side-effects noted in clinical trials include the following:

Cardiovascular system: as with the use of other sustained-release dihydropyridines in patients with ischaemic heart disease, exacerbation of angina pectoris may occur rarely at the start of treatment with Cardene SR. The occurrence of myocardial infarction has been reported although it is not possible to distinguish such an event from the natural course of ischaemic heart disease.

Central nervous system: drowsiness, insomnia, tinnitus, paraesthesiae, functional disorders.

Skin: itching, rashes.

Hepato-renal: impairment, frequency of micturition.

Dyspnoea, gastro-intestinal upset and, rarely, depression, impotence and thrombocytopenia, have also been reported.

Overdose: Symptoms may include marked hypotension, bradycardia, palpitations, flushing, drowsiness, confusion and slurred speech. In laboratory animals, overdosage also resulted in reversible hepatic function abnormalities, sporadic focal hepatic necrosis and progressive atrioventricular conduction block.

Use routine measures (e.g. gastric lavage), including monitoring of cardiac and respiratory functions. Position the patient to avoid cerebral anoxia. Frequent blood pressure determinations are essential. Vasopressors are clinically indicated for patients exhibiting the effects of calcium entry blockade.

Pharmacological properties
Pharmacodynamic properties
Mode of action: Cardene is a potent calcium channel blocker. Pharmacological studies suggest it is highly selective for the peripheral vasculature over the myocardium, accounting for its minimal negative inotropic effects and marked peripheral vasodilatation when used clincally.

In mild to moderate hypertensive patients, Cardene SR has been shown to reduce blood pressure and maintain control over 24 hours, only if the doses are regularly administered exactly 12 hours apart.

Electrophysiological effects: Electrophysiological studies in man show that Cardene does not depress sinus node function or atrial or ventricular conduction in patients with either normal or diseased electrical conduction systems. Refractory periods of the His-Purkinje system were actually shortened slightly by nicardipine and SA conduction time was improved.

Pharmacokinetic properties: Cardene Capsules are completely absorbed with plasma levels detectable 20 minutes following an oral dose. Maximal plasma levels are generally achieved between one and four hours. Cardene SR is subject to saturable first pass metabolism with somewhat lower bioavailability than the standard capsule formulation of nicardipine (about 35% following a 30 mg oral standard capsule at steady state) except at the 60 mg dose. Minimum plasma levels produced by equivalent daily doses are similar. Cardene SR thus exhibits significantly reduced fluctuation in plasma levels in comparison to standard nicardipine capsules.

When Cardene SR is taken with a high fat meal, fluctuation in plasma levels are reduced.

Cardene is extensively metabolised by the liver; none of the metabolites possess significant biological activity.

Preclinical safety data: Please refer to *Pregnancy and lactation.*

Pharmaceutical particulars
List of excipients:
Pregelatinised starch BP, Magnesium stearate BP, Microcrystalline cellulose BP, Starch EP, Lactose EP, Methacrylic acid co-polymer US NF.

Incompatibilities: None known.

Shelf life: 60 months.

Special precautions for storage: Protect from light and excessive humidity. Store below 25°C.

Nature and contents of container:
Blister packs of 56.
Blister packs of 14.
Securitainers of 100.

Instructions for use/handling: No special instructions required.

Administration data
Marketing authorisation holder: Yamanouchi Pharma Ltd, Yamanouchi House, Pyrford Road, West Byfleet, Surrey KT14 6RA.

Marketing authorisation number PL 00166/0184

Date of first authorisation/renewal of authorisation 1 July 1998

Date of (partial) revision of text March 1997.

CONOTRANE* CREAM

Qualitative and quantitative composition A smooth white cream containing benzalkonium chloride 0.1% w/w and Dimethicone 350 BP 22.0% w/w.

Pharmaceutical form Cream for topical administration.

Clinical particulars
Therapeutic indications: Conotrane is used for protection of the skin from moisture, irritants, chafing and contamination with bacteria or yeasts.

It may be used in situations such as in the prevention/treatment of napkin rash, the prevention of pressure sores and in the management of incontinence.

Posology and method of administration: The cream should be applied to the affected area several times a day, as necessary or after every napkin change.

Contra-indications: Known hypersensitivity to benzalkonium chloride.

Special warnings and precautions for use: None stated.

Interaction with other medicaments and other forms of interaction: None stated.

Pregnancy and lactation: Not applicable.

Effects on ability to drive and use machines: None stated.

Undesirable effects: Local hypersensitivity to benzalkonium chloride is rare.

Overdose: Not applicable.

Pharmacological properties
Pharmacodynamic properties: This is a remedy suitable for both prescription and for self medication. It is a cream for topical application containing dimethicone and benzalkonium chloride. The dimethicone is water repellent allowing transpiration of water vapour from the skin. The benzalkonium chloride is a quaternary ammonium compound, active against bacteria and yeasts.

Pharmacokinetic properties: Not applicable.

Preclinical safety data: None stated.

Pharmaceutical particulars
List of excipients: Cetostearyl alcohol, Cetomacrogol 1000, White soft paraffin, Light liquid paraffin, Deionised water, Macrogol 300, Potassium dihydrogen orthophosphate, Geranium SC45

Incompatibilities: None stated.

Shelf life: 3 years.

Special precautions for storage: Store in a cool place.

Nature and contents of container:
(i) 7 g, 15 g, 50 g, and 100 g in white LDPE tubes.
(ii) 500 g white polypropylene pot with screw lid.

Instructions for use/handling: None stated.

Administration data
Marketing authorisation holder: Yamanouchi Pharma Ltd, Yamanouchi House, Pyrford Road, West Byfleet, Surrey KT14 6RA.

Marketing authorisation number PL 00166/0178

Date of first authorisation/renewal of authorisation 1 July 1998

Date of (partial) revision of the text March 1996

Legal category GSL.

DE-NOL*

Presentation De-Nol is presented as a clear red liquid containing 120 mg tri-potassium di-citrato bismuthate (calculated as Bi_2O_3) in each 5 ml. The inactive ingredients in De-Nol include ethanol and sucrose.

Uses Ulcer healing agent. For the treatment of gastric and duodenal ulcers.

Dosage and administration By oral administration. Each dose is to be diluted with 15 ml of water.

Adults and the elderly: Two 5 ml spoonsful twice daily (half an hour before breakfast and half an hour before the evening meal). Alternatively, one 5 ml spoonful four times a day (half an hour before each of the three main meals of the day and two hours after the evening meal). The treatment course should be taken for the full 28-day period and it is important that a dose is not missed. If necessary, one further course of therapy may be given. Maintenance therapy with De-Nol is not indicated, but treatment may be repeated after an interval of one month.

Children: Not recommended.

Milk should not be drunk by itself during the course of treatment as this can prevent the medicine from working properly. Small quantities of milk on breakfast cereal or in tea or coffee taken with meals are permissible. Antacids should not be taken for half an hour before or half an hour after taking a dose of De-Nol as these can interfere with the action of the drug.

Contra-indications, warnings, etc
Contra-indications: De-Nol should not be administered to patients with renal disorders, and on theoretical grounds is contra-indicated in pregnancy.

Interactions: De-Nol may inhibit the efficacy of orally administered tetracyclines.

Side effects: Blackening of the stool usually occurs; darkening of the tongue, nausea and vomiting have been reported.

Overdosage: Extremely few cases of overdosage have occurred; contact the company for further information.

Pharmaceutical precautions Normal pharmaceutical storage and handling are indicated.

Legal category P.

Package quantities Treatment pack of 560 ml as an original pack (OP).

Further information Some patients with an associated gastritis may experience an initial discomfort whilst taking De-Nol. Each 5 ml dose contains ca 100 mg ethanol and 500 mg sucrose.

Product licence number 0166/5024.

DE-NOLTAB*

Qualitative and quantitative composition Tri-potassium di-citrato bismuthate HSE 120 mg (as Bi_2O_3).

Pharmaceutical form Tablet.

Clinical particulars
Therapeutic indications: For the treatment of gastric and duodenal ulcers.

Posology and method of administration:
For adults and the elderly: One tablet to be taken four times a day, half an hour before each of the three main meals and two hours after the last meal of the day, or two tablets to be taken twice daily, half an hour before breakfast and half an hour before the evening meal, or as directed by the physician.

The maximum duration for one course of treatment is two months; De-Noltab should not be used for maintenance therapy.

For children: Not recommended.

Contra-indications: In cases of severe renal insufficiency.

Special warnings and precautions for use: None stated.

Interactions with other medicaments and other forms of interaction: The efficacy of oral tetracyclines may be inhibited.

Pregnancy and lactation: On theoretical grounds De-Noltab is contraindicated in pregnancy. No information is available on excretion in breast milk.

Effects on ability to drive and use machines: None reported.

Undesirable effects: Blackening of the stool usually occurs; nausea and vomiting have been reported.

Overdose: Extremely few cases of overdose have been reported; contact the company for further information.

Pharmacological properties
Pharmacodynamic properties: The active constituent exerts a local healing effect at the ulcer site, and by eradication or reduction of *Helicobacter pylori* defers relapse.

Pharmacokinetic properties: The action is local in the gastro-intestinal tract.

Preclinical safety data: No relevant pre-clinical safety data has been generated.

Pharmaceutical particulars
List of excipients: potassium citrate, ammonium citrate, povidone K 30, amberlite IRP-S8, polyethylene glycol 6000, magnesium stearate, maize starch, hypromellose.

Incompatibilities: None.

Shelf life: Four years.

Special precautions for storage: None.

Nature and contents of container: Amber glass bottles and/or aluminium foil strips, containing 112 tablets.

Instructions for use/handling: None.

Marketing authorisation number 0166/0124.

Date of approval/revision of SPC 20 January 1997.

Legal category P.

DERMAMIST*

Presentation A pressurised aerosol delivering White Soft Paraffin BP 10% as a clear colourless spray. Dermamist also contains Liquid Paraffin BP and Fractionated Coconut Oil BP, with butane/isobutane/propane as propellant.

Uses Dermamist is indicated for the treatment of dry skin conditions including pruritus of the elderly, eczema and ichthyosis by topical application.

Dosage and administration
For adults, children and the elderly: Shake before use. Bathe or shower for not more than ten minutes. Pat dry and apply spray without delay. Do not spray on face. Spray from a distance of approximately 8 inches. Spray away from the face and move the can quickly while spraying to give a very light coverage of the body. Spray sparingly; over application may cause the skin to feel oily.

Contra-indications, warnings, etc Do not use if sensitive to any of the ingredients. For external use only. Keep out of reach of children. Do not spray on face. Use in a ventilated area. Avoid inhalation. Guard against slipping. Do not apply to broken skin. Discontinue use if the condition is made worse. Do not spray on a naked flame or incandescent material.

Pharmaceutical precautions Store below 25°C. Highly flammable; pressurised container. Protect from sunlight. Do not puncture, burn or expose to temperature over 50°C (122°F) even when empty.

Legal category P.

Package quantities 250 ml canister.

Further information Nil.

Product licence number 13147/0001

Product licence holder: Caraderm Ltd, Pine Valley, Rostrevor, Co. Down, Northern Ireland BT34 3DE.

DISIPAL* TABLETS

Qualitative and quantitative composition
Orphenadrine Hydrochloride BP 50 mg.

Pharmaceutical form Tablet.

Clinical particulars
Therapeutic indications: Anti-cholinergic, for the treatment of all forms of Parkinsonism, including drug-induced extra-pyramidal symptoms (neuroleptic syndrome).

Posology and method of administration:
For adults, and the elderly: Initially 150 mg daily in divided doses, increasing by 50 mg every two or three days until maximum benefit is obtained. Optimal dosage is usually 250–300 mg daily in divided doses in idiopathic and post-encephalitic Parkinsonism, 100–300 mg daily in divided doses in the neuroleptic syndrome. Maximal dosage, 400 mg daily in divided doses. The elderly may be more susceptible to side-effects at doses which are clinically optimal.

For children: A dosage for children has not been established.

Contra-indications: Contra-indicated in patients with tardive dyskinesia, glaucoma, or prostatic hypertrophy.

Special warnings and precautions for use: Use with caution in patients with micturition difficulties, in pregnancy, and in the presence of cardiovascular disease and hepatic or renal impairment. Avoid abrupt discontinuation of treatment. For some patients, orphenadrine may be a drug of abuse.

Interactions with other medicaments and other forms of interaction: None stated.

Pregnancy and lactation: No recommendations; if considered necessary, it should be used with caution.

Effects on ability to drive and use machines: None stated.

Undesirable effects: Occasionally dry mouth, disturbances of visual accommodation, gastro-intestinal disturbances, dizziness and micturition difficulties may occur; these usually disappear spontaneously or may be controlled by a slight reduction in dosage. Less commonly, tachycardia, hypersensitivity, nervousness, euphoria and insomnia may be seen.

Overdose: Toxic effects are anti-cholinergic in nature and the treatment is gastric lavage, cholinergics such as carbachol, anti-cholinesterases such as physostigmine, and general non-specific treatment.

Pharmacological properties
Pharmacodynamic properties: Orphenadrine, which is a congener of diphenhydramine without sharing its soporific effect, is an antimuscarinic agent. It also has weak antihistaminic and local anaesthetic properties.

Orphenadrine is used as the hydrochloride in the symptomatic treatment of Parkinsonism. It is also used to alleviate the extrapyramidal syndrome induced by drugs such as the phenothiazine derivatives, but is of no value in tardive dyskinesia, which may be exacerbated.

Pharmacokinetic properties: Orphenadrine is readily absorbed from the gastro-intestinal tract, and very readily absorbed following intramuscular injection. It is rapidly distributed in tissues and most of a dose is metabolised and excreted in the urine along with a small proportion of unchanged drug. A half life of 14 hours has been reported.

Preclinical safety data: No relevant pre-clinical safety data has been generated.

Pharmaceutical particulars
List of excipients: Lactose, Sucrose, Acacia, Maize starch, Tribasic calcium phosphate, Stearic acid, Magnesium stearate, Polyvinylacetatephthalate, Calcium carbonate, Talc, Kaolin, Titanium dioxide, Gelatin, Opalux yellow, White beeswax

Incompatibilities: None.

Shelf life: Three years.

Special precautions for storage: Store at room temperature (15°C–25°C).

Nature and contents of container: Amber glass click-lock bottles and/or securitainers and/or plastic lid-seal containers, containing 100, 250, 1,000, or 10,000 tablets.

Instruction for use/handling: None.

Administrative data
Marketing authorisation holder: Yamanouchi Pharma Ltd, Yamanouchi House, Pyrford Road, West Byfleet, Surrey KT14 6RA.

Marketing authorisation number PL 0166/5001R

Date of first authorisation/renewal of authorisation 6 May 1987/22 May 1997.

Date of (partial) revision of the text 27 January 1997.

FLOMAX* MR

Qualitative and quantitative composition Each capsule contains as active ingredient tamsulosin hydrochloride 400 microgram, equivalent to 367 microgram tamsulosin.

Pharmaceutical form Capsule, modified release.

Clinical particulars
Therapeutic indications: Treatment of functional symptoms of benign prostatic hyperplasia (BPH).

Posology and method of administration: One capsule daily, to be taken after breakfast.

The capsule should be swallowed whole with a drink of water (about 150 ml) in the standing or sitting position.

The capsules should not be crunched or chewed as this will interfere with the modified release of the active ingredient.

Contra-indications: Hypersensitivity to tamsulosin hydrochloride or any other component of the product; a history of orthostatic hypotension; severe hepatic insufficiency.

Special warnings and special precautions for use: As with other $alpha_1$ blockers, a reduction in blood pressure can occur in individual cases during treatment withn Flomax MR., as a result of which, rarely, syncope can occur. At the first signs of orthostatic hypotension (dizziness, weakness) the patient should sit or lie down until the symptoms have disappeared.

Before therapy with Flomax MR is initiated the patient should be examined in order to exclude the presence of other conditions which can cause the same symptoms as benign prostatic hyperplasia. Digital rectal examination and when necessary determination of prostate specific anitigen (PSA) should be performed before treatment and at regular intervals afterwards.

The treatment of severely renally impaired patients (creatinine clearance of less than 10 ml/min) should be approached with caution as these patients have not been studied.

Interactions with other medicaments and other forms of interaction: No interactions have been seen when Flomax MR was given concomitantly with either atenolol, enalapril or nifedrine. Concomitant cimetidine brings about a rise in plasma levels of tamsulosin, and frusemide a fall, but as levels remain within the normal range posology need not be changed.

In vitro neither diazepam nor propanolol, trichlormethiazide, chlormadinon, amitryptyline, diclofenac, glibenclamide, simvastin, and warfarin change the free fraction of tamsulosin in human plasma. Neither does tamsulosin change the free fractions of diazepam, propanolol, trichlormethiazide, and chlormadinon.

No interactions at the level of hepatic metabolism have been seen during *in vitro* studies with liver microsomal fractions (representitave of the cytochrome P_{450}-linked drug metabolising enzyme system), involving amitriptyline, salbutamol, glibenclamide and finasteride. Diclofenac and warfarin, however, may increase the elimination rate of tamsulosin.

Concurrent administration of other α_1-adrenoceptor antagonists could lead to hypotensive effects.

Pregnancy and lactation: Not applicable as Flomax MR is intended for male patients only.

Effects on ability to drive and use machines: No data is available on whether Flomax MR adversely affects the ability to drive or operate machines. However, in this respect patients should be aware of the fact that dizziness can occur.

Undesirable effects: The following adverse reactions have been reported during the use of Flomax MR: dizziness, abnormal ejaculation and, less frequently (1–2%) headache, asthenia, postural hypotension and palpitations.

Gastrointestinal reactions such as nausea, vomiting, diarrhoea, and constipation can occasionally occur. Hypersensitivity reactions such as rash, pruritus, and urticaria can occur occasionally; angiodema has been rarely reported.

Syncope has been reported rarely.

Overdose: No cases of acute overdosage have been reported. However, acute hypotension could theoretically occur after overdosage in which case cardiovascular support should be given. Blood pressure can be restored and heart rate brought back to normal by lying the patient down. If this does not help then volume expanders, and when necessary, vasopressors could be employed. Renal function should be monitored and general supportive measures applied. Dialysis is unlikely to be of help as tamsulosin is very highly bound to plasma proteins.

Measures, such as emesis, can be taken to impede absorption. When large quantities are involved, gastric lavage can be applied and activated charcoal and an osmotic laxative, such as sodium sulphate, can be administered.

Pharmacological properties

Pharmacodynamic properties: Pharmacotherapeutic group: Alpha$_1$-adrenoceptor antagonist. Preparations for the exclusive treatment of prostatic disease.

Mechanism of action: Tamsulosin binds selectively and competitively to postsynaptic alpha$_1$-receptors, in particular to the subtype alpha$_{1A}$, which bring about contraction of the smooth musle of the prostate, whereby tension is reduced.

Pharmacodynamic effects: Flomax MR increases maximum urinary flow rate by reducing smooth muscle tension in prostate and urethra and thereby relieving obstruction.

It also improves the complex of irritative and obstructive symptoms in which bladder instability and tension of the smooth muscles of the lower urinary tract play an important role.

Alpha$_1$-blockers can reduce blood pressure by lowering peripheral resistance. No reduction in blood pressure of any clinical significance was observed during studies with Flomax MR.

Pharmacokinetic properties: Absorption: Tamsulosin is absorbed from the intestine and is almost completely bioavailable.

Absorption of tamsulosin is reduced by a recent meal.

Uniformity of absorption can be promoted by the patient always taking Flomax MR after the usual breakfast.

Tamsulosin shows linear kinetics.

After a single dose of Flomax MR in the fed state, plasma levels of tamsulosin peak at around 6 hours and, in the steady state, which is reached by day 5 of multiple dosing, C_{max} in patients is about two thirds higher than that reached after a single dose. Although this was seen in elderly patients, the same finding would also be expected in young ones.

There is a considerable inter-patient variation in plasma levels both after single and multiple dosing.

Distribution: In man, tamsulosin is about 99% bound to plasma proteins and volume of distribution is small (about 0.2 l/kg).

Biotransformation: Tamsulosin has a low first pass effect, being metabolised slowly. Most tamsulosin is present in plasma in the form of unchanged drug. It is metabolised in the liver.

In rats, hardly any induction of microsomal liver enzymes was seen to be caused by tamsulosin.

No dose adjustment is warranted in hepatic insufficiency.

None of the metabolites are more active than the original compound.

Excretion: Tamsulosin and its metabolites are mainly excreted in the urine with about 9% of a dose being present in the form of unchanged drug.

After a single dose of Flomax MR in the fed state, and in the steady state in patients, elimination half-lives of about 10 and 13 hours respectively have been measured.

The presence of renal impairment does not warrant lowering the dose.

Preclinical safety data: Single and repeat dose toxicity studies were performed in mice, rats and dogs. In addition reproduction toxicity studies were performed in rats, carcinogenicity in mice and rats and *in vivo* and *in vitro* genotoxicity were examined. The general toxicity profile as seen with high doses of tamsulosin is consistent with the known pharmacological actions of the alpha-adrenergic blocking agents. At very high dose levels the ECG was altered in dogs. This response is considered to be not clinically relevant. Tamsulosin showed no relevant genotoxic properties.

Increased incidences of proliferative changes of mammary glands of female rats and mice have been reported. These findings which are probably mediated by hyperprolactinaemia and only occurred at high dose levels are regarded as irrelevant.

Pharmaceutical particulars

List of excipients: Flomax MR modified release capsules contain the following excipients: microcrystalline cellulose, methylacrylic acid copolymer, polysorbate 80, sodium lauryl sulphate, triacetin, calcium stearate, talc, hard gelatin, indigotine E132, titanium dioxide E171, yellow iron oxide E172 and red iron oxide E172.

Incompatibilities: None known.

Shelf life as packaged for sale: Flomax MR modified release capsules can be used up to four years after manufacture. The expiry date is printed on the package.

Special precautions for storage: None.

Nature and contents of container: Strips containing 10 capsules per strip; one, two, or three strips in a cardboard box.

Instructions for use/handling: No special instructions.

Marketing authorisation number MA 0166/0171.

Date of first authorisation/renewal of authorisation 16 April 1996.

Date of (partial) revision of the text 28 July 1998.

HERPID*

Qualitative and quantitative composition A clear, colourless solution containing idoxuridine BP 5% in dimethyl sulphoxide.

Pharmaceutical form Topical Solution.

Clinical particulars

Therapeutic indications: Cutaneous herpes simplex and herpes zoster (shingles).

Posology and method of administration:

Adults and children over 12 years: Herpid should be painted on the lesions and their erythematous bases four times daily for four days. Treatment should start as soon as the condition has been diagnosed, ideally within two to three days after the rash appears. Good results are less likely if treatment is not started within seven days.

Children under 12 years: The use of Herpid in children with malignant disease might be justified but, although not a contra-indication, its use in children under the age of 12 years is not recommended.

No specific information on the use of this product in the elderly is available. Clinical trials have included patients over 65 years and no adverse reactions specific to this age group have been reported.

Contra-indications: Known hypersensitivity to either idoxuridine or dimethyl sulphoxide.

Dermographia.

Special warnings and special precautions for use: Herpid in the eye causes stinging: treat by washing out with water.

Interaction with other medicaments and other forms of interaction: Since the solvent in Herpid can increase the absorption of many substances it is important that no other topical medication be used on the same areas of skin treated with Herpid.

Pregnancy and lactation: Animal studies have shown idoxuridine to be teratogenic. Consequently, Herpid should not be prescribed for women who are pregnant or at risk of becoming pregnant. In a small number of cases of women who used Herpid inadvertently in early pregnancy and who were followed to term, the infant was normal in each case.

Effect on ability to drive and use machines: None.

Undesirable effects: Patients often experience stinging when applying Herpid and a distinctive taste during a course of treatment; both effects are transient.

Skin reactions have occasionally been reported.

Over-usage of the solution may lead to maceration of the skin.

Overdosage: There is no clinical experience of overdosage. Standard supportive measures should be adopted.

Pharmacodynamic properties Idoxuridine is an antiviral agent which act by blocking the uptake of thymidine into the deoxyribonucleic acid (DNA) of the virus and inhibits replication of viruses such as adenovirus, cytomegalovirus, herpes simplex (herpes virus hominus), varicella zoster or herpes zoster (herpes virus varicella) and vaccinia. It has no action against latent forms of the virus. It does not inhibit RNA viruses such as influenza virus or poliovirus.

Pharmacokinetc properties: The idoxuridine dissolves in dimethyl sulphoxide which penetrates the skin and carries the antiviral agent to the deeper levels of the epidermis where the virus is replicating.

Idoxuridine is rapidly metabolised in the body to iodouracil, uracil and iodine which are rapidly excreted in the urine.

Pharmaceutical particulars

List of excipients: Dimethyl sulphoxide.

Incompatibilities: None stated.

Shelf life: 5 years.

Special precautions for storage: Herpid should be stored in its box below 25°C. Do not refrigerate as the contents of the bottle may solidify. If crystals do form, allow to redissolve before use by warming the bottle gently (in the palm of the hand) until the solution is clear. Because the solution is hygroscopic, any remaining after completion of treatment should be discarded.

Nature and contents of container: 5 ml bottle with brush (OP):

Bottle:	Type III amber glass
Cap liner:	high density natural polyethylene
Brush stem:	low density natural polyethylene

Instructions for use/handling:

1) Carefully unscrew the white cap and discard. Replace it with the black cap and brush.

2) Apply the liquid sparingly with the brush 4 times a day to the affected area of skin. It is important to treat only the affected areas.

3) Wash your hands thoroughly after using Herpid.

4) Do not continue a course of treatment on one area of skin for more than four days.

5) Discard any solution remaining in the bottle as soon as the treatment period is complete.

Herpid can damage some synthetic materials (e.g. artificial silk and Terylene) and printed cotton fabrics. Contact between Herpid and these materials should therefore be avoided.

Marketing authorisation number PL 00166/0177

Date of first authorisation/renewal of authorisation
Date of first authorisation: 13.03.74
Date of latest renewal: 29.03.95

Date of partial revision of the text September 1998.

LIPOBASE*

Qualitative and quantitative composition Lipobase contains no active ingredient.

Pharmaceutical form Cream.

Clinical particulars

Therapeutic indications: For use where it is desired by the physician to reduce gradually the topical dosage of Locoid Lipocream. It may also be used where a continuously alternating application of the active product and the base is required e.g. in prophylactic therapy. Application of the Lipobase is also recommended where it is felt by the physician that the use of a bland emollient base is preferable to the cessation of therapy with the active product. Lipobase may also be used as diluent for the active product in those cases where dilution is regarded as necessary by the prescriber. Lipobase may also be used other than in conjunction with a topical corticosteroid for its emollient action, and for the treatment of mild skin lesions such as pruritus or dry, scaly skin, where topical corticosteroid therapy is not warranted.

Posology and method of administration:
For adults, children and the elderly: Lipobase may be used either by replacing an application of the active product or alternating the application of the active product and the base, gradually diminishing the application of active product until therapy ceases, or by the application of the product for its emollient action.

Contra-indications: None stated.

Special warnings and special precautions for use: None stated.

Interaction with other medicaments and other forms of interaction: None stated.

Pregnancy and lactation: None stated.

Effects on ability to drive and use machines: None stated.

Undesirable effects: None stated.

Overdose: None stated.

Pharmacological properties
Pharmacodynamic properties: The product acts topically as an emollient cream.

Pharmacokinetic properties: Topical administration with no pharmacologically active constituents.

Preclinical safety data: No relevant preclinical safety data has been generated.

Pharmaceutical particulars
List of excipients: Cetostearyl alchol BP, Cetomacrogol 1000 BP, Liquid paraffin BP, White soft paraffin BP, Methyl parahydroxybenzoate EP, Sodium citrate (anhydrous) USP, Citric acid (anhydrous) EP, Purified water EP

Incompatibilities: None stated.

Shelf life: 5 years.

Special precautions for storage: Store at room temperature (not more than 25°C).

Nature and contents of container: Collapsible aluminium tube with plastic screw cap containing 30 g, 50 g, 100 g or 200 g, and pump dispenser containing 200 g or 500 g.

Instructions for use/handling: Not applicable.

Administrative data
Marketing authorisation holder: Yamanouchi Pharma Ltd, Yamanouchi House, Pyrford Road, West Byfleet, Surrey KT14 6RA.

Marketing authorisation number PL 0166/0125.

Date of first authorisation/renewal of authorisation
First authorisation granted 19 February 1985.
Renewal granted 27 March 1995.

Date of (partial) revision of the text 21 February 1995.

LOCOID* CREAM LOCOID* OINTMENT

Presentation Locoid Cream, containing 0.1% hydrocortisone 17-butyrate in a cream base. The inactive constituents in Locoid Cream are cetostearyl alcohol, cetomacrogol, liquid paraffin, white soft paraffin, propyl paraben, butyl paraben, citric acid, sodium citrate, and purified water.

Locoid Ointment, containing 0.1% hydrocortisone 17-butyrate in an ointment base. The inactive constituents in Locoid Ointment are liquid paraffin and polyethylene.

Uses Eczema and dermatitis of all types including atopic eczema, photodermatitis, primary irritant and allergic dermatitis, lichen planus, lichen simplex, prurigo nodularis, discoid lupus erythematosus, necrobiosis lipoidica, pretibial myxoedema and erythematosus psoriasis of the scalp, chronic plaque psoriasis of the palms and soles, and other forms of psoriasis (excluding widespread plaque psoriasis).

Dosage and administration Apply a small quantity to the affected part two or three times daily. Application may be made under occlusion in the more resistant lesions such as thickened psoriatic plaques on elbows and knees.

Contra-indications, warnings, etc
Contra-indications: Facial rosacea, acne vulgaris, perioral dermatitis, perianal and genital pruritus, napkin eruptions, bacterial (e.g. impetigo), viral (e.g. herpes simplex) and fungal (e.g. candida or dermatophyte) infections.

Side-effects: Local and systemic toxicity is common especially following long continued use on large areas of damaged skin, in flexures and with polythene occlusion. If used in childhood, or on the face, courses should be limited to 5 days and occlusion should not be used. Local irritation may occur in those with a hypersensitivity to parabens.

Use in pregnancy and lactation: There is inadequate evidence of safety in human pregnancy. Topical administration of corticosteroids to pregnant animals can cause abnormalities of fetal development including cleft plate and intra-uterine growth retardation. There may therefore be a very small risk of such effects in the human fetus.

Other warnings and precautions: Long term continuous therapy should be avoided in all patients irrespective of age. Application under occlusion should be restricted to dermatoses involving limited areas.

Topical corticosteroids may be hazardous in psoriasis for a number of reasons including rebound relapses following development of tolerance, risk of generalised pustular psoriasis and local and systemic toxicity due to impaired barrier function of the skin. Steroids may have a place in psoriasis of the scalp and chronic plaque psoriasis of the hands and feet. Careful patient supervision is important.

Overdosage: Overdosage would result in the topical and systemic signs and symptoms associated with high corticosteroid dosage. If overdosage should occur, treatment should not stop immediately but be gradually withdrawn. Adrenal insufficiency may need therapy with intravenous hydrocortisone. It should be noted that overdosage of this topical corticosteroid product would be unlikely to occur other than as a result of severe and prolonged abuse of product.

Pharmaceutical precautions Store at room temperature (15–25°C).

Legal category POM.

Package quantities *Locoid Cream:* Tubes of 30 g and 100 g as original packs (OP).

Locoid Ointment: Tubes of 30 g and 100 g as original packs (OP).

Further information Locoid is a non-fluorinated topical steroid. Whilst clinical trials have shown it to be as effective as the potent fluorinated steroids, in clinical practice there is a low incidence of reported clinical side-effects.

Product licence numbers
Locoid Cream 0166/0058
Locoid Ointment 0166/0059

LOCOID CRELO*

Qualitative and quantitative composition Hydrocortisone butyrate 0.1% (w/w).

Pharmaceutical form Topical emulsion.

Clinical particulars
Therapeutic indications: The product is recommended for clinical use in the treatment of conditions responsive to topical corticosteroids, e.g. eczema, dermatitis and psoriasis. The product is intended for topical application especially to the scalp, hirsute or facial skin.

Posology and method of administration: Adults, children and the elderly: A small quantity to be applied two or three times a day, only sufficient to cover the affected area. The formulation of the product makes it suitable for use in both scaly lesions and for moist, weeping lesions. Replace the cap firmly after use.

Contra-indications: Contra-indicated in the presence of bacterial (e.g. impetigo), viral (e.g. herpes simplex), fungal (e.g. candida or dermatophyte), infections.

Special warnings and special precautions for use: Avoid contact with the eyes. Although generally regarded as safe, even for long-term administration in adults, there is a potential for overdosage in infancy. Extreme caution is required in dermatoses of infancy including napkin eruption. In such patients, courses of treatment should not normally exceed 7 days.

Interactions with other medicaments and other forms of interaction: None known.

Pregnancy and lactation: There is inadequate evidence of safety in human pregnancy. Topical administration of corticosteroids to pregnant animals can cause abnormalities of fetal development including cleft palate and intra-uterine growth retardation. There may therefore be a very small risk of such effects in the human fetus. The use of topical corticosteroids during lactation is unlikely to present a hazard to infants being breast-fed.

Effects on ability to drive and use machines: None known.

Undesirable effects: Locoid Crelo is usually well tolerated; if signs of hypersensitivity do occur, treatment should be ceased.

In naturally occluded or moist areas of the skin, especially in small children, where absorption may be favoured, unduly prolonged therapy may give rise to systemic side-effects.

Overdose: Overdosage would result in the topical and systemic signs and symptoms associated with high corticosteroid dosage. If overdosage should occur, treatment should not stop immediately but be gradually withdrawn. Adrenal insufficiency may need therapy with intravenous hydrocortisone. It should be noted that overdosage of this topical corticosteroid product would be unlikely to occur other than as a result of severe and prolonged abuse of the product.

Pharmacological properties
Pharmacodynamic properties: The active constituent, hydrocortisone butyrate, is an established topical corticosteroid, equi-efficacious with those corticosteroids classified as potent.

Pharmacokinetic properties: In human in-vivo studies, the potency of this form of active ingredient has been shown to be of the same order as other topical corticosteroids classed as potent. The active ingredient metabolises to hydrocortisone and butyric acid.

Preclinical safety data: The well-established use of hydrocortisone 17-butyrate topical preparations over many years does not warrant further safety evaluation studies in animals.

Pharmaceutical particulars
List of excipients: Cetomacrogol 1000 BP, Cetostearyl Alcohol PhEur, White Soft Paraffin BP, Hard Paraffin HSE, Borage Oil HSE, Butylhydroxytoluene PhEur, Propyleneglycol PhEur, Sodium Citrate HSE, Anhydrous Citric Acid PhEur, Propyl Parahydroxybenzoate PhEur, Butyl Hydroxybenzoate BP, Purified Water PhEur.

Incompatibilities: None known.

Shelf life: 2 years.

Special precautions for storage: Room temperature (15°C–25°C).

Nature and contents of container: White opaque low density polyethylene bottles of 100 g capacity, equipped with a natural low density polyethylene dropper applicator, closed with a white polypropylene screw cap.

Instructions for use/handling: No special instructions.

Marketing authorisation number 0166/0170

Date of approval/revision of SPC April 1995.

Legal category POM.

LOCOID LIPOCREAM*

Qualitative and quantitative composition Hydrocortisone 17-butyrate USP 01.% w/w.

Pharmaceutical form Cream.

Clincial particulars
Therapeutic indications: The product is recommended for topical treatment of corticosteroid sensitive dermatoses, such as eczema, dermatitis and psoriasis.

Posology and method of administration:
For Adults, children and the elderly: Apply a small quantity only sufficient to cover the affected area two or three times a day, or as directed by the prescriber.

Due to the formulation of the base the product may be used both for dry scaly lesions and for moist or weeping lesions.

Contra-indications: This preparation is contra-indicated in the presence of bacterial (e.g. impetigo), viral (e.g. herpes simplex), or fungal (e.g. candida or dermatophyte) infections.

Special warnings and precautions for use: Although generally regarded as safe, even for long-term administration in adults, there is a potential for overdosage in infancy. Extreme caution is required in dermatoses of infancy including napkin eruption. In such patients, courses of treatment should not normally exceed seven days.

Interactions with other medicaments and other forms of interaction: None stated.

Pregnancy and lactation: There is inadequate evidence of safety in human pregnancy. Topical administration of corticosteroids to pregnant animals can cause abnormalities of foetal development including cleft palate and intra-uterine growth retardation. There may therefore be a very small risk of such effects in the human foetus. The use of topical corticosteroids during lactation is unlikely to present a hazard to infants being breast-fed.

Effects on ability to drive and use machines: None stated.

Undesirable effects: Locoid Lipocream is usually well tolerated; if signs of hypersensitivity do occur, treatment should be ceased.

In naturally occluded or moist areas of the skin, especially in small children, where absorption may be favoured, unduly prolonged therapy may give rise to systemic side-effects.

Overdosage: Overdosage would result in the topical

and systemic signs and symptoms associated with high corticosteroid dosage. If overdosage should occur, treatment should not stop immediately but be gradually withdrawn. Adrenal insufficiency may need therapy with intravenous hydrocortisone. It should be noted that overdosage of this topical corticosteroid preparation would be unlikely to occur other than as a result of severe and prolonged abuse of the product.

Pharmacological properties
Pharmacodynamic properties: The active substance, hydrocortisone 17-butyrate, is an established topical corticosteroid, equi-efficacious with those corticosteroids classified as potent.

Pharmacokinetic properties: In human *in-vivo* studies the potency of this formulation has been shown to be of the same order as other topical corticosteroids classified as potent. The active substance metabolises to hydrocortisone and butyric acid.

Preclinical safety data: No relevant pre-clinical safety data have been generated.

Pharmaceutical particulars
List of excipients: Cetomacrogol 1000 BP; Cetostearyl alcohol PhEur; White soft paraffin BP; Light liquid paraffin PhEur; Sodium citrate anhydrous PhEur, except water as USP; Citric acid PhEur; Methyl parahydroxybenzoate PhEur; Purified water PhEur.

Incompatibilites: None stated

Shelf life: Five years

Special precautions for storage: Store at room temperature (not more than 25°C).

Nature and contents of container: Collapsible aluminium tube with plastic screw cap containing 15 g, 30 g, 50 g or 100 g

Instruction for use/handling: None stated

Marketing authorisation number PL 0166/0112.

Date of first authorisation/renewal of authorisation 3 May 1983; renewed 18 September 1998

Date of partial revision of the text September 1998.

LOCOID* SCALP LOTION

Presentation Locoid Scalp Lotion contains 0.1% hydrocortisone 17-butyrate in an alcohol/water base, specially formulated for the treatment of skin disorders of the scalp. The inactive constituents of Locoid Scalp Lotion are glycerin, povidone, citric acid, sodium citrate, iso-propyl alcohol, and purified water.

Uses In the treatment of steroid-responsive dermatoses of the scalp, including seborrhoea capitis with or without an associated severe dandruff; psoriasis of the scalp (excluding widespread plaque psoriasis).

Dosage and administration
Adults, children and the elderly: Apply a small quantity 2 to 3 times daily to the affected area of the scalp, or as directed.

Contra-indications, warnings, etc *Contra-indications:* Facial rosacea, acne vulgaris, perioral dermatitis, perianal and genital pruritus, napkin eruptions, bacterial (e.g. impetigo), viral (e.g. herpes simplex) and fungal (e.g. candida or dermatophyte) infections, known hypersensitivity to the product.

Side-effects: Local and systemic toxicity is common especially following long continued use on large areas. Local irritation may occur.

Use in pregnancy and lactation: There is inadequate evidence of safety in human pregnancy. Topical administration of corticosteroids to pregnant animals can cause abnormalities of fetal development including cleft palate and intra-uterine growth retardation. There may therefore be a very small risk of such effects in the human fetus.

Other warnings and precautions: Long term continuous therapy should be avoided in all patients irrespective of age. Application under occlusion should be restricted to dermatoses involving limited areas.

Topical corticosteroids may be hazardous in psoriasis for a number of reasons including rebound relapses following development of tolerance, risk of generalised pustular psoriasis and local and systemic toxicity due to impaired barrier function of the skin. Steroids may have a place in psoriasis of the scalp and chronic plaque psoriasis of the hands and feet. Careful patient supervision is important.

Overdosage: Overdosage would result in the topical and systemic signs and symptoms associated with high corticosteroid dosage. If overdosage should occur, treatment should not stop immediately but be gradually withdrawn. Adrenal insufficiency may need therapy with intravenous hydrocortisone. It should be noted that overdosage of this topical corticosteroid product would be unlikely to occur other than as a result of severe and prolonged abuse of product.

Pharmaceutical precautions Store at room temperature (15–25°C).

Legal category POM.

Package quantities Plastic squeeze bottles of 100 ml as original packs (OP).

Further information Locoid lotion should be kept away from the eyes, and not used near a fire or naked flame.

Product licence number 0166/0060.

LOCOID* C CREAM

Qualitative and quantitative composition Hydrocortisone 17-butyrate 0.1% and Chlorquinaldol 3%.

Pharmaceutical form Cream.

Clinical particulars
Therapeutic indications: The product is recommended for clinical use in the treatment of conditions responsive to topical corticosteroids, e.g. eczema, dermatitis and psoriasis, where there is concurrent infection by a micro-organism susceptible to chlorquinaldol, or where such infection is to be prevented.

Posology and method of administration: To be applied to the affected part two to four times a day, or as directed by the prescriber. Where necessary, application may be made under an occlusive dressing.

Contra-indications: This preparation is contra-indicated in the presence of viral or fungal infections, tubercular or syphilitic lesions, and in bacterial infections (other than those at the site of inunction responsive to topical chlorquinaldol) unless used in connection with appropriate chemotherapy.

Special warnings and special precautions for use: Contact with the eyes should be avoided.

Interaction with other medicaments and other forms of interaction: None stated.

Pregnancy and lactation: This preparation should not be applied extensively, i.e. in large amounts or for prolonged periods, in pregnancy.

Effects on ability to drive and use machines: None stated.

Undesirable effects: In infants, long-term continuous topical therapy should be avoided. Adrenal suppression can occur, even without occlusion.

Overdose: No details stated.

Pharmacological properties
Pharmacodynamic properties: The active substance is a well-established topical corticosteroid, with an activity classified at potent.

Chlorquinaldol is an established anti-infectious agent with an anti-bacterial and anti-fungal activity.

Pharmacokinetic properties: In-vivo studies have demonstrated the topical activity of the product, e.g. by the McKenzie-Stoughton test.

Chlorquinaldol acts topically at the site of application.

Preclinical safety data: No relevant preclinical safety data has been generated.

Pharmaceutical particulars
List of excipients: Cetostearyl Alcohol BP, Cetomacrogol 1000 BP, Liquid Paraffin BP, White Soft Paraffin BP, Sodium citrate (anhydrous) USP, Citric Acid (anhydrous) PhEur, Purified Water PhEur.

Incompatibilities: None stated.

Shelf life: 4 years.

Special precautions for storage: Store at room temperature (not more than 25°C).

Nature and contents of container: Collapsible aluminium tube with plastic screw cap containing 30 g or 50 g.

Instructions for use/handling: Not applicable.

Marketing authorisation number 0166/0056

Date of approval/revision of SPC 15 March 1995.

Legal category POM.

LOCOID* C OINTMENT

Qualitative and quantitative composition Hydrocortisone 17-butyrate 0.1% and Chlorquinaldol 3%.

Pharmaceutical form Ointment.

Clinical particulars
Therapeutic indications: The product is recommended for clinical use in the treatment of conditions responsive to topical corticosteroids, e.g. eczema, dermatitis and psoriasis, where there is concurrent infection by a micro-organism susceptible to chlorquinaldol, or where such infection is to be prevented.

Posology and method of administration: To be applied to the affected part two to four times a day, or as directed by the prescriber. Where necessary, application may be made under an occlusive dressing.

Contra-indications: This preparation is contra-indicated in the presence of viral or fungal infections, tubercular or syphilitic lesions, and in bacterial infections (other than those at the site of inunction responsive to topical chlorquinaldol) unless used in connection with appropriate chemotherapy.

Special warnings and special precautions for use: Contact with the eyes should be avoided.

Interaction with other medicaments and other forms of interaction: None stated.

Pregnancy and lactation: This preparation should not be applied extensively, i.e. in large amounts or for prolonged periods, in pregnancy.

Effects on ability to drive and use machines: None stated.

Undesirable effects: In infants, long-term continuous topical therapy should be avoided. Adrenal suppression can occur, even without occlusion.

Overdose: No details stated.

Pharmacological properties
Pharmacodynamic properties: The active substance is a well-established topical corticosteroid, with an activity classified at potent.

Chlorquinaldol is an established anti-infectious agent with an anti-bacterial and anti-fungal activity.

Pharmacokinetic properties: In-vivo studies have demonstrated the topical activity of the product, e.g. by the McKenzie-Stoughton test.

Chlorquinaldol acts topically at the site of application.

Preclinical safety data: No relevant preclinical safety data has been generated.

Pharmaceutical particulars
List of excipients: Plastibase 50 W.

Incompatibilities: None stated.

Shelf life: 5 years.

Special precautions for storage: Store at room temperature (not more than 25°C).

Nature and contents of container: Collapsible aluminium tube with plastic screw cap containing 30 g or 50 g.

Instructions for use/handling: Not applicable.

Marketing authorisation number 0166/0057

Date of approval/revision of SPC 15 March 1995.

Legal category POM.

MILDISON* LIPOCREAM

Qualitative and quantitative composition Hydrocortisone PhEur 1% w/w.

Pharmaceutical form Cream.

Clinical particulars
Therapeutic indications: Eczema and dermatitis of all types including atopic eczema, otitis externa, primary irritant and allergic dermatitis, intertrigo, prurigo nodularis, seborrhoeic dermatitis, and insect bite reactions.

Posology and method of administration:
For adults, children and the elderly: Apply a small quantity only sufficient to cover the affected area two or three times a day. Due to the formulation of the base the product may be used both for dry scaly lesions and for moist or weeping lesions.

Contra-indications: Contra-indicated in the presence of bacterial (e.g. impetigo), viral (e.g. herpes simplex), or fungal (e.g. candida or dermatophyte) infections.

Special warnings and precautions for use: Although generally regarded as safe even for long term administration in adults there is a potential for overdosage in infancy. Extreme caution is required in dermatoses of infancy including napkin eruption. In such patients courses of treatment should not normally exceed seven days.

Interactions with other medicaments and other forms of interaction: None stated.

Pregnancy and lactation: There is inadequate evidence of safety in human pregnancy. Topical administration of corticosteroids to pregnant animals can cause abnormalities of foetal development including cleft palate and intra-uterine growth retardation. There may therefore be a very small risk of such effects in the human foetus. The use of topical corticosteroids during lactation is unlikely to present a hazard to infants being breast-fed.

Effects on ability to drive and use machines: None stated.

Undesirable effects: Mildison Lipocream is usually well tolerated; if signs of hypersensitivity do occur treatment should cease.

In naturally occluded or moist areas of the skin,

especially in small children, where absorption may be favoured, unduly prolonged therapy may give rise to systemic side-effects.

Overdose: Overdosage would result on the topical and systemic signs and symptoms associated with high corticosteroid dosage. If overdosage should occur treatment should not stop immediately but should be gradually withdrawn. Adrenal insufficiency may need therapy with intravenous hydrocortisone. It should be noted that overdosage of this topical corticosteroid product would be unlikely to occur other than as a result of severe and prolonged abuse of the product.

Pharmacological properties

Pharmacodynamic properties: The active ingredient, hydrocortisone, is a well-established corticosteroid with the pharmacological actions of a corticosteroid classified as mildly potent.

Pharmacokinetic properties: In human in-vivo studies the potency of this formulation has been demonstrated as being of the same order as other widely available formulations of hydrocortisone 1%.

Preclinical safety data: No relevant pre-clinical safety data has been generated.

Pharmaceutical particulars

List of excipients: Cetostearyl alcohol, Cetomacrogol, Liquid paraffin, White soft paraffin, Methyl parahydroxybenzoate, Sodium citrate, Citric acid, Purified water.

Incompatibilities: None.

Shelf life: Three years.

Special precautions for storage: Store at room temperature (below 25°C).

Nature and contents of container: Collapsible membrane-necked internally coated aluminium tubes with a polyethylene screw cap containing 10 g, 15 g, 30 g, or 100 g.

Instruction for use/handling: None.

Administrative data

Marketing authorisation holder: Yamanouchi Pharma Ltd, Yamanouchi House, Pyrford Road, West Byfleet, Surrey KT14 6RA.

Marketing authorisation number PL 0166/0131.

Date of first authorisation/renewal of authorisation 23 September 1987/30 September 1997

Date of (partial) revision of the text 19 June 1997.

RIDAURA TILTAB TABLETS 3 mg

Qualitative and quantitative composition Auranofin HSE 3 mg.

Pharmaceutical form Tablet.

Clinical particulars

Therapeutic indications: Ridaura is an orally active gold preparation. It is indicated in the management of adults with active progressive rheumatoid arthritis only when non-steroidal anti-inflammatory drugs have been found to be inadequate alone to control the disease, i.e. when second-line therapy is required. In patients with adult rheumatoid arthritis Ridaura has been shown to reduce disease activity reflected by synovitis, associated symptoms, and appropriate laboratory parameters. Gold cannot reverse structural damage to joints caused by previous disease. Ridaura does not produce an immediate response and therapeutic effects may be seen after three to six months of treatment.

Posology and method of administration:

For adults and the elderly only:

Adults: The usual starting dose is 6 mg daily as one 3 mg tablet twice a day, in the morning and the evening. If this is well tolerated a single daily dose may be given as two 3 mg tablets with breakfast or with the evening meal.

Treatment should be continued for a minimum of three to six months to assess response as Ridaura is a slow-acting drug. If the response is inadequate after six months an increase to 9 mg (one tablet three times a day) may be tolerated. If response remains inadequate after a three month trial of 9 mg daily, Ridaura therapy should be discontinued. Safety at dosages exceeding 9 mg daily has not been studied.

Absorption of gold from Ridaura tablets is rapid but incomplete. Although mean blood gold levels are proportional to dose, no correlation between blood gold levels and safety or efficacy has been established. Dosage adjustments should therefore depend on monitoring clinical response and adverse events rather than on monitoring blood gold concentrations.

Anti-inflammatory drugs and analgesics may be prescribed as necessary with Ridaura.

The elderly: Dosage as for adults. As with all drugs extra caution should be exercised in administration to the elderly.

Contra-indications: Contra-indicated in pregnancy.

Although not necessarily reported in association with Ridaura, do not use in patients with a history of any of the following gold-induced disorders: necrotising enterocolitis, pulmonary fibrosis, exfoliate dermatitis, bone marrow aplasia, or other severe blood dyscrasias. Use should also be avoided in progressive renal disease or severe active hepatic disease and in systemic lupus erythromatosus.

Special warnings and precautions for use: Use with caution in patients with any degree of renal impairment or hepatic dysfunction, inflammatory bowel disease, rash, or history of bone marrow depression.

Close monitoring is essential. Full blood count with differential and platelet counts (which should be plotted) and tests for urinary protein must be performed prior to Ridaura therapy and at least monthly thereafter. Patients with gastrointestinal symptoms, with rash, with pruritus (which may precede rash), with stomatitis, or a metallic taste in the mouth (which might precede stomatitis), should also be closely monitored as such symptoms may indicate a need for modification of dosage or withdrawal.

Prior to initiating treatment patients must be advised of the potential side effects associated with Ridaura. They should be warned to report promptly any unusual signs or symptoms during treatment such as pruritus, rash, metallic taste, sore throat or tongue, mouth ulceration, easy bruising, purpura, epistaxis, bleeding gums, menorrhagia, or diarrhoea.

Gold has been shown to be carcinogenic in rodents although there was no evidence of carcinogenicity in a 7-year dog study.

Interactions with other medicaments and other forms of interaction: None stated.

Pregnancy and lactation: Gold is teratogenic in some animal species. Ridaura should not be used in pregnancy. Women of child-bearing potential should not be treated with Ridaura without full consideration of the benefits of treatment against the potential risk of teratogenicity; they should practice effective contraception during treatment and for at least six months after. Patients should be fully informed of the teratogenic risk, and termination of any pregnancy occurring during treatment should be considered in view of the possibility of foetal malformation. If women are to be treated post-partum with Ridaura, breast-feeding should be avoided.

Effects on ability to drive and use machines: None stated.

Undesirable effects: Adverse reactions can occur throughout treatment with Ridaura, although the highest incidence can be expected during the first six months of treatment.

The most common reaction to Ridaura is diarrhoea or loose stools. Nausea may be present and abdominal pain or other gastrointestinal symptoms have been reported alone or in association. These usually resolve if dosage is temporarily reduced, e.g. from 6 mg to 3 mg a day, but if it is necessary to stop treatment it can sometimes be started again at a lower dose without further problem. About one patient in twenty will be unable to tolerate Ridaura because of diarrhoea. Ulcerative enterocolitis has been very rarely reported, as with all gold containing drugs. Therefore patients with gastrointestinal symptoms should be carefully monitored for the appearance of gastrointestinal bleeding and treatment stopped if this occurs.

Rashes, sometimes with pruritus, stomatitis, and oral mucous membrane reactions, alopecia, conjunctivitis, and taste disturbances including a metallic taste, may occur but are usually not persistent and only occasionally require withdrawal of treatment. If however rash is persistent, especially if accompanied by pruritus, treatment should be stopped. Exfoliative dermatitis has been reported with other gold-containing drugs.

Blood dyscrasias including leucopenia, granulocytopenia, and thrombocytopenia can occur separately or in combination at any time during treatment. Agranulocytosis and aplastic anaemia have been reported very rarely. Ridaura should be withdrawn if the platelet count falls below 100,000 per mm^3 or if signs and symptoms suggestive of thrombocytopenia occur.

Transient decreases in haemoglobin or haematocrit early in treatment have been reported but are invariably of no clinical significance.

Gold can produce the nephrotic syndrome or less severe glomerular disease with proteinuria which are usually mild and transient. If however persistent or clinically significant proteinuria develops treatment with Ridaura should be promptly stopped. Treatment may be restarted after the proteinuria has cleared, however under close supervision in patients who have experienced only minimal proteinuria. Minor changes in renal function may also occur.

Pulmonary fibrosis may rarely occur and chest X-ray is recommended at least annually.

Minor transient changes in liver function have been noted.

Overdose: Ridaura overdosage experience is limited. One patient who took 27 mg daily for 10 days developed an encephalopathy and peripheral neuropathy. Ridaura was discontinued and the patient eventually recovered.

In case of acute overdosage immediate induction of vomiting or gastric lavage and appropriate supportive therapy are recommended. Chelating agents such as BAL have been used in injectable gold overdosage, and may be considered, although there has been no specific experience with Ridaura.

Pharmacological properties

Pharmacodynamic properties: Auranofin is a disease-modifying slow-acting immunomodulating agent.

Pharmacokinetic properties: About 20% to 30% of the gold in a dose of Ridaura is absorbed and although there is considerable variation in absorption this is less than that seen with parenteral gold. Steady state blood concentrations are achieved 8 to 12 weeks after starting and are on average 5 to 10 times less than those following parenteral gold, with no correlation with clinical response or adverse events. About 70% of the gold administered in Ridaura appears in the faeces during the first week following a single dose, and at six months after dosing less than 1% of the gold administered remains in the body, in contrast to around 30% of gold given parenterally. In contrast to parenteral gold, which does not become cell-associated, 40% of the gold in the blood of Ridaura-treated patients is associated with blood cells.

The metabolism of Ridaura is not fully understood, although it is clear from both animal and in-vitro studies with human blood that both the sulphur and the phosphorus ligands of Ridaura are rapidly dissociated from the gold.

Preclinical safety data: No relevant pre-clinical safety data has been generated.

Pharmaceutical particulars

List of excipients: Lactose, Microcrystalline cellulose, Maize starch, Sodium starch glycollate, Magnesium stearate, Hydroxypropylmethylcellulose, Propylene glycol, Opaspray M-1-6054.

Incompatibilities: None.

Shelf life: Five years.

Special precautions for storage: None.

Nature and contents of container: Standard SK&F polypropylene securitainers or HDPE containers with wadless polypropylene screw caps containing 60 tablets.

Instruction for use/handling: None.

Administrative data

Marketing authorisation holder: Yamanouchi Pharma Ltd, Yamanouchi House, Pyrford Road, West Byfleet, Surrey KT14 6RA.

Marketing authorisation number PL 0166/0176

Date of first authorisation/renewal of authorisation 1 May 1997

Date of (partial) revision of text 4 August 1997.

ZINERYT*

Qualitative and quantitative composition Erythromycin PhEur 40 mg and Zinc Acetate USP 12 mg per ml on constitution.

Pharmaceutical form Dry powder bottle and solvent bottle to be admixed on dispensing.

Clinical particulars

Therapeutic indications: Topical treatment of acne vulgaris.

Posology and method of administration: For children, adults, and the elderly. Apply twice daily over the whole of the affected area for a period of 10 to 12 weeks.

Contra-indications: Zineryt is contra-indicated in patients who are hypersensitive to erythromycin or other macrolide antibiotics, or to zinc, di-isopropyl sebacate or ethanol.

Special warnings and special precautions for use: Cross resistance may occur with other antibiotics of the macrolide group and also with lincomycin and clindamycin. Contact with the eyes or the mucous membranes of the nose and mouth should be avoided.

Interaction with other medicaments and other forms of interaction: None known.

Pregnancy and lactation: There is no contraindication to the use of Zineryt in pregnancy or lactation.

Effects on ability to drive and use machines: None.

Undesirable effects: Occasionally a burning sensation or a slight redness of the skin may be observed; this is due to the alcohol base of Zineryt and is transient and of minor clinical significance.

Overdose: It is not expected that overdosage would occur in normal use. Patients showing idiosyncratic hypersensitivity should wash the treated area with copious water and simple soap.

Pharmacological properties

Pharmacodynamic properties: Erythromycin is known to be efficacious, at 4%, in the topical treatment of acne vulgaris. Zinc, topically, is established as an aid to wound healing. The zinc acetate is solubilised by complexing with the erythromycin, and delivery of the complex is enhanced by the chosen vehicle.

Pharmacokinetic properties: The complex does not survive in the skin, and erythromycin and zinc penetrate independently. The erythromycin penetrates, and is partially systemically absorbed (0–10% in vitro, 40–50% in animal studies); that portion absorbed is excreted in 24–72 hours. The zinc is not absorbed systemically.

Preclinical safety data: No relevant pre-clinical safety data has been generated.

Pharmaceutical particulars

List of excipients: Di-isopropyl sebacate, ethanol.

Incompatibilities: None known.

Shelf life: 2 years; 5 weeks after constitution.

Special precautions for storage: None. Store at room temperature (15°C–25°C).

Nature and contents of container: Screw-capped HDPE bottles; an applicator cap is fitted when dispensed. When constituted packs are of 30 ml and 90 ml.

Instructions for use/handling: None.

Marketing authorisation number 0166/0109

Date of approval/revision of SPC 27 January 1995.

Legal category POM.

**Trade Mark*

ZENECA Pharma

King's Court
Water Lane
Wilmslow, Cheshire SK9 5AZ

☎ 01625 712712   0800 200123   🗋 01625 712581

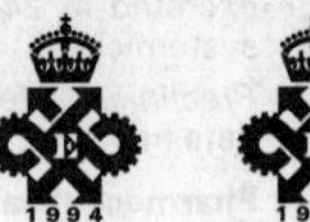

ZENECA

ACCOLATE* ▼

Qualitative and quantitative composition Accolate contains 20 mg zafirlukast in each tablet.

Pharmaceutical form Film coated tablet.

Clinical particulars
Therapeutic indications: Accolate is indicated for the treatment of asthma.

Posology and method of administration: Accolate should be taken continuously.

Adults and children aged 12 years and over: The dosage is one 20 mg tablet twice daily. This dosage should not be exceeded. Higher doses may be associated with elevations of one or more liver enzymes consistent with hepatotoxicity.

As food may reduce the bioavailability of zafirlukast, Accolate should not be taken with meals.

Elderly: The clearance of zafirlukast is significantly reduced in elderly patients (over 65 years old), and C_{max} and AUC are approximately double those of younger adults. However, accumulation of zafirlukast is no greater than that seen in multiple-dose trials conducted in adult subjects with asthma, and the consequences of the altered kinetics in the elderly are unknown.

Clinical experience with Accolate in the elderly (over 65 years) is limited and caution is recommended until further information is available.

Children: There is no clinical experience of the use of Accolate in children under 12 years of age. Until safety information is available, the use of Accolate in children is contra-indicated.

Renal impairment: No dosage adjustment is necessary in patients with mild renal impairment.

Contra-indications: Accolate should not be given to patients who have previously experienced hypersensitivity to the product or any of its ingredients.

Accolate is contra-indicated in patients with a history of moderate or severe renal impairment. Accolate is contra-indicated in patients with hepatic impairment or cirrhosis; it has not been studied in patients with hepatitis or in long term studies of patients with cirrhosis.

Accolate is contra-indicated in children under 12 years of age until safety information is available.

Special warnings and precautions for use: Accolate should be taken regularly to achieve benefit, even during symptom free periods. Accolate therapy should normally be continued during acute exacerbations of asthma.

Accolate does not allow a reduction in existing steroid treatment.

As with inhaled steroids and cromones (disodium cromoglycate, nedocromil sodium), Accolate is not indicated for use in the reversal of bronchospasm in acute asthma attacks.

Accolate has not been evaluated in the treatment of labile (brittle) or unstable asthma.

Cases of Churg-Strauss Syndrome have been reported in association with Accolate usage. A causal relationship has neither been confirmed nor refuted. If a patient develops a Churg-Strauss Syndrome type illness Accolate should be stopped, a rechallenge test should not be performed and treatment should not be restarted.

Elevations in serum transaminases can occur during treatment with Accolate. These are usually asymptomatic and transient but could represent early evidence of hepatotoxicity. (See *Undesirable effects*)

If clinical symptoms or signs suggestive of liver dysfunction occur (e.g. nausea, vomiting, right upper quadrant pain, fatigue, lethargy, flu-like symptoms, enlarged liver, pruritus and jaundice), the serum transaminases, in particular serum ALT, should be measured and the patient managed accordingly. A decision to discontinue Accolate should be individualised to the patient's condition, weighing the risk of hepatic dysfunction against the clinical benefit of Accolate to the patient.

Interactions with other medicaments and other forms of interaction: Accolate may be administered with other therapies routinely used in the management of asthma and allergy. Inhaled steroids, inhaled and oral bronchodilator therapy, antibiotics and antihistamines are examples of agents which have been co-administered with Accolate without adverse interaction.

Accolate may be administered with oral contraceptives without adverse interaction.

Co-administration with warfarin results in an increase in maximum prothrombin time by approximately 35%. It is therefore recommended that if Accolate is co-administered with warfarin, prothrombin time should be closely monitored. The interaction is probably due to an inhibition by zafirlukast of the cytochrome P450 2C9 isoenzyme system.

In clinical trials co-administration with theophylline resulted in decreased plasma levels of zafirlukast, by approximately 30%, but with no effect on plasma theophylline levels. However, during post-marketing surveillance, there have been rare cases of patients experiencing increased theophylline levels when co-administered Accolate.

Co-administration with terfenadine resulted in a 54% decrease in AUC for zafirlukast, but with no effect on plasma terfenadine levels.

Co-administration with acetylsalicylic acid ('aspirin', 650 mg four times a day) may result in increased plasma levels of zafirlukast, by approximately 45%.

Co-administration with erythromycin will result in decreased plasma levels of zafirlukast, by approximately 40%.

The clearance of zafirlukast in smokers may be increased by approximately 20%.

At concentrations of 10 microgram/ml and above, zafirlukast causes increases in the assay value for bilirubin in animal plasma. However, zafirlukast has not been shown to interfere with the 2,5-dichlorophenyl diazonium salt method of bilirubin analysis of human plasma.

Pregnancy and lactation: The safety of Accolate in human pregnancy has not been established. In animal studies, zafirlukast did not have any apparent effect on fertility and did not appear to have any teratogenic or selective toxic effect on the foetus. The potential risks should be weighed against the benefits of continuing therapy during pregnancy and Accolate should be used during pregnancy only if clearly needed.

Zafirlukast is excreted in human breast milk. Accolate should not be administered to mothers who are breast-feeding.

Effects on ability to drive and use machines: There is no evidence that Accolate affects the ability to drive and use machinery.

Undesirable effects: Administration of Accolate in clinical trials against placebo has been associated with headache (9.9% vs 9.0%) or gastrointestinal disturbance (nausea 2.6% vs 2.2%, vomiting 1.2% vs 1.0%, diarrhoea 2.3% vs 1.8%, abdominal pain 1.6% vs 1.2%). These symptoms are usually mild and do not necessitate withdrawal from therapy.

Hypersensitivity reactions, including urticaria and angioedema have been reported. Rashes, including blistering, have also been reported.

Infrequently, elevated serum transaminase levels have been observed in clinical trials against placebo with Accolate (increased ALT 1.0% vs 0.9%, increased AST 0.6% vs 0.6%); at recommended doses the incidence was equivalent to placebo. Rarely the transaminase profile has been consistent with drug-induced hepatitis which resolved following cessation of Accolate therapy.

In placebo-controlled clinical trials, an increased incidence of infection has been observed in elderly patients given Accolate (7.8% vs 1.4%). Infections were usually mild, predominantly affecting the respiratory tract.

Overdose: No information exists with regard to the effects of overdosage of Accolate in humans. Management should be supportive. Removal of excess medication by gastric lavage may be helpful.

Pharmacological properties
Pharmacodynamic properties: The cysteinyl leukotrienes (LTC_4, LTD_4 and LTE_4) are potent inflammatory eicosanoids released from various cells including mast cells and eosinophils. These important proasthmatic mediators bind to cysteinyl leukotriene receptors found in the human airway.

Leukotriene production and receptor occupation has been implicated in the pathophysiology of asthma. Effects include smooth muscle contraction, airway oedema and altered cell activity associated with the inflammatory process, including eosinophil influx to the lung.

Accolate is a competitive highly selective and potent oral peptide leukotriene antagonist of LTC_4, LTD_4 and LTE_4 components of slow reacting substance of anaphylaxis. In vitro studies have shown that Accolate antagonises the contractile activity of all three peptide leukotrienes (leukotriene C_4, D_4, and E_4) in human conducting airway smooth muscle to the same extent. Animal studies have shown Accolate to be effective in preventing peptide leukotriene-induced increases in vascular permeability, which give rise to oedema in the airways, and to inhibit peptide leukotriene-induced influx of eosinophils into airways.

The specificity of Accolate has been shown by its action on leukotriene receptors and not prostaglandin, thromboxane, cholinergic and histamine receptors.

In a placebo-controlled study where segmental bronchoprovocation with allergen was followed by bronchoalveolar lavage 48 hours later, zafirlukast decreased the rise in basophils, lymphocytes and histamine, and reduced the stimulated production of superoxide by alveolar macrophages. Accolate attenuated the increase in bronchial hyperresponsiveness that follows inhaled allergen challenge. Further, methacholine sensitivity was diminished by long-term dosing with Accolate 20 mg twice daily.

Further, in clinical trials evaluating chronic therapy with Accolate, the lung function measured when plasma levels were at trough showed sustained improvements over baseline.

Accolate shows a dose dependent inhibition of bronchoconstriction induced by inhaled LTD_4. Asthmatic patients are approximately 10-fold more sensitive to the bronchoconstricting activity of inhaled LTD_4. A single oral dose of Accolate can enable an asthmatic patient to inhale 100 times more LTD_4 and shows significant protection at 12 and 24 hours.

Accolate inhibits the bronchoconstriction caused by several kinds of challenge, such as the response to sulphur dioxide, exercise and cold air. Accolate attenuates the early and late phase inflammatory reaction caused by various antigens such as grass, cat dander, ragweed and mixed antigens.

In asthmatic patients not adequately controlled by beta-agonist therapy (given as required) Accolate improves symptoms (reducing daytime and nocturnal asthmatic symptoms), improves lung function, reduces the need for concomitant beta-agonist medication and reduces incidence of exacerbations. Similar benefits have been seen in patients with more severe asthma receiving high dose inhaled steroids.

In clinical studies, there was a significant first-dose effect on baseline bronchomotor tone observed within 2 hours of dosing, when peak plasma concentrations had not yet been achieved. Initial improvements in asthma symptoms occurred within the first week, and often the first few days, of treatment with Accolate.

Pharmacokinetic properties: Peak plasma concentrations of zafirlukast are achieved approximately 3 hours after oral administration of Accolate.

Administration of Accolate with food increased the variability in the bioavailability of zafirlukast and reduced bioavailability in most (75%) subjects. The net reduction was approximately 40%.

Following twice-daily administration of Accolate (30 to 80 mg bd), accumulation of zafirlukast in plasma was low (not detectable–2.9 times first dose values; mean 1.45; median 1.27). The terminal half-life of zafirlukast is approximately 10 hours. Steady-state plasma concentrations of zafirlukast were proportional to the dose and predictable from single-dose pharmacokinetic data.

Zafirlukast is extensively metabolised. Following a radiolabelled dose the urinary excretion accounts for approximately 10% dose and faecal excretion for 89%. Zafirlukast is not detected in urine. The metabolites identified in human plasma were found to be at least

90-fold less potent than zafirlukast in a standard in-vitro test of activity.

Zafirlukast is approximately 99% protein bound to human plasma proteins, predominantly albumin, over the concentration range 0.25 to 4.0 microgram/ml.

Pharmacokinetic studies in special populations have been performed in a relatively small number of subjects, and the clinical significance of the following kinetic data is not established.

Pharmacokinetics of zafirlukast in adolescents and adults with asthma were similar to those of healthy adult males. When adjusted for body weight, the pharmacokinetics of zafirlukast are not significantly different between men and women.

Elderly subjects and subjects with stable alcoholic cirrhosis demonstrated an approximately two-fold increase in C_{max} and AUC compared to normal subjects given the same doses of Accolate.

There are no significant differences in the pharmacokinetics of zafirlukast in patients with mild renal impairment and in normal subjects.

Pre-clinical safety data: After multiple doses of greater than 40 mg/kg/day for up to 12 months, liver enlargement associated with degenerative/fatty change or glycogen deposition was seen in rats, mice and dogs. Histiocytic aggregates were seen in a number of tissues of dogs.

Male mice given 300 mg/kg zafirlukast daily had an increased incidence of hepatocellular adenomas compared to control animals. Rats given 2000 mg/kg zafirlukast daily had an increased incidence of urinary bladder papilloma compared to control animals. Zafirlukast was not mutagenic in a range of tests. The clinical significance of these findings during the long term use of Accolate in man is uncertain.

There were no other notable findings from the pre-clinical testing.

Pharmaceutical particulars

List of excipients: Croscarmellose sodium (PhEur); Hypromellose E464 (PhEur); Lactose Monohydrate (PhEur); Magnesium Stearate E572 (PhEur); Microcrystalline Cellulose E460 (PhEur); Povidone (PhEur); Titanium Dioxide E171 (PhEur).

Incompatibilities: None known.

Shelf life: 3 years.

Special precautions for storage: Store below 30°C.

Nature and contents of container: Aluminium laminate/foil blister packs containing 56 or 100 tablets.

Instruction for use/handling: No special precautions.

Marketing authorisation number 12619/0108.

Date of approval/revision of SPC 5 June 1998.

Legal Category POM

AMPHOCIL*

Qualitative and quantitative composition

Ingredient	*Specification reference*	*Quantity (W/W)*
Amphotericin	USP	5.060
Sodium cholesteryl sulphate	House	2.672
Tromethamine	USP	0.571
Disodium edetate	PhEur	0.034
Lactose, monohydrate	PhEur	91.311
Hydrochloric acid	PhEur	0.353[a]
Water for injection	PhEur	[b]
Nitrogen	NF	[c]

[a] HCl qs to a target pH of 7.0±0.5.
[b] Mean NMT 2.0% residual moisture and no individual vial greater than 2.5%.
[c] Used to fill vial headspace.

Pharmaceutical form Amphotericin B USP, 5% (W/W), lyophilisate for reconstitution. Each vial contains either 50 mg (50,000 IU) or 100 mg (100,000 IU) of amphotericin B USP as a complex with sodium cholesteryl sulphate.

Clinical particulars

Therapeutic indications: Amphocil is indicated for the treatment of severe systemic and/or deep mycoses in cases where toxicity or renal failure precludes the use of conventional amphotericin B in effective doses, and in cases where prior systemic antifungal therapy has failed. Fungal infections successfully treated with Amphocil include disseminated candidiasis and aspergillosis. Amphocil has been used successfully in severely neutropenic patients.

Amphocil is not intended for use in common, clinically inapparent fungal diseases diagnosed only by skin tests or serological determinations.

Posology and method of administration:

Dosage: Therapy may begin at a daily dose of 1.0 mg/kg of body weight, increasing to the recommended dose of 3.0–4.0 mg/kg as required. Doses as high as 6 mg/kg have been used in patients. Dosage should be adjusted to the individual requirements of each patient. The median cumulative dose in clinical studies was 3.5 g and the medial treatment duration was 16 days. Ten percent (10%) of patients received 13 g or more of Amphocil over a period of 27 to 409 days.

Administration: Amphocil is administered by intravenous infusion at a rate of 1 to 2 mg/kg/hour. If the patient experiences acute reactions or cannot tolerate the infusion volume, the infusion time may be extended. Pre-medication (e.g. paracetamol, antihistamines, antiemetics) may be administered to patients who have previously suffered infusion related adverse reactions.

Paediatric patients: A limited number of paediatric patients have been treated with Amphocil at daily doses (mg/kg) similar to those in adults. No unusual adverse events were reported.

Elderly patients: A limited number of elderly patients have been treated with Amphocil; available data do not indicate the need for specific dose recommendations or precautions in elderly patients.

Contra-indications, warnings, etc

Contra-indications: Amphocil should not be administered to patients who have documented hypersensitivity to any of its components, unless, in the opinion of the physician, the advantages of using Amphocil outweigh the risks of hypersensitivity.

Special warnings and special precautions for use: A test dose which is advisable when commencing all new courses of treatment should immediately precede the first dose; a small amount of drug (e.g. 20 ml of a solution containing 0.1 g per litre) should be infused over 10 minutes and the patient carefully observed for the next 30 minutes.

In the treatment of diabetic patients: It should be noted that each vial of Amphocil contains lactose monohydrate.

In the treatment of renal dialysis patients: Amphocil should be administered only at the end of each dialysis period. Serum electrolytes, particularly potassium and magnesium, should be regularly monitored.

Interaction with other medicaments and other forms of interaction: There have been no reported interactions between Amphocil and other drugs including cyclosporine. However, caution should be used in patients receiving concomitant therapy with drugs known to interact with conventional amphotericin B such as nephrotoxic drugs (aminoglycosides, cisplatin and pentamidine), corticosteroids and corticotropin (ACTH) that may potentiate hypokalaemia and digitalis glycosides, muscle relaxants and antiarrhythmic agents whose effects may be potentiated in the presence of hypokalaemia.

The use of flucytosine with Amphocil has not been studied. While the synergy between amphotericin B and flucytosine has been reported, amphotericin B may enhance the toxicity of flucytosine by increasing its cellular uptake and impeding its renal excretion.

Pregnancy and use during lactation:

Pregnancy: Animal reproductive toxicology studies with Amphocil have shown no evidence of harm to the foetus. Although the active ingredient, amphotericin B, has been in wide use for many years without apparent ill consequence, there is inadequate evidence of safety of Amphocil in human pregnancy. Therefore it is recommended that administration of Amphocil is avoided in pregnancy unless the anticipated benefit to the patient outweighs the potential risk to the foetus.

Nursing mothers: It is not known whether amphotericin B is excreted in human milk. Consideration should be given to discontinuation of nursing during treatment with Amphocil.

Effects on the ability to drive and use machines: Not applicable to current indication or expected use.

Undesirable effects: In general, the physician should monitor the patient for any type of adverse event associated with conventional amphotericin B. The appearance of adverse reactions does not generally prevent the patient completing the course of treatment. Caution should be exercised when high doses or prolonged therapy is indicated.

Acute reactions including fever, chills and rigours may occur. Anaphylactoid reactions including hypotension, tachycardia, bronchospasm, dyspnoea, hypoxia and hyperventilation have also been reported. Most acute reactions are successfully treated by reducing the rate of infusion and prompt administration of anti-histamines and adrenal corticosteroids. Serious anaphylactoid effects may necessitate discontinuation of Amphocil and treatment with additional supportive therapy (e.g. adrenaline).

Clinical studies conducted so far have shown Amphocil to be less nephrotoxic than conventional amphotericin B. Serum creatinine levels tend to remain consistent throughout the course of therapy even in patients with renal insufficiency. Patients who developed renal insufficiency during treatment with conventional amphotericin B, were stabilised or improved when Amphocil was substituted. Decreases in renal function attributable to Amphocil treatment were rare. However, as with conventional amphotericin B, renal function should be monitored with particular attention to those patients receiving concomitant therapy with nephrotoxic drugs.

There have been no reports of unequivocal hepatic toxicity of Amphocil. Changes in alkaline phosphatase and bilirubin levels were infrequent.

Changes in coagulation, thrombocytopenia and hypomagnesemia were sometimes observed on Amphocil. Anaemia, which is a very common adverse event during treatment with conventional amphotericin B, developed in only 2.5% of the patients treated with Amphocil.

Other reported events include nausea, vomiting, hypertension, headache, backache, diarrhoea and abdominal pain.

Overdose: In case of overdose, stop administration immediately and carefully monitor the patient's clinical status (renal, liver and cardiac function, haematological status, serum electrolytes) and institute symptomatic treatment.

Pharmacological properties

Pharmacodynamic properties: Amphotericin B is a macrocyclic polyene antibiotic isolated from *Streptomyces nodosus*. Amphotericin B has a high affinity for ergosterol, the primary sterol in fungal cell membranes, and a lesser affinity for cholesterol, the predominant sterol of mammalian cell membranes. Binding of amphotericin B to ergosterol results in damage to the fungal cell membrane, enhanced membrane permeability and eventual cell death. Mammalian cell membranes also contain sterols, and it has been suggested that the damage caused by amphotericin B to human cells follows a similar mode of action to that of fungal cells. Amphocil is considered to have the same mode of action as conventional amphotericin B, but with reduced toxicity.

Amphocil is a novel formulation of amphotericin B based on its unique affinity for sterols. Amphocil is a stable complex of amphotericin B and sodium cholesteryl sulphate, a naturally occurring cholesterol metabolite. Amphotericin B and sodium cholesteryl sulphate are complexed in a near equimolar ratio to form uniform disc-shaped microparticles. Amphocil is not a liposomal formulation but a colloidal dispersion of amphotericin B and sodium cholesteryl sulphate.

Pharmacological studies indicated that overall, Amphocil is essentially equivalent, *in vitro*, to conventional amphotericin B against a variety of fungal pathogens. Higher doses of Amphocil are tolerated, thus it is generally more effective in eradicating fungal infections than conventional amphotericin B in several *in vivo* models.

Pharmacokinetic properties: Pharmacokinetic studies in animals demonstrate that the distribution of Amphocil and conventional amphotericin B are notably different. Lower peak plasma levels of amphotericin B and greater total area under the curve values after Amphocil treatment, compared to comparable doses of conventional amphotericin B have been observed. Higher concentrations of amphotericin B measured in the liver, spleen and bone marrow after Amphocil administration were not accompanied by evidence of increased toxicity in these organ systems. Levels in the kidney, a primary site of toxicity of conventional amphotericin B, were 4- to 5-fold lower after treatment with Amphocil and correlated with reduced nephrotoxicity compared to conventional amphotericin B. Maximum plasma concentrations of amphotericin B were lower in Amphocil treated animals. The terminal half-life was longer in the Amphocil treated animals owing to the accumulation of amphotericin B in the liver and its subsequent slow release.

In bone marrow transplant patients administered Amphocil at doses of 0.5 to 8.0 mg/kg/day, there was an increase in both the volume of distribution (V_{ss}) and the total plasma clearance (Cl_t) as the dose escalated. The mean values of V_{ss}, Cl_t and terminal half-life for doses ≤2.0 mg/kg were 2.25 l/kg, 0.0855 l/h/kg and 22.1 hours, respectively. The mean values for doses >2.0 mg/kg were 3.61 l/kg, 0.116 l/h/kg and 27.2 hours respectively. The maximum steady-state concentrations achievable after multiple dosing ranged from 658 to 6212 μg/l for doses of 0.5 to 8.0 mg/kg respectively. There was no evidence of continued accumulation of Amphocil at doses of 8.0 mg/kg/day. There was no net change in renal function over the duration of Amphocil treatment (range from 1 to 108 days, median 28 days).

Preclinical safety data: Amphocil was found to be generally less toxic than conventional amphotericin B in a series of acute and repeat dose studies, with a 4- to 5-fold increased margin of safety. There were no unique toxicities observed following treatment with Amphocil relative to conventional amphotericin B. Nephrotoxicity was diminished during Amphocil treatment even at dose levels 4- to 5-fold higher than toxic doses of conventional amphotericin B. Accumulation of amphotericin B in the liver following Amphocil administration was observed; however, there were no associated signs of increased hepatoxicity relative to conventional amphotericin B. *In-vitro* and *in-vivo* tests on induction of gene and chromosome mutations were negative for amphotericin B. Carcinogenicity studies have not been conducted with amphotericin B or Amphocil. To date there have been no clinical reports of carcinogenicity associated with the use of amphotericin B. Embryo-foetal studies in rats and rabbits, at doses of 2.5 mg/kg/day or greater showed maternal toxicity i.e. reduced weight gain and loss of appetite. There were no adverse effects on embryo-foetal development up to 10 mg/kg/day. There are no specific data for the effect of Amphocil on human fertility, but in multiple dose toxicity studies of up to 13 weeks (in rats and dogs) there was no effect on ovarian or testicular histology. Although amphotericin B has not been associated with peri- or post-natal effects, no studies with Amphocil are available.

Pharmaceutical particulars
List of excipients: The following excipients are contained in each vial of lyophilised product: Sodium cholesteryl sulphate; Tromethamine USP; Edetate Disodium PhEur; Hydrochloric Acid PhEur; Water for Injection PhEur; Lactose Monohydrate PhEur.

Incompatibilities: Do not reconstitute lyophilised powder/cake with saline or dextrose solutions. Do not add saline or electrolytes to the reconstituted concentrate, or mix with other drugs.

If administered through an existing intravenous line, flush with 5% Dextrose for Injection prior to infusion of Amphocil, otherwise administer via a separate line.

The use of any solution other than those recommended, or the presence of a bacteriostatic agent (e.g. benzyl alcohol) in the solution may cause precipitation of Amphocil.

Do not use material that shows evidence of precipitation or any other particulate matter. Strict aseptic technique should always be followed during reconstitution and dilution since no preservatives are present in the lyophilised drug or in the solutions used for reconstitution and dilution.

Shelf life: Unopened vials of lyophilised material have a shelf-life of 36 months and should be stored below 30°C (86°F). After reconstitution, the drug should be refrigerated at 2–8°C (36–46°F) and used within 24 hours. Do not freeze. After further dilution with 5% Dextrose for Injection, the infusion should be stored in a refrigerator (2–8°C) and used within 24 hours. Partially used vials should be discarded.

Special precautions for storage: Store below 30°C (86°F).

Nature and contents of container: The container is a Type I moulded glass vial, the stopper is a grey butyl lyophilisation type stopper, and the cap is an aluminium ring with either a green or yellow polypropylene flip-off top.

Instructions for use/handling: Directions for reconstitution and dilution: Amphocil must be reconstituted by addition of sterile Water for Injection, PhEur, using a sterile syringe and a 20-gauge needle.

Rapidly inject into the vial:

50 mg/vial – 10 ml sterile Water for Injection
100 mg/vial – 20 ml sterile Water for Injection.

Shake gently by hand, rotating the vial, until the yellow fluid becomes clear. Note that the fluid may be opalescent. The liquid in each reconstituted vial will contain 5 mg of amphotericin B per ml. For infusion, further dilute to a final concentration of 0.625 mg/ml by diluting 1 volume of the reconstituted Amphocil with 7 volumes of 5% Dextrose for Injection.

Marketing authorisation holder Sequus Pharmaceuticals Incorporated, 1050 Hamilton Court, Menlo Park, CA 94025, USA.

Marketing authorisation number 11866/0002–3.

Date of approval/revision of SPC 21 December 1995.

Legal category POM.

ARIMIDEX*

Qualitative and quantitative composition Each tablet contains 1 mg anastrozole.

Pharmaceutical form Tablet.

Clinical particulars
Therapeutic indication: Treatment of advanced breast cancer in post-menopausal women whose disease progressed following treatment with tamoxifen or other anti-oestrogens. Efficacy has not been demonstrated in oestrogen receptor negative patients unless they had a previous positive clinical reponse to tamoxifen.

Posology and method of administration:
Adults including the elderly: One 1 mg tablet to be taken orally once a day.

Children: Not recommended for use in children.

Renal impairment: No dose change is recommended in patients with mild or moderate renal impairment.

Hepatic impairment: No dose change is recommended in patients with mild hepatic disease.

Contra-indications: Arimidex is contra-indicated in: pre-menopausal women; pregnant or lactating women; patients with severe renal impairment (creatinine clearance less than 20 ml/min); and patients with moderate or severe hepatic disease; patients with known hypersensitivity to anastrozole or to any of the excipients as referenced in the list of excipients.

Oestrogen-containing therapies should not be co-administered with Arimidex as they would negate its pharmacological action.

Special warnings and special precautions for use: Arimidex is not recommended for use in children as safety and efficacy have not been established in this group of patients.

The menopause should be defined biochemically in any patient where there is doubt about hormonal status.

There are no data to support the safe use of Arimidex in patients with moderate or severe hepatic impairment, or patients with severe impairment of renal function (creatinine clearance less than 20 ml/min).

Interaction with other medicaments and other forms of interaction: Antipyrine and cimetidine clinical interaction studies indicate that the co-administration of Arimidex with other drugs is unlikely to result in clinically significant drug interactions mediated by cytochrome P450.

A review of the clinical trial safety database did not reveal evidence of clinically significant interaction in patients treated with Arimidex who also received other commonly prescribed drugs.

There is no clinical information to date on the use of Arimidex in combination with other anti-cancer agents.

Oestrogen-containing therapies should not be co-administered with Arimidex as they would negate its pharmacological action.

Pregnancy and lactation: Arimidex is contra-indicated in pregnant or lactating women

Effects on ability to drive and use machines: Arimidex is unlikely to impair the ability of patients to drive and operate machinery. However, asthenia and somnolence have been reported with the use of Arimidex and caution should be observed when driving or operating machinery while such symptoms persist.

Undesirable effects: Arimidex has generally been well tolerated. Adverse events have usually been mild to moderate with only few withdrawals from treatment due to undesirable events.

The pharmacological action of Arimidex may give rise to certain expected effects. These include hot flushes, vaginal dryness and hair thinning. Arimidex may also be associated with gastro-intestinal disturbances (anorexia, nausea, vomiting, and diarrhoea), asthenia, somnolence, headache or rash.

Vaginal bleeding has been reported infrequently, mainly in patients during the first few weeks after changing from existing hormonal therapy to treatment with Arimidex. If bleeding persists, further evaluation should be considered.

A causal relationship between anastrozole and thromboembolic events is not established. In clinical trials the frequency of thromboembolic events was not significantly different between anastrozole 1 mg and megestrol acetate, although the incidence with anastrozole 10 mg was lower.

Hepatic changes (elevated gamma-GT or less commonly alkaline phosphatase) have been reported in patients with advanced breast cancer, many of whom had liver and/or bone metastases. A causal relationship for these changes has not been established. Slight increases in total cholesterol have also been observed in clinical trials with Arimidex.

Overdose: There is no clinical experience of accidental overdosage. In animal studies, anastrozole demonstrated low acute toxicity. Clinical trials have been conducted with various dosages of Arimidex, up to 60 mg in a single dose given to healthy male volunteers and up to 10 mg daily given to post-menopausal women with advanced breast cancer; these dosages were well tolerated. A single dose of Arimidex that results in life-threatening symptoms has not been established. There is no specific antidote to overdosage and treatment must be symptomatic.

In the management of an overdose, consideration should be given to the possibility that multiple agents may have been taken. Vomiting may be induced if the patient is alert. Dialysis may be helpful because Arimidex is not highly protein bound. General supportive care, including frequent monitoring of vital signs and close observation of the patient, is indicated.

Pharmacological properties
Pharmacodynamic properties: Arimidex is a potent and highly selective non-steroidal aromatase inhibitor. In post-menopausal women, oestradiol is produced primarily from the conversion of androstenedione to oestrone through the aromatase enzyme complex in peripheral tissues. Oestrone is subsequently converted to oestradiol. Reducing circulating oestradiol levels has been shown to produce a beneficial effect in women with breast cancer. In post-menopausal women, Arimidex at a daily dose of 1 mg produced oestradiol suppression of greater than 80% using a highly sensitive assay.

Current data supports the use of Arimidex as an alternative therapy to megestrol acetate in post-menopausal women with advanced breast cancer which has progressed after previous treatment with tamoxifen or other anti-oestrogens.

Arimidex does not possess any progestogenic, androgenic or oestrogenic activity.

Daily doses of Arimidex up to 10 mg do not have any effect on cortisol or aldosterone secretion, measured before or after standard ACTH challenge testing. Corticoid supplements are therefore not needed.

Pharmacokinetic properties: Absorption of anastrozole is rapid and maximum plasma concentrations typically occur within two hours of dosing (under fasted conditions). Anastrozole is eliminated slowly with a plasma elimination half-life of 40 to 50 hours. Food slightly decreases the rate but not the extent of absorption. The small change in the rate of absorption is not expected to result in a clinically significant effect on steady-state plasma concentrations during once daily dosing of Arimidex tablets. Approximately 90 to 95% of plasma anastrozole steady-state concentrations are attained after 7 daily doses. There is no evidence of time or dose-dependency of anastrozole pharmacokinetic parameters.

Anastrozole pharmacokinetics are independent of age in post-menopausal women.

Pharmacokinetics have not been studied in children.

Anastrozole is only 40% bound to plasma proteins.

Anastrozole is extensively metabolised by post-menopausal women less than 10% of the dose excreted in the urine unchanged within 72 hours of dosing. Metabolism of anastrozole occurs by N-dealkylation, hydroxylation and glucuronidation. The metabolites are excreted primarily via the urine. Triazole, the major metabolite in plasma, does not inhibit aromatase.

The apparent oral clearance of anastrozole in volunteers with stable hepatic cirrhosis or renal impairment was in the range observed in healthy volunteers.

Preclinical safety data:
Acute toxicity: In acute toxicity studies in rodents the median lethal dose of anastrozole was greater than 100 mg/kg/day by the route and greater than 50 mg/kg/day by the intraperitoneal route.

Chronic toxicity: Multiple dose toxicity studies utilised rats and dogs. No no-effect levels were established for anastrozole in the toxicity studies, but those effects that were observed at the low doses (1 mg/kg/day) and mid doses (dog 3 mg/kg/day; rat 5 mg/kg/day) were related to either the pharmacological or enzyme inducing properties of anastrozole and were unaccompanied by toxic or degenerative changes.

Mutagenicity: Genetic toxicology studies with anastrozole show that it is not a mutagen or a clastogen.

Reproductive toxicology: Oral administration of anastrozole to pregnant rats and rabbits caused no teratogenic effects at doses up to 1.0 and 0.2 mg/kg/day respectively. Those effects that were seen (placental enlargement in rats and pregnancy failure in rabbits) were related to the pharmacology of the compound.

Carcinogenicity: No carcinogenicity studies have been conducted using anastrozole.

Pharmaceutical particulars
List of excipients: Lactose PhEur; Polyvidone PhEur; Sodium Starch Glycollate BP; Magnesium Stearate PhEur; Methylhydroxypropylcellulose PhEur; Macrogol 300 PhEur; Titanium Dioxide PhEur.

Incompatibilities: Nil.

Shelf life: The shelf life of Arimidex is 3 years when stored below 30°C.

Special precautions for storage: Nil.

Nature and contents of container: PVC blister/aluminium foil pack of 28 contained in a carton.

Instructions for use/handling: Nil.

Marketing authorisation number 12619/0106.

Date of approval/revision of SPC March 1998.

Legal category POM.

AVLOCLOR* TABLETS

Qualitative and quantitative composition Tablets containing 250 mg chloroquine phosphate which is equivalent to 155 mg chloroquine base.

Pharmaceutical form Tablets.

Clinical particulars

Therapeutic indications:

a) Treatment of malaria.

b) Prophylaxis and suppression of malaria.

c) Treatment of amoebic hepatitis and abscess.

d) Treatment of discoid and systemic lupus erythematosus.

e) Treatment of rheumatoid arthritis.

Dosage and method of administration: The dose should be taken after food.

a) Treatment of malaria

P. falciparum and P. malariae infections

Adults: A single dose of four tablets, followed by two tablets six hours later and then two tablets a day for two days.

Children: A single dose of 10 mg base/kg, followed by 5 mg base/kg six hours later and then 5 mg base/kg a day for two days.

Age (years)	Initial dose	Second dose 6 hrs after first	Dose on each of the two subsequent days
1–4	1 tablet	½ tablet	½ tablet
5–8	2 tablets	1 tablet	1 tablet
9–14	3 tablets	1½ tablets	1½ tablets

P. vivax and P. ovale infections

Adults: A single dose of four tablets, followed by two tablets six hours later and then two tablets a day for two days. Follow with a course of treatment with primaquine if a radical cure is required.

Children: A single dose of 10 mg base/kg, followed by 5 mg base/kg six hours later and then 5 mg base/kg a day for two days. Follow with a course of treatment with primaquine if a radical cure is required.

Elderly patients: There are no special dosage recommendations for the elderly, but it may be advisable to monitor elderly patients so that optimum dosage can be individually determined.

Hepatic or renally impaired patients: Caution is necessary when giving Avloclor to patients with renal disease or hepatic disease.

b) Prophylaxis and suppression of malaria

Adults: Two tablets taken once a week, on the same day each week. Start one week before exposure to risk and continue until four weeks after leaving the malarious area.

Children: A single dose of 5 mg chloroquine base/kg per week on the same day each week. Start one week before exposure to risk and continue until four weeks after leaving the malarious area.

For practical purposes, children aged over 14 years may be treated as adults. The dose given to infants and children should be calculated on their body weight and must not exceed the adult dose regardless of weight.

1–4 years: ½ tablet
5–8 years: 1 tablet
9–15 years: 1½ tablets

Elderly patients: There are no special dosage recommendations for the elderly, but it may be advisable to monitor elderly patients so that optimum dosage can be individually determined.

Hepatic or renally impaired patients: Caution is necessary when giving Avloclor to patients with renal disease or hepatic disease.

c) Amoebic hepatitis

Adults: Four tablets daily for two days followed by one tablet twice daily for two or three weeks.

Elderly patients: There are no special dosage recommendations for the elderly, but it may be advisable to monitor elderly patients so that optimum dosage can be individually determined.

Hepatic or renally impaired patients: Caution is necessary when giving Avloclor to patients with renal disease or hepatic disease.

d) Lupus erythematosus

Adults: One tablet twice daily for one to two weeks followed by a maintenance dosage of one tablet daily.

Elderly patients: There are no special dosage recommendations for the elderly, but it may be advisable to monitor elderly patients so that optimum dosage can be individually determined.

Hepatic or renally impaired patients: Caution is necessary when giving Avloclor to patients with renal disease or hepatic disease.

e) Rheumatoid arthritis

Adults: The usual dosage is one tablet daily.

Elderly patients: There are no special dosage recommendations for the elderly, but it may be advisable to monitor elderly patients so that optimum dosage can be individually determined.

Hepatic or renally impaired patients: Caution is necessary when giving Avloclor to patients with renal disease or hepatic disease.

Contra-indications: There are no absolute contra-indications to the use of Avloclor.

Warnings and precautions for use: In any locality where drug resistant malaria is known or suspected, it is essential to take professional advice on what prophylactic regimen or treatment regimen is appropriate.

Caution is necessary when giving Avloclor to patients with impaired hepatic function, particularly when associated with cirrhosis. Caution is also necessary in patients with porphyria. Avloclor may precipitate severe constitutional symptoms and an increase in the amount of porphyrins excreted in the urine. This reaction is especially apparent in patients with high alcohol intake.

Caution is necessary when giving Avloclor to patients with renal disease.

Avloclor should be used with care in patients with a history of epilepsy.

Prolonged therapy with high doses may lead to occasional development of irreversible retinal damage.

Considerable caution is needed in the use of Avloclor for long-term high dosage therapy and such use should only be considered when no other drug is available.

Patients receiving Avloclor continuously at higher dose levels for periods longer than 12 months should undergo ophthalmic examination before treatment and at three monthly intervals. This also applies to patients receiving Avloclor at weekly intervals for a period of more than 3 years as a prophylactic against malarial attacks or if the total consumption exceeds 1.6 g/kg.

Full blood counts should be carried out regularly during extended treatment as bone marrow suppression may occur rarely.

The use of Avloclor in patients with psoriasis may precipitate a severe attack.

Interactions with other medicaments and other forms of interaction: None have been reported or are known.

Pregnancy and lactation:

Pregnancy: Pregnancy increases the risks from malaria. As with all drugs, the use of Avloclor during pregnancy should be avoided if possible unless, in the case of life threatening infections, in the judgement of the physician, potential benefit outweighs the risk. There is evidence to suggest that Avloclor given to women in high doses throughout pregnancy can give rise to foetal abnormalities including ocular or cochlear damage.

Lactation: Although Avloclor is excreted in breast milk, the amount is insufficient to confer any benefit on the infant. Separate chemoprophylaxis for the infant is required.

Effect on ability to drive and use machinery: Defects in visual accommodation may occur on first taking Avloclor and patients should be warned regarding driving or operating machinery.

Possible adverse reactions: The adverse reactions which may occur at doses used in the prophylaxis or treatment of malaria are generally not of a serious nature. Where prolonged high dosage is required, ie in the treatment of rheumatoid arthritis, adverse reactions can be of a more serious nature.

Adverse reactions reported after Avloclor use are: headache, gastro-intestinal disturbances, skin eruptions, pruritus, occasional depigmentation or loss of hair, difficulty in accommodation, blurring of vision, corneal opacities, retinal degeneration, electrocardiographic changes, neurological and psychiatric changes, including convulsions and psychosis, thrombocytopenia, agranulocytosis, aplastic anaemia, allergic reactions, erythema multiforme, Stevens-Johnson syndrome, cardiomyopathy.

Changes in liver function, including hepatitis and abnormal liver function tests, have been reported rarely.

Overdose: Chloroquine is highly toxic in overdose and children are particularly susceptible. The chief symptoms of overdosage include circulatory collapse due to a potent cardiotoxic effect, respiratory arrest and coma. Symptoms may progress rapidly after initial nausea and vomiting. Cardiac complications may occur without progressively deepening coma.

Death may result from circulatory or respiratory failure or cardiac arrhythmia. If there is no demonstrable cardiac output due to arrhythmias, asystole or electromechanical dissociation, external chest compression should be persisted with for as long as necessary, or until adrenaline and diazepam can be given (see below).

Gastric lavage should be carried out urgently, first protecting the airway and instituting artificial ventilation where necessary. There is a risk of cardiac arrest following aspiration of gastric contents in more serious cases. Activated charcoal left in the stomach may reduce absorption of any remaining chloroquine from the gut. Circulatory status (with central venous pressure measurement), respiration, plasma electrolytes and blood gases should be monitored, with correction of hypokalaemia and acidosis if indicated. Cardiac arrhythmias should not be treated unless life threatening; drugs with quinidine-like effects should be avoided. Intravenous sodium bicarbonate 1-2 mmol/kg over 15 minutes may be effective in conduction disturbances, and DC shock is indicated for ventricular tachycardia and ventricular fibrillation.

Early administration of the following has been shown to improve survival in cases of serious poisoning:

1. Adrenaline infusion 0.25 micrograms/kg/min initially, with increments of 0.25 micrograms/kg/min until adequate systolic blood pressure (more than 100 mm/Hg) is restored; adrenaline reduces the effects of chloroquine on the heart through its inotropic and vasoconstrictor effects.

2. Diazepam infusion (2 mg/kg over 30 minutes as a loading dose, followed by 1-2 mg/kg/day for up to 2-4 days). Diazepam may minimise cardiotoxicity.

Acidification of the urine, haemodialysis, peritoneal dialysis or exchange transfusion have not been shown to be of value in treating chloroquine poisoning. Chloroquine is excreted very slowly, therefore cases of overdosage require observation for several days.

Pharmacological properties

Pharmacodynamic properties: The mode of action of chloroquine on plasmodia has not been fully elucidated. Chloroquine binds to and alters the properties of DNA. Chloroquine also binds to ferriprotoporphyrin IX and this leads to lysis of the plasmodial membrane.

In suppressive treatment, chloroquine inhibits the erythrocytic stage of development of plasmodia. In acute attacks of malaria, it interrupts erythrocytic schizogony of the parasite. Its ability to concentrate in parasitised erythrocytes may account for the selective toxicity against the erythrocytic stages of plasmodial infection.

Pharmacokinetic properties: Studies in volunteers using single doses of chloroquine phosphate equivalent to 300 mg base have found peak plasma levels to be achieved within one to six hours. These levels are in the region of 54-102 microgram/litre, the concentration in erythrocytes being some 4.8 times higher. The elimination half-life of chloroquine is dose dependent and is approximately one hundred hours. Following a single dose, chloroquine may be detected in plasma for more than four weeks. Mean bioavailability from tablets of chloroquine phosphate is 89%. Chloroquine is widely distributed in body tissues such as the eyes, kidneys, liver, and lungs where retention is prolonged.

The principal metabolite is monodesethylchloroquine, which reaches a peak concentration of 10-20 microgram/litre within a few hours. Mean urinary recovery, within 3-13 weeks, is approximately 50% of the administered dose, most being unchanged drug and the remainder as metabolite. Chloroquine may be detected in urine for several months.

Pre-clinical safety data:

Avloclor has been widely used for many years in clinical practice. There is no animal data which adds significant information relevant to the prescriber, to that covered elsewhere in this document.

Pharmaceutical particulars

List of excipients: Magnesium stearate PhEur; Maize starch PhEur.

Incompatibilities: None have been reported or are known.

Shelf life: 5 years.

Special precautions for storage: Store below 30°C. Protect from light and moisture.

Nature and contents of container: HDPE bottle of 100's and PVC/Aluminium Foil Blister Pack of 20's

Instructions for use/handling: No special instructions.

Marketing authorisation number 12619/0002

Date of approval/revision of SPC October 1996

Legal Category POM.

P. for prevention of malaria.

CASODEX* TABLETS 50 mg

Qualitative and quantitative composition Each tablet contains 50 mg bicalutamide (INN)

Pharmaceutical form White film-coated tablet

Clinical particulars

Therapeutic indication: Treatment of advanced prostate cancer in combination with LHRH analogue therapy or surgical castration.

Posology and method of administration:

Adult males including the elderly: one tablet (50 mg) once a day.

Treatment with Casodex should be started at least 3 days before commencing treatment with an LHRH analogue, or at the same time as surgical castration.

Children: Casodex is contra-indicated in children

Renal impairment: no dosage adjustment is necessary for patients with renal impairment.

Hepatic impairment: no dosage adjustment is necessary for patients with mild hepatic impairment. Increased accumulation may occur in patients with moderate to severe hepatic impairment (see *Special warnings and special precautions for use*).

Contra-indications: Casodex is contra-indicated in females and children.

Casodex must not be given to any patient who has shown a hypersensitivity reaction to its use.

Special warnings and special precautions for use: Casodex is extensively metabolised in the liver. Data suggests that its elimination may be slower in subjects with severe hepatic impairment and this could lead to some accumulation of Casodex. Therefore, Casodex should be used with caution in patients with moderate to severe hepatic impairment.

Interaction with other medicaments and other forms of interaction: There is no evidence of any pharmacodynamic or pharmacokinetic interactions between Casodex and LHRH analogues.

Although Casodex does not appear to interact with commonly co-prescribed drugs, formal interaction studies have not been undertaken. Therefore caution should be exercised when prescribing Casodex with other drugs which may inhibit drug oxidation e.g. cimetidine and ketoconazole. In theory, this could result in increased plasma concentrations of Casodex which theoretically could lead to an increase in side effects.

Casodex has shown no evidence of causing enzyme induction during dosing up to 150 mg daily.

In vitro studies have shown that Casodex can displace the coumarin anticoagulant, warfarin, from its protein binding sites. It is therefore recommended that if Casodex is started in patients who are already receiving coumarin anticoagulants, prothrombin time should be closely monitored.

Pregnancy and lactation: Casodex is contra-indicated in females and must not be given to pregnant women or nursing mothers.

Effects on ability to drive and use machines: Casodex is unlikely to impair the ability of patients to drive or operate machinery. However, it should be noted that occasionally somnolence may occur. Any affected patients should exercise caution.

Undesirable effects: Casodex in general, has been well tolerated with few withdrawals due to adverse events.

The pharmacological action of Casodex may give rise to certain expected effects. These include hot flushes, pruritus and in addition, breast tenderness and gynaecomastia which may be reduced by concomitant castration. Casodex may also be associated with the occurrence of diarrhoea, nausea, vomiting, asthenia and dry skin.

Hepatic changes (elevated levels of transaminases, cholestasis and jaundice) have been observed in clinical trials with Casodex. The changes were frequently transient, resolving or improving despite continued therapy or following cessation of therapy. Hepatic failure has occurred very rarely in patients treated with Casodex, but a causal relationship has not been established with certainty. Periodic liver function testing should be considered.

Rare cardiovascular effects such as angina, heart failure, conduction defects including PR and QT interval prolongations, arrhythmias and non-specific ECG changes have been observed.

Thrombocytopenia has been reported rarely.

In addition, the following adverse experiences were reported in clinical trials (as possible adverse drug reactions in the opinion of investigating clinicians, with a frequency of ≥ 1%) during treatment with Casodex plus an LHRH analogue. No causal relationship of these experiences to drug treatment has been made and some of the experiences reported are those that commonly occur in elderly patients:

Cardiovascular system: heart failure.

Gastrointestinal system: anorexia, dry mouth, dyspepsia, constipation, flatulence.

Central nervous system: dizziness, insomnia, somnolence, decreased libido.

Respiratory system: dyspnoea.

Urogenital: impotence, nocturia.

Haematological : anaemia.

Skin and appendages: alopecia, rash, sweating, hirsutism.

Metabolic and nutritional: diabetes mellitus, hyperglycaemia, oedema, weight gain, weight loss.

Whole body: abdominal pain, chest pain, headache, pain, pelvic pain, chills.

Overdose: There is no human experience of overdosage. There is no specific antidote; treatment should be symptomatic. Dialysis may not be helpful, since Casodex is highly protein bound and is not recovered unchanged in the urine. General supportive care, including frequent monitoring of vital signs, is indicated.

Pharmacological properties

Pharmacodynamic properties: Casodex is a non-steroidal anti-androgen, devoid of other endocrine activity. It binds to androgen receptors without activating gene expression, and thus inhibits the androgen stimulus. Regression of prostatic tumours results from this inhibition.

Casodex is a racemate with its antiandrogenic activity being almost exclusively in the (R)-enantiomer.

Pharmacokinetic properties: Casodex is well absorbed following oral administration. There is no evidence of any clinically relevant effect of food on bioavailability.

The (S)-enantiomer is rapidly cleared relative to the (R)-enantiomer, the latter having a plasma elimination half-life of about 1 week.

On daily administration of Casodex, the (R)-enantiomer accumulates about 10 fold in plasma as a consequence of its long half-life.

Steady state plasma concentrations of the (R)-enantiomer of approximately 9 microgram per ml are observed during daily administration of 50 mg doses of Casodex. At steady state the predominantly active (R)-enantiomer accounts for 99% of the total circulating enantiomers.

The pharmacokinetics of the (R)-enantiomer are unaffected by age, renal impairment or mild to moderate hepatic impairment. There is evidence that for subjects with severe hepatic impairment, the (R)-enantiomer is more slowly eliminated from plasma.

Casodex is highly protein bound (96%) and extensively metabolised (via oxidation and glucuronidation): Its metabolites are eliminated via the kidneys and bile in approximately equal proportions.

Preclinical safety data: Casodex is a potent antiandrogen and a mixed function oxidase enzyme inducer in animals. Target organ changes, including tumour induction, in animals, are related to these activities. None of the findings in the preclinical testing is considered to have relevance to the treatment of advanced prostate cancer patients.

Pharmaceutical particulars

List of excipients: Casodex includes the following excipients: Lactose PhEur; Magnesium Stearate PhEur; Methylhydroxypropylcellulose PhEur; Polyethylene Glycol 300 PhEur; Polyvidon PhEur; Sodium Starch Glycollate BP; Titanium Dioxide PhEur.

Incompatibilities: None known.

Shelf life: 3 years

Special precautions for storage: Store below 30°C

Nature and contents of container: PVC blister/aluminium foil packs.

Instructions for use/handling: No special precautions required.

Marketing authorisation number 12619/0102

Date of apporval/revision of SPC March 1996

Legal category POM

CORWIN*

Presentation Corwin tablets containing xamoterol fumarate equivalent to 200 mg xamoterol are round, biconvex, dark yellow, film coated tablets impressed with 'CORWIN' on one face and with an 'S' logo on the reverse. The impressions are highlighted in white. The inactive ingredients are calcium phosphate, gelatin, iron oxide, lactose, macrogol, magnesium carbonate, magnesium stearate, methylhydroxypropylcellulose, sodium starch glycollate and titanium dioxide.

Uses Chronic mild heart failure: Corwin is recommended for the treatment of patients who are not breathless at rest but who are limited by symptoms on exertion (eg breathlessness and fatigue). Treatment with Corwin should be initiated under hospital supervision only after the patient has been fully assessed [see 'Initiation of treatment' below]. After initiation of treatment the appropriate follow-up should be provided by hospital or general practitioners.

Corwin is contra-indicated in patients with moderate to severe heart failure. Some patients with moderate to severe heart failure have shown deterioration on Corwin. See 'Contra-indications' below.

Mode of action: Corwin is a beta$_1$-selective partial agonist. At rest and under conditions of low sympathetic drive Corwin acts predominantly as a beta adrenoceptor agonist. On exercise and under conditions of increased sympathetic drive, eg severe heart failure, Corwin acts as a beta adrenoceptor antagonist. In mild heart failure, Corwin improves cardiac efficiency by modestly increasing myocardial contractility, improving diastolic relaxation and lowering left ventricular filling pressure. The improved ventricular function results in increased cardiac output with no attendant increase in myocardial oxygen demand. This improvement in myocardial performance is maintained on exercise.

Many heart failure patients suffer from concomitant ischaemic heart disease. In patients with angina pectoris, a reduction in myocardial ischaemia on exercise has been demonstrated with Corwin at the dose levels recommended for heart failure.

Dosage and administration

Adults: Treatment should be started with 200 mg once a day for a week; dosage should then be increased to 200 mg twice daily provided that there are no adverse effects. The usual effective dose is 200 mg twice daily (but see renal impairment warning below). Improvement in symptoms of heart failure (eg dyspnoea, fatigue) may be progressive over a period of several weeks.

Elderly patients: No specific dosage reduction is necessary except in those with suspected or established renal impairment (see below).

Initiation of treatment: Treatment should be initiated under hospital supervision after full assessment of the patient who has completed an exercise test which excludes diagnosis of moderate or severe heart failure. In addition to other exclusion criteria under 'Contra-indications' and depending on the method used, the patient should be able to complete one of the following exercise tests (equivalent to 3.6 kilojoules).

- For a bicycle ergometer; two minutes of exercise starting with a load of 20 W for the first minute and at a load of 40 W for the second minute.
- For an exercise treadmill; two minutes of exercise at a treadmill speed of 4 km/h with the treadmill level (ie 0% incline).
- For a corridor walk test; 150 yards on the level in two minutes.
- Alternatively, any other standardised exercise test in which the patient achieves a basal workload equivalent to one of the tests defined above (equivalent to 3.6 kilojoules).

Patients who are unable to complete the minimum of two minutes exercise on the bicycle ergometer or equivalent should not be given Corwin. Assessment of the patient's heart failure status should also include such tests as an ECG and a chest X-ray. Additional investigations such as an echocardiogram may be necessary.

Children: There is no paediatric experience with Corwin and for this reason it is not recommended for use in children.

Contra-indications, warnings, etc

Contra-indications: Corwin is contra-indicated in patients with moderate to severe heart failure because some patients with moderate to severe heart failure have shown deterioration on Corwin.

Corwin should, therefore, not be used in patients with the following features:

- Those who are short of breath or fatigued at rest or limited on minimal exercise.
- Those who have a resting tachycardia (>90 beats per minute) or hypotension (systolic BP<100 mmHg).
- Those who present with acute pulmonary oedema or who have a history of repeated episodes of acute pulmonary oedema.
- Those with peripheral oedema, a raised jugular venous pressure, an enlarged liver or a third heart sound.
- Those who require treatment with doses of diuretics in excess of frusemide 40 mg per day or equivalent.
- Those who require treatment with an ACE inhibitor.

Precautions: Deterioration of disease: Corwin should be withdrawn from patients whose mild heart failure deteriorates whilst on the drug, for example, if the patient develops worsening symptoms (shortness of breath and/or fatigue), diminishing effort tolerance, or the appearance of signs such as peripheral oedema, a raised jugular venous pressure, an enlarged liver or a third heart sound. If Corwin is withdrawn, the patient should be carefully observed.

Renal impairment: Since Corwin is excreted by the kidneys, dosage should be adjusted in cases of severe impairment of renal function. No significant accumulation of Corwin occurs at a GFR greater than 35 ml/min/1.73 m². Significant accumulation of Corwin occurs only when GFR decreases to 15–35 ml/min/1.73 m². This level of renal impairment is usually clinically evident and approximates to a doubling of the serum creatinine (eg greater than 250 micromol/l or 3 mg/dl). The dose of Corwin is 200 mg daily when clinical evidence indicates suspected or established renal impairment (approximate doubling of serum creatinine value or a GFR of 15–35 ml/min/1.73 m²).

Obstructive airways disease: Due to the beta adrenoceptor antagonist effects of Corwin, an increase in airways resistance may be provoked in patients with asthma or chronic obstructive airways disease. In such an event, Corwin should be withdrawn and increased airways resistance may be reversed by the use of inhaled bronchodilator preparations such as salbutamol. Corwin should be used with caution in patients with co-existing obstructive airways disease.

Liver function: Elevations of liver enzymes have been reported rarely in patients receiving Corwin but in such cases no relationship to the drug has been established.

Aortic stenosis/hypertrophic obstructive cardiomyopathy: As with other drugs which increase the force of myocardial contraction, Corwin should be used with caution in patients with outflow obstruction.

Cardiac arrhythmias: Cardiac arrhythmias are common in patients with heart failure. Occasional cases of ventricular arrhythmias have been reported during Corwin therapy and, in some patients, Corwin cannot be excluded as a contributory factor. Ambulatory (Holter) ECG monitoring studies have not shown any evidence that Corwin therapy promotes arrhythmias. In patients with atrial fibrillation, concurrent therapy with a cardiac glycoside must be maintained.

Pregnancy and lactation: There is no evidence for the safety of the drug in human pregnancy. When high doses of Corwin were given to rats and rabbits during the second half of pregnancy, the cardiovascular effects of the drug led to deformations. It is recommended, therefore, that administration of the drug is avoided in pregnancy unless the condition itself carries sufficient risks to the mother and foetus to warrant use.

Studies in rats show that Corwin is excreted in the breast milk of lactating females. Its use in lactating women who are breast feeding should be avoided.

Side-effects: Rarely bronchospasm, worsening of obstructive airways disease and hypotension have been observed after introduction of Corwin.

Adverse experiences in controlled studies showed a small excess in incidence over placebo of gastrointestinal complaints, headache and dizziness.

Although there was also an apparent excess of angina/chest pain such events are not uncommon and are to be expected in heart failure patients. Other controlled studies with Corwin in patients with angina pectoris showed reduced incidence of myocardial ischaemia during exercise.

Rash, palpitations and muscle cramp were also reported.

Overdosage: There is no experience of overdosage with Corwin. Effects are unlikely to be life threatening; symptomatic conservative management is recommended.

Pharmaceutical precautions Corwin tablets should be stored at room temperature.

Legal category POM.

Package quantities Corwin tablets (200 mg) in calendar packs of 56 tablets (OP).

Further information Corwin should not be co-administered with other beta, adrenoceptor agonists or antagonists because of competition between these drugs and Corwin for the beta, adrenoceptor.

Corwin has been co-administered without evidence of incompatibility with a range of other therapies including thiazide and potassium-sparing diuretics, cardiac glycosides, warfarin, antiplatelet drugs and non-steroidal anti-inflammatory drugs.

Product licence number 12619/0009.

DIPRIVAN* 1%

Qualitative and quantitative composition 10 mg propofol per 1 ml.

Pharmaceutical form Oil-in-water emulsion for intravenous injection.

Clinical particulars

Therapeutic Indications: Diprivan 1% is a short-acting intravenous anaesthetic agent suitable for induction and maintenance of general anaesthesia.

Diprivan 1% may also be used for sedation of ventilated patients receiving intensive care. Diprivan 1% may also be used for sedation for surgical and diagnostic procedures.

Posology and method of administration: For specific guidance relating to the administration of Diprivan 1% with a target controlled infusion (TCI) device, which incorporates Diprifusor TCI Software, see *Administration.* Such use is restricted to induction and maintenance of anaesthesia in adults. The Diprifusor TCI system is not recommended for use in ICU sedation or sedation for surgical and diagnostic procedures, or in children.

Induction of general anaesthesia:

Adults: In unpremedicated and premedicated patients, it is recommended that Diprivan 1% should be titrated (approximately 4 ml [40 mg] every 10 seconds in an average healthy adult by bolus injection or infusion) against the response of the patient until the clinical signs show the onset of anaesthesia. Most adult patients aged less than 55 years are likely to require 1.5 to 2.5 mg/kg of Diprivan 1%. The total dose required can be reduced by lower rates of administration (2 to 5 ml/min [20 to 50 mg/min]). Over this age, the requirement will generally be less. In patients of ASA Grades 3 and 4, lower rates of administration should be used (approximately 2 ml [20 mg] every 10 seconds).

Elderly patients: Diprivan 1% should be titrated against the response of the patient. Patients over the age of about 55 years may require lower doses of Diprivan 1% for induction of anaesthesia.

Children: Diprivan 1% is not recommended for induction of anaesthesia in children aged less than 1 month.

When used to induce anaesthesia in children, it is recommended that Diprivan 1% be given slowly until the clinical signs show the onset of anaesthesia. The dose should be adjusted for age and/or weight. Most patients over 8 years of age are likely to require approximately 2.5 mg/kg of Diprivan 1% for induction of anaesthesia. Under this age the requirement may be more. Lower dosage is recommended for children of ASA grades 3 and 4.

Administration of Diprivan 1% by a Diprifusor TCI system is not recommended for induction of general anaesthesia in children.

Maintenance of general anaesthesia:

Adults (including elderly patients): Anaesthesia can be maintained by administering Diprivan 1% either by continuous infusion or by repeat bolus injections to prevent the clinical signs of light anaesthesia. Recovery from anaesthesia is typically rapid and it is therefore important to maintain Diprivan 1% administration until the end of the procedure.

Continuous infusion: The required rate of administration varies considerably between patients, but rates in the region of 4 to 12 mg/kg/h usually maintain satisfactory anaesthesia.

Repeat bolus injections: If a technique involving repeat bolus injections is used, increments of 25 mg (2.5 ml) to 50 mg (5.0 ml) may be given according to clinical need.

Children: Diprivan 1% is not recommended for maintenance of anaesthesia in children less than 3 years of age.

Anaesthesia can be maintained by administering Diprivan 1% by infusion or repeat bolus injection to prevent the clinical signs of light anaesthesia. The required rate of administration varies considerably between patients, but rates in the region of 9 to 15 mg/kg/h usually achieve satisfactory anaesthesia.

Administration of Diprivan 1% by a Diprifusor TCI system is not recommended for maintenance of general anaesthesia in children.

Sedation during intensive care

Adults (including elderly patients): When used to provide sedation for ventilated patients undergoing intensive care, it is recommended that Diprivan 1% be given by continuous infusion.

The infusion rate should be adjusted according to the depth of sedation required, but rates in the region of 0.3 to 4.0 mg/kg/h should achieve satisfactory sedation. Rates of infusion greater than 4.0 mg/kg/h are not recommended. Diprivan 1% may be diluted with 5% Dextrose (see *Dilution and Co-administration* table below).

It is recommended that blood lipid levels be monitored should Diprivan 1% be administered to patients thought to be at particular risk of fat overload.

Administration of Diprivan 1% should be adjusted appropriately if the monitoring indicates that fat is being inadequately cleared from the body. If the patient is receiving other intravenous lipid concurrently, a reduction in quantity should be made in order to take account of the amount of lipid infused as part of the Diprivan 1% formulation; 1.0 ml of Diprivan 1% contains approximately 0.1 g of fat.

If the duration of sedation is in excess of 3 days, lipids should be monitored in all patients.

Administration of Diprivan 1% by a Diprifusor TCI system is not recommended for sedation during intensive care.

Children: Diprivan 1% is not recommended for sedation in children as safety and efficacy have not been demonstrated. Although no causal relationship has been established, serious adverse events (including fatalities) have been observed from spontaneous reports of unlicensed use. These events were seen most often in children with respiratory tract infections given doses in excess of those recommended for adults.

Sedation for surgical and diagnostic procedures:

Adults: To provide sedation for surgical and diagnostic procedures, rates of administration should be individualised and titrated to clinical response.

Most patients will require 0.5 to 1 mg/kg over 1 to 5 minutes for onset of sedation.

Maintenance of sedation may be accomplished by titrating Diprivan 1% infusion to the desired level of sedation–most patients will require 1.5 to 4.5 mg/kg/h. In addition to the infusion, bolus administration of 10 to 20 mg may be used if a rapid increase in the depth of sedation is required. In patients of ASA Grades 3 and 4 the rate of administration and dosage may need to be reduced.

Administration of Diprivan 1% by a Diprifusor TCI system is not recommended for sedation for surgical and diagnostic procedures.

Elderly patients: Diprivan 1% should be titrated against the response of the patient. Patients over the age of about 55 years may require lower doses of Diprivan 1% for sedation for surgical and diagnostic procedures.

Children: Diprivan 1% is not recommended for sedation in children as safety and efficacy have not been demonstrated.

Administration: Diprivan 1% has no analgesic properties and therefore supplementary analgesic agents are generally required in addition to Diprivan 1%. Diprivan 1% has been used in association with spinal and epidural anaesthesia and with commonly used premedicants, neuromuscular blocking drugs, inhalational agents and analgesic agents; no pharmacological incompatibility has been encountered. Lower doses of Diprivan 1% may be required where general anaesthesia is used as an adjunct to regional anaesthetic techniques.

Diprivan 1% can be used for infusion undiluted from glass containers, plastic syringes or Diprivan 1% pre-filled syringes or diluted with 5% Dextrose (Intravenous Infusion BP) only, in PVC infusion bags or glass infusion bottles. Dilutions, which must not exceed 1 in 5 (2 mg propofol per ml) should be prepared aseptically immediately before administration and must be used within 6 hours of preparation.

It is recommended that, when using diluted Diprivan 1%, the volume of 5% Dextrose removed from the infusion bag during the dilution process is totally replaced in volume by Diprivan 1% emulsion. (see *Dilution and Co-administration table below*).

The dilution may be used with a variety of infusion control techniques, but a giving set used alone will not avoid the risk of accidental uncontrolled infusion of large volumes of diluted Diprivan 1%. A burette, drop counter or volumetric pump must be included in the infusion line. The risk of uncontrolled infusion must be taken into account when deciding the maximum amount of Diprivan 1% in the burette.

When Diprivan 1% is used undiluted to maintain anaesthesia, it is recommended that equipment such as syringe pumps or volumetric infusion pumps should always be used to control infusion rates.

Diprivan 1% may be administered via a Y-piece close to the injection site into infusions of the following:

- Dextrose 5% Intravenous Infusion B.P.
- Sodium Chloride 0.9% Intravenous Infusion B.P.
- Dextrose 4% with Sodium Chloride 0.18% Intravenous Infusion B.P.

The glass pre-filled syringe (PFS) has a lower frictional resistance than plastic disposable syringes and operates more easily. Therefore, if Diprivan 1% is administered using a hand held pre-filled syringe, the line between the syringe and the patient must not be left open if unattended.

When the pre-filled syringe presentation is used in a syringe pump appropriate compatibility should be ensured. In particular, the pump should be designed to prevent syphoning and should have an occlusion alarm set no greater than 1000 mm Hg. If using a programmable or equivalent pump that offers options for use of different syringes then choose only the B-D 50/60 ml PLASTIPAK setting when using the Diprivan 1% pre-filled syringe.

Diprivan 1% may be premixed with alfentanil injection containing 500 microgram/ml alfentanil in the ratio of 20:1 to 50:1 v/v. Mixtures should be prepared using sterile technique and used within 6 hours of preparation.

In order to reduce pain on initial injection, Diprivan 1% may be mixed with preservative-free Lignocaine Injection 0.5% or 1%; (see *Dilution and co-administration table below*).

Target controlled infusion–administration of Diprivan 1% by a Diprifusor TCI system: Administration of Diprivan 1% by a Diprifusor TCI system is restricted to induction and maintenance of general anaesthesia in adults. It is not recommended for use in ICU sedation or sedation for surgical and diagnostic procedures, or in children.

To achieve induction and maintenance of anaesthesia in adults, Diprivan 1% may be administered with the assistance of a Target Controlled Infusion (TCI) system. Such systems allow the anaesthetist to achieve and control a desired speed of induction and depth of anaesthesia by setting and adjusting target (predicted) blood concentrations of propofol. Diprivan 1% may be administered by TCI only with a Diprifusor TCI system incorporating Diprifusor TCI software. Such systems will operate only on recognition of electronically tagged pre-filled syringes containing Diprivan 1% or 2% Injection. The Diprifusor TCI system will automatically adjust the infusion rate for the concentration of Diprivan recognised. Users must be familiar with the infusion pump users' manual, and with the administration of Diprivan 1% by TCI and with the correct use of the syringe identification system, all of which are set out in the Diprifusor training manual, available from Zeneca at the address below.

Guidance on propofol target concentrations is given below. In view of interpatient variability in propofol pharmacokinetics and pharmacodynamics, in both premedicated and unpremedicated patients the target propofol concentration should be titrated against the response of the patient in order to achieve the depth of anaesthesia required.

In adult patients under 55 years of age anaesthesia can usually be induced with target propofol concentrations in the region of 4 to 8 microgram/ml. An initial target of 4 microgram/ml is recommended in premedicated patients and in unpremedicated patients an initial target of 6 microgram/ml is advised. Induction time with these targets is generally within the range of 60 to 120 seconds. Higher targets will allow more rapid induction of anaesthesia but may be associated with more pronounced haemodynamic and respiratory depression.

A lower initial target concentration should be used in patients over the age of about 55 years and in patients of ASA grades 3 and 4. The target concentration can then be increased in steps of 0.5 to 1.0 microgram/ml at intervals of 1 minute to achieve a gradual induction of anaesthesia.

Supplementary analgesia will generally be required and the extent to which target concentrations for maintenance of anaesthesia can be reduced will be influenced by the amount of concomitant analgesia administered. Target propofol concentrations in the region of 3 to 6 microgram/ml usually maintain satisfactory anaesthesia.

The predicted propofol concentration on waking is generally in the region of 1.0 to 2.0 microgram/ml and will be influenced by the amount of analgesia given during maintenance.

Dilution and co-administration of Diprivan 1% with other drugs or infusion fluids (see also *Additional precautions section*)

Co-administration Technique	*Additive or Diluent*	*Preparation*	*Precautions*
Pre-mixing.	Dextrose 5% Intravenous Infusion B.P.	Mix 1 part of Diprivan 1% with up to 4 parts of Dextrose 5% Intravenous Infusion B.P in either PVC infusion bags or glass infusion bottles. When diluted in PVC bags it is recommended that the bag should be full and that the dilution be prepared by withdrawing a volume of infusion fluid and replacing it with an equal volume of Diprivan 1%.	Prepare aseptically immediately before administration. The mixture is stable for up to 6 hours.
	Lignocaine Hydro-chloride Injection (0.5% or 1% without preservatives).	Mix 20 parts of Diprivan 1% with up to 1 part of either 0.5% or 1% Lignocaine Hydrochloride Injection.	Prepare mixture aseptically immediately prior to administration. Use for induction only.
	Alfentanil injection (500 microgram/ml).	Mix Diprivan 1% with alfentanil injection in a ratio of 20:1 to 50:1 v/v.	Prepare mixture aseptically; use within 6 hours of preparation.
Co-administration via a Y-piece connector.	Dextrose 5% Intravenous Infusion B.P.	Co-administer via a Y-piece connector.	Place the Y-piece connector close to the injection site.
	Sodium Chloride 0.9% Intravenous Infusion B.P.	As above.	As above.
	Dextrose 4% with Sodium Chloride 0.18% Intravenous Infusion B.P.	As above.	As above.

Contra-indications: Diprivan 1% is contra-indicated in patients with a known allergy to Diprivan 1% or 2%.

Special warnings and special precautions for use: Diprivan 1% should be given by those trained in anaesthesia or, where appropriate, doctors trained in the care of patients in Intensive Care. Patients should be constantly monitored and facilities for maintenance of a patent airway, artificial ventilation, oxygen enrichment and other resuscitative facilities should be readily available at all times. Diprivan 1% should not be administered by the person conducting the diagnostic or surgical procedure.

When Diprivan 1% is administered for sedation for surgical and diagnostic procedures patients should be continually monitored for early signs of hypotension, airway obstruction and oxygen desaturation.

As with other intravenous anaesthetic and sedative agents, patients should be instructed to avoid alcohol before and for at least 8 hours after administration of Diprivan 1%.

Diprivan 1% should be used with caution when used to sedate patients undergoing some procedures where spontaneous movements are particularly undesirable, such as ophthalmic surgery.

As with other intravenous sedative agents, when Diprivan 1% is given along with central nervous system depressants, such as potent analgesics, the sedative effect may be intensified and the possibility of severe respiratory or cardiovascular depression should be considered.

During bolus administration for operative procedures, extreme caution should be exercised in patients with acute pulmonary insufficiency or respiratory depression.

Concomitant use of central nervous system depressants eg, alcohol, general anaesthetics, narcotic analgesics will result in accentuation of their sedative effects. When Diprivan 1% is combined with centrally depressant drugs administered parenterally, severe respiratory and cardiovascular depression may occur. It is recommended that Diprivan 1% is administered following the analgesic and the dose should be carefully titrated to the patient's response.

During induction of anaesthesia, hypotension and transient apnoea may occur depending on the dose and use of premedicants and other agents.

Occasionally, hypotension may require use of intravenous fluids and reduction of the rate of administration of Diprivan 1% during the period of anaesthetic maintenance.

An adequate period is needed prior to discharge of the patient to ensure full recovery after general anaesthesia.

When Diprivan 1% is administered to an epileptic patient, there may be a risk of convulsion.

As with other intravenous anaesthetic agents, caution should be applied in patients with cardiac, respiratory, renal or hepatic impairment or in hypovolaemic, elderly or debilitated patients.

The risk of relative vagal overactivity may be increased because Diprivan 1% lacks vagolytic activity; it has been associated with reports of bradycardia (occasionally profound) and also asystole. The intravenous administration of an anticholinergic agent before induction, or during maintenance of anaesthesia should be considered, especially in situations where vagal tone is likely to predominate, or when Diprivan 1% is used in conjunction with other agents likely to cause a bradycardia.

Appropriate care should be applied in patients with disorders of fat metabolism and in other conditions where lipid emulsions must be used cautiously.

Use is not recommended with electroconvulsive treatment.

As with other anaesthetics, sexual disinhibition may occur during recovery.

Additional precautions: Diprivan 1% contains no antimicrobial preservatives and supports growth of micro-organisms. When Diprivan 1% is to be aspirated, it must be drawn aseptically into a sterile syringe or giving set immediately after opening the ampoule or breaking the vial seal. Administration must commence without delay. Asepsis must be maintained for both Diprivan 1% and infusion equipment throughout the infusion period. Any drugs or fluids added to the Diprivan 1% line must be administered close to the cannula site. Diprivan 1% must not be administered via a microbiological filter.

Diprivan 1% and any syringe containing Diprivan 1% are for single use in an individual patient. For use in long term maintenance of anaesthesia or sedation in intensive care it is recommended that the infusion line and reservoir of Diprivan 1% be discarded and replaced at regular intervals.

Interaction with other medicaments and other forms of interaction: See *Administration.*

Pregnancy and lactation:

Pregnancy: Teratology studies in rats and rabbits showed no teratogenic effects. Diprivan 1% has been used during termination of pregnancy in the first trimester. It should not be used in pregnancy.

Obstetrics: Diprivan 1% crosses the placenta and may be associated with neonatal depression. It should not be used for obstetric anaesthesia.

Lactation: Safety to the neonate has not been established following the use of Diprivan 1% in mothers who are breast feeding.

Effects on ability to drive and use machines: Patients should be advised that performance at skilled tasks, such as driving and operating machinery, may be impaired for some time after general anaesthesia.

Undesirable effects:

General: Induction of anaesthesia is generally smooth with minimal evidence of excitation. Side effects during induction, maintenance and recovery occur uncommonly. Changes in cardiovascular parameters are usually slight but such changes may be important in patients with impaired myocardial oxygen delivery capacity and hypovolaemia. When Diprivan 1% is administered, convulsions, myoclonus and opisthotonos may occur, usually after termination of administration of the product and occasionally delayed. Spontaneous movements and pulmonary oedema have been observed. During the recovery phase nausea, vomiting and headache occur in only a small proportion of patients. Rarely, discolouration of urine has been reported following prolonged administration of Diprivan 1%. Rarely, clinical features of anaphylaxis, which may include angioedema, bronchospasm, erythema and hypotension, occur following Diprivan 1% administration. There have been reports of post-operative fever.

Local: The local pain which may occur during the induction phase of Diprivan 1% anaesthesia can be minimised by the co-administration of lignocaine (see *Dosage and administration*) and by the use of the larger veins of the forearm and antecubital fossa. Thrombosis and phlebitis are rare. Accidental clinical extravasation and animal studies showed minimal tissue reaction. Intra-arterial injection in animals did not induce local tissue effects.

Overdose: Accidental overdosage is likely to cause cardiorespiratory depression. Respiratory depression should be treated by artificial ventilation with oxygen. Cardiovascular depression would require lowering of the patient's head and, if severe, use of plasma expanders and pressor agents.

Pharmacological properties

Pharmacodynamic properties: Propofol (2, 6-diisopropylphenol) is a short-acting general anaesthetic agent with a rapid onset of action of approximately 30 seconds. Recovery from anaesthesia is usually rapid. The mechanism of action, like all general anaesthetics, is poorly understood.

In general, falls in mean arterial blood pressure and slight changes in heart rate are observed when Diprivan 1% is administered for induction and maintenance of anaesthesia. However, the haemodynamic parameters normally remain relatively stable during maintenance and the incidence of untoward haemodynamic changes is low.

Although ventilatory depression can occur following administration of Diprivan 1%, any effects are qualitatively similar to those of other intravenous anaesthetic agents and are readily manageable in clinical practice.

Diprivan 1% reduces cerebral blood flow, intracranial pressure and cerebral metabolism. The reduction in intracranial pressure is greater in patients with an elevated baseline intracranial pressure.

Recovery from anaesthesia is usually rapid and clear headed with a low incidence of headache and post-operative nausea and vomiting.

In general, there is less post-operative nausea and vomiting following anaesthesia with Diprivan 1% than following anaesthesia with inhalational agents. There is evidence that this may be related to a reduced emetic potential of propofol.

Diprivan 1%, at the concentrations likely to occur clinically, does not inhibit the synthesis of adrenocortical hormones.

Pharmacokinetic properties: The decline in propofol concentrations following a bolus dose or following the termination of an infusion can be described by a three compartment open model with very rapid distribution (half-life 2 to 4 minutes), rapid elimination (half-life 30 to 60 minutes), and a slower final phase, representative of redistribution of propofol from poorly perfused tissue.

Propofol is extensively distributed and rapidly cleared from the body (total body clearance 1.5 to 2 litres/minute). Clearance occurs by metabolic processes, mainly in the liver, to form inactive conjugates of propofol and its corresponding quinol, which are excreted in urine.

When Diprivan 1% is used to maintain anaesthesia, blood concentrations asymptotically approach the steady-state value for the given administration rate. The pharmacokinetics are linear over the recommended range of infusion rates of Diprivan 1%.

Preclinical safety data: Propofol is a drug on which

extensive clinical experience has been obtained. All relevant information for the prescriber is provided elsewhere in the Summary of Product Characteristics.

Pharmaceutical particulars

List of excipients: Glycerol PhEur; Purified Egg Phosphatide; Sodium Hydroxide PhEur; Soya-bean Oil PhEur; Water for Injections PhEur

Incompatibilities: The neuromuscular blocking agents, atracurium and mivacurium should not be given through the same intravenous line as Diprivan 1% without prior flushing.

Shelf life:

Shelf life of the product as packaged for sale:

Ampoules	3 years
Vials	3 years
Pre-filled syringe	2 years.

Shelf life after dilution: When diluted, Diprivan 1% must be used within 6 hours of preparation.

Special precautions for storage: Diprivan 1% should be stored between 2°C and 25°C; it must not be frozen.

Nature and contents of container:

(a) Clear neutral glass ampoules of 20 ml in boxes of 5

(b) Clear neutral glass vials of 50 ml and 100 ml

(c) Type 1 glass pre-filled syringe of 50 ml

Instructions for use/handling:

In-use precautions: Containers should be shaken before use.

Any portion of the contents remaining after use should be discarded.

Diprivan 1% should not be mixed prior to administration with injections or infusion fluids other than 5% Dextrose or Lignocaine Injection (see *Administration*).

Marketing authorisation number 12619/0010.

Date of approval/revision of SPC 30 September 1998

Legal category POM

DIPRIVAN* 2%

(Pre-filled syringe and Vial combined)

Qualitative and quantitative composition White, aqueous and isotonic emulsion for intravenous injection containing 20 mg propofol per 1 ml.

Pharmaceutical form Oil-in-water emulsion for intravenous injection.

Clinical particulars

Therapeutic indications: Diprivan 2% is a short-acting intravenous anaesthetic agent suitable for induction and maintenance of general anaesthesia.

Diprivan 2% may also be used for sedation of ventilated patients receiving intensive care.

Posology and method of administration:

For specific guidance relating to the administration of Diprivan 2% with a 'target controlled infusion' (TCI) device, which incorporates Diprifusor TCI Software, see *Administration*. Such use is restricted to induction and maintenance of anaesthesia in adults. The Diprifusor TCI system is not recommended for use in ICU sedation or in children.

Induction of general anaesthesia:

Adults: Diprivan 2% may be used to induce anaesthesia by infusion.

Administration of Diprivan 2% by bolus injection is not recommended.

Diprivan 2% may be used to induce anaesthesia by infusion but only in those patients who will receive Diprivan 2% for maintenance of anaesthesia.

In unpremedicated and premedicated patients, it is recommended that Diprivan 2% should be titrated (approximately 2 ml [40 mg] every 10 seconds in an average healthy adult by infusion) against the response of the patient until the clinical signs show the onset of anaesthesia. Most adult patients aged less than 55 years are likely to require 1.5 to 2.5 mg/kg of Diprivan 2%. The total dose required can be reduced by lower rates of administration (1 to 2.5 ml/min [20 to 50 mg/min]). Over this age, the requirement will generally be less. In patients of ASA Grades 3 and 4, lower rates of administration should be used (approximately 1 ml [20 mg] every 10 seconds).

Elderly patients: Diprivan 2% should be titrated against the response of the patient. Patients over the age of about 55 years may require lower doses of Diprivan 2% for induction of anaesthesia.

Children: Diprivan 2% is not recommended for induction of anaesthesia in children less than 3 years of age.

When used to induce anaesthesia in children, it is recommended that Diprivan 2% be given by slow infusion until the clinical signs show the onset of anaesthesia. The dose should be adjusted for age and/or weight. Most patients over 8 years of age are likely to require approximately 2.5 mg/kg of Diprivan 2% for induction of anaesthesia. Under this age the requirement may be more. Lower dosage is recommended for children of ASA grades 3 and 4.

Administration of Diprivan 2% by a Diprifusor TCI system is not recommended for induction of general anaesthesia in children.

Maintenance of general anaesthesia:

Anaesthesia can be maintained by administering Diprivan 2% by continuous infusion to prevent the clinical signs of light anaesthesia. Administration of Diprivan 2% by bolus injection is not recommended. Recovery from anaesthesia is typically rapid and it is therefore important to maintain Diprivan 2% administration until the end of the procedure.

Adults (including elderly patients): The required rate of administration varies considerably between patients, but rates in the region of 4 to 12 mg/kg/h usually maintain satisfactory anaesthesia.

Children: Diprivan 2% is not recommended for maintenance of anaesthesia in children less than 3 years of age.

The required rate of administration varies considerably between patients but rates in the region of 9 to 15 mg/kg/h usually achieve satisfactory anaesthesia.

Administration of Diprivan 2% by a Diprifusor TCI System is not recommended for maintenance of general anaesthesia in children.

Sedation during intensive care:

Adults (including elderly patients): When used to provide sedation for ventilated patients undergoing intensive care, it is recommended that Diprivan 2% be given by continuous infusion.

The infusion rate should be adjusted according to the depth of sedation required, but rates in the region of 0.3 to 4.0 mg/kg/h should achieve satisfactory sedation. Rates of infusion greater than 4.0 mg/kg/h are not recommended.

It is recommended that blood lipid levels be monitored should Diprivan 2% be administered to patients thought to be at particular risk of fat overload.

Administration of Diprivan 2% should be adjusted appropriately if the monitoring indicates that fat is being inadequately cleared from the body. If the patient is receiving other intravenous lipid concurrently, a reduction in quantity should be made in order to take account of the amount of lipid infused as part of the Diprivan 2% formulation: 1.0 ml of Diprivan 2% contains approximately 0.1 g of fat.

If the duration of sedation is in excess of 3 days, lipids should be monitored in all patients.

Administration of Diprivan 2% by a Diprifusor TCI system is not recommended for sedation during intensive care.

Children: Diprivan 2% is not recommended for sedation in children as safety and efficacy have not been demonstrated. Although no causal relationship has been established, serious adverse events (including fatalities) have been observed from spontaneous reports of unlicensed use of Diprivan. These events were seen most often in children with respiratory tract infections given doses in excess of those recommended for adults.

Administration: Diprivan 2% has no analgesic properties and therefore supplementary analgesic agents are generally required in addition to Diprivan 2%.

Diprivan has been used in association with spinal and epidural anaesthesia and with commonly used premedicants, neuromuscular blocking drugs, inhalational agents and analgesic agents; no pharmacological incompatibility has been encountered. Lower doses of Diprivan 2% may be required where general anaesthesia is used as an adjunct to regional anaesthetic techniques.

Diprivan 2% should not be diluted. Diprivan 2% can be used for infusion undiluted from glass containers, plastic syringes or Diprivan 2% pre-filled syringes.

When Diprivan 2% is used to maintain anaesthesia, it is recommended that equipment such as syringe pumps or volumetric infusion pumps should always be used to control infusion rates.

Diprivan 2% should not be mixed prior to administration with injections or infusion fluids. However, Diprivan 2% may be co-administered via a Y-piece connector close to the injection site with the following:

- Dextrose 5% Intravenous Infusion BP.
- Sodium Chloride 0.9% Intravenous Infusion BP.
- Dextrose 4% with Sodium Chloride 0.18% Intravenous Infusion BP.

The glass pre-filled syringe (PFS) has a lower frictional resistance than plastic disposable syringes and operates more easily. Therefore, if Diprivan 2% is administered using a hand held pre-filled syringe, the line between the syringe and the patient must not be left open if unattended.

When the pre-filled syringe presentation is used in a syringe pump appropriate compatibility should be ensured. In particular, the pump should be designed to prevent syphoning and should have an occlusion alarm set no greater than 1000 mm Hg. If using a programmable or equivalent pump that offers options for use of different syringes then choose only the 'B-D' 50/60 ml 'PLASTIPAK' setting when using the Diprivan 2% pre-filled syringe.

Target controlled infusion–administration of Diprivan 2% by a Diprifusor TCI system:

Administration of Diprivan 2% by a Diprifusor TCI system is restricted to induction and maintenance of general anaesthesia in adults. It is not recommended for use in ICU sedation or in children.

To achieve induction and maintenance of anaesthesia in adults, Diprivan 2% may be administered with the assistance of a Target Controlled Infusion (TCI) system. Such systems allow the anaesthetist to achieve and control a desired speed of induction and depth of anaesthesia by setting and adjusting target (predicted) blood concentrations of propofol. Diprivan 2% may be administered by TCI only with a Diprifusor TCI system incorporating Diprifusor TCI software. Such systems will operate only on recognition of electronically tagged prefilled syringes containing Diprivan 1% or 2% Injection. The Diprifusor TCI system will automatically adjust the infusion rate for the concentration of Diprivan recognised. Users must be familiar with the infusion pump users' manual, and with the administration of Diprivan 2% by TCI and with the correct use of the syringe identification system, all of which are set out in the Diprifusor training manual, available from Zeneca at the address below.

Guidance on propofol target concentrations as given below. In view of interpatient variability in propofol pharmacokinetics and pharmacodynamics, in both premedicated and unpremedicated patients the target propofol concentration should be titrated against the response of the patient in order to achieve the depth of anaesthesia required.

In adult patients under 55 years of age anaesthesia can usually be induced with target propofol concentrations in the region of 4 to 8 microgram/ml. An initial target of 4 microgram/ml is recommended in premedicated patients and in unpremedicated patients an initial target of 6 microgram/ml is advised. Induction time with these targets is generally within the range of 60 to 120 seconds. Higher targets will allow more rapid induction of anaesthesia but may be associated with more pronounced haemodynamic and respiratory depression.

A lower initial target concentration should be used in patients over the age of about 55 years and in patients of ASA Grades 3 and 4. The target concentration can then be increased in steps of 0.5 to 1.0 microgram/ml at intervals of 1 minute to achieve a gradual induction of anaesthesia.

Supplementary analgesia will generally be required and the extent to which target concentrations for maintenance of anaesthesia can be reduced will be influenced by the amount of concomitant analgesia administered. Target propofol concentrations in the region of 3 to 6 microgram/ml usually maintain satisfactory anaesthesia.

The predicted propofol concentration on waking is generally in the region of 1.0 to 2.0 microgram/ml and will be influenced by the amount of analgesia given during maintenance.

Contra-indications: Diprivan 2% is contra-indicated in patients with a known allergy to Diprivan 1% or Diprivan 2%.

Special warnings and special precautions for use: Diprivan 2% should be given by those trained in anaesthesia, or where appropriate, doctors trained in the care of patients in Intensive Care. Facilities for maintenance of a patent airway, artificial ventilation and oxygen enrichment should be available.

During induction of anaesthesia, hypotension and transient apnoea may occur depending on the dose and use of premedicants and other agents.

Occasionally, hypotension may require use of intravenous fluids and reduction of the rate of administration of Diprivan 2% during the period of anaesthetic maintenance.

An adequate period is needed prior to discharge of the patient to ensure full recovery after general anaesthesia.

When Diprivan 2% is administered to an epileptic patient, there may be a risk of convulsion.

As with other intravenous anaesthetic agents, caution should be applied in patients, with cardiac, respiratory, renal or hepatic impairment or in hypovolaemic or debilitated patients.

The risk of relative vagal overactivity may be increased because Diprivan 2% lacks vagolytic activity. Diprivan has been associated with reports of bradycardia (occasionally profound) and also asystole. The intravenous administration of an anticholinergic agent before induction, or during maintenance of anaesthesia should be considered, especially in situations where vagal tone is likely to predominate or when Diprivan 2% is used in conjunction with other agents likely to cause a bradycardia.

Appropriate care should be applied in patients with disorders of fat metabolism and in other conditions where lipid emulsions must be used cautiously.

Use is not recommended with electroconvulsive treatment.

As with other anaesthetics sexual disinhibition may occur during recovery.

Additional precautions: Diprivan 2% contains no antimicrobial preservatives and supports growth of micro-organisms. Asepsis must be maintained for both Diprivan 2% and infusion equipment throughout the infusion period. Any drugs or fluids added to the Diprivan 2% infusion line must be administered close to the cannula site. Diprivan 2% must not be administered via a microbiological filter.

Diprivan 2% and any syringe containing Diprivan 2% are for single use in an individual patient. For use in long-term maintenance of anaesthesia or sedation in intensive care it is recommended that the infusion line and reservoir of Diprivan 2% be discarded and replaced at regular intervals.

Interaction with other medicaments and other forms of interaction: see *Administration.*

Pregnancy and lactation:
Pregnancy: Teratology studies in rats and rabbits showed no teratogenic effects. Diprivan has been used during termination of pregnancy in the first trimester. Diprivan 2% should not be used in pregnancy.

Obstetrics: Diprivan crosses the placenta and may be associated with neonatal depression. It should not be used for obstetric anaesthesia.

Lactation: Safety to the neonate has not been established following the use of Diprivan 2% in mothers who are breast feeding. Diprivan 2% should be avoided, or mothers should stop breast feeding.

Effects on ability to drive and use machines: Patients should be advised that performance at skilled tasks, such as driving and operating machinery, may be impaired for some time after general anaesthesia.

Undesirable effects:
General: Induction of anaesthesia is generally smooth with minimal evidence of excitation. Side effects during induction, maintenance and recovery occur uncommonly. When Diprivan 2% is administered convulsions, myoclonus and opisthotonus may occur, usually after termination of administration of the product and occasionally delayed. Pulmonary oedema has been observed. During the recovery phase, nausea, vomiting and headache occur in only a small proportion of patients. Rarely, discolouration of urine has been reported following prolonged administration with Diprivan. Rarely, clinical features of anaphylaxis, which may include angioedema, bronchospasm, erythema and hypotension, occur following Diprivan administration. There have been reports of post-operative fever.

Local: The local pain which may occur during the induction phase can be minimised by the use of the larger veins of the forearm and anticubital fossa. Thrombosis and phlebitis are rare. Accidental clinical extravasation and animal studies showed minimal tissue reaction. Intra-arterial injection in animals did not induce local tissue effects.

Overdose: Accidental overdosage is likely to cause cardiorespiratory depression. Respiratory depression should be treated by artificial ventilation with oxygen. Cardiovascular depression would require lowering of the patient's head and, if severe, use of plasma expanders and pressor agents.

Pharmacological properties
Pharmacodynamic properties: Propofol (2,6-diisopropylphenol) is a short-acting general anaesthetic agent with a rapid onset of action of approximately 30 seconds. Recovery from anaesthesia is usually rapid. The mechanism of action, like all general anaesthetics, is poorly understood.

In general, falls in mean arterial blood pressure and slight changes in heart rate are observed when Diprivan 2% is administered for induction and maintenance of anaesthesia. However, the haemodynamic parameters normally remain relatively stable during maintenance and the incidence of untoward haemodynamic changes is low.

Although ventilatory depression can occur following administration of Diprivan 2%, any effects are qualitatively similar to those of other intravenous anaesthetic agents and are readily manageable in clinical practice.

Diprivan 2% reduces cerebral blood flow, intracranial pressure and cerebral metabolism. The reduction in intracranial pressure is greater in patients with an elevated baseline intracranial pressure.

Recovery from anaesthesia is usually rapid and clear headed with a low incidence of headache and post-operative nausea and vomiting.

In general, there is less post-operative nausea and vomiting following anaesthesia with Diprivan 2% than following anaesthesia with inhalational agents. There is evidence that this may be related to a reduced emetic potential of propofol.

Diprivan 2%, at the concentrations likely to occur clinically, does not inhibit the synthesis of adrenocortical hormones.

Pharmacokinetic properties: The decline in propofol concentrations following a bolus dose or following the termination of an infusion can be described by a three compartment open model with very rapid distribution (half-life 2 to 4 minutes), rapid elimination (half-life 30 to 60 minutes), and a slower final phase, representative of redistribution of propofol from poorly perfused tissue.

Propofol is extensively distributed and rapidly cleared from the body (total body clearance 1.5 to 2 litres/minute). Clearance occurs by metabolic processes, mainly in the liver, to form inactive conjugates of propofol and its corresponding quinol, which are excreted in urine.

When Diprivan 2% is used to maintain anaesthesia, blood concentrations asymptotically approach the steady-state value for the given administration rate. The pharmacokinetics are linear over the recommended range of infusion rates of Diprivan 2%.

Preclinical safety data: Propofol is a drug on which extensive clinical experience has been obtained. All relevant information for the prescriber is provided elsewhere in the Summary of Product Characteristics.

Pharmaceutical particulars
List of excipients: Glycerol PhEur; Purified Egg Phosphatide; Sodium Hydroxide PhEur; Soya-Bean Oil PhEur; Water for Injections PhEur.

Incompatibilities: The neuromuscular blocking agents, atracurium and mivacurium should not be given through the same intravenous line as Diprivan 2% without prior flushing.

Shelf life:
Shelf life of the product as packaged for sale: 2 years.

Shelf life after dilution: Diprivan 2% should not be diluted.

Special precautions for storage: Storage Precautions: Diprivan 2% should be stored between 2°C and 25°C; it must not be frozen.

Nature and contents of container: 50 ml pre-filled syringe containing propofol 20 mg/ml.; 50 ml vial containing propofol 20 mg/ml.

Instructions for use/handling: In-use precautions: Containers should be shaken before use.

Any portion of the contents remaining after use should be discarded.

Diprivan 2% should not be mixed prior to administration with injections or infusion fluids.

Marketing authorisation numbers
PL 12619/0096 – Pre-filled syringe.
PL 12619/0110 – vial.

Date of approval/revision of SPC November 1997

Legal category POM.

FLUOTHANE*

Presentation Fluothane is a colourless, volatile liquid, non-explosive and non-flammable in the concentrations usually used. Chemically it is 2-bromo-2-chloro-1,1,1-trifluoroethane stabilised with thymol 0.01% w/w (Halothane PhEur).

Uses Fluothane is a volatile anaesthetic which is suitable for the induction and maintenance of anaesthesia for all types of surgery and in patients of all ages.

Mode of action: When inhaled, Fluothane is absorbed through the alveoli into the bloodstream. In the bloodstream Fluothane circulates through the body to the principal site of action, the brain. Here Fluothane causes a progressive depression of the central nervous system, beginning with the higher centres (cerebral cortex) and spreading to the vital centres in the medulla. This depression is reversible. However, its mode of action, like all anaesthetic agents, is unknown.

Fluothane may cause bronchodilation. Bronchial relaxation is usually dose-related and may be due to blockage of pathways, causing bronchoconstriction or depression of bronchial muscular tone.

Fluothane causes a reversible, dose-related decline in renal blood flow, glomerular filtration rate and urinary flow.

Fluothane may be absorbed by the rubber used in some anaesthetic circuits. The rubber/gas partition coefficient at 20°C is 120.

Fluothane has a relatively low solubility in blood and therefore alveoli/blood concentrations equilibrate rapidly. The triexponential decline in Fluothane blood concentrations following the end of administration is thought to represent distribution into three compartments; the vessel rich group (brain/heart/liver), the musculature and adipose tissue. Approximately 80% of the inhaled Fluothane is eliminated unchanged by the lungs. The remaining 20% is metabolised in the liver by oxidative and, under hypoxic conditions, reductive pathways. The main metabolites are trifluoroacetic acid, bromide and chloride salts (via the oxidative pathway) and fluoride salts (via the reductive pathway). The concentrations of metabolites peak 24 hours post-operatively and are eliminated by renal excretion during the following week.

Dosage and administration A number of anaesthetic vaporisers specially designed for use with Fluothane are available. Open, semi-open, semi-closed and closed circuit systems have all been used with good results.

For induction of anaesthesia in the adult patient a concentration of 2–4% Fluothane in oxygen or oxygen/nitrous oxide may be used. In children a concentration of 1.5–2% Fluothane in oxygen or oxygen/nitrous oxide is used. A concentration of 0.5–2% is usually adequate for maintenance of anaesthesia in both adults and children. The lower concentration is usually most suitable for elderly patients.

Contra-indications, warnings, etc Fluothane can induce liver damage; however, the incidence of severe liver damage (jaundice, which may lead to hepatic failure as a consequence of massive hepatic cell necrosis) is unknown. The risk of developing hepatic failure appears to be increased by repeated exposure. Although short intervals of time between exposures are likely to increase the risk of hepatotoxicity, even long intervals between exposure may not eliminate the risks, since some patients have developed severe reactions following Fluothane given many years after the previous exposure. On the information which is available at the present time, it is advised that the following precautions be taken:

(i) A careful anaesthetic history should be taken prior to use, to determine previous exposure and previous reactions following Fluothane anaesthesia.
(ii) Repeated exposure to Fluothane within a period of at least 3 months should be avoided unless there are overriding clinical circumstances.
(iii) History of unexplained jaundice and pyrexia in a patient following exposure to Fluothane is a contra-indication to its future use in that patient unless absolutely essential.
(iv) Fluothane is contra-indicated in patients with a history of malignant hyperthermia, or in whom liver dysfunction, jaundice or unexplained fever, leucocytosis, or eosinophilia has occurred after a previous halogenated anaesthetic administration.
(v) Patients should be informed if they have developed a reaction possibly related to Fluothane anaesthesia; such patients should be provided with a medical alert card stating the problem.

Fluothane is contra-indicated in patients with a previous history of malignant hyperpyrexia or those susceptible to maligant hyperpyrexia.

As Fluothane causes relaxation of the uterine muscle it is advisable that anaesthesia should be maintained in the lightest plane possible during obstetric operations. Obstetric use, especially at high concentrations, may result in post partum haemorrhage.

The role of Fluothane in liver damage occasionally observed after anaesthesia has not been definitely established. However, as such cases appear more frequently after repeated anaesthetic administration, the appearance of unexplained jaundice and pyrexia following exposure to Fluothane should be regarded as a contra-indication to its later use. Repeat exposure within a period of three months should be avoided in all patients. Further risk factors, (other than repeated exposure) appear to be female gender, obesity and middle age.

With the use of halogenated anaesthetics, disruption of the liver function, icterus and fatal liver necrosis have been reported. Such reactions appear to indicate hypersensitivity reactions to anaesthetics. Cirrhosis, viral hepatitis, or other pre-existing liver disease can be a reason to select an anaesthetic other than a halogenated anaesthetic.

Halothane is a potent cerebral vasodilator. Increases in cerebral blood flow and/or intracranial pressure may be observed during anaesthesia with Fluothane. These may be more marked in the presence of intracranial space-occupying lesions. The use of a moderate hyperventilation during neurosurgery is recommended to counteract the rise in intracranial fluid pressure which may occur with Fluothane.

Malignant hyperpyrexia has been reported in some patients receiving Fluothane, more commonly when co-administered with suxamethonium. This syndrome occurs with other anaesthetic agents, and may respond to intravenous dantrolene sodium.

During the induction of Fluothane anaesthesia a moderate fall in blood pressure commonly occurs. (Halothane lowers arterial blood pressure in a dose-dependent manner). The pressure tends to rise when the vapour concentration is reduced to maintenance levels, but it usually remains steady below the pre-operative level. This hypotensive effect is useful in providing a clear operating field and a reduction in haemorrhage. However, if necessary, intravenous doses of methoxamine (5 mg are usually adequate) can be given to counteract the fall in blood pressure.

Anaesthesia with Fluothane may be associated with bradycardia, which may augment its hypotensive effect. The intravenous administration of an anticholinergic agent before induction or during maintenance of anaesthsia should be considered, especially in situations where vagal tone is likely to be predominant or when Fluothane is used in conjunction with other agents likely to cause a bradycardia.

Cardiac arrhythmias have been reported during anaesthesia with Fluothane. Caution is required with regard to the administration of Fluothane to patients with phaeochromocytoma, as it is possible that this may lead to an increased likelihood of intra-operative arrhythmias.

Fluothane may cause respiratory depression, particularly at higher concentrations.

Halothane causes relaxation of skeletal muscle. Caution is required when using Fluothane in patients with myasthenia gravis or those co-administered aminoglycoside antibiotics.

Caution should be exercised during the administration of adrenaline to patients anaesthetised with Fluothane as arrhythmias may be precipitated. For this reason the dose of adrenaline should be restricted and an antiarrhythmic agent administered as appropriate. Caution should also be applied for other sympathomimetics, and for aminophylline, theophylline and tricyclic antidepressants, which may also precipitate arrhythmias.

Fluothane augments the action of non-depolarising muscle relaxants and the muscle relaxant effects of aminoglycosides.

Fluothane may augment the hypotension caused by the ganglionic-blocking effect of tubocurarine.

Bradycardia and/or hypotension may occur during Fluothane anaesthesia. Hypotension may occur particularly during induction.

Shivering may be observed during recovery from anaesthesia, especially if the patient is in cool surroundings.

Post-operative nausea and vomiting may occur after Fluothane anaesthesia.

Ensure adequate room ventilation when Fluothane is being used. Keep the concentration of Fluothane in air as low as possible.

Halothane is absorbed by the rubber used in some anaesthetic circuits. This is of clinical importance when halothane-free circuits are required for patients susceptible to malignant hyperpyrexia, or who have demonstrated hypersensitivity to previous administration of halothane. If rubber circuits are used, and a patient with known sensitivity is next on the list, then a new circuit should be set up.

Pregnancy: Data from animal experiments have indicated that halothane may have teratogenic potential in some species. Although these findings cannot be directly related to man, it would be prudent to avoid general anaesthesia with Fluothane during early pregnancy, except where such use is essential.

Lactation: There are no well controlled studies with Fluothane in lactating women. Fluothane has been detected in breast milk of lactating women, but the effects of Fluothane on breast fed neonates has not been established. However, Fluothane has been in wide use for over 30 years without apparent ill consequence.

Effect on ability to drive or operate machinery: Patients should be advised that performance at skilled tasks, such as driving and operating machinery, may be impaired for some time after general anaesthesia.

Accidental ingestion: Cases of ingestion must be treated symptomatically.

Pharmaceutical precautions Bottles of Fluothane must be securely closed and stored below 25°C, protected from light. Fluothane must be kept in the original container until immediately prior to its use.

Whilst in the liquid phase, Fluothane must not be diluted or contaminated; however, in the vapour phase it may be administered together with oxygen or a mixture of nitrous oxide and oxygen.

Legal category P.

Package quantities Fluothane is supplied in bottles of 250 ml.

Further information *Spillage:* Absorb spillage using a suitable absorbent material and transfer to a closed container for disposal. In case of insufficient ventilation wear suitable respiratory equipment. *Disposal:* Disposal is normally carried out by incineration under carefully controlled conditions.

Product licence number 12619/0014.

FULCIN* 500 TABLETS
FULCIN* 125 TABLETS
FULCIN* ORAL SUSPENSION

Qualitative and quantitative composition Tablets containing 125 mg or 500 mg Griseofulvin PhEur.; Oral suspension containing 2.5% w/v Griseofulvin PhEur. (125 mg griseofulvin in 5 ml).

Pharmaceutical form Tablets; Aqueous suspension.

Clinical particulars

Therapeutic indications: Fulcin is effective against the dermatophytes causing ringworm (tinea) including Microsporum canis, Trichophyton rubrum, Trichophyton verrucosum and Epidermophyton spp.

Fulcin is indicated for the treatment of fungal infections of the skin, hair and nails, when topical therapy has failed or is considered inappropriate.

Posology and method of administration:

Adults: The adult dosage is normally 500 mg daily, but in severe conditions, up to twice this amount may be given, reducing to the lower level when a clinical response has occurred. The normal dosage may be given as one 125 mg tablet or 5 ml suspension four times a day, or as one 500 mg tablet once daily after food.

Children: For children, the most suitable form is the pleasantly flavoured Fulcin Oral Suspension. The daily dosage is 10 mg griseofulvin per kg bodyweight daily i.e. 5 ml of suspension for every 12.5 kg in single or divided doses after food.

Elderly: There are no special dosage recommendations for the elderly, but it may be advisable to monitor elderly patients so that optimum dosage can be individually determined.

The duration of treatment depends on the type of infection and the time required for normal replacement of infected tissues.

For complete eradication of infection, Fulcin treatment should be combined with general measures of care and hygiene. Reservoirs of infection may include clothing, footwear and bedding as well as the patient's hair.

Contra-indications: Fulcin should not be used for prophylaxis.

Fulcin should not be administered to patients who have established porphyria or hepatocellular failure or to patients with lupus erythematosus and related conditions.

Fulcin is contra-indicated in pregnancy (see *Pregnancy and lactation*).

Special warnings and special precautions for use: Griseofulvin is capable of producing aneuploidy (abnormal segregation of chromosomes following cell division) in mammalian cells exposed to the compound in vitro and in vivo. Griseofulvin may damage sperm cells; males should not father children during treatment or within six months of completion of treatment.

A suitable diluent for Fulcin Oral Suspension is syrup BP which has been preserved with methylhydroxybenzoate. The dilution should be used within 14 days of preparation.

Interactions with other medicaments and other forms of interaction: Fulcin may decrease the response to coumarin anticoagulants administered concomitantly.

Liver enzyme inducing drugs, such as barbiturates, may reduce the effectiveness of Fulcin therapy by interfering with gastrointestinal absorption of the drug.

Breakthrough bleeding and amenorrhoea have been reported in patients taking griseofulvin and oral contraceptive steroids. Since failure of oral contraceptive therapy has been reported whilst receiving Fulcin, additional contraceptive precautions should be taken during and one month after treatment.

Patients should be warned that enhancement of the effects of alcohol by griseofulvin has been reported.

Long-term administration of high doses of griseofulvin with food has been reported to induce hepatomas in mice and thyroid tumours in rats. The clinical significance of these findings in man is not known. In view of this data, Fulcin should not be used prophylactically.

Griseofulvin may falsely elevate urinary levels of VMA.

Pregnancy and lactation:

Pregnancy: Fulcin is contra-indicated in pregnancy. Griseofulvin administered to rats during pregnancy has been associated with foetotoxicity and tail deformities at high dosages. Some case reports of human foetal abnormalities have been observed. There is no evidence of safety in human pregnancy and some reports suggest that griseofulvin may produce human foetal abnormalities.

Women should not become pregnant during or within one month of treatment with griseofulvin; if they do, they should seek genetic advice.

Nursing mothers: It is not known if griseofulvin is excreted in breast milk, safety in children of nursing mothers has not been established.

Effects on the ability to drive and use machines: Fulcin may impair the ability of some individuals to drive and operate machinery. There have been occasional reports of dizziness and confusion with impaired coordination and griseofulvin has been reported to enhance the effects of alcohol.

Undesirable effects: Fulcin is generally well tolerated. Urticarial reactions and skin rashes have been noted in a few cases. There have been occasional complaints of headache and gastric discomfort which, in most cases, have regressed during treatment. Dizziness, fatigue, granulocytopenia and leucopenia have also been reported. Photosensitivity associated with griseofulvin therapy has been recorded and there have been rare reports of precipitation of lupus erythematosus and related conditions, erythema multiforme, toxic epidermal necrolysis and related conditions, peripheral neuropathy, confusion with impaired coordination and of oral candidiasis.

Overdose: Treatment of overdosage should be symptomatic.

Pharmacological properties

Pharmacodynamic properties: Griseofulvin inhibits fungal cell mitosis by causing disruption of the mitotic spindle structure, thereby arresting the metaphase of cell division. It is deposited in varying degrees in the keratin precursor cells of skin, hair and nails, rendering the keratin resistant to fungal invasion. As the infected keratin is shed, it is replaced with healthy tissue.

Fulcin is not effective in infections caused by Candida albicans (monilia), Aspergilli, Malassezia furfur (Pityriasis versicolor) and Nocardia species.

Pharmacokinetic properties: Following oral administration, griseofulvin is absorbed principally from the duodenum. Peak plasma concentrations of the drug (approximately 1-2 microgram/ml) occur about 4 hours after dosing. Concentrations of approximately 12- 25 microgram/g are maintained in skin during long term administration, whilst concurrent serum levels remain at 1-2 microgram/ml. When the drug is discontinued, the drug is not detectable after 2 days in the skin and after 4 days in the plasma. The drug has an elimination half-life of 9-24 hours and it is metabolised in the liver, the major metabolite being 6-demethylgriseofulvin which is microbiologically inactive. The metabolites are excreted mainly in the urine whilst unchanged griseofulvin is excreted mainly in the faeces. Griseofulvin is also excreted in perspiration.

Pre-clinical safety data:

See *Special warnings and special precautions for use, Interactions with other medicaments and other forms of interaction and Pregnancy and lactation.*

Pharmaceutical particulars

List of excipients: Tablets: Calcium carboxymethylcellulose USF (125 mg), PhEur (500 mg); Magnesium stearate PhEur; Maize starch PhEur; Povidone BP (125 mg), PhEur (500 mg)

Oral suspension: Calcium chloride hexahydrate PhEur; Chocolate flavour 2606; Cocoa USF; Methylhydroxybenzoate PhEur; Peppermint oil PhEur; Propylhydroxybenzoate PhEur; Sodium alginate; Sodium carboxymethylcellulose PhEur; Sodium citrate PhEur; Sucrose PhEur; Vanillin BP; Purified water PhEur

Incompatibilities: None known.

Shelf life: Tablets–5 years; Oral suspension–4 years.

Special precautions for storage: Tablets–store below 25°C, protect from moisture; Oral suspension - store below 25°C.

Nature and contents of container: Aluminium tubes or HDPE bottles of 100 or 1000 tablets of 125 mg.; Aluminium tubes or HDPE bottles of 25, 100 or 250 tablets of 500 mg; Glass bottles containing 100 ml of suspension.

Instructions for use/handling: Use as directed by the prescriber.

Marketing authorisation numbers
Fulcin Tablets 125 mg PL 12619/0016
Fulcin Tablets 500 mg PL 12619/0017
Fulcin Oral Suspension 2.5% w/v PL 12619/0015

Date of renewal of marketing authorisation
16 June 1997 for 500 mg tablets
21 August 1997 for 125 mg tablets and oral suspension.

Date of approval/revision of the text July 1997.

Legal category POM.

HIBICET* HOSPITAL CONCENTRATE

Qualitative and quantitative composition Chlorhexidine Gluconate 1.5% w/v. (incorporated as Chlorhexidine Gluconate Solution PhEur 7.5% v/v) Cetrimide 15% w/v (incorporated as Strong Cetrimide Solution BP.)

Pharmaceutical form Liquid.

Clinical particulars

Therapeutic indications: Hibicet Hospital Concentrate is an antimicrobial preparation with cleansing properties for general antiseptic purposes.

Posology and method of administration: For external use only.

Dilute as follows:

Method of preparation	*Dilution rate*	*Use*
10 ml made up to 1 litre with water	1 in 100 (1%) Aqueous	Cleansing/antiseptic treatment of wounds and burns.† Swabbing in obstetrics, gynaecology and urology. Cleansing/disinfectant soak for used metal instruments. Clean instrument disinfection where no means of sterilisation is available (30 minutes immersion).‡ Cleansing/disinfection of equipment, furniture and fittings in the vicinity of the patient. Storage of clinical thermometers and sterile instruments.
35 ml made up to 1 litre with water	1 in 30 (approx) Aqueous	Cleansing/antiseptic treatment of wounds and burns where greater cleansing/antisepsis is required. † Cleansing/disinfectant soak for soiled instruments.
35 ml with 200 ml water made up to 1 litre with 95% alcohol	1 in 30 (approx) in 70% Alcohol	Rapid skin antisepsis before operation and other invasive procedures. Disinfection of clean instruments and equipment (two minutes immersion). † Disinfection of clinical thermometers.

† Sterilise the dilution by autoclaving at 115–116°C for 30 minutes or 121–123°C for 15 minutes.

‡ Endoscopes should not be placed in solution of Hibicet.

Children and elderly patients: There are no special dosage recommendations for either elderly patients or children. The normal adult dose is appropriate unless otherwise recommended by the physician.

Contra-indications: Hibicet preparations are contraindicated for patients who have previously shown a hypersensitivity reaction to either chlorhexidine or cetrimide. However, such reactions are extremely rare.

Special warnings and special precautions for use: For external use only. Dilute before use. Avoid contact with the brain, meninges and ears. Not for injection. Do not use in body cavities or as an enema.

The concentrated solution is irritant to eyes and mucous membranes. Keep all solutions out of the eyes. If solutions do come into contact with eyes, wash out promptly and thoroughly with water.

If concentrated cetrimide solutions come into contact with the skin, rinse promptly and thoroughly with water.

Prolonged skin contact with alcoholic solutions should be avoided. Allow to dry before proceeding.

Solutions applied to wounds, burns or broken skin should be sterilised according to BP recommendations.

Syringes and needles which have been immersed in Hibicet solutions should be thoroughly rinsed in sterile water or saline before use.

Hibicet solutions may affect glass cement and therefore are not suitable for the disinfection of endoscopes.

Interactions with other medicaments and other forms of interaction: See Incompatibilities.

Pregnancy and lactation: There is no evidence of any adverse effects on the foetus arising from the use of Hibicet Hospital Concentrate during pregnancy. Therefore no special precautions are recommended.

Effects on ability to drive and use machines: None have been reported or are known.

Undesirable effects: Irritative skin reactions can occasionally occur and rare hypersensitivity to cetrimide preparations, usually developing after repeated application, has been reported.

There have been rare reports of severe burn-like reactions to concentrated cetrimide solutions. Should such a reaction occur treat as a chemical burn.

Generalised allergic reactions to chlorhexidine have also been reported but are extremely rare.

In all these cases, stop application of the product.

Overdose: This has not been reported.

Accidental oral or rectal administration: If the product is swallowed give large quantities of milk, raw egg, gelatin or mild soap. Avoid vomiting or lavage if it is believed that a concentrated solution has been ingested.

Central paralysis cannot be countered by curare antagonists or CNS stimulants but sympathomimetic drugs have been given.

Mechanically assisted ventilation with oxygen may be necessary. Persistent convulsions may be controlled with cautious doses of diazepam or a short-acting barbiturate. Do not give alcohol in any form.

Accidental intravenous infusion: Massive haemolysis can occur which will require blood transfusion.

Accidental intra-uterine administration: Introduction into the uterus can lead to haemolysis and pulmonary embolism.

Pharmacological properties

Pharmacodynamic properties: Hibicet Hospital Concentrate is a topical antiseptic for external use only and is not intended to be administered orally or parenterally. The active agents, chlorhexidine gluconate and cetrimide are strongly cationic, binding to skin, mucosa and exposed tissues, thus percutaneous absorption is poor. There are, as a consequence, no general pharmacological studies available on the effects of Hibicet Hospital Concentrate or other topically administered chlorhexidine/cetrimide formulations.

If chlorhexidine is systemically absorbed there is no evidence of metabolic cleavage of the drug, however, animal studies suggest that systemically absorbed cetrimide may be metabolised to some extent.

Both active agents have a broad spectrum of antimicrobial activity and are bacteriostatic at low concentrations whilst at higher concentrations their activity is rapidly bactericidal. They are both active against dermatophytic fungi (including the yeast *C. Albicans*) and enveloped viruses such as HIV.

Pharmacokinetic properties: Percutaneous absorption of the active agents in Hibicet Hospital Concentrate is poor. Studies in animals using ^{14}C-Labelled cetrimide have shown that even after oral dosing only small amounts were found in the blood plasma and approximately 2% was excreted in the bile during the first 12 hours after treatment: only small amounts of radioactivity were found in the liver, kidneys, spleen, heart, lungs and skeletal muscle and tissue radioactivity declined rapidly.

Similarly, attempts to detect percutaneous absorption of chlorhexidine gluconate in man have shown that, if it occurs at all, the level is exceedingly small and insignificant–the limit of detection used being of the order of 0.005 mg/litre.

Furthermore, it is very unlikely that the pharmacokinetic properties of either chlorhexidine gluconate or cetrimide will be altered significantly in special situations, such as hepatic failure, renal failure, treatment of children, the elderly, in pregnancy or nursing mothers.

Preclinical safety data: Chlorhexidine and cetrimide are drugs on which extensive clinical experience has been obtained. All relevant information for the prescriber is provided elsewhere in the Summary of Product Characteristics.

Pharmaceutical particulars

List of excipients: Benzyl benzoate BP; Industrial methylated spirit; D-gluconolactone; Isopropyl alcohol BP; Liquid deodoriser; Purified water PhEur; Sodium hydroxide BP; Sunset yellow FCF (E110); Terpineol BP.

Incompatibilities: Hypochlorite bleaches may cause brown stains to develop in fabrics which have previously been in contact with preparations containing chlorhexidine.

Chlorhexidine and cetrimide are incompatible with soap and other anionic agents.

Shelf life: 4 years.

Special precautions for storage: Store below 30°C.

Nature and contents of container: White HDPE bottle (5 litres).

Instructions for use/handling: Dilute before use.

Dilute with tap water of an acceptable bacteriological standard or alcohol (ethanol, industrial methylated spirits or isopropanol). Add diluent slowly to prevent excessive foaming.

As a precaution against bacterial contamination, aqueous stock solutions should contain at least 4% v/v of isopropanol or 7% v/v of ethanol which may be denatured (ie industrial methylated spirit).

Hibicet solutions used for instrument storage should contain 0.4% w/v sodium nitrite to inhibit metal corrosion. Such solutions must be changed every 7 days. Prolonged immersion of rubber appliances in Hibicet solutions is undesirable.

As cork may protect certain Gram-negative organisms from the action of antiseptics, Hibicet solutions must be stored in bottles with glass, plastic or rubber closures.

See also *Posology and method of administration* and *Special warnings and special precautions for use.*

Marketing authorisation number 12619/0054.

Date of approval/revision of SPC January 1997

Legal category GSL

HIBISCRUB*

Qualitative and quantitative composition Chlorhexidine Gluconate 4% w/v (incorporated as Chlorhexidine Gluconate Solution PhEur)

Pharmaceutical form Liquid.

Clinical particulars

Therapeutic indications: Hibiscrub is an antimicrobial preparation for pre-operative surgical hand disinfection, antiseptic handwashing on the ward and pre-operative and post-operative skin antisepsis for patients undergoing elective surgery.

Posology and method of administration: For external use only.

Pre-operative surgical hand disinfection: Wet the hands and forearms, apply 5 ml of Hibiscrub and wash for one minute cleaning the fingernails with a brush or scraper. Rinse, apply a further 5 ml of Hibiscrub and continue washing for a further two minutes. Rinse thoroughly and dry.

Antiseptic handwash on the ward: Wet the hands and forearms, apply 5 ml of Hibiscrub and wash for one minute. Rinse thoroughly and dry.

Pre-operative skin antisepsis for the patient: The patient washes his whole body in the bath or shower on at least two occasions, usually the day before and the day of operation, as follows:

The day before operation the patient washes with 25 ml of Hibiscrub beginning with the face and working downwards paying particular attention to areas around the nose, axillae, umbilicus, groin and perineum. The body is then rinsed and the wash repeated with a further 25 ml, this time including the hair. Finally the patient rinses his entire body thoroughly and dries on a clean towel. This procedure should be repeated the following day. Patients confined to bed can be washed with Hibiscrub using a standard bed-bath technique.

Conventional disinfection of the operation site will then be performed when the patient is in theatre.

Post-operative skin antisepsis for the patients: The patient washes his whole body, excluding the operation wound, in the bath or shower usually on the third day after operation using the procedure described above.

Children and elderly patients: There are no special dosage recommendations for either elderly patients or children. The normal adult dose is appropriate unless recommended by the physician.

Contra-indications: Hibitane preparations are contraindicated for patients who have previously shown a hypersensitivity reaction to chlorhexidine. However, such reactions are extremely rare.

Special warnings and special precautions for use: For external use only. Keep out of the eyes and avoid contact with the brain, meninges and middle ear. In patients with head or spinal injuries or perforated ear drum, the benefit of use in pre-operative preparation should be evaluated against the risk of contact. If chlorhexidine solutions come into contact with the eyes, wash out promptly and thoroughly with water.

Do not inject or use in body cavities.

Interaction with other medicaments and other forms of interaction: See *Incompatibilities.*

Pregnancy and lactation: There is no evidence of any adverse effects on the foetus arising from the use of Hibiscrub as a handwash during pregnancy and lactation. Therefore no special precautions are recommended.

Effects on ability to drive and use machines: None have been reported or are known.

Undesirable effects: Irritative skin reactions to chlorhexidine preparations can occasionally occur. Generalised allergic reactions to chlorhexidine have also been reported but are extremely rare.

Overdose: This has not been reported.

Accidental ingestion: Chlorhexidine taken orally is poorly absorbed. Treat with gastric lavage using milk, raw egg, gelatin or mild soap. Employ supportive measures as appropriate.

Pharmacological properties

Pharmacodynamic properties: Mode of action–chlorhexidine has a wide range of antimicrobial activity. Chlorhexidine is effective against a wide range of gram-negative and gram-positive vegetative bacteria, yeasts, dermotophyte fungi and lipophilic viruses. It is inactive against bacterial spores except at elevated temperatures. Because of its cationic nature, chlorhexidine binds strongly to skin, mucosa and other tissues and is thus very poorly absorbed. No detectable blood levels have been found in man following oral use and percutaneous absorption, if it occurs at all, is insignificant.

Pharmacokinetic properties: Retention and uptake kinetics and factors influencing the pharmacokinetics.

Chlorhexidine appears to be very poorly absorbed: No blood levels were detected during a 3-week simulated clinical use of Hibiscrub.

Preclinical safety data: Chlorhexidine is a drug on which extensive clinical experience has been obtained. All relevant information for the prescriber is provided elsewhere in the Summary of Product Characteristics.

Pharmaceutical particulars

List of excipients: D-glucono-delta-lactone; Isopropryl alcohol; Lauryl dimethyl amine oxide; Perfume (Herbacol 15.393/T); Polyoxyethylene-polyoxypropylene block copolymer; Ponceau 4R (E124); Purified water.

Incompatibilities: Chlorhexidine is incompatible with soap and other anionic agents.

Hypochlorite bleaches may cause brown stains to develop in fabrics which have previously been in contact with preparations containing chlorhexidine.

Shelf life: 36 months.

Special precautions for storage: Store below 25°C, protect from light.

Nature and content of containers: HDPE bottles containing 250 ml, 500 ml and 5 litres.

Instructions for use/handling: See *Special warnings and special precautions for use.*

Marketing authorisation number PL 12619/0020.

Date of approval/revision of text June 1997.

Legal Category: GSL

HIBISOL*

Presentation Hibisol is presented as an alcoholic solution containing 0.5% w/v chlorhexidine gluconate (equivalent to 2.5% v/v Chlorhexidine Gluconate Solution PhEur) in 70% w/w Isopropyl Alcohol BP with emollients. Inactive ingredients are castor oil, glycerol, isopropyl alcohol and water.

Uses Hibisol is a rapid-acting antimicrobial preparation for the disinfection of clean intact skin. It is used for pre-operative surgical hand disinfection, hand disinfection on the ward prior to aseptic procedures or after handling contaminated material, and for disinfection of patients' skin prior to surgery or other invasive procedures.

Mode of action: Chlorhexidine is effective against a wide range of Gram negative and Gram positive vegetative bacteria, yeasts, dermatophyte fungi and lipophilic viruses. It is inactive against bacterial spores except at elevated temperatures.

Because of its cationic nature, chlorhexidine binds strongly to skin, mucosa and other tissues and is thus very poorly absorbed. No detectable blood levels have been found in man following oral use and percutaneous absorption, if it occurs at all, is insignificant.

Dosage and administration

Pre-operative surgical hand disinfection: Dispense 5 ml of Hibisol and spread thoroughly over both hands and forearms, rubbing vigorously. When dry apply a further 5 ml and repeat the procedure.

NB. Before the first operation on a list or subsequently when hands are soiled the hands should be cleansed and disinfected with an effective antiseptic/detergent handwash.

Antiseptic hand disinfection on the ward: Dispense 3 ml of Hibisol and spread thoroughly over the hands and wrists rubbing vigorously until dry.

NB. If the hands are soiled, cleanse and *dry* before using Hibisol or alternatively use an effective antiseptic/detergent handwash.

Disinfection of patients' skin: Prior to surgery, apply Hibisol to a sterile swab and rub vigorously over the operation site for a minimum of two minutes. Hibisol is also used for preparation of the skin prior to invasive procedures such as venepuncture.

Contra-indications, warnings, etc Hibisol is contra-indicated for persons who have previously shown a hypersensitivity reaction to chlorhexidine. However, such reactions are extremely rare.

For external use only. Avoid contact with the brain, meninges and middle ear. Not for injection. Do not use in body cavities.

The solution is irritant to eyes and mucous membranes. Keep out of the eyes. If the solution does come into contact with eyes, wash out promptly and thoroughly with water.

Flammable. This preparation contains alcohol. When use is to be followed by diathermy do not allow pooling of the fluid to occur, and ensure that the skin and surrounding drapes are dry.

Prolonged skin contact with alcoholic solutions should be avoided. Allow to dry before proceeding.

Side-effects: Irritative skin reactions can occasionally occur. Generalised allergic reactions to chlorhexidine have also been reported but are extremely rare.

Accidental ingestion: Chlorhexidine taken orally is poorly absorbed. Treat with gastric lavage using milk, raw egg, gelatin or mild soap avoiding pulmonary aspiration. Do not use apomorphine. Assist respiration if necessary and keep patient warm. Intravenous laevulose can accelerate alcohol metabolism. In severe cases, haemodialysis or peritoneal dialysis may be necessary.

Pharmaceutical precautions

Flammable.

Hypochlorite bleaches may cause brown stains to develop in fabrics which have previously been in contact with preparations containing chlorhexidine.

Chlorhexidine is incompatible with soaps and other anionic agents.

Store below 25°C.

Legal category GSL.

Package quantities Containers of 500 ml.

Further information A suitable antiseptic-detergent preparation which is compatible with Hibisol is Hibiscrub.

Product licence number 12619/0021.

HIBITANE* 5% CONCENTRATE

Qualitative and quantitative composition Chlorhexidine gluconate 5% w/v (incorporated as Chlorhexidine Gluconate Solution PhEur).

Pharmaceutical form Liquid.

Clinical particulars

Therapeutic indications: Hibitane 5% Concentrate is an antimicrobial agent for general antiseptic purposes. A surface active agent is present to inhibit precipitation when dilutions are made with hard water.

Posology and method of administration: For external (topical) use only.

No special dosages or indications are specified for use of this product for children or the elderly.

Dilute before use with freshly distilled water, tap water of an acceptable bacteriological standard or alcohol (ethanol, Industrial Methylated Spirit or isopropanol).

Method of preparation	*Concentration of active ingredient required (chlorhexidine gluconate)*	Use
10 ml made up to 1 litre with water (1 in 100)	1 in 2,000 (0.05%) aqueous	Swabbing in obstetrics, wounds and burns.† Storage of sterile instruments
10 ml with 15 ml water made up to 100 ml with 95% alcohol (1 in 10)	1 in 200 (0.5%) in 70% Alcohol	Pre-operative skin disinfection. Emergency instrument disinfection (2 minutes' immersion). (Excluding endoscopes containing cemented glass components)

† Sterilise the dilution by autoclaving at 115–116°C for 30 minutes or 121–123°C for 15 minutes.

Contra-indications: Hibitane preparations are contra-indicated for patients who have previously shown a hypersensitivity reaction to chlorhexidine. However, such reactions are extremely rare.

Special warnings and special precautions for use: For external use only.

Dilute before use.

Solutions applied to wounds, burns or broken skin should be sterile.

Syringes, needles or instruments which have been immersed in Hibitane solutions should be thoroughly rinsed in sterile water or saline before use.

Avoid contact with the brain, meninges and middle ear.

Not for injection.

Do not use in body cavities.

The concentrated solution is irritant to eyes and mucous membranes. Keep all solutions out of the eyes.

If chlorhexidine solutions come into contact with the eyes, wash out promptly and thoroughly with water.

Prolonged skin contact with alcoholic solutions should be avoided. Allow to dry before proceeding.

As with any other antiseptic agent, antimicrobial activity may be diminished through incompatibility or in the presence of significant quantities of organic matter.

Interactions with other medicaments and other forms of interaction: Hibitane 5% Concentrate contains a surfactant and therefore instruments containing cemented glass components should not be disinfected with solutions prepared from Hibitane 5% Concentrate.

The low solubility of inorganic salts of chlorhexidine may cause precipitation and consequent loss of activity if Hibitane 5% Concentrate is diluted with a solution containing inorganic anions, for example, saline or peritoneal dialysis fluid. This precipitation may occur when Hibitane 5% Concentrate is used to disinfect catheters intended for use in peritoneal dialysis. Inadvertent repeated exposure of peritoneal membranes to precipitated material has been claimed as a possible predisposing factor for peritoneal fibrosis.

Pregnancy and lactation: There is no evidence of any adverse effects from the use of Hibitane 5% Concentrate during pregnancy and lactation therefore no special precautions are recommended.

Effects on ability to drive and use machines: None have been reported or are known.

Undesirable effects: Irritative skin reactions can occasionally occur. Generalised allergic reactions to chlorhexidine have also been reported but are extremely rare.

Overdose: This has not been reported.

Accidental ingestion: Chlorhexidine taken orally is poorly absorbed. Treat with gastric lavage with milk, raw egg, gelatin or mild soap. Employ supportive measures as appropriate.

Accidental intravenous infusion: Blood transfusion may be necessary to counteract haemolysis.

Pharmacological properties

Pharmacodynamic properties: Chlorhexidine is effective against a wide range of Gram negative and Gram positive vegetative bacteria, yeasts, dermatophyte fungi and lipophilic viruses. It is inactive against bacterial spores except at elevated temperatures.

Pharmacokinetic properties: Because of its cationic nature, chlorhexidine binds strongly to skin, mucosa and other tissues and is thus very poorly absorbed. No detectable blood levels have been found in man following oral use and percutaneous absorption, if it occurs at all, is insignificant.

Preclinical safety data: Chlorhexidine is a drug on which extensive clinical experience has been obtained. All relevant information for the prescriber is provided elsewhere in the Summary of Product Characteristics.

Pharmaceutical particulars

List of excipients: Carmoisine E122; D-gluconolactone; Isopropyl Alcohol BP; Linalyl acetate; Nonylphenol/ethylene oxide condensate; Purified Water PhEur.

Incompatibilities: Hypochlorite bleaches may cause brown stains to develop in fabrics which have previously been in contact with preparations containing chlorhexidine.

Chlorhexidine is incompatible with soap and other anionic agents.

Shelf life: 4 years

Special precautions for storage: Store below 30°C

Nature and contents of container: HDPE bottle (5 litres)

Instructions for use/handling: As cork may protect certain Gram-negative organisms from the action of antiseptics, Hibitane solutions must be stored in bottles with glass, plastic or rubber closures.

As a precaution against bacterial contamination, stock aqueous solutions should contain at least 4% v/v of isopropanol or 7% v/v of ethanol which may be denatured (for example, Industrial Methylated Spirit).

Aqueous dilutions of Hibitane used for instrument storage should contain 0.1% w/v sodium nitrite to inhibit metal corrosion. Such solutions must be changed every 7 days.

See also *Special warnings and special precautions for use.*

Marketing authorisation number 12619/0022

Date of approval/revision of SPC January 1997

Legal category GSL

INDERAL* TABLETS

Qualitative and quantitative composition Propranolol Hydrochloride PhEur 10 mg.; Propranolol Hydrochloride PhEur 40 mg.; Propranolol Hydrochloride PhEur 80 mg.

Pharmaceutical form Round pink film coated tablets.

Clinical particulars
Therapeutic indications:

a) the control of hypertension;
b) the management of angina pectoris;
c) long term management against re-infarction after recovery from acute myocardial infarction;
d) the control of most forms of cardiac dysrhythmias;
e) the prophylaxis of migraine;
f) the management of essential tremor;
g) relief of situational anxiety and generalised anxiety symptoms, particularly those of somatic type;
h) prophylaxis of upper gastrointestinal bleeding in patients with portal hypertension and oesophageal varices;
i) the adjunctive management of thyrotoxicosis and thyrotoxic crisis;
j) management of hypertrophic obstructive cardiomyopathy;
k) management of phaeochromocytoma peri-operatively (with an alpha-blocker).

Posology and method of administration: For oral administration

Adults:
Hypertension: A starting dose of 80 mg twice a day may be increased at weekly intervals according to response. The usual dose range is 160 to 320 mg per day. With concurrent diuretic or other antihypertensive drugs a further reduction of blood pressure is obtained.

Angina, migraine and essential tremor: A starting dose of 40 mg two or three times daily may be increased by the same amount at weekly intervals according to patient response. An adequate response in migraine and essential tremor is usually seen in the range 80 to 160 mg/day and in angina in the range 120 to 240 mg/day.

Situational and generalised anxiety: A dose of 40 mg daily may provide short term relief of acute situational anxiety. Generalised anxiety, requiring longer term therapy, usually responds adequately to 40 mg twice daily which, in individual cases, may be increased to 40 mg three times daily. Treatment should be continued according to response. Patients should be reviewed after 6 to 12 months treatment.

Dysrhythmias, anxiety tachycardia, hypertrophic obstructive cardiomyopathy and thyrotoxicosis: A dosage range of 10 to 40 mg three or four times a day usually achieves the required response.

Post myocardial infarction: Treatment should start between days 5 and 21 after myocardial infarction, with an initial dose of 40 mg four times a day for 2 or 3 days. In order to improve compliance the total daily dosage may thereafter be given as 80 mg twice a day.

Portal hypertension: Dosage should be titrated to achieve approximately 25% reduction in resting heart rate. Dosage should begin with 40 mg twice daily, increasing to 80 mg twice daily depending on heart rate response. If necessary, the dose may be increased incrementally to a maximum of 160 mg twice daily.

Phaeochromocytoma: (Used only with an alpha-receptor blocking drug).

Pre-operative: 60 mg daily for 3 days is recommended. Non-operable malignant cases: 30 mg daily.

Elderly: Evidence concerning the relation between blood level and age is conflicting. With regard to the elderly, the optimum dose should be individually determined according to clinical response.

Children:
Dysrhythmias, phaeochromocytoma, thyrotoxicosis: Dosage should be individually determined and the following is only a guide: *Oral:* 0.25 to 0.5 mg/kg three or four times daily as required.

Migraine: Oral: Under the age of 12: 20 mg two or three times daily. Over the age of 12: The adult dose.

Fallot's tetralogy: The value of Inderal in this condition is confined mainly to the relief of right-ventricular outflow tract shut-down. It is also useful for treatment of associated dysrhythmias and angina. Dosage should be individually determined and the following is only a guide: *Oral:* Up to 1 mg/kg repeated three or four times daily as required.

Contra-indications: Inderal must not be used if there is a history of bronchial asthma or bronchospasm. The product label states the following warning: "Do not take Inderal if you have a history of asthma or wheezing". A similar warning appears in the patient information leaflet.

Bronchospasm can usually be reversed by beta$_2$-agonist bronchodilators such as salbutamol. Large doses of the beta$_2$- agonist bronchodilator may be required to overcome the beta-blockade produced by propranolol and the dose should be titrated according to the clinical response; both intravenous and inhalational administration should be considered. The use of intravenous aminophylline and/or the use of ipratropium (given by nebuliser) may also be considered. Glucagon (1 to 2 mg given intravenously) has also been reported to produce a bronchodilator effect in asthmatic patients. Oxygen or artificial ventilation may be required in severe cases.

Inderal as with other beta-adrenoceptor blocking drugs must not be used in patients with any of the following: known hypersensitivity to the substance; bradycardia; cardiogenic shock; hypotension; metabolic acidosis; after prolonged fasting; severe peripheral arterial circulatory disturbances; second or third degree heart block; sick sinus syndrome; untreated phaeochromocytoma; uncontrolled heart failure; Prinzmetal's angina.

Special warnings and special precautions for use: Inderal as with other beta-adrenoceptor blocking drugs:

- although contra-indicated in uncontrolled heart failure (see *Contra-indications),* may be used in patients whose signs of heart failure have been controlled. Caution must be exercised in patients whose cardiac reserve is poor.
- although contra-indicated in severe peripheral arterial circulatory disturbances (see *Contra-indications*), may also aggravate less severe peripheral arterial circulatory disturbances.
- due to its negative effect on conduction time, caution must be exercised if it is given to patients with first degree heart block.
- may modify the tachycardia of hypoglycaemia (see *Interactions*).
- may mask the signs of thyrotoxicosis.
- will reduce heart rate as a result of its pharmacological action. In the rare instances when a treated patient develops symptoms which may be attributable to a slow heart rate, the dose may be reduced.
- should not be discontinued abruptly in patients suffering from ischaemic heart disease. Either the equivalent dosage of another beta-adrenoceptor blocking drug may be substituted or the withdrawal of Inderal should be gradual.
- may cause a more severe reaction to a variety of allergens when given to patients with a history of anaphylactic reaction to such allergens. Such patients may be unresponsive to the usual doses of adrenaline used to treat the allergic reactions.

Since the half-life may be increased in patients with significant hepatic or renal impairment, caution must be exercised when starting treatment and selecting the initial dose.

Inderal must be used with caution in patients with decompensated cirrhosis.

In patients with portal hypertension, liver function may deteriorate and hepatic encephalopathy may develop. There have been reports suggesting that treatment with propranolol may increase the risk of developing hepatic encephalopathy.

Interference with laboratory tests. Inderal has been reported to interfere with the estimation of serum bilirubin by the diazo method and with the determination of catecholamines by methods using fluorescence.

Interactions with other medicaments and other forms of interaction: Inderal modifies the tachycardia of hypoglycaemia. Caution must be exercised in the concurrent use of Inderal and hypoglycaemic therapy in diabetic patients. Inderal may prolong the hypoglycaemic response to insulin.

Caution must be exercised in prescribing a beta-adrenoceptor blocking drug with Class I antiarrhythmic agents such as disopyramide.

Digitalis glycosides in association with beta-adrenoceptor blocking drugs may increase atrioventricular conduction time.

Combined use of beta-adrenoceptor blocking drugs and calcium channel blockers with negative inotropic effects (eg, verapamil, diltiazem) can lead to an exaggeration of these effects particularly in patients with impaired ventricular function and/or SA or AV conduction abnormalities. This may result in severe hypotension, bradycardia and cardiac failure. Neither the beta-adrenoceptor blocking drug nor the calcium channel blocker should be administered intravenously within 48 hours of discontinuing the other.

Concomitant therapy with dihydropyridine calcium channel blockers eg, nifedipine, may increase the risk of hypotension, and cardiac failure may occur in patients with latent cardiac insufficiency.

Concomitant use of sympathomimetic agents eg, adrenaline, may counteract the effect of beta-adrenoceptor blocking drugs. Caution must be exercised in the parenteral administration of preparations containing adrenaline to patients taking beta-adrenoceptor blocking drugs as, in rare cases, vasoconstriction, hypertension and bradycardia may result.

Administration of Inderal during infusion of lignocaine may increase the plasma concentration of lignocaine by approximately 30%. Patients already receiving Inderal tend to have higher lignocaine levels than controls. The combination should be avoided.

Concomitant use of cimetidine or hydralazine will increase, whereas concomitant use of alcohol will decrease, the plasma levels of propranolol.

Beta-adrenoceptor blocking drugs may exacerbate the rebound hypertension which can follow the withdrawal of clonidine. If the two drugs are co-administered, the beta-adrenoceptor blocking drug should be withdrawn several days before discontinuing clonidine. If replacing clonidine by beta-adrenoceptor blocking drug therapy, the introduction of beta-adrenoceptor blocking drugs should be delayed for several days after clonidine administration has stopped.

Caution must be exercised if ergotamine, dihydroergotamine or related compounds are given in combination with Inderal since vasospastic reactions have been reported in a few patients.

Concomitant use of prostaglandin synthetase inhibiting drugs eg, ibuprofen and indomethacin, may decrease the hypotensive effects of Inderal.

Concomitant administration of Inderal and chlorpromazine may result in an increase in plasma levels of both drugs. This may lead to an enhanced antipsychotic effect for chlorpromazine and an increased antihypertensive effect for Inderal.

Caution must be exercised when using anaesthetic agents with Inderal. The anaesthetist should be informed and the choice of anaesthetic should be an agent with as little negative inotropic activity as possible. Use of beta-adrenoceptor blocking drugs with anaesthetic drugs may result in attenuation of the reflex tachycardia and increase the risk of hypotension. Anaesthetic agents causing myocardial depression are best avoided.

Pharmacokinetic studies have shown that the following agents may interact with propranolol due to effects on enzyme systems in the liver which metabolise propranolol and these agents: quinidine, propafenone, rifampicin, theophylline, warfarin, thioridazine and dihydropyridine calcium channel blockers such as nifedipine, nisoldipine, nicardipine, isradipine, and lacidipine. Owing to the fact that blood concentrations of either agent may be affected, dosage adjustments may be needed according to clinical judgement. (See also the interaction above concerning the concomitant therapy with dihydropyridine calcium channel blockers).

Pregnancy and lactation:
Pregnancy: As with all drugs Inderal should not be given during pregnancy unless its use is essential. There is no evidence of teratogenicity with Inderal. However beta-adrenoceptor blocking drugs reduce placental perfusion, which may result in intra-uterine foetal death, immature and premature deliveries. In addition, adverse effects (especially hypoglycaemia and bradycardia in the neonate and bradycardia in the foetus) may occur. There is an increased risk of cardiac and pulmonary complications in the neonate in the post-natal period.

Lactation: Most beta-adrenoceptor blocking drugs, particularly lipophilic compounds, will pass into breast milk although to a variable extent. Breast feeding is therefore not recommended following administration of these compounds.

Effects on ability to drive and use machines: Use is unlikely to result in any impairment of the ability of patients to drive or operate machinery. However it should be taken into account that occasionally dizziness or fatigue may occur.

Undesirable effects: Inderal is usually well tolerated. In clinical studies the undesired events reported are usually attributable to the pharmacological actions of propranolol.

The following undesired events, listed by body system, have been reported.

Cardiovascular: bradycardia; heart failure deterioration; postural hypotension which may be associated with syncope; cold extremities. In susceptible patients: precipitation of heart block; exacerbation of intermittent claudication; Raynaud's phenomenon.

CNS: confusion; dizziness; mood changes; nightmares; psychoses and hallucinations; sleep disturbances.

Endocrine: hypoglycaemia in children.
Gastrointestinal: gastrointestinal disturbance.
Haematological: purpura; thrombocytopenia.
Integumentary: alopecia; dry eyes; psoriasiform skin reactions; exacerbation of psoriasis; skin rashes.
Neurological: paraesthesia.
Respiratory: bronchospasm may occur in patients with bronchial asthma or a history of asthmatic complaints, sometimes with fatal outcome (see *Contra-indications*).
Special senses: visual disturbances.
Others: fatigue and/or lassitude (often transient); an increase in ANA (Antinuclear Antibodies) has been observed, however the clinical relevance of this is not clear; isolated reports of myasthenia gravis like syndrome or exacerbation of myasthenia gravis have been reported.

Discontinuance of the drug should be considered if, according to clinical judgement, the well-being of the patient is adversely affected by any of the above reactions. Cessation of therapy with a beta-adrenoceptor blocking drug should be gradual. In the rare event of intolerance, manifested as bradycardia and hypotension, the drug should be withdrawn and, if necessary, treatment for overdosage instituted.

Overdosage: The symptoms of overdosage may include bradycardia, hypotension, acute cardiac insufficiency and bronchospasm.

General treatment should include: close supervision, treatment in an intensive care ward, the use of gastric lavage, activated charcoal and a laxative to prevent absorption of any drug still present in the gastrointestinal tract, the use of plasma or plasma substitutes to treat hypotension and shock.

Excessive bradycardia can be countered with atropine 1 to 2 mg intravenously and/or a cardiac pacemaker. If necessary, this may be followed by a bolus dose of glucagon 10 mg intravenously. If required, this may be repeated or followed by an intravenous infusion of glucagon 1 to 10 mg/hour depending on response. If no response to glucagon occurs or if glucagon is unavailable, a beta-adrenoceptor stimulant such as dobutamine 2.5 to 10 microgram/kg/minute by intravenous infusion may be given. Dobutamine, because of its positive inotropic effect, could also be used to treat hypotension and acute cardiac insufficiency. It is likely that these doses would be inadequate to reverse the cardiac effects of beta-adrenoceptor blockade if a large overdose has been taken. The dose of dobutamine should therefore be increased if necessary to achieve the required response according to the clinical condition of the patient.

Pharmacological properties
Pharmacodynamic properties: Inderal is a competitive antagonist at both the beta$_1$- and beta$_2$ adrenoceptors. It has no agonist activity at the beta-adrenoceptor, but has membrane stabilising activity at concentrations exceeding 1 to 3 mg/litre, though such concentrations are rarely achieved during oral therapy. Competitive beta-adrenoceptor blockade has been demonstrated in man by a parallel shift to the right in the dose-heart rate response curve to beta agonists such as isoprenaline.

Propranolol as with other beta-adrenoceptor blocking drugs, has negative inotropic effects, and is therefore contraindicated in uncontrolled heart failure.

Inderal is a racemic mixture and the active form is the S (-) isomer of propranolol. With the exception of inhibition of the conversion of thyroxine to triiodothyronine, it is unlikely that any additional ancillary properties possessed by R (+) propranolol, in comparison with the racemic mixture, will give rise to different therapeutic effects.

Inderal is effective and well tolerated in most ethnic populations, although the response may be less in black patients.

Pharmacokinetic properties: Following intravenous administration the plasma half-life of propranolol is about 2 hours and the ratio of metabolites to parent drug in the blood is lower than after oral administration. In particular 4-hydroxypropranolol is not present after intravenous administration. Propranolol is completely absorbed after oral administration and peak plasma concentrations occur 1 to 2 hours after dosing in fasting patients. The liver removes up to 90% of an oral dose with an elimination half-life of 3 to 6 hours. Propranolol is widely and rapidly distributed throughout the body with highest levels occurring in the lungs, liver, kidney, brain and heart. Propranolol is highly protein bound (80 to 95%).

Pre-clinical safety data: Propranolol is a drug on which extensive clinical experience has been obtained. Relevant information for the prescriber is provided elsewhere in this Summary of Product Characteristics.

Pharmaceutical particulars
List of excipients: 10 mg, 40 mg and 80 mg; Calcium Carboxymethyl Cellulose USNF; Carmine BPC (E120); Gelatin PhEur; Glycerol PhEur; Lactose PhEur; Light Magnesium Carbonate PhEur; Magnesium Stearate PhEur; Methylhydroxypropylcellulose PhEur; Titanium Dioxide PhEur (E171)

Incompatibilities: None known.

Shelf life: 5 years.

Special precautions for storage: Store below 30°C, protected from light and moisture.

Nature and contents of container: 10 mg & 40 mg: HDPE bottles of 100 tablets; 80 mg: HDPE bottles of 60 tablets.

Instructions for use/handling: None stated.

Market authorisation numbers
10 mg PL 12619/0030
40 mg PL 12619/0031
80 mg PL 12619/0032

Date of approval/revision of the text June 1998

Legal Category POM.

INDERAL* INJECTION

Qualitative and quantitative composition Propranolol Hydrochloride PhEur 0.1% w/v.

Pharmaceutical form Solution for intravenous injection.

Clinical particulars
Therapeutic indications: The emergency treatment of cardiac dysrhythmias and thyrotoxic crisis.

Posology and method of administration: For intravenous injection.

Adults: The initial dose of 'Inderal' is 1 mg (1 ml) injected over 1 minute. This may be repeated at 2-minute intervals until a response is observed or to a maximum dose of 10 mg in conscious patients or 5 mg in patients under anaesthesia.

Elderly: Evidence concerning the relation between blood level and age is conflicting. With regard to the elderly, the optimum dose should be individually determined according to clinical response.

Children:
Dysrhythmias, thyrotoxicosis: Dosage should be individually determined and the following is only a guide:

Intravenous: 0.025 to 0.5 mg/kg injected slowly under ECG control and repeated 3 or 4 times daily as required.

Fallot's tetralogy: The value of Inderal in this condition is confined mainly to the relief of right-ventricular outflow tract shut-down. It is also useful for treatment of associated dysrhythmias and angina. Dosage should be individually determined and the following is only a guide:

Intravenous: Up to 0.1 mg/kg injected slowly under ECG control, repeated 3 or 4 times daily as required.

Contra-indications: Inderal must not be used if there is a history of bronchial asthma or bronchospasm. The product label and patient information leaflet state the following warnings: Label: "Do not use Inderal if the patient has a history of asthma or wheezing". Patient Information Leaflet: "If you have ever had asthma or wheezing, you should not be given Inderal injection. Talk to your doctor".

Bronchospasm can usually be reversed by beta$_2$-agonist bronchodilators such as salbutamol. Large doses of the beta$_2$-agonist bronchodilator may be required to overcome the beta-blockade produced by propranolol and the dose should be titrated according to the clinical response; both intravenous and inhalational administration should be considered. The use of intravenous aminophylline and/or the use of ipratropium (given by nebuliser) may also be considered. Glucagon (1 to 2 mg given intravenously) has also been reported to produce a bronchodilator effect in asthmatic patients. Oxygen or artificial ventilation may be required in severe cases.

Inderal as with other beta-adrenoceptor blocking drugs must not be used in patients with any of the following: known hypersensitivity to the substance; bradycardia; cardiogenic shock; hypotension; metabolic acidosis; after prolonged fasting; severe peripheral arterial circulatory disturbances; second or third degree heart block; sick sinus syndrome; untreated phaeochromocytoma; uncontrolled heart failure; Prinzmetal's angina.

Special warnings and special precautions for use: Inderal as with other beta-adrenoceptor blocking drugs:

- although contra-indicated in uncontrolled heart failure (*Contra-indications*), may be used in patients whose signs of heart failure have been controlled. Caution must be exercised in patients whose cardiac reserve is poor.
- although contra-indicated in severe peripheral arterial circulatory disturbances (see *Contra-indications*), may also aggravate less severe peripheral arterial circulatory disturbances.
- due to its negative effect on conduction time, caution must be exercised if it is given to patients with first degree heart block.
- may modify the tachycardia of hypoglycaemia (see *Interactions*).
- may mask the signs of thyrotoxicosis.
- will reduce heart rate as a result of its pharmacological action. In the rare instances when a treated patient develops symptoms which may be attributable to a slow heart rate, the dose may be reduced.
- should not be discontinued abruptly in patients suffering from ischaemic heart disease. Either the equivalent dosage of another beta-adrenoceptor blocking drug may be substituted or the withdrawal of Inderal should be gradual.
- may cause a more severe reaction to a variety of allergens when given to patients with a history of anaphylactic reaction to such allergens. Such patients may be unresponsive to the usual doses of adrenaline used to treat the allergic reactions.

Since the half-life may be increased in patients with significant hepatic or renal impairment, caution must be exercised when starting treatment and selecting the initial dose.

Inderal must be used with caution in patients with decompensated cirrhosis.

In patients with portal hypertension, liver function may deteriorate and hepatic encephalopathy may develop. There have been reports suggesting that treatment with propranolol may increase the risk of developing hepatic encephalopathy.

Interference with laboratory tests. Inderal has been reported to interfere with the estimation of serum bilirubin by the diazo method and with the determination of catecholamines by methods using fluorescence.

Interactions with other medicaments and other forms of interaction: Inderal modifies the tachycardia of hypoglycaemia. Caution must be exercised in the concurrent use of Inderal and hypoglycaemic therapy in diabetic patients. Inderal may prolong the hypoglycaemic response to insulin.

Caution must be exercised in prescribing a beta-adrenoceptor blocking drug with Class I antiarrhythmic agents such as disopyramide.

Digitalis glycosides in association with beta-adrenoceptor blocking drugs may increase atrioventricular conduction time.

Combined use of beta-adrenoceptor blocking drugs and calcium channel blockers with negative inotropic effects (eg, verapamil, diltiazem) can lead to an exaggeration of these effects particularly in patients with impaired ventricular function and/or SA or AV conduction abnormalities. This may result in severe hypotension, bradycardia and cardiac failure. Neither the beta-adrenoceptor blocking drug nor the calcium channel blocker should be administered intravenously within 48 hours of discontinuing the other.

Concomitant therapy with dihydropyridine calcium channel blockers, eg, nifedipine, may increase the risk of hypotension, and cardiac failure may occur in patients with latent cardiac insufficiency.

Concomitant use of sympathomimetic agents eg, adrenaline, may counteract the effect of beta-adrenoceptor blocking drugs. Caution must be exercised in the parenteral administration of preparations containing adrenaline to patients taking beta-adrenoceptor blocking drugs as, in rare cases, vasoconstriction, hypertension and bradycardia may result.

Administration of Inderal during infusion of lignocaine may increase the plasma concentration of lignocaine by approximately 30%. Patients already receiving Inderal tend to have higher lignocaine levels than controls. The combination should be avoided.

Concomitant use of cimetidine or hydralazine will increase, whereas concomitant use of alcohol will decrease, the plasma levels of propranolol.

Beta-adrenoceptor blocking drugs may exacerbate the rebound hypertension which can follow the withdrawal of clonidine. If the two drugs are co-administered, the beta-adrenoceptor blocking drug should be withdrawn several days before discontinuing clonidine. If replacing clonidine by beta-adrenoceptor blocking drug therapy, the introduction of beta-adrenoceptor blocking drugs should be delayed for several days after clonidine administration has stopped.

Caution must be exercised if ergotamine, dihydroergotamine or related compounds are given in combination with Inderal since vasospastic reactions have been reported in a few patients.

Concomitant use of prostaglandin synthetase inhibiting drugs eg, ibuprofen and indomethacin, may decrease the hypotensive effects of Inderal.

Concomitant administration of Inderal and chlorpromazine may result in an increase in plasma levels of both drugs. This may lead to an enhanced antipsychotic effect for chlorpromazine and an increased antihypertensive effect for Inderal.

Caution must be exercised when using anaesthetic agents with Inderal. The anaesthetist should be informed and the choice of anaesthetic should be an agent with as little negative inotropic activity as possible. Use of beta-adrenoceptor blocking drugs with anaesthetic drugs may result in attenuation of the reflex tachycardia and increase the risk of hypotension. Anaesthetic agents causing myocardial depression are best avoided.

Pharmacokinetic studies have shown that the following agents may interact with propranolol due to effects on enzyme systems in the liver which metabolise propranolol and these agents: quinidine, propafenone, rifampicin, theophylline, warfarin, thioridazine and dihydropyridine calcium channel blockers such as nifedipine, nisoldipine, nicardipine, isradipine, and lacidipine. Owing to the fact that blood concentrations of either agent may be affected, dosage adjustments may be needed according to clinical judgement. (See also the interaction above concerning the concomitant therapy with dihydropyridine calcium channel blockers).

Pregnancy and lactation:

Pregnancy: As with all drugs Inderal should not be given during pregnancy unless its use is essential. There is no evidence of teratogenicity with Inderal. However beta-adrenoceptor blocking drugs reduce placental perfusion, which may result in intra-uterine foetal death, immature and premature deliveries. In addition, adverse effects (especially hypoglycaemia and bradycardia in the neonate and bradycardia in the foetus) may occur. There is an increased risk of cardiac and pulmonary complications in the neonate in the post-natal period.

Lactation: Most beta-adrenoceptor blocking drugs, particularly lipophilic compounds, will pass into breast milk although to a variable extent. Breast feeding is therefore not recommended following administration of these compounds.

Effects on ability to drive and use machines: Use is unlikely to result in any impairment of the ability of patients to drive or operate machinery. However it should be taken into account that occasionally dizziness or fatigue may occur.

Undesirable effects: Inderal is usually well tolerated. In clinical studies the undesired events reported are usually attributable to the pharmacological actions of propranolol.

The following undesired events, listed by body system, have been reported.

Cardiovascular: bradycardia; heart failure deterioration; postural hypotension which may be associated with syncope; cold extremities. In susceptible patients: precipitation of heart block; exacerbation of intermittent claudication; Raynaud's phenomenon.

CNS: confusion; dizziness; mood changes; nightmares; psychoses and hallucinations; sleep disturbances.

Endocrine: hypoglycaemia in children.

Gastrointestinal: gastrointestinal disturbance.

Haematological: purpura; thrombocytopenia.

Integumentary: alopecia; dry eyes; psoriasiform skin reactions; exacerbation of psoriasis; skin rashes.

Neurological: paraesthesia.

Respiratory: bronchospasm may occur in patients with bronchial asthma or a history of asthmatic complaints, sometimes with fatal outcome (see *Contra-indications*).

Special senses: visual disturbances.

Others: fatigue and/or lassitude (often transient); an increase in ANA (Antinuclear Antibodies) has been observed, however the clinical relevance of this is not clear; isolated reports of myasthenia gravis like syndrome or exacerbation of myasthenia gravis have been reported.

Discontinuance of the drug should be considered if, according to clinical judgement, the well-being of the patient is adversely affected by any of the above reactions. Cessation of therapy with a beta-adrenoceptor blocking drug should be gradual. In the rare event of intolerance, manifested as bradycardia and hypotension, the drug should be withdrawn and, if necessary, treatment for overdosage instituted.

Overdosage: The symptoms of overdosage may include bradycardia, hypotension, acute cardiac insufficiency and bronchospasm.

General treatment should include: close supervision, treatment in an intensive care ward, the use of gastric lavage, activated charcoal and a laxative to prevent absorption of any drug still present in the gastrointestinal tract, the use of plasma or plasma substitutes to treat hypotension and shock.

Excessive bradycardia can be countered with atropine 1 to 2 mg intravenously and/or a cardiac pacemaker. If necessary, this may be followed by a bolus dose of glucagon 10 mg intravenously. If required, this may be repeated or followed by an intravenous infusion of glucagon 1 to 10 mg/hour depending on response. If no response to glucagon occurs or if glucagon is unavailable, a beta-adrenoceptor stimulant such as dobutamine 2.5 to 10 microgram/kg/minute by intravenous infusion may be given. Dobutamine, because of its positive inotropic effect, could also be used to treat hypotension and acute cardiac insufficiency. It is likely that these doses would be inadequate to reverse the cardiac effects of beta-adrenoceptor blockade if a large overdose has been taken. The dose of dobutamine should therefore be increased if necessary to achieve the required response according to the clinical condition of the patient.

Pharmacological properties

Pharmacodynamic properties: Inderal is a competitive antagonist at both the $beta_1$- and $beta_2$ adrenoceptors. It has no agonist activity at the beta-adrenoceptor, but has membrane stabilising activity at concentrations exceeding 1 to 3 mg/litre, though such concentrations are rarely achieved during oral therapy. Competitive beta-adrenoceptor blockade has been demonstrated in man by a parallel shift to the right in the dose-heart rate response curve to beta agonists such as isoprenaline.

Propranolol as with other beta-adrenoceptor blocking drugs, has negative inotropic effects, and is therefore contraindicated in uncontrolled heart failure.

Inderal is a racemic mixture and the active form is the S (-) isomer of propranolol. With the exception of inhibition of the conversion of thyroxine to triiodothyronine, it is unlikely that any additional ancillary properties possessed by R (+) propranolol, in comparison with the racemic mixture, will give rise to different therapeutic effects.

Inderal is effective and well tolerated in most ethnic populations, although the response may be less in black patients.

Pharmacokinetic properties: Following intravenous administration the plasma half-life of propranolol is about 2 hours and the ratio of metabolites to parent drug in the blood is lower than after oral administration. In particular 4-hydroxypropranolol is not present after intravenous administration. Propranolol is completely absorbed after oral administration and peak plasma concentrations occur 1 to 2 hours after dosing in fasting patients. The liver removes up to 90% of an oral dose with an elimination half-life of 3 to 6 hours. Propranolol is widely and rapidly distributed throughout the body with highest levels occurring in the lungs, liver, kidney, brain and heart. Propranolol is highly protein bound (80 to 95%).

Pre-clinical safety data: Propranolol is a drug on which extensive clinical experience has been obtained. Relevant information for the prescriber is provided elsewhere in this Summary of Product Characteristics.

Pharmaceutical particulars

List of excipients: Citric acid (anhydrous) PhEur; Water for injections PhEur

Incompatibilities: None known.

Shelf life: 5 years.

Special precautions for storage: Store below 30°C, protected from light.

Nature and contents of container: Ampoule containing 1 ml.

Instructions for use/handling: None stated.

Market authorisation number PL 12619/0027.

Date of first authorisation/renewal of authorisation June 1998.

Legal Category POM.

INDERAL* LA HALF-INDERAL* LA

Presentation Inderal LA and Half-Inderal LA capsules contain spheroids of the beta-adrenoceptor blocking drug propranolol hydrochloride which have a sustained release coating to provide long action.

Inderal LA capsules each contain 160 mg Propranolol Hydrochloride PhEur. Inderal LA is presented as size 1 gelatin capsules with a clear pink body and opaque, lavender cap marked Inderal LA in white.

Half-Inderal LA capsules each contain 80 mg Propranolol Hydrochloride PhEur. Half-Inderal LA is presented as size 3 gelatin capsules with a clear pink body and opaque, pale lavender cap and marked Half-Inderal LA in black.

Inactive ingredients are erythrosine, ethylcellulose, gelatin, glycerol, iron oxide, methylhydroxypropylcellulose, microcrystalline cellulose, and titanium dioxide.

Uses Inderal LA and Half-Inderal LA are indicated in the management of angina, essential tremor, relief of situational anxiety and generalised anxiety symptoms, particularly those of somatic type, prophylaxis of upper gastro-intestinal bleeding in patients with portal hypertension and oesophageal varices, the adjunctive management of thyrotoxicosis, and the prophylaxis of migraine.

Inderal LA is indicated in the control of hypertension. One Half-Inderal LA capsule daily is unlikely on its own to be sufficient to treat hypertension, but it may be used as a starting dose in appropriate patients (e.g. the elderly) or to provide a convenient method of gradual dosage alteration.

Mode of action: Propranolol is a competitive antagonist at both $beta_1$ and $beta_2$-adrenoceptors. It has no agonist activity at the beta-adrenoceptor, but has membrane stabilising activity at concentrations exceeding 1 to 3 mg/litre, though such concentrations are rarely achieved during oral therapy. Competitive beta-adrenoceptor blockade has been demonstrated in man by a parallel shift to the right in the dose-heart rate response curve to beta-agonists such as isoprenaline.

Propranolol, as with other beta-adrenoceptor blocking drugs, has negative inotropic effects, and is therefore contra-indicated in uncontrolled heart failure.

Propranolol is a racemic mixture and the active form is the S(-) isomer. With the exception of inhibition of the conversion of thyroxine to triiodothyronine it is unlikely that any additional ancillary properties possessed by R (+) propranolol, in comparison with the racemic mixture will give rise to different therapeutic effects.

Propranolol is effective and well tolerated in most ethnic populations, although the response may be less in black patients.

The sustained release preparation of propranolol maintains a higher degree of $beta_1$-blockade 24 hours after dosing compared with conventional propranolol.

Propranolol is completely absorbed after oral administration. Following oral dosing with the sustained release preparation of propranolol the blood profile is flatter than after conventional Inderal but the half-life is increased to between 10 and 20 hours. The liver removes up to 90% of an oral dose with an elimination half-life of 3 to 6 hours. Propranolol is widely and rapidly distributed throughout the body with highest levels occurring in the lungs, liver, kidney, brain and heart. Propranolol is highly protein bound (80 to 95%).

Dosage and administration *Adults: Hypertension:* The usual starting dose is one 160 mg Inderal LA capsule daily, taken either morning or evening. An adequate response is seen in most patients at this dosage. If necessary, it can be increased in 80 mg Half-Inderal LA increments until an adequate response is achieved. A further reduction in blood pressure can be obtained if a diuretic or other antihypertensive agent is given in addition to Inderal LA and Half-Inderal LA.

Angina, essential tremor, thyrotoxicosis and the prophylaxis of migraine: One Half-Inderal LA capsule daily taken either morning or evening may be sufficient to provide adequate control in many patients. If necessary the dose may be increased to one Inderal LA capsule per day and an additional Half-Inderal LA increment may be given.

Situational and generalised anxiety: One Half-Inderal LA capsule taken daily should be sufficient to provide short term relief of acute situational anxiety. Generalised anxiety, requiring longer term therapy, usually responds adequately at the same dosage. In individual cases, the dosage may be increased to one Inderal LA capsule per day. Treatment should be continued according to response. Patients should be reviewed after 6 to 12 months' treatment.

Portal hypertension: Dosage should be titrated to achieve approximately 25% reduction in resting heart rate. Dosing should begin with one 80 mg Half-Inderal LA capsule daily, increasing to one 160 mg Inderal LA capsule daily depending on heart rate response. Further 80 mg Half-Inderal LA increments may be added up to a maximum dose of 320 mg once daily.

Patients who are already established on equivalent daily doses of Inderal tablets should be transferred to the equivalent doses of Half-Inderal LA or Inderal LA daily taken either morning or evening.

Children: Inderal LA and Half-Inderal LA are not intended for use in children.

Elderly patients: Evidence concerning the relation between blood level and age is conflicting. It is suggested that treatment should start with one Half-Inderal LA capsule once daily. The dose may be increased to one Inderal LA capsule daily or higher as appropriate.

Contra-indications, warnings, etc Inderal LA and Half-Inderal LA must not be used if there is a history of bronchial asthma or bronchospasm. The product label states the following warning: "Do not take Inderal LA if you have a history of asthma or wheezing". A similar warning appears in the patient information leaflet.

Bronchospasm can usually be reversed by beta$_2$-agonist bronchodilators such as salbutamol. Large doses of the beta$_2$-agonist bronchodilator may be required to overcome the beta-blockade produced by propranolol and the dose should be titrated according to the clinical response; both intravenous and inhalational administration should be considered. The use of intravenous aminophylline and/or the use of ipratropium (given by nebuliser), may also be considered. Glucagon (1 to 2 mg given intravenously) has also been reported to produce a bronchodilator effect in asthmatic patients. Oxygen or artifical ventilation may be required in severe cases.

Inderal LA and Half-Inderal LA, as with other beta-adrenoceptor blocking drugs, must not be used in patients with any of the following conditions: known hypersensitivity to the substance, bradycardia, cardiogenic shock, hypotension, metabolic acidosis, after prolonged fasting, severe peripheral arterial circulatory disturbances, second or third degree heart block, sick sinus syndrome, untreated phaeochromocytoma, uncontrolled heart failure or Prinzmetal's angina.

Inderal LA and Half-Inderal LA as with other beta-adrenoceptor blocking drugs:

- although contra-indicated in uncontrolled heart failure (see *Contra-indications*), may be used in patients whose signs of heart failure have been controlled. Caution must be exercised in patients whose cardiac reserve is poor.
- although contra-indicated in severe peripheral arterial circulatory disturbances (see *Contra-indications*), may also aggravate less severe peripheral arterial circulatory disturbances.
- due to its negative effect on conduction time, caution must be exercised if it is given to patients with first degree heart block.
- may modify the tachycardia of hypoglycaemia.
- may mask the signs of thyrotoxicosis.
- will reduce heart rate, as a result of its pharmacological action. In the rare instances when a treated patient develops symptoms which may be attributable to a slow heart rate, the dose may be reduced.
- should not be discontinued abruptly in patients suffering from ischaemic heart disease. Either the equivalent dosage of another beta-adrenoceptor blocking drug may be substituted or the withdrawal of Inderal LA should be gradual. This can be achieved by first substituting the daily Inderal LA dose by the equivalent in Half-Inderal LA capsules and then gradually reducing the number of capsules.
- may cause a more severe reaction to a variety of allergens, when given to patients with a history of anaphylactic reaction to such allergens. Such patients may be unresponsive to the usual doses of adrenaline used to treat the allergic reactions.

Since the half-life may be increased in patients with significant hepatic or renal impairment, caution must be exercised when starting treatment and selecting the initial dose.

Inderal LA and Half-Inderal LA must be used with caution in patients with decompensated cirrhosis.

In patients with portal hypertension, liver function may deteriorate and hepatic encephalopathy may develop. There have been reports suggesting that treatment with propranolol may increase the risk of developing hepatic encephalopathy.

Inderal LA and Half-Inderal LA modify the tachycardia of hypoglycaemia. Caution must be exercised in the concurrent use of Inderal LA or Half-Inderal LA and hypoglycaemic therapy in diabetic patients. Propranolol may prolong the hypoglycaemic response to insulin.

Caution must be exercised when prescribing a beta-adrenoceptor blocking drug with Class 1 antiarrhythmic agents such as disopyramide.

Combined use of beta-adrenoceptor blocking drugs and calcium channel blockers with negative inotropic effects e.g. verapamil, diltiazem can lead to an exaggeration of these effects, particularly in patients with impaired ventricular function and/or sino-atrial or atrio-ventricular conduction abnormalities. This may result in severe hypotension, bradycardia and cardiac failure. Neither the beta-adrenoceptor blocking drug nor the calcium channel blocker should be administered intravenously within 48 hours of discontinuing the other.

Concomitant therapy with dihydropyridine calcium channel blockers eg, nifedipine, may increase the risk of hypotension, and cardiac failure may occur in patients with latent cardiac insufficiency.

Beta-adrenoceptor blocking drugs may exacerbate the rebound hypertension which can follow the withdrawal of clonidine. If the two drugs are co-administered, the beta-adrenoceptor blocking drug should be withdrawn several days before discontinuing clonidine. If replacing clonidine by beta-adrenoceptor blocking drug therapy, the introduction of beta-adrenoceptor blocking drugs should be delayed for several days after clonidine administration has stopped.

Digitalis glycosides, in association with beta-adrenoceptor blocking drugs, may increase atrio-ventricular conduction time.

Concomitant use of sympathomimetic agents, e.g. adrenaline, may counteract the effect of beta-adrenoceptor blocking drugs. Caution must be exercised in the parenteral administration of preparations containing adrenaline to patients taking beta-adrenoceptor blocking drugs as, in rare cases, vasoconstriction, hypertension and bradycardia may result.

Administration of propranolol during infusion of lignocaine may increase the plasma concentration of lignocaine by approximately 30%. Patients already receiving propranolol tend to have higher lignocaine levels than controls. The combination should be avoided.

Caution must be exercised if ergotamine, dihydroergotamine or related compounds are given in combination with propranolol since vasospastic reactions have been reported in a few patients.

Concomitant use of prostaglandin synthetase inhibiting drugs, e.g. ibuprofen or indomethacin, may decrease the hypotensive effects of propranolol.

Concomitant administration of propranolol and chlorpromazine may result in an increase in plasma levels of both drugs. This may lead to an enhanced antipsychotic effect for chlorpromazine and an increased antihypertensive effect for propranolol.

Concomitant use of cimetidine will increase, whereas concomitant use of alcohol will decrease, the plasma levels of propranolol.

Anaesthesia: Caution must be exercised when using anaesthetic agents with Inderal LA and Half-Inderal LA. The anaesthetist should be informed and the choice of anaesthetic should be the agent with as little negative inotropic activity as possible. Use of beta-adrenoceptor blocking drugs with anaesthetic drugs may result in attenuation of the reflex tachycardia and increase the risk of hypotension. Anaesthetic agents causing myocardial depression are best avoided.

Pharmacokinetic studies have shown that the following agents may interact with propranolol due to effects on enzyme systems in the liver which metabolise propranolol and these agents: quinidine, propafenone, rifampicin, theophylline, warfarin, thioridazine and dihydropyridine calcium channel blockers such as nifedipine, nisoldipine, nicardipine, isradipine and lacidipine. Owing to the fact that blood concentrations of either agent may be affected dosage adjustments may be needed according to clinical judgement. (See also the interaction above concerning the concomitant therapy with dihydropyridine calcium channel blockers).

Interference with laboratory tests: Inderal LA and Half-Inderal LA have been reported to interfere with the estimation of serum bilirubin by the diazo method and with the determination of catecholamines by methods using fluorescence.

Pregnancy: As with all drugs, Inderal LA and Half-Inderal LA should not be given during pregnancy unless their use is essential. There is no evidence of teratogenicity with Inderal. However beta-adrenoceptor blocking drugs reduce placental perfusion, which may result in intra-uterine foetal death, immature and premature deliveries. In addition, adverse effects (especially hypoglycaemia and bradycardia in the neonate and bradycardia in the foetus) may occur. There is an increased risk of cardiac and pulmonary complications in the neonate in the post-natal period.

Lactation: Most beta-adrenoceptor blocking drugs particularly lipophilic compounds, will pass into breast milk although to a variable extent. Breast feeding is therefore not recommended following administration of these compounds.

Effect on ability to drive or operate machinery: The use Inderal LA or Half-Inderal LA is unlikely to result in any impairment of the ability of patients to drive or operate machinery. However, it should be taken into account that occasionally dizziness or fatigue may occur.

Undesirable events: Inderal LA and Half-Inderal LA are usually well tolerated. In clinical studies, the undesired events reported are usually attributable to the pharmacological actions of propranolol.

The following undesired events, listed by body system, have been reported.

Cardiovascular: bradycardia, heart failure deterioration, postural hypotension which may be associated with syncope, cold extremities. In susceptible patients: precipitation of heart block, exacerbation of intermittent claudication, Raynaud's phenomenon.

CNS: confusion, dizziness, mood changes, nightmares, psychoses and hallucinations, sleep disturbance.

Gastrointestinal: gastrointestinal disturbance.

Haematological: purpura, thrombocytopenia.

Integumentary: alopecia, dry eyes, psoriasiform skin reactions, exacerbation of psoriasis, skin rashes.

Neurological: paraesthesia.

Respiratory: bronchospasm may occur in patients with bronchial asthma or a history of asthmatic complaints, sometimes with fatal outcome (see *Contra-indications*).

Special senses: visual disturbances.

Others: fatigue and/or lassitude (often transient), an increase in ANA (antinuclear antibodies) has been observed, however the clinical relevance of this is not clear; isolated reports of myasthenia gravis like syndrome or exacerbation of myasthenia gravis have been reported in patients administered propranolol.

Discontinuance of the drug should be considered if, according to clinical judgement, the well-being of the patient is adversely affected by any of the above reactions. Cessation of therapy with a beta-adrenoceptor blocking drug should be gradual. In the rare event of intolerance manifested as bradycardia and hypotension, the drug should be withdrawn and, if necessary, treatment for overdosage instituted.

Overdosage: The symptoms of overdosage may include bradycardia, hypotension, acute cardiac insufficiency and bronchospasm.

General treatment should include: close supervision, treatment in an intensive care ward, the use of gastric lavage, activated charcoal and a laxative to prevent absorption of any drug still present in the gastrointestinal tract, the use of plasma or plasma substitutes to treat hypotension and shock.

Excessive bradycardia can be countered with atropine 1 to 2 mg intravenously and/or a cardiac pacemaker. If necessary, this may be followed by a bolus dose of glucagon 10 mg intravenously. If required, this may be repeated or followed by an intravenous infusion of glucagon 1 to 10 mg/hour depending on response. If no response to glucagon occurs or if glucagon is unavailable, a beta-adrenoceptor stimulant such as dobutamine 2.5 to 10 microgram/kg/minute by intravenous infusion may be given. Dobutamine, because of its positive inotropic effect could also be used to treat hypotension and acute cardiac insufficiency. It is likely that these doses would be inadequate to reverse the cardiac effects of beta-blockade if a large overdose has been taken. The dose of dobutamine should therefore be increased if necessary to achieve the required response according to the clinical condition of the patient.

Pharmaceutical precautions Store below 30°C, protected from light and moisture.

Legal category POM.

Package quantities Patient Calendar Pack of 28 capsules.

Further information Inderal LA and Half-Inderal LA capsules provide controlled release of propranolol hydrochloride such that blood levels are maintained for over 24 hours following a single oral dose and, unlike therapy with conventional tablets, irregular peaks and troughs of blood level are avoided.

Product licence numbers

Inderal LA	12619/0028
Half-Inderal LA	12619/0029

INDERETIC*

Presentation White, opaque capsules, printed with Inderetic. Each capsule contains 80 mg Propranolol Hydrochloride PhEur and 2.5 mg Bendrofluazide PhEur. Inactive ingredients are gelatin, lactose, magnesium stearate and titanium dioxide.

Uses The management of hypertension.

Mode of action: Propranolol is a competitive antagonist at both the beta$_1$ and beta$_2$-adrenoceptors. It has no agonist activity at the beta-adrenoceptor, but has membrane stabilising activity at concentrations exceeding 1–3 mg/litre, though such concentrations are rarely achieved during oral therapy. Competitive beta-adrenoceptor blockade has been demonstrated in man by a parallel shift to the right in the dose-heart rate response curve to beta-agonists such as isoprenaline.

Propranolol, as with other beta-adrenoceptor blocking drugs, has negative inotropic effects, and is therefore contra-indicated in uncontrolled heart failure.

Propranolol is a racemic mixture and the active form is the S(-) isomer. With the exception of inhibition of the conversion of thyroxine to triiodothyronine it is unlikely that any additional ancillary properties possessed by R (+) propranolol, in comparison with the racemic mixture will give rise to different therapeutic effects.

Bendrofluazide causes diuresis by inhibiting sodium and water reabsorption in the proximal part of the distal tubule of the kidney. The consequences of this are a lowering in plasma volume and therefore cardiac output. However the main mechanism by which bendrofluazide lowers blood pressure is by its vasodilatory property which results in a lowering of peripheral resistance.

Propranolol is effective and well tolerated in most ethnic populations. Black patients respond better to the combination of propranolol and diuretics than to propranolol alone.

Propranolol is completely absorbed after oral administration and peak plasma concentrations occur 1 to 2 hours after dosing in fasting patients. The liver removes up to 90% of an oral dose with an elimination half-life of 3 to 6 hours. Propranolol is widely and rapidly distributed throughout the body with highest levels occurring in the lungs, liver, kidney, brain and heart. Propranolol is highly protein bound (80 to 95%).

Bendrofluazide is readily absorbed after oral administration and peak plasma concentrations occur 2 to 3 hours after dosing. Approximately 70% of the administered dose is metabolised and the remainder is recovered as unchanged drug in the urine. The elimination half-life is between 3 and 9 hours. Bendrofluazide has a high oral bioavailability and the drug distributes to extracellular spaces. Bendrofluazide is 94% bound to human serum albumin. There are no pharmacokinetic interactions between bendrofluazide and propranolol.

Dosage and administration *Adults:* One capsule twice daily should prove effective in most cases. For new patients a maximum response is achieved usually within two weeks. If a greater antihypertensive effect is desired, Inderetic is compatible with most other antihypertensives which may be added (see *Warnings* below).

Children: There is no paediatric experience with Inderetic and for this reason it is not recommended for children.

Elderly patients: Evidence concerning the relation between blood level and age is conflicting. The optimum dose should be individually determined.

Contra-indications, warnings, etc Inderetic must not be used if there is a history of bronchial asthma or bronchospasm. The product label states the following warning: "Do not take Inderetic if you have a history of asthma or wheezing". A similar warning appears in the Patient Information Leaflet.

Bronchospasm can usually be reversed by $beta_2$-agonist bronchodilators such as salbutamol. Large doses of the $beta_2$-agonist bronchodilator may be required to overcome the beta-blockade produced by propranolol and the dose should be titrated according to the clinical response; both intravenous and inhalational administration should be considered. The use of intravenous aminophylline and/or the use of ipratropium (given by nebuliser), may also be considered. Glucagon (1 to 2 mg given intravenously) has also been reported to produce a bronchodilator effect in asthmatic patients. Oxygen or artifical ventilation may be required in severe cases.

Inderetic must not be used in patients with any of the following conditions: known hypersensitivity to either component (or other thiazides), bradycardia, cardiogenic shock, hypotension, metabolic acidosis, after prolonged fasting, severe peripheral arterial circulatory disturbances, second or third degree heart block, sick sinus syndrome, untreated phaeochromocytoma, uncontrolled heart failure, Prinzmetal's angina, anuria or renal failure.

Due to its beta-adrenoceptor blocking drug component, Inderetic:

- although contra-indicated in uncontrolled heart failure (see *Contra-indications*), may be used in patients whose signs of heart failure have been controlled. Caution must be exercised in patients whose cardiac reserve is poor.
- although contra-indicated in severe peripheral arterial circulatory disturbances (see *Contra-indications*), may also aggravate less severe peripheral arterial circulatory disturbances.
- due to its negative effect on conduction time, caution must be exercised if it is given to patients with first degree heart block.
- may modify the tachycardia of hypoglycaemia.
- may mask the signs of thyrotoxicosis.
- will reduce heart rate, as a result of its pharmacological action. In the rare instances when a treated patient develops symptoms which may be attributable to a slow heart rate, the dose may be reduced.
- should not be discontinued abruptly in patients suffering from ischaemic heart disease.
- may cause a more severe reaction to a variety of allergens, when given to patients with a history of anaphylactic reaction to such allergens. Such patients may be unresponsive to the usual doses of adrenaline used to treat the allergic reactions.

Since the half-life may be increased in patients with significant hepatic or renal impairment, caution must be exercised when starting treatment and selecting the initial dose.

Inderetic must be used with caution in patients with decompensated cirrhosis.

In patients with portal hypertension, liver function may deteriorate and hepatic encephalopathy may develop. There have been reports suggesting that treatment with propranolol may increase the risk of developing hepatic encephalopathy.

As with other combinations of beta-adrenoceptor blocking drugs and diuretics and due to it bendrofluazide component, Inderetic:

- may be associated with minor changes in potassium status. Potassium depletion may be dangerous in patients receiving digitalis or those with hepatic cirrhosis with ascites.
- may decrease glucose tolerance. Caution must be exercised when administered to patients with a known predisposition to diabetes.

Inderetic modifies the tachycardia of hypoglycaemia. Caution should be exercised in the concurrent use of Inderetic and hypoglycaemic therapy in diabetic patients. Inderetic may prolong the hypoglycaemic response to insulin.

Caution must be exercised when prescribing a beta-adrenoceptor blocking drug with Class 1 antiarrhythmic agents such as disopyramide.

Combined use of beta-adrenoceptor blocking drugs and calcium channel blockers with negative inotropic effects e.g. verapamil, diltiazem can lead to an exaggeration of these effects, particularly in patients with impaired ventricular function and/or sino-atrial or atrio-ventricular conduction abnormalities. This may result in severe hypotension, bradycardia and cardiac failure. Neither the beta-adrenoceptor blocking drug nor the calcium channel blocker should be administered intravenously within 48 hours of discontinuing the other.

Concomitant therapy with dihydropyridine calcium channel blockers eg, nifedipine, may increase the risk of hypotension, and cardiac failure may occur in patients with latent cardiac insufficiency.

Beta-adrenoceptor blocking drugs may exacerbate the rebound hypertension which can follow the withdrawal of clonidine. If the two drugs are co-administered, the beta-adrenoceptor blocking drug should be withdrawn several days before discontinuing clonidine. If replacing clonidine by beta-adrenoceptor blocking drug therapy, the introduction of beta-adrenoceptor blocking drugs should be delayed for several days after clonidine administration has stopped.

Digitalis glycosides, in association with beta-adrenoceptor blocking drugs, may increase atrio-ventricular conduction time.

Concomitant use of sympathomimetic agents, e.g. adrenaline, may counteract the effect of beta-adrenoceptor blocking drugs. Caution must be exercised in the parenteral administration of preparations containing adrenaline to patients taking beta-adrenoceptor blocking drugs as, in rare cases, vasoconstriction, hypertension and bradycardia may result.

Administration of propranolol during infusion of lignocaine may increase the plasma concentration of lignocaine by approximately 30%. Patients already receiving propranolol tend to have higher lignocaine levels than controls. The combination should be avoided.

Caution must be exercised if ergotamine, dihydroergotamine or related compounds are given in combination with propranolol since vasospastic reactions have been reported in a few patients.

Concomitant use of prostaglandin synthetase inhibiting drugs, e.g. ibuprofen or indomethacin, may decrease the hypotensive effects of propranolol.

Concomitant administration of propranolol and chlorpromazine may result in an increase in plasma levels of both drugs. This may lead to an enhanced antipsychotic effect for chlorpromazine and an increased antihypertensive effect for propranolol.

Concomitant use of cimetidine or hydralazine will increase, whereas concomitant use of alcohol will decrease, the plasma levels of propranolol.

Preparations containing lithium generally should not be given with diuretics because they may reduce its renal clearance.

Anaesthesia: Caution must be exercised when using anaesthetic agents with Inderetic. The anaesthetist should be informed and the choice of anaesthetic should be the agent with as little negative inotropic activity as possible. Use of beta-adrenoceptor blocking drugs with anaesthetic drugs may result in attenuation of the reflex tachycardia and increase the risk of hypotension. Anaesthetic agents causing myocardial depression are best avoided.

Pharmacokinetic studies have shown that the following agents may interact with propranolol due to effects on enzyme systems in the liver which metabolise propranolol and these agents: quinidine, propafenone, rifampicin, theophylline, warfarin, thioridazine and dihydropyridine calcium channel blockers such as nifedipine, nisoldipine, nicardipine, isradipine and lacidipine. Owing to the fact that blood concentrations of either agent may be affected dosage adjustments may be needed according to clinical judgement. (See also the interaction above concerning the concomitant therapy with dihydropyridine calcium channel blockers).

Interference with laboratory tests: Inderetic has been reported to interfere with the estimation of serum bilirubin by the diazo method and with the determination of catecholamines by methods using fluorescence.

Pregnancy: Inderetic must not be given during pregnancy.

Lactation: As diuretics pass into breast milk, they should be avoided in mothers who wish to breast feed. Similarly, breast feeding is not recommended following administration of lipophilic beta-adrenoceptor blocking drugs.

Effect on ability to drive or operate machinery: The use of Inderetic is unlikely to result in any impairment of the ability of patients to drive or operate machinery. Studies to investigate these effects of bendrofluazide have not been carried out. When driving vehicles or operating machinery, it should be taken into account that occasional dizziness or fatigue may occur.

Undesirable events: Inderetic is usually well tolerated. In clinical studies, the undesired events reported are usually attributable to the pharmacological actions of propranolol or bendrofluazide.

Possible undesired events, listed by body system, include:

Cardiovascular: bradycardia, heart failure deterioration, postural hypotension which may be associated with syncope, cold extremities. In susceptible patients: precipitation of heart block, exacerbation of intermittent claudication, Raynaud's phenomenon.

CNS: confusion, dizziness, mood changes, nightmares, psychoses and hallucinations, sleep disturbances.

Gastrointestinal: gastrointestinal disturbance.

Haematological: purpura, thrombocytopenia.

Integumentary: alopecia, dry eyes, psoriasiform skin reactions, exacerbation of psoriasis, skin rashes.

Neurological: paraesthesia.

Respiratory: bronchospasm may occur in patients with bronchial asthma or a history of asthmatic complaints, sometimes with fatal outcome (see *Contra-indications*).

Special senses: visual disturbances.

Others: fatigue and/or lassitude (often transient), an increase in ANA (antinuclear antibodies) has been observed, however the clinical relevance of this is not clear; isolated reports of myasthenia gravis like syndrome or exacerbation of myasthenia gravis have been reported in patients administered propranolol.

Adverse effects of bendrofluazide are uncommon in the dose contained in Inderetic.

Hypokalaemia may occur and may be dangerous in patients receiving digitalis or in those with hepatic cirrhosis when coma may be precipitated.

Hyperuricaemia sometimes occurs, but an attack of gout is rare.

The thiazide diuretics increase blood urea and they should be used with care in patients with renal failure.

Reports of other adverse reactions to thiazides include skin rashes with associated photosensitivity, necrotising vasculitis, acute pancreatitis, blood dyscrasias and aggravation of pre-existing myopia.

Discontinuance of Inderetic should be considered if, according to clinical judgement, the well-being of the patient is adversely affected by any of the above reactions, bearing in mind that cessation of therapy with a beta-adrenoceptor blocking drug should be gradual.

Overdosage: The symptoms of overdosage may include bradycardia, hypotension, acute cardiac insufficiency and bronchospasm.

General treatment should include: close supervision, treatment in an intensive care ward, the use of gastric lavage, activated charcoal and a laxative to prevent absorption of any drug still present in the gastrointestinal tract, the use of plasma or plasma substitutes to treat hypotension and shock.

Excessive bradycardia can be countered with atropine 1 to 2 mg intravenously and/or a cardiac pacemaker. If necessary, this may be followed by a bolus dose of glucagon 10 mg intravenously. If required, this may be repeated or followed by an intravenous infusion of glucagon 1 to 10 mg/hour depending on response. If no response to glucagon occurs or if glucagon is unavailable, a beta-adrenoceptor stimulant such as dobutamine 2.5 to 10 microgram/kg/minute by intravenous infusion may be given. Dobutamine, because of its positive inotropic effect could also be used to treat hypotension and acute cardiac insufficiency. It is likely that these doses would be inadequate to reverse the cardiac effects of beta-blockade if a large overdose has been taken. The dose of dobutamine should therefore be increased if necessary to achieve the required response according to the clinical condition of the patient.

Excessive diuresis should be countered by maintaining normal fluid and electrolyte balance.

Pharmaceutical precautions Store below 25°C, protected from light and moisture.

Legal category POM.

Package quantities Containers of 60 capsules (OP).

Further information Inderetic is designed to aid drug compliance by providing a convenient presentation of the standard beta-adrenoceptor blocking drug Inderal, propranolol hydrochloride, with the diuretic bendrofluazide for the treatment of hypertension. Concurrent use of propranolol and bendrofluazide produces a more pronounced and consistent antihypertensive response than when either component is used alone.

Product licence number 12619/0033.

INDEREX*

Presentation Capsules, having opaque pink caps and opaque grey bodies printed with the name Inderex. Each capsule contains 160 mg Propranolol Hydrochloride PhEur in the form of spheroids having a sustained release coating to provide long action and 5 mg Bendrofluazide PhEur. Inactive ingredients are erythrosine, ethylcellulose, gelatin, iron oxide, lactose, maize starch, methylhydroxypropylcellulose, microcrystalline cellulose, Patent Blue V, stearic acid, talc and titanium dioxide.

Uses The management of hypertension.

Mode of action: Propranolol is a competitive antagonist at both the $beta_1$ and $beta_2$-adrenoceptors. It has no agonist activity at the beta-adrenoceptor, but has membrane stabilising activity at concentrations exceeding 1 to 3 mg/litre, though such concentrations are rarely achieved during oral therapy. Competitive beta-adrenoceptor blockade has been demonstrated in man by a parallel shift to the right in the dose-heart rate response curve to beta-agonists such as isoprenaline. The sustained release preparation of propranolol maintains a higher degree of $beta_1$–blockade 24 hours after dosing compared with conventional propranolol.

Propranolol, as with other beta-adrenoceptor blocking drugs, has negative inotropic effects, and is therefore contra-indicated in uncontrolled heart failure.

Propranolol is a racemic mixture and the active form is the S(-) isomer. With the exception of inhibition of the conversion of thyroxine to triiodothyronine it is unlikely that any additional ancillary properties possessed by R (+) propranolol, in comparison with the racemic mixture will give rise to different therapeutic effects.

Bendrofluazide causes diuresis by inhibiting sodium and water reabsorption in the proximal part of the distal tubule of the kidney. The consequences of this are a lowering in plasma volume and therefore cardiac output. However the main mechanism by which bendrofluazide lowers blood pressure is by its vasodilatory property which results in a lowering of peripheral resistance.

Propranolol is effective and well tolerated in most ethnic populations. Black patients respond better to the combination of propranolol and diuretics than to propranolol alone.

Propranolol is completely absorbed after oral administration. Following oral dosing with the sustained release preparation of propranolol the blood profile is flatter than after conventional Inderal but the half-life is increased to between 10 and 20 hours. The liver removes up to 90% of an oral dose with an elimination half-life of 3 to 6 hours. Propranolol is widely and rapidly distributed throughout the body with highest levels occurring in the lungs, liver, kidney, brain and heart. Propranolol is highly protein bound (80–95%).

Bendrofluazide is readily absorbed after oral administration and peak plasma concentrations occur 2 to 3 hours after dosing. Approximately 70% of the administered dose is metabolised and the remainder is recovered as unchanged drug in the urine. The elimination half-life is between 3 and 9 hours. Bendrofluazide has a high oral bioavailability and the drug distributes to extracellular spaces. Bendrofluazide is 94% bound to human serum albumin. There are no pharmacokinetic interactions between bendrofluazide and propranolol.

Dosage and administration *Adults:* One capsule daily should prove effective in most cases.

For new patients a maximum response is achieved usually within two weeks. If a greater antihypertensive effect is desired, Inderex is compatible with most other antihypertensives which may be added (see *Warnings* below).

Children: There is no paediatric experience with Inderex and for this reason it is not recommended for children.

Elderly patients: Evidence concerning the relation between blood level and age is conflicting. The optimum dose should be individually determined.

Contra-indications, warnings, etc Inderex must not be used if there is a history of bronchial asthma or bronchospasm. The product label states the following warning: "Do not take Inderex if you have a history of asthma or wheezing". A similar warning appears in the patient information leaflet.

Bronchospasm can usually be reversed by $beta_2$-agonist bronchodilators such as salbutamol. Large doses of the $beta_2$-agonist bronchodilator may be required to overcome the beta-blockade produced by propranolol and the dose should be titrated according to the clinical response; both intravenous and inhalational administration should be considered. The use of intravenous aminophylline and/or the use of ipratropium (given by nebuliser), may also be considered. Glucagon (1 to 2 mg given intravenously) has also been reported to produce a bronchodilator effect in asthmatic patients. Oxygen or artifical ventilation may be required in severe cases.

Inderex must not be used in patients with any of the following conditions: known hypersensitivity to either component (or other thiazides), bradycardia, cardiogenic shock, hypotension, metabolic acidosis, after prolonged fasting, severe peripheral arterial circulatory disturbances, second or third degree heart block, sick sinus syndrome, untreated phaeochromocytoma, uncontrolled heart failure, Prinzmetal's angina, anuria or renal failure.

Due to its beta-adrenoceptor blocking drug component, Inderex:

- although contra-indicated in uncontrolled heart failure (see *Contra-indications*), may be used in patients whose signs of heart failure have been controlled. Caution must be exercised in patients whose cardiac reserve is poor.
- although contra-indicated in severe peripheral arterial circulatory disturbances (see *Contra-indications*), may also aggravate less severe peripheral arterial circulatory disturbances.
- due to its negative effect on conduction time, caution must be exercised if it is given to patients with first degree heart block.
- may modify the tachycardia of hypoglycaemia.
- may mask the signs of thyrotoxicosis.
- will reduce heart rate, as a result of its pharmacological action. In the rare instances when a treated patient develops symptoms which may be attributable to a slow heart rate, the dose may be reduced.
- should not be discontinued abruptly in patients suffering from ischaemic heart disease.
- may cause a more severe reaction to a variety of allergens, when given to patients with a history of anaphylactic reaction to such allergens. Such patients may be unresponsive to the usual doses of adrenaline used to treat the allergic reactions.

Since the half-life may be increased in patients with significant hepatic or renal impairment, caution must be exercised when starting treatment and selecting the initial dose.

Inderex must be used with caution in patients with decompensated cirrhosis.

In patients with portal hypertension, liver function may deteriorate and hepatic encephalopathy may develop. There have been reports suggesting that treatment with propranolol may increase the risk of developing hepatic encephalopathy.

As with other combinations of beta-adrenoceptor blocking drugs and diuretics and due to its bendrofluazide component, Inderex:

- may be associated with minor changes in potassium status. Potassium depletion may be dangerous in patients receiving digitalis or those with hepatic cirrhosis with ascites.
- may decrease glucose tolerance. Caution must be exercised when administered to patients with a known predisposition to diabetes.

Inderex modifies the tachycardia of hypoglycaemia. Caution must be exercised in the concurrent use of Inderex and hypoglycaemia therapy in diabetic patients. Inderex may prolong the hypoglycaemic response to insulin.

Caution must be exercised when prescribing a beta-adrenoceptor blocking drug with Class 1 antiarrhythmic agents such as disopyramide.

Combined use of beta-adrenoceptor blocking drugs and calcium channel blockers with negative inotropic effects e.g. verapamil, diltiazem can lead to an exaggeration of these effects, particularly in patients with impaired ventricular function and/or sino-atrial or atrio-ventricular conduction abnormalities. This may result in severe hypotension, bradycardia and cardiac failure. Neither the beta-adrenoceptor blocking drug nor the calcium channel blocker should be administered intravenously within 48 hours of discontinuing the other.

Concomitant therapy with dihydropyridine calcium channel blockers eg, nifedipine, may increase the risk of hypotension, and cardiac failure may occur in patients with latent cardiac insufficiency.

Beta-adrenoceptor blocking drugs may exacerbate the rebound hypertension which can follow the withdrawal of clonidine. If the two drugs are co-administered, the beta-adrenoceptor blocking drug should be withdrawn several days before discontinuing clonidine. If replacing clonidine by beta-adrenoceptor blocking drug therapy, the introduction of beta-adrenoceptor blocking drugs should be delayed for several days after clonidine administration has stopped.

Digitalis glycosides, in association with beta-adrenoceptor blocking drugs, may increase atrio-ventricular conduction time.

Concomitant use of sympathomimetic agents, e.g. adrenaline, may counteract the effect of beta-adrenoceptor blocking drugs. Caution must be exercised in the parenteral administration of preparations containing adrenaline to patients taking beta-adrenoceptor blocking drugs as, in rare cases, vasoconstriction, hypertension and bradycardia may result.

Administration of propranolol during infusion of lignocaine may increase the plasma concentration of lignocaine by approximately 30%. Patients already receiving propranolol tend to have higher lignocaine levels than controls. The combination should be avoided.

Caution must be exercised if ergotamine, dihydroergotamine or related compounds are given in combination with propranolol since vasospastic reactions have been reported in a few patients.

Concomitant use of prostaglandin synthetase inhibiting drugs, e.g. ibuprofen or indomethacin, may decrease the hypotensive effects of propranolol.

Concomitant administration of propranolol and chlorpromazine may result in an increase in plasma levels of both drugs. This may lead to an enhanced antipsychotic effect for chlorpromazine and an increased antihypertensive effect for propranolol.

Concomitant use of cimetidine or hydralazine will increase, whereas concomitant use of alcohol will decrease, the plasma levels of propranolol.

Preparations containing lithium generally should not be given with diuretics because they may reduce its renal clearance.

Anaesthesia: Caution must be exercised when using anaesthetic agents with Inderex. The anaesthetist should be informed and the choice of anaesthetic should be the agent with as little negative inotropic activity as possible. Use of beta-adrenoceptor blocking drugs with anaesthetic drugs may result in attenuation of the reflex tachycardia and increase the risk of hypotension. Anaesthetic agents causing myocardial depression are best avoided.

Pharmacokinetic studies have shown that the following agents may interact with propranolol due to effects on enzyme systems in the liver which metabolise propranolol and these agents: quinidine, propafenone, rifampicin, theophylline, warfarin, thioridazine and dihydropyridine calcium channel blockers such as nifedipine, nisoldipine, nicardipine, isradipine and lacidipine. Owing to the fact that blood concentrations of either agent may be affected dosage adjustments may be needed according to clinical judgement. (See also the interaction above concerning the concomitant therapy with dihydropyridine calcium channel blockers).

Interference with laboratory tests: Inderex has been reported to interfere with the estimation of serum bilirubin by the diazo method and with the determination of catecholamines by methods using fluorescence.

Pregnancy: Inderex must not be given in pregnancy.

Lactation: As diuretics pass into breast milk, they should be avoided in mothers who wish to breast feed. Similarly, breast feeding is not recommended following administration of lipophilic beta-adrenoceptor blocking drugs.

Effect on ability to drive or operate machinery: The use of Inderex is unlikely to result in any impairment of the ability of patients to drive or operate machinery. Studies to investigate the effects of bendrofluazide have not been carried out. When driving vehicles or operating machinery, it should be taken into account that occasional dizziness or fatigue may occur.

Undesirable events: Inderex is usually well tolerated. In clinical studies, the undesired events reported are usually attributable to the pharmacological actions of propranolol or bendrofluazide.

Possible undesired events, listed by body system, include:

Cardiovascular: bradycardia, heart failure deterioration, postural hypotension which may be associated with syncope, cold extremities. In susceptible patients: precipitation of heart block, exacerbation of intermittent claudication, Raynaud's phenomenon.

CNS: confusion, dizziness, mood changes, nightmares, psychoses and hallucinations, sleep disturbance.

Gastrointestinal: gastrointestinal disturbance.

Haematological: purpura, thrombocytopenia.

Integumentary: alopecia, dry eyes, psoriasiform skin reactions, exacerbation of psoriasis, skin rashes.

Neurological: paraesthesia.

Respiratory: bronchospasm may occur in patients with bronchial asthma or a history of asthmatic complaints, sometimes with fatal outcome (see *Contra-indications*).

Special senses: visual disturbances.

Others: fatigue and/or lassitude (often transient), an increase in ANA (antinuclear antibodies) has been observed, however the clinical relevance of this is not clear; isolated reports of myasthenia gravis like syndrome or exacerbation of myasthenia gravis have been reported in patients administered propranolol.

Adverse effects of bendrofluazide are uncommon in the dose contained in Inderex.

Hypokalaemia may occur and may be dangerous in patients receiving digitalis or in those with hepatic cirrhosis when coma may be precipitated.

Hyperuricaemia sometimes occurs, but an attack of gout is rare.

The thiazide diuretics increase blood urea and they should be used with care in patients with renal failure.

Reports of other adverse reactions to thiazides include skin rashes with associated photosensitivity, necrotising vasculitis, acute pancreatitis, blood dyscrasias and aggravation of pre-existing myopia.

Discontinuance of Inderex should be considered if, according to clinical judgement, the well-being of the patient is adversely affected by any of the above reactions, bearing in mind that cessation of therapy with a beta-adrenoceptor blocking drug should be gradual.

Overdosage: The symptoms of overdosage may include bradycardia, hypotension, acute cardiac insufficiency and bronchospasm.

General treatment should include: close supervision, treatment in an intensive care ward, the use of gastric lavage, activated charcoal and a laxative to prevent absorption of any drug still present in the gastrointestinal tract, the use of plasma or plasma substitutes to treat hypotension and shock.

Excessive bradycardia can be countered with atropine 1 to 2 mg intravenously and/or a cardiac pacemaker. If necessary, this may be followed by a bolus dose of glucagon 10 mg intravenously. If required, this may be repeated or followed by an intravenous infusion of glucagon 1 to 10 mg/hour depending on response. If no response to glucagon occurs or if glucagon is unavailable, a beta-adrenoceptor stimulant such as dobutamine 2.5 to 10 microgram/kg/minute by intravenous infusion may be given. Dobutamine, because of its positive inotropic effect could also be used to treat hypotension and acute cardiac insufficiency. It is likely that these doses would be inadequate to reverse the cardiac effects of beta-blockade if a large overdose has been taken. The dose of dobutamine should therefore be increased if necessary to achieve the required response according to the clinical condition of the patient.

Excessive diuresis should be countered by maintaining normal fluid and electrolyte balance.

Pharmaceutical precautions Store below 25°C, protected from light and moisture.

Legal category POM.

Package quantities Patient calendar pack of 28 capsules.

Further information Inderex is designed to aid drug compliance by providing a convenient presentation of a sustained release formulation of propranolol hydrochloride with the diuretic bendrofluazide for the treatment of hypertension. Concurrent use of propranolol and bendrofluazide produces a more pronounced and consistent antihypertensive response than when either component is used alone.

Product licence number 12619/0034.

KALTEN*

Qualitative and quantitative composition Atenolol PhEur 50 mg; Hydrochlorothiazide PhEur 25 mg; Amiloride Hydrochloride PhEur (dihydrate) 2.84 mg (equivalent to Amiloride Hydrochloride 2.5 mg)

Pharmaceutical form Capsules.

Clinical particulars
Therapeutic indications: Management of hypertension.

Posology and method of administration: For oral administration.

Adults: One capsule daily. Kalten is recommended for use in hypertensive patients where monotherapy with a beta-adrenoceptor blocker or diuretic proves inadequate. Where necessary, another anti-hypertensive drug, such as a vasodilator, can be added. Patients can be transferred to preparations containing beta-adrenoceptor blocking drugs from other anti-hypertensive treatments with the exception of clonidine (see *Special warnings and special precautions for use*).

Elderly: One capsule daily. Kalten contains low effective doses of both a beta-adrenoceptor blocking agent and a combination of diuretics with a potassium-sparing action, and may be suited to older patients where higher doses of these drugs may be considered inappropriate.

Children: There is no paediatric experience with Kalten; therefore this preparation is not recommended for use in children.

Contra-indications: Kalten should not be used in patients with any of the following: known hypersensitivity to any of the components; bradycardia; cardiogenic shock; hypotension; metabolic acidosis; severe peripheral arterial circulatory disturbances; second or third degree heart block; sick sinus syndrome; untreated phaeochromocytoma; uncontrolled heart failure; hyperkalaemia (serum potassium greater than 5.5 mmol/l); those receiving concomitant therapy with potassium-sparing diuretics or potassium supplements; anuria; acute renal failure; severe progressive renal disease; diabetic nephropathy; blood urea over 10 mmol/l or serum creatinine over 130 micromol/l in whom serum electrolyte and blood urea levels cannot be monitored carefully and frequently.

In renal impairment, use of a potassium-conserving agent may result in the rapid development of hyperkalaemia (see *Special warnings and special precautions for use*).

Special warnings and special precautions for use: Due to its beta-blocker component, Kalten:

- although contraindicated in uncontrolled heart failure (see *Contra-indications*), may be used in patients whose signs of heart failure have been controlled. Caution must be exercised in patients whose cardiac reserve is poor;
- may increase the number and duration of angina attacks in patients with Prinzmetal's angina due to unopposed alpha receptor mediated coronary artery vasoconstriction. Atenolol is a beta$_1$-selective beta-adrenoceptor blocking drug, consequently the use of Kalten may be considered although utmost caution must be exercised;
- although contra-indicated in severe peripheral arterial circulatory disturbances (see *Contra-indications*) may also aggravate less severe peripheral arterial circulatory disturbances;
- due to its negative effect on conduction time, caution must be exercised if it is given to patients with first degree heart block;
- may modify the tachycardia of hypoglycaemia;
- may mask the signs of thyrotoxicosis;
- will reduce heart rate, as a result of its pharmacological action. In the rare instances when a treated patient develops symptoms which may be attributable to a slow heart rate, the dose may be reduced;
- should not be discontinued abruptly in patients suffering from ischaemic heart disease;
- may cause a more severe reaction to a variety of allergens, when given to patients with a history of anaphylactic reaction to such allergens. Such patients may be unresponsive to the usual doses of adrenaline used to treat the allergic reactions;
- Kalten contains the cardioselective beta-adrenoceptor blocking drug atenolol. Although cardioselective (beta$_1$) beta-adrenoceptor blocking drugs may have less effect on lung function than non-selective beta-adrenoceptor blocking drugs, as with all beta-adrenoceptor blocking drugs, these should be avoided in patients with reversible obstructive airways disease, unless there are compelling clinical reasons for their use. Where such reasons exist, Kalten may be used with caution. Occasionally, some increase in airways resistance may occur in asthmatic patients, however, and this may usually be reversed by commonly used dosage of bronchodilators such as salbutamol or isoprenaline.

The label and patient information leaflet for this product state the following warning: "If you have ever had asthma or wheezing, you should not take this medicine unless you have discussed these symptoms with the prescribing doctor".

Due to its diuretic component, caution must be exercised if Kalten is used in:

- severely ill patients in whom metabolic or respiratory acidosis may occur (eg, decompensated diabetes or cardiopulmonary disease) or in whom fluid and electrolyte balance is critical. Acidosis may be associated with rapid increases in serum potassium;
- patients with hepatic impairment. Amiloride has been reported to precipitate hepatic encephalopathy and deepening jaundice has also occurred in cirrhotic patients;
- diabetic patients, or those with a known predisposition to diabetes, particularly those with abnormal renal function. Hyperkalaemia has commonly occurred in diabetic patients on amiloride, especially those with chronic renal disease or pre-renal azotaemia. The status of renal function should therefore be determined before Kalten is given to known or suspected diabetics. Lowering of glucose tolerance may occur and the insulin dosage of the diabetic patient may require adjustment. Kalten should be discontinued at least 3 days before glucose tolerance testing.
- patients with renal impairment (see also *Contra-indications*), since the use of potassium conserving diuretics may result in the rapid development of hyperkalaemia. Caution is also necessary to avoid the cumulative or toxic effects due to a reduced excretion of the components of Kalten. Azotaemia may be precipitated or increased by hydrochlorothiazide. If increasing azotaemia and oliguria occur, treatment should be discontinued. Changes in plasma potassium have been observed in patients receiving amiloride and hydrochlorothiazide particularly in: the elderly; diabetics; patients with hepatic cirrhosis or congestive heart failure who had known renal impairment, were seriously ill, or were undergoing vigorous diuretic therapy; those receiving digitalis for heart failure; those taking an abnormal (low in potassium) diet and those suffering from gastrointestinal complaints. The measurement of potassium levels are especially appropriate in these patients.

Patients should be carefully observed for clinical, laboratory and ECG evidence of hyperkalaemia (not always associated with an abnormal ECG). Should hyperkalaemia develop, discontinue treatment immediately and if necessary, take active measures to reduce the serum potassium to normal. Hypokalaemia although less likely to occur may predispose to arrhythmias in patients receiving digitalis.

Hyponatraemia and hypochloraemia may occur with Kalten. Any chloride deficiency may be corrected by ammonium chloride (except in hepatic disease) and is largely prevented by a normal salt intake.

Kalten may be associated with hyperuricaemia.

Interactions with other medicaments and other forms of interaction: Combined use of beta-adrenoceptor blocking drugs and calcium channel blockers with negative inotropic effects eg, verapamil, diltiazem can lead to an exaggeration of these effects particularly in patients with impaired ventricular function and/or sino-atrial or atrio-ventricular conduction abnormalities. This may result in severe hypotension, bradycardia and cardiac failure. Neither the beta-adrenoceptor blocking drug nor the calcium channel blocker should be administered intravenously within 48 hours of discontinuing the other.

Concomitant therapy with dihydropyridines eg, nifedipine, may increase the risk of hypotension, and cardiac failure may occur in patients with latent cardiac insufficiency.

Digitalis glycosides, in association with beta-adrenoceptor blocking drugs, may increase atrio-ventricular conduction time.

Beta-adrenoceptor blocking drugs may exacerbate the rebound hypertension which can follow the withdrawal of clonidine. If the two drugs are co-administered, the beta-adrenoceptor blocking drug should be withdrawn several days before discontinuing clonidine. If replacing clonidine by beta-adrenoceptor blocking drug therapy, the introduction of beta-adrenoceptor blocking drugs should be delayed for several days after clonidine administration has stopped.

Caution must be exercised when prescribing a beta-adrenoceptor blocking drug with Class I antiarrhythmic agents such as disopyramide.

Concomitant use of sympathomimetic agents, eg, adrenaline, may counteract the effect of beta-adrenoceptor blocking drugs.

Concomitant use with insulin and oral antidiabetic drugs may lead to the intensification of the blood sugar lowering effects of these drugs.

Concomitant use of prostaglandin synthetase inhibiting drugs (eg, ibuprofen, indomethacin) may decrease the hypotensive effects of beta-adrenoceptor blocking drugs.

Preparations containing lithium should not generally be given with diuretics because they may reduce its renal clearance.

Caution must be exercised when using anaesthetic agents with Kalten. The anaesthetist should be informed and the choice of anaesthetic should be an agent with as little negative inotropic activity as possible. Use of beta-adrenoceptor blocking drugs with anaesthetic drugs may result in attenuation of the reflex tachycardia and increase the risk of hypotension. Anaesthetic agents causing myocardial depression are best avoided.

Pregnancy and lactation: Kalten must not be given during pregnancy.

Kalten must not be given during lactation.

Effects on ability to drive and use machines: Use is unlikely to result in any impairment of the ability of patients to drive or operate machinery. However, it should be taken into account that occasionally dizziness or fatigue may occur.

Undesirable effects: Kalten is well tolerated. In clinical studies, the undesired events reported are usually attributable to the pharmacological actions of its components.

The following undesired events, listed by body system, have been reported:

Atenolol monotherapy:

Cardiovascular: bradycardia; heart failure deterioration; postural hypotension which may be associated with syncope; cold extremities. In susceptible patients: precipitation of heart block; intermittent claudication; Raynaud's phenomenon.

CNS: confusion; dizziness; headache; mood changes; nightmares; psychoses and hallucinations; sleep disturbances of the type noted with other beta-adrenoceptor blocking drugs.

Gastrointestinal: dry mouth, gastrointestinal disturbances. Elevations of transaminase levels have been seen infrequently, rare cases of hepatic toxicity including intrahepatic cholestasis have been reported.

Haematological: purpura; thrombocytopenia.

Integumentary: alopecia; dry eyes; psoriasiform skin reactions; exacerbation of psoriasis; skin rashes.

Neurological: paraesthesia.

Respiratory: bronchospasm may occur in patients with bronchial asthma or a history of asthmatic complaints.

Special senses: visual disturbances.

Others: fatigue; an increase in ANA (Antinuclear Antibodies) has been observed, however the clinical relevance of this is not clear.

Amiloride and hydrochlorothiazide:

Biochemical: electrolyte imbalance; glycosuria; hyperglycaemia; hyperuricaemia.

Cardiovascular: necrotising vasculitis; orthostatic hypotension secondary to diuresis.

CNS: dizziness; headache; vertigo.

Gastrointestinal: acute pancreatitis; anorexia; constipation; cramps; diarrhoea; dry mouth; gastric irritation; jaundice; nausea; pain; salivary gland inflammation; thirst; vomiting.

Haematological: blood dyscrasias; purpura.

Integumentary: skin rashes with associated photosensitivity; urticaria.

Musculoskeletal: muscle cramps.

Neurological: paraesthesia.

Respiratory: pneumonitis; respiratory distress.

Special senses: transient blurred vision; xanthopsia.

Others: fatigue; fever; restlessness. Hypersensitivity reactions, including pulmonary oedema with symptoms of shock, have been reported with hydrochlorothiazide.

Discontinuance of Kalten should be considered if, according to clinical judgement, the well being of the patient is adversely affected by any of the above reactions.

Overdosage: The symptoms of overdosage may include bradycardia, hypotension, and acute cardiac insufficiency and bronchospasm.

General treatment should include: close supervision; treatment in an intensive care ward; the use of gastric lavage; activated charcoal and a laxative to prevent absorption of any drug still present in the gastrointestinal tract, the use of plasma or plasma substitutes to treat hypotension and shock. The possible use of haemodialysis or haemoperfusion can be considered.

Dehydration, electrolyte imbalance and hepatic coma are treated by the established procedures. If hyperkalaemia occurs, active measures should be taken to reduce the serum potassium levels. For respiratory impairment, oxygen or artificial respiration should be administered. Bronchospasm can usually be reversed by bronchodilators.

Excessive diuresis should be countered by maintaining normal fluid and electrolyte balance.

Excessive bradycardia can be countered with atropine 1-2 mg intravenously and/or a cardiac pacemaker. If necessary, this may be followed by a bolus dose of glucagon 10 mg intravenously. If required, this may be repeated or followed by an intravenous infusion of glucagon 1-10 mg/hour depending on response. If no response to glucagon occurs or if glucagon is unavailable, a beta-adrenoceptor stimulant such as dobutamine 2.5 to 10 micrograms/kg/minute by intravenous infusion may be given.

Dobutamine, because of its positive inotropic effect could also be used to treat hypotension and acute cardiac insufficiency. It is likely that these doses would be inadequate to reverse the cardiac effects of beta-adrenoceptor blockade if a large overdose has been taken. The dose of dobutamine should therefore be increased if necessary to achieve the required response according to the clinical condition of the patient.

Pharmacological properties

Pharmacodynamic properties: Kalten combines the antihypertensive activity of a beta-adrenoceptor blocking drug (atenolol) and a potassium sparing diuretic preparation (hydrochlorothiazide and amiloride).

Atenolol is beta$_1$-selective (ie, acts preferentially on beta$_1$-adrenergic receptors in the heart). Selectivity decreases with increasing dose.

Atenolol is without intrinsic sympathomimetic and membrane stabilising activities and, as with other beta-adrenoceptor blocking drugs, has negative inotropic effects (and is therefore contraindicated in uncontrolled heart failure).

As with other beta-adrenoceptor blocking drugs, its mode of action in the treatment of hypertension is unclear.

It is unlikely that any additional ancillary properties possessed by S(-) atenolol, in comparison with the racemic mixture, will give rise to different therapeutic effects.

Atenolol is effective and well tolerated in most ethnic populations although the response may be less in black patients.

Hydrochlorothiazide is a thiazide diuretic acting on the distal tubule. It exerts its effect on sodium and water excretion by inhibiting sodium absorption thereby impeding the capacity of the kidneys to concentrate the urine. It has a relatively flat dose-response curve.

Amiloride is a potassium sparing diuretic which although having a mild antihypertensive effect is used primarily for its potassium conserving effects. It acts on the early distal tubule.

Studies show that the combination of hydrochlorothiazide and amiloride in the ratio of 10 to 1 is optimal to achieve these effects.

Pharmacokinetic properties: Absorption of atenolol following oral dosing is consistent but incomplete (approximately 40-50%) with peak plasma concentrations occurring 2-4 hours after dosing. The atenolol blood levels are consistent and subject to little variability. There is no significant hepatic metabolism of atenolol and more than 90% of that absorbed reaches the systemic circulation unaltered. The plasma half-life is about 6 hours but this may rise in severe renal impairment since the kidney is the major route of elimination. Atenolol penetrates tissues poorly due to its low lipid solubility and its concentration in brain tissue is low. Plasma protein binding is low (approximately 3%).

Absorption of hydrochlorothiazide following oral dosing is rapid but incomplete. The hydrochlorothiazide blood levels are consistent and subject to little variability. There is no significant hepatic metabolism of hydrochlorothiazide. The plasma half-life is between 6 and 10 hours and the kidney is the main route of elimination.

Absorption of amiloride following oral dosing is rapid but incomplete. The amiloride blood levels are inconsistent and subject to moderate variability. There is no significant hepatic metabolism of amiloride and the plasma half-life is about 6 hours.

Thus, atenolol, hydrochlorothiazide and amiloride have compatible pharmacokinetics and when given together, no clinically significant pharmacokinetic interactions occur.

Kalten is effective for at least 24 hours after a single oral daily dose. This simplicity of dosing facilitates compliance by its acceptability to patients.

Pharmaceutical particulars

List of excipients: Lactose PhEur; Maize Starch PhEur; Sodium Starch Glycollate B.P.; Sodium Lauryl Sulphate PhEur; Magnesium Stearate PhEur; Titanium Dioxide PhEur (E171); Red Iron Oxide (E172); Yellow Iron Oxide (E172); Gelatin PhEur.

Incompatibilities: See *Interactions*.

Shelf life: 36 months.

Special precautions for storage: Store below 25°C, protected from light and moisture.

Nature and contents of container: Blister strips of 28.

Instructions for use/handling: Not applicable.

Market authorisation number PL 12619/0035.

Date of approval/revision February 1998.

Legal Category POM

MERONEM*

Qualitative and quantitative composition

Vial for i.v. injection or infusion	*Meronem 250 mg*	*Meronem 500 mg*	*Meronem 1000 mg*
Active ingredient:			
Meropenem trihydrate	285 mg	570 mg	1140 mg
equivalent to anhydrous meropenem	250 mg	500 mg	1000 mg
Excipient:			
Anhydrous sodium carbonate	52 mg	104 mg	208 mg

For each gram of meropenem (anhydrous potency) the vial contains 90 mg (3.9 mmol) of sodium.

Infusion Kits are also available containing either a 500 mg or 1 g vial together with a 100 ml bag of 0.9% w/v sodium chloride intravenous infusion.

Pharmaceutical form Powder for constitution for intravenous administration.

Clinical particulars

Therapeutic indications: Meronem IV is indicated for treatment, in adults and children, of the following infections caused by single or multiple bacteria sensitive to meropenem:

- Pneumonias and nosocomial pneumonias
- Urinary tract infections
- Intra-abdominal infections
- Gynaecological infections, such as endometritis
- Skin and skin structure infections
- Meningitis
- Septicaemia
- Empiric treatment, for presumed infections in adult patients with febrile neutropenia, used as monotherapy or in combination with anti-viral or antifungal agents.

Meronem has proved efficacious alone or in combination with other antimicrobial agents in the treatment of polymicrobial infections.

Intravenous meropenem has been used effectively in patients with cystic fibrosis and chronic lower respiratory tract infections, either as monotherapy or in combination with other antibacterial agents. Eradication of the organism was not always established.

There is no experience in paediatric patients with neutropenia or primary or secondary immunodeficiency.

Posology and method of administration:

Adults: The dosage and duration of therapy shall be established depending on type and severity of infection and the condition of the patient. The recommended daily dosage is as follows:

- 500 mg IV every 8 hours in the treatment of pneumonia, UTI, gynaecological infections such as endometritis, skin and skin structure infections.
- 1 g IV every 8 hours in the treatment of nosocomial pneumonias, peritonitis, presumed infections in neutropenic patients, septicaemia.
- In cystic fibrosis, doses up to 2 g every 8 hours have been used; most patients have been treated with 2 g every 8 hours.
- In meningitis the recommended dosage is 2 g every 8 hours.

As with other antibiotics, particular caution is recommended in using meropenem as monotherapy in critically ill patients with known or suspected Pseudomonas aeruginosa lower respiratory tract infection.

Regular sensitivity testing is recommended when treating Pseudomonas aeruginosa infection.

Dosage schedule for adults with impaired renal function: Dosage should be reduced in patients with creatinine clearance less than 51 ml/min, as scheduled below.

Creatinine clearance (ml/min)	*Dose (based on unit doses of 500 mg, 1 g, 2 g)*	*Frequency*
26 to 50	one unit dose	every 12 hours
10 to 25	one-half unit dose	every 12 hours
<10	one-half unit dose	every 24 hours

Meropenem is cleared by haemodialysis; if continued treatment with Meronem is necessary, it is recommended that the unit dose (based on the type and severity of infection) is administered at the completion of the haemodialysis procedure to restore therapeutically effective plasma concentrations.

There is no experience with the use of Meronem in patients under peritoneal dialysis.

Dosage in adults with hepatic insufficiency: No dosage adjustment is necessary in patients with hepatic insufficiency (see *Warnings and precautions*).

Elderly patients: No dosage adjustment is required for the elderly with normal renal function or creatinine clearance values above 50 ml/min.

Children: For children over 3 months and up to 12 years of age the recommended dose is 10 to 20 mg/kg every 8 hours depending on type and severity of infection, susceptibility of the pathogen and the condition of the patient. In children over 50 kg weight, adult dosage should be used.

For children aged 4 to 18 years with cystic fibrosis, doses ranging from 25 to 40 mg/kg every 8 hours have been used to treat acute exacerbations of chronic lower respiratory tract infections.

In meningitis the recommended dose is 40 mg/kg every 8 hours.

There is no experience in children with renal impairment.

Method of administration: Meronem IV can be given as an intravenous bolus injection over approximately 5 minutes or by intravenous infusion over approximately 15 to 30 minutes using the specific available presentations.

Meronem IV to be used for bolus intravenous injection should be constituted with sterile Water for Injections (5 ml per 250 mg meropenem). This provides an approximate concentration of 50 mg/ml. Constituted solutions are clear, and colourless or pale yellow.

Meronem IV for intravenous infusion may be constituted with compatible infusion fluids (50 to 200 ml) (see *Incompatibilities* and *Special precautions for storage* sections).

Contra-indications: Meronem is contra-indicated in patients who have demonstrated hypersensitivity to this product.

Special warnings and special precautions for use: There is some clinical and laboratory evidence of partial cross-allergenicity between other carbapenems and beta-lactam antibiotics, penicillins and cephalosporins. As with all beta-lactam antibiotics, rare hypersensitivity reactions have been reported (see *Undesirable Effects*). Before initiating therapy with meropenem, careful inquiry should be made concerning previous hypersensitivity reactions to beta-lactam antibiotics. Meronem should be used with caution in patients with such a history. If an allergic reaction to meropenem occurs, the drug should be discontinued and appropriate measures taken.

Use of Meronem in patients with hepatic disease should be made with careful monitoring of transaminase and bilirubin levels.

As with other antibiotics, overgrowth of non-susceptible organisms may occur and, therefore, continuous monitoring of each patient is necessary.

Use in infections caused by methicillin resistant staphylococci is not recommended.

Rarely, pseudomembranous colitis has been reported on Meronem as with practically all antibiotics and may vary in severity from slight to life-threatening. Therefore, antibiotics should be prescribed with care for individuals with a history of gastro-intestinal complaints, particularly colitis.

It is important to consider the diagnosis of pseudomembranous colitis in the case of patients who develop diarrhoea in association with the use of Meronem. Although studies indicate that a toxin produced by *Clostridium difficile* is one of the main causes of antibiotic-associated colitis, other causes should be considered.

The co-administration of Meronem with potentially nephrotoxic drugs should be considered with caution. For dosage see *Posology and method of administration* section.

Paediatric use: Efficacy and tolerability in infants under 3 months old have not been established; therefore, Meronem is not recommended for use below this age. There is no experience in children with altered hepatic or renal function.

Keep all medicines away from children.

Interactions with other medicaments and other forms of interaction: Probenecid competes with meropenem for active tubular secretion and thus inhibits the renal excretion, with the effect of increasing the elimination half-life and plasma concentration of meropenem. As the potency and duration of action of Meronem dosed without probenecid are adequate, the co-administration of probenecid with Meronem is not recommended.

The potential effect of Meronem on the protein binding of other drugs or metabolism has not been studied. The protein binding of Meronem is low (approximately 2%) and, therefore, no interactions with other compounds based on displacement from plasma proteins would be expected.

Meronem may reduce serum valproic acid levels. Subtherapeutic levels may be reached in some patients.

Meronem has been administered concomitantly with other medications without adverse pharmacological interactions. However, no other specific data regarding potential drug interactions is available (apart from probenecid as mentioned above).

Pregnancy and lactation:

Pregnancy: The safety of Meronem in human pregnancy has not been evaluated. Animal studies have not shown any adverse effect on the developing foetus. The only adverse effect observed in animal reproductive studies was an increased incidence of abortions in monkeys at 13 times the expected exposure in man. Meronem should not be used in pregnancy unless the potential benefit justifies the potential risk to the foetus. In every case, it should be used under the direct supervision of the physician.

Lactation: Meropenem is detectable at very low concentrations in animal breast milk. Meronem should not be used in breast-feeding women unless the potential benefit justifies the potential risk to the baby.

Effects on ability to drive and use machines: No data is available, but it is not anticipated that Meronem will affect the ability to drive and use machines.

Undesirable effects: Serious adverse events are rare. During clinical trials the following adverse events have been reported:

Local intravenous injection site reactions: inflammation, thrombophlebitis, pain at the site of injection.

Systemic allergic reactions: rarely, systemic allergic reactions (hypersensitivity) may occur following administration of meropenem. These reactions may include angioedema and manifestations of anaphylaxis;

Skin reactions: rash, pruritus, urticaria. Rarely, severe skin reactions such as erythema multiforme, Stevens-Johnson Syndrome and toxic epidermal necrolysis have been observed;

Gastro-intestinal: abdominal pain, nausea, vomiting, diarrhoea. Pseudomembranous colitis has been reported.

Blood: Reversible thrombocythaemia, eosinophilia, thrombocytopenia, leucopenia and neutropenia (including very rare cases of agranulocytosis). A positive direct or indirect Coombs test may develop in some subjects; there have been reports of reduction in partial thromboplastin time.

Liver function: Increases in serum concentrations of bilirubin, transaminases, alkaline phosphatase and lactic dehydrogenase alone or in combination have been reported.

Central nervous system: headache, paraesthesiae. Convulsions have been reported but a causal link with Meronem has not been established.

Other: Oral and vaginal candidosis.

Overdosage: Accidental overdosage could occur during therapy, particularly in patients with renal impairment. Treatment of overdosage should be symptomatic. In normal individuals rapid renal elimination will occur; in subjects with renal impairment haemodialysis will remove meropenem and its metabolite.

Pharmacological properties

Pharmacodynamic properties: Meropenem is a carbapenem antibiotic for parenteral use, that is relatively stable to human dehydropeptidase-1 (DHP-1) and therefore, does not require the addition of an inhibitor of DHP-1.

Meropenem exerts its bactericidal action by interfering with vital bacterial cell wall synthesis. The ease with which it penetrates bacterial cell walls, its high level of stability to all serine beta-lactamases and its marked affinity for the Penicillin Binding Proteins (PBPs) explain the potent bactericidal action of meropenem against a broad spectrum of aerobic and anaerobic bacteria. Minimum bactericidal concentrations (MBC) are commonly the same as the minimum inhibitory concentrations (MIC). For 76% of the bacteria tested, the MBC:MIC ratios were 2 or less.

Meropenem is stable in susceptibility tests and these tests can be performed using normal routine methods. *In vitro* tests show that meropenem acts synergistically with various antibiotics. It has been demonstrated both *in vitro* and *in vivo* that meropenem has a post-antibiotic effect.

A single set of meropenem susceptibility criteria are recommended based on pharmacokinetics and correlation of clinical and microbiological outcomes with zone diameter and minimum inhibitory concentrations (MIC) of the infecting organisms.

CATEGORISATION	*METHOD OF ASSESSMENT*	
	Zone Diameter (mm)	MIC breakpoints (mg/L)
Susceptible	≥14	≤4
Intermediate	12 to 13	8
Resistant	≤11	≥16

The *in vitro* antibacterial spectrum of meropenem includes the majority of clinically significant Gram-positive and Gram-negative, aerobic and anaerobic strains of bacteria, as shown below:

Gram-positive aerobes: Bacillus spp., *Corynebacterium diphtheriae, Enterococcus liquifaciens, Enterococcus avium, Listeria monocytogenes,* Lactobacillus spp., *Nocardia asteroides, Staphylococcus aureus* (penicillinase negative and positive), Staphylococci-coagulase-negative; including, *Staphylococcus saprophyticus, Staphylococcus capitis, Staphylococcus cohnii, Staphylococcus xylosus, Staphylococcus warneri, Staphylococcus hominis, Staphylococcus simulans, Staphylococcus intermedius, Staphylococcus sciuri, Staphylococcus lugdunensis, Streptococcus pneumoniae* (penicillin susceptible and resistant), *Streptococcus agalactiae, Streptococcus pyogenes, Streptococcus equi, Streptococcus bovis, Streptococcus mitis, Streptococcus mitior, Streptococcus milleri, Streptococcus sanguis, Streptococcus viridans, Streptococcus salivarius, Streptococcus morbillorum,* Streptococcus Group G, Streptococcus Group F, *Rhodococcus equi.*

Gram-negative aerobes: *Achromobacter xylosoxidans, Acinetobacter anitratus, Acinetobacter lwoffii, Acinetobacter baumannii, Aeromonas hydrophila, Aeromonas sorbria, Aeromonas caviae, Alcaligenes faecalis, Bordatella bronchiseptica, Brucella melitensis, Campylobacter coli, Campylobacter jejuni, Citrobacter freundii, Citrobacter diversus, Citrobacter koseri, Citrobacter amalonaticus, Enterobacter aerogenes, Enterobacter (Pantoea) agglomerans, Enterobacter cloacae, Enterobacter sakazakii, Escherichia coli, Escherichia hermannii, Gardnerella vaginalis, Haemophilus influenzae* (including Beta-lactamase positive and ampicillin resistant strains), *Haemophilus parainfluenzae, Haemophilus ducreyi, Helicobacter pylori, Neisseria meningitidis, Neisseria gonorrhoeae* (including Beta-lactamase positive, penicillin resistant and spectinomycin resistant strains), *Hafnia alvei, Klebsiella pneumoniae, Klebsiella aerogenes, Klebsiella ozaenae, Klebsiella oxytoca, Moraxella (Branhamella) catarrhalis, Morganella morganii, Proteus mirabilis, Proteus vulgaris, Proteus penneri, Providencia rettgeri, Providencia stuartii, Providencia alcalifaciens, Pasteurella multocida, Plesiomonas shigelloides, Pseudomonas aeruginosa, Pseudomonas putida, Pseudomonas alcaligenes, Burkholderia (Pseudomonas) cepacia, Pseudomonas fluorescens, Pseudomonas stutzeri, Pseudomonas pseudomallei, Pseudomonas acidovorans, Salmonella spp. including Salmonella enteritidis/typhi, Serratia marcescens, Serratia liquefaciens, Serratia rubidaea, Shigella sonnei, Shigella flexneri, Shigella boydii, Shigella dysenteriae, Vibrio cholerae, Vibrio parahaemolyticus, Vibrio vulnificus, Yersinia enterocolitica.*

Anaerobic bacteria: *Actinomyces odontolyticus, Actinomyces meyeri, Bacteroides-Prevotella-Porphyromonas spp., Bacteroides fragilis, Bacteroides vulgatus, Bacteroides variabilis, Bacteroides pneumosintes, Bacteroides coagulans, Bacteroides uniformis, Bacteroides distasonis, Bacteroides ovatus, Bacteroides thetaiotaomicron, Bacteroides eggerthii, Bacteroides capsillosis, Prevotella buccalis, Prevotella corporis, Bacteroides gracilis, Prevotella melaninogenica, Prevotella intermedia, Prevotella bivia, Prevotella splanchnicus, Prevotella oralis, Prevotella disiens, Prevotella rumenicola, Bacteroides ureolyticus, Prevotella oris, Prevotella buccae, Prevotella denticola, Bacteroides levii, Porphyromonas asaccharolytica,* Bifidobacterium spp., *Bilophila wadsworthia, Clostridium perfringens, Clostridium bifermentans, Clostridium ramosum, Clostridium sporogenes, Clostridium cadaveris, Clostridium sordellii, Clostridium butyricum, Clostridium clostridiiformis, Clostridium innocuum, Clostridium subterminale, Clostridium tertium, Eubacterium lentum, Eubacterium aerofaciens, Fusobacterium mortiferum, Fusobacterium necrophorum, Fusobacterium nucleatum, Fusobacterium varium, Mobiluncus curtisii, Mobiluncus mulieris, Peptostreptococcus anaerobius, Peptostreptococcus micros, Peptostreptococcus saccharolyticus, Peptococcus saccharolyticus, Peptostreptococcus asaccharolyticus, Peptostreptococcus magnus, Peptostreptococcus prevotii, Propionibacterium acnes, Propionibacterium avidium, Propionibacterium granulosum.*

Stenotrophomonas maltophilia, Enterococcus faecium and methicillin-resistant staphylococci have been found to be resistant to meropenem.

Pharmacokinetic properties: A 30 minute intravenous infusion of a single dose of Meronem in healthy volunteers results in peak plasma levels of approximately 11 microgram/ml for the 250 mg dose, 23 microgram/ml for the 500 mg dose and 49 microgram/ml for the 1 g dose.

However, there is no absolute pharmacokinetic proportionality with the administered dose both as regards Cmax and AUC. Furthermore, a reduction in plasma clearance from 287 to 205 ml/min for the range of dosage 250 mg to 2 g has been observed.

A 5 minute intravenous bolus injection of Meronem in healthy volunteers results in peak plasma levels of approximately 52 microgram/ml for the 500 mg dose and 112 microgram/ml for the 1 g dose.

Intravenous infusions of 1 g over 2 minutes, 3 minutes and 5 minutes were compared in a three-way crossover trial. These durations of infusion resulted in peak plasma levels of 110, 91 and 94 microgram/ml, respectively.

After an IV dose of 500 mg, plasma levels of meropenem decline to values of 1 microgram/ml or less, 6 hours after administration.

When multiple doses are administered at 8 hourly intervals to subjects with normal renal function, accumulation of meropenem does not occur.

In subjects with normal renal function, meropenem's elimination half-life is approximately 1 hour.

Plasma protein binding of meropenem is approximately 2%.

Approximately 70% of the administered dose is recovered as unchanged meropenem in the urine over 12 hours, after which little further urinary excretion is detectable. Urinary concentrations of meropenem in excess of 10 microgram/ml are maintained for up to 5 hours after the administration of a 500 mg dose. No accumulation of meropenem in plasma or urine was observed with regimens using 500 mg administered every 8 hours or 1 g administered every 6 hours in volunteers with normal renal function.

The only metabolite of meropenem is microbiologically inactive.

Meropenem penetrates well into most body fluids and tissues including cerebrospinal fluid of patients with bacterial meningitis, achieving concentrations in excess of those required to inhibit most bacteria.

Studies in children have shown that the pharmacokinetics of Meronem in children are similar to those in adults. The elimination half-life for meropenem was approximately 1.5 to 2.3 hours in children under the age of 2 years and the pharmacokinetics are linear over the dose range of 10 to 40 mg/kg.

Pharmacokinetic studies in patients with renal insufficiency have shown the plasma clearance of meropenem correlates with creatinine clearance. Dosage adjustments are necessary in subjects with renal impairment.

Pharmacokinetic studies in the elderly have shown a reduction in plasma clearance of meropenem which correlated with age-associated reduction in creatinine clearance.

Pharmacokinetic studies in patients with liver disease have shown no effects of liver disease on the pharmacokinetics of meropenem.

Pre-clinical safety data: Animal studies indicate that meropenem is well tolerated in the kidney. In animal studies meropenem has shown nephrotoxic effects, only at high dose levels (500 mg/kg).

Effects on the CNS; convulsions in rats and vomiting in dogs, were seen only at high doses (>2000 mg/kg).

For an IV dose the LD_{50} in rodents is greater than 2000 mg/kg. In repeat dose studies (up to 6 months) only minor effects were seen including a small decrease in red cell parameters and an increase in liver weight in dogs treated with doses of 500 mg/kg.

There was no evidence of mutagenic potential in the 5 tests conducted and no evidence of reproductive and teratogenic toxicity in studies at the highest possible doses in rats and monkeys; the no effect dose level of a (small) reduction in F_1 body weight in rat was 120 mg/kg. There was an increased incidence of abortions at 500 mg/kg in a preliminary study in monkeys.

There was no evidence of increased sensitivity to meropenem in juveniles compared to adult animals. The intravenous formulation was well tolerated in animal studies.

The sole metabolite of meropenem had a similar profile of toxicity in animal studies.

Pharmaceutical particulars

List of excipients: Meronem for i.v. injection and infusion includes the excipient anhydrous sodium carbonate.

Incompatibilities: Meronem should not be mixed with or added to other drugs.

Meronem is compatible with the following infusion fluids:

0.9% Sodium Chloride solution
5% or 10% Glucose solution
5% Glucose solution with 0.02% Sodium Bicarbonate
0.9% Sodium Chloride and 5% Glucose solution
5% Glucose with 0.225% Sodium Chloride solution
5% Glucose with 0.15% Potassium Chloride solution
Mannitol 2.5% or 10% solution.

For reconstitution instructions using the Meronem Infusion Kit see leaflet enclosed in the carton.

Shelf life: Meronem has a shelf life of 3 years.

Diluent	*Hours stable up to 25°C*	*4°C*
Solution (1 to 20 mg/ml) prepared with:		
0.9% sodium chloride	8	48
5% glucose	3	14
5% glucose and 0.225% sodium chloride	3	14
5% glucose and 0.9% sodium chloride	3	14
5% glucose and 0.15% potassium chloride	3	14
2.5% or 10% mannitol intravenous infusion	3	14
10% glucose	2	8
5% glucose and 0.02% sodium bicarbonate intravenous infusion	2	8

Solutions of Meronem should not be frozen.

Special precautions for storage: Store below 25°C.

It is recommended to use freshly prepared solutions of Meronem for i.v. injection and infusion. Reconstituted product should be used immediately and must be stored for no longer than 24 hours under refrigeration, only if necessary.

Nature and contents of container: Type 1 glass vials closed with halobutilic rubber stopper and sealed with an aluminium cap.

Packs for intravenous administration: Pack of 10 vials containing 250 mg, 500 mg or 1 g meropenem.

Infusion kits containing one vial of either 500 mg or 1 g meropenem together with a 100 ml bag of 0.9% w/v sodium chloride intravenous infusion.

Instructions for use/handling: Refer to *Posology and method of administration* section above. Standard aseptic technique should be employed during constitution. Shake constituted solution before use. All vials are for single use only.

Marketing authorisation numbers

250 mg	12619/0097
500 mg	12619/0098
1 g	12619/0099

Date of approval/revision of SPC July 1998.

Legal category POM.

MYSOLINE ORAL SUSPENSION

Qualitative and quantitative composition Oral suspension containing Primidone PhEur 250 mg per 5 ml.

Pharmaceutical form Oral suspension

Clinical particulars

Therapeutic indications:

Route of administration: oral.

Mysoline is indicated in the management of grand mal and psychomotor (temporal lobe) epilepsy. It is also of value in the management of focal or Jacksonian seizures, myoclonic jerks and akinetic attacks.

Mysoline is also indicated in the management of essential tremor.

Posology and method of administration: Epilepsy: Treatment must always be planned on an individual basis. In many patients it will be possible to use Mysoline alone, but in some, Mysoline will need to be combined with other anticonvulsants or with supporting therapy.

Mysoline is usually given twice daily. Begin with 125 mg once daily late in the evening. Every 3 days increase the daily dosage by 125 mg until the patient is receiving 500 mg daily. Thereafter, every 3 days increase the daily dosage by 250 mg in adults or 125 mg in children under 9 years–until control is obtained or the maximum tolerated dosage is being given. This may be as much as 1.5 g a day in adults; 1 g a day in children.

Average daily maintenance doses:

	5 ml measures of suspension (250 mg/ 5 ml)	*Milligrams*
Adults and children over 9 years	3 to 6	750 to 1500
Children 6 to 9 years	3 to 4	750 to 1000
Children 2 to 5 years	2 to 3	500 to 750
Children up to 2 years	1 to 2	250 to 500

The total daily dose is usually best divided and given in two equal amounts, one in the morning and the other in the evening. In certain patients, it may be considered advisable to give a larger dose when the seizures are more frequent. For instance: 1) if the attacks are nocturnal then all or most of the day's dose may be given in the evening; 2) if the attacks are associated with some particular event such as menstruation, a slight increase in the appropriate dose is often beneficial.

Elderly patients: It is advisable to monitor elderly patients with reduced renal function who are receiving primidone.

Patients on other anticonvulsants: Where a patient's attacks are not sufficiently well controlled with other anticonvulsants, or disturbing side effects have arisen, Mysoline may be used to augment or replace existing treatment. First add Mysoline to the current anticonvulsant treatment by the method of gradual introduction described previously. When a worthwhile effect has been achieved and the amount of Mysoline being given has been built up to at least half the estimated requirement, withdrawal of the previous treatment can then be attempted. This should be done gradually over a period of 2 weeks, during which time it may be necessary to increase the Mysoline dosage to maintain control.

Withdrawal of previous treatment should not be too rapid or status epilepticus may occur. Where phenobarbitone formed the major part of the previous treatment, however, both its withdrawal and Mysoline substitution should be made earlier, so as to prevent excessive drowsiness from interfering with accurate assessment of the optimum dosage of Mysoline.

Essential tremor: Initially a dose of 50 mg daily should be introduced using Mysoline Suspension. The daily dose should be increased gradually over a 2 to 3 week period until remission of symptoms or the highest dose tolerated up to a maximum of 750 mg daily.

Patients with essential tremor who have not previously been exposed to anticonvulsants, or other drugs known to induce increased hepatic enzyme activity, may experience acute symptoms of tolerance to Mysoline, frequently characterised by vertigo, unsteadiness and nausea. It is, therefore, essential to start such patients at a low dosage (initially 50 mg daily) increasing very slowly up to the maximum tolerated dose or that which produces remission of tremor (up to 750 mg daily).

Contra-indications: Patients who exhibit hypersensitivity or an allergic reaction to primidone should not receive the drug. Primidone should not be administered to patients with acute intermittent porphyria.

Special warnings and special precautions for use: Mysoline should be given with caution and may be required in reduced dosage in children, the elderly, debilitated patients or those with impaired renal, hepatic or respiratory function.

Primidone is a potent CNS depressant and is partially metabolised to phenobarbitone. After prolonged administration there is a potential for tolerance, dependence and a withdrawal reaction on abrupt cessation of treatment.

Exceptionally, as with phenytoin and phenobarbitone, megaloblastic anaemia may develop requiring discontinuation of primidone. This condition may respond to treatment with folic acid and/or Vitamin B_{12}. There have been isolated reports of other blood dyscrasias.

Interactions with other medicaments and other forms of interaction: Both primidone and its major metabolite phenobarbitone induce liver enzyme activity. This may lead to altered pharmacokinetics in concomitantly administered drugs including other anticonvulsants such as phenytoin and coumarin anticoagulants. Blood levels of both Mysoline and any additional anticonvulsant agent may be altered by concomitant administration.

Breakthrough bleeding and failure of contraceptive therapy have been noted in patients taking anticonvulsant drugs and oral contraceptive steroids. This is usually assumed to be due to induction of liver enzymes by the anticonvulsant with accelerated breakdown of the hormones.

The effects of other CNS depressants such as alcohol and barbiturates may be enhanced by the administration of Mysoline.

Pregnancy and lactation:

Pregnancy: There is some evidence of a higher than average incidence of congenital abnormalities in infants born of epileptic mothers. The factors influencing this are unknown, but the possibility that anticonvulsant therapy may be involved and the very slight risk of an abnormal foetus must be weighed against the risk of withholding treatment during pregnancy.

Withdrawal symptoms may occur in the newly born whose mothers have received Mysoline during late pregnancy.

Long-term anticonvulsant therapy can be associated with decreased serum folate levels. As folic acid requirements are also increased during pregnancy, regular screening of patients at risk is advised, and treatment with folic acid and Vitamin B_{12}, although controversial, should be considered.

Anticonvulsant therapy in pregnancy has occasionally been associated with coagulation disorders in the neonates. For this reason pregnant patients should be given Vitamin K_1 through the last month of pregnancy up to the time of delivery. In the absence of such pretreatment, 10 mg Vitamin K_1 may be given to the mother at the time of delivery and 1 mg should be given immediately to the neonate at risk.

Lactation: During breast feeding the baby should be monitored for sedation.

Effects on ability to drive and use machines: As with most other anticonvulsants, patients who drive vehicles or operate machinery should be made aware of the possibility of impaired reaction time.

Undesirable effects: If side effects do appear they are generally confined to the early stages of treatment when patients frequently feel drowsy and listless.

Visual disturbances, nausea, headache, dizziness, vomiting, nystagmus and ataxia have been reported but are usually transient even when pronounced. On occasions an idiosyncratic reaction may occur which involves these symptoms in an acute and severe form necessitating withdrawal of treatment.

Dermatological reactions (including severe skin eruptions) and systemic conditions such as systemic lupus erythematosus (rare) have been reported. Occasional cases of arthralgia have been reported. Rarely personality changes, which may include psychotic reactions, have been reported.

As with phenobarbitone, in rare cases Dupuytren's contracture has been reported in patients administered Mysoline.

Overdose: Primidone is metabolised extensively to phenobarbitone and overdosage leads to varying degrees of CNS depression which, depending on the dose ingested, may include ataxia, loss of consciousness, respiratory depression and coma. Treatment should include aspiration of stomach contents and general supportive measures. There is no specific antidote.

Pharmacological Properties

Pharmacodynamic properties: The activity of Mysoline is due to the anticonvulsant properties of three active moieties, namely primidone itself and its two major metabolites phenobarbitone and phenylethylmalonamide. The relative contribution of these three moieties to the clinical anticonvulsant effect has not been firmly established. Although the precise mode of action of Mysoline is unknown, in common with other anticonvulsants, effects on the neuronal membrane particularly with respect to alteration of ionic fluxes are likely to play a fundamental role.

Mysoline, as with other anticonvulsants, can induce liver enzymes, and although there is insufficient evidence to suggest a causal relationship, there is a theoretical risk of hepatic damage.

Mysoline may also affect vitamin D metabolism, which may predispose to the development of bone disease.

Pharmacokinetic properties: Mysoline is absorbed rapidly from the gastrointestinal tract, peak plasma levels being attained approximately 3 hours after ingestion. Primidone is well distributed in all organs and tissues: it crosses the blood-brain and placental barriers and is excreted in breast milk. The pharmacokinetics of primidone are complex because of biotransformation into two metabolites, phenobarbitone and phenylethylmalonamide, that have anticonvulsant activity and complex pharmacokinetic properties. Primidone has a plasma half-life of approximately 10 hours which is considerably shorter than those of its principal metabolites. Primidone and phenylethylmalonamide are bound to plasma proteins to only a small extent, whereas approximately half of phenobarbitone is bound. Approximately 40% of the drug is excreted unchanged in urine.

Pre-clinical safety data: Primidone is a drug on which extensive clinical experience has been obtained. All relevant information for the prescriber is provided elsewhere in the Summary of Product Characteristics.

Pharmaceutical particulars

List of excipients: Aluminium magnesium silicate; Cetostearyl alcohol/ethyleneoxide condensate; Methyl hydroxybenzoate; Propyl hydroxybenzoate; Purified water; Sodium carboxymethylcellulose; Sucrose; Vanilla flavour

Incompatibilities: None known

Shelf life: 60 months

Special precautions for storage: Store below 25°C.

Nature and contents of containers: Glass bottle (250 ml)

Instructions for use/handling: To be taken as directed by the prescriber.

Marketing authorisation number 12619/0045.

Date of approval/revision of SPC October 1998

Legal category POM

MYSOLINE TABLETS

Qualitative and quantitative composition Oral tablets containing Primidone PhEur 250 mg.

Pharmaceutical form White uncoated oral tablets.

Clinical particulars

Therapeutic indications: Mysoline is indicated in the management of grand mal and psychomotor (temporal lobe) epilepsy. It is also of value in the management of focal or Jacksonian seizures, myoclonic jerks and akinetic attacks.

Management of essential tremor.

Posology and method of administration: Epilepsy: Treatment must always be planned on an individual basis. In many patients it will be possible to use Mysoline alone, but in some, Mysoline will need to be combined with other anticonvulsants or with supporting therapy.

Mysoline is usually given twice daily. Begin with 125 mg once daily late in the evening. Every 3 days increase the daily dosage by 125 mg until the patient is receiving 500 mg daily. Thereafter, every 3 days increase the daily dosage by 250 mg in adults or 125 mg in children under 9 years–until control is obtained or the maximum tolerated dosage is being given. This may be as much as 1.5 g a day in adults; 1 g a day in children.

Average daily maintenance doses:

	Tablets (250 mg) or 5 ml measures of suspension (250 mg/ 5 ml)	*Milligrams*
Adults and children over 9 years	3 to 6	750 to 1500
Children 6 to 9 years	3 to 4	750 to 1000
Children 2 to 5 years	2 to 3	500 to 750
Children up to 2 years	1 to 2	250 to 500

The total daily dose is usually best divided and given in two equal amounts, one in the morning and the other in the evening. In certain patients, it may be considered advisable to give a larger dose when the seizures are more frequent. For instance: 1) if the attacks are nocturnal then all or most of the day's dose may be given in the evening; 2) if the attacks are associated with some particular event such as menstruation, a slight increase in the appropriate dose is often beneficial.

Elderly patients: It is advisable to monitor elderly patients with reduced renal function who are receiving primidone.

Patients on other anticonvulsants: Where a patient's attacks are not sufficiently well controlled with other anticonvulsants, or disturbing side effects have arisen, Mysoline may be used to augment or replace existing treatment. First add Mysoline to the current anticonvulsant treatment by the method of gradual introduction described previously. When a worthwhile effect has been achieved and the amount of Mysoline being given has been built up to at least half the estimated requirement, withdrawal of the previous treatment can then be attempted. This should be done gradually over a period of 2 weeks, during which time it may be necessary to increase the Mysoline dosage to maintain control.

Withdrawal of previous treatment should not be too rapid or status epilepticus may occur. Where phenobarbitone formed the major part of the previous treatment, however, both its withdrawal and Mysoline substitution should be made earlier, so as to prevent excessive drowsiness from interfering with accurate assessment of the optimum dosage of Mysoline.

Essential tremor: Initially a dose of 50 mg daily should be introduced using Mysoline Suspension. The daily dose should be increased gradually over a 2 to 3 week period until remission of symptoms or the highest dose tolerated up to a maximum of 750 mg daily.

Patients with essential tremor who have not previously been exposed to anticonvulsants, or other drugs known to induce increased hepatic enzyme activity, may experience acute symptoms of tolerance to Mysoline, frequently characterised by vertigo, unsteadiness and nausea. It is, therefore, essential to start such patients at a low dosage (initially 50 mg daily) increasing very slowly up to the maximum tolerated dose or that which produces remission of tremor (up to 750 mg daily).

Contra-indications: Patients who exhibit hypersensitivity or an allergic reaction to primidone should not receive the drug. Primidone should not be administered to patients with acute intermittent porphyria.

Special warnings and special precautions for use: Mysoline should be given with caution and may be required in reduced dosage in children, the elderly, debilitated patients or those with impaired renal, hepatic or respiratory function.

Primidone is a potent CNS depressant and is partially metabolised to phenobarbitone. After prolonged administration there is a potential for tolerance, dependence and a withdrawal reaction on abrupt cessation of treatment.

Exceptionally, as with phenytoin and phenobarbitone, megaloblastic anaemia may develop requiring discontinuation of primidone. This condition may respond to treatment with folic acid and/or vitamin B_{12}. There have been isolated reports of other blood dyscrasias.

Interactions with other medicaments and other forms of interaction: Both primidone and its major metabolite phenobarbitone induce liver enzyme activity. This may lead to altered pharmacokinetics in concomitantly administered drugs including other anticonvulsants such as phenytoin and coumarin anticoagulants. Blood levels of both Mysoline and any additional anticonvulsant agent may be altered by concomitant administration.

Breakthrough bleeding and failure of contraceptive therapy have been noted in patients taking anticonvulsant drugs and oral contraceptive steroids. This is usually assumed to be due to induction of liver enzymes by the anticonvulsant with accelerated breakdown of the hormones.

The effects of other CNS depressants such as alcohol and barbiturates may be enhanced by the administration of Mysoline.

Pregnancy and lactation:

Pregnancy: There is some evidence of a higher than average incidence of congenital abnormalities in infants born of epileptic mothers. The factors influencing this are unknown, but the possibility that anticonvulsant therapy may be involved and the very slight risk of an abnormal foetus must be weighed against the risk of withholding treatment during pregnancy.

Withdrawal symptoms may occur in the newly born whose mothers have received Mysoline during late pregnancy.

Long-term anticonvulsant therapy can be associated with decreased serum folate levels. As folic acid requirements are also increased during pregnancy, regular screening of patients at risk is advised, and treatment with folic acid and Vitamin B_{12}, although controversial, should be considered.

Anticonvulsant therapy in pregnancy has occasionally been associated with coagulation disorders in the neonates. For this reason pregnant patients should be given Vitamin K_1 through the last month of pregnancy up to the time of delivery. In the absence of such pretreatment, 10 mg Vitamin K_1 may be given to the mother at the time of delivery and 1 mg should be given immediately to the neonate at risk.

Lactation: During breast feeding the baby should be monitored for sedation.

Effects on ability to drive and use machines: As with most other anticonvulsants, patients who drive vehicles or operate machinery should be made aware of the possibility of impaired reaction time.

Undesirable effects: If side effects do appear they are generally confined to the early stages of treatment when patients frequently feel drowsy and listless.

Visual disturbances, nausea, headache, dizziness, vomiting, nystagmus and ataxia have been reported but are usually transient even when pronounced. On occasions an idiosyncratic reaction may occur which involves these symptoms in an acute and severe form necessitating withdrawal of treatment.

Dermatological reactions (including severe skin eruptions) and systemic conditions such as systemic lupus erythematosus (rare) have been reported. Occasional cases of arthralgia have been reported. Rarely personality changes, which may include psychotic reactions, have been reported. As with phenobarbitone, in rare cases Dupuytren's contracture has been reported in patients administered Mysoline.

Overdose: Primidone is metabolised extensively to phenobarbitone and overdosage leads to varying degrees of CNS depression which, depending on the dose ingested, may include ataxia, loss of consciousness, respiratory depression and coma. Treatment should include aspiration of stomach contents and general supportive measures. There is no specific antidote.

Pharmacological Properties

Pharmacodynamic properties: The activity of Mysoline is due to the anticonvulsant properties of three active moieties, namely primidone itself and its two major metabolites phenobarbitone and phenylethylmalonamide. The relative contribution of these three moieties to the clinical anticonvulsant effect has not been firmly established. Although the precise mode of action of Mysoline is unknown, in common with other anticonvulsants, effects on the neuronal membrane particularly with respect to alteration of ionic fluxes are likely to play a fundamental role.

Mysoline, as with other anticonvulsants, can induce liver enzymes, and although there is insufficient evidence to suggest a causal relationship, there is a theoretical risk of hepatic damage.

Mysoline may also affect vitamin D metabolism,

which may predispose to the development of bone disease.

Pharmacokinetic properties: Mysoline is absorbed rapidly from the gastrointestinal tract, peak plasma levels being attained approximately 3 hours after ingestion. Primidone is well distributed in all organs and tissues: it crosses the blood-brain and placental barriers and is excreted in breast milk. The pharmacokinetics of primidone are complex because of biotransformation into two metabolites, phenobarbitone and phenylethylmalonamide, that have anticonvulsant activity and complex pharmacokinetic properties. Primidone has a plasma half-life of approximately 10 hours which is considerably shorter than those of its principal metabolites. Primidone and phenylethylmalonamide are bound to plasma proteins to only a small extent, whereas approximately half of phenobarbitone is bound. Approximately 40% of the drug is excreted unchanged in urine.

Pre-clinical safety data: Primidone is a drug on which extensive clinical experience has been obtained. All relevant information for the prescriber is provided elsewhere in the Summary of Product Characteristics.

Pharmaceutical particulars
List of excipients: Calcium carboxymethylcellulose USNF; Gelatin PhEur; Magnesium stearate PhEur; Povidone PhEur; Purified water PhEur; Stearic acid BPC.

Incompatibilities: None known

Shelf life: 5 years

Special precautions for storage: Store below 25°C.

Nature and contents of containers: HDPE bottle (100 tablets).

Instructions for use/handling: To be taken as directed by the prescriber.

Marketing authorisation number 12619/0046

Date of approval/revision of SPC August 1998

Legal category POM

NOLVADEX*
NOLVADEX*-D TABLETS
NOLVADEX*-FORTE TABLETS

Presentation *Nolvadex:* White, round, bi-convex tablets, each containing Tamoxifen Citrate PhEur equivalent to 10 mg of tamoxifen, marked with Nolvadex 10 on one face.

Nolvadex-D: White, octagonal, bi-convex tablets, each containing Tamoxifen Citrate PhEur equivalent to 20 mg of tamoxifen, marked with Nolvadex-D on one face.

Nolvadex-Forte: White, elongated octagonal tablets, each containing Tamoxifen Citrate PhEur equivalent to 40 mg of tamoxifen, marked with Nolvadex Forte on one face and bisected on the other side.

Inactive ingredients are croscarmellose sodium, gelatin, lactose, macrogol, magnesium stearate, maize starch, methylhydroxypropylcellulose, and titanium dioxide.

Uses At the recommended dosage Nolvadex has anti-oestrogenic properties and competes with oestrogen for binding sites in target organs. It does not have androgenic properties.

Nolvadex is indicated for:

1. The treatment of breast cancer. The proportion of patients with breast cancer who respond to Nolvadex is similar to that seen with oestrogens or androgens. However, because Nolvadex produces fewer serious undesirable events it is more acceptable to the patient.
2. The treatment of anovulatory infertility.

Mode of action: Nolvadex (tamoxifen) is a non-steroidal, triphenylethylene-based drug which displays a complex spectrum of oestrogen antagonist and oestrogen agonist-like pharmacological effects in different tissues. In breast cancer patients, at the tumour level, tamoxifen acts primarily as an antioestrogen, preventing oestrogen binding to the oestrogen receptor. However, clinical studies have shown some benefit in oestrogen receptor negative tumours which may indicate other mechanisms of action. In the clinical situation, it is recognised that tamoxifen leads to reductions in levels of blood total cholesterol and low density lipoproteins in postmenopausal women of the order of 10 to 20%. Tamoxifen does not adversely affect bone mineral density.

After oral administration, tamoxifen is absorbed rapidly with maximum serum concentrations attained within 4 to 7 hours. Steady state concentrations (about 300 ng/ml) are achieved after 4 weeks treatment with 40 mg daily. The drug is highly protein bound to serum albumin (>99%). Metabolism is by hydroxylation, demethylation and conjugation, giving rise to several metabolites which have a similar pharmacological profile to the parent compound and thus contribute to the therapeutic effect. Excretion occurs primarily via the faeces and an elimination half-life of approximately seven days has been calculated for the drug itself, whereas that for N-desmethyltamoxifen, the principal circulating metabolite, is 14 days.

Dosage and administration
1. *Breast cancer:* The recommended daily dose of tamoxifen is normally 20 mg. No additional benefit, in terms of delayed recurrence or improved survival in patients, has been demonstrated with higher doses. Substantive evidence supporting the use of treatment with 30–40 mg per day is not available, although these doses have been used in some patients with advanced disease.

Elderly patients: Similar dosage regimens of Nolvadex have been used in elderly patients with breast cancer and in some of these patients it has been used as sole therapy.

2. *Infertility:* Before commencing any course of treatment, whether initial or subsequent, the possibility of pregnancy must be excluded. In women who are menstruating regularly, but with anovular cycles, the initial course of treatment consists of 20 mg of Nolvadex daily on the second, third, fourth and fifth days of the menstrual cycle. If unsatisfactory basal temperature records or poor pre-ovulatory cervical mucus indicate that this initial course of treatment has been unsuccessful, further courses may be given during subsequent menstrual periods, increasing the dosage to 40 mg and then to 80 mg daily.

In women who are not menstruating regularly the initial course may begin on any day. If no signs of ovulation are demonstrable then a subsequent course of treatment may start 45 days later, with dosage increased as above. If a patient responds with menstruation, then the next course of treatment is commenced on the second day of the cycle.

Contra-indications, warnings, etc
Pregnancy: Nolvadex must not be administered during pregnancy. There have been a small number of reports of spontaneous abortions, birth defects and foetal deaths after women have taken Nolvadex, although no causal relationship has been established.

Reproductive toxicology studies in rats, rabbits and monkeys have shown no teratogenic potential.

In rodent models of foetal reproductive tract development, tamoxifen was associated with changes similar to those caused by oestradiol, ethynyloestradiol, clomiphene and diethylstilboestrol (DES). Although the clinical relevance of these changes is unknown, some of them, especially vaginal adenosis, are similar to those seen in young women who were exposed to DES *in utero* and who have a 1 in 1000 risk of developing clear-cell carcinoma of the vagina or cervix. Only a small number of pregnant women have been exposed to tamoxifen. Such exposure has not been reported to cause subsequent vaginal adenosis or clear-cell carcinoma of the vagina or cervix in young women exposed *in utero* to tamoxifen.

Women should be advised not to become pregnant whilst taking Nolvadex and should use barrier or other non-hormonal contraceptive methods if sexually active. Pre-menopausal patients must be carefully examined before treatment to exclude pregnancy. Women should be appraised of the potential risks to the foetus, should they become pregnant whilst taking Nolvadex or within 2 months of cessation of therapy.

Menstruation is suppressed in a proportion of premenopausal women receiving Nolvadex for the treatment of breast cancer.

Cystic ovarian swellings have occasionally been observed in premenopausal women receiving Nolvadex.

A small number of patients with bony metastases have developed hypercalcaemia on initiation of therapy.

When Nolvadex is used in combination with coumarin-type anticoagulants, a significant increase in anticoagulant effect may occur. Where such co-administration is initiated, careful monitoring of the patient is recommended.

When Nolvadex is used in combination with cytotoxic agents, there is increased risk of thromboembolic events occurring.

An increased incidence of endometrial changes, including hyperplasia, polyps and cancer, has been reported in association with Nolvadex treatment. The underlying mechanism is unknown but may be related to the oestrogen-like properties of 'Nolvadex'. Any patient receiving or having previously received 'Nolvadex' who reports abnormal gynaecological symptoms, especially vaginal bleeding, or who presents with menstrual irregularities, vaginal discharge and symptoms such as pelvic pain or pressure should be promptly investigated.

Tamoxifen was not mutagenic in a range of *in vitro* and *in vivo* mutagenicity tests. Tamoxifen was genotoxic in some *in vitro* tests and *in vivo* genotoxicity tests in rodents. Gonadal tumours in mice and liver tumours in rats receiving tamoxifen have been reported in long-term studies. The clinical relevance of these findings has not been established.

A number of second primary tumours, occurring at sites other than the endometrium and the opposite breast, have been reported in clinical trials, following the treatment of breast cancer patients with tamoxifen. No causal link has been established and the clinical significance of these observations remains unclear.

Lactation: It is not known if Nolvadex is excreted in human milk and therefore the drug is not recommended during lactation. The decision either to discontinue nursing or discontinue Nolvadex should take into account the importance of the drug to the mother.

Undesirable events: Side effects can be classified as either due to the pharmacological action of the drug, eg, hot flushes, vaginal bleeding, vaginal discharge, pruritus vulvae and tumour flare or as more general effects, eg, gastro-intestinal intolerance, light-headedness, skin rash (including isolated reports of erythema multiforme, Stevens-Johnson syndrome and Bullous Pemphigoid) and, occasionally, fluid retention and alopecia.

When undesirable events are severe it may be possible to control them by a simple reduction of dosage (within the recommended dose range) without loss of control of the disease. If undesirable events do not respond to this measure, it may be necessary to stop the treatment.

Falls in platelet count, usually only to 80,000 to 90,000 per cu mm but occasionally lower, have been reported in patients taking tamoxifen for breast cancer.

A number of cases of visual disturbance including corneal changes, cataracts and retinopathy, have been described in patients receiving Nolvadex.

Uterine fibroids and endometrial changes including hyperplasia and polyps have been reported.

Leucopenia has been observed following the administration of Nolvadex, sometimes in association with anaemia and/or thrombocytopenia. Neutropenia has been reported on rare occasions; this can sometimes be severe.

There have been infrequent reports of venous thromboembolic events occurring during Nolvadex therapy. There is evidence of a small increased risk of these events during Nolvadex therapy, especially when used in combination with cytotoxic agents.

Nolvadex has been associated with changes in liver enzyme levels and on rare occasions with a spectrum of more severe liver abnormalities, including fatty liver, cholestasis and hepatitis.

Overdosage: On theoretical grounds overdosage would be expected to cause enhancement of the pharmacological side-effects mentioned above. Observations in animals show that extreme overdosage (100 to 200 times recommended daily dose) may produce oestrogenic effects.

There is no specific antidote to overdosage, and treatment must be symptomatic.

Pharmaceutical precautions Store below 30°C, protected from light.

Legal category POM.

Package quantities Nolvadex tablets are blister packed in containers of 30 tablets.

Nolvadex-D tablets are blister packed in containers of 30 tablets.

Nolvadex-Forte tablets are blister packed in containers of 30 tablets.

Further information *Effect on ability to drive or operate machinery:* There is no evidence that Nolvadex results in impairment of these activities.

Product licence numbers

Nolvadex	12619/0048
Nolvadex-D	12619/0049
Nolvadex-Forte	12619/0050

PALUDRINE* TABLETS

Qualitative and quantitative composition Proguanil hydrochloride BP 100 mg.

Pharmaceutical form Tablets for oral administration.

Clinical particulars
Therapeutic indications: Paludrine is an effective antimalarial agent. It is recommended for the prevention and suppression of malaria.

Posology and method of administration: Non-immune subjects entering a malarious area are advised to begin treatment with Paludrine 1 week before, or if this is not possible, then at least 24 hours before arrival. The daily dose of Paludrine should be continued throughout exposure to risk and for 4 weeks after leaving the area.

Adults: Two tablets (200 mg) daily
Children: Under 1 year $\frac{1}{4}$ tablet (25 mg) daily

Children:	
1 to 4 years	½ tablet (50 mg) daily
5 to 8 years	1 tablet (100 mg) daily
9 to 14 years	1½ tablets (150 mg) daily
Over 14 years	Adult daily dose

The daily dose is best taken with water, after food, at the same time each day.

Provided the tablet fragment gives the minimum amount specified, precise accuracy in children's dosage is not essential since the drug possesses a wide safety margin.

For a young child, the dose may be administered crushed and mixed with milk, honey or jam.

Elderly patients: There are no special dosage recommendations for the elderly, but it may be advisable to monitor elderly patients so that optimum dosage can be individually determined.

Renal impairment: Based on a theoretical model derived from a single dose pharmacokinetic study, the following guidance is given for adults with renal impairment. (See *Contra-indications* and *Special warnings and special precautions for use.*)

Creatinine clearance ml/min/1.73 m²	*Dosage*
≥60	200 mg once daily (standard dose)
20 to 59	100 mg once daily
10 to 19	50 mg every second day
<10	<50 mg once weekly

The grade of renal impairment and/or the serum creatinine concentration may be approximately equated to creatinine clearance levels as indicated below.

Creatinine clearance ml/min/1.73 m²	*Approx* serum creatinine (micromol/l)*	*Renal impairment grade (arbitrarily divided for dosage purposes)*
≥60	-	-
20 to 59	150 to 300	Mild
10 to 19	300 to 700	Moderate
<10	>700	Severe

* Serum creatinine concentration is only an approximate guide to renal function unless corrected for age, weight and sex.

Contra-indications: Paludrine should be used with caution in patients with severe renal impairment. (See *Posology and method of administration* and *Special warnings and special precautions for use.*)

Special warnings and special precautions for use: Paludrine should be used with caution in patients with severe renal impairment. (See *Posology and method of administration*). There have been rare reports of haematological changes in such patients.

In any locality where drug-resistant malaria is known or suspected, it is essential to take local medical advice on what prophylactic regimen is appropriate. Prophylactic use of Paludrine alone may not be sufficient.

Interactions with other medicaments and other forms of interaction: None have been reported or are known.

Pregnancy and lactation:

Pregnancy: Pregnancy increases the risks from malaria. It is generally accepted that all drug treatment should be avoided if possible during the first trimester of pregnancy. Paludrine has been widely used for over 40 years and a causal connection between its use and any adverse effect on mother or foetus has not been established.

Lactation: Although Paludrine is excreted in breast milk, the amount is insufficient to confer any benefit on the infant. Separate chemoprophylaxis for the infant is required.

Effects on ability to drive and use machines: There is no evidence to suggest that Paludrine causes sedation or is likely to affect concentration.

Undesirable effects: At normal dosage levels the side effect most commonly encountered is mild gastric intolerance. This usually subsides as treatment is continued.

Mouth ulceration and stomatitis have on occasion been reported. Isolated cases of skin reactions and reversible hair loss have been reported in association with the use of proguanil.

Haematological changes in patients with severe renal impairment have been reported.

Overdose: The following effects have been reported in cases of overdosage:

Haematuria, renal irritation, epigastric discomfort and vomiting. There is no specific antidote and symptoms should be treated as they arise.

Pharmacological properties

Pharmacodynamic properties: Proguanil is an antimalarial drug and dihydrofolate reductase inhibitor. It acts like the other antifolate antimalarials by interfering with the folic-folinic acid systems and thus exerts its effect mainly at the time the nucleus is dividing. Since its activity is dependent on its metabolism, proguanil has a slow schizonticidal effect in the blood. It also has some schizonticidal activity in the tissues.

Proguanil is effective against the exoerythrocytic forms of some strains of *Plasmodium falciparum* but it has little or no activity against the exoerythrocytic forms of *P. vivax*. It has a marked sporonticidal effect against some strains *P. falciparum*; it does not kill the gametocytes, but renders them non-infective for the mosquito while the drug is present in the blood. Malaria parasites in the red blood cells are killed more rapidly by chloroquine or quinine than by proguanil, which is therefore not the best drug to use for the treatment of acute malaria.

Soon after proguanil was introduced, it was observed that the drug was inactive as an inhibitor of the in vitro growth of *P.gallinaceum* and *P. cynomolgi*, but that sera from dosed monkeys were active against *P. cynomolgi* in vitro. These findings suggested that proguanil was activated in vivo.

Since that time it has been accepted by most investigators in this field that cycloguanil is the active metabolite of proguanil and that parent compound is inactive per se.

Cycloguanil acts by binding to the enzyme dihydrofolate reductase in the malaria parasite. The effect of this action is to prevent the completion of schizogony. This is seen in the asexual blood stages as an arrest of maturation of the developing schizonts and an accumulation of large, abnormal looking trophozoites.

Proguanil is highly active against the primary exoerythocytic forms of *P. falciparum* and it has a fleeting inhibiting action on those of *P. vivax*. Proguanil is therefore a valuable drug for causal prophylaxis in falciparum malaria.

Pharmacokinetic properties: Proguanil is well absorbed in man with peak plasma concentrations of approximately 140 ng/ml occurring around 4 hours after an oral dose of 200 mg to an adult. The active triazine metabolite cycloguanil peaks at approximately 75 ng/ml 1 hour later. The elimination half-lives for proguanil and cycloguanil are reported to be of the order of 20 hours.

There is a low degree of drug accumulation after repeat doses, leading to steady state conditions after approximately 3 days. When daily doses are not taken, blood levels fall sharply but do not disappear completely until at least 2 or 3 doses are missed.

Pre-clinical safety data: Proguanil is a drug on which extensive clinical experience has been obtained. All relevant information for the prescriber is provided elsewhere in the Summary of Product Characteristics.

Pharmaceutical particulars

List of excipients: Calcium carbonate PhEur; Gelatin PhEur; Magnesium stearate PhEur; Maize starch PhEur

Incompatibilities: None known.

Shelf life: 5 years.

Special precautions for storage: Store below 30°C.

Nature and contents of container: HDPE bottles (100) and blister packs (98).

Instructions for use/handling: Use as directed by the prescriber.

Marketing authorisation number 12619/0051

Date of approval/revision of SPC November 1998

Legal category P

PALUDRINE/AVLOCLOR ANTI-MALARIAL TRAVEL PACK CHLOROQUINE AND PROGUANIL ANTI-MALARIAL TABLETS

Qualitative and quantitative composition Paludrine tablets containing 100 mg proguanil hydrochloride B.P.

Avloclor tablets containing 250 mg chloroquine phosphate PhEur which is equivalent to 155 mg chloroquine base.

Pharmaceutical form Tablets.

Clinical particulars

Therapeutic indication: Prophylaxis and suppression of malaria.

Posology and method of administration: Non-immune subjects entering a malarious area are advised to begin daily treatment with Paludrine 1 week before, or if this is not possible, then at least 24 hours before arrival. The daily dose of Paludrine should be continued throughout exposure to risk and for 4 weeks after leaving the area.

A single dose of Avloclor should be taken each week on the same day each week. Start one week before exposure to risk and continue until 4 weeks after leaving the malarious area.

Each dose should be taken with water after food.

Adults and children over 14 years: Take two Paludrine tablets daily as directed above. Take two Avloclor tablets once a week as directed above.

Children: Do not give to children under 1 year. The following single dose of Paludrine should be taken at the same time each day and the following single dose of Avloclor should be taken once a week on the same day each week.

	Paludrine (at the same time each day)	*Avloclor (on the same day each week)*
1 to 4 years	Half of a tablet	Half of a tablet
5 to 8 years	One tablet	One tablet
9 to 14 years	One and a half tablets	One and a half tablets

For a young child the dose may be administered crushed and mixed with milk, honey or jam.

Provided the Paludrine tablet fragment gives the minimum amount specified, precise accuracy in children's dosage is not essential since the drug possesses a wide safety margin.

The Avloclor dose given to children should be calculated on their body weight (5 mg chloroquine base/kg/week) and must not exceed the adult dose regardless of weight.

Elderly patients: There are no special dosage recommendations for the elderly, but it may be advisable to monitor elderly patients so that optimum dosage can be individually determined.

Paludrine and renal impairment: Based on a theoretical model derived from a single dose pharmacokinetic study, the following guidance is given for adults with renal impairment. (See also *Contra-indications* and *Special warnings and special precautions for use*).

Creatinine clearance ml/min/1.73 m²	Dosage
≥60	200 mg once daily (standard dose)
20 to 59	100 mg once daily
10 to 19	50 mg every second day
<10	50 mg once weekly

The grade of renal impairment and/or the serum creatinine concentration may be approximately equated to creatinine clearance levels as indicated below.

Creatinine clearance ml/min/1.73 m²	*Approx* serum creatinine (micromol/1)*	*Renal Impairment Grade (arbitrarily divided for dosage purposes)*
≥60	-	-
20 to 59	150 to 300	Mild
10 to 19	300 to 700	Moderate
<10	>700	Severe

*Serum creatinine concentration is only an approximate guide to renal function unless corrected for age, weight and sex.

Avloclor and hepatic or renally impaired patients: Caution is necessary when giving Avloclor to patients with renal disease or hepatic disease.

Contra-indications: None known.

Special warnings and special precautions for use:

In any locality where drug resistant malaria is known or suspected, it is essential to take local medical advice on what prophylactic regimen is appropriate.

Paludrine should be used with caution in patients with severe renal impairment. (See also *Posology and method of administration*). There have been rare reports of haematological changes in such patients. Caution is necessary when giving Avloclor to patients with renal disease.

Caution is necessary when giving Avloclor to patients with impaired hepatic function, particularly when associated with cirrhosis. Caution is also necessary in patients with porphyria. Avloclor may precipitate severe constitutional symptoms and an increase in the amount of porphyrins excreted in the urine. This reaction is especially apparent in patients with high alcohol intake.

Avloclor should be used with care in patients with a history of epilepsy.

The use of Avloclor in patients with psoriasis may precipitate a severe attack.

Prolonged or high dose Avloclor therapy:

1. Considerable caution is needed in the use of Avloclor for long-term high dosage therapy and such use should only be considered when no other drug is available.
2. Prolonged therapy with high doses may lead to occasional development of irreversible retinal damage.

3. Patients receiving Avloclor continuously at higher dose levels for periods longer than 12 months should undergo ophthalmic examination before treatment and at three monthly intervals. This also applies to patients receiving Avloclor at weekly intervals for a period of more than 3 years as a prophylactic against malarial attacks or if the total consumption exceeds 1.6 g/kg.
4. Full blood counts should be carried out regularly during extended treatment as bone marrow suppression may occur rarely.

Interactions with other medicaments and other forms of interaction: Antacids may reduce the absorption of proguanil, so should be taken at least 2–3 hours apart.

If you are taking cyclosporin, chloroquine may cause an increase in cyclosporin levels.

When rabies vaccine is injected into the skin, chloroquine may reduce its effectiveness.

Pregnancy and lactation:
Pregnancy: Pregnancy increases the risks from malaria. It is generally accepted that all drug treatment should be avoided if possible during the first trimester of pregnancy.

As with all drugs, the use of Avloclor during pregnancy should be avoided if possible unless, in the case of life threatening situations, in the judgement of the physician, potential benefit outweighs the risk. There is evidence to suggest that Avloclor given to women in high doses throughout pregnancy can give rise to foetal abnormalities including ocular or cochlear damage.

Paludrine has been widely used for over 40 years and a causal connection between its use and any adverse effect on mother or foetus has not been established.

Lactation: Although both Paludrine and Avloclor are excreted in breast milk, the amount is insufficient to confer any benefit on the infant. Separate chemoprophylaxis for the infant is required.

Effects on ability to drive and use machines: Defects in visual accommodation may occur on first taking Avloclor and patients should be warned regarding driving or operating machinery.

There is no evidence to suggest that Paludrine causes sedation or is likely to affect concentration.

Undesirable effects: The adverse reactions which may occur at doses used in the prophylaxis of malaria are generally not of a serious nature.

Paludrine: Mouth ulceration and stomatitis have on occasion been reported. Isolated cases of skin reactions and reversible hair loss have been reported in association with the use of proguanil.

Haematological changes in patients with severe renal impairment have been reported.

At normal dosage levels the side effect most commonly encountered is mild gastric intolerance. This usually subsides as treatment is continued.

Avloclor: Adverse reactions reported after Avloclor use are: headache, gastro-intestinal disturbances, skin eruptions, pruritus, occasional depigmentation or loss of hair, difficulty in accommodation, blurring of vision, corneal opacities, retinal degeneration, electrocardiographic changes, neurological and psychiatric changes, including convulsions and psychosis, thrombocytopenia, agranulocytosis, aplastic anaemia, allergic reactions, erythema multiforme, Stevens-Johnson syndrome, cardiomyopathy.

Changes in liver function, including hepatitis and abnormal liver function tests, have been reported rarely.

Overdose: Paludrine: The following effects have been reported in cases of overdosage:

Haematuria, renal irritation, epigastric discomfort and vomiting. There is no specific antidote and symptoms should be treated as they arise.

Avloclor: Chloroquine is highly toxic in overdose and children are particularly susceptible. The chief symptoms of overdosage include circulatory collapse due to a potent cardiotoxic effect, respiratory arrest and coma. Symptoms may progress rapidly after initial nausea and vomiting. Cardiac complications may occur without progressively deepening coma.

Death may result from circulatory or respiratory failure or cardiac arrhythmia. If there is no demonstrable cardiac output due to arrhythmias, asystole or electromechanical dissociation, external chest compression should be persisted with for as long as necessary, or until adrenaline and diazepam can be given (see below).

Gastric lavage should be carried out urgently, first protecting the airway and instituting artificial ventilation where necessary. There is a risk of cardiac arrest following aspiration of gastric contents in more serious cases. Activated charcoal left in the stomach may reduce absorption of any remaining chloroquine from the gut. Circulatory status (with central venous pressure measurement), respiration, plasma electrolytes and blood gases should be monitored, with correction of hypokalaemia and acidosis if indicated. Cardiac arrhythmias should not be treated unless life threatening; drugs with quinidine-like effects should be avoided. Intravenous sodium bicarbonate 1 to 2 mmol/kg over 15 minutes may be effective in conduction disturbances, and DC shock is indicated for ventricular tachycardia and ventricular fibrillation.

Early administration of the following has been shown to improve survival in cases of serious poisoning:

1. Adrenaline infusion 0.25 micrograms/kg/min initially, with increments of 0.25 micrograms/kg/min until adequate systolic blood pressure (more than 100 mm/Hg) is restored; adrenaline reduces the effects of chloroquine on the heart through its inotropic and vasoconstrictor effects.
2. Diazepam infusion (2 mg/kg over 30 minutes as a loading dose, followed by 1 to 2 mg/kg/day for up to 2 to 4 days). Diazepam may minimise cardiotoxicity.

Acidification of the urine, haemodialysis, peritoneal dialysis or exchange transfusion have not been shown to be of value in treating chloroquine poisoning. Chloroquine is excreted very slowly, therefore cases of overdosage require observation for several days.

Pharmacological properties
Pharmacodynamic properties: Paludrine: Proguanil is an antimalarial drug and dihydrofolate reductase inhibitor. It acts like the other antifolate antimalarials by interfering with the folic-folinic acid systems and thus exerts its effect mainly at the time the nucleus is dividing. Since its activity is dependent on its metabolism, proguanil has a slow schizonticidal effect in the blood. It also has some schizonticidal activity in the tissues.

Proguanil is effective against the exoerythrocytic forms of some strains of *Plasmodium falciparum* but it has little or no activity against the exoerythrocytic forms of *P. vivax*. It has a marked sporonticidal effect against some strains of *P. falciparum;* it does not kill the gametocytes, but renders them non-infective for the mosquito while the drug is present in the blood. Malaria parasites in the red blood cells are killed more rapidly by chloroquine or quinine than by proguanil, which is therefore not the best drug to use for the treatment of acute malaria.

Soon after proguanil was introduced, it was observed that the drug was inactive as an inhibitor of the in vitro growth of *P. gallinaceum* and *P. cynomolgi*, but that sera from dosed monkeys were active against *P. cynomolgi* in vitro. These findings suggested that proguanil was activated in vivo.

Since that time it has been accepted by most investigators in this field that cycloguanil is the active metabolite of proguanil and that parent compound is inactive per se.

Cycloguanil acts by binding to the enzyme dihydrofolate reductase in the malaria parasite. The effect of this action is to prevent the completion of schizogony. This is seen in the asexual blood stages as an arrest of maturation of the developing schizonts and an accumulation of large, abnormal looking trophozoites.

Proguanil is highly active against the primary exoerythocytic forms of *P. falciparum* and it has a fleeting inhibiting action on those of *P. vivax*. Proguanil is therefore a valuable drug for causal prophylaxis in falciparum malaria.

Avloclor: The mode of action of chloroquine on plasmodia has not been fully elucidated. Chloroquine binds to and alters the properties of DNA. Chloroquine also binds to ferriprotoporphyrin IX and this leads to lysis of the plasmodial membrane.

In suppressive treatment, chloroquine inhibits the erythrocytic stage of development of plasmodia. In acute attacks of malaria, it interrupts erythrocytic schizogony of the parasite. Its ability to concentrate in parasitised erythrocytes may account for the selective toxicity against the erythrocytic stages of plasmodial infection.

Pharmacokinetic properties: Paludrine: Proguanil is well absorbed in man with peak plasma concentrations of approximately 140 ng/ml occurring around 4 hours after an oral dose of 200 mg to an adult. The active triazine metabolite cycloguanil peaks at approximately 75 ng/ml 1 hour later. The elimination half-lives for proguanil and cycloguanil are reported to be of the order of 20 hours.

There is a low degree of drug accumulation after repeat doses, leading to steady state conditions after approximately 3 days. When daily doses are not taken, blood levels fall sharply but do not disappear completely until at least 2 or 3 doses are missed.

Avloclor: Studies in volunteers using single doses of chloroquine phosphate equivalent to 300 mg base have found peak plasma levels to be achieved within one to six hours. These levels are in the region of 54 to 102 microgram/litre, the concentration in erythrocytes being some 4.8 times higher. The elimination half-life of chloroquine is dose dependent and is approximately one hundred hours. Following a single dose, chloroquine may be detected in plasma for more than four weeks. Mean bioavailability from tablets of chloroquine phosphate is 89%. Chloroquine is widely distributed in body tissues such as the eyes, kidneys, liver, and lungs where retention is prolonged.

The principal metabolite is monodesethylchloroquine, which reaches a peak concentration of 10 to 20 microgram/litre within a few hours. Mean urinary recovery, within 3 to 13 weeks, is approximately 50% of the administered dose, most being unchanged drug and the remainder as metabolite. Chloroquine may be detected in urine for several months.

Pre-clinical safety data: Both Paludrine and Avloclor have been extensively used for many years in clinical practice. All relevant information for the prescriber is provided elsewhere in this document.

Pharmaceutical particulars
List of excipients:
Paludrine: Calcium carbonate PhEur, Gelatin PhEur, Magnesium stearate PhEur, Maize starch PhEur

Avloclor: Magnesium stearate PhEur, Maize starch PhEur

Incompatibilities: None known.

Shelf life: 5 years.

Special precautions for storage: Store below 30°C. Protect from light and moisture.

Nature and contents of container: PVC/PVDC aluminium foil blister pack of 112's containing 98 Paludrine and 14 Avloclor tablets.

Instructions for use/handling: No special instructions.

Market authorisation number PL 12619/0118

Date of first authorisation/renewal of authorisation 5 November 1997.

Date of (partial) revision of the text November 1998.

SEROQUEL* 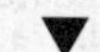

Qualitative and quantitative composition *25 mg tablet:* Each tablet contains 25 mg quetiapine (as 28.78 mg quetiapine fumarate); *100 mg tablet:* Each tablet contains 100 mg quetiapine (as 115.13 mg quetiapine fumarate); *200 mg tablet:* Each tablet contains 200 mg quetiapine (as 230.26 mg quetiapine fumarate).

Pharmaceutical form Film-coated tablets.

Clinical particulars
Therapeutic indication: Seroquel is indicated for the treatment of schizophrenia.

Posology and method of administration: Seroquel should be administered twice daily, with or without food.

Adults: The total daily dose for the first 4 days of therapy is 50 mg (Day 1), 100 mg (Day 2), 200 mg (Day 3) and 300 mg (Day 4).

From Day 4 onwards, the dose should be titrated to the usual effective dose range of 300 to 450 mg/day. Depending on the clinical response and tolerability of the individual patient, the dose may be adjusted within the range 150 to 750 mg/day.

Elderly: As with other antipsychotics, Seroquel should be used with caution in the elderly, especially during the initial dosing period. Elderly patients should be started on Seroquel 25 mg/day. The dose should be increased daily, in increments of 25 to 50 mg, to an effective dose, which is likely to be lower than that in younger patients.

Children and adolescents: The safety and efficacy of Seroquel have not been evaluated in children and adolescents.

Renal and hepatic impairment: The oral clearance of quetiapine is reduced by approximately 25% in patients with renal or hepatic impairment. Quetiapine is extensively metabolised by the liver, and therefore should be used with caution in patients with known hepatic impairment.

Patients with renal or hepatic impairment should be started on Seroquel 25 mg/day. The dose should be increased daily, in increments of 25 to 50 mg, to an effective dose.

Contra-indications: Seroquel is contra-indicated in patients who are hypersensitive to any component of this product.

Special warnings and special precautions for use:
Cardiovascular disease: Seroquel may induce orthostatic hypotension, especially during the initial dose-titration period; this is more common in elderly patients than in younger patients.

In clinical trials, quetiapine was not associated with a persistent increase in QT_c intervals. However, as with other antipsychotics, caution should be exercised when quetiapine is prescribed with drugs known to prolong the QT_c interval, especially in the elderly.

Seroquel should be used with caution in patients with known cardiovascular disease, cerebrovascular disease, or other conditions predisposing to hypotension.

Seizures: In controlled clinical trials there was no difference in the incidence of seizures in patients treated with Seroquel or placebo. As with other antipsychotics, caution is recommended when treating patients with a history of seizures.

Neuroleptic malignant syndrome: Neuroleptic malignant syndrome has been associated with antipsychotic treatment. Clinical manifestations include hyperthermia, altered mental status, muscular rigidity, autonomic instability, and increased creatine phosphokinase. In such an event, Seroquel should be discontinued and appropriate medical treatment given.

Tardive dyskinesia: As with other antipsychotics, there is a potential for Seroquel to cause tardive dyskinesia after long-term treatment. If signs and symptoms of tardive dyskinesia appear, dose reduction or discontinuation of Seroquel should be considered.

Interactions with other medicaments and other forms of interaction: Given the primary central nervous system effects of quetiapine, Seroquel should be used with caution in combination with other centrally acting drugs and alcohol.

The pharmacokinetics of lithium were not altered when co-administered with Seroquel.

Quetiapine did not induce the hepatic enzyme systems involved in the metabolism of antipyrine.

Co-administration of Seroquel and phenytoin (microsomal enzyme inducer) caused increases in clearance of quetiapine. Increased doses of Seroquel may be required to maintain control of psychotic symptoms in patients co-administered Seroquel and phenytoin, or other hepatic enzyme inducers (eg, carbamazepine, barbiturates, rifampicin). The dose of Seroquel may need to be reduced if phenytoin is withdrawn and replaced with a non-inducer (eg, sodium valproate).

The pharmacokinetics of quetiapine were not significantly altered following co-administration with the antipsychotics risperidone or haloperidol. However, co-administration of Seroquel and thioridazine caused increases in clearance of quetiapine.

The pharmacokinetics of quetiapine were not significantly altered following co-administration with the antidepressants imipramine (a known CYP2D6 inhibitor) or fluoxetine (a known CYP3A4 and CYP2D6 inhibitor).

CYP3A4 is the primary enzyme responsible for cytochrome P450 mediated metabolism of quetiapine. The pharmacokinetics of quetiapine were not altered following co-administration with cimetidine or fluoxetine, both of which are known P450 enzyme inhibitors. However, caution is recommended when Seroquel is co-administered with potent CYP3A4 inhibitors (such as systemic ketoconazole or erythromycin).

Pregnancy and lactation: The safety and efficacy of Seroquel during human pregnancy have not been established (see *Pre-clinical safety data, Reproduction studies,* for animal reproductive toxicology data). Therefore, Seroquel should only be used during pregnancy if the benefits justify the potential risks.

The degree to which quetiapine is excreted into human milk is unknown. Women who are breast feeding should therefore be advised to avoid breast feeding while taking Seroquel.

Effect on ability to drive and use machines: Because Seroquel may cause somnolence, patients should be cautioned about operating hazardous machines, including motor vehicles.

Undesirable effects: The most frequent and significant adverse events reported from short-term controlled trials of Seroquel were somnolence (17.5%), dizziness (10%), constipation (9%), postural hypotension (7%), dry mouth (7%), and liver enzyme abnormalities (6%).

Table 1 lists the adverse events that occurred in at least 1% of patients treated with Seroquel in the placebo-controlled phase II/III trials.

Seroquel may be associated with mild asthenia, rhinitis and dyspepsia. As with other antipsychotics, Seroquel may also be associated with limited weight gain, predominantly during the early weeks of treatment.

As with other antipsychotics with alpha$_1$ adrenergic blocking activity, Seroquel may induce orthostatic hypotension (associated with dizziness), tachycardia and, in some patients, syncope; these events occur especially during the initial dose-titration period (see *Special warnings and special precautions for use*).

There have been occasional reports of seizures in patients administered Seroquel, although the frequency was no greater than that observed in patients administered placebo in controlled clinical trials (see *Special warnings and special precautions for use*).

As with other antipsychotic agents, rare cases of possible neuroleptic malignant syndrome have been reported in patients treated with Seroquel (see *Special warnings and special precautions for use*).

Table 1 Adverse events that occurred in at least 1% of patients treated with Seroquel in the placebo-controlled Phase-II/III trials[a]

Body system and COSTART Term	*Number (%) of patients with adverse events*	
	Seroquel (n = 510)	Placebo (n = 206)
Total number (%) of patients with adverse events[b]	406 (79.6)	155 (75.2)
Body as a whole		
Headache	99 (19.4)	36 (17.5)
Asthenia	18 (3.5)	6 (2.9)
Abdominal pain	16 (3.1)	1 (0.5)
Back pain	10 (2.0)	1 (0.5)
Fever	8 (1.6)	2 (1.0)
Chest pain	9 (1.8)	3 (1.5)
Cardiovascular system		
Postural hypotension	36 (7.1)	5 (2.4)
Tachycardia	36 (7.1)	10 (4.9)
Hypertension	9 (1.8)	3 (1.5)
Digestive system		
Constipation	44 (8.6)	10 (4.9)
Dry mouth	33 (6.5)	6 (2.9)
Dyspepsia	32 (6.3)	5 (2.4)
Diarrhoea	10 (2.0)	4 (1.9)
GGT increased	8 (1.6)	1 (0.5)
Haemic and lymphatic system		
Leucopenia	8 (1.6)	0
Metabolic and nutritional disorders		
ALT (SGPT) increased	31 (6.1)	3 (1.5)
AST (SGOT) increased	18 (3.5)	2 (1.0)
Weight gain	10 (2.0)	0
Musculoskeletal system		
Myalgia	6 (1.2)	1 (0.5)
Nervous system		
Somnolence	89 (17.5)	22 (10.7)
Dizziness	49 (9.6)	9 (4.4)
Anxiety	16 (3.1)	6 (2.9)
Respiratory system		
Rhinitis	17 (3.3)	1 (0.5)
Skin and appendages		
Rash	22 (4.3)	6 (2.9)
Dry skin	6 (1.2)	2 (1.0)
Special senses		
Ear pain	6 (1.2)	0
Urogenital system		
Urinary tract infection	7 (1.4)	1 (0.5)

[a] Only adverse events that occurred in a higher proportion of patients treated with Seroquel than with placebo are presented. Adverse events for which the incidence with Seroquel was equal to or less than that with placebo included the following: pain, infection, hostility, accidental injury, hypotension, nausea, vomiting, agitation, insomnia, nervousness, akathisia, hypertonia, tremor, depression, paraesthesia, pharyngitis, amblyopia.
[b] Patients may have had more than one adverse event.

As with other antipsychotic agents, Seroquel has been associated with variations in white blood cell count. Transient asymptomatic leucopenia and/or neutropenia have been observed in patients administered Seroquel, recorded at an incidence of 1.6% in placebo-controlled clinical trials. Occasionally, eosinophilia has been observed.

Asymptomatic elevations in serum transaminase (ALT, AST) or GGT levels have been observed in some patients administered Seroquel. These elevations were usually reversible on continued Seroquel treatment.

Small elevations in non-fasting serum triglyceride levels and total cholesterol have been observed during treatment with Seroquel.

Seroquel treatment was associated with small dose-related decreases in thyroid hormone levels, particularly total T_4 and free T_4. The reduction in total and free T_4 was maximal within the first 2 to 4 weeks of quetiapine treatment, with no further reduction during long-term treatment. There was no evidence of clinically significant changes in TSH concentration over time. In nearly all cases, cessation of quetiapine treatment was associated with a reversal of the effects on total and free T_4, irrespective of the duration of treatment.

As with other antipsychotics, Seroquel may cause prolongation of the QT_c interval, but in clinical trials, this was not associated with a persistent increase (see *Special warnings and special precautions for use*).

Overdose: In clinical trials, experience with Seroquel in overdosage is limited. Estimated doses of Seroquel up to 20 mg have been taken; no fatalities were reported and patients recovered without sequelae.

In general, reported signs and symptoms were those resulting from an exaggeration of the drug's known pharmacological effects, ie, drowsiness and sedation, tachycardia and hypotension.

There is no specific antidote to quetiapine. In cases of severe intoxication, the possibility of multiple drug involvement should be considered, and intensive care procedures are recommended, including establishing and maintaining a patent airway, ensuring adequate oxygenation and ventilation, and monitoring and support of the cardiovascular system.

Close medical supervision and monitoring should be continued until the patient recovers.

Pharmacological properties

Therapeutic classification: N05A

Pharmacodynamic properties: Quetiapine is an atypical antipsychotic agent which interacts with a broad range of neurotransmitter receptors. Quetiapine exhibits a higher affinity for serotonin ($5HT_2$) receptors in the brain than it does for dopamine D_1 and D_2 receptors in the brain. Quetiapine also has high affinity at histaminergic and adrenergic alpha$_1$ receptors, with a lower affinity at adrenergic alpha$_2$ receptors, but no appreciable affinity at cholinergic muscarinic or benzodiazepine receptors. Quetiapine is active in tests for antipsychotic activity, such as conditioned avoidance.

The results of animal studies predictive of EPS liability revealed that quetiapine causes only weak catalepsy at effective dopamine D_2 receptor blocking doses, that quetiapine causes selective reduction in the firing of mesolimbic A10 dopaminergic neurones versus the A9 nigrostriatal neurones involved in motor function, and that quetiapine exhibits minimal dystonic liability in neuroleptic-sensitised monkeys. The results of three placebo-controlled clinical trials, including one that used a dose range of Seroquel of 75 to 750 mg/day, identified no difference between Seroquel and placebo in the incidence of EPS or use of concomitant anticholinergics.

Seroquel does not produce sustained elevations in prolactin. In a multiple fixed-dose clinical trial, there were no differences in prolactin levels at study completion between Seroquel, across the recommended dose range, and placebo.

In clinical trials, Seroquel has been shown to be effective in the treatment of both positive and negative symptoms of schizophrenia. In one trial against chlorpromazine, and two against haloperidol, Seroquel showed similar short-term efficacy.

Pharmacokinetic properties: Quetiapine is well absorbed and extensively metabolised following oral administration. The principal human plasma metabolites do not have significant pharmacological activity. The bioavailability of quetiapine is not significantly affected by administration with food. The elimination half-life of quetiapine is approximately 7 hours. Quetiapine is approximately 83% bound to plasma proteins.

Clinical trials have demonstrated that Seroquel is effective when given twice a day. This is further supported by data from a positron emission tomography (PET) study which identified that $5HT_2$ and D_2 receptor occupancy are maintained for up to 12 hours after dosing with quetiapine.

The pharmacokinetics of quetiapine are linear, and do not differ between men and women.

The mean clearance of quetiapine in the elderly is approximately 30 to 50% lower than that seen in adults aged 18 to 65 years.

The mean plasma clearance of quetiapine was reduced by approximately 25% in subjects with severe renal impairment (creatinine clearance less than 30 ml/min/1.73 m^2) and in subjects with hepatic impairment (stable alcoholic cirrhosis), but the individual clearance values are within the range for normal subjects.

Quetiapine is extensively metabolised, with parent compound accounting for less than 5% of unchanged drug-related material in the urine or faeces, following the administration of radiolabelled quetiapine. Approximately 73% of the radioactivity is excreted in the urine and 21% in the faeces.

In vitro investigations established that CYP3A4 is the primary enzyme responsible for cytochrome P450 mediated metabolism of quetiapine.

Quetiapine and several of its metabolites were found to be weak inhibitors of human cytochrome P450 1A2, 2C9, 2C19, 2D6 and 3A4 activities, but only at concentrations at least 10- to 50-fold higher than those observed in the usual effective dose range of 300 to 450 mg/day in humans. Based on these in vitro results, it is unlikely that co-administration of quetiapine with other drugs will result in clinically significant drug inhibition of cytochrome P450 mediated metabolism of the other drug.

Pre-clinical safety data:
Acute toxicity studies: Quetiapine has low acute toxicity. Findings in mice and rats after oral (500 mg/kg) or intraperitoneal (100 mg/kg) dosing were typical of an effective neuroleptic agent and included decreased motor activity, ptosis, loss of righting reflex, fluid around the mouth and convulsions.

Repeat-dose toxicity studies: In multiple-dose studies in rats, dogs and monkeys, anticipated central nervous system effects of an antipsychotic drug were observed with quetiapine (eg, sedation at lower doses and tremor, convulsions or prostration at higher exposures).

Hyperprolactinaemia, induced through the dopamine D_2 receptor antagonist activity of quetiapine or its metabolites, varied between species but was most marked in the rat, and a range of effects consequent to this were seen in the 12-month study, including mammary hyperplasia, increased pituitary weight, decreased uterine weight and enhanced growth of females.

Reversible morphological and functional effects on the liver, consistent with hepatic enzyme induction, were seen in mouse, rat and monkey.

Thyroid follicular cell hypertrophy and concomitant changes in plasma thyroid hormone levels occurred in rat and monkey.

Pigmentation of a number of tissues, particularly the thyroid, was not associated with any morphological or functional effects.

Transient increases in heart rate, unaccompanied by an effect on blood pressure, occurred in dogs.

Posterior triangular cataracts seen after 6 months in dogs at 100 mg/kg/day were consistent with inhibition of cholesterol biosynthesis in the lens. No cataracts were observed in Cynomolgus monkeys dosed up to 225 mg/kg/day, nor in rodents. Monitoring in clinical studies did not reveal drug-related corneal opacities in man.

No evidence of neutrophil reduction or agranulocytosis was seen in any of the toxicity studies.

Carcinogenicity studies: In the rat study (doses 0, 20, 75 and 250 mg/kg/day) the incidence of mammary adenocarcinomas was increased at all doses in female rats, consequential to prolonged hyperprolactinaemia.

In male rat (250 mg/kg/day) and mouse (250 and 750 mg/kg/day), there was an increased incidence of thyroid follicular cell benign adenomas, consistent with known rodent-specific mechanisms resulting from enhanced hepatic thyroxine clearance.

Reproduction studies: Effects related to elevated prolactin levels (marginal reduction in male fertility and pseudopregnancy, protracted periods of diestrus, increased precoital interval and reduced pregnancy rate) were seen in rats, although these are not directly relevant to humans because of species differences in hormonal control of reproduction.

Quetiapine had no teratogenic effects.

Mutagenicity studies: Genetic toxicity studies with quetiapine show that it is not a mutagen or clastogen.

Pharmaceutical particulars
List of excipients: Core: Povidone (PhEur); Calcium Hydrogen Phosphate (PhEur); Microcrystalline Cellulose (PhEur); Sodium Starch Glycollate Type A (PhEur); Lactose Monohydrate (PhEur); Magnesium Stearate (PhEur).

Coating: Hydroxypropyl Methylcellulose 2910 (PhEur); Macrogol 400 (PhEur); Titanium Dioxide (PhEur, E171); Ferric Oxide, Yellow (PhFr, E172) (25 mg & 100 mg tabs); Ferric Oxide, Red (PhFr, E172) (25 mg tabs).

Incompatibilities: None known.

Shelf life: The shelf life of Seroquel 25 mg tablets and Mixed Pack is 24 months when stored below 30°C.

The shelf life of Seroquel 100 mg and 200 mg tablets is 36 months when stored below 30°C.

Special precautions for storage: None stated.

Nature and contents of container:
25 mg tablet: The tablets are round, 6 mm, peach coloured, bi-convex and film-coated;
100 mg tablet: The tablets are round, 8.5 mm, yellow coloured, bi-convex and film-coated;
200 mg tablet: The tablets are round, 11 mm, white, bi-convex and film-coated.

The tablets are packed into PVC aluminium foil blister strips. The blister strips are themselves packed into cartons.

25 mg tablets, 60 tablets in 6 strips of 10 blisters.

100 mg and 200 mg tablets, 60 tablets in 6 strips of 10 blisters and 90 tablets in 9 strips of 10 blisters.

Mixed pack, 8 tablets 1 strip containing 6 x 25 mg and 2 x 100 mg tablets.

Instructions for use/handling: None stated.

Marketing authorisation numbers
25 mg tablet 12619/0112
100 mg tablet 12619/0113
200 mg tablet 12619/0114

Date of (partial) revision of the text March 1998.

Legal category POM.

SORBICHEW*

Qualitative and quantitative composition Isosorbide Dinitrate 5 mg (incorporated as Diluted Isosorbide Dinitrate USP).

Pharmaceutical form Tablets.

Clinical particulars
Therapeutic indications: The chewable tablets are used to prevent or abort acute attacks of angina pectoris. The chewable tablets may be used for angina pectoris prophylaxis.

Posology and method of administration:
Adults (including the elderly): Treatment of the Acute attack: One or two Sorbichew tablets should be chewed until dissolved completely and swallowed.

Prevention of an expected attack: Immediately prior to the stressful event either one or two Sorbichew tablets should be chewed until dissolved completely and swallowed.

No dosage reduction is necessary in patients with renal or hepatic impairment.

Sorbichew tablets are scored for easier dose adjustment.

Children: The safety and efficacy of Sorbichew in children has not been established.

Contra-indications: Sorbichew is contraindicated in patients with a known sensitivity to the drug or to isosorbide-5-mononitrate and in cases of marked low blood pressure, shock and acute myocardial infarction with low left ventricular filling pressure.

Special warnings and special precautions for use: None stated.

Interaction with other medicaments and other forms of interaction: The hypotensive effects of other drugs may be potentiated.

Beta-adrenoceptor blocking drugs have a different pharmacological action in angina and may have a complementary effect when administered with Sorbichew.

Pregnancy and lactation: Animal studies have shown no adverse effects on the foetus, however, since its safety and efficacy during pregnancy and lactation have not been established, Sorbichew like other drugs, should not be administered to pregnant women and nursing mothers unless considered essential. No data are available on the presence of isosorbide mononitrate in breast milk.

Effects on ability to drive and use machines: The effect of isosorbide dinitrate upon an individual's performance of skilled and potentially dangerous tasks, such as car driving and the operation of machinery, has not been evaluated. However, there have been no published reports of impaired performance of such tasks.

Undesirable effects: A number of nitrate-related adverse effects may occur during treatment including flushing, headache, dizziness and weakness. The incidence of such effects is normally highest at the commencement of treatment and tends to decline with time. If headache is a problem, a temporary lowering of the dose may be necessary. Nausea and vomiting may occur occasionally.

Postural hypotension may occur, especially with high doses.

Dry rash and/or exfoliative dermatitis have been described rarely with isosorbide dinitrate and similar reactions might be expected.

Overdosage: Overdosage should be treated symptomatically. The main symptom is likely to be hypotension and this may be treated by elevation of the legs to promote venous return. Symptomatic and supportive treatment e.g. plasma expanders and if necessary the careful use of vasopressor agents to counterbalance the hypotensive effects may be necessary. Methaemoglobinaemia will normally respond to methylene blue infusion.

Pharmacological properties
Pharmacodynamic properties: The predominant mode of action of isosorbide dinitrate is that of a vasodilator with effects on both arteries and veins.

Pharmacokinetic properties: Following systemic absorption isosorbide dinitrate is metabolised by the liver to isosorbide-2-mononitrate and isosorbide-5-mononitrate. The elimination half-life of isosorbide dinitrate is approximately 0.8 hours. The bioavailability is 22±14% after oral administration because of significant first-pass metabolism. The volume of distribution is 1.5±0.8 l/kg with around 30% binding to plasma proteins. Clearance has been shown to be 45±20 ml/min/kg. Isosorbide-2-mononitrate has a half-life of approximately 2 hours with that of isosorbide-5-mononitrate being 5 hours.

Preclinical safety data: Isosorbide dinitrate is a drug on which extensive clinical experience has been obtained. Relevant information for the prescriber is provided elsewhere in the Summary of Product Characteristics.

Pharmaceutical particulars
List of excipients: Brilliant Blue FCF (Al Lake); Hydrogenated Vegetable Oil USNF; Lime Flavour; Magnesium Stearate USNF; Mannitol USP; Povidone USP; Quinoline Yellow, E104 (Al Lake); Starch USNF; Sugar USNF; Water USP.

Incompatibilities: None known.

Shelf life: 3 years.

Special precautions for storage: Store below 25°C. Protect from moisture.

Nature and contents of container: Square plastic containers containing 12 or 100 tablets.

Instructions for use/handling: Not applicable.

Market authorisation number PL 12619/0056.

Date of approval/revision of SPC May 1998.

Legal Category P

SORBID*-20 SA

Qualitative and quantitative composition Isosorbide Dinitrate 20 mg.

Pharmaceutical form Sustained release capsules.

Clinical particulars
Therapeutic indications: Sorbid-20 SA is indicated in the prophylaxis of angina pectoris.

Posology and method of administration:
Adult: 1–2 Sorbid-20 SA capsules should be swallowed twice daily.

Patients already accustomed to prophylactic nitrate therapy may normally be transferred directly to a therapeutic dose of Sorbid-20 SA. For patients not receiving prophylactic nitrate therapy, it is recommended that they are started with a low dose, which should be increased gradually.

No dosage reduction is necessary in patients with renal or hepatic impairment.

The capsules should be swallowed whole with a little fluid.

Children: The safety and efficacy of Sorbid-20 SA in children has not been established.

Elderly patients: There is no evidence to suggest that an adjustment of dose is necessary. However, caution may be required in elderly patients who are known to be susceptible to the effects of hypotensive medication.

Contra-indications: Sorbid-20 SA is contraindicated in patients with a known sensitivity to the drug or to isosorbide 5-mononitrate and in cases of marked low blood pressure, shock and acute myocardial infarction with low left ventricular filling pressure.

Special warnings and special precautions for use: Sorbid-20 SA is not indicated for the relief of acute anginal attacks. In the event of an acute attack, sublingual or buccal glyceryl trinitrate or sprays should be used.

Interactions with other medicaments and other forms of interaction: The hypotensive effects of other drugs may be potentiated.

Beta-adrenoceptor blocking drugs have a different pharmacological action in angina and may have a complementary effect when administered with Sorbid-20 SA.

Pregnancy and lactation: Animal studies have shown no adverse effects on the foetus, however since its safety and efficacy during pregnancy and lactation have not been established, Sorbid-20 SA like other drugs should not be administered to pregnant women and nursing mothers unless considered essential. No data are available on the presence of isosorbide mononitrate in breast milk.

Effects on ability to drive and use machines: The effect of isosorbide dinitrate upon an individual's performance of skilled and potentially dangerous tasks, such as car driving and the operation of machinery, has not been evaluated. However, there have been no published reports of impaired performance of such tasks.

Undesirable effects: A number of nitrate-related adverse effects may occur during treatment, including flushing, headache, dizziness and weakness. The incidence of such effects is normally highest at the commencement of treatment and tends to decline with time. If headache is a problem, a temporary lowering of the dose may be necessary.

Nausea and vomiting may occur occasionally.

Postural hypotension may occur, especially with high doses.

Dry rash and/or exfoliative dermatitis have been described rarely with isosorbide dinitrate and similar reactions might be expected.

Overdose: Overdosage should be treated symptomatically. The stomach should be aspirated to remove any remaining tablets.

The main symptom is likely to be hypotension and this may be treated by elevation of the legs to promote venous return. Symptomatic and supportive treatment e.g. plasma expanders and if necessary the careful use of vasopressor agents to counterbalance the hypotensive effects may be necessary. Methaemoglobinaemia will normally respond to methylene blue infusion.

Pharmacological properties
Pharmacodynamic properties: Isosorbide dinitrate acts predominantly as a vasodilator with effects on both veins and arteries.

Pharmacokinetic properties: Following oral dosing with Sorbid-20 SA, the peak blood level of isosorbide dinitrate is approximately 8 ng/ml. Isosorbide dinitrate is metabolised by the liver to isosorbide 2-mononitrate and isosorbide 5-mononitrate. The corresponding values for the peak blood level of the 2-mononitrate is approximately 25 ng/ml and for the 5-mononitrate 135 ng/ml. The elimination half-life of isosorbide dinitrate is 2–3 hours, the half-life of isosorbide 2-mononitrate is 4–5 hours and the half-life of isosorbide 5-mononitrate is 5–6 hours.

Preclinical safety data: Isosorbide dinitrate is a drug on which extensive clinical experience has been obtained. Relevant information for the prescriber is provided elsewhere in the Summary of Product Characteristics.

Pharmaceutical particulars
List of excipients: Black Iron Oxide (E172); Erythrosine (E127); Gelatin USNF; Maize Starch PhEur; Quinoline Yellow (E104); Shellac USNF; Sucrose PhEur; Talc PhEur.

Incompatibilities: Nil.

Shelf life: 3 years.

Special precautions for storage: Store below 25°C. Protect from light and moisture.

Nature and contents of container: Blister pack containing 56 capsules.

Instructions for use/handling: Use as directed by the prescriber.

Marketing authorisation number 12619/0057

Date of approval/revision of SPC April 1996

Legal category P

SORBID*-40 SA

Qualitative and quantitative composition Isosorbide Dinitrate 40 mg.

Pharmaceutical form Sustained release capsules.

Clinical particulars
Therapeutic indications: Sorbid-40 SA is indicated in the prophylaxis of angina pectoris.

Posology and method of administration:
Adults: 1–2 Sorbid-40 SA capsules should be swallowed twice daily.

Patients already accustomed to prophylactic nitrate therapy may normally be transferred directly to a therapeutic dose of Sorbid-40 SA. For patients not receiving prophylactic nitrate therapy, it is recommended that they are started with a low dose, which should be increased gradually.

No dosage reduction is necessary in patients with renal or hepatic impairment.

The capsules should be swallowed whole with a little fluid.

Children: The safety and efficacy of Sorbid-40 SA in children has not been established.

Elderly patients: There is no evidence to suggest that an adjustment of dose is necessary. However, caution may be required in elderly patients who are known to be susceptible to the effects of hypotensive medication.

Contra-indications: Sorbid-40 SA is contraindicated in patients with a known sensitivity to the drug or to isosorbide 5-mononitrate and in cases of marked low blood pressure, shock and acute myocardial infarction with low left ventricular filling pressure.

Special warnings and special precautions for use: Sorbid-40 SA is not indicated for the relief of acute anginal attacks. In the event of an acute attack, sublingual or buccal glyceryl trinitrate or sprays should be used.

Interactions with other medicaments and other forms of interaction: The hypotensive effects of other drugs may be potentiated.

Beta-adrenoceptor blocking drugs have a different pharmacological action in angina and may have a complementary effect when administered with Sorbid-40 SA.

Pregnancy and lactation: Animal studies have shown no adverse effects on the foetus, however since its safety and efficacy during pregnancy and lactation have not been established, Sorbid-40 SA like other drugs should not be administered to pregnant women and nursing mothers unless considered essential. No data are available on the presence of isosorbide mononitrate in breast milk.

Effects on ability to drive and use machines: The effect of isosorbide dinitrate upon an individual's performance of skilled and potentially dangerous tasks, such as car driving and the operation of machinery, has not been evaluated. However, there have been no published reports of impaired performance of such tasks.

Undesirable effects: A number of nitrate-related adverse effects may occur during treatment, including flushing, headache, dizziness and weakness. The incidence of such effects is normally highest at the commencement of treatment and tends to decline with time. If headache is a problem a temporary lowering of the dose may be necessary.

Nausea and vomiting may occur occasionally.

Postural hypotension may occur, especially with high doses.

Dry rash and/or exfoliative dermatitis have been described rarely with isosorbide dinitrate and similar reactions might be expected.

Overdose: Overdosage should be treated symptomatically. The stomach should be aspirated to remove any remaining tablets.

The main symptom is likely to be hypotension and this may be treated by elevation of the legs to promote venous return. Symptomatic and supportive treatment e.g. plasma expanders and if necessary the careful use of vasopressor agents to counterbalance the hypotensive effects may be necessary. Methaemoglobinaemia will normally respond to methylene blue infusion.

Pharmacological properties
Pharmacodynamic properties: Isosorbide dinitrate acts predominantly as a vasodilator with effects on both veins and arteries.

Pharmacokinetic properties: Following oral dosing with Sorbid-40 SA, the peak blood level of isosorbide dinitrate is approximately 15 ng/ml. Isosorbide dinitrate is metabolised by the liver to isosorbide 2-mononitrate and isosorbide 5-mononitrate. The corresponding values for the peak blood level of the 2-mononitrate is approximately 45 ng/ml and for the 5-mononitrate 286 ng/ml. The elimination half-life of isosorbide dinitrate is 2–3 hours, the half-life of isosorbide 2-mononitrate is 4–5 hours and the half-life of isosorbide 5-mononitrate is 5–6 hours.

Preclinical safety data: Isosorbide dinitrate is a drug on which extensive clinical experience has been obtained. Relevant information for the prescriber is provided elsewhere in the Summary of Product Characteristics.

Pharmaceutical particulars
List of excipients: Black Iron Oxide (E172); Erythrosine (E127); Gelatin USNF; Maize Starch PhEur; Shellac USNF; Sucrose PhEur; Talc PhEur.

Incompatibilities: Nil.

Shelf life: 3 years.

Special precautions for storage: Store below 25°C. Protect from light and moisture.

Nature and contents of container: Blister pack containing 56 capsules.

Instructions for use/handling: Use as directed by the prescriber.

Marketing authorisation number 12619/0058

Date of approval/revision of SPC April 1996

Legal category P

SORBITRATE* 10

Qualitative and quantitative composition Isosorbide dinitrate 10 mg (incorporated as Diluted Isosorbide Dinitrate USP).

Pharmaceutical form Tablets.

Clinical particulars
Therapeutic indications: Angina prophylaxis.

Congestive cardiac failure - as adjunctive therapy in the management of severe acute or chronic congestive cardiac failure.

Posology and method of administration:
Adults: Angina prophylaxis: 10 to 40 mg, three or four times daily depending on individual requirement.

Patients already accustomed to prophylactic nitrate therapy may normally be transferred directly to a therapeutic dose of Sorbitrate. For patients not receiving prophylactic nitrate therapy, it is recommended that they are started with a low dose, which should be increased gradually.

Congestive cardiac failure: In severe congestive cardiac failure Sorbitrate tablets may be taken in doses of 10 to 40 mg three or four times daily depending on patient requirements. In this situation optimal individual dosage is best determined by continuous haemodynamic monitoring. The use of Sorbitrate in severe congestive cardiac failure should be considered adjunctive therapy to more conventional treatment (eg. digitalis, diuretics etc).

No dosage reduction is necessary in patients with renal or hepatic impairment.

The tablets should be swallowed whole with a little fluid.

Elderly patients: There is no evidence to suggest that an adjustment of dose is necessary. However, caution may be required in elderly patients who are known to be susceptible to the effects of hypotensive medication.

Children: The safety and efficacy of Sorbitrate in children has not been established.

Contra-indications: Sorbitrate is contraindicated in patients with a known sensitivity to the drug or to isosorbide-5-mononitrate and in cases of marked low blood pressure, shock and acute myocardial infarction with low left ventricular filling pressure.

Special warnings and special precautions for use: Sorbitrate is not indicated for the relief of acute anginal attacks. In the event of an acute attack, sublingual or buccal glyceryl trinitrate or sprays should be used.

Interactions with other medicaments and other forms of interaction: The hypotensive effects of other drugs may be potentiated.

Beta-adrenoceptor blocking drugs have a different pharmacological action in angina and may have a complementary effect when administered with Sorbitrate.

Pregnancy and lactation: Animal studies have shown no adverse effects on the foetus, however, since its safety and efficacy during pregnancy and lactation have not been established, Sorbitrate like other drugs, should not be administered to pregnant women and nursing mothers unless considered essential. No data are available on the presence of isosorbide mononitrate in breast milk.

Effects on ability to drive and use machines: The effect of isosorbide dinitrate upon an individual's performance of skilled and potentially dangerous tasks, such as car driving and the operation of machinery, has not been evaluated. However, there have been no published reports of impaired performance of such tasks.

Undesirable effects: A number of nitrate-related adverse effects may occur during treatment including flushing, headache, dizziness and weakness. The incidence of such effects is normally highest at the commencement of treatment and tends to decline with time. If headache is a problem, a temporary lowering of the dose may be necessary. Nausea and vomiting may occur occasionally.

Postural hypotension may occur especially with high doses.

Dry rash and/or exfoliative dermatitis have been described rarely with isosorbide dinitrate and similar reactions might be expected.

Overdosage: Overdosage should be treated symptomatically. The stomach should be aspirated to remove any remaining tablets. The main symptom is likely to be hypotension and this may be treated by elevation of the patient's legs to promote venous return. Symptomatic and supportive treatment eg. plasma expanders and if necessary the careful use of vasopressor agents to counterbalance the hypotensive effects may be necessary. Methaemoglobinaemia will normally respond to methylene blue infusion.

Pharmacological properties

Pharmacodynamic properties: The predominant mode of action of isosorbide dinitrate is that of a vasodilator with effects on both veins and arteries.

Pharmacokinetic properties: Following systemic absorption isosorbide dinitrate is metabolised by the liver to isosorbide-2-mononitrate and isosorbide-5-mononitrate. The elimination half-life of isosorbide dinitrate is approximately 0.8 hours. The bioavailability is 22±14% after oral administration because of significant first-pass metabolism. The volume of distribution is 1.5±0.8 l/kg with around 30% binding to plasma proteins. Clearance has been shown to be 45±20 ml/min/kg. Isosorbide-2-mononitrate has a half-life of approximately 2 hours with that of isosorbide-5-mononitrate being 5 hours.

Preclinical safety data: Isosorbide dinitrate is a drug on which extensive clinical experience has been obtained. Relevant information for the prescriber is provided elsewhere in the Summary of Product Characteristics.

Pharmaceutical particulars

List of excipients: Lactose USNF; Magnesium Stearate USNF; Pre-gelatinised starch USNF; Quinoline yellow E104 (Al lake); Starch USNF; Water USP.

Incompatibilities: None known.

Shelf life: 3 years.

Special precautions for storage: Store below 25°C. Protect from moisture.

Nature and contents of container: HDPE bottle and cap.

Instructions for use/handling: Not applicable.

Market authorisation number PL 12619/0059.

Date of approval/revision of the text November 1997.

Legal category P

SORBITRATE* 20

Qualitative and quantitative composition Isosorbide Dinitrate 20 mg. (Incorporated as Diluted Isosorbide Dinitrate USP).

Pharmaceutical form Tablets.

Clinical particulars

Therapeutic indications: Angina prophylaxis: The tablets are taken orally for protection against angina pectoris.

Congestive cardiac failure: The tablets are taken orally as adjunctive therapy in the management of severe acute or chronic congestive cardiac failure.

Posology and method of administration:

Adults: Angina prophylaxis: 10 to 40 mg, three or four times daily depending on individual requirement.

Patients already accustomed to prophylactic nitrate therapy may normally be transferred directly to a therapeutic dose of Sorbitrate. For patients not receiving prophylactic nitrate therapy, it is recommended that they are started with a low dose, which should be increased gradually.

Congestive cardiac failure: In severe congestive cardiac failure Sorbitrate tablets may be taken in doses of 10–40 mg three or four times daily depending on patient requirements. In this situation optimal individual dose is best determined by continuous haemodynamic monitoring. The use of Sorbitrate in severe congestive cardiac failure should be considered as adjunctive therapy to more conventional treatment (e.g. digitalis, diuretics etc.).

No dosage reduction is necessary in patients with renal or hepatic impairment.

The tablets should be swallowed whole with a little fluid.

Elderly patients: There is no evidence to suggest that an adjustment of dose is necessary. However, caution may be required in elderly patients who are known to be susceptible to the effects of hypotensive medication.

Children: The safety and efficacy of Sorbitrate in children has not been established.

Contra-indications: Sorbitrate is contraindicated in patients with a known sensitivity to the drug and to isosorbide-5-mononitrate and in cases of marked low blood pressure, shock and acute myocardial infarction with low left ventricular filling pressure.

Special warnings and special precautions for use: Sorbitrate is not indicated for the relief of acute anginal attacks. In the event of an acute attack, sublingual or buccal glyceryl trinitrate or sprays should be used.

Interactions with other medicaments and other forms of interaction: The hypotensive effects of other drugs may be potentiated.

Beta-adrenoceptor blocking drugs have a different pharmacological action in angina and may have a complementary effect when administered with Sorbitrate.

Pregnancy and lactation: Animal studies have shown no adverse effects on the foetus, however since its safety and efficacy during pregnancy and lactation have not been established, Sorbitrate like other drugs should not be administered to pregnant women and nursing mothers unless considered essential. No data are available on the presence of isosorbide mononitrate in breast milk.

Effects on ability to drive and use machines: The effect of isosorbide dinitrate upon an individual's performance of skilled and potentially dangerous tasks, such as car driving and the operation of machinery, has not been evaluated. However there have been no published reports of impaired performance of such tasks.

Undesirable effects: A number of nitrate-related adverse effects may occur during treatment, including flushing, headache, dizziness and weakness. The incidence of such effects is normally at the highest at the commencement of treatment and tends to decline with time. If headache is a problem, a temporary lowering of the dose may be necessary. Nausea and vomiting may occur occasionally. Postural hypotension may occur, especially with high doses. Dry rash and/or exfoliative dermatitis have been described rarely with isosorbide dinitrate and similar reactions might be expected.

Overdosage: Overdosage should be treated symptomatically. The stomach should be aspirated to remove any remaining tablets. The main symptom is likely to be hypotension and this may be treated by elevation of the patient's legs to promote venous return. Symptomatic and supportive treatment e.g. plasma expanders and if necessary the careful use of vasopressor agents to counterbalance the hypotensive effects may be necessary. Methaemoglobinaemia will normally respond to methylene blue infusion.

Pharmacological properties

Pharmacodynamic properties: Isosorbide dinitrate relaxes arterial and venous smooth muscle to produce vasodilation. In low doses, the effect is primarily on veins. The resulting venodilatation resulting in a decrease in left and right ventricular end-diastolic pressures. Overall systemic vascular resistance is usually unaffected and heart rate is either unchanged or slightly increased.

Although nitrates do not increase total coronary blood flow in patients with angina due to atherosclerosis, there is evidence that they produce redistribution of blood flow towards the ischaemic subendocardium by selective dilatation of large epicardial vessels. This effect on large vessels may also be responsible for the beneficial effect of nitrates in patients with angina caused by coronary spasm.

Because of the effect of ISDN on veins and arteries, preload and after-load are reduced resulting in a reduction in myocardial oxygen consumption. This is probably the major mechanism of action of ISDN in the treatment of angina.

The reduction in end-diastolic pressure is also responsible for the benefits seen with ISDN in patients with heart failure with doses of ISDN which significantly reduce after-load, an increase in cardiac output may be observed.

Pharmacokinetic properties: Isosorbide dinitrate is readily absorbed following oral administration, peak plasma concentrations occurring 30–60 minutes after dosing. It is rapidly metabolised. The main metabolite being isosorbide-5-mononitrate which has only 1/30 to 1/100 the coronary vasodilating or vasodepressor activity of the parent compound. The other major metabolite is isosorbide-2-mononitrate, which is present in plasma at a concentration of 10–20% of that of the 5-mononitrate. The half-life of the 5-mononitrate and 2-mononitrate is about 5 hours and 2½ hours respectively.

Excretion of ISDN and its metabolite is via the kidneys, principally as glucuronide conjugates.

Preclinical safety data: Isosorbide dinitrate is a drug on which extensive clinical experience has been obtained. Relevant information for the prescriber is provided elsewhere in the Summary of Product Characteristics.

Pharmaceutical particulars

List of excipients: FD & C Blue No. 1 Al Lake; Lactose USNF; Magnesium Stearate USNF; Starch USNF; Pregelatinised Starch Type 1551 USNF.

Incompatibilities: Nil.

Shelf life: 3 Years.

Special precautions for storage: Store below 25°C, protect from moisture.

Nature and contents of container: Glass bottles with plastic cap, HDPE bottle and cap, plastic/aluminium foil strip.

Instructions for use/handling: Use as directed by the prescriber.

Market authorisation number PL 12619/0060.

Date of approval/revision of the text March 1996.

Legal category P

TENIF*

Presentation Tenif is presented as reddish brown capsules bearing the name Tenif and an 'S' logo. Each capsule contains Atenolol PhEur 50 mg and a sustained release formulation of nifedipine 20 mg. The inactive ingredients are gelatin, iron oxide, lactose, macrogol, magnesium carbonate, magnesium stearate, maize starch, methylhydroxypropylcellulose, microcrystalline cellulose, polysorbate, sodium lauryl sulphate and titanium dioxide.

Uses Management of hypertension where therapy with either a calcium channel blocker or a beta-adrenoceptor blocking drug proves inadequate.

Management of chronic stable angina pectoris where therapy with either a calcium channel blocker or a beta-adrenoceptor blocking drug proves inadequate.

Mode of action: Atenolol is a beta-adrenoceptor blocking drug which is $beta_1$-selective (i.e. acts preferentially on $beta_1$-adrenergic receptors in the heart). Selectivity decreases with increasing dose. Atenolol is without intrinsic sympathomimetic and membrane stabilising activities, and, as with other beta-adrenoceptor blocking drugs, has negative inotropic effects (and is therefore contra-indicated in uncontrolled heart failure). As with other beta-adrenoceptor blocking drugs, its mode of action in the treatment of hypertension is unclear. It is probably the action of atenolol in reducing cardiac rate and contractility which makes it effective in eliminating or reducing the symptoms of patients with angina. It is unlikely that any additional ancillary properties possessed by S(-) atenolol, in comparison with the racemic mixture, will give rise to different therapeutic effects.

Atenolol is effective and well tolerated in most ethnic populations although the response may be less in black patients.

Nifedipine is a calcium channel blocker. It is a powerful coronary and peripheral vasodilator which increases myocardial oxygen supply and reduces blood pressure (afterload) and peripheral resistance. Concomitant use of $beta_1$-adrenergic blockade therefore, ameliorates the reflex sympathetic response to nifedipine monotherapy by blocking the rise in heart rate, while atenolol's tendency to increase peripheral resistance is balanced by the vasodilatation and increased sympathetic tone induced by the calcium antagonist. Consequently, greater antihypertensive or antianginal efficacy is achieved by the concomitant use of nifedipine and atenolol than either drug alone. This beneficial pharmacodynamic interaction also results in fewer side effects when lower dosages of the two drugs are used in combination.

Absorption of atenolol following oral dosing is consistent but incomplete (approximately 40 to 50%) with peak plasma concentrations occurring 2 to 4 hours after dosing. Atenolol blood levels are consistent and subject to little variability. There is no significant hepatic metabolism of atenolol and more than 90% of that absorbed reaches the systemic circulation unaltered. The plasma half-life is about 6 hours but this may rise in severe renal impairment since the kidney is the major route of elimination. Atenolol penetrates tissues poorly due to its low lipid solubility and its concentration in brain tissue is low. Plasma protein binding is low (approximately 3%).

Absorption of nifedipine following oral dosing is complete with peak plasma concentrations occurring about every 3 hours after dosing. Nifedipine is > 90% plasma protein bound. There is significant hepatic metabolism of nifedipine. The plasma half-life is between 6 and 11 hours for the sustained formulation of nifedipine.

Co-administration of atenolol and nifedipine has little effect on the pharmacokinetics of either. In the elderly, the systemic bioavailability and elimination half-life of both components are increased.

Dosage and administration
Adults: Hypertension: One capsule daily swallowed with water. If necessary, the dosage may be increased to one capsule dosed every 12 hours. Patients can be transferred to the combination from other antihypertensive treatments with the exception of clonidine (see *'Warnings'* below).

Angina: One capsule every 12 hours swallowed with water. Where additional efficacy is necessary, prophylactic nitrate therapy or additional nifedipine may be of benefit.

Elderly patients: Dosage should not exceed one capsule daily in hypertension or one capsule twice daily in angina.

The pharmacokinetics of nifedipine are altered in the elderly so that lower maintenance doses of nifedipine may be required compared to younger patients.

Children: There is no paediatric experience with Tenif and therefore Tenif should not be used in children.

Contra-indications, warnings, etc Tenif should not be used in patients with any of the following conditions: known hypersensitivity to either component or other dihydropyridines because of the theoretical risk of cross-reactivity; bradycardia; cardiogenic shock; hypotension; metabolic acidosis; severe peripheral arterial circulatory disturbances; second or third degree heart block; sick sinus syndrome; untreated phaeochromocytoma; uncontrolled heart failure; women capable of childbearing or during pregnancy or during lactation; patients with clinically significant aortic stenosis; patients with marked renal impairment (i.e. creatinine clearance below 15 ml/min/1.73 m^2; serum creatinine greater than 600 micromol/litre); patients receiving calcium channel blockers with negative inotropic effects e.g. verapamil and diltiazem; unstable angina; or during or within one month of a myocardial infarction.

Tenif should not be used for the treatment of acute attacks of angina.

The safety of Tenif in malignant hypertension has not been established.

Tenif should not be used for secondary prevention of myocardial infarction.

Tenif should not be administered concomitantly with rifampicin since effective plasma levels of nifedipine may not be achieved owing to enzyme induction.

Due to its beta-adrenoceptor blocking drug component, Tenif:

- although contra-indicated in uncontrolled heart failure (see *Contra-indications*), may be substituted with care in patients already treated with a beta-adrenoceptor blocking drug, and/or whose signs of heart failure have been controlled. Caution must be exercised in patients with conduction defects or whose cardiac reserve is poor, especially as nifedipine also has negative inotropic effects.
- may increase the number and duration of angina attacks in patients with Prinzmetal's angina due to unopposed alpha receptor mediated coronary artery vasoconstriction. Atenolol is a beta$_1$-selective beta-adrenoceptor blocking drug; consequently, the use of Tenif may be considered although utmost caution must be exercised.
- although contra-indicated in severe peripheral arterial circulatory disturbances (see *Contra-indications*), may also aggravate less severe peripheral arterial circulatory disturbances.
- due to its negative effect on conduction time, caution must be exercised if it is given to patients with first degree heart block.
- may modify the tachycardia of hypoglycaemia.
- may mask the signs of thyrotoxicosis.
- will reduce heart rate, as a result of its pharmacological action. In the rare instances when a treated patient develops symptoms which may be attributable to a slow heart rate, the dose may be reduced.
- should not be discontinued abruptly in patients suffering from ischaemic heart disease.
- may cause a more severe reaction to a variety of allergens, when given to patients with a history of anaphylactic reaction to such allergens. Such patients may be unresponsive to the usual doses of adrenaline used to treat the allergic reactions.

Tenif contains the cardioselective beta-adrenoceptor blocking drug atenolol. Although cardioselective (beta$_1$) beta-adrenoceptor blocking drugs may have less effect on lung function than non-selective beta-adrenoceptor blocking drugs, as with all beta-adrenoceptor blocking drugs, these should be avoided in patients with reversible obstructive airways disease, unless there are compelling clinical reasons for their use. Where such reasons exist, Tenif may be used with caution. Occasionally, some increase in airways resistance may occur in asthmatic patients, however, and this may usually be reversed by commonly used dosage of bronchodilators such as salbutamol or isoprenaline.

The label and patient information leaflet for this product state the following warning: "If you have ever had asthma or wheezing, you should not take this medicine unless you have discussed these symptoms with the prescribing doctor".

Due to its nifedipine component it should be noted that:

- in rare cases, a transient increase in blood glucose has been observed with nifedipine in acute studies. This should be considered in patients suffering from diabetes mellitus. Nifedipine has no diabetogenic effect.
- ischaemic pain occurs in a small proportion of patients following introduction of nifedipine monotherapy. Although a 'steal' effect has not been demonstrated, patients experiencing this effect should discontinue nifedipine therapy.
- in single cases of in-vitro fertilisation, calcium antagonists like nifedipine have been associated with reversible biochemical changes in the spermatozoa's head section that may result in impaired sperm function. In those men who are repeatedly unsuccessful in fathering a child by in-vitro fertilisation and where no other explanation can be found, calcium antagonists like nifedipine should be considered as possible causes.

Hypertensive or anginal patients with clinically significant liver disease have not been studied and no dosage adjustment is suggested from the systemic availability of the monocomponents in patients with cirrhosis. However nifedipine is metabolised primarily by the liver and therefore patients with liver dysfunction should be carefully monitored. As a precaution, it is recommended that the dose should not exceed one capsule daily.

Tenif must not be used in conjunction with calcium channel blockers with negative inotropic effects, e.g. verapamil, diltiazem since this can lead to an exaggeration of these effects particularly in patients with impaired ventricular function and/or sino-atrial or atrio-ventricular conduction abnormalities. This may result in severe hypotension, bradycardia and cardiac failure (see *Contra-indications*).

Concomitant therapy with additional dihydropyridines e.g. nifedipine, may increase the risk of hypotension, and cardiac failure may occur in patients with latent cardiac insufficiency.

Atenolol monotherapy: Digitalis glycosides, in association with beta-adrenoceptor blocking drugs, may increase atrio-ventricular conduction time.

Beta-adrenoceptor blocking drugs may exacerbate the rebound hypertension which can follow the withdrawal of clonidine. If the two drugs are co-administered, the beta-adrenoceptor blocking drug should be withdrawn several days before discontinuing clonidine. If replacing clonidine by beta-adrenoceptor blocking drug therapy, the introduction of beta-adrenoceptor blocking drugs should be delayed for several days after clonidine administration has stopped.

Caution must be exercised when prescribing a beta-adrenoceptor blocking drug with Class 1 antiarrhythmic agents such as disopyramide.

Concomitant use of sympathomimetic agents, e.g. adrenaline, may counteract the effect of beta-adrenoceptor blocking drugs.

Concomitant use with insulin and oral antidiabetic drugs may lead to the intensification of the blood sugar lowering effects of these drugs.

Concomitant use of prostaglandin synthetase inhibiting drugs, e.g. ibuprofen or indomethacin, may decrease the hypotensive effects of beta-adrenoceptor blocking drugs.

Anaesthesia: Caution must be exercised when using anaesthetic agents with Tenif. The anaesthetist should be informed and the choice of anaesthetic should be the agent with as little negative inotropic activity as possible. Use of beta-adrenoceptor blocking drugs with anaesthetic drugs may result in attenuation of the reflex tachycardia and increase the risk of hypotension. Anaesthetic agents causing myocardial depression are best avoided.

Nifedipine monotherapy: The antihypertensive effect of nifedipine can be potentiated by simultaneous administration of cimetidine.

The simultaneous administration of nifedipine and quinidine may lead to serum quinidine levels being suppressed regardless of dosage of quinidine.

The simultaneous administration of nifedipine and digoxin may lead to reduced digoxin clearance and hence an increase in the plasma digoxin level. Patients' plasma digoxin levels should be monitored and, if necessary, the digoxin dose reduced.

As with other dihydropyridines, nifedipine should not be taken with grapefruit juice because bioavailability is increased.

Nifedipine should not be administered concomitantly with rifampicin since effective plasma levels of nifedipine may not be achieved owing to enzyme induction.

Other forms of interaction: Nifedipine may cause falsely increased spectrophotometric values of urinary vanillylmandellic acid. However measurement with HPLC was unaffected.

Pregnancy and lactation: Tenif is contra-indicated in women capable of childbearing or during pregnancy or during lactation (see *Contra-indications*).

Effect on ability to drive or operate machinery: The use of Tenif is unlikely to result in any impairment of the ability of patients to drive or operate machinery. However, it should be taken into account that occasionally dizziness or fatigue may occur.

Undesirable events: Tenif is well tolerated. In clinical studies, the undesired events reported are usually attributed to the pharmacological actions of its components.

The following undesired events, listed by body system, have been reported:

Tenif:
Cardiovascular: flushing, oedema.
CNS: dizziness, headache.
Gastrointestinal: gastrointestinal disturbance.
Haematological: purpura.
Others: fatigue.

Atenolol monotherapy:
Cardiovascular: bradycardia, heart failure deterioration, postural hypotension which may be associated with syncope, cold extremities. In susceptible patients: precipitation of heart block, intermittent claudication, Raynaud's phenomenon.
CNS: confusion, mood changes, nightmares, psychoses and hallucinations, sleep disturbances of the type noted with other beta-blockers.
Gastrointestinal: dry mouth. Elevations of transaminase levels have been seen infrequently, rare cases of hepatic toxicity including intrahepatic cholestasis have been reported.
Haematological: thrombocytopenia.
Integumentary: alopecia, dry eyes, psoriasiform skin reactions, exacerbation of psoriasis, skin rashes.
Neurological: paraesthesia.
Respiratory: bronchospasm may occur in patients with bronchial asthma or a history of asthmatic complaints.
Special senses: visual disturbances.
Others: an increase in ANA (antinuclear antibodies) has been observed, however the clinical relevance of this is not clear.

Nifedipine monotherapy:
Cardiovascular: palpitations, tachycardia, gravitational oedema, marked reduction in blood pressure in dialysis patients with malignant hypertension and hypovolaemia.
Neurological: paraesthesia.
Respiratory: dyspnoea.
Gastrointestinal: gingival hyperplasia, hypersensitivity type jaundice and disturbances of liver function such as increased transaminase or intra-hepatic cholestasis which regress after discontinuing therapy.
Haematological: agranulocytosis.
Integumentary: skin reactions such as pruritus, urticaria, photosensitive dermatitis, exanthema and exfoliative dermatitis, erythromelalgia and systemic allergic reactions.
Musculoskeletal: myalgia, tremor (both after high doses).
Urogenital: increased frequency of micturition, gynaecomastia (in older men on long term therapy, which usually regresses on withdrawal of therapy).

As with other sustained release dihydropyridines, exacerbation of angina pectoris may occur rarely at the start of treatment with sustained release formulations of nifedipine. The occurrence of myocardial infarction has been described although it is not possible to distinguish such an event from the natural course of ischaemic heart disease.

Discontinuance of Tenif should be considered if, according to clinical judgement, the well-being of the patient is adversely affected by any of the above reactions.

Overdosage: The symptoms of overdosage may include bradycardia, hypotension, acute cardiac insufficiency and bronchospasm.

General treatment should include: close supervision, treatment in an intensive care ward, the use of gastric lavage, activated charcoal and a laxative to prevent absorption of any drug still present in the gastrointestinal tract, the use of plasma or plasma substitutes to treat hypotension and shock. The possible use of haemodialysis or haemoperfusion may be considered.

Excessive bradycardia can be countered with atropine 1 to 2 mg intravenously and/or a cardiac pacemaker. If necessary, this may be followed by a bolus dose of glucagon 10 mg intravenously. If required, this may be repeated or followed by an intravenous infusion of glucagon 1 to 10 mg/hour depending on response. Intravenous calcium gluconate combined with metaraminol may be beneficial for hypotension induced by nifedipine. If no response to glucagon occurs or if glucagon is unavailable, a beta-adrenoceptor stimulant such as dobutamine 2.5 to 10 microgram/kg/minute by intravenous infusion may be given. Dobutamine, because of its positive inotropic effect could also be used to treat hypotension and acute cardiac insufficiency. It is likely that these doses would be inadequate to reverse the cardiac effects of beta-blockade if a large overdose has been taken. The dose of dobutamine should therefore be increased if necessary to achieve the required response according to the clinical condition of the patient.

In severe cases of hypotension cardiac pacing with appropriate cardiorespiratory support may be necessary.

Bronchospasm can usually be reversed by bronchodilators.

Pharmaceutical precautions Tenif capsules should be stored below 30°C, protected from light and moisture.

Legal category POM

Package quantities Calendar packs of 28 capsules.

Further information When the combined antihypertensive effect or antianginal effect of a beta-adrenoceptor blocking drug and calcium antagonist is required, Tenif is a convenient and acceptable therapy. The combination of atenolol and the slow release formulation of nifedipine, given once daily, provides control of raised blood pressure over a 24 hour period and may be expected to improve patient compliance. Given twice daily the combination provides control of angina.

Product licence number 12619/0071.

TENORETIC*

Qualitative and quantitative composition Atenolol PhEur 100 mg, Chlorthalidone PhEur 25 mg.

Pharmaceutical form Brown film coated tablets.

Clinical particulars

Therapeutic indications: Management of hypertension.

Posology and method of administration:

Adults: One tablet daily. Most patients with hypertension will give a satisfactory response to a single tablet daily of Tenoretic. There is little or no further fall in blood pressure with increased dosage and, where necessary, another antihypertensive drug, such as a vasodilator, can be added.

Elderly: Dosage requirements are often lower in this age group.

Children: There is no paediatric experience with Tenoretic, therefore this preparation is not recommended for children.

Renal impairment: In patients with severe renal impairment, a reduction in the daily dose or in frequency of administration may be necessary.

Contra-indications: Tenoretic should not be used in patients with any of the following: known hypersensitivity to either component; bradycardia; cardiogenic shock; hypotension; metabolic acidosis; severe peripheral arterial circulatory disturbances; second or third degree heart block; sick sinus syndrome; untreated phaeochromocytoma; uncontrolled heart failure.

Tenoretic must not be given during pregnancy or lactation.

Special warnings and special precautions for use: Due to its beta-adrenoceptor blocking drug component Tenoretic:

- although contra-indicated in uncontrolled heart failure (see *Contra-indications*) may be used in patients whose signs of heart failure have been controlled. Caution must be exercised in patients whose cardiac reserve is poor.
- may increase the number and duration of angina attacks in patients with Prinzmetal's angina due to unopposed alpha receptor mediated coronary artery vasoconstriction. Atenolol is a $beta_1$-selective beta-adrenoceptor blocking drug; consequently the use of Tenoretic may be considered although utmost caution must be exercised.
- although contra-indicated in severe peripheral arterial circulatory disturbances (see *Contra-indications*) may also aggravate less severe peripheral arterial circulatory disturbances.
- due to its negative effect on conduction time, caution must be exercised if it is given to patients with first degree heart block.
- may modify the tachycardia of hypoglycaemia.
- may mask the signs of thyrotoxicosis.
- will reduce heart rate, as a result of its pharmacological action. In the rare instances when a treated patient develops symptoms which may be attributable to a slow heart rate, the dose may be reduced.
- should not be discontinued abruptly in patients suffering from ischaemic heart disease.
- may cause a more severe reaction to a variety of allergens, when given to patients with a history of anaphylactic reaction to such allergens. Such patients may be unresponsive to the usual doses of adrenaline used to treat the allergic reactions.

Tenoretic contains the cardioselective beta adrenoceptor blocking drug atenolol. Although cardioselective ($beta_1$) beta-adrenoceptor blocking drugs may have less effect on lung function than non-selective beta-adrenoceptor blocking drugs, as with all beta-adrenoceptor blocking drugs, these should be avoided in patients with reversible obstructive airways disease, unless there are compelling clinical reasons for their use. Where such reasons exist, Tenoretic may be used with caution. Occasionally, some increase in airways resistance may occur in asthmatic patients, however, and this may usually be reversed by commonly used dosage of bronchodilators such as salbutamol or isoprenaline.

The label and patient information leaflet for this product state the following warning: 'If you have ever had asthma or wheezing, you should not take this medicine unless you have discussed these symptoms with the prescribing doctor'.

Due to its chlorthalidone component:

- hypokalaemia may occur. Measurement of potassium levels is appropriate, especially in the older patient, those receiving digitalis preparations for cardiac failure, those taking an abnormal (low in potassium) diet or those suffering from gastrointestinal complaints. Hypokalaemia may predispose to arrhythmias in patients receiving digitalis.
- caution must be exercised in patients with severe renal failure (see *Posology and method of administration*).
- impaired glucose tolerance may occur and caution must be exercised if chlorthalidone is administered to patients with a known pre-disposition to diabetes mellitus.
- hyperuricaemia may occur. Only a minor increase in serum uric acid usually occurs but in cases of prolonged elevation, the concurrent use of a uricosuric agent will reverse the hyperuricaemia.

Interactions with other medicaments and other forms of interaction: Combined use of beta-adrenoceptor blocking drugs and calcium channel blockers with negative inotropic effects eg verapamil, diltiazem, can lead to an exaggeration of these effects particularly in patients with impaired ventricular function and/or sino-atrial or atrio-ventricular conduction abnormalities. This may result in severe hypotension, bradycardia and cardiac failure. Neither the beta-adrenoceptor blocking drug nor the calcium channel blocker should be administered intravenously within 48 hours of discontinuing the other.

Concomitant therapy with dihydropyridines eg nifedipine, may increase the risk of hypotension, and cardiac failure may occur in patients with latent cardiac insufficiency.

Digitalis glycosides, in association with beta-adrenoceptor blocking drugs, may increase atrio-ventricular conduction time.

Beta-adrenoceptor blocking drugs may exacerbate the rebound hypertension which can follow the withdrawal of clonidine. If the two drugs are co-administered, the beta-adrenoceptor blocking drug should be withdrawn several days before discontinuing clonidine. If replacing clonidine by beta-adrenoceptor blocking drug therapy, the introduction of beta-adrenoceptor blocking drugs should be delayed for several days after clonidine administration has stopped.

Caution must be exercised when prescribing a beta-adrenoceptor blocking drug with Class 1 antiarrhythmic agents such as disopyramide.

Concomitant use of sympathomimetic agents, eg adrenaline, may counteract the effect of beta-adrenoceptor blocking drugs.

Concomitant use with insulin and oral antidiabetic drugs may lead to the intensification of the blood sugar lowering effects of these drugs.

Concomitant use of prostaglandin synthetase inhibiting drugs (eg ibuprofen, indomethacin) may decrease the hypotensive effects of beta-adrenoceptor blocking drugs.

Preparations containing lithium should not be given with diuretics because they may reduce its renal clearance.

Caution must be exercised when using anaesthetic agents with Tenoretic. The anaesthetist should be informed and the choice of anaesthetic should be an agent with as little negative inotropic activity as possible. Use of beta-adrenoceptor blocking drugs with anaesthetic drugs may result in attenuation of the reflex tachycardia and increase the risk of hypotension. Anaesthetic agents causing myocardial depression are best avoided.

Pregnancy and lactation:

Pregnancy: Tenoretic must not be given during pregnancy.

Lactation: Tenoretic must not be given during lactation.

Effects on ability to drive and use machines: Use is unlikely to result in any impairment of the ability of patients to drive or operate machinery. However, it should be taken into account that occasionally dizziness or fatigue may occur.

Undesirable effects: Tenoretic is well tolerated. In clinical studies, the undesired events reported are usually attributable to the pharmacological actions of its components.

The following undesired events, listed by body system, have been reported with Tenoretic or either of its components:

Biochemical: hyperuricaemia, hypokalaemia, impaired glucose tolerance (see *Special warnings and special precautions for use*) hyponatraemia related to chlorthalidone.

Cardiovascular: bradycardia; heart failure deterioration; postural hypotension which may be associated with syncope; cold extremities. In susceptible patients: precipitation of heart block; intermittent claudication; Raynaud's phenomenon.

CNS: confusion; dizziness; headache; mood changes; nightmares; psychoses and hallucinations; sleep disturbances of the type noted with other beta-adrenoceptor blocking drugs.

Gastrointestinal: dry mouth, gastrointestinal disturbances; nausea. Elevations of transaminase levels have been seen infrequently, rare cases of hepatic toxicity including intrahepatic cholestasis have been reported.

Haematological: leucopenia; purpura; thrombocytopenia.

Integumentary: alopecia; dry eyes; psoriasiform skin reactions; exacerbation of psoriasis; skin rashes.

Neurological: paraesthesia.

Respiratory: bronchospasm may occur in patients with bronchial asthma or a history of asthmatic complaints.

Special senses: visual disturbances.

Others: fatigue; an increase in ANA (Antinuclear Antibodies) has been observed, however the clinical relevance of this is not clear.

Discontinuance of Tenoretic should be considered if, according to clinical judgement, the well-being of the patient is adversely affected by any of the above reactions.

Overdose: The symptoms of overdosage may include bradycardia, hypotension, acute cardiac insufficiency and bronchospasm.

General treatment should include: close supervision, treatment in an intensive care ward, the use of gastric lavage, activated charcoal and a laxative to prevent absorption of any drug still present in the gastrointestinal tract, the use of plasma or plasma substitutes to treat hypotension and shock. The possible use of haemodialysis or haemoperfusion may be considered.

Excessive bradycardia may be countered with atropine 1 to 2 mg intravenously and/or a cardiac pacemaker. If necessary, this may be followed by a bolus dose of glucagon 10 mg intravenously. If required, this may be repeated or followed by an intravenous infusion of glucagon 1 to 10 mg/hour depending on response. If no response to glucagon occurs or if glucagon is unavailable, a beta-adrenoceptor stimulant such as dobutamine 2.5 to 10 microgram/kg/minute by intravenous infusion may be given. Dobutamine, because of its positive inotropic effects could be used to treat hypotension and acute cardiac insufficiency. It is likely that these doses would be inadequate to reverse the cardiac effects of beta-adrenoceptor blockade if a large overdose has been taken. The dose of dobutamine should therefore be increased if necessary to achieve the required response according to the clinical condition of the patient.

Bronchospasm can usually be reversed by bronchodilators.

Excessive diuresis should be countered by maintaining normal fluid and electolyte balance.

Pharmacological properties

Pharmacodynamic properties: Tenoretic combines the antihypertensive activity of two agents, a beta-adrenoceptor blocking drug (atenolol) and a diuretic (chlorthalidone).

Atenolol is $beta_1$-selective (ie acts preferentially on $beta_1$-adrenergic receptors in the heart). Selectivity decreases with increasing dose.

Atenolol is without intrinsic sympathomimetic and membrane stabilising activities and, as with other beta-adrenoceptor blocking drugs, has negative inotropic effects (and is therefore contraindicated in uncontrolled heart failure).

As with other beta-adrenoceptor blocking drugs, the mode of action of atenolol in the treatment of hypertension is unclear.

It is unlikely that any additional ancillary properties possessed by S (-) atenolol, in comparison with the racemic mixture, will give rise to different therapeutic effects.

Chlorthalidone, a monosulfonamyl diuretic, increases excretion of sodium and chloride. Natriuresis is accompanied by some loss of potassium. The mechanism by which chlorthalidone reduces blood pressure is not fully known but may be related to the excretion and redistribution of body sodium.

Atenolol is effective and well-tolerated in most ethnic populations. Black patients respond better to the combination of atenolol and chlorthalidone, than to atenolol alone.

The combination of atenolol with thiazide-like diuretics has been shown to be compatible and generally more effective than either drug used alone.

Pharmacokinetic properties: Absorption of atenolol following oral dosing is consistent but incomplete (approximately 40 to 50%) with peak plasma concentrations occurring 2 to 4 hours after dosing. The atenolol blood levels are consistent and subject to little variability. There is no significant hepatic metabolism of atenolol and more than 90% of that absorbed reaches the systemic circulation unaltered. The plasma half-life is about 6 hours but this may rise in severe renal impairment since the kidney is the major route of elimination. Atenolol penetrates tissues poorly due to its low lipid solubility and its concentration in brain tissue is low. Plasma protein binding is low (approximately 3%).

Absorption of chlorthalidone following oral dosing is consistent but incomplete (approximately 60%) with peak plasma concentrations occuring about 12 hours after dosing. The chlorthalidone blood levels are consistent and subject to little variability. The plasma half-life is about 50 hours and the kidney is the major route of elimination. Plasma protein binding is high (approximately 75%).

Co-administration of chlorthalidone and atenolol has little effect on the pharmacokinetics of either.

Tenoretic is effective for at least 24 hours after a single oral daily dose. This simplicity of dosing facilitates compliance by its acceptability to patients.

Preclinical safety data: Atenolol and Chlorthalidone are drugs on which extensive clinical experience has been obtained. Relevant information for the prescriber is provided elsewhere in the Summary of Product Characteristics.

Pharmaceutical particulars

List of excipients: Heavy Magnesium Carbonate PhEur; Maize Starch PhEur; Sodium Lauryl Sulphate PhEur; Gelatin PhEur; Magnesium Stearate PhEur; Methylhydroxypropylcellulose PhEur; Macrogol 300 BP; Iron Oxide yellow E172; Iron Oxide red E172; Magnesium Carbonate PhEur.

Incompatibilities: None known.

Shelf life: 4 years.

Special precautions for storage: Store below 25°C. Protect from light and moisture.

Nature and contents of container: Calendar packs of 28 tablets.

Instructions for use/handling: Use as directed by the prescriber.

Market authorisation number 12619/0073

Date of approval/revision of SPC November 1997.

Legal category POM

TENORET 50

Qualitative and quantitative composition Atenolol PhEur 50 mg Chlorthalidone PhEur 12.5 mg.

Pharmaceutical form Tablet.

Clinical particulars

Therapeutic indications: The management of hypertension, particularly suited to the older patients.

Posology and method of administration: Tenoret 50 tablets are administered orally.

Adults: One tablet daily.

Elderly: One tablet daily. Older patients with hypertension who do not respond to low dose therapy with a single agent should have a satisfactory response to a single tablet daily of Tenoret 50. Where hypertensive control is not achieved, addition of a small dose of a third agent eg. as a vasodilator, may be appropriate.

Children: There is no paediatric experience with Tenoret 50, therefore this preparation is not recommended for children.

Renal failure: In patients with renal impairment a reduction in daily dose or in frequency of administration may be necessary.

Contra-indications: Tenoret 50 should not be used in patients with any of the following: known hypersensitivity to either component; bradycardia; cardiogenic shock; hypotension; metabolic acidosis; severe peripheral arterial circulatory disturbances; second or third degree heart block; sick sinus syndrome; untreated phaeochromocytoma; uncontrolled heart failure.

Tenoret 50 must not be given during pregnancy or lactation.

Special warnings and special precautions for use: Due to its beta-adrenoceptor blocking drug component Tenoret 50:

- although contra-indicated in uncontrolled heart failure (see *Contra-indications*), may be used in patients whose signs of heart failure have been controlled. Caution must be exercised in patients whose cardiac reserve is poor.
- may increase the number and duration of angina attacks in patients with Prinzmetal's angina due to unopposed alpha receptor mediated coronary artery vasoconstriction. Atenolol is a $beta_1$-selective beta-adrenoceptor blocking drug; consequently the use of Tenoret 50 may be considered although utmost caution must be exercised.
- although contra-indicated in severe peripheral arterial circulatory disturbances (see *Contra-indications*), may also aggravate less severe peripheral arterial circulatory disturbances.
- due to its negative effect on conduction time, caution must be exercised if it is given to patients with first degree heart block.
- may modify the tachycardia of hypoglycaemia.
- may mask the signs of thyrotoxicosis.
- will reduce heart rate, as a result of its pharmacological action. In the rare instances when a treated patient develops symptoms which may be attributable to a slow heart rate, the dose may be reduced.
- should not be discontinued abruptly in patients suffering from ischaemic heart disease.
- may cause a more severe reaction to a variety of allergens, when given to patients with a history of anaphylactic reactions to such allergens. Such patients may be unresponsive to the usual doses of adrenaline used to treat the allergic reactions.

Tenoret 50 contains the cardioselective beta-adrenoceptor blocking drug atenolol. Although cardioselective ($beta_1$) beta-adrenoceptor blocking drugs may have less effect on lung function than non-selective beta-adrenoceptor blocking drugs, as with all beta-adrenoceptor blocking drugs, these should be avoided in patients with reversible obstructive airways disease, unless there are compelling clinical reasons for their use. Where such reasons exist, Tenoret 50 may be used with caution. Occasionally, some increase in airways resistance may occur in asthmatic patients, however, and this may usually be reversed by commonly used dosage of bronchodilators such as salbutamol or isoprenaline.

The label and patient information leaflet for this product state the following warning: 'If you have ever had asthma or wheezing, you should not take this medicine unless you have discussed these symptoms with the prescribing doctor'.

Due to its chlorthalidone component:

- hypokalaemia may occur. Measurement of potassium levels is appropriate, especially in the older patient, those receiving digitalis preparations for cardiac failure, those taking an abnormal (low in potassium) diet or those suffering from gastrointestinal complaints. Hypokalaemia may predispose to arrhythmias in patients receiving digitalis.
- caution must be exercised in patients with severe renal failure (see *Posology and method of administration*).
- impaired glucose tolerance may occur and caution must be exercised if chlorthalidone is administered to patients with a known pre-disposition to diabetes mellitus.
- hyperuricaemia may occur. Only a minor increase in serum uric acid usually occurs but in cases of prolonged elevation, the concurrent use of a uricosuric agent will reverse the hyperuricaemia.

Interactions with other medicaments and other forms of interaction: Combined use of beta-adrenoceptor blocking drugs and calcium channel blockers with negative inotropic effects eg. verapamil, diltiazem can lead to an exaggeration of these effects particularly in patients with impaired ventricular function and/or sino-atrial or atrio-ventricular conduction abnormalities. This may result in severe hypotension, bradycardia and cardiac failure. Neither the beta-adrenoceptor blocking drug nor the calcium channel blocker should be administered intravenously within 48 hours of discontinuing the other.

Concomitant therapy with dihydropyridines eg. nifedipine, may increase the risk of hypotension, and cardiac failure may occur in patients with latent cardiac insufficiency.

Digitalis glycosides, in association with beta-adrenoceptor blocking drugs, may increase atrio-ventricular conduction time.

Beta-adrenoceptor blocking drugs may exacerbate the rebound hypertension which can follow the withdrawal of clonidine. If the two drugs are co-administered, the beta-adrenoceptor blocking drug should be withdrawn several days before discontinuing clonidine. If replacing clonidine by beta-adrenoceptor blocking drug therapy, the introduction of beta-adrenoceptor blocking drugs should be delayed for several days after clonidine administration has stopped.

Caution must be exercised when prescribing a beta-adrenoceptor blocking drug with Class 1 antiarrhythmic agents such as disopyramide.

Concomitant use of sympathomimetic agents, eg. adrenaline, may counteract the effect of beta-adrenoceptor blocking drugs.

Concomitant use with insulin and oral antidiabetic drugs may lead to the intensification of the blood sugar lowering effects of these drugs.

Concomitant use of prostaglandin synthetase inhibiting drugs eg. ibuprofen and indomethacin, may decrease the hypotensive effects of beta-adrenoceptor blocking drugs.

Preparations containing lithium should not be given with diuretics because they may reduce its renal clearance.

Caution must be exercised when using anaesthetic agents with Tenoret 50. The anaesthetist should be informed and the choice of anaesthetic should be an agent with as little negative inotropic activity as possible. Use of beta-adrenoceptor blocking drugs with anaesthetic drugs may result in attenuation of the reflex tachycardia and increase the risk of hypotension. Anaesthetic agents causing myocardial depression are best avoided.

Pregnancy and lactation:

Pregnancy: Tenoret 50 must not be given during pregnancy.

Lactation: Tenoret 50 must not be given during lactation.

Effect on ability to drive and use machines: Use is unlikely to result in any impairment of the ability of patients to drive or operate machinery. However, it should be taken into account that occasionally dizziness or fatigue may occur.

Undesirable effects: Tenoret 50 is well-tolerated. In clinical studies, the undesired events reported are usually attributable to the pharmacological actions of its components.

The following undesired events, listed by body system, have been reported with Tenoret 50 or either of its components:

Biochemical: hyperuricaemia, hypokalaemia, impaired glucose tolerance (see *Special warnings and special precautions for use*), hyponatraemia related to chlorthalidone.

Cardiovascular: bradycardia; heart failure deterioration; postural hypotension which may be associated with syncope; cold extremities. In susceptible patients; precipitation of heart block; intermittent claudication; Raynaud's phenomenon.

CNS: confusion; dizziness; headache; mood changes; nightmares; psychoses and hallucinations; sleep disturbances of the type noted with other beta-adrenoceptor blocking drugs.

Gastrointestinal: dry mouth; gastrointestinal disturbances; nausea. Elevations of transaminase levels have been seen infrequently, rare cases of hepatic toxicity including intrahepatic cholestasis have been reported.

Haematological: leucopenia; purpura; thrombocytopenia.

Integumentary: alopecia; dry eyes; psoriasiform skin reactions; exacerbation of psoriasis; skin rashes.

Neurological: paraesthesia.

Respiratory: bronchospasm may occur in patients with bronchial asthma or a history of asthmatic complaints.

Special senses: visual disturbances.

Others: fatigue; an increase in ANA (Antinuclear Antibodies) has been observed, however the clinical relevance of this is not clear.

Discontinuance of Tenoret 50 should be considered if, according to clinical judgement, the well-being of the patient is adversely affected by any of the above reactions.

Overdose: The symptoms of overdosage may include bradycardia, hypotension, acute cardiac insufficiency and bronchospasm.

General treatment should include: close supervision, treatment in an intensive care ward, the use of gastric lavage, activated charcoal and a laxative to prevent absorption of any drug still present in the gastrointestinal tract, the use of plasma or plasma substitutes to treat hypotension and shock. The possible use of haemodialysis or haemoperfusion may be considered.

Excessive bradycardia can be countered with atropine 1–2 mg intravenously and/or a cardiac pacemaker. If necessary, this may be followed by a bolus dose of glucagon 10 mg intravenously. If required, this may be repeated or followed by an intravenous infusion of glucagon 1–10 mg/hour depending on response. If no response to glucagon occurs or if glucagon is unavailable, a beta-adrenoceptor stimulant such as dobutamine 2.5 to 10 micrograms/kg/minute by intravenous infusion may be given. Dobutamine, because of its positive inotropic effect, could also be used to treat hypotension and acute cardiac insufficiency. It is likely that these doses would be inadequate to reverse the cardiac effects of beta-adrenoceptor blockade if a large overdose has been taken. The dose of dobutamine should therefore be increased if necessary to achieve the required response according to the clinical condition of the patient.

Bronchospasm can usually be reversed by bronchodilators.

Excessive diuresis should be countered by maintaining normal fluid and electrolyte balance.

Pharmacological properties

Pharmacodynamic properties: Tenoret 50 combines the antihypertensive activity of two agents, a beta-adrenoceptor blocking drug (atenolol) and a diuretic (chlorthalidone).

Atenolol is $beta_1$- selective (ie acts preferentially on $beta_1$-adrenergic receptors in the heart). Selectivity decreases with increasing dose.

Atenolol is without intrinsic sympathomimetic and membrane stabilising activities and, as with other beta-adrenoceptor blocking drugs, has negative inotropic effects (and is therefore contra-indicated in uncontrolled heart failure).

As with other beta-adrenoceptor blocking drugs, the mode of action in the treatment of hypertension is unclear.

It is unlikely that any additional ancillary properties possessed by S (-) atenolol, in comparison with the racemic mixture, will give rise to different therapeutic effects.

Chlorthalidone, a monosulfonamyl diuretic, increases excretion of sodium and chloride. Natriuresis is accompanied by some loss of potassium. The mechanism by which chlorthalidone reduces blood pressure is not fully known but may be related to the excretion and redistribution of body sodium.

Atenolol is effective and well-tolerated in most ethnic populations. Black patients respond better to the combination of atenolol and chlorthalidone, than to atenolol alone.

The combination of atenolol with thiazide-like diuretics has been shown to be compatible and generally more effective than either drug used alone.

Pharmacokinetic properties: Absorption of atenolol following oral dosing is consistent but incomplete (approximately 40–50%) with peak plasma concentrations occurring 2–4 hours after dosing. The atenolol blood levels are consistent and subject to little variability. There is no significant hepatic metabolism of atenolol and more than 90% of that absorbed reaches the systemic circulation unaltered. The plasma half-life is about 6 hours but this may rise in severe renal impairment since the kidney is the major route of elimination. Atenolol penetrates tissues poorly due to its low lipid solubility and its concentration in brain tissue is low. Plasma protein binding is low (approximately 3%).

Absorption of chlorthalidone following oral dosing is consistent but incomplete (approximately 60%) with peak plasma concentrations occurring about 12 hours after dosing. The chlorthalidone blood levels are consistent and subject to little variability. The plasma half-life is about 50 hours and the kidney is the major route of elimination. Plasma protein binding is high (approximately 75%).

Co-administration of chlorthalidone and atenolol has little effect on the pharmacokinetics of either.

Tenoret 50 is effective for at least 24 hours after a single oral daily dose. This simplicity of dosing facilitates compliance by its acceptability to patients.

Pre-clinical safety data relevant to the prescriber: Atenolol and chlorthalidone are drugs on which extensive clinical experience has been obtained. Relevant information for the prescriber is provided elsewhere in the Prescribing Information.

Pharmaceutical particulars

List of excipients: Magnesium Carbonate PhEur; Maize Starch PhEur; Sodium Lauryl Sulphate PhEur; Gelatin PhEur; Magnesium Stearate PhEur; Methylhydroxypropylcellulose PhEur; Macrogol 300 BP; Iron Oxide (E172).

Incompatibilities: None known

Shelf life: 36 months.

Special precautions for storage: Store below 25°C. Protect from light and moisture.

Nature and content of container: Blister packs of 28 tablets contained in a carton.

Instructions for use/handling: Not applicable.

Marketing authorisation number 12619/0072

Date of approval/revision of SPC February 1998.

Legal category POM

TENORMIN* TABLETS
TENORMIN* LS TABLETS
TENORMIN* 25 TABLETS

Presentation Tenormin tablets, containing Atenolol PhEur 100 mg are round, biconvex, orange, film-coated tablets impressed with TENORMIN on one face and an 'S' logo on the reverse. The impressions are highlighted in white.

Tenormin LS tablets, containing Atenolol PhEur 50 mg are round, biconvex, orange, film-coated tablets impressed with TENORMIN LS on one face and bisected on the reverse. The impressions are highlighted in white.

Tenormin 25 tablets, containing Atenolol PhEur 25 mg, are round, biconvex, white, film-coated tablets impressed with TENORMIN 25 on one face and an 'S' logo on the reverse.

The inactive ingredients are gelatin, magnesium carbonate, magnesium stearate, methylhydroxypropylcellulose, sodium lauryl sulphate, maize starch and titanium dioxide. In addition, Tenormin 25 contains glycerol and Tenormin and Tenormin LS contain macrogol, sunset yellow lake and talc.

Uses

i) Management of hypertension
ii) Management of angina pectoris
iii) Management of cardiac arrhythmias
iv) Myocardial infarction: early intervention in the acute phase.

Mode of action: Tenormin (atenolol) is a beta-adrenoceptor blocking drug which is $beta_1$-selective (i.e. acts preferentially on $beta_1$-adrenergic receptors in the heart). Selectivity decreases with increasing dose. It is without intrinsic sympathomimetic and membrane stabilising activities, and, as with other beta-adrenoceptor blocking drugs, has negative inotropic effects (and is therefore contra-indicated in uncontrolled heart failure). As with other beta-adrenoceptor blocking drugs, its mode of action in the treatment of hypertension is unclear. It is probably the action of Tenormin in reducing cardiac rate and contractility which makes it effective in eliminating or reducing the symptoms of patients with angina. It is unlikely that any additional ancillary properties possessed by S(-) atenolol, in comparison with the racemic mixture, will give rise to different therapeutic effects.

Tenormin is effective and well tolerated in most ethnic populations although the response may be less in black patients. Tenormin is compatible with diuretics, other antihypertensive agents and antianginal agents (see *Warnings*).

Early intervention with Tenormin in acute myocardial infarction reduces infarct size and decreases morbidity and mortality. Fewer patients with a threatened infarction progress to frank infarction; the incidence of ventricular arrhythmias is decreased and marked pain relief may result in reduced need of opiate analgesics. Early mortality is decreased. Tenormin is an additional treatment to standard coronary care.

Absorption of atenolol following oral dosing is consistent but incomplete (approximately 40 to 50%) with peak plasma concentrations occurring 2 to 4 hours after dosing. Atenolol blood levels are consistent and subject to little variability. There is no significant hepatic metabolism of atenolol and more than 90% of that absorbed reaches the systemic circulation unaltered. The plasma half-life is about 6 hours but this may rise in severe renal impairment since the kidney is the major route of elimination. Atenolol penetrates tissues poorly due to its low lipid solubility and its concentration in brain tissue is low. Plasma protein binding is low (approximately 3%).

Dosage and administration *Adults: Hypertension:* One tablet daily. Most patients respond to 100 mg daily given orally as a single dose. Some patients, however, will respond to 50 mg given as a single daily dose. The effect will be fully established after one to two weeks. A further reduction in blood pressure may be achieved by combining Tenormin with other antihypertensive agents. For example, co-administration of Tenormin with a diuretic, as in Tenoretic, provides a highly effective and convenient antihypertensive therapy.

Angina: Most patients with angina pectoris will respond to 100 mg given orally once daily or 50 mg given twice daily. It is unlikely that additional benefit will be gained by increasing the dose.

Arrhythmias: A suitable initial dose of Tenormin is 2.5 mg (5 ml) injected intravenously over a 2.5 minute period (i.e. 1 mg/minute). (See also prescribing information for Tenormin Injection.) This may be repeated at 5 minute intervals until a response is observed up to a maximum dosage of 10 mg. If Tenormin is given by infusion, 150 micrograms/kg bodyweight may be administered over a 20 minute period. If required, the injection or infusion may be repeated every 12 hours. Having controlled the arrhythmias with intravenous 'Tenormin', a suitable oral maintenance dosage is 50 to 100 mg daily, given as a single dose.

Myocardial infarction: For patients suitable for treatment with intravenous beta-adrenoceptor blockade and presenting within 12 hours of the onset of the chest pain, Tenormin 5–10 mg should be given by slow intravenous injection (1 mg/minute) followed by Tenormin 50 mg orally about 15 minutes later provided no untoward effects occur from the intravenous dose. This should be followed by a further 50 mg orally 12 hours after the intravenous dose and then 12 hours later by 100 mg orally to be given once daily. If bradycardia and/or hypotension requiring treatment, or any other untoward effects occur, Tenormin should be discontinued.

Elderly patients: Dosage requirements may be reduced, especially in patients with impaired renal function.

Children: There is no paediatric experience with Tenormin and for this reason it is not recommended for use in children.

Renal failure: Since Tenormin is excreted via the kidneys dosage should be adjusted in cases of severe impairment of renal function. No significant accumulation of Tenormin occurs in patients who have a creatinine clearance greater than 35 ml/min/1.73 m² (normal range is 100 to 150 ml/min/1.73 m²). For patients with a creatinine clearance of 15 to 35 ml/min/1.73 m² (equivalent to serum creatinine of 300 to 600 micromol/litre) the oral dose should be 50 mg daily and the intravenous dose should be 10 mg once every two days. For patients with a creatinine clearance of <15 ml/min/1.73 m² (equivalent to serum creatinine of >600 micromol/litre) the oral dose should be 25 mg daily or 50 mg on alternate days and the intravenous dose should be 10 mg once every four days.

Patients on haemodialysis should be given 50 mg orally after each dialysis; this should be done under hospital supervision as marked falls in blood pressure can occur.

Contra-indications, warnings, etc Tenormin as with other beta-adrenoceptor blocking drugs, should not be used in patients with any of the following conditions: known hypersensitivity to the substance, bradycardia, cardiogenic shock, hypotension, metabolic acidosis, severe peripheral arterial circulatory disturbances, second or third degree heart block, sick sinus syndrome, untreated phaeochromocytoma or uncontrolled heart failure.

Tenormin as with other beta-adrenoceptor blocking drugs:

- although contra-indicated in uncontrolled heart failure (see *Contra-indications*), may be used in patients whose signs of heart failure have been controlled. Caution must be exercised in patients whose cardiac reserve is poor.
- may increase the number and duration of angina attacks in patients with Prinzmetal's angina due to unopposed alpha receptor mediated coronary artery vasoconstriction. Tenormin is a $beta_1$-selective beta-adrenoceptor blocking drug; consequently, its use may be considered although utmost caution must be exercised.
- although contra-indicated in severe peripheral arterial circulatory disturbances (see *Contra-indications*), may also aggravate less severe peripheral arterial circulatory disturbances.
- due to its negative effect on conduction time, caution must be exercised if it is given to patients with first degree heart block.
- may modify the tachycardia of hypoglycaemia.
- may mask the signs of thyrotoxicosis.
- will reduce heart rate, as a result of its pharmacological action. In the rare instances when a treated patient develops symptoms which may be attributable to a slow heart rate, the dose may be reduced.
- should not be discontinued abruptly in patients suffering from ischaemic heart disease.
- may cause a more severe reaction to a variety of allergens, when given to patients with a history of anaphylactic reaction to such allergens. Such patients may be unresponsive to the usual doses of adrenaline used to treat the allergic reactions.

Although cardioselective ($beta_1$) beta-adrenoceptor blocking drugs may have less effect on lung function than non-selective beta-adrenoceptor blocking drugs, as with all beta-adrenoceptor blocking drugs, these should be avoided in patients with reversible obstructive airways disease, unless there are compelling clinical reasons for their use. Where such reasons exist, Tenormin may be used with caution. Occasionally, some increase in airways resistance may occur in asthmatic patients, however, and this may usually be reversed by commonly used dosage of bronchodilators such as salbutamol or isoprenaline.

The label and patient information leaflet for this product state the following warning: "If you have ever had asthma or wheezing, you should not take this medicine unless you have discussed these symptoms with the prescribing doctor".

Caution must be exercised when prescribing a beta-adrenoceptor blocking drug with Class 1 antiarrhythmic agents such as disopyramide.

Combined use of beta-adrenoceptor blocking drugs and calcium channel blockers with negative inotropic effects e.g. verapamil, diltiazem can lead to an exaggeration of these effects, particularly in patients with impaired ventricular function and/or sino-atrial or atrio-ventricular conduction abnormalities. This may result in severe hypotension, bradycardia and cardiac failure. Neither the beta-adrenoceptor blocking drug nor the calcium channel blocker should be administered intravenously within 48 hours of discontinuing the other.

Concomitant therapy with dihydropyridines e.g. nifedipine, may increase the risk of hypotension, and cardiac failure may occur in patients with latent cardiac insufficiency.

Beta-adrenoceptor blocking drugs may exacerbate the rebound hypertension which can follow the withdrawal of clonidine. If the two drugs are co-administered, the beta-adrenoceptor blocking drug should be withdrawn several days before discontinuing clonidine. If replacing clonidine by beta-adrenoceptor blocking drug therapy, the introduction of beta-adrenoceptor blocking drugs should be delayed for several days after clonidine administration has stopped.

Digitalis glycosides, in association with beta-adrenoceptor blocking drugs, may increase atrio-ventricular conduction time.

Concomitant use of sympathomimetic agents, e.g. adrenaline, may counteract the effect of beta-adrenoceptor blocking drugs.

Concomitant use with insulin and oral antidiabetic drugs may lead to the intensification of the blood sugar lowering effects of these drugs.

Concomitant use of prostaglandin synthetase inhibiting drugs, e.g. ibuprofen or indomethacin, may decrease the hypotensive effects of beta-adrenoceptor blocking drugs.

Anaesthesia: Caution must be exercised when using anaesthetic agents with Tenormin. The anaesthetist should be informed and the choice of anaesthetic should be the agent with as little negative inotropic activity as possible. Use of beta-adrenoceptor blocking drugs with anaesthetic drugs may result in attenuation of the reflex tachycardia and increase the risk of hypotension. Anaesthetic agents causing myocardial depression are best avoided.

Pregnancy: Tenormin crosses the placental barrier and appears in the cord blood. No studies have been performed on the use of Tenormin in the first trimester and the possibility of foetal injury cannot be excluded. Tenormin has been used under close supervision for the treatment of hypertension in the third trimester. Administration of Tenormin to pregnant women in the management of mild to moderate hypertension has been associated with intra-uterine growth retardation.

The use of Tenormin in women who are, or may become pregnant, requires that the anticipated benefit be weighed against the possible risks, particularly in the first and second trimesters, since beta-adrenoceptor blocking agents, in general, have been associated with a decrease in placental perfusion which may result in intra-uterine deaths, immature and premature deliveries.

Lactation: There is significant accumulation of Tenormin in breast milk. Caution should be exercised when Tenormin is administered to a nursing woman.

Effect on ability to drive or operate machinery: The use of Tenormin is unlikely to result in any impairment of the ability of patients to drive or operate machinery. However, it should be taken into account that occasionally dizziness or fatigue may occur.

Undesirable events: Tenormin is well tolerated. In clinical studies, the undesired events reported are usually attributable to the pharmacological actions of atenolol.

The following undesired events, listed by body system, have been reported.

Cardiovascular: bradycardia, heart failure deterioration, postural hypotension which may be associated with syncope, cold extremities. In susceptible patients: precipitation of heart block, intermittent claudication, Raynaud's phenomenon.

CNS: confusion, dizziness, headache, mood changes, nightmares, psychoses and hallucinations, sleep disturbances of the type noted with other beta-adrenoceptor blocking drugs.

Gastrointestinal: dry mouth, gastrointestinal disturbances. Elevations of transaminase levels have been seen infrequently, rare cases of hepatic toxicity including intrahepatic cholestasis have been reported.

Haematological: purpura, thrombocytopenia.

Integumentary: alopecia, dry eyes, psoriasiform skin reactions, exacerbation of psoriasis, skin rashes.

Neurological: paraesthesia.

Respiratory: bronchospasm may occur in patients with bronchial asthma or a history of asthmatic complaints.

Special senses: visual disturbances.

Others: fatigue, an increase in ANA (antinuclear antibodies) has been observed, however the clinical relevance of this is not clear.

Discontinuance of the drug should be considered if, according to clinical judgement, the well-being of the patient is adversely affected by any of the above reactions.

Overdosage: The symptoms of overdosage may include bradycardia, hypotension, acute cardiac insufficiency and bronchospasm.

General treatment should include: close supervision, treatment in an intensive care ward, the use of gastric lavage, activated charcoal and a laxative to prevent absorption of any drug still present in the gastrointestinal tract, the use of plasma or plasma substitutes to treat hypotension and shock. The possible uses of haemodialysis or haemoperfusion may be considered.

Excessive bradycardia can be countered with atropine 1 to 2 mg intravenously and/or a cardiac pacemaker. If necessary, this may be followed by a bolus dose of glucagon 10 mg intravenously. If required, this may be repeated or followed by an intravenous infusion of glucagon 1 to 10 mg/hour depending on response. If no response to glucagon occurs or if glucagon is unavailable, a beta-adrenoceptor stimulant such as dobutamine 2.5 to 10 microgram/kg/minute by intravenous infusion may be given. Dobutamine, because of its positive inotropic effect could also be used to treat hypotension and acute cardiac insufficiency. It is likely that these doses would be inadequate to reverse the cardiac effects of beta-blockade if a large overdose has been taken. The dose of dobutamine should therefore be increased if necessary to achieve the required response according to the clinical condition of the patient.

Bronchospasm can usually be reversed by bronchodilators.

Pharmaceutical precautions Tenormin, Tenormin LS and Tenormin 25 Tablets should be stored below 30°C, protected from light and moisture.

Legal category POM.

Package quantities Tenormin Tablets: 100 mg in Calendar packs of 28. Tenormin LS Tablets: 50 mg in Calendar packs of 28. Tenormin 25 Tablets: 25 mg in Calendar packs of 28.

Further information Tenormin is effective for at least 24 hours after a single oral dose. The drug facilitates compliance by its acceptability to patients and simplicity of dosing. The narrow dose range and early patient response ensure that the effect of the drug in individual patients is quickly demonstrated. Tenormin is compatible with diuretics, other hypotensive agents and antianginals (but see *Warnings*). Since it acts preferentially on beta-adrenergic receptors in the heart, Tenormin may, with care, be used successfully in the treatment of patients with respiratory disease who cannot tolerate non-selective beta-adrenoceptor blocking drugs.

Product licence numbers

Tenormin Tablets 12619/0078
Tenormin LS Tablets 12619/0077
Tenormin 25 Tablets 12619/0076

TENORMIN* INJECTION

Presentation Tenormin Injection contains 5 mg Atenolol PhEur in 10 ml isotonic, citrate buffered aqueous solution. The inactive ingredients are citric acid/sodium citrate, sodium chloride and water.

Uses Management of arrhythmias and for the early intervention treatment of acute myocardial infarction.

Mode of action: Tenormin (atenolol) is a beta-adrenoceptor blocking drug which is $beta_1$-selective (i.e. acts preferentially on $beta_1$-adrenergic receptors in the heart). Selectivity decreases with increasing dose. Atenolol is without intrinsic sympathomimetic and membrane stabilising activities, and, as with other beta-adrenoceptor blocking drugs, has negative inotropic effects (and is therefore contra-indicated in uncontrolled heart failure). As with other beta-adrenoceptor blocking drugs, its mode of action in the treatment of hypertension is unclear. It is probably the action of Tenormin in reducing cardiac rate and contractility which makes it effective in eliminating or reducing the symptoms of patients with angina. It is unlikely that any additional ancillary properties possessed by S(-) atenolol, in comparison with the racemic mixture, will give rise to different therapeutic effects.

Tenormin is effective and well tolerated in most ethnic populations although the response may be less in black patients. Tenormin is compatible with diuretics, other antihypertensive agents and antianginal agents (see *Warnings*).

Early intervention with Tenormin in acute myocardial infarction reduces infarct size and decreases morbidity and mortality. Fewer patients with a threatened infarction progress to frank infarction; the incidence of ventricular arrhythmias is decreased and marked pain relief may result in reduced need of opiate analgesics. Early mortality is decreased. Tenormin is an additional treatment to standard coronary care.

Following intravenous administration, the blood levels of atenolol decay tri-exponentially with an elimination half-life of about 6 hours. Throughout the intravenous dose range of 5 to 10 mg the blood level profile obeys linear pharmacokinetics and beta-blockade is still measurable 24 hours after a 10 mg intravenous dose. The plasma half-life is about 6 hours but this may rise in severe renal impairment since the kidney is the major route of elimination. Atenolol penetrates tissues poorly due to its low lipid solubility and its concentration in brain tissue is low. Plasma protein binding is low (approximately 3%).

Dosage and administration *Adults: Arrhythmias:* A suitable initial dose of Tenormin is 2.5 mg (5 ml) injected intravenously over a 2.5 minute period (ie 1 mg/minute). This may be repeated at 5 minute intervals until a response is observed up to a maximum dosage of 10 mg. If Tenormin is given by infusion, 150 microgram/kg body weight may be administered over a 20 minute period. If required, the injection or infusion may be repeated every 12 hours. Having controlled the arrhythmias with intravenous Tenormin a suitable oral maintenance dosage is 50 to 100 mg daily (see prescribing information for Tenormin and Tenormin LS Tablets).

Myocardial infarction: For patients suitable for treatment with intravenous beta-adrenoceptor blockade and presenting within 12 hours of the onset of the chest pain, Tenormin 5 to 10 mg should be given by slow intravenous injection (1 mg per minute) followed by Tenormin 50 mg orally about 15 minutes later provided no untoward effects occur from the intravenous dose. This should be followed by a further 50 mg orally 12 hours after the intravenous dose and then 12 hours later by 100 mg orally to be given once daily. If bradycardia and/or hypotension requiring treatment or any other untoward effects occur, Tenormin should be discontinued.

Elderly patients: Dosage requirements may be reduced, especially in patients with impaired renal function.

Children: There is no paediatric experience with Tenormin and for this reason it is not recommended for children.

Renal failure: Since Tenormin is excreted via the kidneys, dosage should be adjusted in cases of severe impairment of renal function. No significant accumulation of Tenormin occurs in patients who have a creatinine clearance greater than 35 ml/min/1.73 m^2 (normal range is 100 to 150 ml/min/1.73 m^2). For patients with a creatinine clearance of 15 to 35 ml/min/1.73 m^2 (equivalent to serum creatinine of 300 to 600 micromol/litre) the oral dose should be 50 mg daily and the intravenous dose should be 10 mg once every two days. For patients with a creatinine clearance of <15 ml/min/1.73 m^2 (equivalent to serum creatinine of >600 micromol/litre) the oral dose should be 25 mg daily or 50 mg on alternate days; and the intravenous dose should be 10 mg once every four days.

Patients on haemodialysis should be given 50 mg orally after each dialysis; this should be done under hospital supervision as marked falls in blood pressure can occur.

Contra-indications, warnings, etc Tenormin as with other beta-adrenoceptor blocking drugs, should not be used in patients with any of the following conditions: known hypersensitivity to the substance, bradycardia, cardiogenic shock, hypotension, metabolic acidosis, severe peripheral arterial circulatory disturbances, second or third degree heart block, sick sinus syndrome, untreated phaeochromocytoma or uncontrolled heart failure.

Tenormin as with other beta-adrenoceptor blocking drugs:

- although contra-indicated in uncontrolled heart failure (see *Contra-indications*), may be used in patients whose signs of heart failure have been controlled. Caution must be exercised in patients whose cardiac reserve is poor.
- may increase the number and duration of angina attacks in patients with Prinzmetal's angina due to unopposed alpha receptor mediated coronary artery vasoconstriction. Tenormin is a $beta_1$-selective beta-adrenoceptor blocking drug; consequently, its use may be considered although utmost caution must be exercised.
- although contra-indicated in severe peripheral arterial circulatory disturbances (see *Contra-indications*), may also aggravate less severe peripheral arterial circulatory disturbances.
- due to its negative effect on conduction time, caution must be exercised if it is given to patients with first degree heart block.
- may modify the tachycardia of hypoglycaemia.
- may mask the signs of thyrotoxicosis.
- will reduce heart rate, as a result of its pharmacological action. In the rare instances when a treated patient develops symptoms which may be attributable to a slow heart rate, the dose may be reduced.
- should not be discontinued abruptly in patients suffering from ischaemic heart disease.
- may cause a more severe reaction to a variety of allergens, when given to patients with a history of anaphylactic reaction to such allergens. Such patients may be unresponsive to the usual doses of adrenaline used to treat the allergic reactions.

Although cardioselective ($beta_1$) beta-adrenoceptor blocking drugs may have less effect on lung function than non-selective beta-adrenoceptor blocking drugs, as with all beta-adrenoceptor blocking drugs, these should be avoided in patients with reversible obstructive airways disease, unless there are compelling clinical reasons for their use. Where such reasons exist, Tenormin may be used with caution. Occasionally, some increase in airways resistance may occur in asthmatic patients, however, and this may usually be reversed by commonly used dosage of bronchodilators such as salbutamol or isoprenaline.

The label and patient information leaflet for this product state the following warnings:

Label: "Tenormin Injection should be used with caution in patients with a history of asthma or wheezing".

Patient Information Leaflet: "If you have ever had asthma or wheezing, you should not be given this medicine unless you have discussed these symptoms with the prescribing doctor".

Caution must be exercised when prescribing a beta-adrenoceptor blocking drug with Class 1 antiarrhythmic agents such as disopyramide.

Combined use of beta-adrenoceptor blocking drugs and calcium channel blockers with negative inotropic effects e.g. verapamil, diltiazem can lead to an exaggeration of these effects, particularly in patients with impaired ventricular function and/or sino-atrial or atrio-ventricular conduction abnormalities. This may result in severe hypotension, bradycardia and cardiac failure. Neither the beta-adrenoceptor blocking drug nor the calcium channel blocker should be administered intravenously within 48 hours of discontinuing the other.

Concomitant therapy with dihydropyridines e.g. nifedipine, may increase the risk of hypotension, and cardiac failure may occur in patients with latent cardiac insufficiency.

Beta-adrenoceptor blocking drugs may exacerbate the rebound hypertension which can follow the withdrawal of clonidine. If the two drugs are co-administered, the beta-adrenoceptor blocking drug should be withdrawn several days before discontinuing clonidine. If replacing clonidine by beta-adrenoceptor blocking drug therapy, the introduction of beta-adrenoceptor blocking drugs should be delayed for several days after clonidine administration has stopped.

Digitalis glycosides, in association with beta-adrenoceptor blocking drugs, may increase atrio-ventricular conduction time.

Concomitant use of sympathomimetic agents, e.g. adrenaline, may counteract the effect of beta-adrenoceptor blocking drugs.

Concomitant use with insulin and oral antidiabetic drugs may lead to the intensification of the blood sugar lowering effects of these drugs.

Concomitant use of prostaglandin synthetase inhibiting drugs, e.g. ibuprofen or indomethacin, may decrease the hypotensive effects of beta-adrenoceptor blocking drugs.

Anaesthesia: Caution must be exercised when using anaesthetic agents with Tenormin. The anaesthetist should be informed and the choice of anaesthetic should be the agent with as little negative inotropic activity as possible. Use of beta-adrenoceptor blocking drugs with anaesthetic drugs may result in attenuation of the reflex tachycardia and increase the risk of hypotension. Anaesthetic agents causing myocardial depression are best avoided.

Pregnancy: Tenormin crosses the placental barrier and appears in the cord blood. No studies have been performed on the use of Tenormin in the first trimester and the possibility of foetal injury cannot be excluded. Tenormin has been used under close supervision for the treatment of hypertension in the third trimester. Administration of Tenormin to pregnant women in the management of mild to moderate hypertension has been associated with intra-uterine growth retardation.

The use of Tenormin in women who are, or may become pregnant, requires that the anticipated benefit be weighed against the possible risks, particularly in the first and second trimesters, since beta-andrenoceptor blocking agents, in general, have been associated with a decrease in placental perfusion which may result in intra-uterine deaths, immature and premature deliveries.

Lactation: There is significant accumulation of Tenormin in breast milk. Caution should be exercised when Tenormin is administered to a nursing woman.

Effect on ability to drive or operate machinery: The use of Tenormin is unlikely to result in any impairment of the ability of patients to drive or operate machinery. However, it should be taken into account that occasionally dizziness or fatigue may occur.

Undesirable events: Tenormin is well tolerated. In clinical studies, the undesired events reported are usually attributable to the pharmacological actions of atenolol.

The following undesired events, listed by body system, have been reported.

Cardiovascular: bradycardia, heart failure deterioration, postural hypotension which may be associated with syncope, cold extremities. In susceptible patients: precipitation of heart block, intermittent claudication, Raynaud's phenomenon.

CNS: confusion, dizziness, headache, mood changes, nightmares, psychoses and hallucinations, sleep disturbances of the type noted with other beta-adrenoceptor blocking drugs.

Gastrointestinal: dry mouth, gastrointestinal disturbances. Elevations of transaminase levels have been seen infrequently, rare cases of hepatic toxicity including intrahepatic cholestasis have been reported.

Haematological: purpura, thrombocytopenia.

Integumentary: alopecia, dry eyes, psoriasiform skin reactions, exacerbation of psoriasis, skin rashes.

Neurological: paraesthesia.

Respiratory: bronchospasm may occur in patients with bronchial asthma or a history of asthmatic complaints.

Special senses: visual disturbances.

Others: fatigue, an increase in ANA (antinuclear antibodies) has been observed, however the clinical relevance of this is not clear.

Discontinuance of the drug should be considered if, according to clinical judgement, the well-being of the patient is adversely affected by any of the above reactions.

Overdosage: The symptoms of overdosage may include bradycardia, hypotension, acute cardiac insufficiency and bronchospasm.

General treatment should include: close supervision, treatment in an intensive care ward, the use of gastric lavage, activated charcoal and a laxative to prevent absorption of any drug still present in the gastrointestinal tract, the use of plasma or plasma substitutes to treat hypotension and shock. The possible use of haemodialysis or haemoperfusion may be considered.

Excessive bradycardia can be countered with atropine 1 to 2 mg intravenously and/or a cardiac pacemaker. If necessary, this may be followed by a bolus dose of glucagon 10 mg intravenously. If required, this may be repeated or followed by an intravenous infusion of glucagon 1 to 10 mg/hour depending on response. If no response to glucagon occurs or if glucagon is unavailable, a beta-adrenoceptor stimulant such as dobutamine 2.5 to 10 microgram/kg/minute by intravenous infusion may be given. Dobutamine, because of its positive inotropic effect could also be used to treat hypotension and acute cardiac insufficiency. It is likely that these doses would be inadequate to reverse the cardiac effects of beta-blockade if a large overdose has been taken. The dose of dobutamine should therefore be increased if necessary to achieve the required response according to the clinical condition of the patient.

Bronchospasm can usually be reversed by bronchodilators.

Pharmaceutical precautions Tenormin Injection should be stored below 25°C, protected from light.

Dilutions of Tenormin Injection in Dextrose Injection BP, Sodium Chloride Injection BP, or Sodium Chloride and Dextrose Injection BP may be used.

Legal category POM.

Package quantities *Injection:* 10 ml ampoules in boxes of 10.

Further information The narrow dose range and early patient response to Tenormin ensure that the effect of the drug in individual patients is quickly demonstrated. Tenormin is fully compatible with diuretics, other hypotensive agents and antianginals (but see *Warnings*). Since it acts preferentially on beta-adrenergic receptors in the heart, Tenormin may, with care, be used successfully in the treatment of patients with respiratory disease who cannot tolerate non selective beta-adrenoceptor blocking drugs.

Product licence number 12619/0074.

TENORMIN SYRUP

Qualitative and quantitative composition Atenolol PhEur 0.5% w/v.

Pharmaceutical form Syrup.

Clinical particulars

Therapeutic indications:

(i) Management of hypertension;
(ii) Management of angina;
(iii) Management of cardiac arrhythmias;
(iv) Myocardial infarction. Early intervention in the acute phase.

Posology and method of administration:

Adults: Hypertension: Two or four 5 ml spoonfuls daily i.e. 50 mg or 100 mg in patients unable to take 50 mg or 100 mg tablets.

Most patients respond to 100 mg once daily. Some patients, however, will respond to 50 mg given as a single daily dose. The effect will be fully established after one to two weeks. A further reduction in blood pressure may be achieved by combining Tenormin with other antihypertensive agents.

Angina: Most patients with angina pectoris will respond to 100 mg (four 5 ml spoonfuls) given orally once a day, or 50 mg (two 5 ml spoonfuls) given twice daily. It is unlikely that additional benefit will be gained by increasing the dose.

Arrhythmias: A suitable initial dose of Tenormin Injection is 2.5 mg (5 ml) given intravenously over a 2.5 minute period (i.e. 1 mg/minute). (See prescribing information for Tenormin Injection). This may be repeated at 5 minute intervals until a response is observed up to a maximum dosage of 10 mg. If Tenormin Injection is given by infusion, 0.15 mg/kg body weight may be administered over a 20 minute period. If required, the injection or infusion may be repeated every 12 hours. Having controlled the arrhythmias, a suitable oral maintenance dosage is 50–100 mg (two to four 5 ml spoonfuls of Tenormin Syrup) daily, given as a single dose.

Myocardial infarction: For patients suitable for treatment with intravenous beta-adrenoceptor blockade and presenting within 12 hours of the onset of the chest pain, Tenormin Injection 5–10 mg should be given by slow intravenous administration (1 mg/minute) followed by Tenormin Syrup 50 mg (two 5 ml spoonfuls) orally about 15 minutes later, provided no untoward effects occur from the intravenous dose. This should be followed by a further 50 mg orally, 12 hours after the intravenous dose and then 12 hours later by 100 mg (four 5 ml spoonfuls) orally, to be given once daily. If bradycardia and/or hypotension requiring treatment, or any other untoward effects occur, Tenormin should be discontinued.

Elderly patients: Dosage requirements may be reduced, especially in patients with impaired renal function.

Children: There is no paediatric experience with Tenormin and for this reason it is not recommended for use in children.

Renal failure: Since Tenormin is excreted via the kidneys, dosage should be adjusted in cases of severe impairment of renal function. No significant accumulation of Tenormin occurs in patients who have a creatinine clearance greater than 35 ml/min/1.73 m^2 (Normal range is 100–150 ml/min/1.73 m^2). For patients with a creatinine clearance of 15–35 ml/min/1.73 m^2 (equivalent to serum creatinine of 300–600 micromol/litre) the oral dose should be 50 mg daily and the intravenous dose should be 10 mg once every two days. For patients with a creatinine clearance of <15 ml/min/1.73 m^2 (equivalent to serum creatinine of >600 micromol/litre) the oral dose should be 25 mg daily or 50 mg on alternate days and the intravenous dose should be 10 mg once every four days.

Patients on haemodialysis should be given 50 mg orally after each dialysis: this should be done under hospital supervision as marked falls in blood pressure can occur.

Contra-indications: Tenormin, as with other beta-adrenoceptor blocking drugs, should not be used in patients with any of the following: known hypersensitivity to the substance; bradycardia; cardiogenic shock; hypotension; metabolic acidosis; severe peripheral arterial circulatory disturbances; second or third degree heart block; sick sinus syndrome; untreated phaeochromocytoma; uncontrolled heart failure.

Special warnings and special precautions for use: Tenormin as with other beta-adrenoceptor blocking agents:

- although contraindicated in uncontrolled heart failure (see *Contraindications*), may be used in patients whose signs of heart failure have been controlled. Caution must be exercised in patients whose cardiac reserve is poor.
- may increase the number and duration of angina attacks in patients with Prinzmetal's angina due to unopposed alpha receptor mediated coronary artery vasoconstriction. Tenormin is a $beta_1$-selective beta-adrenoceptor blocking drug; consequently, its use may be considered although utmost caution must be exercised.
- although contraindicated in severe peripheral arterial circulatory disturbances (see *Contraindications*), may also aggravate less severe peripheral arterial circulatory disturbances.
- due to its negative effect on conduction time, caution must be exercised if it is given to patients with first degree heart block.
- may modify the tachycardia of hypoglycaemia.
- may mask the signs of thyrotoxicosis.
- will reduce heart rate, as a result of its pharmacological action. In the rare instances when a treated patient develops symptoms which may be attributable to a slow heart rate, the dose may be reduced.
- should not be discontinued abruptly in patients suffering from ischaemic heart disease.
- may cause a more severe reaction to a variety of allergens, when given to patients with a history of anaphylactic reaction to such allergens. Such patients may be unresponsive to the usual doses of adrenaline used to treat the allergic reactions.

Although cardioselective ($beta_1$) beta-adrenoceptor blocking drugs may have less effect on lung function than non-selective beta-adrenoceptor blocking drugs, as with all beta-adrenoceptor blocking drugs, these should be avoided in patients with reversible obstructive airways disease, unless there are compelling clinical reasons for their use. Where such reasons exist, Tenormin may be used with caution. Occasionally, some increase in airways resistance may occur in asthmatic patients, however, and this may usually be reversed by commonly used dosage of bronchodilators such as salbutamol or isoprenaline.

The label and patient information leaflet for this product state the following warning: 'If you have ever had asthma or wheezing, you should not take this medicine unless you have discussed these symptoms with the prescribing doctor'.

Interactions with other medicaments and other forms of interaction: Combined use of beta-adrenoceptor blocking drugs and calcium channel blockers with negative inotropic effects e.g. verapamil, diltiazem, can lead to an exaggeration of these effects particularly in patients with impaired ventricular function and/or sino-atrial or atrio-ventricular conduction abnormalities. This may result in severe hypotension, bradycardia and cardiac failure. Neither the beta-adrenoceptor blocking drug nor the calcium channel blocker should be administered intravenously within 48 hours of discontinuing the other.

Concomitant therapy with dihydropyridines e.g. nifedipine, may increase the risk of hypotension, and cardiac failure may occur in patients with latent cardiac insufficiency.

Digitalis glycosides, in association with beta-adrenoceptor blocking drugs, may increase atrioventricular conduction time.

Beta-adrenoceptor blocking drugs may exacerbate the rebound hypertension which can follow the withdrawal of clonidine. If the two drugs are co-administered, the beta-adrenoceptor blocking drug should be withdrawn several days before discontinuing clonidine. If replacing clonidine by beta-adrenoceptor blocking drug therapy, the introduction of beta-adrenoceptor blocking drugs should be delayed for several days after clonidine administration has stopped. (See also prescribing information for clonidine).

Caution must be exercised when prescribing a beta-adrenoceptor blocking drug with Class 1 antiarrhythmic agents such as disopyramide.

Concomitant use of sympathomimetic agents, e.g. adrenaline, may counteract the effect of beta-adrenoceptor blocking drugs.

Concomitant use with insulin and oral antidiabetic drugs may lead to the intensification of the blood sugar lowering effects of these drugs.

Concomitant use of prostaglandin synthetase inhibiting drugs (e.g. ibuprofen, indomethacin), may decrease the hypotensive effects of beta-adrenoceptor blocking drugs.

Caution must be exercised when using anaesthetic agents with Tenormin. The anaesthetist should be informed and the choice of anaesthetic should be an agent with as little negative inotropic activity as possible. Use of beta-adrenoceptor blocking drugs with anaesthetic drugs may result in attenuation of the reflex tachycardia and increase the risk of hypotension. Anaesthetic agents causing myocardial depression are best avoided.

Pregnancy and lactation:
Pregnancy: Tenormin crosses the placental barrier and appears in the cord blood. No studies have been performed on the use of Tenormin in the first trimester and the possibility of foetal injury cannot be excluded. Tenormin has been used under close supervision for the treatment of hypertension in the third trimester. Administration of Tenormin to pregnant women in the management of mild to moderate hypertension has been associated with intra-uterine growth retardation.

The use of Tenormin in women who are, or may become, pregnant requires that the anticipated benefit be weighed against the possible risks, particularly in the first and second trimesters, since beta-adrenoceptor blocking agents, in general, have been associated with a decrease in placental perfusion which may result in intra-uterine deaths, immature and premature deliveries.

Lactation: There is significant accumulation of Tenormin in breast milk. Caution should be exercised when Tenormin is administered to a nursing woman.

Effects on ability to drive and use machines: Use is unlikely to result in any impairment of the ability of patients to drive or operate machinery. However, it should be taken into account that occasionally dizziness or fatigue may occur.

Undesirable effects: Tenormin is well tolerated. In clinical studies, the undesired events reported are usually attributable to the pharmacological actions of atenolol.

The following undesired events, listed by body system, have been reported.

Cardiovascular: bradycardia; heart failure deterioration; postural hypotension which may be associated with syncope; cold extremities. In susceptible patients: precipitation of heart block; intermittent claudication, Raynaud's phenomenon.

CNS: confusion; dizziness; headache; mood changes; nightmares; psychoses and hallucinations; sleep disturbances of the type noted with other beta-adrenoceptor blocking drugs.

Gastrointestinal: dry mouth, gastrointestinal disturbances. Elevations of transaminase levels have been seen infrequently, rare cases of hepatic toxicity including intrahepatic cholestasis have been reported.

Haematological: purpura; thrombocytopenia.

Integumentary: alopecia; dry eyes; psoriasiform skin reactions; exacerbation of psoriasis; skin rashes.

Neurological: paraesthesia.

Respiratory: bronchospasm may occur in patients with bronchial asthma or a history of asthmatic complaints.

Special senses: visual disturbances.

Others: fatigue; an increase in ANA (antinuclear antibodies) has been observed, however the clinical relevance of this is not clear.

Discontinuance of the drug should be considered if, according to clinical judgement, the well-being of the patient is adversely affected by any of the above reactions.

Overdosage: The symptoms of overdosage may include bradycardia, hypotension, acute cardiac insufficiency and bronchospasm.

General treatment should include: close supervision, treatment in an intensive care ward, the use of gastric lavage, activated charcoal and a laxative to prevent absorption of any drug still present in the gastrointestinal tract, the use of plasma or plasma substitutes to treat hypotension and shock. The possible uses of haemodialysis or haemoperfusion may be considered.

Excessive bradycardia may be countered with atropine 1–2 mg intravenously and/or a cardiac pacemaker. If necessary, this may be followed by a bolus dose of glucagon 10 mg intravenously. If required, this may be repeated or followed by an intravenous infusion of glucagon 1–10 mg/hour depending on response. If no response to glucagon occurs or if glucagon is unavailable, a beta-adrenoceptor stimulant such as dobutamine 2.5 to 10 micrograms/kg/minute by intravenous infusion may be given. Dobutamine, because of its positive inotropic effect could also be used to treat hypotension and acute cardiac insufficiency. It is likely that these doses would be inadequate to reverse the cardiac effects of beta-adrenoceptor blockade if a large overdose has been taken. The dose of dobutamine should therefore be increased if necessary to achieve the required response according to the clinical condition of the patient.

Bronchospasm can usually be reversed by bronchodilators.

Pharmacological properties

Pharmacodynamic properties: Atenolol is a beta-adrenoceptor blocking drug which is $beta_1$-selective (i.e. acts preferentially on $beta_1$-adrenergic receptors in the heart). Selectivity decreases with increasing dose.

Atenolol is without intrinsic sympathomimetic and membrane stabilising activities and as with other beta-adrenoceptor blocking drugs, has negative inotropic effects (and is therefore contra-indicated in uncontrolled heart failure).

As with other beta-adrenoceptor blocking drugs, the mode of action of atenolol in the treatment of hypertension is unclear.

It is probably the action of atenolol in reducing cardiac rate and contractility which makes it effective in eliminating or reducing the symptoms of patients with angina.

It is unlikely that any additional ancillary properties possessed by S (-) atenolol, in comparison with the racemic mixture, will give rise to different therapeutic effects.

Tenormin is effective and well-tolerated in most ethnic populations although the response may be less in black patients.

Tenormin is compatible with diuretics, other antihypertensive agents and antianginal agents (see *Interactions with other medicaments and other forms of interaction*).

Early intervention with Tenormin in acute myocardial infarction reduces infarct size and decreases morbidity and mortality. Fewer patients with a threatened infarction progress to frank infarction; the incidence of ventricular arrhythmias is decreased and marked pain relief may result in reduced need of opiate analgesics. Early mortality is decreased. Tenormin is an additional treatment to standard coronary care.

Pharmacokinetic properties: Absorption of atenolol following oral dosing is consistent but incomplete (approximately 40–50%) with peak plasma concentrations occurring 2–4 hours after dosing. The atenolol blood levels are consistent and subject to little variability. There is no significant hepatic metabolism of atenolol and more than 90% of that absorbed reaches the systemic circulation unaltered. The plasma half-life is about 6 hours but this may rise in severe renal impairment since the kidney is the major route of elimination. Atenolol penetrates tissues poorly due to its low lipid solubility and its concentration in brain tissue is low. Plasma protein binding is low (approximately 3%).

Preclinical safety data: Atenolol is a drug on which extensive clinical experience has been obtained. Relevant information for the prescriber is provided elsewhere in the Summary of Product Characteristics.

Pharmaceutical particulars

List of excipients: Citric acid PhEur; Lemon and lime flavour; Methyl hydroxybenzoate PhEur; Propyl hydroxybenzoate PhEur; Purified water PhEur; Saccharin sodium BP; Sodium citrate PhEur; Sorbitol solution BPC.

Incompatibilities: See *Interactions with other medicaments and other forms of interaction.*

Shelf life: 3 years.

Special precautions for storage: Store below 25°C, protected from light.

Nature and contents of container: Amber coloured PET bottles with white polypropylene screw caps containing 300 mls.

Instructions for use/handling: Not applicable.

Additional information: Tenormin syrup is intended for patients unable to swallow Tenormin tablets.

Tenormin is effective for at least 24 hours after once daily dosing with 10 ml or 20 ml Tenormin syrup. Tenormin syrup facilitates compliance by its acceptability to patients and the once daily dosing regimen. The narrow dose range and early patient response ensure that the effect of the drug in individual patients is quickly demonstrated. Tenormin is compatible with diuretics, other hypotensive agents and antianginals (but see *Interactions with other medicaments and other forms of interaction*). Since it acts preferentially on beta-adrenergic receptors in the heart, Tenormin may, with care, be used successfully in the treatment of patients with respiratory disease, who cannot tolerate non-selective beta-adrenoceptor blocking drugs.

Market authorisation number 12619/0075

Date of approval/revision of SPC February 1998

Legal category POM

TOMUDEX* ▼

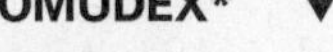

Qualitative and quantitative composition Tomudex contains 2 mg raltitrexed in each vial.

Pharmaceutical form Powder for intravenous injection.

Clinical particulars
Therapeutic indications: The palliative treatment of advanced colorectal cancer where 5-fluorouracil and folinic acid based regimens are either not tolerated or inappropriate.

Posology and method of administration:
Adults: The dose of Tomudex is calculated on the basis of the body surface area. The recommended dose is 3 mg/m² given intravenously, as a single short, intravenous infusion in 50 to 250 ml of either 0.9% sodium chloride solution or 5% dextrose (glucose) solution. It is recommended that the infusion is given over a 15 minute period. Other drugs should not be mixed with Tomudex in the same infusion container. In the absence of toxicity, treatment may be repeated every 3 weeks.

Dose escalation above 3 mg/m² is not recommended, since higher doses have been associated with an increased incidence of life-threatening or fatal toxicity.

Prior to the initiation of treatment and before each subsequent treatment a full blood count (including a differential count and platelets), liver transaminases, serum bilirubin and serum creatinine measurements should be performed. The total white cell count should be greater than 4,000/mm³, the neutrophil count greater than 2,000/mm³ and the platelet count greater than 100,000/mm³ prior to treatment. In the event of toxicity the next scheduled dose should be withheld until signs of toxic effects regress. In particular, signs of gastrointestinal toxicity (diarrhoea or mucositis) and haematological toxicity (neutropenia or thrombocytopenia) should have completely resolved before subsequent treatment is allowed. Patients who develop signs of gastrointestinal toxicity should have their full blood counts monitored at least weekly for signs of haematological toxicity.

Based on the worst grade of gastrointestinal and haematological toxicity observed on the previous treatment and provided that such toxicity has completely resolved, the following dose reductions are recommended for subsequent treatment:

25% dose reduction: in patients with WHO grade 3 haematological toxicity (neutropenia or thrombocytopenia) or WHO grade 2 gastrointestinal toxicity (diarrhoea or mucositis).

50% dose reduction: in patients with WHO grade 4 haematological toxicity (neutropenia or thrombocytopenia) or WHO grade 3 gastrointestinal toxicity (diarrhoea or mucositis).

Once a dose reduction has been made, all subsequent doses should be given at the reduced dose.

Treatment should be discontinued in the event of any WHO grade 4 gastrointestinal toxicity (diarrhoea or mucositis) or in the event of a WHO grade 3 gastrointestinal toxicity associated with WHO grade 4 haematological toxicity. Patients with such toxicity should be managed promptly with standard supportive care measures including i.v. hydration and bone marrow support. In addition pre-clinical data suggest that consideration should be given to the administration of folinic acid. From clinical experience with other antifolates folinic acid may be given at a dose of 25 mg/m² i.v. every 6 hours until the resolution of symptoms. Further use of Tomudex in such patients is not recommended.

It is essential that the dose reduction scheme should be adhered to since the potential for life threatening and fatal toxicity increases if the dose is not reduced or treatment not stopped as appropriate.

Elderly: Dosage and administration as for adults. However, as with other cytotoxics, Tomudex should be used with caution in elderly patients (see *Warnings/Precautions*).

Children: Tomudex is not recommended for use in children as safety and efficacy have not been established in this group of patients.

Renal impairment: For patients with abnormal serum creatinine, before the first or any subsequent treatment, a creatinine clearance should be performed or calculated. For patients with a normal serum creatinine when the serum creatinine may not correlate well with the creatinine clearance due to factors such as age or weight loss, the same procedure should be followed. If creatinine clearance is ≤65 ml/min, the following dose modifications are recommended:

Dose modification in the presence of renal impairment

Creatinine clearance	*Dose as % of 3.0 mg/m²*	*Dosing interval*
>65 ml/min	Full dose	3-weekly
25 to 65 ml/min	50%	4-weekly
55 to 65 ml/min	75%	4-weekly
<25 ml/min	No therapy	Not applicable

See Contra-indications for use in patients with severe renal impairment.

Hepatic impairment: No dosage adjustment is recommended for patients with mild to moderate hepatic impairment. However, given that a proportion of the drug is excreted via the faecal route (see *Pharmacokinetic properties*), and that these patients usually form a poor prognosis group, patients with mild to moderate hepatic impairment need to be treated with caution. (See *Warnings and precautions for use.*) Tomudex has not been studied in patients with severe hepatic impairment, clinical jaundice or decompensated liver disease and its use in such patients is not recommended.

Contra-indications: Tomudex should not be used in pregnant women, in women who may become pregnant during treatment or women who are breast feeding. Pregnancy should be excluded before treatment with Tomudex is commenced (see *Pregnancy* section).

Tomudex is contra-indicated in patients with severe renal impairment.

Special warnings and special precautions for use: It is recommended that Tomudex is only given by or under the supervision of a physician who is experienced in cancer chemotherapy, and in the management of chemotherapy-related toxicity. Patients undergoing therapy should be subject to appropriate supervision so that signs of possible toxic effects or adverse reactions may be detected and treated promptly (see *Posology and method of administration*).

In common with other cytotoxic agents of this type, caution is necessary in patients with depressed bone marrow function, poor general condition, or prior radiotherapy.

Patients whose disease progressed on previous treatment for advanced disease with 5-fluorouracil based regimens may also be resistant to the effects of Tomudex.

Elderly patients are more vulnerable to the toxic effects of Tomudex. Extreme care should be taken to ensure adequate monitoring of adverse reactions especially signs of gastrointestinal toxicity (diarrhoea or mucositis).

A proportion of the Tomudex is excreted via the faecal route (see *Pharmacokinetic properties*), therefore, patients with mild to moderate hepatic impairment should be treated with caution.

Treatment with Tomudex in patients with severe hepatic impairment is not recommended.

It is recommended that pregnancy should be avoided during treatment and for at least 6 months after cessation of treatment if either partner is receiving Tomudex (see also *Pregnancy and lactation*).

There is no clinical experience with extravasation. However, perivascular tolerance studies in animals did not reveal any significant irritant reaction.

Tomudex is a cytotoxic agent and should be handled according to normal procedures adopted for such agents (see *Instructions for use/handling*).

Interaction with other medicaments and other forms of interaction: No specific interaction studies have been conducted in man.

Folinic acid, folic acid or vitamin preparations containing these agents must not be given immediately prior to or during administration of Tomudex, since they may interfere with its action.

There is no experience to date in relation to the combined use of Tomudex with other cytotoxic agents.

Tomudex is 93% protein bound and while it has the potential to interact with similarly highly protein bound drugs, no displacement interaction with warfarin has been observed *in vitro*. Data suggest that active tubular secretion may contribute to the renal excretion of raltitrexed, indicating a potential interaction with other actively secreted drugs such as nonsteroidal anti-inflammatory drugs (NSAIDs). However, a review of the clinical trial safety database did not reveal evidence of clinically significant interaction in patients treated with Tomudex who also received concomitant NSAIDs, warfarin and other commonly prescribed drugs.

Pregnancy and lactation: Pregnancy should be avoided if either partner is receiving Tomudex. It is also recommended that conception should be avoided for at least 6 months after cessation of treatment.

Tomudex should not be used during pregnancy or in women who may become pregnant during treatment (see the *Pre-clinical safety data*). Pregnancy should be excluded before treatment with Tomudex is started. Tomudex should not be given to women who are breast feeding.

Fertility studies in the rat indicate that Tomudex can cause impairment of male fertility. Fertility returned to normal three months after dosing ceased. Tomudex caused embryolethality and foetal abnormalities in pregnant rats.

Effects on ability to drive and use machines: Tomudex may cause malaise or asthenia following infusion and the ability to drive/use machinery could be impaired whilst such symptoms continue.

Undesirable effects: As with other cytotoxic drugs, Tomudex may be associated with certain adverse drug reactions. These mainly include reversible effects on the haemopoietic system, liver enzymes and gastrointestinal tract.

The following effects were reported as possible adverse drug reactions. The incidences represent those that were reported in the colorectal cancer clinical trials irrespective of the clinician's assessment of causality.

Gastrointestinal system: The most frequent effects were nausea in 57% of patients, diarrhoea (37%), vomiting (35%) and anorexia (27%). The incidences of severe (WHO Grade 3 and 4) gastrointestinal adverse events were 12% for nausea and vomiting, 12% for diarrhoea and 2% for mucositis. Other effects include mouth ulceration, dyspepsia and constipation. Severe diarrhoea may be associated with concurrent haematological suppression, especially leucopenia. Subsequent treatment may need to be discontinued or the dose reduced according to the grade of toxicity (see *Posology and method of administration*). Nausea and vomiting are usually responsive to antiemetics.

Haemopoietic system: Leucopenia (23%), anaemia (21%) and thrombocytopenia (4%) have been reported in clinical trials. They are usually mild to moderate, reaching nadir in the first and second week after treatment and recover by the third week. The incidence of severe (WHO Grade 4) leucopenia or thrombocytopenia was 5% and 1% respectively. These may be potentially life-threatening or fatal especially if associated with signs of gastrointestinal toxicity (see *Posology and method of administration*).

Metabolic and nutritional: Reversible increases in AST and ALT have been commonly reported in clinical trials (16% and 13% of patients respectively). Such changes have usually been asymptomatic and self-limiting when not associated with progression of the underlying malignancy. Other effects were weight loss, dehydration, peripheral oedema and increases in alkaline phosphatase.

Musculoskeletal and nervous system: Arthralgia and hypertonia (usually muscular cramps) have each been reported in less than 5% of patients.

Skin, appendages and special senses: Rash was commonly reported in clinical trials (15% of patients) sometimes associated with pruritus. Other effects were desquamation, alopecia, sweating, taste perversion and conjunctivitis each in less than 5% of patients.

Whole body: The most frequent effects were asthenia (45%) and fever (30%) which were usually mild to moderate and reversible. Severe asthenia can occur and may be associated with malaise and a flu-like syndrome. Other effects were abdominal pain (23%), pain (8%), headache (7%) and infection (5%). Cellulitis and sepsis were also reported each in less than 5% of patients.

Overdose: There is no clinically proven antidote available. In the case of inadvertent or accidental administration of an overdose, preclinical data suggest that consideration should be given to the administration of folinic acid. From clinical experience with other antifolates folinic acid may be given at a dose of 25 mg/m² i.v. every 6 hours. As the time interval between Tomudex administration and folinic acid rescue increases, its effectiveness in counteracting toxicity may diminish.

The expected manifestations of overdose are likely to be an exaggerated form of the adverse drug reactions anticipated with the administration of the drug. Patients should, therefore, be carefully monitored for signs of gastrointestinal and haematological toxicity. Symptomatic treatment and standard supportive care measures for the management of this toxicity should be applied.

Pharmacological properties
Pharmacodynamic properties: Raltitrexed is a folate analogue belonging to the family of anti-metabolites and has potent inhibitory activity against the enzyme thymidylate synthase (TS). Compared to other anti-metabolites such as 5-fluorouracil or methotrexate, raltitrexed acts as a direct and specific TS inhibitor. TS is a key enzyme in the *de novo* synthesis of thymidine triphosphate (TTP), a nucleotide required exclusively for deoxyribonuleic acid (DNA) synthesis. Inhibition of TS leads to DNA fragmentation and cell death. Raltitrexed is transported into cells via a reduced folate carrier (RFC) and is then extensively polyglutamated by the enzyme folyl polyglutamate

synthetase (FPGS) to polyglutamate forms that are retained in cells and are even more potent inhibitors of TS. Raltitrexed polyglutamation enhances TS inhibitory potency and increases the duration of TS inhibition in cells which may improve antitumour activity. Polyglutamation could also contribute to increased toxicity due to drug retention in normal tissues.

In clinical trials, Tomudex at the dose of 3 mg/m^2 i.v. every 3 weeks has demonstrated clinical antitumour activity with an acceptable toxicity profile in patients with advanced colorectal cancer.

Four large clinical trials have been conducted with Tomudex in advanced colorectal cancer. Of the three comparative trials, two showed no statistical difference between Tomudex and the combination of 5-fluorouracil plus folinic acid for survival while one trial showed a statistically significant difference in favour of the combination of 5-fluorouracil plus folinic acid. Tomudex as a single agent was as effective as the combination of 5-fluorouracil and folinic acid in terms of objective response rate in all trials.

Pharmacokinetic properties: Following intravenous administration at 3.0 mg/m^2, the concentration-time profile in patients was triphasic: Peak concentrations, found at the end of the infusion, were followed by a rapid initial decline in concentration. This was followed by a slow elimination phase. The key pharmacokinetic parameters are presented below:

Summary of mean pharmacokinetic parameters in patients administered 3.0 mg/m^2 Raltitrexed by intravenous infusion

C_{max} (ng/ml)	$AUC_{0-\infty}$ (ng.h/ml)	CL (ml/min)	CL_r (ml/min)	V_{SS} (l)	$t_{1/2}\beta$ (h)	$t_{1/2}\gamma$ (h)
656	1856	51.6	25.1	548	1.79	198

Key: C_{max}: Peak plasma concentration.
AUC: Area under plasma concentration-time curve.
CL: Clearance. CL_r: Renal clearance.
V_{SS}: Volume of distribution at steady state.
$t_{1/2}\beta$: Half life of the second (β) phase.
$t_{1/2}\gamma$: Terminal half life.

The maximum concentrations of raltitrexed increased linearly with dose over the clinical dose range tested.

During repeated administration at three week intervals, there was no clincally significant plasma accumulation of raltitrexed in patients with normal renal function.

Apart from the expected intracellular polyglutamation, raltitrexed was not metabolised and was excreted unchanged mainly in the urine, 40 to 50%. Raltitrexed was also excreted in the faeces with approximately 15% of the radioactive dose being eliminated over a 10 day period. In the [^{14}C]-raltitrexed trial approximately half of the radiolabel was not recovered during the study period. This suggests that a proportion of the raltitrexed dose is retained within tissues, perhaps as raltitrexed polyglutamates, beyond the end of the measurement period (29 days). Trace levels of radiolabel were detected in red blood cells on Day 29.

Raltitrexed pharmacokinetics are independent of age and gender. Pharmacokinetics have not been evaluated in children.

Mild to moderate hepatic impairment led to a small reduction in plasma clearance of less than 25%.

Mild to moderate renal impairment (creatinine clearance of 25 to 65 ml/min) led to a significant reduction (approximately 50%) in raltitrexed plasma clearance.

Pre-clinical safety data: Perivascular tolerance in studies in animals did not reveal any significant irritant reaction.

Acute toxicity: The approximate LD_{50} values for the mouse and rat are 875 to 1249 mg/kg and >500 mg/kg respectively. In the mouse, levels of 750 mg/kg and above caused death by general intoxication.

Chronic toxicity: In one month continuous and six month intermittent dosing studies in the rat, toxicity was related entirely to the cytotoxic nature of the drug. Principal target organs were the gastrointestinal tract, bone marrow and the testes. In similar studies in the dog, cumulative dose levels similar to that used clinically, elicited only pharmacologically-related changes to proliferating tissue. Target organs in the dog were therefore similar to the rat.

Mutagenicity: Tomudex was not mutagenic in the Ames test or in supplementary tests using *E. coli* or chinese hamster ovary cells. Tomudex caused increased levels of chromosome damage in an *in vitro* assay of human lymphocytes. This effect was ameliorated by the addition of thymidine, thus confirming it to be due to the anti-metabolic nature of the drug. An *in vivo* micronucleus study in the rat indicated that at cytotoxic dose levels, Tomudex is capable of causing chromosome damage in the bone marrow.

Reproductive toxicology: Fertility studies in the rat indicate that Tomudex can cause impairment of male fertility. Fertility returned to normal three months after dosing ceased. Tomudex caused embryolethality and foetal abnormalities in pregnant rats.

Carcinogenicity: The carcinogenic potential of Tomudex has not been evaluated.

Pharmaceutical particulars

List of excipients: Mannitol PhEur, USP; Dibasic Sodium Phosphate Heptahydrate USP; Sodium Hydroxide PhEur, USNF.

Incompatibilities: There is no information on incompatibilities at present and therefore Tomudex should not be mixed with any other drug.

Shelf life: The expiry life of Tomudex is 18 months when stored below 25°C protected from light. Once reconstituted, Tomudex is chemically stable for 24 hours at 25°C exposed to ambient light. For storage recommendation, see Instructions for use/handling.

Special precautions for storage: Unopened vial–Store below 25°C, protected from light. Reconstituted vial–Refrigerate at 2 to 8°C.

Nature and contents of container: Tomudex is packed in 5 ml clear neutral type I glass vials, with a bromobutyl rubber closure and an aluminium crimp seal with a plastic flip-off cover. The vials are packed in individual cartons to protect the product from light.

Instructions for use/handling: Each vial, containing 2 mg of raltitrexed, should be reconstituted with 4 ml of sterile water for injections to produce a 0.5 mg/ml solution.

The appropriate dose of solution is diluted in 50 to 250 ml of either 0.9% sodium chloride or 5% glucose (dextrose) injection and administered by a short intravenous infusion over a period of 15 minutes.

There is no preservative or bacteriostatic agent present in Tomudex or the materials specified for reconstitution or dilution. Tomudex must therefore be reconstituted and diluted under aseptic conditions and it is recommended that solutions of Tomudex should be used as soon as possible. Reconstituted Tomudex solution may be stored refrigerated (2 to 8°C) for up to 24 hours.

In accordance with established guidelines, when diluted in 0.9% sodium chloride of 5% glucose (dextrose) solution, it is recommended that administration of the admixed solution should commence as soon as possible after admixing. The admixed solution must be completely used or discarded within 24 hours of reconstitution of Tomudex intravenous injection.

Reconstituted and diluted solutions do not need to be protected from light.

Do not store partially used vials or admixed solutions for future patient use.

Any unused injection or reconstituted solution should be discarded in a suitable manner for cytotoxics.

Tomudex should be reconstituted for injection by trained personnel in a designated area for the reconstitution of cytotoxic agents. Cytotoxic preparations such as Tomudex should not be handled by pregnant women.

Reconstitution should normally be carried out in a partial containment facility with extraction e.g. a laminar air flow cabinet, and work surfaces should be covered with disposable plastic-backed absorbent paper.

Appropriate protective clothing, including normal surgical disposable gloves and goggles, should be worn. In case of contact with skin, immediately wash thoroughly with water. For splashes in the eye irrigate with clean water, holding the eyelids apart, for at least 10 minutes. Seek medical attention.

Any spillages should be cleared up using standard procedures.

Waste material should be disposed of by incineration in a manner consistent with the handling of cytotoxic agents.

Marketing authorisation number 12619/0107.

Date of approval/revision of SPC October 1998.

Legal category POM.

VIVALAN*

Qualitative and quantitative composition Viloxazine Hydrochloride equivalent to 50 mg Viloxazine

Pharmaceutical form Tablet

Clinical particulars

Therapeutic indications: Vivalan is indicated in the treatment of symptoms of depressive illness especially where sedation is not required.

Posology and method of administration:

Adults: Most patients respond to 300 mg/day preferably taken as 200 mg in the morning and 100 mg at lunchtime. Total daily dose should not exceed 400 mg and the last dose of the day should not be taken later than 6.00 pm.

Elderly: 100 mg/day initially. The initial dose should be increased with caution under close supervision. Half the normal maintenance dose may be sufficient to produce a satisfactory clinical response.

Children: Vivalan is not recommended in children under 14 years of age.

Contra-indications: Mania, severe liver disease, history of peptic ulcer, recent myocardial infarction and during breast feeding.

Special warnings and special precautions for use: Vivalan should be used with caution in patients with ischaemic heart disease and congestive cardiac failure, or any degree of heart block.

Caution is advised when administering Vivalan to patients with epilepsy, especially those receiving phenytoin.

Patients posing a high suicidal risk require close initial supervision.

If surgery is necessary during therapy, the anaesthetist should be informed that the patient has received Vivalan.

In patients taking oral anticoagulants, close monitoring of coagulation tests (e.g. twice weekly) is recommended.

Interactions with other medicaments and other forms of interaction: Vivalan should not be given concurrently with, or within 2 weeks of cessation of therapy with monoamine oxidase inhibitors.

Vivalan may decrease the antihypertensive effect of guanethidine, debrisoquine, bethanidine and possibly clonidine.

When Vivalan is co-administered with drugs which undergo hepatic metabolism via oxidative pathways, there is a possibility of an interaction. It may be necessary therefore to adjust the dose of such coadministered drugs which have narrow therapeutic margins, for example the dosage of phenytoin, carbamazepine, theophylline and oral anticoagulants (such as fluindione, micomalone and warfarin) may need to be reduced.

On theoretical grounds, caution is advised when patients receiving L-DOPA are treated with Vivalan.

Most antidepressants have been shown to potentiate the central nervous depressant action of alcohol, and, therefore, patients should be advised of the risks involved in drinking alcohol whilst on antidepressant medication.

Pregnancy and lactation:

Pregnancy: There is no evidence as to the drug's safety in human pregnancy; do not use during pregnancy, especially during the first and third trimesters, unless there are compelling reasons.

Lactation: Vivalan should not be used during lactation.

Effects on ability to drive and use machines: Vivalan initially may impair alertness, and patients should be advised of the possible hazard when driving or operating machinery.

Undesirable effects: Nausea is frequently observed but may be transient. Headache and vomiting may also occur.

As improvement may not occur during the first 2 weeks of treatment, patients should be closely monitored during this period.

Anticholinergic side effects, such as dry mouth, disturbance of accommodation, tachycardia, constipation and hesitancy of micturition have been reported less frequently with viloxazine than with tricyclic antidepressants.

Cardiac arrhythmias and severe hypotension are less likely to occur with viloxazine than with tricyclic antidepressants in high dosage or in deliberate overdosage.

Adverse effects which have been reported rarely with viloxazine include exacerbation of anxiety and agitation, drowsiness, confusion, ataxia, dizziness, insomnia, tremor, paresthesia, sweating, musculoskeletal pain, mild hypertension and skin rashes.

Psychotic manifestations, including hypomania and aggressive behaviour may be exacerbated.

Two serious adverse effects possibly associated with Vivalan have been reported:

a) Isolated cases of liver damage and jaundice associated with elevated transaminases.

b) Convulsions

Withdrawal symptoms are rare but may include malaise, headache and vomiting.

Overdose: Vivalan is rapidly absorbed and gastric lavage should be carried out with minimum of delay. Overdosage should be treated on general principles with careful monitoring of vital functions, together with intensive supportive therapy where necessary. As the drug is almost exclusively excreted in urine, forced diuresis may be performed to reduce blood levels. There is no specific antidote.

Pharmacological properties

Pharmacodynamic properties: Vivalan belongs to a class of psychotropic agents, the bicyclics. It is well established that Vivalan selectively inhibits noradrenaline uptake at central and peripheral sites and there is some evidence that Vivalan facilitates release of neuronal stores of 5-hydroxytryptamine. However, the precise relationship of these properties to the clinical antidepressant activity of Vivalan is unclear. The overall profile of Vivalan is quite atypical and different from the classical tricyclic antidepressant drugs. In particular, Vivalan produces fewer significant central effects, has little anticholinergic activity and less sympathomimetic activity.

Pharmacokinetic properties: The plasma half-life of viloxazine following administration is in the region of 2 to 5 hours. Viloxazine is rapidly and extensively metabolised by two major metabolic pathways. One involves hydroxylation in the aromatic ring, the other hydroxylation in both aromatic and heterocyclic rings. None of the metabolites identified in man has any significant pharmacological activity in animals. Therefore, it seems likely that the parent compound alone is responsible for the observed antidepressant properties in man. The metabolites of viloxazine are almost exclusively eliminated by the kidneys as glucuronide conjugates. Viloxazine is not highly protein bound.

Preclinical safety data: None stated.

Pharmaceutical particulars
List of excipients: Calcium phosphate BP; Glycerol PhEur; Magnesium stearate PhEur; Maize starch PhEur; Methyl hydroxypropylcellulose PhEur; Microcrystalline cellulose PhEur; Sodium starch glycollate BP; Titanium dioxide PhEur (E171).

Incompatibilities: Vivalan should not be given concurrently with, or within 2 weeks of cessation of therapy with monoamine oxidase inhibitors.

Shelf life: 5 years

Special precautions for storage: Store below 25°C

Nature and contents of container: HDPE bottle (100); Carton containing blister strips (10x10)

Instructions for use/handling: Use as directed by the prescriber.

Marketing authorisation number 12619/0081

Date of approval/revision of SPC October 1998

Legal category POM

ZESTORETIC* 10

Qualitative and quantitative composition Each tablet contains lisinopril dihydrate (equivalent to 10 mg anhydrous lisinopril) and hydrochlorothiazide PhEur 12.5 mg.

Pharmaceutical form Tablet.

Clinical particulars
Therapeutic indications: Zestoretic 10 is indicated in the management of mild to moderate hypertension in patients who have been stabilised on the individual components given in the same proportions.

Posology and method of administration: The usual dosage is one tablet, administered once daily. As with all other medication taken once daily, Zestoretic 10 should be taken at approximately the same time each day.

In general, if the desired therapeutic effect cannot be achieved in a period of 2 to 4 weeks at this dose level, the dose can be increased to two tablets administered once daily.

No adjustment of dosage is required in the elderly.

Safety and effectiveness in children have not been established.

Dosage in renal insufficiency: Thiazides may not be appropriate diuretics for use in patients with renal impairment and are ineffective at creatinine clearance values of 30 ml/min or below (i.e. moderate or severe renal insufficiency).

Zestoretic 10 is not to be used as initial therapy in any patient with renal insufficiency.

In patients with creatinine clearance of >30 and <80 ml/min, Zestoretic 10 may be used, but only after titration of the individual components.

Prior diuretic therapy: Symptomatic hypotension may occur following the initial dose of Zestoretic 10; this is more likely in patients who are volume and/or salt depleted as a result of prior diuretic therapy. The diuretic therapy should be discontinued for 2 to 3 days prior to initiation of therapy with Zestoretic 10. If this is not possible, treatment should be started with lisinopril alone, in a 2.5 mg dose.

Contra-indications: Zestoretic 10 is contra-indicated in pregnancy and treatment should be stopped if pregnancy is suspected (see also *Use in pregnancy*).

Zestoretic 10 is contra-indicated in patients with anuria.

Zestoretic 10 is contra-indicated in patients who are hypersensitive to any component of this product and in patients with a history of angioneurotic oedema relating to previous treatment with an angiotensin-converting enzyme inhibitor and in patients with hereditary or idiopathic angioedema.

Zestoretic 10 is contra-indicated in patients who are hypersensitive to other sulphonamide-derived drugs.

Special warnings and precautions for use:
Hypotension and electrolyte/Fluid imbalance: As with all antihypertensive therapy, symptomatic hypotension may occur in some patients. This was rarely seen in uncomplicated hypertensive patients but is more likely in the presence of fluid or electrolyte imbalance, eg, volume depletion, hyponatraemia, hypochloraemic alkalosis, hypomagnesaemia or hypokalaemia which may occur from prior diuretic therapy, dietary salt restriction, dialysis, or during intercurrent diarrhoea or vomiting. Periodic determination of serum electrolytes should be performed at appropriate intervals in such patients.

In patients at increased risk of symptomatic hypotension, initiation of therapy and dose adjustment should be monitored under close medical supervision.

Particular consideration should be given when therapy is administered to patients with ischaemic heart or cerebrovascular disease because an excessive fall in blood pressure could result in a myocardial infarction or cerebrovascular accident.

If hypotension occurs, the patient should be placed in the supine position and, if necessary, should receive an intravenous infusion of normal saline. A transient hypotensive response is not a contraindication to further doses. Following restoration of effective blood volume and pressure, reinstitution of therapy at reduced dosage may be possible; or either of the components may be used appropriately alone.

As with other vasodilators, 'Zestoretic 10 should be given with caution to patients with aortic stenosis or hypertrophic cardiomyopathy.

Renal function impairment: Thiazides may not be appropriate diuretics for use in patients with renal impairment and are ineffective at creatinine clearance values of 30 ml/min or below (i.e. moderate or severe renal insufficiency).

Zestoretic 10 should not be administered to patients with renal insufficiency (creatinine clearance ≤80 ml/min) until titration of the individual components has shown the need for the doses present in the combination tablet.

In some patients with bilateral renal artery stenosis or stenosis of the artery to a solitary kidney, who have been treated with angiotensin converting enzyme inhibitors, increases in blood urea and serum creatinine, usually reversible upon discontinuation of therapy have been seen. This is especially likely in patients with renal insufficiency. If renovascular hypertension is also present there is an increased risk of severe hypotension and renal insufficiency. In these patients, treatment should be started under close medical supervision with low doses and careful dose titration. Since treatment with diuretics may be a contributory factor to the above, renal function should be monitored during the first few weeks of Zestoretic 10 therapy.

Some hypertensive patients with no apparent pre-existing renal disease have developed usually minor and transient increases in blood urea and serum creatinine when lisinopril has been given concomitantly with a diuretic. If this occurs during therapy with Zestoretic 10, the combination should be discontinued. Reinstitution of therapy at reduced dosage may be possible; or either of the components may be used appropriately alone.

Hepatic disease: Thiazides should be used with caution in patients with impaired hepatic function or progressive liver disease, since minor alterations of fluid and electrolyte balance may precipitate hepatic coma.

Surgery/Anaesthesia: In patients undergoing major surgery or during anaesthesia with agents that produce hypotension, lisinopril may block angiotensin II formation secondary to compensatory renin release. If hypotension occurs and is considered to be due to this mechanism, it can be corrected by volume expansion.

Metabolic and endocrine effects: Thiazide therapy may impair glucose tolerance. Dosage adjustment of antidiabetic agents, including insulin, may be required.

Thiazides may decrease urinary calcium excretion and may cause intermittent and slight elevation of serum calcium. Marked hypercalcaemia may be evidence of hidden hyperparathyroidism. Thiazides should be discontinued before carrying out tests for parathyroid function.

Increases in cholesterol and triglyceride levels may be associated with thiazide diuretic therapy.

Thiazide therapy may precipitate hyperuricaemia and/or gout in certain patients. However, lisinopril may increase urinary uric acid and thus may attenuate the hyperuricaemic effect of hydrochlorothiazide.

Hypersensitivity/Angioneurotic oedema: Angioneurotic oedema of the face, extremities, lips, tongue, glottis and/or larynx has been reported rarely in patients treated with angiotensin converting enzyme inhibitors, including lisinopril. In such cases, Zestoretic 10 should be discontinued promptly and appropriate monitoring should be instituted to ensure complete resolution of symptoms prior to dismissing the patient. In those instances where swelling has been confined to the face and lips, the condition generally resolved without treatment, although antihistamines have been useful in relieving symptoms.

Angioneurotic oedema associated with laryngeal oedema may be fatal. Where there is involvement of the tongue, glottis or larynx, likely to cause airway obstruction, appropriate emergency therapy should be administered promptly. This may include administration of adrenaline and/or the maintenance of a patent airway. The patient should be under close medical supervision until complete and sustained resolution of symptoms has occurred.

Angiotensin converting enzyme inhibitors cause a higher rate of angioedema in black patients than in non-black patients.

Patients with a history of angioedema unrelated to ACE inhibitor therapy may be at increased risk of angioedema while receiving an ACE inhibitor. (See also *Contra-indications*).

In patients receiving thiazides, sensitivity reactions may occur with or without a history of allergy or bronchial asthma. Exacerbation or activation of systemic lupus erythematosus has been reported with the use of thiazides.

Race: Angiotensin converting enzyme inhibitors cause a higher rate of angioedema in black patients than in non-black patients.

Desensitisation: Patients receiving ACE inhibitors during desensitisation treatment (eg. hymenoptera venom) have sustained anaphylactoid reactions. In the same patients, these reactions have been avoided when ACE inhibitors were temporarily withheld but they reappeared upon inadvertent rechallenge.

Haemodialysis membranes: See *Interactions*

Cough: Cough has been reported with the use of ACE inhibitors. Characteristically, the cough is non-productive, persistent and resolves after discontinuation of therapy. ACE inhibitor-induced cough should be considered as part of the differential diagnosis of cough.

Paediatric use: Safety and effectiveness in children have not been established.

Use in the elderly: In clinical studies the efficacy and tolerability of lisinopril and hydrochlorothiazide, administered concomitantly, were similar in both elderly and younger hypertensive patients.

Interaction with other medicaments and other forms of interaction:
Prior diuretic therapy: Symptomatic hypotension may occur following the initial dose of Zestoretic 10; this is more likely in patients who are volume and/or salt depleted as a result of prior diuretic therapy. The diuretic therapy should be discontinued for 2 to 3 days prior to initiation of therapy with Zestoretic 10. If this is not possible, treatment should be started with lisinopril alone, in a 2.5 mg dose.

Haemodialysis membranes: The use of Zestoretic 10 is not indicated in patients requiring dialysis for renal failure. A high incidence of anaphylactoid reactions have been reported in patients dialysed with high-flux membranes (eg. AN 69) and treated concomitantly with an ACE inhibitor. This combination should therefore be avoided.

Serum potassium: The potassium losing effect of thiazide diuretics is usually attenuated by the potassium conserving effect of lisinopril. The use of potassium supplements, potassium-sparing agents or potassium-containing salt substitutes, particularly in patients with impaired renal function, may lead to a significant increase in serum potassium. If concomitant use of Zestoretic 10 and any of these agents is deemed appropriate, they should be used with caution and with frequent monitoring of serum potassium.

Lithium: Lithium generally should not be given with diuretics or ACE inhibitors. Diuretic agents and ACE inhibitors reduce the renal clearance of lithium and add a high risk of lithium toxicity. Refer to the prescribing information for lithium preparations before use of such preparations.

Other agents: Indomethacin may diminish the antihypertensive effect of concomitantly-administered Zestoretic 10. In some patients with compromised renal function who are being treated with non-steroidal anti-inflammatory drugs (NSAIDs), the co-administration of lisinopril may result in a further deterioration of renal function.

The antihypertensive effect of Zestoretic 10 may be potentiated when given concomitantly with other agents likely to cause postural hypotension.

Thiazides may increase the responsiveness to tubocurarine.

Pregnancy and lactation:
Use in pregnancy: Zestoretic 10 is contraindicated in pregnancy and treatment should be stopped if pregnancy is suspected.

ACE inhibitors can cause foetal and neonatal morbidity and mortality when administered to pregnant women during the second and third trimesters. Use of ACE inhibitors during this period has been associated with foetal and neonatal injury including hypotension, renal failure, hyperkalaemia and/or skull hypoplasia in the newborn. Maternal oligohydramnios, presumably representing decreased foetal renal function, has occurred and may result in limb contractures, craniofacial deformations and hypoplastic lung development.

These adverse effects to the embryo and foetus do not appear to have resulted from intrauterine ACE inhibitor exposure limited to the first trimester.

Infants whose mothers have taken lisinopril should be closely observed for hypotension, oliguria and hyperkalaemia. Lisinopril, which crosses the placenta, has been removed from the neonatal circulation by peritoneal dialysis with some clinical benefit, and theoretically may be removed by exchange transfusion. There is no experience with the removal of hydrochlorothiazide, which also crosses the placenta, from the neonatal circulation.

Nursing mothers: It is not known whether lisinopril is secreted in human milk; however, thiazides do appear in human milk. Because of the potential for serious reactions in breast-fed infants, a decision should be made whether to discontinue breast feeding or to discontinue Zestoretic 10, taking into account the importance of the drug to the mother.

Effects on ability to drive and use machines: None known.

Undesirable effects:
Side effects with the combination: Zestoretic 10 is usually well tolerated. In clinical studies, side effects have usually been mild and transient, and in most instances have not required interruption of therapy. The side effects that have been observed have been limited to those reported previously with lisinopril or hydrochlorothiazide.

One of the most common clinical side effects was dizziness, which generally responded to dosage reduction and seldom required discontinuation of therapy.

Other side effects were headache, dry cough, fatigue and hypotension including orthostatic hypotension.

Less common were diarrhoea, nausea, vomiting, dry mouth, rash, gout, palpitations, chest discomfort, muscle cramps and weakness, paraesthesia, asthenia and impotence.

Pancreatitis has been reported rarely with lisinopril and with hydrochlorothiazide and, therefore, is a potential side effect of Zestoretic 10.

Hypersensitivity/Angioneurotic oedema: Angioneurotic oedema of the face, extremities, lips, tongue, glottis and/or larynx has been reported rarely (see *Special warnings and precautions*).

A symptom complex has been reported which may include one or more of the following: fever, vasculitis, myalgia, arthralgia/arthritis, a positive ANA, elevated ESR, eosinophilia and leucocytosis, rash, photosensitivity, or other dermatological manifestations.

Laboratory test findings: Laboratory side effects have rarely been of clinical importance. Occasional hyperglycaemia, hyperuricaemia and hyper- or hypokalaemia have been noted. Usually minor and transient increases in blood urea nitrogen and serum creatinine have been seen in patients without evidence of preexisting renal impairment. If such increases persist, they are usually reversible upon discontinuation of Zestoretic 10. Bone marrow depression, manifest as anaemia and/or thrombocytopenia and/or leucopenia has been reported. Agranulocytosis has been rarely reported. Small decreases in haemoglobin and haematocrit have been reported frequently in hypertensive patients treated with Zestoretic 10 but were rarely of clinical importance unless another cause of anaemia co-existed. Rarely, elevations of liver enzymes and/or serum bilirubin have occurred, but a causal relationship to Zestoretic 10 has not been established.

Other side effects reported with the individual components alone: These may be potential side effects with Zestoretic 10 and include:

Hydrochlorothiazide: anorexia, gastric irritation, constipation, jaundice (intrahepatic cholestatic jaundice), pancreatitis, sialoadenitis, vertigo, xanthopsia, leucopenia, agranulocytosis, thrombocytopenia, aplastic anaemia, haemolytic anaemia, purpura, photosensitivity, urticaria, necrotizing angiitis (vasculitis) (cutaneous vasculitis), fever, respiratory distress including pneumonitis and pulmonary oedema, anaphylactic reactions, hyperglycaemia, glycosuria, hyperuricaemia, electrolyte imbalance including hyponatraemia, muscle spasm, restlessness, transient blurred vision, renal failure, renal dysfunction and interstitial nephritis.

Lisinopril: myocardial infarction or cerebrovascular accident possibly secondary to excessive hypotension in high risk patients, tachycardia, abdominal pain and indigestion, mood alterations, mental confusion, vertigo have occurred; as with other angiotensin converting enzyme inhibitors, taste disturbance and sleep disturbance have been reported; bronchospasm, rhinitis, sinusitis, alopecia, urticaria, diaphoresis, pruritus, psoriasis and severe skin disorders, (including pemphigus, toxic epidermal necrolysis, Stevens-Johnson Syndrome and erythema multiforme), have been reported; hyponatraemia, uraemia, oliguria/anuria, renal dysfunction, acute renal failure, hepatitis (hepatocellular or cholestatic), jaundice and haemolytic anaemia.

Overdose: No specific information is available on the treatment of overdosage with Zestoretic 10. Treatment is symptomatic and supportive. Therapy with Zestoretic 10 should be discontinued and the patient should be kept under very close supervision. Therapeutic measures depend on the nature and severity of the symptoms. Measures to prevent absorption and methods to speed elimination should be employed.

Lisinopril: The most likely features of overdosage would be hypotension, electrolyte disturbance and renal failure. If severe hypotension occurs, the patient should be placed in the shock position and an intravenous infusion of normal saline should be given rapidly. Treatment with angiotensin II (if available) may be considered.

Angiotensin converting enzyme inhibitors may be removed from the general circulation by haemodialysis. The use of high-flux polyacrylonitrile dialysis membranes should be avoided. Serum electrolytes and creatinine should be monitored frequently.

Hydrochlorothiazide: The most common signs and symptoms observed are those caused by electrolyte depletion (hypokalaemia, hypochloraemia, hyponatraemia) and dehydration resulting from excessive diuresis. If digitalis has also been administered hypokalaemia may accentuate cardiac arrhythmias.

Pharmacological properties
Pharmacodynamic properties: Zestoretic 10 is a fixed dose combination product containing lisinopril, an inhibitor of angiotensin converting enzyme (ACE) and hydrochlorothiazide, a thiazide diuretic. Both components have complementary modes of action and exert an additive antihypertensive effect.

Lisinopril is a peptidyl dipeptidase inhibitor. It inhibits the angiotensin converting enzyme (ACE) that catalyses the conversion of angiotensin I to the vasoconstrictor peptide, angiotensin II. Angiotensin II also stimulates aldosterone secretion by the adrenal cortex. Inhibition of ACE results in decreased concentrations of angiotensin II which results in decreased vasopressor activity and reduced aldosterone secretion. The latter decrease may result in an increase in serum potassium concentration.

While the mechanism through which lisinopril lowers blood pressure is believed to be primarily suppression of the renin-angiotensin-aldosterone system, lisinopril is antihypertensive even in patients with low-renin hypertension. ACE is identical to kininase II, an enzyme that degrades bradykinin. Whether increased levels of bradykinin, a potent vasodilatory peptide, play a role in the therapeutic effects of lisinopril remains to be elucidated.

Hydrochlorothiazide is a diuretic and an antihypertensive agent. It affects the distal renal tubular mechanism of electrolyte reabsorption and increases excretion of sodium and chloride in approximately equivalent amounts. Natriuresis may be accompanied by some loss of potassium and bicarbonate. The mechanism of the antihypertensive effect of the thiazides is unknown. Thiazides do not usually affect normal blood pressure.

When combined with other antihypertensive agents, additive falls in blood pressure may occur.

Pharmacokinetic properties: Concomitant administration of lisinopril and hydrochlorothiazide has little or no effect on the bioavailability of either drug. The combination tablet is bioequivalent to concomitant administration of the separate entities.

Lisinopril: Following oral administration of lisinopril, peak serum concentrations occur within about 7 hours. On multiple dosing lisinopril has an effective half life of accumulation of 12.6 hours. Declining serum concentrations exhibit a prolonged terminal phase which does not contribute to drug accumulation. This terminal phase probably represents saturable binding to ACE and is not proportional to dose. Lisinopril does not appear to bind to other serum proteins.

Impaired renal function decreases elimination of lisinopril, which is excreted via the kidneys, but this decrease becomes clinically important only when the glomerular filtration rate is below 30 ml/min. Older patients have higher blood levels and higher values for the area under the plasma concentration time curve than younger patients. Lisinopril can be removed by dialysis.

Based on urinary recovery, the mean extent of absorption of lisinopril is approximately 25%, with interpatient variability (6 to 60%) at all doses tested (5 to 80 mg).

Lisinopril does not undergo metabolism and absorbed drug is excreted unchanged entirely in the urine. Lisinopril absorption is not affected by the presence of food in the gastrointestinal tract.

Studies in rats indicate that lisinopril crosses the blood-brain barrier poorly.

Hydrochlorothiazide: When plasma levels have been followed for at least 24 hours, the plasma half-life has been observed to vary between 5.6 and 14.8 hours. At least 61% of the dose is eliminated unchanged within 24 hours. After oral hydrochlorothiazide, diuresis begins within 2 hours, peaks in about 4 hours and lasts 6 to 12 hours. Hydrochlorothiazide crosses the placental but not the blood-brain barrier.

Preclinical safety data: Lisinopril and hydrochlorthiazide are both drugs on which extensive clinical experience has been obtained, both separately and in combination. All relevant information for the prescriber is provided elsewhere in the Summary of Product Characteristics.

Pharmaceutical particulars
List of excipients: Calcium Hydrogen Phosphate Dihydrate PhEur; Iron Oxide E172; Magnesium Stearate PhEur; Maize Starch PhEur; Mannitol PhEur; Pregelatinised Starch PhEur.

Incompatibilities: None known, but see *Interactions*.

Shelf life: 2.5 years stored in the sales package.

Special precautions for storage: Store below 30°C and protect from light. If blister packs are removed from the carton, they should be protected from light.

Nature and contents of container: Blister packs of 28 tablets.

Instructions for use/handling: Not applicable.

Market authorisation number 12619/0091.

Date of approval/revision of the text June 1998

Legal category POM

ZESTORETIC* 20

Qualitative and quantitative composition Each tablet contains lisinopril dihydrate (equivalent to 20 mg anhydrous lisinopril) and hydrochlorothiazide PhEur 12.5 mg.

Pharmaceutical form Tablet.

Clinical particulars
Therapeutic indication: Zestoretic 20 is indicated in the management of mild to moderate hypertension in patients who have been stabilised on the individual components given in the same proportions.

Posology and method of administration:
The usual dosage is one tablet, administered once daily. As with all other medication taken once daily, Zestoretic 20 should be taken at approximately the same time each day.

In general, if the desired therapeutic effect cannot be achieved in a period of 2 to 4 weeks at this dose level, the dose can be increased to two tablets administered once daily.

Use in the elderly: In clinical studies the efficacy and tolerability of lisinopril and hydrochlorothiazide, administered concomitantly, were similar in both elderly and younger hypertensive patients.

Lisinopril was equally effective in elderly (65 years or older) and non-elderly hypertensive patients. In elderly hypertensive patients, monotherapy with lisinopril was as effective in reducing diastolic blood pressure as monotherapy with either hydrochlorothiazide or atenolol in clinical studies, age did not affect the tolerability of lisinopril.

Safety and effectiveness in children have not been established.

Dosage in renal insufficiency: Thiazides may not be appropriate diuretics for use in patients with renal impairment and are ineffective at creatinine clearance values of 30 ml/min or below (i.e. moderate or severe renal insufficiency).

Zestoretic 20 is not to be used as initial therapy in any patient with renal insufficiency.

In patients with creatinine clearance of >30 and <80 ml/min, Zestoretic 20 may be used, but only after titration of the individual components.

Prior diuretic therapy: Symptomatic hypotension may occur following the initial dose of Zestoretic 20; this is more likely in patients who are volume and/or salt depleted as a result of prior diuretic therapy. The diuretic therapy should be discontinued for 2 to 3 days prior to initiation of therapy with Zestoretic 20. If this is not possible, treatment should be started with lisinopril alone, in a 2.5 mg dose.

Contra-indications: Zestoretic 20 is contra-indicated in pregnancy and treatment should be stopped if pregnancy is suspected (see also *Pregnancy and lactation*).

Zestoretic 20 is contra-indicated in patients with anuria.

Zestoretic 20 is contra-indicated in patients who are hypersensitive to any component of this product and in patients with a history of angioneurotic oedema relating to previous treatment with an angiotensin-converting enzyme inhibitor and in patients with hereditary or idiopathic angioedema.

Zestoretic 20 is contra-indicated in patients who are hypersensitive to other sulphonamide-derived drugs.

Special warnings and special precautions for use:
Hypotension and electrolyte/fluid imbalance:

As with all antihypertensive therapy, symptomatic hypotension may occur in some patients. This was rarely seen in uncomplicated hypertensive patients but is more likely in the presence of fluid or electrolyte imbalance, eg. volume depletion, hyponatraemia, hypochloraemic alkalosis, hypomagnesaemia or hypokalaemia which may occur from prior diuretic therapy, dietary salt restriction, dialysis, or during intercurrent diarrhoea or vomiting. Periodic determination of serum electrolytes should be performed at appropriate intervals in such patients.

In patients at increased risk of symptomatic hypotension, initiation of therapy and dose adjustment should be monitored under close medical supervision.

Particular consideration should be given when therapy is administered to patients with ischaemic heart or cerebrovascular disease because an excessive fall in blood pressure could result in a myocardial infarction or cerebrovascular accident.

If hypotension occurs, the patient should be placed in the supine position and, if necessary, should receive an intravenous infusion of normal saline. A transient hypotensive response is not a contraindication to further doses. Following restoration of effective blood volume and pressure, reinstitution of therapy at reduced dosage may be possible; or either of the components may be used appropriately alone.

As with other vasodilators, Zestoretic 20 should be given with caution to patients with aortic stenosis or hypertrophic cardiomyopathy.

Renal function impairment: Thiazides may not be appropriate diuretics for use in patients with renal impairment and are ineffective at creatinine clearance values of 30 ml/min or below (i.e. moderate or severe renal insufficiency).

Zestoretic 20 should not be administered to patients with renal insufficiency (creatinine clearance ≤80 ml/min) until titration of the individual components has shown the need for the doses present in the combination tablet.

In some patients with bilateral renal artery stenosis or stenosis of the artery to a solitary kidney, who have been treated with angiotensin enzyme inhibitors, increases in blood urea and serum creatinine, usually reversible upon discontinuation of therapy, have been seen. This is especially likely in patients with renal insufficiency. If renovascular hypertension is also present there is an increased risk of severe hypotension and renal insufficiency. In these patients, treatment should be started under close medical supervision with low doses and careful dose titration. Since treatment with diuretics may be a contributory factor to the above, renal function should be monitored during the first few weeks of 'Zestoretic 20 therapy.

Some hypertensive patients with no apparent preexisting renal disease have developed usually minor and transient increases in blood urea and serum creatinine when lisinopril has been given concomitantly with a diuretic. If this occurs during therapy with Zestoretic 20, the combination should be discontinued. Reinstitution of therapy at reduced dosage may be possible; or either of the components may be used appropriately alone.

Hepatic disease: Thiazides should be used with caution in patients with impaired hepatic function or progressive liver disease, since minor alterations of fluid and electrolyte balance may precipitate hepatic coma.

Surgery/anaesthesia: In patients undergoing major surgery or during anaesthesia with agents that produce hypotension, lisinopril may block angiotensin II formation secondary to compensatory renin release. If hypotension occurs and is considered to be due to this mechanism, it can be corrected by volume expansion.

Metabolic and endocrine effects: Thiazide therapy may impair glucose tolerance. Dosage adjustment of antidiabetic agents, including insulin, may be required.

Thiazides may decrease urinary calcium excretion and may cause intermittent and slight elevation of serum calcium. Marked hypercalcaemia may be evidence of hidden hyperparathyroidism. Thiazides should be discontinued before carrying out tests for parathyroid function.

Increases in cholesterol and triglyceride levels may be associated with thiazide diuretic therapy.

Thiazide therapy may precipitate hyperuricaemia and/or gout in certain patients. However, lisinopril may increase urinary uric acid and thus may attenuate the hyperuricaemic effect of hydrochlorothiazide.

Hypersensitivity/angioneurotic oedema: Angioneurotic oedema of the face, extremities, lips, tongue, glottis and/or larynx has been reported rarely in patients treated with angiotensin converting enzyme inhibitors, including lisinopril. In such cases, Zestoretic 20 should be discontinued promptly and appropriate monitoring should be instituted to ensure complete resolution of symptoms prior to dismissing the patient. In those instances where swelling has been confined to the face and lips, the condition generally resolved without treatment, although antihistamines have been useful in relieving symptoms.

Angioneurotic oedema associated with laryngeal oedema may be fatal. Where there is involvement of the tongue, glottis or larynx, likely to cause airway obstruction, appropriate emergency therapy should be administered promptly. This may include administration of adrenaline and/or the maintenance of a patent airway. The patient should be under close medical supervision until complete and sustained resolution of symptoms has occurred.

Angiotensin converting enzyme inhibitors cause a higher rate of angioedema in black patients than in non-black patients.

Patients with a history of angioedema unrelated to ACE inhibitor therapy may be at increased risk of angioedema while receiving an ACE inhibitor. (See *Contra-indications*).

In patients receiving thiazides, sensitivity reactions may occur with or without a history of allergy or bronchial asthma. Exacerbation or activation of systemic lupus erythematosus has been reported with the use of thiazides.

Race: Angiotensin converting enzyme inhibitors cause a higher rate of angioedema in black patients than in non-black patients.

Desensitisation: Patients receiving ACE inhibitors during desensitisation treatment (e.g. hymenoptera venom) have sustained anaphylactoid reactions. In the same patients, these reactions have been avoided when ACE inhibitors were temporarily withheld but they reappeared upon inadvertent rechallenge.

Haemodialysis membranes: (See *Interactions*).

Cough: Cough has been reported with the use of ACE inhibitors. Characteristically, the cough is non-productive, persistent and resolves after discontinuation of therapy.

ACE inhibitor-induced cough should be considered as part of the differential diagnosis of cough.

Paediatric use: Safety and effectiveness in children have not been established.

Use in the elderly: In clinical studies the efficacy and tolerability of lisinopril and hydrochlorothiazide, administered concomitantly, were similar in both elderly and younger hypertensive patients.

Interaction with other medicaments and other forms of interaction:

Prior diuretic therapy: Symptomatic hypotension may occur following the initial dose of Zestoretic 20; this is more likely in patients who are volume and/or salt depleted as a result of prior diuretic therapy. The diuretic therapy should be discontinued for 2 to 3 days prior to initiation of therapy with Zestoretic 20. If this is not possible, treatment should be started with lisinopril alone, in a 2.5 mg dose.

Haemodialysis membranes: The use of Zestoretic 20 is not indicated in patients requiring dialysis for renal failure. A high incidence of anaphylactoid reactions has been reported in patients dialysed with high-flux membranes (e.g. AN 69) and treated concomitantly with an ACE inhibitor. This combination should therefore be avoided.

Serum potassium: The potassium losing effect of thiazide diuretics is usually attenuated by the potassium conserving effect of lisinopril. The use of potassium supplements, potassium-sparing agents or potassium-containing salt substitutes, particularly in patients with impaired renal function, may lead to a significant increase in serum potassium. If concomitant use of Zestoretic 20 and any of these agents is deemed appropriate, they should be used with caution and with frequent monitoring of serum potassium.

Lithium: Lithium generally should not be given with diuretics or ACE inhibitors. Diuretic agents and ACE inhibitors reduce the renal clearance of lithium and add a high risk of lithium toxicity. Refer to the prescribing information for lithium preparations before use of such preparations.

Other agents: Indomethacin may diminish the antihypertensive effect of concomitantly-administered Zestoretic 20. In some patients with compromised renal function who are being treated with nonsteroidal anti-inflammatory drugs (NSAIDs), the co-administration of lisinopril may result in a further deterioration of renal function.

The antihypertensive effect of Zestoretic 20 may be potentiated when given concomitantly with other agents likely to cause postural hypotension.

Thiazides may increase the responsiveness to tubocurarine.

Pregnancy and lactation:

Use in pregnancy: Zestoretic 20 is contraindicated in pregnancy and treatment should be stopped if pregnancy is suspected.

ACE inhibitors can cause foetal and neonatal morbidity and mortality when administered to pregnant women during the second and third trimesters. Use of ACE inhibitors during this period has been associated with foetal and neonatal injury including hypotension, renal failure, hyperkalaemia and/or skull hypoplasia in the newborn. Maternal oligohydramnios, presumably representing decreased foetal renal function, has occurred and may result in limb contractures, craniofacial deformations and hypoplastic lung development.

These adverse effects to the embryo and foetus do not appear to have resulted from intrauterine ACE inhibitor exposure limited to the first trimester.

Infants whose mothers have taken lisinopril should be closely observed for hypotension, oliguria and hyperkalaemia. Lisinopril, which crosses the placenta, has been removed from the neonatal circulation by peritoneal dialysis with some clinical benefit, and theoretically may be removed by exchange transfusion. There is no experience with the removal of hydrochlorothiazide, which also crosses the placenta, from the neonatal circulation.

Nursing mothers: It is not known whether lisinopril is secreted in human milk; however, thiazides do appear in human milk. Because of the potential for serious reactions in breast-fed infants, a decision should be made whether to discontinue breast feeding or to discontinue Zestoretic 20, taking into account the importance of the drug to the mother.

Effects on ability to drive and use machines: None known.

Undesirable effects:

Side effects with the combination: Zestoretic 20 is usually well tolerated. In clinical studies, side effects have usually been mild and transient, and in most instances have not required interruption of therapy. The side effects that have been observed have been limited to those reported previously with lisinopril or hydrochlorothiazide.

One of the most common clinical side effects was dizziness, which generally responded to dosage reduction and seldom required discontinuation of therapy.

Other side effects were headache, dry cough, fatigue and hypotension including orthostatic hypotension.

Less common were diarrhoea, nausea, vomiting, dry mouth, rash, gout, palpitations, chest discomfort, muscle cramps and weakness, paraesthesia, asthenia and impotence.

Pancreatitis has been reported rarely with lisinopril and with hydrochlorothiazide and, therefore, is a potential side effect of Zestoretic 20.

Hypersensitivity/angioneurotic oedema: Angioneurotic oedema of the face, extremities, lips, tongue, glottis and/or larynx has been reported rarely (see *Special warnings and special precautions for use*).

A symptom complex has been reported which may include one or more of the following: fever, vasculitis, myalgia, arthralgia/arthritis, a positive ANA, elevated ESR, eosinophilia and leucocytosis, rash, photosensitivity, or other dermatological manifestations.

Laboratory test findings: Laboratory side effects have rarely been of clinical importance. Occasional hyperglycaemia, hyperuricaemia and hyper- or hypokalaemia have been noted. Usually minor and transient increases in blood urea nitrogen and serum creatinine have been seen in patients without evidence of preexisting renal impairment. If such increases persist, they are usually reversible upon discontinuation of Zestoretic 20. Bone marrow depression, manifest as anaemia and/or thrombocytopenia and/or leucopenia has been reported. Agranulocytosis has been rarely reported. Small decreases in haemoglobin and haematocrit have been reported frequently in hypertensive patients treated with Zestoretic 20 but were rarely of clinical importance unless another cause of anaemia co-existed. Rarely, elevations of liver enzymes and/or serum bilirubin have occurred, but a causal relationship to Zestoretic 20 has not been established.

Other side effects reported with the individual components alone: These may be potential side effects with Zestoretic 20 and include:

Hydrochlorothiazide: anorexia, gastric irritation, constipation, jaundice (intrahepatic cholestatic jaundice), pancreatitis, sialoadenitis, vertigo, xanthopsia, leucopenia, agranulocytosis, thrombocytopenia, aplastic anaemia, haemolytic anaemia, purpura, photosensitivity, urticaria, necrotizing angiitis (vasculitis) (cutaneous vasculitis), fever, respiratory distress including pneumonitis and pulmonary oedema, anaphylactic reactions, hyperglycaemia, glycosuria, hyperuricaemia, electrolyte imbalance including hyponatraemia, muscle spasm, restlessness, transient blurred vision, renal failure, renal dysfunction and interstitial nephritis.

Lisinopril: myocardial infarction or cerebrovascular accident possibly secondary to excessive hypotension in high risk patients, tachycardia, abdominal pain and indigestion, mood alterations, mental confusion, vertigo have occurred; as with other angiotensin converting enzyme inhibitors, taste disturbance and sleep disturbance have been reported; bronchospasm, rhinitis, sinusitis, alopecia, urticaria, diaphoresis, pruritus, psoriasis and severe skin disorders, (including pemphigus, toxic epidermal necrolysis, Stevens-Johnson Syndrome and erythema multiforme), have been reported; hyponatraemia, uraemia, oliguria/anuria, renal dysfunction, acute renal failure, hepatitis (hepatocellular or cholestatic), jaundice and haemolytic anaemia.

Overdose: No specific information is available on the treatment of overdosage with Zestoretic 20. Treatment is symptomatic and supportive. Therapy with Zestoretic 20 should be discontinued and the patient should be kept under very close supervision. Therapeutic measures depend on the nature and severity of the symptoms. Measures to prevent absorption and methods to speed elimination should be employed.

Lisinopril: The most likely features of overdosage would be hypotension, electrolyte disturbance and renal failure. If severe hypotension occurs, the patient should be placed in the shock position and an intravenous infusion of normal saline should be given rapidly. Treatment with angiotensin II (if available) may be considered. Angiotensin converting enzyme inhibitors may be removed from the general circulation by haemodialysis. The use of high-flux polyacrylonitrile dialysis membranes should be avoided. Serum electrolytes and creatinine should be monitored frequently.

Hydrochlorothiazide: The most common signs and symptoms observed are those caused by electrolyte depletion (hypokalaemia, hypochloraemia, hyponatraemia) and dehydration resulting from excessive diuresis. If digitalis has also been administered hypokalaemia may accentuate cardiac arrhythmias.

Pharmacological properties

Pharmacodynamic properties: Zestoretic 20 is a fixed dose combination product containing lisinopril, an inhibitor of angiotensin converting enzyme (ACE) and hydrochlorothiazide, a thiazide diuretic. Both components have complementary modes of action and exert an additive antihypertensive effect.

Lisinopril is a peptidyl dipeptidase inhibitor. It inhibits the angiotensin converting enzyme (ACE) that catalyses the conversion of angiotensin I to the vasoconstrictor peptide, angiotensin II. Angiotensin II also stimulates aldosterone secretion by the adrenal cortex. Inhibition of ACE results in decreased concentrations of angiotensin II which results in decreased vasopressor activity and reduced aldosterone secretion. The latter decrease may result in an increase in serum potassium concentration.

While the mechanism through which lisinopril lowers blood pressure is believed to be primarily suppression of the renin-angiotensin-aldosterone system, lisinopril is antihypertensive even in patients with low-renin hypertension. ACE is identical to kininase II, an enzyme that degrades bradykinin. Whether increased levels of bradykinin, a potent vasodilatory peptide, play a role in the therapeutic effects of lisinopril remains to be elucidated.

Hydrochlorothiazide is a diuretic and an antihypertensive agent. It affects the distal renal tubular mechanism of electrolyte reabsorption and increases excretion of sodium and chloride in approximately equivalent amounts. Natriuresis may be accompanied by some loss of potassium and bicarbonate. The mechanism of the antihypertensive effect of the thiazides is unknown. Thiazides do not usually affect normal blood pressure.

When combined with other antihypertensive agents, additive falls in blood pressure may occur.

Pharmacokinetic properties: Concomitant administration of lisinopril and hydrochlorothiazide has little or no effect on the bioavailability of either drug. The combination tablet is bioequivalent to concomitant administration of the separate entities.

Lisinopril: Following oral administration of lisinopril, peak serum concentrations occur within about 7 hours. On multiple dosing lisinopril has an effective half life of accumulation of 12.6 hours. Declining serum concentrations exhibit a prolonged terminal phase which does not contribute to drug accumulation. This terminal phase probably represents saturable binding to ACE and is not proportional to dose. Lisinopril does not appear to bind to other serum proteins.

Impaired renal function decreases elimination of lisinopril, which is excreted via the kidneys, but this decrease becomes clinically important only when the glomerular filtration rate is below 30 ml/min. Older patients have higher blood levels and higher values for the area under the plasma concentration time curve than younger patients. Lisinopril can be removed by dialysis.

Based on urinary recovery, the mean extent of absorption of lisinopril is approximately 25%, with interpatient variability (6 to 60%) at all doses tested (5 to 80 mg).

Lisinopril does not undergo metabolism and absorbed drug is excreted unchanged entirely in the urine. Lisinopril absorption is not affected by the presence of food in the gastrointestinal tract.

Studies in rats indicate that lisinopril crosses the blood-brain barrier poorly.

Hydrochlorothiazide: When plasma levels have been followed for at least 24 hours, the plasma half-life has been observed to vary between 5.6 and 14.8 hours. At least 61% of the dose is eliminated unchanged within 24 hours. After oral hydrochlorothiazide, diuresis begins within 2 hours, peaks in about 4 hours and lasts 6 to 12 hours. Hydrochlorothiazide crosses the placental but not the blood-brain barrier.

Preclinical safety data: Lisinopril and hydrochlorothiazide are both drugs on which extensive clinical experience has been obtained, both separately and in combination. All relevant information for the prescriber is provided elsewhere in the Summary of Product Characteristics.

Pharmaceutical particulars

List of excipients: Calcium Hydrogen Phosphate Dihydrate PhEur; Magnesium Stearate PhEur; Maize Starch PhEur; Mannitol PhEur; Pregelatinised Maize Starch PhEur.

Incompatibilities: None known, but see *Interactions.*

Shelf life: 2.5 years stored in the sales package.

Special precautions for storage: Store below 30°C, and protect from light.

Nature and contents of container: Blister packs of 28 tablets

Instructions for use/handling: Not applicable.

Market authorisation number PL 12619/0083

Date of first authorisation/renewal of authorisation June 1998.

Legal category POM

ZESTRIL*

Presentation White, round, biconvex uncoated tablets, impressed with a heart shape plus a number denoting tablet strength on one side, containing 2.5 mg lisinopril as the dihydrate. The inactive ingredients are calcium hydrogen phosphate dihydrate, magnesium stearate, maize starch and mannitol.

Pink, round, biconvex uncoated tablets, impressed with a heart shape plus a number denoting the tablet strength on one side and a bisecting line impressed on the other, containing 5 mg lisinopril as the dihydrate. The inactive ingredients are calcium hydrogen phosphate dihydrate, iron oxide, magnesium stearate, maize starch and mannitol.

Pink, round, biconvex uncoated tablets, impressed with a heart shape plus a number denoting the tablet strength and the trademark on one side, containing 10 mg lisinopril as the dihydrate. The inactive ingredients are calcium hydrogen phosphate dihydrate, iron oxide, magnesium stearate, maize starch and mannitol.

Pink, round, biconvex uncoated tablets, impressed with a heart shape plus a number denoting the tablet strength and the trademark on one side, containing 20 mg lisinopril as the dihydrate. The inactive ingredients are calcium hydrogen phosphate dihydrate, iron oxide, magnesium stearate, maize starch and mannitol.

Indications:

Hypertension: Zestril is indicated in the treatment of all grades of essential hypertension and renovascular hypertension. Zestril may be used alone or with other antihypertensive agents.

Congestive heart failure: Zestril is also indicated in the treatment of congestive heart failure as adjunctive therapy with non-potassium sparing diuretics and, where appropriate, digitalis. Treatment with Zestril should be initiated under close medical supervision (in hospital for severe heart failure).

Acute myocardial infarction: Zestril is indicated for the treatment of haemodynamically stable patients, defined as patients who are not in cardiogenic shock and who have a systolic blood pressure greater than 100 mmHg. Zestril may be initiated within 24 hours of the acute myocardial infarction to prevent the subsequent development of left ventricular dysfunction or heart failure and to improve survival. Patients should receive, as appropriate, the standard recommended treatments such as thrombolytics, aspirin and beta-blocker.

Renal complications of diabetes mellitus: In normotensive insulin-dependent and hypertensive non-insulin dependent diabetes mellitus patients who have incipient nephropathy characterised by microalbuminuria, Zestril reduces urinary albumin excretion rate.

Administration is by the oral route.

Mode of action: Lisinopril is a peptidyl dipeptidase inhibitor. It inhibits the angiotensin-converting enzyme (ACE) that catalyses the conversion of angiotensin I to the vasoconstrictor peptide, angiotensin II. Angiotensin II also stimulates aldosterone secretion by the adrenal cortex. Inhibition of ACE results in decreased concentrations of angiotensin II which results in decreased vasopressor activity and reduced aldosterone secretion. The latter decrease may result in an increase in serum potassium concentration.

While the mechanism through which lisinopril lowers blood pressure is believed to be primarily suppression of the renin-angiotensin-aldosterone system, lisinopril is antihypertensive even in patients with low-renin hypertension. ACE is identical to kininase II, an enzyme that degrades bradykinin. Whether increased levels of bradykinin, a potent vasodilatory peptide, play a role in the therapeutic effects of lisinopril remains to be elucidated.

ACE is known to be present in the endothelium and increased ACE activity in diabetic patients, which results in the formation of angiotensin II and destruction of bradykinin, potentiates the damage to the endothelium caused by hyperglycaemia. ACE inhibitors, including lisinopril, inhibit the formation of angiotensin II and breakdown of bradykinin and hence ameliorate endothelial dysfunction.

The effects of lisinopril on urinary albumin excretion rate in diabetic patients is mediated by a reduction in blood pressure as well as a direct mechanism on the renal tissue.

Angiotensin converting enzyme inhibitors may have a lesser effect on blood pressure in black hypertensive patients than in non-black hypertensive patients.

Following oral administration of lisinopril, peak serum concentrations occur within about 7 hours, although there was a trend to a small delay in time taken to reach peak serum concentrations in acute myocardial infarction patients. On multiple dosing lisinopril has an effective half life of accumulation of 12.6 hours.

Declining serum concentrations exhibit a prolonged terminal phase which does not contribute to drug accumulation. This terminal phase probably represents saturable binding to ACE and is not proportional to dose. Lisinopril does not appear to bind to other serum proteins.

Impaired renal function decreases elimination of lisinopril, which is excreted via the kidneys, but this decrease becomes clinically important only when the glomerular filtration rate is below 30 ml/min. Older patients have higher blood levels and higher values for the area under the plasma concentration time curve than younger patients. Lisinopril can be removed by dialysis.

Based on urinary recovery, the mean extent of absorption of lisinopril is approximately 25%, with interpatient variability (6-60%) at all doses tested (5-80 mg).

Lisinopril does not undergo metabolism and absorbed drug is excreted unchanged entirely in the urine. Lisinopril absorption is not affected by the presence of food in the gastrointestinal tract.

Studies in rats indicate that lisinopril crosses the blood-brain barrier poorly.

Dosage and administration Since absorption of Zestril tablets is not affected by food, the tablets may be administered before, during or after meals. Zestril should be administered in a single daily dose. As with all other medication taken once daily, Zestril should be taken at approximately the same time each day.

Hypertension: The need for dosage titration should be determined by measurement of the blood pressure just before the next dose.

Essential and Renovascular Hypertension: Treatment should be started with 2.5 mg once daily and adjusted to achieve optimal blood pressure control. For essential hypertension, in general, if the desired therapeutic effect cannot be achieved in a period of 2 to 4 weeks on a certain dose level, the dose can be further increased.

A 2.5 mg dose seldom achieves a therapeutic response. The usual effective dose range is 10 to 20 mg once daily. The maximum recommended dose is 40 mg once daily.

Diuretic treated patients: If possible, the diuretic should be discontinued, or the dose reduced, 2 to 3 days before beginning therapy with Zestril (see 'Precautions') and may be resumed later if required.

Use in the elderly: Age alone does not appear to affect the efficacy or safety profile of Zestril. Thus, elderly patients should start treatment with Zestril as directed above.

Congestive heart failure: Zestril may be used as adjunctive therapy with non-potassium sparing diuretics with or without digitalis.

Initial dosage: Treatment should be initiated, under close medical supervision, with a recommended starting dose of 2.5 mg with subsequent dose titration.

In the treatment of severe or unstable congestive heart failure, Zestril should always be initiated in hospital under close medical supervision. Other patients who may also be considered to be at higher risk should also have treatment initiated in hospital. These include patients who are on high dose loop diuretics (e.g. > 80 mg frusemide) or on multiple diuretic therapy, have hypovolaemia, hyponatraemia (serum sodium < 130 mEq/l) or systolic blood pressure < 90 mmHg, are on high dose vasodilator therapy, have a serum creatinine >150 micromol/l or are aged 70 years or over.

If possible, the dose of diuretic should be reduced before beginning treatment. Blood pressure and renal function should be monitored closely both before and during treatment because severe hypotension and, more rarely, consequent renal failure have been reported with angiotensin-converting enzyme (ACE) inhibitors. The appearance of hypotension after the initial dose of Zestril does not preclude subsequent careful dose adjustment with the drug, following effective treatment of the hypotension.

Maintenance dosage: The dose should be gradually increased, depending on the patient's response, to the usual maintenance dose (5-20 mg). In clinical trials doses were adjusted at 4 week intervals in patients requiring an additional therapeutic effect. Dose adjustment should be based on the clinical response of individual patients.

Acute myocardial infarction: Treatment with Zestril may be started within 24 hours of the onset of symptoms. The first dose of Zestril is 5 mg given orally, followed by 5 mg after 24 hours, 10 mg after 48 hours and then 10 mg once daily thereafter. Patients with a low systolic blood pressure (120 mmHg or less) should be given a lower dose–2.5 mg orally (see *Precautions*). If hypotension occurs (systolic blood pressure less than or equal to 100 mmHg), a daily maintenance dose of 5 mg may be given with temporary reductions to 2.5 mg if needed. If prolonged hypotension occurs (systolic blood pressure less than 90 mmHg for more than 1 hour), Zestril should be withdrawn.

Dosing should continue for six weeks. The benefit appears to be greatest in patients with large myocardial infarctions and evidence of impaired left ventricular function. Patients who develop symptoms of heart failure, should continue with Zestril (see *Dosage and Administration* for congestive heart failure).

Zestril is compatible with intravenous or transdermal glyceryl trinitrate.

Renal complications of diabetes mellitus: Treatment should be started with 2.5 mg once daily and titrated to achieve the target dose. In normotensive insulin-dependent diabetes mellitus patients, the dose is 10 mg Zestril once daily, which can be increased to 20 mg once daily if necessary to achieve a sitting diastolic blood pressure below 75 mm Hg. In hypertensive non-insulin-dependent diabetes mellitus patients, the dose schedule is as above to achieve a sitting diastolic blood pressure below 90 mm Hg.

Impaired renal function: Zestril is excreted by the kidney and should be used with caution in patients with renal insufficiency.

Zestril is dialysable (see *Precautions*). Dialysis patients may be given the usual dose of Zestril on dialysis days. On the days when patients are not on dialysis the dosage should be tailored to the blood pressure response.

Paediatric use: Zestril has not been studied for use in children.

Contra-indications, warnings, etc

Contra-indications: Zestril is contra-indicated in pregnancy and treatment should be stopped if pregnancy is suspected. ACE inhibitors can cause foetal and neonatal morbidity and mortality when administered to pregnant women during the second and third trimesters. Use of ACE inhibitors during this period has been associated with foetal and neonatal injury including hypotension, renal failure, hyperkalaemia and/or skull hypoplasia in the newborn. Maternal oligohydramnios, presumably representing decreased foetal renal function, has occurred and may result in limb contractures, craniofacial deformations and hypoplastic lung development.

These adverse effects to the embryo and foetus do not appear to have resulted from intrauterine ACE inhibitor exposure limited to the first trimester.

Infants whose mothers have taken lisinopril should be closely observed for hypotension, oliguria and hyperkalaemia. Lisinopril which crosses the placenta, has been removed from the neonatal circulation by peritoneal dialysis with some clinical benefit, and theoretically may be removed by exchange transfusion.

Zestril is contra-indicated in patients who are hypersensitive to any component of this product, in patients with a history of angioneurotic oedema relating to previous ACE-inhibitor therapy and in patients with hereditary or idiopathic angioedema.

Precautions: Assessment of renal function: Evaluation of the patient should include assessment of renal function prior to initiation of therapy and during treatment.

Impaired renal function: Zestril should be used with caution in patients with renal insufficiency, as they may require reduced or less frequent doses (see 'Dosage and Administration'). Close monitoring of renal function during therapy should be performed as deemed appropriate in those with renal insufficiency. In the majority, renal function will not alter, or may improve.

Renal failure has been reported in association with ACE inhibitors and has been mainly in patients with severe congestive heart failure or underlying renal disease, including renal artery stenosis. If recognised promptly and treated appropriately, renal failure is usually reversible.

In some patients with bilateral renal artery stenosis or stenosis of the artery to a solitary kidney, who have been treated with angiotensin converting enzyme inhibitors, increases in blood urea and serum creatinine, usually reversible upon discontinuation of therapy, have been seen. This is especially likely in patients with renal insufficiency. If renovascular hypertension is also present there is an increased risk of severe hypotension and renal insufficiency. In these patients, treatment should be started under close medical supervision with low doses and careful dose titration. Since treatment with diuretics may be a contributary factor to the above, they should be discontinued and renal function should be monitored during the first weeks of Zestril therapy.

Some hypertensive patients, with no apparent pre-existing renal disease, have developed increases in blood urea and creatinine when Zestril has been given concurrently with a diuretic. Dosage reduction of Zestril and/or discontinuation of the diuretic may be required. This situation should raise the possibility of underlying renal artery stenosis.

In acute myocardial infarction: Treatment with lisinopril should not be initiated in patients with evidence of renal dysfunction, defined as serum creatinine concentration exceeding 177 micromol/l and/or proteinuria exceeding 500 mg/24h. If renal dysfunction develops during treatment with Zestril (serum creatinine concentration exceeding 265 micromol/l or a doubling from the pre-treatment value) then the physician should consider withdrawal of Zestril.

Haemodialysis patients: A high incidence of anaphylactoid reactions has been reported in patients dialysed with high-flux membranes (e.g. AN69) and treated concomitantly with an ACE inhibitor. This combination should therefore be avoided.

Symptomatic hypotension: Symptomatic hypotension was seen rarely in uncomplicated hypertensive patients. It is more likely to occur in patients who have been volume-depleted by diuretic therapy, dietary salt restriction, dialysis, diarrhoea, or vomiting. In these patients, by discontinuing diuretic therapy or significantly reducing the diuretic dose 2 to 3 days prior to initiating Zestril, the possibility of this occurrence is reduced.

Severe hypotension has been reported with ACE inhibitors mainly in patients with severe heart failure. Many of these patients were on high doses of loop diuretics, and some had hyponatraemia or functional renal impairment. In patients at risk, initiation of therapy and dose adjustment should be monitored under close medical supervision.

If hypotension develops, the patient should be placed in a supine position. Volume repletion with oral fluids or intravenous normal saline may be required. Intravenous atropine may be necessary if there is associated bradycardia. Treatment with Zestril may be restarted with careful dose titration following restoration of effective blood volume and pressure.

Similar caution and close supervision may apply also to patients with ischaemic heart or cerebrovascular disease in whom severe hypotension could result in a myocardial infarct or cerebrovascular accident.

As with other vasodilators, Zestril should be given with caution to patients with aortic stenosis or hypertrophic cardiomyopathy.

In some patients with congestive heart failure who have normal or low blood pressure, additional lowering of systemic blood pressure may occur with Zestril. If such hypotension becomes symptomatic, a reduction of dose or discontinuation of Zestril may become necessary.

The appearance of hypotension after the initial dose of Zestril does not preclude subsequent careful dose adjustment with the drug after effective management of hypotension.

Hypotension in acute myocardial infarction: Treatment with lisinopril must not be initiated in acute myocardial infarction patients who are at risk of further serious haemodynamic deterioration after treatment with a vasodilator. These are patients with systolic blood pressure of 100 mmHg or lower or cardiogenic shock. During the first 3 days following the infarction, the dose should be reduced if the systolic blood pressure is 120 mmHg or lower. Maintenance doses should be reduced to 5 mg or temporarily to 2.5 mg if systolic blood pressure is 100 mmHg or lower. If hypotension persists (systolic blood pressure less than 90 mmHg for more than 1 hour) then Zestril should be withdrawn.

Angioneurotic oedema: has been reported with ACE inhibitors, including Zestril. In such cases, Zestril should be discontinued immediately and the patient observed. Where swelling is confined to the face, lips and mouth, the condition will usually resolve without further treatment, although antihistamines may be useful in relieving symptoms. These patients should be followed carefully until the swelling has resolved. However, angioedema associated with laryngeal oedema may be fatal. Where there is involvement of the tongue, glottis or larynx, likely to cause airways obstruction, emergency therapy should be administered promptly. This may include the administration of adrenaline and/or the maintenance of a patent airway. The patient should be under close medical supervision until complete and sustained resolution of symptoms has occurred.

Angiotensin converting enzyme inhibitors cause a higher rate of angioedema in black patients than in non-black patients.

Patients with a history of angioedema unrelated to ACE inhibitor therapy may be at increased risk of angioedema while receiving an ACE inhibitor (See also *Contra-indications*).

Race: Angiotensin converting enzyme inhibitors cause a higher rate of angioedema in black patients than in non non-black patients.

Cough: Cough has been reported with the use of ACE inhibitors. Characteristically, the cough is non-productive, persistent and resolves after discontinuation of therapy. ACE inhibitor-induced cough should be considered as part of the differential diagnosis of cough.

Surgery/anaesthesia: In patients undergoing major surgery or during anaesthesia with agents that produce hypotension, Zestril blocks angiotensin II formation secondary to compensatory renin release. This may lead to hypotension which can be corrected by volume expansion.

General: Zestril should not be used in patients with aortic stenosis, cor pulmonale or outflow tract obstruction.

Where Zestril is used as a single agent in hypertension, Afro-Caribbean patients may show a reduced therapeutic response.

Drug interactions: Combination with other antihypertensive agents such as beta-blockers and diuretics may increase the antihypertensive efficacy. Zestril minimises the development of thiazide-induced hypokalaemia and hyperuricaemia.

Indomethacin may reduce the antihypertensive efficacy of Zestril. In some patients with compromised renal function who are being treated with non steroidal anti-inflammatory drugs (NSAIDs), the co-administration of lisinopril may result in a further deterioration in renal function.

ACE inhibitors may potentiate the hypoglycaemic effect of insulin and oral antidiabetic drugs.

Zestril has been used with nitrates without significant clinical interaction.

As Zestril may reduce the elimination of lithium, serum levels of lithium should be monitored if lithium salts are administered.

Plasma potassium: Usually remains within normal

limits. If Zestril is given with a diuretic, the likelihood of diuretic induced hypokalaemia may be lessened. Zestril may elevate plasma potassium levels in patients with renal failure. Potassium supplements, potassium-sparing diuretics and potassium containing salt substitutes are not recommended.

Breast-feeding mothers: Caution should be exercised if Zestril is given to breast feeding mothers because it is not known whether Zestril is excreted in human milk.

Side effects: Hypotension has occurred in association with therapy with Zestril. This appears to occur in certain specific sub-groups (see *Precautions*).

Angioneurotic oedema of the face, extremities, lips, tongue, glottis and/or larynx has been reported rarely. (See *Precautions*).

Other hypersensitivity reactions have been reported.

Other adverse reactions: Dizziness, headache, diarrhoea, cough, nausea and fatigue are the most frequent. Other less frequent side effects include rash and asthenia.

Rare side effects include:
Cardiovascular: Myocardial infarction or cerebrovascular accident possibly secondary to excessive hypotension in high risk patients (See *Precautions*); palpitations; tachycardia.

Digestive: Abdominal pain and indigestion; dry mouth; hepatitis (hepatocellular or cholestatic); jaundice; pancreatitis; vomiting.

Nervous system: Mental confusion; mood alterations; paraesthesia; vertigo. As with other angiotensin converting enzyme inhibitors, taste disturbance and sleep disturbances have been reported.

Respiratory: Bronchospasm; rhinitis; sinusitis.

Skin: Alopecia; diaphoresis; pruritus; urticaria; psoriasis and severe skin disorders have been reported, including pemphigus; toxic epidermal necrolysis; Stevens-Johnson Syndrome and erythema multiforme.

Urogenital: Impotence, oliguria/anuria, acute renal failure, renal dysfunction, uraemia. There have been reports of haemolytic anaemia in patients taking lisinopril although no causal relationship has been established.

A symptom complex has been reported which may include one or more of the following: fever, vasculitis, myalgia, arthralgia/arthritis, a positive ANA, elevated ESR, eosinophilia and leucocytosis. Rash, photosensitivity or other dermatological manifestations may occur.

Laboratory test findings: Clinically important changes in standard laboratory parameters were rarely associated with administration of Zestril. Increases in blood urea, serum creatinine, liver enzymes and serum bilirubin, usually reversible upon discontinuation of Zestril, have been seen.

Bone marrow depression, manifest as anaemia, and/or thrombocytopenia and or leucopenia has been reported. Agranulocytosis has been rarely reported.

Small decreases in haemoglobin and haematocrit, rarely of clinical importance unless another cause of anaemia coexisted, have occurred.

Hyperkalaemia has occurred.

Hyponatraemia has occurred.

Patients receiving ACE inhibitors during desensitisation treatment (e.g. hymenoptera venom) have sustained anaphylactoid reactions. In the same patients, these reactions have been avoided when ACE inhibitors were temporarily withheld but they reappeared on inadvertent rechallenge.

Overdosage: The symptoms of overdosage may include severe hypotension, electrolyte disturbance and renal failure. After ingestion of an overdose, the patient should be kept under very close supervision. Therapeutic measures depend on the nature and severity of the symptoms. Measures to prevent absorption and methods to speed elimination should be employed. If severe hypotension occurs, the patient should be placed in the shock position and an intravenous infusion of normal saline should be given rapidly. Treatment with angiotensin II (if available) may be considered. Angiotensin converting enzyme inhibitors may be removed from the circulation by haemodialysis. The use of high-flux polyacrylonitrile dialysis membranes should be avoided. Serum electrolytes and creatinine should be monitored frequently.

Pharmaceutical precautions Store below 30°C.

Legal category POM.

Package quantities

Tablets 20 mg:	Calendar packs of 28 tablets
Tablets 10 mg:	Calendar packs of 28 tablets
Tablets 5 mg:	Calendar packs of 28 tablets
Tablets 2.5 mg:	Calendar packs of 28 tablets

Further information Nil.

Product licence numbers

Zestril Tablets 2.5 mg	12619/0084
Zestril Tablets 5 mg	12619/0085
Zestril Tablets 10 mg	12619/0086
Zestril Tablets 20 mg	12619/0087

ZOLADEX* 3.6 mg

Qualitative and quantitative composition Goserelin acetate (equivalent to 3.6 mg goserelin).

Pharmaceutical form Sterile depot.

Clinical particulars
Therapeutic indications

(i) Prostate Cancer: Zoladex is indicated in the management of prostate cancer suitable for hormonal manipulation.
(ii) Advanced breast cancer in pre- and peri-menopausal women suitable for hormonal manipulation.
(iii) Endometriosis: In the management of endometriosis, Zoladex alleviates symptoms, including pain, and reduces the size and number of endometrial lesions.
(iv) Endometrial thinning: Zoladex is indicated for the prethinning of the uterine endometrium prior to endometrial ablation or resection.
(v) Uterine fibroids: In conjunction with iron therapy in the haematological improvement of anaemic patients with fibroids prior to surgery.
(vi) Assisted reproduction: Pituitary downregulation in preparation for superovulation.

Posology and method of administration:
Adults: One 3.6 mg depot of Zoladex injected subcutaneously into the anterior abdominal wall, every 28 days. No dosage adjustment is necessary for patients with renal or hepatic impairment or in the elderly.

Endometriosis should be treated for a period of six months only, since at present there are no clinical data for longer treatment periods. Repeat courses should not be given due to concern about loss of bone mineral density. In patients receiving Zoladex for the treatment of endometriosis, the addition of hormone replacement therapy (a daily oestrogenic agent and a progestogenic agent) has been shown to reduce bone mineral density loss and vasomotor symptoms.

For use in endometrial thinning, four or eight weeks treatment. The second depot may be required for the patient with a large uterus or to allow flexible surgical timing.

For women who are anaemic as a result of uterine fibroids, Zoladex 3.6 mg depot with supplementary iron may be administered for up to three months before surgery.

Assisted reproduction: Zoladex 3.6 mg is administered to downregulate the pituitary gland, as defined by serum oestradiol levels similar to those observed in the early follicular phase (approximately 150 pmol/l). This will usually take between 7 and 21 days.

When downregulation is achieved, superovulation (controlled ovarian stimulation) with gonadotrophin is commenced. The downregulation achieved with a depot agonist is more consistent suggesting that, in some cases, there may be an increased requirement for gonadotrophin. At the appropriate stage of follicular development, gonadotrophin is stopped and human chorionic gonadotrophin (hCG) is administered to induce ovulation. Treatment monitoring, oocyte retrieval and fertilisation techniques are performed according to the normal practice of the individual clinic.

Children: Zoladex is not indicated for use in children.

Contra-indications: Zoladex should not be given to patients with a known hypersensitivity to Zoladex or to LHRH analogues. Zoladex should not be used in pregnancy (see *Pregnancy and lactation*).

Special warnings and special precautions for use: Zoladex is not indicated for use in children, as safety and efficacy have not been established in this group of patients.

Males: The use of Zoladex in men at particular risk of developing ureteric obstruction or spinal cord compression should be considered carefully and the patients monitored closely during the first month of therapy. Consideration should be given to the initial use of an anti-androgen (e.g. cyproterone acetate 300 mg daily for three days before and three weeks after commencement of Zoladex) at the start of LHRH analogue therapy since this has been reported to prevent the possible sequelae of the initial rise in serum testosterone. If spinal cord compression or renal impairment due to ureteric obstruction are present or develop, specific standard treatment of these complications should be instituted.

Females: The use of LHRH agonists in women may cause a loss of bone mineral density. Currently available data on Zoladex indicate a mean loss of 4.6% in vertebral bone mineral density following a six month course of treatment with progressive recovery to a mean loss compared to baseline of 2.6% six months after cessation of treatment. In patients receiving Zoladex for the treatment of endometriosis, the addition of hormone replacement therapy (a daily oestrogenic agent and a progestogenic agent) has been shown to reduce bone mineral density loss and vasomotor symptoms.

Zoladex should be used with caution in women with known metabolic bone disease.

Zoladex may cause an increase in uterine cervical resistance, which may result in difficulty in dilating the cervix.

Currently, there are no clinical data on the effect of treating benign gynaecological conditions with Zoladex for periods in excess of six months.

Zoladex should only be administered as part of a regimen for assisted reproduction under the supervision of a specialist experienced in the area.

As with other LHRH agonists, there have been reports of ovarian hyperstimulation syndrome (OHSS), associated with the use of Zoladex 3.6 mg in combination with gonadotrophin. It has been suggested that the downregulation achieved with a depot agonist may lead, in some cases, to an increased requirement for gonadotrophin. The stimulation cycle should be monitored carefully to identify patients at risk of developing OHSS because its severity and incidence may be dependent on the dose regimen of gonadotrophin. Human chorionic gonadotrophin (hCG) should be withheld, if appropriate.

It is recommended that Zoladex is used with caution in assisted reproduction regimens in patients with polycystic ovarian syndrome as follicle recruitment may be increased.

Interactions with other medicaments and other forms of interaction: None known.

Pregnancy and lactation:
Pregnancy: Although reproductive toxicity in animals gave no evidence of teratogenic potential, Zoladex should not be used in pregnancy as there is a theoretical risk of abortion or foetal abnormality if LHRH agonists are used during pregnancy. Potentially fertile women should be examined carefully before treatment to exclude pregnancy. Non hormonal methods of contraception should be employed during therapy and in the case of endometriosis should be continued until menses are resumed.

Pregnancy should be excluded before Zoladex is used for assisted reproduction. The clinical data from use in this setting are limited but the available evidence suggests there is no causal association between Zoladex and any subsequent abnormalities of oocyte development or pregnancy and outcome.

Lactation: The use of Zoladex during breast feeding is not recommended.

Effects on ability to drive and use machines: There is no evidence that Zoladex results in impairment of these activities.

Undesirable events:
General: Rare incidences of hypersensitivity reactions, which may include some manifestations of anaphylaxis have been reported.

Arthralgia has been reported. Skin rashes have been reported which are generally mild, often regressing without discontinuation of therapy.

Changes in blood pressure, manifest as hypotension or hypertension, have been occasionally observed in patients administered Zoladex. These changes are usually transient, resolving either during continued therapy or after cessation of therapy with Zoladex. Rarely, such changes have been sufficent to require medical intervention including withdrawal of treatment from Zoladex.

Occasional local reactions include mild bruising at the subcutaneous injection site.

Males: Pharmacological effects in men include hot flushes and a decrease in libido, seldom requiring withdrawal of therapy. Breast swelling and tenderness have been noted infrequently. Initially, prostate cancer patients may experience a temporary increase in bone pain, which can be managed symptomatically. Isolated cases of ureteric obstruction and spinal cord compression have been recorded.

The use of LHRH agonists in men may cause a loss of bone mineral density.

Females: Pharmacological effects in women include hot flushes and sweating, and loss in libido, seldom requiring withdrawal of therapy. Headaches, mood changes including depression, vaginal dryness and change in breast size have been noted. During early treatment with Zoladex some women may experience vaginal bleeding of variable duration and intensity. If vaginal bleeding occurs it is usually in the first month after starting treatment. Such bleeding probably represents oestrogen withdrawal bleeding and is expected to stop spontaneously.

Initially breast cancer patients may experience a

temporary increase in signs and symptoms, which can be managed symptomatically. In women with fibroids, degeneration of fibroids may occur.

Rarely, breast cancer patients with metastases have developed hypercalcaemia on initiation of therapy.

Rarely, some women may enter the menopause during treatment with LHRH analogues and not resume menses on cessation of therapy. This may simply be a physiological change.

In Assisted Reproduction: As with other LHRH agonists, there have been reports of ovarian hyperstimulation syndrome (OHSS), associated with the use of Zoladex 3.6 mg in combination with gonadotrophin. It has been suggested that the downregulation achieved with a depot agonist may lead, in some cases, to an increased requirement for gonadotrophin. The stimulation cycle should be monitored carefully to identify patients at risk of developing OHSS because its severity and incidence may be dependent on the dose regimen of gonadotrophin. Human chorionic gonadotrophin (hCG) should be withheld, if appropriate.

Follicular and luteal ovarian cysts have been reported to occur following LHRH therapy. Most cysts are asymptomatic, non functional, varying in size and resolve spontaneously.

Overdosage: There is no human experience of overdosage. Animal tests suggest that no effect other than the intended therapeutic effects on sex hormone concentration and on the reproductive tract will be evident with higher doses of Zoladex. If overdosage occurs, this should be managed symptomatically.

Pharmacological properties
Pharmacodynamic properties: Zoladex (D-Ser(Bu^t)^6 Azgly^{10} LHRH) is a synthetic analogue of naturally occurring LHRH. On chronic administration Zoladex results in inhibition of pituitary LH secretion leading to a fall in serum testosterone concentrations in males and serum oestradiol concentrations in females. This effect is reversible on discontinuation of therapy. Initially, Zoladex, like other LHRH agonists, may transiently increase serum testosterone concentration in men and serum oestradiol concentration in women.

In men by around 21 days after the first depot injection testosterone concentrations have fallen to within the castrate range and remain suppressed with continuous treatment every 28 days. This inhibition leads to prostate tumour regression and symptomatic improvement in the majority of patients.

In women serum oestradiol concentrations are suppressed by around 21 days after the first depot injection and, with continuous treatment every 28 days, remain suppressed at levels comparable with those observed in postmenopausal women. This suppression is associated with a response in hormone dependent advanced breast cancer, uterine fibroids, endometriosis and suppression of follicular development within the ovary. It will produce endometrial thinning and will result in amenorrhoea in the majority of patients.

Zoladex in combination with iron has been shown to induce amenorrhoea and improve haemoglobin concentrations and related haematological parameters in women with fibroids who are anaemic. The combination produced a mean haemoglobin concentration 1 g/dl above that achieved by iron therapy alone.

Pharmacokinetic properties: The bioavailability of Zoladex is almost complete. Administration of a depot every four weeks ensures that effective concentrations are maintained with no tissue accumulations. Zoladex is poorly protein bound and has a serum elimination half-life of two to four hours in subjects with normal renal function. The half-life is increased in patients with impaired renal function. For the compound given monthly in a depot formulation, this change will have minimal effect. Hence, no change in dosing is necessary in these patients. There is no significant change in pharmacokinetics in patients with hepatic failure.

Preclinical safety data: Following long-term repeated dosing with Zoladex, an increased incidence of benign pituitary tumours has been observed in male rats. Whilst this finding is similar to that previously noted in this species following surgical castration, any relevance to man has not been established.

In mice, long term repeated dosing with multiples of the human dose produced histological changes in some regions of the digestive system manifested by pancreatic islet cell hyperplasia and a benign proliferative condition in the pyloric region of the stomach, also reported as a spontaneous lesion in this species. The clinical relevance of these findings is unknown.

Pharmaceutical particulars
List of excipients: Lactide/glycolide co-polymer.

Incompatibilities: None known.

Shelf life: 36 months.

Special precautions for storage: Store below 25°C.

Nature and contents of container: Single dose syringe applicator.

Instructions for use handling: Use as directed by the prescriber. Use only if pouch is undamaged. Use immediately after opening pouch.

Marketing authorisation number 12619/0088.

Date of approval/revision of SPC September 1998.

Legal category POM.

ZOLADEX* LA

Qualitative and quantitative composition Each depot contains goserelin acetate equivalent to 10.8 mg goserelin.

Pharmaceutical form Sustained release sterile depot.

Clinical particulars
Therapeutic indication: Zoladex LA is indicated for prostate cancer suitable for hormonal manipulation.

Posology and method of administration:
Adult males (including the elderly): One depot of Zoladex LA injected subcutaneously into the anterior abdominal wall every 12 weeks.

Children: Zoladex LA is not indicated for use in children.

Renal impairment: No dosage adjustment is necessary for patients with renal impairment.

Hepatic impairment: No dosage adjustment for patients with hepatic impairment.

Contra-indications: Zoladex LA should not be given to patients with a known hypersensitivity to Zoladex or to other LHRH analogues.

Special warnings and special precautions for use: Zoladex LA is not indicated for use in females, since there is insufficient evidence of reliable suppression of serum oestradiol. For female patients requiring treatment with goserelin, refer to the prescribing information for Zoladex 3.6 mg.

Zoladex LA is not indicated for use in children, as safety and efficacy have not been established in this group of patients.

The use of Zoladex LA in patients at particular risk of developing ureteric obstruction or spinal cord compression should be considered carefully and the patients monitored closely during the first month of therapy. Consideration should be given to the initial use of an antiandrogen (e.g. cyproterone acetate 300 mg daily for three days before and three weeks after commencement of Zoladex) at the start of LHRH analogue therapy since this has been reported to prevent the possible sequelae of the initial rise in serum testosterone. If spinal cord compression or renal impairment due to ureteric obstruction are present or develop, specific standard treatment of these complications should be instituted.

Interaction with other medicaments and other forms of interaction: None known.

Pregnancy and lactation: Zoladex LA is not indicated for use in females.

Effects on ability to drive and use machinery: There is no evidence that Zoladex LA results in impairment of ability to drive or operate machinery.

Undesirable effects: Rare incidences of hypersensitivity reactions, which may include some manifestations of anaphylaxis, have been reported.

Pharmacological effects in men include hot flushes and a decrease in libido, seldom requiring withdrawal of therapy. Breast swelling and tenderness have been noted infrequently. Initially, prostate cancer patients may experience a temporary increase in bone pain, which can be managed symptomatically. Isolated cases of spinal cord compression have been recorded.

The use of LHRH agonists in men may cause a loss of bone mineral density.

Changes in blood pressure, manifest as hypotension or hypertension, have been occasionally observed in patients administered Zoladex. The changes are usually transient, resolving either during continued therapy or after cessation of therapy with Zoladex. Rarely, such changes have been sufficient to require medical intervention, including withdrawal of treatment from Zoladex.

Although not reported by patients in the clinical trial program of Zoladex LA, following the administration of Zoladex 3.6 mg, arthralgia, skin rashes which are generally mild and often regress without discontinuation of therapy, and isolated cases of ureteric obstruction have been recorded.

Overdose: There is no human experience of overdosage. Animal tests suggest that no effect other than the intended therapeutic effects on sex hormone concentrations and on the reproductive tract will be evident with higher doses of Zoladex LA. If overdosage occurs, this should be managed symptomatically.

Pharmacological properties
Pharmacodynamic properties: Zoladex (D-Ser(Bu^t)^6 Azgly^{10} LHRH) is a synthetic analogue of naturally occurring luteinising-hormone releasing hormone (LHRH). On chronic administration Zoladex LA results in inhibition of pituitary luteinising hormone secretion leading to a fall in serum testosterone concentrations in males. Initially, Zoladex LA like other LHRH agonists transiently increases serum testosterone concentrations.

In men by around 21 days after the first depot injection, testosterone concentrations have fallen to within the castrate range and remain suppressed with treatment every 12 weeks.

Pharmacokinetic properties: Administration of Zoladex LA every 12 weeks ensures that exposure to goserelin is maintained with no clinically significant accumulation. Zoladex is poorly protein bound and has a serum elimination half-life of two to four hours in subjects with normal renal function. The half-life is increased in patients with impaired renal function. For the compound given in a 10.8 mg depot formulation every 12 weeks this change will not lead to any accumulation. Hence, no change in dosing is necessary in these patients. There is no significant change in pharmacokinetics in patients with hepatic failure.

Preclinical safety data: Following long-term repeated dosing with Zoladex, an increased incidence of benign pituitary tumours has been observed in male rats. Whilst this finding is similar to that previously noted in this species following surgical castration, any relevance to humans has not been established.

In mice, long term repeated dosing with multiples of the human dose produced histological changes in some regions of the digestive system. This is manifested by pancreatic islet cell hyperplasia and a benign proliferative condition in the pyloric region of the stomach, also reported as a spontaneous lesion in this species. The clinical relevance of these findings is unknown.

Pharmaceutical particulars
List of excipients: A blend of high and low molecular weight lactide/glycolide copolymers.

Incompatibilities: None known.

Shelf life: 36 months.

Special precautions for storage: Store below 25°C.

Nature and contents of container: Zoladex LA is supplied as a single dose syringe applicator in a sealed pouch which contains a desiccant.

Instructions for use/handling: Use as directed by the prescriber. Use only if pouch is undamaged. Use immediately after opening pouch.

Marketing authorisation number 12619/0103.

Date of approval/revision of SPC September 1998.

Legal category POM.

ZOMIG* ▼

Qualitative and quantitative composition Tablets for oral administration containing 2.5 mg of zolmitriptan.

Pharmaceutical form Tablets.

Clinical particulars
Therapeutic indications: Zomig is indicated for the acute treatment of migraine with or without aura.

Posology and method of administration: The recommended dose of Zomig to treat a migraine attack is 2.5 mg.

If symptoms persist or return within 24 hours, a second dose has been shown to be effective. If a second dose is required, it should not be taken within 2 hours of the initial dose.

If a patient does not achieve satisfactory relief with 2.5 mg doses, subsequent attacks can be treated with 5 mg doses of Zomig.

In those patients who respond, significant efficacy is apparent within 1 hour of dosing.

Zomig is equally effective whenever the tablets are taken during a migraine attack; although it is advisable that Zomig tablets are taken as early as possible after the onset of migraine headache.

In the event of recurrent attacks, it is recommended that the total intake of Zomig in a 24 hour period should not exceed 15 mg.

Zomig is not indicated for prophylaxis of migraine.

Use in children: Safety and efficacy of Zomig in paediatric patients have not been established.

Use in patients aged over 65 years: Safety and efficacy of Zomig in individuals aged over 65 years have not been systematically evaluated.

Patients with hepatic impairment: Metabolism is reduced in patients with hepatic impairment (See *Pharmacokinetic properties*). Therefore for patients with moderate or severe hepatic impairment a maximum dose of 5 mg in 24 hours is recommended.

Patients with renal impairment: No dosage adjustment required (see *Pharmacokinetic properties*).

Contra-indications: Zomig is contra-indicated in patients with known hypersensitivity to any component of the product.

Zomig must not be given to patients with uncontrolled hypertension.

Special warnings and special precautions for use: Zomig should only be used where a clear diagnosis of migraine has been established. Care should be taken to exclude other potentially serious neurological conditions. There are no data on the use of Zomig in hemiplegic or basilar migraine.

Zomig should not be given to patients with symptomatic Wolff-Parkinson-White syndrome or arrhythmias associated with other cardiac accessory conduction pathways.

This class of compounds ($5HT_{1D}$ agonists) has been associated with coronary vasospasm, as a result, patients with ischaemic heart disease were excluded from clinical trials. Zomig is, therefore, not recommended in this patient group. In patients in whom unrecognised coronary artery disease is likely, cardiovascular evaluation prior to commencement of treatment with $5HT_{1D}$ agonists is recommended.

As with other $5HT_{1D}$ agonists, atypical sensations over the precordium (see *Undesirable effects*) have been reported after the administration of zolmitriptan, but in clinical trials these have not been associated with arrhythmias or ischaemic changes on ECG. Zomig may cause mild, transient increases in blood pressure (which may be more pronounced in the elderly), however, this has not been associated with clinical sequelae in the clinical trial programme.

Interactions with other medicaments and other forms of interaction: There is no evidence that concomitant use of migraine prophylactic medications has any effect on the efficacy or unwanted effects of Zomig (for example beta blockers, oral dihydroergotamine, pizotifen).

The pharmacokinetics and tolerability of Zomig were unaffected by acute symptomatic treatments such as paracetamol, metoclopramide and ergotamine. However, it is recommended that patients should leave at least 6 hours between taking an ergotamine preparation and starting Zomig, and vice versa. Concomitant administration of other $5HT_{1D}$ agonists within 12 hours of Zomig treatment should be avoided.

Following administration of moclobemide, a specific MAO-A inhibitor, there was a small increase (26%) in AUC for zolmitriptan and a 3-fold increase in AUC of the active metabolite. Therefore, a maximum intake of 7.5 mg Zomig in 24 hours is recommended in patients taking an MAO-A inhibitor.

Following the administration of cimetidine, a general P450 inhibitor, the half life of zolmitriptan was increased by 44% and the AUC increased by 48%. In addition the half life and AUC of the active N-desmethylated metabolite (183C91) were doubled. A maximum dose of 5 mg Zomig in 24 hours is recommended in patients taking cimetidine. Based on the overall interaction profile, an interaction with inhibitors of the cytochrome P450 isoenzyme CYP1A2 cannot be excluded. Therefore, the same dosage reduction is recommended with compounds of this type, such as fluvoxamine and the quinolone antibiotics (eg, ciprofloxacin).

Fluoxetine does not affect the pharmacokinetic parameters of zolmitriptan. Therapeutic doses of the specific serotonin reuptake inhibitors, fluoxetine, sertraline, paroxetine and citalopram do not inhibit CYPIA2.

Pregnancy and lactation:

Pregnancy: Zomig should be used in pregnancy only if the benefits to the mother justify potential risk to the foetus. There are no studies in pregnant women, but there is no evidence of teratogenicity in animal studies. (See *Preclinical safety data*).

Lactation: Studies have shown that zolmitriptan passes into the milk of lactating animals. No data exist for passage of zolmitriptan into human breast milk. Therefore, caution should be exercised when administering Zomig to women who are breast-feeding.

Effects on ability to drive and use machines: There was no significant impairment of performance of psychomotor tests with doses up to 20 mg Zomig. Use is unlikely to result in an impairment of the ability of patients to drive or operate machinery. However it should be taken into account that somnolence may occur.

Undesirable effects: Zomig is well tolerated. Adverse reactions are typically mild/moderate, transient, not serious and resolve spontaneously without additional treatment. Possible adverse reactions tend to occur within 4 hours of dosing and are no more frequent following repeated dosing.

The following adverse reactions have been the most commonly reported: nausea; dizziness; somnolence; warm sensation; asthenia; dry mouth.

Abnormalities or disturbances of sensation have been reported; heaviness, tightness or pressure may occur in the throat, neck, limbs and chest (with no evidence of ischaemic changes on ECG), as may myalgia, muscle weakness, paraesthesia and dysaesthesia.

Overdose: Volunteers receiving single oral doses of 50 mg commonly experienced sedation.

The elimination half-life of zolmitriptan tablets is 2.5 to 3 hours, (see *Pharmacokinetic properties*) and therefore monitoring of patients after overdose with Zomig tablets should continue for at least 15 hours or while symptoms or signs persist.

There is no specific antidote to zolmitriptan . In cases of severe intoxication, intensive care procedures are recommended, including establishing and maintaining a patent airway, ensuring adequate oxygenation and ventilation, and monitoring and support of the cardiovascular system.

Pharmacological properties

Pharmacodynamic properties: In pre-clinical studies, zolmitriptan has been demonstrated to be a selective agonist for the vascular human recombinant $5HT_{1D\alpha}$ and $5HT_{1D\beta}$ receptor subtypes. Zolmitriptan is a high affinity $5HT_{1D}$ receptor agonist with modest affinity for $5HT_{1A}$ receptors. Zolmitriptan has no significant affinity (as measured by radioligand binding assays) or pharmacological activity at $5HT_2$-, $5HT_3$-, $5HT_4$-, alpha$_1$-, alpha$_2$-, or beta$_1$-, adrenergic; H_1-, H_2-, histaminic; muscarinic; dopaminergic$_1$, or dopaminergic$_2$ receptors. The $5HT_{1D\alpha}$ receptor is predominately located presynaptically at both the peripheral and central synapses of the trigeminal nerve and preclinical studies have shown that zolmitriptan is able to act at both these sites.

Pharmacokinetic properties: Zolmitriptan is rapidly and well absorbed (at least 64%) after oral administration to man. The mean absolute bioavailability of the parent compound is approximately 40%. There is an active metabolite (183C91, the N-desmethyl metabolite) which is also a $5HT_{1D}$ agonist and is 2 to 6 times as potent, in animal models, as zolmitriptan.

In healthy subjects, when given as a single dose, zolmitriptan and its active metabolite 183C91, display dose-proportional AUC and C_{max} over the dose range 2.5 to 50 mg. Absorption is rapid with 75% of C_{max} achieved within 1 hour and plasma concentrations are sustained subsequently for 4 to 6 hours. Zolmitriptan absorption is unaffected by the presence of food. There is no evidence of accumulation on multiple dosing of zolmitriptan.

Zolmitriptan is eliminated largely by hepatic biotransformation followed by urinary excretion of the metabolites. There are three major metabolites: the indole acetic acid, (the major metabolite in plasma and urine), the N-oxide and N-desmethyl analogues. The N-desmethylated metabolite (183C91) is active whilst the others are not. Plasma concentrations of 183C91 are approximately half those of the parent drug, hence it would therefore be expected to contribute to the therapeutic action of Zomig. Over 60% of a single oral dose is excreted in the urine (mainly as the indole acetic acid metabolite) and about 30% in faeces, mainly as unchanged parent compound.

A study to evaluate the effect of liver disease on the pharmacokinetics of zolmitriptan showed that the AUC and Cmax were increased by 94% and 50% respectively in patients with moderate liver disease and by 226% and 47% in patients with severe liver disease compared with healthy volunteers. Exposure to the metabolites, including the active metabolite, was decreased. For the 183C91 metabolite, AUC and Cmax were reduced by 33% and 44% in patients with moderate liver disease and by 82% and 90% in patients with severe liver disease.

The plasma half-life ($T_{\frac{1}{2}}$) of zolmitriptan was 4.7 hours in healthy volunteers, 7.3 hours in patients with moderate liver disease and 12 hours in those with severe liver disease. The corresponding $T_{\frac{1}{2}}$ values for the 183C91 metabolite were 5.7 hours, 7.5 hours and 7.8 hours respectively.

Following intravenous administration, the mean total plasma clearance is approximately 10 ml/min/kg, of which one third is renal clearance. Renal clearance is greater than glomerular filtration rate suggesting renal tubular secretion. The volume of distribution following intravenous administration is 2.4 L/kg. Plasma protein binding is low (approximately 25%). The mean elimination half-life of zolmitriptan is 2.5 to 3 hours. The half-lives of its metabolites are similar, suggesting their elimination is formation-rate limited.

Renal clearance of zolmitriptan and all its metabolites is reduced (7 to 8 fold) in patients with moderate to severe renal impairment compared to healthy subjects, although the AUC of the parent compound and the active metabolite were only slightly higher (16 and 35% respectively) with a 1 hour increase in half-life to 3 to 3.5 hours. These parameters are within the ranges seen in healthy volunteers.

In a small group of healthy individuals there was no pharmacokinetic interaction with ergotamine. Concomitant administration of Zomig with ergotamine/caffeine was well tolerated and did not result in any increase in adverse events or blood pressure changes as compared with Zomig alone.

Selegiline, an MAO-B inhibitor, and fluoxetine (a selective serotonin reuptake inhibitor; SSRI) had no effect on the pharmacokinetic parameters of zolmitriptan.

The pharmacokinetics of zolmitriptan in healthy elderly subjects were similar to those in healthy young volunteers.

Preclinical safety data: An oral teratology study of Zomig has been conducted. At the maximum tolerated doses of Zomig, 1200 mg/kg/day (AUC 605 microgram/ml.h: approx. 3700×AUC of the human maximum recommended daily intake of 15 mg) and 30 mg/kg/day (AUC 4.9 microgram/ml.h: approx. 30×AUC of the human maximum recommended daily intake of 15 mg) in rats and rabbits, respectively, no signs of teratogenicity were apparent.

Five genotoxicity tests have been performed. It was concluded that Zomig is not likely to pose any genetic risk in humans.

Carcinogenicity studies in rats and mice were conducted at the highest feasible doses and gave no suggestion of tumorogenicity.

Reproductive studies in male and female rats, at dose levels limited by toxicity, revealed no effect on fertility.

Pharmaceutical particulars

List of excipients: The following excipients are contained in each tablet as indicated: hydroxypropyl methylcellulose; iron oxide–yellow; lactose; magnesium stearate; microcrystalline cellulose; polyethylene glycol (400 and 8000); sodium starch glycollate; titanium dioxide.

Incompatibilities: None known

Shelf life: 24 months when stored below 30°C.

Special precautions for storage: Store below 30°C.

Nature and contents of container: carton containing 2 strips of 3 tablets; carton containing 2 strips of 3 tablets (with wallet), carton containing 4 strips of 3 tablets.

Instructions for use/handling: No specific instructions.

Marketing authorisation number 12619/0116

Date of approval/revision of SPC July 1998.

Legal category POM

**Trade Mark*

CODE OF PRACTICE FOR THE PHARMACEUTICAL INDUSTRY

Operative Date: 1 January 1998

INTRODUCTION

Promoting Health

The commitment of Britain's pharmaceutical industry to providing high quality effective medicines brings major benefits to both the health of the nation and the country's economy.

The National Health Service spends over £5 billion a year on medicines yet this represents less than 12 per cent of its total expenditure. Medicine exports are worth nearly £5 billion a year – the United Kingdom's second largest foreign exchange earner in manufactured goods. Five of the top twenty prescribed medicines worldwide were discovered in Britain.

Investment into researching and developing new products in the UK is now running at around £2 billion a year and each new medicine takes an average of twelve years to develop before it is authorized for use by doctors, with no guarantee of commercial success. It is vital therefore that the pharmaceutical industry keeps the medical profession informed about its products and promotes their rational use.

The Association of the British Pharmaceutical Industry and its Code of Practice

The Association of the British Pharmaceutical Industry (ABPI) is the trade association representing manufacturers of prescription medicines. It was formed in 1930 and now represents more than one hundred companies which produce 95 per cent of the medicines supplied to the National Health Service.

The ABPI Code of Practice for the Pharmaceutical Industry has been regularly revised since its inception in 1958 and is drawn up in consultation with the British Medical Association, the Royal Pharmaceutical Society of Great Britain and the Medicines Control Agency of the Department of Health.

It is a condition of membership of the ABPI to abide by the Code in both the spirit and the letter. Companies which are not members of the Association may give their formal agreement to abide by the Code and accept the jurisdiction of the Prescription Medicines Code of Practice Authority and about fifty have done so. Thus the Code is accepted by virtually all pharmaceutical companies operating in the UK.

Ensuring High Standards

The aim of the Code of Practice for the Pharmaceutical Industry is to ensure that the promotion of medicines to members of the health professions and to administrative staff is carried out in a responsible, ethical and professional manner. The Code recognises and seeks to achieve a balance between the needs of patients, industry, health professionals and the general public, bearing in mind the political and social environment within which the industry operates and the statutory controls covering medicines.

Strong support is given to the Code by the industry with all companies devoting considerable resources to ensure that their promotional activities comply with it. Any complaint made against a company under the Code is regarded as a serious matter by both that company and the industry as a whole. A number of sanctions may be applied against a company ruled in breach of the Code.

Companies must ensure that all relevant personnel are appropriately trained in the requirements of the Code and have strict internal procedures under which all promotional material and activities are reviewed to ensure compliance with the Code and the appropriate legal requirements. The Code reflects and extends well beyond the legal requirements controlling the advertising of medicines.

The Code incorporates the principles set out in:

- the International Federation of Pharmaceutical Manufacturers Associations' (IFPMA) Code of Pharmaceutical Marketing Practices
- the European Federation of Pharmaceutical Industries' Associations' (EFPIA) European Code of Practice for the Promotion of Medicines
- the European Community Directive on the advertising of medicinal products for human use (92/28/EEC) and
- the World Health Organisation's Ethical criteria for medicinal drug promotion.

Monitoring the Code of Practice

The Code is administered by the Prescription Medicines Code of Practice Authority which is responsible for the provision of advice, guidance and training on the Code as well as for the complaints procedure. Complaints which are made under the Code about promotional material or the promotional activities of companies are considered by the Code of Practice Panel and, where required, by the Code of Practice Appeal Board. Reports on completed cases are published quarterly by the Authority in its Code of Practice Review which is available on request.

Complaints about the promotion of medicines should be submitted to the Director of the Prescription Medicines Code of Practice Authority, 12 Whitehall, London SW1A 2DY, telephone 0171 930 9677, facsimile 0171 930 4554.

Guidance on the interpretation of the Code appears as supplementary information to the text in italics.

PROVISIONS OF THE CODE OF PRACTICE

Clause 1 Scope of Code and Definition of Certain Terms

1.1 This Code applies to the promotion of medicines to members of the United Kingdom health professions and to appropriate administrative staff and to information made available to the general public about medicines so promoted.

It does not apply to the promotion of over-the-counter medicines to members of the health professions when the object of that promotion is to encourage their purchase by members of the general public.

Clause 1.1 Scope of the Code

For the purposes of the application of the Code, the United Kingdom includes the Channel Islands and the Isle of Man.

The Code applies to the promotion of medicines to members of the health professions and to appropriate administrative staff as specified in Clause 1.1. This includes promotion at meetings for UK residents held outside the UK. It also applies to promotion to UK health professionals and to administrative staff at international meetings held outside the UK, except that the promotional material distributed at such meetings will need to comply with local requirements.

The Code does not apply to the promotion of over-the-counter medicines to members of the health professions when the object of that promotion is to encourage their purchase by members of the general public as specified in Clause 1.1. Thus, for example, an advertisement to doctors for an over-the-counter medicine does not come within the scope of the Code if its purpose is to encourage doctors to recommend the purchase of the medicine by patients. Where the advertisement is designed to encourage doctors to prescribe the medicine, then it comes within the scope of the Code.

Advertisements for over-the-counter medicines to pharmacists are outside the scope of the Code. Advertisements to pharmacists for other medicines come within the scope of the Code.

Clause 1.1 Journals with an International Distribution

The Code applies to the advertising of medicines in professional journals which are published in the UK and/or intended for a UK audience.

International journals which are produced in English in the UK are subject to the Code even if only a small proportion of their circulation is to a UK audience. It is helpful in these circumstances to indicate that the information in the advertisement is consistent with the UK marketing authorization.

Where a journal is produced in the UK but intended for distribution solely to overseas countries local requirements and/or the requirements of the International Federation of Pharmaceutical Manufacturers Associations' (IFPMA) Code of Pharmaceutical Marketing Practices should be borne in mind.

Clause 1.1 Advertising to the Public and Advertising Over-the-Counter Medicines to Health Professionals and the Retail Trade

The promotion of medicines to the general public for self medication is covered by the Code of Standards of Advertising Practice for Over-the-Counter Medicines of the Proprietary Association of Great Britain (PAGB). The PAGB also has a Code of Practice for Advertising Over-the-Counter Medicines to Health Professionals and the Retail Trade.

Clause 1.1 Promotion to Administrative Staff

The provisions of the Code apply in their entirety to the promotion of medicines to appropriate administrative staff except where the text indicates otherwise. For example, the prescribing information required under Clause 4 must be included in promotional material provided to administrative staff but it is not permissible to provide samples of medicines to them as this is proscribed by Clause 17.1.

Particular attention is drawn to the provisions of Clause 12.1 and the supplementary information to that clause, which concern the appropriateness of promotional material to those to whom it is addressed.

1.2 The term 'promotion' means any activity undertaken by a pharmaceutical company or with its authority which promotes the prescription, supply, sale or administration of its medicines.

It includes:

- journal and direct mail advertising
- the activities of representatives including detail aids and other printed material used by representatives
- the supply of samples
- the provision of inducements to prescribe, supply or buy medicines by the gift, offer or promise of any benefit or bonus, whether in money or in kind
- the provision of hospitality for promotional purposes
- the sponsorship of promotional meetings
- the sponsorship of scientific meetings including payment of travelling and accommodation expenses in connection therewith
- the provision of information to the general public either directly or indirectly, and
- all other sales promotion in whatever form, such as participation in exhibitions, the use of audio-cassettes, films, records, tapes, video recordings, electronic media, interactive data systems and the like.

It does not include:

- replies made in response to individual enquiries from members of the health professions or in response to specific communications whether of enquiry or comment, including letters published in professional journals, but only if they relate solely to the subject matter of the letter or enquiry, are accurate and do not mislead and are not promotional in nature
- factual, accurate, informative announcements and reference material relating, for example, to pack changes, adverse-reaction warnings, trade catalogues and price lists, provided they include no product claims
- measures or trade practices relating to prices, margins or discounts which were in regular use by a significant proportion of the pharmaceutical industry on 1 January 1993
- data sheets, the contents of which are determined by regulations made under the Medicines Act 1968 and summaries of product characteristics as provided for in EC Directive 65/65
- the labelling on medicines and accompanying package leaflets insofar as they are not promotional for the medicines concerned; the contents of labels and package leaflets are covered by regulations
- statements relating to human health or diseases provided there is no reference, either direct or indirect, to specific medicines.

Clause 1.2 Replies Intended for Use in Response to Individual Enquiries

Replies intended for use in response to enquiries which are received on a regular basis may be drafted in advance provided that they are used only when they directly and solely relate to the particular enquiry. Documents must not have the appearance of promotional material.

1.3 The term 'medicine' means any branded or unbranded medicine intended for use in humans which requires a marketing authorization.

1.4 The term 'health profession' includes members of the medical, dental, pharmacy or nursing professions and any other persons who in the course of their professional activities may prescribe, supply or administer a medicine.

1.5 The term 'over-the-counter medicine' means those medicines or particular packs of medicines which are primarily advertised to the general public for use in self medication.

1.6 The term 'representative' means a representative calling on members of the health professions and administrative staff in relation to the promotion of medicines.

Clause 1.6 Representatives

'Medical representatives' and 'generic sales representatives' are distinguished in Clause 16.3 relating to examinations for representatives.

Clause 2 Discredit to and Reduction of Confidence in the Industry

Activities or materials associated with promotion must never be such as to bring discredit upon, or reduce confidence in, the pharmaceutical industry.

Clause 2 Discredit to and Reduction of Confidence in the Industry

A ruling in breach of this clause is a sign of particular censure and is reserved for such circumstances.

Clause 3 Marketing Authorization.

3.1 A medicine must not be promoted prior to the grant of the marketing authorization which permits its sale or supply.

3.2 The promotion of a medicine must be in accordance with the terms of its marketing authorization and must not be inconsistent with the particulars listed in its summary of product characteristics or data sheet.

Clause 3 Marketing Authorization

The legitimate exchange of medical and scientific information during the development of a medicine is not prohibited provided that any such information or activity does not constitute promotion which is prohibited under this or any other clause.

Clause 3 Promotion at International Conferences

The promotion of medicines at international meetings held in the UK may on occasion pose certain problems with regard to medicines or indications for medicines which do not have a marketing authorization in the UK although they are so authorized elsewhere.

The display and provision of promotional material for such medicines is permitted at international meetings in the UK provided that the following conditions are met:

- *the meeting must be a truly international meeting of high scientific standing with a significant proportion of delegates from outside the UK*
- *any promotional material for medicines or for indications which do not have a UK marketing authorization must be clearly and prominently labelled as such*
- *the material is certified in accordance with Clause 14, except that the signatories need certify only that in their belief the material is a fair and truthful presentation of the facts about the medicine.*

Clause 3.1 Advance Notification of New Products or Product Changes

Health authorities and trust hospitals etc, need to estimate their likely budgets two or three years in advance in order to meet Treasury requirements and there is a need for them to receive advance information about the introduction of new medicines, or changes to existing medicines, which may significantly affect their level of expenditure during future years.

At the time this information is required, the medicines concerned (or the changes to them) will not be the subject of marketing authorizations (though applications will often have been made) and it would thus be contrary to the Code for them to be promoted. Information may, however, be provided on the following basis:

(i) the information must relate to:

(a) a product which contains a new active substance, or

(b) a product which contains an active substance prepared in a new way, such as by the use of biotechnology, or

(c) a product which is to have a significant addition to the existing range of authorized indications, or

(d) a product which has a novel and innovative means of administration

(ii) information should be directed to those responsible for making policy decisions on budgets rather than those expected to prescribe

(iii) the likely cost and budgetary implications must be indicated and must be such that they will make significant differences to the likely expenditure of health authorities and trust hospitals and the like

(iv) only factual information must be provided which should be limited to that sufficient to provide an adequate but succinct account of the product's properties; other products should only be mentioned to put the new product into context in the therapeutic area concerned

(v) the information may be attractively presented and printed but should not be in the style of promotional material – product specific logos should be avoided but company logos may be used; the brand name of the product may be included in moderation but it should not be stylized or used to excess

(vi) the information provided should not include mock up drafts of either summaries of product characteristics or patient information leaflets

(vii) if requested, further information may be supplied or a presentation made.

Clause 3.2 Unauthorized Indications

The promotion of indications not covered by the marketing authorization for a medicine is prohibited by this clause.

Clause 4 Prescribing Information and other Obligatory Information

4.1 The prescribing information listed in Clause 4.2 must be provided in a clear and legible manner in all promotional material for a medicine except for abbreviated advertisements (see Clause 5) and for promotional aids which meet the requirements of Clause 18.3.

The prescribing information must form part of the promotional material and must not be separate from it.

Clause 4.1 Prescribing Information, Summaries of Product Characteristics and Data Sheets

Each promotional item for a medicine must be able to stand alone. For example when a 'Dear Doctor' letter on a medicine is sent in the same envelope with a brochure about the same medicine, each item has to include the prescribing information. It does not suffice to have the prescribing information on only one of the items. The inclusion of a summary of product characteristics or data sheet moreover does not suffice to conform with the provisions of this clause.

The prescribing information must be consistent with the summary of product characteristics or data sheet for the medicine.

Clause 4.1 Advertisements for Devices

Where an advertisement relates to the merits of a device used for administering medicines, such as an inhaler, which is supplied containing a variety of medicines, the prescribing information for one only need be given if the advertisement makes no reference to any particular medicine.

Full prescribing information must, however, be included in relation to each particular medicine which is referred to.

Clause 4.1 Prescribing Information at Exhibitions

The prescribing information for medicines promoted on posters and exhibition panels at meetings must either be provided on the posters or panels themselves or must be available at the company stand. If the prescribing information is made available at the company stand, this should be referred to on the posters or panels.

Clause 4.1 Legibility of Prescribing Information

The prescribing information is the essential information which must be provided in promotional material. It follows therefore that the information must be given in a clear and legible manner which assists readability.

Legibility is not simply a question of type size. The following recommendations will help to achieve clarity:

- *type size should be such that a lower case letter 'x' is no less than 1 mm in height*
- *lines should be no more than 100 characters in length, including spaces*
- *sufficient space should be allowed between lines to facilitate easy reading*
- *a clear style of type should be used*
- *there should be adequate contrast between the colour of the text and the background*
- *dark print on a light background is preferable*
- *emboldening headings and starting each section on a new line aids legibility.*

4.2 The prescribing information consists of the following:

- the name of the medicine (which may be either a brand name or a generic name)
- a quantitative list of the active ingredients, using approved names where such exist, or other non-proprietary names; alternatively, the non-proprietary name of the product if it is the subject of an accepted monograph
- at least one authorized indication for use consistent with the summary of product characteristics or data sheet
- a succinct statement of the information in the summary of product characteristics or data sheet relating to the dosage and method of use relevant to the indications quoted in the advertisement and, where not otherwise obvious, the route of administration
- a succinct statement of the side-effects, precautions and contra-indications relevant to the indications in the advertisement, giving, in an abbreviated form, the substance of the relevant information in the summary of product characteristics or data sheet
- any warning issued by the Medicines Commission, the Committee on Safety of Medicines or the licensing authority, which is required to be included in advertisements
- the cost (excluding VAT) of either a specified package of the medicine to which the advertisement relates, or a specified quantity or recommended daily dose, calculated by reference to any specified package of the product, except in the case of advertisements in journals printed in the UK which have more than 15 per cent of their circulation outside the UK and audio-visual advertisements and prescribing information provided in association with them
- the legal classification of the product
- the number of the relevant marketing authorization and the name and address of the holder of the authorization or the name and address of the part of the business responsible for its sale or supply.

In addition the non-proprietary name of the medicine or a list of the active ingredients using approved names where such exist must appear immediately adjacent to the most prominent display of the brand name in not less than 10 point bold or in a type size which occupies a total area no less than that taken by the brand name.

The information specified above in relation to dosage, method of use, side effects, precautions and contra-indications and any warning which is required to be included in advertisements, must be placed in such a position in the advertisement that its relationship to the claims and indications for the product can be appreciated by the reader.

Clause 4.2 Black Triangle Symbol

Certain newly marketed medicines are required to show an inverted black triangle on their promotional material, other than promotional aids, to denote that special reporting is required in relation to adverse reactions. This is not a Code of Practice or a statutory requirement.

The agreement between the Committee on Safety of Medicines and the ABPI on the use of the black triangle is that:

The symbol should always be black and its size should normally be not less than 5 mm per side but with a smaller size of 3 mm per side for A5 size advertisements and a larger size of 7.5 mm per side for A3 size advertisements:

- *the symbol should appear once and be located adjacent to the most prominent display of the name of the product*
- *no written explanation of the symbol is necessary.*

Clause 4.2 Non-Proprietary Name

'Immediately adjacent to . . .' means immediately before, immediately after, immediately above or immediately below.

4.3 In the case of audio-visual material such as films, video recordings and such like and in the case of interactive data systems, the prescribing information may be provided either:

- by way of a document which is made available to all persons to whom the material is shown or sent, or
- by inclusion on the audio-visual recording or in the interactive data system itself.

When the prescribing information is included in an interactive data system instructions for accessing it must be clearly displayed.

Clause 4.3 Prescribing Information on Audio-Visual Material

Where prescribing information is shown in the audio-visual material as part of the recording, it must be of sufficient clarity and duration so that it is easily readable. The prescribing information must be an integral part of the advertisement and must appear with it. It is not acceptable for the advertisement and the prescribing information to be separated by any other material.

4.4 In the case of audio material, ie. material which consists of sound only, the prescribing information must be provided by way of a document which is made available to all persons to whom the material is played or sent.

4.5 In the case of a journal advertisement where the prescribing information appears overleaf, a reference to where it can be found must appear on the outer edge of the initial page of the advertisement in at least 8 point type.

4.6 In the case of printed promotional material consisting of more than four pages, a clear reference must be given to where the prescribing information can be found.

4.7 Promotional material other than advertisements appearing in professional publications must include the date on which the promotional material was drawn up or last revised.

Clause 4.7 Dates on Loose Inserts

A loose insert is not regarded for this purpose as appearing in the professional publication with which it is sent and must therefore bear the date on which it was drawn up or last revised.

Clause 5 Abbreviated Advertisements

5.1 Abbreviated advertisements are advertisements which are exempt from the requirement to include prescribing information for the advertised medicine, provided that they meet with the requirements of this clause.

5.2 Abbreviated advertisements may only appear in professional publications i.e. publications sent or delivered wholly or mainly to members of the health professions and/or appropriate administrative staff. A loose insert in such a publication cannot be an abbreviated advertisement. Abbreviated advertisements are not permissible in relation to any medicine where the licensing authority has issued a direction that abbreviated advertisements must not be issued.

Clause 5.2 Abbreviated Advertisements–Professional Publications

Abbreviated advertisements are largely restricted to journals and other such professional publications sent or delivered wholly or mainly to members of the health professions etc. A promotional mailing or representative leave piece cannot be an abbreviated advertisement and an abbreviated advertisement cannot appear as part of another promotional item, such as in a brochure consisting of a full advertisement for another of the company's medicines.

Diaries and desk pads bearing a number of advertisements are considered to be professional publications and may include abbreviated advertisements for medicines. Similarly, video programmes and such like sent to doctors etc may be considered professional publications and an abbreviated advertisement may be affixed to the side of the video cassette or included on the box containing the video. The prescribing information must, however, be made available for any advertisement for a medicine appearing on audio-visual material or in an interactive data system. Such advertisements cannot be deemed abbreviated advertisements.

5.3 Abbreviated advertisements must be no larger than 420 square centimetres in size.

5.4 Abbreviated advertisements must contain the following information:

- the name of the medicine (which may be either a brand name or a generic name)
- the non-proprietary name of the medicine or a list of the active ingredients using approved names where such exist
- at least one indication for use consistent with the summary of product characteristics or the data sheet
- the legal classification of the product
- any warning issued by the Medicines Commission, the Committee on Safety of Medicines or the licensing authority which is required to be included in advertisements
- the name and address of the holder of the marketing authorization or the name and address of the part of the business responsible for its sale or supply
- a statement that further information is available on request to the holder of the marketing authorization or that it may be found in the summary of product characteristics or data sheet.

The non-proprietary name of the medicine or the list of the active ingredients, using approved names where such exist, must appear immediately adjacent to the most prominent display of the brand name in not less than 10 point bold or in a type size which occupies a total area no less than that taken by the brand name.

5.5 Abbreviated advertisements may in addition contain a concise statement consistent with the summary of product characteristics or data sheet, giving the reason why the medicine is recommended for the indication or indications given.

Clause 5.4 Non-Proprietary Name

'Immediately adjacent to . . .' means immediately before, immediately after, immediately above or immediately below.

Clauses 5.4 and 5.5 Abbreviated Advertisements–Permitted Information

The contents of abbreviated advertisements are restricted as set out in Clauses 5.4 and 5.5 and the following information should not therefore be included in abbreviated advertisements:

- *marketing authorization numbers*
- *references*
- *dosage particulars*
- *details of pack sizes*
- *cost*
- *quantitative particulars, unless the quantitative information forms part of the licensed name of the medicine.*

There may be exceptions to the above if the information provided, for example the cost of the medicine or the frequency of its dosage or its availability as a patient pack, is given as the reason why the medicine is recommended for the indication or indications referred to in the advertisement.

Artwork used in abbreviated advertisements must not convey any information about a medicine which is additional to that permitted under Clauses 5.4 and 5.5.

Telephone numbers may be included in abbreviated advertisements.

Clause 6 Journal Advertising

6.1 No single advertisement included in a journal may consist of more than two consecutive pages.

6.2 Where the two pages of an advertisement are not facing, neither must be false or misleading when read in isolation.

6.3 No advertisement taking the form of a loose insert in a journal may consist of more than a single sheet of a size no larger than the page size of the journal itself, printed on one or both sides.

6.4 No issue of a journal may bear advertising for a particular product on more than three pages.

Clause 6 Journal Advertisements

See Clause 4 and in particular Clause 4.5 regarding the requirements for prescribing information in journal advertisements

A two page journal advertisement is one where the pages follow on continuously without interruption by intervening editorial text or other copy. Thus, for example, promotional material on two successive right hand pages cannot be a single advertisement. Each such page would need to be treated as a separate advertisement for the purposes of prescribing information.

Similarly, if promotional material appears on the outer edges of the left and right hand pages of a double page spread, and the promotional material is separated by intervening editorial matter then again each page would need to be treated as a separate advertisement.

Clause 6.3 Advertising on the Outside of Journals

Advertising such as cards stapled to a journal and 'wraparounds' must not have a greater surface area than that outlined for loose inserts under Clause 6.3.

Clause 6.4 Limitation on Number of Pages of Advertising

To conform with Clause 6.4 there can be no more than three one page advertisements for a product in a journal. Alternatively there can be one double page advertisement and another separate one page advertisement. Advertisements consisting of three consecutive pages are not permitted. Advertisements taking the form of inserts, whether loose or bound in, count towards the three pages allowed. A loose insert printed on both sides counts as two pages.

A summary of product characteristics or a data sheet is permitted as an insert in addition to the three pages of advertising which is allowed.

Inserts and supplements which are not advertisements as such, though they may be regarded as promotional material, for example reports of conference proceedings, are not subject to the restrictions of Clauses 6.3 and 6.4.

Clause 7 Information, Claims and Comparisons

Clause 7 General

The application of this clause is not limited to information or claims of a medical or scientific nature. It includes, inter alia, information or claims relating to pricing and market share. Thus, for example, any claim relating to the market share of a product must be substantiated without delay upon request as required under Clause 7.4.

7.1 Upon reasonable request, companies must promptly provide members of the health professions and appropriate administrative staff with accurate and relevant information about the medicines which the company markets.

7.2 Information, claims and comparisons must be accurate, balanced, fair, objective and unambiguous and must be based on an up-to-date evaluation of all the evidence and reflect that evidence clearly. They must not mislead either directly or by implication.

Clause 7.2 Misleading Information, Claims and Comparisons

The following are areas where particular care should be taken by companies:

- **claims for superior potency in relation to weight** *are generally meaningless and best avoided unless they can be linked with some practical advantage, for example, reduction in side-effects or cost of effective dosage*
- **the use of data derived from in-vitro studies, studies in healthy volunteers and in animals.** *Care must be taken with the use of such data so as not to mislead as to its significance. The extrapolation of such data to the clinical situation should only be made where there is data to show that it is of direct relevance and significance*
- **economic evaluation of medicines.** *The economic evaluation of medicines is a relatively new science. Care must be taken that any claim involving the economic evaluation of a medicine is borne out by the data available and does not exaggerate its significance.*

  To be acceptable as the basis of promotional claims, the assumptions made in an economic evaluation must be clinically appropriate and consistent with the marketing authorization.

  Attention is drawn to guidance on good practice in the conduct of economic evaluation of medicines which has been given by the Department of Health and the ABPI and which is available upon request from the Prescription Medicines Code of Practice Authority.
- **emerging clinical or scientific opinion.** *Where a clinical or scientific issue exists which has not been resolved in favour of one generally accepted viewpoint, particular care must be taken to ensure that the issue is treated in a balanced manner in promotional material*
- **hanging comparisons** *whereby a medicine is described as being better or stronger or suchlike without stating that with which the medicine is compared must not be made*
- **price comparisons.** *Price comparisons, as with any comparison, must be accurate, fair and must not mislead. Valid comparisons can only be made where like is compared with like. It follows therefore that in making a price comparison it should be made on the basis of the equivalent dosage requirement for the same indications. For example, to compare the cost per ml for topical preparations is likely to mislead unless it can be shown that their usage rates are similar or, where this is not possible, for the comparison to be qualified in such a way as to indicate that usage rates may vary*
- **statistical information.** *Care must be taken to ensure that there is a sound statistical basis for all information, claims and comparisons in promotional material. Differences which do not reach statistical significance must not be presented in such a way as to mislead.*

  Instances have occurred where claims have been based on published papers in which the arithmetic and/or statistical methodology was incorrect. Accordingly, before statistical information is included in promotional material it must have been subjected to statistical appraisal.

7.3 Any information, claim or comparison must be capable of substantiation.

7.4 Substantiation for any information, claim or comparison must be provided without delay at the request of members of the health professions or appropriate administrative staff. It need not be provided, however, in relation to the validity of indications approved in the marketing authorization.

7.5 When promotional material refers to published studies, clear references must be given.

7.6 All artwork including illustrations, graphs and tables must conform to the letter and spirit of the Code. Graphs and tables must be presented in such a way as to give a clear, fair, balanced view of the matters with which they deal, and must not be included unless they are relevant to the claims or comparisons being made.

Clause 7.6 Artwork, Illustrations, Graphs and Tables

Care must be taken to ensure that artwork does not mislead as to the nature of a medicine or any claim or comparison and that it does not detract from any warnings or contra-indications. For example, anatomical drawings used to show results from a study must not exaggerate those results and depictions of children should not be used in relation to products not authorized for use in children in any way which might encourage such use.

Particular care should be taken with graphs and tables to ensure that they do not mislead, for example by their incompleteness or by the use of suppressed zeros or unusual scales. Differences which do not reach statistical significance must not be presented in such a way as to mislead.

Graphs and tables must be adequately labelled so that the information presented can be readily understood. If a graph, table or suchlike is taken from a published paper but has not been reproduced in its entirety, the graph must clearly be labelled as having been adapted from the paper in question (see also Clause 7.5). Any such adaptation must not distort or mislead as to the significance of that graph, table etc. It should also be noted that if a table, graph etc in a paper is unacceptable in terms of the requirements of the Code, because, for example, it gives a visually misleading impression as to the data shown, then it must not be used or reproduced in promotional material.

7.7 Information and claims about side-effects must reflect available evidence or be capable of substantiation by clinical experience. It must not be stated that a product has no side-effects, toxic hazards or risks of addiction. The word 'safe' must not be used without qualification.

Clause 7.7 Use of the Word 'Safe'

The restrictions on the word 'safe' apply equally to grammatical derivatives of the word such as 'safety'. For example, 'demonstrated safety' or 'proven safety' are prohibited under this Clause.

7.8 Exaggerated or all-embracing claims must not be made and superlatives must not be used except for those limited circumstances where they relate to a clear fact about a medicine. Claims should not imply that a medicine or an active ingredient has some special merit, quality or property unless this can be substantiated.

Clause 7.8 Superlatives

Superlatives are those grammatical expressions which denote the highest quality or degree, such as best, strongest, widest etc. A claim that a product was 'the best' treatment for a particular condition, for example could not be substantiated as there are too many variables to enable such a sweeping claim to be proven. The use of a superlative which could be substantiated is a simple statement of fact which can be very clearly demonstrated, such as that a particular medicine is the most widely prescribed in the UK for a certain condition, if this is not presented in a way which misleads as to its significance.

Clause 7.8 Use of the Words 'The' and 'Unique'

In certain circumstances the use of the word 'the' can imply a special merit, quality or property for a medicine which is unacceptable under this clause if it cannot be substantiated. For example, a claim that a product is 'The analgesic' implies that it is in effect the best, and might not be acceptable under this clause.

Similarly, great care needs to be taken with the use of the word 'unique'. Although in some circumstances the word unique may be used to describe some clearly defined special feature of a medicine, in many instances it may simply imply a general superiority. In such instances it is not possible to substantiate the claim as the claim itself is so ill defined.

7.9 The word 'new' must not be used to describe any product or presentation which has been generally available, or any therapeutic indication which has been generally promoted, for more than twelve months in the UK.

7.10 Brand names of other companies' products must not be used unless the prior consent of the proprietors has been obtained.

Clause 8 Disparaging References

8.1 The medicines, products and activities of other pharmaceutical companies must not be disparaged.

Clause 8.1 Disparaging References

Much pharmaceutical advertising contains comparisons with other products and, by the nature of advertising, such comparisons are usually made to show an advantage of the advertised product over its comparator. Provided that such critical references to another company's products are accurate, balanced, fair etc, and can be substantiated, they are acceptable under the Code.

Unjustified knocking copy in which the products or activities of a competitor are unfairly denigrated is prohibited under this clause.

8.2 The health professions and the clinical and scientific opinions of health professionals must not be disparaged.

Clause 9 Format, Suitability and Causing Offence, Sponsorship

9.1 All material and activities must recognise the special nature of medicines and the professional standing of the audience to which they are directed and must not be likely to cause offence. High standards must be maintained at all times.

Clause 9.1 Suitability and Taste

The special nature of medicines and the professional audience to which the material is directed require that the standards set for the promotion of medicines are higher than those which might be acceptable for general commodity advertising.

It follows therefore that certain types, styles and methods of promotion, even where they might be acceptable for the promotion of products other than medicines, are unacceptable. These include:

- *the display of naked or partially naked people for the purpose of attracting attention to the material or the use of sexual imagery for that purpose*
- *'teaser' advertising whereby promotional material is intended to 'tease' the recipient by eliciting an interest in something which will be following or will be available at a later date without providing any actual information about it*
- *the provision of rubber stamps to doctors for use as aids to prescription writing*
- *the provision of private prescription forms preprinted with the name of a medicine.*

9.2 The name or photograph of a member of a health profession must not be used in any way that is contrary to the conventions of that profession.

9.3 Promotional material must not imitate the devices, copy, slogans or general layout adopted by other companies in a way that is likely to mislead or confuse.

9.4 Promotional material must not include any reference to the Medicines Commission, the Committee on Safety of Medicines or the licensing authority, unless this is specifically required by the licensing authority.

9.5 Reproductions of official documents must not be used for promotional purposes unless permission has been given in writing by the appropriate body.

9.6 Extremes of format, size or cost of promotional material must be avoided.

9.7 Postcards, other exposed mailings, envelopes or wrappers must not carry matter which might be regarded as advertising to the general public, contrary to Clause 20.1.

Clause 9.7 Reply Paid Cards

Reply paid cards which are intended to be returned to companies through the post and which relate to a medicine which may not legally be advertised to the general public should not bear both the name of the medicine and information as to its usage but may bear one or the other.

9.8 The telephone, telemessages, e-mail, telex and facsimile machines must not be used for promotional purposes except with the prior permission of the recipient.

9.9 All material relating to medicines and their uses which is sponsored by a pharmaceutical company must clearly indicate that it has been sponsored by that company.

Clause 9.9 Declaration of Sponsorship

The declaration of sponsorship must be sufficiently prominent to ensure that readers of sponsored material are aware of it at the outset.

Clause 10 Disguised Promotion

10.1 Promotional material and activities must not be disguised.

Clause 10.1 Disguised Promotional Material

Promotional material sent in the guise of personal communications, for example by using envelopes or postcards addressed in real or facsimile handwriting is inappropriate. Envelopes must not be used for the dispatch of promotional material if they bear words implying that the contents are non-promotional, for example that the contents provide information relating to safety.

Advertisements in journals must not resemble editorial matter. Care must also be taken with company sponsored reports on meetings and the like to ensure that they are not disguised promotion. Sponsorship must be declared in accordance with Clause 9.9.

10.2 Market research activities, post-marketing surveillance studies, clinical assessments and the like must not be disguised promotion.

Clause 10.2 Guidelines for Company Sponsored Safety Assessment of Marketed Medicines

Attention is drawn to the Guidelines for Company Sponsored Safety Assessment of Marketed Medicines (SAMM) which have been produced jointly by the ABPI, the British Medical Association, the Committee on Safety of Medicines, the Medicines Control Agency and the Royal College of General Practitioners. These state that SAMM studies should not be undertaken for the purposes of promotion.

Clause 10.2 Market Research

Market research is the collection and analysis of information and must be unbiased and non-promotional. The use to which the statistics or information is put may be promotional. The two phases must be kept distinct.

Attention is drawn to the Guidelines on Pharmaceutical Market Research Practice produced by the British Pharmaceutical Market Research Group and the ABPI.

Clause 11 Provision of Reprints and the Use of Quotations

11.1 Reprints of articles in journals must not be provided unsolicited unless the articles have been refereed.

Clause 11.1 Provision of Reprints

The provision of an unsolicited reprint of an article about a medicine constitutes promotion of that medicine and all relevant requirements of the Code must therefore be observed. Particular attention must be paid to the requirements of Clause 3.

When providing an unsolicited reprint of an article about a medicine, it should be accompanied by prescribing information.

11.2 Quotations from medical and scientific literature, or from personal communications must accurately reflect the meaning of the author.

Clause 11.2 Quotations

Any quotation chosen by a company for use in promotional material must comply with the requirements of the Code itself. For example, to quote from a paper which stated that a certain medicine was 'safe and effective' would not be acceptable even if it was an accurate reflection of the meaning of the author of the paper, as it is prohibited under Clause 7.7 of the Code to state without qualification in promotional material that a medicine is safe.

Care should be taken in quoting from any study or the like to ensure that it does not mislead as to its overall significance. (See Clause 7.2 which prohibits misleading information, claims etc in promotional material.) Attention is drawn to the provisions of Clause 7.5 which requires that when promotional material refers to published studies clear references must be given to where they can be found.

11.3 Quotations relating to medicines taken from public broadcasts, for example on radio and television, and from private occasions, such as medical conferences or symposia, must not be used without the formal permission of the speaker.

11.4 The utmost care must be taken to avoid ascribing claims or views to authors when these no longer represent the current views of the authors concerned.

Clause 11.4 Current Views of Authors

If there is any doubt as to the current view of an author, companies should check with the author prior to its use in promotional material.

Clause 12 Distribution of Promotional Material

12.1 Promotional material should only be sent or distributed to those categories of persons whose need for, or interest in, the particular information can reasonably be assumed.

Clause 12.1 Distribution of Promotional Material

Promotional material should be tailored to the audience to whom it is directed. For example, promotional material devised for general practitioners might not be appropriate for hospital doctors and, similarly, material devised for clinicians might not be appropriate for use with National Health Service administrative staff.

12.2 Restraint must be exercised on the frequency of distribution and on the volume of promotional material distributed.

Clause 12.2 Frequency of Mailings

The style of mailings is relevant to their acceptability to doctors and criticism of their frequency is most likely to arise where their informational content is limited or where they appear to be elaborate and expensive. A higher frequency rate will be accepted for mailings on new products than for others.

12.3 Mailing lists must be kept up-to-date. Requests from health professionals to be removed from promotional mailing lists must be complied with promptly and no name may be restored except at their request or with their permission.

Clause 13 Scientific Service Responsible for Information

Companies must have a scientific service to compile and collate all information, whether received from medical representatives or from any other source, about medicines which they market.

Clause 14 Certification of Promotional Material

14.1 Promotional material must not be issued unless its final form, to which no subsequent amendments will be made, has been certified by two persons on behalf of the company in the manner provided by this clause. One of the two persons must be a registered medical practitioner or, in the case of a product for dental use only, a registered medical practitioner or a dentist. The other must be a pharmacist or some other appropriately qualified person or a senior official of the company or an appropriately qualified person whose services are retained for that purpose.

Clause 14.1 Certification

An acceptable way to comply with Clause 14.1 is for the final proof to be certified but this is not obligatory provided that that which is certified is in its final form to which no subsequent amendments will be made.

All promotional material must be certified in this way including promotional aids, audio-visual material, promotional material on databases and representatives' technical briefing materials.

Other material issued by companies which relates to medicines but which is not intended as promotional material for those medicines per se, for example corporate advertising, press releases and educational material for patients etc, should be examined to ensure that it does not contravene the Code or the relevant statutory requirements.

In certifying audio, audio-visual material and material used on interactive data systems, companies must ensure that a written transcript of the material is certified including reproductions of any graphs, tables and the like that appear in the recording. In the event of a complaint, a copy of the written transcript of the material will be requested.

The guidelines on company procedures relating to the Code which are in the Code of Practice booklet give further information on certification.

See also the supplementary information to Clause 3 on promotion at international conferences regarding the certification.

Clause 14.1 Joint Ventures and Co-Promotion

In a joint venture in which a third party provides a service on behalf of a number of pharmaceutical companies, the pharmaceutical companies involved are responsible for any activity carried out by that third party on their behalf.

It follows therefore that the pharmaceutical companies involved should be aware of all aspects of the service carried out on their behalf and take this into account when certifying the material or activity involved. Similarly if two or more pharmaceutical companies organise a joint meeting each company should ensure that the arrangements for the meeting are acceptable.

Under co-promotion arrangements whereby companies jointly promote the same medicine and the promotional material bears both company names, each company should certify the promotional material involved as they will be held jointly responsible for it under the Code.

14.2 The names of those nominated, together with their qualifications, shall be notified in advance to the Product Information and Advertising Unit of the Post Licensing Division of the Medicines Control Agency and to the Prescription Medicines Code of Practice Authority. The names and qualifications of designated alternative signatories must also be given. Changes in the names of nominees must be promptly notified.

14.3 The certificate must certify that the signatories have examined the final form of the material and that in their belief it is in accordance with the requirements of the relevant advertising regulations and this Code, is not inconsistent with the marketing authorization and the summary of product characteristics or data sheet and is a fair and truthful presentation of the facts about the medicine.

Material which is still in use must be recertified at intervals of no more than two years to ensure that it continues to conform with the relevant advertising regulations and the Code.

14.4 Companies shall preserve all certificates, together with the material in the form certified and information indicating the persons to whom it was addressed, the method of dissemination and the date of first dissemination, for not less than three years after its final use and produce them upon request from the Medicines Control Agency or the Prescription Medicines Code of Practice Authority.

Clause 14.4 Retention of Documentation

Companies should note that the Medicines Control Agency is entitled to request particulars of an advertisement, including particulars as to the content and form of the advertisement, the method of dissemination and the date of the first dissemination, and such a request is not subject to any time limit. This does not apply to the certificates themselves in respect of which the three year limit in Clause 14.4 is applicable.

Clause 15 Representatives

Clause 15 Representatives

All provisions in the Code relating to the need for accuracy, balance, fairness, good taste etc apply equally to oral representations as well as printed material. Representatives must not make claims or comparisons which are in any way inaccurate, misleading, disparaging, in poor taste etc, or which are outside the terms of the marketing authorization for the medicine or are inconsistent with the summary of product characteristics or data sheet. Indications for which the medicine does not have a marketing authorization must not be promoted.

Attention is also drawn to the provisions of Clause 9.8 which prohibits the use of the telephone, telemessages, e-mail and telex and facsimile machines for promotional purposes except with the prior permission of the recipient.

Clause 15 Contract Representatives

Companies employing or using contract representatives are responsible for their conduct and must ensure that they comply with the provisions of this and all other relevant clauses in the Code, and in particular the training requirements under Clauses 15.1, 16.1, 16.2 and 16.3.

15.1 Representatives must be given adequate training and have sufficient scientific knowledge to enable them to provide full and accurate information about the medicines which they promote.

15.2 Representatives must at all times maintain a high standard of ethical conduct in the discharge of their duties and must comply with all relevant requirements of the Code.

15.3 Representatives must not employ any inducement or subterfuge to gain an interview. No fee should be paid or offered for the grant of an interview.

Clause 15.3 Hospitality and Payments for Meetings

Attention is drawn to the requirements of Clauses 18 and 19 which prohibit the provision of any financial inducement for the purposes of sales promotion and require that any hospitality provided is secondary to the purpose of a meeting, is not out of proportion to the occasion and does not extend beyond members of the health professions or appropriate administrative staff.

Meetings organised for groups of doctors, other health professionals and/or appropriate administrative staff which are wholly or mainly of a social or sporting nature are unacceptable.

Representatives organising meetings are permitted to provide appropriate hospitality and/or to meet any reasonable, actual costs which may have been incurred. For example, if the refreshments have been organised and paid for by a medical practice the cost may be reimbursed as long as it is reasonable in relation to what was provided and the refreshments themselves were appropriate for the occasion.

Donations in lieu of hospitality are unacceptable as they are inducements for the purpose of holding a meeting. If hospitality is not required at a meeting there is no obligation or right to provide some benefit of an equivalent value.

Clause 15.3 General Medical Council

The General Medical Council is the regulatory body for the medical profession and is responsible for giving guidance on standards of professional conduct and on medical ethics. This guidance is set out in 'Duties of a doctor', a series of four booklets, one of which 'Good medical practice' covers a number of aspects of relationships with the pharmaceutical industry. In relation to representatives, doctors are advised that 'You must not ask for or accept fees for agreeing to meet sales representatives'.

15.4 Representatives must ensure that the frequency, timing and duration of calls on health professionals, administrative staff in hospitals and health authorities and the like, together with the manner in which they are made, do not cause inconvenience. The wishes of individuals on whom representatives wish to call and the arrangements in force at any particular establishment must be observed.

Clause 15.4 Frequency and Manner of Calls on Doctors

The number of calls made on a doctor and the intervals between successive visits are relevant to the determination of frequency.

Companies should arrange that intervals between visits do not cause inconvenience. The number of calls made on a doctor by a representative each year should not normally exceed three on average. This does not include the following which may be additional to those three visits:

- *attendance at group meetings, including audio-visual presentations and the like*
- *a visit which is requested by a doctor or a call which is made in order to respond to a specific enquiry*
- *a visit to follow up a report of an adverse reaction.*

Representatives must always endeavour to treat doctors' time with respect and give them no cause to believe that their time might have been wasted. If for any unavoidable reasons, an appointment cannot be kept, the longest possible notice must be given.

15.5 In an interview, or when seeking an appointment for one, representatives must at the outset take reasonable steps to ensure that they do not mislead as to their identity or that of the company they represent.

15.6 Representatives must transmit forthwith to the scientific service referred to in Clause 13 any information which they receive in relation to the use of the medicines which they promote, particularly reports of side-effects.

15.7 Representatives must be paid a fixed basic salary and any addition proportional to sales of medicines must not constitute an undue proportion of their remuneration.

15.8 Representatives must provide, or have available to provide if requested, a copy of the summary of product characteristics, or where one does not exist, a copy of the data sheet or a document with a similar content, when initiating a discussion on a medicine.

Clause 15.8 Provision of Summary of Product Characteristics/Data Sheet

If discussion on a medicine is initiated by the person or persons on whom a representative calls, the representative is not obliged to have available the information on that medicine referred to in this clause.

15.9 Companies must prepare detailed briefing material for medical representatives on the technical aspects of each medicine which they will promote. A copy of such material must be made available to the Medicines Control Agency and the Prescription Medicines Code of Practice Authority on request. Briefing material must comply with the relevant requirements of the Code, with the exception of Clause 7.10, and, in particular, is subject to the certification requirements of Clause 14.

Briefing material must not advocate, either directly or indirectly, any course of action which would be likely to lead to a breach of the Code.

Clause 15.9 Briefing Material

The detailed briefing material referred to in this clause consists of both the training material used to instruct medical representatives about a medicine and the instructions given to them as to how the product should be promoted.

15.10 Companies are responsible for the activities of their representatives if these are within the scope of their employment even if they are acting contrary to the instructions which they have been given.

Clause 16 Training

16.1 All relevant personnel including members of staff concerned in any way with the preparation or approval of promotional material or of information to be provided to members of the UK health professions and to appropriate administrative staff or of information to be provided to the public, must be fully conversant with the requirements of the Code.

Clause 16.1 Training

Extensive in house training on the Code is carried out by companies and by the Prescription Medicines Code of Practice Authority.

In addition, the Authority runs seminars on the Code which are open to all companies and personnel from advertising agencies, public relations agencies and the like which act for the pharmaceutical industry. Details of these seminars can be obtained from the Authority.

16.2 Representatives must pass the appropriate ABPI representatives examination, as specified in Clause 16.3. Prior to passing the appropriate examination, they may be engaged in such employment for no more than two years, whether continuous or otherwise.

Clause 16.2 Time Allowed to Pass Examination

Prior to passing the appropriate ABPI examination, representatives may be engaged in such employment for no more than two years, whether continuous or otherwise and irrespective of whether those two years have been spent with one company or with more than one company. A representative cannot, for example, do eighteen months with one company and eighteen months with another and so on and thus avoid the examination entirely.

In the event of extenuating circumstances, such as prolonged illness, the Director of the Prescription Medicines Code of Practice Authority may agree to the continued employment of a person as a representative past the end of the two year period, subject to the representative passing the examination within a reasonable time.

Service as a representative prior to 1 January 1996 does not count towards the two year limit on employment as a representative prior to passing the appropriate examination.

16.3 The Medical Representatives Examination is appropriate for, and must be taken by, representatives whose duties comprise or include one or both of:

- calling upon doctors and/or dentists
- the promotion of medicines on the basis, *inter alia*, of their particular therapeutic properties.

The Generic Sales Representatives Examination is appropriate for, and must be taken by, representatives who promote medicines primarily on the basis of price, quality and availability.

Clause 16.3 Medical Representatives and Generic Sales Representatives

The ABPI examinations for medical representatives and generic sales representatives are based on a syllabus published by the ABPI which covers, as appropriate, subjects such as body systems, disease processes and pharmacology, the classification of medicines and pharmaceutical technology. Information on the National Health Service and pharmaceutical industry forms an additional core part of the syllabus. The syllabus is complementary to, and may be incorporated within, the company's induction training which is provided to representatives as a pre-requisite to carrying out their function. Normally representatives should be entered for the appropriate ABPI examination within their first year of employment.

16.4 The following exemptions apply in relation to Clause 16.2:

- persons who were employed as medical representatives on 1 October 1979 are exempt from the need to take the Medical Representatives Examination
- persons with an acceptable professional qualification, for example in pharmacy, medicine or nursing, who were employed as medical representatives at any time before 1 October 1984, are exempt from the need to take the Medical Representatives Examination
- persons who were employed as Generic Sales Representatives on 1 January 1993 are exempt from the need to take the Generic Sales Representatives Examination
- persons who were employed as representatives on 1 January 1996 who had not previously been required to take an examination because they neither promoted generic medicines nor called on doctors and/or dentists are exempt from the need to take either examination.

16.5 Persons who have passed the Medical Representatives Examination whose duties change so as to become those specified in Clause 16.3 as being appropriate to the Generic Sales Representatives Examination are exempt from the need to take that examination.

Persons who have passed the Generic Sales Representatives Examination whose duties change so as to become those specified in Clause 16.3 as being appropriate to the Medical Representatives Examination must pass that examination within two years of their change of duties.

16.6 Details of the numbers of medical and generic sales representatives who have passed the respective examinations above together with the examination status of others, must be provided to the Prescription Medicines Code of Practice Authority on request.

Clause 17 Samples

Clause 17 Definition of Sample

A sample is a small supply of a medicine provided to members of the health professions in order that they may familiarise themselves with it and acquire experience in dealing with it. This includes samples provided for identification purposes for which the provisions of Clause 17 equally apply.

Titration packs, free goods or bonus stock provided to pharmacists and others are not samples. Neither are starter packs classified as samples. This is because they are not for the purposes described above. Starter packs are small packs designed to provide sufficient medicine for a doctor to initiate treatment in such circumstances as a call out in the night or in other instances where there might be some undesirable but unavoidable delay in filling a prescription. It follows therefore that the types of medicines for which starter packs are appropriate are limited.

17.1 Samples may only be provided to health professionals and must not be provided to administrative staff.

17.2 No more than ten samples of a particular medicine may be provided to an individual health professional during the course of a year.

17.3 Samples may only be supplied in response to written requests which have been signed and dated.

Clause 17.3 Sample Requests

This clause does not preclude the provision of a preprinted sample request form bearing the name of the product for signing and dating by the applicant.

All signed and dated written requests for samples should be retained for not less than one year.

17.4 A sample of a medicine must be no larger than the smallest presentation of the medicine on the market.

17.5 Each sample must be marked 'free medical sample–not for resale' or words to that effect and must be accompanied by a copy of the summary of product characteristics, or where one does not exist, a copy of the data sheet or a document with a similar content.

17.6 Samples of medicines which are controlled under the Misuse of Drugs Act 1971 are prohibited except for those medicines coming within Schedule 5 to the Misuse of Drugs Regulations 1985.

17.7 Samples distributed by representatives must be handed direct to the health professionals requesting them or persons authorized to receive them on their behalf.

17.8 The distribution of samples in hospitals must comply with individual hospital requirements.

17.9 Companies must have an adequate system of control and accountability for samples of medicines which they distribute.

17.10 Medicines which are sent by post must be packed so as to be reasonably secure against being opened by young children. No unsolicited medicine must be sent through the post.

17.11 Unsolicited medicines must not be supplied to the general public.

Clause 17.11 Supply of Samples to the General Public

Proposed amendments to the Advertising Regulations under consideration by the Medicines Control Agency at the time of going to press would prohibit the supply of medicines to the general public for promotional purposes, whether solicited or unsolicited.

Clause 18 Gifts and Inducements

18.1 No gift, benefit in kind or pecuniary advantage shall be offered or given to members of the health professions or to administrative staff as an inducement to prescribe, supply, administer or buy any medicine, subject to the provisions of Clause 18.2.

Clause 18.1 Provision of Medical and Educational Goods and Services

Clause 18.1 does not prevent the provision of medical and educational goods and services which will enhance patient care or benefit the National Health Service. The provision of such goods or services must not be done in such a way as to be an inducement to prescribe, supply, administer or buy any medicine. They must not bear the name of any medicine but may bear a corporate name.

Clause 18.1 General Medical Council

In its publication 'Good medical practice' which is referred to in the supplementary information to Clause 15.3, the General Medical Council advises doctors that 'You should not ask for or accept any material rewards, except those of insignificant value, from companies that sell or market drugs or appliances'.

Clause 18.1 Terms of Trade

Measures or trade practices relating to prices, margins and discounts which were in regular use by a significant proportion of the pharmaceutical industry on 1 January 1993 are outside the scope of the Code (see Clause 1.2) and are excluded from the provisions of this clause. Other trade practices are subject to the Code. The terms 'prices', 'margins' and 'discounts' are primarily financial terms.

Schemes which enable health professionals to obtain personal benefits, for example gift vouchers for high street stores, in relation to the purchase of medicines are unacceptable even if they are presented as alternatives to financial discounts.

The Royal Pharmaceutical Society of Great Britain has issued guidance in relation to the acceptance of gifts and inducements to prescribe or supply. The Society states that pharmacists accepting items such as gift vouchers, bonus points, discount holidays, sports equipment etc would be in breach of the Society's Code of Ethics and advises pharmacists not to participate in such offers.

Clause 18.1 Package Deals

Clause 18.1 does not prevent the offer of package deals whereby the purchaser of particular medicines receives with them other associated benefits, such as apparatus for administration, provided that the transaction as a whole is fair and reasonable.

Clause 18.1 Donations to Charities

Donations to charities made by companies in return for health professionals' attendance at company stands at meetings or offered as rewards for completing and returning quiz cards in mailings and such like are not unacceptable under this clause provided that the level of donation for each individual is modest, the money is for a reputable charity and any action required of the health professional is not inappropriate. Any donation to a charity must not constitute a payment that would otherwise be unacceptable under the Code. For example, it would not be acceptable for a representative to pay into a practice equipment fund set up as a charity as this would be a financial inducement prohibited under Clause 18.1. Donations to charities in return for representatives gaining interviews are also prohibited under Clause 15.3 of the Code.

Any offer by a company of a donation to a charity which is conditional upon some action by a health professional must not place undue pressure on the health professional to fulfil that condition. At all times the provisions of Clauses 2 and 9.1 must be kept in mind.

18.2 Gifts in the form of promotional aids and prizes whether related to a particular product or of general utility, may be distributed to members of the health professions and to appropriate administrative staff, provided that the gift or prize is inexpensive and relevant to the practice of their profession or employment.

Clause 18.2 Gifts

Items provided on long term or permanent loan to a doctor or a practice are regarded as gifts and are subject to the requirements of this clause.

Gifts must be inexpensive and relevant to the recipients' work. An 'inexpensive' gift means one which has cost the donor company no more than £5, excluding VAT.

Items of general utility which have been held to be acceptable gifts to doctors as being inexpensive and of relevance to their work include pens, pads, diaries, nail brushes, surgical gloves, desk trays, calendars, a low value phone card, a peak flow whistle, walking sticks and desk clocks.

Items which are for use in the home, and have no use in the ordinary course of the practice of medicine or any other health profession, such as table mats, are unacceptable. Other examples of items which have been found unacceptable are neck cushions, plant seeds, road atlases and compact discs of music which were not considered relevant items and an x-ray light box and an age-sex register on grounds of costs.

Names of medicines should not be used on promotional aids when it would be inappropriate to do so, for example, when it might mislead as to the nature of the item.

Clause 18.2 Competitions and Quizzes

The use of competitions, quizzes and suchlike for the purposes of sales promotion are not necessarily an unacceptable form of promotion. Any competition must, however, be in good taste and must not involve any subject matter which is inappropriate for the promotion of a medicine as required under Clause 9.1. A competition is more likely to be considered acceptable if its subject matter is clearly related to the practice of medicine and pharmacy.

Any competition used for promotional purposes must be a bona fide test of skill and must recognise the professional standing of the recipients.

The provisions of Clause 18.2 apply to the provision of competition prizes. Prizes of a higher value than would ordinarily be acceptable for a promotional aid are acceptable where the competition is a serious one and the prizes are few in number, relevant to the potential recipient's work and not out of proportion to the skill required in the competition. The maximum acceptable cost to the donor of a prize in a promotional competition is £100, excluding VAT.

Gladstone bags, a desk clock and a business card holder are examples of prizes which have been found acceptable in particular competitions or quizzes.

Computer equipment and a substantial travel award offered as a prize in a promotional competition are examples of prizes which have been found unacceptable on grounds of cost.

Attention is drawn to the fact that the items listed above as acceptable competition prizes or gifts are instances where the particular examples in question were found acceptable. It does not mean that any such item is automatically acceptable under the Code.

Clause 18.2 Gifts to or for use by Patients

Some items distributed as promotional aids are intended for use by patients and these are not generally unacceptable provided that they meet the requirements of Clause 18.2; for example, small inexpensive puzzles and toys for a young child to play with during a visit to the doctor.

Other items which may be made available to patients, for example by completing a request card enclosed with a medicine, should meet the relevant principles set out in Clause 18.2, that is they should be inexpensive and related to either the condition under treatment or general health. Care must be taken that any such activity meets all the requirements of the Code and in particular Clause 20.

No gift or promotional aid for use by patients must be given for the purpose of encouraging patients to request a particular medicine.

18.3 The prescribing information for a medicine as required under Clause 4 does not have to be included on a promotional aid if the promotional aid includes no more than the following about the medicine:
- the name of the medicine
- an indication that the name of the medicine is a trade mark
- the name of the company responsible for marketing the product.

Clause 18.3 Promotional Aids–Name of the Medicine

The name of the medicine means the brand name or the non-proprietary name. Both names may be included but it is not obligatory to include both. A promotional aid may bear the names of more than one medicine.

Clause 18.3 Prescribing Information on Note Pads and Calendars

If a promotional aid consists of a note pad or calendar in which the individual pages bear advertising material, there is no need for the individual pages to comply with Clause 4 provided that the information required by that clause is given elsewhere; for example, on the cover.

Clause 19 Hospitality and Meetings

19.1 Companies are permitted to provide appropriate hospitality to members of the health professions and appropriate administrative staff in association with scientific and promotional meetings, scientific congresses and other such meetings. Hospitality must be secondary to the purpose of the meeting. The level of hospitality offered must be appropriate and not out of proportion to the occasion and the costs involved must not exceed that level which the recipients would normally adopt when paying for themselves. It must not extend beyond members of the health professions or appropriate administrative staff.

Clause 19.1 Hospitality and Meetings

The provision of hospitality includes the payment of reasonable, actual travel costs which a company may provide to sponsor a delegate to attend a meeting. The payment of travel expenses and the like for persons accompanying the delegate is not permitted.

The payment of reasonable honoraria and reimbursement of out of pocket expenses, including travel, for speakers, is permissible.

Pharmaceutical companies may appropriately sponsor a wide range of meetings. These range from small lunchtime audio-visual presentations in a group practice, hospital meetings and meetings at postgraduate education centres, launch meetings for new products, management training courses, meetings of clinical trialists, patient support group meetings, satellite symposia through to large international meetings organised by independent bodies with sponsorship from pharmaceutical companies.

With any meeting, certain basic principles apply:
- *the meeting must have a clear educational content*
- *the hospitality associated with the meeting must be secondary to the nature of the meeting, must be appropriate and not out of proportion to the occasion and*
- *any hospitality provided must not extend to spouses and other persons unless that person is a member of the health professions or appropriate administrative staff and qualifies as a proper delegate or participant at the meeting in their own right. It follows therefore that spouses and other such persons must not otherwise be invited to meetings.*

Administrative staff may be invited to meetings where appropriate. For example, receptionists might be invited to a meeting in a general practice when the subject matter related to practice administration.

A useful criterion in determining whether the arrangements for any meeting are acceptable is to apply the question 'would you and your company be willing to have these arrangements generally known?' The impression that is created by the arrangements for any meeting must always be kept in mind.

Meetings organised for groups of doctors, other health professionals and/or for administrative staff which are wholly or mainly of a social or sporting nature are unacceptable.

Clause 19.1 General Medical Council

In its publication 'Good medical practice' which is referred to in the supplementary information to Clause 15.3, the General Medical Council advises doctors that 'You may accept personal travel grants and hospitality from companies for conferences or educational meetings, as long as the main purpose of the event is educational. The amount you receive must not be more than you would normally spend if you were paying for yourself'.

Clause 19.1 Postgraduate Education Allowance (PGEA) Approved Courses

The provisions of this and all other relevant clauses in the Code apply equally to meetings organised or sponsored by pharmaceutical companies which are PGEA approved. The fact that a course is PGEA approved does not mean that the arrangements for the meeting are automatically acceptable under the Code. The relevant provisions of the Code, and in particular, those relating to hospitality, must be observed.

19.2 Payments may not be made to doctors or groups of doctors, either directly or indirectly, for rental for rooms to be used for meetings.

Clause 19.2 Payment of Room Rental

This provision does not preclude the payment of room rental to postgraduate medical centres and the like.

Payment of room rental to doctors or groups of doctors is not permissible even if such payment is made to equipment funds or patients' comforts funds and the like or to charities or companies.

19.3 When meetings are sponsored by pharmaceutical companies, that fact must be disclosed in the papers relating to the meetings and in any published proceedings.

Clause 19.3 Sponsorship and Reports of Meetings

Attention is drawn to Clause 9.9 which requires that all material relating to medicines and their uses which is sponsored by a pharmaceutical company must clearly indicate that it has been sponsored by that company.

It should be noted that where companies are involved in the sponsorship and/or distribution of reports on meetings or symposia etc these reports may constitute promotional material and thus be fully subject to the requirements of the Code.

Clause 20 Relations with the General Public and the Media

20.1 Medicines must not be advertised to the general public if they are prescription only medicines or are medicines which, though not prescription only, may not legally be advertised to the general public. This prohibition does not apply to vaccination campaigns carried out by companies and approved by the health ministers.

Clause 20.1 Advertising of Medicines to the General Public

The advertising of prescription only medicines to the general public is also prohibited by the Advertising Regulations.

The promotion of medicines to the general public for self medication purposes is covered by the Code of Standards of Advertising Practice for Over-the-Counter Medicines of the Proprietary Association of Great Britain (PAGB).

Methods of sale of medicines through pharmacies are also covered by the Code of Ethics of the Royal Pharmaceutical Society of Great Britain.

20.2 Information about medicines which is made available to the general public either directly or indirectly must be factual and presented in a balanced way. It must not raise unfounded hopes of successful treatment or be misleading with respect to the safety of the product.

Statements must not be made for the purpose of encouraging members of the public to ask their doctors to prescribe a specific medicine.

Clause 20.2 Information to the General Public

This clause allows for the provision of non-promotional information about prescription medicines to the general public either in response to a direct inquiry from an individual, including inquiries from journalists, or by dissemination of such information via press conferences, press announcements, television and radio reports, public relations activities and the like. It also includes information provided by means of posters distributed for display in surgery waiting rooms etc.

Any information so provided must observe the principles set out in this clause, that is, it should be factual, balanced and must not be made for the purpose of encouraging members of the public to ask their doctors to prescribe a specific medicine. It must not constitute the advertising of medicines to the general public prohibited under Clause 20.1. The provisions of Clause 20.3 must be observed if an inquiry is from an individual member of the public.

Particular care must be taken in responding to approaches from the media to ensure that the provisions of this clause are upheld.

In the event of a complaint which relates to the provisions of this clause, companies will be asked to provide copies of any information supplied, including copies of any relevant press releases and the like. This information will be assessed to determine whether it fulfils the requirements of this clause.

Summaries of product characteristics, data sheets and package leaflets for medicines may be provided to members of the public on request.

Companies may provide members of the health professions with leaflets concerning a medicine with a view to their provision to patients to whom the medicine has already been prescribed, provided that such a leaflet is factual and non-promotional in nature.

Clause 20.2 Financial Information

Information made available in order to inform shareholders, the Stock Exchange and the like by way of annual reports and announcements etc. may relate to both existing medicines and those not yet marketed. Such information must be factual and presented in a balanced way.

Clause 20.2 Approval of Information

Information on medicines made available under this clause should be examined to ensure that it does not contravene the Code or the relevant statutory requirements.

20.3 Requests from individual members of the public for information or advice on personal medical matters must be refused and the enquirer recommended to consult his or her own doctor.

Clause 20.3 Requests for Information or Advice on Personal Medical Matters

This clause prohibits the provision of information or advice on personal medical matters to individual members of the general public requesting it. The intention behind this prohibition is to ensure that companies do not intervene in the patient/doctor relationship by offering advice or information which properly should be in the domain of the doctor. However, information may be given, including information on medicines prescribed for the enquirer, provided that it complies with the requirements of Clauses 20.1 and 20.2 and does not impinge on the principle behind this clause. For example, answering requests by members of the public as to whether a particular medicine contains sucrose or some other inactive ingredient, or whether there would be problems associated with drinking alcohol whilst taking the medicine or whether the medicine should be taken before or after a meal, is acceptable. The situation with enquiries relating to side-effects, the indications for a medicine and such like is not as clear cut and particular caution is required in dealing with them.

All requests from members of the general public need to be handled with great care and a decision taken as to whether the company can responsibly answer the inquiry.

Requests from patients for information may in some instances best be handled by passing the information to the patients' doctors for discussion with them rather than providing the information direct to the patients concerned.

20.4 The introduction of a new medicine must not be made known to the general public until reasonable steps have been taken to inform the medical and pharmaceutical professions of its availability.

20.5 Companies are responsible for information about their products which is issued by their public relations agencies.

Clause 21 Compliance with Undertakings

When an undertaking has been given in relation to a ruling under the Code, the company concerned must ensure that it complies with that undertaking.

PRESCRIPTION MEDICINES CODE OF PRACTICE AUTHORITY: CONSTITUTION AND PROCEDURE

INTRODUCTION

The Code of Practice for the Pharmaceutical Industry is administered by the Prescription Medicines Code of Practice Authority. The Authority is responsible for the provision of advice, guidance and training on the Code of Practice as well as for the complaints procedure. It is also responsible for arranging for conciliation between companies when requested to do so and for scrutinising journal advertising on a regular basis. Complaints made under the Code about promotional material or the promotional activities of companies are considered by the Code of Practice Panel and, where required, by the Code of Practice Appeal Board. Reports on cases are published quarterly by the Authority and are available on request.

The names of individuals complaining from outside the pharmaceutical industry are kept confidential. In exceptional cases it may be necessary for a company to know the identity of the complainant so that the matter can be properly investigated. Even in these instances, the name of the complainant is only disclosed with the complainant's permission.

Complaints about the promotion of medicines should be submitted to the Director of the Prescription Medicines Code of Practice Authority, 12 Whitehall, London SW1A 2DY; telephone 0171 930 9677; facsimile 0171 930 4554.

STRUCTURE AND RESPONSIBILITIES

1 Prescription Medicines Code of Practice Authority

1.1 The Prescription Medicines Code of Practice Authority is responsible for the administration of the Code of Practice for the Pharmaceutical Industry including the provision of advice, guidance and training on the Code. It is also responsible for arranging for conciliation between companies when requested to do so and for scrutinising journal advertising on a regular basis.

1.2 The Authority also administers the complaints procedure by which complaints made under the Code are considered by the Code of Practice Panel and, where required, by the Code of Practice Appeal Board.

1.3 The Authority is appointed by and reports to the Board of Management of The Association of the British Pharmaceutical Industry (ABPI) and consists of the Director, Secretary and Deputy Secretary.

1.4 The Director has the authority to request copies of any relevant material from a pharmaceutical company, including copies of the certificates authorizing any such material and copies of relevant briefing material for representatives.

1.5 The Authority may consult the Code of Practice Appeal Board upon any matter concerning the Code of Practice or its administration.

2 Code of Practice Panel – Constitution and Procedure

2.1 The Code of Practice Panel consists of members of the Prescription Medicines Code of Practice Authority and meets as business requires to consider complaints made under the Code.

2.2 Two members of the Authority form a quorum for a meeting of the Panel. Decisions are made by majority voting. The Director or, in his absence, the Secretary, acts as Chairman of the Panel and has both an original and a casting vote.

2.3 The Director of the Authority may obtain expert assistance in any field. Expert advisers who are consulted may be invited to attend a meeting of the Panel but have no voting rights.

3 Code of Practice Appeal Board – Constitution

3.1 The Code of Practice Appeal Board and its Chairman are appointed by the Board of Management of the ABPI. The appointment of independent members to the Appeal Board is made following consultation with the Medicines Control Agency.

3.2 The Appeal Board comprises:

- an independent, legally qualified Chairman;
- three independent medical members appointed in consultation with the British Medical Association, one with recent experience as a general practitioner and one with recent experience as a hospital consultant;
- four medical directors or medically qualified senior executives from pharmaceutical companies;
- one independent pharmacist appointed following consultation with the Royal Pharmaceutical Society of Great Britain;
- one member from an independent body involved in providing information on medicines;
- eight directors or senior executives from pharmaceutical companies.

3.3 The Chairman of the Appeal Board is appointed for a term of five years which may be renewed. Members of the Appeal Board are each appointed for a term of three years which may be renewed.

3.4 The Director, Secretary and Deputy Secretary of the Code of Practice Authority comprise the secretariat to the Appeal Board. The secretariat attend meetings of the Appeal Board as observers and provide administrative support to the Appeal Board as appropriate.

4 Code of Practice Appeal Board – Procedure

4.1 The Code of Practice Appeal Board meets as business requires to consider appeals under the Code and any other matter which relates to the Code. The Appeal Board receives reports on all complaints which have been submitted under the Code and details of the action taken on them.

4.2 The Chairman and seven members of the Appeal Board constitute a quorum. Two of those present must be independent members, at least one of whom must be medically qualified, and there must also be present at least one medically qualified member from a pharmaceutical company.

In the event that a quorum cannot be attained for the consideration of a case because of the number of members barred under Paragraph 4.4 below, or for any other reason, the Chairman may co-opt appropriate persons to the Appeal Board so as to enable a quorum to be achieved.

4.3 Decisions are made by majority voting. The Chairman has both an original and a casting vote.

4.4 If a member of the Appeal Board is concerned in a case either as complainant or respondent, that member does not receive copies of the papers circulated in connection with the case and is required to withdraw from the Appeal Board during its consideration.

Members of the Appeal Board are also required to declare any other interest in a case prior to its consideration. The Chairman determines whether it is appropriate for that member to remain for the consideration of the case.

4.5 The Chairman may obtain expert assistance in any field. Expert advisers may be invited to attend a meeting of the Appeal Board but have no voting rights.

4.6 When appeals are considered by the Appeal Board, the respondent company is entitled to have a representative or representatives appear before the Appeal Board to state the company's case.

4.7 Where an appeal is brought which is concerned with an issue of fact between a complainant and the company concerned which cannot be properly resolved without the oral evidence of the persons directly involved, the Chairman may invite such persons to attend and give evidence.

COMPLAINTS PROCEDURE

5 Action on Complaints

5.1 When the Director receives information from which it appears that a company may have contravened the Code, the chief executive of the company concerned is requested to comment on the matters of complaint.

If a complaint concerns a matter closely similar to one which has been the subject of a previous adjudication, it may be allowed to proceed at the discretion of the Director if new evidence is adduced by the complainant or if the passage of time or a change in circumstances raises doubts as to whether the same decision would be made in respect of the current complaint. The Director should normally allow a complaint to proceed if it covers matters similar to those in a decision of the Code of Practice Panel which was not the subject of appeal to the Code of Practice Appeal Board.

If a complainant does not accept a decision of the Director that a complaint should not be proceeded with because a similar complaint has been adjudicated upon previously and nothing has changed in the meantime, then the matter is referred to the Chairman of the Code of Pratice Appeal Board for his decision which is final.

5.2 When the complaint is from a pharmaceutical company, the complaint must be signed or authorized in writing by the company's chief executive and must state those clauses of the Code which are alleged to have been breached.

5.3 Upon receipt of a complaint, the company concerned has ten working days in which to submit its comments in writing.

6 Establishment of *Prima Facie Case* and Consideration by the Code of Practice Panel

6.1 Upon receipt of the comments from the respondent company, the Director must determine whether there is a *prima facie* case to answer under the Code. If, in the view of the Director, no *prima facie* case has been established the complainant and the respondent company are so advised. If the complainant does not accept that view, the matter is referred to the Chairman of the Code of Practice Appeal Board for his decision which is final.

6.2 Once it has been determined that a *prima facie* case exists, the case is referred to the Code of Practice Panel to determine whether or not there has been a breach of the Code.

7 Code of Practice Panel: Rulings

7.1 Where the Code of Practice Panel rules that there is a breach of the Code, the company concerned is so advised and is given the reasons for the decision.

The respondent company has ten working days to provide a written undertaking that the promotional activity or use of the material in question (if not already discontinued or no longer in use) will cease forthwith and that all possible steps will be taken to avoid a similar breach of the Code in the future. This undertaking must be signed by the chief executive of the company or with his or her authority and must be accompanied by details of the actions taken by the company to implement the undertaking, including the date on which the promotional material was finally used or appeared and/or the last date on which the promotional activity took place.

The company must also pay within twenty working days an administrative charge based on the number of matters ruled in breach of the Code.

7.2 Where the Panel rules that there is no breach of the Code, the complainant and respondent company are so advised. Where the complaint is from a pharmaceutical company, the complainant must pay within twenty working days an administrative charge based on the number of matters alleged and ruled not to be in breach of the Code.

When advised of the outcome, the complainant will be sent a copy of the comments and enclosures submitted by the respondent in relation to the complaint. If the respondent objects to this because it regards part of the material as being confidential, and the matter cannot be settled by the Director, then it will be referred to the Chairman of the Code of Practice Appeal Board for his decison which is final.

7.3 The complainant or the respondent company may appeal against rulings of the Panel to the Code of Practice Appeal Board. Appeals must be lodged within ten working days of the notification of the ruling of the Panel and must be accompanied by reasons as to why the Panel's ruling is not accepted. These reasons will be circulated to the Appeal Board.

7.4 Where an appeal is lodged by the complainant, the respondent company has ten working days to comment on the reasons given by the complainant for the appeal and these comments will be circulated to the Appeal Board.

The complainant has five working days to comment on the respondent company's comments upon the reasons given by the complainant for the appeal and these comments also will be circulated to the Appeal Board.

In the event that the respondent objects to certain of its comments being made available to the complainant on the grounds of confidentiality, and the matter cannot be settled by the Director, then the matter will be referred to the Chairman of the Code of Practice Appeal Board who will decide whether those particular comments can be included in the evidence which goes before the Appeal Board.

8 Code of Practice Panel: Reports to the Appeal Board

8.1 Refusal to comply with the procedures set out in Paragraphs 5, 6 and 7 above shall be reported to the Code of Practice Appeal Board for consideration in relation to the provisions of Paragraph 11.1 below.

8.2 The Code of Practice Panel may also report to the Appeal Board any company whose conduct in relation to the Code, or in relation to a particular case before it, warrants consideration by the Appeal Board in relation to the provisions of Paragraphs 10.3 and 11.1 below. Such a report to the Appeal Board may be made notwithstanding the fact that a company has provided an undertaking requested by the Panel.

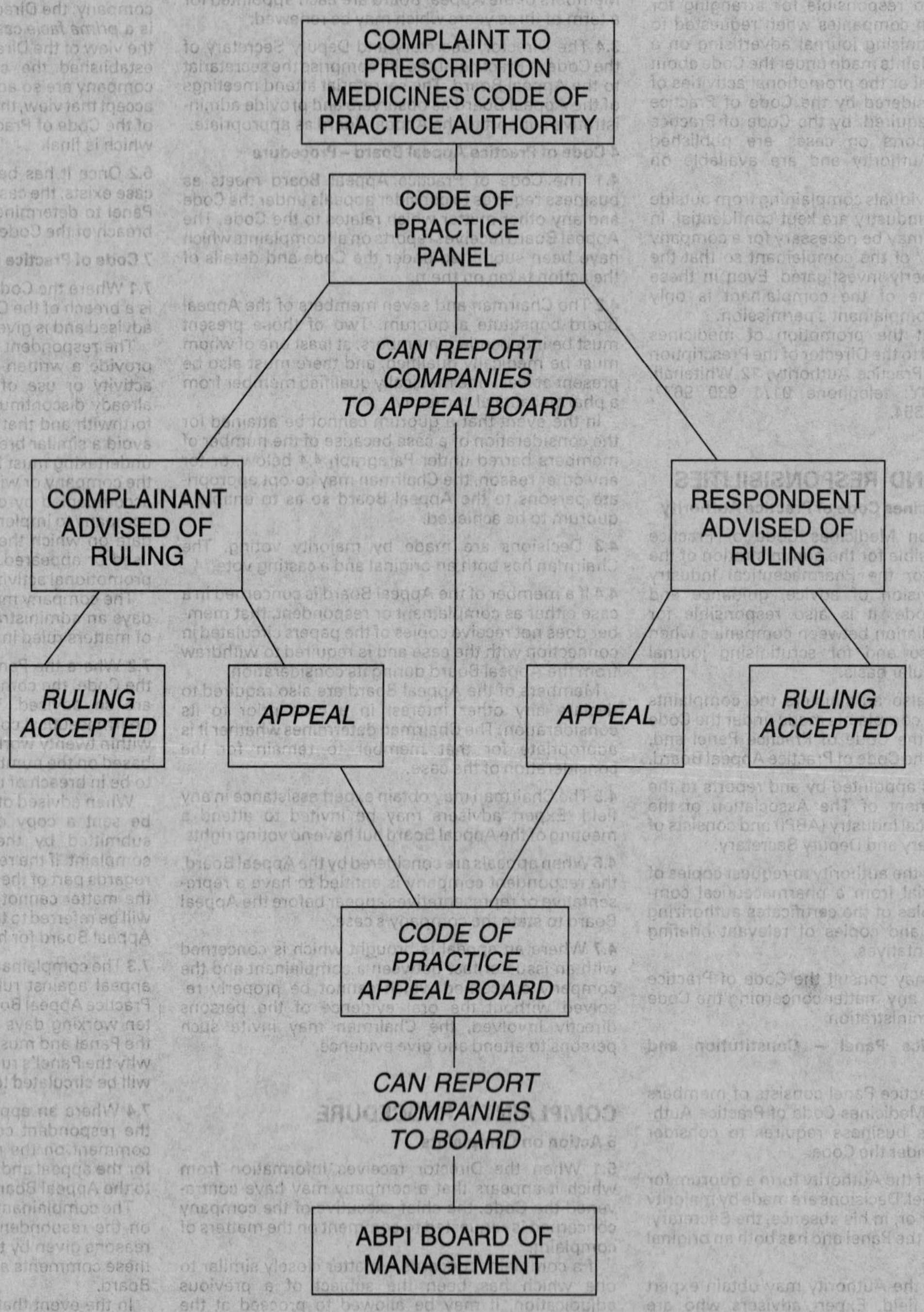
COMPLAINT TO PRESCRIPTION MEDICINES CODE OF PRACTICE AUTHORITY
CODE OF PRACTICE PANEL
CAN REPORT COMPANIES TO APPEAL BOARD
COMPLAINANT ADVISED OF RULING
RESPONDENT ADVISED OF RULING
RULING ACCEPTED
APPEAL
APPEAL
RULING ACCEPTED
CODE OF PRACTICE APPEAL BOARD
CAN REPORT COMPANIES TO BOARD
ABPI BOARD OF MANAGEMENT

8.3 Where the Panel reports a company to the Appeal Board under the provisions of Paragraphs 8.1 and 8.2 above, the company concerned is provided with a copy of the report prior to its consideration and is entitled to have a representative or representatives appear before the Appeal Board to state the company's case.

9 Action on Complaints about Safety from the Medicines Control Agency

9.1 In the event of the Medicines Control Agency making a complaint which relates to the safety or proper use of a medicine, and requesting that an advertisement be withdrawn, the respondent company has five working days to respond with its comments.

9.2 If the Code of Practice Panel upholds the complaint, the company is required to suspend the advertisement or practice forthwith pending the final outcome of the case.

10 Code of Practice Appeal Board: Rulings

10.1 Where the Code of Practice Appeal Board rules that there is no breach of the Code, the complainant and the respondent company are so advised.

Where a complainant pharmaceutical company appeals and the Appeal Board upholds the ruling that there was no breach of the Code, the complainant pharmaceutical company must pay within twenty working days an administrative charge based on the number of matters taken to appeal on which no breach is ruled.

Where a respondent company appeals and the Appeal Board rules that there was no breach of the Code, the complainant pharmaceutical company must pay within twenty working days an administrative charge based on the number of matters taken to appeal on which no breach is ruled.

10.2 Where the Appeal Board rules that there is a breach of the Code, the respondent company is so advised in writing and is given the reasons for the decision. The respondent company then has five working days to provide a written undertaking providing the information specified in Paragraph 7.1.

The company must also pay within twenty working days an administrative charge based on the number of matters ruled in breach of the Code.

10.3 A company ruled in breach of the Code may also be required by the Appeal Board to take steps to recover items given in connection with the promotion of a medicine. Details of the action taken must be provided in writing to the Appeal Board.

10.4 Where a company is ruled in breach of the Code the Appeal Board may require an audit of the company's procedures in relation to the Code to be carried out by the Prescription Medicines Code of Practice Authority.

11 Code of Practice Appeal Board: Reports to the ABPI Board of Management

11.1 Where the Code of Practice Appeal Board considers that the conduct of a company in relation to the Code or a particular case before it warrants such action, it may report the company to the Board of Management of the ABPI for it to consider whether further sanctions should be applied against that company. Such a report may be made notwithstanding the fact that the company has provided an undertaking requested by either the Code of Practice Panel or the Appeal Board.

11.2 Where such a report is made to the Board of Management, the Board of Management may decide:

- to reprimand the company and publish details of that reprimand;
- to require an audit of the company's procedures in relation to the Code to be carried out by the Prescription Medicines Code of Practice Authority and following that audit, decide whether to impose requirements on the company concerned to improve its procedures in relation to the Code;
- to require the company to publish a corrective statement;
- to suspend or expel the company from the ABPI; or
- in the case of companies not in membership of the ABPI, to remove the company from the list of non member companies which have agreed to abide by the Code and to advise the Medicines Control Agency that responsibility for that company under the Code can no longer continue to be accepted.

11.3 Where a report is made to the Board of Management under Paragraph 11.1 above, the company concerned is provided with a copy of the report prior to its consideration and is entitled to have a representative or representatives appear before the Board of Management to state the company's case.

12 Case Reports

12.1 At the conclusion of any case under the Code, the complainant is advised of the outcome and a report is published summarising the details of the case.

12.2 The respondent company and the medicine concerned are named in the report.

In a case where the complaint was initiated by a company or by an organisation or official body, that company or organisation or official body is named in the report. The information given must not, however, be such as to identify any individual person.

12.3 A copy of the report on a case is made available to both the complainant and the respondent company prior to publication. Any amendments to the report suggested by these parties are considered by the Director, consulting with the other party where appropriate. If either party does not accept the Director's decision as to whether or not a report should be amended, the matter is referred to the Chairman of the Code of Practice Appeal Board for his decision which is final.

12.4 Copies of all case reports are submitted to the Code of Practice Appeal Board and the Board of Management of the ABPI for information prior to publication.

Copies of the published reports are sent to the Medicines Control Agency, the Office of Fair Trading, the British Medical Association, the Royal Pharmaceutical Society of Great Britain and the editors of the British Medical Journal and the Pharmaceutical Journal. Copies of the published reports are also available to anyone on request.

GENERAL PROVISIONS

13 Time Periods for Responding to Matters under the Code

The number of working days within which companies or complainants must respond to enquiries etc, from the Prescription Medicines Code of Practice Authority, as referred to in the above procedures, are counted from the date of receipt of the notification in question.

An extension in time to respond to such notifications may be granted at the discretion of the Director of the Authority.

14 Withdrawal of Complaints and Notices of Appeal

14.1 A complaint may be withdrawn by a complainant with the consent of the respondent company up until such time as the respondent company's comments on the complaint have been received by the Prescription Medicines Code of Practice Authority, but not thereafter.

14.2 Notice of appeal may be withdrawn by a complainant with the consent of the respondent company up until such time as the respondent company's comments on the reasons for the appeal have been received by the Authority, but not thereafter.

14.3 Notice of appeal may be withdrawn by a respondent company at any time but if notice is given after the papers relating to its appeal have been circulated to the Code of Practice Appeal Board, then the higher administrative charge will be payable.

15 Code of Practice Levy and Administrative Charges

15.1 An annual Code of Practice levy is paid by members of the ABPI. The levy together with the administrative charges referred to in Paragraphs 7 and 10 above are determined by the Board of Management of the ABPI subject to approval at a General Meeting of the ABPI by a simple majority of those present and voting.

15.2 Administrative charges are payable only by pharmaceutical companies and companies are liable for such charges whether they are members of the ABPI or not.

There are two levels of administrative charge.

The lower level is payable by a company which accepts either a ruling of the Code of Practice Panel that it was in breach of the Code of Practice or a rejection by the Panel of its allegation against another company. The lower level is also payable by a complainant company if a ruling of the Panel that there was a breach of the Code is subsequently overturned by the Code of Practice Appeal Board.

The higher level is paid by a company which unsuccessfully appeals a decision of the Panel.

15.3 Where two or more companies are ruled in breach of the Code in relation to a matter involving co-promotion, each company shall be separately liable to pay an administrative charge.

15.4 The number of administrative charges which apply in a case is determined by the Director of the Prescription Medicines Code of Practice Authority. If a company does not agree with the Director's decision, the matter is referred to the Chairman of the Code of Practice Appeal Board for his decision which is final.

16 Possible Breaches identified by the Code of Practice Panel or Code of Practice Appeal Board

16.1 Where the Code of Practice Panel or Code of Practice Appeal Board identifies a possible breach of the Code of Practice which has not been addressed by the complainant in a case, the respondent company is invited to comment. The company has ten working days to respond in writing.

16.2 If the company accepts there is a breach of the Code of Practice, the company is requested to provide an undertaking providing the information specified in Paragraph 7.1 above. No administrative charge shall be payable in these circumstances and there shall be no case report on the matter in question.

16.3 If the company does not accept there is a breach of the Code of Practice the procedures under Paragraph 6 above onwards shall be followed.

17 Scrutiny of Advertisements

17.1 A sample of advertisements issued by pharmaceutical companies is scrutinised by the Prescription Medicines Code of Practice Authority in relation to the requirements of the Code on a continuing basis.

17.2 Where a *prima facie* breach of the Code is identified under this procedure, the company concerned is requested to comment in writing within ten working days of receipt of the notification.

17.3 If the company accepts there is a breach of the Code, the company is requested to provide an undertaking providing the information specified in Paragraph 7.1 above. No administrative charge is payable in these circumstances.

17.4 If the company does not accept there is a breach of the Code, the procedures under Paragraph 6 above onwards shall be followed.

18 Provision of Advice and Conciliation

18.1 The Prescription Medicines Code of Practice Authority is available to provide informal guidance and advice in relation to the requirements of the Code and, where appropriate, may seek the views of the Code of Practice Appeal Board.

18.2 Companies wishing to seek the assistance of a conciliator with the view to reaching agreement on inter-company differences about promotion may contact the Director of the Authority for advice and assistance.

19 Amendments to the Code of Practice

19.1 The Code of Practice for the Pharmaceutical Industry and this Constitution and Procedure may be amended by a simple majority of those present and voting at a General Meeting of the ABPI.

19.2 The views of the Prescription Medicines Code of Practice Authority, the Code of Practice Panel and the Code of Practice Appeal Board must be sought on any proposal to amend the Code or this Constitution and Procedure. The views of the Medicines Control Agency, the British Medical Association and the Royal Pharmaceutical Society of Great Britain must also be invited.

19.3 The Prescription Medicines Code of Practice Authority, the Code of Practice Panel and the Code of Practice Appeal Board may, in the light of their experience, make recommendations for amendment of the Code and this Constitution and Procedure.

20 Annual Report

An annual report of the Prescription Medicines Code of Practice Authority is published each year with the approval of the Code of Practice Appeal Board. This report includes details of the work of the Authority, the Code of Practice Panel and the Code of Practice Appeal Board during that year.

INDEX

Key
numbers refer to Clauses in the Code
si refers to supplementary information to a clause in the Code
¶ followed by number refers to a paragraph in Constitution and Procedure

Guidelines for company-sponsored safety assessment of marketed medicines (SAMM)

Introduction

It is well-recognised that there is a continuous need to monitor the safety of medicines as they are used in clinical practice. Spontaneous reporting schemes (*e.g.* the UK yellow card system) provide important early warning signals of potential drug hazards and also provide a means of continuous surveillance. Formal studies to evaluate safety may also be necessary, particularly in the confirmation and characterisation of possible hazards identified at an earlier stage of drug development. Such studies may also be useful in identifying previously unsuspected reactions.

Scope of guidelines

These guidelines apply to the conduct of all company-sponsored studies which evaluate the safety of marketed products. They take the place of previous guidelines on post-marketing surveillance which were published in 1988 (BMJ, 296: 399–400). Studies performed under those guidelines were found to have some notable limitations (BMJ, 1992, 304: 1470–1472) and these new guidelines have been prepared in response to the problems identified. The major changes may be summarised as follows:

(1) The scope of the guidelines has been expanded to include all company-sponsored studies which are carried out to evaluate safety of marketed medicines. It should be emphasised that this includes both studies conducted in general practice and in the hospital setting. The name of the guidelines has been changed to reflect the emphasis on safety assessment rather than merely surveillance.

(2) The guidelines have been developed to provide a framework on which a variety of data collection methods can be used to improve the evaluation of the safety of marketed medicines. Whilst it is recognised that the design used needs to be tailored to particular drugs and hazards, the guidelines define the essential principles which may be applied in a variety of situations. The study methods in this field continue to develop and therefore there will be a need to review regularly these guidelines to ensure that they reflect advances made in the assessment of drug safety.

The guidelines have been formulated and agreed by a Working Party which includes representation from the Medicines Control Agency (MCA), Committee on Safety of Medicines (CSM), Association of the British Pharmaceutical Industry (ABPI), British Medical Association (BMA) and the Royal College of General Practitioners (RCGP). Other guidelines exists for the conduct of 'Phase IV clinical trials' where the medication is provided by the sponsoring company (see section 2(b) below). Some of these studies will also meet the definition of a SAMM study (see below) and should therefore also comply with the present guidelines.

1. Definition of Safety Assessment of Marketed Medicines

(a) Safety assessment of marketed medicines (SAMM) is defined as 'a formal investigation conducted for the purpose of assessing the clinical safety of marketed medicine(s) in clinical practice'.

(b) Any study of a marketed drug which has the evaluation of clinical safety as a specific objective should be included. Safety evaluation will be a specific objective in post-marketing studies either when there is a known safety issue under investigation and/or when the numbers of patients to be included will add significantly to the existing safety data for the product(s). Smaller studies conducted primarily for other purposes should not be considered as SAMM studies. However, if a study which is not conducted for the purpose of evaluating safety unexpectedly identifies a hazard, the manufacturer would be expected to inform the MCA immediately and the section of these guidelines covering liaison with regulatory authorities would thereafter apply.

(c) In cases of doubt as to whether or not a study comes under the scope of the guidelines the sponsor should discuss the intended study plan with the MCA.

2. Scope and Objectives of SAMM

(a) SAMM may be conducted for the purpose of identifying previously unrecognised safety issues (hypothesis-generation) or to investigate possible hazards (hypothesis-testing).

(b) A variety of designs may be appropriate including observational cohort studies, case-surveillance or case-control studies. Clinical trials may also be used to evaluate the safety of marketed products, involving systematic allocation of treatment (for example randomisation). Such studies must also adhere to the current guidelines for Phase IV clinical trials.

(c) The design to be used will depend on the objectives of the study, which must be clearly defined in the study plan. Any specific safety concerns to be investigated should be identified in the study plan and explicitly addressed by the proposed methods.

3. Design of studies

Observational cohort studies

(a) The population studied should be as representative as possible of the general population of users, and be unselected unless specifically targeted by the objectives of the study (for example a study of the elderly). Exclusion criteria should be limited to the contraindications stated in the data sheet or summary of product characteristics (SPC). The prescriber should be provided with a data sheet or SPC for all products to be used. Where the product is prescribed outside the indications on the data sheet, such patients should be included in the analysis of the study findings.

(b) Observational cohort studies should normally include appropriate comparator group(s). The comparator group(s) will usually include patients with the disease/indication(s) relevant to the primary study drug and such patients will usually be treated with alternative therapies.

(c) The product(s) should be prescribed in the usual manner, for example on an FP10 form written by the general practitioner or through the usual hospital procedures.

(d) Patients must not be prescribed particular medicines in order to include them in observational cohort studies since this is unethical (see section 15 of the 'Guidelines on the Practices of Ethics Committees in Medical Research involving Human Subjects', Royal College of Physicians, 1990).

(e) The prescribing of a drug and the inclusion of the patient in a study are two issues which must be clearly separated. Drugs must be prescribed solely as a result of a normal clinical evaluation, and since such indications may vary from doctor to doctor a justification for the prescription should be recorded in the study documents. In contrast, the inclusion of the patient in the study must be solely dependent upon the criteria for recruitment which have been specifically identified in the study procedures. Any deviation from the study criteria for recruitment could lead to selection bias.

(f) The study plan should stipulate the maximum number of patients to be entered by a single doctor. No patient should be prospectively entered into more than one study simultaneously.

Case-control studies

(g) Case-control studies are usually conducted retrospectively. In case-control studies comparison is made between the history of drug exposure of cases with the disease of interest and appropriate controls without the disease. The study design should attempt to account for known sources of bias and confounding.

Case-surveillance

(h) The purpose of case-surveillance is to study patients with diseases which are likely to be drug-related and to ascertain drug exposure. Companies who sponsor such studies should liaise particularly closely with the MCA in order to determine the most appropriate arrangements for the reporting of cases.

Clinical trials

(i) Large clinical trials are sometimes useful in the investigation of post-marketing safety issues and these may involve random allocation to treatment. In other respects, an attempt should be made to study patients under as normal conditions as possible. Exclusion criteria should be limited to the contraindications in the data sheet or SPC unless they are closely related to the particular objectives of the study. Clinical trials must also adhere to the current guidelines for Phase IV clinical trials (see 2(b) above). Studies which fulfil the definition of SAMM but are performed under a clinical trial exemption (CTX) or under the clinical trial on a marketed product (CTMP) scheme are within the scope of these guidelines.

4. Conduct of studies

(a) Responsibility for the conduct and quality of company-sponsored studies shall be vested in the company's medical department under the supervision of a named medical practitioner registered in the United Kingdom, and whose name shall be recorded in the study documents.

(b) Where a study is performed for a company by an agent, a named medical practitioner registered in the United Kingdom shall be identified by the agent to supervise the study and liaise with the company's medical department.

(c) Consideration should be given to the appointment of an independent advisory group(s) to monitor the safety information and oversee the study.

5. Liaison with regulatory authorities

(a) Companies proposing to perform a SAMM study are encouraged to discuss the draft study plan with the Medicines Control Agency (MCA) at an early stage. Particular consideration should be given to specific safety issues which may require investigation.

(b) Before the study commences a study plan should be finalised which explains the aims and objectives of the study, the methods to be used (including statistical analysis) and the record keeping which is to be maintained. The company shall submit the study plan plus any proposed initial communications to doctors to the MCA at least one month before the planned start of the study. The MCA will review the proposed study and may comment. The responsibility for the conduct of the study will, however, rest with the sponsoring pharmaceutical company.

(c) The company should inform the MCA when the study has commenced and will normally provide a brief report on its progress at least every six months, or more frequently if requested by MCA.

(d) The regulatory requirements for reporting of suspected adverse reactions must be fulfilled. Companies should endeavour to ensure that they are notified of serious suspected adverse reactions and should report these to the MCA within 15 days of receipt. Events which are not suspected by the investigator to be adverse reactions should not be reported individually as they occur. These and minor adverse reactions should be included in the final report.

(e) A final report on the study should be sent to the MCA within 3 months of follow-up being completed. Ideally this should be a full report but a brief report within 3 months followed by a full report within 6 months of completion of the study would normally be acceptable. The findings of the study should be submitted for publication.

(f) Companies are encouraged to follow MCA guidelines on the content of progress reports and final reports.

6. Promotion of medicines

(a) SAMM studies should not be conducted for the purposes of promotion.

(b) Company representatives should not be involved in SAMM studies in such a way that it could be seen as a promotional exercise.

7. Doctor Participation

(a) Subject to the doctor's terms of service, payment may be offered to the doctor in recompense for his time and any expenses incurred according to the suggested scale of fees published by the BMA.

(b) No inducement for a doctor to participate in a SAMM study should be offered, requested or given.

8. Ethical Issues

(a) The highest possible standards of professional conduct and confidentiality must always be maintained. The patient's right to confidentiality is paramount. The patient's identity in the study documents should be codified and only his or her doctor should be capable of decoding it.

(b) Responsibility for the retrieval of information from personal medical records lies with the consultant or general practitioner responsible for the patient's care. Such information should be directed to the medical practitioner nominated by the company or agent, who is thereafter responsible for the handling of such information.

(c) Reference to a Research Ethics Committee is required if patients are to be approached for information, additional investigations are to be performed or if it is proposed to allocate patients systematically to treatments.

9. Procedure for complaints

A study which gives cause for concern on scientific, ethical or promotional grounds should be referred to the MCA, ABPI and the company concerned. Concerns regarding possible scientific fraud should be referred to the ABPI. They will be investigated and, if appropriate, referred to the General Medical Council.

10. Review of Guidelines

The Working Party will review these guidelines as necessary.

Poisons Information Services

BELFAST
Director: Professor D G Johnson
Address: National Poisons Information Service (Belfast)
Royal Victoria Hospital
Grosvenor Road
Belfast
BT12 6BA
Telephone: 01232 240503 (24-hour service)
01232 248095 (Regional Drug and Poisons Information Service)
Fax: 01232 248030

BIRMINGHAM
Director: Dr J A Vale
Address: National Poisons Information Service (Birmingham Centre)
City Hospital NHS Trust
Dudley Road
Birmingham
B18 7QH
Telephone: 0121 507 5588/5599 (24-hour service)
Fax: 0121 507 5580

CARDIFF
Director: Professor P A Routledge
Address: Welsh National Poisons Unit
Therapeutics and Toxicology Centre,
Academic Centre,
Llandough Hospital
Penarth
Cardiff
CF64 2XX
Telephone: 01222 709901 (24-hour service)
Fax: 01222 704357

DUBLIN
Director: Dr J A Tracey
Address: Poisons Information Centre
Beaumont Hospital
PO Box 1297
Beaumont Road
Dublin 9
Eire
Telephone: 00 353 1 8379966
00 353 1 8379964
Fax: 00 353 1 8376982

EDINBURGH
Director: Dr D N Bateman
Address: Scottish Poisons Information Bureau
The Royal Infirmary
Lauriston Place
Edinburgh
EH3 9YW
Telephone: 0131 536 2300 (24-hour service)
Fax: 0131 536 2304
TOXBASE: For access contact 0131 5362298

LONDON
Director: Dr G N Volans
Address: National Poisons Information Service (London)
Medical Toxicology Unit
Guy's & St Thomas' Hospital Trust
Avonley Road
London SE14 5ER
Telephone: 0171 635 9191 (24-hour emergency service)
0171 771 5370 (laboratory enquiries and Unit Staff)
Fax: 0171 771 5309

NEWCASTLE
Director: Dr S H L Thomas
Address: National Poisons Information Service (Newcastle)
Regional Drug and Therapeutics Centre
Wolfson Unit
Claremont Place
Newcastle upon Tyne
NE2 4HH
Telephone: 0191 232 1525 (Direct line, normal office hours)
0191 232 5131 (24-hour service)
Fax: 0191 261 5733

Monitoring of drug overdoses

The poisons information service monitors reports of drug overdosage in a similar manner to the monitoring of adverse reactions by the Committee on Safety of Medicines. Doctors are encouraged to report unusual or severe cases to this service (whether or not they need to use the service for information or advice). In particular, the service would be keen to hear reports of overdose of those drugs also highlighted by the CSM, using the black triangle, since experience of overdose with these drugs is bound to be limited.

Overdose in pregnancy

All National Poisons Information Service (NPIS) Centres are able to advise on patients who take overdoses while pregnant, however the Newcastle Centre of the NPIS has been designated as the National Co-ordinating Centre for enquiries about poisoning in pregnancy. This service includes the follow up of the outcome of patients exposed to potential overdose in pregnancy. Enquiries about poisoning in pregnancy can, therefore, be directed to any NPIS centre, or to the Newcastle Centre directly on the telephone numbers above, or in writing.

Products new to this edition

The following list comprises products which are the subject of data sheets or summaries of product characteristics (SPCs) in this edition of the Compendium but which were not included in the 1997–98 edition. It does not necessarily follow that they are recently introduced products.

Directory of participants

This directory is included in the Compendium so that doctors and other professional people may obtain additional information about products from participating companies.

Medical Information
Abbott Laboratories Ltd
Abbott House
Norden Road
Maidenhead
Berkshire SL6 4XE
Telephone:
Maidenhead (01628) 773355
Facsimile: (01628) 644185

Akita Pharmaceuticals Limited
33 Moyle House
Churchill Gardens
Westminster
London SW1V 3BE
Telephone: (0870) 6071260
Facsimile: (0870) 6071261

Alcon Laboratories (UK) Ltd
Pentagon Park
Boundary Way
Hemel Hempstead
Hertfordshire HP2 7UD
Telephone: (01442) 341234
Facsimile: (01442) 341200

Medical Information
Allen & Hanburys Ltd
Stockley Park West
Uxbridge
Middlesex UB11 1BT
Telephone: (0181) 990 9000 or FREEFONE 0800 371891 (including 24-hour emergency service)
Facsimile: (0181) 990 4321
Customer Services
Telephone: FREEFONE 0800 221441
Facsimile: (0181) 990 4328

Medical Information
Allergan Ltd
Coronation Road
High Wycombe
Buckinghamshire HP12 3SH
Telephone: (01494) 444722
Facsimile: (01494) 473593/ 436871

Alliance Pharmaceuticals UK Ltd
Avonbridge House
2 Bath Road
Chippenham
Wiltshire SN15 2BB
Telephone: (01249) 466966
Facsimile: (01249) 466977

AMGEN Ltd
240 Cambridge Science Park
Milton Road
Cambridge CB4 0WD
Telephone: (01223) 420305
Facsimile: (01223) 423049/ 420319

Medical Information
Approved Prescription Services Ltd
Brampton Road
Hampden Park
Eastbourne
East Sussex BN22 9AG
Telephone: (01323) 501111
Facsimile: (01323) 520306

ASTA Medica Ltd
168 Cowley Road
Cambridge CB4 0DL
Telephone:
Medical Information (including 24-hour emergency service) (01223) 428811
All other enquiries (01223) 423434
Facsimile: (01223) 420943

Medical Information Department
Astra Pharmaceuticals Ltd
Home Park
Kings Langley
Hertfordshire WD4 8DH
Telephone:
Kings Langley (01923) 266191 (including 24-hour emergency service)
Facsimile: (01923) 260431

Athena Neurosciences
1 Meadway Court
Rutherford Close
Stevenage
Herts SG1 2EF
Telephone: (01438) 730200
Facsimile: (01438) 741452

Baker Norton (Division of Norton Healthcare Ltd)
Albert Basin
Royal Docks
London
E16 2QJ
Telephone: (0990) 020304
Facsimile: (08705) 323334

Bayer plc
Pharmaceutical Division
Bayer House
Strawberry Hill
Newbury
Berkshire RG14 1JA
Telephone: (01635) 563000
Facsimile: (01635) 563393

Beecham Research
See **SmithKline Beecham Pharmaceuticals**

Medical Information Department
Bencard
Welwyn Garden City
Hertfordshire AL7 1EY
Telephone
Welwyn Garden (01707) 325111 or FREEFONE (0800) 616482 (including 24-hour emergency service)
Facsimile: (0181) 913 4560

Medical Information
Berk Pharmaceuticals Limited
Brampton Road
Hampden Park
Eastbourne
East Sussex BN22 9AG
Telephone: (01323) 501111
Facsimile: (01323) 520306

Biogen Europe
55 Avenue des Champs Pierreux
92012 Nanterre
Cedex-France
Telephone: 33 (141) 379595
Facsimile: 33 (141) 372400

Medical Information
Bioglan Laboratories Ltd
5 Hunting Gate
Hitchin
Hertfordshire SG4 0TJ
Telephone:
Hitchin (01462) 438444
Emergency Medical Information:
Dr R. Mason
(01767) 627085
Facsimile: (01462) 421242

Information Services
Boehringer Ingelheim Ltd
Ellesfield Avenue
Bracknell
Berkshire RG12 8YS
Telephone: (01344) 424600 (including 24-hour emergency service)
Facsimile: (01344) 741444

Information Services
Boehringer Ingelheim Hospital Division
Ellesfield Avenue
Bracknell
Berkshire RG12 8YS
Telephone:
Bracknell (01344) 424600 (including 24-hour emergency service)
Facsimile: (01344) 741157

Boehringer Ingelheim Limited Self-Medication Division
Ellesfield Avenue
Bracknell
Berkshire RG12 8YS
Telephone: (01344) 424600
Facsimile: (01344) 741399

Borg Medicare
Dornstauden 15
91233 Neunkirchen-Rollhofen
Germany
Telephone: (9153) 923983
Facsimile: (9153) 923983

Bristol-Myers Pharmaceuticals
Bristol-Myers Squibb House
141-149 Staines Road
Hounslow
Middlesex TW3 3JA
Telephone:
Medical Information Only:
(0181) 754 3740
BMS House and emergencies:
(0181) 572 7422 and FREEFONE 0800 7311736
Facsimile: (0181) 754 3789

Bristol-Myers Squibb Pharmaceuticals Ltd
Bristol-Myers Squibb House
Staines Road
Hounslow TW3 3JA
Telephone:
Medical Information Only:
(0181) 754 3740 and FREEFONE 0800 7311736
BMS House and emergencies:
(0181) 572 7422
Facsimile: (0181) 754 3789

Britannia Pharmaceuticals Ltd
41–51 Brighton Road
Redhill
Surrey RH1 6YS
Telephone:
Redhill (01737) 773741
Facsimile: (01737) 762672

Cambridge Healthcare Supplies Ltd
Francis House
112 Hills Rd
Cambridge CB2 1PH
Telephone: (01202) 734100
Facsimile: (01202) 735100

Cambridge Laboratories
Richmond House
Old Brewery Court
Sandyford Road
Newcastle upon Tyne NE2 1XG
Telephone: (0191) 261 5950
Facsimile: (0191) 222 1006

Castlemead Healthcare Limited
20 Clanwilliam Terrace
Dublin 2
Ireland
Telephone: (278) 0755
Facsimile: (278) 0763

Centeon Ltd
Centeon House
Market Place
Haywards Heath
West Sussex RH16 1DB
Telephone: (01444) 447400
Facsimile: (01444) 447401

Cephalon UK Limited
11/13 Frederick Sanger Road
Surrey Research Park
Guildford GU2 5YD
Telephone: (01483) 453360
Facsimile: (01483) 453324

Chauvin Pharmaceuticals Ltd
Ashton Road
Harold Hill
Romford
Essex RM3 8SL
Telephone: 01708 383838
Facsimile: 01708 371316

Chugai Pharma UK Limited
Mulliner House
Flanders Road
Turnham Green
London W4 1NN
Telephone: (0181) 987 5600
Facsimile: (0181) 987 5660

CIBA Laboratories
See **Novartis Pharmaceuticals UK Ltd**

CIBA Vision Ophthalmics
Flanders Road
Hedge End
Southampton SO30 2LG
Telephone: (01489) 775534
Facsimile: (01489) 798074

Cortecs Healthcare Limited
Abbey Road
Wrexham Industrial Estate
Wrexham LL13 9PW
Telephone: (01244) 288888
Facsimile: (01244) 280299

Technical Department
Cox Pharmaceuticals
A. H. Cox & Co Limited
Whiddon Valley
Barnstaple
North Devon EX32 8NS

Telephone:
Medical information (including 24-hour emergency service) (01271) 311257
All other enquiries (01271) 311200

Facsimile: (01271) 346106

Medical Information
CP Pharmaceuticals Ltd
Ash Road North
Wrexham LL13 9UF

Telephone: (01978) 661261
Direct Line (08.30–16.30 hours): (01978) 666172

Facsimile: (01978) 660130

DBL (David Bull Laboratories)
See **Faulding Pharmaceuticals**

Medical Information
Dermal Laboratories Ltd
Tatmore Place
Gosmore
Hitchin
Hertfordshire SG4 7QR

Telephone:
Hitchin (01462) 458866
Emergency Medical Information
Telephone: Dr M. Whitefield
0181-455 4998

Facsimile: (01462) 420565

DermaPharm Limited
The Old Coach House
34 Elm Road
Chessington
Surrey KT9 1AW

Telephone: (0181) 9742266

Facsimile: (0181) 9742005

E. C. DeWitt & Company Ltd
Tudor Road
Manor Park
Runcorn
Cheshire WA7 1SZ

Telephone: (01928) 579029

Facsimile: (01928) 579712

Medical Information and Drug Surveillance Department
Dista Products Ltd
(a subsidiary of Eli Lilly and Company Limited)
Kingsclere Road
Basingstoke
Hampshire RG21 6XA

Telephone:
Direct Lines (08.30–17.30 hours) for medical information on:
- Antimicrobial and Oncology: (01256) 315246
- Cardiology: (01256) 315244
- Endocrine & Gastroenterology: (01256) 315245
- Neurology: (01256) 315264
- Psychiatric: (01256) 315264, (01256) 315907 or (01256) 315249
- Other products (including 24 hour Emergency Service): Basingstoke (01256) 315000 or Basingstoke (01256) 52011

Facsimile: (01256) 315858

Dominion Pharma Ltd
Dominion House
Lion Lane
Haslemere
Surrey GU27 1JL

Telephone: (01428) 661078

Facsimile: (01428) 661075

Dumex Ltd
at Cox Pharmaceuticals
Whiddon Valley
Barnstaple
North Devon EX32 8NS

Telephone: (01271) 311200

Facsimile: (01271) 346106

Medical Information Department
Du Pont Pharmaceuticals Ltd
Wedgwood Way
Stevenage
Hertfordshire SG1 4QN

Telephone: (01438) 842530

Facsimile: (01438) 842533

Eisai Ltd
3 Shortlands
Hammersmith
London W6 8EE

Telephone: (0181) 600 1400

Facsimile: (0181) 600 1401

Medical Information Department
Elan Pharma
1 Meadway Court
Rutherford Close
Stevenage
Herts SG1 2EF

Telephone: (01438) 730200

Facsimile: (01438) 741452

Ethical Generics Ltd
West Point
46–48 West Street
Newbury
Berkshire RG14 1BD

Telephone: (01635) 568400

Facsimile: (01635) 568401

Evans Medical Ltd
See **Medeva Pharma Ltd**

Exelgyn Laboratoires
6 Rue Christophe Colomb
75008 Paris
France

Telephone: (0800) 7316120

Facsimile: (0800) 7316120

Medical Information
Faulding Pharmaceuticals Plc
Queensway
Royal Leamington Spa
Warwickshire CV31 3RW

Telephone: (01926) 820820

Facsimile: (01926) 821041

Ferring Pharmaceuticals Ltd
The Courtyard
Waterside Drive
Langley
Berkshire SL3 6EZ

Telephone: (01753) 214800

Facsimile: (01753) 214801

Florizel Ltd
15 Kritis Street
10451 Athens
Greece

Forley Ltd
4 Priory Hall
Stillorgan Road
Stillorgan
Co Dublin
Eire

Telephone: (00353) 1 2836665

Facsimile: (00353) 1 2836603

Fournier Pharmaceuticals Ltd
22–23 Progress Business Centre
Whittle Parkway
Slough SL1 6DG

Telephone: (01753) 740400

Facsimile: (01753) 740444

Fujisawa Ltd
8th Floor, CP House
97–107 Uxbridge Road
London W5 5TL

Telephone: (0181) 840 9520 (including 24-hour emergency service)

Facsimile: (0181) 840 9521

Futuna Limited
57 Masonfield
Bamber Bridge
Preston PR5 8HP

Telephone: (0870) 6012037

Facsimile: (0870) 6012036

Galderma (UK) Ltd
Leywood House
Woodside Road
Amersham
Bucks HP6 6AA

Telephone:
(01494) 432606

Facsimile: (01494) 432607

Geigy Pharmaceuticals
See **Novartis Pharmaceuticals UK Ltd**

Glaxo Laboratories
See **Glaxo Wellcome**

Medical Information
Glaxo Wellcome
Stockley Park West
Uxbridge
Middlesex UB11 1BT

Telephone enquiries (including 24-hour emergency service):
Asthma, Allergy and Migraine Products (0181) 990 3001 or FREEPHONE 0800 371891
HIV, Epilepsy, Diabetes and Hospital Products (0181) 990 4877 or FREEPHONE 0800 413524
Other Products (0181) 990 4876 or 4951 or FREEPHONE 0800 413828 or 0800 783 4886

Facsimile: (0181) 990 4372

Customer Services
FREEPHONE 0800 221441

Facsimile: (0181) 990 4328

Telephone: (0181) 990 9000

Facsimile: (0181) 990 4321

Glenwood Laboratories Ltd
Unit D
Jenkins Dale
Chatham
Kent ME4 5RD

Telephone: (01634) 830535

Facsimile: (01634) 831345

Goldshield Healthcare
NLA Tower
12–16 Addiscombe Road
Croydon CR9 6BP

Telephone: (0181) 649 8500

Facsimile: (0181) 686 0807

Grifols UK Ltd
Howlett Way
Thetford
Norfolk
IP24 1HZ

Telephone: (01842) 761942/764260

Facsimile: (01842) 766661

Hawgreen Ltd
4 Priory Hall
Stillorgan Road
Stillorgan
C. Dublin

Telephone: (353) 1 283 6602

Facsimile: (353) 1 283 6658

Helios Healthcare Ltd
11A Ferraidy Street
Peyki
Attikis
Greece

Telephone: (301) 524 6955

Facsimile: (301) 524 5249

HK Pharma Limited
PO Box 105
Hitchin
Herts SG5 2GG

Telephone: (07071) 880292

Facsimile: (07070) 604101

Medical Information Department
Hoechst Marion Roussel Ltd
Broadwater Park
Denham
Uxbridge
Middlesex UB9 5HP

Telephone: (01895) 834343 or FREEFONE 0800 282833
24-hour emergency service (01895) 837586

Facsimile: (01895) 834479

Hyland Immuno
Baxter Healthcare Ltd
Wallingford Road
Compton
nr Newbury
Berkshire
RG20 7QW

Telephone: (01635) 206265

Facsimile: (01635) 206126

ICN Pharmaceuticals Ltd
1 Elmwood
Chineham Business Park
Crockford Lane
Basingstoke
Hampshire RG24 8WG

Telephone: (01256) 707744

Facsimile: (01256) 707334

International Medication Systems (UK) Ltd
Medeva House
Regent Park
Kingston Road
Leatherhead
Surrey KT22 7PQ

Telephone: (01372) 364000

Facsimile: (01372) 364190

Ipsen Ltd
1 Bath Road
Maidenhead
Berkshire SL6 4UH

Telephone: (01628) 771447

Facsimile: (01628) 770199

The Medical Information Department
Janssen-Cilag Ltd
Saunderton
High Wycombe
Buckinghamshire HP14 4HJ

Telephone: (01494) 567567
FREEFONE 0800 7318450 (including 24-hour emergency service)

Facsimile: (01494) 567445

JHC Healthcare Ltd
5 Lower Merrion Street
Dublin 2
Eire

Telephone: 00 3531 283 66 46

Facsimile: 00 3531 283 66 46

Medical Information Department
Knoll Ltd
9 Castle Quay
Castle Boulevard
Nottingham NG7 1FW
Telephone: (0115) 912 5000
Facsimile: (0115) 912 5069

Kyowa Hakko UK Ltd
258 Bath Road
Slough
Berkshire SL1 4DX
Telephone: (01753) 566020
Facsimile: (01753) 566030

Medical Department
Laboratories for Applied Biology Ltd
91 Amhurst Park
London N16 5DR
Telephone: (0181) 800 2252
Facsimile: (0181) 809 6884

Lagap Pharmaceuticals Ltd
Woolmer Way
Bordon
Hampshire GU35 9QE
Telephone:
Bordon (01420) 478301
Facsimile: (01420) 474427

Lederle Laboratories
See **Wyeth Laboratories**

Medical Department
Leo Laboratories Ltd
Longwick Road
Princes Risborough
Buckinghamshire HP27 9RR
Telephone:
Princes Risborough (01844) 347333
Facsimile: (01844) 342278

Medical Information and Drug Surveillance Department
Eli Lilly and Company Limited
Kingsclere Road
Basingstoke
Hampshire RG21 6XA
Telephone:
Direct Lines (08.30–17.30 hours) for medical information on:
- Antimicrobial and Oncology: (01256) 315246
- Cardiology: (01256) 315244
- Endocrinology and Gastroenterology: (01256) 315245
- Neurology: (01256) 315264
- Psychiatric: (01256) 315264, (01256) 315907 or (01256) 315249
- Other products (including 24 hour Emergency Service): Basingstoke (01256) 315000 or Basingstoke (01256) 52011

Facsimile: (01256) 315858

Link Pharmaceuticals Ltd
7/8 Sterling Buildings
Carfax
Horsham
West Sussex RH12 1DR
Telephone: (01403) 272451
Facsimile: (01403) 272455

Lipha Pharmaceuticals Ltd
Harrier House
High Street
West Drayton
Middlesex UB7 7QG
Telephone:
Medical Information Department (09.00 to 17.00 hours): (01895) 452258
24-hour Emergency Service: (01895) 452200
Facsimile: (01895) 420605

The Liposome Company Ltd
3 Shortlands
Hammersmith International Centre
London W6 8EH
Telephone: (0181) 324 0058
Facsimile: (0181) 563 1653

Lorex Synthelabo UK & Ireland Ltd
Foundation Park
Roxborough Way
Maidenhead
Berkshire SL6 3UD
Telephone: (01628) 501200
Facsimile: (01628) 501234

LRC Products Ltd
London International House
Turnford Place
Broxbourne
Hertfordshire EN10 6LN
Telephone: (01992) 451111
Facsimile: (01992) 470133

Medical Department
Lundbeck Ltd
Sunningdale House
Caldecotte Lake Business Park
Caldecotte
Milton Keynes MK7 8LF
Telephone: (01908) 649966
Facsimile: (01908) 647688

Regulatory and Professional Services Department
3M Health Care Limited
3M House
Morley Street
Loughborough
Leicestershire LE11 1EP
Telephone:
Loughborough (01509) 611611 (including 24-hour emergency service)
Facsimile: (01509) 237288

Manx Pharma
Manx House
Spectrum Business Estate
Bircholt Road
Maidstone
Kent ME15 9YP
Telephone: (01622) 766389
Facsimile: (01622) 761435

Marion Merrell Ltd
See **Hoechst Marion Roussel Ltd**

Medical Information Department
Martindale Pharmaceuticals
Bampton Road
Harold Hill
Romford
Essex RM3 8UG
Telephone: (01708) 386660
Facsimile: (01708) 384032

medac Gesellschaft für klinische Spezialpräparate mbH
Fehlandtstrasse 3
20354 Hamburg
Germany
Telephone: +49(0)40 350 91-0
Facsimile: +49(0)40 350 91-300

Medeva Pharma Limited
(formerly Evans Medical Ltd)
Medeva House
Regent Park
Kingston Road
Leatherhead
Surrey KT22 7PQ
Telephone: (01372) 364000
Facsimile: (01372) 364018

Medical Department
E. Merck Pharmaceuticals
(A Division of Merck Ltd)
Harrier House
West Drayton
Middlesex UB7 7QG
Telephone: Medical Information Department (0900 to 1700 hours): (01895) 452258
24-hour Emergency Service: (01895) 452200
Facsimile: (01895) 452296

Medical Department
Merck Sharp & Dohme Ltd
Hertford Road
Hoddesdon
Hertfordshire EN11 9BU
Telephone:
Hoddesdon (01992) 467272 (including 24-hour emergency service)
Facsimile: (01992) 451066

Monmouth Pharmaceuticals Ltd
3 & 4 Huxley Road
Surrey Research Park
Guildford
Surrey GU2 5RE
Telephone: (01483) 565299
Facsimile: (01483) 563658

Medical Information Department
Napp Pharmaceuticals Ltd
(A member of Napp Pharmaceutical Group)
Cambridge Science Park
Milton Road
Cambridge CB4 4GW
Telephone:
Cambridge (01223) 424444 (including 24-hour emergency service)
Telex: 817805
Facsimile: (01223) 424441

Newport Pharmaceuticals Limited
Frans Maas House
Swords Business Park
Swords
Co. Dublin
Ireland
Telephone: 00353 1 890 3011
Facsimile: 00353 1 890 3016

Nexstar Pharmaceuticals Ltd
The Quorum
Barnwell Road
Cambridge CB5 8RE
Telephone: (01223) 571400
Facsimile: (01223) 507047

The Medical Department
Norgine Ltd
Chaplin House
Widewater Place
Moorhall Road
Harefield
Middlesex UB9 6NS
Telephone: (01895) 826600
Facsimile: (01895) 825865

Novartis Consumer Health
Wimblehurst Road
Horsham
West Sussex RH12 5AB
Telephone: (01403) 210211
Facsimile: (01403) 323939

Novartis Pharmaceuticals UK Ltd
Frimley Business Park
Frimley
Camberley
Surrey GU16 5SG
Telephone: (01276) 698370
Facsimile: (01276) 698449

Novex Pharma Ltd
Innovex House
Marlow Park
Marlow
Bucks SL7 1TB
Telephone: (01628) 491500
Facsimile: (01628) 487799

Medical Information
Novo Nordisk Pharmaceuticals Ltd
Novo Nordisk House
Broadfield Park
Brighton Road
Pease Pottage
Crawley
West Sussex RH11 9RT
Telephone: (01293) 613555
Facsimile: (01293) 613535

Medical Department
Nycomed Amersham Plc
Amersham Place
Little Chalfont
Buckinghamshire HP7 9NA
Telephone: (01494) 544000
Facsimile: (01494) 543588

The Medical Information Officer
Organon Laboratories Limited
Cambridge Science Park
Milton Road
Cambridge CB4 0FL
Telephone: Daytime and Emergency Cambridge (01223) 423445
Facsimile: (01223) 424368

Mr C. Ponty
Business Manager
Organon Teknika Ltd
Science Park
Milton Road
Cambridge CB4 0FL
Telephone: Daytime and Emergency Cambridge (01223) 423650
Facsimile: (01223) 420264

Orion Pharma (UK) Ltd
1st Floor, Leat House
Overbridge Square
Hambridge Lane
Newbury
Berkshire RG14 5UX
Telephone: (01635) 520300
Facsimile: (01635) 520319

The Information Department
Paines & Byrne Ltd
Yamanouchi House
Pyrford Road
West Byfleet
Surrey KT14 6RA
Telephone: (01932) 355405
Facsimile: (01932) 353458

Medical Information Department
Parke-Davis
Lambert Court
Chestnut Avenue
Eastleigh
Hampshire SO53 3ZQ
Telephone:
Eastleigh (01703) 620500
Facsimile: (01703) 629819

Pasteur Mérieux MSD Ltd
Mallards Reach
Bridge Avenue
Maidenhead
Berkshire SL6 1QP

Telephone:
Maidenhead (01628) 785291

Facsimile: (01628) 671722

Penn Pharmaceuticals Ltd
Tafarnaubach Industrial Estate
Tredegar
Gwent NP2 3AA

Telephone: (01495) 711222

Facsimile: (01495) 711225/718285

Medical Information
Pfizer Ltd
Ramsgate Road
Sandwich
Kent CT13 9NJ

Telephone:
Sandwich (01304) 616161
(including 24-hour emergency service)
Sandwich (01304) 645210
(medical information only)

Facsimile: (01304) 656221

Pfizer Consumer Healthcare
Wilsom Road
Alton
Hampshire GU34 2TJ

Telephone: (01420) 84801

Facsimile: (01420) 89376

Medical Information Department
Pharmacia & Upjohn
Davy Avenue
Knowlhill
Milton Keynes MK5 8PH

Telephone: (01908) 661101

Facsimile: (01908) 690091

Medical Department
Pharmax Limited
A Division of Forest Laboratories Europe
Bourne Road
Bexley
Kent DA5 1NX

Telephone: (01322) 550550

Facsimile: (01322) 558776

Pierre Fabre Limited
Hyde Abbey House
23 Hyde Street
Winchester
Hampshire SO23 7DR

Telephone: (01962) 856956

Facsimile: (01962) 844014

Procter & Gamble Pharmaceuticals UK Ltd
Lovett House
Lovett Road
Staines
Middlesex TW18 3AZ

Telephone: (01784) 495000

Facsimile: (01784) 495297

Medical Information Department
Quinoderm Ltd
Manchester Road
Oldham
Lancashire OL8 4PB

Telephone: (0161) 624 9307

Facsimile: (0161) 627 0928

Medical Information Unit
Reckitt & Colman Products Ltd
Dansom Lane
Hull HU8 7DS

Telephone: (01482) 326151
(including 24-hour emergency service)

Facsimile: (01482) 582532

Rhône-Poulenc Rorer Ltd
RPR House
50 Kings Hill Avenue
West Malling
Kent ME19 4AH

Telephone: (01732) 584000
(0990) 239604

Facsimile: (01732) 584080

Drug Information
Roche Products Ltd
including Boehringer Mannheim UK Limited
40 Broadwater Road
Welwyn Garden City
Hertfordshire AL7 3AY

Telephone:
Welwyn Garden (01707) 366000
(0800) 3281629

Facsimile: (01707) 390378

Roussel Laboratories Ltd
See **Hoechst Marion Roussel Ltd**

Rybar Laboratories Ltd
East Anton
Andover
Hants SP10 5RG

Telephone: (01264) 333455

Facsimile: (01264) 333460

Sandoz Pharmaceuticals (UK) Ltd
See **Novartis Pharmaceuticals UK Ltd**

Medical Affairs Department
Sankyo Pharma UK Limited
Sankyo House
Repton Place
White Lion Road
Amersham
Buckinghamshire HP7 9LP

Telephone: (01494) 766866

Facsimile: (01494) 766557

Medical Information Services
Sanofi Winthrop Ltd
One Onslow Street
Guildford
Surrey GU1 4YS

Telephone: (01483) 505515
(including 24-hour emergency service)

Facsimile: (01483) 535432

Medical Information Department
Schering Health Care Limited
The Brow
Burgess Hill
West Sussex RH15 9NE

Telephone:
Burgess Hill (01444) 232323

Facsimile: (01444) 246613

Medical Information
Schering-Plough Ltd
Schering-Plough House
Shire Park
Welwyn Garden City
Herts AL7 1TW

Telephone: (01707) 363636

Facsimile: (01707) 363690

Medical Information Department
Schwarz Pharma Limited
Schwarz House
East Street
Chesham
Buckinghamshire HP5 1DG

Telephone:
Chesham (01494) 797500

Facsimile: (01494) 773934

Searle
PO Box 53
Lane End Road
High Wycombe
Buckinghamshire HP12 4HL

Telephone:
High Wycombe (01494) 521124
(including 24-hour emergency service)

Facsimile: (01494) 447872

Serono Laboratories (U.K.) Ltd
99 Bridge Road East
Welwyn Garden City
Hertfordshire AL7 1BG

Telephone:
Welwyn Garden (01707) 331972

Facsimile: (01707) 371873

Medical Department
Servier Laboratories Ltd
Fulmer Hall
Windmill Road
Fulmer
Slough
Buckinghamshire SL3 6HH

Telephone:
Slough (01753) 662744

Facsimile: (01753) 663456

Seton Scholl Healthcare plc
Tubiton House
Medlock Street
Oldham OL1 3HS

Telephone:
Medical information
(9.00–17.00) +24-hour emergency service: (0161) 652 2222
Customer care (sales enquiries): (0161) 654 3000

Facsimile: (0161) 626 9090

Shire Pharmaceuticals Ltd
East Anton
Andover
Hants SP10 5RG

Telephone: (01264) 333455

Facsimile: (01264) 333460

Technical Services Department
Smith & Nephew Healthcare Ltd
Healthcare House
Goulton Street
Hull HU3 4DJ

Telephone: (01482) 222200

Facsimile: (01482) 222211

Medical Information Department
SmithKline Beecham Pharmaceuticals
Welwyn Garden City
Hertfordshire AL7 1EY

Telephone:
Welwyn Garden (01707) 325111
or FREEFONE (0800) 616482
(including 24-hour emergency service)

Facsimile: (01707) 325600

Solvay Healthcare Ltd
Hamilton House
Gaters Hill
West End
Southampton
Hampshire SO18 3JD

Telephone: (01703) 472281

Facsimile: (01703) 465350

E. R. Squibb & Sons Ltd
Bristol-Myers Squibb House
141–149 Staines Road
Hounslow
Middlesex TW3 3JA

Telephone:
Medical Information Only:
(0181) 754 3740 and FREEFONE 0800 7311736
BMS House and emergencies
(0181) 572 7422

Facsimile: (0181) 754 3789

Medical Information
Stafford-Miller Ltd
45 Broadwater Road
Welwyn Garden City
Hertfordshire AL7 3SP

Telephone: (01707) 331001

Facsimile: (01707) 373370

STD Pharmaceutical Products Ltd
Fields Yard
Plough Lane
Hereford HR4 0EL

Telephone:
Hereford (01432) 353684

Facsimile: (01432) 342383

Stiefel Laboratories (UK) Ltd
Holtspur Lane
Wooburn Green
High Wycombe
Buckinghamshire HP10 0AU

Telephone:
Bourne End (01628) 524966

Facsimile: (01628) 810021

Takeda UK Ltd
3 The Courtyard
Meadowbank
Furlong Road
Bourne End
Bucks SL8 5AJ

Telephone: (01628) 537900/526614

Facsimile: (01628) 526615

Medical Information
Trinity Pharmaceuticals Ltd
Tuition House
27/37 St George's Road
London SW19 4EU

Telephone: (0181) 944 9443

Facsimile: (0181) 947 9325

Typharm Ltd
Unit 26
Newtown Business Park
Albion Close
Poole
Dorset BH12 3LL

Telephone:
Poole (01202) 666626

Facsimile: (01202) 666309

UCB Pharma Ltd
Star House
69 Clarendon Road
Watford
Hertfordshire WD1 1DJ

Telephone: (01923) 211811

Facsimile: (01923) 229002

Warner-Lambert Consumer Healthcare
Lambert Court
Chestnut Avenue
Eastleigh
Hampshire SO53 3ZQ

Telephone: (01703) 641400

Facsimile: (01703) 629726

Wellcome UK
The Wellcome Foundation Limited
Stockley Park
Middlesex UB11 1BT

Telephone: (0181) 990 9000

Facsimile: (0181) 990 4321

Medical Information Department
Wyeth Laboratories
incorporating A. H. Robins and Lederle Laboratories
Huntercombe Lane South
Taplow
Maidenhead
Berkshire SL6 0PH

Telephone:
Burnham (Bucks) (01628) 604377 (including 24-hour emergency service)

Facsimile: (01628) 666368

Medical Information Officer
Yamanouchi Pharma Limited
Yamanouchi House
Pyrford Road
West Byfleet
Surrey KT14 6RA

Telephone: (01932) 345535/342291

Facsimile: (01932) 353458

Medical Information
Zeneca Pharma
King's Court
Water Lane
Wilmslow
Cheshire SK9 5AZ

Telephone: (01625) 712712 or FREEFONE 0800 200123 (both include 24-hour emergency service)

Facsimile: (01625) 712581

Index of Products

*Brand names are in ordinary type, generic names in italics. *Under the generic entry, products with an asterisk contain a number of active ingredients and may be available in more than one formulation; products without an asterisk contain a single active ingredient. In certain instances such products may also be available with added constituents and these formulations are often designated by the principal brand name with the addition of a suffix or other mark of distinction. Where several presentations of a product bear the same proprietary name, the page number given below is that of the first of the respective entries. It should be noted that although different products may contain the same active ingredient this does not imply that they are equivalent in regard to bio-availability or therapeutic activity.*

IN CONFIDENCE

COMMITTEE ON SAFETY OF MEDICINES **MEDICINES CONTROL AGENCY**

REPORT ON SUSPECTED ADVERSE DRUG REACTION

(For advice on reporting reactions see The Reporting of Adverse Reactions section in this book)

Do not be put off reporting because some details are not known

NAME OF PATIENT (To allow for linkage with other reports for same patient. Please give record number for hospital patients)	Family name Forename	Sex	AGE or DATE OF BIRTH	WEIGHT (Kg.)

SUSPECT DRUG (Please give brand name and batch number if known)	ROUTE	DAILY DOSE	DATE STARTED	DATE STOPPED	INDICATION

SUSPECTED REACTION

DATE OF ONSET ________ DATE STOPPED ________

OUTCOME (eg fatal, recovered) ________

Was the patient hospitalised because of the reaction ☐ Yes ☐ No

REPORTING DOCTOR (BLOCK LETTERS)

Name: ________

Address: ________

Tel. No. ________ Specialty ________

Signature: Date:

If you would like information about other reports associated with the suspected drug, please tick box ☐

SEND TO CSM, FREEPOST, London SW8 5BR
OR if you are in one of the following NHS regions:
TO CSM West Midlands, FREEPOST, Birmingham B18 7BR
OR CSM Northern, FREEPOST, Newcastle upon Tyne NE1 1BR
OR CSM Wales, FREEPOST, Cardiff CF4 1ZZ
OR CSM Mersey, FREEPOST, Liverpool L3 3AB

IN CONFIDENCE

COMMITTEE ON SAFETY OF MEDICINES **MEDICINES CONTROL AGENCY**

REPORT ON SUSPECTED ADVERSE DRUG REACTION

(For advice on reporting reactions see The Reporting of Adverse Reactions section in this book)

Do not be put off reporting because some details are not known

NAME OF PATIENT (To allow for linkage with other reports for same patient. Please give record number for hospital patients)	Family name Forename	Sex	AGE or DATE OF BIRTH	WEIGHT (Kg.)

SUSPECT DRUG (Please give brand name and batch number if known)	ROUTE	DAILY DOSE	DATE STARTED	DATE STOPPED	INDICATION

SUSPECTED REACTION

DATE OF ONSET ________ DATE STOPPED ________

OUTCOME (eg fatal, recovered) ________

Was the patient hospitalised because of the reaction ☐ Yes ☐ No

REPORTING DOCTOR (BLOCK LETTERS)

Name: ________

Address: ________

Tel. No. ________ Specialty ________

Signature: Date:

If you would like information about other reports associated with the suspected drug, please tick box ☐

SEND TO CSM, FREEPOST, London SW8 5BR
OR if you are in one of the following NHS regions:
TO CSM West Midlands, FREEPOST, Birmingham B18 7BR
OR CSM Northern, FREEPOST, Newcastle upon Tyne NE1 1BR
OR CSM Wales, FREEPOST, Cardiff CF4 1ZZ
OR CSM Mersey, FREEPOST, Liverpool L3 3AB

OTHER DRUGS
(Please record all other drugs, including self-medication, taken during the last 3 months, and give brand name if known)

DRUG	ROUTE	DAILY DOSE	DATE STARTED	DATE STOPPED	INDICATION

ADDITIONAL NOTES (Include relevant medical history, investigations, known allergies, suspected drug interactions. For congenital abnormalities state all other drugs taken during pregnancy and the LMP. Please attach additional pages if necessary.)

OTHER DRUGS
(Please record all other drugs, including self-medication, taken during the last 3 months, and give brand name if known)

DRUG	ROUTE	DAILY DOSE	DATE STARTED	DATE STOPPED	INDICATION

ADDITIONAL NOTES (Include relevant medical history, investigations, known allergies, suspected drug interactions. For congenital abnormalities state all other drugs taken during pregnancy and the LMP. Please attach additional pages if necessary.)

IN CONFIDENCE

COMMITTEE ON SAFETY OF MEDICINES **MEDICINES CONTROL AGENCY**

REPORT ON SUSPECTED ADVERSE DRUG REACTION

(For advice on reporting reactions see The Reporting of Adverse Reactions section in this book)

Do not be put off reporting because some details are not known

NAME OF PATIENT (To allow for linkage with other reports for same patient. Please give record number for hospital patients)	Family name Forename	Sex	AGE or DATE OF BIRTH	WEIGHT (Kg.)

SUSPECT DRUG (Please give brand name and batch number if known)	ROUTE	DAILY DOSE	DATE STARTED	DATE STOPPED	INDICATION

SUSPECTED REACTION

DATE OF ONSET ______ DATE STOPPED ______

OUTCOME (eg fatal, recovered) ______

Was the patient hospitalised because of the reaction ☐ Yes ☐ No

REPORTING DOCTOR (BLOCK LETTERS)

Name: ______

Address: ______

Tel. No. ______ Specialty ______

Signature: Date:

If you would like information about other reports associated with the suspected drug, please tick box ☐

SEND TO CSM, FREEPOST, London SW8 5BR
OR if you are in one of the following NHS regions:
TO CSM West Midlands, FREEPOST, Birmingham B18 7BR
OR CSM Northern, FREEPOST, Newcastle upon Tyne NE1 1BR
OR CSM Wales, FREEPOST, Cardiff CF4 1ZZ
OR CSM Mersey, FREEPOST, Liverpool L3 3AB

IN CONFIDENCE

COMMITTEE ON SAFETY OF MEDICINES **MEDICINES CONTROL AGENCY**

REPORT ON SUSPECTED ADVERSE DRUG REACTION

(For advice on reporting reactions see The Reporting of Adverse Reactions section in this book)

Do not be put off reporting because some details are not known

NAME OF PATIENT (To allow for linkage with other reports for same patient. Please give record number for hospital patients)	Family name Forename	Sex	AGE or DATE OF BIRTH	WEIGHT (Kg.)

SUSPECT DRUG (Please give brand name and batch number if known)	ROUTE	DAILY DOSE	DATE STARTED	DATE STOPPED	INDICATION

SUSPECTED REACTION

DATE OF ONSET ______ DATE STOPPED ______

OUTCOME (eg fatal, recovered) ______

Was the patient hospitalised because of the reaction ☐ Yes ☐ No

REPORTING DOCTOR (BLOCK LETTERS)

Name: ______

Address: ______

Tel. No. ______ Specialty ______

Signature: Date:

If you would like information about other reports associated with the suspected drug, please tick box ☐

SEND TO CSM, FREEPOST, London SW8 5BR
OR if you are in one of the following NHS regions:
TO CSM West Midlands, FREEPOST, Birmingham B18 7BR
OR CSM Northern, FREEPOST, Newcastle upon Tyne NE1 1BR
OR CSM Wales, FREEPOST, Cardiff CF4 1ZZ
OR CSM Mersey, FREEPOST, Liverpool L3 3AB

OTHER DRUGS
(Please record all other drugs, including self-medication, taken during the last 3 months, and give brand name if known)

DRUG	ROUTE	DAILY DOSE	DATE STARTED	DATE STOPPED	INDICATION

ADDITIONAL NOTES (Include relevant medical history, investigations, known allergies, suspected drug interactions. For congenital abnormalities state all other drugs taken during pregnancy and the LMP. Please attach additional pages if necessary.)

OTHER DRUGS
(Please record all other drugs, including self-medication, taken during the last 3 months, and give brand name if known)

DRUG	ROUTE	DAILY DOSE	DATE STARTED	DATE STOPPED	INDICATION

ADDITIONAL NOTES (Include relevant medical history, investigations, known allergies, suspected drug interactions. For congenital abnormalities state all other drugs taken during pregnancy and the LMP. Please attach additional pages if necessary.)

IN CONFIDENCE

COMMITTEE ON SAFETY OF MEDICINES **MEDICINES CONTROL AGENCY**

REPORT ON SUSPECTED ADVERSE DRUG REACTION

(For advice on reporting reactions see The Reporting of Adverse Reactions section in this book)

Do not be put off reporting because some details are not known

NAME OF PATIENT (To allow for linkage with other reports for same patient. Please give record number for hospital patients)	Family name Forename	Sex	AGE or DATE OF BIRTH	WEIGHT (Kg.)

SUSPECT DRUG (Please give brand name and batch number if known)	ROUTE	DAILY DOSE	DATE STARTED	DATE STOPPED	INDICATION

SUSPECTED REACTION

DATE OF ONSET DATE STOPPED

OUTCOME (eg fatal, recovered)

Was the patient hospitalised because of the reaction ☐ Yes ☐ No

REPORTING DOCTOR (BLOCK LETTERS)

Name:

Address:

Tel. No. Specialty

Signature: Date:

If you would like information about other reports associated with the suspected drug, please tick box

SEND TO CSM, FREEPOST, London SW8 5BR
OR if you are in one of the following NHS regions:
TO CSM West Midlands, FREEPOST, Birmingham B18 7BR
OR CSM Northern, FREEPOST, Newcastle upon Tyne NE1 1BR
OR CSM Wales, FREEPOST, Cardiff CF4 1ZZ
OR CSM Mersey, FREEPOST, Liverpool L3 3AB

IN CONFIDENCE

COMMITTEE ON SAFETY OF MEDICINES **MEDICINES CONTROL AGENCY**

REPORT ON SUSPECTED ADVERSE DRUG REACTION

(For advice on reporting reactions see The Reporting of Adverse Reactions section in this book)

Do not be put off reporting because some details are not known

NAME OF PATIENT (To allow for linkage with other reports for same patient. Please give record number for hospital patients)	Family name Forename	Sex	AGE or DATE OF BIRTH	WEIGHT (Kg.)

SUSPECT DRUG (Please give brand name and batch number if known)	ROUTE	DAILY DOSE	DATE STARTED	DATE STOPPED	INDICATION

SUSPECTED REACTION

DATE OF ONSET DATE STOPPED

OUTCOME (eg fatal, recovered)

Was the patient hospitalised because of the reaction ☐ Yes ☐ No

REPORTING DOCTOR (BLOCK LETTERS)

Name:

Address:

Tel. No. Specialty

Signature: Date:

If you would like information about other reports associated with the suspected drug, please tick box

SEND TO CSM, FREEPOST, London SW8 5BR
OR if you are in one of the following NHS regions:
TO CSM West Midlands, FREEPOST, Birmingham B18 7BR
OR CSM Northern, FREEPOST, Newcastle upon Tyne NE1 1BR
OR CSM Wales, FREEPOST, Cardiff CF4 1ZZ
OR CSM Mersey, FREEPOST, Liverpool L3 3AB

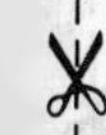

OTHER DRUGS
(Please record all other drugs, including self-medication, taken during the last 3 months, and give brand name if known)

DRUG	ROUTE	DAILY DOSE	DATE STARTED	DATE STOPPED	INDICATION

ADDITIONAL NOTES (Include relevant medical history, investigations, known allergies, suspected drug interactions. For congenital abnormalities state all other drugs taken during pregnancy and the LMP. Please attach additional pages if necessary.)

OTHER DRUGS
(Please record all other drugs, including self-medication, taken during the last 3 months, and give brand name if known)

DRUG	ROUTE	DAILY DOSE	DATE STARTED	DATE STOPPED	INDICATION

ADDITIONAL NOTES (Include relevant medical history, investigations, known allergies, suspected drug interactions. For congenital abnormalities state all other drugs taken during pregnancy and the LMP. Please attach additional pages if necessary.)

IN CONFIDENCE

COMMITTEE ON SAFETY OF MEDICINES **MEDICINES CONTROL AGENCY**

REPORT ON SUSPECTED ADVERSE DRUG REACTION

(For advice on reporting reactions see The Reporting of Adverse Reactions section in this book)

Do not be put off reporting because some details are not known

NAME OF PATIENT (To allow for linkage with other reports for same patient. Please give record number for hospital patients)	Family name Forename	Sex	AGE or DATE OF BIRTH	WEIGHT (Kg.)

SUSPECT DRUG (Please give brand name and batch number if known)	ROUTE	DAILY DOSE	DATE		INDICATION
			STARTED	STOPPED	

SUSPECTED REACTION

DATE OF ONSET ______ DATE STOPPED ______

OUTCOME (eg fatal, recovered) ______

Was the patient hospitalised because of the reaction ☐ Yes ☐ No

REPORTING DOCTOR (BLOCK LETTERS)

Name: ______

Address: ______

Tel. No. ______ Specialty ______

Signature: Date:

If you would like information about other reports associated with the suspected drug, please tick box ☐

SEND TO CSM, FREEPOST, London SW8 5BR
OR if you are in one of the following NHS regions:
TO CSM West Midlands, FREEPOST, Birmingham B18 7BR
OR CSM Northern, FREEPOST, Newcastle upon Tyne NE1 1BR
OR CSM Wales, FREEPOST, Cardiff CF4 1ZZ
OR CSM Mersey, FREEPOST, Liverpool L3 3AB

IN CONFIDENCE

COMMITTEE ON SAFETY OF MEDICINES **MEDICINES CONTROL AGENCY**

REPORT ON SUSPECTED ADVERSE DRUG REACTION

(For advice on reporting reactions see The Reporting of Adverse Reactions section in this book)

Do not be put off reporting because some details are not known

NAME OF PATIENT (To allow for linkage with other reports for same patient. Please give record number for hospital patients)	Family name Forename	Sex	AGE or DATE OF BIRTH	WEIGHT (Kg.)

SUSPECT DRUG (Please give brand name and batch number if known)	ROUTE	DAILY DOSE	DATE		INDICATION
			STARTED	STOPPED	

SUSPECTED REACTION

DATE OF ONSET ______ DATE STOPPED ______

OUTCOME (eg fatal, recovered) ______

Was the patient hospitalised because of the reaction ☐ Yes ☐ No

REPORTING DOCTOR (BLOCK LETTERS)

Name: ______

Address: ______

Tel. No. ______ Specialty ______

Signature: Date:

If you would like information about other reports associated with the suspected drug, please tick box ☐

SEND TO CSM, FREEPOST, London SW8 5BR
OR if you are in one of the following NHS regions:
TO CSM West Midlands, FREEPOST, Birmingham B18 7BR
OR CSM Northern, FREEPOST, Newcastle upon Tyne NE1 1BR
OR CSM Wales, FREEPOST, Cardiff CF4 1ZZ
OR CSM Mersey, FREEPOST, Liverpool L3 3AB

OTHER DRUGS
(Please record all other drugs, including self-medication, taken during the last 3 months, and give brand name if known)

DRUG	ROUTE	DAILY DOSE	DATE STARTED	DATE STOPPED	INDICATION

ADDITIONAL NOTES (Include relevant medical history, investigations, known allergies, suspected drug interactions. For congenital abnormalities state all other drugs taken during pregnancy and the LMP. Please attach additional pages if necessary.)

OTHER DRUGS
(Please record all other drugs, including self-medication, taken during the last 3 months, and give brand name if known)

DRUG	ROUTE	DAILY DOSE	DATE STARTED	DATE STOPPED	INDICATION

ADDITIONAL NOTES (Include relevant medical history, investigations, known allergies, suspected drug interactions. For congenital abnormalities state all other drugs taken during pregnancy and the LMP. Please attach additional pages if necessary.)

IN CONFIDENCE

COMMITTEE ON SAFETY OF MEDICINES **MEDICINES CONTROL AGENCY**

REPORT ON SUSPECTED ADVERSE DRUG REACTION

(For advice on reporting reactions see The Reporting of Adverse Reactions section in this book)

Do not be put off reporting because some details are not known

NAME OF PATIENT (To allow for linkage with other reports for same patient. Please give record number for hospital patients)	Family name / Forename	Sex	AGE or DATE OF BIRTH	WEIGHT (Kg.)

SUSPECT DRUG (Please give brand name and batch number if known)	ROUTE	DAILY DOSE	DATE STARTED	DATE STOPPED	INDICATION

SUSPECTED REACTION

DATE OF ONSET ______ DATE STOPPED ______

OUTCOME (eg fatal, recovered) ______

Was the patient hospitalised because of the reaction ☐ Yes ☐ No

REPORTING DOCTOR (BLOCK LETTERS)

Name: ______

Address: ______

Tel. No. ______ Specialty ______

Signature: Date:

If you would like information about other reports associated with the suspected drug, please tick box ☐

SEND TO CSM, FREEPOST, London SW8 5BR
OR if you are in one of the following NHS regions:
TO CSM West Midlands, FREEPOST, Birmingham B18 7BR
OR CSM Northern, FREEPOST, Newcastle upon Tyne NE1 1BR
OR CSM Wales, FREEPOST, Cardiff CF4 1ZZ
OR CSM Mersey, FREEPOST, Liverpool L3 3AB

IN CONFIDENCE

COMMITTEE ON SAFETY OF MEDICINES **MEDICINES CONTROL AGENCY**

REPORT ON SUSPECTED ADVERSE DRUG REACTION

(For advice on reporting reactions see The Reporting of Adverse Reactions section in this book)

Do not be put off reporting because some details are not known

NAME OF PATIENT (To allow for linkage with other reports for same patient. Please give record number for hospital patients)	Family name / Forename	Sex	AGE or DATE OF BIRTH	WEIGHT (Kg.)

SUSPECT DRUG (Please give brand name and batch number if known)	ROUTE	DAILY DOSE	DATE STARTED	DATE STOPPED	INDICATION

SUSPECTED REACTION

DATE OF ONSET ______ DATE STOPPED ______

OUTCOME (eg fatal, recovered) ______

Was the patient hospitalised because of the reaction ☐ Yes ☐ No

REPORTING DOCTOR (BLOCK LETTERS)

Name: ______

Address: ______

Tel. No. ______ Specialty ______

Signature: Date:

If you would like information about other reports associated with the suspected drug, please tick box ☐

SEND TO CSM, FREEPOST, London SW8 5BR
OR if you are in one of the following NHS regions:
TO CSM West Midlands, FREEPOST, Birmingham B18 7BR
OR CSM Northern, FREEPOST, Newcastle upon Tyne NE1 1BR
OR CSM Wales, FREEPOST, Cardiff CF4 1ZZ
OR CSM Mersey, FREEPOST, Liverpool L3 3AB

OTHER DRUGS
(Please record all other drugs, including self-medication, taken during the last 3 months, and give brand name if known)

DRUG	ROUTE	DAILY DOSE	DATE STARTED	DATE STOPPED	INDICATION

ADDITIONAL NOTES (Include relevant medical history, investigations, known allergies, suspected drug interactions. For congenital abnormalities state all other drugs taken during pregnancy and the LMP. Please attach additional pages if necessary.)

OTHER DRUGS
(Please record all other drugs, including self-medication, taken during the last 3 months, and give brand name if known)

DRUG	ROUTE	DAILY DOSE	DATE STARTED	DATE STOPPED	INDICATION

ADDITIONAL NOTES (Include relevant medical history, investigations, known allergies, suspected drug interactions. For congenital abnormalities state all other drugs taken during pregnancy and the LMP. Please attach additional pages if necessary.)

IN CONFIDENCE

COMMITTEE ON SAFETY OF MEDICINES **MEDICINES CONTROL AGENCY**

REPORT ON SUSPECTED ADVERSE DRUG REACTION

(For advice on reporting reactions see The Reporting of Adverse Reactions section in this book)

Do not be put off reporting because some details are not known

NAME OF PATIENT (To allow for linkage with other reports for same patient. Please give record number for hospital patients)	Family name / Forename	Sex	AGE or DATE OF BIRTH	WEIGHT (Kg.)

SUSPECT DRUG (Please give brand name and batch number if known)	ROUTE	DAILY DOSE	DATE STARTED	DATE STOPPED	INDICATION

SUSPECTED REACTION

DATE OF ONSET ______ DATE STOPPED ______

OUTCOME (eg fatal, recovered) ______

Was the patient hospitalised because of the reaction ☐ Yes ☐ No

REPORTING DOCTOR (BLOCK LETTERS)

Name: ______

Address: ______

Tel. No. ______ Specialty ______

Signature: Date:

If you would like information about other reports associated with the suspected drug, please tick box ☐

SEND TO CSM, FREEPOST, London SW8 5BR
OR if you are in one of the following NHS regions:
TO CSM West Midlands, FREEPOST, Birmingham B18 7BR
OR CSM Northern, FREEPOST, Newcastle upon Tyne NE1 1BR
OR CSM Wales, FREEPOST, Cardiff CF4 1ZZ
OR CSM Mersey, FREEPOST, Liverpool L3 3AB

IN CONFIDENCE

COMMITTEE ON SAFETY OF MEDICINES **MEDICINES CONTROL AGENCY**

REPORT ON SUSPECTED ADVERSE DRUG REACTION

(For advice on reporting reactions see The Reporting of Adverse Reactions section in this book)

Do not be put off reporting because some details are not known

NAME OF PATIENT (To allow for linkage with other reports for same patient. Please give record number for hospital patients) | Family name | Forename | Sex | AGE or DATE OF BIRTH | WEIGHT (Kg.)

SUSPECT DRUG (Please give brand name and batch number if known) | ROUTE | DAILY DOSE | DATE STARTED | STOPPED | INDICATION

SUSPECTED REACTION

DATE OF ONSET ______ DATE STOPPED ______

OUTCOME (eg fatal, recovered) ______

Was the patient hospitalised because of the reaction ☐ Yes ☐ No

REPORTING DOCTOR (BLOCK LETTERS)

Name: ______

Address: ______

Tel. No. ______ Specialty ______

Signature: Date:

If you would like information about other reports associated with the suspected drug, please tick box ☐

SEND TO CSM, FREEPOST, London SW8 5BR
OR if you are in one of the following NHS regions:
TO CSM West Midlands, FREEPOST, Birmingham B18 7BR
OR CSM Northern, FREEPOST, Newcastle upon Tyne NE1 1BR
OR CSM Wales, FREEPOST, Cardiff CF4 1ZZ
OR CSM Mersey, FREEPOST, Liverpool L3 3AB

OTHER DRUGS
(Please record all other drugs, including self-medication, taken during the last 3 months, and give brand name if known)

DRUG	ROUTE	DAILY DOSE	DATE STARTED	DATE STOPPED	INDICATION

ADDITIONAL NOTES (Include relevant medical history, investigations, known allergies, suspected drug interactions. For congenital abnormalities state all other drugs taken during pregnancy and the LMP. Please attach additional pages if necessary.)

OTHER DRUGS
(Please record all other drugs, including self-medication, taken during the last 3 months, and give brand name if known)

DRUG	ROUTE	DAILY DOSE	DATE STARTED	DATE STOPPED	INDICATION

ADDITIONAL NOTES (Include relevant medical history, investigations, known allergies, suspected drug interactions. For congenital abnormalities state all other drugs taken during pregnancy and the LMP. Please attach additional pages if necessary.)

IN CONFIDENCE

COMMITTEE ON SAFETY OF MEDICINES **MEDICINES CONTROL AGENCY**

REPORT ON SUSPECTED ADVERSE DRUG REACTION

(For advice on reporting reactions see The Reporting of Adverse Reactions section in this book)

Do not be put off reporting because some details are not known

NAME OF PATIENT (To allow for linkage with other reports for same patient. Please give record number for hospital patients)	Family name Forename	Sex	AGE or DATE OF BIRTH	WEIGHT (Kg.)

SUSPECT DRUG (Please give brand name and batch number if known)	ROUTE	DAILY DOSE	DATE STARTED	DATE STOPPED	INDICATION

SUSPECTED REACTION

DATE OF ONSET ______ DATE STOPPED ______

OUTCOME (eg fatal, recovered) ______

Was the patient hospitalised because of the reaction ☐ Yes ☐ No

SEND TO CSM, FREEPOST, London SW8 5BR
OR if you are in one of the following NHS regions:
TO CSM West Midlands, FREEPOST, Birmingham B18 7BR
OR CSM Northern, FREEPOST, Newcastle upon Tyne NE1 1BR
OR CSM Wales, FREEPOST, Cardiff CF4 1ZZ
OR CSM Mersey, FREEPOST, Liverpool L3 3AB

REPORTING DOCTOR (BLOCK LETTERS)

Name: ______

Address: ______

Tel. No. ______ Specialty ______

Signature: Date:

If you would like information about other reports associated with the suspected drug, please tick box ☐

IN CONFIDENCE

COMMITTEE ON SAFETY OF MEDICINES **MEDICINES CONTROL AGENCY**

REPORT ON SUSPECTED ADVERSE DRUG REACTION

(For advice on reporting reactions see The Reporting of Adverse Reactions section in this book)

Do not be put off reporting because some details are not known

NAME OF PATIENT (To allow for linkage with other reports for same patient. Please give record number for hospital patients)	Family name Forename	Sex	AGE or DATE OF BIRTH	WEIGHT (Kg.)

SUSPECT DRUG (Please give brand name and batch number if known)	ROUTE	DAILY DOSE	DATE STARTED	DATE STOPPED	INDICATION

SUSPECTED REACTION

DATE OF ONSET ______ DATE STOPPED ______

OUTCOME (eg fatal, recovered) ______

Was the patient hospitalised because of the reaction ☐ Yes ☐ No

SEND TO CSM, FREEPOST, London SW8 5BR
OR if you are in one of the following NHS regions:
TO CSM West Midlands, FREEPOST, Birmingham B18 7BR
OR CSM Northern, FREEPOST, Newcastle upon Tyne NE1 1BR
OR CSM Wales, FREEPOST, Cardiff CF4 1ZZ
OR CSM Mersey, FREEPOST, Liverpool L3 3AB

REPORTING DOCTOR (BLOCK LETTERS)

Name: ______

Address: ______

Tel. No. ______ Specialty ______

Signature: Date:

If you would like information about other reports associated with the suspected drug, please tick box ☐

OTHER DRUGS
(Please record all other drugs, including self-medication, taken during the last 3 months, and give brand name if known)

DRUG	ROUTE	DAILY DOSE	DATE STARTED	DATE STOPPED	INDICATION

ADDITIONAL NOTES (Include relevant medical history, investigations, known allergies, suspected drug interactions. For congenital abnormalities state all other drugs taken during pregnancy and the LMP. Please attach additional pages if necessary.)

OTHER DRUGS
(Please record all other drugs, including self-medication, taken during the last 3 months, and give brand name if known)

DRUG	ROUTE	DAILY DOSE	DATE STARTED	DATE STOPPED	INDICATION

ADDITIONAL NOTES (Include relevant medical history, investigations, known allergies, suspected drug interactions. For congenital abnormalities state all other drugs taken during pregnancy and the LMP. Please attach additional pages if necessary.)

IN CONFIDENCE

COMMITTEE ON SAFETY OF MEDICINES **MEDICINES CONTROL AGENCY**

REPORT ON SUSPECTED ADVERSE DRUG REACTION

(For advice on reporting reactions see The Reporting of Adverse Reactions section in this book)

Do not be put off reporting because some details are not known

NAME OF PATIENT (To allow for linkage with other reports for same patient. Please give record number for hospital patients)	Family name Forename	Sex	AGE or DATE OF BIRTH	WEIGHT (Kg.)

SUSPECT DRUG (Please give brand name and batch number if known)	ROUTE	DAILY DOSE	DATE STARTED	DATE STOPPED	INDICATION

SUSPECTED REACTION

DATE OF ONSET ______ DATE STOPPED ______

OUTCOME (eg fatal, recovered) ______

Was the patient hospitalised because of the reaction ☐ Yes ☐ No

SEND TO CSM, FREEPOST, London SW8 5BR
OR if you are in one of the following NHS regions:
TO CSM West Midlands, FREEPOST, Birmingham B18 7BR
OR CSM Northern, FREEPOST, Newcastle upon Tyne NE1 1BR
OR CSM Wales, FREEPOST, Cardiff CF4 1ZZ
OR CSM Mersey, FREEPOST, Liverpool L3 3AB

REPORTING DOCTOR (BLOCK LETTERS)

Name: ______

Address: ______

Tel. No. ______ Specialty ______

Signature: Date:

If you would like information about other reports associated with the suspected drug, please tick box

IN CONFIDENCE

COMMITTEE ON SAFETY OF MEDICINES **MEDICINES CONTROL AGENCY**

REPORT ON SUSPECTED ADVERSE DRUG REACTION

(For advice on reporting reactions see The Reporting of Adverse Reactions section in this book)

Do not be put off reporting because some details are not known

NAME OF PATIENT (To allow for linkage with other reports for same patient. Please give record number for hospital patients)	Family name Forename	Sex	AGE or DATE OF BIRTH	WEIGHT (Kg.)

SUSPECT DRUG (Please give brand name and batch number if known)	ROUTE	DAILY DOSE	DATE STARTED	DATE STOPPED	INDICATION

SUSPECTED REACTION

DATE OF ONSET ______ DATE STOPPED ______

OUTCOME (eg fatal, recovered) ______

Was the patient hospitalised because of the reaction ☐ Yes ☐ No

SEND TO CSM, FREEPOST, London SW8 5BR
OR if you are in one of the following NHS regions:
TO CSM West Midlands, FREEPOST, Birmingham B18 7BR
OR CSM Northern, FREEPOST, Newcastle upon Tyne NE1 1BR
OR CSM Wales, FREEPOST, Cardiff CF4 1ZZ
OR CSM Mersey, FREEPOST, Liverpool L3 3AB

REPORTING DOCTOR (BLOCK LETTERS)

Name: ______

Address: ______

Tel. No. ______ Specialty ______

Signature: Date:

If you would like information about other reports associated with the suspected drug, please tick box

OTHER DRUGS
(Please record all other drugs, including self-medication, taken during the last 3 months, and give brand name if known)

DRUG	ROUTE	DAILY DOSE	DATE STARTED	DATE STOPPED	INDICATION

ADDITIONAL NOTES (Include relevant medical history, investigations, known allergies, suspected drug interactions. For congenital abnormalities state all other drugs taken during pregnancy and the LMP. Please attach additional pages if necessary.)

OTHER DRUGS
(Please record all other drugs, including self-medication, taken during the last 3 months, and give brand name if known)

DRUG	ROUTE	DAILY DOSE	DATE STARTED	DATE STOPPED	INDICATION

ADDITIONAL NOTES (Include relevant medical history, investigations, known allergies, suspected drug interactions. For congenital abnormalities state all other drugs taken during pregnancy and the LMP. Please attach additional pages if necessary.)

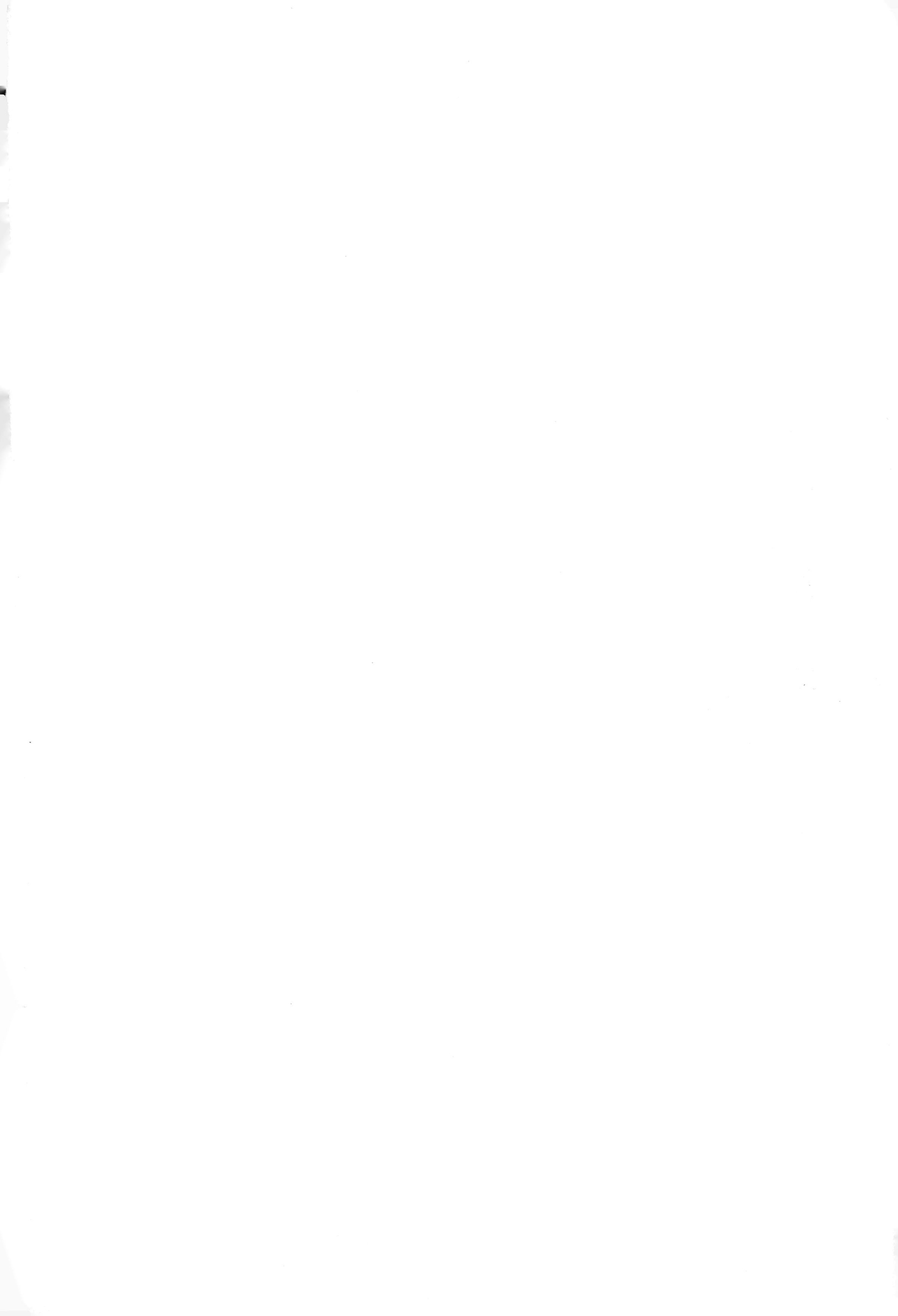